DRUG INFORMATION HANDBOOK

with INTERNATIONAL TRADE NAMES INDEX

Adapted from the *Drug Information Handbook*, 24th Edition, with Canadian and International Drug Monographs

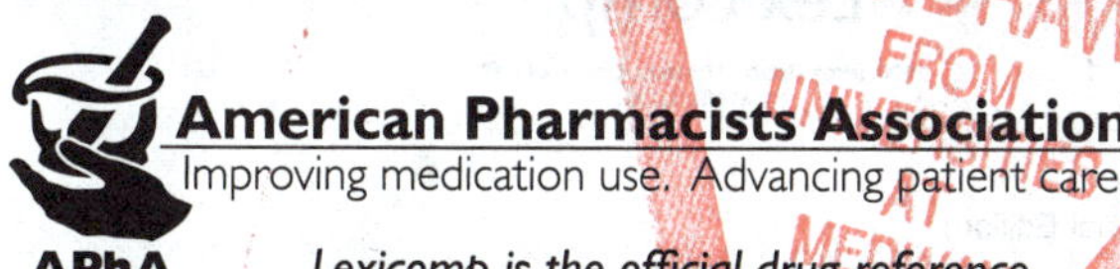

Lexicomp is the official drug reference for the American Pharmacists Association.

24th Edition

Lexicomp®

NOTICE

This data is intended to serve the user as a handy reference and not as a complete drug information resource. It does not include information on every therapeutic agent available. The publication covers over 1,800 commonly used drugs and is specifically designed to present important aspects of drug data in a more concise format than is typically found in medical literature or product material supplied by manufacturers.

The nature of drug information is that it is constantly evolving because of ongoing research and clinical experience and is often subject to interpretation. While great care has been taken to ensure the accuracy of the information and recommendations presented, the reader is advised that the authors, editors, reviewers, contributors, and publishers cannot be responsible for the continued currency of the information or for any errors, omissions, or the application of this information, or for any consequences arising therefrom. Therefore, the author(s) and/or the publisher shall have no liability to any person or entity with regard to claims, loss, or damage caused, or alleged to be caused, directly or indirectly, by the use of information contained herein. Because of the dynamic nature of drug information, readers are advised that decisions regarding drug therapy must be based on the independent judgment of the clinician, changing information about a drug (eg, as reflected in the literature and manufacturer's most current product information), and changing medical practices. Therefore, this data is designed to be used in conjunction with other necessary information and is not designed to be solely relied upon by any user. The user of this data hereby and forever releases the authors and publishers of this data from any and all liability of any kind that might arise out of the use of this data. The editors are not responsible for any inaccuracy of quotation or for any false or misleading implication that may arise due to the text or formulas as used or due to the quotation of revisions no longer official.

Certain of the authors, editors, and contributors have written this book in their private capacities. No official support or endorsement by any federal or state agency or pharmaceutical company is intended or inferred.

The publishers have made every effort to trace any third party copyright holders, if any, for borrowed material. If they have inadvertently overlooked any, they will be pleased to make the necessary arrangements at the first opportunity.

If you have any suggestions or questions regarding any information presented in this data, please contact our drug information pharmacists at 330-650-6506.

This manual was produced using Lexi-Comp's Information Management System™ (LIMS) — a complete publishing service of Lexi-Comp Inc.

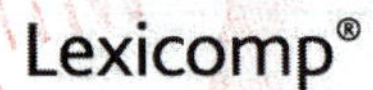

1100 Terex Road • Hudson, Ohio • 44236
(330) 650-6506

ISBN 978-1-59195-343-2 (International Edition)

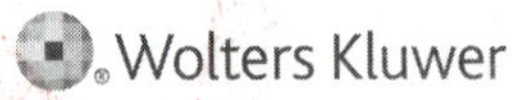

TABLE OF CONTENTS

Drug Information Handbook Editorial Advisory Panel 2
Drug Interactions Editorial Advisory Panel 3
Editorial Advisory Panel 4
Description of Sections and Fields Used in This Handbook 10
Pregnancy Categories 13
Preventing Prescribing Errors 14
FDA Name Differentiation Project: The Use of Tall-Man Letters 16

ALPHABETICAL LISTING OF DRUGS 19

APPENDIX 2223
- Assessment of Liver Function 2224
- Assessment of Renal Function 2225
- Comparative Drug Charts 2228
- Cytochrome P450 and Drug Interactions 2241
- Immunizations and Vaccinations 2250
- Therapy Recommendations 2271
- Miscellaneous 2276

PHARMACOLOGIC CATEGORY INDEX 2287

INTERNATIONAL TRADE NAMES INDEX 2319

DRUG INFORMATION HANDBOOK EDITORIAL ADVISORY PANEL

DRUG INTERACTIONS EDITORIAL ADVISORY PANEL

Kay Burke, PharmD
Senior Clinical Editor
Wolters Kluwer

Jamie Hoffman, PharmD, BCPS
Senior Clinical Editor
Wolters Kluwer

Carrie Nemerovski, PharmD, BCPS
Pharmacotherapy Specialist
Wolters Kluwer

Steve Sklar, PharmD
Senior Clinical Manager
Wolters Kluwer

Stephen M. Stout, PharmD, MS, BCPS
Pharmacotherapy Specialist
Wolters Kluwer

Dan Streetman, PharmD, MS
Pharmacotherapy Specialist
Wolters Kluwer

David M. Weinstein, PhD, RPh
Director, Clinical Content
Wolters Kluwer

EDITORIAL ADVISORY PANEL

Amanda H. Corbett, PharmD, BCPS, FCCP, AAHIVE
Clinical Assistant Professor
Eshelman School of Pharmacy,
University of North Carolina

Susan Cornell, PharmD, CDE, FAPhA, FAADE
Associate Professor
Department of Pharmacy Practice
Assistant Director of Experimental Education
Midwestern University, Chicago College of Pharmacy

Marilyn Cortell, RDH, MS, FAADH
Associate Professor
New York City College of Technology,
City University of New York

Harold L. Crossley, DDS, MS, PhD
Associate Professor of Pharmacology
Baltimore College of Dental Surgery,
University of Maryland

Melanie W. Cucchi, BS, PharmD, RPh
Clinical Manager
Wolters Kluwer

Laura Cummings, PharmD, BCPS
Pharmacotherapy Specialist
Wolters Kluwer

William J. Dana, PharmD, FASHP
Pharmacy Quality Assurance
Harris County Hospital District

Beth Deen, PharmD, BDNSP
Senior Pediatric Clinical Pharmacy Specialist
Cook Children's Medical Center

Julie A. Dopheide, PharmD, BCPP
Associate Professor of Clinical Pharmacy, Psychiatry and the Behavioral Sciences
Schools of Pharmacy and Medicine,
University of Southern California

Mary Duafala, MS
Consultant, Independent Medical Writer
Wolters Kluwer

Kim S. Dufner, PharmD
Clinical Manager
Wolters Kluwer

Teri Dunsworth, PharmD, FCCP, BCPS
Pharmacotherapy Specialist
Wolters Kluwer

Michael S. Edwards, PharmD, MBA, BCOP
Chief, Oncology Pharmacy and *Director, Oncology Pharmacy Residency Program*
Walter Reed Army Medical Center

Vicki L. Ellingrod, PharmD, BCPP
Head, Clinical Pharmacogenomics Laboratory and *Associate Professor*
Department of Psychiatry,
Colleges of Pharmacy and Medicine,
University of Michigan

Kelley K. Engle, BSPharm
Pharmacotherapy Contributor
Stow, Ohio

Christopher Ensor, PharmD, BCPS (AQ-CV)
Clinical Pharmacy Specialist, Thoracic Transplantation
University of Pittsburgh Medical Center

Erin Fabian, PharmD, RPh, BCPS
Pharmacotherapy Specialist
Wolters Kluwer

Elizabeth A. Farrington, PharmD, FCCP, FCCM, FPPAG, BCPS
Pharmacist III - Pediatrics
New Hanover Regional Medical Center

Margaret A. Fitzgerald, MS, APRN, BC, NP-C, FAANP
President
Fitzgerald Health Education Associates, Inc.
Family Nurse Practitioner
Greater Lawrence Family Health Center

Matthew A. Fuller, PharmD, BCPS, BCPP, FASHP
Clinical Pharmacy Specialist, Psychiatry
Cleveland Department of Veterans Affairs Medical Center
Associate Clinical Professor of Psychiatry and *Clinical Instructor of Psychology*
Case Western Reserve University
Adjunct Associate Professor of Clinical Pharmacy
University of Toledo

Carole W. Fuseck, RN, MSN, VA-BC
Registered Nurse, Vascular Access
Fairview Hospital

Jason C. Gallagher, PharmD, BCPS
Clinical Pharmacy Specialist, Infectious Diseases and *Clinical Associate Professor*
Temple University Hospital

Joyce Generali, RPh, MS, FASHP
Director, Synthesized Referential Content
Wolters Kluwer

Meredith D. Girard, MD, FACP
Medical Staff
Department of Internal Medicine, Summa Health Systems
Assistant Professor Internal Medicine
Northeast Ohio Medical University (NEOMED)

Morton P. Goldman, RPh, PharmD, BCPS, FCCP
Health Care Consultant
American Pharmacotherapy, Inc

Julie A. Golembiewski, PharmD
Clinical Associate Professor and *Clinical Pharmacist, Anesthesia/Pain*
Colleges of Pharmacy and Medicine, University of Illinois

Jeffrey P. Gonzales, PharmD, BCPS
Critical Care Clinical Pharmacy Specialist
University of Maryland Medical Center

John Grabenstein, RPh, PhD, FAPhA
Pharmacotherapy Contributor
Wolters Kluwer

Larry D. Gray, PhD, ABMM
Microbiology Contributor
Wolters Kluwer

Tracy Hagemann, PharmD
Associate Professor
College of Pharmacy, The University of Oklahoma

JoEllen L. Hanigosky, PharmD
Clinical Coordinator
Department of Hematology/Oncology/Bone Marrow Transplant, Children's Hospital of Akron

Jason Makii, PharmD, BCPS
Clinical Pharmacy Specialist, Neurosciences Critical Care
University Hospitals Case Medical Center

Melissa Makii, PharmD, BCPS
Clinical Pharmacy Specialist
Pediatric Oncology, Rainbow Babies & Children's Hospital

Vincent F. Mauro, BS, PharmD, FCCP
Professor of Clinical Pharmacy and
Adjunct Professor of Medicine
Colleges of Pharmacy and Medicine,
The University of Toledo

Joseph McGraw, PharmD, MPH, PhD, BCPS
Assistant Professor of Pharmaceutical Science and
Metabolism Laboratory Director
Concordia University Wisconsin, School of Pharmacy

Ann Marie McMullin, MD
Associate Staff
Emergency Services Institute, Cleveland Clinic

Christopher McPherson, PharmD
Clinical Pharmacy Practice Manager
Neonatal Intensive Care Unit, Brigham and
Women's Hospital
Instructor
Department of Pediatric Newborn Medicine,
Harvard Medical School

Timothy F. Meiller, DDS, PhD
Professor
Oncology and Diagnostic Sciences,
Baltimore College of Dental Surgery
Professor of Oncology
Marlene and Stewart Greenebaum Cancer Center,
University of Maryland Medical System

Cathy A. Meives, PharmD
Senior Clinical Manager
Wolters Kluwer

Charla E. Miller Nowak, RPh, PharmD
Neonatal Clinical Pharmacy Specialist
Wolfson Children's Hospital

Julie Miller, PharmD
Pharmacy Clinical Specialist, Cardiology
Columbus Children's Hospital

Katherine Mills, PharmD
Pharmacotherapy Contributor
Bristow, Virginia

Stephanie S. Minich, PharmD, BCOP
Pharmacotherapy Specialist
Wolters Kluwer

Kim Moeller, MSN, RN, ACNS-BC, AOCNS
Unit Manager, Outpatient Infusion
Cooper Cancer Center
Advanced Practice Nurse
Summit Oncology Associates, Summa Health System

Kara M. Morris, DDS, MS
Pediatric Dentist
Olentangy Pediatric Dentistry

Kevin M. Mulieri, BS, PharmD
Pediatric Hematology/Oncology Clinical Specialist
Penn State Milton S. Hershey Medical Center
Instructor of Pharmacology
Penn State College of Medicine

Lynne Nakashima, PharmD
Professional Practice Leader, Clinical Professor
B.C. Cancer Agency, Vancouver Centre, University of BC

Carrie Nemerovski, PharmD, BCPS
Pharmacotherapy Specialist
Wolters Kluwer

Elizabeth A. Neuner, PharmD, BCPS
Infectious Diseases Clinical Specialist
Cleveland Clinic

Carlene N. Oliverio, PharmD, BCPS
Clinical Content Specialist
Wolters Kluwer

Tom Palma, MS, RPh
Medical Science Pharmacist
Wolters Kluwer

Susie H. Park, PharmD, BCPP
Assistant Professor of Clinical Pharmacy
University of Southern Califormia

Nicole Passerrello, PharmD, BCPS
Pharmacotherapy Specialist
Wolters Kluwer

Alpa Patel, PharmD
Antimicrobial Clinical Pharmacist
University of Louisville Hospital

Gayle Pearson, BSPharm, MSA
Drug Information Pharmacist
Peter Lougheed Centre, Alberta Health Services

Jennifer L. Placencia, PharmD
Neonatal Clinical Pharmacy Specialist
Texas Children's Hospital

James A. Ponto, MS, RPh, BCNP
Chief Nuclear Pharmacist
Department of Radiology, University of Iowa,
Hospitals and Clinics
Professor of Clinical Pharmacy
Department of Pharmacy Practice and Science,
University of Iowa College of Pharmacy

Amy L. Potts, PharmD, BCPS
Assistant Director
Department of Pharmacy
PGY1 & PGY2 Residency Program Director
Monroe Carell Jr. Children's Hospital at Vanderbilt

Sally Rafie, PharmD, BCPS
Medical Safety Pharmacist
UC San Diego Health System

Esta Razavi, PharmD
Clinical Editor
Wolters Kluwer

James Reissig, PharmD
Assistant Director, Clinical Services
Akron General Medical Center

A.J. (Fred) Remillard, PharmD
Assistant Dean, Research and Graduate Affairs
College of Pharmacy and Nutrition,
University of Saskatchewan

Elizabeth Rich, RN, BSN, BA
Registered Nurse – Medical Intensive Care Unit
Cleveland Clinic

Sherri J. Willard Argyres, MA, PharmD
Medical Science Pharmacist
Wolters Kluwer

John C. Williamson, PharmD, BCPS
Pharmacy Clinical Coordinator, Infectious Diseases
Wake Forest Baptist Health

Nathan Wirick, PharmD, BCPS
Clinical Specialist in Infectious Diseases and Antibiotic Management
Hillcrest Hospital

Wende Wood, RPh, BSPharm, BCPP
Pharmacotherapy Contributor
Toronto, Ontario, Canada

Richard L. Wynn, BSPharm, PhD
Professor of Pharmacology
Baltimore College of Dental Surgery, University of Maryland

Jessica Zatroch, DDS
Private Practice Dentist
Willoughby Hills, OH

Jennifer Zimmer-Young, PharmD, CCRP
Educator, Clinical Pharmacist
ThedaCare

DESCRIPTION OF SECTIONS AND FIELDS USED IN THIS HANDBOOK

The *Drug Information Handbook with International Trade Names Index, 24th Edition* is divided into four sections.

The first section is a compilation of introductory text pertinent to the use of this book.

The drug information section of the handbook lists all drugs alphabetically by generic name, with extensive cross-referencing provided by U.S. brand names, Canadian brand names, and index terms. This section contains three different types of monographs:

Standard monographs: Based on the *Drug Information Handbook, 24th Edition*, these monographs are developed and reviewed by practitioners within the United States. However, these medications are frequently available for use in many other countries. Since there may be considerable variation in the clinical use of these agents within individual countries, users are encouraged to consult prescribing information for the country of use for additional details concerning contraindications, warnings, and drug interactions, as well as specific dosing.

Canadian international monographs: Designated with a **[CAN/INT]** next to the monograph name, these monographs are developed with input and review from practitioners within Canada. However, these medications are frequently available for use in many other countries. Since there may be considerable variation in the clinical use of these agents within individual countries, users are encouraged to consult the prescribing information for the country of use for additional details concerning contraindications, warnings, and drug interactions, as well as specific dosing.

U.S. and Canadian Monographs

Generic Name	U.S. adopted name
Pronunciation	Phonetic pronunciation guide
Brand Names: U.S.	Trade names (manufacturer-specific) found in the United States. The symbol [DSC] appears after trade names that have been recently discontinued.
Brand Names: Canada	Trade names found in Canada
Index Terms	Other names or accepted abbreviations of the generic drug. May also include common brand names no longer available; this field is used to create cross-references to monographs.
Pharmacologic Category	Unique systematic classification of medications
Additional Appendix Information	Cross-reference to other pertinent drug information found in the appendix section of this handbook
Use	Information pertaining to FDA- or Canadian-approved indications for the drug
Pregnancy Risk Factor	Five categories established by the FDA to indicate the potential of a systemically absorbed drug for causing risk to fetus
Pregnancy Considerations	A summary of human and/or animal information pertinent to or associated with the use of the drug as it relates to clinical effects on the fetus, newborn, or pregnant women
Breast-Feeding Considerations	Information pertinent to or associated with the human use of the drug as it relates to clinical effects on the nursing infant or postpartum woman
Contraindications	Information pertaining to inappropriate use of the drug as dictated by approved labeling
Warnings/Precautions	Precautionary considerations, hazardous conditions related to use of the drug, and disease states or patient populations in which the drug should be cautiously used. Boxed warnings, when present, are clearly identified and are adapted from the FDA-approved labeling. Consult the product labeling for the exact black box warning through the manufacturer's or the FDA website.
Adverse Reactions	Side effects are grouped by body system and include a listing of the more common and/or serious side effects. Due to space limitations, every reported side effect is not listed.
Drug Interactions	
Metabolism/Transport Effects	If a drug has demonstrated involvement with cytochrome P450 enzymes, or other metabolism or transport proteins, this field will identify the drug as an inhibitor, inducer, or substrate of the specific enzyme(s) (eg, CYP1A2 or UGT1A1). CYP450 isoenzymes are identified as substrates (minor or major), inhibitors (weak, moderate, or strong), and inducers (weak or strong).
Avoid Concomitant Use	Designates drug combinations which should not be used concomitantly, due to an unacceptable risk:benefit assessment. Frequently, the concurrent use of the agents is explicitly prohibited or contraindicated by the product labeling.
Increased Effect/Toxicity	Drug combinations that result in a increased or toxic therapeutic effect between the drug listed in the monograph and other drugs or drug classes
Decreased Effect	Drug combinations that result in a decreased therapeutic effect between the drug listed in the monograph and other drugs or drug classes

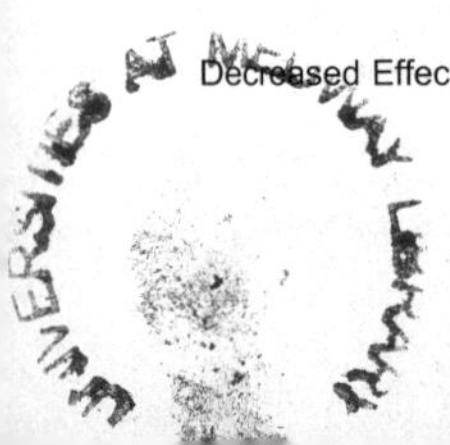

U.S. and Canadian Monographs *(continued)*

Food Interactions	Possible important interactions between the drug listed in the monograph and food, alcohol, or other beverages
Preparation for Administration	Provides information regarding the preparation of drug products prior to administration, including dilution, reconstitution, etc.
Storage/Stability	Information regarding storage and stability of commercially available products and products that have been reconstituted, diluted or otherwise prepared. Provides the time and conditions for which a solution or mixture will maintain potency.
Mechanism of Action	How the drug works in the body to elicit a response
Pharmacodynamics/ Kinetics	The magnitude of a drug's effect depends on the drug concentration at the site of action. The pharmacodynamics are expressed in terms of onset of action and duration of action. Pharmacokinetics are expressed in terms of absorption, distribution, protein binding, metabolism, bioavailability, half-life, time to peak serum concentration, and elimination.
Dosage	The amount of the drug to be typically given or taken during therapy for children and adults; also includes any dosing adjustment/comments for renal impairment or hepatic impairment and other suggested dosing adjustments (eg, hematological toxicity). The following age group definitions are utilized to characterize age-related dosing unless otherwise specified in the monograph: Neonate (0 to 28 days of age), infant (>28 days to 1 year of age), children (1 to 12 years of age), and adolescent (13 to 18 years of age).
Dietary Considerations	Specific dietary modifications and/or restrictions (eg, information about sodium content).
Usual Infusion Concentrations	Information describing the usual concentrations of drugs for continuous infusion administration in the pediatric and adult populations as appropriate. Concentrations are derived from the literature, manufacturer recommendation, or organizational recommendations (eg, the Institute for Safe Medication Practices [ISMP]) and are universally established. Institution-specific standard concentrations may differ from those listed.
Administration	Information regarding the recommended final concentrations, rates of administration for parenteral drugs, or other guidelines or relevant information to properly administer medications
Monitoring Parameters	Laboratory tests and patient physical parameters that should be monitored for safety and efficacy of drug therapy
Reference Range	Therapeutic and toxic serum concentrations listed including peak and trough levels
Additional Information	Information about sodium content and/or pertinent information about specific brands
Product Availability	Provides availability information on products that have been approved by the FDA, but not yet available for use. Estimates for when a product may be available are included, when this information is known. May also provide any unique or critical drug availability issues.
Dosage Forms Considerations	More specific information regarding product concentrations, ingredients, package sizes, amount of doses per container, and other important details pertaining to various formulations of medications
Dosage Forms	Information with regard to form, strength, and availability of the drug in the United States. Please consult labeling for further information.
Dosage Forms: Canada	Information with regard to form, strength, and availability of products that are uniquely available in Canada but currently are not available in the United States
Extemporaneous Preparations	Directions for preparing liquid formulations from solid drug products. May include stability information and references.

International monographs: These monographs are designated by **[INT]** next to the monograph name. These abbreviated monographs are intended to provide a general overview of the use and pharmacologic classification of a drug. Due to variability in the use and availability of specific documentation and review, these monographs are limited in scope. Users are encouraged to consult the prescribing information for the country of use for additional details concerning contraindications, warnings, and drug interactions, as well as specific dosing.

Generic Name	International adopted common name
Pronunciation	Phonetic pronunciation guide
International Brand Names	Common trade names used; abbreviation of country where product is reportedly available is listed in parenthesis behind name (see International Brand Name Index for country abbreviations)
Index Terms	Other names or accepted abbreviations of the generic drug
Pharmacologic Category	Unique systematic classification of medications
Reported Use	Information pertaining to indications or use of the drug. Not country or brand name specific. Individual product labeling should be consulted for appropriate use in a specific country, for a specific indication, or for a specific brand name product.
Dosage Range	Amount of drug used during therapy; reported as a general range. Not indication or country specific. Prior to use, individual product labeling should be consulted.
Product Availability	Product availability varies by country. Product is not available in the United States.
Dosage Forms	Information concerning form and strength. Not country specific; actual availability may vary.

The third section is an invaluable appendix which offers a compilation of tables, guidelines, nomograms, and conversion information which can be helpful when considering patient care. The appendix contains reference to drugs available in the U.S. only.

The last section of this handbook contains two indexes: A **Pharmacologic Category Index** and an **International Trade Names Index**. The Pharmacologic Category Index lists all drugs in this handbook in their unique pharmacologic class.

PREGNANCY CATEGORIES

Pregnancy Categories (sometimes referred to as pregnancy risk factors) are a letter system presented under the *Teratogenic Effects* subsection of the product labeling. The system was initiated in 1979. The categories were required to be part of the package insert for prescription drugs that are systemically absorbed. The Food and Drug Administration (FDA) has updated prescribing labeling requirements and as of June 2015, the pregnancy categories will no longer be part of new product labeling. Prescription products which currently have a pregnancy category letter will be phasing this out of their product information.

The categories are defined as follows:

A — Adequate and well-controlled studies in pregnant women have not shown that the drug increases the risk of fetal abnormalities.

B — Animal reproduction studies show no evidence of impaired fertility or harm to the fetus; however, no adequate and well-controlled studies have been conducted in pregnant women.
or
Animal reproduction studies have shown adverse events; however, studies in pregnant women have not shown that the drug increases the risk of abnormalities.

C — Animal reproduction studies have shown an adverse effect on the fetus. There are no adequate and well-controlled studies in humans and the benefits from the use of the drug in pregnant women may be acceptable, despite its potential risks.
or
Animal reproduction studies have not been conducted.

D — Based on human data, the drug can cause fetal harm when administered to pregnant women, but the potential benefits from the use of the drug may be acceptable, despite its potential risks.

X — Studies in animals or humans have demonstrated fetal abnormalities (or there is positive evidence of fetal risk based on reports and/or marketing experience) and the risk of using the drug in pregnant women clearly outweighs any possible benefit (for example, safer drugs or other forms of therapy are available).

In 2008, the Food and Drug Administration (FDA) proposed new labeling requirements which would eliminate the use of the pregnancy category system and replace it with scientific data and other information specific to the use of the drug in pregnant women. These proposed changes were suggested because the current category system may be misleading. For instance, some practitioners may believe that risk increases from category A to B to C to D to X, which is not the intent. In addition, practitioners may not be aware that some medications are categorized based on animal data, while others are based on human data. The new labeling requirements will contain pregnancy and lactation subsections, each describing a risk summary, clinical considerations, and section for specific data.

For full descriptions of the final rule, refer to the following website: http://www.fda.gov/Drugs/DevelopmentApprovalProcess/DevelopmentResources/Labeling/ucm093307.htm

PREVENTING PRESCRIBING ERRORS

Prescribing errors account for the majority of reported medication errors and have prompted health care professionals to focus on the development of steps to make the prescribing process safer. Prescription legibility has been attributed to a portion of these errors and legislation has been enacted in several states to address prescription legibility. However, eliminating handwritten prescriptions and ordering medications through the use of technology [eg, computerized prescriber order entry (CPOE)] has been the primary recommendation. Whether a prescription is electronic, typed, or hand-printed, additional safe practices should be considered for implementation to maximize the safety of the prescribing process. Listed below are suggestions for safer prescribing:

- Ensure correct patient by using at least 2 patient identifiers on the prescription (eg, full name, birth date, or address). Review prescription with the patient or patient's caregiver.
- If pediatric patient, document patient's birth date or age and most recent weight. If geriatric patient, document patient's birth date or age.
- Prevent drug name confusion: For more information, see http://www.ismp.org/tools/confuseddrugnames.pdf.
  - Use TALLman lettering (eg, buPROPion, busPIRone, predniSONE, prednisoLONE). For more information, see http://www.fda.gov/drugs/drugsafety/medicationerrors/default.htm.
  - Avoid abbreviated drug names (eg, MSO_4, $MgSO_4$, MS, HCT, 6MP, MTX), as they may be misinterpreted and cause error.
  - Avoid investigational names for drugs with FDA approval (eg, FK-506, CBDCA).
  - Avoid chemical names such as 6-mercaptopurine or 6-thioguanine, as sixfold overdoses have been given when these were not recognized as chemical names. The proper names of these drugs are mercaptopurine or thioguanine.
  - Use care when prescribing drugs that look or sound similar (eg, look- alike, sound-alike drugs). Common examples include: Celebrex vs Celexa, hydroxyzine vs hydralazine, Zyprexa vs Zyrtec.
- Avoid dangerous, error-prone abbreviations (eg, regardless of letter-case: U, IU, QD, QOD, µg, cc, @). Do not use apothecary system or symbols. Additionally, text messaging abbreviations (eg, "2Day") should never be used.
  - For more information, see http://www.ismp.org/tools/errorproneabbreviations.pdf.
- Always use a leading zero for numbers less than 1 (0.5 mg is correct and .5 mg is **incorrect**) and never use a trailing zero for whole numbers (2 mg is correct and 2.0 mg is **incorrect**).
- Always use a space between a number and its units as it is easier to read. There should be no periods after the abbreviations mg or mL (10 mg is correct and 10mg is **incorrect**).
- For doses that are greater than 1,000 dosing units, use properly placed commas to prevent 10-fold errors (100,000 units is correct and 100000 units is **incorrect**).
- Do not prescribe drug dosage by the type of container in which the drug is available (eg, do not prescribe "1 amp", "2 vials", etc).
- Do not write vague or ambiguous orders which have the potential for misinterpretation by other health care providers. Examples of vague orders to avoid: "Resume pre-op medications," "give drug per protocol," or "continue home medications."
- Review each prescription with patient (or patient's caregiver) including the medication name, indication, and directions for use.
- Take extra precautions when prescribing *high alert drugs* (drugs that can cause significant patient harm when prescribed in error). Common examples of these drugs include: Anticoagulants, chemotherapy, insulins, opioids, and sedatives.
  - For more information, see http://www.ismp.org/tools/institutionalhighalert.asp or http://www.ismp.org/communityRx/tools/ambulatoryhighalert.asp.

To Err Is Human: Building a Safer Health System, Kohn LT, Corrigan JM, Donaldson MS, eds. Washington, D.C.: National Academy Press. 2000.

A Complete Outpatient Prescription[1]

A complete outpatient prescription can prevent the prescriber, the pharmacist, and/or the patient from making a mistake and can eliminate the need for further clarification. The complete outpatient prescription should contain:

- Patient's full name
- Medication indication
- Allergies
- Prescriber name and telephone or pager number
- For pediatric patients: Their birth date or age and current weight
- For geriatric patients: Their birth date or age
- Drug name, dosage form and strength
- For pediatric patients: Intended daily weight-based dose so that calculations can be checked by the pharmacist (ie, mg/kg/day or units/kg/day)
- Number or amount to be dispensed
- Complete instructions for the patient or caregiver, including the purpose of the medication, directions for use (including dose), dosing frequency, route of administration, duration of therapy, and number of refills.
- Dose should be expressed in convenient units of measure.
- When there are recognized contraindications for a prescribed drug, the prescriber should indicate knowledge of this fact to the pharmacist (ie, when prescribing a potassium salt for a patient receiving an ACE inhibitor, the prescriber should write "K serum leveling being monitored").

Upon dispensing of the final product, the pharmacist should ensure that the patient or caregiver can effectively demonstrate the appropriate administration technique. An appropriate measuring device should be provided or recommended. Household teaspoons and tablespoons should not be used to measure liquid medications due to their variability and inaccuracies in measurement; oral medication syringes are recommended.

For additional information, see http://www.ismp.org/Newsletters/acutecare/articles/20020601.asp

[1]Levine SR, Cohen MR, Blanchard NR, et al. Guidelines for preventing medication errors in pediatrics. *J Pediatr Pharmacol Ther.* 2001;6:426-442.

FDA NAME DIFFERENTIATION PROJECT: THE USE OF TALL-MAN LETTERS

Confusion between similar drug names is an important cause of medication errors. For years, The Institute For Safe Medication Practices (ISMP), has urged generic manufacturers to use a combination of large and small letters as well as bolding (ie, chlorpro**MAZINE** and chlorpro**PAMIDE**) to help distinguish drugs with look-alike names, especially when they share similar strengths. Recently the FDA's Division of Generic Drugs began to issue recommendation letters to manufacturers suggesting this novel way to label their products to help reduce this drug name confusion. Although this project has had marginal success, the method has successfully eliminated problems with products such as diphenhydr**AMINE** and dimenhy**DRINATE**. Hospitals should also follow suit by making similar changes in their own labels, preprinted order forms, computer screens and printouts, and drug storage location labels.

Lexi-Comp, Inc. Medical Publishing will use "Tall-Man" letters for the drugs suggested by the FDA or recommended by ISMP.

The following is a list of generic and brand name product names and recommended revisions.

Drug Product	Recommended Revision
acetazolamide	aceta**ZOLAMIDE**
alprazolam	**ALPRAZ**olam
amiloride	a**MIL**oride
amlodipine	am**LODIP**ine
aripiprazole	**ARIP**iprazole
atomoxetine	ato**MOX**etine
atorvastatin	atorva**STAT**in
Avinza	**AVIN**za
azacitidine	aza**CITID**ine
azathioprine	aza**THIO**prine
bupropion	bu**PROP**ion
buspirone	bus**PIR**one
carbamazepine	car**BAM**azepine
carboplatin	**CARBO**platin
cefazolin	ce**FAZ**olin
cefotetan	cefo**TE**tan
cefoxitin	cef**OX**itin
ceftazidime	cef**TAZ**idime
ceftriaxone	cef**TRIAX**one
Celebrex	Cele**BREX**
Celexa	Cele**XA**
chlordiazepoxide	chlordiaze**POXIDE**
chlorpromazine	chlorpro**MAZINE**
chlorpropamide	chlorpro**PAMIDE**
cisplatin	**CIS**platin
clobazam	clo**BAZ**am
clomiphene	clomi**PHENE**
clomipramine	clomi**PRAMINE**
clonazepam	clonaze**PAM**
clonidine	clo**NID**ine
clozapine	clo**ZAP**ine
cycloserine	cyclo**SERINE**
cyclosporine	cyclo**SPORINE**
dactinomycin	**DACTIN**omycin
daptomycin	**DAPTO**mycin
daunorubicin	**DAUNO**rubicin
dimenhydrinate	dimenhy**DRINATE**
diphenhydramine	diphenhydr**AMINE**
dobutamine	**DOBUT**amine
docetaxel	**DOCE**taxel
dopamine	**DOP**amine
doxorubicin	**DOXO**rubicin
duloxetine	**DUL**oxetine

Drug Product	Recommended Revision
ephedrine	e**PHED**rine
epinephrine	**EPINEPH**rine
epirubicin	**EPI**rubicin
eribulin	eri**BUL**in
fentanyl	fenta**NYL**
flavoxate	flavox**ATE**
fluoxetine	**FLU**oxetine
fluphenazine	flu**PHENAZ**ine
fluvoxamine	fluvoxa**MINE**
glipizide	glipi**ZIDE**
glyburide	gly**BURIDE**
guaifenesin	guai**FEN**esin
guanfacine	guan**FACINE**
Humalog	Huma**LOG**
Humulin	Humu**LIN**
hydralazine	hydr**ALAZINE**
hydrocodone	**HYDRO**codone
hydromorphone	**HYDRO**morphone
hydroxyzine	hydr**OXY**zine
idarubicin	**IDA**rubicin
infliximab	in**FLIX**imab
Invanz	**INV**anz
isotretinoin	**ISO**tretinoin
Klonopin	Klono**PIN**
Lamictal	La**MIC**tal
Lamisil	Lam**ISIL**
lamivudine	lami**VUD**ine
lamotrigine	lamo**TRI**gine
levetiracetam	Lev**ETIRA**cetam
levocarnitine	lev**OCARN**itine
lorazepam	**LOR**azepam
medroxyprogesterone	medroxy**PROGESTER**one
metformin	met**FORMIN**
methylprednisolone	methyl**PREDNIS**olone
methyltestosterone	methyl**TESTOSTER**one
metronidazole	metro**NIDAZOLE**
mitomycin	mito**MY**cin
mitoxantrone	Mito**XAN**trone
Nexavar	Nex**AVAR**
Nexium	Nex**IUM**
nicardipine	ni**CAR**dipine
nifedipine	**NIFE**dipine
nimodipine	ni**MOD**ipine
Novolin	Novo**LIN**
Novolog	Novo**LOG**
olanzapine	**OLANZ**apine
oxcarbazepine	**OX**carbazepine
oxycodone	oxy**CODONE**
Oxycontin	Oxy**CONTIN**
paclitaxel	**PACL**itaxel
paroxetine	**PAR**oxetine
pazopanib	**PAZOP**anib
pemetrexed	**PEME**trexed
penicillamine	penicill**AMINE**
pentobarbital	**PENT**obarbital
phenobarbital	**PHEN**obarbital
ponatinib	**PONAT**inib
pralatrexate	**PRALA**trexate

Drug Product	Recommended Revision
prednisolone	predniso**LONE**
prednisone	predni**SONE**
Prilosec	Pri**LOSEC**
Prozac	**PRO**zac
quetiapine	**QUE**tiapine
quinidine	qui**NID**ine
quinine	qui**NINE**
rabeprazole	**RABE**prazole
Risperdal	Risper**DAL**
risperidone	risperi**DONE**
rituximab	ri**TUX**imab
romidepsin	romi**DEP**sin
romiplostim	romi**PLOS**tim
ropinirole	r**OPINIR**ole
Sandimmune	sand**IMMUNE**
Sandostatin	Sando**STATIN**
Seroquel	**SERO**quel
Sinequan	**SINE**quan
sitagliptin	sita**GLIP**tin
Solu-Cortef	Solu-**CORTEF**
Solu-Medrol	Solu-**MEDROL**
sorafenib	**SORA**fenib
sufentanil	**SUF**entanil
sulfadiazine	sulf**ADIAZINE**
sulfasalazine	sulfa**SALA**zine
sumatriptan	**SUMA**triptan
sunitinib	**SUNI**tinib
Tegretol	**TEG**retol
tiagabine	tia**GAB**ine
tizanidine	ti**ZAN**idine
tolazamide	**TOLAZ**amide
tolbutamide	**TOLBUT**amide
tramadol	tra**MAD**ol
trazodone	tra**ZOD**one
Trental	**TREN**tal
valacyclovir	val**ACY**clovir
valganciclovir	val**GAN**ciclovir
vinblastine	vin**BLAS**tine
vincristine	vin**CRIS**tine
zolmitriptan	**ZOLM**itriptan
Zyprexa	Zy**PREXA**
Zyrtec	Zyr**TEC**

FDA and ISMP lists of look-alike drug names with recommended tall man letter. http://www.ismp.org/tools/tallmanletters.pdf. Accessed January 6, 2011.
Name differentiation project. http://www.fda.gov/Drugs/DrugSafety/MedicationErrors/ucm164587.htm. Accessed January 6, 2011.
U.S. Pharmacopeia. USP quality review: use caution – avoid confusion. March 2001, No. 76. http://www.usp.org

ALPHABETICAL LISTING OF DRUGS

- ◆ **A-25 [OTC]** *see* Vitamin A *on page 2173*
- ◆ **A-200 Lice Treatment Kit [OTC]** *see* Pyrethrins and Piperonyl Butoxide *on page 1746*
- ◆ **A-200 Maximum Strength [OTC]** *see* Pyrethrins and Piperonyl Butoxide *on page 1746*
- ◆ **A+D® Original [OTC]** *see* Vitamin A and Vitamin D (Topical) *on page 2174*
- ◆ **A771726** *see* Teriflunomide *on page 2006*

Abacavir (a BAK a veer)

Brand Names: U.S. Ziagen

Brand Names: Canada Ziagen®

Index Terms Abacavir Sulfate; ABC

Pharmacologic Category Antiretroviral, Reverse Transcriptase Inhibitor, Nucleoside (Anti-HIV)

Use Treatment of HIV infections in combination with other antiretroviral agents

Pregnancy Risk Factor C

Pregnancy Considerations Adverse events have been observed in some animal reproduction studies. Abacavir has a high level of transfer across the human placenta. No increased risk of overall birth defects has been observed following first trimester exposure according to data collected by the antiretroviral pregnancy registry. Cases of lactic acidosis/hepatic steatosis syndrome related to mitochondrial toxicity have been reported in pregnant women with prolonged use of nucleoside analogues. It is not known if pregnancy itself potentiates this known side effect; however, women may be at increased risk of lactic acidosis and liver damage. In addition, these adverse events are similar to other rare but life-threatening syndromes which occur during pregnancy (eg, HELLP syndrome). Hepatic enzymes and electrolytes should be monitored in women receiving nucleoside analogues and clinicians should watch for early signs of the syndrome. In addition, mitochondrial dysfunction may develop in infants following in utero exposure. The pharmacokinetics of abacavir are not significantly changed by pregnancy and dose adjustment is not needed for pregnant women. The DHHS Perinatal HIV Guidelines consider abacavir in combination with lamivudine to be a preferred NRTI backbone for use in antiretroviral-naive pregnant women.

Regardless of CD4 count or HIV RNA copy number, all HIV-infected pregnant women should receive a combination antiretroviral (ARV) drug regimen. A combination of antepartum, intrapartum, and infant ARV prophylaxis is recommended. ARV therapy should be started as soon as possible in women with symptomatic infection. Although earlier initiation may be more effective in reducing the perinatal transmission of HIV, initiation may be delayed until after 12 weeks gestation in women who do not require immediate treatment after careful consideration of maternal conditions (eg, nausea and vomiting) and the potential risks of first trimester fetal exposure for specific agents. A scheduled cesarean delivery at 38 weeks gestation is recommended for all women with HIV RNA >1000 copies/mL or unknown concentrations near delivery in order to decrease transmission. If ARV therapy must be interrupted for <24 hours during the peripartum period, stop then restart all medications simultaneously in order to decrease the chance of developing resistance. Long-term follow-up is recommended for all infants exposed to ARV medications. In couples who want to conceive, the HIV-infected partner should attain maximum viral suppression prior to conception.

Healthcare providers are encouraged to enroll pregnant women exposed to antiretroviral medications in the Antiretroviral Pregnancy Registry (1-800-258-4263 or www.APRegistry.com). Healthcare providers caring for HIV-infected women and their infants may contact the National Perinatal HIV Hotline (888-448-8765) for clinical consultation (HHS [perinatal], 2014).

Breast-Feeding Considerations Abacavir is excreted into breast milk. Maternal or infant antiretroviral therapy does not completely eliminate the risk of postnatal HIV transmission. In addition, multiclass-resistant virus has been detected in breast-feeding infants despite maternal therapy. Therefore, in the United States, where formula is accessible, affordable, safe, and sustainable, and the risk of infant mortality due to diarrhea and respiratory infections is low, complete avoidance of breast-feeding by HIV-infected women is recommended to decrease potential transmission of HIV (HHS [perinatal], 2014).

Contraindications Hypersensitivity to abacavir or any component of the formulation (do not rechallenge patients who have experienced hypersensitivity to abacavir regardless of *HLA-B*5701* status); moderate-to-severe hepatic impairment

Warnings/Precautions Hazardous agent; use appropriate precautions for handling and disposal (NIOSH 2014 [group 2]).

Abacavir should always be used as a component of a multidrug regimen. Use with caution in patients with plasma HIV RNA levels ≥100,000 copies/mL as earlier virologic failure has been observed in one study (HHS [adult], 2014). **[U.S. Boxed Warning]: Serious and sometimes fatal hypersensitivity reactions have occurred.** Patients testing positive for the presence of the *HLA-B*5701* allele are at an increased risk for hypersensitivity reactions. Screening for *HLA-B*5701* allele status is recommended prior to initiating therapy or reinitiating therapy in patients of unknown status, including patients who previously tolerated therapy. Therapy is **not** recommended in patients testing positive for the *HLA-B*5701* allele. An allergy to abacavir should be reported in the patient's medical record (DHHS [adult], 2014). Reactions usually occur within 9 days of starting abacavir; ~90% occur within 6 weeks. Patients exhibiting symptoms from two or more of the following: Fever, skin rash, constitutional symptoms (malaise, fatigue, aches), respiratory symptoms (eg, pharyngitis, dyspnea, cough), and GI symptoms (eg, abdominal pain, diarrhea, nausea, vomiting) should discontinue therapy immediately and call for medical attention. Abacavir should be permanently discontinued if hypersensitivity cannot be ruled out, even when other diagnoses are possible and regardless of *HLA-B*5701* status. Abacavir SHOULD NOT be restarted because more severe symptoms may occur within hours, including LIFE-THREATENING HYPOTENSION AND DEATH. Fatal hypersensitivity reactions have occurred following the reintroduction of abacavir in patients whose therapy was interrupted (ie, interruption in drug supply, temporary discontinuation while treating other conditions). In some cases, signs of hypersensitivity may have been previously present, but attributed to other medical conditions (eg, acute onset respiratory diseases, gastroenteritis, reactions to other medications). If abacavir is restarted following an interruption in therapy, evaluate the patient for previously unsuspected symptoms of hypersensitivity. A higher incidence of severe hypersensitivity reactions may be associated with a 600 mg once daily dosing regimen.

[U.S. Boxed Warning]: Lactic acidosis and severe hepatomegaly with steatosis (sometimes fatal) have occurred with antiretroviral nucleoside analogues. Female gender, prior liver disease, obesity, and prolonged treatment may increase the risk of hepatotoxicity. May be associated with fat redistribution. Immune reconstitution syndrome may develop, resulting in the occurrence of an inflammatory response to an indolent or residual opportunistic infection during initial HIV treatment or activation of autoimmune disorders (eg, Graves disease, polymyositis, Guillain-Barré syndrome) later in therapy; further evaluation and treatment may be required.

Use has been associated with an increased risk of myocardial infarction (MI) in observational studies; however, based on a meta-analysis of 26 randomized trials, the FDA has concluded there is not an increased risk. Consider using with caution in patients with risks for coronary heart disease and minimizing modifiable risk factors (eg, hypertension, hyperlipidemia, diabetes mellitus, and smoking) prior to use. Some dosage forms may contain propylene glycol; large amounts are potentially toxic and have been associated hyperosmolality, lactic acidosis, seizures and respiratory depression; use caution (AAP, 1997; Zar, 2007).

Adverse Reactions Hypersensitivity reactions (which may be fatal) occur in ~5% of patients. Symptoms may include abdominal pain, anaphylaxis, arthralgia, conjunctivitis, diarrhea, edema, fatigue, fever, headache, hepatic failure, lethargy, lymphadenopathy, malaise, mouth ulcerations, myalgia, myolysis, nausea, paresthesia, rash (including erythema multiforme), renal failure, respiratory symptoms (eg, adult respiratory distress syndrome, cough, dyspnea, pharyngitis, respiratory failure), vomiting.

Note: Rates of adverse reactions were defined during combination therapy with other antiretrovirals (lamivudine and efavirenz **or** lamivudine and zidovudine). Only reactions which occurred at a higher frequency in adults (except where noted) than in the comparator group are noted. Adverse reaction rates attributable to abacavir alone are not available.

Central nervous system: Abnormal dreams, anxiety, depression, dizziness, fatigue, fever/chills, headache, malaise

Dermatologic: Rash

Gastrointestinal: Abdominal pain, diarrhea, nausea, vomiting

Hematologic: Thrombocytopenia

Hepatic: AST increased

Neuromuscular & skeletal: Musculoskeletal pain

Miscellaneous: Hypersensitivity reactions, infection

Rare but important or life-threatening: Erythema multiforme, hepatotoxicity, immune reconstitution syndrome, lactic acidosis, MI, pancreatitis, Stevens-Johnson syndrome, toxic epidermal necrolysis

Drug Interactions

Metabolism/Transport Effects None known.

Avoid Concomitant Use There are no known interactions where it is recommended to avoid concomitant use.

Increased Effect/Toxicity

The levels/effects of Abacavir may be increased by: Ganciclovir-Valganciclovir; Ribavirin

Decreased Effect

The levels/effects of Abacavir may be decreased by: Protease Inhibitors

Food Interactions Ethanol decreases the elimination of abacavir and may increase the risk of toxicity. Management: Monitor patients.

Storage/Stability Store oral solution and tablets at controlled room temperature of 20°C to 25°C (68°F to 77°F). Oral solution may be refrigerated; do not freeze.

Mechanism of Action Nucleoside reverse transcriptase inhibitor. Abacavir is a guanosine analogue which is phosphorylated to carbovir triphosphate which interferes with HIV viral RNA-dependent DNA polymerase resulting in inhibition of viral replication.

Pharmacodynamics/Kinetics

Absorption: Rapid and extensive absorption

Distribution: V_d: 0.86 L/kg

Protein binding: 50%

Metabolism: Hepatic via alcohol dehydrogenase and glucuronyl transferase to inactive carboxylate and glucuronide metabolites; intracellulary metabolized to carbovir triphosphate.

Bioavailability: 83%

Half-life elimination: 1.5 hours

Time to peak: 0.7 to 1.7 hours

Excretion: Primarily urine (as metabolites, 1.2% as unchanged drug); feces (16% total dose)

Dosage Oral:

Infants, Children, and Adolescents 3 months to <16 years: 8 mg/kg body weight twice daily (maximum: 300 mg twice daily) in combination with other antiretroviral agents. **Note:** May consider 16 to 20 mg/kg once daily dosing (maximum: 600 mg/day) in stable patients with undetectable viral load and stable CD4 count for more than 6 months (HHS [pediatric], 2014)

U.S. manufacturer labeling: Alternative dosing to be considered for pediatric patients ≥14 kg who are able to swallow tablets:

14 to 21 kg: 150 mg (1/2 tablet) twice daily

>21 kg to <30 kg: 150 mg (1/2 tablet) in the morning and 300 mg (1 tablet) in the evening

≥30 kg: 300 mg (1 tablet) twice daily

Adolescents ≥16 years and Adults: 300 mg twice daily or 600 mg once daily. **Note:** For patients who are HLA-B*5701 negative, abacavir is a component of a recommended regimen (with dolutegravir and lamivudine) for all treatment-naïve patients and a component of a recommended regimen (with efavirenz and lamivudine or with ritonavir boosted atazanavir and lamivudine) in treatment-naïve patients with pre-ART plasma HIV RNA <100,000 copies/mL (HHS [adult], 2014; HHS [pediatric], 2014)

Canadian labeling:

Infants and Children ≥3 months to 12 years: 8 mg/kg body weight twice daily (maximum: 300 mg twice daily) in combination with other antiretroviral agents

Adolescents >12 years and Adults: 300 mg twice daily in combination with other antiretroviral agents

Dosage adjustment in renal impairment: Canadian labeling (not in U.S. labeling): Use in ESRD or use of 600 mg once daily dosing is not recommended.

Dosage adjustment in hepatic impairment:

Mild impairment (Child-Pugh class A): 200 mg twice daily (oral solution is recommended)

Moderate-to-severe impairment (Child-Pugh class B or C): Use is contraindicated (has not been studied).

Dietary Considerations May be taken with or without food.

Administration May be administered with or without food.

Hazardous agent; use appropriate precautions for handling and disposal (NIOSH 2014 [group 2]).

Monitoring Parameters CBC with differential, serum creatine kinase, CD4 count, HIV RNA plasma levels, serum transaminases, triglycerides, serum amylase; *HLA-B*5701* genotype status prior to initiation of therapy and prior to reinitiation of therapy in patients of unknown *HLA-B*5701* status; signs and symptoms of hypersensitivity, particularly in patients untested for the *HLA-B*5701* allele

Additional Information Use regimens of abacavir and nevirapine with caution; both agents cause hypersensitivity reactions early in therapy (HHS, [adult] 2014).

Hypersensitivity testing (*HLA-B*5701*): Prevalence of hypersensitivity reactions has been estimated at 5% to 8% in Caucasians and 2% to 3% in African-Americans. Pretherapy identification of *HLA-B*5701*-positive patients, and subsequent avoidance of abacavir therapy in these patients has been shown to reduce the occurrence of abacavir-mediated hypersensitivity reactions. An allergy to abacavir should be reported in the patient's medical record (HHS, [adult] 2014). A skin patch test is in development for clinical screening purposes; however, only PCR-mediated genotyping methods are currently in clinical practice use for documentation of this susceptibility marker.

Dosage Forms

Solution, Oral:

Ziagen: 20 mg/mL (240 mL)

Tablet, Oral:

Ziagen: 300 mg

Generic: 300 mg

Abacavir and Lamivudine

(a BAK a veer & la MI vyoo deen)

Brand Names: U.S. Epzicom

Brand Names: Canada Kivexa

Index Terms Abacavir Sulfate and Lamivudine; Lamivudine and Abacavir

Pharmacologic Category Antiretroviral, Reverse Transcriptase Inhibitor, Nucleoside (Anti-HIV)

Use Treatment of HIV infections in combination with other antiretroviral agents

Pregnancy Risk Factor C

Dosage HIV treatment: Adolescents ≥16 years weighing >50 kg and Adults: Oral: One tablet (abacavir 600 mg and lamivudine 300 mg) once daily. **Note:** For patients who are HLA-B*5701 negative, abacavir plus lamivudine is a component of a recommended regimen (with dolutegravir) for all treatment-naive patients and a component of a recommended regimen (with efavirenz or ritonavir boosted atazanavir) for patients with pre-ART plasma HIV RNA <100,000 copies/mL (HHS [adult], 2014; HHS [pediatric], 2014)

Dosage adjustment in renal impairment: CrCl <50 mL/minute: Use not recommended

Dosage adjustment in hepatic impairment: Use contraindicated.

Additional Information Complete prescribing information should be consulted for additional detail.

Dosage Forms

Tablet:

Epzicom: Abacavir 600 mg and lamivudine 300 mg

Abacavir, Dolutegravir, and Lamivudine

(a BAK a veer, doe loo TEG ra vir, & la MI vyoo deen)

Brand Names: U.S. Triumeq

Brand Names: Canada Triumeq

Index Terms Abacavir Sulfate, Dolutegravir, and Lamivudine; Dolutegravir, Lamivudine, and Abacavir; Lamivudine, Abacavir, and Dolutegravir

Pharmacologic Category Antiretroviral, Integrase Inhibitor (Anti-HIV); Antiretroviral, Reverse Transcriptase Inhibitor, Nucleoside (Anti-HIV)

Use

HIV infection: Treatment of human immunodeficiency virus type 1 (HIV-1) infection

Limitations of use: Not recommended for use in patients with current or past history of resistance to abacavir, dolutegravir, or lamivudine; not recommended in patients with resistance-associated integrase substitutions or clinically suspected integrase strand transfer inhibitor resistance because the dose of dolutegravir is insufficient in these subpopulations.

Pregnancy Risk Factor C

Dosage

HIV treatment: Adults: Oral: One tablet daily

Dosage adjustment for concomitant therapy with efavirenz, fosamprenavir/ritonavir, tipranavir/ritonavir, or rifampin: One tablet daily, with an additional single-component dolutegravir 50 mg tablet administered daily 12 hours after Triumeq

Dosage adjustment for renal impairment:

CrCl ≥50 mL/minute: No dosage adjustment necessary.

CrCl <50 mL/minute: Use is not recommended (use dose-adjusted individual component drugs).

Dosage adjustment for hepatic impairment:

Mild impairment (Child-Pugh class A): Use is not recommended (use dose-adjusted individual component drugs).

Moderate to severe impairment (Child-Pugh class B or C): Use is contraindicated by the manufacturer.

U.S. labeling: Use is contraindicated.

Canadian labeling: Use is not specifically contraindicated, but is not recommended.

Additional Information Complete prescribing information should be consulted for additional detail.

Dosage Forms

Tablet, Oral:

Triumeq: Abacavir 600 mg, dolutegravir 50 mg, and lamivudine 300 mg

Abacavir, Lamivudine, and Zidovudine

(a BAK a veer, la MI vyoo deen, & zye DOE vyoo deen)

Brand Names: U.S. Trizivir

Brand Names: Canada Trizivir

Index Terms 3TC, Abacavir, and Zidovudine; Azidothymidine, Abacavir, and Lamivudine; AZT, Abacavir, and Lamivudine; Compound S, Abacavir, and Lamivudine; Lamivudine, Abacavir, and Zidovudine; ZDV, Abacavir, and Lamivudine; Zidovudine, Abacavir, and Lamivudine

Pharmacologic Category Antiretroviral, Reverse Transcriptase Inhibitor, Nucleoside (Anti-HIV)

Use HIV infection: Treatment of HIV-1 infection in combination with other antiretroviral agents or alone in patients weighing more than 40 kg.

Pregnancy Risk Factor C

Dosage Oral:

U.S. labeling: Adolescents ≥40 kg and Adults: One tablet twice daily. **Note:** Not recommended for patients <40 kg.

Canadian labeling: Adults ≥50 kg: One tablet twice daily. **Note:** Not recommended for patients <50 kg.

Dosage adjustment in renal impairment: CrCl <50 mL/minute: Avoid use.

Dosage adjustment in hepatic impairment: Use is contraindicated.

Additional Information Complete prescribing information should be consulted for additional detail.

Dosage Forms

Tablet, oral:

Trizivir: Abacavir 300 mg, lamivudine 150 mg, and zidovudine 300 mg

Generic: Abacavir sulfate 300 mg, lamivudine 150 mg, and zidovudine 300 mg

◆ **Abacavir Sulfate** *see* Abacavir *on page* 20

◆ **Abacavir Sulfate and Lamivudine** *see* Abacavir and Lamivudine *on page* 22

◆ **Abacavir Sulfate, Dolutegravir, and Lamivudine** *see* Abacavir, Dolutegravir, and Lamivudine *on page* 22

Abatacept (ab a TA sept)

Brand Names: U.S. Orencia
Brand Names: Canada Orencia
Index Terms BMS-188667; CTLA-4Ig
Pharmacologic Category Antirheumatic, Disease Modifying; Selective T-Cell Costimulation Blocker
Use

Rheumatoid arthritis: Treatment of moderately to severely active adult rheumatoid arthritis (RA); may be used as monotherapy or in combination with other DMARDs

Juvenile idiopathic arthritis: Treatment of moderately to severely active polyarticular juvenile idiopathic arthritis (JIA); may be used as monotherapy or in combination with methotrexate

Note: Abatacept should **not** be used in combination with anakinra or TNF-blocking agents

Pregnancy Risk Factor C

Pregnancy Considerations Adverse effects were not observed in animal studies. Due to the potential risk for development of autoimmune disease in the fetus, use during pregnancy only if clearly needed. A pregnancy registry has been established to monitor outcomes of women exposed to abatacept during pregnancy (1-877-311-8972).

Breast-Feeding Considerations It is not known if abatacept is excreted into human milk. Due to the potential for serious adverse reactions in the nursing infant, a decision should be made to discontinue nursing or to discontinue the drug, taking into account the importance of treatment to the mother.

Contraindications There are no contraindications listed within the manufacturer's U.S. labeling.

Canadian labeling: Hypersensitivity to abatacept or any component of the formulation; patients with, or at risk of sepsis syndrome (eg, immunocompromised, HIV positive)

Warnings/Precautions Serious and potentially fatal infections (including tuberculosis and sepsis) have been reported, particularly in patients receiving concomitant immunosuppressive therapy. RA patients receiving a concomitant TNF antagonist experienced an even higher rate of serious infection. Caution should be exercised when considering the use of abatacept in any patient with a history of recurrent infections, with conditions that predispose them to infections, or with chronic, latent, or localized infections. Patients who develop a new infection while undergoing treatment should be monitored closely. If a patient develops a serious infection, abatacept should be discontinued. Screen patients for latent tuberculosis infection prior to initiating abatacept; safety in tuberculosis-positive patients has not been established. Treat patients testing positive according to standard therapy prior to initiating abatacept. Adult patients receiving abatacept in combination with TNF-blocking agents had higher rates of infections (including serious infections) than patients on TNF-blocking agents alone. Potentially significant drug-drug interactions may exist, requiring dose or frequency adjustment, additional monitoring, and/or selection of alternative therapy. The manufacturer does not recommend concurrent use with anakinra or TNF-blocking agents. Monitor for signs and symptoms of infection when transitioning from TNF-blocking agents to abatacept. Due to the effect of T-cell inhibition on host defenses, abatacept may affect immune responses against infections and malignancies; impact on the development and course of malignancies is not fully defined.

Use caution with chronic obstructive pulmonary disease (COPD), higher incidences of adverse effects (COPD exacerbation, cough, rhonchi, dyspnea) have been observed; monitor closely. Rare cases of hypersensitivity, anaphylaxis, or anaphylactoid reactions have been reported with intravenous administration; may occur with first infusion. Some reactions (hypotension, urticaria, dyspnea) occurred within 24 hours of infusion. Discontinue treatment if anaphylaxis or other serious allergic reaction occurs; medications for the treatment of hypersensitivity reactions should be available for immediate use. Patients should be screened for viral hepatitis prior to use; antirheumatic therapy may cause reactivation of hepatitis B. Patients should be brought up to date with all immunizations before initiating therapy. Live vaccines should not be given concurrently or within 3 months of discontinuation of therapy; there is no data available concerning secondary transmission of live vaccines in patients receiving therapy. Powder for injection may contain maltose, which may result in falsely-elevated serum glucose readings on the day of infusion. Higher incidences of infection and malignancy were observed in the elderly; use with caution.

Adverse Reactions Note: COPD patients experienced a higher frequency of COPD-related adverse reactions (COPD exacerbation, cough, dyspnea, pneumonia, rhonchi)

Cardiovascular: Hypertension
Central nervous system: Dizziness, headache
Dermatologic: Skin rash
Gastrointestinal: Abdominal pain, diarrhea, dyspepsia, nausea
Genitourinary: Urinary tract infection
Immunologic: Immunogenicity
Infection: Herpes simplex infection, influenza
Local: Injection site reaction
Neuromuscular & skeletal: Back pain, limb pain
Respiratory: Bronchitis, cough, nasopharyngitis, pneumonia, rhinitis, sinusitis, upper respiratory tract infection
Miscellaneous: Antibody development, fever, infection, infusion-related reaction
Rare but important or life-threatening: Acute lymphocytic leukemia, anaphylactoid reaction, anaphylaxis, cellulitis, diverticulitis, dyspnea, exacerbation of arthritis, exacerbation of chronic obstructive pulmonary disease, hypersensitivity, hypotension, joint wear, malignant lymphoma, malignant neoplasm (including malignant melanoma, malignant neoplasm of the bile duct, malignant neoplasm of bladder, malignant neoplasm of breast, malignant neoplasm of cervix, malignant neoplasm of kidney, malignant neoplasm of prostate, malignant neoplasm of skin, malignant neoplasm of thyroid, myelodysplastic syndrome, and uterine neoplasm), malignant neoplasm of lung, ovarian cyst, pruritus, pyelonephritis, rhonchi, urticaria, varicella, vasculitis (including hypersensitivity angiitis [cutaneous vasculitis and leukocytoclastic vasculitis]), wheezing

Drug Interactions

Metabolism/Transport Effects None known.

Avoid Concomitant Use

Avoid concomitant use of Abatacept with any of the following: Anakinra; Anti-TNF Agents; BCG; Belimumab; Natalizumab; Pimecrolimus; RiTUXimab; Tacrolimus (Topical); Tocilizumab; Tofacitinib; Vaccines (Live)

Increased Effect/Toxicity

Abatacept may increase the levels/effects of: Belimumab; Leflunomide; Natalizumab; Tofacitinib; Vaccines (Live)

The levels/effects of Abatacept may be increased by: Anakinra; Anti-TNF Agents; Denosumab; Pimecrolimus; RiTUXimab; Roflumilast; Tacrolimus (Topical); Tocilizumab; Trastuzumab

Decreased Effect

Abatacept may decrease the levels/effects of: BCG; Coccidioides immitis Skin Test; Sipuleucel-T; Vaccines (Inactivated); Vaccines (Live)

The levels/effects of Abatacept may be decreased by: Echinacea

Preparation for Administration

IV: Reconstitute each vial with 10 mL SWFI using the provided silicone-free disposable syringe (discard solutions accidentally reconstituted with siliconized syringe as they may develop translucent particles). Inject SWFI down the side of the vial to avoid foaming. The reconstituted solution contains 25 mg/mL abatacept. Further dilute (using a silicone-free syringe) in 100 mL NS to a final concentration of ≤10 mg/mL. Prior to adding abatacept to the 100 mL bag, the manufacturer recommends withdrawing a volume of NS equal to the abatacept volume required, resulting in a final volume of 100 mL. Mix gently; do not shake.

SubQ: Allow prefilled syringe to reach room temperature prior to administration by removing from refrigerator 30-60 minutes prior to administration.

Storage/Stability

Prefilled syringe: Store at 2°C to 8°C (36°F to 46°F); do not freeze. Protect from light.

Powder for injection: Prior to reconstitution, store at 2°C to 8°C (36°F to 46°F); do not freeze. Protect from light. After dilution, may be stored for up to 24 hours at room temperature or refrigerated at 2°C to 8°C (36°F to 46°F). Must be used within 24 hours of reconstitution.

Mechanism of Action Selective costimulation modulator; inhibits T-cell (T-lymphocyte) activation by binding to CD80 and CD86 on antigen presenting cells (APC), thus blocking the required CD28 interaction between APCs and T cells. Activated T lymphocytes are found in the synovium of rheumatoid arthritis patients.

Pharmacodynamics/Kinetics

Bioavailability: SubQ: 78.6% (relative to IV administration)

Distribution: V_{ss}: 0.02-0.13 L/kg

Half-life elimination: 8-25 days

Dosage

Juvenile idiopathic arthritis (JIA): IV:

Children ≥6 years and <75 kg: 10 mg/kg (based on body weight at each administration), repeat dose at 2 weeks and 4 weeks after initial infusion, and every 4 weeks thereafter.

Children ≥6 years and ≥75 kg: **Note:** Dosage is according to body weight. Repeat dose at 2 weeks and 4 weeks after initial dose and every 4 weeks thereafter:

75-100 kg: 750 mg

>100 kg: 1000 mg

Rheumatoid arthritis: Adults:

IV: Dosing is according to body weight. Following the initial IV infusion (using the weight-based dosing), repeat IV infusion (using the same weight-based dosing) at 2 weeks and 4 weeks after the initial infusion, and every 4 weeks thereafter.

<60 kg: 500 mg

60-100 kg: 750 mg

>100 kg: 1000 mg

SubQ: 125 subcutaneously once weekly. **Note:** SubQ dosing may be initiated with or without an IV loading dose.

If initiating with an IV loading dose, administer the initial IV infusion (using the weight-based dosing), then administer 125 mg subcutaneously within 24 hours of the infusion, followed by 125 mg subcutaneously once weekly thereafter.

If transitioning from IV therapy to SubQ therapy, administer the first SubQ dose instead of the next scheduled IV dose.

Elderly: Refer to adult dosing; due to potential for higher rates of infections and malignancies, use caution.

Dosage adjustment for toxicity: Discontinue in patients who develop a serious infection.

Dosage adjustment in renal impairment: No dosage adjustment provided in manufacturer's labeling (has not been studied).

Dosage adjustment in hepatic impairment: No dosage adjustment provided in manufacturer's labeling (has not been studied).

Administration

IV: Infuse over 30 minutes. Administer through a 0.2-1.2 micron low protein-binding filter

SubQ: Allow prefilled syringe to warm to room temperature (for 30-60 minutes) prior to administration. Inject into the front of the thigh (preferred), abdomen (except for 2-inch area around the navel), or the outer area of the upper arms (if administered by a caregiver). Rotate injection sites (≥1 inch apart); do not administer into tender, bruised, red, or hard skin.

Monitoring Parameters Signs and symptoms of infection, signs and symptoms of hypersensitivity reaction; hepatitis and TB screening prior to therapy initiation

Dosage Forms

Solution Prefilled Syringe, Subcutaneous [preservative free]:

Orencia: 125 mg/mL (1 mL)

Solution Reconstituted, Intravenous [preservative free]:

Orencia: 250 mg (1 ea)

- ◆ **Abbott-43818** *see* Leuprolide *on page 1186*
- ◆ **Abbott-Citalopram (Can)** *see* Citalopram *on page 451*
- ◆ **Abbott-Levetiracetam (Can)** *see* LevETIRAcetam *on page 1191*
- ◆ **Abbott-Olanzapine ODT (Can)** *see* OLANZapine *on page 1491*
- ◆ **Abbott-Pantoprazole (Can)** *see* Pantoprazole *on page 1570*
- ◆ **Abbott-Topiramate (Can)** *see* Topiramate *on page 2065*
- ◆ **ABC** *see* Abacavir *on page 20*
- ◆ **ABCD** *see* Amphotericin B Cholesteryl Sulfate Complex *on page 136*

Abciximab (ab SIK si mab)

Brand Names: U.S. ReoPro

Brand Names: Canada ReoPro

Index Terms 7E3; C7E3

Pharmacologic Category Antiplatelet Agent, Glycoprotein IIb/IIIa Inhibitor

Use Prevention of cardiac ischemic complications in patients undergoing percutaneous coronary intervention (PCI); prevention of cardiac ischemic complications in patients with unstable angina (UA)/non-ST-elevation myocardial infarction (NSTEMI) unresponsive to conventional therapy when PCI is scheduled within 24 hours

Note: Intended for use with aspirin and heparin, at a minimum.

Pregnancy Risk Factor C

Pregnancy Considerations Animal reproduction studies have not been conducted. *In vitro* studies have shown only small amounts of abciximab to cross the placenta. It is not known whether abciximab can cause fetal harm when administered to a pregnant woman or can affect reproduction capacity.

Breast-Feeding Considerations It is not known if abciximab is excreted in breast milk. The manufacturer recommends that caution be exercised when administering abciximab to nursing women.

Contraindications Hypersensitivity to abciximab, murine proteins, or any component of the formulation; active internal hemorrhage or recent (within 6 weeks) clinically-significant GI or GU bleeding; history of cerebrovascular accident within 2 years or with significant neurological deficit; clotting abnormalities or administration of oral anticoagulants within 7 days unless prothrombin time (PT) is ≤1.2 times control PT value; thrombocytopenia (<100,000 cells/µL); recent (within 6 weeks) major surgery or trauma; intracranial tumor, arteriovenous malformation, or aneurysm; severe uncontrolled hypertension; history of vasculitis; use of dextran before PTCA or intent to use dextran during PTCA; concomitant use of another parenteral GP IIb/IIIa inhibitor

Warnings/Precautions Administration of abciximab is associated with increased frequency of major bleeding complications, including retroperitoneal bleeding, pulmonary bleeding, spontaneous GI or GU bleeding, and bleeding at the arterial access. Risk may be increased with patients weighing <75 kg, elderly patients (>65 years of age), history of previous GI disease, and recent thrombolytic therapy. When attempting IV access, avoid noncompressible sites (eg, subclavian or jugular veins).

The risk of major bleeds may increase with concurrent use of thrombolytics. Anticoagulation, such as with heparin, may contribute to the risk of bleeding. In serious, uncontrolled bleeding, abciximab and heparin should be stopped. Increased risk of hemorrhage during or following angioplasty is associated with unsuccessful PTCA, PTCA procedure >70 minutes duration, or PTCA performed within 12 hours of symptom onset for acute myocardial infarction. Prior to pulling the sheath, heparin should be discontinued for 3-4 hours and ACT ≤175 seconds or aPTT ≤50 seconds. Use standard compression techniques after sheath removal. Watch the site closely afterwards for further bleeding.

Administration of abciximab may result in human antichimeric antibody formation that can cause hypersensitivity reactions (including anaphylaxis), thrombocytopenia, or diminished efficacy. Readministration of abciximab within 30 days or in patients with human antichimeric antibodies (HACA) increases the incidence and severity of thrombocytopenia.

Adverse Reactions As with all drugs which may affect hemostasis, bleeding is associated with abciximab. Hemorrhage may occur at virtually any site. Risk is dependent on multiple variables, including the concurrent use of multiple agents which alter hemostasis and patient susceptibility.

Cardiovascular: Bradycardia, chest pain, hypotension, peripheral edema

Gastrointestinal: Abdominal pain, nausea

Hematologic & oncologic: Major hemorrhage, minor hemorrhage, thrombocytopenia

Local: Pain at injection site

Neuromuscular & skeletal: Back pain

Miscellaneous: Antibody development

Rare but important or life-threatening: Abnormality in thinking, abscess, allergic reaction (possible), anaphylaxis (possible), arteriovenous fistula, bronchitis, bullous skin disease, cellulitis, cerebrovascular accident, coma, complete atrioventricular block, confusion, diabetes mellitus, edema, embolism, gastroesophageal reflux disease, hyperkalemia, hypertonia, incomplete atrioventricular block, inflammation, intestinal obstruction, intracranial hemorrhage, leukocytosis, nodal arrhythmia, pleural effusion, pleurisy, pneumonia, prostatitis, pseudoaneurysm, pulmonary alveolar hemorrhage, pulmonary embolism, renal insufficiency, thrombophlebitis, urinary retention, ventricular tachycardia

Drug Interactions

Metabolism/Transport Effects None known.

Avoid Concomitant Use

Avoid concomitant use of Abciximab with any of the following: Belimumab; Dextran; Urokinase

Increased Effect/Toxicity

Abciximab may increase the levels/effects of: Agents with Antiplatelet Properties; Anticoagulants; Apixaban; Belimumab; Collagenase (Systemic); Dabigatran Etexilate; Ibritumomab; Obinutuzumab; Rivaroxaban; Salicylates; Thrombolytic Agents; Tositumomab and Iodine I 131 Tositumomab; Urokinase

The levels/effects of Abciximab may be increased by: Dasatinib; Dextran; Glucosamine; Herbs (Anticoagulant/Antiplatelet Properties); Ibrutinib; Limaprost; Multivitamins/Fluoride (with ADE); Multivitamins/Minerals (with ADEK, Folate, Iron); Multivitamins/Minerals (with AE, No Iron); Omega-3 Fatty Acids; Pentosan Polysulfate Sodium; Pentoxifylline; Prostacyclin Analogues; Tipranavir; Vitamin E

Decreased Effect There are no known significant interactions involving a decrease in effect.

Preparation for Administration Bolus dose: Aseptically withdraw the necessary amount of abciximab for the bolus dose into a syringe using a 0.2 or 5 micron low protein-binding syringe filter (or equivalent); the bolus should be administered 10-60 minutes before the procedure.

Continuous infusion: Aseptically withdraw amount required of abciximab for the infusion through a 0.2 or 5 micron low protein-binding syringe filter into a syringe; inject this into 250 mL of NS or D_5W to make solution. If a syringe filter was not used when preparing the infusion, administer using an in-line 0.2 or 0.22 micron low protein-binding filter.

Note: A standard concentration of 7.2 mg in 250 mL of NS or D_5W may also be prepared for all patients and administered at the standard dose (0.125 mcg/kg/minute; maximum: 10 mcg/minute) with a variable rate in mL/hour. Infuse for 12-24 hours via pump after bolus dose; length of therapy dependent on indication. Some institutions use a standard concentration of 9 mg in 250 mL of D_5W or NS.

Storage/Stability Vials should be stored at 2°C to 8°C (36°F to 46°F). Do not freeze or shake. After admixture, the prepared solution is stable for 12 hours.

The following stability information has also been reported: May store intact vials at 24°C to 28°C (76°F to 82°F) for up to 8 days (data on file [Eli Lilly, 2011]). However, the manufacturer recommends storage under refrigeration. Room temperature stability information should only be utilized in situations where the drug has been inadvertently exposed to prolonged room temperature.

Mechanism of Action Fab antibody fragment of the chimeric human-murine monoclonal antibody 7E3; this agent binds to platelet IIb/IIIa receptors, resulting in steric hindrance, thus inhibiting platelet aggregation

Pharmacodynamics/Kinetics

Onset: Rapid; platelet aggregation reduced to <20% of baseline at 10 minutes

Duration: Up to 72 hours for restoration of normal hemostasis (Schror, 2003)

Distribution: V_d: 0.07 L/kg (Schror, 2003)

Protein binding: Mostly bound to GP IIb/IIIa receptors on platelet surface

Metabolism: Unbound abciximab metabolized via proteolytic cleavage (Schror, 2003)

Half-life elimination: Plasma: ~30 minutes; dissociation half-life from GP IIb/IIIa receptors: up to 4 hours (Schror, 2003). **Note:** 29% and 13% of abciximab estimated to remain on GP IIb/IIIa receptors at 8 and 15 days, respectively (Mascelli, 1998). Platelet function may remain abnormal for up to 7 days post infusion (Osende, 2001).

Time to peak: Platelet inhibition: ~30 minutes (Mascelli, 1998)

Dosage

Percutaneous coronary intervention (PCI): IV: 0.25 mg/kg bolus administered 10-60 minutes prior to start of PCI followed by an infusion of 0.125 mcg/kg/minute (maximum: 10 mcg/minute) for 12 hours

Unstable angina/non-ST-elevation MI (UA/NSTEMI) unresponsive to conventional medical therapy with planned PCI within 24 hours: IV: 0.25 mg/kg bolus followed by an 18- to 24-hour infusion of 10 mcg/minute, concluding 1 hour after PCI.

ST-elevation myocardial infarction (STEMI) undergoing primary percutaneous coronary intervention (PCI) (off-label use) (ACCF/AHA [O'Gara, 2013]):

IV:

Loading dose: 0.25 mg/kg bolus administered at the time of PCI

Maintenance infusion: 0.125 mcg/kg/minute (maximum: 10 mcg/minute) continued for up to 12 hours

Intracoronary (off-label route): 0.25 mg/kg bolus administered directly to the site of the infarct lesion; may be followed with an intravenous maintenance infusion if refractory intraprocedural thrombotic complications occur (Stone, 2012).

Dosage adjustment in renal impairment: There are no dosage adjustments provided in the manufacturer's labeling.

Dosage adjustment in hepatic impairment: There are no dosage adjustments provided in the manufacturer's labeling.

Usual Infusion Concentrations: Adult IV infusion: 7.2 mg in 250 mL (concentration: 28.8 **mcg**/mL) **or** 9 mg in 250 mL (concentration: 36 **mcg**/mL) of D_5W or NS

Administration

Abciximab is intended for coadministration with aspirin postangioplasty and heparin infused and weight adjusted to maintain a therapeutic bleeding time (eg, ACT 300 to 500 seconds). Solution must be filtered prior to administration. Do not shake the vial.

Intracoronary administration (off-label route): In select STEMI cases (eg, anterior STEMI), abciximab bolus may be administered through the guiding catheter directly to the culprit lesion site (Stone, 2012; Thiele, 2012)

Monitoring Parameters Prothrombin time, activated partial thromboplastin time (aPTT), hemoglobin, hematocrit, platelet count, fibrinogen, fibrin split products, transfusion requirements, signs of hypersensitivity reactions, guaiac stools, Hemastix® urine. Platelet count should be monitored at baseline, 2-4 hours following bolus infusion, and at 24 hours (or prior to discharge, if before 24 hours). To minimize risk of bleeding:

Abciximab initiated 18-24 hours prior to PCI: Maintain aPTT between 60-85 seconds during the heparin/abciximab infusion period

During PCI: Maintain ACT between 200-300 seconds

Following PCI (if anticoagulation is maintained): Maintain aPTT between 50-75 seconds

Sheath removal should not occur until aPTT is ≤50 seconds or ACT ≤175 seconds.

Maintain bleeding precautions, avoid unnecessary arterial and venous punctures, use saline or heparin lock for blood drawing, assess sheath insertion site and distal pulses of affected leg every 15 minutes for the first hour and then every 1 hour for the next 6 hours. Arterial access site care is important to prevent bleeding. Care should be taken when attempting vascular access that only the anterior wall of the femoral artery is punctured, avoiding a Seldinger (through and through) technique for obtaining sheath access. Femoral vein sheath placement should be avoided unless needed. While the vascular sheath is in place, patients should be maintained on complete bedrest with the head of the bed at a 30° angle and the affected limb restrained in a straight position.

Observe patient for mental status changes, hemorrhage; assess nose and mouth mucous membranes, puncture sites for oozing, ecchymosis, and hematoma formation; and examine urine, stool, and emesis for presence of occult or frank blood; gentle care should be provided when removing dressings.

Dosage Forms

Solution, Intravenous:

ReoPro: 2 mg/mL (5 mL)

◆ **Abelcet** *see* Amphotericin B (Lipid Complex) *on page 138*

◆ **Abelcet® (Can)** *see* Amphotericin B (Lipid Complex) *on page 138*

◆ **Abenol (Can)** *see* Acetaminophen *on page 32*

◆ **ABI-007** *see* PACLitaxel (Protein Bound) *on page 1554*

◆ **Abilify** *see* ARIPiprazole *on page 171*

◆ **Abilify Discmelt** *see* ARIPiprazole *on page 171*

◆ **Abilify Maintena** *see* ARIPiprazole *on page 171*

◆ **Abiraterone** *see* Abiraterone Acetate *on page 26*

Abiraterone Acetate (a bir A ter one AS e tate)

Brand Names: U.S. Zytiga

Brand Names: Canada Zytiga

Index Terms Abiraterone; CB7630

Pharmacologic Category Antiandrogen; Antineoplastic Agent, Antiandrogen

Use Prostate cancer: Treatment of metastatic, castration-resistant prostate cancer (in combination with prednisone)

Pregnancy Risk Factor X

Pregnancy Considerations Adverse effects were observed in animal reproduction studies at doses resulting in less systemic exposure than in humans. Adverse effects were also observed in the reproductive system of animals during toxicology and pharmacology studies. Based on the mechanism of action, abiraterone may cause fetal harm or fetal loss if administered during pregnancy. Abiraterone is not indicated for use in women and is specifically contraindicated in women who are or may become pregnant. It is not known if abiraterone is excreted in semen, therefore, men should use a condom and another method of birth control during treatment and for 1 week following therapy if having intercourse with a woman of reproductive age. Women who are or may become pregnant should wear gloves if contact with tablets may occur.

Breast-Feeding Considerations Not indicated for use in women

Contraindications Women who are or may become pregnant

Canadian labeling: Additional contraindication (not in U.S. labeling): Hypersensitivity to abiraterone acetate or any component of the formulation or container

Warnings/Precautions Hazardous agent - use appropriate precautions for handling and disposal (NIOSH 2014 [group 1]). Significant increases in liver enzymes have been reported (higher likelihood in patients with baseline elevations), generally occurring in the first 3 months of treatment. May require dosage reduction or discontinuation. ALT, AST, and bilirubin should be monitored prior to treatment, every 2 weeks for 3 months and monthly thereafter; patients with hepatic impairment, elevations in liver function tests, or experiencing hepatotoxicity require more frequent monitoring (see Dosage adjustment for hepatic impairment and Monitoring Parameters). Evaluate liver function promptly with signs or symptoms of hepatotoxicity. The safety of retreatment after significant elevations (ALT or AST >20 times the upper limit of normal [ULN] and/or total bilirubin >10 times ULN) has not been evaluated. Avoid use in patients with preexisting severe hepatic impairment; dosage reduction is recommended in patients with baseline moderate impairment. Canadian labeling (not in U.S. labeling) also recommends avoiding use in patients with preexisting moderate hepatic impairment.

Concurrent infection, stress, or interruption of daily corticosteroids is associated with reports of adrenocortical insufficiency. Monitor closely for signs and symptoms of adrenocorticoid insufficiency, which could be masked by adverse events associated with mineralocorticoid excess. Diagnostic testing for adrenal insufficiency may be clinically indicated. Increased corticosteroid doses may be required before, during, and after stress. May cause increased mineralocorticoid levels, which may result in hypertension, hypokalemia and fluid retention (including grades 3 and 4 events). Concomitant administration with corticosteroids reduces the incidence and severity of these adverse events. Due to potential for hypertension, hypokalemia, or fluid retention, use with caution in patients with cardiovascular disease (particularly heart failure, recent MI, or ventricular arrhythmia); patients with left ventricular ejection fraction (LVEF) <50% or NYHA class III or IV heart failure were excluded from clinical trials. Monitor at least monthly for hypertension, hypokalemia, and fluid retention.

Abiraterone must be administered on an empty stomach (administer at least 1 hour before and 2 hours after any food); abiraterone AUC (exposure) may be increased up to 10-fold if administered with food. Potentially significant drug-drug interactions may exist, requiring dose or frequency adjustment, additional monitoring, and/or selection of alternative therapy. Avoid use with concomitant strong CYP3A4 inducers (dose modification is necessary if concomitant use cannot be avoided). Avoid concurrent administration with CYP2D6 substrates with a narrow therapeutic index (eg, thioridazine); if concurrent administration cannot be avoided, consider a dose reduction of the CYP2D6 substrate.

Adverse Reactions Note: Adverse reactions reported for use in combination with prednisone.

Cardiovascular: Cardiac arrhythmia, cardiac failure, chest pain (including chest discomfort), edema, hypertension

Central nervous system: Falling, fatigue, insomnia

Dermatologic: Bruise, skin rash

Endocrine & metabolic: Hot flash, hyperglycemia, hypernatremia, hypertriglyceridemia, hypokalemia, hypophosphatemia

Gastrointestinal: Constipation, diarrhea, dyspepsia

Genitourinary: Groin pain, hematuria, nocturia, polyuria, urinary tract infection

Hematologic & oncologic: Lymphocytopenia

Hepatic: Increased serum ALT, increased serum AST, increased serum bilirubin

Neuromuscular & skeletal: Bone fracture, joint swelling (including joint discomfort), myalgia

Respiratory: Cough, dyspnea, nasopharyngitis, upper respiratory infection

Miscellaneous: Fever

Rare but important or life-threatening: Adrenocortical insufficiency, hypersensitivity pneumonitis, noninfectious pneumonitis

Drug Interactions

Metabolism/Transport Effects Substrate of CYP3A4 (major); **Note:** Assignment of Major/Minor substrate status based on clinically relevant drug interaction potential; **Inhibits** CYP1A2 (weak), CYP2C19 (moderate), CYP2C8 (strong), CYP2C9 (moderate), CYP2D6 (moderate), CYP3A4 (moderate), P-glycoprotein

Avoid Concomitant Use

Avoid concomitant use of Abiraterone Acetate with any of the following: Bosutinib; CYP3A4 Inducers (Strong); Dasabuvir; Enzalutamide; Ibrutinib; Indium 111 Capromab Pendetide; Ivabradine; Lomitapide; Naloxegol; Olaparib; PAZOPanib; Pimozide; Silodosin; Simeprevir; Thioridazine; Tolvaptan; Topotecan; Trabectedin; Ulipristal; VinCRIStine (Liposomal)

Increased Effect/Toxicity

Abiraterone Acetate may increase the levels/effects of: Afatinib; Avanafil; Bosentan; Bosutinib; Brentuximab Vedotin; Budesonide (Systemic, Oral Inhalation); Cannabis; Citalopram; Colchicine; CYP1A2 Substrates; CYP2C19 Substrates; CYP2C8 Substrates; CYP2C9 Substrates; CYP2D6 Substrates; CYP3A4 Substrates; Dabigatran Etexilate; Dapoxetine; Dasabuvir; Dofetilide; DOXOrubicin (Conventional); Dronabinol; Edoxaban; Eliglustat; Enzalutamide; Eplerenone; Everolimus; FentaNYL; Fesoterodine; Halofantrine; Hydrocodone; Ibrutinib; Imatinib; Ivabradine; Ivacaftor; Ledipasvir; Lomitapide; Lurasidone; Metoprolol; Naloxegol; Nebivolol; Nintedanib; Olaparib; OxyCODONE; PAZOPanib; P-glycoprotein/ABCB1 Substrates; Pimecrolimus; Pimozide; Pioglitazone; Propafenone; Prucalopride; Ranolazine; Rifaximin; Rivaroxaban; Salmeterol; Saxagliptin; Silodosin; Simeprevir; Suvorexant; Tetrahydrocannabinol; Thioridazine; Tolvaptan; Topotecan; Trabectedin; Treprostinil; Ulipristal; Vilazodone; VinCRIStine (Liposomal); Zopiclone

The levels/effects of Abiraterone Acetate may be increased by: Propafenone

Decreased Effect

Abiraterone Acetate may decrease the levels/effects of: Clopidogrel; Codeine; Ifosfamide; Indium 111 Capromab Pendetide; Tamoxifen; TraMADol

The levels/effects of Abiraterone Acetate may be decreased by: Bosentan; CYP3A4 Inducers (Moderate); CYP3A4 Inducers (Strong); Dabrafenib; Deferasirox; Siltuximab; Spironolactone; St Johns Wort; Tocilizumab

Food Interactions Taking with food will increase systemic exposure (up to 10-fold). Management: Do not administer with food. Must be taken on an empty stomach, at least 1 hour before and 2 hours after food.

Storage/Stability Store at 20°C to 25°C (68°F to 77°F); excursions are permitted between 15°C and 30°C (59°F and 86°F).

Mechanism of Action Selectively and irreversibly inhibits CYP17 (17 alpha-hydroxylase/C17,20-lyase), an enzyme required for androgen biosynthesis which is expressed in testicular, adrenal, and prostatic tumor tissues. Inhibits the formation of the testosterone precursors dehydroepiandrosterone (DHEA) and androstenedione.

Pharmacodynamics/Kinetics

Distribution: V_{dss}: 19,669 ± 13,358 L

Protein binding: >99%; to albumin and alpha$_1$-acid glycoprotein

Metabolism: Abiraterone acetate is hydrolyzed to the active metabolite abiraterone; further metabolized to inactive metabolites abiraterone sulphate and N-oxide abiraterone sulphate via CYP3A4 and SULT2A1

Bioavailability: Systemic exposure is increased by food

Half-life elimination: 14.4-16.5 hours (Acharya, 2012)

Time to peak: 2 hours (Acharya, 2012)

Excretion: Feces (~88%); urine (~5%)

Dosage Prostate cancer, metastatic, castration-resistant:

Adults: Oral: 1000 mg once daily (in combination with prednisone)

Dosage adjustment for concomitant strong CYP3A4 inducers: Avoid concomitant strong CYP3A4 inducers; if a strong CYP3A4 inducer must be administered concurrently, increase the abiraterone frequency to twice daily (eg, from 1000 mg once daily to 1000 mg twice daily). Upon discontinuation of the strong CYP3A4 inducer, reduce abiraterone back to the prior dose and frequency.

Dosage adjustment in renal impairment: No dosage adjustment necessary.

Dosage adjustment in hepatic impairment:

Hepatic impairment ***prior to*** treatment initiation:

Mild (Child-Pugh class A): No dosage adjustment necessary.

Moderate (Child-Pugh class B):

U.S. labeling: 250 mg once daily. Permanently discontinue if ALT and/or AST >5 times the upper limit of normal (ULN) or total bilirubin >3 times ULN during treatment.

Canadian labeling: Use is not recommended.

Severe (Child-Pugh class C): Avoid use

Hepatotoxicity ***during*** treatment:

U.S. labeling:

ALT and/or AST >5 times ULN or total bilirubin >3 times ULN: Withhold treatment until liver function tests return to baseline or ALT and AST ≤2.5 times ULN and total bilirubin ≤1.5 times ULN, then reinitiate at 750 mg once daily.

Recurrent hepatotoxicity on 750 mg/day: Withhold treatment until liver function tests return to baseline or ALT and AST ≤2.5 times ULN and total bilirubin ≤1.5 times ULN, then reinitiate at 500 mg once daily.

Recurrent hepatotoxicity on 500 mg once daily: Discontinue treatment

Canadian labeling:

ALT or AST >5 times ULN or total bilirubin >3 times ULN:

Withhold treatment until liver function tests normalize, then (when hepatic function returns to baseline) reinitiate at 500 mg once daily

Recurrent hepatotoxicity on 500 mg once daily: Discontinue treatment

ALT >20 times ULN (any time during treatment): Discontinue permanently.

Administration Administer orally on an empty stomach, at least 1 hour before and 2 hours after food. **Note:** The prescribing information describes when to give food with respect to abiraterone; no food should be consumed for at least 2 hours before or for at least 1 hour after the abiraterone dose. Swallow tablets whole with water. Do not crush or chew.

Hazardous agent; use appropriate precautions for handling and disposal (NIOSH 2014 [group 1]). Women who are or may become pregnant should wear gloves if handling the tablets.

Monitoring Parameters ALT, AST, and bilirubin prior to treatment, every 2 weeks for 3 months and monthly thereafter; if baseline moderate hepatic impairment (Child-Pugh class B), monitor ALT, AST, and bilirubin prior to treatment, weekly for the first month, every 2 weeks for 2 months then monthly thereafter. If hepatotoxicity develops during treatment (and only after therapy is interrupted and liver function tests have returned to safe levels), monitor ALT, AST, and bilirubin every 2 weeks for 3 months and monthly thereafter. Monitoring of testosterone levels is not necessary.

Monitor for signs and symptoms of adrenocorticoid insufficiency; if clinically indicated, consider appropriate diagnostics to confirm adrenal insufficiency. Monitor monthly for hypertension, hypokalemia, and fluid retention.

Dosage Forms

Tablet, Oral:

Zytiga: 250 mg

◆ **ABLC** *see* Amphotericin B (Lipid Complex) *on page* 138

AbobotulinumtoxinA

(aye bo BOT yoo lin num TOKS in aye)

Brand Names: U.S. Dysport; Dysport (Glabellar Lines)

Index Terms Botulinum Toxin Type A

Pharmacologic Category Neuromuscular Blocker Agent, Toxin

Use

Cervical dystonia: Treatment of cervical dystonia in adults to decrease the severity of abnormal head position and neck pain in toxin-naive and previously treated patients.

Glabellar lines: Temporary improvement in the appearance of moderate to severe glabellar lines associated with corrugator and procerus muscle activity in adults younger than 65 years.

Pregnancy Risk Factor C

Dosage

Adults:

Cervical dystonia: IM: Initial: 500 units divided among affected muscles in toxin-naïve or toxin-experienced patients. May re-treat at intervals of ≥12 weeks

Dosage adjustments: Adjust dosage in 250-unit increments; do not administer at intervals <12 weeks; dosage range used in studies: 250 to 1000 units

Glabellar lines: Adults <65 years: IM: Inject 10 units (0.05 mL or 0.08 mL) into each of 5 sites (2 injections in each corrugator muscle and 1 injection in the procerus muscle) for a total dose of 50 units; do not administer at intervals <3 months; efficacy has been demonstrated up to 4 repeated administrations

Elderly:

Cervical dystonia: Refer to adult dosing.

Glabellar lines: Not recommended in patients ≥65 years of age

Dosage adjustment in renal impairment: There are no dosage adjustments provided in the manufacturer's labeling.

Dosage adjustment in hepatic impairment: There are no dosage adjustments provided in the manufacturer's labeling.

Additional Information Complete prescribing information should be consulted for additional detail.

Dosage Forms

Solution Reconstituted, Intramuscular:

Dysport: 300 units (1 ea); 500 units (1 ea)

Dysport (Glabellar Lines): 300 units (1 ea)

◆ **Abraxane** *see* PACLitaxel (Protein Bound) *on page* 1554

◆ **Abraxane for Injectable Suspension (Can)** *see* PACLitaxel (Protein Bound) *on page* 1554

◆ **Abreva [OTC]** *see* Docosanol *on page* 661

◆ **Absorica** *see* ISOtretinoin *on page* 1127

◆ **Abstral** *see* FentaNYL *on page* 857

◆ **ABT-335** *see* Fenofibrate and Derivatives *on page* 852

◆ **ABthrax** *see* Raxibacumab *on page* 1786

◆ **ABX-EGF** *see* Panitumumab *on page* 1568

◆ **AC 2993** *see* Exenatide *on page* 830

◆ **ACAM2000®** *see* Smallpox Vaccine *on page* 1900

Acamprosate (a kam PROE sate)

Brand Names: U.S. Campral [DSC]

Brand Names: Canada Campral®

Index Terms Acamprosate Calcium; Calcium Acetylhomotaurinate

Pharmacologic Category GABA Agonist/Glutamate Antagonist

Use Maintenance of alcohol abstinence

Pregnancy Risk Factor C

Dosage Oral: Adults: Alcohol abstinence: 666 mg 3 times/day (a lower dose may be effective in some patients). **Note:** Treatment should be initiated as soon as possible following the period of alcohol withdrawal, when the patient has achieved abstinence and should be maintained if patient relapses.

Dosage adjustment in renal impairment:

CrCl 30-50 mL/minute: 333 mg 3 times/day

CrCl <30 mL/minute: Contraindicated in severe renal impairment.

Dosage adjustment in hepatic impairment:

Mild-to-moderate impairment: No dosage adjustments are recommended

Severe impairment: There are no dosage adjustments provided in manufacturer's labeling.

Additional Information Complete prescribing information should be consulted for additional detail.

Dosage Forms

Tablet Delayed Release, Oral:

Generic: 333 mg

◆ **Acamprosate Calcium** *see* Acamprosate *on page 28*

Acarbose (AY car bose)

Brand Names: U.S. Precose

Brand Names: Canada Glucobay

Pharmacologic Category Antidiabetic Agent, Alpha-Glucosidase Inhibitor

Use Diabetes mellitus, type 2: Adjunct to diet and exercise to lower blood glucose in patients with type 2 diabetes mellitus (noninsulin dependent, NIDDM)

Pregnancy Risk Factor B

Dosage Oral:

Adults: Dosage must be individualized on the basis of effectiveness and tolerance while not exceeding the maximum recommended dose

Initial dose: 25 mg 3 times/day with the first bite of each main meal; to reduce GI effects, some patients may benefit from initiating at 25 mg once daily with gradual titration to 25 mg 3 times/day as tolerated

Maintenance dose: Should be adjusted at 4- to 8-week intervals based on 1-hour postprandial glucose levels and tolerance until maintenance dose is reached. Dosage may be increased from 25 mg 3 times/day to 50 mg 3 times/day. Some patients may benefit from increasing the dose to 100 mg 3 times/day.

Maintenance dose ranges: 50-100 mg 3 times/day.

Maximum dose:

≤60 kg: 50 mg 3 times/day

>60 kg: 100 mg 3 times/day

Patients receiving sulfonylureas or insulin: Acarbose given in combination with a sulfonylurea or insulin will cause a further lowering of blood glucose and may increase the hypoglycemic potential of the sulfonylurea or insulin. If hypoglycemia occurs, appropriate adjustments in the dosage of these agents should be made.

Dosing adjustment in renal impairment:

CrCl ≥25 mL/minute: No dosage adjustment necessary. Although acarbose is primarily excreted unchanged, the increased plasma levels in renal impairment are not expected to affect efficacy (clinical response is localized to the GI tract); however, the effects on adverse effects are unknown.

CrCl <25 mL/minute or S_{cr} >2 mg/dL: Use not recommended (not adequately studied).

Dosing adjustment in hepatic impairment: No dosage adjustment provided in manufacturer's labeling.

Additional Information Complete prescribing information should be consulted for additional detail.

Dosage Forms

Tablet, Oral:

Precose: 25 mg, 50 mg, 100 mg

Generic: 25 mg, 50 mg, 100 mg

◆ **A-Caro-25 [OTC]** *see* Beta-Carotene *on page 251*

◆ **Accel-Amlodipine (Can)** *see* AmLODIPine *on page 123*

◆ **Accel-Clarithromycin (Can)** *see* Clarithromycin *on page 456*

◆ **Accel-Donepezil (Can)** *see* Donepezil *on page 668*

◆ **Accell-Citalopram (Can)** *see* Citalopram *on page 451*

◆ **Accel-Pioglitazone (Can)** *see* Pioglitazone *on page 1654*

◆ **Accolate** *see* Zafirlukast *on page 2192*

◆ **Accolate® (Can)** *see* Zafirlukast *on page 2192*

◆ **AccuNeb [DSC]** *see* Albuterol *on page 69*

◆ **Accupril** *see* Quinapril *on page 1756*

◆ **Accutane** *see* ISOtretinoin *on page 1127*

Acebutolol (a se BYOO toe lole)

Brand Names: U.S. Sectral

Brand Names: Canada Apo-Acebutolol®; Ava-Acebutolol; Mylan-Acebutolol; Mylan-Acebutolol (Type S); Nu-Acebutolol; Rhotral; Sandoz-Acebutolol; Sectral®; Teva-Acebutolol

Index Terms Acebutolol Hydrochloride

Pharmacologic Category Antiarrhythmic Agent, Class II; Antihypertensive; Beta-Blocker With Intrinsic Sympathomimetic Activity

Use Treatment of hypertension; management of ventricular arrhythmias

The 2014 guideline for the management of high blood pressure in adults (Eighth Joint National Committee [JNC 8; James, 2013]) recommends initiation of pharmacologic treatment to lower blood pressure for the following patients:

- Patients ≥60 years of age with systolic blood pressure (SBP) ≥150 mm Hg or diastolic blood pressure (DBP) ≥90 mm Hg. Goal of therapy is SBP <150 mm Hg and DBP <90 mm Hg.
- Patients <60 years of age with SBP ≥140 mm Hg or DBP ≥90 mm Hg. Goal of therapy is SBP <140 mm Hg and DBP <90 mm Hg.
- Patients ≥18 years of age with diabetes and SBP ≥140 mm Hg or DBP ≥90 mm Hg. Goal of therapy is SBP <140 mm Hg and DBP <90 mm Hg.
- Patients ≥18 years of age with chronic kidney disease (CKD) and SBP ≥140 mm Hg or DBP ≥90 mm Hg. Goal of therapy is SBP <140 mm Hg and DBP <90 mm Hg.

In patients with CKD, regardless of race or diabetes status, the use of an ACE inhibitor (ACEI) or angiotensin receptor blocker (ARB) as initial therapy is recommended to improve kidney outcomes. In the general nonblack population (without CKD), including those with diabetes, initial antihypertensive treatment should consist of a thiazide-type diuretic, calcium channel blocker, ACEI, or ARB. In the general black population (without CKD), including those with diabetes, initial antihypertensive treatment should consist of a thiazide-type diuretic or a calcium channel blocker instead of an ACEI or ARB.

Pregnancy Risk Factor B

Dosage Oral:

Adults:

Ventricular arrhythmias: Initial: 400 mg/day in 2 divided doses; maintenance: 600 to 1200 mg/day in divided doses; maximum: 1200 mg/day

Hypertension: Initial: 400 mg in 1 to 2 divided doses; optimal response usually seen at 400 to 800 mg daily (larger doses may be divided) although some patients may respond to as little as 200 mg daily; usual dose range (ASH/ISH [Weber, 2014]): 200 to 400 mg daily; maximum dose: 1200 mg in 2 divided doses

Chronic stable angina (off-label use): Usual dose: 400 to 1200 mg/day in 2 divided doses (Gibbons, 2003); low doses (ie, 400 mg/day) may also be given as once daily (Pina, 1988)

Elderly: Consider dose reduction due to age-related increase in bioavailability; do not exceed 800 mg/day. In the management of hypertension, consider lower initial dose (eg, 200 to 400 mg/day) and titrate to response (Aronow, 2011).

Dosing adjustment in renal impairment:

CrCl 25 to 49 mL/minute: Reduce dose by 50%.

CrCl <25 mL/minute: Reduce dose by 75%.

Dosing adjustment in hepatic impairment: There are no dosage adjustments provided in manufacturer's labeling; use with caution.

Additional Information Complete prescribing information should be consulted for additional detail.

Dosage Forms

Capsule, Oral:

Sectral: 200 mg, 400 mg

Generic: 200 mg, 400 mg

Dosage Forms: Canada

Tablet, Oral:

Sectral: 100 mg, 200 mg, 400 mg

◆ **Acebutolol Hydrochloride** *see* Acebutolol *on page 29*

Aceclofenac [INT] (a se KLO fe nak)

International Brand Names Abdal (IN); ACB (IN); Aceclofar (AE); Aceclonac (CY); Acecpar (VN); Acenac (PK); Acenal (IN); Acer (VN); Aclon (VN); Aflamil (BG, SK); Air-Tal (BE); Airtal (DO, IE, IT, PY, RU, TR); Asec (KR); Barcan (DK, FI, SE); Beofenac (DE); Biofenac (BE, CZ, GR, NL, PT); Bristaflam (CR, GT, HN, NI, PA, SV, VE); Cartrex (FR); Ciaflam (VN); Clanza (PH); Clanza CR (PH); Fornac (IN); Loflam (AE); Mobenac (PH); Preservex (GB, IE); Proflam (BR); Tonec (TW); Tonlief (TW); Urodolox (AR); Zerodol (PE); Zerodol CR (PE)

Pharmacologic Category Analgesic, Nonsteroidal Anti-inflammatory Drug

Reported Use Treatment of pain and inflammation in rheumatoid arthritis, osteoarthritis, and ankylosing spondylitis

Dosage Range Adults: Oral: 100 mg twice daily

Product Availability Product available in various countries; not currently available in the U.S.

Dosage Forms

Tablet: 100 mg

Acemetacin [INT] (ay se MET a sin)

International Brand Names Acemet (MY, PE); Acemetacin Heumann (DE); Acemetacin intermuti (DE); Acemetacin Stada (DE); acemetacin von ct (DE); Acemix (IT); Aceo (TH); Acephlogont (DE); Altren (BE); Analgel (AR); Azeat (DE); Baydol (CO); Baydol LP (CO); Cetacin (KR); Emflex (GB); Espledol (ES); Flamarion (AR); Gynalgia (AR); Mocetasin (VN); Mostanol (DE); Oldan (ES); Pranex (PE); Pranex LP (PE); Rantudal (GR); Rantudil (CN, DE, HU, LU, MX, PL, PT, TR, VN); Rantudil Forte (RO, SA); Rantudil Retard (MX, RO, SA); Rheugasin (VN); Rheumetan (KR); Rheutrop (AT); Shun Song (CN); Solart (IT); Tilur (CH)

Pharmacologic Category Nonsteroidal Anti-inflammatory Drug (NSAID), Oral

Reported Use Treatment of rheumatoid arthritis, osteoarthritis, low back pain, and postoperative pain and inflammation

Dosage Range Adults: Oral: Initial: 120 mg/day in divided doses; may increase to 180 mg/day in divided doses, based on patient response

Product Availability Product available in various countries; not currently available in the U.S.

Dosage Forms

Capsule: 60 mg

Capsule, extended release: 90 mg

◆ **Acenocoumarin** *see* Acenocoumarol [CAN/INT] *on page 30*

Acenocoumarol [CAN/INT] (a see no KOOM a rol)

Brand Names: Canada Sintrom

Index Terms Acenocoumarin; Nicoumalone

Pharmacologic Category Anticoagulant; Anticoagulant, Vitamin K Antagonist

Additional Appendix Information

Reversal of Oral Anticoagulants *on page 2235*

Use Note: Not approved in U.S.

Prophylaxis and treatment of venous thrombosis, pulmonary embolism, and thromboembolic disorders; atrial fibrillation with risk of embolism; adjunct in the prophylaxis of coronary occlusion and transient ischemic attacks

Pregnancy Considerations Acenocoumarol crosses the placenta. Teratogenic effects have been reported with coumarin derivative anticoagulants following first trimester exposure and may include coumarin embryopathy (nasal hypoplasia and/or stippled epiphyses; limb hypoplasia may also be present). Adverse events to the fetus have also been observed following second and third trimester exposure with coumarin derivative anticoagulants and may include CNS abnormalities (including ventral midline dysplasia, dorsal midline dysplasia). Fatal hemorrhage in the fetus has been reported even when the mother's acenocoumarol levels were in the therapeutic range. Acenocoumarol should not be used during pregnancy because of significant risks. Women of childbearing potential are advised to use effective contraception during treatment.

Breast-Feeding Considerations Very small quantities of acenocoumarol can be detected in breast milk and undesirable effects in nursing infants are not anticipated. The manufacturer recommends prophylaxis therapy with phytonadione (1 mg administered once weekly) and monitoring of the infant for signs of bleeding. The American College of Chest Physicians (ACCP) considers acenocoumarol to be safe to use in breast-feeding women (Guyatt, 2012).

Contraindications Hypersensitivity to acenocoumarol, related coumarin derivatives, or any component of the formulation; hemorrhagic tendencies and/or blood dyscrasias (eg, hemophilia, thrombocytopenic purpura, leukemia); recent or potential surgery of the eye or CNS; major regional lumbar block anesthesia or surgery resulting in large, open surfaces; bleeding from the GI, respiratory, or GU tract; aneurysm (cerebral or dissecting aortic); cerebrovascular hemorrhage; recent surgical procedures resulting in increased fibrinolytic activity (eg, surgery of the lung, prostate, uterus); polyarthritis; diverticulitis; emaciation; malnutrition; severe hypertension; severe parenchymal lesions of the liver and kidneys; pericarditis or pericardial effusion; subacute bacterial endocarditis; ascorbic acid deficiency; uncooperative patient (eg, alcoholic, unsupervised senile, or psychotic) intramuscular injections; inadequate laboratory facilities; threatened abortion; eclampsia/pre-eclampsia; pregnancy

Warnings/Precautions Use care in the selection of patients appropriate for this treatment. Use with caution in trauma, acute infection (antibiotics and fever may alter response to acenocoumarol), hepatic impairment, renal impairment, moderate hypertension, polycythemia vera, vasculitis, open wound, active TB, history of PUD, anaphylactic disorders, indwelling catheters, severe diabetes, thyroid disease, and menstruating and postpartum women. Necrosis or gangrene of the skin and other tissues can occur (rarely) due to early hypercoagulability; risk is increased in patients with protein C or S deficiency. "Purple toe" syndrome, due to cholesterol microembolization, has been described with coumarin-type anticoagulants. Women may be at risk of developing ovarian hemorrhage at the time of ovulation. May cause hypersensitivity reactions; cross-reactivity among coumarin anticoagulants has been described.

Hemorrhage is the most serious risk of therapy. Risk factors for bleeding include high intensity anticoagulation (INR >4), age (>65 years), variable INRs, history of GI bleeding, hypertension, cerebrovascular disease, serious heart disease, anemia, severe diabetes, malignancy, trauma, renal insufficiency, polycythemia vera, vasculitis, open wound, history of PUD, indwelling catheters, menstruating and postpartum women, drug-drug interactions and long duration of therapy, known genetic deficiency in CYP2C9 activity or polymorphism of the vitamin K oxidoreductase (VKORC1) gene. Patient must be instructed to report bleeding, accidents, or falls. Patient must also report any new or discontinued medications, herbal or alternative products used, significant changes in smoking or dietary habits. Unrecognized bleeding sites (eg, colon cancer) may be uncovered by anticoagulation. Treatment should be withdrawn at the earliest signs of bleeding.

Use with caution in patients with prolonged dietary insufficiencies (vitamin K deficiency). Use care in the selection of patients appropriate for this treatment. The elderly may be more sensitive to anticoagulant therapy.

Adverse Reactions As with all anticoagulants, bleeding is the major adverse effect of acenocoumarol. Hemorrhage may occur at virtually any site. Risk is dependent on multiple variables, including the intensity of anticoagulation and patient susceptibility.

Dermatologic: Skin necrosis (including hemorrhagic forms) (rare)

Genitourinary: Priapism

Hematologic: Hemorrhage may occur at virtually any site; sites that may be predisposed to bleeding include CNS (brain), eye, GI tract (melena), liver and gall bladder (hematobilia), urogenital tract (hematuria), uterus (metrorrhagia, menorrhagia)

Hepatic: Hepatotoxicity

Reactions observed with similar coumarin derivatives: Alopecia (reversible, rare), appetite decreased, diarrhea, gangrene (rare), hypersensitivity/allergic reactions (dermatitis, fever, urticaria), nausea, purple toe syndrome (rare), vomiting

Drug Interactions

Metabolism/Transport Effects **Substrate** of CYP1A2 (major), CYP2C19 (minor), CYP2C9 (major); **Note:** Assignment of Major/Minor substrate status based on clinically relevant drug interaction potential

Avoid Concomitant Use

Avoid concomitant use of Acenocoumarol with any of the following: Apixaban; Dabigatran Etexilate; Edoxaban; Omacetaxine; Rivaroxaban; Streptokinase; Tamoxifen; Urokinase; Vorapaxar

Increased Effect/Toxicity

Acenocoumarol may increase the levels/effects of: Anticoagulants; Collagenase (Systemic); Deferasirox; Ethotoin; Fosphenytoin; Ibritumomab; Nintedanib; Obinutuzumab; Omacetaxine; Phenytoin; Rivaroxaban; Sulfonylureas; Tositumomab and Iodine I 131 Tositumomab

The levels/effects of Acenocoumarol may be increased by: Abiraterone Acetate; Acetaminophen; Agents with Antiplatelet Properties; Allopurinol; Amiodarone; Amorolfine; Androgens; Apixaban; Bicalutamide; Capecitabine; Cephalosporins; Ceritinib; Chloral Hydrate; Chloramphenicol; Cimetidine; Cloxacillin; Cranberry; CYP1A2 Inhibitors (Moderate); CYP1A2 Inhibitors (Strong); CYP2C9 Inhibitors (Moderate); CYP2C9 Inhibitors (Strong); Dabigatran Etexilate; Dasatinib; Deferasirox; Desvenlafaxine; Dexmethylphenidate; Disulfiram; Dronedarone; Econazole; Edoxaban; Efavirenz; Erythromycin (Ophthalmic); Esomeprazole; Ethacrynic Acid; Ethotoin; Etoposide; Exenatide; Fenugreek; Fibric Acid Derivatives; Fluconazole; Fluorouracil (Systemic); Fluorouracil (Topical); Fosphenytoin; Fusidic Acid (Systemic); Gefitinib; Ginkgo Biloba; Glucagon; Green Tea; Herbs (Anticoagulant/Antiplatelet Properties); HMG-CoA Reductase Inhibitors; Ibrutinib; Ifosfamide; Itraconazole; Ivermectin (Systemic); Ketoconazole (Systemic); Lansoprazole; Leflunomide; Levomilnacipran; Limaprost; Macrolide Antibiotics; Methylphenidate; MetroNIDAZOLE (Systemic); Miconazole (Topical); Mifepristone; Milnacipran; Multivitamins/Fluoride (with ADE); Multivitamins/Minerals (with ADEK, Folate, Iron); Multivitamins/Minerals (with AE, No Iron); Neomycin; Nonsteroidal Anti-Inflammatory Agents; NSAID (COX-2 Inhibitor); NSAID (Nonselective); Omega-3 Fatty Acids; Omeprazole; Oritavancin; Peginterferon Alfa-2b; Penicillins; Pentosan Polysulfate Sodium; Pentoxifylline; Phenytoin; Posaconazole; Propafenone; Prostacyclin Analogues; QuiNIDine; QuiNINE; Quinolone Antibiotics; Salicylates; Selective Serotonin Reuptake Inhibitors; Streptokinase; Sugammadex; Sulfinpyrazone [Off Market]; Sulfonamide Derivatives; Sulfonylureas; Tamoxifen; Tegafur; Tetracycline Derivatives; Thrombolytic Agents; Thyroid Products; Tibolone; Tipranavir; Toremifene; TraMADol; Tricyclic Antidepressants; Urokinase; Vemurafenib; Venlafaxine; Vitamin E; Vorapaxar; Voriconazole; Vorinostat; Zafirlukast

Decreased Effect

The levels/effects of Acenocoumarol may be decreased by: Alcohol (Ethyl); Aminoglutethimide; Antithyroid Agents; AzaTHIOprine; Barbiturates; Bile Acid Sequestrants; Bosentan; Cannabis; CarBAMazepine; Cloxacillin; Coenzyme Q-10; Contraceptives (Estrogens); Contraceptives (Progestins); CYP1A2 Inducers (Strong); CYP2C9 Inducers (Strong); Dabrafenib; Dicloxacillin; Efavirenz; Estrogen Derivatives; Flucloxacillin; Glutethimide; Green Tea; Griseofulvin; Lixisenatide; Mercaptopurine; Multivitamins/Minerals (with ADEK, Folate, Iron); Nafcillin; Phytonadione; Progestins; Rifamycin Derivatives; St Johns Wort; Sucralfate; Teriflunomide

Food Interactions

Ethanol: Acute ethanol ingestion (binge drinking) decreases the metabolism of oral anticoagulants and increases PT/INR. Chronic daily ethanol use increases the metabolism of oral anticoagulants and decreases PT/INR. Management: Avoid ethanol.

Food: Vitamin K can reverse the anticoagulation effects of acenocoumarol; large amounts of food high in vitamin K (such as beef liver, pork liver, green tea, and green leafy vegetables) may reverse acenocoumarol, decrease prothrombin time, and lead to therapeutic failure. Management: Patients should not change dietary habits once stabilized on acenocoumarol therapy. A balanced diet with a consistent intake of vitamin K is essential. High doses of vitamin A, E, or C may alter PT. Cranberry juice or other cranberry products may increase the INR in patients receiving a similar agent (warfarin) and cause severe bleeding (flavonoids found in cranberries may inhibit cytochrome P450 isoenzyme CYP2C9 which metabolize warfarin). Similar risks might be anticipated with acenocoumarol as it also undergoes CYP2C9 metabolism. Management: Use caution with fish oils or omega-3 fatty acids; cranberry juice or other cranberry products.

Storage/Stability Store at 15°C to 30°C (59°F to 86°F).

Mechanism of Action Hepatic synthesis of coagulation factors II, VII, IX, and X, as well as proteins C and S, requires the presence of vitamin K. These clotting factors are biologically activated by the addition of carboxyl groups to key glutamic acid residues within the proteins' structure. In the process, "active" vitamin K is oxidatively converted to an "inactive" form, which is then subsequently reactivated by vitamin K epoxide reductase complex 1 (VKORC1). Coumarins are thought to inhibit VKORC1, thus depleting functional vitamin K reserves and hence reduce synthesis of active clotting factors.

Pharmacodynamics/Kinetics

Onset of action: Peak anticoagulant effect: Oral: 36-48 hours

Absorption: Rapid

Distribution: V_d: 0.16-0.34 L/kg

Protein binding: 99%

Metabolism: Hepatic, via oxidation: R-enantiomer (by CYP2C9 [primary], 1A2, and 2C19; S-enantiomer primarily by CYP2C9) and via keto-reduction to inactive metabolites; also undergoes nitro-reduction via gut flora. (Thijssen, 2000)

Bioavailability: 60%

Half-life elimination: R-enantiomer: ~11 hours; S-enantiomer: <2 hours (Thijssen, 1986)

Time to peak, plasma: 1-3 hours

Excretion: Urine (60% as metabolites; minimal amount as unchanged drug); feces (29% as metabolites)

Dosage Oral: **Note:** Dosage must be individualized. The following information is based on the manufacturer's labeling in Canada.

Adults: Initial: 8-12 mg on day 1, followed by 4-8 mg on day 2. Subsequent dosage should be based on PT/INR measurements. Usual range of maintenance doses: 1-10 mg/day. Tapering of dosage is recommended prior to discontinuation.

Elderly: Lower dosages may be necessary; use with caution

Dosage adjustment in renal impairment: Use with caution; the manufacturer labeling does not provide specific dosing recommendations.

Dosage adjustment in hepatic impairment: Use with caution; the manufacturer labeling does not provide specific dosing recommendations.

Dietary Considerations Foods high in vitamin K (eg, beef liver, pork liver, green tea, and leafy green vegetables) inhibit anticoagulant effect. Do not change dietary habits once stabilized on acenocoumarol therapy. A balanced diet with a consistent intake of vitamin K is essential. Avoid large amounts of alfalfa, asparagus, broccoli, Brussels sprouts, cabbage, cauliflower, green teas, kale, lettuce, spinach, turnip greens, watercress; these decrease efficacy of oral anticoagulants. It is recommended that an adult diet contain a **consistent** vitamin K content of 75-120 mcg/day. Check with healthcare provider before changing diet. Avoid using multivitamins that contain vitamin K.

Administration Administer at the same time each day.

Monitoring Parameters PT/INR (**Note:** To obtain a valid PT in patients receiving heparin, allow 4-5 hours after last IV dose and 12-24 hours after last SubQ dose before blood is drawn); hepatic function, CBC, urinalysis (for albuminuria/proteinuria)

Product Availability Not available in U.S.

Dosage Forms: Canada

Tablet, oral:

Sintrom: 1 mg, 4 mg

◆ **Aceon** *see* Perindopril *on page* 1623

◆ **Acephen [OTC]** *see* Acetaminophen *on page* 32

◆ **Acerola C 500 [OTC]** *see* Ascorbic Acid *on page* 178

◆ **Acetadote** *see* Acetylcysteine *on page* 40

◆ **Aceta-Gesic®** *see* Acetaminophen and Diphenhydramine *on page* 36

Acetaminophen (a seet a MIN oh fen)

Brand Names: U.S. Acephen [OTC]; Aspirin Free Anacin Extra Strength [OTC]; Cetafen Extra [OTC]; Cetafen [OTC]; Excedrin Tension Headache [OTC]; FeverAll Adult [OTC]; FeverAll Childrens [OTC]; FeverAll Infants [OTC]; FeverAll Junior Strength [OTC]; Little Fevers [OTC]; Mapap Arthritis Pain [OTC]; Mapap Children's [OTC]; Mapap Extra Strength [OTC]; Mapap Infant's [OTC]; Mapap Junior Rapid Tabs [OTC]; Mapap [OTC]; Non-Aspirin Pain Reliever [OTC]; Nortemp Children's [OTC]; Ofirmev; Pain & Fever Children's [OTC]; Pain Eze [OTC]; Pharbetol Extra Strength [OTC]; Pharbetol [OTC]; Q-Pap Children's [OTC]; Q-Pap Extra Strength [OTC]; Q-Pap Infant's [OTC]; Q-Pap [OTC]; RapiMed Children's [OTC]; RapiMed Junior [OTC]; Silapap Children's [OTC]; Silapap Infant's [OTC]; Triaminic Children's Fever Reducer Pain Reliever [OTC]; Tylenol 8 Hour [OTC]; Tylenol Arthritis Pain [OTC]; Tylenol Children's Meltaways [OTC]; Tylenol Children's [OTC]; Tylenol Extra Strength [OTC]; Tylenol Jr. Meltaways [OTC]; Tylenol [OTC]; Valorin Extra [OTC]; Valorin [OTC]

Brand Names: Canada Abenol; Apo-Acetaminophen; Atasol; Novo-Gesic; Pediatrix; Tempra; Tylenol

Index Terms APAP (abbreviation is not recommended); N-Acetyl-P-Aminophenol; Paracetamol

Pharmacologic Category Analgesic, Miscellaneous

Use

Pain management:

Injection: Treatment of mild to moderate pain; treatment of moderate to severe pain when combined with opioid analgesia

Oral/Rectal: Temporary relief of minor aches, pains, and headache

Fever: Temporary reduction of fever

Pregnancy Risk Factor C

Pregnancy Considerations Adverse events were observed in some animal reproduction studies. Acetaminophen crosses the placenta and can be detected in cord blood, newborn serum, and urine immediately after delivery (Levy, 1975; Naga Rani, 1989; Wang, 1997). An increased risk of teratogenic effects has not been observed following maternal use of acetaminophen during pregnancy. Prenatal constriction of the ductus arteriosus has been noted in case reports following maternal use during the third trimester (Suhag, 2008; Wood, 2005). The use of acetaminophen in normal doses during pregnancy is not associated with an increased risk of miscarriage or still birth; however, an increase in fetal death or spontaneous abortion may be seen following maternal overdose if treatment is delayed (Li, 2003; Rebordosa, 2009; Riggs, 1989). Frequent maternal use of acetaminophen during pregnancy may be associated with wheezing and asthma in early childhood (Perzanowki, 2010).

Breast-Feeding Considerations Low concentrations of acetaminophen are excreted into breast milk and can be detected in the urine of nursing infants (Notarianni, 1987). Adverse reactions have generally not been observed; however, a rash caused by acetaminophen exposure was reported in one breast-feeding infant (Matheson, 1985). The manufacturer recommends that caution be used if administered to a nursing woman.

Contraindications

Injection: Hypersensitivity to acetaminophen or any component of the formulation; severe hepatic impairment or severe active liver disease

OTC labeling: When used for self-medication, do not use with other drug products containing acetaminophen or if allergic to acetaminophen or any of the inactive ingredients

Warnings/Precautions **[Injection: U.S. Boxed Warning]: Acetaminophen has been associated with acute liver failure, at times resulting in liver transplant and death. Hepatotoxicity is usually associated with excessive acetaminophen intake and often involves more than one product that contains acetaminophen.** Do not exceed the maximum recommended daily dose (>4 g daily in adults). In addition, chronic daily dosing may also result in liver damage in some patients. Limit acetaminophen dose from all sources (prescription, OTC, combination products) and all routes of administration (IV, oral, rectal) to ≤4 g/day (adults). Use with caution in patients with alcoholic liver disease; consuming ≥3 alcoholic drinks/day may increase the risk of liver damage. Use caution in patients with hepatic impairment or active liver disease; use of IV formulation is contraindicated in patients with severe hepatic impairment or severe active liver disease.

[Injection: U.S. Boxed Warning]: Take care to avoid dosing errors with acetaminophen injection, which could result in accidental overdose and death; ensure that the dose in mg is not confused with mL, dosing in patients <50 kg is based on body weight, infusion pumps are properly programmed, and total daily dose of acetaminophen from all sources does not exceed the maximum daily limits.

Hypersensitivity and anaphylactic reactions have been reported including life-threatening anaphylaxis; discontinue immediately if symptoms occur. Serious and potentially fatal skin reactions, including acute generalized exanthematous pustulosis (AGEP), Stevens-Johnson syndrome (SJS), and toxic epidermal necrolysis (TEN), have occurred rarely with acetaminophen use. Discontinue therapy at the first appearance of skin rash.

Some dosage forms may contain propylene glycol; large amounts are potentially toxic and have been associated hyperosmolality, lactic acidosis, seizures, and respiratory depression; use caution (AAP, 1997; Zar, 2007). Some products may contain polysorbate 80 (Tween 80). Some products may contain aspartame which is metabolized to phenylalanine and must be avoided (or used with caution) in patients with phenylketonuria.

Benzyl alcohol and derivatives: Some dosage forms may contain benzyl alcohol and/or sodium benzoate/benzoic acid; benzoic acid (benzoate) is a metabolite of benzyl alcohol; large amounts of benzyl alcohol (≥99 mg/kg/day) have been associated with a potentially fatal toxicity ("gasping syndrome") in neonates; the "gasping syndrome" consists of metabolic acidosis, respiratory distress, gasping respirations, CNS dysfunction (including convulsions, intracranial hemorrhage), hypotension and cardiovascular collapse (AAP, 1997; CDC, 1982); some data suggests that benzoate displaces bilirubin from protein binding sites (Ahlfors, 2001); avoid or use dosage forms containing benzyl alcohol and/or benzyl alcohol derivative with caution in neonates. See manufacturer's labeling.

When used for self-medication (OTC), patients should be instructed to contact healtcare provider if symptoms get worse or new symptoms appear, redness or swelling is present in the painful area, fever lasts >3 days (all ages), or pain (excluding sore throat) lasts longer than: Adults: 10 days, Children and Adolescents: 5 days, Infants: 3 days. When treating children with sore throat, if sore throat is severe, persists for >2 days, or is followed by fever, rash, headache, nausea, or vomiting, consult health care provider immediately.

Use with caution in patients with chronic malnutrition or severe renal impairment; use intravenous formulation with caution in patients with severe hypovolemia. Use with caution in patients with known G6PD deficiency.

Adverse Reactions Oral, Rectal:

Dermatologic: Skin rash

Endocrine & metabolic: Decreased serum bicarbonate, decreased serum calcium, decreased serum sodium, hyperchloremia, hyperuricemia, increased serum glucose

Genitourinary: Nephrotoxicity (with chronic overdose)

Hematologic & oncologic: Anemia, leukopenia, neutropenia, pancytopenia

Hepatic: Increased serum alkaline phosphatase, increased serum bilirubin

Hypersensitivity: Hypersensitivity reaction (rare)

Renal: Hyperammonemia, renal disease (analgesic)

IV:

Cardiovascular: Hypertension, hypotension, peripheral edema, tachycardia

Central nervous system: Agitation (children), anxiety, fatigue, headache (more common in adults), insomnia (more common in adults), trismus

Dermatologic: Pruritus (children), skin rash

Endocrine & metabolic: Hypervolemia, hypoalbuminemia, hypokalemia, hypomagnesemia, hypophosphatemia

Gastrointestinal: Abdominal pain, diarrhea, headache (more common in adults), insomnia (more common in adults), nausea (more common in adults), vomiting (more common in adults)

Genitourinary: Oliguria (children)

Hematologic & oncologic: Anemia

Hepatic: Increased serum transaminases

Local: Infusion site reaction (pain)

Neuromuscular & skeletal: Limb pain, muscle spasm

Ophthalmic: Periorbital edema

Respiratory: Abnormal breath sounds, atelectasis (children), dyspnea, hypoxia, pleural effusion, pulmonary edema, stridor, wheezing

Miscellaneous: Fever

Rare but important or life-threatening: Anaphylaxis, hepatic injury (dose-related), hypersensitivity reaction, severe dermatological reaction (acute generalized exanthematous pustulosis, Stevens-Johnson syndrome, toxic epidermal necrolysis)

Drug Interactions

Metabolism/Transport Effects **Substrate** of CYP1A2 (minor), CYP2A6 (minor), CYP2C9 (minor), CYP2D6 (minor), CYP2E1 (minor), CYP3A4 (minor); **Note:** Assignment of Major/Minor substrate status based on clinically relevant drug interaction potential; **Inhibits** CYP3A4 (weak)

Avoid Concomitant Use

Avoid concomitant use of Acetaminophen with any of the following: Pimozide

Increased Effect/Toxicity

Acetaminophen may increase the levels/effects of: ARIPiprazole; Busulfan; Dasatinib; Dofetilide; Hydrocodone; Imatinib; Lomitapide; Mipomersen; Phenylephrine (Systemic); Pimozide; Prilocaine; Sodium Nitrite; SORAfenib; Vitamin K Antagonists

The levels/effects of Acetaminophen may be increased by: Alcohol (Ethyl); Dasatinib; Isoniazid; Metyrapone; Nitric Oxide; Probenecid; SORAfenib

Decreased Effect

The levels/effects of Acetaminophen may be decreased by: Barbiturates; CarBAMazepine; Cholestyramine Resin; Fosphenytoin-Phenytoin

Food Interactions Rate of absorption may be decreased when given with food. Management: Administer without regard to food.

Preparation for Administration Injectable solution may be administered directly from the vial without further dilution.

Doses <1000 mg (<50 kg): Withdraw appropriate dose from vial and transfer to a separate sterile container (eg, glass bottle, plastic IV container, syringe) for administration. Small volume pediatric doses (up to 600 mg [60 mL]) may be placed in a syringe and infused over 15 minutes via syringe pump.

Doses of 1000 mg (≥50 kg): Insert vented IV set through vial stopper.

Storage/Stability

Injection: Store intact vials at 20°C to 25°C (68°F to 77°F); do not refrigerate or freeze. Use within 6 hours of opening vial or transferring to another container. Discard any unused portion.

Oral formulations: Store at 20°C to 25°C (68°F to 77°F); avoid excessive heat (20°C [104°F]). Avoid high humidity (chewable tablets).

Suppositories: Store at 2°C to 27°C (25°F to 80°F); do not freeze.

Mechanism of Action Although not fully elucidated, believed to inhibit the synthesis of prostaglandins in the central nervous system and work peripherally to block pain impulse generation; produces antipyresis from inhibition of hypothalamic heat-regulating center

Pharmacodynamics/Kinetics

Onset of action:

Oral: <1 hour

IV: Analgesia: 5 to 10 minutes; Antipyretic: Within 30 minutes

Peak effect: IV: Analgesic: 1 hour

Duration:

IV, Oral: Analgesia: 4 to 6 hours

IV: Antipyretic: ≥6 hours

Absorption: Primarily absorbed in small intestine (rate of absorption dependent upon gastric emptying); minimal absorption from stomach; varies by dosage form

Distribution: ~1 L/kg at therapeutic doses

Protein binding: 10% to 25% at therapeutic concentrations; 8% to 43% at toxic concentrations

Metabolism: At normal therapeutic dosages, primarily hepatic metabolism to sulfate and glucuronide conjugates, while a small amount is metabolized by CYP2E1 to a highly reactive intermediate, N-acetyl-p-benzoquinone imine (NAPQI), which is conjugated rapidly with glutathione and inactivated to nontoxic cysteine and mercapturic acid conjugates. At toxic doses (as little as 4 g daily) glutathione conjugation becomes insufficient to meet the metabolic demand causing an increase in NAPQI concentrations, which may cause hepatic cell necrosis. Oral administration is subject to first pass metabolism.

Half-life elimination: Prolonged following toxic doses

Neonates: 7 hours (range: 4 to 10 hours)

Infants: ~4 hours (range: 1 to 7 hours)

Children: 3 hours (range: 2 to 5 hours)

Adolescents: ~3 hours (range: 2 to 4 hours)

Adults: ~2 hours (range: 2 to 3 hours); may be slightly prolonged in severe renal insufficiency (CrCl <30 mL/minute): 2 to 5.3 hours

Time to peak, serum: Oral: Immediate release: 10 to 60 minutes (may be delayed in acute overdoses); IV: 15 minutes

Excretion: Urine (<5% unchanged; 60% to 80% as glucuronide metabolites; 20% to 30% as sulphate metabolites; ~8% cysteine and mercapturic acid metabolites)

Dosage Note: In 2011, McNeil Consumer Healthcare reduced the maximum doses and increased the dosing interval on the labeling of some of their acetaminophen OTC products used in older pediatric patients (usually children ≥12 years and adolescents) and adults in an attempt to protect consumers from inadvertent overdoses. For example, the maximum daily dose of Tylenol Extra Strength and Tylenol Regular Strength was decreased and the dosing interval for Tylenol Extra Strength was increased. Health care professionals may still prescribe or recommend the 4 g daily maximum to patients (but are advised to use their own discretion and clinical judgment) (McNeil Consumer Healthcare, 2014).

When calculating the maximum daily dose, consider all sources of acetaminophen (prescription and OTC) and all routes of administration. Do not exceed the maximum recommended daily dose (see dosing information for further detail).

Oral:

Weight-based dosing: Infants, Children, and Adolescents: 10 to 15 mg/kg/dose every 4 to 6 hours as needed (American Pain Society, 2008; Sullivan, 2011); do **not** exceed 5 doses in 24 hours; maximum daily dose: 75 mg/kg/**day** not to exceed 4 g daily

Fixed dosing: Oral suspension, chewable tablets: Infants and Children <12 years: Consult specific product formulations for appropriate age groups. See table; use of weight to select dose is preferred; if weight is not available, then use age; doses may be repeated every 4 hours; maximum: 5 doses daily

Acetaminophen Pediatric Dosing (Oral)[1]

Weight (kg)	Weight (lbs)	Age	Dosage (mg)
2.7-5.3	6-11	0-3 mo	40
5.4-8.1	12-17	4-11 mo	80
8.2-10.8	18-23	1-2 y	120
10.9-16.3	24-35	2-3 y	160
16.4-21.7	36-47	4-5 y	240
21.8-27.2	48-59	6-8 y	320
27.3-32.6	60-71	9-10 y	400
32.7-43.2	72-95	11 y	480

[1]Manufacturer's recommendations are based on weight in pounds (OTC labeling); weight in kg listed here is derived from pounds and rounded; kg weight listed also is adjusted to allow for continuous weight ranges in kg. OTC labeling instructs consumer to consult with health care provider for dosing instructions in infants and children under 2 years of age.

Immediate release solid dosage formulations: **Note:** Actual OTC dosing recommendations may vary by product and/or manufacturer:

Children 6 to 11 years: 325 mg every 4 to 6 hours; maximum daily dose: 1625 mg **daily**; **Note:** Do not use for more than 5 days unless directed by a health care provider.

Children ≥12 years, Adolescents, and Adults:

Regular strength: 650 mg every 4 to 6 hours; maximum daily dose: 3250 mg **daily** unless directed by health care provider; under physician supervision, daily doses ≤4 g may be used

Extra strength: 1000 mg every 6 hours; maximum daily dose: 3000 mg **daily** unless directed by a health care provider; under physician supervision, daily doses ≤4 g may be used

Extended release: Children ≥12 years, Adolescents, and Adults: 1300 mg every 8 hours; maximum daily dose: 3900 mg **daily**

Rectal:

Infants 6 to 11 months: 80 mg every 6 hours; maximum daily dose: 320 mg **daily**

Infants and Children 12 to 36 months: 80 mg every 4 to 6 hours; maximum daily dose: 400 mg **daily**

Children >3 to 6 years: 120 mg every 4 to 6 hours; maximum daily dose: 600 mg **daily**

Children >6 up to 12 years: 325 mg every 4 to 6 hours; maximum daily dose: 1625 mg **daily**
Children ≥12 years, Adolescents and Adults: 650 mg every 4 to 6 hours; maximum daily dose: 3900 mg **daily**

IV:
Children 2 to 12 years: 15 mg/kg every 6 hours **or** 12.5 mg/kg every 4 hours; maximum single dose: 15 mg/kg/dose (≤750 mg/dose); maximum daily dose: 75 mg/kg/day (≤3.75 g daily)
Adolescents and Adults:
<50 kg: 15 mg/kg every 6 hours or 12.5 mg/kg every 4 hours; maximum single dose: 15 mg/kg/dose (750 mg/dose); maximum daily dose: 75 mg/kg/day (≤3.75 g daily)
≥50 kg: 650 mg every 4 hours or 1000 mg every 6 hours; maximum single dose: 1000 mg/dose; maximum daily dose: 4 g daily

Dosage adjustment in renal impairment:
Oral (Aronoff, 2007):
Infants, Children, and Adolescents:
GFR ≥10 mL/minute/1.73 m^2: No dosage adjustment necessary.
GFR <10 mL/minute/1.73 m^2: Administer every 8 hours
Intermittent hemodialysis or peritoneal dialysis: Administer every 8 hours
CRRT: No dosage adjustment necessary.
Adults:
GFR ≥50 mL/minute/1.73 m^2: No dosage adjustment necessary.
GFR 10 to 50 mL/minute/1.73 m^2: Administer every 6 hours
GFR <10 mL/minute/1.73 m^2: Administer every 8 hours
CRRT: Administer every 6 hours
IV: Children, Adolescents, and Adults: CrCl ≤30 mL/minute: Use with caution; consider decreasing daily dose and extending dosing interval

Dosage adjustment in hepatic impairment:
Oral: Use with caution. Limited, low-dose therapy is usually well tolerated in hepatic disease/cirrhosis. However, cases of hepatotoxicity at daily acetaminophen dosages <4 g daily have been reported.
IV:
Mild to moderate impairment: Use with caution in hepatic impairment or active liver disease; manufacturer's labeling suggests a reduced total daily dosage may be warranted, although no specific dosage adjustments are provided.
Severe impairment: Use is contraindicated.

Dietary Considerations Some products may contain phenylalanine and/or sodium.

Administration
Oral: May administer without regard to food; may administer with food to decrease possible GI upset; shake drops and suspension well before use; do not crush or chew extended release products
Injection: For IV infusion only. Administer undiluted over 15 minutes. Use within 6 hours of opening vial or transferring to another container.
For doses <1000 mg (<50 kg): Withdraw appropriate dose from vial and place into separate empty, sterile container prior to administration.
For doses ≥1000 mg (≥50 kg): Insert vented IV set through vial stopper
Rectal: Remove wrapper; insert suppository well up into the rectum

Monitoring Parameters Serum acetaminophen levels: Where acute overdose suspected and with long-term use in patients with hepatic disease; relief of pain or fever

Dosage Forms
Caplet, oral: 500 mg
Cetafen Extra [OTC]: 500 mg
Mapap Extra Strength [OTC]: 500 mg
Pain Eze [OTC]: 650 mg
Tylenol [OTC]: 325 mg
Tylenol Extra Strength [OTC]: 500 mg
Caplet, extended release, oral:
Mapap Arthritis Pain [OTC]: 650 mg
Tylenol 8 Hour [OTC]: 650 mg
Tylenol Arthritis Pain [OTC]: 650 mg
Capsule, oral:
Mapap Extra Strength [OTC]: 500 mg
Captab, oral: 500 mg
Elixir, oral:
Mapap Children's [OTC]: 160 mg/5 mL (118 mL, 480 mL)
Gelcap, oral: 500 mg
Mapap [OTC]: 500 mg
Gelcap, rapid release, oral: 500 mg
Tylenol Extra Strength [OTC]: 500 mg
Geltab, oral: 500 mg
Excedrin Tension Headache [OTC]: 500 mg
Injection, solution [preservative free]:
Ofirmev: 10 mg/mL (100 mL)
Liquid, oral: 160 mg/5 mL (120 mL, 473 mL); 500 mg/5 mL (240 mL)
Mapap Extra Strength [OTC]: 500 mg/5 mL (237 mL)
Q-Pap Children's [OTC]: 160 mg/5 mL (118 mL, 473 mL)
Silapap Children's [OTC]: 160 mg/5 mL (118 mL, 237 mL, 473 mL)
Tylenol Extra Strength [OTC]: 500 mg/15 mL (240 mL)
Solution, oral: 160 mg/5 mL (5 mL, 10 mL, 20 mL, 118 mL, 473 mL)
Pain & Fever Children's [OTC]: 160 mg/5 mL (118 mL, 473 mL)
Q-Pap Infant's [OTC]: 80 mg/0.8 mL (15 mL)
Silapap Infant's [OTC]: 80 mg/0.8 mL (15 mL, 30 mL)
Suppository, rectal: 120 mg (12s, 50s, 100s); 325 mg (12s); 650 mg (12s, 50s, 100s)
Acephen [OTC]: 120 mg (12s, 50s, 100s); 325 mg (6s, 12s, 50s, 100s); 650 mg (12s, 50s, 100s)
Feverall [OTC]: 80 mg (6s, 50s); 120 mg (6s, 50s); 325 mg (6s, 50s); 650 mg (50s)
Suspension, oral: 160 mg/5 mL (5 mL, 10 mL, 10.15 mL, 20 mL, 20.3 mL)
Mapap Children's [OTC]: 160 mg/5 mL (118 mL)
Mapap Infant's [OTC]: 160 mg/5 mL (59 mL)
Nortemp Children's [OTC]: 160 mg/5 mL (118 mL)
Pain & Fever Children's [OTC]: 160 mg/5 mL (60 mL)
Q-Pap Children's [OTC]: 160 mg/5 mL (118 mL)
Tylenol Children's [OTC]: 160 mg/5 mL (60 mL, 120 mL)
Syrup, oral:
Triaminic Children's Fever Reducer Pain Reliever [OTC]: 160 mg/5 mL (118 mL)
Tablet, oral: 325 mg, 500 mg
Aspirin Free Anacin Extra Strength [OTC]: 500 mg
Cetafen [OTC]: 325 mg
Mapap [OTC]: 325 mg
Non-Aspirin Pain Reliever [OTC]: 325 mg
Pharbetol [OTC]: 325 mg
Pharbetol Extra Strength [OTC]: 500 mg
Q-Pap [OTC]: 325 mg
Q-Pap Extra Strength [OTC]: 500 mg
Tylenol [OTC]: 325 mg
Tylenol Extra Strength [OTC]: 500 mg
Valorin [OTC]: 325 mg
Valorin Extra [OTC]: 500 mg
Tablet, chewable, oral: 80 mg
Mapap Children's [OTC]: 80 mg
Tablet, orally disintegrating, oral: 80 mg, 160 mg
Mapap Children's [OTC]: 80 mg
Mapap Junior Rapid Tabs [OTC]: 160 mg
RapiMed Children's [OTC]: 80 mg
RapiMed Junior [OTC]: 160 mg
Tylenol Children's Meltaways [OTC]: 80 mg
Tylenol Jr. Meltaways [OTC]: 160 mg

- **Acetaminophen and Butalbital** *see* Butalbital and Acetaminophen *on page 314*
- **Acetaminophen and Chlorpheniramine** *see* Chlorpheniramine and Acetaminophen *on page 426*

Acetaminophen and Codeine

(a seet a MIN oh fen & KOE deen)

Brand Names: U.S. Capital® and Codeine; Tylenol® with Codeine No. 3; Tylenol® with Codeine No. 4

Brand Names: Canada ratio-Emtec-30; ratio-Lenoltec; Triatec-30; Triatec-8; Triatec-8 Strong; Tylenol Elixir with Codeine; Tylenol No. 1; Tylenol No. 1 Forte; Tylenol No. 2 with Codeine; Tylenol No. 3 with Codeine; Tylenol No. 4 with Codeine

Index Terms Codeine and Acetaminophen; Emtec; Tylenol #2; Tylenol #3; Tylenol Codeine

Pharmacologic Category Analgesic Combination (Opioid); Analgesic, Opioid

Use Relief of mild-to-moderate pain

Pregnancy Risk Factor C

Dosage Doses should be adjusted according to severity of pain and response of the patient. Adult doses ≥60 mg codeine fail to give commensurate relief of pain but merely prolong analgesia and are associated with an appreciably increased incidence of side effects. Oral:

Children: Analgesic:

Codeine: 0.5-1 mg codeine/kg/dose every 4-6 hours

Acetaminophen: 10-15 mg/kg/dose every 4 hours up to a maximum of 2.6 g/24 hours for children <12 years; **alternatively, the following can be used:**

3-6 years: 5 mL 3-4 times/day as needed of elixir

7-12 years: 10 mL 3-4 times/day as needed of elixir

>12 years: 15 mL every 4 hours as needed of elixir

Adults:

Antitussive: Based on codeine (15-30 mg/dose) every 4-6 hours (maximum: 360 mg/24 hours based on codeine component)

Analgesic: Based on codeine (30-60 mg/dose) every 4-6 hours (maximum: 4000 mg/24 hours based on acetaminophen component)

1-2 tablets every 4 hours to a maximum of 12 tablets/24 hours

Dosing adjustment in renal impairment: See individual agents.

Dosing adjustment in hepatic impairment: Use with caution. Limited, low-dose therapy is usually well tolerated in hepatic disease/cirrhosis; however, cases of hepatotoxicity at daily acetaminophen dosages <4 g/day have been reported. Avoid chronic use in hepatic impairment.

Additional Information Complete prescribing information should be consulted for additional detail.

Dosage Forms

Solution, oral [C-V]: Acetaminophen 120 mg and codeine 12 mg per 5 mL

Suspension, oral [C-V]:

Capital and Codeine [C-V]: Acetaminophen 120 mg and codeine 12 mg per 5 mL

Tablet, oral [C-III]: Acetaminophen 300 mg and codeine 15 mg; acetaminophen 300 mg and codeine 30 mg; acetaminophen 300 mg and codeine 60 mg

Tylenol with Codeine No. 3: Acetaminophen 300 mg and codeine 30 mg

Tylenol with Codeine No. 4: Acetaminophen 300 mg and codeine 60 mg

Dosage Forms: Canada Note: In countries outside of the U.S., some formulations of Tylenol® with Codeine include caffeine.

Caplet:

ratio-Lenoltec No. 1, Tylenol No. 1: Acetaminophen 300 mg, codeine 8 mg, and caffeine 15 mg

Tylenol No. 1 Forte: Acetaminophen 500 mg, codeine 8 mg, and caffeine 15 mg

Solution, oral:

Tylenol Elixir with Codeine: Acetaminophen 160 mg and codeine 8 mg per 5 mL

Tablet:

ratio-Emtec, Triatec-30: Acetaminophen 300 mg and codeine 30 mg

ratio-Lenoltec No. 1: Acetaminophen 300 mg, codeine 8 mg, and caffeine 15 mg

ratio-Lenoltec No. 2, Tylenol No. 2 with Codeine: Acetaminophen 300 mg, codeine 15 mg, and caffeine 15 mg

ratio-Lenoltec No. 3, Tylenol No. 3 with Codeine: Acetaminophen 300 mg, codeine 30 mg, and caffeine 15 mg

ratio-Lenoltec No. 4, Tylenol No. 4 with Codeine: Acetaminophen 300 mg and codeine 60 mg

Triatec-8: Acetaminophen 325 mg, codeine 8 mg, and caffeine 30 mg

Triatec-8 Strong: Acetaminophen 500 mg, codeine 8 mg, and caffeine 30 mg

Acetaminophen and Diphenhydramine

(a seet a MIN oh fen & dye fen HYE dra meen)

Brand Names: U.S. Aceta-Gesic®; Excedrin PM® [OTC]; Goody's PM® [OTC]; Legatrin PM® [OTC]; Mapap PM [OTC]; Percogesic® Extra Strength [OTC]; TopCare® Pain Relief PM [OTC]; Tylenol® PM [OTC]; Tylenol® Severe Allergy [OTC]

Index Terms Diphenhydramine and Acetaminophen

Pharmacologic Category Analgesic, Miscellaneous

Use Aid in the relief of insomnia accompanied by minor pain

Dosage Oral: Adults: 50 mg of diphenhydramine HCl (76 mg diphenhydramine citrate) at bedtime or as directed by physician; do not exceed recommended dosage; not for use in children <12 years of age

Dosing adjustment in hepatic impairment: Use with caution. Limited, low-dose therapy is usually well tolerated in hepatic disease/cirrhosis; however, cases of hepatotoxicity at daily acetaminophen dosages <4 g/day have been reported. Avoid chronic use in hepatic impairment.

Additional Information Complete prescribing information should be consulted for additional detail.

Dosage Forms

Caplet, oral:

Excedrin PM® [OTC]: Acetaminophen 500 mg and diphenhydramine 38 mg

Legatrin PM® [OTC]: Acetaminophen 500 mg and diphenhydramine 50 mg

Mapap PM [OTC], TopCare® Pain Relif PM [OTC], Tylenol® PM [OTC]: Acetaminophen 500 mg and diphenhydramine 25 mg

Percogesic® Extra Strength [OTC]: Acetaminophen 500 mg and diphenhydramine 12.5 mg

Tylenol® Severe Allergy [OTC]: Acetaminophen 500 mg and diphenhydramine 12.5 mg

Captab, oral: Acetaminophen 500 mg and diphenhydramine 25 mg

Gelcap, rapid release, oral:

Tylenol® PM [OTC]: Acetaminophen 500 mg and diphenhydramine 25 mg

Geltab, oral: Acetaminophen 500 mg and diphenhydramine 25 mg

Excedrin® PM [OTC]: Acetaminophen 500 mg and diphenhydramine 38 mg

Tylenol® PM [OTC]: Acetaminophen 500 mg and diphenhydramine 25 mg

Liquid, oral:
Tylenol® PM [OTC]: Acetaminophen 500 mg and diphenhydramine 25 mg per 15 mL
Powder for solution, oral:
Goody's PM® [OTC]: Acetaminophen 500 mg and diphenhydramine 38 mg
Tablet, oral: Acetaminophen 500 mg and diphenhydramine 25 mg
Aceta-Gesic®: Acetaminophen 325 mg and diphenhydramine hydrochloride 12.5 mg
Excedrin® PM [OTC]: Acetaminophen 500 mg and diphenhydramine 38 mg

◆ **Acetaminophen and Hydrocodone** *see* Hydrocodone and Acetaminophen *on page 1012*

◆ **Acetaminophen and Oxycodone** *see* Oxycodone and Acetaminophen *on page 1541*

Acetaminophen and Tramadol
(a seet a MIN oh fen & TRA ma dole)

Brand Names: U.S. Ultracet®
Brand Names: Canada ACT Tramadol/Acet; Apo-Tramadol/Acet®; JAMP-ACET-Tramadol; Mar-Tramadol/Acet; Mint-Tramadol/Acet; Pat-Tramadol/Acet; PMS-Tramadol/Acet; Priva-Tramadol/Acet; RAN-Tramadol/Acet; TEVA-Tramadol/Acetaminophen; Tramacet; Tramaphen-Odan
Index Terms Tramadol Hydrochloride and Acetaminophen
Pharmacologic Category Analgesic Combination (Opioid); Analgesic, Miscellaneous
Use Short-term (≤5 days) management of acute pain
Pregnancy Risk Factor C
Dosage Oral: Adults: Acute pain: Two tablets every 4-6 hours as needed for pain relief (maximum: 8 tablets/day); treatment should not exceed 5 days
Dosage adjustment in renal impairment: CrCl <30 mL/minute: Maximum of 2 tablets every 12 hours; treatment should not exceed 5 days
Dosage adjustment in hepatic impairment: Use is not recommended.
Additional Information Complete prescribing information should be consulted for additional detail.
Dosage Forms
Tablet, oral: Acetaminophen 325 mg and tramadol 37.5 mg
Ultracet®: Acetaminophen 325 mg and tramadol 37.5 mg

Acetaminophen, Aspirin, and Caffeine
(a seet a MIN oh fen, AS pir in, & KAF een)

Brand Names: U.S. Anacin Advanced Headache Formula [OTC]; Excedrin Extra Strength [OTC]; Excedrin Migraine [OTC]; Fem-Prin [OTC]; Goody's Extra Strength Headache Powder [OTC]; Goody's Extra Strength Pain Relief [OTC]; Pain-Off [OTC]; Vanquish Extra Strength Pain Reliever [OTC]
Index Terms Aspirin, Acetaminophen, and Caffeine; Aspirin, Caffeine and Acetaminophen; Caffeine, Acetaminophen, and Aspirin; Caffeine, Aspirin, and Acetaminophen
Pharmacologic Category Analgesic, Miscellaneous
Use
Migraine: Relief of migraine headache
Pain: Relief of minor aches and pain
Dosage
Minor aches and pain: Children >12 years, Adolescents, and Adults: Oral:
Acetaminophen 194 mg/aspirin 227 mg/caffeine 33 mg: Two caplets every 6 hours as needed (maximum: 8 doses per 24 hours)
Acetaminophen 250 mg/aspirin 250 mg/caffeine 65 mg: Two doses every 6 hours as needed (maximum: 8 doses per 24 hours)
Acetaminophen 260 mg/aspirin 520 mg/caffeine 32.5 mg: One powder, placed on tongue or dissolved in water or other liquid, every 6 hours as needed (maximum: 4 powders per 24 hours)
Acetaminophen 325 mg/aspirin 500 mg/caffeine 65 mg: One powder, placed on tongue or dissolved in water or other liquid, every 6 hours as needed (maximum: 4 powders per 24 hours)
Migraine headache:Adults: Oral: Acetaminophen 250 mg/aspirin 250 mg/caffeine 65 mg: Two doses once every 24 hours (maximum: 2 doses per 24 hours)
Dosage adjustment in renal impairment: There are no dosage adjustments provided in the manufacturer's labeling.
Dosage adjustment in hepatic impairment: There are no dosage adjustments provided in the manufacturer's labeling.
Additional Information Complete prescribing information should be consulted for additional detail.
Dosage Forms
Caplet: Acetaminophen 250 mg, aspirin 250 mg, and caffeine 65 mg; acetaminophen 194 mg, aspirin 227 mg, and caffeine 33 mg
Excedrin Extra Strength [OTC], Excedrin® Migraine [OTC]: Acetaminophen 250 mg, aspirin 250 mg, and caffeine 65 mg
Vanquish Extra Strength Pain Reliever [OTC]: Acetaminophen 194 mg, aspirin 227 mg, and caffeine 33 mg
Geltab: Acetaminophen 250 mg, aspirin 250 mg, and caffeine 65 mg
Excedrin Extra Strength [OTC], Excedrin® Migraine [OTC]: Acetaminophen 250 mg, aspirin 250 mg, and caffeine 65 mg
Powder: Acetaminophen 260 mg, aspirin 520 mg, and caffeine 32.5 mg
Goody's Extra Strength Headache Powder [OTC]: Acetaminophen 260 mg, aspirin 520 mg, and caffeine 32.5 mg
Tablet:
Anacin Advanced Headache Formula [OTC], Excedrin® Extra Strength [OTC], Excedrin® Migraine [OTC], Pain-Off [OTC]: Acetaminophen 250 mg, aspirin 250 mg, and caffeine 65 mg
Fem-Prin [OTC]: Acetaminophen 194.4 mg, aspirin 226.8 mg, and caffeine 32.4 mg
Goody's Extra Strength Pain Relief [OTC]: Acetaminophen 130 mg, aspirin 260 mg, and caffeine 16.25 mg

◆ **Acetaminophen, Butalbital, and Caffeine** *see* Butalbital, Acetaminophen, and Caffeine *on page 313*

Acetaminophen, Codeine, and Doxylamine [CAN/INT]
(a seet a MIN oh fen, KOE deen, & dox IL a meen)

Brand Names: Canada Mersyndol® With Codeine
Index Terms Codeine, Doxylamine, and Acetaminophen; Doxylamine Succinate, Codeine Phosphate, and Acetaminophen
Pharmacologic Category Analgesic, Miscellaneous; Analgesic, Opioid; Antitussive; Ethanolamine Derivative; Histamine H_1 Antagonist; Histamine H_1 Antagonist, First Generation
Use Note: Not approved in U.S.
Relief of headache, cold symptoms, neuralgia, and muscular aches/pain
Pregnancy Considerations Refer to individual monographs.

Breast-Feeding Considerations Refer to individual monographs.

Contraindications Hypersensitivity to acetaminophen, codeine, doxylamine, or any component of the formulation; significant respiratory depression (in unmonitored settings); acute or severe bronchial asthma; hypercapnia

Warnings/Precautions Use with caution in patients with hypersensitivity reactions to other phenanthrene-derived opioid agonists (morphine, hydrocodone, hydromorphone, levorphanol, oxycodone, oxymorphone). Tolerance or drug dependence may result from extended use. Avoid use in patients with CNS depression or coma as these patients are susceptible to intracranial effects of CO_2 retention.

Limit total acetaminophen dose to <4 g/day. May cause severe hepatic toxicity on acute overdose; in addition, chronic daily dosing in adults has resulted in liver damage in some patients. Use with caution in patients with alcoholic liver disease; consuming 3 alcoholic drinks/day may increase the risk of liver damage. Have patients avoid ethanol or limit to <3 drinks/day. Use caution in patients with known G6PD deficiency. Use caution in patients with two or more copies of the variant CYP2D6*2 allele; may have extensive conversion to morphine and thus increased opioid-mediated effects. Avoid the use of codeine in these patients; consider alternative analgesics such as morphine or a nonopioid agent (Crews, 2012). The occurrence of this phenotype is seen in 0.5% to 1% of Chinese and Japanese, 0.5% to 1% of Hispanics, 1% to 10% of Caucasians, 3% of African-Americans, and 16% to 28% of North Africans, Ethiopians, and Arabs. Rarely, acetaminophen may cause serious and potentially fatal skin reactions such as acute generalized exanthematous pustulosis, Stevens-Johnson syndrome (SJS), and toxic epidermal necrolysis (TEN). Discontinue treatment if severe skin reactions develop.

After chronic maternal exposure to opioids, neonatal withdrawal syndrome may occur in the newborn; monitor neonate closely. Signs and symptoms include irritability, hyperactivity and abnormal sleep pattern, high pitched cry, tremor, vomiting, diarrhea and failure to gain weight. Onset, duration and severity depend on the drug used, duration of use, maternal dose, and rate of drug elimination by the newborn. Opioid withdrawal syndrome in the neonate, unlike in adults, may be life-threatening and should be treated according to protocols developed by neonatology experts.

This combination should be used with caution in elderly or debilitated patients, angle-closure glaucoma, adrenocortical insufficiency, biliary tract impairment, pancreatitis, cardiovascular disease (including hypertension and tachycardia), hypotension, increased intraocular pressure, thyroid disorders, urinary tract obstruction (including bladder neck obstruction, urethral stricture, and symptomatic prostatic hyperplasia), pyloroduodenal obstruction (including stenotic peptic ulcer), seizure disorder, CNS depression, head injury, or increased intracranial pressure. Use caution in patients with gastrointestinal motility disorders; avoid in paralytic ileus. Also use caution in postoperative patients following thoracotomy or laparotomy due to suppression of cough. Causes sedation; caution must be used in performing tasks which require alertness (eg, operating machinery or driving). Sedative effects of CNS depressants or ethanol are potentiated. Safety and efficacy in pediatric patients <12 years of age have not been established.

Adverse Reactions Also see individual agents.

Rare but important or life-threatening: Hypogonadism (Brennan, 2013; Debono, 2011)

Drug Interactions

Metabolism/Transport Effects Refer to individual components.

Avoid Concomitant Use

Avoid concomitant use of Acetaminophen, Codeine, and Doxylamine with any of the following: Aclidinium; Azelastine (Nasal); Glucagon; Ipratropium (Oral Inhalation); Orphenadrine; Paraldehyde; Pimozide; Potassium Chloride; Thalidomide; Tiotropium; Umeclidinium

Increased Effect/Toxicity

Acetaminophen, Codeine, and Doxylamine may increase the levels/effects of: AbobotulinumtoxinA; Alvimopan; Anticholinergic Agents; ARIPiprazole; Azelastine (Nasal); Buprenorphine; Busulfan; CNS Depressants; Dasatinib; Desmopressin; Diuretics; Dofetilide; Glucagon; Hydrocodone; Imatinib; Lomitapide; Methotrimeprazine; Metyrosine; Mipomersen; Mirabegron; Mirtazapine; OnabotulinumtoxinA; Orphenadrine; Paraldehyde; Phenylephrine (Systemic); Pimozide; Potassium Chloride; Pramipexole; Prilocaine; RimabotulinumtoxinB; ROPINIRole; Rotigotine; Selective Serotonin Reuptake Inhibitors; Sodium Nitrite; SORAfenib; Suvorexant; Thalidomide; Thiazide Diuretics; Tiotropium; Topiramate; Vitamin K Antagonists; Zolpidem

The levels/effects of Acetaminophen, Codeine, and Doxylamine may be increased by: Aclidinium; Alcohol (Ethyl); Amphetamines; Anticholinergic Agents; Brimonidine (Topical); Cannabis; Dasatinib; Doxylamine; Dronabinol; Droperidol; HydrOXYzine; Ipratropium (Oral Inhalation); Isoniazid; Kava Kava; Magnesium Sulfate; MAO Inhibitors; Methotrimeprazine; Metyrapone; Mianserin; Nabilone; Nitric Oxide; Perampanel; Pramlintide; Probenecid; Rufinamide; Sodium Oxybate; Somatostatin Analogs; SORAfenib; Succinylcholine; Tapentadol; Tetrahydrocannabinol; Umeclidinium

Decreased Effect

Acetaminophen, Codeine, and Doxylamine may decrease the levels/effects of: Acetylcholinesterase Inhibitors; Benzylpenicilloyl Polylysine; Betahistine; Hyaluronidase; Itopride; Pegvisomant; Secretin

The levels/effects of Acetaminophen, Codeine, and Doxylamine may be decreased by: Acetylcholinesterase Inhibitors; Ammonium Chloride; Amphetamines; Barbiturates; CarBAMazepine; Cholestyramine Resin; CYP2D6 Inhibitors (Moderate); CYP2D6 Inhibitors (Strong); Fosphenytoin-Phenytoin; Mixed Agonist / Antagonist Opioids; Naltrexone

Storage/Stability Store at 20°C to 25°C (68°F to 77°F).

Mechanism of Action Acetaminophen inhibits the synthesis of prostaglandins in the central nervous system and peripherally blocks pain impulse generation; produces antipyresis from inhibition of hypothalamic heat-regulating center. Codeine binds to opiate receptors in the CNS, causing inhibition of ascending pain pathways, altering the perception of and response to pain; causes cough supression by direct central action in the medulla; produces generalized CNS depression. Doxylamine competes with histamine for H_1-receptor sites on effector cells; blocks chemoreceptor trigger zone, diminishes vestibular stimulation, and depresses labyrinthine function through its central anticholinergic activity.

Pharmacodynamics/Kinetics See individual agents.

Dosage Oral:

Children >12 years and Adults: 1-2 tablets every 4 hours as needed; total dose should not exceed 12 tablets in a 24-hour period

Dosage adjustment in renal impairment: No dosage adjustment required.

Dosage adjustment in hepatic impairment:

Acetaminophen: Use with caution. Limited, low-dose therapy usually well tolerated in hepatic disease/cirrhosis. However, cases of hepatotoxicity at daily acetaminophen dosages <4 g/day have been reported. Avoid chronic use in hepatic impairment.

Codeine: Dosage adjustment of codeine is probably necessary in hepatic insufficiency; no specific guidelines available.

Monitoring Parameters Relief of pain, respiratory and mental status, blood pressure, bowel function; signs or symptoms of hypogonadism or hypoadrenalism (Brennan, 2013)

Product Availability Not available in U.S.

Dosage Forms: Canada

Tablet, oral:

Mersyndol® With Codeine: Acetaminophen 325 mg, codeine 8 mg, and doxylamine 5 mg

- ◆ **Acetasol® HC** *see* Acetic Acid, Propylene Glycol Diacetate, and Hydrocortisone *on page 40*
- ◆ **Acetazolam (Can)** *see* AcetaZOLAMIDE *on page 39*

AcetaZOLAMIDE (a set a ZOLE a mide)

Brand Names: U.S. Diamox Sequels

Brand Names: Canada Acetazolam; Diamox®

Pharmacologic Category Anticonvulsant, Miscellaneous; Carbonic Anhydrase Inhibitor; Diuretic, Carbonic Anhydrase Inhibitor; Ophthalmic Agent, Antiglaucoma

Use Treatment of glaucoma (chronic simple open-angle, secondary glaucoma, preoperatively in acute angle-closure); drug-induced edema or edema due to congestive heart failure (adjunctive therapy; IV and immediate release dosage forms); centrencephalic epilepsies (IV and immediate release dosage forms); prevention or amelioration of symptoms associated with acute mountain sickness (immediate and extended release dosage forms)

Pregnancy Risk Factor C

Dosage Note: IM administration is not recommended because of pain secondary to the alkaline pH

Children:

Altitude illness:

Prevention: Oral: 2.5 mg/kg/dose every 12 hours started either the day before (preferred) or on the day of ascent and may be discontinued after staying at the same elevation for 2-3 days or if descent initiated; maximum dose: 125 mg/dose (Luks, 2010). **Note:** The International Society for Mountain Medicine does not recommend prophylaxis in children except in the rare circumstance of unavoidable rapid ascent or in children with known previous susceptibility to acute mountain sickness (Pollard, 2001).

Treatment: Oral: 2.5 mg/kg/dose every 8-12 hours; maximum dose: 250 mg/dose. **Note:** With high altitude cerebral edema, dexamethasone is the primary treatment; however, acetazolamide may be used adjunctively with the same treatment dose (Luks, 2010; Pollard, 2001).

Epilepsy: Oral: 8-30 mg/kg/day in divided doses. A lower dosing range of 4-16 mg/kg/day in 1-4 divided doses has also been recommended; maximum dose: 30 mg/kg/day or 1 g/day (Oles, 1989; Reiss, 1996). **Note:** Minimal additional benefit with doses >16 mg/kg/day. **Extended release capsule is not recommended for treatment of epilepsy.**

Adults:

Altitude illness: Oral: Manufacturer's labeling: 500-1000 mg/day in divided doses every 8-12 hours (immediate release tablets) or divided every 12-24 hours (extended release capsules). These doses are associated with more frequent and/or increased side effects. Alternative dosing has been recommended:

Prevention: 125 mg twice daily; beginning either the day before (preferred) or on the day of ascent; may be discontinued after staying at the same elevation for 2-3 days or if descent initiated (Basnyat, 2006; Luks, 2010). **Note:** In situations of rapid ascent (such as rescue or military operations), 1000 mg/day is recommended by the manufacturer. The Wilderness Medical Society recommends consideration of using dexamethasone in addition to acetazolamide in these situations (Luks, 2010).

Treatment: 250 mg twice daily. **Note:** With high altitude cerebral edema, dexamethasone is the primary treatment; however, acetazolamide may be used adjunctively with the same treatment dose (Luks, 2010).

Edema: Oral, IV: 250-375 mg once daily

Epilepsy: Oral: 8-30 mg/kg/day in divided doses. A lower dosing range of 4-16 mg/kg/day in 1-4 divided doses has also been recommended; maximum dose: 30 mg/kg/day or 1 g/day (Oles, 1989; Reiss, 1996). **Note:** Minimal additional benefit with doses >16 mg/kg/day. **Extended release capsule is not recommended for treatment of epilepsy.**

Glaucoma:

Chronic simple (open-angle): Oral, IV: 250 mg 1-4 times/day or 500 mg extended release capsule twice daily

Secondary or acute (closed-angle): Oral, IV: Initial: 250-500 mg; maintenance: 125-250 mg every 4 hours (250 mg every 12 hours has been effective in short-term treatment of some patients)

Metabolic alkalosis (off-label use): IV: 500 mg as a single dose; reassess need based upon acid-base status (Marik, 1991; Mazur, 1999)

Respiratory stimulant in stable hypercapnic COPD (off-label use): Oral: 250 mg twice daily (Wagenaar, 2003)

Elderly: Oral: Initial doses should begin at the low end of the dosage range.

Dosage adjustment in renal impairment: Note: Use is contraindicated in marked renal impairment; creatinine clearance cutoff not specified in manufacturer's labeling.

CrCl 10-50 mL/minute: Administer every 12 hours

CrCl <10 mL/minute: Avoid use

Hemodialysis: Moderately dialyzable (20% to 50%)

Peritoneal dialysis: Supplemental dose is not necessary (Schwenk, 1994)

Dosage adjustment in hepatic impairment: Use contraindicated in patients with cirrhosis or marked liver disease or dysfunction.

Additional Information Complete prescribing information should be consulted for additional detail.

Dosage Forms

Capsule Extended Release 12 Hour, Oral:

Diamox Sequels: 500 mg

Generic: 500 mg

Solution Reconstituted, Injection [preservative free]:

Generic: 500 mg (1 ea)

Tablet, Oral:

Generic: 125 mg, 250 mg

Acetic Acid (a SEE tik AS id)

Index Terms Ethanoic Acid

Pharmacologic Category Otic Agent, Anti-infective; Topical Skin Product

Use Irrigation of the bladder; periodic irrigation of indwelling catheters; treatment of superficial bacterial infections of the external auditory canal

Pregnancy Risk Factor C

Dosage

Irrigation: Adults: (**Note:** Dosage of an irrigating solution depends on the capacity or surface area of the structure being irrigated):

For continuous irrigation of the urinary bladder with 0.25% acetic acid irrigation, the rate of administration will approximate the rate of urine flow; usually 500-1500 mL/24 hours

For periodic irrigation of an indwelling urinary catheter to maintain patency, about 50 mL of 0.25% acetic acid irrigation is required

Otic:

Children ≥3 years: Otitis externa: Insert saturated wick; keep moist 24 hours; remove wick and instill 5 drops 3-4 times/day. **Note:** 3-4 drops may be sufficient in children due to the smaller capacity of the ear canal.

Adults: Otitis externa: Insert saturated wick; keep moist 24 hours; remove wick and instill 5 drops 3-4 times/day

Additional Information Complete prescribing information should be consulted for additional detail.

Dosage Forms

Solution, Irrigation:

Generic: 0.25% (250 mL, 500 mL, 1000 mL)

Solution, Otic:

Generic: 2% (15 mL, 60 mL)

◆ **Acetic Acid, Hydrocortisone, and Propylene Glycol Diacetate** *see* Acetic Acid, Propylene Glycol Diacetate, and Hydrocortisone *on page 40*

Acetic Acid, Propylene Glycol Diacetate, and Hydrocortisone

(a SEE tik AS id, PRO pa leen GLY kole dye AS e tate, & hye droe KOR ti sone)

Brand Names: U.S. Acetasol® HC; VoSol® HC [DSC]

Index Terms Acetic Acid, Hydrocortisone, and Propylene Glycol Diacetate; Hydrocortisone, Acetic Acid, and Propylene Glycol Diacetate; Propylene Glycol Diacetate, Acetic Acid, and Hydrocortisone

Pharmacologic Category Otic Agent, Anti-infective

Use Treatment of superficial infections of the external auditory canal caused by organisms susceptible to the action of the antimicrobial, complicated by swelling

Dosage Children ≥3 years and Adults: Otic: Instill 3-5 drops in ear(s) every 4-6 hours

Additional Information Complete prescribing information should be consulted for additional detail.

Dosage Forms

Solution, otic [drops]: Acetic acid 2%, propylene glycol diacetate 3%, and hydrocortisone 1% (10 mL)

Acetasol® HC: Acetic acid 2%, propylene glycol diacetate 3%, and hydrocortisone 1% (10 mL)

◆ **Acetoxymethylprogesterone** *see* MedroxyPROGESTERone *on page 1277*

Acetylcholine (a se teel KOE leen)

Brand Names: U.S. Miochol-E

Brand Names: Canada Miochol®-E

Index Terms Acetylcholine Chloride

Pharmacologic Category Cholinergic Agonist; Ophthalmic Agent, Miotic

Use Produces complete miosis in cataract surgery, keratoplasty, iridectomy, and other anterior segment surgery where rapid miosis is required

Dosage Adults: Intraocular: 0.5-2 mL of 1% injection (5-20 mg) instilled into anterior chamber before or after securing one or more sutures

Dosage adjustment in renal impairment: No dosage adjustment provided in manufacturer's labeling.

Dosage adjustment in hepatic impairment: No dosage adjustment provided in manufacturer's labeling.

Additional Information Complete prescribing information should be consulted for additional detail.

Dosage Forms

Solution Reconstituted, Intraocular:

Miochol-E: 20 mg (1 ea)

◆ **Acetylcholine Chloride** *see* Acetylcholine *on page 40*

Acetylcysteine (a se teel SIS teen)

Brand Names: U.S. Acetadote

Brand Names: Canada Acetylcysteine Injection; Acetylcysteine Solution; Mucomyst®; Parvolex®

Index Terms *N* Acetylcysteine; *N*-Acetyl-L-cysteine; *N*-Acetylcysteine; Acetylcysteine Sodium; Mercapturic Acid; Mucomyst; NAC

Pharmacologic Category Antidote; Mucolytic Agent

Use Antidote for acute acetaminophen poisoning; repeated supratherapeutic ingestion (RSTI) of acetaminophen; adjunctive mucolytic therapy in patients with abnormal or viscid mucous secretions in acute and chronic bronchopulmonary diseases; pulmonary complications of surgery and cystic fibrosis; diagnostic bronchial studies

Pregnancy Risk Factor B

Pregnancy Considerations Adverse events were not observed in animal reproduction studies. Based on limited reports using acetylcysteine to treat acetaminophen poisoning in pregnant women, acetylcysteine has been shown to cross the placenta and may provide protective levels in the fetus.

Acetylcysteine may be used to treat acetaminophen overdose in during pregnancy (Wilkes, 2005). In general, medications used as antidotes should take into consideration the health and prognosis of the mother; antidotes should be administered to pregnant women if there is a clear indication for use and should not be withheld because of fears of teratogenicity (Bailey, 2003).

Breast-Feeding Considerations It is not known if acetylcysteine is excreted in breast milk. The manufacturer recommends that caution be exercised when administering acetylcysteine to nursing women. Based on its pharmacokinetics, the drug should be nearly completely cleared 30 hours after administration; therefore, nursing women may consider resuming nursing 30 hours after dosing is complete.

Contraindications Hypersensitivity to acetylcysteine or any component of the formulation

Warnings/Precautions

Inhalation: Since increased bronchial secretions may develop after inhalation, percussion, postural drainage, and suctioning should follow. If bronchospasm occurs, administer a bronchodilator; discontinue acetylcysteine if bronchospasm progresses.

Intravenous: Acute flushing and erythema have been reported; usually occurs within 30-60 minutes and may resolve spontaneously. Serious anaphylactoid reactions have also been reported and are more commonly associated with IV administration, but may also occur with oral administration (Mroz, 1997). When used for acetaminophen poisoning, the incidence is reduced when the initial loading dose is administered over 60 minutes. The acetylcysteine infusion may be interrupted until treatment of allergic symptoms is initiated; the infusion can then be carefully restarted. Treatment for anaphylactoid reactions should be immediately available. Use caution in patients with asthma or history of bronchospasm as these patients may be at increased risk. Conversely, patients with high acetaminophen levels (>150 mg/dL) may be at a reduced risk for anaphylactoid reactions (Pakravan, 2008; Sandilands, 2009; Waring, 2008).

Acute acetaminophen poisoning: Acetylcysteine is indicated in patients with a serum acetaminophen level that indicates they are at "possible" risk or greater for hepatotoxicity when plotted on the Rumack-Matthew nomogram. There are several situations where the nomogram is of limited use. Serum acetaminophen levels obtained <4 hours postingestion are not interpretable; patients presenting late may have undetectable serum concentrations, despite having received a toxic dose. The nomogram is less predictive of hepatic injury following an acute overdose with an extended release acetaminophen product. The nomogram also does not take into account patients who may be at higher risk of acetaminophen toxicity (eg, alcoholics, malnourished patients, concurrent use of CYP2E1 enzyme-inducing agents [eg, isoniazid]). Nevertheless, acetylcysteine should be administered to any patient with signs of hepatotoxicity, even if the serum acetaminophen level is low or undetectable. Patients who present >24 hours after an acute ingestion or patients who present following an acute ingestion at an unknown time may be candidates for acetylcysteine therapy; consultation with a poison control center or clinical toxicologist is highly recommended.

Repeated supratherapeutic ingestion (RSTI) of acetaminophen: The Rumack-Matthew nomogram is not designed to be used following RSTIs. In general, an accurate past medical history, including a comprehensive acetaminophen ingestion history, in conjunction with AST concentrations and serum acetaminophen levels, may give the clinician insight as to the patient's risk of acetaminophen toxicity. Some experts recommend that acetylcysteine be administered to any patient with "higher than expected" serum acetaminophen levels or serum acetaminophen level >10 mcg/mL, even in the absence of hepatic injury; others recommend treatment for patients with laboratory evidence and/or signs and symptoms of hepatotoxicity (Hendrickson, 2006; Jones, 2000). Consultation with a poison control center or a clinical toxicologist is highly recommended.

Adverse Reactions

Inhalation:

Central nervous system: Chills, drowsiness, fever
Gastrointestinal: Nausea, stomatitis, vomiting
Local: Irritation, stickiness on face following nebulization
Respiratory: Bronchospasm, hemoptysis, rhinorrhea
Miscellaneous: Acquired sensitization (rare), clamminess, unpleasant odor during administration

Intravenous:

Cardiovascular: Edema, flushing, tachycardia
Dermatologic: Pruritus, rash, urticaria
Gastrointestinal: Nausea, vomiting
Respiratory: Pharyngitis, rhinorrhea, rhonchi, throat tightness
Miscellaneous: Anaphylactoid reaction
Rare but important or life-threatening: Anaphylaxis, angioedema, bronchospasm, chest tightness, cough, dizziness, dyspnea, headache, hypotension, respiratory distress, stridor, wheezing

Oral (Bebarta, 2010; Mroz, 1997):

Cardiovascular: Hypotension, tachycardia
Dermatologic: Angioedema, pruritus, urticaria
Gastrointestinal: Nausea, vomiting
Respiratory: Bronchospasm

Drug Interactions

Metabolism/Transport Effects None known.

Avoid Concomitant Use There are no known interactions where it is recommended to avoid concomitant use.

Increased Effect/Toxicity There are no known significant interactions involving an increase in effect.

Decreased Effect There are no known significant interactions involving a decrease in effect.

Preparation for Administration

Oral: Treatment of acetaminophen poisoning: Dilute the 20% solution 1:3 with a cola, orange juice, or other soft drink to prepare a 5% solution. Use within 1 hour of preparation.

Solution for injection (Acetadote): Acetaminophen poisoning: IV:

Loading dose: Dilute 150 mg/kg in D_5W 200 mL.
Second dose: Dilute 50 mg/kg in D_5W 500 mL.
Third dose: Dilute 100 mg/kg in D_5W 1000 mL.
Note: To avoid fluid overload in patients <40 kg and those requiring fluid restriction, decrease volume of D_5W proportionally (see table on next page in dosing section). Discard unused portion.

Solution for inhalation: The 20% solution may be diluted with sodium chloride or sterile water; the 10% solution may be used undiluted.

Intravenous administration of solution for inhalation (off-label route): Using D_5W, dilute acetylcysteine 20% oral solution to a 3% solution.

Storage/Stability

Solution for injection (Acetadote): Store unopened vials at room temperature, 20°C to 25°C (68°F to 77°F). Following reconstitution with D_5W, solution is stable for 24 hours at room temperature. A color change may occur in opened vials (light pink or purple) and does not affect the safety or efficacy.

Solution for inhalation: Store unopened vials at room temperature; once opened, store under refrigeration and use within 96 hours. A color change may occur in opened vials (light purple) and does not affect the safety or efficacy.

Mechanism of Action

Exerts mucolytic action through its free sulfhydryl group which opens up the disulfide bonds in the mucoproteins thus lowering mucous viscosity.

In patients with acetaminophen toxicity, acetylcysteine acts as a hepatoprotective agent by restoring hepatic glutathione, serving as a glutathione substitute, and enhancing the nontoxic sulfate conjugation of acetaminophen.

The presumed mechanism in preventing contrast-induced nephropathy is its ability to scavenge oxygen-derived free radicals and improve endothelium-dependent vasodilation.

Pharmacodynamics/Kinetics

Onset of action: Inhalation: 5-10 minutes
Duration: Inhalation: >1 hour
Distribution: 0.47 L/kg
Protein binding: 83%
Half-life elimination:
Reduced acetylcysteine: 2 hours
Total acetylcysteine: Adults: 5.6 hours; Newborns: 11 hours
Time to peak, plasma: Oral: 1-2 hours
Excretion: Urine

Dosage

Acetaminophen poisoning: **Note:** Only the 72-hour oral and 21-hour IV regimens are FDA-approved. Ideally, in patients with an acute acetaminophen ingestion, treatment should begin within 8 hours of ingestion or as soon as possible after ingestion. In patients who present following RSTI and treatment is deemed appropriate, acetylcysteine should be initiated immediately. Regardless of the treatment regimen selected, serum acetaminophen levels, liver function, and clinical status should be evaluated during and prior to the end of the treatment regimen to determine if treatment discontinuation is appropriate. In patients who continue to experience symptoms of hepatotoxicity or elevated liver function tests at the conclusion of a 72-hour oral or 21-hour IV regimen, extending the treatment course may be appropriate; however, when and to which patients additional doses should be administered is unclear. Possible candidates for extended therapy include patients with a suspected massive overdose, concomitant ingestion of other substances, or patients with preexisting liver disease. In patients with persistently elevated acetaminophen levels, persistently elevated liver function tests, or an elevated INR, additional acetylcysteine should be administered. Typically, an additional "third dose" or "third bag" (IV: 100 mg/kg [maximum: 10 g] infused over 16 hours) is administered; however, this dose may be inadequate in some patients (Rumack, 2012). Consultation with a poison control center or clinical toxicologist is highly recommended to determine optimal patient care.

Children and Adults:

Oral: **Note:** Consultation with a poison control center or clinical toxicologist is highly recommended when considering the discontinuation of oral acetylcysteine prior to the conclusion of a full 18-dose course of therapy.

72-hour regimen: Consists of 18 doses; total dose delivered: 1330 mg/kg

Loading dose: 140 mg/kg

Maintenance dose: 70 mg/kg every 4 hours; repeat dose if emesis occurs within 1 hour of administration

IV (Acetadote):

21-hour regimen: Consists of 3 doses; total dose delivered: 300 mg/kg

Loading dose: 150 mg/kg (maximum: 15 **g**) infused over 60 minutes

Second dose: 50 mg/kg (maximum: 5 **g**) infused over 4 hours

Third dose: 100 mg/kg (maximum: 10 **g**) infused over 16 hours

Note: The fluid volume should be reduced in patients weighing <40 kg according to the following table:

Acetadote Dosing / Fluid Volume Guidelines for Patients ≤40 kg

Body Weight (kg)	Loading Dose 150 mg/kg over 1 h		Second Dose 50 mg/kg over 4 h		Third Dose 100 mg/kg over 16 h	
	Acetadote (mL)	D_5W (mL)	Acetadote (mL)	D_5W (mL)	Acetadote (mL)	D_5W (mL)
40	30	100	10	250	20	500
30	22.5	100	7.5	250	15	500
21	15.75	100	5.25	250	10.5	500
20	15	60	5	140	10	280
15	11.25	45	3.75	105	7.5	210
10	7.5	30	2.5	70	5	140
5	3.75	15	1.25	35	2.5	70

Obesity: In patients who weigh >100 kg, the following dosing regimen is recommended: IV (Acetadote):

21-hour regimen: Consists of 3 doses; total dose delivered: 30 **g**

Loading dose: 15 **g** infused over 60 minutes

Second dose: 5 **g** infused over 4 hours

Third dose: 10 **g** infused over 16 hours

Adjuvant therapy in respiratory conditions: **Note:** Patients should receive an aerosolized bronchodilator 10-15 minutes prior to acetylcysteine.

Inhalation, nebulization (face mask, mouth piece, tracheostomy): Acetylcysteine 10% and 20% solution (dilute 20% solution with sodium chloride or sterile water for inhalation); 10% solution may be used undiluted

Infants: 1-2 mL of 20% solution or 2-4 mL of 10% solution until nebulized given 3-4 times/day

Children and Adults: 3-5 mL of 20% solution or 6-10 mL of 10% solution until nebulized given 3-4 times/day; dosing range: 1-10 mL of 20% solution or 2-20 mL of 10% solution every 2-6 hours

Inhalation, nebulization (tent, croupette): Children and Adults: Dose must be individualized; may require up to 300 mL solution/treatment

Direct instillation: Adults:

Into tracheostomy: 1-2 mL of 10% to 20% solution every 1-4 hours

Through percutaneous intratracheal catheter: 1-2 mL of 20% or 2-4 mL of 10% solution every 1-4 hours via syringe attached to catheter

Diagnostic bronchogram: Nebulization or intratracheal: Adults: 1-2 mL of 20% solution or 2-4 mL of 10% solution administered 2-3 times prior to procedure

Prevention of contrast-induced nephropathy (CIN) (off-label use): Adults: Oral: 600-1200 mg twice daily for 2 days (beginning the day before the procedure); may be given as powder in capsules (some centers use solution, diluted in cola beverage or juice). **Note:** No longer recommended for use prior to percutaneous coronary intervention; instead adequate hydration is preferred (Levine, 2011).

Dosage adjustment in renal impairment: Oral, IV: No dosage adjustment provided in manufacturer's labeling.

Dosage adjustment in hepatic impairment:

Oral: No dosage adjustment provided in manufacturer's labeling.

IV: No dosage adjustment required.

Administration

Inhalation: Acetylcysteine is incompatible with tetracyclines, erythromycin, amphotericin B, iodized oil, chymotrypsin, trypsin, and hydrogen peroxide. Administer separately. Intermittent aerosol treatments are commonly given when patient arises, before meals, and just before retiring at bedtime.

Oral: Treatment of acetaminophen poisoning, administer orally as a 5% solution. Use within 1 hour of preparation. The unpleasant odor (sulfur-like) becomes less noticeable as treatment progresses. If patient vomits within 1 hour of dose, readminister. (**Note:** It is helpful to put the acetylcysteine on ice, in a cup with a cover, and drink through a straw; alternatively, administer via an NG tube).

IV (Acetadote): Acetaminophen poisoning:

Loading dose: Administer over 60 minutes.

Second dose: Administer over 4 hours.

Third dose: Administer over 16 hours.

If the commercial IV form is unavailable, the solution for inhalation has been used; each dose should be infused through a 0.2 micron Millipore filter (in-line) over 60 minutes (Yip, 1998); intravenous administration of the solution for inhalation is not USP 797-compliant.

Note: Undiluted injection, solution (Acetadote) is hyperosmolar (2600 mOsmol/L); when the diluent volume is decreased for patients <40 kg or requiring fluid restriction, the osmolarity of the solution may remain higher than desirable for intravenous infusion. To ensure tolerance of the infusion, osmolarity should be adjusted to a physiologically safe level (eg, ≥150 mOsmol/L in children).

Acetadote concentration: 7 mg/mL

Osmolarity in D_5W: 343 mOsmol/L

Osmolarity in ½NS: 245 mOsmol/L

Osmolarity in SWFI: 91 mOsmol/L

Acetadote concentration: 24 mg/mL

Osmolarity in D_5W: 564 mOsmol/L

Osmolarity in ½NS: 466 mOsmol/L

Osmolarity in SWFI: 312 mOsmol/L

Monitoring Parameters Acetaminophen poisoning: Monitor patient for the development of anaphylaxis or anaphylactoid reactions; monitor serum acetaminophen levels, AST, ALT, bilirubin, PT, INR, serum creatinine, BUN, serum glucose, hemoglobin, hematocrit, and electrolytes. Assess patient for nausea, vomiting, and skin rash following oral administration. Reassess LFTs for possible hepatotoxicity every 4-6 hours. An early elevation in the INR may be related to acetylcysteine therapy (Schmidt, 2002).

Acute ingestion: Obtain the first acetaminophen level 4 hours postingestion (or as soon as possible thereafter); plot on the Rumack-Matthew nomogram. In patients who have ingested an extended release formulation of acetaminophen or have coingested an agent known to delay gastric emptying, obtain a repeat serum acetaminophen measurement 4-6 hours following the first measurement if the original level (taken at 4-8 hours postingestion) when plotted on the Rumack-Matthew nomogram indicated that treatment was not necessary.

Dosage Forms

Injection, solution [preservative free]: 20% (30 mL)
Acetadote: 20% [200 mg/mL] (30 mL)

Solution, for inhalation/oral: 10% [100 mg/mL] (10 mL, 30 mL); 20% [200 mg/mL] (10 mL, 30 mL)

Solution, for inhalation/oral [preservative free]: 10% [100 mg/mL] (4 mL, 10 mL, 30 mL); 20% [200 mg/mL] (4 mL, 10 mL, 30 mL)

- ◆ **Acetylcysteine Injection (Can)** *see* Acetylcysteine *on page 40*
- ◆ **Acetylcysteine, Methylcobalamin, and Methylfolate** *see* Methylfolate, Methylcobalamin, and Acetylcysteine *on page 1334*
- ◆ **Acetylcysteine, Methylfolate, and Methylcobalamin** *see* Methylfolate, Methylcobalamin, and Acetylcysteine *on page 1334*
- ◆ **Acetylcysteine Sodium** *see* Acetylcysteine *on page 40*
- ◆ **Acetylcysteine Solution (Can)** *see* Acetylcysteine *on page 40*
- ◆ **Acetylsalicylic Acid** *see* Aspirin *on page 180*
- ◆ **ACH-Alendronate (Can)** *see* Alendronate *on page 79*
- ◆ **ACH-Anastrozole (Can)** *see* Anastrozole *on page 148*
- ◆ **ACH-Bicalutamide (Can)** *see* Bicalutamide *on page 262*
- ◆ **ACH Candesartan (Can)** *see* Candesartan *on page 335*
- ◆ **ACH-Ezetimibe (Can)** *see* Ezetimibe *on page 832*
- ◆ **ACH-Letrozole (Can)** *see* Letrozole *on page 1181*
- ◆ **ACH-Montelukast (Can)** *see* Montelukast *on page 1392*
- ◆ **Ach-Mycophenolate (Can)** *see* Mycophenolate *on page 1405*
- ◆ **ACH-Pioglitazone (Can)** *see* Pioglitazone *on page 1654*
- ◆ **Achromycin** *see* Tetracycline *on page 2017*
- ◆ **ACH-Telmisartan HCTZ (Can)** *see* Telmisartan and Hydrochlorothiazide *on page 1990*
- ◆ **ACH-Temozolomide (Can)** *see* Temozolomide *on page 1991*
- ◆ **Aciclovir** *see* Acyclovir (Systemic) *on page 47*
- ◆ **Aciclovir** *see* Acyclovir (Topical) *on page 51*

Aciclovir (Ophthalmic) [INT] (ay SYE kloe veer)

International Brand Names Acic-Ophtal (DE); Aciclor (VE); Acivir Eye (IN); Cicloviral (CO); Cusiviral (HK, MY, SG); Cyclovir (IN); Devirus (TW); Dravyr (MY); Geavir (SE); Oftavir (UY); Ophth-cyclovir (PK); Opthavir (MX); Temiral (ID); Virex (CO); Virolex (SK); Zovir (IS); Zovirax (AU, BE, BR, CH, CL, CZ, EE, EG, ES, FI, FR, GB, HK, ID, IE, IL, IN, KR, MX, MY, NO, NZ, RO, SE, SG, TH, TR, UY); Zovirax Eye Ointment (SA)

Pharmacologic Category Antiviral Agent

Reported Use Treatment of herpes simplex keratitis

Dosage Range

Adults: Topical: Apply 1 cm ribbon inside lower eyelid every 4 hours 5 times/day for 14 days or at least 3 days after healing is complete (whichever is shorter)

Children: Refer to adult dosing

Product Availability Product available in various countries; not currently available in the U.S.

Dosage Forms

Ointment, ophthalmic: 3% (4.5 g tube)

- ◆ **Acid Control (Can)** *see* Famotidine *on page 845*
- ◆ **Acid Gone [OTC]** *see* Aluminum Hydroxide and Magnesium Carbonate *on page 103*
- ◆ **Acid Gone Extra Strength [OTC]** *see* Aluminum Hydroxide and Magnesium Carbonate *on page 103*
- ◆ **Acid Reducer [OTC]** *see* Famotidine *on page 845*
- ◆ **Acid Reducer [OTC]** *see* Ranitidine *on page 1777*
- ◆ **Acid Reducer (Can)** *see* Ranitidine *on page 1777*
- ◆ **Acid Reducer Maximum Strength [OTC]** *see* Famotidine *on page 845*
- ◆ **Acid Reducer Maximum Strength [OTC] [DSC]** *see* Ranitidine *on page 1777*
- ◆ **Acidulated Phosphate Fluoride** *see* Fluoride *on page 895*
- ◆ **Aciphex** *see* RABEprazole *on page 1762*
- ◆ **AcipHex Sprinkle** *see* RABEprazole *on page 1762*

Acipimox [INT] (ay CIP e moks)

International Brand Names Olbetam (AT, BE, CH, CL, CN, DK, GB, GR, HK, HN, IL, IT, KR, KW, NL, NO, NZ, QA, SA, SG, SI, TH, TW, ZA); Si LiMeng (CN); YiPing (CN)

Pharmacologic Category Antilipemic Agent, Miscellaneous

Reported Use Alternative or adjunctive treatment for hypertriglyceridemia (Fredrickson type IV hyperlipoproteinemia) and hypercholesterolemia and hypertriglyceridemia (Fredrickson type IIb hyperlipoproteinemia) in patients who have not responded adequately to other treatments such as statins or fibrates.

Dosage Range Adults: Oral: 500-750 mg/day in divided doses with meals

Product Availability Product available in various countries; not currently available in U.S.

Dosage Forms

Capsule, oral: 250 mg

Acitretin (a si TRE tin)

Brand Names: U.S. Soriatane

Brand Names: Canada Soriatane

Pharmacologic Category Retinoid-Like Compound

Use Psoriasis: Treatment of severe psoriasis in adults. Limitations of use: Not for the treatment of acne.

Pregnancy Risk Factor X

Pregnancy Considerations **[U.S. Boxed Warning]: Acitretin is a known teratogen and use is contraindicated in females who are or may become pregnant. Birth defects (including facial, ear, central nervous system, cardiovascular, limb, bone, and joint) have been noted following acitretin exposure during pregnancy. Use only in women with severe psoriasis that is unresponsive to other therapies or with contraindications to the use of alternative treatments. Pregnancy must be avoided for at least 3 years after treatment discontinuation. Two reliable forms of contraception must be used simultaneously for 1 month prior to initiating therapy, during therapy, and for 3 years after discontinuation. Two negative pregnancy tests (sensitivity at least 25 mIU/mL) are required prior to initiating therapy; pregnancy tests must be repeated every month during treatment. In addition, because ethanol forms a teratogenic metabolite and would increase the duration of teratogenic potential, ethanol should not be consumed during treatment or for 2 months after discontinuation.**

Only physicians experienced with the diagnosis and treatment of severe psoriasis, including the use of retinoid treatment, and physicians who understand the risk of teratogenicity should prescribe acitretin. Females of childbearing potential must be able to fulfill all conditions for use prior to initiating therapy, ▶

including a Patient Agreement/Informed Consent (consult manufacturer labeling for further detail). Prescriptions should be written for a limited supply. The Do Your P.A.R.T. (Pregnancy Prevention Actively Required During and After Treatment) program explains teratogenic risks and requirements expected of females of childbearing potential to prevent pregnancies from occurring during use and 3 years following discontinuation; this should be used to educate patients and healthcare providers. Information for the Do Your P.A.R.T. program is available at www.soriatane.com/doyour-part-Program.html or by calling 1-888-784-3335.

Limited amounts of acitretin are found in seminal fluid; although it appears this poses little risk to a fetus, the actual risk of teratogenicity is not known.

Any pregnancy which occurs during treatment, or within 3 years after treatment is discontinued, should be reported to the manufacturer at 1-888-784-3335 or to the FDA at 1-800-FDA-1088.

Breast-Feeding Considerations Acitretin is excreted in breast milk. Due to the potential for serious adverse reactions in the nursing infant, the manufacturer does not recommend acitretin prior to or during nursing (Canadian labeling recommends that women should avoid breast-feeding for at least 3 years after acitretin is discontinued).

Information is available from a woman who started acitretin 40 mg per day, 8 months postpartum. The woman discontinued nursing prior to the study. Milk samples were collected prior to the first dose and twice daily for 9 days; maternal serum samples were also collected. Acitretin and its metabolite were detected in breast milk. Total concentrations of acitretin + metabolite remained relatively stable over the study period (30 to 40 ng/mL) showing no diurnal variation. Because acitretin is primarily distributed into milk fat, actual concentrations in breast milk may vary depending upon the lipid and fat content of the milk (Rollman, 1990).

Current guidelines do not recommend use during lactation due to the potential for cumulative toxicity in a nursing infant (Butler, 2014).

Contraindications Hypersensitivity (eg, angioedema, urticaria) to acitretin, other retinoids, or any component of the formulation; patients who are pregnant or intend on becoming pregnant during therapy or within 3 years after treatment discontinuation; severe hepatic or renal dysfunction; chronic abnormally elevated blood lipid levels; concomitant use with methotrexate or tetracyclines

Acitretin is contraindicated in females of childbearing potential unless all of the following conditions apply.

1) Patient has severe psoriasis unresponsive to other therapy or if clinical condition contraindicates other treatments.
2) Patient must have two negative urine or serum pregnancy tests prior to therapy.
3) Patient must have pregnancy test repeated monthly during therapy. After discontinuation of therapy, a pregnancy test must be repeated every 3 months for at least 3 years.
4) Patient must commit to using two effective forms of birth control starting 1 month prior to acitretin treatment and for 3 years after discontinuation. Prescriber must counsel patient about contraception every month during therapy and every 3 months following discontinuation for at least 3 years.
5) Patient is reliable in understanding and carrying out instructions.
6) Patient has received, and acknowledged, understanding of a careful oral and printed explanation of the hazards of fetal exposure to acitretin and the risk of possible contraception failure. Patient must sign an agreement/informed consent document stating that she understands these risks and that she should not consume ethanol during therapy or for 2 months after discontinuation.

Warnings/Precautions Hazardous agent - use appropriate precautions for handling and disposal (NIOSH 2014 [group 3]).

[U.S. Boxed Warning]: Acitretin is a known teratogen and contraindicated in females who are or may become pregnant. Birth defects (including facial, ear, central nervous system, cardiovascular, limb, bone, and joint) have been noted following acitretin exposure during pregnancy. Use only in women with severe psoriasis that is unresponsive to other therapies or with contraindications to the use of alternative treatments. Pregnancy must be avoided for at least 3 years after treatment discontinuation. Two reliable forms of contraception must be used simultaneously for 1 month prior to initiating therapy, during therapy, and for 3 years after discontinuation. Two negative pregnancy tests (sensitivity at least 25 mIU/mL) are required prior to initiating therapy; pregnancy tests must be repeated every month during treatment. In addition, because ethanol forms a teratogenic metabolite and would increase the duration of teratogenic potential, ethanol should not be consumed during treatment or for 2 months after discontinuation. Any pregnancy which occurs during treatment, or within 3 years after treatment is discontinued, should be reported to the manufacturer at 1-888-784-3335 or to the FDA at 1-800-FDA-1088.

[U.S. Boxed Warning]: Females of childbearing potential must be able to fulfill all conditions for use prior to initiating therapy, including a Patient Agreement/Informed Consent (consult manufacturer labeling for further detail). Prescriptions should be written for a limited supply. The Do Your P.A.R.T. (Pregnancy Prevention Actively Required During and After Treatment) program explains teratogenic risks and requirements expected of females of childbearing potential to prevent pregnancies from occurring during use and 3 years following discontinuation; this should be used to educate patients and healthcare providers. Information for the Do Your P.A.R.T. program is available at www.soriatane.com/doyour-part-Program.html or by calling 1-888-784-3335.

[U.S. Boxed Warning]: Female patients should abstain from ethanol or ethanol-containing products during therapy and for 2 months after discontinuation. [U.S. Boxed Warning]: All patients should be advised not to donate blood during therapy or for 3 years following completion of therapy. [U.S. Boxed Warning]: Changes in transaminases have occurred in up to 1/3 of patients, which generally returned to normal after discontinuation of treatment. Monitor for hepatotoxicity; discontinue if hepatotoxicity is suspected. [U.S. Boxed Warning]: Hepatitis has been reported (including fatalities); some patients received etretinate for ≤1 month before presenting with hepatic signs or symptoms.

Use with caution in patients at risk of hypertriglyceridemias. Lipid changes including, increased triglycerides, increased cholesterol, and decreased HDL are common (up to 66%), which were reversible upon discontinuation of treatment; increased triglycerides may lead to pancreatitis. Consider discontinuation if hypertriglyceridemia and decreased HDL persist. Use is contraindicated in patients with chronic abnormally elevated blood lipid values.

Retinoids, including acitretin, have been associated with pseudotumor cerebri (benign intracranial hypertension). Concurrent use of other drugs associated with this effect (eg, tetracyclines) may increase risk; pseudotumor cerebri has been reported with use of tetracyclines and acitretin independently. Early signs and symptoms include papilledema, headache, nausea, vomiting, and visual disturbances. Discontinue use in patients experiencing papilledema. Impaired glucose control has been reported with retinoid use. Use with caution in patients with diabetes mellitus; new cases of diabetes have been diagnosed. Discontinue if visual changes occur. May cause adverse effects to the eyes and vision, including a decrease in night vision or decreased tolerance to contact lenses. Use caution when operating vehicles at night; discontinue if visual changes occur. Patients receiving long-term treatment should be periodically examined for bony abnormalities; risk versus benefit of therapy should be considered if abnormalities occur. Depression, including aggressive behavior and thoughts of self-harm have been reported; use with caution in patients with a history of mental illness. May be photosensitizing; minimize sun or other UV exposure to treated areas. The risk of burning is increased with phototherapy; decreased doses are required. Capillary leak syndrome, a potential manifestation of retinoic acid syndrome (differentiation syndrome) has been reported with acitretin use. Capillary leak syndrome features may include localized or generalized edema with secondary weight gain, fever, and hypotension; rhabdomyolysis and myalgias have also been reported. Laboratory tests may show neutrophilia, hypoalbuminemia, and an elevated hematocrit. Discontinue use if capillary leak syndrome develops during therapy. Exfoliative dermatitis has been reported with acitretin use; discontinue use if exfoliative dermatitis occurs during therapy. Transient worsening of psoriasis may initially occur; patients should be advised that it may take 2 to 3 months to achieve the full benefits of treatment. Most patients experience relapse of psoriasis after discontinuing therapy. Subsequent courses, when clinically indicated, have produced results similar to the initial course of therapy.

[U.S. Boxed Warning]: All patients must be provided with a medication guide each time acitretin is dispensed. Female patients must also sign an informed consent prior to therapy. [U.S. Boxed Warning]: Only physicians experienced with the diagnosis and treatment of severe psoriasis, including the use of retinoid treatment, and physicians who understand the risk of teratogenicity should prescribe acitretin. Safety and efficacy for pediatric patients have not been established; growth potential may be affected.

Adverse Reactions

Cardiovascular: Edema, flushing

Central nervous system: Central nervous system: Bell's palsy, depression, drowsiness, fatigue, headache, hyperesthesia, hypertonia, insomnia, pain, paresthesia, rigors

Dermatologic: Abnormal hair texture, abnormal skin odor, alopecia, acquired cutaneous adherence, bullous skin disease, cheilitis, cold and clammy skin, dermatitis, diaphoresis (increased), exfoliation of skin, madarosis, nail disease, pruritus, erythematous rash, paronychia, psoriasiform eruption, pyogenic granuloma, seborrhea, skin atrophy, skin fissure, skin rash, sunburn, xeroderma

Endocrine & metabolic: Acetonuria, decreased haptoglobins, decreased HDL cholesterol, decreased serum albumin, decreased serum calcium, decreased serum glucose (fasting), decreased serum iron, decreased serum magnesium, decreased serum potassium, decreased serum sodium, glycosuria, hot flash, hyperchloremia, hypercholesterolemia, hypermagnesemia, hyperphospheremia, hypertriglyceridemia, hypochloremia, hypophosphatemia, increased gamma-glutamyl transferase, increased serum albumin, increased serum calcium, increased serum glucose (fasting), increased serum iron, increased serum potassium, increased serum sodium, increased thirst, increased uric acid, magnesium imbalance (increased/decreased)

Gastrointestinal: Abdominal pain, anorexia, aphthous stomatitis, diarrhea, dysgeusia, gingival hemorrhage, gingivitis, increased appetite, nausea, sialorrhea, stomatitis, tongue disease, xerostomia

Genitourinary: Erythrocyturia, hematuria, proteinuria

Hematologic & oncologic: Change in RBC count, change in WBC count, decreased hematocrit, decreased hemoglobin, decreased neutrophils, increased haptoglobin, increased hematocrit, increased hemoglobin, increased neutrophils, leukocyturia, purpura, reticulocytopenia, reticulocytosis

Hepatic: Increased direct serum bilirubin, increased liver enzymes, increased serum alkaline phosphatase, increased serum bilirubin

Neuromuscular & skeletal: arthralgia, Arthritis, back pain, increased creatine phosphokinase, myalgia, ostealgia, osteoarthritis, peripheral joint hyperostosis, spinal hyperostosis (progression)

Ophthalmic: Blepharitis, blurred vision, cataract, conjunctivitis, diplopia, epithelial keratopathy, eye pain, nocturnal amblyopia, photophobia, xerophthalmia

Otic: Otalgia, tinnitus

Renal: Increased blood urea nitrogen, increased serum creatinine

Respiratory: Epistaxis, rhinitis, sinusitis

Miscellaneous: Ulcer

Rare but important or life-threatening: Abnormal gait, abnormal lacrimation, acne vulgaris, ageusia, aggressive behavior, alcohol intolerance, anal disease, bone disease, bursitis (olecranon), candidiasis, capillary leak syndrome, cerebrovascular accident, chalazion, conjunctival hemorrhage, constipation, corneal lesion, corneal ulcer, cutaneous nodule, cyanosis, cyst, deafness, decreased libido, dyspepsia, dysuria, ectropion, epidermal thinning, exfoliative dermatitis, flu-like symptoms, fungal infection, furunculosis, gastritis, gingival hyperplasia, glossitis, hair discoloration, hepatic cirrhosis, hepatic dysfunction, hepatitis, herpes simplex infection, hordeolum (recurrent), hyperkeratosis, hypersensitivity reaction, hypertrichosis, hypoesthesia, increased bronchial secretions, increased cerumen production, intermittent claudication, laryngitis, leukorrhea, mastalgia, melena, migraine, myasthenia, myocardial infarction, myopathy (with peripheral neuropathy), nail disease (fragility), neuritis, otitis media, pancreatitis, papilledema, peripheral ischemia, pharyngitis, prolonged bleeding time, pseudotumor cerebri, skin hypertrophy, skin photosensitivity, spinal hyperostosis (new lesion), suicidal ideation, tendonitis, tenesmus, thromboembolism, tongue ulcer, vaginitis, voice disorder, warts, weight gain, wound healing impairment

Drug Interactions

Metabolism/Transport Effects

None known.

Avoid Concomitant Use

Avoid concomitant use of Acitretin with any of the following: Alcohol (Ethyl); Methotrexate; Multivitamins/Fluoride (with ADE); Multivitamins/Minerals (with ADEK, Folate, Iron); Multivitamins/Minerals (with AE, No Iron); Tetracycline Derivatives; Vitamin A

Increased Effect/Toxicity

Acitretin may increase the levels/effects of: Methotrexate; Porfimer; Verteporfin; Vitamin A

The levels/effects of Acitretin may be increased by: Alcohol (Ethyl); Multivitamins/Fluoride (with ADE); Multivitamins/Minerals (with ADEK, Folate, Iron); Multivitamins/Minerals (with AE, No Iron); Tetracycline Derivatives

Decreased Effect
Acitretin may decrease the levels/effects of: Contraceptives (Estrogens); Contraceptives (Progestins)

Food Interactions
Ethanol: Use leads to formation of etretinate, a teratogenic metabolite with a prolonged half-life. Management: Female patients must avoid ethanol or ethanol-containing products concomitantly or within 2 months after discontinuing acitretin.
Food: Absorption increased when administered with food. Management: Take with food; avoid ingestion of additional sources of vitamin A (in excess of RDA).

Storage/Stability Store between 15°C to 25°C (59°F to 77°F). Avoid high temperatures and humidity. Protect from light.

Mechanism of Action Binds to and activates all nuclear subtypes (alpha, beta, and gamma) of retinoid X receptors (RXR) and retinoic acid receptors (RAR) to inhibit the expression of the proinflammatory cytokines interleukin-6 (IL-6), migration inhibitory factor-related protein-8 (MRP-8), and interferon-gamma (markers of hyperproliferation and abnormal keratinocyte differentiation). Resulting actions are anti-inflammatory and antiproliferative, and keratinocyte differentiation is normalized in the epithelium.

Pharmacodynamics/Kinetics Etretinate has been detected in serum for up to 3 years following therapy, possibly due to storage in adipose tissue.
Onset of action: May take 2 to 3 months for full effect; improvement may be seen within 8 weeks.
Absorption: Oral: ~72% absorbed when given with food
Protein binding: >99% bound, primarily to albumin
Metabolism: Metabolized to *cis*-acitretin; both compounds are further metabolized. Concomitant ethanol use leads to the formation of etretinate (active).
Half-life elimination: Acitretin: 49 hours (range: 33 to 96); *cis*-acitretin: 63 hours (range: 28 to 157); etretinate: 120 days (range: Up to 168 days)
Time to peak: 2 to 5 hours
Excretion: Feces (34% to 54%); urine (16% to 53%)

Dosage Oral: Adults: Individualization of dosage is required to achieve maximum therapeutic response while minimizing side effects
Initial therapy: Therapy should be initiated at 25 to 50 mg daily, given as a single dose with the main meal
Maintenance doses of 25 to 50 mg daily may be given after initial response to treatment; the maintenance dose should be based on clinical efficacy and tolerability
American Academy of Dermatology recommends: 10 to 50 mg daily as a single dose; doses ≤25 mg daily are used to decrease side effects (Menter, 2009)

Dosing adjustment in renal impairment: There are no dosage adjustments provided in the manufacturer's labeling; use is contraindicated in patients with severely impaired renal function.
Hemodialysis: Not removed by hemodialysis

Dosing adjustment in hepatic impairment: There are no dosage adjustments provided in the manufacturer's labeling; use is contraindicated in patients with severely impaired liver function.

Dietary Considerations Take with food. Avoid ingestion of additional sources of exogenous vitamin A (in excess of RDA); use of ethanol and ethanol-containing products is contraindicated.

Administration Administer with food, preferably with the main meal of the day.

Hazardous agent; use appropriate precautions for handling and disposal (NIOSH 2014 [group 3]).

Monitoring Parameters Lipid profile (baseline and at 1- to 2-week intervals for 4 to 8 weeks); liver function tests (baseline, and at 1- to 2-week intervals until stable, then as clinically indicated); blood glucose in patients with diabetes; bone abnormalities (with long-term use); pregnancy tests (2 negative tests prior to therapy initiation, monthly during treatment, and every 3 months for ≥3 years after discontinuation of therapy)

The American Academy of Dermatology recommends: CBC and renal function tests (baseline and then every 12 weeks); liver function tests (every 2 weeks for the first 8 weeks, then every 6 to 12 weeks thereafter) (Menter, 2009)

Additional Information Female patients are required to use two forms of birth control, at least one of which is a primary form, unless they have undergone a hysterectomy or are postmenopausal. Both forms of birth control must be used simultaneously for at least 1 month prior to therapy and for at least 3 years after discontinuation. Primary forms of birth control include tubal ligation, partner's vasectomy, IUD, or hormonal birth control products. Microdosed progestin products, referred to as "mini-pills," have been shown to be less effective when used with acitretin, and are not recommended. It is not known if other progestin contraceptives (eg, implants or injectables) are adequate methods of contraception during acitretin therapy. Secondary forms of contraception include diaphragms, latex condoms, and cervical caps, all if used with a spermicide.

Dosage Forms
Capsule, Oral:
Soriatane: 10 mg, 17.5 mg, 25 mg
Generic: 10 mg, 17.5 mg, 25 mg

◆ **Aclaro** *see* Hydroquinone *on page* 1020
◆ **Aclaro PD** *see* Hydroquinone *on page* 1020
◆ **Aclasta (Can)** *see* Zoledronic Acid *on page* 2206
◆ **Aclovate** *see* Alclometasone *on page* 72
◆ **ACNU** *see* Nimustine [INT] *on page* 1457

Acrivastine and Pseudoephedrine

(AK ri vas teen & soo doe e FED rin)

Brand Names: U.S. Semprex®-D

Index Terms Pseudoephedrine Hydrochloride and Acrivastine

Pharmacologic Category Alkylamine Derivative; Alpha/Beta Agonist; Decongestant; Histamine H_1 Antagonist; Histamine H_1 Antagonist, Second Generation

Use Relief of symptoms associated with seasonal allergic rhinitis

Pregnancy Risk Factor B

Dosage Oral: Children ≥12 years and Adults: One capsule every 4-6 hours (maximum: 4 doses/24 hours); treatment for >14 days has not been evaluated

Dosing adjustment in renal impairment: Avoid use in patients with CrCl ≤48 mL/minute.

Dosing adjustment in hepatic impairment: There are no dosage adjustments recommended in manufacturer's labeling.

Additional Information Complete prescribing information should be consulted for additional detail.

Dosage Forms
Capsule:
Semprex®-D: Acrivastine 8 mg and pseudoephedrine 60 mg

◆ **Act [OTC]** *see* Fluoride *on page* 895
◆ **ACT-D** *see* DACTINomycin *on page* 551
◆ **ACT-Amlodipine (Can)** *see* AmLODIPine *on page* 123
◆ **ACT Atorvastatin (Can)** *see* AtorvaSTATin *on page* 194
◆ **ACT-Azithromycin (Can)** *see* Azithromycin (Systemic) *on page* 216
◆ **ACT Bosentan (Can)** *see* Bosentan *on page* 280
◆ **ACT Cabergoline (Can)** *see* Cabergoline *on page* 319

- ◆ **ACT Ciprofloxacin (Can)** *see* Ciprofloxacin (Systemic) *on page 441*
- ◆ **ACT Citalopram (Can)** *see* Citalopram *on page 451*
- ◆ **ACT Diltiazem CD (Can)** *see* Diltiazem *on page 634*
- ◆ **ACT Diltiazem T (Can)** *see* Diltiazem *on page 634*
- ◆ **ACT-Donepezil (Can)** *see* Donepezil *on page 668*
- ◆ **ACT-Donepezil ODT (Can)** *see* Donepezil *on page 668*
- ◆ **ACT-Dutasteride (Can)** *see* Dutasteride *on page 702*
- ◆ **Actemra** *see* Tocilizumab *on page 2057*
- ◆ **ACT-Enalapril (Can)** *see* Enalapril *on page 722*
- ◆ **ACT Etidronate (Can)** *see* Etidronate *on page 813*
- ◆ **ACT Ezetimibe (Can)** *see* Ezetimibe *on page 832*
- ◆ **ACT Fluconazole (Can)** *see* Fluconazole *on page 885*
- ◆ **ACT-Fluvoxamine (Can)** *see* FluvoxaMINE *on page 916*
- ◆ **ActHIB** *see Haemophilus* b Conjugate Vaccine *on page 991*
- ◆ **Acthrel** *see* Corticorelin *on page 509*
- ◆ **Acticin** *see* Permethrin *on page 1627*
- ◆ **Acticlate** *see* Doxycycline *on page 689*
- ◆ **Actidose-Aqua [OTC]** *see* Charcoal, Activated *on page 416*
- ◆ **Actidose/Sorbitol [OTC]** *see* Charcoal, Activated *on page 416*
- ◆ **Actifed® (Can)** *see* Triprolidine and Pseudoephedrine *on page 2105*
- ◆ **Actifed Cold/Allergy [OTC]** *see* Chlorpheniramine and Phenylephrine *on page 426*
- ◆ **Actigall** *see* Ursodiol *on page 2116*
- ◆ **ACT-Imatinib (Can)** *see* Imatinib *on page 1047*
- ◆ **Actimmune** *see* Interferon Gamma-1b *on page 1104*
- ◆ **Actimmune® (Can)** *see* Interferon Gamma-1b *on page 1104*
- ◆ **Actinomycin** *see* DACTINomycin *on page 551*
- ◆ **Actinomycin D** *see* DACTINomycin *on page 551*
- ◆ **Actinomycin CI** *see* DACTINomycin *on page 551*
- ◆ **Actiq** *see* FentaNYL *on page 857*
- ◆ **ACT-Irbesartan (Can)** *see* Irbesartan *on page 1110*
- ◆ **ACT Irbesartan/HCT (Can)** *see* Irbesartan and Hydrochlorothiazide *on page 1112*
- ◆ **Activase** *see* Alteplase *on page 99*
- ◆ **Activase rt-PA (Can)** *see* Alteplase *on page 99*
- ◆ **Activated Carbon** *see* Charcoal, Activated *on page 416*
- ◆ **Activated Charcoal** *see* Charcoal, Activated *on page 416*
- ◆ **Activated Ergosterol** *see* Ergocalciferol *on page 753*
- ◆ **Activated Factor XIII** *see* Factor XIII Concentrate (Human) *on page 843*
- ◆ **Activated PCC** *see* Anti-inhibitor Coagulant Complex (Human) *on page 155*
- ◆ **Active-Cyclobenzaprine** *see* Cyclobenzaprine *on page 516*
- ◆ **Active-Ketoprofen** *see* Ketoprofen *on page 1145*
- ◆ **Activella** *see* Estradiol and Norethindrone *on page 781*
- ◆ **Active-Tramadol** *see* TraMADol *on page 2074*
- ◆ **Act Kids [OTC]** *see* Fluoride *on page 895*
- ◆ **ACT Levetiracetam (Can)** *see* LevETIRAcetam *on page 1191*
- ◆ **ACT Levofloxacin (Can)** *see* Levofloxacin (Systemic) *on page 1197*
- ◆ **ACT Losartan (Can)** *see* Losartan *on page 1248*
- ◆ **ACT Losartan/HCT (Can)** *see* Losartan and Hydrochlorothiazide *on page 1250*
- ◆ **ACT Memantine (Can)** *see* Memantine *on page 1286*
- ◆ **ACT Olanzapine (Can)** *see* OLANZapine *on page 1491*
- ◆ **ACT-Olopatadine (Can)** *see* Olopatadine (Ophthalmic) *on page 1500*
- ◆ **Actonel** *see* Risedronate *on page 1816*
- ◆ **Actonel® (Can)** *see* Risedronate *on page 1816*
- ◆ **Actonel® DR (Can)** *see* Risedronate *on page 1816*
- ◆ **Actoplus Met** *see* Pioglitazone and Metformin *on page 1655*
- ◆ **Actoplus Met XR** *see* Pioglitazone and Metformin *on page 1655*
- ◆ **Actos** *see* Pioglitazone *on page 1654*
- ◆ **ACT Oxycodone CR (Can)** *see* OxyCODONE *on page 1538*
- ◆ **ACT Pantoprazole (Can)** *see* Pantoprazole *on page 1570*
- ◆ **ACT-Pramipexole (Can)** *see* Pramipexole *on page 1695*
- ◆ **ACT Pravastatin (Can)** *see* Pravastatin *on page 1700*
- ◆ **ACT Raloxifene (Can)** *see* Raloxifene *on page 1765*
- ◆ **ACT Ramipril (Can)** *see* Ramipril *on page 1771*
- ◆ **ACT Ranitidine (Can)** *see* Ranitidine *on page 1777*
- ◆ **ACT-Repaglinide (Can)** *see* Repaglinide *on page 1791*
- ◆ **Act Restoring [OTC]** *see* Fluoride *on page 895*
- ◆ **ACT Risperidone (Can)** *see* RisperiDONE *on page 1818*
- ◆ **ACT Rizatriptan (Can)** *see* Rizatriptan *on page 1836*
- ◆ **ACT Rizatriptan ODT (Can)** *see* Rizatriptan *on page 1836*
- ◆ **ACT-Ropinirole (Can)** *see* ROPINIRole *on page 1844*
- ◆ **ACT Sertraline (Can)** *see* Sertraline *on page 1878*
- ◆ **ACT-Sildenafil (Can)** *see* Sildenafil *on page 1882*
- ◆ **ACT-Simvastatin (Can)** *see* Simvastatin *on page 1890*
- ◆ **ACT-Sumatriptan (Can)** *see* SUMAtriptan *on page 1953*
- ◆ **ACT Telmisartan (Can)** *see* Telmisartan *on page 1988*
- ◆ **ACT Telmisartan/HCT (Can)** *see* Telmisartan and Hydrochlorothiazide *on page 1990*
- ◆ **ACT Topiramate (Can)** *see* Topiramate *on page 2065*
- ◆ **Act Total Care [OTC]** *see* Fluoride *on page 895*
- ◆ **ACT Tramadol/Acet (Can)** *see* Acetaminophen and Tramadol *on page 37*
- ◆ **ACT Valsartan (Can)** *see* Valsartan *on page 2127*
- ◆ **ACT Venlafaxine XR (Can)** *see* Venlafaxine *on page 2150*
- ◆ **ACT Zopiclone (Can)** *see* Zopiclone [CAN/INT] *on page 2217*
- ◆ **Acular** *see* Ketorolac (Ophthalmic) *on page 1149*
- ◆ **Acular® (Can)** *see* Ketorolac (Ophthalmic) *on page 1149*
- ◆ **Acular LS** *see* Ketorolac (Ophthalmic) *on page 1149*
- ◆ **Acular LS® (Can)** *see* Ketorolac (Ophthalmic) *on page 1149*
- ◆ **Acuvail** *see* Ketorolac (Ophthalmic) *on page 1149*
- ◆ **ACV** *see* Acyclovir (Systemic) *on page 47*
- ◆ **ACV** *see* Acyclovir (Topical) *on page 51*
- ◆ **Acycloguanosine** *see* Acyclovir (Systemic) *on page 47*
- ◆ **Acycloguanosine** *see* Acyclovir (Topical) *on page 51*

Acyclovir (Systemic) (ay SYE kloe veer)

Brand Names: U.S. Zovirax

Brand Names: Canada Apo-Acyclovir; Mylan-Acyclovir; Nu-Acyclovir; ratio-Acyclovir; Teva-Acyclovir; Zovirax

Index Terms Aciclovir; ACV; Acycloguanosine

Pharmacologic Category Antiviral Agent

Use Treatment of genital herpes simplex virus (HSV) and HSV encephalitis

Pregnancy Risk Factor B

Pregnancy Considerations Teratogenic effects were not observed in animal reproduction studies. Acyclovir has been shown to cross the human placenta (Henderson, 1992). Results from a pregnancy registry, established in 1984 and closed in 1999, did not find an increase in the number of birth defects with exposure to acyclovir when compared to those expected in the general population. However, due to the small size of the registry and lack of long-term data, the manufacturer recommends using during pregnancy with caution and only when clearly needed. Acyclovir may be appropriate for the treatment of genital herpes in pregnant women (CDC, 2010).

Breast-Feeding Considerations Acyclovir is excreted in breast milk. The manufacturer recommends that caution be exercised when administering acyclovir to nursing women. Limited data suggest exposure to the nursing infant of ~0.3 mg/kg/day following oral administration of acyclovir to the mother. Nursing mothers with herpetic lesions near or on the breast should avoid breast-feeding (Gartner, 2005).

Contraindications Hypersensitivity to acyclovir, valacyclovir, or any component of the formulation

Warnings/Precautions Use with caution in immunocompromised patients; thrombocytopenic purpura/hemolytic uremic syndrome (TTP/HUS) has been reported. Use caution in the elderly, preexisting renal disease (may require dosage modification), or in those receiving other nephrotoxic drugs. Renal failure (sometimes fatal) has been reported. Maintain adequate hydration during oral or intravenous therapy. Use IV preparation with caution in patients with underlying neurologic abnormalities, serious hepatic or electrolyte abnormalities, or substantial hypoxia.

Varicella-zoster: Treatment should begin within 24 hours of appearance of rash; oral route not recommended for routine use in otherwise healthy children with varicella, but may be effective in patients at increased risk of moderate-to-severe infection (>12 years of age, chronic cutaneous or pulmonary disorders, long-term salicylate therapy, corticosteroid therapy).

Adverse Reactions

Oral:

Central nervous system: Headache, malaise

Gastrointestinal: Diarrhea, nausea, vomiting

Parenteral:

Dermatologic: Hives, itching, rash

Gastrointestinal: Nausea, vomiting

Hepatic: Liver function tests increased

Local: Inflammation at injection site, phlebitis

Renal: Acute renal failure, BUN increased, creatinine increased

All forms: Rare but important or life-threatening: Abdominal pain, aggression, agitation, anemia, anorexia, ataxia, coma, confusion, consciousness decreased, delirium, desquamation, disseminated intravascular coagulopathy (DIC), dizziness, dysarthria, encephalopathy, fatigue, fever, gastrointestinal distress, hallucinations, hematuria, hemolysis, hepatitis, hyperbilirubinemia, hypotension, insomnia, jaundice, leukocytoclastic vasculitis, leukocytosis, leukopenia, lymphadenopathy, mental depression, myalgia, neutrophilia, pain, psychosis, renal failure, renal pain, seizure, somnolence, sore throat, thrombocytopenia, thrombocytopenic purpura/hemolytic uremic syndrome (TTP/HUS), thrombocytosis, visual disturbances

Drug Interactions

Metabolism/Transport Effects None known.

Avoid Concomitant Use

Avoid concomitant use of Acyclovir (Systemic) with any of the following: Foscarnet; Zoster Vaccine

Increased Effect/Toxicity

Acyclovir (Systemic) may increase the levels/effects of: Mycophenolate; Tenofovir; Zidovudine

The levels/effects of Acyclovir (Systemic) may be increased by: Foscarnet; Mycophenolate

Decreased Effect

Acyclovir (Systemic) may decrease the levels/effects of: Zoster Vaccine

Food Interactions Food does not affect absorption of oral acyclovir.

Preparation for Administration Powder for injection: Reconstitute acyclovir 500 mg powder with SWFI 10 mL; do not use bacteriostatic water containing benzyl alcohol or parabens. For intravenous infusion, dilute in D_5W, D_5NS, $D_5{}^{1/4}NS$, $D_5{}^{1/2}NS$, LR, or NS to a final concentration ≤7 mg/mL. Concentrations >10 mg/mL increase the risk of phlebitis.

Storage/Stability

Capsule, oral suspension, tablet: Store at controlled room temperature of 15°C to 25°C (59°F to 77°F); protect from capsule and tablet from moisture.

Injection: Store powder at controlled room temperature of 15°C to 25°C (59°F to 77°F). Reconstituted solutions remain stable for 12 hours at room temperature. Do not refrigerate reconstituted solutions or solutions diluted for infusion as they may precipitate. Once diluted for infusion, use within 24 hours.

Mechanism of Action Acyclovir is converted to acyclovir monophosphate by virus-specific thymidine kinase then further converted to acyclovir triphosphate by other cellular enzymes. Acyclovir triphosphate inhibits DNA synthesis and viral replication by competing with deoxyguanosine triphosphate for viral DNA polymerase and being incorporated into viral DNA.

Pharmacodynamics/Kinetics

Absorption: Oral: 15% to 30%

Distribution: V_d: 0.8 L/kg (63.6 L): Widely (eg, brain, kidney, lungs, liver, spleen, muscle, uterus, vagina, CSF)

Protein binding: 9% to 33%

Metabolism: Converted by viral enzymes to acyclovir monophosphate, and further converted to diphosphate then triphosphate (active form) by cellular enzymes

Bioavailability: Oral: 10% to 20% with normal renal function (bioavailability decreases with increased dose)

Half-life elimination: Terminal: Neonates: 4 hours; Children 1-12 years: 2-3 hours; Adults: 3 hours

Time to peak, serum: Oral: Within 1.5-2 hours

Excretion: Urine (62% to 90% as unchanged drug and metabolite)

Dosage

Genital herpes simplex virus (HSV) infection:

IV: Children ≥12 years, Adolescents, and Adults: Immunocompetent: Initial episode, severe: 5 mg/kg/dose every 8 hours for 5-7 days **or** 5-10 mg/kg/dose every 8 hours for 2-7 days, follow with oral therapy to complete at least 10 days of therapy (CDC, 2010)

Oral:

Infants and Children <12 years: Immunocompetent (off-label use):

Initial episode: 40-80 mg/kg/day divided into 3-4 doses for 5-10 days (maximum: 1000 mg daily) (*Red Book* [AAP], 2012)

Chronic suppression: 40-80 mg/kg/day in 3 divided doses for ≤12 months (maximum: 1000 mg daily) (*Red Book* [AAP], 2009)

Children ≥12 years and Adolescents: Immunocompetent (off-label use):
Initial episode: 200 mg every 4 hours while awake (5 times daily) **or** 400 mg 3 times daily for 7-10 days; treatment can be extended beyond 10 days if healing is not complete (CDC, 2010; *Red Book* [AAP], 2012)
Chronic suppression: 800 mg daily in 2 divided doses for ≤12 continuous months (*Red Book* [AAP], 2012)
Children: HIV-exposed/-positive (off-label use):
Children <45 kg:
Initial episode: 60 mg/kg/day divided into 3 doses daily for 5-14 days (maximum: 1200 mg daily) (CDC, 2009)
Chronic suppression: 20 mg/kg/dose twice daily (maximum dose: 400 mg) (CDC, 2009)
Children ≥45 kg:
Initial episode: 400 mg twice daily for 5-14 days (CDC, 2009)
Chronic suppression: 20 mg/kg/dose twice daily (maximum dose: 400 mg) (CDC, 2009)
Children <12 years: Recurrent infection: Non-HIV-exposed/-positive: 20-25 mg/kg/dose twice daily; maximum dose: 400 mg (Bradley, 2011)
Children ≥12 years: Recurrent infection:
Non-HIV-exposed/-positive: 200 mg every 4 hours while awake (5 times daily) for 5 days **or** 800 mg twice daily for 5 days **or** 800 mg 3 times daily for 2 days (CDC, 2010; *Red Book* [AAP], 2012)
HIV-exposed/-positive: 400 mg 3 times daily for 5-14 days (DHHS [adult], 2013)
Adolescents: Immunocompromised (off-label use):
Initial episode: 400 mg 3 times daily for 5-14 days (DHHS [adult], 2013)
Chronic suppression: 400 mg twice daily (DHHS [adult], 2013)
Adults: Immunocompetent:
Initial episode: 200 mg 5 times daily while awake for 10 days **or** 400 mg 3 times daily for 7-10 days (CDC, 2010)
Recurrence:
Manufacturer's recommendation: **Note:** begin at earliest signs of disease: 200 mg 5 times daily while awake for 5 days
Alternative recommendation: 400 mg 3 times daily for 5 days **or** 800 mg twice daily for 5 days **or** 800 mg 3 times daily for 2 days (CDC, 2010)
Chronic suppression: 400 mg twice daily or 200 mg 3-5 times daily, for up to 12 months followed by re-evaluation

Herpes zoster (shingles):
IV:
Infants: Immunocompetent (off-label use): 10 mg/kg/dose every 8 hours for 7-10 days (*Red Book* [AAP], 2012)
Children ≥1 year and Adolescents: Immunocompetent (off-label use): 500 mg/m^2/dose every 8 hours for 7-10 days; some experts recommend 10 mg/kg/dose every 8 hours. (*Red Book* [AAP], 2012)
Children <12 years: Immunocompromised (off-label use): 10 mg/kg/dose every 8 hours for 7-10 days (*Red Book* [AAP], 2012)
Children ≥12 years, Adolescents, and Adults: Immunocompromised (off-label use): 10 mg/kg/dose or every 8 hours for 7-10 days (*Red Book* [AAP], 2012)
Oral:
Children ≥12 years and Adolescents: Immunocompetent (off-label use): 800 mg 5 times daily for 5-7 days (*Red Book* [AAP], 2012)
Adults: Immunocompetent: 800 mg 5 times daily for 7-10 days

HSV encephalitis: IV:
Infants and Children 3 months to <12 years:
Immunocompetent:
Manufacturer's recommendation: 20 mg/kg/dose every 8 hours for 10 days. **Note:** Doses ≥20 mg/kg may be associated with a higher incidence of nephrotoxicity (*Red Book* [AAP], 2012)
Alternative recommendation: 10-15 mg/kg/dose every 8 hours for 14 to 21 days (*Red Book* [AAP], 2012)
HIV-exposed/-positive: 10 mg/kg/dose every 8 hours for 21 days; do not discontinue therapy until a repeat HSV DNA PCR assay of the cerebrospinal fluid is negative (CDC, 2009)
Children ≥12 years, Adolescents, and Adults: Independent of HIV status:
*Manufacturer's recommendation:*10 mg/kg/dose every 8 hours for 10 days
Alternative recommendation: 10 mg/kg/dose every 8 hours for 14-21 days (*Red Book* [AAP], 2012)

HSV gingivostomatitis (off-label use): HIV-exposed/-positive:
Mild, symptomatic: Oral: Infants and Children: 20 mg/kg/dose 3 times daily for 5-10 days (maximum dose: 400 mg) (CDC, 2009)
Moderate to severe, symptomatic: IV: Infants and Children: 5-10 mg/kg/dose every 8 hours; **Note:** switch to oral therapy once lesions begin to regress (CDC, 2009)

HSV, herpes labialis (cold sore) recurrent, chronic suppressive therapy (off-label use): Oral: Children: 30 mg/kg/day in 3 divided doses for up to 12 months (maximum: 1000 mg/daily). **Note:** Re-evaluate after 12 months (*Red Book* [AAP], 2012)

Mucocutaneous HSV (off-label dose):
IV:
Children and Adolescents: Immunocompromised: Treatment: 10 mg/kg/dose every 8 hours for 7-14 days (Red Book [AAP], 2012)
Children ≥2 years and Adolescents: Immunocompromised, HSV seropositive: Prophylaxis: 5 mg/kg/dose every 8 hours during the period of risk (maximum daily dose: 80 mg/kg/day) (*Red Book* [AAP], 2009; *Red Book* [AAP], 2012)
Adults (immunocompromised): Treatment: 5-10 mg/kg/dose every 8 hours for 7 days (Leflore, 2000)
Oral:
Children ≥2 years and Adolescents: Immunocompromised: Treatment: 1000 mg daily in 3-5 divided doses for 7-14 days (maximum daily dose: 80 mg/kg/day). (*Red Book* [AAP], 2009; *Red Book* [AAP], 2012)
Children ≥2 years and Adolescents: Immunocompromised, HSV seropositive: Prophylaxis: 600-1000 mg daily in 3-5 divided doses during the period of risk (*Red Book* [AAP], 2012)
Adults (immunocompromised): 400 mg 5 times daily for 7 days (Leflore, 2000)

Neonatal HSV: IV: Infants: Birth to 3 months: Treatment:
Manufacturer's recommendations: 10 mg/kg/dose every 8 hours for 10 days
Alternative recommendations: 20 mg/kg/dose every 8 hours for 14 days (skin and mucous membrane disease) to 21 days (CNS disease) (CDC, 2010; Kimberlin, 2013; *Red Book* [AAP], 2012)

Orolabial HSV (off-label use): Oral: Adults: Immunocompetent:
Treatment (episodic/recurrent): 200-400 mg 5 times daily for 5 days (Cernik, 2008; Leflore, 2000; Spruance, 1990)
Chronic suppression: 400 mg 2 times daily (has been clinically evaluated for up to 1 year) (Cernik, 2008; Rooney, 1993)

Varicella-zoster (chickenpox): Begin treatment within the first 24 hours of rash onset:

Oral: **Note:** The CDC HIV guidelines recommended duration of therapy is 7-10 days or until no new lesions for 48 hours (for patients with mild varicella and no or moderate immune suppression) (CDC, 2009)

Children ≥2 years and ≤40 kg: Immunocompetent: 20 mg/kg/dose (maximum: 800 mg per dose) 4 times daily for 5 days

Children >40 kg and Adults: Immunocompetent: 800 mg 4 times daily for 5 days

IV:

Immunocompetent: Children ≥2 years: 10 mg/kg/dose or 500 mg/m^2/dose every 8 hours for 7-10 days (CDC, 2009)

Immunocompromised:

Manufacturer's labeling:

Children <12 years: 10 mg/kg/dose every 8 hours for 7 days

Children ≥12 years, Adolescents, and Adults: 20 mg/kg/dose every 8 hours for 7 days

Alternative recommendations: HIV-exposed/-positive:

Infants: 10 mg/kg/dose every 8 hours for 7-10 days or until no new lesions for 48 hours (CDC, 2009)

Children ≥1 year: 10 mg/kg/dose or 500 mg/m^2/dose every 8 hours for 7-10 days or until no new lesions for 48 hours (CDC, 2009; *Red Book* [AAP], 2012)

Adolescents and Adults: 10-15 mg/kg/dose every 8 hours for 7-10 days (DHHS [adult], 2013)

Varicella-zoster acute retinal necrosis infection in HIV-exposed/-positive (off-label use): IV: Infants and Children: 10 mg/kg/dose every 8 hours for 10-14 days, followed by oral acyclovir or valacyclovir for 4-6 weeks (CDC, 2009)

Prevention of HSV reactivation in HIV-positive patient (off-label use): Oral:

Children: 20 mg/kg/dose twice daily (maximum: 400 mg per dose) (CDC, 2009)

Adults: 400-800 mg 2-3 times daily (CDC, 2010)

Prevention of HSV reactivation in HSCT (off-label use): **Note:** Start at the beginning of conditioning therapy and continue until engraftment or until mucositis resolves (~30 days) (CDC, 2000)

Oral:

Children: 600-1000 mg daily in 3-5 divided doses

Adolescents and Adults: 200 mg 3 times daily

IV:

Children: 250 mg/m^2/dose every 8 hours or 125 mg/m^2/dose every 6 hours

Adolescents and Adults: 250 mg/m^2/dose every 12 hours

Prevention of VZV reactivation in allogeneic HSCT (off-label use): *NCCN guidelines:* Oral: Adults: 800 mg twice daily

Prevention of CMV reactivation in low-risk allogeneic HSCT (off-label use): *NCCN guidelines:* **Note:** Requires close monitoring (due to weak activity); not for use in patients at high risk for CMV disease: Oral: Adults: 800 mg 4 times daily

Treatment of disseminated HSV or VZV or empiric treatment of suspected encephalitis in immunocompromised patients with cancer (off-label use): *NCCN guidelines:* IV: Adults: 10-12 mg/kg/dose every 8 hours

Treatment of episodic HSV infection in HIV-positive patient (off-label use): Oral: Adults: 400 mg 3 times daily for 5-10 days (CDC, 2010)

Dosage adjustment in renal impairment:

Oral:

CrCl 10-25 mL/minute/1.73 m^2: Normal dosing regimen 800 mg 5 times daily: Administer 800 mg every 8 hours

CrCl <10 mL/minute/1.73 m^2:

Normal dosing regimen 200 mg 5 times daily or 400 mg every 12 hours: Administer 200 mg every 12 hours

Normal dosing regimen 800 mg 5 times daily: Administer 800 mg every 12 hours

IV:

CrCl 25-50 mL/minute/1.73 m^2: Administer recommended dose every 12 hours

CrCl 10-25 mL/minute/1.73 m^2: Administer recommended dose every 24 hours

CrCl <10 mL/minute/1.73 m^2: Administer 50% of recommended dose every 24 hours

Intermittent hemodialysis (IHD) (administer after hemodialysis on dialysis days): Dialyzable (60% reduction following a 6-hour session): IV: 2.5-5 mg/kg every 24 hours (Heintz, 2009). **Note:** Dosing dependent on the assumption of 3 times weekly, complete IHD sessions.

Peritoneal dialysis (PD): Administer 50% of normal dose once daily; no supplemental dose needed

Continuous renal replacement therapy (CRRT) (Heintz, 2009; Trotman, 2005): Drug clearance is highly dependent on the method of renal replacement, filter type, and flow rate. Appropriate dosing requires close monitoring of pharmacologic response, signs of adverse reactions due to drug accumulation, as well as drug concentrations in relation to target trough (if appropriate). The following are general recommendations only (based on dialysate flow/ultrafiltration rates of 1-2 L/hour and minimal residual renal function) and should not supersede clinical judgment:

CVVH: IV: 5-10 mg/kg every 24 hours

CVVHD/CVVHDF: IV: 5-10 mg/kg every 12-24 hours

Note: The higher end of dosage range (eg, 10 mg/kg every 12 hours for CVVHDF) is recommended for viral meningoencephalitis and varicella-zoster virus infections.

Dosage adjustment in hepatic impairment: Oral, IV: There are no dosage adjustments provided in manufacturer's labeling; use caution in patients with severe impairment.

Dosing in obesity: Obese patients should be dosed using ideal body weight

Dietary Considerations May be taken with or without food. Some products may contain sodium.

Administration

Oral: May be administered with or without food.

IV: Avoid rapid infusion; infuse over 1 hour to prevent renal damage; maintain adequate hydration of patient; check for phlebitis and rotate infusion sites. Avoid IM or SubQ administration.

Monitoring Parameters Urinalysis, BUN, serum creatinine, liver enzymes, CBC

Dosage Forms

Capsule, Oral:

Zovirax: 200 mg

Generic: 200 mg

Solution, Intravenous:

Generic: 50 mg/mL (10 mL, 20 mL)

Solution Reconstituted, Intravenous:

Generic: 500 mg (1 ea); 1000 mg (1 ea)

Suspension, Oral:

Zovirax: 200 mg/5 mL (473 mL)

Generic: 200 mg/5 mL (473 mL)

Tablet, Oral:

Zovirax: 400 mg, 800 mg

Generic: 400 mg, 800 mg

Acyclovir (Topical) (ay SYE kloe veer)

Brand Names: U.S. Sitavig; Zovirax
Brand Names: Canada Zovirax
Index Terms Aciclovir; ACV; Acycloguanosine
Pharmacologic Category Antiviral Agent, Topical
Use Herpes virus:
Buccal tablet: Treatment of recurrent herpes labialis (cold sores) in immunocompetent adults.
Cream: Treatment of recurrent herpes labialis (cold sores) in immunocompetent children ≥12 years of age, adolescents, and adults.
Ointment: Management of initial genital herpes and in limited non-life-threatening mucocutaneous herpes simplex virus infections in immunocompromised patients.
Pregnancy Risk Factor B
Dosage
Genital HSV: Adults: Topical ointment: Initial episode: 1/2" ribbon of ointment for a 4" square surface area every 3 hours (6 times daily) for 7 days
Herpes labialis (cold sores):
Children ≥12 years, Adolescents, and Adults: Topical cream: Apply 5 times daily for 4 days
Adults: Buccal tablet: Apply one 50 mg tablet as a single dose to the upper gum region (canine fossa).
Mucocutaneous HSV: Adults (non-life-threatening HSV, immunocompromised): Topical ointment: 1/2" ribbon of ointment for a 4" square surface area every 3 hours (6 times daily) for 7 days

Dosage adjustment in renal impairment: There are no dosage adjustments provided in the manufacturer's labeling. However, dosage adjustment is unlikely due to low systemic absorption.
Dosage adjustment in hepatic impairment: There are no dosage adjustments provided in the manufacturer's labeling. However, dosage adjustment is unlikely due to low systemic absorption.
Additional Information Complete prescribing information should be consulted for additional detail.
Dosage Forms
Cream, External:
Zovirax: 5% (5 g)
Ointment, External:
Zovirax: 5% (30 g)
Generic: 5% (5 g, 15 g, 30 g)
Tablet, Buccal:
Sitavig: 50 mg

- **ACZ885** *see* Canakinumab *on page 335*
- **AD32** *see* Valrubicin *on page 2127*
- **Adacel** *see* Diphtheria and Tetanus Toxoids, and Acellular Pertussis Vaccine *on page 649*
- **Adacel®-Polio (Can)** *see* Diphtheria and Tetanus Toxoids, Acellular Pertussis, and Poliovirus Vaccine *on page 646*
- **Adagen** *see* Pegademase Bovine *on page 1588*
- **Adalat XL (Can)** *see* NIFEdipine *on page 1451*
- **Adalat CC** *see* NIFEdipine *on page 1451*

Adalimumab (a da LIM yoo mab)

Brand Names: U.S. Humira; Humira Pediatric Crohns Start; Humira Pen; Humira Pen-Crohns Starter; Humira Pen-Psoriasis Starter
Brand Names: Canada Humira
Index Terms Antitumor Necrosis Factor Alpha (Human); D2E7; Human Antitumor Necrosis Factor Alpha
Pharmacologic Category Antirheumatic, Disease Modifying; Gastrointestinal Agent, Miscellaneous; Monoclonal Antibody; Tumor Necrosis Factor (TNF) Blocking Agent
Use
Ankylosing spondylitis: Treatment of ankylosing spondylitis (may be used in combination with methotrexate or other nonbiologic disease-modifying antirheumatic drugs (DMARDS) in adult patients
Crohn disease: Treatment of active Crohn disease (moderate to severe) in pediatric (≥6 years of age) and adult patients with inadequate response to conventional treatment, or adult patients who have lost response to or are intolerant of infliximab
Juvenile idiopathic arthritis: Treatment of active polyarticular juvenile idiopathic arthritis (moderate to severe) in patients ≥2 years of age; may be used alone or in combination with methotrexate
Plaque psoriasis: Treatment of chronic plaque psoriasis (moderate to severe) in adult patients when systemic therapy is required and other agents are less appropriate
Psoriatic arthritis: Treatment of active psoriatic arthritis in adult patients; may be used alone or in combination with methotrexate or other DMARDs
Rheumatoid arthritis: Treatment of active rheumatoid arthritis (moderate to severe) in adult patients; may be used alone or in combination with methotrexate or other DMARDs
Ulcerative colitis: Treatment of active ulcerative colitis (moderate to severe) in adult patients unresponsive to immunosuppressants (**Note**: Efficacy in patients that are intolerant to or no longer responsive to other TNF blockers has not been established.)
Pregnancy Risk Factor B
Pregnancy Considerations Adverse events were not observed in animal reproduction studies. Adalimumab crosses the placenta and can be detected in cord blood at birth at concentrations higher than those in the maternal serum. In one study of pregnant women with inflammatory bowel disease, adalimumab was found to be measurable in a newborn for up to 11 weeks following delivery. Maternal doses of adalimumab were 40 mg every other week (n=9) or 40 mg weekly (n=1) and the last dose was administered 0.14-8 weeks prior to delivery (median 5.5 weeks) (Mahadevan, 2013). If therapy for inflammatory bowel disease is needed during pregnancy, adalimumab should be discontinued before 30 weeks gestation in order to decrease exposure to the newborn. In addition, the administration of live vaccines should be postponed until anti-TNF concentrations in the infant are negative (Habal, 2012; Mahadeven, 2013; Zelinkova, 2013).

Women exposed to adalimumab during pregnancy for the treatment of an autoimmune disease (eg, inflammatory bowel disease) may contact the OTIS Autoimmune Diseases Study at 877-311-8972.
Breast-Feeding Considerations Low concentrations of adalimumab may be detected in breast milk but are unlikely to be absorbed by a nursing infant. The manufacturer recommends caution be used if administered to a nursing woman.
Contraindications
There are no contraindications listed within the manufacturer's labeling.
Canadian labeling: Hypersensitivity to adalimumab or any component of the formulation; severe infection (eg, sepsis, tuberculosis, opportunistic infection); moderate-to-severe heart failure (NYHA class III/IV)
Warnings/Precautions [U.S. Boxed Warnings]: Patients should be evaluated for latent tuberculosis infection with a tuberculin skin test prior to therapy. Treatment of latent tuberculosis should be initiated before adalimumab is used. Tuberculosis (disseminated or extrapulmonary) has been reactivated while

on adalimumab. Most cases have been reported within the first 8 months of treatment. **Patients with initial negative tuberculin skin tests should receive continued monitoring for tuberculosis throughout treatment; active tuberculosis has developed in this population during treatment.** Rare reactivation of hepatitis B virus (HBV) has occurred in chronic virus carriers; use with caution; evaluate prior to initiation and during treatment.

[U.S. Boxed Warning]: Patients receiving adalimumab are at increased risk for serious infections which may result in hospitalization and/or fatality; infections usually developed in patients receiving concomitant immunosuppressive agents (eg, methotrexate or corticosteroids) and may present as disseminated (rather than local) disease. Active tuberculosis (or reactivation of latent tuberculosis), invasive fungal (including aspergillosis, blastomycosis, candidiasis, coccidioidomycosis, histoplasmosis, and pneumocystosis) and bacterial, viral or other opportunistic infections (including legionellosis and listeriosis) have been reported in patients receiving TNF-blocking agents, including adalimumab. Monitor closely for signs/symptoms of infection. Discontinue for serious infection or sepsis. Consider risks versus benefits prior to use in patients with a history of chronic or recurrent infection. Consider empiric antifungal therapy in patients who are at risk for invasive fungal infection and develop severe systemic illness. Caution should be exercised when considering use in the elderly or in patients with conditions that predispose them to infections (eg, diabetes) or residence/travel from areas of endemic mycoses (blastomycosis, coccidioidomycosis, histoplasmosis), or with latent or localized infections. Do not initiate adalimumab therapy with clinically important active infection. Patients who develop a new infection while undergoing treatment should be monitored closely. There is limited experience with patients undergoing surgical procedures while on therapy; consider long half-life with planned procedures and monitor closely for infection.

[U.S. Boxed Warning]: Lymphoma and other malignancies (some fatal) have been reported in children and adolescent patients receiving TNF-blocking agents, including adalimumab. Half the cases are lymphomas (Hodgkin and non-Hodgkin) and the other cases are varied, but include malignancies not typically observed in this population. Most patients were receiving concomitant immunosuppressants. **[U.S. Boxed Warning]: Hepatosplenic T-cell lymphoma (HSTCL), a rare T-cell lymphoma, has also been reported primarily in patients with Crohn disease or ulcerative colitis treated with adalimumab and who received concomitant azathioprine or mercaptopurine; reports occurred predominantly in adolescent and young adult males.** Rare cases of lymphoma have also been reported in association with adalimumab. A higher incidence of nonmelanoma skin cancers was noted in adalimumab treated patients, when compared to the control group. Impact on the development and course of malignancies is not fully defined. May exacerbate preexisting or recent-onset central or peripheral nervous system demyelinating disorders. Consider discontinuing use in patients who develop peripheral or central nervous system demyelinating disorders during treatment.

May exacerbate preexisting or recent-onset demyelinating CNS disorders. Worsening and new-onset heart failure (HF) has been reported; use caution in patients with decreased left ventricular function. Use caution in patients with HF (Canadian labeling contraindicates use in NYHA III/IV). Patients should be brought up to date with all immunizations before initiating therapy. No data are available concerning the effects of adalimumab on vaccination. Live vaccines should not be given concurrently. No data are available concerning secondary transmission of live vaccines in patients receiving adalimumab. Rare cases of pancytopenia (including aplastic anemia) have been reported with TNF-blocking agents; with significant hematologic abnormalities, consider discontinuing therapy. Positive antinuclear antibody titers have been detected in patients (with negative baselines) treated with adalimumab. Rare cases of autoimmune disorder, including lupus-like syndrome, have been reported; monitor and discontinue adalimumab if symptoms develop. May cause hypersensitivity reactions, including anaphylaxis; monitor. Infection and malignancy has been reported at a higher incidence in elderly patients compared to younger adults; use caution in elderly patients. Potentially significant drug-drug interactions may exist, requiring dose or frequency adjustment, additional monitoring, and/or selection of alternative therapy. The packaging (needle cover of prefilled syringe) may contain latex. Product may contain polysorbate 80. According to the Centers for Disease Control and Prevention (CDC), pen-shaped injection devices should never be used for more than one person (even when the needle is changed) because of the risk of infection. The injection device should be clearly labeled with individual patient information to ensure that the correct pen is used (CDC, 2012).

Adverse Reactions

Cardiovascular: Atrial fibrillation, cardiac arrest, cardiac arrhythmia, cardiac failure, chest pain, coronary artery disease, deep vein thrombosis, hypertension, hypertensive encephalopathy, myocardial infarction, palpitations, pericardial effusion, pericarditis, peripheral edema, subdural hematoma, syncope, tachycardia, vascular disease

Central nervous system: Confusion, headache, myasthenia, paresthesia

Dermatologic: Alopecia, cellulitis, erysipelas, skin rash

Endocrine & metabolic: Dehydration, hypercholesterolemia, hyperlipidemia, ketosis, menstrual disease, parathyroid disease

Gastrointestinal: Abdominal pain, diverticulitis, esophagitis, gastroenteritis, gastrointestinal hemorrhage, nausea, vomiting

Genitourinary: Cholecystitis, cholelithiasis, cystitis, hematuria, pelvic pain, urinary tract infection

Hematologic & oncologic: Adenoma, agranulocytosis, carcinoma (including breast, gastrointestinal, skin, urogenital), granulocytopenia, leukopenia, malignant lymphoma, malignant melanoma, pancytopenia, paraproteinemia, polycythemia, positive ANA titer

Hepatic: Hepatic necrosis, increased serum alkaline phosphatase

Hypersensitivity: Hypersensitivity reaction (more common in children)

Immunologic: Antibody development (significance unknown)

Infection: Herpes zoster, sepsis, serious infection (more common in adults [Burmester, 2012])

Local: Injection site reaction

Neuromuscular & skeletal: Arthralgia, arthritis, arthropathy, back pain, bone fracture, increased creatine phosphokinase, limb pain, multiple sclerosis, muscle cramps, myasthenia, osteonecrosis, septic arthritis, synovitis, systemic lupus erythematosus, tendon disease, tremor

Ophthalmic: Cataract

Renal: Nephrolithiasis, pyelonephritis

Respiratory: Asthma, bronchospasm, dyspnea, flu-like symptoms, pleural effusion, pneumonia, respiratory depression, sinusitis, tuberculosis (including reactivation of latent infection; disseminated, miliary, lymphatic, peritoneal and pulmonary); upper respiratory tract infection

Miscellaneous: Abnormal healing, accidental injury, fever, postoperative complication (infection)

Rare but important or life-threatening: Abscess (limb, perianal), anal fissure, anaphylactoid reaction, anaphylaxis, angioedema, aplastic anemia, appendicitis, bacterial infection, basal cell carcinoma, cerebrovascular accident, cervical dysplasia, circulatory shock, cytopenia, dermal ulcer, endometrial hyperplasia, erythema multiforme, fixed drug eruption, fulminant necrotizing fasciitis, fungal infection, Guillain-Barre syndrome, hepatic failure, hepatitis B (reactivation), hepatosplenic T-cell lymphomas (children, adolescents, and young adults), herpes simplex infection, histoplasmosis, hypersensitivity angiitis, increased serum transaminases, interstitial pulmonary disease (eg, pulmonary fibrosis), intestinal obstruction, intestinal perforation, leukemia, liver metastases, lupus-like syndrome, lymphadenopathy, lymphocytosis, malignant neoplasm of ovary, meningitis (viral), Merkel cell carcinoma, mycobacterium avium complex, myositis (children and adolescents), neutropenia, optic neuritis, pancreatitis, pharyngitis (children and adolescents), protozoal infection, psoriasis (including new onset, palmoplantar, pustular, or exacerbation), pulmonary embolism, respiratory failure, sarcoidosis, septic shock, skin granuloma (annulare; children and adolescents), Stevens-Johnson syndrome, streptococcal pharyngitis (children and adolescents), testicular neoplasm, thrombocytopenia, vasculitis (systemic), viral infection

Drug Interactions

Metabolism/Transport Effects None known.

Avoid Concomitant Use

Avoid concomitant use of Adalimumab with any of the following: Abatacept; Anakinra; BCG; Belimumab; Canakinumab; Certolizumab Pegol; InFLIXimab; Natalizumab; Pimecrolimus; Rilonacept; Tacrolimus (Topical); Tocilizumab; Tofacitinib; Vaccines (Live); Vedolizumab

Increased Effect/Toxicity

Adalimumab may increase the levels/effects of: Abatacept; Anakinra; Belimumab; Canakinumab; Certolizumab Pegol; InFLIXimab; Leflunomide; Natalizumab; Rilonacept; Tofacitinib; Vaccines (Live); Vedolizumab

The levels/effects of Adalimumab may be increased by: Denosumab; Pimecrolimus; Roflumilast; Tacrolimus (Topical); Tocilizumab; Trastuzumab

Decreased Effect

Adalimumab may decrease the levels/effects of: BCG; Coccidioides immitis Skin Test; CycloSPORINE (Systemic); Sipuleucel-T; Theophylline Derivatives; Vaccines (Inactivated); Vaccines (Live); Warfarin

The levels/effects of Adalimumab may be decreased by: Echinacea

Storage/Stability Store under refrigeration at 2°C to 8°C (36°F to 46°F) in original container; do not freeze. Do not use if frozen even if it has been thawed. Protect from light. May be stored at room temperature up to a maximum of 25°C (77°F) for up to 14 days; discard if not used within 14 days.

Mechanism of Action Adalimumab is a recombinant monoclonal antibody that binds to human tumor necrosis factor alpha (TNF-alpha), thereby interfering with binding to TNFα receptor sites and subsequent cytokine-driven inflammatory processes. Elevated TNF levels in the synovial fluid are involved in the pathologic pain and joint destruction in immune-mediated arthritis. Adalimumab decreases signs and symptoms of psoriatic arthritis, rheumatoid arthritis, and ankylosing spondylitis. It inhibits progression of structural damage of rheumatoid and psoriatic arthritis. Reduces signs and symptoms and maintains clinical remission in Crohn disease and ulcerative colitis; reduces epidermal thickness and inflammatory cell infiltration in plaque psoriasis.

Pharmacodynamics/Kinetics

Distribution: V_d: 4.7-6 L; Synovial fluid concentrations: 31% to 96% of serum

Bioavailability: Absolute: 64%

Half-life elimination: Terminal: ~2 weeks (range: 10-20 days)

Time to peak, serum: SubQ: 131 ± 56 hours

Excretion: Clearance increased in the presence of anti-adalimumab antibodies; decreased in patients ≥40 years of age

Dosage SubQ:

Children ≥2 years and Adolescents: Juvenile idiopathic arthritis (JIA):

U.S. labeling:

10 kg to <15 kg: 10 mg every other week

15 kg to <30 kg: 20 mg every other week

≥30 kg: 40 mg every other week

Children ≥4 years and Adolescents: Juvenile idiopathic arthritis (JIA):

Canadian labeling: 24 mg/m^2 (maximum dose: 40 mg) every other week

Children ≥6 years: Crohn disease:

U.S. labeling:

17 kg to <40 kg:

Initial: 80 mg (administered as 2 injections on day 1), then 40 mg 2 weeks later (day 15). **Note:** 40 mg per injection.

Maintenance: 20 mg every other week beginning week 4 (day 29).

≥40 kg:

Initial: 160 mg (administered as 4 injections on day 1 or as 2 injections daily over 2 consecutive days), then 80 mg 2 weeks later (day 15; given as 2 injections on the same day). **Note:** 40 mg per injection.

Maintenance: 40 mg every other week beginning week 4 (day 29).

Adolescents ≥13 years and ≥40 kg: Crohn disease:

Canadian labeling:

Initial: 160 mg (given as 4 injections on day 1 **or** given as 2 injections daily over 2 consecutive days), then 80 mg 2 weeks later (day 15; given as 2 injections on the same day). **Note:** 40 mg per injection.

Maintenance: 20 mg every other week beginning week 4 (day 29); may consider increasing dose to 40 mg every other week for disease flare or inadequate response. Potential benefits of continued therapy should be reassessed if inadequate response at 12 weeks.

Adults:

Ankylosing spondylitis: 40 mg every other week

Crohn disease:

Initial: 160 mg (given as 4 injections on day 1 **or** given as 2 injections daily over 2 consecutive days), then 80 mg 2 weeks later (day 15). **Note:** 40 mg per injection.

Maintenance: 40 mg every other week beginning day 29. **Note:** Some patients may require 40 mg every week as maintenance therapy (Lichtenstein, 2009).

Plaque psoriasis:

Initial: 80 mg as a single dose

Maintenance: 40 mg every other week beginning 1 week after initial dose

Psoriatic arthritis: 40 mg every other week

Rheumatoid arthritis: 40 mg every other week; patients not taking methotrexate may increase dose to 40 mg every week

Ulcerative colitis:

Initial: 160 mg (given as 4 injections on day 1 **or** given as 2 injections daily over 2 consecutive days), then 80 mg 2 weeks later (day 15). **Note:** 40 mg per injection.

Maintenance: 40 mg every other week beginning day 29. **Note:** Only continue maintenance dose in patients demonstrating clinical remission by 8 weeks (day 57) of therapy.

Dosage adjustment in renal impairment: There are no dosage adjustments provided in the manufacturer's labeling (has not been studied).

Dosage adjustment in hepatic impairment: There are no dosage adjustments provided in the manufacturer's labeling (has not been studied).

Administration For SubQ injection at separate sites in the thigh or lower abdomen (avoiding areas within 2 inches of navel); rotate injection sites. May leave at room temperature for ~15 to 30 minutes prior to use; do not remove cap or cover while allowing product to reach room temperature. Do not use if solution is discolored or contains particulate matter. Do not administer to skin which is red, tender, bruised, or hard. Needle cap of the prefilled syringe may contain latex. Prefilled pens and syringes are available for use by patients and the full amount of the syringe should be injected (self-administration); the vial is intended for institutional use only. Vials do not contain a preservative; discard unused portion.

Monitoring Parameters Monitor improvement of symptoms and physical function assessments. Latent TB screening prior to initiating and during therapy; signs/symptoms of infection (prior to, during, and following therapy); CBC with differential; signs/symptoms/worsening of heart failure; HBV screening prior to initiating (all patients), HBV carriers (during and for several months following therapy); signs and symptoms of hypersensitivity reaction; symptoms of lupus-like syndrome; signs/symptoms of malignancy (eg, splenomegaly, hepatomegaly, abdominal pain, persistent fever, night sweats, weight loss), including periodic skin examination.

Dosage Forms

Kit, Subcutaneous [preservative free]:
Humira: 20 mg/0.4 mL, 40 mg/0.8 mL
Humira Pediatric Crohns Start: 40 mg/0.8 mL
Humira Pen: 40 mg/0.8 mL
Humira Pen-Crohns Starter: 40 mg/0.8 mL
Humira Pen-Psoriasis Starter: 40 mg/0.8 mL

Prefilled Syringe Kit, Subcutaneous [preservative free]:
Humira: 10 mg/0.2 mL (1 ea)

Dosage Forms: Canada

Injection, solution [pediatric, preservative free]:
Humira®: 40 mg/0.8 mL (0.8 mL)

◆ **Adamantanamine Hydrochloride** *see* Amantadine *on page 105*

Adapalene (a DAP a leen)

Brand Names: U.S. Differin
Brand Names: Canada Differin®; Differin® XP
Pharmacologic Category Acne Products; Topical Skin Product, Acne
Use Acne vulgaris: Treatment of acne vulgaris.
Pregnancy Risk Factor C
Dosage Acne vulgaris: Children ≥12 years, Adolescents, and Adults: Topical: Apply once daily; use cream and gel in the evening before bedtime

Dosage adjustment in renal impairment: There are no dosage adjustments provided in manufacturer's labeling; however, systemic absorption is not extensive, making the need for a dose adjustment unlikely.

Dosage adjustment in hepatic impairment: There are no dosage adjustments provided in manufacturer's labeling; however, systemic absorption is not extensive, making the need for a dose adjustment unlikely.

Additional Information Complete prescribing information should be consulted for additional detail.

Dosage Forms

Cream, External:
Differin: 0.1% (45 g)
Generic: 0.1% (45 g)

Gel, External:
Differin: 0.1% (45 g); 0.3% (45 g)
Generic: 0.1% (45 g); 0.3% (45 g)

Lotion, External:
Differin: 0.1% (59 mL)

Adapalene and Benzoyl Peroxide
(a DAP a leen & BEN zoe il peer OKS ide)

Brand Names: U.S. Epiduo®
Brand Names: Canada Tactuo™
Index Terms Benzoyl Peroxide and Adapalene
Pharmacologic Category Acne Products; Topical Skin Product; Topical Skin Product, Acne
Use Topical treatment of acne vulgaris
Pregnancy Risk Factor C
Dosage Topical: Children ≥9 years, Adolescents, and Adults: Apply once daily to affected areas after skin has been cleaned and dried
Additional Information Complete prescribing information should be consulted for additional detail.

Dosage Forms

Gel, topical:
Epiduo®: Adapalene 0.1% and benzoyl peroxide 2.5% (45 g)

◆ **Adasuve** *see* Loxapine *on page 1255*
◆ **Adcetris** *see* Brentuximab Vedotin *on page 286*
◆ **Adcirca** *see* Tadalafil *on page 1968*
◆ **ADD 234037** *see* Lacosamide *on page 1154*
◆ **Addaprin [OTC]** *see* Ibuprofen *on page 1032*
◆ **Adderall** *see* Dextroamphetamine and Amphetamine *on page 609*
◆ **Adderall XR** *see* Dextroamphetamine and Amphetamine *on page 609*

Adefovir (a DEF o veer)

Brand Names: U.S. Hepsera
Brand Names: Canada Hepsera
Index Terms Adefovir Dipivoxil; Bis-POM PMEA
Pharmacologic Category Antihepadnaviral, Reverse Transcriptase Inhibitor, Nucleotide (Anti-HBV)
Use Treatment of chronic hepatitis B with evidence of active viral replication (based on persistent elevation of ALT/AST or histologic evidence), including patients with lamivudine-resistant hepatitis B
Pregnancy Risk Factor C
Pregnancy Considerations Adverse events were observed in some animal reproduction studies. Pregnant women exposed to adefovir should be registered with the pregnancy registry (800-258-4263).
Breast-Feeding Considerations It is not known if adefovir is excreted in breast milk. Due to the potential for serious adverse reactions in the nursing infant, a decision should be made whether to discontinue nursing or to discontinue the drug, taking into account the importance of treatment to the mother.
Contraindications Hypersensitivity to adefovir or any component of the formulation
Warnings/Precautions [U.S. Boxed Warning]: Use with caution in patients with renal dysfunction or in patients at risk of renal toxicity (including concurrent nephrotoxic agents or NSAIDs). Chronic administration may result in nephrotoxicity. Dosage adjustment is required in adult patients with renal dysfunction or in patients who develop renal dysfunction during therapy; no data available for use in children ≥12 years or adolescents with renal impairment. Not recommended as first line therapy of chronic HBV due to weak antiviral activity and

high rate of resistance after first year. May be more appropriate as second-line agent in treatment-naïve patients. Combination therapy with lamivudine in nucleoside-naïve patients has not been shown to provide synergistic antiviral effects. In patients with lamivudine-resistant HBV, switching to adefovir monotherapy was associated with a higher risk of adefovir resistance compared to adding adefovir to lamivudine therapy (Lok, 2009).

Calculate creatinine clearance before initiation of therapy. Consider alternative therapy in patients who do not respond to adefovir monotherapy treatment. **[U.S. Boxed Warning]: May cause the development of HIV resistance in patients with unrecognized or untreated HIV infection.** Determine HIV status prior to initiating treatment with adefovir. **[U.S. Boxed Warning]: Fatal cases of lactic acidosis and severe hepatomegaly with steatosis have been reported with the use of nucleoside analogues alone or in combination with other antiretrovirals.** Female gender, obesity, and prolonged treatment may increase the risk of hepatotoxicity. Treatment should be discontinued in patients with lactic acidosis or signs/symptoms of hepatotoxicity (which may occur without marked transaminase elevations). **[U.S. Boxed Warning]: Acute exacerbations of hepatitis may occur (in up to 25% of patients) when antihepatitis therapy is discontinued.** Exacerbations typically occur within 12 weeks and may be self-limited or resolve upon resuming treatment; risk may be increased with advanced liver disease or cirrhosis. Monitor patients following discontinuation of therapy. Ethanol should be avoided in hepatitis B infection due to potential hepatic toxicity. Do not use concurrently with tenofovir (Viread®) or any product containing tenofovir (eg, Truvada®, Atripla®, Complera®).

Adverse Reactions

Central nervous system: Headache
Dermatologic: Pruritus, rash
Endocrine & metabolic: Hypophosphatemia
Gastrointestinal: Abdominal pain, diarrhea, dyspepsia, flatulence, nausea, vomiting
Hepatic: Hepatitis exacerbation
Neuromuscular & skeletal: Back pain, weakness
Renal: Hematuria, renal failure, serum creatinine increased
Respiratory: Cough, rhinitis
Postmarketing and/or case reports: Fanconi syndrome, hepatitis, myopathy, nephrotoxicity, osteomalacia, pancreatitis, proximal renal tubulopathy

Drug Interactions

Metabolism/Transport Effects None known.

Avoid Concomitant Use

Avoid concomitant use of Adefovir with any of the following: Tenofovir

Increased Effect/Toxicity

Adefovir may increase the levels/effects of: Tenofovir

The levels/effects of Adefovir may be increased by: Ganciclovir-Valganciclovir; Ribavirin; Tenofovir

Decreased Effect

Adefovir may decrease the levels/effects of: Tenofovir

Food Interactions Food does not have a significant effect on adefovir absorption. Management: Administer without regard to meals.

Storage/Stability Store controlled room temperature of 25°C (77°F); excursions permitted between 15°C to 30°C (59°F to 86°F).

Mechanism of Action Acyclic nucleotide reverse transcriptase inhibitor (adenosine analog) which interferes with HBV viral RNA-dependent DNA polymerase resulting in inhibition of viral replication.

Pharmacodynamics/Kinetics

Distribution: 0.35-0.39 L/kg
Protein binding: ≤4%
Metabolism: Prodrug; rapidly converted to adefovir (active metabolite) in intestine
Bioavailability: 59%
Half-life elimination: 7.5 hours
Time to peak: 1.75 hours
Excretion: Urine (45% as active metabolite within 24 hours)

Dosage Oral: Children ≥12 years and Adults: 10 mg once daily

Treatment duration (AASLD practice guidelines): Adults:

Hepatitis Be antigen (HBeAg) positive chronic hepatitis: Treat ≥1 year until HBeAg seroconversion and undetectable serum HBV DNA; continue therapy for ≥6 months after HBeAg seroconversion

HBeAg negative chronic hepatitis: Treat >1 year until hepatitis B surface antigen (HBsAg) clearance

Note: Patients not achieving a <2 log decrease in serum HBV DNA after at least 6 months of therapy should either receive additional treatment or be switched to an alternative therapy (Lok, 2009).

Dosage adjustment in renal impairment: Adult recommendations only (no dosage adjustment recommendations available for patients <18 years with renal impairment):

CrCl ≥50 mL/minute: No dosage adjustment necessary
CrCl 20-49 mL/minute: 10 mg every 48 hours
CrCl 10-19 mL/minute: 10 mg every 72 hours

Hemodialysis: 10 mg every 7 days (following dialysis)

Dosage adjustment in hepatic impairment: No adjustment required

Dietary Considerations May be taken without regard to food.

Administration May be administered without regard to food.

Monitoring Parameters HIV status (prior to initiation of therapy); serum creatinine (prior to initiation and during therapy; every 3 months in patients with medical conditions which predispose to renal insufficiency and in all patients treated for >1 year; more frequent monitoring required if preexisting real insufficiency detected [Lok, 2009]); LFTs for several months following discontinuation of adefovir; HBV DNA (every 3-6 months during therapy); HBeAg and anti-HBe

Additional Information Adefovir dipivoxil is a prodrug, rapidly converted to the active component (adefovir). It was previously investigated as a treatment for HIV infections (at dosages substantially higher than the approved dose for hepatitis B). The NDA was withdrawn, and no further studies in the treatment of HIV are anticipated (per manufacturer).

Dosage Forms

Tablet, Oral:

Hepsera: 10 mg
Generic: 10 mg

◆ **Adefovir Dipivoxil** *see* Adefovir *on page 54*
◆ **Adempas** *see* Riociguat *on page 1814*
◆ **Adempas** *see* Riociguat *on page 1814*
◆ **Adenocard** *see* Adenosine *on page 55*
◆ **Adenoscan** *see* Adenosine *on page 55*

Adenosine (a DEN oh seen)

Brand Names: U.S. Adenocard; Adenoscan

Brand Names: Canada Adenocard; Adenosine Injection, USP; PMS-Adenosine

Index Terms 9-Beta-D-Ribofuranosyladenine

Pharmacologic Category Antiarrhythmic Agent, Miscellaneous; Diagnostic Agent

Use

Adenocard: Treatment of paroxysmal supraventricular tachycardia (PSVT) including that associated with accessory bypass tracts (Wolff-Parkinson-White syndrome); when clinically advisable, appropriate vagal maneuvers should be attempted prior to adenosine administration; **not effective for conversion of atrial fibrillation, atrial flutter, or ventricular tachycardia**

Note: While adenosine will not convert atrial fibrillation or atrial flutter, the transient AV-nodal block may aid in the identification of the arrhythmia by exposing the underlying atrial fibrillation or flutter electrocardiographic morphology.

Adenoscan: Pharmacologic stress agent used in myocardial perfusion thallium-201 scintigraphy

Pregnancy Risk Factor C

Pregnancy Considerations Animal reproduction studies have not been conducted. Adenosine is an endogenous substance and adverse fetal effects would not be anticipated. Case reports of administration during pregnancy have indicated no adverse effects on fetus or newborn attributable to adenosine (Blomström-Lundqvist, 2003). ACLS guidelines suggest use is safe and effective in pregnancy (ACLS [Neumar, 2010]).

Breast-Feeding Considerations Adenosine is endogenous in breast milk (Sugawara, 1995). Due to the potential for adverse reactions in the nursing infant, the manufacturer recommends a decision be made to interrupt nursing or not administer adenosine taking into account the importance of treatment to the mother.

Contraindications Hypersensitivity to adenosine or any component of the formulation; second- or third-degree AV block, sick sinus syndrome, or symptomatic bradycardia (except in patients with a functioning artificial pacemaker); known or suspected bronchoconstrictive or bronchospastic lung disease (Adenoscan), asthma (ACLS [Neumar, 2010]; Adenoscan prescribing information, 2014)

Warnings/Precautions ECG monitoring required during use. Equipment for resuscitation and trained personnel experienced in handling medical emergencies should always be immediately available. Adenosine decreases conduction through the AV node and may produce first-, second-, or third-degree heart block. Patients with preexisting S-A nodal dysfunction may experience prolonged sinus pauses after adenosine; use caution in patients with first-degree AV block or bundle branch block. Use is contraindicated in patients with high-grade AV block, sinus node dysfunction or symptomatic bradycardia (unless a functional artificial pacemaker is in place). Rare, prolonged episodes of asystole have been reported, with fatal outcomes in some cases. Discontinue adenosine in any patient who develops persistent or symptomatic high-grade AV block. Use caution in patients receiving other drugs which slow AV node conduction (eg, digoxin, verapamil). Potentially significant interactions may exist, requiring dose or frequency adjustment, additional monitoring, and/or selection of alternative therapy.

There have been reports of atrial fibrillation/flutter after adenosine administration in patients with PSVT associated with accessory conduction pathways; has also been reported in patients with or without a history of atrial fibrillation undergoing myocardial perfusion imaging with adenosine infusion. Adenosine may also produce profound vasodilation with subsequent hypotension. When used as a bolus dose (PSVT), effects are generally self-limiting (due to the short half-life of adenosine). However, when used as a continuous infusion (pharmacologic stress testing), effects may be more pronounced and persistent, corresponding to continued exposure; discontinue infusion in patients who develop persistent or symptomatic hypotension. Adenosine infusions should be used with caution in patients with autonomic dysfunction, stenotic valvular heart disease, pericarditis, pleural effusion, carotid stenosis (with cerebrovascular insufficiency), or uncorrected hypovolemia. Use caution in elderly patients; may be at increased risk of hemodynamic effects, bradycardia, and/or AV block.

Avoid use in patients with bronchoconstriction or bronchospasm (eg, asthma); dyspnea, bronchoconstriction, and respiratory compromise have occurred during use. Per the ACLS guidelines and the manufacturer of Adenoscan, use considered contraindicated in patients with asthma. Use caution in patients with obstructive lung disease not associated with bronchoconstriction (eg, emphysema, bronchitis). Immediately discontinue therapy if severe respiratory difficulty is observed. Appropriate measures for resuscitation should be available during use.

Adenocard: Transient AV block is expected. Administer as a rapid bolus, either directly into a vein or (if administered into an IV line), as close to the patient as possible (followed by saline flush). Dose reduction recommended when administered via central line (ACLS, 2010). When used in PSVT, at the time of conversion to normal sinus rhythm, a variety of new rhythms may appear on the ECG. Watch for proarrhythmic effects (eg, polymorphic ventricular tachycardia) during and shortly after administration/termination of arrhythmia. Benign transient occurrence of atrial and ventricular ectopy is common upon termination of arrhythmia. Adenosine does not convert atrial fibrillation/flutter to normal sinus rhythm; however, may be used diagnostically in these settings if the underlying rhythm is not apparent. Adenosine should not be used in patients with Wolff-Parkinson-White (WPW) syndrome and preexcited atrial fibrillation/flutter since ventricular fibrillation may result (AHA/ACC/HRS [January, 2014]). Use with extreme caution in heart transplant recipients; adenosine may cause prolonged asystole; reduction of initial adenosine dose is recommended (ACLS, 2010); considered by some to be contraindicated in this setting (Delacrétaz, 2006). Avoid use in irregular or polymorphic wide-complex tachycardias; may cause degeneration to ventricular fibrillation (ACLS, 2010). When used for PSVT, dosage reduction recommended when used with concomitant drugs which potentiate the effects of adenosine (carbamazepine, dipyridamole)

Adenoscan: Hypersensitivity reactions (including dyspnea, pharyngeal edema, erythema, flushing, rash, or chest discomfort) have been reported following Adenoscan administration. Seizures (new-onset or recurrent) have been reported following Adenoscan administration; risk may be increased with concurrent use of aminophylline. Use of any methylxanthine (eg, aminophylline, caffeine, theophylline) is not recommended in patients experiencing seizures associated with Adenoscan administration. Drugs which antagonize adenosine (theophylline [includes aminophylline], caffeine) should be withheld for five half-lives prior to adenosine use. Avoid dietary caffeine for at least 12 hours prior to pharmacologic stress testing (Henzlova, 2006). Withhold dipyridamole-containing medications for at least 24 hours prior to pharmacologic stress testing (Henzlova, 2006).

Cardiovascular events: Cardiac arrest (fatal and nonfatal), myocardial infarction (MI), cerebrovascular accident (hemorrhagic and ischemic), and sustained ventricular tachycardia (requiring resuscitation) have occurred following Adenoscan use. Avoid use in patients with signs or symptoms of unstable angina, acute myocardial ischemia, or cardiovascular instability due to possible increased risk of significant cardiovascular consequences. Appropriate measures for resuscitation should be available during use. In addition, systolic and diastolic pressure increases have been observed with Adenoscan infusion. In most instances, blood pressure increases resolved spontaneously within several minutes; occasionally, hypertension lasted for several hours.

Pulmonary artery hypertension: Acute vasodilator testing (not an approved use): Use with extreme caution in patients with concomitant heart failure (LV systolic dysfunction with significantly elevated left heart filling pressures) or pulmonary veno-occlusive disease/pulmonary capillary hemangiomatosis; significant decompensation has occurred with other highly selective pulmonary vasodilators resulting in acute pulmonary edema.

Adverse Reactions

Cardiovascular: Atrioventricular block, cardiac arrhythmia (transient and new arrhythmia after cardioversion; eg, atrial fibrillation, atrial premature contractions, premature ventricular contractions), chest pain, chest pressure (and discomfort), depression of ST segment on ECG, hypotension, palpitations

Central nervous system: Apprehension, dizziness, headache, nervousness, numbness, paresthesia

Dermatologic: Diaphoresis, facial flushing

Gastrointestinal: Gastrointestinal distress, Nausea

Neuromuscular & skeletal: Neck discomfort (includes throat, jaw), upper extremity discomfort

Respiratory: Dyspnea, hyperventilation

Rare but important or life-threatening: Atrial fibrillation, blurred vision, bradycardia, bronchospasm, cardiac arrest, increased intracranial pressure, injection site reaction, myocardial infarction, respiratory arrest, torsades de pointes, transient hypertension, ventricular arrhythmia, ventricular fibrillation, ventricular tachycardia

Drug Interactions

Metabolism/Transport Effects None known.

Avoid Concomitant Use There are no known interactions where it is recommended to avoid concomitant use.

Increased Effect/Toxicity

The levels/effects of Adenosine may be increased by: CarBAMazepine; Digoxin; Dipyridamole; Nicotine

Decreased Effect

The levels/effects of Adenosine may be decreased by: Caffeine and Caffeine Containing Products; Theophylline Derivatives

Storage/Stability Store between 15°C and 30°C (59°F and 86°F). Do **not** refrigerate; crystallization may occur (may dissolve by warming to room temperature).

Mechanism of Action

Antiarrhythmic actions: Slows conduction time through the AV node, interrupting the re-entry pathways through the AV node, restoring normal sinus rhythm

Myocardial perfusion scintigraphy: Adenosine also causes coronary vasodilation and increases blood flow in normal coronary arteries with little to no increase in stenotic coronary arteries; thallium-201 uptake into the stenotic coronary arteries will be less than that of normal coronary arteries revealing areas of insufficient blood flow.

Pharmacodynamics/Kinetics

Onset of action: Rapid

Duration: Very brief

Metabolism: Blood and tissue to inosine then to adenosine monophosphate (AMP) and hypoxanthine

Half-life elimination: <10 seconds

Dosage

Adenocard: **Rapid IV push (over 1 to 2 seconds) via peripheral line, followed by a normal saline flush:**

Infants and Children:

Paroxysmal supraventricular tachycardia: Manufacturer's recommendation: IV:

<50 kg: Initial: 0.05 to 0.1 mg/kg (maximum initial dose: 6 mg). If conversion of PSVT does not occur within 1 to 2 minutes, may increase dose by 0.05 to 0.1 mg/kg. May repeat until sinus rhythm is established or to a maximum single dose of 0.3 mg/kg or 12 mg. Follow each dose with normal saline flush.

≥50 kg: Refer to Adult dosing

Pediatric advanced life support (PALS, 2010): Treatment of SVT: IV, I.O.: Initial: 0.1 mg/kg (maximum initial dose: 6 mg); if not effective within 1 to 2 minutes, administer 0.2 mg/kg (maximum single dose: 12 mg). Follow each dose with ≥5 mL normal saline flush.

Adults: Paroxysmal supraventricular tachycardia: IV (peripheral line; see **Note**): Initial: 6 mg; if not effective within 1 to 2 minutes, 12 mg may be given; may repeat 12 mg bolus if needed (maximum single dose: 12 mg). Follow each dose with 20 mL normal saline flush. **Note:** Initial dose of adenosine should be reduced to 3 mg if patient is currently receiving carbamazepine or dipyridamole, has a transplanted heart or if adenosine is administered via central line (ACLS, 2010).

Adenoscan: Adults:

Pharmacologic stress testing: Continuous IV infusion via peripheral line: 140 mcg/kg/minute for 6 minutes using syringe or volumetric infusion pump; total dose: 0.84 mg/kg. Thallium-201 is injected at midpoint (3 minutes) of infusion.

Acute vasodilator testing in pulmonary artery hypertension (off-label use): IV: Initial: 50 mcg/kg/minute increased by 50 mcg/kg/minute every 2 minutes to a maximum dose of 500 mcg/kg/minute (Schrader, 1992) **or** to a maximum dose of 250 mcg/kg/minute (McLaughlin, 2009); acutely assess vasodilator response

Dosage adjustment in renal impairment: There are no dosage adjustments provided in the manufacturer's labeling. However, adenosine is not renally eliminated.

Dosage adjustment in hepatic impairment: There are no dosage adjustments provided in the manufacturer's labeling. However, adenosine is not hepatically eliminated.

Dietary Considerations Avoid dietary caffeine for at least 12 hours prior to pharmacologic stress testing.

Administration

Adenocard: For rapid bolus IV use only; administer IV push over 1 to 2 seconds at a peripheral IV site as proximal as possible to trunk (not in lower arm, hand, lower leg, or foot); follow each bolus with a rapid normal saline flush (infants and children ≥5 mL; adults 20 mL). Use of 2 syringes (one with adenosine dose and the other with NS flush) connected to a T-connector or stopcock is recommended. If administered via **central line** in adults, reduce initial dose (ACLS, 2010).

Adenoscan: For IV infusion only via peripheral line

Monitoring Parameters ECG, heart rate, blood pressure; consult individual institutional policies and procedures

Dosage Forms

Solution, Intravenous:

Adenocard: 6 mg/2 mL (2 mL); 12 mg/4 mL (4 mL)

Adenoscan: 3 mg/mL (20 mL, 30 mL)

Generic: 3 mg/mL (20 mL, 30 mL); 6 mg/2 mL (2 mL)

Solution, Intravenous [preservative free]:

Generic: 3 mg/mL (20 mL, 30 mL); 6 mg/2 mL (2 mL); 12 mg/4 mL (4 mL)

- ◆ **Adenosine Injection, USP (Can)** *see* Adenosine *on page 55*
- ◆ **Adept** *see* Icodextrin *on page 1037*
- ◆ **ADH** *see* Vasopressin *on page 2142*
- ◆ **Adipex-P** *see* Phentermine *on page 1635*
- ◆ **A&D Jr. [OTC]** *see* Vitamin A and Vitamin D (Systemic) *on page 2174*
- ◆ **ADL-2698** *see* Alvimopan *on page 104*
- ◆ **Ado Trastuzumab** *see* Ado-Trastuzumab Emtansine *on page 58*

Ado-Trastuzumab Emtansine

(a do tras TU zoo mab em TAN seen)

Brand Names: U.S. Kadcyla

Brand Names: Canada Kadcyla

Index Terms Ado Trastuzumab; Adotrastuzumab; T-DM1; Trastuzumab Emtansine; Trastuzumab-DM1; Trastuzumab-MCC-DM1

Pharmacologic Category Antineoplastic Agent, Anti-HER2; Antineoplastic Agent, Antibody Drug Conjugate; Antineoplastic Agent, Antimicrotubular; Antineoplastic Agent, Monoclonal Antibody

Use Breast cancer, metastatic: Treatment (single-agent) of HER2-positive, metastatic breast cancer in patients who previously received trastuzumab and a taxane, separately or in combination, and have either received prior therapy for metastatic disease or developed disease recurrence during or within 6 months of completing adjuvant therapy.

Pregnancy Risk Factor D

Pregnancy Considerations Animal reproduction studies have not been conducted. **[U.S. Boxed Warning]: Exposure to ado-trastuzumab emtansine may cause embryo-fetal death or birth defects. Effective contraception must be used in women of reproductive potential.** Oligohydramnios, pulmonary hypoplasia, skeletal malformations and neonatal death were observed following trastuzumab exposure during pregnancy (trastuzumab is the antibody component of ado-trastuzumab emtansine). The DM1 component of the ado-trastuzumab emtansine formulation is toxic to rapidly dividing cells and is also expected to cause fetal harm. Pregnancy status should be verified prior to therapy. Effective contraception is recommended during therapy and for 6 months (U.S. labeling) or 7 months (Canadian labeling) after treatment for women of childbearing potential.

If ado-trastuzumab emtansine exposure occurs during pregnancy, healthcare providers should report the exposure to the Genentech Adverse Event Line (888-835-2555). Women exposed to ado-trastuzumab emtansine during pregnancy are encouraged to enroll in MotHER Pregnancy Registry (1-800-690-6720).

Breast-Feeding Considerations It is not known if ado-trastuzumab emtansine is excreted into breast milk. Endogenous immunoglobulins are found in breast milk. Due to the potential for serious adverse reactions in the nursing infant, the decision to discontinue ado-trastuzumab emtansine or discontinue breast-feeding during treatment should take in account the benefits of treatment to the mother. Canadian labeling recommends avoiding breast-feeding for 7 months after completion of therapy.

Contraindications

U.S. labeling: There are no contraindications in the manufacturer's labeling.

Canadian labeling: Hypersensitivity to trastuzumab emtansine or any component of the formulation.

Warnings/Precautions Hazardous agent - use appropriate precautions for handling and disposal (NIOSH 2014 [group 1]).

[U.S. Boxed Warning]: May result in left ventricular ejection fraction (LVEF) reductions. Evaluate left ventricular function (in all patients) prior to and at least every 3 months during treatment; withhold for clinically significant left ventricular function decreases. Treatment interruption or dosage reductions are required inpatients who develop decreased LVEF. Use has not been studied in patients with LVEF <50% at baseline, with a history of symptomatic CHF, serious arrhythmia, or recent history (within 6 months) of MI or unstable angina.

[U.S. Boxed Warning]: Serious hepatotoxicity, including liver failure and death, has been reported. Monitor transaminases and bilirubin at baseline and prior to each dose. Increases (transaminases or total bilirubin) may require dose reductions or discontinuation. Hepatotoxicity is typically manifested by asymptomatic and transient increases in transaminases, although fatal cases of drug induced liver injury and hepatic encephalopathy have occurred; may be confounded by comorbidities or concomitant hepatotoxic medications. Use has not been studied in patients with baseline serum transaminases >2.5 times ULN or bilirubin >1.5 times ULN, or in patients with active hepatitis B or C virus. Cases of nodular regenerative hyperplasia (NRH), a rare liver disorder characterized by widespread benign transformation of hepatic parenchyma into small regenerative nodules, have been observed (by biopsy). NRH may develop into noncirrhotic portal hypertension. Consider NRH in patients with clinical symptoms of portal hypertension and/or cirrhosis-like pattern seen on liver CT scan, although without associated transaminase elevations or other manifestations of cirrhosis. Diagnosis of NRH is confirmed by histopathology; permanently discontinue if histopathology confirms NRH.

[U.S. Boxed Warning]: Exposure to ado-trastuzumab emtansine may cause embryo-fetal death or birth defects. Effective contraception must be used in women of reproductive potential. Pregnancy status should be verified prior to therapy; effective contraception is recommended during therapy and for 6 months (U.S. labeling) or 7 months (Canadian labeling) after treatment for women of childbearing potential.

Infusion reactions (flushing, chills, fever, bronchospasm, dyspnea, wheezing, hypotension, and/or tachycardia) have been reported. After termination of infusion, these reactions generally resolved within several hours to a day. Medications for the treatment of reactions should be available for immediate use. Monitor closely for infusion reactions, especially during initial infusion. If reaction occurs, decrease infusion rate; for severe infusion reactions, interrupt infusion; permanently discontinue for life-threatening reactions. Serious allergic/anaphylactic reaction was observed (rare). Use is not recommended in patients who had trastuzumab permanently discontinued due to infusion reaction or hypersensitivity (has not been evaluated).

Thrombocytopenia may occur (nadir achieved: by day 8; generally resolves to ≤ grade 1 by the next scheduled dose); the incidence of thrombocytopenia may be higher in patients of Asian ancestry; monitor platelet count at baseline and prior to each dose; may require treatment interruption or dose reduction. Monitor closely if at bleeding risk due to thrombocytopenia and/or concomitant anticoagulant use. Has not been studied in patients with platelets <100,000/mm^3 at treatment initiation. Neutropenia and anemia have also occurred. Hemorrhagic events, including central nervous system, respiratory, and gastrointestinal hemorrhage, have been observed; some hemorrhages were fatal. Some events occurred in patients who were receiving anticoagulation or antiplatelet therapy, or in patients with thrombocytopenia, although bleeding also occurred in patients without additional risk factors. Use caution when administering with antiplatelet agents or anticoagulants; consider additional monitoring when indicated. Local reactions (erythema, irritation, pain, swelling, or tenderness) secondary to extravasation have been noted; these were generally mild and typically occurred within 24 hours of infusion; monitor infusion site during infusion for possible infiltration. Sensory peripheral neuropathy has been reported, usually grade 1; monitor for signs and symptoms of neuropathy; may require treatment interruption and/or dose reduction. Interstitial lung disease (ILD), including pneumonitis has been reported; some cases resulted in acute respiratory distress syndrome and/or fatalities; permanently discontinue with diagnosis of ILD or pneumonitis. Signs and symptoms of pneumonitis include dyspnea, cough, fatigue, and pulmonary infiltrates; may or may not occur in correlation with infusion reaction. Patients with dyspnea at rest (due to advance malignancy complications or comorbidity) may be at increased risk for pulmonary toxicity.

[U.S. Boxed Warning]: Ado-trastuzumab emtansine and conventional trastuzumab are NOT interchangeable. Do not substitute. In Canada, the generic name for Kadcyla is trastuzumab emtansine (ie, lacks Ado- prefix) and may be confused with conventional trastuzumab. Verify product label prior to reconstitution and administration to prevent medication errors. Potentially significant drug-drug or drug-food interactions may exist, requiring dose or frequency adjustment, additional monitoring, and/or selection of alternative therapy. Establish HER2 overexpression or gene amplification status prior to treatment; has only been studied in patients with evidence of HER2 overexpression, either as 3+ IHC (Dako Herceptest™) or FISH amplification ratio ≥2 (Dako *HER2* FISH pharmDx™ test); there is only limited data on patients with breast cancer positive by FISH and 0 or 1+ by IHC.

Adverse Reactions

Cardiovascular: Hypertension, left ventricular dysfunction, peripheral edema

Central nervous system: Chills, dizziness, fatigue, headache, insomnia, peripheral neuropathy

Dermatologic: Pruritus, skin rash

Endocrine & metabolic: Decreased serum potassium, hypokalemia

Gastrointestinal: Abdominal pain, constipation, diarrhea, dysgeusia, dyspepsia, nausea, stomatitis, vomiting, xerostomia

Genitourinary: Urinary tract infection

Hematologic & oncologic: Anemia, decreased hemoglobin, decreased neutrophils, decreased platelet count, hemorrhage, neutropenia, thrombocytopenia (more common in Asians)

Hepatic: Increased serum alkaline phosphatase, increased serum ALT, increased serum AST, increased serum bilirubin, increased serum transaminases

Hypersensitivity: Hypersensitivity

Immunologic: Antibody development

Neuromuscular & skeletal: Arthralgia, musculoskeletal pain, myalgia, weakness

Ophthalmic: Blurred vision, conjunctivitis, dry eye syndrome, increased lacrimation

Respiratory: Cough, dyspnea, epistaxis, pneumonitis

Miscellaneous: Fever, infusion related reaction

Rare but important or life-threatening: Anaphylactoid reaction, hepatic encephalopathy, hepatotoxicity, nodular regenerative hyperplasia, portal hypertension

Drug Interactions

Metabolism/Transport Effects Substrate of CYP3A4 (major); **Note:** Assignment of Major/Minor substrate status based on clinically relevant drug interaction potential

Avoid Concomitant Use

Avoid concomitant use of Ado-Trastuzumab Emtansine with any of the following: BCG; Belimumab; CloZAPine; Conivaptan; CYP3A4 Inhibitors (Strong); Dipyrone; Fusidic Acid (Systemic); Idelalisib; Natalizumab; Pimecrolimus; Tacrolimus (Topical); Tofacitinib; Vaccines (Live)

Increased Effect/Toxicity

Ado-Trastuzumab Emtansine may increase the levels/effects of: Belimumab; CloZAPine; Leflunomide; Natalizumab; Tofacitinib; Vaccines (Live)

The levels/effects of Ado-Trastuzumab Emtansine may be increased by: Aprepitant; Ceritinib; Conivaptan; CYP3A4 Inhibitors (Moderate); CYP3A4 Inhibitors (Strong); Dasatinib; Denosumab; Dipyrone; Fosaprepitant; Fusidic Acid (Systemic); Idelalisib; Ivacaftor; Luliconazole; Mifepristone; Netupitant; Pimecrolimus; Roflumilast; Simeprevir; Tacrolimus (Topical); Trastuzumab

Decreased Effect

Ado-Trastuzumab Emtansine may decrease the levels/effects of: BCG; Coccidioides immitis Skin Test; Sipuleucel-T; Vaccines (Inactivated); Vaccines (Live)

The levels/effects of Ado-Trastuzumab Emtansine may be decreased by: Echinacea

Preparation for Administration Hazardous agent; use appropriate precautions for handling and disposal (NIOSH 2014 [group 1]). Check vial labels to assure appropriate product is being reconstituted (ado-trastuzumab emtansine and conventional trastuzumab are different products and are **NOT** interchangeable).

Slowly inject sterile water for injection into the vial (5 mL for 100 mg vial or 8 mL for 160 mg vial) to a reconstituted concentration of 20 mg/mL. Gently swirl vial until completely dissolved. Reconstituted solution will be clear or slightly opalescent (there should be no visible particles) and colorless to pale brown. Dilute for infusion by adding to 250 mL sodium chloride 0.9%; gently invert bag to mix (do not shake).

Storage/Stability Store intact vials at 2°C to 8°C (36°F to 46°F). Do not freeze or shake intact vials, reconstituted solution, or solutions diluted for infusion. Reconstituted vials do not contain preservative and should be used immediately, although may be stored for up to 24 hours at 2°C to 8°C (36°F to 46°F). Solutions diluted for infusion should be used immediately, although may be stored at 2°C to 8°C (36°F to 46°F) for up to 24 hours prior to use. This storage time is additional to the time allowed for the reconstituted vials.

Mechanism of Action Ado-trastuzumab emtansine is a HER2-antibody drug conjugate which incorporates the HER2 targeted actions of trastuzumab with the microtubule inhibitor DM1 (a maytansine derivative). The conjugate, which is linked via a stable thioether linker, allows for selective delivery into HER2 overexpressing cells, resulting in cell cycle arrest and apoptosis.

Pharmacodynamics/Kinetics

Distribution: V_d: 3.13 L

Protein binding: DM1: 93%

Metabolism: DM1 undergoes hepatic metabolism via CYP3A4/5

Half-life elimination: ~4 days

Time to peak: Near the end of the infusion

Dosage Note: Do not substitute ado-trastuzumab emtansine (U.S.) or trastuzumab emtansine (Canada) for or with conventional trastuzumab; products are different and are **NOT** interchangeable.

Breast cancer, metastatic, HER2+: Adults: IV: 3.6 mg/kg every 3 weeks until disease progression or unacceptable toxicity; Maximum dose: 3.6 mg/kg

Missed or delayed doses: If a planned dose is missed or delayed, administer as soon as possible (at the dose and rate most recently tolerated), do not wait until the next planned cycle. Then adjust schedule to maintain a 3-week interval between doses.

Dosage adjustment in renal impairment:
CrCl ≥30 mL/minute: No dosage adjustment necessary.
CrCl <30 mL/minute: There are no dosage adjustments provided in the manufacturer's labeling (has not been studied).

Dosage adjustment in hepatic impairment:
Hepatic impairment prior to treatment initiation: There are no dosage adjustments provided in the manufacturer's labeling (has not been studied).
Hepatotoxicity during treatment: Refer to Dosage adjustment for toxicity.

Dosage adjustment for toxicity: Note: After a dose reduction is implemented, do not re-escalate dose.

Infusion-related reaction: Slow infusion rate or interrupt infusion. Permanently discontinue if life-threatening infusion reactions occur.

Dose levels for dosage reductions and/or discontinuation:
Starting dose: 3.6 mg/kg
First dose reduction: Reduce dose to 3 mg/kg
Second dose reduction: Reduce dose to 2.4 mg/kg
Further reductions necessary: Discontinue treatment.

Hematologic toxicity:
Grade 3 thrombocytopenia (platelets 25,000/mm^3 to <50,000/mm^3): Withhold treatment until platelet count recovers to ≤ grade 1 (platelets ≥75,000/mm^3), then resume treatment at the same dose level.
Grade 4 thrombocytopenia (platelets <25,000/mm^3): Withhold treatment until platelet count recovers to ≤ grade 1 (platelets ≥75,000/mm^3), then resume treatment with one dose level reduction.

Cardiotoxicity:
LVEF >45%: Continue treatment.
LVEF 40% to ≤45% and decrease is <10% points from baseline: Continue treatment and repeat LVEF assessment within 3 weeks.
LVEF 40% to ≤45% and decrease is ≥10% points from baseline: Withhold treatment and repeat LVEF assessment within 3 weeks; if repeat LVEF has not recovered to within 10% points from baseline, discontinue treatment.
LVEF <40%: Withhold treatment and repeat LVEF assessment within 3 weeks; if repeat LVEF is confirmed <40%, discontinue treatment.
HF (symptomatic): Discontinue treatment.

Hepatotoxicity:
Grade 2 ALT, AST elevations (>2.5 to ≤5 times ULN): Continue at same dose level.
Grade 3 ALT, AST elevations (>5 to ≤20 times ULN): Withhold until ALT, AST recover to ≤ grade 2, then resume with one dose level reduction.
Grade 4 ALT, AST elevations (>20 times ULN): Permanently discontinue treatment.
Grade 2 hyperbilirubinemia (>1.5 to ≤3 times ULN): Withhold until bilirubin recovers to ≤ grade 1 (≤1.5 times ULN), then resume at the same dose level.
Grade 3 hyperbilirubinemia (>3 to ≤10 times ULN): Withhold until bilirubin recovers to ≤ grade 1, then resume with one dose level reduction.
Grade 4 hyperbilirubinemia (>10 times ULN): Permanently discontinue treatment.
Concomitant ALT, AST >3 times ULN and total bilirubin >2 times ULN: Permanently discontinue treatment.
Nodular regenerative hyperplasia: Permanently discontinue treatment.

Peripheral neuropathy, grade 3 or 4: Temporarily discontinue until resolves to ≤ grade 2.

Pulmonary toxicity: Interstitial lung disease or pneumonitis: Permanently discontinue.

Administration Check label to ensure appropriate product is being administered (ado-trastuzumab emtansine [U.S.] or trastuzumab emtansine [Canada] and conventional trastuzumab are different products and are **NOT** interchangeable).

Infuse over 90 minutes (first infusion) or over 30 minutes (subsequent infusions if prior infusions were well tolerated) through a 0.22 micron inline nonprotein adsorptive polyethersulfone filter. Do not administer IV push or bolus. Do not administer with other medications.

Closely monitor infusion site during administration. Monitor patient during infusion for signs of infusion-related reactions (eg, fever, chills); monitor for at least 90 minutes following initial infusion and (if tolerated) for at least 30 minutes following subsequent infusions.

Hazardous agent; use appropriate precautions for handling and disposal (NIOSH 2014 [group 1]).

Monitoring Parameters Platelet count (at baseline and prior to each dose), transaminases and bilirubin (at baseline and prior to each dose); verify pregnancy status prior to treatment initiation; HER2 expression status. Evaluate left ventricular function (prior to and at least every 3 months during treatment; for LVEF <40% or 40% to 45% with ≥10% absolute decrease below baseline value, reassess within 3 weeks). Monitor infusion site during infusion for possible infiltration; monitor for infusion reactions (during infusion and for 90 minutes after initial infusion and for 30 minutes after subsequent infusions); signs and symptoms of bleeding, neuropathy, and/or pulmonary toxicity

Dosage Forms

Solution Reconstituted, Intravenous [preservative free]:
Kadcyla: 100 mg (1 ea); 160 mg (1 ea)

◆ **Adoxa** *see* Doxycycline *on page 689*

◆ **Adoxa Pak 1/100** *see* Doxycycline *on page 689*

◆ **Adoxa Pak 1/150** *see* Doxycycline *on page 689*

◆ **Adoxa Pak 2/100** *see* Doxycycline *on page 689*

◆ **Adrenaclick** *see* EPINEPHrine (Systemic, Oral Inhalation) *on page 735*

◆ **Adrenalin** *see* EPINEPHrine (Systemic, Oral Inhalation) *on page 735*

◆ **Adrenaline** *see* EPINEPHrine (Systemic, Oral Inhalation) *on page 735*

◆ **Adrenaline Bitartrate** *see* EPINEPHrine (Systemic, Oral Inhalation) *on page 735*

◆ **Adrenaline Hydrochloride** *see* EPINEPHrine (Systemic, Oral Inhalation) *on page 735*

◆ **ADR (error-prone abbreviation)** *see* DOXOrubicin (Conventional) *on page 679*

◆ **Adria** *see* DOXOrubicin (Conventional) *on page 679*

◆ **Adriamycin** *see* DOXOrubicin (Conventional) *on page 679*

◆ **Adriamycin PFS (Can)** *see* DOXOrubicin (Conventional) *on page 679*

◆ **Adrucil** *see* Fluorouracil (Systemic) *on page 896*

◆ **Adsorbent Charcoal** *see* Charcoal, Activated *on page 416*

◆ **Advagraf (Can)** *see* Tacrolimus (Systemic) *on page 1962*

◆ **Advair (Can)** *see* Fluticasone and Salmeterol *on page 912*

◆ **Advair Diskus** *see* Fluticasone and Salmeterol *on page 912*

◆ **Advair HFA** *see* Fluticasone and Salmeterol *on page 912*

- **Advate** *see* Antihemophilic Factor (Recombinant) *on page 152*
- **Advicor** *see* Niacin and Lovastatin *on page 1446*
- **Advil [OTC]** *see* Ibuprofen *on page 1032*
- **Advil (Can)** *see* Ibuprofen *on page 1032*
- **Advil® Cold & Sinus [OTC]** *see* Pseudoephedrine and Ibuprofen *on page 1743*
- **Advil® Cold & Sinus (Can)** *see* Pseudoephedrine and Ibuprofen *on page 1743*
- **Advil® Cold & Sinus Daytime (Can)** *see* Pseudoephedrine and Ibuprofen *on page 1743*
- **Advil Junior Strength [OTC]** *see* Ibuprofen *on page 1032*
- **Advil Migraine [OTC]** *see* Ibuprofen *on page 1032*
- **Advil Pediatric Drops (Can)** *see* Ibuprofen *on page 1032*
- **AEGR-733** *see* Lomitapide *on page 1233*
- **Aerius® (Can)** *see* Desloratadine *on page 594*
- **Aerius® Kids (Can)** *see* Desloratadine *on page 594*

Afatinib (a FA ti nib)

Brand Names: U.S. Gilotrif

Brand Names: Canada Giotrif

Index Terms Afatinib Dimaleate; BIBW 2992

Pharmacologic Category Antineoplastic Agent, Epidermal Growth Factor Receptor (EGFR) Inhibitor; Antineoplastic Agent, Tyrosine Kinase Inhibitor

Use

Non-small cell lung cancer, metastatic: First-line treatment of metastatic non-small cell lung cancer (NSCLC) in patients whose tumors have epidermal growth factor receptor (EGFR) exon 19 deletions or exon 21 (L858R) substitution mutations as detected by an approved test.

Limitations of use: Safety and efficacy have not been established in patients whose tumors express EGFR mutations other than exon 19 deletion or exon 21 (L858R) substitution.

Pregnancy Risk Factor D

Pregnancy Considerations Adverse events were observed in animal reproduction studies. Based on its mechanism of action, afatinib is expected to cause fetal harm if used during pregnancy. Women of reproductive potential should use highly-effective contraception during therapy and for at least 2 weeks after treatment has been discontinued.

Breast-Feeding Considerations It is not known if afatinib is excreted into breast milk. Due to the potential for serious adverse reactions in the nursing infant, the U.S. manufacturer labeling recommends a decision be made whether to discontinue nursing or to discontinue the drug, taking into account the importance of treatment to the mother. The Canadian labeling recommends avoiding breast-feeding during therapy and for at least 2 weeks after treatment has been discontinued.

Contraindications

U.S. labeling: There are no contraindications listed in the manufacturer's labeling.

Canadian labeling: Hypersensitivity to afatinib or any component of the formulation.

Warnings/Precautions Hazardous agent – use appropriate precautions for handling and disposal (meets NIOSH 2014 criteria). Cutaneous reactions (eg, acneiform rash, erythema, and rash) are common; grade 3 reactions (characterized by bullous, blistering, and exfoliating lesions) and palmar-plantar erythrodysesthesia syndrome were also seen in clinical trials. May require therapy interruption and dosage reduction; discontinue if life-threatening cutaneous lesions occur. Patients should be cautioned to avoid sun exposure and/or utilize adequate sun protection. Paronychia requiring dose reduction and discontinuation of therapy has been observed. In clinical trials, diarrhea and stomatitis frequently occurred in patients treated with afatinib; diarrhea was observed in the majority of patients and typically appeared within the first 6 weeks of therapy. Dehydration and renal impairment may occur as a consequence of diarrhea; monitor closely. Patients may require antidiarrheal therapy (eg, loperamide); initiate at the onset of diarrhea and continue until free of loose bowel movements for 12 hours. May necessitate therapy interruption and dosage reduction. The Canadian labeling recommends avoiding use in patients with GI disorders associated with diarrhea (eg, Crohn disease, malabsorption).

Decreases from baseline in left ventricular ejection fraction (LVEF) were noted in some patients receiving afatinib. Patients with abnormal LVEF or a significant cardiac history were excluded from clinical trials; use with caution in patients with cardiac risk factors and/or decreased LVEF. Keratitis was reported rarely in clinical trials; monitor for signs/symptoms of keratitis (eg, acute or worsening eye inflammation, blurred vision, eye pain, lacrimation, light sensitivity, red eye). Interrupt therapy in patients with suspected keratitis and consider discontinuation if diagnosis of ulcerative keratitis is confirmed (permanently discontinue for persistent ulcerative keratitis). Use with caution in patients with a history of keratitis, severe dry eye, ulcerative keratitis, or who wear contact lens (risk factor for keratitis and ulceration). Interstitial lung disease (ILD) or ILD-like reactions occurred in a small percentage of patients treated with afatinib (some fatal). ILD incidence appeared to be higher in Asian as compared to non-Asian patients. Monitor closely for signs/symptoms of ILD (eg, acute respiratory distress syndrome, allergic alveolitis, lung infiltration, pneumonitis). Interrupt therapy for suspected ILD; discontinue therapy with confirmed diagnosis.

Hepatic function test abnormalities (some fatal) were observed in clinical trials. Monitor liver function tests periodically; may require therapy interruption and dosage reduction. Discontinue if severe hepatic impairment occurs during therapy. Closely monitor patients with moderate-to-severe renal impairment, may require dosage adjustments if not tolerated. The Canadian labeling does not recommend use in severe hepatic or severe renal impairment. Potentially significant drug-drug interactions may exist, requiring dose or frequency adjustment, additional monitoring, and/or selection of alternative therapy. Safety and efficacy have not been established in patients with non-small cell lung cancer whose tumors express EGFR mutations other than exon 19 deletion or exon 21 (L858R) substitution. Increased mortality has been observed in a clinical trial evaluating afatinib in combination with vinorelbine for HER2-positive metastatic breast cancer (not an approved use). This combination was also associated with a higher incidence of adverse events (eg, diarrhea, rash), as well as fatalities due to infection and cancer progression. Afatinib should not be used in combination with vinorelbine for the treatment of HER2-positive metastatic breast cancer. Contains lactose; Canadian labeling recommends avoiding use in patients with hereditary conditions of galactose intolerance, Lapp lactase deficiency, or glucose-galactose malabsorption.

Adverse Reactions

Central nervous system: Fatigue

Dermatologic: Acneiform eruption, cheilitis, palmar-plantar erythrodysesthesia, paronychia, pruritus, xeroderma

Endocrine & metabolic: Hypokalemia, weight loss

Gastrointestinal: Decreased appetite, diarrhea, stomatitis, vomiting

Genitourinary: Cystitis

Hepatic: Increased serum transaminases

Ophthalmic: Conjunctivitis
Renal: Renal insufficiency
Respiratory: Epistaxis, pneumonitis (more common in Asian descent), rhinorrhea
Miscellaneous: Fever
Rare but important or life-threatening: Keratitis, pneumonia, sepsis

Drug Interactions

Metabolism/Transport Effects Substrate of BCRP, P-glycoprotein; **Inhibits** BCRP, P-glycoprotein

Avoid Concomitant Use There are no known interactions where it is recommended to avoid concomitant use.

Increased Effect/Toxicity

Afatinib may increase the levels/effects of: Porfimer; Verteporfin

The levels/effects of Afatinib may be increased by: P-glycoprotein/ABCB1 Inhibitors

Decreased Effect

The levels/effects of Afatinib may be decreased by: P-glycoprotein/ABCB1 Inducers

Food Interactions Administration with a high-fat meal decreases C_{max} by 50% and AUC by 39% as compared to the fasted state. Management: Take at least 1 hour before or 2 hours (U.S. labeling) or 3 hours (Canadian labeling) after a meal.

Storage/Stability Store at 25°C (77°F); excursions are permitted between 15°C and 30°C (59°F and 86°F). Dispense in original bottle; protect from high humidity and light.

Mechanism of Action Highly selective blocker of the ErbB family, including EGFR (ErbB1), HER2 (ErbB2), and HER4 (ErbB4); covalently and irreversibly binds to the intracellular tyrosine kinase domain, resulting in tumor growth inhibition and tumor regression

Pharmacodynamics/Kinetics

Absorption: Decreased with high-fat meals
Protein binding: ~95%
Metabolism: Covalently adducted to proteins and nucleophilic small molecules (minimal enzymatic metabolism) (Wind, 2013)
Bioavailability: Tablets: 92% (as compared to an oral solution)
Half-life elimination: 37 hours
Time to peak: 2 to 5 hours
Excretion: Feces (85%); urine (4%); primarily as unchanged drug

Dosage Non-small cell lung cancer (NSCLC), metastatic, with EGFR exon 19 deletions or exon 21 (L858R) substitution mutations: Adults: Oral: 40 mg once daily until disease progression or unacceptable toxicity

Missed doses:

U.S. labeling: Do not take a missed dose within 12 hours of next dose

Canadian labeling: Do not take a missed dose within 8 hours of next dose

Dosage adjustment for concomitant therapy:

U.S. labeling:

P-gp inhibitors: If concomitant therapy is not tolerated, reduce afatinib daily dose by 10 mg. Upon discontinuation of the P-gp inhibitor, resume previous dose as tolerated.

P-gp inducers: Increase afatinib daily dose by 10 mg if on chronic concomitant therapy with a P-gp inducer. Resume previous dose 2 to 3 days after discontinuation of P-gp inducer.

Canadian labeling: Avoid concurrent use with strong P-gp inhibitors or inducers. If concurrent use with a P-gp inhibitor is necessary, administer simultaneously with or after afatinib; monitor closely for adverse effects. The manufacturer labeling does not provide specific recommendations when concurrent use of a P-gp inducer is necessary.

Dosage adjustment for toxicity: Note: Permanently discontinue for intolerability or severe reaction occurring at a dose of 20 mg daily. The Canadian labeling recommends permanently discontinuing therapy for toxicities that do not resolve to ≤ grade 1 within 14 days of therapy interruption.

Cardiovascular: Permanently discontinue for symptomatic left ventricular dysfunction.

Dermatologic: Withhold therapy for prolonged (>7 days) or intolerable grade 2 or higher cutaneous reactions. Upon improvement to baseline or ≤ grade 1, resume therapy at 10 mg per day less than previous dose. Discontinue permanently for life-threatening bullous, blistering, or exfoliative skin lesions.

Gastrointestinal:

Diarrhea: Greater than or equal to grade 2 diarrhea that persists for ≥2 consecutive days despite antidiarrheal therapy: Interrupt therapy until resolution to ≤ grade 1, then resume at 10 mg per day less than previous dose.

Nausea/vomiting: Canadian labeling (not in U.S. labeling): Intolerable grade 2 or persistent (≥7 days) nausea/vomiting despite antiemetic therapy: Interrupt therapy until resolution to ≤ grade 1, then resume at 10 mg per day less than previous dose.

Ocular: Interrupt therapy for suspected keratitis; consider discontinuation if diagnosis of ulcerative keratitis is confirmed. Permanently discontinue for persistent ulcerative keratitis.

Pulmonary: Interrupt therapy for suspected interstitial lung disease (ILD); permanently discontinue if diagnosis is confirmed.

Other toxicity:

Greater than or equal to grade 3 adverse reactions: Withhold therapy for ≥ grade 3 adverse reactions. Upon improvement to baseline or ≤ grade 1, resume therapy at 10 mg per day less than previous dose.

Other poorly tolerated grade 2 adverse reactions persisting ≥7 days: Canadian labeling (not in U.S. labeling): Interrupt therapy until resolution to ≤ grade 1, then resume at 10 mg per day less than previous dose.

Dosage adjustment for renal impairment:

Preexisting mild impairment (CrCl ≥60 mL/minute): No dosage adjustment is necessary.

Preexisting moderate-to-severe impairment (CrCl <60 mL/minute): There are no dosage adjustments provided in the manufacturer's labeling (has not been studied in patients with severe impairment [CrCl <30 mL/minute]); closely monitor and adjust dose if necessary. The Canadian labeling recommends avoiding use if CrCl <30 mL/minute.

Renal toxicity during treatment: If ≥ grade 2 renal toxicity occurs, withhold therapy. Upon improvement to baseline or ≤ grade 1, resume therapy at 10 mg per day less than previous dose.

Dosage adjustment for hepatic impairment:

Preexisting mild-to-moderate impairment (Child-Pugh class A or B): No dosage adjustment is necessary.

Preexisting severe impairment (Child-Pugh class C):

U.S. labeling: There are no dosage adjustments provided in the manufacturer's labeling (has not been studied); closely monitor and adjust dose if necessary.

Canadian labeling: Avoid use.

Hepatotoxicity during treatment: Withhold therapy for ≥ grade 3 hepatic dysfunction. Upon improvement to baseline or ≤ grade 1, resume therapy at 10 mg per day less than previous dose. Permanently discontinue for severe afatinib-induced hepatic impairment.

Dietary Considerations Take at least 1 hour before or 2 hours (U.S. labeling) or 3 hours (Canadian labeling) after a meal.

Administration

U.S. labeling: Administer orally at least 1 hour before or 2 hours after a meal. Do not take a missed dose within 12 hours of the next dose. Hazardous agent; use appropriate precautions for handling and disposal (meets NIOSH 2014 criteria).

Canadian labeling: Administer orally at least 1 hour before or 3 hours after a meal. Do not take a missed dose within 8 hours of the next dose. Swallow whole with water.

Monitoring Parameters EGFR mutation status; liver and renal function (periodically); monitor for skin toxicity, diarrhea, signs/symptoms of dehydration; monitor for signs/symptoms of interstitial lung disease (eg, acute respiratory distress syndrome, allergic alveolitis, lung infiltration, pneumonitis) and keratitis (eg, acute or worsening eye inflammation, blurred vision, eye pain, lacrimation, light sensitivity, red eye). Consider left ventricular ejection fraction assessment prior to and during therapy in patients with cardiac risk factors or conditions that may impair left ventricular function.

Dosage Forms

Tablet, Oral:

Gilotrif: 20 mg, 30 mg, 40 mg

Dosage Forms: Canada

Tablet, Oral:

Giotrif: 20 mg, 30 mg, 40 mg

◆ **Afatinib Dimaleate** *see* Afatinib *on page 61*

◆ **Afeditab CR** *see* NIFEdipine *on page 1451*

◆ **Afinitor** *see* Everolimus *on page 822*

◆ **Afinitor Disperz** *see* Everolimus *on page 822*

◆ **AFirm 1X [OTC]** *see* Vitamin A *on page 2173*

◆ **AFirm 2X [OTC]** *see* Vitamin A *on page 2173*

◆ **AFirm 3X [OTC]** *see* Vitamin A *on page 2173*

Aflibercept (Ophthalmic) (a FLIB er sept)

Brand Names: U.S. Eylea

Brand Names: Canada Eylea

Index Terms AVE 0005; AVE 005; AVE-0005; VEGF Trap; VEGF Trap-Eye

Pharmacologic Category Ophthalmic Agent; Vascular Endothelial Growth Factor (VEGF) Inhibitor

Use

Macular degeneration: Treatment of neovascular (wet) age-related macular degeneration (AMD)

Macular edema: Treatment of macular edema following retinal vein occlusion (RVO) and diabetic macular edema

Pregnancy Risk Factor C

Dosage

Age-related macular degeneration (AMD): Adults: Intravitreal: 2 mg (0.05 mL) once every 4 weeks (monthly) for the first 12 weeks (every 3 months), then 2 mg (0.05 mL) once every 8 weeks (every 2 months) thereafter. Although may be administered every 4 weeks, additional efficacy has not been demonstrated (compared with every 8 week administration).

Diabetic macular edema (DME): Adults: Intravitreal: 2 mg (0.05 mL) once every 4 weeks (monthly) for the first 5 injections, followed by 2 mg (0.05 mL) once every 8 weeks (every 2 months). Although may be administered every 4 weeks, additional efficacy has not been demonstrated (compared with every 8 week administration).

Macular edema following retinal vein occlusion (RVO): Adults: Intravitreal: 2 mg (0.05 mL) once every 4 weeks (monthly)

Dosage adjustment in renal impairment: No dosage adjustment necessary

Dosage adjustment in hepatic impairment: There are no dosage adjustments provided in the manufacturer's labeling (has not been studied); however, no adjustment expected due to minimal systemic absorption

Additional Information Complete prescribing information should be consulted for additional detail.

Dosage Forms

Solution, Intraocular [preservative free]:

Eylea: 2 mg/0.05 mL (0.05 mL)

◆ **Aflibercept I.V.** *see* Ziv-Aflibercept (Systemic) *on page 2204*

◆ **Afluria** *see* Influenza Virus Vaccine (Inactivated) *on page 1075*

◆ **Afluria Preservative Free** *see* Influenza Virus Vaccine (Inactivated) *on page 1075*

◆ **Afrin Saline Nasal Mist [OTC]** *see* Sodium Chloride *on page 1902*

◆ **AG-013736** *see* Axitinib *on page 207*

Agalsidase Alfa [CAN/INT] (aye GAL si days AL fa)

Brand Names: Canada Replagal [DSC]

Index Terms Agalsidase Alpha; Alpha-Galactosidase-A (Gene-Activated)

Pharmacologic Category Enzyme

Use Note: Not approved in U.S.

Replacement therapy for Fabry disease

Pregnancy Considerations Adverse events were not observed in animal reproduction studies. Information related to use in pregnancy is limited (Kalkum, 2009).

Breast-Feeding Considerations It is not known if agalsidase alfa is excreted into breast milk.

Contraindications Hypersensitivity to agalsidase alfa or any component of the formulation; concomitant use with chloroquine, amiodarone, monobenzone, or gentamicin (these agents have the potential to inhibit intracellular agalsidase alfa activity)

Warnings/Precautions Infusion-related reactions are common and rarely may be severe. Mild reactions (chills, facial flushing) may occur during or within 1 hour after infusion. Severe reactions (nausea, pyrexia, rigors, tachycardia, urticaria, vomiting) are rare and most often occur within 2-4 months from the onset of therapy. Patients with a prior history of infusion-related reactions may be premedicated with corticosteroids and antihistamines 1-3 hours before subsequent infusions. Symptoms related to the disease process may be mistaken as an adverse reaction related to therapy. IgG antibodies have been observed in ~55% of treated patients. Approximately 60% of these patients are antibody free within 12-18 months. Use in patients with hepatic impairment has not been studied.

Adverse Reactions Note: The most common and serious adverse reactions are infusion reactions (symptoms may include chills, dyspnea, facial flushing, fever, hypertension, nausea, rigors, tachycardia, urticaria, and vomiting).

Cardiovascular: Chest pain, chest tightness, edema, flushing, hypertension, peripheral coldness, peripheral edema, tachycardia

Central nervous system: Dizziness, fatigue, fatigue aggravated, fever, headache, hypersomnia, hypoesthesia, pain/discomfort, panic attack, somnolence, vertigo

Dermatologic: Acne, dry skin, eczema, erythema, mottled skin, pruritus, rash

Gastrointestinal: Abdominal pain, diarrhea, dyspepsia, dysgeusia, gastrointestinal upset, nausea, stomach cramps, stomach discomfort, vomiting

Neuromuscular & skeletal: Back pain, limb pain, musculoskeletal discomfort, myalgia, neuropathic pain, paresthesia, rigors, tremor, weakness

Ocular: Lacrimation increased, periorbital edema

Respiratory: Cough, dyspnea, hoarseness, nasal congestion, nasopharyngitis, pharyngitis, snoring, throat irritation/tightness

Miscellaneous: Feeling hot, IgG antibody formation, influenza-like syndrome, infusion-related reactions, parosmia

Rare but important or life-threatening: Chills, facial flushing, urticaria

Drug Interactions

Metabolism/Transport Effects None known.

Avoid Concomitant Use

Avoid concomitant use of Agalsidase Alfa with any of the following: Amiodarone; Chloroquine; Gentamicin (Systemic)

Increased Effect/Toxicity There are no known significant interactions involving an increase in effect.

Decreased Effect

The levels/effects of Agalsidase Alfa may be decreased by: Amiodarone; Chloroquine; Gentamicin (Systemic)

Preparation for Administration To make final infusion, add the desired amount of solution (based on patient weight) to 100 mL NS. Mix gently and avoid shaking. Discard unused product.

Storage/Stability Store vials between 2°C to 8°C (36°F to 46°F). Product is preservative free. Administration within 3 hours after dilution is recommended, however, diluted solution is stable for 24 hours at 25°C (77°).

Mechanism of Action Agalsidase alfa is a recombinant form of the enzyme alpha-galactosidase-A, which catalyzes the hydrolysis of globotriaosylceramide (Gb-3) and other glycosphingolipids. These compounds may accumulate (over many years) within the tissues of patients with Fabry disease, leading to renal and cardiovascular complications. Agalsidase has been noted to reduce cellular levels of Gb-3 within the liver, heart, kidney, blood vessels, and in plasma.

Pharmacodynamics/Kinetics

Distribution: V_d: 17% of body weight

Metabolism: Plasma; via peptide hydrolysis

Half-life elimination: ~1.5-2 hours

Dosage Note: Premedication with oral antihistamines and corticosteroids may alleviate infusion-related reactions associated with agalsidase alfa.

IV: Children and Adults: Fabry disease: 0.2 mg/kg every 2 weeks

Dosage adjustment in renal impairment: No dosage adjustment necessary

Dosage adjustment in hepatic impairment: No data available

Administration Infuse over 40 minutes using a dedicated IV line with filter. Do not infuse other agents through same IV line. Interrupt infusion in the presence of infusion-related reactions (eg, chills, flushing, dyspnea, rigors, tachycardia, urticaria). Infusion may be restarted after 5-10 minutes if symptoms subside or after administration of analgesics, antipyretics, antihistamines, and/or corticosteroids.

Monitoring Parameters Globotriaosylceramide (Gb-3) levels (serum and urine)

Product Availability Not available in U.S.

◆ **Agalsidase Alpha** *see* Agalsidase Alfa [CAN/INT] *on page 63*

Agalsidase Beta (aye GAL si days BAY ta)

Brand Names: U.S. Fabrazyme

Brand Names: Canada Fabrazyme®

Index Terms Alpha-Galactosidase-A (Recombinant); r-h α-GAL

Pharmacologic Category Enzyme

Use Replacement therapy for Fabry disease

Pregnancy Risk Factor B

Dosage IV: Children ≥8 years and Adults: 1 mg/kg every 2 weeks

Dosage adjustment in toxicity: Patient with IgE antibodies to agalsidase beta (rechallenge): 0.5 mg/kg every 2 weeks at an initial maximum infusion rate of 0.01 mg/minute; may gradually escalate dose (to maximum of 1 mg/kg every 2 weeks) and/or infusion rate (doubling the infusion rate every 30 minutes to a maximum rate of 0.25 mg/minute) as tolerated.

Dosage adjustment in renal impairment: No dosage adjustment required.

Dosage adjustment in hepatic impairment: No dosage adjustment provided in manufacturer's labeling.

Additional Information Complete prescribing information should be consulted for additional detail.

Dosage Forms

Solution Reconstituted, Intravenous:

Fabrazyme: 5 mg (1 ea); 35 mg (1 ea)

◆ **AG-Citalopram (Can)** *see* Citalopram *on page 451*

◆ **Aggrastat** *see* Tirofiban *on page 2049*

◆ **Aggrenox®** *see* Aspirin and Dipyridamole *on page 185*

◆ **AGN 1135** *see* Rasagiline *on page 1781*

◆ **$AgNO_3$** *see* Silver Nitrate *on page 1886*

◆ **Agriflu (Can)** *see* Influenza Virus Vaccine (Inactivated) *on page 1075*

◆ **Agrylin** *see* Anagrelide *on page 147*

◆ **AHF** *see* Antihemophilic Factor (Recombinant [Porcine Sequence]) *on page 153*

◆ **AHF (Human)** *see* Antihemophilic Factor (Human) *on page 152*

◆ **AHF (Human)** *see* Antihemophilic Factor/von Willebrand Factor Complex (Human) *on page 154*

◆ **AHF (Recombinant)** *see* Antihemophilic Factor (Recombinant) *on page 152*

◆ **AHF (Recombinant)** *see* Antihemophilic Factor (Recombinant [Porcine Sequence]) *on page 153*

◆ **A-hydroCort** *see* Hydrocortisone (Systemic) *on page 1013*

◆ **A-Hydrocort** *see* Hydrocortisone (Systemic) *on page 1013*

◆ **A-hydroCort** *see* Hydrocortisone (Topical) *on page 1014*

◆ **AICC** *see* Anti-inhibitor Coagulant Complex (Human) *on page 155*

◆ **AIDS222089** *see* Bedaquiline *on page 233*

◆ **Airomir (Can)** *see* Albuterol *on page 69*

◆ **AJ-PIP/TAZ (Can)** *see* Piperacillin and Tazobactam *on page 1657*

◆ **AK Cide Oph (Can)** *see* Sulfacetamide and Prednisolone *on page 1944*

◆ **AK-Fluor** *see* Fluorescein *on page 894*

◆ **Akne-Mycin [DSC]** *see* Erythromycin (Topical) *on page 765*

◆ **AK Pentolate Oph Soln (Can)** *see* Cyclopentolate *on page 517*

◆ **AK-Poly-Bac™** *see* Bacitracin and Polymyxin B *on page 222*

◆ **AK Sulf Liq (Can)** *see* Sulfacetamide (Ophthalmic) *on page 1943*

◆ **Akynzeo** *see* Netupitant and Palonosetron *on page 1440*

◆ **ALA** *see* Aminolevulinic Acid *on page 114*

◆ **5-ALA** *see* Aminolevulinic Acid *on page 114*

◆ **Ala Cort** *see* Hydrocortisone (Topical) *on page 1014*

◆ **Alagesic LQ** *see* Butalbital, Acetaminophen, and Caffeine *on page 313*

- ◆ **Alamag [OTC]** *see* Aluminum Hydroxide and Magnesium Hydroxide *on page 103*
- ◆ **Alamag Plus [OTC]** *see* Aluminum Hydroxide, Magnesium Hydroxide, and Simethicone *on page 104*
- ◆ **Ala Scalp** *see* Hydrocortisone (Topical) *on page 1014*
- ◆ **Alavert [OTC]** *see* Loratadine *on page 1241*
- ◆ **Alavert™ Allergy and Sinus [OTC]** *see* Loratadine and Pseudoephedrine *on page 1242*
- ◆ **Alaway [OTC]** *see* Ketotifen (Ophthalmic) *on page 1150*
- ◆ **Alaway Childrens Allergy [OTC]** *see* Ketotifen (Ophthalmic) *on page 1150*

Albendazole (al BEN da zole)

Brand Names: U.S. Albenza

Pharmacologic Category Anthelmintic

Use Treatment of parenchymal neurocysticercosis caused by *Taenia solium* and cystic hydatid disease of the liver, lung, and peritoneum caused by *Echinococcus granulosus*

Pregnancy Risk Factor C

Pregnancy Considerations Adverse events were observed in animal reproduction studies. Albendazole should not be used during pregnancy, if at all possible. The manufacturer recommends a pregnancy test prior to therapy in women of reproductive potential. Women should be advised to avoid pregnancy for at least 1 month following therapy. Discontinue if pregnancy occurs during treatment.

Breast-Feeding Considerations Albendazole excretion into breast milk was studied following a single oral 400 mg dose in breast-feeding women 2 weeks to 6 months postpartum (n=33). Mean albendazole concentrations 6 hours after the dose were 63.7 ± 11.9 ng/mL (maternal serum) and 31.9 ± 9.2 ng/mL (milk). An active and inactive metabolite was also detected in breast milk (Abdel-tawab, 2009). The manufacturer recommends that caution be exercised when administering albendazole to nursing women.

Contraindications Hypersensitivity to albendazole, benzimidazoles, or any component of the formulation

Warnings/Precautions Reversible elevations in hepatic enzymes have been reported; patients with abnormal LFTs and hepatic echinococcosis are at an increased risk of hepatotoxicity. Discontinue therapy if LFT elevations are >2 times the upper limit of normal; may consider restarting treatment with frequent monitoring of LFTs when hepatic enzymes return to pretreatment values. Agranulocytosis, aplastic anemia, granulocytopenia, leukopenia, and pancytopenia have occurred leading to fatalities (rare); use with caution in patients with hepatic impairment (more susceptible to hematologic toxicity). Discontinue therapy in all patients who develop clinically significant decreases in blood cell counts.

Neurocysticercosis: Corticosteroids (eg, dexamethasone or prednisolone) should be administered before or upon initiation of albendazole therapy to minimize inflammatory reactions and prevent cerebral hypertension. Anticonvulsant therapy should be used concurrently during the first week of therapy to prevent seizures. These measures are important to minimize neurological symptoms which may result from uncovering of preexisting neurocysticercosis when using albendazole to treat other conditions. If retinal lesions exist, weigh risk of further retinal damage due to albendazole-induced changes to the retinal lesion vs benefit of disease treatment.

Adverse Reactions

Central nervous system: Dizziness, fever, headache, intracranial pressure increased, meningeal signs, vertigo

Dermatologic: Alopecia

Gastrointestinal: Abdominal pain, nausea, vomiting

Hepatic: LFTs increased

Rare but important or life-threatening: Acute liver failure, acute renal failure, aplastic anemia, agranulocytosis, erythema multiforme, granulocytopenia, hepatitis, hypersensitivity reaction, leukopenia, neutropenia, pancytopenia, rash, Stevens-Johnson syndrome, thrombocytopenia, urticaria

Drug Interactions

Metabolism/Transport Effects **Substrate** of CYP1A2 (minor), CYP3A4 (minor); **Note:** Assignment of Major/Minor substrate status based on clinically relevant drug interaction potential

Avoid Concomitant Use There are no known interactions where it is recommended to avoid concomitant use.

Increased Effect/Toxicity

The levels/effects of Albendazole may be increased by: Grapefruit Juice

Decreased Effect

The levels/effects of Albendazole may be decreased by: Aminoquinolines (Antimalarial); CarBAMazepine; PHENobarbital; Phenytoin

Food Interactions Albendazole serum levels may be increased if taken with a fatty meal (increases the oral bioavailability by up to 5 times). Management: Should be administered with a high-fat meal (peanuts or ice cream).

Storage/Stability Store between 20°C and 25°C (68°F to 77°F)

Mechanism of Action Active metabolite, albendazole sulfoxide, causes selective degeneration of cytoplasmic microtubules in intestinal and tegmental cells of intestinal helminths and larvae; glycogen is depleted, glucose uptake and cholinesterase secretion are impaired, and desecratory substances accumulate intracellulary. ATP production decreases causing energy depletion, immobilization, and worm death.

Pharmacodynamics/Kinetics

Absorption: Poor; may increase up to 5 times when administered with a fatty meal

Distribution: Well inside hydatid cysts and CSF

Protein binding: 70%

Metabolism: Hepatic; extensive first-pass effect; pathways include rapid sulfoxidation to active metabolite (albendazole sulfoxide [major]), hydrolysis, and oxidation

Half-life elimination: 8-12 hours

Time to peak, serum: 2-5 hours

Excretion: Urine (<1% as active metabolite); feces

Dosage Oral:

Infants and Children: Microsporidiosis (other than *Enterocytozoon bienuesi* or *V. corneae*), disseminated or intestinal infection (HIV-positive, off-label use): 15 mg/kg/day (maximum: 800 mg/day) in 2 divided doses continued until immune reconstitution after HAART initiation (CDC, 2009)

Children:

Cysticercus cellulosae (off-label use): 15 mg/kg/day (maximum: 800 mg/day) in 2 divided doses for 8-30 days; may be repeated as necessary

Echinococcus granulosus (tapeworm) (off-label use): 15 mg/kg/day (maximum: 800 mg) divided twice daily for 1-6 months

Giardia duodenalis (giardiasis) (off-label use): 10 mg/kg/day for 5 days (Yereli, 2004)

Children and Adults:

Neurocysticercosis:

<60 kg: 15 mg/kg/day in 2 divided doses (maximum: 800 mg/day) for 8-30 days

≥60 kg: 800 mg/day in 2 divided doses for 8-30 days

Note: Give concurrent anticonvulsant and corticosteroid (eg, dexamethasone or prednisolone) therapy during first week.

Hydatid:

<60 kg: 15 mg/kg/day in 2 divided doses (maximum: 800 mg/day)

≥60 kg: 800 mg/day in 2 divided doses

Note: Administer dose for three 28-day cycles with a 14-day drug-free interval in between each cycle.

Ancylostoma caninum, *Ascaris lumbricoides* (roundworm), *Ancylostoma duodenale* (hookworm), and *Necator americanus* (hookworm) (off-label use): 400 mg as a single dose

Clonorchis sinensis (Chinese liver fluke) (off-label use): 10 mg/kg/day for 7 days

Cutaneous larva migrans (off-label use): 400 mg once daily for 3 days

Enterobius vermicularis (pinworm) (off-label use): 400 mg as a single dose; repeat in 2 weeks

Gnathostoma spinigerum (off-label use): 800 mg/day in 2 divided doses for 21 days

Gongylonemiasis (off-label use): 400 mg once daily for 3 days

Mansonella perstans (off-label use): 800 mg/day in 2 divided doses for 10 days

Oesophagostomum bifurcum (off-label use): 400 mg as a single dose (Ziem, 2004)

Trichinella spiralis (Trichinellosis) (off-label use): 800 mg/day in 2 divided doses for 8-14 days plus corticosteroids for severe symptoms

Visceral larva migrans (toxocariasis) (off-label use): 800 mg/day in 2 divided doses for 5 days

Adults:

Cysticercus cellulosae (off-label use): 800 mg/day in 2 divided doses for 8-30 days; may be repeated as necessary

Disseminated microsporidiosis (off-label use): 800 mg/day in 2 divided doses

Echinococcus granulosus (tapeworm) (off-label use): 800 mg/day in 2 divided doses for 1-6 months

Giardia duodenalis (giardiasis) (off-label use): 400 mg once daily for 5 days

Intestinal microsporidiosis (*E. intestinalis*) (off-label use): 800 mg/day in 2 divided doses for 21 days

Ocular microsporidiosis (off-label use): 800 mg/day in 2 divided doses, in combination with fumagillin

Dosage adjustment in renal impairment: No dosage adjustment provided in the manufacturer's labeling (has not been studied). However, the need for adjustment not likely since albendazole is primarily eliminated by hepatic metabolism.

Dosage adjustment in hepatic impairment: No dosage adjustment provided in manufacturer's labeling. However, patients with underlying liver disease may be more at risk for adverse effects.

Dietary Considerations Should be taken with a high-fat meal.

Administration Should be administered with a high-fat meal. Administer anticonvulsant and corticosteroid therapy during first week of neurocysticercosis therapy. If patients have difficulty swallowing, tablets may be crushed or chewed, then swallowed with a drink of water.

Monitoring Parameters Monitor fecal specimens for ova and parasites for 3 weeks after treatment; if positive, retreat; LFTs and CBC with differential at start of each 28-day cycle and every 2 weeks during therapy (more frequent monitoring for patients with liver disease); ophthalmic exam (patients with neurocysticercosis); pregnancy test

Dosage Forms

Tablet, Oral:

Albenza: 200 mg

◆ **Albenza** *see* Albendazole *on page 65*

Albiglutide (al bi GLOO tide)

Brand Names: U.S. Tanzeum

Index Terms Tanzeum

Pharmacologic Category Antidiabetic Agent, Glucagon-Like Peptide-1 (GLP-1) Receptor Agonist

Use Diabetes mellitus, type 2: Adjunct to diet and exercise to improve glycemic control in the treatment of type 2 diabetes mellitus (noninsulin dependent, NIDDM)

Pregnancy Risk Factor C

Pregnancy Considerations Adverse events have been observed in some animal reproduction studies. Because of the long washout period, consider stopping albiglutide at least 1 month before a planned pregnancy.

In women with diabetes, maternal hyperglycemia can be associated with congenital malformations as well as adverse effects in the fetus, neonate, and the mother (ACOG, 2005; ADA, 2014; Kitzmiller, 2008; Metzger, 2007). To prevent adverse outcomes, prior to conception and throughout pregnancy maternal blood glucose and HbA_{1c} should be kept as close to normal as possible but without causing significant hypoglycemia (ACOG, 2013; ADA, 2014; Blumer, 2013; Kitzmiller, 2008). Prior to pregnancy, effective contraception should be used until glycemic control is achieved (ADA, 2014; Kitzmiller, 2008). Other agents are currently recommended to treat diabetes in pregnant women (ACOG, 2013; Blumer, 2013).

Breast-Feeding Considerations It is not known if albiglutide is excreted in breast milk. The manufacturer recommends a decision be made whether to discontinue nursing or to discontinue the drug, taking into account the importance of treatment to the mother.

Contraindications Severe hypersensitivity to albiglutide or any component of the formulation; history of or family history of medullary thyroid carcinoma (MTC); patients with multiple endocrine neoplasia syndrome type 2 (MEN2)

Warnings/Precautions [U.S. Boxed Warning] Thyroid C-cell tumors have developed in animal studies with glucagon-like peptide-1 (GLP-1) receptor agonists; it is not known if albiglutide causes thyroid C-cell tumor, including medullary thyroid carcinoma (MTC) in humans. Routine serum calcitonin or thyroid ultrasound monitoring is of uncertain value. Patients should be counseled on the risk and symptoms (eg, neck mass, dysphagia, dyspnea, persistent hoarseness) of thyroid tumors. Use is contraindicated in patients with or a family history of MTC and in patients with multiple endocrine neoplasia syndrome type 2 (MEN2). Consultation with an endocrinologist is recommended in patients with thyroid nodules on physical examination or neck imaging and patients who develop elevated calcitonin concentrations. Serious hypersensitivity reactions (including pruritus, rash, and dyspnea) have been reported with use; discontinue therapy in the event of a hypersensitivity reaction; treat appropriately and monitor patients until signs and symptoms resolve. Cases of acute pancreatitis have been reported; monitor for signs and symptoms of pancreatitis (eg, persistent severe abdominal pain which may radiate to the back and which may or may not be accompanied by vomiting). If pancreatitis is suspected, discontinue use. Do not resume unless an alternative etiology of pancreatitis is confirmed. Consider antidiabetic therapies other than albiglutide in patients with a history of pancreatitis.

Not recommended for first-line therapy of type 2 diabetes mellitus in patients inadequately controlled on diet and exercise alone. Do not use in patients with type 1 diabetes mellitus or for the treatment of diabetic ketoacidosis; not a substitute for insulin. Diabetes self-management education (DSME) is essential to maximize the effectiveness of therapy. Use with caution in patients with renal impairment, particularly during initiation of therapy and dose escalation.

Acute renal failure and chronic renal failure exacerbation (sometimes requiring hemodialysis) have been reported; some cases have been reported in patients with no known preexisting renal disease. Reports primarily occurred in patients with nausea/vomiting/diarrhea or dehydration. Use is not recommended in patients with preexisting severe gastrointestinal disease. Potentially significant drug-drug interactions may exist, requiring dose or frequency adjustment, additional monitoring, and/or selection of alternative therapy. Concomitant use of insulin or insulin secretagogues (eg, sulfonylureas) may increase the risk of hypoglycemia; dosage reduction of insulin or insulin secretagogues may be required. Concurrent use with prandial insulin therapy has not been evaluated. Due to its effects on gastric emptying, albiglutide may reduce the rate and extent of absorption of orally-administered drugs; use with caution in patients receiving medications with a narrow therapeutic window or that require rapid absorption from the GI tract.

Adverse Reactions Reactions reported from monotherapy and combination therapy.

Cardiovascular: Atrial fibrillation

Endocrine & metabolic: Hypoglycemia (combination therapy), increased gamma-glutamyl transferase

Gastrointestinal: Diarrhea, gastroesophageal reflux disease, nausea, vomiting

Immunologic: Antibody development (non-neutralizing)

Infection: Influenza

Local: Injection site reaction (including erythema at injection site, hypersensitivity reaction at injection site, itching at injection site, rash at injection site)

Neuromuscular & skeletal: Arthralgia, back pain

Respiratory: Cough, pneumonia, upper respiratory tract infection

Rare but important or life-threatening: Appendicitis, atrial flutter, hypersensitivity, increased serum ALT, increased serum bilirubin, pancreatitis

Drug Interactions

Metabolism/Transport Effects None known.

Avoid Concomitant Use There are no known interactions where it is recommended to avoid concomitant use.

Increased Effect/Toxicity

Albiglutide may increase the levels/effects of: Insulin; Sulfonylureas

The levels/effects of Albiglutide may be increased by: Androgens; Pegvisomant

Decreased Effect

The levels/effects of Albiglutide may be decreased by: Corticosteroids (Orally Inhaled); Corticosteroids (Systemic); Danazol; Luteinizing Hormone-Releasing Hormone Analogs; Somatropin; Thiazide Diuretics

Preparation for Administration Reconstitute powder with the diluent contained in the pen device. Refer to manufacturer's product labeling for full reconstitution instructions. Administer within 8 hours of reconstitution.

Storage/Stability Store unused pens at 2°C to 8°C (36°F to 46°F); may be stored at room temperature (≤30°C [86°F]) for ≤4 weeks prior to reconstitution. Do not freeze. Use within 8 hours of reconstitution.

Mechanism of Action Albiglutide is an agonist of human glucagon-like peptide-1 (GLP-1) receptor and augments glucose-dependent insulin secretion and slows gastric emptying.

Pharmacodynamics/Kinetics

Distribution: V_d: 11 L

Metabolism: Degradation to small peptides and individual amino acids by proteolytic enzymes.

Half-life elimination: ~5 days

Time to peak, plasma: 3 to 5 days

Dosage

Diabetes mellitus, type 2: Adults: SubQ: 30 mg once weekly; may increase to 50 mg once weekly if inadequate glycemic response. Titration to 50 mg once weekly occurred at week 12 in a monotherapy trial and after a minimum of 4 weeks in combination therapy trials.

Missed doses: If a dose is missed, administer as soon as possible within 3 days after the missed dose; dosing can then be resumed on the usual day of administration. If more than 3 days have passed since the dose was missed, omit the missed dose and resume administration at the next regularly scheduled weekly dose.

Dosage adjustment in renal impairment: No dosage adjustment necessary; use caution when initiating or escalating doses.

Dosage adjustment in hepatic impairment: There are no dosage adjustments provided in the manufacturer's labeling (has not been studied); however, changes in hepatic function are not likely to have an effect on elimination.

Dietary Considerations Individualized medical nutrition therapy (MNT) based on ADA recommendations is an integral part of therapy.

Administration Do not inject intravenously or intramuscularly. Inject subcutaneously into the upper arm, thigh, or abdomen; when administering within the same body region, use a different injection site each week. Administer once weekly on the same day each week, without regard to meals or time of day. The day of weekly administration may be changed, as long as the last dose was administered ≥4 days before. Use immediately after attaching and priming the needle; solution can clog the needle if allowed to dry in the primed needle. If using concomitantly with insulin, administer as separate injections (do not mix); may inject in the same body region as insulin, but not adjacent to one another.

Monitoring Parameters Plasma glucose, HbA_{1c}, renal function, signs/symptoms of pancreatitis

Reference Range

Recommendations for glycemic control in nonpregnant adults with diabetes (ADA, 2015):

HbA_{1c}: <7% (a more aggressive [<6.5%] or less aggressive [<8%] HbA_{1c} goal may be targeted based on patient-specific characteristics)

Preprandial capillary plasma glucose: 80 to 130 mg/dL

Peak postprandial capillary blood glucose: <180 mg/dL

Recommendations for glycemic control in pediatric (all age groups) patients with type 1 diabetes (ADA, 2015):

HbA_{1c}: <7.5% (individualization may be appropriate based on patient-specific characteristics; <7% is reasonable if it can be achieved without excessive hypoglycemia)

Preprandial capillary plasma glucose: 90 to 130 mg/dL

Bedtime and overnight capillary blood glucose: 90 to 150 mg/dL

Dosage Forms

Pen-injector, Subcutaneous [preservative free]:

Tanzeum: 30 mg (1 ea); 50 mg (1 ea)

◆ **Albuked 5** *see* Albumin *on page 67*

◆ **Albuked 25** *see* Albumin *on page 67*

Albumin (al BYOO min)

Brand Names: U.S. Albuked 25; Albuked 5; Albumin-ZLB; Albuminar-25; Albuminar-5; AlbuRx; Albutein; Buminate; Flexbumin; Human Albumin Grifols; Kedbumin; Plasbumin-25; Plasbumin-5

Brand Names: Canada Alburex 25; Alburex 5; Albutein 25%; Albutein 5%; Buminate-25%; Buminate-5%; Plasbumin-25; Plasbumin-5

Index Terms Albumin (Human); Normal Human Serum Albumin; Normal Serum Albumin (Human); Salt Poor Albumin; SPA

Pharmacologic Category Blood Product Derivative; Plasma Volume Expander, Colloid

Use Hypovolemia: Plasma volume expansion and maintenance of cardiac output in the treatment of certain types of shock or impending shock; may be useful for burn patients, ARDS, severe nephrosis, hemolytic disease of the newborn, and cardiopulmonary bypass; unless the condition responsible for hypoproteinemia can be corrected, albumin can provide only symptomatic relief or supportive treatment

Note: Nutritional supplementation is not an appropriate indication.

Pregnancy Risk Factor C

Pregnancy Considerations Animal reproduction studies have not been conducted. Albumin is used for the treatment of ovarian hyperstimulation syndrome (ASRM, 2008). Use for other indications may be considered in pregnant women when contraindications to nonprotein colloids exist (Liumbruno, 2009).

Breast-Feeding Considerations Endogenous albumin is found in breast milk. The manufacturer recommends that caution be exercised when administering albumin to nursing women.

Contraindications Hypersensitivity to albumin or any component of the formulation; severe anemia; cardiac failure; dilution with sterile water for injection

Warnings/Precautions Anaphylaxis may occur; discontinue immediately if allergic or anaphylactic reactions are suspected. Cardiac or respiratory failure, renal failure, or increasing intracranial pressure can occur; closely monitor hemodynamic parameters in all patients. Use with caution in conditions where hypervolemia and its consequences or hemodilution may increase the risk of adverse effects (eg, heart failure, pulmonary edema, hypertension, hemorrhagic diathesis, esophageal varices). Adjust rate of administration per hemodynamic status and solution concentration; monitor closely with rapid infusions. Avoid rapid infusions in patients with a history of cardiovascular disease (may cause circulatory overload and pulmonary edema). Discontinue at the first signs of cardiovascular overload (eg, headache, dyspnea, jugular venous distention, rales, abnormal elevations in systemic or central venous blood pressure). All patients should be observed for signs of hypervolemia such as pulmonary edema.

Use with caution in patients with hepatic or renal impairment because of added protein load. Use with caution in those patients for whom sodium restriction is necessary. The parenteral product may contain aluminum (Kelly, 1989); toxic aluminum concentrations may be seen with high doses, prolonged use, or renal dysfunction. Premature neonates are at higher risk due to immature renal function and aluminum intake from other parenteral sources. Parenteral aluminum exposure of >4 to 5 mcg/kg/day is associated with CNS and bone toxicity; tissue loading may occur at lower doses (Federal Register, 2002). See manufacturer's labeling. Albumin is a product of human plasma, may potentially contain infectious agents which could transmit disease. Screening of donors, as well as testing and/or inactivation or removal of certain viruses, reduces the risk. Infections thought to be transmitted by this product should be reported to the manufacturer. Packaging may contain natural latex rubber. Patients with chronic renal insufficiency receiving albumin solution may be at risk for accumulation of aluminum and potential toxicities (eg, hypercalcemia, vitamin D refractory osteodystrophy, anemia, and severe progressive encephalopathy).

Adverse Reactions

Cardiovascular: Congestive heart failure (precipitation), edema, hypertension, hypotension, tachycardia
Central nervous system: Chills, headache
Dermatologic: Pruritus, skin rash, urticaria
Endocrine & metabolic: Hypervolemia
Gastrointestinal: Nausea, vomiting
Hypersensitivity: Anaphylaxis
Respiratory: Bronchospasm, pulmonary edema
Miscellaneous: Fever

Drug Interactions

Metabolism/Transport Effects None known.

Avoid Concomitant Use There are no known interactions where it is recommended to avoid concomitant use.

Increased Effect/Toxicity There are no known significant interactions involving an increase in effect.

Decreased Effect There are no known significant interactions involving a decrease in effect.

Preparation for Administration May dilute 25% albumin solutions with NS or D_5W. Do not use sterile water to dilute albumin solutions, as this has been associated with hypotonic-associated hemolysis. If 5% human albumin is unavailable, it may be prepared by diluting 25% human albumin with 0.9% sodium chloride or 5% dextrose in water. Do not use sterile water to dilute albumin solutions, as this has been associated with hypotonic-associated hemolysis.

Storage/Stability Store at ≤30°C (86°F); do not freeze. Do not use solution if it is turbid or contains a deposit; use within 4 hours after opening vial; discard unused portion.

Mechanism of Action Provides increase in intravascular oncotic pressure and causes mobilization of fluids from interstitial into intravascular space

Dosage IV:

5% should be used in hypovolemic patients or intravascularly-depleted patients

25% should be used in patients in whom fluid and sodium intake must be minimized

Dose depends on condition of patient:

Infants: Hemolytic disease of the newborn: 1 g/kg/dose of 25% albumin prior to or during exchange transfusion

Infants and Younger Children: Hypovolemia: 0.5 to 1 g/kg/dose (10 to 20 mL/kg/dose of albumin 5%); repeat in 30 minute intervals as needed

Older Children and Adolescents: Hypovolemia: 2.5 to 25 g (250 to 500 mL of albumin 5%); repeat in 30 minute intervals as needed.

Adults: Usual dose: 25 g; initial dose may be repeated in 15 to 30 minutes if response is inadequate.

Hypovolemia: 5% albumin: 12.5 to 25 g (250 to 500 mL); repeat as needed. **Note:** May be considered after inadequate response to crystalloid therapy and when nonprotein colloids are contraindicated. The volume administered and the speed of infusion should be adapted to individual response.

Large-volume paracentesis (>5 L) (off-label use): 25% albumin: 5 to 8 g for every liter removed (Garcia-Compeán, 1993; Moore, 2003) **or** 50 g total for paracentesis >5 L (ATS, 2004). **Note:** Administer soon after the procedure to avoid postprocedural complications (eg, hypovolemia, hyponatremia, renal impairment) (Moore, 2003).

SBP in patients with cirrhosis (off-label use): 25% albumin: Initial: 1.5 g/kg, followed by 1 g/kg on day 3 (in conjunction with appropriate antimicrobial therapy) (ATS, 2004; Sort, 1999). **Note:** Clinical trial employed albumin 20%; however, the difference in concentration compared with 25% albumin is deemed to be clinically inconsequential.

Dosage adjustment in renal impairment: There are no dosage adjustments provided in the manufacturer's labeling; use with caution.

Dosage adjustment in hepatic impairment: There are no dosage adjustments provided in the manufacturer's labeling.

Dietary Considerations Some products may contain potassium and/or sodium.

Administration

For IV administration only. Use within 4 hours after opening vial; discard unused portion. In emergencies, may administer as rapidly as necessary to improve clinical condition. After initial volume replacement:

5%: Do not exceed 2 to 4 mL/minute in patients with normal plasma volume; 5 to 10 mL/minute in patients with hypoproteinemia

25%: Do not exceed 1 mL/minute in patients with normal plasma volume; 2 to 3 mL/minute in patients with hypoproteinemia

Rapid infusion may cause vascular overload. Albumin 25% may be given undiluted or diluted in normal saline. May give in combination or through the same administration set as saline or carbohydrates. Do not use with ethanol or protein hydrolysates (precipitation may form).

Monitoring Parameters Hemodynamic parameters, blood pressure, pulmonary edema, hematocrit, electrolytes, infusion rate

Additional Information Albumin 5% and 25% solutions contain 130-160 mEq/L sodium and are considered isotonic with plasma. Dilution of albumin 25% solution with sterile water produces a hypotonic solution; administration of such can cause hemolysis and/or renal failure. An albumin 5% solution is osmotically equivalent to an equal volume of plasma, whereas a 25% solution is osmotically equivalent to 5 times its volume of plasma. Albumin solutions are heated to 60°C for 10 hours, decreasing any possible risk of viral hepatitis transmission. To date, there have been no reports of viral transmission using these products.

Dosage Forms

Solution, Intravenous:

Albumin-ZLB: 5% (250 mL, 500 mL); 25% (50 mL, 100 mL)
Albuminar-5: 5% (250 mL, 500 mL)
Albuminar-25: 25% (50 mL, 100 mL)
AlbuRx: 5% (250 mL, 500 mL)
Albutein: 25% (50 mL, 100 mL)
Buminate: 5% (250 mL, 500 mL); 25% (20 mL)
Plasbumin-5: 5% (50 mL, 250 mL)
Plasbumin-25: 25% (20 mL, 50 mL, 100 mL)
Generic: 5% (50 mL); 25% (50 mL, 100 mL)

Solution, Intravenous [preservative free]:

Albuked 5: 5% (250 mL)
Albuked 25: 25% (50 mL, 100 mL)
Albutein: 5% (250 mL, 500 mL); 25% (50 mL, 100 mL)
Flexbumin: 5% (250 mL); 25% (50 mL, 100 mL)
Human Albumin Grifols: 25% (50 mL, 100 mL)
Kedbumin: 25% (50 mL, 100 mL)
Plasbumin-5: 5% (50 mL, 250 mL)
Plasbumin-25: 25% (20 mL, 50 mL, 100 mL)
Generic: 5% (100 mL, 250 mL, 500 mL); 25% (50 mL, 100 mL)

- ◆ **Albuminar-5** *see* Albumin *on page 67*
- ◆ **Albuminar-25** *see* Albumin *on page 67*
- ◆ **Albumin-Bound Paclitaxel** *see* PACLitaxel (Protein Bound) *on page 1554*
- ◆ **Albumin (Human)** *see* Albumin *on page 67*
- ◆ **Albumin-Stabilized Nanoparticle Paclitaxel** *see* PACLitaxel (Protein Bound) *on page 1554*
- ◆ **Albumin-ZLB** *see* Albumin *on page 67*
- ◆ **Alburex 5 (Can)** *see* Albumin *on page 67*
- ◆ **Alburex 25 (Can)** *see* Albumin *on page 67*
- ◆ **AlbuRx** *see* Albumin *on page 67*
- ◆ **Albutein** *see* Albumin *on page 67*
- ◆ **Albutein 5% (Can)** *see* Albumin *on page 67*
- ◆ **Albutein 25% (Can)** *see* Albumin *on page 67*

Albuterol (al BYOO ter ole)

Brand Names: U.S. AccuNeb [DSC]; ProAir HFA; Proventil HFA; Ventolin HFA; VoSpire ER

Brand Names: Canada Airomir; Apo-Salvent; Apo-Salvent AEM; Apo-Salvent CFC Free; Apo-Salvent Sterules; Dom-Salbutamol; Novo-Salbutamol HFA; PHL-Salbutamol; PMS-Salbutamol; ratio-Ipra-Sal; ratio-Salbutamol; Salbutamol HFA; Sandoz-Salbutamol; Teva-Salbutamol; Teva-Salbutamol Sterinebs P.F.; Ventolin Diskus; Ventolin HFA; Ventolin I.V. Infusion; Ventolin Nebules P.F.

Index Terms Albuterol Sulfate; Salbutamol; Salbutamol Sulphate

Pharmacologic Category Beta$_2$ Agonist

Use Treatment or prevention of bronchospasm in patients with reversible obstructive airway disease; prevention of exercise-induced bronchospasm

Pregnancy Risk Factor C

Pregnancy Considerations Adverse events were observed in some animal reproduction studies. Albuterol crosses the placenta (Boulton, 1997). Congenital anomalies (cleft palate, limb defects) have rarely been reported following maternal use during pregnancy. Multiple medications were used in most cases, no specific pattern of defects has been reported, and no relationship to albuterol has been established. The amount of albuterol available systemically following inhalation is significantly less in comparison to oral doses.

Uncontrolled asthma is associated with adverse events on pregnancy (increased risk of perinatal mortality, preeclampsia, preterm birth, low birth weight infants). Albuterol is the preferred short acting beta agonist when treatment for asthma is needed during pregnancy (NAEPP, 2005; NAEPP, 2007).

Albuterol may affect uterine contractility. Maternal pulmonary edema and other adverse events have been reported when albuterol was used for tocolysis. Albuterol is not approved for use as a tocolytic; use caution when needed to treat bronchospasm in pregnant women. Use of the injection (Canadian product; not available in the U.S.) is specifically contraindicated in women during the first or second trimester who may be at risk of threatened abortion.

Breast-Feeding Considerations It is not known if albuterol is excreted into breast milk. The amount of albuterol available systemically following inhalation is significantly less in comparison to oral doses. According to the manufacturer, the decision to continue or discontinue breast-feeding during therapy should take into account the risk of exposure to the infant and the benefits of treatment to the mother. The use of beta-2-receptor agonists are not considered a contraindication to breast-feeding (NAEPP, 2005).

Contraindications Hypersensitivity to albuterol or any component of the formulation

Injection formulation [Canadian product]: Hypersensitivity to albuterol or any component of the formulation; tachyarrhythmias; risk of abortion during first or second trimester

Warnings/Precautions Optimize anti-inflammatory treatment before initiating maintenance treatment with albuterol. Do not use as a component of chronic therapy without an anti-inflammatory agent. Only the mildest forms of asthma (Step 1 and/or exercise-induced) would not require concurrent use based upon asthma guidelines. Patient must be instructed to seek medical attention in ▶

cases where acute symptoms are not relieved or a previous level of response is diminished. The need to increase frequency of use may indicate deterioration of asthma, and treatment must not be delayed.

Use caution in patients with cardiovascular disease (arrhythmia or hypertension or HF), convulsive disorders, diabetes, glaucoma, hyperthyroidism, or hypokalemia. Beta-agonists may cause elevation in blood pressure, heart rate, and result in CNS stimulation/excitation. Beta$_2$-agonists may increase risk of arrhythmia, increase serum glucose, or decrease serum potassium.

Immediate hypersensitivity reactions (urticaria, angioedema, rash, bronchospasm) have been reported. Do not exceed recommended dose; serious adverse events, including fatalities, have been associated with excessive use of inhaled sympathomimetics. Rarely, paradoxical bronchospasm may occur with use of inhaled bronchodilating agents; this should be distinguished from inadequate response. All patients should utilize a spacer device or valved holding chamber when using a metered-dose inhaler; in addition, use spacer for children <5 years of age and consider adding a face mask for infants and children <4 years of age.

Adverse Reactions Incidence of adverse effects is dependent upon age of patient, dose, and route of administration.

Cardiovascular: Chest discomfort, chest pain, edema, extrasystoles, flushing, hypertension, palpitations, tachycardia

Central nervous system: Anxiety, ataxia, depression, dizziness, drowsiness, emotional lability, excitement (children and adolescents 2 to 14 years), fatigue, headache, hyperactivity (children and adolescents 6 to 14 years), insomnia, malaise, migraine, nervousness, restlessness, rigors, shakiness (children and adolescents 6 to 14 years), vertigo, voice disorder

Dermatologic: Diaphoresis, pallor (children 2 to 6 years), skin rash, urticaria

Endocrine & metabolic: Diabetes mellitus, increased serum glucose

Gastrointestinal: Anorexia (children 2 to 6 years), diarrhea, dyspepsia, eructation, flatulence, gastroenteritis, gastrointestinal symptoms (children 2 to 6 years), glossitis, increased appetite (children and adolescents 6 to 14 years), nausea, unpleasant taste (inhalation site), vomiting, xerostomia

Genitourinary: Difficulty in micturition, urinary tract infection

Hematologic & oncologic: Decreased hematocrit, decreased hemoglobin, decreased white blood cell count, lymphadenopathy

Hepatic: Increased serum ALT, increased serum AST

Hypersensitivity: Hypersensitivity reaction

Infection: Cold symptoms, infection

Local: Application site reaction (HFA inhaler)

Neuromuscular & skeletal: Back pain, hyperkinesia, leg cramps, muscle cramps (frequency increases with age), musculoskeletal pain, tremor (frequency increases with age)

Ophthalmic: Conjunctivitis (children 2 to 6 years)

Otic: Ear disease, otalgia, otitis media, tinnitus

Respiratory: Bronchitis, bronchospasm (exacerbation of underlying pulmonary disease), cough (adolescents and adults), dyspnea, epistaxis (children and adolescents 6 to 14 years), exacerbation of asthma, flu-like symptoms, increased bronchial secretions, laryngitis, nasal congestion, oropharyngeal edema, pharyngitis, pulmonary disease, respiratory tract disease, rhinitis, throat irritation, upper respiratory tract infection, upper respiratory tract inflammation, viral upper respiratory tract infection, wheezing

Miscellaneous: Accidental injury, fever

Rare but important or life-threatening: Anaphylaxis, exacerbation of diabetes mellitus, glossitis, hyperglycemia, hypokalemia, hypotension, ketoacidosis, lactic acidosis, peripheral vasodilation

Drug Interactions

Metabolism/Transport Effects None known.

Avoid Concomitant Use

Avoid concomitant use of Albuterol with any of the following: Beta-Blockers (Nonselective); Iobenguane I 123

Increased Effect/Toxicity

Albuterol may increase the levels/effects of: Atosiban; Loop Diuretics; Sympathomimetics; Thiazide Diuretics

The levels/effects of Albuterol may be increased by: AtoMOXetine; Cannabinoid-Containing Products; Linezolid; MAO Inhibitors; Tedizolid; Tricyclic Antidepressants

Decreased Effect

Albuterol may decrease the levels/effects of: Iobenguane I 123

The levels/effects of Albuterol may be decreased by: Beta-Blockers (Beta1 Selective); Beta-Blockers (Nonselective); Betahistine

Preparation for Administration Solution for nebulization: To prepare a 2.5 mg dose, dilute 0.5 mL of solution to a total of 3 mL with normal saline; also compatible with cromolyn or ipratropium nebulizer solutions.

Storage/Stability

HFA aerosols: Store at 15°C to 25°C (59°F to 77°F).

Ventolin HFA: Discard when counter reads 000 or 12 months after removal from protective pouch, whichever comes first. Store with mouthpiece down.

Infusion solution [Canadian product]: Ventolin IV: Store at 15°C to 30°C (59°F to 86°F). Protect from light. After dilution, discard unused portion after 24 hours.

Solution for nebulization: Store at 2°C to 25°C (36°F to 77°F). Do not use if solution changes color or becomes cloudy. Products packaged in foil should be used within 1 week (or according to the manufacturer's recommendations) if removed from foil pouch.

Syrup: Store at 20°C to 25°C (68°F to 77°F).

Tablet: Store at 20°C to 25°C (68°F to 77°F).

Tablet, extended release: Store at 20°C to 25°C (68°F to 77°F)

Mechanism of Action Relaxes bronchial smooth muscle by action on beta$_2$-receptors with little effect on heart rate

Pharmacodynamics/Kinetics

Onset of action: Peak effect:

Nebulization/oral inhalation: 0.5 to 2 hours

CFC-propelled albuterol: 10 minutes

Ventolin HFA: 25 minutes

Oral: 2 to 3 hours

Duration: Nebulization/oral inhalation: 3 to 4 hours; Oral: 4 to 6 hours

Metabolism: Hepatic to an inactive sulfate

Half-life elimination: Inhalation: 3.8 hours; Oral: 3.7 to 5 hours

Excretion: Urine (30% as unchanged drug)

Dosage

Metered-dose inhaler (90 mcg/puff):

Children ≤4 years *(NAEPP, 2007)*:

Quick relief: 2 puffs every 4 to 6 hours as needed

Exacerbation of asthma (acute, severe): 4 to 8 puffs every 20 minutes for 3 doses, then every 1 to 4 hours as needed

Exercise-induced bronchospasm (prevention): 1 to 2 puffs 5 minutes prior to exercise

Children 5 to 11 years *(NAEPP, 2007)*:

Bronchospasm, quick relief: 2 puffs every 4 to 6 hours as needed

Exacerbation of asthma (acute, severe): 4 to 8 puffs every 20 minutes for 3 doses, then every 1 to 4 hours as needed

Exercise-induced bronchospasm (prevention): 2 puffs 5 to 30 minutes prior to exercise

Children ≥12 years and Adults:

Bronchospasm, quick relief *(NAEPP, 2007)*: 2 puffs every 4 to 6 hours as needed

Exacerbation of asthma (acute, severe) *(NAEPP, 2007)*: 4 to 8 puffs every 20 minutes for up to 4 hours, then every 1 to 4 hours as needed

Exercise-induced bronchospasm (prevention) *(NAEPP, 2007)*: 2 puffs 5 to 30 minutes prior to exercise

Metered-dose inhaler (100 mcg/puff): Airomir [Canadian product]:

Children 6 to 11 years:

Bronchospasm:

Acute treatment: 1 puff; additional puffs may be necessary if inadequate relief however patients should be advised to promptly consult healthcare provider or seek medical attention if no relief from acute treatment

Maintenance: 1 puff; may increase to maximum of 1 puff 4 times daily

Exercise-induced bronchospasm (prevention): 1 puff 30 minutes prior to exercise

Children ≥12 years and Adults:

Bronchospasm:

Acute treatment: 1 to 2 puffs; additional puffs may be necessary if inadequate relief however patients should be advised to promptly consult healthcare provider or seek medical attention if no relief from acute treatment

Maintenance: 1 to 2 puffs 3 to 4 times daily (maximum: 8 puffs daily)

Exercise-induced bronchospasm (prevention): 2 puffs 30 minutes prior to exercise

Nebulization solution:

Children 2 to 12 years: Bronchospasm: 0.63 to 1.25 mg 3 to 4 times daily as needed

Children ≤4 years *(NAEPP, 2007)*:

Quick relief: 0.63 to 2.5 mg every 4 to 6 hours as needed

Exacerbation of asthma (acute, severe): 0.15 mg/kg (minimum: 2.5 mg) every 20 minutes for 3 doses, then 0.15 to 0.3 mg/kg (maximum: 10 mg) every 1 to 4 hours as needed **or** 0.5 mg/kg/hour by continuous nebulization

Children 5 to 11 years *(NAEPP, 2007)*:

Quick relief: 1.25 to 5 mg every 4 to 8 hours as needed

Exacerbation of asthma (acute, severe): 0.15 mg/kg (minimum: 2.5 mg) every 20 minutes for 3 doses, then 0.15 to 0.3 mg/kg (maximum: 10 mg) every 1 to 4 hours as needed **or** 0.5 mg/kg/hour by continuous nebulization

Children ≥12 years and Adults:

Bronchospasm: 2.5 mg 3 to 4 times daily as needed

Quick relief *(NAEPP, 2007)*: 1.25 to 5 mg every 4 to 8 hours as needed

Exacerbation of asthma (acute, severe) *(NAEPP, 2007)*: 2.5 to 5 mg every 20 minutes for 3 doses then 2.5 to 10 mg every 1 to 4 hours as needed, **or** 10 to 15 mg/hour by continuous nebulization

Oral: Note: Oral is not the preferred route for treatment of asthma; inhalation via nebulization or MDI is preferred (NAEPP, 2007).

Children: Bronchospasm:

2 to 6 years: 0.1 to 0.2 mg/kg/dose 3 times daily maximum dose not to exceed 12 mg daily (divided doses)

6 to 12 years: 2 mg/dose 3 to 4 times daily; maximum dose not to exceed 24 mg daily (divided doses)

Extended release: 4 mg every 12 hours; maximum dose not to exceed 24 mg daily (divided doses)

Children >12 years and Adults: Bronchospasm (treatment): 2 to 4 mg/dose 3 to 4 times daily; maximum dose not to exceed 32 mg daily (divided doses)

Extended release: 8 mg every 12 hours; maximum dose not to exceed 32 mg daily (divided doses). A 4 mg dose every 12 hours may be sufficient in some patients, such as adults of low body weight.

Elderly: Bronchospasm (treatment): 2 mg 3 to 4 times daily; maximum: 8 mg 4 times daily

IV continuous infusion: Adults [Canadian product]: Severe bronchospasm and status asthmaticus: Initial: 5 mcg/minute; may increase up to 10 to 20 mcg/minute at 15- to 30-minute intervals if needed

Dosage adjustment in renal impairment: Use with caution in patients with renal impairment. No dosage adjustment required (including patients on hemodialysis, peritoneal dialysis, or CRRT; Aronoff, 2007).

Dosage adjustment in hepatic impairment: No dosage adjustment provided in manufacturer's labeling.

Administration

Metered-dose inhaler: Shake well before use; prime prior to first use, and whenever inhaler has not been used for >2 weeks or when it has been dropped, by releasing 3 to 4 test sprays into the air (away from face). Airomir Canadian product labeling recommends releasing a minimum of 4 test sprays when priming. HFA inhalers should be cleaned with warm water at least once per week; allow to air dry completely prior to use. A spacer device or valved holding chamber is recommended for use with metered-dose inhalers.

Nebulization solution: Concentrated solution should be diluted prior to use. Blow-by administration is not recommended, use a mask device if patient unable to hold mouthpiece in mouth for administration.

Infusion solution [Canadian product]: Do not inject undiluted. Reduce concentration by at least 50% before infusing. Administer as a continuous infusion via infusion pump.

Oral: Do not crush or chew extended release tablets.

Monitoring Parameters FEV_1, peak flow, and/or other pulmonary function tests; blood pressure, heart rate; CNS stimulation; serum glucose, serum potassium; asthma symptoms; arterial or capillary blood gases (if patients condition warrants)

Additional Information The 2007 National Heart, Lung, and Blood Institute Guidelines for the Diagnosis and Management of Asthma do not recommend the use of oral systemic albuterol as a quick-relief medication and do not recommend regularly scheduled daily, chronic use of inhaled beta-agonists for long-term control of asthma.

Dosage Forms Considerations

ProAir HFA 8.5 g canisters and Proventil HFA 6.7 g canisters contain 200 inhalations.

Ventolin HFA 18 g canisters contain 200 inhalations and the 8 g canisters contain 60 inhalations.

Dosage Forms

Aerosol Solution, Inhalation:

ProAir HFA: 90 mcg/actuation (8.5 g)

Proventil HFA: 90 mcg/actuation (6.7 g)

Ventolin HFA: 90 mcg/actuation (8 g, 18 g)

Nebulization Solution, Inhalation:

Generic: 0.63 mg/3 mL (3 mL); 0.083% [2.5 mg/3 mL] (3 mL); 0.5% [2.5 mg/0.5 mL] (20 mL)

Nebulization Solution, Inhalation [preservative free]:

Generic: 0.63 mg/3 mL (3 mL); 1.25 mg/3 mL (3 mL); 0.083% [2.5 mg/3 mL] (3 mL); 0.5% [2.5 mg/0.5 mL] (1 ea)

Syrup, Oral:
Generic: 2 mg/5 mL (473 mL)
Tablet, Oral:
Generic: 2 mg, 4 mg
Tablet Extended Release 12 Hour, Oral:
VoSpire ER: 4 mg, 8 mg
Generic: 4 mg, 8 mg
Dosage Forms: Canada
Aerosol, for oral inhalation:
Airomir: 100 mcg/inhalation (3.7 g, 6.7 g)
Injection, solution:
Ventolin I.V.: 1 mg/1mL (5 mL)

- **Albuterol and Ipratropium** *see* Ipratropium and Albuterol *on page 1109*
- **Albuterol Sulfate** *see* Albuterol *on page 69*
- **Alcaine** *see* Proparacaine *on page 1728*
- **Alcaine® (Can)** *see* Proparacaine *on page 1728*
- **Alcalak [OTC]** *see* Calcium Carbonate *on page 327*

Alclometasone (al kloe MET a sone)

Brand Names: U.S. Aclovate
Index Terms Alclometasone Dipropionate
Pharmacologic Category Corticosteroid, Topical
Additional Appendix Information
Topical Corticosteroids *on page 2230*
Use Treatment of inflammation of corticosteroid-responsive dermatosis (low to medium potency topical corticosteroid)
Pregnancy Risk Factor C
Dosage Note: Therapy should be discontinued when control is achieved; if no improvement is seen within 2 weeks, reassessment of diagnosis may be necessary.
Topical:
Children ≥1 year: Apply thin film to affected area 2-3 times/day; do not use for >3 weeks
Adults: Apply a thin film to the affected area 2-3 times/day
Additional Information Complete prescribing information should be consulted for additional detail.
Dosage Forms
Cream, External:
Aclovate: 0.05% (15 g, 60 g)
Generic: 0.05% (15 g, 45 g, 60 g)
Ointment, External:
Generic: 0.05% (15 g, 45 g, 60 g)

- **Alclometasone Dipropionate** *see* Alclometasone *on page 72*
- **Alcortin A** *see* Iodoquinol and Hydrocortisone *on page 1105*
- **Aldactone** *see* Spironolactone *on page 1931*
- **Aldara** *see* Imiquimod *on page 1055*
- **Aldara P (Can)** *see* Imiquimod *on page 1055*

Aldesleukin (al des LOO kin)

Brand Names: U.S. Proleukin
Brand Names: Canada Proleukin
Index Terms IL-2; Interleukin 2; Interleukin-2; Lymphocyte Mitogenic Factor; Recombinant Human Interleukin-2; T-Cell Growth Factor; TCGF; Thymocyte Stimulating Factor
Pharmacologic Category Antineoplastic Agent, Biological Response Modulator; Antineoplastic Agent, Miscellaneous
Use
Melanoma, metastatic: Treatment of metastatic melanoma
Renal cell cancer, metastatic: Treatment of metastatic renal cell cancer

Limitations of use: Careful patient selection is necessary. Assess performance status (PS); patients with a more favorable PS (Eastern Cooperative Oncology Group [ECOG] PS 0) at treatment initiation respond better to aldesleukin (higher response rate and lower toxicity). Experience in patients with ECOG PS >1 is limited.
Pregnancy Risk Factor C
Pregnancy Considerations Adverse events were observed in animal reproduction studies. Use during pregnancy only if benefits to the mother outweigh potential risk to the fetus. Effective contraception is recommended for fertile males and/or females using this medication.
Breast-Feeding Considerations It is not known if aldesleukin is excreted in breast milk. Due to the potential for serious adverse reactions in the breast-feeding infant, a decision should be made to discontinue breast-feeding or to discontinue the drug, taking into account the importance of treatment to the mother.
Contraindications Hypersensitivity to aldesleukin or any component of the formulation; patients with abnormal thallium stress or pulmonary function tests; patients who have had an organ allograft. **Retreatment is contraindicated** in patients who have experienced sustained ventricular tachycardia (≥5 beats), uncontrolled or unresponsive cardiac arrhythmias, chest pain with ECG changes consistent with angina or MI, cardiac tamponade, intubation >72 hours, renal failure requiring dialysis for >72 hours, coma or toxic psychosis lasting >48 hours, repetitive or refractory seizures, bowel ischemia/perforation, or GI bleeding requiring surgery.
Warnings/Precautions [U.S. Boxed Warning]: Aldesleukin therapy has been associated with capillary leak syndrome (CLS), characterized by vascular tone loss and extravasation of plasma proteins and fluid into extravascular space. CLS results in hypotension and reduced organ perfusion, which may be severe and can result in death. Cardiac arrhythmia, angina, myocardial infarction, respiratory insufficiency (requiring intubation), gastrointestinal bleeding or infarction, renal insufficiency, edema and mental status changes are also associated with CLS. CLS onset is immediately after treatment initiation. Monitor fluid status and organ perfusion status carefully; consider fluids and/or pressor agents to maintain organ perfusion. **[U.S. Boxed Warning]: Therapy should be restricted to patients with normal cardiac and pulmonary functions as defined by thallium stress and formal pulmonary function testing. Extreme caution should be used in patients with a history of prior cardiac or pulmonary disease** and in patients who are fluid-restricted or where edema may be poorly tolerated. Withhold treatment for signs of organ hypoperfusion, including altered mental status, reduced urine output, systolic BP <90 mm Hg or cardiac arrhythmia. Once blood pressure is normalized, may consider diuretics for excessive weight gain/edema. Recovery from CLS generally begins soon after treatment cessation. Perform a thorough clinical evaluation prior to treatment initiation; exclude patients with significant cardiac, pulmonary, renal, hepatic, or central nervous system impairment from treatment. Patients with a more favorable performance status prior to treatment initiation are more likely to respond to aldesleukin treatment, with a higher response rate and generally lower toxicity.

[U.S. Boxed Warning]: Should be administered under the supervision of an experienced cancer chemotherapy physician in a facility with cardiopulmonary or intensive specialists and intensive care facilities available. Adverse effects are frequent and sometimes fatal. May exacerbate preexisting or initial presentation of autoimmune diseases and inflammatory disorders; exacerbation and/or new onset have been reported with aldesleukin and interferon alfa combination therapy. Thyroid disease (hypothyroidism, biphasic thyroiditis, and thyrotoxicosis) may occur; the onset of hypothyroidism is usually 4 to 17 weeks after treatment initiation; may be reversible upon treatment discontinuation (Hamnvik, 2011). Patients should be evaluated and treated for CNS metastases and have a negative scan prior to treatment; new neurologic symptoms and lesions have been reported in patients without preexisting evidence of CNS metastases (symptoms generally improve upon discontinuation, however, cases with permanent damage have been reported). Mental status changes (irritability, confusion, depression) can occur and may indicate bacteremia, sepsis, hypoperfusion, CNS malignancy, or CNS toxicity. May cause seizure; use with caution in patients with seizure disorder. Ethanol use may increase CNS adverse effects.

[U.S. Boxed Warning]: Impaired neutrophil function is associated with treatment; patients are at risk for disseminated infection (including sepsis and bacterial endocarditis), and central line-related gram-positive infections. Treat preexisting bacterial infection appropriately prior to treatment initiation. Antibiotic prophylaxis that has been associated with a reduced incidence of staphylococcal infections in aldesleukin studies includes the use of oxacillin, nafcillin, ciprofloxacin, or vancomycin. Monitor for signs of infection or sepsis during treatment.

[U.S. Boxed Warning]: Withhold treatment for patients developing moderate-to-severe lethargy or somnolence; continued treatment may result in coma. Standard prophylactic supportive care during high-dose aldesleukin treatment includes acetaminophen to relieve constitutional symptoms and an H_2 antagonist to reduce the risk of GI ulceration and/or bleeding. May impair renal or hepatic function; patients must have a serum creatinine ≤1.5 mg/dL prior to treatment. Concomitant nephrotoxic or hepatotoxic agents may increase the risk of renal or hepatic toxicity. Potentially significant drug-drug interactions may exist, requiring dose or frequency adjustment, additional monitoring, and/or selection of alternative therapy. Enhancement of cellular immune function may increase the risk of allograft rejection in transplant patients. An acute array of symptoms resembling aldesleukin adverse reactions (fever, chills, nausea, rash, pruritus, diarrhea, hypotension, edema, and oliguria) were observed within 1 to 4 hours after iodinated contrast media administration, usually when given within 4 weeks after aldesleukin treatment, although has been reported several months after aldesleukin treatment. The incidence of dyspnea and severe urogenital toxicities is potentially increased in elderly patients. Aldesleukin doses >12 to 15 million units/m^2 are associated with a moderate emetic potential; antiemetics are recommended to prevent nausea and vomiting (Dupuis, 2011).

Adverse Reactions

Cardiovascular: Arrhythmia, cardiac arrest, cardiovascular disorder (includes blood pressure and HF and ECG changes), edema, hypotension, MI, peripheral edema, supraventricular tachycardia, tachycardia, vasodilation, ventricular tachycardia

Central nervous system: Anxiety, chills, coma, confusion, dizziness, fever, malaise, pain, psychosis, somnolence, stupor

Dermatologic: Exfoliative dermatitis, pruritus, rash

Endocrine & metabolic: Acidosis, hypocalcemia, hypomagnesemia

Gastrointestinal: Abdomen enlarged, abdominal pain, anorexia, diarrhea, nausea, stomatitis, vomiting, weight gain

Hematologic: Anemia, coagulation disorder (includes intravascular coagulopathy), leukopenia, thrombocytopenia

Hepatic: Alkaline phosphatase increased, AST increased, hyperbilirubinemia

Neuromuscular & skeletal: Weakness

Renal: Acute renal failure, anuria, creatinine increased, oliguria

Respiratory: Apnea, cough, dyspnea; lung disorder (includes pulmonary congestion, rales, and rhonchi); respiratory disorder (includes acute respiratory distress syndrome, infiltrates and pulmonary changes); rhinitis

Miscellaneous: Antibody formation, infection, sepsis

Rare but important or life-threatening: Allergic interstitial nephritis, anaphylaxis, angioedema, asthma, atrial arrhythmia, AV block, blindness (transient or permanent), bowel infarction/necrosis/perforation, bradycardia, bullous pemphigoid, capillary leak syndrome, cardiomyopathy, cellulitis, cerebral edema, cerebral lesions, cerebral vasculitis, cholecystitis, colitis, crescentic IgA glomerulonephritis, Crohn's disease exacerbation, delirium, depression (severe; leading to suicide), diabetes mellitus, duodenal ulcer, encephalopathy, endocarditis, extrapyramidal syndrome, hemorrhage (including cerebral, gastrointestinal, retroperitoneal, subarachnoid, subdural), hepatic failure, hepatitis, hepatosplenomegaly, hypertension, hyperuricemia, hypothermia, hyperthyroidism, inflammatory arthritis, injection site necrosis, insomnia, intestinal obstruction, intestinal perforation, leukocytosis, malignant hyperthermia, meningitis, myocardial ischemia, myocarditis, myopathy, myositis, neuralgia, neuritis, neuropathy, neutropenia, NPN increased, oculobulbar myasthenia gravis, optic neuritis, organ perfusion decreased, pancreatitis, pericardial effusion, pericarditis, peripheral gangrene, phlebitis, pneumonia, pneumothorax, pulmonary edema, pulmonary embolus, respiratory acidosis, respiratory arrest, respiratory failure, rhabdomyolysis, scleroderma, seizure, Stevens-Johnson syndrome, stroke, syncope, thrombosis, thyroiditis, tracheoesophageal fistula, transient ischemic attack, tubular necrosis, ventricular extrasystoles

Drug Interactions

Metabolism/Transport Effects None known.

Avoid Concomitant Use

Avoid concomitant use of Aldesleukin with any of the following: CloZAPine; Corticosteroids; Dipyrone

Increased Effect/Toxicity

Aldesleukin may increase the levels/effects of: CloZAPine; DULoxetine; Hypotensive Agents; Iodinated Contrast Agents; Levodopa; RisperiDONE

The levels/effects of Aldesleukin may be increased by: Barbiturates; Dipyrone; Interferons (Alfa); Nicorandil

Decreased Effect

The levels/effects of Aldesleukin may be decreased by: Corticosteroids

Preparation for Administration Reconstitute vials with 1.2 mL SWFI (preservative free) to a concentration of 18 million units (1.1 mg)/1 mL (sterile water should be injected towards the side of the vial). Gently swirl; do not shake. Further dilute with 50 mL of D_5W. Smaller volumes of D_5W should be used for doses ≤1.5 mg; avoid concentrations <30 **mcg**/mL and >70 **mcg**/mL (an increased variability in drug delivery has been seen). Plastic (polyvinyl chloride) bags result in more consistent drug delivery and are recommended. Filtration may result in loss of bioactivity. Addition of 0.1% albumin has been used to increase stability and decrease the extent of sorption if low final concentrations cannot be avoided.

Avoid bacteriostatic water for injection and NS for reconstitution or dilution; increased aggregation may occur.

Storage/Stability Store intact vials under refrigeration at 2°C to 8°C (36°F to 46°F). Protect from light. Plastic (polyvinyl chloride) bags result in more consistent drug delivery and are recommended. According to the manufacturer, reconstituted vials and solutions diluted for infusion are stable for 48 hours at room temperature or refrigerated although refrigeration is preferred because they do not contain preservatives. Do not freeze.

Mechanism of Action Aldesleukin is a human recombinant interleukin-2 product which promotes proliferation, differentiation, and recruitment of T and B cells, natural killer (NK) cells, and thymocytes; causes cytolytic activity in a subset of lymphocytes and subsequent interactions between the immune system and malignant cells; can stimulate lymphokine-activated killer (LAK) cells and tumor-infiltrating lymphocytes (TIL) cells.

Pharmacodynamics/Kinetics

Metabolism: Renal (metabolized to amino acids)

Half-life elimination: IV: Distribution: 13 minutes; Terminal: 85 minutes

Excretion: Urine (primarily as metabolites)

Dosage Consider premedication with an antipyretic to reduce fever, an H_2 antagonist for prophylaxis of gastrointestinal irritation/bleeding, antiemetics, and antidiarrheals; continue for 12 hours after the last aldesleukin dose. Antibiotic prophylaxis is recommended to reduce the incidence of infection. Aldesleukin doses >12 to 15 million units/m^2 are associated with a moderate emetic potential; antiemetics are recommended to prevent nausea and vomiting.

Neuroblastoma (off-label use): Pediatric: IV: 3 million units/m^2/day continuous infusion over 24 hours daily for 4 days during week 1 and 4.5 million units/m^2/day continuous infusion over 24 hours daily for 4 days during week 2 of cycles 2 and 4 (regimen also includes isotretinoin, anti-GD2 antibody [investigational], and sargramostim) (Yu, 2010).

Renal cell carcinoma, metastatic: Adults: IV: 600,000 units/kg every 8 hours for a maximum of 14 doses; repeat after 9 days for a total of 28 doses per course; re-treat if tumor shrinkage observed (and if no contraindications) at least 7 weeks after hospital discharge date

or

Off-label dosing: 720,000 units/kg every 8 hours for up to 12 doses; repeat with a second cycle 10 to 15 days later (Klapper, 2008)

Melanoma, metastatic: Adults: IV:

Single-agent use: 600,000 units/kg every 8 hours for a maximum of 14 doses; repeat after 9 days for a total of 28 doses per course; re-treat if tumor shrinkage observed (and if no contraindications) at least 7 weeks after hospital discharge date

or

Off-label dosing: 720,000 units/kg every 8 hours for 12 to 15 doses; repeat with a second cycle ~14 days after the first dose of the initial cycle (Smith, 2008)

Combination biochemotherapy (off-label use): 9 million units/m^2/day continuous infusion over 24 hours for 4 days every 3 weeks for up to 4 cycles (Atkins, 2008) **or** 9 million units/m^2/day continuous infusion over 24 hours days 5 to 8, 17 to 20, and 26 to 29 every 42 days for up to 5 cycles (Eton, 2002) **or** 9 million units/m^2/day continuous infusion over 24 hours for 4 days every 3 weeks for 6 cycles (Legha, 1998)

Dosage adjustment in renal impairment: Adults:

Renal impairment prior to treatment initiation:

Serum creatinine ≤1.5 mg/dL: There are no dosage adjustments provided in the manufacturer's labeling.

Serum creatinine >1.5 mg/dL: Do not initiate treatment

Renal toxicity during treatment:

Serum creatinine >4.5 mg/dL (or ≥4 mg/dL with severe volume overload, acidosis, or hyperkalemia): Withhold dose; may resume when <4 mg/dL and fluid/electrolyte status is stable.

Persistent oliguria or urine output <10 mL/hour for 16 to 24 hours with rising serum creatinine: Withhold dose; may resume when urine output >10 mL/hour with serum creatinine decrease of >1.5 mg/dL or normalization.

Hemodialysis: Retreatment is contraindicated in patients with renal failure requiring dialysis for >72 hours.

Dosage adjustment in hepatic impairment: Adults:

Hepatic impairment prior to treatment initiation: There are no dosage adjustments provided in the manufacturer's labeling.

Hepatotoxicity during treatment: Signs of hepatic failure (encephalopathy, increasing ascites, liver pain, hypoglycemia): Withhold dose and discontinue treatment for balance of cycle; may initiate a new course if indicated only after at least 7 weeks past resolution of all signs of hepatic failure (including hospital discharge).

Dosage adjustment for toxicity: Withhold or interrupt a dose for toxicity; do not reduce the dose.

Cardiovascular toxicity:

Atrial fibrillation, supraventricular tachycardia, or bradycardia that is persistent, recurrent, or requires treatment: Withhold dose; may resume when asymptomatic with full recovery to normal sinus rhythm.

Systolic BP <90 mm Hg (with increasing pressor requirements): Withhold dose; may resume treatment when systolic BP ≥90 mm Hg and stable or pressor requirements improve.

Any ECG change consistent with MI, ischemia or myocarditis (with or without chest pain), or suspected cardiac ischemia: Withhold dose; may resume when asymptomatic, MI/myocarditis have been ruled out, suspicion of angina is low, or there is no evidence of ventricular hypokinesia.

CNS toxicity: Mental status change, including moderate confusion or agitation: Withhold dose; may resume when resolved completely.

Dermatologic toxicity: Bullous dermatitis or marked worsening of preexisting skin condition: Withhold dose; may treat with antihistamines or topical products (do not use topical steroids); may resume with resolution of all signs of bullous dermatitis.

Gastrointestinal: Stool guaiac repeatedly >3-4+: Withhold dose; may resume with negative stool guaiac.

Infection: Sepsis syndrome, clinically unstable: Withhold dose; may resume when sepsis syndrome has resolved, patient is clinically stable, and infection is under treatment.

Respiratory toxicity: Oxygen saturation <90%: Withhold dose; may resume when >90%.

Re-treatment with aldesleukin is contraindicated with the following toxicities: Sustained ventricular tachycardia (≥5 beats), uncontrolled or unresponsive cardiac arrhythmias, chest pain with ECG changes consistent with angina or MI, cardiac tamponade, intubation >72 hours, renal failure requiring dialysis for >72 hours, coma or toxic psychosis lasting >48 hours, repetitive or refractory seizures, bowel ischemia/perforation, or GI bleeding requiring surgery

Administration Aldesleukin doses >12 to 15 million units/m^2 are associated with a moderate emetic potential; antiemetics are recommended to prevent nausea and vomiting (Dupuis, 2011).

Administer as IV infusion over 15 minutes (do not administer with an inline filter). Allow solution to reach room temperature prior to administration. Flush before and after with D_5W, particularly if maintenance IV line contains sodium chloride. Some off-label uses/doses are infused as a continuous infusion (Legha, 1998; Yu, 2010). Has also been administered by SubQ injection (off-label route).

Monitoring Parameters

Baseline and periodic: CBC with differential and platelets, blood chemistries including electrolytes, renal and hepatic function tests, and chest x-ray; pulmonary function tests and arterial blood gases (baseline), thallium stress test (prior to treatment). Monitor thyroid function tests (TSH at baseline then every 2-3 months during aldesleukin treatment [Hamnvik, 2011]).

Monitoring during therapy should include daily (hourly if hypotensive) vital signs (temperature, pulse, blood pressure, and respiration rate), weight and fluid intake and output; in a patient with a decreased blood pressure, especially systolic BP <90 mm Hg, cardiac monitoring for rhythm should be conducted. If an abnormal complex or rhythm is seen, an ECG should be performed; vital signs in these hypotension patients should be taken hourly and central venous pressure (CVP) checked; monitor for change in mental status, and for signs of infection.

Additional Information 18 x 10^6 units = 1.1 mg protein

Dosage Forms

Solution Reconstituted, Intravenous [preservative free]:
Proleukin: 22,000,000 units (1 ea)

- ◆ **Aldex® CT [DSC]** *see* Diphenhydramine and Phenylephrine *on page 644*
- ◆ **Aldex GS DM** *see* Guaifenesin, Pseudoephedrine, and Dextromethorphan *on page 989*
- ◆ **Aldomet** *see* Methyldopa *on page 1332*
- ◆ **Aldroxicon I [OTC]** *see* Aluminum Hydroxide, Magnesium Hydroxide, and Simethicone *on page 104*
- ◆ **Aldroxicon II [OTC]** *see* Aluminum Hydroxide, Magnesium Hydroxide, and Simethicone *on page 104*
- ◆ **Aldurazyme** *see* Laronidase *on page 1172*
- ◆ **Aldurazyme® (Can)** *see* Laronidase *on page 1172*

Alemtuzumab (ay lem TU zoo mab)

Brand Names: U.S. Campath; Lemtrada

Brand Names: Canada Lemtrada; MabCampath

Index Terms Anti-CD52 Monoclonal Antibody; Campath; Campath-1H; Humanized IgG1 Anti-CD52 Monoclonal Antibody; MoAb CD52; Monoclonal Antibody Campath-1H; Monoclonal Antibody CD52

Pharmacologic Category Antineoplastic Agent, Anti-CD52; Antineoplastic Agent, Monoclonal Antibody; Monoclonal Antibody

Use

B-cell chronic lymphocytic leukemia: Campath or MabCampath [Canadian product]: Treatment (as a single agent) of B-cell chronic lymphocytic leukemia (B-CLL)

Multiple sclerosis, relapsing: Lemtrada: Treatment of patients with relapsing forms of multiple sclerosis (MS), generally who have had an inadequate response to 2 or more medications indicated for the treatment of MS.

Pregnancy Risk Factor C

Pregnancy Considerations Adverse events were observed in animal reproduction studies. Human IgG is known to cross the placental barrier; therefore, alemtuzumab may also cross the barrier and cause fetal B- and T-lymphocyte depletion. Use during pregnancy only if the benefit to the mother outweighs the potential risk to the fetus. Effective contraception is recommended during and for at least 6 months (Campath) or 4 months (Lemtrada) after treatment for women of childbearing potential and men of reproductive potential.

Breast-Feeding Considerations Human IgG is excreted in breast milk; therefore, alemtuzumab may also be excreted in milk. Due to the potential for serious adverse reactions in the nursing infant, the decision to discontinue alemtuzumab or to discontinue breast-feeding should take into account the importance of treatment to the mother and the half-life of alemtuzumab. The Canadian labeling recommends discontinuing nursing during treatment and for at least 3 months (MabCampath) or 4 months (Lemtrada) after completing treatment course.

Contraindications

U.S. labeling: There are no contraindications listed in the manufacturer's Campath labeling. Lemtrada is contraindicated in patients infected with HIV (due to prolonged reduction in CD4+ lymphocytes).

Canadian labeling:

Lemtrada: Hypersensitivity to alemtuzumab or any component of the formulation; HIV infection; active or latent tuberculosis; severe active infections; active malignancies; concurrent antineoplastic or immunosuppressive therapy; history of progressive multifocal leukoencephalopathy (PML)

MabCampath: Known type 1 hypersensitivity or anaphylactic reactions to alemtuzumab or any component of the formulation; active infections; underlying immunodeficiency (eg, seropositive for HIV); active secondary malignancies; current or history of progressive multifocal leukoencephalopathy (PML)

Warnings/Precautions [U.S. Boxed Warning (Lemtrada)]: Alemtuzumab causes serious, sometimes fatal, autoimmune conditions, such as immune thrombocytopenia and antiglomerular basement membrane disease, in patients receiving alemtuzumab for the treatment of multiple sclerosis (MS). Monitor complete blood counts with differential, serum creatinine levels, and urinalysis with urine cell counts at periodic intervals for 48 months after the last dose of alemtuzumab. Monitor for symptoms of immune thrombocytopenia (easy bruising, petechiae, spontaneous mucocutaneous bleeding, heavy menstrual bleeding) in patients receiving alemtuzumab for MS. Monitor for nephropathy symptoms (eg, elevated serum creatinine, hematuria, proteinuria). Alveolar hemorrhage manifesting as hemoptysis may be present in antiglomerular basement membrane disease. Glomerular nephropathies require urgent evaluation; may lead to renal failure if not treated. Prompt intervention is necessary for autoimmune cytopenias. Idiopathic thrombocytopenic purpura, thyroid disorders, autoimmune hemolytic anemia, autoimmune pancytopenia, undifferentiated connective tissue disorders, acquired hemophilia A, rheumatoid arthritis, vitiligo, retinal pigment epitheliopathy have been reported in patients receiving alemtuzumab for MS. Guillain-Barre syndrome and chronic inflammatory demyelinating polyradiculoneuropathy have been reported in patients receiving alemtuzumab for other uses. Alemtuzumab may increase the risk for other autoimmune conditions. Autoimmune thyroid disorders occurred in over one-third of patients receiving alemtuzumab for MS. In a trial evaluating alemtuzumab versus interferon beta-1a in patients with MS, thyroid dysfunction occurred more frequently in patients taking alemtuzumab (34% versus 6.5%) (Daniels, 2014). The incidence of the first episode of thyroid dysfunction increased annually the first 3 years (year 1: 4.6%; year 2: 13.3%; year 3: 16.1%) then gradually decreased thereafter. Among patients with alemtuzumab-related thyroid dysfunction, Graves' hyperthyroidism occurred most commonly (23%), followed by hypothyroidism and subacute thyroiditis (7% and 4%, respectively). Thyroid dysfunction (thyroiditis, Graves' disease) has also been reported with alemtuzumab use for the treatment of other conditions. For B-CLL treatment, TSH monitoring is recommended; monitor TSH at baseline and every 2 to 3 months during alemtuzumab treatment (Hamnvik, 2011). For MS, monitor TSH at baseline and every 3 months until 48 months after last infusion or longer or at any time during therapy if clinically indicated.

[U.S. Boxed Warning]: Serious and potentially fatal infusion-related reactions may occur; monitor for infusion reaction; carefully monitor during infusion; withhold treatment for serious or grade 3 or 4 infusion reactions. For B-cell chronic lymphocytic leukemia (B-CLL), gradual escalation to the recommended

maintenance dose is required at initiation and with treatment interruptions (for ≥7 days) to minimize infusion-related reactions. For multiple sclerosis, must be administered in a setting with appropriate equipment and personnel to manage anaphylaxis or serious infusion reaction; monitor for 2 hours after each infusion; inform patients that serious infusion reactions may also occur after the 2-hour monitoring period. Infusion reactions have been reported more than 24 hours after infusion. In patients treated for B-CLL, infusion reaction symptoms may include acute respiratory distress syndrome, anaphylactic shock, angioedema, bronchospasm, cardiac arrest, cardiac arrhythmias, chills, dyspnea, fever, hypotension, myocardial infarction, pulmonary infiltrates, rash, rigors, syncope, or urticaria. The incidence of infusion reaction is highest during the first week of B-CLL treatment. Premedicate with acetaminophen and an oral antihistamine. Medications for the treatment of reactions should be available for immediate use. Use caution and carefully monitor blood pressure in patients with ischemic heart disease and patients on antihypertensive therapy. For B-CLL, reinitiate with gradual dose escalation if treatment is withheld ≥7 days. Similar infusion reactions have been observed with use in the treatment of multiple sclerosis; premedication with corticosteroids for initial 3 days of each treatment course is recommended. Antihistamines and/or antipyretics may also be considered. Consider additional monitoring in patients with existing cardiovascular or respiratory compromise (the Canadian labeling recommends obtaining an ECG prior to each treatment course). Observe for infusion-related reactions; advise patients to monitor for signs/symptoms of infusion reaction, particularly during the 24 hours following infusion.

[U.S. Boxed Warning (Campath)]: Serious and fatal cytopenias (including pancytopenia, bone marrow hypoplasia, autoimmune hemolytic anemia, and autoimmune idiopathic thrombocytopenia) have occurred. Single doses >30 mg or cumulative weekly doses >90 mg are associated with an increased incidence of pancytopenia. Severe prolonged myelosuppression, hemolytic anemia, pure red cell aplasia, bone marrow aplasia, and bone marrow hypoplasia have also been reported with use at the normal dose for the treatment of B-CLL. Discontinue for serious hematologic or other serious toxicity (except lymphopenia) until the event resolves. Permanently discontinue if autoimmune anemia or autoimmune thrombocytopenia occurs. Patients receiving blood products should only receive irradiated blood products due to the potential for transfusion-associated GVHD during lymphopenia.

[U.S. Boxed Warning (Campath)]: Serious and potentially fatal infections (bacterial, viral, fungal, and protozoan) have been reported. Administer prophylactic medications against PCP pneumonia and herpes viral infections during treatment and for at least 2 months following last dose or until CD4+ counts are ≥200 cells/mm^3 (whichever is later). Severe and prolonged lymphopenia may occur; CD4+ counts usually return to ≥200 cells/mm^3 within 2 to 6 months; however, CD4+ and CD8+ lymphocyte counts may not return to baseline levels for more than 1 year. Withhold treatment during serious infections; may be reinitiated upon resolution of infection. Monitor for CMV infection (during and for at least 2 months after completion of therapy); initiate appropriate antiviral treatment and withhold alemtuzumab for CMV infection or confirmed CMV viremia (withhold alemtuzumab during CMV antiviral treatment). For patients being treated for MS, initiate antiviral prophylaxis (for herpetic viral infections) beginning on the first day of treatment and continue for at least 2 months or until CD4+ lymphocyte count is ≥200/mm^3. In clinical trials for MS, infections seen more commonly in alemtuzumab-treated patients included nasopharyngitis, urinary tract infection, upper respiratory tract infection, sinusitis, herpetic infections, influenza, and bronchitis; serious cases of appendicitis, gastroenteritis, pneumonia, herpes zoster, and tooth infection also occurred. Consider delaying treatment in patients with active infection until infection is controlled. Patients should be screened for human papilloma virus (HPV) and tuberculosis as clinically necessary. Progressive multifocal leukoencephalopathy (PML) been reported with use (rarely); withhold therapy immediately for signs/symptoms suggestive of PML. According to the Canadian labeling, alemtuzumab is contraindicated in patients with a history of PML.

[U.S. Boxed Warning (Lemtrada)]: Alemtuzumab may cause an increased risk of malignancies, including thyroid cancer, melanoma, and lymphoproliferative disorders, Perform baseline and yearly skin exams. Other malignant neoplasm (breast cancer or basal cell carcinoma) has been observed (rarely) in patients receiving treatment for MS. Use of Lemtrada in patients with active malignancies is contraindicated; use caution if initiating treatment in patients with preexisting malignancy (Canadian labeling).

Pneumonitis (hypersensitivity or fibrosis) has been reported. Monitor for symptoms (dyspnea, cough, wheezing, hemoptysis, chest pain/tightness). Alemtuzumab is associated with a moderate emetic potential in the oncology setting; antiemetics may be recommended to prevent nausea and vomiting (Basch, 2011; Roila, 2010). Potentially significant drug-drug interactions may exist, requiring dose or frequency adjustment, additional monitoring, and/or selection of alternative therapy. If considering Lemtrada treatment for use in a patient who has previously received Campath/MabCampath, consider the additive and long-lasting immune system effects. Patients should not be immunized with live, viral vaccines during or recently after treatment. The ability to respond to any vaccine following therapy is unknown. Testing for antibodies to varicella zoster virus (VZV) is recommended prior to initiation of Lemtrada if history of chickenpox or VZV vaccination status is unknown. When using for the treatment of multiple sclerosis, complete necessary immunizations at least 6 weeks prior to initiating alemtuzumab. Determine if patient has a history varicella or vaccination for VZV; if not, test for VZV antibodies and consider vaccinations for antibody-negative patients; postpone alemtuzumab treatment for 6 weeks following VZV vaccination.

Alemtuzumab is not recommended for use in MS patients with inactive disease or who are stable on other treatment. Patients should commit to at least 48 months of follow-up after the last infusion. Alemtuzumab has not been studied in MS patients infected with HBV or HCV; consider screening patients at increased risk of infection prior to initiating treatment. Use with caution in HBV or HCV carriers; patients may be at risk for viral reactivation. **[U.S. Boxed Warning (Lemtrada)]: Due to the risk of autoimmunity, infusion reactions, and malignancies, alemtuzumab is available only through restricted distribution under a Risk Evaluation Mitigation Strategy (REMS) Program when used for the treatment of MS. Contact 1-855-676-6326 to enroll in the Lemtrada REMS program.** Prescribers and pharmacies must be certified with the REMS program, and patients and healthcare facilities must be enrolled and comply with ongoing monitoring.

Adverse Reactions

Cardiovascular: Bradycardia, chest discomfort, chest pain, cold extremities, flushing, hypotension, palpitations, peripheral edema, tachycardia

Central nervous system: Chills, dizziness, drowsiness, equilibrium disturbance, facial hypoesthesia, fatigue, headache, hyperthermia, hypertonia, increased body temperature, insomnia, pain, paresthesia, vertigo

Dermatologic: Acne vulgaris, allergic dermatitis, alopecia, erythema, erythematous rash, hyperhidrosis, papular rash, pruritic rash, pruritus, pruritus (generalized), skin blister, skin rash, skin rash (generalized), urticaria, xeroderma
Endocrine & metabolic: Chronic lymphocytic thyroiditis, goiter, Graves' disease, hypermenorrhea, hyperthyroidism, hypothyroidism, thyroid stimulating hormone suppression
Gastrointestinal: Abdominal distention, abdominal pain, diarrhea, dyspepsia, gastroenteritis, nausea, oral candidiasis, oral herpes, oral mucosa ulcer, upper abdominal pain, vomiting
Genitourinary: Abnormal urinalysis, cystitis, fungal vaginosis, hematuria, herpes genitalis, increase in urinary protein, irregular menses, occult blood in urine, proteinuria, urinary tract infection, vaginal hemorrhage, vulvovaginal candidiasis
Hematologic & oncologic: Abnormal white blood cell differential, bruise, decreased absolute lymphocyte count, decreased CD-4 cell count, decreased CD-8 cell counts, decreased T cell lymphocytes, hematoma, lymphocytopenia, nonthrombocytopenic purpura, petechia, reduction of B-cells
Hypersensitivity: Cytokine release syndrome
Immunologic: Antibody development (no effect on drug efficacy)
Infection: Bacterial infection, herpes simplex infection, herpes zoster, influenza
Local: Catheter pain
Neuromuscular & skeletal: Arthralgia, back pain, joint sprain, joint swelling, limb pain, musculoskeletal chest pain, myalgia, neck pain, weakness
Ophthalmic: Blurred vision, conjunctivitis
Otic: Otalgia, otic infection
Respiratory: Bronchitis, bronchospasm, cough, dyspnea, epistaxis, nasal congestion, nasopharyngitis, oropharyngeal pain, pharyngitis, rhinitis, sinus congestion, sinusitis, upper respiratory tract infection, wheezing
Miscellaneous: Fever
Rare but important or life-threatening: Abnormal hepatic function tests, acquired blood coagulation disorder, allodynia, altered blood pressure, amenorrhea, anemia, anti-GBM disease, antithyroid antibody positive, aphthous stomatitis, asthma, ataxia, atrial fibrillation, autoimmune hemolytic anemia, autoimmune thrombocytopenia, bacterial vaginosis, candidiasis, cardiac failure, cellulitis, cervical dysplasia, cervicitis, chronic inflammatory demyelinating polyradiculoneuropathy, connective tissue disease (undifferentiated), decreased hematocrit, decreased hemoglobin, decreased monocytes, decreased neutrophils, dehydration, depression, desquamation, eosinopenia, eosinophilia, Epstein-Barr-associated lymphoproliferative disorder, Epstein-Barr infection, esophagitis, furuncle, gastroesophageal reflux disease, gastrointestinal disease, gingival hemorrhage, glycosuria, graft versus host disease (transfusion associated), Guillain-Barre syndrome, hemiparesis, hemophilia A (acquired [anti-Factor VIII antibodies]), hyperemia, hypersensitivity reaction, increased monocytes, infusion site reaction, labyrinthitis, leukocytosis, lymphoproliferative disorder, maculopapular rash, major hemorrhage, malignant lymphoma, malignant melanoma, malignant neoplasm of thyroid, membranous glomerulonephritis, memory impairment, meningitis due to listeria monocytogenes, meningitis (herpes), migraine, mucosal inflammation, multiple sclerosis, muscle spasticity, natural killer cell count increased, neutropenia, night sweats, onychomycosis, optic neuropathy, ostealgia, ovarian cyst, pancytopenia, papule, peripheral neuropathy, photophobia, pleurisy, pneumonia, pneumonitis, positive direct Coombs test, postherpetic neuralgia, progressive multifocal leukoencephalopathy, protozoal infection, psychomotor agitation, pyelonephritis, reactivation of disease, reduced ejection fraction, restless leg syndrome, retinal pigment changes (epitheliopathy), rheumatoid arthritis, serum sickness, skin hyperpigmentation, skin lesion, streptococcal pharyngitis, subacute thyroiditis, suicidal ideation, suicidal tendencies, syncope, tachypnea, thrombocytopenia, tongue discoloration, tonsillitis, tooth abscess, tracheobronchitis, tuberculosis, tumor lysis syndrome, type 1 diabetes mellitus, upper airway symptoms (cough syndrome), urethritis, urinary incontinence, varicella, viral infection, vitiligo, voice disorder, weight gain, weight loss

Drug Interactions

Metabolism/Transport Effects None known.

Avoid Concomitant Use

Avoid concomitant use of Alemtuzumab with any of the following: BCG; Belimumab; CloZAPine; Dipyrone; Natalizumab; Pimecrolimus; Tacrolimus (Topical); Tofacitinib; Vaccines (Live)

Increased Effect/Toxicity

Alemtuzumab may increase the levels/effects of: Belimumab; CloZAPine; Leflunomide; Natalizumab; Tofacitinib; Vaccines (Live)

The levels/effects of Alemtuzumab may be increased by: Denosumab; Dipyrone; Pimecrolimus; Roflumilast; Tacrolimus (Topical); Trastuzumab

Decreased Effect

Alemtuzumab may decrease the levels/effects of: BCG; Coccidioides immitis Skin Test; Sipuleucel-T; Vaccines (Inactivated); Vaccines (Live)

The levels/effects of Alemtuzumab may be decreased by: Echinacea

Preparation for Administration

Campath, MabCampath [Canadian product]: Dilute for infusion in 100 mL NS or D_5W. Compatible in polyvinylchloride (PVC) bags. Gently invert the bag to mix the solution. Do not shake prior to use.

Lemtrada: Withdraw 12 mg (1.2 mL) from vial and add to 100 mL bag of NS or D_5W. Gently invert the bag to mix the solution.

Storage/Stability

Campath: Prior to dilution, store intact (30 mg/1 mL) vials at 2°C to 8°C (36°F to 46°F); do not freeze (if accidentally frozen, thaw in refrigerator prior to administration). Do not shake; protect from light. Following dilution, store at room temperature or refrigerate; protect from light; use within 8 hours. Discard unused portion in the vial.
Lemtrada: Prior to dilution, store intact vials at 2°C to 8°C (36°F to 46°F). Do not freeze. Do not shake; protect from light. Following dilution, store at room temperature or refrigerate; use within 8 hours.
MabCampath [Canadian product]: Prior to dilution, store vials at 2°C to 8°C (36°F to 46°F). Do not freeze (discard vial if frozen). Do not shake. Protect from light. Following dilution, store at room temperature or refrigerate; use within 8 hours.

Mechanism of Action Binds to CD52, a nonmodulating antigen present on the surface of B and T lymphocytes, a majority of monocytes, macrophages, NK cells, and a subpopulation of granulocytes. After binding to $CD52^+$ cells, an antibody-dependent lysis of malignant cells occurs. In multiple sclerosis, alemtuzumab immunomodulatory effects may include alteration in the number, proportions, and properties of some lymphocyte subsets following treatment.

Pharmacodynamics/Kinetics

Distribution: V_d: IV: Campath: 0.18 L/kg (range: 0.1 to 0.4 L/kg); Lemtrada: 14.1 L

Metabolism: Campath: Clearance decreases with repeated dosing (due to loss of CD52 receptors in periphery), resulting in a sevenfold increase in AUC after 12 weeks of therapy.

Half-life elimination: IV: Campath: 11 hours (following first 30 mg dose; range: 2 to 32 hours); 6 days (following the last 30 mg dose; range: 1 to 14 days); Lemtrada: ~2 weeks

Dosage

B-cell chronic lymphocytic leukemia (B-CLL): Campath: Adults: IV: Gradually escalate to a maintenance of 30 mg per dose 3 times weekly on alternate days for a total duration of therapy of up to 12 weeks (Hillmen, 2007; Keating, 2002)

Note: Dose escalation is required; usually accomplished in 3 to 7 days. Single doses >30 mg or cumulative doses >90 mg/week increase the incidence of pancytopenia. Pretreatment (with acetaminophen 500 to 1,000 mg and diphenhydramine 50 mg) is recommended prior to the first dose, with dose escalations, and as clinically indicated; IV glucocorticoids may be used for severe infusion-related reactions. Administer antiviral prophylaxis (for herpetic viral infections) and *Pneumocystis jiroveci* pneumonia (PCP) prophylaxis; continue for at least 2 months after completion of alemtuzumab and until CD4+ lymphocyte count is ≥200/mm^3. Reinitiate with gradual dose escalation if treatment is withheld ≥7 days. Alemtuzumab is associated with a moderate emetic potential in the oncology setting; antiemetics may be recommended to prevent nausea and vomiting (Basch, 2011; Roila, 2010).

Dose escalation: Initial: 3 mg daily beginning on day 1; if tolerated (infusion reaction ≤ grade 2), increase to 10 mg daily; if tolerated (infusion reaction ≤ grade 2), may increase to maintenance of 30 mg per dose 3 times weekly if required for maintenance dose.

B-CLL (off-label route): SubQ: Initial: 3 mg on day 1; if tolerated 10 mg on day 3; if tolerated increase to 30 mg on day 5; maintenance: 30 mg per dose 3 times weekly for a maximum of 18 weeks (Lundin, 2002) **or** 3 mg on day 1; if tolerated 10 mg on day 2; if tolerated 30 mg on day 3, followed by 30 mg per dose 3 times weekly for 4 to 12 weeks (Stilgenbauer, 2009)

Multiple sclerosis, relapsing: Lemtrada: Adults: IV: 12 mg daily for 5 consecutive days (total 60 mg), followed 12 months later by 12 mg daily for 3 consecutive days (total 36 mg); total duration of therapy: 24 months.

Note: Premedicate with corticosteroids (methylprednisolone 1,000 mg or equivalent) immediately prior to alemtuzumab for the first 3 days of each treatment course. Antihistamines and/or antipyretics may also be considered. Administer antiviral prophylaxis (for herpetic viral infections) beginning on the first day of treatment and continue for at least 2 months after completion of alemtuzumab and until CD4+ lymphocyte count is ≥200/mm^3. In some clinical trials patients received an additional 12 mg daily for 3 consecutive days 12 months later (total duration of 36 months) (CAMMS223, 2008; Coles, 2012).

Autoimmune cytopenias, CLL-induced, refractory (off-label use): Adults: IV, SubQ: Gradually escalate to a maintenance of 10 to 30 mg per dose 3 times weekly for 4 to 12 weeks (Karlsson, 2007; Osterborg, 2009).

Graft versus host disease (GVHD), acute, steroid refractory, treatment (off-label use): Adults: IV: 10 mg daily for 5 consecutive days, then 10 mg weekly on days 8, 15, and 22 if CR not achieved (Martinez, 2009) **or** 10 mg weekly until symptom resolution (Schnitzler, 2009)

Renal transplant, induction (off-label use): Adults: IV: 30 mg as a single dose at the time of transplant (Hanaway, 2011)

Stem cell transplant (allogeneic) conditioning regimen (off-label use): Adults: IV: 20 mg daily for 5 days (in combination with fludarabine and melphalan) beginning 8 days prior to transplant (Mead, 2010) **or** beginning 7 days prior to transplant (Van Besien, 2009)

T-cell prolymphocytic leukemia (T-PLL; off-label use): Adults: IV: Initial test dose 3 mg or 10 mg, followed by dose escalation to 30 mg per dose 3 times weekly as tolerated until maximum response (Dearden, 2001) **or** Initial dose: 3 mg day 1, if tolerated increase to 10 mg day 2, if tolerated increase to 30 mg on day 3 (days 1, 2, and 3 are consecutive days), followed by 30 mg per dose every Monday, Wednesday, Friday for a total of 4 to 12 weeks (Keating, 2002)

Dosage adjustment for nonhematologic toxicity:

Treatment of B-CLL: Campath:

Note: If treatment is withheld ≥7 days, reinitiate at 3 mg with re-escalation to 10 mg and then 30 mg.

Grade 3 or 4 infusion reaction: Withhold infusion

Serious infection or other serious adverse reaction: Withhold alemtuzumab until resolution

Autoimmune anemia or autoimmune thrombocytopenia: Discontinue alemtuzumab

Treatment of MS: Lemtrada: Serious infusion reaction: Consider immediate discontinuation

Dosage adjustment for hematologic toxicity (severe neutropenia or thrombocytopenia, not autoimmune):

Treatment of B-CLL: Campath

Note: If treatment is withheld ≥7 days, reinitiate at 3 mg with re-escalation to 10 mg and then 30 mg.

ANC <250/mm^3 and/or platelet count ≤25,000/mm^3:

First occurrence: Withhold treatment; resume at 30 mg per dose when ANC ≥500/mm^3 and platelet count ≥50,000/mm^3

Second occurrence: Withhold treatment; resume at 10 mg per dose when ANC ≥500/mm^3 and platelet count ≥50,000/mm^3

Third occurrence: Discontinue alemtuzumab.

Patients with a baseline ANC ≤250/mm^3 and/or a baseline platelet count ≤25,000/mm^3 at initiation of therapy: If ANC and/or platelet counts decrease to ≤50% of the baseline value:

First occurrence: Withhold treatment; resume at 30 mg per dose upon return to baseline values

Second occurrence: Withhold treatment; resume at 10 mg per dose upon return to baseline values

Third occurrence: Discontinue alemtuzumab.

Dosage adjustment in renal impairment: There are no dosage adjustments provided in the manufacturer's labeling (has not been studied).

Dosage adjustment in hepatic impairment: There are no dosage adjustments provided in the manufacturer's labeling (has not been studied).

Dosing in obesity: *American Society for Blood and Marrow Transplantation (ASBMT) practice guideline committee position statement on chemotherapy dosing in obesity:* Utilize a flat dose based on the regimen selected for hematopoietic stem cell transplant conditioning in adults (Bubalo, 2014).

Administration

Campath or MabCampath [Canadian product]: Administer by IV infusion over 2 hours. Premedicate with diphenhydramine 50 mg and acetaminophen 500 to 1000 mg 30 minutes before each infusion. IV glucocorticoids have been effective in decreasing severe infusion-related events. Start anti-infective prophylaxis. Other drugs should not be added to or simultaneously infused through the same IV line. Do not give IV push or bolus. Compatible in polyvinylchloride (PVC) or polyethylene lined administration sets or low protein binding filters.

Campath: SubQ (off-label route): SubQ administration has been studied (Lundin, 2002; Stilgenbauer, 2009); an increased rate of injection site reactions has been observed, with only rare incidences of chills or infusion-like reactions typically observed with IV infusion. A longer dose escalation time (1 to 2 weeks) may be needed due to injection site reactions (Lundin, 2002). Premedicate with diphenhydramine 50 mg and acetaminophen 500 to 1000 mg 30 minutes before dose. The subQ route should **NOT** be used for the treatment of T-PLL (Deardon, 2011).

Alemtuzumab is associated with a moderate emetic potential in the oncology setting; antiemetics may be recommended to prevent nausea and vomiting (Basch, 2011; Roila, 2010).

Lemtrada: Administer by IV infusion over 4 hours (beginning within 8 hours after dilution); do not administer by IV push or IV bolus. Do not infuse other medications through the same IV line. Premedicate with corticosteroids (methylprednisolone 1,000 mg or equivalent) for first 3 days of each treatment course. Administer in a setting with personnel and equipment appropriate to manage infusion reactions. Monitor vital signs prior to and periodically during the infusion. Infusion reactions should be managed symptomatically; consider discontinuing immediately for severe infusion reaction. Observe for at least 2 hours after each infusion, longer if clinically indicated.

Monitoring Parameters Campath: CBC with differential and platelets (weekly, more frequent if worsening); signs and symptoms of infection; CD4+ lymphocyte counts (after treatment until recovery); CMV antigen (routinely during and for 2 months after treatment); consider TSH at baseline and then every 2 to 3 months during alemtuzumab treatment (Hamnvik, 2011). Monitor closely for infusion reactions (including hypotension, rigors, fever, shortness of breath, bronchospasm, chills, and/or rash); vital signs (prior to and during infusion); carefully monitor BP especially in patients with ischemic heart disease or on antihypertensive medications;

Lemtrada: CBC with differential prior to initiation then monthly until 48 months after last infusion; serum creatinine prior to initiation then monthly until 48 months after last infusion or at any time during therapy if clinically indicated; urinalysis with urine cell counts (prior to initiation then monthly); signs/symptoms of infection; TSH at baseline and every 3 months until 48 months after last infusion or longer or at any time during therapy if clinically indicated; observe for at least 2 hours after each infusion, longer if clinically indicated; ECG prior to each treatment course; annual HPV screening; signs/symptoms of PML; baseline and annual skin exams (for melanoma).

Dosage Forms

Solution, Intravenous [preservative free]:
Campath: 30 mg/mL (1 mL)
Lemtrada: 12 mg/1.2 mL (1.2 mL)

Dosage Forms: Canada

Injection, solution [preservative free]:
MabCampath: 30 mg/mL (1 mL)

Injection, solution [preservative free]:
Lemtrada: 10 mg/mL (1.2 mL)

Alendronate (a LEN droe nate)

Brand Names: U.S. Binosto; Fosamax

Brand Names: Canada ACH-Alendronate; Alendronate-70; Alendronate-FC; Apo-Alendronate; Auro-Alendronate; CO Alendronate; Dom-Alendronate; Fosamax; JAMP-Alendronate; Mint-Alendronate; Mylan-Alendronate; PHL-Alendronate; PMS-Alendronate; PMS-Alendronate-FC; Q-Alendronate; Ran-Alendronate; ratio-Alendronate; Riva-Alendronate; Sandoz-Alendronate; Teva-Alendronate

Index Terms Alendronate Sodium; Alendronic Acid Monosodium Salt Trihydrate; MK-217

Pharmacologic Category Bisphosphonate Derivative

Use

Osteoporosis: Treatment of osteoporosis in postmenopausal females (Fosamax, Binosto); prevention of osteoporosis in postmenopausal females (Fosamax); treatment of osteoporosis in males (Fosamax, Binosto); treatment of Paget disease of the bone in patients who are symptomatic, at risk for future complications, or with alkaline phosphatase ≥2 times the upper limit of normal (Fosamax); treatment of glucocorticoid-induced osteoporosis in males and females with low bone mineral density who are receiving a daily dosage ≥7.5 mg of prednisone (or equivalent) (Fosamax)

Canadian labeling: Additional use (not in U.S. labeling): Prevention of glucocorticoid-induced osteoporosis in males and females

Pregnancy Risk Factor C

Pregnancy Considerations Adverse events were observed in animal reproduction studies. It is not known if bisphosphonates cross the placenta, but fetal exposure is expected (Djokanovic, 2008; Stathopoulos, 2011). Bisphosphonates are incorporated into the bone matrix and gradually released over time. The amount available in the systemic circulation varies by dose and duration of therapy. Theoretically, there may be a risk of fetal harm when pregnancy follows the completion of therapy; however, available data have not shown that exposure to bisphosphonates during pregnancy significantly increases the risk of adverse fetal events (Djokanovic, 2008; Levy, 2009; Stathopoulos, 2011). Until additional data is available, most sources recommend discontinuing bisphosphonate therapy in women of reproductive potential as early as possible prior to a planned pregnancy; use in premenopausal women should be reserved for special circumstances when rapid bone loss is occurring (Bhalla, 2010; Pereira, 2012; Stathopoulos, 2011). Because hypocalcemia has been described following *in utero* bisphosphonate exposure, exposed infants should be monitored for hypocalcemia after birth (Djokanovic, 2008; Stathopoulos, 2011).

Breast-Feeding Considerations It is not known if alendronate is excreted into breast milk. The manufacturer recommends that caution be exercised when administering alendronate to nursing women.

Contraindications

Hypersensitivity to alendronate, other bisphosphonates, or any component of the formulation; hypocalcemia; abnormalities of the esophagus (eg, stricture, achalasia) which delay esophageal emptying; inability to stand or sit upright for at least 30 minutes; increased risk of aspiration (effervescent tablets; oral solution)

Canadian labeling: Additional contraindications (not in U.S. labeling): Renal insufficiency with creatinine clearance <35 mL/min

Warnings/Precautions Use caution in patients with renal impairment (not recommended for use in patients with CrCl <35 mL/minute); hypocalcemia must be corrected before therapy initiation; ensure adequate calcium and vitamin D intake. May cause irritation to upper gastrointestinal mucosa. Esophagitis, dysphagia, esophageal ulcers, esophageal erosions, and esophageal stricture (rare) have been reported; risk increases in patients unable to comply with dosing instructions. Use with caution in patients with dysphagia, esophageal disease, gastritis, duodenitis, or ulcers (may worsen underlying condition). Discontinue use if new or worsening symptoms develop.

Osteonecrosis of the jaw (ONJ) has been reported in patients receiving bisphosphonates. Risk factors include invasive dental procedures (eg, tooth extraction, dental implants, boney surgery); a diagnosis of cancer, with concomitant chemotherapy or corticosteroids; poor oral hygiene, ill-fitting dentures; and comorbid disorders (anemia, coagulopathy, infection, preexisting dental disease); risk may increase with duration of bisphosphonate use. Most reported cases occurred after IV bisphosphonate therapy; however, cases have been reported following oral therapy. A dental exam and preventive dentistry should be performed prior to placing patients with risk factors on chronic bisphosphonate therapy. The manufacturer's labeling states that discontinuing bisphosphonates in patients requiring invasive dental procedures may reduce the risk of ONJ. However, other experts suggest that there is no evidence that discontinuing therapy reduces the risk of developing ONJ (Assael, 2009). The benefit/risk must be assessed by the treating physician and/or dentist/surgeon prior to any invasive dental procedure. Patients developing ONJ while on bisphosphonates should receive care by an oral surgeon.

Atypical femur fractures have been reported in patients receiving bisphosphonates for treatment/prevention of osteoporosis. The fractures include subtrochanteric femur (bone just below the hip joint) and diaphyseal femur (long segment of the thigh bone). Some patients experience prodromal pain weeks or months before the fracture occurs. It is unclear if bisphosphonate therapy is the cause for these fractures, although the majority of cases have been reported in patients taking bisphosphonates. Patients receiving long-term (>3-5 years) therapy may be at an increased risk. Discontinue bisphosphonate therapy in patients who develop a femoral shaft fracture.

Severe (and occasionally debilitating) bone, joint, and/or muscle pain have been reported during bisphosphonate treatment. The onset of pain ranged from a single day to several months. Consider discontinuing therapy in patients who experience severe symptoms; symptoms usually resolve upon discontinuation. Some patients experienced recurrence when rechallenged with same drug or another bisphosphonate; avoid use in patients with a history of these symptoms in association with bisphosphonate therapy. In the management of osteoporosis, re-evaluate the need for continued therapy periodically; the optimal duration of treatment has not yet been determined. Consider discontinuing after 3-5 years of use in patients at low-risk for fracture; following discontinuation, re-evaluate fracture risk periodically.

Potentially significant drug-drug interactions may exist, requiring dose or frequency adjustment, additional monitoring, and/or selection of alternative therapy. Consult drug interactions database for more detailed information. Each effervescent tablet contains 650 mg of sodium (NaCl 1650 mg); use with caution in patients following a sodium-restricted diet.

Adverse Reactions

Central nervous system: Headache

Endocrine & metabolic: Hypocalcemia, hypophosphatemia

Gastrointestinal: Abdominal distension, abdominal pain, acid regurgitation, constipation, diarrhea, dyspepsia, dysphagia, esophageal ulcer, flatulence, gastric ulcer, gastritis, gastroesophageal reflux disease, melena, nausea, vomiting

Neuromuscular & skeletal: Muscle cramps, musculoskeletal pain

Rare but important or life-threatening: Alopecia, anastomotic ulcer, angioedema, atrial fibrillation, dizziness, duodenal ulcer, dysgeusia, episcleritis, erythema, femur fracture (including diaphyseal, low-energy femoral shaft, and subtrochanteric fractures), erosive esophagitis, esophageal perforation, esophageal spasm, esophageal ulcer, esophagitis, exacerbation of asthma, femur fracture (including diaphyseal, low-energy femoral shaft, and subtrochanteric fractures), fever, flu-like symptoms, hypersensitivity reaction, hypocalcemia (symptomatic), joint swelling, lymphocytopenia, malaise, malignant neoplasm of esophagus, myalgia, oropharyngeal ulcer; ostealgia, myalgia, or arthralgia (occasionally severe, considered incapacitating in rare cases); osteonecrosis (jaw), peripheral edema, pruritus, scleritis (rare), skin photosensitivity (rare), skin rash, Stevens-Johnson syndrome, toxic epidermal necrolysis, urticaria, uveitis (rare), vertigo, weakness

Drug Interactions

Metabolism/Transport Effects None known.

Avoid Concomitant Use

Avoid concomitant use of Alendronate with any of the following: Parathyroid Hormone

Increased Effect/Toxicity

Alendronate may increase the levels/effects of: Deferasirox; Phosphate Supplements

The levels/effects of Alendronate may be increased by: Aminoglycosides; Aspirin; Nonsteroidal Anti-Inflammatory Agents; Systemic Angiogenesis Inhibitors

Decreased Effect

Alendronate may decrease the levels/effects of: Parathyroid Hormone

The levels/effects of Alendronate may be decreased by: Antacids; Calcium Salts; Iron Salts; Magnesium Salts; Multivitamins/Minerals (with ADEK, Folate, Iron); Multivitamins/Minerals (with AE, No Iron); Proton Pump Inhibitors

Food Interactions All food and beverages interfere with absorption. Coadministration with dairy products may decrease alendronate absorption. Beverages (especially orange juice, coffee, and mineral water) and food may reduce the absorption of alendronate as much as 60%. Management: Alendronate must be taken first thing in the morning and ≥30 minutes before the first food, beverage (except plain water), or other medication of the day.

Preparation for Administration Tablet, effervescent (Binosto®): Dissolve effervescent tablet in 120 mL of room temperature plain water (not mineral water or flavored water); wait ≥5 minutes after effervescence stops, then stir for 10 seconds and administer.

Storage/Stability

Oral solution: Store at 25°C (77°F), excursions permitted to 15°C to 30°C (59°F to 86°F). Do not freeze.

Tablet (Fosamax®): Store at room temperature of 15°C to 30°C (59°F to 86°F). Keep in well-closed container.

Tablet, effervescent (Binosto®): Store at 20°C to 25°C (68°F to 77°F), excursions permitted to 15°C to 30°C (59°F to 86°F). Protect from moisture. Store in original blister package until use.

Mechanism of Action A bisphosphonate which inhibits bone resorption via actions on osteoclasts or on osteoclast precursors; decreases the rate of bone resorption, leading to an indirect increase in bone mineral density. In Paget's disease, characterized by disordered resorption and formation of bone, inhibition of resorption leads to an indirect decrease in bone formation; but the newly-formed bone has a more normal architecture.

Pharmacodynamics/Kinetics

Distribution: 28 L (exclusive of bone)

Protein binding: ~78%

Metabolism: None

Bioavailability: Fasting: 0.6%; reduced up to 60% with coffee or orange juice

Half-life elimination: Exceeds 10 years

Excretion: Urine; feces (as unabsorbed drug)

Dosage Note: Consider discontinuing after 3 to 5 years of use for osteoporosis in patients at low-risk for fracture. Patients should receive supplemental calcium and vitamin D if dietary intake is inadequate.

Osteoporosis in postmenopausal females: Adults: Oral:

Prophylaxis: 5 mg once daily **or** 35 mg once weekly

Treatment: 10 mg once daily **or** 70 mg once weekly

Osteoporosis in males: Adults: Oral: Treatment: 10 mg once daily **or** 70 mg once weekly

Osteoporosis secondary to glucocorticoids in males and females: Adults: Oral: Treatment (U.S. labeling) or Treatment and prevention (Canadian labeling): 5 mg once daily; a dose of 10 mg once daily should be used in postmenopausal females who are not receiving estrogen.

Paget disease of bone in males and females: Adults: Oral: 40 mg once daily for 6 months

Retreatment: Relapses during the 12 months following therapy occurred in 9% of patients who responded to treatment. Specific retreatment data are not available. Following a 6-month post-treatment evaluation period, retreatment with alendronate may be considered in patients who have relapsed based on increases in serum alkaline phosphatase, which should be measured periodically. Retreatment may also be considered in those who failed to normalize their serum alkaline phosphatase.

Missed doses (once weekly): If a once-weekly dose is missed, it should be given the next morning after remembered; may then return to the original once-weekly schedule (original scheduled day of the week), however, do not give 2 doses on the same day.

Elderly: Refer to adult dosing.

Dosage adjustment in renal impairment:

CrCl ≥35 mL/minute: No dosage adjustment necessary.

CrCl <35 mL/minute: Use not recommended.

Dosage adjustment in hepatic impairment: No dosage adjustment necessary.

Dietary Considerations Ensure adequate calcium and vitamin D intake; if dietary intake is inadequate, dietary supplementation is recommended. Women and men should consume:

Calcium: 1000 mg/day (men: 50-70 years) **or** 1200 mg/day (women ≥51 years and men ≥71 years) (IOM, 2011; NOF, 2013)

Vitamin D: 800-1000 IU/day (men and women ≥50 years) (NOF, 2013). Recommended Dietary Allowance (RDA): 600 IU/day (men and women ≤70 years) **or** 800 IU/day (men and women ≥71 years) (IOM, 2011).

Administration Administer first thing in the morning and ≥30 minutes before the first food, beverage (except plain water), or other medication(s) of the day. Do not take with mineral water or with other beverages. Patients should be instructed to stay upright (not to lie down) for at least 30 minutes **and** until after first food of the day (to reduce esophageal irritation).

Oral solution: Administer oral solution, followed with at least 2 oz of plain water.

Tablet (Fosamax): Must be taken with 6-8 oz of plain water.

Tablet, effervescent (Binosto): Dissolve one tablet in 4 oz of room temperature plain water only; once effervescence stops, wait ≥5 minutes and stir the solution for ~10 seconds and then drink.

Monitoring Parameters

Osteoporosis: Bone mineral density (BMD) should be re-evaluated every 2 years (or more frequently) after initiating therapy (NOF, 2013); in patients with combined alendronate and glucocorticoid treatment, BMD should be made at initiation and repeated after 6-12 months; annual measurements of height and weight, assessment of chronic back pain; serum calcium and 25(OH)D; may consider monitoring biochemical markers of bone turnover

Paget's disease: Alkaline phosphatase; pain; serum calcium and 25(OH)D

Reference Range

Calcium (total): Adults: 9.0-11.0 mg/dL (2.05-2.54 mmol/L), may slightly decrease with aging

Phosphorus: 2.5-4.5 mg/dL (0.81-1.45 mmol/L)

Vitamin D: There is no clear consensus on a reference range for total serum 25(OH)D concentrations or the validity of this level as it relates clinically to bone health. In addition, there is significant variability in the reporting of serum 25(OH)D levels as a result of different assay types in use; however, the following ranges have been suggested:

Adults (IOM, 2011): Sufficient levels in practically all persons: ≥20 ng/mL (50 nmol/L); concern for risk of toxicity: >50 ng/mL (125 nmol/L)

Osteoporosis patients (NOF, 2013): Recommended level to reach and maintain: ~30 ng/mL (75 nmol/L)

Dosage Forms

Solution, Oral:

Generic: 70 mg/75 mL (75 mL)

Tablet, Oral:

Fosamax: 70 mg

Generic: 5 mg, 10 mg, 35 mg, 40 mg, 70 mg

Tablet Effervescent, Oral:

Binosto: 70 mg

Dosage Forms: Canada Refer to Dosage Forms. **Note:** Effervescent tablet and oral solution are not available in Canada.

◆ **Alendronate-70 (Can)** *see* Alendronate *on page* 79

Alendronate and Cholecalciferol

(a LEN droe nate & kole e kal SI fer ole)

Brand Names: U.S. Fosamax Plus D®

Brand Names: Canada Fosavance

Index Terms Alendronate Sodium and Cholecalciferol; Cholecalciferol and Alendronate; Vitamin D_3 and Alendronate

Pharmacologic Category Bisphosphonate Derivative; Vitamin D Analog

Use Treatment of osteoporosis in postmenopausal females; increase bone mass in males with osteoporosis

Pregnancy Risk Factor C

Dosage Osteoporosis: Adults: Oral: One tablet (alendronate 70 mg/cholecalciferol 2800 units **or** alendronate 70 mg/cholecalciferol 5600 units) once weekly. Consider discontinuing after 3-5 years of use for osteoporosis in patients at low-risk for fracture. Supplemental calcium and vitamin D may be necessary if dietary intake is inadequate.

Missed doses: If a once-weekly dose is missed, it should be given the next morning after remembered; may then return to the original once-weekly schedule (original scheduled day of the week), however, do not give 2 doses on the same day.

Dosage adjustment in renal impairment:

CrCl ≥35 mL/minute: No dosage adjustment necessary.

CrCl <35 mL/minute: Use is not recommended.

Dosage adjustment in hepatic impairment: Alendronate: No dosage adjustment necessary. Cholecalciferol: May not be adequately absorbed in patients who have malabsorption due to inadequate bile production.

Additional Information Complete prescribing information should be consulted for additional detail.

Dosage Forms

Tablet:

Fosamax Plus D® 70/2800: Alendronate 70 mg and cholecalciferol 2800 units

Fosamax Plus D® 70/5600: Alendronate 70 mg and cholecalciferol 5600 units

◆ **Alendronate-FC (Can)** *see* Alendronate *on page 79*

◆ **Alendronate Sodium** *see* Alendronate *on page 79*

◆ **Alendronate Sodium and Cholecalciferol** *see* Alendronate and Cholecalciferol *on page 81*

◆ **Alendronic Acid Monosodium Salt Trihydrate** *see* Alendronate *on page 79*

◆ **Aler-Dryl [OTC]** *see* DiphenhydrAMINE (Systemic) *on page 641*

◆ **Alertec (Can)** *see* Modafinil *on page 1386*

◆ **Alesse (Can)** *see* Ethinyl Estradiol and Levonorgestrel *on page 803*

◆ **Alevazol [OTC]** *see* Clotrimazole (Topical) *on page 488*

◆ **Aleve [OTC]** *see* Naproxen *on page 1427*

◆ **Aleve (Can)** *see* Naproxen *on page 1427*

Alfacalcidol [CAN/INT] (Al fa CAL ce dol)

Brand Names: Canada One-Alpha®

Index Terms 1-α-hydroxycholecalciferol; 1-α-hydroxyvitamin D_3; 1alfacalcidol; $_1$alfa-hydroxyvitamin D3

Pharmacologic Category Vitamin D Analog

Use Note: Not approved in U.S.

Management of hypocalcemia, secondary hyperparathyroidism, and osteodystrophy in patients with chronic renal failure

Pregnancy Considerations Adverse events were observed in animal reproduction studies.

Breast-Feeding Considerations Because alfacalcidol may be excreted into breast milk, the manufacturer recommends that breast-feeding be avoided.

Contraindications Hypersensitivity to 1-α-hydroxyvitamin D_3, vitamin D or its analogues and derivatives, or any component of the formulation; hypercalcemia; hyperphosphatemia; evidence of vitamin D toxicity

Warnings/Precautions Avoid use of high or excessive dosing; excessive vitamin D administration may lead to over suppression of PTH, progressive or acute hypercalcemia, hypercalciuria, hyperphosphatemia, and adynamic bone disease. Monitor for hypercalcemia. Dose reductions or discontinuation of therapy and of calcium supplementation may be necessary. Discontinue use if hypercalcemia occurs in dialysis patients; may reinstitute therapy at 50% of previous dose ~1 week after calcium levels have normalized. Hyperphosphatemia may increase the need for phosphate-binding agents. Use with caution in patients receiving digoxin; hypercalcemia may precipitate cardiac arrhythmias in patients taking digoxin. Avoid use with other vitamin D products or derivatives and with magnesium-containing antacids.

Adverse Reactions As associated with Hypervitaminosis D:

Cardiovascular: Cardiac arrhythmia, hypertension

Central nervous system: Headache, hyperthermia, psychosis (rare), somnolence

Dermatologic: Pruritus

Genitourinary: Nocturia

Endocrine & metabolic: Hypercalcemia, hypercholesterolemia, hyperphosphatemia, libido decreased, polydipsia

Gastrointestinal: Anorexia, constipation, nausea, pancreatitis, taste abnormal, vomiting, weight loss, xerostomia

Hepatic: ALT increased, AST increased

Neuromuscular & skeletal: Bone pain, muscle pain, weakness

Ocular: Conjunctivitis, corneal calcification, photophobia

Renal: BUN increased, polyuria

Respiratory: Rhinorrhea

Drug Interactions

Metabolism/Transport Effects None known.

Avoid Concomitant Use

Avoid concomitant use of Alfacalcidol with any of the following: Aluminum Hydroxide; Multivitamins/Fluoride (with ADE); Multivitamins/Minerals (with ADEK, Folate, Iron); Sucralfate; Vitamin D Analogs

Increased Effect/Toxicity

Alfacalcidol may increase the levels/effects of: Aluminum Hydroxide; Cardiac Glycosides; Magnesium Salts; Sucralfate; Vitamin D Analogs

The levels/effects of Alfacalcidol may be increased by: Calcium Salts; Danazol; Multivitamins/Fluoride (with ADE); Multivitamins/Minerals (with ADEK, Folate, Iron); Thiazide Diuretics

Decreased Effect

The levels/effects of Alfacalcidol may be decreased by: Bile Acid Sequestrants; Mineral Oil; Orlistat

Storage/Stability

Oral capsule: Store between 15°C to 25°C (59°F to 77°F). Protect from direct sunlight.

Oral solution: Store between 2°C to 8°C (36°F to 46°F). Protect from direct sunlight.

Injection solution: Store between 2°C to 8°C (36°F to 46°F). Protect from light.

Mechanism of Action Alfacalcidol is rapidly converted to the active metabolite of vitamin D (1,25-dihydroxyvitamin D_3) in the liver, effectively bypassing renal metabolic conversion; promotes intestinal absorption of calcium and phosphorous, resorption of calcium from the bone, and possibly renal reabsorption of calcium

Pharmacodynamics/Kinetics

Onset: 6 hours

Duration of effect on intestinal calcium absorption levels: 1,25-$(OH)_2$ D_3: 48 hours

Protein binding: Extensively to vitamin D-binding protein

Metabolism: Hepatic to 1,25-$(OH)_2$ D_3

Half-life elimination: 3 hours in renal insufficiency

Time to peak of active vitamin D levels: Oral: 12 hours; IV: 4 hours

Dosage Adults: Hypocalcemia, secondary hyperparathyroidism, or osteodystrophy in chronic renal failure:

Oral:

Predialysis patients: **Note:** Limit supplemental calcium to ≤500 mg/day (elemental calcium):

Initial: 0.25 mcg/day for 2 months; if necessary, may titrate dose upward in increments of 0.25 mcg/day every 2 months

Maintenance (usual dose): 0.5 mcg/day; up to 1 mcg/day may be necessary to maintain desired serum calcium concentrations

Dialysis patients:

Initial: 1 mcg/day for up to 4 weeks; if necessary, may titrate dose upward in increments of 0.5 mcg/day every 2-4 weeks. Usual effective dose: 1-2 mcg/day; up to 3 mcg/day may be required in some patients.

Maintenance (usual dose): 0.25-1 mcg/day; dosing interval may be increased (every other day) in patients who develop hypercalcemia

Note: In some studies, intermittent dosing (on dialysis days) in dialysis patients has been shown as efficacious as daily dosing (Tarrass, 2006).

IV: Dialysis patients:

Initial: 1 mcg per dialysis (2-3 times weekly); if inadequate response after 1 week, may titrate dose upward in weekly increments of 1 mcg per dialysis (maximum dose: 12 mcg/week). Total titration period should not exceed 6 weeks.

Maintenance: 1.5-12 mcg per week (divided equally between hemodialysis sessions); usual effective dose: 6 mcg/week.

Dosage adjustment for toxicity:

Predialysis patients: If hypercalcemia develops within the first 2 months of therapy reduce dose to 0.25 mcg every other day; at any other time during therapy, reduce dose by 50% and discontinue all calcium supplements until serum calcium levels normalize.

Dialysis patients: Oral, IV: Discontinue immediately for hypercalcemia; may consider reintroducing therapy at a reduced dose after serum calcium levels normalize.

Dosage adjustment in renal impairment: No dosage adjustment necessary.

Dosage adjustment in hepatic impairment: No dosage adjustment provided in the manufacturer's labeling.

Dietary Considerations Adequate dietary calcium is necessary for clinical response to vitamin D. Recommended daily allowance of calcium in adults: 800-1000 mg (from all sources of calcium intake such as dialysate, diet and calcium supplements).

Administration

Oral: Administer oral solution (drops) and capsules with food.

IV: Shake injection solution well prior to use and administer as bolus IV injection over 30 seconds at the end of each dialysis.

Monitoring Parameters

Serum calcium and phosphorus: Frequency of measurement may be dependent upon the presence and magnitude of abnormalities, the rate of progression of CKD, and the use of treatments for CKD-mineral and bone disorders (KDIGO, 2009):

CKD stage 3: Every 6-12 months

CKD stage 4: Every 3-6 months

CKD stage 5 and 5D: Every 1-3 months

Periodic 24-hour urinary calcium and phosphorus; magnesium; alkaline phosphatase every 12 months or more frequently in the presence of elevated PTH; creatinine, BUN, albumin; intact parathyroid hormone (iPTH) every 3-12 months depending on CKD severity; periodic ophthalmologic exams

Reference Range

Corrected total serum calcium (K/DOQI, 2003): CKD stages 3 and 4: 8.4-10.2 mg/dL (2.1-2.6 mmol/L); CKD stage 5: 8.4-9.5 mg/dL (2.1-2.37 mmol/L); KDIGO guidelines recommend maintaining normal ranges for all stages of CKD (3-5D) (KDIGO, 2009)

Phosphorus (K/DOQI, 2003): CKD stages 3 and 4: 2.7-4.6 mg/dL (0.87-1.48 mmol/L); CKD stage 5 (including those treated with dialysis): 3.5-5.5 mg/dL (1.13-1.78 mmol/L); KDIGO guidelines recommend maintaining normal ranges for CKD stages 3-5 and lowering elevated phosphorus levels toward the normal range for CKD stage 5D (KDIGO, 2009)

Serum calcium-phosphorus product (K/DOQI, 2003): CKD stage 3-5: <55 mg^2/dL^2

PTH: Whole molecule, immunochemiluminometric assay (ICMA): 1.0-5.2 pmol/L; whole molecule, radioimmunoassay (RIA): 10.0-65.0 pg/mL; whole molecule, immunoradiometric, double antibody (IRMA): 1.0-6.0 pmol/L

Target ranges by stage of chronic kidney disease (KDIGO, 2009): CKD stage 3-5: Optimal iPTH is unknown; maintain normal range (assay-dependent); CKD stage 5D: Maintain iPTH within 2-9 times the upper limit of normal for the assay used

Product Availability Not available in the U.S.

Dosage Forms: Canada

Capsule, softgel, oral:

One-Alpha®: 0.25 mcg, 1 mcg [contains sesame oil]

Injection, solution:

One-Alpha®: 2 mcg/mL

Solution, oral [drops]:

One-Alpha®: 2 mcg/mL

◆ **1alfacalcidol** *see* Alfacalcidol [CAN/INT] *on page* 82

◆ **$_1$alfa-hydroxyvitamin D3** *see* Alfacalcidol [CAN/INT] *on page* 82

◆ **Alfenta** *see* Alfentanil *on page* 83

Alfentanil (al FEN ta nil)

Brand Names: U.S. Alfenta

Brand Names: Canada Alfenta; Alfentanil Injection, USP

Index Terms Alfentanil Hydrochloride

Pharmacologic Category Analgesic, Opioid; Anilidopiperidine Opioid

Use

Analgesia: Analgesic adjunct for the maintenance of anesthesia with barbiturate/nitrous oxide/oxygen; analgesic with nitrous oxide/oxygen in the maintenance of general anesthesia; analgesic component for monitored anesthesia care

Anesthetic: Primary anesthetic for induction of anesthesia in general surgery when endotracheal intubation and mechanical ventilation are required

Pregnancy Risk Factor C

Dosage Doses should be titrated to appropriate effects; wide range of doses is dependent upon desired degree of analgesia/anesthesia

Children <12 years: Dose not established

Adults: Base dose on actual body weight unless >20% above ideal body weight, then base dose on lean body weight.

Alfentanil

Indication	Approx Duration of Anesthesia (min)	Induction Period (Initial Dose) (mcg/kg)	Maintenance Period (Increments/ Infusion)	Total Dose (mcg/kg)	Effects
Incremental injection	≤30	8-20	3-5 mcg/kg every 5-20 minutes or 0.5-1 mcg/kg/min	8-40	Spontaneously breathing or assisted ventilation when required.
	30-60	20-50	5-15 mcg/kg every 5-20 minutes	Up to 75	Assisted or controlled ventilation required. Attenuation of response to laryngoscopy and intubation.
Continuous infusion	>45	50-75	0.5-3 mcg/kg/min; average infusion rate 1-1.5 mcg/kg/min	Dependent on duration of procedure	Assisted or controlled ventilation required. Some attenuation of response to intubation and incision, with intraoperative stability.
Anesthetic induction	>45	130-245	0.5-1.5 mcg/kg/min or general anesthetic	Dependent on duration of procedure	Assisted or controlled ventilation required. Administer induction dose slowly (over 3 minutes). Concentration of inhalation agents reduced by 30% to 50% for initial hour.
Monitored Anesthesia Care (MAC)		3-8	3-5 mcg/kg every 5-20 minutes or 0.25-1 mcg/kg/min (may continue infusion until end of procedure)	3-40	Sedation, responsiveness, spontaneously breathing

Dosage adjustment in renal impairment: There are no dosage adjustments provided in the manufacturer's labeling; use with caution. The pharmacokinetics of alfentanil were evaluated in adult patients with chronic renal failure and compared to patients with normal renal function. Although V_{dss} was increased in patients with renal failure, elimination half-life was similar between the 2 groups (Chauvin, 1987). Therefore, prolongation of alfentanil duration of action is not expected and dosage adjustment is not necessary.

Dosage adjustment in hepatic impairment: There are no dosage adjustments provided in the manufacturer's labeling; use with caution.

Dosing in obesity: In patients weighing >20% above ideal body weight, determine dose based on lean body weight.

Additional Information Complete prescribing information should be consulted for additional detail.

Dosage Forms

Injectable, Injection [preservative free]:

Alfenta: 500 mcg/mL (2 mL, 5 mL)

Generic: 500 mcg/mL (2 mL, 5 mL)

◆ **Alfentanil Hydrochloride** *see* Alfentanil *on page 83*

◆ **Alfentanil Injection, USP (Can)** *see* Alfentanil *on page 83*

◆ **Alferon N** *see* Interferon Alfa-n3 *on page 1100*

Alfuzosin (al FYOO zoe sin)

Brand Names: U.S. Uroxatral

Brand Names: Canada Apo-Alfuzosin®; Sandoz-Alfuzosin; Teva-Alfuzosin PR; Xatral

Index Terms Alfuzosin Hydrochloride

Pharmacologic Category Alpha$_1$ Blocker

Use Treatment of the functional symptoms of benign prostatic hyperplasia (BPH)

Pregnancy Risk Factor B

Pregnancy Considerations Adverese effects were not observed in animal reproduction studies.

Contraindications Hypersensitivity to alfuzosin or any component of the formulation; moderate or severe hepatic insufficiency (Child-Pugh class B and C); concurrent use with potent CYP3A4 inhibitors (eg, itraconazole, ketoconazole, ritonavir) or other alpha$_1$-blocking agents

Warnings/Precautions Not intended for use as an antihypertensive drug. May cause significant orthostatic hypotension and syncope, especially with first dose; anticipate a similar effect if therapy is interrupted for a few days, if dosage is rapidly increased, or used with antihypertensives (particularly vasodilators), PDE-5 inhibitors, nitrates or other medications which may result in hypotension. Discontinue if symptoms of angina occur or worsen. Alfuzosin has been shown to prolong the QT interval alone (minimal) and with other drugs with comparable effects on the QT interval (additive); use with caution in patients with known QT prolongation (congenital or acquired). Patients should be cautioned about performing hazardous tasks when starting new therapy or adjusting dosage upward. Discontinue if symptoms of angina occur or worsen. Rule out prostatic carcinoma before beginning therapy. Use caution with severe renal or mild hepatic impairment; contraindicated in moderate-to-severe hepatic impairment. Intraoperative floppy iris syndrome has been observed in cataract surgery patients who were on or were previously treated with alpha$_1$-blockers. Causality has not been established and there appears to be no benefit in discontinuing alpha-blocker therapy prior to surgery. May cause priapism. Contraindicated in patients taking strong CYP3A4 inhibitors or other alpha$_1$-blockers.

Adverse Reactions

Central nervous system: Dizziness, fatigue, headache, pain

Gastrointestinal: Abdominal pain, constipation, dyspepsia, nausea

Genitourinary: Impotence

Respiratory: Bronchitis, pharyngitis, sinusitis, upper respiratory tract infection

Rare but important or life-threatening: Angioedema, atrial fibrillation, chest pain, edema, hepatic injury (including cholestatic), hypotension, intraoperative floppy iris syndrome (with cataract surgery), priapism, pruritus, thrombocytopenia, toxic epidermal necrolysis

Drug Interactions

Metabolism/Transport Effects Substrate of CYP3A4 (major); **Note:** Assignment of Major/Minor substrate status based on clinically relevant drug interaction potential

Avoid Concomitant Use

Avoid concomitant use of Alfuzosin with any of the following: Alpha1-Blockers; Conivaptan; CYP3A4 Inhibitors (Strong); Fusidic Acid (Systemic); Highest Risk QTc-Prolonging Agents; Idelalisib; Ivabradine; Mifepristone; Protease Inhibitors; Telaprevir

Increased Effect/Toxicity

Alfuzosin may increase the levels/effects of: Alpha1-Blockers; Antihypertensives; Highest Risk QTc-Prolonging Agents; Moderate Risk QTc-Prolonging Agents; Nitroglycerin

The levels/effects of Alfuzosin may be increased by: Aprepitant; Beta-Blockers; Conivaptan; CYP3A4 Inhibitors (Moderate); CYP3A4 Inhibitors (Strong); Dapoxetine; Dasatinib; Fosaprepitant; Fusidic Acid (Systemic); Idelalisib; Ivabradine; Ivacaftor; Luliconazole; MAO Inhibitors; Mifepristone; Netupitant; Phosphodiesterase 5 Inhibitors; Protease Inhibitors; QTc-Prolonging Agents (Indeterminate Risk and Risk Modifying); Simeprevir; Telaprevir

Decreased Effect

Alfuzosin may decrease the levels/effects of: Alpha-/Beta-Agonists; Alpha1-Agonists

The levels/effects of Alfuzosin may be decreased by: Bosentan; CYP3A4 Inducers (Moderate); CYP3A4 Inducers (Strong); Dabrafenib; Deferasirox; Mitotane; Siltuximab; St Johns Wort; Tocilizumab

Food Interactions Food increases the extent of absorption. Management: Administer immediately following a meal at the same time each day.

Storage/Stability Store at room temperature of 25°C (77°F); excursions permitted to 15°C to 30°C (59°F to 86°F). Protect from light and moisture.

Mechanism of Action An antagonist of alpha$_1$-adrenoreceptors in the lower urinary tract. Smooth muscle tone is mediated by the sympathetic nervous stimulation of alpha$_1$-adrenoreceptors, which are abundant in the prostate, prostatic capsule, prostatic urethra, and bladder neck. Blockade of these adrenoreceptors can cause smooth muscles in the bladder neck and prostate to relax, resulting in an improvement in urine flow rate and a reduction in BPH symptoms.

Pharmacodynamics/Kinetics

Absorption: Decreased 50% under fasting conditions

Distribution: V_d: 3.2 L/kg

Protein binding: 82% to 90%

Metabolism: Hepatic, primarily via CYP3A4; metabolism includes oxidation, O-demethylation, and N-dealkylation; forms metabolites (inactive)

Bioavailability: 49% following a meal

Half-life elimination: 10 hours

Time to peak, plasma: 8 hours following a meal

Excretion: Feces (69%); urine (24%; 11% as unchanged drug)

Dosage Oral: Adults:

Benign prostatic hyperplasia (BPH): 10 mg once daily

Ureteral stones, expulsion (off-label use): 10 mg once daily, discontinue after successful expulsion (average time to expulsion 1-2 weeks) (Agrawal, 2009; Ahmed, 2010; Gurbuz, 2011). **Note:** Patients with stones >10 mm were excluded from studies.

Dosage adjustment in renal impairment: Bioavailability and maximum serum concentrations are increased with mild (CrCl 60-80 mL/minute), moderate (CrCl 30-59 mL/minute), or severe (CrCl <30 mL/minute) renal impairment.

Note: Safety data is limited in patients with severe renal impairment (CrCl <30 mL/minute). Use with caution.

Dosage adjustment in hepatic impairment:

Mild hepatic impairment: Use has not been studied; use caution

Moderate or severe hepatic impairment (Child-Pugh class B or C): Clearance is decreased and serum concentration is increased; use is contraindicated

Dietary Considerations Take immediately following a meal at the same time each day.

Administration Tablet should be swallowed whole; do not crush or chew. Administer once daily (immediately following a meal); should be taken at the same time each day.

Monitoring Parameters Urine flow, blood pressure, PSA

Dosage Forms

Tablet Extended Release 24 Hour, Oral:

Uroxatral: 10 mg

Generic: 10 mg

◆ **Alfuzosin Hydrochloride** *see* Alfuzosin *on page 84*

◆ **Alglucosidase** *see* Alglucosidase Alfa *on page 85*

Alglucosidase Alfa (al gloo KOSE i dase AL fa)

Brand Names: U.S. Lumizyme; Myozyme

Brand Names: Canada Myozyme

Index Terms Alglucosidase; GAA; rhGAA

Pharmacologic Category Enzyme

Use

Pompe disease: For use in patients with Pompe disease (acid alpha-glucosidase [GAA] deficiency).

Limitations of use: Myozyme: Improves ventilator-free survival in patients with infantile-onset Pompe disease compared with an untreated historical control, whereas use of Myozyme in patients with other forms of Pompe disease has not been adequately studied to ensure safety and efficacy.

Pregnancy Risk Factor C

Dosage Pompe disease: IV:

Infantile-onset (Lumizyme, Myozyme): Infants ≥1 month, Children, and Adolescents: 20 mg/kg every 2 weeks

Noninfantile, late-onset (Lumizyme): Infants ≥1 month, Children, Adolescents, and Adults: 20 mg/kg every 2 weeks

Dosage adjustment in renal impairment: There are no dosage adjustments provided in the manufacturer's labeling.

Dosage adjustment in hepatic impairment: There are no dosage adjustments provided in the manufacturer's labeling.

Additional Information Complete prescribing information should be consulted for additional detail.

Dosage Forms

Solution Reconstituted, Intravenous [preservative free]:

Lumizyme: 50 mg (1 ea)

Myozyme: 50 mg (1 ea)

◆ **Alimta** *see* PEMEtrexed *on page 1606*

◆ **Alinia** *see* Nitazoxanide *on page 1461*

Aliskiren (a lis KYE ren)

Brand Names: U.S. Tekturna

Brand Names: Canada Rasilez

Index Terms Aliskiren Hemifumarate; SPP100

Pharmacologic Category Renin Inhibitor

Use

Hypertension: Treatment of hypertension, alone or in combination with other antihypertensive agents

Note: According to the Eighth Joint National Committee (JNC 8) guidelines, aliskiren is **not** recommended for the initial treatment of hypertension (James, 2013).

Pregnancy Risk Factor D

Pregnancy Considerations **[U.S. Boxed Warning]: Drugs that act on the renin-angiotensin system can cause injury and death to the developing fetus. Discontinue as soon as possible once pregnancy is detected.** The use of drugs which act on the renin-angiotensin system are associated with oligohydramnios. Oligohydramnios, due to decreased fetal renal function, may lead to fetal lung hypoplasia and skeletal malformations. Use is also associated with anuria, hypotension, renal failure, skull hypoplasia, and death in the fetus/neonate. The exposed fetus should be monitored for fetal growth, amniotic fluid volume, and organ formation. Infants exposed *in utero* should be monitored for hyperkalemia, hypotension, and oliguria.

Breast-Feeding Considerations It is not known if aliskiren is excreted in breast milk. Due to the potential for serious adverse reactions in the nursing infant, a decision should be made whether to discontinue nursing or to discontinue the drug, taking into account the importance of treatment to the mother.

Contraindications

U.S. labeling: Concomitant use with an ACE inhibitor or ARB in patients with diabetes mellitus

Canadian labeling: Additional contraindications (not in U.S. labeling): Hypersensitivity to aliskiren or any component of the formulation; history of angioedema with aliskiren, ACE inhibitors, or ARBs; hereditary or idiopathic angioedema; pregnancy, breast-feeding; concomitant use with ACE inhibitors or ARBs in patients with GFR <60 mL/minute/1.73 m^2

Warnings/Precautions [U.S. Boxed Warning]: Drugs that act on the renin-angiotensin system can cause injury and death to the developing fetus. Discontinue as soon as possible once pregnancy is detected. Hypersensitivity reactions, including anaphylaxis and angioedema have been reported; since the effect of aliskiren on bradykinin levels is unknown, the risk of kinin-mediated etiologies of angioedema occurring is also unknown. Use with caution in any patient with a history of angioedema (of any etiology) as angioedema, some cases necessitating hospitalization and intubation, has been observed (rarely) with aliskiren use. Discontinue immediately following the occurrence of anaphylaxis or angioedema; do not readminister. Prolonged frequent monitoring may be required especially if tongue, glottis, or larynx are involved as they are associated with airway obstruction. Patients with a history of airway surgery may have a higher risk of airway obstruction. Early, aggressive, and appropriate management is critical. Hyperkalemia may occur (rarely) during monotherapy; risk may increase in patients with predisposing factors (eg, renal dysfunction, diabetes mellitus or concomitant use with ACE inhibitors, potassium-sparing diuretics, potassium supplements, and/or potassium-containing salts). Symptomatic hypotension may occur (rarely) during the initiation of therapy, particularly in volume or salt-depleted patients or with concomitant use of other agents acting on the renin-angiotensin-aldosterone system. If hypotension does occur, this is not a contraindication for further use; once blood pressure has been stabilized, aliskiren usually can be continued without difficulty. Use with caution or avoid in patients with deteriorating renal function or low renal blood flow (eg, renal artery stenosis, severe heart failure); may increase risk of developing acute renal failure and hyperkalemia. Concomitant use with an ACE inhibitor or ARB may increase risk of developing acute renal failure and should be avoided in patient with GFR <60 mL/minute. Use (monotherapy or combined with ACE inhibitors or ARBs) in patients with type 2 diabetes mellitus has demonstrated an increased incidence of renal impairment, hypotension, and hyperkalemia; use is contraindicated in patients with diabetes mellitus who are taking an ACE inhibitor or ARB. Potentially significant drug-drug interactions may exist, requiring dose or frequency adjustment, additional monitoring, and/or selection of alternative therapy. Serious skins reactions including Stevens Johnson syndrome and toxic epidermal necrolysis (TEN) have been reported.

Adverse Reactions

Dermatologic: Skin rash

Gastrointestinal: Diarrhea

Neuromuscular & skeletal: Increased creatine phosphokinase (>300% increase)

Renal: Increased blood urea nitrogen, increased serum creatinine

Respiratory: Cough

Rare but important or life-threatening: Anaphylaxis, angina pectoris, gastroesophageal reflux disease, hepatic insufficiency, hyperkalemia, increased uric acid, rhabdomyolysis, seizure, severe hypotension, Stevens-Johnson syndrome

Drug Interactions

Metabolism/Transport Effects Substrate of CYP3A4 (minor), P-glycoprotein; **Note:** Assignment of Major/Minor substrate status based on clinically relevant drug interaction potential

Avoid Concomitant Use

Avoid concomitant use of Aliskiren with any of the following: CycloSPORINE (Systemic); Itraconazole

Increased Effect/Toxicity

Aliskiren may increase the levels/effects of: ACE Inhibitors; Amifostine; Angiotensin II Receptor Blockers; Antihypertensives; DULoxetine; Hypotensive Agents; Levodopa; Obinutuzumab; RisperiDONE; RiTUXimab

The levels/effects of Aliskiren may be increased by: Alfuzosin; AtorvaSTATin; Barbiturates; Brimonidine (Topical); Canagliflozin; CycloSPORINE (Systemic); Diazoxide; Heparin; Heparin (Low Molecular Weight); Herbs (Hypotensive Properties); Itraconazole; Ketoconazole (Systemic); MAO Inhibitors; Nicorandil; Nonsteroidal Anti-Inflammatory Agents; Pentoxifylline; P-glycoprotein/ABCB1 Inhibitors; Phosphodiesterase 5 Inhibitors; Potassium Salts; Prostacyclin Analogues; Verapamil

Decreased Effect

Aliskiren may decrease the levels/effects of: Furosemide

The levels/effects of Aliskiren may be decreased by: Grapefruit Juice; Herbs (Hypertensive Properties); Methylphenidate; Nonsteroidal Anti-Inflammatory Agents; P-glycoprotein/ABCB1 Inducers; Yohimbine

Food Interactions High-fat meals decrease absorption. Grapefruit juice may decrease the serum concentration of aliskiren. Management: Administer at the same time each day; may take with or without a meal, but consistent administration with regards to meals is recommended. Avoid concomitant use of aliskiren and grapefruit juice.

Storage/Stability Store at 25°C (77°F); excursions permitted to 15°C to 30°C (59°F to 86°F). Protect from moisture.

Mechanism of Action Aliskiren is a direct renin inhibitor, resulting in blockade of the conversion of angiotensinogen to angiotensin I. Angiotensin I suppression decreases the formation of angiotensin II (Ang II), a potent blood pressure-elevating peptide (via direct vasoconstriction, aldosterone release, and sodium retention). Ang II also functions within the Renin-Angiotensin-Aldosterone System (RAAS) as a negative inhibitory feedback mediator within the renal parenchyma to suppress the further release of renin. Thus, reductions in Ang II levels suppress this feedback loop, leading to further increased plasma renin concentrations (PRC) and subsequent activity (PRA). This disinhibition effect can be potentially problematic for ACE inhibitor and ARB therapy, as increased PRA could partially overcome the pharmacologic inhibition of the RAAS. As aliskiren is a direct inhibitor of renin activity, blunting of PRA despite the increased PRC (from loss of the negative feedback) may be clinically advantageous. The effect of aliskiren on bradykinin levels is unknown.

Pharmacodynamics/Kinetics

Onset of action: Maximum antihypertensive effect: Within 2 weeks

Absorption: Poor; absorption decreased by high-fat meal. Aliskiren is a substrate of P-glycoprotein; concurrent use of P-glycoprotein inhibitors may increase absorption.

Metabolism: Extent of metabolism unknown; *in vitro* studies indicate metabolism via CYP3A4

Bioavailability: ~3%

Half-life elimination: ~24 hours (range: 16 to 32 hours)

Time to peak, plasma: 1 to 3 hours

Excretion: Urine (~25% of absorbed dose excreted unchanged in urine); feces (unchanged via biliary excretion)

Dosage Oral:

Adults: Initial: 150 mg once daily; may increase to 300 mg once daily (maximum: 300 mg daily). Usual dosage range (ASH/ISH [Weber, 2014]): 150 to 300 mg once daily. **Note:** Prior to initiation, correct hypovolemia and/or closely monitor volume status in patients on concurrent diuretics during treatment initiation.

Elderly: No initial dosage adjustment required

Dosage adjustment in renal impairment:

CrCl ≥30 mL/minute: Initial: No dosage adjustment necessary.

CrCl <30 mL/minute: Initial:

U.S. labeling: No dosage adjustment necessary (Vaidyanathan, 2007); however, risk of hyperkalemia and progressive renal dysfunction may occur; use with caution.

Canadian labeling: Avoid use

ESRD (requiring hemodialysis): Initial:

U.S. labeling: No dosage adjustment necessary (Khadzhynov, 2012); however, with chronic therapy, risk of hyperkalemia is increased; use with extreme caution. **Note:** Hemodialysis eliminates a minimal fraction; does not significantly alter overall aliskiren exposure.

Canadian labeling: There are no dosage adjustments provided in the manufacturer's labeling.

Dosage adjustment in hepatic impairment: Mild-to-severe: Initial: No dosage adjustment necessary.

Dietary Considerations May be taken with or without food; however, a high-fat meal reduces absorption. Consistent administration with regards to meals is recommended.

Administration Administer at the same time daily; may take with or without a meal, but consistent administration with regards to meals is recommended.

Monitoring Parameters Blood pressure; serum potassium, BUN, serum creatinine

Dosage Forms

Tablet, Oral:

Tekturna: 150 mg, 300 mg

Aliskiren, Amlodipine, and Hydrochlorothiazide

(a lis KYE ren, am LOE di peen, & hye droe klor oh THYE a zide)

Brand Names: U.S. Amturnide™

Index Terms Aliskiren, Hydrochlorothiazide, and Amlodipine; Amlodipine Besylate, Aliskiren Hemifumarate, and Hydrochlorothiazide; Amlodipine, Aliskiren, and Hydrochlorothiazide; Amlodipine, Hydrochlorothiazide, and Aliskiren; Hydrochlorothiazide, Aliskiren, and Amlodipine; Hydrochlorothiazide, Amlodipine, and Aliskiren

Pharmacologic Category Antianginal Agent; Antihypertensive; Calcium Channel Blocker; Calcium Channel Blocker, Dihydropyridine; Diuretic, Thiazide; Renin Inhibitor

Use Treatment of hypertension (not for initial therapy)

Pregnancy Risk Factor D

Dosage Note: Not for initial therapy. Dose is individualized; combination product may be substituted for individual components in patients currently maintained on all three agents separately, used to switch a patient on any dual combination of the components who is experiencing dose-limiting adverse reactions from an individual component (to a lower dose of that component), or used as add-on therapy in patients not adequately controlled with any two of the following: Aliskiren, dihydropyridine calcium channel blockers, and thiazide diuretics.

Oral: Hypertension: Add-on/switch therapy/replacement therapy:

Adults: Aliskiren 150-300 mg and amlodipine 5-10 mg and hydrochlorothiazide 12.5-25 mg once daily; dose may be titrated after 2 weeks of therapy. Maximum recommended daily dose: Aliskiren 300 mg; amlodipine 10 mg; hydrochlorothiazide 25 mg

Elderly: Use of lower initial doses should be considered (use of individual components may be necessary).

Dosage adjustment in renal impairment:

CrCl ≥30 mL/minute: Initial: No dosage adjustment necessary.

CrCl <30 mL/minute: Initial: No dosage adjustment may be necessary (Vaidyanathan, 2007 [aliskiren]); however, risk of hyperkalemia and progressive renal dysfunction may occur with aliskiren; use with caution; hydrochlorothiazide is usually ineffective when CrCl <30 mL/minute and is contraindicated in patients who are anuric.

ESRD (requiring hemodialysis): Initial: No dosage adjustment may be necessary (Khadzhynov, 2012 [aliskiren]); however, risk of hyperkalemia is increased with chronic aliskiren therapy; use with extreme caution; hydrochlorothiazide is usually ineffective when CrCl <30 mL/minute and is contraindicated in patients who are anuric.

Dosage adjustment in hepatic impairment: Mild-to-severe: Use with caution and titrate slowly; amlodipine elimination prolonged; lower initial dose should be considered (possibly requiring use of the individual agents).

Additional Information Complete prescribing information should be consulted for additional detail.

Dosage Forms

Tablet, oral:

Amturnide: Aliskiren 150 mg, amlodipine 5 mg, and hydrochlorothiazide 12.5 mg; Aliskiren 300 mg, amlodipine 5 mg, and hydrochlorothiazide 12.5 mg; Aliskiren 300 mg, amlodipine 5 mg, and hydrochlorothiazide 25 mg; Aliskiren 300 mg, amlodipine 10 mg, and hydrochlorothiazide 12.5 mg; Aliskiren 300 mg, amlodipine 10 mg, and hydrochlorothiazide 25 mg

Aliskiren and Hydrochlorothiazide

(a lis KYE ren & hye droe klor oh THYE a zide)

Brand Names: U.S. Tekturna HCT

Brand Names: Canada Rasilez HCT

Index Terms Aliskiren Hemifumarate and Hydrochlorothiazide; Hydrochlorothiazide and Aliskiren

Pharmacologic Category Antihypertensive; Diuretic, Thiazide; Renin Inhibitor

Use

Hypertension: Treatment of hypertension, including use as initial therapy in patients likely to need multiple antihypertensives for adequate control

Canadian labeling: Treatment of hypertension when combination therapy is appropriate; not indicated for initial therapy.

Pregnancy Risk Factor D

Dosage Oral: **Note:** Dosage must be individualized. Combination product may be substituted for individual components in patients currently maintained on both agents separately or in patients not adequately controlled with monotherapy (using one of the agents or an agent within same antihypertensive class). The combination product is approved for use as initial therapy in the U.S. labeling but is not approved for this indication in the Canadian labeling.

Adults: Hypertension:

Initial therapy: Aliskiren 150 mg and hydrochlorothiazide 12.5 mg once daily, dose may be titrated at 2- to 4-week intervals; maximum recommended daily doses: Aliskiren 300 mg; hydrochlorothiazide 25 mg

Add-on therapy: Initiate by adding the lowest available dose of the alternative component (aliskiren 150 mg or hydrochlorothiazide 12.5 mg); titrate to effect; maximum recommended daily doses: Aliskiren 300 mg; hydrochlorothiazide 25 mg

Replacement therapy: Substitute for the individually titrated components

Note: Prior to initiation, correct hypovolemia and/or closely monitor volume status in patients on concurrent diuretics during treatment initiation.

Elderly: No initial dosage adjustment required

Dosage adjustment in renal impairment:

CrCl ≥30 mL/minute: Initial: No dosage adjustment necessary.

CrCl <30 mL/minute: Initial: There are no dosage adjustments provided in the manufacturer's labeling (has not been studied); hydrochlorothiazide is usually ineffective when CrCl <30 mL/minute and is contraindicated in anuric patients. The Canadian labeling contraindicates use if GFR <30 mL/minute/1.73 m^2. See also Aliskiren and Hydrochlorothiazide individual monographs.

Dosage adjustment in hepatic impairment:

U.S. labeling: Mild to severe impairment: No dosage adjustment necessary. Use with caution. See also Aliskiren and Hydrochlorothiazide individual monographs.

Canadian labeling:

Mild to moderate impairment: No dosage adjustment necessary. Use with caution.

Severe impairment: Use is not recommended.

Additional Information Complete prescribing information should be consulted for additional detail.

Dosage Forms

Tablet, Oral:

Tekturna HCT: 150/12.5: Aliskiren 150 mg and hydrochlorothiazide 12.5 mg; 150/25: Aliskiren 150 mg and hydrochlorothiazide 25 mg; 300/12.5: Aliskiren 300 mg and hydrochlorothiazide 12.5 mg; 300/25: Aliskiren 300 mg and hydrochlorothiazide 25 mg

Dosage Forms: Canada

Tablet, Oral:

Rasilez HCT: 150/12.5: Aliskiren 150 mg and hydrochlorothiazide 12.5 mg; 150/25: Aliskiren 150 mg and hydrochlorothiazide 25 mg; 300/12.5: Aliskiren 300 mg and hydrochlorothiazide 12.5 mg;300/25: Aliskiren 300 mg and hydrochlorothiazide 25 mg

◆ **Aliskiren Hemifumarate** *see* Aliskiren *on page 85*

◆ **Aliskiren Hemifumarate and Hydrochlorothiazide** *see* Aliskiren and Hydrochlorothiazide *on page 87*

◆ **Aliskiren, Hydrochlorothiazide, and Amlodipine** *see* Aliskiren, Amlodipine, and Hydrochlorothiazide *on page 87*

Alitretinoin (Systemic) [CAN/INT]

(a li TRET i noyn)

Brand Names: Canada Toctino

Index Terms 9-*cis*-Retinoic Acid; 9-*cis*-Tretinoin

Pharmacologic Category Anti-inflammatory Agent; Immunomodulator, Systemic; Retinoic Acid Derivative

Use Note: Not approved in U.S.

Eczema of the hand: Treatment of severe chronic hand eczema refractory to topical corticosteroids

Pregnancy Considerations [Canadian Boxed Warning]: Alitretinoin is a known teratogen and is contraindicated in pregnancy. Females must avoid becoming pregnant while receiving alitretinoin and for at least 1 month after discontinuation of therapy; fetal abnormalities and spontaneous abortion may occur. The risk for severe birth defects is high, with any dose or even with short treatment duration. If treatment with alitretinoin is required in women of childbearing potential, two reliable forms of birth control should be used simultaneously for at least 1 month prior to starting therapy, during therapy, and for 1 month after treatment. Two negative pregnancy tests (sensitivity at least 25 mIU/mL) and onset of next menses for 2 or 3 days are required prior to initiating therapy. Discontinue therapy immediately if pregnancy is discovered during treatment or within 1 month after stopping therapy; patients should be advised of the potential harm to the fetus and the physician and patient should discuss the desire to maintain the pregnancy.

Only physicians familiar with systemic retinoid therapy should prescribe alitretinoin. Females of childbearing potential must be able to fulfill all conditions for use prior to initiating therapy (consult manufacturer labeling for further detail). Physicians are required to use the Toctino Pregnancy Prevention Program, which includes comprehensive information regarding conditions that must be met prior to initiating therapy, birth control options, potential risks of therapy, informed consent, and monthly pregnancy reminders. Even women with amenorrhea, a history of infertility, or those who claim an absence of sexual activity must comply with these conditions.

Minimal amounts of alitretinoin have been detected in the semen of healthy male volunteers. Systemic exposure in female partners is expected to be negligible. The manufacturer labeling suggests that there is no apparent fetal risk in pregnant females whose male partners are receiving alitretinoin.

Breast-Feeding Considerations It is not known if alitretinoin is excreted in breast milk; however, it is highly lipophilic and is likely excreted in human breast milk. Due to the potential for serious adverse reactions in the nursing infant, breast-feeding is contraindicated.

Contraindications Hypersensitivity to alitretinoin, other retinoids, or any component of the formulation (including allergy to peanut or soya); pregnancy; breast-feeding; hepatic impairment; severe renal impairment; uncontrolled hypercholesterolemia; uncontrolled hypertriglyceridemia; uncontrolled hypothyroidism; hypervitaminosis A; fructose intolerance; concurrent use of tetracyclines

Warnings/Precautions Hazardous agent - use appropriate precautions for handling and disposal (NIOSH 2014 [group 3]). Use should be reserved for patients nonresponsive to potent topical corticosteroids and/or other measures (eg, avoidance of irritants/allergens, skin protection). **[Canadian Boxed Warning]: Alitretinoin is a known teratogen and is contraindicated in pregnancy. Females must avoid becoming pregnant while receiving alitretinoin and for at least 1 month after discontinuation of therapy;** fetal abnormalities and spontaneous abortion may occur. The risk for severe birth defects is high, with any dose or even with short treatment duration. **Only physicians familiar with systemic retinoid therapy should prescribe alitretinoin. Females of childbearing potential must be able to fulfill all conditions for use prior to initiating therapy (consult manufacturer labeling for further detail). Physicians are required to use the Toctino Pregnancy Prevention Program, which includes comprehensive information regarding conditions that must be met prior to initiating therapy, birth control options, potential risks of therapy, informed consent, and monthly pregnancy reminders.** Two reliable means of birth control should be used simultaneously for at least 1 month prior to starting therapy. Two negative pregnancy tests (sensitivity at least

25 mIU/mL) and the onset of next menses for 2 or 3 days are required prior to initiating therapy. Refer to Pregnancy Considerations for more detailed discussion. Patients should not donate blood during therapy and for 1 month after discontinuing therapy due to the potential risk to the fetus of a pregnant transfusion recipient.

[Canadian Boxed Warning]: Retinoids (including alitretinoin) have been associated with the development of benign intracranial hypertension, and in some cases involving concomitant tetracycline use. Discontinue use immediately for signs/symptoms of benign intracranial hypertension (eg, headache, abnormal vision, papilledema, nausea, vomiting).

Associated with hypercholesterolemia and hypertriglyceridemia; discontinue use for uncontrollable hypertriglyceridemia or signs/symptoms of pancreatitis. Use with caution in patients with diabetes mellitus; impaired glucose control has been reported with other retinoids. Associated with reversible reductions in thyroid stimulating hormone (TSH) and T_4 (free thyroxine). Transient and reversible transaminase elevations have been observed with other systemic retinoids; consider dose reduction or discontinuation of therapy for persistent clinically relevant effects. Onset of inflammatory bowel disease (IBD) in patients with no history of gastrointestinal disorders has been observed with use of another retinoid; discontinue use immediately for abdominal pain, rectal bleeding, or severe diarrhea. Rule out IBD in patients with severe diarrhea.

Systemic retinoid use may cause depression, psychosis, aggressive or violent behavior, and changes in mood; suicidal thoughts and actions have also been reported (rare). All patients should be observed closely for symptoms of depression or suicidal thoughts. Discontinuation of treatment alone may not be sufficient to relieve symptoms; further evaluation may be necessary. Use with extreme caution in patients with a history of psychiatric disorder.

Use of alitretinoin has been associated with myalgia and arthralgia. Bone changes (eg, premature epiphyseal closure, hyperostosis, calcification of tendons/ligaments) have been observed with other systemic retinoids. Retinoids enhance the effects of ultraviolet (UV) light; avoid excessive exposure to sunlight or sun lamp. Instruct patients to apply sun protectant (≥15 SPF), skin moisturizers, and lip balm when necessary. Dry eyes and/or impaired night vision have been reported with use; may be reversible upon discontinuation of therapy. Caution patients in regards to driving or operating machinery. Intolerance to contact lens (due to dry eyes) may be observed.

Adverse Reactions

Cardiovascular: Flushing, hypertension

Central nervous system: Depression, dizziness, headache

Dermatologic: Alopecia, cheilitis, cheilosis, erythema, xeroderma

Endocrine & metabolic: Decreased HDL cholesterol, decreased serum iron, high total iron binding capacity, hot flash, hypercholesterolemia, increased LDL cholesterol, increased serum triglycerides

Gastrointestinal: Dyspepsia, nausea, upper abdominal pain, vomiting, xerostomia

Hematologic & oncologic: Reticulocytopenia

Infection: Influenza

Neuromuscular & skeletal: Arthralgia, back pain, increased creatine phosphokinase

Ophthalmic: Abnormal sensation in eyes, conjunctivitis, dry eye syndrome

Respiratory: Nasopharyngitis, pharyngitis

Rare but important or life-threatening: Aggressive behavior, ankylosing spondylitis, cataract, decreased thyroid hormones (TSH and T4, reversible), epistaxis, exfoliation of skin, exostosis, nocturnal amblyopia, pseudotumor cerebri, psychotic symptoms, reduced fertility (male), suicidal ideation, suicidal tendencies, vasculitis

Drug Interactions

Metabolism/Transport Effects **Substrate** of CYP3A4 (major); **Note:** Assignment of Major/Minor substrate status based on clinically relevant drug interaction potential

Avoid Concomitant Use

Avoid concomitant use of Alitretinoin (Systemic) with any of the following: Conivaptan; Fusidic Acid (Systemic); Idelalisib; Multivitamins/Fluoride (with ADE); Multivitamins/Minerals (with ADEK, Folate, Iron); Multivitamins/Minerals (with AE, No Iron); Tetracycline Derivatives; Vitamin A

Increased Effect/Toxicity

Alitretinoin (Systemic) may increase the levels/effects of: Methotrexate; Porfimer; Verteporfin; Vitamin A

The levels/effects of Alitretinoin (Systemic) may be increased by: Aprepitant; Ceritinib; Conivaptan; CYP3A4 Inhibitors (Moderate); CYP3A4 Inhibitors (Strong); Dasatinib; Fosaprepitant; Fusidic Acid (Systemic); Idelalisib; Ivacaftor; Luliconazole; Mifepristone; Multivitamins/Fluoride (with ADE); Multivitamins/Minerals (with ADEK, Folate, Iron); Multivitamins/Minerals (with AE, No Iron); Netupitant; Simeprevir; Stiripentol; Tetracycline Derivatives

Decreased Effect

Alitretinoin (Systemic) may decrease the levels/effects of: Contraceptives (Estrogens); Contraceptives (Progestins)

Food Interactions Food significantly enhances systemic exposure and decreases variability in exposure. Management: Administer with a meal.

Storage/Stability Store between 15°C to 30°C (59°F to 86°F) in original packaging. Protect from light.

Mechanism of Action Precise mechanism of alitretinoin in chronic hand eczema is unknown. Binds to both retinoid acid receptor (RAR) and retinoid X receptor (RXR); anti-inflammatory and immunomodulating effects occur through down-regulation of chemokine expression in cytokine-induced dermal cells and suppressed expansion of cytokine-induced leukocytes and antigen presenting cells.

Pharmacodynamics/Kinetics

Duration: Serum concentrations of endogenous alitretinoin return to normal range within 24-72 hours after discontinuation

Absorption: Variable and dose-proportional

Protein binding: 99%

Metabolism: Hepatic via CYP3A4 to metabolites; Major metabolite: 4-oxo-alitretinoin (active)

Bioavailability: Systemic exposure is enhanced by food (Schmitt-Hoffman, 2011)

Half-life elimination: 2-10 hours

Time to peak: 3-4 hours (Weber, 1997)

Excretion: Urine (63% as metabolites); feces (30% as metabolites) (Schmitt-Hoffman, 2012)

Dosage Eczema of the hand (severe, chronic): Adults:

Oral: Initial: 30 mg once daily; usual range: 10-30 mg once daily

Patients at risk for cardiac events: Initiate therapy at 10 mg once daily; monitor closely.

Therapy duration: 12-24 weeks; consider discontinuation of therapy if severe disease is still present after initial 12 weeks of therapy. Patients who relapse may benefit from additional treatment; females who relapse must follow the same contraceptive protocol as when initiating therapy.

Elderly: Refer to adult dosing.

Dosage adjustment for toxicity: Consider dose reduction to 10 mg once daily for intolerable side effects.

Dosage adjustment in renal impairment

Mild to moderate impairment: There are no dosage adjustments provided in the manufacturer's labeling.

Severe impairment: Use is contraindicated.

Dosage adjustment in hepatic impairment: Use is contraindicated.

Dietary Considerations Take with a meal.

Administration Administer once daily with a meal. Missed doses should be taken as soon as possible; 2 doses should not be taken on the same day. Hazardous agent; use appropriate precautions for handling and disposal (NIOSH 2014 [group 3]).

Monitoring Parameters Prior to initiating therapy in female patients, perform two pregnancy tests (sensitivity at least 25 mIU/mL); second test must be performed ≤11 days prior to initiation. Thereafter, perform monthly pregnancy tests during therapy and at 1 month following discontinuation; serum lipids (particularly if at high risk for cardiac events) at baseline and then monthly until lipid response is established and again at discontinuation; hepatic function; serum glucose (periodically in patients with known or suspected diabetes mellitus); thyroid function; signs of depression, mood alteration, psychosis, aggression

Product Availability Not available in the U.S.

Dosage Forms: Canada

Capsule, Oral:

Toctino: 10 mg, 30 mg

- ◆ **Alkeran** *see* Melphalan *on page 1283*
- ◆ **All Day Allergy [OTC]** *see* Cetirizine *on page 411*
- ◆ **All Day Allergy Childrens [OTC]** *see* Cetirizine *on page 411*
- ◆ **All Day Pain Relief [OTC]** *see* Naproxen *on page 1427*
- ◆ **All Day Relief [OTC]** *see* Naproxen *on page 1427*
- ◆ **Allegra 12 Hour (OTC) (Can)** *see* Fexofenadine *on page 873*
- ◆ **Allegra 24 Hour (OTC) (Can)** *see* Fexofenadine *on page 873*
- ◆ **Allegra-D® (Can)** *see* Fexofenadine and Pseudoephedrine *on page 874*
- ◆ **Allegra-D® 12 Hour** *see* Fexofenadine and Pseudoephedrine *on page 874*
- ◆ **Allegra-D® 24 Hour** *see* Fexofenadine and Pseudoephedrine *on page 874*
- ◆ **Allegra Allergy [OTC]** *see* Fexofenadine *on page 873*
- ◆ **Allegra Allergy Childrens [OTC]** *see* Fexofenadine *on page 873*
- ◆ **Allerdryl (Can)** *see* DiphenhydrAMINE (Systemic) *on page 641*
- ◆ **Allerest** *see* Chlorpheniramine and Pseudoephedrine *on page 427*
- ◆ **Allergy [OTC]** *see* Loratadine *on page 1241*
- ◆ **Allergy Relief [OTC]** *see* DiphenhydrAMINE (Systemic) *on page 641*
- ◆ **Allergy Relief [OTC]** *see* Loratadine *on page 1241*
- ◆ **Allergy Relief Childrens [OTC]** *see* DiphenhydrAMINE (Systemic) *on page 641*
- ◆ **Allergy Relief For Kids [OTC]** *see* Loratadine *on page 1241*
- ◆ **Allerject (Can)** *see* EPINEPHrine (Systemic, Oral Inhalation) *on page 735*
- ◆ **Allernix (Can)** *see* DiphenhydrAMINE (Systemic) *on page 641*
- ◆ **Aller-Relief [OTC] (Can)** *see* Cetirizine *on page 411*
- ◆ **Allfen CD** *see* Guaifenesin and Codeine *on page 987*
- ◆ **Allfen CDX** *see* Guaifenesin and Codeine *on page 987*
- ◆ **Alli [OTC]** *see* Orlistat *on page 1520*
- ◆ **Alloprin (Can)** *see* Allopurinol *on page 90*

Allopurinol (al oh PURE i nole)

Brand Names: U.S. Aloprim; Zyloprim

Brand Names: Canada Alloprin; Apo-Allopurinol; JAMP-Allopurinol; Mar-Allopurinol; Novo-Purol; Zyloprim

Index Terms Allopurinol Sodium

Pharmacologic Category Antigout Agent; Xanthine Oxidase Inhibitor

Use

Oral:

Calcium oxalate calculi: Management of recurrent calcium oxalate calculi (with uric acid excretion >800 mg/day in men and >750 mg/day in women)

Gout: Management of primary or secondary gout (acute attack, tophi, joint destruction, uric acid lithiasis, and/or nephropathy)

Lesch-Nyhan syndrome: *Canadian labeling:* Additional use (not in U.S. labeling): Management of hyperuricemia associated with Lesch-Nyhan syndrome

Malignancies: Management of hyperuricemia associated with cancer treatment for leukemia, lymphoma, or solid tumor malignancies

IV: **Malignancies:** Management of hyperuricemia associated with cancer treatment for leukemia, lymphoma, or solid tumor malignancies

Pregnancy Risk Factor C

Pregnancy Considerations Adverse events were observed in some animal reproduction studies. Allopurinol crosses the placenta (Torrance, 2009). An increased risk of adverse fetal events has not been observed (limited data) (Hoeltzenbein, 2013).

Breast-Feeding Considerations Allopurinol and its metabolite are excreted into breast milk; the metabolite was also detected in the serum of the nursing infant (Kamilli, 1993). The U.S. manufacturer recommends caution be used when administering allopurinol to nursing women. The Canadian labeling contraindicates use in nursing women except those with hyperuricemia secondary to malignancy.

Contraindications

Severe hypersensitivity reaction to allopurinol or any component of the formulation

Canadian labeling: Additional contraindications (not in U.S. labeling): Nursing mothers and children (except those with hyperuricemia secondary to malignancy or Lesch-Nyhan syndrome)

Warnings/Precautions Do not use to treat asymptomatic hyperuricemia. Has been associated with a number of hypersensitivity reactions, including severe reactions (vasculitis and Stevens-Johnson syndrome); discontinue at first sign of rash. Consider HLA-B*5801 testing in patients at a higher risk for allopurinol hypersensitivity syndrome (eg, Koreans with stage 3 or worse CKD and Han Chinese and Thai descent regardless of renal function) prior to initiation of therapy (ACR guidelines [Khanna, 2012]). Reversible hepatotoxicity has been reported; use with caution in patients with preexisting hepatic impairment. Bone marrow suppression has been reported; use caution with other drugs causing myelosuppression. Caution in renal impairment, dosage adjustments needed. Full effect on serum uric acid levels in chronic gout may take several weeks to become evident; gradual titration is recommended. Potentially significant drug-drug interactions may exist, requiring dose or frequency adjustment, additional monitoring, and/or selection of alternative therapy.

Adverse Reactions

Dermatologic: Skin rash

Endocrine & metabolic: Gout (acute)

Gastrointestinal: Diarrhea, nausea

Hepatic: Increased liver enzymes, increased serum alkaline phosphatase

Rare but important or life-threatening: Ageusia, agranulocytosis, alopecia, angioedema, aplastic anemia, cataract, cholestatic jaundice, ecchymoses, eczematoid dermatitis, eosinophilia, exfoliative dermatitis, hepatic necrosis, hepatitis, hepatomegaly, hyperbilirubinemia, hypersensitivity reaction, leukocytosis, leukopenia, lichen planus, macular retinitis, myopathy, necrotizing angiitis, nephritis, neuritis, neuropathy, onycholysis, pancreatitis, purpura, renal failure, skin granuloma (annulare), Stevens-Johnson syndrome, thrombocytopenia, toxic epidermal necrolysis, toxic pustuloderma, uremia, vasculitis, vesicobullous dermatitis

Drug Interactions

Metabolism/Transport Effects None known.

Avoid Concomitant Use

Avoid concomitant use of Allopurinol with any of the following: Didanosine; Pegloticase; Tegafur

Increased Effect/Toxicity

Allopurinol may increase the levels/effects of: Amoxicillin; Ampicillin; AzaTHIOprine; Bendamustine; CarBAMazepine; ChlorproPAMIDE; Cyclophosphamide; Didanosine; Mercaptopurine; Pegloticase; Theophylline Derivatives; Vitamin K Antagonists

The levels/effects of Allopurinol may be increased by: ACE Inhibitors; Loop Diuretics; Thiazide Diuretics

Decreased Effect

Allopurinol may decrease the levels/effects of: Tegafur

The levels/effects of Allopurinol may be decreased by: Antacids

Preparation for Administration Reconstitute powder for injection with SWFI. Further dilution with NS or D_5W (50 to 100 mL) to ≤6 mg/mL is recommended.

Storage/Stability

Powder for injection: Store at controlled room temperature of 20°C to 25°C (68°F to 77°F). Following preparation, intravenous solutions should be stored at 20°C to 25°C (68°F to 77°F). Do not refrigerate reconstituted and/or diluted product. Must be administered within 10 hours of solution preparation.

Tablet: Store at controlled room temperature of 20°C to 25°C (68°F to 77°F). Protect from moisture and light.

Mechanism of Action Allopurinol inhibits xanthine oxidase, the enzyme responsible for the conversion of hypoxanthine to xanthine to uric acid. Allopurinol is metabolized to oxypurinol which is also an inhibitor of xanthine oxidase; allopurinol acts on purine catabolism, reducing the production of uric acid without disrupting the biosynthesis of vital purines.

Pharmacodynamics/Kinetics

Onset of action: Peak effect: 1 to 2 weeks

Absorption: Oral: ~80%; Rectal: Poor and erratic

Distribution: V_d: ~1.6 L/kg; V_{ss}: 0.84 to 0.87 L/kg; enters breast milk

Protein binding: <1%

Metabolism: ~75% to active metabolites, chiefly oxypurinol

Bioavailability: 49% to 53%

Half-life elimination:

Normal renal function: Parent drug: 1 to 3 hours; Oxypurinol: 18 to 30 hours

End-stage renal disease: Prolonged

Time to peak, plasma: Oral: 30 to 120 minutes

Excretion: Urine (76% as oxypurinol, 12% as unchanged drug)

Allopurinol and oxypurinol are dialyzable

Dosage

Gout (chronic): Adults: Oral:

Manufacturer's labeling: Initial: 100 mg once daily; increase at weekly intervals in increments of 100 mg/day as needed to achieve desired serum uric acid level. Usual dosage range: 200 to 300 mg/day in mild gout; 400 to 600 mg/day in moderate to severe tophaceous gout. Maximum daily dose: 800 mg/day.

Alternative dosing (off-label): Initial: 100 mg/day, increasing the dose gradually in increments of 100 mg/day every 2 to 5 weeks as needed to achieve desired serum uric acid level of ≤6 mg/dL (ACR guidelines [Khanna, 2012]; EULAR guidelines [Zhang, 2006]; McGill, 2010). Some patients may require therapy targeted at a serum uric acid level <5 mg/dL to control symptoms. Allopurinol may be initiated during an acute gout attack so long as antiinflammatory therapy has been initiated as well (ACR guidelines [Khanna, 2012]).

Management of hyperuricemia associated with chemotherapy and/or radiation therapy:

Oral: **Note:** Doses >300 mg should be given in divided doses.

U.S. labeling:

Children <6 years: 150 mg daily

Children 6 to 10 years: 300 mg daily

Children >10 years and Adults: 600 to 800 mg daily in divided doses

Canadian labeling:

Children 6 to 10 years: 10 mg/kg daily (do not exceed adult dosing); adjust dose as necessary after 48 hours

Adults: 600 to 800 mg daily in 2 to 3 divided doses for 2 to 3 days prior to chemotherapy/radiation therapy then adjust dose per serum uric acid level; for ongoing management, 300 to 400 mg daily is usually sufficient to control serum uric levels.

Alternative dosing (off-label; intermediate risk for tumor lysis syndrome): Children and Adults: Intermediate risk for tumor lysis syndrome: 10 mg/kg daily divided every 8 hours (maximum dose: 800 mg daily) **or** 50 to 100 mg/m^2 every 8 hours (maximum dose: 300 mg/m^2 daily), begin 12 to 24 hours (children) or 1 to 2 days (adults) before initiation of induction chemotherapy; may continue for 3 to 7 days after chemotherapy (Coiffier, 2008)

IV: **Note:** Intravenous daily dose can be given as a single infusion or in equally divided doses at 6-, 8-, or 12-hour intervals.

Manufacturer's labeling:

Children: Starting dose: 200 mg/m^2 daily beginning 1 to 2 days before chemotherapy

Adults: 200 to 400 mg/m^2 daily (maximum dose: 600 mg daily) beginning 1 to 2 days before chemotherapy

Alternative dosing (off-label; intermediate risk for tumor lysis syndrome): Children and Adults: 200 to 400 mg/m^2 daily (maximum dose: 600 mg daily) in 1 to 3 divided doses beginning 1 to 2 days before the start of induction chemotherapy; may continue for 3 to 7 days after chemotherapy (Coiffier, 2008)

Management of hyperuricemia associated with Lesch-Nyhan syndrome: *Canadian labeling (not in U.S. labeling):* Children 6 to 10 years: Oral: 10 mg/kg daily in 1 to 3 divided doses; adjust dose as necessary after 48 hours

Recurrent calcium oxalate stones: Adults: Oral: 200 to 300 mg daily in single or divided doses; may adjust dose as needed to control hyperuricosuria

Dosage adjustment in renal impairment:

Manufacturer's labeling: Oral, IV: Lower doses are required in renal impairment due to potential for accumulation of allopurinol and metabolites.

CrCl 10 to 20 mL/minute: 200 mg daily

CrCl 3 to 10 mL/minute: ≤100 mg daily

CrCl <3 mL/minute: ≤100 mg/dose at extended intervals

Alternative dosing (off-label):

Management of hyperuricemia associated with chemotherapy: Dosage reduction of 50% is recommended in renal impairment (Coiffier, 2008)

Gout: Oral:

Initiate therapy with 50 to 100 mg daily, and gradually increase to a maintenance dose to achieve a serum uric acid level of ≤6 mg/dL (with close monitoring of serum uric acid levels and for hypersensitivity) (Dalbeth, 2007; Sivera, 2013).

or

In patients with stage 4 CKD or worse, initiate therapy at 50 mg/day, increasing the dose every 2-5 weeks to achieve desired uric acid levels of ≤6 mg/dL; doses >300 mg/day are permitted so long as they are accompanied by appropriate patient education and monitoring for toxicity (eg, pruritus, rash, elevated hepatic transaminases). Some patients may require therapy targeted at a serum uric acid level <5 mg/dL to control symptoms (ACR guidelines; Khanna, 2012).

Hemodialysis: Initial: 100 mg alternate days given postdialysis, increase cautiously to 300 mg based on response. If dialysis is on a daily basis, an additional 50% of the dose may be required postdialysis (Dalbeth, 2007)

Dosage adjustment in hepatic impairment: There are no dosage adjustments provided in the U.S. manufacturer's labeling. The Canadian labeling suggests that a dose reduction is necessary but does not provide specific dosing recommendations.

Dietary Considerations Fluid intake should be administered to yield neutral or slightly alkaline urine and an output of ~2 L (in adults).

Administration

Oral: Administer after meals with plenty of fluid.

IV: The rate of infusion depends on the volume of the infusion; infuse maximum single daily doses (600 mg/day) over ≥30 minutes. Whenever possible, therapy should be initiated at 24 to 48 hours before the start of chemotherapy known to cause tumor lysis (including adrenocorticosteroids). IV daily dose can be administered as a single infusion or in equally divided doses at 6-, 8-, or 12-hour interval.

Monitoring Parameters CBC, serum uric acid levels every 2 to 5 weeks during dose titration until desired level is achieved; every 6 months thereafter (ACR guidelines [Khanna, 2012]), I & O, hepatic and renal function, especially at start of therapy; signs and symptoms of hypersensitivity

Reference Range Uric acid, serum: An increase occurs during childhood

Adults:

Males: 3.4 to 7 mg/dL or slightly more

Females: 2.4 to 6 mg/dL or slightly more

Target: ≤6 mg/dL

Values >7 mg/dL are sometimes arbitrarily regarded as hyperuricemia, but there is no sharp line between normals on the one hand, and the serum uric acid of those with clinical gout. Normal ranges cannot be adjusted for purine ingestion, but high purine diet increases uric acid. Uric acid may be increased with body size, exercise, and stress.

Dosage Forms

Solution Reconstituted, Intravenous [preservative free]:

Aloprim: 500 mg (1 ea)

Tablet, Oral:

Zyloprim: 100 mg, 300 mg

Generic: 100 mg, 300 mg

Extemporaneous Preparations A 20 mg/mL oral suspension may be made with tablets and either a 1:1 mixture of Ora-Sweet® and Ora-Plus® or a 1:1 mixture of Ora-Sweet® SF and Ora-Plus® or a 1:4 mixture of cherry syrup concentrate and simple syrup, NF. Crush eight 300 mg tablets in a mortar and reduce to a fine powder. Add small portions of chosen vehicle and mix to a uniform paste; mix while adding the vehicle in incremental proportions to **almost** 120 mL; transfer to a calibrated bottle, rinse mortar with vehicle, and add quantity of vehicle sufficient to make 120 mL. Label "shake well". Stable for 60 days refrigerated or at room temperature (Allen, 1996; Nahata, 2004).

Allen LV Jr and Erickson MA 3rd, "Stability of Acetazolamide, Allopurinol, Azathioprine, Clonazepam, and Flucytosine in Extemporaneously Compounded Oral Liquids," *Am J Health Syst Pharm*, 1996, 53(16):1944-9.

Nahata MC, Pai VB, and Hipple TF, *Pediatric Drug Formulations*, 5th ed, Cincinnati, OH: Harvey Whitney Books Co, 2004.

◆ **Allopurinol Sodium** *see* Allopurinol *on page 90*

◆ **All-*trans* Retinoic Acid** *see* Tretinoin (Systemic) *on page 2096*

◆ **All-*trans* Vitamin A Acid** *see* Tretinoin (Systemic) *on page 2096*

◆ **Almacone [OTC]** *see* Aluminum Hydroxide, Magnesium Hydroxide, and Simethicone *on page 104*

◆ **Almacone Double Strength [OTC]** *see* Aluminum Hydroxide, Magnesium Hydroxide, and Simethicone *on page 104*

Almitrine [INT] (AL mi treen)

International Brand Names Becta (KR); Brecio (KR); Sovarel (ES); Vectarion (BR, EC, ES, FR, NO, VN)

Index Terms Almitrine Dimesylate

Pharmacologic Category Respiratory Stimulant

Reported Use Respiratory stimulant used in acute respiratory failure such as chronic obstructive pulmonary disease (COPD)

Dosage Range Adults:

Oral: 50-100 mg/day in 2 divided doses

I.V.: 1-3 mg/kg/day in divided doses

Product Availability Product available in various countries; not currently available in the U.S.

Dosage Forms

Injection, powder for reconstitution: 15 mg

Tablet, as dimesylate: 50 mg

◆ **Almitrine Dimesylate** *see* Almitrine [INT] *on page 92*

Almotriptan (al moh TRIP tan)

Brand Names: U.S. Axert

Brand Names: Canada Axert; Mylan-Almotriptan; Sandoz-Almotriptan

Index Terms Almotriptan Malate

Pharmacologic Category Antimigraine Agent; Serotonin 5-$HT_{1B,\ 1D}$ Receptor Agonist

Use Acute treatment of migraine with or without aura in adults (with a history of migraine) and adolescents (with a history of migraine lasting ≥4 hours when left untreated)

Pregnancy Risk Factor C

Pregnancy Considerations Adverse events were observed in animal reproduction studies. Information related to almotriptan use in pregnancy is limited (Källén, 2011; Nezvalová-Henriksen, 2010; Nezvalová-Henriksen, 2012). Until additional information is available, other agents are preferred for the initial treatment of migraine in pregnancy (Da Silva, 2012; MacGregor, 2012; Williams, 2012).

Breast-Feeding Considerations It is not known if almotriptan is excreted in breast milk. The manufacturer recommends that caution be exercised when administering almotriptan to nursing women.

Contraindications Hypersensitivity to almotriptan or any component of the formulation; hemiplegic or basilar migraine; known or suspected ischemic heart disease (eg, angina pectoris, MI, documented silent ischemia, coronary artery vasospasm, Prinzmetal's variant angina); cerebrovascular syndromes (eg, stroke, transient ischemic attacks); peripheral vascular disease (eg, ischemic bowel disease); uncontrolled hypertension; use within 24 hours of another 5-HT_1 agonist; use within 24 hours of ergotamine derivatives and/or ergotamine-containing medications (eg, dihydroergotamine, ergotamine)

Warnings/Precautions Almotriptan is only indicated for the treatment of acute migraine headache; not indicated for migraine prophylaxis, or the treatment of cluster headaches, hemiplegic migraine, or basilar migraine. If a patient does not respond to the first dose, the diagnosis of acute migraine should be reconsidered.

Almotriptan should not be given to patients with documented ischemic or vasospastic CAD. Patients with risk factors for CAD (eg, hypertension, hypercholesterolemia, smoker, obesity, diabetes, strong family history of CAD, menopause, male >40 years of age) should undergo adequate cardiac evaluation prior to administration; if the cardiac evaluation is "satisfactory," the first dose of almotriptan should be given in the healthcare provider's office (consider ECG monitoring). All patients should undergo periodic evaluation of cardiovascular status during treatment. Cardiac events (coronary artery vasospasm, transient ischemia, myocardial infarction, ventricular tachycardia/fibrillation, cardiac arrest, and death), cerebral/subarachnoid hemorrhage, stroke, peripheral vascular ischemia, and colonic ischemia have been reported with 5-HT_1 agonist administration. Patients who experience sensations of chest pain/pressure/tightness or symptoms suggestive of angina following dosing should be evaluated for coronary artery disease or Prinzmetal's angina before receiving additional doses; if dosing is resumed and similar symptoms recur, monitor with ECG. Significant elevation in blood pressure, including hypertensive crisis, has also been reported on rare occasions following 5-HT_1 agonist administration in patients with and without a history of hypertension.

Acute migraine agents (eg, triptans, opioids, ergotamine, or a combination of the agents) used for 10 or more days per month may lead to worsening of headaches (medication overuse headache); withdrawal treatment may be necessary in the setting of overuse. Transient and permanent blindness and partial vision loss have been reported (rare) with 5-HT_1 agonist administration. Almotriptan contains a sulfonyl group which is structurally different from a sulfonamide. Cross-reactivity in patients with sulfonamide allergy has not been evaluated; however, the manufacturer recommends that caution be exercised in this patient population. Use with caution in liver or renal dysfunction. Symptoms of agitation, confusion, hallucinations, hyperreflexia, myoclonus, shivering, and tachycardia (serotonin syndrome) may occur with concomitant proserotonergic drugs (ie, SSRIs/SNRIs or triptans) or agents which reduce almotriptan's metabolism. Concurrent use of serotonin precursors (eg, tryptophan) is not recommended. If concomitant administration with SSRIs is warranted, monitor closely, especially at initiation and with dose increases.

Adverse Reactions

Central nervous system: Dizziness, drowsiness, headache

Gastrointestinal: Nausea, vomiting, xerostomia

Neuromuscular & skeletal: Paresthesia

Rare but important or life-threatening: Anaphylactic shock, anaphylaxis, angina pectoris, angioedema, colitis, coronary artery vasospasm, hemiplegia, hypersensitivity reaction, hypertension, ischemic heart disease, mastalgia, myocardial infarction, neuropathy, seizure, skin rash, syncope, tachycardia, ventricular fibrillation, ventricular tachycardia

Drug Interactions

Metabolism/Transport Effects **Substrate** of CYP2D6 (minor), CYP3A4 (minor); **Note:** Assignment of Major/Minor substrate status based on clinically relevant drug interaction potential

Avoid Concomitant Use

Avoid concomitant use of Almotriptan with any of the following: Dapoxetine; Ergot Derivatives; MAO Inhibitors

Increased Effect/Toxicity

Almotriptan may increase the levels/effects of: Antipsychotic Agents; Droxidopa; Ergot Derivatives; Metoclopramide; Serotonin Modulators

The levels/effects of Almotriptan may be increased by: Antiemetics (5HT3 Antagonists); Antipsychotic Agents; CYP3A4 Inhibitors (Strong); Dapoxetine; Ergot Derivatives; MAO Inhibitors

Decreased Effect There are no known significant interactions involving a decrease in effect.

Storage/Stability Store at 25°C (77°F); excursions permitted to 15°C to 30°C (59°F to 86°F).

Mechanism of Action Selective agonist for serotonin (5-HT_{1B} and 5-HT_{1D} receptors) in cranial arteries; causes vasoconstriction and reduces sterile inflammation associated with antidromic neuronal transmission correlating with relief of migraine

Pharmacodynamics/Kinetics

Absorption: Well absorbed

Distribution: V_d: ~180-200 L

Protein binding: ~35%

Metabolism: Via MAO type A oxidative deamination (~27% of dose) and CYP3A4 and 2D6 (~12% of dose) to inactive metabolites

Bioavailability: ~70%

Half-life elimination: 3-4 hours

Time to peak, plasma: 1-3 hours

Excretion: Urine (~75%; ~40% of total dose as unchanged drug); feces (~13% of total dose as unchanged drug and metabolites)

Dosage Oral: Children ≥12 years and Adults: Migraine: Initial: 6.25-12.5 mg in a single dose; if the headache returns, repeat the dose after 2 hours (maximum daily dose: 25 mg)

Note: The safety of treating more than 4 migraines/month has not been established.

Dosage adjustment with concomitant use of an enzyme inhibitor:

Patients receiving a potent CYP3A4 inhibitor: Initial: 6.25 mg in a single dose; maximum daily dose: 12.5 mg

Patients with renal impairment and concomitant use of a potent CYP3A4 inhibitor: Avoid use

Patients with hepatic impairment and concomitant use of a potent CYP3A4 inhibitor: Avoid use

Dosage adjustment in renal impairment: Severe renal impairment (CrCl ≤30 mL/minute): Initial: 6.25 mg in a single dose; maximum daily dose: 12.5 mg

Dosage adjustment in hepatic impairment: Initial: 6.25 mg in a single dose; maximum daily dose: 12.5 mg

Dietary Considerations May be taken without regard to meals.

Administration Administer without regard to meals.

Dosage Forms

Tablet, Oral:

Axert: 6.25 mg, 12.5 mg

◆ **Almotriptan Malate** *see* Almotriptan *on page 92*

◆ **Alocril** *see* Nedocromil *on page 1435*

◆ **Alocril® (Can)** *see* Nedocromil *on page 1435*

◆ **Alodox Convenience** *see* Doxycycline *on page 689*

◆ **Aloe Vesta Antifungal [OTC]** *see* Miconazole (Topical) *on page 1360*

◆ **Alomide** *see* Lodoxamide *on page 1232*

◆ **Alomide® (Can)** *see* Lodoxamide *on page 1232*

◆ **Aloprim** *see* Allopurinol *on page 90*

◆ **Alora** *see* Estradiol (Systemic) *on page 775*

◆ **Aloxi** *see* Palonosetron *on page 1561*

Alpha-Galactosidase (AL fa ga lak TOE si days)

Brand Names: U.S. beano® Meltaways [OTC]; beano® [OTC]

Index Terms *Aspergillus niger*

Pharmacologic Category Enzyme

Use Prevention of flatulence and bloating attributed to a variety of grains, cereals, nuts, and vegetables

Dosage Oral: Children ≥12 years and Adults: Adjust dose according to the number of problem foods per meal:

Tablet, chewable (beano®): Usual dose: 2-3 tablets/meal

Tablet, orally disintegrating (beano® Meltaways): One tablet per meal

Dosage adjustment in renal impairment: No dosage adjustment provided in the manufacturer's labeling.

Dosage adjustment in hepatic impairment: No dosage adjustment provided in the manufacturer's labeling.

Additional Information Complete prescribing information should be consulted for additional detail.

Dosage Forms

Tablet, chewable, oral:

beano® [OTC]: 150 Galactosidase units

Tablet, orally disintegrating, oral:

beano® Meltaways [OTC]: 300 Galactosidase units

◆ **Alpha-Galactosidase-A (Gene-Activated)** *see* Agalsidase Alfa [CAN/INT] *on page 63*

◆ **Alpha-Galactosidase-A (Recombinant)** *see* Agalsidase Beta *on page 64*

◆ **Alphagan (Can)** *see* Brimonidine (Ophthalmic) *on page 288*

◆ **Alphagan P** *see* Brimonidine (Ophthalmic) *on page 288*

◆ **1-α-hydroxycholecalciferol** *see* Alfacalcidol [CAN/INT] *on page 82*

◆ **1α-Hydroxyergocalciferol** *see* Doxercalciferol *on page 679*

◆ **Alpha-Interferon Multi-Subtype** *see* Interferon Alpha, Multi-Subtype [INT] *on page 1100*

◆ **Alphanate** *see* Antihemophilic Factor/von Willebrand Factor Complex (Human) *on page 154*

◆ **AlphaNine SD** *see* Factor IX (Human) *on page 840*

◆ **Alphaquin HP** *see* Hydroquinone *on page 1020*

◆ **AlphaTrex** *see* Betamethasone (Topical) *on page 255*

◆ **Alph-E [OTC]** *see* Vitamin E *on page 2174*

◆ **Alph-E-Mixed [OTC]** *see* Vitamin E *on page 2174*

◆ **Alph-E-Mixed 1000 [OTC]** *see* Vitamin E *on page 2174*

ALPRAZolam (al PRAY zoe lam)

Brand Names: U.S. ALPRAZolam Intensol; ALPRAZolam XR; Niravam; Xanax; Xanax XR

Brand Names: Canada Apo-Alpraz®; Apo-Alpraz® TS; Mylan-Alprazolam; NTP-Alprazolam; Nu-Alpraz; Teva-Alprazolam; Xanax TS™; Xanax®

Pharmacologic Category Benzodiazepine

Additional Appendix Information

Beers Criteria – Potentially Inappropriate Medications for Geriatrics *on page 2271*

Use Treatment of anxiety disorder (GAD); short-term relief of symptoms of anxiety; panic disorder, with or without agoraphobia; anxiety associated with depression

Pregnancy Risk Factor D

Pregnancy Considerations Benzodiazepines have the potential to cause harm to the fetus. Alprazolam and its metabolites cross the human placenta. Teratogenic effects have been observed with some benzodiazepines; however, additional studies are needed. The incidence of premature birth and low birth weights may be increased following maternal use of benzodiazepines; hypoglycemia and respiratory problems in the neonate may occur following exposure late in pregnancy. Neonatal withdrawal symptoms may occur within days to weeks after birth and "floppy infant syndrome" (which also includes withdrawal symptoms) has been reported with some benzodiazepines (Bergman, 1992; Iqbal, 2002; Wikner, 2007).

Breast-Feeding Considerations Benzodiazepines are excreted into breast milk. In a study of eight postpartum women, peak concentrations of alprazolam were found in breast milk ~1 hour after the maternal dose and the half-life was ~14 hours. Samples were obtained over 36 hours following a single oral dose of alprazolam 0.5 mg. Metabolites were not detected in breast milk. In this study, the estimated exposure to the breast-feeding infant was ~3% of the weight-adjusted maternal dose (Oo, 1995). Drowsiness, lethargy, or weight loss in nursing infants have been observed in case reports following maternal use of some benzodiazepines (Iqbal, 2002). Breast-feeding is not recommended by the manufacturer.

Contraindications Hypersensitivity to alprazolam or any component of the formulation (cross-sensitivity with other benzodiazepines may exist); narrow-angle glaucoma; concurrent use with ketoconazole or itraconazole

Warnings/Precautions Rebound or withdrawal symptoms, including seizures, may occur following abrupt discontinuation or large decreases in dose (more common in adult patients receiving >4 mg/day or prolonged treatment); the risk of seizures appears to be greatest 24 to 72 hours following discontinuation of therapy. Breakthrough anxiety may occur at the end of dosing interval. Use with caution in patients receiving concurrent CYP3A4 inhibitors, moderate or strong CYP3A4 inducers, and major CYP3A4 substrates; consider alternative agents that avoid or lessen the potential for CYP-mediated interactions. Use with caution in renal impairment or predisposition to urate nephropathy; has weak uricosuric properties. In older adults, benzodiazepines increase the risk of impaired cognition, delirium, falls, fractures, and motor vehicle accidents. Due to increased sensitivity in this age group, avoid use for treatment of insomnia, agitation, or delirium (Beers Criteria). Use with caution in or debilitated patients, patients with hepatic disease (including alcoholics) or respiratory disease, or obese patients. Cigarette smoking may decrease alprazolam concentrations up to 50%.

Causes CNS depression (dose related) which may impair physical and mental capabilities. Patients must be cautioned about performing tasks that require mental alertness (eg, operating machinery or driving). Effects with other sedative drugs or ethanol may be potentiated. Benzodiazepines have been associated with falls and traumatic injury and should be used with extreme caution in patients who are at risk of these events.

Use caution in patients with depression, particularly if suicidal risk may be present. Episodes of mania or hypomania have occurred in depressed patients treated with alprazolam. May cause physical or psychological dependence. Acute withdrawal may be precipitated in patients after administration of flumazenil. Tolerance does not develop to the anxiolytic effects (Vinkers, 2012). Chronic use of this agent may increase the perioperative benzodiazepine dose needed to achieve desired effect.

Benzodiazepines have been associated with anterograde amnesia. Paradoxical reactions have been reported with benzodiazepines, particularly in adolescent/pediatric or psychiatric patients. Does not have analgesic, antidepressant, or antipsychotic properties.

Adverse Reactions

Central nervous system: Abnormal dreams, agitation, akathisia, altered mental status, ataxia, cognitive dysfunction, confusion, depersonalization, depression, derealization, disinhibition, disorientation, disturbance in attention, dizziness, drowsiness, dysarthria, dystonia, fatigue, fear, hallucination, headache, hypersomnia, hypoesthesia, insomnia, irritability, lethargy, malaise, memory impairment, nervousness, nightmares, paresthesia, restlessness, sedation, seizure, talkativeness, vertigo

Dermatologic: Dermatitis, diaphoresis, skin rash

Endocrine & metabolic: Decreased libido, Increased libido, menstrual disease, weight gain, weight loss

Gastrointestinal: Abdominal pain, anorexia, change in appetite, constipation, diarrhea, dyspepsia, nausea, sialorrhea, vomiting, xerostomia

Genitourinary: Difficulty in micturition, dysmenorrhea, sexual disorder, urinary incontinence

Hepatic: Increased liver enzymes, increased serum bilirubin, jaundice

Neuromuscular & skeletal: Arthralgia, back pain, dyskinesia, muscle cramps, muscle twitching, myalgia, tremor, weakness

Ophthalmic: Blurred vision

Respiratory: Allergic rhinitis, dyspnea, hyperventilation, nasal congestion, upper respiratory tract infection

Rare but important or life-threatening: Amnesia, angioedema, diplopia, falling, galactorrhea, gynecomastia, hepatic failure, hepatitis, homicidal ideation, hyperprolactinemia, hypomania, mania, peripheral edema, sleep apnea, Stevens-Johnson syndrome, suicidal ideation, tinnitus

Drug Interactions

Metabolism/Transport Effects **Substrate** of CYP3A4 (major); **Note:** Assignment of Major/Minor substrate status based on clinically relevant drug interaction potential

Avoid Concomitant Use

Avoid concomitant use of ALPRAZolam with any of the following: Azelastine (Nasal); Conivaptan; Fusidic Acid (Systemic); Idelalisib; Indinavir; Itraconazole; Ketoconazole (Systemic); Methadone; OLANZapine; Orphenadrine; Paraldehyde; Sodium Oxybate; Thalidomide

Increased Effect/Toxicity

ALPRAZolam may increase the levels/effects of: Alcohol (Ethyl); Azelastine (Nasal); Buprenorphine; CloZAPine; CNS Depressants; Hydrocodone; Methadone; Methotrimeprazine; Metyrosine; Mirtazapine; Orphenadrine; Paraldehyde; Pramipexole; ROPINIRole; Rotigotine; Selective Serotonin Reuptake Inhibitors; Sodium Oxybate; Suvorexant; Thalidomide; Zolpidem

The levels/effects of ALPRAZolam may be increased by: Aprepitant; Boceprevir; Brimonidine (Topical); Cannabis; Ceritinib; Conivaptan; CYP3A4 Inhibitors (Moderate); CYP3A4 Inhibitors (Strong); Dasatinib; Doxylamine; Dronabinol; Droperidol; FluvoxaMINE; Fosaprepitant; Fusidic Acid (Systemic); HydrOXYzine; Idelalisib; Indinavir; Itraconazole; Ivacaftor; Kava Kava; Ketoconazole (Systemic); Luliconazole; Macrolide Antibiotics; Magnesium Sulfate; Methotrimeprazine; Mifepristone; Nabilone; Netupitant; OLANZapine; Perampanel; Protease Inhibitors; Rufinamide; Simeprevir; Stiripentol; Tapentadol; Teduglutide; Telaprevir; Tetrahydrocannabinol

Decreased Effect

The levels/effects of ALPRAZolam may be decreased by: Bosentan; CYP3A4 Inducers (Moderate); CYP3A4 Inducers (Strong); Dabrafenib; Deferasirox; Mitotane; Siltuximab; St Johns Wort; Theophylline Derivatives; Tocilizumab; Yohimbine

Food Interactions Alprazolam serum concentration is unlikely to be increased by grapefruit juice because of alprazolam's high oral bioavailability. The C_{max} of the extended release formulation is increased by 25% when a high-fat meal is given 2 hours before dosing. T_{max} is decreased 33% when food is given immediately prior to dose and increased by 33% when food is given ≥1 hour after dose. Management: Administer without regard to food.

Storage/Stability

Immediate release tablets: Store at 20°C to 25°C (68°F to 77°F).

Extended release tablets: Store at 25°C (77°F); excursions permitted to 15°C to 30°C (59°F to 86°F).

Orally-disintegrating tablet: Store at room temperature of 20°C to 25°C (68°F to 77°F). Protect from moisture. Seal bottle tightly and discard any cotton packaged inside bottle.

Mechanism of Action Binds to stereospecific benzodiazepine receptors on the postsynaptic GABA neuron at several sites within the central nervous system, including the limbic system, reticular formation. Enhancement of the inhibitory effect of GABA on neuronal excitability results by increased neuronal membrane permeability to chloride ions. This shift in chloride ions results in hyperpolarization (a less excitable state) and stabilization. Benzodiazepine receptors and effects appear to be linked to the GABA-A receptors. Benzodiazepines do not bind to GABA-B receptors.

Pharmacodynamics/Kinetics

Onset of action: Immediate release and extended release formulations: 1 hour

Duration: Immediate release: 5.1 ± 1.7 hours; Extended release: 11.3 ± 4.2 hours

Absorption: Extended release: Slower relative to immediate release formulation resulting in a concentration that is maintained 5-11 hours after dosing

Distribution: V_d: 0.9-1.2 L/kg

Protein binding: 80%; primarily to albumin

Metabolism: Hepatic via CYP3A4; forms two active metabolites (4-hydroxyalprazolam and α-hydroxyalprazolam)

Bioavailability: 90%

Half-life elimination:

- Adults: 11.2 hours (Immediate release range: 6.3-26.9 hours; Extended release range: 10.7-15.8 hours); Orally-disintegrating tablet range: 7.9-19.2 hours)
- Elderly: 16.3 hours (range: 9-26.9 hours)
- Alcoholic liver disease: 19.7 hours (range: 5.8-65.3 hours)
- Obesity: 21.8 hours (range: 9.9-40.4 hours)
- Race: Asians: Increased by ~25% (as compared to Caucasians)

Time to peak, serum:
Immediate release: 1-2 hours
Extended release: ~9 hours (Glue, 2006); decreased by 1 hour when administered at bedtime (as compared to morning administration); decreased by 33% when administered with a high-fat meal; increased by 33% when administered ≥1 hour after a high-fat meal
Orally-disintegrating tablet: 1.5-2 hours; occurs ~15 minutes earlier when administered with water; increased to ~4 hours when administered with a high-fat meal
Excretion: Urine (as unchanged drug and metabolites)

Dosage Oral: **Note:** Treatment >4 months should be re-evaluated to determine the patient's continued need for the drug
Children: Anxiety (off-label use): Immediate release: Initial: 0.005 mg/kg/dose or 0.125 mg/dose 3 times/day; increase in increments of 0.125-0.25 mg, up to a maximum of 0.02 mg/kg/dose or 0.06 mg/kg/day (range of doses reported in one study: 0.375-3 mg/day) (Pfefferbaum, 1987). See "Dose Reduction" comment below.
Adults:
Anxiety: Immediate release: Initial: 0.25-0.5 mg 3 times/day; titrate dose upward every 3-4 days; usual maximum: 4 mg/day. Patients requiring doses >4 mg/day should be increased cautiously. Periodic reassessment and consideration of dosage reduction is recommended.
Panic disorder:
Immediate release: Initial: 0.5 mg 3 times/day; dose may be increased every 3-4 days in increments ≤1 mg/day. Mean effective dosage: 5-6 mg/day; some patients may require as much as 10 mg/day
Extended release: 0.5-1 mg once daily; may increase dose every 3-4 days in increments ≤1 mg/day (range: 3-6 mg/day)
Switching from immediate release to extended release: Patients may be switched to extended release tablets by taking the total daily dose of the immediate release tablets and giving it once daily using the extended release preparation.
Preoperative anxiety (off-label use): 0.5 mg 60-90 minutes before procedure (De Witte, 2002)
Dose reduction: Abrupt discontinuation should be avoided. Daily dose may be decreased by 0.5 mg every 3 days; however, some patients may require a slower reduction. If withdrawal symptoms occur, resume previous dose and discontinue on a less rapid schedule.
Elderly: **Note:** Elderly patients may be more sensitive to the effects of alprazolam including ataxia and oversedation. The elderly may also have impaired renal function leading to decreased clearance. Titrate gradually, if needed and tolerated.
Immediate release: Initial: 0.25 mg 2-3 times/day
Extended release: Initial: 0.5 mg once daily
Dosing adjustment in renal impairment: No dosage adjustment provided in manufacturer's labeling; however, use caution
Dosing adjustment in hepatic impairment: Advanced liver disease:
Immediate release: 0.25 mg 2-3 times/day; titrate gradually if needed and tolerated
Extended release: 0.5 mg once daily; titrate gradually if needed and tolerated

Dietary Considerations Extended release tablet should be taken once daily in the morning.

Administration
Immediate release preparations: Can be administered sublingually if oral administration is not possible; absorption and onset of effect are comparable to oral administration (Scavone,1987; Scavone, 1992)
Extended release tablet: Should be taken once daily in the morning; do not crush, break, or chew.
Orally-disintegrating tablets: Using dry hands, place tablet on top of tongue and allow to disintegrate. If using one-half of tablet, immediately discard remaining half (may not remain stable). Administration with water is not necessary.

Monitoring Parameters Respiratory and cardiovascular status

Additional Information Not intended for management of anxieties and minor distresses associated with everyday life. Treatment longer than 4 months should be re-evaluated to determine the patient's need for the drug. Patients who become physically dependent on alprazolam tend to have a difficult time discontinuing it; withdrawal symptoms may be severe. To minimize withdrawal symptoms, taper dosage slowly; do not discontinue abruptly. Abrupt discontinuation after sustained use (generally >10 days) may cause withdrawal symptoms.

Dosage Forms
Concentrate, Oral:
ALPRAZolam Intensol: 1 mg/mL (30 mL)
Tablet, Oral:
Xanax: 0.25 mg, 0.5 mg, 1 mg, 2 mg
Generic: 0.25 mg, 0.5 mg, 1 mg, 2 mg
Tablet Dispersible, Oral:
Niravam: 0.25 mg
Generic: 0.25 mg, 0.5 mg, 1 mg, 2 mg
Tablet Extended Release 24 Hour, Oral:
ALPRAZolam XR: 0.5 mg, 1 mg, 2 mg, 3 mg
Xanax XR: 0.5 mg, 1 mg, 2 mg, 3 mg
Generic: 0.5 mg, 1 mg, 2 mg, 3 mg

Extemporaneous Preparations Note: Commercial oral solution is available (Alprazolam Intensol™: 1 mg/mL [dye free, ethanol free, sugar free; contains propylene glycol])

A 1 mg/mL oral suspension may be made with tablets and one of three different vehicles (a 1:1 mixture of Ora-Sweet® and Ora-Plus®, a 1:1 mixture of Ora-Sweet® SF and Ora-Plus®, or a 1:4 mixture of cherry syrup with Simple Syrup, NF). Crush sixty 2 mg tablets in a mortar and reduce to a fine powder. Add 40 mL of vehicle and mix to a uniform paste; mix while adding the vehicle in incremental proportions to **almost** 120 mL; transfer to a calibrated bottle, rinse mortar with vehicle, and add a quantity of vehicle sufficient to make 120 mL. Label "shake well" and "refrigerate". Stable for 60 days.

Nahata MC, Pai VB, and Hipple TF, *Pediatric Drug Formulations*, 5th ed, Cincinnati, OH: Harvey Whitney Books Co, 2004.

- **ALPRAZolam Intensol** *see* ALPRAZolam *on page 94*
- **ALPRAZolam XR** *see* ALPRAZolam *on page 94*
- **Alprolix** *see* Factor IX (Recombinant) *on page 841*

Alprostadil (al PROS ta dill)

Brand Names: U.S. Caverject; Caverject Impulse; Edex; Muse; Prostin VR

Brand Names: Canada Alprostadil Injection USP; Caverject; Muse Pellet; Prostin VR

Index Terms PGE_1; Prostaglandin E_1

Pharmacologic Category Prostaglandin; Vasodilator

Use
Prostin VR Pediatric: Temporary maintenance of patency of ductus arteriosus in neonates with ductal-dependent congenital heart disease until surgery can be performed. These defects include cyanotic (eg, pulmonary atresia, pulmonary stenosis, tricuspid atresia, Fallot's tetralogy, transposition of the great vessels) and acyanotic (eg, interruption of aortic arch, coarctation of aorta, hypoplastic left ventricle) heart disease.
Caverject, Caverject Impulse: Treatment of erectile dysfunction due to vasculogenic, psychogenic, neurogenic, or mixed etiology. May be a useful adjunct to other diagnostic tests in the diagnosis of erectile dysfunction

Edex, Muse: Treatment of erectile dysfunction due to vasculogenic, psychogenic, or neurogenic etiology

Pregnancy Risk Factor C (Muse)

Pregnancy Considerations Adverse events were observed in animal reproduction studies. Alprostadil is not indicated for use in women. The manufacturer of Muse recommends a condom barrier when being used during sexual intercourse with a pregnant woman.

Breast-Feeding Considerations Alprostadil is not indicated for use in women.

Contraindications

Alprostadil (intracavernous): Hypersensitivity to alprostadil, other prostaglandins or any component of the formulation, conditions predisposing patients to priapism (eg, sickle cell anemia or trait, multiple myeloma, leukemia); patients with anatomical deformation of the penis (eg, angulation, cavernosal fibrosis, or Peyronie's disease), or penile implants; use in men for whom sexual activity is inadvisable or contraindicated. Intracavernosal alprostadil is intended for use in adult men only and is not indicated for use in women, children, or newborns.

Alprostadil (transurethral): Hypersensitivity to alprostadil, use in patients with urethral stricture, balanitis (inflammation/infection of the glans penis), severe hypospadias and curvature, and in patients with acute or chronic urethritis; in patients who are prone to venous thrombosis or who have a hyperviscosity syndrome (eg, sickle cell anemia or trait, thrombocythemia, polycythemia, multiple myeloma) and are therefore at increased risk of priapism (rigid erection lasting ≥6 hours). Should not be used in men for whom sexual activity is inadvisable or for sexual intercourse with a pregnant woman unless the couple uses a condom barrier.

Alprostadil (intravenous): There are no contraindications listed in the manufacturer's labeling.

Warnings/Precautions

Prostin VR Pediatric: Use cautiously in neonates with bleeding tendencies. **[U.S. Boxed Warning]: Apnea may occur in 10% to 12% of neonates with congenital heart defects, especially in those weighing <2 kg at birth.** Apnea usually appears during the first hour of drug infusion. When used for patency of ductus arteriosus infuse for the shortest time at the lowest dose consistent with good patient care. Use for >120 hours has been associated with antral hyperplasia and gastric outlet obstruction.

Caverject, Caverject Impulse, Edex, Muse: When used in erectile dysfunction, priapism may occur; treat prolonged priapism (erection persisting for >4 hours) immediately to avoid penile tissue damage and permanent loss of potency; discontinue therapy if signs of penile fibrosis develop (penile angulation, cavernosal fibrosis, or Peyronie disease). Underlying causes of erectile dysfunction should be evaluated and treated prior to therapy. When used in erectile dysfunction (Muse), syncope occurring within 1 hour of administration has been reported. The potential for drug-drug interactions may occur when Muse is prescribed concomitantly with antihypertensives. Instruct patients to avoid ethanol consumption; may have vasodilating effect.

Benzyl alcohol and derivatives: Some dosage forms may contain benzyl alcohol; large amounts of benzyl alcohol (≥99 mg/kg/day) have been associated with a potentially fatal toxicity ("gasping syndrome") in neonates; the "gasping syndrome" consists of metabolic acidosis, respiratory distress, gasping respirations, CNS dysfunction (including convulsions, intracranial hemorrhage), hypotension, and cardiovascular collapse (AAP, 1997; CDC, 1982); some data suggests that benzoate displaces bilirubin from protein binding sites (Ahlfors, 2001); avoid or use dosage forms containing benzyl alcohol with caution in neonates. See manufacturer's labeling.

Adverse Reactions

Intraurethral:

Central nervous system: Dizziness, headache, pain

Genitourinary: Penile pain, testicular pain, urethral bleeding (minor), urethral burning, vulvovaginal pruritus (female partner)

Rare but important or life-threatening: Tachycardia

Intracavernosal injection:

Cardiovascular: Hypertension

Central nervous system: Dizziness, headache

Genitourinary: Penile disease, penile pain, penile rash, penile swelling, prolonged erection (>4 hours), Peyronie's disease

Local: Bruising at injection site, hematoma at injection site

Rare but important or life-threatening: Balanitis, injection site hemorrhage, priapism

Intravenous:

Cardiovascular: Bradycardia, cardiac arrest, edema, flushing, hypertension, hypotension, tachycardia

Central nervous system: Dizziness, headache, seizure

Endocrine & metabolic: Hypokalemia

Gastrointestinal: Diarrhea

Hematologic & oncologic: Disseminated intravascular coagulation

Infection: Sepsis

Local: Local pain (in structures other than the injection site)

Neuromuscular & skeletal: Back pain

Respiratory: Apnea, cough, flu-like symptoms, nasal congestion, sinusitis, upper respiratory infection

Miscellaneous: Fever

Rare but important or life-threatening: Anemia, anuria, bradypnea, cardiac failure, cerebral hemorrhage, gastroesophageal reflux disease, hematuria, hemorrhage, hyperbilirubinemia, hyperemia, hyperirritability, hyperkalemia, hypoglycemia, hypothermia, neck hyperextension, peritonitis, second degree atrioventricular block, shock, supraventricular tachycardia, thrombocytopenia, ventricular fibrillation

Drug Interactions

Metabolism/Transport Effects None known.

Avoid Concomitant Use

Avoid concomitant use of Alprostadil with any of the following: Phosphodiesterase 5 Inhibitors

Increased Effect/Toxicity

The levels/effects of Alprostadil may be increased by: Phosphodiesterase 5 Inhibitors

Decreased Effect There are no known significant interactions involving a decrease in effect.

Preparation for Administration

Caverject Impulse: Provided as a dual-chamber syringe with diluent in one chamber. To mix, hold syringe with needle pointing upward and turn plunger clockwise; turn upside down several times to mix. Device can be set to deliver specified dose, each device can be set at various increments.

Caverject powder: Use only the supplied diluent for reconstitution (ie, bacteriostatic/sterile water with benzyl alcohol 0.945%).

Edex: Reconstitute with NS.

Storage/Stability

Caverject Impulse: Store at or below 25°C (77°F); excursions are permitted between 15°C and 30°C (59°F and 86°F). Following reconstitution, use within 24 hours and discard any unused solution; for single use only.

Caverject powder: The 5 mcg, 10 mcg, and 20 mcg vials should be stored at or below 25°C (77°F). The 40 mcg vial should be stored at 2°C to 8°C (36°F to 46°F) until dispensed. After dispensing, stable for up to 3 months at or below 25°C (77°F). Following reconstitution, all strengths should be stored at or below 25°C (77°F); do not refrigerate or freeze; use within 24 hours.

Edex: Store at 15°C to 30°C (59°F to 86°F); following reconstitution, use immediately and discard any unused solution.

Muse: Refrigerate at 2°C to 8°C (36°F to 46°F); may be stored at room temperature for up to 14 days.

Prostin VR Pediatric: Refrigerate at 2°C to 8°C (36°F to 46°F). The following stability information has also been reported: May be stored at 20°C for up to 34 days or 30°C for up to 26 days (Cohen, 2007). Prior to infusion, dilute with D_5W, $D_{10}W$, or NS; use within 24 hours.

Mechanism of Action Causes vasodilation by means of direct effect on vascular and ductus arteriosus smooth muscle; relaxes trabecular smooth muscle by dilation of cavernosal arteries when injected along the penile shaft, allowing blood flow to and entrapment in the lacunar spaces of the penis (ie, corporeal veno-occlusive mechanism)

Pharmacodynamics/Kinetics

Onset of action: Erectile dysfunction: 5 to 20 minutes

Duration: Erectile dysfunction: Intended duration <1 hour

Distribution: Insignificant following penile injection

Protein binding, plasma: 81% to albumin

Metabolism: ~80% by oxidation in one pass via lungs

Half-life elimination: 5 to 10 minutes

Excretion: Urine (90% as metabolites) within 24 hours

Dosage

Patent ductus arteriosus (Prostin VR Pediatric):

IV continuous infusion into a large vein, or alternatively through an umbilical artery catheter placed at the ductal opening: 0.05-0.1 mcg/kg/minute with therapeutic response, rate is reduced to lowest effective dosage; with unsatisfactory response, rate is increased gradually; maintenance: 0.01-0.4 mcg/kg/minute

Note: Alprostadil is usually given at an infusion rate of 0.1 mcg/kg/minute, but it is often possible to reduce the dosage to 1/2 or even 1/10 without losing the therapeutic effect.

Therapeutic response is indicated by increased pH in those with acidosis or by an increase in oxygenation (PO_2) usually evident within 30 minutes

Erectile dysfunction:

Caverject, Caverject Impulse, Edex: Intracavernous: Individualize dose by careful titration; doses >40 mcg (Edex) or >60 mcg (Caverject, Caverject Impulse) are not recommended: Initial dose must be titrated in physician's office. Patient must stay in the physician's office until complete detumescence occurs; if there is no response, then the next higher dose may be given within 1 hour; if there is still no response, a 1-day interval before giving the next dose is recommended; increasing the dose or concentration in the treatment of impotence results in increasing pain and discomfort.

Initial dose titration:

Vasculogenic, psychogenic, or mixed etiology: Initiate dosage titration at 2.5 mcg.

If there is a partial response, increase dose by 2.5 mcg to a dose of 5 mcg and then, in increments of 5 to 10 mcg (depending on erectile response) until the dose that produces an erection suitable for intercourse and not exceeding a duration of 1 hour is reached.

If there is no response to the initial 2.5 mcg dose, the second dose may be increased to 7.5 mcg and administered within 1 hour, followed by increments of 5 to 10 mcg. According to the prescribing information for Caverject Impulse, no more than 2 doses during the initial titration should be given within a 24 hour period.

If there is a response, then there should be at least a 24 hour interval before the next dose is given.

Neurogenic etiology (eg, spinal cord injury): **Note:** Caverject powder must be used to prepare a 1.25 mcg dose: Initiate dosage titration at 1.25 mcg; may increase to a dose of 2.5 mcg within 1 hour and if necessary, to a dose of 5 mcg; may increase further in increments of 5 mcg until the dose is reached that produces an erection suitable for intercourse, not lasting >1 hour.

Maintenance: Once an appropriate dose has been determined, patient may self-administer injections at a frequency of no more than 3 times/week with at least 24 hours between doses

Muse Pellet: Intraurethral:

Initial: 125 to 250 mcg

Maintenance: Administer as needed to achieve an erection; duration of action is about 30-60 minutes; use only two systems per 24-hour period

Elderly: Elderly patients may have a greater frequency of renal dysfunction; lowest effective dose should be used. In clinical studies with Edex, higher minimally effective doses and a higher rate of lack of effect were noted.

Dosage adjustment in renal impairment: There are no dosage adjustments provided in the manufacturer's labeling.

Dosage adjustment in hepatic impairment: There are no dosage adjustments provided in the manufacturer's labeling.

Usual Infusion Concentrations: Pediatric IV infusion: 10 mcg/mL **or** 20 mcg/mL

Administration

Patent ductus arteriosus (Prostin VR Pediatric): IV continuous infusion into a large vein or alternatively through an umbilical artery catheter placed at the ductal opening; manufacturer recommended maximum concentration for IV infusion: 20 mcg/mL

Erectile dysfunction: Intracavernous:

Caverject, Edex: Use a 1/2 inch, 27- to 30-gauge needle. Inject into the dorsolateral aspect of the proximal third of the penis, avoiding visible veins; alternate side of the penis for injections.

Caverject Impulse consists of a disposable, single dose, dual chamber syringe system. After attaching the provided needle assembly, the dose to be given may be selected and after the site is cleansed with an alcohol swab, injected according to the prescribing information into the dorsolateral aspect of the proximal third of the penis, avoiding visible veins; alternate side of the penis for injections.

Monitoring Parameters Arterial pressure, respiratory rate, heart rate, temperature, degree of penile pain, duration of erection, adequate detumescence after dosing, signs of infection

Dosage Forms

Kit, Intracavernosal:

Caverject Impulse: 10 mcg, 20 mcg

Edex: 10 mcg, 20 mcg, 40 mcg

Pellet, Urethral:

Muse: 125 mcg (1 ea, 6 ea); 250 mcg (1 ea, 6 ea); 500 mcg (1 ea, 6 ea); 1000 mcg (1 ea, 6 ea)

Solution, Injection:

Prostin VR: 500 mcg/mL (1 mL)

Generic: 500 mcg/mL (1 mL)

Solution Reconstituted, Intracavernosal:

Caverject: 20 mcg (1 ea); 40 mcg (1 ea)

◆ **Alprostadil Injection USP (Can)** *see* Alprostadil *on page 96*

◆ **Alrex** *see* Loteprednol *on page 1251*

◆ **Alrex® (Can)** *see* Loteprednol *on page 1251*

◆ **Alsuma** *see* SUMAtriptan *on page 1953*

◆ **Altabax** *see* Retapamulin *on page 1793*

- **Altacaine** *see* Tetracaine (Ophthalmic) *on page 2017*
- **Altace** *see* Ramipril *on page 1771*
- **Altace HCT (Can)** *see* Ramipril and Hydrochlorothiazide [CAN/INT] *on page 1773*
- **Altachlore [OTC]** *see* Sodium Chloride *on page 1902*
- **Altamist Spray [OTC]** *see* Sodium Chloride *on page 1902*
- **Altarussin [OTC]** *see* GuaiFENesin *on page 986*
- **Altaryl [OTC]** *see* DiphenhydrAMINE (Systemic) *on page 641*
- **Altavera** *see* Ethinyl Estradiol and Levonorgestrel *on page 803*

Alteplase (AL te plase)

Brand Names: U.S. Activase; Cathflo Activase

Brand Names: Canada Activase rt-PA; Cathflo Activase

Index Terms Alteplase, Recombinant; Alteplase, Tissue Plasminogen Activator, Recombinant; tPA

Pharmacologic Category Thrombolytic Agent

Use Management of ST-elevation myocardial infarction (STEMI) for the lysis of thrombi in coronary arteries; management of acute ischemic stroke (AIS); management of acute pulmonary embolism (PE)

Recommended criteria for treatment:

STEMI (ACCF/AHA; O'Gara, 2013): Ischemic symptoms within 12 hours of treatment or evidence of ongoing ischemia 12 to 24 hours after symptom onset with a large area of myocardium at risk or hemodynamic instability.

STEMI ECG definition: New ST-segment elevation at the J point in at least 2 contiguous leads of ≥2 mm (0.2 mV) in men or ≥1.5 mm (0.15 mV) in women in leads V_2-V_3 and/or of ≥1 mm (0.1 mV) in other contiguous precordial leads or limb leads. New or presumably new left bundle branch block (LBBB) may interfere with ST-elevation analysis and should not be considered diagnostic in isolation.

At non-PCI-capable hospitals, the ACCF/AHA recommends thrombolytic therapy administration when the anticipated first medical contact (FMC)-to-device time at a PCI-capable hospital is >120 minutes due to unavoidable delays.

AIS: Onset of stroke symptoms within 3 hours of treatment

Acute pulmonary embolism: Age ≤75 years: Documented massive PE (defined as acute PE with sustained hypotension [SBP <90 mm Hg for ≤15 minutes or requiring inotropic support], persistent profound bradycardia [HR <40 bpm with signs or symptoms of shock], or pulselessness); alteplase may be considered for submassive PE with clinical evidence of adverse prognosis (eg, new hemodynamic instability, worsening respiratory insufficiency, severe RV dysfunction, or major myocardial necrosis) and low risk of bleeding complications. **Note:** Not recommended for patients with low-risk PE (eg, normotensive, no RV dysfunction, normal biomarkers) or submassive acute PE with minor RV dysfunction, minor myocardial necrosis, and no clinical worsening (Jaff, 2011).

Cathflo Activase: Restoration of central venous catheter function

Pregnancy Risk Factor C

Pregnancy Considerations Adverse events were observed in animal reproduction studies. The risk of bleeding may be increased in pregnant women. Information related to alteplase use in pregnancy is limited (Leonhardt, 2006; Li, 2012) and most guidelines consider pregnancy to be a relative contraindication for its use (Jaff, 2011; Jauch, 2013; O'Gara, 2013). Alteplase should not be withheld from pregnant women in life-threatening situations but should be avoided when safer alternatives are available (Bates, 2012; Li, 2012; Leonhardt, 2006; Vanden Hoek, 2010).

Breast-Feeding Considerations It is not known if alteplase is excreted in breast milk. The manufacturer recommends that caution be exercised when administering alteplase to nursing women.

Contraindications Hypersensitivity to alteplase or any component of the formulation

Treatment of STEMI or PE: Active internal bleeding; history of CVA; ischemic stroke within 3 months except when within 4.5 hours (Jaff, 2011; O'Gara, 2013); recent intracranial or intraspinal surgery or trauma; intracranial neoplasm; prior intracranial hemorrhage (Jaff, 2011; O'Gara, 2013); arteriovenous malformation or aneurysm; active bleeding (excluding menses) (O'Gara, 2013); known bleeding diathesis; severe uncontrolled hypertension; suspected aortic dissection (Jaff, 2011; O'Gara, 2013); significant closed head or facial trauma (Jaff, 2011; O'Gara, 2013) within 3 months with radiographic evidence of bony fracture or brain injury (Jaff, 2011)

Treatment of acute ischemic stroke: Evidence/history of intracranial hemorrhage or suspicion of subarachnoid hemorrhage on pretreatment evaluation; recent intracranial or intraspinal surgery; stroke or serious head injury within 3 months; uncontrolled hypertension at time of treatment (eg, >185 mm Hg systolic or >110 mm Hg diastolic); seizure at the onset of stroke; active internal bleeding; intracranial neoplasm; arteriovenous malformation or aneurysm; multilobar cerebral infarction (hypodensity >$^1/_3$ cerebral hemisphere); known bleeding diathesis including but not limited to current use of oral anticoagulants with an INR >1.7 (or PT >15 seconds), current use of direct thrombin inhibitors or direct factor Xa inhibitors with elevated sensitive laboratory tests (eg, aPTT, INR, platelet count, and ECT, TT, or appropriate factor Xa activity assays) (See **"Note"**; Jauch, 2013), administration of heparin within 48 hours preceding the onset of stroke with an elevated aPTT at presentation, or platelet count <100,000/mm^3.

Note: The AHA/ASA guidelines do allow the use of direct thrombin inhibitors (eg, dabigatran) or direct factor Xa inhibitors (eg, rivaroxaban) when sensitive laboratory tests (eg, aPTT, INR, platelet count, ECT, TT, or appropriate direct factor Xa activity assays) are normal or the patient has not received a dose of these agents for >2 days (assuming normal renal function).

Additional exclusion criteria within clinical trials:

Presentation <3 hours after initial symptoms (NINDS, 1995): Time of symptom onset unknown, rapidly improving or minor symptoms, major surgery within 2 weeks, GI or urinary tract hemorrhage within 3 weeks, aggressive treatment required to lower blood pressure, glucose level <50 or >400 mg/dL, and arterial puncture at a noncompressible site or lumbar puncture within 1 week.

Presentation 3-4.5 hours after initial symptoms (ECASS-III; Hacke, 2008; Jauch, 2013): Age >80 years, time of symptom onset unknown, rapidly improving or minor symptoms, current use of oral anticoagulants regardless of INR, glucose level <50 or >400 mg/dL, aggressive intravenous treatment required to lower blood pressure, major surgery or severe trauma within 3 months, baseline National Institutes of Health Stroke Scale (NIHSS) score >25 [ie, severe stroke], and history of both stroke and diabetes.

Warnings/Precautions The total dose should not exceed 90 mg for acute ischemic stroke or 100 mg for acute myocardial infarction or pulmonary embolism. Doses ≥150 mg associated with significantly increased risk of intracranial hemorrhage compared to doses ≤100 mg. Concurrent heparin anticoagulation may contribute to bleeding. In the treatment of acute ischemic stroke, concurrent use of anticoagulants was not permitted during the initial 24 hours of the <3 hour window trial (NINDS, 1995). The AHA/ASA does not recommend initiation of anticoagulant therapy within 24 hours of treatment with alteplase (Jauch, 2013). Initiation of SubQ heparin (≤10,000 units) or equivalent doses of low molecular weight heparin for prevention of DVT during the first 24 hours of the 3 to 4.5 hour window trial was permitted and did not increase the incidence of intracerebral hemorrhage (Hacke, 2008). For acute PE, withhold heparin during the 2-hour infusion period. Monitor all potential bleeding sites. Intramuscular injections and nonessential handling of the patient should be avoided. Venipunctures should be performed carefully and only when necessary. If arterial puncture is necessary, use an upper extremity vessel that can be manually compressed. If serious bleeding occurs, the infusion of alteplase and heparin should be stopped. Avoid aspirin for 24 hours following administration of alteplase; administration within 24 hours increases the risk of hemorrhagic transformation.

For the following conditions, the risk of bleeding is higher with use of thrombolytics and should be weighed against the benefits of therapy: Recent major surgery (eg, CABG, obstetrical delivery, organ biopsy, pregnancy, previous puncture of noncompressible vessels), prolonged CPR with evidence of thoracic trauma, lumbar puncture within 1 week, cerebrovascular disease, recent gastrointestinal or genitourinary bleeding, recent trauma, hypertension (adults with systolic BP >175 mm Hg and/or diastolic BP >110 mm Hg), high likelihood of left heart thrombus (eg, mitral stenosis with atrial fibrillation), acute pericarditis, subacute bacterial endocarditis, hemostatic defects including ones caused by severe renal or hepatic dysfunction, significant hepatic dysfunction, pregnancy, diabetic hemorrhagic retinopathy or other hemorrhagic ophthalmic conditions, septic thrombophlebitis or occluded AV cannula at seriously infected site, advanced age (eg, >75 years), any other condition in which bleeding constitutes a significant hazard or would be particularly difficult to manage because of location. When treating acute MI or pulmonary embolism, use with caution in patients receiving oral anticoagulants. In the treatment of acute ischemic stroke (AIS) within 3 hours of symptom onset, the current use of oral anticoagulants is a contraindication per the manufacturer. According to the AHA/ASA, the current use of oral anticoagulants producing an INR >1.7, direct thrombin inhibitors, or direct factor Xa inhibitors with elevated sensitive laboratory tests are contraindications. However, alteplase may be administered to patients with AIS having received direct thrombin inhibitors (eg, dabigatran) or direct factor Xa inhibitors (eg, rivaroxaban) when sensitive laboratory tests (eg, aPTT, INR, platelet count, ECT, TT, or appropriate direct factor Xa activity assays) are normal or the patient has not received a dose of these agents for >2 days (assuming normal renal function). When treating AIS 3 to 4.5 hours after symptom onset, the use of alteplase should be avoided with current use of any oral anticoagulant regardless of INR (Jauch, 2013). In the treatment of STEMI, adjunctive use of parenteral anticoagulants (eg, enoxaparin, heparin, or fondaparinux) is recommended to improve vessel patency and prevent reocclusion and may also contribute to bleeding; monitor for bleeding (ACCF/AHA; O'Gara, 2013).

Coronary thrombolysis may result in reperfusion arrhythmias. Patients who present **within 3 hours** of stroke symptom onset should be treated with alteplase unless contraindications exist. A longer time window (**3 to 4.5 hours** after symptom onset) has been shown to be safe and efficacious for select individuals (Hacke, 2008; Jauch, 2013). Treatment of patients with minor neurological deficit or with rapidly improving symptoms is not recommended. Follow standard management for STEMI while infusing alteplase.

Cathflo Activase: When used to restore catheter function, use Cathflo cautiously in those patients with known or suspected catheter infections. Evaluate catheter for other causes of dysfunction before use. Avoid excessive pressure when instilling into catheter.

Adverse Reactions As with all drugs which may affect hemostasis, bleeding is the major adverse effect associated with alteplase. Hemorrhage may occur at virtually any site. Risk is dependent on multiple variables, including the dosage administered, concurrent use of multiple agents which alter hemostasis, and patient predisposition. Rapid lysis of coronary artery thrombi by thrombolytic agents may be associated with reperfusion-related atrial and/or ventricular arrhythmia. **Note:** Lowest rate of bleeding complications expected with dose used to restore catheter function.

Cardiovascular: Hypotension
Central nervous system: Fever
Dermatologic: Bruising
Gastrointestinal: GI hemorrhage, nausea, vomiting
Genitourinary: GU hemorrhage
Hematologic: Bleeding
Local: Bleeding at catheter puncture site
Rare but important or life-threatening: Angioedema (orolingual), intracranial hemorrhage, retroperitoneal hemorrhage, pericardial hemorrhage, gingival hemorrhage, epistaxis, allergic reaction (anaphylaxis, anaphylactoid reactions, laryngeal edema, rash, and urticaria)
Additional cardiovascular events associated **with use in STEMI:** AV block, asystole, bradycardia, cardiac arrest, cardiac tamponade, cardiogenic shock, cholesterol crystal embolization, electromechanical dissociation, heart failure, hemorrhagic bursitis, mitral regurgitation, myocardial rupture, recurrent ischemia/infarction, pericardial effusion, pericarditis, pulmonary edema, ruptured intracranial AV malformation, seizure, thromboembolism, ventricular tachycardia
Additional events associated **with use in pulmonary embolism:** Pleural effusion, pulmonary re-embolization, pulmonary edema, thromboembolism
Additional events associated **with use in stroke:** Cerebral edema, cerebral herniation, new ischemic stroke, seizure

Drug Interactions

Metabolism/Transport Effects None known.

Avoid Concomitant Use There are no known interactions where it is recommended to avoid concomitant use.

Increased Effect/Toxicity

Alteplase may increase the levels/effects of: Anticoagulants; Dabigatran Etexilate; Prostacyclin Analogues

The levels/effects of Alteplase may be increased by: Agents with Antiplatelet Properties; Herbs (Anticoagulant/Antiplatelet Properties); Limaprost; Salicylates

Decreased Effect

The levels/effects of Alteplase may be decreased by: Aprotinin; Nitroglycerin

Preparation for Administration

Activase:

50 mg vial: Use accompanying diluent; mix by gentle swirling or slow inversion; do not shake. Vacuum is present in 50 mg vial. Final concentration: 1 mg/mL.

100 mg vial: Use transfer set with accompanying diluent (100 mL vial of sterile water for injection). No vacuum is present in 100 mg vial. Final concentration: 1 mg/mL.

Activase: ST-elevation MI: Accelerated infusion: Bolus dose may be prepared by one of three methods:

1) Removal of 15 mL reconstituted (1 mg/mL) solution from vial
2) Removal of 15 mL from a port on the infusion line after priming
3) Programming an infusion pump to deliver a 15 mL bolus at the initiation of infusion

Activase: Acute ischemic stroke: Bolus dose (10% of total dose) may be prepared by one of three methods:

1) Removal of the appropriate volume from reconstituted solution (1 mg/mL)
2) Removal of the appropriate volume from a port on the infusion line after priming
3) Programming an infusion pump to deliver the appropriate volume at the initiation of infusion

Cathflo Activase: Add 2.2 mL SWFI to vial; do not shake. Final concentration: 1 mg/mL.

Storage/Stability

Activase: The lyophilized product may be stored at room temperature (not to exceed 30°C/86°F), or under refrigeration. Once reconstituted, it should be used within 8 hours.

Cathflo Activase: Store lyophilized product under refrigeration. Once reconstituted, it should be used within 8 hours.

Solutions of 0.5 mg/mL, 1 mg/mL, and 2 mg/mL in SWI retained ≥94% of fibrinolytic activity at 48 hours when stored at 2°C in plastic syringes; these solutions retained ≥90% of fibrinolytic activity when stored in plastic syringes at -25°C or -70°C for 7 or 14 days, thawed at room temperature and then stored at 2°C for 48 hours (Davis, 2000). Solutions of 1 mg/mL in SWI were stable for 22 weeks in plastic syringes when stored at -30°C and for ~1 month in glass vials when stored at -20°C; bioactivity remained unchanged for 6 months in propylene containers when stored at -20°C and for 2 weeks in glass vials when stored at -70°C (Generali, 2001).

Mechanism of Action Initiates local fibrinolysis by binding to fibrin in a thrombus (clot) and converts entrapped plasminogen to plasmin

Pharmacodynamics/Kinetics

Duration: >50% present in plasma cleared ~5 minutes after infusion terminated, ~80% cleared within 10 minutes; fibrinolytic activity persists for up to 1 hour after infusion terminated (Semba, 2000)

Excretion: Clearance (in patients with acute MI receiving accelerated regimen): Rapidly from circulating plasma (572 ± 132 mL/minute) (Tanswell, 1992), primarily hepatic; >50% present in plasma is cleared within 5 minutes after the infusion is terminated, ~80% cleared within 10 minutes (Semba, 2000)

Dosage

IV (Activase):

ST-elevation myocardial infarction (STEMI): **Note:** Manufacturer's labeling recommends 3-hour infusion regimen; however, accelerated regimen preferred by the ACCF/AHA (O'Gara, 2013).

Accelerated regimen (weight-based):

Patients >67 kg: Total dose: 100 mg over 1.5 hours; administered as a 15 mg IV bolus over 1 to 2 minutes followed by infusions of 50 mg over 30 minutes, then 35 mg over 1 hour. Maximum total dose: 100 mg

Patients ≤67 kg: Infuse 15 mg IV bolus over 1 to 2 minutes followed by infusions of 0.75 mg/kg (not to exceed 50 mg) over 30 minutes then 0.5 mg/kg (not to exceed 35 mg) over 1 hour. Maximum total dose: 100 mg

Note: Thrombolytic should be administered within 30 minutes of hospital arrival. Generally, there is only a small trend for benefit of therapy after a delay of 12 to 24 hours from symptom onset, but thrombolysis may be considered for selected patients with ongoing ischemic pain and extensive ST elevation; however, primary PCI is preferred in these patients. Administer concurrent aspirin, clopidogrel, and anticoagulant therapy (ie, unfractionated heparin, enoxaparin, or fondaparinux) with alteplase (O'Gara, 2013).

Acute massive or submassive pulmonary embolism (PE): 100 mg over 2 hours; may be administered as a 10 mg bolus followed by 90 mg over 2 hours as was done in patients with submassive PE (Konstantinides, 2002). **Note:** Not recommended for submassive PE with minor RV dysfunction, minor myocardial necrosis, and no clinical worsening or low-risk PE (ie, normotensive, no RV dysfunction, normal biomarkers) (Jaff, 2011).

Acute ischemic stroke: Within 3 hours of the onset of symptom onset (labeled use) **or** within 3 to 4.5 hours of symptom onset (off-label use; Hacke, 2008; Jauch, 2013): **Note:** Perform noncontrast-enhanced CT or MRI prior to administration. Initiation of anticoagulants (eg, heparin) or antiplatelet agents (eg, aspirin) within 24 hours after starting alteplase is not recommended; however, initiation of aspirin within 24 to 48 hours after stroke onset is recommended (Jauch, 2013). Initiation of SubQ heparin (≤10,000 units) or equivalent doses of low molecular weight heparin for prevention of DVT during the first 24 hours of the 3 to 4.5 hour window trial did not increase incidence of intracerebral hemorrhage (Hacke, 2008).

Recommended total dose: 0.9 mg/kg (maximum total dose: 90 mg)

Patients ≤100 kg: Load with 0.09 mg/kg (10% of 0.9 mg/kg dose) as an IV bolus over 1 minute, followed by 0.81 mg/kg (90% of 0.9 mg/kg dose) as a continuous infusion over 60 minutes.

Patients >100 kg: Load with 9 mg (10% of 90 mg) as an IV bolus over 1 minute, followed by 81 mg (90% of 90 mg) as a continuous infusion over 60 minutes.

Prosthetic valve thrombosis, right-sided (any size thrombus) or left-sided (thrombus area <0.8 cm^2, recent onset [<14 days] of NYHA class I to II symptoms), or left-sided (thrombus area ≥0.8 cm^2) when contraindications to surgery exist (off-label use) (ACCP [Guyatt, 2012]; AHA/ACC [Nishimura, 2014]; Alpert, 2003; Roudaut, 2003):

High-dose regimen: Load with 10 mg, followed by 90 mg over 90 to 180 minutes (without heparin during infusion)

Low-dose regimen (preferred for very small adults): Load with 20 mg, followed by 10 mg/hour for 3 hours (without heparin during infusion)

Note: After successful administration of alteplase, heparin infusion should be introduced until warfarin achieves therapeutic INR (aortic: 3.0 to 4.0; mitral: 3.5 to 4.5) (Bonow, 2008). The 2012 ACCP guidelines for antithrombotic therapy make no recommendation regarding INR range after prosthetic valve thrombosis.

Intracatheter: Central venous catheter clearance (Cathflo Activase 1 mg/mL):

Patients <30 kg: 110% of the internal lumen volume of the catheter, not to exceed 2 mg/2 mL; retain in catheter for 0.5 to 2 hours; may instill a second dose if catheter remains occluded

Patients ≥30 kg: 2 mg (2 mL); retain in catheter for 0.5 to 2 hours; may instill a second dose if catheter remains occluded

Intra-arterial: Acute peripheral arterial occlusion (off-label use):

Weight-based regimen: 0.001 to 0.02 mg/kg/hour (maximum dose: 2 mg/hour) (Semba, 2000)

or

Fixed-dose regimen: 0.12 to 2 mg/hour (Semba, 2000)

Note: The ACC/AHA guidelines state that thrombolysis is an effective and beneficial therapy for those with acute limb ischemia (Rutherford categories I and IIa) of <14 days duration (Hirsch, 2006). The optimal dosage and concentration has not been established; a number of intra-arterial delivery techniques are employed with continuous infusion being the most common (Ouriel, 2004). The Advisory Panel to the Society for Cardiovascular and Interventional Radiology on Thrombolytic Therapy recommends dosing of ≤2 mg/hour and concomitant administration of subtherapeutic heparin (aPTT 1.25 to 1.5 times baseline) (Semba, 2000). Duration of alteplase infusion dependent upon size and location of the thrombus; typically between 6 to 48 hours (Disini, 2008).

Intrapleural: Complicated parapneumonic effusion (off-label use):

Children >3 months: 4 mg in 40 mL NS, first dose at time of chest tube placement with 1 hour dwell time, repeat every 24 hours for 3 days (total of 3 doses) **or** 0.1 mg/kg (maximum: 3 mg) in 10 to 30 mL NS, first dose after pigtail catheter (chest tube) placement, 0.75 to 1 hour dwell time, repeat every 8 hours for 3 days (total of 9 doses) (IDSA/PIDS, 2011)

Adults: 10 mg in 30 mL NS administered twice daily with a 1 hour dwell time for a total of 3 days; each dose followed in >2 hours by intrapleural dornase alfa (Rahman, 2011). Some clinicians suggest consideration of fibrinolytic use when patients have failed at least 24 hours of chest tube drainage and are poor surgical candidates (Hamblin, 2010).

Dosage adjustment in renal impairment: There are no dosage adjustment provided in the manufacturer's labeling.

Dosage adjustment in hepatic impairment: There are no dosage adjustment provided in the manufacturer's labeling.

Usual Infusion Concentrations: Pediatric IV infusion: 0.5 mg/mL **or** 1 mg/mL

Usual Infusion Concentrations: Adult IV infusion: 1 mg/mL

Note: Concentrations for some indications (eg, peripheral arterial occlusion) may require further dilution (eg, 0.1 to 0.2 mg/mL [Chan, 2001; Semba, 2000]) and a usual concentration may not be established.

Administration

Activase: ST-elevation MI or acute ischemic stroke: Administer bolus dose (prepared by one of three methods) over 1 minute followed by infusion.

Infusion: Remaining dose for STEMI, AIS, or total dose for acute pulmonary embolism may be administered as follows: Any quantity of drug not to be administered to the patient must be removed from vial(s) prior to administration of remaining dose.

50 mg vial: Either PVC bag or glass vial and infusion set

100 mg vial: Insert spike end of the infusion set through the same puncture site created by transfer device and infuse from vial

If further dilution is desired, may be diluted in equal volume of 0.9% sodium chloride or D_5W to yield a final concentration of 0.5 mg/mL.

Cathflo Activase: Intracatheter: Instill dose into occluded catheter. Do not force solution into catheter. After a 30-minute dwell time, assess catheter function by attempting to aspirate blood. If catheter is functional, aspirate 4 to 5 mL of blood in patients ≥10 kg or 3 mL in patients <10 kg to remove Cathflo Activase and residual clots. Gently irrigate the catheter with NS. If catheter remains nonfunctional, let Cathflo Activase dwell for another 90 minutes (total dwell time: 120 minutes) and reassess function. If catheter function is not restored, a second dose may be instilled.

Parapneumonic effusion (off-label use): Intrapleural: Instill dose into chest tube and clamp drain. Although the optimum dwell time has not been determined, clinical trials more often have used either a 45 minute (Hawkins, 2004) or 1 hour (Rahman, 2011; St. Peter, 2009) dwell time; after dwell period, release clamp and connect chest tube to continuous suction.

Monitoring Parameters

Acute ischemic stroke (AIS): Baseline: Neurologic examination, head CT (without contrast), blood pressure, CBC, aPTT, PT/INR, glucose. During and after initiation: In addition to monitoring for bleeding complications, the 2013 AHA/ASA guidelines for the early management of AIS recommends the following:

Perform neurological assessments every 15 minutes during infusion and every 30 minutes thereafter for the next 6 hours, then hourly until 24 hours after treatment.

If severe headache, acute hypertension, nausea, or vomiting occurs, discontinue the infusion and obtain emergency CT scan.

Measure BP every 15 minutes for the first 2 hours of initiation then every 30 minutes for the next 6 hours, then hourly until 24 hours after initiation of alteplase. Increase frequency if a systolic BP is ≥180 mm Hg or if a diastolic BP is ≥105 mm Hg; administer antihypertensive medications to maintain BP at or below these levels.

Obtain a follow-up CT scan at 24 hours before starting anticoagulants or antiplatelet agents.

Central venous catheter clearance: Assess catheter function by attempting to aspirate blood.

ST-elevation MI: Baseline: Blood pressure, serum cardiac biomarkers, CBC, PT/INR, aPTT. During and after initiation: Assess for evidence of cardiac reperfusion through resolution of chest pain, resolution of baseline ECG changes, preserved left ventricular function, cardiac enzyme washout phenomenon, and/or the appearance of reperfusion arrhythmias; assess for bleeding potential through clinical evidence of GI bleeding, hematuria, gingival bleeding, fibrinogen levels, fibrinogen degradation products, PT and aPTT.

Reference Range Not routinely measured; literature supports therapeutic levels of 0.52 to 1.8 mcg/mL

Fibrinogen: 200 to 400 mg/dL

Activated partial thromboplastin time (aPTT): 22.5 to 38.7 seconds

Prothrombin time (PT): 10.9 to 12.2 seconds

Dosage Forms

Solution Reconstituted, Injection:

Cathflo Activase: 2 mg (1 ea)

Solution Reconstituted, Intravenous:

Activase: 50 mg (1 ea); 100 mg (1 ea)

- **Alteplase, Recombinant** *see* Alteplase *on page 99*
- **Alteplase, Tissue Plasminogen Activator, Recombinant** *see* Alteplase *on page 99*
- **Alti-Flurbiprofen (Can)** *see* Flurbiprofen (Systemic) *on page 906*
- **Alti-Ipratropium (Can)** *see* Ipratropium (Nasal) *on page 1109*
- **Alti-MPA (Can)** *see* MedroxyPROGESTERone *on page 1277*
- **Altoprev** *see* Lovastatin *on page 1252*

Aluminum Hydroxide

(a LOO mi num hye DROKS ide)

Brand Names: U.S. DermaMed [OTC]

Brand Names: Canada Amphojel; Basaljel

Pharmacologic Category Antacid; Antidote; Protectant, Topical

Use

Oral: Antacid: For the temporary relief of heartburn, acid indigestion, and sour stomach)

Topical: Temporary protection of minor cuts, scrapes, and burns

Dosage

Oral:

Antacid: Adults: 640 mg 5 to 6 times daily after meals and at bedtime (maximum: 3840 mg in 24 hours)

Hyperphosphatemia in chronic kidney disease (CKD) (off-label use): **Note:** The use of aluminum hydroxide should be reserved for serum phosphorus levels >7 mg/dL and limited to short-term use (adults: 4 weeks; adolescents: 4 to 6 weeks) given the toxicities associated with long-term use (NKF, 2003; NKF, 2005).

Adolescents and Adults: Initial: 300 to 600 mg 3 times daily with meals (Hudson, 2014).

Topical: Skin protectant: Children, Adolescents, and Adults: Apply to affected area as needed; reapply at least every 12 hours

Dosage adjustment in renal impairment: Aluminum may accumulate in renal impairment.

Additional Information Complete prescribing information should be consulted for additional detail.

Dosage Forms

Ointment, External:

DermaMed [OTC]: (113 g)

Suspension, Oral:

Generic: 320 mg/5 mL (473 mL)

Aluminum Hydroxide and Magnesium Carbonate

(a LOO mi num hye DROKS ide & mag NEE zhum KAR bun nate)

Brand Names: U.S. Acid Gone Extra Strength [OTC]; Acid Gone [OTC]; Gaviscon® Extra Strength [OTC]; Gaviscon® Liquid [OTC]

Index Terms Magnesium Carbonate and Aluminum Hydroxide

Pharmacologic Category Antacid

Use Temporary relief of symptoms associated with gastric acidity

Dosage Oral: Adults:

Liquid:

Gaviscon® Regular Strength: 15-30 mL 4 times/day after meals and at bedtime

Gaviscon® Extra Strength: 15-30 mL 4 times/day after meals

Tablet (Gaviscon® Extra Strength): Chew 2-4 tablets 4 times/day

Dosage adjustment in renal impairment: Aluminum and/or magnesium may accumulate in renal impairment.

Additional Information Complete prescribing information should be consulted for additional detail.

Dosage Forms

Liquid: Aluminum hydroxide 31.7 mg and magnesium carbonate 119.3 mg per 5 mL; aluminum hydroxide 84.6 mg and magnesium carbonate 79.1 mg per 5 mL

Acid Gone [OTC], Gaviscon® [OTC]: Aluminum hydroxide 31.7 mg and magnesium carbonate 119.3 mg per 5 mL

Gaviscon® Extra Strength [OTC]: Aluminum hydroxide 84.6 mg and magnesium carbonate 79.1 mg per 5 mL

Tablet, chewable: Aluminum hydroxide 160 mg and magnesium carbonate 105 mg

Acid Gone Extra Strength [OTC], Gaviscon® Extra Strength [OTC]: Aluminum hydroxide 160 mg and magnesium carbonate 105 mg

Aluminum Hydroxide and Magnesium Hydroxide

(a LOO mi num hye DROKS ide & mag NEE zhum hye DROK side)

Brand Names: U.S. Alamag [OTC]; Mag-Al Ultimate [OTC]; Mag-Al [OTC]

Brand Names: Canada Diovol®; Diovol® Ex; Gelusil® Extra Strength; Mylanta™

Index Terms Magnesium Hydroxide and Aluminum Hydroxide

Pharmacologic Category Antacid

Use Antacid for symptoms related to hyperacidity associated with heartburn, hiatal hernia, upset stomach, peptic ulcer, peptic esophagitis, or gastritis

Dosage Oral: Children ≥12 years and Adults: OTC labeling:

Liquid (aluminum hydroxide 200 mg and magnesium hydroxide 200 mg per 5 mL): 10-20 mL 4 times/day (maximum: 80 mL/day)

Suspension (aluminum hydroxide 500 mg and magnesium hydroxide 500 mg per 5 mL): 10-20 mL 4 times/day, between meals and at bedtime (maximum: 45 mL/day)

Tablet (aluminum hydroxide 300 mg and magnesium hydroxide 150 mg): 1-2 tablets after meals or at bedtime, or as needed (maximum: 16 tablets/day)

Dosage adjustment in renal impairment: Aluminum and/or magnesium may accumulate in severe renal impairment.

Additional Information Complete prescribing information should be consulted for additional detail.

Dosage Forms

Liquid, oral:

Mag-Al [OTC]: Aluminum hydroxide 200 mg and magnesium hydroxide 200 mg per 5 mL

Suspension, oral:

Mag-Al Ultimate [OTC]: Aluminum hydroxide 500 mg and magnesium hydroxide 500 mg per 5 mL

Tablet, chewable:

Alamag [OTC]: Aluminum hydroxide 300 mg and magnesium hydroxide 150 mg

Aluminum Hydroxide and Magnesium Trisilicate

(a LOO mi num hye DROKS ide & mag NEE zhum trye SIL i kate)

Brand Names: U.S. Gaviscon® Tablet [OTC]

Index Terms Magnesium Trisilicate and Aluminum Hydroxide

Pharmacologic Category Antacid

Use Temporary relief of hyperacidity

Dosage Oral: Adults: Chew 2-4 tablets 4 times/day or as directed by healthcare provider

Dosage adjustment in renal impairment: Aluminum and/or magnesium may accumulate in renal impairment.

Additional Information Complete prescribing information should be consulted for additional detail.

Dosage Forms

Tablet, chewable: Aluminum hydroxide 80 mg and magnesium trisilicate 20 mg

Gaviscon® [OTC]: Aluminum hydroxide 80 mg and magnesium trisilicate 20 mg

Aluminum Hydroxide, Magnesium Hydroxide, and Simethicone

(a LOO mi num hye DROKS ide, mag NEE zhum hye DROKS ide, & sye METH i kone)

Brand Names: U.S. Alamag Plus [OTC]; Aldroxicon I [OTC]; Aldroxicon II [OTC]; Almacone Double Strength [OTC]; Almacone [OTC]; Gelusil [OTC]; Geri-Mox [OTC]; Maalox Advanced Maximum Strength [OTC]; Maalox Advanced Regular Strength [OTC]; Mi-Acid Maximum Strength [OTC] [DSC]; Mi-Acid [OTC]; Mintox Plus [OTC]; Mylanta Classic Maximum Strength Liquid [OTC]; Mylanta Classic Regular Strength Liquid [OTC]; Rulox [OTC]

Brand Names: Canada Diovol Plus; Gelusil; Mylanta Double Strength; Mylanta Extra Strength; Mylanta Regular Strength

Index Terms Magnesium Hydroxide, Aluminum Hydroxide, and Simethicone; Simethicone, Aluminum Hydroxide, and Magnesium Hydroxide

Pharmacologic Category Antacid; Antiflatulent

Use Antacid/antigas: Relief of acid indigestion, heartburn, sour stomach, or upset stomach and gas associated with these symptoms

Dosage Antacid/antigas: Children ≥12 years, Adolescents, and Adults: Oral:

Products containing aluminum hydroxide 200 mg, magnesium hydroxide 200 mg, and simethicone 25 mg per tablet: 1 to 4 tablets 4 times daily; may also take as needed, up to 12 to 16 tablets in 24 hours

Products containing aluminum hydroxide 200 mg, magnesium hydroxide 200 mg, and simethicone 20 mg per 5 mL: 10 to 20 mL between meals, at bedtime, or as directed by health care provider; maximum: 80 to 120 mL in 24 hours

Products containing aluminum hydroxide 400 mg, magnesium hydroxide 400 mg, and simethicone 40 mg per 5 mL: 10 to 20 mL between meals, at bedtime, or as directed by health care provider; maximum: 40 to 60 mL in 24 hours

Additional Information Complete prescribing information should be consulted for additional detail.

Dosage Forms

Liquid: Aluminum hydroxide 200 mg, magnesium hydroxide 200 mg, and simethicone 20 mg per 5 mL; aluminum hydroxide 400 mg, magnesium hydroxide 400 mg, and simethicone 40 mg per 5 mL

Aldroxicon I [OTC], Almacone [OTC], Maalox Advanced Regular Strength [OTC], Mi-Acid [OTC], Mylanta Classic Regular Strength [OTC]: Aluminum hydroxide 200 mg, magnesium hydroxide 200 mg, and simethicone 20 mg per 5 mL

Aldroxicon II [OTC], Almacone Double Strength [OTC], Maalox Advanced Maximum Strength [OTC], Mi-Acid Maximum Strength [OTC], Mylanta Classic Maximum Strength [OTC]: Aluminum hydroxide 400 mg, magnesium hydroxide 400 mg, and simethicone 40 mg per 5 mL

Suspension: Aluminum hydroxide 225 mg, magnesium hydroxide 200 mg, and simethicone 25 mg per 5 mL

Geri-Mox [OTC], Rulox [OTC]: Aluminum hydroxide 200 mg, magnesium hydroxide 200 mg, and simethicone 25 mg per 5 mL

Tablet, chewable: Aluminum hydroxide 200 mg, magnesium hydroxide 200 mg, and simethicone 25 mg

Alamag Plus [OTC], Gelusil [OTC], Mintox Plus [OTC]: Aluminum hydroxide 200 mg, magnesium hydroxide 200 mg, and simethicone 25 mg

◆ **Aluminum Sucrose Sulfate, Basic** *see* Sucralfate *on page 1940*

◆ **Alupent** *see* Metaproterenol *on page 1307*

◆ **Aluvea** *see* Urea *on page 2114*

Alverine [INT] (AL ve reen)

International Brand Names Alverix (KR); Audmonal (GB); Audmonal Forte (GB); Averinal (VN); Gastrodog [vet.] (FR); Hepatoum (FR); Profenil (HK, HN); Spasmaverine (FR); Spasmine (BE); Spasmolina (PL); Spasmonal (AE, BE, BH, CN, CY, GB, HK, HN, IE, KW, LB, PK, SA, SG); Spasmonal Forte (CY, GB, IE, LB); Spasmoverine (VN)

Index Terms Alverine Citrate

Pharmacologic Category Antispasmodic Agent, Gastrointestinal

Reported Use Treatment of irritable bowel syndrome and dysmenorrhea

Dosage Range Adults: Oral: 60-120 mg 1-3 times/day

Product Availability Product available in various countries; not currently available in the U.S.

Dosage Forms

Capsule, as citrate: 60 mg, 120 mg

◆ **Alverine Citrate** *see* Alverine [INT] *on page 104*

◆ **Alvesco** *see* Ciclesonide (Systemic) *on page 432*

Alvimopan (al VI moe pan)

Brand Names: U.S. Entereg

Index Terms ADL-2698; LY246736

Pharmacologic Category Gastrointestinal Agent, Miscellaneous; Opioid Antagonist, Peripherally-Acting

Use Postoperative ileus: To accelerate the time to upper and lower GI recovery following surgeries including partial bowel resection with primary anastomosis

Pregnancy Risk Factor B

Pregnancy Considerations Adverse events have not been observed in animal reproduction studies.

Breast-Feeding Considerations It is not known if alvimopan is excreted in breast milk. The manufacturer recommends that caution be exercised when administering alvimopan to nursing women.

Contraindications Patients who have taken therapeutic doses of opioids for more than 7 consecutive days immediately prior to alvimopan

Warnings/Precautions **[U.S. Boxed Warning]: For short-term (≤15 doses) hospital use only. Only hospitals that have registered through the ENTEREG Access Support and Education (E.A.S.E.™) Program and met all requirements may use.** It will not be dispensed to patients who have been discharged from the hospital. Use not recommended in patients with complete bowel obstruction or in patients having gastric or pancreatic anastomosis. Use with caution in patients with hepatic or renal impairment; use not recommended in patients with severe hepatic impairment or ESRD. Use with caution is patients recently exposed to opioids; may be more sensitive to gastrointestinal adverse effects (eg, abdominal pain, diarrhea, nausea and vomiting). Contraindicated in patients who have received therapeutic opioids for >7 consecutive days immediately prior to use. **[U.S. Boxed Warning]: A trend towards an increased incidence of MI was observed in alvimopan (low dose) treated patients compared to placebo in a 12-month study in patients treated with opioids for chronic pain. Other short-term studies have not observed this trend and a causal relationship has not been found.** MI was generally observed more frequently in the initial 1-4 months of treatment. Patients of Japanese descent should be monitored closely for gastrointestinal side effects (eg, abdominal pain, cramping, diarrhea) due to possibility of greater drug exposure; discontinue use if side effects occur.

Adverse Reactions
Cardiovascular: Myocardial infarction
Endocrine & metabolic: Hypokalemia
Gastrointestinal: Dyspepsia
Genitourinary: Urinary retention
Hematologic and oncologic: Anemia
Neuromuscular & skeletal: Back pain

Drug Interactions

Metabolism/Transport Effects None known.

Avoid Concomitant Use

Avoid concomitant use of Alvimopan with any of the following: Methylnaltrexone; Naloxegol

Increased Effect/Toxicity

Alvimopan may increase the levels/effects of: Naloxegol

The levels/effects of Alvimopan may be increased by: Analgesics (Opioid); Methylnaltrexone

Decreased Effect There are no known significant interactions involving a decrease in effect.

Food Interactions When administered with a high-fat meal, extent and rate of absorption may be reduced (C_{max} and AUC decreased by ~38% and 21%, respectively). Management: May administer with or without food.

Storage/Stability Store at 25°C (77°F); excursions permitted to 15°C to 30°C (59°F to 86°F).

Mechanism of Action An opioid receptor antagonist which blocks opioid binding at the mu receptor; alvimopan has restricted ability to cross the blood-brain barrier at therapeutic doses. It selectively and competitively binds to the GI tract mu opioid receptors and antagonizes the peripheral effects of opioids on gastrointestinal motility and secretion. Does not affect opioid analgesic effects or induce opioid withdrawal symptoms.

Pharmacodynamics/Kinetics
Distribution: V_d: 20-40 L
Protein binding: Parent drug: 80%; metabolite: 94% (both primarily to albumin)
Metabolism: Hydrolyzed to an amide hydrolysis compound (active metabolite) by gut microflora; further metabolism of active metabolite to glucuronide conjugates and other minor metabolites.
Bioavailability: ~6% (range: 1% to 19%)
Half-life elimination: 10-17 hours
Time to peak, plasma: Parent drug: ~2 hours; Metabolite: 36 hours
Excretion: Urine (~35% as unchanged drug and metabolites); feces (via biliary excretion)

Dosage Note: For hospital use only
Oral: Adults:
Initial: 12 mg administered 30 minutes to 5 hours prior to surgery
Maintenance: 12 mg twice daily beginning the day after surgery for a maximum of 7 days or until discharged from hospital (maximum total treatment: 15 doses)

Dosage adjustment in renal impairment:
Mild-to-severe impairment: No adjustment needed; use caution
ESRD: Use not recommended

Dosage adjustment in hepatic impairment:
Mild-to-moderate impairment (Child-Pugh class A or B): No adjustment needed; use caution
Severe impairment (Child-Pugh class C): Use not recommended

Dietary Considerations Take with or without food; high-fat meals may decrease the rate and extent of absorption

Administration Patient must be hospitalized. Initial dose should be administered 30 minutes to 5 hours prior to surgery. May be administered with or without food.

Dosage Forms

Capsule, Oral:
Entereg: 12 mg

◆ **ALX-0600** *see* Teduglutide *on page 1982*

◆ **Alyacen 1/35** *see* Ethinyl Estradiol and Norethindrone *on page 808*

◆ **Alyacen 7/7/7** *see* Ethinyl Estradiol and Norethindrone *on page 808*

Amantadine (a MAN ta deen)

Brand Names: Canada Dom-Amantadine; Mylan-Amantadine; PHL-Amantadine; PMS-Amantadine

Index Terms Adamantanamine Hydrochloride; Amantadine Hydrochloride; Symmetrel

Pharmacologic Category Anti-Parkinson's Agent, Dopamine Agonist; Antiviral Agent; Antiviral Agent, Adamantane

Use Prophylaxis and treatment of influenza A viral infection (per manufacturer labeling; also refer to current ACIP guidelines for recommendations during current flu season); treatment of parkinsonism; treatment of drug-induced extrapyramidal symptoms

Pregnancy Risk Factor C

Pregnancy Considerations Teratogenic effects were observed in animal studies and in case reports in humans.

Influenza infection may be more severe in pregnant women. Untreated influenza infection is associated with an increased risk of adverse events to the fetus and an increased risk of complications or death to the mother. Oseltamivir and zanamivir are currently recommended for the treatment or prophylaxis influenza in pregnant women and women up to 2 weeks postpartum. Antiviral agents are currently recommended as an adjunct to vaccination and should not be used as a substitute for vaccination in pregnant women (consult current CDC guidelines).

Healthcare providers are encouraged to refer women exposed to influenza vaccine, or who have taken an antiviral medication during pregnancy to the Vaccines and Medications in Pregnancy Surveillance System (VAMPSS) by contacting The Organization of Teratology Information Specialists (OTIS) at (877) 311-8972

Breast-Feeding Considerations The CDC recommends that women infected with the influenza virus follow general precautions (eg, frequent hand washing) to decrease viral transmission to the child. Mothers with influenza-like illnesses at delivery should consider avoiding close contact with the infant until they have received 48 hours of antiviral medication, fever has resolved, and cough and secretions can be controlled. These measures may help decrease (but not eliminate) the risk of transmitting influenza to the newborn during breast-feeding. During this time, breast milk can be expressed and bottle-fed to the infant by another person who is not infected. Protective measures, such as wearing a face mask, changing into a clean gown or clothing, and strict hand hygiene should be continued by the mother for ≥7 days after the onset of symptoms or until symptom-free for 24 hours. Infant care should be performed by a noninfected person when possible (consult current CDC guidelines).

Contraindications Hypersensitivity to amantadine or any component of the formulation

Warnings/Precautions May cause CNS depression, which may impair physical or mental abilities; patients must be cautioned about performing tasks which require mental alertness (eg, operating machinery or driving). Effects may be potentiated when used with other sedative drugs or ethanol. There have been reports of suicidal ideation/attempt in patients with and without a history of psychiatric illness. Use with caution in patients with liver disease, a history of recurrent and eczematoid dermatitis, uncontrolled psychosis or severe psychoneurosis, seizures and in those receiving CNS stimulant drugs; reduce dose in renal disease; when treating Parkinson's disease, do not discontinue abruptly. In many patients, the therapeutic benefits of amantadine are limited to a few months. Abrupt discontinuation may cause agitation, anxiety, delirium, delusions, depression, hallucinations, paranoia, parkinsonian crisis, slurred speech, or stupor. Upon discontinuation of amantadine therapy, gradually taper dose. Elderly patients may be more susceptible to the CNS effects (using 2 divided daily doses may minimize this effect); may require dosage reductions based on renal function. Use with caution in patients with HF, peripheral edema, or orthostatic hypotension; dosage reduction may be required. Avoid in untreated angle closure glaucoma.

Dopamine agonists have been associated with compulsive behaviors and/or loss of impulse control, which has manifested as pathological gambling, libido increases (hypersexuality), and/or binge eating. Causality has not been established, and controversy exists as to whether this phenomenon is related to the underlying disease, prior behaviors/addictions, and/or drug therapy. Dose reduction or discontinuation of therapy has been reported to reverse these behaviors in some, but not all cases. Risk for melanoma development is increased in Parkinson's disease patients; drug causation or factors contributing to risk have not been established. Patients should be monitored closely and periodic skin examinations should be performed. Tolerance has also been reported with long-term use (Zubenko, 1984).

Due to increased resistance, the ACIP has recommended that rimantadine and amantadine no longer be used for the treatment or prophylaxis of influenza A in the United States until susceptibility has been re-established; consult current guidelines.

Some dosage forms may contain propylene glycol; large amounts are potentially toxic and have been associated hyperosmolality, lactic acidosis, seizures and respiratory depression; use caution (AAP, 1997; Zar, 2007).

Adverse Reactions

Cardiovascular: Livedo reticularis, orthostatic hypotension, peripheral edema

Central nervous system: Abnormal dreams, agitation, anxiety, ataxia, confusion, delirium, depression, dizziness, drowsiness, fatigue, hallucination, headache, insomnia, irritability, nervousness

Gastrointestinal: Anorexia, constipation, diarrhea, nausea, xerostomia

Respiratory: Dry nose

Rare but important or life-threatening: Abnormal gait, acute respiratory tract failure, aggressive behavior, agranulocytosis, amnesia, anaphylaxis, cardiac arrest, cardiac arrhythmia, cardiac failure, coma, decreased libido, delusions, diaphoresis, dysphagia, dyspnea, eczema, EEG pattern changes, euphoria, fever, hyperkinesia, hypersensitivity reaction, hypertension, hypertonia, hypokinesia, hypotension, increased blood urea nitrogen, increased creatine phosphokinase, increased gamma-glutamyl transferase, increased lactate dehydrogenase, increased serum alkaline phosphatase, increased serum ALT, increased serum AST, increased serum bilirubin, increased serum creatinine, keratitis, leukocytosis, leukopenia, mania, muscle spasm, mydriasis, neuroleptic malignant syndrome (associated with dosage reduction or abrupt withdrawal of amantadine), neutropenia, oculogyric crisis, paranoia, paresthesia, pruritus, psychosis, pulmonary edema, seizure, skin photosensitivity, skin rash, slurred speech, stupor, suicidal ideation, suicide, suicide attempt, tachycardia, tachypnea, tremor, urinary retention, visual disturbance, vomiting, weakness

Drug Interactions

Metabolism/Transport Effects Substrate of OCT2

Avoid Concomitant Use

Avoid concomitant use of Amantadine with any of the following: Amisulpride

Increased Effect/Toxicity

Amantadine may increase the levels/effects of: BuPROPion; Glycopyrrolate; Highest Risk QTc-Prolonging Agents; Memantine; Moderate Risk QTc-Prolonging Agents; Trimethoprim

The levels/effects of Amantadine may be increased by: Alcohol (Ethyl); BuPROPion; MAO Inhibitors; Methylphenidate; Mifepristone; Trimethoprim

Decreased Effect

Amantadine may decrease the levels/effects of: Amisulpride; Antipsychotic Agents (First Generation [Typical]); Influenza Virus Vaccine (Live/Attenuated)

The levels/effects of Amantadine may be decreased by: Amisulpride; Antipsychotic Agents (First Generation [Typical]); Antipsychotic Agents (Second Generation [Atypical]); Metoclopramide

Storage/Stability Store at 25°C (77°F); excursions permitted to 15°C to 30°C (59°F to 86°F).

Mechanism of Action

Antiviral:

The mechanism of amantadine's antiviral activity has not been fully elucidated. It appears to primarily prevent the release of infectious viral nucleic acid into the host cell by interfering with the transmembrane domain of the viral M2 protein. Amantadine is also known to prevent viral assembly during replication. Amantadine inhibits the replication of influenza A virus isolates from each of the subtypes (ie, H1N1, H2N2 and H3N2), but has very little or no activity against influenza B virus isolates.

Parkinson disease:

The exact mechanism of amantadine in the treatment of Parkinson disease and drug-induced extrapyramidal reactions is not known. Data from early animal studies suggest that amantadine may have direct and indirect effects on dopamine neurons; however, recent studies have demonstrated that amantadine is a weak, non-competitive NMDA receptor antagonist. Although amantadine has not been shown to possess direct anticholinergic activity, clinically, it exhibits anticholinergic-like side effects (dry mouth, urinary retention, and constipation).

Pharmacodynamics/Kinetics

Onset of action: Antidyskinetic: Within 48 hours

Absorption: Well absorbed

Distribution: V_d: Normal: 1.5-6.1 L/kg; Renal failure: 5.1 ± 0.2 L/kg; in saliva, tear film, and nasal secretions; in animals, tissue (especially lung) concentrations higher than serum concentrations; crosses blood-brain barrier

Protein binding: Normal renal function: ~67%; Hemodialysis: ~59%

Metabolism: Not appreciable; small amounts of an acetyl metabolite identified

Bioavailability: 86% to 90%

Half-life elimination: Normal renal function: 16 ± 6 hours (9-31 hours); Healthy, older (≥60 years) males: 29 hours (range: 20-41 hours); End-stage renal disease: 7-10 days

Time to peak, plasma: 2-4 hours

Excretion: Urine (80% to 90% unchanged) by glomerular filtration and tubular secretion

Dosage Oral:

Children: Influenza A treatment/prophylaxis: **Note:** Due to issues of resistance, amantadine is no longer recommended for the treatment or prophylaxis of influenza A. Please refer to the current ACIP recommendations.

Influenza A treatment:

1-9 years: 5 mg/kg/day in 2 divided doses (manufacturers range: 4.4-8.8 mg/kg/day); maximum dose: 150 mg/day

≥10 years and <40 kg: 5 mg/kg/day in 2 divided doses (CDC, 2011)

≥10 years and ≥40 kg: 100 mg twice daily (CDC, 2011)

Note: Initiate within 24-48 hours after onset of symptoms; continue for 24-48 hours after symptom resolution (duration of therapy is generally 3-5 days)

Influenza A prophylaxis: Refer to "Influenza A treatment" dosing. **Note:** Continue prophylaxis throughout the peak influenza activity in the community or throughout the entire influenza season in patients who cannot be vaccinated. Development of immunity following vaccination takes ~2 weeks; amantadine therapy should be considered for high-risk patients from the time of vaccination until immunity has developed. For children <9 years receiving influenza vaccine for the first time, amantadine prophylaxis should continue for 6 weeks (4 weeks after the first dose and 2 weeks after the second dose).

Adults:

Drug-induced extrapyramidal symptoms: 100 mg twice daily; may increase to 300 mg/day in divided doses, if needed

Parkinson's disease: Usual dose: 100 mg twice daily as monotherapy; may increase to 400 mg/day in divided doses, if needed, with close monitoring. **Note:** Patients with a serious concomitant illness or those receiving high doses of other anti-parkinson drugs should be started at 100 mg/day; may increase to 100 mg twice daily, if needed, after one to several weeks.

Influenza A treatment/prophylaxis: **Note:** Due to issues of resistance, amantadine is no longer recommended for the treatment or prophylaxis of influenza A. Please refer to the current ACIP recommendations. The following is based on the manufacturer's labeling:

Influenza A treatment: 200 mg once daily **or** 100 mg twice daily (may be preferred to reduce CNS effects); **Note:** Initiate within 24-48 hours after onset of symptoms; continue for 24-48 hours after symptom resolution (duration of therapy is generally 3-5 days).

Influenza A prophylaxis: 200 mg once daily **or** 100 mg twice daily (may be preferred to reduce CNS effects). **Note:** Continue prophylaxis throughout the peak influenza activity in the community or throughout the entire influenza season in patients who cannot be vaccinated. Development of immunity following vaccination takes ~2 weeks; amantadine therapy should be considered for high-risk patients from the time of vaccination until immunity has developed.

Elderly (≥65 years): Adjust dose based on renal function; some patients tolerate the drug better when it is given in 2 divided daily doses (to avoid adverse neurologic reactions).

Influenza A treatment/prophylaxis: 100 mg once daily

Dosage adjustment in renal impairment:

CrCl 30-50 mL/minute: Administer 200 mg on day 1, then 100 mg/day

CrCl 15-29 mL/minute: Administer 200 mg on day 1, then 100 mg on alternate days

CrCl <15 mL/minute: Administer 200 mg every 7 days

Hemodialysis: Administer 200 mg every 7 days

Peritoneal dialysis: No supplemental dose is needed

Continuous arteriovenous or venous-venous hemofiltration: No supplemental dose is needed

Dosage adjustment in hepatic impairment: No dosage adjustment provided in manufacturer's labeling; use with caution.

Monitoring Parameters Renal function, Parkinson's symptoms, mental status, influenza symptoms, blood pressure

Dosage Forms

Capsule, Oral:
Generic: 100 mg

Syrup, Oral:
Generic: 50 mg/5 mL (10 mL, 473 mL)

Tablet, Oral:
Generic: 100 mg

- ◆ **Amantadine Hydrochloride** *see* Amantadine *on page 105*
- ◆ **Amaryl** *see* Glimepiride *on page 966*
- ◆ **Amatine (Can)** *see* Midodrine *on page 1365*
- ◆ **Ambi 10PEH/400GFN [OTC]** *see* Guaifenesin and Phenylephrine *on page 988*
- ◆ **AMBI 60PSE/400GFN/20DM** *see* Guaifenesin, Pseudoephedrine, and Dextromethorphan *on page 989*
- ◆ **Ambien** *see* Zolpidem *on page 2212*
- ◆ **Ambien CR** *see* Zolpidem *on page 2212*
- ◆ **Ambifed-G [OTC]** *see* Guaifenesin and Pseudoephedrine *on page 989*
- ◆ **AmBisome** *see* Amphotericin B (Liposomal) *on page 139*
- ◆ **AmBisome® (Can)** *see* Amphotericin B (Liposomal) *on page 139*

Ambrisentan (am bri SEN tan)

Brand Names: U.S. Letairis

Brand Names: Canada Volibris

Index Terms BSF208075

Pharmacologic Category Endothelin Receptor Antagonist; Vasodilator

Use Pulmonary arterial hypertension: Treatment of pulmonary artery hypertension (PAH) World Health Organization (WHO) Group I to improve exercise ability and delay clinical worsening

Pregnancy Risk Factor X

Pregnancy Considerations **[U.S. Boxed Warning]: May cause birth defects; use in pregnancy is contraindicated. Exclude pregnancy prior to initiation of therapy and obtain pregnancy tests monthly during treatment and for 1 month after therapy is complete. Reliable contraception must be used during therapy and for 1 month after stopping treatment.** Based on animal studies, ambrisentan is likely to produce major birth defects if used by pregnant women. Two reliable methods of contraception (eg, hormone method with a barrier method or 2 barrier methods) must be used throughout treatment and for 1 month after stopping treatment. Patients who have undergone a tubal ligation or the insertion of a contraceptive implant or intrauterine device (Copper T 380A or LNg 20) do not require additional contraceptive measures. A missed menses or suspected pregnancy should be reported to a healthcare provider and prompt immediate pregnancy testing. Sperm counts may be reduced in men during treatment (as observed with bosentan). In general, women with pulmonary hypertension should avoid pregnancy (Badesch, 2007; McLaughlin, 2009).

Breast-Feeding Considerations It is not known if ambrisentan is excreted in breast milk. Due to the potential for serious adverse reactions in the nursing infant, the manufacturer recommends a decision be made whether to discontinue nursing or to discontinue the drug, taking into account the importance of treatment to the mother.

Contraindications Pregnancy; idiopathic pulmonary fibrosis, including idiopathic pulmonary fibrosis with pulmonary hypertension (WHO Group 3)

Canadian labeling: Additional contraindications (not in U.S. labeling): Hypersensitivity to ambrisentan or any component of the formulation

Warnings/Precautions Hazardous agent - use appropriate precautions for handling and disposal (NIOSH 2014 [group 3]). **[U.S. Boxed Warning]: May cause birth defects; use in pregnancy is contraindicated. Exclude pregnancy prior to initiation of therapy and obtain**

pregnancy tests monthly during treatment and for 1 month after therapy is complete. Reliable contraception must be used during therapy and for 1 month after stopping treatment. Two reliable methods of contraception (eg, hormone method with a barrier method or 2 barrier methods) must be used throughout treatment and for 1 month after stopping treatment. Patients who have undergone a tubal ligation or the insertion of a contraceptive implant or intrauterine device (Copper T 380A or LNg 20) do not require additional contraceptive measures. A missed menses or suspected pregnancy should be reported to a healthcare provider and prompt immediate pregnancy testing. Women should also be educated on the appropriate use of emergency contraception if failure of contraceptive is known or suspected or in the event of unprotected sex.

[U.S. Boxed Warning]: Because of the high likelihood of teratogenic effects, ambrisentan is only available through the Letairis REMS restricted distribution program. Patients, prescribers, and pharmacies must be registered with and meet conditions of the program. Call 1-866-664-5327 or visit www.letairisrems.com for more information.

Use caution in patients with low hemoglobin levels. May cause decreases in hemoglobin and hematocrit (monitoring of hemoglobin is recommended. Use not recommended in patients with clinically significant anemia. Development of peripheral edema due to treatment and/or disease state (pulmonary arterial hypertension) may occur; a higher incidence is seen in elderly patients. Sperm count may be reduced in men during treatment (as observed with bosentan). No changes in sperm function or hormone levels have been noted. Fertility issues may require discussion with patient. Increases in serum liver aminotransferases have been reported during postmarketing use; however, in the majority of the cases, alternative causes of hepatotoxicity could be identified. Perform liver enzyme testing only when clinically indicated. Discontinue therapy if signs/symptoms of hepatic injury appear, if serum liver aminotransferases >5 times ULN are observed, or if aminotransferases are increased in the presence of bilirubin >2 times ULN. Hepatotoxicity has been reported with other endothelin receptor antagonists (eg, bosentan); however, ambrisentan may be tried in patients that have experienced asymptomatic increases in liver enzymes caused by another endothelin receptor antagonist after the liver enzymes have returned to normal. Use caution in patients with mild hepatic impairment; use not recommended in patients with moderate-to-severe impairment. There have also been postmarketing reports of fluid retention requiring treatment (eg, diuretics, fluid management, hospitalization). Further evaluation may be necessary to determine cause and appropriate treatment or discontinuation of therapy. Discontinue in any patient with pulmonary edema suggestive of pulmonary veno-occlusive disease (PVOD).

Adverse Reactions

Cardiovascular: Flushing, palpitation, peripheral edema

Central nervous system: Headache

Gastrointestinal: Abdominal pain, constipation

Hematologic: Hemoglobin decreased

Hepatic: Liver enzymes increased

Respiratory: Dyspnea, nasal congestion, nasopharyngitis, sinusitis (3%)

Rare but important or life-threatening: Anemia, angioedema, dizziness, fatigue, fluid retention, heart failure, hypersensitivity, liver enzymes increased, nausea, rash, vomiting, weakness

Drug Interactions

Metabolism/Transport Effects Substrate of CYP2C19 (minor), CYP3A4 (minor), P-glycoprotein, UGT1A3, UGT1A9, UGT2B7; **Note:** Assignment of Major/Minor substrate status based on clinically relevant drug interaction potential

Avoid Concomitant Use There are no known interactions where it is recommended to avoid concomitant use.

Increased Effect/Toxicity

The levels/effects of Ambrisentan may be increased by: CycloSPORINE (Systemic)

Decreased Effect There are no known significant interactions involving a decrease in effect.

Storage/Stability Store at 25°C (77°F); excursions are permitted between 15°C and 30°C (59°F and 86°F). Store in original packaging.

Mechanism of Action Blocks endothelin receptor subtypes ET_A and ET_B on vascular endothelium and smooth muscle. Stimulation of ET_A receptors, located primarily in pulmonary vascular smooth muscle cells is associated with vasoconstriction and cellular proliferation. Stimulation of ET_B receptors, located in both pulmonary vascular endothelial cells and smooth muscle cells is associated with vasodilation, antiproliferative effects, and endothelin clearance. Although ambrisentan blocks both ET_A and ET_B receptors, the affinity is greater for the ET_A receptor (>4000 fold higher affinity).

Pharmacodynamics/Kinetics

Protein binding: 99%

Metabolism: Hepatic via CYP3A4, CYP2C19, and uridine 5'-diphosphate glucuronosyltransferases (UGTs) 1A9S, 2B7S, and 1A3S; *in vitro* studies also suggest it is a substrate of organic anion transporting polypeptides (OATP) 1B1 and 1B3 and P-glycoprotein (P-gp)

Half-life elimination: ~9 hours

Time to peak, plasma: ~2 hours

Excretion: Primarily nonrenal

Dosage Oral: Adults: Initial: 5 mg once daily; if tolerated, may increase to maximum 10 mg once daily

Coadministration with cyclosporine: Ambrisentan dose should not exceed 5 mg/day

Dosage adjustment in renal impairment:

Mild-to-moderate renal impairment: No dosage adjustment necessary.

Severe renal impairment: There is no data available for use in severe renal impairment.

Dosage adjustment in hepatic impairment:

Mild hepatic impairment: There is no data available for use in mild hepatic impairment; exposure may be increased.

Moderate-to-severe hepatic impairment: Use not recommended

Dietary Considerations Avoid grapefruit and grapefruit juice.

Administration Swallow tablet whole. Do not split, crush, or chew tablets. May be administered with or without food. Hazardous agent; use appropriate precautions for handling and disposal (NIOSH 2014 [group 3]).

Monitoring Parameters Monitor for significant peripheral edema and evaluate etiology if it occurs; liver enzyme testing when clinically appropriate

A woman of childbearing potential must have a negative pregnancy test prior to the initiation of therapy, monthly during treatment, and 1 month after stopping treatment. Hemoglobin and hematocrit should be measured at baseline, at 1 month, and periodically thereafter (generally stabilizes after the first few weeks of treatment).

Dosage Forms

Tablet, Oral:

Letairis: 5 mg, 10 mg

Ambroxol [INT] (am BROKS ol)

International Brand Names !Ambroxol Basics (DE); Abrolen (GR, LB); Aerobroncol (UY); AGT Ray (IN); Altec (IN); Ambrex (BG); Ambril (AR, VE, VN); Ambrobene (AT, CZ, HU); Ambrocol (KR); Ambrol (BR); Ambrolan (EE); Ambrolar (SA); Ambrolex (AU, PH, TH); Ambron (HK); Ambronox (TH); Ambrosan (CZ, PL); Ambrosia (SA); Ambroten (BR); Ambrotos (PY); Amtuss (MY); Amxol (HK, SG, TH); Ao Gu Li (CN); Atus (IT); Axol (MX, MY, SG); Benflux (PT); Berea (ID); Betalitik (ID); Bisolangin (NL); Branzol (AR); Bromax (PT); Broncot (CL); Brontex (EE); Bronxol (MX, PT); Dinobroxol (ES); Epexol (ID); Flavamed (BG, DK, EE, FI, HR, LT, PL, RU, TR); Fluibron (BR, LB, PK); Fluidin (BR); Lapimuc (ID); Lindoxyl (DE); Lintos (IT); Lo Solvan (CN); Lysopadol (IE); Lysopain (CH); Max (HK, SG); Medroxol (SA); Mucibron (BR); Mucoangin (BE, CH, DE, DK, HU, SE); Mucoclear (SG); Mucodrenol (PT); Mucolin (BR); Muconil (MY); Mucopect (KR); Mucoram (QA); Mucosan (AT, ES); Mucosolvan (AE, AR, AT, BG, BH, BR, CL, CN, CO, CY, CZ, DE, EG, GR, HK, HR, IT, KW, LB, MX, MY, PH, PL, PT, PY, QA, RO, RU, SA, SG, SK, TH, TR, UY, VE, VN); Mucosolvin (IN); Mucosolvon (PK); Mucoxolan (BR); Mucum (AE, BH, SA); Munorm (IN); Muxol (FR, LB, VN); Obroxol (HK); Polibroxol (SG); Propect (ID); Rexambro (NL, SE); Riabroxol (AE, SA); Roxol (KR); Shinoxol (SG); Solvolan (BG, SK); Strepsils Chesty Cough Lozenge (SG); Surbronc (BE, FR); Tabcin (AR); Tavinex (AR); Tocalm (CL); Tosse (GR); Vaksan (AR); Viaxol (MX); Xambrex (PH); Xolvax (VE); Zebron (PY)

Index Terms Ambroxol Hydrochloride

Pharmacologic Category Mucolytic Agent

Reported Use Treatment of acute and chronic respiratory tract disorders associated with viscid mucus

Dosage Range

Oral:

- Children 2 to <6 years: 7.5-15 mg 3 times daily
- Children 6-12 years: 15-30 mg 2-3 times daily
- Children >12 years, Adolescents, Adults, and Elderly: 60-120 mg daily in 2-3 divided doses (immediate release) or 75 mg once daily (extended release capsules; adults only)

Inhalation: Solution for nebulization (7.5 mg/mL):

- Children <6 years: 15 mg (2 mL) 1-2 times daily (or 0.6 mg/kg 1-2 times daily)
- Children ≥6 years, Adolescents, Adults, and Elderly: 15-22.5 mg (2-3 mL) 1-2 times daily

Product Availability Product available in various countries; not currently available in the U.S.

Dosage Forms

Capsule Extended Release, Oral, as hydrochloride: 75 mg

Solution for Nebulization, Inhalation/Oral: 7.5 mg/mL

Syrup, Oral, as hydrochloride: 3 mg/mL [contains sorbitol]; 6 mg/mL [contains sorbitol]

Tablet, Oral, as hydrochloride: 30 mg [contains lactose]

- ◆ **Ambroxol Hydrochloride** *see* Ambroxol [INT] *on page 109*
- ◆ **AMD3100** *see* Plerixafor *on page 1665*
- ◆ **Amdinocillin** *see* Pivmecillinam [INT] *on page 1663*
- ◆ **Amerge** *see* Naratriptan *on page 1430*
- ◆ **A-Methapred** *see* MethylPREDNISolone *on page 1340*
- ◆ **Amethia** *see* Ethinyl Estradiol and Levonorgestrel *on page 803*
- ◆ **Amethia Lo** *see* Ethinyl Estradiol and Levonorgestrel *on page 803*
- ◆ **Amethocaine Hydrochloride** *see* Tetracaine (Ophthalmic) *on page 2017*
- ◆ **Amethocaine Hydrochloride** *see* Tetracaine (Systemic) *on page 2017*
- ◆ **Amethocaine Hydrochloride** *see* Tetracaine (Topical) *on page 2017*
- ◆ **Amethopterin** *see* Methotrexate *on page 1322*
- ◆ **Amethyst** *see* Ethinyl Estradiol and Levonorgestrel *on page 803*
- ◆ **Ametop (Can)** *see* Tetracaine (Topical) *on page 2017*
- ◆ **Amfepramone** *see* Diethylpropion *on page 624*
- ◆ **AMG 073** *see* Cinacalcet *on page 439*
- ◆ **AMG-162** *see* Denosumab *on page 589*
- ◆ **AMG 531** *see* RomiPLOStim *on page 1842*
- ◆ **Amicar** *see* Aminocaproic Acid *on page 113*
- ◆ **Amidate** *see* Etomidate *on page 816*

Amifostine (am i FOS teen)

Brand Names: U.S. Ethyol

Brand Names: Canada Ethyol

Index Terms Ethiofos; Gammaphos; WR-2721; YM-08310

Pharmacologic Category Antidote; Chemoprotective Agent

Use Reduce the incidence of moderate-to-severe xerostomia in patients undergoing postoperative radiation treatment for head and neck cancer, where the radiation port includes a substantial portion of the parotid glands; reduce the cumulative renal toxicity associated with repeated administration of cisplatin

Pregnancy Risk Factor C

Pregnancy Considerations Animal studies have demonstrated embryotoxicity. There are no adequate and well-controlled studies in pregnant women.

Breast-Feeding Considerations Due to the potential for adverse reactions in the nursing infant, breast-feeding should be discontinued.

Contraindications Hypersensitivity to aminothiol compounds or any component of the formulation

Warnings/Precautions Patients who are hypotensive or dehydrated should not receive amifostine. Interrupt antihypertensive therapy for 24 hours before treatment; patients who cannot safely stop their antihypertensives 24 hours before, should not receive amifostine. Adequately hydrated prior to treatment and keep in a supine position during infusion. Monitor blood pressure every 5 minutes during the infusion. If hypotension requiring interruption of therapy occurs, patients should be placed in the Trendelenburg position and given an infusion of normal saline using a separate IV line; subsequent infusions may require a dose reduction. Infusions >15 minutes are associated with a higher incidence of adverse effects. Use caution in patients with cardiovascular and cerebrovascular disease and any other patients in whom the adverse effects of hypotension may have serious adverse events.

Serious cutaneous reactions, including erythema multiforme, Stevens-Johnson syndrome, toxic epidermal necrolysis, toxoderma and exfoliative dermatitis have been reported with amifostine. May be delayed, developing up to weeks after treatment initiation. Cutaneous reactions have been reported more frequently when used as a radioprotectant. Discontinue treatment for severe/serious cutaneous reaction, or with fever. Withhold treatment and obtain dermatologic consultation for rash involving lips or mucosa (of unknown etiology outside of radiation port) and for bullous, edematous or erythematous lesions on hands, feet, or trunk; reinitiate only after careful evaluation.

Amifostine doses >300 mg/m^2 are associated with a moderate emetic potential (Dupuis, 2011). It is recommended that antiemetic medication, including dexamethasone ▶

20 mg IV and a serotonin 5-HT_3 receptor antagonist be administered prior to and in conjunction with amifostine. Rare hypersensitivity reactions, including anaphylaxis and allergic reaction, have been reported; discontinue if allergic reaction occurs; do not rechallenge. Medications for the treatment of hypersensitivity reactions should be available.

Reports of clinically-relevant hypocalcemia are rare, but serum calcium levels should be monitored in patients at risk of hypocalcemia, such as those with nephrotic syndrome; may require calcium supplementation. Should not be used (in patients receiving chemotherapy for malignancies other than ovarian cancer) where chemotherapy is expected to provide significant survival benefit or in patients receiving definitive radiotherapy, unless within the context of a clinical trial.

Adverse Reactions

Cardiovascular: Hypotension

Endocrine & metabolic: Hypocalcemia

Gastrointestinal: Nausea/vomiting

Rare but important or life-threatening: Apnea, anaphylactoid reactions, anaphylaxis, arrhythmia, atrial fibrillation, atrial flutter, back pain, bradycardia, cardiac arrest, chest pain, chest tightness, chills, cutaneous eruptions, dizziness, erythema multiforme, exfoliative dermatitis, extrasystoles, dyspnea, fever, flushing, hiccups, hypersensitivity reactions (fever, rash, hypoxia, dyspnea, laryngeal edema), hypertension (transient), hypoxia, malaise, MI, myocardial ischemia, pruritus, rash (mild), renal failure, respiratory arrest, rigors, seizure, sneezing, somnolence, Stevens-Johnson syndrome, supraventricular tachycardia, syncope, tachycardia, toxic epidermal necrolysis, toxoderma, urticaria

Drug Interactions

Metabolism/Transport Effects None known.

Avoid Concomitant Use There are no known interactions where it is recommended to avoid concomitant use.

Increased Effect/Toxicity

The levels/effects of Amifostine may be increased by: Antihypertensives

Decreased Effect There are no known significant interactions involving a decrease in effect.

Preparation for Administration For IV infusion, reconstitute intact vials with 9.7 mL 0.9% sodium chloride injection and dilute in 0.9% sodium chloride to a final concentration of 5-40 mg/mL. For SubQ administration, reconstitute with 2.5 mL NS or SWFI.

Storage/Stability Store intact vials of lyophilized powder at room temperature of 20°C to 25°C (68°F to 77°F). Reconstituted solutions (500 mg/10 mL) and solutions for infusion are chemically stable for up to 5 hours at room temperature (25°C) or up to 24 hours under refrigeration (2°C to 8°C).

Mechanism of Action Prodrug that is dephosphorylated by alkaline phosphatase in tissues to a pharmacologically-active free thiol metabolite. The free thiol is available to bind to, and detoxify, reactive metabolites of cisplatin; and can also act as a scavenger of free radicals that may be generated (by cisplatin or radiation therapy) in tissues.

Pharmacodynamics/Kinetics

Distribution: V_d: 3.5 L

Metabolism: Hepatic dephosphorylation to two metabolites (active-free thiol and disulfide)

Half-life elimination: ~8 to 9 minutes

Excretion: Urine

Clearance, plasma: 2.17 L/minute

Dosage Note: Amifostine doses >300 mg/m^2 are associated with a moderate emetic potential (Dupuis, 2011). Antiemetic medication, including dexamethasone 20 mg IV and a serotonin 5-HT_3 receptor antagonist, is recommended prior to and in conjunction with amifostine.

Adults:

Cisplatin-induced renal toxicity, reduction: IV: 910 mg/m^2 over 15 minutes once daily 30 minutes prior to cisplatin

For 910 mg/m^2 doses, the manufacturer suggests the following blood pressure-based adjustment schedule:

The infusion of amifostine should be interrupted if the systolic blood pressure decreases significantly from baseline, as defined below:

Decrease of 20 mm Hg if baseline systolic blood pressure <100

Decrease of 25 mm Hg if baseline systolic blood pressure 100-119

Decrease of 30 mm Hg if baseline systolic blood pressure 120-139

Decrease of 40 mm Hg if baseline systolic blood pressure 140-179

Decrease of 50 mm Hg if baseline systolic blood pressure ≥180

If blood pressure returns to normal within 5 minutes (assisted by fluid administration and postural management) and the patient is asymptomatic, the infusion may be restarted so that the full dose of amifostine may be administered. If the full dose of amifostine cannot be administered, the dose of amifostine for subsequent cycles should be 740 mg/m^2.

Xerostomia from head and neck cancer, reduction:

IV: 200 mg/m^2 over 3 minutes once daily 15-30 minutes prior to radiation therapy **or**

SubQ (off-label route): 500 mg once daily prior to radiation therapy

Prevention of radiation proctitis in rectal cancer (off-label use): IV: 340 mg/m^2 once daily prior to radiation therapy (Keefe, 2007; Peterson, 2008)

Dosage adjustment in renal impairment: There are no dosage adjustments provided in the manufacturer's labeling.

Dosage adjustment in hepatic impairment: There are no dosage adjustments provided in the manufacturer's labeling.

Administration Amifostine doses >300 mg/m^2 are associated with a moderate emetic potential; antiemetics are recommended to prevent nausea/vomiting (Dupuis, 2011)

IV: Administer over 3 minutes (prior to radiation therapy) or 15 minutes (prior to cisplatin); administration as a longer infusion is associated with a higher incidence of side effects. Patients should be kept in supine position during infusion. **Note:** SubQ administration (off-label) has been used.

Monitoring Parameters Blood pressure should be monitored every 5 minutes during the infusion and after administration if clinically indicated; serum calcium levels (in patients at risk for hypocalcemia). Evaluate for cutaneous reactions prior to each dose.

Additional Information Oncology Comment: The American Society of Clinical Oncology (ASCO) guidelines for the use of protectants for chemotherapy and radiation (Hensley, 2008) recommend the use of amifostine for prevention of nephrotoxicity due to cisplatin-based chemotherapy and to decrease the incidence of acute and delayed radiation therapy-induced xerostomia. The ASCO guidelines do not recommend the use of amifostine to reduce the incidence of neutropenia or thrombocytopenia associated with chemotherapy or radiation therapy, neurotoxicity or ototoxicity associated with platinum-based chemotherapy, radiation therapy-induced mucositis associated with head and neck cancer, or esophagitis due to chemotherapy in patients with non-small cell lung cancer. Additionally, the guidelines do not support the use of amifostine in patients with head and neck cancer receiving concurrent platinum-based chemotherapy.

Dosage Forms

Solution Reconstituted, Intravenous:

Ethyol: 500 mg (1 ea)

Generic: 500 mg (1 ea)

Solution Reconstituted, Intravenous [preservative free]:

Generic: 500 mg (1 ea)

Amikacin (am i KAY sin)

Brand Names: Canada Amikacin Sulfate Injection, USP; Amikin

Index Terms Amikacin Sulfate

Pharmacologic Category Antibiotic, Aminoglycoside

Use Treatment of serious infections (bone infections, respiratory tract infections, endocarditis, and septicemia) due to organisms resistant to gentamicin and tobramycin, including *Pseudomonas*, *Proteus*, *Serratia*, and other gram-negative bacilli; documented infection of mycobacterial organisms susceptible to amikacin

Pregnancy Risk Factor D

Pregnancy Considerations Adverse events were not observed in the initial animal reproduction studies; however, renal toxicity has been reported in additional studies. Amikacin crosses the placenta, produces detectable serum levels in the fetus, and concentrates in the fetal kidneys. Because of several reports of total irreversible bilateral congenital deafness in children whose mothers received another aminoglycoside (streptomycin) during pregnancy, the manufacturer classifies amikacin as pregnancy risk factor D. Although serious side effects to the fetus have not been reported following maternal use of amikacin, a potential for harm exists.

Due to pregnancy-induced physiologic changes, some pharmacokinetic parameters of amikacin may be altered. Pregnant women have an average-to-larger volume of distribution which may result in lower peak serum levels than for the same dose in nonpregnant women. Serum half-life may also be shorter.

Breast-Feeding Considerations Amikacin is excreted into breast milk in trace amounts; however, it is not absorbed when taken orally. This limited oral absorption may minimize exposure to the nursing infant. Nondose-related effects could include modification of bowel flora. Breast-feeding is not recommended by the manufacturer.

Contraindications Hypersensitivity to amikacin sulfate or any component of the formulation; cross-sensitivity may exist with other aminoglycosides

Warnings/Precautions [U.S. Boxed Warning]: Amikacin may cause neurotoxicity, nephrotoxicity, and/or neuromuscular blockade and respiratory paralysis; usual risk factors include preexisting renal impairment, concomitant neuro-/nephrotoxic medications, advanced age and dehydration. Dose and/or frequency of administration must be monitored and modified in patients with renal impairment. Drug should be discontinued if signs of ototoxicity, nephrotoxicity, or hypersensitivity occur. Ototoxicity is proportional to the amount of drug given and the duration of treatment. Tinnitus or vertigo may be indications of vestibular injury and impending bilateral irreversible damage. Renal damage is usually reversible. Use with caution in patients with neuromuscular disorders, hearing loss and hypocalcemia. Prolonged use may result in fungal or bacterial superinfection, including *C. difficile*-associated diarrhea (CDAD) and pseudomembranous colitis; CDAD has been observed >2 months postantibiotic treatment. Solution contains sodium metabisulfate; use caution in patients with sulfite allergy.

Adverse Reactions

Central nervous system: Neurotoxicity

Genitourinary: Nephrotoxicity

Otic: Auditory ototoxicity, vestibular ototoxicity

Rare but important or life-threatening: Dyspnea, eosinophilia, hypersensitivity reaction

Drug Interactions

Metabolism/Transport Effects None known.

Avoid Concomitant Use

Avoid concomitant use of Amikacin with any of the following: BCG; Foscarnet; Mannitol

Increased Effect/Toxicity

Amikacin may increase the levels/effects of: AbobotulinumtoxinA; Bisphosphonate Derivatives; CARBOplatin; Colistimethate; CycloSPORINE (Systemic); Neuromuscular-Blocking Agents; OnabotulinumtoxinA; RimabotulinumtoxinB; Tenofovir

The levels/effects of Amikacin may be increased by: Amphotericin B; Capreomycin; Cephalosporins (2nd Generation); Cephalosporins (3rd Generation); Cephalosporins (4th Generation); CISplatin; Foscarnet; Loop Diuretics; Mannitol; Nonsteroidal Anti-Inflammatory Agents; Tenofovir; Vancomycin

Decreased Effect

Amikacin may decrease the levels/effects of: BCG; Sodium Picosulfate; Typhoid Vaccine

The levels/effects of Amikacin may be decreased by: Penicillins

Preparation for Administration

Dilute in a compatible solution (eg, NS, D_5W) to a final concentration of 0.25-5 mg/mL.

Storage/Stability Store intact vials at 20°C to 25°C (68°F to 77°F). Following admixture at concentrations of 0.25-5 mg/mL, amikacin is stable for 24 hours at room temperature, 60 days at 4°C (39°F), or 30 days at -15°C (5°F). Previously refrigerated or thawed frozen solutions are stable for 24 hours when stored at 25°C (77°F).

Mechanism of Action Inhibits protein synthesis in susceptible bacteria by binding to 30S ribosomal subunits

Pharmacodynamics/Kinetics

Absorption:

IM: Rapid

Oral: Poorly absorbed

Distribution: V_d: 0.25 L/kg; primarily into extracellular fluid (highly hydrophilic); penetrates blood-brain barrier when meninges inflamed

Relative diffusion of antimicrobial agents from blood into CSF: Good only with inflammation (exceeds usual MICs)

CSF:blood level ratio: Normal meninges: 10% to 20%; Inflamed meninges: 15% to 24%

Protein-binding: 0% to 11%

Half-life elimination (renal function and age dependent):

Infants: Low birth weight (1-3 days): 7-9 hours; Full-term >7 days: 4-5 hours

Children: 1.6-2.5 hours

Adults: Normal renal function: 1.4-2.3 hours; Anuria/end-stage renal disease: 28-86 hours

Time to peak, serum: IM: 45-120 minutes

Excretion: Urine (94% to 98%)

Dosage Note: Individualization is critical because of the low therapeutic index

In underweight and nonobese patients, use of total body weight (TBW) instead of ideal body weight for determining the initial mg/kg/dose is widely accepted (Nicolau, 1995). Ideal body weight (IBW) also may be used to determine doses for patients who are neither underweight nor obese (Gilbert, 2009).

Initial and periodic peak and trough plasma drug levels should be determined, particularly in critically-ill patients with serious infections or in disease states known to significantly alter aminoglycoside pharmacokinetics (eg, cystic fibrosis, burns, or major surgery). Manufacturer recommends a maximum daily dose of 15 mg/kg/day (or 1.5 g/day in heavier patients). Higher doses may be warranted based on therapeutic drug monitoring or susceptibility information.

Usual dosage range:

Infants and Children: IM, IV: 5-7.5 mg/kg/dose every 8 hours

Adults:

IM, IV: 5-7.5 mg/kg/dose every 8 hours; **Note:** Some clinicians suggest a daily dose of 15-20 mg/kg for all patients with normal renal function. This dose is at least as efficacious with similar, if not less, toxicity than conventional dosing.

Intrathecal/intraventricular (off-label route): Meningitis (susceptible gram-negative organisms): 5-50 mg/day

Indication-specific dosing:

Adults:

Endophthalmitis, bacterial (off-label use): Intravitreal: 0.4 mg/0.1 mL NS in combination with vancomycin

Hospital-acquired pneumonia (HAP): IV: 20 mg/kg/day with antipseudomonal beta-lactam or carbapenem (American Thoracic Society/ATS guidelines)

Meningitis (susceptible gram-negative organisms):

IV: 5 mg/kg every 8 hours (administered with another bactericidal drug)

Intrathecal/intraventricular (off-label route): Usual dose: 30 mg/day (IDSA, 2004); Range: 5-50 mg/day (with concurrent systemic antimicrobial therapy) (Gilbert, 1986; Guardado, 2008; IDSA, 2004; Kasiakou, 2005)

***Mycobacterium avium* complex (MAC) (off-label use):** IV: Adjunct therapy (with macrolide, rifamycin, and ethambutol): 8-25 mg/kg 2-3 times weekly for first 2-3 months for severe disease (maximum single dose for age >50 years: 500 mg) (Griffith, 2007)

Mycobacterium fortuitum, M. chelonae, or M. abscessus: IV: 10-15 mg/kg daily for at least 2 weeks with high dose cefoxitin

Dosage adjustment in renal impairment: Some patients may require larger or more frequent doses if serum levels document the need (ie, cystic fibrosis or febrile granulocytopenic patients).

CrCl ≥60 mL/minute: Administer every 8 hours

CrCl 40-60 mL/minute: Administer every 12 hours

CrCl 20-40 mL/minute: Administer every 24 hours

CrCl <20 mL/minute: Loading dose, then monitor levels

Intermittent hemodialysis (IHD) (administer after hemodialysis on dialysis days): Dialyzable (20%; variable; dependent on filter, duration, and type of HD): 5-7.5 mg/kg every 48-72 hours. Follow levels. Redose when pre-HD concentration <10 mg/L; redose when post-HD concentration <6-8 mg/L (Heintz, 2009). **Note:** Dosing dependent on the assumption of 3 times/week, complete IHD sessions.

Peritoneal dialysis (PD): Dose as CrCl <20 mL/minute: Follow levels

Continuous renal replacement therapy (CRRT) (Heintz, 2009; Trotman, 2005): Drug clearance is highly dependent on the method of renal replacement, filter type, and flow rate. Appropriate dosing requires close monitoring of pharmacologic response, signs of adverse reactions due to drug accumulation, as well as drug concentrations in relation to target trough (if appropriate). The following are general recommendations only (based on dialysate flow/ultrafiltration rates of 1-2 L/hour and minimal residual renal function) and should not supersede clinical judgment:

CVVH/CVVHD/CVVHDF: Loading dose of 10 mg/kg followed by maintenance dose of 7.5 mg/kg every 24-48 hours

Note: For severe gram-negative rod infections, target peak concentration of 15-30 mg/L; redose when concentration <10 mg/L (Heintz, 2009).

Dosage adjustment in hepatic impairment: No dosage adjustment provided in manufacturer's labeling.

Dosing in obesity: In moderate obesity (TBW/IBW ≥1.25) or greater, (eg, morbid obesity [TBW/IBW >2]), initial dosage requirement may be estimated using a dosing weight of IBW + 0.4 (TBW - IBW) (Traynor, 1995).

Dietary Considerations Some products may contain sodium.

Administration

IM: Administer IM injection in large muscle mass.

IV: Infuse over 30-60 minutes (children and adults) or over 1-2 hours (infants).

Some penicillins (eg, carbenicillin, ticarcillin, and piperacillin) have been shown to inactivate *in vitro*. This has been observed to a greater extent with tobramycin and gentamicin, while amikacin has shown greater stability against inactivation. Concurrent use of these agents may pose a risk of reduced antibacterial efficacy *in vivo*, particularly in the setting of profound renal impairment. However, definitive clinical evidence is lacking. If combination penicillin/aminoglycoside therapy is desired in a patient with renal dysfunction, separation of doses (if feasible), and routine monitoring of aminoglycoside levels, CBC, and clinical response should be considered.

Intrathecal/Intraventricular (off-label route): Reserved solely for meningitis due to susceptible gram-negative organisms.

Monitoring Parameters Urinalysis, BUN, serum creatinine, appropriately timed peak and trough concentrations, vital signs, temperature, weight, I & O, hearing parameters

Initial and periodic peak and trough plasma drug levels should be determined, particularly in critically-ill patients with serious infections or in disease states known to significantly alter aminoglycoside pharmacokinetics (eg, cystic fibrosis, burns, or major surgery). Aminoglycoside levels measured from blood taken from Silastic® central catheters can sometimes give falsely high readings (draw levels from alternate lumen or peripheral stick, if possible).

Some penicillin derivatives may accelerate the degradation of aminoglycosides *in vitro*. This may be clinically-significant for certain penicillin (ticarcillin, piperacillin, carbenicillin) and aminoglycoside (gentamicin, tobramycin) combination therapy in patients with significant renal impairment. Close monitoring of aminoglycoside levels is warranted.

Reference Range

Therapeutic levels:

Peak:

Life-threatening infections: 25-40 mcg/mL

Serious infections: 20-25 mcg/mL

Urinary tract infections: 15-20 mcg/mL

Trough: <8 mcg/mL

The American Thoracic Society (ATS) recommends trough levels of <4-5 mcg/mL for patients with hospital-acquired pneumonia.

Toxic concentration: Peak: >40 mcg/mL; Trough: >10 mcg/mL

Timing of serum samples: Draw peak 30 minutes after completion of 30-minute infusion or at 1 hour following initiation of infusion or IM injection; draw trough within 30 minutes prior to next dose

Dosage Forms

Solution, Injection:

Generic: 500 mg/2 mL (2 mL); 1 g/4 mL (4 mL)

Solution, Injection [preservative free]:

Generic: 1 g/4 mL (4 mL)

◆ **Amikacin Sulfate** *see* Amikacin *on page 111*

◆ **Amikacin Sulfate Injection, USP (Can)** *see* Amikacin *on page 111*

◆ **Amikin (Can)** *see* Amikacin *on page 111*

AMILoride (a MIL oh ride)

Brand Names: Canada Apo-Amiloride®; Midamor

Index Terms Amiloride Hydrochloride

Pharmacologic Category Antihypertensive; Diuretic, Potassium-Sparing

Use

Counteracts potassium loss induced by other diuretics in the treatment of hypertension or heart failure; usually used in conjunction with more potent diuretics such as thiazides or loop diuretics

According to the Eighth Joint National Committee (JNC 8) guidelines, potassium-sparing diuretics are not recommended for the initial treatment of hypertension (James, 2013). The American Society of Hypertension/International Society of Hypertension (ASH/ISH) suggests that amiloride in combination with other diuretics (eg, hydrochlorothiazide) may be used to prevent hypokalemia associated with diuretics used to manage hypertension (Weber, 2014).

Pregnancy Risk Factor B

Dosage Oral:

Children 1 to 17 years: Hypertension (off-label use): 0.4 to 0.625 mg/kg/day (maximum: 20 mg daily)

Adults: Hypertension, edema (to limit potassium loss): Initial: 5 mg once daily; may increase to 10 mg daily if necessary; doses >10 mg daily are usually not necessary; however, if patient is persistently hypokalemic, the dose may be increased in increments of 5 mg daily up to 20 mg daily with careful monitoring of electrolytes.

Elderly: Initial: 5 mg once daily or every other day

Dosage adjustment in renal impairment:

Manufacturer's recommendations: Use of amiloride in patients with diabetes mellitus or S_{cr} >1.5 mg/dL should be done with caution and is contraindicated in patients with anuria, acute or chronic renal insufficiency, or evidence of diabetic nephropathy.

Alternate recommendations (Aronoff, 2007):

CrCl 10-50 mL/minute: Administer at 50% of normal dose.

CrCl <10 mL/minute: Avoid use.

Dosage adjustment in hepatic impairment: There are no dosage adjustments provided in the manufacturer's labeling; use with caution.

Additional Information Complete prescribing information should be consulted for additional detail.

Dosage Forms

Tablet, Oral:

Generic: 5 mg

◆ **Amiloride Hydrochloride** *see* AMILoride *on page 113*

◆ **2-Amino-6-Mercaptopurine** *see* Thioguanine *on page 2029*

◆ **2-Amino-6-Methoxypurine Arabinoside** *see* Nelarabine *on page 1435*

◆ **2-Amino-6-Trifluoromethoxy-benzothiazole** *see* Riluzole *on page 1812*

◆ **Aminobenzylpenicillin** *see* Ampicillin *on page 141*

Aminocaproic Acid (a mee noe ka PROE ik AS id)

Brand Names: U.S. Amicar

Index Terms EACA; Epsilon Aminocaproic Acid

Pharmacologic Category Antifibrinolytic Agent; Antihemophilic Agent; Hemostatic Agent; Lysine Analog

Use To enhance hemostasis when fibrinolysis contributes to bleeding (causes may include cardiac surgery, hematologic disorders, neoplastic disorders, abruptio placentae, hepatic cirrhosis, and urinary fibrinolysis)

Pregnancy Risk Factor C

Dosage

Acute bleeding: Adults: Oral, IV: Loading dose: 4-5 g during the first hour, followed by 1 g/hour (or 1.25 g/hour using oral solution) for 8 hours or until bleeding controlled (maximum daily dose: 30 g)

Control of bleeding with severe thrombocytopenia (off-label use) (Bartholomew, 1989; Gardner, 1980): Adults:

Initial: IV: 100 mg/kg (maximum dose: 5 g) over 30-60 minutes

Maintenance: Oral, IV: 1-4 g every 4-8 hours or 1 g/hour (maximum daily dose: 24 g)

Control of oral bleeding in congenital and acquired coagulation disorder (off-label use): Adults: Oral: 50-60 mg/kg every 4 hours (Mannucci, 1998)

Prevention of dental procedure bleeding in patients on oral anticoagulant therapy (off-label use): Adults: Oral rinse: Hold 4 g/10 mL in mouth for 2 minutes then spit out. Repeat every 6 hours for 2 days after procedure (Souto, 1996). Concentration and frequency may vary by institution and product availability.

Prevention of perioperative bleeding associated with cardiac surgery (off-label use): IV:

Children: 100 mg/kg given over 20-30 minutes after induction and prior to incision, 100 mg/kg during cardiopulmonary bypass, and 100 mg/kg after heparin reversal over 3 hours (Chauhan, 2004)

Adults: Loading dose of 75-150 mg/kg (typically 5-10 g), followed by 10-15 mg/kg/hour (typically 1 g/hour); may add 2-2.5 g/L of cardiopulmonary bypass circuit priming solution (Gravlee, 2008)

or

Loading dose of 10 g followed by 2 g/hour during surgery; no medication added to the bypass circuit (Fergusson, 2008)

or

10 g over 20-30 minutes prior to skin incision, followed by 10 g after heparin administration then 10 g at discontinuation of cardiopulmonary bypass (Vander Salm, 1996)

Prevention of bleeding associated with extracorporeal membrane oxygenation (ECMO) (off-label use): Children: IV: 100 mg/kg prior to or immediately after cannulation, followed by 25-30 mg/kg/hour for up to 72 hours (Downard, 2003; Horwitz, 1998; Wilson, 1993)

Prevention of perioperative bleeding associated with spinal surgery (eg, idiopathic scoliosis) (off-label use): Children and Adolescents: IV: 100 mg/kg given over 15-20 minutes after induction, followed by 10 mg/kg/hour for the remainder of the surgery; discontinue at time of wound closure (Florentino-Pineda, 2001; Florentino-Pineda, 2004)

Traumatic hyphema (off-label use): Children and Adults: Oral: 50 mg/kg/dose every 4 hours (maximum daily dose: 30 g) for 5 days (Brandt, 2001; Crouch, 1999)

Dosage adjustment in renal impairment: May accumulate in patients with decreased renal function. When used during cardiopulmonary bypass in anephric patients, a normal or slightly reduced loading dose and a continuous infusion rate of 5 mg/kg/hour has been recommended (Gravlee, 2008).

Dosage adjustment in hepatic impairment: No dosage adjustment provided in manufacturer's labeling.

Additional Information Complete prescribing information should be consulted for additional detail.

Dosage Forms

Solution, Intravenous:
Generic: 250 mg/mL (20 mL)

Syrup, Oral:
Amicar: 25% (473 mL)
Generic: 25% (237 mL, 473 mL)

Tablet, Oral:
Amicar: 500 mg, 1000 mg
Generic: 500 mg, 1000 mg

Aminolevulinic Acid (a MEE noh lev yoo lin ik AS id)

Brand Names: U.S. Levulan Kerastick

Brand Names: Canada Levulan Kerastick

Index Terms 5-ALA; 5-Aminolevulinic Acid; ALA; Amino Levulinic Acid; Aminolevulinic Acid HCl; Aminolevulinic Acid Hydrochloride

Pharmacologic Category Photosensitizing Agent, Topical; Topical Skin Product

Use Actinic keratoses: Treatment of minimally to moderately thick actinic keratoses of the face or scalp; to be used in conjunction with blue light illumination

Pregnancy Risk Factor C

Dosage Note: Should only be applied by qualified medical personnel (not intended for application by patients).

Actinic keratoses: Topical: Apply to actinic keratoses (**not** perilesional skin) followed 14 to 18 hours later by blue light illumination. Application/treatment may be repeated at a treatment site (once) after 8 weeks.

Dosage adjustment for renal impairment: There are no dosage adjustments provided in the manufacturer's labeling.

Dosage adjustment for hepatic impairment: There are no dosage adjustments provided in the manufacturer's labeling.

Additional Information Complete prescribing information should be consulted for additional detail.

Dosage Forms

Solution Reconstituted, External:
Levulan Kerastick: 20% (1 ea)

◆ **Amino Levulinic Acid** *see* Aminolevulinic Acid *on page 114*

◆ **5-Aminolevulinic Acid** *see* Aminolevulinic Acid *on page 114*

◆ **Aminolevulinic Acid HCl** *see* Aminolevulinic Acid *on page 114*

◆ **Aminolevulinic Acid Hydrochloride** *see* Aminolevulinic Acid *on page 114*

◆ **4-aminopyridine** *see* Dalfampridine *on page 552*

◆ **5-Aminosalicylic Acid** *see* Mesalamine *on page 1301*

Amiodarone (a MEE oh da rone)

Brand Names: U.S. Cordarone; Nexterone; Pacerone

Brand Names: Canada Amiodarone Hydrochloride For Injection; Apo-Amiodarone; Cordarone; Dom-Amiodarone; Mylan-Amiodarone; PHL-Amiodarone; PMS-Amiodarone; PRO-Amiodarone; Riva-Amiodarone; Sandoz-Amiodarone; Teva-Amiodarone

Index Terms Amiodarone Hydrochloride

Pharmacologic Category Antiarrhythmic Agent, Class III

Additional Appendix Information

Beers Criteria – Potentially Inappropriate Medications for Geriatrics *on page 2271*

Use Management of life-threatening recurrent ventricular fibrillation (VF) or recurrent hemodynamically-unstable ventricular tachycardia (VT) refractory to other antiarrhythmic agents or in patients intolerant of other agents used for these conditions

Pregnancy Risk Factor D

Pregnancy Considerations Adverse events have been observed in some animal reproduction studies. Amiodarone crosses the placenta (~10% to 50%) and may cause fetal harm when administered to a pregnant woman, leading to congenital goiter and hypo- or hyperthyroidism. Growth retardation and premature birth have also been noted (ESG, 2011). Amiodarone should be used in pregnant women only to treat arrhythmias that are life-threatening or refractory to other treatments (Blomström-Lundqvist, 2003; ESG, 2011).

Breast-Feeding Considerations Amiodarone and its active metabolite are excreted into human milk. Breast-feeding may lead to significant infant exposure and potential toxicity. Due to the long half-life, amiodarone may be present in breast milk for several days following discontinuation of maternal therapy (Hall, 2003). The manufacturer recommends that breast-feeding be discontinued if treatment is needed.

Contraindications Hypersensitivity to amiodarone, iodine, or any component of the formulation; severe sinus-node dysfunction causing marked sinus bradycardia; second- and third-degree heart block (except in patients with a functioning artificial pacemaker); bradycardia causing syncope (except in patients with a functioning artificial pacemaker); cardiogenic shock

Warnings/Precautions Note: Although the U.S. Boxed Warnings pertain to the tablet prescribing information, these effects may also be seen with intravenous administration depending on duration of use.

[U.S. Boxed Warning (tablet)]: Only indicated for patients with life-threatening arrhythmias because of risk of substantial toxicity. Alternative therapies should be tried first before using amiodarone. Patients should be hospitalized when amiodarone is initiated. The 2010 ACLS guidelines recommend IV amiodarone as the preferred antiarrhythmic for the treatment of pulseless VT/VF, both life-threatening arrhythmias. In patients with non-life-threatening arrhythmias (eg, atrial fibrillation), amiodarone should be used only if the use of other antiarrhythmics has proven ineffective or are contraindicated.

[U.S. Boxed Warning (tablet)]: Pulmonary toxicity (hypersensitivity pneumonitis or interstitial/alveolar pneumonitis and abnormal diffusion capacity without symptoms) may occur. Reports of acute-onset pulmonary injury (pulmonary infiltrates and/or mass on X-ray, pulmonary alveolar hemorrhage, pleural effusion, bronchospasm, wheezing, fever, dyspnea, cough, hemoptysis, hypoxia) have occurred; some cases have progressed to respiratory failure and/or death. Fatalities due to pulmonary toxicity occur in ~10% of cases; most fatalities due to sudden cardiac death occurred when amiodarone was discontinued; rule out other causes of respiratory impairment before discontinuing amiodarone in patients with life-threatening arrhythmias; use extreme caution if dose is decreased or discontinued. If hypersensitivity pneumonitis occurs, discontinue amiodarone and institute steroid therapy; if interstitial/alveolar pneumonitis occurs, institute steroid therapy and reduce amiodarone dose or preferably, discontinue. Some cases of interstitial/alveolar pneumonitis may resolve following dosage reduction and steroid therapy; rechallenge at a lower dose has not resulted in return of interstitial/alveolar pneumonitis in some patients; however, in some patients the pulmonary lesions have not been reversible. Educate patients about monitoring for symptoms (eg, nonproductive cough, dyspnea, pleuritic pain, hemoptysis, wheezing, weight loss, fever, malaise). Evaluate new respiratory symptoms; preexisting pulmonary disease does not increase risk of developing pulmonary toxicity, but if pulmonary toxicity develops then the prognosis is worse. Use of lower doses may be associated with a decreased incidence, but pulmonary toxicity has been reported in patients treated with low doses. The lowest effective dose should be used as appropriate for the acuity/severity of the arrhythmia being treated. **[U.S. Boxed Warning (tablet)]: Liver toxicity is common, but usually mild with evidence of only increased liver enzymes; severe liver toxicity can occur and has been fatal in a few cases.** Hepatic enzyme levels are frequently elevated in patients exposed to amiodarone; most cases are asymptomatic. If increases >3x ULN (or ≥2x baseline in patients with preexisting elevations), consider dose reduction or discontinuation. Monitor hepatic enzymes regularly in patients on relatively high maintenance doses.

[U.S. Boxed Warning (tablet)]: Amiodarone can exacerbate arrhythmias, by making them more difficult to tolerate or reverse; other types of arrhythmias have occurred, including significant heart block, sinus bradycardia, new ventricular fibrillation, incessant ventricular tachycardia, increased resistance to cardioversion, and polymorphic ventricular tachycardia associated with QTc prolongation (torsades de pointes [TdP]). Risk may be increased with concomitant use of other antiarrhythmic agents or drugs that prolong the QTc interval. Proarrhythmic effects may be prolonged. Amiodarone should not be used in patients with Wolff-Parkinson-White (WPW) syndrome and preexcited atrial fibrillation/flutter since ventricular fibrillation may result (AHA/ACC/HRS [January, 2014]).

Monitor pacing or defibrillation thresholds in patients with implantable cardiac devices (eg, pacemakers, defibrillators). May cause hyper- or hypothyroidism; hyperthyroidism may result in thyrotoxicosis (including fatalities) and/or the possibility of arrhythmia breakthrough or aggravation. If any new signs of arrhythmia appear, consider the possibility of hyperthyroidism. Hypothyroidism (sometimes severe) may be primary or subsequent to resolution of preceding amiodarone-induced hyperthyroidism; myxedema (may be fatal) has been reported. If hyper- or hypothyroidism occurs, reduce dose or discontinue amiodarone. Thyroid nodules and/or thyroid cancer have also been reported. Use caution in patients with thyroid disease; thyroid function should be monitored prior to treatment and periodically thereafter, particularly in the elderly and in patients with underlying thyroid dysfunction. In acute myocardial infarction, beta-blocker therapy should still be initiated even though concomitant amiodarone therapy provides beta-blockade.

Regular ophthalmic examination (including slit lamp and fundoscopy) is recommended. May cause optic neuropathy and/or optic neuritis resulting in visual impairment (peripheral vision loss, changes in acuity) at any time during therapy; permanent blindness has occurred. If symptoms of optic neuropathy and/or optic neuritis occur, prompt ophthalmic evaluation is recommended. If diagnosis of optic neuropathy and/or optic neuritis is confirmed, reevaluate amiodarone therapy. Corneal microdeposits occur in a majority of adults and may cause visual disturbances in up to 10% of patients (blurred vision, halos); asymptomatic microdeposits may be reversible and are not generally considered a reason to discontinue treatment. Corneal refractive laser surgery is generally contraindicated in amiodarone users (from manufacturers of surgical devices).

Peripheral neuropathy has been reported rarely with chronic administration; may resolve when amiodarone is discontinued, but resolution may be slow and incomplete.

Amiodarone is a potent inhibitor of CYP enzymes and transport proteins (including p-glycoprotein), which may lead to increased serum concentrations/toxicity of a number of medications. Particular caution must be used when a drug with QTc-prolonging potential relies on metabolism via these enzymes, since the effect of elevated concentrations may be additive with the effect of amiodarone. Carefully assess risk:benefit of coadministration of other drugs which may prolong QTc interval. Additional potentially significant interactions may exist, requiring dose or frequency adjustment, additional monitoring, and/or selection of alternative therapy. Patients may still be at risk for amiodarone–related drug interactions after the drug has been discontinued. The pharmacokinetics are complex (due to prolonged duration of action and half-life) and difficult to predict. Correct electrolyte disturbances, especially hypokalemia or hypomagnesemia, prior to use and throughout therapy. Use caution when initiating amiodarone in patients on warfarin. Cases of increased INR with or without bleeding have occurred in patients treated with warfarin; monitor INR closely after initiating amiodarone in these patients.

In the treatment of atrial fibrillation in older adults, avoid antiarrhythmics as first-line treatment. In older adults, data suggests rate control may provide more benefits than risks compared to rhythm control for most patients (Beers Criteria).

May cause hypotension and bradycardia (infusion-rate related). May cause life-threatening or fatal cutaneous reactions, including Stevens-Johnson syndrome and toxic epidermal necrolysis (TEN). If symptoms or signs (eg, progressive skin rash often with blisters or mucosal lesions) occur, immediately discontinue. During long-term treatment, a blue-gray discoloration of exposed skin may occur; risk increased in patients with fair complexion or excessive sun exposure; may be related to cumulative dose and duration of therapy. There has been limited experience in patients receiving IV amiodarone for >3 weeks.

Use caution and close perioperative monitoring in surgical patients; may enhance myocardial depressant and conduction effects of halogenated inhalational anesthetics; adult respiratory distress syndrome (ARDS) has been reported postoperatively (fatal in rare cases). Hypotension upon discontinuation of cardiopulmonary bypass during open-heart surgery have been reported (rare); relationship to amiodarone is unknown. Commercially-prepared premixed infusion contains the excipient cyclodextrin (sulfobutyl ether beta-cyclodextrin), which may accumulate in patients with renal insufficiency.

Adverse Reactions In a recent meta-analysis, adult patients taking lower doses of amiodarone (152 to 330 mg daily for at least 12 months) were more likely to develop thyroid, neurologic, skin, ocular, and bradycardic abnormalities than those taking placebo (Vorperian, 1997). Pulmonary toxicity was similar in both the low-dose amiodarone group and in the placebo group, but there was a trend towards increased toxicity in the amiodarone group. Gastrointestinal and hepatic events were seen to a similar extent in both the low-dose amiodarone group and placebo group. As the frequency of adverse events varies considerably across studies as a function of route and dose, a consolidation of adverse event rates is provided by Goldschlager, 2000.

Cardiovascular: Atrioventricular block, bradycardia, cardiac arrhythmia, cardiac conduction disturbance, cardiac failure, CHF, edema, flushing, hypotension (IV, refractory in rare cases), phlebitis (IV, with concentrations >3 mg/mL), sinus node dysfunction. Additional effects associated with IV administration include asystole, atrial fibrillation, atrioventricular dissociation, cardiac arrest, cardiogenic shock, pulseless electrical activity (PEA), torsades de pointes (rare), ventricular fibrillation, and ventricular tachycardia.

Central nervous system: Abnormal gait, altered sense of smell, ataxia, dizziness, fatigue, headache, insomnia, involuntary body movements, malaise, memory impairment, peripheral neuropathy, sleep disorder

Dermatologic: Blue-gray skin pigmentation (oral; with prolonged exposure to amiodarone)

Endocrine & metabolic: Decreased libido, hyperthyroidism (more common in iodine-deficient regions of the world), hypothyroidism

Gastrointestinal: Abdominal pain, altered salivation, anorexia, constipation, dysgeusia, diarrhea, nausea (more common in oral), vomiting

Hematologic & oncologic: Blood coagulation disorder

Hepatic: Increased transaminases (more common in oral)

Neuromuscular & skeletal: Tremor

Ophthalmic: Corneal deposits (may cause visual disturbance), optic neuritis, photophobia, visual disturbance, visual halos

Respiratory: Pulmonary toxicity (toxicity may present as hypersensitivity pneumonitis; pulmonary fibrosis (cough, fever, malaise); pulmonary edema (IV), pneumonitis; interstitial pneumonitis; or alveolar pneumonitis).

Rare but important or life-threatening: Acute renal failure, agranulocytosis, alopecia, anaphylactic shock, angioedema, aplastic anemia, brain disease, bronchiolitis obliterans organizing pneumonia, bronchospasm, cholestatic hepatitis, confusion, delirium, demyelinating polyneuropathy, disorientation, DRESS syndrome, drug-induced Parkinson's disease, dyskinesia, dyspnea, eosinophilic pneumonia, epididymitis (noninfectious), erythema multiforme, exfoliative dermatitis, fever, gynecomastia, hallucination, hemolytic anemia, hemoptysis, hepatic cirrhosis, hepatitis, hypotension, hypoxia, impotence, injection site reaction, intracranial hypertension (IV), leukocytoclastic vasculitis, malignant neoplasm of skin, mass (pulmonary), muscle weakness, myopathy, optic neuropathy, pancreatitis, pancytopenia, pleural effusion, pleurisy, pseudotumor cerebri, pulmonary alveolar hemorrhage, pulmonary infiltrates, prolonged Q-T interval on ECG (associated with worsening of arrhythmia), renal insufficiency, respiratory failure, rhabdomyolysis, SIADH, sinoatrial arrest, skin granuloma, skin rash, spontaneous ecchymosis, Stevens-Johnson syndrome, thrombocytopenia, thyroid cancer, thyroid nodule, thyrotoxicosis, toxic epidermal necrolysis, vasculitis, wheezing

Drug Interactions

Metabolism/Transport Effects Substrate of CYP1A2 (minor), CYP2C19 (minor), CYP2C8 (major), CYP2D6 (minor), CYP3A4 (major), P-glycoprotein; **Note:** Assignment of Major/Minor substrate status based on clinically relevant drug interaction potential; **Inhibits** CYP1A2 (weak), CYP2A6 (moderate), CYP2B6 (weak), CYP2C9 (moderate), CYP2D6 (moderate), CYP3A4 (weak), P-glycoprotein

Avoid Concomitant Use

Avoid concomitant use of Amiodarone with any of the following: Agalsidase Alfa; Agalsidase Beta; Antiarrhythmic Agents (Class Ia); Azithromycin (Systemic); Bosutinib; Ceritinib; Conivaptan; Fingolimod; Fusidic Acid (Systemic); Grapefruit Juice; Highest Risk QTc-Prolonging Agents; Idelalisib; Ivabradine; Mifepristone; Moderate Risk QTc-Prolonging Agents; PAZOPanib; Pimozide; Propafenone; Protease Inhibitors; Silodosin; Tegafur; Thioridazine; Topotecan; VinCRIStine (Liposomal)

Increased Effect/Toxicity

Amiodarone may increase the levels/effects of: Afatinib; Antiarrhythmic Agents (Class Ia); Beta-Blockers; Bosentan; Bosutinib; Bradycardia-Causing Agents; Brentuximab Vedotin; Cannabis; Cardiac Glycosides; Carvedilol; Ceritinib; Colchicine; CycloSPORINE (Systemic); CYP2A6 Substrates; CYP2C9 Substrates; CYP2D6 Substrates; Dabigatran Etexilate; DOXOrubicin (Conventional); Dronabinol; Edoxaban; Everolimus; Fesoterodine; Flecainide; Fosphenytoin; Highest Risk QTc-Prolonging Agents; HMG-CoA Reductase Inhibitors; Hydrocodone; Lacosamide; Ledipasvir; Lidocaine (Systemic); Lidocaine (Topical); Lomitapide; Loratadine; Metoprolol; Mipomersen; Naloxegol; Nebivolol; PAZOPanib; P-glycoprotein/ABCB1 Substrates; Phenytoin; Pimozide; Porfimer; Propafenone; Prucalopride; Rifaximin; Rivaroxaban; Silodosin; Tetrahydrocannabinol; Thioridazine; Topotecan; Verteporfin; VinCRIStine (Liposomal); Vitamin K Antagonists

The levels/effects of Amiodarone may be increased by: Aprepitant; Azithromycin (Systemic); Boceprevir; Bretylium; Calcium Channel Blockers (Nondihydropyridine); Cimetidine; Conivaptan; Cyclophosphamide; CYP2C8 Inhibitors (Moderate); CYP2C8 Inhibitors (Strong); CYP3A4 Inhibitors (Moderate); CYP3A4 Inhibitors (Strong); Deferasirox; Fingolimod; Fosaprepitant; Fosphenytoin; Fusidic Acid (Systemic); Grapefruit Juice; Idelalisib; Ivabradine; Ivacaftor; Lidocaine (Topical); Luliconazole; Mifepristone; Moderate Risk QTc-Prolonging Agents; Netupitant; P-glycoprotein/ABCB1 Inhibitors; Protease Inhibitors; QTc-Prolonging Agents (Indeterminate Risk and Risk Modifying); Simeprevir; Stiripentol; Telaprevir; Tofacitinib

Decreased Effect

Amiodarone may decrease the levels/effects of: Agalsidase Alfa; Agalsidase Beta; Clopidogrel; Codeine; Sodium Iodide I131; Tamoxifen; Tegafur; TraMADol

The levels/effects of Amiodarone may be decreased by: Bile Acid Sequestrants; Bosentan; CYP2C8 Inducers (Strong); CYP3A4 Inducers (Moderate); CYP3A4 Inducers (Strong); Dabrafenib; Deferasirox; Etravirine; Fosphenytoin; Grapefruit Juice; Mitotane; Orlistat; P-glycoprotein/ABCB1 Inducers; Phenytoin; Rifampin; Siltuximab; St Johns Wort; Tocilizumab

Food Interactions Food increases the rate and extent of absorption of amiodarone. Grapefruit juice increases bioavailability of oral amiodarone by 50% and decreases the conversion of amiodarone to N-DEA (active metabolite); altered effects are possible. Management: Take consistently with regard to meals; grapefruit juice should be avoided during therapy.

Storage/Stability

Tablets: Store at 20°C to 25°C (68°F to 77°F); protect from light.

Injection: Store undiluted vials and premixed solutions (Nexterone) at 20°C to 25°C (68°F to 77°F); excursions are permitted between 15°C and 30°C (59°F and 86°F). Protect from light during storage; protect from excessive heat. There is no need to protect solutions from light during administration. When vial contents are admixed in D_5W to a final concentration of 1-6 mg/mL, amiodarone is stable for 24 hours in glass or polyolefin bottles and for 2 hours in polyvinyl chloride (PVC) bags; do not use evacuated glass containers as buffer may cause precipitation. Nexterone is available as premixed solutions. Although amiodarone adsorbs to PVC tubing, all clinical studies used PVC tubing and the recommended doses account for adsorption; in adults, PVC tubing is recommended.

Mechanism of Action Class III antiarrhythmic agent which inhibits adrenergic stimulation (alpha- and beta-blocking properties), affects sodium, potassium, and calcium channels, prolongs the action potential and refractory period in myocardial tissue; decreases AV conduction and sinus node function

Pharmacodynamics/Kinetics

Absorption: Slow and variable

Onset of action: Oral: 2 days to 3 weeks; IV: May be more rapid

Peak effect: 1 week to 5 months

Duration after discontinuing therapy: 7 to 50 days

Note: Mean onset of effect and duration after discontinuation may be shorter in children than adults

Distribution: V_d: 66 L/kg (range: 18 to 148 L/kg)

Protein binding: 96%

Metabolism: Hepatic via CYP2C8 and 3A4 to active N-desethylamiodarone metabolite; possible enterohepatic recirculation

Bioavailability: Oral: 35% to 65%

Half-life elimination: Terminal: 40 to 55 days (range: 26 to 107 days); shorter in children

Time to peak, serum: Oral: 3 to 7 hours

Excretion: Feces; urine (<1% as unchanged drug)

Dosage Note: Lower loading and maintenance doses are preferable in women and all patients with low body weight.

Oral: Adults:

Ventricular arrhythmias:

Prevention of recurrent life-threatening ventricular arrhythmias (eg, VF or hemodynamically unstable VT): 800 to 1600 mg daily in 1 to 2 doses for 1 to 3 weeks, then when adequate arrhythmia control is achieved, decrease to 600 to 800 mg daily in 1 to 2 doses for 1 month; maintenance: 400 mg daily.

Supraventricular arrhythmias:

Atrial fibrillation:

Pharmacologic cardioversion (off-label use): 600 to 800 mg daily in divided doses until 10 g total, then 200 mg daily as maintenance (AHA/ACC/HRS [January, 2014]). Although not supported by clinical evidence, a maintenance dose of 100 mg daily is commonly used especially for the elderly or patients with low body mass (Zimetbaum, 2007). **Note:** Other regimens have been described and may be used clinically:

800 mg daily for 14 days, followed by 600 mg daily for the next 14 days, then 300 mg daily for the remainder of the first year, then 200 mg daily thereafter (Singh, 2005)

or

10 mg/kg/day for 14 days, followed by 300 mg daily for 4 weeks, followed by maintenance dosage of 200 mg daily (Roy, 2000)

Maintenance of sinus rhythm (off-label use): 400 to 600 mg daily in divided doses for 2 to 4 weeks followed by a maintenance dose of 100 to 200 mg once daily (AHA/ACC/HRS [January, 2014])

Prevention of postoperative atrial fibrillation and atrial flutter associated with cardiothoracic surgery (off-label use): 200 mg 3 times daily for 7 days prior to surgery, followed by 200 mg daily until hospital discharge (Daoud, 1997). **Note:** A variety of regimens have been used in clinical trials.

Supraventricular tachycardia (eg, AVNRT, AVRT): **Note:** Amiodarone is an effective therapeutic option with a variety of potential uses in the management of supraventricular tachycardia; however, safety risks limit its therapeutic use. In many cases, amiodarone is reserved for use in patients who have failed other therapies or who have structural heart disease, including left ventricular dysfunction. In general, most patients do not require chronic long-term treatment with antiarrhythmic therapy.

Pharmacologic cardioversion (off-label use): 600 to 800 mg daily in divided doses until 10 g total, then may administer 200 mg daily as maintenance (ACC/AHA/ESC [Blomström-Lundqvist, 2003]; AHA/ACC/HRS [January, 2014]).

IV:

Children:

Pulseless VT or VF: IV, I.O.: 5 mg/kg (maximum: 300 mg per dose) rapid bolus; may repeat twice up to a maximum total dose of 15 mg/kg during acute treatment (PALS, 2010).

Perfusing tachycardias: IV, I.O.: Loading dose: 5 mg/kg (maximum: 300 mg per dose) over 20 to 60 minutes; may repeat twice up to maximum total dose of 15 mg/kg during acute treatment (PALS, 2010).

Adults:

Ventricular arrhythmias:

Pulseless VT or VF (ACLS, 2010): IV push, I.O.: Initial: 300 mg rapid bolus; if pulseless VT or VF continues after subsequent defibrillation attempt or recurs, administer supplemental dose of 150 mg. **Note:** In this setting, administering **undiluted** is preferred (Dager, 2006; Skrifvars, 2004). *The Handbook of Emergency Cardiovascular Care* (Hazinski, 2010) and the 2010 ACLS guidelines do not make any specific recommendations regarding dilution of amiodarone in this setting. Experience limited with I.O. administration of amiodarone. Maximum recommended total daily dose is 2.2 g (ACLS, 2010).

Stable VT: First 24 hours: 1050 mg according to following regimen:

Step 1: 150 mg (100 mL) over first 10 minutes (mix 3 mL in 100 mL D_5W)

Step 2: 360 mg (200 mL) over next 6 hours (mix 18 mL in 500 mL D_5W): 1 mg/minute

Step 3: 540 mg (300 mL) over next 18 hours: 0.5 mg/minute

Note: After the first 24 hours: 0.5 mg/minute utilizing concentration of 1 to 6 mg/mL

Breakthrough stable VT: 150 mg supplemental doses in 100 mL D_5W or NS over 10 minutes (mean daily doses >2.1 g/day have been associated with hypotension)

Supraventricular arrhythmias:

Atrial fibrillation:

Pharmacologic cardioversion (off-label use): 150 mg over 10 minutes, then 1 mg/minute for 6 hours, then 0.5 mg/minute for 18 hours or change to oral maintenance dosing (eg, 100 to 200 mg once daily) (AHA/ACC/HRS [January, 2014]).

Prevention of postoperative atrial fibrillation and atrial flutter associated with cardiothoracic surgery (off-label use): **Note:** A variety of regimens have been used in clinical trials.

Preoperative regimen: 150 mg loading dose, followed by 0.4 mg/**kg**/hour (~0.5 mg/minute for a 70 kg patient) for 3 days prior to surgery and for 5 days postoperative (Lee, 2000).

Postoperative regimen: Starting at postop recovery, 1000 mg infused over 24 hours for 2 days (Guarnieri, 1999).

Rate control (off-label use): 300 mg over 1 hour, then 10 to 50 mg/hour over 24 hours followed by an oral maintenance dose; usual maintenance dose: 100 to 200 mg once daily. **Note:** Amiodarone requires a longer time to achieve rate control as compared to nondihydropyridine calcium channel blockers (eg, diltiazem) (7 hours vs 3 hours, respectively) (AHA/ACC/HRS [January, 2014])

Supraventricular tachycardia (eg, AVNRT, AVRT): **Note:** Amiodarone is an effective therapeutic option with a variety of potential uses in the management of supraventricular tachycardia; however, safety risks limit its therapeutic use. In many cases, amiodarone is reserved for use in patients who have failed other therapies or who have structural heart disease, including left ventricular dysfunction. In general, most patients do not require chronic long-term treatment with antiarrhythmic therapy.

Pharmacologic cardioversion (off-label use): 150 mg over 10 minutes, then 1 mg/minute for 6 hours, then 0.5 mg/minute for 18 hours or may change to oral dosing (ACC/AHA/ESC [Blomström-Lundqvist, 2003]; AHA/ACC/HRS [January, 2014]).

Recommendations for conversion to oral amiodarone after IV administration: Use the following as a guide:

<1-week IV infusion: 800 to 1600 mg daily

1- to 3-week IV infusion: 600 to 800 mg daily

>3-week IV infusion: 400 mg daily

Note: Conversion from IV to oral therapy has not been formally evaluated. Some experts recommend a 1 to 2 day overlap when converting from IV to oral therapy especially when treating ventricular arrhythmias.

Recommendations for conversion to IV amiodarone after oral administration: During long-term amiodarone therapy (ie, ≥4 months), the mean plasma-elimination half-life of the active metabolite of amiodarone is 61 days. Replacement therapy may not be necessary in such patients if oral therapy is discontinued for a period <2 weeks, since any changes in serum amiodarone concentrations during this period may **not** be clinically significant.

Elderly: No specific guidelines available. Dose selection should be cautious, at low end of dosage range, and titration should be slower to evaluate response. Although not supported by clinical evidence, a maintenance dose of 100 mg daily is commonly used especially for the elderly or patients with low body mass (Zimetbaum, 2007).

Dosing adjustment in renal impairment: No dosage adjustment necessary

Hemodialysis: Not dialyzable (0% to 5%); supplemental dose is not necessary.

Peritoneal dialysis: Not dialyzable (0% to 5%); supplemental dose is not necessary.

Dosing adjustment in hepatic impairment: Dosage adjustment is probably necessary in substantial hepatic impairment. No specific guidelines available. If hepatic enzymes exceed 3 times normal or double in a patient with an elevated baseline, consider decreasing the dose or discontinuing amiodarone.

Dietary Considerations Take consistently with regard to meals. Amiodarone is a potential source of large amounts of inorganic iodine; ~3 mg of inorganic iodine per 100 mg of amiodarone is released into the systemic circulation. Recommended daily allowance for iodine in adults is 150 mcg.

Grapefruit juice is not recommended.

Usual Infusion Concentrations: Pediatric Note: Premixed solutions available.

IV infusion: 1.8 mg/mL

Usual Infusion Concentrations: Adult Note: Premixed solutions available.

IV infusion: 450 mg in 250 mL (concentration: 1.8 mg/mL) of D_5W or NS

Administration

Oral: Administer consistently with regard to meals. Take in divided doses with meals if GI upset occurs or if taking large daily dose. If GI intolerance occurs with single-dose therapy, use twice daily dosing.

IV: For infusions >1 hour, use concentrations ≤2 mg/mL unless a central venous catheter is used; commercially-prepared premixed solutions in concentrations of 1.5 mg/mL and 1.8 mg/mL are available. Use only volumetric infusion pump; use of drop counting may lead to underdosage. Administer through an IV line located as centrally as possible. For continuous infusions, an in-line filter has been recommended during administration to reduce the incidence of phlebitis. During pulseless VT/VF, administering **undiluted** is preferred (Dager, 2006; Skrifvars, 2004). *The Handbook of Emergency Cardiovascular Care* (Hazinski, 2010) and the 2010 ACLS guidelines do not make any specific recommendations regarding dilution of amiodarone in this setting.

Adjust administration rate to urgency (give more slowly when perfusing arrhythmia present). Slow the infusion rate if hypotension or bradycardia develops. Infusions >2 hours must be administered in a non-PVC container (eg, glass or polyolefin). PVC tubing is recommended for administration regardless of infusion duration. **Incompatible** with heparin; flush with saline prior to and following infusion. **Note:** IV administration at lower flow rates (potentially associated with use in pediatrics) and higher concentrations than recommended may result in leaching of plasticizers (DEHP) from intravenous tubing. DEHP may adversely affect male reproductive tract development. Alternative means of dosing and administration (1 mg/kg aliquots) may need to be considered.

Monitoring Parameters Blood pressure, heart rate (ECG) and rhythm throughout therapy; assess patient for signs of lethargy, edema of the hands or feet, weight loss, and pulmonary toxicity (baseline pulmonary function tests and chest X-ray; continue monitoring chest X-ray annually during therapy); liver function tests (semiannually); monitor serum electrolytes, especially potassium and magnesium. Assess thyroid function tests before initiation of treatment and then periodically thereafter (some experts suggest every 3-6 months). If signs or symptoms of thyroid disease or arrhythmia breakthrough/exacerbation occur then immediate re-evaluation is necessary. Amiodarone partially inhibits the peripheral conversion of thyroxine (T_4) to triiodothyronine (T_3); serum T_4 and reverse triiodothyronine (rT_3) concentrations may be increased and serum T_3 may be decreased; most patients remain clinically euthyroid, however, clinical hypothyroidism or hyperthyroidism may occur.

Perform regular ophthalmic exams.

Patients with implantable cardiac devices: Monitor pacing or defibrillation thresholds with initiation of amiodarone and during treatment.

Consult individual institutional policies and procedures.

Reference Range Therapeutic: 0.5-2.5 mg/L (SI: 1-4 micromole/L) (parent); desethyl metabolite is active and is present in equal concentration to parent drug

Dosage Forms Considerations

Vials for injection contain benzyl alcohol which has been associated with "gasping syndrome" in neonates. Commercially-prepared premixed solutions do not contain benzyl alcohol.

Dosage Forms

Solution, Intravenous:

Nexterone: 150 mg/100 mL (100 mL); 360 mg/200 mL (200 mL)

Generic: 150 mg/3 mL (3 mL); 450 mg/9 mL (9 mL); 900 mg/18 mL (18 mL)

Tablet, Oral:
Cordarone: 200 mg
Pacerone: 100 mg, 200 mg, 400 mg
Generic: 100 mg, 200 mg, 400 mg

Extemporaneous Preparations A 5 mg/mL oral suspension may be made with tablets and either a 1:1 mixture of Ora-Sweet® and Ora-Plus® or a 1:1 mixture of Ora-Sweet® SF and Ora-Plus® adjusted to a pH between 6-7 using a sodium bicarbonate solution (5 g/100 mL of distilled water). Crush five 200 mg tablets in a mortar and reduce to a fine powder. Add small portions of the chosen vehicle and mix to a uniform paste; mix while adding the vehicle in incremental proportions to **almost** 200 mL; transfer to a calibrated bottle, rinse mortar with vehicle, and add quantity of vehicle sufficient to make 200 mL. Label "shake well" and "protect from light". Stable for 42 days at room temperature or 91 days refrigerated (preferred) (Nahata, 2004).

Nahata MC, Pai VB, and Hipple TF, *Pediatric Drug Formulations*, 5th ed, Cincinnati, OH: Harvey Whitney Books Co, 2004.

◆ **Amiodarone Hydrochloride** *see* Amiodarone *on page 114*

◆ **Amiodarone Hydrochloride For Injection (Can)** *see* Amiodarone *on page 114*

◆ **Amitiza** *see* Lubiprostone *on page 1255*

Amitriptyline (a mee TRIP ti leen)

Brand Names: Canada Apo-Amitriptyline; Bio-Amitriptyline; Elavil; Levate; Novo-Triptyn; PMS-Amitriptyline

Index Terms Amitriptyline Hydrochloride; Elavil

Pharmacologic Category Antidepressant, Tricyclic (Tertiary Amine)

Additional Appendix Information

Beers Criteria – Potentially Inappropriate Medications for Geriatrics *on page 2271*

Use Depression: Treatment of depression

Pregnancy Risk Factor C

Pregnancy Considerations Adverse events have been observed in some animal reproduction studies. Amitriptyline crosses the human placenta; CNS effects, limb deformities, and developmental delay have been noted in case reports (causal relationship not established). Tricyclic antidepressants may be associated with irritability, jitteriness, and convulsions (rare) in the neonate (Yonkers, 2009).

The ACOG recommends that therapy for depression during pregnancy be individualized; treatment should incorporate the clinical expertise of the mental health clinician, obstetrician, primary healthcare provider, and pediatrician (ACOG, 2008). According to the American Psychiatric Association (APA), the risks of medication treatment should be weighed against other treatment options and untreated depression. For women who discontinue antidepressant medications during pregnancy and who may be at high risk for postpartum depression, the medications can be restarted following delivery (APA, 2010). Treatment algorithms have been developed by the ACOG and the APA for the management of depression in women prior to conception and during pregnancy (Yonkers, 2009). Although not a first-line agent, amitriptyline may be used for the treatment of post-traumatic stress disorder in pregnant women (Bandelow, 2008). Migraine prophylaxis should be avoided during pregnancy; if needed, amitriptyline may be used if other agents are ineffective or contraindicated (Pringsheim, 2012).

Breast-Feeding Considerations Amitriptyline is excreted into breast milk. Based on information from six mother/infant pairs, following maternal use of amitriptyline 75-175 mg/day, the estimated exposure to the breast-feeding infant would be 0.2% to 1.9% of the weight-adjusted maternal dose. Adverse events have not been reported in nursing infants (four cases). Infants should be monitored for signs of adverse events; routine monitoring of infant serum concentrations is not recommended (Fortinguerra, 2009). Migraine prophylaxis should be avoided in women who are nursing; if needed, amitriptyline may be used if other agents are ineffective or contraindicated (Pringsheim, 2012). Due to the potential for serious adverse reactions in the nursing infant, the manufacturer recommends a decision be made whether to discontinue nursing or to discontinue the drug, taking into account the importance of treatment to the mother.

Contraindications Hypersensitivity to amitriptyline or any component of the formulation; coadministration with or within 14 days of MAOIs; coadministration with cisapride; acute recovery phase following myocardial infarction

Documentation of allergenic cross-reactivity for tricyclic antidepressants is limited. However, because of similarities in chemical structure and/or pharmacologic actions, the possibility of cross-sensitivity cannot be ruled out with certainty.

Warnings/Precautions [U.S. Boxed Warning]: Antidepressants increase the risk of suicidal thinking and behavior in children, adolescents, and young adults (18-24 years of age) with major depressive disorder (MDD) and other psychiatric disorders; consider risk prior to prescribing. Short-term studies did not show an increased risk in patients >24 years of age and showed a decreased risk in patients ≥65 years. Closely monitor for clinical worsening, suicidality, or unusual changes in behavior, particularly during the initial 1-2 months of therapy or during periods of dosage adjustments (increases or decreases); the patient's family or caregiver should be instructed to closely observe the patient and communicate condition with health care provider. A medication guide should be dispensed with each prescription. **Amitriptyline is not FDA-approved for use in children.**

The possibility of a suicide attempt is inherent in major depression and may persist until remission occurs. Worsening depression and severe abrupt suicidality that are not part of the presenting symptoms may require discontinuation or modification of drug therapy. The patient's family or caregiver should be alerted to monitor patients for the emergence of suicidality and associated behaviors (such as agitation, irritability, hostility, impulsivity, and hypomania) and notify healthcare provider.

May precipitate a shift to mania or hypomania in patients with bipolar disorder. Patients presenting with depressive symptoms should be screened for bipolar disorder. **Amitriptyline is not FDA approved for bipolar depression.**

The degree of sedation, anticholinergic effects, orthostasis, and conduction abnormalities are high relative to other antidepressants. Heart block may be precipitated in patients with preexisting conduction system disease and use is relatively contraindicated in patients with conduction abnormalities. May cause CNS depression, which may impair physical or mental abilities; patients must be cautioned about performing tasks that require mental alertness (eg, operating machinery or driving). Use with caution in patients with a history of cardiovascular disease (including previous MI, stroke, tachycardia, or conduction abnormalities). Use with caution in patients with urinary retention, benign prostatic hyperplasia, increased intraocular pressure (IOP), narrow-angle glaucoma, xerostomia, visual problems, constipation, or a history of bowel obstruction.

TCAs may rarely cause bone marrow suppression; monitor for any signs of infection and obtain CBC if symptoms (eg, fever, sore throat) evident. May alter glucose control - use with caution in patients with diabetes. Recommended by the manufacturer to discontinue prior to elective surgery; risks exist for drug interactions with anesthesia and for cardiac arrhythmias. However, definitive drug interactions have not been widely reported in the literature and continuation of tricyclic antidepressants is generally recommended as long as precautions are taken to reduce the significance of any adverse events that may occur (Pass, 2004). May lower seizure threshold - use caution in patients with a previous seizure disorder or condition predisposing to seizures such as brain damage, alcoholism, or concurrent therapy with other drugs which lower the seizure threshold. May increase the risks associated with electroconvulsive therapy. Bone fractures have been associated with antidepressant treatment. Consider the possibility of a fragility fracture if an antidepressant-treated patient presents with unexplained bone pain, point tenderness, swelling, or bruising (Rabenda, 2013; Rizzoli, 2012). Use with caution in patients with hepatic or renal dysfunction. May cause mild pupillary dilation which in susceptible individuals can lead to an episode of narrow-angle glaucoma. Consider evaluating patients who have not had an iridectomy for narrow-angle glaucoma risk factors. Avoid use in the elderly due to its potent anticholinergic and sedative properties, and potential to cause orthostatic hypotension. Therapy is relatively contraindicated in patients with symptomatic hypotension. In addition, may cause or exacerbate syndrome of inappropriate antidiuretic hormone secretion or hyponatremia; monitor sodium closely with initiation or dosage adjustments in older adults (Beers Criteria).

Abrupt discontinuation or interruption of antidepressant therapy has been associated with a discontinuation syndrome. Symptoms arising may vary with antidepressant however commonly include nausea, vomiting, diarrhea, headaches, light-headedness, dizziness, diminished appetite, sweating, chills, tremors, paresthesias, fatigue, somnolence, and sleep disturbances (eg, vivid dreams, insomnia). Greater risks for developing a discontinuation syndrome have been associated with antidepressants with shorter half-lives, longer durations of treatment, and abrupt discontinuation. For antidepressants of short or intermediate half-lives, symptoms may emerge within 2-5 days after treatment discontinuation and last 7-14 days (APA, 2010; Fava, 2006; Haddad, 2001; Shelton, 2001; Warner, 2006).

Adverse Reactions Anticholinergic effects may be pronounced; moderate to marked sedation can occur (tolerance to these effects usually occurs).

Cardiovascular: Atrioventricular conduction disturbance, cardiac arrhythmia, cardiomyopathy (rare), cerebrovascular accident, ECG changes (nonspecific), edema, facial edema, heart block, hypertension, myocardial infarction, orthostatic hypotension, palpitations, syncope, tachycardia

Central nervous system: Anxiety, ataxia, cognitive dysfunction, coma, confusion, delusions, disorientation, dizziness, drowsiness, drug withdrawal (nausea, headache, malaise, irritability, restlessness, dream and sleep disturbance, mania [rare], and hypomania [rare]), dysarthria, EEG pattern changes, excitement, extrapyramidal reaction (including abnormal involuntary movements and tardive dyskinesia), fatigue, hallucination, headache, hyperpyrexia, insomnia, lack of concentration, nightmares, numbness, paresthesia, peripheral neuropathy, restlessness, sedation, seizure, tingling of extremities

Dermatologic: Allergic skin rash, alopecia, diaphoresis, skin photosensitivity, urticaria

Endocrine & metabolic: Altered serum glucose, decreased libido, galactorrhea, gynecomastia, increased libido, SIADH, weight gain, weight loss

Gastrointestinal: Ageusia, anorexia, constipation, diarrhea, melanoglossia, nausea, paralytic ileus, parotid gland enlargement, stomatitis, unpleasant taste, vomiting, xerostomia

Genitourinary: Breast hypertrophy, impotence, testicular swelling, urinary frequency, urinary retention, urinary tract dilation

Hematologic & oncologic: Bone marrow depression (including agranulocytosis, leukopenia, and thrombocytopenia), eosinophilia, purpura

Hepatic: Hepatic failure, hepatitis (rare; including altered liver function and jaundice)

Hypersensitivity: Tongue edema

Neuromuscular & skeletal: Lupus-like syndrome, tremor, weakness

Ophthalmic: Accommodation disturbance, blurred vision, increased intraocular pressure, mydriasis

Otic: Tinnitus

Rare but important or life-threatening: Angle-closure glaucoma, neuroleptic malignant syndrome (rare; Stevens, 2008), serotonin syndrome (rare)

Drug Interactions

Metabolism/Transport Effects **Substrate** of CYP1A2 (minor), CYP2B6 (minor), CYP2C19 (minor), CYP2C9 (minor), CYP2D6 (major), CYP3A4 (minor); **Note:** Assignment of Major/Minor substrate status based on clinically relevant drug interaction potential; **Inhibits** CYP1A2 (weak), CYP2C19 (weak), CYP2C9 (weak), CYP2D6 (weak), CYP2E1 (weak)

Avoid Concomitant Use

Avoid concomitant use of Amitriptyline with any of the following: Aclidinium; Azelastine (Nasal); Cisapride; Dapoxetine; Glucagon; Iobenguane I 123; Ipratropium (Oral Inhalation); Linezolid; MAO Inhibitors; Methylene Blue; Moxonidine; Orphenadrine; Paraldehyde; Potassium Chloride; Thalidomide; Tiotropium; Umeclidinium

Increased Effect/Toxicity

Amitriptyline may increase the levels/effects of: AbobotulinumtoxinA; Alcohol (Ethyl); Alpha-/Beta-Agonists (Direct-Acting); Alpha1-Agonists; Amphetamines; Analgesics (Opioid); Anticholinergic Agents; Antipsychotic Agents; ARIPiprazole; Aspirin; Azelastine (Nasal); Beta2-Agonists; Buprenorphine; Cisapride; Citalopram; CNS Depressants; Desmopressin; Escitalopram; Fluconazole; Glucagon; Highest Risk QTc-Prolonging Agents; Hydrocodone; Methotrimeprazine; Methylene Blue; Metyrosine; Mirabegron; Moderate Risk QTc-Prolonging Agents; Nicorandil; NSAID (COX-2 Inhibitor); NSAID (Nonselective); OnabotulinumtoxinA; Orphenadrine; Paraldehyde; Potassium Chloride; Pramipexole; QuiNIDine; RimabotulinumtoxinB; ROPINIRole; Rotigotine; Serotonin Modulators; Sodium Phosphates; Sulfonylureas; Suvorexant; Thalidomide; Thiazide Diuretics; Tiotropium; TraMADol; Vitamin K Antagonists; Yohimbine; Zolpidem

The levels/effects of Amitriptyline may be increased by: Abiraterone Acetate; Aclidinium; Altretamine; Antiemetics (5HT3 Antagonists); Antipsychotic Agents; Brimonidine (Topical); BuPROPion; Cannabis; Cimetidine; Cinacalcet; Citalopram; Cobicistat; CYP2D6 Inhibitors (Moderate); CYP2D6 Inhibitors (Strong); Dapoxetine; Darunavir; Dexmethylphenidate; Doxylamine; Dronabinol; Droperidol; DULoxetine; Escitalopram; Fluconazole; FLUoxetine; FluvoxaMINE; HydrOXYzine; Ipratropium (Oral Inhalation); Kava Kava; Linezolid; Lithium; Magnesium Sulfate; MAO Inhibitors; Methotrimeprazine; Methylphenidate; Metoclopramide; Metyrosine; Mianserin; Mifepristone; Nabilone; PARoxetine; Peginterferon Alfa-2b; Perampanel; Pramlintide; Protease Inhibitors; QuiNIDine;

Rufinamide; Sertraline; Sodium Oxybate; Tapentadol; Tedizolid; Terbinafine (Systemic); Tetrahydrocannabinol; Thyroid Products; Topiramate; TraMADol; Umeclidinium; Valproic Acid and Derivatives

Decreased Effect

Amitriptyline may decrease the levels/effects of: Acetylcholinesterase Inhibitors; Alpha1-Agonists; Alpha2-Agonists; Alpha2-Agonists (Ophthalmic); Iobenguane I 123; Itopride; Moxonidine; Secretin

The levels/effects of Amitriptyline may be decreased by: Acetylcholinesterase Inhibitors; Barbiturates; CarBAMazepine; Peginterferon Alfa-2b; St Johns Wort

Storage/Stability Store at 20°C to 25°C (68°F to 77°F). Protect from light.

Mechanism of Action Increases the synaptic concentration of serotonin and/or norepinephrine in the central nervous system by inhibition of their reuptake by the presynaptic neuronal membrane pump.

Pharmacodynamics/Kinetics

Onset of action: Individual responses may vary; however, 4-8 weeks of treatment are needed before determining if a patient with depression is partially or non-responsive; similarly 8-12 weeks are required for an adequate migraine prophylaxis trial (APA, 2010; Prinsheim, 2012)

Absorption: Rapid.

Distribution: V_d: ~18-22 L/kg (Schulz, 1985)

Metabolism: Rapid; hepatic N-demethylation to nortriptyline (active)

Bioavailability: ~43% to 46% (Schulz, 1985)

Half-life elimination: ~13-36 hours (Schulz, 1985)

Time to peak, serum: ~2-5 hours (Schulz, 1985)

Excretion: Urine (glucuronide or sulfate conjugate metabolites; low amounts of unchanged drug)

Special Populations: Elderly: May have increased plasma levels (Schulz, 1985)

Dosage

Children:

Chronic pain management (off-label use): Oral: Initial: 0.1 mg/kg/day at bedtime, may advance as tolerated over 2-3 weeks to 0.5-2 mg/kg/day at bedtime (APS [Miaskowski, 2008]; Freidrichsdorf, 2007; Kliegman, 2011)

Migraine prophylaxis (off-label use): Oral: Initial: 0.25 mg/kg/day, given at bedtime; increase dose by 0.25 mg/kg/day every 2 weeks to 1 mg/kg/day. Reported dosing range: 0.2-1.7 mg/kg/day (Hershey, 2000)

Adolescents: Depressive disorders: Oral: Usual dosage (recommended by the manufacturer): 10 mg 3 times daily and 20 mg at bedtime. In general, lower doses are recommended for adolescent patients. **Note:** Controlled clinical trials have not shown tricyclic antidepressants to be superior to placebo for the treatment of depression in children and adolescents; not recommended as first-line medication; may be beneficial for patient with comorbid conditions (Birmaher, 2007; Dopheide, 2006; Wagner, 2005).

Adults:

Depression: Oral: Initial: 25-50 mg daily single dose at bedtime or in divided doses; initial doses of 100 mg daily may be considered in hospitalized patients. Gradually increase dose to 100-300 mg daily (APA, 2010; Bauer 2013).

Chronic pain management (off-label use): Oral: Initial: 25-50 mg at bedtime; may increase as tolerated to 150 mg daily (McQuay, 1992; Pilowsky, 1982; Zitman, 1990)

Diabetic neuropathy (off-label use): Oral: 25-100 mg daily (Bril, 2011)

Interstitial cystitis (bladder pain syndrome) (off-label use): Oral: 10 to 25 mg daily titrated weekly over several weeks to a target dose of 75 to 100 mg as tolerated (AUA [Hanno, 2014]; Foster, 2010)

Migraine prophylaxis (off-label use): Oral: Initial: 10-25 mg at bedtime; increase at weekly increments of 10-25 mg daily based on response and tolerability up to 150 mg daily (Couch, 1976; Dodick, 2009; Evers, 2009; Keskinbora, 2008)

Post-traumatic stress disorder (PTSD) (off-label use): Oral: Initial: 50 mg daily; increase at 25 mg increments as tolerated to 100 mg within the first week; increase to 150 mg daily, then 200 mg daily before the end of 2 weeks; increase further if necessary and tolerated (Davidson, 1990).

Elderly: Depression: Oral: Usual dosage (recommended by the manufacturer): 10 mg 3 times daily and 20 mg at bedtime. In general, lower doses are recommended for elderly patients.

Dosage adjustment in renal impairment: There are no dosage adjustments provided in manufacturer's labeling; however, renally eliminated; use with caution.

Dosage adjustment in hepatic impairment: There are no dosage adjustments provided in manufacturer's labeling; however, hepatically metabolized; use with caution.

Discontinuation of therapy: Upon discontinuation of antidepressant therapy, gradually taper the dose to minimize the incidence of withdrawal symptoms and allow for the detection of re-emerging symptoms. Evidence supporting ideal taper rates is limited. APA and NICE guidelines suggest tapering therapy over at least several weeks with consideration to the half-life of the antidepressant; antidepressants with a shorter half-life may need to be tapered more conservatively. In addition for long-term treated patients, WFSBP guidelines recommend tapering over 4-6 months. If intolerable withdrawal symptoms occur following a dose reduction, consider resuming the previously prescribed dose and/or decrease dose at a more gradual rate (APA, 2010; Bauer, 2002; Haddad, 2001; NCCMH, 2010; Schatzberg, 2006; Shelton, 2001; Warner, 2006).

MAO inhibitor recommendations:

Switching to or from an MAO inhibitor antidepressant:

Allow 14 days to elapse between discontinuing an MAO inhibitor intended to treat depression and initiation of amitriptyline.

Allow 14 days to elapse between discontinuing amitriptyline and initiation of an MAO inhibitor intended to treat depression.

Use with reversible MAO inhibitors (such as linezolid or IV methylene blue):

Do not initiate amitriptyline in patients receiving linezolid or IV methylene blue; consider other interventions for psychiatric condition.

If urgent treatment with linezolid or IV methylene blue is required in a patient already receiving amitriptyline and potential benefits outweigh potential risks, discontinue amitriptyline promptly and administer linezolid or IV methylene blue. Monitor for serotonin syndrome for 2 weeks or until 24 hours after the last dose of linezolid or IV methylene blue, whichever comes first. May resume amitriptyline 24 hours after the last dose of linezolid or IV methylene blue.

Administration Oral: Administer higher doses preferably at late afternoon or as bedtime doses to minimize daytime sedation.

Monitoring Parameters Evaluate mental status, suicide ideation (especially at the beginning of therapy or when doses are increased or decreased); anxiety, social functioning, mania, panic attacks or other unusual changes in behavior; heart rate, blood pressure and ECG in older adults and patients with preexisting cardiac disease; blood glucose; weight and BMI; blood levels are useful for therapeutic monitoring (APA, 2010).

Reference Range Therapeutic: Amitriptyline plus nortriptyline 80-250 ng/mL (SI: 288-900 nmol/L); amitriptyline plus nortriptyline levels >300 ng/mL are associated with increased side effects; plasma levels do not always correlate with clinical effectiveness (Am J Psychiatry, 1985; Boyer, 1984; Orsulak, 1979)

Dosage Forms

Tablet, Oral:

Generic: 10 mg, 25 mg, 50 mg, 75 mg, 100 mg, 150 mg

Amitriptyline and Chlordiazepoxide

(a mee TRIP ti leen & klor dye az e POKS ide)

Index Terms Chlordiazepoxide and Amitriptyline Hydrochloride; Limbitrol

Pharmacologic Category Antidepressant, Tricyclic (Tertiary Amine); Benzodiazepine

Additional Appendix Information

Beers Criteria – Potentially Inappropriate Medications for Geriatrics *on page 2271*

Use Treatment of moderate-to-severe anxiety and/or agitation and depression

Dosage Initial: 3-4 tablets in divided doses; this may be increased to 6 tablets/day as required; some patients respond to smaller doses and can be maintained on 2 tablets

Discontinuation of therapy: Upon discontinuation of antidepressant therapy, gradually taper the dose to minimize the incidence of withdrawal symptoms and allow for the detection of re-emerging symptoms. Evidence supporting ideal taper rates is limited. APA and NICE guidelines suggest tapering therapy over at least several weeks with consideration to the half-life of the antidepressant; antidepressants with a shorter half-life may need to be tapered more conservatively. In addition for long-term treated patients, WFSBP guidelines recommend tapering over 4-6 months. If intolerable withdrawal symptoms occur following a dose reduction, consider resuming the previously prescribed dose and/or decrease dose at a more gradual rate (APA, 2010; Bauer, 2002; Haddad, 2001; NCCMH, 2010; Schatzberg, 2006; Shelton, 2001; Warner, 2006).

MAO inhibitor recommendations:

Switching to or from an MAO inhibitor intended to treat psychiatric disorders:

Allow 14 days to elapse between discontinuing an MAO inhibitor intended to treat psychiatric disorders and initiation of amitriptyline/chlordiazepoxide.

Allow 14 days to elapse between discontinuing amitriptyline/chlordiazepoxide and initiation of an MAO inhibitor intended to treat psychiatric disorders.

Use with reversible MAO inhibitors (such as linezolid or IV methylene blue):

Do not initiate amitriptyline/chlordiazepoxide in patients receiving linezolid or IV methylene blue; consider other interventions for psychiatric condition.

If urgent treatment with linezolid or IV methylene blue is required in a patient already receiving amitriptyline/chlordiazepoxide and potential benefits outweigh potential risks, discontinue amitriptyline/chlordiazepoxide promptly and administer linezolid or IV methylene blue. Monitor for serotonin syndrome for 2 weeks or until 24 hours after the last dose of linezolid or IV methylene blue, whichever comes first. May resume amitriptyline/chlordiazepoxide 24 hours after the last dose of linezolid or IV methylene blue.

Dosage adjustment in renal impairment: No dosage adjustment provided in manufacturer's labeling; use with caution.

Dosage adjustment in hepatic impairment: No dosage adjustment provided in manufacturer's labeling; use with caution.

Additional Information Complete prescribing information should be consulted for additional detail.

Dosage Forms

Tablet: 12.5/5: Amitriptyline 12.5 mg and chlordiazepoxide 5 mg; 25/10: Amitriptyline 25 mg and chlordiazepoxide 10 mg

Amitriptyline and Perphenazine

(a mee TRIP ti leen & per FEN a zeen)

Brand Names: Canada PMS-Levazine

Index Terms Perphenazine and Amitriptyline Hydrochloride

Pharmacologic Category Antidepressant, Tricyclic (Tertiary Amine); First Generation (Typical) Antipsychotic

Additional Appendix Information

Beers Criteria – Potentially Inappropriate Medications for Geriatrics *on page 2271*

Use Treatment of patients with moderate-to-severe anxiety and/or agitation and depression; schizophrenia with depressive symptoms

Dosage Oral: Adults:

Depression and anxiety:

Initial: One tablet (amitriptyline 25 mg/perphenazine 2 mg or amitriptyline 25 mg/perphenazine 4 mg) 3-4 times/day **or** 1 tablet (amitriptyline 50 mg/perphenazine 4 mg) 2 times/day; initial therapeutic response may be observed after several days or upwards of a few weeks or longer (maximum daily dose: amitriptyline 200 mg/perphenazine 16 mg)

Maintenance: Smallest dose necessary for symptom relief; usually 1 tablet (amitriptyline 25 mg/perphenazine 2 mg or amitriptyline 25 mg/perphenazine 4 mg) 2-4 times/day **or** 1 tablet (amitriptyline 50 mg/perphenazine 4 mg) 2 times/day

Schizophrenia and depression:

Initial: Two tablets (amitriptyline 25 mg/perphenazine 4 mg) 3 times/day; if necessary, a fourth dose may be given at bedtime; initial therapeutic response may be observed after several days or upwards of a few weeks or longer (maximum daily dose: amitriptyline 200 mg/perphenazine 16 mg) (maximum: 64 mg/day of perphenazine)

Maintenance: Smallest dose necessary for symptom relief; usually 1 tablet (amitriptyline 25 mg/perphenazine 2 mg or amitriptyline 25 mg/perphenazine 4 mg) 2-4 times/day **or** 1 tablet (amitriptyline 50 mg/perphenazine 4 mg) 2 times/day

Elderly: One tablet (amitriptyline 10 mg/perphenazine 4 mg) 3-4 times/day

Discontinuation of therapy: Upon discontinuation of antidepressant therapy, gradually taper the dose to minimize the incidence of withdrawal symptoms and allow for the detection of re-emerging symptoms. Evidence supporting ideal taper rates is limited. APA and NICE guidelines suggest tapering therapy over at least several weeks with consideration to the half-life of the antidepressant; antidepressants with a shorter half-life may need to be tapered more conservatively. In addition for long-term treated patients, WFSBP guidelines recommend tapering over 4-6 months. If intolerable withdrawal symptoms occur following a dose reduction, consider resuming the

previously prescribed dose and/or decrease dose at a more gradual rate (APA, 2010; Bauer, 2002; Haddad, 2001; NCCMH, 2010; Schatzberg, 2006; Shelton, 2001; Warner, 2006).

MAO inhibitor recommendations:

Switching to or from an MAO inhibitor intended to treat psychiatric disorders:

Allow 14 days to elapse between discontinuing an MAO inhibitor intended to treat psychiatric disorders and initiation of amitriptyline/perphenazine.

Allow 14 days to elapse between discontinuing amitriptyline/perphenazine and initiation of an MAO inhibitor intended to treat psychiatric disorders.

Use with reversible MAO inhibitors (such as linezolid or IV methylene blue):

Do not initiate amitriptyline/perphenazine in patients receiving linezolid or IV methylene blue; consider other interventions for psychiatric condition.

If urgent treatment with linezolid or IV methylene blue is required in a patient already receiving amitriptyline/perphenazine and potential benefits outweigh potential risks, discontinue amitriptyline/perphenazine promptly and administer linezolid or IV methylene blue. Monitor for serotonin syndrome for 2 weeks or until 24 hours after the last dose of linezolid or IV methylene blue, whichever comes first. May resume amitriptyline/perphenazine 24 hours after the last dose of linezolid or IV methylene blue.

Dosage adjustment in renal impairment: No dosage adjustment provided in manufacturer's labeling.

Dosage adjustment in hepatic impairment: Use caution; no dosage adjustment provided in manufacturer's labeling.

Additional Information Complete prescribing information should be consulted for additional detail.

Dosage Forms

Tablet: 2-10: Amitriptyline 10 mg and perphenazine 2 mg; 2-25: Amitriptyline 25 mg and perphenazine 2 mg; 4-10: Amitriptyline 10 mg and perphenazine 4 mg; 4-25: Amitriptyline 25 mg and perphenazine 4 mg; 4-50: Amitriptyline 50 mg and perphenazine 4 mg

◆ **Amitriptyline Hydrochloride** *see* Amitriptyline *on page 119*

◆ **AMJ 9701** *see* Palifermin *on page 1555*

AmLODIPine (am LOE di peen)

Brand Names: U.S. Norvasc

Brand Names: Canada Accel-Amlodipine; ACT-Amlodipine; Amlodipine-Odan; Apo-Amlodipine; Auro-Amlodipine; Bio-Amlodipine; Dom-Amlodipine; GD-Amlodipine; JAMP-Amlodipine; Mar-Amlodipine; Mint-Amlodipine; Mylan-Amlodipine; Norvasc; PHL-Amlodipine; PMS-Amlodipine; Q-Amlodipine; RAN-Amlodipine; ratio-Amlodipine; Riva-Amlodipine; Sandoz Amlodipine; Septa-Amlodipine; Teva-Amlodipine

Index Terms Amlodipine Besylate

Pharmacologic Category Antianginal Agent; Antihypertensive; Calcium Channel Blocker; Calcium Channel Blocker, Dihydropyridine

Use

Treatment of hypertension; treatment of symptomatic chronic stable angina, vasospastic (Prinzmetal's) angina (confirmed or suspected); prevention of hospitalization due to angina with documented CAD (limited to patients without heart failure or ejection fraction <40%)

The 2014 guideline for the management of high blood pressure in adults (JNC 8) recommends initiation of pharmacologic treatment to lower blood pressure for the following patients (JNC8 [James, 2013]):

- Patients ≥60 years of age, with systolic blood pressure (SBP) ≥150 mm Hg or diastolic blood pressure (DBP) ≥90 mm Hg. Goal of therapy is SBP <150 mm Hg and DBP <90 mm Hg.
- Patients <60 years of age, with SBP ≥140 mm Hg or DBP ≥90 mm Hg. Goal of therapy is SBP <140 mm Hg and DBP <90 mm Hg.
- Patients ≥18 years of age with diabetes, with SBP ≥140 mm Hg or DBP ≥90 mm Hg. Goal of therapy is SBP <140 mm Hg and DBP <90 mm Hg.
- Patients ≥18 years of age with chronic kidney disease (CKD), with SBP ≥140 mm Hg or DBP ≥90 mm Hg. Goal of therapy is SBP <140 mm Hg and DBP <90 mm Hg.

In patients with chronic kidney disease (CKD), regardless of race or diabetes status, the use of an ACE inhibitor (ACEI) or angiotensin receptor blocker (ARB) as initial therapy is recommended to improve kidney outcomes. In the general nonblack population (without CKD) including those with diabetes, initial antihypertensive treatment should consist of a thiazide-type diuretic, calcium channel blocker, ACEI, or ARB. In the general black population (without CKD) including those with diabetes, initial antihypertensive treatment should consist of a thiazide-type diuretic or a calcium channel blocker **instead of** an ACEI or ARB.

The ACCF/AHA 2013 guidelines for management of heart failure state that, with the exception of amlodipine, calcium channel blockers should be avoided and withdrawn whenever possible in patients with heart failure with reduced ejection fraction (HFrEF). While amlodipine, like other calcium channel blockers, has no benefit on functioning or survival, it may be used for the treatment of hypertension or ischemic heart disease in patients with HFrEF (ACCF/AHA [Yancy, 2013]).

Pregnancy Risk Factor C

Pregnancy Considerations Adverse events were observed in some animal reproduction studies. Untreated chronic maternal hypertension is associated with adverse events in the fetus, infant, and mother. If treatment for hypertension during pregnancy is needed, other agents are preferred (ACOG, 2013).

Breast-Feeding Considerations It is not known if amlodipine is excreted into breast milk. The manufacturer recommends nursing be discontinued during treatment.

Contraindications Hypersensitivity to amlodipine or any component of the formulation

Warnings/Precautions Increased angina and/or MI has occurred with initiation or dosage titration of calcium channel blockers. Symptomatic hypotension with or without syncope can rarely occur; blood pressure must be lowered at a rate appropriate for the patient's clinical condition. Use caution in severe aortic stenosis and/or hypertrophic cardiomyopathy with outflow tract obstruction. Use caution in patients with hepatic impairment; may require lower starting dose; titrate slowly with severe hepatic impairment. The most common side effect is peripheral edema; occurs within 2-3 weeks of starting therapy. Reflex tachycardia may occur with use. Peak antihypertensive effect is delayed; dosage titration should occur after 7-14 days on a given dose. Initiate at a lower dose in the elderly.

Adverse Reactions

Cardiovascular: Flushing (more common in females), palpitations, peripheral edema (more common in females)

Central nervous system: Dizziness, drowsiness, fatigue, male sexual disorder

Dermatologic: Pruritus, skin rash

Gastrointestinal: Abdominal pain, nausea
Neuromuscular & skeletal: Muscle cramps, weakness
Respiratory: Dyspnea, pulmonary edema
Rare but important or life-threatening: Acute interstitial nephritis (Ejaz 2000), anorexia, atrial fibrillation, bradycardia, cholestasis, conjunctivitis, depression, diarrhea, difficulty in micturition, diplopia, dysphagia, epistaxis, erythema multiforme, exfoliative dermatitis, eye pain, female sexual disorder, gingival hyperplasia, gynecomastia, hepatitis, hot flash, hyperglycemia, hypersensitivity angiitis, hypersensitivity reaction, hypoesthesia, increased serum transaminases, increased thirst, insomnia, leukopenia, maculopapular rash, myalgia, nocturia, orthostatic hypotension, osteoarthritis, pancreatitis, paresthesia, peripheral ischemia, peripheral neuropathy, phototoxicity, purpura, rigors, tachycardia, thrombocytopenia, tremor, vasculitis, ventricular tachycardia, weight gain

Drug Interactions

Metabolism/Transport Effects **Substrate** of CYP3A4 (major); **Note:** Assignment of Major/Minor substrate status based on clinically relevant drug interaction potential; **Inhibits** CYP1A2 (weak), CYP2A6 (weak), CYP2B6 (weak), CYP2C8 (weak), CYP2C9 (weak), CYP2D6 (weak), CYP3A4 (weak)

Avoid Concomitant Use

Avoid concomitant use of AmLODIPine with any of the following: Conivaptan; Fusidic Acid (Systemic); Idelalisib; Pimozide

Increased Effect/Toxicity

AmLODIPine may increase the levels/effects of: Amifostine; Antihypertensives; ARIPiprazole; Atosiban; Beta-Blockers; Calcium Channel Blockers (Nondihydropyridine); Dofetilide; DULoxetine; Fosphenytoin; Hydrocodone; Hypotensive Agents; Levodopa; Lomitapide; Magnesium Salts; Neuromuscular-Blocking Agents (Nondepolarizing); Nitroprusside; Obinutuzumab; Phenytoin; Pimozide; QuiNIDine; RisperiDONE; RiTUXimab; Simvastatin; Tacrolimus (Systemic)

The levels/effects of AmLODIPine may be increased by: Alfuzosin; Alpha1-Blockers; Antifungal Agents (Azole Derivatives, Systemic); Aprepitant; Barbiturates; Brimonidine (Topical); Calcium Channel Blockers (Nondihydropyridine); Ceritinib; Conivaptan; CycloSPORINE (Systemic); CYP3A4 Inhibitors (Moderate); CYP3A4 Inhibitors (Strong); Dapoxetine; Dasatinib; Diazoxide; Fluconazole; Fosaprepitant; Fusidic Acid (Systemic); Grapefruit Juice; Herbs (Hypotensive Properties); Idelalisib; Ivacaftor; Luliconazole; Macrolide Antibiotics; Magnesium Salts; MAO Inhibitors; Mifepristone; Netupitant; Nicorandil; Pentoxifylline; Phosphodiesterase 5 Inhibitors; Prostacyclin Analogues; Protease Inhibitors; QuiNIDine; Simeprevir; Stiripentol

Decreased Effect

AmLODIPine may decrease the levels/effects of: Clopidogrel; QuiNIDine

The levels/effects of AmLODIPine may be decreased by: Barbiturates; Bosentan; Calcium Salts; CarBAMazepine; CYP3A4 Inducers (Moderate); CYP3A4 Inducers (Strong); Dabrafenib; Deferasirox; Efavirenz; Herbs (Hypertensive Properties); Melatonin; Methylphenidate; Mitotane; Nafcillin; Rifamycin Derivatives; Siltuximab; St Johns Wort; Tocilizumab; Yohimbine

Food Interactions Grapefruit juice may modestly increase amlodipine levels. Management: Monitor closely with concurrent use.

Storage/Stability Store at room temperature of 15°C to 30°C (59°F to 86°F).

Mechanism of Action Inhibits calcium ion from entering the "slow channels" or select voltage-sensitive areas of vascular smooth muscle and myocardium during depolarization, producing a relaxation of coronary vascular smooth muscle and coronary vasodilation; increases myocardial oxygen delivery in patients with vasospastic angina. Amlodipine directly acts on vascular smooth muscle to produce peripheral arterial vasodilation reducing peripheral vascular resistance and blood pressure.

Pharmacodynamics/Kinetics

Duration of antihypertensive effect: 24 hours
Absorption: Oral: Well absorbed
Distribution: V_d: 21 L/kg
Protein binding: 93% to 98%
Metabolism: Hepatic (>90%) to inactive metabolites
Bioavailability: 64% to 90%
Half-life elimination: Terminal: 30-50 hours; increased with hepatic dysfunction
Time to peak, plasma: 6-12 hours
Excretion: Urine (10% of total dose as unchanged drug, 60% of total dose as metabolites)

Dosage Oral:

Children 6-17 years: Hypertension: 2.5-5 mg once daily
Adults:
Hypertension: Initial dose: 5 mg once daily; maximum dose: 10 mg once daily. In general, titrate in 2.5 mg increments over 7-14 days. Usual dosage range (ASH/ISH [Weber, 2014]): 5-10 mg once daily. Target dose (JNC8 [James, 2013]): 10 mg daily.
Angina: Usual dose: 5-10 mg; most patients require 10 mg for adequate effect
Elderly: Dosing should start at the lower end of dosing range and titrated to response due to possible increased incidence of hepatic, renal, or cardiac impairment. Elderly patients also show decreased clearance of amlodipine.
Hypertension: 2.5 mg once daily
Angina: 5 mg once daily

Dosage adjustment in renal impairment: Dialysis: Hemodialysis and peritoneal dialysis do not enhance elimination. Supplemental dose is not necessary.

Dosage adjustment in hepatic impairment:
Angina: Administer 5 mg once daily.
Hypertension: Administer 2.5 mg once daily.

Dietary Considerations May be taken without regard to meals.

Administration May be administered without regard to meals.

Monitoring Parameters Heart rate, blood pressure, peripheral edema

Dosage Forms

Tablet, Oral:
Norvasc: 2.5 mg, 5 mg, 10 mg
Generic: 2.5 mg, 5 mg, 10 mg

Extemporaneous Preparations A 1 mg/mL oral suspension may be made with tablets and either a 1:1 mixture of simple syrup and 1% methylcellulose or a 1:1 mixture of Ora-Plus® and Ora-Sweet®. Crush fifty 5 mg tablets in a mortar and reduce to a fine powder. Add small portions of the chosen vehicle and mix to a uniform paste; mix while adding the vehicle in incremental proportions to **almost** 250 mL; transfer to a calibrated bottle, rinse mortar with vehicle, and add quantity of vehicle sufficient to make 250 mL. Label "shake well" and "refrigerate". Stable for 56 days at room temperature or 91 days refrigerated.

Nahata MC, Morosco RS, and Hipple TF, "Stability of Amlodipine Besylate in Two Liquid Dosage Forms," *J Am Pharm Assoc (Wash)*, 1999, 39(3):375-7.

◆ **Amlodipine, Aliskiren, and Hydrochlorothiazide** *see* Aliskiren, Amlodipine, and Hydrochlorothiazide *on page 87*

Amlodipine and Atorvastatin

(am LOW di peen & a TORE va sta tin)

Brand Names: U.S. Caduet®
Brand Names: Canada Caduet®

Index Terms Atorvastatin and Amlodipine; Atorvastatin Calcium and Amlodipine Besylate

Pharmacologic Category Antianginal Agent; Antihypertensive; Antilipemic Agent, HMG-CoA Reductase Inhibitor; Calcium Channel Blocker; Calcium Channel Blocker, Dihydropyridine

Use For use when treatment with both amlodipine and atorvastatin is appropriate:

Amlodipine: Treatment of hypertension; treatment of chronic stable angina, vasospastic (Prinzmetal's) angina (confirmed or suspected); prevention of hospitalization or to decrease coronary revascularization procedure due to angina with documented CAD (limited to patients without heart failure or ejection fraction <40%)

Atorvastatin: Treatment of dyslipidemias or primary prevention of cardiovascular disease (atherosclerotic) as detailed here:

Primary prevention of cardiovascular disease (high-risk for CVD): To reduce the risk of MI or stroke in patients without evidence of coronary heart disease who have multiple CVD risk factors or type 2 diabetes; also reduces the risk for angina or revascularization procedures in patients with multiple CVD risk factors without evidence of coronary heart disease

Secondary prevention of cardiovascular disease: To reduce the risk of MI, stroke, revascularization procedures, angina, and hospitalization for heart failure

Primary and secondary prevention of atherosclerotic cardiovascular disease (ASCVD) according to the American College of Cardiology/American Heart Association: To reduce the risk of ASCVD in patients with clinical ASCVD (eg, coronary heart disease, stroke/TIA, or peripheral arterial disease presumed to be of atherosclerotic origin); in patients without clinical ASCVD if LDL-C is 190 mg/dL or greater; in patients without clinical ASCVD who have type 1 or type 2 diabetes and are between 40 and 75 years of age; in patients with an estimated 10-year ASCVD risk 7.5% or greater and who are between 40 and 75 years of age (Stone, 2013). Specific recommendations from the Kidney Disease: Improving Global Outcomes (KDIGO) organization have also been released for patients with chronic kidney disease (KDIGO [Tonelli, 2013]).

Treatment of dyslipidemias: To reduce elevations in total cholesterol, LDL-C, apolipoprotein B, and triglycerides in patients with elevations of one or more components, and/or to increase low HDL-C as present in heterozygous familial/nonfamilial hypercholesterolemia and mixed dyslipidemia (Fredrickson type IIa and IIb hyperlipidemias); treatment of primary dysbetalipoproteinemia (Fredrickson type III), elevated serum TG levels (Fredrickson type IV), and homozygous familial hypercholesterolemia

Treatment of heterozygous familial hypercholesterolemia (HeFH) in adolescent patients (10 to 17 years of age, females >1 year postmenarche) having LDL-C ≥190 mg/dL or LDL-C ≥160 mg/dL with positive family history of premature cardiovascular disease (CVD) or with two or more CVD risk factors.

Pregnancy Risk Factor X

Dosage Oral: **Note:** Dose is individualized; combination product may be used as initial therapy or substituted for individual components in patients currently maintained on both agents separately or in patients not adequately controlled with monotherapy (using one of the agents or an agent within same pharmacologic class).

Children 10-17 years (females >1 year postmenarche): Hypertension and hyperlipidemia:

Initial therapy: Amlodipine 2.5 mg and atorvastatin 10 mg once daily; dose may be titrated after 1-2 weeks (amlodipine component) and after 2-4 weeks (atorvastatin component) to a maximum daily dose: Amlodipine 5 mg; atorvastatin 20 mg

Add-on therapy/replacement therapy: Amlodipine 2.5-5 mg and atorvastatin 10-20 mg once daily; dose may be titrated after 1-2 weeks (amlodipine component) and after 2-4 weeks (atorvastatin component) to a maximum daily dose: Amlodipine 5 mg; atorvastatin 20 mg

Adults: Hypertension, angina, and hyperlipidemia:

Initial therapy: Amlodipine 5 mg and atorvastatin 10-20 mg once daily; dose may be titrated after 1-2 weeks (amlodipine component) and after 2-4 weeks (atorvastatin component) to a maximum daily dose: Amlodipine 10 mg; atorvastatin 80 mg

Add-on therapy/replacement therapy: Amlodipine 5-10 mg and atorvastatin 10-80 mg once daily; dose may be titrated after 1-2 weeks (amlodipine component) and after 2-4 weeks (atorvastatin component) to a maximum daily dose: Amlodipine 10 mg; atorvastatin 80 mg

Elderly: Consider starting amlodipine at the lower end of dosing range due to increased incidence of hepatic, renal, or cardiac impairment. Elderly patients also show decreased clearance of amlodipine.

Dosage adjustment for atorvastatin with concomitant medications:

Boceprevir, nelfinavir: Use lowest effective atorvastatin dose (not to exceed 40 mg daily)

Clarithromycin, itraconazole, fosamprenavir, ritonavir (plus darunavir, fosamprenavir, or saquinavir): Use lowest effective atorvastatin dose (not to exceed 20 mg daily)

Dosage adjustment in renal impairment: No dosage adjustment is necessary

Dosage adjustment in hepatic impairment: Contraindicated in patients with active liver disease

Additional Information Complete prescribing information should be consulted for additional detail.

Dosage Forms

Tablet, oral: Amlodipine 2.5 mg and atorvastatin 10 mg; Amlodipine 2.5 mg and atorvastatin 20 mg; Amlodipine 2.5 mg and atorvastatin 40 mg; Amlodipine 5 mg and atorvastatin 10 mg; Amlodipine 5 mg and atorvastatin 20 mg; Amlodipine 5 mg and atorvastatin 40 mg; Amlodipine 5 mg and atorvastatin 80 mg; Amlodipine 10 mg and atorvastatin 10 mg; Amlodipine 10 mg and atorvastatin 20 mg; Amlodipine 10 mg and atorvastatin 40 mg; Amlodipine 10 mg and atorvastatin 80 mg

Caduet®:

2.5/10: Amlodipine 2.5 mg and atorvastatin 10 mg; 2.5/20: Amlodipine 2.5 mg and atorvastatin 20 mg; 2.5/40: Amlodipine 2.5 mg and atorvastatin 40 mg

5/10: Amlodipine 5 mg and atorvastatin 10 mg; 5/20: Amlodipine 5 mg and atorvastatin 20 mg; 5/40: Amlodipine 5 mg and atorvastatin 40 mg; 5/80: Amlodipine 5 mg and atorvastatin 80 mg

10/10: Amlodipine 10 mg and atorvastatin 10 mg; 10/20: Amlodipine 10 mg and atorvastatin 20 mg; 10/40: Amlodipine 10 mg and atorvastatin 40 mg; 10/80: Amlodipine 10 mg and atorvastatin 80 mg

Amlodipine and Benazepril

(am LOE di peen & ben AY ze pril)

Brand Names: U.S. Lotrel®

Index Terms Benazepril Hydrochloride and Amlodipine Besylate

Pharmacologic Category Angiotensin-Converting Enzyme (ACE) Inhibitor; Antianginal Agent; Antihypertensive; Calcium Channel Blocker; Calcium Channel Blocker, Dihydropyridine

Use Treatment of hypertension

Pregnancy Risk Factor D

Dosage Oral: **Note:** Dose is individualized; combination product may be substituted for individual components in patients currently maintained on both agents separately or in patients not adequately controlled with monotherapy (using one of the agents or an agent within same antihypertensive class).

Adults: 2.5-10 mg (amlodipine) and 10-40 mg (benazepril) once daily; maximum: Amlodipine: 10 mg/day; benazepril: 80 mg/day

Elderly: Initial dose: 2.5 mg based on amlodipine component

Dosage adjustment in renal impairment: CrCl ≤30 mL/minute: Use of combination product is not recommended.

Dosage adjustment in hepatic impairment: Initial dose: 2.5 mg based on amlodipine component

Additional Information Complete prescribing information should be consulted for additional detail.

Dosage Forms

Capsule, oral: 2.5/10: Amlodipine 2.5 mg and benazepril 10 mg; 5/10: Amlodipine 5 mg and benazepril 10 mg; 5/20: Amlodipine 5 mg and benazepril 20 mg; 5/40: Amlodipine 5 mg and benazepril hydrochloride 40 mg; 10/20: Amlodipine 10 mg and benazepril 20 mg; 10/40: Amlodipine 10 mg and benazepril hydrochloride 40 mg

Lotrel®: 2.5/10: Amlodipine 2.5 and benazepril 10 mg; 5/10: Amlodipine 5 mg and benazepril 10 mg; 5/20: Amlodipine 5 mg and benazepril 20 mg; 5/40: Amlodipine 5 mg and benazepril 40 mg; 10/20: Amlodipine 10 mg and benazepril 20 mg; 10/40: Amlodipine 10 mg and benazepril 40 mg

Amlodipine and Olmesartan

(am LOE di peen & olme SAR tan)

Brand Names: U.S. Azor

Index Terms Amlodipine Besylate and Olmesartan Medoxomil; Olmesartan and Amlodipine

Pharmacologic Category Angiotensin II Receptor Blocker; Antianginal Agent; Antihypertensive; Calcium Channel Blocker; Calcium Channel Blocker, Dihydropyridine

Use Hypertension: Treatment of hypertension

Pregnancy Risk Factor D

Dosage Dose is individualized; combination product may be substituted for individual components in patients currently maintained on both agents separately or in patients not adequately controlled with monotherapy (using one of the agents or an agent the within same antihypertensive class). May also be used as initial therapy in patients who are likely to need >1 antihypertensive to control blood pressure.

Hypertension: Oral:

Adults:

Initial therapy (antihypertensive naive): Amlodipine 5 mg/olmesartan 20 mg once daily; dose may be increased after 1 to 2 weeks of therapy. Maximum dose: Amlodipine 10 mg/olmesartan 40 mg once daily.

Add-on/replacement therapy: Amlodipine 5 to 10 mg and olmesartan 20 to 40 mg once daily depending upon previous doses, current control, and goals of therapy; dose may be titrated after 2 weeks of therapy. Maximum dose: Amlodipine 10 mg/olmesartan 40 mg once daily.

Elderly: Initial therapy is not recommended in patients ≥75 years.

Dosage adjustment in renal impairment: Moderate to severe impairment (CrCl <40 mL/minute): No initial dosage adjustment necessary.

Dosage adjustment in hepatic impairment: Initial therapy is not recommended

Additional Information Complete prescribing information should be consulted for additional detail.

Dosage Forms

Tablet:

Azor: 5/20: Amlodipine 5 mg and olmesartan medoxomil 20 mg; 5/40: Amlodipine 5 mg and olmesartan medoxomil 40 mg; 10/20: Amlodipine 10 mg and olmesartan medoxomil 20 mg; 10/40: Amlodipine 10 mg and olmesartan medoxomil 40 mg

◆ **Amlodipine and Telmisartan** *see* Telmisartan and Amlodipine *on page 1989*

Amlodipine and Valsartan

(am LOE di peen & val SAR tan)

Brand Names: U.S. Exforge®

Index Terms Amlodipine Besylate and Valsartan; Valsartan and Amlodipine

Pharmacologic Category Angiotensin II Receptor Blocker; Antianginal Agent; Antihypertensive; Calcium Channel Blocker; Calcium Channel Blocker, Dihydropyridine

Use Treatment of hypertension

Pregnancy Risk Factor D

Dosage Oral: Dose is individualized; combination product may be used as initial therapy or substituted for individual components in patients currently maintained on both agents separately or in patients not adequately controlled with monotherapy (using one of the agents or an agent within same antihypertensive class).

Adults: Hypertension:

Initial therapy: Amlodipine 5 mg and valsartan 160 mg once daily, dose may be titrated after 1-2 weeks of therapy. Maximum recommended doses: Amlodipine 10 mg daily; valsartan 320 mg daily

Add-on/replacement therapy: Amlodipine 5-10 mg and valsartan 160-320 mg once daily; dose may be titrated after 3-4 weeks of therapy. Maximum recommended doses: Amlodipine 10 mg daily; valsartan 320 mg daily

Elderly: Use of lower initial doses should be considered.

Dosing adjustment in renal impairment:

CrCl ≥30 mL/minute: No dosage adjustment necessary.

CrCl <30 mL/minute: No dosage adjustment provided in manufacturer's labeling; safety and efficacy has not been established.

Dosing adjustment in hepatic impairment:

Mild-to-moderate impairment: Use with caution; amlodipine elimination prolonged and valsartan exposure doubled in patients with mild-to-moderate chronic disease compared to healthy volunteers. No dosage adjustment for valsartan is necessary; however, a lower initial amlodipine dose may be required (possibly requiring use of the individual agents).

Severe impairment: No dosage adjustment provided in manufacturer's labeling; however, similar to patients with mild to moderate impairment, a lower initial amlodipine dose may be required (possibly requiring use of the individual agents); titrate slowly.

Additional Information Complete prescribing information should be consulted for additional detail.

Dosage Forms

Tablet:

Exforge®: 5/160: Amlodipine 5 mg and valsartan 160 mg; 5/320: Amlodipine 5 mg and valsartan 320 mg; 10/160: Amlodipine 10 mg and valsartan 160 mg; 10/320: Amlodipine 10 mg and valsartan 320 mg

◆ **Amlodipine Besylate** *see* AmLODIPine *on page 123*

◆ **Amlodipine Besylate, Aliskiren Hemifumarate, and Hydrochlorothiazide** *see* Aliskiren, Amlodipine, and Hydrochlorothiazide *on page 87*

◆ **Amlodipine Besylate and Olmesartan Medoxomil** *see* Amlodipine and Olmesartan *on page 126*

◆ **Amlodipine Besylate and Telmisartan** *see* Telmisartan and Amlodipine *on page 1989*

◆ **Amlodipine Besylate and Valsartan** *see* Amlodipine and Valsartan *on page 126*

◆ **Amlodipine Besylate, Olmesartan Medoxomil, and Hydrochlorothiazide** *see* Olmesartan, Amlodipine, and Hydrochlorothiazide *on page 1498*

◆ **Amlodipine Besylate, Valsartan, and Hydrochlorothiazide** *see* Amlodipine, Valsartan, and Hydrochlorothiazide *on page 127*

◆ **Amlodipine, Hydrochlorothiazide, and Aliskiren** *see* Aliskiren, Amlodipine, and Hydrochlorothiazide *on page 87*

◆ **Amlodipine, Hydrochlorothiazide, and Olmesartan** *see* Olmesartan, Amlodipine, and Hydrochlorothiazide *on page 1498*

◆ **Amlodipine, Hydrochlorothiazide, and Valsartan** *see* Amlodipine, Valsartan, and Hydrochlorothiazide *on page 127*

◆ **Amlodipine-Odan (Can)** *see* AmLODIPine *on page 123*

Amlodipine, Valsartan, and Hydrochlorothiazide

(am LOE di peen, val SAR tan, & hye droe klor oh THYE a zide)

Brand Names: U.S. Exforge HCT®

Index Terms Amlodipine Besylate, Valsartan, and Hydrochlorothiazide; Amlodipine, Hydrochlorothiazide, and Valsartan; Hydrochlorothiazide, Amlodipine, and Valsartan; Valsartan, Hydrochlorothiazide, and Amlodipine

Pharmacologic Category Angiotensin II Receptor Blocker; Antianginal Agent; Antihypertensive; Calcium Channel Blocker; Calcium Channel Blocker, Dihydropyridine; Diuretic, Thiazide

Use Treatment of hypertension (not for initial therapy)

Pregnancy Risk Factor D

Dosage Oral: **Note:** Not for initial therapy. Dose is individualized; combination product may be substituted for individual components in patients currently maintained on all three agents separately or in patients not adequately controlled with any two of the following antihypertensive classes: Calcium channel blockers, angiotensin II receptor blockers, and diuretics.

Adults: Hypertension: Add-on/switch/replacement therapy: Amlodipine 5-10 mg and valsartan 160-320 mg and hydrochlorothiazide 12.5-25 mg once daily; dose may be titrated after 2 weeks of therapy. Maximum recommended daily dose: Amlodipine 10 mg/valsartan 320 mg/ hydrochlorothiazide 25 mg

Elderly: Use of lower initial doses should be considered.

Dosage adjustment in renal impairment:

CrCl ≥30 mL/minute: No dosage adjustment necessary.

CrCl <30 mL/minute: No dosage adjustment provided in manufacturer's labeling; safety and efficacy has not been established; hydrochlorothiazide is usually ineffective when CrCl <30 mL/minute and is contraindicated in patients who are anuric.

Dosage adjustment in hepatic impairment:

Mild-to-moderate impairment: Use with caution; amlodipine elimination prolonged and valsartan exposure doubled in patients with mild-to-moderate chronic disease compared to healthy volunteers. No dosage adjustment for valsartan is necessary; however, a lower initial amlodipine dose may be required (possibly requiring use of the individual agents).

Severe impairment: No dosage adjustment provided in manufacturer's labeling; however, similar to patients with mild to moderate impairment, a lower initial amlodipine dose may be required (possibly requiring use of the individual agents); titrate slowly.

Additional Information Complete prescribing information should be consulted for additional detail.

Dosage Forms

Tablet, oral:

Exforge HCT®: Amlodipine 5 mg, valsartan 160 mg, and hydrochlorothiazide 12.5 mg; Amlodipine 5 mg, valsartan 160 mg, and hydrochlorothiazide 25 mg; Amlodipine 10 mg, valsartan 160 mg, and hydrochlorothiazide 12.5 mg; Amlodipine 10 mg, valsartan 160 mg, and hydrochlorothiazide 25 mg; Amlodipine 10 mg, valsartan 320 mg, and hydrochlorothiazide 25 mg

◆ **Ammens® Original Medicated [OTC]** *see* Zinc Oxide *on page 2200*

◆ **Ammens® Shower Fresh [OTC]** *see* Zinc Oxide *on page 2200*

◆ **Ammonapse** *see* Sodium Phenylbutyrate *on page 1908*

Ammonium Chloride (a MOE nee um KLOR ide)

Pharmacologic Category Electrolyte Supplement, Parenteral

Use Treatment of hypochloremic states or metabolic alkalosis

Pregnancy Risk Factor C

Dosage Metabolic alkalosis: The following equations represent different methods of correction utilizing either the serum HCO_3^-, the serum chloride, or the base excess

Dosing of mEq NH_4 Cl via the chloride-deficit method (hypochloremia):

Dose of mEq NH_4Cl = [0.2 L/kg x body weight (kg)] x [103 - observed serum chloride]; administer 50% of dose over 12 hours, then re-evaluate

Note: 0.2 L/kg is the estimated chloride volume of distribution and 103 is the average normal serum chloride concentration (mEq/L)

Dosing of mEq NH_4 Cl via the bicarbonate-excess method (refractory hypochloremic metabolic alkalosis):

Dose of NH_4Cl = [0.5 L/kg x body weight (kg)] x (observed serum HCO_3^- - 24); administer 50% of dose over 12 hours, then re-evaluate

Note: 0.5 L/kg is the estimated bicarbonate volume of distribution and 24 is the average normal serum bicarbonate concentration (mEq/L)

These equations will yield different requirements of ammonium chloride

Dosage adjustment in renal impairment: Severe impairment: use is contraindicated.

Dosage adjustment in hepatic impairment: Severe impairment: use is contraindicated.

Additional Information Complete prescribing information should be consulted for additional detail.

Dosage Forms

Injection, solution: Ammonium 5 mEq/mL and chloride 5 mEq/mL (20 mL)

◆ **Ammonul®** *see* Sodium Phenylacetate and Sodium Benzoate *on page 1908*

◆ **AMN107** *see* Nilotinib *on page 1454*

◆ **Amnesteem** *see* ISOtretinoin *on page 1127*

Amobarbital (am oh BAR bi tal)

Brand Names: U.S. Amytal Sodium
Brand Names: Canada Amytal®
Index Terms Amobarbital Sodium; Amylobarbitone
Pharmacologic Category Barbiturate
Additional Appendix Information
Beers Criteria – Potentially Inappropriate Medications for Geriatrics *on page 2271*
Use Hypnotic in short-term treatment of insomnia; reduce anxiety and provide sedation preoperatively
Pregnancy Risk Factor D
Dosage
Children:
Sedative: IM, IV: 6 to 12 years: Manufacturer's dosing range: 65 to 500 mg
Hypnotic (off-label use): IM: 2 to 3 mg/kg (maximum: 500 mg)
Adults:
Hypnotic: IM, IV: 65 to 200 mg at bedtime (maximum single dose: 1000 mg)
Sedative: IM, IV: 30 to 50 mg 2 to 3 times/day (maximum single dose: 1000 mg)
"Amytal interview" (off-label use): IV: 50 to 100 mg/minute for total dose of 200 to 1000 mg or until patient experiences drowsiness, impaired attention, slurred speech, or nystagmus (Kavirajan 1999)
Wada test (off-label use): Intra-carotid: 60 to 200 mg (usual dose: 125 mg) over 2 to 5 seconds via percutaneous transfemoral catheter; after 30 to 45 minutes has elapsed since completion of first injection, may repeat dose for evaluation of contralateral hemisphere (Acharya, 1997; Patel, 2011). **Note:** Due to the adverse effects associated with intra-carotid amobarbital and questionable reliability and validity, other less invasive tests (eg, functional MRI) may be recommended (Sharan, 2011).
Dosing adjustment in renal/hepatic impairment: Dosing should be reduced; specific recommendations not available.
Additional Information Complete prescribing information should be consulted for additional detail.
Dosage Forms
Solution Reconstituted, Injection:
Amytal Sodium: 500 mg (1 ea)

◆ **Amobarbital Sodium** *see* Amobarbital *on page 128*
◆ **Amoclan** *see* Amoxicillin and Clavulanate *on page 133*

Amorolfine [INT] (a MOE role fen)

International Brand Names Amocoat (TW); Ariva (HR); Curanail (FR); Curanel (CH); Finail (DK, SE); Fungilac (HR); Laquifun (AR); Loceryl (AE, AR, AT, BE, BH, BR, CH, CL, CN, CO, CR, CY, CZ, DE, DK, DO, EC, EE, FI, FR, GB, GR, GT, HK, HN, HU, IE, IL, IN, IS, KR, KW, LB, LT, MY, NI, NO, NZ, PA, PE, PL, QA, RU, SA, SE, SG, SI, SK, SV, TH, TR, TW, UY, VE, ZA); Loceryl Nail Lacquer (AU); Locetar (ES, IT, PH, PT); Micobutina (AR); Odenil (ES); Pekiron (TW)
Index Terms Amorolfine Hydrochloride
Pharmacologic Category Antifungal Agent, Topical
Reported Use Topical treatment of nail infections caused by a variety of fungi (onychomycosis)
Dosage Range Topical: Apply to affected toenails or fingernails once or twice weekly. Treatment may be needed for ~6 months for fingernails or 9-12 months for toenails.
Product Availability Product available in various countries; not currently available in the U.S.
Dosage Forms
Liquid, topical, as hydrochloride: 250 mg/5 mL (5 mL) [packaged with 10 spatulas, 30 cleaning pads, and 30 nail files]

◆ **Amorolfine Hydrochloride** *see* Amorolfine [INT] *on page 128*

Amoxapine (a MOKS a peen)

Index Terms Asendin [DSC]
Pharmacologic Category Antidepressant, Tricyclic (Secondary Amine)
Additional Appendix Information
Beers Criteria – Potentially Inappropriate Medications for Geriatrics *on page 2271*
Use Depression: For the relief of symptoms of depression in patients with neurotic or reactive depressive disorders as well as endogenous and psychotic depressions; for depression accompanied by anxiety or agitation.
Pregnancy Risk Factor C
Pregnancy Considerations Adverse events were observed in some animal reproduction studies. Tricyclic antidepressants may be associated with irritability, jitteriness, and convulsions (rare) in the neonate (Yonkers, 2009).

The ACOG recommends that therapy for depression during pregnancy be individualized; treatment should incorporate the clinical expertise of the mental health clinician, obstetrician, primary healthcare provider, and pediatrician (ACOG, 2008). According to the American Psychiatric Association (APA), the risks of medication treatment should be weighed against other treatment options and untreated depression. For women who discontinue antidepressant medications during pregnancy and who may be at high risk for postpartum depression, the medications can be restarted following delivery (APA, 2010). Treatment algorithms have been developed by the ACOG and the APA for the management of depression in women prior to conception and during pregnancy (Yonkers, 2009).
Breast-Feeding Considerations Amoxapine is excreted into breast milk. A case report notes low concentrations of amoxapine and its active metabolite in the milk of a nonnursing woman who developed galactorrhea during therapy (Gelenberg, 1979). The manufacturer recommends that caution be used if administered to a nursing woman.
Contraindications Hypersensitivity to amoxapine, any component of the formulation, or dibenzoxazepine compounds; use with or within 14 days of MAO inhibitors; acute recovery phase following myocardial infarction
Warnings/Precautions [U.S. Boxed Warning]: Antidepressants increase the risk of suicidal thinking and behavior in children, adolescents, and young adults (18 to 24 years of age) with major depressive disorder (MDD) and other psychiatric disorders; consider risk prior to prescribing. Short-term studies did not show an increased risk in patients >24 years of age and showed a decreased risk in patients ≥65 years. Closely monitor for clinical worsening, suicidality, or unusual changes in behavior, particularly during the initial 1 to 2 months of therapy or during periods of dosage adjustments (increases or decreases); the patient's family or caregiver should be instructed to closely observe the patient and communicate condition with healthcare provider. A medication guide should be dispensed with each prescription. **Amoxapine is not FDA approved for use in pediatric patients.**

The possibility of a suicide attempt is inherent in major depression and may persist until remission occurs. Use caution in high-risk patients. Worsening depression and severe abrupt suicidality that are not part of the presenting symptoms may require discontinuation or modification of drug therapy. The patient's family or caregiver should be alerted to monitor patients for the emergence of suicidality and associated behaviors (such as agitation, irritability, hostility, impulsivity, and hypomania) and notify the healthcare provider.

May precipitate a shift to mania or hypomania in patients with bipolar disorder. Patients presenting with depressive symptoms should be screened for bipolar disorder. Monotherapy in patients with bipolar disorder should be avoided. Patients presenting with depressive symptoms should be screened for bipolar disorder, including details regarding family history of suicide, bipolar disorder, and depression. **Amoxapine is not FDA approved for bipolar depression.** May cause extrapyramidal symptoms, including pseudoparkinsonism, acute dystonic reactions, akathisia, and tardive dyskinesia (risk of these reactions is low). Risk of dystonia (and possibly other EPS) may be greater with increased doses, use of conventional antipsychotics, males, and younger patients (APA, 2004). Risk of tardive dyskinesia (potentially irreversible) is often associated with total cumulative dose, therapy duration, and may also be increased in elderly patients (particularly elderly women); antipsychotics may also mask signs/symptoms of tardive dyskinesia. Therapy should be discontinued in any patient if signs/symptoms of tardive dyskinesia appear. May be associated with neuroleptic malignant syndrome.

May cause anticholinergic effects (constipation, xerostomia, blurred vision, urinary retention); use with caution in patients with decreased gastrointestinal motility, paralytic ileus, urinary retention, BPH, xerostomia, or visual problems. The degree of anticholinergic blockade produced by this agent is high relative to other antidepressants (Bauer, 2013). May cause CNS depression, which may impair physical or mental abilities; patients must be cautioned about performing tasks that require mental alertness (eg, operating machinery or driving). The degree of sedation is moderate relative to other antidepressants (Bauer, 2013). Use with caution in patients with a history of cardiovascular disease (including previous MI, stroke, tachycardia, or conduction abnormalities). May lower seizure threshold; use caution in patients with a previous seizure disorder or condition predisposing to seizures such as brain damage, alcoholism, or concurrent therapy with other drugs which lower the seizure threshold (APA, 2010). May increase the risks associated with electroconvulsive therapy. Bone fractures have been associated with antidepressant treatment. Consider the possibility of a fragility fracture if an antidepressant-treated patient presents with unexplained bone pain, point tenderness, swelling, or bruising (Rabenda, 2013; Rizzoli, 2012). Use with caution in patients with diabetes mellitus; may alter glucose regulation (APA, 2010).

May cause mild pupillary dilation which in susceptible individuals can lead to an episode of narrow-angle glaucoma. Consider evaluating patients who have not had an iridectomy for narrow-angle glaucoma risk factors. Use caution in elderly patients; may cause or exacerbate syndrome of inappropriate antidiuretic hormone secretion or hyponatremia; monitor sodium closely with initiation or dosage adjustments in older adults. May be inappropriate in older adults depending on comorbidities (eg, dementia, delirium) or in patients with a history of falls and fractures due to its potent anticholinergic effects (Beers Criteria). May also have increased risk of adverse events, including tardive dyskinesia (particularly older women) and sedation. Potentially significant interactions may exist, requiring dose or frequency adjustment, additional monitoring, and/or selection of alternative therapy.

Abrupt discontinuation or interruption of antidepressant therapy has been associated with a discontinuation syndrome. Symptoms arising may vary with antidepressant however commonly include nausea, vomiting, diarrhea, headaches, lightheadedness, dizziness, diminished appetite, sweating, chills, tremors, paresthesias, fatigue, somnolence, and sleep disturbances (eg, vivid dreams, insomnia). Greater risks for developing a discontinuation syndrome have been associated with antidepressants with shorter half-lives, longer durations of treatment, and abrupt discontinuation. For antidepressants of short or intermediate half-lives, symptoms may emerge within 2 to 5 days after treatment discontinuation and last 7 to 14 days (APA, 2010; Fava, 2006; Haddad, 2001; Shelton, 2001; Warner, 2006).

Adverse Reactions

Cardiovascular: Edema, palpitations

Central nervous system: Anxiety, ataxia, confusion, dizziness, drowsiness, EEG pattern changes, excitement, fatigue, headache, insomnia, nervousness, nightmares, restlessness

Dermatologic: Diaphoresis, skin rash

Endocrine & metabolic: Increased serum prolactin

Gastrointestinal: Constipation, increased appetite, nausea, xerostomia

Neuromuscular & skeletal: Tremor, weakness

Ophthalmic: Blurred vision

Rare but important or life-threatening: Accommodation disturbance, agranulocytosis, alopecia, altered serum glucose, anorexia, atrial arrhythmia, diarrhea, extrapyramidal reaction, galactorrhea, hallucination, heart block, hepatic insufficiency, hepatitis, hypersensitivity reaction, hypomania, impotence, increased intraocular pressure, lack of concentration, menstrual disease, mydriasis, myocardial infarction, neuroleptic malignant syndrome, numbness, painful ejaculation, pancreatitis, paralytic ileus, paresthesia, parotid swelling, petechia, purpura, SIADH, skin photosensitivity, syncope, tardive dyskinesia, testicular swelling, thrombocytopenia, tingling sensation, tinnitus, urinary retention, vasculitis, vomiting, weight gain

Drug Interactions

Metabolism/Transport Effects Substrate of CYP2D6 (major); **Note:** Assignment of Major/Minor substrate status based on clinically relevant drug interaction potential

Avoid Concomitant Use

Avoid concomitant use of Amoxapine with any of the following: Aclidinium; Azelastine (Nasal); Dapoxetine; Glucagon; Iobenguane I 123; Ipratropium (Oral Inhalation); Linezolid; MAO Inhibitors; Methylene Blue; Moxonidine; Orphenadrine; Paraldehyde; Potassium Chloride; Thalidomide; Tiotropium; Umeclidinium

Increased Effect/Toxicity

Amoxapine may increase the levels/effects of: AbobotulinumtoxinA; Alcohol (Ethyl); Alpha-/Beta-Agonists (Direct-Acting); Alpha1-Agonists; Amphetamines; Analgesics (Opioid); Anticholinergic Agents; Antipsychotic Agents; Azelastine (Nasal); Beta2-Agonists; Buprenorphine; Citalopram; CNS Depressants; Desmopressin; Escitalopram; Glucagon; Highest Risk QTc-Prolonging Agents; Hydrocodone; Methotrimeprazine; Methylene Blue; Metyrosine; Mirabegron; Moderate Risk QTc-Prolonging Agents; Nicorandil; OnabotulinumtoxinA; Orphenadrine; Paraldehyde; Potassium Chloride; Pramipexole; QuiNIDine; RimabotulinumtoxinB; ROPINIRole; Rotigotine; Serotonin Modulators; Sodium Phosphates; Sulfonylureas; Suvorexant; Thalidomide; Thiazide Diuretics; Tiotropium; Topiramate; TraMADol; Vitamin K Antagonists; Yohimbine; Zolpidem

The levels/effects of Amoxapine may be increased by: Abiraterone Acetate; Aclidinium; Altretamine; Antiemetics (5HT3 Antagonists); Antipsychotic Agents; Brimonidine (Topical); Cannabis; Cimetidine; Cinacalcet; Citalopram;

Cobicistat; CYP2D6 Inhibitors (Moderate); CYP2D6 Inhibitors (Strong); Dapoxetine; Darunavir; Dexmethylphenidate; Doxylamine; Dronabinol; Droperidol; DULoxetine; Escitalopram; FLUoxetine; FluvoxaMINE; HydrOXYzine; Ipratropium (Oral Inhalation); Kava Kava; Linezolid; Lithium; Magnesium Sulfate; MAO Inhibitors; Methotrimeprazine; Methylphenidate; Metoclopramide; Metyrosine; Mianserin; Mifepristone; Nabilone; PARoxetine; Peginterferon Alfa-2b; Perampanel; Pramlintide; Protease Inhibitors; QuiNIDine; Rufinamide; Sertraline; Sodium Oxybate; Tapentadol; Tedizolid; Terbinafine (Systemic); Tetrahydrocannabinol; Thyroid Products; TraMADol; Umeclidinium; Valproic Acid and Derivatives

Decreased Effect

Amoxapine may decrease the levels/effects of: Acetylcholinesterase Inhibitors; Alpha1-Agonists; Alpha2-Agonists; Alpha2-Agonists (Ophthalmic); Iobenguane I 123; Ioflupane I 123; Itopride; Moxonidine; Secretin

The levels/effects of Amoxapine may be decreased by: Acetylcholinesterase Inhibitors; Barbiturates; CarBAMazepine; Peginterferon Alfa-2b; St Johns Wort

Storage/Stability Store at 20°C to 25°C (68°F to 77°F).

Mechanism of Action Reduces the reuptake of serotonin and norepinephrine. The metabolite, 7-OH-amoxapine has significant dopamine receptor blocking activity similar to antipsychotic agents.

Pharmacodynamics/Kinetics

Onset of antidepressant effect: Usually occurs after 1 to 2 weeks, but may require 4 to 6 weeks

Absorption: Rapid and well absorbed

Distribution: V_d: 0.9 to 1.2 L/kg

Protein binding: ~90%

Metabolism: Extensively metabolized; hepatic hydroxylation produces two active metabolites, 7-hydroxyamoxapine (7-OH-amoxapine) and 8-hydroxyamoxapine (8-OH-amoxapine); metabolites undergo conjugation to form glucuronides

Half-life elimination: 8 hours; 8-hydroxyamoxapine metabolite: 30 hours

Time to peak, serum: ~90 minutes

Excretion: Urine

Dosage

Depression: Oral:

Adults: Initial: 50 mg once to 3 times daily. Doses may be increased to 100 mg 2 to 3 times daily by the end of the first week based on response and tolerability; if 300 mg daily has been reached and maintained for at least 2 weeks and no response is observed, may further increase to 400 mg daily. Hospitalized patients refractory to antidepressant therapy (and no history of seizures) may be cautiously titrated to 600 mg daily in divided doses. Usual dosage: 100 to 400 mg daily (Bauer, 2013). Once an effective dose is reached, doses ≤300 mg may be given once daily at bedtime and doses >300 mg daily should be divided. Maximum daily dose: 400 mg outpatient; 600 mg hospitalized patients.

Elderly: Initial: 25 mg 2 to 3 times daily. Dose may be increased to 50 mg 2 to 3 times daily by the end of the first week based on response and tolerability; if dose is ineffective, may further increase cautiously to 300 mg daily. Usual dosage: 100 to 150 mg daily. Once an effective dose is reached, doses ≤300 mg may be given once daily at bedtime. Maximum daily dose: 300 mg.

Discontinuation of therapy: Upon discontinuation of antidepressant therapy, gradually taper the dose to minimize the incidence of withdrawal symptoms and allow for the detection of re-emerging symptoms. Evidence supporting ideal taper rates is limited. APA and NICE guidelines suggest tapering therapy over at least several weeks with consideration to the half-life of the antidepressant; antidepressants with a shorter half-life may need to be tapered more conservatively. In addition for long-term treated patients, WFSBP guidelines recommend tapering over 4 to 6 months. If intolerable withdrawal symptoms occur following a dose reduction, consider resuming the previously prescribed dose and/or decrease dose at a more gradual rate (APA, 2010; Bauer, 2002; Haddad, 2001; NCCMH, 2010; Schatzberg, 2006; Shelton, 2001; Warner, 2006).

MAO inhibitor recommendations:

Switching to or from an MAO inhibitor intended to treat psychiatric disorders:

Allow 14 days to elapse between discontinuing an MAO inhibitor intended to treat psychiatric disorders and initiation of amoxapine.

Allow 14 days to elapse between discontinuing amoxapine and initiation of an MAO inhibitor intended to treat psychiatric disorders.

Use with reversible MAO inhibitors (such as linezolid or IV methylene blue):

Do not initiate amoxapine in patients receiving linezolid or IV methylene blue; consider other interventions for psychiatric condition.

If urgent treatment with linezolid or IV methylene blue is required in a patient already receiving amoxapine and potential benefits outweigh potential risks, discontinue amoxapine promptly and administer linezolid or IV methylene blue. Monitor for serotonin syndrome for 2 weeks or until 24 hours after the last dose of linezolid or IV methylene blue, whichever comes first. May resume amoxapine 24 hours after the last dose of linezolid or IV methylene blue.

Dosage adjustment in renal impairment: There are no dosage adjustments provided in the manufacturer's labeling. However, amoxapine is primarily eliminated renally, and renal failure may develop in overdoses; use with caution.

Dosage adjustment in hepatic impairment: There are no dosage adjustments provided in the manufacturer's labeling.

Monitoring Parameters Evaluate mental status, suicide ideation (especially at the beginning of therapy or when doses are increased or decreased); anxiety, social functioning, mania, panic attacks, or other unusual changes in behavior; heart rate, blood pressure, and ECG in older adults and patients with preexisting cardiac disease; blood glucose; weight and BMI (APA, 2010).

Additional Information Extrapyramidal reactions and tardive dyskinesia may occur.

Dosage Forms

Tablet, Oral:

Generic: 25 mg, 50 mg, 100 mg, 150 mg

Amoxicillin (a moks i SIL in)

Brand Names: U.S. Moxatag

Brand Names: Canada Apo-Amoxi®; Mylan-Amoxicillin; Novamoxin®; NTP-Amoxicillin; Nu-Amoxi; PHL-Amoxicillin; PMS-Amoxicillin; Pro-Amox-250; Pro-Amox-500

Index Terms *p*-Hydroxyampicillin; Amoxicillin Trihydrate; Amoxil; Amoxycillin

Pharmacologic Category Antibiotic, Penicillin

Use Treatment of otitis media, sinusitis, and infections caused by susceptible organisms involving the upper and lower respiratory tract, skin, and urinary tract; as part of a multidrug regimen for *H. pylori* eradication; periodontitis

Pregnancy Risk Factor B

Pregnancy Considerations Adverse events have not been observed in animal reproduction studies. Maternal use of amoxicillin has generally not resulted in an increased risk of adverse fetal effects; however, an increased risk of cleft lip with cleft palate has been observed in some studies. It is the drug of choice for the treatment of chlamydial infections in pregnancy and for anthrax prophylaxis when penicillin susceptibility is documented. Amoxicillin may be used in certain situations prior to vaginal delivery in women at high risk for endocarditis.

Due to pregnancy-induced physiologic changes, oral amoxicillin clearance is increased during pregnancy resulting in lower concentrations and smaller AUCs. Oral ampicillin-class antibiotics are poorly absorbed during labor.

Breast-Feeding Considerations Very small amounts of amoxicillin are excreted in breast milk. The manufacturer recommends that caution be exercised when administering amoxicillin to nursing women. Nondose-related effects could include modification of bowel flora and allergic sensitization of the infant.

Contraindications Hypersensitivity to amoxicillin, penicillin, other beta-lactams, or any component of the formulation

Warnings/Precautions In patients with renal impairment, doses and/or frequency of administration should be modified in response to the degree of renal impairment; in addition, use of certain dosage forms (eg, extended release 775 mg tablet and immediate release 875 mg tablet) should be avoided in patients with CrCl <30 mL/minute or patients requiring hemodialysis. A high percentage of patients with infectious mononucleosis have developed rash during therapy with amoxicillin; ampicillin-class antibiotics not recommended in these patients. Serious and occasionally severe or fatal hypersensitivity (anaphylactoid) reactions have been reported in patients on penicillin therapy, especially with a history of beta-lactam hypersensitivity, history of sensitivity to multiple allergens, or previous IgE-mediated reactions (eg, anaphylaxis, angioedema, urticaria). Use with caution in asthmatic patients. Prolonged use may result in fungal or bacterial superinfection, including *C. difficile*-associated diarrhea (CDAD) and pseudomembranous colitis; CDAD has been observed >2 months postantibiotic treatment.

Chewable tablets contain phenylalanine.

Benzyl alcohol and derivatives: Some dosage forms may contain sodium benzoate/benzoic acid; benzoic acid (benzoate) is a metabolite of benzyl alcohol; large amounts of benzyl alcohol (≥99 mg/kg/day) have been associated with a potentially fatal toxicity ("gasping syndrome") in neonates; the "gasping syndrome" consists of metabolic acidosis, respiratory distress, gasping respirations, CNS dysfunction (including convulsions, intracranial hemorrhage), hypotension, and cardiovascular collapse (AAP, 1997; CDC, 1982); some data suggests that benzoate displaces bilirubin from protein binding sites (Ahlfors, 2001); avoid or use dosage forms containing benzyl alcohol derivative with caution in neonates. See manufacturer's labeling.

Adverse Reactions

Cardiovascular: Hypersensitivity angiitis

Central nervous system: Agitation, anxiety, behavioral changes, confusion, dizziness, headache, hyperactivity (reversible), insomnia, seizure

Dermatologic: Acute generalized exanthematous pustulosis, erythematous maculopapular rash, erythema multiforme, exfoliative dermatitis, Stevens-Johnson syndrome, toxic epidermal necrolysis, urticaria

Gastrointestinal: Dental discoloration (brown, yellow, or gray; rare), diarrhea, hemorrhagic colitis, melanoglossia, mucocutaneous candidiasis, nausea, pseudomembranous colitis, vomiting

Genitourinary: Crystalluria

Hematologic & oncologic: Agranulocytosis, anemia, eosinophilia, hemolytic anemia, leukopenia,thrombocytopenia, thrombocytopenia purpura

Hepatic: Cholestatic hepatitis, cholestatic jaundice, hepatitis (acute cytolytic), increased serum ALT, increased serum AST

Hypersensitivity: Anaphylaxis

Immunologic: Serum sickness-like reaction

Drug Interactions

Metabolism/Transport Effects None known.

Avoid Concomitant Use

Avoid concomitant use of Amoxicillin with any of the following: BCG; Probenecid

Increased Effect/Toxicity

Amoxicillin may increase the levels/effects of: Methotrexate; Vitamin K Antagonists

The levels/effects of Amoxicillin may be increased by: Allopurinol; Probenecid

Decreased Effect

Amoxicillin may decrease the levels/effects of: BCG; Mycophenolate; Sodium Picosulfate; Typhoid Vaccine

The levels/effects of Amoxicillin may be decreased by: Tetracycline Derivatives

Storage/Stability

Amoxil®: Oral suspension remains stable for 14 days at room temperature or if refrigerated (refrigeration preferred). Unit-dose antibiotic oral syringes are stable at room temperature for at least 72 hours (Tu, 1988).

Moxatag™: Store at 25°C (77°F); excursions permitted to 15°C to 30°C (59°F to 86°F).

Mechanism of Action Inhibits bacterial cell wall synthesis by binding to one or more of the penicillin-binding proteins (PBPs) which in turn inhibits the final transpeptidation step of peptidoglycan synthesis in bacterial cell walls, thus inhibiting cell wall biosynthesis. Bacteria eventually lyse due to ongoing activity of cell wall autolytic enzymes (autolysins and murein hydrolases) while cell wall assembly is arrested.

Pharmacodynamics/Kinetics

Absorption: Oral: Rapid and nearly complete; food does not interfere

Extended-release tablet: Rate of absorption is slower compared to immediate-release formulations; food decreases the rate but not extent of absorption

Distribution: Readily into liver, lungs, prostate, muscle, middle ear effusions, maxillary sinus secretions, bone, gallbladder, bile, and into ascitic and synovial fluids; poor CSF penetration (except when meninges are inflamed)

CSF:blood level ratio: Normal meninges: <1%; Inflamed meninges: 8% to 90%

Protein binding: 17% to 20%

Metabolism: Partially hepatic

Half-life elimination:

Neonates, full-term: 3.7 hours

Infants and Children: 1-2 hours

Adults: Normal renal function: 0.7-1.4 hours

CrCl <10 mL/minute: 7-21 hours

Time to peak: Capsule: 2 hours; Extended-release tablet: 3.1 hours; Suspension: 1 hour

Excretion: Urine (60% as unchanged drug); lower in neonates

Note: Extended-release tablets: In healthy volunteers, serum drug concentrations were below 0.25 mcg/mL and undetectable at 16 hours following dosing.

Dosage

Usual dosage range:

Children ≤3 months: Oral: 20-30 mg/kg/day divided every 12 hours

Children >3 months and <40 kg: Oral: 20-100 mg/kg/day in divided doses every 8-12 hours

Children >3 months and ≥40 kg: Refer to adult dosing

Children ≥12 years: Oral: Extended-release tablet: 775 mg once daily

Adults: Oral: 250-500 mg every 8 hours or 500-875 mg twice daily

Extended-release tablet: 775 mg once daily

Indication-specific dosing:

Children >3 months and <40 kg: Oral: **Note:** In general, children >3 months and ≥40 kg should be dosed according to the adult recommendations except where indicated.

Acute otitis media: 80-90 mg/kg/day divided every 12 hours

Community-acquired pneumonia (CAP) (IDSA/PIDS, 2011): Note: In children ≥5 years, a macrolide antibiotic should be added if atypical pneumonia cannot be ruled out.

Empiric treatment or *S. pneumoniae* (MICs to penicillin ≤2.0 mcg/mL) (preferred): 90 mg/kg/day in 2-3 divided doses (maximum: 4 g/day). **Note:** Dividing in 3 doses is recommended for MIC = 2 mcg/mL.

Group A *Streptococcus* (moderate-to-severe) (preferred): 50-75 mg/kg/day in 2 divided doses (maximum: 4 g/day)

H. influenzae (beta-lactamase negative) mild infection (preferred): 75-100 mg/kg/day in 3 divided doses (maximum: 4 g/day)

Ear, nose, throat, genitourinary tract, or skin/skin structure infections: Note: Amoxicillin-clavulanate is preferred for first-line treatment of acute bacterial rhinosinusitis (Chow, 2012):

Mild-to-moderate: 25 mg/kg/day in divided doses every 12 hours **or** 20 mg/kg/day in divided doses every 8 hours

Severe: 45 mg/kg/day in divided doses every 12 hours **or** 40 mg/kg/day in divided doses every 8 hours

Tonsillitis and/or pharyngitis: Children ≥12 years: Extended-release tablet: 775 mg once daily

Lower respiratory tract infections: 45 mg/kg/day in divided doses every 12 hours **or** 40 mg/kg/day in divided doses every 8 hours

Lyme disease: 25-50 mg/kg/day divided every 8 hours (maximum: 500 mg)

Pharyngitis, group A streptococci (IDSA guidelines): 50 mg/kg once daily or alternatively, 25 mg/kg twice daily (maximum total daily dose: 1000 mg) for 10 days (Shulman, 2012)

Postexposure inhalational anthrax prophylaxis (ACIP recommendations): Children <40 kg: 45 mg/kg/day divided into 3 daily doses (maximum: 500 mg/dose) (ACIP, 2010). **Note:** The AAP recommends a higher dose (80 mg/kg/day divided into 3 daily doses [maximum: 500 mg/dose]) due to the lack of data on amoxicillin dosages for treating anthrax and the high mortality rate.

Note: Use **only** if isolates of the specific *B. anthracis* are sensitive to amoxicillin (MIC ≤0.125 mcg/mL). Duration of antibiotic postexposure prophylaxis (PEP) is ≥60 days in a previously-unvaccinated exposed person. Antimicrobial therapy should continue for 14 days after the third dose of PEP vaccine. Those who are partially or fully vaccinated should receive at least a 30-day course of antimicrobial PEP and continue with licensed vaccination regimen. Unvaccinated workers, even those wearing personal protective equipment with adequate respiratory protection, should receive antimicrobial PEP. Antimicrobial PEP is not required for fully-vaccinated people (five-dose IM vaccination series with a yearly booster) who enter an anthrax area clothed in personal protective equipment. If respiratory protection is disrupted, a 30-day course of antimicrobial therapy is recommended (ACIP, 2010).

Prophylaxis against infective endocarditis (off-label use): 50 mg/kg 30-60 minutes before procedure. **Note:** American Heart Association (AHA) guidelines now recommend prophylaxis only in patients undergoing invasive procedures and in whom underlying cardiac conditions may predispose to a higher risk of adverse outcomes should infection occur. As of April 2007, routine prophylaxis for GI/GU procedures is no longer recommended by the AHA.

Adults: Oral:

Chlamydial infection during pregnancy (off-label use): 500 mg 3 times/day for 7 days (CDC, 2010)

Ear, nose, throat, genitourinary tract, or skin/skin structure infections: Note: Amoxicillin-clavulanate is preferred for first-line treatment of acute bacterial rhinosinusitis (Chow, 2012):

Mild-to-moderate: 500 mg every 12 hours **or** 250 mg every 8 hours

Severe: 875 mg every 12 hours **or** 500 mg every 8 hours

Tonsillitis and/or pharyngitis: Extended-release tablet: 775 mg once daily

***Helicobacter pylori* eradication:** 1000 mg twice daily; requires combination therapy with at least one other antibiotic and an acid-suppressing agent (proton pump inhibitor or H_2 blocker)

Lower respiratory tract infections: 875 mg every 12 hours **or** 500 mg every 8 hours

Lyme disease: 500 mg every 6-8 hours (depending on size of patient) for 21-30 days

Periodontitis (aggressive) (in combination with metronidazole) associated with presense of *Actinobacillus actinomycetemcomitans* (AA): Oral: 500 mg every 8 hours for 10 days used in addition to scaling and root planing (Varela, 2011)

Pharyngitis, group A streptococci (IDSA guidelines): 1000 mg once daily or 500 mg twice daily (maximum daily dose: 1000 mg) for 10 days (Shulman, 2012)

Postexposure inhalational anthrax prophylaxis (ACIP recommendations): 500 mg every 8 hours. **Note:** Use **only** if isolates of the specific *B. anthracis* are sensitive to amoxicillin (MIC ≤0.125 mcg/mL); may be administered to pregnant and breast-feeding women. Duration of antibiotic postexposure prophylaxis (PEP) is ≥60 days in a previously unvaccinated exposed person. Antimicrobial therapy should continue for 14 days after the third dose of PEP vaccine. Those who are partially or fully vaccinated should receive at least a 30-day course of antimicrobial PEP and continue with licensed vaccination regimen. Unvaccinated workers, even those wearing personal protective equipment with adequate respiratory protection, should receive antimicrobial PEP. Antimicrobial PEP is not required for fully vaccinated people (five-dose IM vaccination series with a yearly booster) who enter an anthrax area clothed in personal protective equipment. If respiratory protection is disrupted, a 30-day course of antimicrobial therapy is recommended (ACIP, 2010).

Prophylaxis against infective endocarditis: Oral: 2 g 30-60 minutes before procedure. **Note:** American Heart Association (AHA) guidelines now recommend prophylaxis only in patients undergoing invasive procedures and in whom underlying cardiac conditions may predispose to a higher risk of adverse outcomes should infection occur. As of April 2007, routine prophylaxis for GI/GU procedures is no longer recommended by the AHA.

Prophylaxis in total joint replacement patients undergoing dental procedures which produce bacteremia: 2 g 1 hour prior to procedure

Prosthetic joint infection, chronic antimicrobial suppression of prosthetic joint infection associated with beta-hemolytic streptococci, penicillin-susceptible *Enterococcus* spp, or *Propionibacterium* spp (off-label use): Oral: 500 mg 3 times daily (Osmon, 2013)

Dosage adjustment in renal impairment: Use of certain dosage forms (eg, extended-release 775 mg tablet and immediate-release 875 mg tablet) should be avoided in patients with CrCl <30 mL/minute or patients requiring hemodialysis.

CrCl 10-30 mL/minute: 250-500 mg every 12 hours

CrCl <10 mL/minute: 250-500 mg every 24 hours

Dialysis: Moderately dialyzable (20% to 50%) by hemo- or peritoneal dialysis; approximately 50 mg of amoxicillin per liter of filtrate is removed by continuous arteriovenous or venovenous hemofiltration; dose as per CrCl <10 mL/minute guidelines

Dosage adjustment in hepatic impairment: No dosage adjustment provided in manufacturer's labeling.

Dietary Considerations May be taken with food. Some products may contain phenylalanine.

Moxatag™: Take within 1 hour of finishing a meal.

Administration Administer around-the-clock to promote less variation in peak and trough serum levels. The appropriate amount of suspension may be mixed with formula, milk, fruit juice, water, ginger ale, or cold drinks; administer dose immediately after mixing.

Moxatag™ extended release tablet: Administer within 1 hour of finishing a meal.

Some penicillins (eg, carbenicillin, ticarcillin, and piperacillin) have been shown to inactivate aminoglycosides *in vitro*. This has been observed to a greater extent with tobramycin and gentamicin, while amikacin has shown greater stability against inactivation. Concurrent use of these agents may pose a risk of reduced antibacterial efficacy *in vivo*, particularly in the setting of profound renal impairment. However, definitive clinical evidence is lacking. If combination penicillin/aminoglycoside therapy is desired in a patient with renal dysfunction, separation of doses (if feasible), and routine monitoring of aminoglycoside levels, CBC, and clinical response should be considered.

Monitoring Parameters With prolonged therapy, monitor renal, hepatic, and hematologic function periodically; assess patient at beginning and throughout therapy for infection; monitor for signs of anaphylaxis during first dose

Dosage Forms

Capsule, Oral:

Generic: 250 mg, 500 mg

Suspension Reconstituted, Oral:

Generic: 125 mg/5 mL (80 mL, 100 mL, 150 mL); 200 mg/5 mL (50 mL, 75 mL, 100 mL); 250 mg/5 mL (80 mL, 100 mL, 150 mL); 400 mg/5 mL (50 mL, 75 mL, 100 mL)

Tablet, Oral:

Generic: 500 mg, 875 mg

Tablet Chewable, Oral:

Generic: 125 mg, 250 mg

Tablet Extended Release 24 Hour, Oral:

Moxatag: 775 mg

Generic: 775 mg

Amoxicillin and Clavulanate

(a moks i SIL in & klav yoo LAN ate)

Brand Names: U.S. Amoclan; Augmentin; Augmentin ES-600; Augmentin XR

Brand Names: Canada Amoxi-Clav; Apo-Amoxi-Clav; Clavulin; Novo-Clavamoxin; ratio-Aclavulanate

Index Terms Amoxicillin and Clavulanate Potassium; Amoxicillin and Clavulanic Acid; Amoxycillin and Clavulanate Potassium; Amoxycillin and Clavulanic Acid; Clavulanic Acid and Amoxicillin; Clavulanic Acid and Amoxycillin; Co-Amoxiclav

Pharmacologic Category Antibiotic, Penicillin

Use Treatment of otitis media, sinusitis, and infections caused by susceptible organisms involving the lower respiratory tract, skin and skin structure, and urinary tract; spectrum same as amoxicillin with additional coverage of beta-lactamase producing *B. catarrhalis*, *H. influenzae*, *N. gonorrhoeae*, and *S. aureus* (not MRSA). The expanded coverage of this combination makes it a useful alternative when amoxicillin resistance is present and patients cannot tolerate alternative treatments.

Pregnancy Risk Factor B

Pregnancy Considerations Adverse events have not been observed in animal reproduction studies. Both amoxicillin and clavulanic acid cross the placenta. Maternal use of amoxicillin/clavulanate has generally not resulted in an increased risk of birth defects. A possible increased risk of necrotizing enterocolitis in neonates or bowel disorders in children exposed to amoxicillin/clavulanate *in utero* has been observed. In women with acute infections during pregnancy, amoxicillin/clavulanate may be given if an antibiotic is required and appropriate based on bacterial sensitivity; however, use is not recommended in the management of preterm premature rupture of membranes. Oral ampicillin-class antibiotics are poorly absorbed during labor. When used during pregnancy, pharmacokinetic changes have been observed with amoxicillin alone (refer to the Amoxicillin monograph for details).

Breast-Feeding Considerations Amoxicillin is found in breast milk. The manufacturer recommends that caution be used if administered to breast-feeding women. The use of amoxicillin/clavulanate may be safe while breast-feeding. However, the risk of adverse events in the infant may be increased when compared to the use of amoxicillin alone and the risk may be related to maternal dose. Nondose-related effects could include modification of bowel flora and allergic sensitization of the infant.

Contraindications Hypersensitivity to amoxicillin, clavulanic acid, penicillin, or any component of the formulation; history of cholestatic jaundice or hepatic dysfunction with amoxicillin/clavulanate potassium therapy; Augmentin XR: severe renal impairment (CrCl <30 mL/minute) and hemodialysis patients

Canadian labeling: Additional contraindications (not in U.S. labeling): Hypersensitivity to cephalosporins; suspected or confirmed mononucleosis

Warnings/Precautions Hypersensitivity reactions, including anaphylaxis (some fatal), have been reported. Prolonged use may result in fungal or bacterial superinfection, including *C. difficile*-associated diarrhea (CDAD) and pseudomembranous colitis; CDAD has been observed >2 months postantibiotic treatment. In patients with renal impairment, doses and/or frequency of administration should be modified in response to the degree of renal impairment. High percentage of patients with infectious mononucleosis have developed rash during therapy; ampicillin-class antibiotics not recommended in these patients. Incidence of diarrhea is higher than with amoxicillin alone. Due to differing content of clavulanic acid, not all formulations are interchangeable; use of an inappropriate product for a specific dosage could result in either diarrhea (which may be severe) or subtherapeutic clavulanic acid concentrations leading to decreased clinical efficacy. Low incidence of cross-allergy with cephalosporins exists. Some products contain phenylalanine.

Adverse Reactions

Dermatologic: Diaper rash, skin rash, urticaria

Gastrointestinal: Abdominal distress, diarrhea, loose stools, nausea, vomiting

Genitourinary: Vaginitis

Infection: Candidiasis, vaginal mycosis

Rare but important or life-threatening: Cholestatic jaundice, flatulence, headache, hepatic insufficiency, hepatitis, increased liver enzymes, increased serum alkaline phosphatase, prolonged prothrombin time, thrombocythemia, vasculitis (hypersensitivity)

Additional adverse reactions seen with **ampicillin-class antibiotics:** Acute generalized exanthematous pustulosis, agitation, agranulocytosis, anaphylaxis, anemia, angioedema, anxiety, behavioral changes, confusion, convulsions, crystalluria, dental discoloration, dizziness, dyspepsia, enterocolitis, eosinophilia, erythema multiforme, exfoliative dermatitis, gastritis, glossitis, hematuria, hemolytic anemia, hemorrhagic colitis, hyperactivity, immune thrombocytopenia, increased serum bilirubin, increased serum transaminases, insomnia, interstitial nephritis, leukopenia, melanoglossia, mucocutaneous candidiasis, pruritus, pseudomembranous colitis, serum sickness-like reaction, Stevens-Johnson syndrome, stomatitis, thrombocytopenia, toxic epidermal necrolysis

Drug Interactions

Metabolism/Transport Effects None known.

Avoid Concomitant Use

Avoid concomitant use of Amoxicillin and Clavulanate with any of the following: BCG; Probenecid

Increased Effect/Toxicity

Amoxicillin and Clavulanate may increase the levels/effects of: Methotrexate; Vitamin K Antagonists

The levels/effects of Amoxicillin and Clavulanate may be increased by: Allopurinol; Probenecid

Decreased Effect

Amoxicillin and Clavulanate may decrease the levels/effects of: BCG; Mycophenolate; Sodium Picosulfate; Typhoid Vaccine

The levels/effects of Amoxicillin and Clavulanate may be decreased by: Tetracycline Derivatives

Preparation for Administration Reconstitute powder for oral suspension with appropriate amount of water as specified on the bottle. Shake vigorously until suspended.

Storage/Stability

Powder for oral suspension: Store dry powder at room temperature of 25°C (77°F). Reconstituted oral suspension should be kept in refrigerator. Discard unused suspension after 7-10 days (consult manufacturer labeling for specific recommendations). Unit-dose antibiotic oral syringes are stable under refrigeration for 24 hours (Tu, 1988).

Tablet: Store at room temperature of 25°C (77°F).

Mechanism of Action Clavulanic acid binds and inhibits beta-lactamases that inactivate amoxicillin resulting in amoxicillin having an expanded spectrum of activity. Amoxicillin inhibits bacterial cell wall synthesis by binding to one or more of the penicillin-binding proteins (PBPs) which in turn inhibits the final transpeptidation step of peptidoglycan synthesis in bacterial cell walls, thus inhibiting cell wall biosynthesis. Bacteria eventually lyse due to ongoing activity of cell wall autolytic enzymes (autolysins and murein hydrolases) while cell wall assembly is arrested.

Pharmacodynamics/Kinetics Amoxicillin pharmacokinetics are not affected by clavulanic acid.

Amoxicillin: See Amoxicillin monograph.

Clavulanic acid:

Protein binding: ~25%

Metabolism: Hepatic

Half-life elimination: 1 hour

Time to peak: 1 hour

Excretion: Urine (30% to 40% as unchanged drug)

Dosage Note: Dose is based on the amoxicillin component; see "Augmentin Product-Specific Considerations" table on next page.

Usual dosage range:

Infants <3 months: Oral: 30 mg/kg/day divided every 12 hours using the 125 mg/5 mL suspension

Children ≥3 months and <40 kg: Oral: 20-90 mg/kg/day divided every 8-12 hours

Children >40 kg and Adults: Oral: 250-500 mg every 8 hours or 875 mg every 12 hours

Indication-specific dosing:

Children ≥3 months and <40 kg: Oral:

Community-acquired pneumonia (CAP) (IDSA/PIDS, 2011): Note: In children ≥5 years, a macrolide antibiotic should be added if atypical pneumonia cannot be ruled out.

Presumed bacterial (mild-to-moderate infection) (alternative to amoxicillin): 90 mg/kg/day divided every 12 hours

H. influenzae (typeable or nontypeable; beta-lactamase producing), step-down therapy or mild infection (preferred): 45 mg/kg/day divided every 8 hours **or** 90 mg/kg/day divided every 12 hours

Group A streptococci, chronic carrier treatment (IDSA guidelines): Refer to adult dosing.

Lower respiratory tract infections, severe infections, sinusitis: 45 mg/kg/day divided every 12 hours **or** 40 mg/kg/day divided every 8 hours

Mild-to-moderate infections: 25 mg/kg/day divided every 12 hours or 20 mg/kg/day divided every 8 hours

Otitis media (amoxicillin 600 mg and clavulanate potassium 42.9 mg per 5 mL): 90 mg/kg/day divided every 12 hours for 10 days in children with severe illness and when coverage for β-lactamase-positive *H. influenzae* and *M. catarrhalis* is needed.

Children <16 years: Oral:

Acute bacterial rhinosinusitis: 45 mg/kg/day divided every 12 hours (preferred) for 10-14 days. **Note:** May use high-dose therapy (90 mg/kg/day divided every 12 hours) if initial therapy fails, in areas with high endemic rates of penicillin-nonsusceptible *S. pneumoniae*, those with severe infections, daycare attendance, age <2 years, recent hospitalization, antibiotic use within the past month, or who are immunocompromised (Chow, 2012).

Children ≥16 years and Adults: Oral:

Acute bacterial rhinosinusitis: Extended release tablet: 2000 mg every 12 hours for 10 days or 500 mg every 8 hours or 875 mg every 12 hours for 5-7 days **Note:** May use high-dose therapy (extended release: 2000 mg every 12 hours) if initial therapy fails, in areas with high endemic rates of penicillin-nonsusceptible *S. pneumoniae*, those with severe infections, age >65 years, recent hospitalization, antibiotic use within the past month, or who are immunocompromised (Chow, 2012).

Bite wounds (animal/human): 875 mg every 12 hours **or** 500 mg every 8 hours

Chronic obstructive pulmonary disease: 875 mg every 12 hours **or** 500 mg every 8 hours

Diabetic foot: Extended release tablet: Two 1000 mg tablets every 12 hours for 7-14 days

Erysipelas: 875 mg every 12 hours **or** 500 mg every 8 hours

Febrile neutropenia: 875 mg every 12 hours

Group A streptococci, chronic carrier treatment (IDSA guidelines): 40 mg/kg/day divided every 8 hours (maximum: 2000 mg daily) for 10 days (Shulman, 2012)

Pneumonia:

Aspiration: 875 mg every 12 hours

Community-acquired: Extended release tablet: Two 1000 mg tablets every 12 hours for 7-10 days

Prosthetic joint infection, chronic antimicrobial suppression, oxacillin-susceptible *Staphylococci* (alternative to cephalexin or cefadroxil) (off-label use): 500 mg 3 times daily (Osmon, 2013)

Pyelonephritis (acute, uncomplicated): 875 mg every 12 hours **or** 500 mg every 8 hours

Skin abscess: 875 mg every 12 hours

Dosage adjustment in renal impairment:

CrCl <30 mL/minute: Do not use 875 mg tablet or extended release tablets

CrCl 10-30 mL/minute: 250-500 mg every 12 hours

CrCl <10 mL/minute: 250-500 mg every 24 hours

Hemodialysis: Moderately dialyzable (20% to 50%)

250-500 mg every 24 hours; administer dose during and after dialysis. Do not use extended release tablets.

Peritoneal dialysis: Moderately dialyzable (20% to 50%)

Amoxicillin: Administer 250 mg every 12 hours

Clavulanic acid: Dose for CrCl <10 mL/minute

Continuous arteriovenous or venovenous hemofiltration effects:

Amoxicillin: ~50 mg of amoxicillin/L of filtrate is removed

Clavulanic acid: Dose for CrCl <10 mL/minute

Augmentin Product-Specific Considerations

Strength	Form	Consideration
125 mg	S	q8h dosing
	S	For adults having difficulty swallowing tablets, 125 mg/5 mL suspension may be substituted for 500 mg tablet.
200 mg	CT, S	q12h dosing
	CT	Contains phenylalanine
	S	For adults having difficulty swallowing tablets, 200 mg/5 mL suspension may be substituted for 875 mg tablet.
250 mg	S, T	q8h dosing
	T	Not for use in patients <40 kg
	S	For adults having difficulty swallowing tablets, 250 mg/5 mL suspension may be substituted for 500 mg tablet.
400 mg	CT, S	q12h dosing
	CT	Contains phenylalanine
	S	For adults having difficulty swallowing tablets, 400 mg/5 mL suspension may be substituted for 875 mg tablet.
500 mg	T	q8h or q12h dosing
600 mg	S	q12h dosing
		Not for use in adults or children ≥40 kg
		600 mg/5 mL suspension is not equivalent to or interchangeable with 200 mg/5 mL or 400 mg/5 mL due to differences in clavulanic acid.
875 mg	T	q12h dosing; not for use in CrCl <30 mL/minute
1000 mg	XR	q12h dosing
		Not for use in children <16 years of age
		Not interchangeable with two 500 mg tablets
		Not for use if CrCl <30 mL/minute or hemodialysis

Legend: CT = chewable tablet, S = suspension, T = tablet, XR = extended release.

Dosage adjustment in hepatic impairment: There are no dosage adjustments provided in manufacturer's labeling; use with caution. Use contraindicated in patients with a history of amoxicillin and clavulanate-associated hepatic dysfunction.

Dietary Considerations May be taken with meals or on an empty stomach; take with meals to increase absorption and decrease GI upset; may mix with milk, formula, or juice. Extended release tablets should be taken with food. Some products may contain sodium. Some products contain phenylalanine; if you have phenylketonuria or PKU, avoid use. All dosage forms contain potassium.

Administration Administer around-the-clock to promote less variation in peak and trough serum levels. Administer with food to increase absorption and decrease stomach upset; shake suspension well before use. Extended release tablets should be administered with food.

Some penicillins (eg, carbenicillin, ticarcillin, and piperacillin) have been shown to inactivate aminoglycosides *in vitro*. This has been observed to a greater extent with tobramycin and gentamicin, while amikacin has shown greater stability against inactivation. Concurrent use of these agents may pose a risk of reduced antibacterial efficacy *in vivo*, particularly in the setting of profound renal impairment. However, definitive clinical evidence is lacking. If combination penicillin/aminoglycoside therapy is desired in a patient with renal dysfunction, separation of doses (if feasible), and routine monitoring of aminoglycoside levels, CBC, and clinical response should be considered.

Monitoring Parameters Assess patient at beginning and throughout therapy for infection; with prolonged therapy, monitor renal, hepatic, and hematologic function periodically; monitor for signs of anaphylaxis during first dose

Additional Information Two 250 mg tablets are not equivalent to a 500 mg tablet (both tablet sizes contain equivalent clavulanate). Two 500 mg tablets are not equivalent to a single 1000 mg extended release tablet.

Dosage Forms

Powder for suspension, oral:

Generic: 200: Amoxicillin 200 mg and clavulanate potassium 28.5 mg per 5 mL; 250: Amoxicillin 250 mg and clavulanate potassium 62.5 mg per 5 mL; 400: Amoxicillin 400 mg and clavulanate potassium 57 mg per 5 mL; 600: Amoxicillin 600 mg and clavulanate potassium 42.9 mg per 5 mL

Amoclan:

200: Amoxicillin 200 mg and clavulanate potassium 28.5 mg per 5 mL

400: Amoxicillin 400 mg and clavulanate potassium 57 mg per 5 mL

600: Amoxicillin 600 mg and clavulanate potassium 42.9 mg per 5 mL

Augmentin:

125: Amoxicillin 125 mg and clavulanate potassium 31.25 mg per 5 mL

250: Amoxicillin 250 mg and clavulanate potassium 62.5 mg per 5 mL

Augmentin ES-600:

600: Amoxicillin 600 mg and clavulanate potassium 42.9 mg per 5 mL (75 mL, 125 mL, 200 mL) [contains phenylalanine 7 mg/5 mL, potassium 0.23 mEq/5 mL; strawberry cream flavor]

Tablet, oral:

Generic: 250: Amoxicillin 250 mg and clavulanate potassium 125 mg; 500: Amoxicillin 500 mg and clavulanate potassium 125 mg; 875: Amoxicillin 875 mg and clavulanate potassium 125 mg

Augmentin:

500: Amoxicillin 500 mg and clavulanate potassium 125 mg

875: Amoxicillin 875 mg and clavulanate potassium 125 mg

Tablet, chewable, oral: Generic: 200: Amoxicillin 200 mg and clavulanate potassium 28.5 mg; 400: Amoxicillin 400 mg and clavulanate potassium 57 mg

Tablet, extended release, oral:

Generic: Amoxicillin 1000 mg and clavulanate acid 62.5 mg

Augmentin XR: 1000: Amoxicillin 1000 mg and clavulanate acid 62.5 mg

Dosage Forms: Canada Note: Also refer to Dosage Forms.

Powder for suspension, oral:

Clavulin:

125: Amoxicillin 125 mg and clavulanate potassium 31.25 mg per 5 mL

200: Amoxicillin 200 mg and clavulanate potassium 28.5 mg per 5 mL

250: Amoxicillin 250 mg and clavulanate potassium 62.5 mg per 5 mL

400: Amoxicillin 400 mg and clavulanate potassium 57 mg per 5 mL

Tablet, oral:

Clavulin:

500: Amoxicillin 500 mg and clavulanate potassium 125 mg

875: Amoxicillin 875 mg and clavulanate potassium 125 mg

◆ **Amoxicillin and Clavulanate Potassium** *see* Amoxicillin and Clavulanate *on page 133*

◆ **Amoxicillin and Clavulanic Acid** *see* Amoxicillin and Clavulanate *on page 133*

Amoxicillin and Cloxacillin [INT]

(a moks i SIL in & kloks a SIL in)

International Brand Names Amclo (IN); Megamox (IN); Moxiclox (IN)

Index Terms Cloxacillin and Amoxicillin

Pharmacologic Category Antibiotic, Penicillin

Reported Use Treatment of susceptible infections

Dosage Range Note: Dosage expressed as combined amount of amoxicillin plus cloxacillin

Children 2-10 years: IV, IM: 250-500 mg every 6-8 hours

Adults:

Oral: 1000-2000 mg 3 times/day

IV, IM: 500-1000 mg every 6-8 hours

Product Availability Product available in various countries; not currently available in the U.S.

Dosage Forms

Capsule: 250 mg: amoxicillin 125 mg and cloxacillin sodium 125 mg; 500 mg: amoxicillin 250 mg and cloxacillin sodium 250 mg; 1 g: amoxicillin 500 mg and cloxacillin sodium 500 mg

◆ **Amoxicillin, Clarithromycin, and Lansoprazole** *see* Lansoprazole, Amoxicillin, and Clarithromycin *on page 1169*

◆ **Amoxicillin, Clarithromycin, and Omeprazole** *see* Omeprazole, Clarithromycin, and Amoxicillin *on page 1511*

◆ **Amoxicillin Trihydrate** *see* Amoxicillin *on page 130*

◆ **Amoxi-Clav (Can)** *see* Amoxicillin and Clavulanate *on page 133*

◆ **Amoxil** *see* Amoxicillin *on page 130*

◆ **Amoxycillin** *see* Amoxicillin *on page 130*

◆ **Amoxycillin and Clavulanate Potassium** *see* Amoxicillin and Clavulanate *on page 133*

◆ **Amoxycillin and Clavulanic Acid** *see* Amoxicillin and Clavulanate *on page 133*

◆ **Amphetamine and Dextroamphetamine** *see* Dextroamphetamine and Amphetamine *on page 609*

◆ **Amphojel (Can)** *see* Aluminum Hydroxide *on page 103*

◆ **Amphotec** *see* Amphotericin B Cholesteryl Sulfate Complex *on page 136*

◆ **Amphotec® (Can)** *see* Amphotericin B Cholesteryl Sulfate Complex *on page 136*

Amphotericin B Cholesteryl Sulfate Complex

(am foe TER i sin bee kole LES te ril SUL fate KOM plecks)

Brand Names: U.S. Amphotec

Brand Names: Canada Amphotec®

Index Terms ABCD; Amphotericin B Colloidal Dispersion

Pharmacologic Category Antifungal Agent, Parenteral

Use Treatment of invasive aspergillosis in patients who have failed amphotericin B deoxycholate treatment, or who have renal impairment or experience unacceptable toxicity which precludes treatment with amphotericin B deoxycholate in effective doses.

Pregnancy Risk Factor B

Dosage Children and Adults: IV: *Usual dosage range:* 3-4 mg/kg/day. **Note:** 6 mg/kg/day has been used for treatment of life-threatening invasive aspergillosis in immunocompromised patients (Bowden, 2002).

Premedication: For patients who experience chills, fever, hypotension, nausea, or other nonanaphylactic infusion-related immediate reactions, premedicate with the following drugs 30-60 minutes prior to drug administration: A nonsteroidal with or without diphenhydramine **or** acetaminophen with diphenhydramine **or** hydrocortisone 50-100 mg with or without a nonsteroidal and diphenhydramine (Paterson, 2008).

Test dose: For patients receiving their first dose in a new treatment course, a small amount (10 mL of the final preparation, containing between 1.6-8.3 mg) infused over 15-30 minutes is recommended. The patient should then be observed for an additional 30 minutes.

Dosage adjustment in renal impairment:

Mild to moderate impairment: No dosage adjustment provided in manufacturer's labeling. However, no pharmacokinetic changes were noted in patients with mild-to-moderate impairment.

Severe impairment: No dosage adjustment provided in manufacturer's labeling (has not been studied).

Dosage adjustment in hepatic impairment: No dosage adjustment provided in manufacturer's labeling (has not been studied).

Additional Information Complete prescribing information should be consulted for additional detail.

Dosage Forms

Suspension Reconstituted, Intravenous:

Amphotec: 50 mg (1 ea); 100 mg (1 ea)

◆ **Amphotericin B Colloidal Dispersion** *see* Amphotericin B Cholesteryl Sulfate Complex *on page 136*

Amphotericin B (Conventional)

(am foe TER i sin bee con VEN sha nal)

Brand Names: Canada Fungizone

Index Terms Amphotericin B Deoxycholate; Amphotericin B Desoxycholate; Conventional Amphotericin B

Pharmacologic Category Antifungal Agent, Parenteral

Use

Life-threatening fungal infections: Treatment of patients with progressive, potentially life-threatening fungal infections: Aspergillosis, cryptococcosis (torulosis), North American blastomycosis, systemic candidiasis, coccidioidomycosis, histoplasmosis, zygomycosis (including mucormycosis due to susceptible species of the genera *Absidia, Mucor,* and *Rhizopus*), and infections due to related susceptible species of *Conidiobolus, Basidiobolus,* and sporotrichosis.

Leishmaniasis: May be useful in the treatment of American mucocutaneous leishmaniasis, but it is not the drug of choice as primary therapy.

Pregnancy Risk Factor B

Dosage Premedication: For patients who experience infusion-related immediate reactions, premedicate with the following drugs 30 to 60 minutes prior to drug administration: NSAID and/or diphenhydramine **or** acetaminophen with diphenhydramine **or** hydrocortisone. If the patient experiences rigors during the infusion, meperidine may be administered.

Usual dosage ranges:

Infants and Children:

Test dose: IV: 0.1 mg/kg/dose to a maximum of 1 mg; infuse over 30 to 60 minutes. Many clinicians believe a test dose is unnecessary.

Maintenance dose: 0.25 to 1 mg/kg/day given once daily; infuse over 2 to 6 hours. Once therapy has been established, amphotericin B can be administered on an every-other-day basis at 1 to 1.5 mg/kg/dose; cumulative dose: 1.5 to 2 g over 6 to 10 weeks.

Duration of therapy: Varies with nature of infection, usual duration is 4 to 12 weeks or cumulative dose of 1 to 4 g

Adults:

Test dose: 1 mg infused over 20 to 30 minutes. Many clinicians believe a test dose is unnecessary.

Maintenance dose: Usual: 0.3 to 1.5 mg/kg/day; 1 to 1.5 mg/kg over 4 to 6 hours every other day may be given once therapy is established; aspergillosis, rhinocerebral mucormycosis, often require 1 to 1.5 mg/kg/day; do not exceed 1.5 mg/kg/day

Indication-specific dosing:

Infants and Children:

Aspergillosis (HIV-exposed/-positive): IV: 1 to 1.5 mg/kg/day once daily (CDC, 2009)

Candidiasis (HIV-exposed/-positive):

Invasive: IV: 0.5 to 1.5 mg/kg/day once daily (CDC, 2009)

Esophageal: IV: 0.3 to 0.5 mg/kg/day once daily (CDC, 2009)

Oropharyngeal, refractory: IV: 0.3 to 0.5 mg/kg/day (CDC, 2009)

Coccidioidomycosis (HIV-exposed/-positive): IV: 0.5 to 1 mg/kg/day (CDC, 2009)

***Cryptococcus,* CNS disease (HIV-exposed/-positive):** IV: 0.7 to 1 mg/kg/day plus flucytosine; **Note:** Minimum 2 week induction followed by consolidation and chronic suppressive therapy; may increase amphotericin dose to 1.5 mg/kg/day if flucytosine is not tolerated.

***Cryptococcus,* disseminated (non-CNS disease) or severe pulmonary disease (HIV-exposed/-positive):** IV: 0.7 to 1 mg/kg/day once daily with or without flucytosine

Histoplasma, CNS or severe disseminated: IV: 1 mg/kg/day once daily (CDC, 2009)

Adults:

Aspergillosis, disseminated: IV: 0.6 to 0.7 mg/kg/day for 3 to 6 months

Bone marrow transplantation (prophylaxis): IV: Low-dose amphotericin B 0.1 to 0.25 mg/kg/day has been administered after bone marrow transplantation to reduce the risk of invasive fungal disease.

Candidemia (neutropenic or non-neutropenic): IV: 0.5 to 1 mg/kg/day until 14 days after first negative blood culture and resolution of signs and symptoms (Pappas, 2009)

Candidiasis, chronic, disseminated: IV: 0.5 to 0.7 mg/kg/day for 3 to 6 months and resolution of radiologic lesions (Pappas, 2009)

Dematiaceous fungi: IV: 0.7 mg/kg/day in combination with an azole

Endocarditis: IV: 0.6 to 1 mg/kg/day (with or without flucytosine) for 6 weeks after valve replacement; **Note:** If isolates susceptible and/or clearance demonstrated, guidelines recommend step-down to fluconazole; also for long-term suppression therapy if valve replacement is not possible (Pappas, 2009)

Endophthalmitis, fungal (off-label use):

Intravitreal: 5 to 12.5 mcg (with or without concomitant systemic therapy) (Brod, 1990)

IV: 0.7 to 1 mg/kg/day (with flucytosine) for at least 4 to 6 weeks (Pappas, 2009)

Esophageal candidiasis: IV: 0.3 to 0.7 mg/kg/day for 14 to 21 days after clinical improvement (Pappas, 2009)

Histoplasmosis: Chronic, severe pulmonary or disseminated: IV: 0.5 to 1 mg/kg/day for 7 days, then 0.8 mg/kg every other day (or 3 times/week) until total dose of 10 to 15 mg/kg; may continue itraconazole as suppressive therapy (lifelong for immunocompromised patients)

Meningitis:

Candidal: IV: 0.7 to 1 mg/kg/day (with or without flucytosine) for at least 4 weeks; **Note:** Liposomal amphotericin favored by IDSA guidelines based on decreased risk of nephrotoxicity and potentially better CNS penetration (Pappas, 2009)

Cryptococcal or Coccidioides: Intrathecal: Initial: 0.01 to 0.05 mg as single daily dose; may increase daily in increments of 0.025 to 0.1 mg as tolerated (maximum: 1.5 mg/day; most patients will tolerate a maximum dose of ~0.5 mg/treatment). Once titration to a maximum tolerated dose is achieved, that dose is administered daily. Once CSF improvement noted, may decrease frequency on a weekly basis (eg, 5 times/week, then 3 times/week, then 2 times/week, then once weekly, then once every other week, then once every 2 weeks, etc) until administration occurs once every 6 weeks. Typically, concurrent oral azole therapy is maintained (Stevens, 2001). **Note:** IDSA notes that the use of intrathecal amphotericin for cryptococcal meningitis is generally discouraged and rarely necessary (Perfect, 2010).

Histoplasma: IV: 0.5 to 1 mg/kg/day for 7 days, then 0.8 mg/kg every other day (or 3 times/week) for 3 months total duration; follow with fluconazole suppressive therapy for up to 12 months

Meningoencephalitis, cryptococcal (Perfect, 2010):

IV:

HIV positive: Induction: 0.7 to 1 mg/kg/day (plus flucytosine 100 mg/kg/day) for 2 weeks, then change to oral fluconazole for at least 8 weeks; alternatively, amphotericin (0.7 to 1 mg/kg/day) may be continued uninterrupted for 4 to 6 weeks; maintenance: amphotericin 1 mg/kg/week for ≥1 year may be considered, but inferior to use of azoles

HIV negative: Induction: 0.7 to 1 mg/kg/day (plus flucytosine 100 mg/kg/day) for 2 weeks (low-risk patients), ≥4 weeks (non-low-risk, but without neurologic complication, immunosuppression, underlying disease, and negative CSF culture at 2 weeks), >6 weeks (neurologic complication or patients intolerant of flucytosine) Follow with azole consolidation/maintenance treatment.

Oropharyngeal candidiasis: IV: 0.3 mg/kg/day for 7 to 14 days (Pappas, 2009)

Osteoarticular candidiasis: IV: 0.5 to 1 mg/kg/day for several weeks, followed by fluconazole for 6 to 12 months (osteomyelitis) or 6 weeks (septic arthritis) (Pappas, 2009)

Penicillium marneffei: IV: 0.6 mg/kg/day for 2 weeks

Pneumonia: Cryptococcal (mild-to-moderate): IV:
HIV positive: 0.5 to 1 mg/kg/day
HIV negative: 0.5 to 0.7 mg/kg/day (plus flucytosine) for 2 weeks

Sporotrichosis: Pulmonary, meningeal, osteoarticular, or disseminated: IV: Total dose of 1 to 2 g, then change to oral itraconazole or fluconazole for suppressive therapy

Urinary tract candidiasis (IDSA [Pappas, 2009]):
Fungus balls: IV: 0.5 to 0.7 mg/kg/day with or without flucytosine 25 mg/kg 4 times daily
Pyelonephritis: IV: 0.5 to 0.7 mg/kg/day with or without flucytosine 25 mg/kg 4 times daily for 2 weeks
Symptomatic cystitis: IV: 0.3 to 0.6 mg/kg/day for 1 to 7 days
Bladder irrigation in patients with C. krusei or fluconazole-resistant C. glabrata: Irrigate with 50 mcg/mL solution instilled periodically or continuously for 5 to 7 days or until cultures are clear. **Note:** Recommended for use in conjunction with other treatment modalities (Fisher, 2011).

Dosage adjustment in renal impairment: If renal dysfunction is due to the drug, the daily total can be decreased by 50% or the dose can be given every other day; IV therapy may take several months

Renal replacement therapy: Poorly dialyzed; no supplemental dose or dosage adjustment necessary, including patients on intermittent hemodialysis or CRRT.

Peritoneal dialysis (PD): Administration in dialysate: 1 to 2 mg/L of peritoneal dialysis fluid either with or without low-dose IV amphotericin B (a total dose of 2 to 10 mg/kg given over 7 to 14 days). Precipitate may form in ionic dialysate solutions.

Dosage adjustment in hepatic impairment: No dosage adjustment provided in manufacturer's labeling.

Additional Information Complete prescribing information should be consulted for additional detail.

Dosage Forms

Solution Reconstituted, Injection:
Generic: 50 mg (1 ea)

- **Amphotericin B Deoxycholate** *see* Amphotericin B (Conventional) *on page 136*
- **Amphotericin B Desoxycholate** *see* Amphotericin B (Conventional) *on page 136*

Amphotericin B (Lipid Complex)

(am foe TER i sin bee LIP id KOM pleks)

Brand Names: U.S. Abelcet

Brand Names: Canada Abelcet®

Index Terms ABLC

Pharmacologic Category Antifungal Agent, Parenteral

Use Treatment of invasive fungal infection in patients who are refractory to or intolerant of conventional amphotericin B (amphotericin B deoxycholate) therapy

Pregnancy Risk Factor B

Dosage IV: **Note:** Premedication: For patients who experience infusion-related immediate reactions, premedicate with the following drugs 30-60 minutes prior to drug administration: A nonsteroidal anti-inflammatory agent ± diphenhydramine **or** acetaminophen with diphenhydramine **or** hydrocortisone. If the patient experiences rigors during the infusion, meperidine may be administered.

Children and Adults:

Usual dose: 5 mg/kg once daily

Manufacturer's labeling: Invasive fungal infections (when patients are intolerant or refractory to conventional amphotericin B): 5 mg/kg/day

Indication-specific dosing:

Infants and Children:

Aspergillosis (HIV-positive patients) (alternative to preferred therapy): 5 mg/kg/day for ≥12 weeks (CDC, [pediatric], 2009)

Candidiasis, invasive (HIV-positive patients) (alternative to preferred therapy): 5 mg/kg/day; treatment duration based on clinical response, treat until 2-3 weeks after last positive blood culture (CDC [pediatric], 2009)

***Cryptococcus neoformans*, disseminated disease (non-CNS disease) (HIV-positive patients):** 5 mg/kg/day (with or without flucytosine); treatment duration of non-CNS disease varies by clinical response and site/severity of infection (CDC [pediatric], 2009)

Adults:

Aspergillosis, invasive (HIV-positive or HIV-negative patients) (alternative to preferred therapy): 5 mg/kg/day; duration of treatment in HIV-negative patients depends on site of infection, extent of disease and level of immunosuppression; in HIV-positive patients, treat until CD4 count >200 cells/mm^3 and evidence of clinical response (CDC [adults], 2009; Walsh, 2008)

Blastomycosis, moderately-severe-to-severe (off-label dose): 3-5 mg/kg/day for 1-2 weeks or until improvement, followed by oral itraconazole (Chapman, 2008)

Candidiasis (off-label dose):
Chronic disseminated candidiasis, pericarditis or myocarditis due to Candida, suppurative thrombophlebitis: 3-5 mg/kg/day. **Note:** In chronic disseminated candidiasis, transition to fluconazole after several weeks in stable patients is preferred (Pappas, 2009)
CNS candidiasis: 3-5 mg/kg/day (with or without flucytosine) for several weeks, followed by fluconazole (Pappas, 2009)
Endocarditis due to Candida, infected pacemaker, ICD, or VAD: 3-5 mg/kg/day (with or without flucytosine); continue to treat for 4-6 weeks after device removal unless device cannot be removed then chronic suppression with fluconazole is recommended (Pappas, 2009)

Coccidioidomycosis (off-label dose):
Progressive, disseminated: (alternative to preferred therapy): 2-5 mg/kg/day (Galgiani, 2005)
HIV-positive patients with severe, nonmeningeal infection: 4-6 mg/kg/day until clinical improvement, then switch to fluconazole or itraconazole (CDC, 2009)

Cryptococcosis:
Cryptococcal meningoencephalitis in HIV-positive patients (as an alternative to conventional amphotericin B in patients with renal concerns): Induction therapy: 4-6 mg/kg/day (off-label dose; CDC [adult], 2009) or 5 mg/kg/day (Perfect, 2010) with flucytosine for at least 2 weeks, followed by oral fluconazole. **Note:** If flucytosine is not given due to intolerance, duration of amphotericin B lipid complex therapy should be 4-6 weeks (Perfect, 2010).
Cryptococcal meningoencephalitis in HIV-negative patients and nontransplant patients (as an alternative to conventional amphotericin B): Induction therapy: 5 mg/kg/day (with flucytosine if possible) for ≥4 weeks followed by oral fluconazole. **Note:** If flucytosine is not given or treatment is interrupted, consider prolonging induction therapy for an additional 2 weeks (Perfect, 2010).

Cryptococcal meningoencephalitis in transplant recipients: Induction therapy: 5 mg/kg/day (with flucytosine) for at least 2 weeks, followed by oral fluconazole **Note:** If flucytosine is not given, duration of amphotericin B lipid complex therapy should be 4-6 weeks (Perfect, 2010).

Nonmeningeal cryptococcosis: Induction therapy: 5 mg/kg/day (with flucytosine if possible) for ≥4 weeks may be used for severe pulmonary cryptococcosis or for cryptococcemia with evidence of high fungal burden, followed by oral fluconazole. **Note:** If flucytosine is not given or treatment is interrupted, consider prolonging induction therapy for an additional 2 weeks (Perfect, 2010).

Histoplasmosis:

Acute pulmonary (moderately-severe-to-severe): 5 mg/kg/day for 1-2 weeks, followed by oral itraconazole (Wheat, 2007)

Progressive disseminated (alternative to preferred therapy): 5 mg/kg/day for 1-2 weeks, followed by oral itraconazole (Wheat, 2007)

Sporotrichosis (off-label dose):

Meningeal: 5 mg/kg/day for 4-6 weeks, followed by oral itraconazole (Kauffman, 2007)

Pulmonary, osteoarticular, and disseminated: 3-5 mg/kg/day, followed by oral itraconazole after a favorable response is seen with amphotericin initial therapy (Kauffman, 2007)

Dosing adjustment in renal impairment:

Manufacturer's recommendations: No dosage adjustment provided in manufacturer's labeling (has not been studied).

Alternate recommendations (Aronoff, 2007):

Intermittent hemodialysis: No supplemental dosage necessary.

Peritoneal dialysis: No supplemental dosage necessary.

Continuous renal replacement therapy (CRRT): No supplemental dosage necessary.

Dosing adjustment in hepatic impairment: No dosage adjustment provided in manufacturer's labeling (has not been studied).

Additional Information Complete prescribing information should be consulted for additional detail.

Dosage Forms

Suspension, Intravenous:

Abelcet: 5 mg/mL (20 mL)

Amphotericin B (Liposomal)

(am foe TER i sin bee lye po SO mal)

Brand Names: U.S. AmBisome

Brand Names: Canada AmBisome®

Index Terms Amphotericin B Liposome; L-AmB

Pharmacologic Category Antifungal Agent, Parenteral

Use Empirical therapy for presumed fungal infection in febrile, neutropenic patients; treatment of patients with *Aspergillus* species, *Candida* species, and/or *Cryptococcus* species infections refractory to amphotericin B desoxycholate (conventional amphotericin), or in patients where renal impairment or unacceptable toxicity precludes the use of amphotericin B desoxycholate; treatment of cryptococcal meningitis in HIV-infected patients; treatment of visceral leishmaniasis

Pregnancy Risk Factor B

Pregnancy Considerations Adverse events were not observed in animal reproduction studies. Amphotericin crosses the placenta and enters the fetal circulation. Amphotericin B is recommended for the treatment of serious systemic fungal diseases in pregnant women; refer to current guidelines (King, 1998).

Breast-Feeding Considerations It is not known if amphotericin is excreted into breast milk. Due to its poor oral absorption, systemic exposure to the nursing infant is expected to be decreased; however, because of the potential for toxicity, breast-feeding is not recommended (Mactal-Haaf, 2001).

Contraindications Hypersensitivity to amphotericin B deoxycholate or any component of the formulation

Warnings/Precautions Patients should be under close clinical observation during initial dosing. As with other amphotericin B-containing products, anaphylaxis has been reported. Facilities for cardiopulmonary resuscitation should be available during administration. Acute infusion reactions (including fever and chills) may occur 1-2 hours after starting infusions; reactions are more common with the first few doses and generally diminish with subsequent doses. Immediately discontinue infusion if severe respiratory distress occurs; the patient should not receive further infusions. Concurrent use of amphotericin B with other nephrotoxic drugs may enhance the potential for drug-induced renal toxicity. Concurrent use with antineoplastic agents may enhance the potential for renal toxicity, bronchospasm or hypotension. Acute pulmonary toxicity has been reported in patients receiving simultaneous leukocyte transfusions and amphotericin B. Safety and efficacy have not been established in patients <1 month of age.

Adverse Reactions Nephrotoxicity and infusion-related hyperpyrexia, rigor, and chilling are reduced relative to amphotericin deoxycholate.

Cardiovascular: Atrial fibrillation, bradycardia, cardiac arrest, cardiac arrhythmia, cardiomegaly, chest pain, edema, facial edema, flushing, heart valve disease, hypertension, hypotension, localized phlebitis, orthostatic hypotension, peripheral edema, tachycardia, vascular disorder, vasodilatation

Central nervous system: Abnormality in thinking, agitation, anxiety, chills, coma, confusion, depression, dizziness, drowsiness, dysesthesia, dystonia, hallucination, headache, insomnia, malaise, nervousness, pain, paresthesia, rigors, seizure

Dermatologic: Alopecia, cellulitis, dermal ulcer, dermatological reaction, diaphoresis, maculopapular rash, pruritus, skin discoloration, skin rash, urticaria, vesiculobullous dermatitis, xeroderma

Endocrine & metabolic: Acidosis, hyperchloremia, hyperglycemia, hyperkalemia, hypermagnesemia, hypernatremia, hyperphosphatemia, hypervolemia, hypocalcemia, hypokalemia, hypomagnesemia, hyponatremia, hypophosphatemia, increased lactate dehydrogenase, increased nonprotein nitrogen

Gastrointestinal: Abdominal pain, anorexia, aphthous stomatitis, constipation, diarrhea, dyspepsia, dysphagia, enlargement of abdomen, eructation, fecal incontinence, flatulence, gastrointestinal hemorrhage, gingival hemorrhage, hematemesis, hemorrhoids, hiccups, increased serum amylase, intestinal obstruction, mucositis, nausea, rectal disease, stomatitis, vomiting, xerostomia

Genitourinary: Dysuria, hematuria, nephrotoxicity, toxic nephrosis, urinary incontence, vaginal hemorrhage

Hematologic & oncologic: Anemia, blood coagulation disorder, bruise, decreased prothrombin time, hemophthalmos, hemorrhage, hypoproteinemia, increased prothrombin time, leukopenia, oral hemorrhage, petechia, purpura, thrombocytopenia

Hepatic: Abnormal hepatic function tests (not specified), hepatic injury, hepatic veno-occlusive disease, hepatomegaly, hyperbilirubinemia, increased serum alkaline phosphatase, increased serum ALT, increased serum AST

Hypersensitivity: Delayed hypersensitivity, hypersensitivity reaction, transfusion reaction

Immunologic: Graft versus host disease

Infection: Infection, herpes simplex infection, sepsis

Local: Inflammation at injection site
Neuromuscular & skeletal: Arthralgia, back pain, myalgia, neck pain, ostealgia, tremor, weakness
Ophthalmic: Conjunctivitis, dry eyes
Renal: Acute renal failure, increased blood urea nitrogen, increased serum creatinine, renal failure, renal function abnormality
Respiratory: Asthma, atelectasis, cough, dry nose, dyspnea, epistaxis, flu-like symptoms, hemoptysis, hyperventilation, hypoxia, pharyngitis, pleural effusion, pneumonia, pulmonary disease, pulmonary edema, respiratory alkalosis, respiratory failure, respiratory insufficiency, rhinitis, sinusitis
Miscellaneous: Infusion related reactions (fever, chills, vomiting, nausea, dyspnea, tachycardia, hypertension, vasodilation, hypotension, hyperventilation, hypoxia), procedural complication
Rare but important or life-threatening: Agranulocytosis, angioedema, cyanosis, hemorrhagic cystitis, hypoventilation, rhabdomyolysis

Drug Interactions

Metabolism/Transport Effects None known.

Avoid Concomitant Use

Avoid concomitant use of Amphotericin B (Liposomal) with any of the following: Foscarnet; Saccharomyces boulardii

Increased Effect/Toxicity

Amphotericin B (Liposomal) may increase the levels/effects of: Aminoglycosides; Cardiac Glycosides; Colistimethate; CycloSPORINE (Systemic); Flucytosine

The levels/effects of Amphotericin B (Liposomal) may be increased by: Corticosteroids (Orally Inhaled); Corticosteroids (Systemic); Foscarnet

Decreased Effect

Amphotericin B (Liposomal) may decrease the levels/effects of: Saccharomyces boulardii

The levels/effects of Amphotericin B (Liposomal) may be decreased by: Antifungal Agents (Azole Derivatives, Systemic)

Preparation for Administration Reconstitute with 12 mL SWFI to a concentration of 4 mg/mL. The use of any solution other than those recommended, or the presence of a bacteriostatic agent in the solution, may cause precipitation. **Shake the vial vigorously** for 30 seconds, until dispersed into a translucent yellow suspension.

Filtration and dilution: Withdraw appropriate amount of reconstituted solution into a syringe, attach a 5-micron filter, and inject contents of syringe through filter needle into an appropriate amount of D_5W. Dilute to a final concentration of 1-2 mg/mL (0.2-0.5 mg/mL for infants and small children).

Storage/Stability Store intact vials at ≤25°C (≤77°F). Reconstituted vials are stable refrigerated at 2°C to 8°C (36°F to 46°F) for 24 hours. Do not freeze. Manufacturer's labeling states infusion should begin within 6 hours of dilution with D_5W; data on file with Astellas Pharma shows extended formulation stability when admixed in D_5W at 0.2-2 mg/mL (in polyolefin or PVC bags) for up to 11 days when stored refrigerated at 2°C to 8°C (36°F to 46°F).

Mechanism of Action Binds to ergosterol altering cell membrane permeability in susceptible fungi and causing leakage of cell components with subsequent cell death. Proposed mechanism suggests that amphotericin causes an oxidation-dependent stimulation of macrophages (Lyman, 1992).

Pharmacodynamics/Kinetics Half-life elimination: 7-10 hours (following a single 24-hour dosing interval); Terminal half-life: 100-153 hours (following multiple dosing up to 49 days)

Dosage

Usual dosage range:

Children ≥1 month: IV: 3-6 mg/kg/day

Adults: IV: 3-6 mg/kg/day; **Note:** Higher doses (7.5-15 mg/kg/day) have been used clinically in special cases (CDC [parameningeal], 2012; Kauffman, 2012; Walsh, 2001)

Note: Premedication: For patients who experience non-anaphylactic infusion-related immediate reactions, premedicate with the following drugs 30-60 minutes prior to drug administration: A nonsteroidal anti-inflammatory agent ± diphenhydramine; **or** acetaminophen with diphenhydramine; **or** hydrocortisone. If the patient experiences rigors during the infusion, meperidine may be administered.

Indication-specific dosing:

Children ≥1 month: IV:

Empiric therapy: 3 mg/kg/day

Systemic fungal infections *(Aspergillus, Candida, Cryptococcus)*: 3-5 mg/kg/day

Systemic fungal infections (HIV-exposed/-positive [CDC, 2009; off-label use]):

Aspergillosis: 5 mg/kg/day once daily

Candida, invasive: 5 mg/kg/day once daily (may consider addition of oral flucytosine for severe disease)

Cryptococcal meningitis: 4-6 mg/kg/day once daily plus oral flucytosine

Cryptococcus, disseminated (non-CNS): 3-5 mg/kg/day (may consider addition of oral flucytosine)

Histoplasmosis: 3-5 mg/kg/day once daily

Visceral leishmaniasis:

Immunocompetent: 3 mg/kg/day on days 1-5, and 3 mg/kg/day on days 14 and 21; a repeat course may be given in patients who do not achieve parasitic clearance

Note: Alternate regimen of 10 mg/kg/day for 2 days has been reportedly effective.

Immunocompromised: 4 mg/kg/day on days 1-5, and 4 mg/kg/day on days 10, 17, 24, 31, and 38

Adults: IV:

Cryptococcal meningitis (HIV-positive): 6 mg/kg/day or 4-6 mg/kg/day in combination with addition of oral flucytosine 25 mg/kg 4 times daily (off-label combination; CDC, 2009)

Empiric candidiasis therapy: 3-5 mg/kg/day (Pappas, 2009)

Endocarditis: IV: 3-5 mg/kg/day (with or without flucytosine 25 mg/kg 4 times daily) for 6 weeks after valve replacement; **Note:** If isolates susceptible and/or clearance demonstrated, guidelines recommend step-down to fluconazole; also for long-term suppression therapy if valve replacement is not possible (Pappas, 2009)

Fungal sinusitis: Limited data in immunocompromised patients have shown efficacy with 3-10 mg/kg/day (Barron, 2005; Pagano, 2004; Rokicka, 2006). **Note:** An azole antifungal is recommended if causative organism is *Aspergillus* spp or *Pseudallescheria boydii* (*Scedosporium* sp).

Meningitis (secondary to contaminated [eg, *Exserohilum rostratum*] steroid products), severe or in patients not improving with voriconazole monotherapy (off-label use) (CDC [parameningeal], 2012; Kauffman, 2012): IV: 5-6 mg/kg/day in combination with voriconazole for ≥3 months; a higher dose (7.5 mg/kg/day) may be considered in patients who are not improving. **Note:** Consult an infectious disease specialist and current CDC guidelines for specific treatment recommendations.

Osteoarticular candidiasis: IV: 3-5 mg/kg/day for several weeks, followed by fluconazole for 6-12 months (osteomyelitis) or 6 weeks (septic arthritis) (Pappas, 2009)

Osteoarticular infection (secondary to contaminated [eg, *Exserohilum rostratum*] steroid products), severe or in patients with clinical instability (off-label use) (CDC [osteoarticular], 2012; Kauffman, 2012): IV: 5 mg/kg/day in combination with voriconazole for ≥3 months. **Note:** Consult an infectious disease specialist and current CDC guidelines for specific treatment recommendations.

Systemic fungal infections *(Aspergillus, Candida, Cryptococcus)*: 3-5 mg/kg/day

General invasive Candidal disease: 3-5 mg/kg/day with oral flucytosine 25 mg/kg 4 times daily (off-label combination; Pappas, 2009)

Candidal meningitis: 3-5 mg/kg/day with or without oral flucytosine 25 mg/kg 4 times daily (off-label combination; Pappas, 2009)

Histoplasmosis (off-label use): 3-5 mg/kg/day (CDC, 2009)

Visceral leishmaniasis:

Immunocompetent: 3 mg/kg/day on days 1-5, and 3 mg/kg/day on days 14 and 21; a repeat course may be given in patients who do not achieve parasitic clearance

Note: Alternate regimen of 2 mg/kg/day for 5 days has been reportedly effective.

Immunocompromised: 4 mg/kg/day on days 1-5, and 4 mg/kg/day on days 10, 17, 24, 31, and 38

Dosage adjustment in renal impairment: None necessary; effects of renal impairment are not currently known

Poorly dialyzed; no supplemental dose or dosage adjustment necessary, including patients on intermittent hemodialysis, peritoneal dialysis, or continuous renal replacement therapy (eg, CVVHD).

Dosage adjustment in hepatic impairment: No dosage adjustment provided in manufacturer's labeling (has not been studied).

Dietary Considerations If on parenteral nutrition, may need to adjust the amount of lipid infused. The lipid portion of amphotericin B (liposomal) formulation contains 0.27 kcal per 5 mg (Sacks, 1997).

Administration Administer via intravenous infusion, over a period of approximately 2 hours. Infusion time may be reduced to approximately 1 hour in patients in whom the treatment is well-tolerated. If the patient experiences discomfort during infusion, the duration of infusion may be increased. Administer at a rate of 2.5 mg/kg/hour. Existing intravenous line should be flushed with D_5W prior to infusion (if not feasible, administer through a separate line). An in-line membrane filter (not less than 1 micron) may be used.

For a patient who experiences chills, fever, hypotension, nausea, or other nonanaphylactic infusion-related reactions, premedicate with the following drugs, 30-60 minutes prior to drug administration: A nonsteroidal (eg, ibuprofen, choline magnesium trisalicylate) ± diphenhydramine **or** acetaminophen with diphenhydramine **or** hydrocortisone. If the patient experiences rigors during the infusion, meperidine may be administered.

Monitoring Parameters BUN and serum creatinine levels should be determined every other day while therapy is increased and at least weekly thereafter. Renal function (monitor frequently during therapy), electrolytes (especially potassium and magnesium), liver function tests, temperature, hematocrit, PT/PTT, CBC; monitor input and output; monitor for signs of hypokalemia (muscle weakness, cramping, drowsiness, ECG changes, etc); monitor cardiac function if used concurrently with corticosteroids

Additional Information Amphotericin B (liposomal) is a true single bilayer liposomal drug delivery system. Liposomes are closed, spherical vesicles created by mixing specific proportions of amphophilic substances such as phospholipids and cholesterol so that they arrange themselves into multiple concentric bilayer membranes when hydrated in aqueous solutions. Single bilayer liposomes are then formed by microemulsification of multilamellar vesicles using a homogenizer. Amphotericin B (liposomal) consists of these unilamellar bilayer liposomes with amphotericin B intercalated within the membrane. Due to the nature and quantity of amphophilic substances used, and the lipophilic moiety in the amphotericin B molecule, the drug is an integral part of the overall structure of the amphotericin B liposomal liposomes. Amphotericin B (liposomal) contains true liposomes that are <100 nm in diameter.

Dosage Forms

Suspension Reconstituted, Intravenous:

AmBisome: 50 mg (1 ea)

◆ **Amphotericin B Liposome** *see* Amphotericin B (Liposomal) *on page* 139

Ampicillin (am pi SIL in)

Brand Names: Canada Ampicillin for Injection; Apo-Ampi; Novo-Ampicillin; Nu-Ampi

Index Terms Aminobenzylpenicillin; Ampicillin Sodium; Ampicillin Trihydrate

Pharmacologic Category Antibiotic, Penicillin

Use

Oral:

Genitourinary tract infections: Treatment of genitourinary tract infections caused by *Esherichia coli*, *Proteus mirabilis*, enterococci, *Shigella*, *Salmonella typhosa* and other *Salmonella*, and nonpenicillinase-producing *N. gonorrhoeae*. **Note:** Ampicillin is **not** recommended by the CDC as a first-line agent in the treatment of gonorrhea (CDC, 2010).

GI tract infections: Treatment of GI tract infections caused by *Shigella*, *S. typhosa* and other *Salmonella*, *E. coli*, *P. mirabilis*, and enterococci. **Note:** Ampicillin is not recommended as a first-line agent for Shigellosis, Salmonellosis (nontyphoid), or *Salmonella enterica* species (typhoid fever) due to development of resistance (CDC, 2014).

Respiratory tract infections: Treatment of respiratory tract infections caused by nonpenicillinase-producing *H. influenzae* and staphylococci, and streptococci, including *Streptococcus pneumoniae*.

Injection:

Bacterial meningitis: Treatment of bacterial meningitis caused by *E. coli*, group B streptococci, and other gram-negative bacteria (*Listeria monocytogenes, N. meningitidis*).

Gastrointestinal infections: Treatment of GI infections caused by *S. typhosa* (typhoid fever), other *Salmonella* species and *Shigella* species (dysentery). **Note:** Ampicillin is **not** recommended as a first-line agent for Shigellosis, Salmonellosis (nontyphoid), or *S. enterica* species (typhoid fever) due to development of resistance (CDC, 2014).

Respiratory tract infections: Treatment of respiratory tract infections caused by *S. pneumoniae*, *Staphylococcus aureus* (penicillinase and nonpenicillinase producing), *H. influenzae*, and group A beta-hemolytic streptococci.

Septicemia and endocarditis: Treatment of septicemia and endocarditis caused by susceptible gram-positive organisms, including Streptococcus species, penicillin G-susceptible staphylococci, and enterococci; gram-negative sepsis caused by *E. coli*, *P. mirabilis*, and *Salmonella* species.

Urinary tract infections: Treatment of urinary tract infections caused by sensitive strains of *E. coli* and *P. mirabilis*.

Pregnancy Risk Factor B

Pregnancy Considerations Adverse events have not been observed in animal reproduction studies. Ampicillin crosses the placenta, providing detectable concentrations in the cord serum and amniotic fluid (Bolognese, 1968; Fisher, 1967; MacAulay, 1966). Maternal use of ampicillin has generally not resulted in an increased risk of birth defects (Aselton, 1985; Czeizel, 2001b; Heinonen, 1977; Jick, 1981; Puhó, 2007). Ampicillin is recommended for use in pregnant women for the management of preterm premature rupture of membranes (PPROM) and for the prevention of early-onset group B streptococcal (GBS) disease in newborns. Ampicillin may also be used in certain situations prior to vaginal delivery in women at high risk for endocarditis (ACOG, 2013; ACOG No. 120, 2011; ACOG No. 485, 2011; CDC [RR-10], 2010).

The volume of distribution of ampicillin is increased during pregnancy and the half-life is decreased. As a result, serum concentrations in pregnant patients are approximately 50% of those in nonpregnant patients receiving the same dose. Higher doses may be needed during pregnancy. Although oral absorption is not altered during pregnancy, oral ampicillin is poorly absorbed during labor (Philipson, 1977; Philipson, 1978; Wasz-Höckert, 1970).

Breast-Feeding Considerations Ampicillin is excreted in breast milk. The manufacturer recommends that caution be exercised when administering ampicillin to nursing women. Due to the low concentrations in human milk, minimal toxicity would be expected in the nursing infant. Nondose-related effects could include modification of bowel flora and allergic sensitization.

Contraindications Clinically significant hypersensitivity (eg, anaphylaxis) to ampicillin, any component of the formulation, or other penicillins; infections caused by penicillinase-producing organisms

Warnings/Precautions Dosage adjustment may be necessary in patients with renal impairment. Serious and occasionally severe or fatal hypersensitivity (anaphylactoid) reactions have been reported in patients on penicillin therapy, especially with a history of beta-lactam hypersensitivity, history of sensitivity to multiple allergens, or previous IgE-mediated reactions (eg, anaphylaxis, angioedema, urticaria). Serious anaphylactoid reactions require emergency treatment and airway management. Appropriate treatments must be readily available. Use with caution in asthmatic patients. Appearance of any rash should be carefully evaluated to differentiate a nonallergic ampicillin rash from a hypersensitivity reaction. High percentage of patients with infectious mononucleosis have developed rash during therapy with ampicillin; ampicillin-class antibiotics not recommended in these patients This rash (generalized maculopapular and pruritic) usually appears 7 to 10 days after initiation and usually resolves within a week of discontinuation. It is not known whether these patients are truly allergic to ampicillin. Ampicillin rash occurs in 5% to 10% of children receiving ampicillin and is a generalized dull red, maculopapular rash, generally appearing 3 to 14 days after the start of therapy. It normally begins on the trunk and spreads over most of the body. It may be most intense at pressure areas, elbows, and knees. Prolonged use may result in fungal or bacterial superinfection, including *Clostridium difficile*-associated diarrhea (CDAD) and pseudomembranous colitis; CDAD has been observed >2 months postantibiotic treatment.

Adverse Reactions

Central nervous system: Brain disease (penicillin-induced), glossalgia, seizure, sore mouth

Dermatologic: Erythema multiforme, exfoliative dermatitis, skin rash, urticaria

Note: Appearance of a rash should be carefully evaluated to differentiate (if possible) nonallergic ampicillin rash from hypersensitivity reaction. Incidence is higher in patients with viral infection, *Salmonella* infection, lymphocytic leukemia, or patients that have hyperuricemia.

Gastrointestinal: Diarrhea, enterocolitis, glossitis, melanoglossia, nausea, oral candidiasis, pseudomembranous colitis, stomatitis, vomiting

Hematologic & oncologic: Agranulocytosis, anemia, eosinophilia, hemolytic anemia, immune thrombocytopenia, leukopenia

Hepatic: Increased serum AST

Hypersensitivity: Anaphylaxis

Immunologic: Serum sickness-like reaction

Renal: Interstitial nephritis (rare)

Respiratory: Stridor

Miscellaneous: Fever

Drug Interactions

Metabolism/Transport Effects None known.

Avoid Concomitant Use

Avoid concomitant use of Ampicillin with any of the following: BCG; Probenecid

Increased Effect/Toxicity

Ampicillin may increase the levels/effects of: Methotrexate; Vitamin K Antagonists

The levels/effects of Ampicillin may be increased by: Allopurinol; Probenecid

Decreased Effect

Ampicillin may decrease the levels/effects of: Atenolol; BCG; Mycophenolate; Sodium Picosulfate; Typhoid Vaccine

The levels/effects of Ampicillin may be decreased by: Chloroquine; Lanthanum; Tetracycline Derivatives

Food Interactions Food decreases ampicillin absorption rate; may decrease ampicillin serum concentration. Management: Take at equal intervals around-the-clock, preferably on an empty stomach (30 minutes before or 2 hours after meals). Maintain adequate hydration, unless instructed to restrict fluid intake.

Preparation for Administration

IM: Dissolve contents of vial in sterile water for injection or bacteriostatic water for injection; final concentration for IM injection is 125 mg/mL or 250 mg/mL. Solutions for IM injection. Should be freshly prepared and used within 1 hour.

IV:

Direct IV use: Dissolve contents of 125 mg, 250 mg, or 500 mg vial in 5 mL SWFI. Alternatively, dissolve contents of 1 g or 2 g vial in 7.4 or 14.8 mL SWFI, respectively.

Intermittent infusion: Minimum volume: Concentration should not exceed 30 mg/mL due to concentration-dependent stability restrictions. Standard diluent: 500 mg/50 mL NS; 1 g/50 mL NS; 2 g/100 mL NS.

Storage/Stability

Oral:

Capsules: Store at 20°C to 25°C (68°F to 77°F).

Oral suspension: Store dry powder at 20°C to 25°C (68°F to 77°F). Once reconstituted, oral suspension is stable for 14 days under refrigeration.

IV:

Solutions for IM or direct IV should be used within 1 hour. Stability of parenteral admixture (20 mg/mL) in NS at 25°C (77°F) is 8 hours and at 4°C (39°F) is 2 days.

Mechanism of Action Inhibits bacterial cell wall synthesis by binding to one or more of the penicillin-binding proteins (PBPs) which in turn inhibits the final transpeptidation step of peptidoglycan synthesis in bacterial cell walls, thus inhibiting cell wall biosynthesis. Bacteria eventually lyse due to ongoing activity of cell wall autolytic enzymes (autolysins and murein hydrolases) while cell wall assembly is arrested.

Pharmacodynamics/Kinetics

Absorption: Oral: 50%

Distribution: Penetration into CSF occurs with inflamed meninges only

Protein binding: ~20%

Half-life elimination: Adults: 1-1.8 hours (Bergan, 1979)

Dosage

Usual dosage range:

Infants and Children:

Oral: 50 to 100 mg/kg/day divided every 6 hours (maximum: 2 to 4 g/day)

IM, IV: 25 to 200 mg/kg/day divided every 3 to 4 hours (maximum: 12 g/day)

Adults:

Oral: 250 to 500 mg every 6 hours

IM, IV: 1 to 2 g every 4 to 6 hours or 50 to 250 mg/kg/day in divided doses (maximum: 12 g/day)

Indication-specific dosing:

Infants, Children, and Adolescents:

Community-acquired pneumonia (CAP) (IDSA/PIDS, 2011): Infants >3 months and Children: IV: **Note:** May consider addition of vancomycin or clindamycin to empiric therapy if community-acquired MRSA suspected. In children ≥5 years, a macrolide antibiotic should be added if atypical pneumonia cannot be ruled out. Maximum daily dose of ampicillin: 12 g/day (Red Book [AAP 2012]).

Empiric treatment or *S. pneumoniae* (moderate to severe; MICs to penicillin ≤2.0 mcg/mL) or *H. influenzae* (beta-lactamase negative) (preferred): 150 to 200 mg/kg/day divided every 6 hours

Group A *Streptococcus* (moderate to severe) (preferred): 200 mg/kg/day divided every 6 hours

S. pneumoniae (moderate-to-severe; MICs to penicillin ≥4.0 mcg/mL) (alternative to ceftriaxone): 300 to 400 mg/kg/day divided every 6 hours

Endocarditis prophylaxis (off-label use):

Dental, oral, or respiratory tract procedures: IM, IV: 50 mg/kg within 30 to 60 minutes prior to procedure in patients not allergic to penicillin and unable to take oral amoxicillin. Maximum single dose of ampicillin: 2 g. Intramuscular injections should be avoided in patients who are receiving anticoagulant therapy. In these circumstances, orally administered regimens should be given whenever possible. Intravenously administered antibiotics should be used for patients who are unable to tolerate or absorb oral medications (Wilson, 2007).

Note: American Heart Association (AHA) guidelines now recommend prophylaxis only in patients undergoing invasive procedures and in whom underlying cardiac conditions may predispose to a higher risk of adverse outcomes should infection occur.

Genitourinary and gastrointestinal tract procedures: **Note:** Routine prophylaxis for GI/GU procedures is no longer recommended by the AHA. Consider only in patients with the highest risk of adverse outcome from endocarditis (eg, prosthetic heart valve, previous endocarditis, some categories of congenital heart disease, valvulopathy in cardiac transplant patients) who have an established GI or GU enterococcal infection or for those already receiving antibiotic therapy to prevent a wound infection or sepsis associated with a GI or GU procedure in which enterococcal coverage is desired (Wilson, 2007)

IM, IV:

High-risk patients: 50 mg/kg (maximum: 2 g) within 30 minutes prior to procedure, followed by ampicillin 25 mg/kg (or amoxicillin 25 mg/kg orally) 6 hours later; must be used in combination with gentamicin. Maximum single dose of ampicillin: 2 g (Dajani, 1997). **Note:** Routine prophylaxis for GI/GU procedures is no longer recommended by the AHA (Wilson, 2007).

Moderate-risk patients: 50 mg/kg within 30 minutes prior to procedure. Maximum single dose of ampicillin: 2 g (Dajani, 1997).

Endocarditis treatment (off-label dose): IV: 300 mg/kg/day in divided doses every 4 to 6 hours in combination with other antibiotics (maximum: 12 g/day) (Baddour, 2005)

Genitourinary or gastrointestinal infections:

Oral:

Infants and Children ≤20 kg: 100 mg/kg/day in divided doses 4 times daily

Children and Adolescents >20 kg: 500 mg 4 times daily

IM, IV:

Infants and Children <40 kg: 50 mg/kg/day in divided doses every 6 to 8 hours

Children and Adolescents ≥40 kg: 500 mg every 6 hours

Mild to moderate infections:

Oral: 50 to 100 mg/kg/day divided every 6 hours (maximum: 2 to 4 g/day) (*Red Book* [AAP 2012])

IM, IV: 100 to 150 mg/kg/day divided every 6 hours (maximum: 2 to 4 g/day) (*Red Book* [AAP 2012])

Respiratory tract infections:

Oral:

Infants and Children ≤20 kg: 50 mg/kg/day in divided doses 3 to 4 times daily

Children and Adolescents >20 kg: 250 mg 4 times daily

IM, IV:

Infants and Children <40 kg: 25 to 50 mg/kg/day in divided doses every 6 to 8 hours

Children and Adolescents ≥40 kg: 250 to 500 mg every 6 hours

Severe infections, meningitis, septicemia: IM, IV: **Note:** Treatment should be initiated with IV infusion therapy and may be continued with IM injections if preferred

Manufacturer recommendation: 150 to 200 mg/kg/day in divided doses every 3 to 4 hours

Alternative recommendation: 200 to 400 mg/kg/day in divided doses every 6 hours (maximum: 6 to 12 g/day) (Red Book [AAP 2012])

Surgical (perioperative) prophylaxis in liver transplantation (off-label use): Children ≥1 year: IV: 50 mg/kg within 60 minutes prior to surgery (maximum: 2,000 mg/dose) in combination with cefotaxime. Doses may be repeated in 2 hours if procedure is lengthy or if there is excessive blood loss (Bratzler, 2013).

Adults:

Endocarditis:

Treatment (off-label dose): IV: 2 g every 4 hours in combination with other antibiotics (Baddour, 2005)

Prophylaxis (off-label use):

Dental, oral, or respiratory tract procedures: IM, IV: 2 g within 30 to 60 minutes prior to procedure in patients not allergic to penicillin and unable to take oral amoxicillin. Intramuscular injections should be avoided in patients who are receiving anticoagulant therapy. In these circumstances, orally administered regimens should be given whenever possible. Intravenously administered antibiotics should be used for patients who are unable to tolerate or absorb oral medications. (Wilson, 2007)

Note: American Heart Association (AHA) guidelines now recommend prophylaxis only in patients undergoing invasive procedures and in whom underlying cardiac conditions may predispose to a higher risk of adverse outcomes should infection occur.

Genitourinary and gastrointestinal tract procedures: **Note:** Routine prophylaxis for GI/GU procedures is no longer recommended by the AHA. Consider only in patients with the highest risk of adverse outcome from endocarditis (eg, prosthetic heart valve, previous endocarditis, some categories of congenital heart disease, cardiac valvulopathy in cardiac transplant patients) who have an established GI or GU enterococcal infection or for those already receiving antibiotic therapy to prevent a wound infection or sepsis associated with a GI or GU procedure in which enterococcal coverage is desired (Wilson, 2007).

High-risk patients: IM, IV: 2 g within 30 minutes prior to procedure, followed by ampicillin 1 g (or amoxicillin 1 g orally) 6 hours later; must be used in combination with gentamicin (Dajani, 1997)

Moderate-risk patients: IM, IV: 2 g within 30 minutes prior to procedure (Dajani, 1997)

Genitourinary or gastrointestinal infections: Oral, IM, IV: 500 mg every 6 hours

Group B streptococcus (maternal dose for neonatal prophylaxis) (off-label use): IV: 2 g initial dose, then 1 g every 4 hours until delivery (CDC, 2010)

***Listeria* infections (off-label dosing; Lorber, 1997):** IV:

Bacteremia: 200 mg/kg/day divided every 6 hours for ≥2 weeks

Brain abscess or rhombencephalitis: 200 mg/kg/day divided every 4 hours with concomitant aminoglycoside for ≥6 weeks

Endocarditis: 200 mg/kg/day divided every 6 hours with concomitant aminoglycoside for ≥4 to 6 weeks

Meningitis: 200 mg/kg/day divided every 4 hours with concomitant aminoglycoside for ≥3 weeks

Mild to moderate infections: Oral: 250 to 500 mg every 6 hours

Prosthetic joint infection, *Enterococcus* spp (penicillin-susceptible) (off-label use): IV: 12 g continuous infusion every 24 hours **or** 2 g every 4 hours for 4 to 6 weeks; consider addition of aminoglycoside (Osmon, 2013)

Respiratory tract infections:

Oral: 250 mg 4 times daily

IM, IV: 250 to 500 mg every 6 hours

Sepsis/meningitis: IM, IV: **Note:** administer doses IV initially; IM may be used later in therapy course: 150 to 200 mg/kg/day divided every 3 to 4 hours (range: 6 to 12 g/day)

Surgical (perioperative) prophylaxis in liver transplantation (off-label use): IV: 2 g within 60 minutes prior to surgery in combination with cefotaxime. Doses may be repeated in 2 hours if procedure is lengthy or if there is excessive blood loss (Bratzler, 2013).

Urinary tract infections (ampicillin-susceptible *Enterococcus*) (off-label use): IV: 1 to 2 g every 4 to 6 hours with or without an aminoglycoside (Heintz, 2010)

Dosage adjustment in renal impairment: There are no dosage adjustments provided in the manufacturer's labeling; however, the following adjustments have been recommended (Aronoff, 2007):

CrCl >50 mL/minute: Administer every 6 hours

CrCl 10 to 50 mL/minute: Administer every 6 to 12 hours

CrCl <10 mL/minute: Administer every 12 to 24 hours

End stage renal disease (ESRD) on intermittent hemodialysis (IHD): Dialyzable (20% to 50%): IV: 1 to 2 g every 12 to 24 hours (administer after hemodialysis on dialysis days) (Heintz, 2009). **Note:** Dosing dependent on the assumption of 3 times/week, complete IHD sessions.

Peritoneal dialysis (PD): IV: 250 mg every 12 hours (Aronoff, 2007)

Continuous renal replacement therapy (CRRT) (Heintz, 2009): Drug clearance is highly dependent on the method of renal replacement, filter type, and flow rate. Appropriate dosing requires close monitoring of pharmacologic response, signs of adverse reactions due to drug accumulation, as well as drug concentrations in relation to target trough (if appropriate). The following are general recommendations only (based on dialysate flow/ultrafiltration rates of 1 to 2 L/hour and minimal residual renal function) and should not supersede clinical judgment: IV:

CVVH: Loading dose of 2 g followed by 1 to 2 g every 8 to 12 hours

CVVHD: Loading dose of 2 g followed by 1 to 2 g every 8 hours

CVVHDF: Loading dose of 2 g followed by 1 to 2 g every 6 to 8 hours

Dosage adjustment in hepatic impairment: There are no dosage adjustments provided in the manufacturer's labeling.

Dietary Considerations Take on an empty stomach 30 minutes before or 2 hours after meals. Some products may contain sodium.

Administration Administer around-the-clock to promote less variation in peak and trough serum levels.

Oral: Administer on an empty stomach with a full glass (8 oz) of water (ie, 30 minutes prior to or 2 hours after meals) to increase total absorption.

IM.: Inject deep IM into a large muscle mass

IV: Direct IV bolus: Administer over 3 to 5 minutes (125 to 500 mg) or over 10 to 15 minutes (1 to 2 g). More rapid infusion may cause seizures.

Infusion: Rapid infusion may cause seizures. Adjust rate of infusion so that the total dose is administered before admixture stability expires.

Monitoring Parameters With prolonged therapy, monitor renal, hepatic, and hematologic function periodically; observe signs and symptoms of anaphylaxis during first dose

Dosage Forms

Capsule, Oral:

Generic: 250 mg, 500 mg

Solution Reconstituted, Injection:

Generic: 125 mg (1 ea); 250 mg (1 ea); 500 mg (1 ea); 1 g (1 ea); 2 g (1 ea); 10 g (1 ea)

Solution Reconstituted, Injection [preservative free]:

Generic: 250 mg (1 ea); 500 mg (1 ea)

Solution Reconstituted, Intravenous:

Generic: 1 g (1 ea); 2 g (1 ea); 10 g (1 ea)

Solution Reconstituted, Intravenous [preservative free]:

Generic: 10 g (1 ea)

Suspension Reconstituted, Oral:

Generic: 125 mg/5 mL (100 mL, 200 mL); 250 mg/5 mL (100 mL, 200 mL)

Ampicillin and Cloxacillin [INT]

(am pi SIL in & kloks a SIL in)

International Brand Names Ampiclox (AE, EG, PK); Amplium (IT); Apoclox (PK); Cloxapene (IN); Cloxipen

(AE); Jielite (CN); Kaifa (CN); Lampicin Fort (HK); Megapen (IN); Ultracloxam (LB)

Index Terms Ampicillin Trihydrate and Cloxacillin Sodium; Cloxacillin and Ampicillin

Pharmacologic Category Antibiotic, Penicillin

Reported Use Treatment of susceptible infections

Dosage Range Note: Dosage expressed as combined ampicillin and cloxacillin

Children 2-10 years: IV: 250-500 mg every 6 hours

Children >10 years and Adults:

IM, IV: 250-1000 mg every 6 hours

Oral: 500-1500 mg 4 times daily

Product Availability Product available in various countries; not currently available in the U.S.

Dosage Forms

Capsule: 500 mg [contains ampicillin 250 mg and cloxacillin 250 mg]

Injection, powder for reconstitution, neonatal: 75 mg [contains ampicillin 50 mg and cloxacillin 25 mg]

Injection, powder for reconstitution: 500 mg [contains ampicillin 250 mg and cloxacillin 250 mg]

Powder for neonatal drops: 90 mg/0.6 mL (8 mL) [contains ampicillin 60 mg and cloxacillin 30 mg; sodium benzoate; packaged with pipette]

Powder for oral suspension: 250 mg/5 mL (100 mL) [contains ampicillin 125 mg and cloxacillin; sodium benzoate; fruit flavor]

Ampicillin and Sulbactam

(am pi SIL in & SUL bak tam)

Brand Names: U.S. Unasyn

Brand Names: Canada Unasyn

Index Terms Sulbactam and Ampicillin

Pharmacologic Category Antibiotic, Penicillin

Use Bacterial infections: Treatment of susceptible bacterial infections involved with skin and skin structure, intra-abdominal infections, gynecological infections; spectrum is that of ampicillin plus organisms producing beta-lactamases such as *S. aureus*, *H. influenzae*, *E. coli*, *Klebsiella*, *Acinetobacter*, *Enterobacter*, and anaerobes

Pregnancy Risk Factor B

Pregnancy Considerations Adverse events have not been observed in animal reproduction studies. Both ampicillin and sulbactam cross the placenta. Maternal use of penicillins has generally not resulted in an increased risk of birth defects. When used during pregnancy, pharmacokinetic changes have been observed with ampicillin alone (refer to the Ampicillin monograph for details). Ampicillin/sulbactam may be considered for prophylactic use prior to cesarean delivery (consult current guidelines).

Breast-Feeding Considerations Ampicillin and sulbactam are both excreted into breast milk in low concentrations. The manufacturer recommends that caution be used if administering to lactating women. Nondose-related effects could include modification of bowel flora and allergic sensitization of the infant. The maternal dose of sulbactam does not need altered in the postpartum period. Also refer to the Ampicillin monograph.

Contraindications Hypersensitivity (eg, anaphylaxis or Stevens-Johnson syndrome) to ampicillin, sulbactam, or to other beta-lactam antibacterial drugs (eg, penicillins, cephalosporins), or any component of the formulations; history of cholestatic jaundice or hepatic dysfunction associated with ampicillin/sulbactam

Warnings/Precautions Dosage adjustment may be necessary in patients with renal impairment. Serious and occasionally severe or fatal hypersensitivity (anaphylactic) reactions have been reported in patients on penicillin therapy, especially with a history of beta-lactam hypersensitivity, history of sensitivity to multiple allergens. Patients with a history of penicillin hypersensitivity have experienced severe reactions when treated with cephalosporins. Before initiating therapy, carefully investigate previous penicillin, cephalosporin, or other allergen hypersensitivity. If an allergic reaction occurs, discontinue and institute appropriate therapy. Hepatitis and cholestatic jaundice have been reported (including fatalities). Toxicity is usually reversible. Monitor hepatic function at regular intervals in patients with hepatic impairment. High percentage of patients with infectious mononucleosis have developed rash during therapy with ampicillin; ampicillin-class antibacterials are not recommended in these patients. Appearance of a rash should be carefully evaluated to differentiate a nonallergic ampicillin rash from a hypersensitivity reaction. Prolonged use may result in fungal or bacterial superinfection, including *C. difficile*-associated diarrhea (CDAD) and pseudomembranous colitis; CDAD has been observed >2 months postantibiotic treatment.

Adverse Reactions Also see Ampicillin.

Cardiovascular: Thrombophlebitis

Dermatologic: Skin rash

Gastrointestinal: Diarrhea

Local: Pain at injection site (IM/IV)

Rare but important or life-threatening: Acute generalized exanthematous pustulosis, agranulocytosis, anemia, basophilia, candidiasis, casts in urine (hyaline), chest pain, chills, cholestasis, cholestatic hepatitis, *clostridium difficile* associated diarrhea, convulsions, decreased neutrophils, decreased serum albumin, decreased serum total protein, dysuria, edema, eosinophilia, erythema, erythema multiforme, erythrocyturia, exfoliative dermatitis, gastritis, glossitis, hairy tongue, headache, hemolytic anemia, hepatic insufficiency, hepatitis, hyperbilirubinemia, hypersensitivity reaction, immune thrombocytopenia, increased blood urea nitrogen, increased lactate dehydrogenase, increased liver enzymes, increased monocytes, increased serum creatinine, injection site reaction,interstitial nephritis, jaundice, leukopenia, lymphocytopenia, lymphocytosis (abnormal), nausea, positive direct Coombs test, pruritus, pseudomembranous colitis, Stevens-Johnson syndrome, stomatitis, thrombocythemia, thrombocytopenia, urinary retention, urticaria

Drug Interactions

Metabolism/Transport Effects None known.

Avoid Concomitant Use

Avoid concomitant use of Ampicillin and Sulbactam with any of the following: BCG; Probenecid

Increased Effect/Toxicity

Ampicillin and Sulbactam may increase the levels/effects of: Methotrexate; Vitamin K Antagonists

The levels/effects of Ampicillin and Sulbactam may be increased by: Allopurinol; Probenecid

Decreased Effect

Ampicillin and Sulbactam may decrease the levels/effects of: Atenolol; BCG; Mycophenolate; Sodium Picosulfate; Typhoid Vaccine

The levels/effects of Ampicillin and Sulbactam may be decreased by: Chloroquine; Lanthanum; Tetracycline Derivatives

Preparation for Administration

Direct IV administration and IV infusion: Reconstitute with sterile water for injection (SWFI). Sodium chloride 0.9% (NS) is the diluent of choice for IV infusion use.

IM administration: Reconstitute with SWFI **or** 0.5% or 2% lidocaine hydrochloride injection.

Storage/Stability

Prior to reconstitution, store at 20°C to 25°C (68°F to 77°F).

IM: Concentration of 375 mg/mL (250 mg ampicillin/125 mg sulbacatam) should be used within 1 hour after reconstitution.

Intermittent IV infusion: Solutions made in NS are stable up to 72 hours when refrigerated whereas dextrose solutions (same concentration) are stable for only 4 hours. For stability related to specific concentrations and temperatures, see prescribing information.

Mechanism of Action Inhibits bacterial cell wall synthesis by binding to one or more of the penicillin-binding proteins (PBPs) which in turn inhibits the final transpeptidation step of peptidoglycan synthesis in bacterial cell walls, thus inhibiting cell wall biosynthesis. Bacteria eventually lyse due to ongoing activity of cell wall autolytic enzymes (autolysins and murein hydrolases) while cell wall assembly is arrested. The addition of sulbactam, a beta-lactamase inhibitor, to ampicillin extends the spectrum of ampicillin to include some beta-lactamase-producing organisms.

Pharmacodynamics/Kinetics

Ampicillin: See Ampicillin monograph.

Sulbactam:

Distribution: Widely distributed to bile, blister, and tissue fluids; distributed to cerebrospinal fluid in the presence of inflamed meninges

Protein binding: 38%

Half-life elimination: Normal renal function: 1 to 1.3 hours; **Note:** Elimination kinetics of both ampicillin and sulbactam are similarly affected in patients with renal impairment, therefore, the blood concentration ratio is expected to remain constant regardless of renal function.

Excretion: Urine (~75% to 85% as unchanged drug) within 8 hours

Dosage Note: Unasyn (ampicillin/sulbactam) is a combination product.

Usual dosage range:

Children and Adolescents: IV: 100 to 200 mg **ampicillin/**kg/day divided every 6 hours (maximum: 8 g ampicillin daily or 12 g ampicillin/sulbactam daily)

Adults: IM, IV: 1.5 to 3 g **ampicillin/sulbactam** every 6 hours (maximum: 12 g ampicillin/sulbactam daily)

Indication-specific dosing:

Infants, Children, and Adolescents: **Note:** Dosage recommendations are expressed as mg of the **ampicillin** component.

Infective endocarditis (off-label use) (AHA/IDSA [Baddour, 2005])

Bartonella spp. (Native valve): IV: 200 mg ampicillin/kg/day in 4 or 6 divided doses with concomitant gentamicin for 4 to 6 weeks.

Enterococcus organism (resistant to penicillin/susceptible to aminoglycoside and vancomycin): IV: 200 mg ampicillin/kg/day in 4 divided doses with concomitant gentamicin for 6 weeks. **Note:** If enterococcus is gentamicin resistant, then >6 weeks of ampicillin-sulbactam therapy needed.

HACEK organism: 200 mg ampicillin/kg/day in 4 or 6 divided doses for 4 weeks.

Intravascular catheter-associated bloodstream infection (off-label use) (IDSA, 2009):

Infants: IV: 100 to 150 mg ampicillin/kg/day in 4 divided doses

Children and Adolescents: IV: 100 to 200 mg ampicillin/kg/day in 4 divided doses

Children and Adolescents: **Note:** Dosage recommendations are expressed as mg of the **ampicillin** component.

Epiglottitis: IV: 100 to 200 mg ampicillin/kg/day divided in 4 doses

Mild to moderate infections: IV: 100 to 200 mg ampicillin/kg/day divided every 6 hours (maximum: 8 g ampicillin daily or 12 g ampicillin/sulbactam daily)

Peritonsillar and retropharyngeal abscess: IV: 200 mg ampicillin/kg/day in 4 divided doses

Severe infections: IV: 200 mg ampicillin/kg/day divided every 6 hours (maximum: 8 g ampicillin daily or 12 g ampicillin/sulbactam daily)

Surgical (perioperative) prophylaxis (off-label use): Children ≥1 year: IV: 50 mg ampicillin/kg within 60 minutes prior to surgical incision (maximum dose: 2000 mg ampicillin or 3 g ampicillin/sulbactam daily). Doses may be repeated in 2 hours if procedure is lengthy or if there is excessive blood loss (Bratzler, 2013).

Adults: **Note:** Dosage recommendations are expressed as grams of **ampicillin/sulbactam** combination:

Acute bacterial rhinosinusitis, severe infection requiring hospitalization (off-label use): IV: 1.5 to 3 g every 6 hours for 5 to 7 days (Chow, 2012)

Amnionitis, cholangitis, diverticulitis, endomyometritis (with doxycycline), endophthalmitis, epididymitis/orchitis, liver abscess (with metronidazole), or peritonitis: IV: 3 g every 6 hours

Bite (human, canine/feline): *Pasteurella multocida:* IV: 1.5 to 3 g every 6 hours

Infective endocarditis (off-label use) (AHA/IDSA [Baddour, 2005]):

Bartonella spp. (Native valve): IV: 3 g every 6 hours with concomitant gentamicin for 4 to 6 weeks.

Enterococcus organism (resistant to penicillin/susceptible to aminoglycoside and vancomycin): IV: 3 g every 6 hours with concomitant gentamicin for 6 weeks. **Note:** If enterococcus is gentamicin resistant, then >6 weeks of ampicillin-sulbactam therapy needed.

HACEK organism: IV: 3 g every 6 hours for 4 weeks

Intravascular catheter-associated bloodstream infection, *Acinetobacter* spp (off-label use) (IDSA, 2009): IV: 3 g every 6 hours

Orbital cellulitis: IV: 3 g every 6 hours

Osteomyelitis (diabetic foot) (Lipsky, 2004): IV: 3 g every 6 hours

Pelvic inflammatory disease (off-label use): IV: 3 g every 6 hours (for 24 hours after clinical improvement is noted) with doxycycline (continued for a total of 14 days) (CDC, 2010)

Peritonitis associated with CAPD: Intraperitoneal:

Intermittent: 3 g added to one exchange every 12 hours; allow to dwell for at least 6 hours (Blackwell, 1990; Li, 2010)

Continuous: Loading dose: 1.5 g per liter of dialysate; maintenance dose: 150 mg per liter of dialysate (Li, 2010)

Pneumonia (off-label use):

Aspiration or community-acquired: IV: 1.5 to 3 g every 6 hours for ≥5 days (Geckler, 1994; Majcher-Peszynska, 2014; Mandell, 2007; Rossoff, 1995). **Note:** In ICU patients, give with azithromycin or a fluoroquinolone (Mandell, 2007).

Hospital-acquired (empiric, early onset, no known risk factors for multidrug-resistant pathogens): IV: 3 g every 6 hours for ≥5 days (ATS, 2005; Jauregui, 1995)

Surgical (perioperative) prophylaxis (off-label use): IV: 3 g within 60 minutes prior to surgical incision. Doses may be repeated in 2 hours if procedure is lengthy or if there is excessive blood loss (Bratzler, 2013).

Urinary tract infections, pyelonephritis: IV: 3 g every 6 hours for 14 days

Dosage adjustment in renal impairment: Note: Estimation of renal function for the purpose of drug dosing should be done using the Cockcroft-Gault formula. Dosage recommendations are expressed as grams of **ampicillin/sulbactam** combination:

CrCl ≥30 mL/minute/1.73 m^2: No dosage adjustment necessary.

CrCl 15 to 29 mL/minute/1.73 m^2: 1.5 to 3 g every 12 hours

CrCl 5 to 14 mL/minute/1.73 m^2: 1.5 to 3 g every 24 hours

End stage renal disease (ESRD) on intermittent hemodialysis (IHD) (administer after hemodialysis on dialysis days): 1.5 to 3 g every 12 to 24 hours (Heintz, 2009). **Note:** Dosing dependent on the assumption of 3 times weekly, complete IHD sessions.

Continuous renal replacement therapy (CRRT): Drug clearance is highly dependent on the method of renal replacement, filter type, and flow rate. Appropriate dosing requires close monitoring of pharmacologic response, signs of adverse reactions due to drug accumulation, as well as drug levels in relation to target trough (if appropriate). The following are general recommendations only (based on dialysate flow/ultrafiltration rates of 1 to 2 L/hour and minimal residual renal function) and should not supersede clinical judgment (Heintz, 2009; Trotman, 2005):

CVVH: Initial: 3 g; maintenance: 1.5 to 3 g every 8 to 12 hours

CVVHD: Initial: 3 g; maintenance: 1.5 to 3 g every 8 hours

CVVHDF: Initial: 3 g; maintenance: 1.5 to 3 g every 6 to 8 hours

Dosage adjustment in hepatic impairment: There is no dosage adjustment provided in the manufacturer's labeling.

Dietary Considerations Some products may contain sodium.

Administration Administer around-the-clock to promote less variation in peak and trough serum levels.

IV: Administer by slow injection over 10 to 15 minutes or as an IV infusion over 15 to 30 minutes. Ampicillin and gentamicin should not be mixed in the same IV tubing.

Some penicillins (eg, ampicillin, carbenicillin, ticarcillin, and piperacillin) have been shown to inactivate aminoglycosides *in vitro*. This has been observed to a greater extent with tobramycin and gentamicin, while amikacin has shown greater stability against inactivation. Concurrent Y-site administration should be avoided.

IM: Inject deep I.M. into large muscle mass; a concentration of 375 mg/mL ampicillin/sulbactam (250 mg ampicillin/125 mg sulbactam per mL) is recommended; may be diluted in sterile water or lidocaine 0.5% or lidocaine 2% for I.M. administration.

Monitoring Parameters With prolonged therapy, monitor hematologic, renal, and hepatic function; monitor for signs of anaphylaxis during first dose. In patients with preexisting hepatic impairment, monitor hepatic function at regular intervals.

Dosage Forms

Injection, powder for reconstitution: 1.5 g [ampicillin 1 g and sulbactam 0.5 g]; 3 g [ampicillin 2 g and sulbactam 1 g]; 15 g [ampicillin 10 g and sulbactam 5 g]

Unasyn®: 1.5 g [ampicillin 1 g and sulbactam 0.5 g]; 3 g [ampicillin 2 g and sulbactam 1 g]; 15 g [ampicillin 10 g and sulbactam 5 g]; 15 g [ampicillin 10 g and sulbactam 5 g

- ◆ **Ampicillin for Injection (Can)** *see* Ampicillin *on page 141*
- ◆ **Ampicillin Sodium** *see* Ampicillin *on page 141*
- ◆ **Ampicillin Trihydrate** *see* Ampicillin *on page 141*
- ◆ **Ampicillin Trihydrate and Cloxacillin Sodium** *see* Ampicillin and Cloxacillin [INT] *on page 144*
- ◆ **AMPT** *see* Metyrosine *on page 1359*
- ◆ **Ampyra** *see* Dalfampridine *on page 552*
- ◆ **AMR101** *see* Omega-3 Fatty Acids *on page 1507*
- ◆ **Amrix** *see* Cyclobenzaprine *on page 516*
- ◆ **Amturnide™** *see* Aliskiren, Amlodipine, and Hydrochlorothiazide *on page 87*
- ◆ **Amvisc** *see* Hyaluronate and Derivatives *on page 1006*
- ◆ **Amvisc Plus** *see* Hyaluronate and Derivatives *on page 1006*
- ◆ **Amylase, Lipase, and Protease** *see* Pancrelipase *on page 1566*

Amyl Nitrite (AM il NYE trite)

Index Terms Isoamyl Nitrite

Pharmacologic Category Antianginal Agent; Antidote; Vasodilator

Use Coronary vasodilator in angina pectoris

Note: Given the widespread use of newer nitrate compounds, the use of amyl nitrite for patients experiencing angina pectoris has fallen out of favor.

Pregnancy Risk Factor C

Dosage Inhalation:

Angina: Adults: 2 to 6 nasal inhalations from 1 crushed ampul; may repeat in 3 to 5 minutes

Cyanide toxicity (off-label use): Children, Adolescents, and Adults: 0.3 mL ampul crushed into a gauze pad and placed in front of the patient's mouth (or endotracheal tube if patient is intubated) to inhale over 15 to 30 seconds; repeat every minute until sodium nitrite can be administered (Mokhlesi, 2003). **Note:** Must separate administrations by at least 30 seconds to allow for adequate oxygenation; each ampul will last for ~3 minutes. Amyl nitrite is a temporary intervention that should only be used until IV sodium nitrite infusion is ready for administration (ATSDR).

Pharmacologic provocation of latent left ventricular outflow tract (LVOT) gradient in hypertrophic cardiomyopathy (HCM) (off-label use): Adults: 3-4 deep inhalations from 1 crushed ampul over a 10-15 second period (Gersh, 2011; Nagueh, 2011; Reagan, 2005). **Note:** The use of more physiologic testing (eg, treadmill testing with Doppler echocardiography) may be preferred over amyl nitrite inhalation (Maron, 2003; Nagueh, 2011).

Additional Information Complete prescribing information should be consulted for additional detail.

Dosage Forms

Liquid, for inhalation: USP: 85% to 103% (0.3 mL)

- ◆ **Amylobarbitone** *see* Amobarbital *on page 128*
- ◆ **Amytal® (Can)** *see* Amobarbital *on page 128*
- ◆ **Amytal Sodium** *see* Amobarbital *on page 128*
- ◆ **AN100226** *see* Natalizumab *on page 1432*
- ◆ **Anacaine** *see* Benzocaine *on page 246*
- ◆ **Anacin Advanced Headache Formula [OTC]** *see* Acetaminophen, Aspirin, and Caffeine *on page 37*
- ◆ **Anadrol-50** *see* Oxymetholone *on page 1546*
- ◆ **Anafranil** *see* ClomiPRAMINE *on page 475*
- ◆ **Anafranil® (Can)** *see* ClomiPRAMINE *on page 475*

Anagrelide (an AG gre lide)

Brand Names: U.S. Agrylin

Brand Names: Canada Agrylin; Dom-Anagrelide; Mylan-Anagrelide; PMS-Anagrelide; Sandoz-Anagrelide

Index Terms Anagrelide Hydrochloride; BL4162A

Pharmacologic Category Antiplatelet Agent; Phosphodiesterase-3 Enzyme Inhibitor

Use Thrombocythemia: Treatment of thrombocythemia associated with myeloproliferative disorders to reduce the risk of thrombosis and reduce associated symptoms (including thrombohemorrhagic events)

Pregnancy Risk Factor C

Dosage Note: Maintain initial dose for ≥1 week, then adjust to the lowest effective dose to reduce and maintain platelet count <600,000/mm^3 ideally to the normal range; the dose must not be increased by >0.5 mg per day in any 1 week; maximum single dose: 2.5 mg; maximum daily dose: 10 mg

Thrombocythemia:

Children: Oral: Initial: 0.5 mg once daily (range: 0.5 mg 1 to 4 times daily)

Adults: Oral: Initial: 0.5 mg 4 times daily or 1 mg twice daily (most patients will experience adequate response at dose ranges of 1.5 to 3 mg per day)

Thrombocythemia, essential (off-label dosing): Adults: Oral: 0.5 mg twice daily for 1 week, then adjust dose to maintain platelet counts at normal (≤450,000/mm^3) or near normal (450,000/mm^3 to 600,000/mm^3) levels (Gisslinger, 2013).

Elderly: There are no special requirements for dosing in the elderly

Dosage adjustment in renal impairment: No dosage adjustment necessary; monitor closely.

Dosage adjustment in hepatic impairment:

Moderate impairment (Child-Pugh score 7 to 9): Initial: 0.5 mg once daily; maintain for at least 1 week with careful monitoring of cardiovascular status; the dose must not be increased by >0.5 mg per day in any 1 week.

Severe impairment (Child-Pugh score ≥10): Avoid use.

Additional Information Complete prescribing information should be consulted for additional detail.

Dosage Forms

Capsule, Oral:

Agrylin: 0.5 mg

Generic: 0.5 mg, 1 mg

◆ **Anagrelide Hydrochloride** *see* Anagrelide *on page 147*

Anakinra (an a KIN ra)

Brand Names: U.S. Kineret

Brand Names: Canada Kineret

Index Terms IL-1Ra; Interleukin-1 Receptor Antagonist

Pharmacologic Category Antirheumatic, Disease Modifying; Interleukin-1 Receptor Antagonist

Use Treatment of moderately- to severely-active rheumatoid arthritis (RA) in adult patients who have failed one or more disease-modifying antirheumatic drugs (DMARDs; may be used alone or in combination with DMARDs [other than tumor necrosis factor-blocking agents]); treatment of neonatal-onset multisystem inflammatory disease (NOMID), which is a cryopyrin-associated periodic syndrome (CAPS)

Pregnancy Risk Factor B

Dosage

Neonatal-onset multisystem inflammatory disease (NOMID): Infants, Children, Adolescents, and Adults: SubQ: Initial: 1 to 2 mg/kg daily in 1 to 2 divided doses; adjust dose in 0.5 to 1 mg/kg increments as needed; usual maintenance dose: 3 to 4 mg/kg daily (maximum: 8 mg/kg daily). **Note:** The prefilled syringe does not allow doses lower than 20 mg to be administered.

Rheumatoid arthritis (RA): Adults: SubQ: 100 mg once daily (administer at approximately the same time each day)

Juvenile idiopathic arthritis, systemic (off-label use): Children and Adolescents: SubQ: Initial: 1 to 2 mg/kg once daily; maximum initial dose: 100 mg; if no response after 1 to 2 weeks, may titrate up to 4 mg/kg once daily (maximum daily dose: 200 mg) (Dewitt, 2012; Hedrich, 2012; Lequerré, 2008; Nigrovic, 2011; Quartier, 2011; Ringold, 2013).

Dosage adjustment in renal impairment:

CrCl ≥30 mL/minute: No dosage adjustment necessary.

CrCl <30 mL/minute:

NOMID: Infants, Children, Adolescents, and Adults: No dosage adjustment necessary; however, decrease frequency of administration to every other day.

RA: Adults: 100 mg every other day

ESRD (**Note:** <2.5% of the dose is removed by hemodialysis or CAPD):

NOMID: Infants, Children, Adolescents, and Adults: No dosage adjustment necessary; however, decrease frequency of administration to every other day.

RA: Adults: 100 mg every other day

Dosage adjustment in hepatic impairment: No dosage adjustments provided in the manufacturer's labeling (has not been studied).

Additional Information Complete prescribing information should be consulted for additional detail.

Dosage Forms

Solution Prefilled Syringe, Subcutaneous [preservative free]:

Kineret: 100 mg/0.67 mL (0.67 mL)

◆ **Analpram E™** *see* Pramoxine and Hydrocortisone *on page 1698*

◆ **Analpram HC®** *see* Pramoxine and Hydrocortisone *on page 1698*

◆ **Anandron® (Can)** *see* Nilutamide *on page 1455*

◆ **Anapen (Can)** *see* EPINEPHrine (Systemic, Oral Inhalation) *on page 735*

◆ **Anapen Junior (Can)** *see* EPINEPHrine (Systemic, Oral Inhalation) *on page 735*

◆ **Anaprox** *see* Naproxen *on page 1427*

◆ **Anaprox DS** *see* Naproxen *on page 1427*

◆ **Anascorp** *see Centruroides* Immune $F(ab')_2$ (Equine) *on page 405*

◆ **Anaspaz** *see* Hyoscyamine *on page 1026*

Anastrozole (an AS troe zole)

Brand Names: U.S. Arimidex

Brand Names: Canada ACH-Anastrozole; Apo-Anastrozole; Arimidex; Auro-Anastrozole; Bio-Anastrozole; JAMP-Anastrozole; Mar-Anastrozole; Med-Anastrozole; Mint-Anastrozole; Mylan-Anastrozole; PMS-Anastrozole; RAN-Anastrozole; Riva-Anastrozole; Sandoz-Anastrozole; Taro-Anastrozole; Teva-Anastrozole; Zinda-Anastrozole

Index Terms ICI-D1033; ZD1033

Pharmacologic Category Antineoplastic Agent, Aromatase Inhibitor

Use Breast cancer:

First-line treatment of locally-advanced or metastatic breast cancer (hormone receptor-positive or unknown) in postmenopausal women

Adjuvant treatment of early hormone receptor-positive breast cancer in postmenopausal women

Treatment of advanced breast cancer in postmenopausal women with disease progression following tamoxifen therapy

Pregnancy Risk Factor X

Pregnancy Considerations Adverse events were observed in animal reproduction studies. Anastrozole is contraindicated in women who are or may become pregnant (may cause fetal harm if administered during pregnancy). Use in premenopausal women with breast cancer does not provide any clinical benefit.

Breast-Feeding Considerations It is not known if anastrozole is excreted in breast milk. Due to the potential for serious adverse reactions in the nursing infant, a decision should be made whether to discontinue nursing or to discontinue the drug, taking into account the importance of treatment to the mother. The Canadian labeling contraindicates use in lactating women.

Contraindications Hypersensitivity to anastrozole or any component of the formulation; use in women who are or may become pregnant

Canadian labeling: Additional contraindications (not in U.S. labeling): Lactating women

Warnings/Precautions Hazardous agent - use appropriate precautions for handling and disposal (NIOSH 2014 [group 1]). Use is contraindicated in women who are or may become pregnant. Anastrozole offers no clinical benefit in premenopausal women with breast cancer. Patients with preexisting ischemic cardiac disease have an increased risk for ischemic cardiovascular events.

Due to decreased circulating estrogen levels, anastrozole is associated with a reduction in bone mineral density (BMD); decreases (from baseline) in total hip and lumbar spine BMD have been reported. Patients with preexisting osteopenia are at higher risk for developing osteoporosis (Eastell, 2008). When initiating anastrozole treatment, follow available guidelines for bone mineral density management in postmenopausal women with similar fracture risk; concurrent use of bisphosphonates may be useful in patients at risk for fractures.

Elevated total cholesterol levels (contributed to by LDL cholesterol increases) have been reported in patients receiving anastrozole; use with caution in patients with hyperlipidemias; cholesterol levels should be monitored/managed in accordance with current guidelines for patients with LDL elevations. Plasma concentrations in patients with stable hepatic cirrhosis were within the range of concentrations seen in normal subjects across all clinical trials; use has not been studied in patients with severe hepatic impairment.

Adverse Reactions

Cardiovascular: Angina pectoris, chest pain, edema, hypertension, ischemic heart disease, myocardial infarction, peripheral edema, vasodilatation, venous thrombosis (including pulmonary embolism, thrombophlebitis, retinal vein thrombosis)

Central nervous system: Anxiety, carpal tunnel syndrome, cerebrovascular insufficiency, confusion, depression, dizziness, drowsiness, fatigue, headache, hypertonia, insomnia, lethargy, malaise, mood disorder, nervousness, pain, paresthesia

Dermatologic: Alopecia, diaphoresis, pruritus, skin rash

Endocrine & metabolic: Hot flash, hypercholesterolemia, increased gamma-glutamyl transferase, increased serum cholesterol, weight gain, weight loss

Gastrointestinal: Abdominal pain, anorexia, constipation, diarrhea, dyspepsia, gastrointestinal disease, gastrointestinal distress, nausea, vomiting, xerostomia

Genitourinary: Leukorrhea, mastalgia, pelvic pain, urinary tract infection, vaginal discharge, vaginal dryness, vaginal hemorrhage, vaginitis, vulvovaginitis

Hematologic & oncologic: Anemia, breast neoplasm, leukopenia, lymphedema, neoplasm, tumor flare

Hepatic: Increased serum alkaline phosphatase, increased serum ALT, increased serum AST

Infection: Infection

Neuromuscular & skeletal: Arthralgia, arthritis, arthrosis, back pain, bone fracture, myalgia, neck pain, ostealgia, osteoporosis, pathological fracture, weakness

Ophthalmic: Cataract

Respiratory: Bronchitis, dyspnea, flu-like symptoms, increased cough, pharyngitis, rhinitis, sinusitis

Miscellaneous: Accidental injury, cyst, fever

Rare but important or life-threatening: Anaphylaxis, angioedema, cerebral infarction, cerebral ischemia, dermal ulcer, endometrial carcinoma, erythema multiforme, hepatitis, hepatomegaly, hypercalcemia, hypersensitivity angiitis (including anaphylactoid purpura [IgA vasculitis]), jaundice, joint stiffness, pulmonary embolism, retinal thrombosis, skin blister, skin lesion, Stevens-Johnson syndrome, tenosynovitis (stenosing), urticaria

Drug Interactions

Metabolism/Transport Effects Inhibits CYP1A2 (weak), CYP2C8 (weak), CYP2C9 (weak), CYP3A4 (weak)

Avoid Concomitant Use

Avoid concomitant use of Anastrozole with any of the following: Estrogen Derivatives; Pimozide

Increased Effect/Toxicity

Anastrozole may increase the levels/effects of: ARIPiprazole; Dofetilide; Hydrocodone; Lomitapide; Methadone; Pimozide

Decreased Effect

The levels/effects of Anastrozole may be decreased by: Estrogen Derivatives; Tamoxifen

Storage/Stability Store at 20°C to 25°C (68°F to 77°F).

Mechanism of Action Potent and selective nonsteroidal aromatase inhibitor. By inhibiting aromatase, the conversion of androstenedione to estrone, and testosterone to estradiol, is prevented, thereby decreasing tumor mass or delaying progression in patients with tumors responsive to hormones. Anastrozole causes an 85% decrease in estrone sulfate levels.

Pharmacodynamics/Kinetics

Onset of estradiol reduction: 70% reduction after 24 hours; 80% after 2 weeks of therapy

Duration of estradiol reduction: 6 days

Absorption: Well absorbed; extent of absorption not affected by food

Protein binding, plasma: 40%

Metabolism: Extensively hepatic (~85%) via N-dealkylation, hydroxylation, and glucuronidation; primary metabolite (triazole) inactive

Half-life elimination: ~50 hours

Time to peak, plasma: ~2 hours without food; 5 hours with food

Excretion: Feces; urine (urinary excretion accounts for ~10% of total elimination, mostly as metabolites)

Dosage

Breast cancer, advanced: Adults: Postmenopausal females: Oral: 1 mg once daily; continue until tumor progression

Breast cancer, early (adjuvant treatment): Adults: Postmenopausal females: Oral: 1 mg once daily. **Note:** The American Society of Clinical Oncology (ASCO) guidelines for Adjuvant Endocrine Therapy of Hormone-Receptor Positive Breast Cancer (Focused Update) recommend a maximum duration of 5 years of aromatase inhibitor (AI) therapy for postmenopausal women; AIs may be combined with tamoxifen for a total duration of up to 10 years of endocrine therapy. Refer to the guidelines for specific recommendations based on menopausal status and tolerability (Burstein, 2014).

Breast cancer, risk reduction (off-label use): Postmenopausal females ≥40 years: Oral: 1 mg once daily for 5 years (Cuzick, 2014)

Dosage adjustment in renal impairment: No dosage adjustment necessary.

Dosage adjustment in hepatic impairment:

Mild to moderate impairment or stable hepatic cirrhosis: No dosage adjustment necessary.

Severe hepatic impairment: There are no dosage adjustments provided in the manufacturer's labeling (has not been studied).

Administration May be administered with or without food. Hazardous agent; use appropriate precautions for handling and disposal (NIOSH 2014 [group 1]).

Monitoring Parameters

Bone mineral density; total cholesterol and LDL

Breast cancer risk reduction (off-label use): Bone mineral density at baseline, mammograms, and clinical breast exam at baseline and at least every 2 years (Cuzick, 2014)

Dosage Forms

Tablet, Oral:

Arimidex: 1 mg

Generic: 1 mg

- ◆ **Anbesol [OTC]** *see* Benzocaine *on page* 246
- ◆ **Anbesol® Baby (Can)** *see* Benzocaine *on page* 246
- ◆ **Anbesol Cold Sore Therapy [OTC]** *see* Benzocaine *on page* 246
- ◆ **Anbesol JR [OTC]** *see* Benzocaine *on page* 246
- ◆ **Anbesol Maximum Strength [OTC]** *see* Benzocaine *on page* 246
- ◆ **Ancef** *see* CeFAZolin *on page* 373

Ancestim [INT] (an SES tim)

International Brand Names Stemgen (ZA)

Pharmacologic Category Stem Cell Factor, Human

Reported Use For use in combination with filgrastim in patients requiring peripheral blood progenitor cell (PBPC) transplantation who are at risk of poor PBPC mobilization.

Dosage Range Adults: SubQ: **Note:** Ancestim should be given with filgrastim, as separate injection and at separate sites, 24 hours before to 24 hours after chemotherapy

Cytokine only mobilization: 20 mcg/kg/day until completion of apheresis

Post chemotherapy mobilization: 20 mcg/kg/day, starting 24 hours after chemotherapy until completion of apheresis

Product Availability Product available in various countries; not currently available in the U.S.

Dosage Forms

Injection, powder for reconstitution [preservative free]: 1500 mcg/mL (1.2 mL)

- ◆ **Anchoic Acid** *see* Azelaic Acid *on page* 213
- ◆ **Ancobon** *see* Flucytosine *on page* 889
- ◆ **Andriol (Can)** *see* Testosterone *on page* 2010
- ◆ **Androcur® (Can)** *see* Cyproterone [CAN/INT] *on page* 530
- ◆ **Androcur® Depot (Can)** *see* Cyproterone [CAN/INT] *on page* 530
- ◆ **Androderm** *see* Testosterone *on page* 2010
- ◆ **AndroGel** *see* Testosterone *on page* 2010
- ◆ **AndroGel Pump** *see* Testosterone *on page* 2010
- ◆ **Android** *see* MethylTESTOSTERone *on page* 1345
- ◆ **Andropository (Can)** *see* Testosterone *on page* 2010
- ◆ **Androxy [DSC]** *see* Fluoxymesterone *on page* 903
- ◆ **AneCream [OTC]** *see* Lidocaine (Topical) *on page* 1211
- ◆ **AneCream5 [OTC]** *see* Lidocaine (Topical) *on page* 1211
- ◆ **Anectine** *see* Succinylcholine *on page* 1939
- ◆ **Aneurine Hydrochloride** *see* Thiamine *on page* 2028
- ◆ **Anexate (Can)** *see* Flumazenil *on page* 892
- ◆ **Angiomax** *see* Bivalirudin *on page* 268

Anidulafungin (ay nid yoo la FUN jin)

Brand Names: U.S. Eraxis

Brand Names: Canada Eraxis

Index Terms LY303366

Pharmacologic Category Antifungal Agent, Parenteral; Echinocandin

Use Treatment of candidemia and other forms of *Candida* infections (including those of intra-abdominal, peritoneal, and esophageal locus)

Pregnancy Risk Factor B

Dosage IV: Adults:

Candidemia, intra-abdominal or peritoneal candidiasis: Initial dose: 200 mg on day 1; subsequent dosing: 100 mg daily; treatment should continue until 14 days after last positive culture

Esophageal candidiasis: Initial dose: 100 mg on day 1; subsequent dosing: 50 mg daily; treatment should continue for a minimum of 14 days and for at least 7 days after symptom resolution

Dosage adjustment in renal impairment: No dosage adjustment necessary, including dialysis patients.

Dosage adjustment in hepatic impairment: No dosage adjustment necessary.

Additional Information Complete prescribing information should be consulted for additional detail.

Dosage Forms

Solution Reconstituted, Intravenous [preservative free]: Eraxis: 50 mg (1 ea); 100 mg (1 ea)

Aniracetam [INT] (a ni RA se tam)

International Brand Names Ampamet (IT); Bi Si Ling (CN); Bo Bang Lin (CN); Draganon (IT, JP); Pergamid (AR); Reset (IT); Sarpul (JP); Shuntan (CN)

Pharmacologic Category Nootropic

Reported Use Attention and memory disorders of a degenerative or vascular origin in the elderly

Dosage Range Adults: Oral: 1500 mg/day in divided doses

Product Availability Product available in various countries; not currently available in the U.S.

Dosage Forms

Granules [sachet]: 750 mg, 1500 mg

Tablet: 750 mg

- ◆ **Ansaid (Can)** *see* Flurbiprofen (Systemic) *on page* 906
- ◆ **Ansamycin** *see* Rifabutin *on page* 1803
- ◆ **Antabuse** *see* Disulfiram *on page* 654
- ◆ **Antacid [OTC]** *see* Calcium Carbonate *on page* 327
- ◆ **Antacid Calcium [OTC]** *see* Calcium Carbonate *on page* 327
- ◆ **Antacid Extra Strength [OTC]** *see* Calcium Carbonate *on page* 327
- ◆ **Antagon** *see* Ganirelix *on page* 949
- ◆ **Antara** *see* Fenofibrate and Derivatives *on page* 852
- ◆ **Anthraforte® (Can)** *see* Anthralin *on page* 150

Anthralin (AN thra lin)

Brand Names: U.S. Dritho-Creme HP; Zithranol; Zithranol-RR

Brand Names: Canada Anthraforte®; Anthranol®; Anthrascalp®; Micanol®

Index Terms Dithranol

Pharmacologic Category Antipsoriatic Agent; Keratolytic Agent

Use Treatment of psoriasis (quiescent or chronic psoriasis)

Pregnancy Risk Factor C

Dosage Children (off-label) and Adults: Topical: Generally, apply once a day or as directed. The irritant potential of anthralin is directly related to the strength being used and each patient's individual tolerance. Always commence treatment using a short, daily contact time (5-10 minutes) for at least 1 week using the lowest strength possible. Contact time may be gradually increased (to 20-30 minutes) as tolerated.

Skin application: Apply sparingly only to psoriatic lesions and rub gently and carefully into the skin until absorbed. Avoid applying an excessive quantity which may cause unnecessary soiling and staining of the clothing or bed linen.

Scalp application: Comb hair to remove scalar debris, wet hair and, after suitably parting, rub cream well into the lesions, taking care to prevent the cream from spreading onto the forehead.

Remove by washing or showering; optimal period of contact will vary according to the strength used and the patient's response to treatment. Continue treatment until the skin is entirely clear (ie, when there is nothing to feel with the fingers and the texture is normal).

Additional Information Complete prescribing information should be consulted for additional detail.

Dosage Forms

Cream, External:

Dritho-Creme HP: 1% (50 g)

Zithranol-RR: 1.2% (45 g)

Shampoo, External:

Zithranol: 1% (85 g)

◆ **Anthranol® (Can)** *see* Anthralin *on page 150*

◆ **Anthrascalp® (Can)** *see* Anthralin *on page 150*

Anthrax Vaccine Adsorbed

(AN thraks vak SEEN ad SORBED)

Brand Names: U.S. BioThrax

Index Terms AVA

Pharmacologic Category Vaccine, Inactivated (Bacterial)

Additional Appendix Information

Immunization Administration Recommendations *on page 2250*

Immunization Recommendations *on page 2255*

Use Immunization against *Bacillus anthracis* in persons 18 to 65 years of age at high risk for exposure.

The Advisory Committee on Immunization Practices (ACIP) recommends routine vaccination (preexposure vaccination) for the following (CDC [Wright 2010]):

- Persons who work directly with the organism in the laboratory
- Persons who handle animals or animal products only when
  - potentially infected in research settings;
  - in areas of high incidence of enzootic anthrax; or
  - where standards and restrictions are not sufficient to prevent exposure
- Military personnel deployed to areas with high risk of exposure as recommended by the Department of Defense (DoD)
- Persons engaged in environmental investigations or remediation efforts

Routine immunization for the general population is not recommended. Routine vaccination may be offered to emergency and other responders (police and fire departments, the National Guard, etc.) on a voluntary basis under the direction of a comprehensive occupational health and safety program (CDC [Wright 2010]).

The ACIP recommends postexposure prophylaxis after inhalation exposure to aerosolized *Bacillus anthracis* spores for the following (in the absence of completing a preexposure, routine vaccination schedule) (CDC [Wright 2010]):

- The general public, including pregnant and breastfeeding women
- Medical professionals
- Children ages 0 to 18 years as determined on an event-by-event basis
- Persons engaged in handling certain animals or animal products
- Persons who work directly with the organism in the laboratory (postexposure vaccination dependent upon pre-event vaccination status)
- Military personnel as recommended by the DoD
- Persons engaged in environmental investigations or remediation efforts (postexposure vaccination dependent upon pre-event vaccination status)
- Emergency and other responders (police and fire departments, the National Guard, etc.)
- Persons working in postal facilities

Pregnancy Risk Factor D

Dosage

Children <18 years: Safety and efficacy have not been established. **Note:** Use in children is recommended by the ACIP as determined on an event-by-event basis; refer to adult dosing for postexposure prophylaxis.

Adults:

Preexposure prophylaxis: Adults ≤65 years:

IM:

Primary immunization: Three injections of 0.5 mL each given at day 0, 1 month, and 6 months. Booster injections of 0.5 mL each should be given at 12 and 18 months after the initiation of the series.

Subsequent booster injections: 0.5 mL at 1-year intervals are recommended in persons who remain at risk

SubQ:

Primary immunization: Four injections of 0.5 mL each given at day 0, 2 weeks, 4 weeks, and 6 months. Booster injections of 0.5 mL each should be given at 12 months and 18 months.

Subsequent booster injections: 0.5 mL at 1-year intervals are recommended in persons who remain at risk.

Note: SubQ administration is only to be used for primary immunization in persons who are at risk for hematoma formation following IM injection.

Postexposure prophylaxis (inhalation exposure) (CDC [Wright 2010]): Three injections of 0.5 mL each given at day 0, week 2, and week 4. Administer with a 60-day course of antibiotics. (Vaccination should begin within 10 days of exposure. Refer to guidelines provided as part of emergency use authorization [EUA] or investigational new drug [IND] application at the time of the event). **Note:** Additional considerations for postexposure prophylaxis following occupational exposures:

Fully vaccinated: Personnel who have completed the primary vaccination series and booster injections do not require postexposure prophylaxis if wearing protective equipment. If respiratory protection is disrupted, a 30-day course of antimicrobial therapy is recommended.

Previously unvaccinated: Workers should receive the vaccine as directed per postexposure prophylaxis along with the 60-day course of antimicrobial therapy (antimicrobial therapy should continue for 14 days after the third dose of PEP vaccine), then switch to the licensed regimen at the 6-month dose.

Partially vaccinated: Any person who started but did not complete the primary vaccination series should receive a 30-day course of antimicrobial therapy and continue with the primary vaccination schedule.

Elderly: Safety and efficacy have not been established for patients >65 years of age

Additional Information Complete prescribing information should be consulted for additional detail.

Dosage Forms

Injection, suspension:

BioThrax: *Bacillus anthracis* proteins (5 mL)

◆ **Anti-4 Alpha Integrin** *see* Natalizumab *on page 1432*

◆ **Anti-D Immunoglobulin** *see* Rh_o(D) Immune Globulin *on page 1794*

◆ **Antibody-Drug Conjugate SGN-35** *see* Brentuximab Vedotin *on page 286*

◆ **Anti-CD20 Monoclonal Antibody** *see* RiTUXimab *on page 1825*

◆ **Anti-CD30 ADC SGN-35** *see* Brentuximab Vedotin *on page 286*

◆ **Anti-CD30 Antibody-Drug Conjugate SGN-35** *see* Brentuximab Vedotin *on page 286*

◆ **Anti-CD52 Monoclonal Antibody** *see* Alemtuzumab *on page 75*

◆ **anti-c-erB-2** *see* Trastuzumab *on page 2085*

◆ **Anti-Dandruff [OTC]** *see* Selenium Sulfide *on page 1877*

◆ **Anti-Diarrheal [OTC]** *see* Loperamide *on page 1236*

◆ **Antidigoxin Fab Fragments, Ovine** *see* Digoxin Immune Fab *on page 630*

◆ **Antidiuretic Hormone** *see* Vasopressin *on page 2142*

◆ **anti-ERB-2** *see* Trastuzumab *on page 2085*

◆ **Antifungal [OTC]** *see* Miconazole (Topical) *on page 1360*

◆ **Anti-Fungal [OTC]** *see* Tolnaftate *on page 2063*

Antihemophilic Factor (Human)

(an tee hee moe FIL ik FAK tor HYU man)

Brand Names: U.S. Hemofil M; Koate-DVI; Monoclate-P

Brand Names: Canada Hemofil M

Index Terms AHF (Human); Factor VIII (Human); Kaote DVI

Pharmacologic Category Antihemophilic Agent; Blood Product Derivative

Use Prevention and treatment of hemorrhagic episodes in patients with hemophilia A (classic hemophilia); perioperative management of hemophilia A; can be of significant therapeutic value in patients with acquired factor VIII inhibitors not exceeding 10 Bethesda units/mL

Pregnancy Risk Factor C

Dosage Children and Adults: IV: Individualize dosage based on coagulation studies performed prior to treatment and at regular intervals during treatment. In general, administration of factor VIII 1 unit/kg will increase circulating factor VIII levels by ~2 units/dL. (General guidelines presented; consult individual product labeling for specific dosing recommendations.)

Dosage based on desired factor VIII increase (%):

To calculate dosage needed based on desired factor VIII increase (%):

Body weight (kg) x 0.5 units/kg x desired factor VIII increase (%) = units factor VIII required

For example:

50 kg x 0.5 units/kg x 30 (% increase) = 750 units factor VIII

Dosage based on expected factor VIII increase (%):

It is also possible to calculate the **expected** % factor VIII increase:

(# units administered x 2%/units/kg) divided by body weight (kg) = expected % factor VIII increase

For example:

(1400 units x 2%/units/kg) divided by 70 kg = 40%

General guidelines:

Minor hemorrhage: 10-20 units/kg as a single dose to achieve FVIII plasma level ~20% to 40% of normal. Mild superficial or early hemorrhages may respond to a single dose; may repeat dose every 12-24 hours for 1-3 days until bleeding is resolved or healing achieved.

Moderate hemorrhage/minor surgery: 15-25 units/kg to achieve FVIII plasma level 30% to 50% of normal. If needed, may continue with a maintenance dose of 10-15 units/kg every 8-12 hours.

Major to life-threatening hemorrhage: Initial dose 40-50 units/kg, followed by a maintenance dose of 20-25 units/kg every 8-12 hours until threat is resolved, to achieve FVIII plasma level 80% to 100% of normal.

Major surgery: 50 units/kg given preoperatively to raise factor VIII level to 100% before surgery begins. May repeat as necessary after 6-12 hours initially and for a total of 10-14 days until healing is complete. Intensity of therapy may depend on type of surgery and postoperative regimen.

Bleeding prophylaxis: May be administered on a regular basis for bleeding prophylaxis. Doses of 24-40 units/kg 3 times/week have been reported in patients with severe hemophilia to prevent joint bleeding.

If bleeding is not controlled with adequate dose, test for presence of inhibitor. It may not be possible or practical to control bleeding if inhibitor titers are >10 Bethesda units/mL.

Elderly: Response in the elderly is not expected to differ from that of younger patients; dosage should be individualized

Dosage adjustment in renal impairment: No dosage adjustment provided in manufacturer's labeling.

Dosage adjustment in hepatic impairment: No dosage adjustment provided in manufacturer's labeling.

Additional Information Complete prescribing information should be consulted for additional detail.

Dosage Forms Considerations

Strengths expressed with approximate values. Consult individual vial labels for exact potency within each vial.

Hemofil M packaged contents may contain natural rubber latex.

Dosage Forms

Kit, Intravenous:

Monoclate-P: ~250 units, ~500 units, ~1000 units, ~1500 units

Solution Reconstituted, Intravenous [preservative free]:

Hemofil M: ~250 units (1 ea); ~500 units (1 ea); ~1000 units (1 ea); ~1700 units (1 ea)

Koate-DVI: ~250 units (1 ea); ~1000 units (1 ea)

Antihemophilic Factor (Recombinant)

(an tee hee moe FIL ik FAK tor ree KOM be nant)

Brand Names: U.S. Advate; Eloctate; Helixate FS; Kogenate FS; Kogenate FS Bio-Set; Recombinate; Xyntha; Xyntha Solofuse

Brand Names: Canada Advate; Helixate FS; Kogenate FS; Xyntha; Xyntha Solofuse

Index Terms AHF (Recombinant); Efraloctocog Alfa; Factor VIII (Recombinant); Moroctocog Alfa; Novoeight; Octacog Alfa; rAHF

Pharmacologic Category Antihemophilic Agent

Use Hemophilia A:

Control and prevention of bleeding episodes: For the prevention and control of bleeding episodes in adults and children with hemophilia A.

Perioperative management: For surgical prophylaxis in adults and children with hemophilia A.

Routine prophylaxis to prevent or reduce the frequency of bleeding (Advate, Eloctate, Kogenate FS, Xyntha [Canadian labeling; not in U.S. labeling]): For routine prophylactic treatment to prevent or reduce the frequency of bleeding episodes in adults and children with hemophilia A.

Routine prophylaxis to prevent bleeding episodes and joint damage (Helixate FS, Kogenate FS): For routine prophylactic treatment to reduce the frequency of bleeding episodes and the risk of joint damage in children without preexisting joint damage.

Pregnancy Risk Factor C

Dosage IV:

Hemophilia A: Children, Adolescents, and Adults: Individualize dosage based on coagulation studies performed prior to treatment and at regular intervals during treatment. In general, administration of factor VIII 1 unit/kg will increase circulating factor VIII levels by ~2 units/dL. (General guidelines presented; consult individual product labeling for specific dosing recommendations.)

Dosage based on desired factor VIII increase (%):

To calculate dosage needed based on desired factor VIII increase (%):

[Body weight (kg) x desired factor VIII increase (%)] divided by 2 (%/units/kg) = units factor VIII required

For example:

50 kg x 30 (% increase) divided by 2 = 750 units factor VIII

Dosage based on expected factor VIII increase (%):

It is also possible to calculate the **expected** % factor VIII increase:

[# units administered x 2(%/units/kg)] divided by body weight (kg) = expected % factor VIII increase

For example:

[1,400 units x 2] divided by 70 kg = 40%

General guidelines (consult individual product labeling for specific dosage recommendations): Note: Children <6 years may require higher doses and/or more frequent administration.

Minor hemorrhage: 10 to 20 units/kg as a single dose to achieve FVIII plasma level ~20% to 40% of normal. Mild superficial or early hemorrhages may respond to a single dose; may repeat dose every 12 to 24 hours for 1 to 3 days until bleeding is resolved or healing achieved.

Moderate hemorrhage/minor surgery: 15 to 30 units/kg to achieve FVIII plasma level 30% to 60% of normal. May repeat 1 dose at 12 to 24 hours if needed. Some products suggest continuing for ≥3 days until pain and disability are resolved.

Major to life-threatening hemorrhage: Initial dose 30 to 50 units/kg followed by a maintenance dose of 20 to 50 units/kg every 8 to 24 hours until threat is resolved, to achieve FVIII plasma level 60% to 100% of normal.

Minor surgery (including tooth extraction): 15 to 50 units/kg to raise factor VIII level to ~30% to 100% before procedure/surgery. May repeat every 12 to 24 hours until bleeding is resolved.

Major surgery: 40 to 60 units/kg given preoperatively to raise factor VIII level to ~60% to 120% before surgery begins. May repeat as necessary after 6 to 24 hours until wound healing. Intensity of therapy may depend on type of surgery and postoperative regimen.

If bleeding is not controlled with adequate dose, test for presence of inhibitor. It may not be possible or practical to control bleeding if inhibitor titers >10 Bethesda units/mL.

Routine prophylaxis to prevent bleeding episodes and joint damage (Helixate FS, Kogenate FS): Children (without preexisting joint damage): 25 units/kg every other day

Routine prophylaxis to prevent or reduce the frequency of bleeding episodes:

Advate: Children, Adolescents, and Adults: 20 to 40 units/kg every other day (3 to 4 times weekly). Alternatively, an every-third-day dosing regimen may be used to target factor VIII trough levels of ≥1%.

Eloctate: Children, Adolescents, and Adults: 50 units/kg every 4 days; may adjust within the range of 25 to 65 units/kg at 3- to 5-day intervals based on patient response. More frequent or higher doses up to 80 units/kg may be required in children <6 years.

Kogenate FS: Adults: 25 units/kg 3 times weekly

Xyntha (Canadian labeling; not in U.S. labeling): Adolescents and Adults (treatment experienced): 25 to 35 units/kg 3 times weekly

Elderly: Response in the elderly is not expected to differ from that of younger patients; dosage should be individualized

Dosage adjustment in renal impairment: There are no dosage adjustments provided in the manufacturer's labeling.

Dosage adjustment in hepatic impairment: There are no dosage adjustments provided in the manufacturer's labeling.

Additional Information Complete prescribing information should be consulted for additional detail.

Product Availability

Novoeight: FDA approved October 2013; availability anticipated in the second quarter of 2015.

Novoeight is indicated for use in children and adults with hemophilia A (congenital factor VIII deficiency or classic hemophilia) for control and prevention of bleeding episodes, perioperative management, and routine prophylaxis to prevent or reduce the frequency of bleeding episodes.

Dosage Forms Considerations

Strengths expressed with approximate values. Consult individual vial labels for exact potency within each vial.

Dosage Forms

Kit, Intravenous:

Kogenate FS: 250 units, 500 units, 1000 units

Kit, Intravenous [preservative free]:

Helixate FS: 250 units, 500 units, 1000 units, 2000 units, 3000 units

Kogenate FS: 2000 units, 3000 units

Kogenate FS Bio-Set: 250 units, 500 units, 1000 units, 2000 units, 3000 units

Xyntha: 250 units, 500 units, 1000 units, 2000 units

Xyntha Solofuse: 250 units, 500 units, 1000 units, 2000 units, 3000 units

Solution Reconstituted, Intravenous [preservative free]:

Advate: 250 units (1 ea); 500 units (1 ea); 1000 units (1 ea); 1500 units (1 ea); 2000 units (1 ea); 3000 units (1 ea); 4000 units (1 ea)

Eloctate: 250 units (1 ea); 500 units (1 ea); 750 units (1 ea); 1000 units (1 ea); 1500 units (1 ea); 2000 units (1 ea); 3000 units (1 ea)

Recombinate: 220-400 units (1 ea); 401-800 units (1 ea); 801-1240 units (1 ea); 1241-1800 units (1 ea); 1801-2400 units (1 ea)

Antihemophilic Factor (Recombinant [Porcine Sequence])

(an tee hee moe FIL ik FAK tor ree KOM be nant POR sine SEE kwens)

Brand Names: U.S. Obizur

Index Terms AHF; AHF (Recombinant); Factor VIII; Factor VIII (Recombinant); pFVIII; rAHF; rpFVIII

Pharmacologic Category Antihemophilic Agent

Use

Acquired hemophilia A: Treatment of bleeding episodes in adults with acquired hemophilia A

Limitations of use: Not indicated for the treatment of congenital hemophilia A or von Willebrand disease; safety and efficacy of has not been established in patients with baseline anti- porcine factor VIII inhibitor titer >20 BU.

Pregnancy Risk Factor C

Dosage

Acquired hemophilia A: Adults: IV: **Note:** Dose, dosing frequency, and duration based on location and severity of bleeding, target factor VIII levels, and clinical condition of the patient. Plasma levels of factor VIII should not exceed 200% of normal or 200 units/dL.

Minor to moderate hemorrhage: 200 units/kg initially to achieve factor VIII plasma level 50% to 100% of normal; titrate subsequent doses to maintain recommended factor VIII trough levels and individual clinical response; dose every 4 to 12 hours (frequency may be adjusted based on clinical response/factor VIII levels).

Major hemorrhage: 200 units/kg initially to achieve factor VIII plasma level 100% to 200% (for acute bleed) or 50% to 100% (after acute bleed is controlled, if required) of normal; titrate subsequent doses to maintain recommended factor VIII trough levels and individual clinical response; dose every 4 to 12 hours (frequency may be adjusted based on clinical response/factor VIII levels).

Dosage adjustment in renal impairment: There are no dosage adjustments provided in the manufacturer's labeling.

Dosage adjustment in hepatic impairment: There are no dosage adjustments provided in the manufacturer's labeling.

Additional Information Complete prescribing information should be consulted for additional detail.

Dosage Forms

Solution Reconstituted, Intravenous:

Obizur: 500 units (1 ea)

Antihemophilic Factor/von Willebrand Factor Complex (Human)

(an tee hee moe FIL ik FAK tor von WILL le brand FAK tor KOM plex HYU man)

Brand Names: U.S. Alphanate; Humate-P; Wilate

Brand Names: Canada Humate-P

Index Terms AHF (Human); Factor VIII (Human)/von Willebrand Factor; Factor VIII Concentrate; FVIII/vWF; von Willebrand Factor/Factor VIII Complex; VWF/FVIII Concentrate; VWF:RCo; vWF:RCof

Pharmacologic Category Antihemophilic Agent; Blood Product Derivative

Use

Factor VIII deficiency: Alphanate, Humate-P: Prevention and treatment of hemorrhagic episodes in patients with hemophilia A (classical hemophilia); **Note:** Wilate is not approved for use in patients with hemophilia A or acquired factor VIII deficiency

von Willebrand disease (VWD):

Alphanate: Prophylaxis with surgical and/or invasive procedures in patients with VWD when desmopressin is either ineffective or contraindicated; **Note:** Not indicated for patients with severe VWD (type 3) undergoing major surgery

Humate-P: Treatment of spontaneous or trauma-induced bleeding, as well as prevention of excessive bleeding during and after surgery in patients with severe VWD, including mild or moderate disease where use of desmopressin is known or suspected to be inadequate; **Note:** Not indicated for the prophylaxis of spontaneous bleeding episodes

Wilate: Treatment of spontaneous and trauma-induced bleeding in patients with severe VWD, including mild or moderate disease where use of desmopressin is known or suspected to be inadequate or contraindicated; **Note:** Not indicated for prophylaxis of spontaneous bleeding or prevention of excessive bleeding during and after surgery

Pregnancy Risk Factor C

Dosage

Factor VIII deficiency: General guidelines (consult specific product labeling for Alphanate or Humate-P): Children and Adults: IV:

Individualize dosage based on coagulation studies performed prior to treatment and at regular intervals during treatment; in general, administration of factor VIII 1 unit/kg will increase circulating factor VIII levels by ~2 units/dL.

Minor hemorrhage: Loading dose: FVIII:C 15 units/kg to achieve FVIII:C plasma level ~30% of normal. If second infusion is needed, half the loading dose may be given once or twice daily for 1 to 2 days.

Moderate hemorrhage: Loading dose: FVIII:C 25 units/kg to achieve FVIII:C plasma level ~50% of normal; Maintenance: FVIII:C 15 units/kg every 8 to 12 hours for 1 to 2 days in order to maintain FVIII:C plasma levels at 30% of normal. Repeat the same dose once or twice daily for up to 7 days or until adequate wound healing.

Life-threatening hemorrhage/major surgery: Loading dose: FVIII:C 40 to 50 units/kg; Maintenance: FVIII:C 20 to 25 units/kg every 8 to 12 hours to maintain FVIII:C plasma levels at 80% to 100% of normal for 7 days. Continue same dose once or twice daily for another 7 days in order to maintain FVIII:C levels at 30% to 50% of normal.

von Willebrand disease (VWD): Treatment:

Humate-P: Children and Adults: IV: Individualize dosage based on coagulation studies performed prior to treatment and at regular intervals during treatment; in general, administration of factor VIII 1 unit/kg would be expected to raise circulating VWF:RCo ~5 units/dL

Type 1, mild VWD: Minor hemorrhage (if desmopressin is not appropriate) or major hemorrhage:

Loading dose: VWF:RCo 40 to 60 units/kg

Maintenance dose: VWF:RCo 40 to 50 units/kg every 8 to 12 hours for 3 days, keeping VWF:RCo nadir >50%; follow with 40 to 50 units/kg daily for up to 7 days

Type 1, moderate or severe VWD:

Minor hemorrhage: VWF:RCo 40 to 50 units/kg for 1 to 2 doses

Major hemorrhage:

Loading dose: VWF:RCo 50 to 75 units/kg

Maintenance dose: VWF:RCo 40 to 60 units/kg every 8 to 12 hours for 3 days to keep the VWF:RCo nadir >50%, then 40 to 60 units/kg daily for a total of up to 7 days

Types 2 and 3 VWD:

Minor hemorrhage: VWF:RCo 40 to 50 units/kg for 1 to 2 doses

Major hemorrhage:

Loading dose: VWF:RCo 60 to 80 units/kg

Maintenance dose: VWF:RCo 40 to 60 units/kg every 8 to 12 hours for 3 days, keeping the VWF:RCo nadir >50%; follow with 40 to 60 units/kg daily for a total of up to 7 days

Wilate: Children and Adults: IV:

Minor hemorrhage:

Loading dose: VWF:RCo: 20 to 40 units/kg

Maintenance dose: 20 to 30 units/kg every 12 to 24 hours for ≤3 days, keeping the VWF:RCo nadir >30%

Major hemorrhage:
Loading dose: VWF:RCo: 40 to 60 units/kg
Maintenance dose: 20 to 40 units/kg every 12 to 24 hours for 5 to 7 days, keeping the VWF:RCo nadir >50%

von Willebrand disease (VWD): Prophylaxis:
Alphanate: Surgery/invasive procedure prophylaxis (except patients with type 3 undergoing major surgery):
Children: IV:
Preoperative dose: VWF:RCo: 75 units/kg 1 hour prior to surgery
Maintenance dose: VWF:RCo: 50 to 75 units/kg every 8 to 12 hours as clinically needed. For minor procedures, maintain FVIII:C activity level of 40 to 50 units/dL during postoperative days 1 to 3; for major procedures, maintain FVIII:C activity level of 100 units/dL for 3 to 7 days. Do not exceed FVIII:C activity level of 150 units/dL.
Adults: IV:
Preoperative dose: VWF:RCo: 60 units/kg 1 hour prior to surgery
Maintenance dose: VWF:RCo: 40 to 60 units/kg every 8 to 12 hours as clinically needed. For minor procedures, maintain FVIII:C activity level of 40 to 50 units/dL during postoperative days 1 to 3; for major procedures, maintain VFIII:C activity level of 100 units/dL for 3 to 7 days. Do not exceed FVIII:C activity level of 150 units/dL.
Humate-P: Surgery/procedure prevention of bleeding: Children and Adults: IV:
Emergency surgery: Administer VWF:RCo 50 to 60 units/kg; monitor trough coagulation factor levels for subsequent doses
Surgical management (nonemergency):
Loading dose calculation based on baseline target VWF:RCo: (Target peak VWF:RCo - Baseline VWF:RCo) x weight (in kg) / IVR = units VWF:RCo required. Administer loading dose 1 to 2 hours prior to surgery. **Note:** If *in vivo* recovery (IVR) not available, assume 2 units/dL per units/kg of VWF:RCo product administered.
Target concentrations for VWF:RCo following loading dose:
Major surgery: 100 units/dL
Minor surgery: 50 to 60 units/dL
Maintenance dose: Initial: One-half loading dose, followed by subsequent dosing determined by target trough concentrations, generally every 8-12 hours. Patients with shorter half-lives may require dosing every 6 hours.
Target maintenance trough VWF:RCo concentrations:
Major surgery: >50 units/dL for up to 3 days, followed by >30 units/dL for a minimum total treatment of 72 hours
Minor surgery: ≥30 units/dL for a minimum duration of 48 hours
Oral surgery: ≥30 units/dL for a minimum duration of 8 to 12 hours

Elderly: Response in the elderly is not expected to differ from that of younger patients; dosage should be individualized

Dosage adjustment in renal impairment: There are no dosage adjustments provided in the manufacturer's labeling.
Dosage adjustment in hepatic impairment: There are no dosage adjustments provided in the manufacturer's labeling.
Additional Information Complete prescribing information should be consulted for additional detail.

Dosage Forms Considerations
Strengths expressed with approximate values. Consult individual vial labels for exact potency within each vial.
Dosage Forms
Injection, powder for reconstitution [human derived]:
Alphanate:
250 units [Factor VIII and VWF:RCo ratio varies by lot]
500 units [Factor VIII and VWF:RCo ratio varies by lot]
1000 units [Factor VIII and VWF:RCo ratio varies by lot]
1500 units [Factor VIII and VWF:RCo ratio varies by lot]
2000 units [Factor VIII and VWF:RCo ratio varies by lot]
Humate-P:
FVIII 250 units and VWF:RCo 600 units
FVIII 500 units and VWF:RCo 1200 units
FVIII 1000 units and VWF:RCo 2400 units
Wilate:
FVIII 500 units and VWF:RCo 500 units
FVIII 1000 units and VWF:RCo 1000 units

◆ **Anti-Hist Allergy [OTC]** *see* DiphenhydrAMINE (Systemic) *on page 641*

Anti-inhibitor Coagulant Complex (Human)

(an TEE in HI bi tor coe AG yoo lant KOM pleks HYU man)

Brand Names: U.S. Feiba
Brand Names: Canada FEIBA NF
Index Terms Activated PCC; AICC; aPCC; Coagulant Complex Inhibitor; Factor Eight Inhibitor Bypassing Activity; Factor VIII Inhibitor Bypassing Activity; FEIBA NF; FEIBA VH
Pharmacologic Category Activated Prothrombin Complex Concentrate (aPCC); Antihemophilic Agent; Blood Product Derivative
Use
Hemorrhage in patients with hemophilia: For use in patients with hemophilia A and B with inhibitors for control and prevention of bleeding episodes.
Perioperative bleeding management in patients with hemophilia: For use in patients with hemophilia A and B with inhibitors for perioperative management.
Routine prophylaxis of bleeding events in patients with hemophilia: For use in patients with hemophilia A and B for routine prophylaxis to prevent or reduce the frequency of bleeding episodes.
Pregnancy Risk Factor C
Dosage
Control and prevention of bleeding episodes: Children, Adolescents, and Adults: IV: **Note:** Considered a first-line treatment when factor VIII inhibitor titer is >5 Bethesda units (BU) (antihemophilic factor may be preferred when titer <5 BU)
General dosing guidelines: 50-100 units/kg per dose (maximum: 100 units/kg [single dose], 200 units/kg/day [total daily dose]). Dosage and duration of treatment depend on the location and extent of bleeding and clinical condition of the patient. If total single dose exceeds 100 units/kg or total daily dose exceeds 200 units/kg/day, monitor closely for DIC, coronary ischemia, and signs/symptoms of other thromboembolic events.
Joint hemorrhage: 50-100 units/kg every 12 hours until pain and acute disabilities are improved (maximum: 200 units/kg/day)
Mucous membrane bleeding: 50-100 units/kg every 6 hours for at least 1 day or until bleeding is resolved (maximum: 200 units/kg/day)
Soft tissue hemorrhage (eg, retroperitoneal bleed): 100 units/kg every 12 hours until resolution of bleed (maximum: 200 units/kg/day)

Other severe hemorrhage (eg, intracranial hemorrhage): 100 units/kg every 6-12 hours; continue until resolution of bleed (maximum: 200 units/kg/day).

Perioperative management:

Preoperative: 50-100 units/kg (single dose) administered immediately prior to surgery.

Postoperative: 50-100 units/kg every 6-12 hours until resolution of bleed and healing is achieved (maximum: 200 units/kg/day)

Routine prophylaxis: 85 units/kg every other day.

Hemorrhage (moderate-to-severe) due to acquired hemophilia (off-label use): Adults: IV: **Optimal dosing has not been established:** 50-100 units/kg every 8-12 hours until bleeding controlled has been suggested; may continue for 24-72 hours based on site, type, and severity of bleeding (maximum: 200 units/kg/day) (Huth-Kuhne, 2009; Sallah, 2004).

Life-threatening hemorrhage associated with dabigatran (off-label use): Adults: IV: **Optimal dosing has not been established.** Based on multiple case reports with various types of hemorrhage, a dosage range of 25 to 100 units/kg has been used (Dager, 2013; Faust, 2013; Kiraly, 2013; Neyens, 2014; Schulman, 2013). In one case study, after administration of 26 units/kg, an additional dose of 16 units/kg was administered for a concern of rebleeding (Dager, 2013). Others, including the European Heart Rhythm Association (EHRA), have recommended the use of 50 units/kg (EHRA [Heidbuchel, 2013]; Weitz, 2012). **Note:** The use of anti-inhibitor coagulant complex (FEIBA, activated 4-factor PCC) may be associated with a higher risk of thrombosis compared to nonactivated PCCs especially with higher doses; monitor closely for arterial and venous thrombosis.

Dosage adjustment in renal impairment: No dosage adjustment provided in manufacturer's labeling.

Dosage adjustment in hepatic impairment: No dosage adjustment provided in manufacturer's labeling.

Additional Information Complete prescribing information should be consulted for additional detail.

Dosage Forms Considerations

FEIBA strengths expressed in terms of Factor VIII inhibitor bypassing activity with nominal strength values. Consult individual vial labels for exact potency within each vial.

Dosage Forms

Solution Reconstituted, Intravenous [preservative free]: FEIBA: 500 units (1 ea); 1000 units (1 ea); 2500 units (1 ea)

◆ **Anti-Itch Maximum Strength [OTC]** *see* Hydrocortisone (Topical) *on page* 1014

◆ **Anti-PD-1 human monoclonal antibody MDX-1106** *see* Nivolumab *on page* 1469

◆ **Anti-PD-1 Monoclonal Antibody MK-3475** *see* Pembrolizumab *on page* 1604

Antipyrine and Benzocaine

(an tee PYE reen & BEN zoe kane)

Brand Names: U.S. Aurodex® [DSC]

Brand Names: Canada Auralgan®

Index Terms Benzocaine and Antipyrine

Pharmacologic Category Otic Agent, Analgesic; Otic Agent, Cerumenolytic

Use Temporary relief of pain and reduction of swelling associated with acute congestive and serous otitis media; facilitates ear wax removal

Pregnancy Risk Factor C

Dosage Otic: Children and Adults:

Otitis media: Fill ear canal with solution; moisten cotton pledget with antipyrine and benzocaine solution, place in external ear, repeat every 1-2 hours until pain and congestion are relieved

Ear wax removal: Instill drops 3 times/day for 2-3 days; before and after ear wax removal, moisten cotton pledget with antipyrine and benzocaine solution and place in external ear after solution instillation.

Dosage adjustment in renal impairment: No dosage adjustment provided in manufacturer's labeling.

Dosage adjustment in hepatic impairment: No dosage adjustment provided in manufacturer's labeling.

Additional Information Complete prescribing information should be consulted for additional detail.

Dosage Forms

Solution, otic [drops]: Antipyrine 5.4% and benzocaine 1.4% (10 mL, 15 mL), Antipyrine 5.5% and benzocaine 1.4% (14 mL)

Antithrombin (an tee THROM bin)

Brand Names: U.S. ATryn; Thrombate III

Brand Names: Canada Antithrombin III NF; Thrombate III®

Index Terms Antithrombin Alfa; Antithrombin III; AT; AT-III; hpAT; rhAT; rhATIII

Pharmacologic Category Anticoagulant; Blood Product Derivative

Use

Treatment of antithrombin deficiency: Thrombate III: Antithrombin III (human) is indicated for the treatment of patients with hereditary antithrombin (AT) deficiency in connection with surgical or obstetrical procedures or when they suffer from thromboembolism.

Prevention of thromboembolic events: ATryn: Recombinant antithrombin is indicated for the prevention of perioperative and peripartum thromboembolic events in patients with hereditary antithrombin deficiency.

Limitations of use: ATryn is not indicated for treatment of thromboembolic events in patients with hereditary antithrombin deficiency.

Pregnancy Risk Factor B (Thrombate III); C (ATryn)

Dosage IV: Adults: Antithrombin deficiency:

ATryn: Prophylaxis of thrombosis during perioperative and peripartum procedures:

Dosing is individualized based on pretherapy antithrombin (AT) activity levels. Therapy should begin before delivery or ~24 hours prior to surgery to obtain target AT activity levels. Dosing should be targeted to keep levels between 80% to 120% of normal. Loading dose should be given as a 15-minute infusion, followed by maintenance dose as a continuous infusion. Doses may be calculated based on the following formulas:

Surgical patients (nonpregnant):

Loading dose: [(100 - baseline AT activity level) **divided** by 2.3] x body weight (kg) = units of antithrombin required

Maintenance infusion: [(100 - baseline AT activity level) **divided** by 10.2] x body weight (kg) = units of antithrombin required/hour

Pregnant patients: **Note:** Pregnant women undergoing surgical procedures (other than a Cesarean section) should also be dosed according to the formula below.

Loading dose: [(100 - baseline AT activity level) **divided** by 1.3] x body weight (kg) = units of antithrombin required

Maintenance infusion: [(100 - baseline AT activity level) **divided** by 5.4] x body weight (kg) = units of antithrombin required/hour

Dosing adjustments: Adjustments should be made based on AT activity levels to maintain levels between 80% to 120% of normal. Surgery or delivery may rapidly decrease AT levels; check AT level just after surgery or delivery. The first AT level should be obtained 2 hours after initiation and adjusted as follows:

AT activity level <80%: Increase dose by 30%; recheck AT level 2 hours after adjustment. Alternatively, an additional bolus dose (using loading dose formula) may be needed to rapidly restore AT levels. Calculate the additional bolus/loading dose using the last available AT activity result. After additional loading/bolus dose given, resume maintenance infusion at the same rate prior to bolus administration.

AT activity level 80% to 120%: No dosage adjustment needed; recheck AT level in 6 hours

AT activity level >120%: Decrease dose by 30%; recheck AT level 2 hours after adjustment

Thrombate III: Prophylaxis of thrombosis during surgical or obstetrical procedures or treatment of thromboembolism:

Initial loading dose: Dosing is individualized based on pretherapy antithrombin (AT) levels. The initial dose should raise AT levels to 80% to 120% and may be calculated based on the following formula:

[(desired AT level % - baseline AT level %) x body weight (kg)] **divided** by 1.4 = units of antithrombin required

For example, if a 70 kg adult patient had a baseline AT level of 57%, the initial dose would be

[(120% - 57%) x 70] divided by 1.4 = 3150 units

Maintenance dose: In general, subsequent dosing should be targeted to keep levels between 80% to 120% which may be achieved by administering 60% of the initial loading dose every 24 hours. Adjustments may be made by adjusting dose or interval. Maintain level within normal range for 2-8 days depending on type of procedure/situation.

Dosage adjustment in renal impairment: There are no dosage adjustments provided in the manufacturer's labeling.

Dosage adjustment in hepatic impairment: There are no dosage adjustments provided in the manufacturer's labeling.

Additional Information Complete prescribing information should be consulted for additional detail.

Dosage Forms

Solution Reconstituted, Intravenous:

Thrombate III: 500 units (1 ea); 1000 units (1 ea)

ATryn: 1750 units (1 ea)

◆ **Antithrombin III** *see* Antithrombin *on page 156*

◆ **Antithrombin III NF (Can)** *see* Antithrombin *on page 156*

◆ **Antithrombin Alfa** *see* Antithrombin *on page 156*

Antithymocyte Globulin (Equine)

(an te THY moe site GLOB yu lin, E kwine)

Brand Names: U.S. Atgam

Brand Names: Canada Atgam

Index Terms Antithymocyte Immunoglobulin; ATG; Horse Antihuman Thymocyte Gamma Globulin; Lymphocyte Immune Globulin

Pharmacologic Category Immune Globulin; Immunosuppressant Agent; Polyclonal Antibody

Use

Aplastic anemia: Treatment of moderate-to-severe aplastic anemia in patients not considered suitable candidates for bone marrow transplantation

Limitations of use: The usefulness of antithymocyte globulin (equine) has not be demonstrated in patients with aplastic anemia who are suitable candidates for transplantation, or in aplastic anemia secondary to neoplastic disease, storage disease, myelofibrosis, Fanconi syndrome, or in patients with known prior treatment with myelotoxic agents or radiation therapy

Renal transplantation: Management of allograft rejection in renal transplantation, either in combination with conventional treatments for the management of acute rejection, or as an adjunct treatment in the prevention of rejection

Pregnancy Risk Factor C

Dosage Test dose: A skin test is recommended prior to administration of the initial dose Test initially with an epicutaneous prick of undiluted antithymocyte globulin (ATG); if no wheal in 10 minutes, then use 0.02 mL intradermally of a 1:1000 dilution of ATG in normal saline along with a separate saline control of 0.02 mL; observe in 10 minutes. A positive skin reaction consists of a wheal with the initial prick test (undiluted) or ≥3 mm in diameter larger than the saline control with the diluted intradermal test. Alternatively, a 0.1 mL test dose (5 mg/mL concentration) may be administered intradermally along with a separate saline control; erythema larger than 5 mm in diameter (compared to the control) is considered a positive test (Molldrem, 2002). A positive skin test is suggestive of an increased risk for systemic allergic reactions with an infusion, although anaphylaxis may occur in patients who display negative skin tests. If ATG treatment is deemed appropriate following a positive skin test, the first infusion should be administered in a controlled environment with intensive life support immediately available. A systemic reaction precludes further administration of the drug.

Consider premedication with an antihistamine, corticosteroids, hydrocortisone, and/or an antipyretic.

Aplastic anemia protocol: Pediatrics and Adults: IV: 10 to 20 mg/kg/day for 8 to 14 days; then if needed, may administer every other day for 7 more doses for a total of 21 doses in 28 days **or**

Off-label dosing (in combination with cyclosporine):

Children >10 kg, Adolescents, and Adults: IV: 40 mg/kg/day for 4 days (Rosenfeld, 1995)

Children >2 years, Adolescents, and Adults: IV: 40 mg/kg/day for 4 days (Scheinberg, 2011)

Renal transplantation:

Pediatrics: IV:

Rejection prophylaxis: 15 mg/kg/day for 14 days, then give every other day for 7 more doses for a total of 21 doses in 28 days; the initial dose should be administered within 24 hours before or after transplantation (range: 5 to 25 mg/kg/day)

Rejection treatment: 10 to 15 mg/kg/day for 14 days, then if needed, may administer every other day for 7 more doses for a total of 21 doses in 28 days (range: 5 to 25 mg/kg/day)

Adults: IV:

Rejection prophylaxis: 15 mg/kg/day for 14 days, then give every other day for 7 more doses for a total of 21 doses in 28 days; the initial dose should be administered within 24 hours before or after transplantation (range: 10 to 30 mg/kg/day)

Rejection treatment: 10 to 15 mg/kg/day for 14 days, then if needed, may administer every other day for 7 more doses for a total of 21 doses in 28 days (range: 10 to 30 mg/kg/day)

Acute GVHD treatment (off-label use): Pediatrics and Adults: IV: 30 mg/kg/dose every other day for 6 doses (MacMillan, 2007) **or** 15 mg/kg/dose twice daily for 10 doses (MacMillan, 2002)

Myelodysplastic syndromes, refractory, lower-risk disease (off-label use): Adults: IV: 40 mg/kg/dose once daily for 4 days; an intradermal test dose was administered prior to treatment (Molldrem, 2002)

Dosage adjustment for toxicity:

Anaphylaxis: Discontinue infusion immediately; administer epinephrine. May require corticosteroids, respiration assistance, and/or other resuscitative measures. Do not resume infusion.

Hemolysis (severe and unremitting): May require discontinuation of treatment.

Leukopenia (severe and unremitting) in renal transplant patients: Discontinue treatment.

Thrombocytopenia (severe and unremitting) in renal transplant patients: Discontinue treatment.

Dosage adjustment in renal impairment: There are no dosage adjustments provided in the manufacturer's labeling.

Dosage adjustment in hepatic impairment: There are no dosage adjustments provided in the manufacturer's labeling.

Dosing in obesity: *American Society for Blood and Marrow Transplantation (ASBMT) practice guideline committee position statement on chemotherapy dosing in obesity:* Utilize actual body weight (full weight) to calculate mg/kg dosing for hematopoietic stem cell transplant conditioning regimens (Bubalo, 2014).

Additional Information Complete prescribing information should be consulted for additional detail.

Dosage Forms

Injectable, Intravenous:

Atgam: 50 mg/mL (5 mL)

Antithymocyte Globulin (Rabbit)

(an te THY moe site GLOB yu lin RAB bit)

Brand Names: U.S. Thymoglobulin

Brand Names: Canada Thymoglobulin

Index Terms Antithymocyte Immunoglobulin; rATG

Pharmacologic Category Immune Globulin; Immunosuppressant Agent; Polyclonal Antibody

Use Renal transplant rejection: Treatment of acute rejection of renal transplant; used in conjunction with concomitant immunosuppression

Pregnancy Risk Factor C

Dosage Treatment of acute renal transplant rejection: Pediatric and Adults: IV: 1.5 mg/kg/day for 7 to 14 days

Dosage adjustment for toxicity:

WBC count 2,000 to 3,000 cells/mm^3 or platelet count 50,000 to 75,000 cells/mm^3: Reduce dose by 50%.

WBC count <2,000 cells/mm^3 or platelet count <50,000 cells/mm^3: Consider discontinuing treatment.

Dosing in obesity: *American Society for Blood and Marrow Transplantation (ASBMT) practice guideline committee position statement on chemotherapy dosing in obesity:* Utilize actual body weight (full weight) to calculate mg/kg dosing for hematopoietic stem cell transplant conditioning regimens (Bubalo, 2014).

Additional Information Complete prescribing information should be consulted for additional detail.

Dosage Forms

Solution Reconstituted, Intravenous:

Thymoglobulin: 25 mg (1 ea)

- ◆ **Antithymocyte Immunoglobulin** *see* Antithymocyte Globulin (Equine) *on page 157*
- ◆ **Antithymocyte Immunoglobulin** *see* Antithymocyte Globulin (Rabbit) *on page 158*
- ◆ **Antitumor Necrosis Factor Alpha (Human)** *see* Adalimumab *on page 51*
- ◆ **Anti-VEGF Monoclonal Antibody** *see* Bevacizumab *on page 257*
- ◆ **Anti-VEGF rhuMAb** *see* Bevacizumab *on page 257*
- ◆ **Antivenin (*Centruroides*) Immune F(ab')$_2$ (Equine)** *see* *Centruroides* Immune F(ab')$_2$ (Equine) *on page 405*
- ◆ **Antivenin Scorpion** *see* *Centruroides* Immune F(ab')$_2$ (Equine) *on page 405*
- ◆ **Antivenom (*Centruroides*) Immune F(ab')$_2$ (Equine)** *see* *Centruroides* Immune F(ab')$_2$ (Equine) *on page 405*
- ◆ **Antivenom Scorpion** *see* *Centruroides* Immune F(ab')$_2$ (Equine) *on page 405*
- ◆ **Antivert** *see* Meclizine *on page 1277*
- ◆ **Antizol** *see* Fomepizole *on page 922*
- ◆ **Anucort-HC** *see* Hydrocortisone (Topical) *on page 1014*
- ◆ **Anusol-HC** *see* Hydrocortisone (Topical) *on page 1014*
- ◆ **Anuzinc (Can)** *see* Zinc Sulfate *on page 2200*
- ◆ **Anzemet** *see* Dolasetron *on page 663*
- ◆ **4-AP** *see* Dalfampridine *on page 552*
- ◆ **AP24534** *see* PONATinib *on page 1680*
- ◆ **APAP (abbreviation is not recommended)** *see* Acetaminophen *on page 32*
- ◆ **APC8015** *see* Sipuleucel-T *on page 1893*
- ◆ **aPCC** *see* Anti-inhibitor Coagulant Complex (Human) *on page 155*
- ◆ **ApexiCon** *see* Diflorasone *on page 625*
- ◆ **ApexiCon E** *see* Diflorasone *on page 625*
- ◆ **Apidra** *see* Insulin Glulisine *on page 1086*
- ◆ **Apidra® (Can)** *see* Insulin Glulisine *on page 1086*
- ◆ **Apidra SoloStar** *see* Insulin Glulisine *on page 1086*

Apixaban

(a PIX a ban)

Brand Names: U.S. Eliquis

Brand Names: Canada Eliquis

Pharmacologic Category Anticoagulant; Anticoagulant, Factor Xa Inhibitor

Additional Appendix Information

Oral Anticoagulant Comparison Chart *on page 2233*

Reversal of Oral Anticoagulants *on page 2235*

Use

Deep vein thrombosis: Treatment of deep vein thrombosis; to reduce the risk of recurrent deep vein thrombosis following initial therapy

Nonvalvular atrial fibrillation: To reduce the risk of stroke and systemic embolism in patients with nonvalvular atrial fibrillation (AF)

Note: The 2014 American Heart Association/American College of Cardiology/Heart Rhythm Society guidelines for the management of AF recommend oral anticoagulation for patients with nonvalvular AF or atrial flutter with prior stroke, TIA, or a CHA_2DS_2-VASc score ≥2. As an alternative to warfarin, apixaban may also be used for 3 weeks prior and 4 weeks after cardioversion in patients with AF or atrial flutter of ≥48 hours duration or when the duration is unknown (January, 2014)

Postoperative venous thromboprophylaxis following hip or knee replacement surgery: Prophylaxis of deep vein thrombosis, which may lead to pulmonary embolism, in patients who have undergone hip or knee replacement surgery

Pulmonary embolism: Treatment of pulmonary embolism; to reduce the risk of recurrent pulmonary embolism following initial therapy

Pregnancy Risk Factor B

Pregnancy Considerations Adverse events were not observed in animal reproduction studies. Data are insufficient to evaluate the safety of oral factor Xa inhibitors during pregnancy; use during pregnancy should be avoided (Bates, 2012).

Breast-Feeding Considerations It is not known if apixaban is excreted in breast milk. Apixaban is not recommended for use in breast-feeding women; use of alternative anticoagulants is preferred (Bates, 2012)

Contraindications

U.S. labeling: Severe hypersensitivity reaction (ie, anaphylaxis) to apixaban or any component of the formulation; active pathological bleeding

Canadian labeling: Hypersensitivity to apixaban or any component of the formulation; clinically-significant active bleeding (including gastrointestinal bleeding); lesions or conditions at increased risk of clinically-significant bleeding (eg, cerebral infarct [ischemic or hemorrhagic], active peptic ulcer disease with recent bleeding; patients with spontaneous or acquired impairment of hemostasis); hepatic disease associated with coagulopathy and clinically-relevant bleeding risk; concomitant systemic treatment with agents that are strong inhibitors of both CYP3A4 and P-glycoprotein (P-gp); concomitant treatment with any other anticoagulant including unfractionated heparin (except at doses used to maintain patency of central venous or arterial catheter), low molecular weight heparins, heparin derivatives (eg, fondaparinux), and oral anticoagulants including warfarin, dabigatran, rivaroxaban except when transitioning to or from apixaban therapy

Warnings/Precautions [U.S. Boxed Warning]: Premature discontinuation of any oral anticoagulant, including apixaban, in the absence of adequate alternative anticoagulation increases the risk of thrombotic events. When used to prevent stroke in patients with nonvalvular atrial fibrillation, an increased risk of stroke was observed upon transition from apixaban to warfarin in clinical trials. If apixaban must be discontinued for reasons other than bleeding or completion of a course of therapy, consider the use of another anticoagulant to prevent stroke from occurring.

May increase the risk of bleeding; serious, potentially fatal bleeding may occur. Concomitant use of drugs that affect hemostasis increases the risk of bleeding. Monitor for signs and symptoms of bleeding. Discontinue therapy with active pathological hemorrhage and promptly evaluate for bleeding source. No specific antidote exists for apixaban reversal; hemodialysis does not appear to have a substantial impact on apixaban exposure. Although not evaluated in clinical trials, in the event of apixaban-related hemorrhage, the use of prothrombin complex concentrate (PCC), activated prothrombin complex concentrate, or recombinant factor VIIa may be considered. The use of activated oral charcoal may be considered if ingestion occurred within 2 to 6 hours of presentation.

[U.S. Boxed Warning]: Spinal or epidural hematomas resulting in long-term or permanent paralysis may occur with neuraxial anesthesia (epidural or spinal anesthesia) or spinal/epidural puncture; the risk is increased by the use of indwelling epidural catheters, with concomitant administration of other drugs that affect hemostasis (eg, NSAIDS, platelet inhibitors, other anticoagulants), in patients with a history of traumatic or repeated epidural or spinal punctures, a history of spinal deformity or surgery, or if optimal timing between the administration of apixaban and neuraxial procedures is not known. Consider the potential benefit versus risk prior to neuraxial intervention in patients who are anticoagulated or scheduled to be anticoagulated for thromboprophylaxis. In patients who receive both apixaban and neuraxial anesthesia, avoid removal of epidural or intrathecal catheter for at least 24 hours following last apixaban dose; avoid apixaban administration for at least 5 hours following catheter removal. If traumatic puncture occurs, delay administration of apixaban for at least 48 hours. **Monitor for signs of neurologic impairment (eg, numbness/weakness of legs, bowel/bladder dysfunction). If neurologic impairment is noted, prompt treatment is necessary.**

In hemodynamically unstable patients with acute PE or patients with PE requiring thrombolysis or pulmonary embolectomy, the use of apixaban is not recommended as an alternative to unfractionated heparin for initial treatment. In a clinical trial of high-risk, post-acute coronary syndrome (ACS) patients (off-label use), use of apixaban in addition to standard antiplatelet therapy increased the incidence of major bleeding (including intracranial and fatal bleeding) without any significant clinical benefit (Alexander, 2011). In acutely ill patients (eg, heart failure, respiratory failure) at risk for venous thromboembolism (VTE) receiving apixaban for extended VTE prophylaxis, an increased incidence of major bleeding without greater efficacy was observed with extended apixaban therapy (eg, 30 days) versus low molecular weight heparin (enoxaparin) therapy for 1 to 2 weeks (Goldhaber, 2011). Canadian labeling: Use in patients undergoing hip fracture surgery has not been studied; avoid use in these patients.

Use with caution in moderate impairment (Child-Pugh class B) as there is limited clinical experience in these patients; dosing recommendations cannot be provided. Use in severe hepatic impairment (Child-Pugh class C) is not recommended. Systemic exposure increases with worsening renal function. Bleeding risk may be increased in severe renal impairment (CrCl <15 to 29 mL/minute); use with caution. Patients with ESRD with or without hemodialysis have not been studied. Dosage reduction is recommended for patients with nonvalvular atrial fibrillation with a serum creatinine ≥1.5 mg/dL **and** are *either* ≥80 years of age or weigh ≤60 kg. Safety and efficacy have not been established in patients with prosthetic heart valves or significant rheumatic heart disease (eg, mitral stenosis); use is not recommended. Non-valvular atrial fibrillation is defined as atrial fibrillation that occurs in the absence of rheumatic mitral valve disease, mitral valve repair, or prosthetic heart valve (AHA/ACC/HRS [January, 2014]).

Potentially significant drug-drug interactions may exist, requiring dose or frequency adjustment, additional monitoring, and/or selection of alternative therapy. Systemic exposure is increased ~32% in patients >65 years of age and may be increased by 20% to 30% in patients <50 kg and decreased by 20% to 30% in patients >120 kg; dosage reduction is recommended for patients with nonvalvular atrial fibrillation with any 2 of the following: ≥80 years of age, weight ≤60 kg, or serum creatinine ≥1.5 mg/dL

Discontinue apixaban at least 24 to 48 hours prior to elective surgery or invasive procedures depending on risk or location of bleeding.

Adverse Reactions Note: Includes adverse reactions from nonvalvular atrial fibrillation and hip/knee replacement surgery clinical trials.

Endocrine & metabolic: Increased gamma-glutamyl transferase

Gastrointestinal: Nausea

Hematologic & oncologic: Anemia, bruise, hemorrhage, postprocedural hemorrhage

Hepatic: Increased serum transaminases

Rare but important or life-threatening: Anaphylaxis, gastrointestinal hemorrhage, hematuria, hemophthalmos, hypersensitivity, hypotension, incision site hemorrhage, increased serum alkaline phosphatase, increased serum AST, increased serum bilirubin, intracranial hemorrhage, muscle hemorrhage, perioperative blood loss, postoperative hematoma (incision site), rectal hemorrhage, syncope, thrombocytopenia, wound secretion

Drug Interactions

Metabolism/Transport Effects Substrate of BCRP, CYP1A2 (minor), CYP2C19 (minor), CYP2C8 (minor), CYP2C9 (minor), CYP3A4 (major), P-glycoprotein; **Note:** Assignment of Major/Minor substrate status based on clinically relevant drug interaction potential; **Inhibits** CYP2C19 (weak)

Avoid Concomitant Use

Avoid concomitant use of Apixaban with any of the following: Anticoagulants; Conivaptan; CYP3A4 Inducers (Strong); CYP3A4 Inhibitors (Strong); Dabigatran Etexilate; Edoxaban; Idelalisib; Omacetaxine; Rivaroxaban; St Johns Wort; Urokinase; Vorapaxar

Increased Effect/Toxicity

Apixaban may increase the levels/effects of: Anticoagulants; Collagenase (Systemic); Deferasirox; Ibritumomab; Nintedanib; Obinutuzumab; Omacetaxine; Rivaroxaban; Tositumomab and Iodine I 131 Tositumomab

The levels/effects of Apixaban may be increased by: Agents with Antiplatelet Properties; Aprepitant; Ceritinib; Conivaptan; CYP3A4 Inhibitors (Moderate); CYP3A4 Inhibitors (Strong); Dabigatran Etexilate; Dasatinib; Edoxaban; Fosaprepitant; Fusidic Acid (Systemic); Herbs (Anticoagulant/Antiplatelet Properties); Ibrutinib; Idelalisib; Ivacaftor; Limaprost; Luliconazole; Mifepristone; Naproxen; Netupitant; Nonsteroidal Anti-Inflammatory Agents; Omega-3 Fatty Acids; Pentosan Polysulfate Sodium; P-glycoprotein/ABCB1 Inhibitors; Prostacyclin Analogues; Salicylates; Simeprevir; Sugammadex; Thrombolytic Agents; Tibolone; Tipranavir; Urokinase; Vitamin E; Vorapaxar

Decreased Effect

The levels/effects of Apixaban may be decreased by: Bosentan; CYP3A4 Inducers (Moderate); CYP3A4 Inducers (Strong); Dabrafenib; Deferasirox; Estrogen Derivatives; P-glycoprotein/ABCB1 Inducers; Progestins; Siltuximab; St Johns Wort; Tocilizumab

Food Interactions Grapefruit juice may increase levels/effects of apixaban. Management: Advise patients who consume grapefruit juice during therapy to use caution; monitor for increased effects (eg, bleeding).

Storage/Stability Store at 20°C to 25°C (68°F to 77°F); excursions are permitted between 15°C and 30°C (59°F and 86°F).

Mechanism of Action Inhibits platelet activation and fibrin clot formation via direct, selective and reversible inhibition of free and clot-bound factor Xa (FXa). FXa, as part of the prothrombinase complex consisting also of factor Va, calcium ions, and phospholipid, catalyzes the conversion of prothrombin to thrombin. Thrombin both activates platelets and catalyzes the conversion of fibrinogen to fibrin.

Pharmacodynamics/Kinetics

Onset: 3 to 4 hours

Distribution: V_{ss}: ~21 L

Protein binding: ~87%

Metabolism: Hepatic predominantly via CYP3A4/5 and to a lesser extent via CYP1A2, 2C8, 2C9, 2C19, and 2J2 to inactive metabolites; substrate of P-glycoprotein (P-gp) and breast cancer resistant protein (BCRP)

Bioavailability: ~50%

Half-life elimination: ~12 hours

Time to peak: 3 to 4 hours

Excretion: Urine (~27% as parent drug); feces

Dosage Oral:

Adults:

Deep venous thrombosis:

Treatment: 10 mg twice daily for 7 days followed by 5 mg twice daily

Reduction in the risk of recurrence: 2.5 mg twice daily after at least 6 months of treatment for DVT

Nonvalvular atrial fibrillation (to prevent stroke and systemic embolism): 5 mg twice daily **unless** patient has any 2 of the following: Age ≥80 years, body weight ≤60 kg, or serum creatinine ≥1.5 mg/dL, then reduce dose to 2.5 mg twice daily.

Postoperative venous thromboprophylaxis:

Hip replacement surgery: 2.5 mg twice daily beginning 12 to 24 hours postoperatively; duration: 35 days

Knee replacement surgery: 2.5 mg twice daily beginning 12 to 24 hours postoperatively; duration: 12 days

Pulmonary embolism (PE):

Treatment: 10 mg twice daily for 7 days followed by 5 mg twice daily

Reduction in the risk of recurrence: 2.5 mg twice daily after at least 6 months of treatment for PE

Elderly: Refer to adult dosing. Nonvalvular atrial fibrillation (to prevent stroke and systemic embolism): If patient is ≥80 years of age **and** *either* weighs ≤60 kg or has a serum creatinine ≥1.5 mg/dL, then reduce dose to 2.5 mg twice daily

Conversion from warfarin to apixaban: Discontinue warfarin and initiate apixaban when INR is <2

Conversion from apixaban to warfarin: **Note:** Apixaban affects the INR; measuring the INR during coadministration with warfarin therapy may not be useful for determining an appropriate dose of warfarin

U.S. labeling: If continuous anticoagulation is necessary, discontinue apixaban and begin both a parenteral anticoagulant with warfarin when the next dose of apixaban is due; discontinue parenteral anticoagulant when INR reaches an acceptable range

Canadian labeling: Initiate warfarin or other vitamin K antagonist (VKA) at usual starting doses and continue apixaban until INR ≥2, then discontinue apixaban. During concomitant therapy, manufacturer recommends initiating INR testing on day 3 and just prior to each dose of apixaban.

Conversion between apixaban and other non-warfarin anticoagulants: Discontinue anticoagulant being taken and begin the other at the next scheduled dose

Dosage adjustment of apixaban with concomitant medications:

U.S. labeling: For patients receiving dual strong CYP3A4 and P-glycoprotein inhibitors (eg, clarithromycin, ketoconazole, itraconazole, ritonavir) and apixaban doses greater than 2.5 mg twice daily, reduce apixaban dose by 50%: **Note:** Avoid concomitant use with dual strong CYP3A4 and P-glycoprotein inhibitors if patient is already taking apixaban 2.5 mg twice daily or patient meets 2 of the following criteria: Age ≥80 years, body weight ≤60 kg, or serum creatinine ≥1.5 mg/dL.

Canadian labeling: Dual CYP3A4 and P-glycoprotein inhibitors: No dosage adjustment necessary for moderate dual inhibitors. Use is contraindicated with strong dual inhibitors.

Dosage adjustment in renal impairment:

U.S. labeling:

Deep vein thrombosis (DVT), pulmonary embolism (PE), reduction in the risk of recurrent DVT and PE: No dosage adjustment necessary; however, patients with a serum creatinine >2.5 mg/dL or CrCl <25 mL/minute (as determined by Cockcroft-Gault equation) were excluded from the clinical trials (Agnelli, 2013a; Agnelli, 2013b)

Nonvalvular atrial fibrillation (to prevent stroke and systemic embolism):

Serum creatinine <1.5 mg/dL: No dosage adjustment necessary *unless* age ≥80 years and body weight ≤60 kg, then reduce dose to 2.5 mg twice daily (also refer to adult dosing).

Serum creatinine ≥1.5 mg/dL **and** *either* age ≥80 years **or** body weight ≤60 kg: 2.5 mg twice daily. **Note:** In patients with severe or end-stage chronic kidney disease, warfarin remains the anticoagulant of choice (AHA/ACC/HRS [January, 2014]).

ESRD requiring hemodialysis: 5 mg twice daily; reduce to 2.5 mg twice daily if age ≥80 years or body weight ≤60 kg. **Note:** In patients with severe or end-stage chronic kidney disease, warfarin remains the anticoagulant of choice (AHA/ACC/HRS [January, 2014]).

Postoperative (hip or knee replacement) venous thromboprophylaxis: No dosage adjustment necessary; however, patients with either clinically significant renal impairment (ADVANCE-1 [Lassen, 2009]), impaired renal function (ADVANCE-2 [Lassen, 2010b]), or CrCl <30 mL/minute (as determined by Cockcroft-Gault equation) (ADVANCE-3 [Lassen 2010a]) were excluded from the respective clinical trials.

Canadian labeling: **Note:** Estimated creatinine clearance (eCrCl) may be calculated using Cockcroft-Gault equation.

Nonvalvular atrial fibrillation (to prevent stroke and systemic embolism):

eCrCl ≥25 mL/minute: No dosage adjustment necessary. Patients with serum creatinine ≥1.5 mg/dL (SI: ≥133 micromole/L) **and** either age ≥80 years **or** body weight ≤60 kg: 2.5 mg twice daily

eCrCl 15 to 24 mL/minute: There are no dosage adjustments provided in manufacturer's labeling (very limited data).

eCrCl <15 mL/minute: Use is not recommended.

Dialysis: Use is not recommended.

Postoperative (hip or knee replacement) venous thromboprophylaxis:

eCrCl ≥30 mL/minute): No dosage adjustment required.

eCrCl 15 to 29 mL/minute: There are no dosage adjustments provided in manufacturer's labeling; use with caution as bleeding risk may be increased.

eCrCl <15 mL/minute: Use is not recommended.

Dialysis: Use is not recommended.

Dosage adjustment in hepatic impairment:

U.S. labeling:

Mild impairment (Child-Pugh class A): No dosage adjustment required.

Moderate impairment (Child-Pugh class B): There are no dosage adjustments provided in manufacturer's labeling; use with caution (limited clinical experience in these patients).

Severe impairment (Child-Pugh class C): Use is not recommended.

Canadian labeling:

Mild or moderate impairment (Child-Pugh class A or B): No dosage adjustment required; use with caution.

Severe impairment (Child-Pugh class C): Use is not recommended.

Note: Use is contraindicated in patients with hepatic disease associated with coagulopathy and clinically-relevant bleeding risk.

Administration Administer without regard to meals. After hip/knee replacement, initial dose should be administered 12 to 24 hours postoperatively. If patient unable to swallow whole tablets, may crush 5 mg or 2.5 mg tablets and suspend in 60 mL of D_5W followed by immediate delivery through a nasogastric tube. No information regarding administration of suspension by mouth is available.

Monitoring Parameters Renal function prior to initiation, when clinically indicated, and at least annually in all patients (AHA/ACC/HRS [January, 2014]), hepatic function; signs of bleeding. Routine monitoring of coagulation tests is not required. Although not recommended to assess effectiveness, the prothrombin time (PT), INR, and aPTT are prolonged with apixaban. Anti-FXa assay may be helpful (plasma concentrations and anti-FXa activity exhibit linear relationship) in guiding clinical decisions.

When converting from apixaban to a vitamin K antagonist (VKA), Canadian labeling recommends INR testing just prior to each dose of apixaban beginning on day 3 of concurrent therapy with the VKA.

Reference Range Predicted steady state anti-FXa activity: Peak: 1.3 units/mL; trough: 0.84 units/mL

Dosage Forms

Tablet, Oral:

Eliquis: 2.5 mg, 5 mg

- **Aplenzin** *see* BuPROPion *on page 305*
- **Aplisol** *see* Tuberculin Tests *on page 2110*
- **Aplonidine** *see* Apraclonidine *on page 165*
- **APO-066** *see* Deferiprone *on page 585*
- **Apo-Acebutolol® (Can)** *see* Acebutolol *on page 29*
- **Apo-Acetaminophen (Can)** *see* Acetaminophen *on page 32*
- **Apo-Acyclovir (Can)** *see* Acyclovir (Systemic) *on page 47*
- **Apo-Alendronate (Can)** *see* Alendronate *on page 79*
- **Apo-Alfuzosin® (Can)** *see* Alfuzosin *on page 84*
- **Apo-Allopurinol (Can)** *see* Allopurinol *on page 90*
- **Apo-Alpraz® (Can)** *see* ALPRAZolam *on page 94*
- **Apo-Alpraz® TS (Can)** *see* ALPRAZolam *on page 94*
- **Apo-Amiloride® (Can)** *see* AMILoride *on page 113*
- **Apo-Amiodarone (Can)** *see* Amiodarone *on page 114*
- **Apo-Amitriptyline (Can)** *see* Amitriptyline *on page 119*
- **Apo-Amlodipine (Can)** *see* AmLODIPine *on page 123*
- **Apo-Amoxi® (Can)** *see* Amoxicillin *on page 130*
- **Apo-Amoxi-Clav (Can)** *see* Amoxicillin and Clavulanate *on page 133*
- **Apo-Ampi (Can)** *see* Ampicillin *on page 141*
- **Apo-Anastrozole (Can)** *see* Anastrozole *on page 148*
- **Apo-Atenol (Can)** *see* Atenolol *on page 189*
- **Apo-Atomoxetine (Can)** *see* AtoMOXetine *on page 191*
- **Apo-Atorvastatin (Can)** *see* AtorvaSTATin *on page 194*
- **Apo-Azathioprine (Can)** *see* AzaTHIOprine *on page 210*
- **Apo-Azithromycin (Can)** *see* Azithromycin (Systemic) *on page 216*
- **Apo-Azithromycin Z (Can)** *see* Azithromycin (Systemic) *on page 216*
- **Apo-Baclofen (Can)** *see* Baclofen *on page 223*
- **Apo-Beclomethasone (Can)** *see* Beclomethasone (Nasal) *on page 232*
- **Apo-Benzydamine (Can)** *see* Benzydamine [CAN/INT] *on page 249*
- **Apo-Bicalutamide (Can)** *see* Bicalutamide *on page 262*
- **Apo-Bisacodyl [OTC] (Can)** *see* Bisacodyl *on page 265*
- **Apo-Bisoprolol (Can)** *see* Bisoprolol *on page 266*
- **Apo-Brimonidine (Can)** *see* Brimonidine (Ophthalmic) *on page 288*
- **Apo-Brimonidine P (Can)** *see* Brimonidine (Ophthalmic) *on page 288*

- ◆ **Apo-Bromazepam® (Can)** *see* Bromazepam [CAN/INT] *on page 290*
- ◆ **Apo-Buspirone (Can)** *see* BusPIRone *on page 311*
- ◆ **Apo-Butorphanol (Can)** *see* Butorphanol *on page 314*
- ◆ **Apo-Cal (Can)** *see* Calcium Carbonate *on page 327*
- ◆ **Apo-Candesartan (Can)** *see* Candesartan *on page 335*
- ◆ **Apo-Candesartan HCTZ (Can)** *see* Candesartan and Hydrochlorothiazide *on page 338*
- ◆ **Apo-Capto (Can)** *see* Captopril *on page 342*
- ◆ **Apo-Carbamazepine (Can)** *see* CarBAMazepine *on page 346*
- ◆ **Apo-Carvedilol (Can)** *see* Carvedilol *on page 367*
- ◆ **Apo-Cefaclor® (Can)** *see* Cefaclor *on page 372*
- ◆ **Apo-Cefadroxil (Can)** *see* Cefadroxil *on page 372*
- ◆ **Apo-Cefprozil® (Can)** *see* Cefprozil *on page 389*
- ◆ **Apo-Cefuroxime (Can)** *see* Cefuroxime *on page 399*
- ◆ **Apo-Cephalex (Can)** *see* Cephalexin *on page 405*
- ◆ **Apo-Cetirizine [OTC] (Can)** *see* Cetirizine *on page 411*
- ◆ **Apo-Chlorhexidine Oral Rinse (Can)** *see* Chlorhexidine Gluconate *on page 422*
- ◆ **Apo-Chlorpropamide® (Can)** *see* ChlorproPAMIDE *on page 429*
- ◆ **Apo-Chlorthalidone (Can)** *see* Chlorthalidone *on page 430*
- ◆ **Apo-Ciclopirox (Can)** *see* Ciclopirox *on page 433*
- ◆ **Apo-Cilazapril (Can)** *see* Cilazapril [CAN/INT] *on page 434*
- ◆ **Apo-Cilazapril/Hctz (Can)** *see* Cilazapril and Hydrochlorothiazide [CAN/INT] *on page 436*
- ◆ **Apo-Cimetidine (Can)** *see* Cimetidine *on page 438*
- ◆ **Apo-Ciproflox (Can)** *see* Ciprofloxacin (Systemic) *on page 441*
- ◆ **Apo-Citalopram (Can)** *see* Citalopram *on page 451*
- ◆ **Apo-Clarithromycin (Can)** *see* Clarithromycin *on page 456*
- ◆ **Apo-Clarithromycin XL (Can)** *see* Clarithromycin *on page 456*
- ◆ **Apo-Clindamycin (Can)** *see* Clindamycin (Systemic) *on page 460*
- ◆ **Apo-Clobazam (Can)** *see* CloBAZam *on page 465*
- ◆ **Apo-Clomipramine® (Can)** *see* ClomiPRAMINE *on page 475*
- ◆ **Apo-Clonazepam (Can)** *see* ClonazePAM *on page 478*
- ◆ **Apo-Clonidine® (Can)** *see* CloNIDine *on page 480*
- ◆ **Apo-Clopidogrel (Can)** *see* Clopidogrel *on page 484*
- ◆ **Apo-Clorazepate® (Can)** *see* Clorazepate *on page 487*
- ◆ **Apo-Cloxi (Can)** *see* Cloxacillin [CAN/INT] *on page 488*
- ◆ **Apo-Clozapine (Can)** *see* CloZAPine *on page 490*
- ◆ **Apo-Cromolyn Nasal Spray [OTC] (Can)** *see* Cromolyn (Nasal) *on page 514*
- ◆ **Apo-Cyclobenzaprine (Can)** *see* Cyclobenzaprine *on page 516*
- ◆ **Apo-Cyclosporine (Can)** *see* CycloSPORINE (Systemic) *on page 522*
- ◆ **Apo-Desmopressin (Can)** *see* Desmopressin *on page 594*
- ◆ **Apo-Dexamethasone (Can)** *see* Dexamethasone (Systemic) *on page 599*
- ◆ **Apo-Diazepam® (Can)** *see* Diazepam *on page 613*
- ◆ **Apo-Diclo (Can)** *see* Diclofenac (Systemic) *on page 617*
- ◆ **Apo-Diclo Rapide (Can)** *see* Diclofenac (Systemic) *on page 617*
- ◆ **Apo-Diclo SR (Can)** *see* Diclofenac (Systemic) *on page 617*
- ◆ **Apo-Diflunisal (Can)** *see* Diflunisal *on page 626*
- ◆ **Apo-Digoxin (Can)** *see* Digoxin *on page 627*
- ◆ **Apo-Diltiaz (Can)** *see* Diltiazem *on page 634*
- ◆ **Apo-Diltiaz CD (Can)** *see* Diltiazem *on page 634*
- ◆ **Apo-Diltiaz SR (Can)** *see* Diltiazem *on page 634*
- ◆ **Apo-Diltiaz TZ (Can)** *see* Diltiazem *on page 634*
- ◆ **Apo-Dimenhydrinate [OTC] (Can)** *see* DimenhyDRINATE *on page 637*
- ◆ **Apo-Dipyridamole FC® (Can)** *see* Dipyridamole *on page 652*
- ◆ **Apo-Divalproex (Can)** *see* Valproic Acid and Derivatives *on page 2123*
- ◆ **Apo-Docusate Calcium [OTC] (Can)** *see* Docusate *on page 661*
- ◆ **Apo-Docusate Sodium [OTC] (Can)** *see* Docusate *on page 661*
- ◆ **Apo-Domperidone (Can)** *see* Domperidone [CAN/INT] *on page 666*
- ◆ **Apo-Donepezil (Can)** *see* Donepezil *on page 668*
- ◆ **Apo-Dorzo-Timop (Can)** *see* Dorzolamide and Timolol *on page 673*
- ◆ **Apo-Doxazosin (Can)** *see* Doxazosin *on page 674*
- ◆ **Apo-Doxepin (Can)** *see* Doxepin (Systemic) *on page 676*
- ◆ **Apo-Doxy (Can)** *see* Doxycycline *on page 689*
- ◆ **Apo-Doxy Tabs (Can)** *see* Doxycycline *on page 689*
- ◆ **Apo-Dutasteride (Can)** *see* Dutasteride *on page 702*
- ◆ **Apo-Enalapril (Can)** *see* Enalapril *on page 722*
- ◆ **Apo-Enalapril Maleate/Hctz (Can)** *see* Enalapril and Hydrochlorothiazide *on page 725*
- ◆ **Apo-Entecavir (Can)** *see* Entecavir *on page 731*
- ◆ **Apo-Erythro Base (Can)** *see* Erythromycin (Systemic) *on page 762*
- ◆ **Apo-Erythro E-C (Can)** *see* Erythromycin (Systemic) *on page 762*
- ◆ **Apo-Erythro-ES (Can)** *see* Erythromycin (Systemic) *on page 762*
- ◆ **Apo-Erythro-S (Can)** *see* Erythromycin (Systemic) *on page 762*
- ◆ **Apo-Escitalopram (Can)** *see* Escitalopram *on page 765*
- ◆ **Apo-Esomeprazole (Can)** *see* Esomeprazole *on page 771*
- ◆ **Apo-Etodolac (Can)** *see* Etodolac *on page 815*
- ◆ **Apo-Ezetimibe (Can)** *see* Ezetimibe *on page 832*
- ◆ **Apo-Famciclovir® (Can)** *see* Famciclovir *on page 843*
- ◆ **Apo-Famotidine (Can)** *see* Famotidine *on page 845*
- ◆ **Apo-Fenofibrate (Can)** *see* Fenofibrate and Derivatives *on page 852*
- ◆ **Apo-Feno-Micro (Can)** *see* Fenofibrate and Derivatives *on page 852*
- ◆ **Apo-Feno-Super (Can)** *see* Fenofibrate and Derivatives *on page 852*
- ◆ **Apo-Fentanyl Matrix (Can)** *see* FentaNYL *on page 857*
- ◆ **Apo-Ferrous Gluconate® (Can)** *see* Ferrous Gluconate *on page 870*
- ◆ **Apo-Ferrous Sulfate® (Can)** *see* Ferrous Sulfate *on page 871*
- ◆ **Apo-Finasteride (Can)** *see* Finasteride *on page 878*

- **Apo-Flavoxate® (Can)** *see* FlavoxATE *on page 881*
- **Apo-Flecainide® (Can)** *see* Flecainide *on page 882*
- **Apo-Fluconazole (Can)** *see* Fluconazole *on page 885*
- **Apo-Flunisolide® (Can)** *see* Flunisolide (Nasal) *on page 893*
- **Apo-Fluoxetine (Can)** *see* FLUoxetine *on page 899*
- **Apo-Fluphenazine® (Can)** *see* FluPHENAZine *on page 905*
- **Apo-Fluphenazine Decanoate® (Can)** *see* FluPHENAZine *on page 905*
- **Apo-Flurazepam (Can)** *see* Flurazepam *on page 906*
- **Apo-Flurbiprofen (Can)** *see* Flurbiprofen (Systemic) *on page 906*
- **Apo-Flutamide (Can)** *see* Flutamide *on page 907*
- **Apo-Fluticasone (Can)** *see* Fluticasone (Nasal) *on page 910*
- **Apo-Fluvoxamine (Can)** *see* FluvoxaMINE *on page 916*
- **Apo-Folic® (Can)** *see* Folic Acid *on page 919*
- **Apo-Fosinopril (Can)** *see* Fosinopril *on page 932*
- **Apo-Furosemide (Can)** *see* Furosemide *on page 940*
- **Apo-Gabapentin (Can)** *see* Gabapentin *on page 943*
- **Apo-Gain® (Can)** *see* Minoxidil (Topical) *on page 1374*
- **Apo-Gemfibrozil (Can)** *see* Gemfibrozil *on page 956*
- **Apo-Gliclazide (Can)** *see* Gliclazide [CAN/INT] *on page 964*
- **Apo-Glimepiride (Can)** *see* Glimepiride *on page 966*
- **Apo-Glyburide (Can)** *see* GlyBURIDE *on page 972*
- **Apo-Haloperidol (Can)** *see* Haloperidol *on page 993*
- **Apo-Haloperidol LA (Can)** *see* Haloperidol *on page 993*
- **Apo-Hydralazine (Can)** *see* HydrALAZINE *on page 1007*
- **Apo-Hydro (Can)** *see* Hydrochlorothiazide *on page 1009*
- **Apo-Hydromorphone (Can)** *see* HYDROmorphone *on page 1016*
- **Apo-Hydroxyquine (Can)** *see* Hydroxychloroquine *on page 1021*
- **Apo-Hydroxyurea (Can)** *see* Hydroxyurea *on page 1021*
- **Apo-Hydroxyzine (Can)** *see* HydrOXYzine *on page 1024*
- **Apo-Ibuprofen (Can)** *see* Ibuprofen *on page 1032*
- **Apo-Imatinib (Can)** *see* Imatinib *on page 1047*
- **Apo-Imiquimod (Can)** *see* Imiquimod *on page 1055*
- **Apo-Indapamide (Can)** *see* Indapamide *on page 1065*
- **Apo-Indomethacin (Can)** *see* Indomethacin *on page 1067*
- **Apo-Ipravent® (Can)** *see* Ipratropium (Nasal) *on page 1109*
- **Apo-Irbesartan (Can)** *see* Irbesartan *on page 1110*
- **Apo-Irbesartan/HCTZ (Can)** *see* Irbesartan and Hydrochlorothiazide *on page 1112*
- **Apo-ISMN (Can)** *see* Isosorbide Mononitrate *on page 1126*
- **Apo-K (Can)** *see* Potassium Chloride *on page 1687*
- **Apo-Ketoconazole (Can)** *see* Ketoconazole (Systemic) *on page 1144*
- **Apo-Ketorolac® (Can)** *see* Ketorolac (Systemic) *on page 1146*
- **Apo-Ketorolac Injectable® (Can)** *see* Ketorolac (Systemic) *on page 1146*
- **Apo-Ketorolac® Ophthalmic (Can)** *see* Ketorolac (Ophthalmic) *on page 1149*
- **APO-Ketotifen® (Can)** *see* Ketotifen (Systemic) [CAN/INT] *on page 1149*
- **Apo-Labetalol (Can)** *see* Labetalol *on page 1151*
- **Apo-Lactulose (Can)** *see* Lactulose *on page 1156*
- **Apo-Lamivudine (Can)** *see* LamiVUDine *on page 1157*
- **Apo-Lamivudine HBV (Can)** *see* LamiVUDine *on page 1157*
- **Apo-Lamotrigine (Can)** *see* LamoTRIgine *on page 1160*
- **Apo-Lansoprazole (Can)** *see* Lansoprazole *on page 1166*
- **Apo-Latanoprost (Can)** *see* Latanoprost *on page 1172*
- **Apo-Leflunomide (Can)** *see* Leflunomide *on page 1174*
- **Apo-Letrozole (Can)** *see* Letrozole *on page 1181*
- **Apo-Levetiracetam (Can)** *see* LevETIRAcetam *on page 1191*
- **Apo-Levobunolol® (Can)** *see* Levobunolol *on page 1194*
- **Apo-Levocarb (Can)** *see* Carbidopa and Levodopa *on page 351*
- **Apo-Levocarb CR (Can)** *see* Carbidopa and Levodopa *on page 351*
- **APO-Levofloxacin (Can)** *see* Levofloxacin (Systemic) *on page 1197*
- **Apo-Linezolid (Can)** *see* Linezolid *on page 1217*
- **Apo-Lisinopril (Can)** *see* Lisinopril *on page 1226*
- **Apo-Lisinopril/Hctz (Can)** *see* Lisinopril and Hydrochlorothiazide *on page 1229*
- **Apo-Lithium Carbonate (Can)** *see* Lithium *on page 1230*
- **Apo-Loperamide® (Can)** *see* Loperamide *on page 1236*
- **Apo-Loratadine (Can)** *see* Loratadine *on page 1241*
- **Apo-Lorazepam (Can)** *see* LORazepam *on page 1243*
- **Apo-Losartan (Can)** *see* Losartan *on page 1248*
- **Apo-Losartan/HCTZ (Can)** *see* Losartan and Hydrochlorothiazide *on page 1250*
- **Apo-Lovastatin (Can)** *see* Lovastatin *on page 1252*
- **Apo-Loxapine (Can)** *see* Loxapine *on page 1255*
- **Apo-Medroxy (Can)** *see* MedroxyPROGESTERone *on page 1277*
- **Apo-Meloxicam (Can)** *see* Meloxicam *on page 1283*
- **Apo-Memantine (Can)** *see* Memantine *on page 1286*
- **Apo-Metformin (Can)** *see* MetFORMIN *on page 1307*
- **Apo-Methazolamide® (Can)** *see* Methazolamide *on page 1317*
- **Apo-Methoprazine (Can)** *see* Methotrimeprazine [CAN/INT] *on page 1329*
- **Apo-Methotrexate (Can)** *see* Methotrexate *on page 1322*
- **Apo-Methylphenidate (Can)** *see* Methylphenidate *on page 1336*
- **Apo-Methylphenidate SR (Can)** *see* Methylphenidate *on page 1336*
- **Apo-Metoclop (Can)** *see* Metoclopramide *on page 1345*
- **Apo-Metoprolol (Can)** *see* Metoprolol *on page 1350*
- **Apo-Metoprolol SR (Can)** *see* Metoprolol *on page 1350*
- **Apo-Metoprolol (Type L) (Can)** *see* Metoprolol *on page 1350*
- **Apo-Midodrine (Can)** *see* Midodrine *on page 1365*
- **Apo-Minocycline (Can)** *see* Minocycline *on page 1371*
- **Apo-Mirtazapine (Can)** *see* Mirtazapine *on page 1376*

- ◆ **Apo-Moclobemide (Can)** *see* Moclobemide [CAN/INT] *on page* 1384
- ◆ **Apo-Modafinil (Can)** *see* Modafinil *on page* 1386
- ◆ **Apo-Mometasone® (Can)** *see* Mometasone (Nasal) *on page* 1391
- ◆ **Apo-Montelukast (Can)** *see* Montelukast *on page* 1392
- ◆ **Apo-Mycophenolate (Can)** *see* Mycophenolate *on page* 1405
- ◆ **Apo-Nabumetone (Can)** *see* Nabumetone *on page* 1411
- ◆ **Apo-Nadol (Can)** *see* Nadolol *on page* 1411
- ◆ **Apo-Napro-Na (Can)** *see* Naproxen *on page* 1427
- ◆ **Apo-Napro-Na DS (Can)** *see* Naproxen *on page* 1427
- ◆ **Apo-Naproxen (Can)** *see* Naproxen *on page* 1427
- ◆ **Apo-Naproxen EC (Can)** *see* Naproxen *on page* 1427
- ◆ **Apo-Naproxen SR (Can)** *see* Naproxen *on page* 1427
- ◆ **Apo-Nifed PA (Can)** *see* NIFEdipine *on page* 1451
- ◆ **Apo-Nitrazepam (Can)** *see* Nitrazepam [CAN/INT] *on page* 1461
- ◆ **Apo-Nitrofurantoin (Can)** *see* Nitrofurantoin *on page* 1463
- ◆ **Apo-Nizatidine (Can)** *see* Nizatidine *on page* 1471
- ◆ **Apo-Norflox® (Can)** *see* Norfloxacin *on page* 1475
- ◆ **Apo-Nortriptyline (Can)** *see* Nortriptyline *on page* 1476
- ◆ **Apo-Oflox (Can)** *see* Ofloxacin (Systemic) *on page* 1490
- ◆ **Apo-Olanzapine (Can)** *see* OLANZapine *on page* 1491
- ◆ **Apo-Olanzapine ODT (Can)** *see* OLANZapine *on page* 1491
- ◆ **Apo-Olopatadine (Can)** *see* Olopatadine (Ophthalmic) *on page* 1500
- ◆ **Apo-Omeprazole (Can)** *see* Omeprazole *on page* 1508
- ◆ **Apo-Ondansetron (Can)** *see* Ondansetron *on page* 1513
- ◆ **Apo-Orciprenaline® (Can)** *see* Metaproterenol *on page* 1307
- ◆ **Apo-Oxaprozin (Can)** *see* Oxaprozin *on page* 1532
- ◆ **Apo-Oxazepam® (Can)** *see* Oxazepam *on page* 1532
- ◆ **Apo-Oxcarbazepine (Can)** *see* OXcarbazepine *on page* 1532
- ◆ **Apo-Oxybutynin (Can)** *see* Oxybutynin *on page* 1536
- ◆ **Apo-Oxycodone/Acet (Can)** *see* Oxycodone and Acetaminophen *on page* 1541
- ◆ **Apo-Oxycodone CR (Can)** *see* OxyCODONE *on page* 1538
- ◆ **APOP [DSC]** *see* Sulfacetamide (Topical) *on page* 1943
- ◆ **Apo-Paclitaxel (Can)** *see* PACLitaxel (Conventional) *on page* 1550
- ◆ **Apo-Pantoprazole (Can)** *see* Pantoprazole *on page* 1570
- ◆ **Apo-Paroxetine (Can)** *see* PARoxetine *on page* 1579
- ◆ **Apo-Pen VK (Can)** *see* Penicillin V Potassium *on page* 1614
- ◆ **Apo-Perphenazine® (Can)** *see* Perphenazine *on page* 1627
- ◆ **Apo-Pimozide® (Can)** *see* Pimozide *on page* 1651
- ◆ **Apo-Pindol (Can)** *see* Pindolol *on page* 1652
- ◆ **Apo-Pioglitazone (Can)** *see* Pioglitazone *on page* 1654
- ◆ **Apo-Piroxicam (Can)** *see* Piroxicam *on page* 1662
- ◆ **Apo-Pramipexole (Can)** *see* Pramipexole *on page* 1695
- ◆ **Apo-Pravastatin (Can)** *see* Pravastatin *on page* 1700
- ◆ **Apo-Prazo (Can)** *see* Prazosin *on page* 1703
- ◆ **Apo-Prednisone (Can)** *see* PredniSONE *on page* 1706
- ◆ **Apo-Pregabalin (Can)** *see* Pregabalin *on page* 1710
- ◆ **Apo-Primidone® (Can)** *see* Primidone *on page* 1714
- ◆ **Apo-Procainamide (Can)** *see* Procainamide *on page* 1716
- ◆ **Apo-Prochlorperazine (Can)** *see* Prochlorperazine *on page* 1718
- ◆ **Apo-Propafenone (Can)** *see* Propafenone *on page* 1725
- ◆ **Apo-Propranolol (Can)** *see* Propranolol *on page* 1731
- ◆ **Apo-Quetiapine (Can)** *see* QUEtiapine *on page* 1751
- ◆ **Apo-Quinapril (Can)** *see* Quinapril *on page* 1756
- ◆ **Apo-Quinidine (Can)** *see* QuiNIDine *on page* 1759
- ◆ **Apo-Quinine® (Can)** *see* QuiNINE *on page* 1761
- ◆ **Apo-Rabeprazole (Can)** *see* RABEprazole *on page* 1762
- ◆ **Apo-Raloxifene (Can)** *see* Raloxifene *on page* 1765
- ◆ **Apo-Ramipril (Can)** *see* Ramipril *on page* 1771
- ◆ **Apo-Ranitidine (Can)** *see* Ranitidine *on page* 1777
- ◆ **Apo-Repaglinide (Can)** *see* Repaglinide *on page* 1791
- ◆ **Apo-Riluzole® (Can)** *see* Riluzole *on page* 1812
- ◆ **Apo-Risedronate® (Can)** *see* Risedronate *on page* 1816
- ◆ **Apo-Risperidone (Can)** *see* RisperiDONE *on page* 1818
- ◆ **Apo-Rivastigmine (Can)** *see* Rivastigmine *on page* 1833
- ◆ **Apo-Rizatriptan (Can)** *see* Rizatriptan *on page* 1836
- ◆ **Apo-Rizatriptan RPD (Can)** *see* Rizatriptan *on page* 1836
- ◆ **Apo-Rosuvastatin (Can)** *see* Rosuvastatin *on page* 1848
- ◆ **Apo-Salvent (Can)** *see* Albuterol *on page* 69
- ◆ **Apo-Salvent AEM (Can)** *see* Albuterol *on page* 69
- ◆ **Apo-Salvent CFC Free (Can)** *see* Albuterol *on page* 69
- ◆ **Apo-Salvent-Ipravent Sterules (Can)** *see* Ipratropium and Albuterol *on page* 1109
- ◆ **Apo-Salvent Sterules (Can)** *see* Albuterol *on page* 69
- ◆ **Apo-Selegiline (Can)** *see* Selegiline *on page* 1873
- ◆ **Apo-Sertraline (Can)** *see* Sertraline *on page* 1878
- ◆ **Apo-Sildenafil (Can)** *see* Sildenafil *on page* 1882
- ◆ **Apo-Simvastatin (Can)** *see* Simvastatin *on page* 1890
- ◆ **Apo-Sotalol (Can)** *see* Sotalol *on page* 1927
- ◆ **Apo-Sucralfate (Can)** *see* Sucralfate *on page* 1940
- ◆ **Apo-Sulfasalazine (Can)** *see* SulfaSALAzine *on page* 1950
- ◆ **Apo-Sulfatrim (Can)** *see* Sulfamethoxazole and Trimethoprim *on page* 1946
- ◆ **Apo-Sulfatrim DS (Can)** *see* Sulfamethoxazole and Trimethoprim *on page* 1946
- ◆ **Apo-Sulfatrim Pediatric (Can)** *see* Sulfamethoxazole and Trimethoprim *on page* 1946
- ◆ **Apo-Sulin (Can)** *see* Sulindac *on page* 1953
- ◆ **Apo-Sumatriptan (Can)** *see* SUMAtriptan *on page* 1953
- ◆ **Apo-Tamox (Can)** *see* Tamoxifen *on page* 1971
- ◆ **Apo-Tamsulosin CR (Can)** *see* Tamsulosin *on page* 1974
- ◆ **Apo-Temazepam (Can)** *see* Temazepam *on page* 1990
- ◆ **Apo-Terazosin (Can)** *see* Terazosin *on page* 2001
- ◆ **Apo-Terbinafine (Can)** *see* Terbinafine (Systemic) *on page* 2002
- ◆ **Apo-Tetra (Can)** *see* Tetracycline *on page* 2017
- ◆ **Apo-Theo LA® (Can)** *see* Theophylline *on page* 2026

- ◆ **Apo-Tiaprofenic (Can)** *see* Tiaprofenic Acid [CAN/INT] *on page 2034*
- ◆ **Apo-Ticlopidine (Can)** *see* Ticlopidine *on page 2040*
- ◆ **Apo-Timol® (Can)** *see* Timolol (Systemic) *on page 2042*
- ◆ **Apo-Timop® (Can)** *see* Timolol (Ophthalmic) *on page 2043*
- ◆ **Apo-Tizanidine (Can)** *see* TiZANidine *on page 2051*
- ◆ **Apo-Tobramycin (Can)** *see* Tobramycin (Systemic, Oral Inhalation) *on page 2052*
- ◆ **Apo-Tolbutamide® (Can)** *see* TOLBUTamide *on page 2062*
- ◆ **Apo-Topiramate (Can)** *see* Topiramate *on page 2065*
- ◆ **Apo-Tramadol (Can)** *see* TraMADol *on page 2074*
- ◆ **Apo-Tramadol/Acet® (Can)** *see* Acetaminophen and Tramadol *on page 37*
- ◆ **Apo-Travoprost Z (Can)** *see* Travoprost *on page 2089*
- ◆ **Apo-Trazodone (Can)** *see* TraZODone *on page 2091*
- ◆ **Apo-Trazodone D (Can)** *see* TraZODone *on page 2091*
- ◆ **Apo-Triazide (Can)** *see* Hydrochlorothiazide and Triamterene *on page 1012*
- ◆ **Apo-Trifluoperazine® (Can)** *see* Trifluoperazine *on page 2102*
- ◆ **Apo-Trimethoprim® (Can)** *see* Trimethoprim *on page 2104*
- ◆ **Apo-Valacyclovir (Can)** *see* ValACYclovir *on page 2119*
- ◆ **Apo-Valganciclovir (Can)** *see* ValGANciclovir *on page 2121*
- ◆ **Apo-Valproic (Can)** *see* Valproic Acid and Derivatives *on page 2123*
- ◆ **Apo-Valsartan (Can)** *see* Valsartan *on page 2127*
- ◆ **Apo-Valsartan/HCTZ (Can)** *see* Valsartan and Hydrochlorothiazide *on page 2129*
- ◆ **Apo-Venlafaxine XR (Can)** *see* Venlafaxine *on page 2150*
- ◆ **Apo-Verap (Can)** *see* Verapamil *on page 2154*
- ◆ **Apo-Verap SR (Can)** *see* Verapamil *on page 2154*
- ◆ **Apo-Voriconazole (Can)** *see* Voriconazole *on page 2176*
- ◆ **Apo-Warfarin (Can)** *see* Warfarin *on page 2186*
- ◆ **Apo-Zidovudine (Can)** *see* Zidovudine *on page 2196*
- ◆ **Apo-Zopiclone (Can)** *see* Zopiclone [CAN/INT] *on page 2217*
- ◆ **APPG** *see* Penicillin G Procaine *on page 1613*
- ◆ **Apprilon (Can)** *see* Doxycycline *on page 689*

Apraclonidine (a pra KLOE ni deen)

Brand Names: U.S. Iopidine

Brand Names: Canada Iopidine

Index Terms Aplonidine; Apraclonidine Hydrochloride; p-Aminoclonidine

Pharmacologic Category Alpha$_2$ Agonist, Ophthalmic

Use

0.5% solution: Short-term, adjunctive therapy in patients who require additional reduction of IOP

1% solution: Prevention and treatment of postsurgical intraocular pressure (IOP) elevation following argon laser trabeculoplasty, argon laser iridotomy or Nd:YAG posterior capsulotomy

Pregnancy Risk Factor C

Dosage Intraocular pressure reduction: Adults: Ophthalmic:

0.5%: Instill 1 to 2 drops in the affected eye(s) 3 times daily

1%: Instill 1 drop in operative eye 1 hour prior to anterior segment laser surgery, second drop in same eye immediately upon completion of procedure

Dosage adjustment in renal impairment: There are no dosage adjustments provided in the manufacturer's labeling; monitor cardiovascular parameters closely.

Dosage adjustment in hepatic impairment: There are no dosage adjustments provided in the manufacturer's labeling; monitor cardiovascular parameters closely.

Additional Information Complete prescribing information should be consulted for additional detail.

Dosage Forms

Solution, Ophthalmic:

Iopidine: 0.5% (5 mL, 10 mL); 1% (1 ea)

Generic: 0.5% (5 mL, 10 mL)

- ◆ **Apraclonidine Hydrochloride** *see* Apraclonidine *on page 165*

Apremilast (a PRE mi last)

Brand Names: U.S. Otezla

Brand Names: Canada Otezla

Index Terms CC-10004

Pharmacologic Category Phosphodiesterase-4 Enzyme Inhibitor

Use

Psoriasis: Treatment of patients with moderate to severe plaque psoriasis who are candidates for phototherapy or systemic therapy

Psoriatic arthritis: Treatment of adult patients with active psoriatic arthritis (PsA)

Pregnancy Risk Factor C

Pregnancy Considerations Adverse events were observed in some animal reproduction studies. A registry is available for women exposed to apremilast during pregnancy (877-311-8972). The Canadian labeling contraindicates use during pregnancy and recommends women attempting to conceive avoid use.

Breast-Feeding Considerations It is not known if apremilast is excreted into breast milk. The U.S. labeling recommends that caution be used if administered to a nursing woman. The Canadian labeling contraindicates use in nursing women.

Contraindications

Hypersensitivity to apremilast or any component of the formulation

Canadian labeling: Additional contraindications (not in US labeling): Pregnancy; breast-feeding

Warnings/Precautions Use caution in patients with latent infections such as tuberculosis, viral hepatitis, herpes viral infection and herpes zoster (limited experience). Use in patients with severe immunological diseases, severe acute infectious diseases, or psoriasis patients treated with immunosuppressive therapy has not been evaluated. May cause weight loss; monitor weight regularly. Discontinuation of therapy should be considered with unexplained or significant weight loss. Neuropsychiatric effects (eg, depression, suicidal ideation, mood changes) have been reported. Use with caution in patients with a history of depression and/or suicidal thoughts/behavior. Instruct patients/caregivers to report worsening psychiatric symptoms and consider risks/benefits of continuation of therapy in such patients. Use with caution in renal impairment. Systemic exposure is increased in patients with severe renal impairment (CrCl <30 mL/minute); dosage reduction is recommended. Potentially significant drug-drug interactions may exist, requiring dose or frequency adjustment, additional monitoring, and/or selection of alternative therapy.

Adverse Reactions

Central nervous system: Depression, fatigue, headache, insomnia, migraine, tension headache

Dermatologic: Folliculitis, skin rash

Endocrine & metabolic: Weight loss

Gastrointestinal: Abdominal pain, decreased appetite, diarrhea, dyspepsia, frequent bowel movements, gastroesophageal reflux disease, nausea, upper abdominal pain, vomiting

Hypersensitivity: Hypersensitivity

Infection: Tooth abscess

Neuromuscular & skeletal: Back pain

Respiratory: Bronchitis, cough, nasopharyngitis, upper respiratory tract infection

Rare but important or life-threatening: Exacerbation of psoriasis (rebound following discontinuation), suicidal ideation

Drug Interactions

Metabolism/Transport Effects Substrate of CYP3A4 (major), P-glycoprotein; **Note:** Assignment of Major/Minor substrate status based on clinically relevant drug interaction potential

Avoid Concomitant Use

Avoid concomitant use of Apremilast with any of the following: CYP3A4 Inducers (Strong)

Increased Effect/Toxicity

Apremilast may increase the levels/effects of: Riociguat

Decreased Effect

The levels/effects of Apremilast may be decreased by: Bosentan; CYP3A4 Inducers (Moderate); CYP3A4 Inducers (Strong); Dabrafenib; Deferasirox; Siltuximab; St Johns Wort; Tocilizumab

Storage/Stability Store below 30°C (86°F).

Mechanism of Action Apremilast inhibits phosphodiesterase 4 (PDE4) specific for cyclic adenosine monophosphate (cAMP) which results in increased intracellular cAMP levels and regulation of numerous inflammatory mediators (eg, decreased expression of nitric oxide synthase, TNF-α, and interleukin [IL]-23, as well as increased IL-10) (Schafer, 2012).

Pharmacodynamics/Kinetics

Absorption: Well absorbed

Distribution: V_d: 87 L

Protein binding: ~68%

Metabolism: Hepatic, primarily via CYP3A4: minor pathways include CYP1A2 and CYP2A6

Bioavailability: ~73%

Half-life elimination: ~6 to 9 hours

Time to peak: ~2.5 hours

Excretion: Urine (58%; 3% unchanged drug); feces (39%; 7% unchanged drug)

Dosage Active psoriatic arthritis or plaque psoriasis (moderate to severe):

Adults: Oral: Initial: 10 mg in the morning. Titrate upward by additional 10 mg per day on days 2 to 5 as follows: Day 2: 10 mg twice daily; Day 3: 10 mg in the morning and 20 mg in the evening; Day 4: 20 mg twice daily; Day 5: 20 mg in the morning and 30 mg in the evening. Maintenance dose: 30 mg twice daily starting on day 6

Elderly: Refer to adult dosing

Dosage adjustment for renal impairment: CrCl <30 mL/minute: Initial: 10 mg in the morning on days 1 to 3; titrate using morning doses only (skip evening doses) to 20 mg on days 4 and 5. Maintenance dose: 30 mg once daily in the morning starting on day 6.

Dosage adjustment for hepatic impairment: No dosage adjustment necessary.

Administration Oral: Administer without regard to food. Do not crush, chew, or split tablets.

Monitoring Parameters Monitor weight regularly during therapy; renal function; signs or symptoms of mood changes, depression, or suicidal thoughts

Dosage Forms

Tablet, Oral:

Otezla: 30 mg

Tablet Therapy Pack, Oral:

Otezla: 10 & 20 & 30 mg (27 ea)

Aprepitant (ap RE pi tant)

Brand Names: U.S. Emend

Brand Names: Canada Emend

Index Terms L 754030; MK 869

Pharmacologic Category Antiemetic; Substance P/Neurokinin 1 Receptor Antagonist

Use

Chemotherapy-induced nausea and vomiting: Prevention of acute and delayed nausea and vomiting associated with moderately- and highly-emetogenic chemotherapy (in combination with other antiemetics).

Postoperative nausea and vomiting: Prevention of postoperative nausea and vomiting (PONV).

Pregnancy Risk Factor B

Pregnancy Considerations Adverse events were not observed in animal reproduction studies. Use during pregnancy only if clearly needed. Efficacy of hormonal contraceptive may be reduced; alternative or additional methods of contraception should be used both during treatment with fosaprepitant or aprepitant and for at least 1 month following the last fosaprepitant/aprepitant dose.

Breast-Feeding Considerations It is not known if aprepitant is excreted in breast milk. Due to the potential for adverse reactions in the nursing infant, the decision to discontinue aprepitant or to discontinue breast-feeding should take into account the benefits of treatment to the mother.

Contraindications Hypersensitivity to aprepitant or any component of the formulation; concurrent use with cisapride or pimozide

Warnings/Precautions Potentially significant drug-drug interactions may exist, requiring dose or frequency adjustment, additional monitoring, and/or selection of alternative therapy. Use caution with severe hepatic impairment (Child-Pugh class C); has not been studied. Not studied for treatment of existing nausea and vomiting. Chronic continuous administration is not recommended.

Adverse Reactions Note: Adverse reactions reported as part of a combination chemotherapy regimen or with general anesthesia.

Cardiovascular: Bradycardia, hypotension

Central nervous system: Dizziness, fatigue

Endocrine & metabolic: Dehydration

Gastrointestinal: Abdominal pain, constipation, diarrhea, dyspepsia, epigastric distress, gastritis, hiccups, nausea, stomatitis

Genitourinary Proteinuria

Hepatic: Increased serum ALT, increased serum AST

Neuromuscular & skeletal: Weakness

Renal: Increased blood urea nitrogen

Rare but important or life-threatening: Acid regurgitation, acne vulgaris, anaphylaxis, anemia, angioedema, anxiety, arthralgia, back pain, candidiasis, confusion, conjunctivitis, cough, decreased appetite, decreased serum albumin, decreased visual acuity, deep vein thrombosis, depression, diabetes mellitus, diaphoresis, disorientation, dysarthria, dysgeusia, dysphagia, dyspnea, dysuria, edema, enterocolitis, eructation, erythrocyturia, febrile neutropenia, flatulence, flushing, glycosuria, herpes simplex infection, hyperglycemia, hypersensitivity reaction, hypertension, hypoesthesia, hypokalemia, hyponatremia, hypothermia, hypovolemia, hypoxia, increased serum alkaline phosphatase, increased serum bilirubin, leukocytosis, leukocyturia, malaise, miosis, musculoskeletal pain, myalgia, myasthenia, myocardial infarction, neutropenic sepsis, obstipation, pain, palpitations, pelvic pain, perforated duodenal ulcer, peripheral neuropathy, peripheral sensory neuropathy, pharyngitis, pharyngolaryngeal pain, pneumonia, pneumonitis, pruritus, pulmonary embolism, renal insufficiency, respiratory insufficiency, respiratory tract infection, rhinorrhea, rigors, sensory disturbance, septic shock, sialorrhea, skin rash, Stevens-Johnson syndrome, syncope, tachycardia, thrombocytopenia, toxic epidermal necrolysis, tremor, urinary tract infection, urticaria, voice disorder, weight loss, wheezing, xerostomia

Drug Interactions

Metabolism/Transport Effects Substrate of CYP1A2 (minor), CYP2C19 (minor), CYP3A4 (major); **Note:** Assignment of Major/Minor substrate status based on clinically relevant drug interaction potential; **Inhibits** CYP2C19 (weak), CYP2C9 (weak), CYP3A4 (moderate); **Induces** CYP2C9 (strong), CYP3A4 (weak)

Avoid Concomitant Use

Avoid concomitant use of Aprepitant with any of the following: Bosutinib; Cisapride; Conivaptan; Fusidic Acid (Systemic); Ibrutinib; Idelalisib; Ivabradine; Lomitapide; Naloxegol; Olaparib; Pimozide; Simeprevir; Tolvaptan; Trabectedin; Ulipristal

Increased Effect/Toxicity

Aprepitant may increase the levels/effects of: Avanafil; Bosentan; Bosutinib; Budesonide (Systemic, Oral Inhalation); Cannabis; Cisapride; Colchicine; Corticosteroids (Systemic); CYP3A4 Substrates; Dapoxetine; Diltiazem; Dofetilide; DOXOrubicin (Conventional); Dronabinol; Eliglustat; Eplerenone; Everolimus; FentaNYL; Halofantrine; Hydrocodone; Ibrutinib; Ifosfamide; Imatinib; Ivabradine; Ivacaftor; Lomitapide; Lurasidone; Naloxegol; Olaparib; OxyCODONE; Pimecrolimus; Pimozide; Propafenone; Ranolazine; Rivaroxaban; Salmeterol; Saxagliptin; Simeprevir; Sirolimus; Suvorexant; Tetrahydrocannabinol; Tolvaptan; Trabectedin; Ulipristal; Vilazodone; Zopiclone; Zuclopenthixol

The levels/effects of Aprepitant may be increased by: Ceritinib; Conivaptan; CYP3A4 Inhibitors (Moderate); CYP3A4 Inhibitors (Strong); Dasatinib; Diltiazem; Fosaprepitant; Fusidic Acid (Systemic); Idelalisib; Luliconazole; Mifepristone; Netupitant; Stiripentol

Decreased Effect

Aprepitant may decrease the levels/effects of: ARIPiprazole; Contraceptives (Estrogens); Contraceptives (Progestins); CYP2C9 Substrates; Diclofenac (Systemic); Hydrocodone; PARoxetine; Saxagliptin; TOLBUTamide; Warfarin

The levels/effects of Aprepitant may be decreased by: Bosentan; CYP3A4 Inducers (Moderate); CYP3A4 Inducers (Strong); Dabrafenib; Deferasirox; Mitotane; PARoxetine; Rifampin; Siltuximab; St Johns Wort; Tocilizumab

Food Interactions Aprepitant serum concentration may be increased when taken with grapefruit juice. Management: Avoid concurrent use.

Storage/Stability Store at room temperature of 20°C to 25°C (68°F to 77°F).

Mechanism of Action Prevents acute and delayed vomiting by inhibiting the substance P/neurokinin 1 (NK_1) receptor; augments the antiemetic activity of 5-HT_3 receptor antagonists and corticosteroids to inhibit acute and delayed phases of chemotherapy-induced emesis.

Pharmacodynamics/Kinetics

Distribution: V_d: ~70 L; crosses the blood-brain barrier

Protein binding: >95%

Metabolism: Extensively hepatic via CYP3A4 (major); CYP1A2 and CYP2C19 (minor); forms 7 metabolites (weakly active)

Bioavailability: ~60% to 65%

Half-life elimination: Terminal: ~9 to 13 hours

Time to peak, plasma: ~3 to 4 hours

Dosage

Prevention of chemotherapy-induced nausea/vomiting:

Manufacturer labeling:

Prevention of nausea/vomiting associated with highly-emetogenic chemotherapy: Adults: Oral: 125 mg 1 hour prior to chemotherapy on day 1, followed by 80 mg once daily on days 2 and 3 (in combination with a 5-HT_3 antagonist antiemetic on day 1 and dexamethasone on days 1 to 4)

Prevention of nausea/vomiting associated with moderately-emetogenic chemotherapy: Adults: Oral: 125 mg 1 hour prior to chemotherapy on day 1, followed by 80 mg once daily on days 2 and 3 (in combination with a 5-HT_3 antagonist antiemetic and dexamethasone on day 1)

Pediatric guideline recommendations: Prevention of nausea/vomiting associated with highly-emetogenic chemotherapy (off-label use): Children ≥12 years and Adolescents: Oral:

Pediatric Oncology Group of Ontario (POGO; Dupuis, 2013): 125 mg prior to chemotherapy on day 1, followed by 80 mg once daily on days 2 and 3. The antiemetic regimen also includes a 5-HT_3 antagonist and dexamethasone.

Adult guideline recommendations: Prevention of nausea/vomiting associated with highly-emetogenic chemotherapy (including anthracycline and cyclophosphamide [AC] regimens): Adults: Oral:

American Society of Clinical Oncology (ASCO; Basch, 2011): 125 mg prior to chemotherapy on day 1, followed by 80 mg once daily on days 2 and 3 (in combination with a 5-HT_3 antagonist antiemetic on day 1 and dexamethasone on days 1 to 4 or days 1 to 3)

Multinational Association of Supportive Care in Cancer (MASCC) and European Society of Medical Oncology (ESMO) (Roila, 2010): 125 mg prior to chemotherapy on day 1, followed by 80 mg once daily on days 2 and 3 (in combination with a 5-HT_3 antagonist antiemetic on day 1 and dexamethasone on days 1 to 4 **or** day 1 only [AC regimen])

Prevention of postoperative nausea/vomiting (PONV): Adults: Oral: 40 mg within 3 hours prior to induction

Dosage adjustment in renal impairment: No dosage adjustment necessary.

ESRD undergoing dialysis: No dosage adjustment necessary.

Dosage adjustment in hepatic impairment:

Mild-to-moderate impairment (Child-Pugh class A or B): No dosage adjustment necessary.

Severe impairment (Child-Pugh class C): Use with caution; no data available.

Dietary Considerations May be taken with or without food.

Administration

Chemotherapy-induced nausea/vomiting: Administer with or without food. First dose should be given 1 hour prior to antineoplastic therapy; subsequent doses should be given in the morning.

PONV: Administer within 3 hours prior to induction; follow health care provider instructions about food/drink restrictions prior to surgery.

Dosage Forms

Capsule, Oral:

Emend: 40 mg, 80 mg, 125 mg, 80 mg & 125 mg

Extemporaneous Preparations A 20 mg/mL oral aprepitant suspension may be prepared with capsules and a 1:1 combination of Ora-Sweet® and Ora-Plus® (or Ora-Blend®). Empty the contents of four 125 mg capsules into a mortar and reduce to a fine powder (process will take 10-15 minutes). Add small portions of vehicle and mix to a uniform paste. Add sufficient vehicle to form a liquid; transfer to a graduated cylinder, rinse mortar with vehicle, and add quantity of vehicle sufficient to make 25 mL. Label "shake well" and "refrigerate". Stable for 90 days refrigerated.

Dupuis LL, Lingertat-Walsh K, and Walker SE, "Stability of an Extemporaneous Oral Liquid Aprepitant Formulation," *Support Care Cancer*, 2009, 17(6):701-6.

- **Aprepitant Injection** *see* Fosaprepitant *on page 929*
- **Apresoline** *see* HydrALAZINE *on page 1007*
- **Apri** *see* Ethinyl Estradiol and Desogestrel *on page 799*
- **Apriso** *see* Mesalamine *on page 1301*
- **Aprodine [OTC]** *see* Triprolidine and Pseudoephedrine *on page 2105*

Aprotinin (a proe TYE nin)

Brand Names: U.S. Trasylol [DSC]
Brand Names: Canada Trasylol
Pharmacologic Category Blood Product Derivative; Hemostatic Agent
Use Prevention of perioperative blood loss in patients who are at increased risk for blood loss and blood transfusions in association with cardiopulmonary bypass in coronary artery bypass graft (CABG) surgery

Note: Aprotinin has been withdrawn from the worldwide market due to evidence demonstrating an increased risk of renal dysfunction, myocardial infarction, and mortality in patients undergoing cardiac surgery (Canada has lifted this suspension); use limited to investigational use in the U.S. only according to a special treatment protocol allowing for treatment in select patients at increased risk of blood loss and transfusion during CABG surgery when alternative therapies are unacceptable.

Pregnancy Risk Factor B
Dosage Adults: Test dose: **All** patients should receive a 1 mL (1.4 mg) IV test dose at least 10 minutes prior to the loading dose to assess the potential for allergic reactions.

Notes:

The loading dose should be given after induction of anesthesia but prior to sternotomy. In patients with previous exposure to aprotinin, administer loading dose just prior to cannulation. A constant infusion is continued until surgery is complete.

To avoid physical incompatibility with heparin when adding to pump-prime solution, each agent should be added during recirculation to assure adequate dilution.

Regimen A (standard dose):

2 million KIU (280 mg; 200 mL) loading dose IV over 20-30 minutes
2 million KIU (280 mg; 200 mL) into pump prime volume
500,000 KIU/hour (70 mg/hour; 50 mL/hour) IV during operation

Regimen B (low dose):

1 million KIU (140 mg; 100 mL) loading dose IV over 20-30 minutes
1 million KIU (140 mg; 100 mL) into pump prime volume
250,000 KIU/hour (35 mg/hour; 25 mL/hour) IV during operation

Dosage adjustment in renal impairment: No adjustment required, but increased risk of worsening renal dysfunction with use; monitor closely

Dosage adjustment in hepatic impairment: No information available

Additional Information Complete prescribing information should be consulted for additional detail.

- **Aptivus** *see* Tipranavir *on page 2047*
- **Aquacort® (Can)** *see* Hydrocortisone (Topical) *on page 1014*
- **AquaMEPHYTON® (Can)** *see* Phytonadione *on page 1647*
- **Aquanil HC [OTC]** *see* Hydrocortisone (Topical) *on page 1014*
- **Aquaphilic/Carbamide [OTC]** *see* Urea *on page 2114*
- **Aquasol A** *see* Vitamin A *on page 2173*
- **Aquasol E [OTC]** *see* Vitamin E *on page 2174*
- **Aquavit-E [OTC]** *see* Vitamin E *on page 2174*
- **Aqueous Procaine Penicillin G** *see* Penicillin G Procaine *on page 1613*
- **Aqueous Selenium [OTC]** *see* Selenium *on page 1876*
- **Aqueous Vitamin E [OTC]** *see* Vitamin E *on page 2174*
- **Ara-C** *see* Cytarabine (Conventional) *on page 535*
- **Arabinosylcytosine** *see* Cytarabine (Conventional) *on page 535*
- **Aralen** *see* Chloroquine *on page 424*
- **Aranelle** *see* Ethinyl Estradiol and Norethindrone *on page 808*
- **Aranesp (Can)** *see* Darbepoetin Alfa *on page 565*
- **Aranesp (Albumin Free)** *see* Darbepoetin Alfa *on page 565*
- **Arava** *see* Leflunomide *on page 1174*
- **Arbinoxa** *see* Carbinoxamine *on page 356*
- **Arcalyst** *see* Rilonacept *on page 1810*
- **Arcapta Neohaler** *see* Indacaterol *on page 1063*
- **Aredia (Can)** *see* Pamidronate *on page 1563*
- **Arestin Microspheres (Can)** *see* Minocycline *on page 1371*

Arformoterol (ar for MOE ter ol)

Brand Names: U.S. Brovana
Index Terms (R,R)-Formoterol L-Tartrate; Arformoterol Tartrate
Pharmacologic Category $Beta_2$-Adrenergic Agonist; $Beta_2$-Adrenergic Agonist, Long-Acting
Use Chronic obstructive pulmonary disease: Long-term maintenance treatment of bronchoconstriction in patients with chronic obstructive pulmonary disease (COPD), including chronic bronchitis and emphysema
Pregnancy Risk Factor C
Dosage COPD: Adults: Nebulization: 15 mcg twice daily; maximum: 30 mcg daily

Dosage adjustment in renal impairment: No dosage adjustment necessary.

Dosage adjustment in hepatic impairment: No dosage adjustment necessary. Use with caution; systemic drug exposure prolonged.

Additional Information Complete prescribing information should be consulted for additional detail.
Dosage Forms

Nebulization Solution, Inhalation:
Brovana: 15 mcg/2 mL (2 mL)

- **Arformoterol Tartrate** *see* Arformoterol *on page 168*

Argatroban (ar GA troh ban)

Pharmacologic Category Anticoagulant; Anticoagulant, Direct Thrombin Inhibitor

Additional Appendix Information

Reversal of Oral Anticoagulants *on page 2235*

Use

Heparin-induced thrombocytopenia: Prophylaxis or treatment of thrombosis in adult patients with heparin-induced thrombocytopenia (HIT)

Percutaneous coronary intervention: As an anticoagulant for percutaneous coronary intervention (PCI) in adult patients who have or are at risk of developing HIT

Pregnancy Risk Factor B

Pregnancy Considerations Adverse events were not observed in animal studies. Information related to argatroban in pregnancy is limited. Use of parenteral direct thrombin inhibitors in pregnancy should be limited to those women who have severe allergic reactions to heparin, including heparin-induced thrombocytopenia, and who cannot receive danaparoid (Guyatt, 2012).

Breast-Feeding Considerations It is not known if argatroban is excreted in human milk. Because of the serious potential of adverse effects to the nursing infant, a decision to discontinue nursing or discontinue argatroban should be considered.

Contraindications Hypersensitivity to argatroban or any component of the formulation; major bleeding

Warnings/Precautions Hemorrhage can occur at any site in the body. Extreme caution should be used when there is an increased danger of hemorrhage, such as severe hypertension, immediately following lumbar puncture, spinal anesthesia, major surgery (including brain, spinal cord, or eye surgery), congenital or acquired bleeding disorders, and gastrointestinal ulcers. Use caution in critically-ill patients; reduced clearance may require dosage reduction. Use caution with hepatic dysfunction. Argatroban prolongs the PT/INR. Concomitant use with warfarin will cause increased prolongation of the PT and INR greater than that of warfarin alone. If warfarin is initiated concurrently with argatroban, initial PT/INR goals while on argatroban may require modification; alternative guidelines for monitoring therapy should be followed. Safety and efficacy for use with other thrombolytic agents has not been established. Discontinue all parenteral anticoagulants prior to starting therapy. Allow reversal of heparin's effects before initiation. Patients with hepatic dysfunction may require >4 hours to achieve full reversal of argatroban's anticoagulant effect following treatment. Avoid use during PCI in patients with clinically significant hepatic disease or elevations of ALT/AST (≥3 times ULN); use in these patients has not been evaluated. Limited pharmacokinetic and dosing information is available from use in critically-ill children with heparin-induced thrombocytopenia (HIT).

Adverse Reactions As with all anticoagulants, bleeding is the major adverse effect of argatroban. Hemorrhage may occur at virtually any site. Risk is dependent on multiple variables, including the intensity of anticoagulation and patient susceptibility.

Cardiovascular: Angina pectoris, bradycardia, cardiac arrest, chest pain (PCI related), coronary occlusion, hypotension, ischemic heart disease, myocardial infarction (PCI), thrombosis, vasodilation, ventricular tachycardia

Central nervous system: Headache, intracranial hemorrhage, pain

Dermatologic: Dermatological reaction (bullous eruption, rash)

Gastrointestinal: Abdominal pain, diarrhea, gastrointestinal hemorrhage, nausea, vomiting

Genitourinary: Genitourinary tract hemorrhage (including hematuria)

Hematologic & oncologic: Brachial bleeding, decreased hematocrit, decreased hemoglobin, groin bleeding, minor hemorrhage (CABG related)

Neuromuscular & skeletal: Back pain (PCI related)

Respiratory: Cough, dyspnea, hemoptysis

Miscellaneous: Fever

Rare but important or life-threatening: Aortic valve stenosis, bleeding at injection site (or access site; minor), hypersensitivity reaction, local hemorrhage (limb and below-the-knee stump), pulmonary edema, retroperitoneal bleeding

Drug Interactions

Metabolism/Transport Effects None known.

Avoid Concomitant Use

Avoid concomitant use of Argatroban with any of the following: Apixaban; Dabigatran Etexilate; Edoxaban; Omacetaxine; Rivaroxaban; Urokinase; Vorapaxar

Increased Effect/Toxicity

Argatroban may increase the levels/effects of: Anticoagulants; Collagenase (Systemic); Deferasirox; Ibritumomab; Nintedanib; Obinutuzumab; Omacetaxine; Rivaroxaban; Tositumomab and Iodine I 131 Tositumomab

The levels/effects of Argatroban may be increased by: Agents with Antiplatelet Properties; Apixaban; Dabigatran Etexilate; Dasatinib; Edoxaban; Herbs (Anticoagulant/Antiplatelet Properties); Ibrutinib; Limaprost; Nonsteroidal Anti-Inflammatory Agents; Omega-3 Fatty Acids; Pentosan Polysulfate Sodium; Prostacyclin Analogues; Salicylates; Sugammadex; Thrombolytic Agents; Tibolone; Tipranavir; Urokinase; Vitamin E; Vorapaxar

Decreased Effect

The levels/effects of Argatroban may be decreased by: Estrogen Derivatives; Progestins

Preparation for Administration

Vials for injection, 2.5 mL (100 mg/mL) concentrate: Prior to administration, each vial must be diluted to a final concentration of 1 mg/mL. Solution may be mixed with sodium chloride 0.9% injection, dextrose 5% injection, or lactated Ringer's injection. Do not mix with other medications prior to dilution. To prepare solution for IV administration, dilute each 250 mg vial with 250 mL of diluent or dilute 500 mg per 500 mL of diluent. Mix by repeated inversion for 1 minute. A slight but brief haziness may occur upon mixing; use of diluent at room temperature is recommended.

Premixed vials for infusion, 50 mL or 125 mL (1 mg/mL): No further dilution is required.

Storage/Stability

Vials for injection, 2.5 mL (100 mg/mL) concentrate: Prior to use, store vial in original carton at 25°C (77°F); excursions permitted to 15°C to 30°C (59°F to 86°F). Do not freeze. Retain in the original carton to protect from light. The diluted, prepared solution is stable for 24 hours at 20°C to 25°C (68°F to 77°F) in ambient indoor light. Do not expose to direct sunlight. Prepared solutions that are protected from light and kept at 20°C to 25°C (68°F to 77°F) or under refrigeration at 2°C to 8°C (36°F to 46°F) are stable for up to 96 hours.

Premixed vials for infusion, 50 mL or 125 mL (1 mg/mL): Store at controlled room temperature of 20°C to 25°C (68°F to 77°F). Keep in original container to protect from light.

Mechanism of Action A direct, highly-selective thrombin inhibitor. Reversibly binds to the active thrombin site of free and clot-associated thrombin. Inhibits fibrin formation; activation of coagulation factors V, VIII, and XIII; activation of protein C; and platelet aggregation.

Pharmacodynamics/Kinetics

Onset of action: Immediate

Distribution: 174 mL/kg

Protein binding: Albumin: 20%; alpha$_1$-acid glycoprotein: 35%

Metabolism: Hepatic via hydroxylation and aromatization (major route). Metabolism via CYP3A4/5 (minor route) to four known metabolites. Unchanged argatroban is the major plasma component. Plasma concentration of metabolite M1 is 0% to 20% of the parent drug and is three- to five-fold weaker.

Half-life elimination: 39-51 minutes; Hepatic impairment: ≤181 minutes

Time to peak: Steady-state: 1-3 hours

Excretion: Feces (65%); urine (22%); low quantities of metabolites M2-4 in urine

Clearance is decreased in critically-ill pediatric patients

Dosage IV:

Children: **Heparin-induced thrombocytopenia (HIT)** (dosing based on limited data from critically-ill patients):

Initial dose: 0.75 mcg/kg/minute

Maintenance dose: Patient may not be at steady-state but measure aPTT after 2 hours; adjust dose until the steady-state aPTT is 1.5 to 3 times the initial baseline value, not exceeding 100 seconds; dosage may be adjusted in increments of 0.1 to 0.25 mcg/kg/minute. **Note:** Frequent dosage adjustments may be required to maintain desired anticoagulant activity.

Adults:

Heparin-induced thrombocytopenia (HIT):

Initial dose: 2 mcg/kg/minute

Obesity: Pharmacokinetics and pharmacodynamics have not been evaluated prospectively in obese patients; however, retrospective data suggest using actual body weight to dose and that adjustment of initial dose is unnecessary in obesity (BMI up to 51 kg/m^2) (Rice, 2007).

Maintenance dose: Patient may not be at steady-state but measure aPTT after 2 hours; adjust dose until the steady-state aPTT is 1.5 to 3 times the initial baseline value, not exceeding 100 seconds; dosage should not exceed 10 mcg/kg/minute

Note: Critically-ill patients with normal hepatic function have become excessively anticoagulated with FDA-approved or lower starting doses of argatroban. Doses between 0.15 to 1.3 mcg/kg/minute were required to maintain aPTTs in the target range (Reichert, 2003). In a prospective observational study of critically-ill patients with multiple organ dysfunction (MODS) and suspected or proven HIT, an initial infusion dose of 0.2 mcg/kg/minute was found to be sufficient and safe in this population (Beiderlinden, 2007). Consider reducing starting dose to 0.2 mcg/kg/minute in critically-ill patients with MODS defined as a minimum number of two organ failures. Another report of a cardiac patient with anasarca secondary to acute renal failure had a reduction in argatroban clearance similar to patients with hepatic dysfunction. Reduced clearance may have been due to reduced liver perfusion (de Denus, 2003). The American College of Chest Physicians has recommended an initial infusion rate of 0.5 to 1.2 mcg/kg/minute for patients with heart failure, MODS, severe anasarca, or postcardiac surgery (Linkins, 2012).

Conversion to oral anticoagulant: Because there may be a combined effect on the INR when argatroban is combined with warfarin, loading doses of warfarin should not be used. Warfarin therapy should be started at the expected daily dose.

Patients receiving ≤2 mcg/kg/minute of argatroban: Argatroban therapy can be stopped when the INR is >4 on combined warfarin and argatroban therapy; repeat INR measurement in 4 to 6 hours; if INR is below therapeutic level, argatroban therapy may be restarted. Repeat procedure daily until desired INR on warfarin alone is obtained.

Patients receiving >2 mcg/kg/minute of argatroban: In order to predict the INR on warfarin alone, reduce dose of argatroban to 2 mcg/kg/minute; measure INR for argatroban and warfarin 4 to 6 hours after dose reduction; argatroban therapy can be stopped when the INR on warfarin and argatroban combined therapy is >4. Repeat INR measurement in 4 to 6 hours; if INR is below therapeutic level, argatroban therapy may be restarted. Repeat procedure daily until desired INR on warfarin alone is obtained.

Note: The American College of Chest Physicians suggests monitoring chromogenic factor X assay when transitioning from argatroban to warfarin (Garcia, 2012) or overlapping administration of warfarin for a minimum of 5 days until INR is within target range; recheck INR after anticoagulant effect of argatroban has dissipated (Guyatt, 2012). Factor X levels <45% have been associated with INR values >2 after the effects of argatroban have been eliminated (Arpino, 2005).

Prefilter administration for continuous renal replacement therapy (CRRT) in critically-ill patients with HIT (off-label use; Link, 2009): 0.1 to 1.5 mcg/kg/minute. **Note:** Loading dose of 100 mcg/kg was administered during clinical trial; however, this may be unnecessary.

Percutaneous coronary intervention (PCI):

Initial: Begin infusion of 25 mcg/kg/minute and administer bolus dose of 350 mcg/kg (over 3 to 5 minutes). ACT should be checked 5 to 10 minutes after bolus infusion; proceed with procedure if ACT >300 seconds.

Obesity: Pharmacokinetics and pharmacodynamics have not been evaluated prospectively in obese patients; however, retrospective data suggest using actual body weight to dose and that adjustment of initial dose is unnecessary in obesity (BMI up to 51 kg/m^2) (Hursting, 2008).

Following initial bolus:

ACT <300 seconds: Give an additional 150 mcg/kg bolus, and increase infusion rate to 30 mcg/kg/minute (recheck ACT in 5 to 10 minutes)

ACT >450 seconds: Decrease infusion rate to 15 mcg/kg/minute (recheck ACT in 5 to 10 minutes)

Once a therapeutic ACT (300 to 450 seconds) is achieved, infusion should be continued at this dose for the duration of the procedure.

If dissection, impending abrupt closure, thrombus formation during PCI, or inability to achieve ACT >300 seconds: An additional bolus of 150 mcg/kg, followed by an increase in infusion rate to 40 mcg/kg/minute may be administered.

Note: Post-PCI anticoagulation, if required, may be achieved by continuing infusion at a reduced dose of 2 mcg/kg/minute with close monitoring of aPTT; adjust infusion rate as needed.

Elderly: No initial dose adjustment is necessary for elderly patients with normal liver function

Dosage adjustment in renal impairment: Removal during hemodialysis and continuous venovenous hemofiltration is clinically insignificant (Tang, 2005). No dosage adjustment necessary.

Dosage adjustment in hepatic impairment: Decreased clearance and increased elimination half-life are seen with hepatic impairment; dose reduction and careful titration are required.

Children: Initial dose: 0.2 mcg/kg/minute; adjust dose in increments of ≤0.05 mcg/kg/minute

Adults: Per manufacturer labeling, the initial dose for moderate-to-severe hepatic impairment (Child-Pugh classes B and C) is 0.5 mcg/kg/minute; monitor aPTT closely and adjust dose as necessary. However, patients with severe hepatic impairment (Child-Pugh class C) may require further reduction of the initial dose.

One case report describes a dose of 0.05 mcg/kg/minute required to maintain a stable, therapeutic aPTT in a patient with severe hepatic impairment (Yarbrough, 2012). **Note:** During PCI, avoid use in patients with elevations of ALT/AST (≥3 times ULN); the use of argatroban in these patients has not been evaluated.

Usual Infusion Concentrations: Pediatric Note: Premixed solutions available.

IV infusion: 1000 **mcg**/mL

Usual Infusion Concentrations: Adult Note: Premixed solutions available.

IV infusion: 250 mg in 250 mL (concentration: 1000 **mcg**/mL) in D_5W or NS

Administration The 2.5 mL (100 mg/mL) **concentrated** vial **must be diluted to 1 mg/mL** prior to administration. The premixed 50 mL or 125 mL (1 mg/mL) vial requires no further dilution. The premixed 1 mg/mL vial may be inverted for use with an infusion set.

Administer bolus dose over 3 to 5 minutes through a large bore intravenous line.

Monitoring Parameters Monitor hemoglobin, hematocrit, signs and symptoms of bleeding.

HIT: Obtain baseline aPTT prior to start of therapy. Patient may not be at steady-state but check aPTT 2 hours after start of therapy to adjust dose, keeping the steady-state aPTT 1.5 to 3 times the initial baseline value (not exceeding 100 seconds).

PCI: Monitor ACT before dosing, 5 to 10 minutes after bolus dosing, and after any change in infusion rate and at the end of the procedure. Additional ACT assessments should be made every 20 to 30 minutes during extended PCI procedures.

Additional Information Platelet counts recovered by day 3 in 53% of patients with heparin-induced thrombocytopenia and in 58% of patients with heparin-induced thrombocytopenia with thrombosis syndrome.

Dosage Forms

Solution, Intravenous:

Generic: 125 mg/125 mL (125 mL); 100 mg/mL (2.5 mL)

Solution, Intravenous [preservative free]:

Generic: 50 mg/50 mL (50 mL)

Arginine (AR ji neen)

Brand Names: U.S. R-Gene 10

Index Terms Arginine HCl; Arginine Hydrochloride; L-Arginine; L-Arginine Hydrochloride

Pharmacologic Category Diagnostic Agent

Use Pituitary function test (growth hormone)

Pregnancy Risk Factor B

Dosage IV: Pituitary function test:

Children: 0.5 g/kg/dose administered over 30 minutes

Adults: 30 g (300 mL) administered over 30 minutes

Additional Information Complete prescribing information should be consulted for additional detail.

Dosage Forms

Solution, Intravenous [preservative free]:

R-Gene 10: 10% (300 mL)

◆ **Arginine HCl** *see* Arginine *on page* *171*

◆ **Arginine Hydrochloride** *see* Arginine *on page* *171*

◆ **8-Arginine Vasopressin** *see* Vasopressin *on page* *2142*

◆ **Aricept** *see* Donepezil *on page* *668*

◆ **Aricept ODT** *see* Donepezil *on page* *668*

◆ **Aricept RDT (Can)** *see* Donepezil *on page* *668*

◆ **Aridol** *see* Mannitol *on page* *1269*

◆ **Arimidex** *see* Anastrozole *on page* *148*

ARIPiprazole (ay ri PIP ray zole)

Brand Names: U.S. Abilify; Abilify Discmelt; Abilify Maintena

Brand Names: Canada Abilify; Abilify Maintena

Index Terms BMS 337039; OPC-14597

Pharmacologic Category Second Generation (Atypical) Antipsychotic

Additional Appendix Information

Beers Criteria – Potentially Inappropriate Medications for Geriatrics *on page 2271*

Use

Oral:

Bipolar I disorder: Acute treatment of manic and mixed episodes associated with bipolar I disorder.

Irritability associated with autistic disorder: Treatment of irritability associated with autistic disorder.

Major depressive disorder: Adjunctive treatment of major depressive disorder.

Schizophrenia: Treatment of schizophrenia.

Tourette disorder: Treatment of Tourette disorder.

Injection:

Agitation associated with schizophrenia or bipolar mania (immediate-release injection only): Treatment of agitation associated with schizophrenia or bipolar mania.

Schizophrenia (extended-release injection only): Treatment of schizophrenia.

Pregnancy Risk Factor C

Pregnancy Considerations Adverse events were observed in animal reproduction studies. Aripiprazole crosses the placenta; aripiprazole and dehydro-aripiprazole can be detected in the cord blood at delivery (Nguyen, 2011; Wantanabe, 2011). Antipsychotic use during the third trimester of pregnancy has a risk for abnormal muscle movements (extrapyramidal symptoms [EPS]) and/or withdrawal symptoms in newborns following delivery. Symptoms in the newborn may include agitation, feeding disorder, hypertonia, hypotonia, respiratory distress, somnolence, and tremor; these effects may be self-limiting or require hospitalization.

Treatment algorithms have been developed by the ACOG and the APA for the management of depression in women prior to conception and during pregnancy (Yonkers, 2009). The ACOG recommends that therapy during pregnancy be individualized; treatment with psychiatric medications during pregnancy should incorporate the clinical expertise of the mental health clinician, obstetrician, primary healthcare provider, and pediatrician. Safety data related to atypical antipsychotics during pregnancy is limited and routine use is not recommended. However, if a woman is inadvertently exposed to an atypical antipsychotic while pregnant, continuing therapy may be preferable to switching to a typical antipsychotic that the fetus has not yet been exposed to; consider risk:benefit (ACOG, 2008).

Healthcare providers are encouraged to enroll women exposed to aripiprazole during pregnancy in the National Pregnancy Registry for Atypical Antipsychotics (866-961-2388 or http://www.womensmentalhealth.org/clinical-and-research-programs/pregnancyregistry/).

Breast-Feeding Considerations Aripiprazole is excreted in breast milk (Schlotterbeck, 2007; Watanabe, 2011). In one case report, milk concentrations were ~20% of the maternal plasma concentration (maternal dose: 15 mg/day; ~6 months postpartum) (Schlotterbeck, 2007); however, aripiprazole was not detected in the breast milk in a second case (limit of detection 10 ng/mL; maternal dose: 15 mg/day; ~1 month postpartum) (Lutz, 2010). Aripiprazole was also detected in the neonatal blood 6 days after delivery in a breast-fed infant also exposed during pregnancy. In this case report, the authors suggest *in utero* exposure could have contributed to the findings due to the long elimination half-life of aripiprazole (Watanabe, 2011). In one report, lactation was not able to be established, possibly due to changes in maternal prolactin potentially caused by aripiprazole (Mendhekar, 2006). The manufacturer recommends a decision be made whether to discontinue nursing or to discontinue the drug, taking into account the importance of treatment to the mother.

Contraindications Hypersensitivity (eg, anaphylaxis, pruritus, urticaria) to aripiprazole or any component of the formulation.

Warnings/Precautions [U.S. Boxed Warning]: Elderly patients with dementia-related psychosis treated with antipsychotics are at an increased risk of death compared to placebo. Most deaths appeared to be either cardiovascular (eg, heart failure, sudden death) or infectious (eg, pneumonia) in nature. In addition, an increased incidence of cerebrovascular effects (eg, transient ischemic attack, cerebrovascular accidents) has been reported in studies of placebo-controlled trials of aripiprazole in elderly patients with dementia-related psychosis. **Aripiprazole is not approved for the treatment of dementia-related psychosis.**

[U.S. Boxed Warning]: Antidepressants increase the risk of suicidal thinking and behavior in children, adolescents, and young adults (18 to 24 years of age) with major depressive disorder (MDD) and other psychiatric disorders; consider risk prior to prescribing. The possibility of a suicide attempt is inherent in major depression and may persist until remission occurs. Patients treated with antidepressants should be observed for clinical worsening and suicidality, especially during the initial few months of a course of drug therapy, or at times of dose changes, either increases or decreases. Prescriptions should be written for the smallest quantity consistent with good patient care. The patient's family or caregiver should be alerted to monitor patients for the emergence of suicidality and associated behaviors; patients should be instructed to notify their healthcare provider if any of these symptoms or worsening depression or psychosis occur.

Leukopenia, neutropenia, and agranulocytosis (sometimes fatal) have been reported in clinical trials and postmarketing reports with antipsychotic use; presence of risk factors (eg, preexisting low WBC/ANC or history of drug-induced leuko-/neutropenia) should prompt periodic blood count assessment. Discontinue therapy at first signs of blood dyscrasias or if absolute neutrophil count <1,000/mm^3.

A medication guide concerning the use of antidepressants should be dispensed with each prescription. Aripiprazole is not FDA approved for adjunctive treatment of depression in children.

May cause extrapyramidal symptoms (EPS), including pseudoparkinsonism, acute dystonic reactions, akathisia, and tardive dyskinesia (risk of these reactions is very low relative to typical/conventional antipsychotics, frequencies reported are similar to placebo). Risk of dystonia (and probably other EPS) may be greater with increased doses, use of conventional antipsychotics, males, and younger patients. May be associated with neuroleptic malignant syndrome (NMS).

May cause CNS depression, which may impair physical or mental abilities; patients must be cautioned about performing tasks that require mental alertness (eg, operating machinery, driving). May cause orthostatic hypotension (although reported rates are similar to placebo); use caution in patients at risk of this effect or those who would not tolerate transient hypotensive episodes (cerebrovascular disease, cardiovascular disease, or other medications which may predispose). Use caution in patients with Parkinson disease (Lehman [APA], 2004); predisposition to seizures; and severe cardiac disease. May alter cardiac conduction; life-threatening arrhythmias have occurred with therapeutic doses of antipsychotics. Esophageal dysmotility and aspiration have been associated with antipsychotic use; use caution in patients at risk for aspiration pneumonia (eg, Alzheimer dementia). May alter temperature regulation. Potentially significant interactions may exist, requiring dose or frequency adjustment, additional monitoring, and/or selection of alternative therapy.

Atypical antipsychotics have been associated with metabolic changes including loss of glucose control, lipid changes, and weight gain (risk profile varies with product). Development of hyperglycemia in some cases, may be extreme and associated with ketoacidosis, hyperosmolar coma, or death. Reports of hyperglycemia with aripiprazole therapy have been few and specific risk associated with this agent is not known. Use caution in patients with diabetes or other disorders of glucose regulation; monitor for worsening of glucose control.

Use in elderly patients with dementia-related psychosis is associated with an increased risk of mortality and cerebrovascular accidents; aripiprazole is not approved for the treatment of dementia-related psychosis; avoid antipsychotic use for behavioral problems associated with dementia unless alternative nonpharmacologic therapies have failed and patient may harm self or others. In addition, use may cause or exacerbate syndrome of inappropriate antidiuretic hormone secretion or hyponatremia; monitor sodium closely with initiation or dosage adjustments in older adults (Beers Criteria).

Tablets may contain lactose; avoid use in patients with galactose intolerance or glucose-galactose malabsorption.

Orally disintegrating tablets may contain phenylalanine.

There are two formulations available for intramuscular administration: Abilify is an immediate-release short-acting formulation and Abilify Maintena is an extended-release formulation. These products are **not** interchangeable.

Adverse Reactions

Cardiovascular: Chest pain, hypertension, orthostatic hypotension, peripheral edema, tachycardia

Central nervous system: Agitation, akathisia (dose-related; more common in adults), anxiety, ataxia, cognitive dizziness, drooling (children), drowsiness (more common in children), dysfunction (more common in children), dystonia (children), extrapyramidal reaction (dose-related), fatigue (dose-related; more common in children), headache (more common in adults), hypersomnia (children), insomnia, lethargy (children), nervousness, pain, restlessness, sedation (dose-related; more common in children)

Dermatologic: Skin rash (children)

Endocrine & metabolic: Increased thirst (children), weight gain (≥7% body weight), weight loss

Gastrointestinal: Abdominal distress, constipation (more common in adults), decreased appetite (children), diarrhea (children), dyspepsia, gastric distress, increased appetite (children), nausea, sialorrhea (dose-related), toothache, upper abdominal pain (children), vomiting, xerostomia (more common in adults)

Genitourinary: Dysmenorrhea (children)

Local: Injection site reaction (injection)

Neuromuscular & skeletal: Arthralgia (more common in adults), dyskinesia (children), increased creatine phosphokinase, limb pain, muscle cramps, muscle spasm, myalgia, stiffness (more common in adults), tremor (dose-related), weakness

Ophthalmic: Accommodation disturbance, blurred vision

Respiratory: Aspiration pneumonia, cough, dyspnea, nasal congestion, nasopharyngitis (children), pharyngolaryngeal pain, rhinorrhea (children), upper respiratory tract infection

Miscellaneous: Fever (children)

Rare but important or life-threatening: Abnormal bilirubin levels, agranulocytosis, akinesia, alopecia, amenorrhea, anaphylaxis, angina pectoris, angioedema, anorexia, anorgasmia, atrial fibrillation, atrial flutter, atrioventricular block, bradycardia, cardiorespiratory arrest, catatonia, cerebrovascular accident, choreoathetosis, cogwheel rigidity, delirium, depression, diabetes mellitus, diabetic ketoacidosis, diplopia, disruption of body temperature regulation, edema, erectile dysfunction, esophagitis, extrasystoles, gynecomastia, hepatitis, homicidal ideation, hostility, hyperglycemia, hyperlipidemia, hypersensitivity, hypertonia, hypoglycemia, hypokalemia, hypokinesia, hyponatremia, hypotension, hypothermia, hypotonia, increased blood urea nitrogen, increased creatinine clearance, increased gamma-glutamyl transferase, increased lactate dehydrogenase, increased serum prolactin, intentional injury, ischemic heart disease, jaundice, leukopenia, mastalgia, memory impairment, myocardial infarction, myoclonus, neuroleptic malignant syndrome, neutropenia, nocturia, pancreatitis, Parkinson's disease, priapism, prolonged Q-T interval on ECG, rhabdomyolysis, seizure (including injection), suicidal ideation, suicidal tendencies, supraventricular tachycardia, syncope, tardive dyskinesia, thrombocytopenia, tics, tonic-clonic seizures, uncontrolled diabetes mellitus, urinary retention, ventricular tachycardia

Drug Interactions

Metabolism/Transport Effects **Substrate** of CYP2D6 (major), CYP3A4 (major); **Note:** Assignment of Major/Minor substrate status based on clinically relevant drug interaction potential

Avoid Concomitant Use

Avoid concomitant use of ARIPiprazole with any of the following: Amisulpride; Azelastine (Nasal); Conivaptan; Fusidic Acid (Systemic); Idelalisib; Metoclopramide; Orphenadrine; Paraldehyde; Sulpiride; Thalidomide

Increased Effect/Toxicity

ARIPiprazole may increase the levels/effects of: Alcohol (Ethyl); Amisulpride; Azelastine (Nasal); Buprenorphine; CNS Depressants; DULoxetine; FLUoxetine; Haloperidol; Highest Risk QTc-Prolonging Agents; Hydrocodone; Methadone; Methotrimeprazine; Methylphenidate; Metyrosine; Mirtazapine; Moderate Risk QTc-Prolonging Agents; Orphenadrine; Paraldehyde; PARoxetine; Ritonavir; Selective Serotonin Reuptake Inhibitors; Serotonin Modulators; Sulpiride; Suvorexant; Thalidomide; Zolpidem

The levels/effects of ARIPiprazole may be increased by: Abiraterone Acetate; Acetylcholinesterase Inhibitors (Central); Brimonidine (Topical); Cannabis; Ceritinib; Conivaptan; CYP2D6 Inhibitors (Moderate); CYP2D6 Inhibitors (Strong); CYP2D6 Inhibitors (Weak); CYP3A4 Inhibitors (Moderate); CYP3A4 Inhibitors (Strong); CYP3A4 Inhibitors (Weak); Dasatinib; Doxylamine; Dronabinol; Droperidol; DULoxetine; FLUoxetine; Fusidic Acid (Systemic); Haloperidol; HydrOXYzine; Idelalisib; Ivacaftor; Kava Kava; Lithium; Luliconazole; Magnesium Sulfate; Methadone; Methotrimeprazine; Methylphenidate; Metoclopramide; Metyrosine; Mifepristone; Nabilone; Netupitant; PARoxetine; Peginterferon Alfa-2b; Perampanel; Ritonavir; Serotonin Modulators; Sertraline; Simeprevir; Sodium Oxybate; Stiripentol; Tapentadol; Tetrahydrocannabinol

Decreased Effect

ARIPiprazole may decrease the levels/effects of: Amphetamines; Anti-Parkinson's Agents (Dopamine Agonist); Haloperidol; Quinagolide

The levels/effects of ARIPiprazole may be decreased by: CYP3A4 Inducers; Dabrafenib; Lithium; Mitotane; Peginterferon Alfa-2b; Siltuximab; St Johns Wort; Tocilizumab

Food Interactions Ingestion with a high-fat meal delays time to peak plasma level. Management: Administer without regard to meals.

Preparation for Administration

Injection, powder (extended release):

Prefilled syringe: Rotate the syringe plunger rod to release diluent. Shake vigorously for 20 seconds or until the suspension is uniform; the resulting suspension will be milky white and opaque. (Refer to manufacturer's labeling for full preparation technique.) Inject full syringe contents immediately following reconstitution.

Vial for reconstitution: Reconstitute using 1.5 mL sterile water for injection (SWFI) (provided) for the 300 mg vial or 1.9 mL SWFI (provided) for the 400 mg vial to a final concentration of 200 mg/mL; residual SWFI should be discarded after reconstitution. Shake vigorously for 30 seconds or until the suspension is uniform; the resulting suspension will be milky white and opaque. If the suspension is not administered immediately after reconstitution, shake vigorously for 60 seconds prior to administration.

Storage/Stability

Injection, powder (extended release):

Prefilled syringe: Store below 30°C (86°F). Do not freeze. Protect from light and store in original package.

Vial for reconstitution: Store unused vials at 25°C (77°F); excursions permitted to 15°C to 30°C (59°F to 86°F). If the suspension is not administered immediately after reconstitution, store at room temperature in the vial (do not store in a syringe).

Injection, solution (immediate release): Store at 25°C (77°F); excursions permitted to 15°C to 30°C (59°F to 86°F). Protect from light. Retain in carton until time of use.

Oral solution and tablets: Store at 25°C (77°F); excursions permitted to 15°C to 30°C (59°F to 86°F). Use oral solution within 6 months after opening.

Mechanism of Action Aripiprazole is a quinolinone antipsychotic which exhibits high affinity for D_2, D_3, 5-HT_{1A}, and 5-HT_{2A} receptors; moderate affinity for D_4, 5-HT_{2C}, 5-HT_7, $alpha_1$ adrenergic, and H_1 receptors. It also possesses moderate affinity for the serotonin reuptake transporter; has no affinity for muscarinic (cholinergic) receptors. Aripiprazole functions as a partial agonist at the D_2 and 5-HT_{1A} receptors, and as an antagonist at the 5-HT_{2A} receptor.

Pharmacodynamics/Kinetics

Onset of action: Initial: 1 to 3 weeks

Absorption: Well absorbed

Distribution: V_d: 4.9 L/kg

Protein binding: ≥99%, primarily to albumin

Metabolism: Hepatic, via CYP2D6, CYP3A4 (dehydro-aripiprazole metabolite has affinity for D_2 receptors similar to the parent drug and represents 40% of the parent drug exposure in plasma)

Bioavailability: IM: 100%; Tablet: 87%

Half-life elimination: Aripiprazole: 75 hours; dehydro-aripiprazole: 94 hours; IM, extended release (terminal): ~30 to 47 days (dose-dependent)

CYP2D6 poor metabolizers: Aripiprazole: 146 hours

Time to peak, plasma:

IM:

Immediate release: 1 to 3 hours

Extended release: 5 to 7 days

Tablet: 3 to 5 hours

With high-fat meal: Aripiprazole: Delayed by 3 hours; dehydro-aripiprazole: Delayed by 12 hours

Excretion: Feces (55%, ~18% of the total dose as unchanged drug); urine (25%, <1% of the total dose as unchanged drug)

Dosage Note: Oral solution may be substituted for the oral tablet on a mg-per-mg basis, up to 25 mg. Patients receiving 30 mg tablets should be given 25 mg oral solution. Orally disintegrating tablets (Abilify Discmelt) are bioequivalent to the immediate-release tablets (Abilify).

Acute agitation (schizophrenia/bipolar mania): Adults: IM, immediate release: 9.75 mg as a single dose (range: 5.25 to 15 mg; a lower dose of 5.25 mg IM may be considered when clinical factors warrant); repeated doses may be given at ≥2-hour intervals to a maximum of 30 mg/day. **Note:** If ongoing therapy with aripiprazole is necessary, transition to oral therapy as soon as possible.

Bipolar I disorder (acute manic or mixed episodes):

Children ≥10 years and Adolescents (U.S. labeling): Oral: Initial: 2 mg once daily for 2 days, followed by 5 mg once daily for 2 days with a further increase to target dose of 10 mg once daily as monotherapy or as adjunct to lithium or valproic acid; subsequent dose increases may be made in 5 mg increments, up to a maximum of 30 mg/day.

Adolescents ≥13 years (Canadian labeling): Oral: Initial: 2 mg once daily for 2 days, followed by 5 mg once daily for 2 days with a further increase to target dose of 10 mg once daily as monotherapy; subsequent dose increases may be made in 5 mg increments, up to a maximum of 30 mg/day. **Note:** Not approved for maintenance or as adjunctive therapy.

Adults: Oral:

Monotherapy: Initial: 15 mg once daily. May increase to 30 mg once daily if clinically indicated (maximum: 30 mg/day); safety of doses >30 mg/day has not been evaluated

Adjunct to lithium or valproic acid: Initial: 10 to 15 mg once daily. May increase to 30 mg once daily if clinically indicated (maximum: 30 mg/day); safety of doses >30 mg/day has not been evaluated.

Depression (adjunctive with antidepressants): Adults: Oral: Initial: 2 to 5 mg/day (range: 2 to 15 mg/day); dose adjustments of up to 5 mg/day may be made in intervals of ≥1 week, up to a maximum of 15 mg/day. **Note:** Dosing based on patients already receiving antidepressant therapy.

Irritability associated with autistic disorder: Children ≥6 years and Adolescents: Oral: Initial: 2 mg once daily for 7 days, followed by an increase to 5 mg once daily; subsequent dose increases may be made in 5 mg increments at intervals of ≥1 week, up to a maximum of 15 mg/day. Assess the need for ongoing treatment periodically.

Schizophrenia:

Adolescents ≥13 years (U.S. labeling) or ≥15 years (Canadian labeling): Oral: Initial: 2 mg once daily for 2 days, followed by 5 mg once daily for 2 days with a further increase to target dose of 10 mg once daily; subsequent dose increases may be made in 5 mg increments up to a maximum of 30 mg/day (30 mg/day not shown to be more efficacious than 10 mg/day).

Adults:

Oral: 10 or 15 mg once daily; may be increased to a maximum of 30 mg once daily (efficacy at dosages above 10 to 15 mg has not been shown to be increased). Dosage titration should not be more frequent than every 2 weeks.

IM, extended release: 400 mg once monthly (doses should be separated by ≥26 days); **Note:** Tolerability should be established using oral aripiprazole prior to initiation of parenteral therapy; due to the half-life of oral aripiprazole, it may take up to 2 weeks to fully assess tolerability. Continue oral aripiprazole (or other oral antipsychotic) for 14 days during initiation of parenteral therapy.

Missed doses:

Second or third doses missed:

>4 weeks but <5 weeks since last dose: Administer next dose as soon as possible

>5 weeks since last dose: Administer oral aripiprazole for 14 days with next injection

Fourth or subsequent doses missed:

>4 weeks but <6 weeks since last dose: Administer next dose as soon as possible

>6 weeks since last dose: Administer oral aripiprazole for 14 days with next injection

Dosage adjustment for adverse effects: Consider reducing dose to 300 mg once monthly

Tourette syndrome: Children ≥6 years and Adolescents: Oral:

<50 kg: Initial: 2 mg/day for 2 days then increase to a target dose of 5 mg/day; may increase dose up to a maximum of 10 mg/day based on response and tolerability; dosage adjustments should occur gradually at intervals of no less than 1 week. Assess the need for ongoing treatment periodically.

≥50 kg: Initial: 2 mg/day for 2 days, then increase to 5 mg/day for 5 days with a target dose of 10 mg/day on day 8; may increase dose up to a maximum of 20 mg/day, based on response and tolerability, in 5 mg/day increments at intervals no less than 1 week. Assess the need for ongoing treatment periodically.

Dosage adjustment with concurrent CYP450 inducer or inhibitor therapy:

Oral and IM, immediate release: **Note:** Dose reduction does not apply when adjunctive aripiprazole is administered to patients with major depressive disorder; follow usual dosing recommendations.

CYP3A4 inducers (eg, carbamazepine, rifampin): Aripiprazole dose should be doubled over 1 to 2 weeks; dose should be subsequently reduced to the original level over 1 to 2 weeks if concurrent inducer agent is discontinued.

Strong CYP3A4 inhibitors (eg, itraconazole, clarithromycin): Aripiprazole dose should be reduced to 50% of the usual dose, and proportionally increased upon discontinuation of the inhibitor agent.

Strong CYP2D6 inhibitors (eg, quinidine, fluoxetine, paroxetine): Aripiprazole dose should be reduced to 50% of the usual dose, and proportionally increased upon discontinuation of the inhibitor agent.

CYP3A4 and CYP2D6 inhibitors: Aripiprazole dose should be reduced to 25% of the usual dose. In patients receiving inhibitors of differing (eg, moderate 3A4/strong 2D6) or same (eg, moderate 3A4/moderate 2D6) potencies (excluding concurrent strong inhibitors), further dosage adjustments can be made to achieve the desired clinical response. In patients receiving strong CYP3A4 and 2D6 inhibitors, aripiprazole dose is proportionally increased upon discontinuation of one or both inhibitor agents.

IM, extended release: **Note:** Dosage adjustments are not recommended for concomitant use of CYP3A4 inhibitors, CYP2D6 inhibitors or CYP3A4 inducers for <14 days. In patients who had their aripiprazole dose adjusted for concomitant therapy, the aripiprazole dose may need to be increased if the CYP3A4 and/or CYP2D6 inhibitor is withdrawn.

CYP3A4 inducers: Avoid use; aripiprazole serum concentrations may fall below effective levels.

Strong CYP3A4 or CYP2D6 inhibitors:

Current aripiprazole dose of 300 mg once monthly: Reduce aripiprazole dose to 200 mg once monthly

Current aripiprazole dose of 400 mg once monthly: Reduce aripiprazole dose to 300 mg once monthly

Strong CYP3A4 inhibitors **and** CYPD2D6 inhibitors:
Current aripiprazole dose of 300 mg once monthly: Reduce aripiprazole dose to 160 mg once monthly
Current aripiprazole dose of 400 mg once monthly: Reduce aripiprazole dose to 200 mg once monthly

Dosage adjustment based on CYP2D6 metabolizer status:
Oral and IM, immediate release: Aripiprazole dose should be reduced to 50% of the usual dose in CYP2D6 poor metabolizers and to 25% of the usual dose in poor metabolizers receiving a concurrent strong CYP3A4 inhibitor (eg, itraconazole, clarithromycin); subsequently adjust dose for favorable clinical response.
IM, extended release: Reduce aripiprazole dose to 300 mg once monthly in CYP2D6 poor metabolizers; reduce dose to 200 mg once monthly in CYP2D6 poor metabolizers receiving a concurrent CYP3A4 inhibitor for >14 days.

Dosage adjustment in renal impairment: No dosage adjustment necessary.

Dosage adjustment in hepatic impairment: No dosage adjustment necessary.

Dietary Considerations Some products may contain phenylalanine.

Administration
Injection: For IM use only; do not administer SubQ or IV; **Note:** Immediate-release and extended-release parenteral products are **not** interchangeable.
Immediate release: Inject slowly into deep muscle mass
Extended release: Inject slowly into gluteal muscle using the provided 1.5 inch (38 mm) needle for nonobese patients or the provided 2 inch (50 mm) needle for obese patients. Do not massage muscle after administration. Rotate injection sites between the two gluteal muscles. Administer monthly (doses should be separated by ≥26 days).
Oral: Administer with or without food. Tablet and oral solution may be interchanged on a mg-per-mg basis, up to 25 mg. Doses using 30 mg tablets should be exchanged for 25 mg oral solution. Orally disintegrating tablets (Abilify Discmelt) are bioequivalent to the immediate-release tablets (Abilify).
Orally disintegrating tablet: Remove from foil blister by peeling back (do not push tablet through the foil). Place tablet in mouth immediately upon removal. Tablet dissolves rapidly in saliva and may be swallowed without liquid. If needed, can be taken with liquid. Do not split tablet.

Monitoring Parameters Mental status; vital signs (as clinically indicated); blood pressure (baseline; repeat 3 months after antipsychotic initiation, then yearly); weight, height, BMI, waist circumference (baseline; repeat at 4, 8, and 12 weeks after initiating or changing therapy, then quarterly; consider switching to a different antipsychotic for a weight gain ≥5% of initial weight); CBC (as clinically indicated; monitor frequently during the first few months of therapy in patients with preexisting low WBC or history of drug-induced leukopenia/neutropenia); electrolytes and liver function (annually and as clinically indicated); personal and family history of obesity, diabetes, dyslipidemia, hypertension, or cardiovascular disease (baseline; repeat annually); fasting plasma glucose level/HbA_{1c} (baseline; repeat 3 months after starting antipsychotic, then yearly); fasting lipid panel (baseline; repeat 3 months after initiation of antipsychotic; if LDL level is normal repeat at 2- to 5-year intervals or more frequently if clinical indicated); changes in menstruation, libido, development of galactorrhea, erectile and ejaculatory function (yearly); abnormal involuntary movements or parkinsonian signs (baseline; repeat weekly until dose stabilized for at least 2 weeks after introduction and for 2 weeks after any significant dose increase); tardive dyskinesia (every 12 months; high-risk patients every 6 months); ocular examination (yearly in patients >40 years; every 2 years in younger patients) (ADA, 2004; Lehman, 2004; Marder, 2004).

Product Availability Abilify Maintena prefilled dual-chamber syringe: FDA approved September 2014; availability anticipated in January 2015. The Abilify Maintena dual-chamber syringe will be available in 300 mg and 400 mg doses for deep intramuscular gluteal injection only by health care professionals. Consult prescribing information for additional information.

Dosage Forms Considerations Oral solution contains fructose 200 mg and sucrose 400 mg per mL.

Dosage Forms
Solution, Intramuscular:
Abilify: 9.75 mg/1.3 mL (1.3 mL)
Solution, Oral:
Abilify: 1 mg/mL (150 mL)
Suspension Reconstituted, Intramuscular:
Abilify Maintena: 300 mg (1 ea); 400 mg (1 ea)
Tablet, Oral:
Abilify: 2 mg, 5 mg, 10 mg, 15 mg, 20 mg, 30 mg
Tablet Dispersible, Oral:
Abilify Discmelt: 10 mg, 15 mg

Dosage Forms: Canada Note: Refer to Dosage Forms. Dispersible tablet, oral solution, and IM preparations are not available in Canada.

◆ **Aristospan (Can)** *see* Triamcinolone (Systemic) *on page 2099*

◆ **Aristospan Intra-Articular** *see* Triamcinolone (Systemic) *on page 2099*

◆ **Aristospan Intralesional** *see* Triamcinolone (Systemic) *on page 2099*

◆ **Arixtra** *see* Fondaparinux *on page 924*

Armodafinil (ar moe DAF i nil)

Brand Names: U.S. Nuvigil

Index Terms R-modafinil

Pharmacologic Category Central Nervous System Stimulant

Use Improve wakefulness in patients with excessive daytime sleepiness associated with narcolepsy and shift work sleep disorder (SWSD); adjunctive therapy for obstructive sleep apnea/hypopnea syndrome (OSAHS)

Pregnancy Risk Factor C

Pregnancy Considerations Adverse events have been observed in animal reproduction studies, including visceral and skeletal abnormalities and decreased fetal weight. Efficacy of steroidal contraceptives may be decreased; alternate means of contraception should be considered during therapy and for 1 month after armodafinil is discontinued. A pregnancy registry has been established for patients exposed to armodafinil; healthcare providers are encouraged to register pregnant patients or pregnant women may register themselves by calling 1-866-404-4106.

Breast-Feeding Considerations It is not known if armodafinil or its metabolite is excreted into breast milk. The manufacture recommends caution be used if administered to a nursing woman.

Contraindications Hypersensitivity to armodafinil, modafinil, or any component of the formulation

Warnings/Precautions For use following complete evaluation of sleepiness and in conjunction with other standard treatments (eg, CPAP). The degree of sleepiness should be reassessed frequently; some patients may not return to a normal level of wakefulness. Patients with excessive sleepiness should be advised to avoid driving or any other potentially dangerous activity. Use >12 weeks has not been studied; patient should be reevaluated to determine effectiveness if use exceeds 12 weeks. Use is not recommended in patients with a history of angina or myocardial infarction, left ventricular hypertrophy, or patients with mitral valve prolapse who have developed mitral valve prolapse syndrome with previous CNS stimulant use. Patients with these conditions may also experience chest pain, palpitations, dyspnea, and transient ischemic T-wave changes on ECG. Increased blood pressure monitoring may be required in patients taking armodafinil. New or additional antihypertensive therapy may be needed.

Serious and life-threatening rashes including Stevens-Johnson syndrome, toxic epidermal necrolysis, and drug rash with eosinophilia and systemic symptoms (DRESS) have been reported. In modafinil clinical trials, rashes were more likely to occur in children; serious, postmarketing reactions have occurred with modafinil in adults and children as well as with armodafinil in adults. Most cases have been reported within the first 5 weeks of initiating therapy; however, rare cases have occurred after prolonged therapy. No risk factors have been identified to predict occurrence or severity of these reactions. Patients should be advised to discontinue use at first sign of rash (unless the rash is clearly not drug-related). Rare cases of multiorgan hypersensitivity reactions (with modafinil) and cases of angioedema and anaphylactoid reactions (armodafinil) have been reported. Signs and symptoms of multiorgan hypersensitivity reactions are diverse. Patients typically present with fever and rash associated with other organ system involvement. Patients should be advised to discontinue therapy and promptly report any signs or symptoms related to these adverse effects.

Caution should be exercised when modafinil is given to patients with a history of psychosis, depression, or mania; use may worsen symptoms (eg, mania, hallucinations, suicidal thoughts) of these disease; discontinue therapy if psychiatric symptoms develop. Use may impair the ability to engage in potentially hazardous activities; patients must be cautioned about performing tasks which require mental alertness (eg, operating machinery or driving). Stimulants may unmask tics in individuals with coexisting Tourette's syndrome. Use caution with hepatic impairment; consider use of a reduced dosage in patients with hepatic impairment or elderly patients. Safety and efficacy have not been established in patients with severe renal impairment. Use with caution in patients with a history of drug abuse; potential for drug dependency exists. Instruct patients to avoid concomitant ethanol consumption.

Adverse Reactions

Cardiovascular: Increased heart rate, palpitations

Central nervous system: Agitation, anxiety, depressed mood, depression (dose related), dizziness, fatigue, headache (dose related), insomnia (dose related), lack of concentration, migraine, nervousness, pain, paresthesia

Dermatologic: Contact dermatitis, diaphoresis, skin rash (dose related)

Endocrine & metabolic: Increased gamma-glutamyl transferase, increased thirst

Gastrointestinal: Abdominal pain, anorexia, appetite decreased, constipation, diarrhea, loose stools, nausea (dose related), vomiting, xerostomia (dose related)

Hepatic: GGT increased

Hypersensitivity: Seasonal allergy

Neuromuscular & skeletal: Tremor

Renal: Polyuria

Respiratory: Dyspnea, flu-like symptoms

Miscellaneous: Fever

Rare but important or life-threatening: Anaphylactoid reaction, angioedema, hypersensitivity, increased liver enzymes, pancytopenia, systolic hypertension

Drug Interactions

Metabolism/Transport Effects Substrate of CYP3A4 (major); **Note:** Assignment of Major/Minor substrate status based on clinically relevant drug interaction potential; **Inhibits** CYP2C19 (moderate); **Induces** CYP3A4 (weak)

Avoid Concomitant Use

Avoid concomitant use of Armodafinil with any of the following: Conivaptan; Fusidic Acid (Systemic); Idelalisib; Iobenguane I 123

Increased Effect/Toxicity

Armodafinil may increase the levels/effects of: Citalopram; CYP2C19 Substrates; Sympathomimetics

The levels/effects of Armodafinil may be increased by: Aprepitant; AtoMOXetine; Cannabinoid-Containing Products; Ceritinib; Conivaptan; CYP3A4 Inhibitors (Moderate); CYP3A4 Inhibitors (Strong); Dasatinib; Fosaprepitant; Fusidic Acid (Systemic); Idelalisib; Ivacaftor; Linezolid; Luliconazole; Mifepristone; Netupitant; Simeprevir; Stiripentol; Tedizolid

Decreased Effect

Armodafinil may decrease the levels/effects of: ARIPiprazole; Clopidogrel; Contraceptives (Estrogens); CycloSPORINE (Systemic); Hydrocodone; Iobenguane I 123; Saxagliptin

The levels/effects of Armodafinil may be decreased by: Bosentan; CYP3A4 Inducers (Moderate); CYP3A4 Inducers (Strong); Dabrafenib; Deferasirox; Mitotane; Siltuximab; St Johns Wort; Tocilizumab

Food Interactions Food delays absorption, but minimal effects on bioavailability. Food may affect the onset and time course of armodafinil. Management: Administer without regard to meals.

Storage/Stability Store at 20°C to 25°C (68°F to 77°F).

Mechanism of Action The exact mechanism of action of armodafinil is unknown. It is the R-enantiomer of modafinil. Armodafinil binds to the dopamine transporter and inhibits dopamine reuptake, which may result in increased extracellular dopamine levels in the brain. However, it does not appear to be a dopamine receptor agonist and also does not appear to bind to or inhibit the most common receptors or enzymes that are relevant for sleep/wake regulation.

Pharmacodynamics/Kinetics

Absorption: Readily absorbed

Distribution: V_d: 42 L

Protein binding: ~60% (based on modafinil; primarily albumin)

Metabolism: Hepatic, multiple pathways, including amine hydrolysis and CYP3A4/5; metabolites include R-modafinil acid and modafinil sulfone

Half-life elimination: 15 hours; Steady state: ~7 days

Time to peak, plasma: 2 hours (fasted)

Excretion: Urine (based on modafinil: 80% predominantly as metabolites; <10% as unchanged drug)

Dosage Oral:

Adults:

Narcolepsy: 150-250 mg once daily in the morning

Obstructive sleep apnea/hypopnea syndrome (OSAHS): 150-250 mg once daily in the morning; doses >150 mg have not been shown to have an increased benefit

Shift work sleep disorder (SWSD): 150 mg given once daily ~1 hour prior to work shift

Elderly: Consider lower initial dosage. Concentrations were almost doubled in clinical trials (based on modafinil)

Dosage adjustment in renal impairment: Safety and efficacy have not been established in severe renal impairment.

Dosage adjustment in hepatic impairment: Severe hepatic impairment: The manufacturer recommends a reduced dose; based on modafinil pharmacokinetics, a dose reduction of one-half the normal dose should be considered.

Dietary Considerations Take with or without meals.
Administration May be administered without regard to food.
Monitoring Parameters Signs of hypersensitivity, rash, psychiatric symptoms, levels of sleepiness, blood pressure, and drug abuse
Dosage Forms
Tablet, Oral:
Nuvigil: 50 mg, 150 mg, 200 mg, 250 mg

◆ **Armour Thyroid** *see* Thyroid, Desiccated *on page 2031*

◆ **Arnuity Ellipta** *see* Fluticasone (Oral Inhalation) *on page 907*

◆ **Aromasin** *see* Exemestane *on page 828*

◆ **Arranon** *see* Nelarabine *on page 1435*

Arsenic Trioxide (AR se nik tri OKS id)

Brand Names: U.S. Trisenox
Brand Names: Canada Trisenox
Index Terms As_2O_3
Pharmacologic Category Antineoplastic Agent, Miscellaneous
Use Remission induction and consolidation in patients with relapsed or refractory acute promyelocytic leukemia (APL) characterized by t(15;17) translocation or PML/RAR-alpha gene expression
Pregnancy Risk Factor D
Dosage Note: Arsenic trioxide is associated with a moderate emetic potential; antiemetics are recommended to prevent nausea and vomiting (Dupuis, 2011)
IV:
Acute promyelocytic leukemia (APL), relapsed or refractory: Children ≥4 years (U.S. labeling) or ≥5 years (Canadian labeling) and Adults:
Induction: 0.15 mg/kg/day; administer daily until bone marrow remission; maximum induction: 60 doses
Consolidation: 0.15 mg/kg/day starting 3-6 weeks after completion of induction therapy; maximum consolidation: 25 doses over a period of up to 5 weeks
APL initial treatment (off-label use):
Children: Induction, consolidation, and maintenance (Mathews, 2006):
Induction: 0.15 mg/kg/day (maximum dose: 10 mg); administer daily until bone marrow remission; maximum induction: 60 doses
Consolidation: 0.15 mg/kg/day (maximum dose: 10 mg) for 4 weeks, starting 4 weeks after completion of induction therapy
Maintenance: 0.15 mg/kg/dose (maximum dose: 10 mg) administered 10 days per month for 6 months, starting 4 weeks after completion of consolidation therapy
Adults:
Induction, consolidation, and maintenance (Mathews, 2006):
Induction: 10 mg/day; administer daily until bone marrow remission; maximum induction: 60 doses
Consolidation: 10 mg/day for 4 weeks, starting 4 weeks after completion of induction therapy
Maintenance: 10 mg/dose administered 10 days per month for 6 months, starting 4 weeks after completion of consolidation therapy
Consolidation therapy after remission induction with tretinoin, daunorubicin and cytarabine (Powell, 2007; Powell, 2010): Two consolidation courses (2 weeks apart): 0.15 mg/kg/day 5 days/week for 5 weeks
In combination with tretinoin (Estey, 2006; Ravandi, 2009):
Induction (beginning 10 days after initiation of tretinoin): 0.15 mg/kg/day until bone marrow remission; maximum induction: 75 doses
Consolidation: 0.15 mg/kg/day Monday through Friday for 4 weeks every 8 weeks for 4 cycles (weeks 1 to 4, 9 to 12, 17 to 20, and 25 to 28)
Myelodysplastic syndromes (MDS; off-label use): Adults: 0.25 mg/kg/day 5 consecutive days/week for 2 weeks, followed by a 2-week rest period (Schiller, 2006)

Dosage adjustment in renal impairment:
Mild-to-moderate impairment (CrCl ≥30 mL/minute): No dosage adjustment provided in manufacturer's labeling.
Severe renal impairment (CrCl <30 mL/minute): Use with caution (systemic exposure to metabolites may be higher); may require dosage reduction; monitor closely for toxicity
Dialysis patients: Has not been studied
Dosage adjustment in hepatic impairment: No dosage adjustment provided in manufacturer's labeling; use with caution. Patients with severe impairment (Child-Pugh class C) should be monitored closely for toxicity.

Dosing in obesity: *ASCO Guidelines for appropriate chemotherapy dosing in obese adults with cancer:* Utilize patient's actual body weight (full weight) for calculation of body surface area- or weight-based dosing, particularly when the intent of therapy is curative; manage regimen-related toxicities in the same manner as for nonobese patients; if a dose reduction is utilized due to toxicity, consider resumption of full weight-based dosing with subsequent cycles, especially if cause of toxicity (eg, hepatic or renal impairment) is resolved (Griggs, 2012).
Note: The Canadian labeling recommends dosing obese pediatric patients based on ideal body weight.
Additional Information Complete prescribing information should be consulted for additional detail.
Dosage Forms
Solution, Intravenous:
Trisenox: 10 mg/10 mL (10 mL)

◆ **Artane** *see* Trihexyphenidyl *on page 2103*

◆ **Artemether and Benflumetol** *see* Artemether and Lumefantrine *on page 177*

Artemether and Lumefantrine
(ar TEM e ther & loo me FAN treen)

Brand Names: U.S. Coartem
Index Terms Artemether and Benflumetol; Benflumetol and Artemether; Lumefantrine and Artemether
Pharmacologic Category Antimalarial Agent
Use Treatment of acute, uncomplicated malaria infections due to *Plasmodium falciparum*, including geographical regions where chloroquine resistance has been reported
Pregnancy Risk Factor C
Dosage Oral: Three-day schedule for the treatment of uncomplicated malaria (chloroquine-resistant uncomplicated *P. falciparum*):
Children 2 months to ≤16 years:
5 to <15 kg: One tablet at hour 0 and hour 8 on the first day, then 1 tablet twice daily on day 2 and day 3 (total of 6 tablets per treatment course)
15 to <25 kg: Two tablets at hour 0 and hour 8 on the first day, then 2 tablets twice daily on day 2 and day 3 (total of 12 tablets per treatment course)
25 to <35 kg: Three tablets at hour 0 and hour 8 on the first day, then 3 tablets twice daily on day 2 and day 3 (total of 18 tablets per treatment course)
≥35 kg: Four tablets at hour 0 and hour 8 on the first day, then 4 tablets twice daily on day 2 and day 3 (total of 24 tablets per treatment course)
Children >16 years and Adults:
25 to <35 kg: Three tablets at hour 0 and hour 8 on the first day, then 3 tablets twice daily on day 2 and day 3 (total of 18 tablets per treatment course)

≥35 kg: Four tablets at hour 0 and hour 8 on the first day, then 4 tablets twice daily on day 2 and day 3 (total of 24 tablets per treatment course)

Dosage adjustment in renal impairment: Dosage adjustment not recommended in mild or moderate impairment. Use caution in severe renal impairment (has not been studied).

Dosage adjustment in hepatic impairment: Dosage adjustments are not recommended in mild or moderate impairment. Use caution in severe impairment (has not been studied).

Additional Information Complete prescribing information should be consulted for additional detail.

Dosage Forms

Tablet:

Coartem: Artemether 20 mg and lumefantrine 120 mg

◆ **Artemisinin Derivative** *see* Artesunate *on page* 178

Artesunate (ar TES oo nate)

Index Terms Artemisinin Derivative; Artesunic Acid; Dihydroartemisinin Hemisuccinate Sodium; Dihydroqinghaosu Hemisuccinate Sodium; Nuartez; P01BE03; Qinghao Derivative; Qinghaosu Derivative; Sodium Artesunate

Pharmacologic Category Antimalarial Agent; Artemisinin Derivative

Dosage IV: Children and Adults: 2.4 mg/kg/dose initially, followed by 2.4 mg/kg/dose at 12 hours, 24 hours, and 48 hours after the initial dose for a total of 4 doses over a period of 3 days; longer treatment duration (eg, an additional 4 days [Hess, 2010]) may be required in severely-ill patients or in patients unable to transition to oral therapy (Hess, 2010; Rosenthal, 2008). **Note:** Because of the short half-life of artesunate and a high risk of recrudescence, oral antimalarial therapy must begin ≤4 hours after the last dose of IV artesunate. Appropriate oral therapies include atovaquone-proguanil, doxycycline (in patients >8 years of age and nonpregnant adults), clindamycin, **or** mefloquine (CDC, 2009, Hess, 2010; Rosenthal, 2008).

Dosage adjustment in renal impairment: No dosage adjustment necessary (Rosenthal, 2008).

Dosage adjustment in hepatic impairment: No dosage adjustment necessary (Rosenthal, 2008).

Additional Information Complete prescribing information should be consulted for additional detail.

◆ **Artesunic Acid** *see* Artesunate *on page* 178
◆ **Arthrotec** *see* Diclofenac and Misoprostol *on page* 621
◆ **Arzerra** *see* Ofatumumab *on page* 1488
◆ **As_2O_3** *see* Arsenic Trioxide *on page* 177
◆ **ASA** *see* Aspirin *on page* 180
◆ **5-ASA** *see* Mesalamine *on page* 1301
◆ **ASA and Diphenhydramine** *see* Aspirin and Diphenhydramine *on page* 185
◆ **Asacol (Can)** *see* Mesalamine *on page* 1301
◆ **Asacol 800 (Can)** *see* Mesalamine *on page* 1301
◆ **Asacol HD** *see* Mesalamine *on page* 1301
◆ **Asaphen (Can)** *see* Aspirin *on page* 180
◆ **Asaphen E.C. (Can)** *see* Aspirin *on page* 180
◆ **Asclera** *see* Polidocanol *on page* 1672
◆ **Ascocid [OTC]** *see* Ascorbic Acid *on page* 178
◆ **Ascocid-ISO-pH [OTC]** *see* Ascorbic Acid *on page* 178
◆ **Ascor L 500** *see* Ascorbic Acid *on page* 178
◆ **Ascor L NC** *see* Ascorbic Acid *on page* 178

Ascorbic Acid (a SKOR bik AS id)

Brand Names: U.S. Acerola C 500 [OTC]; Asco-Tabs-1000 [OTC]; Ascocid [OTC]; Ascocid-ISO-pH [OTC]; Ascor L 500; Ascor L NC; BProtected Vitamin C [OTC]; C-500 [OTC]; C-Time [OTC]; Cemill SR [OTC]; Cemill [OTC]; Chew-C [OTC]; Fruit C 500 [OTC]; Fruit C [OTC]; Fruity C [OTC]; Mega-C/A Plus; Ortho-CS 250; Vita-C [OTC]

Brand Names: Canada Ascor L 500; Vitamin C

Index Terms Vitamin C

Pharmacologic Category Vitamin, Water Soluble

Use

Ascorbic acid deficiency: Treatment of symptoms of mild deficiency; use in conditions requiring an increased intake (eg, burns, wound healing)

Dietary supplement: As a dietary vitamin C supplement

Scurvy: Prevention and treatment of scurvy

Pregnancy Risk Factor C

Dosage

Recommended adequate intake (AI) (IOM, 2000):
- 0 to 6 months: 40 mg daily
- 7 to 12 months: 50 mg daily

Recommended daily allowance (RDA) (IOM, 2000):
- 1 to 3 years: 15 mg daily; upper limit of intake should not exceed 400 mg daily
- 4 to 8 years: 25 mg daily; upper limit of intake should not exceed 650 mg daily
- 9 to 13 years: 45 mg daily; upper limit of intake should not exceed 1,200 mg daily
- 14 to 18 years: Upper limit of intake should not exceed 1,800 mg daily
  - Males: 75 mg daily
  - Females: 65 mg daily
- Adults: Upper limit of intake should not exceed 2,000 mg daily
  - Males: 90 mg daily
  - Females: 75 mg daily
- Pregnant females:
  - 14 to 18 years: 80 mg daily; upper limit of intake should not exceed 1,800 mg daily
  - 19 to 50 years: 85 mg daily; upper limit of intake should not exceed 2,000 mg daily
- Lactating females:
  - 14 to 18 years: 115 mg daily; upper limit of intake should not exceed 1,800 mg daily
  - 19 to 50 years: 120 mg daily; upper limit of intake should not exceed 2,000 mg daily
- Adult smoker: Add an additional 35 mg daily

Infants, Children, and Adolescents:

Scurvy: Oral: 100 to 300 mg daily until body stores are replenished; dose and duration of therapy should be individualized; doses as low as 10 mg daily may be effective (Popovich, 2009; Weinstein, 2001)

Adults: IM, IV, SubQ:

Ascorbic acid deficiency: 70 to 150 mg daily is an average protective dose; doses 3 to 5 times the RDA may be adequate for conditions with increased requirements.

Burns: 1 to 2 g daily for severe burns; dose may be determined by extent of tissue injury.

Wound healing: 300 to 500 mg daily for 7 to 10 days pre- and post-operatively; larger doses have also been used.

Scurvy: 300 to 1,000 mg daily; dose and duration of therapy should be individualized; doses up to 6 g per day have been administered (per manufacturer)

Adults, oral:

Scurvy: 100 to 300 mg daily until body stores are replenished; dose and duration of therapy should be individualized; doses as low as 10 mg may be effective (Hirschmann, 1999; Popovich, 2009; Weinstein, 2001).

Additional Information Complete prescribing information should be consulted for additional detail.

Dosage Forms

Capsule Extended Release, Oral:
C-Time [OTC]: 500 mg
Generic: 500 mg

Capsule Extended Release, Oral [preservative free]:
Generic: 500 mg

Crystals, Oral:
Vita-C [OTC]: (120 g, 480 g)

Liquid, Oral:
BProtected Vitamin C [OTC]: 500 mg/5 mL (236 mL)
Generic: 500 mg/5 mL (473 mL)

Powder, Oral:
Ascocid [OTC]: (227 g)
Generic: (113 g, 120 g, 480 g)

Powder Effervescent, Oral:
Ascocid-ISO-pH [OTC]: (150 g)

Solution, Injection:
Generic: 500 mg/mL (50 mL)

Solution, Injection [preservative free]:
Ascor L 500: 500 mg/mL (50 mL)
Ascor L NC: 500 mg/mL (50 mL)
Mega-C/A Plus: 500 mg/mL (50 mL)
Ortho-CS 250: 250 mg/mL (100 mL)
Generic: 250 mg/mL (30 mL)

Syrup, Oral:
Generic: 500 mg/5 mL (118 mL, 473 mL)

Tablet, Oral:
Asco-Tabs-1000 [OTC]: 1000 mg
Generic: 100 mg, 250 mg, 500 mg, 1000 mg

Tablet, Oral [preservative free]:
Generic: 250 mg, 500 mg

Tablet Chewable, Oral:
Chew-C [OTC]: 500 mg
Fruit C [OTC]: 100 mg
Fruit C 500 [OTC]: 500 mg
Fruity C [OTC]: 250 mg
Generic: 100 mg, 250 mg, 500 mg

Tablet Chewable, Oral [preservative free]:
C-500 [OTC]: 500 mg
Generic: 500 mg

Tablet Extended Release, Oral:
Cemill [OTC]: 500 mg
Cemill SR [OTC]: 1000 mg
Generic: 500 mg, 1000 mg, 1500 mg

Wafer, Oral [preservative free]:
Acerola C 500 [OTC]: 500 mg (50 ea)

◆ **Asco-Tabs-1000 [OTC]** *see* Ascorbic Acid *on page 178*

◆ **Ascriptin Maximum Strength [OTC]** *see* Aspirin *on page 180*

◆ **Ascriptin Regular Strength [OTC]** *see* Aspirin *on page 180*

Asenapine (a SEN a peen)

Brand Names: U.S. Saphris

Brand Names: Canada Saphris

Pharmacologic Category Antimanic Agent; Second Generation (Atypical) Antipsychotic

Additional Appendix Information

Beers Criteria – Potentially Inappropriate Medications for Geriatrics *on page 2271*

Use

Bipolar disorder: Treatment of acute mania or mixed episodes associated with bipolar I disorder (as monotherapy or in combination with lithium or valproate)

Schizophrenia: Acute and maintenance treatment of schizophrenia

Pregnancy Risk Factor C

Dosage Sublingual: Adults: **Note:** Safety of doses >20 mg/day has not been evaluated:

Schizophrenia:

Acute treatment: Initial: 5 mg twice daily. Daily doses >20 mg/day in clinical trials did not appear to offer any additional benefits and increased risk of adverse effects.

Maintenance treatment: Initial: 5 mg twice daily; may increase to 10 mg twice daily after 1 week based on tolerability

Bipolar disorder:

Monotherapy: Initial: 10 mg twice daily; decrease to 5 mg twice daily if dose not tolerated

Combination therapy (with lithium or valproate): 5 mg twice daily; may increase to 10 mg twice daily based on tolerability

Dosing adjustment in renal impairment: No dosage adjustment is necessary

Dosing adjustment in hepatic impairment:

Mild-to-moderate hepatic impairment (Child-Pugh class A or B): No dosage adjustment is necessary

Severe hepatic impairment (Child-Pugh class C): Use is not recommended

Additional Information Complete prescribing information should be consulted for additional detail.

Dosage Forms

Tablet Sublingual, Sublingual:
Saphris: 5 mg, 10 mg

◆ **Asendin [DSC]** *see* Amoxapine *on page 128*

◆ **Asmanex 7 Metered Doses** *see* Mometasone (Oral Inhalation) *on page 1389*

◆ **Asmanex 14 Metered Doses** *see* Mometasone (Oral Inhalation) *on page 1389*

◆ **Asmanex 30 Metered Doses** *see* Mometasone (Oral Inhalation) *on page 1389*

◆ **Asmanex 60 Metered Doses** *see* Mometasone (Oral Inhalation) *on page 1389*

◆ **Asmanex 120 Metered Doses** *see* Mometasone (Oral Inhalation) *on page 1389*

◆ **Asmanex HFA** *see* Mometasone (Oral Inhalation) *on page 1389*

◆ **Asmanex Twisthaler (Can)** *see* Mometasone (Oral Inhalation) *on page 1389*

◆ **ASNase** *see* Asparaginase (*E. coli*) *on page 179*

◆ **Asparaginase** *see* Asparaginase (*E. coli*) *on page 179*

Asparaginase (*E. coli*) (a SPEAR a ji nase e ko lye)

Brand Names: U.S. Elspar [DSC]

Brand Names: Canada Kidrolase

Index Terms *E. coli* Asparaginase; ASNase; Asparaginase; L-ASP; L-asparaginase (*E. coli*)

Pharmacologic Category Antineoplastic Agent, Enzyme; Antineoplastic Agent, Miscellaneous

Use Acute lymphoblastic leukemia (ALL): Treatment (in combination with other chemotherapy) of ALL

Pregnancy Risk Factor C

Dosage Note: Dose, frequency, number of doses, and start date may vary by protocol and treatment phase.

Acute lymphoblastic leukemia (ALL): Manufacturer's U.S. labeling: Children and Adults: IV, IM: 6000 units/m^2/dose 3 times weekly

CCG 1922 protocol (off-label dosing): Children: IM: 6000 units/m^2/dose 3 times weekly for 9 doses beginning either on day 2, 3, or 4 (induction phase) and 6000 units/m^2/dose on Monday, Wednesday, and Friday for 6 doses beginning day 3 (delayed intensification phase) (Bostrom, 2004)

DFCI-ALL Consortium protocol 00-01 (off-label dosing): Children: IM: 25,000 units/m^2 for 1 dose (induction phase) and 25,000 units/m^2/dose weekly for 30 weeks (intensification phase) (Vrooman, 2013)

DFCI-ALL Consortium protocol 95-01 (off-label dosing): Children: IM: 25,000 units/m^2 for 1 dose on day 4 (induction phase) and 25,000 units/m^2/dose weekly for 20 weeks (intensification phase) (Moghrabi, 2007)

Hyper-CVAD regimen (off-label dosing): Adolescents ≥13 years and Adults: IV 20,000 units weekly for 4 doses (starting on day 2) during either months 7 and 19 or months 7 and 11 of intensification phase (Thomas, 2010)

Larson regimen (off-label dosing): Adults: SubQ: 6000 units/m^2/dose on days 5, 8, 11, 15, 18, and 22 (induction phase) and on days 15, 18, 22, and 25 (early intensification phase) (Larson, 1995)

Linker regimen (off-label dosing): Adults: IM:

Remission induction: 6000 units/m^2/dose on days 17-28; if bone marrow on day 28 is positive for residual leukemia: 6000 units/m^2/dose on days 29-35 (Linker, 1991)

Consolidation (Treatment A; cycles 1, 3, 5, and 7): 12,000 units/m^2/dose on days 2, 4, 7, 9, 11, and 14 (Linker, 1991)

Lymphoblastic lymphoma (off-label use): Adolescents >15 years and Adults: Hyper-CVAD regimen: IV: 20,000 units weekly for 4 doses (starting on day 2) for 2 cycles (months 7 and 11) during maintenance phase (Thomas, 2004)

Dosage adjustment for toxicity:

Allergic reaction/hypersensitivity: Discontinue for severe reactions.

Neurotoxicity (posterior reversible encephalopathy syndrome; PRES): Interrupt therapy for suspected PRES; control blood pressure and closely monitor for seizure activity.

Pancreatitis: Discontinue permanently (per manufacturer).

Thrombotic event: Discontinue for serious reactions.

Dosage adjustment in renal impairment: No dosage adjustment provided in manufacturer's labeling.

Dosage adjustment in hepatic impairment: No dosage adjustment provided in manufacturer's labeling.

Dosing in obesity: *ASCO Guidelines for appropriate chemotherapy dosing in obese adults with cancer:* Utilize patient's actual body weight (full weight) for calculation of body surface area- or weight-based dosing, particularly when the intent of therapy is curative; manage regimen-related toxicities in the same manner as for nonobese patients; if a dose reduction is utilized due to toxicity, consider resumption of full weight-based dosing with subsequent cycles, especially if cause of toxicity (eg, hepatic or renal impairment) is resolved (Griggs, 2012).

Additional Information Complete prescribing information should be consulted for additional detail.

Product Availability Elspar: Manufacturing of asparaginase (*E. coli*) was discontinued by Lundbeck at the end of 2012. Elspar was acquired by Recordati Rare Diseases; availability information is currently unavailable.

Asparaginase (*Erwinia*)

(a SPEAR a ji nase er WIN i ah)

Brand Names: U.S. Erwinaze

Brand Names: Canada Erwinase

Index Terms *Erwinia chrysanthemi*; Asparaginase *Erwinia chrysanthemi*; L-asparaginase (*Erwinia*)

Pharmacologic Category Antineoplastic Agent, Enzyme; Antineoplastic Agent, Miscellaneous

Use Acute lymphoblastic leukemia: Treatment (in combination with other chemotherapy) of acute lymphoblastic leukemia (ALL) in patients with hypersensitivity to *E. coli*-derived asparaginase

Pregnancy Risk Factor C

Dosage Note: If administering IV, consider monitoring nadir serum asparaginase activity (NSAA) levels; if desired levels are not achieved, change to IM administration.

Acute lymphoblastic leukemia (ALL): Children ≥1 year, Adolescents, and Adults: IM, IV:

As a substitute for pegaspargase: 25,000 units/m^2 3 times weekly (Mon, Wed, Fri) for 6 doses for each planned pegaspargase dose

As a substitute for asparaginase (E. coli): 25,000 units/m^2 for each scheduled asparaginase (*E. coli*) dose

Canadian labeling (not in the U.S. labeling): ALL induction:

Children <14 years: IM: 6000 units/m^2 3 times weekly for 9 doses beginning day 4 of week 1 (in combination with vincristine, prednisone, methotrexate, and daunorubicin)

Children >14 years and Adults: SubQ: 10,000 units/m^2 days 1, 3, and 5 of week 4 and day 1 of week 5 (in combination with prednisolone, vincristine, mercaptopurine, and methotrexate) **or** 10,000 units/m^2 3 times weekly (starting week 4) for 4 weeks (in combination with prednisolone, vincristine, and daunorubicin)

Dosage adjustment for toxicity:

Hemorrhagic or thrombotic event: Discontinue treatment; may resume treatment upon symptom resolution

Pancreatitis:

Mild pancreatitis: Withhold treatment until signs and symptoms subside and amylase levels return to normal; may resume after resolution

Severe or hemorrhagic pancreatitis (abdominal pain >72 hours and amylase ≥2 x ULN): Discontinue treatment; further use is contraindicated.

Serious hypersensitivity reaction: Discontinue treatment

Dosage adjustment in renal impairment: There are no dosage adjustments provided in the manufacturer's labeling.

Dosage adjustment in hepatic impairment: There are no dosage adjustments provided in the manufacturer's labeling.

Dosing in obesity: *ASCO Guidelines for appropriate chemotherapy dosing in obese adults with cancer:* Utilize patient's actual body weight (full weight) for calculation of body surface area- or weight-based dosing, particularly when the intent of therapy is curative; manage regimen-related toxicities in the same manner as for nonobese patients; if a dose reduction is utilized due to toxicity, consider resumption of full weight-based dosing with subsequent cycles, especially if cause of toxicity (eg, hepatic or renal impairment) is resolved (Griggs, 2012).

Additional Information Complete prescribing information should be consulted for additional detail.

Dosage Forms

Solution Reconstituted, Intramuscular:

Erwinaze: 10,000 units (1 ea)

◆ **Asparaginase *Erwinia chrysanthemi*** *see* Asparaginase (*Erwinia*) *on page 180*

◆ **Aspart Insulin** *see* Insulin Aspart *on page 1083*

◆ **Aspercin [OTC]** *see* Aspirin *on page 180*

◆ ***Aspergillus niger*** *see* Alpha-Galactosidase *on page 94*

◆ **Aspergum [OTC]** *see* Aspirin *on page 180*

Aspirin (AS pir in)

Brand Names: U.S. Ascriptin Maximum Strength [OTC]; Ascriptin Regular Strength [OTC]; Aspercin [OTC];

Aspergum [OTC]; Aspir-low [OTC]; Aspirtab [OTC]; Bayer Aspirin Extra Strength [OTC]; Bayer Aspirin Regimen Adult Low Strength [OTC]; Bayer Aspirin Regimen Children's [OTC]; Bayer Aspirin Regimen Regular Strength [OTC]; Bayer Genuine Aspirin [OTC]; Bayer Plus Extra Strength [OTC]; Bayer Women's Low Dose Aspirin [OTC]; Buffasal [OTC]; Bufferin Extra Strength [OTC]; Bufferin [OTC]; Buffinol [OTC]; Ecotrin Arthritis Strength [OTC]; Ecotrin Low Strength [OTC]; Ecotrin [OTC]; Halfprin [OTC]; St Joseph Adult Aspirin [OTC]; Tri-Buffered Aspirin [OTC]

Brand Names: Canada Asaphen; Asaphen E.C.; Entrophen; Novasen; Praxis ASA EC 81 Mg Daily Dose; Pro-AAS EC-80

Index Terms Acetylsalicylic Acid; ASA; Baby Aspirin

Pharmacologic Category Antiplatelet Agent; Salicylate

Additional Appendix Information

Beers Criteria - Potentially Inappropriate Medications for Geriatrics *on page 2271*

Oral Antiplatelet Comparison Chart *on page 2239*

Use Treatment of mild-to-moderate pain, inflammation, and fever; prevention and treatment of acute coronary syndromes (ST-elevation MI, non-ST-elevation MI, unstable angina), acute ischemic stroke, and transient ischemic episodes; management of rheumatoid arthritis, juvenile idiopathic arthritis (formerly called juvenile rheumatoid arthritis), rheumatic fever, osteoarthritis; adjunctive therapy in revascularization procedures (coronary artery bypass graft [CABG], percutaneous transluminal coronary angioplasty [PTCA], carotid endarterectomy), stent implantation

Pregnancy Considerations Salicylates have been noted to cross the placenta and enter fetal circulation. Adverse effects reported in the fetus include mortality, intrauterine growth retardation, salicylate intoxication, bleeding abnormalities, and neonatal acidosis. Use of aspirin close to delivery may cause premature closure of the ductus arteriosus. Adverse effects reported in the mother include anemia, hemorrhage, prolonged gestation, and prolonged labor (Østensen, 1998). Low-dose aspirin may be used to prevent preeclampsia in women with a history of early-onset preeclampsia and preterm delivery (<34 0/7 weeks), or preeclampsia in ≥1 prior pregnancy (ACOG, 2013). Low-dose aspirin is used to treat complications resulting from antiphospholipid syndrome in pregnancy (either primary or secondary to SLE) (ACCP [Guyatt, 2012]; Carp, 2004; Tincani, 2003). Low-dose aspirin to prevent thrombosis may also be used during the second and third trimesters in women with prosthetic valves (mechanical or bioprosthetic). The use of warfarin is recommended, along with low dose aspirin, in those with mechanical prosthetic valves (Nishimura, 2014). In general, low doses during pregnancy needed for the treatment of certain medical conditions have not been shown to cause fetal harm; however, discontinuing therapy prior to delivery is recommended (Østensen, 2006). Use of safer agents for routine management of pain or headache should be considered.

Breast-Feeding Considerations Low amounts of aspirin can be found in breast milk. Milk/plasma ratios ranging from 0.03 to 0.3 have been reported. Peak levels in breast milk are reported to be at ~9 hours after a dose. Metabolic acidosis was reported in one infant following an aspirin dose of 3.9 g/day in the mother. The WHO considers occasional doses of aspirin to be compatible with breast-feeding, but to avoid long-term therapy and consider monitoring the infant for adverse effects (WHO, 2002). Other sources suggest avoiding aspirin while breast-feeding due to the theoretical risk of Reye's syndrome (Bar-Oz, 2003; Spigset, 2000). When used for vascular indications, breast-feeding may be continued during low-dose aspirin therapy (ACCP [Guyatt, 2012]).

Contraindications OTC labeling: When used for self-medication, do not use if allergic to aspirin or other pain reliever/fever reducer or for at least 7 days after tonsillectomy or oral surgery.

Warnings/Precautions Use with caution in patients with platelet and bleeding disorders, renal dysfunction, dehydration, erosive gastritis, or peptic ulcer disease. Heavy ethanol use (>3 drinks/day) can increase bleeding risks. Avoid use in severe renal failure or in severe hepatic failure. Low-dose aspirin for cardioprotective effects is associated with a two- to fourfold increase in UGI events (eg, symptomatic or complicated ulcers); risks of these events increase with increasing aspirin dose; during the chronic phase of aspirin dosing, doses >81 mg are not recommended unless indicated (Bhatt, 2008). Use of safer agents for routine management of pain or headache throughout pregnancy should be considered. If possible, avoid use during the third trimester of pregnancy.

Discontinue use if tinnitus or impaired hearing occurs. Caution in mild-to-moderate renal failure (only at high dosages). Patients with sensitivity to tartrazine dyes, nasal polyps, and asthma may have an increased risk of salicylate sensitivity. In the treatment of acute ischemic stroke, avoid aspirin for 24 hours following administration of alteplase; administration within 24 hours increases the risk of hemorrhagic transformation (Jauch, 2013). Concurrent use of aspirin and clopidogrel is not recommended for secondary prevention of ischemic stroke or TIA in patients unable to take oral anticoagulants due to hemorrhagic risk (Furie, 2011). Surgical patients should avoid ASA if possible, for 1 to 2 weeks prior to surgery, to reduce the risk of excessive bleeding (except in patients with cardiac stents that have not completed their full course of dual antiplatelet therapy [aspirin, clopidogrel]; patient-specific situations need to be discussed with cardiologist; AHA/ACC/SCAI/ACS/ADA Science Advisory provides recommendations). When used concomitantly with ≤325 mg of aspirin, NSAIDs (including selective COX-2 inhibitors) substantially increase the risk of gastrointestinal complications (eg, ulcer); concomitant gastroprotective therapy (eg, proton pump inhibitors) is recommended (Bhatt, 2008). Potentially significant drug-drug interactions may exist, requiring dose or frequency adjustment, additional monitoring, and/or selection of alternative therapy.

Elderly: Avoid chronic use of doses >325 mg/day (unless alternative agents ineffective and patient can receive concomitant gastroprotective agent); nonselective oral NSAID use is associated with an increased risk of GI bleeding and peptic ulcer disease in older adults in high risk category (eg, >75 years or age or receiving concomitant oral/parenteral corticosteroids, anticoagulants, or antiplatelet agents) (Beers Criteria).

When used for self-medication (OTC labeling): Children and teenagers who have or are recovering from chickenpox or flu-like symptoms should not use this product. Changes in behavior (along with nausea and vomiting) may be an early sign of Reye's syndrome; patients should be instructed to contact their healthcare provider if these occur.

Aspirin resistance is defined as measurable, persistent platelet activation that occurs in patients prescribed a therapeutic dose of aspirin. Clinical aspirin resistance, the recurrence of some vascular event despite a regular therapeutic dose of aspirin, is considered aspirin treatment failure. Estimates of biochemical aspirin resistance range from 5.5% to 60% depending on the population studied and the assays used (Gasparyan, 2008). Patients with aspirin resistance may have a higher risk of cardiovascular events compared to those who are aspirin sensitive (Gum, 2003).

Adverse Reactions As with all drugs which may affect hemostasis, bleeding is associated with aspirin. Hemorrhage may occur at virtually any site. Risk is dependent on multiple variables including dosage, concurrent use of multiple agents which alter hemostasis, and patient susceptibility. Many adverse effects of aspirin are dose related, and are extremely rare at low dosages. Other serious reactions are idiosyncratic, related to allergy or individual sensitivity.

Cardiovascular: Cardiac arrhythmia, edema, hypotension, tachycardia

Central nervous system: Agitation, cerebral edema, coma, confusion, dizziness, fatigue, headache, hyperthermia, insomnia, lethargy, nervousness, Reye's syndrome

Dermatologic: Skin Rash, urticaria

Endocrine & metabolic: Acidosis, dehydration, hyperglycemia, hyperkalemia, hypernatremia (buffered forms), hypoglycemia (children)

Gastrointestinal: Duodenal ulcer, dyspepsia, epigastric distress, gastritis, gastrointestinal erosion, gastrointestinal ulcer, heartburn, nausea, stomach pain, vomiting

Genitourinary: Postpartum hemorrhage, prolonged gestation, prolonged labor, proteinuria, stillborn infant

Hematologic & oncologic: Anemia, blood coagulation disorder, disseminated intravascular coagulation, hemolytic anemia, hemorrhage, iron deficiency anemia, prolonged prothrombin time, thrombocytopenia

Hepatic: Hepatitis (reversible), hepatotoxicity, increased serum transaminases

Hypersensitivity: Anaphylaxis, angioedema

Neuromuscular & skeletal: Acetabular bone destruction, rhabdomyolysis, weakness

Otic: Hearing loss, tinnitus

Renal: Increased blood urea nitrogen, increased serum creatinine, interstitial nephritis, renal failure (including cases caused by rhabdomyolysis), renal insufficiency, renal papillary necrosis

Respiratory: Asthma, bronchospasm, dyspnea, hyperventilation, laryngeal edema, noncardiogenic pulmonary edema, respiratory alkalosis, tachypnea

Miscellaneous: Low birth weight

Rare but important or life-threatening: Anorectal stenosis (suppository), atrial fibrillation (toxicity), cardiac conduction disturbance (toxicity), cerebral infarction (ischemic), cholestatic jaundice, colitis, colonic ulceration, coronary artery vasospasm, delirium, esophageal obstruction, esophagitis (with esophageal ulcer), hematoma (esophageal), oral mucosa ulcer (aspirin-containing chewing gum), periorbital edema, rhinosinusitis

Drug Interactions

Metabolism/Transport Effects Substrate of CYP2C9 (minor); **Note:** Assignment of Major/Minor substrate status based on clinically relevant drug interaction potential; **Induces** CYP2C19 (moderate)

Avoid Concomitant Use

Avoid concomitant use of Aspirin with any of the following: Dexketoprofen; Floctafenine; Influenza Virus Vaccine (Live/Attenuated); Ketorolac (Nasal); Ketorolac (Systemic); Omacetaxine; Urokinase

Increased Effect/Toxicity

Aspirin may increase the levels/effects of: Agents with Antiplatelet Properties; Alendronate; Anticoagulants; Apixaban; Carbonic Anhydrase Inhibitors; Carisoprodol; Collagenase (Systemic); Corticosteroids (Systemic); Dabigatran Etexilate; Dexketoprofen; Heparin; Hypoglycemic Agents; Ibritumomab; Methotrexate; NSAID (COX-2 Inhibitor); Obinutuzumab; Omacetaxine; PRALAtrexate; Rivaroxaban; Salicylates; Thrombolytic Agents; Ticagrelor; Tositumomab and Iodine I 131 Tositumomab; Urokinase; Valproic Acid and Derivatives; Varicella Virus-Containing Vaccines; Vitamin K Antagonists

The levels/effects of Aspirin may be increased by: Agents with Antiplatelet Properties; Ammonium Chloride; Antidepressants (Tricyclic, Tertiary Amine); Calcium Channel Blockers (Nondihydropyridine); Dasatinib; Floctafenine; Ginkgo Biloba; Glucosamine; Herbs (Anticoagulant/Antiplatelet Properties); Ibrutinib; Influenza Virus Vaccine (Live/Attenuated); Ketorolac (Nasal); Ketorolac (Systemic); Limaprost; Loop Diuretics; Multivitamins/Fluoride (with ADE); Multivitamins/Minerals (with ADEK, Folate, Iron); Multivitamins/Minerals (with AE, No Iron); NSAID (Nonselective); Omega-3 Fatty Acids; Pentosan Polysulfate Sodium; Pentoxifylline; Potassium Acid Phosphate; Prostacyclin Analogues; Selective Serotonin Reuptake Inhibitors; Serotonin/Norepinephrine Reuptake Inhibitors; Tipranavir; Treprostinil; Vitamin E

Decreased Effect

Aspirin may decrease the levels/effects of: ACE Inhibitors; Carisoprodol; Dexketoprofen; Hyaluronidase; Loop Diuretics; Multivitamins/Fluoride (with ADE); Multivitamins/Minerals (with ADEK, Folate, Iron); Multivitamins/Minerals (with AE, No Iron); NSAID (Nonselective); Probenecid; Ticagrelor; Tiludronate

The levels/effects of Aspirin may be decreased by: Corticosteroids (Systemic); Dexketoprofen; Floctafenine; Ketorolac (Nasal); Ketorolac (Systemic); NSAID (Nonselective)

Food Interactions Food may decrease the rate but not the extent of oral absorption. Benedictine liqueur, prunes, raisins, tea, and gherkins have a potential to cause salicylate accumulation. Fresh fruits containing vitamin C may displace drug from binding sites, resulting in increased urinary excretion of aspirin. Curry powder, paprika, licorice; may cause salicylate accumulation. These foods contain 6 mg salicylate/100 g. An ordinary American diet contains 10-200 mg/day of salicylate. Management: Administer with food or large volume of water or milk to minimize GI upset. Limit curry powder, paprika, licorice.

Storage/Stability Store oral dosage forms (caplets, tablets) at room temperature; protect from moisture; see product-specific labeling for details. Keep suppositories in refrigerator; do not freeze. Hydrolysis of aspirin occurs upon exposure to water or moist air, resulting in salicylate and acetate, which possess a vinegar-like odor. Do not use if a strong odor is present.

Mechanism of Action Irreversibly inhibits cyclooxygenase-1 and 2 (COX-1 and 2) enzymes, via acetylation, which results in decreased formation of prostaglandin precursors; irreversibly inhibits formation of prostaglandin derivative, thromboxane A_2, via acetylation of platelet cyclooxygenase, thus inhibiting platelet aggregation; has antipyretic, analgesic, and anti-inflammatory properties

Pharmacodynamics/Kinetics

Duration: 4 to 6 hours

Absorption: Rapid

Distribution: V_d: 10 L; readily into most body fluids and tissues

Metabolism: Hydrolyzed to salicylate (active) by esterases in GI mucosa, red blood cells, synovial fluid, and blood; metabolism of salicylate occurs primarily by hepatic conjugation; metabolic pathways are saturable

Bioavailability: 50% to 75% reaches systemic circulation

Half-life elimination: Parent drug: 15 to 20 minutes; Salicylates (dose dependent): 3 hours at lower doses (300 to 600 mg), 5 to 6 hours (after 1 g), 10 hours with higher doses

Time to peak, serum: ~1 to 2 hours

Excretion: Urine (75% as salicyluric acid, 10% as salicylic acid)

Dosage

Children:

Analgesic and antipyretic: Oral, rectal: 10 to 15 mg/kg/dose every 4 to 6 hours, up to a total of 4 g/day

Anti-inflammatory: Oral: Initial: 60 to 90 mg/kg/day in divided doses; usual maintenance: 80 to 100 mg/kg/day divided every 6 to 8 hours; monitor serum concentrations

Antiplatelet effects: Adequate pediatric studies have not been performed; pediatric dosage is derived from adult studies and clinical experience and is not well established. Doses are typically rounded to a convenient amount (eg, 1/2 of 81 mg tablet).

Acute ischemic stroke (AIS): Oral:

Noncardioembolic: 1 to 5 mg/kg/dose once daily for ≥2 years; patients with recurrent AIS or TIAs should be transitioned to clopidogrel, LMWH, or warfarin (Monagle, 2012)

Secondary to Moyamoya and non-Moyamoya vasculopathy: 1 to 5 mg/kg/dose once daily. **Note:** In non-Moyamoya vasculopathy, continue aspirin for 3 months, with subsequent use guided by repeat cerebrovascular imaging (Monagle, 2012).

Blalock-Taussig shunts, primary prophylaxis (off-label use): Oral: 1 to 5 mg/kg/dose once daily (Monagle, 2012)

Fontan surgery, primary prophylaxis: Oral: 5 mg/kg/dose once daily (Monagle, 2011)

Prosthetic heart valve: Oral:

Bioprosthetic aortic valve (in normal sinus rhythm): 1 to 5 mg/kg/dose once daily (ACCP [Guyatt, 2012]; Monagle, 2012)

Mechanical aortic and/or mitral valve: Low-dose aspirin (eg, 1 to 5 mg/kg/day) combined with vitamin K antagonist (eg, warfarin) is recommended as first-line antithrombotic therapy (ACCP [Guyatt, 2012]). Alternative regimens: 6 to 20 mg/kg/dose once daily in combination with dipyridamole (Bradley, 1985; El Makhlouf, 1987; LeBlanc, 1993; Serra, 1987; Solymar, 1991)

Ventricular assist device (VAD) placement: Oral: 1 to 5 mg/kg/dose once daily initiated within 72 hours of VAD placement; should be used with heparin (initiated between 8 to 48 hours following implantation) (Monagle, 2012)

Kawasaki disease (off-label use): Oral: 80 to 100 mg/kg/day divided every 6 hours for up to 14 days (until fever resolves for at least 48 hours); then decrease dose to 3 to 5 mg/kg/day once daily; in patients without coronary artery abnormalities, give lower dose (ie, 3 to 5 mg/kg/day) for at least 6 to 8 weeks. In patients with coronary artery abnormalities, low-dose aspirin should be continued indefinitely (in combination with warfarin). **Note:** Combine with IV immune globulin treatment within 10 days of symptom onset (Newburger, 2004).

Adults: **Note:** For most cardiovascular uses, typical maintenance dosing of aspirin is 81 mg once daily.

Acute coronary syndrome (ST- elevation myocardial infarction [STEMI], unstable angina (UA)/non-ST-elevation myocardial infarction [NSTEMI]): Oral: Initial: 162 to 325 mg given on presentation (patient should chew nonenteric-coated aspirin especially if not taking before presentation); for patients unable to take oral, may use a rectal suppository dose of 600 mg (Maalouf, 2009). Maintenance (secondary prevention): 81 mg once daily preferred. When aspirin is used with ticagrelor, the recommended maintenance dose of aspirin is 81 mg/day (ACCF/AHA [Anderson, 2013]; ACCF/AHA [O'Gara, 2013]).

UA/NSTEMI: Concomitant antiplatelet therapy (ACCF/AHA [Anderson, 2013]):

If invasive strategy chosen: Aspirin is recommended in combination with either clopidogrel, ticagrelor, (or prasugrel if at the time of PCI) or an IV GP IIb/IIIa inhibitor (if given before PCI, eptifibatide and tirofiban are preferred agents).

If noninvasive strategy chosen: Aspirin is recommended in combination with clopidogrel or ticagrelor and anticoagulant therapy.

Analgesic and antipyretic:

Oral: 325 to 650 mg every 4 to 6 hours up to 4 g/day

Rectal: 300 to 600 mg every 4 to 6 hours up to 4 g/day

Anti-inflammatory: Oral: Initial: 2.4 to 3.6 g/day in divided doses; usual maintenance: 3.6 to 5.4 g/day; monitor serum concentrations

Aortic valve repair (off-label use): Oral: 50 to 100 mg once daily (ACCP [Guyatt, 2012], 2012)

Atrial fibrillation (to prevent thromboembolism in patients not candidates for oral anticoagulation or at low risk of ischemic stroke [CHA_2DS_2-VASc score of 1]) (off-label use): Oral: 75 to 325 mg once daily (AHA/ACC/HRS [January, 2014]; AHA/ASA [Furie, 2011]). **Note:** Combination therapy with clopidogrel has been suggested over aspirin alone for those patients who are unsuitable for or choose not to take oral anticoagulant for reasons other than concerns for bleeding (ACCP [Guyatt, 2012]).

As an alternative to adjusted-dose warfarin in patients with atrial fibrillation and mitral stenosis: 75 to 325 mg once daily with (preferred) or without clopidogrel (ACCP [Guyatt, 2012])

CABG: Oral: 100 to 325 mg once daily initiated either preoperatively or within 6 hours postoperatively; continue indefinitely (ACCF/AHA [Hillis, 2011]). For secondary prevention in patients with prior CABG surgery, the American College of Chest Physicians recommends the use of 75 to 100 mg daily (ACCP [Vandvik, 2012]).

Carotid artery stenosis (off-label use): Oral: 75 to 100 mg once daily. **Note:** When symptomatic (including recent carotid endarterectomy), the use of clopidogrel or aspirin/extended-release dipyridamole has been suggested over aspirin alone (ACCP [Guyatt, 2012]).

Colorectal cancer risk reduction (unlabeled use): **Note:** The optimal dose and duration of therapy for colorectal cancer risk reduction are unknown. Consider risk versus benefit ratio when initiating aspirin for this indication.

Primary/Secondary prevention: Oral: 75 to 325 mg once daily (Rothwell, 2010; Sandler, 2003; Ye, 2013).

Hereditary nonpolyposis colon cancer (HNPCC; Lynch Syndrome) carriers: Oral: 600 mg once daily for at least 2 years (ASCO [Stoffel, 2014]; Burn, 2011).

Coronary artery disease (CAD), established (off-label use): Oral: 75 to 100 mg once daily (ACCP [Guyatt, 2012])

PCI: Oral:

Non-emergent PCI: Preprocedure: 81 to 325 mg (325 mg [nonenteric coated] in aspirin-naive patients) starting at least 2 hours (preferably 24 hours) before procedure. Postprocedure: 81 mg once daily continued indefinitely (in combination with a $P2Y_{12}$ inhibitor [eg, clopidogrel, prasugrel, ticagrelor] up to 12 months) (ACCF/AHA/SCAI [Levine, 2011])

Primary PCI: Preprocedure: 162 to 325 mg as early as possible prior to procedure; 325 mg preferred followed by a maintenance dose of 81 mg once daily even when a stent is deployed (ACCF/AHA [O'Gara, 2013]).

Alternatively, in patients who have undergone elective PCI with either bare metal or drug-eluting stent placement: The American College of Chest Physicians recommends the use of 75 to 325 mg once daily (in combination with clopidogrel) for 1 month (BMS) or 3 to 6 months (dependent upon DES type) followed by 75 to 100 mg once daily (in combination with clopidogrel) for up to12 months. For patients who underwent PCI but did not have stent placement, 75 to 325 mg once daily (in combination with clopidogrel) for 1 month is recommended. In either case, single antiplatelet therapy (either aspirin or clopidogrel) is recommended indefinitely (ACCP [Guyatt, 2012]).

Pericarditis (off-label use): Oral: Initial: 2.4 to 3.6 g daily in 3 to 4 divided doses; usual maintenance: 3.6 to 5.4 g daily in divided doses; gradually taper over 2- to 3-week period as appropriate (Imazio, 2004; Imazio, 2009).

Pericarditis in association with myocardial infarction (off-label use): Initial: 650 mg 4 times daily; may increase after 24 hours to 975 mg 4 times daily if necessary (ACCF/AHA [O'Gara, 2013]; Berman, 1981).

Peripheral arterial disease (off-label use): Oral: 75 to 100 mg once daily (ACCP [Guyatt, 2012]) **or** 75 to 325 mg once daily; may use in conjunction with clopidogrel in those who are not at an increased risk of bleeding but are of high cardiovascular risk. **Note:** These recommendations also pertain to those with intermittent claudication or critical limb ischemia, prior lower extremity revascularization, or prior amputation for lower extremity ischemia (Rooke, 2011).

Peripheral artery percutaneous transluminal angioplasty (with or without stenting) or peripheral artery bypass graft surgery, postprocedure (off-label use): Oral: 75 to 100 mg once daily (ACCP [Guyatt, 2012]). **Note:** For below-knee bypass graft surgery with prosthetic grafts, combine with clopidogrel (ACCP [Guyatt, 2012]).

Preeclampsia prevention (women at risk) (off-label use): Oral: 75 to 100 mg once daily starting in the second trimester (ACCP [Guyatt, 2012]; USPSTF [LeFevre, 2014]) **or** 60 to 80 mg once daily beginning late in the first trimester (ACOG, 2013).

Primary prevention: Oral:

American College of Chest Physicians: Prevention of myocardial infarction and stroke: Select individuals ≥50 years of age (without symptomatic cardiovascular disease): 75 to 100 mg once daily (ACCP [Vandvik, 2012])

Prosthetic heart valve: Oral:

Bioprosthetic aortic valve (patient in normal sinus rhythm) (off-label use): 50 to 100 mg once daily; usual dose: 81 mg once daily. **Note:** If mitral bioprosthetic valve, oral anticoagulation with warfarin (instead of aspirin) is recommended for the first 3 months postoperatively, followed by aspirin alone (ACCP [Guyatt, 2012]).

Mechanical aortic or mitral valve (off-label use):

Low risk of bleeding: 50 to 100 mg once daily (in combination with warfarin) (ACCP [Guyatt, 2012])

History of thromboembolism while receiving oral anticoagulants: 75 to 100 mg once daily (in combination with warfarin) (Furie, 2011)

Transcatheter aortic bioprosthetic valve (off-label use): 50 to 100 mg once daily (in combination with clopidogrel) (ACCP [Guyatt, 2012])

Pregnant women, mechanical prosthesis or bioprosthesis (off-label use): 75 to 100 mg once daily during the second and third trimesters (when used for mechanical prosthetic valve, combine with warfarin) (AHA/ACC [Nishimura, 2014]).

Stroke/TIA: Oral:

Acute ischemic stroke/TIA: Initial: 160 to 325 mg within 48 hours of stroke/TIA onset, followed by 75 to 100 mg once daily (ACCP [Guyatt, 2012]). The AHA/ASA recommends an initial dose of 325 mg within 24 to 48 hours after stroke; do not administer aspirin within 24 hours after administration of alteplase (Jauch, 2013).

Cardioembolic, secondary prevention (oral anticoagulation unsuitable): 75 to 100 mg once daily (in combination with clopidogrel) (ACCP [Guyatt, 2012]; The ACTIVE Investigators [Connolly, 2009])

Cryptogenic with patent foramen ovale (PFO) or atrial septal aneurysm: 50 to 100 mg once daily (ACCP [Guyatt, 2012])

Noncardioembolic, secondary prevention: 75 to 325 mg once daily (Smith, 2011) **or** 75 to 100 mg once daily (ACCP [Guyatt, 2012]). **Note:** Combination aspirin/extended release dipyridamole or clopidogrel is preferred over aspirin alone (ACCP [Guyatt, 2012]).

Women at high risk, primary prevention: 81 mg once daily **or** 100 mg every other day (Goldstein, 2010)

Dosing adjustment in renal impairment: CrCl <10 mL/minute: Avoid use.

Hemodialysis: Dialyzable (50% to 100%)

Dosing adjustment in hepatic disease: Avoid use in severe liver disease.

Administration

Oral: Do not crush enteric coated tablet. Administer with food or a full glass of water to minimize GI distress. For acute myocardial infarction, have patient chew tablet.

Rectal: Remove suppository from plastic packet and insert into rectum as far as possible.

Reference Range Timing of serum samples: Peak levels usually occur 2 hours after ingestion. Salicylate serum concentrations correlate with the pharmacological actions and adverse effects observed. The serum salicylate concentration (mcg/mL) and the corresponding clinical correlations are as follows: See table.

Serum Salicylate: Clinical Correlations

Serum Salicylate Concentration (mcg/mL)	Desired Effects	Adverse Effects / Intoxication
~100	Antiplatelet Antipyresis Analgesia	GI intolerance and bleeding, hypersensitivity, hemostatic defects
150-300	Anti-inflammatory	Mild salicylism
250-400	Treatment of rheumatic fever	Nausea/vomiting, hyperventilation, salicylism, flushing, sweating, thirst, headache, diarrhea, and tachycardia
>400-500		Respiratory alkalosis, hemorrhage, excitement, confusion, asterixis, pulmonary edema, convulsions, tetany, metabolic acidosis, fever, coma, cardiovascular collapse, renal and respiratory failure

Dosage Forms

Caplet, oral: 500 mg

Ascriptin Maximum Strength [OTC]: 500 mg
Bayer Aspirin Extra Strength [OTC]: 500 mg
Bayer Genuine Aspirin [OTC]: 325 mg
Bayer Plus Extra Strength [OTC]: 500 mg
Bayer Women's Low Dose Aspirin [OTC]: 81 mg

Caplet, enteric coated, oral:

Bayer Aspirin Regimen Regular Strength [OTC]: 325 mg

Gum, chewing, oral:

Aspergum [OTC]: 227 mg (12s)

Suppository, rectal: 300 mg (12s); 600 mg (12s)

Tablet, oral: 325 mg

Ascriptin Regular Strength [OTC]: 325 mg
Aspercin [OTC]: 325 mg
Aspirtab [OTC]: 325 mg
Bayer Genuine Aspirin [OTC]: 325 mg
Buffasal [OTC]: 325 mg
Bufferin [OTC]: 325 mg
Bufferin Extra Strength [OTC]: 500 mg
Buffinol [OTC]: 324 mg
Tri-Buffered Aspirin [OTC]: 325 mg

Tablet, chewable, oral: 81 mg

Bayer Aspirin Regimen Children's [OTC]: 81 mg
St Joseph Adult Aspirin [OTC]: 81 mg

Tablet, enteric coated, oral: 81 mg, 325 mg, 650 mg
Aspir-low [OTC]: 81 mg
Bayer Aspirin Regimen Adult Low Strength [OTC]: 81 mg
Ecotrin [OTC]: 325 mg
Ecotrin Arthritis Strength [OTC]: 500 mg
Ecotrin Low Strength [OTC]: 81 mg
Halfprin [OTC]: 81 mg
St Joseph Adult Aspirin [OTC]: 81 mg

- **Aspirin, Acetaminophen, and Caffeine** *see* Acetaminophen, Aspirin, and Caffeine *on page 37*
- **Aspirin and Carisoprodol** *see* Carisoprodol and Aspirin *on page 364*

Aspirin and Diphenhydramine

(AS pir in & dye fen HYE dra meen)

Brand Names: U.S. Bayer® PM [OTC]

Index Terms ASA and Diphenhydramine; Aspirin and Diphenhydramine Citrate; Diphenhydramine and ASA; Diphenhydramine and Aspirin; Diphenhydramine Citrate and Aspirin

Pharmacologic Category Analgesic, Miscellaneous

Use Aid in the relief of insomnia accompanied by minor pain or headache

Dosage Oral: Children ≥12 years and Adults: Pain-associated insomnia: Two caplets (1000 mg aspirin/77 mg diphenhydramine citrate) at bedtime if needed or as directed by physician; do not exceed recommended dosage; not for use in children <12 years of age

Additional Information Complete prescribing information should be consulted for additional detail.

Dosage Forms

Caplet, oral:
Bayer® PM [OTC]: Aspirin 500 mg and diphenhydramine 38.3 mg

- **Aspirin and Diphenhydramine Citrate** *see* Aspirin and Diphenhydramine *on page 185*

Aspirin and Dipyridamole

(AS pir in & dye peer ID a mole)

Brand Names: U.S. Aggrenox®

Brand Names: Canada Aggrenox®

Index Terms Aspirin and Extended-Release Dipyridamole; Dipyridamole and Aspirin

Pharmacologic Category Antiplatelet Agent

Use Reduction in the risk of stroke in patients who have had transient ischemia of the brain or ischemic stroke due to thrombosis

Pregnancy Risk Factor D

Dosage Oral: Adults:
Stroke prevention: One capsule (dipyridamole 200 mg, aspirin 25 mg) twice daily
Alternative regimen for patients with intolerable headache: One capsule at bedtime and low-dose aspirin in the morning. Return to usual dose (1 capsule twice daily) as soon as tolerance to headache develops (usually within a week).
Carotid artery stenosis, symptomatic (including recent carotid endarterectomy) (off-label use): One capsule (dipyridamole 200 mg, aspirin 25 mg) twice daily (Guyatt, 2012)
Hemodialysis graft patency (off-label use): One capsule (dipyridamole 200 mg, aspirin 25 mg) twice daily

Dosage adjustment in renal impairment: Avoid use in patients with severe renal dysfunction (CrCl <10 mL/minute). Studies have not been done in patients with renal impairment.

Dosage adjustment in hepatic impairment: Avoid use in patients with severe hepatic impairment. Studies have not been done in patients with varying degrees of hepatic impairment.
Elderly: Plasma concentrations were 40% higher, but specific dosage adjustments have not been recommended.

Additional Information Complete prescribing information should be consulted for additional detail.

Dosage Forms

Capsule:
Aggrenox®: Aspirin 25 mg [immediate release] and dipyridamole 200 mg [extended release]

- **Aspirin and Extended-Release Dipyridamole** *see* Aspirin and Dipyridamole *on page 185*
- **Aspirin and Oxycodone** *see* Oxycodone and Aspirin *on page 1542*
- **Aspirin, Caffeine and Acetaminophen** *see* Acetaminophen, Aspirin, and Caffeine *on page 37*
- **Aspirin, Caffeine, and Butalbital** *see* Butalbital, Aspirin, and Caffeine *on page 314*
- **Aspirin, Caffeine, and Orphenadrine** *see* Orphenadrine, Aspirin, and Caffeine *on page 1522*
- **Aspirin, Carisoprodol, and Codeine** *see* Carisoprodol, Aspirin, and Codeine *on page 364*
- **Aspirin, Dihydrocodeine, and Caffeine** *see* Dihydrocodeine, Aspirin, and Caffeine *on page 632*
- **Aspirin Free Anacin Extra Strength [OTC]** *see* Acetaminophen *on page 32*
- **Aspirin, Orphenadrine, and Caffeine** *see* Orphenadrine, Aspirin, and Caffeine *on page 1522*
- **Aspir-low [OTC]** *see* Aspirin *on page 180*
- **Aspirtab [OTC]** *see* Aspirin *on page 180*
- **Astagraf XL** *see* Tacrolimus (Systemic) *on page 1962*
- **Astelin [DSC]** *see* Azelastine (Nasal) *on page 213*
- **Astelin (Can)** *see* Azelastine (Nasal) *on page 213*
- **Astepro** *see* Azelastine (Nasal) *on page 213*
- **Asthmanefrin Refill [OTC]** *see* EPINEPHrine (Systemic, Oral Inhalation) *on page 735*
- **Asthmanefrin Starter Kit [OTC]** *see* EPINEPHrine (Systemic, Oral Inhalation) *on page 735*
- **Astramorph** *see* Morphine (Systemic) *on page 1394*
- **AT** *see* Antithrombin *on page 156*
- **AT-III** *see* Antithrombin *on page 156*
- **Atacand** *see* Candesartan *on page 335*
- **Atacand HCT** *see* Candesartan and Hydrochlorothiazide *on page 338*
- **Atacand Plus (Can)** *see* Candesartan and Hydrochlorothiazide *on page 338*
- **Atarax (Can)** *see* HydrOXYzine *on page 1024*
- **Atasol (Can)** *see* Acetaminophen *on page 32*

Atazanavir (at a za NA veer)

Brand Names: U.S. Reyataz

Brand Names: Canada Reyataz

Index Terms Atazanavir Sulfate; ATV; BMS-232632

Pharmacologic Category Antiretroviral, Protease Inhibitor (Anti-HIV)

Use HIV-1 Infection: Treatment of HIV-1 infections in combination with other antiretroviral agents in patients ≥3 months weighing ≥10 kg
Limitations of use:
Not recommended for use in pediatric patients younger than 3 months due to the risk of kernicterus

Use in treatment-experienced patients should be guided by the number of baseline primary protease inhibitor resistance substitutions

Pregnancy Risk Factor B

Pregnancy Considerations Adverse events were not observed in animal reproduction studies. Atazanavir has a low level of transfer across the human placenta with cord blood concentrations reported as 13% to 21% of maternal serum concentrations at delivery. An increased risk of teratogenic effects has not been observed based on information collected by the antiretroviral pregnancy registry. A small increased risk of preterm birth has been associated with maternal use of protease inhibitor-based combination antiretroviral (ARV) therapy during pregnancy; however, the benefits of use generally outweigh this risk and protease inhibitors (PIs) should not be withheld if otherwise recommended. Hyperglycemia, new onset of diabetes mellitus, or diabetic ketoacidosis have been reported with PIs; it is not clear if pregnancy increases this risk. Hyperbilirubinemia or hypoglycemia may occur in neonates following *in utero* exposure to atazanavir, although data are conflicting.

The DHHS Perinatal HIV Guidelines recommend atazanavir as a preferred PI in antiretroviral-naive pregnant women when combined with low-dose ritonavir boosting. Pharmacokinetic studies suggest that standard dosing during pregnancy may provide decreased plasma concentrations and some experts recommend increased doses during the second and third trimesters. However, the manufacturer notes that dose adjustment is not required unless using concomitant H_2-receptor blockers or tenofovir or for ARV-naive pregnant women taking efavirenz. May give as once-daily dosing.

Regardless of CD4 count or HIV RNA copy number, all HIV-infected pregnant women should receive a combination antiretroviral (ARV) drug regimen. A combination of antepartum, intrapartum, and infant ARV prophylaxis is recommended. ARV therapy should be started as soon as possible in women with symptomatic infection. Although earlier initiation may be more effective in reducing the perinatal transmission of HIV, initiation may be delayed until after 12 weeks gestation in women who do not require immediate treatment after careful consideration of maternal conditions (eg, nausea and vomiting) and the potential risks of first trimester fetal exposure for specific agents. A scheduled cesarean delivery at 38 weeks gestation is recommended for all women with HIV RNA >1000 copies/mL or unknown concentrations near delivery in order to decrease transmission. If ARV therapy must be interrupted for <24 hours during the peripartum period, stop then restart all medications simultaneously in order to decrease the chance of developing resistance. Long-term follow-up is recommended for all infants exposed to ARV medications. In couples who want to conceive, the HIV-infected partner should attain maximum viral suppression prior to conception.

Healthcare providers are encouraged to enroll pregnant women exposed to antiretroviral medications in the Antiretroviral Pregnancy Registry (1-800-258-4263 or www.APRegistry.com). Healthcare providers caring for HIV-infected women and their infants may contact the National Perinatal HIV Hotline (888-448-8765) for clinical consultation (DHHS [perinatal], 2014).

Breast-Feeding Considerations Atazanavir is excreted into breast milk. Maternal or infant antiretroviral therapy does not completely eliminate the risk of postnatal HIV transmission. In addition, multiclass-resistant virus has been detected in breast-feeding infants despite maternal therapy. Therefore, in the United States, where formula is accessible, affordable, safe, and sustainable, and the risk of infant mortality due to diarrhea and respiratory infections is low, complete avoidance of breast-feeding by HIV-infected women is recommended to decrease potential transmission of HIV (DHHS [perinatal], 2014).

Contraindications

Hypersensitivity (eg, Stevens-Johnson syndrome, erythema multiforme, or toxic skin eruptions) to atazanavir or any component of the formulation; concurrent therapy with alfuzosin, cisapride, ergot derivatives (dihydroergotamine, ergonovine, ergotamine, methylergonovine), indinavir, irinotecan, lovastatin, midazolam (oral), nevirapine, pimozide, rifampin, sildenafil (when used for pulmonary artery hypertension [eg, Revatio]), simvastatin, St John's wort, or triazolam; coadministration with drugs that strongly induce CYP3A and may lead to lower atazanavir exposure and loss of efficacy.

Canadian labeling: Additional contraindications (not in U.S. labeling): Concomitant use of quinidine or bepridil (currently not marketed in Canada)

Warnings/Precautions Atazanavir may prolong PR interval; ECG monitoring should be considered in patients with preexisting conduction abnormalities or with medications which prolong AV conduction (dosage adjustment required with some agents); rare cases of second-degree AV block have been reported. May cause or exacerbate preexisting hepatic dysfunction; use caution in patients with transaminase elevations prior to therapy or underlying hepatic disease, such as hepatitis B or C or cirrhosis; monitor closely at baseline and during treatment. Not recommended in patients with severe hepatic impairment. In combination with ritonavir, is not recommended in patients with any degree of hepatic impairment.

Asymptomatic elevations in bilirubin (unconjugated) occur commonly during therapy with atazanavir; consider alternative therapy if bilirubin is >5 times ULN. Evaluate alternative etiologies if transaminase elevations also occur.

Cases of nephrolithiasis have been reported in postmarketing surveillance; temporary or permanent discontinuation of therapy should be considered if symptoms develop. Not recommended for use in treatment-experienced patients with end stage renal disease (ESRD) on hemodialysis.

Protease inhibitors have been associated with a variety of hypersensitivity events (some severe), including rash, anaphylaxis (rare), angioedema, bronchospasm, erythema multiforme, Stevens-Johnson syndrome (rare) and/or toxic skin eruptions (including DRESS [drug rash, eosinophilia and systemic symptoms] syndrome). It is generally recommended to discontinue treatment if severe rash or moderate symptoms accompanied by other systemic symptoms occur.

Use with caution in patients with hemophilia A or B; increased bleeding during protease inhibitor therapy has been reported. Changes in glucose tolerance, hyperglycemia, exacerbation of diabetes, DKA, and new-onset diabetes mellitus have been reported in patients receiving protease inhibitors. May be associated with fat redistribution (buffalo hump, increased abdominal girth, breast engorgement, facial atrophy). Immune reconstitution syndrome may develop resulting in the occurrence of an inflammatory response to an indolent or residual opportunistic infection during initial HIV treatment or activation of autoimmune disorders (eg, Graves' disease, polymyositis, Guillain-Barré syndrome) later in therapy; further evaluation and treatment may be required. Oral powder contains phenylalanine; avoid or use with caution in patients with phenylketonuria. Oral powder is not recommended for use in children <10 kg or ≥25 kg. Do not use in children <3 months of age due to potential for kernicterus. Potentially significant drug-drug interactions may exist, requiring dose or frequency adjustment, additional monitoring, and/or selection of alternative therapy.

Adverse Reactions Includes data from both treatment-naive and treatment-experienced patients; listed for adults unless otherwise specified.

Cardiovascular: First degree atrioventricular block, second degree atrioventricular block, peripheral edema

Central nervous system: Depression, dizziness, headache (more common in children), insomnia, peripheral neuropathy

Dermatologic: Skin rash (more common in adults)

Endocrine & metabolic: Hyperglycemia, hypoglycemia (children), increased amylase (children and adults), increased serum cholesterol (≥240 mg/dL), increased serum triglycerides

Gastrointestinal: Abdominal pain, diarrhea (more common in children), increased serum lipase (children and adults), nausea, vomiting (more common in children)

Hematologic & oncologic: Decreased hemoglobin (children and adults), neutropenia (more common in children), thrombocytopenia

Hepatic: Increased serum ALT (children and adults; more common in patients seropositive for hepatitis B and/or C), increased serum AST (more common in patients seropositive for hepatitis B and/or C), increased serum bilirubin (children and adults), jaundice

Neuromuscular & skeletal: Increased creatine phosphokinase, limb pain (children), myalgia

Respiratory: Cough (children), nasal congestion (children), oropharyngeal pain (children), rhinorrhea (children), wheezing (children)

Miscellaneous: Fever (more common in children)

Rare but important or life-threatening: Cholecystitis, cholelithiasis, cholestasis, complete atrioventricular block (rare), diabetes mellitus, DRESS syndrome, edema, erythema multiforme, immune reconstitution syndrome, interstitial nephritis, left bundle branch block, maculopapular rash, nephrolithiasis, pancreatitis, prolongation P-R interval on ECG, prolonged Q-T interval on ECG, Stevens-Johnson syndrome, torsades de pointes

Drug Interactions

Metabolism/Transport Effects Substrate of CYP3A4 (major); **Note:** Assignment of Major/Minor substrate status based on clinically relevant drug interaction potential; **Inhibits** CYP1A2 (weak), CYP2C8 (weak), CYP2C9 (weak), CYP3A4 (strong), UGT1A1

Avoid Concomitant Use

Avoid concomitant use of Atazanavir with any of the following: Ado-Trastuzumab Emtansine; Alfuzosin; Amiodarone; Apixaban; Astemizole; Avanafil; Axitinib; Belinostat; Bosutinib; Buprenorphine; Cabozantinib; Ceritinib; Cisapride; Conivaptan; Crizotinib; Dapoxetine; Dronedarone; Eplerenone; Ergot Derivatives; Everolimus; Fusidic Acid (Systemic); Halofantrine; Ibrutinib; Idelalisib; Indinavir; Irinotecan; Ivabradine; Lapatinib; Lercanidipine; Lomitapide; Lovastatin; Lurasidone; Macitentan; Midazolam; Naloxegol; Nevirapine; Nilotinib; Nisoldipine; Olaparib; PACLitaxel; Pimozide; QuiNIDine; Ranolazine; Red Yeast Rice; Regorafenib; Repaglinide; Rifampin; Rivaroxaban; Salmeterol; Silodosin; Simeprevir; Simvastatin; St Johns Wort; Suvorexant; Tamsulosin; Terfenadine; Ticagrelor; Tipranavir; Tolvaptan; Toremifene; Trabectedin; Triazolam; Ulipristal; Vemurafenib; VinCRIStine (Liposomal); Vorapaxar; Voriconazole

Increased Effect/Toxicity

Atazanavir may increase the levels/effects of: Ado-Trastuzumab Emtansine; Alfuzosin; Almotriptan; Alosetron; ALPRAZolam; Amiodarone; Apixaban; ARIPiprazole; Astemizole; AtorvaSTATin; Avanafil; Axitinib; Bedaquiline; Belinostat; Bortezomib; Bosentan; Bosutinib; Brentuximab Vedotin; Brinzolamide; Budesonide (Nasal); Budesonide (Systemic, Oral Inhalation); Buprenorphine; Cabazitaxel; Cabozantinib; Calcium Channel Blockers (Dihydropyridine); Calcium Channel Blockers (Nondihydropyridine); Cannabis; CarBAMazepine; Ceritinib; Cisapride; Clarithromycin; Colchicine; Conivaptan; Contraceptives (Progestins); Corticosteroids (Orally Inhaled); Corticosteroids (Systemic); Crizotinib; Cyclophosphamide; CycloSPORINE (Systemic); CYP3A4 Substrates; Dapoxetine; Dasatinib; Digoxin; DOXOrubicin (Conventional); Dronabinol; Dronedarone; Dutasteride; Eliglustat; Enfuvirtide; Eplerenone; Ergot Derivatives; Erlotinib; Etizolam; Etravirine; Everolimus; FentaNYL; Fesoterodine; Fluticasone (Nasal); Fluticasone (Oral Inhalation); Fluvastatin; GuanFACINE; Halofantrine; Highest Risk QTc-Prolonging Agents; Hydrocodone; Ibrutinib; Iloperidone; Imatinib; Imidafenacin; Indinavir; Irinotecan; Ivabradine; Ivacaftor; Ixabepilone; Lacosamide; Lapatinib; Lercanidipine; Levobupivacaine; Levomilnacipran; Lomitapide; Lovastatin; Lurasidone; Macitentan; Maraviroc; Meperidine; MethylPREDNISolone; Midazolam; Mifepristone; Moderate Risk QTc-Prolonging Agents; Naloxegol; Nefazodone; Nevirapine; Nilotinib; Nisoldipine; Olaparib; Ospemifene; OxyCODONE; PACLitaxel; Paricalcitol; PAZOPanib; Pimecrolimus; Pimozide; Pitavastatin; PONATinib; Pranlukast; PrednisoLONE (Systemic); PredniSONE; Propafenone; Protease Inhibitors; QUEtiapine; QuiNIDine; Ranolazine; Red Yeast Rice; Regorafenib; Repaglinide; Retapamulin; Rifabutin; Rilpivirine; Riociguat; Rivaroxaban; RomiDEPsin; Rosiglitazone; Rosuvastatin; Ruxolitinib; Salmeterol; Saxagliptin; Sildenafil; Silodosin; Simeprevir; Simvastatin; SORAfenib; Suvorexant; Tacrolimus (Systemic); Tacrolimus (Topical); Tadalafil; Tamsulosin; Temsirolimus; Tenofovir; Terfenadine; Tetrahydrocannabinol; Ticagrelor; Tofacitinib; Tolterodine; Tolvaptan; Toremifene; Trabectedin; TraZODone; Triazolam; Tricyclic Antidepressants; Ulipristal; Vardenafil; Vemurafenib; Vilazodone; VinCRIStine (Liposomal); Vorapaxar; Voriconazole; Warfarin; Zopiclone; Zuclopenthixol

The levels/effects of Atazanavir may be increased by: Clarithromycin; Conivaptan; CycloSPORINE (Systemic); CYP3A4 Inhibitors (Moderate); CYP3A4 Inhibitors (Strong); Delavirdine; Enfuvirtide; Fusidic Acid (Systemic); Idelalisib; Indinavir; Luliconazole; Mifepristone; Netupitant; Posaconazole; Simeprevir; Stiripentol; Telaprevir

Decreased Effect

Atazanavir may decrease the levels/effects of: Abacavir; Boceprevir; Clarithromycin; Contraceptives (Estrogens); Delavirdine; Didanosine; Disulfiram; Ifosfamide; LamoTRIgine; Meperidine; Prasugrel; Telaprevir; Ticagrelor; Valproic Acid and Derivatives; Voriconazole; Zidovudine

The levels/effects of Atazanavir may be decreased by: Antacids; Boceprevir; Bosentan; Buprenorphine; CarBAMazepine; CYP3A4 Inducers (Moderate); CYP3A4 Inducers (Strong); Dabrafenib; Deferasirox; Didanosine; Efavirenz; Etravirine; Garlic; H2-Antagonists; Minocycline; Mitotane; Nevirapine; Proton Pump Inhibitors; Rifampin; Siltuximab; St Johns Wort; Tenofovir; Tipranavir; Tocilizumab; Voriconazole

Food Interactions Bioavailability of atazanavir increased when taken with food. Management: Administer with food.

Preparation for Administration

Oral powder: It is preferable to mix oral powder with food such as applesauce or yogurt. Mixing oral powder with a beverage (eg, milk, infant formula, water) may be used for infants who can drink from a cup. For young infants (less than 6 months) who cannot eat solid food or drink from a cup, oral powder should be mixed with infant formula and given using an oral dosing syringe. Administration of atazanavir and infant formula using an infant bottle is not recommended because full dose may not be delivered.

Determine the number of packets (4 or 5 packets) needed. Mix with a small amount (one tablespoon) of soft food (preferred [eg, applesauce, yogurt]) or beverage (milk, formula, water). After administration, add an additional small amount of soft food or beverage to the container, mix, and feed the residual amount to insure that the entire dose has been consumed.

Storage/Stability

Store capsules at 25°C (77°F); excursions are permitted between 15°C and 30°C (59°F and 86°F).

Store oral powder below 30°C (86°F). Store oral powder in the original packet and do not open until ready to use. Once the oral powder is mixed with food or beverage, it may be kept at 20°C to 30°C (68°F to 86°F) for up to 1 hour prior to administration.

Mechanism of Action Binds to the site of HIV-1 protease activity and inhibits cleavage of viral Gag-Pol polyprotein precursors into individual functional proteins required for infectious HIV. This results in the formation of immature, noninfectious viral particles.

Pharmacodynamics/Kinetics

Absorption: Rapid; enhanced with food

Protein binding: 86%

Metabolism: Hepatic, via multiple pathways including CYP3A4; forms two metabolites (inactive)

Half-life elimination: Unboosted therapy: 7 to 8 hours; Boosted therapy (with ritonavir): 9 to 18 hours

Time to peak, plasma: 2 to 3 hours

Excretion: Feces (79%, 20% of total dose as unchanged drug); urine (13%, 7% of total dose as unchanged drug)

Dosage Treatment of HIV-1 infection: Oral:

Infants ≥3 months, Children, and Adolescents <18 years:

Antiretroviral-naive patients: Note: Ritonavir-boosted atazanavir dosing regimen is preferred:

Ritonavir-unboosted regimen:

Children 6 years to <13 years: Dose not established; use not recommended

Adolescents <40 kg **who are not able to tolerate ritonavir**: No dosage recommendations provided in the manufacturer's labeling.

Adolescents ≥40 kg **who are not able to tolerate ritonavir**: Atazanavir 400 mg once daily (without ritonavir). **Note:** Ritonavir-boosted atazanavir dosing regimen is preferred; data indicate that higher atazanavir dosing (ie, higher on a mg/kg or mg/m2 basis than predicted by adult dosing guidelines) may be needed when atazanavir is used without ritonavir boosting in children and adolescents (DHHS [pediatric], 2014).

Ritonavir-boosted regimen: **Note:** An increase to atazanavir 300 mg once daily for patients ≥35 kg, especially when given with tenofovir, may be considered (DHHS [pediatric] 2014)

Antiretroviral-naive and experienced patients:

Oral powder: Infants ≥3 months and Children weighing 10 kg to <25 kg:

10 to <15 kg: Atazanavir 200 mg (4 packets) **plus** ritonavir 80 mg once daily

15 to <25 kg: Atazanavir 250 mg (5 packets) **plus** ritonavir 80 mg once daily

Oral capsules: Children ≥6 years and Adolescents <18 years:

15 to <20 kg: Atazanavir 150 mg once daily **plus** ritonavir 100 mg once daily

20 to <40 kg: Atazanavir 200 mg once daily **plus** ritonavir 100 mg once daily

≥40 kg: Atazanavir 300 mg once daily **plus** ritonavir 100 mg once daily

Dosing adjustment for concomitant therapy: Antiretroviral-experienced or antiretroviral-naive patients: Coadministration with H_2 antagonists, proton pump inhibitors, or other antiretroviral agents (eg, efavirenz, tenofovir, didanosine):

Infants ≥3 months and Children weighing 10 kg to <25 kg: There are no specific atazanavir dosage adjustments provided in the manufacturer's labeling; refer to adult dosing for recommendations regarding the timing and maximum doses of concomitant proton pump inhibitors, H_2 antagonists, and other antiretroviral agents.

Infants ≥3 months and Children 6 to <13 years: Use not recommended.

Adolescents <40 kg: Use not recommended.

Adolescents ≥40 kg:

Ritonavir-unboosted regimen: Use not recommended.

Ritonavir-boosted regimen: Refer to adult dosing.

Adults:

Antiretroviral-naive patients: Atazanavir 300 mg once daily **plus** ritonavir 100 mg once daily **or** atazanavir 400 mg once daily in patients unable to tolerate ritonavir. **Note:** Recommended (with ritonavir) as a first-line therapy with tenofovir/emtricitabine in all nonpregnant antiretroviral-naive patients and with abacavir/lamivudine in nonpregnant antiretroviral-naive patients with pre-ART plasma HIV RNA <100,000 copies/mL who are HLA-B*5701 negative (DHHS [adult], 2013). Do not use tenofovir with unboosted atazanavir (DHHS [adult], 2014).

Antiretroviral-experienced patients: Atazanavir 300 mg once daily **plus** ritonavir 100 mg once daily. **Note:** Atazanavir without ritonavir is not recommended in antiretroviral-experienced patients with prior virologic failure.

Pregnant patients, antiretroviral-naive or -experienced: Atazanavir 300 mg once daily **plus** ritonavir 100 mg once daily. **Note:** Preferred regimen for pregnant patients who are antiretroviral-naive (DHHS [perinatal], 2014). Postpartum dosage adjustment not needed. Observe patient for adverse events, especially within 2 months after delivery. Dose adjustments required for treatment-experienced patients during their second and third trimester if concomitant tenofovir *or* H_2 antagonist use (insufficient information for dose adjustment if *both* tenofovir and an H_2 antagonist are used). Some experts recommend atazanavir 400 mg plus ritonavir 100 mg in all pregnant women during the second and third trimesters due to decreased plasma concentrations (DHHS [perinatal], 2014).

Dosage adjustments for concomitant therapy:

Coadministration with efavirenz:

Antiretroviral-naive patients: Atazanavir 400 mg plus ritonavir 100 mg given with efavirenz 600 mg (all once daily but administered at different times; atazanavir and ritonavir with food and efavirenz on an empty stomach).

Antiretroviral-experienced patients: Concurrent use not recommended due to decreased atazanavir exposure.

Coadministration with didanosine buffered or enteric-coated formulations: Administer atazanavir 2 hours before or 1 hour after didanosine buffered or enteric coated formulations

Coadministration with H_2 antagonists:

Antiretroviral-naive patients: Atazanavir 300 mg plus ritonavir 100 mg given simultaneously with, or at least 10 hours after an H_2 antagonist equivalent dose of ≤80 mg famotidine/day

Patients unable to tolerate ritonavir: Atazanavir 400 mg once daily given at least 2 hours before or at least 10 hours after an H_2 antagonist equivalent daily dose of ≤40 mg famotidine (single dose ≤20 mg)

Antiretroviral-experienced patients: Atazanavir 300 mg plus ritonavir 100 mg given simultaneously with, or at least 10 hours after an H_2 antagonist equivalent dose of ≤40 mg famotidine/day

Antiretroviral-experienced pregnant patients in the second or third trimester: Atazanavir 400 mg plus ritonavir 100 mg simultaneously with, or at least 10 hours after an H_2 antagonist. **Note:** Insufficient information for dose adjustment if tenofovir **and** an H_2 antagonist are used.

Coadministration with proton pump inhibitors:

U.S. labeling:

Antiretroviral-naive patients: Atazanavir 300 mg plus ritonavir 100 mg given 12 hours after a proton pump inhibitor equivalent dose of ≤20 mg omeprazole/day

Antiretroviral-experienced patients: Concurrent use not recommended. (**Note:** One study noted adequate serum concentrations when atazanavir 400 mg plus ritonavir 100 mg was given at the same time or 12 hours after omeprazole 20 mg.)

Canadian labeling: Concurrent use is not recommended; however, if unavoidable, administer atazanavir 400 mg plus ritonavir 100 mg once daily with proton pump inhibitor equivalent dose of ≤20 mg omeprazole/day. **Note:** Manufacturer labeling does not specify patient population (antiretroviral- naive and/or experienced) to which dosing recommendation applies.

Coadministration with tenofovir:

Antiretroviral-naive patients: Atazanavir 300 mg plus ritonavir 100 mg given with tenofovir 300 mg (all as a single daily dose)

Antiretroviral-experienced patients: Atazanavir 300 mg plus ritonavir 100 mg given with tenofovir 300 mg (all as a single daily dose); if H_2 antagonist coadministered (not to exceed equivalent daily dose of ≤40 mg famotidine), increase atazanavir to 400 mg (plus ritonavir 100 mg) once daily

Antiretroviral-experienced pregnant patients in the second or third trimester: Atazanavir 400 mg plus ritonavir 100 mg. **Note:** Insufficient information for dose adjustment if tenofovir **and** an H_2 antagonist are used

Dosage adjustment in renal impairment:

End stage renal disease (ESRD) not on intermittent hemodialysis (IHD): No dosage adjustment necessary

ESRD receiving IHD:

Antiretroviral-naive patients: Use boosted therapy of atazanavir 300 mg with ritonavir 100 mg once daily

Antiretroviral-experienced patients: Not recommended

Dosage adjustment in hepatic impairment:

Atazanavir:

Mild-to-moderate hepatic insufficiency: Use with caution; if moderate insufficiency (Child-Pugh class B) and no prior virologic failure, reduce dose to 300 mg once daily.

Severe hepatic insufficiency (Child-Pugh class C): Not recommended

Note: Patients with underlying hepatitis B or C may be at increased risk of hepatic decompensation.

Atazanavir/ritonavir: Use not recommended in hepatic impairment (has not been studied).

Dietary Considerations Must be taken with food; enhances absorption.

Administration Administer with food. Administer atazanavir 2 hours before or 1 hour after didanosine buffered formulations, didanosine enteric-coated capsules, other buffered medications, or antacids. Administer atazanavir (with ritonavir) simultaneously with, or at least 10 hours after, H_2-receptor antagonists; administer atazanavir (without ritonavir) at least 2 hours before or at least 10 hours after H_2-receptor antagonist. Administer atazanavir (with ritonavir) 12 hours after proton pump inhibitor.

Additional formulation specific information:

Oral capsules: Swallow capsules whole, do not open.

Oral powder: Mixing with food: Using a spoon, mix the recommended number of oral powder packets with a minimum of one tablespoon of food (such as applesauce or yogurt) in a small container. Feed the mixture to the infant or young child. Add an additional one tablespoon of food to the container, mix, and feed the child the residual mixture.

Mixing with a beverage such as milk or water in a small drinking cup: Using a spoon, mix the recommended number of oral powder packets with a minimum of 30 mL of the beverage in a drinking cup. Have the child drink the mixture. Add an additional 15 mL more of beverage to the cup, mix, and have the child drink the residual mixture. If water is used, food should also be taken at the same time.

Mixing with liquid infant formula using an oral dosing syringe and a small medicine cup: Using a spoon, mix the recommended number of oral powder packets with 10 mL of prepared liquid infant formula in the medicine cup. Draw up the full amount of the mixture into an oral syringe and administer into either right or left inner cheek of infant. Pour another 10 mL of formula into the medicine cup to rinse off remaining oral powder in cup. Draw up residual mixture into the syringe and administer into either right or left inner cheek of infant.

Administer the entire dosage of oral powder (mixed in the food or beverage) within one hour of preparation (may leave the mixture at room temperature during this one hour period). Ensure that the patient eats or drinks all the food or beverage that contains the powder. Additional food may be given after consumption of the entire mixture. Administer ritonavir immediately following oral powder administration.

Monitoring Parameters Viral load, CD4, serum glucose; liver function tests, bilirubin, drug levels (with certain concomitant medications), ECG monitoring in patients with preexisting prolonged PR interval or with concurrent AV nodal blocking drugs

Additional Information A listing of medications that should not be used concurrently is available with each bottle and patients should be provided with this information.

Dosage Forms

Capsule, Oral:

Reyataz: 150 mg, 200 mg, 300 mg

Packet, Oral:

Reyataz: 50 mg (30 ea)

◆ **Atazanavir Sulfate** *see* Atazanavir *on page 185*

◆ **Atelvia** *see* Risedronate *on page 1816*

Atenolol (a TEN oh lole)

Brand Names: U.S. Tenormin

Brand Names: Canada Apo-Atenol; Ava-Atenolol; CO Atenolol; Dom-Atenolol; JAMP-Atenolol; Mint-Atenolol; Mylan-Atenolol; Nu-Atenol; PMS-Atenolol; RAN-Atenolol; ratio-Atenolol; Riva-Atenolol; Sandoz-Atenolol; Septa-Atenolol; Tenormin; Teva-Atenolol

Pharmacologic Category Antianginal Agent; Antihypertensive; Beta-Blocker, Beta-1 Selective

Use Treatment of hypertension, alone or in combination with other agents; management of angina pectoris; secondary prevention postmyocardial infarction

The 2014 guideline for the management of high blood pressure in adults (Eighth Joint National Committee [JNC 8]) recommends initiation of pharmacologic treatment to lower blood pressure for the following patients (JNC8 [James, 2013]):

- Patients ≥60 years of age with systolic blood pressure (SBP) ≥150 mm Hg or diastolic blood pressure (DBP) ≥90 mm Hg. Goal of therapy is SBP <150 mm Hg and DBP <90 mm Hg.
- Patients <60 years of age with SBP ≥140 mm Hg or DBP is ≥90 mm Hg. Goal of therapy is SBP <140 mm Hg and DBP <90 mm Hg.
- Patients ≥18 years of age with diabetes and SBP ≥140 mm Hg or DBP ≥90 mm Hg. Goal of therapy is SBP <140 mm Hg and DBP <90 mm Hg.
- Patients ≥18 years of age with chronic kidney disease (CKD) and SBP ≥140 mm Hg or DBP ≥90 mm Hg. Goal of therapy is SBP <140 mm Hg and DBP <90 mm Hg.

In patients with CKD, regardless of race or diabetes status, the use of an ACE inhibitor (ACEI) or angiotensin receptor blocker (ARB) as initial therapy is recommended to improve kidney outcomes. In the general nonblack population (without CKD) including those with diabetes, initial antihypertensive treatment should consist of a thiazide-type diuretic, calcium channel blocker, ACEI, or ARB. In the general black population (without CKD) including those with diabetes, initial antihypertensive treatment should consist of a thiazide-type diuretic or a calcium channel blocker **instead of** an ACEI or ARB.

Pregnancy Risk Factor D

Pregnancy Considerations Studies in pregnant women have demonstrated a risk to the fetus; therefore, the manufacturer classifies atenolol as pregnancy category D. Atenolol crosses the placenta and is found in cord blood. In a cohort study, an increased risk of cardiovascular defects was observed following maternal use of beta-blockers during pregnancy. Intrauterine growth restriction (IUGR), small placentas, as well as fetal/neonatal bradycardia, hypoglycemia, and/or respiratory depression have been observed following *in utero* exposure to beta-blockers as a class. Adequate facilities for monitoring infants at birth should be available. Untreated chronic maternal hypertension and pre-eclampsia are also associated with adverse events in the fetus, infant, and mother. The maternal pharmacokinetic parameters of atenolol during the second and third trimesters are within the ranges reported in nonpregnant patients. Although atenolol has shown efficacy in the treatment of hypertension in pregnancy, it is not the drug of choice due to potential IUGR in the infant.

Breast-Feeding Considerations Atenolol is excreted in breast milk and has been detected in the serum and urine of nursing infants. Peak concentrations in breast milk have been reported to occur between 2 to 8 hours after the maternal dose and in some cases are higher than the peak maternal serum concentration. Although most studies have not reported adverse events in nursing infants, avoiding maternal use while nursing infants with renal dysfunction or infants <44 weeks postconceptual age has been suggested. Beta-blockers with less distribution into breast milk may be preferred. The manufacturer recommends that caution be exercised when administering atenolol to nursing women.

Contraindications Hypersensitivity to atenolol or any component of the formulation; sinus bradycardia; sinus node dysfunction; heart block greater than first-degree (except in patients with a functioning artificial pacemaker); cardiogenic shock; uncompensated cardiac failure; pulmonary edema; pregnancy

Warnings/Precautions Consider preexisting conditions such as sick sinus syndrome before initiating. Administer cautiously in compensated heart failure and monitor for a worsening of the condition (efficacy of atenolol in heart failure has not been established). **[U.S. Boxed Warning]: Beta-blocker therapy should not be withdrawn abruptly (particularly in patients with CAD), but gradually tapered to avoid acute tachycardia, hypertension, and/or ischemia.** Beta-blockers without alpha1-adrenergic receptor blocking activity should be avoided in patients with Prinzmetal variant angina (Mayer, 1998). Chronic beta-blocker therapy should not be routinely withdrawn prior to major surgery. Beta-blockers should be avoided in patients with bronchospastic disease (asthma). Atenolol, with B_1 selectivity, has been used cautiously in bronchospastic disease with close monitoring. May precipitate or aggravate symptoms of arterial insufficiency in patients with PVD and Raynaud's disease; use with caution and monitor for progression of arterial obstruction. Use cautiously in patients with diabetes - may mask hypoglycemic symptoms. May mask signs of hyperthyroidism (eg, tachycardia); use caution if hyperthyroidism is suspected, abrupt withdrawal may precipitate thyroid storm. Alterations in thyroid function tests may be observed. Use cautiously in the renally impaired (dosage adjustment required). Caution in myasthenia gravis or psychiatric disease (may cause CNS depression). Bradycardia may be observed more frequently in elderly patients (>65 years of age); dosage reductions may be necessary. Adequate alpha-blockade is required prior to use of any beta-blocker for patients with untreated pheochromocytoma. May induce or exacerbate psoriasis. Use caution with history of severe anaphylaxis to allergens; patients taking beta-blockers may become more sensitive to repeated challenges. Treatment of anaphylaxis (eg, epinephrine) in patients taking beta-blockers may be ineffective or promote undesirable effects. Use with caution in patients on concurrent digoxin, verapamil, or diltiazem; bradycardia or heart block can occur. Use with caution in patients receiving inhaled anesthetic agents known to depress myocardial contractility.

Adverse Reactions

Cardiovascular: Bradycardia (persistent), cardiac failure, chest pain, cold extremities, complete atrioventricular block, edema, hypotension, Raynaud's phenomenon, second degree atrioventricular block

Central nervous system: Confusion, decreased mental acuity, depression, dizziness, fatigue, headache, insomnia, lethargy, nightmares

Gastrointestinal: Constipation, diarrhea, nausea

Genitourinary: Impotence

Rare but important or life-threatening: Alopecia, dyspnea (especially with large doses), hallucination, increased liver enzymes, lupus-like syndrome, Peyronie's disease, positive ANA titer, psoriasiform eruption, psychosis, thrombocytopenia, wheezing

Drug Interactions

Metabolism/Transport Effects None known.

Avoid Concomitant Use

Avoid concomitant use of Atenolol with any of the following: Ceritinib; Floctafenine; Methacholine

Increased Effect/Toxicity

Atenolol may increase the levels/effects of: Alpha-/Beta-Agonists (Direct-Acting); Alpha1-Blockers; Alpha2-Agonists; Amifostine; Antihypertensives; Bradycardia-Causing Agents; Bupivacaine; Cardiac Glycosides; Ceritinib; Cholinergic Agonists; Disopyramide; DULoxetine; Ergot Derivatives; Fingolimod; Grass Pollen Allergen Extract (5 Grass Extract); Hypotensive Agents; Insulin; Lacosamide; Levodopa; Lidocaine (Systemic); Lidocaine (Topical); Mepivacaine; Methacholine; Midodrine; Obinutuzumab; RisperiDONE; RiTUXimab; Sulfonylureas

The levels/effects of Atenolol may be increased by: Acetylcholinesterase Inhibitors; Alpha2-Agonists; Amiodarone; Anilidopiperidine Opioids; Barbiturates; Bretylium; Brimonidine (Topical); Calcium Channel Blockers (Dihydropyridine); Calcium Channel Blockers (Nondihydropyridine); Diazoxide; Dipyridamole; Disopyramide; Dronedarone; Floctafenine; Glycopyrrolate; Herbs (Hypotensive Properties); MAO Inhibitors; Nicorandil; Pentoxifylline; Phosphodiesterase 5 Inhibitors; Prostacyclin Analogues; Regorafenib; Reserpine; Tofacitinib

Decreased Effect

Atenolol may decrease the levels/effects of: Beta2-Agonists; Theophylline Derivatives

The levels/effects of Atenolol may be decreased by: Ampicillin; Herbs (Hypertensive Properties); Methylphenidate; Nonsteroidal Anti-Inflammatory Agents; Yohimbine

Food Interactions Atenolol serum concentrations may be decreased if taken with food. Management: Administer without regard to meals.

Storage/Stability Store at 20°C to 25°C (68°F to 77°F).

Mechanism of Action Competitively blocks response to beta-adrenergic stimulation, selectively blocks $beta_1$-receptors with little or no effect on $beta_2$-receptors except at high doses

Pharmacodynamics/Kinetics

Onset of action: Peak effect: Oral: 2 to 4 hours

Duration: Normal renal function: 12 to 24 hours

Absorption: Oral: Rapid, incomplete (~50%)

Distribution: Low lipophilicity; does not cross blood-brain barrier

Protein binding: 6% to 16%

Metabolism: Limited hepatic

Half-life elimination: Beta:

Neonates: ≤35 hours; Mean: 16 hours

Children: 4.6 hours; children >10 years may have longer half-life (>5 hours) compared to children 5 to 10 years (<5 hours)

Adults: Normal renal function: 6 to 7 hours, prolonged with renal impairment; End-stage renal disease: 15 to 35 hours

Time to peak, plasma: Oral: 2 to 4 hours

Excretion: Feces (50%); urine (40% as unchanged drug)

Dosage Oral:

Children: Hypertension: 0.5 to 1 mg/kg/dose given daily; range of 0.5 to 1.5 mg/kg/day; maximum dose: 2 mg/kg/day up to 100 mg daily

Adults:

Hypertension: Initial: 25 to 50 mg once daily; after 1 to 2 weeks, may increase to 100 mg once daily; usual dose (ASH/ISH [Weber, 2014]): 100 mg once daily; target dose (JNC 8 [James, 2013]): 100 mg once daily. Doses >100 mg are unlikely to produce any further benefit.

Angina pectoris: 50 mg once daily, may increase to 100 mg/day. Some patients may require 200 mg daily.

Postmyocardial infarction: 100 mg daily or 50 mg twice daily for 6 to 9 days postmyocardial infarction.

Atrial fibrillation (rate control) (off-label use): Usual maintenance dose: 25 to 100 mg once daily (AHA/ACC/HRS [January, 2014])

Thyrotoxicosis (off-label use): 25 to 100 mg once or twice daily (Bahn, 2011)

Elderly: Hypertension: Consider lower initial doses and titrate to response (Aronow, 2011).

Dosage adjustment in renal impairment:

CrCl >35 mL/minute/1.73 m^2: No dosage adjustment necessary.

CrCl 15 to 35 mL/minute/1.73 m^2: Maximum dose: 50 mg daily

CrCl <15 mL/minute/1.73 m^2: Maximum dose: 25 mg daily

Hemodialysis: Moderately dialyzable (20% to 50%) via hemodialysis; administer dose postdialysis or administer 25 to 50 mg supplemental dose.

Peritoneal dialysis: Elimination is not enhanced; supplemental dose is not necessary.

Dosage adjustment in hepatic impairment: There are no dosage adjustments provided in the manufacturer's labeling; however, atenolol undergoes minimal hepatic metabolism.

Dietary Considerations May be taken without regard to meals.

Administration When administered acutely for cardiac treatment, monitor ECG and blood pressure. May be administered without regard to meals.

Monitoring Parameters Acute cardiac treatment: Monitor ECG and blood pressure

Dosage Forms

Tablet, Oral:

Tenormin: 25 mg, 50 mg, 100 mg

Generic: 25 mg, 50 mg, 100 mg

Extemporaneous Preparations A 2 mg/mL oral suspension may be made with tablets. Crush four 50 mg tablets in a mortar and reduce to a fine powder. Add a small amount of glycerin and mix to a uniform paste. Mix while adding Ora-Sweet® SF vehicle in incremental proportions to **almost** 100 mL; transfer to a calibrated bottle, rinse mortar with vehicle, and add quantity of vehicle sufficient to make 100 mL. Label "shake well" and "refrigerate". Stable for 90 days.

Nahata MC, Pai VB, and Hipple TF, *Pediatric Drug Formulations*, 5th ed, Cincinnati, OH: Harvey Whitney Books Co, 2004.

- **ATG** *see* Antithymocyte Globulin (Equine) *on page 157*
- **Atgam** *see* Antithymocyte Globulin (Equine) *on page 157*
- **Athletes Foot Spray [OTC]** *see* Tolnaftate *on page 2063*
- **Ativan** *see* LORazepam *on page 1243*
- **Atlizumab** *see* Tocilizumab *on page 2057*
- **ATNAA** *see* Atropine and Pralidoxime *on page 203*

AtoMOXetine (AT oh mox e teen)

Brand Names: U.S. Strattera

Brand Names: Canada Apo-Atomoxetine; DOM-Atomoxetine; Mylan-Atomoxetine; PMS-Atomoxetine; RIVA-Atomoxetine; Sandoz-Atomoxetine; Strattera; Teva-Atomoxetine

Index Terms Atomoxetine Hydrochloride; LY139603; Methylphenoxy-Benzene Propanamine; Tomoxetine

Pharmacologic Category Norepinephrine Reuptake Inhibitor, Selective

Use Attention deficit hyperactivity disorder: Treatment of attention deficit hyperactivity disorder (ADHD)

Pregnancy Risk Factor C

Pregnancy Considerations Adverse events have been observed in animal reproduction studies. Information related to atomoxetine use in pregnancy is limited; appropriate contraception is recommended for sexually active women of childbearing potential (Heiligenstein, 2003).

Breast-Feeding Considerations It is not known if atomoxetine is excreted in breast milk. The manufacturer recommends that caution be exercised when administering atomoxetine to nursing women.

Contraindications Hypersensitivity to atomoxetine or any component of the formulation; use with or within 14 days of MAO inhibitors; narrow-angle glaucoma; current or past history of pheochromocytoma; severe cardiac or vascular disorders in which the condition would be expected to deteriorate with clinically important increases in blood pressure (eg, 15 to 20 mm Hg) or heart rate (eg, 20 beats/minute).

Canadian labeling: Additional contraindications (not in U.S. labeling): Symptomatic cardiovascular diseases, moderate-to-severe hypertension; advanced arteriosclerosis; uncontrolled hyperthyroidism

Warnings/Precautions [U.S. Boxed Warning]: Use caution in pediatric patients; may be an increased risk of suicidal ideation. Closely monitor for clinical worsening, suicidality, or unusual changes in behavior; especially during the initial few months of a course of drug therapy, or at times of dose changes, either increases or decreases. The family or caregiver should be instructed to closely observe the patient and communicate condition with healthcare provider. New or worsening symptoms of hostility or aggressive behaviors have been associated with atomoxetine, particularly with the initiation of therapy. Treatment-emergent psychotic or manic symptoms (eg, hallucinations, delusional thinking, mania) may occur in children and adolescents without a prior history of psychotic illness or mania; consider discontinuation of treatment if symptoms occur. Use caution in patients with comorbid bipolar disorder; therapy may induce mixed/manic episode. Atomoxetine is not approved for major depressive disorder. Patients presenting with depressive symptoms should be screened for bipolar disorder. Recommended to be used as part of a comprehensive treatment program for attention deficit disorders. Atomoxetine does not worsen anxiety in patients with existing anxiety disorders or tics related to Tourette's disorder.

Use caution with hepatic disease (dosage adjustments necessary in moderate and severe hepatic impairment). Use may be associated with rare but severe hepatotoxicity, including hepatic failure; discontinue and do not restart if signs or symptoms of hepatotoxic reaction (eg, jaundice, pruritus, flu-like symptoms, dark urine, right upper quadrant tenderness) or laboratory evidence of liver disease are noted. Use caution in patients who are poor metabolizers of CYP2D6 metabolized drugs ("poor metabolizers"), bioavailability increases; dosage adjustments are recommended in patients known to be CYP2D6 poor metabolizers.

Orthostasis can occur; use caution in patients predisposed to hypotension or those with abrupt changes in heart rate or blood pressure. Atomoxetine has been associated with serious cardiovascular events including sudden death in patients with preexisting structural cardiac abnormalities or other serious heart problems (sudden death in children and adolescents; sudden death, stroke, and MI in adults). Atomoxetine should be avoided in patients with known serious structural cardiac abnormalities, cardiomyopathy, serious heart rhythm abnormalities, or other serious cardiac problems that could increase the risk of sudden death that these conditions alone carry. Patients should be carefully evaluated for cardiac disease prior to initiation of therapy. Perform a prompt cardiac evaluation in patients who develop symptoms of exertional chest pain, unexplained syncope, or other symptoms suggestive of cardiac disease during treatment. May cause increased heart rate or blood pressure; use caution with hypertension or other cardiovascular or cerebrovascular disease; CYP2D6 poor metabolizers may experience greater increases in blood pressure and heart rate effects. Use caution in patients with a history of urinary retention or bladder outlet obstruction; may cause urinary retention/hesitancy; use caution in patients with history of urinary retention or bladder outlet obstruction. Prolonged and painful erections (priapism), sometimes requiring surgical intervention, have been reported with stimulant and atomoxetine use in pediatric and adult patients. Priapism has been reported to develop after some time on the drug, often subsequent to an increase in dose and also during a period of drug withdrawal (drug holidays or discontinuation). Patients with certain hematological dyscrasias (eg, sickle cell disease), malignancies, perineal trauma, or concomitant use of alcohol, illicit drugs, or other medications associated with priapism may be at increased risk. Patients who develop abnormally sustained or frequent and painful erections should discontinue therapy and seek immediate medical attention. An emergent urological consultation should be obtained in severe cases. Use has been associated with different dosage forms and products; it is not known if rechallenge with a different formulation will risk recurrence. Avoidance of stimulants and atomoxetine may be preferred in patients with severe cases that were slow to resolve and/or required detumescence (Eiland, 2014). Allergic reactions (including anaphylactic reactions, angioneurotic edema, urticaria, and rash) may occur (rare).

Growth in pediatric patients should be monitored during treatment. Height and weight gain may be reduced during the first 9 to 12 months of treatment, but should recover by 3 years of therapy.

Adverse Reactions

Cardiovascular: Cold extremities, flushing, increased diastolic blood pressure, orthostatic hypotension, palpitations, syncope, systolic hypertension, tachycardia

Central nervous system: Abnormal dreams, agitation, anxiety, chills, depression, disturbed sleep, dizziness, drowsiness, emotional lability, fatigue, headache, insomnia, irritability, jitteriness, paresthesia (higher in adults; postmarketing observation in children), restlessness

Dermatologic: Excoriation, hyperhidrosis, skin rash

Endocrine & metabolic: Decreased libido, hot flash, increased thirst, menstrual disease, weight loss

Gastrointestinal: Abdominal pain, anorexia, constipation, decreased appetite, diarrhea, dysgeusia, dyspepsia, flatulence, nausea, vomiting, xerostomia

Genitourinary: Dysmenorrhea, dysuria, ejaculatory disorder, erectile dysfunction, orgasm abnormal, pollakiuria, prostatitis, urinary frequency, urinary retention

Neuromuscular & skeletal: Back pain, muscle spasm, tremor, weakness

Ophthalmic: Blurred vision, conjunctivitis, mydriasis

Respiratory: Oropharyngeal pain, pharyngolaryngeal pain, sinus headache

Miscellaneous: Therapeutic response unexpected

Rare but important or life-threatening: Aggressive behavior, allergy disorder, anaphylaxis, angioedema, cerebrovascular accident, delusions, growth suppression (children), hallucination, hepatotoxicity, hostility, hypersensitivity reaction, hypomania, impulsivity, jaundice, mania, myocardial infarction, panic attack, pelvic pain, peripheral vascular disease, priapism, prolonged Q-T interval on ECG, Raynaud's phenomenon, seizure (including patients with no prior history or known risk factors for seizure), severe hepatic disease, suicidal ideation, testicular pain, tics

Drug Interactions

Metabolism/Transport Effects Substrate of CYP2C19 (minor), CYP2D6 (major); **Note:** Assignment of Major/Minor substrate status based on clinically relevant drug interaction potential; **Inhibits** CYP2D6 (weak), CYP3A4 (weak)

Avoid Concomitant Use

Avoid concomitant use of AtoMOXetine with any of the following: Iobenguane I 123; MAO Inhibitors; Pimozide

Increased Effect/Toxicity

AtoMOXetine may increase the levels/effects of: ARIPiprazole; Beta2-Agonists; Dofetilide; Hydrocodone; Lomitapide; Pimozide; Sympathomimetics

The levels/effects of AtoMOXetine may be increased by: Abiraterone Acetate; Cobicistat; CYP2D6 Inhibitors (Moderate); CYP2D6 Inhibitors (Strong); Darunavir; MAO Inhibitors; Peginterferon Alfa-2b

Decreased Effect

AtoMOXetine may decrease the levels/effects of: Iobenguane I 123

The levels/effects of AtoMOXetine may be decreased by: Peginterferon Alfa-2b

Storage/Stability Store at 25°C (77°F); excursions are permitted between 15°C and 30°C (59°F and 86°F).

Mechanism of Action Selectively inhibits the reuptake of norepinephrine (Ki 4.5 nM) with little to no activity at the other neuronal reuptake pumps or receptor sites.

Pharmacodynamics/Kinetics

Absorption: Rapid

Distribution: V_d: IV: 0.85 L/kg

Protein binding: 98%, primarily albumin

Metabolism: Hepatic, via CYP2D6 and CYP2C19; forms metabolites (4-hydroxyatomoxetine, active, equipotent to atomoxetine; N-desmethylatomoxetine, limited activity)

Bioavailability: 63% in extensive metabolizers; 94% in poor metabolizers

Half-life elimination: Atomoxetine: 5 hours (up to 24 hours in poor metabolizers); Active metabolites: 4-hydroxyatomoxetine: 6-8 hours; N-desmethylatomoxetine: 6-8 hours (34-40 hours in poor metabolizers)

Time to peak, plasma: 1-2 hours

Excretion: Urine (80%, as conjugated 4-hydroxy metabolite); feces (17%)

Dosage Oral: **Note:** Atomoxetine may be discontinued without the need for tapering dose.

ADHD treatment:

U.S. labeling:

Children ≥6 years and ≤70 kg:

Initial: 0.5 mg/kg/day, increase after minimum of 3 days to ~1.2 mg/kg/day; may administer as either a single daily dose or 2 evenly divided doses in morning and late afternoon/early evening. Maximum daily dose: 1.4 mg/kg or 100 mg, whichever is less.

Dosage adjustment in patients receiving strong CYP2D6 inhibitors (eg, paroxetine, fluoxetine, quinidine) or patients known to be CYP2D6 poor metabolizers: Initial: 0.5 mg/kg/day; if tolerating therapy but inadequate response, may increase after minimum of 4 weeks to 1.2 mg/kg/day.

Children ≥6 years and >70 kg and Adults:

Initial: 40 mg/day, increased after minimum of 3 days to ~80 mg/day; may administer as either a single daily dose or two evenly divided doses in morning and late afternoon/early evening. May increase to 100 mg/day in 2-4 additional weeks to achieve optimal response. Maximum daily dose: 100 mg/day.

Dosage adjustment in patients receiving strong CYP2D6 inhibitors (eg, paroxetine, fluoxetine, quinidine) or patients known to be CYP2D6 poor metabolizers: Initial: 40 mg/day; if tolerating therapy but inadequate response, may increase after minimum of 4 weeks to 80 mg/day.

Canadian labeling:

Children ≥6 years and ≤70 kg:

Initial: ~0.5 mg/kg/day for 7-14 days (Step 1); if tolerated, may increase to ~0.8 mg/kg/day for 7-14 days (Step 2), then to ~1.2 mg/kg/day (Step 3); reevaluate after ≥30 days and adjust for response if necessary. Maximum daily dose: 1.4 mg/kg or 100 mg, whichever is less. **Note:** Children should weigh at least 20 kg at the time of initiation as 10 mg is the lowest available capsule strength and capsules are to be swallowed whole.

Dosing recommendations according to weight:

Initial (Step 1):

20-29 kg: 10 mg/day

30-44 kg: 18 mg/day

45-64 kg: 25 mg/day

65-70 kg: 40 mg/day

First titration (Step 2):

20-29 kg: 18 mg/day

30-44 kg: 25 mg/day

45-64 kg: 40 mg/day

65-70 kg: 60 mg/day

Second titration (Step 3):

20-29 kg: 25 mg/day

30-44 kg: 40 mg/day

45-64 kg: 60 mg/day

65-70 kg: 80 mg/day

Dosage adjustment in patients receiving strong CYP2D6 inhibitors: Initial: 0.5 mg/kg/day; may increase to next dosage level after 14 days if previous dose is well tolerated but response is inadequate. **Note:** Canadian labeling does not include specific dosing recommendations in regards to patients who are poor CYP2D6 metabolizers although similar dose reductions would appear necessary.

Children ≥6 years and >70 kg and Adults:

Initial: 40 mg/day for 7-14 days (Step 1); if tolerated, may increase dose at 7-14 day intervals to 60 mg/day (Step 2) then to 80 mg/day (Step 3). If optimal response is not obtained after 2-4 additional weeks, may increase to a maximum dose of 100 mg/day.

Dosage adjustment in patients receiving strong CYP2D6 inhibitors: Initial: 40 mg/day; may increase to next dosage level after 14 days if previous dose is well tolerated but response is inadequate. **Note:** Canadian labeling does not include specific dosing recommendations in regards to patients who are poor CYP2D6 metabolizers although similar dose reductions would appear necessary.

Elderly: Use has not been evaluated in the elderly.

Dosage adjustment in renal impairment: No dosage adjustment necessary

Dosage adjustment in hepatic impairment:

Mild impairment (Child-Pugh class A): No dosage adjustment provided in manufacturer's labeling.

Moderate impairment (Child-Pugh class B): All doses should be reduced to 50% of normal.

Severe impairment (Child-Pugh class C): All doses should be reduced to 25% of normal.

Administration Administer with or without food as a single daily dose in the morning or as two evenly divided doses in morning and late afternoon/early evening. Swallow capsules whole; do not open capsules. If opened accidentally, do not touch eyes; wash hands immediately (product is an ocular irritant).

Monitoring Parameters Patient growth (weight/height gain in children); attention, hyperactivity, anxiety, worsening of aggressive behavior or hostility; blood pressure and pulse (baseline and following dose increases and periodically during treatment)

Family members and caregivers need to monitor patient daily for emergence of irritability, agitation, unusual changes in behavior, and suicide ideation. Pediatric patients should be monitored closely for suicidality, clinical worsening, or unusual changes in behavior, especially during the initial for months of therapy or at times of dose changes. Appearance of symptoms needs to be immediately reported to healthcare provider.

Thoroughly evaluate for cardiovascular risk. Monitor heart rate, blood pressure, and consider obtaining ECG prior to initiation (Martinez-Raga, 2013; Vetter, 2008). Periodically reevaluate the long-term usefulness of the drug for the individual patient.

Dosage Forms

Capsule, Oral:

Strattera: 10 mg, 18 mg, 25 mg, 40 mg, 60 mg, 80 mg, 100 mg

◆ **Atomoxetine Hydrochloride** *see* AtoMOXetine *on page 191*

AtorvaSTATin (a TORE va sta tin)

Brand Names: U.S. Lipitor

Brand Names: Canada ACT Atorvastatin; Apo-Atorvastatin; Auro-Atorvastatin; Ava-Atorvastatin; Dom-Atorvastatin; GD-Atorvastatin; JAMP-Atorvastatin; Lipitor; Mylan-Atorvastatin; Novo-Atorvastatin; PMS-Atorvastatin; RAN-Atorvastatin; ratio-Atorvastatin; Riva-Atorvastatin; Sandoz-Atorvastatin

Index Terms Atorvastatin Calcium

Pharmacologic Category Antilipemic Agent, HMG-CoA Reductase Inhibitor

Use Treatment of dyslipidemias or primary prevention of cardiovascular disease (atherosclerotic) as detailed below:

Prevention of cardiovascular disease:

Primary prevention of cardiovascular disease (high-risk for CVD): To reduce the risk of MI or stroke in patients without evidence of heart disease who have multiple CVD risk factors or type 2 diabetes. Treatment reduces the risk for angina or revascularization procedures in patients with multiple risk factors.

Secondary prevention of cardiovascular disease: To reduce the risk of nonfatal MI, nonfatal stroke, revascularization procedures, hospitalization for heart failure, and angina in patients with evidence of coronary heart disease.

Primary and secondary prevention of atherosclerotic cardiovascular disease (ASCVD) according to the American College of Cardiology/American Heart Association: To reduce the risk of ASCVD in patients with clinical ASCVD (eg, coronary heart disease, stroke/TIA, or peripheral arterial disease presumed to be of atherosclerotic origin); in patients without clinical ASCVD if LDL-C is 190 mg/dL or greater; in patients without clinical ASCVD who have type 1 or type 2 diabetes and are between 40 and 75 years of age; in patients with an estimated 10-year ASCVD risk 7.5% or greater and who are between 40 and 75 years of age (Stone, 2013). Specific recommendations from the Kidney Disease: Improving Global Outcomes (KDIGO) organization have also been released for patients with chronic kidney disease (KDIGO [Tonelli, 2013]).

Treatment of dyslipidemias: To reduce elevations in total cholesterol (C), LDL-C, apolipoprotein B, and triglycerides in patients with elevations of one or more components, and/or to increase low HDL-C as present in Fredrickson type IIa, IIb, III, and IV hyperlipidemias, heterozygous familial and nonfamilial hypercholesterolemia, and homozygous familial hypercholesterolemia

Treatment of heterozygous familial hypercholesterolemia (HeFH) in adolescent patients (10 to 17 years of age, females >1 year postmenarche) having LDL-C ≥190 mg/dL or LDL-C ≥160 mg/dL with positive family history of premature cardiovascular disease (CVD) or with two or more CVD risk factors.

Pregnancy Risk Factor X

Pregnancy Considerations Adverse events were observed in animal reproductions studies. There are reports of congenital anomalies following maternal use of HMG-CoA reductase inhibitors in pregnancy; however, maternal disease, differences in specific agents used, and the low rates of exposure limit the interpretation of the available data (Godfrey, 2012; Lecarpentier, 2012). Cholesterol biosynthesis may be important in fetal development; serum cholesterol and triglycerides increase normally during pregnancy. The discontinuation of lipid lowering medications temporarily during pregnancy is not expected to have significant impact on the long term outcomes of primary hypercholesterolemia treatment.

Use of atorvastatin is contraindicated in pregnancy or those who may become pregnant. HMG-CoA reductase inhibitors should be discontinued prior to pregnancy (ADA, 2013). If treatment of dyslipidemias is needed in pregnant women or in women of reproductive age, other agents are preferred (Berglund, 2012; Stone, 2013). The manufacturer recommends administration to women of childbearing potential only when conception is highly unlikely and patients have been informed of potential hazards.

Breast-Feeding Considerations It is not known if atorvastatin is excreted into breast milk. Due to the potential for serious adverse reactions in a nursing infant, use while breast-feeding is contraindicated by the manufacturer.

Contraindications Hypersensitivity to atorvastatin or any component of the formulation; active liver disease; unexplained persistent elevations of serum transaminases; pregnancy (or those who may become pregnant); breast-feeding

Note: Telaprevir Canadian product monograph contraindicates use with atorvastatin.

Warnings/Precautions Secondary causes of hyperlipidemia should be ruled out prior to therapy. Atorvastatin has not been studied when the primary lipid abnormality is chylomicron elevation (Fredrickson types I and V). Liver function tests must be obtained prior to initiating therapy, repeat if clinically indicated thereafter. May cause hepatic dysfunction. Use with caution in patients who consume large amounts of ethanol or have a history of liver disease; monitoring is recommended. Use is contraindicated in patients with active liver disease or unexplained persistent elevations of serum transaminases; monitoring is recommended. Use high-dose atorvastatin with caution in patients with prior stroke or TIA; the risk of hemorrhagic stroke may be increased.

Rhabdomyolysis with acute renal failure has occurred. Risk is dose related and is increased with concurrent use of lipid-lowering agents which may cause rhabdomyolysis (fibric acid derivatives or niacin at doses ≥1 g/day) or during concurrent use with potent CYP3A4 inhibitors (including amiodarone, clarithromycin, erythromycin, itraconazole, ketoconazole, nefazodone, grapefruit juice in large quantities, verapamil, or protease inhibitors such as indinavir, nelfinavir, or ritonavir). Ensure patient is on the lowest effective atorvastatin dose. If concurrent use of clarithromycin or combination protease inhibitors (eg, lopinavir/ritonavir or ritonavir/saquinavir) is warranted consider dose adjustment of atorvastatin. Do not use with cyclosporine, gemfibrozil, tipranavir plus ritonavir, or telaprevir. Monitor closely if used with other drugs associated with myopathy. Weigh the risk versus benefit when combining any of these drugs with atorvastatin. Discontinue in any patient in which CPK levels are markedly elevated (>10 times ULN) or if myopathy is suspected/diagnosed. The manufacturer recommends temporary discontinuation for elective major surgery, acute medical or surgical conditions, or in any patient experiencing an acute or serious condition predisposing to renal failure (eg, sepsis, hypotension, trauma, uncontrolled seizures). Based on current research and clinical guidelines (Fleisher, 2009), HMG-CoA reductase inhibitors should be continued in the perioperative period. Use with caution in patients with advanced age, these patients are predisposed to myopathy. Immune-mediated necrotizing myopathy (IMNM), an autoimmune-mediated myopathy, has been reported (rarely) with HMG-CoA reductase inhibitor therapy. IMNM presents as proximal muscle weakness with elevated CPK levels, which persists despite discontinuation of HMG-CoA reductase inhibitor therapy; additionally, muscle biopsy may show necrotizing myopathy with limited inflammation; immunosuppressive therapy (eg, corticosteroids, azathioprine) may be used for treatment.

Adverse Reactions

Central nervous system: Insomnia

Gastrointestinal: Diarrhea, dyspepsia, nausea

Genitourinary: Urinary tract infection

Hepatic: Increased serum transaminases (with 80 mg/day dosing)

Neuromuscular & skeletal: Arthralgia, limb pain, muscle spasm, musculoskeletal pain, myalgia

Respiratory: Nasopharyngitis, pharyngolaryngeal pain

Rare but important or life-threatening: Abnormal uterine bleeding, ageusia, alopecia, altered sense of smell, amnesia (reversible), anaphylaxis, anemia, angioedema, anorexia, ataxia, biliary colic, blurred vision, bullous rash, bursitis, cholestasis, cholestatic jaundice, cognitive impairment (reversible), colitis, confusion (reversible), depression, diabetes mellitus (new onset), dizziness, duodenal ulcer, dysgeusia, dysphagia, ecchymoses, elevated glycosylated hemoglobin (Hb A_{1c}), emotional lability, epistaxis, eructation, erythema multiforme, esophagitis, fatigue, flatulence, gastritis, gastroenteritis, gingival hemorrhage, glossitis, hematuria, hepatic failure, hepatitis, hyperglycemia, hypoglycemia, increased creatine phosphokinase, increased serum alkaline phosphatase, increased serum glucose, jaundice, joint swelling, leg cramps, malaise, melena, memory impairment (reversible), migraine, muscle fatigue, myasthenia, myopathy, myositis, neck pain, neck stiffness, nephritis, nightmares, pancreatitis, paresthesia, peripheral neuropathy, petechia, pruritus, rectal hemorrhage, rhabdomyolysis, rupture of tendon, skin photosensitivity, Stevens-Johnson syndrome, stomatitis, syncope, tendinous contracture, tenesmus, thrombocytopenia, tinnitus, torticollis, toxic epidermal necrolysis, urticaria, vaginal hemorrhage, vomiting

Additional class-related events or case reports (not necessarily reported with atorvastatin therapy): Cataract, dermatomyositis, eosinophilia, erectile dysfunction, fulminant hepatic necrosis, gynecomastia, hemolytic anemia, hepatic cirrhosis, immune-mediated necrotizing myopathy, impairment of extraocular movement, interstitial pulmonary disease, lupus-like syndrome, ophthalmoplegia, peripheral nerve palsy, polymyalgia rheumatica, positive ANA titer, renal failure (secondary to rhabdomyolysis), thyroid dysfunction, tremor, vasculitis, vertigo

Drug Interactions

Metabolism/Transport Effects Substrate of CYP3A4 (major), P-glycoprotein, SLCO1B1; **Note:** Assignment of Major/Minor substrate status based on clinically relevant drug interaction potential; **Inhibits** CYP3A4 (weak), P-glycoprotein

Avoid Concomitant Use

Avoid concomitant use of AtorvaSTATin with any of the following: Bosutinib; Conivaptan; CycloSPORINE (Systemic); Fusidic Acid (Systemic); Gemfibrozil; Idelalisib; PAZOPanib; Pimozide; Posaconazole; Red Yeast Rice; Silodosin; Telaprevir; Tipranavir; Topotecan; VinCRIStine (Liposomal)

Increased Effect/Toxicity

AtorvaSTATin may increase the levels/effects of: Afatinib; Aliskiren; ARIPiprazole; Bosutinib; Brentuximab Vedotin; Cimetidine; Colchicine; DAPTOmycin; Digoxin; Diltiazem; Dofetilide; DOXOrubicin (Conventional); Edoxaban; Everolimus; Hydrocodone; Ketoconazole (Systemic); Ledipasvir; Lomitapide; Midazolam; Naloxegol; PAZOPanib; P-glycoprotein/ABCB1 Substrates; Pimozide; Prucalopride; Rifaximin; Rivaroxaban; Silodosin; Spironolactone; Topotecan; Trabectedin; Verapamil; VinCRIStine (Liposomal)

The levels/effects of AtorvaSTATin may be increased by: Acipimox; Amiodarone; Aprepitant; Azithromycin (Systemic); Bezafibrate; Boceprevir; Ceritinib; Ciprofibrate; Clarithromycin; Cobicistat; Colchicine; Conivaptan; CycloSPORINE (Systemic); CYP3A4 Inhibitors (Moderate); CYP3A4 Inhibitors (Strong); Cyproterone; Danazol; Dasatinib; Diltiazem; Dronedarone; Eltrombopag; Erythromycin (Systemic); Fenofibrate and Derivatives; Fluconazole; Fosaprepitant; Fusidic Acid (Systemic); Gemfibrozil; Grapefruit Juice; Idelalisib; Itraconazole; Ivacaftor; Ketoconazole (Systemic); Luliconazole; Mifepristone; Netupitant; Niacin; Niacinamide; P-glycoprotein/ABCB1 Inhibitors; Posaconazole; Protease Inhibitors; QuiNINE; Raltegravir; Ranolazine; Red Yeast Rice; Sildenafil; Simeprevir; Stiripentol; Telaprevir; Telithromycin; Teriflunomide; Tipranavir; Verapamil; Voriconazole

Decreased Effect

AtorvaSTATin may decrease the levels/effects of: Dabigatran Etexilate; Lanthanum

The levels/effects of AtorvaSTATin may be decreased by: Antacids; Bexarotene (Systemic); Bile Acid Sequestrants; Bosentan; CYP3A4 Inducers (Moderate); CYP3A4 Inducers (Strong); Dabrafenib; Deferasirox; Efavirenz; Etravirine; Fosphenytoin; Mitotane; P-glycoprotein/ABCB1 Inducers; Phenytoin; Rifamycin Derivatives; Siltuximab; St Johns Wort; Tocilizumab

Food Interactions Atorvastatin serum concentrations may be increased by grapefruit juice. Management: Avoid concurrent intake of large quantities of grapefruit juice (>1 quart/day).

Storage/Stability Store at controlled room temperature of 20°C to 25°C (68°F to 77°F).

Mechanism of Action Inhibitor of 3-hydroxy-3-methylglutaryl coenzyme A (HMG-CoA) reductase, the rate-limiting enzyme in cholesterol synthesis (reduces the production of mevalonic acid from HMG-CoA); this then results in a compensatory increase in the expression of LDL receptors on hepatocyte membranes and a stimulation of LDL catabolism

Pharmacodynamics/Kinetics

Onset of action: Initial changes: 3-5 days; Maximal reduction in plasma cholesterol and triglycerides: 2 weeks

Absorption: Rapid

Distribution: V_d: ~381 L

Protein binding: ≥98%

Metabolism: Hepatic; forms active ortho- and parahydroxylated derivatives and an inactive beta-oxidation product

Bioavailability: ~14% (parent drug); ~30% (parent drug and equipotent metabolites)

Half-life elimination: Parent drug: 14 hours; Equipotent metabolites: 20-30 hours

Time to peak, serum: 1-2 hours

Excretion: Bile; urine (<2% as unchanged drug)

Dosage Oral:

Primary prevention: Note: Doses should be individualized according to the baseline LDL-cholesterol concentrations and patient response; adjustments should be made at intervals of 2 to 4 weeks (4 weeks for children)

Children 10 to 17 years (females >1 year postmenarche):

HeFH: 10 mg once daily (maximum: 20 mg/day)

Adults:

Hypercholesterolemia (heterozygous familial and nonfamilial) and mixed hyperlipidemia (Fredrickson types IIa and IIb): Initial: 10 to 20 mg once daily; patients requiring >45% reduction in LDL-C may be started at 40 mg once daily; range: 10 to 80 mg once daily

Homozygous familial hypercholesterolemia: 10 to 80 mg once daily

ACC/AHA Blood Cholesterol Guideline recommendations to reduce the risk of atherosclerotic cardiovascular disease (ASCVD) (Stone, 2013): Adults ≥21 years:

Primary Prevention:

LDL-C ≥190 mg/dL: High intensity therapy: 80 mg once daily; if unable to tolerate, may reduce dose to 40 mg once daily

Type 1 or 2 diabetes and age 40 to 75 years: Moderate intensity therapy: 10 to 20 mg once daily

Type 1 or 2 diabetes, age 40 to 75 years, and an estimated 10-year ASCVD risk ≥7.5%: High intensity therapy: 80 mg once daily; if unable to tolerate, may reduce dose to 40 mg once daily

Age 40 to 75 years and an estimated 10-year ASCVD risk ≥7.5%: Moderate to high intensity therapy: 10 to 80 mg once daily

Secondary prevention:

Patient has clinical ASCVD (eg, coronary heart disease, stroke/TIA, or peripheral arterial disease presumed to be of atherosclerotic origin) **and:**

Age ≤75 years: High-intensity therapy: 80 mg once daily; if unable to tolerate, may reduce dose to 40 mg once daily

Age >75 years or not a candidate for high intensity therapy: Moderate intensity therapy: 10 to 20 mg once daily

Intensive lipid-lowering after an ACS event regardless of baseline LDL (off-label use): Initial: 80 mg once daily; adjust based on patient tolerability (Cannon, 2004; Pederson, 2005; Schwartz, 2001). **Note:** Currently, the ACC/AHA guidelines for UA/NSTEMI do not specify which statin to use (ACCF/AHA [Anderson, 2013]). Also consider the ACC/AHA Blood Cholesterol Guideline recommendations (Stone, 2013).

Noncardioembolic stroke/TIA (off-label use): Initial: 80 mg once daily; adjust based on patient tolerability (Adams, 2008; Amarenco, 2006). Also consider the ACC/AHA Blood Cholesterol Guideline recommendations (Stone, 2013).

Dosage adjustment for atorvastatin with concomitant medications:

Boceprevir, nelfinavir: Use lowest effective atorvastatin dose (not to exceed 40 mg daily)

Clarithromycin, itraconazole, fosamprenavir, ritonavir (plus darunavir, fosamprenavir, or saquinavir): Use lowest effective atorvastatin dose (not to exceed 20 mg daily)

Lomitapide: Consider atorvastatin dose reduction (per lomitapide manufacturer).

Dosing adjustment for toxicity:

Severe muscle symptoms or fatigue: Promptly discontinue use; evaluate CPK, creatinine, and urinalysis for myoglobinuria (Stone, 2013).

Mild to moderate muscle symptoms: Discontinue use until symptoms can be evaluated; evaluate patient for conditions that may increase the risk for muscle symptoms (eg, hypothyroidism, reduced renal or hepatic function, rheumatologic disorders such as polymyalgia rheumatica, steroid myopathy, vitamin D deficiency, or primary muscle diseases). Upon resolution, resume the original or lower dose of atorvastatin. If muscle symptoms recur, discontinue atorvastatin use. After muscle symptom resolution, may then use a low dose of a different statin; gradually increase if tolerated. In the absence of continued statin use, if muscle symptoms or elevated CPK continues after 2 months, consider other causes of muscle symptoms. If determined to be due to another condition aside from statin use, may resume statin therapy at the original dose (Stone, 2013).

Dosage adjustment in renal impairment: No dosage adjustment necessary.

Dosage adjustment in hepatic impairment: Contraindicated in active liver disease or in patients with unexplained persistent elevations of serum transaminases.

Dietary Considerations May take with food if desired; may take without regard to time of day. Before initiation of therapy, patients should be placed on a standard cholesterol-lowering diet for 3 to 6 months and the diet should be continued during drug therapy. Atorvastatin serum concentration may be increased when taken with grapefruit juice; avoid concurrent intake of large quantities (>1 quart/day).

Red yeast rice contains variable amounts of several compounds that are structurally similar to HMG-CoA reductase inhibitors, primarily monacolin K (or mevinolin) which is structurally identical to lovastatin; concurrent use of red yeast rice with HMG-CoA reductase inhibitors may increase the incidence of adverse and toxic effects (Lapi, 2008; Smith, 2003).

Administration May be administered with food if desired; may take without regard to time of day. Swallow whole; do not break, crush, or chew.

Monitoring Parameters

2013 ACC/AHA Blood Cholesterol Guideline recommendations (Stone, 2013):

Lipid panel (total cholesterol, HDL, LDL, triglycerides): Baseline lipid panel; fasting lipid profile within 4-12 weeks after initiation or dose adjustment and every 3-12 months (as clinically indicated) thereafter. If 2 consecutive LDL levels are <40 mg/dL, consider decreasing the dose.

Hepatic transaminase levels: Baseline measurement of hepatic transaminase levels (ie, ALT); measure hepatic function if symptoms suggest hepatotoxicity (eg, unusual fatigue or weakness, loss of appetite, abdominal pain, dark-colored urine or yellowing of skin or sclera) during therapy.

CPK: CPK should not be routinely measured. Baseline CPK measurement is reasonable for some individuals (eg, family history of statin intolerance or muscle disease, clinical presentation, concomitant drug therapy that may increase risk of myopathy). May measure CPK in any patient with symptoms suggestive of myopathy (pain, tenderness, stiffness, cramping, weakness, or generalized fatigue).

Evaluate for new-onset diabetes mellitus during therapy; if diabetes develops, continue statin therapy and encourage adherence to a heart-healthy diet, physical activity, a healthy body weight, and tobacco cessation.

If patient develops a confusional state or memory impairment, may evaluate patient for nonstatin causes (eg, exposure to other drugs), systemic and neuropsychiatric causes, and the possibility of adverse effects associated with statin therapy.

Manufacturer recommendation: Liver enzyme tests at baseline and repeated when clinically indicated. Measure CPK when myopathy is being considered or may measure CPK periodically in high risk patients (eg, drug-drug interaction). Upon initiation or titration, lipid panel should be analyzed within 2-4 weeks.

Dosage Forms

Tablet, Oral:

Lipitor: 10 mg, 20 mg, 40 mg, 80 mg

Generic: 10 mg, 20 mg, 40 mg, 80 mg

◆ **Atorvastatin and Amlodipine** *see* Amlodipine and Atorvastatin *on page* *124*

◆ **Atorvastatin and Ezetimibe** *see* Ezetimibe and Atorvastatin *on page* *833*

◆ **Atorvastatin Calcium** *see* AtorvaSTATin *on page* *194*

◆ **Atorvastatin Calcium and Amlodipine Besylate** *see* Amlodipine and Atorvastatin *on page 124*

Atosiban [INT] (a TOE si ban)

International Brand Names Tractocile (AE, AR, AT, BE, BH, CH, CN, CY, CZ, DE, DK, EE, FI, FR, GB, GR, HK, HR, HU, IE, IS, IT, JO, KR, LB, LT, MY, NL, NO, NZ, PH, PL, PT, QA, RO, SA, SE, SI, SK, TH, TR, VN, ZA)

Index Terms Atosiban Acetate

Pharmacologic Category Tocolytic Agent

Reported Use Inhibit uncomplicated premature labor

Dosage Range Adults: Females: IV: Initial: 6.75 **mg** bolus injection followed by continuous infusion at 100-300 **mcg**/minute; maximum: 330.75 **mg** in 48 hours

Product Availability Product available in various countries; not currently available in the U.S.

Dosage Forms

Injection, solution: 7.5 mg/mL (0.9 mL [6.75 mg], 5 mL)

◆ **Atosiban Acetate** *see* Atosiban [INT] *on page 197*

Atovaquone (a TOE va kwone)

Brand Names: U.S. Mepron

Brand Names: Canada Mepron®

Pharmacologic Category Antiprotozoal

Use

Pneumocystis jirovecii pneumonia (PCP) prophylaxis: Prevention of PCP in patients who are intolerant to trimethoprim-sulfamethoxazole (TMP-SMZ)

Pneumocystis jirovecii pneumonia (PCP) treatment: Acute oral treatment of mild-to-moderate PCP in patients who are intolerant to TMP-SMZ

Pregnancy Risk Factor C

Pregnancy Considerations Adverse events were observed in animal reproduction studies. Diagnosis and treatment of *Pneumocystis jirovecii* pneumonia (PCP) in pregnant women is the same as in nonpregnant women; however, information specific to the use of atovaquone in pregnancy is limited (DHHS [OI], 2013).

Breast-Feeding Considerations It is not known if atovaquone is excreted in breast milk. The manufacturer recommends that caution be exercised when administering atovaquone to nursing women.

Contraindications Patients who have or develop potentially life-threatening allergic reaction to atovaquone or any component of the formulation

Warnings/Precautions When used for *Pneumocystis jirovecii* pneumonia (PCP) treatment, has only been indicated in mild-to-moderate PCP; not studied for use in severe PCP; atovaquone has less adverse effects than trimethoprim-sulfamethoxazole (TMP-SMZ; the treatment of choice for mild-to-moderate PCP), although atovaquone is less effective than TMP-SMZ (DHHS [OI], 2013). Use with caution in elderly patients. Absorption may be decreased in patients who have diarrhea or vomiting; monitor closely and consider use of an antiemetic; if severe, consider use of an alternative antiprotozoal. Consider parenteral therapy with alternative agents in patients who have difficulty taking atovaquone with food; gastrointestinal disorders may limit absorption of oral medications; may not achieve adequate plasma levels. Use with caution in patients with severe hepatic impairment; monitor closely; rare cases of hepatitis, elevated liver function tests, and liver failure have been reported. Potentially significant drug-drug interactions may exist, requiring dose or frequency adjustment, additional monitoring, and/or selection of alternative therapy.

Benzyl alcohol and derivatives: Some dosage forms may contain benzyl alcohol; large amounts of benzyl alcohol (≥99 mg/kg/day) have been associated with a potentially fatal toxicity ("gasping syndrome") in neonates; the "gasping syndrome" consists of metabolic acidosis, respiratory distress, gasping respirations, CNS dysfunction (including convulsions, intracranial hemorrhage), hypotension and cardiovascular collapse (AAP, 1997; CDC, 1982); some data suggests that benzoate displaces bilirubin from protein binding sites (Ahlfors, 2001); avoid or use dosage forms containing benzyl alcohol with caution in neonates. See manufacturer's labeling.

Adverse Reactions

Cardiovascular: Hypotension

Central nervous system: Anxiety, depression, dizziness, headache, insomnia, pain

Dermatologic: Diaphoresis, pruritus, skin rash

Endocrine & metabolic: Hyperglycemia, hypoglycemia, hyponatremia, increased amylase

Gastrointestinal: Abdominal pain, amylase increased, anorexia, constipation, diarrhea, dysgeusia, dyspepsia, heartburn, nausea, oral candidiasis, vomiting

Hematologic & oncologic: Anemia, neutropenia

Hepatic: Increased liver enzymes

Infection: Infection

Neuromuscular & skeletal: Myalgia, weakness

Renal: Increased blood urea nitrogen, increased serum creatinine

Respiratory: Bronchospasm, cough, dyspnea, flu-like symptoms, rhinitis, sinusitis

Miscellaneous: Fever

Rare but important or life-threatening: Acute renal failure, angioedema, constriction of the pharynx, corneal disease (vortex keratopathy), desquamation, erythema multiforme, hepatic failure (rare), hepatitis (rare), hypersensitivity reaction, methemoglobinemia, pancreatitis, Stevens-Johnson syndrome, thrombocytopenia, urticaria

Drug Interactions

Metabolism/Transport Effects None known.

Avoid Concomitant Use

Avoid concomitant use of Atovaquone with any of the following: Efavirenz; Rifamycin Derivatives; Ritonavir

Increased Effect/Toxicity

Atovaquone may increase the levels/effects of: Etoposide

Decreased Effect

Atovaquone may decrease the levels/effects of: Indinavir

The levels/effects of Atovaquone may be decreased by: Efavirenz; Metoclopramide; Rifamycin Derivatives; Ritonavir; Tetracycline

Food Interactions Ingestion with a fatty meal increases absorption. Management: Administer with food, preferably high-fat meals (peanuts or ice cream).

Storage/Stability Store at 15°C to 25°C (59°F to 77°F). Do not freeze. Dispense in tight container.

Mechanism of Action Inhibits electron transport in mitochondria resulting in the inhibition of key metabolic enzymes responsible for the synthesis of nucleic acids and ATP

Pharmacodynamics/Kinetics

Absorption: Significantly increased with a high-fat meal

Distribution: V_{dss}: 0.6 ± 0.17 L/kg

Protein binding: >99%

Metabolism: Undergoes enterohepatic recirculation

Bioavailability: 32% to 62%

Half-life elimination: 1.5-4 days

Excretion: Feces (>94% as unchanged drug); urine (<1%)

Dosage

Pneumocystis jirovecii pneumonia (PCP), prevention:

Infants and Children <13 years (off-label use; CDC, 2009): Oral:

1-3 months: 30 mg/kg once daily with food

4-24 months: 45 mg/kg once daily with food

>24 months: 30 mg/kg once daily with food

Adolescents ≥13 years and Adults: Oral: 1500 mg once daily with food

PCP, mild-to-moderate, treatment:

Infants and Children <13 years (off-label use; CDC, 2009): Oral:

Birth to 3 months: 30-40 mg/kg/day in 2 divided doses with food (maximum: 1500 mg daily)

3-24 months: 45 mg/kg/day in 2 divided doses with food (maximum: 1500 mg daily)

≥24 months: 30-40 mg/kg/day in 2 divided doses with food (maximum: 1500 mg daily)

Adolescents ≥13 years and Adults: Oral: 750 mg twice daily with food for 21 days

Babesiosis (off-label use): Oral:

Children: 40 mg/kg/day in 2 divided doses with azithromycin for 7-10 days (maximum: 1500 mg daily). **Note:** Relapsing infection may require at least 6 weeks of therapy (Vannier, 2012).

Adults: 750 mg twice daily with azithromycin for 7-10 days; **Note:** Relapsing infection may require at least 6 weeks of therapy (Krauss, 2000; Vannier, 2012).

Toxoplasma gondii prophylaxis (CDC, 2009): Infants and Children <13 years (off-label use; either as monotherapy or with pyrimethamine plus leucovorin): Oral:

1-3 months: 30 mg/kg once daily with food

4-24 months: 45 mg/kg once daily with food

>24 months: 30 mg/kg once daily with food

Toxoplasma gondii encephalitis (off-label use) (DHHS [OI], 2013): Adolescents ≥13 years and Adults: Oral:

Prophylaxis: 1500 mg once daily with food (either as monotherapy or with pyrimethamine plus leucovorin)

Treatment: 1500 mg twice daily with food (either with pyrimethamine plus leucovorin, or with sulfadiazine, or as monotherapy) for at least 6 weeks (longer if extensive disease or incomplete response)

Chronic maintenance: 750-1500 mg twice daily with food (either with pyrimethamine plus leucovorin, or with sulfadiazine, or as monotherapy); may discontinue when asymptomatic and CD4 count >200/mm^3 for 6 months

Dosage adjustment in renal impairment: No dosage adjustment provided in manufacturer's labeling (has not been studied). However, atovaquone is not appreciably renally excreted.

Dosage adjustment in hepatic impairment: No dosage adjustment provided in manufacturer's labeling (has not been studied). However, atovaquone undergoes enterohepatic cycling and primarily hepatic excretion.

Dietary Considerations Must be taken with meals.

Administration Must be administered with meals. Shake suspension gently before use. Once opened, the foil pouch can be emptied on a dosing spoon, in a cup, or directly into the mouth.

Monitoring Parameters Hepatic function, CD4 count (for chronic maintenance treatment in toxoplasmosis)

Dosage Forms

Suspension, Oral:

Mepron: 750 mg/5 mL (5 mL, 210 mL)

Generic: 750 mg/5 mL (210 mL)

Atovaquone and Proguanil

(a TOE va kwone & pro GWA nil)

Brand Names: U.S. Malarone®

Brand Names: Canada Malarone®; Malarone® Pediatric

Index Terms Atovaquone and Proguanil Hydrochloride; Proguanil and Atovaquone; Proguanil Hydrochloride and Atovaquone

Pharmacologic Category Antimalarial Agent

Use

Malaria prevention: Prophylaxis of *Plasmodium falciparum* malaria, including areas where chloroquine resistance has been reported

Malaria treatment: Treatment of acute, uncomplicated *P. falciparum* malaria

Pregnancy Risk Factor C

Dosage Oral:

Children and Adolescents (dosage based on body weight):

Prevention of malaria: Start 1-2 days prior to entering a malaria-endemic area, continue throughout the stay and for 7 days after returning. Take as a single dose, once daily.

5-8 kg (off-label dosing): Atovaquone/proguanil 31.25 mg/12.5 mg (Boggild, 2007)

9-10 kg (off-label dosing): Atovaquone/proguanil 46.8 mg/18.75 mg (Boggild, 2007)

11-20 kg: Atovaquone/proguanil 62.5 mg/25 mg

21-30 kg: Atovaquone/proguanil 125 mg/50 mg

31-40 kg: Atovaquone/proguanil 187.5 mg/75 mg

>40 kg: Atovaquone/proguanil 250 mg/100 mg

Treatment of acute malaria: Take as a single dose, once daily for 3 consecutive days.

5-8 kg: Atovaquone/proguanil 125 mg/50 mg

9-10 kg: Atovaquone/proguanil 187.5 mg/75 mg

11-20 kg: Atovaquone/proguanil 250 mg/100 mg

21-30 kg: Atovaquone/proguanil 500 mg/200 mg

31-40 kg: Atovaquone/proguanil 750 mg/300 mg

>40 kg: Atovaquone/proguanil 1000 mg/400 mg

Adults:

Prevention of malaria: Atovaquone/proguanil 250 mg/100 mg once daily; start 1-2 days prior to entering a malaria-endemic area, continue throughout the stay and for 7 days after returning

Treatment of acute malaria: Atovaquone/proguanil 1000 mg/400 mg as a single dose, once daily for 3 consecutive days

Elderly: Use with caution.

Dosage adjustment in renal impairment:

CrCl ≥30 mL/minute: No dosage adjustment necessary.

CrCl <30 mL/minute:

Prophylaxis: Use is contraindicated.

Treatment: No dosage adjustment necessary; however, use with extreme caution and only if the benefits outweigh the risks.

Dosage adjustment in hepatic impairment:

Mild-to-moderate impairment: No dosage adjustment necessary.

Severe impairment; No dosage adjustment provided in manufacturer's labeling (has not been studied).

Additional Information Complete prescribing information should be consulted for additional detail.

Dosage Forms

Tablet: Atovaquone 250 mg and proguanil hydrochloride 100 mg

Malarone®: Atovaquone 250 mg and proguanil 100 mg

Tablet [pediatric]:

Malarone®: Atovaquone 62.5 mg and proguanil 25 mg

◆ **Atovaquone and Proguanil Hydrochloride** *see* Atovaquone and Proguanil *on page 198*

◆ **ATRA** *see* Tretinoin (Systemic) *on page 2096*

◆ **Atrac-Tain [OTC]** *see* Urea *on page 2114*

Atracurium (a tra KYOO ree um)

Brand Names: Canada Atracurium Besylate Injection

Index Terms Atracurium Besylate

Pharmacologic Category Neuromuscular Blocker Agent, Nondepolarizing

Use Adjunct to general anesthesia to facilitate endotracheal intubation and to relax skeletal muscles during surgery; to facilitate mechanical ventilation in ICU patients; does not relieve pain or produce sedation

Pregnancy Risk Factor C

Pregnancy Considerations Adverse events were observed in animal reproduction studies. Small amounts of atracurium have been shown to cross the placenta when given to women during cesarean section.

Breast-Feeding Considerations It is not known if atracurium is excreted in breast milk. The manufacturer recommends that caution be exercised when administering atracurium to nursing women.

Contraindications Hypersensitivity to atracurium besylate or any component of the formulation

Warnings/Precautions Reduce initial dosage and inject slowly (over 1-2 minutes) in patients in whom substantial histamine release would be potentially hazardous (eg, patients with clinically-important cardiovascular disease). Maintenance of an adequate airway and respiratory support is critical. Certain clinical conditions may result in potentiation or antagonism of neuromuscular blockade:

Potentiation: Electrolyte abnormalities, severe hyponatremia, severe hypocalcemia, severe hypokalemia, hypermagnesemia, neuromuscular diseases, acidosis, acute intermittent porphyria, renal failure, hepatic failure

Antagonism: Alkalosis, hypercalcemia, demyelinating lesions, peripheral neuropathies, diabetes mellitus

Increased sensitivity in patients with myasthenia gravis, Eaton-Lambert syndrome; resistance in burn patients (>30% of body) for period of 5-70 days postinjury; resistance in patients with muscle trauma, denervation, immobilization, infection, chronic treatment with atracurium. Cross-sensitivity with other neuromuscular-blocking agents may occur; use extreme caution in patients with previous anaphylactic reactions. Use caution in the elderly. Bradycardia may be more common with atracurium than with other neuromuscular-blocking agents since it has no clinically-significant effects on heart rate to counteract the bradycardia produced by anesthetics. Should be administered by adequately trained individuals familiar with its use.

Benzyl alcohol and derivatives: Some dosage forms may contain benzyl alcohol; large amounts of benzyl alcohol (≥99 mg/kg/day) have been associated with a potentially fatal toxicity ("gasping syndrome") in neonates; the "gasping syndrome" consists of metabolic acidosis, respiratory distress, gasping respirations, CNS dysfunction (including convulsions, intracranial hemorrhage), hypotension and cardiovascular collapse (AAP, 1997; CDC, 1982); some data suggests that benzoate displaces bilirubin from protein binding sites (Ahlfors, 2001); avoid or use dosage forms containing benzyl alcohol with caution in neonates. See manufacturer's labeling.

Adverse Reactions Mild, rare, and generally suggestive of histamine release

Cardiovascular: Flushing

Rare but important or life-threatening: Bronchial secretions, erythema, hives, itching, wheezing

Postmarketing and/or case reports: Acute quadriplegic myopathy syndrome (prolonged use), allergic reaction, bradycardia, bronchospasm, dyspnea, hypotension, injection site reaction, laryngospasm, myositis ossificans (prolonged use), seizure, tachycardia, urticaria

Causes of prolonged neuromuscular blockade: Accumulation of active metabolites; cumulative drug effect, metabolism/excretion decreased (hepatic and/or renal impairment); electrolyte imbalance (hypokalemia, hypocalcemia, hypermagnesemia, hypernatremia); excessive drug administration; hypothermia

Drug Interactions

Metabolism/Transport Effects None known.

Avoid Concomitant Use

Avoid concomitant use of Atracurium with any of the following: QuiNINE

Increased Effect/Toxicity

Atracurium may increase the levels/effects of: Cardiac Glycosides; Corticosteroids (Systemic); OnabotulinumtoxinA; RimabotulinumtoxinB

The levels/effects of Atracurium may be increased by: AbobotulinumtoxinA; Aminoglycosides; Calcium Channel Blockers; Capreomycin; Clindamycin (Topical); Colistimethate; CycloSPORINE (Systemic); Fosphenytoin-Phenytoin; Inhalational Anesthetics; Ketorolac (Nasal); Ketorolac (Systemic); Lincosamide Antibiotics; Lithium; Loop Diuretics; Magnesium Salts; Polymyxin B; Procainamide; QuiNIDine; QuiNINE; Spironolactone; Tetracycline Derivatives; Vancomycin

Decreased Effect

The levels/effects of Atracurium may be decreased by: Acetylcholinesterase Inhibitors; Fosphenytoin-Phenytoin; Loop Diuretics

Preparation for Administration Atracurium should not be mixed with alkaline solutions.

Storage/Stability Refrigerate intact vials at 2°C to 8°C (36°F to 46°F); protect from freezing. Use vials within 14 days upon removal from the refrigerator to room temperature of 25°C (77°F). Dilutions of 0.2 mg/mL or 0.5 mg/mL in 0.9% sodium chloride, dextrose 5% in water, or 5% dextrose in sodium chloride 0.9% are stable for up to 24 hours at room temperature or under refrigeration.

Mechanism of Action Blocks neural transmission at the myoneural junction by binding with cholinergic receptor sites

Pharmacodynamics/Kinetics

Onset of action (dose dependent): 2-3 minutes

Duration: Recovery begins in 20-35 minutes following initial dose of 0.4-0.5 mg/kg under balanced anesthesia; recovery to 95% of control takes 60-70 minutes

Metabolism: Undergoes ester hydrolysis and Hofmann elimination (nonbiologic process independent of renal, hepatic, or enzymatic function); metabolites have no neuromuscular blocking properties; laudanosine, a product of Hofmann elimination, is a CNS stimulant and can accumulate with prolonged use. Laudanosine is hepatically metabolized.

Half-life elimination: Biphasic: Adults: Initial (distribution): 2 minutes; Terminal: 20 minutes

Excretion: Urine (<5%)

Dosage IV (not to be used IM): Dose to effect; doses must be individualized due to interpatient variability

Adjunct to surgical anesthesia (neuromuscular blockade):

Children 1 month to 2 years: Initial: 0.3-0.4 mg/kg followed by maintenance doses as needed to maintain neuromuscular blockade

Children >2 years, Adolescents, and Adults: 0.4-0.5 mg/kg, then 0.08-0.1 mg/kg administered 20-45 minutes after initial dose to maintain neuromuscular block; repeat dose at 15- to 25-minute intervals

Initial dose after succinylcholine for intubation (balanced anesthesia): Adults: 0.3-0.4 mg/kg

Pretreatment/priming: 10% of intubating dose (eg, 0.04-0.05 mg/kg) given 2-4 minutes before the larger second dose (Mehta, 1985; Miller, 2010). **Note:** Although priming has been advocated by some, priming may either be uncomfortable for the patient, increase the risk of aspiration and difficulty swallowing, or intubating conditions after priming may not be as good as that seen with succinylcholine (Miller, 2010).

Maintenance infusion for continued surgical relaxation during extended surgical procedures: At initial signs of recovery from bolus dose, a continuous infusion may be initiated at a rate of 9-10 **mcg**/kg/**minute** (0.54-0.6 **mg**/kg/**hour**); block usually maintained by a rate of 5-9 **mcg**/kg/**minute** (0.3-0.54 **mg**/kg/**hour**) under balanced anesthesia; range: 2-15 **mcg**/kg/**minute** (0.12-0.9 **mg**/kg/**hour**)

ICU paralysis (eg, facilitate mechanical ventilation) in selected adequately sedated patients (off-label dosing): Adults: Initial bolus of 0.4-0.5 mg/kg, followed by 4-20 **mcg**/kg/**minute** (0.24-1.2 **mg**/kg/**hour**) (Greenberg, 2013; Murray, 2002)

Dosage adjustment in renal impairment: No dosage adjustment necessary.

Dosage adjustment in hepatic impairment: No dosage adjustment necessary.

Dosing in obesity: Morbidly-obese patients should be dosed using ideal body weight or an adjusted body weight (ie, between IBW and total body weight [TBW]) (Erstad, 2004). In a bariatric surgical population of morbidly-obese patients who were administered an induction dose of atracurium based on TBW as compared to IBW, time to recovery of twitch response was prolonged (Kralingen, 2011).

Administration May be given undiluted as a bolus injection; not for IM injection due to tissue irritation; administration via infusion requires the use of an infusion pump; use infusion solutions within 24 hours of preparation

Monitoring Parameters Vital signs (heart rate, blood pressure, respiratory rate); degree of muscle relaxation (via peripheral nerve stimulator and presence of spontaneous movement); renal function (serum creatinine, BUN) and liver function when in ICU

In the ICU setting, prolonged paralysis and generalized myopathy, following discontinuation of agent, may be minimized by appropriately monitoring degree of blockade.

Additional Information Atracurium is classified as an intermediate-duration neuromuscular-blocking agent. It does not appear to have a cumulative effect on the duration of blockade. It does not relieve pain or produce sedation.

Dosage Forms

Solution, Intravenous:

Generic: 50 mg/5 mL (5 mL); 100 mg/10 mL (10 mL)

Solution, Intravenous [preservative free]:

Generic: 50 mg/5 mL (5 mL)

- ◆ **Atracurium Besylate** *see* Atracurium *on page 198*
- ◆ **Atracurium Besylate Injection (Can)** *see* Atracurium *on page 198*
- ◆ **Atralin** *see* Tretinoin (Topical) *on page 2099*
- ◆ **Atriance™ (Can)** *see* Nelarabine *on page 1435*
- ◆ **Atripla** *see* Efavirenz, Emtricitabine, and Tenofovir *on page 709*
- ◆ **AtroPen** *see* Atropine *on page 200*

Atropine (A troe peen)

Brand Names: U.S. AtroPen; Atropine-Care [DSC]; Isopto Atropine

Brand Names: Canada Dioptic's Atropine Solution; Isopto® Atropine

Index Terms Atropine Sulfate

Pharmacologic Category Anticholinergic Agent; Anticholinergic Agent, Ophthalmic; Antidote; Antispasmodic Agent, Gastrointestinal; Ophthalmic Agent, Mydriatic

Additional Appendix Information

Beers Criteria – Potentially Inappropriate Medications for Geriatrics *on page 2271*

Use

Injection: Preoperative medication to inhibit salivation and secretions; treatment of symptomatic sinus bradycardia, AV block (nodal level); antidote for anticholinesterase poisoning (carbamate insecticides, nerve agents, organophosphate insecticides); adjuvant use with anticholinesterases (eg, edrophonium, neostigmine) to decrease their side effects during reversal of neuromuscular blockade

Note: Use is no longer recommended in the management of asystole or pulseless electrical activity (PEA) (ACLS, 2010).

Ophthalmic: Produce mydriasis and cycloplegia for examination of the retina and optic disc and accurate measurement of refractive errors; produce papillary dilation in inflammatory conditions (eg, uveitis)

Pregnancy Risk Factor B/C (manufacturer specific)

Pregnancy Considerations Animal reproduction studies have not been conducted. Atropine has been found to cross the human placenta.

Breast-Feeding Considerations Trace amounts of atropine are excreted into breast milk. Anticholinergic agents may suppress lactation.

Contraindications Hypersensitivity to atropine or any component of the formulation; narrow-angle glaucoma; adhesions between the iris and lens (ophthalmic product); pyloric stenosis; prostatic hypertrophy

Note: No contraindications exist in the treatment of life-threatening organophosphate or carbamate insecticide or nerve agent poisoning.

Warnings/Precautions Heat prostration may occur in the presence of high environmental temperatures. Psychosis may occur in sensitive individuals or following use of excessive doses. Avoid use if possible in patients with obstructive uropathy or in other conditions resulting in urinary retention; use is contraindicated in patients with prostatic hypertrophy. Avoid use in patients with paralytic ileus, intestinal atony of the elderly or debilitated patient, severe ulcerative colitis, and toxic megacolon complicating ulcerative colitis. Use with caution in patients with autonomic neuropathy, hyperthyroidism, renal or hepatic impairment, myocardial ischemia, HF, tachyarrhythmias (including sinus tachycardia), hypertension, and hiatal hernia associated with reflux esophagitis. Treatment-related blood pressure increases and tachycardia may lead to ischemia, precipitate an MI, or increase arrhythmogenic potential. In heart transplant recipients, atropine will likely be ineffective in treatment of bradycardia due to lack of vagal innervation of the transplanted heart; cholinergic reinnervation may occur over time (years), so atropine may be used cautiously; however, some may experience paradoxical slowing of the heart rate and high-degree AV block upon administration (ACLS, 2010; Bernheim, 2004).

Avoid relying on atropine for effective treatment of type II second-degree or third-degree AV block (with or without a new wide QRS complex). Asystole or bradycardic pulseless electrical activity (PEA): Although no evidence exists for significant detrimental effects, routine use is unlikely to have a therapeutic benefit and is no longer recommended (ACLS, 2010).

AtroPen®: There are no absolute contraindications for the use of atropine in severe organophosphate or carbamate insecticide or nerve agent poisonings; however in mild poisonings, use caution in those patients where the use of atropine would be otherwise contraindicated. Formulation for use by trained personnel only. Clinical symptoms consistent with highly-suspected organophosphate or carbamate insecticides or nerve agent poisoning should be treated with antidote immediately; administration should not be delayed for confirmatory laboratory tests. Signs of atropinization include flushing, mydriasis, tachycardia, and dryness of the mouth or nose. Monitor effects closely when administering subsequent injections as necessary. The presence of these effects is not indicative of the success of therapy; inappropriate use of mydriasis as an indicator of successful treatment has resulted in atropine toxicity. Reversal of bronchial secretions is the preferred indicator of success. Adjunct treatment with a cholinesterase reactivator (eg, pralidoxime) may be required in patients with toxicity secondary to organophosphorus insecticides or nerve agents. Treatment should always include proper evacuation and decontamination procedures; medical personnel should protect themselves from inadvertent contamination. Antidotal administration is intended only for initial management; definitive and more extensive medical care is required following administration. Individuals should not rely solely on antidote for treatment, as other supportive measures (eg, artificial respiration) may still be required. Atropine reverses the muscarinic but not the nicotinic effects associated with anticholinesterase toxicity.

Children may be more sensitive to the anticholinergic effects of atropine; use with caution in children with spastic paralysis. May be inappropriate in older adults depending on comorbidities (eg, dementia, delirium) due to its potent anticholinergic effects (Beers Criteria).

Adverse Reactions Severity and frequency of adverse reactions are dose related and vary greatly; listed reactions are limited to significant and/or life-threatening.

Cardiovascular: Cardiac arrhythmia, flushing, hypotension, palpitations, tachycardia

Central nervous system: Ataxia, coma, delirium, disorientation, dizziness, drowsiness, excitement, hallucination, headache, insomnia, nervousness

Dermatologic: Anhidrosis, scarlatiniform rash, skin rash, urticaria

Gastrointestinal: Ageusia, bloating, constipation, delayed gastric emptying, nausea, paralytic ileus, vomiting, xerostomia

Genitourinary: Urinary hesitancy, urinary retention

Hypersensitivity: Anaphylaxis

Neuromuscular & skeletal: Laryngospasm, weakness

Ocular: Angle-closure glaucoma, blurred vision, cycloplegia, dry eye syndrome, increased intraocular pressure, mydriasis

Respiratory: Dry nose, dry throat, dyspnea, pulmonary edema

Miscellaneous: Fever

Drug Interactions

Metabolism/Transport Effects None known.

Avoid Concomitant Use

Avoid concomitant use of Atropine with any of the following: Aclidinium; Glucagon; Ipratropium (Oral Inhalation); Potassium Chloride; Tiotropium; Umeclidinium

Increased Effect/Toxicity

Atropine may increase the levels/effects of: AbobotulinumtoxinA; Analgesics (Opioid); Anticholinergic Agents; Cannabinoid-Containing Products; Glucagon; Mirabegron; OnabotulinumtoxinA; Potassium Chloride; RimabotulinumtoxinB; Thiazide Diuretics; Tiotropium; Topiramate

The levels/effects of Atropine may be increased by: Aclidinium; Ipratropium (Oral Inhalation); Mianserin; Pramlintide; Umeclidinium

Decreased Effect

Atropine may decrease the levels/effects of: Acetylcholinesterase Inhibitors; Itopride; Secretin

The levels/effects of Atropine may be decreased by: Acetylcholinesterase Inhibitors

Preparation for Administration Preparation of bulk atropine solution for mass chemical terrorism: Add atropine sulfate powder to 100 mL NS in polyvinyl chloride bags to yield a final concentration of 1 mg/mL (Dix, 2003).

Storage/Stability

Injection: Store injection at controlled room temperature of 15°C to 30°C (59°F to 86°F); avoid freezing. In addition, AtroPen® should be protected from light. Preparation of bulk atropine solution for mass chemical terrorism at a concentration of 1 mg/mL is stable for 72 hours at 4°C to 8°C (39°F to 46°F); 20°C to 25°C (68°F to 77°F); 32°C to 36°C (90°F to 97°F) (Dix, 2003).

Ophthalmic products: Store at 20°C to 25°C (68°F to 77°F); keep tightly closed.

Mechanism of Action Blocks the action of acetylcholine at parasympathetic sites in smooth muscle, secretory glands, and the CNS; increases cardiac output, dries secretions. Atropine reverses the muscarinic effects of cholinergic poisoning due to agents with acetylcholinesterase inhibitor activity by acting as a competitive antagonist of acetylcholine at muscarinic receptors. The primary goal in cholinergic poisonings is reversal of bronchorrhea and bronchoconstriction. Atropine has no effect on the nicotinic receptors responsible for muscle weakness, fasciculations, and paralysis.

Pharmacodynamics/Kinetics

Onset of action: IM, IV: Rapid

Absorption: IM: Rapid and well absorbed

Distribution: Widely throughout the body; crosses blood-brain barrier

Metabolism: Hepatic via enzymatic hydrolysis

Half-life elimination: 2-3 hours; Children <2 years of age: 7 hours; Elderly 65-75 years of age: 10 hours

Time to peak: IM: 3 minutes

Excretion: Urine (30% to 50% as unchanged drug and metabolites)

Dosage

Infants and Children: Doses <0.1 mg have been associated with paradoxical bradycardia.

Inhibit salivation and secretions (preanesthesia): IM, IV, SubQ:

<5 kg: 0.02 mg/kg/dose 30-60 minutes preop then every 4-6 hours as needed. Use of a minimum dosage of 0.1 mg in neonates <5 kg will result in dosages >0.02 mg/kg. There is no documented minimum dosage in this age group.

>5 kg: 0.01-0.02 mg/kg/dose to a maximum 0.4 mg/dose 30-60 minutes preop; minimum dose: 0.1 mg

Alternate dosing:

3-7 kg (7-16 lb): 0.1 mg

8-11 kg (17-24 lb): 0.15 mg

11-18 kg (24-40 lb): 0.2 mg

18-29 kg (40-65 lb): 0.3 mg

>30 kg (>65 lb): 0.4 mg

Bradycardia:

IV, I.O.: 0.02 mg/kg, minimum dose recommended by PALS: 0.1 mg; however, use of a minimum dosage of 0.1 mg in patients <5 kg will result in dosages >0.02 mg/kg and is not recommended (Barrington, 2011); there is no documented minimum dosage in this age group; maximum single dose: 0.5 mg; may repeat once in 3-5 minutes; maximum total dose: 1 mg (PALS, 2010).

Endotracheal: 0.04-0.06 mg/kg; may repeat once if needed (PALS, 2010)

Children: Organophosphate or carbamate insecticide or nerve agent poisoning: **Note:** The dose of atropine required varies considerably with the severity of poisoning. The total amount of atropine used for carbamate poisoning is usually less than with organophosphate insecticide or nerve agent poisoning. Severely poisoned patients may exhibit significant tolerance to atropine; ≥2 times the suggested doses may be needed. Titrate to pulmonary status (decreased bronchial secretions); consider administration of atropine via continuous IV infusion in patients requiring large doses of atropine. Once patient is stable for a period of time, the dose/dosing frequency may be decreased. Pralidoxime is a component of the management of organophosphate insecticide and nerve agent toxicity; refer to Pralidoxime monograph for the specific route and dose.

IV, IM (off-label dose): Initial: 0.05-0.1 mg/kg; repeat every 5-10 minutes as needed, doubling the dose if previous dose does not induce atropinization (Hegenbarth, 2008; Rotenberg, 2003). Maintain atropinization by administering repeat doses as needed for ≥2-12 hours based on recurrence of symptoms (Reigart, 1999).

IV infusion (off-label dose): Following atropinization, administer 10% to 20% of the total loading dose required to induce atropinization as a continuous IV infusion per hour; adjust as needed to maintain adequate atropinization without atropine toxicity (Eddleston, 2004b; Roberts, 2007).

IM (AtroPen®):

Mild symptoms (≥2 mild symptoms): Administer the weight-based dose listed below as soon as an exposure is known or strongly suspected. If severe symptoms develop after the first dose, 2 additional doses should be repeated in rapid succession 10 minutes after the first dose; do not administer more than 3 doses. If profound anticholinergic effects occur in the absence of excessive bronchial secretions, further doses of atropine should be withheld.

Severe symptoms (≥1 severe symptoms): Immediately administer **three** weight-based doses in rapid succession.

Weight-based dosing:

<6.8 kg (15 lb): 0.25 mg/dose
6.8-18 kg (15-40 lb): 0.5 mg/dose
18-41 kg (40-90 lb): 1 mg/dose
>41 kg (>90 lb): 2 mg/dose

Symptoms of insecticide or nerve agent poisoning, as provided by manufacturer in the AtroPen® product labeling, to guide therapy:

Mild symptoms: Blurred vision, bradycardia, breathing difficulties, chest tightness, coughing, drooling, miosis, muscular twitching, nausea, runny nose, salivation increased, stomach cramps, tachycardia, teary eyes, tremor, vomiting, or wheezing

Severe symptoms: Breathing difficulties (severe), confused/strange behavior, defecation (involuntary), muscular twitching/generalized weakness (severe), respiratory secretions (severe), seizure, unconsciousness, urination (involuntary); **Note:** Infants may become drowsy or unconscious with muscle floppiness as opposed to muscle twitching.

Endotracheal (off-label route): Increase the dose by 2-3 times the usual IV dose. Mix with 3-5 mL of normal saline and administer. Flush with 3-5 mL of NS and follow with 5 assisted manual ventilations (Rotenberg, 2003).

Adults (doses <0.5 mg have been associated with paradoxical bradycardia):

Inhibit salivation and secretions (preanesthesia): IM, IV, SubQ: 0.4-0.6 mg 30-60 minutes preop and repeat every 4-6 hours as needed

Bradycardia: **Note:** Atropine may be ineffective in heart transplant recipients: IV: 0.5 mg every 3-5 minutes, not to exceed a total of 3 mg or 0.04 mg/kg (ACLS, 2010)

Neuromuscular blockade reversal: IV: 25-30 mcg/kg 30-60 seconds before neostigmine or 7-10 mcg/kg 30-60 seconds before edrophonium

Organophosphate or carbamate insecticide or nerve agent poisoning: **Note:** The dose of atropine required varies considerably with the severity of poisoning. The total amount of atropine used for carbamate poisoning is usually less than with organophosphate insecticide or nerve agent poisoning. Severely poisoned patients may exhibit significant tolerance to atropine; ≥2 times the suggested doses may be needed. Titrate to pulmonary status (decreased bronchial secretions); consider administration of atropine via continuous IV infusion in patients requiring large doses of atropine. Once patient is stable for a period of time, the dose/dosing frequency may be decreased. Pralidoxime is a component of the management of organophosphate insecticide and nerve agent toxicity; refer to Pralidoxime monograph for the specific route and dose.

IV, IM (off-label dose): Initial: 1-6 mg (ATSDR, 2011; Roberts, 2007); repeat every 3-5 minutes as needed, doubling the dose if previous dose did not induce atropinization (Eddleston, 2004b; Roberts, 2007). Maintain atropinization by administering repeat doses as needed for ≥2-12 hours based on recurrence of symptoms (Reigart, 1999).

IV Infusion (off-label dose): Following atropinization, administer 10% to 20% of the total loading dose required to induce atropinization as a continuous IV infusion per hour; adjust as needed to maintain adequate atropinization without atropine toxicity (Eddleston, 2004b; Roberts, 2007)

IM (AtroPen®):

Mild symptoms (≥2 mild symptoms): Administer 2 mg as soon as an exposure is known or strongly suspected. If severe symptoms develop after the first dose, 2 additional doses should be repeated in rapid succession 10 minutes after the first dose; do not administer more than 3 doses. If profound anticholinergic effects occur in the absence of excessive bronchial secretions, further doses of atropine should be withheld.

Severe symptoms (≥1 severe symptoms): Immediately administer **three** 2 mg doses in rapid succession.

Symptoms of insecticide or nerve agent poisoning, as provided by manufacturer in the AtroPen® product labeling, to guide therapy:

Mild symptoms: Blurred vision, bradycardia, breathing difficulties, chest tightness, coughing, drooling, miosis, muscular twitching, nausea, runny nose, salivation increased, stomach cramps, tachycardia, teary eyes, tremor, vomiting, or wheezing

Severe symptoms: Breathing difficulties (severe), confused/strange behavior, defecation (involuntary), muscular twitching/generalized weakness (severe), respiratory secretions (severe), seizure, unconsciousness, urination (involuntary)

Mydriasis, cycloplegia (preprocedure): Ophthalmic (1% solution): Instill 1-2 drops 1 hour before procedure.

Uveitis: Ophthalmic:

1% solution: Instill 1-2 drops up to 4 times/day

Ointment: Apply a small amount in the conjunctival sac up to 3 times/day; compress the lacrimal sac by digital pressure for 1-3 minutes after instillation

Dosage adjustment in renal impairment: No dosage adjustment provided in manufacturer's labeling.

Dosage adjustment in hepatic impairment: No dosage adjustment provided in manufacturer's labeling.

Administration

IM: AtroPen®: Administer to the outer thigh. Firmly grasp the autoinjector with the green tip (0.5 mg, 1 mg, and 2 mg autoinjector) or black tip (0.25 mg autoinjector) pointed down; remove the yellow safety release (0.5 mg, 1 mg, and 2 mg autoinjector) or gray safety release (0.25 autoinjector). Jab the green tip at a 90° angle against the outer thigh; may be administered through clothing as long as pockets at the injection site are empty. In thin patients or patients <6.8 kg (15 lb), bunch up the thigh prior to injection. Hold the autoinjector in place for 10 seconds following the injection; remove the autoinjector and massage the injection site. After administration, the needle will be visible; if the needle is not visible, repeat the above steps. After use, bend the needle against a hard surface (needle does not retract) to avoid accidental injury.

IV: Administer undiluted by rapid IV injection; slow injection may result in paradoxical bradycardia. In bradycardia, atropine administration should not delay treatment with external pacing.

Endotracheal: Dilute in NS or sterile water. Absorption may be greater with sterile water. Stop compressions (if using for cardiac arrest), spray the drug quickly down the tube. Follow immediately with several quick insufflations and continue chest compressions.

Monitoring Parameters Heart rate, blood pressure, pulse, mental status; intravenous administration requires a cardiac monitor

Organophosphate or carbamate insecticide or nerve agent poisoning: Heart rate, blood pressure, respiratory status, oxygenation secretions. Maintain atropinization with repeated dosing as indicated by clinical status. Crackles in lung bases, or continuation of cholinergic signs, may be signs of inadequate dosing. Pulmonary improvement may not parallel other signs of atropinization. Monitor for signs and symptoms of atropine toxicity (eg, fever, muscle fasciculations, delirium); if toxicity occurs, discontinue atropine and monitor closely.

Consult individual institutional policies and procedures.

Dosage Forms

Device, Intramuscular:

AtroPen: 0.25 mg/0.3 mL (0.3 mL); 0.5 mg/0.7 mL (0.7 mL); 1 mg/0.7 mL (0.7 mL); 2 mg/0.7 mL (0.7 mL)

Ointment, Ophthalmic:

Generic: 1% (3.5 g)

Solution, Injection:

Generic: 0.05 mg/mL (5 mL); 0.1 mg/mL (5 mL, 10 mL); 0.4 mg/mL (1 mL, 20 mL); 1 mg/mL (1 mL)

Solution, Injection [preservative free]:

Generic: 0.4 mg/mL (1 mL); 0.8 mg/mL (0.5 mL); 1 mg/mL (1 mL)

Solution, Ophthalmic:

Isopto Atropine: 1% (5 mL, 15 mL)

Generic: 1% (2 mL, 5 mL, 15 mL)

◆ **Atropine and Diphenoxylate** *see* Diphenoxylate and Atropine *on page 644*

Atropine and Pralidoxime

(A troe peen & pra li DOKS eem)

Brand Names: U.S. ATNAA; Duodote

Index Terms Atropine and Pralidoxime Chloride; Mark 1; NAAK; Nerve Agent Antidote Kit; Pralidoxime and Atropine

Pharmacologic Category Anticholinergic Agent; Antidote

Use

ATNAA: Treatment of poisoning in patients who have been exposed to organophosphate nerve agents (eg, tabun, sarin, soman) that have acetylcholinesterase-inhibiting activity for self- or buddy-administration by military personnel

Duodote™: Treatment of poisoning by organophosphate nerve agents (eg, tabun, sarin, soman) or organophosphate insecticides for use by trained emergency medical services personnel

Pregnancy Risk Factor C

Dosage IM: Adults: Organophosphate insecticide or nerve agent poisoning: **Note:** If exposure is suspected, antidotal therapy should be given immediately as soon as symptoms appear (critical to administer immediately in case of soman exposure). Definitive medical care should be sought after any injection given. One injection only may be given as self-aid. If repeat injections needed, administration must be done by another trained individual. Emergency medical personnel who have self-administered a dose must determine capacity to continue to provide care.

ATNAA:

Mild symptoms (some or all mild symptoms): Self-Aid or Buddy-Aid: 1 injection (wait 10-15 minutes for effect); if the patient is able to ambulate, and knows who and where they are, then no further injections are needed. If symptoms still present: Buddy-Aid: May repeat 1-2 more injections

Severe symptoms (if most or all): Buddy-Aid: If no self-aid given, 3 injections in rapid succession; if 1 self-aid injection given, 2 injections in rapid succession

Maximum cumulative dose: 3 injections

Symptoms of organophosphate insecticide or nerve agent poisoning, as provided by the manufacturer in the ATNAA product labeling to guide therapy:

Mild symptoms: Breathing difficulties, chest tightness, coughing, difficulty in seeing, drooling, headache, localized sweating and muscular twitching, miosis, nausea (with or without vomiting), runny nose, stomach cramps, tachycardia (followed by bradycardia), wheezing

Severe symptoms: Bradycardia, confused/strange behavior, convulsions, increased wheezing and breathing difficulties, involuntary urination/defecation, miosis (severe), muscular twitching/generalized weakness (severe), red/teary eyes, respiratory failure, unconsciousness, vomiting

Duodote™:

Mild symptoms (≥2 mild symptoms): 1 injection (wait 10-15 minutes for effect); if after 10-15 minutes no severe symptoms emerge, no further injections are indicated; if any severe symptoms emerge at any point following the initial injection, repeat dose by giving 2 additional injections in rapid succession. Transport to medical care facility.

Severe symptoms (≥1 severe symptom): 3 injections in rapid succession. Transport to medical care facility.

Maximum cumulative dose: 3 injections unless medical care support (eg, hospital, respiratory support) is available

Symptoms of organophosphate insecticide or nerve agent poisoning, as provided by manufacturer in the Duodote™ product labeling to guide therapy:

Mild symptoms: Airway secretions increased, blurred vision, bradycardia, breathing difficulties, chest tightness, drooling miosis, nausea, vomiting, runny nose, salivation, stomach cramps (acute onset), tachycardia, teary eyes, tremors/muscular twitching, wheezing/coughing

Severe symptoms: Breathing difficulties (severe), confused/strange behavior, convulsions, copious secretions from lung or airway, involuntary urination/defecation, muscular twitching/generalized weakness (severe)

Dosage adjustment in renal impairment: Use caution in renal impairment; pralidoxime is renally eliminated.

Dosage adjustment in hepatic impairment: No dosage adjustment provided in manufacturer's labeling.

Additional Information Complete prescribing information should be consulted for additional detail.

Dosage Forms

Injection, solution:

ATNAA, Duodote™: Atropine 2.1 mg/0.7 mL and pralidoxime chloride 600 mg/2 mL [contains benzyl alcohol; prefilled autoinjector]

- **Atropine and Pralidoxime Chloride** *see* Atropine and Pralidoxime *on page 203*
- **Atropine-Care [DSC]** *see* Atropine *on page 200*
- **Atropine, Hyoscyamine, Phenobarbital, and Scopolamine** *see* Hyoscyamine, Atropine, Scopolamine, and Phenobarbital *on page 1027*
- **Atropine Sulfate** *see* Atropine *on page 200*
- **Atropine Sulfate and Edrophonium Chloride** *see* Edrophonium and Atropine *on page 706*
- **Atrovent** *see* Ipratropium (Nasal) *on page 1109*
- **Atrovent® (Can)** *see* Ipratropium (Nasal) *on page 1109*
- **Atrovent HFA** *see* Ipratropium (Systemic) *on page 1108*
- **ATryn** *see* Antithrombin *on page 156*

Attapulgite [CAN/INT] (at a PULL gite)

Brand Names: Canada Kaopectate Children's [OTC]; Kaopectate Extra Strength [OTC]; Kaopectate [OTC]

Pharmacologic Category Antidiarrheal

Use Note: Not approved in U.S.

Symptomatic treatment of diarrhea and cramps

Contraindications Hypersensitivity to attapulgite or any component of the formulation

Warnings/Precautions Consult health care provider before initiating therapy if high fever or bloody stools are present. Do not use for >2 days. If diarrhea persists, consult health care provider.

Drug Interactions

Metabolism/Transport Effects None known.

Avoid Concomitant Use There are no known interactions where it is recommended to avoid concomitant use.

Increased Effect/Toxicity There are no known significant interactions involving an increase in effect.

Decreased Effect There are no known significant interactions involving a decrease in effect.

Mechanism of Action Nonselectively absorbs excess intestinal fluid, thereby reducing stool liquidity. May interfere with absorption of nutrients and other drugs as well.

Pharmacodynamics/Kinetics Absorption: Not absorbed

Dosage Oral: Give after each bowel movement

Children:

3-6 years: 300 mg/dose; maximum dose: 2100 mg/day

6-12 years: 600-750 mg/dose; maximum dose: 4500 mg/day

Children >12 years and Adults: 1200-1500 mg/dose; maximum dose: 8400 mg/day

Administration Shake liquid well before administering. Do not administer within 2-3 hours of other medications.

Monitoring Parameters Signs of fluid and electrolyte loss

Additional Information Attapulgite has been removed from the U.S. market. The U.S. Food and Drug Administration (FDA) found controlled studies documenting the efficacy of attapulgite to be inadequate.

Product Availability Not available in U.S.

Dosage Forms: Canada

Suspension, oral:

Kaopectate®: 600 mg/15 mL

Kaopectate® Children's: 600 mg/15 mL

Kaopectate® Extra Strength: 750 mg/15 mL

- **ATV** *see* Atazanavir *on page 185*
- **Aubagio** *see* Teriflunomide *on page 2006*
- **Aubra** *see* Ethinyl Estradiol and Levonorgestrel *on page 803*
- **Augmentin** *see* Amoxicillin and Clavulanate *on page 133*
- **Augmentin ES-600** *see* Amoxicillin and Clavulanate *on page 133*
- **Augmentin XR** *see* Amoxicillin and Clavulanate *on page 133*
- **Auralgan® (Can)** *see* Antipyrine and Benzocaine *on page 156*

Auranofin (au RANE oh fin)

Brand Names: U.S. Ridaura

Brand Names: Canada Ridaura®

Pharmacologic Category Gold Compound

Use Management of active stage classic or definite rheumatoid arthritis in patients who do not respond to or tolerate other agents

Pregnancy Risk Factor C

Dosage Oral: Adults: 6 mg/day in 1-2 divided doses; after 6 months may be increased to 9 mg/day in 3 divided doses; discontinue therapy if no response after 3 months at 9 mg/day

Note: Signs of clinical improvement may not be evident until after 3 months of therapy.

Dosage adjustment in renal impairment: There are no dosage adjustments provided in the manufacturer's labeling. The following guidelines have been used by some clinicians (Aronoff, 2007):

CrCl 50-80 mL/minute: Reduce dose to 50%

CrCl <50 mL/minute: Avoid use

Dosage adjustment in hepatic impairment: No dosage adjustment provided in manufacturer's labeling.

Additional Information Complete prescribing information should be consulted for additional detail.

Dosage Forms

Capsule, Oral:

Ridaura: 3 mg

- **Auraphene-B [OTC]** *see* Carbamide Peroxide *on page 350*
- **Auro-Alendronate (Can)** *see* Alendronate *on page 79*
- **Auro-Amlodipine (Can)** *see* AmLODIPine *on page 123*
- **Auro-Anastrozole (Can)** *see* Anastrozole *on page 148*
- **Auro-Atorvastatin (Can)** *see* AtorvaSTATin *on page 194*
- **Auro-Carvedilol (Can)** *see* Carvedilol *on page 367*
- **Auro-Cefixime (Can)** *see* Cefixime *on page 380*
- **Auro-Cefprozil (Can)** *see* Cefprozil *on page 389*
- **Auro-Cefuroxime (Can)** *see* Cefuroxime *on page 399*
- **Auro-Ciprofloxacin (Can)** *see* Ciprofloxacin (Systemic) *on page 441*
- **Auro-Citalopram (Can)** *see* Citalopram *on page 451*
- **Auro-Cyclobenzaprine (Can)** *see* Cyclobenzaprine *on page 516*
- **Aurodex® [DSC]** *see* Antipyrine and Benzocaine *on page 156*
- **Auro-Donepezil (Can)** *see* Donepezil *on page 668*
- **Auro-Finasteride (Can)** *see* Finasteride *on page 878*
- **Auro-Gabapentin (Can)** *see* Gabapentin *on page 943*
- **Auro-Galantamine ER (Can)** *see* Galantamine *on page 946*
- **Auro-Irbesartan (Can)** *see* Irbesartan *on page 1110*
- **Auro-Lamotrigine (Can)** *see* LamoTRIgine *on page 1160*
- **Auro-Letrozole (Can)** *see* Letrozole *on page 1181*
- **Auro-Levetiracetam (Can)** *see* LevETIRAcetam *on page 1191*
- **Auro-Lisinopril (Can)** *see* Lisinopril *on page 1226*
- **Auro-Losartan (Can)** *see* Losartan *on page 1248*
- **Auro-Losartan HCT (Can)** *see* Losartan and Hydrochlorothiazide *on page 1250*
- **Auro-Meloxicam (Can)** *see* Meloxicam *on page 1283*

- ◆ **Auro-Mirtazapine (Can)** *see* Mirtazapine *on page 1376*
- ◆ **Auro-Mirtazapine OD (Can)** *see* Mirtazapine *on page 1376*
- ◆ **Auro-Montelukast (Can)** *see* Montelukast *on page 1392*
- ◆ **Auro-Montelukast Chewable Tablets (Can)** *see* Montelukast *on page 1392*
- ◆ **Auro-Nevirapine (Can)** *see* Nevirapine *on page 1440*
- ◆ **Auro-Omeprazole (Can)** *see* Omeprazole *on page 1508*
- ◆ **Auro-Paroxetine (Can)** *see* PARoxetine *on page 1579*
- ◆ **Auro-Pioglitazone (Can)** *see* Pioglitazone *on page 1654*
- ◆ **Auro-Pramipexole (Can)** *see* Pramipexole *on page 1695*
- ◆ **Auro-Quetiapine (Can)** *see* QUEtiapine *on page 1751*
- ◆ **Auro-Ramipri (Can)** *see* Ramipril *on page 1771*
- ◆ **Auro-Repaglinide (Can)** *see* Repaglinide *on page 1791*
- ◆ **Auro-Sertraline (Can)** *see* Sertraline *on page 1878*
- ◆ **Auro-Simvastatin (Can)** *see* Simvastatin *on page 1890*
- ◆ **Auro-Terbinafine (Can)** *see* Terbinafine (Systemic) *on page 2002*
- ◆ **AURO-Topiramate (Can)** *see* Topiramate *on page 2065*
- ◆ **Auro-Valsartan (Can)** *see* Valsartan *on page 2127*
- ◆ **Auryxia** *see* Ferric Citrate *on page 869*
- ◆ **Auvi-Q** *see* EPINEPHrine (Systemic, Oral Inhalation) *on page 735*
- ◆ **AVA** *see* Anthrax Vaccine Adsorbed *on page 151*
- ◆ **Ava-Acebutolol (Can)** *see* Acebutolol *on page 29*
- ◆ **Ava-Atenolol (Can)** *see* Atenolol *on page 189*
- ◆ **Ava-Atorvastatin (Can)** *see* AtorvaSTATin *on page 194*
- ◆ **Ava-Bisoprolol (Can)** *see* Bisoprolol *on page 266*
- ◆ **Ava-Bupropion SR (Can)** *see* BuPROPion *on page 305*
- ◆ **Ava-Cefprozil (Can)** *see* Cefprozil *on page 389*
- ◆ **Ava-Clindamycin (Can)** *see* Clindamycin (Systemic) *on page 460*
- ◆ **Ava-Cyclobenzaprine (Can)** *see* Cyclobenzaprine *on page 516*
- ◆ **Ava-Diltiazem (Can)** *see* Diltiazem *on page 634*
- ◆ **Ava-Famciclovir (Can)** *see* Famciclovir *on page 843*
- ◆ **Ava-Fenofibrate Micro (Can)** *see* Fenofibrate and Derivatives *on page 852*
- ◆ **Ava-Fluoxetine (Can)** *see* FLUoxetine *on page 899*
- ◆ **Ava-Fluvoxamine (Can)** *see* FluvoxaMINE *on page 916*
- ◆ **Ava-Fosinopril (Can)** *see* Fosinopril *on page 932*
- ◆ **AVA-Furosemide (Can)** *see* Furosemide *on page 940*
- ◆ **Avage** *see* Tazarotene *on page 1980*
- ◆ **AVA-Gliclazide (Can)** *see* Gliclazide [CAN/INT] *on page 964*
- ◆ **Ava-Glyburide (Can)** *see* GlyBURIDE *on page 972*
- ◆ **Ava-Hydrochlorothiazide (Can)** *see* Hydrochlorothiazide *on page 1009*
- ◆ **Ava-Irbesartan (Can)** *see* Irbesartan *on page 1110*
- ◆ **Avakine** *see* InFLIXimab *on page 1070*
- ◆ **Avalide** *see* Irbesartan and Hydrochlorothiazide *on page 1112*
- ◆ **Ava-Lisinopril/Hctz (Can)** *see* Lisinopril and Hydrochlorothiazide *on page 1229*
- ◆ **Ava-Lovastatin (Can)** *see* Lovastatin *on page 1252*
- ◆ **Ava-Meloxicam (Can)** *see* Meloxicam *on page 1283*
- ◆ **Ava-Metformin (Can)** *see* MetFORMIN *on page 1307*
- ◆ **Ava-Metoprolol (Can)** *see* Metoprolol *on page 1350*
- ◆ **Ava-Metoprolol (Type L) (Can)** *see* Metoprolol *on page 1350*
- ◆ **Ava-Mirtazapine (Can)** *see* Mirtazapine *on page 1376*
- ◆ **Avamys (Can)** *see* Fluticasone (Nasal) *on page 910*

Avanafil (a VAN a fil)

Brand Names: U.S. Stendra

Index Terms Stendra

Pharmacologic Category Phosphodiesterase-5 Enzyme Inhibitor

Use Erectile dysfunction: Treatment of erectile dysfunction

Pregnancy Risk Factor C

Pregnancy Considerations Based on data from animal reproduction studies, avanafil is predicted to have a low risk for major developmental abnormalities in humans. This product is not indicated for use in women.

Breast-Feeding Considerations This product is not indicated for use in women.

Contraindications Coadministration with any form of organic nitrates, either regularly and/or intermittently; hypersensitivity to avanafil or any component of the formulation.

Warnings/Precautions There is a degree of cardiac risk associated with sexual activity; therefore, physicians may wish to consider the patient's cardiovascular status prior to initiating any treatment for erectile dysfunction. Use caution in patients with anatomical deformation of the penis (angulation, cavernosal fibrosis, or Peyronie's disease) and in patients who have conditions which may predispose them to priapism (sickle cell anemia, multiple myeloma, leukemia). Priapism, painful erection >6 hours in duration has been reported (rarely). Instruct patients to seek immediate medical attention if erection persists >4 hours.

Use is not recommended in patients with hypotension (<90/50 mm Hg); uncontrolled hypertension (>170/100 mm Hg); unstable angina or angina during intercourse; life-threatening arrhythmias, stroke, or MI within the last 6 months; cardiac failure or coronary artery disease causing unstable angina. Safety and efficacy have not been studied in these patients. Use caution in patients with left ventricular outflow obstruction (eg, aortic stenosis, idiopathic hypertrophic subaortic stenosis). Use caution with alpha-blockers; dosage adjustment is needed. Patients should avoid or limit concurrent substantial alcohol consumption as this may increase the risk of symptomatic hypotension.

Rare cases of nonarteritic ischemic optic neuropathy (NAION) have been reported; patients who have already experienced NAION are at an increased risk of recurrence. Other risk factors for NAION include heart disease, diabetes, hypertension, smoking, age >50 years, or history of certain eye problems. Use with caution in these patients only when the benefits outweigh the risks. Sudden decrease or loss of hearing has been reported rarely; hearing changes may be accompanied by tinnitus and dizziness.

Safety and efficacy have not been studied in patients with the following conditions, therefore, use in these patients is not recommended at this time: Severe hepatic impairment (Child-Pugh class C); severe renal impairment; end-stage renal disease requiring dialysis; retinitis pigmentosa or other degenerative retinal disorders. Potentially significant drug-drug interactions may exist, requiring dose or frequency adjustment, additional monitoring, and/or selection of alternative therapy. Use of avanafil is contraindicated in patients currently taking nitrate preparations. According to the manufacturer, when nitrate administration is deemed medically necessary in a life-threatening situation, may administer nitrates only if 12 hours has elapsed after avanafil use. Of note, the elimination half-life of avanafil is similar to that of sildenafil and vardenafil which both require 24 hours to elapse prior to administration of nitrates (ACCF/AHA [Anderson, 2013]; ACCF/AHA [O'Gara, 2013]). Potential underlying causes of erectile dysfunction should be evaluated prior to treatment.

Adverse Reactions

Cardiovascular: ECG abnormality, flushing

Central nervous system: Dizziness, headache

Gastrointestinal: Viral gastroenteritis

Neuromuscular & skeletal: Back pain

Respiratory: Nasal congestion, nasopharyngitis, upper respiratory tract infection

Rare but important or life-threatening: Angina pectoris, anterior ischemic optic neuropathy (nonarteritic), balanitis, deep vein thrombosis, depression, gastritis, gastroesophageal reflux disease, hearing loss, hematuria, hyperglycemia, hypertension, hypoglycemia, hypotension, increased serum ALT, myalgia, nausea, nephrolithiasis, palpitations, peripheral edema, pollakiuria, priapism, skin rash, urinary tract infection, vision color changes, vision loss (temporary or permanent), wheezing

Drug Interactions

Metabolism/Transport Effects Substrate of CYP3A4 (major); **Note:** Assignment of Major/Minor substrate status based on clinically relevant drug interaction potential

Avoid Concomitant Use

Avoid concomitant use of Avanafil with any of the following: Alprostadil; Amyl Nitrite; Conivaptan; CYP3A4 Inhibitors (Strong); Dapoxetine; Fusidic Acid (Systemic); Idelalisib; Itraconazole; Ketoconazole (Systemic); Phosphodiesterase 5 Inhibitors; Posaconazole; Riociguat; Vasodilators (Organic Nitrates); Voriconazole

Increased Effect/Toxicity

Avanafil may increase the levels/effects of: Alpha1-Blockers; Alprostadil; Amyl Nitrite; Antihypertensives; Bosentan; Phosphodiesterase 5 Inhibitors; Riociguat; Vasodilators (Organic Nitrates)

The levels/effects of Avanafil may be increased by: Alcohol (Ethyl); Conivaptan; CYP3A4 Inhibitors (Moderate); CYP3A4 Inhibitors (Strong); Dapoxetine; Dasatinib; Fluconazole; Fusidic Acid (Systemic); Idelalisib; Itraconazole; Ivacaftor; Ketoconazole (Systemic); Lorcaserin; Luliconazole; Mifepristone; Posaconazole; Sapropterin; Simeprevir; Voriconazole

Decreased Effect

The levels/effects of Avanafil may be decreased by: Bosentan; CYP3A4 Inducers (Moderate); CYP3A4 Inducers (Strong); Dabrafenib; Deferasirox; Etravirine; Mitotane; Siltuximab; St Johns Wort; Tocilizumab

Food Interactions Grapefruit juice may increase serum levels/toxicity of avanafil. Management: Avoid grapefruit juice.

Storage/Stability Store at 20°C to 25°C (68°F to 77°F); excursions are permitted to 30°C (86°F). Protect from light.

Mechanism of Action Does not directly cause penile erections, but affects the response to sexual stimulation. The physiologic mechanism of erection of the penis involves release of nitric oxide (NO) in the corpus cavernosum during sexual stimulation. NO then activates the enzyme guanylate cyclase, which results in increased levels of cyclic guanosine monophosphate (cGMP), producing smooth muscle relaxation and inflow of blood to the corpus cavernosum. Avanafil enhances the effect of NO by inhibiting phosphodiesterase type 5 (PDE-5), which is responsible for degradation of cGMP in the corpus cavernosum; when sexual stimulation causes local release of NO, inhibition of PDE-5 by avanafil causes increased levels of cGMP in the corpus cavernosum, resulting in smooth muscle relaxation and inflow of blood to the corpus cavernosum; at recommended doses, it has no effect in the absence of sexual stimulation.

Pharmacodynamics/Kinetics

Absorption: Rapid

Protein binding: ~99%

Metabolism: Hepatic via CYP3A4 (major), CYP2C (minor); forms metabolites (active and inactive)

Half-life elimination: Terminal: ~5 hours

Time to peak, plasma: 30 to 45 minutes (fasting); 1.12 to 1.25 hours (high-fat meal)

Excretion: Feces (~62%); urine (~21%)

Dosage Oral: Erectile dysfunction:

Adults: Initial: 100 mg taken ~15 minutes prior to sexual activity; taken as one single dose and not more than once daily; dose may be increased to 200 mg ~15 minutes prior to sexual activity or decreased to 50 mg ~30 minutes prior to sexual activity using the lowest dose that provides benefit; maximum: 200 mg daily

Elderly ≥65 years: Refer to adult dosing.

Dosing adjustment with concomitant medications:

Alpha-blocker (dose should be stable at time of avanafil initiation): Initial avanafil dose: 50 mg taken as one single dose and not more than once daily.

Moderate CYP34A inhibitors (including amprenavir, aprepitant, diltiazem, erythromycin, fluconazole, fosamprenavir, verapamil): Maximum avanafil dose: 50 mg taken as one single dose and not more than once daily.

Strong CYP3A4 inhibitors (including atazanavir, clarithromycin, indinavir, itraconazole, ketoconazole, nefazodone, nelfinavir, saquinavir, ritonavir, telithromycin): Avoid concomitant use of avanafil.

Dosage adjustment in renal impairment:

CrCl ≥30 mL/minute: No dosage adjustment necessary.

CrCl <30 mL/minute: Has not been studied; use is not recommended by the manufacturer.

ESRD requiring hemodialysis: Has not been studied; use is not recommended by the manufacturer.

Dosage adjustment in hepatic impairment:

Mild-to-moderate hepatic impairment (Child-Pugh class A or B): No dosage adjustment required

Severe hepatic impairment (Child-Pugh class C): Has not been studied; use is not recommended by the manufacturer

Dietary Considerations Avoid grapefruit juice.

Administration May be administered with or without food, ~15 to 30 minutes prior to sexual activity.

Monitoring Parameters Monitor for response, adverse reactions, blood pressure, and heart rate.

Dosage Forms

Tablet, Oral:

Stendra: 50 mg, 100 mg, 200 mg

◆ **Ava-Naproxen EC (Can)** *see* Naproxen *on page 1427*

◆ **Avandamet** *see* Rosiglitazone and Metformin *on page 1847*

◆ **Avandaryl** *see* Rosiglitazone and Glimepiride *on page 1847*

◆ **Avandia** *see* Rosiglitazone *on page 1847*

◆ **Ava-Nortriptyline (Can)** *see* Nortriptyline *on page 1476*

◆ **Ava-Omeprazole (Can)** *see* Omeprazole *on page 1508*

◆ **Ava-Ondansetron (Can)** *see* Ondansetron *on page 1513*

◆ **Ava-Pantoprazole (Can)** *see* Pantoprazole *on page 1570*

◆ **Ava-Pramipexole (Can)** *see* Pramipexole *on page 1695*

◆ **Avapro** *see* Irbesartan *on page 1110*

◆ **Avapro HCT** *see* Irbesartan and Hydrochlorothiazide *on page 1112*

◆ **Ava-Quetiapine (Can)** *see* QUEtiapine *on page 1751*

- **AVAR** *see* Sulfur and Sulfacetamide *on page 1953*
- **AVAR-e** *see* Sulfur and Sulfacetamide *on page 1953*
- **AVAR-e Green** *see* Sulfur and Sulfacetamide *on page 1953*
- **AVAR-e LS** *see* Sulfur and Sulfacetamide *on page 1953*
- **Ava-Risperidone (Can)** *see* RisperiDONE *on page 1818*
- **AVAR LS** *see* Sulfur and Sulfacetamide *on page 1953*
- **Ava-Simvastatin (Can)** *see* Simvastatin *on page 1890*
- **Avastin** *see* Bevacizumab *on page 257*
- **Ava-Sumatriptan (Can)** *see* SUMAtriptan *on page 1953*
- **Ava-Valsartan (Can)** *see* Valsartan *on page 2127*
- **Ava-Valsartan/HCT (Can)** *see* Valsartan and Hydrochlorothiazide *on page 2129*
- **Avaxim (Can)** *see* Hepatitis A Vaccine *on page 1001*
- **Avaxim-Pediatric (Can)** *see* Hepatitis A Vaccine *on page 1001*
- **AVC Vaginal** *see* Sulfanilamide *on page 1950*
- **AVE 0005** *see* Aflibercept (Ophthalmic) *on page 63*
- **Aveed** *see* Testosterone *on page 2010*
- **Avelox** *see* Moxifloxacin (Systemic) *on page 1401*
- **Avelox ABC Pack** *see* Moxifloxacin (Systemic) *on page 1401*
- **Avelox I.V. (Can)** *see* Moxifloxacin (Systemic) *on page 1401*
- **Aventyl (Can)** *see* Nortriptyline *on page 1476*
- **Aviane** *see* Ethinyl Estradiol and Levonorgestrel *on page 803*
- **Avian Influenza Virus Vaccine** *see* Influenza A Virus Vaccine (H5N1) *on page 1074*
- **Avidoxy** *see* Doxycycline *on page 689*
- **AVINza** *see* Morphine (Systemic) *on page 1394*
- **Avita** *see* Tretinoin (Topical) *on page 2099*
- **Avodart** *see* Dutasteride *on page 702*
- **Avonex** *see* Interferon Beta-1a *on page 1100*
- **Avonex Pen** *see* Interferon Beta-1a *on page 1100*
- **AVP** *see* Vasopressin *on page 2142*
- **Axert** *see* Almotriptan *on page 92*
- **Axid** *see* Nizatidine *on page 1471*
- **Axid AR [OTC]** *see* Nizatidine *on page 1471*
- **Axiron** *see* Testosterone *on page 2010*

Axitinib (ax I ti nib)

Brand Names: U.S. Inlyta

Brand Names: Canada Inlyta

Index Terms AG-013736

Pharmacologic Category Antineoplastic Agent, Tyrosine Kinase Inhibitor; Antineoplastic Agent, Vascular Endothelial Growth Factor (VEGF) Inhibitor

Use **Renal cell carcinoma, advanced:** Treatment of advanced renal cell carcinoma after failure of one prior systemic therapy.

Pregnancy Risk Factor D

Pregnancy Considerations Teratogenic, embryotoxic, and fetotoxic events were observed in animal reproduction studies when administered in doses less than the normal human dose. Based on its mechanism of action and because axitinib inhibits angiogenesis (a critical component of fetal development), adverse effects on pregnancy would be expected. Women of childbearing potential should be advised to avoid pregnancy during therapy.

Breast-Feeding Considerations It is not known if axitinib is excreted in breast milk. Due to the potential for serious adverse reactions in the nursing infant, the manufacturer recommends a decision be made whether to discontinue nursing or to discontinue the drug, taking into account the importance of treatment to the mother.

Contraindications There are no contraindications listed within the manufacturer's labeling.

Warnings/Precautions Hazardous agent - use appropriate precautions for handling and disposal (meets NIOSH 2014 criteria). May cause hypertension; the median onset is within the first month, and has been observed as early as 4 days after treatment initiation. Hypertensive crisis has been reported. Blood pressure should be well-controlled prior to treatment initiation. Monitor blood pressure and treat with standard antihypertensive therapy. Persistent hypertension (despite antihypertensive therapy) may require dose reduction; discontinue if severe and persistent despite concomitant antihypertensives (or dose reduction), or with evidence of hypertensive crisis. Monitor for hypotension if on antihypertensive therapy and axitinib is withheld or discontinued. Cardiac failure, including fatal events, has been observed rarely. Monitor for signs/symptoms of cardiac failure throughout therapy; management may require permanent therapy discontinuation.

Gastrointestinal perforation and fistulas (including a fatality) have been reported. Monitor for signs/symptoms throughout treatment. Has not been studied in patients with recent active gastrointestinal bleeding; use is not recommended.

Arterial thrombotic events (cerebrovascular accident, MI, retinal artery occlusion, and transient ischemic attack), with fatalities, have been reported. Venous thrombotic events, including pulmonary embolism, deep vein thrombosis, retinal vein occlusion and retinal vein thrombosis, have been observed (with some fatalities). Use with caution in patients with a history of or risks for arterial or venous thrombotic events; has not been studied in patients within 12 months of an arterial thrombotic event or within 6 months of a venous thrombotic event. Hemorrhagic events (cerebral hemorrhage, gastrointestinal hemorrhage, hematuria, hemoptysis, and melena) have been reported (with some fatalities). Temporarily interrupt treatment with any hemorrhage requiring medical intervention.

Cases of reversible posterior leukoencephalopathy syndrome (RPLS) have been reported. Symptoms of RPLS include confusion, headache, hypertension (mild-to-severe), lethargy, seizure, blindness and/or other vision, or neurologic disturbances; interrupt treatment and manage hypertension. MRI is recommended to confirm RPLS diagnosis. Discontinue axitinib if RPLS is confirmed. The safety of reinitiating axitinib in patients previously experiencing RPLS is unknown.

Hypothyroidism occurs commonly with tyrosine kinase inhibitors, including axitinib. Hyperthyroidism has also been reported. Monitor thyroid function at baseline and periodically throughout therapy. Thyroid disorders should be treated according to standard practice to achieve/maintain euthyroid state. Proteinuria is associated with use. Monitor for proteinuria at baseline and periodically throughout therapy. If moderate or severe proteinuria occurs, reduce dose or temporarily withhold treatment. Although the effect on wound healing has not been studied with axitinib, vascular endothelial growth factor (VEGF) receptor inhibitors are associated with impaired wound healing. Discontinue treatment at least 24 hours prior to scheduled surgery; treatment reinitiation should be guided by clinical judgment and wound assessment. Has not been studied in patients with evidence of untreated brain metastases; use is not recommended. Systemic exposure to axitinib is increased in patients with moderate hepatic impairment;

dose reductions are recommended. Has not been studied in patients with severe hepatic impairment. Increases in ALT have been observed during treatment; monitor liver function tests. Potentially significant drug-drug interactions may exist, requiring dose or frequency adjustment, additional monitoring, and/or selection of alternative therapy.

Adverse Reactions

Cardiovascular: Arterial thrombotic events, deep vein thrombosis, hypertension, transient ischemic attack, venous thrombotic events

Central nervous system: Dizziness, dysphonia, fatigue, headache

Dermatologic: Alopecia, dry skin, erythema, palmar-plantar erythrodysesthesia syndrome, pruritus, rash

Endocrine & metabolic: Bicarbonate decreased, dehydration, hyper-/hypoglycemia, hyperkalemia, hypernatremia, hyper-/hypothyroidism, hypoalbuminemia, hypocalcemia, hyponatremia, hypophosphatemia

Gastrointestinal: Abdominal pain, amylase increased, appetite decreased, constipation, diarrhea, dyspepsia, fistula, gastrointestinal perforation, hemorrhoids, lipase increased, mucosal inflammation, nausea, rectal hemorrhage, stomatitis, taste alteration, vomiting, weight loss

Hematologic: Anemia, hemoglobin increased, hemorrhage, leukopenia, lymphopenia, polycythemia, thrombocytopenia

Hepatic: Alkaline phosphatase increased, ALT increased, AST increased

Neuromuscular & skeletal: Arthralgia, limb pain, myalgia, weakness

Ocular: Retinal vein occlusion/thrombosis

Otic: Tinnitus

Renal: Creatinine increased, hematuria, proteinuria

Respiratory: Cough, dyspnea, epistaxis, hemoptysis, pulmonary embolism

Rare but important or life-threatening: Cerebral bleeding, cerebrovascular accident, fever, hypertensive crisis, heart failure, neutropenia, reversible posterior leukoencephalopathy syndrome (RPLS)

Drug Interactions

Metabolism/Transport Effects Substrate of CYP1A2 (minor), CYP2C19 (minor), CYP3A4 (major), UGT1A1; **Note:** Assignment of Major/Minor substrate status based on clinically relevant drug interaction potential

Avoid Concomitant Use

Avoid concomitant use of Axitinib with any of the following: Conivaptan; CYP3A4 Inducers (Moderate); CYP3A4 Inducers (Strong); CYP3A4 Inhibitors (Strong); Fusidic Acid (Systemic); Grapefruit Juice; Idelalisib; St Johns Wort

Increased Effect/Toxicity

Axitinib may increase the levels/effects of: Bisphosphonate Derivatives

The levels/effects of Axitinib may be increased by: Aprepitant; Ceritinib; Conivaptan; CYP3A4 Inhibitors (Moderate); CYP3A4 Inhibitors (Strong); Dasatinib; Fosaprepitant; Fusidic Acid (Systemic); Grapefruit Juice; Idelalisib; Ivacaftor; Luliconazole; Mifepristone; Netupitant; Simeprevir

Decreased Effect

The levels/effects of Axitinib may be decreased by: CYP3A4 Inducers (Moderate); CYP3A4 Inducers (Strong); Deferasirox; Siltuximab; St Johns Wort; Tocilizumab

Food Interactions Axitinib serum concentrations may be increased when taken with grapefruit or grapefruit juice. Management: Avoid concurrent use.

Storage/Stability Store at 20°C to 25°C (68°F to 77°F); excursions permitted to 15°C to 30°C (59°F to 86°F).

Mechanism of Action Axitinib is a selective second generation tyrosine kinase inhibitor which blocks angiogenesis and tumor growth by inhibiting vascular endothelial growth factor receptors (VEGFR-1, VEGFR-2, and VEGFR-3).

Pharmacodynamics/Kinetics

Absorption: Rapid (Rugo, 2005)

Distribution: V_d: 160 L

Protein binding: >99%; to albumin (primarily) and to alpha$_1$ acid glycoprotein (AAG)

Metabolism: Hepatic; primarily via CYP3A4/5 and to a lesser extend via CYP1A2, CYP2C19 and UGT1A1

Bioavailability: 58%

Half-life elimination: 2.5 to 6 hours

Time to peak: 2.5 to 4 hours

Excretion: Feces (~41%; 12% as unchanged drug); urine (~23%; as metabolites)

Dosage Renal cell cancer, advanced: Adults: Oral: Initial: 5 mg twice daily (approximately every 12 hours)

Dose increases: If dose is tolerated (no adverse events above grade 2, blood pressure is normal and no antihypertensive use) for at least 2 consecutive weeks, may increase the dose to 7 mg twice daily, and then further increase (using the same tolerance criteria) to 10 mg twice daily.

Dose decreases: For adverse events, reduce dose from 5 mg twice daily to 3 mg twice daily; further reduce to 2 mg twice daily if adverse events persist.

Dosage adjustment for strong CYP3A4 inhibitors: Avoid concomitant administration with strong CYP3A4 inhibitors (eg, clarithromycin, itraconazole, ketoconazole, nefazodone, protease inhibitors, telithromycin, voriconazole, grapefruit juice); if concomitant administration with a strong CYP3A4 inhibitor cannot be avoided, ~50% dosage reduction is recommended; adjust dose based on individual tolerance and safety. When the strong CYP3A4 inhibitor is discontinued, resume previous axitinib dose after 3-5 half-lives of the inhibitor have passed.

Dosing adjustment for toxicity:

Adverse events: May require temporary interruption, dose decreases (reduce dose from 5 mg twice daily to 3 mg twice daily; further reduce to 2 mg twice daily) or discontinuation

Cardiac failure: May require permanent discontinuation

Hypertension: Treat with standard antihypertensive therapy.

Persistent hypertension: May require dose reduction

Severe, persistent (despite antihypertensives and dose reduction), or evidence of hypertensive crisis: Discontinue treatment

Hemorrhage: Any bleeding requiring medical intervention: Temporarily interrupt treatment.

Proteinuria (moderate-to-severe): Reduce dose or temporarily interrupt treatment.

Dosage adjustment in renal impairment:

Mild to severe renal impairment (CrCl 15 to <89 mL/minute): No initial dosage adjustment necessary.

End-stage renal disease (ESRD) There are no dosage adjustments provided in the manufacturer's labeling; use with caution.

Dosage adjustment in hepatic impairment:

Mild impairment (Child-Pugh class A): No starting dosage adjustment necessary.

Moderate impairment (Child-Pugh class B): Reduce starting dose by ~50%; increase or decrease based on individual tolerance.

Severe impairment (Child-Pugh class C): There are no dosage adjustments provided in the manufacturer's labeling (has not been studied).

Dietary Considerations May be taken without regard to food. Avoid grapefruit and grapefruit juice.

Administration Oral: Swallow tablet whole with a glass of water. May be taken with or without food. If a dose is missed or vomited, do not make up; resume dosing with the next scheduled dose. A suspension may be prepared for nasogastric administration (refer to Extemporaneous Preparations information).

Hazardous agent; use appropriate precautions for handling and disposal (meets NIOSH 2014 criteria).

Monitoring Parameters Hepatic function (ALT, AST, and bilirubin; baseline and periodic), thyroid function (baseline and periodic), urinalysis (for proteinuria; baseline and periodically); blood pressure, signs/symptoms of RPLS, gastrointestinal bleeding/perforation/fistula, signs/symptoms cardiac failure

Thyroid function testing recommendations (Hamnvik, 2011):

Preexisting levothyroxine therapy: Obtain baseline TSH levels, then monitor every 4 weeks until levels and levothyroxine dose are stable, then monitor every 2 months

Without preexisting thyroid hormone replacement: TSH at baseline, then monthly for 4 months, then every 2-3 months

Dosage Forms

Tablet, Oral:

Inlyta: 1 mg, 5 mg

Extemporaneous Preparations Hazardous agent – use appropriate precautions for handling and disposal (meets NIOSH 2014 criteria). For patients unable to swallow tablets whole, a suspension may be prepared for nasogastric tube administration (for doses of 2 to 10 mg). Place a 20 mL tightly capped amber syringe in a small drinking glass, with the open end of the syringe pointing up. Place the appropriate axitinib dose in the open syringe barrel; add 15 mL of USP grade water (do not use tap water or bottled water) to the syringe. Allow at least 10 minutes to dissolve the tablets; avoid direct light. Place the plunger of the syringe into the barrel, invert the syringe so the tip is pointing upward and remove the cap. Expel excess air; replace the cap until ready for use (keep syringe tip facing up). Prior to administration, gently invert the syringe several times to ensure a uniform suspension. Flush the nasogastric feeding tube with 15 mL of USP grade water before administration. After administering the dose, draw up 10 mL of USP grade water (into the same syringe which contained the dose) and flush the feeding tube; repeat this step 5 additional times to ensure the entire dose has been administered. Lastly, flush the feeding tube with a separate syringe containing 15 mL of USP grade water. Administer within 15 minutes of preparation.

Borst DL, Arruda LS, MacLean E, Pithavala YK, Morgado JE. Common questions regarding clinical use of axitinib in advanced renal cell carcinoma. *Am J Health Syst Pharm*. 2014;71(13):1092-1096.

◆ **AY-25650** *see* Triptorelin *on page* 2107

◆ **Aygestin** *see* Norethindrone *on page* 1473

◆ **Ayr [OTC]** *see* Sodium Chloride *on page* 1902

◆ **Ayr Nasal Mist Allergy/Sinus [OTC]** *see* Sodium Chloride *on page* 1902

◆ **Ayr Saline Nasal [OTC]** *see* Sodium Chloride *on page* 1902

◆ **Ayr Saline Nasal Drops [OTC]** *see* Sodium Chloride *on page* 1902

◆ **Ayr Saline Nasal Gel [OTC]** *see* Sodium Chloride *on page* 1902

◆ **Ayr Saline Nasal No-Drip [OTC]** *see* Sodium Chloride *on page* 1902

◆ **AYR Saline Nasal Rinse [OTC]** *see* Sodium Chloride *on page* 1902

◆ **5-Aza-2'-deoxycytidine** *see* Decitabine *on page* 581

AzaCITIDine (ay za SYE ti deen)

Brand Names: U.S. Vidaza

Brand Names: Canada Vidaza

Index Terms 5-Azacytidine; 5-AZC; AZA-CR; Azacytidine; Ladakamycin

Pharmacologic Category Antineoplastic Agent, Antimetabolite; Antineoplastic Agent, DNA Methylation Inhibitor

Use Myelodysplastic syndromes: Treatment of myelodysplastic syndrome (MDS) in patients with the following subtypes: Refractory anemia or refractory anemia with ringed sideroblasts (if accompanied by neutropenia or thrombocytopenia or requiring transfusions), refractory anemia with excess blasts, refractory anemia with excess blasts in transformation, and chronic myelomonocytic leukemia

Pregnancy Risk Factor D

Dosage Note: Azacitidine is associated with a moderate emetic potential (Basch, 2011; Roila, 2010); antiemetics are recommended to prevent nausea and vomiting.

Myelodysplastic syndromes (MDS): Adults: IV, SubQ: Initial cycle: 75 mg/m^2/day for 7 days. Subsequent cycles: 75 mg/m^2/day for 7 days every 4 weeks; dose may be increased to 100 mg/m^2/day if no benefit is observed after 2 cycles and no toxicity other than nausea and vomiting have occurred. Patients should be treated for a minimum of 4-6 cycles; treatment may be continued as long as patient continues to benefit.

Note: Alternate (off-label) schedules (which have produced hematologic response) have been used for convenience in community oncology centers (Lyons, 2009): SubQ:

75 mg/m^2/day for 5 days (Mon-Fri), 2 days rest (Sat, Sun), then 75 mg/m^2/day for 2 days (Mon, Tues); repeat cycle every 28 days **or**

50 mg/m^2/day for 5 days (Mon-Fri), 2 days rest (Sat, Sun), then 50 mg/m^2/day for 5 days (Mon-Fri); repeat cycle every 28 days **or**

75 mg/m^2/day for 5 days (Mon-Fri), repeat cycle every 28 days

Acute myeloid leukemia (AML; off-label use): SubQ: 75 mg/m^2/day for 7 days every 4 weeks for at least 6 cycles (Fenaux, 2010)

Elderly: Refer to adult dosing; due to the potential for decreased renal function in the elderly, select dose carefully and closely monitor renal function

Dosage adjustment based on hematology: MDS:

For baseline WBC ≥3 x 10^9/L, ANC ≥1.5 x 10^9/L, and platelets ≥75 x 10^9/L:

Nadir count: ANC <0.5 x 10^9/L or platelets <25 x 10^9/L: Administer 50% of dose during next treatment course

Nadir count: ANC 0.5-1.5 x 10^9/L or platelets 25-50 x 10^9/L: Administer 67% of dose during next treatment course

Nadir count: ANC >1.5 x 10^9/L or platelets >50 x 10^9/L: Administer 100% of dose during next treatment course

For baseline WBC <3 x 10^9/L, ANC <1.5 x 10^9/L, or platelets <75 x 10^9/L: Adjust dose as follows based on nadir counts and bone marrow biopsy cellularity at the time of nadir, unless clear improvement in differentiation at the time of the next cycle:

WBC or platelet nadir decreased 50% to 75% from baseline and bone marrow biopsy cellularity at time of nadir 30% to 60%: Administer 100% of dose during next treatment course

WBC or platelet nadir decreased 50% to 75% from baseline and bone marrow biopsy cellularity at time of nadir 15% to 30%: Administer 50% of dose during next treatment course

WBC or platelet nadir decreased 50% to 75% from baseline and bone marrow biopsy cellularity at time of nadir <15%: Administer 33% of dose during next treatment course

WBC or platelet nadir decreased >75% from baseline and bone marrow biopsy cellularity at time of nadir 30% to 60%: Administer 75% of dose during next treatment course

WBC or platelet nadir decreased >75% from baseline and bone marrow biopsy cellularity at time of nadir 15% to 30%: Administer 50% of dose during next treatment course

WBC or platelet nadir decreased >75% from baseline and bone marrow biopsy cellularity at time of nadir <15%: Administer 33% of dose during next treatment course

Note: If a nadir defined above occurs, administer the next treatment course 28 days after the start of the preceding course as long as WBC and platelet counts are >25% above the nadir and rising. If a >25% increase above the nadir is not seen by day 28, reassess counts every 7 days. If a 25% increase is not seen by day 42, administer 50% of the scheduled dose.

Dosage adjustment based on serum electrolytes: If serum bicarbonate falls to <20 mEq/L (unexplained decrease): Reduce dose by 50% for next treatment course

Dosage adjustment in renal impairment:

Renal impairment at *baseline*:

Mild to moderate impairment (CrCl ≥30 mL/minute): No dosage adjustment necessary (Douvali, 2012).

Severe impairment (CrCl <30 mL/minute): No dosage adjustment necessary for cycle 1; due to renal excretion of azacitidine and metabolites, monitor closely for toxicity.

Renal toxicity *during* treatment: Unexplained increases in BUN or serum creatinine: Delay next cycle until values reach baseline or normal, then reduce dose by 50% for next treatment course.

Dosage adjustment in hepatic impairment: No dosage adjustment provided in the manufacturer's labeling (has not been studied). Use is contraindicated in patients with advanced malignant hepatic tumors.

Dosing in obesity: *ASCO Guidelines for appropriate chemotherapy dosing in obese adults with cancer:* Utilize patient's actual body weight (full weight) for calculation of body surface area- or weight-based dosing, particularly when the intent of therapy is curative; manage regimen-related toxicities in the same manner as for nonobese patients; if a dose reduction is utilized due to toxicity, consider resumption of full weight-based dosing with subsequent cycles, especially if cause of toxicity (eg, hepatic or renal impairment) is resolved (Griggs, 2012).

Additional Information Complete prescribing information should be consulted for additional detail.

Dosage Forms

Suspension Reconstituted, Injection:

Generic: 100 mg (1 ea)

Suspension Reconstituted, Injection [preservative free]:

Vidaza: 100 mg (1 ea)

Generic: 100 mg (1 ea)

◆ **AZA-CR** *see* AzaCITIDine *on page* *209*

◆ **Azactam** *see* Aztreonam *on page* *220*

◆ **Azactam in Dextrose** *see* Aztreonam *on page* *220*

◆ **Azacytidine** *see* AzaCITIDine *on page* *209*

◆ **5-Azacytidine** *see* AzaCITIDine *on page* *209*

◆ **5-Aza-dCyd** *see* Decitabine *on page* *581*

◆ **Azaepothilone B** *see* Ixabepilone *on page* *1138*

Azapropazone [INT] (ay za PRO pa zone)

International Brand Names Cinnamin (JP); Debelex (AR); Prolixan (AT, CH, CZ, HU, IT, NL, PT); Rheumox (GB, IE); Tolyprin (DE)

Pharmacologic Category Analgesic, Nonsteroidal Anti-inflammatory Drug

Reported Use Treatment of rheumatoid arthritis, ankylosing spondylitis, and acute gout

Dosage Range Oral:

Rheumatoid arthritis and ankylosing spondylitis:

Adults ≤60 years: 1200 mg daily in 2-4 divided doses

Adults >60 years: 600 mg daily in 2 divided doses

Acute gout:

Adults ≤60 years: 1200-1800 mg daily in 2-4 divided doses

Adults >60 years: 600-1800 mg daily in 2-4 divided doses

Dosage adjustment in renal impairment:

CrCl 50-75 mL/minute: Reduce dose by 1/3 to 1/2

CrCl <50 mL/minute: Reduce dose by 1/2 to 2/3

Product Availability Product available in various countries; not currently available in the U.S.

Dosage Forms

Capsule: 300 mg

Tablet: 600 mg

◆ **Azarga™ (Can)** *see* Brinzolamide and Timolol [CAN/INT] *on page* *289*

◆ **Azasan** *see* AzaTHIOprine *on page* *210*

◆ **AzaSite** *see* Azithromycin (Ophthalmic) *on page* *219*

AzaTHIOprine (ay za THYE oh preen)

Brand Names: U.S. Azasan; Imuran

Brand Names: Canada Apo-Azathioprine; Imuran; Mylan-Azathioprine; Teva-Azathioprine

Index Terms Azathioprine Sodium

Pharmacologic Category Immunosuppressant Agent

Use

Renal transplantation: Adjunctive therapy in prevention of rejection of kidney transplants

Rheumatoid arthritis: Treatment of active rheumatoid arthritis (RA), to reduce signs and symptoms

Pregnancy Risk Factor D

Pregnancy Considerations Adverse events have been observed in animal reproduction studies. Azathioprine crosses the placenta in humans; congenital anomalies, immunosuppression, hematologic toxicities (lymphopenia, pancytopenia), and intrauterine growth retardation have been reported. Azathioprine should not be used to treat rheumatoid arthritis during pregnancy. Women of childbearing potential should avoid becoming pregnant during treatment.

The National Transplantation Pregnancy Registry (NTPR, Temple University) is a registry for pregnant women taking immunosuppressants following any solid organ transplant. The NTPR encourages reporting of all immunosuppressant exposures during pregnancy in transplant recipients at 877-955-6877.

Breast-Feeding Considerations Azathioprine is excreted in breast milk. Due to potential for serious adverse reactions in the nursing infant, breast-feeding is not recommended by the manufacturer.

Contraindications Hypersensitivity to azathioprine or any component of the formulation; pregnancy (in patients with rheumatoid arthritis); patients with rheumatoid arthritis and a history of treatment with alkylating agents (eg, cyclophosphamide, chlorambucil, melphalan) may have a prohibitive risk of malignancy with azathioprine treatment

Warnings/Precautions Hazardous agent - use appropriate precautions for handling and disposal (NIOSH 2014 [group 2]).

[U.S. Boxed Warning]: Immunosuppressive agents, including azathioprine, increase the risk of development of malignancy; lymphoma (in post-transplant patients) and hepatosplenic T-cell lymphoma (HSTCL) (in patients with inflammatory bowel disease) have been reported. Patients should be informed of the risk for malignancy development. HSTCL is a rare white blood cell cancer that is usually fatal and has predominantly occurred in adolescents and young adults treated for Crohn disease or ulcerative colitis and receiving TNF blockers (eg, adalimumab, certolizumab pegol, etanercept, golimumab), azathioprine, and/or mercaptopurine. Most cases of HSTCL have occurred in patients treated with a combination of immunosuppressant agents, although there have been reports of HSTCL in patients receiving azathioprine or mercaptopurine monotherapy. Renal transplant patients are also at increased risk for malignancy (eg, skin cancer, lymphoma); limit sun and ultraviolet light exposure and use appropriate sun protection.

Dose-related hematologic toxicities (leukopenia, thrombocytopenia, and anemias, including macrocytic anemia, or pancytopenia) may occur; may be severe and/or delayed. Patients with intermediate thiopurine methyltransferase (TPMT) activity may be at increased risk for hematologic toxicity at conventional azathioprine doses; patients with low or absent TPMT activity are at risk for severe, life-threatening myelotoxicity. Myelosuppression may be more severe with renal transplants undergoing rejection. Monitor CBC with differential and platelets weekly during the first month, then twice a month for 2 months, then monthly (or more frequently if clinically indicated). May require treatment interruption or dose reduction.

Chronic immunosuppression increases the risk of serious, sometimes fatal, infections (bacterial, viral, fungal, protozoal, and opportunistic). Progressive multifocal leukoencephalopathy (PML), an opportunistic CNS infection caused by reactivation of the JC virus, has been reported in patients receiving immunosuppressive therapy, including azathioprine; promptly evaluate any patient presenting with neurological changes. Consider decreasing the degree of immunosuppression with consideration to the risk of organ rejection in transplant patients.

Use with caution in patients with liver disease or renal impairment; monitor hematologic function closely. Azathioprine is metabolized to mercaptopurine; concomitant use may result in profound myelosuppression and should be avoided. Patients with genetic deficiency of thiopurine methyltransferase (TPMT) or concurrent therapy with drugs which may inhibit TPMT are more sensitive to myelosuppressive effects. Patients with intermediate TPMT activity may be at risk for increased myelosuppression; those with low or absent TPMT activity are at risk for developing severe myelotoxicity. TPMT genotyping or phenotyping may assist in identifying patients at risk for developing toxicity. Consider TPMT testing in patients with abnormally low CBC unresponsive to dose reduction. TPMT testing does not substitute for CBC monitoring. Potentially significant drug-drug interactions may exist, requiring dose or frequency adjustment, additional monitoring, and/or selection of alternative therapy. Xanthine oxidase inhibitors may increase risk for hematologic toxicity; reduce azathioprine dose when used concurrently with allopurinol; patients with low or absent TPMT activity may require further dose reductions or discontinuation.

Hepatotoxicity (transaminase, bilirubin, and alkaline phosphatase elevations) may occur, usually in renal transplant patients and generally within 6 months of transplant; normally reversible with discontinuation; monitor liver function periodically. Rarely, hepatic sinusoidal obstruction syndrome (SOS; formerly called veno-occlusive disease) has been reported; discontinue if hepatic SOS is suspected. Severe nausea, vomiting, diarrhea, rash, fever, malaise, myalgia, hypotension, and liver enzyme abnormalities may occur within the first several weeks of treatment and are generally reversible upon discontinuation. **[U.S. Boxed Warning]: Should be prescribed by physicians familiar with the risks, including hematologic toxicities and mutagenic potential.** Immune response to vaccines may be diminished.

Adverse Reactions

Central nervous system: Malaise

Gastrointestinal: Diarrhea, nausea and vomiting (rheumatoid arthritis)

Hematologic and oncologic: Leukopenia (more common in renal transplant), neoplasia (renal transplant), thrombocytopenia

Hepatic: Hepatotoxicity, increased serum alkaline phosphatase, increased serum bilirubin, increased serum transaminases

Infection: Increased susceptibility to infection (more common in renal transplant; includes bacterial, fungal, protozoal, viral, opportunistic, and reactivation of latent infections)

Neuromuscular & skeletal: Myalgia

Miscellaneous: Fever

Rare but important or life-threatening: Abdominal pain, acute myelocytic leukemia, alopecia, anemia, arthralgia, bone marrow depression, hemorrhage, hepatic veno-occlusive disease, hepatosplenic T-cell lymphomas, hypersensitivity, hypotension, interstitial pneumonitis (reversible), JC virus infection, macrocytic anemia, malignant lymphoma, malignant neoplasm of skin, negative nitrogen balance, pancreatitis, pancytopenia, progressive multifocal leukoencephalopathy, skin rash, steatorrhea, Sweet's syndrome (acute febrile neutrophilic dermatosis)

Drug Interactions

Metabolism/Transport Effects None known.

Avoid Concomitant Use

Avoid concomitant use of AzaTHIOprine with any of the following: BCG; Febuxostat; Mercaptopurine; Natalizumab; Pimecrolimus; Tacrolimus (Topical); Tofacitinib; Vaccines (Live)

Increased Effect/Toxicity

AzaTHIOprine may increase the levels/effects of: Cyclophosphamide; Leflunomide; Mercaptopurine; Natalizumab; Tofacitinib; Vaccines (Live)

The levels/effects of AzaTHIOprine may be increased by: 5-ASA Derivatives; ACE Inhibitors; Allopurinol; Denosumab; Febuxostat; Pimecrolimus; Ribavirin; Roflumilast; Sulfamethoxazole; Tacrolimus (Topical); Trastuzumab; Trimethoprim

Decreased Effect

AzaTHIOprine may decrease the levels/effects of: BCG; Coccidioides immitis Skin Test; Sipuleucel-T; Vaccines (Inactivated); Vaccines (Live); Vitamin K Antagonists

The levels/effects of AzaTHIOprine may be decreased by: Echinacea

Preparation for Administration Hazardous agent; use appropriate precautions for handling and disposal (NIOSH 2014 [group 2]).

Powder for injection [Canadian product]: Reconstitute each vial with 5 to 10 mL sterile water for injection (adding 5 mL will result in a 10 mg/mL solution); gently swirl to dissolve. May further dilute in NS for infusion.

Storage/Stability

Tablet: Store at 15°C to 25°C (59°F to 77°F). Protect from light and moisture.

Powder for injection [Canadian product]: Store intact vials at 15°C to 25°C (59°F to 77°F). Protect from light. Use immediately after preparation; discard unused portion.

Mechanism of Action Azathioprine is an imidazolyl derivative of mercaptopurine; metabolites are incorporated into replicating DNA and halt replication; also block the pathway for purine synthesis (Taylor, 2005). The 6-thioguanine nucleotide metabolites appear to mediate the majority of azathioprine's immunosuppressive and toxic effects.

Pharmacodynamics/Kinetics

Absorption: Oral: Well absorbed

Protein binding: ~30%

Metabolism: Hepatic; metabolized to 6-mercaptopurine via glutathione S-transferase (GST) reduction. Further metabolized (in the liver and GI tract) via three major pathways: Hypoxanthine guanine phosphoribosyltransferase (to active metabolites: 6-thioguanine-nucleotides, or 6-TGNs), xanthine oxidase (to inactive metabolite: 6-thiouric acid), and thiopurine methyltransferase (TPMT) (to inactive metabolite: 6-methylmercaptopurine)

Half-life elimination: Azathioprine and mercaptopurine: Variable: ~2 hours (Taylor, 2005)

Time to peak: Oral: 1-2 hours (including metabolites)

Excretion: Urine (primarily as metabolites)

Dosage Note: Patients with intermediate TPMT activity may be at risk for increased myelosuppression; those with low or absent TPMT activity receiving conventional azathioprine doses are at risk for developing severe, life-threatening myelotoxicity. Dosage reductions are recommended for patients with reduced TPMT activity; consider discontinuing in patients with abnormal blood counts that do not respond to dose reduction.

Renal transplantation (treatment usually started the day of transplant, however, has been initiated [rarely] 1 to 3 days prior to transplant): Adults:

Oral: Initial: 3 to 5 mg/kg daily usually given as a single daily dose, then 1 to 3 mg/kg daily maintenance

IV [Canadian product]: Initial: 3 to 5 mg/kg daily; Maintenance: dose reduction to 1 to 3 mg/kg daily is usually possible. **Note:** IV is indicated only in patients unable to tolerate oral medications (dosing should be transitioned from IV to oral as soon as tolerated)

Rheumatoid arthritis: Adults:

Oral:

Initial: 1 mg/kg/day (50 to 100 mg) given once daily or divided twice daily for 6 to 8 weeks; may increase by 0.5 mg/kg every 4 weeks until response or up to 2.5 mg/kg/day; an adequate trial should be a minimum of 12 weeks

Maintenance dose: Reduce dose by 0.5 mg/kg (~25 mg daily) every 4 weeks until lowest effective dose is reached; optimum duration of therapy not specified; may be discontinued abruptly (monitor for delayed toxicities)

IV [Canadian product]: **Note:** IV is indicated only in patients unable to tolerate oral medications (dosing should be transitioned from IV to oral as soon as tolerated):

Initial: ~1 mg/kg/day (50 to 100 mg) given once daily or divided twice daily for 6 to 8 weeks; may increase by 0.5 mg/kg every 4 weeks until response or up to 2.5 mg/kg/day; an adequate trial should be a minimum of 12 weeks

Maintenance dose: Reduce dose by 0.5 mg/kg (~25 mg daily) every 4 weeks until lowest effective dose is reached; optimum duration of therapy not specified; may be discontinued abruptly (monitor for delayed toxicities)

Crohn disease, remission maintenance or reduction of steroid use (off-label use): Adults: Oral: 2 to 3 mg/kg/day (Lichtenstein, 2009)

Dermatomyositis/polymyositis, adjunctive management (off-label use): Adults: Oral: 50 mg/day in conjunction with prednisone; increase by 50 mg/week to total dose of 2 to 3 mg/kg/day (Briemberg, 2003); **Note:** Onset of beneficial effects may take 3 to 6 months; however, may be preferred over methotrexate in patients with pulmonary or hepatic toxicity.

Immune thrombocytopenia (ITP), chronic refractory (off-label use): Adults: Oral: Maintenance: 100 to 200 mg/day (Boruchov, 2007)

Lupus nephritis, maintenance (off-label use): Adults: Oral: Initial: 2 mg/kg/day; may reduce to 1.5 mg/kg/day after 1 month (if proteinuria <1 g/day and serum creatinine stable) (Moroni, 2006) **or** target dose: 2 mg/kg/day (Hahn, 2012; Houssiau, 2010)

Ulcerative colitis, remission maintenance or reduction of steroid use (off-label use): Adults: Oral: 1.5 to 2.5 mg/kg/day (Kornbluth, 2010)

Dosage adjustment for concomitant use with allopurinol: Reduce azathioprine dose to one-third or one-fourth the usual dose when used concurrently with allopurinol. Patients with low or absent TPMT activity may require further dose reductions or discontinuation.

Dosage adjustment for toxicity:

Rapid WBC count decrease, persistently low WBC count, or serious infection: Reduce dose or temporarily withhold treatment

Severe toxicity (hematologic or other) in renal transplantation: May require discontinuation

Hepatic sinusoidal obstruction syndrome (SOS; veno-occlusive disease): Permanently discontinue

Dosage adjustment in renal impairment: There are no specific dosage adjustments provided in the manufacturer's labeling; however, oliguric patients, particularly those with tubular necrosis in the immediate post-transplant period (cadaveric transplant) may have delayed clearance and typically receive lower doses. The following adjustments have been recommended (Aronoff, 2007):

CrCl >50 mL/minute: No adjustment recommended

CrCl 10-50 mL/minute: Administer 75% of normal dose

CrCl <10 mL/minute: Administer 50% of normal dose

Hemodialysis (dialyzable; ~45% removed in 8 hours): Administer 50% of normal dose; supplement: 0.25 mg/kg

CRRT: Administer 75% of normal dose

Dosage adjustment in hepatic impairment: There are no dosage adjustments provided in the manufacturer's labeling.

Administration

Oral: Administering tablets after meals or in divided doses may decrease adverse GI events.

IV [Canadian product]: Infusion is usually administered over 30 to 60 minutes, although may be infused over 5 minutes up to over 8 hours.

Hazardous agent; use appropriate precautions for handling and disposal (NIOSH 2014 [group 2]).

Monitoring Parameters CBC with differential and platelets (weekly during first month, twice monthly for months 2 and 3, then monthly; monitor more frequently with dosage modifications), total bilirubin, liver function tests, creatinine clearance, TPMT genotyping or phenotyping (consider TPMT testing in patients with abnormally low CBC unresponsive to dose reduction); monitor for symptoms of infection

For use as immunomodulatory therapy in CD or UC, monitor CBC with differential weekly for 1 month, then biweekly for 1 month, followed by monitoring every 1-2 months throughout the course of therapy; monitor more frequently if symptomatic. LFTs should be assessed every 3 months. Monitor for signs/symptoms of malignancy (eg, splenomegaly, hepatomegaly, abdominal pain, persistent fever, night sweats, weight loss).

Dosage Forms

Tablet, Oral:

Azasan: 75 mg, 100 mg

Imuran: 50 mg

Generic: 50 mg

Dosage Forms: Canada Note: Refer also to Dosage Forms.

Injection, powder for reconstitution [preservative free]:

Imuran: 50 mg

Extemporaneous Preparations Hazardous agent: Use appropriate precautions for handling and disposal (NIOSH 2014 [group 2]).

A 50 mg/mL oral suspension may be prepared with tablets. Crush one-hundred-twenty 50 mg tablets in a mortar and reduce to a fine powder. Add 40 mL of either cherry syrup (diluted 1:4 with Simple Syrup, USP); a 1:1 mixture of Ora-Sweet® and Ora-Plus®; or a 1:1 mixture of Ora-Sweet® SF and Ora-Plus®, and mix to a uniform paste. Mix while adding the vehicle in incremental proportions to **almost** 120 mL; transfer to a calibrated bottle, rinse mortar with vehicle, and add quantity of vehicle sufficient to make 120 mL. Label "shake well", "refrigerate", and "protect from light". Stable for 60 days refrigerated.

Allen LV Jr and Erickson MA 3rd, "Stability of Acetazolamide, Allopurinol, Azathioprine, Clonazepam, and Flucytosine in Extemporaneously Compounded Oral Liquids," *Am J Health Syst Pharm*, 1996, 53(16):1944-9.

- **Azathioprine Sodium** *see* AzaTHIOprine *on page 210*
- **5-AZC** *see* AzaCITIDine *on page 209*
- **AZD6140** *see* Ticagrelor *on page 2035*
- **AZD6474** *see* Vandetanib *on page 2135*

Azelaic Acid (a zeh LAY ik AS id)

Brand Names: U.S. Azelex; Finacea

Brand Names: Canada Finacea

Index Terms Anchoic Acid; Lepargylic Acid

Pharmacologic Category Topical Skin Product, Acne

Use

Acne vulgaris (cream): Treatment of mild to moderate inflammatory acne vulgaris.

Rosacea (gel): Treatment of inflammatory papules and pustules of mild to moderate rosacea.

Limitations of use: Efficacy for treatment of erythema in rosacea in the absence of papules and pustules has not been evaluated.

Pregnancy Risk Factor B

Dosage

Acne vulgaris: Children ≥12 years, Adolescents, and Adults: Topical: Cream 20%: Apply a thin film to the affected area(s) twice daily, in the morning and evening; may reduce to once daily if persistent skin irritation occurs. Improvement in condition is usually seen within 4 weeks.

Rosacea: Adults: Topical: Gel 15%: Apply a thin layer to the affected area(s) of the face twice daily, in the morning and evening; reassess if no improvement after 12 weeks of therapy.

Dosage adjustment in renal impairment: There are no dosage adjustments provided in the manufacturer's labeling. However, dosage adjustment unlikely due to low systemic absorption.

Dosage adjustment in hepatic impairment: There are no dosage adjustments provided in the manufacturer's labeling. However, dosage adjustment unlikely due to low systemic absorption.

Additional Information Complete prescribing information should be consulted for additional detail.

Dosage Forms

Cream, External:

Azelex: 20% (30 g, 50 g)

Gel, External:

Finacea: 15% (50 g)

Azelastine (Nasal) (a ZEL as teen)

Brand Names: U.S. Astelin [DSC]; Astepro

Brand Names: Canada Astelin

Index Terms Azelastine Hydrochloride

Pharmacologic Category Histamine H_1 Antagonist; Histamine H_1 Antagonist, Second Generation

Use Treatment of the symptoms of seasonal or perennial allergic rhinitis such as rhinorrhea, sneezing, and nasal pruritus; treatment of the symptoms of vasomotor rhinitis

Pregnancy Risk Factor C

Dosage

Perennial allergic rhinitis: Intranasal (Astepro):

Children 6 to <12 years: One spray in each nostril twice daily

Children ≥12 years, Adolescents, and Adults: Two sprays in each nostril twice daily

Seasonal allergic rhinitis: Intranasal:

Children 5 to <12 years (Astelin): One spray in each nostril twice daily

Children 6 to <12 years (Astepro): One spray in each nostril twice daily

Children ≥12 years, Adolescents, and Adults (Astelin, Astepro): 1-2 sprays in each nostril twice daily; alternatively, Astepro (azelastine 0.15%) may be administered as 2 sprays in each nostril once daily

Vasomotor rhinitis: Intranasal: Children ≥12 years, Adolescents, and Adults (Astelin): Two sprays in each nostril twice daily

Dosage adjustment in renal impairment: No dosage adjustment provided in manufacturer's labeling.

Dosage adjustment in hepatic impairment: No dosage adjustment necessary.

Additional Information Complete prescribing information should be consulted for additional detail.

Dosage Forms Considerations Astelin and Astepro 30 mL bottles contain 200 sprays each.

Dosage Forms

Solution, Nasal:

Astepro: 0.15% (30 mL)

Generic: 137 mcg/spray (30 mL); 0.15% (30 mL)

Azelastine (Ophthalmic) (a ZEL as teen)

Brand Names: U.S. Optivar [DSC]

Index Terms Azelastine Hydrochloride

Pharmacologic Category Histamine H_1 Antagonist; Histamine H_1 Antagonist, Second Generation

Use Treatment of itching of the eye associated with seasonal allergic conjunctivitis

Pregnancy Risk Factor C

Dosage Ophthalmic: Children ≥3 years and Adults: Instill 1 drop into affected eye(s) twice daily.

Dosage adjustment in renal impairment: No dosage adjustment provided in manufacturer's labeling.

Dosage adjustment in hepatic impairment: No dosage adjustment provided in manufacturer's labeling.

Additional Information Complete prescribing information should be consulted for additional detail.

Dosage Forms

Solution, Ophthalmic:

Generic: 0.05% (6 mL)

Azelastine and Fluticasone
(a ZEL as teen & floo TIK a sone)

Brand Names: U.S. Dymista™

Index Terms Fluticasone Propionate and Azelastine Hydrochloride

Pharmacologic Category Corticosteroid, Nasal; Histamine H_1 Antagonist, Second Generation

Use Symptomatic relief of seasonal allergic rhinitis

Pregnancy Risk Factor C

Dosage Intranasal: Seasonal allergic rhinitis: Children ≥12 years and Adults: 1 spray (137 mcg azelastine/50 mcg fluticasone) per nostril twice daily

Dosage adjustment in renal impairment: No dosage adjustment provided in manufacturer's labeling.

Dosage adjustment in hepatic impairment: No dosage adjustment necessary.

Additional Information Complete prescribing information should be consulted for additional detail.

Dosage Forms

Suspension, intranasal [spray]:

Dymista™: Azelastine hydrochloride 0.1% [137 mcg/spray] and fluticasone propionate 0.037% [50 mcg/spray] (23 g)

◆ **Azelastine Hydrochloride** *see* Azelastine (Nasal) *on page 213*

◆ **Azelastine Hydrochloride** *see* Azelastine (Ophthalmic) *on page 213*

◆ **Azelex** *see* Azelaic Acid *on page 213*

Azelnidipine [INT] (a zel NID e peen)

International Brand Names Beiqi (CN); Calblock (JP)

Pharmacologic Category Calcium Channel Blocker

Reported Use Management of hypertension

Dosage Range Adults: Oral: Hypertension: 8-16 mg/day

Product Availability Product available in various countries; not currently available in the U.S.

Dosage Forms

Tablet: 8 mg, 16 mg

◆ **Azidothymidine** *see* Zidovudine *on page 2196*

◆ **Azidothymidine, Abacavir, and Lamivudine** *see* Abacavir, Lamivudine, and Zidovudine *on page 22*

◆ **Azilect** *see* Rasagiline *on page 1781*

Azilsartan (ay zil SAR tan)

Brand Names: U.S. Edarbi

Brand Names: Canada Edarbi

Index Terms Azilsartan Medoxomil; AZL-M

Pharmacologic Category Angiotensin II Receptor Blocker; Antihypertensive

Use Hypertension: Treatment of hypertension; may be used alone or in combination with other antihypertensives

The 2014 guideline for the management of high blood pressure in adults (Eighth Joint National Committee [JNC 8]) recommends initiation of pharmacologic treatment to lower blood pressure for the following patients:

- Patients ≥60 years of age with systolic blood pressure (SBP) ≥150 mm Hg or diastolic blood pressure (DBP) ≥90 mm Hg. Goal of therapy is SBP <150 mm Hg and DBP <90 mm Hg.
- Patients <60 years of age with SBP ≥140 mm Hg or DBP is ≥90 mm Hg. Goal of therapy is SBP <140 mm Hg and DBP <90 mm Hg.
- Patients ≥18 years of age with diabetes and SBP ≥140 mm Hg or DBP ≥90 mm Hg. Goal of therapy is SBP <140 mm Hg and DBP <90 mm Hg.
- Patients ≥18 years of age with chronic kidney disease (CKD) and SBP ≥140 mm Hg or DBP ≥90 mm Hg. Goal of therapy is SBP <140 mm Hg and DBP <90 mm Hg.

In patients with CKD, regardless of race or diabetes status, the use of an ACE inhibitor (ACEI) or angiotensin receptor blocker (ARB) as initial therapy is recommended to improve kidney outcomes. In the general nonblack population (without CKD) including those with diabetes, initial antihypertensive treatment should consist of a thiazide-type diuretic, calcium channel blocker, ACEI, or ARB. In the general black population (without CKD) including those with diabetes, initial antihypertensive treatment should consist of a thiazide-type diuretic or a calcium channel blocker instead of an ACEI or ARB.

Pregnancy Risk Factor D

Pregnancy Considerations [U.S. Boxed Warning]: Drugs that act on the renin-angiotensin system can cause injury and death to the developing fetus. Discontinue as soon as possible once pregnancy is detected. The use of drugs which act on the renin-angiotensin system are associated with oligohydramnios. Oligohydramnios, due to decreased fetal renal function, may lead to fetal lung hypoplasia and skeletal malformations. Use is also associated with anuria, hypotension, renal failure, skull hypoplasia, and death in the fetus/neonate. The exposed fetus should be monitored for fetal growth, amniotic fluid volume, and organ formation. Infants exposed *in utero* should be monitored for hyperkalemia, hypotension, and oliguria (exchange transfusions or dialysis may be needed). These adverse events are generally associated with maternal use in the second and third trimesters.

Untreated chronic maternal hypertension is also associated with adverse events in the fetus, infant, and mother. The use of angiotensin II receptor blockers is not recommended to treat chronic uncomplicated hypertension in pregnant women and should generally be avoided in women of reproductive potential (ACOG, 2013).

Breast-Feeding Considerations It is not known if azilsartan is excreted into breast milk. Due to the potential for serious adverse reactions in the nursing infant, the manufacturer recommends a decision be made whether to discontinue nursing or to discontinue the drug, taking into account the importance of treatment to the mother.

Contraindications

U.S. labeling: Concomitant use with aliskiren in patients with diabetes mellitus

Canadian labeling: Hypersensitivity to azilsartan medoxomil or any component of the formulation; concomitant use with aliskiren in patients with diabetes or moderate-to-severe renal impairment (GFR <60 mL/minute/1.73 m^2).

Warnings/Precautions [U.S. Boxed Warning]: Drugs that act on the renin-angiotensin system can cause injury and death to the developing fetus. Discontinue as soon as possible once pregnancy is detected. Angiotensin II receptor blockers may cause hyperkalemia; avoid potassium supplementation unless specifically required by healthcare provider. Avoid use or use a smaller dose in patients who are volume depleted; correct depletion first. May be associated with deterioration of renal function and/or increases in serum creatinine, particularly in patients with low renal blood flow (eg, renal artery stenosis, heart failure, volume depletion) whose glomerular filtration rate (GFR) is dependent on efferent arteriolar vasoconstriction by angiotensin II. Use with caution in unstented unilateral/bilateral renal artery stenosis. When unstented bilateral renal artery stenosis is present, use is generally avoided due to the elevated risk of deterioration in renal function unless possible benefits outweigh risks. Use with caution in preexisting renal insufficiency; significant aortic/mitral stenosis. Potentially significant drug-drug interactions may exist, requiring dose or frequency adjustment, additional monitoring, and/or selection of alternative therapy. In surgical patients on chronic angiotensin receptor blocker (ARB) therapy, intraoperative hypotension may occur with induction and maintenance of general anesthesia.

Angioedema has been reported rarely with some angiotensin II receptor antagonists (ARBs) and may occur at any time during treatment (especially following first dose). It may involve the head and neck (potentially compromising airway) or the intestine (presenting with abdominal pain). Patients with idiopathic or hereditary angioedema or previous angioedema associated with ACE-inhibitor therapy may be at an increased risk. Prolonged frequent monitoring may be required, especially if tongue, glottis, or larynx are involved, as they are associated with airway obstruction. Patients with a history of airway surgery may have a higher risk of airway obstruction. Discontinue therapy immediately if angioedema occurs. Aggressive early management is critical. Intramuscular (IM) administration of epinephrine may be necessary. Do not readminister to patients who have had angioedema with ARBs.

Adverse Reactions

Cardiovascular: Hypotension, orthostatic hypotension

Central nervous system: Dizziness, fatigue

Gastrointestinal: Diarrhea, nausea

Hematologic & oncologic: Decreased hemoglobin, decreased hematocrit, decreased red blood cells, leukopenia (rare), thrombocytopenia (rare)

Neuromuscular & skeletal: Muscle spasm, weakness

Renal: Increased serum creatinine

Respiratory: Cough

Rare but important or life-threatening: Angioedema, pruritus, skin rash

Drug Interactions

Metabolism/Transport Effects Substrate of CYP2C9 (minor); **Note:** Assignment of Major/Minor substrate status based on clinically relevant drug interaction potential

Avoid Concomitant Use There are no known interactions where it is recommended to avoid concomitant use.

Increased Effect/Toxicity

Azilsartan may increase the levels/effects of: ACE Inhibitors; Amifostine; Antihypertensives; CycloSPORINE (Systemic); DULoxetine; Hypotensive Agents; Levodopa; Lithium; Nonsteroidal Anti-Inflammatory Agents; Obinutuzumab; Potassium-Sparing Diuretics; RisperiDONE; RiTUXimab; Sodium Phosphates

The levels/effects of Azilsartan may be increased by: Alfuzosin; Aliskiren; Barbiturates; Brimonidine (Topical); Canagliflozin; Dapoxetine; Diazoxide; Eplerenone; Heparin; Heparin (Low Molecular Weight); Herbs (Hypotensive Properties); MAO Inhibitors; Nicorandil; Pentoxifylline; Phosphodiesterase 5 Inhibitors; Potassium Salts; Prostacyclin Analogues; Tolvaptan; Trimethoprim

Decreased Effect

The levels/effects of Azilsartan may be decreased by: Herbs (Hypertensive Properties); Methylphenidate; Nonsteroidal Anti-Inflammatory Agents; Yohimbine

Storage/Stability Store at 25°C (77°F); excursions permitted to 15°C to 30°C (59°F to 86°F). Protect from moisture and light. Dispense and store in original container.

Mechanism of Action Angiotensin II (which is formed by enzymatic conversion from angiotensin I) is the primary pressor agent of the renin-angiotensin system. Effects of angiotensin II include vasoconstriction, stimulation of aldosterone synthesis/release, cardiac stimulation, and renal sodium reabsorption. Azilsartan inhibits angiotensin II's vasoconstrictor and aldosterone-secreting effects by selectively blocking the binding of angiotensin II to the AT_1 receptor in vascular smooth muscle and adrenal gland tissues (azilsartan has a stronger affinity for the AT_1 receptor than the AT_2 receptor). The action is independent of the angiotensin II synthesis pathways. Azilsartan does not inhibit ACE (kininase II), therefore it does not affect the response to bradykinin (the clinical relevance of this is unknown) and does not bind to or inhibit other receptors or ion channels of importance in cardiovascular regulation.

Pharmacodynamics/Kinetics

Distribution: V_d: ~16 L

Protein binding: >99%; primarily to serum albumin

Metabolism: Gut: prodrug hydrolyzed to active metabolite; Hepatic: primarily via CYP2C9 to inactive metabolites

Bioavailability: ~60%

Half-life elimination: ~11 hours

Time to peak, serum: 1.5-3 hours

Excretion: Feces (~55%); urine (~42%, 15% as unchanged drug)

Clearance: 2.3 mL/minute

Dosage Oral: Adults:

U.S. labeling: 80 mg once daily; consider initial dose of 40 mg once daily in patients with volume depletion (eg, patients receiving high-dose diuretics); usual dosage (ASH/ISH [Weber, 2014]): 80 mg daily

Canadian labeling: Initial: 40 mg once daily; may increase to 80 mg once daily if necessary

Dosage adjustment in renal impairment:

U.S. labeling: No dosage adjustment necessary; however, carefully monitor the patient.

Canadian labeling:

Mild-to-moderate impairment: No dosage adjustment is necessary; however, carefully monitor the patient.

Severe impairment or end stage renal disease (ESRD): No dosage adjustment provided in manufacturer's labeling (has not been studied). Use with caution.

Dosage adjustment in hepatic impairment:

U.S. labeling:

Mild-to-moderate impairment: No dosage adjustment necessary; however, carefully monitor the patient.

Severe impairment: No dosage adjustment provided in manufacturer's labeling (has not been studied).

Canadian labeling:

Mild-to-moderate moderate impairment: There is no specific dosage adjustment provided in manufacturer's labeling; however, a reduced initial dose is recommended. Do not exceed daily dose of 80 mg.

Severe impairment: Use is not recommended.

Dietary Considerations May be taken with or without food.

Administration Administer without regard to food.

Monitoring Parameters Electrolytes, serum creatinine, BUN; blood pressure

Dosage Forms

Tablet, Oral:

Edarbi: 40 mg, 80 mg

Azilsartan and Chlorthalidone

(ay zil SAR tan & klor THAL i done)

Brand Names: U.S. Edarbyclor

Brand Names: Canada Edarbyclor™

Index Terms Azilsartan Medoxomil and Chlorthalidone; Chlorthalidone and Azilsartan

Pharmacologic Category Angiotensin II Receptor Blocker; Antihypertensive; Diuretic, Thiazide

Use Treatment of hypertension

Pregnancy Risk Factor D

Dosage Dose is individualized; combination product may be substituted for individual components in patients currently maintained on both agents separately or in patients not adequately controlled with monotherapy (using one of the agents or an agent within the same antihypertensive class). May also be used as initial therapy in patients who are likely to need >1 antihypertensive to control blood pressure.

Oral: Adults: Hypertension: *Initial therapy:* Azilsartan 40 mg/chlorthalidone 12.5 mg once daily; dose may be increased after 2-4 weeks of therapy to azilsartan 40 mg/ chlorthalidone 25 mg once daily. Maximum recommended dose: Azilsartan 40 mg/day; chlorthalidone 25 mg/day

Dosage adjustment in renal impairment:

Mild-to-moderate renal impairment (eGFR 30-90 mL/ minute/1.73 m^2): No dosage adjustment necessary.

Severe renal impairment (eGFR <30 mL/minute/1.73 m^2): No dosage adjustment provided in manufacturer's labeling (has not been studied); use with caution.

Dosage adjustment in hepatic impairment:

U.S. labeling:

Mild-to-moderate hepatic impairment: No initial dosage adjustment necessary; monitor patient carefully.

Severe hepatic impairment: No dosage adjustment provided in manufacturer's labeling (has not been studied); use with caution.

Canadian labeling:

Mild-to-moderate hepatic impairment: Initial dosage reduction is recommended although specific adjustments are not provided in the manufacturer labeling; monitor patient carefully.

Severe hepatic impairment: Use is not recommended (has not been studied).

Additional Information Complete prescribing information should be consulted for additional detail.

Dosage Forms

Tablet, Oral:

Edarbyclor: 40/25: Azilsartan medoxomil 40 mg and chlorthalidone 25 mg, 40/12.5: Azilsartan medoxomil 40 mg and chlorthalidone 12.5 mg

◆ **Azilsartan Medoxomil** *see* Azilsartan *on page 214*

◆ **Azilsartan Medoxomil and Chlorthalidone** *see* Azilsartan and Chlorthalidone *on page 215*

Azithromycin (Systemic) (az ith roe MYE sin)

Brand Names: U.S. Zithromax; Zithromax Tri-Pak; Zithromax Z-Pak; Zmax

Brand Names: Canada ACT-Azithromycin; Apo-Azithromycin; Apo-Azithromycin Z; Azithromycin for Injection; Azithromycin for Injection, USP; Dom-Azithromycin; GD-Azithromycin; Mylan-Azithromycin; Novo-Azithromycin; PHL-Azithromycin; PMS-Azithromycin; PRO-Azithromycine; Riva-Azithromycin; Sandoz-Azithromycin; Zithromax; Zithromax For Intravenous Injection; Zmax SR

Index Terms Azithromycin Dihydrate; Azithromycin Monohydrate; Z-Pak; Zithromax TRI-PAK; Zithromax Z-PAK

Pharmacologic Category Antibiotic, Macrolide

Use Oral, IV: Treatment of acute otitis media due to *H. influenzae, M. catarrhalis*, or *S. pneumoniae*; pharyngitis/ tonsillitis due to *S. pyogenes*, community-acquired pneumonia due to *Chlamydia pneumonia, H. influenzae, M. pneumoniae*, or *S. pneumoniae*; pelvic inflammatory disease (PID) due to *C. trachomatis, N. gonorrhoeae*, or *M. hominis*; genital ulcer disease (in men) due to *H. ducreyi* (chancroid); acute bacterial exacerbations of chronic obstructive pulmonary disease (COPD) due to *H. influenzae, M. catarrhalis*, or *S. pneumoniae*; acute bacterial sinusitis due to *H. influenzae, M. catarrhalis*, or *S. pneumoniae*; prevention of *Mycobacterium avium* complex (MAC) (alone or in combination with rifabutin) in patients with advanced HIV infection; treatment of disseminated MAC (in combination with ethambutol) in patients with advanced HIV infection; skin and skin structure infections (uncomplicated) due to *S. aureus, S. pyogenes*, or *S. agalactiae*; urethritis and cervicitis due to *C. trachomatis* or *N. gonorrhoeae*

Pregnancy Risk Factor B

Pregnancy Considerations Adverse events were not observed in animal reproduction studies. Azithromycin crosses the placenta (Ramsey, 2003). The maternal serum half-life of azithromycin is unchanged in early pregnancy and decreased at term; however, high concentrations of azithromycin are sustained in the myometrium and adipose tissue (Fischer, 2012; Ramsey, 2003). Azithromycin is recommended for the treatment of several infections, including chlamydia, gonococcal infections, and *Mycobacterium avium* complex (MAC) in pregnant patients (consult current guidelines) (CDC, 2010; DHHS, 2013).

Breast-Feeding Considerations Azithromycin is excreted in low amounts into breast milk (Kelsey, 1994). Decreased appetite, diarrhea, rash, and somnolence have been reported in nursing infants exposed to macrolide antibiotics (Goldstein, 2009). The manufacturer recommends that caution be exercised when administering azithromycin to breast-feeding women.

Contraindications Hypersensitivity to azithromycin, other macrolide (eg, azalide or ketolide) antibiotics, or any component of the formulation; history of cholestatic jaundice/hepatic dysfunction associated with prior azithromycin use

Note: The manufacturer does not list concurrent use of pimozide as a contraindication; however, azithromycin is listed as a contraindication in the manufacturer's labeling for pimozide.

Warnings/Precautions Use with caution in patients with preexisting liver disease; hepatocellular and/or cholestatic hepatitis, with or without jaundice, hepatic necrosis, failure and death have occurred. Discontinue immediately if symptoms of hepatitis occur (malaise, nausea, vomiting, abdominal colic, fever). Allergic reactions have been reported (rare); reappearance of allergic reaction may occur shortly after discontinuation without further azithromycin exposure. May mask or delay symptoms of incubating gonorrhea or syphilis, so appropriate culture and susceptibility tests should be performed prior to initiating a treatment regimen. Prolonged use may result in fungal or bacterial superinfection, including *C. difficile*-associated diarrhea (CDAD); CDAD has been observed >2 months postantibiotic treatment. Use caution with renal dysfunction. Macrolides (especially erythromycin) have been associated with rare QTc prolongation and ventricular arrhythmias, including torsade de pointes; consider avoiding use in patients with prolonged QT interval, congenital long QT syndrome, history of torsade de pointes, bradyarrhythmias, uncorrected hypokalemia or hypomagnesemia, clinically significant bradycardia, uncompensated heart failure, or concurrent use of Class IA (eg, quinidine, procainamide) or Class III (eg, amiodarone, dofetilide, sotalol) antiarrhythmic agents or other drugs known to prolong the QT interval. Use with caution in patients with myasthenia gravis.

Oral suspensions (immediate release and extended release) are not interchangeable.

Adverse Reactions

Dermatologic: Pruritus, skin rash

Gastrointestinal: Abdominal pain, anorexia, diarrhea, nausea, stomach cramps, vomiting

Genitourinary: Vaginitis

Local: (with IV administration): Local inflammation, pain at injection site

Rare but important or life-threatening: Acute renal failure, ageusia, aggressive behavior, anaphylaxis, anemia, angioedema, anosmia, auditory disturbance, candidiasis, cardiac arrhythmia (including ventricular tachycardia), chest pain, cholestatic jaundice, conjunctivitis (pediatric patients), deafness, DRESS syndrome, eczema, edema, enteritis, erythema multiforme (rare), fungal dermatitis, fungal infection, gastritis, hearing loss, hepatic failure, hepatic necrosis, hepatitis, hyperactivity, hyperkinesia, hypotension, increased liver enzymes, insomnia, interstitial nephritis, jaundice, leukopenia, melena, mucositis, nephritis, neutropenia (mild), oral candidiasis, pancreatitis, pharyngitis, pleural effusion, prolonged Q-T interval on ECG (rare), pseudomembranous colitis, pyloric stenosis, seizure, skin photosensitivity, Stevens-Johnson syndrome (rare), syncope, taste perversion, thrombocytopenia, tongue discoloration (rare), torsades de pointes (rare), toxic epidermal necrolysis (rare), vesiculobullous rash

Drug Interactions

Metabolism/Transport Effects **Substrate** of CYP3A4 (minor); **Note:** Assignment of Major/Minor substrate status based on clinically relevant drug interaction potential; **Inhibits** CYP1A2 (weak), P-glycoprotein

Avoid Concomitant Use

Avoid concomitant use of Azithromycin (Systemic) with any of the following: Amiodarone; BCG; Bosutinib; Highest Risk QTc-Prolonging Agents; Ivabradine; Mifepristone; PAZOPanib; Pimozide; QuiNINE; Silodosin; Terfenadine; Topotecan; VinCRIStine (Liposomal)

Increased Effect/Toxicity

Azithromycin (Systemic) may increase the levels/effects of: Afatinib; Amiodarone; AtorvaSTATin; Bosutinib; Brentuximab Vedotin; Cardiac Glycosides; Colchicine; CycloSPORINE (Systemic); Dabigatran Etexilate; DOXOrubicin (Conventional); Edoxaban; Everolimus; Highest Risk QTc-Prolonging Agents; Ivermectin (Systemic); Ledipasvir; Lovastatin; Moderate Risk QTc-Prolonging Agents; Naloxegol; PAZOPanib; P-glycoprotein/ABCB1 Substrates; Pimozide; Prucalopride; QuiNINE; Rifaximin; Rilpivirine; Rivaroxaban; Silodosin; Simvastatin; Tacrolimus (Systemic); Tacrolimus (Topical); Terfenadine; Topotecan; VinCRIStine (Liposomal); Vitamin K Antagonists

The levels/effects of Azithromycin (Systemic) may be increased by: Ivabradine; Mifepristone; Nelfinavir; QTc-Prolonging Agents (Indeterminate Risk and Risk Modifying)

Decreased Effect

Azithromycin (Systemic) may decrease the levels/effects of: BCG; Sodium Picosulfate; Typhoid Vaccine

Food Interactions Rate and extent of GI absorption may be altered depending upon the formulation. Azithromycin suspension, not tablet form, has significantly increased absorption (46%) with food. Management: Immediate release suspension and tablet may be taken without regard to food; extended release suspension should be taken on an empty stomach (at least 1 hour before or 2 hours following a meal).

Preparation for Administration Injection (Zithromax®): Prepare initiation solution by adding 4.8 mL of sterile water for injection to the 500 mg vial (resulting concentration: 100 mg/mL). Use of a standard syringe is recommended due to the vacuum in the vial (which may draw additional solution through an automated syringe).

The initial solution should be further diluted to a concentration of 1 mg/mL (500 mL) to 2 mg/mL (250 mL) in 0.9% sodium chloride, 5% dextrose in water, or lactated Ringer's.

Storage/Stability

Injection (Zithromax): Store intact vials of injection at room temperature. Reconstituted solution is stable for 24 hours when stored below 30°C (86°F). The diluted solution is stable for 24 hours at or below room temperature (30°C [86°F]) and for 7 days if stored under refrigeration (5°C [41°F]).

Suspension, immediate release (Zithromax): Store dry powder below 30°C (86°F). Store reconstituted suspension at 5°C to 30°C (41°F to 86°F) and use within 10 days.

Suspension, extended release (Zmax): Store dry powder ≤30°C (86°F). Following reconstitution, store at 25°C (77°F); excursions permitted to 15°C to 30°C (59°F to 86°F); do not refrigerate or freeze. Should be consumed within 12 hours following reconstitution.

Tablet (Zithromax): Store between 15°C to 30°C (59°F to 86°F).

Mechanism of Action Inhibits RNA-dependent protein synthesis at the chain elongation step; binds to the 50S ribosomal subunit resulting in blockage of transpeptidation

Pharmacodynamics/Kinetics

Absorption: Oral: Rapid

Distribution: Extensive tissue; distributes well into skin, lungs, sputum, tonsils, and cervix; penetration into CSF is poor; V_d: 31-33 L/kg

Protein binding (concentration dependent): Oral, IV: 7% to 51%

Metabolism: Hepatic

Bioavailability: Oral: 38%, decreased by 17% with extended release suspension; variable effect with food (increased with immediate or delayed release oral suspension, unchanged with tablet)

Half-life elimination: Oral, IV: Terminal: Immediate release: 68-72 hours; Extended release: 59 hours

Time to peak, serum: Oral: Immediate release: 2-3 hours; Extended release: 5 hours

Excretion: Oral, IV: Biliary (major route); urine (6%)

Dosage Note: Extended release suspension (Zmax) is not interchangeable with immediate release formulations. Use should be limited to approved indications. All doses are expressed as immediate release azithromycin unless otherwise specified.

Usual dosage range:

Children ≥6 months: Oral: 5-12 mg/kg given once daily (maximum: 500 mg daily) **or** 30 mg/kg as a single dose (maximum: 1500 mg)

Extended release suspension (Zmax): 60 mg/kg as a single dose; **Note:** Extended release suspension (Zmax): Dose in mL is equal to the weight in lbs for patients <75 lbs (34 kg). Pediatric patients ≥75 lbs should receive the adult dose.

Adolescents ≥16 years and Adults:

Oral: 250-600 mg once daily **or** 1-2 g as a single dose

Extended release suspension (Zmax): 2 g as a single dose

IV: 250-500 mg once daily

Indication-specific dosing:

Children:

Bacterial sinusitis: Oral: 10 mg/kg once daily for 3 days (maximum: 500 mg daily)

Cat scratch disease (off-label use; Bass, 1998; Stevens, 2005): Oral:

<45.5 kg: 10 mg/kg as a single dose, then 5 mg/kg once daily for 4 additional days

>45.5 kg: 500 mg as a single dose, then 250 mg once daily for 4 additional days

***Chlamydia trachomatis* infection (off-label use):** Oral: Children ≥45 kg: 1 g as a single dose (CDC, 2010)

Community-acquired pneumonia (CAP) (IDSA/PIDS, 2011): Infants >3 months and Children: **Note:** A beta-lactam antibiotic should be added if typical bacterial pneumonia cannot be ruled out

Presumed mild infection or step-down therapy, atypical *(M. pneumoniae, C. pneumoniae, C. trachomatis)* (preferred): Oral: 10 mg/kg (maximum dose: 500 mg) as a single dose on the first day, followed by 5 mg/kg/day (maximum dose: 250 mg) on days 2 through 5.

Presumed moderate-to-severe infection, atypical *(M. pneumoniae, C. pneumoniae, C. trachomatis)*: IV: 10 mg/kg/day on days 1 and 2, then switch to oral azithromycin therapy if possible to finish the 5-day course

Alternative regimens for community-acquired pneumonia: Oral: 10 mg/kg (maximum dose: 500 mg) once daily for 3 days (Kogan, 2003)

Extended release suspension (Zmax):

<75 lbs (34 kg): 60 mg/kg as a single dose

≥75 lbs (34 kg): Refer to adult dosing

Disseminated *M. avium* complex disease in patients with advanced HIV infection (off-label use; DHHS, 2013): Oral:

Treatment: 10-12 mg/kg/day (maximum: 500 mg) in combination with ethambutol; patients with severe disease should also receive rifabutin

Primary prophylaxis: 20 mg/kg (maximum: 1200 mg) once weekly (preferred) or alternatively, 5 mg/kg/day once daily (maximum: 250 mg daily)

Secondary prophylaxis: 5 mg/kg/day once daily (maximum: 250 mg daily) in combination with ethambutol, with or without rifabutin

Otitis media: Oral:

1-day regimen: 30 mg/kg as a single dose (maximum: 1500 mg)

3-day regimen: 10 mg/kg once daily for 3 days (maximum: 500 mg daily)

5-day regimen: 10 mg/kg on day 1 (maximum: 500 mg daily) followed by 5 mg/kg/day once daily on days 2-5 (maximum: 250 mg daily)

Pertussis (off-label use; CDC, 2005): Oral:

Children <6 months: 10 mg/kg/day for 5 days

Children ≥6 months: 10 mg/kg on day 1 (maximum: 500 mg daily) followed by 5 mg/kg/day once daily on days 2-5 (maximum: 250 mg daily)

Pharyngitis (including susceptible group A streptococci), tonsillitis (as an alternative agent in penicillin-allergic patients):

Manufacturer's labeling and AHA/AAP recommendations: Children ≥2 years and Adolescents: Oral: 12 mg/kg/dose once daily for 5 days (maximum: 500 mg daily) (AHA guidelines [Gerber, 2009]; Red Book [AAP, 2012])

Alternative recommendations: Children and Adolescents: Oral: 12 mg/kg (maximum: 500 mg) on day 1 followed by 6 mg/kg/dose (maximum: 250 mg) once daily on days 2 through 5 (IDSA guidelines [Shulman, 2012])

Prophylaxis against infective endocarditis (off-label use): Oral: 15 mg/kg 30-60 minutes before procedure (maximum: 500 mg). **Note:** American Heart Association (AHA) guidelines now recommend prophylaxis only in patients undergoing invasive procedures and in whom underlying cardiac conditions may predispose to a higher risk of adverse outcomes should infection occur. As of April 2007, routine prophylaxis for GI/GU procedures is no longer recommended by the AHA.

Shigella dysentery type 1 (off-label use): Oral: 6-20 mg/kg/day for 1-5 days (WHO, 2005)

Adolescents ≥16 years and Adults:

Babesiosis (off-label use): Oral: 500-1000 mg on day 1, followed by 250 mg once daily for 7-10 days with atovaquone; higher doses may be required in immunocompromised patients (600-1000 mg daily). **Note:** Relapsing infection may require at least 6 weeks of therapy (Krause, 2000; Vannier, 2012; IDSA [Wormser, 2006]).

Bacterial sinusitis: Oral: 500 mg daily for a total of 3 days

Extended release suspension (Zmax): 2 g as a single dose

Cat scratch disease (off-label use): Oral: >45.5 kg: 500 mg as a single dose, then 250 mg once daily for 4 additional days (Bass, 1998; Stevens, 2005)

Chancroid due to *H. ducreyi*: Oral: 1 g as a single dose (CDC, 2010)

***Chlamydia trachomatis* infection:** Oral: 1 g as a single dose

Community-acquired pneumonia:

Oral: 500 mg on day 1 followed by 250 mg once daily on days 2-5

Extended release suspension (Zmax): 2 g as a single dose

IV: 500 mg as a single dose for at least 2 days, follow IV therapy by the oral route with a single daily dose of 500 mg to complete a 7- to 10-day course of therapy.

Disseminated *M. avium* complex disease in patients with advanced HIV infection: Oral:

Treatment: 600 mg daily in combination with ethambutol

Primary prophylaxis: 1200 mg once weekly (preferred), with or without rifabutin **or** alternatively, 600 mg twice weekly (DHHS, 2013)

Secondary prophylaxis: 500-600 mg daily in combination with ethambutol (DHHS, 2013)

Gonococcal infection, uncomplicated (cervix, rectum, urethra) (off-label regimen): Oral: 1 g as a single dose in combination with ceftriaxone (preferred) or cefixime (only if ceftriaxone unavailable); if cefixime is used, test-of-cure in 7 days is recommended (CDC, 2012). **Note:** Monotherapy with azithromycin single dose of 2 g has been associated with resistance and/or treatment failure; however, may be appropriate for treatment of a gonococcal infection in pregnant women who cannot tolerate a cephalosporin (CDC, 2010).

Patients with severe cephalosporin allergy: 2 g as a single dose and test-of-cure in 7 days (CDC, 2012)

Gonococcal infection, uncomplicated (pharynx) (off-label use): Oral: 1 g as a single dose in combination with ceftriaxone (CDC, 2012)

Gonococcal infection, expedited partner therapy (off-label use): Oral: 1 g as a single dose in combination with cefixime (CDC, 2012). **Note:** Only used if a heterosexual partner cannot be linked to evaluation and treatment in a timely manner; dose delivered to partner by patient, collaborating pharmacy, or disease investigation specialist.

Granuloma inguinale (donovanosis) (off-label use): Oral: 1 g once a week for at least 3 weeks (and until lesions have healed) (CDC, 2010)

Mild-to-moderate respiratory tract, skin, and soft tissue infections: Oral: 500 mg in a single loading dose on day 1 followed by 250 mg daily as a single dose on days 2-5

Alternative regimen: Bacterial exacerbation of COPD: 500 mg daily for a total of 3 days

***M. genitalium* infections (off-label use)** (confirmed cases in males or females or clinically significant persistent urethritis in males): Oral: 1 g as a single dose or 500 mg on day 1, followed by 250 mg daily on days 2-5 (Manhart, 2011):

Note: Follow up patients on either regimen in 3-4 weeks for test of cure; consider moxifloxacin for treatment failures (Manhart, 2011)

Pelvic inflammatory disease (PID): IV: 500 mg as a single dose for 1-2 days, follow IV therapy by the oral route with a single daily dose of 250 mg to complete a 7-day course of therapy

Pertussis (off-label use; CDC, 2005): Oral: 500 mg on day 1 followed by 250 mg daily on days 2-5 (maximum: 500 mg daily)

Pharyngitis (including susceptible group A streptococci), tonsillitis (as an alternative agent in penicillin-allergic patients): Oral: 12 mg/kg (maximum: 500 mg) on day 1 followed by 6 mg/kg (maximum: 250 mg) once daily on days 2 through 5. **Note:** Regimen is also recommended by the Infectious Disease Society of America (IDSA) (Shulman, 2012).

Prophylaxis against infective endocarditis (off-label use): Oral: 500 mg 30-60 minutes prior to the procedure. **Note:** American Heart Association (AHA) guidelines now recommend prophylaxis only in patients undergoing invasive procedures and in whom underlying cardiac conditions may predispose to a higher risk of adverse outcomes should infection occur. As of April 2007, routine prophylaxis for GI/GU procedures is no longer recommended by the AHA.

Prophylaxis against sexually-transmitted diseases following sexual assault (off-label use): Oral: 1 g as a single dose (in combination with a cephalosporin and metronidazole) (CDC, 2010)

Shigella dysentery type 1 (off-label use): Oral: 1000-1500 mg once daily for 1-5 days (WHO, 2005)

Adults:

Prevention of pulmonary exacerbations in patients with noncystic fibrosis bronchiectasis (off-label use): Oral: 500 mg 3 days per week. **Note:** Duration of treatment in clinical trial was 6 months; durations >6 months have not been evaluated. Trial patients had ≥1 exacerbation in the past year, no macrolide treatment for >3 months in the past 6 months, and were screened for nontuberculous mycobacterial infection prior to treatment (Wong, 2012). A more selective approach for patients with functionally mild disease has been suggested (Wilson, 2012).

Dosage adjustment in renal impairment: Use with caution in patients with GFR <10 mL/minute (AUC increased by 35% compared to patients with normal renal function); however, no dosage adjustment is provided in the manufacturer's labeling.

No supplemental dose or dosage adjustment necessary, including patients on intermittent hemodialysis, peritoneal dialysis, or continuous renal replacement therapy (eg, CVVHD) (Aronoff, 2007; Heintz, 2009).

Dosage adjustment in hepatic impairment: Azithromycin is predominantly hepatically eliminated; however, there is no dosage adjustment provided in the manufacturer's labeling, Use with caution due to potential for hepatotoxicity (rare); discontinue immediately for signs or symptoms of hepatitis.

Dietary Considerations

Some products may contain sodium and/or sucrose.

Oral suspension, immediate release, may be administered with or without food.

Oral suspension, extended release, should be taken on an empty stomach (at least 1 hour before or 2 hours following a meal).

Tablet may be administered with food to decrease GI effects.

Administration

IV: Infuse over 1 hour (2 mg/mL infusion) or over 3 hours (1 mg/mL infusion). Not for IM or IV bolus administration.

Oral: Immediate release suspension and tablet may be taken without regard to food; extended release suspension should be taken on an empty stomach (at least 1 hour before or 2 hours following a meal), within 12 hours of reconstitution.

Monitoring Parameters Liver function tests, CBC with differential; when used as part of alternative treatment for gonococcal infection, test-of-cure 7 days after dose (CDC, 2012)

Additional Information Zithromax® tablets and immediate release suspension may be interchanged (eg, two Zithromax® 250 mg tablets may be substituted for one Zithromax® 500 mg tablet or the tablets may be substituted with the immediate release suspension); however, the extended release suspension (Zmax®) is not bioequivalent with Zithromax® and therefore should not be interchanged.

Azithromycin is not recommended for treatment of early syphilis; the 23S rRNA mutation, which has been associated with macrolide resistance, has been documented in multiple geographic areas and in the MSM population. If a penicillin allergic patient cannot take doxycycline (preferred alternative to penicillin), azithromycin (single 2 g dose orally) may be considered but close clinical follow-up is needed (Ghanem, 2011).

Dosage Forms

Packet, Oral:

Zithromax: 1 g (3 ea, 10 ea)

Generic: 1 g (3 ea, 10 ea)

Solution Reconstituted, Intravenous:

Zithromax: 500 mg (1 ea)

Generic: 500 mg (1 ea); 2.5 g (1 ea)

Solution Reconstituted, Intravenous [preservative free]:

Generic: 500 mg (1 ea)

Suspension Reconstituted, Oral:

Zithromax: 100 mg/5 mL (15 mL); 200 mg/5 mL (15 mL, 22.5 mL, 30 mL)

Zmax: 2 g (1 ea)

Generic: 100 mg/5 mL (15 mL); 200 mg/5 mL (15 mL, 22.5 mL, 30 mL)

Tablet, Oral:

Zithromax: 250 mg, 500 mg, 600 mg

Zithromax Tri-Pak: 500 mg

Zithromax Z-Pak: 250 mg

Generic: 250 mg, 500 mg, 600 mg

Azithromycin (Ophthalmic) (az ith roe MYE sin)

Brand Names: U.S. AzaSite

Pharmacologic Category Antibiotic, Macrolide; Antibiotic, Ophthalmic

Use Treatment of bacterial conjunctivitis caused by susceptible microorganisms

Pregnancy Risk Factor B

Dosage Ophthalmic: **Usual dosage range:** Bacterial conjunctivitis: Children ≥1 year and Adults: Instill 1 drop into affected eye(s) twice daily (8-12 hours apart) for 2 days, then 1 drop into affected eye(s) once daily for 5 days

Additional Information Complete prescribing information should be consulted for additional detail.

Dosage Forms

Solution, Ophthalmic:

AzaSite: 1% (2.5 mL)

◆ **Azithromycin Dihydrate** *see* Azithromycin (Systemic) *on page 216*

◆ **Azithromycin for Injection (Can)** *see* Azithromycin (Systemic) *on page 216*

◆ **Azithromycin for Injection, USP (Can)** *see* Azithromycin (Systemic) *on page 216*

◆ **Azithromycin Monohydrate** *see* Azithromycin (Systemic) *on page 216*

◆ **AZL-M** *see* Azilsartan *on page 214*

◆ **Azo-Gesic [OTC]** *see* Phenazopyridine *on page 1629*

◆ **Azolen Tincture [OTC]** *see* Miconazole (Topical) *on page 1360*

◆ **Azopt** *see* Brinzolamide *on page 288*

◆ **Azopt® (Can)** *see* Brinzolamide *on page 288*

◆ **Azor** *see* Amlodipine and Olmesartan *on page 126*

Azosemide [INT] (AY zoe se mide)

International Brand Names Diat (JP); Luret (DE); Uretin (KR); Ya Li (CN)

Pharmacologic Category Diuretic, Loop

Reported Use Management of edema associated with congestive heart failure and hepatic or renal disease; treatment of hypertension

Dosage Range Adults: Oral: 30-120 mg/day reported in clinical studies

Product Availability Product available in various countries; not currently available in the U.S.

Dosage Forms

Tablet: 30 mg, 60 mg

◆ **AZT (Can)** *see* Zidovudine *on page 2196*

◆ **AZT + 3TC (error-prone abbreviation)** *see* Lamivudine and Zidovudine *on page 1160*

◆ **AZT, Abacavir, and Lamivudine** *see* Abacavir, Lamivudine, and Zidovudine *on page 22*

◆ **AZT (error-prone abbreviation)** *see* Zidovudine *on page 2196*

◆ **Azthreonam** *see* Aztreonam *on page 220*

Aztreonam (AZ tree oh nam)

Brand Names: U.S. Azactam; Azactam in Dextrose; Cayston

Brand Names: Canada Cayston

Index Terms Azthreonam

Pharmacologic Category Antibiotic, Miscellaneous

Use

Injection: Treatment of patients with urinary tract infections, lower respiratory tract infections, septicemia, skin/skin structure infections, intra-abdominal infections, and gynecological infections caused by susceptible gram-negative bacilli

Inhalation: Improve respiratory symptoms in cystic fibrosis (CF) patients with *Pseudomonas aeruginosa*

Pregnancy Risk Factor B

Pregnancy Considerations Adverse events have not been observed in animal reproduction studies; therefore, the manufacturer classifies aztreonam as pregnancy category B. Aztreonam crosses the placenta and enters cord blood during middle and late pregnancy. Distribution to the fetus is minimal in early pregnancy. The amount of aztreonam available systemically following inhalation is significantly less in comparison to doses given by injection.

Breast-Feeding Considerations Very small amounts of aztreonam are excreted in breast milk. The poor oral absorption of aztreonam (<1%) may limit adverse effects to the infant. Nondose-related effects could include modification of bowel flora. Maternal use of aztreonam inhalation is not likely to pose a risk to breast-feeding infants.

Contraindications Hypersensitivity to aztreonam or any component of the formulation

Warnings/Precautions Rare cross-allergenicity to penicillins, cephalosporins, or carbapenems may occur; use with caution in patients with a history of hypersensitivity to beta-lactams. Use caution in renal impairment; dosing adjustment required for the injectable formulation. Prolonged use may result in fungal or bacterial superinfection, including *C. difficile*-associated diarrhea (CDAD) and pseudomembranous colitis; CDAD has been observed >2 months postantibiotic treatment. Use with caution in bone marrow transplant patients with multiple risk factors for toxic epidermal necrolysis (TEN) (eg, sepsis, radiation therapy, drugs known to cause TEN); rare cases of TEN in this population have been reported. Patients colonized with *Burkholderia cepacia* have not been studied. Potentially significant interactions may exist, requiring dose or frequency adjustment, additional monitoring, and/or selection of alternative therapy. Safety and efficacy has not been established in patients with FEV_1 <25% or >75% predicted. To reduce the development of resistant bacteria and maintain efficacy reserve use for CF patients with known *Pseudomonas aeruginosa*. Bronchospasm may occur occur following nebulization; administer a bronchodilator prior to treatment.

Adverse Reactions

Inhalation:

Cardiovascular: Chest discomfort

Dermatologic: Skin rash

Gastrointestinal: Abdominal pain, sore throat, vomiting

Respiratory: Bronchospasm, cough, nasal congestion, wheezing

Miscellaneous: Fever (more common in children)

Rare but important or life-threatening: Arthralgia, facial edema, hypersensitivity reaction, joint swelling, tightness in chest and throat

Injection:

Dermatologic: Rash (more common in children)

Gastrointestinal: Diarrhea, nausea, vomiting

Hematologic & oncologic: Eosinophilia (more common in children), neutropenia (more common in children), thrombocythemia (more common in children)

Hepatic: Increased serum transaminases (ALT/AST; children)

Local: Inflammation at injection site, injection site reaction (erythema, induration; more common in children), pain at injection site (more common in children)

Renal: Increased serum creatinine (children)

Miscellaneous: Fever

Rare but important or life-threatening: Anaphylaxis, anemia, angioedema, aphthous stomatitis, *Clostridium difficile* associated diarrhea, erythema multiforme, exfoliative dermatitis, gastrointestinal hemorrhage, hepatitis, leukocytosis, leukopenia, oral mucosa ulcer, pancytopenia, positive direct Coombs test, prolonged partial thromboplastin time, prolonged prothrombin time, pseudomembranous colitis, seizure, thrombocytopenia, toxic epidermal necrolysis, vaginitis, ventricular bigeminy (transient), ventricular premature contractions (transient), vulvovaginal candidiasis

Drug Interactions

Metabolism/Transport Effects None known.

Avoid Concomitant Use

Avoid concomitant use of Aztreonam with any of the following: BCG

Increased Effect/Toxicity There are no known significant interactions involving an increase in effect.

Decreased Effect

Aztreonam may decrease the levels/effects of: BCG; Sodium Picosulfate; Typhoid Vaccine

Preparation for Administration

Inhalation: Reconstitute immediately prior to use. Squeeze diluent into opened glass vial. Replace rubber stopper and gently swirl vial until contents have completely dissolved.

IM: Reconstitute vial with at least 3 mL SWFI, sterile bacteriostatic water for injection, NS, or bacteriostatic sodium chloride per gram of aztreonam; immediately shake vigorously.

IV:

Bolus injection: Reconstitute vial with 6-10 mL SWFI; immediately shake vigorously.

Infusion: Reconstitute vial with at least 3 mL SWFI per gram of aztreonam; immediately shake vigorously. Reconstituted solutions are colorless to light yellow straw and may turn pink upon standing without affecting potency. Further dilute in an appropriate solution for infusion to a final concentration ≤2% (ie, final concentration should not exceed 20 mg/mL).

Storage/Stability

Inhalation: Prior to reconstitution, store at 2°C to 8°C (36°F to 46°F). Once removed from refrigeration, aztreonam and the diluent may be stored at room temperature (up to 25°C [77°F]) for ≤28 days. Protect from light. Use immediately after reconstitution.

Vials: Prior to reconstitution, store at room temperature; avoid excessive heat. After reconstitution, solutions for infusion with a final concentration of ≤20 mg/mL should be used within 48 hours if stored at room temperature or within 7 days if refrigerated. Solutions for infusion with a final concentration of >20 mg/mL (if prepared with SWFI or NS **only**) should also be used within 48 hours if stored at room temperature or within 7 days if refrigerated; all other solutions for infusion with a final concentration >20 mg/mL must be used immediately after preparation (unless prepared with SWFI or NS).

Premixed frozen containers: Store unused container frozen at ≤ -20°C (-4°F). Frozen container can be thawed at room temperature of 25°C (77°F) or in a refrigerator, 2°C to 8°C (36°F to 46°F). Thawed solution should be used within 48 hours if stored at room temperature or within 14 days if stored under refrigeration. **Do not freeze.**

Mechanism of Action Inhibits bacterial cell wall synthesis by binding to one or more of the penicillin-binding proteins (PBPs) which in turn inhibits the final transpeptidation step of peptidoglycan synthesis in bacterial cell walls, thus inhibiting cell wall biosynthesis. Bacteria eventually lyse due to ongoing activity of cell wall autolytic enzymes (autolysins and murein hydrolases) while cell wall assembly is arrested. Monobactam structure makes cross-allergenicity with beta-lactams unlikely.

Pharmacodynamics/Kinetics

Absorption: IM: Well absorbed; IM and IV doses produce comparable serum concentrations; Inhalation: Low systemic absorption

Distribution: Injection: Widely to most body fluids and tissues

V_d: Children: 0.2-0.29 L/kg; Adults: 0.2 L/kg

Relative diffusion of antimicrobial agents from blood into CSF: Good only with inflammation (exceeds usual MICs)

CSF:blood level ratio: Meninges: Inflamed: 8% to 40%; Normal: ~1%

Protein binding: 56%

Metabolism: Injection: Hepatic (minor %)

Half-life elimination: Injection:

Children 2 months to 12 years: 1.7 hours

Adults: Normal renal function: 1.7-2.9 hours

End-stage renal disease: 6-8 hours

Time to peak: IM, IV push: Within 60 minutes; IV infusion: 1.5 hours

Excretion: Injection: Urine (60% to 70% as unchanged drug); feces (~13% to 15%)

Dosage

Children ≥9 months and Adolescents: IV:

Mild-to-moderate infections: 30 mg/kg/dose every 8 hours; maximum: 120 mg/kg/day (8 g daily)

Moderate-to-severe infections: 30 mg/kg/dose every 6-8 hours; maximum: 120 mg/kg/day (8 g daily)

Cystic fibrosis: 50 mg/kg/dose every 6-8 hours (ie, up to 200 mg/kg/day); maximum: 8 g daily. **Note:** Higher doses (8-12 g daily) may be needed for patients with cystic fibrosis (Zobell, 2013).

Children ≥1 year: Surgical (perioperative) prophylaxis (off-label use): IV: 30 mg/kg within 60 minutes prior to surgery (maximum: 2000 mg per dose). Doses may be repeated in 4 hours if procedure is lengthy or if there is excessive blood loss (Bratzler, 2013).

Children ≥7 years, Adolescents, and Adults: Inhalation (nebulizer): Cystic fibrosis: 75 mg 3 times daily (at least 4 hours apart) for 28 days; do not repeat for 28 days after completion

Adults:

Urinary tract infection: IM, IV: 500 mg to 1 g every 8-12 hours

Moderately severe systemic infections: 1 g IV or IM or 2 g IV every 8-12 hours. **Note:** IV route preferred for septicemia, intra-abdominal abscess, or peritonitis; higher doses (8-12 g daily) may be needed for patients with cystic fibrosis (Zobell, 2013) or other infections (Solomkin, 2010).

Severe systemic or life-threatening infections (eg, *Pseudomonas aeruginosa*): IV: 2 g every 6-8 hours; maximum: 8 g daily. **Note:** Higher doses (8-12 g daily) may be needed for patients with cystic fibrosis (Zobell, 2013) or other infections (Solomkin, 2010).

Surgical (perioperative) prophylaxis (off-label use): IV: 2 g within 60 minutes prior to surgery. Doses may be repeated in 4 hours if procedure is lengthy or if there is excessive blood loss (Bratzler, 2013).

Dosage adjustment in renal impairment:

Oral inhalation: Dosage adjustment not required for mild, moderate, or severe renal impairment

IM, IV: Adults: Following initial dose, maintenance doses should be given as follows:

CrCl 10-30 mL/minute: 50% of usual dose at the usual interval

CrCl <10 mL/minute: 25% of usual dosage at the usual interval

Intermittent hemodialysis (IHD): Dialyzable (20% to 50%): Loading dose of 500 mg, 1 g, or 2 g, followed by 25% of initial dose at usual interval; for serious/life-threatening infections, administer 12.5% of initial dose after each hemodialysis session (given in addition to the maintenance doses). Alternatively, may administer 500 mg every 12 hours (Heintz, 2009). **Note:** Dosing dependent on the assumption of 3 times/week, complete IHD sessions.

Peritoneal dialysis (PD): Administer as for CrCl <10 mL/minute (Aronoff, 2007)

Continuous renal replacement therapy (CRRT) (Heintz, 2009; Trotman, 2005): Drug clearance is highly dependent on the method of renal replacement, filter type, and flow rate. Appropriate dosing requires close monitoring of pharmacologic response, signs of adverse reactions due to drug accumulation, as well as drug concentrations in relation to target trough (if appropriate). The following are general recommendations only (based on dialysate flow/ultrafiltration rates of 1-2 L/hour and minimal residual renal function) and should not supersede clinical judgment:

CVVH: Loading dose of 2 g followed by 1-2 g every 12 hours

CVVHD/CVVHDF: Loading dose of 2 g followed by either 1 g every 8 hours **or** 2 g every 12 hours (Heintz, 2009)

Dosage adjustment in hepatic impairment: No dosage adjustment provided in manufacturer's labeling. Use with caution (minor hepatic elimination occurs).

Administration

Inhalation: Administer using only an Altera nebulizer system; **administer alone; do not mix with other nebulizer medications.** Administer a bronchodilator before administration of aztreonam (short-acting: 15 minutes to 4 hours before; long-acting: 30 minutes to 12 hours before). For patients on multiple inhaled therapies, administer bronchodilator first, then mucolytic, and lastly, aztreonam. To administer Cayston, pour reconstituted solution into the handset of the nebulizer system, turn unit on. Place the mouthpiece in the patient's mouth and encourage to breath normally through the mouth. Administration time is usually 2-3 minutes. Administer doses ≥4 hours apart.

Injection: Doses >1 g should be administered IV

IM: Administer by deep injection into large muscle mass, such as upper outer quadrant of gluteus maximus or the lateral part of the thigh

IV: Administer by slow IV push over 3-5 minutes or by intermittent infusion over 20-60 minutes.

Monitoring Parameters

Injection: Periodic liver function test; monitor for signs of anaphylaxis during first dose

Inhalation: Consider measuring FEV_1 prior to initiation of therapy

Additional Information Although marketed as an agent similar to aminoglycosides, aztreonam is a monobactam antimicrobial with almost pure gram-negative aerobic activity. It cannot be used for gram-positive infections.

Dosage Forms

Solution, Intravenous:

Azactam in Dextrose: 1 g (50 mL); 2 g (50 mL)

Solution Reconstituted, Inhalation [preservative free]:

Cayston: 75 mg (84 mL)

Solution Reconstituted, Injection:

Azactam: 1 g (1 ea); 2 g (1 ea)

Generic: 1 g (1 ea); 2 g (1 ea)

- ◆ **Azulfidine** *see* SulfaSALAzine *on page 1950*
- ◆ **Azulfidine EN-tabs** *see* SulfaSALAzine *on page 1950*
- ◆ **Azurette** *see* Ethinyl Estradiol and Desogestrel *on page 799*
- ◆ **B-2-400 [OTC]** *see* Riboflavin *on page 1803*
- ◆ **B6** *see* Pyridoxine *on page 1747*
- ◆ **B-663** *see* Clofazimine [INT] *on page 473*
- ◆ **B1939** *see* Eribulin *on page 755*
- ◆ **B2036-PEG** *see* Pegvisomant *on page 1604*
- ◆ **Baby Anbesol [OTC]** *see* Benzocaine *on page 246*
- ◆ **Baby Aspirin** *see* Aspirin *on page 180*
- ◆ **Baby Ayr Saline [OTC]** *see* Sodium Chloride *on page 1902*
- ◆ **BabyBIG®** *see* Botulism Immune Globulin (Intravenous-Human) *on page 284*
- ◆ **BACiiM** *see* Bacitracin (Systemic) *on page 222*
- ◆ **BaciJect (Can)** *see* Bacitracin (Systemic) *on page 222*
- ◆ **Bacillus Calmette-Guérin (BCG) Live** *see* BCG *on page 229*
- ◆ **Bacitin (Can)** *see* Bacitracin (Topical) *on page 222*

Bacitracin (Systemic) (bas i TRAY sin)

Brand Names: U.S. BACiiM

Brand Names: Canada BaciJect

Pharmacologic Category Antibiotic, Miscellaneous

Use Pneumonia and empyema: Treatment of pneumonia and empyema in infants caused by susceptible staphylococci; due to toxicity risks, systemic uses of bacitracin should be limited to situations where less toxic alternatives would not be effective

Dosage Do not administer IV:

Infants: IM:

≤2.5 kg: 900 units/kg/day in 2 to 3 divided doses

>2.5 kg: 1000 units/kg/day in 2 to 3 divided doses

Additional Information Complete prescribing information should be consulted for additional detail.

Dosage Forms

Solution Reconstituted, Intramuscular:

BACiiM: 50,000 units (1 ea)

Generic: 50,000 units (1 ea)

Solution Reconstituted, Intramuscular [preservative free]:

Generic: 50,000 units (1 ea)

Bacitracin (Ophthalmic) (bas i TRAY sin)

Pharmacologic Category Antibiotic, Ophthalmic

Use Superficial ocular infections: Treatment of superficial ocular infections involving the conjunctiva or cornea due to susceptible organisms

Dosage Ophthalmic infection: Children, Adolescents, and Adults: Ophthalmic: Apply 1 to 3 times daily

Additional Information Complete prescribing information should be consulted for additional detail.

Dosage Forms

Ointment, Ophthalmic:

Generic: 500 units/g (1 g, 3.5 g)

Bacitracin (Topical) (bas i TRAY sin)

Brand Names: Canada Bacitin

Pharmacologic Category Antibiotic, Topical

Use Topical infection prevention: Prevention of infection in minor cuts, scrapes, or burns.

Dosage Prevention of infection: Children, Adolescents, and Adults: Topical: Apply 1 to 3 times daily

Additional Information Complete prescribing information should be consulted for additional detail.

Dosage Forms

Ointment, External:

Generic: 500 units/g (1 ea, 1 g, 14 g, 14.2 g, 15 g, 28 g, 28.35 g, 28.4 g, 30 g, 120 g, 453.9 g, 454 g)

Bacitracin and Polymyxin B

(bas i TRAY sin & pol i MIKS in bee)

Brand Names: U.S. AK-Poly-Bac™; Polycin™; Polysporin® [OTC]

Brand Names: Canada LID-Pack®; Optimyxin®

Index Terms Polymyxin B and Bacitracin

Pharmacologic Category Antibiotic, Ophthalmic; Antibiotic, Topical

Use Treatment of superficial infections caused by susceptible organisms

Pregnancy Risk Factor C

Dosage Children and Adults:

Ophthalmic ointment: Instill 1/2" ribbon in the affected eye(s) every 3-4 hours for acute infections or 2-3 times/day for mild-to-moderate infections for 7-10 days

Topical ointment/powder: Apply to affected area 1-4 times/day; may cover with sterile bandage if needed

Additional Information Complete prescribing information should be consulted for additional detail.

Dosage Forms

Ointment, ophthalmic: Bacitracin 500 units and polymyxin B 10,000 units per g (3.5 g)

AK-Poly-Bac™: Bacitracin 500 units and polymyxin B 10,000 units per g (3.5 g)

Polycin™: Bacitracin 500 units and polymyxin B 10,000 units per g (3.5 g)

Ointment, topical: Bacitracin 500 units and polymyxin B 10,000 units per g (15 g, 30 g)

Polysporin®: Bacitracin 500 units and polymyxin B 10,000 units per g (0.9 g, 15 g, 30 g)

Powder, topical:

Polysporin®: Bacitracin 500 units and polymyxin B 10,000 units per g (10 g)

Bacitracin, Neomycin, and Polymyxin B

(bas i TRAY sin, nee oh MYE sin, & pol i MIKS in bee)

Brand Names: U.S. Neo-Polycin™; Neosporin® Neo To Go® [OTC]; Neosporin® Topical [OTC]

Index Terms Neomycin, Bacitracin, and Polymyxin B; Polymyxin B, Bacitracin, and Neomycin; Triple Antibiotic

Pharmacologic Category Antibiotic, Ophthalmic; Antibiotic, Topical

Use Helps prevent infection in minor cuts, scrapes, and burns; short-term treatment of superficial external ocular infections caused by susceptible organisms

Pregnancy Risk Factor C

Dosage Children and Adults:

Ophthalmic: Ointment: Instill 1/2" into the conjunctival sac every 3-4 hours for 7-10 days for acute infections

Topical: Apply 1-3 times/day to infected area; may cover with sterile bandage as needed

Additional Information Complete prescribing information should be consulted for additional detail.

Dosage Forms

Ointment, ophthalmic: Bacitracin 400 units, neomycin 3.5 mg, and polymyxin B 10,000 units per g (3.5 g)

Neo-Polycin™: Bacitracin 400 units, neomycin 3.5 mg, and polymyxin B 10,000 units per g (3.5 g)

Ointment, topical: Bacitracin 400 units, neomycin 3.5 mg, and polymyxin B 5000 units per g (0.9 g, 15 g, 30 g, 454 g)

Neosporin® [OTC]: Bacitracin 400 units, neomycin 3.5 mg, and polymyxin B 5000 units per g (15 g, 30 g)

Neosporin® Neo To Go® [OTC]: Bacitracin 400 units, neomycin 3.5 mg, and polymyxin B 5000 units per g (0.9 g)

Bacitracin, Neomycin, Polymyxin B, and Hydrocortisone

(bas i TRAY sin, nee oh MYE sin, pol i MIKS in bee, & hye droe KOR ti sone)

Brand Names: U.S. Cortisporin® Ointment; Neo-Polycin™ HC

Brand Names: Canada Cortisporin® Topical Ointment

Index Terms Hydrocortisone, Bacitracin, Neomycin, and Polymyxin B; Neomycin, Bacitracin, Polymyxin B, and Hydrocortisone; Polymyxin B, Bacitracin, Neomycin, and Hydrocortisone

Pharmacologic Category Antibiotic, Ophthalmic; Antibiotic, Topical; Corticosteroid, Ophthalmic; Corticosteroid, Topical

Use Prevention and treatment of susceptible inflammatory conditions where bacterial infection (or risk of infection) is present

Pregnancy Risk Factor C

Dosage Children and Adults:

Ophthalmic: Ointment: Instill 1/2 inch ribbon to inside of lower lid every 3-4 hours until improvement occurs

Topical: Apply sparingly 2-4 times/day. Therapy should be discontinued when control is achieved; if no improvement is seen, reassessment of diagnosis may be necessary.

Additional Information Complete prescribing information should be consulted for additional detail.

Dosage Forms

Ointment, ophthalmic: Bacitracin 400 units, neomycin sulfate 3.5 mg, polymyxin B 10,000 units, and hydrocortisone 10 mg per g (3.5 g)

Neo-Polycin™ HC: Bacitracin 400 units, neomycin 3.5 mg, polymyxin B 10,000 units, and hydrocortisone 10 mg per g (3.5 g)

Ointment, topical:

Cortisporin®: Bacitracin 400 units, neomycin 3.5 mg, polymyxin B 5000 units, and hydrocortisone 10 mg per g (15 g)

Baclofen (BAK loe fen)

Brand Names: U.S. EnovaRX-Baclofen; Gablofen; Lioresal

Brand Names: Canada Apo-Baclofen; Dom-Baclofen; Lioresal; Lioresal D.S.; Lioresal Intrathecal; Mylan-Baclofen; Novo-Baclofen; PHL-Baclofen; PMS-Baclofen; ratio-Baclofen; Riva-Baclofen; VPI-Baclofen Intrathecal

Pharmacologic Category Skeletal Muscle Relaxant

Use

Spasticity:

Oral: Management of reversible spasticity associated with multiple sclerosis or spinal cord lesions

Intrathecal: Management of severe spasticity of spinal cord origin (eg, spinal cord injury, multiple sclerosis) or cerebral origin (eg, cerebral palsy, traumatic brain injury). May be considered as an alternative to destructive neurosurgical procedures.

Pregnancy Risk Factor C

Pregnancy Considerations Adverse events were observed in animal reproduction studies. Withdrawal symptoms in the neonate were noted in a case report following the maternal use of oral baclofen 20 mg 4 times/day throughout pregnancy (Ratnayaka, 2001). Plasma concentrations following administration of intrathecal baclofen are significantly less than those with oral doses; exposure to the fetus is expected to be limited (Morton, 2009).

Breast-Feeding Considerations Baclofen is excreted into breast milk. Very small amounts were found in the breast milk of a woman 14 days postpartum after oral use. Following a single oral dose of baclofen 20 mg, the total amount of baclofen excreted in breast milk within 26 hours was 22 mcg (Eriksson, 1981). Adverse events were not observed in a nursing infant following maternal use of intrathecal baclofen 200 mcg/day throughout pregnancy and while nursing (Morton, 2009). Due to the potential for adverse events in the nursing infant, breast-feeding is not recommended by the manufacturer.

Contraindications Hypersensitivity to baclofen or any component of the formulation

Warnings/Precautions **[U.S. Boxed Warning]: Abrupt withdrawal of intrathecal baclofen has resulted in severe sequelae (hyperpyrexia, obtundation, rebound/exaggerated spasticity, muscle rigidity, and rhabdomyolysis), leading to organ failure and some fatalities. Prevention of abrupt discontinuation requires careful attention to programming and monitoring of infusion system, refill scheduling and procedures, and pump alarms. Risk may be higher in patients with injuries at T-6 or above, history of baclofen withdrawal, or limited ability to communicate.** Abrupt withdrawal of oral therapy has been associated with hallucinations and seizures; gradual dose reductions (over ~1 to 2 weeks) are recommended in the absence of severe adverse reactions.

Patients receiving intrathecal baclofen should be infection-free prior to the test dose and pump implantation. Clinicians should be experienced with chronic intrathecal infusion therapy. Pump should only be implanted if patients' response to bolus intrathecal baclofen was adequately evaluated and found to be safe and effective. Resuscitative equipment should be readily available. Monitor closely during the initial phase of pump use and when adjusting the dosing rate and/or the concentration in the reservoir. Educate patients and caregivers on proper home care of the pump and insertion site; early symptoms of baclofen withdrawal (eg, return of baseline spasticity, hypotension, paresthesia, pruritus); signs/symptoms of overdose (eg, dizziness, somnolence, respiratory depression, seizures); and appropriate actions in the event of an overdose. Cases (most from pharmacy compounded preparations) of intrathecal mass formation at the implanted catheter tip have been reported; may lead to loss of clinical response, pain or new/worsening neurological effects. Neurosurgical evaluation and/or an appropriate imaging study should be considered if a mass is suspected. Use caution with history of autonomic dysreflexia; presence of nociceptive stimuli or abrupt baclofen withdrawal may cause an autonomic dysreflexia episode.

May cause CNS depression, which may impair physical or mental abilities; patients must be cautioned about performing tasks which require mental alertness (eg, operating machinery or driving). Elderly patients are more sensitive to the effects of baclofen and are more likely to experience adverse CNS effects at higher doses. Use with caution in patients with seizure disorder, renal impairment, respiratory disease, psychiatric disease, peptic ulcer disease, decreased GI motility, and/or gastrointestinal obstructive disorders.

Efficacy of oral baclofen has not been established in patients with stroke, Parkinson disease, or cerebral palsy; therefore, use is not recommended. Not indicated for spasticity associated with rheumatic disorders. Use with caution when spasticity is utilized to sustain upright posture and balance in locomotion, or when spasticity is necessary to obtain increased function. Adverse effects are more likely in patients with spastic states of cerebral origin; cautious dosing and careful monitoring are necessary.

Animal studies have shown an increased incidence in ovarian cysts; however, incidence observed in multiple sclerosis patients treated with baclofen for up to one year was similar to the estimated incidence in healthy females. Spontaneous resolution occurred in most of these MS patients while continuing treatment. May cause acute urinary retention (may be related to underlying disease); use with caution in patients with urinary obstruction. Potentially significant drug-drug interactions may exist, requiring dose or frequency adjustment, additional monitoring, and/or selection of alternative therapy.

Adverse Reactions

Cardiovascular: Hypotension

Central nervous system: Ataxia, confusion, drowsiness, fatigue, headache, hypotonia, insomnia, psychiatric disturbance, slurred speech, vertigo

Dermatologic: Skin rash

Gastrointestinal: Constipation, nausea

Genitourinary: Polyuria

Neuromuscular & skeletal: Weakness

Rare but important or life-threatening: Chest pain, dyspnea, dysuria, hematuria, impotence, inhibited ejaculation, nocturia, palpitations, syncope, urinary incontinence, urinary retention

Withdrawal reactions have occurred with abrupt discontinuation (particularly severe with intrathecal use).

Drug Interactions

Metabolism/Transport Effects None known.

Avoid Concomitant Use

Avoid concomitant use of Baclofen with any of the following: Azelastine (Nasal); Orphenadrine; Paraldehyde; Thalidomide

Increased Effect/Toxicity

Baclofen may increase the levels/effects of: Alcohol (Ethyl); Azelastine (Nasal); Buprenorphine; CNS Depressants; Hydrocodone; Methotrimeprazine; Metyrosine; Mirtazapine; Orphenadrine; Paraldehyde; Pramipexole; ROPINIRole; Rotigotine; Selective Serotonin Reuptake Inhibitors; Suvorexant; Thalidomide; Zolpidem

The levels/effects of Baclofen may be increased by: Brimonidine (Topical); Cannabis; Doxylamine; Dronabinol; Droperidol; HydrOXYzine; Kava Kava; Magnesium Sulfate; Methotrimeprazine; Nabilone; Perampanel; Rufinamide; Sodium Oxybate; Tapentadol; Tetrahydrocannabinol

Decreased Effect There are no known significant interactions involving a decrease in effect.

Preparation for Administration Intrathecal: Screening doses should be a 50 mcg/mL concentration and withdrawn from the 1 mL screening ampul (50 mcg/mL); do not further dilute. Maintenance infusions for patients who require concentrations other than 500 mcg/mL or 2,000 mcg/mL must be diluted with preservative-free sodium chloride.

Storage/Stability

Injection: Do not store above 30°C (86°F). Does not require refrigeration. Do not freeze.

Tablets: Store at 20°C to 25°C (68°F to 77°F).

Mechanism of Action Inhibits the transmission of both monosynaptic and polysynaptic reflexes at the spinal cord level, possibly by hyperpolarization of primary afferent fiber terminals, with resultant relief of muscle spasticity

Pharmacodynamics/Kinetics

Onset of action: Intrathecal bolus: 30 minutes to 1 hour; Continuous infusion: 6 to 8 hours after infusion initiation

Peak effect: Intrathecal bolus: 4 hours (effects may last 4 to 8 hours); Continuous infusion: 24 to 48 hours

Absorption (dose dependent): Oral: Rapid

Protein binding: 30%

Metabolism: Hepatic (15% of dose)

Half-life elimination: Oral: 2 to 4 hours; Intrathecal: CSF elimination half-life: 1.5 hours over first 4 hours

Time to peak, serum: Oral: Within 2 hours

Excretion: Urine (85% as unchanged drug) and feces

Dosage

Oral: **Note:** Use the lowest effective dose; patients who fail to respond within a reasonable amount of time should be slowly withdrawn from therapy (avoid abrupt withdrawal of drug).

Spasticity:

Children ≥12 years, Adolescents, and Adults: *Manufacturer labeling:* Initial: 5 mg 3 times daily; may increase by 5 mg per dose every 3 days (ie, 5 mg 3 times daily for 3 days, then 10 mg 3 times daily for 3 days, etc.) until optimal response is reached. Usual dosage range: 40 to 80 mg daily. Do not exceed 80 mg daily (20 mg 4 times daily).

Children <12 years (off-label): Caution: Limited published data in children; the following is a compilation of small prospective studies (Albright, 1996; Milla, 1977; Scheinberg, 2006) and one large retrospective study (Lubsch, 2006):

<2 years: 10 to 20 mg daily divided every 8 hours; titrate dose every 3 days in increments of 5 to 15 mg daily to a maximum of 40 mg daily

2 to 7 years: Initial: 20 to 30 mg daily divided every 8 hours; titrate dose every 3 days in increments of 5 to 15 mg daily to a maximum of 60 mg daily

≥8 years: 30 to 40 mg daily divided every 8 hours; titrate dose every 3 days in increments of 5 to 15 mg daily to a maximum of 120 mg daily

Note: Lubsch retrospective analysis noted that higher daily dosages of baclofen were needed as the time increased from injury onset, as age increased, and as the number of concomitant antispasticity medications increased. Each of these variables may represent drug tolerance or progressive spasticity. In this review, doses as high as 200 mg daily were used.

Hiccups (off-label use): Adults: 5 to 10 mg 3 times daily (maximum: 75 mg daily in divided doses) (Guelaud, 1995; Zhang, 2014)

Intrathecal: Spasticity: Children ≥4 years, Adolescents, and Adults (U.S. labeling) or Adults (Canadian labeling):

Screening dose: Initial: 50 mcg (1 mL) for 1 dose; following administration, observe patient for 4 to 8 hours. A positive response consists of a significant decrease in muscle tone and/or frequency and/or severity of spasms. If response is inadequate, may give 75 mcg as a second screening dose 24 hours after the first screening dose; observe patient for 4 to 8 hours. If response is still inadequate, may repeat a final screening dose of 100 mcg given 24 hours after the second screening dose. Patients not responding to screening dose of 100 mcg should not be considered for chronic infusion/implanted pump. **Note:** A 25 mcg initial screening dose may be considered in very small pediatric patients. Canadian labeling suggests that a 10 mcg dose may be administered if adverse reactions occur with a 25 mcg dose.

Dose titration following pump implant: After positive response to screening dose, a maintenance intrathecal infusion can be administered via an implanted intrathecal pump.

Initial total daily dose via pump: Double the screening dose that gave a positive response and administer over 24 hours, unless efficacy of the bolus dose was maintained for >8 hours (U.S. labeling) or >12 hours (Canadian labeling), then infuse a dose equivalent to the screening dose over 24 hours. Do not increase dose in first 24 hours (to allow steady state to be achieved); thereafter, dosage adjustments may be made as follows:

U.S. labeling:

Children ≥4 years and Adolescents: Increase daily dose slowly by 5% to 15% once every 24 hours until satisfactory response

Adults: Increase daily dose slowly by 10% to 30% (spasticity of spinal cord origin) or 5% to 15% (spasticity of cerebral origin) once every 24 hours until satisfactory response

Canadian labeling: Adults: Increase daily dose slowly by 10% to 30% once every 24 hours (if using a programmable pump) or once every 48 hours (if using a nonprogrammable pump)

Maintenance:

U.S. labeling:

Children ≥4 years and Adolescents: Daily dose may be increased 5% to 20% (maximum increase: 20%). Dose may also be decreased 10% to 20% for adverse effects. Patients <12 years required lower daily doses in clinical trials (average dose: 274 mcg daily; dosage range: 24 mcg to 1,199 mcg/day); dose requirements of patients >12 years were similar to that of adults.

Adults: Daily dose may be increased 5% to 20% (maximum increase: 20%) (spasticity of cerebral origin) or by 10% to 40% (maximum increase: 40%) (spasticity of spinal cord origin). Dose may also be decreased 10% to 20% for adverse effects. Most patients have been adequately maintained on 90 mcg to 703 mcg daily (spasticity of cerebral origin) or 300 mcg to 800 mcg daily (spasticity of spinal cord origin). Experience with doses >1,000 mcg daily is limited.

Canadian labeling: Adults: Daily dose may be increased 10% to 30%. Dose may also be decreased 10% to 20% for adverse effects. Most patients have been adequately maintained on 300 mcg to 800 mcg daily

Note: Dosage adjustments may be required often during the first few months of therapy to adjust for life style changes due to alleviation of spasticity. Maintain lowest dose that produces adequate response. Most patients require gradual increases over time to maintain optimal response. Sudden large requirements for a dose increase may indicate a catheter complication (eg, kink, dislodgement).Titrate dose to allow sufficient muscle tone and occasional spasms to optimize activities of daily living, support circulation, and possibly prevent DVT formation. **Use extreme caution when filling the pump; follow manufacturer instructions carefully;** 5% to 10% of patients receiving chronic therapy become refractory to dose adjustments; may consider a drug holiday (hospitalized patients only) with a gradual withdrawal over 2 to 4 weeks and use of alternative spasticity management methods. Following the drug holiday intrathecal baclofen may be resumed at the initial continuous infusion dose.

Elderly: Oral: Refer to adult dosing; use with caution. If benefits are not observed, withdraw the drug slowly.

Dosage adjustment in renal impairment: There are no dosage adjustments provided in the manufacturer's labeling. However, baclofen is primarily renally eliminated; use with caution; dosage reduction may be necessary.

Hemodialysis: Oral:

U.S. labeling: There are no dosage adjustments provided in the manufacturer's labeling.

Canadian labeling: 5 mg once daily

Dosage adjustment in hepatic impairment: Oral:

U.S. labeling: There are no dosage adjustments provided in the manufacturer's labeling.

Canadian labeling: No dosage adjustment necessary; use with caution.

Administration

Intrathecal: For screening dosages, administer as a bolus injection (50 mcg/mL concentration) by barbotage into the subarachnoid space over at least 1 minute, followed by maintenance infusion.

Oral: The Canadian labeling recommends administering with food or milk in patients with persistent nausea despite dose reductions.

Monitoring Parameters Regular electroencephalogram (EEG) in patients with epilepsy (loss of seizure control has been reported).

Dosage Forms Considerations

EnovaRX-Baclofen is a compounding kit. Refer to manufacturer's labeling for compounding instructions.

Dosage Forms

Cream, External:

EnovaRX-Baclofen: 1% (60 g, 120 g)

Solution, Intrathecal [preservative free]:

Gablofen: 50 mcg/mL (1 mL); 10,000 mcg/20 mL (20 mL); 20,000 mcg/20 mL (20 mL); 40,000 mcg/20 mL (20 mL)

Lioresal: 0.05 mg/mL (1 mL); 10 mg/20 mL (20 mL); 10 mg/5 mL (5 mL); 40 mg/20 mL (20 mL)

Tablet, Oral:

Generic: 10 mg, 20 mg

Extemporaneous Preparations A 5 mg/mL oral suspension may be made with tablets. Crush thirty 20 mg tablets in a mortar and reduce to a fine powder. Add a small amount of glycerin and mix to a uniform paste. Mix while adding Simple Syrup, NF in incremental proportions to

almost 120 mL; transfer to a calibrated bottle, rinse mortar with vehicle, and add a sufficient quantity of vehicle to make 120 mL. Label "shake well" and "refrigerate". Stable for 35 days (Johnson, 1993).

A 10 mg/mL oral suspension may be made with tablets. Crush one-hundred-twenty 10 mg tablets in a mortar and reduce to a fine powder. Add small portions (60 mL) of a 1:1 mixture of Ora-Sweet® and Ora-Plus® and mix to a uniform paste; mix while adding the vehicle in incremental proportions to **almost** 120 mL; transfer to a calibrated bottle, rinse mortar with vehicle, and add quantity of vehicle sufficient to make 120 mL. Label "shake well" and "refrigerate". Stable for 60 days (Allen, 1996).

Allen LV Jr and Erickson MA 3rd, "Stability of Baclofen, Captopril, Diltiazem Hydrochloride, Dipyridamole, and Flecainide Acetate in Extemporaneously Compounded Oral Liquids," *Am J Health Syst Pharm*, 1996, 53(18):2179-84.

Johnson CE and Hart SM, "Stability of an Extemporaneously Compounded Baclofen Oral Liquid," *Am J Hosp Pharm*, 1993, 50 (11):2353-5.

◆ **Bactocill in Dextrose** *see* Oxacillin *on page 1528*

◆ **Bactrim** *see* Sulfamethoxazole and Trimethoprim *on page 1946*

◆ **Bactrim DS** *see* Sulfamethoxazole and Trimethoprim *on page 1946*

◆ **Bactroban** *see* Mupirocin *on page 1404*

◆ **Bactroban Nasal** *see* Mupirocin *on page 1404*

◆ **Baking Soda** *see* Sodium Bicarbonate *on page 1901*

◆ **BAL** *see* Dimercaprol *on page 638*

◆ **Bal in Oil** *see* Dimercaprol *on page 638*

◆ **Balmex® [OTC]** *see* Zinc Oxide *on page 2200*

◆ **Balminil Decongestant (Can)** *see* Pseudoephedrine *on page 1742*

◆ **Balminil DM D (Can)** *see* Pseudoephedrine and Dextromethorphan *on page 1743*

◆ **Balminil DM + Decongestant + Expectorant (Can)** *see* Guaifenesin, Pseudoephedrine, and Dextromethorphan *on page 989*

◆ **Balminil DM + Decongestant + Expectorant Extra Strength (Can)** *see* Guaifenesin, Pseudoephedrine, and Dextromethorphan *on page 989*

◆ **Balminil DM E (Can)** *see* Guaifenesin and Dextromethorphan *on page 987*

◆ **Balminil Expectorant (Can)** *see* GuaiFENesin *on page 986*

Balsalazide (bal SAL a zide)

Brand Names: U.S. Colazal; Giazo

Index Terms Balsalazide Disodium

Pharmacologic Category 5-Aminosalicylic Acid Derivative; Anti-inflammatory Agent

Use Treatment of mildly- to moderately-active ulcerative colitis

Giazo™: Only approved in males ≥18 years; effectiveness in females was not demonstrated

Pregnancy Risk Factor B

Pregnancy Considerations Teratogenic effects were not observed in animal reproduction studies. Mesalamine (5-aminosalicylic acid) is the active metabolite of balsalazide; mesalamine is known to cross the placenta.

Breast-Feeding Considerations Mesalamine, 5-aminosalicylic acid, is the active metabolite of balsalazide. Low levels of mesalamine enter breast milk; a case of bloody diarrhea in a breast-fed infant has been reported.

Contraindications Hypersensitivity to balsalazide or its metabolites, salicylates, or any component of the formulation

Warnings/Precautions Pyloric stenosis may prolong gastric retention of balsalazide. Renal toxicity and hepatic failure have been observed with other mesalamine (5-aminosalicylic acid) products; use with caution in patients with known renal or hepatic disease. Symptomatic worsening of ulcerative colitis may occur following initiation of treatment. May cause an acute intolerance syndrome (cramping, acute abdominal pain, bloody diarrhea; sometimes fever, headache, rash); discontinue if this occurs. May cause staining of teeth or tongue if capsule is opened and sprinkled on food.

Adverse Reactions

Central nervous system: Fatigue, fever, headache (more common in children than adults), insomnia

Endocrine & metabolic: Dysmenorrhea

Gastrointestinal: Abdominal pain (more common in children than adults), anorexia, cramps, constipation, diarrhea, dyspepsia, flatulence, hematochezia, nausea, stomatitis, ulcerative colitis exacerbation, vomiting, xerostomia

Genitourinary: Urinary tract infection

Hematologic: Anemia

Neuromuscular & skeletal: Arthralgia, musculoskeletal pain, myalgia

Respiratory: Cough, pharyngolaryngeal pain, pharyngitis, respiratory infection, rhinitis

Miscellaneous: Flu-like syndrome

Rare but important or life-threatening: Alopecia, alveolitis, AST increased, back pain, blood pressure increased, cholestatic jaundice, cirrhosis, defecation urgency, dizziness, dyspnea, edema, erythema nodosum, facial edema, fever, gastroenteritis, gastroesophageal reflux, hard stool, heart rate increased, hepatocellular damage, hepatotoxicity, hyperbilirubinemia, hypersensitivity, interstitial nephritis, jaundice, Kawasaki-like syndrome, lethargy, liver failure, liver necrosis, liver function tests increased, malaise, myocarditis, pain, pancreatitis, pericarditis, pleural effusion, pneumonia (with and without eosinophilia), pruritus, rash, renal failure, vasculitis

Drug Interactions

Metabolism/Transport Effects None known.

Avoid Concomitant Use There are no known interactions where it is recommended to avoid concomitant use.

Increased Effect/Toxicity

Balsalazide may increase the levels/effects of: Heparin; Heparin (Low Molecular Weight); Thiopurine Analogs; Varicella Virus-Containing Vaccines

The levels/effects of Balsalazide may be increased by: Nonsteroidal Anti-Inflammatory Agents

Decreased Effect

Balsalazide may decrease the levels/effects of: Cardiac Glycosides

Storage/Stability Store at controlled room temperature of 20°C to 25°C (68°F to 77°F); excursions permitted to 15°C to 30°C (59°F to 86°F).

Mechanism of Action Balsalazide is a prodrug, converted by bacterial azoreduction to 5-aminosalicylic acid (mesalamine, active), 4-aminobenzoyl-β-alanine (inert), and their metabolites. 5-aminosalicylic acid may decrease inflammation by blocking the production of arachidonic acid metabolites topically in the colon mucosa.

Pharmacodynamics/Kinetics

Onset of action: Delayed; may require several days to weeks

Absorption: Very low and variable

Protein binding: Balsalazide: ≥99%

Metabolism: Azoreduced in the colon to 5-aminosalicylic acid (active), 4-aminobenzoyl-β-alanine (inert), and N-acetylated metabolites

Half-life elimination: Primary effect is topical (colonic mucosa); therapeutic effect appears not to be influenced by the systemic half-life of balsalazide (1.9 hours) or its metabolites (5-ASA [9.5 hours], N-Ac-5-ASA [10.4 hours])

Time to peak: Balsalazide: Capsule: 1-2 hours; Tablet: 0.5 hours

Excretion: Feces (65% as 5-aminosalicylic acid, 4-aminobenzoyl-β-alanine, and N-acetylated metabolites); urine (<16% as N-acetylated metabolites); Parent drug: Urine or feces (<1%)

Dosage Oral:

Capsule:

Children 5-17 years: 750 mg 3 times daily for up to 8 weeks **or** 2.25 g (three 750 mg capsules) 3 times daily for up to 8 weeks

Adults: 2.25 g (three 750 mg capsules) 3 times daily for up to 8-12 weeks

Tablet (Giazo™): Adults: Males: 3.3 g (three 1.1 g tablets) twice daily for up to 8 weeks

Elderly: Refer to adult dosing.

Dosage adjustment in renal impairment: No dosage adjustment provided in manufacturer's labeling. Renal toxicity has been observed with other 5-aminosalicylic acid products; use with caution.

Dosage adjustment in hepatic impairment: No dosage adjustment provided in manufacturer's labeling.

Dietary Considerations Some products may contain sodium. Take tablets with or without food.

Administration

Capsule: Should be swallowed whole or may be opened and sprinkled on applesauce. Applesauce mixture may be chewed; swallow immediately, do not store mixture for later use. When sprinkled on food, may cause staining of teeth or tongue.

Tablet: Administer with or without food.

Monitoring Parameters Improvement or worsening of symptoms; renal function (prior to initiation, then periodically); liver function tests

Additional Information Balsalazide 750 mg is equivalent to mesalamine 267 mg

Dosage Forms

Capsule, Oral:

Colazal: 750 mg

Generic: 750 mg

Tablet, Oral:

Giazo: 1.1 g

◆ **Balsalazide Disodium** *see* Balsalazide *on page 226*

◆ **Balsam Peru, Castor Oil, and Trypsin** *see* Trypsin, Balsam Peru, and Castor Oil *on page 2109*

◆ **Balziva** *see* Ethinyl Estradiol and Norethindrone *on page 808*

Bambuterol [INT] (bam BYOO ter ol)

International Brand Names A-Terol (KR); Abel (IN); Asthterol (KR); Baburol (TW); Bambec (AT, BH, BR, CN, DE, DK, EG, GB, KR, NO, PH, PK, QA, SE, SG, TH, TW, VN); Bambudil (IN); Lungtec (TW, VN); Oxeol (DK, FR); Roburol (IN)

Index Terms Bambuterol Hydrochloride

Pharmacologic Category $Beta_2$-Adrenergic Agonist

Reported Use Treatment of bronchospasm in bronchial asthma, chronic bronchitis, and emphysema

Dosage Range Oral:

Children 2-5 years: 10 mg/day

Children 6-12 years: See Adult dose; due to differences in kinetics, doses >10 mg are not recommended in Asian children

Adults: Initial: 10 mg/day; may be increased to 20 mg/day after 1-2 weeks based on clinical effect. Patients previously treated with oral $beta_2$ agonists may be started at 20 mg/day.

Dosing adjustment in renal impairment: CrCl ≤50 mL/minute: 5 mg/day

Product Availability Product available in various countries; not currently available in the U.S.

Dosage Forms

Solution, oral: 1 mg/mL [contains sodium benzoate]

Tablet: 10 mg, 20 mg

◆ **Bambuterol Hydrochloride** *see* Bambuterol [INT] *on page 227*

Bamifylline [INT] (bam IF i lin)

International Brand Names Airest (IT); Bami-med (BE, CH); Bamifix (BR, IT); Bamiphil (KR); Baphil (KR); Briofil (IT); Trentadil (BE, FR, KR, LU)

Index Terms Bamifylline Hydrochloride

Pharmacologic Category Antiasthmatic

Reported Use Treatment of asthma

Dosage Range Adults:

Oral: 600-900 mg/day in 2-3 divided doses, increase to 2800 mg/day in 3 divided doses if needed

IM, IV: 600 mg/day in 2 doses

Product Availability Product available in various countries; not currently available in the U.S.

Dosage Forms

Tablet: 300 mg, 600 mg

◆ **Bamifylline Hydrochloride** *see* Bamifylline [INT] *on page 227*

◆ **Banophen [OTC]** *see* DiphenhydrAMINE (Systemic) *on page 641*

◆ **Banzel** *see* Rufinamide *on page 1854*

◆ **Baraclude** *see* Entecavir *on page 731*

Barbexaclone [INT] (bar BEKS a klone)

International Brand Names Maliasin (AT, CH, DE, IT, PY, TR)

Pharmacologic Category Anticonvulsant, Miscellaneous

Reported Use Treatment of epilepsy

Dosage Range Adults: Oral: 200-400 mg/day in divided doses

Product Availability Product available in various countries; not currently available in the U.S.

Dosage Forms

Tablet: 25 mg, 100 mg

◆ **Baridium [OTC]** *see* Phenazopyridine *on page 1629*

Barnidipine [INT] (bar NID a peen)

International Brand Names Barnix (ES); Cypress (NL); Dilacor (AR); Hypoca (CN, JP, TW); Libradin (ES, IT, NL); Oldeca (KR); Vasexten (BE, CZ, GR, NL, SA)

Index Terms Barnidipine Hydrochloride

Pharmacologic Category Calcium Channel Blocker, Dihydropyridine

Reported Use Management of hypertension

Dosage Range Adults: Oral: Hypertension: 5-20 mg/day

Product Availability Product available in various countries; not currently available in the U.S.

Dosage Forms

Capsule, sustained release: 10 mg, 15 mg

◆ **Barnidipine Hydrochloride** *see* Barnidipine [INT] *on page 227*

- ◆ **Basaljel (Can)** *see* Aluminum Hydroxide *on page 103*
- ◆ **Base Ointment** *see* Zinc Oxide *on page 2200*

Basiliximab (ba si LIK si mab)

Brand Names: U.S. Simulect

Brand Names: Canada Simulect

Pharmacologic Category Immunosuppressant Agent; Monoclonal Antibody

Use Renal transplant rejection: Prophylaxis of acute organ rejection in renal transplantation in combination with cyclosporine (modified) and corticosteroids

Pregnancy Risk Factor B

Pregnancy Considerations Adverse effects were not observed in animal reproduction studies. IL-2 receptors play an important role in the development of the immune system. Women of childbearing potential should use effective contraceptive measures before beginning treatment, during, and for 4 months after completion of basiliximab treatment. The National Transplantation Pregnancy Registry (NTPR, Temple University) is a registry for pregnant women taking immunosuppressants following any solid organ transplant. The NTPR encourages reporting of all immunosuppressant exposures during pregnancy in transplant recipients at 877-955-6877.

Breast-Feeding Considerations It is not known if basiliximab is excreted in human milk. Because many immunoglobulins are secreted in milk and the potential for serious adverse reactions exists, a decision should be made to discontinue nursing or discontinue the drug, taking into account the importance of the drug to the mother. The Canadian labeling recommends women avoid nursing for 4 months following the last dose.

Contraindications Known hypersensitivity to basiliximab or any component of the formulation

Warnings/Precautions To be used as a component of an immunosuppressive regimen which includes cyclosporine and corticosteroids. The incidence of lymphoproliferative disorders and/or opportunistic infections may be increased by immunosuppressive therapy. Severe hypersensitivity reactions, occurring within 24 hours, have been reported. Reactions, including anaphylaxis, have occurred both with the initial exposure and/or following re-exposure after several months. Use caution during re-exposure to a subsequent course of therapy in a patient who has previously received basiliximab; patients in whom concomitant immunosuppression was prematurely discontinued due to abandoned transplantation or early graft loss are at increased risk for developing a severe hypersensitivity reaction upon re-exposure. Discontinue permanently if a severe reaction occurs. Medications for the treatment of hypersensitivity reactions should be available for immediate use. Treatment may result in the development of human antimurine antibodies (HAMA); however, limited evidence suggesting the use of muromonab-CD3 or other murine products is not precluded. **[U.S. Boxed Warning]: Should be administered under the supervision of a physician experienced in immunosuppression therapy and organ transplant management.** In renal transplant patients receiving basiliximab plus prednisone, cyclosporine, and mycophenolate, new-onset diabetes, glucose intolerance, and impaired fasting glucose were observed at rates significantly higher than observed in patients receiving prednisone, cyclosporine, and mycophenolate without basiliximab (Aasebo, 2010). Potentially significant drug-drug interactions may exist, requiring dose or frequency adjustment, additional monitoring, and/or selection of alternative therapy.

Adverse Reactions

Cardiovascular: Abnormal heart sounds, angina, arrhythmia, atrial fibrillation, chest pain, generalized edema, heart failure, hyper-/hypotension,peripheral edema, tachycardia

Central nervous system: Agitation, anxiety, depression, dizziness, fatigue, fever, headache, hypoesthesia, insomnia, malaise, pain

Dermatologic: Acne, cyst, hypertrichosis, pruritus, rash, skin disorder, skin ulceration, wound complications

Endocrine & metabolic: Acidosis, dehydration, diabetes mellitus, fluid overload, glucocorticoids increased, hyper-/hypocalcemia, hypercholesterolemia, hyperglycemia, hyper-/hypokalemia, hyperlipemia, hypertriglyceridemia, hyperuricemia, hypoglycemia, hypomagnesemia, hyponatremia, hypophosphatemia, hypoproteinemia

Gastrointestinal: Abdomen enlarged, abdominal pain, constipation, diarrhea, dyspepsia esophagitis, flatulence, gastroenteritis, GI hemorrhage, gingival hyperplasia, melena, moniliasis, nausea, stomatitis (including ulcerative), vomiting, weight gain

Genitourinary: Bladder disorder, dysuria, genital edema (male), impotence, ureteral disorder, urinary frequency, urinary retention, urinary tract infection

Hematologic: Anemia, hematoma, hemorrhage, leukopenia, polycythemia, purpura, thrombocytopenia, thrombosis

Neuromuscular & skeletal: Arthralgia, arthropathy, back pain, cramps, fracture, hernia, leg pain, myalgia, neuropathy, paresthesia, rigors, tremor, weakness

Ocular: Abnormal vision, cataract, conjunctivitis

Renal: Albuminuria, hematuria, nonprotein nitrogen increased, oliguria, renal function abnormal, renal tubular necrosis

Respiratory: Bronchitis, bronchospasm, cough, dyspnea, infection (upper respiratory), pharyngitis, pneumonia, pulmonary edema, rhinitis, sinusitis

Miscellaneous: Accidental trauma, cytomegalovirus (CMV) infection, herpes infection (simplex and zoster), infection, sepsis

Rare but important or life-threatening: Anaphylaxis, capillary leak syndrome, cytokine release syndrome, diabetes (new onset), fasting glucose impaired, glucose intolerance, hypersensitivity reaction (including heart failure, hypotension, tachycardia, bronchospasm, dyspnea, pulmonary edema, respiratory failure, sneezing, pruritus, rash, urticaria), lymphoproliferative disease

Drug Interactions

Metabolism/Transport Effects None known.

Avoid Concomitant Use

Avoid concomitant use of Basiliximab with any of the following: BCG; Belimumab; Natalizumab; Pimecrolimus; Tacrolimus (Topical); Tofacitinib; Vaccines (Live)

Increased Effect/Toxicity

Basiliximab may increase the levels/effects of: Belimumab; Hypoglycemic Agents; Leflunomide; Natalizumab; Tofacitinib; Vaccines (Live)

The levels/effects of Basiliximab may be increased by: Denosumab; Herbs (Hypoglycemic Properties); MAO Inhibitors; Pimecrolimus; Roflumilast; Salicylates; Selective Serotonin Reuptake Inhibitors; SGLT2 Inhibitors; Tacrolimus (Topical); Trastuzumab

Decreased Effect

Basiliximab may decrease the levels/effects of: BCG; Coccidioides immitis Skin Test; Sipuleucel-T; Vaccines (Inactivated); Vaccines (Live)

The levels/effects of Basiliximab may be decreased by: Echinacea; Loop Diuretics

Preparation for Administration Reconstitute with preservative-free sterile water for injection (reconstitute 10 mg vial with 2.5 mL, 20 mg vial with 5 mL). Shake gently to dissolve. May further dilute reconstituted solution with 25 mL (10 mg) or 50 mL (20 mg) 0.9% sodium chloride or dextrose 5% in water. When mixing the solution, gently invert the bag to avoid foaming. Do not shake solutions diluted for infusion.

Storage/Stability Store intact vials refrigerated at 2°C to 8°C (36°F to 46°F). Should be used immediately after reconstitution; however, if not used immediately, reconstituted solution may be stored at 2°C to 8°C for up to 24 hours or at room temperature for up to 4 hours. Discard the reconstituted solution if not used within 24 hours.

Mechanism of Action Chimeric (murine/human) immunosuppressant monoclonal antibody which blocks the alpha-chain of the interleukin-2 (IL-2) receptor complex; this receptor is expressed on activated T lymphocytes and is a critical pathway for activating cell-mediated allograft rejection

Pharmacodynamics/Kinetics

Duration: Mean: 36 days (determined by IL-2R alpha saturation)

Distribution: Mean: V_d: Children 1 to 11 years: 4.8 ± 2.1 L; Adolescents 12 to 16 years: 7.8 ± 5.1 L; Adults: 8.6 ± 4.1 L

Half-life elimination: Children 1 to 11 years: 9.5 days; Adolescents 12 to 16 years: 9.1 days; Adults: Mean: 7.2 days

Dosage Note: Patients previously administered basiliximab should only be re-exposed to a subsequent course of therapy with extreme caution.

Acute renal transplant rejection prophylaxis: **Note:** Use in pediatric patients is not approved in the Canadian labeling (limited pharmacokinetic data available).

Children <35 kg: IV: 10 mg within 2 hours prior to transplant surgery, followed by a second 10 mg dose 4 days after transplantation; the second dose should be withheld if complications occur (including severe hypersensitivity reactions or graft loss)

Children ≥35 kg and Adults: IV: 20 mg within 2 hours prior to transplant surgery, followed by a second 20 mg dose 4 days after transplantation; the second dose should be withheld if complications occur (including severe hypersensitivity reactions or graft loss)

Acute cardiac transplant rejection prophylaxis (off-label use): Adults: IV: 20 mg on the day of transplant, followed by a second dose 4 days after transplantation (Mehra, 2005); usually given within the first hour postoperatively

Acute liver transplant rejection prophylaxis (off-label use): Adults: IV: 20 mg within 6 hours of organ reperfusion, followed by a second 20 mg dose 4 days after transplantation (Neuhaus, 2002)

Treatment of refractory acute GVHD (off-label use): Adults: IV: 20 mg on days 1 and 4; may repeat for recurrent acute GVHD (Schmidt-Hieber, 2005). Additional data may be necessary to further define the role of basiliximab in this condition.

Dosage adjustment in renal impairment: There are no dosage adjustments provided in the manufacturer's labeling.

Dosage adjustment in hepatic impairment: There are no dosage adjustments provided in the manufacturer's labeling.

Administration For intravenous administration only. Infuse as a bolus or IV infusion over 20-30 minutes. (Bolus dosing is associated with nausea, vomiting, and local pain at the injection site.) Administer only after assurance that patient will receive renal graft and immunosuppression. For the treatment of acute GVHD (off-label use), the dose was diluted in 250 mL NS and administered over 30 minutes (Schmidt-Hieber, 2005).

Monitoring Parameters Signs and symptoms of acute rejection; hypersensitivity, infection

Dosage Forms

Solution Reconstituted, Intravenous [preservative free]:
Simulect: 10 mg (1 ea); 20 mg (1 ea)

- ◆ **BAY 43-9006** *see* SORAfenib *on page 1923*
- ◆ **BAY 59-7939** *see* Rivaroxaban *on page 1830*
- ◆ **BAY 63-2521** *see* Riociguat *on page 1814*
- ◆ **BAY 73-4506** *see* Regorafenib *on page 1787*
- ◆ **Baycadron** *see* Dexamethasone (Systemic) *on page 599*
- ◆ **Bayer Aspirin Extra Strength [OTC]** *see* Aspirin *on page 180*
- ◆ **Bayer Aspirin Regimen Adult Low Strength [OTC]** *see* Aspirin *on page 180*
- ◆ **Bayer Aspirin Regimen Children's [OTC]** *see* Aspirin *on page 180*
- ◆ **Bayer Aspirin Regimen Regular Strength [OTC]** *see* Aspirin *on page 180*
- ◆ **Bayer Genuine Aspirin [OTC]** *see* Aspirin *on page 180*
- ◆ **Bayer Plus Extra Strength [OTC]** *see* Aspirin *on page 180*
- ◆ **Bayer® PM [OTC]** *see* Aspirin and Diphenhydramine *on page 185*
- ◆ **Bayer Women's Low Dose Aspirin [OTC]** *see* Aspirin *on page 180*
- ◆ **Baza Antifungal [OTC]** *see* Miconazole (Topical) *on page 1360*
- ◆ **Baza® Clear [OTC]** *see* Vitamin A and Vitamin D (Topical) *on page 2174*
- ◆ **Bazedoxifene and Estrogens (Conjugated/Equine)** *see* Estrogens (Conjugated/Equine) and Bazedoxifene *on page 782*
- ◆ **B-Caro-T [OTC]** *see* Beta-Carotene *on page 251*

BCG (bee see jee)

Brand Names: U.S. TheraCys; Tice BCG

Brand Names: Canada BCG Vaccine; ImmuCyst; Oncotice

Index Terms Bacillus Calmette-Guérin (BCG) Live; BCG Vaccine U.S.P. *(percutaneous use product)*; BCG, Live

Pharmacologic Category Antineoplastic Agent, Biological Response Modulator; Vaccine, Live (Bacterial)

Additional Appendix Information

Immunization Administration Recommendations *on page 2250*

Immunization Recommendations *on page 2255*

Use

BCG intravesical: Treatment and prophylaxis of carcinoma *in situ* of the bladder; prophylaxis of primary or recurrent superficial or minimally invasive papillary tumors following transurethral resection

BCG vaccine: Immunization against *Mycobacterium tuberculosis* in persons not previously infected and who are at high risk for exposure

BCG vaccine is not routinely administered for the prevention of *M. tuberculosis* in the United States. The Advisory Committee on Immunization Practices (ACIP) recommends vaccination be considered for the following:

- Children with a negative tuberculin skin test who are continually exposed to (and cannot be separated from) adults who are untreated or ineffectively treated for TB disease when the child cannot be given long-term treatment for infection **or** if the adult has TB caused by strains resistant to isoniazid and rifampin.

- Healthcare workers with a high percentage of patients with *M. tuberculosis* strains resistant to both isoniazid and rifampin, if there is ongoing transmission of the resistant strains and subsequent infection is likely, or if comprehensive infection-control precautions have not been successful. In addition, healthcare workers should be counseled on the risks and benefits of vaccination and treatment of latent TB infection

Pregnancy Risk Factor C

Dosage

Immunization against tuberculosis: Percutaneous: **Note:** Initial lesion usually appears after 10 to 14 days consisting of small, red papule at injection site and reaches maximum diameter of 3 mm in 4 to 6 weeks.

Children <1 month: 0.2 to 0.3 mL (half-strength dilution). Administer tuberculin test (5 TU) after 2 to 3 months; repeat vaccination after 1 year of age for negative tuberculin test if indications persist.

Children >1 month and Adults: 0.2 to 0.3 mL (full strength dilution); conduct postvaccinal tuberculin test (5 TU of PPD) in 2 to 3 months; if test is negative, repeat vaccination.

Immunotherapy for bladder cancer: Intravesicular: Adults: **Note:** Treatment should begin 7 to 14 days after biopsy or TUR. The contents of one vial is used for each dose.

TheraCys: One dose instilled into bladder (retain for 2 hours) once weekly for 6 weeks followed by 1 treatment at 3, 6, 12, 18, and 24 months after initial treatment

TICE BCG: One dose instilled into the bladder (retain for 2 hours) once weekly for 6 weeks (may repeat cycle 1 time) followed by approximately once monthly for at least 6 to 12 months

Dosage adjustment in renal impairment: There are no dosage adjustments provided in the manufacturer's labeling.

Dosage adjustment in hepatic impairment: There are no dosage adjustments provided in the manufacturer's labeling.

Additional Information Complete prescribing information should be consulted for additional detail.

Dosage Forms

Injectable, Injection:
Generic: 50 mg (1 ea)

Suspension Reconstituted, Intravesical:
Tice BCG: 50 mg (1 ea)

Suspension Reconstituted, Intravesical [preservative free]:
TheraCys: 81 mg (1 ea)

- ◆ **BCG, Live** *see* BCG *on page 229*
- ◆ **BCG Vaccine (Can)** *see* BCG *on page 229*
- ◆ **BCG Vaccine U.S.P.** ***(percutaneous use product)*** *see* BCG *on page 229*
- ◆ **BCNU** *see* Carmustine *on page 364*
- ◆ **BCX-1812** *see* Peramivir *on page 1619*
- ◆ **BCX 2600** *see* Stiripentol [CAN/INT] *on page 1935*
- ◆ **beano® [OTC]** *see* Alpha-Galactosidase *on page 94*
- ◆ **beano® Meltaways [OTC]** *see* Alpha-Galactosidase *on page 94*
- ◆ **Bebulin** *see* Factor IX Complex (Human) [(Factors II, IX, X)] *on page 838*
- ◆ **Bebulin VH** *see* Factor IX Complex (Human) [(Factors II, IX, X)] *on page 838*

Becaplermin (be KAP ler min)

Brand Names: U.S. Regranex

Index Terms Recombinant Human Platelet-Derived Growth Factor B; rPDGF-BB

Pharmacologic Category Growth Factor, Platelet-Derived; Topical Skin Product

Use Adjunctive treatment of diabetic neuropathic ulcers occurring on the lower limbs and feet that extend into subcutaneous tissue (or beyond) and have adequate blood supply

Pregnancy Risk Factor C

Dosage Topical: Adults: Diabetic ulcers: Apply appropriate amount of gel once daily with a cotton swab or similar tool, as a coating over the ulcer. The amount of becaplermin to be applied will vary depending on the size of the ulcer area.

Note: If the ulcer does not decrease in size by ~30% after 10 weeks of treatment or complete healing has not occurred in 20 weeks, continued treatment with becaplermin gel should be reassessed.

To calculate the length of gel applied to the ulcer, measure the greatest length of the ulcer by the greatest width of the ulcer. Tube size and unit of measure will determine the formula used in the calculation. Recalculate amount of gel needed every 1-2 weeks, depending on the rate of change in ulcer area.

Centimeters:

15 g tube: [ulcer length (cm) x width (cm)] divided by 4 = length of gel (cm)

2 g tube: [ulcer length (cm) x width (cm)] divided by 2 = length of gel (cm)

Inches:

15 g tube: [length (in) x width (in)] x 0.6 = length of gel (in)

2 g tube: [length (in) x width (in)] x 1.3 = length of gel (in)

Additional Information Complete prescribing information should be consulted for additional detail.

Dosage Forms

Gel, External:
Regranex: 0.01% (15 g)

Beclomethasone (Systemic)

(be kloe METH a sone)

Brand Names: U.S. Qvar

Brand Names: Canada QVAR

Index Terms Vanceril

Pharmacologic Category Corticosteroid, Inhalant (Oral)

Additional Appendix Information

Inhaled Corticosteroids *on page 2229*

Use

Asthma: Maintenance and prophylactic treatment of asthma in patients ≥5 years (including those who require corticosteroids and those who may benefit from a dose reduction/elimination of systemically administered corticosteroids).

Limitations of use: Not for relief of acute bronchospasm.

Pregnancy Risk Factor C

Pregnancy Considerations Adverse events have been observed in animal reproduction studies. Hypoadrenalism may occur in newborns following maternal use of corticosteroids in pregnancy. Based on available data, an overall increased risk of congenital malformations or a decrease in fetal growth has not been associated with maternal use of inhaled corticosteroids during pregnancy (Bakhireva, 2005; NAEPP, 2005; Namazy, 2004). Uncontrolled asthma is associated with adverse events in pregnancy (increased risk of perinatal mortality, pre-eclampsia, preterm birth, low birth weight infants). Inhaled corticosteroids are recommended for the treatment of asthma during pregnancy (most information available using budesonide) (ACOG, 2008; NAEPP, 2005).

Breast-Feeding Considerations Other corticosteroids have been found in breast milk; however, information for beclomethasone is not available. Due to the potential for serious adverse reactions in the nursing infant, the manufacturer recommends a decision be made whether to discontinue nursing or to discontinue the drug, taking into account the importance of treatment to the mother. Use of inhaled corticosteroids is not a contraindication to breast-feeding (NAEPP, 2005).

Contraindications

Hypersensitivity to beclomethasone or any component of the formulation; status asthmaticus, or other acute asthma episodes requiring intensive measures

Documentation of allergenic cross-reactivity for corticosteroids is limited. However, because of similarities in chemical structure and/or pharmacologic actions, the possibility of cross-sensitivity cannot be ruled out with certainty.

Canadian labeling: Additional contraindications (not in U.S. labeling): Moderate to severe bronchiectasis requiring intensive measures; untreated fungal, bacterial, or tubercular infections of the respiratory tract

Warnings/Precautions May cause hypercorticism or suppression of hypothalamic-pituitary-adrenal (HPA) axis, particularly in younger children or in patients receiving high doses for prolonged periods. HPA axis suppression may lead to adrenal crisis. Withdrawal and discontinuation of a corticosteroid should be done slowly and carefully. Particular care is required when patients are transferred from systemic corticosteroids to inhaled products due to possible adrenal insufficiency or withdrawal from steroids, including an increase in allergic symptoms. Patients receiving >20 mg per day of prednisone (or equivalent) may be most susceptible. Fatalities have occurred due to adrenal insufficiency in asthmatic patients during and after transfer from systemic corticosteroids to aerosol steroids; aerosol steroids do **not** provide the systemic steroid needed to treat patients having trauma, surgery, or infections (particularly gastroenteritis), or other conditions with severe electrolyte loss.

Bronchospasm may occur with wheezing after inhalation (possibly life-threatening); if bronchospasm occurs, discontinue steroid and treat with a fast-acting bronchodilator. Supplemental steroids (oral or parenteral) may be needed during stress or severe asthma attacks. Not to be used in status asthmaticus or for the relief of acute bronchospasm. Immediate hypersensitivity reactions may occur, including angioedema, bronchospasm, rash, and urticaria; discontinue use if reaction occurs. Corticosteroid use may cause psychiatric disturbances, including depression, euphoria, insomnia, mood swings, and personality changes. Preexisting psychiatric conditions may be exacerbated by corticosteroid use. Prolonged use of corticosteroids may also increase the incidence of secondary infection, mask acute infection (including fungal infections), prolong or exacerbate viral infections, or limit response to vaccines. Avoid use, if possible, in patients with ocular herpes, active or quiescent respiratory or untreated viral, fungal, parasitic or bacterial systemic infections (Canadian labeling contraindicates use with untreated respiratory infections). Exposure to chickenpox or measles should be avoided. Close observation is required in patients with latent tuberculosis and/or TB reactivity; restrict use in active TB. Prolonged treatment with corticosteroids has been associated with the development of Kaposi sarcoma (case reports); if noted, discontinuation of therapy should be considered. *Candida albicans* infections may occur in the mouth and pharynx; rinsing (and spitting) with water after inhaler use may decrease risk. Rare cases of vasculitis (Churg-Strauss syndrome) or other systemic eosinophilic conditions can occur; often associated with decrease and/or withdrawal of oral corticosteroid therapy following initiation of inhaled corticosteroid.

Use with caution in patients with major risk factors for decreased bone mineral count. Use with caution in patients with thyroid disease, hepatic impairment, renal impairment, cardiovascular disease, diabetes, glaucoma, cataracts, myasthenia gravis, patients at risk for seizures, or GI diseases (diverticulitis, peptic ulcer, ulcerative colitis). Use caution following acute MI (corticosteroids have been associated with myocardial rupture). Because of the risk of adverse effects, systemic corticosteroids should be used cautiously in elderly patients in the smallest possible effective dose for the shortest duration.

Orally inhaled corticosteroids may cause a reduction in growth velocity in pediatric patients (~1 centimeter per year [range: 0.3 to 1.8 cm per year] and related to dose and duration of exposure). To minimize the systemic effects of orally inhaled corticosteroids, each patient should be titrated to the lowest effective dose. Growth should be routinely monitored in pediatric patients. A gradual tapering of dose may be required prior to discontinuing therapy; there have been reports of systemic corticosteroid withdrawal symptoms (eg, joint/muscle pain, lassitude, depression) when withdrawing oral inhalation therapy. When transferring to oral inhalation therapy from systemic corticosteroid therapy; previously suppressed allergic conditions (rhinitis, conjunctivitis, eczema, arthritis, and eosinophilic conditions) may be unmasked; during transition monitor pulmonary function tests (FEV_1 or PEF), beta-agonist use, and asthma symptoms and observe for signs and symptoms of adrenal insufficiency.

Adverse Reactions

Central nervous system: Headache, pain, voice disorder

Gastrointestinal: Nausea

Genitourinary: Dysmenorrhea

Neuromuscular & skeletal: Back pain

Respiratory: Cough, pharyngitis, rhinitis, sinusitis, upper respiratory tract infection

Rare but important or life-threatening: Anaphylactoid reaction, anaphylaxis, behavioral changes (such as aggressiveness, depression, sleep disturbances, psychomotor hyperactivity, suicidal ideation; more common in children), decreased linear skeletal growth rate (in children/adolescents), hypersensitivity reaction (immediate and delayed; including angioedema, bronchospasm, rash, urticaria), HPA-axis suppression; rarely glaucoma, increased intraocular pressure, and cataracts have been reported with inhaled corticosteroids

Drug Interactions

Metabolism/Transport Effects None known.

Avoid Concomitant Use

Avoid concomitant use of Beclomethasone (Oral Inhalation) with any of the following: Aldesleukin; BCG; Natalizumab; Pimecrolimus; Tacrolimus (Topical); Tofacitinib

Increased Effect/Toxicity

Beclomethasone (Oral Inhalation) may increase the levels/effects of: Amphotericin B; Ceritinib; Deferasirox; Leflunomide; Loop Diuretics; Natalizumab; Thiazide Diuretics; Tofacitinib

The levels/effects of Beclomethasone (Oral Inhalation) may be increased by: Denosumab; Pimecrolimus; Tacrolimus (Topical); Telaprevir; Trastuzumab

Decreased Effect

Beclomethasone (Oral Inhalation) may decrease the levels/effects of: Aldesleukin; Antidiabetic Agents; BCG; Coccidioides immitis Skin Test; Corticorelin; Hyaluronidase; Sipuleucel-T; Telaprevir; Vaccines (Inactivated)

The levels/effects of Beclomethasone (Oral Inhalation) may be decreased by: Echinacea

Storage/Stability Store at 25°C (77°F); excursions are permitted between 15°C and 30°C (59°F and 86°F). Do not use or store near heat or open flame. Do not puncture canisters. Store on concave end of canister with actuator on top.

Mechanism of Action Controls the rate of protein synthesis; depresses the migration of polymorphonuclear leukocytes, fibroblasts; reverses capillary permeability and lysosomal stabilization at the cellular level to prevent or control inflammation

Pharmacodynamics/Kinetics

Onset of action: Therapeutic effect: 1 to 4 weeks

Absorption: Readily; quickly hydrolyzed by pulmonary esterases to active metabolite (beclomethasone-17-monoproprionate [17-BMP]) during absorption

Protein binding: 17-BMP: 94% to 96%

Metabolism: Pro-drug; undergoes rapid conversion to 17-BMP during absorption; followed by additional metabolism via CYP3A4 to other, less active metabolites (beclomethasone-21-monopropionate [21-BMP] and beclomethasone [BOH])

Half-life elimination: 17-BMP: 2.8 hours

Time to peak, plasma: Oral inhalation: BDP: 0.5 hours; 17-BMP: 0.7 hours

Excretion: Mainly in feces; urine (<10%)

Dosage Inhalation, oral:

Asthma (doses should be titrated to the lowest effective dose once asthma is controlled):

U.S. labeling:

Children 5 to 11 years: Initial: 40 mcg twice daily; maximum dose: 80 mcg twice daily

Children ≥12 years and Adults:

Patients previously on bronchodilators only: Initial dose 40 to 80 mcg twice daily; maximum dose: 320 mcg twice day

Patients previously on inhaled corticosteroids: Initial dose 40 to 160 mcg twice daily; maximum dose: 320 mcg twice daily

Asthma Guidelines (NAEPP, 2007):

Children 5 to 11 years:

"Low" dose: 80 to 160 mcg daily

"Medium" dose: >160 to 320 mcg daily

"High" dose: >320 mcg daily

Children ≥12 years and Adults:

"Low" dose: 80 to 240 mcg daily

"Medium" dose: >240 to 480 mcg daily

"High" dose: >480 mcg daily

Canadian labeling:

Children 5 to 11 years: Initial: 50 mcg twice daily; maximum dose: 100 mcg twice daily

Children ≥12 years and Adults:

Mild asthma: 50 to 100 mcg twice daily; maximum dose: 100 mcg twice daily

Moderate asthma: 100 to 250 mcg twice daily; maximum dose: 250 mcg twice daily

Severe asthma: 300 to 400 mcg twice daily; maximum dose: 400 mcg twice daily

Conversion from oral systemic corticosteroid to orally inhaled corticosteroid: Initiation of oral inhalation therapy should begin in patients whose asthma is reasonably stabilized on oral corticosteroids (OCS). A gradual dose reduction of OCS should begin ~7 days after starting inhaled therapy. U.S. labeling recommends reducing prednisone dose no more rapidly than ≤2.5 mg/day (or equivalent of other OCS) every 1 to 2 weeks. The Canadian labeling recommends decreasing the daily dose of prednisone by 1 mg (or equivalent of other OCS) every 7 days or more in closely monitored patients. If adrenal insufficiency occurs, temporarily increase the OCS dose and follow with a more gradual withdrawal. **Note:** When transitioning from systemic to inhaled corticosteroids, supplemental systemic corticosteroid therapy may be necessary during periods of stress or during severe asthma attacks.

Chronic obstructive pulmonary disease (stable) (off-label use): Adults: 50 to 400 mcg daily in combination with a long-acting bronchodilator (GOLD, 2014)

Dosage adjustment in renal impairment: There are no dosage adjustments provided in the manufacturer's labeling.

Dosage adjustment in hepatic impairment: There are no dosage adjustments provided in the manufacturer's labeling.

Administration Canister does not need shaken prior to use. Prime canister by spraying twice into the air prior to initial use or if not in use for >10 days. Avoid spraying in face or eyes. Exhale fully prior to bringing inhaler to mouth. Place inhaler in mouth, close lips around mouthpiece, and inhale slowly and deeply. Remove inhaler and hold breath for approximately 5 to 10 seconds. Rinse mouth and throat with water (and spit) after use to prevent *Candida* infection. Do not wash or put inhaler in water; mouth piece may be cleaned with a dry tissue or cloth. Discard the inhaler when the dose counter displays "0". Patients using a spacer should inhale immediately due to decreased amount of medication that is delivered with a delayed inspiration.

Monitoring Parameters Growth (adolescents) and signs/symptoms of HPA axis suppression/adrenal insufficiency; signs/symptoms of oral candidiasis; ocular effects (eg, cataracts, increased intraocular pressure, glaucoma)

Additional Information Effects of inhaled steroids on growth have been observed in the absence of laboratory evidence of HPA axis suppression, suggesting that growth velocity is a more sensitive indicator of systemic corticosteroid exposure in pediatric patients than some commonly used tests of HPA axis function. The long-term effects of this reduction in growth velocity associated with orally-inhaled corticosteroids, including the impact on final adult height, are unknown. The potential for "catch up" growth following discontinuation of treatment with inhaled corticosteroids has not been adequately studied.

Dosage Forms Considerations

QVAR 8.7 g canisters contain 120 inhalations.

Dosage Forms

Aerosol Solution, Inhalation:

Qvar: 40 mcg/actuation (8.7 g); 80 mcg/actuation (8.7 g)

Dosage Forms: Canada

Aerosol, for oral inhalation:

QVAR: 50 mcg/inhalation (6.5 g, 12.4 g); 100 mcg/inhalation (6.5 g, 12.4 g)

Beclomethasone (Nasal) (be kloe METH a sone)

Brand Names: U.S. Beconase AQ; Qnasl; Qnasl Childrens

Brand Names: Canada Apo-Beclomethasone; Mylan-Beclo AQ; Rivanase AQ

Index Terms Beclomethasone Dipropionate

Pharmacologic Category Corticosteroid, Nasal

Additional Appendix Information

Inhaled Corticosteroids *on page 2229*

Use

Nasal polyps Beconase AQ only: Prevention of recurrence of nasal polyps following surgical removal

Rhinitis:

Beconase AQ: Relief of symptoms of seasonal or perennial allergic rhinitis and nonallergic (vasomotor) rhinitis

Qnasl: Treatment of the nasal symptoms associated with seasonal or perennial allergic rhinitis in patients 4 years and older.

Pregnancy Risk Factor C

Dosage Inhalation, nasal:

Beconase AQ: Rhinitis, nasal polyps (postsurgical prophylaxis):

Children 6 to 11 years: Initial: One inhalation (42 mcg) in each nostril twice daily (total dose: 168 mcg daily). If response is inadequate, may increase to 2 inhalations (84 mcg) in each nostril twice daily (total dose: 336 mcg daily); once adequate control is achieved, decrease to 1 inhalation (42 mcg) in each nostril twice daily (total dose: 168 mcg daily). Maximum dose: 336 mcg daily.

Children ≥12 years, Adolescents, and Adults: One or two (42 or 84 mcg) inhalations in each nostril twice daily (total dose: 168 to 336 mcg daily; maximum dose: 336 mcg daily)

Qnasl: Allergic rhinitis:

Children 4 to 11 years: Qnasl 40 mcg: One inhalation (40 mcg) in each nostril once daily (maximum: 80 mcg daily)

Children ≥12 years, Adolescents, and Adults: Qnasl 80 mcg: Two inhalations (160 mcg) in each nostril once daily (maximum: 320 mcg daily)

Dosage adjustment in renal impairment: There are no dosage adjustments provided in the manufacturer's labeling.

Dosage adjustment in hepatic impairment: There are no dosage adjustments provided in the manufacturer's labeling.

Additional Information Complete prescribing information should be consulted for additional detail.

Dosage Forms Considerations

Beconase AQ 25 g bottles contain 180 sprays.

Qnasl 8.7 g bottles contain 120 actuations.

Dosage Forms

Aerosol Solution, Nasal:

Qnasl: 80 mcg/actuation (8.7 g)

Qnasl Childrens: 40 mcg/actuation (4.9 g)

Suspension, Nasal:

Beconase AQ: 42 mcg/spray (25 g)

◆ **Beclomethasone Dipropionate** *see* Beclomethasone (Nasal) *on page 232*

◆ **Beconase AQ** *see* Beclomethasone (Nasal) *on page 232*

Bedaquiline (bed AK wi leen)

Brand Names: U.S. Sirturo

Index Terms AIDS222089; R207910; TMC207

Pharmacologic Category Antitubercular Agent

Use Multidrug-resistant tuberculosis: Treatment of pulmonary multidrug-resistant tuberculosis (MDR-TB) in combination therapy in adults (≥18 years of age) when other alternatives are not available

Pregnancy Risk Factor B

Dosage Note: Use with ≥3 drugs also active against the patient's *M. tuberculosis* isolate.

Usual dosage range: Adults: Oral: Directly observed therapy (DOT):

Weeks 1-2: 400 mg once daily. **Note:** If a dose is missed during weeks 1-2, do not make up the missed dose, and continue the usual dosing schedule.

Weeks 3-24: 200 mg 3 times weekly (total weekly dose: 600 mg). **Note:** Space doses at least 48 hours apart. If a dose is missed during weeks 3-24, administer the missed dose as soon as possible, and resume the 3-times-weekly schedule.

Dosage adjustment in renal impairment:

Mild-to-moderate renal impairment: No dosage adjustment necessary.

Severe renal impairment: No dosage adjustment provided in manufacturer's labeling; use with caution.

Intermittent hemodialysis (IHD) or peritoneal dialysis (PD): No dosage adjustment provided in manufacturer's labeling. Use with caution (CDC, 2013); bedaquiline is highly protein bound and not likely to be removed by dialysis.

Dosage adjustment in hepatic impairment:

Mild or moderate impairment (Child-Pugh class A or B): No dosage adjustment necessary.

Severe impairment (Child-Pugh class C): No dosage adjustment provided in manufacturer's labeling; use should be avoided (CDC, 2013).

Additional Information Complete prescribing information should be consulted for additional detail.

Dosage Forms

Tablet, Oral:

Sirturo: 100 mg

Befunolol [INT] (be FYU noe lol)

International Brand Names Bentos (FR, JP, KR); Betaclar (IT); Glauconex (AT, BE, DE, LU, NL); Thilonium (GR)

Index Terms Befunolol Hydrochloride

Pharmacologic Category Beta Blocker, Intrinsic Sympathomimetic Activity (ISA)

Reported Use Management of ocular hypertension and open-angle glaucoma

Dosage Range Adults: Ophthalmic: One drop in affected eye(s) twice daily

Product Availability Product available in various countries; not currently available in the U.S.

Dosage Forms

Solution, ophthalmic, as hydrochloride: 0.25%, 0.5%, 1%

◆ **Befunolol Hydrochloride** *see* Befunolol [INT] *on page 233*

◆ **Behenyl Alcohol** *see* Docosanol *on page 661*

Belatacept (bel AT a sept)

Brand Names: U.S. Nulojix

Index Terms BMS-224818; LEA29Y

Pharmacologic Category Selective T-Cell Costimulation Blocker

Use

Kidney transplant: Prophylaxis of organ rejection concomitantly with basiliximab induction, mycophenolate, and corticosteroids in adult Epstein-Barr virus (EBV) seropositive kidney transplant recipients

Limitations of use: Use only in EBV seropositive patients; use for prophylaxis of organ rejection in transplanted organs other than the kidney has not been established.

Pregnancy Risk Factor C

Pregnancy Considerations Adverse events have been observed in animal reproduction studies. According to the manufacturer, do not use belatacept in pregnancy unless the potential benefit to the mother outweighs the potential risk to the fetus. A pregnancy registry has been established to monitor outcomes of women exposed to belatacept during pregnancy (1-877-955-6877).

Breast-Feeding Considerations It is not known if belatacept is excreted in breast milk. Due to the potential for serious adverse reactions in the nursing infant, the manufacturer recommends a decision be made whether to discontinue nursing or to discontinue the drug, taking into account the importance of treatment to the mother.

Contraindications Transplant patients who are Epstein-Barr virus (EBV) seronegative or with unknown EBV serostatus

Warnings/Precautions [U.S. Boxed Warning]: Risk of post-transplant lymphoproliferative disorder (PTLD) is increased, primarily involving the CNS, in patients receiving belatacept compared to patients receiving cyclosporine-based regimens. Degree of immunosuppression is a risk factor for PTLD developing; do not exceed recommended dosing. Patients who are Epstein-Barr virus seronegative (EBV) are at an even higher risk; use is contraindicated in patients without evidence of immunity to EBV. Therapy is only appropriate in patients who are EBV seropositive via evidence of acquired immunity, such as presence of IgG antibodies to viral capsid antigen [VCA] and EBV nuclear antigen [EBNA]. Cytomegalovirus (CMV) infection and T-cell depleting therapy also increases the risk for PTLD; T-cell depleting therapies to treat acute rejection should be used with caution. Although CMV disease is a risk for PTLD and CMV seronegative patients are at an increased risk for CMV disease, the clinical role, if any, of determining CMV serology to determine risk of PTLD development has not been determined.

[U.S. Boxed Warning]: Risk for infection is increased. Immunosuppressive therapy may lead to bacterial, viral (CMV and herpes), fungal, and protozoal infections, including opportunistic infections (may be fatal). Tuberculosis (TB) is increased; test patients for latent TB prior to initiation, and treat latent TB infection prior to use. Prophylaxis for CMV is recommended for at least 3 months after transplantation; prophylaxis for *Pneumocystis jiroveci* is recommended after transplantation. Patients receiving immunosuppressive therapy are at an increased risk of activation of latent viral infections, including John Cunningham virus (JCV) and BK virus infection. Activation of JCV may result in progressive multifocal leukoencephalopathy (PML), a rare and potentially fatal condition affecting the CNS. Symptoms of PML include apathy, ataxia, cognitive deficiencies, confusion, and hemiparesis. Polyoma virus-associated nephropathy (PVAN), primarily from activation of BK virus, may also occur and lead to the deterioration of renal function and/or renal graft loss. Risk factors for the development of PML and PVAN include immunosuppression and treatment with immunosuppressant therapy. The onset of PML or PVAN may warrant a reduction in immunosuppressive therapy; however, in transplant recipients, the risk of reduced immunosuppression and graft rejection should be considered.

[U.S. Boxed Warning]: Risk for malignancy is increased. Malignancy, including skin malignancy and PTLD, is associated with the use of belatacept; higher than recommended doses or more frequent dosing is not recommended; patients should be advised to limit their exposure to sunlight/UV light.

[U.S. Boxed Warning]: Therapy is not recommended in liver transplant patients due to increased risk of graft loss and death. [U.S. Boxed Warning]: Should be administered under the supervision of a physician experienced in immunosuppressive therapy. Increased rate and grade of acute rejection, particularly grade 3 rejection, and graft loss has been observed with belatacept when corticosteroids were minimized to 5 mg daily between day 3 and week 6 post-transplant; corticosteroid dosing should be consistent with clinical trial experience (ie, tapered to ~15 mg [10 to 20 mg] daily by the first 6 weeks post-transplant and remain at ~10 mg [5 to 10 mg] daily for the first 6 months post-transplant). Immunization with live vaccines should be avoided during treatment. Potentially significant drug-drug interactions may exist, requiring dose or frequency adjustment, additional monitoring, and/or selection of alternative therapy.

Adverse Reactions Reported during clinical trials using belatacept compared to a cyclosporine control regimen. All patients also received basiliximab induction, mycophenolate mofetil, and corticosteroids, and were followed up to 3 years.

Cardiovascular: Arteriovenous fistula site complication (thrombosis), atrial fibrillation, hyper-/hypotension, peripheral edema
Central nervous system: Anxiety, dizziness, fever, Guillain-Barré syndrome, headache, insomnia
Dermatologic: Acne vulgaris, alopecia, hyperhidrosis
Endocrine & metabolic: Diabetes mellitus (new onset), hypercholesterolemia, hyperglycemia, hyper-/hypokalemia, hyperuricemia, hypocalcemia, hypomagnesemia, hypophosphatemia, lipid metabolism disorder
Gastrointestinal: Abdominal pain, constipation, diarrhea, nausea, stomatitis, upper abdominal pain, vomiting
Genitourinary: Dysuria, urinary incontinence, urinary tract infection
Hematologic & oncologic: Anemia, hematoma, leukopenia, lymphocele, malignant neoplasm, malignant neoplasm of skin (nonmelanoma), neutropenia
Immunologic: Antibody development
Infection: Cytomegalovirus disease, herpes, increased susceptibility to infection (including serious infection), influenza, polyoma virus
Neuromuscular & skeletal: Arthralgia, back pain, musculoskeletal pain, tremor
Renal: Acute renal failure, chronic allograft nephropathy, hematuria, hydronephrosis, increased serum creatinine, proteinuria, renal artery stenosis, renal disease (BK virus-associated), renal graft dysfunction, renal insufficiency, renal tubular necrosis
Respiratory: Bronchitis, cough, dyspnea, nasopharyngitis, tuberculosis, upper respiratory tract infection
Miscellaneous: Infusion related reaction
Rare but important or life-threatening: Aspergillosis (cerebral; higher dosing regimen), encephalitis (Chagas, West Nile; higher dosing regimen), lymphoproliferative disorder (post-transplant; incidence is 9-fold higher in non-EBV seropositive patients), meningitis (cryptococcal), progressive multifocal leukoencephalopathy (higher dosing regimen), renal graft rejection

Drug Interactions

Metabolism/Transport Effects None known.

Avoid Concomitant Use

Avoid concomitant use of Belatacept with any of the following: BCG; Belimumab; Natalizumab; Pimecrolimus; Tacrolimus (Topical); Tofacitinib; Vaccines (Live)

Increased Effect/Toxicity

Belatacept may increase the levels/effects of: Belimumab; Leflunomide; Natalizumab; Tofacitinib; Vaccines (Live)

The levels/effects of Belatacept may be increased by: Denosumab; Pimecrolimus; Roflumilast; Tacrolimus (Topical); Trastuzumab

Decreased Effect

Belatacept may decrease the levels/effects of: BCG; Coccidioides immitis Skin Test; Sipuleucel-T; Vaccines (Inactivated); Vaccines (Live)

The levels/effects of Belatacept may be decreased by: Echinacea

Preparation for Administration Reconstitute each vial with 10.5 mL of diluent (SWFI, NS, or D_5W only) using the provided silicone-free disposable syringe, and an 18- to 21-gauge needle. Reconstitute using **only** the silicone-free syringe provided; if the provided silicone-free syringe is dropped or becomes contaminated, use a new silicone-free disposable syringe from inventory (contact the manufacturer on obtaining additional silicone-free disposable syringes). If powder is inadvertently mixed using a siliconized syringe, discard solution; translucent particles may develop. Inject the diluent down the side of the vial to avoid foaming. Rotate the vial and invert with gentle swirling until completely dissolved; do **not** shake vial. Immediately transfer the reconstituted solution using the same silicone-free syringe to an infusion bag or bottle with NS or D_5W (if NS or D_5W were used to reconstitute, the same fluid should be used to further dilute). Gently rotate the infusion bag or bottle; do not shake. The final concentration should range from 2 mg/mL and 10 mg/mL (typical infusion volume is 100 mL; volumes ranging from 50 mL to 250 mL may be used). Prior to adding belatacept to the infusion solution, the manufacturer recommends withdrawing a volume equal to the amount of belatacept to be added.

Storage/Stability Prior to use, store refrigerated at 2°C to 8°C (36°F to 46°F). Protect from light. After dilution, the reconstituted solution should be transferred from the vial to infusion bag or bottle immediately; infusion solution may be stored refrigerated for up to 24 hours, with a maximum of 4 hours of the 24 hours at room temperature, 20°C to 25°C (68°F to 77°F), and room light. Infusion must be completed within 24 hours of reconstitution. Discard unused solution in vials.

Mechanism of Action Fusion protein which acts as a selective T-cell (lymphocyte) costimulation blocker by binding to CD80 and CD86 receptors on antigen presenting cells (APC), blocking the required CD28 mediated interaction between APCs and T cells needed to activate T lymphocytes. T-cell stimulation results in cytokine production and proliferation, mediators in immunologic rejection associated with kidney transplantation.

Pharmacodynamics/Kinetics

Distribution: V_{ss}: 0.11 L/kg (transplant patients)

Half-life elimination: ~10 days (healthy patients and kidney transplant patients)

Dosage Note: Dosing is based on actual body weight at the time of transplantation; do not modify weight-based dosing during course of therapy unless the change in body weight is >10%. The prescribed dose must be evenly divisible by 12.5 mg to allow accurate preparation of the reconstituted solution using the required disposable syringe provided by the manufacturer. For example, the calculated dose for a 64 kg patient: 64 kg x 10 mg per kg = 640 mg. The nearest doses to 640 mg that are evenly divisible by 12.5 mg would be 637.5 mg or 650 mg; the closest dose to the calculated dose is 637.5 mg, therefore, 637.5 should be the actual prescribed dose for the patient.

Kidney transplant, prophylaxis of organ rejection: Adults: IV: **Note:** Use in combination with basiliximab induction, mycophenolate mofetil, and corticosteroids.

Initial phase: 10 mg/kg on Day 1 (day of transplant, prior to implantation) and on Day 5 (~96 hours after Day 1 dose), followed by 10 mg/kg at the end of Week 2, Week 4, Week 8, and Week 12 following transplantation

Maintenance phase: 5 mg/kg every 4 weeks (plus or minus 3 days) beginning at the end of Week 16 following transplantation

Elderly: Refer to adult dosing

Dosage adjustment in renal impairment: There are no dosage adjustments provided in the manufacturer's labeling; however, renal function did not affect clearance in pharmacokinetic studies of kidney transplant patients.

Dosage adjustment in hepatic impairment: There are no dosage adjustments provided in the manufacturer's labeling; however, hepatic function did not affect clearance in pharmacokinetic studies of kidney transplant patients.

Administration Administer as an IV infusion over 30 minutes using an infusion set with a 0.2 to 1.2 micron low protein-binding filter. The infusion must be completed within 24 hours of reconstitution of the lyophilized powder. Infuse in a separate line from other infused agents.

Monitoring Parameters New-onset or worsening neurological, cognitive, or behavioral signs/symptoms; signs/symptoms of infection or malignancy; TB screening prior to therapy initiation; EBV seropositive verification prior to therapy initiation

Additional Information If additional silicone-free disposable syringes are needed, contact Bristol-Myers Squibb at 1-888-NULOJIX.

Dosage Forms

Solution Reconstituted, Intravenous:

Nulojix: 250 mg (1 ea)

◆ **Beleodaq** *see* Belinostat *on page 236*

Belimumab (be LIM yoo mab)

Brand Names: U.S. Benlysta

Brand Names: Canada Benlysta

Pharmacologic Category Monoclonal Antibody

Use

Systemic lupus erythematosus: Treatment of adult patients with active, autoantibody-positive systemic lupus erythematosus (SLE) who are receiving standard therapy.

Limitations of use: Use is not recommended in patients with severe active lupus nephritis, severe active CNS lupus, or in combination with other biologics, including B-cell targeted therapies or intravenous (IV) cyclophosphamide.

Pregnancy Risk Factor C

Pregnancy Considerations Adverse events were observed in some animal reproduction studies. IgG molecules are known to cross the placenta (belimumab is an engineered IgG molecule). Effective contraception should be used during and for at least 4 months following treatment in women of childbearing potential. Healthcare providers are encouraged to enroll women exposed to belimumab during pregnancy in a pregnancy registry (877-681-6296); patients may also enroll themselves.

Breast-Feeding Considerations It is not known if belimumab is excreted in breast milk. Because IgG molecules are excreted in breast milk, a decision should be made whether to discontinue nursing or to discontinue the drug, taking into account the importance of treatment to the mother.

Contraindications Hypersensitivity (anaphylaxis) to belimumab or any component of the formulation

Warnings/Precautions Deaths due to infection, cardiovascular disease, and suicide were higher in belimumab patients compared to placebo during clinical trials. Serious and potentially fatal infections may occur during treatment. Use with caution in patients with chronic infections; treatment should not be undertaken if receiving therapy for chronic infection. Consider interrupting belimumab in patients who develop new infections and initiate appropriate anti-infective treatment; monitor closely. Cases of progressive multifocal leukoencephalopathy (PML) associated with JC virus (some fatal) have been reported in patients with SLE receiving immunosuppressants, including belimumab. Risk factors for PML include immunosuppressant therapies and impaired immune function. Consider diagnosis of PML in any patient presenting with new-onset or deteriorating neurologic signs/symptoms; consult a neurologist (or other appropriate specialist). If PML is confirmed, consider discontinuing immunosuppressant treatment, including belimumab.

Acute hypersensitivity reactions including anaphylaxis (with fatalities) and infusion-related reactions (eg, bradycardia, hypotension, myalgia, headache, rash, and urticaria) have been reported, including patients who had previously tolerated infusions of belimumab; onset may occur within hours of the infusion or may be delayed. ▶

Monitor for an appropriate time following administration. Discontinue for severe reactions (anaphylaxis, angioedema); infusion may be slowed or temporarily interrupted for other infusion-related reactions. Risk for hypersensitivity reactions may be increased with history of multiple drug allergies or significant hypersensitivity. Immunosuppressants may increase risk of malignancy. May cause psychiatric adverse effects, including anxiety, insomnia, or new/worsening depression. Potentially significant drug-drug interactions may exist, requiring dose or frequency adjustment, additional monitoring, and/or selection of alternative therapy. Live vaccines should not be given within 30 days before or concurrently with belimumab. Black/African-American patients may have a lower response rate; use with caution.

Adverse Reactions

Central nervous system: Anxiety, depression, headache, insomnia, migraine

Dermatologic: Dermatological reaction

Gastrointestinal: Diarrhea, nausea, viral gastroenteritis

Genitourinary: Cystitis, urinary tract infection (site not specified)

Hematologic & oncologic: Leukopenia

Hypersensitivity: Hypersensitivity

Infection: Influenza

Neuromuscular & skeletal: Limb pain

Respiratory: Bronchitis, nasopharyngitis, pharyngitis, sinusitis, upper respiratory tract infection

Miscellaneous: Fever, infusion related reaction

Rare but important or life-threatening: Anaphylaxis (including fatalities), antibody development, bradycardia, cellulitis, myalgia, pneumonia, progressive multifocal leukoencephalopathy (immune compromised), suicidal tendencies

Drug Interactions

Metabolism/Transport Effects None known.

Avoid Concomitant Use

Avoid concomitant use of Belimumab with any of the following: Abatacept; BCG; Belatacept; Cyclophosphamide; Etanercept; Monoclonal Antibodies; Natalizumab; Pimecrolimus; Tacrolimus (Topical); Tofacitinib; Vaccines (Live)

Increased Effect/Toxicity

Belimumab may increase the levels/effects of: Cyclophosphamide; Leflunomide; Natalizumab; Tofacitinib; Vaccines (Live)

The levels/effects of Belimumab may be increased by: Abatacept; Belatacept; Etanercept; Monoclonal Antibodies; Pimecrolimus; Roflumilast; Tacrolimus (Topical)

Decreased Effect

Belimumab may decrease the levels/effects of: BCG; Coccidioides immitis Skin Test; Sipuleucel-T; Vaccines (Inactivated)

The levels/effects of Belimumab may be decreased by: Echinacea

Preparation for Administration To reconstitute, remove vial from the refrigerator and allow to stand 10 to 15 minutes to reach room temperature. Reconstitute 120 mg vial with 1.5 mL of sterile water for injection (SWFI). Reconstitute 400 mg vial with 4.8 mL of SWFI. To minimize foaming, direct SWFI toward the side of the vial. Gently swirl for 60 seconds every 5 minutes until powder has dissolved (usual reconstitution time is 10-15 minutes, but may take up to 30 minutes); do not shake. If utilizing a mechanical reconstitution device, do not exceed 500 rpm or 30 minutes. Further dilute reconstituted solution in 250 mL of 0.9% sodium chloride (dilute only in 0.9% sodium chloride) by first removing and discarding the volume equivalent to the volume of the reconstituted solution to be added to prepare the appropriate dose; add the appropriate volume of the reconstituted solution to the infusion container and gently invert to mix solution. Protect from light. Solution may be stored refrigerated or at room temperature.

Storage/Stability Prior to reconstitution, store unused vials between 2°C and 8°C (36°F and 46°F); do not freeze. Protect from light. Avoid exposure to heat. Prior to further dilution, the reconstituted solution must be stored under refrigeration. The diluted solution may be stored refrigerated or at room temperature. Infusion must be completed within 8 hours of reconstitution.

Mechanism of Action Belimumab is an IgG1-lambda monoclonal antibody that prevents the survival of B lymphocytes by blocking the binding of soluble human B lymphocyte stimulator protein (BLyS) to receptors on B lymphocytes. This reduces the activity of B-cell mediated immunity and the autoimmune response.

Pharmacodynamics/Kinetics

Onset of action: B cells: 8 weeks; Clinical improvement (SLE Responder Index and flare reduction): 16 weeks (Navarra, 2011)

Distribution: V_d: 5.29 L

Half-life elimination: 19.4 days

Dosage Systemic lupus erythematosus (SLE): Adults: IV: Initial: 10 mg/kg every 2 weeks for 3 doses; Maintenance: 10 mg/kg every 4 weeks

Dosage adjustment in renal impairment:

CrCl ≥15 mL/minute: No dosage adjustment necessary.

CrCl <15 mL/minute: There are no dosage adjustments provided in the manufacturer's labeling (has not been studied).

Dosage adjustment in hepatic impairment: There are no dosage adjustments provided in the manufacturer's labeling (has not been studied).

Administration Administer intravenously over 1 hour through a dedicated IV line. Do **NOT** administer as an IV push or bolus. Discontinue infusion for severe hypersensitivity reaction (eg, anaphylaxis, angioedema). The infusion may be slowed or temporarily interrupted for minor reactions. Consider premedicating with an antihistamine and antipyretic for prophylaxis against hypersensitivity or infusion reactions.

Monitoring Parameters Monitor for hypersensitivity and/or infusion reactions; infections; worsening of depression, mood changes, or suicidal thoughts

Dosage Forms

Solution Reconstituted, Intravenous [preservative free]:

Benlysta: 120 mg (1 ea); 400 mg (1 ea)

Belinostat (be LIN oh stat)

Brand Names: U.S. Beleodaq

Index Terms PXD101

Pharmacologic Category Antineoplastic Agent, Histone Deacetylase Inhibitor

Use Peripheral T-cell lymphoma: Treatment of relapsed or refractory peripheral T-cell lymphoma (PTCL)

Pregnancy Risk Factor D

Pregnancy Considerations Animal reproduction studies have not been conducted. Belinostat is a genotoxic drug that targets dividing cells; embryofetal toxicity is expected if exposure occurs during pregnancy. Based on animal data, belinostat may also impair male fertility. Women of reproductive potential should avoid pregnancy during treatment with belinostat.

Breast-Feeding Considerations It is not known if belinostat is excreted in breast milk. Due to the potential for serious adverse reactions in the nursing infant, the manufacturer recommends that a decision be made whether to discontinue nursing or to discontinue the drug, taking into account the importance of treatment to the mother.

Contraindications There are no contraindications listed in the manufacturer's labeling.

Warnings/Precautions Hazardous agent – Use appropriate precautions for handling and disposal (meets NIOSH 2014 criteria).

May cause thrombocytopenia, leukopenia (neutropenia and lymphopenia), and/or anemia. Monitor blood counts at baseline and weekly during treatment. May require dosage reduction, treatment delay, or discontinuation. Serious infections (occasionally fatal), including pneumonia and sepsis, have occurred with treatment. Do not administer in patients with an active infection. Heavily pretreated patients (history of extensive or intensive prior chemotherapy) may be at higher risk for life-threatening infections.

May cause liver function test abnormalities and fatal hepatotoxicity. Monitor liver function tests at baseline and prior to each cycle. May require dosage reduction, treatment delay, or permanent discontinuation (based on the severity of the hepatotoxicity). Belinostat is metabolized hepatically and increased exposure is expected to occur in patients with hepatic impairment. Patients with moderate to severe hepatic impairment (total bilirubin >1.5 times ULN) were excluded from clinical studies. Tumor lysis syndrome (TLS) has been observed; closely monitor patients with advanced disease and/or high tumor burden. If TLS occurs, initiate appropriate treatment. Nausea, vomiting, and diarrhea occur with belinostat; may require management with antiemetic and antidiarrheal medications. In a phase 1 study, nausea/vomiting generally occurred at the end of the infusion each day (rarely persisting beyond day 5 each cycle) and was managed with standard antiemetics (Steele, 2011).

Belinostat is primarily metabolized by UGT1A1; the initial dose should be reduced in patients known to be homozygous for UGT1A1*28 allele. Potentially significant drug-drug interactions may exist, requiring dose or frequency adjustment, additional monitoring, and/or selection of alternative therapy.

Adverse Reactions

Cardiovascular: Hypotension, peripheral edema, phlebitis, prolonged Q-T interval on ECG

Central nervous system: Chills, dizziness, fatigue, headache

Dermatologic: Pruritus, skin rash

Endocrine & metabolic: Hypokalemia, increased lactate dehydrogenase

Gastrointestinal: Abdominal pain, constipation, decreased appetite, diarrhea, nausea, vomiting

Hematologic & oncologic: Anemia, thrombocytopenia

Infection: Infection

Local: Pain at injection site

Renal: Increased serum creatinine

Respiratory: Cough, dyspnea, pneumonia

Miscellaneous: Fever, multi-organ failure

Rare but important or life-threatening: Hepatic failure, leukopenia, sepsis, tumor lysis syndrome, ventricular fibrillation

Drug Interactions

Metabolism/Transport Effects **Substrate** of CYP2A6 (minor), CYP2C9 (minor), CYP3A4 (minor), P-glycoprotein, UGT1A1; **Note:** Assignment of Major/Minor substrate status based on clinically relevant drug interaction potential; **Inhibits** CYP2C8 (weak), CYP2C9 (weak)

Avoid Concomitant Use

Avoid concomitant use of Belinostat with any of the following: Atazanavir; CloZAPine; Dipyrone

Increased Effect/Toxicity

Belinostat may increase the levels/effects of: CloZAPine

The levels/effects of Belinostat may be increased by: Atazanavir; Dipyrone

Decreased Effect There are no known significant interactions involving a decrease in effect.

Preparation for Administration Hazardous agent; use appropriate precautions for handling and disposal (meets NIOSH 2014 criteria). Reconstitute each 500 mg vial with SWFI 9 mL to a concentration of 50 mg/mL. Swirl vial contents until there are no visible particles in the reconstituted solution. Further dilute the appropriate dose in NS 250 mL; do not use if cloudy or precipitate is present.

Storage/Stability Store intact vials at 20°C to 25°C (68°F to 77°F); excursions are permitted between 15°C and 30°C (59°F and 86°F). Retain in original package until use. The reconstituted solution may be stored for 12 hours at 15°C to 25°C (59°F to 77°F). Solutions diluted for infusion may be stored for up to 36 hours (including infusion time) at 15°C to 25°C (59°F to 77°F).

Mechanism of Action Histone deacetylase (HDAC) inhibitor which catalyzes acetyl group removal from protein lysine residues (of histone and some nonhistone proteins). Inhibition of histone deacetylase results in accumulation of acetyl groups, leading to cell cycle arrest and apoptosis. Belinostat has preferential cytotoxicity toward tumor cells versus normal cells.

Pharmacodynamics/Kinetics

Distribution: ~114 L/m^2 (Steele, 2011); mean volume of distribution approaches total body water

Protein binding: 93% to 96%

Metabolism: Hepatic; predominantly via UGT1A1, also by CYP2A6, CYP2C9, and CYP3A4 to the amide and acid metabolites

Half-life elimination: 1.1 hours

Time to peak: At end of infusion (Steele, 2011)

Excretion: Urine (~40%, predominantly as metabolites; <2% as unchanged drug)

Dosage Note: ANC should be ≥1000/mm^3 and platelets should be ≥50,000/mm^3 prior to each cycle

Peripheral T-cell lymphoma, relapsed or refractory: Adults: IV: 1000 mg/m^2 daily on days 1 to 5 of a 21-day cycle; repeat every 21 days until disease progression or unacceptable toxicity (O'Connor, 2013)

Dosage adjustment for patients with reduced UGT1A1 activity: Reduce initial dose to 750 mg/m^2 for patients known to be homozygous for UGT1A1*28 allele.

Dosage adjustment for toxicity:

Hematologic toxicity: ANC should be ≥1000/mm^3 and platelets should be ≥50,000/mm^3 prior to each cycle and prior to resuming treatment following a delay due to toxicity. Resume subsequent treatment according to the following parameters:

- Platelets ≥25,000/mm^3 and nadir ANC ≥500/mm^3: No dosage adjustment necessary (continue treatment without modification).
- Nadir ANC <500/mm^3 and any platelet count: Reduce dose by 25% (to 750 mg/m^2).
- Platelets <25,000/mm^3 and any nadir ANC: Reduce dose by 25% (to 750 mg/m^2).
- Recurrent nadir ANC <500/mm^3 and/or recurrent nadir platelets <25,000/mm^3 following 2 dosage reductions: Discontinue treatment.

Nonhematologic toxicity: Nonhematologic toxicities should be grade 2 or lower prior to retreatment. Resume subsequent treatment according to the following parameters:

- Any grade 3 or 4 toxicity (except nausea, vomiting, or diarrhea): Reduce dose by 25% (to 750 mg/m^2).
- Recurrent grade 3 or 4 toxicity following 2 dosage reductions: Discontinue treatment.
- Grade 3 or 4 nausea, vomiting, or diarrhea: Manage with supportive care; reduce the dose only if duration is >7 days with supportive management.

Dosage adjustment in renal impairment:

CrCl >39 mL/minute: Exposure is not altered (dosage adjustment is not likely necessary).

CrCl ≤39 mL/minute: There are no dosage adjustments provided in the manufacturer's labeling (data is insufficient to recommend a dose).

Dosage adjustment in hepatic impairment:

Mild hepatic impairment: There are no dosage adjustments provided in the manufacturer's labeling (exposure is expected to be increased in hepatic impairment).

Moderate to severe hepatic impairment (total bilirubin >1.5 times ULN): There are no dosage adjustments provided in the manufacturer's labeling (data is insufficient to recommend a dose).

Dosing in obesity: *ASCO Guidelines for appropriate chemotherapy dosing in obese adults with cancer:* Utilize patient's actual body weight (full weight) for calculation of body surface area- or weight-based dosing, particularly when the intent of therapy is curative; manage regimen-related toxicities in the same manner as for nonobese patients; if a dose reduction is utilized due to toxicity, consider resumption of full weight-based dosing with subsequent cycles, especially if cause of toxicity (eg, hepatic or renal impairment) is resolved (Griggs, 2012).

Administration IV: Infuse over 30 minutes using a 0.22-micron inline filter; if infusion site pain or other symptoms associated with infusion occur, may increase infusion time to 45 minutes.

Hazardous agent; use appropriate precautions for handling and disposal (meets NIOSH 2014 criteria).

Monitoring Parameters Monitor CBC with platelets and differential at baseline and weekly; serum chemistries (including renal and hepatic functions tests) at baseline and before each cycle; monitor for signs/symptoms of gastrointestinal toxicity (eg, nausea, vomiting, diarrhea), tumor lysis syndrome, and infection.

Dosage Forms

Solution Reconstituted, Intravenous:

Beleodaq: 500 mg (1 ea)

◆ **Belladonna Alkaloids With Phenobarbital** *see* Hyoscyamine, Atropine, Scopolamine, and Phenobarbital *on page 1027*

Belladonna and Opium (bel a DON a & OH pee um)

Index Terms B&O; Opium and Belladonna

Pharmacologic Category Analgesic Combination (Opioid); Analgesic, Opioid; Antispasmodic Agent, Urinary

Additional Appendix Information

Beers Criteria – Potentially Inappropriate Medications for Geriatrics *on page 2271*

Use Relief of moderate-to-severe pain associated with ureteral spasms not responsive to nonopioid analgesics and to space intervals between injections of opioids

Pregnancy Risk Factor C

Dosage Rectal: Children >12 years and Adults: 1 suppository 1-2 times/day, up to 4 doses/day

Additional Information Complete prescribing information should be consulted for additional detail.

Dosage Forms

Suppository: Belladonna extract 16.2 mg and opium 30 mg; belladonna extract 16.2 mg and opium 60 mg

◆ **Belsomra** *see* Suvorexant *on page 1961*

◆ **Belviq** *see* Lorcaserin *on page 1246*

◆ **Benadryl [OTC]** *see* DiphenhydrAMINE (Systemic) *on page 641*

◆ **Benadryl (Can)** *see* DiphenhydrAMINE (Systemic) *on page 641*

◆ **Benadryl-D® Allergy & Sinus [OTC]** *see* Diphenhydramine and Phenylephrine *on page 644*

◆ **Benadryl-D® Children's Allergy & Sinus [OTC]** *see* Diphenhydramine and Phenylephrine *on page 644*

◆ **Benadryl Allergy [OTC]** *see* DiphenhydrAMINE (Systemic) *on page 641*

◆ **Benadryl Allergy Childrens [OTC]** *see* DiphenhydrAMINE (Systemic) *on page 641*

◆ **Benadryl Dye-Free Allergy [OTC]** *see* DiphenhydrAMINE (Systemic) *on page 641*

Benazepril (ben AY ze pril)

Brand Names: U.S. Lotensin

Brand Names: Canada Lotensin

Index Terms Benazepril Hydrochloride

Pharmacologic Category Angiotensin-Converting Enzyme (ACE) Inhibitor; Antihypertensive

Use Hypertension: Treatment of hypertension, either alone or in combination with other antihypertensive agents

The 2014 guideline for the management of high blood pressure in adults (Eighth Joint National Committee [JNC 8]) recommends initiation of pharmacologic treatment to lower blood pressure for the following patients:

- Patients ≥60 years of age with systolic blood pressure (SBP) ≥150 mm Hg or diastolic blood pressure (DBP) ≥90 mm Hg. Goal of therapy is SBP <150 mm Hg and DBP <90 mm Hg.
- Patients <60 years of age with SBP ≥140 mm Hg or DBP is ≥90 mm Hg. Goal of therapy is SBP <140 mm Hg and DBP <90 mm Hg.
- Patients ≥18 years of age with diabetes and SBP ≥140 mm Hg or DBP ≥90 mm Hg. Goal of therapy is SBP <140 mm Hg and DBP <90 mm Hg.
- Patients ≥18 years of age with chronic kidney disease (CKD) and SBP ≥140 mm Hg or DBP ≥90 mm Hg. Goal of therapy is SBP <140 mm Hg and DBP <90 mm Hg.

In patients with CKD, regardless of race or diabetes status, the use of an ACE inhibitor (ACEI) or angiotensin receptor blocker (ARB) as initial therapy is recommended to improve kidney outcomes. In the general nonblack population (without CKD) including those with diabetes, initial antihypertensive treatment should consist of a thiazide-type diuretic, calcium channel blocker, ACEI, or ARB. In the general black population (without CKD) including those with diabetes, initial antihypertensive treatment should consist of a thiazide-type diuretic or a calcium channel blocker **instead of** an ACEI or ARB.

Pregnancy Risk Factor D

Pregnancy Considerations [U.S. Boxed Warning]: Drugs that act on the renin-angiotensin system can cause injury and death to the developing fetus. Discontinue as soon as possible once pregnancy is detected. Benazepril crosses the placenta; teratogenic effects may occur following maternal use during pregnancy. Drugs that act on the renin-angiotensin system are associated with oligohydramnios. Oligohydramnios, due to decreased fetal renal function, may lead to fetal lung hypoplasia and skeletal malformations. Their use in pregnancy is also associated with anuria, hypotension, renal failure, skull hypoplasia, and death in the fetus/neonate. Chronic maternal hypertension itself is also associated with adverse events in the fetus/infant. ACE inhibitors are not recommended during pregnancy to treat maternal hypertension or heart failure. Use of an ACE inhibitor should also be avoided in any woman of reproductive age. Women who are planning a pregnancy should be considered for other medication options if an ACE inhibitor is currently prescribed or the ACE inhibitor should be discontinued as soon as possible once pregnancy is detected. The exposed fetus should be monitored for fetal growth, amniotic fluid volume, and organ formation. Infants exposed to an ACE inhibitor *in utero* should be monitored for hyperkalemia, hypotension, and oliguria (exchange transfusions or dialysis may be needed). These adverse events are generally associated with maternal use in the second and third trimesters.

Untreated chronic maternal hypertension is also associated with adverse events in the fetus, infant, and mother. The use of ACE inhibitors is not recommended to treat chronic uncomplicated hypertension in pregnant women and should generally be avoided in women of reproductive potential (ACOG, 2013).

Breast-Feeding Considerations Small amounts of benazepril and benazeprilat are found in breast milk.

Contraindications Hypersensitivity to benazepril or any component of the formulation; patients with a history of angioedema (with or without prior ACE inhibitor therapy); concomitant use with aliskiren in patients with diabetes mellitus

Canadian labeling: Additional contraindications (not in U.S. labeling): Concomitant use with aliskiren in patients with moderate to severe renal impairment (GFR <60 mL/minute/1.73 m^2); pregnancy; breast-feeding; rare hereditary problems of galactose intolerance (eg, galactosemia, Lapp Lactase deficiency or glucose-galactose malabsorption)

Warnings/Precautions Anaphylactic reactions may occur rarely with ACE inhibitors. At any time during treatment (especially following first dose) angioedema may occur rarely with ACE inhibitors. It may involve the head and neck (potentially compromising airway) or the intestine (presenting with abdominal pain). African-Americans and patients with idiopathic or hereditary angioedema may be at an increased risk. Prolonged frequent monitoring may be required especially if tongue, glottis, or larynx are involved as they are associated with airway obstruction. Patients with a history of airway surgery may have a higher risk of airway obstruction. Aggressive early and appropriate management is critical. Contraindicated in patients with history of angioedema with or without prior ACE inhibitor therapy. Hypersensitivity reactions may be seen during hemodialysis (eg, CVVHD) with high-flux dialysis membranes (eg, AN69), and rarely, during low density lipoprotein apheresis with dextran sulfate cellulose. Rare cases of anaphylactoid reactions have been reported in patients undergoing sensitization treatment with hymenoptera (bee, wasp) venom while receiving ACE inhibitors.

Symptomatic hypotension with or without syncope can occur with ACE inhibitors (usually with the first several doses); effects are most often observed in volume depleted patients; close monitoring of patient is required especially with initial dosing and dosing increases; blood pressure must be lowered at a rate appropriate for the patient's clinical condition. Initiation of therapy in patients with ischemic heart disease or cerebrovascular disease warrants close observation due to the potential consequences posed by falling blood pressure (eg, MI, stroke). **[U.S. Boxed Warning]: Drugs that act on the renin-angiotensin system can cause injury and death to the developing fetus. Discontinue as soon as possible once pregnancy is detected.** Use with caution in hypertrophic cardiomyopathy with outflow tract obstruction, severe aortic stenosis, or before, during, or immediately after major surgery.

Hyperkalemia may occur with ACE inhibitors; risk factors include renal dysfunction, diabetes mellitus, concomitant use of potassium-sparing diuretics, potassium supplements and/or potassium-containing salts. Use cautiously, if at all, with these agents and monitor potassium periodically. Cough may occur with ACE inhibitors. Other causes of cough should be considered (eg, pulmonary congestion in patients with heart failure) and excluded prior to discontinuation. Use with caution in patients with diabetes receiving insulin or oral antidiabetic agents; may be at increased risk for episodes of hypoglycemia.

May be associated with deterioration of renal function and/or increases in serum creatinine, particularly in patients with low renal blood flow (eg, renal artery stenosis, heart failure) whose glomerular filtration rate (GFR) is dependent on efferent arteriolar vasoconstriction by angiotensin II; deterioration may result in oliguria, acute renal failure, and progressive azotemia. Small increases in serum creatinine may occur following initiation; consider discontinuation only in patients with progressive and/or significant deterioration in renal function. Use with caution in patients with unstented unilateral/bilateral renal artery stenosis. When unstented bilateral renal artery stenosis is present, use is generally avoided due to the elevated risk of deterioration in renal function unless possible benefits outweigh risks. Potentially significant drug-drug interactions may exist, requiring dose or frequency adjustment, additional monitoring, and/or selection of alternative therapy.

Rare toxicities associated with ACE inhibitors include cholestatic jaundice (which may progress to fulminant hepatic necrosis), agranulocytosis, neutropenia, or leukopenia with myeloid hypoplasia. Patients with collagen vascular diseases (especially with concomitant renal impairment) or renal impairment alone may be at increased risk for hematologic toxicity; periodically monitor CBC with differential in these patients.

Adverse Reactions

Central nervous system: Dizziness, drowsiness, headache, orthostatic dizziness

Renal: Increased serum creatinine, renal insufficiency (may occur in patients with bilateral renal artery stenosis or hypovolemia)

Respiratory: Cough

Rare but important or life-threatening: Agranulocytosis, alopecia, anaphylactoid reaction, angina pectoris, angioedema (includes head, neck, and intestinal angioedema), arthralgia, arthritis, asthma, dermatitis, dyspnea, ECG changes, eosinophilia, flushing, gastritis, hemolytic anemia, hyperbilirubinemia, hyperglycemia, hyperkalemia, hypersensitivity, hypertonia, hyponatremia, hypotension, impotence, increased blood urea nitrogen (transient), increased serum transaminases, increased uric acid, insomnia, leukopenia, myalgia, neutropenia, orthostatic hypotension, palpitations, pancreatitis, paresthesia, pemphigus, peripheral edema, proteinuria, pruritus, shock, skin photosensitivity, skin rash, Stevens-Johnson syndrome, syncope, thrombocytopenia, vomiting

Anaphylaxis, eosinophilic pneumonitis, neutropenia, agranulocytosis, renal failure, and renal insufficiency have been reported with other ACE inhibitors. In addition, a syndrome including arthralgia, elevated ESR, eosinophilia, fever, interstitial nephritis, myalgia, rash, and vasculitis has been reported to be associated with ACE inhibitors.

Drug Interactions

Metabolism/Transport Effects None known.

Avoid Concomitant Use There are no known interactions where it is recommended to avoid concomitant use.

Increased Effect/Toxicity

Benazepril may increase the levels/effects of: Allopurinol; Amifostine; Antihypertensives; AzaTHIOprine; DULoxetine; Ferric Gluconate; Gold Sodium Thiomalate; Grass Pollen Allergen Extract (5 Grass Extract); Hypotensive Agents; Iron Dextran Complex; Levodopa; Lithium; Nonsteroidal Anti-Inflammatory Agents; Obinutuzumab; RisperiDONE; RiTUXimab; Sodium Phosphates

The levels/effects of Benazepril may be increased by: Alfuzosin; Aliskiren; Angiotensin II Receptor Blockers; Barbiturates; Brimonidine (Topical); Canagliflozin; Dapoxetine; Diazoxide; DPP-IV Inhibitors; Eplerenone; Everolimus; Heparin; Heparin (Low Molecular Weight); Herbs (Hypotensive Properties); Hydrochlorothiazide; Loop Diuretics; MAO Inhibitors; Nicorandil; Pentoxifylline; Phosphodiesterase 5 Inhibitors; Potassium Salts; Potassium-Sparing Diuretics; Prostacyclin Analogues; Sirolimus; Temsirolimus; Thiazide Diuretics; TiZANidine; Tolvaptan; Trimethoprim

Decreased Effect

Benazepril may decrease the levels/effects of: Hydrochlorothiazide

The levels/effects of Benazepril may be decreased by: Aprotinin; Herbs (Hypertensive Properties); Icatibant; Lanthanum; Methylphenidate; Nonsteroidal Anti-Inflammatory Agents; Salicylates; Yohimbine

Storage/Stability Store at ≤30°C (86°F). Protect from moisture.

Mechanism of Action Competitive inhibition of angiotensin I being converted to angiotensin II, a potent vasoconstrictor, through the angiotensin I-converting enzyme (ACE) activity, with resultant lower levels of angiotensin II which causes an increase in plasma renin activity and a reduction in aldosterone secretion

Pharmacodynamics/Kinetics

Reduction in plasma angiotensin-converting enzyme (ACE) activity:

Onset of action: Peak effect: 1-2 hours after 2-20 mg dose

Duration: >90% inhibition for 24 hours after 5-20 mg dose

Reduction in blood pressure:

Peak effect: Single dose: 2-4 hours; Continuous therapy: 2 weeks

Absorption: Rapid (37%); food does not alter significantly; metabolite (benazeprilat) itself unsuitable for oral administration due to poor absorption

Distribution: V_d: ~8.7 L

Protein binding:

Benazepril: ~97%

Benazeprilat: ~95%

Metabolism: Rapidly and extensively hepatic to its active metabolite, benazeprilat, via enzymatic hydrolysis; extensive first-pass effect

Half-life elimination: Benazeprilat: Effective: 10-11 hours; Terminal: Children: 5 hours, Adults: 22 hours

Time to peak: Parent drug: 0.5-1 hour

Excretion:

Urine (trace amounts as benazepril; 20% as benazeprilat; 12% as other metabolites)

Clearance: Nonrenal clearance (ie, biliary, metabolic) appears to contribute to the elimination of benazeprilat (11% to 12%), particularly patients with severe renal impairment; hepatic clearance is the main elimination route of unchanged benazepril

Dialysis: ~6% of metabolite removed within 4 hours of dialysis following 10 mg of benazepril administered 2 hours prior to procedure; parent compound not found in dialysate

Dosage Oral: Hypertension:

Children ≥6 years: Initial: 0.2 mg/kg/day (up to 10 mg daily) as monotherapy; dosing range: 0.1 to 0.6 mg/kg/day (maximum dose: 40 mg daily)

Adults: Initial: 10 mg/day in patients not receiving a diuretic; 20 to 80 mg daily as a single dose or 2 divided doses; the need for twice-daily dosing should be assessed by monitoring peak (2 to 6 hours after dosing) and trough responses. Usual dosage (ASH/ISH [Weber, 2014]): 10 to 40 mg daily.

Note: Patients taking diuretics should have them discontinued 2 to 3 days prior to starting benazepril. If they cannot be discontinued, then initial dose should be 5 mg; restart after blood pressure is stabilized if needed.

Elderly: Oral: Initial: 5 to 10 mg daily in single or divided doses; usual range: 20 to 40 mg daily; adjust for renal function; also see **Note** in adult dosing.

Dosage adjustment in renal impairment: CrCl <30 mL/minute:

Children: Use is not recommended.

Adults: Administer 5 mg/day initially; maximum daily dose: 40 mg.

Hemodialysis: Moderately dialyzable (20% to 50%); administer dose postdialysis or administer 25% to 35% supplemental dose.

Peritoneal dialysis: Supplemental dose is not necessary.

Dosage adjustment in hepatic impairment: No dosage adjustment provided in manufacturer's labeling (has not been studied); use with caution.

Monitoring Parameters Blood pressure; serum creatinine and potassium; if patient has collagen vascular disease and/or renal impairment, periodically monitor CBC with differential

Dosage Forms

Tablet, Oral:

Lotensin: 10 mg, 20 mg, 40 mg

Generic: 5 mg, 10 mg, 20 mg, 40 mg

Extemporaneous Preparations A 2 mg/mL oral suspension may be made with tablets. Mix fifteen benazepril 20 mg tablets in an amber polyethylene terephthalate bottle with Ora-Plus® 75 mL. Shake for 2 minutes, allow suspension to stand for ≥1 hour, then shake again for at least 1 additional minute. Add Ora-Sweet® 75 mL to suspension and shake to disperse. Will make 150 mL of a 2 mg/mL suspension. Label "shake well" and "refrigerate". Stable for 30 days.

Lotensin® prescribing information, Novartis Pharmaceuticals Corporation, Suffern, NY, 2009.

Benazepril and Hydrochlorothiazide

(ben AY ze pril & hye droe klor oh THYE a zide)

Brand Names: U.S. Lotensin HCT®

Index Terms Benazepril Hydrochloride and Hydrochlorothiazide; Hydrochlorothiazide and Benazepril

Pharmacologic Category Angiotensin-Converting Enzyme (ACE) Inhibitor; Antihypertensive; Diuretic, Thiazide

Use Treatment of hypertension

Pregnancy Risk Factor D

Dosage Note: Not for initial therapy; dose should be individualized.

Oral: Range: Benazepril: 5-20 mg; Hydrochlorothiazide: 6.25-25 mg/day

Add-on therapy:

Patients not adequately controlled on benazepril monotherapy: Initiate benazepril 10-20 mg/hydrochlorothiazide 12.5 mg; titrate to effect at 2- to 3-week intervals

Patients controlled on hydrochlorothiazide 25 mg/day but experience significant potassium loss with this regimen: Initiate benazepril 5 mg/hydrochlorothiazide 6.25 mg

Replacement therapy: Substitute for the individually titrated components

Dosage adjustment in renal impairment: CrCl ≤30 mL/minute: Not recommended; loop diuretics are preferred.

Dosage adjustment in hepatic impairment: No dosage adjustment provided in manufacturer's labeling (has not been studied); use with caution.

Additional Information Complete prescribing information should be consulted for additional detail.

Dosage Forms

Tablet:

Generics:

5/6.25: Benazepril 5 mg and hydrochlorothiazide 6.25 mg

10/12.5: Benazepril 10 mg and hydrochlorothiazide 12.5 mg

20/12.5: Benazepril 20 mg and hydrochlorothiazide 12.5 mg

20/25: Benazepril 20 mg and hydrochlorothiazide 25 mg

Brands:

Lotensin HCT® 10/12.5: Benazepril 10 mg and hydrochlorothiazide 12.5 mg

Lotensin HCT® 20/12.5: Benazepril 20 mg and hydrochlorothiazide 12.5 mg

Lotensin HCT® 20/25: Benazepril 20 mg and hydrochlorothiazide 25 mg

◆ **Benazepril Hydrochloride** *see* Benazepril *on page 238*

◆ **Benazepril Hydrochloride and Amlodipine Besylate** *see* Amlodipine and Benazepril *on page 125*

◆ **Benazepril Hydrochloride and Hydrochlorothiazide** *see* Benazepril and Hydrochlorothiazide *on page 240*

Bencyclane [INT] (ben CY clane)

International Brand Names Diacyclan (GR); Fludilat (BR, DE, GR, ID, PT, TH, VE); Furudin (KR); Halidor (HU, PL, RU, TR); Ludilat (AT)

Index Terms Benzacyclane Fumarate

Pharmacologic Category Vasodilator

Reported Use Management of peripheral and cerebral vascular disorders

Dosage Range Oral: Adults: 100-200 mg 3 times/day

Product Availability Product available in various countries; not currently available in the U.S.

Dosage Forms

Tablet: 100 mg

Bendamustine (ben da MUS teen)

Brand Names: U.S. Treanda

Brand Names: Canada Treanda

Index Terms Bendamustine Hydrochloride; Cytostasan; SDX-105

Pharmacologic Category Antineoplastic Agent, Alkylating Agent; Antineoplastic Agent, Alkylating Agent (Nitrogen Mustard)

Use

Chronic lymphocytic leukemia: Treatment of chronic lymphocytic leukemia (CLL)

Non-Hodgkin lymphoma: Treatment of indolent B-cell non-Hodgkin lymphoma (NHL) which has progressed during or within 6 months of rituximab treatment or a rituximab-containing regimen

Pregnancy Risk Factor D

Pregnancy Considerations Adverse events were observed in animal reproduction studies. May cause fetal harm if administered during pregnancy. For women and men of reproductive potential, the U.S. labeling recommends effective contraception during and for 3 months after treatment. The Canadian labeling recommends effective contraception beginning 2 weeks prior to treatment and for ≥1 month after treatment.

Breast-Feeding Considerations It is not known if bendamustine is excreted in breast milk. Due to the potential for serious adverse reactions in the nursing infant, the decision to discontinue bendamustine or discontinue breast-feeding should take into account the benefits of treatment to the mother.

Contraindications Hypersensitivity (eg, anaphylactic or anaphylactoid reactions) to bendamustine or any component of the formulation

Warnings/Precautions Hazardous agent - use appropriate precautions for handling and disposal (NIOSH 2014 [group 1]). Myelosuppression (neutropenia, thrombocytopenia, and anemia) is a common toxicity; may require therapy delay and/or dose reduction; monitor blood counts frequently (nadirs typically occurred in the third week of treatment). Complications due to febrile neutropenia and severe thrombocytopenia have been reported (some fatal). ANC should recover to ≥1000/mm^3 and platelets to ≥75,000/mm^3 prior to cycle initiation. Pneumonia, sepsis, and septic shock have been reported; fatalities due to infection have occurred; patients with myelosuppression are more susceptible to infection; monitor closely.

Infusion reactions, including chills, fever, pruritus, and rash are common; rarely, anaphylactic and anaphylactoid reactions have occurred, particularly with the second or subsequent cycle(s). Patients who experienced grade 3 or higher allergic reactions should not be rechallenged. Consider premedication with antihistamines, antipyretics, and corticosteroids for patients with a history of grade 1 or 2 infusion reaction. Discontinue for severe allergic reaction or grade 4 infusion reaction; consider discontinuation with grade 3 infusion reaction. Rash, toxic skin reactions and bullous exanthema have been reported with monotherapy and in combination with other antineoplastics; may be progressive or worsen with continued treatment; discontinue bendamustine treatment for severe or progressive skin reaction; monitor closely; withhold or discontinue bendamustine treatment for severe or progressive skin reaction. The risk for severe skin toxicity is increased with concurrent use of allopurinol and other medications known to cause skin toxicity; Stevens-Johnson syndrome (SJS) and toxic epidermal necrolysis (TEN) have been reported. TEN has also been reported when used in combination with rituximab. Bendamustine is an irritant with vesicant-like properties; ensure proper needle or catheter placement prior to and during infusion; avoid extravasation; erythema, marked swelling, and pain have been reported with extravasation. Bendamustine is associated with a moderate emetic potential (Basch, 2011; Dupuis, 2011; Roila, 2010); antiemetics are recommended to prevent nausea and vomiting.

Tumor lysis syndrome (usually occurring in the first treatment cycle) may occur as a consequence of antineoplastic treatment, including treatment with bendamustine. May lead to life-threatening acute renal failure; vigorous hydration and prophylactic measures (eg, antihyperuricemic therapy) should be instituted prior to treatment in high-risk patients; monitor closely. **Note:** Allopurinol may increase the risk for bendamustine skin toxicity. May cause hypokalemia; monitor potassium closely during therapy, particularly in patients with cardiac disease.

Per manufacturer's labeling, use with caution in patients with mild hepatic impairment. However, a pharmacokinetic study showed only slight differences in bendamustine AUC and C_{max} in patients with mild hepatic impairment (defined in the study as total bilirubin 1 to 1.5 times ULN or AST greater than ULN), as compared to patients with normal hepatic function (Owen, 2010). Use is not recommended in patients with moderate (AST or ALT 2.5 to 10 times ULN and total bilirubin 1.5 to 3 times ULN) or severe (total bilirubin >3 times ULN) hepatic impairment.

Use with caution in patients with mild-to-moderate renal impairment. The U.S. and Canadian product labels do not recommend use in patients with CrCl <40 mL/minute. A pharmacokinetic study illustrated only slight differences in bendamustine AUC and C_{max} in patients with mild (CrCl >50 to ≤80 mL/minute) and moderate (CrCl >30 to ≤50 mL/minute) renal dysfunction, compared to patients with normal renal function (Owen, 2010). A retrospective safety study found no significant difference in lab toxicities between CLL patients with renal impairment (CrCl <40 mL/minute) compared to those without renal impairment, although an increase in grades 3/4 thrombocytopenia and grades 3/4 BUN increases were detected in patients with renal impairment (Nordstrom, 2012); monitor blood counts and renal function. **Note:** UK labeling (Levact prescribing information, October, 2010) recommends no dosage adjustment for patients with CrCl >10 mL/minute. Secondary malignancies (including myelodysplastic syndrome, myeloproliferative disorders, acute myeloid leukemia and bronchial cancer) and premalignant diseases have been reported in patients who have received bendamustine. Potentially significant drug-drug interactions may exist, requiring dose or frequency adjustment, additional monitoring, and/or selection of alternative therapy.

Adverse Reactions

Cardiovascular: Chest pain, exacerbation of hypertension, hypotension, peripheral edema, tachycardia

Central nervous system: Anxiety, chills, depression, dizziness, fatigue, headache, insomnia, pain

Dermatologic: Hyperhidrosis, night sweats, pruritus, skin rash, xeroderma

Endocrine & metabolic: Dehydration, hyperglycemia, hyperuricemia, hypocalcemia, hypokalemia, hyponatremia, weight loss

Gastrointestinal: Abdominal distention, abdominal pain, anorexia, constipation, decreased appetite, diarrhea, dysgeusia, dyspepsia, gastroesophageal reflux disease, nausea, oral candidiasis, stomatitis, vomiting, xerostomia

Genitourinary: Urinary tract infection

Hematologic & oncologic: Bone marrow depression (nadir: In week 3), decreased hemoglobin, decreased neutrophils, febrile neutropenia, leukopenia, lymphocytopenia, thrombocytopenia

Hepatic: Increased serum ALT, increased serum AST, increased serum bilirubin

Hypersensitivity: Hypersensitivity

Infection: Herpes simplex infection, herpes zoster, infection

Local: Catheter pain, infusion site reaction

Neuromuscular & skeletal: Arthralgia, back pain, limb pain, ostealgia, weakness

Renal: Increased serum creatinine

Respiratory: Cough, dyspnea, nasal congestion, nasopharyngitis, pharyngolaryngeal pain, pneumonia, sinusitis, upper respiratory tract infection, wheezing

Miscellaneous: Fever

Rare but important or life-threatening: Acute renal failure, alopecia, anaphylaxis, bronchogenic carcinoma, bullous rash, cardiac failure, dermatitis, dermatological reaction (toxic), drowsiness, erythema, exacerbation of hepatitis B, hemolysis, infusion related reaction, mucositis, myelodysplastic syndrome, myeloid leukemia (acute), myeloproliferative disease, pneumonitis, pulmonary fibrosis, sepsis, septic shock, skin necrosis, Stevens-Johnson syndrome, toxic epidermal necrolysis, tumor lysis syndrome

Drug Interactions

Metabolism/Transport Effects **Substrate** of BCRP, CYP1A2 (minor), P-glycoprotein; **Note:** Assignment of Major/Minor substrate status based on clinically relevant drug interaction potential

Avoid Concomitant Use

Avoid concomitant use of Bendamustine with any of the following: CloZAPine; Dipyrone

Increased Effect/Toxicity

Bendamustine may increase the levels/effects of: CloZAPine

The levels/effects of Bendamustine may be increased by: Allopurinol; CYP1A2 Inhibitors (Strong); Dipyrone

Decreased Effect

The levels/effects of Bendamustine may be decreased by: CYP1A2 Inducers (Strong)

Preparation for Administration Hazardous agent; use appropriate precautions for handling and disposal (NIOSH 2014 [group 1]).

Powder for solution: Reconstitute 25 mg vial with 5 mL and 100 mg vial with 20 mL of sterile water for injection to a concentration of 5 mg/mL; powder usually dissolves within 5 minutes. Prior to administration, dilute appropriate dose in 500 mL NS (or $D_{2.5}$½NS) to a final concentration of 0.2 to 0.6 mg/mL; mix thoroughly.

Solution: Prior to administration, dilute appropriate dose in 500 mL NS (or $D_{2.5}$½NS) to a final concentration of 0.2 to 0.7 mg/mL; resulting solution should be colorless to yellow. Some closed system transfer devices may not be compatible with undiluted bendamustine.

Storage/Stability

Powder for solution: Prior to reconstitution, store intact vials up to 25°C (77°F); excursions are permitted up to 30°C (86°F). Protect from light. The solution in the vial (reconstituted with SWFI) is stable for 30 minutes (transfer to 500 mL infusion bag within that 30 minutes). The solution diluted in 500 mL for infusion is stable for 24 hours refrigerated or 3 hours at room temperature and room light. Infusion must be completed within these time frames.

Solution: Store intact vials between 2°C to 8°C (36°F to 46°F); protect from light. Solutions diluted for infusion are stable for up to 24 hours when stored at 2°C to 8°C (36°F to 46°F) or for up to 2 hours when stored at 15°C to 30°C (59°F to 86°F) and room light. Infusion must be completed within these time frames.

Mechanism of Action Bendamustine is an alkylating agent (nitrogen mustard derivative) with a benzimidazole ring (purine analog) which demonstrates only partial cross-resistance (*in vitro*) with other alkylating agents. It leads to cell death via single and double strand DNA cross-linking. Bendamustine is active against quiescent and dividing cells. The primary cytotoxic activity is due to bendamustine (as compared to metabolites).

Pharmacodynamics/Kinetics

Distribution: V_{ss}: ~20 to 25 L

Protein binding: 94% to 96%

Metabolism: Hepatic (extensive), via CYP1A2 to active (minor) metabolites gamma-hydroxy bendamustine (M3) and N-desmethyl-bendamustine (M4); also via hydrolysis to low cytotoxic metabolites, monohydroxy bendamustine (HP1) and dihydroxy bendamustine (HP2)

Half-life elimination: Bendamustine: ~40 minutes; M3: ~3 hours; M4: ~30 minutes

Time to peak, serum: At end of infusion

Excretion: Feces (~25%); urine (~50%; ~3% as active parent drug)

Dosage Note: Bendamustine is associated with a moderate emetic potential (Basch, 2011; Roila, 2010); antiemetics are recommended to prevent nausea and vomiting.

Chronic lymphocytic leukemia (CLL): Adults: IV: 100 mg/m² over 30 minutes on days 1 and 2 of a 28-day treatment cycle (as a single agent) for up to 6 cycles (Knauf, 2009; Knauf, 2012)

CLL, first-line treatment (off-label dosing): Adults: IV: 90 mg/m^2 on days 1 and 2 of a 28-day treatment cycle (in combination with rituximab) for up to 6 cycles (Fischer, 2012)

CLL, relapsed/refractory (off-label dosing): Adults: IV: 70 mg/m^2 on days 1 and 2 of a 28-day treatment cycle (in combination with rituximab) for up to 6 cycles (Fischer, 2011)

Non-Hodgkin lymphomas: Adults: IV:

Lymphoma, indolent B-cell, refractory: 120 mg/m^2 over 60 minutes on days 1 and 2 of a 21-day treatment cycle (as a single agent) for up to 8 cycles (Kahl, 2010)

Lymphoma, indolent B-cell, follicular, or mantle cell, first-line (off-label use): 90 mg/m^2 on days 1 and 2 of a 28-day treatment cycle (in combination with rituximab) for up to 6 cycles (Rummel, 2009)

Lymphoma, follicular, relapsed or refractory (off-label use): 90 mg/m^2 on days 1 and 2 of a 35-day treatment cycle (in combination with bortezomib and rituximab) for 5 cycles (Fowler, 2011)

Lymphoma, mantle cell, relapsed or refractory (off-label use): 90 mg/m^2 over 30 minutes on days 2 and 3 of a 28-day treatment cycle (in combination with rituximab) for up to 4 cycles (Rummel, 2005)

Hodgkin lymphoma, relapsed or refractory (off-label use): Adults: IV: 120 mg/m^2 on days 1 and 2 of a 28-day treatment cycle for up to 6 cycles (Moskowitz, 2013)

Multiple myeloma, salvage therapy (off-label use): Adults: IV: 90 to 100 mg/m^2 on days 1 and 2 of a 28-day treatment cycle for at least 2 cycles (Knop, 2005)

Waldenström macroglobulinemia, refractory (off-label use): Adults: IV: 90 mg/m^2 on days 1 and 2 of a 28-day treatment cycle (in combination with rituximab) for 6 cycles (Treon, 2011) **or** 90 mg/m^2 over 30 minutes on days 2 and 3 of a 28-day treatment cycle (in combination with rituximab) for 4 cycles (Rummel, 2005)

Dosage adjustment for toxicity:

Infusion reactions:

Grade 1 or 2: Consider premedication with antihistamines, antipyretics, and corticosteroids in subsequent cycles

Grade 3: Consider discontinuing treatment

Grade 4: Discontinue treatment

Skin reaction, severe or progressive: Withhold or discontinue treatment

Treatment delay:

Hematologic toxicity ≥ grade 4: Delay treatment until resolves (ANC ≥1000/mm^3, platelets ≥75,000/mm^3)

Nonhematologic toxicity ≥ grade 2 (clinically significant): Delay treatment until resolves to ≤ grade 1

Dose modification in CLL:

Hematologic toxicity ≥ grade 3: Reduce dose to 50 mg/m^2 on days 1 and 2 of each treatment cycle. For recurrent hematologic toxicity (≥ grade 3), further reduce dose to 25 mg/m^2 on days 1 and 2 of the treatment cycle. May cautiously re-escalate dose in subsequent cycles.

Nonhematologic toxicity ≥ grade 3 (clinically significant): Reduce dose to 50 mg/m^2 on days 1 and 2 of the treatment cycle with discretion. May cautiously re-escalate dose in subsequent cycles.

Dose modification in NHL:

Hematologic toxicity grade 4: Reduce dose to 90 mg/m^2 on days 1 and 2 of each treatment cycle. For recurrent hematologic toxicity (grade 4), further reduce dose to 60 mg/m^2 on days 1 and 2 of each treatment cycle.

Nonhematologic toxicity ≥ grade 3: Reduce dose to 90 mg/m^2 on days 1 and 2 of the treatment cycle with discretion. For recurrent toxicity ≥ grade 3, further reduce dose to 60 mg/m^2 on days 1 and 2 of each treatment cycle.

Dosage adjustment in renal impairment:

CrCl <40 mL/minute: Use is not recommended in the U.S. and Canadian manufacturers' labeling.

Study data suggest minor changes in systemic exposure may occur with mild-to-moderate renal impairment. Based on a pharmacokinetic study (patients receiving 120 mg/m^2 for 2 days every 21 days), only slight differences in bendamustine AUC and C_{max} were demonstrated in patients with mild (CrCl >50 to ≤80 mL/minute) and moderate (CrCl >30 to ≤50 mL/minute) renal dysfunction, compared to patients with normal renal function (Owen, 2010). A retrospective study of bendamustine in CLL and NHL patients with renal impairment (CrCl <40 mL/minute) compared to those without (CrCl ≥60 mL/minute) found no significant difference in lab toxicities in CLL patients with renal impairment compared to those without renal impairment, although an increase in grades 3/4 thrombocytopenia was noted in NHL patients and grades 3/4 BUN increases were higher when combining data for CLL and NHL (Nordstrom, 2012).

Note: UK manufacturer's labeling (Levact [prescribing information], October, 2010) recommends no dosage adjustment for patients with CrCl >10 mL/minute.

Dosage adjustment in hepatic impairment:

Mild impairment: Per U.S. and Canadian manufacturers' labeling, use with caution. However, a pharmacokinetic study showed only slight differences in bendamustine AUC and C_{max} in patients with mild hepatic impairment (defined in the study as total bilirubin 1 to 1.5 times ULN or AST greater than ULN), compared to patients with normal hepatic function (Owen, 2010).

Moderate impairment (AST or ALT 2.5 to 10 times ULN and total bilirubin 1.5 to 3 times ULN): Use is not recommended.

Severe impairment (total bilirubin >3 times ULN): Use is not recommended.

Dosing in obesity: *American Society of Clinical Oncology (ASCO) Guidelines for appropriate chemotherapy dosing in obese adults with cancer:* Utilize patient's actual body weight (full weight) for calculation of body surface area- or weight-based dosing, particularly when the intent of therapy is curative; manage regimen-related toxicities in the same manner as for nonobese patients; if a dose reduction is utilized due to toxicity, consider resumption of full weight-based dosing with subsequent cycles, especially if cause of toxicity (eg, hepatic or renal impairment) is resolved (Griggs, 2012).

Administration Infuse over 30 minutes for the treatment of CLL and over 60 minutes for NHL; administration times for off-label uses/doses vary by protocol. Consider premedication with antihistamines, antipyretics, and corticosteroids for patients with a previous grade 1 or 2 infusion reaction to bendamustine. Bendamustine is associated with a moderate emetic potential (Basch, 2011; Dupuis, 2011; Roila, 2010); antiemetics are recommended to prevent nausea and vomiting.

Irritant with vesicant-like properties; ensure proper needle or catheter placement prior to and during infusion. Avoid extravasation; monitor IV site for redness, swelling, or pain.

Extravasation management: If extravasation occurs, stop infusion immediately and disconnect (leave cannula/needle in place); gently aspirate extravasated solution (do **NOT** flush the line); remove needle/cannula; elevate extremity. Apply dry cold compresses for 20 minutes 4 times daily (Perez Fildago, 2012). May be managed with sodium thiosulfate in the same manner as mechlorethamine extravasation (Schulmeister, 2011).

Sodium thiosulfate 1/6 M solution (instructions for mechlorethamine): Inject subcutaneously into extravasation area using 2 mL for each mg of drug suspected to have extravasated (Perez Fidalgo, 2012; Polovich, 2009).

Hazardous agent; use appropriate precautions for handling and disposal (NIOSH 2014 [group 1]).

Monitoring Parameters CBC with differential and platelets (monitored weekly [initially] in clinical trials); serum creatinine; ALT, AST, and total bilirubin; monitor potassium and uric acid levels in patients at risk for tumor lysis syndrome; monitor for infusion reactions anaphylaxis, infection, and dermatologic toxicity; monitor IV site during and after infusion.

Canadian labeling also recommends periodic monitoring of blood pressure, serum glucose, and ECG (in patients with cardiac disease particularly if concomitant electrolyte disturbances).

Dosage Forms

Solution, Intravenous:

Treanda: 45 mg/0.5 mL (0.5 mL); 180 mg/2 mL (2 mL)

Solution Reconstituted, Intravenous:

Treanda: 25 mg (1 ea); 100 mg (1 ea)

- ◆ **Bendamustine Hydrochloride** *see* Bendamustine *on page 241*
- ◆ **Benefiber [OTC]** *see* Wheat Dextrin *on page 2190*
- ◆ **Benefiber Drink Mix [OTC]** *see* Wheat Dextrin *on page 2190*
- ◆ **Benefiber For Children [OTC]** *see* Wheat Dextrin *on page 2190*
- ◆ **Benefiber Plus Calcium [OTC]** *see* Wheat Dextrin *on page 2190*
- ◆ **BeneFIX** *see* Factor IX (Recombinant) *on page 841*
- ◆ **BeneFix (Can)** *see* Factor IX (Recombinant) *on page 841*
- ◆ **Benemid [DSC]** *see* Probenecid *on page 1716*
- ◆ **Benflumetol and Artemether** *see* Artemether and Lumefantrine *on page 177*
- ◆ **BenGay [OTC]** *see* Methyl Salicylate and Menthol *on page 1344*
- ◆ **Benicar** *see* Olmesartan *on page 1496*
- ◆ **Benicar HCT** *see* Olmesartan and Hydrochlorothiazide *on page 1498*
- ◆ **Benlysta** *see* Belimumab *on page 235*
- ◆ **Benoxinate Hydrochloride and Fluorescein Sodium** *see* Fluorescein and Benoxinate *on page 895*

Benperidol [INT] (ben PER i dole)

International Brand Names Anquil (GB, IE); Benperidol-neuraxpharm (DE); Concilium (AR); Frenactil (BE, LU, NL); Glianimon (DE, GR)

Pharmacologic Category Antipsychotic Agent, Typical, Phenothiazine

Reported Use Treatment of psychotic conditions including control of deviant antisocial sexual behavior

Dosage Range Adults: Oral: 0.25-1.5 mg/day in divided doses

Product Availability Product available in various countries; not currently available in the U.S.

Dosage Forms

Tablet: 0.25 mg

Benserazide and Levodopa [CAN/INT]

(ben SER a zide & lee voe DOE pa)

Brand Names: Canada Prolopa®

Index Terms Levodopa and Benserazide

Pharmacologic Category Anti-Parkinson's Agent, Dopamine Agonist

Use Note: Not approved in U.S.

Treatment of Parkinson's disease (except drug-induced Parkinsonism)

Pregnancy Considerations Adverse events have been observed with levodopa in animal reproduction studies; use of this combination is contraindicated in pregnant women and women of childbearing age without proper contraception. Levodopa crosses the placenta and can be metabolized by the fetus and detected in fetal tissue (Merchant, 1995). The incidence of Parkinson's disease in pregnancy is relatively rare and information related to the use of benserazide/levodopa in pregnant women is limited (Hagell, 1998; von Graevenitz, 1996).

Breast-Feeding Considerations Levodopa is excreted into breast milk (based on a study using carbidopa/levodopa) (Thulin, 1998); excretion of benserazide is not known. Breast-feeding is not recommended by the manufacturer since occurrence of skeletal malformations in infants cannot be excluded.

Contraindications Hypersensitivity to benserazide, levodopa, sympathomimetics, or any component of the formulation; use with or within 14 days of MAO inhibitors; patients with clinical laboratory evidence of uncompensated cardiovascular, endocrine, renal, hepatic, hematologic, or pulmonary disease; patients with decompensated endocrine, renal, hepatic, cardiac disorders, psychiatric disorders, narrow-angle glaucoma, or closed-angle glaucoma; patients <25 years of age (due to possibility of skeletal abnormalities from benserazide); pregnancy or use in women of childbearing potential without adequate contraception

Warnings/Precautions If patient is already receiving levodopa, discontinue levodopa at least 12 hours before starting benserazide/levodopa and begin at 15% of previous amount of levodopa. Not indicated in management of intention tremor, Huntington's chorea, or drug-induced extrapyramidal symptoms. Administer in careful increments and observe closely for development of abnormal involuntary movements. May be associated with depression and suicidal thoughts/behavior. Use extreme caution in patients with psychotic disorders or patients receiving phenothiazines or TCAs. May increase human growth hormone levels. Use caution in patients with cardiovascular disease (MI, atrial, nodal, or ventricular arrhythmias); initiate in a monitored setting. Use caution in patients with ulcers, seizure disorders, and diabetes. Monitor IOP carefully in patients with wide-angle glaucoma. Use caution in patients with renal or hepatic impairment; use is contraindicated in decompensated renal or hepatic disease. Do not withdraw abruptly (may cause neuroleptic malignant syndrome [NMS]). Patient must be instructed to resume normal activities gradually (rapid mobilization may increase risk of injury). Dopamine agonists used for Parkinson's disease or restless legs syndrome have been associated with compulsive behaviors and/or loss of impulse control, which has manifested as pathological gambling, libido increases (hypersexuality), and/or binge eating. Causality has not been established, and controversy exists as to whether this phenomenon is related to the underlying disease, prior behaviors/addictions and/or drug therapy. Dose reduction or discontinuation of therapy has been reported to reverse these behaviors in some, but not all cases. Risk for melanoma development is increased in Parkinson's disease patients; drug causation or factors contributing to risk have not been established. Patients should be monitored closely and periodic skin examinations should be performed.

Patients must be cautioned about performing tasks which require mental alertness. **[Canadian Boxed Warning]:** Patients have reported falling asleep while engaging in activities of daily living and sometimes without significant warning signs. Monitor for daytime somnolence or preexisting sleep disorder; discontinue if significant daytime sleepiness or episodes of falling asleep occur. Use with caution in patients receiving other CNS depressants or psychoactive agents; effects with other sedative drugs or ethanol may be potentiated.

Distribute dietary protein throughout the day to avoid fluctuations of levodopa absorption. Use with caution in the elderly; may be more sensitive to CNS effects of levodopa.

Adverse Reactions

Cardiovascular: Arrhythmias, chest pain, edema, ECG changes (nonspecific), flushing, hypertension, orthostatic hypotension, pallor, phlebitis

Central nervous system: Agitation, anxiety, ataxia, bruxism, confusion, delusions, dementia, depression, euphoria, faintness, fatigue, fever, gait abnormalities, hallucinations (mostly visual), headache, impulse control symptoms (including pathological gambling), insomnia, lethargy, malaise, neuroleptic malignant-like syndrome, nightmares, oculogyric crisis, on-off phenomena, paranoid ideation, psychotic episodes, sedation, seizures, somnolence, suicidal tendencies/behavior, temporal disorientation, trismus

Dermatological: Alopecia, pruritus, rash

Endocrine & metabolic: Libido increased, protein-bound iodine increased, uric acid increased

Gastrointestinal: Abdominal distress or pain, anorexia, burning sensation on tongue, constipation, diarrhea, duodenal ulcer, dysphagia, epigastric pain, eructation, flatulence, GI bleeding, nausea, sialorrhea, taste alterations, vomiting, weight gain/loss, xerostomia

Genitourinary: Discoloration of urine, hematuria, nocturia, urinary frequency, urinary retention or incontinence

Hematologic: Agranulocytosis, hemolytic anemia (rare), leukopenia (transient), Positive Coombs' test, thrombocytopenia

Hepatic: Alkaline phosphatase increased, bilirubin increased, LDH increased, transaminases increased

Neuromuscular & skeletal: Akinesia paradoxica, choreiform and involuntary movements, dystonia, end-of-dose akinesia, hand tremor, low back pain, muscle spasm and twitching, musculoskeletal pain, numbness, torticollis, weakness

Ocular: Activation of latent Horner's syndrome, blepharospasm, blurred vision, diplopia, diluted pupils

Renal: BUN increased

Respiratory: Bizarre breathing pattern, cough, hoarseness, postnasal drip

Miscellaneous: Diaphoresis, discoloration of sweat, hiccups, hypersensitivity reactions, lip/mouth/tongue tightness

Drug Interactions

Metabolism/Transport Effects None known.

Avoid Concomitant Use

Avoid concomitant use of Benserazide and Levodopa with any of the following: Amisulpride; Sulpiride

Increased Effect/Toxicity

Benserazide and Levodopa may increase the levels/effects of: BuPROPion; MAO Inhibitors

The levels/effects of Benserazide and Levodopa may be increased by: Hypotensive Agents; Methylphenidate; Papaverine; Sapropterin

Decreased Effect

Benserazide and Levodopa may decrease the levels/effects of: Amisulpride; Antipsychotic Agents (First Generation [Typical]); Sulpiride

The levels/effects of Benserazide and Levodopa may be decreased by: Amisulpride; Antipsychotic Agents (First Generation [Typical]); Antipsychotic Agents (Second Generation [Atypical]); Fosphenytoin; Glycopyrrolate; Iron Salts; Isoniazid; Methionine; Metoclopramide; Multivitamins/Fluoride (with ADE); Multivitamins/Minerals (with ADEK, Folate, Iron); Multivitamins/Minerals (with AE, No Iron); Papaverine; Phenytoin; Pyridoxine; Sulpiride

Food Interactions High-protein diets may decrease effect of levodopa; food impairs or reduces the rate and extent of levodopa absorption (15% to 30%). Iron salts (ferrous sulfate) may decrease the absorption of levodopa. Management: Administer with or immediately after meals.

Storage/Stability Store at 15°C to 30°C (59°F to 86°F). Protect from light.

Mechanism of Action Symptoms of Parkinson's disease are due to a lack of striatal dopamine. Levodopa crosses into the blood-brain barrier (BBB) and is converted to dopamine by striatal enzymes. Benserazide inhibits the peripheral plasma breakdown of levodopa by inhibiting its decarboxylation and therefore increases levodopa availability at the BBB.

Pharmacodynamics/Kinetics

Absorption: Benserazide: 66% to 74% from GI tract

Distribution:

- Benserazide: Does not cross the blood-brain barrier; mainly concentrated in kidneys, liver, lungs, and small intestine
- Levodopa: 57 L; crosses the blood-brain barrier and not bound to plasma proteins

Metabolism:

- Benserazide: Hydroxylated to trihydroxybenzylhydrazine, a potent inhibitor of decarboxylase
- Levodopa: Major pathways: Decarboxylation and O-methylation; Minor pathways; Transamination and oxidation

Bioavailability: Levodopa: 98% (range: 74% to 112%)

Half-life elimination: Levodopa: 1.5 hours; 3-O-methyldopa (major metabolite): 15 hours

Time to peak, serum: ~1 hour

Excretion: Benserazide: Urine (64%); feces (24%)

Dosage Oral: Adults: **Note:** Dosage expressed as levodopa/benserazide. Dosage should be introduced gradually, individualized, and continued for 3-6 weeks before assessing benefit.

Patients currently receiving levodopa therapy: Discontinue levodopa ≥12 hours prior to the initiation of therapy; start at 15% of previous levodopa dose.

Patients **NOT** on levodopa therapy: Initial: 100/25 mg 1-2 times/day; increase dose by 100/25 mg every 3-4 days until therapeutic effect; usual optimal dosage: 400/100 mg to 800/200 mg divided into 4-6 doses

Note: The 200/50 mg capsules should be used only when maintenance therapy is reached. The 50/12.5 mg capsules should be used to decrease adverse effects when adjusting dose. Total daily dose during the first year of therapy should not exceed 1000-1200 mg of levodopa. After 1 year of therapy, the maximum recommended daily dose of levodopa is 600 mg/day.

Patients experiencing dystonia: Dosage reduction is recommended

Brief interruption of therapy: Reinitiate therapy at previous dose when patient is able to resume treatment.

Extended interruption of therapy: Reinitiate therapy at a lower dose and adjust gradually when patient is able to resume treatment

Dosage adjustment in renal impairment: There are no dosage adjustments provided in manufacturer's labeling. Use in decompensated renal disease is contraindicated.

Dosage adjustment in hepatic impairment: There are no dosage adjustments provided in manufacturer's labeling. Use in decompensated hepatic disease is contraindicated.

Dietary Considerations High-protein diets may decrease effect of levodopa.

Administration Administer with or immediately after meals. Capsules should be swallowed whole; do not crush, chew, open, or dissolve in liquid.

Monitoring Parameters Regular assessment of cardiovascular, hepatic, hematopoietic, and renal function; monitor blood glucose in patients with diabetes; symptoms of psychosis and dystonia

Additional Information Not available in U.S.

"On-off" (a clinical syndrome characterized by sudden periods of drug activity/inactivity) can be managed by giving smaller, more frequent doses or adding a dopamine agonist or selegiline. Protein in the diet should be distributed throughout the day to avoid fluctuations in levodopa absorption.

Product Availability Not available in U.S.

Dosage Forms: Canada

Capsule:

Prolopa®: 50-12.5: Levodopa 50 mg and benserazide 12.5 mg; 100-25: Levodopa 100 mg and benserazide 25 mg; 200-50: Levodopa 200 mg and benserazide 50 mg

Bentoquatam (BEN toe kwa tam)

Brand Names: U.S. Ivy Block [OTC]

Index Terms Quaternium-18 Bentonite

Pharmacologic Category Topical Skin Product

Use Skin protectant for the prevention of poison ivy, poison oak, and poison sumac

Dosage Skin protectant: Children ≥6 years and Adults: Topical: Apply to skin 15 minutes prior to potential exposure to poison ivy, poison oak, or poison sumac; may reapply every 4 hours

Additional Information Complete prescribing information should be consulted for additional detail.

Dosage Forms

Lotion, topical:

Ivy Block [OTC]: 5% (30 mL, 120 mL)

- ◆ **Bentyl** *see* Dicyclomine *on page 622*
- ◆ **Bentylol (Can)** *see* Dicyclomine *on page 622*
- ◆ **Benuryl (Can)** *see* Probenecid *on page 1716*
- ◆ **Benylin® 3.3 mg-D-E (Can)** *see* Guaifenesin, Pseudoephedrine, and Codeine *on page 989*
- ◆ **Benylin® D for Infants (Can)** *see* Pseudoephedrine *on page 1742*
- ◆ **Benylin Cough and Chest Congestion (Can)** *see* Guaifenesin, Pseudoephedrine, and Dextromethorphan *on page 989*
- ◆ **Benylin Cough Plus Cold Relief (Can)** *see* Guaifenesin, Pseudoephedrine, and Dextromethorphan *on page 989*
- ◆ **Benylin® DM-D (Can)** *see* Pseudoephedrine and Dextromethorphan *on page 1743*
- ◆ **Benylin DM-E (Can)** *see* Guaifenesin and Dextromethorphan *on page 987*
- ◆ **Benylin® E Extra Strength (Can)** *see* GuaiFENesin *on page 986*
- ◆ **Benzacyclane Fumarate** *see* Bencyclane [INT] *on page 241*
- ◆ **Benzamycin®** *see* Erythromycin and Benzoyl Peroxide *on page 765*
- ◆ **Benzamycin® Pak** *see* Erythromycin and Benzoyl Peroxide *on page 765*
- ◆ **Benzathine Benzylpenicillin** *see* Penicillin G Benzathine *on page 1609*
- ◆ **Benzathine Penicillin G** *see* Penicillin G Benzathine *on page 1609*
- ◆ **Benzene Hexachloride** *see* Lindane *on page 1217*
- ◆ **Benzhexol Hydrochloride** *see* Trihexyphenidyl *on page 2103*
- ◆ **Benzmethyzin** *see* Procarbazine *on page 1717*

Benzocaine (BEN zoe kane)

Brand Names: U.S. Anacaine; Anbesol Cold Sore Therapy [OTC]; Anbesol JR [OTC]; Anbesol Maximum Strength [OTC]; Anbesol [OTC]; Baby Anbesol [OTC]; Benz-O-Sthetic [OTC]; Benzocaine Oral Anesthetic [OTC]; Bi-Zets/Benzotroches [OTC]; Cepacol Dual Relief [OTC]; Cepacol Sensations Hydra [OTC]; Cepacol Sensations Warming [OTC]; Cepacol Sore Throat + Coating [OTC]; Cepacol Sore Throat Max Numb [OTC]; Cepacol Sore Throat [OTC]; Chiggerex [OTC]; Chiggertox [OTC]; Dent-O-Kain/20 [OTC]; Dentapaine [OTC]; Foille [OTC]; Hurri-Caine One [OTC]; Hurricaine [OTC]; Ivy-Rid [OTC]; Kank-A Mouth Pain [OTC]; Ora-film [OTC]; Oral Pain Relief Max St [OTC]; Pinnacaine Otic; Sore Throat Relief [OTC]; Topex Topical Anesthetic; Trocaine Throat [OTC]; Zilactin Baby [OTC]

Brand Names: Canada Anbesol® Baby; Zilactin Baby®; Zilactin-B®

Index Terms Ethyl Aminobenzoate

Pharmacologic Category Antihemorrhoidal Agent; Local Anesthetic

Use Temporary relief of pain associated with pruritic dermatosis, pruritus, minor burns, acute congestive, bee stings, and insect bites; mouth and gum irritations (toothache, minor sore throat pain, canker sores, dentures, orthodontia, teething, mucositis, stomatitis); sunburn; hemorrhoids; anesthetic lubricant for passage of catheters and endoscopic tubes

Pregnancy Risk Factor C

Dosage Note: These are general dosing guidelines; refer to specific product labeling for dosing instructions.

Children ≥4 months: Topical (oral): Teething pain: 7.5% to 10%: Apply to affected gum area up to 4 times daily

Children ≥2 years and Adults:

Topical:

Bee stings, insect bites, minor burns, sunburn: 5% to 20%: Apply to affected area 3-4 times daily as needed. In cases of bee stings, remove stinger before treatment.

Boils: 20%: Apply to affected area up to 2 times daily (maximum: 2 times/day)

Lubricant for passage of catheters and instruments: 20%: Apply evenly to exterior of instrument prior to use.

Topical (oral): Mouth and gum irritation: 10% to 20%: Apply thin layer to affected area up to 4 times daily

Children ≥5 years and Adults: Oral: Sore throat: Allow 1 lozenge (10-15 mg) to dissolve slowly in mouth; may repeat every 2 hours as needed

Children ≥6 years and Adults: Topical (oral) spray: 5%: Sore throat or mouth: One spray to affected area, then wait ≥1 minute and spit; may repeat up to 4 times daily. **Note:** Children 6-11 years should only use under adult supervision.

Children ≥12 years and Adults: Rectal: Hemorrhoids: 5% to 20%: Apply externally to affected area up to 6 times daily

Additional Information Complete prescribing information should be consulted for additional detail.

Dosage Forms

Aerosol, External:

Ivy-Rid [OTC]: 2% (82.5 mL)

Gel, Mouth/Throat:
Anbesol [OTC]: 10% (9 g)
Anbesol JR [OTC]: 10% (9 g)
Anbesol Maximum Strength [OTC]: 20% (9 g)
Baby Anbesol [OTC]: 7.5% (9 g)
Benz-O-Sthetic [OTC]: 20% (15 g, 29 g)
Dentapaine [OTC]: 20% (11 g)
Hurricaine [OTC]: 20% (5.25 g, 28.4 g, 30 g)
Zilactin Baby [OTC]: 10% (9.4 g)
Liquid, External:
Chiggertox [OTC]: 2.1% (30 mL)
Liquid, Mouth/Throat:
Anbesol [OTC]: 10% (12 mL)
Anbesol Maximum Strength [OTC]: 20% (12 mL)
Benz-O-Sthetic [OTC]: 20% (56 g)
Cepacol Dual Relief [OTC]: 5% (22.2 mL)
Dent-O-Kain/20 [OTC]: 20% (9 mL)
Oral Pain Relief Max St [OTC]: 20% (15 mL)
Lozenge, Mouth/Throat:
Bi-Zets/Benzotroches [OTC]: 15 mg (10 ea)
Cepacol Sensations Hydra [OTC]: 3 mg (20 ea)
Cepacol Sensations Warming [OTC]: 4 mg (20 ea)
Cepacol Sore Throat [OTC]: 15 mg (576 ea); 15% (16 ea); 15 mg (16 ea)
Cepacol Sore Throat + Coating [OTC]: 15 mg (16 ea)
Cepacol Sore Throat Max Numb [OTC]: 15 mg (16 ea)
Sore Throat Relief [OTC]: 10 mg (2 ea)
Trocaine Throat [OTC]: 10 mg (1 ea)
Ointment, External:
Anacaine: 10% (30 g)
Anbesol Cold Sore Therapy [OTC]: 20% (9 g)
Chiggerex [OTC]: 2% (52.5 g)
Foille [OTC]: 5% (28 g)
Solution, Mouth/Throat:
Benz-O-Sthetic [OTC]: 20% (30 mL)
Benzocaine Oral Anesthetic [OTC]: 20% (59.7 g)
Hurricaine [OTC]: 20% (57 g, 30 mL)
HurriCaine One [OTC]: 20% (2 ea, 25 ea)
Kank-A Mouth Pain [OTC]: 20% (9.75 mL)
Topex Topical Anesthetic: 20% (57 g)
Solution, Otic:
Pinnacaine Otic: 20% (15 mL)
Strip, Mouth/Throat:
Ora-film [OTC]: 6% (12 ea)
Swab, Mouth/Throat:
Benz-O-Sthetic [OTC]: 20% (2 ea)
Hurricaine [OTC]: 20% (72 ea)

◆ **Benzocaine and Antipyrine** *see* Antipyrine and Benzocaine *on page 156*

◆ **Benzocaine and Cetylpyridinium** *see* Cetylpyridinium and Benzocaine [CAN/INT] *on page 415*

◆ **Benzocaine and Cetylpyridinium Chloride** *see* Cetylpyridinium and Benzocaine [CAN/INT] *on page 415*

Benzocaine, Butamben, and Tetracaine

(BEN zoe kane, byoo TAM ben, & TET ra kane)

Brand Names: U.S. Cetacaine

Index Terms Benzocaine, Butamben, and Tetracaine Hydrochloride; Benzocaine, Butyl Aminobenzoate, and Tetracaine; Butamben, Tetracaine, and Benzocaine; Exactacain; Tetracaine, Benzocaine, and Butamben

Pharmacologic Category Local Anesthetic

Use Topical anesthetic to control pain in surgical or endoscopic procedures, or other procedures in the ear, nose, mouth, pharynx, larynx, trachea, bronchi, and esophagus (may also be used for vaginal or rectal procedure, when feasible); anesthetic for accessible mucous membranes except for the eyes; to control pain or gagging (spray only)

Dosage Topical anesthetic: **Note:** Decrease dose in the acutely-ill patient.
Children: Dose has not been established; dose reduction is suggested
Adults: Cetacaine:
Spray: Apply for ≤1 second; use of sprays >2 seconds is contraindicated. **Note:** Spray provides ~200 mg/second
Gel: Apply 200 mg (~1/4 to 1/2 inch); application of >400 mg (>1 inch) is contraindicated
Liquid: Apply 200 mg (~0.2 mL); application of >400 mg (~0.4 mL) is contraindicated
Elderly: Dose reduction is suggested

Dosage adjustment in renal impairment: No dosage adjustment provided in manufacturer's labeling.
Dosage adjustment in hepatic impairment: No dosage adjustment provided in manufacturer's labeling.

Additional Information Complete prescribing information should be consulted for additional detail.

Dosage Forms
Aerosol, spray, topical [kit]:
Cetacaine: Benzocaine 14%, butamben 2%, and tetracaine 2% (56 g)
Aerosol, spray, topical:
Cetacaine: Benzocaine 14%, butamben 2%, and tetracaine 2% (56 g)
Cetacaine: Benzocaine 14%, butamben 2%, and tetracaine 2% (32 g)
Liquid, topical, kit:
Cetacaine: Benzocaine 14%, butamben 2%, and tetracaine 2% (14 g)
Liquid, topical:
Cetacaine: Benzocaine 14%, butamben 2%, and tetracaine 2% (14 g, 30 g)

◆ **Benzocaine, Butamben, and Tetracaine Hydrochloride** *see* Benzocaine, Butamben, and Tetracaine *on page 247*

◆ **Benzocaine, Butyl Aminobenzoate, and Tetracaine** *see* Benzocaine, Butamben, and Tetracaine *on page 247*

◆ **Benzocaine Oral Anesthetic [OTC]** *see* Benzocaine *on page 246*

◆ **Benzoic Acid, Hyoscyamine, Methenamine, Methylene Blue, and Phenyl Salicylate** *see* Methenamine, Phenyl Salicylate, Methylene Blue, Benzoic Acid, and Hyoscyamine *on page 1318*

◆ **Benzoic Acid, Methenamine, Methylene Blue, Phenyl Salicylate, and Hyoscyamine** *see* Methenamine, Phenyl Salicylate, Methylene Blue, Benzoic Acid, and Hyoscyamine *on page 1318*

Benzonatate (ben ZOE na tate)

Brand Names: U.S. Tessalon Perles; Zonatuss

Index Terms Tessalon Perles

Pharmacologic Category Antitussive

Use Symptomatic relief of nonproductive cough

Pregnancy Risk Factor C

Dosage Children >10 years and Adults: Oral: 100-200 mg 3 times/day as needed for cough; maximum dose: 600 mg/day
Dosage adjustment in renal impairment: No dosage adjustment provided in manufacturer's labeling.
Dosage adjustment in hepatic impairment: No dosage adjustment provided in manufacturer's labeling.

Additional Information Complete prescribing information should be consulted for additional detail.

Dosage Forms
Capsule, Oral:
Tessalon Perles: 100 mg
Zonatuss: 150 mg
Generic: 100 mg, 200 mg

◆ **Benz-O-Sthetic [OTC]** *see* Benzocaine *on page 246*

◆ **Benzoyl Peroxide and Adapalene** *see* Adapalene and Benzoyl Peroxide *on page 54*

◆ **Benzoyl Peroxide and Erythromycin** *see* Erythromycin and Benzoyl Peroxide *on page 765*

Benzoyl Peroxide and Hydrocortisone

(BEN zoe il peer OKS ide & hye droe KOR ti sone)

Brand Names: U.S. Vanoxide-HC®

Brand Names: Canada Vanoxide-HC®

Index Terms Hydrocortisone and Benzoyl Peroxide

Pharmacologic Category Acne Products; Topical Skin Product; Topical Skin Product, Acne

Use Treatment of acne vulgaris and oily skin

Pregnancy Risk Factor C

Dosage Adolescents ≥12 years and Adults: Topical: Apply thin film 1-3 times/day

Additional Information Complete prescribing information should be consulted for additional detail.

Dosage Forms

Lotion, topical:

Vanoxide-HC®: Benzoyl peroxide 5% and hydrocortisone 0.5% (25 mL)

Benztropine (BENZ troe peen)

Brand Names: U.S. Cogentin

Brand Names: Canada Benztropine Omega; Kynesia; PMS-Benztropine

Index Terms Benztropine Mesylate

Pharmacologic Category Anti-Parkinson's Agent, Anticholinergic; Anticholinergic Agent

Additional Appendix Information

Beers Criteria – Potentially Inappropriate Medications for Geriatrics *on page 2271*

Use

Extrapyramidal disorders: Aid in the control of extrapyramidal disorders (except tardive dyskinesia) due to neuroleptic drugs (eg, phenothiazines).

Parkinsonism: Adjunctive therapy of all forms of parkinsonism.

Pregnancy Considerations Animal reproduction studies have not been conducted. Paralytic ileus (which resolved rapidly) was reported in two newborns exposed to a combination of benztropine and chlorpromazine during the second and third trimesters and the last 6 weeks of pregnancy, respectively (Falterman, 1980).

Breast-Feeding Considerations It is not known if benztropine is excreted in breast milk. Anticholinergic agents may suppress lactation.

Contraindications Hypersensitivity to benztropine or any component of the formulation; children <3 years of age (due to atropine-like adverse effects)

Warnings/Precautions May cause anticholinergic effects (constipation, xerostomia, blurred vision, urinary retention). Use with caution in children >3 years of age due to its anticholinergic effects (dose has not been established). Use is contraindicated in children <3 years of age. Use with caution in hot weather or during exercise. May cause anhydrosis and hyperthermia, which may be severe. The risk is increased in hot environments, particularly in the elderly, alcoholics, patients with CNS disease, and those with prolonged outdoor exposure. If there is evidence of anhidrosis, consider decreasing dose so the ability to maintain body heat equilibrium by perspiration is not impaired.

Use with caution in patients >65 years of age; response in elderly may be altered. Initiate at low doses in the elderly and increase as needed while monitoring for adverse events. Avoid use of oral benztropine in older adults for prevention of extrapyramidal symptoms with antipsychotics and alternative agents preferred in the treatment of Parkinson's disease. May be inappropriate in older adults depending on comorbidities (eg, dementia, delirium) due to its potent anticholinergic effects (Beers Criteria). Avoid use in angle-closure glaucoma.

Use with caution in patients with tachycardia, glaucoma, prostatic hyperplasia (especially in the elderly), any tendency toward urinary retention, and obstructive disease of the GI or GU tracts. When given in large doses or to susceptible patients, may cause weakness and inability to move particular muscle groups.

May be associated with confusion, visual hallucinations, or excitement (generally at higher dosages). Intensification of symptoms or toxic psychosis may occur in patients with mental disorders. May cause CNS depression, which may impair physical or mental abilities; patients must be cautioned about performing tasks which require mental alertness (eg, operating machinery or driving). Benztropine does not relieve symptoms of tardive dyskinesia and may potentially exacerbate symptoms.

Potentially significant drug-drug interactions may exist, requiring dose or frequency adjustment, additional monitoring, and/or selection of alternative therapy.

Adverse Reactions

Cardiovascular: Tachycardia

Central nervous system: Confusion, depression, disorientation, heatstroke, hyperthermia, lethargy, memory impairment, nervousness, numbness of fingers, psychotic symptoms (exacerbation of preexisting symptoms), toxic psychosis, visual hallucination

Dermatologic: Skin rash

Gastrointestinal: Constipation, nausea, paralytic ileus, vomiting, xerostomia

Genitourinary: Dysuria, urinary retention

Ophthalmic: Blurred vision, mydriasis

Drug Interactions

Metabolism/Transport Effects Substrate of CYP2D6 (minor); **Note:** Assignment of Major/Minor substrate status based on clinically relevant drug interaction potential

Avoid Concomitant Use

Avoid concomitant use of Benztropine with any of the following: Aclidinium; Glucagon; Ipratropium (Oral Inhalation); Potassium Chloride; Tiotropium; Umeclidinium

Increased Effect/Toxicity

Benztropine may increase the levels/effects of: AbobotulinumtoxinA; Analgesics (Opioid); Anticholinergic Agents; Cannabinoid-Containing Products; Glucagon; Mirabegron; OnabotulinumtoxinA; Potassium Chloride; RimabotulinumtoxinB; Thiazide Diuretics; Tiotropium; Topiramate

The levels/effects of Benztropine may be increased by: Aclidinium; Ipratropium (Oral Inhalation); Mianserin; Pramlintide; Umeclidinium

Decreased Effect

Benztropine may decrease the levels/effects of: Acetylcholinesterase Inhibitors; Ioflupane I 123; Itopride; Secretin

The levels/effects of Benztropine may be decreased by: Acetylcholinesterase Inhibitors

Storage/Stability Store at 20°C to 25°C (68°F to 77°F).

Mechanism of Action Possesses both anticholinergic and antihistaminic effects. *In vitro* anticholinergic activity approximates that of atropine; *in vivo* it is only about half as active as atropine. Animal data suggest its antihistaminic activity and duration of action approach that of pyrilamine maleate.

Pharmacodynamics/Kinetics

Onset of action: IM, IV: Within a few minutes; there is no significant difference between onset of effect after intravenous or intramuscular injection

Metabolism: Hepatic (N-oxidation, N-dealkylation, and ring hydroxylation) (from animal studies only) (Brocks, 1999)
Time to peak, plasma: Oral: 7 hours (Brocks, 1999)

Dosage

Drug-induced extrapyramidal symptoms: Oral, IM, IV:
Children ≥3 years (off-label dose): 0.02 to 0.05 mg/kg/dose 1 to 2 times daily (Bellman, 1974; Habre, 1999; Joseph, 1995; Teoh, 2002)
Adolescents (off-label dose): 1 to 4 mg every 12 to 24 hours (Nelson, 1996)
Adults:
Initial: 1 to 2 mg 2 to 3 times daily for reactions developing soon after initiation of antipsychotic medication. Usually provides relief within 1 to 2 days. Titrate gradually at 0.5 mg increments at 5- to 6-day intervals based on response and tolerability. Usual dosage is 1 to 4 mg once or twice daily up to a maximum daily dose of 6 mg. Treatment may be continued for 1 to 2 weeks, after which treatment should be withdrawn to reassess continued need for therapy. May reinitiate benztropine if symptoms recur (Holloman, 1997; Tonda, 1994). **Note:** Certain drug-induced extrapyramidal disorders that develop slowly may not respond to benztropine.
Acute dystonic reactions: 1 to 2 mg to treat acute reactions followed by 1 to 2 mg (orally) 1 to 2 times daily for up to 7 to 28 days to prevent recurrence. **Note:** IM/IV administration is preferred over oral administration for severe acute reactions due to the faster onset of action (Holloman, 1997; Tonda, 1994).

Parkinsonism: Adults: Oral, IM, IV:
Idiopathic parkinsonism: Initial: 0.5 to 1 mg daily at bedtime or in 2 to 4 divided doses. Titrate in 0.5 mg increments every 5 to 6 days based on response and tolerability. Usual dose: 1 to 2 mg daily (range: 0.5 to 6 mg daily) although some patients may need 4 to 6 mg daily; maximum: 6 mg daily
Postencephalitic parkinsonism: Initial: 2 mg daily as a single dose at bedtime or in 2 to 4 divided doses; a lower initial dose of 0.5 mg at bedtime may be considered in highly sensitive patients. Titrate in 0.5 mg increments every 5 to 6 days based on response and tolerability. Usual dose: 1 to 2 mg daily (range: 0.5 to 6 mg daily); maximum: 6 mg daily.
Note: Lower initial doses may be appropriate for older and thinner patients.

Elderly: Use caution or avoid; anticholinergics generally not tolerated in older adults. If used, start at low end of dosing range and increase only as needed and as tolerated.

Dosage adjustment in renal impairment: There are no dosage adjustments provided in the manufacturer's labeling.

Dosage adjustment in hepatic impairment: There are no dosage adjustments provided in the manufacturer's labeling.

Dietary Considerations Tablet may be taken with or without food.

Administration

Oral: Administer with or without food.
Injectable: Administer IM or IV if oral route is unacceptable. Manufacturer's labeling states there is no difference in onset of effect after IV or IM injection and therefore there is usually no need to use the IV route. No specific instructions on administering benztropine IV are provided in the labeling. The IV route has been reported in the literature (slow IV push when reported), although specific instructions are lacking (Duncan, 2001; Lydon, 1998; Sachdev, 1993; Schramm, 2002).

Monitoring Parameters Pulse, anticholinergic effects

Dosage Forms

Solution, Injection:
Cogentin: 1 mg/mL (2 mL)
Generic: 1 mg/mL (2 mL)

Tablet, Oral:
Generic: 0.5 mg, 1 mg, 2 mg

◆ **Benztropine Mesylate** *see* Benztropine *on page 248*
◆ **Benztropine Omega (Can)** *see* Benztropine *on page 248*

Benzydamine [CAN/INT] (ben ZID a meen)

Brand Names: Canada Apo-Benzydamine; Dom-Benzydamine; Novo-Benzydamine; Pharixia; Tantum

Index Terms Benzydamine Hydrochloride

Pharmacologic Category Local Anesthetic, Oral

Use Note: Not approved in U.S.
Symptomatic treatment of pain associated with acute pharyngitis; treatment of pain associated with radiation-induced oropharyngeal mucositis

Pregnancy Considerations Safety has not been established in pregnant women. Use only when potential benefit outweighs possible risk to the fetus.

Breast-Feeding Considerations It is not known if benzydamine is excreted in breast milk. The manufacturer recommends that caution be exercised when administering benzydamine peroxide to nursing women.

Contraindications Hypersensitivity to benzydamine or any component of the formulation

Warnings/Precautions May cause local irritation and/or burning sensation in patients with altered mucosal integrity. Dilution (1:1 in warm water) may attenuate this effect. Use caution in renal impairment.

Adverse Reactions

Central nervous system: Drowsiness, headache
Gastrointestinal: Nausea, vomiting, xerostomia
Local: Burning/stinging sensation, numbness
Respiratory: Cough, pharyngeal irritation

Drug Interactions

Metabolism/Transport Effects None known.

Avoid Concomitant Use There are no known interactions where it is recommended to avoid concomitant use.

Increased Effect/Toxicity There are no known significant interactions involving an increase in effect.

Decreased Effect There are no known significant interactions involving a decrease in effect.

Storage/Stability Store at 15°C to 30°C; protect from freezing.

Mechanism of Action Local anesthetic and anti-inflammatory, reduces local pain and inflammation. Does not interfere with arachidonic acid metabolism.

Pharmacodynamics/Kinetics

Absorption: Oral rinse may be absorbed, at least in part, through the oral mucosa
Excretion: Urine (primarily as unchanged drug)

Dosage Oral rinse: Adults:
Acute pharyngitis: Gargle with 15 mL of undiluted solution every 1½-3 hours until symptoms resolve. Patient should expel solution from mouth following use; solution should not be swallowed.
Mucositis: 15 mL of undiluted solution as a gargle or rinse 3-4 times/day; contact should be maintained for at least 30 seconds, followed by expulsion from the mouth
Dosage adjustment in renal impairment: No adjustment required.

Administration Patient should not swallow the liquid. Begin treatment 1 day prior to initiation of radiation therapy and continue daily during treatment. Continue oral rinse treatments after the completion of radiation therapy until desired result/healing is achieved.

Product Availability Not available in U.S.

Dosage Forms: Canada

Oral rinse: 0.15% (100 mL, 250 mL)

◆ **Benzydamine Hydrochloride** *see* Benzydamine [CAN/INT] *on page 249*

Benzyl Alcohol (BEN zill AL koe hol)

Brand Names: U.S. Ulesfia; Zilactin [OTC]

Pharmacologic Category Analgesic, Topical; Antiparasitic Agent, Topical; Pediculocide; Topical Skin Product

Use

Oral pain (gel only): Temporary relief of pain from cold sores/fever blisters, canker sores, mouth sores, and/or gum irritations

Head lice (lotion only): Treatment of head lice infestation in patients 6 months and older

Pregnancy Risk Factor B

Dosage Topical:

Gel: Oral pain: Children ≥2 years, Adolescents, and Adults: Apply to affected area up to 4 times daily

Lotion: Head lice: Infants ≥6 months, Children, Adolescents, and Adults: Apply appropriate volume for hair length to dry hair and completely saturate the scalp; leave on for 10 minutes; rinse thoroughly with water; repeat in 7 days

Hair length 0 to 2 inches: 4 to 6 ounces
Hair length 2 to 4 inches: 6 to 8 ounces
Hair length 4 to 8 inches: 8 to 12 ounces
Hair length 8 to 16 inches: 12 to 24 ounces
Hair length 16 to 22 inches: 24 to 32 ounces
Hair length >22 inches: 32 to 48 ounces

Dosage adjustment in renal impairment: There are no dosage adjustments provided in the manufacturer's labeling.

Dosage adjustment in hepatic impairment: There are no dosage adjustments provided in the manufacturer's labeling.

Additional Information Complete prescribing information should be consulted for additional detail.

Dosage Forms

Gel, Mouth/Throat:

Zilactin [OTC]: 10% (7.1 g)

Lotion, External:

Ulesfia: 5% (227 g)

◆ **Benzylpenicillin Benzathine** *see* Penicillin G Benzathine *on page 1609*

◆ **Benzylpenicillin Potassium** *see* Penicillin G (Parenteral/Aqueous) *on page 1611*

◆ **Benzylpenicillin Sodium** *see* Penicillin G (Parenteral/Aqueous) *on page 1611*

Benzylthiouracil [INT] (BEN zil thye oh YOOR a sil)

International Brand Names Basdene (FR)

Pharmacologic Category Antithyroid Agent

Reported Use Treatment of hyperthyroidism

Dosage Range Adults: Oral: Initial: 150-200 mg/day in 3-4 divided doses; may decrease to 100 mg/day after several weeks

Product Availability Product available in various countries; not currently available in the U.S.

Dosage Forms

Tablet: 25 mg

Bepotastine (be poe TAS teen)

Brand Names: U.S. Bepreve

Index Terms Bepotastine Besilate

Pharmacologic Category Histamine H_1 Antagonist; Histamine H_1 Antagonist, Second Generation; Mast Cell Stabilizer

Use Treatment of itching associated with allergic conjunctivitis

Pregnancy Risk Factor C

Dosage Ophthalmic: Children ≥2 years and Adults: Allergic conjunctivitis: Instill 1 drop into the affected eye(s) twice daily

Additional Information Complete prescribing information should be consulted for additional detail.

Dosage Forms

Solution, Ophthalmic:

Bepreve: 1.5% (5 mL, 10 mL)

◆ **Bepotastine Besilate** *see* Bepotastine *on page 250*

◆ **Bepreve** *see* Bepotastine *on page 250*

Beractant (ber AKT ant)

Brand Names: U.S. Survanta

Brand Names: Canada Survanta®

Index Terms Bovine Lung Surfactant; Natural Lung Surfactant

Pharmacologic Category Lung Surfactant

Use Prevention and treatment of respiratory distress syndrome (RDS) in premature infants

Prophylactic therapy: Body weight <1250 g in infants at risk for developing, or with evidence of, surfactant deficiency (administer within 15 minutes of birth)

Rescue therapy: Treatment of infants with RDS confirmed by x-ray and requiring mechanical ventilation (administer as soon as possible - within 8 hours of age)

Pregnancy Considerations Beractant is only indicated for use in premature infants.

Contraindications There are no contraindications listed within the FDA-approved labeling

Warnings/Precautions For endotracheal administration only. Rapidly affects oxygenation and lung compliance; restrict use to a highly-supervised clinical setting with immediate availability of clinicians experienced in intubation and ventilatory management of premature infants. Transient episodes of bradycardia and decreased oxygen saturation occur. Discontinue dosing procedure and initiate measures to alleviate the condition; may reinstitute after the patient is stable. Produces rapid improvements in lung oxygenation and compliance that may require frequent adjustments to oxygen delivery and ventilator settings.

Adverse Reactions During the dosing procedure:

Cardiovascular: Transient bradycardia

Respiratory: Oxygen desaturation

Rare but important or life-threatening: Apnea, endotracheal tube blockage, hypercarbia, hyper-/hypotension, post-treatment nosocomial sepsis probability increased, pulmonary air leaks, pulmonary interstitial emphysema, vasoconstriction

Drug Interactions

Metabolism/Transport Effects None known.

Avoid Concomitant Use

Avoid concomitant use of Beractant with any of the following: Ceritinib

Increased Effect/Toxicity

Beractant may increase the levels/effects of: Bradycardia-Causing Agents; Ceritinib; Lacosamide

The levels/effects of Beractant may be increased by: Bretylium; Tofacitinib

Decreased Effect There are no known significant interactions involving a decrease in effect.

Storage/Stability **Refrigerate**; protect from light. Prior to administration, warm by standing at room temperature for 20 minutes or held in hand for 8 minutes. **Artificial warming methods should not be used.** Unused, unopened vials warmed to room temperature may be returned to the refrigerator within 24 hours of warming only once.

Mechanism of Action Replaces deficient or ineffective endogenous lung surfactant in neonates with respiratory distress syndrome (RDS) or in neonates at risk of developing RDS. Surfactant prevents the alveoli from collapsing during expiration by lowering surface tension between air and alveolar surfaces.

Pharmacodynamics/Kinetics Excretion: Clearance: Alveolar clearance is rapid

Dosage

Endotracheal: Premature infants:

Prophylactic treatment: Administer 4 mL/kg (100 mg phospholipids/kg) as soon as possible; as many as 4 doses may be administered during the first 48 hours of life, no more frequently than 6 hours apart. The need for additional doses is determined by evidence of continuing respiratory distress; if the infant is still intubated and requiring at least 30% inspired oxygen to maintain a PaO_2 ≤80 torr.

Rescue treatment: Administer 4 mL/kg (100 mg phospholipids/kg) as soon as the diagnosis of RDS is made; may repeat if needed, no more frequently than every 6 hours to a maximum of 4 doses

Dosage adjustment in renal impairment: No dosage adjustment provided in manufacturer's labeling.

Dosage adjustment in hepatic impairment: No dosage adjustment provided in manufacturer's labeling.

Administration For endotracheal administration only

Suction infant prior to administration. Inspect solution to verify complete mixing of the suspension (may swirl gently, but DO NOT SHAKE). Do not filter dose and avoid shaking.

Administer endotracheally by instillation through a 5-French end-hole catheter inserted into the infant's endotracheal tube.

Administer the dose in four 1 mL/kg aliquots. Each quarter-dose is instilled over 2-3 seconds followed by at least 30 seconds of manual ventilation or until stable; each quarter-dose is administered with the infant in a different position. Slightly downward inclination with head turned to the right, then repeat with head turned to the left; then slightly upward inclination with head turned to the right, then repeat with head turned to the left. Following administration of one full dose, withhold suctioning for 1 hour unless signs of significant airway obstruction.

Monitoring Parameters Continuous ECG and transcutaneous O_2 saturation should be monitored during administration; frequent arterial blood gases are necessary to prevent postdosing hyperoxia and hypocarbia

Additional Information Each mL contains 25 mg phospholipids suspended in 0.9% sodium chloride solution. Contents of 1 mL: 0.5-1.75 mg triglycerides, 1.4-3.5 mg free fatty acids, and <1 mg protein.

Dosage Forms

Suspension, Inhalation:

Survanta: Phospholipids 25 mg/mL (4 mL, 8 mL)

Beraprost [INT] (BER a prost)

International Brand Names Bedoz (KR); Belnarl (JP); Beracle (KR); Berasil (KR); Berast (KR); Berasus (JP); Dorner (CN, ID, JP, PH, TH)

Index Terms Beraprost Sodium

Pharmacologic Category Prostaglandin

Reported Use Treatment of pulmonary hypertension

Dosage Range Adults: Oral: Primary pulmonary hypertension: 60-180 mcg/day in 3 divided doses

Product Availability Product available in various countries; not currently available in the U.S.

Dosage Forms

Tablet: 20 mcg

- ◆ **Beraprost Sodium** *see* Beraprost [INT] *on page 251*
- ◆ **Berinert** *see* C1 Inhibitor (Human) *on page 315*
- ◆ **Beriplex P/N** *see* Prothrombin Complex Concentrate (Human) [(Factors II, VII, IX, X), Protein C, and Protein S] *on page 1738*

Besifloxacin (be si FLOX a sin)

Brand Names: U.S. Besivance

Brand Names: Canada Besivance™

Index Terms Besifloxacin Hydrochloride; BOL-303224-A; SS734

Pharmacologic Category Antibiotic, Fluoroquinolone; Antibiotic, Ophthalmic

Use Treatment of bacterial conjunctivitis

Pregnancy Risk Factor C

Dosage Ophthalmic: Children ≥1 year and Adults: Bacterial conjunctivitis: Instill 1 drop into affected eye(s) 3 times/day (4-12 hours apart) for 7 days

Additional Information Complete prescribing information should be consulted for additional detail.

Dosage Forms

Suspension, Ophthalmic:

Besivance: 0.6% (5 mL)

- ◆ **Besifloxacin Hydrochloride** *see* Besifloxacin *on page 251*
- ◆ **Besivance** *see* Besifloxacin *on page 251*
- ◆ **Besivance™ (Can)** *see* Besifloxacin *on page 251*
- ◆ **β,β-Dimethylcysteine** *see* PenicillAMINE *on page 1608*
- ◆ **9-Beta-D-Ribofuranosyladenine** *see* Adenosine *on page 55*
- ◆ **Betacaine (Can)** *see* Lidocaine (Topical) *on page 1211*
- ◆ **Beta Care Betamide [OTC]** *see* Urea *on page 2114*

Beta-Carotene (BAY ta KARE oh teen)

Brand Names: U.S. A-Caro-25 [OTC]; B-Caro-T [OTC]; Caroguard [OTC]

Pharmacologic Category Vitamin, Fat Soluble

Use Prophylaxis against photosensitivity reactions in erythropoietic protoporphyria (EPP)

Dosage Oral: EPP (Lumitene™):

Children <14 years: 30-150 mg/day

Adults: 30-300 mg/day

Dosage adjustment in renal impairment: No dosage adjustment provided in manufacturer's labeling (has not been studied); use with caution.

Dosage adjustment in hepatic impairment: No dosage adjustment provided in manufacturer's labeling (has not been studied); use with caution.

Additional Information Complete prescribing information should be consulted for additional detail.

Dosage Forms

Capsule, Oral:

A-Caro-25 [OTC]: 25,000 units

Generic: 25,000 units

Capsule, Oral [preservative free]:

B-Caro-T [OTC]: 15 mg

Caroguard [OTC]: 15 mg

Generic: 25,000 units

- ◆ **Betaderm (Can)** *see* Betamethasone (Topical) *on page 255*
- ◆ **Betagan** *see* Levobunolol *on page 1194*
- ◆ **Betagan® (Can)** *see* Levobunolol *on page 1194*
- ◆ **Beta HC [OTC]** *see* Hydrocortisone (Topical) *on page 1014*

Betahistine [CAN/INT] (bay ta HISS teen)

Brand Names: Canada CO Betahistine; Serc; Teva-Betahistine

Index Terms Betahistine Dihydrochloride

Pharmacologic Category Histamine H_3 Antagonist; Histamine H_1 Agonist

Use Note: Not approved in U.S.

Ménière disease: Treatment of Ménière disease (to decrease episodes of vertigo)

Pregnancy Considerations There are no adequate and well-controlled studies in pregnant women. Should be used only when potential benefit to the woman outweighs possible risk to fetus.

Breast-Feeding Considerations It is not known if betahistine is excreted in breast milk. The manufacturer recommends that caution be exercised when administering betahistine to nursing women.

Contraindications Hypersensitivity to betahistine or any component of the formulation; peptic ulcer disease; pheochromocytoma

Warnings/Precautions Use caution in patients with asthma, hepatic impairment, or cardiovascular disease. Use is contraindicated in the presence or history of peptic ulcer.

Adverse Reactions

Central nervous system: Confusion, convulsions, drowsiness (case reports), hallucination, headache, paraesthesia

Cardiovascular: Hypotension (including orthostatic and postural hypotension), tachycardia, ventricular premature contractions (case reports)

Dermatologic: Pruritus, skin rash, Stevens-Johnson syndrome, urticaria

Gastrointestinal: Abdominal distension, abdominal pain, bloating, dyspepsia, nausea, peptic ulcer (including exacerbation of previous disease), vomiting

Hypersensitivity: Anaphylaxis, angioedema, hypersensitivity reaction

Respiratory: Dyspnea

Drug Interactions

Metabolism/Transport Effects None known.

Avoid Concomitant Use There are no known interactions where it is recommended to avoid concomitant use.

Increased Effect/Toxicity

The levels/effects of Betahistine may be increased by: MAO Inhibitors

Decreased Effect

Betahistine may decrease the levels/effects of: Beta2-Agonists

The levels/effects of Betahistine may be decreased by: Antihistamines

Storage/Stability Store at 15°C to 30°C (59°F to 86°F). Protect from moisture.

Mechanism of Action Agonist of histamine at H_1 receptor and antagonist at H_3 receptor; relatively inactive at H_2 receptor. Animal studies suggest that betahistine may increase cochlear blood flow and produce excitatory effects on neuronal activity of cortical and subcortical structures via H_1-receptor agonism and decrease vestibular sensory input and increase synthesis and release of histamine from the hypothalamus via H_3-receptor antagonism (Ihler, 2012; Lacour, 2007).

Pharmacodynamics/Kinetics

Absorption: Rapid, complete; delayed by food

T_{max}: 1 hour to reach peak levels of inactive metabolite

Protein binding: <5%

Metabolism: Rapid and almost complete hepatic metabolism to 2-pyridylacetic acid (inactive metabolite)

Half-life elimination: ~3.5 hours (inactive metabolite)

Excretion: Urine (~91%; primarily as inactive metabolite)

Dosage Ménière disease (to decrease episodes of vertigo):

Adults: Oral: 8-16 mg 3 times daily or 24 mg twice daily; usual dosage range: 24-48 mg daily in divided doses. Doses slowly titrated (ie, approximately every 3 months) up to 480 mg daily (off-label dosing) have been reported in a small number of cases with severe, resistant disease (Lezius, 2011).

Elderly: Refer to adult dosing; use with caution due to likelihood of decreased hepatic/renal function.

Dosage adjustment in renal impairment: No dosage adjustment provided in manufacturer's labeling (has not been studied); use with caution.

Dosage adjustment in hepatic impairment: No dosage adjustment provided in manufacturer's labeling (has not been studied). Betahistine primarily undergoes hepatic metabolism; use with caution.

Dietary Considerations May be taken with food to avoid adverse gastrointestinal effects.

Administration Administration with meals is recommended to avoid adverse gastrointestinal effects.

Product Availability Not available in U.S.

Dosage Forms: Canada

Tablet, oral: 8 mg, 16 mg, 24 mg

- ◆ **Betahistine Dihydrochloride** *see* Betahistine [CAN/INT] *on page 252*

Betaine (BAY ta een)

Brand Names: U.S. Cystadane

Brand Names: Canada Cystadane

Index Terms Betaine Anhydrous

Pharmacologic Category Homocystinuria, Treatment Agent

Use Homocystinuria: Treatment of homocystinuria including deficiencies or defects in cystathionine beta-synthase (CBS), 5,10-methylene tetrahydrofolate reductase (MTHFR), and cobalamin cofactor metabolism (CBL).

Pregnancy Risk Factor C

Dosage Homocystinuria: Oral:

Infants and Children <3 years: Initial dose: 100 mg/kg/day in 2 divided doses; increase weekly by 50 mg/kg increments, as needed

Children ≥3 years, Adolescents, and Adults: Usual dose: 3 g twice daily; dosages of up to 20 g/day have been necessary to control homocysteine levels in some patients

Note: Dosage in all patients can be gradually increased until plasma total homocysteine is undetectable or present only in small amounts. One in vitro study indicated minimal benefit from exceeding a twice daily dosing schedule and a 150 mg/kg/day dosage.

Dosage adjustment in renal impairment: There are no dosage adjustments provided in the manufacturer's labeling.

Dosage adjustment in hepatic impairment: There are no dosage adjustments provided in the manufacturer's labeling.

Additional Information Complete prescribing information should be consulted for additional detail.

Dosage Forms

Powder, Oral:

Cystadane: 1 g/scoop (180 g)

Tablet, Oral:

Generic: 300 mg

- ◆ **Betaine Anhydrous** *see* Betaine *on page 252*
- ◆ **Betaject (Can)** *see* Betamethasone (Systemic) *on page 253*
- ◆ **Betaloc (Can)** *see* Metoprolol *on page 1350*

Betamethasone (Systemic) (bay ta METH a sone)

Brand Names: U.S. Celestone Soluspan; Celestone [DSC]

Brand Names: Canada Betaject; Celestone Soluspan

Index Terms Betamethasone Acetate; Betamethasone Sodium Phosphate; Flubenisolone

Pharmacologic Category Corticosteroid, Systemic

Additional Appendix Information

Corticosteroids Systemic Equivalencies *on page 2228*

Use

Intramuscular:

Allergic states: Control of severe or incapacitating allergic conditions intractable to adequate trials of conventional treatment in asthma, atopic dermatitis, contact dermatitis, drug hypersensitivity reactions, perennial or seasonal allergic rhinitis, serum sickness, transfusion reactions

Dermatologic diseases: Bullous dermatitis herpetiformis, exfoliative erythroderma, mycosis fungoides, pemphigus, severe erythema multiforme (Stevens-Johnson syndrome)

Endocrine disorders: Congenital adrenal hyperplasia, hypercalcemia associated with cancer, nonsuppurative thyroiditis. Hydrocortisone or cortisone is the drug of choice in primary or secondary adrenocortical insufficiency. Synthetic analogs may be used in conjunction with mineralocorticoids where applicable; in infancy mineralocorticoid supplementation is of particular importance

Gastrointestinal diseases: To tide the patient over a critical period of the disease in regional enteritis and ulcerative colitis

Hematologic disorders: Acquired (autoimmune) hemolytic anemia, Diamond-Blackfan anemia, pure red cell aplasia, selected cases of secondary thrombocytopenia

Neoplastic diseases: Palliative management of leukemias and lymphomas

Nervous system: Acute exacerbations of multiple sclerosis; cerebral edema associated with primary or metastatic brain tumor or craniotomy

Ophthalmic diseases: Sympathetic ophthalmia, temporal arteritis, uveitis and ocular inflammatory conditions unresponsive to topical corticosteroids

Renal diseases: To induce diuresis or remission of proteinuria in idiopathic nephrotic syndrome or that due to lupus erythematosus

Respiratory diseases: Berylliosis, fulminating or disseminated pulmonary tuberculosis when used concurrently with appropriate antituberculous chemotherapy, idiopathic eosinophilic pneumonias, symptomatic sarcoidosis

Rheumatic disorders: Adjunctive therapy for short-term administration (to tide the patient over an acute episode or exacerbation) in acute gouty arthritis; acute rheumatic carditis; ankylosing spondylitis; psoriatic arthritis; rheumatoid arthritis, including juvenile rheumatoid arthritis (selected cases may require low-dose maintenance therapy); treatment of dermatomyositis, polymyositis, and systemic lupus erythematosus.

Miscellaneous: Trichinosis with neurologic or myocardial involvement, tuberculous meningitis with subarachnoid block or impending block when used with appropriate antituberculous chemotherapy

Intra-articular or soft tissue administration:

Adjunctive therapy for short-term administration (to tide the patient over an acute episode or exacerbation) in acute gouty arthritis, acute and subacute bursitis, acute nonspecific tenosynovitis, epicondylitis, rheumatoid arthritis, synovitis of osteoarthritis

Intralesional:

Treatment of alopecia areata; discoid lupus erythematosus; keloids; localized hypertrophic, infiltrated, inflammatory lesions of granuloma annulare, lichen planus, lichen simplex chronicus (neurodermatitis), and psoriatic plaques; necrobiosis lipoidica diabeticorum

Pregnancy Risk Factor C

Pregnancy Considerations Adverse events have been observed with corticosteroids in animal reproduction studies. Betamethasone crosses the placenta (Brownfoot, 2013); and is partially metabolized by placental enzymes to an inactive metabolite (Murphy, 2007). Some studies have shown an association between first trimester systemic corticosteroid use and oral clefts (Park-Wyllie, 2000; Pradat, 2003). Systemic corticosteroids may have an effect on fetal growth (decreased birth weight); however, information is conflicting (Lunghi, 2010). Hypoadrenalism may occur in newborns following maternal use of corticosteroids during pregnancy; monitor.

Because antenatal corticosteroid administration may reduce the incidence of intraventricular hemorrhage, necrotizing enterocolitis, neonatal mortality, and respiratory distress syndrome, the injection is often used in patients with preterm premature rupture of membranes (membrane rupture between 24 0/7 weeks and 34 0/7 weeks of gestation) who are at risk of preterm delivery (ACOG, 2013). When systemic corticosteroids are needed in pregnancy, it is generally recommended to use the lowest effective dose for the shortest duration of time, avoiding high doses during the first trimester (Leachman, 2006; Lunghi, 2010; Makol, 2011; Østensen, 2009).

Women exposed to betamethasone during pregnancy for the treatment of an autoimmune disease may contact the OTIS Autoimmune Diseases Study at 877-311-8972.

Breast-Feeding Considerations Corticosteroids are excreted in human milk. The onset of milk secretion after birth may be delayed and the volume of milk produced may be decreased by antenatal betamethasone therapy; this affect was seen when delivery occurred 3-9 days after the betamethasone dose in women between 28 and 34 weeks gestation. Antenatal betamethasone therapy did not affect milk production when birth occurred <3 days or >10 days of treatment (Henderson, 2008).

The manufacturer notes that when used systemically, maternal use of corticosteroids have the potential to cause adverse events in a nursing infant (eg, growth suppression, interfere with endogenous corticosteroid production) and therefore recommends that caution be exercised when administering betamethasone to nursing women. If there is concern about exposure to the infant, some guidelines recommend waiting 4 hours after the maternal dose of an oral systemic corticosteroid before breast-feeding in order to decrease potential exposure to the infant (based on a study using prednisolone) (Bae, 2011; Leachman, 2006; Makol, 2011; Ost, 1985).

Contraindications

Hypersensitivity to any component of the formulation; IM administration contraindicated in idiopathic thrombocytopenic purpura.

Documentation of allergenic cross-reactivity for glucocorticoids is limited. However, because of similarities in chemical structure and/or pharmacologic actions, the possibility of cross-sensitivity cannot be ruled out with certainty.

Warnings/Precautions Avoid concurrent use of other corticosteroids.

May cause hypercorticism or suppression of hypothalamic-pituitary-adrenal (HPA) axis, particularly in younger children or in patients receiving high doses for prolonged periods. HPA axis suppression may lead to adrenal crisis. Withdrawal and discontinuation of a corticosteroid should be done slowly and carefully. Particular care is required when patients are transferred from systemic corticosteroids to inhaled products due to possible adrenal insufficiency or withdrawal from steroids, including an increase in allergic symptoms. Patients receiving >20 mg per day of prednisone (or equivalent) may be most susceptible. Fatalities have occurred due to adrenal insufficiency in asthmatic patients during and after transfer from systemic corticosteroids to aerosol steroids; aerosol steroids do not provide the systemic steroid needed to treat patients having trauma, surgery, or infections. In stressful situations, HPA axis-suppressed patients should receive adequate supplementation with natural glucocorticoids (hydrocortisone or cortisone) rather than betamethasone (due to lack of mineralocorticoid activity).

Acute myopathy has been reported with high-dose corticosteroids, usually in patients with neuromuscular transmission disorders; may involve ocular and/or respiratory muscles; monitor creatine kinase; recovery may be delayed. Corticosteroid use may cause psychiatric disturbances, including depression, euphoria, insomnia, mood swings, and personality changes. Preexisting psychiatric conditions may be exacerbated by corticosteroid use. Prolonged use of corticosteroids may also increase the incidence of secondary infection, mask acute infection (including fungal infections), prolong or exacerbate viral infections, or limit response to killed or inactivated vaccines. Special pathogens (*Amoeba, Candida, Cryptococcus, Mycobacterium, Nocardia, Pneumocystis, Strongyloides*, or *Toxoplasma*) may be activated or an infection exacerbation may occur (may be fatal). Amebiasis or *Strongyloides* infections should be particularly ruled out. Exposure to varicella zoster (chickenpox) should be avoided; corticosteroids should not be used to treat ocular herpes simplex. Corticosteroids should not be used for cerebral malaria or viral hepatitis. Close observation is required in patients with latent tuberculosis and/or TB reactivity; restrict use in active TB (only in conjunction with antituberculosis treatment). Prolonged treatment with corticosteroids has been associated with the development of Kaposi sarcoma (case reports); if noted, discontinuation of therapy should be considered. High-dose corticosteroids should not be used to manage acute head injury. Rare cases of anaphylactoid reactions have been observed in patients receiving corticosteroids.

Use with caution in patients with thyroid disease, hepatic impairment, renal impairment, cardiovascular disease, diabetes, glaucoma, cataracts, myasthenia gravis, patients at risk for osteoporosis, patients at risk for seizures, or GI diseases (diverticulitis, fresh intestinal anastomoses, peptic ulcer, ulcerative colitis) due to perforation risk. Use caution following acute MI (corticosteroids have been associated with myocardial rupture). Use with caution in patients with HF and/or hypertension; long-term use has been associated with fluid retention and electrolyte disturbances. Dietary modifications may be necessary. Use with caution in patients with a recent history of myocardial infarction (MI); left ventricular free wall rupture has been reported after the use of corticosteroids. Use with caution in patients with renal impairment; fluid and sodium retention and increased potassium and calcium excretion may occur. Dietary modifications may be necessary. Not recommended for the treatment of optic neuritis; may increase frequency of new episodes. Intra-articular injection may result in joint tissue damage. Injection into an infected site should be avoided. Injection into a previously infected join is usually not recommended. If infection is suspected, joint fluid examination is recommended. If septic arthritis occurs after injection, institute appropriate antimicrobial therapy. Suspension for injection is for intramuscular, intra-articular or intralesional use only, do not administer intravenously. Corticosteroids are not approved for epidural injection. Serious neurologic events (eg, spinal cord infarction, paraplegia, quadriplegia, cortical blindness, stroke), some resulting in death, have been reported with epidural injection of corticosteroids, with and without use of fluoroscopy. Intra-articular injected corticosteroids may be systemically absorbed. May produce systemic as well as local effects. Appropriate examination of any joint fluid present is necessary to exclude a septic process. Avoid injection into an infected site. Do not inject into unstable joints. Intra-articular injection may result in damage to joint tissues. Potentially significant drug-drug interactions may exist, requiring dose or frequency adjustment, additional monitoring, and/or selection of alternative therapy. Because of the risk of adverse effects, systemic corticosteroids should be used cautiously in the elderly in the smallest possible effective dose for the shortest duration. Withdraw therapy with gradual tapering of dose.

Prolonged use in children may affect growth velocity; growth should be routinely monitored in pediatric patients.

Adverse Reactions

Cardiovascular: Congestive heart failure, edema, hyper-/hypotension

Central nervous system: Dizziness, headache, insomnia, intracranial pressure increased, lightheadedness, nervousness, pseudotumor cerebri, seizure, vertigo

Dermatologic: Ecchymoses, facial erythema, fragile skin, hirsutism, hyper-/hypopigmentation, perioral dermatitis (oral), petechiae, striae, wound healing impaired

Endocrine & metabolic: Amenorrhea, Cushing's syndrome, diabetes mellitus, growth suppression, hyperglycemia, hypokalemia, menstrual irregularities, pituitary-adrenal axis suppression, protein catabolism, sodium retention, water retention

Local: Injection site reactions (intra-articular use), sterile abscess

Neuromuscular & skeletal: Arthralgia, muscle atrophy, fractures, muscle weakness, myopathy, osteoporosis, necrosis (femoral and humeral heads)

Ocular: Cataracts, glaucoma, intraocular pressure increased

Miscellaneous: Anaphylactoid reaction, diaphoresis, hypersensitivity, secondary infection

Drug Interactions

Metabolism/Transport Effects None known.

Avoid Concomitant Use

Avoid concomitant use of Betamethasone (Systemic) with any of the following: Aldesleukin; BCG; Indium 111 Capromab Pendetide; Mifepristone; Natalizumab; Pimecrolimus; Tacrolimus (Topical); Tofacitinib

Increased Effect/Toxicity

Betamethasone (Systemic) may increase the levels/effects of: Acetylcholinesterase Inhibitors; Amphotericin B; Androgens; Ceritinib; Deferasirox; Leflunomide; Loop Diuretics; Natalizumab; Nicorandil; NSAID (COX-2 Inhibitor); NSAID (Nonselective); Quinolone Antibiotics; Thiazide Diuretics; Tofacitinib; Vaccines (Live); Warfarin

The levels/effects of Betamethasone (Systemic) may be increased by: Aprepitant; CYP3A4 Inhibitors (Strong); Denosumab; Estrogen Derivatives; Fosaprepitant;

Indacaterol; Mifepristone; Neuromuscular-Blocking Agents (Nondepolarizing); Pimecrolimus; Roflumilast; Salicylates; Tacrolimus (Topical); Telaprevir; Trastuzumab

Decreased Effect

Betamethasone (Systemic) may decrease the levels/effects of: Aldesleukin; Antidiabetic Agents; BCG; Calcitriol; Coccidioides immitis Skin Test; Corticorelin; Hyaluronidase; Indium 111 Capromab Pendetide; Isoniazid; Salicylates; Sipuleucel-T; Telaprevir; Urea Cycle Disorder Agents; Vaccines (Inactivated)

The levels/effects of Betamethasone (Systemic) may be decreased by: Aminoglutethimide; Barbiturates; Echinacea; Mifepristone; Mitotane; Primidone; Rifamycin Derivatives

Storage/Stability Store at 25°C (77°F); excursions are permitted between 15°C and 30°C (59°F and 86°F). Protect from light.

Mechanism of Action Controls the rate of protein synthesis; depresses the migration of polymorphonuclear leukocytes, fibroblasts; reverses capillary permeability and lysosomal stabilization at the cellular level to prevent or control inflammation

Dosage Note: Dosages expressed as combined amount of betamethasone sodium phosphate and betamethasone acetate; 1 mg is equivalent to betamethasone sodium phosphate 0.5 mg and betamethasone acetate 0.5 mg. Base dosage on severity of disease and patient response.

Infants, Children, and Adolescents: IM: 0.02 to 0.3 mg/kg/day (0.6 to 9 mg/m^2/day) in 3 or 4 divided doses.

Adults: Usual dosage range: IM: Initial: 0.25 to 9 mg daily

Indication-specific dosing: Adults:

Antenatal fetal maturation (off-label use): IM: In women with preterm premature rupture of membranes (membrane rupture between 24 0/7 weeks and 34 0/7 weeks of gestation), a single course of corticosteroids is recommended if there is a risk of preterm delivery (ACOG, 2013). Although the optimal corticosteroid and dose have not been determined, betamethasone 12 mg every 24 hours for a total of 2 doses has been used in most studies (Brownfoot, 2013).

Bursitis (other than of foot), tenosynovitis, peritendinitis: Intrabursal: 3 to 6 mg (0.5 to 1 mL) for one dose; several injections may be required for acute exacerbations or chronic conditions; reduced doses may be warranted for repeat injections.

Dermatologic: Intralesional: 1.2 mg/cm^2 (0.2 mL/cm^2) for one dose (maximum: 6 mg [1 mL] weekly)

Foot disorders: Intra-articular: 1.5 to 6 mg (0.25 to 1 mL) per dose at 3- to 7-day intervals. Dose is based upon condition:

Bursitis: 1.5 to 3 mg (0.25 to 0.5 mL)

Tenosynovitis: 3 mg (0.5 mL)

Acute gouty arthritis: 3 to 6 mg (0.5 to 1 mL)

Multiple sclerosis: IM: 30 mg daily for 1 week, followed by 12 mg every other day for 4 weeks.

Rheumatoid and osteoarthritis: Intra-articular: 3 to 12 mg (0.5 to 2 mL) for one dose. Dose is based upon the joint size:

Very large (eg, hip): 6 to 12 mg (1 to 2 mL)

Large (eg, knee, ankle, shoulder): 6 mg (1 mL)

Medium (eg, elbow, wrist): 3 to 6 mg (0.5 to 1 mL)

Small (eg, inter- or metacarpophalangeal, sternoclavicular): 1.5 to 3 mg (0.25 to 0.5 mL)

Dosage adjustment in renal impairment: There are no dosage adjustments provided in the manufacturer's labeling.

Dosage adjustment in hepatic impairment: There are no dosage adjustments provided in the manufacturer's labeling.

Administration If suspension is coadministered with a local anesthetic, it may be mixed in syringe with 1% or 2% lidocaine HCl (without parabens) or similar parabens-free local anesthetic. Withdraw the dose of betamethasone suspension from the vial into the syringe, then draw up the local anesthetic into the syringe and shake the syringe briefly. Do not inject the local anesthetic directly into the suspension vial.

IM: Do **not** give injectable sodium phosphate/acetate suspension IV or epidurally

Intrabursal: Tendinitis, tenosynovitis: Inject into affected tendon sheaths (not directly into tendons).

Intradermal: Using a 25-gauge 1 mL (eg, tuberculin) syringe with 1/2-inch needle inject a uniform depot. Do **not** inject subcutaneously

Monitoring Parameters Growth in children

Dosage Forms

Suspension, Injection:

Celestone Soluspan: Betamethasone sodium phosphate 3 mg and betamethasone acetate 3 mg per 1 mL (5 mL)

Generic: Betamethasone sodium phosphate 3 mg and betamethasone acetate 3 mg per 1 mL (5 mL)

Betamethasone (Topical) (bay ta METH a sone)

Brand Names: U.S. AlphaTrex; Diprolene; Diprolene AF; Luxiq

Brand Names: Canada Betaderm; Betnesol; Celestoderm V; Celestoderm V/2; Diprolene; Diprosone; Luxiq; Prevex B; ratio-Ectosone; Ratio-Topilene; Ratio-Topisone; Rivasone; Rolene; Rosone; Taro-Sone; Valisone Scalp Lotion

Index Terms Betamethasone Dipropionate; Betamethasone Dipropionate, Augmented; Betamethasone Valerate

Pharmacologic Category Corticosteroid, Topical

Additional Appendix Information

Corticosteroids Systemic Equivalencies *on page 2228*

Topical Corticosteroids *on page 2230*

Use Inflammatory dermatoses: Treatment of corticosteroid-responsive dermatoses, such as seborrheic or atopic dermatitis, neurodermatitis, anogenital pruritus, psoriasis, or the inflammatory phase of xerosis

Pregnancy Risk Factor C

Dosage Topical: Base dosage on severity of disease and patient response. Use lowest dose possible.

Children: Use minimal amount for shortest period of time to avoid HPA axis suppression.

Cream, lotion, or ointment: Unaugmented formulations: Refer to adult dosing.

Adolescents: Use minimal amount for shortest period of time to avoid HPA axis suppression.

Cream, augmented formulation: Apply once or twice daily (maximum: 45 g weekly). **Note:** Reassess if no improvement after 2 weeks of treatment.

Gel, augmented formulation: Apply once or twice daily; rub in gently (maximum: 50 g weekly). **Note:** Reassess if no improvement after 2 weeks of treatment.

Lotion, augmented formulation: Apply a few drops once or twice daily; rub in gently (maximum: 50 mL weekly). **Note:** Reassess if no improvement after 2 weeks of treatment.

Ointment, augmented formulation: Apply once or twice daily (maximum: 50 g weekly). **Note:** Reassess if no improvement after 2 weeks of treatment.

Adults:

Cream, unaugmented formulation: Apply 1 to 3 times daily. **Note:** Twice daily application is usually effective.

Cream, augmented formulation: Apply once or twice daily (maximum: 45 g weekly). **Note:** Reassess if no improvement after 2 weeks of treatment.

Foam: Apply to the scalp twice daily, once in the morning and once at night

Gel, augmented formulation: Apply once or twice daily; rub in gently (maximum: 50 g weekly). **Note:** Reassess if no improvement after 2 weeks of treatment.

Lotion, unaugmented formulation: Apply a few drops twice daily

Lotion, augmented formulation: Apply a few drops once or twice daily; rub in gently (maximum: 50 mL weekly). **Note:** Reassess if no improvement after 2 weeks of treatment.

Ointment, unaugmented formulation: Apply 1 to 3 times daily. **Note:** Twice daily application is usually effective.

Ointment, augmented formulation: Apply once or twice daily (maximum: 50 g weekly). **Note:** Reassess if no improvement after 2 weeks of treatment.

Dosage adjustment in renal impairment: There are no dosage adjustments provided in the manufacturer's labeling.

Dosage adjustment in hepatic impairment: There are no dosage adjustments provided in the manufacturer's labeling.

Additional Information Complete prescribing information should be consulted for additional detail.

Dosage Forms

Cream, External:

Diprolene AF: 0.05% (15 g, 50 g)

Generic: 0.05% (15 g, 45 g, 50 g); 0.1% (15 g, 45 g)

Foam, External:

Luxiq: 0.12% (50 g, 100 g)

Generic: 0.12% (50 g, 100 g)

Gel, External:

AlphaTrex: 0.05% (15 g, 50 g)

Generic: 0.05% (15 g, 50 g)

Lotion, External:

Diprolene: 0.05% (30 mL, 60 mL)

Generic: 0.05% (30 mL, 60 mL); 0.1% (60 mL)

Ointment, External:

Diprolene: 0.05% (15 g, 50 g)

Generic: 0.05% (15 g, 45 g, 50 g); 0.1% (15 g, 45 g)

◆ **Betamethasone Acetate** *see* Betamethasone (Systemic) *on page 253*

Betamethasone and Clotrimazole

(bay ta METH a sone & kloe TRIM a zole)

Brand Names: U.S. Lotrisone

Brand Names: Canada Lotriderm

Index Terms Clotrimazole and Betamethasone

Pharmacologic Category Antifungal Agent, Topical; Corticosteroid, Topical

Use

Fungal infections: Topical treatment of symptomatic inflammatory tinea pedis, tinea cruris, and tinea corporis caused by *Trichophyton rubrum*, *T. mentagrophytes*, and *Epidermophyton floccosum* in patients ≥17 years

Limitations of use: Efficacy of betamethasone/clotrimazole lotion in the treatment of zoophilic dermatophytes (eg, Microsporum canis) has not been established.

Pregnancy Risk Factor C

Dosage

Infants, Children, and Adolescents <17 years: Do not use.

Adolescents ≥17 years and Adults:

Tinea corporis, tinea cruris: Topical:

Cream: Massage into affected area twice daily, morning and evening for 1 week; re-evaluate after 1 week if no clinical improvement; do not exceed 45 g cream per week; maximum duration: 2 weeks

Lotion: Massage into affected area twice daily, morning and evening; re-evaluate after 1 week if no clinical improvement; do not exceed 45 mL lotion per week; maximum duration: 2 weeks

Tinea pedis: Topical:

Cream: Massage into affected area twice daily, morning and evening for 2 weeks; re-evaluate after 2 weeks if no clinical improvement; do not exceed 45 g cream per week; maximum duration: 4 weeks

Lotion: Massage into affected area twice daily, morning and evening; re-evaluate after 2 weeks if no clinical improvement; do not exceed 45 mL lotion per week; maximum duration: 4 weeks.

Elderly: Use with caution; skin atrophy and skin ulceration (rare) have been reported in patients with thinning skin; do not use for diaper dermatitis or under occlusive dressings

Dosage adjustment in renal impairment: There are no dosage adjustments provided in the manufacturer's labeling.

Dosage adjustment in hepatic impairment: There are no dosage adjustments provided in the manufacturer's labeling.

Additional Information Complete prescribing information should be consulted for additional detail.

Dosage Forms

Cream: Betamethasone 0.05% and clotrimazole 1% (15 g, 45 g)

Lotrisone: Betamethasone 0.05% and clotrimazole 1% (15 g, 45 g)

Lotion: Betamethasone 0.05% and clotrimazole 1% (30 mL)

Lotrisone: Betamethasone 0.05% and clotrimazole 1% (30 mL)

◆ **Betamethasone Dipropionate** *see* Betamethasone (Topical) *on page 255*

◆ **Betamethasone Dipropionate and Calcipotriene Hydrate** *see* Calcipotriene and Betamethasone *on page 321*

◆ **Betamethasone Dipropionate, Augmented** *see* Betamethasone (Topical) *on page 255*

◆ **Betamethasone Sodium Phosphate** *see* Betamethasone (Systemic) *on page 253*

◆ **Betamethasone Valerate** *see* Betamethasone (Topical) *on page 255*

◆ **Betapace** *see* Sotalol *on page 1927*

◆ **Betapace AF** *see* Sotalol *on page 1927*

◆ **Betasept Surgical Scrub [OTC]** *see* Chlorhexidine Gluconate *on page 422*

◆ **Betaseron** *see* Interferon Beta-1b *on page 1103*

◆ **Betaxin (Can)** *see* Thiamine *on page 2028*

Betaxolol (Systemic) (be TAKS oh lol)

Brand Names: U.S. Kerlone

Index Terms Betaxolol Hydrochloride

Pharmacologic Category Antihypertensive; Beta-Blocker, Beta-1 Selective

Use Hypertension: Management of hypertension

The 2014 guideline for the management of high blood pressure in adults (Eighth Joint National Committee [JNC 8]) recommends initiation of pharmacologic treatment to lower blood pressure for the following patients (JNC8 [James, 2013]):

- Patients ≥60 years of age, with systolic blood pressure (SBP) ≥150 mm Hg or diastolic blood pressure (DBP) ≥90 mm Hg. Goal of therapy is SBP <150 mm Hg and DBP <90 mm Hg.

- Patients <60 years of age, with SBP ≥140 mm Hg or DBP ≥90 mm Hg. Goal of therapy is SBP <140 mm Hg and DBP <90 mm Hg.
- Patients ≥18 years of age with diabetes, with SBP ≥140 mm Hg or DBP ≥90 mm Hg. Goal of therapy is SBP <140 mm Hg and DBP <90 mm Hg.
- Patients ≥18 years of age with chronic kidney disease (CKD), with SBP ≥140 mm Hg or DBP ≥90 mm Hg. Goal of therapy is SBP <140 mm Hg and DBP <90 mm Hg.

In patients with CKD, regardless of race or diabetes status, the use of an ACE inhibitor (ACEI) or angiotensin receptor blocker (ARB) as initial therapy is recommended to improve kidney outcomes. In the general nonblack population (without CKD) including those with diabetes, initial antihypertensive treatment should consist of a thiazide-type diuretic, calcium channel blocker, ACEI, or ARB. In the general black population (without CKD) including those with diabetes, initial antihypertensive treatment should consist of a thiazide-type diuretic or a calcium channel blocker **instead of** an ACEI or ARB.

Pregnancy Risk Factor C

Dosage Oral:

Adults: Initial: 10 mg once daily; may increase dose to 20 mg daily after 7 to14 days if desired response is not achieved. Increasing the dose beyond 20 mg daily has not been shown to produce further antihypertensive effect.

Elderly: Refer to adult dosing; initial dose: 5 mg daily

Dosage adjustment in renal impairment: Severe impairment: Initial dose: 5 mg daily; may increase every 2 weeks up to a maximum of 20 mg daily

Hemodialysis: Initial dose: 5 mg daily; may increase every 2 weeks up to a maximum of 20 mg daily. Supplemental dose not required.

Dosage adjustment in hepatic impairment: Dosage adjustments are not routinely required.

Additional Information Complete prescribing information should be consulted for additional detail.

Dosage Forms

Tablet, Oral:

Kerlone: 10 mg, 20 mg

Generic: 10 mg, 20 mg

Betaxolol (Ophthalmic) (be TAKS oh lol)

Brand Names: U.S. Betoptic-S

Brand Names: Canada Betoptic S; Sandoz-Betaxolol

Index Terms Betaxolol Hydrochloride

Pharmacologic Category Ophthalmic Agent, Antiglaucoma

Use Treatment of chronic open-angle glaucoma or ocular hypertension

Pregnancy Risk Factor C

Dosage

Children and Adults: Ophthalmic suspension (Betoptic® S): Instill 1 drop into affected eye(s) twice daily.

Adults: Ophthalmic solution: Instill 1-2 drops into affected eye(s) twice daily.

Elderly: Ophthalmic: Refer to adult dosing.

Additional Information Complete prescribing information should be consulted for additional detail.

Dosage Forms

Solution, Ophthalmic:

Generic: 0.5% (5 mL, 10 mL, 15 mL)

Suspension, Ophthalmic:

Betoptic-S: 0.25% (10 mL, 15 mL)

◆ **Betaxolol Hydrochloride** *see* Betaxolol (Ophthalmic) *on page 257*

◆ **Betaxolol Hydrochloride** *see* Betaxolol (Systemic) *on page 256*

Bethanechol (be THAN e kole)

Brand Names: U.S. Urecholine

Brand Names: Canada Duvoid®; PHL-Bethanechol; PMS-Bethanechol

Index Terms Bethanechol Chloride

Pharmacologic Category Cholinergic Agonist

Use Treatment of acute postoperative and postpartum nonobstructive (functional) urinary retention; treatment of neurogenic atony of the urinary bladder with retention

Pregnancy Risk Factor C

Dosage Oral:

Children:

Urinary retention (off-label use): 0.3-0.6 mg/kg/day in 3-4 divided doses

Adults:

Urinary retention, neurogenic bladder: Initial: 10-50 mg 3-4 times/day (some patients may require dosages of 50-100 mg 4 times/day). To determine effective dose, may initiate at a dose of 5-10 mg, with additional doses of 5-10 mg hourly until an effective cumulative dose is reached. Cholinergic effects at higher oral dosages may be cumulative.

Elderly: Use the lowest effective dose

Dosage adjustment in renal impairment: No dosage adjustment provided in manufacturer's labeling.

Dosage adjustment in hepatic impairment: No dosage adjustment provided in manufacturer's labeling.

Additional Information Complete prescribing information should be consulted for additional detail.

Dosage Forms

Tablet, Oral:

Urecholine: 5 mg, 10 mg, 25 mg, 50 mg

Generic: 5 mg, 10 mg, 25 mg, 50 mg

Dosage Forms: Canada

Tablet:

Duvoid®: 10 mg, 25 mg, 50 mg

◆ **Bethanechol Chloride** *see* Bethanechol *on page 257*

◆ **Bethkis** *see* Tobramycin (Systemic, Oral Inhalation) *on page 2052*

◆ **Betimol** *see* Timolol (Ophthalmic) *on page 2043*

◆ **Betnesol (Can)** *see* Betamethasone (Topical) *on page 255*

◆ **Betoptic-S** *see* Betaxolol (Ophthalmic) *on page 257*

◆ **Betoptic S (Can)** *see* Betaxolol (Ophthalmic) *on page 257*

Bevacizumab (be vuh SIZ uh mab)

Brand Names: U.S. Avastin

Brand Names: Canada Avastin

Index Terms Anti-VEGF Monoclonal Antibody; Anti-VEGF rhuMAb; rhuMAb-VEGF

Pharmacologic Category Antineoplastic Agent, Monoclonal Antibody; Antineoplastic Agent, Vascular Endothelial Growth Factor (VEGF) Inhibitor; Vascular Endothelial Growth Factor (VEGF) Inhibitor

Use

Cervical cancer, persistent/recurrent/metastatic: Treatment of persistent, recurrent, or metastatic cervical cancer (in combination with paclitaxel and either cisplatin or topotecan). **Note:** Not an approved use in Canada.

Colorectal cancer, metastatic: First- or second-line treatment of metastatic colorectal cancer (CRC) (in combination with fluorouracil-based chemotherapy); second-line treatment of metastatic CRC (in combination with fluoropyrimidine-irinotecan- or fluoropyrimidine-oxaliplatin-based chemotherapy) after progression on a first-line treatment containing bevacizumab.

Limitations of use: Not indicated for the adjuvant treatment of colon cancer.

Glioblastoma: Treatment of progressive glioblastoma (as a single agent).

Limitations of use: Effectiveness is based on improvement in objective response rate.

Non-small cell lung cancer, nonsquamous: First-line treatment of unresectable, locally advanced, recurrent or metastatic nonsquamous non-small cell lung cancer (NSCLC) (in combination with carboplatin and paclitaxel).

Ovarian (epithelial), fallopian tube, or primary peritoneal cancer (platinum-resistant recurrent): Treatment of platinum-resistant recurrent epithelial ovarian, fallopian tube, or primary peritoneal cancer (in combination with paclitaxel, doxorubicin [liposomal], or topotecan) in patients who received no more than 2 prior chemotherapy regimens. **Note:** Not an approved use in Canada.

Renal cell carcinoma, metastatic: Treatment of metastatic renal cell carcinoma (RCC) (in combination with interferon alfa). **Note:** Not an approved use in Canada.

Pregnancy Risk Factor C

Pregnancy Considerations Teratogenic effects have been observed in animal reproduction studies. Angiogenesis is of critical importance to human fetal development, and bevacizumab inhibits angiogenesis. Adequate contraception during therapy is recommended (and for ≥6 months following last dose of bevacizumab). Patients should also be counseled regarding prolonged exposure following discontinuation of therapy due to the long half-life of bevacizumab.

Based on animal studies, bevacizumab may disrupt normal menstrual cycles and impair fertility by several effects, including reduced endometrial proliferation and follicular developmental arrest. Some parameters do not recover completely, or recover very slowly following discontinuation.

Breast-Feeding Considerations It is not known if bevacizumab is excreted in breast milk. Immunoglobulins are excreted in breast milk, and it is assumed that bevacizumab may appear in breast milk. Because of the potential for serious adverse reactions in the nursing infant, the decision to discontinue bevacizumab or to discontinue breast-feeding during therapy should take into account the benefits of treatment to the mother. The half-life of bevacizumab is up to 50 days (average 20 days), and this should be considered when decisions are made concerning breast-feeding resumption.

Note: Canadian labeling recommends to discontinue breast-feeding during treatment and to avoid breast-feeding a minimum of 6 months following discontinuation of treatment.

Contraindications

There are no contraindications listed in the manufacturer's labeling.

Canadian labeling: Hypersensitivity to bevacizumab, any component of the formulation, Chinese hamster ovary cell products or other recombinant human or humanized antibodies; untreated CNS metastases

Warnings/Precautions [U.S. Boxed Warning]: Gastrointestinal (GI) perforation (sometimes fatal) has occurred in 0.3 to 3.2% of clinical study patients receiving bevacizumab; discontinue (permanently) if GI perforation occurs. All cervical cancer patients with GI perforation had a history of prior pelvic radiation. GI perforation was observed in patients with platinum-resistant ovarian cancer, although patients with evidence of recto-sigmoid involvement (by pelvic exam), bowel involvement (on CT scan), or clinical symptoms of bowel obstruction were excluded from the study; avoid bevacizumab use in these ovarian cancer patient populations. Most cases occur within 50 days of treatment initiation; monitor patients for signs/symptoms (eg, fever, abdominal pain with constipation and/or nausea/vomiting). GI fistula (including enterocutaneous, esophageal, duodenal, and rectal fistulas), and intra-abdominal abscess have been reported in patients receiving bevacizumab for colorectal cancer, ovarian cancer, and other cancers (not related to treatment duration). Non-GI fistula formation (including tracheoesophageal, bronchopleural, biliary, vaginal, vesical, renal, bladder, and female tract fistulas) has been observed (rarely fatal), most commonly within the first 6 months of treatment. Gastrointestinal-vaginal fistulas have been reported in cervical cancer patients, all of whom had received prior pelvic radiation; patients may also have bowel obstructions requiring surgical intervention and diverting ostomies. Permanently discontinue in patients who develop internal organ fistulas, tracheoesophageal (TE) fistula, or any grade 4 fistula. **[U.S. Boxed Warning]: The incidence of wound healing and surgical complications, including serious and fatal events, is increased in patients who have received bevacizumab; discontinue with wound dehiscence. Although the appropriate interval between withholding bevacizumab and elective surgery has not been defined, bevacizumab should be discontinued at least 28 days prior to surgery and should not be reinitiated for at least 28 days after surgery and until wound is fully healed.** In a retrospective review of central venous access device placements, a greater risk of wound dehiscence was observed when port placement and bevacizumab administration were separated by <14 days (Erinjeri, 2011).

[U.S. Boxed Warning]: Severe or fatal hemorrhage, including hemoptysis, gastrointestinal bleeding, central nervous system hemorrhage, epistaxis, and vaginal bleeding have been reported (up to 5 times more frequently if receiving bevacizumab). Avoid use in patients with serious hemorrhage or recent hemoptysis (≥2.5 mL blood). Serious or fatal pulmonary hemorrhage has been reported in patients receiving bevacizumab (primarily in patients with non–small cell lung cancer with squamous cell histology [not an FDA-approved indication]). Intracranial hemorrhage, including cases of grade 3 or 4 hemorrhage, has occurred in patients with previously treated glioblastoma. Treatment discontinuation is recommended in all patients with intracranial or other serious hemorrhage. Use with caution in patients with CNS metastases; once case of CNS hemorrhage was observed in an ongoing study of NSCLC patients with CNS metastases. Use in patients with untreated CNS metastases is contraindicated in the Canadian labeling. Use with caution in patients at risk for thrombocytopenia.

Bevacizumab is associated with an increased risk for arterial thromboembolic events (ATE), including cerebral infarction, stroke, MI, TIA, angina, and other ATEs, when used in combination with chemotherapy. History of ATE, diabetes, or ≥65 years of age may present an even greater risk. Although patients with cancer are already at risk for venous thromboembolism (VTE), a meta-analysis of 15 controlled trials has demonstrated an increased risk for VTE in patients who received bevacizumab (Nalluri, 2008). Cervical cancer patients receiving bevacizumab plus chemotherapy may be at increased risk of grade 3 or higher VTE compared to those patients who received chemotherapy alone. Permanently discontinue therapy in patients with severe ATE or life-threatening (grade 4) VTE, including pulmonary embolism; the safety of treatment reinitiation after ATE has not been studied.

Use with caution in patients with cardiovascular disease. Among approved and nonapproved uses evaluated thus far, the incidence of heart failure (HF) and/or left ventricular dysfunction (including LVEF decline), is higher in patients receiving bevacizumab plus chemotherapy when compared to chemotherapy alone. Bevacizumab may potentiate the cardiotoxic effects of anthracyclines. HF is more common with prior anthracycline exposure and/or left chest wall irradiation. The safety of therapy resumption or continuation in patients with cardiac dysfunction has not been studied. In studies of patients with metastatic breast cancer (an off-label use), the incidence of grades 3 or 4 HF was increased in patients receiving bevacizumab plus paclitaxel, compared to the control arm. Patients with metastatic breast cancer who had received prior anthracycline therapy had a higher rate of HF compared to those receiving paclitaxel alone (3.8% vs 0.6% respectively). A meta-analysis of 5 studies which enrolled patients with metastatic breast cancer who received bevacizumab suggested an association with an increased risk of heart failure; all trials included in the analysis enrolled patients who either received prior or were receiving concurrent anthracycline therapy (Choueiri, 2011).

Bevacizumab may cause and/or worsen hypertension; the incidence of severe hypertension in increased with bevacizumab. Use caution in patients with preexisting hypertension and monitor BP closely (every 2 to 3 weeks during treatment; regularly after discontinuation if bevacizumab-induced hypertension occurs or worsens). Permanent discontinuation is recommended in patients who experience a hypertensive crisis or hypertensive encephalopathy. Temporarily discontinue in patients who develop uncontrolled hypertension. An increase in diastolic and systolic blood pressures were noted in a retrospective review of patients with renal insufficiency (CrCl ≤60 mL/minute) who received bevacizumab for renal cell cancer (Gupta, 2011). Cases of posterior reversible encephalopathy syndrome (PRES) have been reported. Symptoms (which include headache, seizure, confusion, lethargy, blindness and/or other vision, or neurologic disturbances) may occur from 16 hours to 1 year after treatment initiation. Resolution of symptoms usually occurs within days after discontinuation; however, neurologic sequelae may remain. PRES may be associated with hypertension; discontinue bevacizumab and begin management of hypertension, if present. The safety of treatment reinitiation after PRES is not known.

Infusion reactions (eg, hypertension, hypertensive crisis, wheezing, oxygen desaturation, hypersensitivity [including anaphylactic/anaphylactoid reactions], chest pain, rigors, headache, diaphoresis) may occur with the first infusion (uncommon); interrupt therapy in patients experiencing severe infusion reactions and administer appropriate therapy; there are no data to address routine premedication use or reinstitution of therapy in patients who experience severe infusion reactions. Cases of necrotizing fasciitis, including fatalities, have been reported (rarely); usually secondary to wound healing complications, GI perforation or fistula formation. Discontinue in patients who develop necrotizing fasciitis. Proteinuria and/or nephrotic syndrome have been associated with bevacizumab; risk may be increased in patients with a history of hypertension; thrombotic microangiopathy has been associated with bevacizumab-induced proteinuria. Withhold treatment for ≥2 g proteinuria/24 hours and resume when proteinuria is <2 g/24 hours; discontinue in patients with nephrotic syndrome. Elderly patients (≥65 years of age) are at higher risk for adverse events, including thromboembolic events and proteinuria; serious adverse events occurring more frequently in the elderly also include weakness, deep thrombophlebitis, sepsis, hyper-/hypotension, MI, CHF, diarrhea, constipation, anorexia, leukopenia, anemia, dehydration, hypokalemia, and hyponatremia. Potentially significant drug-drug interactions may exist, requiring dose or frequency adjustment, additional monitoring, and/or selection of alternative therapy. Microangiopathic hemolytic anemia (MAHA) has been reported when bevacizumab has been used in combination with sunitinib. Concurrent therapy with sunitinib and bevacizumab is also associated with dose-limiting hypertension in patients with metastatic renal cell cancer. The incidence of hand-foot syndrome is increased in patients treated with bevacizumab plus sorafenib in comparison to those treated with sorafenib monotherapy. When used in combination with myelosuppressive chemotherapy, increased rates of severe or febrile neutropenia and neutropenic infection were reported. Bevacizumab, in combination with chemotherapy (or biologic therapy), is associated with an increased risk of treatment-related mortality; a higher risk of fatal adverse events was identified in a meta-analysis of 16 trials in which bevacizumab was used for the treatment of various cancers (breast cancer, colorectal cancer, non–small cell lung cancer, pancreatic cancer, prostate cancer, and renal cell cancer) and compared to chemotherapy alone (Ranpura, 2011). When bevacizumab is used in combination with myelosuppressive chemotherapy, increased rates of severe or febrile neutropenia and neutropenic infection have been reported. In premenopausal women receiving bevacizumab in combination with mFOLFOX (fluorouracil/oxaliplatin based chemotherapy) the incidence of ovarian failure (amenorrhea ≥3 months) was higher (34%) compared to women who received mFOLFOX alone (2%); ovarian function recovered in some patients after treatment was discontinued; premenopausal women should be informed of the potential risk of ovarian failure. Serious eye infections and vision loss due to endophthalmitis have been reported from intravitreal administration (off-label use/route).

Adverse Reactions Reported monotherapy and as part of combination chemotherapy regimens.

Cardiovascular: Arterial thrombosis, deep vein thrombosis, hypertension, hypotension, intra-abdominal thrombosis (venous), left ventricular dysfunction, peripheral edema, pulmonary embolism, syncope, thrombosis, venous thromboembolism, venous thromboembolism (secondary; with oral anticoagulants)

Central nervous system: Anxiety, dizziness, fatigue, headache, pain, peripheral sensory neuropathy, taste disorder, voice disorder

Dermatologic: Acne vulgaris, alopecia, cellulitis, dermal ulcer, exfoliative dermatitis, palmar-plantar erythrodysesthesia, xeroderma

Endocrine & metabolic: Dehydration, hyperglycemia, hypoalbuminemia, hypokalemia, hypomagnesemia, hyponatremia, ovarian failure, weight loss

Gastrointestinal: Abdominal pain, anorexia, colitis, constipation, decreased appetite, diarrhea, dyspepsia, gastritis, gastrointestinal fistula, gastrointestinal hemorrhage, gastrointestinal perforation, gastroesophageal reflux disease, gingival hemorrhage (minor), gingival pain, gingivitis, intestinal obstruction, nausea, oral mucosa ulcer, rectal pain, stomatitis, vomiting, xerostomia

Genitourinary: Pelvic pain, proteinuria (median onset: 5.6 months; median time to resolution: 6.1 months), urinary tract infection, vaginal hemorrhage

Hematologic & oncologic: Febrile neutropenia, hemorrhage (CNS), leukopenia, lymphocytopenia, neutropenia, neutropenic infection, pulmonary hemorrhage, thrombocytopenia

Infection: Abscess (tooth), infection (serious; pneumonia, catheter infection, or wound infection)

Neuromuscular & skeletal: Back pain, dysarthria, myalgia, weakness

Ophthalmic: Blurred vision

Otic: Deafness, tinnitus

Renal: Increased serum creatinine

Respiratory: Dyspnea, epistaxis, pneumonitis, rhinitis, upper respiratory tract infection

Miscellaneous: Fistula (anal, gastrointestinal-vaginal), infusion related reaction, postoperative wound complication (including dehiscence)

Rare but important or life-threatening: Angina pectoris, antibody development (anti-bevacizumab and neutralizing), bladder fistula, bronchopleural fistula, cerebral infarction, conjunctival hemorrhage, endophthalmitis (infectious and sterile), fistula of bile duct, fulminant necrotizing fasciitis, gallbladder perforation, gastrointestinal ulcer, hemolytic anemia (microangiopathic; when used in combination with sunitinib), hemoptysis, hemorrhagic stroke, hypersensitivity, hypertensive crisis, hypertensive encephalopathy, increased intraocular pressure, intestinal necrosis, intraocular inflammation (iritis, vitritis), mesenteric thrombosis, myocardial infarction, nasal septum perforation, ocular hyperemia, osteonecrosis of the jaw, ovarian failure, pancytopenia, polyserositis, pulmonary hypertension, rectal fistula, renal failure, renal fistula, renal thrombotic microangiopathy, retinal detachment, retinal hemorrhage, reversible posterior leukoencephalopathy syndrome, sepsis, tracheoesophageal fistula, vaginal fistula, vitreous hemorrhage, vitreous opacity

Drug Interactions

Metabolism/Transport Effects None known.

Avoid Concomitant Use

Avoid concomitant use of Bevacizumab with any of the following: Belimumab; CloZAPine; Dipyrone; SUNItinib

Increased Effect/Toxicity

Bevacizumab may increase the levels/effects of: Antineoplastic Agents (Anthracycline, Systemic); Belimumab; Bisphosphonate Derivatives; CloZAPine; Irinotecan; SORAfenib; SUNItinib

The levels/effects of Bevacizumab may be increased by: Dipyrone; SUNItinib

Decreased Effect There are no known significant interactions involving a decrease in effect.

Preparation for Administration Dilute in 100 mL NS prior to infusion (the manufacturer recommends a total volume of 100 mL). Do not mix with dextrose-containing solutions.

Storage/Stability Store intact vials at 2°C to 8°C (36°F to 46°F); do not freeze. Protect from light; do not shake. Diluted solutions are stable for up to 8 hours under refrigeration. Discard unused portion of vial.

Mechanism of Action Bevacizumab is a recombinant, humanized monoclonal antibody which binds to, and neutralizes, vascular endothelial growth factor (VEGF), preventing its association with endothelial receptors, Flt-1 and KDR. VEGF binding initiates angiogenesis (endothelial proliferation and the formation of new blood vessels). The inhibition of microvascular growth is believed to retard the growth of all tissues (including metastatic tissue).

Pharmacodynamics/Kinetics

Distribution: V_d: 46 mL/kg

Half-life elimination: ~20 days (range: 11 to 50 days)

Dosage

Cervical cancer, persistent/recurrent/metastatic: IV: 15 mg/kg every 3 weeks (in combination with paclitaxel and either cisplatin or topotecan) until disease progression or unacceptable toxicity (Tewari, 2014)

Colorectal cancer, metastatic, in combination with fluorouracil-based chemotherapy: Adults: IV: 5 mg/kg every 2 weeks (in combination with bolus-IFL) **or** 10 mg/kg every 2 weeks (in combination with FOLFOX4)

Canadian labeling: IV: 5 mg/kg every 2 weeks (in combination with fluorouracil-based chemotherapy)

Colorectal cancer, metastatic, following first-line therapy containing bevacizumab: Adults: IV: 5 mg/kg every 2 weeks **or** 7.5 mg/kg every 3 weeks (in combination with fluoropyrimidine-irinotecan or fluoropyrimidine-oxaliplatin based regimen)

Glioblastoma: Adults: IV: 10 mg/kg every 2 weeks as monotherapy **or** (off-label dosing) 10 mg/kg every 2 weeks (in combination with irinotecan) (Vredenburgh, 2007)

Non-small cell lung cancer (nonsquamous cell histology): Adults: IV: 15 mg/kg every 3 weeks (in combination with carboplatin and paclitaxel) for 6 cycles followed by maintenance treatment (off-label use) of bevacizumab 15 mg/kg every 3 weeks as monotherapy until disease progression or unacceptable toxicity (Sandler, 2006)

Ovarian (epithelial), fallopian tube, or primary peritoneal cancer (platinum-resistant recurrent): Adults: IV: 10 mg/kg every 2 weeks (in combination with weekly paclitaxel, every 4 week doxorubicin [liposomal], or days 1, 8, and 15 topotecan) **or** 15 mg/kg every 3 weeks (in combination with every 3 week topotecan) (Pujade-Lauraine, 2014)

Renal cell cancer, metastatic: Adults: IV: 10 mg/kg every 2 weeks (in combination with interferon alfa) **or** (off-label dosing) 10 mg/kg every 2 weeks as monotherapy (Yang, 2003)

Age-related macular degeneration (off-label use/route): Adults: Intravitreal: 1.25 mg (0.05 mL) monthly for 3 months, then may be given scheduled (monthly) or as needed based on monthly ophthalmologic assessment (Chakravarthy, 2013; Martin, 2012)

Breast cancer, metastatic (off-label use): Adults: IV: 10 mg/kg every 2 weeks (in combination with paclitaxel) (Miller, 2007)

Endometrial cancer, recurrent or persistent (off-label use): Adults: IV: 15 mg/kg every 3 weeks (as monotherapy) until disease progression or unacceptable toxicity (Aghajanian, 2011)

Soft tissue sarcoma, angiosarcoma, metastatic or locally advanced (off-label use): Adults: IV: 15 mg/kg every 3 weeks until disease progression or unacceptable toxicity (Agulnik, 2013). Additional data may be necessary to further define the role of bevacizumab in this condition.

Dosage adjustment for toxicity: IV administration (systemic): There are no recommended dosage reductions. Temporary suspension is recommended for severe infusion reactions, at least 4 weeks prior to (and after) elective surgery, in moderate to severe proteinuria (in most studies, treatment was withheld for ≥2 g proteinuria/24 hours), or in patients with severe hypertension which is not controlled with medical management. Permanent discontinuation is recommended (by the manufacturer) in patients who develop wound dehiscence and wound healing complications requiring intervention, necrotizing fasciitis, fistula (GI and non-GI), GI perforation, intra-abdominal abscess, hypertensive crisis, hypertensive encephalopathy, serious bleeding/hemorrhage, severe arterial thromboembolic event, life-threatening (grade 4) venous thromboembolic events (including pulmonary embolism), nephrotic syndrome, or PRES.

Dosage adjustment in renal impairment: There are no dosage adjustments provided in the manufacturer's labeling.

Dosage adjustment in hepatic impairment: There are no dosage adjustments provided in the manufacturer's labeling.

Administration

IV: Infuse the initial dose over 90 minutes. The second infusion may be shortened to 60 minutes if the initial infusion is well tolerated. The third and subsequent infusions may be shortened to 30 minutes if the 60-minute infusion is well tolerated. Monitor closely during the infusion for signs/symptoms of an infusion reaction. After tolerance at the 90-, 60-, and 30-minute infusion rates has been established, some institutions use an off-label 10-minute infusion rate (0.5 mg/kg/minute) for bevacizumab dosed at 5 mg/kg (Reidy, 2007). In a study evaluating the safety of the 0.5 mg/kg/minute infusion rate, proteinuria and hypertension incidences were not increased with the shorter infusion time (Shah, 2013). Do not administer IV push. Do not administer with dextrose solutions. Temporarily withhold bevacizumab for 4 weeks prior to elective surgery and for at least 4 weeks (and until the surgical incision is fully healed) after surgery.

Intravitreal injection (off-label use/route): Adequate local anesthesia and a topical broad-spectrum antimicrobial agent should be administered prior to the procedure.

Monitoring Parameters Monitor closely during the infusion for signs/symptoms of an infusion reaction. Monitor CBC with differential; signs/symptoms of gastrointestinal perforation, fistula, or abscess (including abdominal pain, constipation, vomiting, and fever); signs/symptoms of bleeding, including hemoptysis, gastrointestinal, and/or CNS bleeding, and/or epistaxis. Monitor blood pressure every 2 to 3 weeks; more frequently if hypertension develops during therapy. Continue to monitor blood pressure after discontinuing due to bevacizumab-induced hypertension. Monitor for proteinuria/nephrotic syndrome with urine dipstick; collect 24-hour urine in patients with ≥2+ reading. Monitor for signs/symptoms of thromboembolism (arterial and venous).

AMD (off-label use): Monitor intraocular pressure and retinal artery perfusion

Dosage Forms

Solution, Intravenous [preservative free]:

Avastin: 100 mg/4 mL (4 mL); 400 mg/16 mL (16 mL)

Bexarotene (Systemic) (beks AIR oh teen)

Brand Names: U.S. Targretin

Pharmacologic Category Antineoplastic Agent, Retinoic Acid Derivative

Use Treatment of cutaneous manifestations of cutaneous T-cell lymphoma in patients who are refractory to at least one prior systemic therapy

Pregnancy Risk Factor X

Dosage Oral: Adults:

Cutaneous T-cell lymphoma, refractory: Initial: 300 mg/m^2/day taken as a single daily dose; if well tolerated, but no response after 8 weeks of therapy, may increase to 400 mg/m^2/day; continue as long as clinical benefit is demonstrated.

Cutaneous T-cell lymphomas, relapsed/refractory (off-label dose): 150 mg daily (in combination with denileukin diftitox) (Foss, 2005)

Mycosis fungoides/Sezary syndrome, refractory/resistant (off-label dose): 75-150 mg daily in combination with PUVA; maximum dose: 300 mg daily (Rupoli, 2010; Singh, 2004)

Dosage adjustment for toxicity: If necessitated by toxicity, may decrease dose from 300 mg/m^2/day to 200 mg/m^2/day, then to 100 mg/m^2/day, or temporarily hold. Upon recovery, may titrate dose upward with careful monitoring.

Hepatotoxicity: If AST, ALT, or bilirubin >3 times ULN, consider holding or discontinuing therapy.

Hypertriglyceridemia: Consider reducing dose or suspending therapy.

Dosage adjustment in renal impairment: No dosage adjustment provided in manufacturer's labeling (has not been studied); however, renal insufficiency may result in significant protein binding changes and alter pharmacokinetics of bexarotene.

Dosage adjustment in hepatic impairment: No dosage adjustment provided in manufacturer's labeling (has not been studied); however, hepatic impairment would be expected to result in decreased clearance of bexarotene due to the extensive hepatic contribution to elimination.

Dosing in obesity: *ASCO Guidelines for appropriate chemotherapy dosing in obese adults with cancer:* Utilize patient's actual body weight (full weight) for calculation of body surface area- or weight-based dosing, particularly when the intent of therapy is curative; manage regimen-related toxicities in the same manner as for nonobese patients; if a dose reduction is utilized due to toxicity, consider resumption of full weight-based dosing with subsequent cycles, especially if cause of toxicity (eg, hepatic or renal impairment) is resolved (Griggs, 2012).

Additional Information Complete prescribing information should be consulted for additional detail.

Dosage Forms

Capsule, Oral:

Targretin: 75 mg

Bexarotene (Topical) (beks AIR oh teen)

Brand Names: U.S. Targretin

Pharmacologic Category Antineoplastic Agent, Retinoic Acid Derivative

Use Treatment of cutaneous lesions in patients with refractory cutaneous T-cell lymphoma (stage 1A and 1B) or who have not tolerated other therapies

Pregnancy Risk Factor X

Dosage Topical: Adults: Apply once every other day for first week, then increase on a weekly basis to once daily, 2 times/day, 3 times/day, and finally 4 times/day, according to tolerance

Dosing adjustment in renal impairment: No studies have been conducted; however, renal insufficiency may result in significant protein binding changes and alter pharmacokinetics of bexarotene

Dosing adjustment in hepatic impairment: No studies have been conducted; however, hepatic impairment would be expected to result in decreased clearance of bexarotene due to the extensive hepatic contribution to elimination

Additional Information Complete prescribing information should be consulted for additional detail.

Dosage Forms

Gel, External:

Targretin: 1% (60 g)

◆ **Beyaz** *see* Ethinyl Estradiol, Drospirenone, and Levomefolate *on page 812*

Bezafibrate [CAN/INT] (be za FYE brate)

Brand Names: Canada Bezalip SR

Pharmacologic Category Antilipemic Agent, Fibric Acid

Use Note: Not approved in U.S.

Adjunct to diet and other therapeutic measures for treatment of type IIa and IIb mixed hyperlipidemia, to regulate lipid and apoprotein levels (reduce serum TG, LDL-cholesterol, and apolipoprotein B, increase HDL-cholesterol and apolipoprotein A); treatment of adult patients with high to very high triglyceride levels (Fredrickson classification type IV and V hyperlipidemias) who are at high risk of sequelae and complications from their dyslipidemia

Pregnancy Considerations Use is contraindicated in pregnant women. Embryotoxicity has occurred in animals at toxic doses. Therapy should be discontinued in women who become pregnant during therapy. Women planning pregnancy should discontinue bezafibrate several months before conception and women of childbearing potential should employ effective birth control methods.

Breast-Feeding Considerations Do not use during lactation due to absence of data concerning the presence of bezafibrate in human breast milk.

Contraindications Hypersensitivity to bezafibrate, fibrates, or any component of the formulation; photoallergic or phototoxic reactions to fibrates; hepatic impairment; primary biliary cirrhosis; renal impairment (serum creatinine >1.5 mg/dL, CrCl <60 mL/minute, or patients undergoing dialysis); preexisting gallbladder disease; concomitant use with HMG CoA reductase inhibitors in patients predisposed to myopathy (eg, preexisting renal impairment, hormonal or electrolyte imbalance, severe infection, trauma, surgery); pregnancy or breast-feeding; not indicated for the treatment of type I hyperlipoproteinemia

Warnings/Precautions Secondary causes of hyperlipidemia should be ruled out prior to therapy. Has been shown to be hepatotoxic and possibly tumorigenic (animal models); discontinue if response is not obtained in 3 months. Use is contraindicated in hepatic impairment, including primary biliary cirrhosis. Abnormal liver function tests have been observed (reversible when discontinued). May increase risk for cholelithiasis. Use is contraindicated in renal impairment (serum creatinine >1.5 mg/dL, CrCl <60 mL/minute, or patients undergoing dialysis). Bezafibrate has been associated with rare myositis or rhabdomyolysis; risk may be increased by concurrent therapy with HMG-CoA reductase inhibitors or cyclosporine. Mild decreases in WBCs, platelets, and hemoglobin may occur following initiation of therapy; levels tend to stabilize with prolonged therapy. Use with caution in patient taking warfarin; adjustments in warfarin therapy may be required. Use is not recommended in patients >70 years of age. Limited experience is available in children; therefore, caution should be used when treating children.

Adverse Reactions

Central nervous system: Dizziness, headache, insomnia, migraine, pain

Dermatologic: Eczema, erythema, pruritus, urticaria

Gastrointestinal: Constipation, diarrhea, dyspepsia, epigastric distress, flatulence, gastritis, nausea

Hematologic: Anemia

Hepatic: ALT increased, AST increased

Neuromuscular & skeletal: CPK increased

Respiratory: Bronchitis, pharyngitis

Miscellaneous: Allergic reaction

Rare but important or life-threatening): Acute renal failure, cholelithiasis, creatinine increased, hypersensitivity, myopathy, pancytopenia, rhabdomyolysis, rhabdomyolysis, Stevens-Johnson syndrome, thrombocytopenia purpura, toxic epidermal necrolysis, WBC decreased

Drug Interactions

Metabolism/Transport Effects **Substrate** of CYP3A4 (minor); **Note:** Assignment of Major/Minor substrate status based on clinically relevant drug interaction potential

Avoid Concomitant Use

Avoid concomitant use of Bezafibrate with any of the following: Ciprofibrate; Ezetimibe; MAO Inhibitors

Increased Effect/Toxicity

Bezafibrate may increase the levels/effects of: Colchicine; Ezetimibe; HMG-CoA Reductase Inhibitors; Sulfonylureas; Vitamin K Antagonists

The levels/effects of Bezafibrate may be increased by: Acipimox; Ciprofibrate; CycloSPORINE (Systemic); MAO Inhibitors; Raltegravir

Decreased Effect

Bezafibrate may decrease the levels/effects of: Chenodiol; CycloSPORINE (Systemic); Ursodiol

The levels/effects of Bezafibrate may be decreased by: Bile Acid Sequestrants

Storage/Stability Store at room temperature of 15°C to 30°C (59°F to 86°F). Protect from moisture.

Mechanism of Action Mechanism not definitely established; may increase VLDL catabolism by increasing lipoprotein and hepatic triglyceride lipase activities; attenuation of triglyceride biosynthesis by inhibition of acetyl-CoA carboxylase; decreased cholesterol biosynthesis by inhibition of 3-hydroxy-3-methyglutaryl-coenzyme A reductase

Pharmacodynamics/Kinetics

Distribution: ~17 L

Protein binding: 94% to 96%

Half-life elimination: 1-2 hours

Time to peak, serum: 3-4 hours

Excretion: Urine (95%); feces (3%)

Dosage Oral:

Children ≥20 kg (limited experience available; use caution): 10-20 mg/kg/day (maximum: 400 mg). **Note:** Based on child's weight, dosing may not be possible as the manufacturer recommends administering the sustained release tablet whole.

Adults: 400 mg once daily

Elderly: Manufacturer labeling recommends avoiding use in patients >70 years of age due to declining renal function and the likelihood of CrCl <60 mL/minute in this population.

Dosing interval in renal impairment:

CrCl ≥60 mL/minute: No dosage adjustment required

CrCl <60 mL/minute **or** S_{cr} >1.5 mg/dL: Use is contraindicated

Dialysis: Use is contraindicated.

Dosage adjustment in hepatic impairment: Use is contraindicated in hepatic impairment

Dietary Considerations Should be taken with or after meals. Before initiation of therapy, patients should be placed on a standard lipid-lowering diet for 6 weeks and the diet should be continued during drug therapy.

Administration Do not crush or chew; tablet should be swallowed whole with sufficient fluid. Take in morning or evening with or after meals.

Monitoring Parameters Periodic evaluation of serum lipids, cholesterol, and triglycerides (especially in the first few months of therapy). LFTs after 3-6 months; then at least annually. CBC (periodically during the first 12 months). Fasting glucose, creatinine, and CPK periodically.

Product Availability Not available in U.S.

Dosage Forms: Canada

Tablet, sustained release, oral:

Bezalip® SR: 400 mg

◆ **Bezalip SR (Can)** *see* Bezafibrate [CAN/INT] *on page* 261

◆ **BG-12** *see* Dimethyl Fumarate *on page* 639

◆ **BI 397** *see* Dalbavancin *on page* 551

◆ **BI-1356** *see* Linagliptin *on page* 1215

◆ **BI10773** *see* Empagliflozin *on page* 718

◆ **Biaxin** *see* Clarithromycin *on page* 456

◆ **Biaxin XL** *see* Clarithromycin *on page* 456

◆ **Biaxin XL Pac** *see* Clarithromycin *on page* 456

◆ **Biaxin BID (Can)** *see* Clarithromycin *on page* 456

◆ **BIBF1120** *see* Nintedanib *on page* 1458

◆ **BIBW 2992** *see* Afatinib *on page* 61

Bicalutamide (bye ka LOO ta mide)

Brand Names: U.S. Casodex

Brand Names: Canada ACH-Bicalutamide; Apo-Bicalutamide; Casodex; CO Bicalutamide; Dom-Bicalutamide;

JAMP-Bicalutamide; Mylan-Bicalutamide; Novo-Bicalutamide; PHL-Bicalutamide; PMS-Bicalutamide; PRO-Bicalutamide; RAN-Bicalutamide; Sandoz-Bicalutamide

Index Terms CDX; ICI-176334

Pharmacologic Category Antineoplastic Agent, Antiandrogen

Use

Prostate cancer, metastatic: Treatment of stage D_2 metastatic prostate cancer (in combination with an LHRH agonist)

Limitation of use: Bicalutamide 150 mg daily is not approved for use alone or with other treatments

Pregnancy Risk Factor X

Pregnancy Considerations Adverse events were observed in animal reproduction studies. Bicalutamide use is contraindicated in women. Androgen receptor inhibition during pregnancy may affect fetal development.

Breast-Feeding Considerations Bicalutamide is not indicated for use in women.

Contraindications Hypersensitivity to bicalutamide or any component of the formulation; use in women, especially women who are or may become pregnant

Warnings/Precautions Hazardous agent - use appropriate precautions for handling and disposal (NIOSH 2014 [group 1]). Rare cases of death or hospitalization due to hepatitis have been reported postmarketing. Use with caution in moderate-to-severe hepatic dysfunction. Hepatotoxicity generally occurs within the first 3 to 4 months of use; patients should be monitored for signs and symptoms of liver dysfunction. Bicalutamide should be discontinued if patients have jaundice or ALT is >2 times the upper limit of normal. Androgen-deprivation therapy may increase the risk for cardiovascular disease (Levine, 2010). May cause gynecomastia, breast pain, or lead to spermatogenesis inhibition. When used in combination with LHRH agonists, a loss of glycemic control and decrease in glucose tolerance has been reported in patients with diabetes; monitor. May cause gynecomastia or breast pain (at higher, off-label doses), or lead to spermatogenesis inhibition. Potentially significant drug-drug interactions may exist, requiring dose or frequency adjustment, additional monitoring, and/or selection of alternative therapy.

Adverse Reactions

Cardiovascular: Angina pectoris, cardiac arrest, cardiac failure, chest pain, coronary artery disease, edema, hypertension, myocardial infarction, peripheral edema, syncope

Central nervous system: Anxiety, chills, confusion, depression, dizziness, drowsiness, headache, hypertonia, insomnia, myasthenia, nervousness, neuropathy, pain, paresthesia

Dermatologic: Alopecia, diaphoresis, pruritus, skin rash, xeroderma

Endocrine & metabolic: Decreased libido, dehydration, gout, gynecomastia (more common in monotherapy), hot flash, hypercholesterolemia, hyperglycemia, weight gain, weight loss

Gastrointestinal: Abdominal pain, anorexia, constipation, diarrhea, dyspepsia, dysphagia, flatulence, hernia, melena, nausea, periodontal abscess, vomiting, xerostomia

Genitourinary: Difficulty in micturition, dysuria, hematuria, impotence, mastalgia (more common in monotherapy), nocturia, pelvic pain, urinary incontinence, urinary retention, urinary tract infection, urinary urgency

Hematologic & oncologic: Anemia, gastrointestinal carcinoma, rectal hemorrhage, skin carcinoma

Hepatic: Increased liver enzymes, increased serum alkaline phosphatase

Infection: Herpes zoster, infection, sepsis

Neuromuscular & skeletal: Arthritis, back pain, leg cramps, myalgia, neck pain, ostealgia, pathological fracture, weakness

Ophthalmic: Cataract

Renal: Hydronephrosis, increased blood urea nitrogen, increased serum creatinine, polyuria

Respiratory: Asthma, bronchitis, cough, dyspnea, epistaxis, flu-like symptoms, pharyngitis, pneumonia, rhinitis, sinusitis

Miscellaneous: Cyst, fever

Rare but important or life-threatening: Decreased glucose tolerance, decreased hemoglobin, decreased white blood cell count, hepatitis, hepatotoxicity, hypersensitivity (including angioneurotic edema and urticaria), increased serum bilirubin, interstitial pneumonitis, pulmonary fibrosis

Drug Interactions

Metabolism/Transport Effects Inhibits CYP3A4 (moderate)

Avoid Concomitant Use

Avoid concomitant use of Bicalutamide with any of the following: Astemizole; Bosutinib; Cisapride; Ibrutinib; Indium 111 Capromab Pendetide; Ivabradine; Lomitapide; Naloxegol; Olaparib; Pimozide; Simeprevir; Terfenadine; Tolvaptan; Trabectedin; Ulipristal

Increased Effect/Toxicity

Bicalutamide may increase the levels/effects of: ARIPiprazole; Astemizole; Avanafil; Bosentan; Bosutinib; Budesonide (Systemic, Oral Inhalation); Cannabis; Cisapride; Colchicine; CYP3A4 Substrates; Dapoxetine; Dofetilide; DOXOrubicin (Conventional); Dronabinol; Eliglustat; Eplerenone; Everolimus; FentaNYL; Halofantrine; Hydrocodone; Ibrutinib; Imatinib; Ivabradine; Ivacaftor; Lomitapide; Lurasidone; Naloxegol; Olaparib; OxyCODONE; Pimecrolimus; Pimozide; Propafenone; Ranolazine; Rivaroxaban; Salmeterol; Saxagliptin; Simeprevir; Suvorexant; Terfenadine; Tetrahydrocannabinol; Tolvaptan; Trabectedin; Ulipristal; Vilazodone; Vitamin K Antagonists; Zopiclone; Zuclopenthixol

Decreased Effect

Bicalutamide may decrease the levels/effects of: Ifosfamide; Indium 111 Capromab Pendetide

Storage/Stability Store at room temperature of 20°C to 25°C (68°F to 77°F).

Mechanism of Action Androgen receptor inhibitor; pure nonsteroidal antiandrogen that binds to androgen receptors; specifically a competitive inhibitor for the binding of dihydrotestosterone and testosterone; prevents testosterone stimulation of cell growth in prostate cancer

Pharmacodynamics/Kinetics

Absorption: Well absorbed; unaffected by food

Protein binding: 96%

Metabolism: Extensively hepatic; glucuronidation and oxidation of the R (active) enantiomer to inactive metabolites; the S enantiomer is inactive

Half-life elimination: Active enantiomer: ~6 days

Time to peak, plasma: Active enantiomer: ~31 hours

Excretion: Urine and feces

Dosage

Prostate cancer, metastatic: Adults: Oral: 50 mg once daily (in combination with an LHRH analogue)

Prostate cancer, locally advanced, high recurrence risk (off-label use): Adults: Oral: 150 mg once daily (as monotherapy) (McLeod, 2006). Additional trials may be necessary to further define the role of bicalutamide in this condition.

Dosage adjustment in renal impairment: No dosage adjustment necessary.

Dosage adjustment in hepatic impairment:

Hepatic impairment at treatment initiation: Mild, moderate, or severe impairment: No dosage adjustment is necessary. Use with caution in patients with moderate-to-severe impairment; clearance may be delayed in severe impairment (based on a limited number of patients).

Hepatic impairment during treatment: ALT >2 times ULN or jaundice develops: Discontinue immediately.

Administration Dose should be taken at the same time each day, either in the morning or in the evening. May be administered with or without food. Treatment for metastatic cancer should be started concomitantly with an LHRH analogue.

Hazardous agent; use appropriate precautions for handling and disposal (NIOSH 2014 [group 1]).

Monitoring Parameters Periodically monitor CBC, ECG, echocardiograms, serum testosterone, luteinizing hormone, and prostate specific antigen (PSA). Liver function tests should be obtained at baseline and repeated regularly during the first 4 months of treatment, and periodically thereafter; monitor for signs and symptoms of liver dysfunction (discontinue if jaundice is noted or ALT is >2 times the upper limit of normal). Monitor blood glucose in patients with diabetes. If initiating bicalutamide in patients who are on warfarin, closely monitor prothrombin time.

Dosage Forms

Tablet, Oral:

Casodex: 50 mg

Generic: 50 mg

- ◆ **Bicillin L-A** *see* Penicillin G Benzathine *on page 1609*
- ◆ **Bicillin® C-R** *see* Penicillin G Benzathine and Penicillin G Procaine *on page 1611*
- ◆ **Bicillin® C-R 900/300** *see* Penicillin G Benzathine and Penicillin G Procaine *on page 1611*
- ◆ **Bicitra** *see* Sodium Citrate and Citric Acid *on page 1905*
- ◆ **BiCNU** *see* Carmustine *on page 364*
- ◆ **Bidex [OTC]** *see* GuaiFENesin *on page 986*
- ◆ **BiDil** *see* Isosorbide Dinitrate and Hydralazine *on page 1126*

Bifonazole [INT] (BYE fone a zole)

International Brand Names Amycor (FR); Azolmen (IT); Bifazol (IT); Bifokey (ES); Bifomyk (DE); Bifon (DE); Bifonal (AR); Bifonazol R.O. (AR); Bimicot (AR); Canesten (AU, DE); Canesten Extra Bifonazol (DE); Fungiderm (AT); Micofun (CO); Moldina (ES); Monostop (ES); Mycospor (AR, AU, BE, CZ, DE, ES, GR, HR, LU, MX, NL, NO, PT, ZA); Mycosporan (SE); Mycosporin (AT)

Pharmacologic Category Antifungal Agent, Topical

Reported Use Topical treatment of fungal infections of skin and nails

Dosage Range Adults: Topical: Apply to affected area once daily, preferably before going to bed. Duration of treatment is 2-4 weeks depending on the indication.

Product Availability Product available in various countries; not currently available in the U.S.

Dosage Forms

Cream: 1%

Gel: 1%

Powder: 1%

Solution, topical: 1%

Spray: 1%

- ◆ **BIG-IV** *see* Botulism Immune Globulin (Intravenous-Human) *on page 284*
- ◆ **Biltricide** *see* Praziquantel *on page 1702*

Bimatoprost (bi MAT oh prost)

Brand Names: U.S. Latisse; Lumigan

Brand Names: Canada Latisse; Lumigan; Lumigan RC

Pharmacologic Category Ophthalmic Agent, Antiglaucoma; Prostaglandin, Ophthalmic

Use

Elevated intraocular pressure (Lumigan only): Reduction of elevated intraocular pressure (IOP) in patients with open-angle glaucoma or ocular hypertension

Hypotrichosis of the eyelashes (Latisse only): Treatment of hypotrichosis of the eyelashes

Pregnancy Risk Factor C

Dosage

Elevated intraocular pressure (Lumigan): Adolescents ≥16 years and Adults: Ophthalmic: Instill 1 drop into affected eye(s) once daily in the evening; do not exceed once-daily dosing (may decrease IOP-lowering effect). If used with other topical ophthalmic agents, separate administration by at least 5 minutes.

Hypotrichosis of the eyelashes (Latisse): Children ≥5 years, Adolescents, and Adults: Ophthalmic, topical: Place one drop on applicator and apply evenly along the skin of the upper eyelid at base of eyelashes once daily at bedtime; repeat procedure for second eye (use a clean applicator).

Dosage in renal impairment: There are no dosage adjustments provided in the manufacturer's labeling.

Dosage in hepatic impairment: There are no dosage adjustments provided in the manufacturer's labeling.

Additional Information Complete prescribing information should be consulted for additional detail.

Dosage Forms

Solution, External:

Latisse: 0.03% (3 mL, 5 mL)

Solution, Ophthalmic:

Lumigan: 0.01% (2.5 mL, 5 mL, 7.5 mL)

Bimatoprost and Timolol [INT]

(bi MAT oh prost & TIM oh lol)

International Brand Names Bimat-T (VN); Ganfort (AE, AR, AT, AU, BE, BR, CH, CL, CN, CO, CY, CZ, DE, DK, EC, EE, ES, FI, FR, GB, GR, HK, HR, HU, IE, IL, IN, IS, IT, KR, KW, LB, LT, LU, MT, MY, NL, NO, NZ, PE, PH, PL, PT, RO, SA, SE, SG, SI, SK, TH, VN); Ganforti (MX)

Index Terms Timolol and Bimatoprost

Pharmacologic Category Beta Blocker, Nonselective; Ophthalmic Agent, Antiglaucoma; Prostaglandin, Ophthalmic

Reported Use Decrease of intraocular pressure (IOP) in patients with open-angle glaucoma or ocular hypertension who are insufficiently responsive to topical beta-blockers or prostaglandin analogues

Dosage Range Ophthalmic: Adults: Instill 1 drop into affected eye(s) once daily

Product Availability Product available in various countries; not currently available in the U.S.

Dosage Forms

Solution, ophthalmic: Bimatoprost 0.03% and timolol maleate 0.5% (3 mL) [contains benzalkonium chloride]

- ◆ **Binosto** *see* Alendronate *on page 79*
- ◆ **Bio-Amitriptyline (Can)** *see* Amitriptyline *on page 119*
- ◆ **Bio-Amlodipine (Can)** *see* AmLODIPine *on page 123*
- ◆ **Bio-Anastrozole (Can)** *see* Anastrozole *on page 148*
- ◆ **Bio-Diazepam (Can)** *see* Diazepam *on page 613*
- ◆ **Bio-Donepezil (Can)** *see* Donepezil *on page 668*
- ◆ **Bio-Ezetimibe (Can)** *see* Ezetimibe *on page 832*
- ◆ **Bio-Flurazepam (Can)** *see* Flurazepam *on page 906*
- ◆ **Bio-Furosemide (Can)** *see* Furosemide *on page 940*
- ◆ **Bio Glo** *see* Fluorescein *on page 894*
- ◆ **Bio-Hydrochlorothiazide (Can)** *see* Hydrochlorothiazide *on page 1009*
- ◆ **Bio-Letrozole (Can)** *see* Letrozole *on page 1181*

◆ **Bionect** *see* Hyaluronate and Derivatives *on page 1006*
◆ **Bioniche Promethazine (Can)** *see* Promethazine *on page 1723*
◆ **Bio-Oxazepam (Can)** *see* Oxazepam *on page 1532*
◆ **BioQuin Durules (Can)** *see* QuiNIDine *on page 1759*
◆ **Bio-Statin** *see* Nystatin (Oral) *on page 1481*
◆ **BioThrax** *see* Anthrax Vaccine Adsorbed *on page 151*
◆ **Biphentin (Can)** *see* Methylphenidate *on page 1336*
◆ **Bird Flu Vaccine** *see* Influenza A Virus Vaccine (H5N1) *on page 1074*
◆ **Bisac-Evac [OTC]** *see* Bisacodyl *on page 265*

Bisacodyl (bis a KOE dil)

Brand Names: U.S. Bisac-Evac [OTC]; Bisacodyl EC [OTC]; Bisacodyl Laxative [OTC]; Biscolax [OTC]; Correct [OTC]; Ducodyl [OTC]; Dulcolax [OTC]; Ex-Lax Ultra [OTC]; Fleet Bisacodyl [OTC]; Fleet Laxative [OTC]; Gentle Laxative [OTC]; Laxative [OTC]; Stimulant Laxative [OTC]; The Magic Bullet [OTC]; Womens Laxative [OTC]

Brand Names: Canada Apo-Bisacodyl [OTC]; Bisacodyl-Odan [OTC]; Bisacolax [OTC]; Carter's Little Pills [OTC]; Codulax [OTC]; Dulcolax For Women [OTC]; Dulcolax [OTC]; PMS-Bisacodyl [OTC]; ratio-Bisacodyl [OTC]; Silver Bullet Suppository [OTC]; Soflax EX [OTC]; The Magic Bullett [OTC]; Woman's Laxative [OTC]

Pharmacologic Category Laxative, Stimulant

Use Treatment of constipation; colonic evacuation prior to procedures or examination

Dosage

Children:

Oral: >6 years: 5-10 mg (0.3 mg/kg) at bedtime or before breakfast

Rectal suppository:

<2 years: 5 mg as a single dose

>2 years: 10 mg

Adults:

Oral: 5-15 mg as single dose (up to 30 mg when complete evacuation of bowel is required)

Rectal suppository: 10 mg as single dose

Dosage adjustment in renal impairment: No dosage adjustment provided in manufacturer's labeling. Use with caution in patients with impaired renal function.

Dosage adjustment in hepatic impairment: No dosage adjustment provided in manufacturer's labeling.

Additional Information Complete prescribing information should be consulted for additional detail.

Dosage Forms

Enema, Rectal:

Fleet Bisacodyl [OTC]: 10 mg/30 mL (37 mL)

Suppository, Rectal:

Bisac-Evac [OTC]: 10 mg (1 ea, 8 ea, 12 ea, 50 ea, 100 ea, 500 ea, 1000 ea)

Bisacodyl Laxative [OTC]: 10 mg (12 ea)

Biscolax [OTC]: 10 mg (12 ea, 100 ea)

Dulcolax [OTC]: 10 mg (4 ea, 8 ea, 16 ea, 28 ea, 50 ea)

Gentle Laxative [OTC]: 10 mg (4 ea, 8 ea, 12 ea)

Laxative [OTC]: 10 mg (12 ea, 100 ea)

The Magic Bullet [OTC]: 10 mg (10 ea, 100 ea)

Generic: 10 mg (12 ea, 50 ea, 100 ea)

Tablet Delayed Release, Oral:

Bisacodyl EC [OTC]: 5 mg

Correct [OTC]: 5 mg

Ducodyl [OTC]: 5 mg

Dulcolax [OTC]: 5 mg

Ex-Lax Ultra [OTC]: 5 mg

Fleet Laxative [OTC]: 5 mg

Gentle Laxative [OTC]: 5 mg

Stimulant Laxative [OTC]: 5 mg

Womens Laxative [OTC]: 5 mg

◆ **Bisacodyl EC [OTC]** *see* Bisacodyl *on page 265*
◆ **Bisacodyl Laxative [OTC]** *see* Bisacodyl *on page 265*
◆ **Bisacodyl-Odan [OTC] (Can)** *see* Bisacodyl *on page 265*
◆ **Bisacolax [OTC] (Can)** *see* Bisacodyl *on page 265*
◆ **bis(chloroethyl) nitrosourea** *see* Carmustine *on page 364*
◆ **bis-chloronitrosourea** *see* Carmustine *on page 364*
◆ **Biscolax [OTC]** *see* Bisacodyl *on page 265*
◆ **Bismatrol** *see* Bismuth *on page 265*
◆ **Bismatrol [OTC]** *see* Bismuth *on page 265*
◆ **Bismatrol Maximum Strength [OTC]** *see* Bismuth *on page 265*

Bismuth (BIZ muth)

Brand Names: U.S. Bismatrol Maximum Strength [OTC]; Bismatrol [OTC]; Diotame [OTC]; Geri-Pectate [OTC]; Kao-Tin [OTC]; Peptic Relief [OTC]; Pepto-Bismol To-Go [OTC]; Pepto-Bismol [OTC]; Pink Bismuth [OTC]; Stomach Relief Max St [OTC]; Stomach Relief Plus [OTC]; Stomach Relief [OTC]

Index Terms Bismatrol; Bismuth Subsalicylate; Pink Bismuth

Pharmacologic Category Antidiarrheal

Use Subsalicylate formulation: Symptomatic treatment of mild, nonspecific diarrhea; control of traveler's diarrhea (enterotoxigenic *Escherichia coli*); as part of a multidrug regimen for *H. pylori* eradication to reduce the risk of duodenal ulcer recurrence

Dosage Oral:

Treatment of nonspecific diarrhea, control/relieve traveler's diarrhea: Subsalicylate: Children >12 years and Adults: 524 mg every 30 minutes to 1 hour as needed up to 8 doses/24 hours

Helicobacter pylori eradication: Subsalicylate: Adults: 524 mg 4 times/day with meals and at bedtime; requires combination therapy

Dosing adjustment in renal impairment: Bismuth has been associated with nephrotoxicity in overdose (Leussnik, 2002); although there are no specific recommendations by the manufacturer, consider using with caution in patients with renal impairment.

Additional Information Complete prescribing information should be consulted for additional detail.

Dosage Forms

Suspension, Oral:

Bismatrol [OTC]: 262 mg/15 mL (236 mL)

Bismatrol Maximum Strength [OTC]: 525 mg/15 mL (236 mL)

Geri-Pectate [OTC]: 262 mg/15 mL (355 mL)

Kao-Tin [OTC]: 262 mg/15 mL (236 mL, 473 mL)

Peptic Relief [OTC]: 262 mg/15 mL (237 mL)

Pepto-Bismol [OTC]: 262 mg/15 mL (473 mL)

Pink Bismuth [OTC]: 262 mg/15 mL (236 mL, 237 mL)

Stomach Relief [OTC]: 262 mg/15 mL (237 mL, 355 mL); 527 mg/30 mL (240 mL, 480 mL)

Stomach Relief Max St [OTC]: 525 mg/15 mL (237 mL)

Stomach Relief Plus [OTC]: 525 mg/15 mL (240 mL, 480 mL)

Tablet Chewable, Oral:

Bismatrol [OTC]: 262 mg

Diotame [OTC]: 262 mg

Peptic Relief [OTC]: 262 mg

Pepto-Bismol To-Go [OTC]: 262 mg

Pink Bismuth [OTC]: 262 mg

Stomach Relief [OTC]: 262 mg

Generic: 262 mg

◆ **Bismuth Subsalicylate** *see* Bismuth *on page 265*

Bisoprolol (bis OH proe lol)

Brand Names: U.S. Zebeta

Brand Names: Canada Apo-Bisoprolol; Ava-Bisoprolol; Mylan-Bisoprolol; Novo-Bisoprolol; PHL-Bisoprolol; PMS-Bisoprolol; PRO-Bisoprolol; Sandoz-Bisoprolol; Teva-Bisoprolol

Index Terms Bisoprolol Fumarate

Pharmacologic Category Antihypertensive; Beta-Blocker, Beta-1 Selective

Use Hypertension: Treatment of hypertension, alone or in combination with other agents

The 2014 guideline for the management of high blood pressure in adults (Eighth Joint National Committee [JNC 8]) recommends initiation of pharmacologic treatment to lower blood pressure for the following patients (JNC8 [James, 2013]):

- Patients ≥60 years of age, with systolic blood pressure (SBP) ≥150 mm Hg or diastolic blood pressure (DBP) ≥90 mm Hg. Goal of therapy is SBP <150 mm Hg and DBP <90 mm Hg.
- Patients <60 years of age, with SBP ≥140 mm Hg or DBP ≥90 mm Hg. Goal of therapy is SBP <140 mm Hg and DBP <90 mm Hg.
- Patients ≥18 years of age with diabetes, with SBP ≥140 mm Hg or DBP ≥90 mm Hg. Goal of therapy is SBP <140 mm Hg and DBP <90 mm Hg.
- Patients ≥18 years of age with chronic kidney disease (CKD), with SBP ≥140 mm Hg or DBP ≥90 mm Hg. Goal of therapy is SBP <140 mm Hg and DBP <90 mm Hg.

In patients with CKD, regardless of race or diabetes status, the use of an ACE inhibitor (ACEI) or angiotensin receptor blocker (ARB) as initial therapy is recommended to improve kidney outcomes. In the general nonblack population (without CKD) including those with diabetes, initial antihypertensive treatment should consist of a thiazide-type diuretic, calcium channel blocker, ACEI, or ARB. In the general black population (without CKD) including those with diabetes, initial antihypertensive treatment should consist of a thiazide-type diuretic or a calcium channel blocker **instead of** an ACEI or ARB.

Pregnancy Risk Factor C

Pregnancy Considerations Adverse events were observed in animal reproduction studies; therefore, the manufacturer classifies bisoprolol as pregnancy category C. In a cohort study, an increased risk of cardiovascular defects was observed following maternal use of beta-blockers during pregnancy. Intrauterine growth restriction (IUGR), small placentas, as well as fetal/neonatal bradycardia, hypoglycemia, and/or respiratory depression have been observed following *in utero* exposure to beta-blockers as a class. Adequate facilities for monitoring infants at birth should be available. Untreated chronic maternal hypertension and pre-eclampsia are also associated with adverse events in the fetus, infant, and mother. Limited information is available related to the use of bisoprolol for the treatment of hypertension in pregnancy; other agents may be more appropriate for use.

Breast-Feeding Considerations It is not known if bisoprolol is excreted into breast milk. The manufacturer recommends that caution be exercised when administering bisoprolol to nursing women.

Contraindications Cardiogenic shock; overt cardiac failure; marked sinus bradycardia or heart block greater than first-degree (except in patients with a functioning artificial pacemaker)

Warnings/Precautions Consider preexisting conditions such as sick sinus syndrome before initiating. Use caution in patients with heart failure; use gradual and careful titration; monitor for symptoms of congestive heart failure. Beta-blockers without alpha1-adrenergic receptor blocking activity should be avoided in patients with Prinzmetal variant angina (Mayer, 1998). Use with caution in patients with myasthenia gravis, psychiatric disease (may cause CNS depression), bronchospastic disease, undergoing anesthesia; and in those with impaired hepatic function. Bradycardia may be observed more frequently in elderly patients (>65 years of age); dosage reductions may be necessary. Beta-blocker therapy should not be withdrawn abruptly (particularly in patients with CAD), but gradually tapered to avoid acute tachycardia, hypertension, and/or ischemia. Chronic beta-blocker therapy should not be routinely withdrawn prior to major surgery. Can precipitate or aggravate symptoms of arterial insufficiency in patients with PVD and Raynaud's disease; use with caution and monitor for progression of arterial obstruction. Use caution with concurrent use of digoxin, verapamil, or diltiazem; bradycardia or heart block may occur. Use with caution in patients receiving inhaled anesthetic agents known to depress myocardial contractility. Bisoprolol, with beta$_1$-selectivity, may be used cautiously in bronchospastic disease with close monitoring. Use cautiously in patients with diabetes because it can mask prominent hypoglycemic symptoms. May mask signs of hyperthyroidism (eg, tachycardia); use caution if hyperthyroidism is suspected, abrupt withdrawal may precipitate thyroid storm. Dosage adjustment is required in patients with significant hepatic or renal dysfunction. Adequate alpha-blockade is required prior to use of any beta-blocker for patients with untreated pheochromocytoma. May induce or exacerbate psoriasis. Use caution with history of severe anaphylaxis to allergens; patients taking beta-blockers may become more sensitive to repeated challenges. Treatment of anaphylaxis (eg, epinephrine) in patients taking beta-blockers may be ineffective or promote undesirable effects.

Adverse Reactions

Cardiovascular: Chest pain

Central nervous system: Fatigue, insomnia, hypoesthesia

Gastrointestinal: Diarrhea, nausea, vomiting

Neuromuscular & skeletal: Arthralgia, weakness

Respiratory: Dyspnea, rhinitis, sinusitis, upper respiratory infection

Rare but important or life-threatening: Abdominal pain, abnormal lacrimation, acne vulgaris, alopecia, amnesia, angioedema, anxiety, asthma, back pain, bradycardia (dose related), bronchitis, bronchospasm, cardiac arrhythmia, claudication, cold extremities, confusion (especially in the elderly), congestive heart failure, constipation, cough, cystitis, decreased libido, depression, dermatitis, dizziness, drowsiness, dysgeusia, dyspepsia, dyspnea on exertion, eczema, edema, exfoliative dermatitis, eye pain, flushing, gastritis, gout, hallucination, headache, hearing loss, hyperesthesia, hyperglycemia, hyperkalemia, hyperphosphatemia, hypersensitivity angiitis, hypertriglyceridemia, hypotension, impotence, increased blood urea nitrogen, increased serum creatinine, increased serum transaminases, increased uric acid, insomnia, leukopenia, malaise, muscle cramps, myalgia, neck pain, nervousness, orthostatic hypotension, palpitations, paresthesia, peptic ulcer, Peyronie's disease, pharyngitis, polyuria, positive ANA titer, pruritus, psoriasiform eruption, psoriasis, purpura, renal colic, restlessness, sensation of eye pressure, skin rash, syncope, thrombocytopenia, tinnitus, tremor, twitching, vasculitis, vertigo, visual disturbance, weight gain, xerostomia

Drug Interactions

Metabolism/Transport Effects Substrate of CYP2D6 (minor), CYP3A4 (major); **Note:** Assignment of Major/Minor substrate status based on clinically relevant drug interaction potential

Avoid Concomitant Use

Avoid concomitant use of Bisoprolol with any of the following: Ceritinib; Conivaptan; Floctafenine; Fusidic Acid (Systemic); Idelalisib; Methacholine

Increased Effect/Toxicity

Bisoprolol may increase the levels/effects of: Alpha-/Beta-Agonists (Direct-Acting); Alpha1-Blockers; Alpha2-Agonists; Amifostine; Antihypertensives; Antipsychotic Agents (Phenothiazines); Bradycardia-Causing Agents; Bupivacaine; Cardiac Glycosides; Ceritinib; Cholinergic Agonists; Disopyramide; DULoxetine; Ergot Derivatives; Fingolimod; Grass Pollen Allergen Extract (5 Grass Extract); Hypotensive Agents; Insulin; Lacosamide; Levodopa; Lidocaine (Systemic); Lidocaine (Topical); Mepivacaine; Methacholine; Midodrine; Obinutuzumab; RisperiDONE; RiTUXimab; Sulfonylureas

The levels/effects of Bisoprolol may be increased by: Acetylcholinesterase Inhibitors; Alpha2-Agonists; Aminoquinolines (Antimalarial); Amiodarone; Anilidopiperidine Opioids; Antipsychotic Agents (Phenothiazines); Aprepitant; Barbiturates; Bretylium; Brimonidine (Topical); Calcium Channel Blockers (Dihydropyridine); Calcium Channel Blockers (Nondihydropyridine); Conivaptan; CYP3A4 Inhibitors (Moderate); CYP3A4 Inhibitors (Strong); Dasatinib; Diazoxide; Dipyridamole; Disopyramide; Dronedarone; Floctafenine; Fosaprepitant; Fusidic Acid (Systemic); Herbs (Hypotensive Properties); Idelalisib; Ivacaftor; Luliconazole; MAO Inhibitors; Mifepristone; Netupitant; Nicorandil; Pentoxifylline; Phosphodiesterase 5 Inhibitors; Propafenone; Prostacyclin Analogues; Regorafenib; Reserpine; Simeprevir; Stiripentol; Tofacitinib

Decreased Effect

Bisoprolol may decrease the levels/effects of: Beta2-Agonists; Theophylline Derivatives

The levels/effects of Bisoprolol may be decreased by: Barbiturates; Bosentan; CYP3A4 Inducers (Moderate); CYP3A4 Inducers (Strong); Dabrafenib; Deferasirox; Herbs (Hypertensive Properties); Methylphenidate; Mitotane; Nonsteroidal Anti-Inflammatory Agents; Siltuximab; St Johns Wort; Tocilizumab; Yohimbine

Storage/Stability Store at controlled room temperature 20°C to 25°C (68°F to 77°F). Protect from moisture.

Mechanism of Action Selective inhibitor of beta$_1$-adrenergic receptors; competitively blocks beta$_1$-receptors, with little or no effect on beta$_2$-receptors at doses ≤20 mg

Pharmacodynamics/Kinetics

Onset of action: 1 to 2 hours

Absorption: Rapid and almost complete

Distribution: Widely; highest concentrations in heart, liver, lungs, and saliva; crosses blood-brain barrier

Protein binding: ~30%

Metabolism: Extensively hepatic; significant first-pass effect (~20%)

Bioavailability: ~80%

Half-life elimination: Normal renal function: 9 to 12 hours; CrCl <40 mL/minute: 27 to 36 hours; Hepatic cirrhosis: 8 to 22 hours

Time to peak: 2 to 4 hours

Excretion: Urine (50% as unchanged drug, remainder as inactive metabolites); feces (<2%)

Dosage Oral:

Adults:

Hypertension: Initial: 2.5 to 5 mg once daily; may be increased to 10 mg and then up to 20 mg once daily, if necessary; usual dose range (ASH/ISH [Weber, 2014]): 5 to 10 mg once daily

Atrial fibrillation (rate control) (off-label use): Usual maintenance dose: 2.5 to 10 mg once daily (AHA/ACC/HRS [January, 2014])

Heart failure (off-label use): Initial: 1.25 mg once daily; maximum dose: 10 mg once daily. **Note:** Initiate only in stable patients or hospitalized patients after volume status has been optimized and IV diuretics, vasodilators, and inotropic agents have all been successfully discontinued. Caution should be used when initiating in patients who required inotropes during their hospital course. Increase dose gradually and monitor for congestive signs and symptoms of HF making every effort to achieve target dose shown to be effective (ACCF/AHA [Yancy, 2013]; CIBIS-II Investigators and Committees, 1999; HFSA [Lindenfeld, 2010]).

Elderly: Refer to adult dosing.

Dosage adjustment in renal impairment:

Hypertension: CrCl <40 mL/minute: Initial: 2.5 mg daily; increase cautiously.

Heart failure (off-label use): In clinical trials, the initial recommended dosage (ie, 1.25 mg once daily) was not reduced further based on CrCl; however, patients with serum creatinine ≥3.4 mg/dL were excluded in one trial (CIBIS-II Investigators and Committees, 1999) and those with a serum creatinine ≥2.5 mg/dL were excluded in another trial (Willenheimer, 2005).

Hemodialysis: Not dialyzable

Dosage adjustment in hepatic impairment: Hepatitis or cirrhosis: Initial: 2.5 mg daily; increase cautiously.

Dietary Considerations May be taken without regard to meals.

Administration May be administered without regard to meals.

Monitoring Parameters Blood pressure, heart rate, ECG; serum glucose regularly (in patients with diabetes)

Dosage Forms

Tablet, Oral:

Zebeta: 5 mg, 10 mg

Generic: 5 mg, 10 mg

Bisoprolol and Hydrochlorothiazide

(bis OH proe lol & hye droe klor oh THYE a zide)

Brand Names: U.S. Ziac®

Brand Names: Canada Ziac®

Index Terms Bisoprolol Fumarate and Hydrochlorothiazide; Hydrochlorothiazide and Bisoprolol

Pharmacologic Category Antihypertensive; Beta-Blocker, Beta-1 Selective; Diuretic, Thiazide

Use Treatment of hypertension

Pregnancy Risk Factor C

Dosage Oral: Hypertension:

Children (off-label use): Initial: Bisoprolol 2.5 mg/hydrochlorothiazide 6.25 mg once daily; up to a maximum of bisoprolol 10 mg/hydrochlorothiazide 6.25 mg daily

Adults: Initial: Bisoprolol 2.5 mg and hydrochlorothiazide 6.25 mg once daily; dose may be titrated at ≥2-week intervals. Maximum dose (manufacturer recommended): Bisoprolol 20 mg/hydrochlorothiazide 12.5 mg once daily

Add-on/replacement therapy: Bisoprolol 2.5-20 mg and hydrochlorothiazide 6.25-12.5 mg once daily

Dosage adjustment in renal impairment: Caution should be used in dosing/titrating patients with renal impairment. Discontinue use with progressive renal impairment; use is contraindicated in patients with anuria.

Dosage adjustment in hepatic impairment: Caution should be used in dosing/titrating patients. Dosage adjustment necessary with severe impairment. Specific dosing recommendations are not provided in manufacturer labeling.

Additional Information Complete prescribing information should be consulted for additional detail.

Dosage Forms

Tablet, oral: 2.5/6.25: Bisoprolol 2.5 mg and hydrochlorothiazide 6.25 mg; 5/6.25: Bisoprolol 5 mg and hydrochlorothiazide 6.25 mg; 10/6.25: Bisoprolol 10 mg and hydrochlorothiazide 6.25 mg

Ziac®: 2.5/6.25: Bisoprolol 2.5 mg and hydrochlorothiazide 6.25 mg; 5/6.25: Bisoprolol 5 mg and hydrochlorothiazide 6.25 mg; 10/6.25: Bisoprolol 10 mg and hydrochlorothiazide 6.25 mg

◆ **Bisoprolol Fumarate** *see* Bisoprolol *on page 266*

◆ **Bisoprolol Fumarate and Hydrochlorothiazide** *see* Bisoprolol and Hydrochlorothiazide *on page 267*

◆ **Bis-POM PMEA** *see* Adefovir *on page 54*

◆ **Bistropamide** *see* Tropicamide *on page 2108*

◆ **Bivalent Human Papillomavirus Vaccine** *see* Papillomavirus (Types 16, 18) Vaccine (Human, Recombinant) *on page 1574*

Bivalirudin (bye VAL i roo din)

Brand Names: U.S. Angiomax

Brand Names: Canada Angiomax

Index Terms Hirulog

Pharmacologic Category Anticoagulant; Anticoagulant, Direct Thrombin Inhibitor

Use Anticoagulant used in conjunction with aspirin for patients with unstable angina undergoing percutaneous transluminal coronary angioplasty (PTCA) or percutaneous coronary intervention (PCI) with provisional glycoprotein IIb/IIIa inhibitor; anticoagulant used in conjunction with aspirin for patients undergoing PCI with (or at risk of) heparin-induced thrombocytopenia (HIT) / thrombosis syndrome (HITTS)

Canadian labeling: Additional uses (not in U.S. labeling): In conjunction with aspirin for treatment of patients with ST-elevation myocardial infarction (STEMI) undergoing primary PCI; anticoagulant with or without aspirin in patients undergoing cardiac surgery with (or at risk of) heparin-induced thrombocytopenia (HIT) / thrombosis syndrome (HITTS)

Pregnancy Risk Factor B

Pregnancy Considerations Adverse events have not been observed in animal reproduction studies. Bivalirudin is used in conjunction with aspirin, which may lead to maternal or fetal adverse effects, especially during the third trimester. Use of parenteral direct thrombin inhibitors in pregnancy should be limited to those women who have severe allergic reactions to heparin, including heparin-induced thrombocytopenia, and who cannot receive danaparoid (Guyatt, 2012).

Breast-Feeding Considerations It is not known if bivalirudin is excreted in breast milk. The manufacturer recommends that caution be exercised when administering bivalirudin to nursing women.

Contraindications Hypersensitivity to bivalirudin or any component of the formulation; active major bleeding

Canadian labeling: Additional contraindications (not in U.S. labeling): Major blood clotting disorders; acute gastric or duodenal ulcer; cerebral hemorrhage; severe cerebro-spinal trauma; bacterial endocarditis; severe uncontrolled hypertension; diabetic or hemorrhagic retinopathy; proximal use of spinal/epidural anesthesia

Warnings/Precautions Not for intramuscular use. Safety and efficacy have not been established in patients with unstable angina or acute coronary syndromes who are not undergoing PTCA or PCI. Increased risk of thrombus formation (some fatal) has been reported with bivalirudin use in gamma brachytherapy. As with all anticoagulants, bleeding may occur at any site and should be considered following an unexplained fall in blood pressure or hematocrit, or any unexplained symptom. Use with caution in patients with disease states associated with increased risk of bleeding. Use with caution in patients with renal impairment; dosage reduction required.

Adverse Reactions As with all anticoagulants, bleeding is the major adverse effect of bivalirudin. Hemorrhage may occur at virtually any site. Risk is dependent on multiple variables, including the intensity of anticoagulation, concurrent use of a glycoprotein IIb/IIIa inhibitor, and patient susceptibility. Additional adverse effects are often related to idiosyncratic reactions, and the frequency is difficult to estimate. Adverse reactions reported were generally less than those seen with heparin.

Cardiovascular: Angina pectoris, bradycardia, hypertension, hypotension

Central nervous system: Anxiety, headache, insomnia, nervousness, pain

Gastrointestinal: Abdominal pain, dyspepsia, nausea, vomiting

Genitourinary: Pelvic pain, urinary retention

Hematologic & oncologic: Major hemorrhage, minor hemorrhage

Local: Pain at injection site

Neuromuscular & skeletal: Back pain

Miscellaneous: Fever

Rare but important or life-threatening: Cerebral ischemia, confusion, facial paralysis, hemorrhage (fatal), hypersensitivity reaction (including anaphylaxis), increased susceptibility to infection, intracranial hemorrhage, oliguria, pulmonary edema, renal failure, retroperitoneal hemorrhage, sepsis, syncope, thrombocytopenia, vascular disease, venous thrombosis (during PCI, including intracoronary brachytherapy), ventricular fibrillation

Drug Interactions

Metabolism/Transport Effects None known.

Avoid Concomitant Use

Avoid concomitant use of Bivalirudin with any of the following: Apixaban; Dabigatran Etexilate; Edoxaban; Omacetaxine; Rivaroxaban; Urokinase; Vorapaxar

Increased Effect/Toxicity

Bivalirudin may increase the levels/effects of: Anticoagulants; Collagenase (Systemic); Deferasirox; Ibritumomab; Nintedanib; Obinutuzumab; Omacetaxine; Rivaroxaban; Tositumomab and Iodine I 131 Tositumomab

The levels/effects of Bivalirudin may be increased by: Agents with Antiplatelet Properties; Apixaban; Dabigatran Etexilate; Dasatinib; Edoxaban; Herbs (Anticoagulant/Antiplatelet Properties); Ibrutinib; Limaprost; Nonsteroidal Anti-Inflammatory Agents; Omega-3 Fatty Acids; Pentosan Polysulfate Sodium; Prostacyclin Analogues; Salicylates; Sugammadex; Thrombolytic Agents; Tibolone; Tipranavir; Urokinase; Vitamin E; Vorapaxar

Decreased Effect

The levels/effects of Bivalirudin may be decreased by: Estrogen Derivatives; Progestins

Preparation for Administration Reconstitute each 250 mg with 5 mL SWFI. Gently swirl to dissolve. Further dilution in D_5W or NS (50 mL to make 5 mg/mL solution **or** 500 mL to make 0.5 mg/mL solution) is required prior to infusion.

Storage/Stability Store unopened vials at 20°C to 25°C (68°F to 77°F); excursions permitted between 15°C to 30°C. Following reconstitution, vials should be stored at 2°C to 8°C for up to 24 hours. Do not freeze. Final dilutions of 0.5 mg/mL or 5 mg/mL are stable at room temperature for up to 24 hours.

Mechanism of Action Bivalirudin acts as a specific and reversible direct thrombin inhibitor; it binds to the catalytic and anionic exosite of both circulating and clot-bound thrombin. Catalytic binding site occupation functionally inhibits coagulant effects by preventing thrombin-mediated cleavage of fibrinogen to fibrin monomers, and activation of factors V, VIII, and XIII. Shows linear dose- and concentration-dependent prolongation of ACT, aPTT, PT, and TT.

Pharmacodynamics/Kinetics

Onset of action: Immediate

Duration: Coagulation times return to baseline ~1 hour following discontinuation of infusion

Distribution: 0.2 L/kg

Protein binding, plasma: Does not bind other than thrombin

Metabolism: Blood proteases

Half-life elimination: Normal renal function (CrCl ≥90 mL/minute): 25 minutes

Excretion: Urine (20%), proteolytic cleavage

Dosage IV: Adults: **Note:** If clinically indicated, provisional glycoprotein (GP) IIb/IIIa inhibition (eg, abciximab, eptifibatide, tirofiban) may be concomitantly administered during percutaneous coronary intervention (PCI). In addition to aspirin, concomitant administration of clopidogrel, prasugrel, or ticagrelor is also recommended for patients undergoing PCI (ACCF/AHA/SCAI [Levine, 2011]).

PTCA/PCI with or without HIT/HITTS: Initial: 0.75 mg/kg bolus immediately prior to procedure, followed by 1.75 mg/kg/hour for the duration of procedure and up to 4 hours postprocedure if needed (according to the manufacturer); may determine ACT 5 minutes after bolus dose; may administer additional bolus of 0.3 mg/kg if necessary. If continued anticoagulation is needed after the initial 4-hour postprocedure infusion, the infusion may be continued at 0.2 mg/kg/hour for up to an additional 20 hours (U.S. labeling) or 0.25 mg/kg/hour for 4 to 12 hours post procedure (Canadian labeling).

Unstable angina/non-ST-elevation myocardial infarction (UA/NSTEMI) (moderate-high risk) undergoing early invasive strategy:

During PCI: 0.75 mg/kg bolus prior to procedure, followed by 1.75 mg/kg/hour (ACCF/AHA [Anderson, 2013]).

Prior to PCI (U.S. off-label dose): Alternatively, may administer an initial 0.1 mg/kg bolus prior to diagnostic angiography, followed by 0.25 mg/kg/hour. Once PCI is determined to be necessary, give an additional bolus of 0.5 mg/kg and increase infusion rate to 1.75 mg/kg/hour; may discontinue at end of procedure or continue for up to 4 hours postprocedure if necessary (Stone, 2006). If, after angiography, cardiac surgery is deemed necessary, discontinue bivalirudin 3 hours prior to surgery and dose with unfractionated heparin per institutional practice. If medical management is the decided treatment approach, may either discontinue bivalirudin or continue at 0.25 mg/kg/hour for up to 72 hours (ACCF/AHA [Anderson, 2013]).

Canadian labeling: Initial: 0.1 mg/kg bolus, followed by 0.25 mg/kg/hour for up to 72 hours if patient is medically managed. If PCI is determined to be necessary, give an additional bolus of 0.5 mg/kg and increase infusion rate to 1.75 mg/kg/hour; may resume infusion at 0.25 mg/kg/hour for 4-12 hours following PCI if necessary. If coronary artery bypass graft (CABG) surgery is deemed necessary, discontinue bivalirudin infusion 1 hour prior to CABG (on-pump) surgery and dose with unfractionated heparin or continue infusion until time of CABG (off-pump) surgery, then give 0.5 mg/kg bolus and increase infusion rate to 1.75 mg/kg/hour until end of surgery.

STEMI undergoing primary PCI *(U.S. off-label use)*: Initial: 0.75 mg/kg bolus, followed by 1.75 mg/kg/hour for the duration of procedure; may continue postprocedure at a reduced dose if clinically indicated (ACCF/AHA [O'Gara, 2013]; Stone, 2008). In STEMI patients who are at a high risk of bleeding, it is reasonable to use bivalirudin monotherapy in preference to the combination of unfractionated heparin and a GP IIb/IIIa receptor antagonist (ACCF/AHA [O'Gara, 2013]). Of note, a single-center, open-label, randomized controlled trial comparing heparin to bivalirudin in patients with STEMI undergoing primary PCI (mostly with a radial approach) demonstrated that heparin reduces the incidence of major adverse cardiovascular events with no increase in bleeding as compared to bivalirudin (Shahzad, 2014).

If patient received unfractionated heparin (UFH) prior to procedure and bivalirudin is the desired anticoagulant: Discontinue heparin if infusing; without measurement of ACT, may initiate bivalirudin ≥30 minutes after the last UFH bolus but before PCI occurs (Stone, 2008). Switching patients from UFH to bivalirudin has been shown to be safe compared to continuing with UFH and as needed glycoprotein IIb/IIIa inhibition; median time from prerandomization UFH bolus to bivalirudin administration within the HORIZONS-AMI trial was 64 ± 61 minutes (Dangas, 2011).

Canadian labeling: Initial: 0.75 mg/kg bolus, followed by 1.75 mg/kg/hour for the duration of procedure or for up to 4 hours postprocedure if needed; determine ACT 5 minutes after bolus dose; may administer additional bolus of 0.3 mg/kg if necessary. If continued anticoagulation is needed after the initial 4-hour postprocedure infusion, the infusion may be continued at 0.25 mg/kg/hour for 4-12 hours.

Cardiac surgery in patients with acute or subacute heparin-induced thrombocytopenia, urgent surgery required: *U.S. off-label use* (Linkins, 2012): Intraoperative:

Off-pump: Initial bolus: 0.75 mg/kg, followed by continuous infusion 1.75 mg/kg/hour to maintain ACT >300 seconds (Dyke, 2007). If patient needs to go on-pump, Canadian labeling recommends an additional 0.25 mg/kg bolus and increasing the infusion rate to 2.5 mg/kg/hour.

On-pump: Initial bolus: 1 mg/kg, followed by continuous infusion 2.5 mg/kg/hour; 50 mg bolus added to priming solution of cardiopulmonary bypass (CPB) circuit. Additional boluses of 0.1-0.5 mg/kg may be given to maintain ACT >2.5 times baseline ACT. **Note:** Special maneuvers needed to prevent stasis and consequent clotting within CPB circuit during or after surgery (Koster, 2007). Per Canadian labeling, after completion of CPB, provision to allow recirculation of the circuit may be done by administering 50 mg **into the circuit** followed by a continuous infusion of 50 mg/hour **into the circuit.**

Canadian labeling: Pre -and post-cardiac surgery administration: Initial bolus: 0.1 mg/kg, followed by continuous infusion 0.2 mg/kg/hour for up to 48 hours prior to surgery or for up to 14 days after surgery; maintain aPTT 1.5-2.5 times baseline aPTT.

Heparin-induced thrombocytopenia (HIT) (off-label use): Initial dose: 0.15-0.2 mg/kg/hour; adjust to aPTT 1.5-2.5 times baseline value (Linkins, 2012). **Note:** Although the use of bivalirudin is not a currently recommended treatment for HIT due to insufficient evidence, the American College of Chest Physicians recommends overlapping administration of warfarin for a minimum of 5 days until INR is within target range; recheck INR after the non-heparin anticoagulant effect has dissipated (Linkins, 2012).

Elderly: No dosage adjustment is needed in elderly patients with normal renal function. Puncture site hemorrhage and catheterization site hemorrhage were seen more often in patients ≥65 years of age.

Dosage adjustment in renal impairment: Infusion dose should be reduced based on degree of renal impairment; initial bolus dose remains unchanged; monitor activated coagulation time (ACT) or aPTT depending on indication.

For use in PCI:

U.S. labeling:

CrCl ≥30 mL/minute: No adjustment required.

CrCl 10-29 mL/minute: Decrease infusion rate to 1 mg/kg/hour

Dialysis-dependent patients (off dialysis during administration): Decrease infusion rate to 0.25 mg/kg/hour

Hemodialysis: Approximately 25% removed during hemodialysis

Canadian labeling: **Note:** Check ACT following dose alterations at 5 and 45 minutes in renally impaired patients. If ACT ≤250 seconds give additional bolus 0.3 mg/kg and double infusion rate to maintain ACT ~350 seconds; if ACT 250-300 seconds give additional bolus 0.3 mg/kg to maintain ACT ~350 seconds.

CrCl ≥30 mL/minute: No adjustment required.

CrCl 10-29 mL/minute: Decrease infusion rate to 1 mg/kg/hour

Dialysis-dependent patients (off dialysis during administration): Decrease infusion rate to 0.25 mg/kg/hour

For use in cardiac surgery:

Canadian labeling:

CrCl ≥30 mL/minute: No adjustment required; monitor ACT.

CrCl <30 mL/minute: There are no dosage adjustments provided in the manufacturer's labeling; has not been studied; monitor ACT.

For use in HIT: There are no dosage adjustments provided in the manufacturer's labeling for this population; however, the following dose ranges have been observed in small retrospective observational studies (Kiser 2006; Kiser, 2008; Tsu, 2011). Of note, critically-ill patients comprised a significant proportion of patients in these observational studies. The following dose recommendations are based on the mean dose achieving aPTT goal within these studies; overlaps may exist; **Note:** The Cockcroft-Gault equation was used in all studies to define creatinine clearance:

CrCl >60 mL/minute: 0.13 mg/kg/hour

CrCl 30-60 mL/minute: 0.08-0.1 mg/kg/hour

CrCl <30 mL/minute: 0.04-0.05 mg/kg/hour

Intermittent hemodialysis (IHD): 0.07 mg/kg/hour (Tsu, 2011)

CRRT (eg, CVVH or CVVHDF): 0.03-0.07 mg/kg/hour (Kiser, 2006; Tsu, 2011)

Sustained low-efficiency daily diafiltration (SLEDD): 0.09 mg/kg/hour (Tsu, 2011)

Dosage adjustment in hepatic impairment: No dosage adjustment necessary.

Usual Infusion Concentrations: Adult IV infusion: 250 mg in 500 mL (concentration: 0.5 mg/mL) **or** 250 mg in 50 mL (concentration: 5 mg/mL) of D_5W or NS

Administration For IV administration only.

Monitoring Parameters Depends upon indication for use of bivalirudin: ACT or aPTT

Dosage Forms

Solution Reconstituted, Intravenous:

Angiomax: 250 mg (1 ea)

◆ **Bivigam** *see* Immune Globulin *on page 1056*

◆ **Bi-Zets/Benzotroches [OTC]** *see* Benzocaine *on page 246*

◆ **BL4162A** *see* Anagrelide *on page 147*

◆ **Blenoxane** *see* Bleomycin *on page 270*

◆ **Bleo** *see* Bleomycin *on page 270*

Bleomycin (blee oh MYE sin)

Brand Names: Canada Blenoxane; Bleomycin Injection, USP

Index Terms Blenoxane; Bleo; Bleomycin Sulfate; BLM

Pharmacologic Category Antineoplastic Agent, Antibiotic

Use

Head and neck cancers: Treatment of squamous cell carcinomas of the head and neck

Hodgkin lymphoma: Treatment of Hodgkin lymphoma

Malignant pleural effusion: Sclerosing agent for malignant pleural effusion

Testicular cancer: Treatment of testicular cancer

Pregnancy Risk Factor D

Dosage Note: The risk for pulmonary toxicity increases with age >70 years and cumulative lifetime dose of >400 units. **International considerations:** Dosages below expressed as USP units; 1 USP unit = 1 mg (by potency) = 1,000 international units (Stefanou, 2001).

Children and Adults: Test dose for lymphoma patients: IM, IV, SubQ: Because of the possibility of an anaphylactoid reaction, the manufacturer recommends administering 1 to 2 units of bleomycin before the first 1 to 2 doses; monitor vital signs every 15 minutes; wait a minimum of 1 hour before administering remainder of dose; if no acute reaction occurs, then the regular dosage schedule may be followed. **Note:** Test doses may not be predictive of a reaction (Lam, 2005) and/or may produce false-negative results.

Hodgkin lymphoma (off-label dosing): Children IV: ABVD: 10 units/m^2 days 1 and 15 of a 28-day treatment cycle (in combination with doxorubicin, vinblastine, and dacarbazine) (Hutchinson, 1998)

Hodgkin lymphoma (off-label dosing): Adults: IV:

ABVD: 10 units/m^2 days 1 and 15 of a 28-day treatment cycle (in combination with doxorubicin, vinblastine, and dacarbazine) (Straus, 2004)

BEACOPP: 10 units/m^2 day 8 of a 21-day treatment cycle (in combination with etoposide, doxorubicin, cyclophosphamide, vincristine, procarbazine, and prednisone) (Dann, 2007; Diehl, 2003)

Stanford V: 5 units/m^2/dose in weeks 2, 4, 6, 8, 10 and 12 (in combination with mechlorethamine, vinblastine, vincristine, doxorubicin, etoposide, and prednisone) (Horning, 2000; Horning, 2002)

Testicular cancer (off-label dosing): Adults: IV: BEP: 30 units/dose days 1, 8, and 15 of a 21-day treatment cycle for 4 cycles (in combination with etoposide and cisplatin) (Culine, 2008; Nichols, 1998)

Ovarian germ cell cancer (off-label use): Adults: IV: BEP: 30 units/dose days 1, 8, and 15 of a 21-day treatment cycle for 3 cycles (Williams, 1994) **or** 15 units/m^2 day 1 of a 21-day treatment cycle for 4 cycles (Cushing, 2004); in combination with etoposide and cisplatin

Malignant pleural effusion: Adults: Intrapleural: 60 units as a single instillation; mix in 50 to 100 mL of NS

Elderly: Refer to adult dosing; the incidence of pulmonary toxicity is higher in patients older than 70 years.

Dosage adjustment for toxicity:

Pulmonary changes: Discontinue until determined not to be drug-related.

Pulmonary diffusion capacity for carbon monoxide (DL_{CO}) <30% to 35% of baseline: Discontinue treatment.

Dosage adjustment in renal impairment:

The U.S. labeling recommends the following adjustments (creatinine clearance should be estimated using the Cockcroft-Gault formula):

CrCl >50 mL/minute: No dosage adjustment necessary.

CrCl 40-50 mL/minute: Administer 70% of normal dose

CrCl 30-40 mL/minute: Administer 60% of normal dose

CrCl 20-30 mL/minute: Administer 55% of normal dose

CrCl 10-20 mL/minute: Administer 45% of normal dose

CrCl 5-10 mL/minute: Administer 40% of normal dose

The Canadian labeling recommends the following adjustment: CrCl ≤40 mL/minute: Reduce dose by 40% to 75%.

The following adjustments have also been recommended:

Aronoff, 2007: Adults: Continuous renal replacement therapy (CRRT): Administer 75% of dose

Kintzel, 1995: Adults:

CrCl 46-60 mL/minute: Administer 70% of dose

CrCl 31-45 mL/minute: Administer 60% of dose

CrCl <30 mL/minute: Consider use of alternative drug

Dosage adjustment in hepatic impairment: There are no dosage adjustments provided in the manufacturer's labeling (has not been studied); however, adjustment for hepatic impairment is not necessary (King, 2001).

Dosing in obesity: *ASCO Guidelines for appropriate chemotherapy dosing in obese adults with cancer:* Fixed doses (dosing which is independent of body weight or BSA), are used in some protocols (eg, testicular cancer); due to toxicity concerns, the same fixed dose should also be considered for obese patients (Griggs, 2012).

Additional Information Complete prescribing information should be consulted for additional detail.

Dosage Forms

Solution Reconstituted, Injection:

Generic: 15 units (1 ea); 30 units (1 ea)

Solution Reconstituted, Injection [preservative free]:

Generic: 15 units (1 ea); 30 units (1 ea)

◆ **Bleomycin Injection, USP (Can)** *see* Bleomycin *on page 270*

◆ **Bleomycin Sulfate** *see* Bleomycin *on page 270*

◆ **Bleph-10** *see* Sulfacetamide (Ophthalmic) *on page 1943*

◆ **Bleph 10 DPS (Can)** *see* Sulfacetamide (Ophthalmic) *on page 1943*

◆ **Blephamide®** *see* Sulfacetamide and Prednisolone *on page 1944*

◆ **BLES (Can)** *see* Bovine Lipid Extract Surfactant [CAN/INT] *on page 285*

Blinatumomab (blin a TOOM oh mab)

Brand Names: U.S. Blincyto

Index Terms MT103

Pharmacologic Category Antineoplastic Agent, Anti-CD19/CD3; Antineoplastic Agent, Monoclonal Antibody

Use Acute lymphoblastic leukemia: Treatment of Philadelphia chromosome-negative (Ph-) relapsed or refractory B-cell precursor acute lymphoblastic leukemia (ALL)

Pregnancy Risk Factor C

Pregnancy Considerations Animal reproductions studies have not been conducted.

Breast-Feeding Considerations It is not known if blinatumomab is excreted in breast milk. Due to the potential for serious adverse reactions in the nursing infant, the manufacturer recommends a decision be made to discontinue nursing or to discontinue the drug, taking into account the importance of treatment to the mother.

Contraindications Known hypersensitivity to blinatumomab or any component of the formulation

Warnings/Precautions [U.S. Boxed Warning]: Cytokine release syndrome (CRS), which may be life-threatening or fatal, has occurred. Interrupt or discontinue therapy as recommended. Infusion reactions have also occurred, and may be difficult to distinguish from CRS. CRS symptoms may include pyrexia, headache, nausea, weakness, hypotension, increased transaminases, and elevated total bilirubin. In some patients, disseminated intravascular coagulation (DIC), capillary leak syndrome (CLS), and hemophagocytic lymphohistiocytosis/macrophage activation syndrome (HLH/MAS) have been reported in the setting of CRS. Monitor closely for signs/symptoms of these conditions; may require therapy interruption or discontinuation. CRS which was life-threatening or fatal occurred rarely. **[U.S. Boxed Warning]: Neurological toxicities, which may be severe, life-threatening, or fatal, have occurred. Interrupt or discontinue therapy as recommended.** Neurotoxicity has occurred in approximately half of patients in clinical trials. The median time to onset was 7 days. Grade 3 or higher neurotoxicity (eg, encephalopathy, convulsions, speech disorders, disturbances in consciousness, confusion and disorientation, and coordination and balance disorders) has also been observed. Patients are at risk for loss of consciousness due to neurologic events while taking blinatumomab; advise patients to avoid driving, participating in hazardous occupations, or operating heavy or dangerous machinery during treatment. Monitor patients for signs/symptoms of neurotoxicity; may require therapy interruption or discontinuation. The majority of symptoms resolved after interrupting therapy. Leukoencephalopathy (as seen on MRI) has been reported, particularly in those patients who received prior treatment with cranial irradiation and antileukemia chemotherapy (eg, high dose methotrexate or intrathecal cytarabine).

Neutropenia and neutropenic fever, including life-threatening episodes, have been reported. Monitor blood counts throughout therapy; may require therapy interruption if prolonged neutropenia occurs. Anemia and thrombocytopenia may also occur. Serious infections such as sepsis, pneumonia, bacteremia, opportunistic infections, and catheter-related infections have been reported in approximately one-fourth of patients in clinical trials (may be life-threatening or fatal). Consider prophylactic antibiotics if appropriate, and monitor closely for signs/symptoms of infection. Treat promptly if infection occurs. Transient increases in liver enzymes (associated both with and without CRS) may occur during therapy. The median time to enzyme elevation was 15 days; grade 3 or higher elevations were observed in a small percentage of patients. Monitor ALT, AST, GGT, and total bilirubin at baseline and during treatment. Interrupt therapy if transaminases are >5 times ULN or if bilirubin is >3 times ULN. Life-threatening or fatal tumor lysis syndrome (TLS) has been observed. Administer measures to prevent TLS (eg, pretreatment nontoxic cytoreduction, and hydration during treatment). Monitor for signs/symptoms of TLS (eg, acute renal failure, hyperkalemia, hypocalcemia, hyperuricemia, and/or hyperphosphatemia); may require treatment interruption or discontinuation. Elderly patients experienced an increased rate of neurotoxicity (including cognitive disorder), encephalopathy, confusion, and serious infections as compared to patients less than 65 years. Preparation and administration errors have occurred. Do not flush infusion line, particularly when changing infusion bags or at completion of infusion; may result in overdose and complications. IV bag volume will be more than the volume administered to the patient (240 mL) to account for IV line priming and to ensure that the full dose is administered. Follow preparation and administration instructions carefully. Refer to manufacturer labeling for further information.

Adverse Reactions

Cardiovascular: Chest pain, edema, hypertension, hypotension, peripheral edema, tachycardia

Central nervous system: Aphasia, brain disease, chills, confusion, cognitive dysfunction, convulsions, disorientation, dizziness, fatigue, headache, insomnia, loss of consciousness, memory impairment, neurotoxicity (incidence increased in older adults), paresthesia

Dermatologic: Skin rash

Endocrine & metabolic: Hyperglycemia, hypoalbuminemia, hypokalemia, hypomagnesemia, hypophosphatemia, increased gamma-glutamyl transferase, weight gain

Gastrointestinal: Abdominal pain, constipation, decreased appetite, diarrhea, nausea, vomiting

Hematologic & oncologic: Anemia, decreased serum immunoglobulins, febrile neutropenia, leukocytosis, leukopenia, lymphocytopenia, neutropenia, thrombocytopenia, tumor lysis syndrome

Hepatic: Increased liver enzymes, increased serum ALT, increased serum AST, increased serum bilirubin

Hypersensitivity: Cytokine release syndrome (including cytokine storms, cytokine storm, hypersensitivity

Infection: Bacterial infection, infection, fungal infection, sepsis, viral infection

Neuromuscular & skeletal: Arthralgia, back pain, limb pain, ostealgia, tremor

Respiratory: Cough, dyspnea, pneumonia

Miscellaneous: Fever

Rare but important or life-threatening: Bronchospasm, capillary leak syndrome, leukoencephalopathy, speech disturbance

Drug Interactions

Metabolism/Transport Effects None known.

Avoid Concomitant Use

Avoid concomitant use of Blinatumomab with any of the following: BCG; CloZAPine; Dipyrone; Natalizumab; Pimecrolimus; Tacrolimus (Topical); Tofacitinib; Vaccines (Live)

Increased Effect/Toxicity

Blinatumomab may increase the levels/effects of: CloZAPine; Leflunomide; Natalizumab; Tofacitinib; Vaccines (Live)

The levels/effects of Blinatumomab may be increased by: Denosumab; Dipyrone; Pimecrolimus; Roflumilast; Tacrolimus (Topical); Trastuzumab

Decreased Effect

Blinatumomab may decrease the levels/effects of: BCG; Coccidioides immitis Skin Test; Sipuleucel-T; Vaccines (Inactivated); Vaccines (Live)

The levels/effects of Blinatumomab may be decreased by: Echinacea

Preparation for Administration All doses should be prepared in a prefilled 250 mL NS bag. Prefilled 250 mL NS bags typically contain overfill to a volume of 265 to 275 mL and dose calculations are based on a starting volume of 265 to 275 mL (if necessary, adjust the bag volume to achieve a starting volume between 265 and 275 mL). Final bag volume will be more than the volume administered to the patient (240 mL) to account for IV line priming and to ensure that the full dose is administered. Use only polyolefin, PVC non-di-ethylhexylphthalate (non-DEHP), or ethyl vinyl acetate (EVA) infusion bags or pump cassettes. IV solution stabilizer provided is used to coat the prefilled NS bag prior to addition of reconstituted blinatumomab. Therefore, the IV solution stabilizer is added to the NS bag; do NOT use IV solution stabilizer for reconstitution of blinatumomab. Preparation and administration errors have occurred; follow preparation instructions carefully. Refer to manufacturer labeling for further information.

9 mcg daily dose infused over 24 hours at a rate of 10 mL/hour: Transfer **5.5 mL** of IV solution stabilizer to the prefilled 250 mL NS bag using a 10 mL syringe; gently mix to avoid foaming. Reconstitute **one** vial of lyophilized powder with 3 mL of preservative-free SWFI; direct stream toward the side of the vial and gently swirl to avoid excess foaming. Do not shake; final reconstituted concentration is 12.5 **mcg**/mL. Reconstituted solution should be clear to slightly opalescent, colorless to slightly yellow; do not use if cloudy or if precipitation occurs. Transfer **0.83 mL** of reconstituted solution into the prefilled NS bag; gently mix. Remove air from the IV bag; prime IV line with the prepared infusion solution only (do not prime with NS). If not used immediately, store at 2°C to 8°C (36°F to 46°F) for up to 8 days (infusion must be completed within this time frame).

9 mcg daily dose infused over 48 hours at a rate of 5 mL/hour: Transfer **5.5 mL** of IV solution stabilizer to the prefilled 250 mL NS bag using a 10 mL syringe; gently mix to avoid foaming. Reconstitute **one** vial of lyophilized powder with 3 mL of preservative-free SWFI; direct stream toward the side of the vial and gently swirl to avoid excess foaming. Do not shake; final reconstituted concentration is 12.5 **mcg**/mL. Reconstituted solution should be clear to slightly opalescent, colorless to slightly yellow; do not use if cloudy or if precipitation occurs. Transfer **1.7 mL** of reconstituted solution into the prefilled NS bag; gently mix. Remove air from the IV bag; prime IV line with the prepared infusion solution only (do not prime with NS). If not used immediately, store at 2°C to 8°C (36°F to 46°F) for up to 8 days (infusion must be completed within this time frame).

28 mcg daily dose infused over 24 hours at a rate of 10 mL/hour: Transfer **5.6 mL** of IV solution stabilizer to the prefilled 250 mL NS bag using a 10 mL syringe; gently mix to avoid foaming. Reconstitute **one** vial of lyophilized powder with 3 mL of preservative-free SWFI; direct stream toward the side of the vial and gently swirl to avoid excess foaming. Do not shake; final reconstituted concentration is 12.5 **mcg**/mL. Reconstituted solution should be clear to slightly opalescent, colorless to slightly yellow; do not use if cloudy or if precipitation occurs. Transfer **2.6 mL** of reconstituted solution into the prefilled NS bag; gently mix. Remove air from the IV bag; prime IV line with the prepared infusion solution only (do not prime with NS). If not used immediately, store at 2°C to 8°C (36°F to 46°F) for up to 8 days (infusion must be completed within this time frame).

28 mcg daily dose infused over 48 hours at a rate of 5 mL/hour: Transfer **5.6 mL** of IV solution stabilizer to the prefilled 250 mL NS bag using a 10 mL syringe; gently mix to avoid foaming. Use 2 vials of lyophilized powder; reconstitute each vial with 3 mL of preservative-free SWFI; direct stream toward the side of the vial and gently swirl to avoid excess foaming. Do not shake; final reconstituted concentration in each vial is 12.5 **mcg**/mL. Reconstituted solution should be clear to slightly opalescent, colorless to slightly yellow; do not use if cloudy or if precipitation occurs. Transfer **5.2 mL** (2.7 mL from one vial and the remaining 2.5 mL from the second vial) of reconstituted solution into the prefilled NS bag; gently mix. Remove air from the IV bag; prime IV line with the prepared infusion solution only (do not prime with NS). If not used immediately, store at 2°C to 8°C (36°F to 46°F) for up to 8 days (infusion must be completed within this time frame).

Storage/Stability Store intact vials (drug and solution stabilizer) in the original package at 2°C to 8°C (36°F to 46°F); protect from light. Do not freeze. Intact vials of both drug and stabilizer may be stored for up to 8 hours at room temperature. Reconstituted solution is stable for up to 4 hours at 23°C to 27°C (73°F to 81°F) or up to 24 hours at 2°C to 8°C (36°F to 46°F). Solutions diluted for infusion are stable for up to 48 hours at 23°C to 27°C (73°F to 81°F) or up to 8 days at 2°C to 8°C (36°F to 46°F). Infusion should be completed within these time frames; if IV bag of solution for infusion is not administered within the time frames and temperatures indicated, discard; do not refrigerate again.

Mechanism of Action Blinatumomab is a bispecific CD19-directed CD3 T-cell engager which binds to CD19 expressed on B-cells and CD3 expressed on T-cells. It activates endogenous T cells by connecting CD3 in the T-cell receptor complex with CD19 on B-cells (malignant and benign), thus forming a cytolytic synapse between a cytotoxic T-cell and the cancer target B-cell (Topp, 2014). Blinatumomab mediates the production of cytolytic proteins, release of inflammatory cytokines, and proliferation of T cells, which result in lysis of CD19-positive cells.

Pharmacodynamics/Kinetics

Distribution: 4.52 L

Half-life elimination: 2.11 hours

Excretion: Urine (negligible amounts)

Dosage Note: Hospitalization is recommended for the first 9 days of cycle 1, and the first 2 days of cycle 2. Close observation by a healthcare professional (or hospitalization) is recommended for initiation of all subsequent cycles or for therapy reinitiation (eg, treatment is interrupted for 4 or more hours). Do **not** flush infusion line, particularly when changing infusion bags or at completion of infusion; may result in overdose and complications. Premedicate with dexamethasone 20 mg IV one hour prior to the first dose of each cycle, prior to a step dose (eg, cycle 1 day 8), or when restarting therapy after an interruption of ≥4 hours.

Acute lymphoblastic leukemia (B-cell precursor), Philadelphia chromosome-negative, relapsed/refractory: Adults ≥45 kg: IV: Each treatment cycle consists of 4 weeks of continuous infusion followed by a 2-week treatment-free interval (allow at least 2 weeks treatment-free between cycles). Therapy involves 2 induction cycles followed by 3 additional cycles for consolidation (total of up to 5 cycles).

Cycle 1: 9 **mcg** daily administered as a continuous infusion on days 1 to 7, followed by 28 **mcg** daily as a continuous infusion on days 8 to 28 of a 6-week treatment cycle

Cycles 2 through 5: 28 **mcg** daily administered as a continuous infusion on days 1 to 28 of a 6-week treatment cycle

Dosage adjustment for toxicity: If the interruption after an adverse event is no longer than 7 days, continue the same cycle to a total of 28 days of infusion inclusive of days before and after the interruption in that cycle. If an interruption due to an adverse event is longer than 7 days, start a new cycle.

Cytokine release syndrome (CRS):

Grade 3: Interrupt therapy until resolved, then resume dosing at 9 **mcg** daily. Increase dose to 28 **mcg** daily after 7 days if toxicity does not recur.

Grade 4: Discontinue permanently

Neurologic toxicity:

Grade 3: Interrupt therapy for at least 3 days and until toxicity is ≤ grade 1 (mild), then resume dosing at 9 **mcg** daily. Increase dose to 28 **mcg** daily after 7 days if toxicity does not recur. If toxicity occurred at the 9 **mcg** daily dose, or if it takes more than 7 days to resolve, discontinue permanently.

Grade 4: Discontinue permanently

Seizure: Discontinue permanently if more than 1 seizure occurs.

Other clinically relevant toxicity:

Grade 3: Interrupt therapy until toxicity is ≤ grade 1 (mild), then resume dosing at 9 mcg daily. Increase dose to 28 mcg daily after 7 days if toxicity does not recur. If toxicity takes more than 14 days to resolve, discontinue permanently.

Grade 4: Discontinue permanently

Dosage adjustment for renal impairment:

CrCl ≥30 mL/minute: No dosage adjustment necessary.

CrCl <30 mL/minute: There are no dosage adjustments provided in the manufacturer's labeling (has not been studied).

Hemodialysis: There are no dosage adjustments provided in the manufacturer's labeling (has not been studied).

Dosage adjustment for hepatic impairment:

There are no dosage adjustments provided in the manufacturer's labeling (has not been studied).

Hepatotoxicity during treatment: Interrupt therapy if transaminases are >5 times ULN or if bilirubin is >3 times ULN.

Administration IV: Administer 240 mL as a continuous IV infusion at a constant flow rate of 10 mL/hour for 24 hours or 5 mL/hour for 48 hours (depending on dose, duration, and/or concentration) through a dedicated lumen. Use a programmable, lockable, non-elastomeric infusion pump with an alarm; IV tubing should include a sterile, non-pyrogenic, low protein-binding, 0.2 micron in-line filter. Only use polyolefin, PVC non-di-ethylhexylphthalate (non-DEHP), or ethyl vinyl acetate (EVA) infusion bags, pump cassettes and IV tubing. IV tubing should be primed with prepared infusion solution, not NS. Premedicate with dexamethasone 20 mg IV one hour prior to the first dose of each cycle, prior to a step dose (such as cycle 1 day 8), or when restarting therapy after an interruption of ≥4 hours.

Do not flush infusion line, particularly when changing infusion bags or at completion of infusion; may result in excess dosage and complications. Do not infuse other medications through the same line.

Monitoring Parameters CBC with differential, liver function tests (ALT, AST, GGT, and total bilirubin) at baseline and throughout therapy; signs/symptoms of cytokine release syndrome, neurotoxicity, infection, and tumor lysis syndrome

Dosage Forms

Solution Reconstituted, Intravenous [preservative free]:

Blincyto: 35 mcg (1 ea)

◆ **Blincyto** *see* Blinatumomab *on page 271*

◆ **BLM** *see* Bleomycin *on page 270*

◆ **Bloxiverz** *see* Neostigmine *on page 1438*

◆ **BMS-188667** *see* Abatacept *on page 23*

◆ **BMS 201038** *see* Lomitapide *on page 1233*

◆ **BMS-224818** *see* Belatacept *on page 233*

◆ **BMS-232632** *see* Atazanavir *on page 185*

◆ **BMS-247550** *see* Ixabepilone *on page 1138*

◆ **BMS 337039** *see* ARIPiprazole *on page 171*

◆ **BMS-354825** *see* Dasatinib *on page 574*

◆ **BMS-477118** *see* Saxagliptin *on page 1867*

◆ **BMS-936558** *see* Nivolumab *on page 1469*

◆ **B&O** *see* Belladonna and Opium *on page 238*

Boceprevir (boe SE pre vir)

Brand Names: U.S. Victrelis

Brand Names: Canada Victrelis

Index Terms SCH503034

Pharmacologic Category Antihepaciviral, Protease Inhibitor (Anti-HCV)

Use Chronic hepatitis C: Treatment of chronic hepatitis C (CHC) genotype 1 (in combination with peginterferon alfa and ribavirin) in adult patients with compensated liver disease (including cirrhosis) who were previously untreated or have failed prior therapy with peginterferon alfa and ribavirin therapy including prior null responders, partial responders, and relapsers

Pregnancy Risk Factor B / X (in combination with ribavirin and peginterferon alfa)

Pregnancy Considerations Adverse events were not observed with boceprevir in animal reproduction studies; however, boceprevir must not be used as monotherapy (must be used in combination with peginterferon alfa and ribavirin). Adverse events have been observed with ribavirin and interferons (specific studies with peginterferon alfa-2a have not been conducted) in animal reproduction studies. Use of ribavirin in combination with peginterferon alfa-2a is contraindicated in pregnant women and males whose female partners are pregnant. A negative pregnancy test is required before initiation of therapy and pregnancy testing should be conducted monthly during treatment and for 6 months after therapy has ended. Women of childbearing potential and males must use at least 2 effective forms of contraception during treatment and continue contraceptive measures for at least 6 months after completion of therapy. One of the two forms of effective contraception may be a combined oral contraceptive product with at least 1 mg of norethindrone; oral contraceptives with <1 mg of norethindrone and other forms of hormonal contraception are contraindicated because they have not been studied. If patient or female partner becomes pregnant during treatment, she should be counseled about potential risks of exposure. Health care providers and patients are encouraged to enroll women exposed to ribavirin during pregnancy or within 6 months after treatment in the Ribavirin Pregnancy Registry (800-593-2214).

Breast-Feeding Considerations It is not known if boceprevir is excreted into breast milk. According to the manufacturer, due to the potential for serious adverse reactions in the nursing infant, a decision should be made whether to discontinue nursing or to discontinue the drug, taking into account the importance of treatment to the mother.

Breast-feeding is not linked to the spread of hepatitis C virus; however, if nipples are cracked or bleeding, breastfeeding is not recommended (CDC, 2010).

Contraindications

Hypersensitivity to boceprevir or any component of the formulation; pregnancy; male partners of pregnant women

Coadministration with CYP3A4/5 highly-dependent substrates (alfuzosin, cisapride, doxazosin, drospirenone, ergot derivatives [dihydroergotamine, ergonovine, ergotamine, methylergonovine], lovastatin, midazolam [oral], pimozide, sildenafil/tadalafil [when used for treatment of pulmonary arterial hypertension], silodosin, simvastatin, tamsulosin, triazolam) or strong CYP3A4/5 inducers (carbamazepine, phenobarbital, phenytoin, rifampin, St John's wort)

Refer to Peginterferon Alfa and Ribavirin monographs for individual product contraindications.

Canadian labeling: Additional contraindications (not in U.S. labeling): Autoimmune hepatitis, hepatic decompensation (Child-Pugh class B or C); coadministration with amiodarone, astemizole, propafenone, quinidine, terfenadine

Warnings/Precautions Combination therapy with ribavirin and interferons may cause birth defects; avoid pregnancy in females and female partners of male patients during therapy and for 6 months following treatment; two forms of effective contraception should be used. Combination therapy with ribavirin and peginterferon alfa-2a is contraindicated in pregnancy. Serious acute hypersensitivity reactions, angioedema and urticaria have been reported with boceprevir, peginterferon alfa, and ribavirin combination therapy. Discontinuation of combination therapy and institution of supportive measures may be necessary. Safety and efficacy have not been established in patients who have uncompensated cirrhosis or have received organ transplants. Monotherapy is not effective for chronic hepatitis C infection. Patients who have less than 0.5-$\log_{10}$ HCV-RNA decline at treatment week 4 with peginterferon alfa and ribavirin when **initiating** boceprevir therapy are predicted to have less than a 2-$\log_{10}$ HCV-RNA decline by treatment week 12. Those poor responders treated with boceprevir will likely not have a sustained virologic response (SVR) and have a predisposition to viral resistance at treatment failure.

Anemia has been reported with peginterferon alfa and ribavirin; addition of boceprevir is associated with further hemoglobin decreases. With anemia management, average hemoglobin decrease in clinical trials was ~1 g/dL. Dose reduction of ribavirin therapy is recommended for the initial management of anemia if hemoglobin <10 g/dL; permanent discontinuation of ribavirin treatment is recommended if hemoglobin <8.5 g/dL. The addition of boceprevir to peginterferon alfa and ribavirin therapy is also associated with a higher incidence of neutropenia. May be severe or life-threatening (rare); discontinuation of therapy may be necessary. Dose reductions of peginterferon alfa and ribavirin were needed more often in patients also taking boceprevir. Serious cases of pancytopenia have been reported in patients receiving boceprevir in combination with peginterferon alfa and ribavirin. Complete blood counts with differential should be obtained pretreatment and at weeks 2, 4, 8, and 12, as well as other times during treatment. If ribavirin is permanently discontinued, boceprevir and peginterferon alfa must also be discontinued.

Adverse Reactions

Central nervous system: Chills, dizziness, fatigue, headache, insomnia, irritability

Dermatologic: Alopecia, dry skin, rash

Gastrointestinal: Abnormal taste, appetite decreased, diarrhea, nausea, vomiting, xerostomia

Hematologic: Anemia, neutropenia, thrombocytopenia

Neuromuscular & skeletal: Arthralgia, weakness

Respiratory: Dyspnea

Rare but important or life-threatening: Agranulocytosis, angioedema, drug rash with eosinophilia and systemic symptoms (DRESS) syndrome, exfoliative dermatitis, exfoliative rash, mouth ulceration, pancytopenia, pneumonia, sepsis, Stevens-Johnson syndrome, stomatitis, thromboembolic events, toxic skin eruption, toxicoderma, urticaria

Drug Interactions

Metabolism/Transport Effects Substrate of BCRP, CYP3A4 (major), P-glycoprotein; **Note:** Assignment of Major/Minor substrate status based on clinically relevant drug interaction potential; **Inhibits** CYP3A4 (strong), P-glycoprotein

Avoid Concomitant Use

Avoid concomitant use of Boceprevir with any of the following: Ado-Trastuzumab Emtansine; Alfuzosin; Apixaban; Astemizole; Avanafil; Axitinib; Bosutinib; Cabozantinib; CarBAMazepine; Ceritinib; Cisapride; Cobicistat; Conivaptan; Crizotinib; CYP3A4 Inducers (Strong); Dapoxetine; Dihydroergotamine; Doxazosin; Dronedarone; Drospirenone; Efavirenz; Eplerenone; Ergoloid Mesylates; Ergonovine; Ergotamine; Etravirine; Everolimus; Fosphenytoin; Halofantrine; Ibrutinib; Irinotecan; Ivabradine; Lapatinib; Lercanidipine; Lomitapide; Lovastatin; Lurasidone; Macitentan; Methylergonovine; Midazolam; Naloxegol; Nilotinib; Nisoldipine; Olaparib; PHENobarbital; Phenytoin; Pimozide; Primidone; Ranolazine; Red Yeast Rice; Regorafenib; Rifabutin; Rifampin; Rivaroxaban; Salmeterol; Sildenafil; Silodosin; Simeprevir; Simvastatin; St Johns Wort; Suvorexant; Tamsulosin; Terfenadine; Ticagrelor; Tipranavir; Tolvaptan; Toremifene; Trabectedin; Triazolam; Ulipristal; Vemurafenib; VinCRIStine (Liposomal); Vorapaxar

Increased Effect/Toxicity

Boceprevir may increase the levels/effects of: Ado-Trastuzumab Emtansine; Alfuzosin; Almotriptan; Alosetron; ALPRAZolam; Amiodarone; Apixaban; ARIPiprazole; Astemizole; AtorvaSTATin; Avanafil; Axitinib; Bedaquiline; Bepridil [Off Market]; Bortezomib; Bosentan; Bosutinib; Brentuximab Vedotin; Brinzolamide; Budesonide (Nasal); Budesonide (Systemic, Oral Inhalation); Buprenorphine; Cabazitaxel; Cabozantinib; Cannabis; Ceritinib; Cisapride; Clarithromycin; Colchicine; Conivaptan;

Contraceptives (Progestins); Corticosteroids (Orally Inhaled); Corticosteroids (Systemic); Crizotinib; CycloSPORINE (Systemic); CYP3A4 Substrates; Dapoxetine; Dasatinib; Desipramine; Digoxin; Dihydroergotamine; Dofetilide; Doxazosin; DOXOrubicin (Conventional); Dronabinol; Dronedarone; Drospirenone; Dutasteride; Efavirenz; Eliglustat; Eplerenone; Ergoloid Mesylates; Ergonovine; Ergotamine; Erlotinib; Etizolam; Everolimus; FentaNYL; Fesoterodine; Flecainide; Fluticasone (Nasal); Fluticasone (Oral Inhalation); Fluvastatin; GuanFACINE; Halofantrine; Hydrocodone; Ibrutinib; Idelalisib; Iloperidone; Imatinib; Imidafenacin; Irinotecan; Itraconazole; Ivabradine; Ivacaftor; Ixabepilone; Ketoconazole (Systemic); Lacosamide; Lapatinib; Lercanidipine; Levobupivacaine; Levomilnacipran; Lomitapide; Lovastatin; Lumefantrine; Lurasidone; Macitentan; Maraviroc; Methadone; Methylergonovine; MethylPREDNISolone; Midazolam; Mifepristone; Naloxegol; Nilotinib; Nisoldipine; Olaparib; Ospemifene; OxyCODONE; Paricalcitol; PAZOPanib; Pimecrolimus; Pimozide; Pitavastatin; PONATinib; Posaconazole; Pranlukast; Pravastatin; PrednisoLONE (Systemic); PredniSONE; Propafenone; QUEtiapine; QuiNIDine; Ranolazine; Red Yeast Rice; Regorafenib; Repaglinide; Retapamulin; Rifabutin; Rilpivirine; Rivaroxaban; RomiDEPsin; Rosuvastatin; Ruxolitinib; Salmeterol; Saxagliptin; Sildenafil; Silodosin; Simeprevir; Simvastatin; Sirolimus; SORAfenib; Suvorexant; Tacrolimus (Systemic); Tadalafil; Tamsulosin; Terfenadine; Tetrahydrocannabinol; Ticagrelor; Tofacitinib; Tolterodine; Tolvaptan; Toremifene; Trabectedin; TraZODone; Triazolam; Ulipristal; Vardenafil; Vemurafenib; Vilazodone; VinCRIStine (Liposomal); Vorapaxar; Voriconazole; Warfarin; Zopiclone; Zuclopenthixol

The levels/effects of Boceprevir may be increased by: Clarithromycin; Cobicistat; CycloSPORINE (Systemic); Itraconazole; Ketoconazole (Systemic); Posaconazole; Voriconazole

Decreased Effect

Boceprevir may decrease the levels/effects of: Buprenorphine; Contraceptives (Estrogens); Escitalopram; Etravirine; Ifosfamide; Methadone; Prasugrel; Protease Inhibitors; Ritonavir; Ticagrelor; Tipranavir; Warfarin

The levels/effects of Boceprevir may be decreased by: Bosentan; CarBAMazepine; CYP3A4 Inducers (Moderate); CYP3A4 Inducers (Strong); Dabrafenib; Deferasirox; Efavirenz; Fosphenytoin; PHENobarbital; Phenytoin; Primidone; Protease Inhibitors; Rifabutin; Rifampin; Ritonavir; Siltuximab; St Johns Wort; Tipranavir; Tocilizumab

Storage/Stability Store refrigerated at 2°C to 8°C (36°F to 46°F). After dispensing, may be stored at room temperature of up to 25°C (77°F) for 3 months; keep container closed tightly; avoid excessive heat.

Mechanism of Action Binds reversibly to nonstructural protein 3 (NS 3) serine protease and inhibits replication of the hepatitis C virus. Considered a direct-acting antiviral treatment for HCV, also called a specifically targeted antiviral therapy for HCV (STAT-C).

Pharmacodynamics/Kinetics

Absorption: Food (type or timing is not important) enhances absorption by up to 65%

Distribution: V_d: ~772 L

Protein binding: ~75%

Metabolism: Primarily hepatic via aldo-ketoreductase pathway to inactive metabolites. Also some oxidative CYP 3A4/5 metabolism.

Half-life elimination: Plasma: Adults: ~3.4 hours

Time to peak, serum: 2 hours

Excretion: Feces (79%); urine (9%)

Dosage Oral: Adults: 800 mg 3 times daily (in combination with peginterferon alfa and ribavirin). *Missed doses:* If a dose is missed, skip dose if it is <2 hours before the next dose; if ≥2 hours before next dose is due, take dose with food and resume normal dosing schedule. **Note:** Boceprevir-containing regimens are **not** recommended for treatment-naive patients or for prior relapse patients nonresponsive to peginterferon/ribavirin regimens with or without an HCV protease inhibitor (AASLD/IDSA, 2014)

Treatment-naive patients without cirrhosis (interferon-responsive [≥1-log_{10} HCV-RNA decline in viral load] at week 4):

Weeks 1-4: Peginterferon alfa with concomitant ribavirin only

Weeks 5-8: Boceprevir 800 mg 3 times daily with continued peginterferon alfa and ribavirin

Weeks 9-24 (based on HCV-RNA results at week 8):

HCV-RNA **undetectable** or **detectable** at a level of <100 units/mL: Boceprevir 800 mg 3 times daily with continued peginterferon alfa and ribavirin

HCV-RNA ≥100 units/mL but <1000 units/mL: Boceprevir 800 mg 3 times daily with continued peginterferon alfa and ribavirin. Recheck HCV-RNA at week 12. If HCV-RNA ≥100 units/mL at week 12, discontinue treatment (boceprevir, peginterferon alfa, and ribavirin).

HCV-RNA ≥1000 units/mL: Discontinue treatment (boceprevir, peginterferon alfa, and ribavirin)

Weeks ≥24:

HCV-RNA **undetectable** at week 8 and week 24: Boceprevir 800 mg 3 times daily with continued peginterferon alfa and ribavirin for 4 additional weeks (through week 28)

HCV-RNA **detectable** (≥100 units/mL but <1000 units/mL) at Week 8 and **undetectable** at week 24:

U.S. labeling: Boceprevir 800 mg 3 times daily with continued peginterferon alfa and ribavirin for 12 additional weeks (through week 36), followed by peginterferon alfa and ribavirin for additional 12 weeks (through week 48)

Canadian labeling: Boceprevir 800 mg 3 times daily with continued peginterferon alfa and ribavirin for 4 additional weeks (through week 28), followed by peginterferon alfa and ribavirin for additional 20 weeks (through week 48)

HCV-RNA **detectable** at week 24: Discontinue treatment (boceprevir, peginterferon alfa, and ribavirin)

Treatment-naive patients (interferon nonresponsive [<0.5-log_{10} HCV-RNA decline in viral load] at week 4): **Note:** Manufacturer also recommends consideration of treatment of poor responders [<1-log_{10} HCV-RNA decline in viral load at week 4] in order to maximize rate of sustained virologic response (SVR):

Weeks 1-4: Peginterferon alfa with concomitant ribavirin only

Weeks 5-48: Boceprevir 800 mg 3 times daily with continued peginterferon alfa and ribavirin

Previously-treated patients without cirrhosis (partial response or relapser): **Note:** Previously treated does not include prior treatment with boceprevir. "Partial response" includes patients with a ≥2-log_{10} HCV-RNA decrease by week 12, but a nonsustained virologic response thereafter. "Relapser" includes patients with an undetectable HCV-RNA upon completion of previous treatment, but with detectable HCV-RNA during the follow-up period.

Weeks 1-4: Peginterferon alfa with concomitant ribavirin only

Weeks 5-8: Boceprevir 800 mg 3 times daily with continued peginterferon alfa and ribavirin

Weeks 9-24 (based on HCV-RNA results at week 8):
HCV-RNA **undetectable** or <100 units/mL: Boceprevir 800 mg 3 times daily with continued peginterferon alfa and ribavirin
HCV-RNA ≥100 units/mL but <1000 units/mL: Boceprevir 800 mg 3 times daily with continued peginterferon alfa and ribavirin. Recheck HCV-RNA at week 12. If HCV-RNA ≥100 units/mL at week 12, discontinue treatment (boceprevir, peginterferon alfa, and ribavirin)
HCV-RNA ≥1000 units/mL: Discontinue treatment (boceprevir, peginterferon alfa, and ribavirin)
Weeks ≥24:
HCV-RNA **undetectable** at week 8 and week 24: Boceprevir 800 mg 3 times daily with continued peginterferon alfa and ribavirin for 12 additional weeks (through week 36)
HCV-RNA **detectable** (≥100 units/mL but <1000 units/mL) at Week 8 and **undetectable** at week 24: Boceprevir 800 mg 3 times daily with continued peginterferon alfa and ribavirin for 12 additional weeks (through week 36), followed by peginterferon alfa and ribavirin for additional 12 weeks (through week 48)
HCV-RNA **detectable** at week 24: Discontinue treatment (boceprevir, peginterferon alfa, and ribavirin)
Previously treated patients with <2-log$_{10}$ HCV-RNA decline by week 12 (prior null responders):
Weeks 1-4: Peginterferon alfa with concomitant ribavirin only
Weeks 5-8: Boceprevir 800 mg 3 times daily with continued peginterferon alfa and ribavirin
Weeks 9-24 (based on HCV-RNA results at week 8):
HCV-RNA **undetectable** or <100 units/mL: Boceprevir 800 mg 3 times daily with continued peginterferon alfa and ribavirin
HCV-RNA ≥100 units/mL but <1000 units/mL: Boceprevir 800 mg 3 times daily with continued peginterferon alfa and ribavirin. Recheck HCV-RNA at week 12. If HCV-RNA ≥100 units/mL at week 12, discontinue treatment (boceprevir, peginterferon alfa, and ribavirin).
HCV-RNA ≥1000 units/mL: Discontinue treatment (boceprevir, peginterferon alfa, and ribavirin)
Weeks ≥24:
HCV-RNA **undetectable** at week 24: Boceprevir 800 mg 3 times daily with continued peginterferon alfa and ribavirin for 24 additional weeks (through week 48)
HCV-RNA **detectable** at week 24: Discontinue treatment (boceprevir, peginterferon alfa, and ribavirin)
Cirrhosis, compensated:
Weeks 1-4: Peginterferon alfa with concomitant ribavirin only
Weeks 5-48: Boceprevir 800 mg 3 times daily with continued peginterferon alfa and ribavirin

Dosage adjustment in renal impairment:
Mild-to-severe impairment: No dosage adjustment necessary.
ESRD requiring hemodialysis: No dosage adjustment necessary. Not removed by hemodialysis.

Dosage adjustment in hepatic impairment:
Mild, moderate, or severe impairment: No dosage adjustment necessary.
Compensated cirrhosis: Consider risks and benefits before initiating therapy in patients with compensated cirrhosis who have platelet count less than 100,000/mm^3 and serum albumin less than 3.5 g/dL at baseline. Monitor closely for signs of infection and worsening of liver function. Also refer to Peginterferon Alfa and Ribavirin individual monographs.
Decompensated cirrhosis: No dosage adjustment provided in manufacturer's labeling (has not been studied); not approved for use in decompensated cirrhosis (safety/efficacy not established). Also refer to Peginterferon Alfa and Ribavirin individual monographs.

Dietary Considerations Take with food. The type or timing of a meal is not important as long as dose is taken with food.

Administration Administer with food (a meal or light snack). Doses should be taken approximately every 7-9 hours. Administer concurrently with peginterferon alfa and ribavirin.

Monitoring Parameters
CBC with differential and platelet count at baseline and at weeks 2, 4, 8 and 12, then periodically (and when clinically indicated)
Baseline serum albumin (patients with compensated cirrhosis)
Serum HCV RNA at baseline, weeks 4, 8, 12 and 24, end of treatment, during treatment follow up, and when clinically indicated
Pretreatment and monthly pregnancy test up to 6 months following discontinuation of therapy for women of childbearing age
Signs of infection and worsening of liver function (especially in compensated cirrhosis)

Reference Range
Treatment futility: HCV-RNA ≥1000 units/mL at treatment week 8, ≥100 units/mL at treatment week 12, or confirmed, detectable HCV-RNA at treatment week 24
Rapid virological response (RVR): Absence of detectable HCV RNA after 4 weeks of treatment
Early viral response (EVR): ≥2-log decrease in HCV RNA after 8-12 weeks of treatment
End of treatment response (ETR): Absence of detectable HCV RNA at end of the recommended treatment period
Sustained treatment response (STR): Absence of HCV RNA in the serum 6 months following completion of full treatment course
Sustained virologic response (SVR): Plasma HCV RNA <25 units/mL at follow up week 24

Additional Information In clinical studies of treatment-naive patients, a sustained virologic response (SVR) with peginterferon alfa, ribavirin, and boceprevir was achieved in ~68% of non-African-American patients versus 40% of controls (peginterferon alfa and ribavirin only). African-American patients had a lower rate of SVR compared to controls (42% to 53% dependent upon treatment duration versus 23% of controls). Rapid virologic response (RVR) at week 4 of lead-in treatment with peginterferon alfa and ribavirin can predict patient success after the addition of boceprevir and guide treatment duration. Patients who have marginal response during the lead-in treatment phase have a lower SVR after the addition of boceprevir; these patients may need close monitoring for regimen adherence and resistance development.

Dosage Forms
Capsule, Oral:
Victrelis: 200 mg

◆ **BOL-303224-A** *see* Besifloxacin *on page 251*

◆ **Bonefos® (Can)** *see* Clodronate [CAN/INT] *on page 469*

◆ **Boniva** *see* Ibandronate *on page 1028*

◆ **Boostrix** *see* Diphtheria and Tetanus Toxoids, and Acellular Pertussis Vaccine *on page 649*

Bortezomib (bore TEZ oh mib)

Brand Names: U.S. Velcade
Brand Names: Canada Velcade
Index Terms LDP-341; MLN341; PS-341
Pharmacologic Category Antineoplastic Agent; Proteasome Inhibitor

Use

Mantle cell lymphoma: Treatment of mantle cell lymphoma

Multiple myeloma: Treatment of multiple myeloma

Pregnancy Risk Factor D

Pregnancy Considerations Adverse effects (fetal loss and decreased fetal weight) were observed in animal reproduction studies at doses less than the equivalent human dose (based on BSA). Women of reproductive potential should avoid becoming pregnant and should use effective contraception during treatment.

Breast-Feeding Considerations It is not known if bortezomib is excreted in breast milk. Due to the potential for serious adverse reactions in the nursing infant, the decision to discontinue bortezomib or to discontinue breast-feeding should take into account the benefits of treatment to the mother.

Contraindications Hypersensitivity (excluding local reactions) to bortezomib, boron, mannitol, or any component of the formulation; administration via the intrathecal route

Warnings/Precautions Hazardous agent - use appropriate precautions for handling and disposal (NIOSH 2014 [group 1]). May cause or worsen peripheral neuropathy (usually sensory but may be mixed sensorimotor); risk may be increased with previous use of neurotoxic agents or preexisting peripheral neuropathy (patients with preexisting neuropathy should use only after risk versus benefit assessment); monitor for signs and symptoms; adjustment of dose and/or schedule may be required. The incidence of grades 2 and 3 peripheral neuropathy may be lower with SubQ route (compared to IV); consider SubQ administration in patients with preexisting or at high risk for peripheral neuropathy; the majority of patients with ≥ grade 2 peripheral neuropathy have improvement in or resolution of symptoms with dose adjustments or discontinuation; in a study of elderly patients receiving a weekly bortezomib schedule with combination chemotherapy, the incidence of peripheral neuropathy was significantly reduced without an effect on outcome (Boccadoro, 2010; Palumbo, 2009). May cause hypotension (including postural and orthostatic); use caution with dehydration, history of syncope, or medications associated with hypotension (may require adjustment of antihypertensive medication, hydration, and mineralocorticoids and/or sympathomimetics). Has been associated with the development or exacerbation of heart failure (HF) and decreased left ventricular ejection fraction (LVEF); monitor closely in patients with risk factors for HF or existing heart disease, although HF and decreased LVEF have been observed in patients without risk factors. Has also been associated with isolated reports of QTc prolongation.

Pulmonary disorders (some fatal) including pneumonitis, interstitial pneumonia, lung infiltrates, and acute respiratory distress syndrome (ARDS) have been reported. Pulmonary hypertension (without left heart failure or significant pulmonary disease has been reported rarely). Promptly evaluate with new or worsening cardiopulmonary symptoms; therapy interruption may be required. Tumor lysis syndrome has been reported; risk is increased in patients with high tumor burden prior to treatment. Posterior reversible leukoencephalopathy syndrome (PRES, formerly RPLS) has been reported (rarely). Promptly evaluate with new or worsening cardiopulmonary symptoms. Symptoms of PRES include confusion, headache, hypertension, lethargy, seizure, blindness and/or other vision, or neurologic disturbances; discontinue bortezomib if PRES occurs. MRI is recommended to confirm PRES diagnosis. The safety of reinitiating bortezomib in patients previously experiencing PRES is unknown. Herpes (zoster and simplex) reactivation has been reported with bortezomib; consider antiviral prophylaxis during therapy. Hematologic toxicity, including grade 3 and 4 neutropenia and severe thrombocytopenia, may occur (nadirs generally occur following the last dose of a cycle and recover prior to the next cycle); risk is increased in patients with pretreatment platelet counts <75,000/µL; frequent monitoring is required throughout treatment; may require dosage or schedule adjustments; withhold treatment for platelets <30,000/µL. Management with platelet transfusions and supportive care may be necessary. Hemorrhage (gastrointestinal and intracerebral) due to low platelet count has been observed. Acute liver failure has been reported (rarely) in patients receiving multiple concomitant medications and with serious underlying conditions. Hepatitis, transaminase increases, and hyperbilirubinemia have also been reported; interrupt therapy to assess reversibility. Use caution in patients with hepatic dysfunction; reduced initial doses are recommended for moderate and severe hepatic impairment (exposure is increased); closely monitor for toxicities. Hyper- and hypoglycemia may occur in diabetic patients receiving oral hypoglycemics; may require adjustment of diabetes medications. Nausea, vomiting, diarrhea or constipation may occur; may require antiemetics or antidiarrheals; ileus may occur; administer fluid and electrolytes to prevent dehydration (monitor closely); interrupt therapy for severe symptoms.

Potentially significant drug-drug/drug-food interactions may exist, requiring dose or frequency adjustment, additional monitoring, and/or selection of alternative therapy. Coadministration of strong CYP3A4 inhibitors may increase bortezomib exposure; monitor for toxicity and consider dose reduction if concurrent therapy cannot be avoided. Efficacy may be reduced when administered with strong CYP3A4 inducers; concomitant use is not recommended.

For IV or SubQ administration only. Intrathecal administration is contraindicated; inadvertent intrathecal administration has resulted in death. Bortezomib should **NOT** be prepared during the preparation of any intrathecal medications. After preparation, keep bortezomib in a location **away** from the separate storage location recommended for intrathecal medications. Bortezomib should **NOT** be delivered to the patient at the same time with any medications intended for central nervous system administration. The reconstituted concentrations for IV and SubQ administration are different; use caution when calculating the volume for each route and dose. The manufacturer provides stickers to facilitate identification of the route for reconstituted vials.

Adverse Reactions Incidences reported are associated with monotherapy. Additional adverse reactions reported with mono- or combination therapy.

Cardiovascular: Acute pulmonary edema, aggravated atrial fibrillation, angina pectoris, atrial flutter, atrioventricular block, bradycardia, cardiac disease (treatment emergent), cardiac failure, cardiogenic shock, cerebrovascular accident, deep vein thrombosis, edema, embolism (peripheral), facial edema, hemorrhagic stroke, hypertension, hypotension, ischemic heart disease, myocardial infarction, pericardial effusion, pericarditis, peripheral edema, phlebitis, portal vein thrombosis, pulmonary edema, pulmonary embolism, septic shock, sinoatrial arrest, subdural hematoma, torsades de pointes, transient ischemic attacks, ventricular tachycardia

Central nervous system: Agitation, anxiety, ataxia, brain disease, cerebral hemorrhage, chills, coma, confusion, cranial nerve palsy, dizziness (excludes vertigo), dysarthria, dysautonomia, dysesthesia, fatigue, headache, insomnia, malaise, mental status changes, motor dysfunction, neuralgia, paralysis, paresthesia, peripheral neuropathy, psychosis, seizure, spinal cord compression, suicidal ideation, vertigo

Dermatologic: Pruritus, skin rash, urticaria

Endocrine & metabolic: Amyloid heart disease, dehydration, hyperglycemia (diabetic patients), hyperkalemia, hypernatremia, hyperuricemia, hypocalcemia, hypoglycemia (diabetic patients), hypokalemia, hyponatremia, weight loss

Gastrointestinal: Abdominal pain, anorexia, cholestasis, constipation, decreased appetite, diarrhea, duodenitis (hemorrhagic), dysphagia, fecal impaction, gastritis (hemorrhagic), gastroenteritis, gastroesophageal reflux disease, hematemesis, intestinal obstruction, intestinal perforation, melena, nausea, oral candidiasis, pancreatitis, paralytic ileus, peritonitis, stomatitis, vomiting

Genitourinary: Bladder spasm, hematuria, hemorrhagic cystitis, urinary incontinence, urinary retention, urinary tract infection

Hematologic & oncologic: Anemia, disseminated intravascular coagulation, febrile neutropenia, hemorrhage, leukopenia, lymphocytopenia, neutropenia, oral mucosal petechiae, thrombocytopenia

Hepatic: Ascites, hepatic failure, hepatic hemorrhage, hepatitis, hyperbilirubinemia

Hypersensitivity: Anaphylaxis, angioedema, hypersensitivity, hypersensitivity angiitis

Infection: Aspergillosis, bacteremia, herpes simplex infection, herpes zoster, herpes zoster (reactivation), listeriosis, toxoplasmosis

Local: Catheter infection, injection site reaction (mostly redness SubQ), irritation at injection site (IV)

Neuromuscular & skeletal: Arthralgia, back pain, bone fracture, limb pain, myalgia, ostealgia, weakness

Ophthalmic: Blurred vision, conjunctival infection, conjunctival irritation, diplopia

Otic: Auditory impairment

Renal: Bilateral hydronephrosis, nephrolithiasis, proliferative glomerulonephritis, renal failure

Respiratory: Adult respiratory distress syndrome, aspiration pneumonia, atelectasis, bronchitis, chronic obstructive pulmonary disease (exacerbation), cough, dyspnea, epistaxis, hemoptysis, hypoxia, laryngeal edema, nasopharyngitis, pleural effusion, pneumonia, pneumonitis, pulmonary hypertension, pulmonary infiltrates (including diffuse), respiratory tract infection, sinusitis

Miscellaneous: Fever

Rare but important or life-threatening: Acute ischemic stroke, amyloidosis, blindness, cardiac arrest, cardiac tamponade, deafness (bilateral), decreased left ventricular ejection fraction, dysgeusia, dyspepsia, herpes meningoencephalitis, increased gamma-glutamyl transferase, increased serum alkaline phosphatase, increased serum transaminases, interstitial pneumonitis, ischemic colitis, ocular herpes simplex, optic neuritis, progressive multifocal leukoencephalopathy, prolonged QT interval on ECG, respiratory failure, reversible posterior leukoencephalopathy syndrome, sepsis, SIADH, Stevens-Johnson syndrome, subarachnoid hemorrhage, Sweet syndrome, syncope, tachycardia, toxic epidermal necrolysis, tumor lysis syndrome

Drug Interactions

Metabolism/Transport Effects **Substrate** of CYP1A2 (minor), CYP2C19 (major), CYP2C9 (minor), CYP2D6 (minor), CYP3A4 (major); **Note:** Assignment of Major/Minor substrate status based on clinically relevant drug interaction potential; **Inhibits** CYP1A2 (weak), CYP2C19 (moderate), CYP2C9 (weak), CYP2D6 (weak), CYP3A4 (weak)

Avoid Concomitant Use

Avoid concomitant use of Bortezomib with any of the following: CloZAPine; CYP3A4 Inducers (Strong); Dipyrone; Green Tea; Pimozide; St Johns Wort

Increased Effect/Toxicity

Bortezomib may increase the levels/effects of: ARIPiprazole; Citalopram; CloZAPine; CYP2C19 Substrates; Highest Risk QTc-Prolonging Agents; Hydrocodone; Lomitapide; Moderate Risk QTc-Prolonging Agents; Pimozide

The levels/effects of Bortezomib may be increased by: CYP3A4 Inhibitors (Strong); Dipyrone; Mifepristone

Decreased Effect

Bortezomib may decrease the levels/effects of: Clopidogrel

The levels/effects of Bortezomib may be decreased by: Ascorbic Acid; Bosentan; CYP2C19 Inducers (Strong); CYP3A4 Inducers (Moderate); CYP3A4 Inducers (Strong); Dabrafenib; Deferasirox; Green Tea; Multivitamins/Fluoride (with ADE); Multivitamins/Minerals (with ADEK, Folate, Iron); Multivitamins/Minerals (with AE, No Iron); Siltuximab; St Johns Wort; Tocilizumab

Preparation for Administration Note: The reconstituted concentrations for IV and SubQ administration are different; the manufacturer provides stickers to facilitate identification of the route for reconstituted vials. The amount contained in each vial may exceed the prescribed dose; use care with dosage and volume calculations.

Hazardous agent; use appropriate precautions for handling and disposal (NIOSH 2014 [group 1]). Reconstitute only with normal saline (NS). Reconstituted solutions should be clear and colorless.

IV: Reconstitute each 3.5 mg vial with 3.5 mL NS to a concentration of 1 mg/mL.

SubQ: Reconstitute each 3.5 mg vial with 1.4 mL NS to a concentration of 2.5 mg/mL (Moreau, 2011). If injection site reaction occurs, the more dilute 1 mg/mL concentration may be used SubQ.

Storage/Stability Prior to reconstitution, store intact vials at 25°C (77°F); excursions are permitted between 15°C and 30°C (59°F and 86°F). Once reconstituted, the manufacturer recommends use within 8 hours of reconstitution. However, stability studies have demonstrated solutions of 1 mg/mL (vial or syringe) may be stored at room temperature for up to 3 days, or under refrigeration for up to 5 days (Andre, 2005); or refrigerated in the original vial for up to 15 days (Vanderloo, 2010). Protect from light. After preparation, keep bortezomib in a location away from the separate storage location recommended for intrathecal medications.

Mechanism of Action Bortezomib inhibits proteasomes, enzyme complexes which regulate protein homeostasis within the cell. Specifically, it reversibly inhibits chymotrypsin-like activity at the 26S proteasome, leading to activation of signaling cascades, cell-cycle arrest, and apoptosis.

Pharmacodynamics/Kinetics

Distribution: 498 to 1884 L/m^2; distributes widely to peripheral tissues

Protein binding: ~83%

Metabolism: Hepatic primarily via CYP2C19 and 3A4 and to a lesser extent CYP1A2; forms metabolites (inactive) via deboronization followed by hydroxylation

Half-life elimination: Single dose: IV: 9 to 15 hours; Multiple dosing: 1 mg/m^2: 40 to 193 hours; 1.3 mg/m^2: 76 to 108 hours

Dosage Note: Consecutive doses should be separated by at least 72 hours.

Multiple myeloma (first-line therapy; in combination with melphalan and prednisone): Adults: IV, SubQ: 1.3 mg/m^2 days 1, 4, 8, 11, 22, 25, 29, and 32 of a 42-day treatment cycle for 4 cycles, followed by 1.3 mg/m^2 days 1, 8, 22, and 29 of a 42-day treatment cycle for 5 cycles.

Retreatment may be considered for multiple myeloma patients who had previously responded to bortezomib (either as monotherapy or in combination) and who have relapsed at least 6 months after completing prior bortezomib therapy; initiate at the last tolerated dose.

Alternative first-line therapy (off-label dosing): Adults:

CyBorD regimen: IV: 1.5 mg/m^2 days 1, 8, 15, and 22 of a 28-day treatment cycle for 4 cycles (may continue beyond 4 cycles) in combination with cyclophosphamide and dexamethasone (Khan, 2012)

PAD regimen: IV: Induction: 1.3 mg/m^2 days 1, 4, 8, and 11 of a 28-day treatment cycle for 3 cycles (in combination with doxorubicin and dexamethasone), followed by conditioning/stem cell transplantation, and then maintenance bortezomib 1.3 mg/m^2 once every 2 weeks for 2 years (Sonneveld, 2012)

VRd regimen: IV: 1.3 mg/m^2 days 1, 4, 8, and 11 of a 21-day treatment cycle for 8 cycles (in combination with lenalidomide and dexamethasone) (Kumar, 2012; Richardson, 2010)

Patients ≥65 years: IV: 1.3 mg/m^2 days 1, 8, 15, and 22 of a 35-day treatment cycle, in combination with **either** melphalan and prednisone or melphalan, prednisone, and thalidomide (Boccadoro, 2010; Bringhen, 2010; Palumbo, 2009)

Multiple myeloma (relapsed): Adults: IV, SubQ: 1.3 mg/m^2 twice weekly for 2 weeks on days 1, 4, 8, and 11 of a 21-day treatment cycle. Therapy extending beyond 8 cycles may be administered by the standard schedule or may be given once weekly for 4 weeks (days 1, 8, 15, and 22), followed by a 13-day rest (days 23 through 35).

Retreatment may be considered for multiple myeloma patients who had previously responded to bortezomib (either as monotherapy or in combination) and who have relapsed at least 6 months after completing prior bortezomib therapy; initiate at the last tolerated dose. Administer twice weekly for 2 weeks on days 1, 4, 8, and 11 of a 21-day treatment cycle (either as a single-agent or in combination with dexamethasone) for a maximum of 8 cycles.

Alternative relapsed therapy (off-label dosing): Adults: IV: 1.3 mg/m^2 days 1, 4, 8, and 11 of a 21-day treatment cycle for at least 8 cycles or until disease progression or unacceptable toxicity (in combination with liposomal doxorubicin) (Orlowski, 2007)

Mantle cell lymphoma (first-line therapy; in combination with rituximab, cyclophosphamide, doxorubicin, and prednisone [VcR-CAP]): Adults: IV: 1.3 mg/m^2 days 1, 4, 8, 11 of a 21-day treatment cycle for 6 cycles. If response first documented at cycle 6, treatment for an additional 2 cycles is recommended.

Mantle cell lymphoma (relapsed): Adults: IV, SubQ: 1.3 mg/m^2 twice weekly for 2 weeks on days 1, 4, 8, and 11 of a 21-day treatment cycle. Therapy extending beyond 8 cycles may be administered by the standard schedule or may be given once weekly for 4 weeks (days 1, 8, 15, and 22), followed by a 13-day rest (days 23 through 35).

Cutaneous and peripheral T-cell lymphoma, relapsed/refractory (off-label use): Adults: IV: 1.3 mg/m^2 twice weekly for 2 weeks on days 1, 4, 8, and 11 of a 21-day treatment cycle (Zinzani, 2007); additional data may be necessary to further define the role of bortezomib in this condition.

Follicular lymphoma, relapsed/refractory (off-label use): Adults: IV: 1.3 mg/m^2 days 1, 4, 8, and 11 of a 28-day treatment cycle, in combination with bendamustine and rituximab for 6 cycles (Friedberg, 2011) **or** 1.6 mg/m^2 days 1, 8, 15, and 22 of a 35-day treatment cycle, in combination with bendamustine and rituximab for 5 cycles (Fowler, 2011)

Systemic light-chain amyloidosis (off-label use): Adults: IV: 1.3 mg/m^2 days 1, 4, 8, and 11 of a 21-day treatment cycle (with or without dexamethasone) (Kastritis, 2010)

Waldenström's macroglobulinemia, relapsed/refractory (off-label use): Adults: IV: 1.3 mg/m^2 days 1, 4, 8, and 11 of a 21-day treatment cycle (Chen, 2007) **or** 1.3 mg/m^2 days 1, 4, 8, and 11 of a 21-day treatment cycle (in combination with dexamethasone and rituximab) (Treon, 2009) **or** 1.6 mg/m^2 days 1, 8, and 15 of a 28-day treatment cycle (in combination with rituximab) (Ghobrial, 2010)

Dosage adjustment for toxicity:

Myeloma (first-line therapy):

Platelets should be ≥70,000/mm^3, ANC should be ≥1000/mm^3, and nonhematologic toxicities should resolve to grade 1 or baseline prior to therapy initiation.

Platelets ≤30,000/mm^3 or ANC ≤750/mm^3 on bortezomib day(s) (except day 1): Withhold bortezomib; if several bortezomib doses in consecutive cycles are withheld, reduce dose 1 level (1.3 mg/m^2/dose reduced to 1 mg/m^2/dose; 1 mg/m^2/dose reduced to 0.7 mg/m^2/dose)

Grade ≥3 nonhematological toxicity (other than neuropathy): Withhold bortezomib until toxicity resolves to grade 1 or baseline. May reinitiate bortezomib at 1 dose level reduction (1.3 mg/m^2/dose reduced to 1 mg/m^2/dose; 1 mg/m^2/dose reduced to 0.7 mg/m^2/dose).

Neuropathic pain and/or peripheral sensory or motor neuropathy: See "Neuropathic pain and/or peripheral sensory or motor neuropathy" toxicity adjustment guidelines below.

Mantle cell lymphoma (first-line therapy):

Platelets should be ≥100,000/mm^3, ANC should be ≥1,500/mm^3, hemoglobin should be ≥8 g/dL, and nonhematologic toxicities should resolve to grade 1 or baseline prior to each cycle (cycle 2 and beyond).

Platelets <25,000/mm^3 or ≥ grade 3 neutropenia on bortezomib day(s) (except day 1): Withhold bortezomib for up to 2 weeks until platelets are ≥25,000/mm^3 and/or ANC ≥750/mm^3, then reduce dose 1 level (1.3 mg/m^2/dose reduced to 1 mg/m^2/dose; 1 mg/m^2/dose reduced to 0.7 mg/m^2/dose). If hematologic toxicity does not resolve after withholding therapy, discontinue bortezomib.

Grade ≥3 nonhematological toxicity (other than neuropathy): Withhold bortezomib until toxicity resolves to ≤ grade 2. May reinitiate bortezomib at 1 dose level reduction (1.3 mg/m^2/dose reduced to 1 mg/m^2/dose; 1 mg/m^2/dose reduced to 0.7 mg/m^2/dose).

Neuropathic pain and/or peripheral sensory or motor neuropathy: See "Neuropathic pain and/or peripheral sensory or motor neuropathy" toxicity adjustment guidelines below.

Relapsed multiple myeloma and mantle cell lymphoma:

Grade 3 nonhematological (excluding neuropathy) or grade 4 hematological toxicity: Withhold until toxicity resolved; may reinitiate with a 25% dose reduction (1.3 mg/m^2/dose reduced to 1 mg/m^2/dose; 1 mg/m^2/dose reduced to 0.7 mg/m^2/dose)

Neuropathic pain and/or peripheral sensory or motor neuropathy:

Note: Consider subQ administration in patients with preexisting or at high risk for peripheral neuropathy.

Grade 1 (asymptomatic; deep tendon reflex loss or paresthesia) without pain or loss of function: No action needed

Grade 1 with pain or grade 2 (moderate symptoms; limiting instrumental activities of daily living): Reduce dose to 1 mg/m^2

Grade 2 with pain or grade 3 (severe symptoms; limiting self-care activities of daily living): Withhold until toxicity resolved, may reinitiate at 0.7 mg/m^2 once weekly

Grade 4 (life-threatening consequences with urgent intervention indicated): Discontinue therapy

Dosage adjustment in renal impairment: No dosage adjustment is necessary. Dialysis may reduce bortezomib concentrations; administer postdialysis (Leal, 2011).

Dosage adjustment in hepatic impairment:

Mild impairment (bilirubin ≤1 times ULN and AST >ULN or bilirubin >1 to 1.5 times ULN): No initial dose adjustment is necessary (LoRusso, 2012).

Moderate (bilirubin >1.5 to 3 times ULN) and severe impairment (bilirubin >3 times ULN): Reduce initial dose to 0.7 mg/m^2 in the first cycle; based on patient tolerance, may consider dose escalation to 1 mg/m^2 (LoRusso, 2012) or further dose reduction to 0.5 mg/m^2 in subsequent cycles.

Dosing in obesity: *ASCO Guidelines for appropriate chemotherapy dosing in obese adults with cancer:* Utilize patient's actual body weight (full weight) for calculation of body surface area- or weight-based dosing, particularly when the intent of therapy is curative; manage regimen-related toxicities in the same manner as for nonobese patients; if a dose reduction is utilized due to toxicity, consider resumption of full weight-based dosing with subsequent cycles, especially if cause of toxicity (eg, hepatic or renal impairment) is resolved (Griggs, 2012).

Dietary Considerations Green tea and green tea extracts may diminish the therapeutic effect of bortezomib and should be avoided (Golden, 2009). Avoid grapefruit juice. Avoid additional, nondietary sources of ascorbic acid supplements, including multivitamins containing ascorbic acid (may diminish bortezomib activity) during treatment, especially 12 hours before and after bortezomib treatment (Perrone, 2009).

Administration Note: The reconstituted concentrations for IV and SubQ administration are different; use caution when calculating the volume for each route and dose. Consider SubQ administration in patients with preexisting or at high risk for peripheral neuropathy.

IV: Administer via rapid IV push (3-5 seconds). When administering in combination with rituximab for first-line therapy of mantle cell lymphoma, administer bortezomib prior to rituximab.

SubQ: Subcutaneous administration of bortezomib 1.3 mg/m^2 days 1, 4, 8, and 11 of a 21-day treatment cycle has been studied in a limited number of patients with relapsed multiple myeloma; doses were administered subcutaneously (concentration of 2.5 mg/mL) into the thigh or abdomen, rotating the injection site with each dose; injections at the same site within a single cycle were avoided (Moreau, 2010; Moreau, 2011). Response rates were similar to IV administration; decreased incidence of grade 3 or higher adverse events were observed with SubQ administration. Administer at least 1 inch from an old site and never administer to tender, bruised, erythematous, or indurated sites. If injection site reaction occurs, the more dilute 1 mg/mL concentration may be used SubQ (or IV administration of 1 mg/mL concentration may be considered).

For IV or SubQ administration only; fatalities have been reported with inadvertent intrathecal administration. Bortezomib should **NOT** be delivered to the patient at the same time with any medications intended for central nervous system administration.

Hazardous agent; use appropriate precautions for handling and disposal (NIOSH 2014 [group 1]).

Monitoring Parameters CBC with differential and platelets (monitor frequently throughout therapy); liver function tests (in patients with existing hepatic impairment); signs/symptoms of peripheral neuropathy, dehydration, hypotension, or PRES; renal function, pulmonary function (with new or worsening pulmonary symptoms)

Dosage Forms

Solution Reconstituted, Injection:

Velcade: 3.5 mg (1 ea)

Bosentan (boe SEN tan)

Brand Names: U.S. Tracleer

Brand Names: Canada ACT Bosentan; Mylan-Bosentan; PMS-Bosentan; Sandoz-Bosentan; Teva-Bosentan; Tracleer

Pharmacologic Category Endothelin Receptor Antagonist; Vasodilator

Use Treatment of pulmonary artery hypertension (PAH) (WHO Group I) in patients with NYHA Class II, III, or IV symptoms to improve exercise capacity and decrease the rate of clinical deterioration

Pregnancy Risk Factor X

Pregnancy Considerations [U.S. Boxed Warning]: May cause birth defects; use in pregnancy is contraindicated. Exclude pregnancy prior to initiation of therapy and obtain pregnancy tests monthly during treatment. Reliable contraception must be used during therapy and for 1 month after stopping treatment. Hormonal contraceptives (oral, injectable, transdermal, or implantable) may not be effective and a second method of contraception (nonhormonal) is required. Patients with tubal ligation or an implanted IUD (Copper T 380A or LNg 20) do not need additional contraceptive measures. When a hormonal or barrier contraceptive is used, one additional method of contraception is still needed if a male partner has had a vasectomy. When initiating treatment for women of reproductive potential, a negative pregnancy test should be documented within the first 5 days of a normal menstrual period and ≥11 days after the last unprotected intercourse. A missed menses or suspected pregnancy should be reported to a healthcare provider and prompt immediate pregnancy testing. Sperm counts may be reduced in men during treatment. Women of childbearing potential should avoid splitting, crushing, or handling broken tablets and exposure to the generated dust (tablet splitting is currently outside of product labeling).

Breast-Feeding Considerations Due to the potential risk of adverse events in a nursing infant, a decision should be made to discontinue nursing or discontinue therapy.

Contraindications Hypersensitivity to bosentan or any component of the formulation; concurrent use of cyclosporine or glyburide; pregnancy

Canadian labeling: Additional contraindications (not in U.S. labeling): Moderate-to-severe hepatic impairment and/or baseline ALT or AST >3 times the upper limit of normal (ULN), particularly when total bilirubin >2 times ULN

Warnings/Precautions Hazardous agent - use appropriate precautions for handling and disposal (NIOSH 2014 [group 3]). **[U.S. Boxed Warning]: May cause hepatotoxicity; has been associated with a high incidence (~11%) of significant transaminase elevations (ALT or AST ≥3 times ULN) with or without elevations in bilirubin and rare cases of unexplained hepatic cirrhosis (after >12 months of therapy) or hepatic failure. Monitor transaminases at baseline then monthly thereafter. Adjust dosage if elevations in liver enzymes occur without symptoms of hepatic injury or elevated bilirubin. Treatment should be stopped in patients who develop elevated transaminases either in combination with symptoms of hepatic injury (unusual fatigue, jaundice, nausea, vomiting, abdominal pain, and/or fever) or elevated bilirubin (≥2 times ULN); safety of reintroduction is unknown. Avoid use in patients with baseline serum transaminases >3 times ULN or moderate-to-severe hepatic impairment.** Transaminase elevations are dose dependent, generally asymptomatic, occur both early and late in therapy, progress slowly, and are usually reversible after treatment interruption or discontinuation. Consider the benefits of treatment versus the risk of hepatotoxicity when initiating therapy in patients with WHO Class II symptoms.

[U.S. Boxed Warning]: May cause birth defects; use in pregnancy is contraindicated. Exclude pregnancy prior to initiation of therapy and obtain pregnancy tests monthly during treatment. Reliable contraception must be used during therapy and for 1 month after stopping treatment. Hormonal contraceptives (oral, injectable, transdermal, or implantable) may not be effective and a second method of contraception (nonhormonal) is required. Patients with tubal ligation or an implanted IUD (Copper T 380A or LNg 20) do not need additional contraceptive measures. (See Pregnancy Considerations.)

[U.S. Boxed Warning]: Because of the risks of hepatic impairment and the high likelihood of teratogenic effects, bosentan is only available through the T.A.P. restricted distribution program. Patients, prescribers, and pharmacies must be registered with and meet conditions of T.A.P. Call 1-866-228-3546 or visit http://www.tracleer.com/hcp/prescribing-tracleer.asp for more information.

A reduction in hematocrit/hemoglobin may be observed within the first few weeks of therapy with subsequent stabilization of levels. Hemoglobin reductions >15% have been observed in some patients. Measure hemoglobin prior to initiating therapy, at 1 and 3 months, and every 3 months thereafter. Significant decreases in hemoglobin in the absence of other causes may warrant the discontinuation of therapy.

Development of peripheral edema due to treatment and/or disease state (pulmonary arterial hypertension) may occur. There have also been postmarketing reports of fluid retention requiring treatment (eg, diuretics, fluid management, hospitalization). Further evaluation may be necessary to determine cause and appropriate treatment or discontinuation of therapy. Bosentan should be discontinued in any patient with pulmonary edema suggestive of pulmonary veno-occlusive disease (PVOD). Bosentan may interact with many medications, resulting in potentially serious and/or life-threatening adverse events (see Drug Interactions).

Adverse Reactions

Cardiovascular: Chest pain, edema, flushing, hypotension, palpitations, syncope

Central nervous system: Headache

Dermatologic: Pruritus

Genitourinary: Spermatogenesis inhibition

Hematologic & oncologic: Anemia, decreased hemoglobin (typically in first 6 weeks of therapy)

Hepatic: Hepatic insufficiency, increased serum transaminases (≥3 times ULN; dose-related)

Neuromuscular & skeletal: Arthralgia

Respiratory: Respiratory tract infection, sinusitis

Rare but important or life-threatening: Anaphylaxis, angioedema, hepatic cirrhosis (prolonged therapy), hepatic failure (rare), hyperbilirubinemia, hypersensitivity, hypersensitivity angiitis, jaundice, leukopenia, neutropenia, peripheral edema, skin rash, thrombocytopenia, weight gain, worsening of heart failure

Drug Interactions

Metabolism/Transport Effects Substrate of CYP2C9 (minor), CYP3A4 (minor), SLCO1B1; **Note:** Assignment of Major/Minor substrate status based on clinically relevant drug interaction potential; **Induces** CYP2C9 (moderate), CYP3A4 (moderate)

Avoid Concomitant Use

Avoid concomitant use of Bosentan with any of the following: Axitinib; Bosutinib; CycloSPORINE (Systemic); Enzalutamide; GlyBURIDE; Nisoldipine; Olaparib; Simeprevir; Ulipristal

Increased Effect/Toxicity

Bosentan may increase the levels/effects of: Clarithromycin; Ifosfamide

The levels/effects of Bosentan may be increased by: Atazanavir; Boceprevir; Cobicistat; CycloSPORINE (Systemic); CYP2C9 Inhibitors (Moderate); CYP2C9 Inhibitors (Strong); CYP3A4 Inhibitors (Moderate); CYP3A4 Inhibitors (Strong); Darunavir; Eltrombopag; Fosamprenavir; GlyBURIDE; Indinavir; Lopinavir; Nelfinavir; Phosphodiesterase 5 Inhibitors; Rifampin; Ritonavir; Saquinavir; Telaprevir; Teriflunomide; Tipranavir

Decreased Effect

Bosentan may decrease the levels/effects of: ARIPiprazole; Atazanavir; Axitinib; Boceprevir; Bosutinib; Clarithromycin; Contraceptives (Estrogens); Contraceptives (Progestins); CycloSPORINE (Systemic); CYP3A4 Substrates; Darunavir; Dasabuvir; Enzalutamide; FentaNYL; Fosamprenavir; GlyBURIDE; HMG-CoA Reductase Inhibitors; Hydrocodone; Ibrutinib; Ifosfamide; Indinavir; Lopinavir; Nelfinavir; Nisoldipine; Olaparib; Ombitasvir; Paritaprevir; Phosphodiesterase 5 Inhibitors; Saquinavir; Saxagliptin; Simeprevir; Telaprevir; Tipranavir; Ulipristal; Vitamin K Antagonists

The levels/effects of Bosentan may be decreased by: GlyBURIDE; Rifampin

Food Interactions Bioavailability of bosentan is not affected by food. Bosentan serum concentrations may be increased by grapefruit juice. Management: Avoid grapefruit/grapefruit juice.

Storage/Stability Store at 20°C to 25°C (68°F to 77°F); excursions permitted to 15°C to 30°C (59°F to 86°F).

Mechanism of Action Blocks endothelin receptors on vascular endothelium and smooth muscle. Stimulation of these receptors is associated with vasoconstriction. Although bosentan blocks both ET_A and ET_B receptors, the affinity is higher for the A subtype.

Pharmacodynamics/Kinetics

Distribution: V_d: ~18 L

Protein binding, plasma: >98% primarily to albumin

Metabolism: Hepatic via CYP2C9 and 3A4 to three primary metabolites (one contributing ~10% to 20% pharmacologic activity); autoinduction may occur with chronic dosing

Bioavailability: ~50%

Half-life elimination: 5 hours; prolonged with heart failure, possibly in PAH

Time to peak, plasma: 3-5 hours

Excretion: Feces (as metabolites); urine (<3% as unchanged drug)

Dosage Oral:

Adolescents >12 years and Adults: Pulmonary artery hypertension:

<40 kg: Initial and maintenance: 62.5 mg twice daily

≥40 kg: Initial: 62.5 mg twice daily for 4 weeks; increase to maintenance dose of 125 mg twice daily. Doses >125 mg twice daily do not appear to confer additional clinical benefit, but may increase risk of liver toxicity.

Note: When discontinuing treatment, consider a reduction in dosage to 62.5 mg twice daily for 3-7 days (to avoid clinical deterioration).

Canadian labeling (not in U.S. labeling): Children 3-18 years:

10-20 kg: Initial: 31.25 mg once daily for 4 weeks; increase to maintenance dose of 31.25 mg twice daily

>20-40 kg: Initial: 31.25 mg twice daily for 4 weeks; increase to maintenance dose of 62.5 mg twice daily

>40 kg: Initial: 62.5 mg twice daily for 4 weeks; increase to maintenance dose of 125 mg twice daily

Coadministration with protease inhibitor regimen:

Dosage adjustment for concurrent use with atazanavir/ritonavir, darunavir/ritonavir, fosamprenavir, lopinavir/ritonavir, ritonavir, saquinavir/ritonavir, tipranavir/ritonavir:

Coadministration of bosentan in patients currently receiving one of these protease inhibitor regimens for at least 10 days: Begin with bosentan 62.5 mg once daily or every other day based on tolerability

Coadministration of one of these protease inhibitor regimens in patients currently receiving bosentan: Discontinue bosentan 36 hours prior to the initiation of an above regimen. After at least 10 days of the protease inhibitor regimen, resume bosentan 62.5 mg once daily or every other day based on tolerability.

Dosage adjustment for concurrent use with indinavir or nelfinavir:

Coadministration of bosentan in patients currently receiving indinavir or nelfinavir: Begin with bosentan 62.5 mg once daily or every other day based on tolerability

Coadministration of indinavir or nelfinavir in patients currently receiving bosentan: Adjust bosentan to 62.5 mg once daily or every other day based on tolerability

Dosage adjustment in renal impairment: No dosage adjustment necessary.

Dosage adjustment in hepatic impairment:

Mild impairment (Child-Pugh class A): No dosage adjustment necessary.

Moderate-to-severe impairment (Child-Pugh class B and C) and/or baseline transaminase >3 times ULN: Use not recommended; systemic exposure significantly increased in patients with moderate impairment (not studied in patients with severe impairment).

Modification based on transaminase elevation:

If any elevation, regardless of degree, is accompanied by clinical symptoms of hepatic injury (unusual fatigue, nausea, vomiting, abdominal pain, fever, or jaundice) or a serum bilirubin ≥2 times ULN, treatment should be stopped.

AST/ALT >3 times but ≤5 times ULN: Confirm with additional test; if confirmed, reduce dose to 62.5 mg twice daily or interrupt treatment and monitor every 2 weeks. If transaminase levels return to pretreatment values, may continue or reintroduce treatment at the starting dose, as appropriate. When reintroducing treatment, recheck transaminases within 3 days and at least every 2 weeks thereafter.

AST/ALT >5 times but ≤8 times ULN: Confirm with additional test; if confirmed, stop treatment. Monitor transaminase levels at least every 2 weeks. May reintroduce treatment, as appropriate, at starting dose, following return to pretreatment values. Recheck within 3 days and at least every 2 weeks thereafter following reinitiation.

AST/ALT >8 times ULN: Stop treatment and do not reintroduce.

Dietary Considerations May be taken with or without food. Avoid grapefruit and grapefruit juice.

Administration May be administered with or without food, once in the morning and once in the evening. Women of childbearing potential should avoid excessive handling of broken tablets.

Hazardous agent; use appropriate precautions for handling and disposal (NIOSH 2014 [group 3]).

Monitoring Parameters Serum transaminase (AST and ALT) and bilirubin should be determined prior to the initiation of therapy and at monthly intervals thereafter. Monitor for clinical signs and symptoms of liver injury (eg, abdominal pain, fatigue, fever, jaundice, nausea, vomiting). Hemoglobin and hematocrit should be measured at baseline, at 1 month and 3 months of treatment, and every 3 months thereafter (generally stabilizes after 4-12 weeks of treatment).

A woman of childbearing potential must have a negative pregnancy test prior to the initiation of therapy and monthly thereafter (prior to shipment of monthly refill).

Dosage Forms

Tablet, Oral:

Tracleer: 62.5 mg, 125 mg

Extemporaneous Preparations Hazardous agent; use appropriate precautions for handling and disposal (NIOSH 2014 [group 3]).

Note: Tablets are not scored; a commercial pill cutter should be used to prepare a 31.25 mg dose from the 62.5 mg tablet; the half-cut 62.5 mg tablets are stable for up to 4 weeks when stored at room temperature in the high-density polyethylene plastic bottle provided by the manufacturer. Since bosentan is classified as a teratogen (Pregnancy Risk Factor X), individuals should avoid exposure to bosentan powder (dust) by taking appropriate measures (eg, using gloves and mask); women of childbearing potential should avoid exposure to dust generated from broken or split tablets.

Crushing of the tablets is not recommended; bosentan tablets will disintegrate rapidly (within 5 minutes) in 5-25 mL of water to create a suspension. An appropriate aliquot of the suspension can be used to deliver the prescribed dose. Any remaining suspension should be discarded. Bosentan should not be mixed or dissolved in liquids with a low (acidic) pH (eg, fruit juices) due to poor solubility; the drug is most soluble in solutions with a pH >8.5.

◆ **Bosulif** *see* Bosutinib *on page* 282

Bosutinib (boe SUE ti nib)

Brand Names: U.S. Bosulif

Brand Names: Canada Bosulif

Index Terms Bosutinib Monohydrate; SKI-606

Pharmacologic Category Antineoplastic Agent, BCR-ABL Tyrosine Kinase Inhibitor; Antineoplastic Agent, Tyrosine Kinase Inhibitor

Use Chronic myelogenous leukemia (CML):

U.S. labeling: Treatment of chronic, accelerated or blast phase Philadelphia chromosome-positive (Ph+) CML in patients resistant or intolerant to prior therapy

Canadian labeling: Treatment of chronic, accelerated or blast phase Philadelphia chromosome-positive (Ph+) CML in patients resistant or intolerant to prior therapy and for whom subsequent treatment with imatinib, nilotinib, and dasatinib is not appropriate

Pregnancy Risk Factor D

Pregnancy Considerations Adverse events were observed in animal reproduction studies. Based on the mechanism of action, bosutinib may cause fetal harm if administered in pregnancy. Females of reproductive potential should use effective contraception during bosutinib treatment and for at least 30 days after completion of treatment. The Canadian labeling suggests that semen from male patients (including those who have undergone successful vasectomy) receiving bosutinib may pose a risk to a developing fetus and recommends that male patients use effective contraception while receiving treatment, during any treatment interruptions, and for at least 4 weeks after discontinuation of treatment.

Breast-Feeding Considerations It is not known if bosutinib is excreted in breast milk. Due to the potential for serious adverse reactions in the nursing infant, the decision to discontinue bosutinib or discontinue breast-feeding should take into account the benefits of treatment to the mother.

Contraindications

Hypersensitivity to bosutinib or any component of the formulation

Canadian labeling: Additional contraindications (not in U.S. labeling): History of long QT syndrome or with persistent QT interval >480 milliseconds; uncorrected hypokalemia or hypomagnesemia; hepatic impairment

Warnings/Precautions Hazardous agent - use appropriate precautions for handling and disposal (meets NIOSH 2014 criteria).

Diarrhea, nausea, vomiting, and abdominal pain may occur. Monitor; may require treatment interruption, dose reduction, or discontinuation. For patients experiencing diarrhea (all grades), the median time to onset was 2 days; median duration (per event) was 1 day; manage diarrhea with antidiarrheals and/or fluid replacement. Nausea and vomiting may be managed with antiemetics and fluid replacement. Acute pancreatitis has been reported; use caution in patients with a prior history of pancreatitis. The Canadian labeling recommends interruption of therapy in patients with elevated amylase/lipase accompanied by abdominal symptoms and evaluation to rule out pancreatitis.

Bleeding events (eg, GI, ophthalmic, pericardial, cerebral, vaginal) have been reported. Anemia, neutropenia, and thrombocytopenia may also occur. May require treatment interruption, dose reduction, or discontinuation. Monitor blood counts weekly during first month, then monthly thereafter (or as clinically indicated). Fluid retention, manifesting as pericardial effusion, pleural effusion, pulmonary edema and/or peripheral edema may occur; may be severe. Monitor for fluid retention (eg, weight gain) and manage appropriately; may require treatment interruption, dose reduction, or discontinuation. QTcF >500 milliseconds was observed rarely (≤0.8%) in clinical trials (Abbas, 2012; Cortes, 2012); patients with significant or uncontrolled cardiovascular disease (including prolonged QT interval at baseline) were not studied. The Canadian labeling recommends obtaining an ECG (baseline and as clinically indicated thereafter), correction of preexisting hypokalemia and/or hypomagnesemia and periodic monitoring of serum potassium and magnesium.

Bosutinib exposure is increased in patients with hepatic impairment; dose reduction is recommended (Canadian labeling contraindicates use in patients with hepatic impairment at baseline). Hepatotoxicity has been reported during treatment; dose reductions may be necessary. Monitor liver function. ALT and AST elevations may occur, usually with an onset in the first 3 months of treatment (median onset was ~30 to 33 days; median duration was 21 days). One case of drug-induced liver injury has been reported; full recovery occurred after discontinuation. Bosutinib exposure is increased in patients with moderate or severe renal impairment. Declines in glomerular filtration rates throughout bosutinib treatment have been observed in clinical studies; monitor renal function at baseline and during therapy, particularly in patients with preexisting impairment or other risk factors for renal dysfunction. Consider dosage adjustment in patients with renal dysfunction at baseline or with treatment emergent impairment. Bone fracture and mineral abnormalities (eg, hypophosphatemia) has been reported (Bosulif Canadian product monograph, 2014); monitor patients with severe osteoporosis or endocrine disease (eg, hyperparathyroidism) for mineral abnormalities and/or changes in bone density.

Potentially significant drug-drug interactions may exist, requiring dose or frequency adjustment, additional monitoring, and/or selection of alternative therapy. Proton pump inhibitors (PPIs) may decrease bosutinib effects; consider using short acting antacids or H_2 antagonists instead of PPIs; separate administration of antacids or H_2 antagonists from bosutinib by at least 2 hours.

Adverse Reactions

Cardiovascular: Chest pain, edema, pericardial effusion, prolonged Q-T interval on ECG

Central nervous system: Dizziness, fatigue, headache, pain

Dermatologic: Acne vulgaris, pruritus, skin rash, urticaria

Endocrine & metabolic: Dehydration, hypokalemia, hypophosphatemia, hyperkalemia

Gastrointestinal: abdominal pain, decreased appetite, diarrhea, dysgeusia, gastritis, increase serum lipase, nausea, vomiting

Hematologic & oncologic: Anemia, febrile neutropenia, neutropenia, thrombocytopenia

Hepatic: Hepatic insufficiency, hepatotoxicity, increased serum ALT, increased serum AST, increased serum bilirubin

Hypersensitivity: Hypersensitivity reaction

Infection: Influenza

Neuromuscular & skeletal: Arthralgia, back pain, increased creatine phosphokinase, myalgia, weakness

Otic: Tinnitus

Renal: Increased serum creatinine, renal failure

Respiratory: Bronchitis, cough, dyspnea, nasopharyngitis, pleural effusion, pneumonia, respiratory tract infection

Miscellaneous: Fever

Rare but important or life-threatening: Anaphylactic shock, erythema multiforme, exfoliative dermatitis, gastrointestinal hemorrhage, pancreatitis, pericarditis, pulmonary edema, pulmonary hypertension, respiratory failure

Drug Interactions

Metabolism/Transport Effects **Substrate** of CYP3A4 (major), P-glycoprotein; **Note:** Assignment of Major/Minor substrate status based on clinically relevant drug interaction potential; **Inhibits** P-glycoprotein

Avoid Concomitant Use

Avoid concomitant use of Bosutinib with any of the following: CloZAPine; Conivaptan; CYP3A4 Inducers (Moderate); CYP3A4 Inducers (Strong); CYP3A4 Inhibitors (Moderate); CYP3A4 Inhibitors (Strong); Dipyrone; Fusidic Acid (Systemic); Idelalisib; P-glycoprotein/ABCB1 Inhibitors; St Johns Wort

Increased Effect/Toxicity

Bosutinib may increase the levels/effects of: CloZAPine; Highest Risk QTc-Prolonging Agents; Moderate Risk QTc-Prolonging Agents

The levels/effects of Bosutinib may be increased by: Conivaptan; CYP3A4 Inhibitors (Moderate); CYP3A4 Inhibitors (Strong); Dasatinib; Dipyrone; Fusidic Acid (Systemic); Idelalisib; Luliconazole; Mifepristone; P-glycoprotein/ABCB1 Inhibitors

Decreased Effect

The levels/effects of Bosutinib may be decreased by: Antacids; CYP3A4 Inducers (Moderate); CYP3A4 Inducers (Strong); Deferasirox; H2-Antagonists; P-glycoprotein/ABCB1 Inducers; Proton Pump Inhibitors; Siltuximab; St Johns Wort; Tocilizumab

Food Interactions Grapefruit juice may increase bosutinib plasma concentration. Management: Avoid grapefruit juice.

Storage/Stability Store at room temperature of 20°C to 25°C (68°F to 77°F); excursions permitted to 15°C to 30°C (59°F to 86°F).

Mechanism of Action BCR-ABL tyrosine kinase inhibitor (TKI); inhibits BCR-ABL kinase that promotes CML. Also inhibits SRC family (including SRC, LYN, and HCK). Bosutinib has minimal activity against c-KIT and platelet-derived growth factor receptor (PDGFR), which are non-specific targets associated with toxicity in other TKIs (Cortes, 2012). Bosutinib has activity in 16 of 18 imatinib-resistant BCR-ABL mutations, with the exceptions of the T315I and V299L mutants (Cortes, 2011).

Pharmacodynamics/Kinetics

Onset:

Median time to complete hematologic response (in responders): 2 weeks (Cortes, 2011)

Median time to major cytogenetic response (in responders): 12.3 weeks (Cortes, 2011)

Median time to first complete cytogenic response: 12.9 weeks (Cortes, 2012)

Absorption: Slow (Abbas, 2012)

Distribution: V_d: 6,080 ± 1,230 L

Protein binding: 94% to plasma proteins

Metabolism: Hepatic via CYP3A4, primarily to inactive metabolites oxydechlorinated (M2) bosutinib and *N*-desmethylated (M5) bosutinib, also to bosutinib *N*-oxide (M6)

Half-life elimination: 22 to 27 hours (Cortes, 2011)

Time to peak: 4 to 6 hours

Excretion: Feces (91%); urine (3%)

Dosage Philadelphia chromosome-positive chronic myelogenous leukemia (Ph+CML): Adults: Oral: 500 mg once daily; continue until disease progression or unacceptable toxicity. **Note:** If complete hematologic response is not achieved by week 8 or complete cytogenetic response is not achieved by week 12, in the absence of grade 3 or higher adverse reactions, consider increasing the dose from 500 mg once daily to 600 mg once daily.

Missed doses: If a dose is missed beyond 12 hours, skip the dose and resume the usual dose the following day.

Dosage adjustment for toxicity:

Hematologic toxicity: ANC <1,000/mm³ or platelets <50,000/mm³: Withhold treatment until ANC ≥1,000/mm³ **and** platelets ≥50,000/mm³; if recovery occurs within 2 weeks, resume treatment at the same dose. If ANC and platelets remain low for >2 weeks, upon recovery, resume treatment with the dose reduced by 100 mg. If cytopenia recurs, withhold until recovery and resume treatment with the dose reduced by an additional 100 mg. Doses <300 mg daily have not been evaluated.

Nonhematologic toxicity:

Diarrhea: Grade 3 or 4 (≥7 stools/day increase over baseline): Withhold treatment until recovery to ≤ grade 1; may resume at 400 mg once daily.

Other clinically significant nonhematologic toxicity, moderate or severe: Withhold treatment until resolved, then consider resuming at 400 mg once daily; may re-escalate dose to 500 mg once daily if clinically appropriate.

Dosage adjustment in renal impairment:

Preexisting impairment:

Mild impairment (CrCl >50 to 80 mL/minute): There are no dosage adjustments provided in manufacturer's labeling, however, based on the pharmacokinetics, the need for dosage adjustment is not likely.

Moderate impairment (CrCl 30 to 50 mL/minute): Initial: 400 mg once daily.

Severe impairment (CrCl <30 mL/minute): Reduce dose to 300 mg once daily (this dose is predicted to result in an AUC similar to that of patients with normal renal function, however, there is no efficacy data for this dose in CML patients with renal impairment).

Renal toxicity during treatment: If unable to tolerate initial dose, reduce dose per adjustment recommendations for toxicity (withhold treatment until resolved, then consider resuming at 400 mg once daily; if clinically appropriate may re-escalate dose to 500 mg once daily).

Hemodialysis: There are no dosage adjustments provided in the manufacturer's labeling (has not been studied).

Dosage adjustment in hepatic impairment:

Preexisting impairment (mild, moderate, or severe):

U.S. labeling: Reduce dose to 200 mg once daily (this dose is predicted to result in an AUC similar to that of patients with normal hepatic function, however, there is no efficacy data for this dose in CML patients with hepatic impairment).

Canadian labeling: Use is contraindicated in hepatic impairment.

Hepatotoxicity during treatment:

ALT or AST >5 times ULN: Withhold treatment until recovery to ≤2.5 times ULN and resume at 400 mg once daily thereafter. If recovery to ≤2.5 times ULN takes >4 weeks: Discontinue bosutinib.

ALT or AST ≥3 times ULN in conjunction with bilirubin elevation >2 times ULN and alkaline phosphatase <2 times ULN: Discontinue bosutinib.

Dietary Considerations Take with food.

Administration Oral: Administer with food. Swallow tablet whole; do not crush or break. Hazardous agent; use appropriate precautions for handling and disposal (meets NIOSH 2014 criteria).

Monitoring Parameters CBC with differential and platelets (weekly during first month, then monthly thereafter, or as clinically indicated); hepatic enzymes (monthly for first 3 months or as clinically indicated; monitor more frequently with transaminase elevations); renal function (at baseline and throughout therapy); diarrhea episodes; fluid/edema status (eg, weight gain)

Canadian labeling: Additional recommendations (not in U.S. labeling): ECG (baseline then as clinically indicated); serum electrolytes and lipase/amylase (baseline, frequently during treatment, and as clinically indicated); bone density (patients with severe osteoporosis or endocrine disease)

Dosage Forms

Tablet, Oral:

Bosulif: 100 mg, 500 mg

◆ **Bosutinib Monohydrate** *see* Bosutinib *on page 282*

◆ **Botox** *see* OnabotulinumtoxinA *on page 1512*

◆ **Botox Cosmetic** *see* OnabotulinumtoxinA *on page 1512*

◆ **Botulinum Toxin Type A** *see* AbobotulinumtoxinA *on page 28*

◆ **Botulinum Toxin Type A** *see* IncobotulinumtoxinA *on page 1062*

◆ **Botulinum Toxin Type A** *see* OnabotulinumtoxinA *on page 1512*

◆ **Botulinum Toxin Type B** *see* RimabotulinumtoxinB *on page 1813*

Botulism Immune Globulin (Intravenous-Human)

(BOT yoo lism i MYUN GLOB you lin, in tra VEE nus, YU man)

Brand Names: U.S. BabyBIG®

Index Terms BIG-IV

Pharmacologic Category Blood Product Derivative; Immune Globulin

Use Treatment of infant botulism caused by toxin type A or B

Dosage IV: Infants <1 year: Infant botulism: 50 mg/kg as a single dose as soon as diagnosis of infant botulism is made. **Note:** The recommended dose may vary with each manufactured sublot; verify dose with the prescribing information and guidance provided with each product shipment.

Dosage adjustment for toxicity: *Infusion reactions:* Slow the infusion rate or temporarily interrupt infusion for minor reaction (ie, flushing). Discontinue infusion and administer epinephrine for anaphylactic reaction or significant hypotension.

Dosage adjustment in renal impairment: Use with caution; the rate of infusion and concentration of solution should be minimized in patients with renal impairment or those at risk for renal dysfunction.

Dosage adjustment in hepatic impairment: No dosage adjustment provided in manufacturer's labeling.

Additional Information Complete prescribing information should be consulted for additional detail.

Dosage Forms

Injection, powder for reconstitution [preservative free]:
BabyBIG®: ~100 mg

◆ **Boudreaux's® Butt Paste [OTC]** *see* Zinc Oxide *on page 2200*

Bovine Lipid Extract Surfactant [CAN/INT] (BOH vine LIP id EK strakt ser FAK tunt)

Brand Names: Canada BLES

Pharmacologic Category Lung Surfactant

Use Note: Not approved in U.S.

Treatment of neonatal respiratory distress syndrome (NRDS)

Breast-Feeding Considerations Bovine lipid extract surfactant is only indicated for use in premature infants.

Contraindications Active pulmonary hemorrhage

Warnings/Precautions Restrict use to a highly-supervised clinical setting with immediate availability of clinicians experienced in intubation and ventilatory management of premature infants. For intratracheal administration only. Correct acidosis, hypoglycemia, hypothermia, or hypotension prior to administration. Marked impairment of ventilation during or shortly after dosing may indicate mucous plugs within endotracheal tube (ETT); suction patient prior to administration and monitor closely. Transient episodes of bradycardia and decreased oxygen saturation may occur. Discontinue administration; assess and treat underlying cause; may reinstitute after the patient is stable.

Hyperoxia may occur within minutes of administration; assess and adjust ventilator and oxygen delivery as necessary. Therapy may be associated with increased incidence of sepsis.

Adverse Reactions

Cardiovascular: Bradycardia, hypotension

Central nervous system: Hydrocephalus, periventricular leukomalacia, seizures

Respiratory: Apnea, endotracheal tube complications, pneumonia, pneumothorax, pulmonary function decreased (defined as decreased oxygen saturation or increased CO_2), pulmonary hemorrhage, pulmonary interstitial emphysema, respiratory acidosis

Miscellaneous: Sepsis

Rare but important or life-threatening: Acidosis, hypertension, hypoxia

Drug Interactions

Metabolism/Transport Effects None known.

Avoid Concomitant Use

Avoid concomitant use of Bovine Lipid Extract Surfactant with any of the following: Ceritinib

Increased Effect/Toxicity

Bovine Lipid Extract Surfactant may increase the levels/effects of: Bradycardia-Causing Agents; Ceritinib; Lacosamide

The levels/effects of Bovine Lipid Extract Surfactant may be increased by: Bretylium; Tofacitinib

Decreased Effect There are no known significant interactions involving a decrease in effect.

Preparation for Administration Does not require reconstitution prior to use.

Storage/Stability Store frozen at -10°C (14°F). May also be stored under refrigeration at 2°C to 8°C (36°F to 46°F) for up to 2 weeks, and then may return to freezer until packaging expiration date. Unopened vials kept at room temperature for <6 hours may be returned to freezer or refrigerator up to maximum of 2 times. Bring vial(s) to room temperature by gently rolling in hand (5-15 minutes), placing at room temperature (20-60 minutes), or in a water bath at 37°C (99°F) (2-5 minutes). Gently swirl or invert vial to suspend the lipid and disperse any agglomerates. Suspension should appear off-white to yellow and may contain an even dispersion of fine flecks of lipid. Discard vial if suspension is dark or does not disperse evenly.

Mechanism of Action Replaces deficient or ineffective endogenous lung surfactant in neonates with respiratory distress syndrome (RDS). Surfactant prevents the alveoli from collapsing during expiration by lowering surface tension between air and alveolar surfaces.

Pharmacodynamics/Kinetics Onset of action: 5-30 minutes

Dosage Intratracheal: Infants: Rescue treatment: Administer 5 mL/kg/dose (equals phospholipids 135 mg/kg/dose); may repeat if needed, to a maximum of 4 doses within the first 5 days of life

Administration For intratracheal administration only. Suction infant prior to administration. Inspect solution to verify complete mixing of the suspension (may swirl gently, but **DO NOT SHAKE**). Do not filter dose. After proper placement of ETT has been established, administer intratracheally by instillation through a #5-French feeding tube inserted into the infant's ETT.

Administer as a single bolus dose or administer dose in up to 3 aliquots as tolerated. Each dose or aliquot is instilled over 2-3 seconds followed by at least 30 seconds of manual ventilation. Avoid administering as a slow drip or in small aliquots as this may lead to poor distribution and uneven lung compliance.

Infant should be supine for the first aliquot, than turned to the left and right for subsequent aliquots. Allow 1-2 minute recovery periods after each aliquot; oxygen saturation should be ~95% before administration of next aliquot. Following administration of one full dose, withhold suctioning for 2 hours unless clinically necessary.

Monitoring Parameters Continuous ECG and transcutaneous O_2 saturation should be monitored during administration; after administration, frequent arterial blood gas sampling is necessary to prevent postdosing hyperoxia and hypocarbia; tidal volume after dosing

Product Availability Not available in U.S.

Dosage Forms: Canada

Suspension, intratracheal [preservative free]:
BLES®: Phospholipids 27 mg/mL (3 mL, 4 mL, 5 mL)

◆ **Bovine Lung Surfactant** *see* Beractant *on page 250*

◆ **Bovine Lung Surfactant** *see* Calfactant *on page 334*

◆ **BP 8 Cough [OTC]** *see* Guaifenesin, Pseudoephedrine, and Dextromethorphan *on page 989*

◆ **BP 10-1** *see* Sulfur and Sulfacetamide *on page 1953*
◆ **BP Cleansing Wash** *see* Sulfur and Sulfacetamide *on page 1953*
◆ **BProtected Pedia Iron [OTC]** *see* Ferrous Sulfate *on page 871*
◆ **BProtected Vitamin C [OTC]** *see* Ascorbic Acid *on page 178*
◆ **BRAF(V600E) Kinase Inhibitor RO5185426** *see* Vemurafenib *on page 2148*
◆ **Bravelle** *see* Urofollitropin *on page 2116*
◆ **Brentuximab** *see* Brentuximab Vedotin *on page 286*

Brentuximab Vedotin (bren TUX i mab ve DOE tin)

Brand Names: U.S. Adcetris
Brand Names: Canada Adcetris
Index Terms Anti-CD30 ADC SGN-35; Anti-CD30 Antibody-Drug Conjugate SGN-35; Antibody-Drug Conjugate SGN-35; Brentuximab; SGN-35
Pharmacologic Category Antineoplastic Agent, Anti-CD30; Antineoplastic Agent, Antibody Drug Conjugate; Antineoplastic Agent, Monoclonal Antibody
Use
Hodgkin lymphoma: Treatment of Hodgkin lymphoma after failure of at least 2 prior chemotherapy regimens (in patients ineligible for transplant) or after autologous stem cell transplant failure.
Anaplastic large cell lymphoma: Treatment of systemic anaplastic large cell lymphoma (sALCL) after failure of at least 1 prior chemotherapy regimen.
Pregnancy Risk Factor D
Pregnancy Considerations Adverse events were observed in animal reproduction studies. Based on the mechanism of action, may cause fetal harm if administered to a pregnant woman.
Breast-Feeding Considerations It is not known if brentuximab vedotin is excreted in breast milk. According to the manufacturer, the decision to continue or discontinue breast-feeding during therapy should take into account the risk of exposure to the infant and the benefits of treatment to the mother.
Contraindications U.S. labeling: Concurrent use with bleomycin

Canadian labeling: Hypersensitivity to brentuximab or any component of the formulation; concurrent use with bleomycin; patients who have or have history of progressive multifocal leukoencephalopathy
Warnings/Precautions Hazardous agent - use appropriate precautions for handling and disposal (NIOSH 2014 [group 1]).

[U.S. Boxed Warning]: Cases of progressive multifocal leukoencephalopathy (PML) and death due to JC virus infection have been reported. Immunosuppression due to prior chemotherapy treatments or underlying disease may also contribute to PML development. New-onset signs/symptoms of central nervous system abnormalities (eg, changes in mood, memory, cognition, motor incoordination and/or weakness, speech and/or visual disturbances) should receive prompt evaluation with neurology consultation, brain MRI, and lumbar puncture or brain biopsy. Withhold treatment with new-onset symptoms suggestive of PML; discontinue if diagnosis of PML is confirmed.

Peripheral neuropathy is common and is generally cumulative; usually sensory neuropathy, although motor neuropathy has also been observed; neuropathy completely resolved in nearly half of patients; almost one-third had partial improvement. Monitor for symptoms of neuropathy (hypoesthesia, hyperesthesia, paresthesia, discomfort, burning sensation, neuropathic pain, or weakness); dose interruption, reduction or discontinuation may be recommended for new or worsening neuropathy.

Grade 3 or 4 neutropenia, thrombocytopenia, and anemia may occur; neutropenia may be severe and/or prolonged (≥1 week); neutropenic fever also has been reported; monitor blood counts prior to each dose and consider more frequent monitoring for patients with Grade 3 or 4 neutropenia; may require growth factor support, dose interruption, reduction or discontinuation. Serious infections, including opportunistic infections (eg, pneumonia, bacteremia, sepsis/septic shock) have been reported (some fatal); monitor for signs or symptoms of bacterial, fungal, or viral infections. Infusion reactions, including anaphylaxis have been reported; monitor during infusion. For anaphylaxis, immediately and permanently discontinue and administer appropriate medical intervention. For infusion-related reaction, interrupt infusion and administer appropriate medical intervention; premedicate for subsequent infusions (with acetaminophen, an antihistamine, and/or a corticosteroid).

Potentially significant drug-drug interactions may exist, requiring dose or frequency adjustment, additional monitoring, and/or selection of alternative therapy. Due to the risk for pulmonary injury, concurrent use with bleomycin is contraindicated. In a study comparing brentuximab combined with ABVD (doxorubicin, bleomycin, vinblastine, and dacarbazine) to brentuximab combined with AVD (doxorubicin, vinblastine, and dacarbazine), the occurrence of pulmonary toxicity was 40% in the brentuximab/ABVD group compared to a literature-based frequency of ≤25% for other bleomycin-containing regimens. There were no cases of pulmonary toxicity documented with brentuximab in combination with AVD. Pulmonary symptoms/toxicities reported with brentuximab in combination with ABVD consisted of cough, dyspnea, and interstitial infiltration/inflammation; most patients responded to corticosteroids.

Serious hepatotoxicity, including fatalities, has occurred; cases were consistent with hepatocellular injury, with elevations of transaminases and/or bilirubin. Some have occurred after the initial dose or after rechallenge. The risk for hepatotoxicity may be increased with preexisting liver disease, elevated baseline liver enzymes, and concurrent medications. Monitor liver enzymes and bilirubin. Treatment delay, dose reduction or discontinuation may be required for new, worsening, or recurrent hepatotoxicity. Avoid use in patients with moderate to severe hepatic impairment (Child-Pugh classes B and C). The frequency of grade 3/4 toxicities (and deaths) was increased in patients with severe impairment (compared to patients with normal hepatic function). A component of brentuximab vedotin, the microtubule-disrupting agent monomethylauristatin E (MMAE) is excreted hepatically. MMAE exposure is increased ~2.2-fold in patients with hepatic impairment.

Avoid use in patients with severe renal impairment (CrCl <30 mL/minute). The frequency of grade 3/4 toxicities (and deaths) was increased in patients with severe impairment (compared to patients with normal renal function). A component of brentuximab vedotin, the microtubule-disrupting agent MMAE is excreted renally; MMAE exposure is increased in patients with severe impairment. Stevens-Johnson syndrome (SJS) and toxic epidermal necrolysis (TEN) have been reported (some fatal). Discontinue (and begin appropriate management) if SJS or TEN occur. Tumor lysis syndrome (TLS) may occur; risk of TLS is higher in patients with a high tumor burden or with rapid tumor proliferation; monitor closely.
Adverse Reactions
Cardiovascular: Peripheral edema, pulmonary embolism, septic shock, supraventricular cardiac arrhythmia

Central nervous system: Anxiety, chills, dizziness, fatigue, headache, insomnia, pain, peripheral motor neuropathy, peripheral sensory neuropathy
Dermatologic: Alopecia, night sweats, pruritus, skin rash, xeroderma
Endocrine & metabolic: Weight loss
Gastrointestinal: Abdominal pain, constipation, decreased appetite, diarrhea, nausea, vomiting
Genitourinary: Urinary tract infection
Hematologic & oncologic: Anemia, lymphadenopathy, neutropenia, thrombocytopenia
Immunologic: Antibody development (antibrentuximab)
Neuromuscular & skeletal: Arthralgia, back pain, limb pain, muscle spasm, myalgia
Renal: Pyelonephritis
Respiratory: Cough, dyspnea, oropharyngeal pain, pneumonitis, pneumothorax, upper respiratory tract infection
Miscellaneous: Fever, infusion related reaction (grades 1/2)
Rare but important or life-threatening: Anaphylaxis, febrile neutropenia, hepatotoxicity, hyperglycemia, infection (including pneumonia, bacteremia, sepsis), pancreatitis, progressive multifocal leukoencephalopathy, Stevens-Johnson syndrome, tumor lysis syndrome

Drug Interactions

Metabolism/Transport Effects **Substrate** of CYP3A4 (minor), P-glycoprotein; **Note:** Assignment of Major/Minor substrate status based on clinically relevant drug interaction potential

Avoid Concomitant Use

Avoid concomitant use of Brentuximab Vedotin with any of the following: BCG; Belimumab; Bleomycin; Natalizumab; Pimecrolimus; Tacrolimus (Topical); Tofacitinib; Vaccines (Live)

Increased Effect/Toxicity

Brentuximab Vedotin may increase the levels/effects of: Belimumab; Bleomycin; Leflunomide; Natalizumab; Tofacitinib; Vaccines (Live)

The levels/effects of Brentuximab Vedotin may be increased by: CYP3A4 Inhibitors (Strong); Denosumab; P-glycoprotein/ABCB1 Inhibitors; Pimecrolimus; Roflumilast; Tacrolimus (Topical); Trastuzumab

Decreased Effect

Brentuximab Vedotin may decrease the levels/effects of: BCG; Coccidioides immitis Skin Test; Sipuleucel-T; Vaccines (Inactivated); Vaccines (Live)

The levels/effects of Brentuximab Vedotin may be decreased by: CYP3A4 Inducers (Strong); Echinacea; P-glycoprotein/ABCB1 Inducers

Preparation for Administration Hazardous agent: Use appropriate precautions for handling and disposal (NIOSH 2014 [group 1]). Reconstitute each 50 mg vial with 10.5 mL sterile water for injection (SWFI), resulting in a concentration of 5 mg/mL. Direct SWFI toward the vial wall; do not direct toward the cake or powder. Swirl gently to dissolve, do not shake. Reconstituted solution should be clear to slightly opalescent without visible particles. Further dilute in at least 100 mL of either NS, D_5W, or lactated Ringer's to a final concentration of 0.4 to 1.8 mg/mL; gently invert bag to mix. Do not mix with other medications. Use within 24 hours of initial reconstitution.

Storage/Stability Store intact vials refrigerated at 2°C to 8°C (36°F to 46°F) in the original carton. Protect from light. Reconstituted solution should be diluted immediately; however, may be stored refrigerated for up to 24 hours; do not freeze. Solutions diluted for infusion should be used immediately after preparation; however, may be stored for 24 hours refrigerated (do not freeze); use within 24 hours of initial reconstitution.

Mechanism of Action Brentuximab vedotin is an antibody drug conjugate (ADC) directed at CD30 consisting of 3 components: 1) a CD30-specific chimeric IgG1 antibody cAC10; 2) a microtubule-disrupting agent, monomethylauristatin E (MMAE); and 3) a protease cleavable dipeptide linker (which covalently conjugates MMAE to cAC10). The conjugate binds to cells which express CD30, and forms a complex which is internalized within the cell and releases MMAE. MMAE binds to the tubules and disrupts the cellular microtubule network, inducing cell cycle arrest (G2/M phase) and apoptosis.

Pharmacodynamics/Kinetics

Distribution: V_{dss}: ADC: 6 to 10 L
Metabolism: MMAE: Minimal, primarily via oxidation by CYP3A4/5
Half-life elimination: Terminal: ADC: ~4 to 6 days
Time to peak: ADC: At end of infusion; MMAE: ~1 to 3 days
Excretion: MMAE: Feces (~72%, primarily unchanged); urine

Dosage

Hodgkin lymphoma, refractory: Adults: IV: 1.8 mg/kg (maximum dose: 180 mg) every 3 weeks, continue until disease progression or unacceptable toxicities
Systemic anaplastic large cell lymphoma (sALCL), refractory: Adults: IV: 1.8 mg/kg (maximum dose: 180 mg) every 3 weeks, continue until disease progression or unacceptable toxicities

Dosage adjustment for toxicity:

Hematologic toxicity:

Grade 3 or 4 neutropenia: Withhold treatment until resolves to baseline or ≤ grade 2, consider growth factor support in subsequent cycles.
Recurrent grade 4 neutropenia (despite the use of growth factor support): Consider reducing the dose to 1.2 mg/kg or discontinuing treatment
Grade 3 or 4 thrombocytopenia (Canadian labeling): Monitor closely; dose delays or platelet transfusions may be considered.

Nonhematologic toxicities:

Anaphylaxis: Discontinue immediately and permanently
Infusion reaction: Interrupt infusion and administer appropriate medical intervention. Premedicate subsequent infusions with acetaminophen, an antihistamine, and/or a corticosteroid.
Peripheral neuropathy, new or worsening grade 2 or 3: Withhold treatment until improves or returns to grade 1 or baseline; then resume with dose reduced to 1.2 mg/kg
Peripheral neuropathy, grade 4: Discontinue treatment
Progressive multifocal leukoencephalopathy (PML): Withhold treatment with new-onset symptoms suggestive of PML; discontinue if PML diagnosis confirmed
Stevens-Johnson syndrome or toxic epidermal necrolysis: Discontinue and administer appropriate medical intervention

Dosage adjustment in renal impairment:

CrCl ≥30 mL/minute: Initial: No dosage adjustment necessary.
CrCl <30 mL/minute: Initial: Avoid use.

Dosage adjustment in hepatic impairment:

Mild impairment (Child-Pugh class A): Initial: 1.2 mg/kg (maximum dose: 120 mg) every 3 weeks.
Moderate to severe impairment (Child-Pugh class B or C): Avoid use.

Administration Infuse over 30 minutes. Do not administer as IV push or bolus; do not mix or infuse with other medications. Hazardous agent; use appropriate precautions for handling and disposal (NIOSH 2014 [group 1]).

Monitoring Parameters CBC with differential prior to each dose (more frequently if clinically indicated); liver and renal function tests. Monitor for infusion reaction, tumor lysis syndrome, signs/symptoms of progressive multifocal leukoencephalopathy (PML), and for signs of neuropathy (hypoesthesia, hyperesthesia, paresthesia, discomfort, burning sensation, or neuropathic pain or weakness), dermatologic toxicity, or infection.

Dosage Forms

Solution Reconstituted, Intravenous [preservative free]:
Adcetris: 50 mg (1 ea)

◆ **Breo Ellipta** *see* Fluticasone and Vilanterol *on page 914*

◆ **Brethaire** *see* Terbutaline *on page 2004*

◆ **Brethine** *see* Terbutaline *on page 2004*

◆ **Brevibloc** *see* Esmolol *on page 769*

◆ **Brevibloc in NaCl** *see* Esmolol *on page 769*

◆ **Brevibloc Premixed (Can)** *see* Esmolol *on page 769*

◆ **Brevicon** *see* Ethinyl Estradiol and Norethindrone *on page 808*

◆ **Brevicon 0.5/35 (Can)** *see* Ethinyl Estradiol and Norethindrone *on page 808*

◆ **Brevicon 1/35 (Can)** *see* Ethinyl Estradiol and Norethindrone *on page 808*

◆ **Brevital (Can)** *see* Methohexital *on page 1321*

◆ **Brevital Sodium** *see* Methohexital *on page 1321*

◆ **Bricanyl** *see* Terbutaline *on page 2004*

◆ **Bricanyl® Turbuhaler® (Can)** *see* Terbutaline *on page 2004*

◆ **Briellyn** *see* Ethinyl Estradiol and Norethindrone *on page 808*

◆ **Brilinta** *see* Ticagrelor *on page 2035*

Brimonidine (Ophthalmic) (bri MOE ni deen)

Brand Names: U.S. Alphagan P

Brand Names: Canada Alphagan; Apo-Brimonidine; Apo-Brimonidine P; PMS-Brimonidine Tartrate; ratio-Brimonidine; Sandoz-Brimonidine

Index Terms Brimonidine Tartrate

Pharmacologic Category Alpha$_2$ Agonist, Ophthalmic; Ophthalmic Agent, Antiglaucoma

Use Lowering of intraocular pressure (IOP) in patients with open-angle glaucoma or ocular hypertension

Pregnancy Risk Factor B

Dosage Ophthalmic: Children ≥2 years and Adults: Glaucoma, ocular hypertension: Instill 1 drop in affected eye(s) 3 times/day (approximately every 8 hours)

Additional Information Complete prescribing information should be consulted for additional detail.

Dosage Forms

Solution, Ophthalmic:
Alphagan P: 0.1% (5 mL, 10 mL, 15 mL); 0.15% (5 mL, 10 mL, 15 mL)
Generic: 0.15% (5 mL, 10 mL, 15 mL); 0.2% (5 mL, 10 mL, 15 mL)

Brimonidine (Topical) (bri MOE ni deen)

Brand Names: U.S. Mirvaso

Index Terms Brimonidine Tartrate

Pharmacologic Category Alpha$_2$-Adrenergic Agonist

Use Rosacea: Topical treatment of persistent (nontransient) facial erythema of rosacea in adults

Pregnancy Risk Factor B

Dosage Rosacea: Adults: Topical: Apply a pea-size amount once daily as a thin layer across the entire face covering the central forehead, each cheek, nose, and chin. Do not apply to eyes or lips.

Additional Information Complete prescribing information should be consulted for additional detail.

Dosage Forms

Gel, External:
Mirvaso: 0.33% (30 g)

Brimonidine and Timolol
(bri MOE ni deen & TIM oh lol)

Brand Names: U.S. Combigan

Brand Names: Canada Combigan

Index Terms Brimonidine Tartrate and Timolol Maleate; Timolol and Brimonidine

Pharmacologic Category Alpha$_2$ Agonist, Ophthalmic; Beta-Blocker, Nonselective; Ophthalmic Agent, Antiglaucoma

Use Reduction of intraocular pressure (IOP) in patients with glaucoma or ocular hypertension

Pregnancy Risk Factor C

Dosage Ophthalmic: Children ≥2 years and Adults: Instill 1 drop into affected eye(s) twice daily

Note: In the Canadian labeling, use in children (at any age) is not recommended

Additional Information Complete prescribing information should be consulted for additional detail.

Dosage Forms

Solution, ophthalmic [drops]:
Combigan: Brimonidine 0.2% and timolol 0.5% (5 mL,10 mL)

Dosage Forms: Canada

Solution, ophthalmic [drops]:
Combigan: Brimonidine 0.2% and timolol 0.5% (2.5 mL, 5 mL,10 mL)

◆ **Brimonidine Tartrate** *see* Brimonidine (Ophthalmic) *on page 288*

◆ **Brimonidine Tartrate** *see* Brimonidine (Topical) *on page 288*

◆ **Brimonidine Tartrate and Timolol Maleate** *see* Brimonidine and Timolol *on page 288*

◆ **Brintellix** *see* Vortioxetine *on page 2183*

Brinzolamide (brin ZOH la mide)

Brand Names: U.S. Azopt

Brand Names: Canada Azopt®

Pharmacologic Category Carbonic Anhydrase Inhibitor (Ophthalmic); Ophthalmic Agent, Antiglaucoma

Use Treatment of elevated intraocular pressure in patients with ocular hypertension or open-angle glaucoma

Pregnancy Risk Factor C

Dosage Ophthalmic: Adults: Ocular hypertension or open-angle glaucoma: Instill 1 drop in affected eye(s) 3 times/day

Dosage adjustment in renal impairment: Severe renal impairment (CrCl <30 mL/minute): Use is not recommended (has not been studied; brinzolamide and metabolite are excreted predominately by the kidney).

Dosage adjustment in hepatic impairment: No dosage adjustment provided in manufacturer's labeling.

Additional Information Complete prescribing information should be consulted for additional detail.

Dosage Forms

Suspension, Ophthalmic:
Azopt: 1% (10 mL, 15 mL)

Brinzolamide and Timolol [CAN/INT]

(brin ZOH la mide & TIM oh lol)

Brand Names: Canada Azarga™

Index Terms Brinzolamide and Timolol Maleate; Timolol Maleate and Brinzolamide

Pharmacologic Category Beta-Blocker, Nonselective; Carbonic Anhydrase Inhibitor (Ophthalmic); Ophthalmic Agent, Antiglaucoma

Use Note: Not approved in U.S.

Treatment of elevated intraocular pressure in patients with ocular hypertension or open-angle glaucoma

Pregnancy Considerations There are no adequate and well-controlled studies in pregnant women with the combination product. Use only if benefit outweighs risk. Bradycardia and arrhythmia have been reported in an infant following ophthalmic administration of timolol during pregnancy. See individual agents.

Breast-Feeding Considerations Timolol is excreted in breast milk following oral and ophthalmic administration, though clinical beta blockade is not likely at recommended ophthalmologic doses. It is unknown whether brinzolamide is excreted in breast milk. Use of the combination product during lactation is not recommended.

Contraindications Hypersensitivity to brinzolamide, timolol, other beta-blockers, sulfonamides, or any component of the formulation; current or history of bronchial asthma; severe chronic obstructive pulmonary disease (COPD); severe allergic rhinitis and bronchial hyper-reactivity; sinus bradycardia, second-/third degree atrioventricular (AV) block, overt cardiac failure, cardiogenic shock; hyperchloremic acidosis; severe renal impairment

Warnings/Precautions See individual agents.

Adverse Reactions Also see individual agents.

Gastrointestinal: Taste perversion

Ocular: Blurred vision, eye irritation, eye pain, foreign body sensation in eyes

Rare but important or life-threatening: Abnormal eye sensation, anterior chamber flare, asthenopia, blepharitis, blepharitis allergic, conjunctival hyperemia, conjunctivitis allergic, COPD, corneal disorder, corneal erosion, cough, eye discharge, eye pruritus, eyelid erythema, eyelid margin crusting, eyelid pruritus, hypotension, insomnia, lacrimation increased, lichen planus, ocular hyperemia, pharyngolaryngeal pain, photophobia, punctuate keratitis, rhinorrhea, scleral hyperemia, xerophthalmia

Drug Interactions

Metabolism/Transport Effects Refer to individual components.

Avoid Concomitant Use

Avoid concomitant use of Brinzolamide and Timolol with any of the following: Beta2-Agonists; Carbonic Anhydrase Inhibitors; Ceritinib; Floctafenine; Methacholine

Increased Effect/Toxicity

Brinzolamide and Timolol may increase the levels/effects of: Alpha-/Beta-Agonists (Direct-Acting); Alpha-/Beta-Agonists (Indirect-Acting); Alpha1-Blockers; Alpha2-Agonists; Antipsychotic Agents (Phenothiazines); ARIPiprazole; Bradycardia-Causing Agents; Bupivacaine; Carbonic Anhydrase Inhibitors; Cardiac Glycosides; Ceritinib; Cholinergic Agonists; Disopyramide; DULoxetine; Ergot Derivatives; Fingolimod; Grass Pollen Allergen Extract (5 Grass Extract); Hypotensive Agents; Insulin; Lacosamide; Levodopa; Lidocaine (Systemic); Lidocaine (Topical); Mepivacaine; Methacholine; Midodrine; RisperiDONE; Sulfonylureas

The levels/effects of Brinzolamide and Timolol may be increased by: Abiraterone Acetate; Acetylcholinesterase Inhibitors; Alpha2-Agonists; Aminoquinolines (Antimalarial); Amiodarone; Anilidopiperidine Opioids; Antipsychotic Agents (Phenothiazines); Barbiturates; Bretylium; Calcium Channel Blockers (Dihydropyridine); Calcium Channel Blockers (Nondihydropyridine); Cobicistat; CYP2D6 Inhibitors (Moderate); CYP2D6 Inhibitors (Strong); CYP3A4 Inhibitors (Strong); Darunavir; Dipyridamole; Disopyramide; Dronedarone; Floctafenine; MAO Inhibitors; Nicorandil; Peginterferon Alfa-2b; Propafenone; Regorafenib; Reserpine; Selective Serotonin Reuptake Inhibitors; Tofacitinib

Decreased Effect

Brinzolamide and Timolol may decrease the levels/effects of: Beta2-Agonists; Theophylline Derivatives

The levels/effects of Brinzolamide and Timolol may be decreased by: Barbiturates; Nonsteroidal Anti-Inflammatory Agents; Peginterferon Alfa-2b; Rifamycin Derivatives

Storage/Stability Store at 2°C to 30°C (36°F to 86°F). Discard 60 days after opening.

Mechanism of Action

Brinzolamide inhibits carbonic anhydrase, leading to decreased aqueous humor secretion. This results in a reduction of intraocular pressure.

Timolol: Blocks both $beta_1$- and $beta_2$-adrenergic receptors, reduces intraocular pressure by reducing aqueous humor production or possibly outflow.

Pharmacodynamics/Kinetics See individual agents.

Dosage Ophthalmic: Adults: Instill 1 drop in affected eye(s) twice daily

Administration If using additional topical ophthalmic preparations, separate administration by at least 5 minutes. Remove contact lens prior to administration and wait 15 minutes before reinserting. Shake bottle well prior to administration. Gently close eyelid after instillation. Instruct patients to avoid allowing the tip of the dispensing container to contact the eye or surrounding structures. Ocular solutions can become contaminated by common bacteria known to cause ocular infections. Serious damage to the eye and subsequent loss of vision may occur from using contaminated solutions. If changing from another ophthalmic antiglaucoma agent, discontinue use of first agent and initiate brinzolamide/timolol the following day.

Monitoring Parameters Ophthalmic exams and IOP periodically; heart rate/signs of cardiac failure (patients with severe cardiac disease)

Product Availability Not available in U.S.

Dosage Forms: Canada

Solution, ophthalmic [drops]:

Azarga™: Brinzolamide 1% and timolol maleate 0.5% (5 mL)

◆ **Brinzolamide and Timolol Maleate** *see* Brinzolamide and Timolol [CAN/INT] *on page 289*

◆ **Brisdelle** *see* PARoxetine *on page 1579*

◆ **British Anti-Lewisite** *see* Dimercaprol *on page 638*

Brivudine [INT] (BRI vu deen)

International Brand Names Bridic (PT); Brival (RO); Brivex (CH); Brivir (BG, GR); Brivirac (IT); Brivox (CR, DO, GT, HN, NI, PA, SV); Brivozost (HR); Brivumen (EE); Helpin (CZ, DE); Mevir (AT); Nervinex (ES); Zecovir (IT); Zerpex (BE); Zostevir (CZ); Zostex (CN, DE, TR); Zostydol (AR)

Pharmacologic Category Antiviral Agent

Reported Use Treatment of herpes zoster and herpes simplex

Dosage Range Adults: Oral: 125 mg daily

Product Availability Product available in various countries; not currently available in the U.S.

Dosage Forms

Tablet: 125 mg

◆ **BRL 43694** *see* Granisetron *on page 983*

Bromazepam [CAN/INT] (broe MA ze pam)

Brand Names: Canada Apo-Bromazepam®; Lectopam®; Mylan-Bromazepam; Novo-Bromazepam; Nu-Bromazepam; PRO-Doc Limitee Bromazepam

Pharmacologic Category Benzodiazepine

Use Note: Not approved in U.S.

Short-term, symptomatic treatment of anxiety

Pregnancy Considerations Adverse events were observed in animal reproduction studies. Benzodiazepines have the potential to cause harm to the fetus. An increased risk of fetal malformations may be associated with first trimester exposure (malformations of the heart, cleft lip/palate). Maternal use later in pregnancy may be associated with adverse events in the fetus (irregular heart beat) and neonate (hypothermia, hypotonia, respiratory depression, poor feeding, withdrawal).

Breast-Feeding Considerations Bromazepam and metabolites are expected to be found in breast milk, therefore, use while breast-feeding is not recommended by the manufacturer. Drowsiness, lethargy, or weight loss in nursing infants have been observed in case reports following maternal use of some benzodiazepines (Iqbal, 2002).

Contraindications Hypersensitivity to bromazepam or any component of the formulation (cross-sensitivity with other benzodiazepines may exist); myasthenia gravis; narrow-angle glaucoma; severe hepatic or respiratory disease; sleep apnea

Warnings/Precautions Benzodiazepines have been associated with anterograde amnesia; paradoxical reactions, including hyperactive or aggressive behavior, have also been reported. Tolerance, psychological and physical dependence may occur with prolonged use. Use with caution in patients with a history of drug abuse or acute alcoholism; potential for drug dependency exists. May cause CNS depression, which may impair physical or mental abilities; effects may be potentiated by other CNS depressants, psychoactive medication, or ethanol. Patients must be cautioned about performing tasks which require mental alertness (eg, operating machinery or driving). Use is not recommended in patients with depressive disorders or psychosis. May cause respiratory depression; use with caution particularly in patients with preexisting or chronic respiratory disease and concomitantly with other respiratory depressive agents. Use is contraindicated with severe disease. Use with extreme caution in patients who are at risk of falls (elderly); benzodiazepines have been associated with falls and traumatic injury. Use with caution in debilitated patients, patients with an impaired gag reflex, patients with hepatic or renal impairment.

Bromazepam does not have analgesic, antidepressant, or antipsychotic properties. Rebound or withdrawal symptoms may occur following abrupt discontinuation or large decreases in dose. Use caution when reducing dose or withdrawing therapy; decrease slowly and monitor for withdrawal symptoms. Flumazenil may cause withdrawal in patients receiving long-term benzodiazepine therapy.

May contain lactose; do not use with galactose intolerance, Lapp lactase deficiency, or glucose-galactose malabsorption syndromes.

Adverse Reactions

Cardiovascular: Cardiac arrest, hypotension, palpitation, tachycardia

Central nervous system: Anterograde amnesia, ataxia, confusion, depression, dizziness, drowsiness, euphoria, headache, lethargy, physical and psychological dependence, seizure. In addition, paradoxical reactions (including aggression, agitation, excitation, hallucinations, nightmares, release of hostility, restlessness, and psychosis) are known to occur with benzodiazepines.

Dermatologic: Pruritus, rash

Endocrine & metabolic: Hyperglycemia, hypoglycemia, libido changes

Gastrointestinal: Gastritis (rare), nausea, vomiting, xerostomia

Genitourinary: Incontinence

Hematologic: Hemoglobin decreased, hematocrit decreased, WBCs increased/decreased

Hepatic: Transaminases increased, alkaline phosphatase increased, bilirubin increased

Neuromuscular & skeletal: Weakness, muscle spasm

Ocular: Blurred vision, diplopia

Respiratory: Respiratory depression

Miscellaneous: Allergic reactions including anaphylaxis have been reported with benzodiazepines

Drug Interactions

Metabolism/Transport Effects **Substrate** of CYP1A2 (major), CYP3A4 (minor); **Note:** Assignment of Major/Minor substrate status based on clinically relevant drug interaction potential; **Inhibits** CYP2E1 (weak)

Avoid Concomitant Use

Avoid concomitant use of Bromazepam with any of the following: Azelastine (Nasal); Methadone; OLANZapine; Orphenadrine; Paraldehyde; Sodium Oxybate; Thalidomide

Increased Effect/Toxicity

Bromazepam may increase the levels/effects of: Alcohol (Ethyl); Azelastine (Nasal); Buprenorphine; CloZAPine; CNS Depressants; Fosphenytoin; Hydrocodone; Methadone; Methotrimeprazine; Metyrosine; Mirtazapine; Orphenadrine; Paraldehyde; Phenytoin; Pramipexole; ROPINIRole; Rotigotine; Selective Serotonin Reuptake Inhibitors; Sodium Oxybate; Suvorexant; Thalidomide; Zolpidem

The levels/effects of Bromazepam may be increased by: Abiraterone Acetate; Brimonidine (Topical); Cannabis; Cimetidine; CYP1A2 Inhibitors (Moderate); CYP1A2 Inhibitors (Strong); Deferasirox; Doxylamine; Dronabinol; Droperidol; FluvoxaMINE; HydrOXYzine; Kava Kava; Magnesium Sulfate; Methotrimeprazine; Nabilone; OLANZapine; Peginterferon Alfa-2b; Perampanel; Rufinamide; Tapentadol; Teduglutide; Tetrahydrocannabinol; Vemurafenib

Decreased Effect

The levels/effects of Bromazepam may be decreased by: Theophylline Derivatives; Yohimbine

Food Interactions Food may decrease systemic exposure and delay onset of clinical effects. Serum concentration may be increased by grapefruit juice. Management: Administer without regard to meals. Avoid grapefruit juice.

Storage/Stability Store at room temperature of 15°C to 30°C (59°F to 86°F).

Mechanism of Action Binds to stereospecific benzodiazepine receptors on the postsynaptic GABA neuron at several sites within the central nervous system, including the limbic system, reticular formation. Enhancement of the inhibitory effect of GABA on neuronal excitability results by increased neuronal membrane permeability to chloride ions. This shift in chloride ions results in hyperpolarization (a less excitable state) and stabilization. Benzodiazepine receptors and effects appear to be linked to the GABA-A receptors. Benzodiazepines do not bind to GABA-B receptors.

Pharmacodynamics/Kinetics

Protein binding: 70%

Metabolism: Hepatic

Bioavailability: 60%

Half-life elimination: 20 hours

Time to peak, serum: ≤2 hours (may be delayed by food)

Excretion: Urine (69%), as metabolites

Dosage Oral:

Adults: Initial: 6-18 mg/day in equally divided doses; initial course of treatment should not last longer than 1 week; optimal dosage range: 6-30 mg/day

Elderly/debilitated: Initial dose: 3 mg/day in divided doses; may adjust dose cautiously based on response and tolerance

Dosage adjustment in renal impairment: No dosage adjustment provided in manufacturer's labeling; initiate therapy conservatively, titrate cautiously.

Dosage adjustment in hepatic impairment: Mild to moderate impairment: Initiate therapy conservatively; titrate cautiously. Severe impairment: Use contraindicated.

Dietary Considerations May be taken with or without food. Avoid grapefruit juice.

Administration May be administered with or without food. Serum concentration may be decreased by food.

Monitoring Parameters Respiratory, cardiovascular, and mental status; periodic CBC and liver function tests

Product Availability Not available in U.S.

Dosage Forms: Canada

Tablet: 1.5 mg, 3 mg, 6 mg

Lectopam®: 3 mg, 6 mg

◆ **Bromday [DSC]** *see* Bromfenac *on page* 291

Bromfenac (BROME fen ak)

Brand Names: U.S. Bromday [DSC]; Prolensa

Index Terms Bromfenac Sodium

Pharmacologic Category Nonsteroidal Anti-inflammatory Drug (NSAID), Ophthalmic

Use Treatment of postoperative inflammation and reduction in ocular pain following cataract removal

Pregnancy Risk Factor C

Dosage Ophthalmic (0.07%, 0.09%): Adults: Instill 1 drop into affected eye(s) once daily beginning 1 day prior to surgery and continuing on the day of surgery and for 2 weeks postoperatively

Dosage adjustment in renal impairment: There are no dosage adjustments provided in the manufacturer's labeling. However, dosage adjustment unlikely due to low systemic absorption.

Dosage adjustment in hepatic impairment: There are no dosage adjustments provided in the manufacturer's labeling. However, dosage adjustment unlikely due to low systemic absorption.

Additional Information Complete prescribing information should be consulted for additional detail.

Dosage Forms

Solution, Ophthalmic:

Prolensa: 0.07% (3 mL)

Generic: 0.09% (1.7 mL, 2.5 mL, 5 mL)

◆ **Bromfenac Sodium** *see* Bromfenac *on page* 291

Bromhexine [INT] (brom HEKS een)

International Brand Names Amiorel (AR); An Bu (CN); Aparsonin (DE); Asthamxine (SG); Axel Bromhexine (SG); Basiflux (PT); Bexedan (UY); Bi Li (CN); Bislan (MY, SG); Bisofan (HK); Bisolex (HR); Bisolvex (PH); Bisolvon (AE, AR, AT, AU, BE, BH, BR, CH, CL, CO, CY, CZ, DE, DK, EG, ES, FI, FR, GR, HN, HR, ID, IE, IN, IT, JO, KR, KW, LB, LU, MX, NL, NO, NZ, PE, PH, PK, PT, PY, QA, SA, SE, SI, TH, UY, VE, VN); Bisolvon Chesty (AU); Bisolvon[vet.] (CH); Bisuran (BR); Bontoss (BR); Brom (HK); Bromex (BE, IN, LU, TH); Bromexidryl (AR); Bromexin (PY); Bromexina-ratiopharm (PT); Bromfluex (RO); Bromhex (SE); Bromhexin (DE, DK); Bromhexin ACO (SE); Bromhexin BC (DE); Bromhexin Berlin-Chemie (DE); Bromhexin Eu Rho (DE); Bromhexin Funcke (DE); Bromhexin Losung Funcke (DE); bromhexin von ct (DE, LU); Bromhexin "Dak" (DK); Bromhexin-ratiopharm (DE); Bromhexina Austral (AR); Bromhexina Lafedar (AR); Bromhexina Sintesina (AR); Bromhexina Vannier (AR); Bromhexine EG (BE); Bromhexine-Eurogenerics (LU); Bromhexine-ratiopharm (BE); Bromicof (MX); Bromika (ID); Bromox (VE); Bromxine (GR, HN, SG); Bronair (EC); Bronchosan (SK); Broncocalmine (AR); Broncokin (IT); Bronkese (ZA); Bronquisedan Elixir (AR); Brontol (CO); Bropavol (CL); Brotussol (DE); Catarrosine (AR); Darolan (NL); Dexolut (ID); Disol (HK); Dur-Elix (AU); Extovon (TH); Ezipect (SA); Ezolvin (SA); Famel Broomhexine (NL); Flecoxin (CY); Flegamina (CZ, PL); Flubron[vet.] (FR); Flumed (CL); Fulpen A (JP); Hosolvon (SG); Hostlos (DK); Hustentabs-ratiopharm (DE, LU); Hustosol (CH); Icubron (UY); Lisomucin (PT); Lorbi (AR); Lubrirhin (DE); Lupotus (HR); Medex (AR); Medipekt (FI); Metasolvens (CH); Movex (IL); Muco-Sol (KR); Mucofree (SA); Mucolan (AE); Mucoless (IL); Mucolex (MY); Mucolix (HN, SG); Mucolyte (SA); Mucosol (SG); Mucotrop (CO); Mucovin (FI); Namir (AR); Neosolvon (AE); No-Tos (AR); Omniapharm (DE); Paxirasol (CZ, HU); Pulmitropic (SA); Pulmo-Rest (ID); Quentan [vet.] (FR); Reosil (VE); Riaxine (AE, SA); Romilar rood (NL); Silbron (AR); Solubron (PE); Solvex (IL, QA, SA); Solvexin (JO, KW); Solvinex (ID); Solvolin (CH); SP-Mucosov (SG); Tesacof (MX); Tosseque (PT); Tossimex (CH); Tostop (AR, PY); Tussine (JO); Vasican (HN, SG); Viscolyt (DK)

Index Terms Bromhexine Hydrochloride

Pharmacologic Category Mucolytic Agent

Reported Use Acute and chronic bronchopulmonary diseases associated with abnormal mucous secretion and impaired mucous transport

Dosage Range

Oral:

Children 2 to <6 years: 8 mg daily in 2-3 divided doses

Children 6 to <12 years: 4-8 mg 3 times daily (maximum: 8 mg 3 times daily)

Children ≥12 years, Adolescents, and Adults: 8 mg 3 times daily (maximum: 48 mg daily in 3-4 divided doses)

Inhalation: Solution for nebulization (2 mg/mL):

Children 2 to <6 years: 1.3 mg (10 drops) twice daily

Children 6 to <12 years: 2 mg (1 mL) twice daily

Children ≥12 years and Adolescents: 4 mg (2 mL) twice daily

Adults: 8 mg (4 mL) twice daily

Product Availability Product available in various countries; not currently available in the U.S.

Dosage Forms

Solution for Nebulization, Inhalation/Oral, as hydrochloride: 2 mg/mL

Solution, Oral, as hydrochloride: 0.8 mg/mL, 1.6 mg/mL

Tablet, Oral, as hydrochloride: 8 mg

◆ **Bromhexine Hydrochloride** *see* Bromhexine [INT] *on page* 291

Bromocriptine (broe moe KRIP teen)

Brand Names: U.S. Cycloset; Parlodel

Brand Names: Canada Dom-Bromocriptine; PMS-Bromocriptine

Index Terms Bromocriptine Mesylate; Cycloset

Pharmacologic Category Anti-Parkinson's Agent, Dopamine Agonist; Antidiabetic Agent, Dopamine Agonist; Ergot Derivative

Use

Acromegaly (excluding Cycloset): Treatment of acromegaly

Hyperprolactinemia (excluding Cycloset): Treatment of prolactin-secreting pituitary adenoma or disorders associated with hyperprolactinemia including amenorrhea with or without galactorrhea, hypogonadism, or infertility

Parkinson disease (excluding Cycloset): Treatment of the signs and symptoms of idiopathic or postencephalitic Parkinson disease; as adjunctive treatment to levodopa (alone or with a peripheral decarboxylase inhibitor)

Type 2 diabetes mellitus (Cycloset only): To improve glycemic control in adults with type 2 diabetes mellitus (noninsulin dependent, NIDDM) as an adjunct to diet and exercise

Pregnancy Risk Factor B

Dosage Oral:

Children and Adolescents: Hyperprolactinemia:

11 to 15 years (based on limited information): Initial: 1.25 to 2.5 mg daily; dosage may be increased as tolerated to achieve a therapeutic response (range: 2.5 to 10 mg daily).

≥16 years: Refer to adult dosing

Adults:

Acromegaly: Initial: 1.25 to 2.5 mg daily increasing by 1.25 to 2.5 mg daily as necessary every 3 to 7 days; usual dose: 20 to 30 mg/day (maximum: 100 mg/day)

Hyperprolactinemia: Initial: 1.25 to 2.5 mg daily; may be increased by 2.5 mg daily as tolerated every 2 to 7 days until optimal response (range: 2.5 to 15 mg/day)

Parkinsonism: 1.25 mg twice daily, increased by 2.5 mg daily in 2- to 4-week intervals as needed (maximum: 100 mg daily)

Type 2 diabetes (Cycloset only): Initial: 0.8 mg once daily; may increase at weekly intervals in 0.8 mg increments as tolerated; usual dose: 1.6 to 4.8 mg daily (maximum: 4.8 mg daily)

Neuroleptic malignant syndrome (off-label use): 2.5 mg (orally or via gastric tube) every 8 to 12 hours, increased to a maximum of 45 mg daily, if needed; continue therapy until NMS is controlled, then taper slowly (Gortney, 2009; Strawn, 2007)

Dosage adjustment in renal impairment: There are no dosage adjustments provided in the manufacturer's labeling (has not been studied).

Dosage adjustment in hepatic impairment: There are no dosage adjustment provided in the manufacturer's labeling. However, adjustment may be necessary due to extensive hepatic metabolism; use with caution.

Additional Information Complete prescribing information should be consulted for additional detail.

Dosage Forms

Capsule, Oral:

Parlodel: 5 mg

Generic: 5 mg

Tablet, Oral:

Cycloset: 0.8 mg

Generic: 2.5 mg

◆ **Bromocriptine Mesylate** *see* Bromocriptine *on page 291*

◆ **Bromoprida** *see* Bromopride [INT] *on page 292*

Bromopride [INT] (BRAHM o pride)

International Brand Names Bentril (KR); Bilenzima (BR); Bromopan (BR); Digerex (BR); Digesan (BR); Digesprid (BR); Digestil (BR); Digestina (BR); Pangest (BR); Plamet (BR); Pridecil (BR); Procirex (IT); Puraid (KR); Valopride (IT)

Index Terms Bromoprida; Bromopride Hydrochloride; VAL-13081

Pharmacologic Category Antiemetic; Gastrointestinal Agent, Prokinetic

Reported Use Treatment of nausea and vomiting, including postoperative nausea and vomiting (PONV); gastroesophageal reflux disease (GERD); as preparation for endoscopy and GI radiographic studies

Dosage Range Adults:

Oral: 20-60 mg/day in divided doses

IM, IV: 10-20 mg/day

Product Availability Product available in various countries; not currently available in the U.S.

◆ **Bromopride Hydrochloride** *see* Bromopride [INT] *on page 292*

Bromperidol [INT] (brom PER i dole)

International Brand Names Brom (KR); Bromidol (DK); Bromidol Depot (DK); Bromodol (AR, GR); Bromodol Decanoato (AR); Erodium (AR); Impromen (BE, DE, IT, LU, NL); Impromen decanoas (BE, LU, NL); Impromen Tropfen (DE); Tesoprel (DE, KR); Tesoprel Tropfen (DE)

Index Terms Bromperidol Decanoate

Pharmacologic Category Antipsychotic Agent, Typical, Phenothiazine

Reported Use Treatment of schizophrenia and other psychoses

Dosage Range Adults:

Oral: 1-15 mg/day, up to 50 mg/day

IM: 300 mg every 4 weeks

Product Availability Product available in various countries; not currently available in the U.S.

Dosage Forms

Injection, solution, as decanoate: 50 mg/mL (1 mL, 3 mL)

Solution, oral: 30 mg/mL (10 mL)

Tablet: 5 mg, 10 mg

◆ **Bromperidol Decanoate** *see* Bromperidol [INT] *on page 292*

Brompheniramine (brome fen IR a meen)

Brand Names: U.S. J-Tan PD [OTC]; Respa-BR

Index Terms Brompheniramine Maleate; Brompheniramine Tannate

Pharmacologic Category Alkylamine Derivative; Histamine H_1 Antagonist; Histamine H_1 Antagonist, First Generation

Additional Appendix Information

Beers Criteria – Potentially Inappropriate Medications for Geriatrics *on page 2271*

Use Upper respiratory allergies: Temporary relief of sneezing; itchy, watery eyes; itchy nose or throat; and runny nose caused by hay fever (allergic rhinitis) or other upper respiratory allergies.

Dosage Upper respiratory allergies: Oral:

Children 2 to <6 years: 1 mg (1 mL) every 4 to 6 hours (maximum: 6 mg [6 mL] per 24 hours)

Children 6 to <12 years: 2 mg (2 mL) every 4 to 6 hours (maximum: 12 mg [12 mL] per 24 hours)

Additional Information Complete prescribing information should be consulted for additional detail.

Dosage Forms

Liquid, Oral:

J-Tan PD [OTC]: 1 mg/mL (30 mL)

Tablet Extended Release 12 Hour, Oral:

Respa-BR: 11 mg

◆ **Brompheniramine Maleate** *see* Brompheniramine *on page 292*

◆ **Brompheniramine Tannate** *see* Brompheniramine *on page 292*

◆ **Broncho Saline [OTC]** *see* Sodium Chloride *on page 1902*

Brotizolam [INT] (broe TYE zoe lam)

International Brand Names Bondormin (IL); Dormex (CL); Lendorm (AT, DE, DK); Lendormin (BE, CH, CN, DE, GR, HU, IE, IT, JP, KR, LU, NL, PT, VE); Lindormin (MX); Mederantil[vet.] (CH, DE, FR); Nimbisan (IT); Noctilan (CL); Sintonal (ES)

Pharmacologic Category Benzodiazepine

Reported Use Short-term management of insomnia

Dosage Range Adults: Oral: 0.25 mg at bedtime

Product Availability Product available in various countries; not currently available in the U.S.

Dosage Forms

Tablet: 0.25 mg

- ◆ **Brovana** *see* Arformoterol *on page 168*
- ◆ **BSF208075** *see* Ambrisentan *on page 107*
- ◆ **BTK inhibitor PCI-32765** *see* Ibrutinib *on page 1030*
- ◆ **BTX-A** *see* OnabotulinumtoxinA *on page 1512*
- ◆ **B-type Natriuretic Peptide (Human)** *see* Nesiritide *on page 1439*
- ◆ **Buckleys Chest Congestion [OTC]** *see* GuaiFENesin *on page 986*
- ◆ **Budeprion SR [DSC]** *see* BuPROPion *on page 305*

Budesonide (Systemic) (byoo DES oh nide)

Brand Names: U.S. Entocort EC; Pulmicort; Pulmicort Flexhaler; Uceris

Brand Names: Canada Entocort; Pulmicort Turbuhaler

Pharmacologic Category Corticosteroid, Inhalant (Oral); Corticosteroid, Systemic

Additional Appendix Information

Inhaled Corticosteroids *on page 2229*

Use

Nebulization: Maintenance and prophylactic treatment of asthma

Oral capsule: Treatment of active Crohn disease (mild-to-moderate) involving the ileum and/or ascending colon; maintenance of remission (for up to 3 months) of Crohn disease (mild-to-moderate) involving the ileum and/or ascending colon

Oral inhalation: Maintenance and prophylactic treatment of asthma; includes patients who require oral corticosteroids and those who may benefit from systemic dose reduction/elimination

Oral tablet: Induction of remission in patients with active ulcerative colitis (mild-to-moderate)

Pregnancy Risk Factor C (capsule, tablet)/B (inhalation)

Pregnancy Considerations Adverse events have been observed with corticosteroids in animal reproduction studies. Some studies have shown an association between first trimester systemic corticosteroid use and oral clefts (Park-Wyllie, 2000; Pradat, 2003). Systemic corticosteroids may also influence fetal growth (decreased birth weight); however, information is conflicting (Lunghi, 2010). Hypoadrenalism may occur in newborns following maternal use of corticosteroids in pregnancy; monitor. When systemic corticosteroids are needed in pregnancy, it is generally recommended to use the lowest effective dose for the shortest duration of time, avoiding high doses during the first trimester (Leachman, 2006; Lunghi, 2010). Budesonide may be used for the induction of remission in pregnant women with inflammatory bowel disease (Habal, 2012).

Based on available data, an overall increased risk of congenital malformations or a decrease in fetal growth has not been associated with maternal use of inhaled corticosteroids during pregnancy (Bakhireva, 2005; NAEPP, 2005; Namazy, 2004). In addition, studies of pregnant women specifically using inhaled budesonide have not demonstrated an increased risk of congenital abnormalities. Uncontrolled asthma is associated with adverse events on pregnancy (increased risk of perinatal mortality, pre-eclampsia, preterm birth, low birth weight infants). Inhaled corticosteroids are recommended for the treatment of asthma during pregnancy; budesonide is preferred (ACOG, 2008; NAEPP, 2005).

Breast-Feeding Considerations Following use of the powder for oral inhalation, ~0.3% to 1% of the maternal dose was found in breast milk. The maximum concentration appeared within 45 minutes of dosing. Plasma budesonide levels obtained from infants ~90 minutes after breast-feeding (~140 minutes after maternal dose) were below the limit of quantification. Concentrations of budesonide in breast milk are expected to be higher following administration of oral capsules/tablets than after an inhaled dose.

Due to the potential for serious adverse reactions in the nursing infant, the manufacturers of the oral tablets and capsules recommend a decision be made whether to discontinue nursing or to discontinue the drug, taking into account the importance of treatment to the mother. If there is concern about exposure to the infant, some guidelines recommend waiting 4 hours after the maternal dose of an oral systemic corticosteroid before breast-feeding in order to decrease potential exposure to the nursing infant (based on a study using prednisolone) (Habal, 2012; Ost, 1985).

According to the manufacturer of the product for inhalation, the decision to continue or discontinue breast-feeding during therapy should take into account the risk of minimal exposure to the infant and the benefits of breast-feeding to the mother. The use of inhaled corticosteroids is not considered a contraindication to breast-feeding (NAEPP, 2005).

Contraindications Hypersensitivity to budesonide or any component of the formulation; primary treatment of status asthmaticus, acute episodes of asthma; not for relief of acute bronchospasm

Canadian labeling: Additional contraindications (not in U.S. labeling): Moderate-to-severe bronchiectasis, pulmonary tuberculosis (active or quiescent), untreated respiratory infection (bacterial, fungal, or viral)

Warnings/Precautions May cause hypercorticism or suppression of hypothalamic-pituitary-adrenal (HPA) axis, particularly in younger children, in patients receiving high doses for prolonged periods, or with concomitant CYP3A4 inhibitor use. HPA axis suppression may lead to adrenal crisis. Withdrawal and discontinuation of a corticosteroid should be done slowly and carefully. Particular care is required when patients are transferred from systemic corticosteroids to inhaled products or corticosteroids with lower systemic effect due to possible adrenal insufficiency or withdrawal from steroids, including an increase in allergic symptoms. Adult patients receiving >20 mg per day of prednisone (or equivalent) may be most susceptible. Fatalities have occurred due to adrenal insufficiency in asthmatic patients during and after transfer from systemic corticosteroids to aerosol steroids; aerosol steroids do not provide the systemic steroid needed to treat patients having trauma, surgery, or infections. Do not use this product to transfer patients directly from oral corticosteroid therapy.

Bronchospasm may occur with wheezing after inhalation; if this occurs stop steroid and treat with a fast-acting bronchodilator (eg, albuterol). Supplemental steroids (oral or parenteral) may be needed during stress or severe asthma attacks. Not to be used in status asthmaticus or for the relief of acute bronchospasm. Acute myopathy has been reported with high-dose corticosteroids, usually in patients with neuromuscular transmission disorders; may involve ocular and/or respiratory muscles; monitor creatine kinase; recovery may be delayed. Corticosteroid use may cause psychiatric disturbances, including depression, euphoria, insomnia, mood swings, and personality changes. Preexisting psychiatric conditions may be exacerbated by corticosteroid use. Prolonged use of corticosteroids may also increase the incidence of secondary infection, mask acute infection (including fungal infections), prolong or exacerbate viral infections, or limit response to vaccines. Exposure to chickenpox should be avoided; corticosteroids should not be used to treat ocular herpes simplex. Corticosteroids should not be used for viral hepatitis. Close observation is required in patients with latent tuberculosis and/or TB reactivity; restrict use in active TB (only in conjunction with antituberculosis treatment). *Candida albicans* infections may occur in the mouth and pharynx; rinsing (and spitting) with water after inhaler use may decrease risk. Prolonged treatment with corticosteroids has been associated with the development of Kaposi's sarcoma (case reports); if noted, discontinuation of therapy should be considered.

Use with caution in patients with thyroid disease, hepatic impairment, renal impairment, cardiovascular disease, diabetes, glaucoma, cataracts, myasthenia gravis, patients at risk for osteoporosis, patients at risk for seizures, or GI diseases (diverticulitis, peptic ulcer, ulcerative colitis) due to perforation risk. Use caution following acute MI (corticosteroids have been associated with myocardial rupture). Because of the risk of adverse effects, systemic corticosteroids should be used cautiously in the elderly in the smallest possible effective dose for the shortest duration.

Potentially significant interactions may exist, requiring dose or frequency adjustment, additional monitoring, and/or selection of alternative therapy. Consult drug interactions database for more detailed information.

Orally-inhaled corticosteroids may cause a reduction in growth velocity in pediatric patients (~1 centimeter per year [range: 0.3-1.8 cm per year] and related to dose and duration of exposure). To minimize the systemic effects of orally-inhaled corticosteroids, each patient should be titrated to the lowest effective dose. Growth should be routinely monitored in pediatric patients. Withdraw systemic therapy with gradual tapering of dose. There have been reports of systemic corticosteroid withdrawal symptoms (eg, joint/muscle pain, lassitude, depression) when withdrawing oral inhalation therapy. Pulmicort Flexhaler contains lactose; very rare anaphylactic reactions have been reported in patients with severe milk protein allergy.

Adverse Reactions

Oral capsules:

Cardiovascular: Chest pain, edema, facial edema, flushing, hypertension, palpitations, tachycardia

Central nervous system: Agitation, amnesia, confusion, dizziness, drowsiness, headache, insomnia, malaise, nervousness, paresthesia, sleep disorder, vertigo

Dermatologic: Acne vulgaris, alopecia, atrophic striae, dermatitis, dermatological disease, eczema

Endocrine & metabolic: Adrenocortical insufficiency, hirsutism, hypokalemia, intermenstrual bleeding, menstrual disease, redistribution of body fat (moon face, buffalo hump), weight gain

Gastrointestinal: Anus disease, dental disease, diarrhea, dyspepsia, enteritis, epigastric pain, exacerbation of Crohn's disease, gastrointestinal fistula, glossitis, hemorrhoids, increased appetite, intestinal obstruction, nausea, oral candidiasis

Genitourinary: Dysuria, hematuria, nocturia, pyuria, urinary frequency, urinary tract infection

Hematologic & oncologic: Abnormal neutrophils, anemia, bruise, C-reactive protein increased, increased erythrocyte sedimentation rate, leukocytosis, purpura

Hepatic: Increased serum alkaline phosphatase

Hypersensitivity: Tongue edema

Infection: Abscess, viral infection

Neuromuscular & skeletal: Arthralgia, arthritis, hyperkinesia, muscle cramps, myalgia, tremor, weakness

Ophthalmic: Eye disease, visual disturbance

Otic: Otic infection

Respiratory: Bronchitis, dyspnea, flu-like symptoms, pharyngeal disease, respiratory tract infection, rhinitis, sinusitis

Miscellaneous: Abscess, C-reactive protein increased, diaphoresis, fat redistribution (moon face, buffalo hump), flu-like syndrome, erythrocyte sedimentation rate increased, viral infection

Rare but important or life-threatening: Anaphylaxis, intracranial hypertension (benign)

Oral inhaler (Pulmicort Flexhaler):

Cardiovascular: Syncope

Central nervous system: Headache, hypertonia, insomnia, pain, voice disorder

Endocrine & metabolic: Weight gain

Gastrointestinal: Abdominal pain, dysgeusia, dyspepsia, nausea, oral candidiasis, viral gastroenteritis, vomiting, xerostomia

Hematologic & oncologic: Bruise

Infection: Infection

Neuromuscular & skeletal: Arthralgia, back pain, bone fracture, myalgia, neck pain, weakness

Otic: Otitis media

Respiratory: Allergic rhinitis, cough, nasal congestion, nasopharyngitis, pharyngitis, respiratory tract infection, rhinitis, sinusitis, viral upper respiratory tract infection

Miscellaneous: Fever

Rare but important or life-threatening: Adrenocortical insufficiency, aggressive behavior, cataract, depression, glaucoma, hypercorticoidism, hypersensitivity (immediate and delayed [includes rash, contact dermatitis, angioedema, bronchospasm, urticaria]), increased intraocular pressure, psychosis, wheezing (patients with severe milk allergy)

Oral tablets:

Central nervous system: Emotional lability, fatigue, headache

Dermatologic: Acne vulgaris

Endocrine & metabolic: Decreased cortisol, hirsutism

Gastrointestinal: Abdominal distension, constipation, flatulence, nausea, upper abdominal pain

Genitourinary: Urinary tract infection

Neuromuscular & skeletal: Arthralgia

Rare but important or life-threatening: Anaphylaxis, intracranial hypertension (benign)

Suspension for nebulization:

Cardiovascular: Chest pain

Central nervous system: Emotional lability, fatigue, voice disorder

Dermatologic: Contact dermatitis, eczema, pruritus, pustular rash, skin rash

Gastrointestinal: Abdominal pain, anorexia, diarrhea, gastroenteritis, vomiting

Hematologic & oncologic: Cervical lymphadenopathy, purpura

Hypersensitivity: Hypersensitivity reaction

Infection: Candidiasis, herpes simplex infection, infection, viral infection

Neuromuscular & skeletal: Bone fracture, hyperkinesia, myalgia

Ophthalmic: Conjunctivitis, eye infection

Otic: Otalgia, otic infection, otitis externa, otitis media

Respiratory: Cough, epistaxis, flu-like symptoms, respiratory tract infection, rhinitis, stridor

Rare but important or life-threatening: Adrenocortical insufficiency, aggressive behavior, avascular necrosis of femoral head, bronchitis, cataract, depression, glaucoma, growth suppression, hypercorticoidism, hypersensitivity (immediate and delayed [includes angioedema, bronchospasm, urticaria]), increased intraocular pressure, osteoporosis, psychosis

Drug Interactions

Metabolism/Transport Effects Substrate of CYP3A4 (major); **Note:** Assignment of Major/Minor substrate status based on clinically relevant drug interaction potential

Avoid Concomitant Use

Avoid concomitant use of Budesonide (Systemic, Oral Inhalation) with any of the following: Aldesleukin; BCG; Conivaptan; Fusidic Acid (Systemic); Grapefruit Juice; Idelalisib; Natalizumab; Pimecrolimus; Tacrolimus (Topical); Tofacitinib

Increased Effect/Toxicity

Budesonide (Systemic, Oral Inhalation) may increase the levels/effects of: Amphotericin B; Deferasirox; Leflunomide; Loop Diuretics; Natalizumab; Thiazide Diuretics; Tofacitinib

The levels/effects of Budesonide (Systemic, Oral Inhalation) may be increased by: Conivaptan; CYP3A4 Inhibitors (Moderate); CYP3A4 Inhibitors (Strong); Dasatinib; Denosumab; Fusidic Acid (Systemic); Grapefruit Juice; Idelalisib; Ivacaftor; Luliconazole; Mifepristone; Pimecrolimus; Simeprevir; Stiripentol; Tacrolimus (Topical); Telaprevir; Trastuzumab

Decreased Effect

Budesonide (Systemic, Oral Inhalation) may decrease the levels/effects of: Aldesleukin; Antidiabetic Agents; BCG; Coccidioides immitis Skin Test; Corticorelin; Hyaluronidase; Sipuleucel-T; Vaccines (Inactivated)

The levels/effects of Budesonide (Systemic, Oral Inhalation) may be decreased by: Antacids; Bile Acid Sequestrants; Echinacea

Food Interactions Grapefruit juice may double systemic exposure of orally administered budesonide. Administration of capsules with a high-fat meal delays peak concentration, but does not alter the extent of absorption; administration of tablets with a high-fat meal decreases peak concentration (~27%). Management: Avoid grapefruit juice when using oral capsules or tablets.

Storage/Stability

Oral capsules and tablets: Store at 25°C (77°F); excursions permitted to 15°C to 30°C (59°F to 86°F); keep container tightly closed.

Oral inhaler (Pulmicort Flexhaler): Store at controlled room temperature of 20°C to 25°C (68°F to 77°F). Protect from moisture.

Suspension for nebulization: Store upright at 20°C to 25°C (68°F to 77°F). Protect from light. Do not refrigerate or freeze. Once aluminum package is opened, solution should be used within 2 weeks. Continue to protect from light.

Mechanism of Action Controls the rate of protein synthesis; depresses the migration of polymorphonuclear leukocytes, fibroblasts; reverses capillary permeability and lysosomal stabilization at the cellular level to prevent or control inflammation. Has potent glucocorticoid activity and weak mineralocorticoid activity.

Pharmacodynamics/Kinetics

Onset of action: Nebulization: 2-8 days; Inhalation: 24 hours

Peak effect: Nebulization: 4-6 weeks; Inhalation: 1-2 weeks

Distribution: 2.2-3.9 L/kg

Protein binding: 85% to 90%

Metabolism: Hepatic via CYP3A4 to two metabolites: 16 alpha-hydroxyprednisolone and 6 beta-hydroxybudesonide; minor activity

Bioavailability: Limited by high first-pass effect; Capsule: 9% to 21%; Nebulization: 6%; Inhalation: 6% to 13%

Half-life elimination: 2-3.6 hours

Time to peak: Capsule: 0.5-10 hours (variable in Crohn disease); Nebulization: 10-30 minutes; Inhalation: 1-2 hours; Tablet: 7.4-19.2 hours

Excretion: Urine (60%) and feces as metabolites

Dosage

Nebulization: Asthma: Pulmicort Respules: Children 12 months to 8 years: Titrate to lowest effective dose once patient is stable; start at 0.25 mg/day or use as follows:

Previous therapy of bronchodilators alone: 0.5 mg/day administered as a single dose or divided twice daily (maximum daily dose: 0.5 mg)

Previous therapy of inhaled corticosteroids: 0.5 mg/day administered as a single dose or divided twice daily (maximum daily dose: 1 mg)

Previous therapy of oral corticosteroids: 1 mg/day administered as a single dose or divided twice daily (maximum daily dose: 1 mg)

Asthma Guidelines (NAEPP, 2007):

Children 0 to 4 years:

"Low" dose: 0.25 to 0.5 mg/day

"Medium" dose: >0.5 to 1 mg/day

"High" dose: >1 mg/day

Children 5 to 11 years:

"Low" dose: 0.5 mg/day

"Medium" dose: 1 mg/day

"High" dose: 2 mg/day

Oral inhalation: Asthma: Titrate to lowest effective dose once patient is stable.

U.S. labeling: Pulmicort Flexhaler: **Note:** May increase dose after 1 to 2 weeks of therapy in patients who are not adequately controlled.

Children ≥6 years: Initial: 180 mcg twice daily (some patients may be initiated at 360 mcg twice daily); maximum: 360 mcg twice daily

Asthma Guidelines (NAEPP, 2007) (administer in divided doses twice daily):

Children 5 to 11 years:

"Low" dose: 180 to 400 mcg/day

"Medium" dose: >400 to 800 mcg/day

"High" dose: >800 mcg/day

Children ≥12 years: Refer to adult dosing.

Adults: Initial: 360 mcg twice daily (selected patients may be initiated at 180 mcg twice daily); maximum: 720 mcg twice daily

Asthma Guidelines (NAEPP, 2007) (administer in divided doses twice daily):

"Low" dose: 180 to 600 mcg/day

"Medium" dose: >600 to 1200 mcg/day

"High" dose: >1200 mcg/day

Canadian labeling: Pulmicort Turbuhaler:

Children 6 to 11 years:

Initial (or during periods of severe asthma or when switching from oral corticosteroid therapy): 200 to 400 mcg daily in 2 divided doses

Maintenance: Individualized, lowest effective dose in 2 divided doses

Children ≥12 years and Adults:

Initial (or during periods of severe asthma or when switching from oral corticosteroid therapy): 400 to 2400 mcg daily in 2 to 4 divided doses

Maintenance: 200 to 400 mcg twice daily (higher doses may be needed for some patients). Patients taking 400 mcg/day may take as a single daily dose.

Conversion from oral systemic corticosteroid to orally inhaled corticosteroid: Initiation of oral inhalation therapy should begin in patients whose asthma is reasonably stabilized on oral corticosteroids (OCS). A gradual dose reduction of OCS should begin ~7 to 10 days after starting inhaled therapy. U.S. labeling recommends reducing prednisone dose by 2.5 mg/day (or equivalent of other OCS) on a weekly basis (patients using oral inhaler) or by ≤25% every 1 to 2 weeks (patients using respules). The Canadian labeling recommends decreasing the daily dose of prednisone by 2.5 mg (or equivalent of other OCS) every 4 days in closely monitored patients or every 10 days if not closely monitored. If adrenal insufficiency occurs, temporarily increase the OCS dose and follow with a more gradual withdrawal. **Note:** When transitioning from systemic to inhaled corticosteroids, supplemental systemic corticosteroid therapy may be necessary during periods of stress or during severe asthma attacks.

Oral:

Capsule: Crohn disease (active): Adults: 9 mg once daily in the morning for up to 8 weeks; recurring episodes may be treated with a repeat 8-week course of treatment

Maintenance of remission: Following treatment of active disease (control of symptoms with CDAI <150), treatment may be continued at a dosage of 6 mg once daily for up to 3 months. If symptom control is maintained for 3 months, tapering of the dosage to complete cessation is recommended. Continued dosing beyond 3 months has not been demonstrated to result in substantial benefit.

Tablet: Ulcerative colitis (active): Adults: 9 mg once daily in the morning for up to 8 weeks

Dosage adjustment in renal impairment: Inhalation, Nebulization, Oral: No dosage adjustment provided in manufacturer's labeling (has not been studied).

Dosage adjustment in hepatic impairment: Inhalation, Nebulization, Oral: No specific dosage adjustment provided in the manufacturer's labeling (has not been studied). Manufacturer labeling for oral budesonide suggests a dosage reduction may be necessary with moderate to severe impairment. Budesonide undergoes hepatic metabolism; bioavailability increased in cirrhosis; monitor closely for signs and symptoms of hypercorticism.

Dietary Considerations Oral capsules, tablets: Avoid grapefruit juice.

Administration

Oral capsule, tablet: May be administered without regard to meals. Swallow whole; do not crush, chew, or break.

Powder for inhalation:

Pulmicort Flexhaler: Hold inhaler in upright position (mouthpiece up) to load dose. Do not shake prior to use. Unit should be primed prior to first use only. It will not need primed again, even if not used for a long time. Place mouthpiece between lips and inhale forcefully and deeply. Do not exhale through inhaler; do not use a spacer. Dose indicator does not move with every dose, usually only after 5 doses. Discard when dose indicator reads "0". Rinse mouth with water after each use to reduce incidence of candidiasis.

Pulmicort Turbuhaler [CAN, not available in the U.S.]: Hold inhaler in upright position (mouthpiece up) to load dose. Do not shake inhaler after dose is loaded. Unit should be primed prior to first use. Place mouthpiece between lips and inhale forcefully and deeply; mouthpiece should face up. Do not exhale through inhaler; do not use a spacer. When a red mark appears in the dose indicator window, 20 doses are left. When the red mark reaches the bottom of the window, the inhaler should be discarded. Rinse mouth with water after use to reduce incidence of candidiasis.

Suspension for nebulization: Shake well before using. Use Pulmicort Respules with jet nebulizer connected to an air compressor; administer with mouthpiece or facemask. Do not use ultrasonic nebulizer. Do not mix with other medications in nebulizer. Rinse mouth following treatments to decrease risk of oral candidiasis (wash face if using face mask).

Monitoring Parameters Monitor growth in pediatric patients; blood pressure, serum glucose, weight with high-dose or long-term oral use; signs and symptoms of hypercorticism or adrenal suppression

Asthma: FEV_1, peak flow, and/or other pulmonary function tests

Additional Information Effects of inhaled steroids on growth have been observed in the absence of laboratory evidence of HPA axis suppression, suggesting that growth velocity is a more sensitive indicator of systemic corticosteroid exposure in pediatric patients than some commonly used tests of HPA axis function. The long-term effects of this reduction in growth velocity associated with orally-inhaled corticosteroids, including the impact on final adult height, are unknown. The potential for "catch up" growth following discontinuation of treatment with inhaled corticosteroids has not been adequately studied.

Dosage Forms Considerations Pulmicort Flexhaler 180 mcg/actuation canisters contain 120 actuations and the 90 mcg/actuation canisters contain 60 inhalations.

Dosage Forms

Aerosol Powder Breath Activated, Inhalation:

Pulmicort Flexhaler: 90 mcg/actuation (1 ea); 180 mcg/actuation (1 ea)

Capsule Extended Release 24 Hour, Oral:

Entocort EC: 3 mg

Generic: 3 mg

Suspension, Inhalation:

Pulmicort: 0.25 mg/2 mL (2 mL); 0.5 mg/2 mL (2 mL); 1 mg/2 mL (2 mL)

Generic: 0.25 mg/2 mL (2 mL); 0.5 mg/2 mL (2 mL)

Tablet Extended Release 24 Hour, Oral:

Uceris: 9 mg

Dosage Forms: Canada

Powder for oral inhalation:

Pulmicort Turbuhaler: 100 mcg/inhalation, 200 mcg/inhalation, 400 mcg/inhalation

Budesonide (Nasal) (byoo DES oh nide)

Brand Names: U.S. Rhinocort Aqua

Brand Names: Canada Mylan-Budesonide AQ; Rhinocort® Aqua®; Rhinocort® Turbuhaler®

Pharmacologic Category Corticosteroid, Nasal

Additional Appendix Information

Inhaled Corticosteroids *on page 2229*

Use Management of symptoms of seasonal or perennial rhinitis

Canadian labeling: Additional use (not in U.S. labeling): Prevention and treatment of nasal polyps

Pregnancy Risk Factor B

Dosage Nasal inhalation:

U.S. labeling (Rhinocort® Aqua®): Rhinitis: Children ≥6 years and Adults: 64 mcg/day as a single 32 mcg spray in each nostril. Some patients who do not achieve adequate control may benefit from increased dosage. A reduced dosage may be effective after initial control is achieved.

Maximum dose: Children <12 years: 128 mcg/day; Adults: 256 mcg/day

Canadian labeling:

Rhinocort® Aqua®: Children ≥6 years and Adults:

Nasal polyps: 256 mcg/day administered as a single 64 mcg spray in each nostril twice daily

Rhinitis: Initial: 256 mcg/day administered as two 64 mcg sprays in each nostril once daily or a single 64 mcg spray in each nostril twice daily; Maintenance: Individualize, lowest effective dose

Maximum dose: 256 mcg/day

Rhinocort® Turbuhaler®: Children ≥6 years and Adults:

Nasal polyps: 100 mcg into each nostril twice daily (maximum: 400 mcg/day)

Rhinitis: Initial: 200 mcg into each nostril once daily; Maintenance: Individualize, lowest effective dose (maximum: 400 mcg/day)

Dosage adjustment in renal impairment: No dosage adjustment provided in manufacturer's labeling (has not been studied).

Dosage adjustment in hepatic impairment: No dosage adjustment provided in manufacturer's labeling. Systemic availability of budesonide may be increased in patients with cirrhosis; monitor closely for signs and symptoms of hypercorticism; dosage reduction may be required.

Additional Information Complete prescribing information should be consulted for additional detail.

Dosage Forms Considerations

Rhinocort Aqua 8.6 g bottles contain 120 sprays.

Dosage Forms

Suspension, Nasal:

Rhinocort Aqua: 32 mcg/actuation (8.6 g)

Generic: 32 mcg/actuation (8.6 g)

Dosage Forms: Canada

Powder for nasal inhalation:

Rhinocort® Turbuhaler®: 100 mcg/inhalation

Suspension, intranasal [spray]:

Rhinocort® Aqua®: 64 mcg/inhalation

◆ **Budesonide and Eformoterol** *see* Budesonide and Formoterol *on page 297*

Budesonide and Formoterol

(byoo DES oh nide & for MOH te rol)

Brand Names: U.S. Symbicort

Brand Names: Canada Symbicort

Index Terms Budesonide and Eformoterol; Eformoterol and Budesonide; Formoterol and Budesonide; Formoterol Fumarate Dihydrate and Budesonide

Pharmacologic Category $Beta_2$ Agonist; $Beta_2$-Adrenergic Agonist, Long-Acting; Corticosteroid, Inhalant (Oral)

Use Treatment of asthma in patients ≥12 years of age where combination therapy is indicated; maintenance treatment of airflow obstruction associated with chronic obstructive pulmonary disease (COPD; including chronic bronchitis and emphysema)

Pregnancy Risk Factor C

Dosage Oral inhalation:

Asthma:

Children 5 to 11 years (off-label): Symbicort 80/4.5: Two inhalations twice daily. Do not exceed 4 inhalations per day (Morice, 2008; NAEPP, 2007).

Children ≥12 years and Adults:

U.S. labeling: Symbicort 80/4.5, Symbicort 160/4.5: Two inhalations twice daily (maximum: 4 inhalations/day). Recommended starting dose combination is determined according to asthma severity. In patients not adequately controlled on the lower combination dose following 1 to 2 weeks of therapy, consider the higher dose combination.

Canadian labeling:

Symbicort 100 Turbuhaler [CAN; not available in U.S.], Symbicort 200 Turbuhaler [CAN; not available in U.S.]: Initial: 1 to 2 inhalations twice daily until symptom control, then titrate to lowest effective dosage to maintain control

Maintenance: 1 to 2 inhalations once or twice daily (maximum: 8 inhalations/day as temporary treatment in periods of worsening asthma)

Symbicort Maintenance and Reliever Therapy (Symbicort SMART): **Note:** Not approved in the U.S.:

Maintenance: Symbicort 100 Turbuhaler [CAN] **or** Symbicort 200 Turbuhaler [CAN]: 1 to 2 inhalations twice daily **or** 2 inhalations once daily

Reliever therapy: Symbicort 100 Turbuhaler [CAN] **or** Symbicort 200 Turbuhaler [CAN]: One additional inhalation as needed, may repeat if no relief for up to 6 inhalations total (maximum: 8 inhalations/day)

COPD: Adults:

U.S. labeling: Symbicort 160/4.5: Two inhalations twice daily (maximum: 4 inhalations/day)

Canadian labeling: Symbicort 200 Turbuhaler [CAN; not available in U.S.]: Two inhalations twice daily (maximum: 4 inhalations/day)

Dosage adjustment in renal impairment: No dosage adjustment provided in the manufacturer's labeling (has not been studied).

Dosing adjustment in hepatic impairment: No dosage adjustment provided in manufacturer's labeling (has not been studied). However, close monitoring of patients with hepatic disease may be warranted due to hepatic metabolism of both agents.

Additional Information Complete prescribing information should be consulted for additional detail.

Dosage Forms

Aerosol for oral inhalation:

Symbicort 80/4.5: Budesonide 80 mcg and formoterol fumarate dihydrate 4.5 mcg per actuation (6.9 g) [60 metered inhalations]; budesonide 80 mcg and formoterol fumarate dihydrate 4.5 mcg per actuation (10.2 g) [120 metered inhalations]

Symbicort 160/4.5: Budesonide 160 mcg and formoterol fumarate dihydrate 4.5 mcg per actuation (6 g) [60 metered inhalations]; budesonide 160 mcg and formoterol fumarate dihydrate 4.5 mcg per actuation (10.2 g) [120 metered inhalations]

Dosage Forms: Canada

Powder for oral inhalation:

Symbicort 100 Turbuhaler: Budesonide 100 mcg and formoterol dihydrate 6 mcg per inhalation (available in 60 or 120 metered doses) [delivers ~80 mcg budesonide and 4.5 mcg formoterol per inhalation]

Symbicort 200 Turbuhaler: Budesonide 200 mcg and formoterol dihydrate 6 mcg per inhalation (available in 60 or 120 metered doses) [delivers ~160 mcg budesonide and 4.5 mcg formoterol per inhalation]

◆ **Buffasal [OTC]** *see* Aspirin *on page 180*

◆ **Bufferin [OTC]** *see* Aspirin *on page 180*

◆ **Bufferin Extra Strength [OTC]** *see* Aspirin *on page 180*

◆ **Buffinol [OTC]** *see* Aspirin *on page 180*

Bumetanide (byoo MET a nide)

Brand Names: Canada Burinex

Index Terms Bumex

Pharmacologic Category Antihypertensive; Diuretic, Loop

Use Management of edema secondary to heart failure or hepatic or renal disease (including nephrotic syndrome)

Pregnancy Risk Factor C

Pregnancy Considerations Adverse events have been observed in some animal reproduction studies.

Breast-Feeding Considerations It is not known if bumetanide is excreted in breast milk. Breast-feeding is not recommended by the manufacturer. Diuretics have the potential to decrease milk volume and suppress lactation.

Contraindications Hypersensitivity to bumetanide or any component of the formulation; anuria; patients with hepatic coma or in states of severe electrolyte depletion until the condition improves or is corrected

Warnings/Precautions [U.S. Boxed Warning]: Excessive amounts can lead to profound diuresis with fluid and electrolyte loss; close medical supervision and dose evaluation are required. Potassium supplementation and/or use of potassium-sparing diuretics may be necessary to prevent hypokalemia. In cirrhosis, initiate bumetanide therapy with conservative dosing and close monitoring of electrolytes; avoid sudden changes in fluid and electrolyte balance and acid/base status which may lead to hepatic encephalopathy. *In vitro* studies using pooled sera from critically-ill neonates have shown bumetanide to be a potent displacer of bilirubin; avoid use in neonates at risk for kernicterus. Coadministration of antihypertensives may increase the risk of hypotension.

Monitor fluid status and renal function in an attempt to prevent oliguria, azotemia, and reversible increases in BUN and creatinine; close medical supervision of aggressive diuresis required. Bumetanide-induced ototoxicity (usually transient) may occur with rapid IV administration, renal impairment, excessive doses, and concurrent use of other ototoxins (eg, aminoglycosides). Asymptomatic hyperuricemia has been reported with use.

Chemical similarities are present among sulfonamides, sulfonylureas, carbonic anhydrase inhibitors, thiazides, and loop diuretics (except ethacrynic acid); the manufacturer's labeling states that bumetanide may be used in patients allergic to furosemide. Use in patients with sulfonylurea allergy is not specifically contraindicated in product labeling; however, a risk of cross-reaction exists in patients with allergy to any of these compounds; avoid use when previous reaction has been severe. Discontinue if signs of hypersensitivity are noted.

Benzyl alcohol and derivatives: Some dosage forms may contain benzyl alcohol; large amounts of benzyl alcohol (≥99 mg/kg/day) have been associated with a potentially fatal toxicity ("gasping syndrome") in neonates; the "gasping syndrome" consists of metabolic acidosis, respiratory distress, gasping respirations, CNS dysfunction (including convulsions, intracranial hemorrhage), hypotension and cardiovascular collapse (AAP, 1997; CDC, 1982); some data suggests that benzoate displaces bilirubin from protein binding sites (Ahlfors, 2001); avoid or use dosage forms containing benzyl alcohol with caution in neonates. See manufacturer's labeling.

Adverse Reactions

Central nervous system: Dizziness

Endocrine & metabolic: abnormal serum calcium, abnormal lactate dehydrogenase, hyponatremia, hyperglycemia, phosphorus change, variations in bicarbonate

Genitourinary: Azotemia

Neuromuscular & skeletal: Muscle cramps

Renal: Increased serum creatinine

Respiratory: Variations in CO_2 content

Rare but important or life-threatening: Abdominal pain, abnormal alkaline phosphatase, abnormal bilirubin levels, abnormal hematocrit, abnormal hemoglobin level, abnormal transaminase, arthritic pain, asterixis, auditory impairment, blood cholesterol abnormal, brain disease (in patients with preexisting liver disease), change in creatinine clearance, change in prothrombin time, change in WBC count, chest pain, dehydration, diaphoresis, diarrhea, dyspepsia, ECG changes, erectile dysfunction, fatigue, glycosuria, headache, hyperventilation, hypotension, musculoskeletal pain, nausea, nipple tenderness, orthostatic hypotension, otalgia, ototoxicity, premature ejaculation, proteinuria, pruritus, renal failure, skin rash, Stevens-Johnson syndrome, thrombocytopenia, toxic epidermal necrolysis, urticaria, vertigo, vomiting, weakness, xerostomia

Drug Interactions

Metabolism/Transport Effects None known.

Avoid Concomitant Use There are no known interactions where it is recommended to avoid concomitant use.

Increased Effect/Toxicity

Bumetanide may increase the levels/effects of: ACE Inhibitors; Allopurinol; Amifostine; Aminoglycosides; Antihypertensives; Cardiac Glycosides; CISplatin; Dofetilide; DULoxetine; Foscarnet; Hypotensive Agents; Ivabradine; Levodopa; Lithium; Methotrexate; Neuromuscular-Blocking Agents; Obinutuzumab; RisperiDONE; RiTUXimab; Salicylates; Sodium Phosphates; Topiramate

The levels/effects of Bumetanide may be increased by: Alfuzosin; Analgesics (Opioid); Barbiturates; Beta2-Agonists; Brimonidine (Topical); Canagliflozin; Corticosteroids (Orally Inhaled); Corticosteroids (Systemic); CycloSPORINE (Systemic); Diazoxide; Herbs (Hypotensive Properties); Licorice; MAO Inhibitors; Methotrexate; Nicorandil; Pentoxifylline; Phosphodiesterase 5 Inhibitors; Probenecid; Prostacyclin Analogues

Decreased Effect

Bumetanide may decrease the levels/effects of: Hypoglycemic Agents; Lithium; Neuromuscular-Blocking Agents

The levels/effects of Bumetanide may be decreased by: Bile Acid Sequestrants; Fosphenytoin; Herbs (Hypertensive Properties); Methotrexate; Methylphenidate; Nonsteroidal Anti-Inflammatory Agents; Phenytoin; Probenecid; Salicylates; Yohimbine

Food Interactions Bumetanide serum levels may be decreased if taken with food. Management: It has been recommended that bumetanide be administered without food (Bard, 2004).

Storage/Stability

IV: Store vials at 15°C to 30°C (59°F to 86°F). Infusion solutions should be used within 24 hours after preparation. Light sensitive; discoloration may occur when exposed to light.

Tablet: Store at 15°C to 30°C (59°F to 86°F); protect from light.

Mechanism of Action Inhibits reabsorption of sodium and chloride in the ascending loop of Henle and proximal renal tubule, interfering with the chloride-binding cotransport system, thus causing increased excretion of water, sodium, chloride, magnesium, phosphate, and calcium; it does not appear to act on the distal tubule

Pharmacodynamics/Kinetics

Onset of action: Oral, IM: 0.5-1 hour; IV: 2-3 minutes

Peak effect: Oral: 1-2 hours; IV: 15-30 minutes

Duration: 4-6 hours

Distribution: V_d: Neonates and Infants: 0.26-0.39 L/kg; Adults: 9-25 L

Protein binding: 94% to 96%

Metabolism: Partially hepatic

Bioavailability: 59% to 89% (median: 80%)

Half-life elimination: Neonates: ~6 hours; Infants (1 month): ~2.4 hours; Adults: 1-1.5 hours

Excretion: Urine (81% of total dose; 45% of which is unchanged drug); feces (2% of total dose)

Dosage

Infants and Children: Oral, IM, IV: 0.015-0.1 mg/kg/dose every 6-24 hours (maximum dose: 10 mg/day)

Adults: Edema, heart failure:

Oral: 0.5-2 mg/dose 1-2 times daily; if diuretic response to initial dose is not adequate, may repeat in 4-5 hours for up to 2 doses (maximum dose: 10 mg daily). ACCF/AHA 2013 heart failure guidelines recommend initial dosing of 0.5- 1 mg once or twice daily and a maximum total daily dose of 10 mg (Yancy, 2013).

IM, IV: 0.5-1 mg/dose; if diuretic response to initial dose is not adequate, may repeat in 2-3 hours for up to 2 doses (maximum dose: 10 mg daily)

Continuous IV infusion (off-label dose): Initial: 1 mg IV load then 0.5-2 mg/hour; repeat loading dose before increasing infusion rate (ACCF/AHA [Yancy, 2013]; Brater, 1998). **Note:** With lower baseline CrCl (eg, CrCl <25 mL/minute), the upper end of the initial infusion dosage range should be considered.

Dosage adjustment in renal impairment: Use is contraindicated in anuria. Use with caution in renal insufficiency due to increased risk of adverse effects.

Dosage adjustment in hepatic impairment: Use is contraindicated in hepatic coma. Use with caution in cirrhosis and ascites due to increased risk of precipitating hepatic coma; initiate with conservative doses and monitoring.

Dietary Considerations Administration with food slows the rate and reduces the extent of absorption and may reduce diuretic efficacy (Bard, 2004). May require increased intake of potassium-rich foods.

Administration

IV: Administer slowly, over 1-2 minutes.

Oral: An alternate-day schedule or a 3-4 daily dosing regimen with rest periods of 1-2 days in between may be the most tolerable and effective regimen for the continued control of edema.

Monitoring Parameters Blood pressure; serum electrolytes, renal function; fluid status (weight and I & O), blood pressure

Dosage Forms

Solution, Injection:

Generic: 0.25 mg/mL (2 mL, 4 mL, 10 mL)

Tablet, Oral:

Generic: 0.5 mg, 1 mg, 2 mg

Dosage Forms: Canada Note: Solution for injection is not available in Canada.

Tablet, Oral:

Burinex: 1 mg, 5 mg

◆ **Bumex** *see* Bumetanide *on page 297*

◆ **Buminate** *see* Albumin *on page 67*

◆ **Buminate-5% (Can)** *see* Albumin *on page 67*

◆ **Buminate-25% (Can)** *see* Albumin *on page 67*

◆ **Bunavail** *see* Buprenorphine and Naloxone *on page 304*

◆ **Bupap** *see* Butalbital and Acetaminophen *on page 314*

◆ **Buphenyl** *see* Sodium Phenylbutyrate *on page 1908*

Bupivacaine (byoo PIV a kane)

Brand Names: U.S. Bupivacaine Spinal; Marcaine; Marcaine Preservative Free; Marcaine Spinal; Sensorcaine; Sensorcaine-MPF; Sensorcaine-MPF Spinal

Brand Names: Canada Marcaine®; Sensorcaine®

Index Terms Bupivacaine Hydrochloride

Pharmacologic Category Local Anesthetic

Use Local or regional anesthesia; spinal anesthesia; diagnostic and therapeutic procedures; obstetrical procedures (only 0.25% and 0.5% concentrations)

0.25%: Local infiltration, peripheral nerve block, sympathetic block, caudal or epidural block

0.5%: Peripheral nerve block, caudal and epidural block

0.75% **(not for obstetrical anesthesia)**: Retrobulbar block, epidural block. **Note:** Reserve for surgical procedures where a high degree of muscle relaxation and prolonged effect are necessary

Pregnancy Risk Factor C

Dosage Dose varies with procedure, depth of anesthesia, vascularity of tissues, duration of anesthesia, and condition of patient. Do not use solutions containing preservatives for caudal or epidural block.

Children >12 years and Adults:

Local anesthesia: Infiltration: 0.25% infiltrated locally; maximum: 175 mg

Caudal block (preservative free): 15-30 mL of 0.25% or 0.5%

Epidural block (other than caudal block; preservative free): Administer in 3-5 mL increments, allowing sufficient time to detect toxic manifestations of inadvertent IV or intrathecal administration: 10-20 mL of 0.25% or 0.5%

Surgical procedures requiring a high degree of muscle relaxation and prolonged effects **only**: 10-20 mL of 0.75% (**Note:** Not to be used in obstetrical cases)

Peripheral nerve block: 5 mL of 0.25% or 0.5%; maximum: 400 mg/day

Sympathetic nerve block: 20-50 mL of 0.25%

Retrobulbar anesthesia: 2-4 mL of 0.75%

Adults: Spinal anesthesia: Preservative free solution of 0.75% bupivacaine in 8.25% dextrose:

Lower extremity and perineal procedures: 1 mL

Lower abdominal procedures: 1.6 mL

Normal vaginal delivery: 0.8 mL (higher doses may be required in some patients)

Cesarean section: 1-1.4 mL

Dosage adjustment in renal impairment: No dosage adjustments provided in manufacturer's labeling; use with caution.

Dosage adjustment in hepatic impairment: No dosage adjustments provided in manufacturer's labeling; use with caution.

Additional Information Complete prescribing information should be consulted for additional detail.

Dosage Forms

Solution, Injection:

Marcaine: 0.25% (50 mL); 0.5% (50 mL)

Sensorcaine: 0.25% (50 mL); 0.5% (50 mL)

Sensorcaine-MPF: 0.25% (10 mL, 30 mL); 0.5% (10 mL, 30 mL); 0.75% (10 mL, 30 mL)

Generic: 0.25% (10 mL, 30 mL, 50 mL); 0.5% (10 mL, 30 mL, 50 mL); 0.75% (10 mL, 30 mL)

Solution, Injection [preservative free]:

Marcaine: 0.75% (10 mL, 30 mL)

Marcaine Preservative Free: 0.25% (10 mL, 30 mL); 0.5% (10 mL, 30 mL)

Generic: 0.25% (10 mL, 20 mL, 30 mL); 0.5% (10 mL, 20 mL, 30 mL); 0.75% (10 mL, 20 mL, 30 mL)

Solution, Intrathecal [preservative free]:

Bupivacaine Spinal: 0.75% [7.5 mg/mL] (2 mL)

Marcaine Spinal: 0.75% [7.5 mg/mL] (2 mL)

Sensorcaine-MPF Spinal: 0.75% [7.5 mg/mL] (2 mL)

◆ **(-)-bupivacaine** *see* Levobupivacaine [INT] *on page 1194*

◆ **Bupivacaine Hydrochloride** *see* Bupivacaine *on page 299*

Bupivacaine (Liposomal)

(byoo PIV a kane lye po SO mal)

Brand Names: U.S. Exparel

Index Terms Bupivacaine Liposome; DepoFoam Bupivacaine; Exparel; Liposomal Bupivacaine

Pharmacologic Category Analgesic, Nonopioid

Use Injected into the surgical site (eg, bunionectomy, hemorrhoidectomy) to provide postoperative analgesia

Pregnancy Risk Factor C

Dosage Infiltration (local): Adults: Postoperative analgesia: Dose is based on surgical site and volume required to cover the area (in general, the maximum total dose is 266 mg).

Bunionectomy: 7 mL into the tissues surrounding the osteotomy and 1 mL into the subcutaneous tissue of the surgical site (total dose = 8 mL [106 mg])

Hemorrhoidectomy: 30 mL (20 mL vial diluted with 10 mL NS or LR) divided and administered as 6 injections of 5 mL each (total dose = 30 mL [266 mg])

Dosage adjustment in renal impairment: There are no dosage adjustments provided in manufacturer's labeling; however, renal impairment may reduce bupivacaine elimination increasing systemic exposure and the risk of adverse effects or toxicities; use with caution.

Dosage adjustment in hepatic impairment: There are no dosage adjustments provided in manufacturer's labeling; however, moderate-to-severe impairment may reduce bupivacaine metabolism increasing systemic exposure and the risk of adverse effects or toxicities; use with caution.

Additional Information Complete prescribing information should be consulted for additional detail.

Dosage Forms

Suspension, Injection:

Exparel: 1.3% (20 mL)

◆ **Bupivacaine Liposome** *see* Bupivacaine (Liposomal) *on page 299*

◆ **Bupivacaine Spinal** *see* Bupivacaine *on page 299*

Bupranolol [INT] (byoo PRAN oh lole)

International Brand Names Adomed (AT); Betadran (FR); betadrenol (DE, IT); Betadrenol (SG); Monobeltin (ES); Ophtorenin (DE)

Index Terms Bupranolol Hydrochloride

Pharmacologic Category Beta-Adrenergic Blocker, Nonselective; Beta-Adrenergic Blocker, Ophthalmic

Reported Use

Ophthalmic: Management of glaucoma

Oral: Management of cardiovascular disorders

Dosage Range Adults:

Oral: 100-400 mg/day

Ophthalmic: 0.05% to 0.5%

Product Availability Product available in various countries; not currently available in the U.S.

Dosage Forms

Capsule, extended release: 160 mg

Solution, ophthalmic: 0.25%

Tablet: 10 mg, 40 mg, 80 mg

◆ **Bupranolol Hydrochloride** *see* Bupranolol [INT] *on page 300*

◆ **Buprenex** *see* Buprenorphine *on page 300*

Buprenorphine (byoo pre NOR feen)

Brand Names: U.S. Buprenex; Butrans

Brand Names: Canada Butrans

Index Terms Buprenorphine Hydrochloride

Pharmacologic Category Analgesic, Opioid; Analgesic, Opioid Partial Agonist

Additional Appendix Information

Opioid Conversion Table *on page 2232*

Use

Injection: Management of moderate-to-severe pain

Sublingual tablet: Treatment of opioid dependence

Transdermal patch: Management of pain severe enough to require around-the-clock, long-term, opioid treatment and for which alternative treatment options are inadequate

Pregnancy Risk Factor C

Pregnancy Considerations Adverse effects have been observed in some animal reproduction studies. Buprenorphine crosses the placenta; buprenorphine and norbuprenorphine can be detected in newborn serum, urine, and meconium following in utero exposure (CSAT, 2004). **[U.S. Boxed Warning]: Prolonged use can result in neonatal opioid withdrawal syndrome. If not recognized and treated, this may be life-threatening and require management according to protocols developed by neonatology experts.** Following chronic opioid therapy in pregnancy, adverse events in the newborn (including withdrawal) may occur; monitoring of the neonate is recommended. The minimum effective dose should be used if opioids are needed (Chou, 2009). The onset of withdrawal in infants of women receiving buprenorphine during pregnancy ranged from day 1 to day 8 of life, most occurring on day 1. Symptoms of withdrawal may include agitation, apnea, bradycardia, convulsions, hypertonia, myoclonus, respiratory depression, and tremor.

Buprenorphine is currently considered an alternate treatment for pregnant women who need therapy for opioid addiction (CSAT, 2004; Dow, 2012); however, use in pregnancy for this purpose is increasing (ACOG, 2012; Soyka, 2013). Buprenorphine should not be used to treat pain during labor. Women receiving buprenorphine for the treatment of addiction should be maintained on their daily dose of buprenorphine in addition to receiving the same pain management options during labor and delivery as opioid-naive women; maintenance doses of buprenorphine will not provide adequate pain relief. Narcotic agonist-antagonists should be avoided for the treatment of labor pain in women maintained on buprenorphine due to the risk of precipitating acute withdrawal. In addition, buprenorphine should not be given to women in labor taking methadone (ACOG, 2012).

Amenorrhea may develop secondary to substance abuse; pregnancy may occur following the initiation of buprenorphine maintenance treatment. Contraception counseling is recommended to prevent unplanned pregnancies (Dow, 2012). Long-term opioid use may cause secondary hypogonadism, which may lead to sexual dysfunction or infertility (Brennan, 2013).

Breast-Feeding Considerations Buprenorphine is excreted in breast milk. Breast-feeding is not recommended by the manufacturer. Nursing infants exposed to large doses of opioids should be monitored for apnea and sedation (Montgomery, 2012).

When buprenorphine is used to treat opioid addiction in nursing women, most guidelines do not contraindicate breast-feeding as long as the infant is tolerant to the dose and other contraindications do not exist; caution should be used when nursing infants not previously exposed (ACOG, 2012; CSAT, 2004; Montgomery, 2012). If additional illicit substances are being abused, women treated with buprenorphine should pump and discard breast milk until sobriety is established (ACOG, 2012; Dow, 2012).

Contraindications Hypersensitivity to buprenorphine or any component of the formulation

Transdermal patch: Additional contraindications: Significant respiratory depression; acute or severe asthma; known or suspected paralytic ileus

Documentation of allergenic cross-reactivity for morphine and related drugs in this class is limited. However, because of similarities in chemical structure and/or pharmacologic actions, the possibility of cross-sensitivity cannot be ruled out with certainty.

Warnings/Precautions An opioid-containing analgesic regimen should be tailored to each patient's needs and based upon the type of pain being treated (acute versus chronic), the route of administration, degree of tolerance for opioids (naive versus chronic user), age, weight, and medical condition. The optimal analgesic dose varies widely among patients. Doses should be titrated to pain relief/prevention.

May cause CNS depression, which may impair physical or mental abilities; patients must be cautioned about performing tasks which require mental alertness (eg, operating machinery or driving). Elderly may be more sensitive to CNS depressant and constipating effects. May cause respiratory depression - use caution in patients with respiratory disease or preexisting respiratory depression. Hypersensitivity reactions, including bronchospasm, angioneurotic edema, and anaphylactic shock, have also been reported. Potential for drug dependency exists, abrupt cessation may precipitate withdrawal. Use caution in elderly, debilitated, cachectic, pediatric patients, depression or suicidal tendencies. Tolerance, psychological and physical dependence may occur with prolonged use. Partial antagonist activity may precipitate acute opioid withdrawal in opioid-dependent individuals.

Hepatitis has been reported with buprenorphine use; hepatic events ranged from transient, asymptomatic transaminase elevations to hepatic failure; in many cases, patients had preexisting hepatic dysfunction. Monitor liver function tests in patients at increased risk for hepatotoxicity (eg, history of alcohol abuse, preexisting hepatic dysfunction, IV drug abusers) prior to and during therapy. Use with caution in patients with moderate hepatic impairment; dosage adjustment recommended in severe hepatic impairment.

Use with caution in patients with pulmonary or renal function impairment. Also use caution in patients with head injury or increased ICP, biliary tract dysfunction, pancreatitis, patients with history of hyperthyroidism, morbid obesity, adrenal insufficiency, prostatic hyperplasia, urinary stricture, toxic psychosis, pancreatitis, alcoholism, delirium tremens, or kyphoscoliosis. Avoid use in patients with CNS depression or coma as these patients are susceptible to intracranial effects of CO_2 retention. May cause severe hypotension, including orthostatic hypotension and syncope; use with caution in patients with hypovolemia, cardiovascular disease (including acute MI), or drugs which may exaggerate hypotensive effects (including phenothiazines or general anesthetics). May obscure diagnosis or clinical course of patients with acute abdominal conditions. Use with caution in patients with a history of ileus or bowel obstruction; use of transdermal patch is contraindicated in patients with known or suspected paralytic ileus. Opioid therapy may lower seizure threshold; use caution in patients with a history of seizure disorders. Potentially significant drug-drug interactions may exist, requiring dose or frequency adjustment, additional monitoring, and/or selection of alternative therapy.

Transdermal patch: Indicated for the management of pain severe enough to require daily, around the clock, long-term opioid treatment; should not be used for as-needed pain relief. **[U.S. Boxed Warning]: May cause potentially life-threatening respiratory depression; monitor for respiratory depression, especially during initiation or dose escalation. Misuse or abuse by chewing, swallowing, snorting, or injecting buprenorphine extracted from the transdermal system will result in the uncontrolled delivery of buprenorphine and pose a significant risk of overdose and death. Accidental exposure to even one dose, especially in children, can result in a fatal overdose.** Do not exceed one 20 **mcg**/hour transdermal patch due to the risk of QTc-interval prolongation. Avoid using in patients with a personal or family history of long QT syndrome or in patients with predisposing factors increasing the risk of QT abnormalities (eg, concurrent medications such as antiarrhythmics, hypokalemia, unstable heart failure, unstable atrial fibrillation). **[U.S. Boxed Warning]: Abuse, misuse, and addiction, which can lead to overdose and death, may occur.** Risk of opioid abuse is increased in patients with a history or family history of alcohol or drug abuse or mental illness (eg, major depression). Assess each patient's risk before prescribing, and monitor all patients for the development of these behaviors or conditions. The misuse of transdermal buprenorphine by placing it in the mouth, chewing it, swallowing it, or using it in ways other than indicated may cause choking, overdose, and death. To properly dispose of Butrans patch, fold it over on itself and flush down the toilet; alternatively, seal the used patch in the provided Patch-Disposal Unit and dispose of in the trash. Avoid exposure of application site and surrounding area to direct external heat sources (eg, heating pads, electric blankets, heating lamps, saunas, hot water, or direct sunlight). Buprenorphine release from the patch is temperature-dependent and may result in overdose. Patients who experience fever or increase in core temperature should be monitored closely and adjust dose if signs or respiratory depression or central nervous system depression occur. Application site reactions, including rare cases of severe reactions (eg, vesicles, discharge, "burns"), have been observed with use; onset varies from days to months after initiation; patients should be instructed to report severe reactions promptly. Therapy with the transdermal patch is not appropriate for use in the management of addictions. **[U.S. Boxed Warning]: Prolonged use during pregnancy may result in neonatal abstinence syndrome (NAS) in neonates and infants. If not recognized and treated, this may be life-threatening and require management according to protocols developed by neonatology experts.** Monitor neonate closely. Signs and symptoms include irritability, hyperactivity and abnormal sleep pattern, high pitched cry, tremor, vomiting, diarrhea and failure to gain weight. Onset, duration and severity depend on the drug used, duration of use, maternal dose, and rate of drug elimination by the newborn.

Concurrent use of agonist/antagonist analgesics may precipitate withdrawal symptoms and/or reduced analgesic efficacy in patients following prolonged therapy with mu opioid agonists. Abrupt discontinuation following prolonged use may also lead to withdrawal symptoms and is not recommended; taper dose gradually when discontinuing.

Sublingual tablets, which are used for induction treatment of opioid dependence, should not be started until effects of withdrawal are evident.

Adverse Reactions

Injection:

Cardiovascular: Hypotension
Central nervous system: Dizziness, headache, sedation
Dermatologic: Diaphoresis
Gastrointestinal: Nausea, vomiting
Ophthalmic: Miosis
Respiratory: Respiratory depression
Rare but important or life-threatening: Amblyopia, anaphylactic shock, apnea, bradycardia, conjunctivitis, coma, cyanosis, depersonalization, depression, diplopia, euphoria, hallucination, hypersensitivity, hypertension, hypogonadism (Brennan, 2013; Debono, 2011), injection site reaction, psychosis, seizure, slurred speech, tachycardia, urinary retention, Wenckebach period on ECG

Tablet:

Central nervous system: Anxiety, chills, depression, dizziness, drowsiness, headache, insomnia, nervousness, pain, withdrawal syndrome
Dermatologic: Diaphoresis
Gastrointestinal: Abdominal pain, constipation, diarrhea, dyspepsia, nausea, vomiting
Infection: Abscess, infection
Neuromuscular & skeletal: Back pain, weakness
Ophthalmic: Lacrimation
Respiratory: Cough, flu-like symptoms, pharyngitis, rhinitis

Miscellaneous: Fever

Rare but important or life-threatening: Anaphylactic shock, angioedema, hepatic encephalopathy, hepatic failure, hepatic necrosis, hepatitis (including cytolytic), hepatorenal syndrome, hypersensitivity, hypogonadism (Brennan, 2013; Debono, 2011), increased serum transaminases

Transdermal patch:

Cardiovascular: Chest pain, hypertension, peripheral edema

Central nervous system: Anxiety, depression, dizziness, drowsiness, fatigue, headache, hypoesthesia, insomnia, migraine, paresthesia

Dermatologic: Diaphoresis, pruritus, rash

Gastrointestinal: Abdominal distress, anorexia, constipation, diarrhea, dyspepsia, nausea, upper abdominal pain, vomiting, xerostomia

Genitourinary: Urinary tract infection

Local: Application site erythema, application site irritation, application site rash, local pruritus

Neuromuscular & skeletal: Arthralgia, back pain, joint swelling, limb pain, muscle spasm, musculoskeletal pain, myalgia, neck pain, tremor, weakness

Respiratory: Bronchitis, cough, dyspnea, flu-like symptoms, nasopharyngitis, pharyngolaryngeal pain, sinusitis, upper respiratory tract infection

Miscellaneous: Fever

Rare but important or life-threatening: Angina pectoris, angioedema, application site dermatitis, bradycardia, contact dermatitis, diverticulitis, exacerbation of asthma, hallucination, hyperventilation, hypersensitivity reaction, hypogonadism (Brennan, 2013; Debono, 2011), hypotension, hypoventilation, increased serum ALT, intestinal obstruction, loss of consciousness, memory impairment, mental deficiency, mental status changes, miosis (dose-related), orthostatic hypotension, psychosis, respiratory depression, respiratory distress, respiratory failure, syncope, tachycardia, urinary incontinence, urinary retention, vasodilatation, visual disturbance, withdrawal syndrome

Drug Interactions

Metabolism/Transport Effects Substrate of CYP3A4 (major); **Note:** Assignment of Major/Minor substrate status based on clinically relevant drug interaction potential; **Inhibits** CYP1A2 (weak), CYP2A6 (weak), CYP2C19 (weak), CYP2D6 (weak)

Avoid Concomitant Use

Avoid concomitant use of Buprenorphine with any of the following: Atazanavir; Azelastine (Nasal); Conivaptan; Fusidic Acid (Systemic); Idelalisib; MAO Inhibitors; Orphenadrine; Paraldehyde; Thalidomide

Increased Effect/Toxicity

Buprenorphine may increase the levels/effects of: Alvimopan; Azelastine (Nasal); Desmopressin; Diuretics; Hydrocodone; MAO Inhibitors; Methotrimeprazine; Metyrosine; Orphenadrine; Paraldehyde; Pramipexole; ROPINIRole; Rotigotine; Selective Serotonin Reuptake Inhibitors; Suvorexant; Thalidomide; Zolpidem

The levels/effects of Buprenorphine may be increased by: Alcohol (Ethyl); Amphetamines; Anticholinergic Agents; Aprepitant; Atazanavir; Boceprevir; Brimonidine (Topical); Cannabis; Ceritinib; CNS Depressants; Cobicistat; Conivaptan; CYP3A4 Inhibitors (Moderate); CYP3A4 Inhibitors (Strong); Dasatinib; Dronabinol; Droperidol; Fosaprepitant; Fusidic Acid (Systemic); Idelalisib; Ivacaftor; Kava Kava; Luliconazole; Magnesium Sulfate; Methotrimeprazine; Mifepristone; Nabilone; Netupitant; Perampanel; Rufinamide; Simeprevir; Sodium Oxybate; Stiripentol; Succinylcholine; Tapentadol; Tetrahydrocannabinol

Decreased Effect

Buprenorphine may decrease the levels/effects of: Atazanavir; Pegvisomant

The levels/effects of Buprenorphine may be decreased by: Ammonium Chloride; Boceprevir; Bosentan; CYP3A4 Inducers (Moderate); CYP3A4 Inducers (Strong); Dabrafenib; Deferasirox; Efavirenz; Etravirine; Mitotane; Naltrexone; Siltuximab; St Johns Wort; Tocilizumab

Storage/Stability

Injection: Protect from excessive heat >40°C (>104°F). Protect from light.

Patch, tablet: Store at room temperature of 25°C (77°F); excursions permitted between 15°C to 30°C (59°F to 86°F).

Mechanism of Action Buprenorphine exerts its analgesic effect via high affinity binding to μ opiate receptors in the CNS; displays partial mu agonist and weak kappa antagonist activity

Pharmacodynamics/Kinetics

Onset of action: Analgesic: IM: Within 15 minutes

Peak effect: IM: ~1 hour; Transdermal patch: Steady state achieved by day 3

Duration: IM: ≥6 hours

Absorption: IM, SubQ: 30% to 40%. Application of a heating pad onto the transdermal system may increase blood concentrations of buprenorphine 26% to 55%

Distribution: V_d: 97 to 187 L/kg

Protein binding: High (~96%, primarily to alpha- and beta globulin)

Metabolism: Primarily hepatic via N-dealkylation by CYP3A4 to norbuprenorphine (active metabolite), and to a lesser extent via glucuronidation by UGT1A1 and 2B7 to buprenorphine 3-O-glucuronide; the major metabolite, norbuprenorphine, also undergoes glucuronidation via UGT1A3; extensive first-pass effect

Bioavailability (relative to IV administration): IM: 70%; Sublingual tablet: 29%; Transdermal patch: ~15%

Half-life elimination: IV: 2.2 to 3 hours; Apparent terminal half-life: Sublingual tablet: ~37 hours; Transdermal patch: ~26 hours. **Note:** Extended elimination half-life for sublingual administration may be due to depot effect (Kuhlman, 1996).

Time to peak, plasma: Sublingual: 30 minutes to 1 hour (Kuhlman, 1996)

Excretion: Feces (~70%); urine (27% to 30%)

Dosage

IM, IV: Acute pain (moderate-to-severe): **Note: Long-term use is not recommended.** The following recommendations are guidelines and do not represent the maximum doses that may be required in all patients. Doses should be titrated to pain relief/prevention. In high-risk patients (eg, elderly, debilitated, presence of respiratory disease) and/or concurrent CNS depressant use, reduce dose by one-half. Buprenorphine has an analgesic ceiling.

Children 2 to 12 years: IM, slow IV: 2 to 6 **mcg**/kg every 4 to 6 hours

Children ≥13 years and Adults:

IM: Initial: Opioid-naive: 0.3 mg every 6 to 8 hours as needed; initial dose (up to 0.3 mg) may be repeated once in 30 to 60 minutes after the initial dose if needed; usual dosage range: 0.15 to 0.6 mg every 4 to 8 hours as needed

Slow IV: Initial: Opioid-naive: 0.3 mg every 6 to 8 hours as needed; initial dose (up to 0.3 mg) may be repeated once in 30 to 60 minutes after the initial dose if needed

Adults: IV infusion: Opioid withdrawal in heroin-dependent hospitalized patients (off-label): 0.3 to 0.9 mg (diluted in 50 to 100 mL of NS) over 20 to 30 minutes every 6 to 12 hours (Welsh, 2002)

Sublingual tablet: Children ≥16 years and Adults: Opioid dependence: **Note:** The combination product, buprenorphine and naloxone, is preferred therapy over buprenorphine monotherapy for induction treatment (and stabilization/maintenance treatment) for short-acting opioid dependence (U.S. Department of Health and Human Services, 2005).

Manufacturer's labeling:

Induction: Day 1: 8 mg; Day 2 and subsequent induction days: 16 mg; usual induction dosage range: 12 to 16 mg/day (induction usually accomplished over 3 to 4 days). Treatment should begin at least 4 hours after last use of heroin or other short-acting opioids, preferably when first signs of withdrawal appear. Titrating dose to clinical effectiveness should be done as rapidly as possible to prevent undue withdrawal symptoms and patient drop-out during the induction period. There is little controlled experience with induction in patients on methadone or other long-acting opioids; consult expert physician experienced with this procedure.

Maintenance: Target dose: 16 mg daily; in some patients 12 mg daily may be effective; patients should be switched to the buprenorphine/naloxone combination product for maintenance and unsupervised therapy

Transdermal patch: Adults: Chronic pain (moderate-to-severe):

Opioid-naive patients: Initial: 5 **mcg**/hour applied once every 7 days

Opioid-experienced patients (conversion from other opioids to buprenorphine): Discontinue all other around-the-clock opioid drugs when buprenorphine therapy is initiated. Short-acting analgesics as needed may be continued until analgesia with transdermal buprenorphine is attained. There is a potential for buprenorphine to precipitate withdrawal in patients already receiving opioids.

Patients who were receiving daily dose of <30 mg of oral morphine equivalents: Initial: 5 **mcg**/hour applied once every 7 days

Patients who were receiving daily dose of 30 to 80 mg of oral morphine equivalents: Taper the current around-the-clock opioid for up to 7 days to ≤30 mg/day of oral morphine or equivalent before initiating therapy. Initial: 10 **mcg**/hour applied once every 7 days

Patient who were receiving daily dose of >80 mg of oral morphine equivalents: Buprenorphine transdermal patch, even at the maximum dose of 20 **mcg**/hour applied once every 7 days, may not provide adequate analgesia; **consider the use of an alternate analgesic.**

Dose titration (opioid-naive or opioid-experienced patients): May increase dose, based on patient's supplemental short-acting analgesic requirements, with a minimum titration interval of 72 hours (maximum dose: 20 **mcg**/hour applied once every 7 days; risk for QTc prolongation increases with doses ≥20 **mcg**/hour patch).

Discontinuation of therapy: Taper dose gradually every 7 days to prevent withdrawal in the physically dependent patient; consider initiating immediate-release opioids, if needed.

Elderly:

IM, slow IV: 0.15 mg every 6 hours; elderly patients are more likely to suffer from confusion and drowsiness compared to younger patients

Transdermal patch: Chronic pain (moderate-to-severe): No specific dosage adjustments required; use caution due to potential for increased risk of adverse events. Refer to adult dosing.

Dosage adjustment in renal impairment: Injection, sublingual, transdermal: There are no dosage adjustments provided in the manufacturer's labeling (has not been adequately studied); use with caution.

Dosage adjustment in hepatic impairment:

Injection: There are no dosage adjustments provided in the manufacturer's labeling; undergoes extensive hepatic metabolism; use with caution, especially in severe impairment.

Sublingual:

Mild impairment: No dosage adjustment necessary.

Moderate impairment: No dosage adjustment necessary; use caution and monitor for signs and symptoms of toxicity or overdose.

Severe impairment: Consider reducing initial and titration incremental dose by 50%; monitor for signs and symptoms of toxicity or overdose.

Transdermal patch: Severe impairment: There are no dosage adjustments provided in the manufacturer's labeling (has not been studied); consider alternative therapy with more flexibility for dosing adjustments.

Administration

IM: Administer via deep IM injection

IV: Administer slowly, over at least 2 minutes. Administration over 20 to 30 minutes preferred when managing opioid withdrawal in heroin-dependent hospitalized patients (Welsh, 2002).

Oral: Sublingual tablet: Tablet should be placed under the tongue until dissolved; should not be swallowed. If two or more tablets are needed per dose, all may be placed under the tongue at once, or two at a time. To ensure consistent bioavailability, subsequent doses should always be taken the same way.

Transdermal patch: Apply patch to intact, nonirritated skin only. Apply to a hairless or nearly hairless skin site. If hairless site is not available, do not shave skin; hair at application site should be clipped. Prior to application, if the site must be cleaned, clean with clear water and allow to dry completely; do not use soaps, alcohol, oils, lotions, or abrasives due to potential for increased skin absorption. Do not use any patch that has been damaged, cut or manipulated in any way. Remove patch from protective pouch immediately before application. Remove the protective backing, and apply the sticky side of the patch to one of eight possible application sites (upper outer arm, upper chest, upper back or the side of the chest [each site on either side of the body]). Up to 2 patches may be applied at the same time adjacent to one another at the same application site. Firmly press patch in place and hold for ~15 seconds. Change patch every 7 days. Rotate patch application sites; wait ≥21 days before reapplying another patch to the same skin site. Avoid exposing application site to external heat sources (eg, heating pad, electric blanket, heat lamp, hot tub). Incidental exposure to water while bathing or showering is acceptable based on experience during clinical studies. If there is difficulty with patch adhesion, the edges of the system may be taped in place with first-aid tape. If ineffective, the system may be covered with waterproof or semipermeable adhesive dressings suitable for 7 days of wear. If the patch falls off during the 7-day dosing interval, dispose of the patch and apply a new patch to a different skin site. Dispose of patches using the Patch-Disposal Unit or by folding the adhesive sides of the patch together and then flushing down the toilet.

Monitoring Parameters Pain relief, respiratory and mental status, CNS depression (especially in elderly, debilitated or cachectic patients particularly during treatment initiation or titration, or when using concomitant CNS depressants), blood pressure (monitor for hypotension during initiation and titration); LFTs (prior to initiation and during therapy); signs of addiction, abuse, or misuse; symptoms of withdrawal; patients with biliary tract disease for worsening symptoms; application site reactions (transdermal patch); signs or symptoms of hypogonadism or hypoadrenalism (Brennan, 2013); signs and symptoms of toxicity or overdose (especially in patients with hepatic impairment).

Dosage Forms

Patch Weekly, Transdermal:

Butrans: 5 mcg/hr (4 ea); 7.5 mcg/hr (4 ea); 10 mcg/hr (4 ea); 15 mcg/hr (4 ea); 20 mcg/hr (4 ea)

Solution, Injection:

Buprenex: 0.3 mg/mL (1 mL)

Generic: 0.3 mg/mL (1 mL)

Tablet Sublingual, Sublingual:

Generic: 2 mg, 8 mg

Extemporaneous Preparations A 0.075 mg/mL solution can be made using the 0.3 mg/mL injection, 95% ethanol, and simple syrup. Add 1.26 mL of 95% ethanol to 0.3 mg buprenorphine obtained from an 0.3 mg/1 mL ampule, mix well, and add quantity of simple syrup sufficient to obtain 4 mL (final volume). Solution is stable under refrigeration and at room temperature for 30 days when stored in amber glass bottles and for 7 days when stored in oral syringes (Anagnostis, 2011; Anagnostis, 2013).

Anagnostis EA, Sadaka RE, Sailor LA, et al, "Formulation of Buprenorphine for Sublingual Use in Neonates," *J Pediatr Pharmacol Ther*, 2011, 16(4):281-4.

Anagnostis EA, personal communication, March 2013.

Buprenorphine and Naloxone

(byoo pre NOR feen & nal OKS one)

Brand Names: U.S. Bunavail; Suboxone; Zubsolv

Brand Names: Canada Suboxone

Index Terms Buprenorphine Hydrochloride and Naloxone Hydrochloride Dihydrate; Naloxone and Buprenorphine; Naloxone Hydrochloride Dihydrate and Buprenorphine Hydrochloride

Pharmacologic Category Analgesic, Opioid; Analgesic, Opioid Partial Agonist

Use

Opioid dependence: Treatment of opioid dependence.

General information: Buprenorphine/naloxone should be used as part of a complete treatment plan to include counseling and psychosocial support

Pregnancy Risk Factor C

Dosage Opioid dependence: Sublingual:

Adolescents ≥16 years and Adults:

Manufacturer's labeling: Induction:

Notes:

Buprenorphine/naloxone is not recommended for use during the induction period for long-acting opioids or methadone; initial treatment should begin using buprenorphine monotherapy under supervision. Patients should be switched to the combination product for maintenance and unsupervised therapy.

Buprenorphine/naloxone sublingual film product may be used during the induction period for short-acting opioids or heroin; initial treatment may begin using buprenorphine/naloxone sublingual film or buprenorphine sublingual monotherapy when signs of moderate opioid withdrawal appear and not less than 6 hours after last opioid use. Titrate to adequate maintenance dose as rapidly as possible based on control of acute withdrawal symptoms.

Sublingual film: Heroin or short-acting opioid dependency:

Day 1 induction dose: Initial: Buprenorphine 2 mg/naloxone 0.5 mg or buprenorphine 4 mg/naloxone 1 mg; may titrate dose, based on control of acute withdrawal symptoms, in increments of buprenorphine 2 mg/naloxone 0.5 mg or buprenorphine 4 mg/naloxone 1 mg approximately every 2 hours up to a total dose of buprenorphine 8 mg/naloxone 2 mg.

Day 2 induction dose: Up to buprenorphine 16 mg/naloxone 4 mg once daily

Manufacturer's labeling: Maintenance:

Buccal film (Bunavail: buprenorphine 2.1 mg/naloxone 0.3 mg, buprenorphine 4.2 mg/naloxone 0.7 mg, buprenorphine 6.3 mg/naloxone 1 mg): Target dose: Buprenorphine 8.4 mg/naloxone 1.4 mg once daily; dosage should be adjusted in increments/decrements of buprenorphine 2.1 mg/naloxone 0.3 mg to a level which maintains treatment and suppresses opioid withdrawal symptoms; usual range: Buprenorphine 2.1 to 12.6 mg/naloxone 0.3 to 2.1 mg once daily

Sublingual film and sublingual tablet (buprenorphine 2 mg/naloxone 0.5 mg and buprenorphine 8 mg/naloxone 2 mg): Target dose: Buprenorphine 16 mg/naloxone 4 mg once daily; dosage should be adjusted in increments/decrements of buprenorphine 2 mg/naloxone 0.5 mg or buprenorphine 4 mg/naloxone 1 mg to a level which maintains treatment and suppresses opioid withdrawal symptoms; usual range: Buprenorphine 4 to 24 mg/naloxone 1 to 6 mg once daily

Sublingual tablet (Zubsolv: buprenorphine 1.4 mg/naloxone 0.36 mg, buprenorphine 5.7 mg/naloxone 1.4 mg, buprenorphine 8.6 mg/naloxone 2.1 mg, or buprenorphine 11.4 mg/naloxone 2.9 mg): Target dose: buprenorphine 11.4 mg/naloxone 2.9 mg once daily; dosage should be adjusted in increments/decrements of buprenorphine 1.4 mg or 2.8 mg/naloxone 0.36 or 0.72 mg to a level which maintains treatment and suppresses opioid withdrawal symptoms; usual range: buprenorphine 2.8 to 17.2 mg/naloxone 0.72 to 4.2 mg once daily. The corresponding doses going from induction with buprenorphine sublingual tablets to maintenance treatment with Zubsolv are:

Final sublingual buprenorphine dose during induction: 8 mg: Zubsolv maintenance dose: Buprenorphine 5.7 mg/naloxone 1.4 mg once daily

Final sublingual buprenorphine dose during induction: 12 mg: Zubsolv maintenance dose: Buprenorphine 8.6 mg/naloxone 2.1 mg once daily

Final sublingual buprenorphine dose during induction: 16 mg: Zubsolv maintenance dose: Buprenorphine 11.4 mg/naloxone 2.9 mg once daily

Off-label dosing recommendations (U.S. Department of Health and Human Services, 2004): Doses provided based on buprenorphine content.

Induction (only administer combination product for induction in patients who are dependent on **short-acting** opioids and whose last dose of opioids was >12-24 hours prior to induction):

Day 1 induction dose: Initial: 4 mg; may repeat dose after >2 hours if withdrawal symptoms not relieved; maximum daily dose on day 1: 8 mg daily

Day 2 induction dose: Previous dose from day 1 if no withdrawal symptoms present; if symptoms of withdrawal present, increase day 1 dose by 4 mg. If withdrawal symptoms not relieved after >2 hours, may administer 4 mg; maximum daily dose on day 2: 16 mg daily

Subsequent induction days: If withdrawal symptoms are not present, daily dose is established. If withdrawal symptoms are present, increase dose in increments of 2 mg or 4 mg each day as needed for symptom relief. Target daily dose by the end of the first week: 12 mg or 16 mg daily; maximum daily dose: 32 mg daily

Stabilization: Usual dose: 16-24 mg daily; maximum dose: 32 mg daily

Switching between sublingual tablets and sublingual film: Same dosage should be used as the previous administered product. **Note:** Potential for greater bioavailability with certain sublingual film strengths compared to the same strength of the sublingual tablet; monitor closely for either over- or underdosing when switching patients from one formulation to another.

Switching between buccal film and sublingual tablets or films: Due to differences in the bioavailability of Bunavail buccal films compared to other buprenorphine/naloxone sublingual tablets, different strengths must be given to achieve equivalent doses. When switching between Bunavail and other sublingual tablets or films, corresponding dosage strengths are as follows:

Bunavail buprenorphine 2.1 mg/naloxone 0.3 mg = buprenorphine 4 mg/naloxone 1 mg sublingual tablets or films

Bunavail buprenorphine 4.2 mg/naloxone 0.7 mg = buprenorphine 8 mg/naloxone 2 mg sublingual tablets or films

Bunavail buprenorphine 6.3 mg/naloxone 1 mg = buprenorphine 12 mg/naloxone 3 mg sublingual tablets or films

Switching between sublingual film strengths: Systemic exposure may be different with various combinations of sublingual film strengths; pharmacists should not substitute one or more film strengths for another (eg, switching from three buprenorphine 4 mg/naloxone 1 mg films to a single buprenorphine 12 mg/naloxone 3 mg film, or vice-versa) without health care provider approval, and patients should be monitored closely for either over- or underdosing when switching between film strengths.

Switching between sublingual tablet products: Due to differences in the bioavailability of Zubsolv sublingual tablets compared to other buprenorphine/naloxone sublingual tablets, different strengths must be given to achieve equivalent doses. When switching between Zubsolv and other sublingual tablets, corresponding dosage strengths are as follows:

Zubsolv buprenorphine 1.4 mg/naloxone 0.36 mg sublingual tablets = buprenorphine 2 mg/naloxone 0.5 mg sublingual tablets

Zubsolv buprenorphine 5.7 mg/naloxone 1.4 mg sublingual tablets = buprenorphine 8 mg/naloxone 2 mg sublingual tablets

Zubsolv buprenorphine 8.6 mg/naloxone 2.1 mg sublingual tablet = buprenorphine 12 mg/naloxone 3 mg sublingual tablets (as one buprenorphine 8 mg/naloxone 2 mg sublingual tablet and two buprenorphine 2 mg/naloxone 0.5 mg sublingual tablets)

Zubsolv buprenorphine 11.4 mg/naloxone 2.9 mg sublingual tablet = buprenorphine 16 mg/naloxone 4 mg sublingual tablets (as two buprenorphine 8 mg/naloxone 2 mg sublingual tablets)

Dosage adjustment in renal impairment: There are no dosage adjustments provided in the manufacturer's labeling (has not been adequately studied). Use with caution.

Dosing adjustment in hepatic impairment:

Mild hepatic impairment: No dosage adjustment necessary.

Moderate hepatic impairment: Use with caution during maintenance treatment (due to extensive metabolism of buprenorphine and naloxone, use may not be appropriate). Suboxone use is not recommended during induction therapy.

Severe hepatic impairment: Use is not recommended.

Additional Information Complete prescribing information should be consulted for additional detail.

Product Availability Zubsolv new SL tablet strengths (8.6 mg/2.1 mg; 11.4 mg/2.9 mg): FDA approved December 2014; availability of the 8.6 mg/2.1 mg strength is anticipated in early 2015 and availability of the 11.4 mg/2.9 mg strength is anticipated later in 2015.

Dosage Forms

Film, buccal:

Bunavail: Buprenorphine 2.1 mg and naloxone 0.3 mg; buprenorphine 4.2 mg and naloxone 0.7 mg; buprenorphine 6.3 mg and naloxone 1 mg

Film, sublingual:

Suboxone: Buprenorphine 2 mg and naloxone 0.5 mg; buprenorphine 4 mg and naloxone 1 mg; buprenorphine 8 mg and naloxone 2 mg; buprenorphine 12 mg and naloxone 3 mg

Tablet, sublingual: Buprenorphine 2 mg and naloxone 0.5 mg; buprenorphine 8 mg and naloxone 2 mg

Zubsolv: Buprenorphine 1.4 mg and naloxone 0.36 mg; buprenorphine 5.7 mg and naloxone 1.4 mg

◆ **Buprenorphine Hydrochloride** *see* Buprenorphine *on page 300*

◆ **Buprenorphine Hydrochloride and Naloxone Hydrochloride Dihydrate** *see* Buprenorphine and Naloxone *on page 304*

◆ **Buproban** *see* BuPROPion *on page 305*

BuPROPion (byoo PROE pee on)

Brand Names: U.S. Aplenzin; Budeprion SR [DSC]; Buproban; Forfivo XL; Wellbutrin; Wellbutrin SR; Wellbutrin XL; Zyban

Brand Names: Canada Ava-Bupropion SR; Bupropion SR; Mylan-Bupropion XL; Novo-Bupropion SR; PMS-Bupropion SR; ratio-Bupropion SR; Sandoz-Bupropion SR; Wellbutrin SR; Wellbutrin XL; Zyban

Index Terms Bupropion Hydrobromide; Bupropion Hydrochloride

Pharmacologic Category Antidepressant, Dopamine/Norepinephrine-Reuptake Inhibitor; Smoking Cessation Aid

Use

Major depressive disorder (Aplenzin, Forfivo XL, Wellbutrin, Wellbutrin SR, Wellbutrin XL): Treatment of major depressive disorder (MDD).

Seasonal affective disorder (Aplenzin, Wellbutrin XL): Prevention of seasonal major depressive episodes in patients with a diagnosis of seasonal affective disorder (SAD).

Smoking cessation (Buproban and Zyban): As an aid to smoking cessation treatment.

Pregnancy Risk Factor C

Pregnancy Considerations Adverse events have been observed in some animal reproduction studies. Bupropion and its metabolites were found to cross the placenta in *in vitro* studies (Earhart, 2012). An increased risk of congenital malformations has not been observed following maternal use of bupropion during pregnancy; however, data specific to cardiovascular malformations is inconsistent. The long-term effects on development and behavior have not been studied. The ACOG recommends that antidepressant therapy during pregnancy be individualized; treatment of depression during pregnancy should incorporate the clinical expertise of the mental health clinician, obstetrician, primary healthcare provider, and pediatrician. According to the American Psychiatric Association (APA), the risks of medication treatment should be weighed against other treatment options and untreated depression. For women who discontinue antidepressant medications during pregnancy and who may be at high risk for postpartum depression, the medications can be restarted following delivery. Treatment algorithms have been developed by the ACOG and the APA for the management of depression in women prior to conception and during pregnancy (ACOG, 2008; APA, 2010; Yonkers, 2009). There is insufficient information related to the use of bupropion to recommend use in pregnancy (ACOG, 2010).

Breast-Feeding Considerations Bupropion and its metabolites are excreted into breast milk. The estimated dose to a nursing infant varies by study and has been reported as ~2% of the weight-adjusted maternal dose (range: 1.4% to 10.6%) (Davis, 2009; Haas, 2004). Adverse events have been reported with some antidepressants and a seizure was noted in one 6-month old nursing infant exposed to bupropion (a causal effect could not be confirmed) (Chaudron, 2004; Hale, 2010). Recommendations for use in nursing women vary by manufacturer labeling.

Contraindications Hypersensitivity to bupropion or any component of the formulation; seizure disorder; history of anorexia/bulimia; patients undergoing abrupt discontinuation of ethanol or sedatives, including benzodiazepines, barbiturates, or antiepileptic drugs; use of MAO inhibitors or MAO inhibitors intended to treat psychiatric disorders (concurrently or within 14 days of discontinuing either bupropion or the MAO inhibitor); initiation of bupropion in a patient receiving linezolid or intravenous methylene blue; patients receiving other dosage forms of bupropion

Aplenzin, Wellbutrin XL: Additional contraindications: Other conditions that increase seizure risk, including arteriovenous malformation, severe head injury, severe stroke, CNS tumor, CNS infection

Warnings/Precautions [U.S. Boxed Warning]: Use in treating psychiatric disorders: Antidepressants increase the risk of suicidal thinking and behavior in children, adolescents, and young adults (18 to 24 years of age) with major depressive disorder (MDD) and other psychiatric disorders; consider risk prior to prescribing. Short-term studies did not show an increased risk in patients >24 years of age and showed a decreased risk in patients ≥65 years. All patients must be closely monitored for clinical worsening, suicidality, or unusual changes in behavior, especially during the initiation of therapy (generally first 1 to 2 months) or following an increase or decrease in dosage. The patient's family or caregiver should be instructed to closely observe the patient and communicate condition with healthcare provider. A medication guide should be dispensed with each prescription.

[U.S. Boxed Warning]: Use in smoking cessation: Serious neuropsychiatric events have occurred in patients taking bupropion for smoking cessation, including changes in mood (eg, depression, mania), psychosis, hallucinations, paranoia, delusions, homicidal ideation, hostility, agitation, aggression, anxiety, panic, suicidal ideation, suicide attempt and completed suicide. **The majority occurred during bupropion treatment; some occurred during treatment discontinuation. A causal relationship is uncertain as depressed mood may be a symptom of nicotine withdrawal. Some cases also occurred in patients taking bupropion who continued to smoke. Observe all patients taking bupropion for neuropsychiatric reactions. Instruct patients to contact a health care provider if neuropsychiatric reactions occur.**

The possibility of a suicide attempt is inherent in major depression and may persist until remission occurs. Worsening depression and severe abrupt suicidality that are not part of the presenting symptoms may require discontinuation or modification of drug therapy. Use caution in high-risk patients during initiation of therapy. Prescriptions should be written for the smallest quantity consistent with good patient care. The patient's family or caregiver should be alerted to monitor patients for the emergence of suicidality and associated behaviors such as anxiety, agitation, panic attacks, insomnia, irritability, hostility, impulsivity, akathisia, hypomania, and mania; patients should be instructed to notify their healthcare provider if any of these symptoms or worsening depression or psychosis occur.

May cause delusions, hallucinations, psychosis, concentration disturbance, paranoia, and confusion; most common in depressed patients and patients with a diagnosis of bipolar disorder. Symptoms may abate with dose reduction and/or withdrawal of treatment. May precipitate a manic, mixed, or hypomanic episode; risk is increased in patients with bipolar disorder or who have risk factors for bipolar disorder. Screen patients for a history of bipolar disorder and the presence of risk factors including a family history of bipolar disorder, suicide, or depression. **Bupropion is not FDA approved for bipolar depression.**

May cause a dose-related risk of seizures. Use is contraindicated in patients with a history of seizures or certain conditions with high seizure risk (eg, arteriovenous malformation, severe head injury, severe stroke, CNS tumor, or CNS infection, history of anorexia/bulimia, or patients undergoing abrupt discontinuation of ethanol, benzodiazepines, barbiturates, or antiepileptic drugs). Use caution with concurrent use of antipsychotics, antidepressants, theophylline, systemic corticosteroids, stimulants (including cocaine), anorectants, or hypoglycemic agents, or with excessive use of ethanol, benzodiazepines, sedative/hypnotics, or opioids. Use with caution in seizure-potentiating metabolic disorders (hypoglycemia, hyponatremia, severe hepatic impairment, and hypoxia). The dose-dependent risk of seizures may be reduced by gradual dose increases and by not exceeding the maximum daily dose. Use of multiple bupropion formulations is contraindicated. Permanently discontinue if seizure occurs during therapy. Chewing, crushing, or dividing long-acting products may increase seizure risk.

May cause CNS stimulation (restlessness, anxiety, insomnia) or anorexia. May increase the risks associated with electroconvulsive therapy (ECT). Consider discontinuing, when possible, prior to ECT. May cause weight loss; use caution in patients where weight loss is not desirable. The incidence of sexual dysfunction with bupropion is generally lower than with SSRIs.

May elevate blood pressure and cause hypertension. Events have been observed in patients with or without evidence of preexisting hypertension. The risk is increased when used concomitantly with monoamine oxidase inhibitors, nicotine replacement, or other drugs that increase dopaminergic or noradrenergic activity. Assess blood pressure before treatment and monitor periodically. Use caution in patients with cardiovascular disease. All children diagnosed with ADHD who may be candidates for stimulant medications should have a thorough cardiovascular assessment to identify risk factors for sudden cardiac death prior to initiation of drug therapy. Use with caution in patients with hepatic or renal dysfunction and in elderly patients; reduced dose and/or frequency may be recommended; Forfivo XL is not recommended in patients with hepatic or renal impairment. Elderly patients may be at greater risk of accumulation during chronic dosing. May cause motor or cognitive impairment in some patients; use with caution if tasks requiring alertness such as operating machinery or driving are undertaken. May cause mild pupillary dilation, which in susceptible individuals can lead to an episode of narrow-angle glaucoma. Consider evaluating patients who have not had an iridectomy for narrow-angle glaucoma risk factors. Anaphylactoid/anaphylactic reactions have occurred, with symptoms of pruritus, urticaria, angioedema, and dyspnea. Serious reactions have been (rarely) reported, including erythema multiforme,

Stevens-Johnson syndrome and anaphylactic shock. Arthralgia, myalgia, and fever with rash and other symptoms suggestive of delayed hypersensitivity resembling serum sickness have been reported. Potentially significant drug-drug interactions may exist, requiring dose or frequency adjustment, additional monitoring, and/or selection of alternative therapy.

Extended release tablet: Insoluble tablet shell may remain intact and be visible in the stool.

Adverse Reactions

Cardiovascular: Cardiac arrhythmia, chest pain, flushing, hypertension, hypotension, palpitations, tachycardia

Central nervous system: Abnormal dreams, agitation, akathisia, anxiety, central nervous system stimulation, confusion, depression, dizziness, drowsiness, headache, hostility, insomnia, irritability, memory impairment, migraine, nervousness, pain, paresthesia, sensory disturbance, sleep disorder, twitching

Dermatologic: Diaphoresis, pruritus, skin rash, urticaria

Endocrine & metabolic: Decreased libido, hot flash, menstrual disease, weight gain, weight loss

Gastrointestinal: Abdominal pain, anorexia, increased appetite, constipation, diarrhea, dysgeusia, dyspepsia, dysphagia, flatulence, nausea, vomiting, xerostomia

Genitourinary: Urinary tract infection, urinary urgency, vaginal hemorrhage

Hypersensitivity: Hypersensitivity reaction (including anaphylaxis, pruritus, urticaria)

Infection: Infection

Neuromuscular & skeletal: Arthralgia, arthritis, myalgia, neck pain, tremor, weakness

Ophthalmic: Amblyopia, blurred vision

Otic: Auditory disturbance, tinnitus

Renal: Polyuria

Respiratory: Cough, pharyngitis, sinusitis, upper respiratory infection

Miscellaneous: Fever

Rare but important or life-threatening:Abnormal accommodation, akinesia, alopecia, amnesia, anaphylactic shock, anaphylactoid reaction, anemia, angioedema, aphasia, ataxia, atrioventricular block, cerebrovascular accident, colitis, coma, cystitis, deafness, delayed hypersensitivity, delirium, delusions, depersonalization, derealization, diplopia, dysarthria, dyskinesia, dyspareunia, dysphoria, dystonia, dysuria, edema, EEG pattern changes, erythema multiforme, esophagitis, euphoria, exfoliative dermatitis, extrapyramidal reaction, extrasystoles, facial edema, gastric ulcer, gastroesophageal reflux disease, gastrointestinal hemorrhage, gingival hemorrhage, glossitis, glycosuria, gynecomastia, hallucination, hepatic injury, hepatic insufficiency, hepatitis, hirsutism, hyperglycemia, hyperkinesia, hypertonia, hypoglycemia, hypokinesia, hypomania, impotence, increased intraocular pressure, increased libido, intestinal perforation, jaundice, leukocytosis, leukopenia, lymphadenopathy, manic behavior, myasthenia, mydriasis, myocardial infarction, myoclonus, neuralgia, neuropathy, orthostatic hypotension, painful erection, pancreatitis, pancytopenia, paranoia, pneumonia, psychiatric signs and symptoms, pulmonary embolism, rhabdomyolysis, salpingitis, sciatica, seizure (dose-related), SIADH, skin photosensitivity, Stevens-Johnson syndrome, stomatitis, suicidal ideation, syncope, tardive dyskinesia, thrombocytopenia, tongue edema, urinary incontinence, urinary retention, vasodilatation

Drug Interactions

Metabolism/Transport Effects **Substrate** of CYP1A2 (minor), CYP2A6 (minor), CYP2B6 (major), CYP2C9 (minor), CYP2D6 (minor), CYP2E1 (minor), CYP3A4 (minor); **Note:** Assignment of Major/Minor substrate status based on clinically relevant drug interaction potential; **Inhibits** CYP2D6 (strong), OCT2

Avoid Concomitant Use

Avoid concomitant use of BuPROPion with any of the following: MAO Inhibitors; Pimozide; Tamoxifen; Thioridazine

Increased Effect/Toxicity

BuPROPion may increase the levels/effects of: Alcohol (Ethyl); ARIPiprazole; AtoMOXetine; Citalopram; CYP2D6 Substrates; DOXOrubicin (Conventional); Eliglustat; Fesoterodine; FLUoxetine; FluvoxaMINE; Iloperidone; Lorcaserin; Metoprolol; Nebivolol; OCT2 Substrates; PARoxetine; Pimozide; Propafenone; Tetrabenazine; Thioridazine; Tricyclic Antidepressants; Vortioxetine

The levels/effects of BuPROPion may be increased by: Alcohol (Ethyl); Anti-Parkinson's Agents (Dopamine Agonist); CYP2B6 Inhibitors (Moderate); MAO Inhibitors; Mifepristone; Quazepam

Decreased Effect

BuPROPion may decrease the levels/effects of: Codeine; Iloperidone; Ioflupane I 123; Tamoxifen; TraMADol

The levels/effects of BuPROPion may be decreased by: CYP2B6 Inducers (Strong); Dabrafenib; Efavirenz; Lopinavir; Ritonavir

Storage/Stability

Store at 15°C to 30°C (59°F to 86°F).

Wellbutrin, Wellbutrin XL, Zyban: Protect from light and moisture.

Mechanism of Action Aminoketone antidepressant structurally different from all other marketed antidepressants; like other antidepressants the mechanism of bupropion's activity is not fully understood. Bupropion is a relatively weak inhibitor of the neuronal uptake of norepinephrine and dopamine, and does not inhibit monoamine oxidase or the reuptake of serotonin. Metabolite inhibits the reuptake of norepinephrine. The primary mechanism of action is thought to be dopaminergic and/or noradrenergic.

Pharmacodynamics/Kinetics

Absorption: Rapid

Distribution: V_d: ~20 to 47 L/kg (Laizure, 1985)

Protein binding: 84%

Metabolism: Extensively hepatic via CYP2B6 to hydroxybupropion; non-CYP-mediated metabolism to erythrohydrobupropion and threohydrobupropion. Metabolite activity ranges from 20% to 50% potency of bupropion.

Half-life:

Distribution: 3 to 4 hours

Elimination: ~21 hours after chronic dosing (range: 12 to 30 hours); Metabolites (after a single dose): Hydroxybupropion: 20 ± 5 hours; Erythrohydrobupropion: 33 ± 10 hours; Threohydrobupropion: 37 ± 13 hours

Extended release (Aplenzin): 21 ± 7 hours; Metabolites: Hydroxybupropion: 24 ± 5 hours; Erythrohydrobupropion: 31 ± 8 hours; Threohydrobupropion: 51 ± 9 hours

Time to peak, serum:

Bupropion: Immediate release: Within 2 hours; Sustained release: Within 3 hours; Extended release: ~5 hours (Forfivo XL: 5 hours [fasting]; 12 hours [fed])

Metabolite: Hydroxybupropion: Immediate release: ~3 hours; Extended release, sustained release: ~6 to 7 hours

Excretion: Urine (87%, primarily as metabolites); feces (10%, primarily as metabolites)

Dosage Oral:

Children and Adolescents: ADHD (off-label use): Hydrochloride salt: 1.4 to 6 mg/kg/day (Barrickman, 1995; Conners, 1996)

Adults:

Depression: **Note:** Treatment should be periodically evaluated at appropriate intervals to ensure lowest effective dose is used.

Immediate release hydrochloride salt: Initial: 100 mg twice daily; after 3 days may increase to the usual dose of 100 mg 3 times a day; if no clinical improvement after several weeks, may increase to a maximum dose of 450 mg daily in 3 or 4 divided doses; do not exceed 150 mg in a single dose

Sustained release hydrochloride salt: Initial: 150 mg daily in the morning; if tolerated, after 3 days, may increase to a target dose of 150 mg twice daily; if no clinical improvement after several weeks, may increase to a maximum dose of 200 mg twice daily

Extended release:

Hydrochloride salt (Wellbutrin XL): Initial: 150 mg once daily in the morning; if tolerated, as early as day 4, may increase to a maximum of 300 mg once daily. **Note:** Forfivo XL may only be used after initial dose titration with other bupropion products.

Hydrochloride salt (Forfivo XL): *Switching from Wellbutrin immediate release, SR, or XL to Forfivo XL:* Patients receiving 300 mg daily of bupropion hydrochloride for at least 2 weeks and requiring a dose increase or patients already taking 450 mg daily of bupropion hydrochloride may switch to Forfivo XL 450 mg once daily.

Hydrobromide salt (Aplenzin): Initial: 174 mg once daily in the morning; may increase as early as day 4 of dosing to 348 mg once daily (target dose); maximum dose: 522 mg daily.

Switching from hydrochloride salt formulation (eg, Wellbutrin immediate release, SR, XL, or Forfivo XL) to hydrobromide salt formulation (Aplenzin):

Bupropion hydrochloride 150 mg daily is equivalent to bupropion hydrobromide 174 mg once daily

Bupropion hydrochloride 300 mg daily is equivalent to bupropion hydrobromide 348 mg once daily

Bupropion hydrochloride 450 mg daily is equivalent to bupropion hydrobromide 522 mg once daily

SAD: Initial: 150 mg once daily (Wellbutrin XL) or 174 mg once daily (Aplenzin) in the morning; if tolerated, may increase after 1 week to 300 mg once daily (Wellbutrin XL) or 348 mg once daily (Aplenzin) in the morning.

Note: Prophylactic treatment should be reserved for those patients with frequent depressive episodes and/or significant impairment. Initiate treatment in the Autumn prior to symptom onset, and discontinue in early Spring with dose tapering. Doses >300 mg daily (Wellbutrin XL) or >348 mg daily (Aplenzin) have not been studied in SAD (maximum dose: Wellbutrin XL 300 mg daily; Aplenzin 522 mg daily).

Smoking cessation (Zyban, Buproban): Initial: 150 mg once daily; increase to 150 mg twice daily with at least 8 hours between doses; treatment should continue for 7 to 12 weeks (maximum dose: 300 mg daily).

Note: Therapy should begin at least 1 week before target quit date. Target quit dates are generally in the second week of treatment. If patient successfully quits smoking after 7 to 12 weeks, may consider ongoing maintenance therapy based on individual patient risk:benefit. Efficacy of maintenance therapy (300 mg daily) has been demonstrated for up to 6 months. Conversely, if significant progress has not been made by the seventh week of therapy, success is unlikely and treatment discontinuation should be considered.

Elderly:

Depression: Oral (hydrochloride salt): Initial: 37.5 mg of immediate release tablets twice daily or 100 mg daily of sustained release tablets; increase by 37.5 to 100 mg every 3 to 4 days as tolerated to a maximum dose of 300 mg daily (in divided doses). There is evidence that the elderly respond at 150 mg daily in divided doses, but some may require a higher dose. **Note:** Patients with Alzheimer's dementia-related depression may require a lower starting dosage of 37.5 mg once or twice daily (100 mg daily sustained release), increased as needed up to 300 mg daily in divided doses (300 mg daily for sustained release) (Rabins, 2007).

Smoking cessation: Refer to adult dosing.

Dosing conversion between hydrochloride salt immediate (Wellbutrin), sustained (Wellbutrin SR), and extended release (Wellbutrin XL, Forfivo XL) products: Convert using same total daily dose (up to the maximum recommended dose for a given dosage form), but adjust frequency as indicated for sustained (twice daily) or extended (once daily) release products.

Discontinuation of therapy: Upon discontinuation of antidepressant therapy, gradually taper the dose to allow for the detection of re-emerging symptoms. Withdrawal symptoms resulting from abrupt discontinuation are unlikely because bupropion has minimal serotonergic activity (APA, 2010).

Manufacturer recommendations:

Aplenzin: In patients receiving 348 mg once daily, taper dose down to 174 mg once daily for 2 weeks prior to discontinuing.

Wellbutrin XL: In patients receiving 300 mg once daily, taper dose down to 150 mg once daily for 2 weeks prior to discontinuing.

MAO inhibitor recommendations:

Switching to or from an MAO inhibitor antidepressant:

Allow 14 days to elapse between discontinuing an MAO inhibitor intended to treat depression and initiation of bupropion.

Allow 14 days to elapse between discontinuing bupropion and initiation of an MAO inhibitor intended to treat depression.

Use with reversible MAO inhibitors (such as linezolid or IV methylene blue):

Do not initiate bupropion in patients receiving linezolid or IV methylene blue; consider other interventions for psychiatric condition.

If urgent treatment with linezolid or IV methylene blue is required in a patient already receiving bupropion and potential benefits outweigh potential risks, discontinue bupropion promptly and administer linezolid or IV methylene blue. Monitor for increased risk of hypertensive reactions for 2 weeks or until 24 hours after the last dose of linezolid or IV methylene blue, whichever comes first. May resume bupropion 24 hours after the last dose of linezolid or IV methylene blue.

Dosage adjustment in renal impairment: Use with caution; manufacturer's labeling suggests a reduction in dose and/or frequency be considered but does not provide specific dosing recommendations. Aplenzin, Wellbutrin, Wellbutrin SR, Wellbutrin XL, and Zyban product labeling defines renal impairment as GFR <90 mL/minute.

Forfivo XL: Use is not recommended.

Dosage adjustment in hepatic impairment:

Mild impairment (Child-Pugh score 5 to 6): Use with caution; manufacturer's labeling suggests a reduction in dose and/or frequency be considered but does not provide specific dosing recommendations.

Forfivo XL: Use is not recommended.

Moderate to severe impairment, including severe hepatic cirrhosis (Child-Pugh score 7 to 15): Use with extreme caution; maximum dose:

Aplenzin: 174 mg every other day

Buproban: Severe hepatic cirrhosis: 150 mg every other day

Forfivo XL: Use is not recommended.
Wellbutrin: 75 mg once daily
Wellbutrin SR: 100 mg once daily or 150 mg every other day
Wellbutrin XL, Zyban: 150 mg every other day

Administration

May be taken without regard to meals. The manufacturer states that tablets should be swallowed whole; do not crush, chew, or divide.

Extended release: Administer once daily with at least 24 hours between successive doses.

Immediate release: Administer 3 to 4 times daily with at least 6 hours between successive doses; do not exceed 150 mg in a single dose.

Sustained release: Administer 2 times daily with at least 8 hours between successive doses.

Monitoring Parameters Body weight; mental status for depression, suicidal ideation (especially at the beginning of therapy or when doses are increased or decreased), anxiety, social functioning, mania, panic attacks; blood pressure (baseline and periodically especially when used in conjunction with nicotine transdermal replacement); renal and hepatic function

When used for the treatment of ADHD, thoroughly evaluate for cardiovascular risk. Monitor heart rate, blood pressure, and consider obtaining ECG prior to initiation (Vetter, 2008).

Reference Range Therapeutic levels (trough, 12 hours after last dose): 50 to 100 ng/mL

Additional Information Risk of seizures: When using bupropion hydrochloride immediate release tablets, seizure risk is increased at total daily dosage >450 mg, individual dosages >150 mg, or by sudden, large increments in dose. Data for the immediate-release formulation of bupropion revealed a seizure incidence of 0.4% in patients treated at doses in the 300-450 mg/day range. The estimated seizure incidence increases almost 10-fold between 450 mg and 600 mg per day. Data for the sustained release dosage form revealed a seizure incidence of 0.1% in patients treated at a dosage range of 100-300 mg/day, and increases to ~0.4% at the maximum recommended dose of 400 mg/day.

Dosage Forms

Tablet, Oral:
Wellbutrin: 75 mg, 100 mg
Generic: 75 mg, 100 mg

Tablet Extended Release 12 Hour, Oral:
Buproban: 150 mg
Wellbutrin SR: 100 mg, 150 mg, 200 mg
Zyban: 150 mg
Generic: 100 mg, 150 mg, 200 mg

Tablet Extended Release 24 Hour, Oral:
Aplenzin: 174 mg, 348 mg, 522 mg
Forfivo XL: 450 mg
Wellbutrin XL: 150 mg, 300 mg
Generic: 150 mg, 300 mg

Dosage Forms: Canada Refer to Dosage Forms. **Note:** Aplenzin, Buproban, and Forfivo XL are not available in Canada.

- ◆ **Bupropion and Naltrexone** *see* Naltrexone and Bupropion *on page 1423*
- ◆ **Bupropion Hydrobromide** *see* BuPROPion *on page 305*
- ◆ **Bupropion Hydrochloride** *see* BuPROPion *on page 305*
- ◆ **Bupropion Hydrochloride and Naltrexone Hydrochloride** *see* Naltrexone and Bupropion *on page 1423*
- ◆ **Bupropion SR (Can)** *see* BuPROPion *on page 305*
- ◆ **Burinex (Can)** *see* Bumetanide *on page 297*
- ◆ **Buscopan (Can)** *see* Scopolamine (Systemic) *on page 1870*

Buserelin [CAN/INT] (BYOO se rel in)

Brand Names: Canada Suprefact; Suprefact Depot

Index Terms Buserelin Acetate

Pharmacologic Category Gonadotropin Releasing Hormone Agonist

Use Note: Not approved in U.S.

Prostate cancer: Palliative treatment in patients with hormone-dependent advanced prostate cancer (stage D)

Endometriosis: Treatment of endometriosis in women who do not require surgical intervention as first-line therapy (length of therapy is usually 6 months, but no longer than 9 months)

Pregnancy Considerations Buserelin is contraindicated in pregnant women. Patients should employ a nonhormonal method of contraception during therapy. To exclude preexisting pregnancy, begin treatment on the first or second day of menses; if there is doubt, a pregnancy test is recommended. Ovulation may occur with a missed dose; in the event a patient conceives, therapy should be discontinued.

Breast-Feeding Considerations Small amounts of buserelin can be detected in breast milk. Contains benzyl alcohol, which has been associated with gasping syndrome in premature infants. Breast-feeding is contraindicated by the manufacturer.

Contraindications Hypersensitivity to buserelin or any component of the formulation; patients with nonhormone-dependent prostate cancer; patients who have undergone orchiectomy; patients with undiagnosed abnormal vaginal bleeding; pregnancy; breast-feeding

Warnings/Precautions Hazardous agent - use appropriate precautions for handling and disposal (meets NIOSH 2014 criteria). Reactions including allergic asthma with dyspnea, as well as anaphylactic/anaphylactoid shock, have been observed in buserelin treated patients. Transient worsening of signs and symptoms may develop during the first few weeks of treatment. Adjunctive anti-androgen therapy is recommended for patients with prostate cancer to minimize exacerbations. Caution and close monitoring should be used in patients with vertebral metastases who are at risk for lesion exacerbation with possible spinal cord compression; initiate antiandrogen therapy 7 days prior to beginning buserelin therapy and continue for 5 weeks with buserelin therapy. Reversal of hypogonadism induced by therapy has not been established in this patient population. Testosterone suppression is associated with the development of anemia. Monitor for signs of urinary obstruction or retention. Androgen-deprivation therapy may increase the risk for cardiovascular disease (Levine, 2010). Androgen deprivation may increase the QT interval (on ECG); consider benefit/risk ratio in patients with congenital long QT syndrome, concomitant antiarrhythmic therapy, or heart failure. Oral contraceptives should be discontinued prior to starting therapy; use of a nonhormonal contraceptive is recommended. Bone density changes may occur; patients at risk for reduced bone density include those with chronic alcohol and/or tobacco use, family history of osteoporosis, and chronic treatment with anticonvulsants or corticosteroids. Use of buserelin for >6 months or in association with other risk factors may contribute to additional bone loss. Use with caution in patients with hypertension, diabetes, or depression. Patients must be cautioned about performing tasks which require mental alertness (eg, operating machinery or driving). The development of pituitary adenomas may rarely be seen with long-term therapy.

Adverse Reactions Note: Adverse reaction profile differs based on population/medication and route of administration.

Cardiovascular: Edema, hypertension, palpitations, peripheral edema

Central nervous system: Anxiety, depression, dizziness, emotional lability, headache, hostility, insomnia, malaise, nervousness, pain, sleep disorder

Dermatologic: Acne vulgaris (endometriosis), dermatological reaction, diaphoresis, pruritus, urticaria at injection site (subcutaneous), xeroderma

Endocrine & metabolic: Decreased libido (more common in endometriosis), gynecomastia (prostatic cancer), hirsutism (endometriosis), hot flash, hypermenorrhea (endometriosis), increased testosterone level (clinical flare; prostatic cancer), loss of libido (prostatic cancer), menstrual disease (endometriosis), premenstrual syndrome (endometriosis), weight gain, weight loss

Gastrointestinal: Constipation, diarrhea, dysgeusia, flatulence, gastrointestinal distress, gastrointestinal fullness, increased appetite, nausea, sore throat, vomiting, xerostomia

Genitourinary: Dyspareunia (endometriosis), impotence (prostatic cancer), leukorrhea (endometriosis), mastalgia (endometriosis), pelvic pain (endometriosis), vaginal discharge (endometriosis), vaginal discomfort (endometriosis), vaginal dryness (endometriosis), vaginitis (endometriosis)

Hematologic & oncologic: Purpura

Infection: Infection

Local: Application site irritation (intranasal), application site reaction (intranasal), injection site reaction (subcutaneous), irritation at injection site (subcutaneous), pain at injection site (subcutaneous), swelling at injection site (subcutaneous)

Neuromuscular & skeletal: Arthralgia, back pain, limb pain, myalgia, neck stiffness, weakness

Respiratory: Dry nose (intranasal), nasal mucosa irritation (intranasal), rhinitis, upper respiratory tract infection

Rare but important or life-threatening: Accommodation disturbance, amnesia, anemia, anorexia, arthritis, bleeding at injection site, breast atrophy (endometriosis), breast hypertrophy (endometriosis), cardiac failure, dyslipidemia, ejaculatory disorder (prostatic cancer), extrinsic asthma, fecal incontinence, feminization (prostatic cancer), hyperalgesia, hyperglycemia, hypersensitivity reaction, increased acid phosphatase (transient), increased plasma estradiol concentration (endometriosis; transient), increased serum bilirubin, increased serum transaminases, lactation (endometriosis; female), leukopenia, myelofibrosis, ovarian cyst (endometriosis; during initial phase of therapy), pituitary neoplasm, skin photosensitivity, suicidal tendencies, syncope, tachycardia, testicular atrophy (prostatic cancer), thrombocytopenia, thrombosis, transient blindness (one eye), urinary retention, vaginal hemorrhage (endometriosis)

Drug Interactions

Metabolism/Transport Effects None known.

Avoid Concomitant Use

Avoid concomitant use of Buserelin with any of the following: Corifollitropin Alfa; Highest Risk QTc-Prolonging Agents; Indium 111 Capromab Pendetide; Ivabradine; Mifepristone

Increased Effect/Toxicity

Buserelin may increase the levels/effects of: Corifollitropin Alfa; Highest Risk QTc-Prolonging Agents; Moderate Risk QTc-Prolonging Agents

The levels/effects of Buserelin may be increased by: Ivabradine; Mifepristone; QTc-Prolonging Agents (Indeterminate Risk and Risk Modifying)

Decreased Effect

Buserelin may decrease the levels/effects of: Antidiabetic Agents; Indium 111 Capromab Pendetide

Storage/Stability Store in original container. Do not freeze. Protect from light.

Injection: Store at 15°C to 25°C (59°F to 77°F); protect from heat; After opening, may keep for up to 14 days at room temperature.

Depot: Store at 15°C to 30°C (59°F to 86°F); protect from excessive heat.

Nasal solution: Store at 15°C to 25°C (59°F to 77°F); protect from heat. Store in upright position. After opening, may keep for up to 5 weeks at room temperature.

Mechanism of Action Synthetic peptide analog of Gonadotropin hormone releasing hormone (GnRH) with substitutions at positions 6 and 10; altered peptide structure results in a significantly magnified GnRH agonist effect with an extended duration of activity. Following an initial rise in the pituitary gonadotropins luteinizing hormone (LH) and follicle-stimulating hormone (FSH), chronic administration of buserelin results in a sustained suppression of LH and FSH and an interference with the production of ovarian and testicular steroids. Eventually, a decline in gonadal steroids to castration levels is observed.

Pharmacodynamics/Kinetics

Protein binding: ~15%

Metabolism: Plasma; inactive metabolites

Half-life elimination: SubQ: Immediate release: 80 minutes; Depot implants: 20-30 days; Nasal: 1-2 hours

Time to peak, plasma: Depot: <1 day

Excretion: Urine (50% as unchanged drug)

Dosage

Prostate cancer, advanced: Adults: **Note:** Administration of an antiandrogen agent beginning 7 days prior to initiation of buserelin therapy and continuing for ~5 weeks with buserelin therapy is recommended in patients with prostate cancer.

SubQ:

Suprefact: Initial: 500 mcg every 8 hours for 7 days. Maintenance: 200 mcg once daily

Suprefact Depot

2-month: 6.3 mg implant every 2 months (dosage interval may be shortened or extended by a few days if needed)

3-month: 9.45 mg implant every 3 months (dosage interval may be shortened or extended by a few days if needed)

Intranasal (Suprefact): Maintenance: 400 mcg (200 mcg into each nostril) 3 times daily

Endometriosis: Adults: Intranasal (Suprefact): 400 mcg (200 mcg into each nostril) 3 times daily; treatment duration is usually 6 months; maximum duration: 9 months

Missed doses: Non-depot formulations: If a dose is missed, take as soon as remembered; if it is almost time for the next dose, skip the missed dose and continue with regular dosing schedule.

Dosage adjustment in renal impairment: No dosage adjustment provided in the manufacturer's labeling (has not been studied)

Dosage adjustment in hepatic impairment: No dosage adjustment provided in the manufacturer's labeling (has not been studied)

Administration

Intranasal: Administer at equal time intervals; before first application pump bottle several times in upright position until a uniform mist is released; priming may need to be repeated between uses

SubQ: Rotate injection sites; administer at equal time intervals.

Depot formulation: Administer into lateral abdominal wall; a local anesthetic may be administered to injection site prior to implantation.

Hazardous agent; use appropriate precautions for handling and disposal (meets NIOSH 2014 criteria).

Monitoring Parameters Blood glucose levels (in patients with diabetes); blood pressure (in hypertensive patients); mood changes

Prostate cancer: Serum testosterone levels (4-6 weeks after initiation of therapy and every 3 months thereafter), prostate-specific antigen (PSA), prostatic acid phosphatase (PAP), bone scan, CT scan, ultrasound; digital rectal exam; ECG (in patients at risk for QT prolongation)

Endometriosis: Serum estradiol levels

Product Availability Not available in U.S.

Dosage Forms: Canada

Implant, subcutaneous:

Suprefact Depot: 6.3 mg, 9.45 mg

Injection, solution:

Suprefact: 1 mg/mL (5.5 mL, 10 mL)

Solution, intranasal:

Suprefact: 1mg/1mL (10 mL)

◆ **Buserelin Acetate** *see* Buserelin [CAN/INT] *on page 309*

◆ **BuSpar** *see* BusPIRone *on page 311*

BusPIRone (byoo SPYE rone)

Brand Names: Canada Apo-Buspirone; Bustab; Dom-Buspirone; Novo-Buspirone; PMS-Buspirone; Riva-Buspirone

Index Terms BuSpar; Buspirone Hydrochloride

Pharmacologic Category Antianxiety Agent, Miscellaneous

Use Management of generalized anxiety disorder (GAD)

Pregnancy Risk Factor B

Pregnancy Considerations Adverse events have not been observed in animal reproduction studies.

Breast-Feeding Considerations It is not known if buspirone is excreted in breast milk. Breast-feeding is not recommended by the manufacturer.

Contraindications Hypersensitivity to buspirone or any component of the formulation

Warnings/Precautions Use in severe hepatic or renal impairment is not recommended. Low potential for cognitive or motor impairment; until effects on patient known, patients should be warned to use caution when performing tasks which require mental alertness (eg, operating machinery or driving). Effects may be potentiated when used with other sedative drugs or ethanol. Use with MAO inhibitors may result in hypertensive reactions; concurrent use is not recommended. Restlessness syndrome has been reported in small number of patients; may be attributable to buspirone's antagonism of central dopamine receptors. Monitor for signs of any dopamine-related movement disorders (eg, dystonia, akathisia, pseudo-parkinsonism). Buspirone does not exhibit cross-tolerance with benzodiazepines or other sedative/hypnotic agents. If substituting buspirone for any of these agents, gradually withdraw the drug(s) prior to initiating buspirone.

Adverse Reactions

Cardiovascular: Chest pain

Central nervous system: Abnormal dreams, ataxia, confusion, dizziness, drowsiness, excitement, headache, nervousness, numbness, outbursts of anger, paresthesia

Dermatologic: Diaphoresis, skin rash

Gastrointestinal: Diarrhea, nausea, sore throat

Neuromuscular & skeletal: Musculoskeletal pain, tremor, weakness

Ophthalmic: Blurred vision

Otic: Tinnitus

Respiratory: Nasal congestion

Rare but important or life-threatening: Alcohol abuse, alopecia, amenorrhea, angioedema, anorexia, bradycardia, bruise, cardiac failure, cardiomyopathy, cerebrovascular accident, claustrophobia, cogwheel rigidity, conjunctivitis, dyskinesia, dystonia, edema, eosinophilia, epistaxis, extrapyramidal reaction, galactorrhea, hallucination, hemorrhagic diathesis, hypersensitivity reaction, hypertension, hyperventilation, hypotension, increased intraocular pressure, increased serum ALT, increased serum AST, increased serum transaminases, irritable bowel syndrome, leukopenia, memory impairment, menstrual disease, myocardial infarction, parkinsonian-like syndrome, pelvic inflammatory disease, personality disorder, photophobia, psychosis, rectal hemorrhage, restless leg syndrome, seizure, serotonin syndrome, slowed reaction time, slurred speech, suicidal ideation, syncope, thrombocytopenia, thyroid disease, urinary incontinence, visual disturbance (tunnel vision)

Drug Interactions

Metabolism/Transport Effects **Substrate** of CYP2D6 (minor), CYP3A4 (major); **Note:** Assignment of Major/Minor substrate status based on clinically relevant drug interaction potential

Avoid Concomitant Use

Avoid concomitant use of BusPIRone with any of the following: Azelastine (Nasal); Conivaptan; Dapoxetine; Fusidic Acid (Systemic); Idelalisib; MAO Inhibitors; Methylene Blue; Orphenadrine; Paraldehyde; Thalidomide

Increased Effect/Toxicity

BusPIRone may increase the levels/effects of: Alcohol (Ethyl); Antidepressants (Serotonin Reuptake Inhibitor/Antagonist); Antipsychotic Agents; Azelastine (Nasal); Buprenorphine; CNS Depressants; Hydrocodone; MAO Inhibitors; Methotrimeprazine; Methylene Blue; Metoclopramide; Metyrosine; Orphenadrine; Paraldehyde; Pramipexole; ROPINIRole; Rotigotine; Selective Serotonin Reuptake Inhibitors; Serotonin Modulators; Suvorexant; Thalidomide; Zolpidem

The levels/effects of BusPIRone may be increased by: Antiemetics (5HT3 Antagonists); Antifungal Agents (Azole Derivatives, Systemic); Antipsychotic Agents; Aprepitant; Brimonidine (Topical); Calcium Channel Blockers (Nondihydropyridine); Cannabis; Ceritinib; Conivaptan; CYP3A4 Inhibitors (Moderate); CYP3A4 Inhibitors (Strong); Dapoxetine; Dasatinib; Doxylamine; Dronabinol; Droperidol; Fosaprepitant; Fusidic Acid (Systemic); Grapefruit Juice; HydrOXYzine; Idelalisib; Ivacaftor; Kava Kava; Luliconazole; Macrolide Antibiotics; Magnesium Sulfate; Methotrimeprazine; Mifepristone; Nabilone; Netupitant; Perampanel; Rufinamide; Selective Serotonin Reuptake Inhibitors; Simeprevir; Sodium Oxybate; Stiripentol; Tapentadol; Tetrahydrocannabinol

Decreased Effect

BusPIRone may decrease the levels/effects of: Ioflupane I 123

The levels/effects of BusPIRone may be decreased by: Bosentan; CYP3A4 Inducers (Moderate); CYP3A4 Inducers (Strong); Dabrafenib; Deferasirox; Mitotane; Rifamycin Derivatives; Siltuximab; St Johns Wort; Tocilizumab; Yohimbine

Food Interactions Food may decrease the absorption of buspirone, but it may also decrease the first-pass metabolism, thereby increasing the bioavailability of buspirone. Grapefruit juice may cause increased buspirone concentrations. Management: Administer with or without food, but must be consistent. Avoid intake of large quantities of grapefruit juice.

Storage/Stability Store at 25°C (77°F); excursions permitted between 15°C to 30°C (59°F to 86°F). Protect from light.

Mechanism of Action The mechanism of action of buspirone is unknown. Buspirone has a high affinity for serotonin 5-HT_{1A} and 5-HT_2 receptors, without affecting benzodiazepine-GABA receptors. Buspirone has moderate affinity for dopamine D_2 receptors.

Pharmacodynamics/Kinetics

Absorption: Rapid

Distribution: V_d: 5.3 L/kg

Protein binding: 86%

Metabolism: Hepatic oxidation, primarily via CYP3A4 to several metabolites including an active metabolite, 1-pyrimidinylpiperazine (1-PP; exhibits about 25% of the activity of buspirone); extensive first-pass effect

Half-life elimination: 2-3 hours

Time to peak, serum: 40-90 minutes

Excretion: Urine: 29% to 63% (primarily as metabolites); feces: 18% to 38%

Dosage

Generalized anxiety disorder (GAD): Adults: Oral: Initial: 7.5 mg twice daily; may increase every 2-3 days in increments of 2.5 mg twice daily to a maximum of 30 mg twice daily; a dose of 10-15 mg twice daily was most often used in clinical trials that allowed for dose titration

Augmentation agent for antidepressants (off-label use): Adults: Oral: Initial: 7.5 mg twice daily; may increase weekly in increments of 7.5 mg twice daily to a maximum of 30 mg twice daily (Trivedi, 2006).

Dosing adjustment in renal impairment: Patients with impaired renal function demonstrated increased plasma levels and a prolonged half-life of buspirone. Use in patients with severe renal impairment not recommended.

Dosing adjustment in hepatic impairment: Patients with impaired hepatic function demonstrated increased plasma levels and a prolonged half-life of buspirone. Use in patients with severe hepatic impairment not recommended.

Dietary Considerations May be taken with or without food, but must be consistent. Avoid large quantities of grapefruit juice.

Administration May be administered with or without food, but must be consistent.

Monitoring Parameters Mental status, symptoms of anxiety

Additional Information Has shown little potential for abuse; needs continuous use. Because of slow onset, not appropriate for "as needed" (prn) use or for brief, situational anxiety. Ineffective for treatment of benzodiazepine or ethanol withdrawal.

Dosage Forms

Tablet, Oral:

Generic: 5 mg, 7.5 mg, 10 mg, 15 mg, 30 mg

◆ **Buspirone Hydrochloride** *see* BusPIRone *on page 311*

◆ **Bussulfam** *see* Busulfan *on page 312*

◆ **Bustab (Can)** *see* BusPIRone *on page 311*

Busulfan (byoo SUL fan)

Brand Names: U.S. Busulfex; Myleran

Brand Names: Canada Busulfex; Myleran

Index Terms Bussulfam; Busulfanum; Busulphan

Pharmacologic Category Antineoplastic Agent, Alkylating Agent

Use

Chronic myeloid leukemia (CML):

Injection: Conditioning regimen prior to allogeneic hematopoietic progenitor cell transplantation for CML (in combination with cyclophosphamide)

Tablets: Palliative treatment of CML

Pregnancy Risk Factor D

Dosage Note: Premedicate with prophylactic anticonvulsant therapy (eg, phenytoin) prior to high-dose busulfan treatment. Busulfan is associated with a moderate emetic potential (depending on dose and/or administration route); antiemetics may be recommended to prevent nausea and vomiting (Dupuis, 2011).

Children:

CML, palliation (manufacturer's labeling): Oral:

Remission induction: 60 mcg/kg/day or 1.8 mg/m²/day; titrate dose (or withhold) to maintain leukocyte counts ≥15,000/mm³ (doses >4 mg/day should be reserved for patients with the most compelling symptoms)

Maintenance: When leukocyte count ≥50,000/mm³: Resume induction dose **or** (if remission <3 months) 1 to 3 mg/day (to control hematologic status and prevent relapse)

HSCT conditioning regimens:

IV:

≤12 kg: 1.1 mg/kg/dose (actual body weight) every 6 hours for 16 doses (over 4 days)

>12 kg: 0.8 mg/kg/dose (actual body weight) every 6 hours for 16 doses (over 4 days)

Adjust dose to desired AUC (1125 micromolar•minute) using the following formula:

Adjusted dose (mg) = Actual dose (mg) x [target AUC (micromolar•minute) / actual AUC (micromolar•minute)]

Reduced intensity conditioning regimen (off-label dosing): 0.8 mg/kg/dose for 1 dose 7 to 10 days prior to transplant, followed by ~0.8 mg/kg/dose (busulfan kinetics calculated after initial dose) every 6 hours for 7 doses beginning 3 to 6 days prior to transplant (in combination with fludarabine and antithymocyte globulin) (Pulsipher, 2009)

Oral (off-label use): 1 mg/kg/dose every 6 hours for 16 doses beginning 9 days prior to transplant (in combination with cyclophosphamide) (Cassileth, 1998)

Adults:

CML, palliation (manufacturer's labeling): Oral:

Remission induction: 60 mcg/kg/day or 1.8 mg/m²/day; usual range: 4 to 8 mg/day; titrate dose (or withhold) to maintain leukocyte counts ≥15,000/mm³ (doses >4 mg/day should be reserved for patients with the most compelling symptoms)

Maintenance: When leukocyte count ≥50,000/mm³: Resume induction dose **or** (if remission <3 months) 1 to 3 mg/day (to control hematologic status and prevent relapse)

HSCT conditioning regimen:

IV: 0.8 mg/kg every 6 hours for 4 days (a total of 16 doses); **Note:** Use ideal body weight or actual body weight, (whichever is lower) for dosing.

Obesity: For obese or severely-obese patients, use of an adjusted body weight [IBW + 0.25 x (actual – IBW)] is recommended (by the manufacturer).

Reduced intensity conditioning regimen (off-label dosing): 0.8 mg/kg/day for 4 days starting 5 days prior to transplant (in combinations with fludarabine) (Ho, 2009)

Oral (off-label use): 1 mg/kg/dose every 6 hours for 16 doses (in combination with cyclophosphamide) (Socié, 2001) **or** 1 mg/kg/dose every 6 hours for 16 doses beginning 9 days prior to transplant (in combination with cyclophosphamide) (Cassileth, 1993) **or** 0.44 mg/kg/dose every 6 hours for 16 doses (in combination with cyclophosphamide) (Anderson, 1996) **or** 1 mg/kg/dose every 6 hours for 16 doses beginning 6 days prior to transplant (in combination with melphalan) (Fermand, 2005)

Essential thrombocythemia (off-label use): Oral: 2 to 4 mg daily (Fabris, 2009; Tefferi, 2011)

Polycythemia vera, refractory (off-label uses): Oral: 2 to 4 mg daily (Tefferi, 2011)

Dosing adjustment in renal impairment:

IV: There are no dosage adjustments provided in the manufacturer's labeling (has not been studied).

Oral: There are no dosage adjustments provided in the manufacturer's labeling (elimination appears to be independent of renal function); however, it has been suggested that adjustment is not necessary (Aronoff, 2007).

Dosing adjustment in hepatic impairment:

IV: There are no dosage adjustments provided in the manufacturer's labeling (has not been studied).

Oral: There are no dosage adjustments provided in the manufacturer's labeling.

Dosing in obesity:

*American Society of Clinical Oncology (ASCO) Guidelines for appropriate chemotherapy dosing in obese adults with cancer (**Note:** Excludes HSCT dosing):* Utilize patient's actual body weight (full weight) for calculation of body surface area- or weight-based dosing, particularly when the intent of therapy is curative; manage regimen-related toxicities in the same manner as for nonobese patients; if a dose reduction is utilized due to toxicity, consider resumption of full weight-based dosing with subsequent cycles, especially if cause of toxicity (eg, hepatic or renal impairment) is resolved (Griggs, 2012).

American Society for Blood and Marrow Transplantation (ASBMT) practice guideline committee position statement on chemotherapy dosing in obesity (Bubalo, 2014):

Busulfan (oral): **Note:** For doses over 12 mg/kg utilize pharmacokinetically targeted dosage (as appropriate for disease state). When busulfan and cyclophosphamide are used in combination for HSCT conditioning, the maximum tolerated busulfan dose is 4 mg/kg/day for 4 days. The maximum tolerated busulfan dose has not been determined when used in combination with other agents.

Body surface area (BSA) dosing: Adults and pediatrics: Utilize actual body weight (ABW) to calculate BSA

Weight based dosing (mg/kg): Adults: Utilize ABW25 for obese and nonobese patients; Pediatric: Utilize actual body weight (ABW)

ABW25: Adjusted wt (kg) = Ideal body weight (kg) + 0.25 [actual wt (kg) - ideal body weight (kg)]

Additional Information Complete prescribing information should be consulted for additional detail.

Dosage Forms

Solution, Intravenous:

Busulfex: 6 mg/mL (10 mL)

Tablet, Oral:

Myleran: 2 mg

◆ **Busulfanum** *see* Busulfan *on page 312*

◆ **Busulfex** *see* Busulfan *on page 312*

◆ **Busulphan** *see* Busulfan *on page 312*

Butabarbital (byoo ta BAR bi tal)

Brand Names: U.S. Butisol Sodium

Pharmacologic Category Barbiturate

Additional Appendix Information

Beers Criteria – Potentially Inappropriate Medications for Geriatrics *on page 2271*

Use Sedative; hypnotic

Pregnancy Risk Factor D

Dosage Oral:

Children: Preoperative sedation: 2-6 mg/kg/dose (maximum: 100 mg)

Adults:

Sedative: 15-30 mg 3-4 times/day

Hypnotic: 50-100 mg at bedtime. When used for insomnia, treatment should be limited since barbiturates lose effectiveness for sleep induction and maintenance after 2 weeks.

Preop: 50-100 mg 1-1½ hours before surgery

Elderly: Use with caution; reduce dose if use is needed

Dosage adjustment in renal impairment: Reduce dose if use is needed

Dosage adjustment in hepatic impairment: Reduce dose if use is needed

Additional Information Complete prescribing information should be consulted for additional detail.

Dosage Forms

Tablet, Oral:

Butisol Sodium: 30 mg, 50 mg

Butalbital, Acetaminophen, and Caffeine
(byoo TAL bi tal, a seet a MIN oh fen, & KAF een)

Brand Names: U.S. Alagesic LQ; Dolgic Plus; Esgic; Esgic-Plus; Fioricet; Margesic; Zebutal

Index Terms Acetaminophen, Butalbital, and Caffeine

Pharmacologic Category Barbiturate

Use Tension or muscle contraction headache: Relief of symptom complex of tension or muscle contraction headache

Pregnancy Risk Factor C

Dosage

Adults: Oral: 1-2 tablets or capsules (or 15-30 mL solution) every 4 hours; not to exceed 6 tablets or capsules (or 90 mL solution) daily

Elderly: Not recommended for use in the elderly

Dosage adjustment in renal impairment: No dosage adjustment provided in the manufacturer's labeling; use with caution, especially with severe impairment.

Dosage adjustment in hepatic impairment: No dosage adjustment provided in the manufacturer's labeling; use with caution, especially with severe impairment.

Additional Information Complete prescribing information should be consulted for additional detail.

Dosage Forms

Capsule, oral: Butalbital 50 mg, acetaminophen 300 mg, and caffeine 40 mg

Esgic: Butalbital 50 mg, acetaminophen 325 mg, and caffeine 40 mg

Fioricet: Butalbital 50 mg, acetaminophen 300 mg, and caffeine 40 mg

Margesic: Butalbital 50 mg, acetaminophen 325 mg, and caffeine 40 mg

Zebutal: Butalbital 50 mg, acetaminophen 325 mg, and caffeine 40 mg; Butalbital 50 mg, acetaminophen 500 mg, and caffeine 40 mg

Liquid, oral:

Alagesic LQ: Butalbital 50 mg, acetaminophen 325 mg, and caffeine 40 mg per 15 mL

Tablet, oral: Butalbital 50 mg, acetaminophen 325 mg, and caffeine 40 mg

Dolgic Plus: Butalbital 50 mg, acetaminophen 750 mg, and caffeine 40 mg

Esgic: Butalbital 50 mg, acetaminophen 325 mg, and caffeine 40 mg

Butalbital and Acetaminophen
(byoo TAL bi tal & a seet a MIN oh fen)

Brand Names: U.S. Bupap; Orviban CF; Phrenilin Forte; Promacet
Index Terms Acetaminophen and Butalbital
Pharmacologic Category Analgesic, Miscellaneous; Barbiturate
Use Relief of the symptomatic complex of tension or muscle contraction headache
Pregnancy Risk Factor C
Dosage Oral:
Children ≥12 years and Adults:
Butalbital 50 mg and acetaminophen 300-325 mg: 1-2 tablets every 4 hours as needed (maximum: 6 tablets/ 24 hours)
Butalbital 50 mg and acetaminophen 650 mg: One tablet/ capsule every 4 hours as needed (maximum: 6 doses/ 24 hours)
Elderly: Use with caution; see adult dosing

Dosage adjustment in renal impairment: No dosage adjustment provided in the manufacturer's labeling; however, use with caution; dose reduction or alternate therapy should be considered, especially with severe impairment.
Dosage adjustment in hepatic impairment: No dosage adjustment provided in the manufacturer's labeling; however, use with caution; dose reduction or alternate therapy should be considered, especially with severe impairment.
Additional Information Complete prescribing information should be consulted for additional detail.
Dosage Forms
Tablet, oral: Butalbital 50 mg and acetaminophen 325 mg
Promacet: Butalbital 50 mg and acetaminophen 650 mg
Bupap, Orbivan CF: Butalbital 50 mg and acetaminophen 300 mg
Capsule, oral:
Phrenilin Forte: Butalbital 50 mg and acetaminophen 650 mg

Butalbital, Aspirin, and Caffeine
(byoo TAL bi tal, AS pir in, & KAF een)

Brand Names: U.S. Fiorinal®
Brand Names: Canada Fiorinal®
Index Terms Aspirin, Caffeine, and Butalbital; Butalbital Compound
Pharmacologic Category Barbiturate
Use Relief of the symptomatic complex of tension or muscle contraction headache
Pregnancy Risk Factor C
Dosage
Oral: Adults: 1-2 tablets or capsules every 4 hours; not to exceed 6 tablets or capsules/day
Elderly: Not recommended for use in the elderly
Dosing adjustment in renal/hepatic impairment: Dosage should be reduced
Additional Information Complete prescribing information should be consulted for additional detail.
Dosage Forms
Capsule: Butalbital 50 mg, aspirin 325 mg, and caffeine 40 mg
Fiorinal®: Butalbital 50 mg, aspirin 325 mg, and caffeine 40 mg

◆ **Butalbital Compound** *see* Butalbital, Aspirin, and Caffeine *on page 314*
◆ **Butamben, Tetracaine, and Benzocaine** *see* Benzocaine, Butamben, and Tetracaine *on page 247*

Butenafine (byoo TEN a feen)

Brand Names: U.S. Lotrimin Ultra [OTC]; Mentax
Index Terms Butenafine Hydrochloride
Pharmacologic Category Antifungal Agent, Topical
Use Topical treatment of tinea pedis (athlete's foot), tinea cruris (jock itch), tinea corporis (ringworm), and tinea versicolor
Pregnancy Risk Factor C
Dosage Children >12 years and Adults: Topical:
Tinea corporis, tinea cruris (Lotrimin® ultra™): Apply once daily for 2 weeks to affected area and surrounding skin
Tinea versicolor (Mentax®): Apply once daily for 2 weeks to affected area and surrounding skin
Tinea pedis (Lotrimin® ultra™): Apply to affected skin between and around the toes, twice daily for 1 week, or once daily for 4 weeks
Additional Information Complete prescribing information should be consulted for additional detail.
Dosage Forms
Cream, External:
Lotrimin Ultra [OTC]: 1% (30 g)
Mentax: 1% (15 g, 30 g)

◆ **Butenafine Hydrochloride** *see* Butenafine *on page 314*
◆ **Butisol Sodium** *see* Butabarbital *on page 313*

Butoconazole (byoo toe KOE na zole)

Brand Names: U.S. Gynazole-1
Brand Names: Canada Femstat® One; Gynazole-1®
Index Terms Butoconazole Nitrate
Pharmacologic Category Antifungal Agent, Imidazole Derivative; Antifungal Agent, Vaginal
Use Local treatment of vulvovaginal candidiasis
Pregnancy Risk Factor C
Dosage Adults: Females: Gynazole-1®: Insert 1 applicatorful (~5 g) intravaginally as a single dose
Additional Information Complete prescribing information should be consulted for additional detail.
Dosage Forms
Cream, Vaginal:
Gynazole-1: 2% (5.8 g)

◆ **Butoconazole Nitrate** *see* Butoconazole *on page 314*

Butorphanol (byoo TOR fa nole)

Brand Names: Canada Apo-Butorphanol; PMS-Butorphanol
Index Terms Butorphanol Tartrate; Stadol
Pharmacologic Category Analgesic, Opioid; Analgesic, Opioid Partial Agonist
Additional Appendix Information
Opioid Conversion Table *on page 2232*
Use
Parenteral: Management of pain when the use of an opioid analgesic is appropriate; preoperative or preanesthetic medication; supplement to balanced anesthesia; management of pain during labor.
Nasal spray: Management of pain when the use of an opioid analgesic is appropriate.
Pregnancy Risk Factor C
Dosage Note: These are guidelines and do not represent the maximum doses that may be required in all patients. Doses should be titrated to pain relief/prevention. Butorphanol has an analgesic ceiling.

Adults:

Parenteral:

Acute pain (moderate-to-severe):

IM: Initial: 2 mg, may repeat every 3-4 hours as needed; usual range: 1-4 mg every 3-4 hours as needed

IV: Initial: 1 mg, may repeat every 3-4 hours as needed; usual range: 0.5-2 mg every 3-4 hours as needed

Preoperative medication: IM: 2 mg 60-90 minutes before surgery

Supplement to balanced anesthesia: IV: 2 mg shortly before induction and/or an incremental dose of 0.5-1 mg (up to 0.06 mg/kg), depending on previously administered sedative, analgesic, and hypnotic medications

Pain during labor (fetus >37 weeks gestation and no signs of fetal distress):

IM, IV: 1-2 mg; may repeat in 4 hours

Note: Alternative analgesia should be used for pain associated with delivery or if delivery is anticipated within 4 hours

Nasal spray:

Pain: Initial: 1 spray (~1 mg per spray) in 1 nostril; if adequate pain relief is not achieved within 60-90 minutes, an additional 1 spray in 1 nostril may be given; may repeat initial dose sequence in 3-4 hours after the last dose as needed

Alternatively, an initial dose of 2 mg (1 spray in each nostril) may be used in patients who will be able to remain recumbent (in the event drowsiness or dizziness occurs); additional 2 mg doses should not be given for 3-4 hours

Elderly:

IM, IV: Initial dosage should generally be 1/2 of the recommended dose; repeated dosing must be based on initial response rather than fixed intervals, but generally should be at least 6 hours apart

Nasal spray: Initial dose should not exceed 1 mg; a second dose may be given after 90-120 minutes if needed. In Canadian labeling, repeated dosing must be based on initial response rather than fixed intervals, but generally should be at least 6 hours apart.

Dosage adjustment in renal impairment:

IM, IV: Initial dosage should generally be 1/2 of the recommended dose; repeated dosing must be based on initial response rather than fixed intervals, but generally should be at least 6 hours apart

Nasal spray: Initial dose should not exceed 1 mg; a second dose may be given after 90-120 minutes if needed. Repeated dosing must be based on initial response rather than fixed intervals, but generally should be at least 6 hours apart.

Canadian labeling: CrCl <30 mL/minute: Increase initial dosing interval to 6-8 hours.

Dosage adjustment in hepatic impairment:

IM, IV: Initial dosage should generally be 1/2 of the recommended dose; repeated dosing must be based on initial response rather than fixed intervals, but generally should be at least 6 hours apart

Nasal spray: Initial dose should not exceed 1 mg; a second dose may be given after 90-120 minutes if needed. Repeated dosing must be based on initial response rather than fixed intervals, but generally should be at least 6 hours apart.

Canadian labeling: Increase interval of repeat dosing to 6-12 hours.

Additional Information Complete prescribing information should be consulted for additional detail.

Dosage Forms

Solution, Injection:

Generic: 1 mg/mL (1 mL); 2 mg/mL (1 mL, 2 mL, 10 mL)

Solution, Injection [preservative free]:

Generic: 1 mg/mL (1 mL); 2 mg/mL (1 mL)

Solution, Nasal:

Generic: 10 mg/mL (2.5 mL)

- ◆ **Butorphanol Tartrate** *see* Butorphanol *on page 314*
- ◆ **Butrans** *see* Buprenorphine *on page 300*
- ◆ **BW-430C** *see* LamoTRIgine *on page 1160*
- ◆ **BW524W91** *see* Emtricitabine *on page 720*
- ◆ **Bydureon** *see* Exenatide *on page 830*
- ◆ **Byetta (Can)** *see* Exenatide *on page 830*
- ◆ **Byetta 5 MCG Pen** *see* Exenatide *on page 830*
- ◆ **Byetta 10 MCG Pen** *see* Exenatide *on page 830*
- ◆ **Bystolic** *see* Nebivolol *on page 1434*
- ◆ **C1 Esterase Inhibitor** *see* C1 Inhibitor (Human) *on page 315*
- ◆ **C1 Esterase Inhibitor** *see* C1 Inhibitor (Recombinant) *on page 316*
- ◆ **C1-INH** *see* C1 Inhibitor (Human) *on page 315*
- ◆ **C1-INH** *see* C1 Inhibitor (Recombinant) *on page 316*
- ◆ **C1-Inhibitor** *see* C1 Inhibitor (Human) *on page 315*
- ◆ **C1-Inhibitor** *see* C1 Inhibitor (Recombinant) *on page 316*
- ◆ **C1INHRP** *see* C1 Inhibitor (Human) *on page 315*
- ◆ **C2B8 Monoclonal Antibody** *see* RiTUXimab *on page 1825*
- ◆ **2C4 Antibody** *see* Pertuzumab *on page 1627*
- ◆ **C7E3** *see* Abciximab *on page 24*
- ◆ **311C90** *see* ZOLMitriptan *on page 2210*
- ◆ **C225** *see* Cetuximab *on page 413*
- ◆ **C-500 [OTC]** *see* Ascorbic Acid *on page 178*

C1 Inhibitor (Human) (cee won in HIB i ter HYU man)

Brand Names: U.S. Berinert; Cinryze

Brand Names: Canada Berinert

Index Terms C1 Esterase Inhibitor; C1-INH; C1-Inhibitor; C1INHRP; Human C1 Inhibitor

Pharmacologic Category Blood Product Derivative; C1 Esterase Inhibitor

Use

Hereditary angioedema:

Berinert: Treatment of acute abdominal, facial, or laryngeal attacks of hereditary angioedema (HAE) in adult and adolescent patients

Cinryze: Routine prophylaxis against angioedema attacks in adult and adolescent patients with HAE

Pregnancy Risk Factor C

Dosage IV: Adolescents and Adults:

Routine prophylaxis against hereditary angioedema (HAE) attacks (Cinryze): 1000 units every 3-4 days

Treatment of abdominal, facial, or laryngeal HAE attacks (Berinert): 20 units/kg

Dosage adjustment in renal impairment: No dosage adjustment provided in manufacturer's labeling (has not been studied).

Dosage adjustment in hepatic impairment: No dosage adjustment provided in manufacturer's labeling (has not been studied).

Additional Information Complete prescribing information should be consulted for additional detail.

Dosage Forms

Kit, Intravenous:

Berinert: 500 units

Solution Reconstituted, Intravenous [preservative free]:

Cinryze: 500 units (1 ea)

C1 Inhibitor (Recombinant)

(cee won in HIB i ter ree KOM be nant)

Brand Names: U.S. Ruconest

Index Terms C1 Esterase Inhibitor; C1-INH; C1-Inhibitor; Conestat Alfa; Recombinant C1 Inhibitor

Pharmacologic Category C1 Esterase Inhibitor

Use

Hereditary angioedema: Treatment of acute attacks of hereditary angioedema (HAE) in adult and adolescent patients

Limitations of use: Effectiveness not established in HAE patients with laryngeal attacks.

Pregnancy Risk Factor B

Pregnancy Considerations Adverse events were not observed in animal reproduction studies. Human C1 inhibitor concentrate is the preferred treatment for HAE during pregnancy; recombinant C1 inhibitor should be avoided until more data is available. Current guidelines recommend discontinuing the recombinant product 1 week prior to conception. Women with HAE should be monitored closely during pregnancy and for at least 72 hours after delivery (Caballero, 2012).

Breast-Feeding Considerations It is not known if C1 Inhibitor (recombinant) is excreted into breast milk. The manufacturer recommends that caution be used if administered to a nursing woman. Until more data is available, current guidelines recommend plasma-derived human C1 inhibitor concentrate as the preferred treatment for HAE during lactation (Caballero, 2012).

Contraindications Life-threatening immediate hypersensitivity reactions, including anaphylaxis, to C1 esterase inhibitor preparations or any component of the formulation; allergy to rabbits or rabbit-derived products

Warnings/Precautions Severe hypersensitivity reactions (eg, urticaria, hives, tightness of the chest, wheezing, hypotension, anaphylaxis) may occur during or after administration. Signs/symptoms of hypersensitivity reactions may be similar to the attacks associated with hereditary angioedema, therefore, consideration should be given to treatment methods. In the event of acute hypersensitivity reactions C1 inhibitor therapy should be discontinued and appropriate treatment should be instituted. Serious arterial and venous thromboembolic events have been reported at recommended doses in patients with risk factors (eg, presence of an indwelling venous catheter/ access device, prior history of thrombosis, underlying atherosclerosis, use of oral contraceptives or certain androgens, morbid obesity, immobility). Closely monitor patients with preexisting risks for thrombotic events during and after administration.

Adverse Reactions

Central nervous system: Headache (more common in adolescents than in adults), vertigo

Dermatologic: Burning sensation of skin, erythema (marginatum)

Gastrointestinal: Abdominal pain (adolescent), diarrhea, nausea

Hematologic & oncologic: C-reactive protein increased, increased fibrin, lipoma

Hypersensitivity: Angioedema

Immunologic: Antibody development (after repeat therapy exposure, non-neutralizing)

Neuromuscular & skeletal: Back pain

Respiratory: Sneezing

Respiratory: Oropharyngeal pain (adolescents)

Rare but important or life-threatening: Abdominal pain, arterial thromboembolism, hypersensitivity reaction, venous thromboembolism

Drug Interactions

Metabolism/Transport Effects None known.

Avoid Concomitant Use There are no known interactions where it is recommended to avoid concomitant use.

Increased Effect/Toxicity

The levels/effects of C1 Inhibitor (Recombinant) may be increased by: Androgens; Estrogen Derivatives; Progestins

Decreased Effect There are no known significant interactions involving a decrease in effect.

Preparation for Administration Allow diluent and C1 inhibitor to warm to room temperature. Reconstitute with 14 mL SWFI. Slowly add SWFI and swirl slowly to mix; avoid foaming. Resulting concentration is 150 units/mL. If patient requires contents of ≥1 vial, contents of multiple vials may be pooled into a single syringe.

Storage/Stability Store intact vials at 2°C to 25°C (36°F to 77°F) for up to 48 months; do not freeze. Protect from light. Reconstituted solution may be stored at 2°C to 8°C (36°F to 46°F) for ≤8 hours; do not freeze. Discard unused portion.

Mechanism of Action C1 inhibitor, a serine protease inhibitor (serpin), regulates the activation of the complement and contact system pathways by irreversibly binding target proteases. Suppression of contact system activation by C1 inhibitor through the inactivation of plasma kallikrein and factor XIIa is thought to modulate vascular permeability that leads to clinical manifestations of hereditary angioedema (HAE) attacks by preventing the generation of bradykinin.

Pharmacodynamics/Kinetics

Onset of action: Onset of symptom relief: Median: 90 minutes

Distribution: V_{ss}: ~3 L

Half-life elimination: ~2.5 hours

Time to peak: ~0.3 hours

Dosage Hereditary angioedema (HAE): Adolescents and Adults: IV: 50 units/kg as a single dose for patients weighing <84 kg; 4,200 units as a single dose for patients weighing ≥84 kg. Maximum dose: 4,200 units. If attack symptoms persist, one additional dose may be administered; no more than 2 doses may be administered per 24 hours.

Dosage adjustment for renal impairment: There are no dosage adjustments provided in the manufacturer's labeling (has not been studied).

Dosage adjustment for hepatic impairment: There are no dosage adjustments provided in the manufacturer's labeling (has not been studied).

Administration Administer by a separate infusion line as a slow IV injection over ~5 minutes. Appropriately trained patients may self-administer upon recognition of an HAE attack.

Monitoring Parameters Monitor for signs/symptoms of hypersensitivity reactions and thrombotic events.

Dosage Forms

Solution Reconstituted, Intravenous [preservative free]: Ruconest: 2100 units (1 ea)

Cabazitaxel (ca baz i TAKS el)

Brand Names: U.S. Jevtana

Brand Names: Canada Jevtana

Index Terms RPR-116258A; XRP6258

Pharmacologic Category Antineoplastic Agent, Antimicrotubular; Antineoplastic Agent, Taxane Derivative

Use Prostate cancer: Treatment of hormone-refractory metastatic prostate cancer (in combination with prednisone) in patients previously treated with a docetaxel-containing regimen

Pregnancy Risk Factor D

Pregnancy Considerations Adverse events have been observed in animal reproduction studies. May cause fetal harm if administered during pregnancy. Pregnant women should avoid exposure to cabazitaxel.

Breast-Feeding Considerations It is not known if cabazitaxel is excreted in breast milk. Due to the potential for serious adverse reactions in the nursing infant, the manufacturer recommends a decision be made whether to discontinue nursing or to discontinue the drug, taking into account the importance of treatment to the mother.

Contraindications Hypersensitivity to cabazitaxel, polysorbate 80, or any component of the formulation; neutrophil count ≤1500/mm^3

Warnings/Precautions Hazardous agent - use appropriate precautions for handling and disposal (NIOSH 2014 [group 1]). **[U.S. Boxed Warning]: Severe hypersensitivity reactions, including generalized rash, erythema, hypotension, and bronchospasm may occur; immediate discontinuation is required if hypersensitivity is severe; administer appropriate supportive medications. Premedicate with an IV antihistamine, corticosteroid and H_2 antagonist prior to infusion. Use in patients with history of severe hypersensitivity to cabazitaxel or polysorbate 80 is contraindicated.** Observe closely during infusion, especially during the first and second infusions; reaction may occur within minutes. Do not rechallenge after severe hypersensitivity reactions.

[U.S. Boxed Warning]: Deaths due to neutropenia have been reported. Do not administer in patients with neutrophil count ≤1500/mm^3; monitor blood counts frequently. Dose reductions are recommended following neutropenic fever or prolonged neutropenia. Administration of WBC growth factors may reduce the risk of complications due to neutropenia; consider primary WBC growth factor prophylaxis in high-risk patients (eg, >65 years of age, poor performance status, history of neutropenic fever, extensive prior radiation, poor nutrition status, or other serious comorbidities); secondary prophylaxis and therapeutic WBC growth factors should be considered in all patients with increased risk for neutropenic complications. Monitor complete blood counts weekly during cycle 1 and prior to subsequent treatment cycles, or as clinically indicated. Patients ≥65 years of age are more likely to experience certain adverse reactions, including neutropenia and neutropenic fever. Fatigue, asthenia, pyrexia, dizziness, urinary tract infection, and dehydration also occurred more frequently in elderly patients compared to younger patients.

Use is not recommended in patients with hepatic impairment (total bilirubin ≥ULN or AST and/or ALT ≥1.5 times ULN). Due to extensive hepatic metabolism, cabazitaxel exposure is increased in patients with hepatic impairment. Renal failure (including rare fatalities) has been reported from clinical trials; generally associated with dehydration, sepsis, or obstructive uropathy; use with caution in patients with severe renal impairment (CrCl <30 mL/minute) and end-stage renal disease. Nausea, vomiting and diarrhea may occur. Diarrhea may be severe and may result in dehydration and electrolyte imbalance; fatalities have been reported. Antiemetics, antidiarrheal medication, and fluid and electrolyte replacement may be necessary. Diarrhea ≥ grade 3 may require treatment delay and or dosage reduction. Gastrointestinal hemorrhage and perforation, enterocolitis, neutropenic enterocolitis, and ileus (some fatal) have also been observed. Use with caution in patients at risk of developing gastrointestinal complications (eg, elderly patients, those with neutropenia or a prior history of pelvic radiation, adhesions, GI ulceration or bleeding, concomitant use of steroids, NSAIDs, antiplatelet or anticoagulant medications). Evaluate promptly if symptoms such as abdominal pain and tenderness, fever, persistent constipation, and diarrhea (with or without neutropenia) occur. May require treatment interruption and/or therapy discontinuation.

Failure to properly reconstitute the concentrated vial of cabazitaxel with the correct amount of diluent may lead to higher dosage being administered and increased risk of toxicity. Follow manufacturer instructions carefully. Potentially significant drug-drug interactions may exist, requiring dose or frequency adjustment, additional monitoring, and/or selection of alternative therapy.

Some dosage forms may contain polysorbate 80 (also known as Tweens). Hypersensitivity reactions, usually a delayed reaction, have been reported following exposure to pharmaceutical products containing polysorbate 80 in certain individuals (Isaksson, 2002; Lucente 2000; Shelley, 1995). Thrombocytopenia, ascites, pulmonary deterioration, and renal and hepatic failure have been reported in premature neonates after receiving parenteral products containing polysorbate 80 (Alade, 1986; CDC, 1984). See manufacturer's labeling.

Adverse Reactions Note: Adverse reactions reported for combination therapy with prednisone.

Cardiovascular: Arrhythmias, hypotension, peripheral edema

Central nervous system: Dizziness, fatigue, fever, headache, pain

Dermatologic: Alopecia

Endocrine & metabolic: Dehydration

Gastrointestinal: Abdominal pain, anorexia, constipation, diarrhea, dyspepsia, mucosal inflammation, nausea, taste alteration, vomiting, weight loss

Genitourinary: Dysuria, urinary tract infection

Hematologic: Anemia, leukopenia, neutropenia (nadir: 12 days [range: 4-17 days]), neutropenic fever, thrombocytopenia

Hepatic: ALT increased, AST increased, bilirubin increased

Neuromuscular & skeletal: Arthralgia, back pain, muscle spasm, peripheral neuropathy, weakness

Renal: Hematuria

Respiratory: Cough, dyspnea

Rare but important or life-threatening: Colitis, electrolyte imbalance, enterocolitis, gastritis, gastrointestinal hemorrhage, gastrointestinal perforation, hypersensitivity (eg, rash, erythema, hypotension, bronchospasm), intestinal obstruction, neutropenic enterocolitis, renal failure, sepsis, septic shock

Drug Interactions

Metabolism/Transport Effects Substrate of CYP2C8 (minor), CYP3A4 (major); **Note:** Assignment of Major/Minor substrate status based on clinically relevant drug interaction potential

Avoid Concomitant Use

Avoid concomitant use of Cabazitaxel with any of the following: BCG; CloZAPine; Conivaptan; Dipyrone; Fusidic Acid (Systemic); Idelalisib; Natalizumab; Pimecrolimus; Tacrolimus (Topical); Tofacitinib; Vaccines (Live)

Increased Effect/Toxicity

Cabazitaxel may increase the levels/effects of: Antineoplastic Agents (Anthracycline, Systemic); CloZAPine; DOXOrubicin (Conventional); Leflunomide; Natalizumab; Tofacitinib; Vaccines (Live)

The levels/effects of Cabazitaxel may be increased by: Aprepitant; Ceritinib; Conivaptan; CYP3A4 Inhibitors (Moderate); CYP3A4 Inhibitors (Strong); Dasatinib; Denosumab; Dipyrone; Fosaprepitant; Fusidic Acid (Systemic); Idelalisib; Ivacaftor; Luliconazole; Mifepristone; Netupitant; Pimecrolimus; Platinum Derivatives; Roflumilast; Simeprevir; Stiripentol; Tacrolimus (Topical); Trastuzumab

Decreased Effect

Cabazitaxel may decrease the levels/effects of: BCG; Coccidioides immitis Skin Test; Sipuleucel-T; Vaccines (Inactivated); Vaccines (Live)

The levels/effects of Cabazitaxel may be decreased by: Bosentan; CYP3A4 Inducers (Moderate); CYP3A4 Inducers (Strong); Dabrafenib; Deferasirox; Echinacea; Mitotane; Siltuximab; St Johns Wort; Tocilizumab

Food Interactions Grapefruit juice may increase the levels/effects of cabazitaxel. Management: Avoid grapefruit juice.

Preparation for Administration Hazardous agent; use appropriate precautions for handling and disposal (NIOSH 2014 [group 1]). Do not prepare or administer in PVC-containing infusion containers. Cabazitaxel and diluent vials contain overfill. **Preparation requires 2 steps.** Slowly inject the **entire contents** of the provided diluent vial into the 60 mg/1.5 mL cabazitaxel vial, directing the diluent down the vial wall. Mix gently by inverting the vial for at least 45 seconds; do not shake. Allow vial to sit so that foam dissipates and solution appears homogeneous. This results in an intermediate reconstituted concentration of 10 mg/mL. The U.S. labeling recommends to further dilute within 30 minutes into a 250 mL D_5W or NS non-PVC infusion container to final concentration of 0.1 to 0.26 mg/mL (total doses >65 mg will require a larger infusion volume; final concentration should not exceed 0.26 mg/mL). The Canadian labeling recommends further dilution of the reconstituted vial occur within 60 minutes. Gently invert container to mix. Do not use infusion solutions if crystals or precipitate appear; discard if this occurs. Infusion should be completed within 8 hours if stored at room temperature. For infusion solutions stored under refrigeration, the U.S. labeling recommends that the infusion be completed within 24 hours. The Canadian labeling recommends that the infusion be completed within 48 hours.

Storage/Stability Store intact vials at 25°C (77°F); excursions permitted between 15°C and 30°C (59°F and 86°F). Do not refrigerate. Do not prepare or administer in PVC-containing infusion containers. The U.S. labeling indicates the initial reconstituted solution (at 10 mg/mL) is stable for 30 minutes in the vial and that solutions for infusion are stable for up to 8 hours at room temperature (includes the 1 hour infusion) or 24 hours refrigerated (includes the 1 hour infusion). The Canadian labeling indicates the initial reconstituted solution (at 10 mg/mL) is stable for 1 hour in the vial and that solutions for infusion are stable for up to 8 hours at room temperature (includes the 1 hour infusion) or 48 hours refrigerated (includes the 1 hour infusion).

Mechanism of Action Cabazitaxel is a taxane derivative which is a microtubule inhibitor; it binds to tubulin promoting assembly into microtubules and inhibiting disassembly which stabilizes microtubules. This inhibits microtubule depolymerization and cell division, arresting the cell cycle and inhibiting tumor proliferation. Unlike other taxanes, cabazitaxel has a poor affinity for multidrug resistance (MDR) proteins, therefore conferring activity in resistant tumors.

Pharmacodynamics/Kinetics

Distribution: V_{dss}: 4864 L; has greater CNS penetration than other taxanes

Protein binding: 89% to 92%; primarily to serum albumin and lipoproteins

Metabolism: Extensively hepatic; primarily via CYP3A4 and 3A5; also via CYP2C8 (minor)

Half-life elimination: Terminal: 95 hours

Excretion: Feces (76% as metabolites); Urine (~4%)

Dosage Note: Premedicate at least 30 minutes prior to each dose of cabazitaxel with an antihistamine (eg, diphenhydramine IV 25 mg or equivalent), a corticosteroid (eg, dexamethasone 8 mg IV or equivalent), and an H_2 antagonist (eg, ranitidine 50 mg IV or equivalent). Antiemetic prophylaxis is also recommended.

Prostate cancer, metastatic: Adults: IV: 25 mg/m^2/dose once every 3 weeks (in combination with prednisone)

Dosage adjustment for concomitant use with strong CYP3A inhibitors: Concomitant use with strong CYP3A inhibitors (eg, ketoconazole, itraconazole, clarithromycin, protease inhibitors, nefazodone, telithromycin, voriconazole) may increase cabazitaxel plasma concentrations; avoid concurrent use. If concomitant use cannot be avoided, consider reducing cabazitaxel dose by 25%.

Dosage adjustment for toxicity:

Hematologic toxicity:

Neutropenia ≥ grade 3 for >1 week despite WBC growth factors: Delay treatment until ANC >1500/mm^3 and then reduce dose to 20 mg/m^2 with continued WBC growth factor secondary prophylaxis

Neutropenic fever or neutropenic infection: Delay treatment until improvement/resolution and ANC >1500/mm^3 and then reduce dose to 20 mg/m^2 with continued WBC growth factor secondary prophylaxis

Persistent hematologic toxicity (despite dosage reduction): Discontinue treatment

Nonhematologic toxicity:

Severe hypersensitivity: Discontinue immediately

Diarrhea ≥ grade 3 or persistent despite appropriate medication, fluids, and electrolyte replacement: Delay treatment until improves or resolves and then reduce dose to 20 mg/m^2

Persistent diarrhea (despite dosage reduction): Discontinue treatment

Peripheral neuropathy (grade 2): Delay treatment until improves or resolves and then reduce dose to 20 mg/m^2

Persistent peripheral neuropathy (despite dosage reduction) or ≥ grade 3 peripheral neuropathy: Discontinue treatment

Dosage adjustment in renal impairment:

Mild to moderate renal impairment (CrCl ≥30 mL/minute): No dosage adjustment necessary.

Severe renal impairment (CrCl <30 mL/minute) or end-stage renal disease (ESRD): Use with caution.

Dosage adjustment in hepatic impairment: Hepatic impairment (total bilirubin ≥ULN or AST and/or ALT ≥1.5 times ULN): Use is not recommended

Dosing in obesity: ASCO Guidelines for appropriate chemotherapy dosing in obese adults with cancer: Utilize patient's actual body weight (full weight) for calculation of body surface area- or weight-based dosing, particularly when the intent of therapy is curative; manage regimen-related toxicities in the same manner as for nonobese patients; if a dose reduction is utilized due to toxicity, consider resumption of full weight-based dosing with subsequent cycles, especially if cause of toxicity (eg, hepatic or renal impairment) is resolved (Griggs, 2012).

Dietary Considerations Avoid grapefruit juice.

Administration IV: Infuse over 1 hour using a 0.22 micron inline filter. Do not use polyurethane-containing infusion sets for administration. Allow to reach room temperature prior to infusion. Premedicate with an antihistamine, a corticosteroid, and an H_2 antagonist at least 30 minutes prior to infusion. Observe closely during infusion (for hypersensitivity). Antiemetic prophylaxis (oral or IV) is also recommended.

Hazardous agent; use appropriate precautions for handling and disposal (NIOSH 2014 [group 1]).

Monitoring Parameters CBC with differential and platelets (weekly during first cycle, then prior to each treatment cycle and as clinically indicated); hepatic/renal function; monitor for hypersensitivity reactions and gastrointestinal disorders (eg, nausea, vomiting, diarrhea, gastrointestinal hemorrhage and perforation, ileus, colitis, abdominal pain/tenderness)

Dosage Forms

Solution, Intravenous:

Jevtana: 60 mg/1.5 mL (1.5 mL)

Cabergoline (ca BER goe leen)

Brand Names: Canada ACT Cabergoline; Dostinex

Pharmacologic Category Ergot Derivative

Use

Hyperprolactinemic disorders: Treatment of hyperprolactinemic disorders, either idiopathic or caused by pituitary adenomas.

Limitations of use: Not indicated for inhibition or suppression of physiologic lactation.

Canadian labeling: Additional use (not in U.S. labeling): Prevention of the onset of physiological lactation in the puerperium when clinically indicated (eg, still born baby or neonatal death, conditions that interfere with suckling, severe acute or chronic mental illness, maternal disease which may be transmitted to the baby that require medications which are excreted in the milk).

Limitations of use: Not indicated for suppression of already established postpartum lactation.

Pregnancy Risk Factor B

Dosage Oral: Adults:

Hyperprolactinemia:

U.S. labeling: Initial dose: 0.25 mg twice weekly; the dose may be increased by 0.25 mg twice weekly up to a maximum of 1 mg twice weekly according to the patient's serum prolactin level. Dosage increases should not occur more rapidly than every 4 weeks. Once a normal serum prolactin level is maintained for 6 months, discontinue cabergoline and monitor prolactin levels to determine if cabergoline should be reinstituted. The durability of efficacy beyond 24 months of therapy has not been established.

Canadian labeling: Initial dose: 0.5 mg once weekly or 0.25 mg twice weekly; weekly dose may be increased by 0.5 mg per week at 4 week intervals until optimal therapeutic response. Therapeutic dose: Usual: 1 mg/week (range: 0.25 to 2 mg/week). Once a normal serum prolactin level is maintained for 6 months, discontinue cabergoline and monitor prolactin levels to determine if cabergoline should be reinstituted. **Note:** May divide weekly dose into 2 or more divided doses per week (recommended for doses >1 mg/week) based on tolerability.

Lactation inhibition *(Canadian labeling; not in U.S. labeling)*: 1 mg single dose on first day postpartum

Elderly: Refer to adult dosing; start at the low end of the dosage range.

Dosage adjustment in renal impairment: There are no dosage adjustments provided in the manufacturer's labeling; however, cabergoline pharmacokinetics are not altered in patients with moderate to severe renal impairment.

Dosage adjustment in hepatic impairment: There are no dosage adjustments provided in the manufacturer's labeling; however, use caution in patients with severe hepatic impairment (Child-Pugh class C) (cabergoline bioavailability is increased).

Additional Information Complete prescribing information should be consulted for additional detail.

Dosage Forms

Tablet, Oral:

Generic: 0.5 mg

- ◆ **Caduet®** *see* Amlodipine and Atorvastatin *on page 124*
- ◆ **CaEDTA** *see* Edetate CALCIUM Disodium *on page 705*
- ◆ **Caelyx (Can)** *see* DOXOrubicin (Liposomal) *on page 684*
- ◆ **Cafcit®** *see* Caffeine *on page 319*
- ◆ **CAFdA** *see* Clofarabine *on page 470*

Caffeine (KAF een)

Brand Names: U.S. Cafcit®; Enerjets [OTC]; No Doz® Maximum Strength [OTC]; Vivarin® [OTC]

Index Terms Caffeine and Sodium Benzoate; Caffeine Citrate; Caffeine Sodium Benzoate; Sodium Benzoate and Caffeine

Pharmacologic Category Central Nervous System Stimulant; Phosphodiesterase Enzyme Inhibitor, Nonselective

Use

Caffeine citrate: Treatment of idiopathic apnea of prematurity

Caffeine and sodium benzoate: Treatment of acute respiratory depression (not a preferred agent)

Caffeine [OTC labeling]: Restore mental alertness or wakefulness when experiencing fatigue

Pregnancy Risk Factor C

Pregnancy Considerations Adverse events were observed in animal reproduction studies. Caffeine crosses the placenta; serum concentrations in the fetus are similar to those in the mother (Grosso, 2005). Based on current studies, usual dietary exposure to caffeine is unlikely to cause congenital malformations (Brent, 2011). However, available data shows conflicting results related to maternal caffeine use and the risk of other adverse events, such as spontaneous abortion or growth retardation (Brent, 2011; Jahanfar, 2013). The half-life of caffeine is prolonged during the second and third trimesters of pregnancy and maternal and fetal exposure is also influenced by maternal smoking or drinking (Brent, 2011; Koren, 2000). Current guidelines recommend limiting caffeine intake from all sources to ≤200 mg/day (ACOG, 2010).

Breast-Feeding Considerations Caffeine is detected in breast milk (Berlin, 1981; Hildebrant, 1983; Ryu, 1985a); concentrations may be dependent upon maternal consumption and her ability to metabolize (eg, smoker versus nonsmoker) (Brent, 2011). The ability of the breast-feeding child to metabolize caffeine is age-dependent (Hildebrant, 1983). Irritability and jitteriness have been reported in the nursing infant exposed to high concentrations of caffeine in breast milk (Martin, 2007). Infant heart rates and sleep patterns were not found to be affected in normal, full-term infants exposed to lesser amounts of caffeine (Ryu, 1985b).

Contraindications Hypersensitivity to caffeine or any component of the formulation; sodium benzoate is not for use in neonates

Warnings/Precautions Use with caution in patients with a history of peptic ulcer, gastroesophageal reflux, impaired renal or hepatic function, seizure disorders, or cardiovascular disease. Avoid use in patients with symptomatic cardiac arrhythmias, agitation, anxiety, or tremor. Over-the-counter [OTC] products contain an amount of caffeine similar to one cup of coffee; limit the use of other caffeine-containing beverages or foods.

Caffeine citrate should not be interchanged with caffeine and sodium benzoate. Avoid use of products containing sodium benzoate in neonates; has been associated with a potentially fatal toxicity ("gasping syndrome"). Neonates receiving caffeine citrate should be closely ▶

monitored for the development of necrotizing enterocolitis. Caffeine serum levels should be closely monitored to optimize therapy and prevent serious toxicity.

Adverse Reactions Primarily serum-concentration related.

Cardiovascular: Angina pectoris, chest pain, flushing, palpitations, sinus tachycardia, supraventricular tachycardia, vasodilatation, ventricular arrhythmia

Central nervous system: Agitation, delirium, dizziness, hallucination, headache, insomnia, irritability, psychosis, restlessness

Dermatologic: Urticaria

Gastrointestinal: Esophageal motility disorder (sphincter tone decreased), gastritis

Genitourinary: Diuresis

Neuromuscular & skeletal: Fasciculations

Ophthalmic: Increased intraocular pressure (>180 mg caffeine), miosis

Drug Interactions

Metabolism/Transport Effects Substrate of CYP1A2 (major), CYP2C9 (minor), CYP2D6 (minor), CYP2E1 (minor), CYP3A4 (minor); **Note:** Assignment of Major/Minor substrate status based on clinically relevant drug interaction potential; **Inhibits** CYP1A2 (weak)

Avoid Concomitant Use

Avoid concomitant use of Caffeine with any of the following: Iobenguane I 123; Stiripentol

Increased Effect/Toxicity

Caffeine may increase the levels/effects of: Formoterol; Indacaterol; Olodaterol; Sympathomimetics

The levels/effects of Caffeine may be increased by: Abiraterone Acetate; AtoMOXetine; Cannabinoid-Containing Products; CYP1A2 Inhibitors (Moderate); CYP1A2 Inhibitors (Strong); Deferasirox; Linezolid; Norfloxacin; Peginterferon Alfa-2b; Stiripentol; Tedizolid; Vemurafenib

Decreased Effect

Caffeine may decrease the levels/effects of: Adenosine; Iobenguane I 123; Lithium; Regadenoson

The levels/effects of Caffeine may be decreased by: Teriflunomide

Preparation for Administration Parenteral:

Caffeine citrate: May administer without dilution or diluted with D_5W to 10 mg caffeine citrate/mL.

Caffeine and sodium benzoate: For spinal headaches, dilute in 1000 mL NS.

Storage/Stability Store at 20°C to 25°C (68°F to 77°F).

Caffeine citrate: Injection and oral solution contain no preservatives; injection is chemically stable for at least 24 hours at room temperature when diluted to 10 mg/mL (as caffeine citrate) with D_5W, $D_{50}W$, Intralipid® 20%, and Aminosyn® 8.5%; also compatible with dopamine (600 mcg/mL), calcium gluconate 10%, heparin (1 unit/mL), and fentanyl (10 mcg/mL) at room temperature for 24 hours.

Mechanism of Action Increases levels of 3'5' cyclic AMP by inhibiting phosphodiesterase; CNS stimulant which increases medullary respiratory center sensitivity to carbon dioxide, stimulates central inspiratory drive, and improves skeletal muscle contraction (diaphragmatic contractility); prevention of apnea may occur by competitive inhibition of adenosine

Pharmacodynamics/Kinetics

Distribution: V_d:

Neonates: 0.8-0.9 L/kg

Children >9 months to Adults: 0.6 L/kg

Protein binding: 17% (children) to 36% (adults)

Metabolism: Hepatic, via demethylation by CYP1A2. **Note:** In neonates, interconversion between caffeine and theophylline has been reported (caffeine levels are ~25% of measured theophylline after theophylline administration and ~3% to 8% of caffeine would be expected to be converted to theophylline)

Half-life elimination:

Neonates: 72-96 hours (range: 40-230 hours)

Children >9 months and Adults: 5 hours

Time to peak, serum: Oral: Within 30 minutes to 2 hours

Excretion:

Neonates ≤1 month: 86% excreted unchanged in urine

Infants >1 month and Adults: In urine, as metabolites

Dosage Note: Caffeine citrate should not be interchanged with the caffeine sodium benzoate formulation.

Caffeine citrate: Neonates: Apnea of prematurity: Oral, IV:

Loading dose: 10-20 mg/kg as caffeine citrate (5-10 mg/kg as caffeine base). If theophylline has been administered to the patient within the previous 3 days, a full or modified loading dose (50% to 75% of a loading dose) may be given.

Maintenance dose: 5 mg/kg/day as caffeine citrate (2.5 mg/kg/day as caffeine base) once daily starting 24 hours after the loading dose. Maintenance dose is adjusted based on patient's response and serum caffeine concentrations.

Caffeine and sodium benzoate:

Children: Stimulant: IM, IV, SubQ: 8 mg/kg every 4 hours as needed

Children ≥12 years and Adults: OTC labeling (stimulant): Oral: 100-200 mg every 3-4 hours as needed

Adults:

Electroconvulsive therapy: IV: 300-2000 mg

Respiratory depression: IM, IV: 250 mg as a single dose; may repeat as needed. Maximum single dose should be limited to 500 mg; maximum amount in any 24-hour period should generally be limited to 2500 mg.

Spinal puncture headache (off-label use):

IV: 500 mg in 1000 mL NS infused over 1 hour, followed by 1000 mL NS infused over 1 hour; a second course of caffeine can be given for unrelieved headache pain in 4 hours.

Oral: 300 mg as a single dose

Stimulant/diuretic (off-label use): IM, IV: 500 mg, maximum single dose: 1 g

Dosage adjustment in renal impairment: No dosage adjustment required.

Dietary Considerations Oral formulations may be taken without regard to feedings or meals.

Administration

Oral: May be administered without regard to feedings or meals. May administer injectable formulation (caffeine citrate) orally.

Parenteral:

Caffeine citrate: Infuse loading dose over at least 30 minutes; maintenance dose may be infused over at least 10 minutes. May administer without dilution.

Caffeine and sodium benzoate: IV as slow direct injection. For spinal headaches, infuse diluted solution over 1 hour. Follow with 1000 mL NS; infuse over 1 hour. May administer IM undiluted.

Reference Range

Therapeutic: Apnea of prematurity: 8-20 mcg/mL

Potentially toxic: >20 mcg/mL

Toxic: >50 mcg/mL

Dosage Forms

Caplet:

No Doz® Maximum Strength [OTC]: 200 mg

Injection, solution [preservative free]: 20 mg/mL (3 mL)

Cafcit®: 20 mg/mL (3 mL)

Lozenge:

Enerjets® [OTC]: 75 mg

Solution, oral [preservative free]: 20 mg/mL (3 mL)
Cafcit®: 20 mg/mL
Tablet: 200 mg
Vivarin® [OTC]: 200 mg

Extemporaneous Preparations A 10 mg/mL oral solution of caffeine (as citrate) may be prepared from 10 g citrated caffeine powder combined with 10 g citric acid USP and dissolved in 1000 mL sterile water. Label "shake well". Stable for 3 months at room temperature (Nahata, 2004).

A 20 mg/mL oral solution of caffeine (as citrate) may be made from 10 g citrated caffeine powder and dissolved in 250 mL sterile water for irrigation. Stir solution until completely clear, then add a 2:1 mixture of simple syrup and cherry syrup in sufficient quantity to make 500 mL. Label "shake well" and "refrigerate". Stable for 90 days (Eisenberg, 1984).

Eisenberg MG and Kang N, "Stability of Citrated Caffeine Solutions for Injectable and Enteral Use," *Am J Hosp Pharm*, 1984, 41(11):2405-6.
Nahata MC, Pai VB, and Hipple TF, *Pediatric Drug Formulations*, 5th ed, Cincinnati, OH: Harvey Whitney Books Co, 2004.

◆ **Caffeine, Acetaminophen, and Aspirin** *see* Acetaminophen, Aspirin, and Caffeine *on page* 37
◆ **Caffeine and Sodium Benzoate** *see* Caffeine *on page* 319
◆ **Caffeine, Aspirin, and Acetaminophen** *see* Acetaminophen, Aspirin, and Caffeine *on page* 37
◆ **Caffeine Citrate** *see* Caffeine *on page* 319
◆ **Caffeine, Dihydrocodeine, and Aspirin** *see* Dihydrocodeine, Aspirin, and Caffeine *on page* 632
◆ **Caffeine, Orphenadrine, and Aspirin** *see* Orphenadrine, Aspirin, and Caffeine *on page* 1522
◆ **Caffeine Sodium Benzoate** *see* Caffeine *on page* 319
◆ **CAL-101** *see* Idelalisib *on page* 1038

Calamine (KAL a meen)

Index Terms Calamine Lotion
Pharmacologic Category Topical Skin Product
Use Employed primarily as an astringent, protectant, and soothing agent for conditions such as poison ivy, poison oak, poison sumac, sunburn, insect bites, or minor skin irritations
Dosage Topical: Children and Adults: Apply to affected area as often as needed
Additional Information Complete prescribing information should be consulted for additional detail.
Dosage Forms
Lotion, External:
Generic: 8% (120 mL, 177 mL, 180 mL, 240 mL)

◆ **Calamine Lotion** *see* Calamine *on page* 321
◆ **Calan** *see* Verapamil *on page* 2154
◆ **Calan SR** *see* Verapamil *on page* 2154
◆ **Calax [OTC] (Can)** *see* Docusate *on page* 661
◆ **Calcarb 600 [OTC]** *see* Calcium Carbonate *on page* 327
◆ **Cal-Carb Forte [OTC]** *see* Calcium Carbonate *on page* 327
◆ **Calcet Petites [OTC]** *see* Calcium and Vitamin D *on page* 326
◆ **Calci-Chew [OTC]** *see* Calcium Carbonate *on page* 327
◆ **Calcidol [OTC]** *see* Ergocalciferol *on page* 753
◆ **Calciferol [OTC]** *see* Ergocalciferol *on page* 753
◆ **Calcijex (Can)** *see* Calcitriol *on page* 323
◆ **Calcimar (Can)** *see* Calcitonin *on page* 322
◆ **Calci-Mix [OTC]** *see* Calcium Carbonate *on page* 327
◆ **Calcionate [OTC]** *see* Calcium Glubionate *on page* 330

Calcipotriene (kal si POE try een)

Brand Names: U.S. Calcitrene; Dovonex; Sorilux
Brand Names: Canada Dovonex
Index Terms Calcipotriol
Pharmacologic Category Topical Skin Product; Vitamin D Analog
Use Treatment of plaque psoriasis of the body (cream, foam, ointment) or of the scalp (foam, solution)
Pregnancy Risk Factor C
Dosage Plaque psoriasis: Topical: Adults:
Cream: Apply a thin film to the affected skin twice daily
Foam: Apply a thin film to the affected skin or scalp twice daily
Ointment: Apply a thin film to the affected skin once or twice daily
Solution: Apply to the affected scalp twice daily
Additional Information Complete prescribing information should be consulted for additional detail.
Dosage Forms
Cream, External:
Dovonex: 0.005% (60 g, 120 g)
Generic: 0.005% (60 g, 120 g)
Foam, External:
Sorilux: 0.005% (60 g, 120 g)
Ointment, External:
Calcitrene: 0.005% (60 g, 120 g)
Generic: 0.005% (60 g, 120 g)
Solution, External:
Generic: 0.005% (60 mL)

Calcipotriene and Betamethasone
(kal si POE try een & bay ta METH a sone)

Brand Names: U.S. Taclonex
Brand Names: Canada Dovobet
Index Terms Betamethasone Dipropionate and Calcipotriene Hydrate; Calcipotriol and Betamethasone Dipropionate
Pharmacologic Category Corticosteroid, Topical; Vitamin D Analog
Use Plaque psoriasis:
Ointment: Treatment of plaque psoriasis in patients 12 years and older.
Suspension: Treatment of plaque psoriasis of the scalp (patients 12 years and older) and body (adults).
Pregnancy Risk Factor C
Dosage Plaque psoriasis: Topical:
Ointment: **Note:** Application to >30% of body surface area is not recommended
Children ≥12 years and Adolescents: Apply to affected area of skin once daily for up to 4 weeks (maximum dose: 60 g weekly).
Adults: Apply to affected area of skin once daily for up to 4 weeks (maximum dose: 100 g weekly).
Suspension:
Children ≥12 years and Adolescents: Apply to affected area of scalp once daily for up to 8 weeks (maximum dose: 60 g weekly).
Adults: Apply to affected area of skin or scalp once daily for up to 8 weeks (maximum dose: 100 g weekly)

Dosage adjustment in renal impairment: There are no dosage adjustments provided in the manufacturer's labeling.
Dosage adjustment in hepatic impairment: There are no dosage adjustments provided in the manufacturer's labeling.
Additional Information Complete prescribing information should be consulted for additional detail.

Dosage Forms

Ointment, topical:

Taclonex: Calcipotriene 0.005% and betamethasone 0.064% (60 g, 100 g)

Generic: Calcipotriene 0.005% and betamethasone dipropionate 0.064% (60 g, 100 g)

Suspension, topical:

Taclonex: Calcipotriene 0.005% and betamethasone 0.064%

Dosage Forms: Canada

Ointment, topical:

Dovobet: Calcipotriol 50 mcg/g and betamethasone 0.5 mg/g (30 g, 60 g, 120 g)

◆ **Calcipotriol** *see* Calcipotriene *on page 321*

◆ **Calcipotriol and Betamethasone Dipropionate** *see* Calcipotriene and Betamethasone *on page 321*

◆ **Calcite-500 (Can)** *see* Calcium Carbonate *on page 327*

Calcitonin (kal si TOE nin)

Brand Names: U.S. Fortical; Miacalcin

Brand Names: Canada Calcimar

Index Terms Calcitonin (Salmon); Salcatonin

Pharmacologic Category Antidote; Hormone

Use

Injection:

Hypercalcemia: Adjunctive therapy for hypercalcemia

Paget disease: Treatment of symptomatic Paget disease of bone (osteitis deformans) in patients who are nonresponsive or intolerant to alternative therapy

Postmenopausal osteoporosis: Treatment of osteoporosis in women more than 5 years postmenopause

Intranasal:

Postmenopausal osteoporosis: Treatment of postmenopausal osteoporosis in women more than 5 years postmenopause

Pregnancy Risk Factor C

Pregnancy Considerations Adverse events have been observed in animal reproduction studies. Calcitonin does not cross the placenta.

Breast-Feeding Considerations It is not known if calcitonin is excreted in human breast milk. Calcitonin has been shown to decrease milk production in animals. The manufacturer recommends that caution be exercised when administering calcitonin to nursing women.

Contraindications Hypersensitivity to calcitonin salmon or any component of the formulation

Warnings/Precautions A skin test should be performed prior to initiating therapy of calcitonin salmon in patients with suspected sensitivity; anaphylactic shock, anaphylaxis, bronchospasm, and swelling of the tongue or throat have been reported; have epinephrine immediately available for a possible hypersensitivity reaction. A detailed skin testing protocol is available from the manufacturers. Rhinitis and epistaxis have been reported; mucosal alterations may occur. Perform nasal examinations with visualization of the nasal mucosa, turbinates, septum and mucosal blood vessels prior to initiation of therapy, periodically during therapy, and at any time nasal symptoms occur. Temporarily withdraw use if ulceration of nasal mucosa occurs. Discontinue for severe ulcerations >1.5 mm, those that penetrate below the mucosa, or those associated with heavy bleeding. Patients >65 years of age may experience a higher incidence of nasal adverse events with calcitonin nasal spray.

Hypocalcemia with tetany and seizure activity has been reported. Hypocalcemia and other disorders affecting mineral metabolism (eg, vitamin D deficiency) should be corrected before initiating therapy; monitor serum calcium and symptoms of hypocalcemia during therapy. Administer in conjunction with calcium and vitamin D. Fracture reduction efficacy has not been demonstrated; use has not been shown to increase spinal bone mineral density in early postmenopausal women. Use should be reserved for patients for whom alternative treatments are not suitable (eg, patients for whom other therapies are contraindicated or for patients who are intolerant or unwilling to use other therapies). Analyses of randomized controlled trials (in osteoporosis and osteoarthritis) using the nasal spray and oral formulations have demonstrated a statistically significant increase in the risk of the development of cancer in calcitonin-treated patients (compared to placebo). The risk for malignancies is associated with long-term use of calcitonin (trials ranged from 6 months to 5 years in duration). Periodically reassess continued use of calcitonin therapy, carefully considering the risks versus benefits. Similar risk for other routes (subcutaneous, IM, IV) cannot be ruled out. Definitive efficacy of calcitonin-salmon in decreasing fractures is lacking compared to other agents approved for osteoporosis treatment; consider potential benefits of therapy against risks in osteoporosis treatment, including the potential risk for malignancy with long-term use.

Adverse Reactions

Cardiovascular: Angina pectoris, flushing (more common with injection), hypertension

Central nervous system: Depression, dizziness, fatigue, paresthesia

Dermatologic: Erythematous rash

Gastrointestinal: Abdominal pain, constipation, diarrhea, dyspepsia, nausea (more common with injection)

Genitourinary: Cystitis

Hematologic & oncologic: Lymphadenopathy

Infection: Increased susceptibility to infection

Local: Injection site reaction

Neuromuscular & skeletal: Back pain, myalgia, osteoarthritis

Ophthalmic: Abnormal lacrimation, conjunctivitis

Respiratory: Bronchospasm, flu-like symptoms, nasal mucosa ulcer, rhinitis (including ulcerative), sinusitis, upper respiratory tract infection

Rare but important or life-threatening): Alopecia, altered sense of smell, anaphylactic shock, anaphylactoid reaction, anaphylaxis, anemia, anorexia, arthritis, bronchitis, bundle branch block, cerebrovascular accident, cholelithiasis, dermal ulcer, eczema, edema, excoriation (nasal mucosa), gastritis, goiter, hearing loss, hematuria, hepatitis, hypersensitivity reaction, hyperthyroidism, malignant neoplasm, migraine, myocardial infarction, nephrolithiasis, neuralgia, nocturia, palpitations, periorbital edema, pneumonia, polymyalgia rheumatica, polyuria, pyelonephritis, tachycardia, thrombophlebitis, vitreous opacity, weight gain

Drug Interactions

Metabolism/Transport Effects None known.

Avoid Concomitant Use There are no known interactions where it is recommended to avoid concomitant use.

Increased Effect/Toxicity

Calcitonin may increase the levels/effects of: Zoledronic Acid

Decreased Effect

Calcitonin may decrease the levels/effects of: Lithium

Preparation for Administration Injection: NS has been recommended for the dilution to prepare a skin test in patients with suspected sensitivity.

Storage/Stability

Injection: Store under refrigeration at 2°C to 8°C (36°F to 46°F); protect from freezing. The following stability information has also been reported: May be stored at room temperature for up to 14 days (Cohen, 2007).

Nasal: Store unopened bottle under refrigeration at 2°C to 8°C (36°F to 46°F); do not freeze.

Fortical: After opening, store for up to 30 days at 20°C to 25°C (68°F to 77°F); excursions permitted to 15°C to 30°C (59°F to 86°F). Store in upright position.

Miacalcin: After opening, store for up to 35 days at room temperature of 15°C to 30°C (59°F to 86°F). Store in upright position.

Mechanism of Action Peptide sequence similar to human calcitonin; functionally antagonizes the effects of parathyroid hormone. Directly inhibits osteoclastic bone resorption; promotes the renal excretion of calcium, phosphate, sodium, magnesium, and potassium by decreasing tubular reabsorption; increases the jejunal secretion of water, sodium, potassium, and chloride

Pharmacodynamics/Kinetics

Onset of action:

Hypercalcemia: IM, SubQ: ~2 hours

Paget's disease: Within a few months; may take up to 1 year for neurologic symptom improvement

Duration: Hypercalcemia: IM, SubQ: 6 to 8 hours

Distribution: V_d: 0.15 to 0.3 L/kg

Metabolism: Metabolized in kidneys, blood and peripheral tissue

Bioavailability: IM: 66%; SubQ: 71%; Nasal: ~3% to 5% (relative to IM)

Half-life elimination (terminal): IM 58 minutes; SubQ 59 to 64 minutes; Nasal: ~18 to 23 minutes

Time to peak, plasma: SubQ ~23 minutes; Nasal: ~10 to 13 minutes

Excretion: Urine (as inactive metabolites)

Dosage Adults:

Paget's disease, symptomatic (Miacalcin): IM, SubQ: 100 units daily. **Note:** Due to the risk of malignancy associated with prolonged calcitonin use, the Canadian labeling recommends limiting therapy in most patients to ≤3 months; under exceptional circumstances (eg, impending pathologic fracture), therapy may be extended to ≤6 months

Hypercalcemia (Miacalcin): Initial: IM, SubQ: 4 units/kg every 12 hours; after 1 to 2 days, may increase up to 8 units/kg every 12 hours; if the response remains unsatisfactory after 2 more days, may further increase up to a maximum of 8 units/kg every 6 hours

Postmenopausal osteoporosis:

IM, SubQ: Miacalcin: 100 units daily

Intranasal: Fortical, Miacalcin: 200 units (1 spray) in one nostril once daily

Dosage adjustment in renal impairment: There are no dosage adjustments provided in the manufacturer's labeling.

Dosage adjustment in hepatic impairment: There are no dosage adjustments provided in the manufacturer's labeling.

Dietary Considerations Patients with Paget's disease and hypercalcemia should follow a low calcium diet as prescribed. Recommended amounts of vitamin D and calcium intake is essential for preventing/treating osteoporosis. If dietary intake is inadequate, dietary supplementation is recommended. Women and men should consume:

Calcium: 1000 mg/day (men: 50 to 70 years) **or** 1200 mg/day (women ≥51 years and men ≥71 years) (IOM, 2011; NOF, 2013)

Vitamin D: 800 to 1000 units/day (men and women ≥50 years) (NOF, 2013). Recommended Dietary Allowance (RDA): 600 units/day (men and women ≤70 years) **or** 800 units/day (men and women ≥71 years) (IOM, 2011).

Administration

Injection: May be administered IM or SubQ. IM route is preferred if the injection volume is >2 mL (use multiple injection sites if dose volume is >2 mL). SubQ route is preferred for outpatient self-administration unless the injection volume is >2 mL.

Nasal spray: Before first use, allow bottle to reach room temperature, then prime pump by releasing at least 5 sprays until full spray is produced. To administer, place nozzle into nostril with head in upright position. Alternate nostrils daily. Do not prime pump before each daily use. Discard after 30 doses.

Monitoring Parameters

Osteoporosis: Bone mineral density (BMD) should be reevaluated every 2 years (or more frequently) after initiating therapy (NOF, 2013); annual measurements of height and weight, assessment of chronic back pain; serum calcium and 25(OH)D; consider measuring biochemical markers of bone turnover

Paget's disease: Alkaline phosphatase; pain; serum calcium and 25(OH)D

Nasal formulation: Visualization of nasal mucosa, turbinate, septum, and mucosal blood vessels (at baseline and with nasal complaints)

Consider periodic examinations of urine sediment

Reference Range

Calcium (total): Adults: 9.0 to 11.0 mg/dL (2.05 to 2.54 mmol/L), may slightly decrease with aging

Phosphorus: 2.5 to 4.5 mg/dL (0.81 to 1.45 mmol/L)

Vitamin D: There is no clear consensus on a reference range for total serum 25(OH)D concentrations or the validity of this level as it relates clinically to bone health. In addition, there is significant variability in the reporting of serum 25(OH)D levels as a result of different assay types in use; however, the following ranges have been suggested:

Adults (IOM, 2011): Sufficient levels in practically all persons: ≥20 ng/mL (50 nmol/L); concern for risk of toxicity: >50 ng/mL (125 nmol/L)

Osteoporosis patients (NOF, 2013): Recommended level to reach and maintain: ~30 ng/mL (75 nmol/L)

Dosage Forms

Solution, Injection:

Miacalcin: 200 units/mL (2 mL)

Solution, Nasal:

Fortical: 200 units/actuation (3.7 mL)

Miacalcin: 200 units/actuation (3.7 mL)

Generic: 200 units/actuation (3.7 mL)

Dosage Forms: Canada Refer to Dosage Forms. Intranasal solution is not available in Canada.

◆ **Calcitonin (Salmon)** *see* Calcitonin *on page 322*

◆ **Calcitrate [OTC]** *see* Calcium and Vitamin D *on page 326*

◆ **Cal-Citrate [OTC]** *see* Calcium Citrate *on page 330*

◆ **Calcitrene** *see* Calcipotriene *on page 321*

Calcitriol (kal si TRYE ole)

Brand Names: U.S. Rocaltrol; Vectical

Brand Names: Canada Calcijex; Calcitriol Injection; Calcitriol-Odan; Rocaltrol; Silkis

Index Terms 1,25 Dihydroxycholecalciferol

Pharmacologic Category Vitamin D Analog

Use

Management of hypocalcemia in patients on chronic renal dialysis (oral, injection); management of secondary hyperparathyroidism in patients with chronic kidney disease (CKD) not yet on dialysis (predialysis patients) (oral); management of hypocalcemia in patients with hypoparathyroidism and pseudohypoparathyroidism (oral); management of mild-to-moderate plaque psoriasis (topical)

Canadian labeling: Additional uses (not in U.S. labeling): Vitamin D-resistant rickets (oral)

Pregnancy Risk Factor C

Pregnancy Considerations Teratogenic effects have been observed in some animal reproduction studies. Mild hypercalcemia has been reported in a newborn following maternal use of calcitriol during pregnancy. Adverse effects on fetal development were not observed with use of calcitriol during pregnancy in women (N=9) with pseudovitamin D-dependent rickets. Doses were adjusted every 4 weeks to keep calcium concentrations within normal limits (Edouard, 2011). If calcitriol is used for the management of hypoparathyroidism in pregnancy, dose adjustments may be needed as pregnancy progresses and again following delivery. Vitamin D and calcium levels should be monitored closely and kept in the lower normal range.

Breast-Feeding Considerations Low levels are found in breast milk (~2 pg/mL)

Contraindications

U.S. labeling:

Oral, injection: Hypersensitivity to calcitriol or any component of the formulation; hypercalcemia, vitamin D toxicity

Topical: There are no contraindications listed in the manufacturer's labeling.

Canadian labeling:

Oral, injection: Hypersensitivity to calcitriol, vitamin D or its analogues or derivatives, or any component of the formulation or container; hypercalcemia, vitamin D toxicity

Topical: Ophthalmic or internal use; hypercalcemia or a history of abnormal calcium metabolism; concurrent systemic treatment of calcium homeostasis; severe renal impairment or end-stage renal disease (ESRD)

Warnings/Precautions Oral, injection: Adequate dietary (supplemental) calcium is necessary for clinical response to vitamin D. Excessive vitamin D may cause severe hypercalcemia, hypercalciuria, and hyperphosphatemia. Discontinue use immediately in adult patients with a calcium-phosphate product (serum calcium times phosphorus) >70 mg^2/dL^2, may resume therapy at decreased doses when levels are appropriate. Other forms of vitamin D should be withheld during therapy to avoid the potential for hypercalcemia to develop. In addition, several months may be required for ergocalciferol levels to return to baseline in patients switching from ergocalciferol therapy to calcitriol. Monitor calcium levels closely with initiation of therapy and with dose adjustments; discontinue use promptly in patients who develop hypercalcemia. Avoid abrupt dietary modifications (eg, increased intake of dairy products) which may lead to hypercalcemia; adjust calcium intake if indicated and maintain adequate hydration. Chronic hypercalcemia can result in generalized vascular and soft tissue calcification. Immobilized patients may be at a higher risk for hypercalcemia.

Use oral calcitriol with caution in patients with malabsorption syndromes (efficacy may be limited and/or response may be unpredictable). Use of calcitriol for the treatment of secondary hyperparathyroidism associated with CKD is not recommended in patients with rapidly worsening kidney function or in noncompliant patients. Increased serum phosphate levels in patients with renal failure may lead to calcification; the use of an aluminum-containing phosphate binder is recommended along with a low phosphate diet in these patients. Use with caution in patients taking cardiac glycosides; digitalis toxicity is potentiated by hypocalcemia. Concomitant use with magnesium-containing products such as antacids may lead to hypermagnesemia in patients receiving chronic renal dialysis. Products may contain coconut (capsule) or palm seed oil (oral solution). Some products may contain tartrazine.

Topical: May cause hypercalcemia; if alterations in calcium occur, discontinue treatment until levels return to normal. For external use only; not for ophthalmic, oral, or intravaginal use. Do not apply to facial skin, eyes, or lips. Absorption may be increased with occlusive dressings. Avoid or limit excessive exposure to natural or artificial sunlight, or phototherapy. The safety and effectiveness has not been evaluated in patients with erythrodermic, exfoliative, or pustular psoriasis. Canadian labeling does not recommend use in patients with hepatic or renal impairment.

Adverse Reactions

Oral, IV:

Cardiovascular: Cardiac arrhythmia, hypertension

Central nervous system: Apathy, drowsiness, headache, hyperthermia, metallic taste, psychosis, sensory disturbance

Dermatologic: Erythema, erythema multiforme, pruritus, skin rash, urticaria

Endocrine & metabolic: Albuminuria, calcinosis, decreased libido, dehydration, growth suppression, hypercalcemia, hypercholesterolemia, polydipsia, weight loss

Gastrointestinal: Abdominal pain, anorexia, constipation, nausea, pancreatitis, stomach pain, vomiting, xerostomia

Genitourinary: Hypercalciuria, nocturia, urinary tract infection

Hepatic: Increased serum ALT, increased serum AST

Hypersensitivity: Hypersensitivity reaction

Local: Pain at injection site (mild)

Neuromuscular & skeletal: Dystrophy, myalgia, ostealgia, weakness

Ophthalmic: Conjunctivitis, photophobia

Renal: Calcium nephrolithiasis, increased blood urea nitrogen, increased serum creatinine, polyuria

Respiratory: Rhinorrhea

Rare but important or life-threatening: Anaphylaxis

Topical:

Dermatologic: Pruritus, psoriasis, skin discomfort

Endocrine & metabolic: Hypercalcemia

Genitourinary: Urine abnormality, hypercalciuria

Rare but important or life-threatening: Kidney stones

Drug Interactions

Metabolism/Transport Effects **Substrate** of CYP3A4 (major); **Note:** Assignment of Major/Minor substrate status based on clinically relevant drug interaction potential; **Induces** CYP3A4 (weak)

Avoid Concomitant Use

Avoid concomitant use of Calcitriol with any of the following: Aluminum Hydroxide; Conivaptan; Fusidic Acid (Systemic); Idelalisib; Multivitamins/Fluoride (with ADE); Multivitamins/Minerals (with ADEK, Folate, Iron); Sucralfate; Vitamin D Analogs

Increased Effect/Toxicity

Calcitriol may increase the levels/effects of: Aluminum Hydroxide; Cardiac Glycosides; Magnesium Salts; Sucralfate; Vitamin D Analogs

The levels/effects of Calcitriol may be increased by: Aprepitant; Calcium Salts; Ceritinib; Conivaptan; CYP3A4 Inhibitors (Moderate); CYP3A4 Inhibitors (Strong); Danazol; Dasatinib; Fosaprepitant; Fusidic Acid (Systemic); Idelalisib; Ivacaftor; Luliconazole; Mifepristone; Multivitamins/Fluoride (with ADE); Multivitamins/Minerals (with ADEK, Folate, Iron); Netupitant; Simeprevir; Stiripentol; Thiazide Diuretics

Decreased Effect

Calcitriol may decrease the levels/effects of: ARIPiprazole; Hydrocodone; Saxagliptin

The levels/effects of Calcitriol may be decreased by: Bile Acid Sequestrants; Bosentan; Corticosteroids (Systemic); CYP3A4 Inducers (Moderate); CYP3A4 Inducers (Strong); Dabrafenib; Deferasirox; Mineral Oil; Mitotane; Orlistat; Sevelamer; Siltuximab; St Johns Wort; Tocilizumab

Storage/Stability

Oral capsule, injection, solution: Store at room temperature of 15°C to 30°C (59°F to 86°F). Protect from light.

Topical: Store at room temperature of 25°C (77°F); excursions permitted to 15°C to 30°C (59°F to 86°F); do not refrigerate; do not freeze.

Mechanism of Action Calcitriol, the active form of vitamin D (1,25 hydroxyvitamin D_3), binds to and activates the vitamin D receptor in kidney, parathyroid gland, intestine, and bone, stimulating intestinal calcium transport and absorption. It reduces PTH levels and improves calcium and phosphate homeostasis by stimulating bone resorption of calcium and increasing renal tubular reabsorption of calcium. Decreased renal conversion of vitamin D to its primary active metabolite (1,25 hydroxyvitamin D) in chronic renal failure leads to reduced activation of vitamin D receptor, which subsequently removes inhibitory suppression of parathyroid hormone (PTH) release; increased serum PTH (secondary hyperparathyroidism) reduces calcium excretion and enhances bone resorption.

The mechanism by which calcitriol is beneficial in the treatment of psoriasis has not been established.

Pharmacodynamics/Kinetics

Duration: Oral, IV: 3 to 5 days

Absorption: Oral: Rapid

Protein binding: 99.9%

Metabolism: Primarily to calcitroic acid and a lactone metabolite

Half-life elimination: Children ~27 hours; Healthy adults: 5 to 8 hours; Hemodialysis: 16 to 22 hours

Time to peak, serum: Oral: 3 to 6 hours; Hemodialysis: 8 to 12 hours

Excretion: Primarily feces; urine

Dosage

Hypocalcemia in patients on chronic renal dialysis:

Adults:

Oral: Initial: 0.25 mcg daily; may increase dose by 0.25 mcg daily at 4- to 8-week intervals, up to 0.5-1 mcg daily; patients with normal or mildly decreased serum calcium levels may respond to 0.25 mcg every other day

IV:

U.S. labeling: Initial: 1-2 mcg 3 times weekly approximately every other day. Adjust dose by 0.5-1 mcg at 2- to 4-week intervals; dosing range: 0.5-4 mcg 3 times weekly. Gradual dose reduction and discontinuation of therapy may be necessary as PTH levels decrease below target of (1.5-3 x ULN) in response to therapy.

Canadian labeling: Initial: 0.5 mcg 3 times weekly, approximately every other day. Adjust dose by 0.25-0.5 mcg at 2- to 4-week intervals; dosing range: 0.5-3 mcg 3 times weekly

Hypocalcemia in hypoparathyroidism/pseudohypoparathyroidism:

U.S. labeling: Oral:

Children 1-5 years: Usual dosage range: 0.25-0.75 mcg once daily (may adjust dose at 2- to 4-week intervals)

Children ≥6 years and Adults: Initial: 0.25 mcg daily (may adjust dose at 2- to 4-week intervals); range: 0.5-2 mcg once daily

Canadian labeling: Oral:

Children: Initial: 0.03-0.05 mcg/kg/day; evaluate response after 2 weeks and increase dose by 25% if response is inadequate. Dose may be increased or decreased by 25% every 2 weeks thereafter until therapeutic response is achieved. **Note:** May consider initial dose of 0.05 mcg/kg/day for severe hypocalcemia/ symptoms (hospitalization recommended with close monitoring and dose reduction as soon as clinically possible). Maintenance dose: 0.014-0.04 mcg/kg/day

Adults: Initial: 0.25 mcg daily; may increase dose by 0.25 mcg daily at 2- to 4-week intervals. Discontinue use immediately for hypercalcemia; may resume therapy after calcium levels normalize.

Psoriasis: Adults: Topical: Apply twice daily to affected areas (maximum: 200 g weekly); Canadian labeling recommends maximum of 30 g daily

Secondary hyperparathyroidism associated with moderate-to-severe CKD in patients not yet on dialysis:

U.S. labeling: Oral:

Children <3 years: Initial dose: 0.01-0.015 mcg/kg/day

Children ≥3 years, Adolescents, and Adults: Initial: 0.25 mcg daily; may increase to 0.5 mcg daily

Note: KDIGO guidelines do not recommend routine vitamin D therapy (with vitamin D supplements or a vitamin D analog [eg, calcitriol]) for progressive or persistently elevated PTH concentrations in CKD patients (stages 3-5) not on dialysis in the absence of suspected/documented Vitamin D deficiency. Caution is advised to avoid hypercalcemia or elevated phosphate levels (KDIGO, 2009; KDIGO, 2012; Uhlig, 2010).

Vitamin D-dependent rickets type 1/pseudovitamin D deficiency rickets (PDDR):

U.S. off-label use: Children and Adults: Oral: Initial: 0.5 mcg twice daily; subsequent dosing adjusted to maintain normal serum calcium and PTH levels; median dose after 2 years: 0.25 mcg daily (range: 0.1-0.5 mcg daily) (Edouard, 2011)

Canadian labeling: Children: Oral: Initial: 0.01-0.025 mcg/kg/day; evaluate response after two weeks and increase dose by 25% if response is inadequate. Dose may be increased or decreased by 25% every 2 weeks thereafter until therapeutic response is achieved. **Note:** May consider initial dose of 0.05 mcg/kg/day for severe hypocalcemia/ symptoms (hospitalization recommended with close monitoring and dose reduction as soon as clinically possible). Maintenance dose: 0.0046-0.015 mcg/kg/day.

Vitamin D-resistant rickets: *Canadian labeling (not in U.S. labeling):* Adults: Oral: Initial: 0.25 mcg daily; may increase dose by 0.25 mcg daily at 2- to 4-week intervals if response is inadequate; discontinue use immediately for hypercalcemia and do not resume until calcium levels normalize.

X-linked hypophosphatemic rickets: *Canadian labeling (not in U.S. labeling):* Children: Oral: Initial: 0.01-0.02 mcg/kg/day; evaluate response after 2 weeks and increase dose by 25% if response is inadequate. Dose may be increased or decreased by 25% every two weeks thereafter until therapeutic response is achieved. **Note:** May consider initial dose of 0.05 mcg/kg/day for severe hypocalcemia/ symptoms (hospitalization recommended with close monitoring and dose reduction as soon as clinically possible). Maintenance dose: 0.01-0.05 mcg/kg/day.

Elderly: Start at the lower end of the dosage range. Refer to adult dosing.

Dosage adjustment in renal impairment: No dosage adjustment necessary.

Dosage adjustment in hepatic impairment: There are no dosage adjustments provided in the manufacturer's labeling.

Dietary Considerations May be taken without regard to food. Give with meals to reduce GI problems. Adequate calcium intake should be maintained during therapy; dietary phosphorous may need to be restricted.

Administration

IV: May be administered as a bolus dose IV through the catheter at the end of hemodialysis.

Oral: May be administered without regard to food. Administer with meals to reduce GI problems.

Topical: Apply externally; not for ophthalmic, oral, or intravaginal use. Do not apply to eyes, lips, or facial skins. Rub in gently so that no medication remains visible. Limit application to only the areas of skin affected by psoriasis.

Monitoring Parameters

Manufacturer's labeling:

Oral therapy:

Dialysis patients: Serum calcium, phosphorus, magnesium, and alkaline phosphate monitored periodically

Hypoparathyroid patients: Serum calcium, phosphorus, 24 hour urinary calcium monitored periodically

Predialysis patients: Serum calcium, phosphorus, alkaline phosphatase, creatinine, and intact PTH, initially; then serum calcium, phosphorus, alkaline phosphatase, and creatinine monthly x 6 months, then periodically. Intact PTH should be monitored every 3-4 months.

During titration periods (all patients), monitor serum calcium levels at least twice weekly.

IV therapy: Serum calcium and phosphorus twice weekly (following initiation and during dosage adjustments) and periodically during therapy; periodic magnesium, alkaline phosphatase, 24 hour urinary calcium and phosphorous

KDIGO guidelines (2009):

Serum calcium, phosphorus, and PTH: CKD stages 3-5D: Frequency of monitoring should be based on the presence and magnitude of abnormalities, as well as the rate of CKD progression. Reasonable intervals are:

CKD stage 3: Serum calcium and phosphorus, every 6 to 12 months; PTH: monitor based on baseline level and CKD progression

CKD stage 4: Serum calcium and phosphorus every 3 to 6 months; PTH every 6 to 12 months

CKD stage 5 (includes 5D): Serum calcium and phosphorus every 1 to 3 months; PTH every 3 to 6 months

Alkaline phosphatase: CKD stages 4-5D: Monitor every 12 months or more frequently in the presence of increased PTH levels

Reference Range

Corrected total serum calcium: KDIGO guidelines recommend maintaining normal ranges for all stages of CKD (3-5D) (KDIGO, 2009)

Phosphorus: KDIGO guidelines recommend maintaining normal ranges for CKD stages 3-5 and lowering elevated phosphorus levels toward the normal range for CKD stage 5D (KDIGO, 2009)

PTH: Whole molecule, immunochemiluminometric assay (ICMA): 1 to 5.2 pmol/L; whole molecule, radioimmunoassay (RIA): 10 to 65 pg/mL; whole molecule, immunoradiometric, double antibody (IRMA): 1 to 6 pmol/L

Target ranges by stage of chronic kidney disease (KDIGO, 2009): CKD stage 3-5: Optimal iPTH is unknown; maintain normal range (assay-dependent); CKD stage 5D: Maintain iPTH within 2-9 times the upper limit of normal for the assay used

Dosage Forms

Capsule, Oral:

Rocaltrol: 0.25 mcg, 0.5 mcg

Generic: 0.25 mcg, 0.5 mcg

Ointment, External:

Vectical: 3 mcg/g (100 g)

Generic: 3 mcg/g (100 g)

Solution, Intravenous:

Generic: 1 mcg/mL (1 mL)

Solution, Oral:

Rocaltrol: 1 mcg/mL (15 mL)

Generic: 1 mcg/mL (15 mL)

Dosage Forms: Canada

Ointment, topical:

Silkis™: 3 mcg/g (5 g, 30 g, 100 g)

◆ **Calcitriol Injection (Can)** *see* Calcitriol *on page 323*

◆ **Calcitriol-Odan (Can)** *see* Calcitriol *on page 323*

◆ **Calcium 600 [OTC]** *see* Calcium Carbonate *on page 327*

Calcium Acetate (KAL see um AS e tate)

Brand Names: U.S. Calphron [OTC]; Eliphos; PhosLo; Phoslyra

Brand Names: Canada PhosLo®

Pharmacologic Category Antidote; Calcium Salt; Phosphate Binder

Use Control of hyperphosphatemia in end-stage renal failure; does not promote aluminum absorption

Pregnancy Risk Factor C

Dosage Oral: Adults, on dialysis: Initial: 1334 mg with each meal, can be increased gradually (ie, every 2-3 weeks) to bring the serum phosphate value to <6 mg/dL as long as hypercalcemia does not develop (usual dose: 2001-2668 mg calcium acetate with each meal); do not give additional calcium supplements

Dosage adjustment in renal impairment: No dosage adjustment necessary.

Dosage adjustment in hepatic impairment: No dosage adjustment provided in manufacturer's labeling.

Additional Information Complete prescribing information should be consulted for additional detail.

Dosage Forms Considerations

Calcium acetate is approximately 25% elemental calcium

Calcium acetate 667 mg = elemental calcium 169 mg = calcium 8.45 mEq = calcium 4.23 mmol

Dosage Forms

Capsule, Oral:

PhosLo: 667 mg

Generic: 667 mg

Solution, Oral:

Phoslyra: 667 mg/5 mL (473 mL)

Tablet, Oral:

Calphron [OTC]: 667 mg

Eliphos: 667 mg

Generic: 667 mg, 668 mg

◆ **Calcium Acetylhomotaurinate** *see* Acamprosate *on page 28*

Calcium and Vitamin D

(KAL see um & VYE ta min dee)

Brand Names: U.S. Cal-CYUM [OTC]; Calcet Petites [OTC]; Calcitrate [OTC]; Caltrate 600+D [OTC]; Caltrate 600+Soy [OTC]; Caltrate ColonHealth [OTC]; Caltrate Gummy Bites [OTC]; Chew-Cal [OTC]; Citracal Maximum [OTC]; Citracal Petites [OTC]; Citracal Regular [OTC]; Liqua-Cal [OTC]; Os-Cal 500+D [OTC]; Oysco 500+D [OTC]; Oysco D [OTC]

Index Terms Calcium Citrate and Vitamin D; Vitamin D and Calcium Carbonate

Pharmacologic Category Calcium Salt; Electrolyte Supplement, Oral; Vitamin, Fat Soluble

Use Dietary supplement, antacid

Dosage Oral: Adults: Refer to individual monographs for dietary reference intake.

Dosage adjustment in renal impairment: Use caution in severe renal impairment

Additional Information Complete prescribing information should be consulted for additional detail.

Dosage Forms

Caplet, oral:

Citracal Maximum [OTC]: Calcium 315 mg and vitamin D 250 units

Os-Cal [OTC]: Calcium 500 mg and vitamin D 200 units

Os-Cal Extra D [OTC]: Calcium 500 mg and vitamin D 600 units

Capsule, softgel, oral: Calcium 500 mg and vitamin D 500 units; calcium 600 mg and vitamin D 100 units; calcium 600 mg and vitamin D 200 units

Liqua-Cal [OTC]: Calcium 600 mg and vitamin D 200 units

Tablet, oral: Calcium 250 mg and vitamin D 125 units; calcium 315 mg and vitamin D 200 units; calcium 500 mg and vitamin D 125 units; calcium 500 mg and vitamin D 200 units; calcium 600 mg and vitamin D 125 units; calcium 600 mg and vitamin D 200 units; calcium 600 mg and vitamin D 400 units

Calcet Petites [OTC]: Calcium 200 mg and vitamin D 250 units

Calcitrate [OTC]: Calcium 315 mg and vitamin D 250 units

Caltrate 600+D [OTC]: Calcium 600 mg and vitamin D 200 units

Caltrate 600+Soy [OTC]: Calcium 600 mg and vitamin D 200 units

Caltrate ColonHealth [OTC]: Calcium 600 mg and vitamin D 200 units

Citracal Petites [OTC]: Calcium 200 mg and vitamin D 250 units

Citracal Regular [OTC]: Calcium 250 mg and vitamin D 200 units

Oysco D [OTC]: Calcium 250 mg and vitamin D 125 units

Oysco 500+D [OTC]: Calcium 500 mg and vitamin D 200 units

Tablet, chewable: Calcium 500 mg and vitamin D 100 units; calcium 500 mg and vitamin D 200 units; calcium 500 mg and vitamin D 600 units; calcium 600 mg and vitamin D 400 units

Caltrate Gummy Bites [OTC]: Calcium 250 mg and vitamin D 400 units

Os-Cal [OTC]: Calcium 500 mg and vitamin D 600 units

Wafer, chewable:

Cal-CYUM [OTC]: Calcium 519 mg and vitamin D 150 units (50s)

Chew-Cal [OTC]: Calcium 333 mg and vitamin D 40 units (100s, 250s)

◆ **Calcium Antacid [OTC]** *see* Calcium Carbonate *on page 327*

◆ **Calcium Antacid Extra Strength [OTC]** *see* Calcium Carbonate *on page 327*

◆ **Calcium Antacid Ultra Max St [OTC]** *see* Calcium Carbonate *on page 327*

Calcium Carbonate (KAL see um KAR bun ate)

Brand Names: U.S. Alcalak [OTC]; Antacid Calcium [OTC]; Antacid Extra Strength [OTC]; Antacid [OTC]; Cal-Carb Forte [OTC]; Cal-Gest Antacid [OTC]; Cal-Mint [OTC]; Calcarb 600 [OTC]; Calci-Chew [OTC]; Calci-Mix [OTC]; Calcium 600 [OTC]; Calcium Antacid Extra Strength [OTC]; Calcium Antacid Ultra Max St [OTC]; Calcium Antacid [OTC]; Calcium High Potency [OTC]; Caltrate 600 [OTC]; Florical [OTC]; Maalox Childrens [OTC]; Maalox [OTC]; Os-Cal [OTC] [DSC]; Oysco 500 [OTC]; Titralac [OTC]; Tums E-X 750 [OTC]; Tums Freshers [OTC]; Tums Kids [OTC]; Tums Lasting Effects [OTC]; Tums Smoothies [OTC]; Tums Ultra 1000 [OTC]; Tums [OTC]

Brand Names: Canada Apo-Cal; Calcite-500; Caltrate; Caltrate Select; Os-Cal; Tums Chews Extra Strength; Tums Extra Strength; Tums Regular Strength; Tums Smoothies; Tums Ultra Strength

Index Terms Oscal

Pharmacologic Category Antacid; Antidote; Calcium Salt; Electrolyte Supplement, Oral

Use

Antacid: For the relief of acid indigestion, heartburn, sour stomach, and GI upset associated with these symptoms

Calcium supplementation: For use as a dietary supplement when calcium intake may be inadequate (eg, osteoporosis, osteomalacia, hypocalcemic rickets) (IOM, 2011)

Dosage Oral (dosage is in terms of calcium **carbonate** except where noted; calcium carbonate generally provides approximately 40% elemental calcium):

Dietary Reference Intake for Calcium:

0 to <6 months: Adequate intake: 200 mg **elemental calcium** daily

6 to 12 months: Adequate intake: 260 mg **elemental calcium** daily

1 to 3 years: RDA: 700 mg **elemental calcium** daily

4 to 8 years: RDA: 1000 mg **elemental calcium** daily

9 to 18 years: RDA: 1300 mg **elemental calcium** daily

Adults, Females/Males: RDA:

19 to 50 years: 1000 mg **elemental calcium** daily

≥51 years, females: 1200 mg **elemental calcium** daily

51 to 70 years, males: 1000 mg **elemental calcium** daily

>70 years, males: 1200 mg **elemental calcium** daily

Females: Pregnancy/Lactating: RDA: Requirements are the same as in nonpregnant or nonlactating females (IOM, 2011)

Antacid:

Children 2 to 4 years (10.9 to 21.3 kg): 375 to 400 mg as symptoms occur; maximum: 1500 mg daily for up to 2 weeks; OTC dosing recommendations may vary by product and/or manufacturer; specific product labeling should be consulted

Children 5 to 11 years (≥21.8 kg): 750 to 800 mg as symptoms occur; maximum: 3000 mg daily for up to 2 weeks; OTC dosing recommendations may vary by product and/or manufacturer; specific product labeling should be consulted

Children ≥12 years, Adolescents, and Adults: Generally, 1 to 4 tablets as symptoms occur; maximum: 8000 mg daily for up to 2 weeks; OTC dosing recommendations may vary by product and/or manufacturer; specific product labeling should be consulted

Calcium supplementation:

Children 2 to 4 years: 750 mg twice daily

Children ≥4 years: 750 mg 3 times daily

Adolescents and Adults: 500 mg to 4 g daily in 1 to 3 divided doses; OTC dosing recommendations may vary by product and/or manufacturer; specific product labeling should be consulted

Hyperphosphatemia in chronic kidney disease (off-label use): Adults: Total dose of elemental calcium (including dietary sources and calcium-based phosphate binders) should not exceed 2000 mg daily (Eknoyan, 2003).

Dosing adjustment in renal impairment: CrCl <25 mL/minute: Dosage adjustments may be necessary depending on the serum calcium levels

Dosing adjustment in hepatic impairment: There are no dosage adjustments provided in the manufacturer's labeling (has not been studied).

Additional Information Complete prescribing information should be consulted for additional detail.

Dosage Forms Considerations 1 g calcium carbonate = elemental calcium 400 mg = calcium 20 mEq = calcium 10 mmol

Dosage Forms

Capsule, Oral:
Calci-Mix [OTC]: 1250 mg
Florical [OTC]: 364 mg

Powder, Oral:
Generic: 800 mg/2 g (480 g)

Suspension, Oral:
Generic: 1250 mg/5 mL (5 mL, 473 mL, 500 mL)

Tablet, Oral:
Cal-Carb Forte [OTC]: 1250 mg
Calcarb 600 [OTC]: 1500 mg
Calcium 600 [OTC]: 600 mg
Calcium High Potency [OTC]: 600 mg
Caltrate 600 [OTC]: 1500 mg
Florical [OTC]: 364 mg
Oysco 500 [OTC]: 500 mg
Generic: 500 mg, 600 mg, 1250 mg

Tablet, Oral [preservative free]:
Calcium 600 [OTC]: 600 mg
Generic: 500 mg, 600 mg, 1250 mg

Tablet Chewable, Oral:
Alcalak [OTC]: 420 mg
Antacid [OTC]: 420 mg, 500 mg
Antacid Calcium [OTC]: 500 mg
Antacid Extra Strength [OTC]: 750 mg
Cal-Gest Antacid [OTC]: 500 mg
Cal-Mint [OTC]: 260 mg
Calci-Chew [OTC]: 1250 mg
Calcium Antacid [OTC]: 500 mg
Calcium Antacid Extra Strength [OTC]: 750 mg
Calcium Antacid Ultra Max St [OTC]: 1000 mg
Maalox [OTC]: 600 mg
Maalox Childrens [OTC]: 400 mg
Titralac [OTC]: 420 mg
Tums [OTC]: 500 mg
Tums E-X 750 [OTC]: 750 mg
Tums Freshers [OTC]: 500 mg
Tums Kids [OTC]: 750 mg
Tums Lasting Effects [OTC]: 500 mg
Tums Smoothies [OTC]: 750 mg
Tums Ultra 1000 [OTC]: 1000 mg
Generic: 260 mg, 500 mg, 750 mg

Tablet Chewable, Oral [preservative free]:
Generic: 500 mg

◆ **Calcium Carbonate and Etidronate Disodium** *see* Etidronate and Calcium Carbonate [CAN/INT] *on page 814*

Calcium Carbonate and Magnesium Hydroxide

(KAL see um KAR bun ate & mag NEE zhum hye DROKS ide)

Brand Names: U.S. Mi-Acid Double Strength [OTC]; Mylanta Supreme [OTC]; Mylanta Ultra [OTC]

Index Terms Magnesium Hydroxide and Calcium Carbonate; Rolaids

Pharmacologic Category Antacid

Use Hyperacidity

Dosage Adults: Oral: 2-4 tablets between meals, at bedtime, or as directed by health care provider

Additional Information Complete prescribing information should be consulted for additional detail.

Dosage Forms

Liquid:
Mylanta Supreme [OTC]: Calcium carbonate 400 mg and magnesium hydroxide 135 mg per 5 mL

Tablet, chewable: Calcium carbonate 550 mg and magnesium hydroxide 110 mg; calcium carbonate 675 mg and magnesium hydroxide 135 mg; calcium carbonate 700 mg and magnesium hydroxide 300 mg
Mi-Acid Double Strength [OTC], Mylanta Ultra [OTC]: Calcium carbonate 700 mg and magnesium hydroxide 300 mg

Calcium Chloride (KAL see um KLOR ide)

Pharmacologic Category Calcium Salt; Electrolyte Supplement, Parenteral

Use Treatment of hypocalcemia and conditions secondary to hypocalcemia (eg, tetany, seizures, arrhythmias); emergent treatment of severe hypermagnesemia

Pregnancy Risk Factor C

Pregnancy Considerations Animal reproduction studies have not been conducted. Calcium crosses the placenta. The amount of calcium reaching the fetus is determined by maternal physiological changes. Calcium requirements are the same in pregnant and nonpregnant females (IOM, 2011). Information related to use as an antidote in pregnancy is limited. In general, medications used as antidotes should take into consideration the health and prognosis of the mother; antidotes should be administered to pregnant women if there is a clear indication for use and should not be withheld because of fears of teratogenicity (Bailey, 2003).

Breast-Feeding Considerations Calcium is excreted in breast milk. The amount of calcium in breast milk is homeostatically regulated and not altered by maternal calcium intake. Calcium requirements are the same in lactating and nonlactating females (IOM, 2011).

Contraindications Known or suspected digoxin toxicity; not recommended as routine treatment in cardiac arrest (includes asystole, ventricular fibrillation, pulseless ventricular tachycardia, or pulseless electrical activity)

Warnings/Precautions For IV use only; do not inject SubQ or IM; avoid rapid IV administration (do not exceed 100 mg/minute except in emergency situations). Vesicant; ensure proper catheter or needle position prior to and during infusion; avoid extravasation; extravasation may result in severe necrosis and sloughing. Monitor the IV site closely. Use with caution in patients with hyperphosphatemia, respiratory acidosis, renal impairment, or respiratory failure; acidifying effect of calcium chloride may potentiate acidosis. Use with caution in patients with chronic renal failure to avoid hypercalcemia; frequent monitoring of serum calcium and phosphorus is necessary. Use with caution in hypokalemic or digitalized patients since acute rises in serum calcium levels may precipitate cardiac arrhythmias; use is contraindicated with known or suspected digoxin toxicity. Hypomagnesemia is a common cause of hypocalcemia; therefore, correction of hypocalcemia may be difficult in patients with concomitant hypomagnesemia. Evaluate serum magnesium and correct hypomagnesemia (if necessary), particularly if initial treatment of hypocalcemia is refractory. The parenteral product may contain aluminum; toxic aluminum concentrations may be seen with high doses, prolonged use, or renal dysfunction. Premature neonates are at higher risk due to immature renal function and aluminum intake from other parenteral sources. Parenteral aluminum exposure of >4 to 5 mcg/kg/day is associated with CNS and bone toxicity; tissue loading may occur at lower doses (Federal Register, 2002). See manufacturer's labeling. Avoid metabolic acidosis (ie, administer only up to 2 to 3 days then change to another calcium salt).

Ceftriaxone may complex with calcium causing precipitation. Fatal lung and kidney damage associated with calcium-ceftriaxone precipitates has been observed in premature and term neonates. Due to reports of precipitation reaction in neonates, do not coadminister ceftriaxone with calcium-containing solutions, even via separate infusion lines/sites or at different times in any neonate. Ceftriaxone should not be administered simultaneously with any calcium-containing solution via a Y-site in any patient. However, ceftriaxone and calcium-containing solutions may be administered sequentially of one another for use in patients **other than neonates** if infusion lines are thoroughly flushed (with a compatible fluid) between infusions. Multiple salt forms of calcium exist; close attention must be paid to the salt form when ordering and administering calcium; incorrect selection or substitution of one salt for another without proper dosage adjustment may result in serious over or under dosing.

Adverse Reactions IV:

Cardiovascular (following rapid IV injection): Bradycardia, cardiac arrest, cardiac arrhythmia, hypotension, syncope, vasodilatation

Central nervous system: Feeling abnormal (sense of oppression; with rapid IV injection), tingling sensation (with rapid IV injection)

Endocrine & metabolic: Hot flash (with rapid IV injection), hypercalcemia

Gastrointestinal: Dysgeusia (chalky taste), gastrointestinal irritation, increased serum amylase

Local: Local tissue necrosis (following extravasation)

Renal: Nephrolithiasis

Rare but important or life-threatening: Cutaneous calcification

Drug Interactions

Metabolism/Transport Effects None known.

Avoid Concomitant Use

Avoid concomitant use of Calcium Chloride with any of the following: Calcium Acetate

Increased Effect/Toxicity

Calcium Chloride may increase the levels/effects of: Calcium Acetate; Cardiac Glycosides; CefTRIAXone; Vitamin D Analogs

The levels/effects of Calcium Chloride may be increased by: Multivitamins/Fluoride (with ADE); Multivitamins/Minerals (with ADEK, Folate, Iron); Thiazide Diuretics

Decreased Effect

Calcium Chloride may decrease the levels/effects of: Bisphosphonate Derivatives; Calcium Channel Blockers; Deferiprone; DOBUTamine; Dolutegravir; Eltrombopag; Multivitamins/Fluoride (with ADE); Phosphate Supplements; Tetracycline Derivatives; Thyroid Products; Trientine

The levels/effects of Calcium Chloride may be decreased by: Trientine

Preparation for Administration IV: For intermittent IV infusion, dilute to a maximum concentration of 20 mg/mL.

Storage/Stability Store intact vials at 20°C to 25°C (68°F to 77°F); excursions permitted to 15°C to 30°C (59°F to 86°F). Do not refrigerate solutions; IV infusion solutions are stable for 24 hours at room temperature.

Although calcium chloride is not routinely used in the preparation of parenteral nutrition, it is important to note that phosphate salts may precipitate when mixed with calcium salts. Solubility is improved in amino acid parenteral nutrition solutions. Check with a pharmacist to determine compatibility.

Mechanism of Action Moderates nerve and muscle performance via action potential excitation threshold regulation

Pharmacodynamics/Kinetics

Protein binding: ~40%, primarily to albumin (Wills, 1971)

Excretion: Primarily feces (80% as insoluble calcium salts); urine (20%)

Dosage Note: One gram of calcium chloride salt is equal to 270 mg of elemental calcium.

Dosages are expressed in terms of the calcium chloride salt based on a solution concentration of 100 mg/mL (10%) containing 1.4 mEq (27 mg)/mL elemental calcium.

Hypocalcemia: IV: **Note:** In general, IV calcium gluconate is preferred over IV calcium chloride in nonemergency settings due to the potential for extravasation with calcium chloride.

Acute, symptomatic: Manufacturer's recommendations:

Children: 2.7-5 mg/kg/dose every 4-6 hours

Adults: 200-1000 mg every 1-3 days

Severe, symptomatic (eg, seizure, tetany): Adults: 1000 mg over 10 minutes; repeat every 60 minutes until symptoms resolve (French, 2012)

Cardiac arrest or cardiotoxicity in the presence of hyperkalemia, hypocalcemia, or hypermagnesemia: **Note:** Routine use in cardiac arrest is not recommended due to the lack of improved survival (Kleinman, 2010; Neumar, 2010).

Infants and Children: IV, I.O.: 20 mg/kg (maximum: 2000 mg/dose); may repeat as necessary (Hegenbarth, 2008; Kleinman, 2010)

Adults: IV: 500-1000 mg over 2-5 minutes; may repeat as necessary (Vanden Hoek, 2010)

Beta-blocker overdose, refractory to glucagon and high-dose vasopressors (off-label use): **Note:** Optimal dose has not been established (DeWitt, 2004)

Adults: IV: 20 mg/kg over 5-10 minutes followed by an infusion of 20 mg/kg/hour titrated to adequate hemodynamic response (Vanden Hoek, 2010)

Calcium channel blocker overdose (off-label use): **Note:** Optimal dose has not been established (DeWitt, 2004).

Infants and Children:

IV, I.O.: Initial: 10-20 mg/kg (maximum: 2000 mg/dose) over 10-15 minutes; may repeat every 10-15 minutes (Arroyo, 2009; Kleinman, 2010); if favorable response obtained, consider IV infusion

IV infusion: 20-50 mg/kg/hour (Arroyo, 2009)

Adults:

IV: Initial: 1000-2000 mg over 5 minutes; may repeat every 10-20 minutes with 3-4 additional doses **or** 1000 mg every 2-3 minutes until clinical effect is achieved (DeWitt, 2004); if favorable response obtained, consider IV infusion

IV infusion: 20-40 mg/kg/hour (DeWitt, 2004; Salhanick, 2003)

Dosage adjustment in renal impairment: No initial dosage adjustment necessary; however, accumulation may occur with renal impairment and subsequent doses may require adjustment based on serum calcium concentrations.

Dosage adjustment in hepatic impairment: No initial dosage adjustment necessary; subsequent doses should be guided by serum calcium concentrations.

Administration For IV administration only. Not for IM or SubQ administration (severe necrosis and sloughing may occur). Avoid rapid administration (do not exceed 100 mg/minute except in emergency situations). For intermittent IV infusion, infuse diluted solution over 1 hour or no greater than 45-90 mg/kg/hour (0.6-1.2 mEq/kg/hour); administration via a central or deep vein is preferred; do not use scalp, small hand or foot veins for IV administration (severe necrosis and sloughing may occur). Monitor ECG if calcium is infused faster than 2.5 mEq/minute; **stop the infusion if the patient complains of pain or discomfort.** Warm solution to body temperature prior to administration. **Do not infuse calcium chloride in the same IV line as phosphate-containing solutions.**

Vesicant; ensure proper needle or catheter placement prior to and during IV infusion. Avoid extravasation.

Extravasation management: If extravasation occurs, stop infusion immediately and disconnect (leave needle/cannula in place); gently aspirate extravasated solution (do **NOT** flush the line); initiate hyaluronidase antidote; remove needle/cannula; apply dry cold compresses (Hurst, 2004); elevate extremity.

Hyaluronidase: Intradermal or SubQ: Inject a total of 1 mL (15 units/mL) as five separate 0.2 mL injections (using a 25-gauge needle) into area of extravasation at the leading edge in a clockwise manner (MacCara, 1983; Zenk, 1981).

Monitoring Parameters Monitor infusion site, ECG when appropriate; serum calcium and ionized calcium (normal: 8.5-10.2 mg/dL [total]; 4.5-5.0 mg/dL [ionized]), albumin, serum phosphate; magnesium (to facilitate calcium repletion)

Calcium channel blocker overdose, beta-blocker overdose: Hemodynamic response, serum ionized calcium concentration

Reference Range

Serum total calcium: 8.4-10.2 mg/dL (2.1-2.55 mmol/L). **Note:** Due to a poor correlation between the serum ionized calcium (free) and total serum calcium, particularly in states of low albumin or acid/base imbalances, direct measurement of ionized calcium is recommended.

In low albumin states, the corrected **total** serum calcium may be estimated by the following equation (assuming a normal albumin of 4 g/dL [40 g/L]).

Corrected total calcium (mg/dL) = measured total calcium (mg/mL) + 0.8 [4 - measured serum albumin(g/dL)]

or

Corrected total calcium (mmol/L) = measured total calcium (mmol/L) + 0.02 [40-measured serum albumin (g/L)]

Additional Information 14 mEq calcium/g (10 mL); 270 mg elemental calcium/g calcium chloride (27% elemental calcium)

Dosage Forms Considerations 1 g calcium chloride = elemental calcium 273 mg = calcium 13.6 mEq = calcium 6.8 mmol

Dosage Forms

Solution, Intravenous:
Generic: 10% (10 mL)

Solution, Intravenous [preservative free]:
Generic: 10% (10 mL)

Calcium Citrate (KAL see um SIT rate)

Brand Names: U.S. Cal-Citrate [OTC]; Calcitrate [OTC]

Brand Names: Canada Osteocit®

Pharmacologic Category Calcium Salt

Use Dietary supplement

Dosage Oral: Dosage is in terms of **elemental** calcium

Dietary Reference Intake for Calcium:
- 1-6 months: Adequate intake: 200 mg/day
- 7-12 months: Adequate intake: 260 mg/day
- 1-3 years: RDA: 700 mg/day
- 4-8 years: RDA: 1000 mg/day
- 9-18 years: RDA: 1300 mg/day
- Adults, Females/Males: RDA:
  - 19-50 years: 1000 mg/day
  - ≥51 years, females: 1200 mg/day
  - 51-70 years, males: 1000 mg/day
  - >70 years, males: 1200 mg/day
- Female: Pregnancy/Lactating: RDA: Requirements are the same as in nonpregnant or nonlactating females

Additional Information Complete prescribing information should be consulted for additional detail.

Dosage Forms Considerations 1 g calcium citrate = elemental calcium 211 mg = calcium 10.5 mEq = calcium 5.25 mmol

Dosage Forms

Capsule, Oral [preservative free]:
Cal-Citrate [OTC]: 150 mg

Granules, Oral:
Generic: 760 mg/3.5 g (480 g)

Tablet, Oral:
Generic: 250 mg, 950 mg, 1040 mg

Tablet, Oral [preservative free]:
Calcitrate [OTC]: 950 mg

◆ **Calcium Citrate and Vitamin D** *see* Calcium and Vitamin D *on page 326*

◆ **Calcium Disodium Edetate** *see* Edetate CALCIUM Disodium *on page 705*

◆ **Calcium Disodiumethylenediaminetetraacetic Acid** *see* Edetate CALCIUM Disodium *on page 705*

◆ **Calcium Folinate** *see* Leucovorin Calcium *on page 1183*

Calcium Glubionate (KAL see um gloo BYE oh nate)

Brand Names: U.S. Calcionate [OTC]

Pharmacologic Category Calcium Salt

Use Dietary supplement

Dosage Dosage is in terms of **elemental** calcium

Dietary Reference Intake for Calcium: Oral:
- 1-6 months: Adequate intake: 200 mg/day
- 7-12 months: Adequate intake: 260 mg/day
- 1-3 years: RDA: 700 mg/day
- 4-8 years: RDA: 1000 mg/day
- 9-18 years: RDA: 1300 mg/day
- Adults, Females/Males: RDA:
  - 19-50 years: 1000 mg/day
  - ≥51 years, females: 1200 mg/day
  - 51-70 years, males: 1000 mg/day
  - >70 years, males: 1200 mg/day
- Females: Pregnancy/Lactating: RDA: Requirements are the same as in nonpregnant or nonlactating females

Dietary supplement: Oral:
- Infants <12 months: 5 mL 5 times/day; may mix with juice or formula
- Children <4 years: 10 mL 3 times/day
- Children ≥4 years and Adults: 15 mL 3 times/day

Additional Information Complete prescribing information should be consulted for additional detail.

Dosage Forms Considerations 1 g calcium glubionate = elemental calcium 63.8 mg = calcium 3.2 mEq = calcium 1.6 mmol

Dosage Forms

Syrup, Oral:
Calcionate [OTC]: 1.8 g/5 mL (473 mL)

Calcium Gluconate (KAL see um GLOO koe nate)

Brand Names: U.S. Cal-Glu [OTC]

Pharmacologic Category Calcium Salt; Electrolyte Supplement, Oral; Electrolyte Supplement, Parenteral

Use

IV: Treatment of hypocalcemia and conditions secondary to hypocalcemia (eg, tetany, seizures, arrhythmias); treatment of cardiac disturbances secondary to hyperkalemia; adjunctive treatment of rickets, osteomalacia, and magnesium sulfate overdose; decrease capillary permeability in allergic conditions, nonthrombocytopenic purpura, and exudative dermatoses (eg, dermatitis herpetiformis, pruritus secondary to certain drugs); treatment of black widow spider bites to relieve muscle cramping

Oral: Dietary calcium supplementation

Pregnancy Risk Factor C

Pregnancy Considerations Animal reproduction studies have not been conducted. Calcium crosses the placenta. The amount of calcium reaching the fetus is determined by maternal physiological changes. Calcium requirements are the same in pregnant and nonpregnant females (IOM, 2011). Information related to use as an antidote in pregnancy is limited. In general, medications used as antidotes should take into consideration the health and prognosis of the mother; antidotes should be administered to pregnant women if there is a clear indication for use and should not be withheld because of fears of teratogenicity (Bailey, 2003).

Breast-Feeding Considerations Calcium is excreted in breast milk. The amount of calcium in breast milk is homeostatically regulated and not altered by maternal calcium intake. Calcium requirements are the same in lactating and nonlactating females (IOM, 2011).

Contraindications Ventricular fibrillation; hypercalcemia; concomitant use of IV calcium gluconate and ceftriaxone in neonates

Warnings/Precautions Multiple salt forms of calcium exist; close attention must be paid to the salt form when ordering and administering calcium; incorrect selection or substitution of one salt for another without proper dosage adjustment may result in serious over or under dosing. Avoid too rapid IV administration (do not exceed 200 mg/minute except in emergency situations);may result in vasodilation, hypotension, bradycardia, arrhythmias, and cardiac arrest. Parenteral calcium is a vesicant; ensure proper catheter or needle position prior to and during infusion. Avoid extravasation; may result in necrosis. Monitor the IV site closely. Use with caution in severe hyperphosphatemia or severe hypokalemia. Hypercalcemia may occur in patients with renal failure; frequent determination of serum calcium is necessary. Use caution with chronic renal disease. Use caution when administering calcium supplements to patients with a history of kidney stones. Hypomagnesemia is a common cause of hypocalcemia; therefore, correction of hypocalcemia may be difficult in patients with concomitant hypomagnesemia. Evaluate serum magnesium and correct hypomagnesemia (if necessary), particularly if initial treatment of hypocalcemia is refractory.

The parenteral product may contain aluminum; toxic aluminum concentrations may be seen with high doses, prolonged use, or renal dysfunction. Premature neonates are at higher risk due to immature renal function and aluminum intake from other parenteral sources. Parenteral aluminum exposure of >4 to 5 mcg/kg/day is associated with CNS and bone toxicity; tissue loading may occur at lower doses (Federal Register, 2002). See manufacturer's labeling.

Constipation, bloating, and gas are common with oral calcium supplements (especially carbonate salt). Administering oral calcium with food and vitamin D will optimize calcium absorption. Some products may contain tartrazine, which may cause allergic reactions in susceptible individuals.

Potentially significant drug-drug interactions may exist, requiring dose or frequency adjustment, additional monitoring, and/or selection of alternative therapy.

Adverse Reactions

IV:

Cardiovascular (with rapid IV injection): Arrhythmia, bradycardia, cardiac arrest, hypotension, syncope, vasodilation

Central nervous system: Sense of oppression (with rapid IV injection)

Endocrine & metabolic: Hypercalcemia

Gastrointestinal: Chalky taste

Neuromuscular & skeletal: Tingling sensation (with rapid IV injection)

Miscellaneous: Heat waves (with rapid IV injection)

Postmarketing and/or case reports: Calcinosis cutis

Oral: Gastrointestinal: Constipation

Drug Interactions

Metabolism/Transport Effects None known.

Avoid Concomitant Use

Avoid concomitant use of Calcium Gluconate with any of the following: Calcium Acetate

Increased Effect/Toxicity

Calcium Gluconate may increase the levels/effects of: Calcium Acetate; Cardiac Glycosides; CefTRIAXone; Vitamin D Analogs

The levels/effects of Calcium Gluconate may be increased by: Multivitamins/Fluoride (with ADE); Multivitamins/Minerals (with ADEK, Folate, Iron); Thiazide Diuretics

Decreased Effect

Calcium Gluconate may decrease the levels/effects of: Bisphosphonate Derivatives; Calcium Channel Blockers; Deferiprone; DOBUTamine; Dolutegravir; Eltrombopag; Estramustine; Multivitamins/Fluoride (with ADE); Phosphate Supplements; Quinolone Antibiotics; Strontium Ranelate; Tetracycline Derivatives; Thyroid Products; Trientine

The levels/effects of Calcium Gluconate may be decreased by: Trientine

Preparation for Administration

IV: Observe the vial for the presence of particulates. If particulates are observed, place vial in a 60°C to 80°C water bath for 15 to 30 minutes (or until solution is clear); occasionally shake to dissolve; cool to body/room temperature before use. Do not use vial if particulates do not dissolve. **Note:** Due to the potential presence of particulates, American Regent, Inc recommends the use of a 5 micron filter when preparing calcium gluconate-containing IV solutions (Important Drug Administration Information, American Regent, 2013); a similar recommendation has not been noted by other manufacturers. Usual concentrations: 1 g/100 mL D_5W or NS; 2 g/100 mL D_5W or NS. Maximum concentration in parenteral nutrition solutions is variable depending upon concentration and solubility (consult detailed reference).

Inhalation: Treatment of hydrofluoric acid burns (off-label use): Mix 1 mL of 10% calcium gluconate solution with 4 mL NS to make a 2.5% solution.

Storage/Stability

IV: Store intact vials at 20°C to 25°C (68°F to 77°F); excursions are permitted between 15°C and 30°C (59°F and 86°F). Do not freeze. Calcium-phosphate stability in parenteral nutrition solutions is dependent upon the pH of the solution, temperature, and relative concentration of each ion. The pH of the solution is primarily dependent upon the amino acid concentration. The higher the percentage amino acids the lower the pH, the more soluble the calcium and phosphate. Individual commercially available amino acid solutions vary significantly with respect to pH lowering potential and consequent calcium phosphate compatibility.

Oral: Store at room temperature; consult product labeling for specific requirements.

Mechanism of Action Moderates nerve and muscle performance via action potential threshold regulation.

In hydrogen fluoride exposures, calcium gluconate provides a source of calcium ions to complex free fluoride ions and prevent or reduce toxicity; administration also helps to correct fluoride-induced hypocalcemia.

Pharmacodynamics/Kinetics

Absorption: Oral: Requires vitamin D; calcium is absorbed in soluble, ionized form; solubility of calcium is increased in an acid environment

Protein binding: ~40%, primarily to albumin (Wills, 1971)

Excretion: Primarily feces (as unabsorbed calcium salts); urine (20%)

Dosage Note: One gram of calcium gluconate salt is equal to 93 mg of elemental calcium.

Dosages are expressed in terms of the calcium gluconate salt (unless otherwise specified as elemental calcium). Dosages expressed in terms of the calcium gluconate salt are based on a solution concentration of 100 mg/mL (10%) containing 0.465 mEq (9.3 mg)/mL elemental calcium, except where noted.

Dietary Reference Intake for Calcium (IOM, 2011): Oral: **Note:** Dose expressed as elemental calcium:

1 to 6 months: Adequate intake: 200 mg **elemental calcium** daily

7 to 12 months: Adequate intake: 260 mg **elemental calcium** daily

1 to 3 years: RDA: 700 mg **elemental calcium** daily

4 to 8 years: RDA: 1000 mg **elemental calcium** daily

9 to 18 years: RDA: 1300 mg **elemental calcium** daily

Adults, Females/Males: RDA:

19 to 50 years: 1000 mg **elemental calcium** daily

≥51 years, females: 1200 mg **elemental calcium** daily

51 to 70 years, males: 1000 mg **elemental calcium** daily

>70 years, males: 1200 mg **elemental calcium** daily

Females: Pregnancy/Lactating: RDA: Requirements are the same as in nonpregnant or nonlactating females

Hypocalcemia: IV:

Infants, Children, and Adolescents:

General dosing: IV: 200 to 500 mg/kg/day as a continuous infusion or in 4 divided doses (maximum dose: 1000 mg/dose [Infants, Children]; 2000 to 3000 mg/dose [Adolescents]) (Edmondson, 1990; Zhou, 2009)

Symptomatic (ie, seizures, tetany): IV: 100 to 200 mg/kg/dose over 5 to 10 minutes; usual adult dose: 1000 to 2000 mg/dose; may repeat after 6 hours or follow with a continuous infusion of 200 to 800 mg/kg/day (Edmondson, 1990; Kelly, 2013; Misra, 2008; Nelson, 1996; Zhou, 2009)

Adults:

Mild (ionized calcium: 4 to 5 mg/dL [1 to 1.2 mmol/L]): 1000 to 2000 mg over 2 hours; asymptomatic patients may be given oral calcium (Ariyan, 2004; French, 2012)

Moderate-to-severe (without seizure or tetany; ionized calcium: <4 mg/dL [<1 mmol/L]): 4000 mg over 4 hours (French, 2012)

Severe symptomatic (eg, seizure, tetany): 1000 to 2000 mg over 10 minutes; repeat every 60 minutes until symptoms resolve (French, 2012)

Note: Repeat ionized calcium measurement 6 to 10 hours after completion of administration. Check for hypomagnesemia and correct if present. Consider continuous infusion if hypocalcemia is likely to recur due to ongoing losses (French, 2012).

Continuous infusion: 5 to 20 mg/kg/hour (Pai, 2011)

Cardiac arrest or cardiotoxicity in the presence of hyperkalemia, hypocalcemia, or hypermagnesemia: IV, intraosseous:

Infants, Children, and Adolescents: 60 to 100 mg/kg/dose (maximum: 3000 mg/dose); may repeat in 10 minutes if necessary; if effective, consider IV infusion (Hegenbarth, 2008)

Adults: 1500 to 3000 mg over 2 to 5 minutes (Vanden Hoek, 2010)

Note: Routine use in cardiac arrest is not recommended due to the lack of improved survival (Kleinman, 2010; Neumar, 2010):

Parenteral nutrition, maintenance requirement: IV (Mirtallo, 2004): **Note:** Dose expressed as **elemental calcium:**

Infants and Children (≤50 kg): 0.5 to 4 **mEq elemental calcium**/kg/day

Children (>50 kg), Adolescents, and Adults: 10 to 20 **mEq elemental calcium** daily

Calcium channel blocker overdose (off-label use): Hypotension/conduction disturbances:

Infants, Children, and Adolescents: IV, intraosseous: 60 mg/kg/dose administered over 30 to 60 minutes (Hegenbarth, 2008). **Note:** Calcium chloride may provide a more rapid increase of ionized calcium in critically-ill children. Calcium gluconate may be substituted if calcium chloride is not available.

Adults: IV: 60 to 120 mg/kg/**hour** (Salhanick, 2003) **or** 60 mg/kg/dose over 5 minutes (maximum: 3000 to 6000 mg/dose) every 10 to 20 minutes; may repeat for 3 to 4 additional doses (Vanden Hoek, 2010; DeWitt, 2004). In life-threatening situations, 1000 mg has been administered every 2 to 3 minutes until clinical effect is achieved (Buckley, 1994). In one report, 18 **g** was administered over a 3-hour period (Luscher, 1994).

Hydrofluoric acid burns, treatment (off-label route/use): Children, Adolescents, and Adults:

SubQ (off-label route/use): 5% to 10% solution: 0.5 **mL**/cm^2 of burned tissue (Dibbell, 1970; Hatzifotis, 2004; Kirkpatrick, 1995; Krenzelok, 1999). Infiltration should be carried 0.5 cm away from the margin of the injured tissue into the surrounding uninjured areas. Repeat if pain recurs. Local anesthesia may be required to perform procedure; pain resolution is the therapeutic endpoint and if a local anesthetic is utilized, it may be difficult to determine the success of therapy (**Note: Never** use calcium chloride for subcutaneous injection).

Intra-arterial (off-label route/use): Add 10 **mL** of a 10% solution to 50 mL of D_5W. Infuse over 4 hours into the artery that provides the vascular supply to the affected area (Hatzifotis, 2004; Kirkpatrick, 1995). Pain usually resolves by the end of the infusion; repeat if pain recurs. **This intervention should be used only by those accustomed to this technique. Extreme care should be taken to avoid the extravasation.** A poison information center or clinical toxicologist should be consulted prior to implementation.

Inhalation (off-label route/use): 2.5% nebulization solution: Mix 1 **mL** of 10% calcium gluconate solution with 4 mL NS to make a 2.5% solution and administer via nebulization (Hatzifotis, 2004).

Dosing adjustment in renal impairment: No initial dosage adjustment necessary; however, accumulation may occur with renal impairment and subsequent doses may require adjustment based on serum calcium concentrations.

Dosing adjustment in hepatic impairment: No initial dosage adjustment necessary; subsequent doses should be guided by serum calcium concentrations. In patients in the anhepatic stage of liver transplantation, equal rapid increases in ionized concentrations occur suggesting that calcium gluconate does not require hepatic metabolism for release of ionized calcium (Martin, 1990).

Administration

Oral: Administer with plenty of fluids with or following meals. The 10% calcium gluconate injection may be administered orally in young pediatric patients (Mimouni, 1994).

IV: Administer slowly (~1.5 mL calcium gluconate 10% per minute; not to exceed 200 mg/minute except in emergency situations) through a small needle into a large vein in order to avoid too rapid increases in the serum calcium and extravasation. **Note:** Due to the potential presence of particulates, American Regent, Inc recommends the use of a 0.22 micron inline filter for IV administration (1.2 micron filter if admixture contains lipids) (Important Drug Administration Information, American Regent, 2013); a similar recommendation has not been noted by other manufacturers. Not for IM administration. In acute situations of symptomatic hypocalcemia, infusions over 5 to 10 minutes have been described in pediatric patients (Kelly, 2013; Misra, 2008).

Vesicant; ensure proper needle or catheter placement prior to and during IV infusion. Avoid extravasation.

Extravasation management: If extravasation occurs, stop infusion immediately and disconnect (leave needle/cannula in place); gently aspirate extravasated solution (do **NOT** flush the line); initiate hyaluronidase antidote; remove needle/cannula; apply dry cold compresses (Hurst, 2004); elevate extremity.

Hyaluronidase: Intradermal or SubQ: Inject a total of 1 mL (15 units/mL) as five separate 0.2 mL injections (using a 25-gauge needle) into area of extravasation at the leading edge in a clockwise manner (MacCara, 1983; Zenk, 1981).

Treatment of hydrofluoric acid burns (off-label use):

SubQ infiltration (off-label route): Using a 27- or 30-gauge needle, approach the wound from the distal point of injury and infiltrate directly into the affected dermis and subcutaneous tissue. The infiltration should be carried 0.5 cm away from the margin of the injured tissue into the surrounding uninjured areas (Dibbell, 1970). Avoid excessive administration as it can cause compartment syndrome and further exacerbate tissue damage. Following subungual exposure, administer to the affected area via the lateral or volar route through the fat pad (under digital nerve block); administration may also require removal of the nailbed, splitting the distal nail from the nailbed, or trimming the nail to the nailbed to reach the affected area (Kirkpatrick, 1995; Roberts, 1989).

Intra-arterial (off-label route): Requires radiology to place an arterial catheter in an artery supplying blood to the area of exposure; infuse over four hours (Vance, 1986). **This intervention should be used only by those accustomed to this technique. Care should be taken to avoid the extravasation.** A poison information center or clinical toxicologist should be consulted prior to implementation.

Inhalation: Dilute 10% calcium gluconate solution to a 2.5% solution and administer via nebulization.

Reference Range

Serum total calcium: 8.4 to 10.2 mg/dL (2.1 to 2.55 mmol/L). **Note:** Due to a poor correlation between the serum ionized calcium (free) and total serum calcium, particularly in states of low albumin or acid/base imbalances, direct measurement of ionized calcium is recommended.

In low albumin states, the corrected **total** serum calcium may be estimated by the following equation (assuming a normal albumin of 4 g/dL [40 g/L]).

Corrected total calcium (mg/dL) = measured total calcium (mg/mL) + 0.8 [4 - measured serum albumin(g/dL)]

or

Corrected total calcium (mmol/L) = measured total calcium (mmol/L) + 0.02 [40-measured serum albumin (g/L)]

Dosage Forms Considerations 1 g calcium gluconate = elemental calcium 93 mg = calcium 4.65 mEq = calcium 2.33 mmol

Dosage Forms

Capsule, Oral [preservative free]:
Cal-Glu [OTC]: 500 mg

Solution, Intravenous:
Generic: 10% (10 mL, 50 mL, 100 mL)

Solution, Intravenous [preservative free]:
Generic: 10% (100 mL)

Tablet, Oral:
Generic: 50 mg, 500 mg

◆ **Calcium High Potency [OTC]** *see* Calcium Carbonate *on page 327*

◆ **Calcium Leucovorin** *see* Leucovorin Calcium *on page 1183*

◆ **Calcium Levoleucovorin** *see* LEVOleucovorin *on page 1200*

Calcium Polystyrene Sulfonate [CAN/INT] (KAL see um pol i STI reen sul fo NATE)

Brand Names: Canada Resonium Calcium®

Index Terms Calcium Polystyrene Sulphonate; Polystyrene Sulfonate Calcium

Pharmacologic Category Antidote

Use Note: Not approved in U.S.
Treatment of hyperkalemia

Pregnancy Considerations Does not undergo GI absorption. There are no adequate and well-controlled studies in pregnant women. In general, medications used as antidotes should take into consideration the health and prognosis of the mother; antidotes should be administered to pregnant women if there is a clear indication for use and should not be withheld because of fears of teratogenicity (Bailey, 2003).

Breast-Feeding Considerations Does not undergo GI absorption

Contraindications Hypersensitivity to polystyrene sulfonate resins or any component of the formulation; potassium <5 mmol/L (5 mEq/L); conditions associated with hypercalcemia (eg, metastatic carcinoma, hyperparathyroidism); obstructive bowel disease; oral administration in neonates; use in neonates with reduced gut motility (postoperative, drug induced)

Warnings/Precautions Use may be associated with electrolyte disturbances including hypokalemia, hypercalcemia, and/or hypomagnesemia. Closely monitor electrolytes during therapy and discontinue if potassium ≤5 mmol/L (5 mEq/L). Sudden increases in calcium may be observed with use in renal impairment and/or dialysis patients. Monitor calcium weekly (or more frequently if clinically indicated). Dosage adjustments may be necessary. Discontinue use for clinically significant constipation. May resume therapy with return of normal bowel function. Avoid magnesium containing laxatives.

Use of a similar agent (sodium polystyrene sulfonate) has rarely been associated with concretion formation and colonic necrosis/intestinal obstruction. May be related to use of sorbitol enema with inadequate or absence of lavage after resin use. Avoid concomitant use of oral/rectal sorbitol. Avoid excess dosing or inadequate dilution with rectal administration to avoid resin impaction. Premature/low-birth-weight infants may be at risk for GI hemorrhage or colonic necrosis. Avoid oral administration in neonates.

Adverse Reactions

Endocrine & metabolic: Hypercalcemia, hypokalemia, hypomagnesemia

Gastrointestinal: Anorexia, concretions (bezoars; oral administration), constipation, diarrhea, fecal impaction (rectal administration), gastric irritation, GI necrosis/ulceration, ischemic colitis, nausea, obstruction (rare), rectal hemorrhage, vomiting

Respiratory: Acute bronchitis, bronchopneumonia

Drug Interactions

Metabolism/Transport Effects None known.

Avoid Concomitant Use

Avoid concomitant use of Calcium Polystyrene Sulfonate with any of the following: Laxatives (Magnesium Containing); Meloxicam; Sorbitol

Increased Effect/Toxicity

Calcium Polystyrene Sulfonate may increase the levels/effects of: Aluminum Hydroxide; Cardiac Glycosides

The levels/effects of Calcium Polystyrene Sulfonate may be increased by: Antacids; Laxatives (Magnesium Containing); Meloxicam; Sorbitol

Decreased Effect

Calcium Polystyrene Sulfonate may decrease the levels/effects of: Lithium; Thyroid Products

Preparation for Administration

Oral: Prepare a suspension or paste by mixing each 1 gram of resin with 3-4 mL of water or sweetened beverage (avoid fruit juices or other beverages with high potassium content).

Rectal:

Neonates: Mix appropriate dose with 2% methylcellulose (100 mL) and water (100 mL)

Children: Mix appropriate dose in a proportional amount of 10% dextrose in water

Adults: Mix 30 g of resin with 2% methylcellulose (100 mL) and water (100 mL)

Storage/Stability Store between 15°C to 30°C (59°F to 86°F).

Mechanism of Action Removes potassium by exchanging calcium ions for potassium ions in the intestine before the resin is passed from the body

Pharmacodynamics/Kinetics

Onset of action: May be delayed 2-3 days due to GI transit time

Absorption: None

Excretion: Feces (100%)

Dosage Note: Initiate treatment if potassium level >6 mmol/L (6 mEq/L); discontinue when potassium ≤5 mmol/L (5 mEq/L). In small children and infants, employ lower doses by using the practical exchange ratio of 1 mEq potassium/g of resin as the basis for calculation.

Hyperkalemia:

Neonates: Rectal: 0.5-1 g/kg/dose

Children: Oral, rectal (**Note:** Oral route preferred): Initial: 1 g/kg/day in divided doses; Maintenance: May reduce dose to 0.5 g/kg/day in divided doses

Adults:

Oral: 15 g 3-4 times/day

Rectal: 30 g once daily

Dietary Considerations May administer orally with honey, jam, or liquids with low potassium content. Do **not** mix in fruit juices (eg, orange juice) or other beverages with high potassium content. Some products may contain sodium.

Administration

Oral: Administer orally (via nasogastric tube if unable to swallow) as suspension or paste **Note:** More rapid lowering of potassium may be achieved with concomitant oral and rectal administration. Rectal route may be discontinued once orally administered resin has reached rectum.

Rectal: Enema route is less effective than oral administration. Administer rectally as suspension. Enema should be retained as long as possible (product labeling suggests for at least 9 hours in adults or as long as possible) as greater amounts of potassium are excreted as retention time increases. Follow enema with irrigation to remove resin. **Note:** More rapid lowering of potassium may be achieved with concomitant oral and rectal administration. Rectal route may be discontinued once orally administered resin has reached rectum.

Monitoring Parameters Close monitoring of serum electrolytes (potassium, sodium, calcium, magnesium) is necessary; ECG

Reference Range Serum potassium: Adults: 3.5-5.2 mEq/L

Additional Information *In vitro* exchange capacity is 1.3-2 mmol/g of potassium, while *in vivo* potassium binding capacity is less,

Product Availability Not available in U.S.

Dosage Forms: Canada

Powder for suspension, oral/rectal:

Resonium Calcium®: 300 g

◆ **Calcium Polystyrene Sulphonate** *see* Calcium Polystyrene Sulfonate [CAN/INT] *on page 333*

◆ **Cal-CYUM [OTC]** *see* Calcium and Vitamin D *on page 326*

◆ **Caldolor** *see* Ibuprofen *on page 1032*

Calfactant (kaf AKT ant)

Brand Names: U.S. Infasurf

Index Terms Bovine Lung Surfactant

Pharmacologic Category Lung Surfactant

Use Prevention of respiratory distress syndrome (RDS) in premature infants at high risk for RDS and for the treatment ("rescue") of premature infants who develop RDS

Prophylaxis: Therapy at birth with calfactant is indicated for premature infants <29 weeks of gestational age at significant risk for RDS. Should be administered as soon as possible, preferably within 30 minutes after birth.

Treatment: For infants ≤72 hours of age with RDS (confirmed by clinical and radiologic findings) and requiring endotracheal intubation.

Dosage Intratracheal administration **only**: Each dose is 3 mL/kg body weight at birth; should be administered every 12 hours for a total of up to 3 doses

Dosage adjustment in renal impairment: No dosage adjustment provided in manufacturer's labeling.

Dosage adjustment in hepatic impairment: No dosage adjustment provided in manufacturer's labeling.

Additional Information Complete prescribing information should be consulted for additional detail.

Dosage Forms

Suspension, Inhalation:

Infasurf: 35 mg phospholipids and 0.7 mg protein per mL (3 mL, 6 mL)

◆ **Cal-Gest Antacid [OTC]** *see* Calcium Carbonate *on page 327*

◆ **Cal-Glu [OTC]** *see* Calcium Gluconate *on page 330*

◆ **Cal-Mint [OTC]** *see* Calcium Carbonate *on page 327*

◆ **Calmylin with Codeine (Can)** *see* Guaifenesin, Pseudoephedrine, and Codeine *on page 989*

◆ **Calphron [OTC]** *see* Calcium Acetate *on page 326*

◆ **Caltrate (Can)** *see* Calcium Carbonate *on page 327*

◆ **Caltrate 600 [OTC]** *see* Calcium Carbonate *on page 327*

◆ **Caltrate 600+D [OTC]** *see* Calcium and Vitamin D *on page 326*

◆ **Caltrate 600+Soy [OTC]** *see* Calcium and Vitamin D *on page 326*

- **Caltrate ColonHealth [OTC]** *see* Calcium and Vitamin D *on page 326*
- **Caltrate Gummy Bites [OTC]** *see* Calcium and Vitamin D *on page 326*
- **Caltrate Select (Can)** *see* Calcium Carbonate *on page 327*
- **Cambia** *see* Diclofenac (Systemic) *on page 617*
- **Camila** *see* Norethindrone *on page 1473*
- **Campath** *see* Alemtuzumab *on page 75*
- **Campath-1H** *see* Alemtuzumab *on page 75*
- **Camphorated Tincture of Opium (error-prone synonym)** *see* Paregoric *on page 1577*
- **Campral [DSC]** *see* Acamprosate *on page 28*
- **Campral® (Can)** *see* Acamprosate *on page 28*
- **Camptosar** *see* Irinotecan *on page 1112*
- **Camptothecin-11** *see* Irinotecan *on page 1112*
- **camrese** *see* Ethinyl Estradiol and Levonorgestrel *on page 803*

Canakinumab (can a KIN ue mab)

Brand Names: U.S. Ilaris

Brand Names: Canada Ilaris

Index Terms ACZ885

Pharmacologic Category Interleukin-1 Beta Inhibitor; Interleukin-1 Inhibitor; Monoclonal Antibody

Use

Cryopyrin-associated periodic syndromes:

U.S. labeling: Treatment of cryopyrin-associated periodic syndromes (CAPS) in adults and children 4 years and older, including familial cold autoinflammatory syndrome (FCAS) and Muckle-Wells syndrome (MWS).

Canadian labeling: Treatment of cryopyrin-associated periodic syndromes (CAPS) in adults and children 2 years and older, including familial cold autoinflammatory syndrome (FCAS) and Muckle-Wells syndrome (MWS). May also be used in Neonatal-Onset Multisystem Inflammatory Disease (NOMID) although clinical data has not confirmed improvement of CNS symptoms in this patient population.

Systemic juvenile idiopathic arthritis: Treatment of active systemic juvenile idiopathic arthritis (SJIA) in patients 2 years and older.

Pregnancy Risk Factor C

Dosage

Cryopyrin-associated periodic syndromes (CAPS): SubQ:

U.S. labeling:

Children ≥4 years and Adolescents:

15 to 40 kg: 2 mg/kg every 8 weeks; may increase to 3 mg/kg if response inadequate

>40 kg: 150 mg every 8 weeks

Adults >40 kg: 150 mg every 8 weeks

Canadian labeling:

Children ≥2 years and Adolescents:

15 to 40 kg: Initial: 2 mg/kg every 8 weeks; if inadequate response after 7 days may consider further titration by 2 mg/kg every 7 days up to a maximum dose of 8 mg/kg (do not exceed 600 mg). The dose at which a satisfactory response is achieved should be maintained and administered every 8 weeks.

>40 kg: 150 mg every 8 weeks; if inadequate response after 7 days may consider further titration by 150 mg every 7 days up to a maximum dose of 600 mg. The dose at which a satisfactory response is achieved should be maintained and administered every 8 weeks.

Adults: >40 kg: 150 mg every 8 weeks; if inadequate response after 7 days may consider further titration by 150 mg every 7 days up to a maximum dose of 600 mg. The dose at which a satisfactory response is achieved should be maintained and administered every 8 weeks.

Systemic juvenile idiopathic arthritis (SJIA): SubQ: Children ≥2 years and ≥7.5 kg (U.S. labeling) or >9 kg (Canadian labeling) and Adolescents: 4 mg/kg every 4 weeks (maximum: 300 mg per dose)

Dosage adjustment in renal impairment:

U.S. labeling: There are no dosage adjustments provided in the manufacturer's labeling.

Canadian labeling: No dosage adjustment necessary; limited data in this population.

Dosage adjustment in hepatic impairment: There are no dosage adjustments provided in the manufacturer's labeling (has not been studied).

Additional Information Complete prescribing information should be consulted for additional detail.

Dosage Forms

Solution Reconstituted, Subcutaneous [preservative free]:

Ilaris: 180 mg (1 ea)

Dosage Forms: Canada

Injection, powder for reconstitution:

Ilaris: 150 mg

- **Canasa** *see* Mesalamine *on page 1301*
- **Cancidas** *see* Caspofungin *on page 370*
- **Cancidas® (Can)** *see* Caspofungin *on page 370*

Candesartan (kan de SAR tan)

Brand Names: U.S. Atacand

Brand Names: Canada ACH Candesartan; Apo-Candesartan; Atacand; CO Candesartan; DOM-Candesartan; JAMP-Candesartan; Mylan-Candesartan; PMS-Candesartan; Ran-Candesartan; Sandoz-Candesartan; Teva-Candesartan

Index Terms Candesartan Cilexetil

Pharmacologic Category Angiotensin II Receptor Blocker; Antihypertensive

Use

Heart failure: Treatment of heart failure (NYHA class II-IV)

Note: The ACCF/AHA 2013 heart failure guidelines recommend the use of ARBs (ie, candesartan, losartan, and valsartan) in patients with HF with reduced ejection fraction who cannot tolerate ACE inhibitors (due to cough) to reduce morbidity and mortality. They also suggest that ARBs are reasonable first-line alternatives to ACE inhibitors in patients already maintained on an ARB for other indications (ACCF/AHA [Yancy, 2013]).

Hypertension: Alone or in combination with other antihypertensive agents in treating hypertension

The 2014 guideline for the management of high blood pressure in adults (Eighth Joint National Committee [JNC 8; James, 2013]) recommends initiation of pharmacologic treatment to lower blood pressure for the following patients:

- Patients ≥60 years of age with systolic blood pressure (SBP) ≥150 mm Hg or diastolic blood pressure (DBP) ≥90 mm Hg. Goal of therapy is SBP <150 mm Hg and DBP <90 mm Hg.
- Patients <60 years of age with SBP ≥140 mm Hg or DBP ≥90 mm Hg. Goal of therapy is SBP <140 mm Hg and DBP <90 mm Hg.
- Patients ≥18 years of age with diabetes and SBP ≥140 mm Hg or DBP ≥90 mm Hg. Goal of therapy is SBP <140 mm Hg and DBP <90 mm Hg.

- Patients ≥18 years of age with chronic kidney disease (CKD) and SBP ≥140 mm Hg or DBP ≥90 mm Hg. Goal of therapy is SBP <140 mm Hg and DBP <90 mm Hg.

In patients with CKD, regardless of race or diabetes status, the use of an ACE inhibitor (ACEI) or angiotensin receptor blocker (ARB) as initial therapy is recommended to improve kidney outcomes. In the general nonblack population (without CKD), including those with diabetes, initial antihypertensive treatment should consist of a thiazide-type diuretic, calcium channel blocker, ACEI, or ARB. In the general black population (without CKD), including those with diabetes, initial antihypertensive treatment should consist of a thiazide-type diuretic or a calcium channel blocker instead of an ACEI or ARB.

Pregnancy Risk Factor D

Pregnancy Considerations [U.S. Boxed Warning]: Drugs that act on the renin-angiotensin system can cause injury and death to the developing fetus. Discontinue as soon as possible once pregnancy is detected. The use of drugs which act on the renin-angiotensin system are associated with oligohydramnios. Oligohydramnios, due to decreased fetal renal function, may lead to fetal lung hypoplasia and skeletal malformations. Use is also associated with anuria, hypotension, renal failure, skull hypoplasia, and death in the fetus/neonate. The exposed fetus should be monitored for fetal growth, amniotic fluid volume, and organ formation. Infants exposed *in utero* should be monitored for hyperkalemia, hypotension, and oliguria (exchange transfusions or dialysis may be needed). These adverse events are generally associated with maternal use in the second and third trimesters.

Untreated chronic maternal hypertension is also associated with adverse events in the fetus, infant, and mother. The use of angiotensin II receptor blockers is not recommended to treat chronic uncomplicated hypertension in pregnant women and should generally be avoided in women of reproductive potential (ACOG, 2013).

Breast-Feeding Considerations It is not known if candesartan is excreted into breast milk. Due to the potential for serious adverse reactions in the nursing infant, the manufacturer recommends a decision be made whether to discontinue nursing or to discontinue the drug, taking into account the importance of treatment to the mother. The Canadian labeling contraindicates use in breast-feeding women.

Contraindications

Hypersensitivity to candesartan or any component of the formulation; concomitant use with aliskiren in patients with diabetes mellitus

Canadian labeling: Additional contraindications (not in U.S. labeling): Concomitant use with aliskiren in patients with moderate-to-severe renal impairment (GFR <60 mL/minute/1.73 m^2); pregnancy; breast-feeding; children <1 year of age; rare hereditary problems of galactose intolerance, Lapp lactase deficiency or glucose-galactose malabsorption

Warnings/Precautions [U.S. Boxed Warning]: Drugs that act on the renin-angiotensin system can cause injury and death to the developing fetus. Discontinue as soon as possible once pregnancy is detected. May cause hyperkalemia; avoid potassium supplementation unless specifically required by healthcare provider. Avoid use or use a smaller dose in patients who are volume depleted; correct depletion first. May be associated with deterioration of renal function and/or increases in serum creatinine, particularly in patients with low renal blood flow (eg, renal artery stenosis, heart failure) whose glomerular filtration rate (GFR) is dependent on efferent arteriolar vasoconstriction by angiotensin II; deterioration may result in oliguria, acute renal failure, and progressive azotemia. Small increases in serum creatinine may occur following initiation; consider discontinuation only in patients with progressive and/or significant deterioration in renal function. Use with caution in unstented unilateral/bilateral renal artery stenosis, preexisting renal insufficiency, or significant aortic/mitral stenosis. Systemic exposure increases in hepatic impairment. U.S. manufacturer labeling recommends a dosage adjustment in patients with moderate hepatic impairment; pharmacokinetics have not been studied in severe hepatic impairment. Use caution when initiating in heart failure; may need to adjust dose, and/or concurrent diuretic therapy, because of candesartan-induced hypotension. In surgical patients on chronic angiotensin receptor blocker (ARB) therapy, intraoperative hypotension may occur with induction and maintenance of general anesthesia Potentially significant drug-drug interactions may exist, requiring dose or frequency adjustment, additional monitoring, and/or selection of alternative therapy. Pediatric patients with a GFR <30 mL/minute/1.73 m^2 should not receive candesartan; has not been evaluated. Avoid use in infants <1 year of age due to potential effects on the development of immature kidneys.

Angioedema has been reported rarely with some angiotensin II receptor antagonists (ARBs) and may occur at any time during treatment (especially following first dose). It may involve the head and neck (potentially compromising airway) or the intestine (presenting with abdominal pain). Patients with idiopathic or hereditary angioedema or previous angioedema associated with ACE-inhibitor therapy may be at an increased risk. Prolonged frequent monitoring may be required, especially if tongue, glottis, or larynx are involved, as they are associated with airway obstruction. Patients with a history of airway surgery may have a higher risk of airway obstruction. Discontinue therapy immediately if angioedema occurs. Aggressive early management is critical. Intramuscular (IM) administration of epinephrine may be necessary. Do not readminister to patients who have had angioedema with ARBs.

Adverse Reactions

Cardiovascular: Angina pectoris, hypotension, myocardial infarction, palpitations, tachycardia

Central nervous system: Anxiety, depression, dizziness, drowsiness, headache, paresthesia, vertigo

Dermatologic: Diaphoresis, skin rash

Endocrine & metabolic: Hyperglycemia, hyperkalemia, hypertriglyceridemia, hyperuricemia

Gastrointestinal: Dyspepsia, gastroenteritis

Genitourinary: Hematuria

Neuromuscular & skeletal: Back pain, increased creatine phosphokinase, myalgia, weakness

Renal: Increased serum creatinine

Respiratory: Dyspnea, epistaxis, pharyngitis, rhinitis, upper respiratory tract infection

Miscellaneous: Fever

Rare but important or life-threatening: Atrial fibrillation, bradycardia, cardiac failure, cerebrovascular accident, confusion, hepatic insufficiency, hepatitis, hypersensitivity, leukopenia, loss of consciousness, pancreatitis, pneumonia, presyncope, pulmonary edema, renal failure, rhabdomyolysis, thrombocytopenia

Drug Interactions

Metabolism/Transport Effects Substrate of CYP2C9 (minor); **Note:** Assignment of Major/Minor substrate status based on clinically relevant drug interaction potential; **Inhibits** CYP2C8 (weak), CYP2C9 (weak)

Avoid Concomitant Use There are no known interactions where it is recommended to avoid concomitant use.

Increased Effect/Toxicity

Candesartan may increase the levels/effects of: ACE Inhibitors; Amifostine; Antihypertensives; CycloSPORINE (Systemic); DULoxetine; Hypotensive Agents;

Levodopa; Lithium; Nonsteroidal Anti-Inflammatory Agents; Obinutuzumab; Potassium-Sparing Diuretics; RisperiDONE; RiTUXimab; Sodium Phosphates

The levels/effects of Candesartan may be increased by: Alfuzosin; Aliskiren; Barbiturates; Brimonidine (Topical); Canagliflozin; Dapoxetine; Diazoxide; Eplerenone; Heparin; Heparin (Low Molecular Weight); Herbs (Hypotensive Properties); MAO Inhibitors; Nicorandil; Pentoxifylline; Phosphodiesterase 5 Inhibitors; Potassium Salts; Prostacyclin Analogues; Tolvaptan; Trimethoprim

Decreased Effect

The levels/effects of Candesartan may be decreased by: Herbs (Hypertensive Properties); Methylphenidate; Nonsteroidal Anti-Inflammatory Agents; Yohimbine

Storage/Stability Store at 25°C (77°F); excursions permitted to 15°C to 30°C (59°F to 86°F).

Mechanism of Action Candesartan is an angiotensin receptor antagonist. Angiotensin II acts as a vasoconstrictor. In addition to causing direct vasoconstriction, angiotensin II also stimulates the release of aldosterone. Once aldosterone is released, sodium as well as water are reabsorbed. The end result is an elevation in blood pressure. Candesartan binds to the AT1 angiotensin II receptor. This binding prevents angiotensin II from binding to the receptor thereby blocking the vasoconstriction and the aldosterone secreting effects of angiotensin II.

Pharmacodynamics/Kinetics

Onset of action: 2-3 hours

Peak effect: 6-8 hours

Duration: >24 hours

Distribution: V_d: 0.13 L/kg

Protein binding: >99%

Metabolism: Parent compound bioactivated during absorption via ester hydrolysis within intestinal wall to candesartan

Bioavailability: 15%

Half-life elimination (dose dependent): 5-9 hours

Time to peak: 3 to 4 hours

Excretion: Urine (26%)

Dosage

Hypertension: **Note:** Antihypertensive effect usually observed within 2 weeks; maximum antihypertensive effect seen within 4 to 6 weeks. Consider lower initial dosages in volume depleted patients; if possible, correct volume depletion prior to administration. Use in children <6 years is not approved in the Canadian labeling.

Children 1 to <6 years: Oral: Initial: 0.2 mg/kg/day in 1 to 2 divided doses; titrate to response; usual range: 0.05 to 0.4 mg/kg/day; maximum daily dose: 0.4 mg/kg/day

Children ≥6 years and Adolescents <17 years: Oral:

U.S. labeling:

<50 kg: Initial: 4 to 8 mg daily in 1 to 2 divided doses; titrate to response; usual range: 2 to 16 mg daily; maximum daily dose: 32 mg daily

≥50 kg: Initial: 8 to 16 mg daily in 1 to 2 divided doses; titrate to response; usual range: 4 to 32 mg daily; maximum daily dose: 32 mg daily

Children ≥6 years and Adolescents ≤17 years: Oral:

Canadian labeling:

<50 kg: Initial: 4 mg once daily; titrate to response; maximum dose: 8 mg daily

≥50 kg: Initial: 8 mg once daily; titrate to response; maximum dose: 16 mg daily

Adults: Oral: Dosage must be individualized. Initial: 16 mg once daily; titrate to response; usual range: 8 to 32 mg daily in 1 to 2 divided doses; target dose (JNC 8 [James, 2013]): 12 to 32 mg daily; maximum daily dose: 32 mg daily.

Heart failure: Adults: Oral: Initial: 4 mg once daily (U.S. labeling) or alternatively 4 to 8 mg once daily (ACCF/AHA [Yancy, 2013]; double the dose at 2-week intervals as tolerated; target dose: 32 mg once daily (ACCF/AHA [Yancy, 2013])

Note: Concurrent therapy with an ACE inhibitor may provide additional benefit in patients with HF with reduced EF who remain symptomatic on standard therapy and are unable to receive an aldosterone antagonist (ACCF/AHA [Yancy, 2013]).

Canadian labeling: Initial: 4 mg once daily; double the dose at 2-week intervals as tolerated; target dose: 32 mg once daily

Elderly: No initial dosage adjustment is necessary for elderly patients (although higher concentrations (C_{max}) and AUC were observed in this population).

Dosage adjustment in renal impairment:

U.S. labeling:

Children ≥1 year and Adolescents <17 years: There are no dosage adjustments provided in the manufacturer's labeling (has not been studied). Children with GFR <30 mL/minute/1.73 m^2 should not receive candesartan.

Adults: No initial dosage adjustment necessary; however, in patients with severe renal impairment (CrCl <30 mL/minute/1.73 m^2) AUC and C_{max} were approximately doubled after repeated dosing.

Canadian labeling:

Children ≥6 and Adolescents ≤17 years: There are no dosage adjustments provided in manufacturer's labeling (has not been studied).

Adults:

Mild impairment: No dosage adjustment necessary.

Moderate or severe impairment: Consider initial dose of 4 mg once daily in patients with hypertension.

Dialysis: Consider initial dose of 4 mg once daily in patients with hypertension.

Dosage adjustment in hepatic impairment:

U.S. labeling:

Mild impairment (Child-Pugh class A): No initial dosage adjustment necessary.

Moderate impairment (Child-Pugh class B): Initial: 8 mg daily (AUC increased by 145%) in adult patients with hypertension. There are no dosage adjustments provided in the manufacturer's labeling for pediatric patients.

Severe impairment (Child-Pugh class C): There are no dosage adjustments provided in the manufacturer's labeling (has not been studied); however, systemic exposure increases significantly in moderate impairment.

Canadian labeling:

Children: There are no dosage adjustments provided in the manufacturer's labeling (has not been studied).

Adults:

Mild to moderate impairment: No dosage adjustment necessary.

Severe impairment: Limited experience; consider initial dose of 4 mg once daily in adult patients with hypertension.

Administration Administer without regard to meals. An oral suspension may be prepared for children unable to swallow tablets (refer to Extemporaneous Preparations information).

Monitoring Parameters Supine blood pressure, electrolytes, serum creatinine, BUN, urinalysis, symptomatic hypotension, and tachycardia; in heart failure, serum potassium during dose escalation and periodically thereafter

2013 ACCF/AHA Heart Failure guideline recommendations: Within 1-2 weeks after initiation, reassess blood pressure (including postural blood pressure changes), renal function, and serum potassium; follow closely after dose changes. Patients with systolic blood pressure <80 mm Hg, low serum sodium, diabetes mellitus, and impaired renal function should be closely monitored (ACCF/AHA [Yancy, 2013]).

Additional Information May have an advantage over losartan due to minimal metabolism requirements and consequent use in mild-to-moderate hepatic impairment

Dosage Forms

Tablet, Oral:

Atacand: 4 mg, 8 mg, 16 mg, 32 mg

Generic: 4 mg, 8 mg, 16 mg, 32 mg

Extemporaneous Preparations Oral suspension may be made in concentrations ranging from 0.1 to 2 mg/mL; typically 1 mg/mL oral suspension suitable for majority of prescribed doses; any strength tablet may be used. A 1 mg/mL (total volume: 160 mL) oral suspension may be made with tablets and a 1:1 mixture of Ora-Plus® and Ora-Sweet SF®. Prepare the vehicle by adding 80 mL of Ora-Plus® and 80 mL of Ora-Sweet SF® or, alternatively, use 160 mL of Ora-Blend SF®. Add a small amount of vehicle to five 32 mg tablets and grind into a smooth paste using a mortar and pestle. Transfer the paste to a calibrated amber PET bottle, rinse the mortar and pestle clean using the vehicle, add this to the bottle, and then add a quantity of vehicle sufficient to make 160 mL. The suspension is stable at room temperature for 100 days unopened or 30 days after the first opening; do not freeze; label "shake well before use." (Atacand prescribing information, 2013).

Candesartan and Hydrochlorothiazide

(kan de SAR tan & hye droe klor oh THYE a zide)

Brand Names: U.S. Atacand HCT

Brand Names: Canada Apo-Candesartan HCTZ; Atacand Plus; Candesartan HCT; Candesartan-HCTZ; Co-Candesartan/HCT; Mylan-Candesartan HCTZ; PMS-Candesartan HCTZ; Sandoz-Candesartan Plus; Teva-Candesartan/HCTZ

Index Terms Candesartan Cilexetil and Hydrochlorothiazide; Hydrochlorothiazide and Candesartan

Pharmacologic Category Angiotensin II Receptor Blocker; Antihypertensive; Diuretic, Thiazide

Use Hypertension: Treatment of hypertension; combination product should not be used for initial therapy

Pregnancy Risk Factor D

Dosage Hypertension, replacement therapy: Adults: Oral: Combination product can be substituted for individual agents; maximum therapeutic effect would be expected within 4 weeks

Usual dosage range:

Candesartan: 8-32 mg daily, given once daily or twice daily in divided doses

Hydrochlorothiazide: 12.5-50 mg once daily

Elderly: No initial dosage adjustment is recommended.

Dosage adjustment in renal impairment:

CrCl ≥30 mL/minute: No dosage adjustment necessary.

CrCl <30 mL/minute: No dosage adjustment provided in manufacturer's labeling (safety and efficacy not established); however, AUC and serum levels of candesartan are increased, and the half-life of hydrochlorothiazide is prolonged in severe renal impairment. Use is contraindicated in anuric patients.

Dosage adjustment in hepatic impairment:

Mild impairment (Child-Pugh class A): No dosage adjustment necessary.

Moderate-to-severe impairment (Child-Pugh classes B and C): Not recommended for initiation since an appropriate adjusted dose is not commercially available.

Additional Information Complete prescribing information should be consulted for additional detail.

Dosage Forms

Tablet, oral: 16/12.5: Candesartan cilexetil 16 mg and hydrochlorothiazide 12.5 mg; 32/12.5: Candesartan cilexetil 32 mg and hydrochlorothiazide 12.5 mg; 32/25: Candesartan cilexetil 32 mg and hydrochlorothiazide 25 mg

Atacand HCT: 16/12.5: Candesartan 16 mg and hydrochlorothiazide 12.5 mg; 32/12.5: Candesartan 32 mg and hydrochlorothiazide 12.5 mg; 32/25: Candesartan 32 mg and hydrochlorothiazide 25 mg

- ◆ **Candesartan Cilexetil** *see* Candesartan *on page 335*
- ◆ **Candesartan Cilexetil and Hydrochlorothiazide** *see* Candesartan and Hydrochlorothiazide *on page 338*
- ◆ **Candesartan HCT (Can)** *see* Candesartan and Hydrochlorothiazide *on page 338*
- ◆ **Candesartan-HCTZ (Can)** *see* Candesartan and Hydrochlorothiazide *on page 338*
- ◆ **Candistatin (Can)** *see* Nystatin (Topical) *on page 1482*
- ◆ **CanesOral (Can)** *see* Fluconazole *on page 885*
- ◆ **Canesten® Topical (Can)** *see* Clotrimazole (Topical) *on page 488*
- ◆ **Canesten® Vaginal (Can)** *see* Clotrimazole (Topical) *on page 488*
- ◆ **Cannabidiol and Tetrahydrocannabinol** *see* Tetrahydrocannabinol and Cannabidiol [CAN/INT] *on page 2018*
- ◆ **Canthacur® (Can)** *see* Cantharidin [CAN/INT] *on page 338*

Cantharidin [CAN/INT] (kan THAR e din)

Brand Names: Canada Canthacur®; Cantharone®

Pharmacologic Category Keratolytic Agent

Use Note: Not approved in U.S.

Removal of common warts, molluscum contagiosum, and periungual warts

Pregnancy Considerations Use is not recommended during pregnancy.

Contraindications

Canthacur®: Hypersensitivity to cantharidin or any component of the formulation; alcoholic beverages for several hours after treatment; use on mosaic warts

Cantharone®: Use in diabetics or in individuals with impaired peripheral circulation; use near eyes or on face or mucous membranes; in anogenital, intertriginous, or axilla areas

Warnings/Precautions Strong vesicant that may cause blistering of normal skin or mucous membranes; reactions may be more severe in patients with fair complexion and/or blue eyes. Do not apply to irritated or inflamed skin. Residual pigmentation has been reported (rarely) with use. **For external use only.** Not for use near the eyes, on mucous membranes, in anogenital, intertriginous or axilla areas. Avoid treating multiple lesions during the first visit to determine patient tolerability. Should be applied only by a physician; not recommended for dispensing to patient.

Adverse Reactions

Dermatologic: Annular warts, depigmentation (temporary)

Local: Blisters, burning, pain, tenderness, tingling

Miscellaneous: Chemical lymphangitis

Drug Interactions

Metabolism/Transport Effects None known.

Avoid Concomitant Use There are no known interactions where it is recommended to avoid concomitant use.

Increased Effect/Toxicity There are no known significant interactions involving an increase in effect.

Decreased Effect There are no known significant interactions involving a decrease in effect.

Storage/Stability Highly flammable; protect from heat, fire, and flame.

Mechanism of Action Cantharidin is a vesicant thought to cause wart exfoliation via its acantholytic actions.

Dosage Topical: Children ≥3 years, Adolescents, and Adults: **Note:** Canthacur® product insert does not specify minimum age requirement for use in children.

Common or periungual warts: Apply to lesion and to 1-3 mm surrounding margin; once dry, cover with nonporous tape; remove tape in 24 hours. Treat once weekly for new or resistant lesions (2-3 treatments may be necessary). Patients scheduled for curettage should return 24 hours after treatment for procedure; reassess in 4 weeks for resolution and/or healing.

Molluscum contagiosum: Apply directly to lesion; once dry, cover large or resistant lesions with nonporous tape for 4-6 hours (Cantharone®) or 6-8 hours (Canthacur®). May retreat once weekly for new or resistant lesions.

Palpebral warts: Canthacur®: Apply directly to lesion and leave uncovered. Avoid touching normal skin or applying inside eyelash; may repeat in 7-10 days

Plantar warts: Apply to lesion and to 1-3 mm surrounding margin; once dry, cover with nonporous tape for up to 1 week; may retreat in 1-2 weeks if necessary

Dosage adjustment in renal impairment: No dosage adjustment provided in manufacturer's labeling.

Dosage adjustment in hepatic impairment: No dosage adjustment provided in manufacturer's labeling.

Administration For external use only; apply to clean skin. No cutting or prior treatment is required. Occasionally, nails must be trimmed to expose subungual warts to medication. Using a wooden applicator stick, apply to lesion(s). Allow to dry for a few minutes. Palpebral warts treated with Canthacur® should be left uncovered. Avoid touching normal skin or applying inside eyelash; instruct patients not to touch eyelid. Large or resistant lesions due to molluscum contagiosum should be covered with a piece of nonporous adhesive tape for 4-6 hours (Cantharone®) or 6-8 hours (Canthacur®). Other lesions should be covered with a piece of nonporous adhesive tape for 4-6 hours for up to 1 week. Within 24 hours, a blister forms and healing is typically evident within 7 days. Additional treatment may be necessary for resistant lesions. Medication may be used for pain and itching at night.

Monitoring Parameters Treated areas for adequate healing; pain and tolerability of treatment

Product Availability Not available in U.S.

Dosage Forms: Canada Excipient information presented when available (limited, particularly for generics); consult specific product labeling.

Liquid:

Canthacur®, Cantharone®: Cantharidin 0.7% in a film-forming vehicle (7.5 mL)

◆ **Cantharone® (Can)** *see* Cantharidin [CAN/INT] *on page 338*

◆ **CAPE** *see* Capecitabine *on page 339*

Capecitabine (ka pe SITE a been)

Brand Names: U.S. Xeloda

Brand Names: Canada Teva-Capecitabine; Xeloda

Index Terms CAPE

Pharmacologic Category Antineoplastic Agent, Antimetabolite; Antineoplastic Agent, Antimetabolite (Pyrimidine Analog)

Use

Breast cancer, metastatic:

Monotherapy: Treatment of metastatic breast cancer resistant to both paclitaxel and an anthracycline-containing regimen or resistant to paclitaxel in patients for whom further anthracycline therapy is not indicated

Combination therapy: Treatment of metastatic breast cancer (in combination with docetaxel) after failure of a prior anthracycline-containing regimen

Colorectal cancer: First-line treatment of metastatic colorectal cancer when treatment with a fluoropyrimidine alone is preferred; adjuvant therapy of Dukes' C colon cancer after complete resection of the primary tumor when fluoropyrimidine therapy alone is preferred

Pregnancy Risk Factor D

Pregnancy Considerations Adverse effects were observed in animal reproduction studies. Fetal harm may occur if administered during pregnancy. Women of childbearing potential should use effective contraceptives to avoid pregnancy during treatment.

Breast-Feeding Considerations It is not known if capecitabine is excreted in breast milk. Due to the potential for serious adverse reactions in the nursing infant, the decision to discontinue capecitabine or to discontinue breast-feeding should take into account the importance of treatment to the mother.

Contraindications Hypersensitivity to capecitabine, fluorouracil, or any component of the formulation; known deficiency of dihydropyrimidine dehydrogenase (DPD); severe renal impairment (CrCl <30 mL/minute)

Warnings/Precautions Hazardous agent - use appropriate precautions for handling and disposal (NIOSH 2014 [group 1]). Bone marrow suppression may occur, hematologic toxicity is more common when used in combination therapy; use with caution; dosage adjustments may be required. Product labeling recommends that patients with baseline platelets <100,000/mm^3 and/or neutrophils <1,500/mm^3 not receive capecitabine therapy and also to withhold for grade 3 or 4 hematologic toxicity during treatment. Rare and unexpected severe toxicity (stomatitis, diarrhea, neutropenia, neurotoxicity) may be attributed to dihydropyrimidine dehydrogenase (DPD) deficiency.

Capecitabine may cause diarrhea (may be severe); median time to first occurrence of grade 2 to 4 diarrhea was 34 days; median duration of grades 3 or 4 diarrhea was 5 days. Withhold treatment for grades 2 to 4 diarrhea; subsequent doses should be reduced after grade 3 or 4 diarrhea or recurrence of grade 2 diarrhea. Antidiarrheal therapy (eg, loperamide) is recommended. Necrotizing enterocolitis (typhlitis) has been reported. Dehydration may occur rapidly in patients with diarrhea, nausea, vomiting, anorexia, and/or weakness; adequately hydrate prior to treatment initiation. Elderly patients may be a higher risk for dehydration. **Note:** Canadian labeling recommends treatment interruption for dehydration requiring IV hydration lasting <24 hours and dosage reduction if IV hydration required for ≥24 hours; correct precipitating factors and ensure rehydration prior to resuming therapy.

Hand-and-foot syndrome is characterized by numbness, dysesthesia/paresthesia, tingling, painless or painful swelling, erythema, desquamation, blistering, and severe pain; median onset is 79 days (range: 11 to 360 days). If grade 2 or 3 hand-and-foot syndrome occurs, interrupt administration of capecitabine until decreases to grade 1. Following grade 3 hand-and-foot syndrome, decrease subsequent doses of capecitabine. In patients with colorectal cancer, treatment with capecitabine immediately following 6 weeks of fluorouracil/leucovorin (FU/LV) therapy has been associated with an increased incidence of grade ≥3 toxicity, when compared to patients receiving the reverse sequence, capecitabine (two 3-week courses) followed by FU/LV (Hennig, 2008).

Grade 3 and 4 hyperbilirubinemia have been observed in patients with and without hepatic metastases at baseline (median onset: 64 days). Transaminase and alkaline phosphatase elevations have also been reported. If capecitabine-related grade 3 or 4 hyperbilirubinemia occurs, Interrupt treatment until bilirubin ≤3 times ULN. Use with caution in patients with mild to moderate hepatic impairment due to liver metastases; effect of severe hepatic impairment has not been studied. Dehydration may occur, resulting in acute renal failure (may be fatal); concomitant use with nephrotoxic agents and baseline renal dysfunction may increase the risk. Use with caution in patients with mild to moderate renal impairment; reduce dose with moderate impairment (exposure to capecitabine and metabolites is increased) and carefully monitor and reduce subsequent dose (with any grade 2 or higher adverse effect) with mild to moderate impairment; use is contraindicated in severe impairment. Use with caution in patients ≥60 years of age, the incidence of treatment-related adverse events may be higher.

Cardiotoxicity has been observed with capecitabine, including myocardial infarction, ischemia, angina, dysrhythmias, cardiac arrest, cardiac failure, sudden death, ECG changes, and cardiomyopathy; may be more common in patients with a history of coronary artery disease. **[U.S. Boxed Warning]: Capecitabine may increase the anticoagulant effects of warfarin; bleeding events, including death, have occurred with concomitant use. Increases in prothrombin time (PT) and INR may occur within several days to months after capecitabine initiation, and may continue up to 1 month after capecitabine discontinuation; may occur in patients with or without liver metastases. Monitor frequently and adjust anticoagulation dosing accordingly. An increased risk of coagulopathy is correlated with a cancer diagnosis and age >60 years.** Other potentially significant drug-drug interactions may exist, requiring dose or frequency adjustment, additional monitoring, and/or selection of alternative therapy.

Adverse Reactions Derived from monotherapy trials.

Cardiovascular: Chest pain, edema, venous thrombosis

Central nervous system: Depression, dizziness, fatigue, headache, insomnia, lethargy, mood changes, mouth pain, neuropathy, pain, paresthesia

Dermatologic: Alopecia, dermatitis, erythema, nail disease, palmar-plantar erythrodysesthesia (hand-and-foot syndrome; may be dose limiting), skin discoloration, skin rash

Endocrine & metabolic: Dehydration

Gastrointestinal: Abdominal pain, anorexia, constipation, decreased appetite, diarrhea (may be dose limiting), dysgeusia (colorectal cancer), dyspepsia, gastrointestinal hemorrhage, gastrointestinal motility disorder, GI inflammation (upper; colorectal cancer), intestinal obstruction, nausea, sore throat, stomatitis, vomiting

Hematologic & oncologic: Anemia, lymphocytopenia, neutropenia, thrombocytopenia

Hepatic: Increased serum bilirubin

Infection: Viral infection (colorectal cancer)

Neuromuscular & skeletal: Arthralgia, back pain, limb pain, myalgia, neuropathy, weakness

Ophthalmic: Conjunctivitis, eye irritation, visual disturbance (colorectal cancer)

Respiratory: Cough, dyspnea, epistaxis

Miscellaneous: Fever

Rare but important or life-threatening (from monotherapy or combination therapy): Abnormal gait, angina pectoris, arthritis, ascites, asthma, atrial fibrillation, blood coagulation disorder, bradycardia, brain disease, bronchitis, bronchopneumonia, bronchospasm, cachexia, cardiac arrhythmia, cardiac failure, cardiomyopathy, cerebrovascular accident, cholestatic hepatitis, colitis, confusion, decreased prothrombin time, duodenitis, dysphagia, ecchymoses, esophagitis, fibrosis, fungal infection, gastric ulcer, gastroenteritis, gastrointestinal perforation, hemorrhage, hepatic failure, hepatic fibrosis, hepatitis, hypersensitivity, hypertension, hypertriglyceridemia, hypokalemia, hypomagnesemia, hypotension, immune thrombocytopenia, intestinal obstruction, keratoconjunctivitis, lacrimal stenosis, laryngitis, leukopenia, loss of consciousness, lymphedema, myocardial infarction, myocarditis, necrotizing enterocolitis (typhlitis), nocturia, ostealgia, pancytopenia, pericardial effusion, phlebitis (venous), pneumonia, pruritus, pulmonary embolism, radiation recall phenomenon, rectal pain, renal insufficiency, respiratory distress, sedation, sepsis, skin changes (fingerprint distortion; secondary to hand-and-foot syndrome), skin photosensitivity, Stevens-Johnson syndrome, syncope, tachycardia, toxic epidermal necrolysis, toxic megacolon, ventricular premature contractions

Drug Interactions

Metabolism/Transport Effects Inhibits CYP2C9 (strong)

Avoid Concomitant Use

Avoid concomitant use of Capecitabine with any of the following: BCG; CloZAPine; Dipyrone; Gimeracil; Natalizumab; Pimecrolimus; Tacrolimus (Topical); Tofacitinib; Vaccines (Live)

Increased Effect/Toxicity

Capecitabine may increase the levels/effects of: Bosentan; Carvedilol; CloZAPine; CYP2C9 Substrates; Diclofenac (Systemic); Dronabinol; Fosphenytoin; Lacosamide; Leflunomide; Natalizumab; Ospemifene; Phenytoin; Tetrahydrocannabinol; Tofacitinib; Vaccines (Live); Vitamin K Antagonists

The levels/effects of Capecitabine may be increased by: Cannabis; Cimetidine; Denosumab; Dipyrone; Gimeracil; Leucovorin Calcium-Levoleucovorin; Pimecrolimus; Roflumilast; Tacrolimus (Topical); Trastuzumab

Decreased Effect

Capecitabine may decrease the levels/effects of: BCG; Coccidioides immitis Skin Test; Sipuleucel-T; Vaccines (Inactivated); Vaccines (Live)

The levels/effects of Capecitabine may be decreased by: Echinacea

Food Interactions Food reduced the rate and extent of absorption of capecitabine. Management: Administer within 30 minutes after a meal.

Storage/Stability Store at room temperature of 25°C (77°F); excursions permitted between 15°C and 30°C (59°F and 86°F). Keep bottle tightly closed.

Mechanism of Action Capecitabine is a prodrug of fluorouracil. It undergoes hydrolysis in the liver and tissues to form fluorouracil which is the active moiety. Fluorouracil is a fluorinated pyrimidine antimetabolite that inhibits thymidylate synthetase, blocking the methylation of deoxyuridylic acid to thymidylic acid, interfering with DNA, and to a lesser degree, RNA synthesis. Fluorouracil appears to be phase specific for the G_1 and S phases of the cell cycle.

Pharmacodynamics/Kinetics

Absorption: Rapid and extensive (rate and extent reduced by food)

Protein binding: <60%; ~35% to albumin

Metabolism:

Hepatic: Inactive metabolites: 5′-deoxy-5-fluorocytidine, 5′-deoxy-5-fluorouridine

Tissue: Enzymatically metabolized to fluorouracil, which is then metabolized to active metabolites, 5-fluoroxyuridine monophosphate (F-UMP) and 5-5-fluoro-2'-deoxyuridine-5'-O-monophosphate (F-dUMP)

Half-life elimination: 0.5 to 1 hour

Time to peak: 1.5 hours; Fluorouracil: 2 hours

Excretion: Urine (96%, 57% as α-fluoro-β-alanine; <3% as unchanged drug); feces (<3%)

Dosage

Breast cancer, metastatic: Adults: Oral: 1,250 mg/m^2 twice daily for 2 weeks, every 21 days (as either monotherapy or in combination with docetaxel)

Colorectal cancer, metastatic: Adults: Oral: 1,250 mg/m^2 twice daily for 2 weeks, every 21 days. **Note:** Capecitabine toxicities, particularly hand-foot syndrome, may be higher in North American populations; therapy initiation at doses of 1,000 mg/m^2 twice daily (for 2 weeks every 21 days) may be considered (Haller, 2008).

Dukes' C colon cancer, adjuvant therapy: Adults: Oral: 1,250 mg/m^2 twice daily for 2 weeks, every 21 days, for a recommended total duration of 24 weeks (8 cycles of 2 weeks of drug administration and 1-week rest period).

Off-label uses:

Breast cancer, metastatic (off-label dosing): Adults: Oral: 1,000 mg/m^2 twice daily (in combination with ixabepilone) on days 1 to 14 of a 3-week cycle until disease progression or unacceptable toxicity (Thomas, 2007)

Breast cancer, metastatic, HER2+ (off-label dosing): Adults: Oral: 1,000 mg/m^2 twice daily (in combination with lapatinib) on days 1 to 14 of a 3-week cycle until disease progression or unacceptable toxicity (Geyer, 2006) **or** 1,250 mg/m^2 twice daily (in combination with trastuzumab) on days 1 to 14 of a 3-week cycle (Bartsch, 2007)

Breast cancer, metastatic, HER2+ with brain metastases, first-line therapy (off-label dosing): Adults: Oral: 1,000 mg/m^2 twice daily (in combination with lapatinib) on days 1 to 14 of a 3-week cycle until disease progression or unacceptable toxicity (Bachelot, 2012)

Colorectal cancer (off-label dosing): Adults: Oral: 1,000 mg/m^2 twice daily (in combination with oxaliplatin) on days 1 to 14 of a 3-week cycle for 8 or 16 cycles (Cassidy, 2008; Haller, 2011; Schmoll, 2007)

Esophageal and gastric cancers (off-label uses): Adults: Oral:

Preoperative or definitive chemoradiation: 800 mg/m^2 twice daily (in combination with cisplatin and radiation) on days 1 to 5 weekly for 5 weeks (Lee, 2007) **or** 625 mg/m^2 twice daily (in combination with oxaliplatin and radiation) on days 1 to 5 weekly for 5 weeks (Javle, 2009)

Postoperative chemoradiation: 625 to 825 mg/m^2 twice daily during radiation therapy (Lee, 2006)

Locally advanced or metastatic (chemoradiation not indicated): 1,000 to 1,250 mg/m^2 twice daily (monotherapy or in combination with cisplatin with or without trastuzumab) on days 1 to 14 of a 3-week cycle (Bang, 2010; Hong, 2004; Kang, 2009) **or** 625 mg/m^2 twice daily (in combination with epirubicin and cisplatin or oxaliplatin) on days 1 to 21 of a 3-week cycle for up to 8 cycles (Cunningham, 2008; Sumpter, 2005)

Hepatobiliary cancers, advanced (off-label use): Adults: Oral: 650 mg/m^2 twice daily (in combination with gemcitabine) on days 1 to 14 of a 3-week cycle (Knox, 2005) **or** 1,000 mg/m^2 twice daily (in combination with oxaliplatin) on days 1 to 14 of a 3-week cycle (Nehls, 2008) **or** 1,250 mg/m^2 twice daily (in combination with cisplatin) on days 1 to 14 of a 3-week cycle (Kim, 2003); all regimens continued until disease progression or unacceptable toxicity

Neuroendocrine (pancreatic/islet cell) tumors, metastatic or unresectable: Adults: Oral: 750 mg/m^2 twice daily (in combination with temozolomide) on days 1 to 14 of a 4-week cycle (Strosberg, 2011)

Ovarian, fallopian tube, or peritoneal cancer, platinum-refractory: Adults: Oral: 1,000 mg/m^2 twice daily on days 1 to 14 of a 3-week cycle until disease progression or unacceptable toxicity (Wolf, 2006)

Pancreatic cancer, metastatic (off-label use): Adults: Oral: 1,250 mg/m^2 twice daily on days 1 to 14 of a 3-week cycle (Cartwright, 2002) **or** 830 mg/m^2 twice daily (in combination with gemcitabine) on days 1 to 21 of a 4-week cycle until disease progression or unacceptable toxicity (Cunningham, 2009)

Unknown primary cancer (off-label use): Adults: Oral: 1,000 mg/m^2 twice daily (in combination with oxaliplatin) on days 1 to 14 of a 3-week cycle for up to 6 cycles or until disease progression (Hainsworth, 2010) **or** 800 mg/m^2 twice daily (in combination with carboplatin and gemcitabine) on days 1 to 14 of a 3-week cycle for up to 8 cycles or until disease progression or unacceptable toxicity (Schneider, 2007)

Elderly: The elderly may be more sensitive to the toxic effects of fluorouracil. Insufficient data are available to provide dosage modifications.

Dosing adjustment in renal impairment: Note: Renal function may be estimated using the Cockcroft-Gault formula for dosage adjustment purposes.

Renal impairment at treatment initiation:

CrCl ≥51 mL/minute: Initial: No dosage adjustment necessary.

CrCl 30 to 50 mL/minute: Initial: Administer 75% of usual dose (Cassidy, 2002; Poole, 2002; Xeloda prescribing information, 2014)

CrCl <30 mL/minute: Use is contraindicated (Poole, 2002; Xeloda prescribing information, 2014)

Renal toxicity during treatment: Refer to Dosage adjustment for toxicity.

Dosing adjustment in hepatic impairment:

Hepatic impairment at treatment initiation:

Mild to moderate impairment: No starting dose adjustment necessary (Ecklund, 2005; Superfin, 2007); however, carefully monitor patients.

Severe hepatic impairment: There are no dosage adjustments provided in the manufacturer's labeling (has not been studied).

Hepatotoxicity during treatment: Hyperbilirubinemia, grade 3 or 4: Interrupt treatment until bilirubin ≤3 times ULN.

Dosing in obesity: *ASCO Guidelines for appropriate chemotherapy dosing in obese adults with cancer:* Utilize patient's actual body weight (full weight) for calculation of body surface area- or weight-based dosing, particularly when the intent of therapy is curative; manage regimen-related toxicities in the same manner as for nonobese patients; if a dose reduction is utilized due to toxicity, consider resumption of full weight-based dosing with subsequent cycles, especially if cause of toxicity (eg, hepatic or renal impairment) is resolved (Griggs, 2012).

Dosage adjustment for toxicity: See table on next page (**Note:** Capecitabine dosing recommendations apply to both monotherapy and when used in combination therapy with docetaxel).

Monitor carefully for toxicity and adjust dose as necessary. Doses reduced for toxicity should not be increased at a later time. For combination therapy, also refer to docetaxel product labeling for docetaxel dose modifications. If treatment delay is required for either capecitabine or docetaxel, withhold both agents until appropriate to resume combination treatment.

Recommended Capecitabine Dose Modifications

Toxicity Grades	During a Course of Therapy	Dose Adjustment for Next Cycle (% of starting dose)
Grade 1	Maintain dose level	Maintain dose level
Grade 2		
1st appearance	Interrupt until resolved to grade 0 to 1	100%
2nd appearance	Interrupt until resolved to grade 0 to 1	75%
3rd appearance	Interrupt until resolved to grade 0 to 1	50%
4th appearance	Discontinue treatment permanently	
Grade 3		
1st appearance	Interrupt until resolved to grade 0 to 1	75%
2nd appearance	Interrupt until resolved to grade 0 to 1	50%
3rd appearance	Discontinue treatment permanently	
Grade 4		
1st appearance	Discontinue permanently **or** If in the patient's best interest to continue, interrupt until resolved to grade 0 to 1	50%

Dosage adjustments for hematologic toxicity in combination therapy with ixabepilone:

Neutrophils <500/mm³ for ≥7 days or neutropenic fever: Hold for concurrent diarrhea or stomatitis until neutrophils recover to >1,000/mm³, then continue at same dose

Platelets <25,000/mm³ (or <50,000/mm³ with bleeding): Hold for concurrent diarrhea or stomatitis until platelets recover to >50,000/mm³, then continue at same dose

Administration Usually administered in 2 divided doses taken 12 hours apart. Doses should be taken with water within 30 minutes after a meal. Swallow tablets whole; do not cut or crush.

Hazardous agent; use appropriate precautions for handling and disposal (NIOSH 2014 [group 1]).

Monitoring Parameters Renal function should be estimated at baseline to determine initial dose. During therapy, CBC with differential, hepatic function, and renal function should be monitored. Monitor for diarrhea, dehydration, hand/foot syndrome, stomatitis, and cardiotoxicity. Monitor INR closely if receiving concomitant warfarin.

Additional Information Oncology Comment: An investigational uridine prodrug, uridine triacetate (formerly called vistonuridine), has been studied in a limited number of cases of fluorouracil overdose. Of 17 patients receiving uridine triacetate beginning within 8 to 96 hours after fluorouracil overdose, all patients fully recovered (von Borstel, 2009). Updated data has described a total of 28 patients treated with uridine triacetate for fluorouracil overdose (including overdoses related to continuous infusions delivering fluorouracil at rates faster than prescribed), all of whom recovered fully (Bamat, 2010). An additional case report describes accidental capecitabine ingestion by a 22 month old child; uridine triacetate was initiated approximately 7 hours after exposure. The patient received uridine triacetate every 6 hours for a total of 20 doses through nasogastric tube administration; he was asymptomatic throughout his course and was discharged with normal laboratory values (Kanie, 2011). Refer to Uridine Triacetate monograph.

Dosage Forms

Tablet, Oral:

Xeloda: 150 mg, 500 mg

Generic: 150 mg, 500 mg

Extemporaneous Preparations Hazardous agent: Use appropriate precautions for handling and disposal (NIOSH 2014 [group 1]).

A 10 mg/mL oral solution may be made with tablets. Crush four 500 mg tablets in a mortar and reduce to a fine powder; add to 200 mL water. Capecitabine tablets are water soluble (data on file from Roche). Administer immediately after preparation, 30 minutes after a meal.

Judson IR, Beale PJ, Trigo JM, et al, "A Human Capecitabine Excretion Balance and Pharmacokinetic Study After Administration of a Single Oral Dose of ^{14}C-Labelled Drug," *Invest New Drugs*, 1999, 17 (1):49-56.

- **Capex** *see* Fluocinolone (Topical) *on page 893*
- **Capex® (Can)** *see* Fluocinolone (Topical) *on page 893*
- **Capital® and Codeine** *see* Acetaminophen and Codeine *on page 36*
- **Capmist DM [OTC]** *see* Guaifenesin, Pseudoephedrine, and Dextromethorphan *on page 989*
- **Capoten** *see* Captopril *on page 342*
- **Caprelsa** *see* Vandetanib *on page 2135*

Captopril (KAP toe pril)

Brand Names: Canada Apo-Capto; Dom-Captopril; Mylan-Captopril; PMS-Captopril

Index Terms Capoten

Pharmacologic Category Angiotensin-Converting Enzyme (ACE) Inhibitor; Antihypertensive

Use

Diabetic nephropathy: Treatment of diabetic nephropathy (proteinuria more than 500 mg daily) in patients with type 1 insulin-dependent diabetes mellitus and retinopathy

Heart failure: Treatment of congestive heart failure

The American College of Cardiology Foundation/American Heart Association (ACCF/AHA) 2013 heart failure guidelines recommend the use of angiotensin-converting enzyme (ACE) inhibitors, along with other guideline directed medical therapies, to prevent heart failure in patients with a reduced ejection fraction who have a history of myocardial infarction (stage B heart failure), to prevent heart failure in any patient with a reduced ejection fraction (stage B heart failure), or to treat those with heart failure and reduced ejection fraction (stage C heart failure) (Yancy, 2013).

Hypertension: Management of hypertension

The 2014 guideline for the management of high blood pressure in adults (Eighth Joint National Committee [JNC 8]) recommends initiation of pharmacologic treatment to lower blood pressure for the following patients:

- Patients ≥60 years of age with systolic blood pressure (SBP) ≥150 mm Hg or diastolic blood pressure (DBP) ≥90 mm Hg. Goal of therapy is SBP <150 mm Hg and DBP <90 mm Hg.
- Patients <60 years of age with SBP ≥140 mm Hg or DBP is ≥90 mm Hg. Goal of therapy is SBP <140 mm Hg and DBP <90 mm Hg.
- Patients ≥18 years of age with diabetes and SBP ≥140 mm Hg or DBP ≥90 mm Hg. Goal of therapy is SBP <140 mm Hg and DBP <90 mm Hg.
- Patients ≥18 years of age with chronic kidney disease (CKD) and SBP ≥140 mm Hg or DBP ≥90 mm Hg. Goal of therapy is SBP <140 mm Hg and DBP <90 mm Hg.

In patients with CKD, regardless of race or diabetes status, the use of an ACE inhibitor (ACEI) or angiotensin receptor blocker (ARB) as initial therapy is recommended to improve kidney outcomes. In the general nonblack population (without CKD) including those with diabetes, initial antihypertensive treatment should consist of a thiazide-type diuretic, calcium channel blocker, ACEI, or ARB. In the general black population (without CKD) including those with diabetes, initial antihypertensive treatment should consist of a thiazide-type diuretic or a calcium channel blocker **instead of** an ACEI or ARB.

Left ventricular dysfunction after myocardial infarction: To improve survival following myocardial infarction in clinically stable patients with left ventricular dysfunction manifested as an ejection fraction of 40% or less, and to reduce the incidence of overt heart failure and subsequent hospitalizations for congestive heart failure in these patients.

Note: The 2013 American College of Cardiology Foundation/American Heart Association guidelines for the management of patients with ST-elevation myocardial infarction (STEMI) states that an ACE inhibitor (eg, captopril) should be initiated within the first 24 hours after STEMI in patients with anterior MI, heart failure, or left ventricular ejection fraction ≤40%. It is also reasonable to initiate an ACE inhibitor in all patients with STEMI (ACCF/AHA [O'Gara, 2013]).

Pregnancy Risk Factor D

Pregnancy Considerations **[U.S. Boxed Warning]: Drugs that act on the renin-angiotensin system can cause injury and death to the developing fetus. Discontinue as soon as possible once pregnancy is detected.** Captopril crosses the placenta; teratogenic effects may occur following maternal use during pregnancy. Drugs that act on the renin-angiotensin system are associated with oligohydramnios. Oligohydramnios, due to decreased fetal renal function, may lead to fetal lung hypoplasia and skeletal malformations. Their use in pregnancy is also associated with anuria, hypotension, renal failure, skull hypoplasia, and death in the fetus/neonate. Chronic maternal hypertension itself is also associated with adverse events in the fetus/infant. ACE inhibitors are not recommended during pregnancy to treat maternal hypertension or heart failure. Use of an ACE inhibitor should also be avoided in any woman of reproductive age. Women who are planning a pregnancy should be considered for other medication options if an ACE inhibitor is currently prescribed or the ACE inhibitor should be discontinued as soon as possible once pregnancy is detected. The exposed fetus should be monitored for fetal growth, amniotic fluid volume, and organ formation. Infants exposed to an ACE inhibitor *in utero* should be monitored for hyperkalemia, hypotension, and oliguria (exchange transfusions or dialysis may be needed). These adverse events are generally associated with maternal use in the second and third trimesters.

Untreated chronic maternal hypertension is also associated with adverse events in the fetus, infant, and mother. The use of ACE inhibitors is not recommended to treat chronic uncomplicated hypertension in pregnant women and should generally be avoided in women of reproductive potential (ACOG, 2013).

Breast-Feeding Considerations Captopril is excreted in breast milk. Breast-feeding is not recommended by the manufacturer.

Contraindications Hypersensitivity to captopril, any other ACE inhibitor, or any component of the formulation; angioedema related to previous treatment with an ACE inhibitor; concomitant use with aliskiren in patients with diabetes mellitus

Warnings/Precautions Anaphylactic reactions may occur rarely with ACE inhibitors. At any time during treatment (especially following first dose) angioedema may occur rarely with ACE inhibitors; may involve the head and neck (potentially compromising airway) or the intestine (presenting with abdominal pain). African-Americans and patients with idiopathic or hereditary angioedema may be at an increased risk. Prolonged frequent monitoring may be required especially if tongue, glottis, or larynx are involved as they are associated with airway obstruction. Patients with a history of airway surgery may have a higher risk of airway obstruction. Aggressive early and appropriate management is critical. Use in patients with previous angioedema associated with ACE inhibitor therapy is contraindicated. Severe anaphylactoid reactions may be seen during hemodialysis (eg, CVVHD) with high-flux dialysis membranes (eg, AN69), and rarely, during low density lipoprotein apheresis with dextran sulfate cellulose. Rare cases of anaphylactoid reactions have been reported in patients undergoing sensitization treatment with hymenoptera (bee, wasp) venom while receiving ACE inhibitors.

Symptomatic hypotension with or without syncope can occur with ACE inhibitors (usually with the first several doses); effects are most often observed in volume depleted patients; close monitoring of patient is required especially with initial dosing and dosing increases; blood pressure must be lowered at a rate appropriate for the patient's clinical condition. Initiation of therapy in patients with ischemic heart disease or cerebrovascular disease warrants close observation due to the potential consequences posed by falling blood pressure (eg, MI, stroke). Use with caution in hypertrophic cardiomyopathy with outflow tract obstruction, aortic stenosis, or before, during, or immediately after major surgery. Extemporaneous preparations of liquid formulations may vary; this may affect the rate and extent of absorption causing intrapatient variability regarding dosing and safety profile for the patient; use with caution and monitor closely if dosage formulations are changed (Bhatt, 2011; Mulla, 2007). **[U.S. Boxed Warning]: Drugs that act on the renin-angiotensin system can cause injury and death to the developing fetus. Discontinue as soon as possible once pregnancy is detected.**

Hyperkalemia may occur with ACE inhibitors; risk factors include renal dysfunction, diabetes mellitus, concomitant use of potassium-sparing diuretics, potassium supplements and/or potassium containing salts. Use cautiously, if at all, with these agents and monitor potassium closely. Cough may occur with ACE inhibitors. Other causes of cough should be considered (eg, pulmonary congestion in patients with heart failure) and excluded prior to discontinuation.

May be associated with deterioration of renal function and/or increases in BUN and serum creatinine, particularly in patients with low renal blood flow (eg, renal artery stenosis, heart failure) whose glomerular filtration rate (GFR) is dependent on efferent arteriolar vasoconstriction by angiotensin II; deterioration may result in oliguria, acute renal failure, and progressive azotemia. Small benign increases in serum creatinine may occur following initiation; consider discontinuation only in patients with progressive and/or significant deterioration in renal function (Bakris, 2000). Use with caution in patients with unstented unilateral/bilateral renal artery stenosis. When unstented bilateral renal artery stenosis is present, use is generally avoided due to the elevated risk of deterioration in renal function unless possible benefits outweigh risks. ACE inhibitors effectiveness is less in black patients than in non-blacks. In addition, ACE inhibitors cause a higher rate of angioedema in black than in non-black patients. Potentially significant drug-drug interactions may exist, requiring dose or frequency adjustment, additional monitoring, and/or selection of alternative therapy.

Rare toxicities associated with ACE inhibitors include cholestatic jaundice (which may progress to fulminant hepatic necrosis, some fatal), agranulocytosis, neutropenia with myeloid hypoplasia; anemia and thrombocytopenia have also occurred. If neutropenia develops (neutrophil count <1,000/mm^3), discontinue therapy. Patients with collagen vascular diseases (especially with concomitant renal impairment) or renal impairment alone may be at increased risk for hematologic toxicity; closely monitor CBC with differential for the first 3 months of therapy and periodically thereafter in these patients. Total urinary proteins greater than 1 g per day have been reported (<1%); nephrotic syndrome occurred in about one-fifth of proteinuric patients. In most cases, proteinuria subsided or cleared within six months (whether or not captopril was continued).

Adverse Reactions

Cardiovascular: Angina pectoris, cardiac arrest, cardiac arrhythmia, cardiac failure, chest pain, flushing, hypotension, myocardial infarction, orthostatic hypotension, palpitations, Raynaud's phenomenon, syncope, tachycardia

Central nervous system: Ataxia, cerebrovascular insufficiency, confusion, depression, drowsiness, myasthenia, nervousness

Dermatologic: Bullous pemphigoid, erythema multiforme, exfoliative dermatitis, pallor, pruritus, skin rash (maculopapular or urticarial; in patients with rash, a positive ANA and/or eosinophilia has been noted), Stevens-Johnson syndrome

Endocrine & metabolic: Gynecomastia, hyperkalemia, hyponatremia (symptomatic)

Gastrointestinal: Cholestasis, dysgeusia (loss of taste or diminished perception), dyspepsia, glossitis, pancreatitis

Genitourinary: Impotence, nephrotic syndrome, oliguria, proteinuria, urinary frequency

Hematologic: Agranulocytosis, anemia, neutropenia (in patients with renal insufficiency or collagen-vascular disease), pancytopenia, thrombocytopenia

Hepatic: Hepatic necrosis (rare), hepatitis, increased serum alkaline phosphatase, increased serum bilirubin, increased serum transaminases, jaundice

Hypersensitivity: Anaphylactoid reaction, angioedema, hypersensitivity reaction (rash, pruritus, fever, arthralgia, and eosinophilia; depending on dose and renal function)

Neuromuscular & skeletal: Myalgia, weakness

Ophthalmic: Blurred vision

Renal: Increased serum creatinine, polyuria, renal failure, renal insufficiency, renal insufficiency (worsening; may occur in patients with bilateral renal artery stenosis or hypovolemia)

Respiratory: Bronchospasm, cough, eosinophilic pneumonitis, rhinitis

Rare but important or life-threatening: Alopecia, angina pectoris, anorexia, aphthous stomatitis, aplastic anemia, cholestatic jaundice, eosinophilia, glomerulonephritis, Guillain-Barre syndrome, hemolytic anemia, Huntington's chorea (exacerbation), hyperthermia, increased erythrocyte sedimentation rate, insomnia, interstitial nephritis, Kaposi's sarcoma, peptic ulcer, pericarditis, psoriasis, seizure (in premature infants), systemic lupus erythematosus, vasculitis, visual hallucination (Doane, 2013)

Drug Interactions

Metabolism/Transport Effects **Substrate** of CYP2D6 (major); **Note:** Assignment of Major/Minor substrate status based on clinically relevant drug interaction potential

Avoid Concomitant Use There are no known interactions where it is recommended to avoid concomitant use.

Increased Effect/Toxicity

Captopril may increase the levels/effects of: Allopurinol; Amifostine; Antihypertensives; AzaTHIOprine; DULoxetine; Ferric Gluconate; Gold Sodium Thiomalate; Grass Pollen Allergen Extract (5 Grass Extract); Hypotensive Agents; Iron Dextran Complex; Levodopa; Lithium; Nonsteroidal Anti-Inflammatory Agents; Obinutuzumab; RisperiDONE; RiTUXimab; Sodium Phosphates

The levels/effects of Captopril may be increased by: Abiraterone Acetate; Alfuzosin; Aliskiren; Angiotensin II Receptor Blockers; Barbiturates; Brimonidine (Topical); Canagliflozin; Cobicistat; CYP2D6 Inhibitors (Moderate); CYP2D6 Inhibitors (Strong); Dapoxetine; Darunavir; Diazoxide; DPP-IV Inhibitors; Eplerenone; Everolimus; Heparin; Heparin (Low Molecular Weight); Herbs (Hypotensive Properties); Loop Diuretics; MAO Inhibitors; Nicorandil; Peginterferon Alfa-2b; Pentoxifylline; Phosphodiesterase 5 Inhibitors; Potassium Salts; Potassium-Sparing Diuretics; Prostacyclin Analogues; Sirolimus; Temsirolimus; Thiazide Diuretics; TiZANidine; Tolvaptan; Trimethoprim

Decreased Effect

The levels/effects of Captopril may be decreased by: Antacids; Aprotinin; Herbs (Hypertensive Properties); Icatibant; Lanthanum; Methylphenidate; Nonsteroidal Anti-Inflammatory Agents; Peginterferon Alfa-2b; Salicylates; Yohimbine

Food Interactions Captopril serum concentrations may be decreased if taken with food. Long-term use of captopril may lead to a zinc deficiency which can result in altered taste perception. Management: Take on an empty stomach 1 hour before or 2 hours after meals.

Storage/Stability Store at 20°C to 25°C (68°F to 77°F); protect from moisture.

Mechanism of Action Competitive inhibitor of angiotensin-converting enzyme (ACE); prevents conversion of angiotensin I to angiotensin II, a potent vasoconstrictor; results in lower levels of angiotensin II which causes an increase in plasma renin activity and a reduction in aldosterone secretion

Pharmacodynamics/Kinetics

Onset of action: Peak effect: Blood pressure reduction: 1 to 1.5 hours after dose

Duration: Dose related, may require several weeks of therapy before full hypotensive effect

Absorption: Rapid

Distribution: V_{dss}: 0.7 L/kg (Duchun, 1982)

Bioavailability: ~60% to 75% (Cody, 1985); reduced 30% to 40% by food

Protein binding: 25% to 30%

Half-life elimination:

Adults, healthy volunteers: ~1.7 hours (Duchin, 1982). In two studies, patients with chronic renal failure demonstrated approximately 2-fold longer half-lives as compared to normal subjects (Giudicelli 1984; Onoyama, 1981). Half-life was up to 21 hours in patients with severe renal impairment and up to 32 hours in patients on chronic hemodialysis in another study (Duchin, 1984)

Time to peak: ~1 hour

Excretion: Urine (>95%) within 24 hours (40% to 50% as unchanged drug)

Dosage Note: Titrate dose according to patient's response; use lowest effective dose.

Children ≤1 year and Adolescents ≤17 years: Hypertension: Oral: Initial: 0.3 to 0.5 mg/kg/dose every 8 hours; titrate upward to maximum of 6 mg/kg/day in 2 to 4 divided doses (NHBPEP, 2004; NHLBI, 2011); maximum daily dose: 450 mg daily.

Adults:

Acute hypertension (urgency/emergency): Oral, sublingual: 25 mg, may repeat as needed; consider alternative therapy if blood pressure is nonresponsive within 20 to 30 minutes (Angeli, 1991; Castro del Castillo, 1988; Ceyhan, 1990; Damasceno, 1997; Tschollar, 1985). **Note:** May be given sublingually, but therapeutic advantage has not been demonstrated over oral administration (Karakilic, 2012).

Heart failure with reduced ejection fraction (HFrEF) (ACCF/AHA [Yancy, 2013]): Oral:

Initial dose: 6.25 mg 3 times daily

Target dose: 50 mg 3 times daily

Hypertension: Oral:

Initial dose: 25 mg 2 to 3 times daily (a lower initial dose of 12.5 mg 3 times daily may also be considered [VA Cooperative Study Group, 1984]); may increase at 1- to 2-week intervals up to 50 mg 3 times daily; add thiazide diuretic, unless severe renal impairment coexists then consider loop diuretic, before further dosage increases or consider other treatment options; maximum dose: 150 mg 3 times daily

Target dose (JNC 8 [James, 2013]): 75 to 100 mg twice daily

Usual dose range (ASH/ISH [Weber, 2014]): 50 to 100 mg twice daily

LV dysfunction after MI: Oral: Initial: 6.25 mg; if tolerated, follow with 12.5 mg 3 times daily; then increase to 25 mg 3 times daily during next several days and then gradually increase over next several weeks to target dose of 50 mg 3 times daily (some dose schedules are more aggressive to achieve an increased goal dose within the first few days of initiation). **Note:** In those patients with STEMI in the anterior location, heart failure, or LV ejection fraction ≤ 0.4, an ACE inhibitor (eg, captopril) should be initiated within the first 24 hours after MI (ACCF/AHA [O'Gara, 2013]).

Diabetic nephropathy: Oral: Initial: 25 mg 3 times daily. May be taken with other antihypertensive therapy if required to further lower blood pressure.

Elderly: Hypertension: Consider lower initial doses and titrate to response (Aronow, 2011)

Dosage adjustment in renal impairment:

Manufacturers recommendations: Reduce initial daily dose and titrate slowly (1- to 2-week intervals) with smaller increments. Slowly back titrate to determine the minimum effective dose once the desired therapeutic effect has been reached.

Alternative recommendations (Aronoff, 2007):

Infants, Children, and Adolescents: **Note:** Renally adjusted dose recommendations are based on doses of 0.1 to 0.5 mg/kg/dose every 6 to 8 hours; maximum daily dose: 6 mg/kg/day.

GFR 10 to 50 mL/minute/1.73 m^2: Administer 75% of dose

GFR <10 mL/minute/1.73 m^2: Administer 50% of dose

Intermittent hemodialysis: Administer 50% of dose

Peritoneal dialysis (PD): Administer 50% of dose

Adults:

CrCl 10 to 50 mL/minute: Administer at 75% of normal dose every 12-18 hours.

CrCl <10 mL/minute: Administer at 50% of normal dose every 24 hours.

Intermittent hemodialysis (IHD): Administer after hemodialysis on dialysis days

Peritoneal dialysis: Dose for CrCl 10-50 mL/minute; supplemental dose is not necessary

Dosage adjustment in hepatic impairment: There are no dosage adjustments provided in the manufacturer's labeling (has not been studied).

Dietary Considerations Should be taken at least 1 hour before eating.

Administration Administer at least 1 hour before meals. Unstable in aqueous solutions; to prepare solution for oral administration, mix prior to administration and use within 10 minutes (Allen, 1996).

Monitoring Parameters BUN, electrolytes, serum creatinine; blood pressure. In patients with renal impairment and/or collagen vascular disease, closely monitor CBC with differential for the first 3 months of therapy and periodically thereafter.

2013 ACCF/AHA Heart Failure guideline recommendations: Within 1-2 weeks after initiation and periodically thereafter, reassess renal function and serum potassium especially in patients with preexisting hypotension, hyponatremia, diabetes mellitus, azotemia, or those taking potassium supplements (ACCF/AHA [Yancy, 2013]).

Dosage Forms

Tablet, Oral:

Generic: 12.5 mg, 25 mg, 50 mg, 100 mg

Dosage Forms: Canada Note: Also refer to Dosage Forms.

Tablet, Oral: 6.25 mg

Extemporaneous Preparations A 1 mg/mL oral solution may be made by allowing two 50 mg tablets to dissolve in 50 mL of distilled water. Add the contents of one 500 mg sodium ascorbate injection ampul or one 500 mg ascorbic acid tablet and allow to dissolve. Add quantity of distilled water sufficient to make 100 mL. Label "shake well" and "refrigerate". Stable for 56 days refrigerated.

Nahata MC, Pai VB, and Hipple TF, *Pediatric Drug Formulations*, 5th ed, Cincinnati, OH: Harvey Whitney Books Co, 2004.

Captopril and Hydrochlorothiazide

(KAP toe pril & hye droe klor oh THYE a zide)

Index Terms Hydrochlorothiazide and Captopril

Pharmacologic Category Angiotensin-Converting Enzyme (ACE) Inhibitor; Antihypertensive; Diuretic, Thiazide

Use Management of hypertension

Pregnancy Risk Factor D

Dosage Oral: Adults: Hypertension, CHF: May be substituted for previously titrated dosages of the individual components; alternatively, may initiate as follows:

Initial: Single tablet (captopril 25 mg/hydrochlorothiazide 15 mg) taken once daily; daily dose of captopril should not exceed 150 mg; daily dose of hydrochlorothiazide should not exceed 50 mg

Dosage adjustment in renal impairment: May respond to smaller or less frequent doses.

Dosage adjustment in hepatic impairment: No dosage adjustments provided in manufacturer's labeling; use with caution.

Additional Information Complete prescribing information should be consulted for additional detail.

Dosage Forms

Tablet, oral: 25/15: Captopril 25 mg and hydrochlorothiazide 15 mg; 25/25: Captopril 25 mg and hydrochlorothiazide 25 mg; 50/15: Captopril 50 mg and hydrochlorothiazide 15 mg; 50/25: Captopril 50 mg and hydrochlorothiazide 25 mg

◆ **Carac** *see* Fluorouracil (Topical) *on page 899*

◆ **Carafate** *see* Sucralfate *on page 1940*

Carbachol (KAR ba kole)

Brand Names: U.S. Isopto Carbachol; Miostat

Brand Names: Canada Isopto® Carbachol; Miostat®

Index Terms Carbacholine; Carbamylcholine Chloride

Pharmacologic Category Cholinergic Agonist; Ophthalmic Agent, Antiglaucoma; Ophthalmic Agent, Miotic

Use Lowers intraocular pressure in the treatment of glaucoma; cause miosis during surgery

Pregnancy Risk Factor C

Dosage Adults:

Ophthalmic: Instill 1-2 drops up to 3 times/day

Intraocular: 0.5 mL instilled into anterior chamber before or after securing sutures

Dosage adjustment in renal impairment: No dosage adjustment provided in manufacturer's labeling.

Dosage adjustment in hepatic impairment: No dosage adjustment provided in manufacturer's labeling.

Additional Information Complete prescribing information should be consulted for additional detail.

Dosage Forms

Solution, Intraocular:

Miostat: 0.01% (1.5 mL)

Solution, Ophthalmic:

Isopto Carbachol: 1.5% (15 mL); 3% (15 mL)

◆ **Carbacholine** *see* Carbachol *on page 346*

◆ **Carbaglu** *see* Carglumic Acid *on page 362*

CarBAMazepine (kar ba MAZ e peen)

Brand Names: U.S. Carbatrol; Epitol; Equetro; TEGretol; TEGretol-XR

Brand Names: Canada Apo-Carbamazepine; Dom-Carbamazepine; Mapezine; Mylan-Carbamazepine CR; Nu-Carbamazepine; PMS-Carbamazepine; Sandoz-Carbamazepine; Taro-Carbamazepine Chewable; Tegretol; Teva-Carbamazepine

Index Terms CBZ; SPD417

Pharmacologic Category Anticonvulsant, Miscellaneous

Additional Appendix Information

Beers Criteria – Potentially Inappropriate Medications for Geriatrics *on page 2271*

Use

Carbatrol, Tegretol, Tegretol-XR: Partial seizures with complex symptomatology (psychomotor, temporal lobe), generalized tonic-clonic seizures (grand mal), mixed seizure patterns, trigeminal neuralgia, glossopharyngeal neuralgia

Equetro: Acute manic or mixed episodes associated with bipolar 1 disorder

Pregnancy Risk Factor D

Pregnancy Considerations Studies in pregnant women have demonstrated a risk to the fetus. Carbamazepine and its metabolites can be found in the fetus and may be associated with teratogenic effects, including spina bifida, craniofacial defects, cardiovascular malformations, and hypospadias. The risk of teratogenic effects is higher with anticonvulsant polytherapy than monotherapy. Developmental delays have also been observed following *in utero* exposure to carbamazepine (per manufacturer); however, socioeconomic factors, maternal and paternal IQ, and polytherapy may contribute to these findings. Pregnancy may cause small decreases of carbamazepine plasma concentrations in the second and third trimesters; monitoring should be considered. When used for the treatment of bipolar disorder, use of carbamazepine should be avoided during the first trimester of pregnancy if possible. The use of a single medication for the treatment of bipolar disorder or epilepsy in pregnancy is preferred. Carbamazepine may decrease plasma concentrations of hormonal contraceptives; breakthrough bleeding or unintended pregnancy may occur and alternate or back-up methods of contraception should be considered.

Patients exposed to carbamazepine during pregnancy are encouraged to enroll themselves into the AED Pregnancy Registry by calling 1-888-233-2334. Additional information is available at www.aedpregnancyregistry.org.

Breast-Feeding Considerations Carbamazepine and its active epoxide metabolite are found in breast milk. Carbamazepine can also be detected in the serum of nursing infants. Transient hepatic dysfunction has been observed in some case reports. Nursing should be discontinued if adverse events are observed. According to the manufacturer, the decision to continue or discontinue breast-feeding during therapy should take into account the risk of exposure to the infant and the benefits of treatment to the mother. Respiratory depression, seizures, nausea, vomiting, diarrhea, and/or decreased feeding have been observed in neonates exposed to carbamazepine *in utero* and may represent a neonatal withdrawal syndrome.

Contraindications Hypersensitivity to carbamazepine, tricyclic antidepressants, or any component of the formulation; bone marrow depression; with or within 14 days of MAO inhibitor use; concurrent use of nefazodone; concomitant use of delavirdine or other non-nucleoside reverse transcriptase inhibitors

Warnings/Precautions Hazardous agent - use appropriate precautions for handling and disposal (NIOSH 2014 [group 2]).

[U.S. Boxed Warning]: The risk of developing aplastic anemia or agranulocytosis is increased during treatment. Monitor CBC, platelets, and differential prior to and during therapy; discontinue if significant bone marrow suppression occurs. A spectrum of hematologic effects has been reported with use (eg, agranulocytosis, aplastic anemia, neutropenia, leukopenia, thrombocytopenia, pancytopenia, and anemias); patients with a previous history of adverse hematologic reaction to any drug may be at increased risk. Early detection of hematologic change is important; advise patients of early signs and symptoms including fever, sore throat, mouth ulcers, infections, easy bruising, and petechial or purpuric hemorrhage.

[U.S. Boxed Warning]: Severe and sometimes fatal dermatologic reactions, including toxic epidermal necrolysis (TENS) and Stevens-Johnson syndrome (SJS), may occur during therapy. The risk is increased in patients with the variant *HLA-B*1502* allele, found almost exclusively in patients of Asian ancestry. Patients of Asian descent should be screened prior to initiating therapy. Avoid use in patients testing positive for the allele; discontinue therapy in patients who have a serious dermatologic reaction. The risk of SJS or TENS may also be increased if carbamazepine is used in combination with other antiepileptic drugs associated with these reactions. Presence of the *HLA-B*1502* allele has not been found to predict the risk of less serious dermatologic reactions such as anticonvulsant hypersensitivity syndrome or nonserious rash. The risk of developing a hypersensitivity reaction may be increased in patients with the variant *HLA-A*3101* allele. These hypersensitivity reactions include SJS/TEN, maculopapular eruptions, and drug reaction with eosinophilia and systemic symptoms (DRESS/multiorgan hypersensitivity). The *HLA-A*3101* allele may occur more frequently patients of African-American, Arabic, Asian, European, Indian, Latin American, and Native American ancestry. Hypersensitivity has also been reported in patients experiencing reactions to other anticonvulsants; the history of hypersensitivity reactions in the patient or their immediate family members should be reviewed. Approximately 25% to 30% of patients allergic to carbamazepine will also have reactions with oxcarbazepine. Potentially serious, sometimes fatal multiorgan hypersensitivity reactions (also known as drug reaction with eosinophilia and systemic symptoms [DRESS]) have been reported with some antiepileptic drugs including carbamazepine; monitor for signs and symptoms of possible disparate manifestations associated with lymphatic, hepatic, renal, and/or hematologic organ systems; gradual discontinuation and conversion to alternate therapy may be required.

Antiepileptics are associated with an increased risk of suicidal behavior/thoughts with use (regardless of indication); patients should be monitored for signs/symptoms of depression, suicidal tendencies, and other unusual behavior changes during therapy and instructed to inform their healthcare provider immediately if symptoms occur.

Administer carbamazepine with caution to patients with history of cardiac damage, ECG abnormalities (or at risk for ECG abnormalities), hepatic or renal disease. Rare cases of a hepatic failure and vanishing bile duct syndrome involving destruction and disappearance of the intrahepatic bile ducts have been reported. Clinical courses of vanishing bile duct syndrome have been variable ranging from fulminant to indolent. Some cases have also had features associated with other immunoallergenic syndromes such as multiorgan hypersensitivity (DRESS syndrome) and serious dermatologic reactions including Stevens-Johnson syndrome. May activate latent psychosis and/or cause confusion or agitation; elderly patients may be at an increased risk for psychiatric effects.

Carbamazepine is not effective in absence, myoclonic, or akinetic seizures; exacerbation of certain seizure types have been seen after initiation of carbamazepine therapy in children with mixed seizure disorders. Abrupt discontinuation is not recommended in patients being treated for seizures. Dizziness or drowsiness may occur; caution should be used when performing tasks which require alertness until the effects are known. Potentially significant interactions may exist, requiring dose or frequency adjustment, additional monitoring, and/or selection of alternative therapy. Carbamazepine has mild anticholinergic activity; use with caution in patients with increased intraocular pressure, or sensitivity to anticholinergic effects. Hyponatremia caused by the syndrome of inappropriate antidiuretic hormone secretion (SIADH) may occur during therapy. Risk may be increased in the elderly or in patients also taking diuretics and may be dose-dependent. Use caution in elderly patients; may cause or exacerbate syndrome of inappropriate antidiuretic hormone secretion or hyponatremia; monitor sodium closely with initiation or dosage adjustments in older adults (Beers Criteria).

Administration of the suspension will yield higher peak and lower trough serum levels than an equal dose of the tablet form; consider a lower starting dose given more frequently (same total daily dose) when using the suspension. The suspension may contain sorbitol; avoid use in patents with hereditary fructose intolerance.

Adverse Reactions

Cardiovascular: Aggravation of coronary artery disease, atrioventricular block, cardiac arrhythmia, cardiac failure, edema, hypertension, hypotension, syncope, thromboembolism, thrombophlebitis

Central nervous system: Abnormality in thinking, agitation, amnesia, ataxia, chills, confusion, depression, dizziness, drowsiness, fatigue, hallucinations, headache, hyperacusis, neuroleptic malignant syndrome (NMS), paresthesia, peripheral neuritis, slurred speech, speech disturbance, talkativeness, twitching, vertigo

Dermatologic: Acute generalized exanthematous pustulosis, alopecia, diaphoresis, dyschromia, erythema multiforme, erythema nodosum, exfoliative dermatitis, onychomadesis, pruritus, skin photosensitivity, skin rash, Stevens-Johnson syndrome, toxic epidermal necrolysis, urticaria

Endocrine & metabolic: Abnormal thyroid function test, albuminuria, glycosuria, hypocalcemia, hyponatremia, porphyria, SIADH

Gastrointestinal: Abdominal pain, anorexia, constipation, diarrhea, gastric distress, glossitis, nausea, pancreatitis, stomatitis, vanishing bile duct syndrome, vomiting, xerostomia

Genitourinary: Azotemia, impotence, oliguria, urinary frequency, urinary retention

Hematologic & oncologic: Agranulocytosis, anemia, aplastic anemia, bone marrow depression, eosinophilia, leukocytosis, leukopenia, lymphadenopathy, pancytopenia, purpura, thrombocytopenia

Hepatic: Abnormal hepatic function tests, hepatic failure, hepatitis, jaundice

Hypersensitivity: Hypersensitivity reaction, multi-organ hypersensitivity

Neuromuscular & skeletal: Arthralgia, exacerbation of systemic lupus erythematosus, leg cramps, myalgia, osteoporosis, tremor, weakness

Ophthalmic: Blurred vision, cataract, conjunctivitis, diplopia, increased intraocular pressure, nystagmus, oculomotor disturbances

Otic: Tinnitus

Renal: Increased blood urea nitrogen, renal failure

Respiratory: Dry throat, pneumonia

Miscellaneous: Fever

Rare but important or life-threatening: Aseptic meningitis, defective spermatogenesis, hirsutism, lupus-like syndrome, maculopapular rash, paralysis, reduced fertility (male), suicidal ideation

Drug Interactions

Metabolism/Transport Effects Substrate of CYP2C8 (minor), CYP3A4 (major); **Note:** Assignment of Major/Minor substrate status based on clinically relevant drug interaction potential; **Induces** CYP1A2 (strong), CYP2B6 (strong), CYP2C19 (strong), CYP2C8 (strong), CYP2C9 (strong), CYP3A4 (strong), P-glycoprotein

Avoid Concomitant Use

Avoid concomitant use of CarBAMazepine with any of the following: Abiraterone Acetate; Apixaban; Apremilast; Artemether; Axitinib; Azelastine (Nasal); Bedaquiline; Boceprevir; Bortezomib; Bosutinib; Cabozantinib; Ceritinib; CloZAPine; Conivaptan; Crizotinib; Dabigatran Etexilate; Dasabuvir; Dienogest; Dipyrone; Dolutegravir; Dronedarone; Eliglustat; Enzalutamide; Everolimus; Fusidic Acid (Systemic); Ibrutinib; Idelalisib; Irinotecan; Itraconazole; Ivacaftor; Lapatinib; Ledipasvir; Lumefantrine; Lurasidone; Macitentan; MAO Inhibitors; Mifepristone; Naloxegol; Nefazodone; Netupitant; NIFEdipine; Nilotinib; Nintedanib; Nisoldipine; Olaparib; Ombitasvir; Orphenadrine; Paraldehyde; Paritaprevir; PAZOPanib; Pirfenidone; Pomalidomide; PONATinib; Praziquantel; Ranolazine; Regorafenib; Reverse Transcriptase Inhibitors (Non-Nucleoside); Rivaroxaban; Roflumilast; RomiDEPsin; Simeprevir; Sofosbuvir; SORAfenib; Stiripentol;

Suvorexant; Tasimelteon; Telaprevir; Thalidomide; Ticagrelor; Tofacitinib; Tolvaptan; Toremifene; Trabectedin; TraMADol; Ulipristal; Vandetanib; Vemurafenib; VinCRIStine (Liposomal); Vorapaxar; Voriconazole

Increased Effect/Toxicity

CarBAMazepine may increase the levels/effects of: Adenosine; Alcohol (Ethyl); Azelastine (Nasal); Buprenorphine; Clarithromycin; ClomiPRAMINE; CloZAPine; CNS Depressants; Desmopressin; Eslicarbazepine; Fosphenytoin; Hydrocodone; Lacosamide; Lithium; MAO Inhibitors; Methotrimeprazine; Metyrosine; Orphenadrine; Paraldehyde; Phenytoin; Pramipexole; Rotigotine; Thalidomide

The levels/effects of CarBAMazepine may be increased by: Allopurinol; Brimonidine (Topical); Calcium Channel Blockers (Nondihydropyridine); Cannabis; Carbonic Anhydrase Inhibitors; Cimetidine; Ciprofloxacin (Systemic); Clarithromycin; Conivaptan; CYP3A4 Inhibitors (Moderate); CYP3A4 Inhibitors (Strong); Danazol; Darunavir; Dipyrone; Doxylamine; Dronabinol; Droperidol; Fluconazole; Fusidic Acid (Systemic); Grapefruit Juice; HydrOXYzine; Idelalisib; Isoniazid; Kava Kava; LamoTRIgine; Loxapine; Luliconazole; Macrolide Antibiotics; Magnesium Sulfate; Methotrimeprazine; Nabilone; Nefazodone; Protease Inhibitors; QUEtiapine; QuiNINE; Selective Serotonin Reuptake Inhibitors; Sodium Oxybate; Stiripentol; Tapentadol; Telaprevir; Tetrahydrocannabinol; Thiazide Diuretics; TraMADol; Valproic Acid and Derivatives; Zolpidem

Decreased Effect

CarBAMazepine may decrease the levels/effects of: Abiraterone Acetate; Acetaminophen; Afatinib; Albendazole; Apixaban; Apremilast; ARIPiprazole; Artemether; Axitinib; Bazedoxifene; Bedaquiline; Bendamustine; Boceprevir; Bortezomib; Bosutinib; Brentuximab Vedotin; Cabozantinib; Calcium Channel Blockers (Dihydropyridine); Calcium Channel Blockers (Nondihydropyridine); Canagliflozin; Cannabidiol; Cannabis; Caspofungin; Ceritinib; Clarithromycin; CloZAPine; Cobicistat; Contraceptives (Estrogens); Contraceptives (Progestins); Crizotinib; CycloSPORINE (Systemic); CYP1A2 Substrates; CYP2B6 Substrates; CYP2C19 Substrates; CYP2C8 Substrates; CYP2C9 Substrates; CYP3A4 Substrates; Dabigatran Etexilate; Dasabuvir; Dasatinib; Diclofenac (Systemic); Dienogest; Dolutegravir; DOXOrubicin (Conventional); Doxycycline; Dronabinol; Dronedarone; Eliglustat; Elvitegravir; Enzalutamide; Erlotinib; Eslicarbazepine; Everolimus; Exemestane; Ezogabine; Felbamate; FentaNYL; Fingolimod; Flunarizine; Fosphenytoin; Gefitinib; GuanFACINE; Haloperidol; Ibrutinib; Idelalisib; Imatinib; Irinotecan; Itraconazole; Ivacaftor; Ixabepilone; Lacosamide; LamoTRIgine; Lapatinib; Ledipasvir; Linagliptin; Lopinavir; Lumefantrine; Lurasidone; Macitentan; Maraviroc; Mebendazole; Methadone; MethylPREDNISolone; Mianserin; Mifepristone; Naloxegol; Nefazodone; Netupitant; NIFEdipine; Nilotinib; Nintedanib; Nisoldipine; Olaparib; Ombitasvir; OXcarbazepine; Paliperidone; Paritaprevir; PAZOPanib; Perampanel; P-glycoprotein/ABCB1 Substrates; Phenytoin; Pirfenidone; Pomalidomide; PONATinib; Praziquantel; Protease Inhibitors; QUEtiapine; QuiNINE; Ranolazine; Regorafenib; Reverse Transcriptase Inhibitors (Non-Nucleoside); RisperiDONE; Rivaroxaban; Roflumilast; RomiDEPsin; Rufinamide; Saxagliptin; Selective Serotonin Reuptake Inhibitors; Simeprevir; Sofosbuvir; SORAfenib; SUNItinib; Suvorexant; Tadalafil; Tasimelteon; Telaprevir; Temsirolimus; Tetrahydrocannabinol; Theophylline Derivatives; Thyroid Products; Ticagrelor; Tofacitinib; Tolvaptan; Topiramate; Toremifene; Trabectedin; TraMADol; Treprostinil; Tricyclic Antidepressants; Ulipristal; Valproic Acid and Derivatives; Vandetanib; Vecuronium; Vemurafenib; Vilazodone; VinCRIStine (Liposomal); Vitamin K Antagonists; Vorapaxar; Voriconazole; Vortioxetine; Ziprasidone; Zolpidem; Zuclopenthixol

The levels/effects of CarBAMazepine may be decreased by: Bosentan; CYP3A4 Inducers (Moderate); CYP3A4 Inducers (Strong); Dabrafenib; Deferasirox; Felbamate; Fosphenytoin; Mefloquine; Methylfolate; Mianserin; Mitotane; Orlistat; Phenytoin; Reverse Transcriptase Inhibitors (Non-Nucleoside); Rufinamide; Siltuximab; St Johns Wort; Theophylline Derivatives; Tocilizumab; TraMADol

Food Interactions Carbamazepine serum levels may be increased if taken with food and/or grapefruit juice. Management: Avoid concurrent ingestion of grapefruit juice. Maintain adequate hydration, unless instructed to restrict fluid intake.

Storage/Stability

Carbatrol®, Equetro®: Store at controlled room temperature (25°C [77°F]); excursions permitted to 15°C to 30°C (59°F to 86°F); protect from light and moisture.

Tegretol®-XR: Store at controlled room temperature, 15°C to 30°C (59°F to 86°F); protect from moisture.

Tegretol® tablets and chewable tablets: Store at ≤30°C (86°F); protect from light and moisture.

Tegretol® suspension: Store at ≤30°C (86°F); shake well before using.

Mechanism of Action In addition to anticonvulsant effects, carbamazepine has anticholinergic, antineuralgic, antidiuretic, muscle relaxant, antimanic, antidepressive, and antiarrhythmic properties; may depress activity in the nucleus ventralis of the thalamus or decrease synaptic transmission or decrease summation of temporal stimulation leading to neural discharge by limiting influx of sodium ions across cell membrane or other unknown mechanisms; stimulates the release of ADH and potentiates its action in promoting reabsorption of water; chemically related to tricyclic antidepressants

Pharmacodynamics/Kinetics

Absorption: Slow

Distribution: V_d: Neonates: 1.5 L/kg; Children: 1.9 L/kg; Adults: 0.59-2 L/kg

Protein binding: Carbamazepine: 75% to 90%, may be decreased in newborns; Epoxide metabolite: 50%

Metabolism: Hepatic via CYP3A4 to active epoxide metabolite; induces hepatic enzymes to increase metabolism

Bioavailability: 85%

Half-life elimination: **Note:** Half-life is variable because of autoinduction which is usually complete 3-5 weeks after initiation of a fixed carbamazepine regimen.

- Carbamazepine: Initial: 25-65 hours; Extended release: 35-40 hours; Multiple doses: Children: 8-14 hours; Adults: 12-17 hours
- Epoxide metabolite: Initial: 25-43 hours

Time to peak, serum: Unpredictable:

- Immediate release: Suspension: 1.5 hour; tablet: 4-5 hours
- Extended release: Carbatrol®, Equetro®: 12-26 hours (single dose), 4-8 hours (multiple doses); Tegretol®-XR: 3-12 hours

Excretion: Urine 72% (1% to 3% as unchanged drug); feces (28%)

Dosage Dosage must be adjusted according to patient's response and serum concentrations. Administer tablets (chewable or conventional) in 2-3 divided doses daily and suspension in 4 divided doses daily. Oral:

Epilepsy:

Children:

- <6 years: Initial: 10-20 mg/kg/day divided twice or 3 times daily as tablets or 4 times/day as suspension; increase dose every week until optimal response and therapeutic levels are achieved
  - Maintenance dose: Divide into 3-4 doses daily (tablets or suspension); maximum recommended dose: 35 mg/kg/day

6-12 years: Initial: 200 mg/day in 2 divided doses (tablets or extended release tablets) or 4 divided doses (oral suspension); increase by up to 100 mg/day at weekly intervals using a twice daily regimen of extended release tablets or 3-4 times daily regimen of other formulations until optimal response and therapeutic levels are achieved

Maintenance: Usual: 400-800 mg/day; maximum recommended dose: 1000 mg/day

Note: Children <12 years who receive ≥400 mg/day of carbamazepine may be converted to extended release capsules (Carbatrol®) using the same total daily dosage divided twice daily

Children >12 years and Adults: Initial: 400 mg/day in 2 divided doses (tablets or extended release tablets) or 4 divided doses (oral suspension); increase by up to 200 mg/day at weekly intervals using a twice daily regimen of extended release tablets or capsules, or a 3-4 times/day regimen of other formulations until optimal response and therapeutic levels are achieved; usual dose: 800-1200 mg/day

Maximum recommended doses:

Children 12-15 years: 1000 mg/day

Children >15 years: 1200 mg/day

Adults: 1600 mg/day; however, some patients have required up to 1.6-2.4 g/day

Trigeminal or glossopharyngeal neuralgia: Adults: Initial: 200 mg/day in 2 divided doses (tablets, extended release tablets, or extended release capsules) or 4 divided doses (oral suspension) with food, gradually increasing in increments of 200 mg/day as needed

Maintenance: Usual: 400-800 mg daily in 2 divided doses (tablets, extended release tablets, or extended release capsules) or 4 divided doses (oral suspension); maximum dose: 1200 mg/day

Bipolar disorder: Adults: Initial: 400 mg/day in 2 divided doses (tablets, extended release tablets, or extended release capsules) or 4 divided doses (oral suspension), may adjust by 200 mg/day increments; maximum dose: 1600 mg/day.

Note: Equetro® is the only formulation specifically approved by the FDA for the management of bipolar disorder.

Neuropathic pain, critically-ill patients (off-label use): Initial: 50-100 mg twice daily in combination with IV opioids; Maintenance: 100-200 mg every 4-6 hours; maximum dose: 1200 mg daily (Barr, 2013)

Dosing adjustment in renal impairment: Dosage adjustments are not required or recommended in the manufacturer's labeling; however, the following guidelines have been used by some clinicians (Aronoff, 2007):

Children and Adults:

GFR <10 mL/minute: Administer 75% of dose

Hemodialysis, peritoneal dialysis: Administer 75% of dose (postdialysis)

Continuous renal replacement therapy (CRRT):

Children: Administer 75% of dose

Adults: No dosage adjustment recommended

Dosing adjustment in hepatic impairment: Use with caution in hepatic impairment; metabolized primarily in the liver

Dietary Considerations Drug may cause GI upset, take with large amount of water or food to decrease GI upset. May need to split doses to avoid GI upset.

Administration

Suspension: Must be given on a 3-4 times/day schedule versus tablets which can be given 2-4 times/day. Since a given dose of suspension will produce higher peak and lower trough levels than the same dose given as the tablet form, patients given the suspension should be started on lower doses given more frequently (same total daily dose) and increased slowly to avoid unwanted side effects. When carbamazepine suspension has been combined with chlorpromazine or thioridazine solutions, a precipitate forms which may result in loss of effect. Therefore, it is recommended that the carbamazepine suspension dosage form not be administered at the same time with other liquid medicinal agents or diluents. Should be administered with meals.

Extended release capsule (Carbatrol®, Equetro®): Consists of three different types of beads: Immediate release, extended-release, and enteric release. The bead types are combined in a ratio to allow twice daily dosing. May be opened and contents sprinkled over food such as a teaspoon of applesauce; may be administered with or without food; do not crush or chew.

Extended release tablet: Should be inspected for damage. Damaged extended release tablets (without release portal) should not be administered. Should be administered with meals; swallow whole, do not crush or chew.

Hazardous agent; use appropriate precautions for handling and disposal (NIOSH 2014 [group 2]).

Monitoring Parameters CBC with platelet count and differential, reticulocytes, serum iron, lipid panel, liver function tests, urinalysis, BUN, serum carbamazepine levels, thyroid function tests, serum sodium; pregnancy test; ophthalmic exams (intraocular pressure, pupillary reflexes); observe patient for excessive sedation, especially when instituting or increasing therapy; signs of rash; *HLA-B*1502* genotype screening prior to therapy initiation in patients of Asian descent; suicidality (eg, suicidal thoughts, depression, behavioral changes)

Reference Range

Timing of serum samples: Absorption is slow, peak levels occur 8-65 hours after ingestion of the first dose; the half-life ranges from 8-60 hours, therefore, steady-state is achieved in 2-5 days

Epilepsy: Therapeutic levels: 4-12 mcg/mL (SI: 17-51 micromole/L)

Toxic concentration: >15 mcg/mL; patients who require higher levels of 8-12 mcg/mL (SI: 34-51 micromole/L) should be watched closely. Side effects including CNS effects occur commonly at higher dosage levels. If other anticonvulsants are given therapeutic range is 4-8 mcg/mL.

Dosage Forms

Capsule Extended Release 12 Hour, Oral:

Carbatrol: 100 mg, 200 mg, 300 mg

Equetro: 100 mg, 200 mg, 300 mg

Generic: 100 mg, 200 mg, 300 mg

Suspension, Oral:

TEGretol: 100 mg/5 mL (450 mL)

Generic: 100 mg/5 mL (450 mL)

Tablet, Oral:

Epitol: 200 mg

TEGretol: 200 mg

Generic: 200 mg

Tablet Chewable, Oral:

Generic: 100 mg

Tablet Extended Release 12 Hour, Oral:

TEGretol-XR: 100 mg, 200 mg, 400 mg

Generic: 200 mg, 400 mg

Extemporaneous Preparations Hazardous agent: Use appropriate precautions for handling and disposal (NIOSH 2014 [group 2]).

Note: Commercial oral suspension is available (20 mg/mL)

A 40 mg/mL oral suspension may be made with tablets. Crush twenty 200 mg tablets in a mortar and reduce to a fine powder. Add small portions of Simple Syrup, NF and mix to a uniform paste; mix while adding the vehicle in incremental proportions to **almost** 100 mL; transfer to a calibrated bottle, rinse mortar with vehicle, and add sufficient quantity of vehicle to make 100 mL. Label "shake well" and "refrigerate". Stable for 90 days.

Nahata MC, Pai VB, and Hipple TF, *Pediatric Drug Formulations*, 5th ed, Cincinnati, OH: Harvey Whitney Books Co, 2004.

- ◆ **Carbamide** *see* Urea *on page* 2114

Carbamide Peroxide (KAR ba mide per OKS ide)

Brand Names: U.S. Auraphene-B [OTC]; Debrox [OTC]; E-R-O Ear Drops [OTC]; E-R-O Ear Wax Removal System [OTC]; Ear Drops Earwax Aid [OTC]; Ear Wax Remover [OTC] [DSC]; Earwax Treatment Drops [OTC]; Gly-Oxide [OTC]; Thera-Ear [OTC]

Index Terms Urea Peroxide

Pharmacologic Category Anti-inflammatory, Locally Applied; Otic Agent, Cerumenolytic

Use Relief of minor inflammation of gums, oral mucosal surfaces, and lips including canker sores and dental irritation; emulsify and disperse ear wax

Dosage Children and Adults:

Oral: Inflammation/dental irritation: Solution (should not be used for >7 days): Oral preparation should not be used in children <2 years of age; apply several drops undiluted on affected area 4 times/day after meals and at bedtime; expectorate after 2-3 minutes **or** place 10 drops onto tongue, mix with saliva, swish for several minutes, expectorate

Otic:

Children <12 years: Tilt head sideways and individualize the dose according to patient size; 3 drops (range: 1-5 drops) twice daily for up to 4 days, tip of applicator should not enter ear canal; keep drops in ear for several minutes by keeping head tilted and placing cotton in ear

Children ≥12 years and Adults: Tilt head sideways and instill 5-10 drops twice daily up to 4 days, tip of applicator should not enter ear canal; keep drops in ear for several minutes by keeping head tilted and placing cotton in ear

Additional Information Complete prescribing information should be consulted for additional detail.

Dosage Forms

Solution, Mouth/Throat:

Gly-Oxide [OTC]: 10% (15 mL, 60 mL)

Solution, Otic:

Auraphene-B [OTC]: 6.5% (15 mL)
Debrox [OTC]: 6.5% (15 mL)
E-R-O Ear Drops [OTC]: 6.5% (15 mL)
E-R-O Ear Wax Removal System [OTC]: 6.5% (15 mL)
Ear Drops Earwax Aid [OTC]: 6.5% (15 mL)
Earwax Treatment Drops [OTC]: 6.5% (15 mL)
Thera-Ear [OTC]: 6.5% (15 mL)

- ◆ **Carbamylcholine Chloride** *see* Carbachol *on page* 346
- ◆ **Carbatrol** *see* CarBAMazepine *on page* 346

Carbenoxolone [INT] (kar ben OKS oh lone)

International Brand Names Bioplex (GB); Bioral (AU, GB); Carbosan (IE); Herpesan (HK, MY, SG); Rowadermat (AT); Sanodin (ES)

Index Terms Carbenoxolone Sodium

Pharmacologic Category Gastrointestinal Agent, Miscellaneous

Reported Use Treatment of esophageal inflammation and ulceration

Dosage Range Adults: Oral: One chewable tablet 3 times/day after meals and 2 tablets at bedtime for 6-12 weeks

Product Availability Product available in various countries; not currently available in the U.S.

Dosage Forms

Tablet, chewable: 20 mg [contains alginic acid 600 mg, aluminum hydroxide 240 mg, magnesium trisilicate 60 mg, and sodium bicarbonate 210 mg]

- ◆ **Carbenoxolone Sodium** *see* Carbenoxolone [INT] *on page* 350

Carbetocin [CAN/INT] (kar BE toe sin)

Brand Names: Canada Duratocin™

Pharmacologic Category Oxytocic Agent

Use Note: Not approved in U.S.

Prevention of uterine atony and postpartum hemorrhage following elective cesarean section under anesthesia (epidural or spinal)

Pregnancy Considerations Use in pregnancy prior to delivery is contraindicated. Carbetocin induced contractions are of a longer duration than those observed with oxytocin and are not stopped by discontinuation of therapy. Improper use during pregnancy may produce symptoms similar to those observed with oxytocin overdosage (eg, hyperstimulation of uterus, uterine rupture).

Breast-Feeding Considerations Small amounts of carbetocin were detected in the breast milk of 5 healthy nursing women approximately 7-14 weeks postpartum though peak levels observed were 50 times lower than in plasma. Exposure to the breast-feeding infant is expected to be minimal and not expected to pose significant health risks as carbetocin in breast milk is rapidly degraded in the GI tract of a nursing infant. Ability of carbetocin to stimulate breast milk ejection (milk letdown) has not been determined.

Contraindications Hypersensitivity to carbetocin, oxytocin, or any component of the formulation; administration prior to delivery of infant for any reason (including elective or medical induction of labor); vascular disease; use in children

Warnings/Precautions Use in pregnancy prior to delivery is contraindicated. Carbetocin induced contractions are of a longer duration than those observed with oxytocin and are not stopped by discontinuation of therapy. Improper use during pregnancy may produce symptoms similar to those observed with oxytocin overdosage (eg, hyperstimulation of uterus, uterine rupture). Therapy should not be repeated if response to initial dose is inadequate; aggressive therapy with alternative agents (eg, oxytocin, ergonovine) should be utilized.

Persistent bleeding warrants further evaluation to rule out coagulopathy, genital tract trauma, or the presence of retained placental fragments. Use has not been studied in patients with significant heart disease, hypertension, or history of coagulopathy. Use in patients with vascular disease (especially coronary artery disease) should be avoided or employed with extreme caution. Use in endocrine (excluding gestational diabetes), hepatic, and/or renal disease has not been studied. Use in elderly women is not recommended. Use in children is contraindicated.

Adverse Reactions

Cardiovascular: Chest pain, flushing, hypotension, tachycardia

Central nervous system: Anxiety, chills, dizziness, headache

Dermatologic: Pruritus

Gastrointestinal: Abdominal pain, metallic taste, nausea, vomiting

Hematologic: Anemia
Neuromuscular & skeletal: Back pain, tremor
Respiratory: Dyspnea
Miscellaneous: Diaphoresis, feeling of warmth

Drug Interactions

Metabolism/Transport Effects None known.

Avoid Concomitant Use

Avoid concomitant use of Carbetocin with any of the following: Carboprost Tromethamine; Dinoprostone; Misoprostol

Increased Effect/Toxicity

The levels/effects of Carbetocin may be increased by: Carboprost Tromethamine; Dinoprostone; Misoprostol

Decreased Effect There are no known significant interactions involving a decrease in effect.

Storage/Stability Store under refrigeration at 2°C to 8°C (36°F to 46°F); do not freeze. Use immediately after opening.

Mechanism of Action Binds oxytocin receptors located in uterine smooth muscle producing rhythmic uterine contractions characteristic to deliver, as well as increasing both the frequency of existing contractions and uterine tone. Enhances uterine involution early in postpartum.

Pharmacodynamics/Kinetics

Onset of action: ~2 minutes
Duration: ~60 minutes
Half-life elimination: ~29-53 minutes
Excretion: Urine (<1%, as unchanged drug)

Dosage IV: Adults: Prevention of uterine atony and postpartum bleeding: 100 mcg (single dose only)

Dosage adjustment in renal impairment: No dosage adjustment provided in manufacturer's labeling (has not been studied).

Dosage adjustment in hepatic impairment: No dosage adjustment provided in manufacturer's labeling (has not been studied).

Administration Administer as bolus IV injection over 1 minute only after delivery of infant has been completed by cesarean section. May administer before or after delivery of placenta.

Monitoring Parameters Persistent postpartum bleeding; blood pressure

Product Availability Not available in U.S.

Dosage Forms: Canada

Injection, solution:

Duratocin™: 100 mcg/mL (1 mL)

Carbidopa (kar bi DOE pa)

Brand Names: U.S. Lodosyn

Pharmacologic Category Anti-Parkinson's Agent, Decarboxylase Inhibitor

Use Given with carbidopa-levodopa in the treatment of parkinsonism to enable a lower dosage of levodopa to be used and a more rapid response to be obtained and to decrease side effects; use with carbidopa-levodopa in patients requiring additional carbidopa; has no effect without levodopa

Pregnancy Risk Factor C

Dosage Oral: Adults: **Note:** Optimal daily dosage determined by careful titration; generally if carbidopa is ≥70 mg/day, a 1:10 proportion of carbidopa:levodopa provides the most patient response.

Carbidopa augmentation in patients receiving carbidopa-levodopa:

Patients receiving Sinemet® 10/100: 25 mg carbidopa daily with first daily dose of Sinemet® 10/100; if necessary, 12.5-25 mg carbidopa may be given with each subsequent dose of Sinemet® 10/100; maximum: 200 mg carbidopa/day (including carbidopa from Sinemet®)

Patients receiving Sinemet® 25/250 or Sinemet® 25/100: 25 mg carbidopa with any dose of Sinemet® 25/250 or Sinemet® 25/100 throughout the day; maximum: 200 mg carbidopa/day (including carbidopa from Sinemet®)

Individual titration of carbidopa and levodopa: Initial: 25 mg carbidopa 3-4 times/day; administer at the same time as levodopa, initial dose of levodopa should be 20% to 25% of the previous levodopa dose in carbidopa-naive patients; first dose of carbidopa should be taken ≥12 hours after the last dose of levodopa in carbidopa-naive patients; increase or decrease dose by 1/2 or 1 tablet/day

Additional Information Complete prescribing information should be consulted for additional detail.

Dosage Forms

Tablet, Oral:

Lodosyn: 25 mg
Generic: 25 mg

Carbidopa and Levodopa

(kar bi DOE pa & lee voe DOE pa)

Brand Names: U.S. Parcopa [DSC]; Rytary; Sinemet; Sinemet CR

Brand Names: Canada Apo-Levocarb; Apo-Levocarb CR; Dom-Levo-Carbidopa; Duodopa; Levocarb CR; PMS-Levocarb CR; PRO-Levocarb; Sinemet; Sinemet CR; Teva-Levocarbidopa

Index Terms Duopa; Levodopa and Carbidopa; Rytary

Pharmacologic Category Anti-Parkinson's Agent, Decarboxylase Inhibitor; Anti-Parkinson's Agent, Dopamine Precursor

Additional Appendix Information

Oral Dosages That Should Not Be Crushed *on page 2276*

Use Parkinson disease: Treatment of Parkinson disease, postencephalitic parkinsonism, and symptomatic parkinsonism that may follow carbon monoxide and/or manganese intoxication; treatment of motor fluctuations in advanced Parkinson disease (intestinal suspension [Duopa] only).

Pregnancy Risk Factor C

Pregnancy Considerations Adverse events have been observed in some animal reproduction studies using this combination. Carbidopa can be detected in the umbilical cord, but absorption in fetal tissue is minimal. Levodopa crosses the placenta and can be metabolized by the fetus and detected in fetal tissue (Merchant, 1995). The incidence of Parkinson disease in pregnancy is relatively rare, and information related to the use of carbidopa/levodopa in pregnant women is limited (Ball, 1995; Cook, 1985; Golbe, 1987; Serikawa, 2011; Shulman, 2000). Current guidelines note that the available information is insufficient to make a recommendation for the treatment of restless legs syndrome in pregnant women (Aurora, 2012).

Breast-Feeding Considerations Levodopa is excreted in breast milk. A study was done in one lactating woman at 4.5 months postpartum who had been taking carbidopa/levodopa for several years. Regardless of the formulation (sustained release or immediate release) peak levodopa concentrations in the breast milk were found ~3 hours after the maternal dose and returned to baseline ~6 hours after the dose. The highest milk concentration (3.47 nmol/L) was found following the immediate-release tablet and this was 27% of the peak maternal plasma concentration (occurring 30 minutes after the dose) and ~40% of the simultaneous plasma concentration. Carbidopa was not evaluated (Thulin, 1998). The manufacturer recommends that caution be exercised when administering carbidopa/levodopa to nursing women.

Contraindications

Hypersensitivity to levodopa, carbidopa, or any component of the formulation; concurrent use with nonselective monoamine oxidase inhibitors (MAOIs) or use within the last 14 days

Tablets: Additional contraindications: Narrow angle glaucoma

Canadian labeling: Additional contraindications: Clinical or laboratory evidence of uncompensated cardiovascular, endocrine, hepatic, hematologic or pulmonary disease (eg, including bronchial asthma), or renal disease; when administration of a sympathomimetic amine (eg, epinephrine, norepinephrine, isoproterenol) is contraindicated; in the presence of a suspicious, undiagnosed skin lesion or history of melanoma; intestinal gel therapy in patients with any condition preventing the required placement of a PEG tube for administration (ie, pathological changes of gastric wall, inability to bring gastric and abdominal wall together, blood coagulation disorders, peritonitis, acute pancreatitis, paralytic ileus).

Warnings/Precautions Use with caution in patients with history of cardiovascular disease (including a history of myocardial infarction who have residual atrial, nodal, or ventricular arrhythmias), pulmonary diseases (such as asthma), psychosis, glaucoma, endocrine disease, and in severe renal and hepatic dysfunction. Use oral products with caution in patients with peptic ulcer disease. Use with caution when interpreting plasma/urine catecholamine levels; falsely diagnosed pheochromocytoma has been rarely reported. Dopaminergic agents have been associated with a syndrome resembling neuroleptic malignant syndrome on abrupt withdrawal, rapid dose reduction, significant dosage reduction after long-term use, or changes in dopaminergic therapy. Avoid sudden discontinuation or rapid dose reduction; taper dose to reduce the risk of hyperpyrexia and confusion. Elderly patients may be more sensitive to CNS effects (eg, hallucinations) of levodopa. May cause or exacerbate dyskinesias. May cause orthostatic hypotension; Parkinson disease patients appear to have an impaired capacity to respond to a postural challenge; use with caution in patients at risk of hypotension (such as those receiving antihypertensive drugs) or where transient hypotensive episodes would be poorly tolerated (cardiovascular disease or cerebrovascular disease). Observe patients closely for development of depression with concomitant suicidal tendencies.

Dopamine agonists have been associated with compulsive behaviors and/or loss of impulse control, which has manifested as pathological gambling, increased sexual urges, intense urges to spend money, binge or compulsive eating; and/or other intense urges. Dose reduction or discontinuation of therapy has been reported to reverse these behaviors in some, but not all cases. Risk for melanoma development is increased in Parkinson disease patients; drug causation or factors contributing to risk have not been established. Patients should be monitored closely and periodic skin examinations should be performed. A symptom complex resembling neuroleptic malignant syndrome (NMS) has been reported in association with rapid dose reduction, or abrupt withdrawal. Identification of more severe NMS-like reactions (eg, altered consciousness, hyperthermia, involuntary movements, muscle rigidity, autonomic instability, mental status changes) can be complex; monitor patients closely for this reaction and when the dosage of levodopa is reduced abruptly or discontinued. Discontinue treatment immediately if signs/symptoms arise. Protein in the diet should be distributed throughout the day to avoid fluctuations in levodopa absorption. A high-protein diet may reduce the effectiveness of the enteral formulations. Urine, saliva, or sweat may appear dark in color (red, brown, black) during therapy.

Abnormal thinking and behavior changes have been reported and may include aggressive behavior, agitation, confusion, delirium, delusions, disorientation, paranoid ideation, and psychotic-like behavior. Hallucinations may occur and be accompanied by confusion and to a lesser extent sleep disorder and excessive dreaming; typically presents shortly after initiation of therapy and may require dose reduction. Somnolence and falling asleep while engaged in activities of daily living (including operation of motor vehicles) have been reported; some cases reported that there were no warning signs for the onset of symptoms. Symptom onset may occur well after initiation of treatment; some events have occurred more than 1 year after start of therapy. Prior to treatment initiation, evaluate for factors that may increase these risks such as concomitant sedating medications, and the presence of sleep disorders. Monitor for drowsiness or sleepiness. If significant daytime sleepiness or episodes of falling asleep during activities that require active participation occurs (eg, driving, conversations, eating), discontinue the medication. There is insufficient information to suggest that dose reductions will eliminate these symptoms. Peripheral neuropathy has been reported with use; prior to initiation, evaluate patients for history of neuropathy and known risk factors (eg, deficiency of vitamin B_6 and/or B_{12}, diabetes mellitus, hypothyroidism). Assess patients for peripheral neuropathy periodically during therapy. Potentially significant interactions may exist, requiring dose or frequency adjustment, additional monitoring, and/or selection of alternative therapy.

Intestinal suspension (Duopa): GI complications (eg, bezoar, ileus, implant site erosion/ulcer, intestinal hemorrhage, intestinal ischemia, intestinal obstruction, intestinal perforation, pancreatitis, peritonitis, pneumoperitoneum, postoperative wound infection) may occur (may be fatal). Patients should notify their health care provider immediately if abdominal pain, prolonged constipation, nausea, vomiting, fever, and/or melanotic stool occur.

Intestinal gel (Duodopa [Canadian product]): Product should be prescribed only by neurologists experienced in the treatment of Parkinson disease and who have completed the Duodopa Education Program. Response to levodopa/carbidopa intestinal gel therapy should be assessed with a short term test period of administration via a temporary nasojejunal tube prior to placement of a percutaneous endoscopic gastrostomy-jejunostomy (PEG-J) tube for permanent access and administration. Sudden deterioration in therapy response with recurring motor symptoms may indicate PEG-J tube complications (eg, displacement) or obstruction of the infusion device. Tube or infusion device complications may require initiation of oral levodopa/carbidopa therapy until complications are resolved.

Adverse Reactions

Cardiovascular: Cardiac arrhythmia, chest pain, edema, flushing, hypertension, hypotension, myocardial infarction, orthostatic hypotension, palpitations, phlebitis, syncope

Central nervous system: Abnormal dreams, abnormal gait, agitation, anxiety, ataxia, confusion, decreased mental acuity, delusions, dementia, depression (with or without suicidal tendencies), disorientation, dizziness, drowsiness, euphoria, extrapyramidal reaction, falling, fatigue, glossopyrosis, hallucination, headache, Horner's syndrome (reactivation), impulse control disorder, insomnia, malaise, memory impairment, nervousness, neuroleptic malignant syndrome, nightmares, numbness, on-off phenomenon, paranoia, paresthesia, pathological gambling, peripheral neuropathy, psychosis, seizure (causal relationship not established), trismus

Dermatologic: Alopecia, diaphoresis, discoloration of sweat, skin rash

Endocrine & metabolic: Abnormal alanine aminotransferase, abnormal alkaline phosphatase, abnormal aspartate transaminase, abnormal lactate dehydrogenase, glycosuria, hot flash, hyperglycemia, hypokalemia, increased libido (including hypersexuality), increased uric acid, weight gain, weight loss

Gastrointestinal: Abdominal distress, abdominal pain, anorexia, bruxism, constipation, diarrhea, discoloration of saliva, duodenal ulcer, dysgeusia, dyspepsia, dysphagia, flatulence, gastrointestinal hemorrhage, heartburn, hiccups, nausea, sialorrhea, sore throat, vomiting, xerostomia

Genitourinary: Difficulty in micturition, priapism, proteinuria, urinary frequency, urinary incontinence, urinary retention, urinary tract infection, urine discoloration

Hematologic & oncologic: Agranulocytosis, anemia, decreased hematocrit, decreased hemoglobin, hemolytic anemia, IgA vasculitis, leukopenia, malignant melanoma

Hepatic: Abnormal bilirubin levels

Hypersensitivity: Hypersensitivity reaction (angioedema, pruritus, urticaria, bullous lesions [including pemphigus-like reactions])

Immunologic: Abnormal Coombs' test

Neuromuscular & skeletal: Back pain, dyskinesia (including choreiform, dystonic and other involuntary movements), excessive tremors, leg pain, muscle cramps, muscle twitching, shoulder pain, weakness

Ophthalmic: Blepharospasm, blurred vision, diplopia, mydriasis, oculogyric crisis (may be associated with acute dystonic reactions)

Respiratory: Cough, dyspnea, hoarseness, upper respiratory tract infection

Drug Interactions

Metabolism/Transport Effects None known.

Avoid Concomitant Use

Avoid concomitant use of Carbidopa and Levodopa with any of the following: Amisulpride; Sulpiride

Increased Effect/Toxicity

Carbidopa and Levodopa may increase the levels/effects of: BuPROPion; Droxidopa; MAO Inhibitors

The levels/effects of Carbidopa and Levodopa may be increased by: Hypotensive Agents; Methylphenidate; Papaverine; Sapropterin

Decreased Effect

Carbidopa and Levodopa may decrease the levels/effects of: Amisulpride; Antipsychotic Agents (First Generation [Typical]); Droxidopa; Sulpiride

The levels/effects of Carbidopa and Levodopa may be decreased by: Amisulpride; Antipsychotic Agents (First Generation [Typical]); Antipsychotic Agents (Second Generation [Atypical]); Fosphenytoin; Glycopyrrolate; Iron Salts; Isoniazid; Methionine; Metoclopramide; Multivitamins/Fluoride (with ADE); Multivitamins/Minerals (with ADEK, Folate, Iron); Multivitamins/Minerals (with AE, No Iron); Papaverine; Phenytoin; Pyridoxine; Sulpiride

Food Interactions High protein diets have the potential to impair levodopa absorption; levodopa competes with certain amino acids for transport across the gut wall or across the blood-brain barrier. Management: Avoid high protein diets.

Preparation for Administration Intestinal suspension (Duopa): Fully thaw in refrigerator prior to use. To ensure controlled thawing, take the cartons containing the seven individual cassettes out of the transport box and separate the cartons from each other. Assign a 12-week, use-by date based on the time the cartons are put into the refrigerator to thaw (may take up to 96 hours to thaw). Once thawed, the individual cartons may be packed in a closer configuration within the refrigerator. Remove one cassette from refrigerator 20 minutes prior to administration (failure to use at room temperature may result in inaccurate dosage).

Storage/Stability

Oral formulations: Store at 25°C (77°F); excursions permitted between 15°C to 30°C (59°F to 86°F). Protect from light and moisture.

Intestinal suspension (Duopa): Store in freezer at -20°C (-4°F). Fully thaw in refrigerator at 2°C to 8°C (36°F to 46°F) prior to use; protect from light. To ensure controlled thawing, remove the cartons containing the seven individual cassettes from the transport box and separate the cartons from each other. Assign a 12-week, use-by date based on the time the cartons are put in the refrigerator to thaw (may take up to 96 hours to thaw). Once thawed, the individual cartons may be packed in a closer configuration within the refrigerator. Cassettes are for single use only and should be discarded daily following infusion (up to 16 hours). Do not re-use opened cassettes.

Intestinal gel (Duodopa [Canadian product]): Store in refrigerator at 2°C to 8°C (36°F to 46°F). Keep in outer carton to protect from light. Cassettes are for single use only and should be discarded daily following infusion (up to 16 hours).

Mechanism of Action Parkinson disease symptoms are due to a lack of striatal dopamine; levodopa circulates in the plasma to the blood-brain-barrier (BBB), where it crosses, to be converted by striatal enzymes to dopamine; carbidopa inhibits the peripheral plasma breakdown of levodopa by inhibiting its decarboxylation, and thereby increases available levodopa at the BBB

Pharmacodynamics/Kinetics

Absorption: Absorption of levodopa may be decreased with high-fat, high-calorie or high-protein meal.

Distribution: Levodopa: 0.9 to 1.6 L/kg (in presence of carbidopa), crosses the blood-brain barrier; Carbidopa: Does not cross the blood-brain barrier

Metabolism: Levodopa has two major pathways (decarboxylation and O-methylation) and two minor pathways (transamination and oxidation) of metabolism; Carbidopa inhibits the decarboxylation of levodopa to dopamine in the peripheral tissue to allow greater levodopa distribution into the CNS

Bioavailability:

Controlled and extended release: Levodopa: Bioavailability is ~70% to 75% relative to availability from immediate release formulation; Carbidopa: Bioavailability is ~50% to 58% relative to availability from immediate release formulation

Intestinal gel [Canadian product]: Levodopa: Similar bioavailability relative to oral administration of tablet formulations (81% to 98%)

Intestinal suspension: Levodopa: 97% relative to oral immediate release tablets

Half-life elimination: Immediate release: Levodopa (in presence of carbidopa): 1.5 hours; Half-life may be prolonged with controlled and extended release formulations due to continuous absorption

Time to peak: Immediate release: 0.5 hours; Controlled and extended release: 2 hours; Intestinal gel [Canadian product]: Therapeutic plasma levels reached 10 to 30 minutes following morning bolus dose; Intestinal suspension: 2.5 hours

Excretion: Urine

Dosage

Parkinson disease: Adults:

Oral:

Immediate release tablet, orally disintegrating tablet: **Note:** Carbidopa/levodopa tablets are available in a 1:4 ratio of carbidopa to levodopa as well as 1:10 ratio. Tablets of the two ratios may be given separately or combined as needed to provide the optimum dosage.

Initial: Carbidopa 25 mg/levodopa 100 mg 3 times daily (preferred) or carbidopa 10 mg/levodopa 100 mg 3 to 4 times daily (typically does not provide an adequate amount of carbidopa for most patients)

Patients previously treated with levodopa <1,500 mg daily: Carbidopa 25 mg/levodopa 100 mg 3 or 4 times daily

Patients previously treated with levodopa >1,500 mg daily: Carbidopa 25 mg/levodopa 250 mg 3 or 4 times daily

Note: Discontinue levodopa at least 12 hours before starting therapy with carbidopa/levodopa. Substitute the combination drug at a dosage that will provide approximately 25% (~20% [Canadian labeling]) of the previous levodopa dosage.

Dosage adjustment: Alternate tablet strengths may be substituted according to individual carbidopa/levodopa requirements. Use of more than 1 dosage strength or dosing 4 times daily may be required (maximum: 8 tablets of any strength daily or 200 mg of carbidopa and 2,000 mg of levodopa)

Carbidopa 10 mg/levodopa 100 mg:

U.S. labeling: Increase by 1 tablet daily or every other day, as necessary, to 2 tablets 4 times daily

Canadian labeling: Increase by 1 tablet every 3 days

Carbidopa 25 mg/levodopa 100 mg:

U.S. labeling: Increase by 1 tablet daily or every other day

Canadian labeling: Increase by 1 tablet every 3 days

Carbidopa 25 mg/levodopa 250 mg:

U.S. labeling: Increase by 1/2 or 1 tablet daily or every other day

Canadian labeling: Increase by 1 tablet every day or every other day

Controlled-release tablet:

Patients not currently receiving levodopa: Initial:

U.S. labeling: Carbidopa 50 mg/levodopa 200 mg 2 times daily, at intervals not <6 hours

Canadian labeling: Carbidopa 25 to 50 mg/levodopa 100 to 200 mg 2 times daily, at intervals not <6 hours; initial dosing should not exceed levodopa 600 mg daily

Patients currently receiving levodopa: **Note:** Discontinue levodopa at least 12 hours (at least 8 hours [Canadian labeling]) before starting carbidopa/levodopa therapy. Initial: Substitute at a dosage that will provide approximately 25% of the previous levodopa dosage; usual initial dose in mild to moderate disease is carbidopa 50 mg/levodopa 200 mg 2 times daily

Patients converting from immediate-release formulation to controlled release: Initial: Dosage should be substituted at an amount that provides ~10% more of levodopa/day; total calculated dosage is administered in divided doses 2 to 3 times/day (or ≥3 times/day for patients maintained on levodopa ≥700 mg). Intervals between doses should be 4 to 8 hours while awake; when divided doses are not equal, smaller doses should be given toward the end of the day. Depending on clinical response, dosage may need to be increased to provide up to 30% more levodopa/day.

Dosage adjustment: May adjust every 3 days; intervals should be >4 hours during the waking day (maximum dose: 8 tablets/day)

Extended-release capsule: **Note:** Carbidopa/levodopa extended-release capsules are not interchangeable with other carbidopa/levodopa products.

Patients not currently receiving levodopa: Initial: Carbidopa 23.75 mg/levodopa 950 mg 3 times daily for 3 days; on day 4, increase to carbidopa 36.25 mg/levodopa 145 mg 3 times daily. May increase dose up to carbidopa 97.5 mg//levodopa 390 mg 3 times a day; frequency of dosing may be increased to a maximum of 5 times daily if needed and tolerated (maximum: carbidopa 612.5 mg /levodopa 2,450 mg per day).

Patients converting from immediate-release formulation to extended-release capsules: Initial: Initial dose based off of total current daily dose of levodopa in immediate-release carbidopa/levodopa as follows (frequency of dosing may be increased to a maximum of 5 times daily if needed and tolerated):

If total daily dose of levodopa is between 400 mg to 549 mg: 3 capsules of carbidopa 23.75 mg/levodopa 95 mg 3 times daily (levodopa total daily dose: 855 mg).

If total daily dose of levodopa is between 550 mg to 749 mg: 4 capsules of carbidopa 23.75 mg/levodopa 95 mg 3 times daily (levodopa total daily dose: 1,140 mg).

If total daily dose of levodopa is between 750 mg to 949 mg: 3 capsules of carbidopa 36.25 mg/levodopa 145 mg 3 times daily (levodopa total daily dose: 1,305 mg).

If total daily dose of levodopa is between 950 mg to 1,249 mg: 3 capsules of carbidopa 48.75 mg/levodopa 195 mg 3 times daily (levodopa total daily dose: 1,755 mg).

If total daily dose of levodopa is ≥1,250 mg: 4 capsules of carbidopa 48.75 mg/levodopa 195 mg 3 times daily (levodopa total daily dose: 2,340 mg) **or** 3 capsules of carbidopa 61.25/levodopa 245 mg 3 times daily (levodopa total daily dose: 2,205 mg).

Dosage adjustment: Adjust dose as needed (maximum dose: carbidopa 612.5 mg/levodopa 2,450 mg per day)

Concomitant therapy: For patients currently treated with carbidopa/levodopa plus catechol-O-methyl transferase (COMT) inhibitors (eg, entacapone), the initial total daily dose of carbidopa/levodopa may need to be increased. Use of carbidopa/levodopa extended-release capsules in combination with other levodopa products has not been studied.

Intestinal infusion via PEG-J tube:

Intestinal suspension (Duopa): Initial: **Note:** Prior to initiation of therapy, convert patients from all forms of levodopa to oral immediate-release carbidopa/levodopa tablets (1:4 ratio). Total daily dose (expressed in terms of levodopa) consists of a morning dose, a continuous dose, and extra doses. Maximum dose is 2,000 mg of the levodopa component (ie, one cassette per day) over 16 hours. Patients should receive their routine nighttime dosage of oral immediate-release carbidopa/levodopa after discontinuation of daily infusion.

Morning dose and continuous dose: Refer to manufacturer's labeling for morning dose and continuous dose calculations and titration instructions.

Extra doses: Can be used to manage acute "off" symptoms that are not controlled by the morning and continuous dose. Set extra dose function at 1 mL (20 mg of levodopa) initially; adjust in 0.2 mL increments if needed. Maximum: One extra dose every 2 hours. **Note:** Frequent extra doses may cause or worsen dyskinesias.

Discontinuation: Avoid sudden discontinuation or rapid dose reduction; taper dose or switch patients to oral immediate-release carbidopa/levodopa.

Intestinal gel (Duodopa [Canadian product]): **Note:** Conversion to/from oral levodopa tablet formulations and the intestinal gel formulation can be done on a 1:1 ratio. Total daily dose (expressed in terms of levodopa) consists of a morning bolus dose, a continuous maintenance dose, and additional bolus doses when necessary. Nighttime dosing may be necessary in certain rare situations (eg, nocturnal akinesia). Dosage adjustments should be carried out over a period of a few weeks. Patients should receive their routine night-time dosage of oral levodopa/carbidopa after discontinuation of daily infusion

Morning bolus dose:

Day 1: Based on a percentage of the previous morning levodopa intake and volume to fill intestinal tubing:

Previous morning dose of levodopa ≤200 mg: Administer Duodopa at 80% of dose

Previous morning dose of levodopa 201 to 399 mg: Administer Duodopa at 70% of dose

Previous morning dose of levodopa ≥400 mg: Administer Duodopa at 60% of dose

Day 2 and beyond till dose is stable: Adjust dose based on response to the previous morning levodopa intake and volume to fill intestinal tubing): Usual: Levodopa 100 to 200 mg (5 to 10 mL); Maximum: Levodopa 300 mg (15 mL)

Continuous maintenance dose: Adjustable in increments of 2 mg/hour (0.1 mL/hour) and based on previous daily intake of levodopa: Usual: Levodopa 40 to 120 mg/hour (2 to 6 mL/hour) infused up to 16 hours; Range: Levodopa 20 to 200 mg/hour (1 to 10 mL/hour). Higher doses may be necessary in exceptional cases.

Additional bolus doses: Usual: Levodopa: 10 to 40 mg (0.5 to 2 mL), if needed for rapid deterioration of motor functions (eg, hypokinesia); may give additional doses hourly until stable dose is established then give every 2 hours as needed. In patients requiring >5 additional boluses/day, consider increasing the maintenance dose

Restless leg syndrome (RLS) (off-label use; Silber, 2004): Adults: Oral:

Immediate release tablet: Carbidopa 25 mg/levodopa 100 mg (0.5 to 1 tablet) given in the evening, at bedtime, or upon waking during the night with RLS symptoms

Controlled release tablet: Carbidopa 25 mg/levodopa 100 mg (1 tablet) before bedtime for RLS symptoms that awaken patient during the night

Elderly: Refer to adult dosing

Dosage adjustment for toxicity: Intestinal suspension (Duopa):

Dyskinesias or levodopa-related adverse reactions within 1 hour of morning dose on preceding day: Decrease morning dose by 1 mL.

Dyskinesias or adverse reactions lasting ≥1 hour on the preceding day: Decrease the continuous dose by 0.3 mL per hour.

Dyskinesias or adverse reactions lasting for 2 or more periods of ≥1 hour on the preceding day: Decrease the continuous dose by 0.6 mL per hour.

Dosage adjustment in renal impairment:

U.S. labeling: There are no dosage adjustments provided in the manufacturer's labeling; use with caution.

Canadian labeling: There are no dosage adjustments provided in the manufacturer's labeling; titrate dose cautiously in severe impairment. Use is contraindicated in uncompensated renal disease.

Dosage adjustment in hepatic impairment:

U.S. labeling: There are no dosage adjustments provided in the manufacturer's labeling; use with caution.

Canadian labeling: There are no dosage adjustments provided in the manufacturer's labeling; titrate dose cautiously in severe impairment. Use is contraindicated in uncompensated hepatic disease.

Dietary Considerations Avoid high protein diets (>2 g/kg) which may decrease the efficacy of levodopa via competition with amino acids in crossing the blood-brain barrier. Some products may contain phenylalanine.

Administration

Intestinal suspension (Duopa): Remove one cassette from refrigerator 20 minutes prior to use (failure to use at room temperature may result in inaccurate dosage). Administer as a 16-hour infusion through either a naso-jejunal tube (temporary administration) or through a percutaneous endoscopic gastrostomy-jejunostomy (PEG-J) tube (long-term administration) connected to the CADD-Legacy 1400 pump. At the end of administration, disconnect the tube from the pump at the end of the infusion and flush with room-temperature drinking water with a syringe. Following discontinuation of the daily infusion, patients should administer their routine night-time dosage of oral immediate-release carbidopa/levodopa.

Intestinal gel (Duodopa [Canadian product]): Gel is administered directly to the jejunum via a portable infusion pump (CADD-legacy Duodopa pump). Administer through a temporary nasojejunal tube for a short-term test period to evaluate patient response and for dose optimization. Long-term administration requires placement of PEG-J tube for intestinal infusion. Continuous maintenance dose is infused throughout the day for up to 16 hours if necessary, may administer at night (eg, nocturnal akinesia). Disconnect PEG-J tube from infusion pump at end of infusion and flush with room temperature water to prevent occlusion of tubing. Following discontinuation of the daily infusion, patients should administer their routine night-time dosage of oral levodopa/carbidopa.

Extended-release capsule: Administer with or without food; a high-fat, high-calorie meal may delay the absorption of levodopa by ~2 hours. Swallow capsules whole; do not chew, divide, or crush capsules. Patients who have difficulty swallowing intact capsules may open the capsule, sprinkle entire contents on a small amount of applesauce (1 to 2 tablespoons) and consume immediately (do not store for future use).

Oral tablet formulations: Space doses evenly over the waking hours. Administer with meals to decrease GI upset. Controlled release product should not be chewed or crushed. Orally disintegrating tablets do not require water; the tablet should disintegrate on the tongue's surface before swallowing.

Monitoring Parameters Signs and symptoms of Parkinson disease; periodic hepatic function tests, BUN, creatinine, and CBC; periodic skin examinations; blood pressure, standing and sitting/supine; symptoms of dyskinesias, mental status changes; cardiac function (particularly during initial dosage adjustment), IOP (in patients with glaucoma); signs and symptoms of neuroleptic malignant syndrome if abrupt discontinuation required (as with surgery); drowsiness or sleepiness; signs of depression (including suicidal thoughts); signs and symptoms of peripheral neuropathy prior to therapy and periodically during therapy.

Additional Canadian labeling recommendations include vitamin B_{12}, vitamin B_6, folic acid, homocysteine, and methylmalonic acid levels prior to initiation and regularly thereafter (Duodopa Canadian product monograph, 2014).

Additional Information To block the peripheral conversion of levodopa to dopamine, ≥70 mg/day of carbidopa is needed. "On-off" (a clinical syndrome characterized by sudden periods of drug activity/inactivity), can be managed by giving smaller, more frequent doses of Sinemet or adding a dopamine agonist or selegiline; when adding a new agent, doses of Sinemet can usually be decreased. Protein in the diet should be distributed throughout the day to avoid fluctuations in levodopa absorption. Levodopa is the drug of choice when rigidity is the predominant presenting symptom.

Conversion from levodopa to carbidopa/levodopa: **Note:** Levodopa must be discontinued at least 12 hours prior to initiation of levodopa/carbidopa:

Initial dose: Levodopa portion of carbidopa/levodopa should be at least 25% of previous levodopa therapy.

Levodopa <1,500 mg/day: Sinemet or Parcopa (levodopa 25 mg/carbidopa 100 mg) 3-4 times/day

Levodopa ≥1,500 mg/day: Sinemet or Parcopa (levodopa 25 mg/carbidopa 250 mg) 3-4 times/day

Conversion from immediate release carbidopa/levodopa (Sinemet or Parcopa) to Sinemet CR (50/200):

Sinemet or Parcopa [total daily dose of levodopa]/Sinemet CR:

Sinemet or Parcopa (levodopa 300-400 mg/day): Sinemet CR (50/200) 1 tablet twice daily

Sinemet or Parcopa (levodopa 500-600 mg/day): Sinemet CR (50/200) 1½ tablets twice daily or 1 tablet 3 times/day

Sinemet or Parcopa (levodopa 700-800 mg/day): Sinemet CR (50/200) 4 tablets in 3 or more divided doses

Sinemet or Parcopa (levodopa 900-1,000 mg/day): Sinemet CR (50/200) 5 tablets in 3 or more divided doses

Intervals between doses of Sinemet CR should be 4-8 hours while awake; when divided doses are not equal, smaller doses should be given toward the end of the day

Product Availability

Rytary extended-release capsules: FDA approved January 2015; availability anticipated in February 2015. Rytary is indicated for the treatment of Parkinson's disease, postencephalitic parkinsonism, and parkinsonism that may follow carbon monoxide intoxication or manganese intoxication.

Duopa: FDA approved January 2015; anticipated availability is currently unknown. Duopa is an enteral suspension indicated for the treatment of motor fluctuations in patients with advanced Parkinson disease.

Dosage Forms

Capsule, extended release:

Rytary:

23.75/95: Carbidopa 23.75 mg and levodopa 95 mg

36.25/145: Carbidopa 36.25 mg and levodopa 145 mg

48.75/195: Carbidopa 48.75 mg and levodopa 195 mg

61.25/245: Carbidopa 61.25 mg and levodopa 245 mg

Tablet: 10/100: Carbidopa 10 mg and levodopa 100 mg; 25/100: Carbidopa 25 mg and levodopa 100 mg; 25/250: Carbidopa 25 mg and levodopa 250 mg

Sinemet:

10/100: Carbidopa 10 mg and levodopa 100 mg

25/100: Carbidopa 25 mg and levodopa 100 mg

25/250: Carbidopa 25 mg and levodopa 250 mg

Tablet, extended release: 25/100: Carbidopa 25 mg and levodopa 100 mg; 50/200: Carbidopa 50 mg and levodopa 200 mg

Tablet, orally disintegrating: 10/100: Carbidopa 10 mg and levodopa 100 mg; 25/100: Carbidopa 25 mg and levodopa 100 mg; 25/250: Carbidopa 25 mg and levodopa 250 mg

Tablet, sustained release: 25/100: Carbidopa 25 mg and levodopa 100 mg; 50/200: Carbidopa 50 mg and levodopa 200 mg

Sinemet CR:

25/100: Carbidopa 25 mg and levodopa 100 mg

50/200: Carbidopa 50 mg and levodopa 200 mg

Dosage Forms: Canada

Intestinal gel:

Duodopa: Carbidopa 5 mg and levodopa 20 mg/1 mL (100 mL)

Extemporaneous Preparations An oral suspension containing carbidopa 1.25 mg and levodopa 5 mg per mL may be made with tablets. Crush ten tablets each containing carbidopa 25 mg and levodopa 100 mg and reduce to a fine powder. Add small portions of a 1:1 mixture of Ora-Sweet® and Ora-Plus® and mix to a uniform paste; mix while adding the vehicle in equal proportions to **almost** 200 mL; transfer to a calibrated bottle, rinse mortar with vehicle, and add sufficient quantity of vehicle to make 200 mL. Label "shake well" and "refrigerate". Stable 42 days under refrigeration. Also stable 28 days at room temperature.

Nahata MC, Morosco RS, and Leguire LE, "Development of Two Stable Oral Suspensions of Levodopa-Carbidopa for Children With Amblyopia," *J Pediatr Ophthalmol Strabismus*, 2000, 37(6):333-7.

◆ **Carbidopa, Entacapone, and Levodopa** *see* Levodopa, Carbidopa, and Entacapone *on page 1196*

◆ **Carbidopa, Levodopa, and Entacapone** *see* Levodopa, Carbidopa, and Entacapone *on page 1196*

Carbimazole [INT] (kar BI ma zol)

International Brand Names Anti-Thyrox (IN); Basolest (NL); Bimaz (VN); Camazol (MY, SG); Camen (KR); Carbimazol Aliud (AT); Carbimazol Henning (DE); Carbizole (PK); Neo-Mercazole (AE, AU, CH, DK, FR, GB, HN, ID, IE, IN, KW, NO, NZ, SA, VN, ZA); Neo-Thyreostat (DE); Neo-Tomizol (ES); Neomercazol (JO); Neomercazole (CY, HK, PH, PK, QA, TR); Neomerdin (PH); Neotrox (PH); Thymazole (MY); Thyrostat (GR); Tyrazol (FI)

Pharmacologic Category Antithyroid Agent

Reported Use Treatment of hyperthyroidism, thyrotoxicosis, and preparation of patients for radioactive iodine therapy or thyroidectomy.

Dosage Range Hyperthyroidism:

Children: Oral: Initial: 15 mg daily

Adults: Oral: Initial: 20-60 mg daily given in 2-3 divided doses; maintenance: 5-15 mg daily or alternatively 20-60 mg daily when receiving concurrent thyroid replacement therapy

Product Availability Product available in various countries; not currently available in the U.S.

Dosage Forms

Tablet: 5 mg, 20 mg

Carbinoxamine (kar bi NOKS a meen)

Brand Names: U.S. Arbinoxa; Karbinal ER; Palgic [DSC]

Index Terms Carbinoxamine Maleate; Karbinal™ ER

Pharmacologic Category Ethanolamine Derivative; Histamine H_1 Antagonist; Histamine H_1 Antagonist, First Generation

Additional Appendix Information

Beers Criteria – Potentially Inappropriate Medications for Geriatrics *on page 2271*

Use Allergies: For the symptomatic treatment of seasonal and perennial allergic rhinitis; vasomotor rhinitis; allergic conjunctivitis caused by inhalant allergens and foods; mild, uncomplicated allergic skin manifestations of urticaria and angioedema; dermatographism; as therapy for anaphylactic reactions adjunctive to epinephrine and other standard measures after the acute manifestations have been controlled; amelioration of the severity of allergic reactions to blood or plasma.

Pregnancy Risk Factor C

Dosage Allergies: Oral:

Extended release:

Children 2 to <4 years: 3-4 mg every 12 hours

Children 4 to <6 years: 3-8 mg every 12 hours

Children 6 to <12 years: 6-12 mg every 12 hours

Children ≥12 years, Adolescents, and Adults: 6-16 mg every 12 hours

Immediate release:

Children 2 to <6 years: 0.2-0.4 mg/kg/day divided into 3-4 doses (weight-based dosing preferred) **or** 1-2 mg 3-4 times daily

Children 6 to <12 years: 2-4 mg 3-4 times daily

Children ≥12 years, Adolescents, and Adults: 4-8 mg 3-4 times daily

Dosage adjustment in renal impairment: No dosage adjustment provided in manufacturer's labeling.

Dosage adjustment in hepatic impairment: No dosage adjustment provided in manufacturer's labeling.

Additional Information Complete prescribing information should be consulted for additional detail.

Product Availability Karbinal ER (extended release) oral suspension: FDA approved March 2013; availability anticipated is January 2015. Consult the prescribing information for additional information.

Dosage Forms

Liquid Extended Release, Oral:

Karbinal ER: 4 mg/5 mL (480 mL)

Solution, Oral:

Arbinoxa: 4 mg/5 mL (473 mL)

Generic: 4 mg/5 mL (118 mL, 473 mL)

Tablet, Oral:

Arbinoxa: 4 mg

Generic: 4 mg

- ◆ **Carbinoxamine Maleate** *see* Carbinoxamine *on page 356*
- ◆ **Carbocaine** *see* Mepivacaine *on page 1295*
- ◆ **Carbocaine® (Can)** *see* Mepivacaine *on page 1295*
- ◆ **Carbocaine Preservative-Free** *see* Mepivacaine *on page 1295*
- ◆ **Carbocisteina** *see* Carbocisteine [INT] *on page 357*

Carbocisteine [INT] (kar boe SIS tee een)

International Brand Names Acuphlem (ZA); Aflem (PH); Anatac (ES); Arbistin (MX); Bai Yue (CN); Bocytin (TH); Bronchathiol (FR); Broncholit (ID); Broquial-PM (PE); Cabotin (TW); Carbocin (BR); Carboflem (PH); Carbotos (CL); Carsemex (TH); Cicough (TH); Co-Flem (ZA); Coldin (CL); Drill (HU); Estival (GR); Expelin (MX); Expetan (HK); Expetan Kids (HK); Exputex (IE); Fenorin (CZ); Finatux (PT); Flemex (VN); Fluditec (EE); Fluifort (HK); Griflux (PT); Humexcough (BG); Jintum (TW); Kai Yin (CN); Medibronc (FR); Mephathiol (CH); Mical (IL); Muciclar (AE, QA); Muco Rhinathiol (BE); Muco-Treat (IL); Mucocis (IT); Mucodin (SG); Mucodyne (GB, IN, JP); Mucofar (VE); Mucoflux (BR); Mucolase (AE); Mucolit (IL, UY); Mucolitic (AR); Mucopront (BH, EG, PY, QA, VE); Mucotablets (QA); Mucotal (LB); Pectodrill (CZ, ES, PL); Pectox (AR, CH); Reodyn (FI); Rhinathiol (AE, BH, CY, HU, ID, KR, KW, LB, NL, QA, SA); Siroxyl (BE, GR); Solmux (HK); Solucis (IT); Solvex (AE); Zoradine (MY)

Index Terms Carbocisteina; Carbocysteina; Carbocysteine; Carboxymethylcysteine; S-Carboxymethyl L-Cysteine; S-Carboxymethylcysteine; S-CMC

Pharmacologic Category Mucolytic Agent

Reported Use Adjunctive mucolytic therapy in respiratory tract disorders characterized by excessive or viscous mucous secretions

Dosage Range Oral:

Children 2-5 years: 200-500 mg daily in 2-4 divided doses

Children 6-12 years: 300-750 mg daily in 3 divided doses

Adults: 1500-2250 mg daily in 3-4 divided doses

Product Availability Product available in various countries; not currently available in the U.S.

Dosage Forms

Capsule: 375 mg

Syrup: 2 g/100 mL; 2.5g/100 mL; 5 g/100 mL

- ◆ **Carbocysteina** *see* Carbocisteine [INT] *on page 357*
- ◆ **Carbocysteine** *see* Carbocisteine [INT] *on page 357*
- ◆ **Carb-O-Lac5 [OTC]** *see* Urea *on page 2114*
- ◆ **Carb-O-Lac HP [OTC]** *see* Urea *on page 2114*
- ◆ **Carbolith (Can)** *see* Lithium *on page 1230*
- ◆ **Carb-O-Philic/20 [OTC]** *see* Urea *on page 2114*
- ◆ **Carb-O-Philic/40** *see* Urea *on page 2114*

CARBOplatin (KAR boe pla tin)

Brand Names: Canada Carboplatin Injection; Carboplatin Injection BP

Index Terms CBDCA; Paraplatin

Pharmacologic Category Antineoplastic Agent, Alkylating Agent; Antineoplastic Agent, Platinum Analog

Additional Appendix Information

Beers Criteria – Potentially Inappropriate Medications for Geriatrics *on page 2271*

Use Ovarian cancer: Initial treatment of advanced ovarian cancer in combination with other established chemotherapy agents; palliative treatment of recurrent ovarian cancer after prior chemotherapy, including cisplatin-based treatment

Pregnancy Risk Factor D

Pregnancy Considerations Embryotoxicity and teratogenicity have been observed in animal reproduction studies. May cause fetal harm if administered during pregnancy. Women of childbearing potential should avoid becoming pregnant during treatment.

Breast-Feeding Considerations It is not known if carboplatin is excreted in breast milk. Due to the potential for toxicity in nursing infants, breast-feeding is not recommended.

Contraindications History of severe allergic reaction to carboplatin, cisplatin, other platinum-containing formulations, mannitol, or any component of the formulation; should not be used in patients with severe bone marrow depression or significant bleeding

Warnings/Precautions Hazardous agent - use appropriate precautions for handling and disposal (NIOSH 2014 [group 1]). High doses have resulted in severe abnormalities of liver function tests. **[U.S. Boxed Warning]: Bone marrow suppression, which may be severe, is dose related; may result in infection (due to neutropenia) or bleeding (due to thrombocytopenia); anemia may require blood transfusion;** reduce dosage in patients with bone marrow suppression; cycles should be delayed until WBC and platelet counts have recovered. Patients who have received prior myelosuppressive therapy and patients with renal dysfunction are at increased risk for bone marrow suppression. Anemia is cumulative.

When calculating the carboplatin dose using the Calvert formula and an estimated glomerular filtration rate (GFR), the laboratory method used to measure serum creatinine may impact dosing. Compared to other methods, standardized isotope dilution mass spectrometry (IDMS) may underestimate serum creatinine values in patients with low creatinine values (eg, ≤0.7 mg/dL) and may overestimate GFR in patients with normal renal function. This may result in higher calculated carboplatin doses and increased toxicities. If using IDMS, the Food and Drug Administration (FDA) recommends that clinicians consider capping estimated GFR at a maximum of 125 mL/minute to avoid potential toxicity.

[U.S. Boxed Warning]: Anaphylactic-like reactions have been reported with carboplatin; may occur within minutes of administration. Epinephrine, corticosteroids and antihistamines have been used to treat symptoms. The risk of allergic reactions (including anaphylaxis) is increased in patients previously exposed to platinum therapy. Skin testing and desensitization protocols have been reported (Confina-Cohen, 2005; Lee, 2004; Markman, 2003). When administered as sequential infusions, taxane derivatives (docetaxel, paclitaxel) should be administered before the platinum derivatives (carboplatin, cisplatin) to limit myelosuppression and to enhance efficacy. Ototoxicity may occur when administered concomitantly with aminoglycosides. Clinically significant hearing loss has been reported to occur in pediatric patients when carboplatin was administered at higher than recommended doses in combination with other ototoxic agents (eg, aminoglycosides). In a study of children receiving carboplatin for the treatment of retinoblastoma, those <6 months of age at treatment initiation were more likely to experience ototoxicity; long-term audiology monitoring is recommended (Qaddoumi, 2012). Loss of vision (usually reversible within weeks of discontinuing) has been reported with higher than recommended doses.

Use caution in elderly patients; may cause or exacerbate syndrome of inappropriate antidiuretic hormone secretion or hyponatremia; monitor sodium closely with initiation or dosage adjustments in older adults (Beers Criteria). Peripheral neuropathy occurs infrequently, the incidence of peripheral neuropathy is increased in patients >65 years of age and those who have previously received cisplatin treatment. Patients >65 years of age are more likely to develop severe thrombocytopenia.

Limited potential for nephrotoxicity unless administered concomitantly with aminoglycosides. **[U.S. Boxed Warning]: Vomiting may occur.** Carboplatin is associated with a moderate emetic potential in adult patients and a high emetic potential in pediatric patients; antiemetics are recommended to prevent nausea and vomiting (Basch, 2011; Dupuis, 2011; Roila, 2010). May be severe in patients who have received prior emetogenic therapy. **[U.S. Boxed Warning]: Should be administered under the supervision of an experienced cancer chemotherapy physician.**

Adverse Reactions

Central nervous system: Neurotoxicity, pain, peripheral neuropathy

Dermatologic: Alopecia

Endocrine & metabolic: Hypocalcemia, hypokalemia, hypomagnesemia, hyponatremia

Gastrointestinal: Abdominal pain, constipation, diarrhea, dysgeusia, mucositis, nausea (without vomiting), stomatitis, vomiting

Hematologic & oncologic: Anemia, bleeding complications, bone marrow depression (dose related and dose limiting; nadir at ~21 days with single-agent therapy), hemorrhage, leukopenia, neutropenia, thrombocytopenia

Hepatic: Increased serum alkaline phosphatase, increased serum AST, increased serum bilirubin

Hypersensitivity: Hypersensitivity

Infection: Infection

Neuromuscular & skeletal: Weakness

Ophthalmic: Visual disturbance

Otic: Ototoxicity

Renal: Decreased creatinine clearance, increased blood urea nitrogen, increased serum creatinine

Rare but important or life-threatening: Anaphylaxis, anorexia, bronchospasm, cardiac failure, cerebrovascular accident, dehydration, embolism, erythema, febrile neutropenia, hemolytic anemia (acute), hemolytic-uremic syndrome, hypertension, hypotension, injection site reaction (pain, redness, swelling), limb ischemia (acute), malaise, metastases, pruritus, skin rash, tissue necrosis (associated with extravasation), urticaria, vision loss

Drug Interactions

Metabolism/Transport Effects None known.

Avoid Concomitant Use

Avoid concomitant use of CARBOplatin with any of the following: BCG; CloZAPine; Dipyrone; Natalizumab; Pimecrolimus; SORAfenib; Tacrolimus (Topical); Tofacitinib; Vaccines (Live)

Increased Effect/Toxicity

CARBOplatin may increase the levels/effects of: Bexarotene (Systemic); CloZAPine; Leflunomide; Natalizumab; Taxane Derivatives; Tofacitinib; Topotecan; Vaccines (Live)

The levels/effects of CARBOplatin may be increased by: Aminoglycosides; Denosumab; Dipyrone; Pimecrolimus; Roflumilast; SORAfenib; Tacrolimus (Topical); Trastuzumab

Decreased Effect

CARBOplatin may decrease the levels/effects of: BCG; Coccidioides immitis Skin Test; Fosphenytoin-Phenytoin; Sipuleucel-T; Vaccines (Inactivated); Vaccines (Live)

The levels/effects of CARBOplatin may be decreased by: Echinacea

Preparation for Administration Hazardous agent; use appropriate precautions for handling and disposal (NIOSH 2014 [group 1]).

Solution for injection: Manufacturer's labeling states solution can be further diluted to concentrations as low as 0.5 mg/mL in NS or D_5W; however, most clinicians generally dilute dose in either 100 mL or 250 mL of NS or D_5W.

Concentrations used for desensitization vary based on protocol.

Needles or IV administration sets that contain aluminum should not be used in the preparation or administration of carboplatin; aluminum can react with carboplatin resulting in precipitate formation and loss of potency.

Storage/Stability Store intact vials at room temperature at 25°C (77°F); excursions permitted to 15°C to 30°C (59°F to 86°F). Protect from light. Further dilution to a concentration as low as 0.5 mg/mL is stable at room temperature (25°C) for 8 hours in NS or D_5W. Stability has also been demonstrated for dilutions in D_5W in PVC bags at room temperature for 9 days (Benaji, 1994); however, the manufacturer recommends use within 8 hours due to lack of preservative. Multidose vials are stable for up to 14 days after opening when stored at 25°C (77°F) following multiple needle entries.

Mechanism of Action Carboplatin is a platinum compound alkylating agent which covalently binds to DNA; interferes with the function of DNA by producing interstrand DNA cross-links

Pharmacodynamics/Kinetics

Distribution: V_d: 16 L (based on a dose of 300 to 500 mg/m^2); into liver, kidney, skin, and tumor tissue

Protein binding: Carboplatin: 0%; Platinum (from carboplatin): Irreversibly binds to plasma proteins

Metabolism: Minimally hepatic to aquated and hydroxylated compounds

Half-life elimination: CrCl >60 mL/minute: Carboplatin: 2.6 to 5.9 hours (based on a dose of 300 to 500 mg/m^2); Platinum (from carboplatin): ≥5 days

Excretion: Urine (~70% as carboplatin within 24 hours; 3% to 5% as platinum within 1 to 4 days)

Dosage Note: Doses for adults are commonly calculated by the target AUC using the Calvert formula, where **Total dose (mg) = Target AUC x (GFR + 25)**. If estimating glomerular filtration rate (GFR) instead of a measured GFR, the Food and Drug Administration (FDA) recommends that clinicians consider capping estimated GFR at a maximum of 125 mL/minute to avoid potential toxicity. Carboplatin is associated with a moderate emetic potential in adult patients and a high emetic potential in pediatric patients; antiemetics are recommended to prevent nausea and vomiting (Basch, 2011; Dupuis, 2011; Roila, 2010).

Ovarian cancer, advanced: *Manufacturer's labeling:* Adults: IV: 360 mg/m^2 every 4 weeks (as a single agent) **or** 300 mg/m^2 every 4 weeks (in combination with cyclophosphamide) **or** Target AUC 4 to 6 (single agent; in previously treated patients)

Off-label dosing: Target AUC 5 to 7.5 every 3 weeks (in combination with paclitaxel) (Ozols, 2003; Parmar, 2003) **or** Target AUC 5 every 3 weeks (in combination with docetaxel) (Vasey, 2004)

Bladder cancer (off-label use): Adults: IV: Target AUC 5 every 3 weeks (in combination with gemcitabine) (Bamias, 2006) **or** Target AUC 6 every 3 weeks (in combination with paclitaxel) (Vaughn, 2002)

Breast cancer, metastatic (off-label use): Adults: IV: Target AUC 6 every 3 weeks (in combination with trastuzumab and paclitaxel) (Robert, 2006) **or** Target AUC 6 every 3 weeks (in combination with trastuzumab and docetaxel) (Pegram, 2004; Valero, 2011)

Central nervous system tumors (off-label use):

Glioma: Children: IV: 175 mg/m^2 weekly for 4 weeks every 6 weeks, with a 2-week recovery period between courses (in combination with vincristine) (Packer, 1997)

Neuroblastoma, localized and unresectable: IV: Children ≥10 kg: 200 mg/m^2/day days 1, 2, and 3 every 21 days for 2 cycles (in combination with etoposide for 2 cycles then followed by cyclophosphamide, doxorubicin and vincristine) (Rubie, 1998) **or** Children <1 year: 6.6 mg/kg/day days 1, 2, and 3 (in combination with etoposide for 2 cycles, then followed by cyclophosphamide, doxorubicin, and vincristine) (Rubie, 2001)

Cervical cancer, recurrent or metastatic (off-label use): Adults: IV: Target AUC 5 every 3 weeks (in combination with paclitaxel) (Pectasides, 2009) **or** Target AUC 5-6 every 4 weeks (in combination with paclitaxel) (Tinker, 2005) **or** 400 mg/m^2 every 28 days (as a single agent) (Weiss, 1990)

Endometrial cancer (off-label use): Adults: IV: Target AUC 5 every 3 weeks (in combination with paclitaxel) (Pectasides, 2008) **or** Target AUC 2 on days 1, 8, and 15 every 28 days (in combination with paclitaxel) (Secord, 2007)

Esophageal cancer (off-label use): Adults: IV: Target AUC 2 on days 1, 8, 15, 22, and 29 for 1 cycle (in combination with paclitaxel) (van Meerten, 2006) **or** Target AUC 5 every 3 weeks (in combination with paclitaxel) (El-Rayes, 2004)

Head and neck cancer (off-label use): Adults: IV: Target AUC 5 every 3 weeks (in combination with cetuximab) (Chan, 2005) **or** Target AUC 5 every 3 weeks (in combination with cetuximab and fluorouracil) (Vermorken, 2008) **or** 300 mg/m^2 every 4 weeks (in combination with fluorouracil) (Forastiere, 1992) **or** Target AUC 6 every 3 weeks (in combination with paclitaxel) (Clark, 2001)

Hodgkin lymphoma, relapsed or refractory (off-label use): Adults: IV: Target AUC 5 (maximum dose: 800 mg) for 2 cycles (in combination with ifosfamide and etoposide) (Moskowitz, 2001)

Malignant pleural mesothelioma (off-label use): Adults: IV: Target AUC 5 every 3 weeks (in combination with pemetrexed) (Castagneto, 2008; Ceresoli, 2006)

Melanoma, advanced or metastatic (off-label use): Adults: IV: Target AUC 2 on days 1, 8, and 15 every 4 weeks (in combination with paclitaxel) (Rao, 2006)

Non-Hodgkin lymphomas, relapsed or refractory (off-label use): Adults: IV: Target AUC 5 (maximum dose: 800 mg) per cycle for 3 cycles (in combination with rituximab, ifosfamide and etoposide) (Kewalramani, 2004)

Non-small cell lung cancer (off-label use): Adults: IV: Target AUC 6 every 3 to 4 weeks (in combination with paclitaxel) (Ramalingam, 2008; Schiller, 2002; Strauss, 2008) **or** Target AUC 6 every 3 weeks (in combination with bevacizumab and paclitaxel) (Sandler, 2006) **or** Target AUC 5 every 3 weeks (in combination with pemetrexed) (Gronberg, 2009) **or** in combination with radiation therapy and paclitaxel (Belani, 2005):

Target AUC 6 every 3 weeks for 2 cycles **or**

Target AUC 6 every 3 weeks for 2 cycles; then target AUC 2 weekly for 7 weeks **or**

Target AUC 2 every week for 7 weeks; then target AUC 6 every 3 weeks for 2 cycles

Sarcomas: Ewing sarcoma, osteosarcoma (off-label uses): Children and Adults: IV: 400 mg/m^2/day for 2 days every 21 days (in combination with ifosfamide and etoposide) (van Winkle, 2005)

Small cell lung cancer (off-label use): Adults: IV: Target AUC 6 every 3 weeks (in combination with etoposide) (Skarlos, 2001) **or** Target AUC 5 every 3 weeks (in combination with irinotecan) (Hermes, 2008) **or** Target AUC 5 every 28 days (in combination with irinotecan) (Schmittel, 2006)

Testicular cancer (off-label use): Adults: IV: Target AUC 7 as a one-time dose (Oliver, 2011) **or** 700 mg/m^2/day for 3 days beginning 5 days prior to peripheral stem cell infusion (in combination with etoposide) for 2 cycles (Einhorn, 2007)

Thymic malignancies (off-label use): Adults: IV: Target AUC 5 every 3 weeks (in combination with paclitaxel) (Lemma, 2008)

Unknown primary adenocarcinoma (off-label use): Adults: IV: Target AUC 6 every 3 weeks (in combination with paclitaxel) (Briasoulis, 2000) **or** Target AUC 6 every 3 weeks (in combination with docetaxel) (Greco, 2000) **or** Target AUC 6 every 3 weeks (in combination with paclitaxel and etoposide) (Hainsworth, 2006) **or** Target AUC 5 every 3 weeks (in combination with paclitaxel and gemcitabine) (Greco, 2002)

Elderly: The Calvert formula should be used to calculate dosing for elderly patients.

Dosage adjustment for toxicity: Platelets <50,000 cells/mm^3 or ANC <500 cells/mm^3: Administer 75% of dose

Dosage adjustment in renal impairment: Note: Dose determination with Calvert formula uses GFR and, therefore, inherently adjusts for renal dysfunction.

The manufacturer's labeling recommends the following dosage adjustments for single-agent therapy: Adults:

Baseline CrCl 41 to 59 mL/minute: Initiate at 250 mg/m^2 and adjust subsequent doses based on bone marrow toxicity

Baseline CrCl 16 to 40 mL/minute: Initiate at 200 mg/m^2 and adjust subsequent doses based on bone marrow toxicity

Baseline CrCl ≤15 mL/minute: There are no dosage adjustments provided in the manufacturer's labeling.

The following dosage adjustments have also been recommended:

Aronoff, 2007:

Children:

GFR <50 mL/minute: Use Calvert formula incorporating patient's GFR

Hemodialysis, peritoneal dialysis, continuous renal replacement therapy (CRRT): Use Calvert formula incorporating patient's GFR

Adults (**Note:** For dosing based on **mg/m²**):
GFR >50 mL/minute: No dosage adjustment is necessary
GFR 10 to 50 mL/minute: Administer 50% of the dose
GFR <10 mL/minute: Administer 25% of the dose
Hemodialysis: Administer 50% of dose
Continuous ambulatory peritoneal dialysis (CAPD): Administer 25% of dose
Continuous renal replacement therapy (CRRT): 200 mg/m²
Janus, 2010: Hemodialysis: Carboplatin dose (mg) = Target AUC x 25; administer on a nondialysis day, hemodialysis should occur between 12-24 hours after carboplatin dose

Dosage adjustment in hepatic impairment: There are no dosage adjustments provided in the manufacturer's labeling; however, carboplatin undergoes minimal hepatic metabolism therefore dosage adjustment may not be needed.

Dosing in obesity:
American Society of Clinical Oncology (ASCO) Guidelines for appropriate chemotherapy dosing in obese adults with cancer: Dosing based on GFR should be considered in obese patients; GFR should not exceed 125 mL/minute (Griggs, 2012).
American Society for Blood and Marrow Transplantation (ASBMT) practice guideline committee position statement on chemotherapy dosing in obesity: Utilize actual body weight (full weight) for calculation of body surface area (when applicable) in carboplatin dosing for hematopoietic stem cell transplant conditioning regimens in adults. Based on the literature, there is no consensus for carboplatin dosing based on AUC in transplant conditioning regimens or dosing adjustments during transplant for obese patients (Bubalo, 2014).

Administration Carboplatin is associated with a moderate emetic potential in adult patients and a high emetic potential in pediatric patients; antiemetics are recommended to prevent nausea and vomiting (Basch, 2011; Dupuis, 2011; Roila, 2010).

Infuse over at least 15 minutes; usually infused over 15 to 60 minutes, although some protocols may require infusions up to 24 hours. When administered as a part of a combination chemotherapy regimen, sequence of administration may vary by regimen; refer to specific protocol for sequence recommendation.

Needles or IV administration sets that contain aluminum should not be used in the preparation or administration of carboplatin; aluminum can react with carboplatin resulting in precipitate formation and loss of potency.

Hazardous agent; use appropriate precautions for handling and disposal (NIOSH 2014 [group 1]).

Monitoring Parameters CBC (with differential and platelet count), serum electrolytes, serum creatinine and BUN, creatinine clearance, liver function tests; audiology evaluations (children <6 months of age)

Dosage Forms
Solution, Intravenous:
Generic: 50 mg/5 mL (5 mL); 150 mg/15 mL (15 mL); 450 mg/45 mL (45 mL); 600 mg/60 mL (60 mL)
Solution, Intravenous [preservative free]:
Generic: 50 mg/5 mL (5 mL); 150 mg/15 mL (15 mL); 450 mg/45 mL (45 mL); 600 mg/60 mL (60 mL)
Solution Reconstituted, Intravenous:
Generic: 150 mg (1 ea)

◆ **Carboplatin Injection (Can)** *see* CARBOplatin *on page 357*
◆ **Carboplatin Injection BP (Can)** *see* CARBOplatin *on page 357*
◆ **Carboprost** *see* Carboprost Tromethamine *on page 360*

Carboprost Tromethamine
(KAR boe prost tro METH a meen)

Brand Names: U.S. Hemabate
Brand Names: Canada Hemabate
Index Terms Carboprost; Prostaglandin F_2 Alpha Analog; Prostaglandin F_2 Analog
Pharmacologic Category Abortifacient; Prostaglandin
Use
Termination of pregnancy: For aborting pregnancy between week 13 and 20 of gestation as calculated from the first day of the last normal menstrual period and in the following conditions related to second trimester abortion: Failure of expulsion of the fetus during the course of treatment by another method; premature rupture of membranes in intrauterine methods with loss of drug and insufficient or absent uterine activity; requirement of a repeat intrauterine instillation of drug for expulsion of the fetus; inadvertent or spontaneous rupture of membranes in the presence of a previable fetus and absence of adequate activity for expulsion.
Refractory postpartum uterine hemorrhage: Treatment of postpartum hemorrhage due to uterine atony that has not responded to conventional methods of management. Prior treatment should include the use of intravenously (IV) administered oxytocin, manipulative techniques such as uterine massage and, unless contraindicated, intramuscular ergot preparations.

Pregnancy Risk Factor C

Dosage IM: Adults:
Refractory postpartum uterine bleeding: Initial: 250 mcg; if needed, may repeat at 15- to 90-minute intervals; maximum total dose: 2 mg (8 doses)
Termination of pregnancy: Initial: 250 mcg, then 250 mcg at 1.5- to 3.5-hour intervals, depending on uterine response; a 500 mcg dose may be given if uterine response is not adequate after several 250 mcg doses; do not exceed 12 mg total dose or continuous administration for >2 days. **Note:** A 100 mcg test dose may be considered.

Dosage adjustment in renal impairment: Use with caution in patients with a history of renal disease; use is contraindicated in patients with active renal disease.
Dosage adjustment in hepatic impairment: Use with caution in patients with a history of hepatic disease; use is contraindicated in patients with active hepatic disease.

Additional Information Complete prescribing information should be consulted for additional detail.

Dosage Forms
Solution, Intramuscular:
Hemabate: 250 mcg/mL (1 mL)

◆ **Carboxymethylcysteine** *see* Carbocisteine [INT] *on page 357*
◆ **Carboxypeptidase-G2** *see* Glucarpidase *on page 971*
◆ **Cardec™ DM [OTC]** *see* Chlorpheniramine, Phenylephrine, and Dextromethorphan *on page 428*
◆ **Cardene IV** *see* NiCARdipine *on page 1446*
◆ **Cardene SR [DSC]** *see* NiCARdipine *on page 1446*
◆ **Cardizem** *see* Diltiazem *on page 634*
◆ **Cardizem CD** *see* Diltiazem *on page 634*
◆ **Cardizem LA** *see* Diltiazem *on page 634*
◆ **Cardura** *see* Doxazosin *on page 674*
◆ **Cardura-1 (Can)** *see* Doxazosin *on page 674*
◆ **Cardura-2 (Can)** *see* Doxazosin *on page 674*
◆ **Cardura-4 (Can)** *see* Doxazosin *on page 674*

◆ **Cardura XL** *see* Doxazosin *on page 674*

Carfilzomib (kar FILZ oh mib)

Brand Names: U.S. Kyprolis

Index Terms PR-171

Pharmacologic Category Antineoplastic Agent; Proteasome Inhibitor

Use Treatment of multiple myeloma in patients who have received at least 2 prior treatment regimens (including a proteasome inhibitor and an immunomodulator) with disease progression within 60 days after the most recent treatment

Pregnancy Risk Factor D

Pregnancy Considerations Adverse events were observed in animal reproduction studies at doses less than the recommended human dose (based on BSA). Based on the mechanism of action, adverse fetal events would be expected to occur with use in pregnant women. Females of reproductive potential are advised to avoid pregnancy during therapy.

Breast-Feeding Considerations Due to the potential for adverse reactions in nursing infants, the manufacturer recommends avoiding breast-feeding during therapy.

Contraindications There are no contraindications listed in the manufacturer's labeling.

Warnings/Precautions Hazardous agent - use appropriate precautions for handling and disposal (meets NIOSH 2014 criteria). Thrombocytopenia (including grade 4) was observed in patients receiving carfilzomib, with platelet nadirs occurring around day 8 of each 28-day treatment cycle, and recovery to baseline by the start of the next cycle. Monitor platelets closely and adjust dose or withhold therapy if necessary. Anemia, lymphopenia, and neutropenia were also observed. Death caused by cardiac arrest has occurred within 24 hours of drug administration. Carfilzomib has been associated with the development or worsening of congestive heart failure (HF) and decreased left ventricular ejection fraction (LVEF). HF, pulmonary edema, and decreased LVEF were observed in clinical trials; monitor closely for cardiac complications; withhold therapy for grade 3 or 4 cardiac events until recovery. Patients with New York Heart Association Class III and IV heart failure, recent myocardial infarction (within 6 months), and conduction abnormalities not managed by medication were excluded from clinical trials. Pulmonary arterial hypertension (PAH) was observed (including grade 3) in studies; perform cardiac imaging or other testing as appropriate, and withhold carfilzomib until PAH is resolved or returns to baseline. Dyspnea (including 1 death) has been reported; monitor closely, and withhold carfilzomib until symptom resolution or return to baseline.

Infusion reactions such as chills, fever, arthralgia, myalgia, shortness of breath, hypotension, facial flushing, facial edema, vomiting, weakness, syncope, chest tightness, or angina may occur immediately following or within 24 hours of carfilzomib infusion. To lessen the incidence and intensity of infusion reactions, administer dexamethasone prior to drug administration. Tumor lysis syndrome (TLS) risk is increased in multiple myeloma patients with a high tumor burden. Adequately hydrate patients prior to carfilzomib therapy and monitor closely for signs and symptoms of tumor lysis syndrome. If TLS occurs, interrupt treatment until resolved.

Hepatic failure, including fatal cases, has been reported rarely (<1%). Increased transaminases and hyperbilirubinemia have also been observed. Interrupt carfilzomib therapy in patients with grade 3 or higher hepatic toxicity until resolved or recovered to baseline; monitor liver enzymes closely and for signs of toxicity.

Adverse Reactions

Cardiovascular: Cardiac failure (includes CHF, pulmonary edema, ejection fraction decreased); chest wall pain, hypertension, peripheral edema

Central nervous system: Chills, dizziness, fatigue, fever, headache, hypoesthesia, insomnia, pain

Endocrine & metabolic: Hypercalcemia, hyperglycemia, hypokalemia, hypomagnesemia, hyponatremia, hypophosphatemia

Gastrointestinal: Anorexia, constipation, diarrhea, nausea, vomiting

Hematologic: Anemia, leukopenia, lymphopenia, neutropenia, thrombocytopenia

Hepatic: AST increased

Neuromuscular & skeletal: Arthralgia, back pain, limb pain, muscle spasms, peripheral neuropathy, weakness

Renal: Creatinine increased, renal failure

Respiratory: Cough, dyspnea, pneumonia, pulmonary artery hypertension, upper respiratory tract infection

Miscellaneous: Herpes zoster reactivation

Rare but important or life-threatening: Bilirubin increased, hepatic failure, infusion reaction, intracranial hemorrhage, multiorgan failure, myocardial ischemia, neutropenic fever, sepsis, tumor lysis syndrome

Drug Interactions

Metabolism/Transport Effects Substrate of P-glycoprotein; **Inhibits** CYP3A4 (weak), P-glycoprotein

Avoid Concomitant Use

Avoid concomitant use of Carfilzomib with any of the following: CloZAPine; Dipyrone; Pimozide

Increased Effect/Toxicity

Carfilzomib may increase the levels/effects of: ARIPiprazole; CloZAPine; Dofetilide; Hydrocodone; Lomitapide; Pimozide

The levels/effects of Carfilzomib may be increased by: Dipyrone; P-glycoprotein/ABCB1 Inhibitors

Decreased Effect

The levels/effects of Carfilzomib may be decreased by: P-glycoprotein/ABCB1 Inducers

Preparation for Administration Hazardous agent; use appropriate precautions for handling and disposal (meets NIOSH 2014 criteria). Reconstitute with 29 mL sterile water for injection to a concentration of 2 mg/mL (directing solution onto the inside wall of the vial to avoid foaming). Gently invert and/or swirl vial slowly for ~1 minute to mix; do not shake. If foaming results, allow solution to sit for 2-5 minutes until foaming resolves. Reconstituted solution should be clear and colorless. May further dilute dose in 50 mL D_5W. The amount contained in each vial may exceed the prescribed dose; use care with dosage and volume calculations. Discard unused portion of the vial.

Storage/Stability Store intact vials refrigerated at 2°C to 8°C (36°F to 46°F). Do not shake; store in original carton until use to protect from light. Reconstituted drug (in the vial or in a syringe) and preparations diluted for infusion are stable for 4 hours at room temperature or for 24 hours refrigerated at 2°C to 8°C (36°F to 46°F).

Mechanism of Action Carfilzomib inhibits proteasomes, which are responsible for intracellular protein homeostasis. Specifically, it is a potent, selective, and irreversible inhibitor of chymotrypsin-like activity of the 20S proteasome, leading to cell cycle arrest and apoptosis.

Pharmacodynamics/Kinetics

Distribution: V_{dss}: 28 L

Protein binding: 97%

Metabolism: Rapid and extensive; peptidase cleavage and epoxide hydrolysis; minimal metabolism through cytochrome P450-mediated mechanisms

Half-life elimination: Doses ≥15 mg/m^2: <1 hour on day 1 of cycle 1

Dosage IV: Adults: **Note:** Hydrate with 250-500 mL normal saline (or other appropriate IV fluid) predose (recommended) and postdose (if needed) during cycle 1 (continue in subsequent cycles if necessary). Premedicate with dexamethasone (4 mg orally or IV) prior to all doses in cycle 1, all doses during first dose escalation cycle, and as needed with future cycles to reduce the incidence and severity of infusion reaction.

Multiple myeloma, relapsed/refractory: **Note:** Patients with a body surface area (BSA) >2.2 m^2 should be dosed based upon a maximum BSA of 2.2 m^2. Dose adjustments for weight changes of ≤20% are not necessary, per manufacturer labeling.

Cycle 1: 20 mg/m^2 on 2 consecutive days, each week for 3 weeks (days 1, 2, 8, 9, 15, and 16) of a 28-day treatment cycle

Cycle 2 and subsequent cycles (if cycle 1 is tolerated): 27 mg/m^2 on 2 consecutive days, each week for 3 weeks (days 1, 2, 8, 9, 15, and 16) of a 28-day treatment cycle. Continue until disease progression or occurrence of unacceptable toxicity.

Dosage adjustment for toxicity:

Hematologic toxicity:

ANC: Grade 3 or 4 neutropenia: Withhold dose; continue at same dose level if fully recovered before next scheduled dose. If recovered to grade 2, reduce dose by one dose level (from 27 mg/m^2 to 20 mg/m^2 or from 20 mg/m^2 to 15 mg/m^2). Consider escalating to the previous dose if reduced dose is tolerated.

Platelets: Grade 4 thrombocytopenia: Withhold dose; continue at same dose level if fully recovered before next scheduled dose. If recovered to grade 3 thrombocytopenia, reduce dose by one dose level (from 27 mg/m^2 to 20 mg/m^2 or from 20 mg/m^2 to 15 mg/m^2). Consider escalating to the previous dose if reduced dose is tolerated.

Nonhematologic toxicity:

Cardiac: Grade 3 or 4, new onset or worsening of congestive heart failure, decreased left ventricular function, or myocardial ischemia: Withhold dose until resolved or at baseline. After resolution, if appropriate to reinitiate, consider restarting at a reduced dose level (from 27 mg/m^2 to 20 mg/m^2 or from 20 mg/m^2 to 15 mg/m^2). Consider escalating to the previous dose if reduced dose is tolerated.

Hepatic: Grade 3 or 4 elevation of bilirubin, transaminases, or other liver abnormalities: Withhold dose until resolved or at baseline. After resolution, if appropriate to reinitiate, consider restarting at a reduced dose level (from 27 mg/m^2 to 20 mg/m^2 or from 20 mg/m^2 to 15 mg/m^2). Consider escalating to the previous dose if reduced dose is tolerated.

Peripheral neuropathy: Grade 3 or 4: Withhold dose until resolved or at baseline. After resolution, if appropriate to reinitiate, restart at prior dose or at a reduced dose level (from 27 mg/m^2 to 20 mg/m^2 or from 20 mg/m^2 to 15 mg/m^2). Consider escalating to the previous dose if reduced dose is tolerated.

Pulmonary toxicity

Pulmonary hypertension: Withhold dose until resolved or at baseline. After resolution, if appropriate to reinitiate, restart at prior dose or at a reduced dose level (from 27 mg/m^2 to 20 mg/m^2 or from 20 mg/m^2 to 15 mg/m^2). Consider escalating to the previous dose if reduced dose is tolerated.

Grade 3 or 4 pulmonary complications: Withhold dose until resolved or at baseline. After resolution, consider restarting (at next scheduled treatment) at a reduced dose level (from 27 mg/m^2 to 20 mg/m^2 or from 20 mg/m^2 to 15 mg/m^2). Consider escalating to the previous dose if reduced dose is tolerated.

Renal: Serum creatinine ≥2 times baseline: Withhold dose until renal function has improved to grade 1 or baseline. If renal toxicity due to carfilzomib, reduce dose at the next scheduled treatment (from 27 mg/m^2 to 20 mg/m^2 or from 20 mg/m^2 to 15 mg/m^2). Consider escalating to the previous dose if reduced dose is tolerated. If toxicity not due to carfilzomib, restart at previous dose.

Tumor lysis syndrome: Interrupt treatment until resolved.

Other grade 3 or 4 nonhematologic toxicities: Withhold dose until resolved or at baseline. After resolution, consider restarting (at next scheduled treatment) at a reduced dose level (from 27 mg/m^2 to 20 mg/m^2 or from 20 mg/m^2 to 15 mg/m^2). Consider escalating to the previous dose if reduced dose is tolerated.

Dosage adjustment in renal impairment: No dosage adjustment provided in manufacturer's labeling; however, results from a phase 2 trial in patients with renal impairment indicate that the pharmacokinetics and safety of carfilzomib were unchanged in this patient population; no dosage adjustment is necessary in patients with baseline dysfunction, including hemodialysis (Harvey, 2012; Niesvizky, 2011). **Note:** Dialysis clearance of carfilzomib has not been studied; per manufacturer labeling, administer postdialysis.

Dosage adjustment in hepatic impairment: No dosage adjustment provided in manufacturer's labeling (has not been studied; patients with ALT or AST ≥3 times ULN and bilirubin ≥2 times ULN were excluded from clinical trials).

Dosing in obesity: *ASCO Guidelines for appropriate chemotherapy dosing in obese adults with cancer:* In general, utilize patient's actual body weight (full weight) for calculation of body surface area- or weight-based dosing, particularly when the intent of therapy is curative; manage regimen-related toxicities in the same manner as for nonobese patients; if a dose reduction is utilized due to toxicity, consider resumption of full weight-based dosing with subsequent cycles, especially if cause of toxicity (eg, hepatic or renal impairment) is resolved (Griggs, 2012). **Note:** According to the manufacturer, patients with a body surface area (BSA) >2.2 m^2 should be dosed based upon a maximum BSA of 2.2 m^2; dose adjustments for weight changes of ≤20% are not necessary.

Administration IV: Administer over 2-10 minutes. Flush line before and after carfilzomib with NS or D_5W. Hazardous agent; use appropriate precautions for handling and disposal (meets NIOSH 2014 criteria).

Hazardous agent; use appropriate precautions for handling and disposal.

Monitoring Parameters CBC with differential and platelets (monitor frequently throughout therapy); renal function, pulmonary function (with new or worsening pulmonary symptoms), liver function tests, serum creatinine. Signs/symptoms of infusion-related reactions, congestive heart failure, tumor lysis syndrome, and peripheral neuropathy.

Dosage Forms

Solution Reconstituted, Intravenous:

Kyprolis: 60 mg (1 ea)

Carglumic Acid (kar GLU mik AS id)

Brand Names: U.S. Carbaglu

Index Terms N-Carbamoyl-L-Glutamic Acid; N-Carbamylglutamate

Pharmacologic Category Antidote; Metabolic Alkalosis Agent; Urea Cycle Disorder (UCD) Treatment Agent

Use Hyperammonemia: Adjunctive treatment of acute hyperammonemia and maintenance therapy of chronic hyperammonemia due to the deficiency of the hepatic enzyme N-acetylglutamate synthase (NAGS) in adult and pediatric patients

Pregnancy Risk Factor C

Dosage Oral: Infants, Children, Adolescents, and Adults:

Acute hyperammonemia: 100 to 250 mg/kg/day given in 2 or 4 divided doses (rounded to the nearest 100 mg for adults); titrate to age-appropriate plasma ammonia levels. Concomitant adjunctive ammonia-lowering therapy recommended.

Chronic hyperammonemia: Usual dose (based on limited data): <100 mg/kg/day given in 2 or 4 divided doses; titrate to age-appropriate plasma ammonia levels

Dosage adjustment in renal impairment: There are no dosage adjustments provided in the manufacturer's labeling.

Dosage adjustment in hepatic impairment: There are no dosage adjustments provided in the manufacturer's labeling.

Additional Information Complete prescribing information should be consulted for additional detail.

Dosage Forms

Tablet, Oral:

Carbaglu: 200 mg

- ◆ **Carimune NF** *see* Immune Globulin *on page 1056*
- ◆ **Caripul (Can)** *see* Epoprostenol *on page 746*
- ◆ **Carisoprodate** *see* Carisoprodol *on page 363*

Carisoprodol (kar eye soe PROE dole)

Brand Names: U.S. Soma

Index Terms Carisoprodate; Isobamate

Pharmacologic Category Skeletal Muscle Relaxant

Additional Appendix Information

Beers Criteria - Potentially Inappropriate Medications for Geriatrics *on page 2271*

Use Short-term (2-3 weeks) treatment of acute musculoskeletal pain

Pregnancy Risk Factor C

Pregnancy Considerations Animal data suggests that carisoprodol crosses placenta and adverse events have been observed in animal studies. Limited postmarketing data with meprobamate (the active metabolite) demonstrate a possible risk for congenital malformations. Use only if benefit outweighs the risk.

Breast-Feeding Considerations Carisoprodol and its active metabolite, meprobamate are excreted into breast milk. Carisoprodol levels in breast milk may be 2-4 times that of maternal plasma levels. The estimated dose to the infant was reported as 6.9% of the weight adjusted maternal dose in one case report (Briggs, 2008) and ~4% of the weight-adjusted maternal dose in another (Nordeng, 2001). In both cases, breast milk production was decreased requiring supplemental formula or cessation of breast-feeding. Other than slight sedation reported in one infant, no symptoms of withdrawal or other adverse events were noted in these two cases. Effects on long-term development are not known. The manufacturer recommends caution be used if carisoprodol is administered to a nursing woman.

Contraindications Hypersensitivity to carisoprodol, carbamates (eg, meprobamate), or any component of the formulation; history of acute intermittent porphyria

Warnings/Precautions Can cause CNS depression, which may impair physical or mental abilities. Concomitant use of other CNS depressants may enhance these effects. Patients must be cautioned about performing tasks which require mental alertness (eg, operating machinery or driving); postmarketing reports of motor vehicle accidents have been associated with use. Effects with other CNS-depressant drugs or ethanol may be potentiated. Use with caution in patients with hepatic/renal dysfunction. Tolerance or drug dependence may result from extended use. Limit use to 2-3 weeks; use caution in patients who may be prone to addiction. May precipitate withdrawal after abrupt cessation of prolonged use. Has been associated (rarely) with seizures in patients with and without seizure history.

Carisoprodol should be used with caution in patients who are poor CYP2C19 metabolizers; poor metabolizers have been shown to have a fourfold increase in exposure to carisoprodol and a 50% reduced exposure to the metabolite meprobamate compared to normal metabolizers. Prevalence of poor metabolizers in the Asian population is ~15% to 20% while that of Caucasians and African-Americans is ~3% to 5%. Potentially significant drug-drug interactions may exist, requiring dose or frequency adjustment, additional monitoring, and/or selection of alternative therapy. Muscle relaxants are poorly tolerated by the elderly due to potent anticholinergic effects, sedation, and risk of fracture. Efficacy is questionable at dosages tolerated by elderly patients; avoid use (Beers Criteria).

Adverse Reactions

Central nervous system: Dizziness, drowsiness

Rare but important or life-threatening: Abdominal cramps, agitation, allergic dermatitis, anaphylaxis, angioedema, ataxia, burning sensation of eyes, depression, drug dependence, dyspnea, epigastric pain, eosinophilia, erythema multiforme, exacerbation of asthma, fixed drug eruption, hallucination, headache, hiccups, hypersensitivity reaction, idiosyncratic reaction (symptoms may include agitation, ataxia, confusion, diplopia, disorientation, dysarthria, euphoria, extreme weakness, muscle twitching, mydriasis, temporary vision loss, and/or transient quadriplegia); insomnia, irritability, leukopenia, nausea, orthostatic hypotension, pancytopenia, paradoxical central nervous system stimulation, pruritus, psychosis, seizure, skin rash, syncope, tachycardia, transient flushing of face, tremor, urticaria, vertigo, vomiting, weakness, withdrawal syndrome (abdominal cramps, headache, insomnia, nausea, seizure)

Drug Interactions

Metabolism/Transport Effects Substrate of CYP2C19 (major); **Note:** Assignment of Major/Minor substrate status based on clinically relevant drug interaction potential

Avoid Concomitant Use

Avoid concomitant use of Carisoprodol with any of the following: Azelastine (Nasal); Orphenadrine; Paraldehyde; Thalidomide

Increased Effect/Toxicity

Carisoprodol may increase the levels/effects of: Alcohol (Ethyl); Azelastine (Nasal); Buprenorphine; CNS Depressants; Hydrocodone; Methotrimeprazine; Metyrosine; Mirtazapine; Orphenadrine; Paraldehyde; Pramipexole; ROPINIRole; Rotigotine; Selective Serotonin Reuptake Inhibitors; Suvorexant; Thalidomide; Zolpidem

The levels/effects of Carisoprodol may be increased by: Aspirin; Brimonidine (Topical); Cannabis; CYP2C19 Inhibitors (Moderate); CYP2C19 Inhibitors (Strong); Doxylamine; Dronabinol; Droperidol; HydrOXYzine; Kava Kava; Luliconazole; Magnesium Sulfate; Methotrimeprazine; Nabilone; Perampanel; Rufinamide; Sodium Oxybate; St Johns Wort; Tapentadol; Tetrahydrocannabinol

Decreased Effect

The levels/effects of Carisoprodol may be decreased by: Aspirin; CYP2C19 Inducers (Strong); Dabrafenib; St Johns Wort

Storage/Stability Store at 20°C to 25°C (68°F to 77°F).

Mechanism of Action Precise mechanism is not yet clear, but many effects have been ascribed to its central depressant actions. In animals, carisoprodol blocks interneuronal activity and depresses polysynaptic neuron transmission in the spinal cord and reticular formation of the brain. It is also metabolized to meprobamate, which has anxiolytic and sedative effects.

Pharmacodynamics/Kinetics
Onset of action: Rapid
Duration: 4-6 hours
Protein binding: Carisoprodol: <70%; Meprobamate: <25% (Olsen, 1994)
Metabolism: Hepatic, via CYP2C19 to active metabolite (meprobamate)
Half-life elimination: Carisoprodol: ~2 hours; Meprobamate: ~10 hours
Time to peak, plasma: 1.5-2 hours
Excretion: Urine, as metabolite

Dosage Note: Carisoprodol should only be used for short periods (2-3 weeks) due to lack of evidence of effectiveness with prolonged use.
Oral: Adolescents ≥16 years and Adults: 250-350 mg 3 times daily and at bedtime
Dosing adjustment in renal impairment: No dosage adjustment provided in manufacturer's labeling (has not been studied); carisoprodol undergoes renal excretion and should be used with caution.
Dialysis: Removed by hemo- and peritoneal dialysis
Dosing adjustment in hepatic impairment: No dosage adjustment provided in manufacturer's labeling (has not been studied); carisoprodol undergoes hepatic metabolism and should be used with caution.

Dietary Considerations May be taken with or without food.

Administration Administer with or without food.

Monitoring Parameters CNS effects (eg, mental status, excessive drowsiness); relief of pain and/or muscle spasm; signs of misuse, abuse, and addiction

Dosage Forms
Tablet, Oral:
Soma: 250 mg, 350 mg
Generic: 250 mg, 350 mg

Carisoprodol and Aspirin
(kar eye soe PROE dole & AS pir in)

Index Terms Aspirin and Carisoprodol; Soma Compound

Pharmacologic Category Skeletal Muscle Relaxant

Use Relief of discomfort associated with acute, painful skeletal muscle conditions

Pregnancy Risk Factor C

Dosage Oral:
Children ≥16 years and Adults: Acute skeletal muscle pain: 1-2 tablets 4 times/day for 2-3 weeks (maximum: 8 tablets/24 hours)
Elderly: Avoid use in the elderly due to risk of orthostatic hypotension and CNS depression
Dosing adjustment in renal impairment: Use in renal impairment has not been studied; use with caution
Dosing adjustment in hepatic impairment: Use in hepatic impairment has not been studied; use with caution

Additional Information Complete prescribing information should be consulted for additional detail.

Dosage Forms
Tablet: Carisoprodol 200 mg and aspirin 325 mg

Carisoprodol, Aspirin, and Codeine
(kar eye soe PROE dole, AS pir in, and KOE deen)

Index Terms Aspirin, Carisoprodol, and Codeine; Codeine, Aspirin, and Carisoprodol; Soma Compound w/Codeine

Pharmacologic Category Skeletal Muscle Relaxant

Use Skeletal muscle relaxant

Pregnancy Risk Factor C

Dosage Oral:
Adults: 1 or 2 tablets 4 times daily (maximum: 8 tablets per day); treatment should be temporary (2-3 weeks)
Elderly: Avoid or use with caution in the elderly (>65 years of age); adverse effects (eg, orthostatic hypotension and CNS depression) may be potentiated.
Dosage adjustment in renal impairment: No dosage adjustment provided in manufacturer's labeling.
Dosage adjustment in hepatic impairment: No dosage adjustment provided in manufacturer's labeling.

Additional Information Complete prescribing information should be consulted for additional detail.

Dosage Forms
Tablet: Carisoprodol 200 mg, aspirin 325 mg, and codeine 16 mg

- **Carmol [OTC]** *see* Urea *on page 2114*
- **Carmol 10 [OTC]** *see* Urea *on page 2114*
- **Carmol 20 [OTC]** *see* Urea *on page 2114*
- **Carmol-HC® [DSC]** *see* Urea and Hydrocortisone *on page 2115*

Carmustine (kar MUS teen)

Brand Names: U.S. BiCNU; Gliadel Wafer

Brand Names: Canada BiCNU; Gliadel Wafer

Index Terms BCNU; bis(chloroethyl) nitrosourea; bis-chloronitrosourea; Carmustine Polymer Wafer; Carmustinum; WR-139021

Pharmacologic Category Antineoplastic Agent, Alkylating Agent; Antineoplastic Agent, Alkylating Agent (Nitrosourea)

Use
Injection: Treatment of brain tumors (glioblastoma, brainstem glioma, medulloblastoma, astrocytoma, ependymoma, and metastatic brain tumors), multiple myeloma, Hodgkin lymphoma (relapsed or refractory), non-Hodgkin lymphomas (relapsed or refractory)
Wafer (implant): Adjunct to surgery in patients with recurrent glioblastoma multiforme; adjunct to surgery and radiation in patients with newly-diagnosed high-grade malignant glioma

Pregnancy Risk Factor D

Pregnancy Considerations Adverse events have been observed in animal reproduction studies. Carmustine can cause fetal harm if administered to a pregnant woman. Women of childbearing potential should avoid becoming pregnant while on treatment.

Breast-Feeding Considerations It is not known if carmustine is excreted in breast milk. Due to the potential for serious adverse reactions in the nursing infant, the manufacturer recommends breast-feeding be discontinued during treatment.

Contraindications Hypersensitivity to carmustine or any component of the formulation

Warnings/Precautions Hazardous agent - use appropriate precautions for handling and disposal (NIOSH 2014 [group 1]).

[U.S. Boxed Warning]: Injection: Bone marrow suppression (primarily thrombocytopenia and leukopenia) is the major carmustine toxicity; generally is delayed. Monitor blood counts weekly for at least 6 weeks after administration. Myelosuppression is cumulative. When given at the FDA-approved doses, treatment should not be administered less than 6 weeks apart. Consider nadir blood counts from prior dose for dosage adjustment. May cause bleeding (due to thrombocytopenia) or infections (due to neutropenia); monitor closely. Patients must have platelet counts >100,000/mm^3 and leukocytes >4000/mm^3 for a repeat dose. Anemia may occur (less common and less severe than leukopenia or thrombocytopenia). Long-term use is associated with the development of secondary malignancies (acute leukemias and bone marrow dysplasias).

[U.S. Boxed Warnings]: Injection: Dose-related pulmonary toxicity may occur; patients receiving cumulative doses >1400 mg/m^2 are at higher risk. Delayed onset of pulmonary fibrosis (may be fatal) has occurred in children up to 17 years after treatment; this occurred in ages 1 to 16 for the treatment of intracranial tumors; cumulative doses ranged from 770-1800 mg/m^2 (in combination with cranial radiotherapy). Pulmonary toxicity is characterized by pulmonary infiltrates and/or fibrosis and has been reported from 9 days to 43 months after nitrosourea treatment (including carmustine). Although pulmonary toxicity generally occurs in patients who have received prolonged treatment, pulmonary fibrosis has been reported with cumulative doses <1400 mg/m^2. In addition to high cumulative doses, other risk factors for pulmonary toxicity include history of lung disease and baseline predicted forced vital capacity (FVC) or carbon monoxide diffusing capacity (DL_{CO}) <70%. Baseline and periodic pulmonary function tests are recommended. For high-dose treatment (transplant; off-label dose), acute lung injury may occur ~1 to 3 months post transplant; advise patients to contact their transplant physician for dyspnea, cough, or fever; interstitial pneumonia may be managed with a course of corticosteroids. Children are at higher risk for delayed pulmonary toxicity.

Carmustine is associated with a moderate to high emetic potential (dose-related); antiemetics are recommended to prevent nausea and vomiting (Basch, 2011; Dupuis, 2011). Potentially significant drug-drug interactions may exist, requiring dose or frequency adjustment, additional monitoring, and/or selection of alternative therapy. Injection site burning and local tissue reactions, including swelling, pain, erythema, and necrosis have been reported. Monitor infusion site closely for infiltration or injection site reactions. Reversible increases in transaminases, bilirubin and alkaline phosphatase have been reported (rare); monitor liver function tests periodically during treatment. Renal failure, progressive azotemia, and decreased kidney size have been reported in patients who have received large cumulative doses or prolonged treatment (renal toxicity has also been reported in patients who have received lower cumulative doses); monitor renal function tests periodically during treatment. Off-label administration (intraarterial intracarotid route) has been associated with ocular toxicity. Consider initiating treatment at the lower end of the dose range in the elderly. Diluent contains ethanol. With wafer implantation, monitor closely for known craniotomy-related complications (seizure, intracranial infection, abnormal wound healing, brain edema); intracerebral mass effect (unresponsive to corticosteroids) has been reported; may lead to brain herniation; avoid communication between the resection cavity and the ventricular system to prevent wafer migration; communications larger than the wafer should be closed prior to implantation; wafer migration may cause obstructive hydrocephalus. **[U.S. Boxed Warning]: Injection: Should be administered under the supervision of an experienced cancer chemotherapy physician.**

Adverse Reactions

IV:

Cardiovascular: Arrhythmia (with high doses), chest pain, flushing (with rapid infusion), hypotension, tachycardia
Central nervous system: Ataxia, dizziness
Central nervous system: Ethanol intoxication (with high doses), headache
Dermatologic: Hyperpigmentation/skin burning (after skin contact)
Gastrointestinal: Nausea (common; dose related), vomiting (common; dose related), mucositis (with high doses), toxic enterocolitis (with high doses)
Hematologic: Leukopenia (common; onset: 5-6 weeks; recovery: after 1-2 weeks), thrombocytopenia (common: onset: ~4 weeks; recovery: after 1-2 weeks), anemia, neutropenic fever, secondary malignancies (acute leukemia, bone marrow dysplasias)
Hepatic: Alkaline phosphatase increased, bilirubin increased, hepatic sinusoidal obstruction syndrome (SOS; veno-occlusive disease; with high doses), transaminases increased
Local: Injection site reactions (burning, erythema, necrosis, pain, swelling)
Ocular: Conjunctival suffusion (with rapid infusion), neuroretinitis
Renal: Kidney size decreased, progressive azotemia, renal failure
Respiratory: Interstitial pneumonitis (with high doses), pulmonary fibrosis, pulmonary hypoplasia, pulmonary infiltrates
Miscellaneous: Allergic reaction, infection (with high doses)

Wafer:

Cardiovascular: Chest pain, deep thrombophlebitis, facial edema
Central nervous system: Anxiety, ataxia, brain edema, confusion, depression, facial paralysis, fever, hallucination, headache, hypesthesia, intracranial hypertension, meningitis, pain, seizure (grand mal), somnolence, speech disorder
Dermatologic: Abnormal wound healing, rash
Endocrine: Diabetes
Gastrointestinal: Abdominal pain, constipation, diarrhea, nausea, vomiting
Genitourinary: Urinary tract infection
Hematologic: Hemorrhage
Local: Abscess
Neuromuscular & skeletal: Back pain, weakness

Rare but important or life-threatening: Abnormal thinking, allergic reaction, amnesia, aspiration pneumonia, cerebral hemorrhage, cerebral infarction, coma, cyst formation, diplopia, dizziness, dysphagia, eye pain, fecal incontinence, gastrointestinal hemorrhage, hydrocephalus, hyperglycemia, hyper-/hypotension, hypokalemia, hyponatremia, insomnia, leukocytosis, monoplegia, neck pain, paranoia, peripheral edema, sepsis, thrombocytopenia, urinary incontinence, visual field defect

Drug Interactions

Metabolism/Transport Effects None known.

Avoid Concomitant Use

Avoid concomitant use of Carmustine with any of the following: BCG; CloZAPine; Dipyrone; Natalizumab; Pimecrolimus; Tacrolimus (Topical); Tofacitinib; Vaccines (Live)

Increased Effect/Toxicity

Carmustine may increase the levels/effects of: CloZAPine; Leflunomide; Natalizumab; Tofacitinib; Vaccines (Live)

The levels/effects of Carmustine may be increased by: Cimetidine; Denosumab; Dipyrone; Melphalan; Pimecrolimus; Roflumilast; Tacrolimus (Topical); Trastuzumab

Decreased Effect

Carmustine may decrease the levels/effects of: BCG; Coccidioides immitis Skin Test; Sipuleucel-T; Vaccines (Inactivated); Vaccines (Live)

The levels/effects of Carmustine may be decreased by: Echinacea

Preparation for Administration Hazardous agent; use appropriate precautions for handling and disposal (NIOSH 2014 [group 1]).

Injection: Reconstitute initially with 3 mL of supplied diluent (dehydrated alcohol injection, USP); then further dilute with SWFI (27 mL), this provides a concentration of 3.3 mg/mL in ethanol 10%; protect from light; further dilute for infusion with D_5W using a non-PVC container (eg, glass or polyolefin).

Storage/Stability

Injection: Store intact vials and provided diluent under refrigeration at 2°C to 8°C (36°F to 46°F).

Reconstituted solutions are stable for 24 hours refrigerated (2°C to 8°C) and protected from light. Examine reconstituted vials for crystal formation prior to use. If crystals are observed, they may be redissolved by warming the vial to room temperature with agitation.

Solutions diluted to a concentration of 0.2 mg/mL in D_5W are stable for 8 hours at room temperature (25°C) in glass and protected from light. Although the manufacturer recommends only glass containers be used, stability of a 1 mg/mL solution in D_5W has also been demonstrated for up to 6 hours (with a 6% to 7% loss of potency) in polyolefin containers (Trissel, 2006).

Wafer: Store at or below -20°C (-4°F). Unopened foil pouches may be kept at room temperature for up to 6 hours.

Mechanism of Action Interferes with the normal function of DNA and RNA by alkylation and cross-linking the strands of DNA and RNA, and by possible protein modification; may also inhibit enzyme processes by carbamylation of amino acids in protein

Pharmacodynamics/Kinetics

Distribution: 3.3 L/kg; readily crosses blood-brain barrier producing CSF levels >50% of blood plasma levels; highly lipid soluble

Metabolism: Rapidly hepatic; forms active metabolites

Half-life elimination: Biphasic: Initial: 1.4 minutes; Secondary: 20 minutes (active metabolites: Plasma half-life of 67 hours)

Excretion: Urine (~60% to 70%) within 96 hours; lungs (6% to 10% as CO_2)

Dosage Note: Carmustine is associated with a moderate to high emetic potential (dose-related); antiemetics are recommended to prevent nausea and vomiting (Basch, 2011; Dupuis, 2011).

IV: Adults: Brain tumors, Hodgkin lymphoma, multiple myeloma, non-Hodgkin's lymphoma (per manufacturer labeling): 150-200 mg/m^2 every 6 weeks or 75 to 100 mg/m^2/day for 2 days every 6 weeks

Indication-specific dosing: IV:

Brain tumor, primary (off-label doses):

80 mg/m^2/day for 3 days every 8 weeks for 6 cycles (Brandes, 2004)

200 mg/m^2 every 8 weeks [maximum cumulative dose: 1500 mg/m^2] (Selker, 2002)

Hodgkin lymphoma, relapsed or refractory (off-label dose): Mini-BEAM regimen: 60 mg/m^2 day 1 every 4 to 6 weeks (in combination with etoposide, cytarabine, and melphalan) (Colwill, 1995; Martin, 2001)

Multiple myeloma, relapsed, refractory (off-label dose): VBMCP regimen: 20 mg/m^2 day 1 every 35 days (in combination with vincristine, melphalan, cyclophosphamide, and prednisone) (Kyle, 2006; Oken, 1997)

Stem cell or bone marrow transplant, autologous (off-label use):

BEAM regimen: 300 mg/m^2 6 days prior to transplant (in combination with etoposide, cytarabine, and melphalan) (Chopra, 1993; Linch, 2010)

CBV regimen: 600 mg/m^2 3 days prior to transplant (in combination with cyclophosphamide and etoposide) (Reece, 1991)

Implantation (wafer): Adults: Recurrent glioblastoma multiforme, newly-diagnosed high-grade malignant glioma: 8 wafers placed in the resection cavity (total dose 61.6 mg); should the size and shape not accommodate 8 wafers, the maximum number of wafers allowed (up to 8) should be placed

Topical: Mycosis fungoides, early stage (off-label use; Zackheim, 2003):

Ointment (10 mg/100 grams petrolatum): Apply (with gloves) once daily to affected areas

Solution (0.2% solution in alcohol; dilute 5 mL in 60 mL water): Apply (with gloves) once daily to affected areas

Dosing adjustments for hematologic toxicity: Based on nadir counts with previous dose (manufacturer's labeling). IV:

If leukocytes >3000/mm^3 and platelets >75,000/mm^3: Administer 100% of dose

If leukocytes 2000-2999/mm^3 or platelets 25,000-74,999/mm^3: Administer 70% of dose

If leukocytes <2000/mm^3 or platelets <25,000/mm^3: Administer 50% of dose

Dosing adjustment in renal impairment: IV: There are no dosage adjustments provided in the manufacturer's labeling. The following dosage adjustments have been used by some clinicians (Kintzel, 1995):

CrCl 46 to 60 mL/minute: Administer 80% of dose

CrCl 31 to 45 mL/minute: Administer 75% of dose

CrCl ≤30 mL/minute: Consider use of alternative drug

Dosing adjustment in hepatic impairment: Dosage adjustment may be necessary; however, no specific guidelines are available.

Dosing in obesity:

*American Society of Clinical Oncology (ASCO) Guidelines for appropriate chemotherapy dosing in obese adults with cancer (**Note:** Excludes HSCT dosing):* Utilize patient's actual body weight (full weight) for calculation of body surface area- or weight-based dosing, particularly when the intent of therapy is curative; manage regimen-related toxicities in the same manner as for nonobese patients; if a dose reduction is utilized due to toxicity, consider resumption of full weight-based dosing with subsequent cycles, especially if cause of toxicity (eg, hepatic or renal impairment) is resolved (Griggs, 2012).

American Society for Blood and Marrow Transplantation (ASBMT) practice guideline committee position statement on chemotherapy dosing in obesity: Utilize actual body weight (full weight) for calculation of body surface area in carmustine dosing for hematopoietic stem cell transplant conditioning regimens in adult patients weighing ≤120% of their ideal body weight (IBW). In patients weighing >120% IBW, utilize adjusted body weight 25% (ABW25) to calculate BSA (Bubalo, 2014).

ABW25: Adjusted wt (kg) = Ideal body weight (kg) + 0.25 [actual wt (kg) - ideal body weight (kg)]

Administration

Carmustine is associated with a moderate to high emetic potential (dose-related); antiemetics are recommended to prevent nausea and vomiting (Basch, 2011; Dupuis, 2011).

Injection: Irritant (alcohol-based diluent). Significant absorption to PVC containers; should be prepared in either glass or polyolefin containers. Infuse over 2 hours (infusions <2 hours may lead to injection site pain or burning); infuse through a free-flowing saline or dextrose infusion, or administer through a central catheter to alleviate venous pain/irritation.

High-dose carmustine (transplant dose; off-label use): Infuse over a least 2 hours to avoid excessive flushing, agitation, and hypotension; was infused over 1 hour in some trials (Chopra, 1993). **High-dose carmustine may be fatal if not followed by stem cell rescue.** Monitor vital signs frequently during infusion; patients should be supine during infusion and may require the Trendelenburg position, fluid support, and vasopressor support.

Implant: Double glove before handling; outer gloves should be discarded as chemotherapy waste after handling wafers. Any wafer or remnant that is removed upon repeat surgery should be discarded as chemotherapy waste. The outer surface of the external foil pouch is not sterile. Open pouch gently; avoid pressure on the wafers to prevent breakage. Wafer that are broken in half may be used, however, wafers broken into more than 2 pieces should be discarded in a biohazard container. Oxidized regenerated cellulose (Surgicel) may be placed over the wafer to secure; irrigate cavity prior to closure.

Topical (off-label use): Apply solution with brush or gauze pads; ointment and solution should be applied while wearing gloves to involved areas only; avoid contact with eyes or mouth (Zackheim, 2003).

Hazardous agent; use appropriate precautions for handling and disposal (NIOSH 2014 [group 1]).

Monitoring Parameters CBC with differential and platelet count (weekly for at least 6 weeks after a dose), pulmonary function tests (FVC, DL_{CO}; at baseline and frequently during treatment), liver function (periodically), renal function tests (periodically); monitor blood pressure and vital signs during administration, monitor infusion site for possible infiltration

Wafer: Complications of craniotomy (seizures, intracranial infection, brain edema)

Dosage Forms

Solution Reconstituted, Intravenous:

BiCNU: 100 mg (1 ea)

Wafer, Implant:

Gliadel Wafer: 7.7 mg (8 ea)

◆ **Carmustine Polymer Wafer** *see* Carmustine *on page 364*

◆ **Carmustinum** *see* Carmustine *on page 364*

◆ **Caroguard [OTC]** *see* Beta-Carotene *on page 251*

Carpipramine [INT] (kar PI pra meen)

International Brand Names Prazinil (FR)

Index Terms Carpipramine Hydrochloride

Pharmacologic Category Antianxiety Agent

Reported Use Management of anxiety disorders and psychosis

Dosage Range Adults: Oral: 50 mg 3 times/day; range: 50-400 mg/day

Product Availability Product available in various countries; not currently available in the U.S.

Dosage Forms

Tablet, as hydrochloride: 50 mg

◆ **Carpipramine Hydrochloride** *see* Carpipramine [INT] *on page 367*

◆ **Carrington Antifungal [OTC]** *see* Miconazole (Topical) *on page 1360*

◆ **Carter's Little Pills [OTC] (Can)** *see* Bisacodyl *on page 265*

◆ **Cartia XT** *see* Diltiazem *on page 634*

Carvedilol (KAR ve dil ole)

Brand Names: U.S. Coreg; Coreg CR

Brand Names: Canada Apo-Carvedilol; Auro-Carvedilol; Dom-Carvedilol; JAMP-Carvedilol; Mylan-Carvedilol; Novo-Carvedilol; PMS-Carvedilol; RAN-Carvedilol; ratio-Carvedilol

Pharmacologic Category Antihypertensive; Beta-Blocker With Alpha-Blocking Activity

Use

Hypertension: Management of hypertension.

The 2014 guideline for the management of high blood pressure in adults (Eighth Joint National Committee [JNC 8]) recommends initiation of pharmacologic treatment to lower blood pressure for the following patients (JNC 8 [James, 2013]):

- Patients ≥60 years of age, with systolic blood pressure (SBP) ≥150 mm Hg or diastolic blood pressure (DBP) ≥90 mm Hg. Goal of therapy is SBP <150 mm Hg and DBP <90 mm Hg.
- Patients <60 years of age, with SBP ≥140 mm Hg or DBP ≥90 mm Hg. Goal of therapy is SBP <140 mm Hg and DBP <90 mm Hg.
- Patients ≥18 years of age with diabetes, with SBP ≥140 mm Hg or DBP ≥90 mm Hg. Goal of therapy is SBP <140 mm Hg and DBP <90 mm Hg.
- Patients ≥18 years of age with chronic kidney disease (CKD), with SBP ≥140 mm Hg or DBP ≥90 mm Hg. Goal of therapy is SBP <140 mm Hg and DBP <90 mm Hg.

In patients with CKD, regardless of race or diabetes status, the use of an ACE inhibitor (ACEI) or angiotensin receptor blocker (ARB) as initial therapy is recommended to improve kidney outcomes. In the general non-black population (without CKD) including those with diabetes, initial antihypertensive treatment should consist of a thiazide-type diuretic, calcium channel blocker, ACEI, or ARB. In the general black population (without CKD) including those with diabetes, initial antihypertensive treatment should consist of a thiazide-type diuretic or a calcium channel blocker **instead of** an ACEI or ARB.

Heart failure: Mild to severe chronic heart failure of ischemic or cardiomyopathic origin (usually in addition to standard therapy [eg, diuretics, ACE inhibitors]).

The ACCF/AHA 2013 heart failure guidelines recommend the use of 1 of the 3 beta blockers (ie, bisoprolol, carvedilol, or extended-release metoprolol succinate) for all patients with recent or remote history of MI or ACS and reduced ejection fraction (rEF) to reduce mortality, for all patients with rEF to prevent symptomatic HF (even if no history of MI), and for all patients with current or prior symptoms of HF with reduced ejection fraction (HFrEF), unless contraindicated, to reduce morbidity and mortality (Yancy, 2013).

Left ventricular dysfunction following myocardial infarction (MI): Left ventricular dysfunction following MI (clinically stable with LVEF ≤40%)

Pregnancy Risk Factor C

Pregnancy Considerations Adverse events have been observed in animal reproduction studies. In a cohort study, an increased risk of cardiovascular defects was observed following maternal use of beta-blockers during pregnancy (Lennestål, 2009). Intrauterine growth restriction (IUGR), small placentas, as well as fetal/neonatal bradycardia, hypoglycemia, and/or respiratory depression have been observed following *in utero* exposure to beta-blockers as a class. Adequate facilities for monitoring infants at birth should be available. Untreated chronic maternal hypertension and pre-eclampsia are also associated with adverse events in the fetus, infant, and mother. Carvedilol is not currently recommended for the initial treatment of maternal hypertension during pregnancy (ACOG, 2001; ACOG, 2002).

Breast-Feeding Considerations It is not known if carvedilol is excreted in breast milk. Due to the potential for serious adverse reactions in the nursing infant, the manufacturer recommends a decision be made whether to discontinue nursing or to discontinue the drug, taking into account the importance of treatment to the mother.

Contraindications

Serious hypersensitivity to carvedilol or any component of the formulation; decompensated cardiac failure requiring intravenous inotropic therapy; bronchial asthma or related bronchospastic conditions; second- or third-degree AV block, sick sinus syndrome, and severe bradycardia (except in patients with a functioning artificial pacemaker); cardiogenic shock; severe hepatic impairment

Documentation of allergenic cross-reactivity for drugs alpha/beta adrenergic blocking agents is limited. However, because of similarities in chemical structure and/or pharmacologic actions, the possibility of cross-sensitivity cannot be ruled out with certainty.

Warnings/Precautions Heart failure patients may experience a worsening of renal function (rare); risk factors include ischemic heart disease, diffuse vascular disease, underlying renal dysfunction, and/or systolic BP <100 mm Hg. Initiate cautiously and monitor for possible deterioration in patient status (eg, symptoms of HF). Worsening heart failure or fluid retention may occur during upward titration; dose reduction or temporary discontinuation may be necessary. Adjustment of other medications (ACE inhibitors and/or diuretics) may also be required. Bradycardia may occur; reduce dosage if heart rate drops to <55 beats/minute. Bradycardia may be observed more frequently in elderly patients (>65 years of age); dosage reductions may be necessary.

Symptomatic hypotension with or without syncope may occur with carvedilol (usually within the first 30 days of therapy); close monitoring of patient is required especially with initial dosing and dosing increases; blood pressure must be lowered at a rate appropriate for the patient's clinical condition. Initiation with a low dose, gradual up-titration, and administration with food may help to decrease the occurrence of hypotension or syncope. Advise patients to avoid driving or other hazardous tasks during initiation of therapy due to the risk of syncope. Beta-blocker therapy should not be withdrawn abruptly (particularly in patients with CAD), but gradually tapered to avoid acute tachycardia, hypertension, and/or ischemia. Chronic beta-blocker therapy should not be routinely withdrawn prior to major surgery.

In general, patients with bronchospastic disease should not receive beta-blockers; if used at all, should be used cautiously with close monitoring. May precipitate or aggravate symptoms of arterial insufficiency in patients with PVD; use with caution and monitor for progression of arterial obstruction. Use with caution in patients with diabetes; may potentiate hypoglycemia and/or mask signs and symptoms (eg, sweating, anxiety, tachycardia). In patients with heart failure and diabetes, use of carvedilol may worsen hyperglycemia; may require adjustment of antidiabetic agents. May mask signs of hyperthyroidism (eg, tachycardia); if hyperthyroidism is suspected, carefully manage and monitor; abrupt withdrawal may exacerbate symptoms of hyperthyroidism or precipitate thyroid storm. May induce or exacerbate psoriasis. Use with caution in patients suspected of having Prinzmetal variant angina. Use with caution in patients with myasthenia gravis. Use with caution in patients with mild to moderate hepatic impairment; use is contraindicated in patients with severe impairment. Use with caution in patients with pheochromocytoma; adequate alpha-blockade is required prior to use. Use caution with history of severe anaphylaxis to allergens; patients taking beta-blockers may become more sensitive to repeated challenges. Treatment of anaphylaxis (eg, epinephrine) in patients taking beta-blockers may be ineffective or promote undesirable effects.

Intraoperative floppy iris syndrome has been observed in cataract surgery patients who were on or were previously treated with alpha$_1$-blockers; there appears to be no benefit in discontinuing alpha-blocker therapy prior to surgery. Instruct patients to inform ophthalmologist of carvedilol use when considering eye surgery. Potentially significant interactions may exist, requiring dose or frequency adjustment, additional monitoring, and/or selection of alternative therapy.

Adverse Reactions

Cardiovascular: Angina, AV block, bradycardia, cerebrovascular accident, edema (including generalized, dependent, and peripheral), hyper-/hypotension, hyper-/hypovolemia, orthostatic hypotension, palpitation, syncope

Central nervous system: Depression, dizziness, fatigue, fever, headache, hypoesthesia, hypotonia, insomnia, malaise, somnolence, vertigo, weakness

Endocrine & metabolic: Diabetes mellitus, gout, hypercholesterolemia, hyper-/hypoglycemia, hyponatremia, hyperkalemia, hypertriglyceridemia, hyperuricemia

Gastrointestinal: Abdominal pain, diarrhea, melena, nausea, periodontitis, vomiting, weight gain/loss

Genitourinary: Impotence

Hematologic: Anemia, prothrombin decreased, purpura, thrombocytopenia

Hepatic: Alkaline phosphatase increased, GGT increased, transaminases increased

Neuromuscular & skeletal: Arthralgia, arthritis, back pain, muscle cramps, paresthesia

Ocular: Blurred vision

Renal: Albuminuria, BUN increased, creatinine increased, glycosuria, hematuria, nonprotein nitrogen increased, renal insufficiency

Respiratory: Cough, dyspnea, nasopharyngitis, dyspnea, nasal congestion, pulmonary edema, rales, rhinitis, sinus congestion

Miscellaneous: Allergy, flu-like syndrome, injury, sudden death

Rare but important or life-threatening: Anaphylactoid reaction, alopecia, angioedema, aplastic anemia, amnesia, asthma, bronchospasm, bundle branch block, cholestatic jaundice, concentration decreased, diaphoresis, erythema multiforme, exfoliative dermatitis, GI hemorrhage, HDL decreased, hearing decreased, hyperbilirubinemia, hypersensitivity reaction, hypokalemia, hypokinesia, interstitial pneumonitis, leukopenia, libido decreased, migraine, myocardial ischemia, nervousness, neuralgia, nightmares, pancytopenia, paresis, peripheral ischemia, photosensitivity, pruritus, rash (erythematous, maculopapular, and psoriaform), respiratory alkalosis, seizure, Stevens-Johnson syndrome, tachycardia, tinnitus, toxic epidermal necrolysis, urinary incontinence, urticaria, xerostomia

Drug Interactions

Metabolism/Transport Effects **Substrate** of CYP1A2 (minor), CYP2C9 (minor), CYP2D6 (major), CYP2E1 (minor), CYP3A4 (minor), P-glycoprotein; **Note:** Assignment of Major/Minor substrate status based on clinically relevant drug interaction potential; **Inhibits** P-glycoprotein

Avoid Concomitant Use

Avoid concomitant use of Carvedilol with any of the following: Beta2-Agonists; Bosutinib; Ceritinib; Floctafenine; Methacholine; PAZOPanib; Silodosin; Topotecan; VinCRIStine (Liposomal)

Increased Effect/Toxicity

Carvedilol may increase the levels/effects of: Afatinib; Alpha-/Beta-Agonists (Direct-Acting); Alpha1-Blockers; Alpha2-Agonists; Amifostine; Antihypertensives; Antipsychotic Agents (Phenothiazines); Bosutinib; Bradycardia-Causing Agents; Brentuximab Vedotin; Bupivacaine; Cardiac Glycosides; Ceritinib; Cholinergic Agonists; Colchicine; CycloSPORINE (Systemic); Dabigatran Etexilate; Digoxin; Disopyramide; DOXOrubicin (Conventional); DULoxetine; Edoxaban; Ergot Derivatives; Everolimus; Fingolimod; Grass Pollen Allergen Extract (5 Grass Extract); Hypotensive Agents; Insulin; Lacosamide; Ledipasvir; Levodopa; Lidocaine (Systemic); Lidocaine (Topical); Mepivacaine; Methacholine; Midodrine; Naloxegol; Obinutuzumab; PAZOPanib; P-glycoprotein/ABCB1 Substrates; Prucalopride; Rifaximin; RisperiDONE; RiTUXimab; Rivaroxaban; Silodosin; Sulfonylureas; Topotecan; VinCRIStine (Liposomal)

The levels/effects of Carvedilol may be increased by: Abiraterone Acetate; Acetylcholinesterase Inhibitors; Alpha2-Agonists; Aminoquinolines (Antimalarial); Amiodarone; Anilidopiperidine Opioids; Antipsychotic Agents (Phenothiazines); Barbiturates; Bretylium; Brimonidine (Topical); Calcium Channel Blockers (Dihydropyridine); Calcium Channel Blockers (Nondihydropyridine); Cimetidine; Cobicistat; CYP2C9 Inhibitors (Moderate); CYP2C9 Inhibitors (Strong); CYP2D6 Inhibitors (Moderate); CYP2D6 Inhibitors (Strong); Darunavir; Diazoxide; Digoxin; Dipyridamole; Disopyramide; Dronedarone; Floctafenine; Herbs (Hypotensive Properties); MAO Inhibitors; NiCARdipine; Nicorandil; Peginterferon Alfa-2b; Pentoxifylline; P-glycoprotein/ABCB1 Inhibitors; Phosphodiesterase 5 Inhibitors; Propafenone; Prostacyclin Analogues; Regorafenib; Reserpine; Selective Serotonin Reuptake Inhibitors; Tofacitinib

Decreased Effect

Carvedilol may decrease the levels/effects of: Beta2-Agonists; Theophylline Derivatives

The levels/effects of Carvedilol may be decreased by: Barbiturates; Herbs (Hypertensive Properties); Methylphenidate; Nonsteroidal Anti-Inflammatory Agents; Peginterferon Alfa-2b; P-glycoprotein/ABCB1 Inducers; Rifamycin Derivatives; Yohimbine

Food Interactions Food decreases rate but not extent of absorption. Management: Administration with food minimizes risks of orthostatic hypotension.

Storage/Stability

Coreg: Store at <30°C (<86°F). Protect from moisture.

Coreg CR: Store at 25°C (77°F); excursions permitted to 15°C to 30°C (59°F to 86°F). Protect from light.

Mechanism of Action As a racemic mixture, carvedilol has nonselective beta-adrenoreceptor and alpha-adrenergic blocking activity. No intrinsic sympathomimetic activity has been documented. Associated effects in hypertensive patients include reduction of cardiac output, exercise- or beta-agonist-induced tachycardia, reduction of reflex orthostatic tachycardia, vasodilation, decreased peripheral vascular resistance (especially in standing position), decreased renal vascular resistance, reduced plasma renin activity, and increased levels of atrial natriuretic peptide. In CHF, associated effects include decreased pulmonary capillary wedge pressure, decreased pulmonary artery pressure, decreased heart rate, decreased systemic vascular resistance, increased stroke volume index, and decreased right arterial pressure (RAP).

Pharmacodynamics/Kinetics

Onset of action: Antihypertensive effect: 30 minutes

Peak antihypertensive effect: ~1 to 2 hours

Absorption: Rapid and extensive; delayed with food

Distribution: V_d: 115 L

Protein binding: >98%, primarily to albumin

Metabolism: Extensively hepatic, via CYP2C9, 2D6, 3A4, 2C19, 1A2, and 2E1 (2% excreted unchanged); three active metabolites (4-hydroxyphenyl metabolite is 13 times more potent than parent drug for beta-blockade); first-pass effect; plasma concentrations in the elderly and those with cirrhotic liver disease are 50% and 4 to 7 times higher, respectively

Bioavailability: Immediate release: ~25% to 35% (due to significant first-pass metabolism); Extended release: ~85% of immediate release; high-fat meal increases AUC and C_{max} ~20%

Half-life elimination: 7 to 10 hours

Time to peak, plasma: Extended release: ~5 hours

Excretion: Primarily feces

Dosage Oral: Adults: Reduce dosage if heart rate drops to <55 beats/minute.

Hypertension:

Immediate release: 6.25 mg twice daily; if tolerated, dose should be maintained for 1 to 2 weeks, then increased to 12.5 mg twice daily. If necessary, dosage may be increased to a maximum of 25 mg twice daily after 1 to 2 weeks. Usual dosage range (ASH/ISH [Weber, 2014]): 6.25 to 25 mg twice daily.

Extended release: Initial: 20 mg once daily, if tolerated, dose should be maintained for 1 to 2 weeks then increased to 40 mg once daily if necessary; if this dose is tolerated, maintain for 1 to 2 weeks and then if necessary increase to 80 mg once daily; maximum dose: 80 mg once daily

Heart failure: **Note:** Initiate only in stable patients or hospitalized patients after volume status has been optimized and IV diuretics, vasodilators, and inotropic agents have all been successfully discontinued. Caution should be used when initiating in patients who required inotropes during their hospital course. Increase dose gradually and monitor for congestive signs and symptoms of HF making every effort to achieve target dose shown to be effective (ACCF/AHA [Yancy, 2013]; HFSA [Lindenfeld, 2010]; Packer, 1996)

Immediate release: 3.125 mg twice daily for 2 weeks; if this dose is tolerated, may increase to 6.25 mg twice daily. Double the dose every 2 weeks to the highest dose tolerated by patient. (Prior to initiating therapy, other heart failure medications should be stabilized and fluid retention minimized.)

Maximum recommended dose:

Mild-to-moderate heart failure:

<85 kg: 25 mg twice daily

>85 kg: 50 mg twice daily

Severe heart failure: 25 mg twice daily (Packer, 2001)

Extended release: Initial: 10 mg once daily for 2 weeks; if the dose is tolerated, increase dose to 20 mg, 40 mg, and 80 mg over successive intervals of at least 2 weeks. Maintain on lower dose if higher dose is not tolerated. **Note:** The 2013 ACCF/AHA heart failure guidelines recommend a maximum dose of 80 mg once daily (Yancy, 2013).

Left ventricular dysfunction following MI: **Note**: Should be initiated only after patient is hemodynamically stable and fluid retention has been minimized.

Immediate release: Initial 3.125 to 6.25 mg twice daily; increase dosage incrementally (ie, from 6.25 to 12.5 mg twice daily) at intervals of 3 to 10 days, based on tolerance, to a target dose of 25 mg twice daily. **Note:** The 2013 ACCF/AHA heart failure guidelines recommend a maximum dose of 50 mg twice daily (Yancy, 2013).

Extended release: Initial: 10 to 20 mg once daily; increase dosage incrementally at intervals of 3 to 10 days, based on tolerance, to a target dose of 80 mg once daily.

Angina pectoris (off-label use): Immediate release: 25 to 50 mg twice daily

Atrial fibrillation (rate control) (off-label use): Usual maintenance dose: 3.125 to 25 mg twice daily (AHA/ACC/HRS [January, 2014]). In patients with heart failure, the initial dose of 3.125 mg twice daily may be increased at 2-week intervals to a target dose of 25 mg twice daily (50 mg twice daily for patients weighing >85 kg) (Khand, 2003)

Elderly: Hypertension: Consider lower initial dose and titrate to response (Aronow, 2011)

Conversion from immediate release to extended release (Coreg CR):

Current dose immediate release tablets 3.125 mg twice daily: Convert to extended release capsules 10 mg once daily

Current dose immediate release tablets 6.25 mg twice daily: Convert to extended release capsules 20 mg once daily

Current dose immediate release tablets 12.5 mg twice daily: Convert to extended release capsules 40 mg once daily

Current dose immediate release tablets 25 mg twice daily: Convert to extended release capsules 80 mg once daily

Dosage adjustment in renal impairment: No dosage adjustment necessary

Dosage adjustment in hepatic impairment:

Mild to moderate impairment: There are no dosage adjustments provided in the manufacturer's labeling.

Severe impairment: Use is contraindicated.

Dietary Considerations Should be taken with food to minimize the risk of orthostatic hypotension.

Administration Administer with food to minimize the risk of orthostatic hypotension. Extended-release capsules and its contents should not be crushed, chewed, or divided. Capsules may be opened and its contents sprinkled on applesauce for immediate use.

Monitoring Parameters Heart rate, blood pressure (base need for dosage increase on trough blood pressure measurements and for tolerance on standing systolic pressure 1 hour after dosing); renal studies, BUN, liver function; blood glucose in diabetics; in patients with increased risk for developing renal dysfunction, monitor during dosage titration.

Dosage Forms

Capsule Extended Release 24 Hour, Oral:

Coreg CR: 10 mg, 20 mg, 40 mg, 80 mg

Tablet, Oral:

Coreg: 3.125 mg, 6.25 mg, 12.5 mg, 25 mg

Generic: 3.125 mg, 6.25 mg, 12.5 mg, 25 mg

Dosage Forms: Canada Note: Refer to Dosage Forms. Extended-release capsules are not available in Canada.

Extemporaneous Preparations A 1.25 mg/mL carvedilol oral suspension may be made with tablets and one of two different vehicles (Ora-Blend or 1:1 mixture of Ora-Sweet and Ora-Plus). Crush five 25 mg tablets in a mortar and reduce to a fine powder; add 15 mL of purified water and mix to a uniform paste. Mix while adding chosen vehicle in incremental proportions to almost 100 mL; transfer to a calibrated amber bottle, rinse mortar with vehicle, and add quantity of vehicle sufficient to make 100 mL. Label "shake well". Stable for 84 days when stored in amber prescription bottles at room temperature (Loyd, 2006).

Carvedilol oral liquid suspensions (0.1 mg/mL and 1.67 mg/mL) made from tablets, water, Ora-Plus, and Ora-Sweet were stable for 12 weeks when stored in glass amber bottles at room temperature (25°C). Use one 3.125 mg tablet for the 0.1 mg/mL suspension or two 25 mg tablets for the 1.67 mg/mL suspension; grind the tablet(s) and compound a mixture with 5 mL of water, 15 mL Ora-Plus, and 10 mL Ora-Sweet. Final volume of each suspension: 30 mL; label "shake well" (data on file, GlaxoSmithKline, Philadelphia, PA: DOF #132 [**Note:** Manufacturer no longer disseminates this document]).

Loyd A Jr, "Carvedilol 1.25 mg/mL Oral Suspension," *Int J Pharm Compounding*, 2006, 10(3):220.

◆ **Casodex** *see* Bicalutamide *on page 262*

Caspofungin (kas poe FUN jin)

Brand Names: U.S. Cancidas

Brand Names: Canada Cancidas®

Index Terms Caspofungin Acetate

Pharmacologic Category Antifungal Agent, Parenteral; Echinocandin

Use Treatment of invasive *Aspergillus* infections in patients who are refractory or intolerant of other therapies; treatment of candidemia and other *Candida* infections (intra-abdominal abscesses, peritonitis, pleural space); treatment of esophageal candidiasis; empirical treatment for presumed fungal infections in febrile neutropenic patients

Pregnancy Risk Factor C

Pregnancy Considerations Adverse events have been observed in animal reproduction studies. When treatment of invasive *Aspergillus* or *Candida* infections is needed during pregnancy, other agents are preferred (DHHS [adult] 2014; Pappas 2009). Use may be considered in HIV-infected pregnant women with invasive *Aspergillus* or *Candida* infections when refractory to other agents (DHHS [adult] 2014)

Breast-Feeding Considerations It is not known if caspofungin is excreted in breast milk. The manufacturer recommends that caution be exercised when administering caspofungin to nursing women.

Contraindications Hypersensitivity to caspofungin or any component of the formulation

Warnings/Precautions Anaphylaxis and histamine-related reactions (eg, angioedema, facial swelling, bronchospasm, rash, sensation of warmth) have been reported. Discontinue if anaphylaxis occurs; consider discontinuation if histamine-related reactions occur. Administer supportive treatment if needed. Concurrent use of cyclosporine should be limited to patients for whom benefit outweighs risk, due to a high frequency of hepatic transaminase elevations observed during concurrent use. Potentially significant drug-drug interactions may exist, requiring dose or frequency adjustment, additional monitoring, and/or selection of alternative therapy. Use caution in hepatic impairment; increased transaminases and rare cases of liver impairment (including failure and hepatitis) have been reported in pediatric and adult patients. Monitor liver function tests during therapy; if tests become abnormal or worsen, consider discontinuation. Dosage reduction required in adults with moderate hepatic impairment; safety and efficacy have not been established in children with any degree of hepatic impairment and adults with severe hepatic impairment.

Adverse Reactions

Cardiovascular: Hypertension, hypotension, peripheral edema, tachycardia

Central nervous system: Chills, headache

Dermatologic: Erythema, pruritus, skin rash

Endocrine & metabolic: Hyperglycemia, hypokalemia, hypomagnesemia

Gastrointestinal: Abdominal pain, diarrhea, gastric irritation, nausea, vomiting

Hematologic & oncologic: Anemia, decreased hematocrit, decreased hemoglobin, decreased white blood cell count

Hepatic: Decreased serum albumin, increased serum alkaline phosphatase increased, increased serum ALT, increased serum AST, increased serum bilirubin

Immunologic: Graft versus host disease (infants, children, and adolescents

Infection: Sepsis
Local: Catheter infection, localized phlebitis
Renal: Hematuria, increased blood urea nitrogen, increased serum creatinine
Respiratory: Cough, dyspnea, pleural effusion, pneumonia, rales, respiratory distress, respiratory failure
Miscellaneous: Fever, infusion related reaction, septic shock
Rare but important or life-threatening: Abdominal distention, adult respiratory distress syndrome, anaphylaxis, anorexia, anxiety, arthralgia, atrial fibrillation, back pain, bacteremia, blood coagulation disorder, cardiac arrest, confusion, constipation, decreased appetite, decubitus ulcer, depression, dizziness, drowsiness, dyspepsia, dystonia, edema, epistaxis, erythema multiforme, fatigue, febrile neutropenia, flushing, hematuria, hepatic failure, hepatitis, hepatomegaly, hepatotoxicity, histamine release (including facial swelling, bronchospasm, sensation of warmth), hypercalcemia, hyperkalemia, hypervolemia, hypoxia, increased gamma-glutamyl transferase, infusion site reaction (pain/pruritus/swelling), insomnia, limb pain, myocardial infarction, nephrotoxicity (serum creatinine ≥2 x baseline value or ≥1 mg/dL in patients with serum creatinine above ULN range), pancreatitis, pulmonary edema, pulmonary infiltrates, renal failure, seizure, Stevens-Johnson syndrome, tachypnea, thrombocytopenia, tremor, urinary tract infection, urticaria, weakness

Drug Interactions

Metabolism/Transport Effects None known.

Avoid Concomitant Use

Avoid concomitant use of Caspofungin with any of the following: Saccharomyces boulardii

Increased Effect/Toxicity

The levels/effects of Caspofungin may be increased by: CycloSPORINE (Systemic)

Decreased Effect

Caspofungin may decrease the levels/effects of: Saccharomyces boulardii; Tacrolimus (Systemic)

The levels/effects of Caspofungin may be decreased by: Inducers of Drug Clearance; Rifampin

Preparation for Administration Bring refrigerated vial to room temperature. Reconstitute vials using 10.8 mL 0.9% sodium chloride for injection, SWFI, or bacteriostatic water for injection, resulting in a concentration of 5 mg/mL for the 50 mg vial, and 7 mg/mL for the 70 mg vial (vials contain overfill). Mix gently to dissolve until clear solution is formed; do not use if cloudy or contains particles. Solution should be further diluted with 0.9%, 0.45%, or 0.225% sodium chloride or LR (do not exceed final concentration of 0.5 mg/mL).

Storage/Stability Store intact vials at 2°C to 8°C (36°F to 46°F). Reconstituted solution may be stored at ≤25°C (≤77°F) for 1 hour prior to preparation of infusion solution. Solutions diluted for infusion should be used within 24 hours when stored at ≤25°C (≤77°F) or within 48 hours when stored at 2°C to 8°C (36°F to 46°F).

Mechanism of Action Inhibits synthesis of β(1,3)-D-glucan, an essential component of the cell wall of susceptible fungi. Highest activity is in regions of active cell growth. Mammalian cells do not require β(1,3)-D-glucan, limiting potential toxicity.

Pharmacodynamics/Kinetics

Protein binding: ~97% to albumin
Metabolism: Slowly, via hydrolysis and *N*-acetylation as well as by spontaneous degradation, with subsequent metabolism to component amino acids. Overall metabolism is extensive.
Half-life elimination: Beta (distribution): 9-11 hours; Terminal: 40-50 hours
Excretion: Urine (41%; primarily as metabolites, ~1% of total dose as unchanged drug); feces (35%; primarily as metabolites)

Dosage Note: Duration of caspofungin treatment should be determined by patient status and clinical response.

Aspergillosis (invasive), candidemia, esophageal candidiasis, empiric therapy: Infants ≥3 months, Children, and Adolescents ≤17 years: IV: Initial dose: 70 mg/m^2 on day 1, subsequent dosing: 50 mg/m^2 once daily, if clinical response inadequate, may increase to 70 mg/m^2 once daily if tolerated, but increased efficacy not demonstrated (maximum dose: 70 mg daily). Refer to adult dosing for indication-specific recommended durations.

Aspergillosis (invasive): Adults: IV: Initial dose: 70 mg on day 1; subsequent dosing: 50 mg once daily. Duration of therapy should be a minimum of 6-12 weeks or throughout period of immunosuppression and until lesions have resolved (Walsh, 2008). Salvage treatment with 70 mg once daily (off-label dosing) has been reported (Maertens, 2006).

Candidemia: Adults: IV: Initial dose: 70 mg on day 1; subsequent dosing: 50 mg once daily; generally continue for at least 14 days after the last positive culture or longer if neutropenia warrants. Higher doses (150 mg once daily infused over ~2 hours) compared to the standard adult dosing regimen (50 mg once daily) have not demonstrated additional benefit or toxicity in patients with invasive candidiasis (Betts, 2009).

Esophageal candidiasis: Adults: IV: 50 mg once daily; continue for 7-14 days after symptom resolution. **Note:** The majority of patients studied for this indication also had oropharyngeal involvement.

Empiric therapy: Adults: IV: Initial dose: 70 mg on day 1; subsequent dosing: 50 mg once daily; continue until resolution of neutropenia; if fungal infection confirmed, continue for a minimum of 14 days (continue for at least 7 days after resolution of both neutropenia and clinical symptoms); if clinical response inadequate, may increase up to 70 mg once daily if tolerated, but increased efficacy not demonstrated.

Concomitant use of an enzyme inducer:

Children: Patients receiving carbamazepine, dexamethasone, efavirenz, nevirapine, phenytoin, or rifampin (and possibly other enzyme inducers): Consider 70 mg/m^2 once daily (maximum: 70 mg daily)

Adults:

Patients receiving rifampin: 70 mg caspofungin once daily

Patients receiving carbamazepine, dexamethasone, efavirenz, nevirapine, **or** phenytoin (and possibly other enzyme inducers): May require an increased dose of caspofungin 70 mg once daily.

Elderly: The number of patients >65 years of age in clinical studies was not sufficient to establish whether a difference in response may be anticipated.

Dosage adjustment in renal impairment: No dosage adjustment necessary.

End-stage renal disease (ESRD) requiring hemodialysis: Poorly dialyzed; no supplemental dose or dosage adjustment necessary, including patients on intermittent hemodialysis (IHD), peritoneal dialysis, or continuous renal replacement therapy (eg, CVVHD).

Dosage adjustment in hepatic impairment:

Children: Mild-to-severe insufficiency (Child-Pugh classes A, B, or C): No dosage adjustment provided in manufacturer's labeling (has not been studied).

Adults:

Mild insufficiency (Child-Pugh class A): No dosage adjustment necessary.

Moderate insufficiency (Child-Pugh class B): 70 mg on day 1 (where recommended), followed by 35 mg once daily

Severe insufficiency (Child-Pugh class C): No dosage adjustment provided in manufacturer's labeling (has not been studied).

Administration Infuse slowly, over ~1 hour. Monitor during infusion; isolated cases of possible histamine-related reactions have occurred during clinical trials (rash, flushing, pruritus, facial edema).

Monitoring Parameters Liver function; anaphylaxis or histamine-related reactions (eg, facial swelling, bronchospasm, sensation of warmth)

Dosage Forms

Solution Reconstituted, Intravenous:

Cancidas: 50 mg (1 ea); 70 mg (1 ea)

◆ **Caspofungin Acetate** *see* Caspofungin *on page 370*

◆ **Castor Oil, Trypsin, and Balsam Peru** *see* Trypsin, Balsam Peru, and Castor Oil *on page 2109*

◆ **Cataflam [DSC]** *see* Diclofenac (Systemic) *on page 617*

◆ **Catapres** *see* CloNIDine *on page 480*

◆ **Catapres® (Can)** *see* CloNIDine *on page 480*

◆ **Catapres-TTS-1** *see* CloNIDine *on page 480*

◆ **Catapres-TTS-2** *see* CloNIDine *on page 480*

◆ **Catapres-TTS-3** *see* CloNIDine *on page 480*

◆ **Cathflo Activase** *see* Alteplase *on page 99*

◆ **Caverject** *see* Alprostadil *on page 96*

◆ **Caverject Impulse** *see* Alprostadil *on page 96*

◆ **CaviRinse** *see* Fluoride *on page 895*

◆ **Cayston** *see* Aztreonam *on page 220*

◆ **Caziant** *see* Ethinyl Estradiol and Desogestrel *on page 799*

◆ **CB-1348** *see* Chlorambucil *on page 419*

◆ **CB7630** *see* Abiraterone Acetate *on page 26*

◆ **CBDCA** *see* CARBOplatin *on page 357*

◆ **CBZ** *see* CarBAMazepine *on page 346*

◆ **CC-4047** *see* Pomalidomide *on page 1677*

◆ **CC-5013** *see* Lenalidomide *on page 1177*

◆ **CC-10004** *see* Apremilast *on page 165*

◆ **CCI-779** *see* Temsirolimus *on page 1994*

◆ **ccIIV3 [Flucelvax]** *see* Influenza Virus Vaccine (Inactivated) *on page 1075*

◆ **CCNU** *see* Lomustine *on page 1235*

◆ **2-CdA** *see* Cladribine *on page 455*

◆ **CDB-2914** *see* Ulipristal *on page 2113*

◆ **CDCA** *see* Chenodiol *on page 417*

◆ **CDDP** *see* CISplatin *on page 448*

◆ **CDP870** *see* Certolizumab Pegol *on page 409*

◆ **CDX** *see* Bicalutamide *on page 262*

◆ **CE** *see* Estrogens (Conjugated/Equine, Systemic) *on page 787*

◆ **CE** *see* Estrogens (Conjugated/Equine, Topical) *on page 790*

◆ **Ceclor® (Can)** *see* Cefaclor *on page 372*

◆ **Cedax** *see* Ceftibuten *on page 394*

◆ **CEE** *see* Estrogens (Conjugated/Equine, Systemic) *on page 787*

◆ **CEE** *see* Estrogens (Conjugated/Equine, Topical) *on page 790*

◆ **CeeNU** *see* Lomustine *on page 1235*

Cefaclor (SEF a klor)

Brand Names: Canada Apo-Cefaclor®; Ceclor®; Novo-Cefaclor; Nu-Cefaclor; PMS-Cefaclor

Pharmacologic Category Antibiotic, Cephalosporin (Second Generation)

Use Treatment of susceptible bacterial infections including otitis media, lower respiratory tract infections, acute exacerbations of chronic bronchitis, pharyngitis and tonsillitis, urinary tract infections, skin and skin structure infections

Pregnancy Risk Factor B

Dosage

Usual dosage range:

Children >1 month: Oral: 20-40 mg/kg/day divided every 8-12 hours (maximum dose: 1 g/day)

Adults: Oral: 250-500 mg every 8 hours

Indication-specific dosing:

Children: Oral:

Otitis media: 40 mg/kg/day divided every 12 hours

Pharyngitis: 20 mg/kg/day divided every 12 hours

Dosage adjustment in renal impairment:

CrCl 10-50 mL/minute: Administer 50% to 100% of dose

CrCl <10 mL/minute: Administer 50% of dose

Hemodialysis: Moderately dialyzable (20% to 50%)

Dosage adjustment in hepatic impairment: No dosage adjustment provided in manufacturer's labeling.

Additional Information Complete prescribing information should be consulted for additional detail.

Dosage Forms

Capsule, Oral:

Generic: 250 mg, 500 mg

Suspension Reconstituted, Oral:

Generic: 125 mg/5 mL (150 mL); 250 mg/5 mL (150 mL); 375 mg/5 mL (100 mL)

Tablet Extended Release 12 Hour, Oral:

Generic: 500 mg

Cefadroxil (sef a DROKS il)

Brand Names: Canada Apo-Cefadroxil; PRO-Cefadroxil; Teva-Cefadroxil

Index Terms Cefadroxil Monohydrate; Duricef

Pharmacologic Category Antibiotic, Cephalosporin (First Generation)

Use

Pharyngitis and/or tonsillitis: Treatment of pharyngitis and/or tonsillitis caused by *Streptococcus pyogenes* (group A beta-hemolytic streptococci).

Skin and skin structure infections: Treatment of skin and skin structure infections caused by staphylococci and/or streptococci.

Urinary tract infection: Treatment of urinary tract infections caused by *Escherichia coli*, *Proteus mirabilis*, and *Klebsiella* species.

Pregnancy Risk Factor B

Pregnancy Considerations Adverse events have not been observed in animal reproduction studies. Cefadroxil crosses the placenta. Limited data is available concerning the use of cefadroxil in pregnancy; however, adverse fetal effects were not noted in a small clinical trial.

Breast-Feeding Considerations Very small amounts of cefadroxil are excreted in breast milk. The manufacturer recommends that caution be exercised when administering cefadroxil to nursing women. Nondose-related effects could include modification of bowel flora.

Contraindications Hypersensitivity to cefadroxil, any component of the formulation, or other cephalosporins

Warnings/Precautions Modify dosage in patients with renal impairment (CrCl <50 mL/minute/1.73 m^2). Use with caution in patients with a history of penicillin allergy, especially IgE-mediated reactions (eg, anaphylaxis, angioedema, urticaria). Use with caution in patients with a history of gastrointestinal disease, particularly colitis. Prolonged use may result in fungal or bacterial superinfection, including *C. difficile*-associated diarrhea (CDAD) and pseudomembranous colitis; CDAD has been observed >2 months postantibiotic treatment. Only IM penicillin has been shown to be effective in the prophylaxis of rheumatic fever. Cefadroxil is generally effective in the eradication of streptococci from the oropharynx; efficacy data for cefadroxil in the prophylaxis of subsequent rheumatic fever episodes are not available.

Suspension may contain sulfur dioxide (sulfite); hypersensitivity reactions, including anaphylaxis and/or asthmatic exacerbations, may occur (may be life threatening).

Benzyl alcohol and derivatives: Some dosage forms may contain sodium benzoate/benzoic acid; benzoic acid (benzoate) is a metabolite of benzyl alcohol; large amounts of benzyl alcohol (≥99 mg/kg/day) have been associated with a potentially fatal toxicity ("gasping syndrome") in neonates; the "gasping syndrome" consists of metabolic acidosis, respiratory distress, gasping respirations, CNS dysfunction (including convulsions, intracranial hemorrhage), hypotension, and cardiovascular collapse (AAP, 1997; CDC, 1982); some data suggests that benzoate displaces bilirubin from protein binding sites (Ahlfors, 2001); avoid or use dosage forms containing benzyl alcohol derivative with caution in neonates. See manufacturer's labeling.

Adverse Reactions

Gastrointestinal: Diarrhea

Rare but important or life-threatening: Agranulocytosis, anaphylaxis, angioedema, cholestasis, *Clostridium difficile* associated diarrhea, dyspepsia, erythema multiforme, erythematous rash, genital candidiasis, hepatic failure, increased serum transaminases, maculopapular rash, neutropenia, pseudomembranous colitis, serum sickness, Stevens-Johnson syndrome, thrombocytopenia, vaginitis

Drug Interactions

Metabolism/Transport Effects None known.

Avoid Concomitant Use

Avoid concomitant use of Cefadroxil with any of the following: BCG

Increased Effect/Toxicity

Cefadroxil may increase the levels/effects of: Vitamin K Antagonists

The levels/effects of Cefadroxil may be increased by: Probenecid

Decreased Effect

Cefadroxil may decrease the levels/effects of: BCG; Sodium Picosulfate; Typhoid Vaccine

Food Interactions Concomitant administration with food, infant formula, or cow's milk does **not** significantly affect absorption.

Preparation for Administration Powder for suspension: Refer to manufacturer's product labeling for reconstitution instructions. Shake vigorously until suspended.

Storage/Stability Store capsules, tablets and un-reconstituted oral suspension at 20°C to 25°C (68°F to 77F); excursions are permitted to 15°C to 30°C (59°F to 86°F). After reconstitution, oral suspension may be stored for 14 days under refrigeration (4°C).

Mechanism of Action Inhibits bacterial cell wall synthesis by binding to one or more of the penicillin-binding proteins (PBPs) which in turn inhibits the final transpeptidation step of peptidoglycan synthesis in bacterial cell walls, thus inhibiting cell wall biosynthesis. Bacteria eventually lyse due to ongoing activity of cell wall autolytic enzymes (autolysins and murein hydrolases) while cell wall assembly is arrested.

Pharmacodynamics/Kinetics

Absorption: Rapid and well absorbed

Excretion: Urine (>90% as unchanged drug)

Dosage

Usual dosage range: Oral:

Children: 30 mg/kg/day divided every 12 hours (maximum: 2000 mg daily)

Adults: 1-2 g daily in a single dose or 2 divided doses

Indication-specific dosing: Oral:

Pharyngitis, group A streptococci (IDSA guidelines): Children and Adults: 30 mg/kg once daily (maximum: 1 g daily) for 10 days (Shulman, 2012). **Note:** Recommended as an alternative agent in penicillin-allergic patients; however, avoid in patients with immediate type hypersensitivity to penicillin.

Prosthetic joint infection, chronic oral antimicrobial suppression, staphylococci (oxacillin-susceptible) (preferred) (off-label use): Adults: 500 mg every 12 hours (Osmon, 2013)

Skin and skin structure infections: Adults: 1 g daily in a single or 2 divided doses

Tonsillitis: Adults: 1 g daily in a single or 2 divided doses for 10 days

Urinary tract infections: Adults: 1 g twice daily. For uncomplicated infections: 1 or 2 g daily in a single or 2 divided doses

Dosage adjustment in renal impairment:

CrCl 25-50 mL/minute: Administer every 12 hours

CrCl 10-25 mL/minute: Administer every 24 hours

CrCl <10 mL/minute: Administer every 36 hours

Dosage adjustment in hepatic impairment: No dosage adjustment provided in manufacturer's labeling.

Administration Administer around-the-clock to promote less variation in peak and trough serum levels. Administer without regards to meals; administration with food may diminish GI complaints.

Monitoring Parameters Monitor renal function. Observe for signs and symptoms of anaphylaxis during first dose.

Dosage Forms

Capsule, Oral:

Generic: 500 mg

Suspension Reconstituted, Oral:

Generic: 250 mg/5 mL (100 mL); 500 mg/5 mL (75 mL, 100 mL)

Tablet, Oral:

Generic: 1 g

◆ **Cefadroxil Monohydrate** *see* Cefadroxil *on page 372*

CeFAZolin (sef A zoe lin)

Brand Names: Canada Cefazolin For Injection; Cefazolin For Injection, USP

Index Terms Ancef; Cefazolin Sodium; Kefzol

Pharmacologic Category Antibiotic, Cephalosporin (First Generation)

Use

Biliary tract infections: Due to *Escherichia coli*, various strains of streptococci, *Proteus mirabilis*, *Klebsiella* species and *Staphylococcus aureus*.

Bone and joint infections: Due to *S. aureus*.

Endocarditis: Due to *S. aureus* (penicillin-sensitive and penicillin-resistant) and group A beta-hemolytic streptococci.

Genital infections (ie, prostatitis, epididymitis): Due to *E. coli*, *P. mirabilis*, and *Klebsiella* species.

Perioperative prophylaxis: The prophylactic administration of cefazolin preoperatively, intraoperatively, and postoperatively may reduce the incidence of certain postoperative infections in patients undergoing surgical procedures.

Respiratory tract infections: Due to *S. pneumoniae*, *Klebsiella* species, *Haemophilus influenzae*, *S. aureus* (penicillin-sensitive and penicillin-resistant) and group A beta-hemolytic streptococci.

Septicemia: Due to *Streptococcus pneumoniae*, *S. aureus* (penicillin-sensitive and penicillin-resistant), *P. mirabilis*, *E. coli* and *Klebsiella* species.

Skin and skin structure infections: Due to *S. aureus* (penicillin-sensitive and penicillin-resistant), group A beta-hemolytic streptococci and other strains of streptococci.

Urinary tract infections: Due to *E. coli*, *P. mirabilis*, *Klebsiella* species and some strains of enterobacter.

Pregnancy Risk Factor B

Pregnancy Considerations Adverse effects were not observed in animal reproduction studies. Cefazolin crosses the placenta. Adverse events have not been reported in the fetus following administration of cefazolin prior to cesarean section. Cefazolin is recommended for group B streptococcus prophylaxis in pregnant patients with a nonanaphylactic penicillin allergy. It is also one of the antibiotics recommended for prophylactic use prior to cesarean delivery and may be used in certain situations prior to vaginal delivery in women at high risk for endocarditis.

Due to pregnancy-induced physiologic changes, the pharmacokinetics of cefazolin are altered. The half-life is shorter, the AUC is smaller, and the clearance and volume of distribution are increased.

Breast-Feeding Considerations Small amounts of cefazolin are excreted in breast milk. The manufacturer recommends that caution be exercised when administering cefazolin to nursing women. Nondose-related effects could include modification of bowel flora.

Contraindications Known allergy to the cephalosporin group of antibiotics

Warnings/Precautions Modify dosage in patients with severe renal impairment. Use with caution in patients with a history of penicillin allergy, especially IgE-mediated reactions (eg, anaphylaxis, angioedema, urticaria). Prolonged use may result in fungal or bacterial superinfection, including *C. difficile*-associated diarrhea (CDAD) and pseudomembranous colitis; CDAD has been observed >2 months postantibiotic treatment. May be associated with increased INR, especially in nutritionally-deficient patients, prolonged treatment, hepatic or renal disease. Use with caution in patients with a history of seizure disorder; high levels, particularly in the presence of renal impairment, may increase risk of seizures. Potentially significant drug-drug interactions may exist, requiring dose or frequency adjustment, additional monitoring, and/or selection of alternative therapy.

Adverse Reactions

Cardiovascular: Localized phlebitis

Central nervous system: Seizure

Dermatologic: Pruritus, skin rash, Stevens-Johnson syndrome

Gastrointestinal: Abdominal cramps, anorexia, diarrhea, nausea, oral candidiasis, pseudomembranous colitis, vomiting

Genitourinary: Vaginitis

Hepatic: Hepatitis, increased serum transaminases

Hematologic: Eosinophilia, leukopenia, neutropenia, thrombocythemia, thrombocytopenia

Hypersensitivity: Anaphylaxis

Local: Pain at injection site

Renal: Increased blood urea nitrogen, increased serum creatinine, renal failure

Miscellaneous: Fever

Drug Interactions

Metabolism/Transport Effects None known.

Avoid Concomitant Use

Avoid concomitant use of CeFAZolin with any of the following: BCG

Increased Effect/Toxicity

CeFAZolin may increase the levels/effects of: Fosphenytoin; Phenytoin; Vitamin K Antagonists

The levels/effects of CeFAZolin may be increased by: Probenecid

Decreased Effect

CeFAZolin may decrease the levels/effects of: BCG; Sodium Picosulfate; Typhoid Vaccine

Preparation for Administration Dilute 500 mg vial with 2 mL SWFI and 1 g vial with 2.5 mL SWFI; reconstituted solution may be directly injected after further dilution with 5 mL SWFI or further diluted for IV administration in 50-100 mL compatible solution; 10 g vial may be diluted with 45 mL to yield 1 g/5 mL or 96 mL to yield 1 g/10 mL.

Storage/Stability Store intact vials at room temperature and protect from temperatures exceeding 40°C. Reconstituted solutions of cefazolin are light yellow to yellow. Protection from light is recommended for the powder and for the reconstituted solutions. Reconstituted solutions are stable for 24 hours at room temperature and for 10 days under refrigeration. Stability of parenteral admixture at room temperature (25°C) is 48 hours. Stability of parenteral admixture at refrigeration temperature (4°C) is 14 days.

DUPLEX: Store at 20°C to 25°C (68°F to 77°F); excursions permitted to 15°C to 30°C (59°F to 86°F) prior to activation. Following activation, stable for 24 hours at room temperature and for 7 days under refrigeration.

Mechanism of Action Inhibits bacterial cell wall synthesis by binding to one or more of the penicillin-binding proteins (PBPs) which in turn inhibits the final transpeptidation step of peptidoglycan synthesis in bacterial cell walls, thus inhibiting cell wall biosynthesis. Bacteria eventually lyse due to ongoing activity of cell wall autolytic enzymes (autolysins and murein hydrolases) while cell wall assembly is arrested.

Pharmacodynamics/Kinetics

Distribution: Widely into most body tissues and fluids including gallbladder, liver, kidneys, bone, sputum, bile, pleural, and synovial; CSF penetration is poor

Protein binding: 74% to 86%

Metabolism: Minimally hepatic

Half-life elimination: IM or IV: ~2 hours; prolonged with renal impairment

Time to peak, serum: IM: 0.5-2 hours

Excretion: Urine (80% to 100% as unchanged drug)

Dosage

Usual dosage range: IM, IV:

Children >1 month: 25-100 mg/kg/day divided every 6-8 hours; maximum: 6 **g** daily

Adults: 250-1500 mg every 6-12 (usually 8) hours, depending on severity of infection; maximum dose: 12 **g** daily

Indication-specific dosing:

Infants and Children: IM, IV:

Community-acquired pneumonia (CAP) (IDSA/PIDS, 2011), moderate-to-severe infection, *S. aureus* (methicillin-susceptible) (preferred): Infants >3 months and Children: 150 mg/kg/day divided every 8 hours

Perioperative prophylaxis (off-label use): Children ≥1 year: IV: **Note:** For most surgical procedures, joint clinical practice guidelines from the American Society of Health-System Pharmacists, Infectious Diseases Society of America, Surgical Infection Society, and Society for Healthcare Epidemiology of America

(ASHP/IDSA/SIS/SHEA) recommend a dose of 30 mg/kg (maximum dose: 2000 mg) administered within 60 minutes prior to surgical incision. For procedures requiring anaerobic coverage (eg, appendectomy, small bowel surgery with intestinal obstruction, colon procedures), combine cefazolin with metronidazole as an alternative to a second generation cephalosporin with anaerobic activity (eg, cefoxitin or cefotetan). Cefazolin doses may be repeated intraoperatively in 4 hours if procedure is lengthy or if there is excessive blood loss (Bratzler, 2013)

Prophylaxis against infective endocarditis (off-label use): 50 mg/kg 30-60 minutes before procedure; maximum dose: 1000 mg. Intramuscular injections should be avoided in patients who are receiving anticoagulant therapy. In these circumstances, orally administered regimens should be given whenever possible. Intravenously administered antibiotics should be used for patients who are unable to tolerate or absorb oral medications.

Note: American Heart Association (AHA) guidelines now recommend prophylaxis only in patients undergoing invasive procedures and in whom underlying cardiac conditions may predispose to a higher risk of adverse outcomes should infection occur. As of April 2007, routine prophylaxis for GI/GU procedures is no longer recommended by the AHA.

Infants, Children, and Adolescents: Intraperitoneal:

Peritonitis, treatment (off-label route; Warady, 2012):

Intermittent exchange: 20 mg/kg every 24 hours in the long dwell

Continuous exchange: Loading dose: 500 mg per liter of dialysate; maintenance: 125 mg per liter of dialysate

Adults: IM, IV:

Cholecystitis, mild-to-moderate: IV: 1-2 g every 8 hours for 4-7 days (provided source controlled)

Endocarditis due to MSSA (without prosthesis) (off-label use): IV: 2 g every 8 hours for 6 weeks with or without gentamicin for the initial 3-5 days; **Note:** Recommended for penicillin-allergic (nonanaphylactoid) patients (Baddour, 2005)

Group B streptococcus (neonatal prophylaxis): IV: 2 g once, then 1 g every 8 hours until delivery (CDC, 2010)

Intra-abdominal infection, complicated, community-acquired, mild-to-moderate (in combination with metronidazole): IV: 1-2 g every 8 hours for 4-7 days (provided source controlled)

Moderate-to-severe infections: IV: 500 mg to 1 g every 6-8 hours

Mild infection with gram-positive cocci: 250-500 mg every 8 hours

Prophylaxis against infective endocarditis (off-label use): 1 g 30-60 minutes before procedure. Intramuscular injections should be avoided in patients who are receiving anticoagulant therapy. In these circumstances, orally administered regimens should be given whenever possible. Intravenously administered antibiotics should be used for patients who are unable to tolerate or absorb oral medications.

Note: American Heart Association (AHA) guidelines now recommend prophylaxis only in patients undergoing invasive procedures and in whom underlying cardiac conditions may predispose to a higher risk of adverse outcomes should infection occur. As of April 2007, routine prophylaxis for GI/GU procedures is no longer recommended by the AHA.

Perioperative prophylaxis:

Manufacturer's labeling: 1 g initiated 30-60 minutes prior to surgery; may repeat after 2 hours if procedure is lengthy with 500 mg to 1 g intraoperatively, followed by 500 mg to 1 g every 6-8 hours for 24 hours postoperatively.

Guideline recommendations (off-label): IV: **Note:** For most surgical procedures, joint clinical practice guidelines from the American Society of Health-System Pharmacists, Infectious Diseases Society of America, Surgical Infection Society, and Society for Healthcare Epidemiology of America (ASHP/IDSA/SIS/SHEA) recommend a dose of 2 g within 60 minutes prior to surgical incision (for nonobese patients weighing <120 kg). For procedures requiring anaerobic coverage (eg, appendectomy, small bowel surgery with intestinal obstruction, colon procedures), combine cefazolin with metronidazole as an alternative to a second generation cephalosporin with anaerobic activity (eg, cefoxitin or cefotetan). Cefazolin doses may be repeated intraoperatively in 4 hours if procedure is lengthy or if there is excessive blood loss (Bratzler, 2013).

Obesity: The ASHP/IDSA/SIS/SHEA guidelines recommend that for patients weighing ≥120 kg, a dose of 3 g within 60 minutes prior to surgical incision should be administered (Bratzler, 2013). Alternatively, for patients with BMI >40 kg/m^2, a single 2 g dose may be sufficient for common general surgical procedures lasting <5 hours; patients enrolled in this multigroup study had a BMI up to a group mean of 55.7 kg/m^2 (Ho, 2012).

Cardiothoracic surgery: IV: 1 g (see **"Note"**) initiated 30-60 minutes prior to surgery (usually at the time of anesthetic induction); repeat dose if the duration of operation exceeds 3 hours (Hillis, 2011). The ASHP/IDSA/SIS/SHEA guidelines recommend the use of 2 g (single dose) administered within 60 minutes prior to surgical incision (Bratzler, 2013). May either continue for ≤48 hours postoperatively or administer as a single dose preoperatively (may be preferred due to reduced cost and potential for antimicrobial resistance) (Bratzler, 2013; Bucknell, 2000; Douglas, 2011; Edwards, 2006; Hillis, 2011).

Note: For patients weighing >60 kg, the Society of Thoracic Surgeons recommends a preoperative dose of 2 g administered within 60 minutes of skin incision. If the surgical incision remains open in the operating room, follow with 1 g every 3-4 hours unless cardiopulmonary bypass is to be discontinued within 4 hours then delay administration (Engelman, 2007).

Peritonitis, treatment (off-label route; Li, 2010): Intraperitoneal:

Intermittent exchange: 15 mg/kg per exchange every 24 hours in the long dwell (≥6 hours)

Continuous exchange: Loading dose: 500 mg per liter of dialysate. Maintenance: 125 mg per liter of dialysate.

Note: If patient has residual renal function (eg, >100 mL/day urine output), empirically increase each dose by 25%.

Automated peritoneal dialysis: 20 mg/kg every 24 hours in the long day dwell; **Note:** Guidelines suggest nighttime levels of intraperitoneal cefazolin may fall below the MIC of most organisms and adding cefazolin to each exchange may be warranted

Pneumococcal pneumonia: IV: 500 mg every 12 hours

Prosthetic joint infection, *Staphylococcal* (oxacillin-susceptible): IV: 1-2 g every 8 hours for 2-6 weeks (in combination with rifampin) followed by oral antibiotic treatment and suppressive regimens (Osmon, 2013)

Severe infection: IV: 1-1.5 g every 6 hours

UTI (uncomplicated): 1 g every 12 hours

Dosage adjustment in renal impairment:

CrCl 35-54 mL/minute: Administer full dose in intervals of ≥8 hours

CrCl 11-34 mL/minute: Administer 50% of usual dose every 12 hours

CrCl ≤10 mL/minute: Administer 50% of usual dose every 18-24 hours

Intermittent hemodialysis (IHD) (administer after hemodialysis on dialysis days): Dialyzable (20% to 50%): 500 mg to 1 g every 24 hours **or** use 1-2 g every 48-72 hours (Heintz, 2009) **or** 15-20 mg/kg (maximum dose: 2 g) after dialysis 3 times weekly (Ahern, 2003; Sowinski, 2001) **or** 2 g after dialysis if next dialysis expected in 48 hours or 3 g after dialysis if next dialysis is expected in 72 hours (Stryjewski, 2007).

Note: Dosing dependent on the assumption of 3 times weekly, complete IHD sessions.

Peritoneal dialysis (PD): IV: 500 mg every 12 hours

Continuous renal replacement therapy (CRRT) (Heintz, 2009; Trotman, 2005): Drug clearance is highly dependent on the method of renal replacement, filter type, and flow rate. Appropriate dosing requires close monitoring of pharmacologic response, signs of adverse reactions due to drug accumulation, as well as drug concentrations in relation to target trough (if appropriate). The following are general recommendations only (based on dialysate flow/ultrafiltration rates of 1-2 L/hour and minimal residual renal function) and should not supersede clinical judgment:

CVVH: Loading dose of 2 g followed by 1-2 g every 12 hours

CVVHD/CVVHDF: Loading dose of 2 g followed by either 1 g every 8 hours **or** 2 g every 12 hours. **Note:** Dosage of 1 g every 8 hours results in similar steady-state concentrations as 2 g every 12 hours and is more cost effective (Heintz, 2009).

Dosage adjustment in hepatic impairment: No dosage adjustment provided in manufacturer's labeling.

Dietary Considerations Some products may contain sodium.

Administration

IM: Inject deep IM into large muscle mass.

IV: Inject direct IV over 5 minutes or may infuse as an intermittent infusion over 30-60 minutes.

Some penicillins (eg, carbenicillin, ticarcillin and piperacillin) have been shown to inactivate aminoglycosides *in vitro*. This has been observed to a greater extent with tobramycin and gentamicin, while amikacin has shown greater stability against inactivation. Concurrent use of these agents may pose a risk of reduced antibacterial efficacy *in vivo*, particularly in the setting of profound renal impairment. However, definitive clinical evidence is lacking. If combination penicillin/aminoglycoside therapy is desired in a patient with renal dysfunction, separation of doses (if feasible), and routine monitoring of aminoglycoside levels, CBC, and clinical response should be considered.

Monitoring Parameters Renal function periodically when used in combination with other nephrotoxic drugs, hepatic function tests, CBC; monitor for signs of anaphylaxis during first dose

Dosage Forms

Solution, Intravenous:

Generic: 1 g (50 mL)

Solution Reconstituted, Injection:

Generic: 500 mg (1 ea); 1 g (1 ea); 10 g (1 ea); 20 g (1 ea); 100 g (1 ea); 300 g (1 ea)

Solution Reconstituted, Injection [preservative free]:

Generic: 500 mg (1 ea); 1 g (1 ea); 10 g (1 ea); 20 g (1 ea)

Solution Reconstituted, Intravenous:

Generic: 1 g (1 ea); 2 g (1 ea)

◆ **Cefazolin For Injection (Can)** *see* CeFAZolin *on page 373*

◆ **Cefazolin For Injection, USP (Can)** *see* CeFAZolin *on page 373*

◆ **Cefazolin Sodium** *see* CeFAZolin *on page 373*

Cefdinir (SEF di ner)

Index Terms CFDN; Omnicef

Pharmacologic Category Antibiotic, Cephalosporin (Third Generation)

Use

Acute bacterial otitis media: Treatment of acute bacterial otitis media in pediatric patients caused by *Haemophilus influenzae* (including beta-lactamase-producing strains), *Streptococcus pneumoniae* (penicillin-susceptible strains only) and *Moraxella catarrhalis* (including beta-lactamase-producing strains).

Acute exacerbations of chronic bronchitis: Treatment of acute exacerbations of chronic bronchitis in adults and adolescents caused by *H. influenzae* (including beta-lactamase producing strains), *H. parainfluenzae* (including beta-lactamase-producing strains), *S. pneumoniae* (penicillin-susceptible strains only) and *M. catarrhalis* (including beta-lactamase-producing strains).

Acute maxillary sinusitis: Treatment of acute maxillary sinusitis in adults and adolescents caused by *H. influenzae* (including beta-lactamase-producing strains), *S. pneumoniae* (penicillin-susceptible strains only) and *M. catarrhalis* (including beta-lactamase-producing strains). **Note:** Limitations of use: According to the IDSA guidelines for acute bacterial rhinosinusitis, cefdinir is no longer recommended as monotherapy for initial empiric treatment (Chow, 2012).

Community-acquired pneumonia: Treatment of community-acquired pneumonia in adults and adolescents caused by *H. influenzae* (including beta-lactamase-producing strains), H. parainfluenzae (including beta-lactamase-producing strains), *S. pneumoniae* (penicillin-susceptible strains only) and *M. catarrhalis* (including beta-lactamase-producing strains).

Pharyngitis/Tonsillitis: Treatment of pharyngitis/tonsillitis in adults, adolescents, and pediatric patients caused by *S. pyogenes*.

Uncomplicated skin and skin structure infections: Treatment of uncomplicated skin and skin structure infections in adults, adolescents, and pediatric patients caused by *Staphylococcus aureus* (including beta-lactamase-producing strains) and *S. pyogenes*.

Pregnancy Risk Factor B

Pregnancy Considerations Teratogenic events have not been observed in animal reproduction studies. An increase in most types of birth defects was not found following first trimester exposure to cephalosporins.

Breast-Feeding Considerations Cefdinir is not detectable in breast milk following a single cefdinir 600 mg dose. If present in breast milk, nondose-related effects could include modification of bowel flora.

Contraindications Hypersensitivity to cefdinir, any component of the formulation, or other cephalosporins.

Warnings/Precautions Administer cautiously to penicillin-sensitive patients, especially IgE-mediated reactions (eg, anaphylaxis, urticaria). Prolonged use may result in fungal or bacterial superinfection, including *C. difficile*-associated diarrhea (CDAD) and pseudomembranous colitis; CDAD has been observed >2 months postantibiotic treatment. Use with caution in patients with a history of colitis. Use caution with renal dysfunction (CrCl <30 mL/minute); dose adjustment may be required. Potentially significant drug-drug interactions may exist, requiring dose or frequency adjustment, additional monitoring, and/or selection of alternative therapy.

Adverse Reactions

Central nervous system: Headache

Dermatologic: Skin rash

Endocrine & metabolic: Decreased serum bicarbonate, glycosuria, hyperglycemia, hyperphosphatemia, increased gamma-glutamyl transferase, increased lactate dehydrogenase

Gastrointestinal: Abdominal pain, diarrhea, nausea, vomiting

Genitourinary: Proteinuria, occult blood in urine, urine alkalinization, vaginitis, vulvovaginal candidiasis

Hematologic: Change in WBC count, elevated urine leukocytes, eosinophilia, functional disorder of polymorphonuclear neutrophils, lymphocytopenia, lymphocytosis, thrombocythemia

Hepatic: Increased serum alkaline phosphatase, increased serum ALT

Renal: Increased urine specific gravity

Rare but important or life-threatening: Abnormal stools, anaphylaxis, anorexia, asthma, blood coagulation disorder, bloody diarrhea, candidiasis, cardiac failure, chest pain, cholestasis, conjunctivitis, constipation, cutaneous candidiasis, decreased hemoglobin, decreased urine specific gravity, disseminated intravascular coagulation, dizziness, drowsiness, dyspepsia, enterocolitis (acute), eosinophilic pneumonitis, erythema multiforme, erythema nodosum, exfoliative dermatitis, facial edema, fever, flatulence, fulminant hepatitis, granulocytopenia, hemolytic anemia, hemorrhagic colitis, hemorrhagic diathesis, hepatic failure, hepatitis (acute), hyperkalemia, hyperkinesia, hypersensitivity angiitis, hypertension, hypocalcemia, hypophosphatemia, immune thrombocytopenia, increased amylase, increased blood urea nitrogen, increased monocytes, increased serum AST, increased serum bilirubin, insomnia, interstitial pneumonitis (idiopathic), intestinal obstruction, involuntary body movements, jaundice, laryngeal edema, leukopenia, leukorrhea, loss of consciousness, maculopapular rash, melena, myocardial infarction, pancytopenia, peptic ulcer, pneumonia (drug-induced), pruritus, pseudomembranous colitis, renal disease, renal failure (acute), respiratory failure (acute), rhabdomyolysis, serum sickness, shock, Stevens-Johnson syndrome, stomatitis, thrombocytopenia, toxic epidermal necrolysis, upper gastrointestinal hemorrhage, weakness, xerostomia

Drug Interactions

Metabolism/Transport Effects None known.

Avoid Concomitant Use

Avoid concomitant use of Cefdinir with any of the following: BCG

Increased Effect/Toxicity

Cefdinir may increase the levels/effects of: Aminoglycosides; Vitamin K Antagonists

The levels/effects of Cefdinir may be increased by: Probenecid

Decreased Effect

Cefdinir may decrease the levels/effects of: BCG; Sodium Picosulfate; Typhoid Vaccine

The levels/effects of Cefdinir may be decreased by: Iron Salts; Multivitamins/Minerals (with ADEK, Folate, Iron)

Preparation for Administration Refer to manufacturer's product labeling for reconstitution instructions.

Storage/Stability Store at 20°C to 25°C (68°F to 77°F). Store reconstituted suspension at room temperature 20°C to 25°C (68°F to 77°F) for 10 days.

Mechanism of Action Inhibits bacterial cell wall synthesis by binding to one or more of the penicillin-binding proteins (PBPs) which in turn inhibits the final transpeptidation step of peptidoglycan synthesis in bacterial cell walls, thus inhibiting cell wall biosynthesis. Bacteria eventually lyse due to ongoing activity of cell wall autolytic enzymes (autolysins and murein hydrolases) while cell wall assembly is arrested.

Pharmacodynamics/Kinetics

Distribution: V_d:

Children 6 months to 12 years: 0.67 L/kg

Adults: 0.35 L/kg

Protein binding: 60% to 70%

Metabolism: Minimal

Bioavailability: Capsule: 16% to 21%; suspension 25%

Half-life elimination: ~100 minutes

Time to peak, plasma: 2 to 4 hours

Excretion: Primarily urine (~12% to 18% as unchanged drug)

Dosage

Usual dosage range:

Infants ≥6 months and Children: Oral: 7 mg/kg/dose twice daily or 14 mg/kg/dose once daily (maximum: 600 mg/day)

Adolescents and Adults: Oral: 300 mg twice daily or 600 mg once daily

Indication-specific dosing:

Infants ≥6 months and Children: Oral:

Acute bacterial otitis media, pharyngitis/tonsillitis: 7 mg/kg/dose twice daily for 5 to 10 days **or** 14 mg/kg/dose once daily for 10 days (maximum: 600 mg/day)

Acute maxillary sinusitis: 7 mg/kg/dose twice daily **or** 14 mg/kg/dose once daily for 10 days (maximum: 600 mg/day). **Note:** According to the IDSA guidelines for acute bacterial rhinosinusitis, cefdinir is no longer recommended as monotherapy for initial empiric treatment (Chow, 2012).

Uncomplicated skin and skin structure infections: 7 mg/kg/dose twice daily for 10 days (maximum: 600 mg/day)

Adolescents and Adults: Oral:

Acute exacerbations of chronic bronchitis, pharyngitis/tonsillitis: 300 mg twice daily for 5 to 10 days **or** 600 mg once daily for 10 days

Acute maxillary sinusitis: 300 mg twice daily **or** 600 mg once daily for 10 days. **Note:** According to the IDSA guidelines for acute bacterial rhinosinusitis, cefdinir is no longer recommended as monotherapy for initial empiric treatment (Chow, 2012).

Community-acquired pneumonia, uncomplicated skin and skin structure infections: 300 mg twice daily for 10 days

Dosing adjustment in renal impairment:

CrCl ≥30 mL/minute: No dosage adjustment necessary.

CrCl <30 mL/minute:

Infants ≥6 months and Children: 7 mg/kg once daily (maximum: 300 mg/day)

Adolescents and Adults: 300 mg once daily

ESRD requiring intermittent hemodialysis (IHD): Dialyzable: Initial dose: 300 mg (or 7 mg/kg/dose) every other day. Postdialysis, 300 mg (or 7 mg/kg/dose) should be given. Subsequent doses (300 mg or 7 mg/kg/dose) should be administered every other day.

Dosing adjustment in hepatic impairment: No dosage adjustment necessary.

Administration Twice daily doses should be given every 12 hours. May be administered with or without food. Manufacturer recommends administering at least 2 hours before or after antacids or iron supplements. Shake suspension well before use.

Monitoring Parameters Monitor renal function. Observe for signs and symptoms of anaphylaxis during first dose.

Dosage Forms

Capsule, Oral:

Generic: 300 mg

Suspension Reconstituted, Oral:

Generic: 125 mg/5 mL (60 mL, 100 mL); 250 mg/5 mL (60 mL, 100 mL)

Cefditoren (sef de TOR en)

Brand Names: U.S. Spectracef

Index Terms Cefditoren Pivoxil

Pharmacologic Category Antibiotic, Cephalosporin (Third Generation)

Use Treatment of acute bacterial exacerbation of chronic bronchitis or community-acquired pneumonia (due to susceptible organisms including *Haemophilus influenzae*, *Haemophilus parainfluenzae*, *Streptococcus pneumoniae*-penicillin susceptible only, *Moraxella catarrhalis*); pharyngitis or tonsillitis (*Streptococcus pyogenes*); and uncomplicated skin and skin-structure infections (*Staphylococcus aureus* - not MRSA, *Streptococcus pyogenes*)

Pregnancy Risk Factor B

Dosage

Usual dosage range:

Children ≥12 years and Adults: Oral: 200-400 mg twice daily

Indication-specific dosing:

Children ≥12 years and Adults: Oral:

Acute bacterial exacerbation of chronic bronchitis: 400 mg twice daily for 10 days

Dental infections (off-label use): 400 mg twice daily for 10 days

Community-acquired pneumonia: 400 mg twice daily for 14 days

Pharyngitis, tonsillitis, uncomplicated skin and skin structure infections: 200 mg twice daily for 10 days

Dosage adjustment in renal impairment:

CrCl 30-49 mL/minute/1.73 m^2: Maximum dose: 200 mg twice daily

CrCl <30 mL/minute/1.73 m^2: Maximum dose: 200 mg once daily

End-stage renal disease: Appropriate dosing not established

Dosage adjustment in hepatic impairment:

Mild-to-moderate impairment: Adjustment not required

Severe impairment (Child-Pugh Class C): Specific guidelines not available

Additional Information Complete prescribing information should be consulted for additional detail.

Dosage Forms

Tablet, Oral:

Spectracef: 200 mg, 400 mg

Generic: 200 mg, 400 mg

◆ **Cefditoren Pivoxil** *see* Cefditoren *on page 378*

Cefepime (SEF e pim)

Brand Names: U.S. Maxipime

Brand Names: Canada Maxipime

Index Terms Cefepime Hydrochloride

Pharmacologic Category Antibiotic, Cephalosporin (Fourth Generation)

Use

Febrile neutropenia: Treatment (empiric monotherapy) of febrile neutropenic patients.

Intra-abdominal infections: Treatment of complicated intra-abdominal infections, in combination with metronidazole, caused by *Escherichia coli*, viridans group streptococci, *Pseudomonas aeruginosa*, *Klebsiella pneumoniae*, *Enterobacter* species, or *Bacteroides fragilis*.

Pneumonia (moderate to severe): Treatment of moderate to severe pneumonia caused by *Streptococcus pneumoniae*, including cases associated with concurrent bacteremia, *P. aeruginosa*, *K. pneumoniae*, or *Enterobacter* species.

Skin and skin structure infections: Treatment of moderate to severe uncomplicated skin and skin structure infections caused by *Staphylococcus aureus* (methicillin-susceptible isolates only) or *Streptococcus pyogenes*.

Urinary tract infections (including pyelonephritis): Treatment of complicated and uncomplicated urinary tract infections (UTIs), including pyelonephritis, caused by *E. coli* or *K. pneumoniae*, when the infection is severe, or caused by *E. coli*, *K. pneumoniae*, or *Proteus mirabilis*, when the infection is mild to moderate, including cases associated with concurrent bacteremia with these microorganisms.

Pregnancy Risk Factor B

Pregnancy Considerations Adverse events were not observed in animal reproduction studies. Cefepime crosses the placenta.

Breast-Feeding Considerations Small amounts of cefepime are excreted in breast milk. The manufacturer recommends that caution be exercised when administering cefepime to nursing women. Nondose-related effects could include modification of bowel flora.

Contraindications Hypersensitivity to cefepime, other cephalosporins, penicillins, other beta-lactam antibiotics, or any component of the formulation

Warnings/Precautions Severe neurological reactions (some fatal) have been reported, including encephalopathy, myoclonus, seizures, and nonconvulsive status epilepticus; risk may be increased in the presence of renal impairment (CrCl ≤60 mL/minute); ensure dose adjusted for renal function or discontinue therapy if patient develops neurotoxicity; effects are often reversible upon discontinuation of cefepime. Serious adverse reactions have occurred in elderly patients with renal insufficiency given unadjusted doses of cefepime, including life-threatening or fatal occurrences of the following: encephalopathy, myoclonus, and seizures. Use with caution in patients with a history of penicillin or cephalosporin allergy, especially IgE-mediated reactions (eg, anaphylaxis, urticaria). Prolonged use may result in fungal or bacterial superinfection, including *C. difficile*-associated diarrhea (CDAD) and pseudomembranous colitis; CDAD has been observed >2 months postantibiotic treatment. Use with caution in patients with a history of gastrointestinal disease, especially colitis. May be associated with increased INR, especially in nutritionally-deficient patients, prolonged treatment, hepatic or renal disease. Use with caution in patients with a history of seizure disorder; high levels, particularly in the presence of renal impairment, may increase risk of seizures.

Adverse Reactions

Cardiovascular: Localized phlebitis

Central nervous system: Headache

Dermatologic: Pruritus, skin rash

Endocrine & metabolic: Hypophosphatemia

Gastrointestinal: Diarrhea, nausea, vomiting

Hematologic & oncologic: Eosinophilia, positive direct Coombs test (without hemolysis)

Hepatic: Abnormal partial thromboplastin time, abnormal prothrombin time, increased serum ALT, increased serum AST

Local: Local pain

Miscellaneous: Fever

Rare but important or life-threatening: Agranulocytosis, anaphylactic shock, anaphylaxis, brain disease, colitis, coma, confusion, decreased hematocrit, hallucination, hypercalcemia, hyperkalemia, hyperphosphatemia, hypocalcemia, increased blood urea nitrogen, increased serum alkaline phosphatase, increased serum bilirubin, increased serum creatinine, leukopenia, neutropenia, oral candidiasis, pseudomembranous colitis, seizure, status epilepticus (nonconvulsive), stupor, thrombocytopenia, urticaria, vaginitis

Drug Interactions

Metabolism/Transport Effects None known.

Avoid Concomitant Use

Avoid concomitant use of Cefepime with any of the following: BCG

Increased Effect/Toxicity

Cefepime may increase the levels/effects of: Aminoglycosides; Vitamin K Antagonists

The levels/effects of Cefepime may be increased by: Probenecid

Decreased Effect

Cefepime may decrease the levels/effects of: BCG; Sodium Picosulfate; Typhoid Vaccine

Preparation for Administration

IV: Reconstitute 1 or 2 g vial with 10 mL of a compatible diluent (resulting concentration of 100 mg/mL for 1 g vial and 160 mg/mL for 2 g vial) and further dilute in a compatible IV infusion fluid.

IM: Reconstitute 1 g vial with 2.4 mL of SWFI, NS, D_5W, lidocaine 0.5% or 1%, or bacteriostatic water for injection; resulting concentration is 280 mg/mL.

Storage/Stability

Vials: Store intact vials at 20°C to 25°C (68°F to 77°F). Protect from light. After reconstitution, stable in NS and D_5W for 24 hours at room temperature and 7 days refrigerated. Refer to the manufacturer's product labeling for other acceptable reconstitution solutions.

Dual chamber containers: Store unactivated containers at 20°C to 25°C (68°F to 77°F); excursions permitted to 15°C to 30°C (59°F to 85°F). Do not freeze. Following reconstitution, use within 12 hours if stored at room temperature or within 5 days if stored under refrigeration.

Premixed solution: Store frozen at -20°C (-4°F). Thawed solution is stable for 24 hours at room temperature or 7 days under refrigeration; do not refreeze.

Mechanism of Action Inhibits bacterial cell wall synthesis by binding to one or more of the penicillin-binding proteins (PBPs) which in turn inhibits the final transpeptidation step of peptidoglycan synthesis in bacterial cell walls, thus inhibiting cell wall biosynthesis. Bacteria eventually lyse due to ongoing activity of cell wall autolytic enzymes (autolysis and murein hydrolases) while cell wall assembly is arrested.

Pharmacodynamics/Kinetics

Absorption: IM: Rapid and complete

Distribution: V_d: Adults: 16 to 20 L; crosses blood-brain barrier

Protein binding, plasma: ~20%

Metabolism: Minimally hepatic

Half-life elimination: 2 hours

Time to peak: IM: 1 to 2 hours; IV: 0.5 hours

Excretion: Urine (85% as unchanged drug)

Dosage

Usual dosage range:

Infants ≥2 months, Children, and Adolescents ≤16 years (≤40 kg): IV: 50 mg/kg/dose every 8 to 12 hours (maximum: 2 g/dose); IM: 50 mg/kg/dose every 12 hours (maximum: 1 g/dose)

Children >40 kg, Adolescents >16 years, and Adults: IV: 1 to 2 g every 8 to 12 hours; IM: 0.5 to 1 g every 12 hours

Indication-specific dosing:

Infants ≥2 months, Children, and Adolescents ≤16 years (≤40 kg):

Febrile neutropenia: IV: 50 mg/kg/dose every 8 hours for 7 days or until neutropenia resolves (maximum: 2 g/dose)

Pneumonia: IV:

Due to *P. aeruginosa*: 50 mg/kg/dose every 8 hours for 10 days (maximum: 2 g/dose)

Not due to *P. aeruginosa*: 50 mg/kg/dose every 12 hours for 10 days (maximum: 2 g/dose)

Skin and skin structure infections (uncomplicated): IV: 50 mg/kg/dose every 12 hours for 10 days (maximum: 2 g/dose)

Urinary tract infections, complicated and uncomplicated: IM, IV: 50 mg/kg/dose every 12 hours for 7 to 10 days (maximum: 2 g/dose); **Note:** IM may be considered for mild-to-moderate infection only

Intra-abdominal infection, complicated (off-label use): IV: **Note:** IDSA 2010 guidelines recommend duration of 4 to 7 days (provided source controlled): 50 mg/kg/dose every 12 hours in combination with metronidazole (Solomkin [IDSA], 2010)

Children >40 kg, Adolescents >16 years, and Adults:

Febrile neutropenia, monotherapy: IV: 2 g every 8 hours for 7 days or until the neutropenia resolves

Intra-abdominal infections, complicated, severe (in combination with metronidazole): IV: **Note:** IDSA 2010 guidelines recommend duration of 4 to 7 days (provided source controlled). Not recommended for hospital-acquired intra-abdominal infections (IAI) associated with multidrug-resistant gram negative organisms or in mild-to-moderate community-acquired IAIs due to risk of toxicity and the development of resistant organisms (Solomkin, [IDSA] 2010).

Due to *P. aeruginosa*: 2 g every 8 hours for 7 to 10 days

Not due to *P. aeruginosa*: 2 g every 8 to 12 hours for 7 to 10 days

Pneumonia: IV: **Note:** Duration of therapy may vary considerably for healthcare associated pneumonia (7 to 21 days). In absence of *Pseudomonas*, and if appropriate empiric treatment used and patient responsive, it may be clinically appropriate to reduce duration of therapy to 7 to 10 days (American Thoracic Society Guidelines, 2005).

Due to *P. aeruginosa*: 1 to 2 g every 8 hours for 10 days; **Note:** Longer courses (eg, 14 to 21 days) may be required (American Thoracic Society Guidelines, 2005).

Not due to *P. aeruginosa*: 1 to 2 g every 8 to 12 hours for 10 days

Skin and skin structure infections, uncomplicated: IV: 2 g every 12 hours for 10 days

Urinary tract infections, complicated and uncomplicated:

Mild-to-moderate: IM, IV: 0.5 to 1 g every 12 hours for 7 to 10 days

Severe: IV: 2 g every 12 hours for 10 days

Adults:

Brain abscess, postneurosurgical prevention (off-label use): IV: 2 g every 8 hours with vancomycin (Tunkel, 2004)

Prosthetic joint infection, *Enterobacter spp.* or *Pseudomonas aeruginosa* (off-label use): IV: 2 g every 12 hours for 4 to 6 weeks; **Note:** When treating *P. aeruginosa*, consider addition of an aminoglycoside (Osmon, 2013)

Dosage adjustment in renal impairment:

Children: No dosage adjustment provided in the manufacturer's labeling; however, similar dosage adjustments to adults would be anticipated based on comparable pharmacokinetics between children and adults.

Adults: Recommended maintenance schedule based on creatinine clearance (may be estimated using the Cockcroft-Gault formula), compared to normal dosing schedule: See table.

Cefepime Hydrochloride

Creatinine Clearance (mL/minute)	Recommended Maintenance Schedule			
>60 (normal recommended dosing schedule)	500 mg every 12 hours	1 g every 12 hours	2 g every 12 hours	2 g every 8 hours
30-60	500 mg every 24 hours	1 g every 24 hours	2 g every 24 hours	2 g every 12 hours
11-29	500 mg every 24 hours	500 mg every 24 hours	1 g every 24 hours	2 g every 24 hours
<11	250 mg every 24 hours	250 mg every 24 hours	500 mg every 24 hours	1 g every 24 hours

Intermittent hemodialysis (IHD) (administer after hemodialysis on dialysis days): IV: Initial: 1 g (single dose) on day 1. Maintenance: 0.5-1 g every 24 hours **or** 1-2 g every 48-72 hours (Heintz, 2009) **or** 2 g 3 times weekly after dialysis (Perez, 2012). **Note:** Dosing dependent on the assumption of 3 times weekly, complete IHD sessions.

Peritoneal dialysis (PD): Removed to a lesser extent than hemodialysis; administer normal recommended dose every 48 hours

Continuous renal replacement therapy (CRRT) (Heintz, 2009; Trotman, 2005): Drug clearance is highly dependent on the method of renal replacement, filter type, and flow rate. Appropriate dosing requires close monitoring of pharmacologic response, signs of adverse reactions due to drug accumulation, as well as drug concentrations in relation to target trough (if appropriate). The following are general recommendations only (based on dialysate flow/ultrafiltration rates of 1-2 L/hour and minimal residual renal function) and should not supersede clinical judgment:

CVVH: Loading dose of 2 g followed by 1-2 g every 12 hours

CVVHD/CVVHDF: Loading dose of 2 g followed by either 1 g every 8 hours **or** 2 g every 12 hours. **Note:** Dosage of 1 g every 8 hours results in similar steady-state concentrations as 2 g every 12 hours and is more cost effective (Heintz, 2009).

Note: Consider higher dosage of 4 g/day if treating *Pseudomonas* or life-threatening infections in order to maximize time above MIC (Trotman, 2005). Dosage of 2 g every 8 hours may be needed for gram-negative rods with MIC ≥4 mg/L (Heintz, 2009).

Dosage adjustment in hepatic impairment: No dosage adjustment necessary.

Administration May be administered either IM or IV

Inject deep IM into large muscle mass. Inject direct IV over 5 minutes (Garrelts, 1999). Infuse intermittent infusion over 30 minutes.

Monitoring Parameters Monitor renal function. Observe for signs and symptoms of anaphylaxis during first dose.

Dosage Forms

Solution, Intravenous:

Generic: 1 g/50 mL (50 mL); 2% (100 mL)

Solution Reconstituted, Injection:

Maxipime: 1 g (1 ea); 2 g (1 ea)

Generic: 1 g (1 ea); 2 g (1 ea)

Solution Reconstituted, Intravenous:

Maxipime: 1 g (1 ea); 2 g (1 ea)

Generic: 1 g/50 mL (1 ea); 2 g/50 mL (1 ea)

◆ **Cefepime Hydrochloride** *see* Cefepime *on page 378*

Cefixime (sef IKS eem)

Brand Names: U.S. Suprax

Brand Names: Canada Auro-Cefixime; Suprax

Index Terms Cefixime Trihydrate

Pharmacologic Category Antibiotic, Cephalosporin (Third Generation)

Use Treatment of uncomplicated urinary tract infections (due to *Escherichia coli* and *Proteus mirabilis*), otitis media (due to *Haemophilus influenzae, Moraxella catarrhalis,* and *Streptococcus pyogenes*), pharyngitis and tonsillitis (due to *Streptococcus pyogenes*), acute exacerbations of chronic bronchitis (due to *Streptococcus pneumoniae* and *Haemophilus influenzae*); uncomplicated cervical/urethral gonorrhea (due to *N. gonorrhoeae* [penicillinase- and non-penicillinase-producing])

Note: Due to concerns of resistance, the CDC no longer recommends use of cefixime as a first-line regimen in the treatment of uncomplicated gonorrhea in the U.S.; ceftriaxone is the preferred cephalosporin (CDC, 2012).

Pregnancy Risk Factor B

Pregnancy Considerations Teratogenic effects were not observed in animal reproduction studies. Cefixime crosses the placenta and can be detected in the amniotic fluid. An increase in most types of birth defects was not found following first trimester exposure to cephalosporins. Cefixime may be used for the treatment of gonococcal infections in pregnant women in certain situations (refer to current guidelines).

Breast-Feeding Considerations It is not known if cefixime is excreted in breast milk. The manufacturer recommends that consideration be given to discontinuing nursing temporarily during treatment. If present in breast milk, nondose-related effects could include modification of bowel flora.

Contraindications Hypersensitivity to cefixime, any component of the formulation, or other cephalosporins

Warnings/Precautions Prolonged use may result in fungal or bacterial superinfection, including *C. difficile*-associated diarrhea (CDAD) and pseudomembranous colitis; CDAD has been observed >2 months postantibiotic treatment. Modify dosage in patients with renal impairment. Use with caution in patients with a history of penicillin allergy, especially IgE-mediated reactions (eg, anaphylaxis, urticaria).

Chewable tablets contain phenylalanine.

Benzyl alcohol and derivatives: Some dosage forms may contain sodium benzoate/benzoic acid; benzoic acid (benzoate) is a metabolite of benzyl alcohol; large amounts of benzyl alcohol (≥99 mg/kg/day) have been associated with a potentially fatal toxicity ("gasping syndrome") in neonates; the "gasping syndrome" consists of metabolic acidosis, respiratory distress, gasping respirations, CNS dysfunction (including convulsions, intracranial hemorrhage), hypotension, and cardiovascular collapse (AAP, 1997; CDC, 1982); some data suggests that benzoate displaces bilirubin from protein binding sites (Ahlfors, 2001); avoid or use dosage forms containing benzyl alcohol derivative with caution in neonates. See manufacturer's labeling.

Adverse Reactions

Gastrointestinal: Abdominal pain, diarrhea, dyspepsia, flatulence, loose stools, nausea

Rare but important or life-threatening: Acute renal failure, anaphylactoid reaction, anaphylaxis, angioedema, candidiasis, dizziness, drug fever, eosinophilia, erythema multiforme, facial edema, fever, headache, hepatitis, hyperbilirubinemia, increased blood urea nitrogen, increased serum creatinine, increased serum transaminases, jaundice, leukopenia, neutropenia, prolonged prothrombin time, pruritus, pseudomembranous colitis, seizure, serum sickness-like reaction, skin rash, Stevens-Johnson syndrome, thrombocytopenia, toxic epidermal necrolysis, urticaria, vaginitis, vomiting

Drug Interactions

Metabolism/Transport Effects None known.

Avoid Concomitant Use

Avoid concomitant use of Cefixime with any of the following: BCG

Increased Effect/Toxicity

Cefixime may increase the levels/effects of: Aminoglycosides; Vitamin K Antagonists

The levels/effects of Cefixime may be increased by: Probenecid

Decreased Effect

Cefixime may decrease the levels/effects of: BCG; Sodium Picosulfate; Typhoid Vaccine

Food Interactions Food delays cefixime absorption. Management: May administer with or without food.

Preparation for Administration Powder for suspension: Refer to manufacturer's product labeling for reconstitution instructions.

Storage/Stability

Capsule, chewable tablet, tablet: Store at 20°C to 25°C (68°F to 77°F).

Powder for suspension: Prior to reconstitution, store at 20°C to 25°C (68°F to 77°F). After reconstitution, suspension may be stored for 14 days at room temperature or under refrigeration.

Mechanism of Action Inhibits bacterial cell wall synthesis by binding to one or more of the penicillin-binding proteins (PBPs); which in turn inhibits the final transpeptidation step of peptidoglycan synthesis in bacterial cell walls, thus inhibiting cell wall biosynthesis. Bacteria eventually lyse due to ongoing activity of cell wall autolytic enzymes (autolysins and murein hydrolases) while cell wall assembly is arrested.

Pharmacodynamics/Kinetics **Note:** Chewable tablets and oral suspension are bioequivalent. However, oral suspension and tablet (nonchewable)/capsule formulations are **not** considered bioequivalent (oral suspension AUC ~10% to 25% greater compared with tablet after doses of 100-400 mg in normal adult volunteers).

Absorption: 40% to 50%; **Note:** Capsule AUC reduced by ~15% and C_{max} by ~25% when taken with food.

Distribution: Widely throughout the body and reaches therapeutic concentration in most tissues and body fluids, including synovial, pericardial, pleural, peritoneal; bile, sputum, and urine; bone, myocardium, gallbladder, and skin and soft tissue

Protein binding: 65%

Half-life elimination: Normal renal function: 3-4 hours; Renal failure: Up to 11.5 hours

Time to peak, serum: Tablet, suspension: 2-6 hours; Capsule: 3-8 hours; Delayed with food

Excretion: Urine (50% of absorbed dose as active drug); feces (10%)

Dosage

Usual dosage range: Note: Otitis media should be treated using the chewable tablets or suspension **only**. Chewable tablets and suspension achieve higher peak blood levels compared to an equivalent dose using the tablet or capsule.

Children ≥6 months and ≤45 kg: Oral: 8 mg/kg/day divided every 12-24 hours (maximum: 400 mg daily)

Dosing recommendations based on body weight (doses are rounded for use of oral suspension or chewable tablet):

5 to <7.6 kg: 50 mg daily
7.6 to <10.1 kg: 80 mg daily
10.1 to <12.6 kg: 100 mg daily
12.6 to <20.6 kg: 150 mg daily
20.6 to <28.1 kg: 200 mg daily
28.1 to <33.1 kg: 250 mg daily
33.1 to <40.1 kg: 300 mg daily
40.1 to ≤45 kg: 350 mg daily

Children >45 kg or >12 years, Adolescents, and Adults: Oral: 400 mg daily divided every 12-24 hours

Indication-specific dosing:

Children: Oral:

Acute bacterial rhinosinusitis (off-label use): 8 mg/kg/day divided every 12 hours with concomitant clindamycin for 10-14 days. **Note:** Recommended in patients with non-type I penicillin allergy, after failure of initial therapy or in patients at risk for antibiotic resistance (eg, daycare attendance, age <2 years, recent hospitalization, antibiotic use within the past month) (Chow, 2012).

S. pyogenes **infections:**

Children ≥6 months and ≤45 kg: 8 mg/kg/day divided every 12-24 hours for ≥10 days (maximum: 400 mg daily)

Children >45 kg or >12 years and Adolescents: 400 mg daily divided every 12-24 hours for ≥10 days

Typhoid fever (off-label use): 15-20 mg/kg/day divided every 12 hours for 7-14 days; maximum 400 mg daily (Girgis, 1995; Stephens, 2002)

Gonococcal infection, uncomplicated: Children >45 kg: 400 mg as a single dose in combination with oral azithromycin (preferred) or oral doxycycline (CDC, 2010). **Note:** CDC no longer recommends cefixime as a first-line agent, only use as an alternative agent with test-of-cure follow up in 7 days (CDC, 2012). In Canada, due to increased antimicrobial resistance, the Public Health Agency of Canada recommends 800 mg as a single dose (off-label dose) for treatment of uncomplicated gonococcal infections in children ≥9 years of age.

Adults: Oral:

Gonococcal infection, uncomplicated cervical/urethral/rectal (rectal off-label use) gonorrhea due to *N. gonorrhoeae:* 400 mg as a single dose in combination with oral azithromycin (preferred) or oral doxycycline (CDC, 2010). **Note:** CDC no longer recommends cefixime as a first-line agent (ceftriaxone is the preferred cephalosporin), if cefixime is used as an alternative agent, test-of-cure follow up in 7 days is recommended; in addition, cefixime is **not** an option for the treatment of uncomplicated gonorrhea of the pharynx (CDC, 2012). In Canada, due to increased antimicrobial resistance, the Public Health Agency of Canada recommends 800 mg as a single dose (off-label dose) for treatment of uncomplicated gonococcal infections.

Gonococcal infection, expedited partner therapy: 400 mg as a single dose in combination with oral azithromycin (CDC, 2012). **Note:** Only used if a heterosexual partner cannot be linked to evaluation and treatment in a timely manner; dose delivered to partner by patient, collaborating pharmacy, or disease investigation specialist.

S. pyogenes **infections:** 400 mg daily divided every 12-24 hours for ≥10 days

Typhoid fever (off-label use): 15-20 mg/kg/day in 2 divided doses for 7-14 days (Parry, 2002; WHO, 2003)

Dosage adjustment in renal impairment: Adults:
CrCl ≥60 mL/minute: No dosage adjustment necessary.
CrCl 21-59 mL/minute: 260 mg once daily
CrCl ≤20 mL/minute:
Chewable tablet, tablet: 200 mg once daily
100 mg/5 mL suspension: 172 mg once daily
200 mg/5 mL suspension: 176 mg once daily
500 mg/5 mL suspension: 180 mg once daily
Intermittent hemodialysis (not significantly removed by hemodialysis): 260 mg once daily
CAPD (not significantly removed by peritoneal dialysis):
Chewable tablet, tablet: 200 mg once daily
100 mg/5 mL suspension: 172 mg once daily
200 mg/5 mL suspension: 176 mg once daily
500 mg/5 mL suspension: 180 mg once daily

Dosage adjustment in hepatic impairment: No dosage adjustment provided in manufacturer's labeling.

Dietary Considerations Chewable tablets contain phenylalanine.

Administration May be administered with or without food. Shake oral suspension well before use. Chewable tablets must be chewed or crushed before swallowing.

Monitoring Parameters Renal function; with prolonged therapy, monitor renal and hepatic function periodically. Observe for signs and symptoms of anaphylaxis during first dose. When used as part of alternative treatment for gonococcal infection, test-of-cure 7 days after dose (CDC, 2012).

Dosage Forms

Capsule, Oral:
Suprax: 400 mg

Suspension Reconstituted, Oral:
Suprax: 100 mg/5 mL (50 mL); 200 mg/5 mL (50 mL, 75 mL); 500 mg/5 mL (10 mL, 20 mL)

Tablet Chewable, Oral:
Suprax: 100 mg, 200 mg

◆ **Cefixime Trihydrate** *see* Cefixime *on page 380*

Cefoperazone and Sulbactam [INT]

(sef oh PER a zone & SUL bak tam)

International Brand Names Alzone-S (IN); Bacperazone (RU); Bactazon (ID); Bacticep (TH); Cebactam (CO); Cefactam (PY, UY); Cefanozix (PY); Cefmate (IN); Cefobacatam (PH); Cefobactam DI (ID); Cefobeta (IN); Cefolatam (KR); Cefpar SB (TH); Cefper (MY, TH); Cefratam (ID); Dalipaitan (CN); Fanlin (CN); Linglanxin (CN); Peratam (KR); Prazone-S (TH); Simextam (ID); Soperam (ID); Sulbazon (PH); Sulbazone (KR); Sulcef (RO); Sulimax (PY); Sulperason (RU); Sulperazon (BG, CL, CO, CZ, HK, LT, MY, PE, PL, SK, TH, TR, UY, VE, VN); Sulperazone (PH); Vaxcel Cefobactam (MY)

Index Terms Sulbactam and Cefoperazone

Pharmacologic Category Antibiotic, Cephalosporin

Reported Use Upper and lower respiratory and urinary tract infections; skin, soft tissue, bone and joint infections; septicemia, meningitis, peritonitis, cholecystitis, cholangitis, pelvic inflammatory disease, endometritis, gonorrhea, and other abdominal and genital tract infections

Dosage Range Note: For severe infections additional cefoperazone (without sulbactam), administered separately, may be required (depending on available dosage forms)

IM, IV: Adults: 1-2 g (cefoperazone) every 12 hours; maximum daily dose: 4 g (sulbactam)

Product Availability Product available in various countries; not currently available in the U.S.

Dosage Forms

Injection, powder for reconstitution: 1 g: cefoperazone sodium 0.5 g and sulbactam sodium 0.5 g; 1.5 g: cefoperazone sodium 1 g and sulbactam sodium 0.5 g; 2 g: cefoperazone sodium 1 g and sulbactam sodium 1 g

◆ **Cefotan** *see* CefoTEtan *on page 385*

Cefotaxime (sef oh TAKS eem)

Brand Names: U.S. Claforan; Claforan in D5W

Brand Names: Canada Cefotaxime Sodium For Injection; Claforan

Index Terms Cefotaxime Sodium

Pharmacologic Category Antibiotic, Cephalosporin (Third Generation)

Use

Bacteremia/Septicemia: Treatment of bacteremia/septicemia caused by *Escherichia coli*, *Klebsiella* species, and *Serratia marcescens*, *Staphylococcus aureus* and *Streptococcus* species (including *Streptococcus pneumoniae*).

Bone or joint infections: Treatment of bone or joint infections caused by *S. aureus* (penicillinase and non-penicillinase producing strains), *Streptococcus* species (including *Streptococcus pyogenes*), *Pseudomonas* species (including *Pseudomonas aeruginosa*), and *Proteus mirabilis*.

CNS infections: Treatment of CNS infections (eg, meningitis, ventriculitis) caused by *Neisseria meningitidis*, *Haemophilus influenzae*, *S. pneumoniae*, *Klebsiella pneumoniae*, and *E. coli*.

Genitourinary infections: Treatment of genitourinary infections, including urinary tract infections (UTIs), caused by *Enterococcus* species, *Staphylococcus epidermidis*, *S. aureus* (penicillinase and nonpenicillinase producing), *Citrobacter* species, *Enterobacter* species, *E. coli*, *Klebsiella* species, *P. mirabilis*, *Proteus vulgaris*, *Providencia stuartii*, *Morganella morganii*, *Providencia rettgeri*, *S. marcescens*, and *Pseudomonas* species (including *P. aeruginosa*). Also, uncomplicated gonorrhea (cervical/urethral and rectal) caused by *Neisseria gonorrhoeae*, including penicillinase-producing strains.

Gynecologic infections: Treatment of gynecologic infections, including pelvic inflammatory disease, endometritis, and pelvic cellulitis, caused by *S. epidermidis*, *Streptococcus* species, *Enterococcus* species, *Enterobacter* species, *Klebsiella* species, *E. coli*, *P. mirabilis*, *Bacteroides* species (including *Bacteroides fragilis*), *Clostridium* species, and anaerobic cocci (including *Peptostreptococcus* and *Peptococcus* species) and *Fusobacterium* species (including *Fusobacterium nucleatum*).

Intra-abdominal infections: Treatment of intra-abdominal infections, including peritonitis caused by *Streptococcus* species, *E. coli*, *Klebsiella* species, *Bacteroides* species, and anaerobic cocci (including *Peptostreptococcus* species and *Peptococcus* species), *P. mirabilis*, and *Clostridium* species.

Lower respiratory tract infections: Treatment of lower respiratory tract infections, including pneumonia, caused by *S. pneumoniae*, *S. pyogenes* (group A streptococci) and other streptococci (excluding enterococci, [eg, *Enterococcus faecalis*]), *S. aureus* (penicillinase and nonpenicillinase producing), *E. coli*, *Klebsiella* species, *H. influenzae* (including ampicillin-resistant strains), *H. parainfluenzae*, *P. mirabilis*, *S. marcescens*, *Enterobacter* species, and indole-positive *Proteus* and *Pseudomonas* species (including *P. aeruginosa*).

Skin and skin structure infections: Treatment of skin and skin structure infections caused by *S. aureus* (penicillinase and nonpenicillinase producing), *S. epidermidis*, *S. pyogenes* (group A streptococci) and other streptococci, *Enterococcus* species, *Acinetobacter* species, *E. coli*, *Citrobacter* species (including *Citrobacter freundii*), *Enterobacter* species, *Klebsiella* species, *P. mirabilis*, *P. vulgaris*, *M. morganii*, *P. rettgeri*, *Pseudomonas* species, *S. marcescens*, *Bacteroides* species, and anaerobic cocci (including *Peptostreptococcus* species and *Peptococcus* species).

Surgical prophylaxis: Reduce the incidence of certain infections in patients undergoing surgical procedures (eg, abdominal or vaginal hysterectomy, GI and GU tract surgery) that may be classified as contaminated or potentially contaminated; reduce the incidence of certain postoperative infections in patients undergoing cesarean section.

Pregnancy Risk Factor B

Pregnancy Considerations Adverse events have not been observed in animal reproduction studies. Cefotaxime crosses the human placenta and can be found in fetal tissue. An increase in most types of birth defects was not found following first trimester exposure to cephalosporins. During pregnancy, peak cefotaxime serum concentrations are decreased and the serum half-life is shorter. Cefotaxime is approved for use in women undergoing cesarean section (consult current guidelines for appropriate use).

Breast-Feeding Considerations Low concentrations of cefotaxime are found in breast milk. The manufacturer recommends that caution be exercised when administering cefotaxime to nursing women. Nondose-related effects could include modification of bowel flora. The pregnancy-related changes in cefotaxime pharmacokinetics continue into the early postpartum period.

Contraindications Hypersensitivity to cefotaxime, any component of the formulation, or other cephalosporins

Warnings/Precautions A potentially life-threatening arrhythmia has been reported in patients who received a rapid (<1 minute) bolus injection via central venous catheter. Granulocytopenia and more rarely agranulocytosis may develop during prolonged treatment (>10 days). Minimize tissue inflammation by changing infusion sites when needed. Use with caution in patients with a history of penicillin allergy, especially IgE-mediated reactions (eg, anaphylaxis, urticaria). Prolonged use may result in fungal or bacterial superinfection, including *C. difficile*-associated diarrhea (CDAD) and pseudomembranous colitis; CDAD has been observed >2 months postantibiotic treatment. Use with caution in patients with renal impairment; dosage adjustment may be required. Use with caution in patients with a history of colitis. Potentially significant drug-drug interactions may exist, requiring dose or frequency adjustment, additional monitoring, and/or selection of alternative therapy.

Adverse Reactions

Dermatologic: Pruritus, skin rash

Gastrointestinal: Colitis, diarrhea, nausea, vomiting

Local: Pain at injection site

Rare but important or life-threatening: Agranulocytosis, anaphylaxis, brain disease, candidiasis, cardiac arrhythmia (after rapid IV injection via central catheter), cholestasis, eosinophilia, erythema multiforme, fever, headache, hemolytic anemia, hepatitis, increased blood urea nitrogen, increased gamma-glutamyl transferase, increased lactate dehydrogenase, increased serum alkaline phosphatase, increased serum ALT, increased serum AST, increased serum bilirubin, increased serum creatinine, increased serum transaminases, interstitial nephritis, jaundice, leukopenia, neutropenia, phlebitis, positive direct Coombs test, pseudomembranous colitis, Stevens-Johnson syndrome, thrombocytopenia, toxic epidermal necrolysis, urticaria, vaginitis

Drug Interactions

Metabolism/Transport Effects None known.

Avoid Concomitant Use

Avoid concomitant use of Cefotaxime with any of the following: BCG

Increased Effect/Toxicity

Cefotaxime may increase the levels/effects of: Aminoglycosides; Vitamin K Antagonists

The levels/effects of Cefotaxime may be increased by: Probenecid

Decreased Effect

Cefotaxime may decrease the levels/effects of: BCG; Sodium Picosulfate; Typhoid Vaccine

Preparation for Administration

IM: Reconstitute vials with SWFI or bacteriostatic water for injection; dilute with 2 mL for the 500 mg vial (resulting concentration ~230 mg/mL), 3 mL for the 1 g vial (resulting concentration ~300 mg/mL), and 5 mL for the 2 g vial (resulting concentration 330 mg/mL). Shake to dissolve.

IV: Reconstitute vials with ≥10 mL SWFI; resulting concentration: 50 mg/mL (500 mg vial), 95 mg/mL (1 g vial), or 180 mg/mL (2 g vial). Shake to dissolve. May be further diluted up to 1000 mL with NS, D_5W, $D_{10}W$, D_5NS, $D_5{}^1/_2NS$, $D_5{}^1/_4NS$, or LR.

Storage/Stability Store intact vials below 30°C (86°F). Protect from light. Reconstituted solution is stable for 12 to 24 hours at room temperature, 7 to 10 days when refrigerated, for 13 weeks when frozen. For IV infusion in NS or D_5W, solution is stable for 24 hours at room temperature, 5 days when refrigerated, or 13 weeks when frozen in Viaflex plastic containers. Thawed solutions of frozen premixed bags are stable for 24 hours at room temperature or 10 days when refrigerated.

Mechanism of Action Inhibits bacterial cell wall synthesis by binding to one or more of the penicillin-binding proteins (PBPs) which in turn inhibits the final transpeptidation step of peptidoglycan synthesis in bacterial cell walls, thus inhibiting cell wall biosynthesis. Bacteria eventually lyse due to ongoing activity of cell wall autolytic enzymes (autolysins and murein hydrolases) while cell wall assembly is arrested. Cefotaxime has activity in the presence of some beta-lactamases, both penicillinases and cephaolsporinases, of gram-negative and gram-positive bacteria. *Enterococcus* species may be intrinsically resistant to cefotaxime. Most extended-spectrum beta-lactamase (ESBL)-producing and carbapenemase-producing isolates are resistant to cefotaxime.

Pharmacodynamics/Kinetics

Distribution: Widely to body tissues and fluids including aqueous humor, ascitic and prostatic fluids, bone; penetrates CSF best when meninges are inflamed

Metabolism: Partially hepatic to active metabolite, desacetylcefotaxime

Half-life elimination:

Cefotaxime: Infants ≤1500 g: 4.6 hours; Infants >1500 g: 3.4 hours; Adults: ~1 hour; prolonged with renal and/or hepatic impairment

Desacetylcefotaxime: 1.3 to 1.9 hours; prolonged with renal impairment (Ings, 1982)

Time to peak, serum: IM: Within 30 minutes

Excretion: Urine (~60% as unchanged drug and metabolites)

Dosage

Usual dosage range:

Infants, Children, and Adolescents:

Manufacturer's recommendations:

<50 kg: IM, IV: 50 to 180 mg/kg/day in divided doses every 4 to 6 hours (maximum dose: 12 g daily)

≥50 kg: Refer to adult dosing

Alternate recommendations (Red Book [AAP], 2012): IM, IV:

Mild to moderate infection: 50 to 180 mg/kg/day in divided doses every 6 to 8 hours (maximum dose: 6 g daily)

Severe infection: 200 to 225 mg/kg/day in divided doses every 4 to 6 hours; up to 300 mg/kg/day has been used for meningitis (maximum dose: 12 g daily)

Adults: IM, IV: 1 to 2 g every 4 to 12 hours (maximum dose, 12 g daily)

Uncomplicated infections: IM, IV: 1 g every 12 hours

Moderate to severe infections: IM, IV: 1 to 2 g every 8 hours

Life-threatening infections: IV: 2 g every 4 hours

Indication-specific dosing:

Infants and Children:

Acute bacterial rhinosinusitis, severe infection requiring hospitalization (off-label use): Children: IV: 100 to 200 mg/kg/day divided every 6 hours for 10 to 14 days (Chow, 2012)

Community-acquired pneumonia (CAP) (IDSA/PIDS, 2011): Infants >3 months and Children: IV: **Note:** May consider addition of vancomycin or clindamycin to empiric therapy if community-acquired MRSA suspected. In children ≥5 years, a macrolide antibiotic should be added if atypical pneumonia cannot be ruled out.

Empiric treatment, *Haemophilus influenzae*, group A *Streptococcus*, or *S. pneumoniae* (MICs to penicillin ≤2.0 mcg/mL), patient fully immunized for *H. influenzae* type b and *S. pneumoniae*, or minimal local resistance to penicillin in invasive pneumococcal strains (alternative to ampicillin or penicillin): 50 mg/kg/dose every 8 hours

Moderate-to-severe infection, patient not fully immunized for *H. influenzae* type b and *S. pneumoniae*, or significant local resistance to penicillin in invasive pneumococcal strains (preferred): 50 mg/kg/dose every 8 hours

Moderate-to-severe infection, *H. influenzae* (beta-lactamase producing) (preferred): 50 mg/kg/dose every 8 hours

Complicated community-acquired intra-abdominal infection (in combination with metronidazole): IV: 150 to 200 mg/kg/day divided every 6 to 8 hours (Solomkin, 2010)

Lyme disease (as an alternative to ceftriaxone): *Cardiac or CNS manifestations:* IV: 150 to 200 mg/kg/day in divided doses every 6 to 8 hours for 14 to 28 days; maximum daily dose: 6 g daily (Halperin, 2007; Wormser, 2006)

Meningitis (in combination with vancomycin): IV: 225 to 300 mg/kg/day in divided doses every 6 to 8 hours (Tunkel, 2004)

Sepsis: IV: 150 mg/kg/day divided every 8 hours

Surgical (perioperative) prophylaxis (off-label use): Children ≥1 year: IV: 50 mg/kg within 60 minutes prior to surgery (maximum: 1000 mg per dose). Doses may be repeated in 3 hours if procedure is lengthy or if there is excessive blood loss. **Note:** preferred agent (with ampicillin) in liver transplantation (Bratzler, 2013).

Infants and Children ≤12 years:

Typhoid fever: IM, IV: 150 to 200 mg/kg/day in 3 to 4 divided doses (maximum: 12 g daily); fluoroquinolone resistant: 80 mg/kg/day in 3 to 4 divided doses (maximum: 12 g daily)

Children ≥50 kg, Adolescents, and Adults:

Arthritis (septic): IV: 1 g every 8 hours

Brain abscess, meningitis: IV: 2 g every 4 to 6 hours in combination with other antimicrobial therapy as warranted (Kowlessar, 2006; Tunkel, 2004)

Cesarean section: IM, IV: 1 g IV as soon as the umbilical cord is clamped, then 1 g IV or IM at 6 and 12 hours after the first dose

Lyme disease (as an alternative to ceftriaxone):

Cardiac manifestations: IV: 2 g every 8 hours for 14 to 21 days (Wormser, 2006)

CNS manifestations: IV: 2 g every 8 hours for 10 to 28 days (Halperin, 2007; Wormser, 2006)

Peritonitis (spontaneous): IV: 2 g every 8 hours, unless life-threatening then 2 g every 4 hours (Gilbert, 2011; Runyon, 2009)

Sepsis: IV: 2 g every 6 to 8 hours

Skin and soft tissue:

Bite wounds (animal): IV: 2 g every 6 hours

Mixed, necrotizing: IV: 2 g every 6 hours, with metronidazole or clindamycin (Stevens, 2005)

Children ≥45 kg, Adolescents ≥45 kg, and Adults:

Gonorrhea (CDC, 2010) (as an alternative to ceftriaxone):

Uncomplicated gonorrhea of the cervix, urethra, or rectum (off-label regimen): IM: 0.5 g as a single dose in combination with oral azithromycin (preferred) or oral doxycycline (alternative to preferred)

Note: May also administer 1 g as a single dose for rectal gonorrhea in adult males (per the manufacturer)

Disseminated: IV: 1 g every 8 hours continue for 24 to 48 hours after improvement begins then switch to oral therapy. Total duration of therapy at least 7 days

Adults:

Acute bacterial rhinosinusitis, severe infection requiring hospitalization: IV: 2 g every 4 to 6 hours for 5 to 7 days (Chow, 2012)

Complicated community-acquired intra-abdominal infection of mild-to-moderate severity, including hepatic abscess (in combination with metronidazole): IV: 1 to 2 g every 6 to 8 hours for 4 to 7 days (provided source controlled). **Note:** For severe infections, consider other antimicrobial agents (Bradley, 1987; Kim, 2010; Solomkin, 2010).

Surgical (perioperative) prophylaxis (off-label use): IV: 1 g within 60 minutes prior to surgical incision. Doses may be repeated in 3 hours if procedure is lengthy or if there is excessive blood loss. **Note:** preferred agent (with ampicillin) in liver transplantation (Bratzler, 2013).

Obesity: The ASHP/IDSA/SIS/SHEA guidelines recommend that for patients weighing ≥120 kg (or alternatively defined as BMI >30 kg/m^2), a dose of 2 g within 60 minutes prior to surgical incision should be administered (Bratzler, 2013).

Dosage adjustment in renal impairment:

Manufacturer's labeling: **Note:** Renal function may be estimated using Cockcroft-Gault formula for dosage adjustment purposes.

CrCl <20 mL/minute/1.73 m^2: Dose should be decreased by 50%.

Alternate recommendations:

Children: **Note:** Glomerular filtration rate (GFR) should be estimated using an acceptable pediatric method (eg, Schwartz equation, Traub-Johnson equation, or a height/weight nomogram):

The following dosage adjustments have been used by some clinicians (Aronoff, 2007):

GFR 30 to 50 mL/minute/1.73 m^2: 35 to 70 mg/kg/dose every 8 to 12 hours

GFR 10 to 29 mL/minute/1.73 m^2: 35 to 70 mg/kg/dose every 12 hours

GFR <10 mL/minute/1.73 m^2: 35 to 70 mg/kg/dose every 24 hours

Intermittent hemodialysis (IHD): 35 to 70 mg/kg/dose every 24 hours

Peritoneal dialysis: 35 to 70 mg/kg/dose every 24 hours

Continuous renal replacement therapy (CRRT): 35 to 70 mg/kg/dose every 12 hours

Adults: The following dosage adjustments have been used by some clinicians (Aronoff, 2007; Heintz, 2009; Trotman, 2005):

GFR >50 mL/minute: Administer every 6 hours (Aronoff, 2007)

GFR 10 to 50 mL/minute: Administer every 6 to 12 hours (Aronoff, 2007)

GFR <10 mL/minute: Administer every 24 hours **or** decrease the dose by 50% (and administer at usual intervals) (Aronoff, 2007)

Intermittent hemodialysis (IHD): Administer 1 to 2 g every 24 hours (on dialysis days, administer after hemodialysis). **Note:** Dosing dependent on the assumption of 3 times/week, complete IHD sessions (Heintz, 2009).

Peritoneal dialysis (PD): 1 g every 24 hours (Aronoff, 2007)

Continuous renal replacement therapy (CRRT) (Heintz, 2009; Trotman, 2005): Drug clearance is highly dependent on the method of renal replacement, filter type, and flow rate. Appropriate dosing requires close monitoring of pharmacologic response, signs of adverse reactions due to drug accumulation, as well as drug concentrations in relation to target trough (if appropriate). The following are general recommendations only (based on dialysate flow/ultrafiltration rates of 1 to 2 L/hour and minimal residual renal function) and should not supersede clinical judgment:

CVVH: 1 to 2 g every 8 to 12 hours

CVVHD: 1 to 2 g every 8 hours

CVVHDF: 1 to 2 g every 6 to 8 hours

Dosage adjustment in hepatic impairment: There are no dosage adjustments provided in the manufacturer's labeling.

Dietary Considerations Some products may contain sodium.

Administration

IM: Inject deep IM into large muscle mass. Individual doses of 2 g may be given if the dose is divided and administered in different IM sites.

IV: Can be administered IV bolus over at least 3 to 5 minutes or as an IV intermittent infusion over 15 to 30 minutes.

Monitoring Parameters Observe for signs and symptoms of anaphylaxis during first dose; CBC with differential (especially with long courses [>10 days]); renal function

Dosage Forms

Solution, Intravenous:

Claforan in D_5W: 1 g/50 mL (50 mL); 2 g/50 mL (50 mL)

Solution Reconstituted, Injection:

Claforan: 500 mg (1 ea); 1 g (1 ea); 2 g (1 ea); 10 g (1 ea)

Generic: 500 mg (1 ea); 1 g (1 ea); 2 g (1 ea); 10 g (1 ea)

Solution Reconstituted, Intravenous:

Claforan: 1 g (1 ea); 2 g (1 ea)

◆ **Cefotaxime Sodium** *see* Cefotaxime *on page 382*

◆ **Cefotaxime Sodium For Injection (Can)** *see* Cefotaxime *on page 382*

CefoTEtan (SEF oh tee tan)

Index Terms Cefotan; Cefotetan Disodium

Pharmacologic Category Antibiotic, Cephalosporin (Second Generation)

Use Surgical (perioperative) prophylaxis; intra-abdominal infections and other mixed infections; respiratory tract, skin and skin structure, bone and joint, urinary tract and gynecologic infections as well as septicemia; active against gram-negative enteric bacilli including *E. coli*, *Klebsiella*, and *Proteus*; less active against staphylococci and streptococci than first generation cephalosporins, but active against anaerobes including *Bacteroides fragilis*

Pregnancy Risk Factor B

Pregnancy Considerations Adverse events have not been observed in animal reproduction studies. Cefotetan crosses the placenta and produces therapeutic concentrations in the amniotic fluid and cord serum. Cefotetan is one of the antibiotics recommended for prophylactic use prior to cesarean delivery.

Breast-Feeding Considerations Very small amounts of cefotetan are excreted in human milk. The manufacturer recommends caution when giving cefotetan to a breast-feeding mother. Nondose-related effects could include modification of bowel flora.

Contraindications Hypersensitivity to cefotetan, any component of the formulation, or other cephalosporins; previous cephalosporin-associated hemolytic anemia

Warnings/Precautions Modify dosage in patients with severe renal impairment. Although cefotetan contains the methyltetrazolethiol side chain, bleeding has not been a significant problem. Use with caution in patients with a history of penicillin allergy, especially IgE-mediated reactions (eg, anaphylaxis, urticaria). Cefotetan has been associated with a higher risk of hemolytic anemia relative to other cephalosporins (approximately threefold); monitor carefully during use and consider cephalosporin-associated immune anemia in patients who have received cefotetan within 2-3 weeks (either as treatment or prophylaxis). Prolonged use may result in fungal or bacterial superinfection, including *C. difficile*-associated diarrhea (CDAD) and pseudomembranous colitis; CDAD has been observed >2 months postantibiotic treatment. May be associated with increased INR, especially in nutritionally-deficient patients, prolonged treatment, hepatic or renal disease.

Adverse Reactions

Gastrointestinal: Diarrhea

Hepatic: Transaminases increased

Miscellaneous: Hypersensitivity reactions

Rare but important or life-threatening: Agranulocytosis, anaphylaxis, bleeding, BUN increased, creatinine increased, eosinophilia, fever, hemolytic anemia, leukopenia, nausea, nephrotoxicity, phlebitis, prolonged PT, pruritus, pseudomembranous colitis, rash, thrombocytopenia, thrombocytosis, urticaria, vomiting

Reactions reported with other cephalosporins: Agranulocytosis, aplastic anemia, cholestasis, colitis, hemolytic anemia, hemorrhage, pancytopenia, renal dysfunction, seizure, Stevens-Johnson syndrome, superinfection, toxic epidermal necrolysis, toxic nephropathy

Drug Interactions

Metabolism/Transport Effects None known.

Avoid Concomitant Use

Avoid concomitant use of CefoTEtan with any of the following: BCG

Increased Effect/Toxicity

CefoTEtan may increase the levels/effects of: Alcohol (Ethyl); Aminoglycosides; Carbocisteine; Vitamin K Antagonists

The levels/effects of CefoTEtan may be increased by: Probenecid

Decreased Effect

CefoTEtan may decrease the levels/effects of: BCG; Sodium Picosulfate; Typhoid Vaccine

Food Interactions Concurrent use with ethanol may cause a disulfiram-like reaction. Management: Monitor patients.

Storage/Stability Reconstituted solution is stable for 24 hours at room temperature and 96 hours when refrigerated. For IV infusion in NS or D_5W solution and after freezing, thawed solution is stable for 24 hours at room temperature or 96 hours when refrigerated. Frozen solution is stable for 12 weeks. Thawed solutions of the commercially available frozen cefotetan injections are stable for 48 hours at room temperature or 21 days when refrigerated.

Mechanism of Action Inhibits bacterial cell wall synthesis by binding to one or more of the penicillin-binding proteins (PBPs) which in turn inhibits the final transpeptidation step of peptidoglycan synthesis in bacterial cell walls, thus inhibiting cell wall biosynthesis. Bacteria eventually lyse due to ongoing activity of cell wall autolytic enzymes (autolysins and murein hydrolases) while cell wall assembly is arrested.

Pharmacodynamics/Kinetics

Distribution: Widely to body tissues and fluids including bile, sputum, prostatic, peritoneal; low concentrations enter CSF

Protein binding: 76% to 90%

Half-life elimination: 3-5 hours

Time to peak, serum: IM: 1.5-3 hours

Excretion: Primarily urine (as unchanged drug); feces (20%)

Dosage

Usual dosage range:

Children (off-label use): IM, IV: 20-40 mg/kg/dose every 12 hours (maximum: 6 **g** daily)

Adults: IM, IV: 1-6 g daily in divided doses every 12 hours

Indication-specific dosing:

Children (off-label use):

Surgical (perioperative) prophylaxis: Children ≥1 year: IV: 40 mg/kg 30-60 minutes prior to surgery (maximum: 2000 mg/dose). Doses may be repeated in 6 hours if procedure is lengthy or if there is excessive blood loss (Bratzler, 2013).

Adolescents and Adults:

Pelvic inflammatory disease: IV: 2 g every 12 hours; used in combination with doxycycline (CDC, 2010)

Adults:

Orbital cellulitis, odontogenic infections: IV: 2 g every 12 hours (Bailey, 2007; Quayle, 1987)

Surgical (perioperative) prophylaxis:

Manufacturer recommendations: IV: 1-2 g 30-60 minutes prior to surgery. **Note:** When used for cesarean section, dose should be given as soon as umbilical cord is clamped.

Alternative recommendations: IV: 2 g within 60 minutes prior to surgery. Doses may be repeated in 6 hours if procedure is lengthy or if there is excessive blood loss (Bratzler, 2013).

Susceptible infections: IM, IV: 1-6 g daily in divided doses every 12 hours; usual dose: 1-2 g every 12 hours for 5-10 days; 1-2 g may be given every 24 hours for urinary tract infection; **Note:** Due to high rates of *B. fragilis* group resistance, not recommended for the treatment of community-acquired intra-abdominal infections (Solomkin, 2010)

Urinary tract infection: IM, IV: 500 mg every 12 hours or 1-2 g every 12-24 hours

Dosage adjustment in renal impairment:

CrCl 10-30 mL/minute: Administer every 24 hours

CrCl <10 mL/minute: Administer every 48 hours

Hemodialysis: Dialyzable (5% to 20%); administer 1/4 the usual dose every 24 hours on days between dialysis; administer 1/2 the usual dose on the day of dialysis.

Continuous arteriovenous or venovenous hemodiafiltration effects: Administer 750 mg every 12 hours

Dosage adjustment in hepatic impairment: No dosage adjustment provided in manufacturer's labeling.

Dietary Considerations Some products may contain sodium.

Administration

IM: Inject deep IM into large muscle mass.

IV: Inject direct IV over 3-5 minutes. Infuse intermittent infusion over 30 minutes.

Monitoring Parameters Monitor renal, hepatic, and hematologic function periodically with prolonged therapy. Monitor prothrombin time in patients at risk of prolongation during cephalosporin therapy (nutritionally-deficient, prolonged treatment, renal or hepatic disease). Monitor for signs and symptoms of hemolytic anemia, including hematologic parameters where appropriate.

Dosage Forms

Solution Reconstituted, Injection:

Generic: 1 g (1 ea); 2 g (1 ea); 10 g (1 ea)

Solution Reconstituted, Intravenous:

Generic: 1 g (1 ea); 2 g (1 ea)

◆ **Cefotetan Disodium** *see* CefoTEtan *on page 385*

CefOXitin (se FOKS i tin)

Brand Names: U.S. Mefoxin

Brand Names: Canada Cefoxitin For Injection

Index Terms Cefoxitin Sodium

Pharmacologic Category Antibiotic, Cephalosporin (Second Generation)

Use

Bone and joint infections: Treatment of bone and joint infections caused by *Staphylococcus aureus* (including penicillinase-producing strains).

Gynecological infections: Treatment of endometritis, pelvic cellulitis, and pelvic inflammatory disease caused by *Escherichia coli*, *Neisseria gonorrhoeae* (including penicillinase-producing strains), *Bacteroides* species including *Bacteroides fragilis*, *Clostridium* species, *P. niger*, *Peptostreptococcus* species, and *Streptococcus agalactiae*.

Intra-abdominal infections: Treatment of peritonitis and intra-abdominal infections or abscess, caused by *E. coli*, *Klebsiella* species, *Bacteroides* species (including *B. fragilis*), and *Clostridium* species.

Lower respiratory tract infections: Treatment of pneumonia and lung abscess, caused by *Streptococcus pneumoniae*, other streptococci (excluding enterococci; eg, *Enterococcus faecalis* [formerly *Streptococcus faecalis*]), *S. aureus* (including penicillinase-producing strains), *E. coli*, *Klebsiella* species, *Haemophilus influenzae*, and *Bacteroides* species.

Perioperative prophylaxis: Prophylaxis of infection in patients undergoing uncontaminated GI surgery, abdominal or vaginal hysterectomy, or cesarean section.

Septicemia: Treatment of septicemia caused by *S. pneumoniae*, *S. aureus* (including penicillinase-producing strains), *E. coli*, *Klebsiella* species, and *Bacteroides* species including *B. fragilis*.

Skin and skin structure infections: Treatment of skin and skin structure infections caused by *S. aureus* (including penicillinase-producing strains), *Staphylococcus epidermidis*, *Streptococcus pyogenes* and other streptococci (excluding enterococci [eg, *E. faecalis*] [formerly *S. faecalis*]), *E. coli*, *Proteus mirabilis*, *Klebsiella* species, *Bacteroides* species including *B. fragilis*, *Clostridium* species, *P. niger*, and *Peptostreptococcus* species.

Urinary tract infections: Treatment of UTIs caused by *E. coli*, *Klebsiella* species, *P. mirabilis*, *Morganella morganii*, *Proteus vulgaris*, and *Providencia* species (including *Providencia rettgeri*).

Limitations of use: Cefoxitin does not have activity against *Chlamydia trachomatis*. When cefoxitin is used to treat pelvic inflammatory disease, add appropriate antichlamydial coverage.

Pregnancy Risk Factor B

Pregnancy Considerations Adverse events have not been observed in animal reproduction studies. Cefoxitin crosses the placenta and reaches the cord serum and amniotic fluid.

Peak serum concentrations of cefoxitin during pregnancy may be similar to or decreased compared to nonpregnant values. Maternal half-life may be shorter at term. Pregnancy-induced hypertension increases trough concentrations in the immediate postpartum period. Cefoxitin is one of the antibiotics recommended for prophylactic use prior to cesarean delivery.

Breast-Feeding Considerations Very small amounts of cefoxitin are excreted in breast milk. The manufacturer recommends that caution be exercised when administering cefoxitin to nursing women. Nondose-related effects could include modification of bowel flora. Cefoxitin pharmacokinetics may be altered immediately postpartum.

Contraindications Hypersensitivity to cefoxitin, any component of the formulation, or other cephalosporins

Warnings/Precautions Modify dosage in patients with severe renal impairment. Prolonged use may result in superinfection. Use with caution in patients with a history of penicillin allergy, especially IgE-mediated hypersensitivity reactions (eg, anaphylaxis, urticaria). If a hypersensitivity reaction occurs, discontinue immediately. Use with caution in patients with a history of seizures or gastrointestinal disease (particularly colitis). Prolonged use may result in fungal or bacterial superinfection, including *C. difficile*-associated diarrhea (CDAD) and pseudomembranous colitis; CDAD has been observed >2 months postantibiotic treatment. For group A beta-hemolytic streptococcal infections, antimicrobial therapy should be given for at least 10 days to guard against the risk of rheumatic fever or glomerulonephritis. In pediatric patients ≥3 months of age, higher doses have been associated with an increased incidence of eosinophilia and elevated AST. Elderly patients are more likely to have decreased renal function; use care in dose selection and monitor renal function.

Adverse Reactions

Gastrointestinal: Diarrhea

Rare but important or life-threatening: Anaphylaxis, angioedema, bone marrow depression, dyspnea, eosinophilia, exacerbation of myasthenia gravis, exfoliative dermatitis, fever, hemolytic anemia, hypotension, increased blood urea nitrogen, increased serum creatinine, increased serum transaminases, interstitial nephritis, jaundice, leukopenia, nausea, nephrotoxicity (increased; with aminoglycosides), phlebitis, prolonged prothrombin time, pruritus, pseudomembranous colitis, skin rash, thrombocytopenia, thrombophlebitis, toxic epidermal necrolysis, urticaria, vomiting

Drug Interactions

Metabolism/Transport Effects None known.

Avoid Concomitant Use

Avoid concomitant use of CefOXitin with any of the following: BCG

Increased Effect/Toxicity

CefOXitin may increase the levels/effects of: Aminoglycosides; Vitamin K Antagonists

The levels/effects of CefOXitin may be increased by: Probenecid

Decreased Effect

CefOXitin may decrease the levels/effects of: BCG; Sodium Picosulfate; Typhoid Vaccine

Preparation for Administration Reconstitute vials with SWFI, bacteriostatic water for injection, NS, or D_5W. For IV infusion, solutions may be further diluted in NS, $D_5{}^1/_4$NS, $D_5{}^1/_2$NS, D_5NS, D_5W, $D_{10}W$, LR, D_5LR, mannitol 5% or 10%, or sodium bicarbonate 5%.

Storage/Stability Prior to reconstitution store between 2°C and 25°C (36°F and 77°F). Avoid exposure to temperatures >50°C (122°F). Cefoxitin tends to darken depending on storage conditions; however, product potency is not adversely affected.

Reconstituted solutions of 1 g per 10 mL in sterile water for injection, bacteriostatic water for injection, sodium chloride 0.9% injection, or dextrose 5% injection are stable for 6 hours at room temperature or for 7 days under refrigeration (<5°C [43°F]).

DUPLEX container: Store unactivated container at 20°C to 25°C (68°F to 77°F); excursions permitted to 15°C to 30°C (59°F to 86°F); do not freeze. Following activation, solution is stable for 12 hours at room temperature and 7 days refrigerated.

Mechanism of Action Inhibits bacterial cell wall synthesis by binding to one or more of the penicillin-binding proteins (PBPs) which in turn inhibits the final transpeptidation step of peptidoglycan synthesis in bacterial cell walls, thus inhibiting cell wall biosynthesis. Bacteria eventually lyse due to ongoing activity of cell wall autolytic enzymes (autolysins and murein hydrolases) while cell wall assembly is arrested.

Pharmacodynamics/Kinetics

Distribution: Widely to body tissues and fluids including pleural, synovial, bile; poorly penetrates into CSF even with inflammation of the meninges (Landesman, 1981)

Protein binding: 65% to 79%

Half-life elimination: 41-59 minutes; prolonged with renal impairment

Excretion: Urine (85% as unchanged drug)

Dosage

Usual dosage range:

Infants >3 months, Children, and Adolescents: IV: 80-160 mg/kg/day in divided doses every 4-6 hours (maximum dose: 12 **g daily**)

Adults: IV: 1-2 g every 6-8 hours (maximum dose: 12 g daily)

Note: IM injection is painful

Indication-specific dosing: Note: For group A beta-hemolytic streptococcal infections, antimicrobial therapy should be given for at least 10 days to guard against the risk of rheumatic fever or glomerulonephritis

Infants >3 months, Children, and Adolescents:

Manufacturer's labeling: IV: 80-160 mg/kg/day divided every 4-6 hours (maximum daily dose: 12 **g daily**)

Alternative recommendations (Redbook [AAP, 2012]):

Mild-to-moderate infection: IV: 80 mg/kg/day in divided doses every 6-8 hours (maximum daily dose: 4000 mg daily)

Severe infection: IV: 160 mg/kg/day in divided doses every 6 hours (maximum daily dose: 12 **g daily**)

Surgical (perioperative) prophylaxis:

Manufacturer recommendations: IV: 30-40 mg/kg 30-60 minutes prior to surgical incision followed by 30-40 mg/kg/dose every 6 hours for no more than 24 hours after surgery depending on the procedure

Alternative recommendations:

Children ≥1 year: IV: 40 mg/kg within 60 minutes prior to surgical incision (maximum: 2000 mg per dose). Doses may be repeated in 2 hours if procedure is lengthy or if there is excessive blood loss (Bratzler, 2013).

Adolescents: Refer to adult dosing.

Adults:

Gas gangrene: IV: 2 g every 4 hours or 3 g every 6 hours (maximum daily dosage: 12 g daily)

Intra-abdominal infection, complicated, community acquired, mild-to-moderate (Solomkin, 2010): IV: 2 g every 6 hours for 4-7 days (provided source controlled)

Moderately severe or severe infections: IV: 1 g every 4 hours or 2 g every 6-8 hours (maximum daily dosage: 8 g daily)

***Mycobacterium abscessus*, not MTB or MAI (off-label use; Griffith, 2007):** IV: 12 g daily in divided doses with concomitant amikacin for ≥14 days

Pelvic inflammatory disease (CDC, 2010):

Inpatients: IV: 2 g every 6 hours **plus** doxycycline for at least 24 hours after clinical improvement, followed by doxycycline to complete 14 days

Outpatients: IM: 2 g **plus** oral probenecid as a single dose, followed by doxycycline (with or without concomitant metronidazole) for 14 days

Surgical (perioperative) prophylaxis:

Manufacturer recommendations (procedures other than Cesarian section): IV: 2 g 30-60 minutes prior to surgical incision, followed by 2 g every 6 hours for no more than 24 hours after surgery depending on the procedure

Cesarean section: IV: 2 g as soon as umbilical cord is clamped as a single dose **or** 2 g as soon as umbilical cord is clamped followed by 2 g at 4 and 8 hours after the initial dose.

Alternative recommendations: 2 g within 60 minutes prior to surgical incision. Doses may be repeated in 2 hours if procedure is lengthy or if there is excessive blood loss (Bratzler, 2013).

Uncomplicated cutaneous, urinary tract, lung infections: IV: 1 g every 6-8 hours (maximum daily dosage: 4 g daily)

Dosage adjustment in renal impairment:

CrCl 30-50 mL/minute: 1-2 g every 8-12 hours
CrCl 10-29 mL/minute: 1-2 g every 12-24 hours
CrCl 5-9 mL/minute: 0.5-1 g every 12-24 hours
CrCl <5 mL/minute: 0.5-1 g every 24-48 hours

Hemodialysis: Loading dose: 1-2 g after each hemodialysis; maintenance dose as noted above based on creatinine clearance

Dosage adjustment in hepatic impairment: There are no dosage adjustments provided in manufacturer's labeling.

Dietary Considerations Some products may contain sodium.

Administration

IM: Inject deep IM into large muscle mass. **Note:** IM injection is painful and this route of administration is not described in the prescribing information.

IV: Can be administered IVP over 3-5 minutes or by IV intermittent infusion over 10-60 minutes

Monitoring Parameters Monitor renal function periodically when used in combination with other nephrotoxic drugs; prothrombin time. Observe for signs and symptoms of anaphylaxis during first dose.

Dosage Forms

Solution, Intravenous:
Mefoxin: 1 g (50 mL); 2 g (50 mL)

Solution Reconstituted, Injection:
Generic: 10 g (1 ea)

Solution Reconstituted, Injection [preservative free]:
Generic: 10 g (1 ea)

Solution Reconstituted, Intravenous:
Generic: 1 g (1 ea); 2 g (1 ea)

Solution Reconstituted, Intravenous [preservative free]:
Generic: 1 g (1 ea); 2 g (1 ea)

◆ **Cefoxitin For Injection (Can)** *see* CefOXitin *on page 386*

◆ **Cefoxitin Sodium** *see* CefOXitin *on page 386*

Cefpirome [INT] (SEF pir ome)

International Brand Names Abirom (ID); Allard (IN); Ceferom (TW); Cefire (VN); Cefrin (PH); Cefrom (AT, CN, FR, GR, ID, IN, KW, PK, SA, TW, ZA); Ferome (TH); Givincef (ID); Hancerom (KR); Luobang (CN); Medtol (VN); Ucerom (KR); Unipiren (VN); Yarox (ID); Zeferom (PH)

Index Terms Cefpirome sulphate

Pharmacologic Category Antibiotic, Cephalosporin (Fourth Generation)

Reported Use Lower respiratory tract infections, complicated upper and lower urinary tract infections, septicemia, bacteremia, and neutropenic fever caused by susceptible organisms

Dosage Range Adults: I.V.: 1-2 g every 12 hours; maximum daily dose: 4 g

Dosage adjustment in renal impairment: Decrease dose if CrCl is <50 mL/minute

Product Availability Product available in various countries; not currently available in the U.S.

Dosage Forms

Injection, powder for reconstitution: 0.5 g, 1 g, 2 g

◆ **Cefpirome sulphate** *see* Cefpirome [INT] *on page 388*

Cefpodoxime (sef pode OKS eem)

Index Terms Cefpodoxime Proxetil; Vantin

Pharmacologic Category Antibiotic, Cephalosporin (Third Generation)

Use Treatment of susceptible acute, community-acquired pneumonia caused by *S. pneumoniae* or nonbeta-lactamase producing *H. influenzae*; acute uncomplicated gonorrhea caused by *N. gonorrhoeae*; uncomplicated skin and skin structure infections caused by *S. aureus* or *S. pyogenes*; acute otitis media caused by *S. pneumoniae*, *H. influenzae*, or *M. catarrhalis*; pharyngitis or tonsillitis; and uncomplicated urinary tract infections caused by *E. coli*, *Klebsiella*, and *Proteus*

Pregnancy Risk Factor B

Pregnancy Considerations Teratogenic events were not observed in animal reproduction studies. An increase in most types of birth defects was not found following first trimester exposure to cephalosporins.

Breast-Feeding Considerations Cefpodoxime is excreted in breast milk. The manufacturer recommends discontinuing nursing or discontinuing the medication in breast-feeding women. Nondose-related effects could include modification of bowel flora.

Contraindications Hypersensitivity to cefpodoxime, any component of the formulation, or other cephalosporins

Warnings/Precautions Modify dosage in patients with severe renal impairment. Prolonged use may result in fungal or bacterial superinfection, including *C. difficile*-associated diarrhea (CDAD) and pseudomembranous colitis; CDAD has been observed >2 months postantibiotic treatment. Use with caution in patients with a history of penicillin allergy, especially IgE-mediated reactions (eg, anaphylaxis, urticaria).

Benzyl alcohol and derivatives: Some dosage forms may contain sodium benzoate/benzoic acid; benzoic acid (benzoate) is a metabolite of benzyl alcohol; large amounts of benzyl alcohol (≥99 mg/kg/day) have been associated with a potentially fatal toxicity ("gasping syndrome") in neonates; the "gasping syndrome" consists of metabolic acidosis, respiratory distress, gasping respirations, CNS dysfunction (including convulsions, intracranial hemorrhage), hypotension, and cardiovascular collapse (AAP, 1997; CDC, 1982); some data suggests that benzoate displaces bilirubin from protein binding sites (Ahlfors, 2001); avoid or use dosage forms containing benzyl alcohol derivative with caution in neonates. See manufacturer's labeling.

Adverse Reactions

Central nervous system: Headache

Dermatologic: Diaper rash, skin rash

Gastrointestinal: Abdominal pain, diarrhea, nausea, vomiting

Genitourinary: Vaginal infection

Rare but important or life-threatening: Anaphylaxis, anxiety, chest pain, cough, decreased appetite, dizziness, dysgeusia, epistaxis, eye pruritus, fatigue, fever, flatulence, flushing, fungal skin infection, hypotension, insomnia, malaise, nightmares, pruritus, pseudomembranous colitis, purpuric nephritis, tinnitus, vulvovaginal candidiasis, weakness, xerostomia

Drug Interactions

Metabolism/Transport Effects None known.

Avoid Concomitant Use

Avoid concomitant use of Cefpodoxime with any of the following: BCG

Increased Effect/Toxicity

Cefpodoxime may increase the levels/effects of: Aminoglycosides; Vitamin K Antagonists

The levels/effects of Cefpodoxime may be increased by: Probenecid

Decreased Effect

Cefpodoxime may decrease the levels/effects of: BCG; Sodium Picosulfate; Typhoid Vaccine

The levels/effects of Cefpodoxime may be decreased by: Antacids; H2-Antagonists

Food Interactions Food and/or low gastric pH delays absorption and may increase serum levels. Management: Take with or without food at regular intervals on an around-the-clock schedule to promote less variation in peak and trough serum levels.

Storage/Stability

Granules for suspension: Store at 20°C to 25°C (68°F to 77°F); after reconstitution, suspension may be stored in refrigerator for 14 days.

Tablet: Store at 20°C to 25°C (68°F to 77°F); protect from light.

Mechanism of Action Inhibits bacterial cell wall synthesis by binding to one or more of the penicillin-binding proteins (PBPs) which in turn inhibits the final transpeptidation step of peptidoglycan synthesis in bacterial cell walls, thus inhibiting cell wall biosynthesis. Bacteria eventually lyse due to ongoing activity of cell wall autolytic enzymes (autolysins and murein hydrolases) while cell wall assembly is arrested.

Pharmacodynamics/Kinetics

Absorption: Rapid and well absorbed (50%), acid stable; enhanced in the presence of food or low gastric pH

Distribution: Good tissue penetration, including lung and tonsils; penetrates into pleural fluid

Protein binding: 18% to 23%

Metabolism: De-esterified in GI tract to active metabolite, cefpodoxime

Half-life elimination: 2.2 hours; prolonged with renal impairment

Time to peak: Within 1 hour

Excretion: Urine (80% as unchanged drug) in 24 hours

Dosage

Usual dosage range:

Children 2 months to 12 years: Oral: 10 mg/kg/day divided every 12 hours (maximum: 200 mg/dose)

Children ≥12 years and Adults: Oral: 100-400 mg every 12 hours

Indication-specific dosing:

Children 2 months to 12 years: Oral:

Acute bacterial rhinosinusitis (off-label use): Children: 10 mg/kg/day divided every 12 hours (maximum: 200 mg/dose) with concomitant clindamycin for 10-14 days. **Note:** Recommended in patients with non-type I penicillin allergy, after failure of initial therapy or in patients at risk for antibiotic resistance (eg, daycare attendance, age <2 years, recent hospitalization, antibiotic use within the past month) (Chow, 2012)

Acute maxillary sinusitis: 10 mg/kg/day divided every 12 hours for 10 days (maximum: 200 mg/dose)

Acute otitis media: 10 mg/kg/day divided every 12 hours for 5 days (maximum: 200 mg/dose)

Pharyngitis/tonsillitis: 10 mg/kg/day in 2 divided doses for 5-10 days (maximum: 100 mg/dose)

Children ≥12 years and Adults: Oral:

Acute community-acquired pneumonia and bacterial exacerbations of chronic bronchitis: 200 mg every 12 hours for 14 days and 10 days, respectively

Acute maxillary sinusitis: 200 mg every 12 hours for 10 days

Pharyngitis/tonsillitis: 100 mg every 12 hours for 5-10 days

Skin and skin structure: 400 mg every 12 hours for 7-14 days

Uncomplicated gonorrhea (male and female) and rectal gonococcal infections (female): 200 mg as a single dose

Uncomplicated urinary tract infection: 100 mg every 12 hours for 7 days

Dosing adjustment in renal impairment: CrCl <30 mL/minute: Administer every 24 hours

Hemodialysis: Administer dose 3 times/week following hemodialysis

Dietary Considerations May be taken with food.

Administration Administer around-the-clock to promote less variation in peak and trough serum levels. Shake suspension well before using.

Monitoring Parameters Monitor renal function. Observe for signs and symptoms of anaphylaxis during first dose.

Dosage Forms

Suspension Reconstituted, Oral:

Generic: 50 mg/5 mL (50 mL, 100 mL); 100 mg/5 mL (50 mL, 100 mL)

Tablet, Oral:

Generic: 100 mg, 200 mg

◆ **Cefpodoxime Proxetil** *see* Cefpodoxime *on page 388*

Cefprozil (sef PROE zil)

Brand Names: Canada Apo-Cefprozil®; Auro-Cefprozil; Ava-Cefprozil; Cefzil®; RAN™-Cefprozil; Sandoz-Cefprozil

Index Terms Cefzil

Pharmacologic Category Antibiotic, Cephalosporin (Second Generation)

Use Treatment of otitis media and infections involving the respiratory tract and skin and skin structure; active against methicillin-sensitive staphylococci, many streptococci, and various gram-negative bacilli including *E. coli*, some *Klebsiella*, *P. mirabilis*, *H. influenzae*, and *Moraxella*.

Pregnancy Risk Factor B

Pregnancy Considerations Adverse events were not observed in animal reproduction studies.

Breast-Feeding Considerations Small amounts of cefprozil are excreted in breast milk. The manufacturer recommends that caution be exercised when administering cefprozil to nursing women. Nondose-related effects could include modification of bowel flora.

Contraindications Hypersensitivity to cefprozil, any component of the formulation, or other cephalosporins

Warnings/Precautions Modify dosage in patients with severe renal impairment. Use with caution in patients with a history of penicillin allergy, especially IgE-mediated reactions (eg, anaphylaxis, urticaria). Prolonged use may result in fungal or bacterial superinfection, including *C. difficile*-associated diarrhea (CDAD) and pseudomembranous colitis; CDAD has been observed >2 months postantibiotic treatment. Some products may contain phenylalanine.

Benzyl alcohol and derivatives: Some dosage forms may contain sodium benzoate/benzoic acid; benzoic acid (benzoate) is a metabolite of benzyl alcohol; large amounts of benzyl alcohol (≥99 mg/kg/day) have been associated with a potentially fatal toxicity ("gasping syndrome") in neonates; the "gasping syndrome" consists of metabolic acidosis, respiratory distress, gasping respirations, CNS dysfunction (including convulsions, intracranial hemorrhage), hypotension, and cardiovascular collapse (AAP, 1997; CDC, 1982); some data suggests that benzoate displaces bilirubin from protein binding sites (Ahlfors, 2001); avoid or use dosage forms containing benzyl alcohol derivative with caution in neonates. See manufacturer's labeling.

Some dosage forms may contain polysorbate 80 (also known as Tweens). Hypersensitivity reactions, usually a delayed reaction, have been reported following exposure to pharmaceutical products containing polysorbate 80 in certain individuals (Isaksson, 2002; Lucente 2000; Shelley, 1995). Thrombocytopenia, ascites, pulmonary deterioration, and renal and hepatic failure have been reported in premature neonates after receiving parenteral products containing polysorbate 80 (Alade, 1986; CDC, 1984). See manufacturer's labeling.

Adverse Reactions

Central nervous system: Dizziness

Dermatologic: Diaper rash

Gastrointestinal: Abdominal pain, diarrhea, nausea, vomiting

Genitourinary: Genital pruritus, vaginitis

Hepatic: Transaminases increased

Miscellaneous: Superinfection

Rare but important or life-threatening: Anaphylaxis, angioedema, arthralgia, BUN increased, cholestatic jaundice, confusion, creatinine increased, eosinophilia, erythema multiforme, fever, headache, hyperactivity, insomnia, leukopenia, pseudomembranous colitis, rash, serum sickness, somnolence, Stevens-Johnson syndrome, thrombocytopenia, urticaria

Reactions reported with other cephalosporins: Agranulocytosis, aplastic anemia, colitis, hemolytic anemia, hemorrhage, interstitial nephritis, pancytopenia, renal dysfunction, seizure, superinfection, toxic epidermal necrolysis, toxic nephropathy, vaginitis

Drug Interactions

Metabolism/Transport Effects None known.

Avoid Concomitant Use

Avoid concomitant use of Cefprozil with any of the following: BCG

Increased Effect/Toxicity

Cefprozil may increase the levels/effects of: Aminoglycosides; Vitamin K Antagonists

The levels/effects of Cefprozil may be increased by: Probenecid

Decreased Effect

Cefprozil may decrease the levels/effects of: BCG; Sodium Picosulfate; Typhoid Vaccine

Food Interactions Food delays cefprozil absorption. Management: May administer with food.

Storage/Stability Store at 20°C to 25°C (68°F to 77°F); excursions permitted to 15°C to 30°C (59°F to 86°F). Refrigerate suspension after reconstitution; discard after 14 days.

Mechanism of Action Inhibits bacterial cell wall synthesis by binding to one or more of the penicillin-binding proteins (PBPs) which in turn inhibits the final transpeptidation step of peptidoglycan synthesis in bacterial cell walls, thus inhibiting cell wall biosynthesis. Bacteria eventually lyse due to ongoing activity of cell wall autolytic enzymes (autolysins and murein hydrolases) while cell wall assembly is arrested.

Pharmacodynamics/Kinetics

Absorption: Well absorbed (94%)

Protein binding: 35% to 45%

Half-life elimination: Normal renal function: 1.3 hours

Time to peak, serum: Fasting: 1.5 hours

Excretion: Urine (61% as unchanged drug)

Dosage

Usual dosage range:

Infants and Children >6 months to 12 years: Oral: 7.5-15 mg/kg/day divided every 12 hours

Children >12 years and Adults: Oral: 250-500 mg every 12 hours or 500 mg every 24 hours

Indication-specific dosing:

Infants and Children >6 months to 12 years: Oral:

Otitis media: 15 mg/kg every 12 hours for 10 days

Children 2-12 years: Oral:

Pharyngitis/tonsillitis: 7.5-15 mg/kg/day divided every 12 hours for 10 days (administer for >10 days if due to *S. pyogenes*); maximum: 1 g/day

Uncomplicated skin and skin structure infections: 20 mg/kg every 24 hours for 10 days; maximum: 1 g/day

Children >12 years and Adults: Oral:

Pharyngitis/tonsillitis: 500 mg every 24 hours for 10 days

Secondary bacterial infection of acute bronchitis or acute bacterial exacerbation of chronic bronchitis: 500 mg every 12 hours for 10 days

Uncomplicated skin and skin structure infections: 250 mg every 12 hours or 500 mg every 12-24 hours for 10 days

Dosage adjustment in renal impairment: CrCl <30 mL/minute: Reduce dose by 50%

Hemodialysis: Reduced by hemodialysis; administer dose after the completion of hemodialysis

Dosage adjustment in hepatic impairment: No dosage adjustment necessary.

Dietary Considerations May be taken with food. Oral suspension may contain phenylalanine; consult product labeling.

Administration Administer around-the-clock to promote less variation in peak and trough serum levels. Chilling the reconstituted oral suspension improves flavor (do not freeze).

Monitoring Parameters Monitor renal function. Assess patient at beginning and throughout therapy for infection; monitor for signs of anaphylaxis during first dose.

Dosage Forms

Suspension Reconstituted, Oral:

Generic: 125 mg/5 mL (50 mL, 75 mL, 100 mL); 250 mg/5 mL (50 mL, 75 mL, 100 mL)

Tablet, Oral:

Generic: 250 mg, 500 mg

Cefsulodin [INT] (sef SUL oh din)

International Brand Names Monaspor (AT, CZ, NL); Pseudocef (AT, DE, JP); Pyocefal (FR); Takesulin (JP); Ulfaret (ES, GR)

Index Terms Cefsulodin Sodium

Pharmacologic Category Antibiotic, Cephalosporin (Third Generation)

Reported Use Treatment of susceptible bacterial infections caused by *Pseudomonas aeruginosa*

Dosage Range Adults: IM, IV: 3-6 g/day in 4 divided doses

Product Availability Product available in various countries; not currently available in the U.S.

Dosage Forms

Injection, powder for reconstitution, as sodium: 1 g

◆ **Cefsulodin Sodium** *see* Cefsulodin [INT] *on page 391*

Ceftaroline Fosamil (sef TAR oh leen FOS a mil)

Brand Names: U.S. Teflaro

Index Terms PPI-0903; PPI-0903M; T-91825; TAK-599

Pharmacologic Category Antibiotic, Cephalosporin (Fifth Generation)

Use

Acute bacterial skin and skin structure infections: Treatment of acute bacterial skin and skin structure infections caused by susceptible isolates of the following gram-positive and gram-negative microorganisms: *Staphylococcus aureus* (including methicillin-susceptible and methicillin-resistant isolates), *Streptococcus pyogenes*, *Streptococcus agalactiae*, *Escherichia coli*, *Klebsiella pneumoniae*, and *Klebsiella oxytoca*.

Community-acquired bacterial pneumonia: Treatment of community-acquired bacterial pneumonia caused by susceptible isolates of the following gram-positive and gram-negative microorganisms: *Streptococcus pneumoniae* (including cases with concurrent bacteremia), *S. aureus* (methicillin-susceptible isolates only), *Haemophilus influenzae*, *K. pneumoniae*, *K. oxytoca*, and *E. coli*.

Pregnancy Risk Factor B

Pregnancy Considerations Adverse events have been observed in some animal reproduction studies.

Breast-Feeding Considerations It is not known if ceftaroline fosamil is excreted in breast milk. The manufacturer recommends that caution be exercised when administering ceftaroline fosamil to nursing women.

Contraindications Known serious hypersensitivity to ceftaroline, other members of the cephalosporin class, or any component of the formulation

Warnings/Precautions Use with caution in patients with a history of penicillin cephalosporin, or carbapenem allergy, especially IgE-mediated reactions (eg, anaphylaxis, angioedema, urticaria). Seroconversion from a negative to a positive direct Coombs' test has been reported. Hemolytic anemia was not reported in clinical studies; however, if anemia develops during or after treatment, diagnostic tests should include a direct Coombs' test. If drug-induced hemolytic anemia is considered, discontinue the drug and institute supportive care as clinically indicated. Prolonged use may result in fungal or bacterial superinfection, including *C. difficile*-associated diarrhea (CDAD) and pseudomembranous colitis (including fatalities); CDAD has been observed >2 months postantibiotic treatment. Use with caution in patients with renal impairment (CrCl ≤50 mL/minute); dosage adjustments recommended. Use with caution in the elderly; dosage adjustment should be based on renal function. Potentially significant drug-drug interactions may exist, requiring dose or frequency adjustment, additional monitoring, and/or selection of alternative therapy.

Adverse Reactions

Cardiovascular: Phlebitis

Central nervous system: Headache, insomnia

Dermatologic: Pruritus, skin rash

Endocrine & metabolic: Hypokalemia

Gastrointestinal: Constipation, diarrhea, nausea, vomiting

Hematologic & oncologic: Positive Coombs' test (without hemolysis)

Hepatic: Increased serum transaminases

Rare but important or life-threatening: Agranulocytosis, anemia, *Clostridium difficile* associated diarrhea, dizziness, eosinophilia, fever, hepatitis, hyperglycemia, hyperkalemia, hypersensitivity, neutropenia, palpitations, renal failure, seizures, thrombocytopenia

Drug Interactions

Metabolism/Transport Effects None known.

Avoid Concomitant Use

Avoid concomitant use of Ceftaroline Fosamil with any of the following: BCG

Increased Effect/Toxicity

Ceftaroline Fosamil may increase the levels/effects of: Vitamin K Antagonists

The levels/effects of Ceftaroline Fosamil may be increased by: Probenecid

Decreased Effect

Ceftaroline Fosamil may decrease the levels/effects of: BCG; Sodium Picosulfate; Typhoid Vaccine

Preparation for Administration Reconstitute 400 mg or 600 mg vial with 20 mL SWFI, NS, D_5W, or LR; mix gently. Reconstituted solution should be further diluted for IV administration in 50-250 mL of a compatible solution. Use the same solution as used for reconstitution (**Note:** If SWFI was used for reconstitution, then appropriate infusion solutions include NS, 1/2NS, D_5W, $D_{2.5}W$, or LR). Color of infusion solutions ranges from clear and light to dark yellow depending on concentration and storage conditions; potency is not affected.

Storage/Stability Store unused vials at 25°C (77°F); excursions permitted between 15°C and 30°C (59°F and 86°F). Per the manufacturer, unused vials can also be stored at 2°C to 8°C (36°F to 46°F). Diluted solutions should be used within 6 hours when stored at room temperature or within 24 hours if refrigerated at 2°C to 8°C (36°F to 46°F).

Mechanism of Action Inhibits bacterial cell wall synthesis by binding to penicillin-binding proteins (PBPs) 1 through 3. This action blocks the final transpeptidation step of peptidoglycan synthesis in bacterial cell walls and inhibits cell wall biosynthesis. Bacteria eventually lyse due to ongoing activity of cell wall autolytic enzymes (autolysis and murein hydrolases) while cell wall assembly is arrested. Ceftaroline has a strong affinity for PBP2a, a modified PBP in MRSA, and PBP2x in *S. pneumoniae*, contributing to its spectrum of activity against these bacteria.

Pharmacodynamics/Kinetics

Distribution: V_d: 18.3-21.6 L

Protein binding: ~20%

Metabolism: Ceftaroline fosamil (inactive prodrug) undergoes rapid conversion to bioactive ceftaroline in plasma by phosphatase enzyme; ceftaroline is hydrolyzed to form inactive ceftaroline M-1 metabolite

Half-life elimination: 2.7 hours

Time to peak: 1 hour

Excretion: Urine (~88%); feces (~6%)

Dosage IV: Adults:

Usual dosage range: 600 mg every 12 hours

Indication-specific dosage:

Pneumonia, community-acquired: 600 mg every 12 hours for 5-7 days

Skin and skin structure, complicated: 600 mg every 12 hours for 5-14 days

Dosage adjustment in renal impairment: Note: Renal function may be estimated using the Cockcroft-Gault formula for dosage adjustment purposes.

CrCl >50 mL/minute: No dosage adjustment necessary.

CrCl >30-50 mL/minute: 400 mg every 12 hours

CrCl 15-30 mL/minute: 300 mg every 12 hours

CrCl <15 mL/minute: 200 mg every 12 hours

ESRD patients receiving hemodialysis: 200 mg every 12 hours; dose should be given after hemodialysis on dialysis days

Dosage adjustment in hepatic impairment: No dosage adjustment provided in manufacturer's labeling (has not been studied). However, ceftaroline is primarily renally eliminated.

Administration Administer by slow IV infusion over 60 minutes.

Monitoring Parameters Obtain specimen for culture and susceptibility prior to the first dose. Monitor for signs of anaphylaxis during first dose. Monitor renal function.

Additional Information Considered to be ineffective against *Pseudomonas aeruginosa*, *Enterococcus* species (including vancomycin-susceptible and -resistant isolates), extended-spectrum beta-lactamase (ESBL) producing or AmpC overexpressing Enterobacteriaceae.

Dosage Forms

Solution Reconstituted, Intravenous:

Teflaro: 400 mg (1 ea); 600 mg (1 ea)

CefTAZidime (SEF tay zi deem)

Brand Names: U.S. Fortaz; Fortaz in D5W; Tazicef

Brand Names: Canada Ceftazidime For Injection; Fortaz

Pharmacologic Category Antibiotic, Cephalosporin (Third Generation)

Use

Bacterial septicemia: Treatment of septicemia caused by *Pseudomonas aeruginosa*, *Klebsiella* spp., *Haemophilus influenzae*, *Escherichia coli*, *Serratia* spp., *Streptococcus pneumoniae*, and *Staphylococcus aureus* (methicillin-susceptible strains).

Bone and joint infections: Treatment of bone and joint infections caused by *Pseudomonas aeruginosa*, *Klebsiella* spp., *Enterobacter* spp., and *Staphylococcus aureus* (methicillin-susceptible strains).

CNS infections: Treatment of meningitis, caused by *Haemophilus influenzae* and *Neisseria meningitidis*. Ceftazidime has also been used successfully in cases of meningitis due to Pseudomonas aeruginosa and Streptococcus pneumoniae.

Empiric therapy in the immunocompromised patient: Empiric treatment of infections in immunocompromised patients.

Gynecologic infections: Treatment of endometritis, pelvic cellulitis, and other infections of the female genital tract caused by *Escherichia coli*.

Intra-abdominal infections: Treatment of peritonitis caused by *Escherichia coli*, *Klebsiella* spp., and *Staphylococcus aureus* (methicillin-susceptible strains) and polymicrobial intra-abdominal infections caused by aerobic and anaerobic organisms and some *Bacteroides* spp. (many strains of *Bacteroides fragilis* are resistant).

Lower respiratory tract infections: Treatment of lower respiratory tract infections, including pneumonia, caused by *Pseudomonas aeruginosa* and other *Pseudomonas* spp.; *Haemophilus influenzae*, including ampicillin-resistant strains; *Klebsiella* spp.; *Enterobacter* spp.; *Proteus mirabilis*; *Escherichia coli*; *Serratia* spp.; *Citrobacter* spp.; *Streptococcus pneumoniae*; and *Staphylococcus aureus* (methicillin-susceptible strains).

Skin and skin-structure infections: Treatment of skin and skin-structure infections caused by *Pseudomonas aeruginosa*; *Klebsiella* spp.; *Escherichia coli*; *Proteus* spp.; including *Proteus mirabilis* and indole-positive *Proteus*; *Enterobacter* spp.; *Serratia* spp.; *Staphylococcus aureus* (methicillin-susceptible strains); and *Streptococcus pyogenes* (group A beta-hemolytic streptococci).

Urinary tract infections (UTI): Treatment of complicated and uncomplicated UTIs caused by *Pseudomonas aeruginosa*; *Enterobacter* spp.; *Proteus* spp., including *Proteus mirabilis* and indole-positive *Proteus*; *Klebsiella* spp.; and *Escherichia coli*.

Pregnancy Risk Factor B

Pregnancy Considerations Adverse events have not been observed in animal reproduction studies. Ceftazidime crosses the placenta and reaches the cord serum and amniotic fluid. An increase in most types of birth defects was not found following first trimester exposure to cephalosporins. Maternal peak serum concentration is unchanged in the first trimester. After the first trimester, serum concentrations decrease by approximately 50% of those in nonpregnant patients. Renal clearance is increased during pregnancy.

Breast-Feeding Considerations Very small amounts of ceftazidime are excreted in breast milk. The manufacturer recommends that caution be exercised when administering ceftazidime to nursing women. Ceftazidime in not absorbed when given orally; therefore, any medication that is distributed to human milk should not result in systemic concentrations in the nursing infant. Nondose-related effects could include modification of bowel flora.

Contraindications Clinically significant hypersensitivity to ceftazidime, other cephalosporins, or any component of the formulation

Warnings/Precautions Modify dosage in patients with severe renal impairment. Use with caution in patients with a history of penicillin allergy, especially IgE-mediated reactions (eg, anaphylaxis, urticaria). High ceftazidime levels in patients with renal insufficiency can lead to seizures, encephalopathy, coma, asterixis, myoclonia, and neuromuscular excitability. Reduce total daily dosage. Prolonged use may result in fungal or bacterial superinfection, including *C. difficile*-associated diarrhea (CDAD) and pseudomembranous colitis; CDAD has been observed >2 months postantibiotic treatment. May be associated with increased INR, especially in nutritionally-deficient patients, prolonged treatment, hepatic or renal disease. Use with caution in patients with a history of seizure disorder; high levels may increase risk of seizures.

Adverse Reactions

Cardiovascular: Phlebitis

Endocrine & metabolic: Increased gamma-glutamyl transferase, increased lactate dehydrogenase

Gastrointestinal: Diarrhea

Hematologic & oncologic: Eosinophilia, positive direct Coombs test (without hemolysis), thrombocythemia

Hepatic: Increased serum alkaline phosphatase, increased serum ALT, increased serum AST

Hypersensitivity: Hypersensitivity reactions

Local: Inflammation at injection site, pain at injection site

Rare but important or life-threatening: Agranulocytosis, anaphylaxis, angioedema, asterixis, brain disease, candidiasis, *Clostridium difficile* associated diarrhea, erythema multiforme, hemolytic anemia, hyperbilirubinemia, increased lactate dehydrogenase, leukopenia, lymphocytosis, myoclonus, nausea, neuromuscular excitability, neutropenia, paresthesia, pseudomembranous colitis, renal disease (may be severe, including renal failure), renal insufficiency, seizure, skin rash, Stevens-Johnson syndrome, thrombocytopenia, toxic epidermal necrolysis, vaginitis

Drug Interactions

Metabolism/Transport Effects None known.

Avoid Concomitant Use

Avoid concomitant use of CefTAZidime with any of the following: BCG

Increased Effect/Toxicity

CefTAZidime may increase the levels/effects of: Aminoglycosides; Vitamin K Antagonists

The levels/effects of CefTAZidime may be increased by: Probenecid

Decreased Effect

CefTAZidime may decrease the levels/effects of: BCG; Sodium Picosulfate; Typhoid Vaccine

Preparation for Administration

IM: Using SWFI, bacteriostatic water, lidocaine 0.5%, or lidocaine 1%, reconstitute the 500 mg vials with 1.5 mL or the 1 g vials with 3 mL; final concentration of *~280 mg/mL*

IV: Using SWFI, reconstitute as follows (**Note:** After reconstitution, may dilute further with a compatible solution to administer via IV infusion):

Fortaz, Tazicef:

~100 mg/mL solution:

500 mg vial: 5.3 mL SWFI (withdraw 5 mL from the reconstituted vial to obtain a 500 mg dose)

1 g vial: 10 mL SWFI (withdraw 10 mL from the reconstituted vial to obtain a 1 g dose)

6 g vial: 56 mL SWFI (withdraw 10 mL from the reconstituted vial to obtain a 1 g dose)

~170 mg/mL solution: 2 g vial: 10 mL SWFI (withdraw 11.5 mL from the reconstituted vial to obtain a 2 g dose)

~200 mg/mL solution: 6 g vial: 26 mL SWFI (withdraw 5 mL from the reconstituted vial to obtain a 1 g dose)

Storage/Stability

Store intact vials at 20°C to 25°C (68°F to 77°F). Protect from light. Reconstituted solution and solution further diluted for IV infusion are stable for 24 weeks when immediately frozen at -20°C (-4°F). After freezing, thawed solution in NS in a Viaflex small volume container for IV administration is stable for 24 hours at room temperature or for 7 days when refrigerated. Do not refreeze the thawed solution. Ceftazidime solutions (concentrations 1 to 40 mg/mL) in NS, D_5W, D_5NS, LR, $D_{10}W$, Ringer's injection, or SWFI are stable for 24 hours at room temperature (20°C to 25°C [68°F to 77°F]) and for 7 days if refrigerated (4°C [39°F]). Consult detailed reference regarding stability of ceftazidime in other solutions.

Premixed frozen solution: Store frozen at -20°C (-4°F). Thawed solution is stable for 8 hours at room temperature or for 3 days under refrigeration; do not refreeze.

Mechanism of Action Inhibits bacterial cell wall synthesis by binding to one or more of the penicillin-binding proteins (PBPs) which in turn inhibits the final transpeptidation step of peptidoglycan synthesis in bacterial cell walls, thus inhibiting cell wall biosynthesis. Bacteria eventually lyse due to ongoing activity of cell wall autolytic enzymes (autolysins and murein hydrolases) while cell wall assembly is arrested.

Pharmacodynamics/Kinetics

Distribution: Widely throughout the body including bone, bile, skin, CSF (higher concentrations achieved when meninges are inflamed), endometrium, heart, pleural and lymphatic fluids

Protein binding: <10%

Half-life elimination: 1 to 2 hours, prolonged with renal impairment

Time to peak, serum: IM: ~1 hour

Excretion: Urine (80% to 90% as unchanged drug)

Dosage

Usual dosage range:

Infants and Children 1 month to 12 years: IV: 30 to 50 mg/kg/dose every 8 hours (maximum dose: 6 g daily)

Adolescents and Adults: IM, IV: 500 mg to 2 g every 8 to 12 hours

Indication-specific dosing:

Infants, Children, and Adolescents:

Cystic fibrosis:

Manufacturer recommendations: 150 mg/kg/day divided every 8 hours (maximum: 6 g daily)

Alternative recommendations: 200 to 300 mg/kg/day divided every 8 hours (maximum: 6 g daily) (*Red Book* [AAP] 2012)

Infants, Children, Adolescents, and Adults:

Melioidosis (off-label use): IV: Note: Switching to meropenem therapy is indicated if patient condition worsens (eg, organ failure, new infection focus development, repeat blood cultures remained positive). Oral eradication therapy is recommended after the intensive (acute) phase treatment is complete (Lipsitz, 2012).

Severe, acute phase: Infants >3 months, Children, Adolescents, and Adults: 50 mg/kg/dose every 8 hours (maximum dose: 2 g) or 2 g for one dose, followed by 6 g daily by continuous infusion for ≥10 days with or without TMP/SMX (Lipsitz, 2012). **Note:** Depending on infection severity, the dose for patients ≥3 months can be ≤40 mg/kg (maximum dose: 2 g) (Lipsitz, 2012).

Adults:

Cystic fibrosis: IV:

Manufacturer recommendations: 90 to 150 mg/kg/day divided every 8 hours (maximum: 6 g daily)

Alternative recommendations: Intermittent IV infusion: 200 to 400 mg/kg/day divided every 6 to 8 hours (maximum: 8 to 12 g daily); or by continuous IV infusion: 100 to 200 mg//kg/day (maximum: 12 g daily) (Zobell, 2013).

Empiric therapy in immunocompromised patients: IV: 2 g every 8 hours.

Endophthalmitis, bacterial (off-label use): Intravitreal: 2 to 2.25 mg/0.1 mL NS in combination with vancomycin (Jackson, 2003; Roth, 1997)

Intra-abdominal infection, severe (in combination with metronidazole): IV: 2 g every 8 hours for 4 to 7 days (provided source controlled). Not recommended for hospital-acquired intra-abdominal infections (IAI) associated with multidrug-resistant gram negative organisms or in mild-to-moderate community-acquired IAIs due to risk of toxicity and the development of resistant organisms (Solomkin, 2010).

Peritonitis (CAPD) (off-label route; Li, 2010): Intraperitoneal:

Intermittent: 1 to 1.5 g every 24 hours per exchange in the long dwell (≥6 hours)

Continuous (per liter exchange): Loading dose: 500 mg; maintenance dose: 125 mg. **Note:** If patient has residual renal function (eg, >100 mL/day urine output), empirically increase each dose by 25%.

Pneumonia:

Uncomplicated: IM, IV: 500 mg to 1 g every 8 hours

Hospital-acquired pneumonia (off-label dose): IV: 2 g every 8 hours (ATS/IDSA, 2005)

Prosthetic joint infection, *Pseudomonas aeruginosa* (alternative to cefepime or meropenem): IV: 2 g every 8 hours for 4 to 6 weeks (consider addition of an aminoglycoside) (Osmon, 2013)

Severe infections, including meningitis, CNS infection, osteomyelitis, gynecological: IV: 2 g every 8 hours

Dosage adjustment in renal impairment: Note: If the dose recommended in the dosing section is lower than that recommended for patients with renal insufficiency as outlined below, the lower dose should be used:

CrCl 31 to 50 mL/minute: 1 g every 12 hours
CrCl 16 to 30 mL/minute: 1 g every 24 hours
CrCl 6 to 15 mL/minute: 500 mg every 24 hours
CrCl <5 mL/minute: 500 mg every 48 hours

Intermittent hemodialysis (IHD) (administer after hemodialysis on dialysis days): Dialyzable (50% to 100%): 500 mg to 1 g every 24 hours **or** 1 to 2 g every 48 to 72 hours (Heintz, 2009). **Note:** Dosing dependent on the assumption of 3 times per week, complete IHD sessions.

Peritoneal dialysis (PD): IV:

Intermittent: Loading dose of 1 g, followed by 500 mg every 24 hours

Continuous: Loading dose of 1 g, followed by 500 mg every 24 hours. **Note:** an additional 125 mg per liter of exchange fluid may be added to the dialysate if clinically warranted.

Continuous renal replacement therapy (CRRT) (Heintz, 2009; Trotman, 2005): Drug clearance is highly dependent on the method of renal replacement, filter type, and flow rate. Appropriate dosing requires close monitoring of pharmacologic response, signs of adverse reactions due to drug accumulation, as well as drug concentrations in relation to target trough (if appropriate). The following are general recommendations only (based on dialysate flow/ultrafiltration rates of 1 to 2 L/hour and minimal residual renal function) and should not supersede clinical judgment:

CVVH: Loading dose of 2 g followed by 1 to 2 g every 12 hours

CVVHD/CVVHDF: Loading dose of 2 g followed by either 1 g every 8 hours **or** 2 g every 12 hours. **Note:** Dosage of 1 g every 8 hours results in similar steady-state concentrations as 2 g every 12 hours and is more cost effective. Dosage of 2 g every 8 hours may be needed for gram-negative rods with MIC ≥4 mg/L (Heintz, 2009).

Note: For patients receiving CVVHDF, some recommend giving a loading dose of 2 g followed by 3 g over 24 hours as a continuous IV infusion to maintain concentrations ≥4 times the MIC for susceptible pathogens (Heintz, 2009).

Dosage adjustment in hepatic impairment: No dosage adjustment necessary

Dietary Considerations Some products may contain sodium.

Administration Administer around-the-clock to promote less variation in peak and trough serum levels. Ceftazidime can be administered deep IM into large mass muscle, IVP over 3 to 5 minutes, or IV intermittent infusion over 15 to 30 minutes. Do not admix with aminoglycosides in same bottle/bag. Ceftazidime may be administered intravitreally as 2 to 2.25 mg/0.1 mL NS in combination with vancomycin (separate syringes) (Jackson, 2003; Roth, 1997).

Intraperitoneal administration may be used **in conjunction with** IV use for systemic infections if continuous peritoneal dialysis is used (added to the dialysate in each exchange). Intraperitoneal administration alone may also be used for the treatment of peritonitis and added to the dialysate in intermittent (added to the longest dwell time per day) or continuous (loading dose, followed by a maintenance dose per liter of exchange) peritoneal dialysis.

Monitoring Parameters Monitor renal function. Observe for signs and symptoms of anaphylaxis during first dose.

Additional Information With some organisms, resistance may develop during treatment (including *Enterobacter* spp and *Serratia* spp). Consider combination therapy or periodic susceptibility testing for organisms with inducible resistance.

Dosage Forms

Solution, Intravenous:
Fortaz in D5W: 1 g (50 mL); 2 g (50 mL)
Tazicef: 1 g/50 mL (50 mL)

Solution Reconstituted, Injection:
Fortaz: 500 mg (1 ea); 1 g (1 ea); 2 g (1 ea); 6 g (1 ea)
Tazicef: 1 g (1 ea); 2 g (1 ea); 6 g (1 ea)
Generic: 1 g (1 ea); 2 g (1 ea); 6 g (1 ea); 100 g (1 ea)

Solution Reconstituted, Injection [preservative free]:
Generic: 1 g (1 ea); 2 g (1 ea); 6 g (1 ea)

Solution Reconstituted, Intravenous:
Fortaz: 1 g (1 ea); 2 g (1 ea)
Tazicef: 1 g (1 ea); 2 g (1 ea)
Generic: 1 g/50 mL (1 ea); 2 g/50 mL (1 ea)

◆ **Ceftazidime For Injection (Can)** *see* CefTAZidime *on page 392*

Ceftibuten (sef TYE byoo ten)

Brand Names: U.S. Cedax

Pharmacologic Category Antibiotic, Cephalosporin (Third Generation)

Use Treatment of acute exacerbations of chronic bronchitis, acute bacterial otitis media, and pharyngitis/tonsillitis

Pregnancy Risk Factor B

Dosage

Usual dosage range:

Children 6 months to <12 years: Oral: 9 mg/kg/day for 10 days (maximum dose: 400 mg/day)

Children ≥12 years and Adults: Oral: 400 mg once daily for 10 days

Dosage adjustment in renal impairment:

CrCl ≥50 mL//minute: No adjustment needed

CrCl 30-49 mL//minute: Administer 4.5 mg/kg or 200 mg every 24 hours

CrCl 5-29 mL/minute: Administer 2.25 mg/kg or 100 mg every 24 hours.

Hemodialysis: Administer 400 mg or 9 mg/kg (maximum: 400 mg) after each hemodialysis session

Dosage adjustment in hepatic impairment: No dosage adjustment provided in manufacturer's labeling.

Additional Information Complete prescribing information should be consulted for additional detail.

Dosage Forms

Capsule, Oral:
Cedax: 400 mg
Generic: 400 mg

Suspension Reconstituted, Oral:
Cedax: 90 mg/5 mL (60 mL, 90 mL, 120 mL); 180 mg/5 mL (30 mL, 60 mL)
Generic: 180 mg/5 mL (60 mL)

◆ **Ceftin** *see* Cefuroxime *on page 399*

Ceftolozane and Tazobactam

(sef TOL oh zane & taz oh BAK tam)

Brand Names: U.S. Zerbaxa

Index Terms CXA 201; Tazobactam and Ceftolozane

Pharmacologic Category Antibiotic, Cephalosporin (Fifth Generation)

Use

Intra-abdominal infections: Treatment of complicated intra-abdominal infections in adults, in combination with metronidazole, caused by *Enterobacter cloacae*, *Escherichia coli*, *Klebsiella oxytoca*, *K. pneumoniae*, *Proteus mirabilis*, *Pseudomonas aeruginosa*, *Bacteroides fragilis*, *Streptococcus anginosus*, *Streptococcus constellatus*, and *Streptococcus salivarius*.

Urinary tract infections: Treatment of complicated urinary tract infections, including pyelonephritis, in adults caused by *Escherichia coli, Klebsiella pneumoniae, Proteus mirabilis*, and *Pseudomonas aeruginosa*.

Pregnancy Risk Factor B

Pregnancy Considerations Adverse events were observed in some animal reproduction studies. Tazobactam crosses the placenta (Bourget, 1998).

Breast-Feeding Considerations It is not known if ceftolozane or tazobactam are excreted into breast milk. The manufacturer recommends that caution be used if administered to a nursing woman.

Contraindications Serious hypersensitivity to ceftolozane/tazobactam, piperacillin/tazobactam, other members of the beta-lactam class, or any component of the formulation.

Warnings/Precautions Hypersensitivity and anaphylaxis (serious and sometimes fatal) have been reported in patients receiving beta-lactam drugs. Question patient about previous hypersensitivity reactions to other cephalosporins, penicillins or other beta-lactams. Cross-sensitivity has been established. If administered, use with caution and if anaphylaxis occurs, discontinue and institute appropriate supportive therapy. Use may result in fungal or bacterial superinfection, including *C. difficile*-associated diarrhea (CDAD) and pseudomembranous colitis; CDAD has been observed >2 months postantibiotic treatment. Exposure to ceftolozane is increased with increasing degrees of renal impairment; monitor creatinine clearance (CrCl) at least daily in patients with changing renal function and adjust the dose. In clinical trials, cure rates were lower in patients with a baseline CrCl of 30 to 50 mL/minute.

Adverse Reactions

Cardiovascular: Atrial fibrillation, hypotension

Central nervous system: Anxiety, dizziness, headache, insomnia

Dermatologic: Skin rash

Endocrine: Hypokalemia

Gastrointestinal: Abdominal pain, constipation, diarrhea, nausea, vomiting

Hematologic & oncologic: Anemia, thrombocythemia

Hepatic: Increased serum ALT, increased serum AST

Miscellaneous: Fever

Rare but important or life-threatening: Abdominal distention, angina pectoris, candidiasis, *Clostridium difficile* associated diarrhea, dyspnea, dyspepsia, flatulence, fungal urinary tract infection, gastritis, hyperglycemia, hypomagnesemia, hypophosphatemia, increased gamma-glutamyl transferase, increased serum alkaline phosphatase, infusion site reaction, intestinal obstruction, nonhemorrhagic stroke, oropharyngeal candidiasis, paralytic ileus, positive direct Coombs test, renal failure, renal insufficiency, tachycardia, urticaria, venous thrombosis

Drug Interactions

Metabolism/Transport Effects None known.

Avoid Concomitant Use

Avoid concomitant use of Ceftolozane and Tazobactam with any of the following: BCG

Increased Effect/Toxicity

Ceftolozane and Tazobactam may increase the levels/effects of: Vitamin K Antagonists

The levels/effects of Ceftolozane and Tazobactam may be increased by: Probenecid

Decreased Effect

Ceftolozane and Tazobactam may decrease the levels/effects of: BCG; Sodium Picosulfate; Typhoid Vaccine

Preparation for Administration

Constitute the vial with 10 mL SWFI or NS and gently shake to dissolve. The final volume is approximately 11.4 mL and contains ceftolozane/tazobactam 1.5 g (ceftolozane 1 g and tazobactam 500 mg).

To prepare the required dose, withdraw the appropriate volume from the reconstituted vial. Add the withdrawn volume to an infusion bag containing 100 mL of NS or D_5W.

Infusions range from clear, colorless solutions to solutions that are clear and slightly yellow. Variations in color within this range do not affect the potency of the product.

Storage/Stability Store intact vials at 2°C to 8°C (36°F to 46°F); protect from light. Reconstituted solution may be held for 1 hour prior to transfer and further dilution in an infusion bag. Diluted solution may be stored for 24 hours at room temperature or for 7 days at 2°C to 8°C (36°F to 46°F); do not freeze.

Mechanism of Action Ceftolozane inhibits bacterial cell wall synthesis by binding to one or more of the penicillin-binding proteins (PBPs); which in turn inhibits the final transpeptidation step of peptidoglycan synthesis in bacterial cell walls, thus inhibiting cell wall biosynthesis. Ceftolozane is an inhibitor of PBPs of *Pseudomonas aeruginosa* (eg, PBP1b, PBP1c, and PBP3) and *Escherichia coli* (eg, PBP3). Tazobactam irreversibly inhibits many beta-lactamases (eg, certain penicillinases and cephalosporinases), and can covalently bind to some plasmid-mediated and chromosomal bacterial beta-lactamases.

Pharmacodynamics/Kinetics

Distribution: V_d: Ceftolozane: 13.5 L; Tazobactam: 18.2 L

Protein binding: Ceftolozane: 16% to 20%; Tazobactam: 30%

Metabolism: Ceftolozane: Not metabolized; Tazobactam: Hydrolyzed to inactive metabolite

Half-life elimination: Ceftolozane: ~3 hours; Tazobactam: ~1 hour

Time to peak, plasma: Immediately following completion of 60-minute infusion

Excretion: Ceftolozane: Urine (>95% as unchanged drug); Tazobactam: urine (>80% as unchanged drug)

Dosage Note: Zerbaxa (ceftolozane/tazobactam) is a combination product. Dosage recommendations are expressed as grams of ceftolozane/tazobactam combination.

Intra-abdominal infections (complicated): Adult: IV: 1.5 g every 8 hours for 4 to 14 days in combination with metronidazole

Urinary tract infections (complicated, includes pyelonephritis): Adult: IV: 1.5 g every 8 hours for 7 days

Dosage adjustment in renal impairment: Note: Estimation of renal function for the purpose of drug dosing should be done using the Cockcroft-Gault formula.

CrCl >50 mL/minute: No dosage adjustment necessary.

CrCl 30 to 50 mL/minute: 750 mg every 8 hours

CrCl 15 to 29 mL/minute: 375 mg every 8 hours

CrCl <15 mL/minute not on dialysis: There are no dosage adjustments provided in the manufacturer's labeling (has not been studied).

End-stage renal disease (ESRD) requiring intermittent hemodialysis (IHD): Dialyzable (~66%). Initial: 750 mg for one dose, followed by 150 mg every 8 hours. Administer dose immediately after dialysis on dialysis days.

Dosage adjustment in hepatic impairment: No dosage adjustment necessary.

Dietary Considerations Some products may contain sodium.

Administration Intravenous: Administer by intermittent infusion over 60 minutes.

Monitoring Parameters Serum creatinine and CrCl at baseline and daily in patients with changing renal function,

Dosage Forms

Solution Reconstituted, Intravenous [preservative free]:

Zerbaxa: 1.5 g: Ceftolozane 1 g and tazobactam 0.5 g (1 ea)

CefTRIAXone (sef trye AKS one)

Brand Names: U.S. Rocephin

Brand Names: Canada Ceftriaxone for Injection USP; Ceftriaxone Sodium for Injection; Ceftriaxone Sodium for Injection BP

Index Terms Ceftriaxone Sodium

Pharmacologic Category Antibiotic, Cephalosporin (Third Generation)

Use Treatment of lower respiratory tract infections, acute bacterial otitis media, skin and skin structure infections, bone and joint infections, intra-abdominal and urinary tract infections, pelvic inflammatory disease (PID), uncomplicated gonorrhea, bacterial septicemia, and meningitis; used in surgical (perioperative) prophylaxis

Pregnancy Risk Factor B

Pregnancy Considerations Teratogenic effects have not been observed in animal reproduction studies. Ceftriaxone crosses the placenta and distributes to amniotic fluid. An increase in most types of birth defects was not found following first trimester exposure to cephalosporins. Pregnancy was found to influence the single dose pharmacokinetics of ceftriaxone when administered prior to delivery. The pharmacokinetics of ceftriaxone following multiple doses in the third trimester are similar to those of non-pregnant patients. Ceftriaxone is recommended for use in pregnant women for the treatment of gonococcal infections, Lyme disease, and may be used in certain situations prior to vaginal delivery in women at high risk for endocarditis (consult current guidelines).

Breast-Feeding Considerations Low concentrations of ceftriaxone are excreted in breast milk. The manufacturer recommends that caution be exercised when administering ceftriaxone to nursing women. Nondose-related effects could include modification of bowel flora.

Contraindications Hypersensitivity to ceftriaxone sodium, any component of the formulation, or other cephalosporins; **do not use in hyperbilirubinemic neonates**, particularly those who are premature since ceftriaxone is reported to displace bilirubin from albumin binding sites; concomitant use with intravenous calcium-containing solutions/products in neonates (≤28 days)

Warnings/Precautions Use with caution in patients with a history of penicillin allergy, especially IgE-mediated reactions (eg, anaphylaxis, urticaria). Abnormal gallbladder sonograms have been reported, possibly due to cetriaxone-calcium precipitates; discontinue in patients who develop signs and symptoms of gallbladder disease. Secondary to biliary obstruction, pancreatitis has been reported rarely. Use with caution in patients with a history of GI disease, especially colitis. Severe cases (including some fatalities) of immune-related hemolytic anemia have been reported in patients receiving cephalosporins, including ceftriaxone. Prolonged use may result in fungal or bacterial superinfection, including *C. difficile*-associated diarrhea (CDAD) and pseudomembranous colitis; CDAD has been observed >2 months postantibiotic treatment.

Potentially significant interactions may exist, requiring dose or frequency adjustment, additional monitoring, and/or selection of alternative therapy. May be associated with increased INR (rarely), especially in nutritionally-deficient patients, prolonged treatment, hepatic or renal disease. No adjustment is generally necessary in patients with renal impairment; use with caution in patients with concurrent hepatic dysfunction and significant renal disease, dosage should not exceed 2 g/day. Ceftriaxone may complex with calcium causing precipitation. Fatal lung and kidney damage associated with calcium-ceftriaxone precipitates has been observed in premature and term neonates. Do not reconstitute, admix, or coadminister with calcium-containing solutions, even via separate infusion lines/sites or at different times in any neonatal patient. Ceftriaxone should not be diluted or administered simultaneously with any calcium-containing solution via a Y-site in any patient. However, ceftriaxone and calcium-containing solution may be administered sequentially of one another for use in patients **other than neonates** if infusion lines are thoroughly flushed, with a compatible fluid, between infusions

Adverse Reactions

Dermatologic: Local skin tightening (IM), skin rash

Gastrointestinal: Diarrhea

Hematologic & oncologic: Eosinophilia, leukopenia, thrombocythemia

Hepatic: Increased serum transaminases

Local: Induration at injection site (I.M), pain at injection site, tenderness at injection site (IV), warm sensation at injection site (IM)

Renal: Increased blood urea nitrogen

Rare but important or life-threatening: Abdominal pain, agranulocytosis, allergic dermatitis, anaphylaxis, anemia, basophilia, bronchospasm, candidiasis, casts in urine, chills, choledocholithiasis, cholelithiasis, colitis, decreased prothrombin time, diaphoresis, dizziness, dysgeusia, dyspepsia, edema, epistaxis, erythema multiforme, fever, flatulence, flushing, gallbladder sludge, glossitis, glycosuria, headache, hematuria, hemolytic anemia, hypersensitivity pneumonitis, increased monocytes, increased serum alkaline phosphatase, increased serum bilirubin, increased serum creatinine, jaundice, leukocytosis, lymphocytopenia, lymphocytosis, nausea, nephrolithiasis, neutropenia, oliguria, palpitations, pancreatitis, phlebitis, prolonged prothrombin time, pruritus, pseudomembranous colitis, seizure, serum sickness, Stevens-Johnson syndrome, stomatitis, thrombocytopenia, toxic epidermal necrolysis, urticaria, vaginitis, vomiting

Drug Interactions

Metabolism/Transport Effects None known.

Avoid Concomitant Use

Avoid concomitant use of CefTRIAXone with any of the following: BCG

Increased Effect/Toxicity

CefTRIAXone may increase the levels/effects of: Aminoglycosides; Vitamin K Antagonists

The levels/effects of CefTRIAXone may be increased by: Calcium Salts (Intravenous); Probenecid; Ringer's Injection (Lactated)

Decreased Effect

CefTRIAXone may decrease the levels/effects of: BCG; Sodium Picosulfate; Typhoid Vaccine

Preparation for Administration

IM injection: Vials should be reconstituted with appropriate volume of diluent (including D_5W, NS, SWFI, bacteriostatic water, or 1% lidocaine) to make a final concentration of 250 mg/mL or 350 mg/mL.

Volume to add to create a **250 mg/mL** solution:
- 250 mg vial: 0.9 mL
- 500 mg vial: 1.8 mL
- 1 g vial: 3.6 mL
- 2 g vial: 7.2 mL

Volume to add to create a **350 mg/mL** solution:
- 500 mg vial: 1.0 mL
- 1 g vial: 2.1 mL
- 2 g vial: 4.2 mL

IV infusion: Infusion is prepared in two stages: Initial reconstitution of powder, followed by dilution to final infusion solution.

Vials: Reconstitute powder with appropriate IV diluent (including SWFI, D_5W, $D_{10}W$, NS) to create an initial solution of ~100 mg/mL. Recommended volume to add:

250 mg vial: 2.4 mL

500 mg vial: 4.8 mL

1 g vial: 9.6 mL

2 g vial: 19.2 mL

Note: After reconstitution of powder, further dilution into a volume of compatible solution (eg, 50-100 mL of D_5W or NS) is recommended.

Piggyback bottle: Reconstitute powder with appropriate IV diluent (D_5W or NS) to create a resulting solution of ~100 mg/mL. Recommended initial volume to add:

1 g bottle:10 mL

2 g bottle: 20 mL

Note: After reconstitution, to prepare the final infusion solution, further dilution to 50 mL or 100 mL volumes with the appropriate IV diluent (including D_5W or NS) is recommended.

Storage/Stability

Powder for injection: Prior to reconstitution, store at room temperature ≤25°C (≤77°F). Protect from light.

Premixed solution (manufacturer premixed): Store at -20°C; once thawed, solutions are stable for 3 days at room temperature of 25°C (77°F) or for 21 days refrigerated at 5°C (41°F). Do not refreeze.

Stability of reconstituted solutions:

10-40 mg/mL: Reconstituted in D_5W, $D_{10}W$, NS, or SWFI: Stable for 2 days at room temperature of 25°C (77°F) or for 10 days when refrigerated at 4°C (39°F). Stable for 26 weeks when frozen at -20°C when reconstituted with D_5W or NS. Once thawed (at room temperature), solutions are stable for 2 days at room temperature of 25°C (77°F) or for 10 days when refrigerated at 4°C (39°F); does not apply to manufacturer's premixed bags. Do not refreeze.

100 mg/mL:

Reconstituted in D_5W, SWFI, or NS: Stable for 2 days at room temperature of 25°C (77°F) or for 10 days when refrigerated at 4°C (39°F).

Reconstituted in lidocaine 1% solution or bacteriostatic water: Stable for 24 hours at room temperature of 25°C (77°F) or for 10 days when refrigerated at 4°C (39°F).

250-350 mg/mL: Reconstituted in D_5W, NS, lidocaine 1% solution, bacteriostatic water, or SWFI: Stable for 24 hours at room temperature of 25°C (77°F) or for 3 days when refrigerated at 4°C (39°F).

Mechanism of Action Inhibits bacterial cell wall synthesis by binding to one or more of the penicillin-binding proteins (PBPs) which in turn inhibits the final transpeptidation step of peptidoglycan synthesis in bacterial cell walls, thus inhibiting cell wall biosynthesis. Bacteria eventually lyse due to ongoing activity of cell wall autolytic enzymes (autolysins and murein hydrolases) while cell wall assembly is arrested.

Pharmacodynamics/Kinetics

Absorption: IM: Well absorbed

Distribution: V_d: 6-14 L; widely throughout the body including gallbladder, lungs, bone, bile, CSF (higher concentrations achieved when meninges are inflamed)

Protein binding: 85% to 95%

Half-life elimination: Normal renal and hepatic function: 5-9 hours; Renal impairment (mild-to-severe): 12-16 hours

Time to peak, serum: IM: 2-3 hours

Excretion: Urine (33% to 67% as unchanged drug); feces (as inactive drug)

Dosage

Usual dosage range:

Infants and Children: IM, IV: 50-100 mg/kg/day in 1-2 divided doses (maximum: 4000 mg daily [meningitis]; 2000 mg daily [nonmeningeal infections])

Adults: IM, IV: 1-2 g every 12-24 hours

Indication-specific dosing:

Infants and Children:

Acute bacterial rhinosinusitis, severe infection requiring hospitalization (off-label use): Children: IV: 50 mg/kg/day divided every 12 hours for 10-14 days (Chow, 2012)

Community-acquired pneumonia (CAP) (IDSA/PIDS [Bradley, 2011]): Infants >3 months and Children: IV: 50-100 mg/kg/day once daily or divided every 12 hours. **Note:** May consider addition of vancomycin or clindamycin to empiric therapy if community-acquired MRSA suspected. Use the higher end of the range for penicillin-resistant *S. pneumoniae*; in children ≥5 years, a macrolide antibiotic should be added if atypical pneumonia cannot be ruled out; preferred in patients not fully immunized for *H. influenzae* type b and *S. pneumoniae*, or significant local resistance to penicillin in invasive pneumococcal strains

Epiglottitis (off-label use): IM, IV: 50-100 mg/kg once daily; reported duration of treatment ranged from 2-14 days

Gonococcal infections:

Arthritis (CDC, 2010): IM, IV:

≤45 kg: 50 mg/kg/dose once daily (maximum: 1000 mg) for 7 days

>45 kg: 50 mg/kg/dose once daily (maximum: 2000 mg) for 7 days

Bacteremia (CDC, 2010): IM, IV:

≤45 kg: 50 mg/kg/dose once daily (maximum: 1000 mg) for 7 days

>45 kg: 50 mg/kg/dose once daily (maximum: 2000 mg) for 7 days

Conjunctivitis, complicated (off-label use): IM, IV:

<45 kg: 50 mg/kg in a single dose (maximum: 1000 mg)

≥45 kg: 1000 mg in a single dose

Disseminated (off-label use): IM, IV:

Infants: 25-50 mg/kg/dose once daily for 7 days (10-14 days for meningitis) (CDC, 2010); **Note**: Use contraindicated in hyperbilirubinemic neonates.

Children <45 kg: 25-50 mg/kg/dose once daily (maximum: 1000 mg) for 7 days (CDC, 2010)

Children >45 kg: Refer to adult dosing.

Endocarditis (off-label use):

≤45 kg: IM, IV: 50 mg/kg/day every 12 hours (maximum: 2000 mg daily) for at least 28 days

>45 kg: IV: 1000-2000 mg every 12 hours, for at least 28 days

Meningitis:

≤45 kg: IV: 50 mg/kg/day given every 12 hours (maximum: 2000 mg daily); usual duration of treatment is 10-14 days (Red Book, 2012)

>45 kg: IV: 1000-2000 mg every 12 hours; usual duration of treatment is 10-14 days (CDC, 2010)

Prophylaxis (due to maternal gonococcal infection): IM, IV: 25-50 mg/kg as a single dose (maximum: 125 mg) (CDC, 2010)

Uncomplicated cervicitis, pharyngitis, proctitis, urethritis, vulvovaginitis (off-label use) (CDC, 2010):

≤45 kg: IM: 125 mg as a single dose

>45 kg: Refer to adult dosing

Infective endocarditis: IM, IV:

Native valve: 100 mg/kg once daily for 2-4 weeks; **Note:** If using 2-week regimen, concurrent gentamicin is recommended

Prosthetic valve: 100 mg/kg once daily for 6 weeks (with or without 2 weeks of gentamicin [dependent on penicillin MIC]); **Note:** For HACEK organisms, duration of therapy is 4 weeks

Enterococcus faecalis (resistant to penicillin, aminoglycoside, and vancomycin), native or prosthetic valve: 100 mg/kg/day divided every 12 hours for ≥8 weeks administered concurrently with ampicillin

Prophylaxis: 50 mg/kg 30-60 minutes before procedure; maximum dose: 1000 mg. Intramuscular injections should be avoided in patients who are receiving anticoagulant therapy. In these circumstances, orally administered regimens should be given whenever possible. Intravenously administered antibiotics should be used for patients who are unable to tolerate or absorb oral medications.

Note: American Heart Association (AHA) guidelines now recommend prophylaxis only in patients undergoing invasive procedures and in whom underlying cardiac conditions may predispose to a higher risk of adverse outcomes should infection occur. As of April 2007, routine prophylaxis for GI/GU procedures is no longer recommended by the AHA.

Lyme disease, persistent arthritis (off-label use): IM, IV: 75-100 mg/kg (maximum: 2000 mg) for 2-4 weeks

Mild-to-moderate infections: IM, IV: 50-75 mg/kg/day in 1-2 divided doses every 12-24 hours (maximum: 2000 mg daily); continue until at least 2 days after signs and symptoms of infection have resolved

Meningitis (empiric treatment): IM, IV: Loading dose of 100 mg/kg (maximum: 4000 mg), followed by 100 mg/kg/day divided every 12-24 hours (maximum: 4000 mg daily); usual duration of treatment is 7-14 days

Otitis media:

Acute: IM: 50 mg/kg in a single dose (maximum: 1000 mg)

Persistent or relapsing (off-label use): IM, IV: 50 mg/kg once daily for 3 days

Pneumonia: IV: 50-75 mg/kg once daily

Prophylaxis against sexually-transmitted diseases following sexual assault (off-label use):

≤45 kg: IM: 125 mg in a single dose (in combination with azithromycin and metronidazole) (CDC, 2010)

>45 kg: Refer to adult dosing

Serious infections: IV: 80-100 mg/kg/day in 1-2 divided doses (maximum: 4000 mg daily)

Shigella dysentery type 1 (off-label dose): IM: 50-100 mg/kg/day for 2-5 days (WHO, 2005)

Skin/skin structure infections: IM, IV: 50-75 mg/kg/day in 1-2 divided doses (maximum: 2000 mg daily)

Surgical (perioperative) prophylaxis (off-label dose): Children ≥ 1year: IV: 50-75 mg/kg within 60 minutes prior to surgery (maximum dose: 2000 mg) (Bratzler, 2013).

Typhoid fever (off-label use): IV: 75-80 mg/kg once daily for 5-14 days

Children >8 years (≥45 kg) and Adolescents:

Epididymitis, acute (off-label use): IM: 125 mg in a single dose

Children <15 years:

Chemoprophylaxis for high-risk contacts (close exposure to patients with invasive meningococcal disease) (off-label use): IM: 125 mg in a single dose. Children ≥15 years: Refer to adult dosing.

Adults:

Acute bacterial rhinosinusitis, severe infection requiring hospitalization (off-label use): IV: 1-2 g every 12-24 hours for 5-7 days (Chow, 2012)

Arthritis, septic (off-label use): IV: 1-2 g once daily

Brain abscess (off-label use): IV: 2 g every 12 hours with metronidazole

Cavernous sinus thrombosis (off-label use): IV: 2 g once daily with vancomycin or linezolid

Chancroid (off-label use): IM: 250 mg as single dose (CDC, 2010)

Chemoprophylaxis for high-risk contacts (close exposure to patients with invasive meningococcal disease) (off-label use): IM: 250 mg in a single dose

Cholecystitis, mild-to-moderate: 1-2 g every 12-24 hours for 4-7 days (provided source controlled)

Gonococcal infections:

Uncomplicated gonorrhea of the cervix, pharynx, urethra, or rectum (off-label regimen): IM: 250 mg in a single dose with oral azithromycin (preferred) or oral doxycycline (alternative to preferred) (CDC, 2012)

Conjunctivitis, complicated (off-label use): IM: 1 g in a single dose (CDC, 2010)

Disseminated (off-label use): IM, IV: 1 g once daily for 24-48 hours may switch to cefixime (after improvement noted) to complete a total of 7 days of therapy (CDC, 2010)

Endocarditis (off-label use): IV: 1-2 g every 12 hours for at least 28 days (CDC, 2010)

Epididymitis, acute (off-label use): IM: 250 mg in a single dose with doxycycline (CDC, 2010)

Meningitis: IV: 1-2 g every 12 hours for 10-14 days (CDC, 2010)

Infective endocarditis: IM, IV:

Native valve: 2 g once daily for 2-4 weeks; **Note:** If using 2-week regimen, concurrent gentamicin is recommended

Prosthetic valve: IM, IV: 2 g once daily for 6 weeks (with or without 2 weeks of gentamicin [dependent on penicillin MIC]); **Note:** For HACEK organisms, duration of therapy is 4 weeks

Enterococcus faecalis (resistant to penicillin, aminoglycoside, and vancomycin), native or prosthetic valve: 2 g twice daily for ≥8 weeks administered concurrently with ampicillin

Prophylaxis: IM, IV: 1 g 30-60 minutes before procedure. Intramuscular injections should be avoided in patients who are receiving anticoagulant therapy. In these circumstances, orally administered regimens should be given whenever possible. Intravenously administered antibiotics should be used for patients who are unable to tolerate or absorb oral medications.

Note: American Heart Association (AHA) guidelines now recommend prophylaxis only in patients undergoing invasive procedures and in whom underlying cardiac conditions may predispose to a higher risk of adverse outcomes should infection occur. As of April 2007, routine prophylaxis for GI/GU procedures is no longer recommended by the AHA.

Intra-abdominal infection, complicated, community-acquired, mild-to-moderate (in combination with metronidazole): 1-2 g every 12-24 hours for 4-7 days (provided source controlled)

Lyme disease (off-label use): IV: 2 g once daily for 14-28 days

Mastoiditis (hospitalized; off-label use): IV: 2 g once daily; >60 years old: 1 g once daily

Meningitis (empiric treatment): IV: 2 g every 12 hours for 7-14 days (longer courses may be necessary for selected organisms)

Orbital cellulitis (off-label use) and endophthalmitis: IV: 2 g once daily

Pelvic inflammatory disease: IM: 250 mg in a single dose plus doxycycline (with or without metronidazole) (CDC, 2010)

Pneumonia, community-acquired: IV: 1 g once daily, usually in combination with a macrolide; consider 2 g daily for patients at risk for more severe infection and/or resistant organisms (ICU status, age >65 years, disseminated infection)

Prophylaxis against sexually-transmitted diseases following sexual assault: IM: 250 mg as a single dose (in combination with azithromycin and metronidazole) (CDC, 2010)

Prosthetic joint infection: IV:

Staphylococci, oxacillin-susceptible: 1-2 g every 24 hours for 2-6 weeks (in combination with rifampin) followed by oral antibiotic treatment and suppressive regimens (Osmon, 2013)

Streptococci, beta-hemolytic: 2 g every 24 hours for 4-6 weeks (Osmon, 2013)

Pyelonephritis (acute, uncomplicated): Females: IV: 1-2 g once daily (Stamm, 1993). Many physicians administer a single parenteral dose before initiating oral therapy (Warren, 1999).

Septic/toxic shock/necrotizing fasciitis (off-label use): IV: 2 g once daily; with clindamycin for toxic shock

Surgical (perioperative) prophylaxis: IV: 1 g 30 minutes to 2 hours before surgery

Manufacturers recommendation: 1 g 30 minutes to 2 hours before surgery

Alternative recommendation: 1-2 g within 60 minutes prior to surgery (Bratzler, 2013).

Alternative recommendation for colorectal procedures: 2 g within 60 minutes prior to surgery with concomitant metronidazole (Bratzler, 2013).

Cholecystectomy: 1-2 g every 12-24 hours, discontinue within 24 hours unless infection outside gallbladder suspected

Syphilis (off-label use): IM, IV: 1 g once daily for 10-14 days; **Note:** Alternative treatment for early syphilis, optimal dose, and duration have not been defined (CDC, 2010)

Typhoid fever (off-label use): IV: 2 g once daily for 14 days

Whipple's disease (off-label use): Initial: 2 g once daily for 10-14 days, then oral therapy for ~1 year.

Dosage adjustment in renal impairment: No dosage adjustment is generally necessary in renal impairment; **Note:** Concurrent renal and hepatic dysfunction: Maximum dose: ≤2 g daily

Poorly dialyzed; no supplemental dose or dosage adjustment necessary, including patients on intermittent hemodialysis, peritoneal dialysis, or continuous renal replacement therapy (eg, CVVHD).

Dosage adjustment in hepatic impairment: No adjustment necessary unless there is concurrent renal dysfunction (see Dosage adjustment in renal impairment).

Dietary Considerations Some products may contain sodium.

Administration Do not admix with aminoglycosides in same bottle/bag. Do not reconstitute, admix, or coadminister with calcium-containing solutions. Infuse intermittent infusion over 30 minutes.

IM: Inject deep IM into large muscle mass; a concentration of 250 mg/mL or 350 mg/mL is recommended for all vial sizes except the 250 mg size (250 mg/mL is suggested); can be diluted with 1:1 water or 1% lidocaine for IM administration.

IV: Infuse as an intermittent infusion over 30 minutes. IV push administration over 1-4 minutes has been reported in children ≥12 years, adolescents, and adults (concentration: 100 mg/mL), primarily in patients outside the hospital setting (Baumgartner, 1983; Garrelts, 1988; Poole, 1999), although a 2 g dose administered IV push over 5 minutes resulted in tachycardia, restlessness, diaphoresis, and palpitations in one patient (Lossos, 1994). IV push administration in young infants may also have been a contributing factor in risk of cardiopulmonary events occurring from interactions between ceftriaxone and calcium (Bradley, 2009).

Monitoring Parameters Prothrombin time. Observe for signs and symptoms of anaphylaxis.

Dosage Forms

Solution, Intravenous:

Generic: 20 mg/mL (50 mL); 40 mg/mL (50 mL)

Solution Reconstituted, Injection:

Rocephin: 500 mg (1 ea); 1 g (1 ea)

Generic: 250 mg (1 ea); 500 mg (1 ea); 1 g (1 ea); 2 g (1 ea)

Solution Reconstituted, Intravenous:

Generic: 1 g (1 ea); 2 g (1 ea); 10 g (1 ea)

◆ **Ceftriaxone for Injection USP (Can)** *see* CefTRIAXone *on page 396*

◆ **Ceftriaxone Sodium** *see* CefTRIAXone *on page 396*

◆ **Ceftriaxone Sodium for Injection (Can)** *see* CefTRIAXone *on page 396*

◆ **Ceftriaxone Sodium for Injection BP (Can)** *see* CefTRIAXone *on page 396*

Cefuroxime (se fyoor OKS eem)

Brand Names: U.S. Ceftin; Zinacef; Zinacef in Sterile Water

Brand Names: Canada Apo-Cefuroxime; Auro-Cefuroxime; Ceftin; Cefuroxime For Injection; Cefuroxime For Injection, USP; PRO-Cefuroxime; ratio-Cefuroxime

Index Terms Cefuroxime Axetil; Cefuroxime Sodium

Pharmacologic Category Antibiotic, Cephalosporin (Second Generation)

Use Treatment of infections caused by staphylococci, group B streptococci, *H. influenzae* (type A and B), *E. coli*, *Enterobacter*, *Salmonella*, and *Klebsiella*; treatment of susceptible infections of the upper and lower respiratory tract, otitis media, urinary tract, uncomplicated skin and soft tissue, bone and joint, sepsis, uncomplicated gonorrhea and early lyme disease; surgical (perioperative) prophylaxis

Pregnancy Risk Factor B

Pregnancy Considerations Adverse events were not observed in animal reproduction studies. Cefuroxime crosses the placenta and reaches the cord serum and amniotic fluid. Placental transfer is decreased in the presence of oligohydramnios. Several studies have failed to identify an increased teratogenic risk to the fetus following maternal cefuroxime use.

During pregnancy, mean plasma concentrations of cefuroxime are 50% lower, the AUC is 25% lower, and the plasma half-life is shorter than nonpregnant values. At term, plasma half-life is similar to nonpregnant values and peak maternal concentrations after IM administration are slightly decreased. Pregnancy does not alter the volume of distribution. Cefuroxime is one of the antibiotics recommended for prophylactic use prior to cesarean delivery.

Breast-Feeding Considerations Cefuroxime is excreted in breast milk. Manufacturer recommendations vary; caution is recommended if cefuroxime IV is given to a nursing woman and it is recommended to consider discontinuing nursing temporarily during treatment following oral cefuroxime. Nondose-related effects could include modification of bowel flora.

Contraindications Hypersensitivity to cefuroxime, any component of the formulation, or other cephalosporins

Warnings/Precautions Modify dosage in patients with severe renal impairment. Use with caution in patients with a history of penicillin allergy, especially IgE-mediated reactions (eg, anaphylaxis, urticaria). Prolonged use may result in fungal or bacterial superinfection, including *C. difficile*-associated diarrhea (CDAD) and pseudomembranous colitis; CDAD has been observed >2 months postantibiotic treatment. Use with caution in patients with a history of colitis or with gastrointestinal malabsorption (not studied). Use with caution in patients with a history of seizure disorder; cephalosporins have been associated with seizure activity, particularly in patients with renal impairment not receiving dose adjustments. Discontinue if seizures occur. May be associated with increased INR, especially in nutritionally deficient patients, prolonged treatment, hepatic or renal disease. Tablets and oral suspension are not bioequivalent (do not substitute on a mg-per-mg basis). Tablets should not be crushed or chewed due to a strong, persistent bitter taste. Patients unable to swallow whole tablets should be prescribed the oral suspension. Potentially significant drug-drug interactions may exist, requiring dose or frequency adjustment, additional monitoring, and/or selection of alternative therapy.

Benzyl alcohol and derivatives: Some dosage forms may contain sodium benzoate/benzoic acid; benzoic acid (benzoate) is a metabolite of benzyl alcohol; large amounts of benzyl alcohol (≥99 mg/kg/day) have been associated with a potentially fatal toxicity ("gasping syndrome") in neonates; the "gasping syndrome" consists of metabolic acidosis, respiratory distress, gasping respirations, CNS dysfunction (including convulsions, intracranial hemorrhage), hypotension, and cardiovascular collapse (AAP, 1997; CDC, 1982); some data suggests that benzoate displaces bilirubin from protein binding sites (Ahlfors, 2001); avoid or use dosage forms containing benzyl alcohol derivative with caution in neonates. See manufacturer's labeling.

Phenylalanine: Some products may contain phenylalanine.

Adverse Reactions

Cardiovascular: Local thrombophlebitis

Dermatologic: Diaper rash (children)

Endocrine & metabolic: Increased lactate dehydrogenase

Gastrointestinal: Diarrhea (duration-dependent), nausea and vomiting, unpleasant taste

Genitourinary: Vaginitis

Hematologic: Decreased hematocrit, decreased hemoglobin, eosinophilia

Hepatic: Increased serum alkaline phosphatase, increased serum transaminases

Immunologic: Jarisch-Herxheimer reaction

Rare but important or life-threatening: Anaphylaxis, angioedema, anorexia, brain disease, candidiasis, chest tightness, cholestasis, *Clostridium difficile* associated diarrhea, colitis, decreased creatinine clearance, drug fever, dyspepsia, dysuria, erythema, erythema multiforme, gastrointestinal hemorrhage, gastrointestinal infection, glossitis, headache, hearing loss, hemolytic anemia, hepatitis, hyperactivity, hyperbilirubinemia, hypersensitivity, hypersensitivity angiitis, increased blood urea nitrogen, increased liver enzymes, increased serum creatinine, increased thirst, interstitial nephritis, irritability, joint swelling, leukopenia, muscle cramps, muscle rigidity, muscle spasm (neck), neutropenia, oral mucosa ulcer, pancytopenia, positive direct Coombs test, prolonged prothrombin time, pseudomembranous colitis, renal insufficiency, renal pain, seizure, serum sickness-like reaction, sialorrhea, sinusitis, Stevens-Johnson syndrome, swollen tongue, tachycardia, thrombocytopenia (rare), toxic epidermal necrolysis, trismus, upper respiratory tract infection, urethral bleeding, urethral pain, urinary tract infection, vaginal discharge, vaginal irritation, viral infection, vulvovaginal candidiasis, vulvovaginal pruritus

Drug Interactions

Metabolism/Transport Effects None known.

Avoid Concomitant Use

Avoid concomitant use of Cefuroxime with any of the following: BCG

Increased Effect/Toxicity

Cefuroxime may increase the levels/effects of: Aminoglycosides; Vitamin K Antagonists

The levels/effects of Cefuroxime may be increased by: Probenecid

Decreased Effect

Cefuroxime may decrease the levels/effects of: BCG; Sodium Picosulfate; Typhoid Vaccine

The levels/effects of Cefuroxime may be decreased by: Antacids; H2-Antagonists

Food Interactions Bioavailability is increased with food; cefuroxime serum levels may be increased if taken with food or dairy products. Management: Administer tablet without regard to meals; suspension must be administered with food.

Storage/Stability

Injection: Store intact vials at 15°C to 30°C (59°F to 86°F); protect from light. Reconstituted solution is stable for 24 hours at room temperature and 48 hours when refrigerated. IV infusion in NS or D_5W solution is stable for 24 hours at room temperature, 7 days when refrigerated, or 26 weeks when frozen. After freezing, thawed solution is stable for 24 hours at room temperature or 21 days when refrigerated.

ADD-Vantage vials: Joined, but not activated, vials are stable for 14 days. Once activated, stable for 24 hours at room temperature and 7 days refrigerated. Do not freeze.

Premix Galaxy plastic containers: Store frozen at -20°C. Thaw container at room temperature or under refrigeration; do not force thaw. Thawed solution is stable for 24 hours at room temperature and 28 days refrigerated; do not refreeze.

Oral suspension: Prior to reconstitution, store at 2°C to 30°C (36°F to 86°F). Reconstituted suspension is stable for 10 days at 2°C to 8°C (36°F to 46°F).

Tablet: Store at 15°C to 30°C (59°F to 86°F).

Mechanism of Action Inhibits bacterial cell wall synthesis by binding to one or more of the penicillin-binding proteins (PBPs) which in turn inhibits the final transpeptidation step of peptidoglycan synthesis in bacterial cell walls, thus inhibiting cell wall biosynthesis. Bacteria eventually lyse due to ongoing activity of cell wall autolytic enzymes (autolysins and murein hydrolases) while cell wall assembly is arrested.

Pharmacodynamics/Kinetics

Absorption: Oral (cefuroxime axetil): Increases with food

Distribution: Widely to body tissues and fluids; crosses blood-brain barrier; therapeutic concentrations achieved in CSF even when meninges are not inflamed

Protein binding: 33% to 50%

Bioavailability: Tablet: Fasting: 37%; Following food: 52%

Half-life elimination: Children: 1 to 2 hours; Adults: 1 to 2 hours; prolonged with renal impairment

Time to peak, serum: IM: ~15 to 60 minutes; IV: 2 to 3 minutes; Oral: Children: 3 to 4 hours; Adults: 2 to 3 hours

Excretion: Urine (66% to 100% as unchanged drug)

Dosage Note: Cefuroxime axetil film-coated tablets and oral suspension are not bioequivalent and are not substitutable on a mg/mg basis

Usual dosage range:

Children 3 months to 12 years:

Oral: 20-30 mg/kg/day in 2 divided doses

IM, IV: 75-150 mg/kg/day divided every 8 hours (maximum dose: 6 g daily)

Children ≥13 years and Adults:

Oral: 250-500 mg twice daily

IM, IV: 750 mg to 1.5 g every 6-8 hours or 100-150 mg/kg/day in divided doses every 6-8 hours (maximum: 6 g daily)

Indication-specific dosing:

Children ≥1 year:

Surgical (perioperative) prophylaxis: IV: 50 mg/kg within 60 minutes prior to surgical incision (maximum dose: 1500 mg). Doses may be repeated in 4 hours if procedure is lengthy or if there is excessive blood loss (Bratzler, 2013).

Children ≥3 months to 12 years:

Acute bacterial maxillary sinusitis, acute otitis media:

Oral: Suspension: 30 mg/kg/day in 2 divided doses for 10 days (maximum dose: 1000 mg daily); tablet: 250 mg twice daily for 10 days

IM, IV: 75-150 mg/kg/day divided every 8 hours (maximum dose: 6 g daily)

Impetigo: Oral: Suspension: 30 mg/kg/day in 2 divided doses for 10 days (maximum dose: 1000 mg daily)

Pharyngitis/tonsillitis:

Oral: Suspension: 20 mg/kg/day (maximum: 500 mg daily) in 2 divided doses for 10 days

IM, IV: 75-150 mg/kg day divided every 8 hours (maximum: 6 g daily)

Urinary tract infection, uncomplicated (off-label dosing):

Children ≥2 months to 2 years: Oral: 20-30 mg/kg/day divided twice daily for 7-14 days (AAP, 2011)

Children ≥2 years: Moderate to severe disease (possible pyelonephritis): Oral: 20-30 mg/kg/day divided twice daily (maximum dose: 1000 mg daily) (Bradley, 2012; Red Book [AAP, 2012])

Adolescents: Refer to adult dosing.

Adults (all oral doses listed are for tablet formulation):

Bronchitis (acute and exacerbations of chronic bronchitis):

Oral: 250-500 mg every 12 hours for 10 days

IV: 500-750 mg every 8 hours (complete therapy with oral dosing)

Cellulitis, orbital: IV: 1.5 g every 8 hours

Cholecystitis, mild-to-moderate: IV: 1.5 g every 8 hours for 4-7 days (provided source controlled)

Gonorrhea:

Disseminated: IM, IV: 750 mg every 8 hours

Uncomplicated:

Oral: 1 g as a single dose

IM: 1.5 g as single dose (administer in 2 different sites with probenecid)

Intra-abdominal infection, complicated, community-acquired, mild-to-moderate (in combination with metronidazole): IV: 1.5 g every 8 hours for 4-7 days (provided source controlled)

Lyme disease (early): Oral: 500 mg twice daily for 20 days

Pharyngitis/tonsillitis and sinusitis: Oral: 250 mg twice daily for 10 days

Pneumonia (uncomplicated): IV: 750 mg every 8 hours

Severe or complicated infections: IM, IV: 1.5 g every 8 hours (up to 1.5 g every 6 hours in life-threatening infections)

Skin/skin structure infection (uncomplicated):

Oral: 250-500 mg every 12 hours for 10 days

IM, IV: 750 mg every 8 hours

Surgical (perioperative) prophylaxis: IV:

Manufacturer's recommendation: 1.5 g 30 minutes to 1 hour prior to procedure (if procedure is prolonged can give 750 mg every 8 hours IV or IM)

Open heart: IV: 1.5 g every 12 hours for a total of 4 doses starting at anesthesia induction

Alternative recommendation: 1.5 g within 60 minutes prior to surgical incision. Doses may be repeated in 4 hours if procedure is lengthy or if there is excessive blood loss (Bratzler, 2013).

Urinary tract infection (uncomplicated):

Oral: 250 mg every 12 hours for 7-10 days

IM, IV: 750 mg every 8 hours

Dosage adjustment in renal impairment:

Oral:

Manufacturer's labeling:

CrCl ≥30 mL/minute: No dosage adjustment necessary

CrCl 10 to <30 mL/minute: Administer full dose every 24 hours

CrCl <10 mL/minute: Administer full dose every 48 hours

ESRD requiring intermittent hemodialysis (IHD): Additional full dose should be given at the end of each dialysis session

Alternate dosing (Aronoff, 2007): Children: **Note:** Renally adjusted dose recommendations are based on doses of 30 mg/kg/day divided every 12 hours:

CrCl ≥30 mL/minute/1.73 m^2: No dosage adjustment necessary

CrCl ≥10 to 29 mL/minute/1.73 m^2: 15 mg/kg/dose every 12 hours

CrCl <10 mL/minute/1.73 m^2: 15 mg/kg/dose every 24 hours

Hemodialysis: Dialyzable: 15 mg/kg/dose every 24 hours.

Peritoneal dialysis: 15 mg/kg/dose every 24 hours.

IV: Children and Adults:

Manufacturer's labeling:

CrCl >20 mL/minute: No dosage adjustment necessary

CrCl 10 to 20 mL/minute: Administer full dose every 12 hours

CrCl <10 mL/minute: Administer full dose every 24 hours

Hemodialysis: Administer additional dose at the end of dialysis

Alternate dosing (Aronoff, 2007):

Peritoneal dialysis:

Children: 25 to 50 mg/kg dose every 24 hours

Adults: Administer full dose every 24 hours

Continuous renal replacement therapy (CRRT):

Children: 25 to 50 mg/kg every 8 hours

Adults: 1 g every 12 hours

Dosage adjustment in hepatic impairment: There are no dosage adjustments provided in the manufacturer's labeling.

Dietary Considerations Some products may contain phenylalanine and/or sodium.

Oral suspension: Should be taken with food.

Administration

Oral suspension: Administer with food. Shake well before use.

Oral tablet: May administer without regard to meals. Swallow tablet whole (crushed tablet has strong, persistent, bitter taste).

IM: Inject deep IM into large muscle mass.

IV: Inject direct IV over 3-5 minutes. Infuse intermittent infusion over 15-30 minutes.

Monitoring Parameters Monitor renal, hepatic, and hematologic function periodically with prolonged therapy. Monitor prothrombin time in patients at risk of prolongation during cephalosporin therapy (nutritionally-deficient, prolonged treatment, renal or hepatic disease). Observe for signs and symptoms of anaphylaxis during first dose.

Dosage Forms

Solution, Intravenous:

Zinacef in Sterile Water: 1.5 g (50 mL)

Solution Reconstituted, Injection:

Zinacef: 750 mg (1 ea); 1.5 g (1 ea); 7.5 g (1 ea)

Generic: 750 mg (1 ea); 1.5 g (1 ea); 7.5 g (1 ea); 75 g (1 ea); 225 g (1 ea)

Solution Reconstituted, Intravenous:
Zinacef: 750 mg (1 ea); 1.5 g (1 ea)
Generic: 750 mg (1 ea); 1.5 g (1 ea); 7.5 g (1 ea)
Suspension Reconstituted, Oral:
Ceftin: 125 mg/5 mL (100 mL); 250 mg/5 mL (50 mL, 100 mL)
Generic: 125 mg/5 mL (100 mL)
Tablet, Oral:
Ceftin: 250 mg, 500 mg
Generic: 250 mg, 500 mg

- ◆ **Cefuroxime Axetil** *see* Cefuroxime *on page 399*
- ◆ **Cefuroxime For Injection (Can)** *see* Cefuroxime *on page 399*
- ◆ **Cefuroxime For Injection, USP (Can)** *see* Cefuroxime *on page 399*
- ◆ **Cefuroxime Sodium** *see* Cefuroxime *on page 399*
- ◆ **Cefzil** *see* Cefprozil *on page 389*
- ◆ **Cefzil® (Can)** *see* Cefprozil *on page 389*
- ◆ **CeleBREX** *see* Celecoxib *on page 402*
- ◆ **Celebrex (Can)** *see* Celecoxib *on page 402*

Celecoxib (se le KOKS ib)

Brand Names: U.S. CeleBREX

Brand Names: Canada Celebrex

Pharmacologic Category Nonsteroidal Anti-inflammatory Drug (NSAID), COX-2 Selective

Use Relief of the signs and symptoms of osteoarthritis, ankylosing spondylitis, juvenile idiopathic arthritis (JIA), and rheumatoid arthritis; management of acute pain; treatment of primary dysmenorrhea

Pregnancy Risk Factor C (prior to 30 weeks gestation)/D (≥30 weeks gestation)

Pregnancy Considerations Teratogenic effects have been observed in some animal studies; therefore, celecoxib is classified as pregnancy category C. Celecoxib is a NSAID that primarily inhibits COX-2 whereas other currently available NSAIDs are nonselective for COX-1 and COX-2. The effects of this selective inhibition to the fetus have not been well studied and limited information is available specific to celecoxib. NSAID exposure during the first trimester is not strongly associated with congenital malformations; however, cardiovascular anomalies and cleft palate have been observed following NSAID exposure in some studies. The use of a NSAID close to conception may be associated with an increased risk of miscarriage. Nonteratogenic effects have been observed following NSAID administration during the third trimester including: Myocardial degenerative changes, prenatal constriction of the ductus arteriosus, fetal tricuspid regurgitation, failure of the ductus arteriosus to close postnatally; renal dysfunction or failure, oligohydramnios; gastrointestinal bleeding or perforation, increased risk of necrotizing enterocolitis; intracranial bleeding (including intraventricular hemorrhage), platelet dysfunction with resultant bleeding; pulmonary hypertension. Because it may cause premature closure of the ductus arteriosus, the use of celecoxib is not recommended ≥30 weeks gestation. The chronic use of NSAIDs in women of reproductive age may be associated with infertility that is reversible upon discontinuation of the medication. A registry is available for pregnant women exposed to autoimmune medications including celecoxib. For additional information contact the Organization of Teratology Information Specialists, OTIS Autoimmune Diseases Study, at 877-311-8972.

Breast-Feeding Considerations Small amounts of celecoxib are found in breast milk. The manufacturer recommends that caution be exercised when administering celecoxib to nursing women.

Contraindications

Hypersensitivity to celecoxib, sulfonamides, aspirin, other NSAIDs, or any component of the formulation; patients who have demonstrated allergic-type reactions to sulfonamides; patients who have experienced asthma, urticaria, or allergic-type reactions after taking aspirin or other NSAIDs; treatment of perioperative pain in the setting of CABG surgery.

Canadian labeling: Additional contraindications (not in U.S. labeling): Pregnancy (third trimester); women who are breast-feeding; severe, uncontrolled heart failure; active gastrointestinal ulcer (gastric, duodenal, peptic) or bleeding; inflammatory bowel disease; cerebrovascular bleeding; severe liver impairment or active hepatic disease; severe renal impairment (CrCl <30 mL/minute) or deteriorating renal disease; known hyperkalemia; use in children

Warnings/Precautions **[U.S. Boxed Warning]: NSAIDs are associated with an increased risk of serious (and potentially fatal) adverse cardiovascular thrombotic events, including MI and stroke.** Risk may be increased with duration of use or preexisting cardiovascular risk factors or disease. Carefully evaluate individual cardiovascular risk profiles prior to prescribing. New-onset or exacerbation of hypertension may occur (NSAIDS may impair response to thiazide or loop diuretics); may contribute to cardiovascular events; monitor blood pressure; use with caution in patients with hypertension. May cause sodium and fluid retention; use with caution in patients with edema, cerebrovascular disease, or ischemic heart disease. Avoid use in patients with heart failure (ACCF/AHA [Yancy, 2013]). Long-term cardiovascular risk in children has not been evaluated.

[U.S. Boxed Warning]: Celecoxib is contraindicated for treatment of perioperative pain in the setting of coronary artery bypass graft (CABG) surgery. Risk of MI and stroke may be increased with use following CABG surgery.

[U.S. Boxed Warning]: NSAIDs may increase risk of serious gastrointestinal ulceration, bleeding, and perforation (may be fatal). These events may occur at any time during therapy and without warning. Use caution with a history of GI disease (bleeding or ulcers), concurrent therapy with aspirin, anticoagulants and/or corticosteroids, smoking, use of alcohol, the elderly or debilitated patients. When used concomitantly with aspirin, a substantial increase in the risk of gastrointestinal complications (eg, ulcer) occurs; concomitant gastroprotective therapy (eg, proton pump inhibitors) is recommended (Bhatt, 2008).

Use the lowest effective dose for the shortest duration of time, consistent with individual patient goals, to reduce risk of cardiovascular or GI adverse events. Alternate therapies should be considered for patients at high risk.

NSAIDs may cause serious skin adverse events including exfoliative dermatitis, Stevens-Johnson syndrome (SJS), and toxic epidermal necrolysis (TEN); may occur without warning and in patients without prior known sulfa allergy. Anaphylactoid reactions may occur, even without prior exposure; patients with "aspirin triad" (bronchial asthma, aspirin intolerance, rhinitis) may be at increased risk. Do not use in patients who have experienced an anaphylactic reaction with NSAID or aspirin therapy. The manufacturer's labeling states to not administer to patients with aspirin-sensitive asthma due to severe and potentially fatal bronchospasm that has been reported in such patients having received aspirin and the potential for cross reactivity with other NSAIDs. The manufacturer also states to use with caution in patients with other forms of asthma. However, in patients with known aspirin-exacerbated respiratory disease (AERD), the use of celecoxib initiated at a low dose with gradual titration in patients with stable, mild-to-moderate persistent asthma has been used without incident (Morales, 2013).

Use with caution in patients with decreased hepatic (dosage adjustments are recommended for moderate hepatic impairment; not recommended for patients with severe hepatic impairment) or renal function. Transaminase elevations have been reported with use; closely monitor patients with any abnormal LFT. Severe hepatic reactions (eg, fulminant hepatitis, liver failure) have occurred with NSAID use, rarely; discontinue if signs or symptoms of liver disease develop, if systemic manifestations occur, or with persistent or worsening abnormal hepatic function tests. NSAID use may compromise existing renal function; dose-dependent decreases in prostaglandin synthesis may result from NSAID use, causing a reduction in renal blood flow which may cause renal decompensation (usually reversible). Patients with impaired renal function, dehydration, heart failure, liver dysfunction, those taking diuretics, ACE inhibitors, angiotensin II receptor blockers, and the elderly are at greater risk for renal toxicity. Rehydrate patient before starting therapy; monitor renal function closely. Not recommended for use in patients with advanced renal disease or severe renal insufficiency; discontinue use with persistent or worsening abnormal renal function tests. Long-term NSAID use may result in renal papillary necrosis. Should not be considered a treatment or replacement of corticosteroid-dependent diseases.

Anaphylactoid reactions may occur, even with no prior exposure to celecoxib. Use with caution in patients with known or suspected deficiency of cytochrome P450 isoenzyme 2C9; poor metabolizers may have higher plasma levels due to reduced metabolism; consider reduced initial doses. Alternate therapies should be considered in patients with JIA who are poor metabolizers of CYP2C9.

Anemia may occur with use; monitor hemoglobin or hematocrit in patients on long-term treatment. Celecoxib does not affect PT, PTT or platelet counts; does not inhibit platelet aggregation at approved doses.

Use with caution in pediatric patients with systemic-onset juvenile idiopathic arthritis (JIA); serious adverse reactions, including disseminated intravascular coagulation, may occur.

Adverse Reactions

Cardiovascular: Angina pectoris, aortic insufficiency, chest pain, coronary artery disease, edema, facial edema, hypertension (aggravated), myocardial infarction, palpitations, peripheral edema, sinus bradycardia, tachycardia, ventricular hypertrophy

Central nervous system: Anxiety, depression, dizziness, drowsiness, fatigue, headache, hypertonia, hypoesthesia, insomnia, migraine, nervousness, pain, paresthesia, vertigo

Dermatologic: Alopecia, cellulitis, dermatitis, diaphoresis, erythematous rash, maculopapular rash, pruritus, skin photosensitivity, skin rash, urticaria, xeroderma

Endocrine & metabolic: Albuminuria, decreased plasma testosterone, hot flash, hypercholesterolemia, hyperglycemia, hypokalemia, increased nonprotein nitrogen, ovarian cyst, weight gain

Gastrointestinal: Abdominal pain, anorexia, constipation, diarrhea, diverticulitis, dyspepsia, dysphagia, eructation, esophagitis, flatulence, gastritis, gastroenteritis, gastroesophageal reflux disease, gastrointestinal ulcer, hemorrhoids, hiatal hernia, increased appetite, melena, nausea, stomatitis, tenesmus, vomiting, xerostomia

Genitourinary: Cystitis, dysuria, hematuria, urinary frequency

Hematologic & oncologic: Anemia, bruise, thrombocythemia

Hepatic: Increased serum alkaline phosphatase, increased serum transaminases

Hypersensitivity: Hypersensitivity exacerbation, hypersensitivity reaction

Neuromuscular & skeletal: Arthralgia, back pain, increased creatine phosphokinase, leg cramps, myalgia, osteoarthritis, synovitis, tendonitis

Ophthalmic: Conjunctival hemorrhage, vitreous opacity

Otic: Deafness, labyrinthitis, tinnitus

Renal: Increased blood urea nitrogen, increased serum creatinine, nephrolithiasis

Respiratory: Bronchitis, bronchospasm, cough, dyspnea, epistaxis, flu-like symptoms, laryngitis, nasopharyngitis, pharyngitis, pneumonia, rhinitis, sinusitis, upper respiratory tract infection

Miscellaneous: Cyst, fever

Rare but important or life-threatening: Acute renal failure, agranulocytosis, anaphylactoid reaction, angioedema, anosmia, aplastic anemia, aseptic meningitis, cardiac failure, cerebrovascular accident, cholelithiasis, colitis, deep vein thrombosis, dysgeusia, erythema multiforme, esophageal perforation, exfoliative dermatitis, gangrene of skin or other tissue, gastrointestinal hemorrhage, hepatic failure, hepatic necrosis, hepatitis (including fulminant), hypoglycemia, hyponatremia, interstitial nephritis, intestinal obstruction, intestinal perforation, intracranial hemorrhage, jaundice, leukopenia, pancreatitis, pancytopenia, pulmonary embolism, renal papillary necrosis, sepsis, Stevens-Johnson syndrome, syncope, thrombocytopenia, thrombophlebitis, toxic epidermal necrolysis, vasculitis, ventricular fibrillation

Drug Interactions

Metabolism/Transport Effects Substrate of CYP2C9 (major), CYP3A4 (minor); **Note:** Assignment of Major/Minor substrate status based on clinically relevant drug interaction potential; **Inhibits** CYP2C8 (moderate), CYP2D6 (moderate)

Avoid Concomitant Use

Avoid concomitant use of Celecoxib with any of the following: Dexketoprofen; Floctafenine; Ketorolac (Nasal); Ketorolac (Systemic); Nonsteroidal Anti-Inflammatory Agents; NSAID (COX-2 Inhibitor); Omacetaxine; Thioridazine

Increased Effect/Toxicity

Celecoxib may increase the levels/effects of: 5-ASA Derivatives; Aliskiren; Aminoglycosides; Anticoagulants; ARIPiprazole; Bisphosphonate Derivatives; CycloSPORINE (Systemic); CYP2C8 Substrates; CYP2D6 Substrates; Deferasirox; Desmopressin; Digoxin; DOXOrubicin (Conventional); Eliglustat; Eplerenone; Estrogen Derivatives; Fesoterodine; Haloperidol; Lithium; Methotrexate; Metoprolol; Nebivolol; NSAID (COX-2 Inhibitor); Omacetaxine; Porfimer; Potassium-Sparing Diuretics; PRALAtrexate; Prilocaine; Quinolone Antibiotics; Sodium Nitrite; Tacrolimus (Systemic); Tenofovir; Thioridazine; Vancomycin; Verteporfin; Vitamin K Antagonists

The levels/effects of Celecoxib may be increased by: ACE Inhibitors; Angiotensin II Receptor Blockers; Antidepressants (Tricyclic, Tertiary Amine); Aspirin; Ceritinib; Corticosteroids (Systemic); CycloSPORINE (Systemic); CYP2C9 Inhibitors (Moderate); CYP2C9 Inhibitors (Strong); Dexketoprofen; Floctafenine; Herbs (Anticoagulant/Antiplatelet Properties); Ketorolac (Nasal); Ketorolac (Systemic); Mifepristone; Nitric Oxide; Nonsteroidal Anti-Inflammatory Agents; Probenecid; Propafenone; Selective Serotonin Reuptake Inhibitors; Sodium Phosphates; Treprostinil

Decreased Effect

Celecoxib may decrease the levels/effects of: ACE Inhibitors; Aliskiren; Angiotensin II Receptor Blockers; Beta-Blockers; Codeine; Eplerenone; HydrALAZINE; Loop Diuretics; Potassium-Sparing Diuretics; Prostaglandins (Ophthalmic); Selective Serotonin Reuptake Inhibitors; Tamoxifen; Thiazide Diuretics; TraMADol

The levels/effects of Celecoxib may be decreased by: Bile Acid Sequestrants; CYP2C9 Inducers (Strong); Dabrafenib

Food Interactions Peak concentrations are delayed and AUC is increased by 10% to 20% when taken with a high-fat meal. Management: Administer without regard to meals.

Storage/Stability Store at 25°C (77°F); excursions permitted to 15°C to 30°C (59°F to 86°F).

Mechanism of Action Inhibits prostaglandin synthesis by decreasing the activity of the enzyme, cyclooxygenase-2 (COX-2), which results in decreased formation of prostaglandin precursors; has antipyretic, analgesic, and anti-inflammatory properties. Celecoxib does not inhibit cyclooxygenase-1 (COX-1) at therapeutic concentrations.

Pharmacodynamics/Kinetics

Distribution: V_d (apparent): ~400 L

Protein binding: ~97% primarily to albumin

Metabolism: Hepatic via CYP2C9; forms inactive metabolites

Bioavailability: Absolute: Unknown

Half-life elimination: ~11 hours (fasted)

Time to peak: ~3 hours

Excretion: Feces (~57% as metabolites, <3% as unchanged drug); urine (27% as metabolites, <3% as unchanged drug)

Dosage Note: Use the lowest effective dose for the shortest duration of time, consistent with individual patient treatment goals. Oral:

Children ≥2 years: Juvenile idiopathic arthritis (JIA):

≥10 kg to ≤25 kg: 50 mg twice daily

>25 kg: 100 mg twice daily

Adults:

Acute pain or primary dysmenorrhea: Initial dose: 400 mg, followed by an additional 200 mg if needed on day 1; maintenance dose: 200 mg twice daily as needed.

Canadian labeling: Recommended maximum dose for treatment of acute pain: 400 mg/day up to 7 days

Ankylosing spondylitis: 200 mg/day as a single dose or in divided doses twice daily; if no effect after 6 weeks, may increase to 400 mg/day. If no response following 6 weeks of treatment with 400 mg/day, consider discontinuation and alternative treatment.

Canadian labeling: Recommended maximum dose: 200 mg/day

Osteoarthritis: 200 mg/day as a single dose or in divided doses twice daily

Rheumatoid arthritis: 100-200 mg twice daily

Acute gout (off-label use): 800 mg once followed by 400 mg on day 1; then 400 mg twice daily for one week (ACR guidelines [Khanna, 2012]; Schumacker, 2012)

Elderly: No specific adjustment based on age is recommended. However, the AUC in elderly patients may be increased by 50% as compared to younger subjects. Initiate at the lowest recommended dose in patients weighing <50 kg.

*Dosing adjustment in poor CYP2C9 metabolizers (eg, CYP2C9*3/*3):* Consider reducing initial dose by 50%; consider alternative treatment in patients with JIA who are poor CYP2C9 metabolizers.

Canadian labeling: Recommended maximum dose: 100 mg/day

Dosing adjustment in renal impairment:

Advanced renal disease: Use is not recommended; however, if celecoxib treatment cannot be avoided, monitor renal function closely

Severe renal insufficiency: Use is not recommended.

Canadian labeling: CrCl <30 mL/minute: Use is contraindicated.

Abnormal renal function tests (persistent or worsening): Discontinue use

Dosing adjustment in hepatic impairment:

Moderate hepatic impairment (Child-Pugh class B): Reduce dose by 50%

Severe hepatic impairment (Child-Pugh class C): Use is not recommended

Canadian labeling: Use is contraindicated.

Abnormal liver function tests (persistent or worsening): Discontinue use

Dietary Considerations May be taken without regard to meals.

Administration May be administered without regard to meals. Capsules may be swallowed whole or the entire contents emptied onto a teaspoon of cool or room temperature applesauce. The contents of the capsules sprinkled onto applesauce may be stored under refrigeration for up to 6 hours.

Monitoring Parameters CBC; blood chemistry profile; occult blood loss and periodic liver function tests; monitor renal function (urine output, serum BUN and creatinine; monitor response (pain, range of motion, grip strength, mobility, ADL function), inflammation; blood pressure (baseline and during treatment); observe for weight gain, edema; observe for bleeding, bruising; evaluate gastrointestinal effects (abdominal pain, bleeding, dyspepsia)

JIA: Monitor for development of abnormal coagulation tests with systemic onset JIA

Dosage Forms

Capsule, Oral:

CeleBREX: 50 mg, 100 mg, 200 mg, 400 mg

Generic: 50 mg, 100 mg, 200 mg, 400 mg

◆ **Celestoderm V (Can)** *see* Betamethasone (Topical) *on page 255*

◆ **Celestoderm V/2 (Can)** *see* Betamethasone (Topical) *on page 255*

◆ **Celestone [DSC]** *see* Betamethasone (Systemic) *on page 253*

◆ **Celestone Soluspan** *see* Betamethasone (Systemic) *on page 253*

◆ **CeleXA** *see* Citalopram *on page 451*

◆ **Celexa (Can)** *see* Citalopram *on page 451*

Celiprolol [INT] (SEE li proe lole)

International Brand Names Cardem (ES); Celectol (CZ, FR, GB, PL, VN); Celipres (PL); Celipro-Lich (DE); Celiprol (RU); Cordiax (IT); Delaien (CN); Dilanorm (NL); Selectol (AE, AT, BE, CH, CL, CY, DE, FI, GR, HR, IE, KR, LU, TR); Selecturon (AT); Su Ya (CN); Tenoloc (CZ, SK)

Index Terms Celiprolol Hydrochloride

Pharmacologic Category Beta Blocker With Intrinsic Sympathomimetic Activity

Reported Use Treatment of angina, hypertension

Dosage Range Oral: 200-400 mg once daily; no dosage alteration needed the in elderly

Dosage adjustment in renal impairment: Adjustment may be needed; for CrCl 15-40 mL/minute: 100-200 mg daily

Product Availability Product available in various countries; not currently available in the U.S.

Dosage Forms

Tablet: 200 mg

- ◆ **Celiprolol Hydrochloride** *see* Celiprolol [INT] *on page 404*
- ◆ **CellCept** *see* Mycophenolate *on page 1405*
- ◆ **CellCept Intravenous** *see* Mycophenolate *on page 1405*
- ◆ **CellCept I.V. (Can)** *see* Mycophenolate *on page 1405*
- ◆ **Cell Culture Inactivated Influenza Vaccine, Trivalent [Flucelvax]** *see* Influenza Virus Vaccine (Inactivated) *on page 1075*
- ◆ **Celontin** *see* Methsuximide *on page 1331*
- ◆ **Celontin® (Can)** *see* Methsuximide *on page 1331*
- ◆ **Celsentri (Can)** *see* Maraviroc *on page 1272*
- ◆ **Cemill [OTC]** *see* Ascorbic Acid *on page 178*
- ◆ **Cemill SR [OTC]** *see* Ascorbic Acid *on page 178*
- ◆ **CEM-Urea** *see* Urea *on page 2114*
- ◆ **Cenestin [DSC]** *see* Estrogens (Conjugated A/Synthetic) *on page 782*
- ◆ **Cenestin (Can)** *see* Estrogens (Conjugated A/Synthetic) *on page 782*
- ◆ **Centany** *see* Mupirocin *on page 1404*
- ◆ **Centany AT** *see* Mupirocin *on page 1404*
- ◆ ***Centruroides* Immune FAB2 (Equine)** *see Centruroides* Immune F(ab')$_2$ (Equine) *on page 405*

Centruroides Immune F(ab')$_2$ (Equine)

(sen tra ROY dez i MYUN fab too E kwine)

Brand Names: U.S. Anascorp

Index Terms *Centruroides* Immune FAB2 (Equine); Antivenin (*Centruroides*) Immune F(ab')$_2$ (Equine); Antivenin Scorpion; Antivenom (*Centruroides*) Immune F(ab')$_2$ (Equine); Antivenom Scorpion; Scorpion Antivenin; Scorpion Antivenom

Pharmacologic Category Antivenin

Use Treatment of scorpion envenomation

Pregnancy Risk Factor C

Dosage IV: Children and Adults: **Note:** Initiate therapy as soon as possible after scorpion sting. Initial: 3 vials (containing ≤360 mg total protein and ≥450 LD50 [mouse] neutralizing units); may administer additional vials in 1-vial increments every 30-60 minutes as needed.

Dosing adjustment in renal impairment: There are no dosage adjustments provided in manufacturer's labeling.

Dosing adjustment in hepatic impairment: There are no dosage adjustments provided in manufacturer's labeling.

Additional Information Complete prescribing information should be consulted for additional detail.

Dosage Forms

Solution Reconstituted, Intravenous [preservative free]:
Anascorp: (1 ea)

- ◆ **Cepacol® (Can)** *see* Cetylpyridinium and Benzocaine [CAN/INT] *on page 415*
- ◆ **Cepacol Dual Relief [OTC]** *see* Benzocaine *on page 246*
- ◆ **Cepacol Sensations Hydra [OTC]** *see* Benzocaine *on page 246*
- ◆ **Cepacol Sensations Warming [OTC]** *see* Benzocaine *on page 246*
- ◆ **Cepacol Sore Throat [OTC]** *see* Benzocaine *on page 246*
- ◆ **Cepacol Sore Throat + Coating [OTC]** *see* Benzocaine *on page 246*
- ◆ **Cepacol Sore Throat Max Numb [OTC]** *see* Benzocaine *on page 246*

Cephalexin (sef a LEKS in)

Brand Names: U.S. Keflex

Brand Names: Canada Apo-Cephalex; Dom-Cephalexin; Keflex; PMS-Cephalexin; Teva-Cephalexin

Index Terms Cephalexin Monohydrate

Pharmacologic Category Antibiotic, Cephalosporin (First Generation)

Use Treatment of susceptible bacterial infections including respiratory tract infections, otitis media, skin and skin structure infections, bone infections, and genitourinary tract infections, including acute prostatitis; alternative therapy for acute infective endocarditis prophylaxis

Pregnancy Risk Factor B

Pregnancy Considerations Adverse events were not observed in animal reproduction studies. Cephalexin crosses the placenta and produces therapeutic concentrations in the fetal circulation and amniotic fluid. An increased risk of teratogenic effects has not been observed following maternal use of cephalexin. Peak concentrations in pregnant patients are similar to those in nonpregnant patients. Prolonged labor may decrease oral absorption.

Breast-Feeding Considerations Small amounts of cephalexin are excreted in breast milk. The manufacturer recommends that caution be exercised when administering cephalexin to nursing women. Maximum milk concentration occurs ~4 hours after a single oral dose and gradually disappears by 8 hours after administration. Nondose-related effects could include modification of bowel flora.

Contraindications Hypersensitivity to cephalexin, any component of the formulation, or other cephalosporins

Warnings/Precautions Modify dosage in patients with severe renal impairment. Use with caution in patients with a history of penicillin allergy, especially IgE-mediated reactions (eg, anaphylaxis, urticaria). Prolonged use may result in fungal or bacterial superinfection, including *C. difficile*-associated diarrhea (CDAD) and pseudomembranous colitis; CDAD has been observed >2 months postantibiotic treatment. May be associated with increased INR, especially in nutritionally-deficient patients, prolonged treatment, hepatic or renal disease.

Adverse Reactions

Central nervous system: Agitation, confusion, dizziness, fatigue, hallucination, headache

Dermatologic: Erythema multiforme (rare), genital pruritus, skin rash, Stevens-Johnson syndrome (rare), toxic epidermal necrolysis (rare), urticaria

Gastrointestinal: Abdominal pain, diarrhea, dyspepsia, gastritis, nausea (rare), pseudomembranous colitis, vomiting (rare)

Genitourinary: Genital candidiasis, vaginal discharge, vaginitis

Hematologic & oncologic: Eosinophilia, hemolytic anemia, neutropenia, thrombocytopenia

Hepatic: Cholestatic jaundice (rare), hepatitis (transient, rare), increased serum ALT, increased serum AST

Hypersensitivity: Anaphylaxis, angioedema, hypersensitivity reaction

Neuromuscular & skeletal: Arthralgia, arthritis, arthropathy

Renal: Interstitial nephritis (rare)

Drug Interactions

Metabolism/Transport Effects None known.

Avoid Concomitant Use

Avoid concomitant use of Cephalexin with any of the following: BCG

Increased Effect/Toxicity

Cephalexin may increase the levels/effects of: MetFORMIN; Vitamin K Antagonists

The levels/effects of Cephalexin may be increased by: Probenecid

Decreased Effect

Cephalexin may decrease the levels/effects of: BCG; Sodium Picosulfate; Typhoid Vaccine

The levels/effects of Cephalexin may be decreased by: Multivitamins/Minerals (with ADEK, Folate, Iron); Multivitamins/Minerals (with AE, No Iron); Zinc Salts

Food Interactions Peak antibiotic serum concentration is lowered and delayed, but total drug absorbed is not affected. Cephalexin serum levels may be decreased if taken with food. Management: Administer without regard to food.

Storage/Stability

Capsule: Store at 15°C to 30°C (59°F to 86°F).

Powder for oral suspension: Refrigerate suspension after reconstitution; discard after 14 days.

Tablet: Store at 20°C to 25°C (68°F to 77°F).

Mechanism of Action Inhibits bacterial cell wall synthesis by binding to one or more of the penicillin-binding proteins (PBPs) which in turn inhibits the final transpeptidation step of peptidoglycan synthesis in bacterial cell walls, thus inhibiting cell wall biosynthesis. Bacteria eventually lyse due to ongoing activity of cell wall autolytic enzymes (autolysins and murein hydrolases) while cell wall assembly is arrested.

Pharmacodynamics/Kinetics

Absorption: Rapid (90%); delayed in young children

Distribution: Widely into most body tissues and fluids, including gallbladder, liver, kidneys, bone, sputum, bile, and pleural and synovial fluids; CSF penetration is poor

Protein binding: 6% to 15%

Half-life elimination: Adults: 0.5-1.2 hours; prolonged with renal impairment

Time to peak, serum: ~1 hour

Excretion: Urine (80% to 100% as unchanged drug) within 8 hours

Dosage

Usual dosage range:

Children >1 year: Oral: 25-100 mg/kg/day every 6-8 hours (maximum: 4 g/day)

Adults: Oral: 250-1000 mg every 6 hours; maximum: 4 g/day

Indication-specific dosing:

Infants >3 months and Children: Oral:

Community-acquired pneumonia (CAP) (IDSA/PIDS, 2011), *S. aureus* (methicillin-susceptible), mild infection or step-down therapy (preferred): 75-100 mg/kg/day in 3-4 divided doses

Children: Oral:

Furunculosis: 25-50 mg/kg/day in 4 divided doses

Impetigo: 25 mg/kg/day in 4 divided doses

Otitis media: 75-100 mg/kg/day in 4 divided doses

Prophylaxis against infective endocarditis (dental, oral, or respiratory tract procedures): 50 mg/kg 30-60 minutes prior to procedure (maximum: 2 g). **Note:** American Heart Association (AHA) guidelines now recommend prophylaxis only in patients undergoing invasive procedures and in whom underlying cardiac conditions may predispose to a higher risk of adverse outcomes should infection occur.

Severe infections: 50-100 mg/kg/day in divided doses every 6-8 hours

Skin abscess: 50 mg/kg/day in 4 divided doses (maximum: 4 g)

Skin and skin structure infections: Children >1 year: 25-50 mg/kg/day divided every 12 hours

Streptococcal pharyngitis: Children >1 year: 25-50 mg/kg/day divided every 12 hours. **Note:** Recommended by the Infectious Disease Society of America (IDSA) as an alternative agent for group A streptococcal pharyngitis in penicillin-allergic patients (avoid in patients with immediate-type hypersensitivity to penicillin) at a dose of 40 mg/kg/day divided twice daily (maximum: 1000 mg daily) for 10 days (Shulman, 2012).

Adolescents >15 years and Adults: Oral:

Cellulitis and mastitis: 500 mg every 6 hours

Furunculosis/skin abscess: 250 mg 4 times/day

Prophylaxis against infective endocarditis (dental, oral, or respiratory tract procedures): 2 g 30-60 minutes prior to procedure. **Note:** American Heart Association (AHA) guidelines now recommend prophylaxis only in patients undergoing invasive procedures and in whom underlying cardiac conditions may predispose to a higher risk of adverse outcomes should infection occur.

Prophylaxis in total joint replacement patients undergoing dental procedures which produce bacteremia: 2 g 1 hour prior to procedure

Prosthetic joint infection, chronic oral antimicrobial suppression (off-label use): Oral:

Propionibacterium spp (alternative to penicillin or amoxicillin): 500 mg every 6-8 hours (Osmon, 2013)

Staphylococci, oxacillin-susceptible (preferred): 500 mg every 6-8 hours (Osmon, 2013)

Streptococci, beta-hemolytic (alternative to penicillin or amoxicillin): 500 mg every 6-8 hours (Osmon, 2013)

Skin and skin structure infections: 500 mg every 12 hours

Streptococcal pharyngitis: 500 mg every 12 hours. **Note:** Recommended by the Infectious Disease Society of America (IDSA) as an alternative agent for group A streptococcal pharyngitis in penicillin-allergic patients (avoid in patients with immediate-type hypersensitivity to penicillin) with a duration of 10 days (Shulman, 2012).

Uncomplicated cystitis: 500 mg every 12 hours for 7-14 days

Dosage adjustment in renal impairment: Adults:

CrCl 10-50 mL/minute: 500 mg every 8-12 hours

CrCl <10: 250-500 mg every 12-24 hours

Hemodialysis: 250 mg every 12-24 hours; moderately dialyzable (20% to 50%); give dose after dialysis session

Dosage adjustment in hepatic impairment: No dosage adjustment provided in manufacturer's labeling.

Dietary Considerations Take without regard to food. If GI distress, take with food.

Administration Take without regard to food. If GI distress, take with food. Give around-the-clock to promote less variation in peak and trough serum levels.

Monitoring Parameters With prolonged therapy monitor renal, hepatic, and hematologic function periodically; monitor for signs of anaphylaxis during first dose

Dosage Forms

Capsule, Oral:

Keflex: 250 mg, 500 mg, 750 mg

Generic: 250 mg, 500 mg, 750 mg

Suspension Reconstituted, Oral:

Generic: 125 mg/5 mL (100 mL, 200 mL); 250 mg/5 mL (100 mL, 200 mL)

Tablet, Oral:

Generic: 250 mg, 500 mg

◆ **Cephalexin Monohydrate** *see* Cephalexin *on page 405*

◆ **Ceprotin** *see* Protein C Concentrate (Human) *on page 1738*

◆ **Cerdelga** *see* Eliglustat *on page 712*

◆ **Cerebyx** *see* Fosphenytoin *on page 934*

◆ **Cerefolin® NAC** *see* Methylfolate, Methylcobalamin, and Acetylcysteine *on page 1334*

◆ **Cerezyme** *see* Imiglucerase *on page 1051*

Ceritinib (se RI ti nib)

Brand Names: U.S. Zykadia

Index Terms LDK378; Zykadia

Pharmacologic Category Antineoplastic Agent, Anaplastic Lymphoma Kinase Inhibitor; Antineoplastic Agent, Tyrosine Kinase Inhibitor

Use Non-small cell lung cancer, metastatic: Treatment of patients with anaplastic lymphoma kinase (ALK)-positive metastatic non-small cell lung cancer (NSCLC) who have progressed on or are intolerant to crizotinib

Pregnancy Risk Factor D

Pregnancy Considerations Adverse events were observed in animal reproduction studies. Based on its mechanism of action, ceritinib may cause fetal harm if administered to a pregnant woman. Women of reproductive potential should use effective contraception during and for at least 2 weeks following therapy discontinuation.

Breast-Feeding Considerations It is not known if ceritinib is excreted in breast milk. Due to the potential for serious adverse reactions in the nursing infant, breast-feeding is not recommended by the manufacturer.

Contraindications There are no contraindications listed in the manufacturer's labeling.

Warnings/Precautions Hazardous agent – use appropriate precautions for handling and disposal (meets NIOSH 2014 criteria). Symptomatic bradycardia may occur; heart rate <50 beats/minute has occurred. If possible, avoid concurrent use with other agents known to cause bradycardia (eg, beta blockers, nondihydropyridine calcium channel blockers, clonidine, digoxin). Monitor heart rate and blood pressure regularly. If symptomatic bradycardia (not life-threatening) occurs, withhold treatment until recovery to asymptomatic bradycardia or to a heart rate of ≥60 beats/minute, evaluate concurrent medications, and adjust ceritinib dose. Permanently discontinue for life-threatening bradycardia due to ceritinib; if life-threatening bradycardia occurs and concurrent medications associated with bradycardia can be discontinued or dose adjusted, restart ceritinib at a reduced dose (with frequent monitoring). QTc interval prolongation has occurred in clinical studies, and may be concentration-dependent. Periodically monitor ECG and electrolytes in patients with heart failure, bradyarrhythmias, electrolyte abnormalities, or who are taking medications known to prolong the QTc interval. May require treatment interruption, dosage reduction, or discontinuation. Avoid use in patients with congenital long QTc syndrome. Permanently discontinue in patients who develop QTc interval prolongation in combination with torsades de pointes or polymorphic ventricular tachycardia or signs/symptoms of serious arrhythmia.

Diarrhea, nausea, vomiting, or abdominal pain occurred in the majority of patients in clinical trials; over one-third of patients required dose reductions due to severe or persistent gastrointestinal toxicity. Manage symptoms medically with appropriate therapy (eg, antidiarrheals, antiemetics, fluid replacement) as indicated. May require therapy interruption and dosage reduction. Hepatotoxicity has been observed in patients treated with ceritinib in clinical trials, including ALT levels >5 times ULN in over one-quarter of patients. Monitor liver function tests (eg, ALT, AST, total bilirubin) monthly and as clinically necessary, more frequently in patients who develop transaminase abnormalities. May require therapy interruption, dosage reduction, and/or discontinuation. Use with caution in patients with hepatic impairment (has not been studied in patients with moderate or severe impairment). Ceritinib is metabolized and eliminated hepatically; systemic exposure and toxicities may be increased in patients with hepatic dysfunction. Hyperglycemia, including grade 3 and 4 toxicity, has been observed in ceritinib-treated patients. The risk of grade 3 or 4 hyperglycemia increases significantly in diabetic patients or those with glucose intolerance; risk is also increased in patients receiving corticosteroids. Monitor blood glucose levels as clinically necessary, particularly in patients with diabetes. May require initiation or optimization of antihyperglycemic therapy. Temporarily interrupt therapy for hyperglycemia until adequately controlled; reduce dose upon recovery. If adequate glycemic control is not possible with medical management, permanently discontinue ceritinib. Severe and life-threatening interstitial lung disease (ILD)/pneumonitis (some fatal) may occur. Monitor for signs/symptoms of pulmonary toxicity; permanently discontinue in patients diagnosed with treatment related ILD/pneumonitis. Potentially significant interactions may exist, requiring dose or frequency adjustment, additional monitoring, and/or selection of alternative therapy. In vitro studies indicate that cetirinib solubility and bioavailability may be decreased at higher pH; concurrent use with proton pump inhibitors, H_2-receptor antagonists, or antacids has not been evaluated.

Adverse Reactions

Cardiovascular: Bradycardia, prolonged Q-T interval on ECG, sinus bradycardia

Central nervous system: Fatigue, neuropathy (including paresthesia, muscular weakness, gait disturbance, peripheral neuropathy, hypoesthesia, peripheral sensory neuropathy, dysesthesia, neuralgia, peripheral motor neuropathy, hypotonia, polyneuropathy)

Dermatologic: Skin rash (including maculopapular rash, acneiform dermatitis)

Endocrine & metabolic: Decreased serum phosphate, increased serum glucose

Gastrointestinal: Abdominal pain, constipation, decreased appetite, diarrhea, disease of esophagus (including dyspepsia, gastroesophageal reflux disease, dysphagia), increased serum lipase, nausea, vomiting

Hematologic & oncologic: Decreased hemoglobin

Hepatic: Increased serum ALT, increased serum AST, increased serum bilirubin

Ophthalmic: Visual disturbance (including vision impairment, blurred vision, photopsia, accommodation disorder, presbyopia, reduced visual acuity)

Renal: Increased serum creatinine

Respiratory: Interstitial pulmonary disease

Drug Interactions

Metabolism/Transport Effects Substrate of CYP3A4 (major), P-glycoprotein; **Note:** Assignment of Major/Minor substrate status based on clinically relevant drug interaction potential; **Inhibits** CYP2C9 (moderate), CYP3A4 (moderate)

Avoid Concomitant Use

Avoid concomitant use of Ceritinib with any of the following: Bosutinib; Bradycardia-Causing Agents; Conivaptan; CYP3A4 Inducers (Strong); CYP3A4 Inhibitors (Strong); Fusidic Acid (Systemic); Grapefruit Juice; Highest Risk QTc-Prolonging Agents; Ibrutinib; Idelalisib; Ivabradine; Lomitapide; Mifepristone; Naloxegol; Olaparib; Pimozide; Simeprevir; St Johns Wort; Tolvaptan; Trabectedin; Ulipristal

Increased Effect/Toxicity

Ceritinib may increase the levels/effects of: ARIPiprazole; Avanafil; Bosentan; Bosutinib; Budesonide (Systemic, Oral Inhalation); Cannabis; Colchicine; CYP2C9 Substrates; CYP3A4 Substrates; Dapoxetine; DOXOrubicin (Conventional); Dronabinol; Eplerenone; Everolimus; FentaNYL; Highest Risk QTc-Prolonging Agents; Hydrocodone; Ibrutinib; Imatinib; Ivabradine; Ivacaftor; Lacosamide; Lomitapide; Lurasidone; Moderate Risk QTc-Prolonging Agents; Naloxegol; Olaparib; OxyCODONE; Pimecrolimus; Pimozide; Ranolazine; Rivaroxaban; Salmeterol; Saxagliptin; Simeprevir; Suvorexant;

Tetrahydrocannabinol; Tolvaptan; Trabectedin; Ulipristal; Vilazodone; Zopiclone

The levels/effects of Ceritinib may be increased by: Aprepitant; Bradycardia-Causing Agents; Bretylium; Conivaptan; Corticosteroids; CYP3A4 Inhibitors (Moderate); CYP3A4 Inhibitors (Strong); Dasatinib; Fosaprepitant; Fusidic Acid (Systemic); Grapefruit Juice; Idelalisib; Ivabradine; Luliconazole; Mifepristone; Netupitant; P-glycoprotein/ABCB1 Inhibitors; QTc-Prolonging Agents (Indeterminate Risk and Risk Modifying); Tofacitinib

Decreased Effect

Ceritinib may decrease the levels/effects of: Ifosfamide

The levels/effects of Ceritinib may be decreased by: Bosentan; CYP3A4 Inducers (Moderate); CYP3A4 Inducers (Strong); Dabrafenib; Deferasirox; P-glycoprotein/ABCB1 Inducers; Siltuximab; St Johns Wort; Tocilizumab

Food Interactions A high-fat meal increases AUC and C_{max} by 73% and 41%, respectively and a low-fat meal increases AUC and C_{max} by 58% and 43%, respectively; systemic exposure when administered with a meal may exceed that of a typical dose, and may result in increased toxicity. Management: Administer on an empty stomach, at least 2 hours before or after a meal.

Storage/Stability Store at 25°C (77°F); excursions are permitted between 15°C and 30°C (59°F and 86°F).

Mechanism of Action Potent inhibitor of anaplastic lymphoma kinase (ALK), a tyrosine kinase involved in the pathogenesis of non-small cell lung cancer. ALK gene abnormalities due to mutations or translocations may result in expression of oncogenic fusion proteins (eg, ALK fusion protein) which alter signaling and expression and result in increased cellular proliferation and survival in tumors which express these fusion proteins. ALK inhibition reduces proliferation of cells expressing the genetic alteration. Ceritinib also inhibits insulin-like growth factor 1 receptor (IGF-1R), insulin receptor (InsR), and ROS1. Ceritinib has demonstrated activity in crizotinib-resistant tumors in NSCLC xenograft models.

Pharmacodynamics/Kinetics

Absorption: AUC and C_{max} increased 73% and 41%, respectively, when administered with a high-fat meal, and 58% and 43%, respectively when taken with a low-fat meal (when compared to fasting)

Distribution: 4230 L (following a single dose), with a small preferential distribution to red blood cells versus plasma

Protein binding: 97% to human plasma proteins

Metabolism: Primarily hepatic via CYP3A

Half-life elimination: 41 hours

Time to peak: ~4 to 6 hours

Excretion: Feces (~92% with 68% as unchanged drug); urine (~1%)

Dosage

Non-small cell lung cancer (ALK-positive), metastatic:

Adults: Oral: 750 mg once daily; continue until disease progression or unacceptable toxicity.

Missed doses: If a dose is missed, take the missed dose unless the next dose is due within 12 hours.

Dosage adjustment for toxicity:

Note: Over half of patients initiating treatment required at least 1 dose reduction; the median time to the first dose reduction was 7 weeks. Discontinue if patients are unable to tolerate 300 mg daily.

Cardiac:

Bradycardia:

Symptomatic bradycardia (not life-threatening): Interrupt therapy and evaluate concomitant medications known to cause bradycardia. Upon recovery to asymptomatic bradycardia or to a heart rate ≥60 beats per minute, adjust the dose.

Symptomatic bradycardia (life-threatening or requiring intervention) in patients taking concomitant medications known to cause bradycardia/hypotension: Interrupt therapy until recovery to asymptomatic bradycardia or to a heart rate ≥60 beats per minute. If the concomitant medication can be adjusted or discontinued, resume ceritinib therapy with the dose reduced by 150 mg.

Symptomatic bradycardia (life-threatening) in patients not taking concomitant medications known to cause bradycardia/hypotension: Permanently discontinue therapy.

QTc prolongation:

QTc interval >500 msec on at least 2 separate ECGs: Interrupt therapy until QTc interval is <481 msec or recovers to baseline if baseline QTc is ≥481 msec, then resume therapy with a 150 mg dose reduction.

QTc prolongation in combination with torsades de pointes, polymorphic ventricular tachycardia, or signs/symptoms of serious arrhythmia: Permanently discontinue therapy.

Gastrointestinal: Severe or intolerable nausea, vomiting, or diarrhea (despite appropriate management): Interrupt therapy until improved, then resume treatment with a 150 mg dose reduction.

Metabolic: Persistent hyperglycemia >250 mg/dL (despite optimal antihyperglycemic therapy): Interrupt therapy until hyperglycemia is adequately controlled, then resume therapy with a 150 mg dose reduction. If hyperglycemia cannot be controlled, discontinue ceritinib permanently.

Pulmonary: Treatment-related interstitial lung disease/pneumonitis (any grade): Permanently discontinue therapy.

Dosage adjustment for concomitant therapy:

Strong CYP3A4 inhibitors: Avoid concomitant use of strong CYP3A inhibitors; if concurrent administration cannot be avoided, reduce ceritinib dose by approximately one-third (rounded to the nearest 150 mg dose). After discontinuation of the strong CYP3A inhibitor, resume ceritinib therapy at the dose used prior to initiation of the CYP3A4 inhibitor.

Strong CYP3A4 inducers: Avoid concurrent use of strong CYP3A inducers (eg, carbamazepine, phenytoin, rifampin, and St John's wort) during treatment with ceritinib.

Dosage adjustment for renal impairment: There are no dosage adjustments provided in the manufacturer's labeling (has not been studied). However, renal excretion is limited, and dosage adjustment is likely not necessary.

Dosage adjustment for hepatic impairment:

Preexisting mild impairment (total bilirubin ≤ULN and AST >ULN **or** total bilirubin >1 to 1.5 times ULN and any AST): No dosage adjustment is necessary.

Preexisting moderate or severe impairment: There are no dosage adjustments provided in the manufacturer's labeling (has not been studied). Ceritinib is primarily metabolized and eliminated hepatically; exposure is likely increased in patients with hepatic impairment.

Hepatotoxicity during treatment:

ALT or AST >5 times ULN with total bilirubin ≤2 times ULN: Interrupt therapy until recovery to baseline or ALT/AST ≤3 times ULN, then resume with a 150 mg dose reduction.

ALT or AST >3 times ULN with total bilirubin >2 times ULN in the absence of cholestasis or hemolysis: Permanently discontinue therapy.

Administration Administer orally on an empty stomach (at least 2 hours before or 2 hours after a meal). Hazardous agent; use appropriate precautions for handling and disposal (meets NIOSH 2014 criteria).

Monitoring Parameters CBC, renal function, liver function, blood glucose; cardiac monitoring (heart rate and QTc interval); signs/symptoms of gastrointestinal and pulmonary toxicity

Product Availability Zykadia: FDA approved April 2014; anticipated availability is currently undetermined.

Dosage Forms

Capsule, Oral:

Zykadia: 150 mg

◆ **Cerovel** *see* Urea *on page 2114*

Certolizumab Pegol (cer to LIZ u mab PEG ol)

Brand Names: U.S. Cimzia; Cimzia Prefilled; Cimzia Starter Kit

Brand Names: Canada Cimzia

Index Terms CDP870

Pharmacologic Category Antirheumatic, Disease Modifying; Gastrointestinal Agent, Miscellaneous; Tumor Necrosis Factor (TNF) Blocking Agent

Use

Ankylosing spondylitis: Treatment of adults with active ankylosing spondylitis (AS)

Crohn disease: Treatment of moderately to severely active Crohn disease in patients who have inadequate response to conventional therapy

Psoriatic arthritis: Treatment of adult patients with active psoriatic arthritis

Rheumatoid arthritis: Treatment of adults with moderately to severely active rheumatoid arthritis (RA) (as monotherapy or in combination with nonbiological disease-modifying antirheumatic drugs [DMARDS])

Pregnancy Risk Factor B

Pregnancy Considerations Adverse effects were not observed in animal reproduction studies. Certolizumab pegol was found to cross the human placenta. Serum concentrations in 12 infants of 10 mothers were ≥75% lower than the maternal serum at delivery (last maternal dose of 400 mg given 5-42 days prior to birth). Although placental transfer was low, infants may have a slower rate of elimination than adults. In one infant, certolizumab pegol serum concentrations decreased from 1.02 to 0.84 mcg/mL over 4 weeks. Adverse events were not reported. The safety of administering live or live-attenuated vaccines to exposed infants is not known. If a biologic agent such as certolizumab pegol is needed to treat inflammatory bowel disease during pregnancy, it is recommended to hold therapy after 30 weeks gestation (Habal, 2012).

Healthcare providers are encouraged to enroll women exposed to certolizumab pegol during pregnancy in the MotherToBaby Autoimmune Diseases Study by contacting the Organization of Teratology Information Specialists (OTIS) (877-311-8972). The Canadian labeling recommends that women of childbearing potential use reliable contraception during therapy and for at least 5 months after the last dose of certolizumab.

Breast-Feeding Considerations It is not known if certolizumab pegol is excreted in breast milk. Due to the potential for serious adverse reactions in the nursing infant, the manufacturer recommends a decision be made whether to discontinue nursing or to discontinue the drug, taking into account the importance of treatment to the mother.

Contraindications There are no contraindications listed within the manufacturer's U.S. labeling.

Canadian labeling: Hypersensitivity to certolizumab pegol or any component of the formulation; active tuberculosis or other severe infections (eg, sepsis, abscesses, opportunistic infections); moderate to severe heart failure (NYHA Class III/IV)

Warnings/Precautions [U.S. Boxed Warning]: Patients receiving certolizumab are at increased risk for serious infections which may result in hospitalization and/or fatality; infections usually developed in patients receiving concomitant immunosuppressive agents (eg, methotrexate or corticosteroids) and may present as disseminated (rather than local) disease. Active tuberculosis (or reactivation of latent tuberculosis), invasive fungal (including aspergillosis, blastomycosis, candidiasis, coccidioidomycosis, histoplasmosis, and pneumocystosis) and bacterial, viral or other opportunistic infections (including legionellosis and listeriosis) have been reported in patients receiving TNF-blocking agents, including certolizumab. Monitor closely for signs/symptoms of infection. Discontinue for serious infection or sepsis. Consider risks versus benefits prior to use in patients with a history of chronic or recurrent infection. Consider empiric antifungal therapy in patients who are at risk for invasive fungal infection and develop severe systemic illness. Caution should be exercised when considering use in the elderly or in patients with conditions that predispose them to infections (eg, diabetes) or residence/travel from areas of endemic mycoses (blastomycosis, coccidioidomycosis, histoplasmosis), or with latent or localized infections. Do not initiate certolizumab therapy with active infection, including clinically important localized infection. Patients who develop a new infection while undergoing treatment should be monitored closely. **[U.S. Boxed Warning]: Lymphoma and other malignancies (some fatal) have been reported in children and adolescent patients receiving other TNF-blocking agents.** Approximately half of the malignancies reported in children were lymphomas (Hodgkin and non-Hodgkin) while other cases varied and included malignancies not typically observed in this population. The onset of malignancy was after a median of 30 months (range: 1-84 months) after the initiation of the TNF-blocking agent. Use of TNF blockers may affect defenses against malignancies; impact on the development and course of malignancies is not fully defined. Chronic immunosuppressant therapy use may be a predisposing factor for malignancy development; rheumatoid arthritis alone has been previously associated with an increased rate of lymphoma. Hepatosplenic T-cell lymphoma (HSTCL), a rare T-cell lymphoma, has also been associated with TNF-blocking agents, primarily reported in adolescent and young adult males with Crohn disease or ulcerative colitis, most of whom had received concurrent treatment with azathioprine and/or 6-mercaptopurine. Melanoma and Merkel cell carcinoma have been reported with TNF-blocking agents including certolizumab. Perform periodic skin examinations in all patients during therapy, particularly those at increased risk for skin cancer.

Tuberculosis has been reported with certolizumab treatment. **[U.S. Boxed Warnings]: Patients should be evaluated for tuberculosis risk factors and for latent tuberculosis infection (with a tuberculin skin test) prior to therapy. Treatment of latent tuberculosis should be initiated before use. Patients with initial negative tuberculin skin tests should receive continued monitoring for tuberculosis throughout treatment;** active tuberculosis has developed in this population during treatment. Use with caution in patients who have resided in regions where tuberculosis is endemic. Consider antituberculosis treatment (prior to certolizumab treatment) in patients with a history of latent or active tuberculosis if adequate treatment course cannot be confirmed, and for patients with risk factors for tuberculosis despite a negative test. Carefully consider benefits and risks of initiating certolizumab treatment in patients who have been exposed to tuberculosis.

Rare reactivation of hepatitis B virus (HBV) has occurred in chronic carriers of the virus, usually in patients receiving concomitant immunosuppressants; evaluate for HBV prior to initiation in all patients. Patients who test positive for HBV surface antigen should be referred for hepatitis B evaluation/treatment prior to certolizumab initiation. Monitor for clinical and laboratory signs of active infection during and for several months following discontinuation of treatment in HBV carriers; interrupt therapy if reactivation occurs and treat appropriately with antiviral therapy; if resumption of therapy is deemed necessary, exercise caution and monitor patient closely.

Hypersensitivity reactions, including angioedema, dyspnea, hypotension, rash, serum sickness and urticaria have been reported (rarely) with treatment; discontinue and do not resume therapy if hypersensitivity occurs. Some of these reactions have occurred after the first dose. Use with caution in patients who have experienced hypersensitivity with other TNF blockers. Use with caution in heart failure patients; worsening heart failure and new onset heart failure have been reported with TNF blockers, including certolizumab pegol; monitor closely. The Canadian labeling contraindicates use in moderate-to-severe heart failure (NYHA Class III/IV).

Rare cases of pancytopenia and other significant cytopenias, including aplastic anemia and have been reported with TNF-blocking agents. Leukopenia and thrombocytopenia have occurred with certolizumab; use with caution in patients with underlying hematologic disorders; consider discontinuing therapy with significant hematologic abnormalities. Autoantibody formation may develop; rarely resulting in autoimmune disorder, including lupus-like syndrome; monitor and discontinue if symptoms develop. A small number of patients (8%) develop antibodies to certolizumab during therapy. Antibody-positive patients may have an increased incidence of adverse events (including injection site pain/erythema, abdominal pain and erythema nodosum). Use with caution in patients with preexisting or recent-onset CNS demyelinating disorders; rare cases of optic neuritis, seizure, peripheral neuropathy, and demyelinating disease (eg, multiple sclerosis, Guillain-Barré syndrome; new onset or exacerbation) have been reported.

Potentially significant drug-drug interactions may exist, requiring dose or frequency adjustment, additional monitoring, and/or selection of alternative therapy. Use caution when switching between biological disease modifying antirheumatic drugs (DMARDs); overlapping of biological activity may increase the risk for infection.

Patients should be up to date with all immunizations before initiating therapy; patients may receive vaccines other than live or live attenuated vaccines during therapy. There is no data available concerning the effects of therapy on vaccination or secondary transmission of live vaccines in patients receiving therapy. Use has not been studied in patients with renal impairment; however, the pharmacokinetics of the pegylated (polyethylene glycol) component may be dependent on renal function. Use with caution in the elderly, may be at higher risk for infections.

Adverse Reactions

Cardiovascular: Angina pectoris, atrial fibrillation, cardiac arrhythmia, cardiac failure (new or worsening), cerebrovascular accident, hypertension, hypertensive heart disease, ischemic heart disease, myocardial infarction, pericardial effusion, pericarditis, transient ischemic attack, vasculitis

Central nervous system: Anxiety, bipolar mood disorder, fatigue, headache, suicidal tendencies

Dermatologic: Alopecia, dermatitis, erythema nodosum, skin rash, urticaria

Endocrine & metabolic: Menstrual disease

Gastrointestinal: Nausea (Schreiber, 2005)

Genitourinary: Nephrotic syndrome, urinary tract infection

Hematologic & oncologic: Anemia, hemorrhage, hypercoagulability state, leukopenia, lymphadenopathy, pancytopenia, positive ANA titer, thrombophlebitis

Hepatic: Hepatitis, increased serum transaminases

Immunologic: Antibody development

Infection: Infection

Neuromuscular & skeletal: Arthralgia, back pain

Ophthalmic: Optic neuritis, retinal hemorrhage, uveitis

Renal: Renal failure

Respiratory: Bronchitis, cough, nasopharyngitis, pharyngitis, tuberculosis (peritoneal, pulmonary, and disseminated), upper respiratory tract infection

Miscellaneous: Fever

Rare but important or life-threatening: Aplastic anemia, cytopenia, demyelinating disease (exacerbation), fistula, hepatosplenic T-cell lymphoma, herpes virus infection, hypersensitivity reaction (eg, dyspnea, hot flush, hypotension, malaise, serum sickness, syncope), intestinal obstruction, leukemia, lupus erythematosus, lupus-like syndrome, lymphoma, malignant melanoma, malignant neoplasm, Merkel cell carcinoma, opportunistic infection (rare), peripheral edema, peripheral neuropathy, pneumonia, psoriasis (including new onset, palmoplantar, pustular, or exacerbation), pyelonephritis, reactivation of HBV, sarcoidosis, seizure, thrombocytopenia, viral infection

Drug Interactions

Metabolism/Transport Effects None known.

Avoid Concomitant Use

Avoid concomitant use of Certolizumab Pegol with any of the following: Abatacept; Anakinra; Anti-TNF Agents; BCG; Canakinumab; Natalizumab; Pimecrolimus; Rilonacept; RiTUXimab; Tacrolimus (Topical); Tocilizumab; Tofacitinib; Vaccines (Live); Vedolizumab

Increased Effect/Toxicity

Certolizumab Pegol may increase the levels/effects of: Abatacept; Anakinra; Canakinumab; Leflunomide; Natalizumab; Rilonacept; Tofacitinib; Vaccines (Live); Vedolizumab

The levels/effects of Certolizumab Pegol may be increased by: Anti-TNF Agents; Denosumab; Pimecrolimus; RiTUXimab; Roflumilast; Tacrolimus (Topical); Tocilizumab; Trastuzumab

Decreased Effect

Certolizumab Pegol may decrease the levels/effects of: BCG; Coccidioides immitis Skin Test; Sipuleucel-T; Vaccines (Inactivated); Vaccines (Live)

The levels/effects of Certolizumab Pegol may be decreased by: Echinacea; Pegloticase

Preparation for Administration Vials: Allow to reach room temperature prior to reconstitution. Using aseptic technique, reconstitute each vial with 1 mL sterile water for injection (provided) to a concentration of ~200 mg/mL; the manufacturer recommends using a 20-gauge needle (provided). Gently swirl to facilitate wetting of powder; do not shake. Allow vials to set undisturbed (may take up to 30 minutes) until fully reconstituted. Reconstituted solutions should not contain visible particles or gels in the solution.

Storage/Stability

Store intact vials and syringes at 2°C to 8°C (36°F to 46°F); do not freeze. Do not separate contents of carton prior to use. Protect from light. Bring to room temperature prior to administration.

Reconstituted vials may be retained at room temperature for up to 2 hours or refrigerated (do not freeze) for up to 24 hours prior to administration. Discard unused portion of vial or syringe.

Mechanism of Action Certolizumab pegol is a pegylated humanized antibody Fab' fragment of tumor necrosis factor alpha (TNF-alpha) monoclonal antibody. Certolizumab pegol binds to and selectively neutralizes human TNF-alpha activity. (Elevated levels of TNF-alpha have a role in the inflammatory process associated with Crohn disease and in joint destruction associated with rheumatoid arthritis.) Since it is not a complete antibody (lacks Fc region), it does not induce complement activation, antibody-dependent cell-mediated cytotoxicity, or apoptosis. Pegylation of certolizumab allows for delayed elimination and therefore an extended half-life.

Pharmacodynamics/Kinetics

Distribution: V_{ss}: 6-8 L

Bioavailability: SubQ: ~80% (range: 76% to 88%)

Half-life elimination: ~14 days

Time to peak, plasma: 54-171 hours

Dosage Note: Each 400 mg dose should be administered as 2 injections of 200 mg each

Ankylosing spondylitis: Adults: SubQ: Initial: 400 mg, repeat dose 2 and 4 weeks after initial dose; Maintenance: 200 mg every 2 weeks or 400 mg every 4 weeks

Crohn disease: Adults: SubQ: Initial: 400 mg, repeat dose 2 and 4 weeks after initial dose; Maintenance: 400 mg every 4 weeks

Psoriatic arthritis: Adults: SubQ: Initial: 400 mg, repeat dose 2 and 4 weeks after initial dose; Maintenance: 200 mg every other week. May consider maintenance dose of 400 mg every 4 weeks.

Rheumatoid arthritis: Adults: SubQ: Initial: 400 mg, repeat dose 2 and 4 weeks after initial dose; Maintenance: 200 mg every other week. May consider maintenance dose of 400 mg every 4 weeks. May be administered alone or in combination with methotrexate.

Dosage adjustment for toxicity: Hypersensitivity, lupus-like syndrome, serious infection, sepsis, or hepatitis B reactivation: Discontinue treatment.

Dosage adjustment in renal impairment: There are no dosage adjustments provided in the manufacturer's labeling (has not been studied); pharmacokinetics of the pegylated (polyethylene glycol) component of certolizumab pegol is expected to be dependent on renal function.

Dosage adjustment in hepatic impairment: There are no dosage adjustments provided in the manufacturer's labeling.

Administration SubQ: Bring to room temperature prior to administration. After reconstitution (of vials), draw each vial into separate syringes (using 20-gauge needles).

Administer each syringe subcutaneously (using provided 23-gauge needle) to separate sites on abdomen or thigh. Rotate injections sites; do not administer to areas where skin is tender, bruised, red, or hard.

Missed doses (Canadian labeling): Wait until the next scheduled dose if within 1 week; if the next scheduled dose is ≥1 week administer as soon as possible then follow with next scheduled dose.

Monitoring Parameters Monitor improvement of symptoms and physical function assessments. Latent TB screening prior to initiating and during therapy; signs/symptoms of infection (prior to, during, and following therapy); CBC with differential; signs/symptoms/worsening of heart failure; HBV screening prior to initiating (all patients), HBV carriers (during and for several months following therapy); signs and symptoms of hypersensitivity reaction; symptoms of lupus-like syndrome; signs/symptoms of malignancy (eg, splenomegaly, hepatomegaly, abdominal pain, persistent fever, night sweats, weight loss) including periodic skin examinations.

Dosage Forms

Kit, Subcutaneous:

Cimzia: 200 mg

Kit, Subcutaneous [preservative free]:

Cimzia Prefilled: 200 mg/mL

Cimzia Starter Kit: 6 X 200 mg/mL

◆ **Cerubidine** *see* DAUNOrubicin (Conventional) *on page 577*

◆ **Cervarix** *see* Papillomavirus (Types 16, 18) Vaccine (Human, Recombinant) *on page 1574*

◆ **Cervidil** *see* Dinoprostone *on page 640*

◆ **Cervidil® (Can)** *see* Dinoprostone *on page 640*

◆ **C.E.S.** *see* Estrogens (Conjugated/Equine, Systemic) *on page 787*

◆ **C.E.S.** *see* Estrogens (Conjugated/Equine, Topical) *on page 790*

◆ **C.E.S.® (Can)** *see* Estrogens (Conjugated/Equine, Systemic) *on page 787*

◆ **Cetacaine** *see* Benzocaine, Butamben, and Tetracaine *on page 247*

◆ **Cetafen [OTC]** *see* Acetaminophen *on page 32*

◆ **Cetafen Extra [OTC]** *see* Acetaminophen *on page 32*

Cetirizine (se TI ra zeen)

Brand Names: U.S. All Day Allergy Childrens [OTC]; All Day Allergy [OTC]; Cetirizine HCl Allergy Child [OTC]; Cetirizine HCl Childrens Alrgy [OTC]; Cetirizine HCl Childrens [OTC]; Cetirizine HCl Hives Relief [OTC]; ZyrTEC Allergy Childrens [OTC]; ZyrTEC Allergy [OTC]; ZyrTEC Childrens Allergy [OTC]; ZyrTEC Childrens Hives Relief [OTC]; ZyrTEC Hives Relief [OTC]

Brand Names: Canada Aller-Relief [OTC]; Apo-Cetirizine [OTC]; Extra Strength Allergy Relief [OTC]; PMS-Cetirizine; Reactine; Reactine [OTC]

Index Terms Cetirizine Hydrochloride; P-071; UCB-P071

Pharmacologic Category Histamine H_1 Antagonist; Histamine H_1 Antagonist, Second Generation; Piperazine Derivative

Use

Upper respiratory allergies: Temporarily relieves symptoms of upper respiratory allergies.

Urticaria: Relieves itching due to urticaria.

Pregnancy Considerations Maternal use of cetirizine has not been associated with an increased risk of major malformations. The use of antihistamines for the treatment of rhinitis during pregnancy is generally considered to be safe at recommended doses. Although safety data is limited, cetirizine may be a preferred second generation antihistamine for the treatment of rhinitis during pregnancy.

Breast-Feeding Considerations Cetirizine is excreted into breast milk.

Contraindications Hypersensitivity to cetirizine, hydroxyzine, or any component of the formulation

Warnings/Precautions Cetirizine should be used cautiously in patients with hepatic or renal impairment; consider dosage adjustment in patients with renal impairment. Use with caution in elderly patients; may be more sensitive to adverse effects. May cause drowsiness; use caution performing tasks which require alertness (eg, operating machinery or driving). Potentially significant drug-drug interactions may exist, requiring dose or frequency adjustment, additional monitoring, and/or selection of alternative therapy. Effects may be potentiated when used with other sedative drugs or ethanol.

Adverse Reactions

Central nervous system: Dizziness (adults), drowsiness (more common in adults), headache (children), fatigue (adults), insomnia (more common in children), malaise

Gastrointestinal: Abdominal pain (children), diarrhea, nausea, vomiting, xerostomia (adults)

Respiratory: Bronchospasm (children), epistaxis (epistaxis), pharyngitis (children)

Rare but important or life-threatening (as reported in adults and/or children): Aggressive behavior, anaphylaxis, angioedema, ataxia, chest pain, confusion, convulsions, depersonalization, depression, dysgeusia, edema, fussiness, hallucination, hemolytic anemia, hepatic insufficiency, hepatitis, hypertension, hypotension (severe), irritability, nervousness, ototoxicity, palpitations, paralysis, paresthesia, skin photosensitivity, skin rash, suicidal ideation, tongue discoloration, tongue edema, tremor, visual field defect, weakness

Drug Interactions

Metabolism/Transport Effects Substrate of CYP3A4 (minor), P-glycoprotein; **Note:** Assignment of Major/Minor substrate status based on clinically relevant drug interaction potential

Avoid Concomitant Use

Avoid concomitant use of Cetirizine with any of the following: Aclidinium; Azelastine (Nasal); Glucagon; Ipratropium (Oral Inhalation); Orphenadrine; Paraldehyde; Potassium Chloride; Thalidomide; Tiotropium; Umeclidinium

Increased Effect/Toxicity

Cetirizine may increase the levels/effects of: AbobotulinumtoxinA; Alcohol (Ethyl); Analgesics (Opioid); Anticholinergic Agents; Azelastine (Nasal); Buprenorphine; CNS Depressants; Glucagon; Hydrocodone; Methotrimeprazine; Metyrosine; Mirabegron; Mirtazapine; OnabotulinumtoxinA; Orphenadrine; Paraldehyde; Potassium Chloride; Pramipexole; RimabotulinumtoxinB; ROPINIRole; Rotigotine; Selective Serotonin Reuptake Inhibitors; Suvorexant; Thalidomide; Thiazide Diuretics; Tiotropium; Topiramate; Zolpidem

The levels/effects of Cetirizine may be increased by: Aclidinium; Brimonidine (Topical); Cannabis; Doxylamine; Dronabinol; Droperidol; HydrOXYzine; Ipratropium (Oral Inhalation); Kava Kava; Magnesium Sulfate; Methotrimeprazine; Mianserin; Nabilone; Perampanel; P-glycoprotein/ABCB1 Inhibitors; Pramlintide; Rufinamide; Sodium Oxybate; Tapentadol; Tetrahydrocannabinol; Umeclidinium

Decreased Effect

Cetirizine may decrease the levels/effects of: Acetylcholinesterase Inhibitors; Benzylpenicilloyl Polylysine; Betahistine; Hyaluronidase; Itopride; Secretin

The levels/effects of Cetirizine may be decreased by: Acetylcholinesterase Inhibitors; Amphetamines; P-glycoprotein/ABCB1 Inducers

Food Interactions Cetirizine's absorption and maximal concentration are reduced when taken with food. Management: May be taken without regard to meals.

Storage/Stability Store at 20°C to 25°C (68°F to 77°F); excursions are permitted between 15°C and 30°C (59°F and 86°F).

Mechanism of Action Competes with histamine for H_1-receptor sites on effector cells in the gastrointestinal tract, blood vessels, and respiratory tract

Pharmacodynamics/Kinetics

Onset of action: Suppression of skin wheal and flare: 0.7 hours (Simons, 1999)

Duration of action: Suppression of skin wheal and flare: ≥24 hours (Simons, 1999)

Absorption: Rapid

Distribution: 0.56 L/kg (Simons, 1999)

Protein binding, plasma: Mean: 93%

Metabolism: Limited hepatic

Half-life elimination: 8 hours

Time to peak, serum: 1 hour

Excretion: Urine (70%); feces (10%)

Dosage Upper respiratory allergies, urticaria: Oral:

Infants and Children:

6 to <12 months: 2.5 mg once daily

12 months to <2 years: 2.5 mg once daily; may increase to a maximum dose of 2.5 mg every 12 hours if needed

2 to 5 years: Initial: 2.5 mg once daily; may be increased to a maximum dose of 2.5 mg every 12 hours **or** 5 mg once daily

Children ≥6 years, Adolescents, and Adults: 5 to 10 mg once daily, depending upon symptom severity (maximum dose: 10 mg daily)

Elderly: 5 mg once daily (maximum dose: 5 mg daily)

Dosage adjustment in renal impairment: There are no dosage adjustments provided in the manufacturer's labeling; however, the following adjustments have been recommended (Aronoff, 2007):

Infants, Children, and Adolescents:

GFR ≥30 mL/minute/1.73 m^2: No dosage adjustment necessary.

GFR 10 to 29 mL/minute/1.73 m^2: Decrease dose by 50%.

GFR <10 mL/minute/1.73 m^2: Not recommended.

Intermittent hemodialysis or peritoneal dialysis: Decrease dose by 50%.

Adults:

GFR >50 mL/minute: No dosage adjustment necessary.

GFR ≤50 mL/minute: 5 mg once daily

Intermittent hemodialysis: 5 mg once daily; 5 mg 3 times per week may also be effective.

Peritoneal dialysis: 5 mg once daily.

Dosage adjustment in hepatic impairment: There are no dosage adjustments provided in the manufacturer's labeling.

Administration

May be administered with or without food.

Chewable tablet: Chew tablet before swallowing; may be taken with or without water.

Monitoring Parameters Relief of symptoms, sedation and anticholinergic effects

Dosage Forms

Capsule, Oral:

ZyrTEC Allergy [OTC]: 10 mg

Solution, Oral:

All Day Allergy Childrens [OTC]: 5 mg/5 mL (118 mL)

Cetirizine HCl Allergy Child [OTC]: 5 mg/5 mL (120 mL)

Cetirizine HCl Childrens [OTC]: 1 mg/mL (118 mL)

Cetirizine HCl Hives Relief [OTC]: 5 mg/5 mL (120 mL)

Generic: 1 mg/mL (120 mL, 473 mL)

Syrup, Oral:

Cetirizine HCl Childrens Alrgy [OTC]: 1 mg/mL (118 mL, 120 mL)

ZyrTEC Childrens Allergy [OTC]: 1 mg/mL (118 mL); 5 mg/5 mL (5 mL, 118 mL)

ZyrTEC Childrens Hives Relief [OTC]: 1 mg/mL (118 mL)

Generic: 1 mg/mL (120 mL, 473 mL, 480 mL); 5 mg/5 mL (5 mL, 120 mL)

Tablet, Oral:

All Day Allergy [OTC]: 10 mg

ZyrTEC Allergy [OTC]: 10 mg

ZyrTEC Hives Relief [OTC]: 10 mg

Generic: 5 mg, 10 mg

Tablet Chewable, Oral:

All Day Allergy Childrens [OTC]: 5 mg, 10 mg

ZyrTEC Childrens Allergy [OTC]: 5 mg, 10 mg

Generic: 5 mg, 10 mg

Tablet Dispersible, Oral:

ZyrTEC Allergy Childrens [OTC]: 10 mg

◆ **Cetirizine HCl Allergy Child [OTC]** *see* Cetirizine *on page 411*

◆ **Cetirizine HCl Childrens [OTC]** *see* Cetirizine *on page 411*

◆ **Cetirizine HCl Childrens Alrgy [OTC]** *see* Cetirizine *on page 411*

◆ **Cetirizine HCl Hives Relief [OTC]** *see* Cetirizine *on page 411*

◆ **Cetirizine Hydrochloride** *see* Cetirizine *on page 411*

◆ **Cetraxal** *see* Ciprofloxacin (Otic) *on page 446*

Cetrorelix (set roe REL iks)

Brand Names: U.S. Cetrotide

Brand Names: Canada Cetrotide®

Index Terms Cetrorelix Acetate

Pharmacologic Category Gonadotropin Releasing Hormone Antagonist

Use Inhibits premature luteinizing hormone (LH) surges in women undergoing controlled ovarian stimulation

Pregnancy Risk Factor X

Dosage

Adults: Females: SubQ: Used in conjunction with controlled ovarian stimulation therapy using gonadotropins (FSH, hMG):

Single-dose regimen: 3 mg given when serum estradiol levels show appropriate stimulation response, usually stimulation day 7 (range: days 5-9). If hCG is not administered within 4 days, continue cetrorelix at 0.25 mg/day until hCG is administered.

Multiple-dose regimen: 0.25 mg morning or evening of stimulation day 5, or morning of stimulation day 6; continue until hCG is administered.

Elderly: Not intended for use in women ≥65 years of age (Phase 2 and Phase 3 studies included women 19-40 years of age)

Dosing adjustment in renal impairment:

Severe impairment: Use is contraindicated

Mild-to-moderate impairment: No dosage adjustment provided in manufacturer's labeling.

Dosing adjustment in hepatic impairment: No dosage adjustment provided in manufacturer's labeling.

Additional Information Complete prescribing information should be consulted for additional detail.

Dosage Forms

Kit, Subcutaneous:

Cetrotide: 0.25 mg

◆ **Cetrorelix Acetate** *see* Cetrorelix *on page 413*

◆ **Cetrotide** *see* Cetrorelix *on page 413*

◆ **Cetrotide® (Can)** *see* Cetrorelix *on page 413*

Cetuximab (se TUK see mab)

Brand Names: U.S. Erbitux

Brand Names: Canada Erbitux

Index Terms C225; IMC-C225; MOAB C225

Pharmacologic Category Antineoplastic Agent, Epidermal Growth Factor Receptor (EGFR) Inhibitor; Antineoplastic Agent, Monoclonal Antibody

Use

Colorectal cancer, metastatic: Treatment of *KRAS* mutation-negative (wild-type), EGFR-expressing metastatic colorectal cancer (in combination with FOLFIRI [irinotecan, fluorouracil, and leucovorin] as first-line treatment, in combination with irinotecan [in patients refractory to irinotecan-based chemotherapy], or as a single agent in patients who have failed oxaliplatin and irinotecan based chemotherapy or who are intolerant to irinotecan).

Limitation of use: Cetuximab is not indicated for the treatment of KRAS mutation-positive colorectal cancer.

Head and neck cancer, squamous cell: Treatment of squamous cell cancer of the head and neck (as a single agent for recurrent or metastatic disease after platinum-based chemotherapy failure; in combination with radiation therapy as initial treatment of locally or regionally advanced disease; in combination with platinum and fluorouracil-based chemotherapy as first-line treatment of locoregional or metastatic disease).

Pregnancy Risk Factor C

Pregnancy Considerations Adverse events were observed in animal reproduction studies. Human IgG is known to cross the placenta. Because cetuximab inhibits epidermal growth factor (EGF), a component of fetal development, adverse effects on pregnancy would be expected. The manufacturer recommends that males and females use effective contraception during therapy and for 6 months following the last dose of cetuximab.

Breast-Feeding Considerations It is not known if cetuximab is excreted in breast milk. IgG antibodies can be detected in breast milk. Due to the potential for serious adverse reactions in the nursing infant, the manufacturer recommends that the decision to discontinue cetuximab or discontinue breast-feeding should take into account the benefits of treatment to the mother. If breast-feeding is interrupted for cetuximab treatment, based on the half-life, breast-feeding should not be resumed for at least 60 days following the last cetuximab dose.

Contraindications There are no contraindications listed in the manufacturer's U.S. product labeling.

Canadian labeling: Severe hypersensitivity to cetuximab or any component of the formulation

Warnings/Precautions **[U.S. Boxed Warning]: In clinical trials, serious infusion reactions have been reported in ~3% of patients; fatal outcome has been reported rarely (<1 in 1,000); interrupt infusion promptly and permanently discontinue for serious infusion reactions.** Reactions have included airway obstruction (bronchospasm, stridor, hoarseness), hypotension, loss of consciousness, shock, MI, and/or cardiac arrest. Premedicate with an IV H_1 antagonist 30-60 minutes prior to the first dose; premedication for subsequent doses is based on clinical judgement and with consideration of prior reaction to the initial infusion. The use of nebulized albuterol-based premedication to prevent infusion reaction has been reported (Tra, 2008). Approximately 90% of reactions occur with the first infusion despite the use of prophylactic antihistamines. Immediate treatment for anaphylactic/anaphylactoid reactions should be available during administration. The manufacturer recommends monitoring patients for at least 1 hour following completion of infusion, or longer if a reaction occurs. Mild-to-moderate infusion reactions are managed by slowing the infusion rate (by 50%) and administering antihistamines. Patients with preexisting IgE antibody against cetuximab (specific for galactose-α-1,3-galactose) are reported to have a higher incidence of severe hypersensitivity reaction. Severe hypersensitivity reaction has been reported more frequently in patients living in the middle south area of the United States, including North Carolina and Tennessee (Chung, 2008; O'Neil, 2007).

[U.S. Boxed Warning]: In patients with squamous cell head and neck cancer, cardiopulmonary arrest and/or sudden death has occurred in 2% of patients receiving radiation therapy in combination with cetuximab and in 3% of patients receiving combination chemotherapy (platinum and fluorouracil-based) with cetuximab. Closely monitor serum electrolytes (magnesium, potassium, calcium) during and after cetuximab treatment (monitor for at least 8 weeks after treatment). Use with caution in patients with history of coronary artery disease, HF, and arrhythmias; fatalities have been reported. Interstitial lung disease (ILD) has been reported;

use with caution in patients with preexisting lung disease; interrupt treatment for acute onset or worsening of pulmonary symptoms; permanently discontinue with confirmed ILD.

Acneiform rash has been reported in 76% to 88% of patients (severe in 1% to 17%), usually developing within the first 2 weeks of therapy; may require dose modification; generally resolved after discontinuation in most patients, although persisted beyond 28 days in some patients; monitor for dermatologic toxicity and corresponding infections. Acneiform rash should be treated with topical and/or oral antibiotics; topical corticosteroids are not recommended. In colorectal cancer, the presence of acneiform rash correlates with treatment response and prolonged survival (Cunningham, 2004). Other dermatologic toxicities, including dry skin, fissures, hypertrichosis, paronychial inflammation, and skin infections have been reported; related ocular toxicities (blepharitis, conjunctivitis, keratitis, ulcerative keratitis with decreased visual acuity) may also occur. Sunlight may exacerbate skin reactions (limit sun exposure). Hypomagnesemia is common (may be severe); the onset of electrolyte disturbance may occur within days to months after initiation of treatment; monitor magnesium, calcium, and potassium during treatment and for at least 8 weeks after completion; may require electrolyte replacement. Non-neutralizing anti-cetuximab antibodies were detected in 5% of evaluable patients. In a study of radiation therapy **and** cisplatin with or without cetuximab in patients with squamous cell head and neck cancer, an increase in the incidence of adverse reactions (eg, grade 3/4 mucositis, radiation recall, acneiform rash, electrolyte abnormalities, and cardiac events including ischemia) was noted in patients receiving cetuximab, including fatal reactions; there was no improvement in the primary endpoint of progression-free survival.

In patients with colorectal cancer, cetuximab is only indicated for EGFR-expressing, *KRAS* mutation-negative metastatic colorectal cancer. Determine *KRAS* mutation status prior to treatment (the therascreen KRAS RGQ PCR Kit is approved in the U.S. to determine *KRAS* gene mutation information). Patients with a codon 12 or 13 (exon 2) *KRAS* mutation are unlikely to benefit from EGFR inhibitor therapy and should not receive cetuximab treatment; cetuximab is not effective for *KRAS* mutation-positive colorectal cancer. Cetuximab is also reported to be ineffective in patients with *BRAF* V600E mutation (Di Nicolantonio, 2008). In trials for colorectal cancer, evidence of EGFR expression was required, although the response rate did not correlate with either the percentage of cells positive for EGFR or the intensity of expression. EGFR expression has been detected in nearly all patients with head and neck cancer, therefore laboratory evidence of EGFR expression is not necessary for head and neck cancers.

Adverse Reactions Except where noted, reactions reported for studies with cetuximab monotherapy.

Cardiovascular: Cardiorespiratory arrest (with radiation therapy)

Central nervous system: Anxiety, chills, confusion, depression, fatigue, headache, insomnia, pain, peripheral sensory neuropathy, taste disorder

Dermatologic: Acneiform eruption (all studies; onset: ≤14 days), nail disease, pruritus, skin rash (including desquamation), xeroderma

Endocrine & metabolic: Dehydration, hypomagnesemia (all studies)

Gastrointestinal: Abdominal pain, constipation, diarrhea, nausea, stomatitis, taste disturbance, vomiting, xerostomia

Immunologic: Antibody development

Infection: Infection (all studies), sepsis (all studies

Neuromuscular & skeletal: Arthralgia, ostealgia

Renal: Renal failure (all studies)

Respiratory: Cough, dyspnea

Miscellaneous: Fever, infusion related reaction (all studies; 90% of severe reactions occurred with first infusion)

Rare but important or life-threatening (all studies): Abscess, aseptic meningitis, blepharitis, cardiac arrest, cardiac arrhythmia, cellulitis, cheilitis, conjunctivitis, corneal ulcer, hypertrichosis, hypotension, interstitial pulmonary disease (occurred between the fourth and eleventh doses), keratitis, leukopenia, loss of consciousness, myocardial infarction, pulmonary embolism, radiodermatitis, shock, skin fissure, skin infection, stridor

Drug Interactions

Metabolism/Transport Effects None known.

Avoid Concomitant Use There are no known interactions where it is recommended to avoid concomitant use.

Increased Effect/Toxicity There are no known significant interactions involving an increase in effect.

Decreased Effect There are no known significant interactions involving a decrease in effect.

Preparation for Administration Reconstitution is not required. Appropriate dose should be added to empty sterile container (may contain a small amount of visible white, amorphous cetuximab particles); do not shake or dilute. Discard unused portion of the vial.

Storage/Stability Store intact vials refrigerated at 2°C to 8°C (36°F to 46°F); do not freeze. Preparations in infusion containers are stable for up to 12 hours refrigerated at 2°C to 8°C (36°F to 46°F) and up to 8 hours at room temperature of 20°C to 25°C (68°F to 77°F).

Mechanism of Action Recombinant human/mouse chimeric monoclonal antibody which binds specifically to the epidermal growth factor receptor (EGFR, HER1, c-ErbB-1) and competitively inhibits the binding of epidermal growth factor (EGF) and other ligands. Binding to the EGFR blocks phosphorylation and activation of receptor-associated kinases, resulting in inhibition of cell growth, induction of apoptosis, and decreased matrix metalloproteinase and vascular endothelial growth factor production. EGFR signal transduction results in *KRAS* wild-type activation; cells with *KRAS* mutations appear to be unaffected by EGFR inhibition.

Pharmacodynamics/Kinetics

Distribution: V_d: ~2 to 3 L/m^2

Half-life elimination: ~112 hours (range: 63 to 230 hours)

Dosage Note: Premedicate with an H_1 antagonist (eg, diphenhydramine 50 mg) IV 30 to 60 minutes prior to the first dose; premedication for subsequent doses is based on clinical judgement.

Colorectal cancer, metastatic, *KRAS* mutation-negative (wild-type): Adults: IV:

Initial loading dose: 400 mg/m^2 infused over 120 minutes

Maintenance dose: 250 mg/m^2 infused over 60 minutes weekly until disease progression or unacceptable toxicity

Note: If given in combination with FOLFIRI (irinotecan, fluorouracil, and leucovorin), complete cetuximab infusion 1 hour prior to FOLFIRI.

Head and neck cancer (squamous cell): Adults: IV:

Initial loading dose: 400 mg/m^2 infused over 120 minutes

Maintenance dose: 250 mg/m^2 infused over 60 minutes weekly

Note: If given in combination with radiation therapy, administer loading dose 1 week prior to initiation of radiation course; weekly maintenance dose should be completed 1 hour prior to radiation for the duration of radiation therapy (6 to 7 weeks). If given in combination with chemotherapy, administer loading dose on the day of initiation of platinum and fluorouracil-based chemotherapy, cetuximab infusion should be completed 1 hour prior to initiation of chemotherapy; weekly maintenance dose should be completed 1 hour prior to chemotherapy; continue until disease progression or unacceptable toxicity. Monotherapy weekly doses should be continued until disease progression or unacceptable toxicity.

Colorectal cancer, advanced, biweekly administration (off-label dosing): Adults: IV: 500 mg/m^2 every 2 weeks (initial dose infused over 120 minutes, subsequent doses infused over 60 minutes) in combination with irinotecan (Pfeiffer, 2008)

Non-small cell lung cancer (NSCLC), EGFR-expressing, advanced (off-label use): Adults: IV: Initial loading dose: 400 mg/m^2, followed by maintenance dose: 250 mg/m^2 weekly in combination with cisplatin and vinorelbine for up to 6 cycles, then as monotherapy until disease progression or unacceptable toxicity (Pirker, 2009; Pirker, 2012)

Squamous cell skin cancer, unresectable (off-label use): Adults: IV: Initial loading dose: 400 mg/m^2, followed by maintenance dose: 250 mg/m^2 weekly until disease progression (Maubec, 2011)

Dosage adjustment for toxicity:

Infusion reactions, grade 1 or 2 and nonserious grade 3: Reduce the infusion rate by 50% and continue to use prophylactic antihistamines

Infusion reactions, severe: Immediately and permanently discontinue treatment

Pulmonary toxicity:

Acute onset or worsening pulmonary symptoms: Hold treatment

Interstitial lung disease: Permanently discontinue

Skin toxicity, mild-to-moderate: No dosage modification required

Acneiform rash, severe (grade 3 or 4):

First occurrence: Delay cetuximab infusion 1 to 2 weeks

If improvement, continue at 250 mg/m^2

If no improvement, discontinue therapy

Second occurrence: Delay cetuximab infusion 1 to 2 weeks

If improvement, continue at reduced dose of 200 mg/m^2

If no improvement, discontinue therapy

Third occurrence: Delay cetuximab infusion 1 to 2 weeks

If improvement, continue at reduced dose of 150 mg/m^2

If no improvement, discontinue therapy

Fourth occurrence: Discontinue therapy

Note: Dose adjustments are not recommended for severe **radiation** dermatitis.

Dosage adjustment in renal impairment: There are no dosage adjustments provided in the manufacturer's labeling.

Dosage adjustment in hepatic impairment: There are no dosage adjustments provided in the manufacturer's labeling.

Administration Administer via IV infusion; loading dose over 2 hours, weekly maintenance dose over 1 hour. Do not administer as IV push or bolus. Do not shake or dilute. Administer via infusion pump or syringe pump. Following the infusion, an observation period (1 hour) is recommended; longer observation time (following an infusion reaction) may be required. Premedication with an H_1 antagonist prior to the initial dose is recommended. The maximum infusion rate is 10 mg/minute. Administer through a low protein-binding 0.22 micrometer in-line filter. Use 0.9% NaCl to flush line at the end of infusion.

For biweekly administration (off-label frequency and dose), the initial dose was infused over 120 minutes and subsequent doses infused over 60 minutes (Pfeiffer, 2007; Pfeiffer, 2008).

Monitoring Parameters Vital signs during infusion and observe for at least 1 hour postinfusion. Patients developing dermatologic toxicities should be monitored for the development of complications. Periodic monitoring of serum magnesium, calcium, and potassium are recommended to continue over an interval consistent with the half-life (8 weeks); monitor closely (during and after treatment) for cetuximab plus radiation therapy. *KRAS* genotyping of tumor tissue in patients with colorectal cancer (the therascreen *KRAS* RGQ PCR Kit is approved in the U.S. to determine *KRAS* gene mutation status [codon 12 or 13]).

Additional Information Oncology Comment: The American Society of Clinical Oncology (ASCO) provisional clinical opinion (Allegra, 2009) recommend genotyping tumor tissue for *KRAS* mutation in all patients with metastatic colorectal cancer (genotyping may be done on archived specimens). Patients with known codon 12 or 13 *KRAS* gene mutations are unlikely to respond to EGFR inhibitors and should not receive cetuximab. Favorable progression-free survival and overall survival has been demonstrated with cetuximab in patients with *KRAS* wild-type (Karapetis, 2008; Van Cutsem, 2008). Cetuximab is also reported to be ineffective in patients with *BRAF* V600E mutation (Di Nicolantonio, 2008). Dermatologic toxicity with cetuximab is predictive for response; the presence of acneiform rash correlates with treatment response and prolonged survival (Cunningham, 2004).

Dosage Forms

Solution, Intravenous [preservative free]:

Erbitux: 100 mg/50 mL (50 mL); 200 mg/100 mL (100 mL)

Cetylpyridinium and Benzocaine [CAN/INT] (SEE til peer i DI nee um & BEN zoe kane)

Brand Names: Canada Cepacol®; Kank-A®

Index Terms Benzocaine and Cetylpyridinium; Benzocaine and Cetylpyridinium Chloride; Cetylpyridinium Chloride and Benzocaine

Pharmacologic Category Local Anesthetic

Use Note: Not approved in U.S.

Symptomatic relief of sore throat

Drug Interactions

Metabolism/Transport Effects None known.

Avoid Concomitant Use There are no known interactions where it is recommended to avoid concomitant use.

Increased Effect/Toxicity

Cetylpyridinium and Benzocaine may increase the levels/effects of: Prilocaine; Sodium Nitrite

The levels/effects of Cetylpyridinium and Benzocaine may be increased by: Nitric Oxide

Decreased Effect There are no known significant interactions involving a decrease in effect.

Dosage Antiseptic/anesthetic: Oral: Dissolve in mouth as needed for sore throat

Product Availability Not available in U.S.

Dosage Forms: Canada Excipient information presented when available (limited, particularly for generics); consult specific product labeling.

◆ **Cetylpyridinium Chloride and Benzocaine** *see* Cetylpyridinium and Benzocaine [CAN/INT] *on page 415*

Cevimeline (se vi ME leen)

Brand Names: U.S. Evoxac

Brand Names: Canada Evoxac®

Index Terms Cevimeline Hydrochloride

Pharmacologic Category Cholinergic Agonist

Use Treatment of symptoms of dry mouth in patients with Sjögren's syndrome

Pregnancy Risk Factor C

Dosage Oral:

Adults: 30 mg 3 times/day

Elderly: No specific dosage adjustment is recommended; however, use caution when initiating due to potential for increased sensitivity

Dosage adjustment in renal impairment: No dosage adjustment provided in the manufacturer's labeling.

Dosage adjustment in hepatic impairment: No dosage adjustment provided in the manufacturer's labeling.

Additional Information Complete prescribing information should be consulted for additional detail.

Dosage Forms

Capsule, Oral:

Evoxac: 30 mg

Generic: 30 mg

- ◆ **Cevimeline Hydrochloride** *see* Cevimeline *on page 415*
- ◆ **CFDN** *see* Cefdinir *on page 376*
- ◆ **CG** *see* Chorionic Gonadotropin (Human) *on page 431*
- ◆ **CG5503** *see* Tapentadol *on page 1975*
- ◆ **CGP 33101** *see* Rufinamide *on page 1854*
- ◆ **CGP-39393** *see* Desirudin *on page 593*
- ◆ **CGP-42446** *see* Zoledronic Acid *on page 2206*
- ◆ **CGP-57148B** *see* Imatinib *on page 1047*
- ◆ **CGS-20267** *see* Letrozole *on page 1181*
- ◆ **CGX-625** *see* Omacetaxine *on page 1501*
- ◆ **Champix® (Can)** *see* Varenicline *on page 2139*
- ◆ **Chantix** *see* Varenicline *on page 2139*
- ◆ **Chantix Continuing Month Pak** *see* Varenicline *on page 2139*
- ◆ **Chantix Starting Month Pak** *see* Varenicline *on page 2139*
- ◆ **Charac-25 [OTC] (Can)** *see* Charcoal, Activated *on page 416*
- ◆ **Charac-50 [OTC] (Can)** *see* Charcoal, Activated *on page 416*
- ◆ **Charactol-25 [OTC] (Can)** *see* Charcoal, Activated *on page 416*
- ◆ **Charactol-50 [OTC] (Can)** *see* Charcoal, Activated *on page 416*

Charcoal, Activated (CHAR kole AK tiv ay ted)

Brand Names: U.S. Actidose-Aqua [OTC]; Actidose/Sorbitol [OTC]; Char-Flo with Sorbitol [OTC]; EZ Char [OTC]; Kerr Insta-Char in Sorbitol [OTC]; Kerr Insta-Char [OTC]

Brand Names: Canada Charac-25 [OTC]; Charac-50 [OTC]; Charactol-25 [OTC]; Charactol-50 [OTC]; Charcodote Susp [OTC]; Charcodote TFS [OTC]; Charcodote-Aqueous Sus; Premium Activated Charcoal [OTC]

Index Terms Activated Carbon; Activated Charcoal; Adsorbent Charcoal; Liquid Antidote; Medicinal Carbon; Medicinal Charcoal

Pharmacologic Category Antidote

Use

Suspension: Activated charcoal is a nonabsorbable adsorbent that may be considered in the management of poisonings when gastrointestinal decontamination of drugs or chemicals is indicated (eg, presentation to a treatment facility within 1 hour of ingestion). Activated charcoal is generally an effective adsorbent of drugs and chemicals with a molecular weight range of 100-1000 daltons. Multidose activated charcoal may be considered if a patient has ingested a life-threatening amount of carbamazepine, dapsone, phenobarbital, quinine, or theophylline (Vale, 1999).

Capsules, tablets: Digestive aid

Pregnancy Considerations Activated charcoal is not absorbed systemically following oral administration. Systemic absorption would be required in order for activated charcoal to cross the placenta and reach the fetus. In general, medications used as antidotes should take into consideration the health and prognosis of the mother; antidotes should be administered to pregnant women if there is a clear indication for use and should not be withheld because of fears of teratogenicity (Bailey, 2003).

Breast-Feeding Considerations Activated charcoal is not absorbed systemically following oral administration.

Contraindications There are no absolute contraindications listed within the manufacturer's labeling.

Note: The American Academy of Clinical Toxicology (AACT) and European Association of Poisons Centres and Clinical Toxicologists (EAPCCT) consider the following to be contraindications to the use of charcoal (Chyka, 2005; Vale, 1999): Presence of intestinal obstruction or GI tract not anatomically intact; patients at risk of GI hemorrhage or perforation; patients with an unprotected airway (eg, CNS depression without intubation); if use would increase the risk and severity of aspiration

Warnings/Precautions Charcoal may cause vomiting; the risk appears to be greater when charcoal is administered with sorbitol (Chyka, 2005). IV antiemetics may be required to reduce the risk of vomiting or to control vomiting to facilitate administration (Vale, 1999). Due to the risk of vomiting, avoid the use of charcoal in hydrocarbon and caustic ingestions. Use caution with decreased peristalsis. Some products may contain sorbitol. Coadministration of a cathartic is **not** recommended; cathartics (eg, sorbitol, mannitol, magnesium sulfate) have not been demonstrated to change patient outcome and have no role in the management of the poisoned patient. Cathartics subject the patient to the risk of developing significant fluid and electrolyte abnormalities (AACT, 2004a). Do not use products containing sorbitol in persons with a genetic intolerance to fructose or in patients who are dehydrated; may cause excessive diarrhea. Ipecac should not be administered routinely in the management of poisoned patients (AACT, 2004b).

Not effective in the treatment of poisonings due to the ingestion of low molecular weight compounds such as cyanide, iron, ethanol, methanol, or lithium. Most effective when administered within 30-60 minutes of ingestion. Based on experimental and clinical studies, multidose activated charcoal, in most acute poisonings, has not been shown to reduce morbidity or mortality (Vale, 1999). It may be considered if a patient has ingested a life-threatening amount of carbamazepine, dapsone, phenobarbital, quinine, or theophylline, although no controlled studies have demonstrated clinical benefit.

Benzyl alcohol and derivatives: Some dosage forms may contain sodium benzoate/benzoic acid; benzoic acid (benzoate) is a metabolite of benzyl alcohol; large amounts of benzyl alcohol (≥99 mg/kg/day) have been associated with a potentially fatal toxicity ("gasping syndrome") in neonates; the "gasping syndrome" consists of metabolic acidosis, respiratory distress, gasping respirations, CNS dysfunction (including convulsions, intracranial hemorrhage), hypotension, and cardiovascular collapse (AAP, 1997; CDC, 1982); some data suggests that benzoate displaces bilirubin from protein binding sites (Ahlfors, 2001); avoid or use dosage forms containing benzyl alcohol derivative with caution in neonates. See manufacturer's labeling.

Some dosage forms may contain propylene glycol; large amounts are potentially toxic and have been associated hyperosmolality, lactic acidosis, seizures and respiratory depression; use caution (AAP, 1997; Zar, 2007). Capsules and tablets should not be used for the treatment of poisoning.

Adverse Reactions

Gastrointestinal: Abdominal distention, appendicitis, bowel obstruction, constipation, vomiting

Ocular: Corneal abrasion (with direct contact)

Respiratory: Aspiration, respiratory failure

Miscellaneous: Fecal discoloration (black)

Drug Interactions

Metabolism/Transport Effects None known.

Avoid Concomitant Use There are no known interactions where it is recommended to avoid concomitant use.

Increased Effect/Toxicity There are no known significant interactions involving an increase in effect.

Decreased Effect

Charcoal, Activated may decrease the levels/effects of: Leflunomide; Teriflunomide

Food Interactions The addition of some flavoring agents (eg, milk, ice cream, sherbet, marmalade) are known to reduce the adsorptive capacity, and therefore the efficacy, of activated charcoal and should be avoided in preference to activated charcoal-water slurries; nevertheless, these flavoring agents do not completely compromise the effectiveness of activated charcoal and may be necessary in some circumstances (eg, administration in pediatric patients) to enhance compliance (Cooney, 1995; Dagnone, 2002).

Preparation for Administration Powder: Dilute with at least 8 mL of water per 1 g of charcoal, or mix in a charcoal to water ratio of 1:4 to 1:8; mix to form a slurry (eg, mix 25 g with sufficient tap water to create a 4-ounce slurry or mix 50 g with sufficient tap water to create an 8-ounce slurry).

Storage/Stability Adsorbs gases from air, store in a closed container.

Mechanism of Action Adsorbs toxic substances, thus inhibiting GI absorption

Pharmacodynamics/Kinetics Excretion: Feces (as charcoal)

Dosage Oral, NG: **Note:** Some products may contain sorbitol; coadministration of a cathartic, including sorbitol, is **not** recommended. Some clinicians still recommend dosing activated charcoal in a 10:1 (charcoal:poison) ratio for optimal efficacy (Gude, 2009); however, the amount of poison ingested is commonly unknown, which makes this approach challenging and often impractical (Chyka, 2005).

Single dose (Chyka, 2005):

Infants <1 year: 10-25 g; **Note:** Although dosing by body weight is reported in children (0.5-1 g/kg) and published in many resources, there are no data or scientific rationale to support this recommendation.

Children 1-12 years: 25-50 g

Children >12 years and Adults: 25-100 g

Multidose:

Children: Initial dose: 25-50 g followed by multiple doses of 10-25 g every 4 hours

Adults: Initial dose: 50-100 g followed by 25-50 g every 4 hours

Administration Flavoring agents (eg, chocolate, concentrated fruit juice) or thickening agents (eg, bentonite, carboxymethylcellulose) can enhance charcoal's palatability. Check for presence of bowel sounds before administration. IV antiemetics may be required to reduce the risk of vomiting. The activated charcoal container should be agitated thoroughly before administration. The container should be rinsed with a small quantity of water to insure that the patient has received all of the activated charcoal (Krenzelok, 1991).

Capsules and tablets should not be used for the treatment of poisoning.

Dosage Forms

Liquid, Oral:

Actidose-Aqua [OTC]: 15 g/72 mL (72 mL); 25 g/120 mL (120 mL); 50 g/240 mL (240 mL)

Actidose/Sorbitol [OTC]: 25 g/120 mL (120 mL); 50 g/240 mL (240 mL)

Kerr Insta-Char [OTC]: 25 g/120 mL (120 mL); 50 g/240 mL (240 mL)

Kerr Insta-Char in Sorbitol [OTC]: 25 g/120 mL (120 mL); 50 g/240 mL (240 mL)

Suspension, Oral:

Char-Flo with Sorbitol [OTC]: 25 g (120 mL)

Suspension Reconstituted, Oral:

EZ Char [OTC]: 25 g (1 ea)

- ◆ **Charcodote-Aqueous Sus (Can)** *see* Charcoal, Activated *on page 416*
- ◆ **Charcodote Susp [OTC] (Can)** *see* Charcoal, Activated *on page 416*
- ◆ **Charcodote TFS [OTC] (Can)** *see* Charcoal, Activated *on page 416*
- ◆ **Char-Flo with Sorbitol [OTC]** *see* Charcoal, Activated *on page 416*
- ◆ **Chateal** *see* Ethinyl Estradiol and Levonorgestrel *on page 803*
- ◆ **Chemet** *see* Succimer *on page 1939*
- ◆ **Chenodal** *see* Chenodiol *on page 417*
- ◆ **Chenodeoxycholic Acid** *see* Chenodiol *on page 417*

Chenodiol (kee noe DYE ole)

Brand Names: U.S. Chenodal

Index Terms CDCA; Chenodeoxycholic Acid

Pharmacologic Category Bile Acid

Use Oral dissolution of radiolucent cholesterol gallstones in selected patients as an alternative to surgery

Pregnancy Risk Factor X

Dosage Oral:

Cerebrotendinous xanthomatosis (off-label use): Adults: 750 mg daily in 3 divided doses (Beringer, 1984)

Gallstone dissolution (monotherapy): Adults: Initial: 250 mg twice daily for the first 2 weeks and increasing by 250 mg daily each week thereafter until the recommended or maximum tolerated dose is achieved; maintenance: 13-16 mg/kg/day in 2 divided doses. **Note:** Dosages <10 mg/kg are usually ineffective and may increase the risk of cholecystectomy.

Gallstone dissolution (combination therapy; off-label dose): Adults: 5-7.5 mg/kg/day once daily at bedtime, in combination with ursodeoxycholic acid, with or without adjuvant lithotripsy (Jazrawi, 1992; Pereira, 1997; Petroni, 2001)

Dosage adjustment in renal impairment: No dosage adjustment provided in manufacturer's labeling.

Dosage adjustment in hepatic impairment: Use extreme caution; contraindicated for use in presence of known hepatocyte dysfunction or bile duct abnormalities

Additional Information Complete prescribing information should be consulted for additional detail.

Dosage Forms

Tablet, Oral:

Chenodal: 250 mg

- ◆ **Cheracol D [OTC]** *see* Guaifenesin and Dextromethorphan *on page 987*
- ◆ **Cheracol Plus [OTC]** *see* Guaifenesin and Dextromethorphan *on page 987*
- ◆ **Cheratussin** *see* GuaiFENesin *on page 986*

◆ **Cheratussin® DAC** *see* Guaifenesin, Pseudoephedrine, and Codeine *on page 989*

◆ **Chew-C [OTC]** *see* Ascorbic Acid *on page 178*

◆ **Chew-Cal [OTC]** *see* Calcium and Vitamin D *on page 326*

◆ **CHG** *see* Chlorhexidine Gluconate *on page 422*

◆ **Chickenpox Vaccine** *see* Varicella Virus Vaccine *on page 2141*

◆ **Chiggerex [OTC]** *see* Benzocaine *on page 246*

◆ **Chiggertox [OTC]** *see* Benzocaine *on page 246*

◆ **Childrens Advil [OTC]** *see* Ibuprofen *on page 1032*

◆ **Children's Advil® Cold (Can)** *see* Pseudoephedrine and Ibuprofen *on page 1743*

◆ **Childrens Ibuprofen [OTC]** *see* Ibuprofen *on page 1032*

◆ **Childrens Loratadine [OTC]** *see* Loratadine *on page 1241*

◆ **Childrens Motrin [OTC]** *see* Ibuprofen *on page 1032*

◆ **Childrens Motrin Jr Strength [OTC]** *see* Ibuprofen *on page 1032*

◆ **Childrens Silfedrine [OTC]** *see* Pseudoephedrine *on page 1742*

◆ **Children's Advil (Can)** *see* Ibuprofen *on page 1032*

◆ **Children's Europrofen (Can)** *see* Ibuprofen *on page 1032*

◆ **Children's Motion Sickness Liquid [OTC] (Can)** *see* DimenhyDRINATE *on page 637*

◆ **Chloditan** *see* Mitotane *on page 1382*

◆ **Chlodithane** *see* Mitotane *on page 1382*

◆ **Chloral** *see* Chloral Hydrate [CAN/INT] *on page 418*

Chloral Hydrate [CAN/INT] (KLOR al HYE drate)

Brand Names: Canada PMS-Chloral Hydrate

Index Terms Chloral; Hydrated Chloral; Trichloroacetaldehyde Monohydrate

Pharmacologic Category Hypnotic, Miscellaneous

Additional Appendix Information

Beers Criteria – Potentially Inappropriate Medications for Geriatrics *on page 2271*

Use Note: Not approved in U.S.

Pain control: Adjunct to opiates and analgesics for postoperative pain control

Sedation: Short-term sedative and hypnotic (<2 weeks); sedative/hypnotic for diagnostic procedures; sedative prior to EEG evaluations

Withdrawal: Monotherapy or concomitant with paraldehyde for prevention of alcohol withdrawal symptoms and/or to suppress syndrome once it develops; reduction of anxiety associated with withdrawal of opiates or barbiturates

Pregnancy Considerations Animal reproduction studies have not been conducted. Chloral hydrate crosses the placenta, and long-term use may lead to withdrawal symptoms in the neonate.

Breast-Feeding Considerations Chloral hydrate is excreted in breast milk; use by breast-feeding women may cause sedation in the infant.

Contraindications Hypersensitivity to chloral hydrate or any component of the formulation; marked hepatic or renal impairment

Warnings/Precautions May cause CNS depression, which may impair physical or mental abilities; patients must be cautioned about performing tasks that require mental alertness (eg, operating machinery or driving). Effects may be potentiated when used with other sedative drugs or ethanol. Use with caution in patients with porphyria, cardiac disease, gastrointestinal disease, or respiratory disorders. Excessive sedation or other adverse effects may be more likely to occur in elderly patients; dose reduction may be necessary. Life-threatening respiratory obstruction and deaths have been reported with use in children; use with extreme caution. Use with caution in neonates; prolonged use in neonates is associated with direct hyperbilirubinemia (active metabolite [TCE] competes with bilirubin for glucuronide conjugation in the liver). Tolerance to hypnotic effect develops; therefore, not recommended for use >2 weeks. Taper dosage to avoid withdrawal with prolonged use. Health care provider should be alert to problems of abuse and misuse. Patients should be assessed for risk of abuse or addiction prior to therapy and all patients should be monitored for signs of abuse or misuse.

Benzyl alcohol and derivatives: Some dosage forms may contain sodium benzoate/benzoic acid; benzoic acid (benzoate) is a metabolite of benzyl alcohol; large amounts of benzyl alcohol (≥99 mg/kg/day) have been associated with a potentially fatal toxicity ("gasping syndrome") in neonates; the "gasping syndrome" consists of metabolic acidosis, respiratory distress, gasping respirations, CNS dysfunction (including convulsions, intracranial hemorrhage), hypotension, and cardiovascular collapse (AAP, 1997; CDC, 1982); some data suggests that benzoate displaces bilirubin from protein binding sites (Ahlfors, 2001); avoid or use dosage forms containing benzyl alcohol derivative with caution in neonates. See manufacturer's labeling.

Adverse Reactions

Cardiovascular: Atrial arrhythmia, depression of myocardial contractility, hypotension, shortening of refractory periods, torsades de pointes, ventricular arrhythmia

Central nervous system: Abnormal gait, ataxia, confusion, delirium, dizziness, drowsiness, drug dependence (physical and psychological; with prolonged use or large doses), hallucinations, hangover effect, malaise, nightmares, paradoxical excitation, somnambulism, vertigo

Dermatologic: Skin rash (including erythema, eczematoid dermatitis, urticaria, scarlatiniform exanthems)

Endocrine & metabolic: Acute porphyria, ketonuria

Gastrointestinal: Diarrhea, flatulence, gastric irritation, nausea, vomiting

Hematologic & oncologic: Acute porphyria, eosinophilia, leukopenia

Ophthalmic: Allergic conjunctivitis, blepharoptosis, keratoconjunctivitis

Otic: Increased middle ear pressure (infants and children)

Respiratory: Airway obstruction (young children), laryngeal edema (children)

Miscellaneous: Drug tolerance

Drug Interactions

Metabolism/Transport Effects None known.

Avoid Concomitant Use

Avoid concomitant use of Chloral Hydrate with any of the following: Azelastine (Nasal); Furosemide; Orphenadrine; Paraldehyde; Sodium Oxybate; Thalidomide

Increased Effect/Toxicity

Chloral Hydrate may increase the levels/effects of: Alcohol (Ethyl); Azelastine (Nasal); Buprenorphine; CNS Depressants; Highest Risk QTc-Prolonging Agents; Hydrocodone; Methotrimeprazine; Metyrosine; Mirtazapine; Moderate Risk QTc-Prolonging Agents; Orphenadrine; Paraldehyde; Pramipexole; ROPINIRole; Rotigotine; Selective Serotonin Reuptake Inhibitors; Sodium Oxybate; Suvorexant; Thalidomide; Vitamin K Antagonists; Zolpidem

The levels/effects of Chloral Hydrate may be increased by: Brimonidine (Topical); Cannabis; Doxylamine; Dronabinol; Droperidol; Furosemide; HydrOXYzine; Kava Kava; Magnesium Sulfate; Methotrimeprazine; Mifepristone; Nabilone; Perampanel; Rufinamide; Tapentadol; Tetrahydrocannabinol

Decreased Effect

The levels/effects of Chloral Hydrate may be decreased by: Flumazenil

Storage/Stability Store syrup and capsules at controlled room temperature. Store syrup in a light-resistant, airtight container; protect from freezing.

Mechanism of Action Central nervous system depressant effects are due to its active metabolite trichloroethanol, mechanism unknown

Pharmacodynamics/Kinetics

Onset of action: Time to sleep: 0.5-1 hour

Duration: 4-8 hours

Absorption: Oral: Well absorbed

Metabolism: Rapidly hepatic to trichloroethanol (active metabolite); variable amounts hepatically and renally to trichloroacetic acid (inactive)

Half-life elimination: Active metabolite: 8-10 hours

Excretion: Urine (as metabolites); feces (small amounts)

Dosage

Children: Oral:

Hypnotic: 50 mg/kg/day in 1 or more divided doses; maximum single dose: 1000 mg

Sedation or anxiety: 25 mg/kg/day in 1 or more divided doses; maximum single dose: 500 mg

Procedural sedation: 25-50 mg/kg/dose 30 minutes prior to procedure; may repeat in 30 minutes using half the dose

Adults: Oral:

Sedation, anxiety: 250 mg 3 times daily

Hypnotic: 500-1000 mg 15-30 minutes before bedtime or 30 minutes prior to procedure, not to exceed 2000 mg per 24 hours

Elderly: Oral: Hypnotic: Usual dose: 250 mg 15-30 minutes before bedtime

Dosage adjustment/comments in renal impairment: Contraindicated in patients with marked renal impairment.

Dosage adjustment/comments in hepatic impairment: Contraindicated in patients with marked hepatic impairment.

Administration May dilute syrup in water or other oral liquid (eg, fruit juice or ginger ale) to minimize gastric irritation. Administer capsules after meals (when used as sedative).

Monitoring Parameters Vital signs, O_2 saturation and blood pressure with doses used for conscious sedation

Additional Information Not an analgesic

Product Availability Not available in U.S.

Dosage Forms: Canada

Capsule, Oral: 500 mg

Syrup, Oral: 100 mg/mL

Chlorambucil (klor AM byoo sil)

Brand Names: U.S. Leukeran

Brand Names: Canada Leukeran®

Index Terms CB-1348; Chlorambucilum; Chloraminophene; Chlorbutinum; WR-139013

Pharmacologic Category Antineoplastic Agent, Alkylating Agent; Antineoplastic Agent, Alkylating Agent (Nitrogen Mustard)

Use

Chronic lymphocytic leukemia (CLL): Management of CLL

Lymphomas: Management of Hodgkin lymphoma and non-Hodgkin lymphomas (NHL)

Canadian labeling: Additional uses (not in U.S. labeling): Management of Waldenström's macroglobulinemia

Pregnancy Risk Factor D

Pregnancy Considerations Animal reproduction studies have demonstrated teratogenicity. Chlorambucil crosses the human placenta. Following exposure during the first trimester, case reports have noted adverse renal effects (unilateral agenesis). Women of childbearing potential should avoid becoming pregnant while receiving treatment. **[U.S. Boxed Warning]: Affects human fertility; probably mutagenic and teratogenic as well**; chromosomal damage has been documented. Reversible and irreversible sterility (when administered to prepubertal and pubertal males), azoospermia (in adult males) and amenorrhea (in females) have been observed. Fibrosis, vasculitis and depletion of primordial follicles have been noted on autopsy of the ovaries.

Breast-Feeding Considerations It is not known if chlorambucil is excreted in breast milk. Due to the potential for serious adverse reactions in the nursing infant, the decision to discontinue chlorambucil or to discontinue breastfeeding should take into account the benefits of treatment to the mother.

Contraindications Hypersensitivity to chlorambucil or any component of the formulation; hypersensitivity to other alkylating agents (may have cross-hypersensitivity); prior (demonstrated) resistance to chlorambucil

Canadian labeling: Additional contraindications (not in U.S. labeling): Use within 4 weeks of a full course of radiation or chemotherapy

Warnings/Precautions Hazardous agent - use appropriate precautions for handling and disposal (NIOSH 2014 [group 1]). Seizures have been observed; use with caution in patients with seizure disorder or head trauma; history of nephrotic syndrome and high pulse doses are at higher risk of seizures. **[U.S. Boxed Warning]: May cause severe bone marrow suppression;** neutropenia may be severe. Reduce initial dosage if patient has received myelosuppressive or radiation therapy within the previous 4 weeks, or has a depressed baseline leukocyte or platelet count. Irreversible bone marrow damage may occur with total doses approaching 6.5 mg/kg. Progressive lymphopenia may develop (recovery is generally rapid after discontinuation). Avoid administration of live vaccines to immunocompromised patients. Rare instances of severe skin reactions (eg, erythema multiforme, Stevens-Johnson syndrome, toxic epidermal necrolysis) have been reported; discontinue promptly if skin reaction occurs.

Chlorambucil is primarily metabolized in the liver. Dosage reductions should be considered in patients with hepatic impairment. **[U.S. Boxed Warning]: Affects human fertility; carcinogenic in humans and probably mutagenic and teratogenic as well;** chromosomal damage has been documented. Reversible and irreversible sterility (when administered to prepubertal and pubertal males), azoospermia (in adult males) and amenorrhea (in females) have been observed. **[U.S. Boxed Warning]: Carcinogenic;** acute myelocytic leukemia and secondary malignancies may be associated with chronic therapy. Duration of treatment and higher cumulative doses are associated with a higher risk for development of leukemia. Potentially significant drug-drug interactions may exist, requiring dose or frequency adjustment, additional monitoring, and/or selection of alternative therapy.

Adverse Reactions

Central nervous system: Agitation (rare), ataxia (rare), confusion (rare), drug fever, fever, focal/generalized seizure (rare), hallucinations (rare)

Dermatologic: Angioneurotic edema, erythema multiforme (rare), rash, skin hypersensitivity, Stevens-Johnson syndrome (rare), toxic epidermal necrolysis (rare), urticaria
Endocrine & metabolic: Amenorrhea, infertility, SIADH (rare)
Gastrointestinal: Diarrhea (infrequent), nausea (infrequent), oral ulceration (infrequent), vomiting (infrequent)
Genitourinary: Azoospermia, cystitis (sterile)
Hematologic: Neutropenia (onset: 3 weeks; recovery: 10 days after last dose), bone marrow failure (irreversible), bone marrow suppression, anemia, leukemia (secondary), leukopenia, lymphopenia, pancytopenia, thrombocytopenia
Hepatic: Hepatotoxicity, jaundice
Neuromuscular & skeletal: Flaccid paresis (rare), muscular twitching (rare), myoclonia (rare), peripheral neuropathy, tremor (rare)
Respiratory: Interstitial pneumonia, pulmonary fibrosis
Miscellaneous: Allergic reactions, malignancies (secondary)

Drug Interactions

Metabolism/Transport Effects None known.

Avoid Concomitant Use

Avoid concomitant use of Chlorambucil with any of the following: BCG; CloZAPine; Dipyrone; Natalizumab; Pimecrolimus; Tacrolimus (Topical); Tofacitinib; Vaccines (Live)

Increased Effect/Toxicity

Chlorambucil may increase the levels/effects of: CloZAPine; Leflunomide; Natalizumab; Tofacitinib; Vaccines (Live)

The levels/effects of Chlorambucil may be increased by: Denosumab; Dipyrone; Pimecrolimus; Roflumilast; Tacrolimus (Topical); Trastuzumab

Decreased Effect

Chlorambucil may decrease the levels/effects of: BCG; Coccidioides immitis Skin Test; Sipuleucel-T; Vaccines (Inactivated); Vaccines (Live)

The levels/effects of Chlorambucil may be decreased by: Echinacea

Food Interactions Absorption is decreased when administered with food. Management: Administer preferably on an empty stomach.

Storage/Stability Store in refrigerator at 2°C to 8°C (36°F to 46°F).

Mechanism of Action Alkylating agent; interferes with DNA replication and RNA transcription by alkylation and cross-linking the strands of DNA

Pharmacodynamics/Kinetics

Absorption: Rapid and complete (>70%); reduced with food
Distribution: V_d: ~0.3 L/kg
Protein binding: ~99%; primarily to albumin
Metabolism: Hepatic (extensively); primarily to active metabolite, phenylacetic acid mustard
Half-life elimination: ~1.5 hours; Phenylacetic acid mustard: ~1.8 hours
Time to peak, plasma: Within 1 hour; Phenylacetic acid mustard: 1.2-2.6 hours
Excretion: Urine (~20% to 60%, primarily as inactive metabolites, <1% as unchanged drug or phenylacetic acid mustard)

Dosage

Children: Nephrotic syndrome, steroid sensitive (off-label use): Oral: 0.2 mg/kg once daily for 8 weeks (Hodson, 2010)

Adults: **Note:** With bone marrow lymphocytic infiltration involvement (in CLL, Hodgkin lymphoma, or NHL), the maximum dose is 0.1 mg/kg/day. While short treatment courses are preferred, if maintenance therapy is required, the maximum dose is 0.1 mg/kg/day.

Chronic lymphocytic leukemia (CLL): Oral:

U.S. labeling: 0.1 mg/kg/day for 3-6 weeks **or** 0.4 mg/kg pulsed doses administered intermittently, biweekly, or monthly (increased by 0.1 mg/kg/dose until response/toxicity observed)

Canadian labeling: Initial: 0.15 mg/kg/day until WBC is 10,000/mm^3; interrupt treatment for 4 weeks, then may resume at 0.1 mg/kg/day until response (generally ~2 years)/toxicity observed

Off-label dosing for CLL: 0.4 mg/kg day 1 every 2 weeks; if tolerated may increase by 0.1 mg/kg with each treatment course to a maximum dose of 0.8 mg/kg and maximum of 24 cycles (Eichhorst, 2009) **or** 30 mg/m^2 day 1 every 2 weeks (in combination with prednisone) (Raphael, 1991) **or** 40 mg/m^2 day 1 every 4 weeks until disease progression or complete remission or response plateau for up to a maximum of 12 cycles (Rai, 2000)

Hodgkin lymphoma: Oral:

U.S. labeling: 0.2 mg/kg/day for 3-6 weeks

Canadian labeling: 0.2 mg/kg/day for 4-8 weeks

Non-Hodgkin lymphomas (NHL): Oral:

U.S. labeling: 0.1 mg/kg/day for 3-6 weeks

Canadian labeling: Initial: 0.1-0.2 mg/kg/day for 4-8 weeks; for maintenance treatment, reduce dose or administer intermittently

Waldenström's macroglobulinemia (U.S. off-label use): Oral: 0.1 mg/kg/day (continuously) for at least 6 months **or** 0.3 mg/kg/day for 7 days every 6 weeks for at least 6 months (Kyle, 2000)

Elderly: Refer to adult dosing; begin at the lower end of dosing range(s)

Dosage adjustment for toxicity:

Skin reactions: Discontinue treatment
Hematologic:
WBC or platelets below normal: Reduce dose
Severely depressed WBC or platelet counts: Discontinue
Persistently low neutrophil or platelet counts or peripheral lymphocytosis: May be suggestive of bone marrow infiltration; if infiltration confirmed, do not exceed 0.1 mg/kg/day.
Concurrent or within 4 weeks (before or after) of chemotherapy/radiotherapy: Initiate treatment cautiously; reduce dose; monitor closely.

Dosage adjustment in renal impairment: No dosage adjustment provided in manufacturer's labeling; however, renal elimination of unchanged chlorambucil and active metabolite (phenylacetic acid mustard) is minimal and renal impairment is not likely to affect elimination. The following adjustments have been recommended: Adults: Aronoff, 2007:

CrCl >50 mL/minute: No adjustment necessary
CrCl 10-50 mL/minute: Administer 75% of dose
CrCl <10 mL/minute: Administer 50% of dose
Peritoneal dialysis (PD): Administer 50% of dose

Kintzel, 1995: Based on the pharmacokinetics, dosage adjustment is not indicated

Dosage adjustment in hepatic impairment: Chlorambucil undergoes extensive hepatic metabolism. Although dosage reduction should be considered in patients with hepatic impairment, no dosage adjustment is provided in the manufacturer's labeling (data is insufficient).

Dosing in obesity: *ASCO Guidelines for appropriate chemotherapy dosing in obese adults with cancer:* Utilize patient's actual body weight (full weight) for calculation of body surface area- or weight-based dosing, particularly when the intent of therapy is curative; manage regimen-related toxicities in the same manner as for nonobese patients; if a dose reduction is utilized due to toxicity, consider resumption of full weight-based dosing with subsequent cycles, especially if cause of toxicity (eg, hepatic or renal impairment) is resolved (Griggs, 2012). **Note:** The manufacturer recommends the maximum dose should not exceed 0.1 mg/kg/day if maintenance therapy is required and with bone marrow infiltration.

Administration May be administered as a single daily dose; preferably on an empty stomach.

Hazardous agent; use appropriate precautions for handling and disposal (NIOSH 2014 [group 1]).

Monitoring Parameters Liver function tests, CBC with differential (weekly, with WBC monitored twice weekly during the first 3-6 weeks of treatment)

Dosage Forms

Tablet, Oral:

Leukeran: 2 mg

Extemporaneous Preparations Hazardous agent: Use appropriate precautions for handling and disposal (NIOSH 2014 [group 1]).

A 2 mg/mL oral suspension may be prepared with tablets. Crush sixty 2 mg tablets in a mortar and reduce to a fine powder. Add small portions of methylcellulose 1% and mix to a uniform paste (total methylcellulose: 30 mL); mix while adding simple syrup in incremental proportions to **almost** 60 mL; transfer to a graduated cylinder, rinse mortar and pestle with simple syrup, and add quantity of vehicle sufficient to make 60 mL. Transfer contents of graduated cylinder to an amber prescription bottle. Label "shake well", "refrigerate", and "protect from light". Stable for 7 days refrigerated.

Dressman JB and Poust RI, "Stability of Allopurinol and of Five Antineoplastics in Suspension," *Am J Hosp Pharm*, 1983, 40(4):616-8.

Nahata MC, Pai VB, and Hipple TF, *Pediatric Drug Formulations*, 5th ed, Cincinnati, OH: Harvey Whitney Books Co, 2004.

◆ **Chlorambucilum** *see* Chlorambucil *on page 419*

◆ **Chloraminophene** *see* Chlorambucil *on page 419*

Chloramphenicol (klor am FEN i kole)

Brand Names: Canada Chloromycetin®; Chloromycetin® Succinate; Diochloram®; Pentamycetin®

Pharmacologic Category Antibiotic, Miscellaneous

Use Treatment of serious infections due to organisms resistant to other less toxic antibiotics or when its penetrability into the site of infection is clinically superior to other antibiotics to which the organism is sensitive; useful in infections caused by *Bacteroides*, *H. influenzae*, *Neisseria meningitidis*, *Salmonella*, and *Rickettsia*; active against many vancomycin-resistant enterococci

Pregnancy Considerations Chloramphenicol crosses the placenta producing cord concentrations approaching maternal serum concentrations. An increased risk of teratogenic effects has not been associated with the use of chloramphenicol in pregnancy (Czeizel, 2000; Heinonen, 1977). "Gray Syndrome" has occurred in premature infants and newborns receiving chloramphenicol. The manufacturer recommends caution if used in a pregnant patient near term or during labor. Chloramphenicol may be used for the treatment of Rocky Mountain spotted fever in pregnant women although caution should be used when administration occurs during the third trimester (CDC, 2006).

Breast-Feeding Considerations Chloramphenicol and its inactive metabolites are excreted in breast milk. Chloramphenicol is well absorbed following oral administration; however, metabolism and excretion are highly variable in infants and children. The half-life is also significantly prolonged in low birth weight infants (Powell, 1982). Due to the potential for serious adverse reactions in the nursing infant, the manufacturer recommends that caution be exercised when administering chloramphenicol to nursing women. Other sources recommended avoiding use while breast-feeding, especially infants <34 weeks postconceptual age or when unusually large doses are needed (Atkinson, 1988; Matsuda, 1984; Plomp, 1983). Non-dose-related effects could include modification of bowel flora.

Contraindications Hypersensitivity to chloramphenicol or any component of the formulation; treatment of trivial or viral infections; bacterial prophylaxis

Warnings/Precautions Hazardous agent - use appropriate precautions for handling and disposal (NIOSH 2014 [group 2]).

Use in neonates (including premature) has resulted in "gray-baby syndrome" characterized by circulatory collapse, cyanosis, acidosis, abdominal distention (with or without emesis), myocardial depression, coma, and death; progression of symptoms is rapid; prompt termination of therapy required. Reaction result from drug accumulation possibly caused by the impaired neonatal hepatic or renal function. Reduce dose with impaired liver function. Use with care in patients with glucose 6-phosphate dehydrogenase deficiency. **[U.S. Boxed Warning]: Serious and fatal blood dyscrasias (aplastic anemia, hypoplastic anemia, thrombocytopenia, and granulocytopenia) have occurred after both short-term and prolonged therapy. Monitor CBC frequently in all patients;** discontinue if evidence of myelosuppression. Irreversible bone marrow suppression may occur weeks or months after therapy. Avoid repeated courses of treatment. Should not be used for minor infections or when less potentially toxic agents are effective. Prolonged use may result in fungal or bacterial superinfection, including *C. difficile*-associated diarrhea (CDAD) and pseudomembranous colitis; CDAD has been observed >2 months postantibiotic treatment.

Adverse Reactions

Central nervous system: Confusion, delirium, depression, fever, headache

Dermatologic: Angioedema, rash, urticaria

Gastrointestinal: Diarrhea, enterocolitis, glossitis, nausea, stomatitis, vomiting

Hematologic: Aplastic anemia, bone marrow suppression, granulocytopenia, hypoplastic anemia, pancytopenia, thrombocytopenia

Ocular: Optic neuritis

Miscellaneous: Anaphylaxis, hypersensitivity reactions, Gray syndrome

Drug Interactions

Metabolism/Transport Effects Inhibits CYP2C19 (strong), CYP2C9 (weak)

Avoid Concomitant Use

Avoid concomitant use of Chloramphenicol with any of the following: BCG; CloZAPine; Dipyrone

Increased Effect/Toxicity

Chloramphenicol may increase the levels/effects of: Alcohol (Ethyl); Barbiturates; Carbocisteine; Citalopram; CloZAPine; CycloSPORINE (Systemic); CYP2C19 Substrates; Sulfonylureas; Tacrolimus (Systemic); Vitamin K Antagonists; Voriconazole

The levels/effects of Chloramphenicol may be increased by: Dipyrone

Decreased Effect

Chloramphenicol may decrease the levels/effects of: BCG; Clopidogrel; Cyanocobalamin; Sodium Picosulfate; Typhoid Vaccine

The levels/effects of Chloramphenicol may be decreased by: Barbiturates; Rifampin

Storage/Stability Store at room temperature prior to reconstitution. Reconstituted solutions remain stable for 30 days. Use only clear solutions. Frozen solutions remain stable for 6 months.

Mechanism of Action Reversibly binds to 50S ribosomal subunits of susceptible organisms preventing amino acids from being transferred to growing peptide chains thus inhibiting protein synthesis

Pharmacodynamics/Kinetics

Distribution: To most tissues and body fluids

Chloramphenicol: V_d: 0.5-1 L/kg

Chloramphenicol succinate: V_d: 0.2-3.1 L/kg; decreased with hepatic or renal dysfunction

Protein binding: Chloramphenicol: ~60%; decreased with hepatic or renal dysfunction and in newborn infants

Metabolism:

Chloramphenicol: Hepatic to metabolites (inactive)

Chloramphenicol succinate: Hydrolyzed in the liver, kidney and lungs to chloramphenicol (active)

Bioavailability:

Chloramphenicol: Oral: ~80%

Chloramphenicol succinate: IV: ~70%; highly variable, dependent upon rate and extent of metabolism to chloramphenicol

Half-life elimination:

Normal renal function:

Chloramphenicol: Adults: ~4 hours; Children 4-6 hours; Infants: Significantly prolonged

Chloramphenicol succinate: Adults: ~3 hours

End-stage renal disease: Chloramphenicol: 3-7 hours

Hepatic disease: Prolonged

Excretion: Urine (~30% as unchanged chloramphenicol succinate in adults, 6% to 80% in children; 5% to 15% as chloramphenicol)

Dosage

Children: Usual dosing range: IV: 50-100 mg/kg/day in divided doses every 6 hours; maximum daily dose: 4 g/day

Meningitis: IV: Infants >30 days and Children: 75-100 mg/kg/day divided every 6 hours

Adults: 50-100 mg/kg/day in divided doses every 6 hours; maximum daily dose: 4 g/day

Dosing adjustment in renal impairment: Use with caution; monitor serum concentrations

Dosing adjustment/comments in hepatic impairment: Use with caution; monitor serum concentrations.

Dietary Considerations May have increased dietary need for riboflavin, pyridoxine, and vitamin B_{12}. Some products may contain sodium.

Administration Do not administer IM; can be administered IVP over at least 1 minute at a concentration of 100 mg/mL, or IV intermittent infusion over 15-30 minutes at a final concentration for administration of ≤20 mg/mL.

Hazardous agent; use appropriate precautions for handling and disposal (NIOSH 2014 [group 2]).

Monitoring Parameters CBC with differential (baseline and every 2 days during therapy), periodic liver and renal function tests, serum drug concentration

Reference Range

Therapeutic levels:

Meningitis:

Peak: 15-25 mcg/mL; toxic concentration: >40 mcg/mL

Trough: 5-15 mcg/mL

Other infections:

Peak: 10-20 mcg/mL

Trough: 5-10 mcg/mL

Timing of serum samples: Draw levels 0.5-1.5 hours after completion of IV dose

Dosage Forms

Solution Reconstituted, Intravenous:

Generic: 1 g (1 ea)

◆ **ChloraPrep One Step [OTC]** *see* Chlorhexidine Gluconate *on page 422*

◆ **Chlorax (Can)** *see* Clidinium and Chlordiazepoxide *on page 460*

◆ **Chlorbutinum** *see* Chlorambucil *on page 419*

ChlordiazePOXIDE (klor dye az e POKS ide)

Index Terms Librium; Methaminodiazepoxide Hydrochloride

Pharmacologic Category Benzodiazepine

Additional Appendix Information

Beers Criteria – Potentially Inappropriate Medications for Geriatrics *on page 2271*

Use Management of anxiety disorder or for the short-term relief of symptoms of anxiety; withdrawal symptoms of acute alcoholism; preoperative apprehension and anxiety

Pregnancy Risk Factor D

Dosage Oral:

Children <6 years: Not recommended

Children ≥6 years and Adolescents: Anxiety: Usual daily dose: 5 mg 2-4 times daily. Dose may be increased to 10 mg 2-3 times daily in some patients, if necessary.

Adults:

Anxiety:

Mild-moderate anxiety: Usual daily dose: 5-10 mg 3-4 times daily

Severe anxiety: Usual daily dose: 20-25 mg 3-4 times daily

Preoperative anxiety: 5-10 mg 3-4 times daily on the days preceding surgery

Ethanol withdrawal symptoms: Initial dose: 50-100 mg; dose may be repeated as necessary to a maximum of 300 mg per 24 hours. **Note:** Frequency of repeat doses is often based on institution-specific protocols. Once agitation is under control, maintain therapy at lowest effective dose.

Elderly or debilitated patients: Usual daily dose: 5 mg 2-4 times daily. Avoid use if possible due to long-acting metabolite.

Dosage adjustment in renal impairment: Dosage adjustments are not provided in the manufacturer's labeling; however, the following guidelines have been used by some clinicians (Aronoff, 2007): Adults: CrCl <10 mL/minute: Administer 50% of dose

Peritoneal dialysis: Administer 50% of the dose (Aronoff, 2007).

Dosage adjustment/comments in hepatic impairment: There are no specific hepatic dosage adjustments provided in the manufacturer's labeling; however, chlordiazepoxide undergoes hepatic metabolism and should be used with caution.

Additional Information Complete prescribing information should be consulted for additional detail.

Dosage Forms

Capsule, Oral:

Generic: 5 mg, 10 mg, 25 mg

◆ **Chlordiazepoxide and Amitriptyline Hydrochloride** *see* Amitriptyline and Chlordiazepoxide *on page 122*

◆ **Chlordiazepoxide and Clidinium** *see* Clidinium and Chlordiazepoxide *on page 460*

◆ **Chlorethazine** *see* Mechlorethamine (Systemic) *on page 1276*

◆ **Chlorethazine Mustard** *see* Mechlorethamine (Systemic) *on page 1276*

Chlorhexidine Gluconate

(klor HEKS i deen GLOO koe nate)

Brand Names: U.S. Betasept Surgical Scrub [OTC]; ChloraPrep One Step [OTC]; Hibiclens [OTC]; Hibistat [OTC]; Paroex; Peridex; Periogard; Tegaderm CHG Dressing [OTC]

Brand Names: Canada Apo-Chlorhexidine Oral Rinse; Denti-Care Chlorhexidine Gluconate Oral Rinse; GUM Paroex; ORO-Clense; Perichlor; Peridex Oral Rinse; Periogard; X-Pur Chlorhexidine

Index Terms 3M Avagard [OTC]; CHG

Pharmacologic Category Antibiotic, Oral Rinse; Antibiotic, Topical

Use

Topical: Skin cleanser for preoperative skin preparation, skin wound and general skin cleanser for patients; surgical scrub and antiseptic hand rinse for healthcare personnel

Oral rinse: Antibacterial dental rinse for gingivitis treatment

Periodontal chip: Adjunctive therapy to reduce pocket depth in patients with periodontitis

Pregnancy Risk Factor B/C (manufacturer specific)

Dosage Adults:

Oral rinse: Treatment of gingivitis: Swish for 30 seconds with 15 mL (one capful) of undiluted oral rinse after toothbrushing, then expectorate; repeat twice daily (morning and evening). Therapy should be initiated immediately following a dental prophylaxis. Patient should be reevaluated and given a dental prophylaxis at intervals no longer than every 6 months.

Periodontal chip: Periodontitis: One chip is inserted into a periodontal pocket with a probing pocket depth ≥5 mm. Up to 8 chips may be inserted in a single visit. Treatment is recommended every 3 months in pockets with a remaining depth ≥5 mm. If dislodgment occurs 7 days or more after placement, the subject is considered to have had the full course of treatment. If dislodgment occurs within 48 hours, a new chip should be inserted. The chip biodegrades completely and does not need to be removed. Patients should avoid dental floss at the site of periodontal chip insertion for 10 days after placement because flossing might dislodge the chip.

Insertion of periodontal chip: Pocket should be isolated and surrounding area dried prior to chip insertion. The chip should be grasped using forceps with the rounded edges away from the forceps. The chip should be inserted into the periodontal pocket to its maximum depth. It may be maneuvered into position using the tips of the forceps or a flat instrument.

Topical: Skin cleanser for preoperative skin preparation, skin wound and general skin cleanser for patients; surgical scrub and antiseptic hand rinse for healthcare personnel:

Surgical scrub: Scrub hands and forearms for 3 minutes paying close attention to nails, cuticles, and interdigital spaces, and rinse thoroughly, wash for an additional 3 minutes, rinse, and dry thoroughly.

Surgical hand antiseptic: Lotion: Dispense 1 pumpful in palm of 1 hand; dip fingertips of opposite hand into solution and work it under nails. Spread remainder evenly over hand and just above elbow, covering all surfaces. Repeat on other hand. Dispense another pumpful in each hand and reapply to each hand up to the wrist. Allow to dry before gloving.

Healthcare personnel hand antiseptic:

Liquid or solution: Wash with ~5 mL for 15 seconds; rinse thoroughly with water and dry.

Lotion: Apply to clean, dry hands and nails. Dispense 1 pumpful (2 mL) into the palm of 1 hand; apply evenly to cover both hands up to the wrists; allow to dry without wiping.

Towelette: Rub 15 seconds paying close attention to nails and interdigital spaces; no watering or toweling necessary

Preoperative skin preparation:

Solution: Apply liberally to surgical site and swab for at least 2 minutes. Dry with sterile towel. Repeat procedure (swab for additional 2 minutes and dry with sterile towel).

Applicator (ChloraPrep One-Step):

Dry surgical sites (eg, abdomen, arm): Completely wet treatment area; use gentle back and forth strokes for ~30 seconds. Allow solution to air dry for ~30 seconds. If using an ignition source (eg, electrocautery), allow solution to completely dry for a minimum of 3 minutes for hairless skin and up to 1 hour in hair; do not blot or wipe away. **Note:** Prior to use with electrocautery procedures, consult specific product labeling to determine if the ChloraPrep product may be used near an ignition source.

Moist surgical sites (eg, inguinal area): Completely wet treatment area; use gentle back and forth strokes for ~2 minutes. Allow solution to air dry for ~1 minute. If using an ignition source (eg, electrocautery), allow solution to completely dry for a minimum of 3 minutes for hairless skin and up to 1 hour in hair; do not blot or wipe away. **Note:** Prior to use with electrocautery procedures, consult specific product labeling to determine if the ChloraPrep product may be used near an ignition source.

Preparation of skin prior to an injection: Swab: Apply swab to procedure site for 15 seconds; allow to air dry for 30 seconds (do not blot or wipe dry). **Note:** Maximum treatment area for 1 swab is ~2.5 inches x 2.5 inches.

Wound care and general skin cleansing: Rinse area with water, then apply minimum amount necessary to cover skin or wound area and wash gently. Rinse again thoroughly.

Additional Information Complete prescribing information should be consulted for additional detail.

Dosage Forms

Liquid, External:

Betasept Surgical Scrub [OTC]: 4% (118 mL, 237 mL, 473 mL, 946 mL, 3780 mL)

Hibiclens [OTC]: 4% (15 mL, 118 mL, 236 mL, 473 mL, 946 mL, 3790 mL)

Generic: 2% (118 mL); 4% (118 mL, 237 mL, 473 mL, 946 mL, 3800 mL)

Miscellaneous, External:

Hibistat [OTC]: 0.5% (50 ea)

Tegaderm CHG Dressing [OTC]: (Dressing) (1 ea)

Pad, External:

Generic: 2% (2 ea, 6 ea)

Solution, External:

ChloraPrep One Step [OTC]: 2% (3 mL, 10.5 mL)

Solution, Mouth/Throat:

Paroex: 0.12% (473 mL)

Peridex: 0.12% (118 mL, 473 mL)

Periogard: 0.12% (473 mL)

Generic: 0.12% (15 mL, 473 mL)

◆ **Chlormeprazine** *see* Prochlorperazine *on page 1718*

◆ **2-Chlorodeoxyadenosine** *see* Cladribine *on page 455*

◆ **Chloromag** *see* Magnesium Chloride *on page 1261*

◆ **Chloromycetin® (Can)** *see* Chloramphenicol *on page 421*

◆ **Chloromycetin® Succinate (Can)** *see* Chloramphenicol *on page 421*

Chloroprocaine (klor oh PROE kane)

Brand Names: U.S. Nesacaine; Nesacaine-MPF

Brand Names: Canada Nesacaine®-CE

Index Terms Chloroprocaine Hydrochloride

Pharmacologic Category Local Anesthetic

Use Infiltration anesthesia, peripheral nerve block, epidural anesthesia

Pregnancy Risk Factor C

Dosage Dosage varies with anesthetic procedure, the area to be anesthetized, the vascularity of the tissues, depth of anesthesia required, degree of muscle relaxation required, and duration of anesthesia; range.

Children >3 years (normally developed): Maximum dose (without epinephrine): 11 mg/kg; for infiltration, concentrations of 0.5% to 1% are recommended; for nerve block, concentrations of 1% to 1.5% are recommended

Adults:

Maximum single dose (without epinephrine): 11 mg/kg; maximum dose: 800 mg

Maximum single dose (with epinephrine): 14 mg/kg; maximum dose: 1000 mg

Infiltration and peripheral nerve block:

Mandibular: 2%: 2-3 mL; total dose 40-60 mg

Infraorbital: 2%: 0.5-1 mL; total dose 10-20 mg

Brachial plexus: 2%; 30-40 mL; total dose 600-800 mg

Digital (without epinephrine): 1%; 3-4 mL; total dose: 30-40 mg

Pudendal: 2%; 10 mL each side; total dose: 400 mg

Paracervical: 1%; 3 mL per each of four sites

Caudal block: Preservative-free: 2% or 3%: 15-25 mL; may repeat at 40-60 minute intervals

Lumbar epidural block: Preservative-free: 2% or 3%: 2-2.5 mL per segment; usual total volume: 15-25 mL; may repeat with doses that are 2-6 mL less than initial dose every 40-50 minutes.

Dosage adjustment in renal impairment: No dosage adjustments provided in manufacturer's labeling. Use with caution due to increased risk of adverse effects.

Dosage adjustment in hepatic impairment: No dosage adjustments provided in manufacturer's labeling. Use with caution due to increased risk of adverse effects.

Additional Information Complete prescribing information should be consulted for additional detail.

Dosage Forms

Solution, Injection:

Nesacaine: 1% (30 mL); 2% (30 mL)

Solution, Injection [preservative free]:

Nesacaine-MPF: 2% (20 mL); 3% (20 mL)

Generic: 2% (20 mL); 3% (20 mL)

◆ **Chloroprocaine Hydrochloride** *see* Chloroprocaine *on page 423*

Chloroquine (KLOR oh kwin)

Brand Names: U.S. Aralen

Brand Names: Canada Aralen; Novo-Chloroquine

Index Terms Chloroquine Phosphate

Pharmacologic Category Aminoquinoline (Antimalarial)

Use

Malaria: Suppressive treatment and acute attacks of malaria due to *Plasmodium vivax*, *P. malariae*, *P. ovale*, and susceptible strains of *P. falciparum*.

Extraintestinal amebiasis: Treatment of extraintestinal amebiasis.

Pregnancy Considerations In animal reproduction studies, drug accumulated in fetal ocular tissues and remained for several months following drug elimination from the rest of the body. Chloroquine and its metabolites cross the placenta and can be detected in the cord blood and urine of the newborn infant (Akintonwa, 1988; Essien, 1982; Law, 2008). In one study, chloroquine and its metabolites were measurable in the cord blood 89 days (mean) after the last maternal dose (Law, 2008).

Malaria infection in pregnant women may be more severe than in nonpregnant women and has a high risk of maternal and perinatal morbidity and mortality. Therefore, pregnant women and women who are likely to become pregnant are advised to avoid travel to malaria-risk areas. Chloroquine is recommended for the treatment of pregnant women for uncomplicated malaria in chloroquine-sensitive regions; when caused by chloroquine-sensitive *P. vivax* or *P. ovale*, pregnant women should be maintained on chloroquine prophylaxis for the duration of their pregnancy (refer to current guidelines) (CDC, 2011; CDC, 2012).

Breast-Feeding Considerations Chloroquine and its metabolite can be detected in breast milk. Per product labeling, 11 lactating women with malaria were given a single oral dose of chloroquine 600 mg. The maximum daily dose to the breast-feeding infant was calculated to be 0.7% of the maternal dose. Additional information has been published and results are variable. In one study, the relative dose to the nursing infant was calculated to be 2.3% (chloroquine) and 1% (metabolite) of the weight-adjusted maternal dose with the samples obtained a median of 17 days after the last dose. Women in this study received chloroquine phosphate 750 mg daily for 3 days. This report also provides data from other studies, listing relative infant doses of chloroquine ranging from 0.9% to 9.5% of the maternal dose (Law, 2008). Due to the potential for serious adverse reactions in the nursing infant, the manufacturer recommends a decision be made whether to discontinue nursing or to discontinue the drug, taking into account the importance of treatment to the mother. Other sources consider the amount of chloroquine exposure to the nursing infant to be safe when normal maternal doses for malaria are used. However, the amount of chloroquine obtained by a nursing infant from breast milk would not provide adequate protection if therapy for malaria in the infant is needed (CDC, 2012).

Contraindications Hypersensitivity to 4-aminoquinoline compounds or any component of the formulation; the presence of retinal or visual field changes either attributable to 4-aminoquinoline compounds or to any other etiology

Warnings/Precautions Use with caution in patients with hepatic impairment, alcoholism or in conjunction with hepatotoxic drugs. May exacerbate psoriasis or porphyria. Use caution in patients with seizure disorders. Use caution in G6PD deficiency; 4-aminoquinolines such as chloroquine has been associated with hemolysis and renal impairment. Use with caution in patients with preexisting auditory damage; discontinue immediately if hearing defects are noted. Retinopathy, maculopathy, and macular degeneration have occurred; irreversible retinal damage has occurred with prolonged or high dose 4-aminoquinoline therapy; risk factors include age, duration of therapy, and/or high doses. Monitoring is required, especially with prolonged therapy. Discontinue immediately if signs/symptoms occur; visual changes may progress even after therapy is discontinued. Use has been associated with ECG changes, AV block, and cardiomyopathy. May cause QT prolongation and subsequent torsade de pointes; avoid use in patients with diagnosed or suspected congenital long QT syndrome. Rare hematologic reactions including agranulocytosis, aplastic anemia, neutropenia, pancytopenia, and thrombocytopenia; monitor CBC during prolonged therapy. Consider discontinuation if severe blood disorders occur that are unrelated to disease. Acute extrapyramidal disorders may occur, usually resolving after discontinuation of therapy and/or symptomatic treatment. Skeletal muscle myopathy or neuromyopathy, leading to progressive weakness and atrophy of proximal muscle groups have been reported; muscle strength (especially proximal muscles) should be assessed periodically during prolonged therapy; discontinue therapy if weakness occurs. Potentially significant drug-drug interactions may exist, requiring dose or frequency adjustment, additional monitoring, and/or selection of alternative therapy.

Certain strains of *P. falciparum* are resistant to 4-aminoquinoline compounds. Prior to initiation of therapy, it should be determined if chloroquine is appropriate for use in the region to be visited; do not use for the treatment of *P. falciparum* acquired in areas of chloroquine resistance or where chloroquine prophylaxis has failed. Patients should be treated with another antimalarial if patient is infected with a resistant strain of plasmodia. Chloroquine does not prevent relapses in patients with vivax or malariae malaria; will not prevent vivax or malariae infection when administered as a prophylactic. Also consult current CDC guidelines for treatment recommendations.

Adverse Reactions

Cardiovascular: Cardiomyopathy, ECG changes (rare; including prolonged QRS and QTc intervals, T wave inversion or depression), hypotension (rare), torsades de pointes (rare)

Central nervous system: Agitation, anxiety, confusion, decreased deep tendon reflex, delirium, depression, extrapyramidal reaction (dystonia, dyskinesia, protrusion of the tongue, torticollis), hallucination, headache, insomnia, personality changes, polyneuropathy, psychosis, seizure

Dermatologic: Alopecia, bleaching of hair, blue gray skin pigmentation, erythema multiforme (rare), exacerbation of psoriasis, exfoliative dermatitis (rare), lichen planus, pleomorphic rash, pruritus, skin photosensitivity, Stevens-Johnson syndrome (rare), toxic epidermal necrolysis (rare), urticaria

Gastrointestinal: Abdominal cramps, anorexia, diarrhea, nausea, vomiting

Hematologic & oncologic: Agranulocytosis (rare; reversible), aplastic anemia, neutropenia, pancytopenia, thrombocytopenia

Hepatic: Hepatitis, increased liver enzymes

Hypersensitivity: Anaphylactoid reaction, anaphylaxis, angioedema

Immunologic: DRESS syndrome

Neuromuscular & skeletal: Myopathy, neuromuscular disease, proximal myopathy

Ophthalmic: Accommodation disturbances, blurred vision, corneal opacity (reversible), macular degeneration (may be irreversible), maculopathy (may be irreversible), nocturnal amblyopia, retinopathy (including irreversible changes in some patients long-term or high-dose therapy), visual field defects

Otic: Deafness (nerve), hearing loss (risk increased in patients with preexisting auditory damage), tinnitus

Drug Interactions

Metabolism/Transport Effects Substrate of CYP2D6 (major), CYP3A4 (major); **Note:** Assignment of Major/Minor substrate status based on clinically relevant drug interaction potential; **Inhibits** CYP2D6 (moderate)

Avoid Concomitant Use

Avoid concomitant use of Chloroquine with any of the following: Agalsidase Alfa; Agalsidase Beta; Artemether; Conivaptan; Fusidic Acid (Systemic); Highest Risk QTc-Prolonging Agents; Idelalisib; Ivabradine; Lumefantrine; Mefloquine; Mifepristone; Thioridazine

Increased Effect/Toxicity

Chloroquine may increase the levels/effects of: Antipsychotic Agents (Phenothiazines); ARIPiprazole; Beta-Blockers; Cardiac Glycosides; CYP2D6 Substrates; Dapsone (Systemic); Dapsone (Topical); DOXOrubicin (Conventional); Fesoterodine; Highest Risk QTc-Prolonging Agents; Lumefantrine; Mefloquine; Metoprolol; Moderate Risk QTc-Prolonging Agents; Nebivolol; Prilocaine; Sodium Nitrite; Thioridazine

The levels/effects of Chloroquine may be increased by: Abiraterone Acetate; Aprepitant; Artemether; Conivaptan; CYP2D6 Inhibitors (Moderate); CYP2D6 Inhibitors (Strong); CYP3A4 Inhibitors (Moderate); CYP3A4 Inhibitors (Strong); Dapsone (Systemic); Dasatinib; Fosaprepitant; Fusidic Acid (Systemic); Idelalisib; Ivabradine; Ivacaftor; Luliconazole; Mefloquine; Mifepristone; Netupitant; Nitric Oxide; Peginterferon Alfa-2b; QTc-Prolonging Agents (Indeterminate Risk and Risk Modifying); Simeprevir; Stiripentol

Decreased Effect

Chloroquine may decrease the levels/effects of: Agalsidase Alfa; Agalsidase Beta; Ampicillin; Anthelmintics; Codeine; Rabies Vaccine; Tamoxifen; TraMADol

The levels/effects of Chloroquine may be decreased by: Antacids; Bosentan; CYP3A4 Inducers (Moderate); CYP3A4 Inducers (Strong); Dabrafenib; Deferasirox; Kaolin; Lanthanum; Mitotane; Peginterferon Alfa-2b; Siltuximab; St Johns Wort; Tocilizumab

Storage/Stability Store at 25°C (77°F); excursions are permitted between 15°C and 30°C (59°F and 86°F); protect from light.

Mechanism of Action Binds to and inhibits DNA and RNA polymerase; interferes with metabolism and hemoglobin utilization by parasites; inhibits prostaglandin effects; chloroquine concentrates within parasite acid vesicles and raises internal pH resulting in inhibition of parasite growth; may involve aggregates of ferriprotoporphyrin IX acting as chloroquine receptors causing membrane damage; may also interfere with nucleoprotein synthesis

Pharmacodynamics/Kinetics

Absorption: Rapid and almost complete

Distribution: Widely in body tissues

Protein binding: 55%

Metabolism: Partially hepatic to main metabolite, desethylchloroquine

Excretion: Urine (≥50% as unchanged drug); acidification of urine increases elimination

Dosage Oral: **Note:** Each 250 mg of chloroquine phosphate is equivalent to 150 mg of chloroquine base

Malaria chemoprophylaxis:

Children: 8.3 mg/kg/week (5 mg/kg base) on the same day each week (not to exceed 500 mg/dose [300 mg base/dose]); begin 1-2 weeks prior to exposure; continue while in endemic area and for 4 weeks after leaving endemic area (CDC, 2014)

Adults: 500 mg (300 mg base) weekly on the same day each week; begin 1-2 weeks prior to exposure; continue while in endemic area and for 4 weeks after leaving endemic area (CDC, 2014)

Malaria treatment:

Children: 16.6 mg/kg (10 mg/kg base) on day 1 (maximum: 1000 mg [600 mg base]), followed by 8.3 mg/kg (5 mg/kg base) (maximum: 500 mg [300 mg base]) 6-, 24-, and 48 hours after first dose (CDC, 2009)

Adults: 1 g (600 mg base) on day 1, followed by 500 mg (300 mg base) 6-, 24-, and 48 hours after first dose (CDC, 2009)

Extraintestinal amebiasis: Adults: 1 g (600 mg base) daily for 2 days followed by 500 mg daily (300 mg base) for at least 2-3 weeks; may be combined with an intestinal amebicide.

Lupus erythematosus (off-label use): Adults: 250 mg (150 mg base) once daily for ≥3 months (Bezerra, 2005; Lesiak, 2008)

Rheumatoid arthritis (off-label use): Adults: 250 mg (150 mg base) once daily for ≥1 year. **Note:** Not considered first-line agent. (Fowler, 1984; Freedman, 1960)

Dosage adjustment in renal impairment: The FDA-approved labeling does not contain renal dosing adjustment guidelines; the following guidelines have been used by some clinicians (Aronoff, 2007):

CrCl ≥10 mL/minute: No dosage adjustment necessary.

CrCl <10 mL/minute: Administer 50% of dose

Hemodialysis effects: Minimally removed by hemodialysis

Hemodialysis, peritoneal dialysis: Administer 50% of dose

Continuous renal replacement therapy (CRRT): No dosage adjustment necessary.

Dosage adjustment in hepatic impairment: No dosage adjustment provided in manufacturer's labeling; use with caution.

Monitoring Parameters Ophthalmic exams at baseline and periodically thereafter during prolonged therapy; visual acuity, expert slit-lamp, fundoscopic and visual field tests are recommended. Evaluate neuromuscular function periodically during prolonged therapy. Periodic CBC in patients receiving prolonged therapy

Dosage Forms

Tablet, Oral:

Aralen: 500 mg [equivalent to chloroquine base 300 mg]

Generic: 250 mg [equivalent to chloroquine base 150 mg], 500 mg [equivalent to chloroquine base 300 mg]

Extemporaneous Preparations A 15 mg chloroquine phosphate/mL oral suspension (equivalent to 9 mg chloroquine base/mL) may be made from tablets and a 1:1 mixture of Ora-Sweet® and Ora-Plus®. Crush three 500 mg chloroquine phosphate tablets (equivalent to 300 mg base/tablet) in a mortar and reduce to a fine powder. Add 15 mL of the vehicle and mix to a uniform paste; mix while adding the vehicle in incremental proportions to **almost** 100 mL; transfer to a calibrated bottle, rinse mortar with vehicle, and add quantity of vehicle sufficient to make 100 mL. Label "shake well before using" and "protect from light". Stable for up to 60 days when stored in the dark at room temperature or refrigerated (preferred).

Allen LV Jr and Erickson MA 3rd, "Stability of Alprazolam, Chloroquine Phosphate, Cisapride, Enalapril Maleate, and Hydralazine Hydrochloride in Extemporaneously Compounded Oral Liquids," *Am J Health Syst Pharm*, 1998, 55(18):1915-20.

◆ **Chloroquine Phosphate** *see* Chloroquine *on page 424*

Chlorothiazide (klor oh THYE a zide)

Brand Names: U.S. Diuril; Sodium Diuril

Pharmacologic Category Antihypertensive; Diuretic, Thiazide

Use Management of hypertension; adjunctive treatment of edema

The 2014 guideline for the management of high blood pressure in adults (Eighth Joint National Committee [JNC 8]) recommends initiation of pharmacologic treatment to lower blood pressure for the following patients:

- Patients ≥60 years of age with systolic blood pressure (SBP) ≥150 mm Hg or diastolic blood pressure (DBP) ≥90 mm Hg. Goal of therapy is SBP <150 mm Hg and DBP <90 mm Hg.
- Patients <60 years of age with SBP ≥140 mm Hg or DBP is ≥90 mm Hg. Goal of therapy is SBP <140 mm Hg and DBP <90 mm Hg.
- Patients ≥18 years of age with diabetes and SBP ≥140 mm Hg or DBP ≥90 mm Hg. Goal of therapy is SBP <140 mm Hg and DBP <90 mm Hg.
- Patients ≥18 years of age with chronic kidney disease (CKD) and SBP ≥140 mm Hg or DBP ≥90 mm Hg. Goal of therapy is SBP <140 mm Hg and DBP <90 mm Hg.

In patients with CKD, regardless of race or diabetes status, the use of an ACE inhibitor (ACEI) or angiotensin receptor blocker (ARB) as initial therapy is recommended to improve kidney outcomes. In the general nonblack population (without CKD) including those with diabetes, initial antihypertensive treatment should consist of a thiazide-type diuretic, calcium channel blocker, ACEI, or ARB. In the general black population (without CKD), including those with diabetes, initial antihypertensive treatment should consist of a thiazide-type diuretic or a calcium channel blocker **instead of** an ACEI or ARB.

Pregnancy Risk Factor C

Dosage Note: The manufacturer states that IV and oral dosing are equivalent. Some clinicians may use lower IV doses; however, because of chlorothiazide's poor oral absorption. IV dosing in infants and children has not been well established.

Infants <6 months: Oral: 10 to 30 mg/kg/day in 2 divided doses (maximum dose: 375 mg daily)

Infants >6 months and Children: Oral: 10 to 20 mg/kg/day in 1 to 2 divided doses (maximum dose: 375 mg daily in children <2 years or 1000 mg daily in children 2 to 12 years)

Infants and Children: IV (off-label): 5 to 10 mg/kg/day in 2 divided doses (Costello, 2007)

Adults:

Hypertension: Oral: 500 to 2000 mg daily divided in 1 to 2 doses

Edema: Oral, IV: 500 to 1000 mg once or twice daily; intermittent treatment (eg, therapy on alternative days) may be appropriate for some patients

ACCF/AHA 2013 heart failure guidelines:

Oral: 250 to 500 mg once or twice daily (maximum daily dose: 1000 mg)

IV: 500 to 1000 mg once daily in combination with a loop diuretic for sequential nephron blockade

Dosage adjustment in renal impairment: CrCl <10 mL/minute: Avoid use. Ineffective with CrCl <30 mL/minute unless in combination with a loop diuretic (Aronoff, 2007)

Dosage adjustment in hepatic impairment: No dosage adjustments provided in manufacturer's labeling; use with caution.

Additional Information Complete prescribing information should be consulted for additional detail.

Dosage Forms

Solution Reconstituted, Intravenous:

Sodium Diuril: 500 mg (1 ea)

Generic: 500 mg (1 ea)

Suspension, Oral:

Diuril: 250 mg/5 mL (237 mL)

Tablet, Oral:

Generic: 250 mg, 500 mg

Chlorpheniramine and Acetaminophen

(klor fen IR a meen & a seet a MIN oh fen)

Brand Names: U.S. Coricidin HBP® Cold and Flu [OTC]

Index Terms Acetaminophen and Chlorpheniramine

Pharmacologic Category Alkylamine Derivative; Analgesic, Miscellaneous; Histamine H_1 Antagonist; Histamine H_1 Antagonist, First Generation

Use Symptomatic relief of congestion, headache, aches and pains of colds and flu

Dosage Adults: Oral: 2 tablets every 4 hours

Additional Information Complete prescribing information should be consulted for additional detail.

Dosage Forms

Tablet:

Coricidin HBP® Cold and Flu [OTC]: Chlorpheniramine 2 mg and acetaminophen 325 mg

◆ **Chlorpheniramine and Dextromethorphan** *see* Dextromethorphan and Chlorpheniramine *on page 610*

Chlorpheniramine and Phenylephrine

(klor fen IR a meen & fen il EF rin)

Brand Names: U.S. Actifed Cold/Allergy [OTC]; Dallergy Drops [OTC]; Ed ChlorPed D [OTC]; Ed-A-Hist™ [OTC]; Maxichlor PEH [OTC] [DSC]; nasohist™ [OTC] [DSC]; NoHist LQ [OTC]; Sudafed PE® Sinus + Allergy [OTC]; Triaminic® Children's Cold & Allergy [OTC]; Virdec [OTC]

Index Terms Chlorpheniramine Maleate and Phenylephrine Hydrochloride; Phenylephrine and Chlorpheniramine

Pharmacologic Category Alkylamine Derivative; Alpha-Adrenergic Agonist; Decongestant; Histamine H_1 Antagonist; Histamine H_1 Antagonist, First Generation

Use Temporary relief of upper respiratory conditions such as nasal congestion, runny nose, and sneezing due to the common cold, hay fever, or allergic or vasomotor rhinitis

Dosage Antihistamine/decongestant: Oral: **Note:** Chlorpheniramine dosing in terms of chlorpheniramine maleate; phenylephrine dosing in terms of phenylephrine hydrochloride:

Children 2-5 years:

Liquid:

Chlorpheniramine 1 mg and phenylephrine 2.5 mg per 1 mL: 1 mL every 4-6 hours (maximum: 4 mL/24 hours)

Chlorpheniramine 2 mg and phenylephrine 5 mg per 1 mL: 0.5 mL every 4 hours (maximum: 3 mL/24 hours)

Children 6-11 years:

Liquid:

Chlorpheniramine 1 mg and phenylephrine 2-2.5 mg per 1 mL: 2 mL every 4-6 hours (maximum: 8 mL/24 hours)

Chlorpheniramine 1-2 mg and phenylephrine 3.5-5 mg per 1 mL: 1 mL every 4-6 hours (maximum: 6 mL/24 hours)

Chlorpheniramine 1 mg and phenylephrine 2.5 mg per 5 mL: 10 mL every 4 hours (maximum: 60 mL/24 hours)

Chlorpheniramine 4 mg and phenylephrine 10 mg per 5 mL: 2.5 mL every 4-6 hours (maximum: 15 mL/24 hours)

Tablet: Chlorpheniramine 3-4 mg and phenylephrine 10 mg: One-half tablet every 4-6 hours (maximum: 3 tablets/24 hours)

Children ≥12 years and Adults:

Liquid: Chlorpheniramine 4 mg and phenylephrine 10 mg per 5 mL: 5 mL every 4-6 hours (maximum: 30 mL/24 hours)

Tablet: Chlorpheniramine 3-4 mg and phenylephrine 10 mg: One tablet every 4-6 hours (maximum: 6 tablets/24 hours)

Additional Information Complete prescribing information should be consulted for additional detail.

Dosage Forms

Liquid, oral:

Ed-A-Hist™ [OTC], NoHist LQ [OTC]: Chlorpheniramine 4 mg and phenylephrine 10 mg per 5 mL (473 mL)

Liquid, oral [drops]:

Cardec Drops [OTC]: Chlorpheniramine 1 mg and phenylephrine 3.5 mg per 1 mL (30 mL)

Dallergy Drops [OTC]: Chlorpheniramine 1 mg and phenylephrine 2.5 mg per 1 mL (30 mL)

Ed ChlorPed D [OTC]: Chlorpheniramine 2 mg and phenylephrine 5 mg per 1 mL (60 mL)

Virdec [OTC]: Chlorpheniramine 1 mg and phenylephrine 3.5 mg per 1 mL (30 mL)

Syrup, oral:

Triaminic® Children's Cold & Allergy [OTC]: Chlorpheniramine 1 mg and phenylephrine 2.5 mg per 5 mL (118 mL)

Tablet, oral: Chlorpheniramine 4 mg and phenylephrine 10 mg

Actifed Cold/Allergy [OTC], Ed A-Hist™ [OTC], Sudafed PE® Sinus + Allergy [OTC]: Chlorpheniramine 4 mg and phenylephrine 10 mg

Chlorpheniramine and Pseudoephedrine

(klor fen IR a meen & soo doe e FED rin)

Brand Names: U.S. Dicel® Chewable [OTC]; LoHist-D [OTC]; Maxichlor PSE [OTC]; Neutrahist Pediatric [OTC]; SudoGest™ Sinus & Allergy [OTC]

Brand Names: Canada Triaminic® Cold & Allergy

Index Terms Allerest; Chlorpheniramine Maleate and Pseudoephedrine Hydrochloride; Chlorpheniramine Tannate and Pseudoephedrine Tannate; Pseudoephedrine and Chlorpheniramine

Pharmacologic Category Alkylamine Derivative; Alpha/Beta Agonist; Decongestant; Histamine H_1 Antagonist; Histamine H_1 Antagonist, First Generation

Use Relief of nasal congestion associated with the common cold, hay fever, allergic rhinitis, and other allergies

Pregnancy Risk Factor C

Dosage Rhinitis/decongestant: Oral: **Note:** All dosing is presented in terms of chlorpheniramine maleate and pseudoephedrine hydrochloride.

Children: 6-11 years:

Liquid:

Chlorpheniramine 0.8 mg and pseudoephedrine 9 mg per 1 mL: 2 mL every 4-6 hours (maximum: 8 mL/24 hours)

Chlorpheniramine 2 mg and pseudoephedrine 30 mg per 5 mL: 5 mL every 4-6 hours (maximum: 30 mL/24 hours)

Tablet:

Chlorpheniramine 2 mg and pseudoephedrine 30 mg: One tablet every 4-6 hours (maximum: 4 tablets/24 hours)

Chlorpheniramine 4 mg and pseudoephedrine 60 mg: One-half tablet every 4-6 hours (maximum: 2 tablets/24 hours)

Children ≥12 years and Adults:

Liquid: Chlorpheniramine 2 mg and pseudoephedrine 30 mg per 5 mL: 10 mL every 4-6 hours (maximum: 60 mL/24hours)

Tablet:

Chlorpheniramine 2 mg and pseudoephedrine 30 mg: Two tablets every 4-6 hours (maximum: 8 tablets/24 hours)

Chlorpheniramine 4 mg and pseudoephedrine 60 mg: One tablet every 4-6 hours (maximum: 4 tablets/24 hours)

Additional Information Complete prescribing information should be consulted for additional detail.

Dosage Forms

Liquid, oral:

LoHist-D [OTC]: Chlorpheniramine 2 mg and pseudoephedrine 30 mg per 5 mL (473 mL)

Liquid, oral [drops]:

Neutrahist Pediatric [OTC]: Chlorpheniramine 0.8 mg and pseudoephedrine 9 mg per 1 mL (30 mL)

Tablet, oral: Chlorpheniramine 4 mg and pseudoephedrine 60 mg

Maxichlor PSE [OTC], SudoGest™ Sinus & Allergy [OTC]: Chlorpheniramine 4 mg and pseudoephedrine 60 mg

Tablet, chewable, oral:

Dicel® Chewables [OTC]: Chlorpheniramine 2 mg and pseudoephedrine 30 mg

◆ **Chlorpheniramine, Dextromethorphan, and Pseudoephedrine** *see* Chlorpheniramine, Pseudoephedrine, and Dextromethorphan *on page 428*

◆ **Chlorpheniramine Maleate and Dextromethorphan Hydrobromide** *see* Dextromethorphan and Chlorpheniramine *on page 610*

◆ **Chlorpheniramine Maleate and Hydrocodone Bitartrate** *see* Hydrocodone and Chlorpheniramine *on page 1012*

◆ **Chlorpheniramine Maleate and Phenylephrine Hydrochloride** *see* Chlorpheniramine and Phenylephrine *on page 426*

◆ **Chlorpheniramine Maleate and Pseudoephedrine Hydrochloride** *see* Chlorpheniramine and Pseudoephedrine *on page 427*

◆ **Chlorpheniramine Maleate, Dihydrocodeine Bitartrate, and Phenylephrine Hydrochloride** *see* Dihydrocodeine, Chlorpheniramine, and Phenylephrine *on page 633*

◆ **Chlorpheniramine Maleate, Pseudoephedrine Hydrochloride, and Dextromethorphan Hydrobromide** *see* Chlorpheniramine, Pseudoephedrine, and Dextromethorphan *on page 428*

Chlorpheniramine, Phenylephrine, and Dextromethorphan

(klor fen IR a meen, fen il EF rin, & deks troe meth OR fan)

Brand Names: U.S. Cardec™ DM [OTC]; Corfen-DM [OTC]; De-Chlor DM [OTC]; Ed A-Hist DM [OTC]; Father John's® Plus [OTC]; Maxichlor PEH DM [OTC] [DSC]; nasohist™ DM pediatric [OTC] [DSC]; Neo DM [OTC] [DSC]; NoHist DM [OTC]; Norel CS [OTC]; PE-Hist-DM [OTC]; Trigofen DM [OTC]; Virdec DM [OTC]

Index Terms Dextromethorphan, Chlorpheniramine, and Phenylephrine; Phenylephrine, Chlorpheniramine, and Dextromethorphan

Pharmacologic Category Alkylamine Derivative; Alpha-Adrenergic Agonist; Antitussive; Decongestant; Histamine H_1 Antagonist; Histamine H_1 Antagonist, First Generation

Use Temporary relief of cough and upper respiratory symptoms associated with allergies or the common cold

Dosage Note: All dosing is presented in terms of chlorpheniramine maleate, phenylephrine hydrochloride, and dextromethorphan hydrobromide.

Oral: Relief of cough and cold symptoms:

Children: 2-5 years: Liquid: Chlorpheniramine 1 mg, phenylephrine 2.5 mg, and dextromethorphan 2.5 mg per 1 mL: 1 mL every 4-6 hours (maximum: 4 mL/24 hours)

Children: 6-11 years:

Liquid:

Chlorpheniramine 0.75 mg, phenylephrine 1.75 mg, and dextromethorphan 2.75 mg per 1 mL: 2 mL every 4-6 hours (maximum: 12 mL/24 hours)

Chlorpheniramine 1 mg, phenylephrine 2-2.5 mg, and dextromethorphan 2.5-3 mg per 1 mL: 2 mL every 4-6 hours (maximum: 8 mL/24 hours)

Chlorpheniramine 1 mg, phenylephrine 3.5 mg, and dextromethorphan 3 mg per 1 mL: 1 mL every 4-6 hours (maximum: 6 mL/24 hours)

Chlorpheniramine 2-4 mg, phenylephrine 5-10 mg, and dextromethorphan 15 mg per 5 mL: 2.5 mL every 4-6 hours (maximum: 15 mL/24 hours)

Tablet: Chlorpheniramine 4 mg, phenylephrine 10 mg, and dextromethorphan 20 mg: One-half tablet every 4-6 hours (maximum: 3 tablets/24 hours)

Children ≥12 years and Adults:

Liquid:

Chlorpheniramine 2 mg, phenylephrine 5 mg, and dextromethorphan 5 mg per 15 mL: 30 mL every 4 hours (maximum: 180 mL/24 hours)

Chlorpheniramine 2-4 mg, phenylephrine 5-10 mg, and dextromethorphan 15 mg per 5 mL: 5 mL every 4-6 hours (maximum: 30 mL/24 hours)

Tablet: Chlorpheniramine 4 mg, phenylephrine 10 mg, and dextromethorphan 20 mg: One tablet every 4-6 hours (maximum: 6 tablets/24 hours)

Additional Information Complete prescribing information should be consulted for additional detail.

Dosage Forms

Liquid, oral:

Corfen-DM [OTC], Ed A-Hist DM [OTC], NoHist DM [OTC]: Chlorpheniramine 4 mg, phenylephrine 10 mg, and dextromethorphan 15 mg per 5 mL

De-Chlor DM [OTC]: Chlorpheniramine 2 mg, phenylephrine 10 mg, and dextromethorphan 15 mg per 5 mL

Father John's® Plus [OTC]: Chlorpheniramine 2 mg, phenylephrine 5 mg, and dextromethorphan 5 mg per 15 mL

Norel CS [OTC]: Chlorpheniramine maleate 4 mg, phenylephrine hydrochloride 10 mg, and dextromethorphan hydrobromide 12.5 mg per 5 mL

Liquid, oral [drops]:

Cardec™ DM [OTC], Virdec DM [OTC]: Chlorpheniramine 1 mg, phenylephrine 3.5 mg, and dextromethorphan 3 mg per 1 mL

Trigofen DM [OTC]: Chlorpheniramine 1 mg, phenylephrine 2 mg, and dextromethorphan 3 mg per 1 mL

Tablet, oral: Chlorpheniramine 4 mg, phenylephrine 10 mg, and dextromethorphan 20 mg

Chlorpheniramine, Pseudoephedrine, and Dextromethorphan

(klor fen IR a meen, soo doe e FED rin, & deks troe meth OR fan)

Brand Names: U.S. Dicel® DM Chewables [OTC]; Kidkare Children's Cough/Cold [OTC]; M-END DM [OTC] [DSC]; Maxichlor PSE DM [OTC] [DSC]; Neutrahist PDX [OTC] [DSC]; Pedia Relief™ Cough-Cold [OTC]; Pediatric Cough & Cold [OTC]; Rescon DM [OTC]

Index Terms Chlorpheniramine Maleate, Pseudoephedrine Hydrochloride, and Dextromethorphan Hydrobromide; Chlorpheniramine Tannate, Pseudoephedrine Tannate, and Dextromethorphan Tannate; Chlorpheniramine, Dextromethorphan, and Pseudoephedrine; Dexchlorpheniramine Tannate, Pseudoephedrine Tannate, and Dextromethorphan Tannate; Dextromethorphan, Chlorpheniramine, and Pseudoephedrine; Pseudoephedrine, Chlorpheniramine, and Dextromethorphan

Pharmacologic Category Alkylamine Derivative; Alpha/Beta Agonist; Antitussive; Decongestant; Histamine H_1 Antagonist; Histamine H_1 Antagonist, First Generation

Use Temporarily relieves nasal congestion, runny nose, cough, and sneezing due to the common cold, hay fever, or allergic rhinitis

Dosage Relief of cold symptoms: Oral: **Note:** All dosing is presented in terms of chlorpheniramine maleate, pseudoephedrine hydrochloride, and dextromethorphan hydrobromide.

Children 6-11 years:

Liquid:

Chlorpheniramine 0.8 mg, pseudoephedrine 9 mg, and dextromethorphan 3 mg per 1 mL: 2 mL every 4-6 hours (maximum: 8 mL/24 hours)

Chlorpheniramine 1 mg, pseudoephedrine 15 mg, and dextromethorphan 5 mg per 5 mL: 10 mL every 4-6 hours (maximum: 40 mL/24 hours)

Chlorpheniramine 2 mg, pseudoephedrine 15 mg, and dextromethorphan 15 mg per 5 mL: 5 mL every 6 hours (maximum: 20 mL/24 hours)

Chlorpheniramine 2 mg, pseudoephedrine 30 mg, and dextromethorphan 10 mg per 5 mL: 5 mL every 4-6 hours (maximum: 20 mL/24 hours)

Chlorpheniramine 4 mg, pseudoephedrine 20 mg, and dextromethorphan 20 mg per 5 mL: 2.5 mL every 4-6 hours (maximum: 15 mL/24 hours)

Tablet:
Chlorpheniramine 2 mg, pseudoephedrine 30 mg, and dextromethorphan 10 mg: One tablet every 4-6 hours (maximum: 4 tablets/24 hours)
Chlorpheniramine 4 mg, pseudoephedrine 60 mg, and dextromethorphan 20 mg: One-half tablet every 4-6 hours (maximum: 2 tablets/24 hours)
Children ≥12 years and Adults:
Liquid:
Chlorpheniramine 2 mg, pseudoephedrine 15 mg, and dextromethorphan 15 mg per 5 mL: 10 mL every 6 hours (maximum: 40 mL/24 hours)
Chlorpheniramine 2 mg, pseudoephedrine 30 mg, and dextromethorphan 10 mg per 5 mL: 10 mL every 4-6 hours (maximum: 40 mL/24 hours)
Chlorpheniramine 4 mg, pseudoephedrine 20 mg, and dextromethorphan 20 mg per 5 mL: 5 mL every 4-6 hours (maximum: 30 mL/24 hours)
Tablet:
Chlorpheniramine 2 mg, pseudoephedrine 30 mg, and dextromethorphan 10 mg: Two tablets every 4-6 hours (maximum: 8 tablets/24 hours)
Chlorpheniramine 4 mg, pseudoephedrine 60 mg, and dextromethorphan 20 mg: One tablet every 4-6 hours (maximum: 4 tablets/24 hours)

Additional Information Complete prescribing information should be consulted for additional detail.

Dosage Forms

Liquid, oral: Chlorpheniramine 1 mg, pseudoephedrine 15 mg, and dextromethorphan 5 mg per 5 mL
Kidkare Children's Cough/Cold [OTC], Pedia Relief™ [OTC], Pediatric Cough & Cold [OTC]: Chlorpheniramine 1 mg, pseudoephedrine 15 mg, and dextromethorphan 5 mg per 5 mL (120 mL)
Maxichlor PSE DM [OTC]: Chlorpheniramine 4 mg, pseudoephedrine 20 mg, and dextromethorphan 20 mg per 5 mL (473 mL)
Rescon DM [OTC]: Chlorpheniramine 2 mg, pseudoephedrine 30 mg, and dextromethorphan 10 mg per 5 mL (120 mL, 480 mL)

Tablet, oral: Chlorpheniramine 4 mg, pseudoephedrine 60 mg, and dextromethorphan 20 mg

Tablet, chewable, oral:
Dicel® DM Chewables [OTC]: Chlorpheniramine 2 mg, pseudoephedrine 30 mg, and dextromethorphan 10 mg

◆ **Chlorpheniramine Tannate and Pseudoephedrine Tannate** *see* Chlorpheniramine and Pseudoephedrine *on page 427*

◆ **Chlorpheniramine Tannate, Pseudoephedrine Tannate, and Dextromethorphan Tannate** *see* Chlorpheniramine, Pseudoephedrine, and Dextromethorphan *on page 428*

ChlorproMAZINE (klor PROE ma zeen)

Brand Names: Canada Chlorpromazine Hydrochloride Inj; Teva-Chlorpromazine

Index Terms Chlorpromazine Hydrochloride; CPZ; Thorazine

Pharmacologic Category Antimanic Agent; First Generation (Typical) Antipsychotic

Additional Appendix Information
Beers Criteria – Potentially Inappropriate Medications for Geriatrics *on page 2271*

Use Management of psychotic disorders (control of mania, treatment of schizophrenia); control of nausea and vomiting; relief of restlessness and apprehension before surgery; acute intermittent porphyria; adjunct in the treatment of tetanus; intractable hiccups; combativeness and/or explosive hyperexcitable behavior in children 1-12 years of age and in short-term treatment of hyperactive children

Dosage
Children ≥6 months:
Schizophrenia/psychoses:
Oral: 0.5-1 mg/kg/dose every 4-6 hours; older children may require 200 mg/day or higher
IM, IV: 0.5-1 mg/kg/dose every 6-8 hours
<5 years (<22.7 kg): Maximum: 40 mg/day
5-12 years (22.7-45.5 kg): Maximum: 75 mg/day
Nausea and vomiting:
Oral: 0.5-1 mg/kg/dose every 4-6 hours as needed
IM, IV: 0.5-1 mg/kg/dose every 6-8 hours
<5 years (<22.7 kg): Maximum: 40 mg/day
5-12 years (22.7-45.5 kg): Maximum: 75 mg/day
Adults:
Schizophrenia/psychoses:
Oral: Range: 30-800 mg/day in 1-4 divided doses, initiate at lower doses and titrate as needed; usual dose: 200-600 mg/day; some patients may require 1-2 g/day
IM, IV: Initial: 25 mg, may repeat (25-50 mg) in 1-4 hours, gradually increase to a maximum of 400 mg/dose every 4-6 hours until patient is controlled; usual dose: 300-800 mg/day
Intractable hiccups:
Oral, IM: 25-50 mg 3-4 times/day
IV (refractory to oral or IM treatment): 25-50 mg via slow IV infusion
Nausea and vomiting:
Oral: 10-25 mg every 4-6 hours
IM, IV: 25-50 mg every 4-6 hours
Elderly: Behavioral symptoms associated with dementia (off-label use): Initial: 10-25 mg 1-2 times/day; increase at 4- to 7-day intervals by 10-25 mg/day. Increase dose intervals (bid, tid, etc) as necessary to control behavior response or side effects; maximum daily dose: 800 mg; gradual increases (titration) may prevent some side effects or decrease their severity.
Dosing comments in renal impairment: Hemodialysis: Not dialyzable (0% to 5%)
Dosing adjustment/comments in hepatic impairment: Avoid use in severe hepatic dysfunction

Additional Information Complete prescribing information should be consulted for additional detail.

Dosage Forms

Solution, Injection:
Generic: 25 mg/mL (1 mL, 2 mL)

Tablet, Oral:
Generic: 10 mg, 25 mg, 50 mg, 100 mg, 200 mg

◆ **Chlorpromazine Hydrochloride** *see* ChlorproMAZINE *on page 429*

◆ **Chlorpromazine Hydrochloride Inj (Can)** *see* ChlorproMAZINE *on page 429*

ChlorproPAMIDE (klor PROE pa mide)

Brand Names: Canada Apo-Chlorpropamide®

Pharmacologic Category Antidiabetic Agent, Sulfonylurea

Additional Appendix Information
Beers Criteria – Potentially Inappropriate Medications for Geriatrics *on page 2271*

Use Management of blood sugar in type 2 diabetes mellitus (noninsulin dependent, NIDDM) as an adjunct to diet and exercise to lower blood glucose

Pregnancy Risk Factor C

Dosage Oral: The dosage of chlorpropamide is variable and should be individualized based upon the patient's response
Initial dose:
Adults: 250 mg daily in mild-to-moderate diabetes in middle-aged, stable diabetic patients

Elderly: 100-125 mg daily

Note: After 5-7 days of initiation, subsequent daily dosages may be increased or decreased by 50-125 mg at 3- to 5-day intervals (slower upward titration may be appropriate in older patients)

Maintenance dose: 100-250 mg daily; severe diabetics may require 500 mg daily; avoid doses >750 mg daily

Dosage adjustment in renal impairment: No specific dosage adjustment provided in manufacturer's labeling; conservative initial and maintenance doses are recommended.

Alternate recommendations (Aronoff, 2007):

CrCl >50 mL/minute: Reduce dose by 50%.

CrCl <50 mL/minute: Avoid use.

Hemodialysis: Avoid use.

Peritoneal dialysis: Avoid use.

Continuous renal replacement therapy (CRRT): Avoid use.

Dosage adjustment in hepatic impairment: No specific dosage adjustment provided in manufacturer's labeling; conservative initial and maintenance doses are recommended in patients with liver impairment since chlorpropamide undergoes extensive hepatic metabolism.

Additional Information Complete prescribing information should be consulted for additional detail.

Dosage Forms

Tablet, Oral:

Generic: 100 mg, 250 mg

Chlorthalidone (klor THAL i done)

Brand Names: Canada Apo-Chlorthalidone

Index Terms Hygroton

Pharmacologic Category Antihypertensive; Diuretic, Thiazide

Use Management of mild-to-moderate hypertension when used alone or in combination with other agents; treatment of edema associated with heart failure, renal dysfunction, hepatic cirrhosis, or corticosteroid and estrogen therapy.

The 2014 guideline for the management of high blood pressure in adults (Eighth Joint National Committee [JNC 8]) recommends initiation of pharmacologic treatment to lower blood pressure for the following patients:

- Patients ≥60 years of age with systolic blood pressure (SBP) ≥150 mm Hg or diastolic blood pressure (DBP) ≥90 mm Hg. Goal of therapy is SBP <150 mm Hg and DBP <90 mm Hg.
- Patients <60 years of age with SBP ≥140 mm Hg or DBP is ≥90 mm Hg. Goal of therapy is SBP <140 mm Hg and DBP <90 mm Hg.
- Patients ≥18 years of age with diabetes and SBP ≥140 mm Hg or DBP ≥90 mm Hg. Goal of therapy is SBP <140 mm Hg and DBP <90 mm Hg.
- Patients ≥18 years of age with chronic kidney disease (CKD) and SBP ≥140 mm Hg or DBP ≥90 mm Hg. Goal of therapy is SBP <140 mm Hg and DBP <90 mm Hg.

In patients with CKD, regardless of race or diabetes status, the use of an ACE inhibitor (ACEI) or angiotensin receptor blocker (ARB) as initial therapy is recommended to improve kidney outcomes. In the general nonblack population (without CKD) including those with diabetes, initial antihypertensive treatment should consist of a thiazide-type diuretic, calcium channel blocker, ACEI, or ARB. In the general black population (without CKD), including those with diabetes, initial antihypertensive treatment should consist of a thiazide-type diuretic or a calcium channel blocker **instead of** an ACEI or ARB.

Pregnancy Risk Factor B

Dosage Oral:

Children and Adolescents: Hypertension (off-label use): Initial: 0.3 mg/kg once daily, up to 2 mg/kg/day; maximum: 50 mg daily (NHBPEP, 2004; NHLBI, 2011)

Adults:

Edema: Initial: 50 to 100 mg once daily or 100 mg on alternate days; maximum dose: 200 mg daily

Heart failure-associated edema: Initial: 12.5 to 25 mg once daily; maximum daily dose: 100 mg (ACCF/AHA [Yancy, 2013])

Hypertension: Initial: 25 mg once daily **or** 12.5 mg once daily (JNC 8 [James, 2013]); may increase after a suitable trial to 50 mg once daily; maximum: 100 mg daily; usual dosage range (ASH/ISH [Weber, 2014]): 12.5 to 25 mg daily. Target dose range (JNC 8 [James, 2013]): 12.5 to 25 mg daily.

Calcium nephrolithiasis (off-label use): 25 mg once daily (AUA Guidelines [Pearle, 2014])

Elderly: Initial: 12.5 to 25 mg once daily or every other day; there is little advantage to using doses >25 mg daily

Dosage adjustment in renal impairment:

CrCl ≥10 mL/minute: No dosage adjustment necessary (Aronoff, 2007)

CrCl <10 mL/minute: Avoid use. Ineffective with low GFR (Aronoff, 2007)

Dosage adjustment in hepatic impairment: There are no dosage adjustments provided in manufacturer's labeling; use with caution.

Additional Information Complete prescribing information should be consulted for additional detail.

Dosage Forms

Tablet, Oral:

Generic: 25 mg, 50 mg, 100 mg

◆ **Chlorthalidone and Azilsartan** *see* Azilsartan and Chlorthalidone *on page 215*

◆ **Chlor-Tripolon ND® (Can)** *see* Loratadine and Pseudoephedrine *on page 1242*

Chlorzoxazone (klor ZOKS a zone)

Brand Names: U.S. Lorzone; Parafon Forte DSC

Pharmacologic Category Skeletal Muscle Relaxant

Additional Appendix Information

Beers Criteria – Potentially Inappropriate Medications for Geriatrics *on page 2271*

Use Symptomatic treatment of muscle spasm and pain associated with acute musculoskeletal conditions

Dosage Muscle spasm:

Adults: Oral: 500 mg 3-4 times daily, may increase up to 750 mg 3-4 times daily. May consider dose reductions as symptoms improve.

Elderly: In general, avoid use or use cautiously at lower doses. Refer to adult dosing.

Dosage adjustment in renal impairment: No dosage adjustment provided in manufacturer's labeling.

Dosage adjustment in hepatic impairment: No dosage adjustment provided in manufacturer's labeling.

Additional Information Complete prescribing information should be consulted for additional detail.

Dosage Forms

Tablet, Oral:

Lorzone: 375 mg, 750 mg

Parafon Forte DSC: 500 mg

Generic: 500 mg

◆ **Cholecalciferol and Alendronate** *see* Alendronate and Cholecalciferol *on page 81*

◆ **Cholera and Traveler's Diarrhea Vaccine** *see* Travelers' Diarrhea and Cholera Vaccine [CAN/INT] *on page 2088*

◆ **Cholera Vaccine** *see* Travelers' Diarrhea and Cholera Vaccine [CAN/INT] *on page 2088*

Cholestyramine Resin (koe LES teer a meen REZ in)

Brand Names: U.S. Prevalite; Questran; Questran Light

Brand Names: Canada Novo-Cholamine; Novo-Cholamine Light; Olestyr; PMS-Cholestyramine; Questran; Questran Light Sugar Free; ZYM-Cholestyramine-Light; ZYM-Cholestyramine-Regular

Pharmacologic Category Antilipemic Agent, Bile Acid Sequestrant

Use Adjunct in the management of primary hypercholesterolemia; pruritus associated with elevated levels of bile acids; regression of arteriolosclerosis

Pregnancy Risk Factor C

Dosage Oral (dosages are expressed in terms of anhydrous resin):

Children (off-label use): 240 mg/kg/day in 2-3 divided doses; need to titrate dose depending on indication, response and tolerance; maximum: 8 g/day

Adults: Initial: 4 g 1-2 times/day; increase gradually over ≥1-month intervals; maintenance: 8-16 g/day divided in 2 doses; maximum: 24 g/day

Dosage adjustment in renal impairment: No dosage adjustment provided in manufacturer's labeling; however, use with caution in renal impairment; may cause hyperchloremic acidosis.

Dosage adjustment in hepatic impairment: No dosage adjustment necessary; not absorbed from the gastrointestinal tract.

Additional Information Complete prescribing information should be consulted for additional detail.

Dosage Forms

Packet, Oral:
- Prevalite: 4 g (1 ea, 42 ea, 60 ea)
- Questran: 4 g (1 ea, 60 ea)
- Generic: 4 g (1 ea, 60 ea)

Powder, Oral:
- Prevalite: 4 g/dose (231 g)
- Questran: 4 g/dose (378 g)
- Questran Light: 4 g/dose (210 g)
- Generic: 4 g/dose (210 g, 239.4 g, 378 g)

◆ **Choline Fenofibrate** *see* Fenofibrate and Derivatives *on page 852*

Choline Magnesium Trisalicylate
(KOE leen mag NEE zhum trye sa LIS i late)

Index Terms Tricosal; Trilisate

Pharmacologic Category Salicylate

Use

Acute painful shoulder: Management of acute painful shoulder

Analgesia: Relief of mild to moderate pain

Antipyresis: Management of pyrexia

Arthritis: Relief of signs/symptoms of osteoarthritis, rheumatoid arthritis, and other arthritis (long-term management and acute flares)

Juvenile rheumatoid arthritis: Anti-inflammatory or analgesic management (in children) of juvenile rheumatoid arthritis and other appropriate conditions

Pregnancy Risk Factor C

Dosage Note: Dosing is based on salicylate content. Individualize dose based on response; may require 2 to 3 weeks to achieve optimal effect.

Juvenile rheumatoid arthritis: Oral:

Children and Adolescents ≤37 kg: 50 mg/kg daily in 2 divided doses

Children and Adolescents >37 kg: 2250 mg daily in 2 divided doses

Acute painful shoulder, osteoarthritis, rheumatoid arthritis, or other severe arthritis: Adults: Oral: Initial: 1500 mg twice daily or 3000 mg once daily at bedtime

Analgesia (mild to moderate pain) or pyrexia: Adults: Oral: 2000 mg to 3000 mg daily in 2 or 3 divided doses; adjust dose to obtain optimal therapeutic response

Elderly: 750 mg 3 times daily; adjust dose to obtain optimum therapeutic response

Dosage adjustment in renal impairment: There are no dosage adjustments provided in the manufacturer's labeling; use with caution in acute or chronic renal impairment. Avoid use in severe renal impairment; monitor salicylate levels and adjust dose accordingly.

Dosage adjustment in hepatic impairment: There are no dosage adjustments provided in the manufacturer's labeling; use with caution in acute or chronic hepatic impairment; monitor salicylate levels and adjust dose accordingly.

Additional Information Complete prescribing information should be consulted for additional detail.

Dosage Forms

Liquid, Oral:
- Generic: 500 mg/5 mL (240 mL)

Tablet, Oral:
- Generic: 1000 mg

◆ **Chondroitin Sulfate and Sodium Hyaluronate** *see* Sodium Chondroitin Sulfate and Sodium Hyaluronate *on page 1905*

◆ **Choriogonadotropin Alfa** *see* Chorionic Gonadotropin (Recombinant) *on page 432*

◆ **Chorionic Gonadotropin for Injection (Can)** *see* Chorionic Gonadotropin (Human) *on page 431*

Chorionic Gonadotropin (Human)
(kor ee ON ik goe NAD oh troe pin, HYU man)

Brand Names: U.S. Novarel; Pregnyl

Brand Names: Canada Chorionic Gonadotropin for Injection; Pregnyl®

Index Terms CG; hCG

Pharmacologic Category Gonadotropin; Ovulation Stimulator

Use Induces ovulation and pregnancy in anovulatory, infertile females; treatment of hypogonadotropic hypogonadism, prepubertal cryptorchidism; spermatogenesis induction with follitropin alfa

Pregnancy Risk Factor X

Dosage IM:

Children: Various regimens:

Prepubertal cryptorchidism:

4000 units 3 times/week for 3 weeks **or**
5000 units every second day for 4 injections **or**
500 units 3 times/week for 4-6 weeks **or**
15 injections of 500-1000 units given over 6 weeks

Hypogonadotropic hypogonadism: Males:

500-1000 units 3 times/week for 3 weeks, followed by the same dose twice weekly for 3 weeks **or**
4000 units 3 times/week for 6-9 months, then reduce dosage to 2000 units 3 times/week for additional 3 months

Adults:

Induction of ovulation: Females: 5000-10,000 units one day following last dose of menotropins

Spermatogenesis induction associated with hypogonadotropic hypogonadism: Males: Treatment regimens vary (range: 1000-2000 units 2-3 times a week). Administer hCG until serum testosterone levels are normal (may require 2-3 months of therapy), then may add follitropin alfa or menopausal gonadotropin if needed to induce spermatogenesis; continue hCG at the dose required to maintain testosterone levels.

Dosage adjustment in renal impairment: No dosage adjustment provided in manufacturer's labeling; use with caution.

Dosage adjustment in hepatic impairment: No dosage adjustment provided in manufacturer's labeling.

Additional Information Complete prescribing information should be consulted for additional detail.

Dosage Forms

Solution Reconstituted, Intramuscular:

Novarel: 10,000 units (1 ea)
Pregnyl: 10,000 units (1 ea)
Generic: 10,000 units (1 ea)

Chorionic Gonadotropin (Recombinant)

(kor ee ON ik goe NAD oh troe pin ree KOM be nant)

Brand Names: U.S. Ovidrel

Brand Names: Canada Ovidrel®

Index Terms Choriogonadotropin Alfa; r-hCG

Pharmacologic Category Gonadotropin; Ovulation Stimulator

Use As part of an assisted reproductive technology (ART) program, induces ovulation in infertile females who have been pretreated with follicle stimulating hormones (FSH); induces ovulation and pregnancy in infertile females when the cause of infertility is functional

Pregnancy Risk Factor X

Dosage SubQ:

Adults: Females:

Assisted reproductive technologies (ART) and ovulation induction: 250 mcg given 1 day following the last dose of follicle stimulating agent. Use only after adequate follicular development has been determined. Hold treatment when there is an excessive ovarian response.

Elderly: Safety and efficacy have not been established

Dosage adjustment in renal impairment: Safety and efficacy have not been established

Dosage adjustment in hepatic impairment: Safety and efficacy have not been established

Additional Information Complete prescribing information should be consulted for additional detail.

Dosage Forms

Injectable, Subcutaneous:

Ovidrel: 250 mcg/0.5 mL (0.5 mL)

◆ **CI-1008** *see* Pregabalin *on page 1710*

◆ **Cialis** *see* Tadalafil *on page 1968*

Ciclesonide (Systemic) (sye KLES oh nide)

Brand Names: U.S. Alvesco

Brand Names: Canada Alvesco

Pharmacologic Category Corticosteroid, Inhalant (Oral)

Use Prophylactic management of bronchial asthma

Pregnancy Risk Factor C

Dosage Oral inhalation (Alvesco®):

Asthma: **Note:** Titrate to the lowest effective dose once asthma stability is achieved:

U.S. labeling: Children ≥12 years and Adults:

Prior therapy with bronchodilators alone: Initial: 80 mcg twice daily (maximum dose: 320 mcg/day)

Prior therapy with inhaled corticosteroids: Initial: 80 mcg twice daily (maximum dose: 640 mcg/day)

Prior therapy with oral corticosteroids: Initial: 320 mcg twice daily (maximum dose: 640 mcg/day)

Canadian labeling:

Children 6-11 years: Initial: 100-200 mcg once daily; maintenance: 100-200 mcg/day (1-2 puffs once daily)

Children ≥12 years and Adults: Initial: 400 mcg once daily; maintenance: 100-800 mcg/day (1-2 puffs once daily; more severe asthma may require 400 mcg twice daily)

Note: Canadian Thoracic Society 2010 Asthma Management guidelines recommend dose titration in children 6-11 years who fail to achieve an adequate response in spite of adherence to therapy and/or lack of alternative factors (eg, environmental triggers) which might impair response. In children ≥12 years and adults, doses >200 mcg/day may provide minimal additional benefit while increasing risks for adverse events; add-on therapy should be considered prior to dose increases >200 mcg/day (Lougheed, 2010).

Global Strategy for Asthma Management and Prevention, 2011: Children >5 years and Adults:

"Low" dose: 80-160 mcg/day
"Medium" dose: >160-320 mcg/day
"High" dose: >320 mcg/day

Conversion from oral to orally-inhaled steroid: Initiation of oral inhalation therapy should begin in patients who have previously been stabilized on oral corticosteroids (OCS). A gradual dose reduction of OCS should begin ~7-10 days after starting inhaled therapy. U.S. labeling recommends reducing prednisone dose no more rapidly than ≤2.5 mg/day on a weekly basis. The Canadian labeling recommends decreasing the daily dose of prednisone by 1 mg (or equivalent of other OCS) every 7 days in closely monitored patients, and every 10 days in patients whom close monitoring is not possible. In the presence of withdrawal symptoms, resume previous OCS dose for 1 week before attempting further dose reductions.

Dosage adjustment in renal impairment: There are no dosage adjustments provided in the manufacturer labeling (has not been studied); however, dose adjustments may not be necessary as ≤20% of drug is eliminated renally.

Dosage adjustment in hepatic impairment: Dosage adjustments are not necessary.

Additional Information Complete prescribing information should be consulted for additional detail.

Dosage Forms Considerations Alvesco 6.1 g canisters contain 60 inhalations.

Dosage Forms

Aerosol Solution, Inhalation:

Alvesco: 80 mcg/actuation (6.1 g); 160 mcg/actuation (6.1 g)

Dosage Forms: Canada

Aerosol for oral inhalation:

Alvesco®: 100 mcg/inhalation; 200 mcg/inhalation

Ciclesonide (Nasal) (sye KLES oh nide)

Brand Names: U.S. Omnaris; Zetonna

Brand Names: Canada Drymira; Omnaris; Omnaris HFA

Pharmacologic Category Corticosteroid, Nasal

Use Management of seasonal and perennial allergic rhinitis

Pregnancy Risk Factor C

Dosage Intranasal:

Seasonal allergic rhinitis:

Omnaris®:

U.S. labeling: Children ≥6 years and Adults: 2 sprays (50 mcg/spray) per nostril once daily; maximum: 200 mcg/day

Canadian labeling: Children ≥12 years and Adults: 2 sprays (50 mcg/spray) per nostril once daily; maximum: 200 mcg/day

Zetonna™: Children ≥12 years and Adults: 1 spray (37 mcg/spray) per nostril once daily; maximum: 74 mcg/day

Perennial allergic rhinitis: Children ≥12 years and Adults:

Omnaris®: 2 sprays (50 mcg/spray) per nostril once daily; maximum: 200 mcg/day

Zetonna™: 1 spray (37 mcg/spray) per nostril once daily; maximum: 74 mcg/day

Dosage adjustment in renal impairment: No dosage adjustment provided in manufacturer's labeling (has not been studied).

Dosage adjustment in hepatic impairment: No dosage adjustment necessary.

Additional Information Complete prescribing information should be consulted for additional detail.

Dosage Forms Considerations

Omnaris 12.5 g bottles contain 120 actuations.

Zetonna 6.1 g canisters contain 60 actuations.

Dosage Forms

Aerosol Solution, Nasal:

Zetonna: 37 mcg/actuation (6.1 g)

Suspension, Nasal:

Omnaris: 50 mcg/actuation (12.5 g)

◆ **Ciclodan** *see* Ciclopirox *on page 433*

◆ **Ciclodan Cream** *see* Ciclopirox *on page 433*

◆ **Ciclodan Solution** *see* Ciclopirox *on page 433*

Ciclopirox (sye kloe PEER oks)

Brand Names: U.S. Ciclodan; Ciclodan Cream; Ciclodan Solution; Ciclopirox Treatment; CNL8 Nail; Loprox; Pedipirox-4 Nail [DSC]; Penlac

Brand Names: Canada Apo-Ciclopirox; Loprox; Penlac; PMS-Ciclopirox; Stieprox; Taro-Ciclopirox

Index Terms Ciclopirox Olamine

Pharmacologic Category Antifungal Agent, Topical

Use

Cream/suspension: Treatment of tinea pedis (athlete's foot), tinea cruris (jock itch), tinea corporis (ringworm), cutaneous candidiasis, and tinea versicolor (pityriasis)

Gel: Treatment of tinea pedis (athlete's foot), tinea corporis (ringworm); seborrheic dermatitis of the scalp

Lacquer (solution): Topical treatment of mild-to-moderate onychomycosis of the fingernails and toenails due to *Trichophyton rubrum* (not involving the lunula) and the immediately-adjacent skin

Shampoo: Treatment of seborrheic dermatitis of the scalp

Pregnancy Risk Factor B

Dosage Topical:

Children >10 years and Adults: Tinea pedis, tinea cruris, tinea corporis, cutaneous candidiasis, and tinea versicolor: Cream/suspension: Apply twice daily, gently massage into affected areas; if no improvement after 4 weeks of treatment, re-evaluate the diagnosis.

Children ≥12 years and Adults: Onychomycosis of the fingernails and toenails: Lacquer (solution): Apply to adjacent skin and affected nails daily (as a part of a comprehensive management program for onychomycosis). Remove with alcohol every 7 days.

Children >16 years and Adults:

Tinea pedis, tinea corporis: Gel: Apply twice daily, gently massage into affected areas and surrounding skin; if no improvement after 4 weeks of treatment, re-evaluate diagnosis

Seborrheic dermatitis of the scalp:

Gel: Apply twice daily, gently massage into affected areas and surrounding skin; if no improvement after 4 weeks of treatment, re-evaluate diagnosis.

Shampoo: Apply ~5 mL to wet hair; lather, and leave in place ~3 minutes; rinse. May use up to 10 mL for longer hair. Repeat twice weekly for 4 weeks; allow a minimum of 3 days between applications; if no improvement after 4 weeks of treatment, re-evaluate diagnosis.

Dosage adjustment in renal impairment: No dosage adjustment provided in manufacturer's labeling.

Dosage adjustment in hepatic impairment: No dosage adjustment provided in manufacturer's labeling.

Additional Information Complete prescribing information should be consulted for additional detail.

Dosage Forms

Cream, External:

Ciclodan: 0.77% (90 g)

Generic: 0.77% (15 g, 30 g, 90 g)

Gel, External:

Generic: 0.77% (30 g, 45 g, 100 g)

Kit, External:

Ciclodan Cream: 0.77%

Ciclodan Solution: 8%

Ciclopirox Treatment: 8%

CNL8 Nail: 8%

Generic: 8%

Shampoo, External:

Loprox: 1% (120 mL)

Generic: 1% (120 mL)

Solution, External:

Ciclodan: 8% (6.6 mL)

Penlac: 8% (6.6 mL)

Generic: 8% (6.6 mL)

Suspension, External:

Generic: 0.77% (30 mL, 60 mL)

◆ **Ciclopirox Olamine** *see* Ciclopirox *on page 433*

◆ **Ciclopirox Treatment** *see* Ciclopirox *on page 433*

◆ **Ciclosporin** *see* CycloSPORINE (Ophthalmic) *on page 529*

◆ **Ciclosporin** *see* CycloSPORINE (Systemic) *on page 522*

◆ **Cidecin** *see* DAPTOmycin *on page 563*

Cidofovir (si DOF o veer)

Brand Names: U.S. Vistide

Pharmacologic Category Antiviral Agent

Use Treatment of cytomegalovirus (CMV) retinitis in patients with acquired immunodeficiency syndrome (AIDS). **Note:** Should be administered with probenecid.

Pregnancy Risk Factor C

Pregnancy Considerations [U.S. Boxed Warning]: Possibly carcinogenic and teratogenic based on animal data. May cause hypospermia. Cidofovir was shown to be teratogenic and embryotoxic in animal studies, some at doses which also produced maternal toxicity. Reduced testes weight and hypospermia were also noted in animal studies. There are no adequate and well-controlled studies in pregnant women; use during pregnancy only if the potential benefit to the mother outweighs the possible risk to the fetus. Women of childbearing potential should use effective contraception during therapy and for 1 month following treatment. Males should use a barrier contraceptive during therapy and for 3 months following treatment.

Breast-Feeding Considerations The CDC recommends **not** to breast-feed if diagnosed with HIV to avoid postnatal transmission of the virus.

Contraindications Hypersensitivity to cidofovir; history of clinically-severe hypersensitivity to probenecid or other sulfa-containing medications; serum creatinine >1.5 mg/dL; CrCl <55 mL/minute; urine protein ≥100 mg/dL (≥2+ proteinuria); use with or within 7 days of nephrotoxic agents; direct intraocular injection

Warnings/Precautions Hazardous agent - use appropriate precautions for handling and disposal (NIOSH 2014 [group 2]).

[U.S. Boxed Warning]: Dose-dependent nephrotoxicity requires dose adjustment or discontinuation if changes in renal function occur during therapy (eg, proteinuria, glycosuria, decreased serum phosphate, uric acid or bicarbonate, and elevated creatinine). Neutropenia has been reported; monitor counts during therapy. Cases of ocular hypotony have also occurred; monitor intraocular pressure. Monitor for signs of metabolic acidosis. Safety and efficacy have not been established in the elderly. Administration must be accompanied by oral probenecid and intravenous saline prehydration. **[U.S. Boxed Warning]: Indicated only for CMV retinitis treatment in HIV patients; possibly carcinogenic and teratogenic based on animal data. May cause hypospermia.**

Adverse Reactions

Cardiovascular: Cardiomyopathy, cardiovascular disorder, CHF, edema, orthostatic hypotension, shock, syncope, tachycardia

Central nervous system: Agitation, amnesia, anxiety, chills, confusion, convulsion, dizziness, fever, hallucinations, headache, insomnia, malaise, pain, vertigo

Dermatologic: Alopecia, photosensitivity reaction, skin discoloration, urticaria

Endocrine & metabolic: Adrenal cortex insufficiency

Gastrointestinal: Abdominal pain, anorexia, aphthous stomatitis, colitis, constipation, diarrhea, dysphagia, fecal incontinence, gastritis, GI hemorrhage, gingivitis, melena, nausea, proctitis, splenomegaly, stomatitis, tongue discoloration, vomiting

Genitourinary: Urinary incontinence

Hematologic: Anemia, hypochromic anemia, leukocytosis, leukopenia, lymphadenopathy, lymphoma-like reaction, neutropenia, pancytopenia, thrombocytopenia, thrombocytopenic purpura

Local: Injection site reaction

Neuromuscular & skeletal: Tremor, weakness

Ocular: Amblyopia, blindness, cataract, conjunctivitis, corneal lesion, diplopia, intraocular pressure decreased, iritis, ocular hypotony, uveitis, vision abnormal

Otic: Hearing loss

Renal: Creatinine increased, Fanconi syndrome, proteinuria, renal toxicity

Respiratory: Cough, dyspnea, pneumonia

Rare but important or life-threatening: Hepatic failure, metabolic acidosis, pancreatitis

Miscellaneous: Allergic reaction, infection, oral moniliasis, sepsis, serum bicarbonate decreased

Drug Interactions

Metabolism/Transport Effects None known.

Avoid Concomitant Use There are no known interactions where it is recommended to avoid concomitant use.

Increased Effect/Toxicity

Cidofovir may increase the levels/effects of: Tenofovir

Decreased Effect There are no known significant interactions involving a decrease in effect.

Preparation for Administration Hazardous agent; use appropriate precautions for handling and disposal (NIOSH 2014 [group 2]).

Dilute dose in NS 100 mL prior to infusion.

Storage/Stability Store at controlled room temperature 20°C to 25°C (68°F to 77°F). Store admixtures under refrigeration for ≤24 hours. Cidofovir infusion admixture should be administered within 24 hours of preparation at room temperature or refrigerated. Admixtures should be allowed to equilibrate to room temperature prior to use.

Mechanism of Action Cidofovir is converted to cidofovir diphosphate which is the active intracellular metabolite; cidofovir diphosphate suppresses CMV replication by selective inhibition of viral DNA synthesis. Incorporation of cidofovir into growing viral DNA chain results in reductions in the rate of viral DNA synthesis.

Pharmacodynamics/Kinetics The following pharmacokinetic data is based on a combination of cidofovir administered with probenecid:

Distribution: V_d: 0.54 L/kg; does not cross significantly into CSF

Protein binding: <6%

Metabolism: Minimal; phosphorylation occurs intracellularly

Half-life elimination, plasma: ~2.6 hours

Excretion: Urine

Dosage Adults:

Induction: 5 mg/kg IV over 1 hour once weekly for 2 consecutive weeks

Maintenance: 5 mg/kg over 1 hour once every other week

Note: Administer with probenecid 2 g orally 3 hours prior to each cidofovir dose and 1 g at 2 hours and 8 hours after completion of the infusion (total: 4 g)

Hydrate with at least 1 L of 0.9% NS IV prior to each cidofovir infusion; infuse saline over a 1- to 2-hour period immediately prior to cidofovir infusion. A second liter may be administered over a 1- to 3-hour period at the start of cidofovir infusion or immediately following infusion, if tolerated

Dosage adjustment in renal impairment:

Changes in renal function during therapy: If the creatinine increases by 0.3-0.4 mg/dL, reduce the cidofovir dose to 3 mg/kg; discontinue therapy for increases ≥0.5 mg/dL or development of ≥3+ proteinuria

Preexisting renal impairment: Use is contraindicated with serum creatinine >1.5 mg/dL, CrCl <55 mL/minute, or urine protein ≥100 mg/dL (≥2+ proteinuria)

Dosage adjustment in hepatic impairment: No dosage adjustment provided in manufacturer's labeling.

Administration For IV infusion only. Infuse over 1 hour. Hydrate with 1 L of 0.9% NS IV prior to cidofovir infusion. A second liter may be administered over a 1- to 3-hour period immediately following infusion, if tolerated.

Hazardous agent; use appropriate precautions for handling and disposal (NIOSH 2014 [group 2]).

Monitoring Parameters Serum creatinine and urine protein (within 48 hours of each dose), WBCs (prior to each dose); intraocular pressure and visual acuity, signs and symptoms of uveitis/iritis

Dosage Forms

Solution, Intravenous:

Vistide: 75 mg/mL (5 mL)

Solution, Intravenous [preservative free]:

Generic: 75 mg/mL (5 mL)

◆ **Cilastatin and Imipenem** *see* Imipenem and Cilastatin *on page 1051*

Cilazapril [CAN/INT] (sye LAY za pril)

Brand Names: Canada Apo-Cilazapril; CO Cilazapril; Inhibace; Mylan-Cilazapril; Novo-Cilazapril; PHL-Cilazapril; PMS-Cilazapril

Index Terms Cilazapril Monohydrate

Pharmacologic Category Angiotensin-Converting Enzyme (ACE) Inhibitor; Antihypertensive

Use Note: Not approved in U.S.

Management of hypertension; adjunctive treatment of heart failure (HF)

Note: The ACCF/AHA 2013 heart failure guidelines recommend the use of ACE inhibitors, along with other guideline directed medical therapies, to prevent heart failure in patients with a reduced ejection fraction who have a history of MI (Stage B HF), to prevent heart failure in any patient with a reduced ejection fraction (Stage B HF), or to treat those with heart failure and reduced ejection fraction (Stage C HFrEF) (ACCF/AHA [Yancy, 2013]).

Pregnancy Considerations **[Canadian Boxed Warning]: Use of cilazapril is contraindicated during pregnancy. Drugs that act on the renin-angiotensin system can cause injury and death to the developing fetus. Discontinue as soon as possible once pregnancy is detected. Females planning pregnancy should be switched to alternative therapy that has been proven safe during pregnancy.** Teratogenic effects may occur following maternal use during pregnancy. Drugs that act on the renin-angiotensin system are associated with oligohydramnios. Oligohydramnios, due to decreased fetal renal function, may lead to fetal lung hypoplasia and skeletal malformations. Their use in pregnancy is also associated with anuria, hypotension, renal failure, skull hypoplasia, and death in the fetus/neonate. Chronic maternal hypertension itself is also associated with adverse events in the mother and fetus/infant. However, ACE inhibitors are not recommended during pregnancy to treat maternal hypertension or heart failure. Use of an ACE inhibitor should also be avoided in any woman of reproductive age. The exposed fetus should be monitored for fetal growth, amniotic fluid volume, and organ formation. Infants exposed to an ACE inhibitor *in utero* should be monitored for hyperkalemia, hypotension, and oliguria.

Breast-Feeding Considerations It is not known if cilazapril is excreted into breast milk. Use is contraindicated in nursing women.

Contraindications Hypersensitivity to cilazapril, any other ACE inhibitor, or any component of the formulation; angioedema related to previous treatment with an ACE inhibitor; hereditary or idiopathic angioedema; ascites; concomitant use with aliskiren-containing drugs in patients with diabetes mellitus (type 1 or 2) or moderate-to-severe renal impairment (GFR <60 mL/minute/1.73 m^2); pregnancy; breast-feeding

Warnings/Precautions **[Canadian Boxed Warning]: Use is contraindicated during pregnancy. Drugs that act on the renin-angiotensin system can cause injury and death to the developing fetus. Discontinue as soon as possible once pregnancy is detected.**

Anaphylactic reactions may occur rarely with ACE inhibitors. At any time during treatment (especially following first dose) angioedema may occur rarely with ACE inhibitors; it may involve the head and neck (potentially compromising the airway) or the intestine (presenting with abdominal pain). Black-skinned patients of African descent and patients with idiopathic or hereditary angioedema may be at an increased risk. Prolonged frequent monitoring may be required especially if tongue, glottis, or larynx are involved as they are associated with airway obstruction. Patients with a history of airway surgery may have a higher risk of airway obstruction. Aggressive early and appropriate management is critical. Use in patients with previous angioedema associated with ACE inhibitor therapy or hereditary or idiopathic angioedema is contraindicated. Severe anaphylactoid reactions may be seen during hemodialysis (eg, CVVHD) with high-flux dialysis membranes (eg, AN69). Rare cases of anaphylactoid reactions have been reported in patients undergoing sensitization treatment with hymenoptera (bee, wasp) venom while receiving ACE inhibitors.

Symptomatic hypotension with or without syncope can occur with ACE inhibitors (usually with the first several doses); effects are most often observed in volume depleted patients; correct volume depletion prior to initiation; close monitoring of patient is required especially with initial dosing and dosing increases; blood pressure must be lowered at a rate appropriate for the patient's clinical condition. Initiation of therapy in patients with ischemic heart disease or cerebrovascular disease warrants close observation due to the potential consequences posed by falling blood pressure (eg, MI, stroke). Use with caution in hypertrophic cardiomyopathy with outflow tract obstruction, severe aortic stenosis, or before, during, or immediately after major surgery.

Hyperkalemia may occur with ACE inhibitors; risk factors include renal dysfunction, diabetes mellitus, concomitant use of potassium-sparing diuretics, potassium supplements and/or potassium-containing salts. Use cautiously, if at all, with these agents and monitor potassium closely. Cough may occur with ACE inhibitors. Other causes of cough should be considered (eg, pulmonary congestion in patients with heart failure) and excluded prior to discontinuation.

May be associated with deterioration of renal function and/or increases in serum creatinine, particularly in patients with low renal blood flow (eg, renal artery stenosis, heart failure) whose glomerular filtration rate (GFR) is dependent on efferent arteriolar vasoconstriction by angiotensin II; deterioration may result in oliguria, acute renal failure, and progressive azotemia. Small increases in serum creatinine may occur following initiation; consider discontinuation only in patients with progressive and/or significant deterioration in renal function. Use with caution in patients with unstented unilateral/bilateral renal artery stenosis. When unstented bilateral renal artery stenosis is present, use is generally avoided due to the elevated risk of deterioration in renal function unless possible benefits outweigh risks.

Antihypertensive effect of ACE inhibitors is reduced in black-skinned patients of African descent. Use with caution in patients with preexisting liver dysfunction and/or cirrhosis without ascites (contraindicated in patients with ascites); close monitoring is required and a dose reduction may be necessary. Rare toxicities associated with ACE inhibitors include cholestatic jaundice (which may progress to fulminant hepatic necrosis), agranulocytosis, neutropenia, or leukopenia with myeloid hypoplasia. Patients with collagen vascular diseases (especially with concomitant renal impairment) or renal impairment alone may be at increased risk for hematologic toxicity; periodically monitor CBC with differential in these patients. Contains lactose; avoid use in patients with galactose intolerance, Lapp lactase deficiency, or glucose-galactose malabsorption.

Adverse Reactions

Cardiovascular: Hypotension (symptomatic), orthostatic hypotension, palpitation

Central nervous system: Dizziness, fatigue, headache

Gastrointestinal: Nausea

Neuromuscular & skeletal: Weakness

Renal: Increased serum creatinine

Respiratory: Cough

Rare but important or life-threatening: Angina, angioedema, arrhythmia, atrial fibrillation, AV block, bradycardia, bronchospasm, cardiac decompensation, cardiac failure, depression, extrasystoles, GI bleed, hemolytic anemia, hyperglycemia, hyperkalemia, MI, neutropenia, pancreatitis, paresthesia, renal failure, Stevens-Johnson syndrome, syncope, tachycardia, thrombocytopenic purpura, visual hallucinations (Doane, 2013)

Drug Interactions

Metabolism/Transport Effects None known.

Avoid Concomitant Use There are no known interactions where it is recommended to avoid concomitant use.

Increased Effect/Toxicity

Cilazapril may increase the levels/effects of: Allopurinol; Amifostine; Antihypertensives; AzaTHIOprine; DULoxetine; Ferric Gluconate; Gold Sodium Thiomalate; Grass Pollen Allergen Extract (5 Grass Extract); Hypotensive Agents; Iron Dextran Complex; Levodopa; Lithium; Nonsteroidal Anti-Inflammatory Agents; Obinutuzumab; RisperiDONE; RiTUXimab; Sodium Phosphates

The levels/effects of Cilazapril may be increased by: Alfuzosin; Aliskiren; Angiotensin II Receptor Blockers; Barbiturates; Brimonidine (Topical); Canagliflozin; Dapoxetine; Diazoxide; DPP-IV Inhibitors; Eplerenone; Everolimus; Heparin; Heparin (Low Molecular Weight); Herbs (Hypotensive Properties); Loop Diuretics; MAO Inhibitors; Nicorandil; Pentoxifylline; Phosphodiesterase 5 Inhibitors; Potassium Salts; Potassium-Sparing Diuretics; Prostacyclin Analogues; Sirolimus; Temsirolimus; Thiazide Diuretics; TiZANidine; Tolvaptan; Trimethoprim

Decreased Effect

The levels/effects of Cilazapril may be decreased by: Aprotinin; Herbs (Hypertensive Properties); Icatibant; Lanthanum; Methylphenidate; Nonsteroidal Anti-Inflammatory Agents; Salicylates; Yohimbine

Food Interactions Cilazapril serum concentrations may be decreased if taken with food (no apparent effect on activity). Management: Administer without regard to food.

Storage/Stability Store at 15°C to 30°C (59°F to 86°F).

Mechanism of Action Cilazapril is a prodrug that is rapidly converted to cilazaprilat (active metabolite), a competitive inhibitor of angiotensin-converting enzyme (ACE); prevents conversion of angiotensin I to angiotensin II, a potent vasoconstrictor; results in lower levels of angiotensin II which causes an increase in plasma renin activity and a reduction in aldosterone secretion.

Pharmacodynamics/Kinetics

Onset of action: ~1-2 hours

Peak effect: Antihypertensive effect: 3-7 hours; Heart failure (reduction of systemic vascular resistance and pulmonary capillary wedge pressure): 2-4 hours

Duration: Therapeutic effect: Up to 24 hours

Absorption: Rapid

Metabolism: Cilazapril (prodrug) hydrolyzed to active metabolite (cilazaprilat)

Bioavailability: Cilazaprilat: 57%

Half-life elimination: Cilazaprilat: Terminal: Single dose: 36-49 hours; Multidose: ~54 hours

Time to peak: Cilazaprilat: Within 2 hours

Excretion: Cilazaprilat: Urine (53% unchanged)

Dosage Oral:

Heart failure:

Adults: Initial: 0.5 mg once daily; if tolerated, after 5 days increase to 1 mg/day (lowest maintenance dose); may increase to usual maximum of 2.5 mg once daily. (**Note:** Some additional benefit has been observed with doses up to 5 mg/day in a few patients.)

Elderly: Initial: 0.5 mg once daily; if tolerated, after 5 days increase to 1 mg/day (lowest maintenance dose); may increase to maximum of 2.5 mg once daily

Hypertension:

Adults: Initial: 2.5 mg once daily; titrate to response at intervals of at least 2 weeks. Usual dose: 2.5-5 mg once daily (maximum dose: 10 mg/day). **Note:** May administer total daily dose in 2 divided doses if antihypertensive effect diminishes over 24-hour dosing interval.

Combination therapy with diuretic: Initial: 0.5 mg once daily; titrate slowly as tolerated

Elderly: Initial: ≤1.25 mg once daily; titrate slowly as tolerated

Combination therapy with diuretic: Initial: 0.5 mg once daily; titrate slowly as tolerated

Dosage adjustment in renal impairment:

Heart failure:

CrCl >40 mL/minute: Initial 0.5 mg once daily (maximum dose: 2.5 mg once daily). **Note:** The manufacturer labeling does not define the estimated creatinine clearance value at which a dosage adjustment is not required.

CrCl 10-40 mL/minute: Initial: 0.25-0.5 mg once daily (maximum dose: 2.5 mg once daily)

CrCl <10 mL/minute: Use is not recommended.

Hypertension:

CrCl >40 mL/minute: Initial: 1 mg once daily (maximum dose: 5 mg once daily). **Note:** The manufacturer labeling does not define the estimated creatinine clearance value at which a dosage adjustment is not required.

CrCl 10-40 mL/minute: Initial: 0.5 mg once daily (maximum dose: 2.5 mg once daily)

CrCl <10 mL/minute: Use is not recommended.

Dosage adjustment in hepatic impairment: Cirrhotic patients (without ascites): Hypertension: Initial: ≤0.5 mg once daily (use with caution)

Dietary Considerations May be taken with or without food.

Administration May be administered with or without food.

Monitoring Parameters Serum creatinine, BUN, electrolytes, LFT (at baseline and periodically thereafter in patients with preexisting hepatic impairment), CBC with differential (in patients with renal impairment and/or collagen vascular disease); serum glucose (patients with diabetes); blood pressure

Product Availability Not available in U.S.

Dosage Forms: Canada

Tablet, Oral: 1 mg, 2.5 mg, 5 mg

Cilazapril and Hydrochlorothiazide [CAN/INT] (sye LAY za pril & hye droe klor oh THYE a zide)

Brand Names: Canada Apo-Cilazapril/Hctz; Inhibace Plus; Novo-Cilazapril/HCTZ

Index Terms Cilazapril Monohydrate and Hydrochlorothiazide; Hydrochlorothiazide and Cilazapril

Pharmacologic Category Angiotensin-Converting Enzyme (ACE) Inhibitor; Diuretic, Thiazide

Use Note: Not approved in U.S.

Treatment of mild-to-moderate hypertension; not indicated for initial treatment of hypertension

Pregnancy Considerations [Canadian Boxed Warning]: Drugs that act on the renin-angiotensin system can cause injury and death to the developing fetus. Discontinue as soon as possible once pregnancy is detected. Use is contraindicated in pregnant women. See individual agents.

Breast-Feeding Considerations Hydrochlorothiazide is excreted into breast milk; use of this combination is contraindicated in nursing women

Contraindications Hypersensitivity to cilazapril, hydrochlorothiazide, or any component of the formulation; hypersensitivity to other ACE inhibitors, thiazides or sulfonamide-derived drugs; history of angioedema related to previous treatment with an ACE inhibitor; hereditary or idiopathic angioedema; anuria; patients with ascites; concomitant use with aliskiren-containing drugs in patients with diabetes mellitus (type 1 or type 2) or moderate-to-severe renal impairment (GFR <60 mL/minute/1.73 m^2); pregnancy; breast-feeding

Warnings/Precautions See individual agents.

Adverse Reactions

Cardiovascular: Palpitation

Central nervous system: Dizziness, fatigue, somnolence

Gastrointestinal: Nausea

Genitourinary: Polyuria

Hematologic: Transient neutropenia

Hepatic: Transaminases increased

Respiratory: Cough

Rare but important or life-threatening: Acute interstitial pneumonitis, acute pulmonary edema, acute renal failure, agranulocytosis, alkaline phosphatase increased, angina, angioedema, arthralgia, atrial fibrillation, bleeding time increased, bradycardia, BUN increased, cerebrovascular disorder, cholestatic hepatitis (with or without necrosis), depression, dermatitis, diaphoresis, diplopia, dyspepsia, dyspnea, erythema multiforme, extrasystoles, facial edema, GGT increased, gout, hemolytic anemia, hyperbilirubinemia, hyponatremia, hypotension (including postural), hypothermia, insomnia, leukorrhea, malaise, melena, MI, myalgia, neurosis, pancreatitis, paresthesia, paroniria, pemphigus, peripheral edema, peripheral ischemia, pruritus, pseudoporphyria, purpura, rash, Stevens-Johnson syndrome, stroke, tachycardia, thrombocytopenia, tinnitus, toxic epidermal necrolysis, transaminases increased, vertigo, vision abnormal, vomiting, xerostomia

Drug Interactions

Metabolism/Transport Effects None known.

Avoid Concomitant Use

Avoid concomitant use of Cilazapril and Hydrochlorothiazide with any of the following: Dofetilide

Increased Effect/Toxicity

Cilazapril and Hydrochlorothiazide may increase the levels/effects of: ACE Inhibitors; Allopurinol; Amifostine; Antihypertensives; AzaTHIOprine; Benazepril; Calcium Salts; CarBAMazepine; Cardiac Glycosides; Cyclophosphamide; Diazoxide; Dofetilide; DULoxetine; Ferric Gluconate; Gold Sodium Thiomalate; Grass Pollen Allergen Extract (5 Grass Extract); Hypotensive Agents; Iron Dextran Complex; Ivabradine; Levodopa; Lithium; Multivitamins/Minerals (with ADEK, Folate, Iron); Multivitamins/Minerals (with AE, No Iron); Nonsteroidal Anti-Inflammatory Agents; Obinutuzumab; OXcarbazepine; Porfimer; RisperiDONE; RiTUXimab; Sodium Phosphates; Topiramate; Toremifene; Verteporfin; Vitamin D Analogs

The levels/effects of Cilazapril and Hydrochlorothiazide may be increased by: Alcohol (Ethyl); Alfuzosin; Aliskiren; Analgesics (Opioid); Angiotensin II Receptor Blockers; Anticholinergic Agents; Barbiturates; Beta2-Agonists; Brimonidine (Topical); Canagliflozin; Corticosteroids (Orally Inhaled); Corticosteroids (Systemic); Dapoxetine; Dexketoprofen; Diazoxide; DPP-IV Inhibitors; Eplerenone; Everolimus; Heparin; Heparin (Low Molecular Weight); Herbs (Hypotensive Properties); Licorice; Loop Diuretics; MAO Inhibitors; Multivitamins/Fluoride (with ADE); Nicorandil; Pentoxifylline; Phosphodiesterase 5 Inhibitors; Potassium Salts; Potassium-Sparing Diuretics; Prostacyclin Analogues; Selective Serotonin Reuptake Inhibitors; Sirolimus; Temsirolimus; Thiazide Diuretics; TiZANidine; Tolvaptan; Trimethoprim

Decreased Effect

Cilazapril and Hydrochlorothiazide may decrease the levels/effects of: Antidiabetic Agents

The levels/effects of Cilazapril and Hydrochlorothiazide may be decreased by: Aprotinin; Benazepril; Bile Acid Sequestrants; Herbs (Hypertensive Properties); Icatibant; Lanthanum; Methylphenidate; Nonsteroidal Anti-Inflammatory Agents; Salicylates; Yohimbine

Storage/Stability Store at 15°C to 30°C (59°F to 86°F).

Pharmacodynamics/Kinetics See individual agents.

Dosage Oral:

Adults: See individual agents. Initiate therapy with combination product only after successful titration of individual agents to adequate blood pressure control. Dose is individualized; range: Cilazapril: 2.5-10 mg; Hydrochlorothiazide: 6.25-25 mg daily

Elderly: Reduction of initial dose may be necessary.

Dosage adjustment in renal impairment:

CrCl ≥10 mL/minute: Cilazapril dose reduction is necessary; see individual agents

CrCl <10 mL/minute: Use is not recommended. Hydrochlorothiazide is usually ineffective with a GFR <30 mL/minute. With severe renal impairment, a loop diuretic is preferred for use with cilazapril.

Dosage adjustment in hepatic impairment: Cirrhotic patients (without ascites): Cilazapril dose reduction is necessary; see individual agents

Dietary Considerations May be taken with or without food.

Administration Oral: Administer with or without food in the morning to avoid nocturia.

Monitoring Parameters Blood pressure; BUN, serum creatinine, and electrolytes; liver function tests (at baseline and then periodically thereafter in patients with preexisting hepatic dysfunction); if patient has collagen vascular disease and/or renal impairment, periodically monitor CBC with differential

Product Availability Not available in U.S.

Dosage Forms: Canada

Tablet: 5/12.5: Cilazapril 5 mg and hydrochlorothiazide 12.5 mg

Inhibace® Plus 5/12.5: Cilazapril 5 mg and hydrochlorothiazide 12.5 mg

- **Cilazapril Monohydrate** *see* Cilazapril [CAN/INT] *on page 434*
- **Cilazapril Monohydrate and Hydrochlorothiazide** *see* Cilazapril and Hydrochlorothiazide [CAN/INT] *on page 436*

Cilostazol (sil OH sta zol)

Brand Names: U.S. Pletal

Index Terms OPC-13013

Pharmacologic Category Antiplatelet Agent; Phosphodiesterase-3 Enzyme Inhibitor

Additional Appendix Information

Oral Antiplatelet Comparison Chart *on page 2239*

Use Symptomatic management of peripheral vascular disease, primarily intermittent claudication

Pregnancy Risk Factor C

Pregnancy Considerations Adverse events have been observed in animal reproduction studies.

Breast-Feeding Considerations It is not known if cilostazol is excreted in human milk. According to the manufacturer, the decision to continue or discontinue breast-feeding during therapy should take into account the risk of exposure to the infant and the benefits of treatment to the mother.

Contraindications Hypersensitivity to cilostazol or any component of the formulation; heart failure (HF) of any severity; hemostatic disorders or active bleeding

Warnings/Precautions [U.S. Boxed Warning]: The use of this drug is contraindicated in patients with heart failure. Use with caution in severe underlying heart disease. Use with caution in patients receiving other platelet aggregation inhibitors or in patients with thrombocytopenia. Discontinue therapy if thrombocytopenia or leukopenia occur; progression to agranulocytosis (reversible) has been reported when cilostazol was not immediately stopped. Withhold for at least 4-6 half-lives prior to elective surgical procedures. Use caution in moderate-to-severe hepatic impairment. Use cautiously in severe renal impairment (CrCl <25 mL/minute). Potentially significant drug-drug interactions may exist, requiring dose or frequency adjustment, additional monitoring, and/or selection of alternative therapy.

Adverse Reactions

Cardiovascular: Palpitation, peripheral edema, tachycardia

Central nervous system: Dizziness, headache

Gastrointestinal: Abdominal pain, abnormal stools, diarrhea, dyspepsia, flatulence, nausea

Infection: Increased susceptibility to infection

Neuromuscular & skeletal: Back pain, myalgia

Respiratory: Cough, pharyngitis, rhinitis

Rare but important or life-threatening: Agranulocytosis, anemia, aplastic anemia, asthma, atrial fibrillation, atrial flutter, blindness, blood pressure increased, bursitis, cardiac arrest, cardiac failure, cerebral hemorrhage, cerebral infarction, cerebrovascular accident, chest pain, cholelithiasis, colitis, coronary stent thrombosis, cystitis, diabetes mellitus, duodenal ulcer, duodenitis, ecchymoses, esophageal hemorrhage, esophagitis, gastrointestinal hemorrhage, gout, granulocytopenia, hematoma (extradural), hemorrhage, hemorrhage (eye), hepatic insufficiency, hot flash, hyperglycemia, hypotension, interstitial pneumonitis, intracranial hemorrhage, jaundice, leukopenia, myocardial infarction, neuralgia, nodal arrhythmia, orthostatic hypotension, pain, peptic ulcer, periodontal abscess, pneumonia, polycythemia, prolonged Q-T interval on ECG, pruritus, pulmonary hemorrhage, rectal hemorrhage, retinal hemorrhage, retroperitoneal hemorrhage, skin hypertrophy, Stevens-Johnson syndrome, subdural hematoma, supraventricular tachycardia, syncope, thrombocytopenia, thrombosis, torsades de pointes, vaginal hemorrhage, ventricular tachycardia

Drug Interactions

Metabolism/Transport Effects Substrate of CYP1A2 (minor), CYP2C19 (major), CYP2D6 (minor), CYP3A4 (major); **Note:** Assignment of Major/Minor substrate status based on clinically relevant drug interaction potential

Avoid Concomitant Use

Avoid concomitant use of Cilostazol with any of the following: Conivaptan; Fusidic Acid (Systemic); Idelalisib; Urokinase

Increased Effect/Toxicity

Cilostazol may increase the levels/effects of: Agents with Antiplatelet Properties; Anticoagulants; Apixaban; Collagenase (Systemic); Dabigatran Etexilate; Ibritumomab; Obinutuzumab; Riociguat; Rivaroxaban; Salicylates; Thrombolytic Agents; Tositumomab and Iodine I 131 Tositumomab; Urokinase

The levels/effects of Cilostazol may be increased by: Anagrelide; Antifungal Agents (Azole Derivatives, Systemic); Aprepitant; Ceritinib; Conivaptan; CYP2C19 Inhibitors (Moderate); CYP2C19 Inhibitors (Strong); CYP3A4 Inhibitors (Moderate); CYP3A4 Inhibitors (Strong); Dasatinib; Esomeprazole; Fosaprepitant; Fusidic Acid (Systemic); Glucosamine; Herbs (Anticoagulant/Antiplatelet Properties); Ibrutinib; Idelalisib; Ivacaftor; Limaprost; Luliconazole; Macrolide Antibiotics; Mifepristone; Multivitamins/Fluoride (with ADE); Multivitamins/Minerals (with ADEK, Folate, Iron); Multivitamins/Minerals (with AE, No Iron); Netupitant; Omega-3 Fatty Acids; Omeprazole; Pentosan Polysulfate Sodium; Pentoxifylline; Prostacyclin Analogues; Simeprevir; Stiripentol; Tipranavir; Vitamin E

Decreased Effect

The levels/effects of Cilostazol may be decreased by: Bosentan; CYP3A4 Inducers (Moderate); CYP3A4 Inducers (Strong); Dabrafenib; Deferasirox; Mitotane; Siltuximab; St Johns Wort; Tocilizumab

Food Interactions Taking cilostazol with a high-fat meal may increase peak concentration by 90%. Grapefruit juice may increase serum levels of cilostazol and enhance toxic effects. Management: Administer cilostazol on an empty stomach 30 minutes before or 2 hours after meals. Avoid concurrent ingestion of grapefruit juice.

Storage/Stability Store at 20°C to 25°C (68°F to 77°F); protect from light.

Mechanism of Action Cilostazol and its metabolites are inhibitors of phosphodiesterase III. As a result, cyclic AMP is increased leading to reversible inhibition of platelet aggregation, vasodilation, and inhibition of vascular smooth muscle cell proliferation.

Pharmacodynamics/Kinetics

Onset of action: 2-4 weeks; may require up to 12 weeks

Protein binding: Cilostazol 95% to 98%; active metabolites 66% to 97%

Metabolism: Hepatic via CYP3A4 (primarily), 1A2, 2C19, and 2D6; 2 active metabolites

Half-life elimination: 11-13 hours

Excretion: Urine (74%) and feces (20%) as metabolites

Dosage Adults: Oral:

Intermittent claudication: 100 mg twice daily (when refractory to exercise therapy and smoking cessation, use in combination with either aspirin or clopidogrel) (Guyatt, 2012)

PCI (following elective stent placement) (off-label use): 100 mg twice daily in combination with aspirin or clopidogrel. **Note:** Only recommended in patients with an allergy or intolerance to either aspirin or clopidogrel (Guyatt, 2012).

Secondary prevention of noncardioembolic stroke or TIA (off-label use): 100 mg twice daily. **Note:** Clopidogrel or aspirin/extended release dipyridamole recommended over the use of cilostazol (Guyatt, 2012).

Dosage adjustment for cilostazol with concomitant medications:

CYP2C19 inhibitors (eg, omeprazole): Dosage of cilostazol should be reduced to 50 mg twice daily

CYP3A4 inhibitors (eg, ketoconazole, itraconazole, erythromycin, diltiazem): Dosage of cilostazol should be reduced to 50 mg twice daily

Dosage adjustment in renal impairment: No dosage adjustment provided in the manufacturer's labeling; use with caution.

Dosage adjustment in hepatic impairment: No dosage adjustment provided in manufacturer's labeling (has not been studied in moderate-to-severe hepatic impairment); use with caution.

Dietary Considerations It is best to take cilostazol 30 minutes before or 2 hours after meals (breakfast and dinner).

Administration Administer cilostazol 30 minutes before or 2 hours after meals (breakfast and dinner).

Dosage Forms

Tablet, Oral:

Pletal: 50 mg, 100 mg

Generic: 50 mg, 100 mg

◆ **Ciloxan** *see* Ciprofloxacin (Ophthalmic) *on page 446*

Cimetidine (sye MET i deen)

Brand Names: U.S. Cimetidine Acid Reducer [OTC]; Tagamet HB [OTC]

Brand Names: Canada Apo-Cimetidine; Dom-Cimetidine; Mylan-Cimetidine; Novo-Cimetidine; Nu-Cimet; PMS-Cimetidine

Pharmacologic Category Histamine H_2 Antagonist

Use Short-term treatment of active duodenal ulcers and benign gastric ulcers; maintenance therapy of duodenal ulcer; treatment of gastric hypersecretory states; treatment of gastroesophageal reflux disease (GERD)

OTC labeling: Prevention or relief of heartburn, acid indigestion, or sour stomach

Pregnancy Risk Factor B

Dosage Oral:

Children: 20-40 mg/kg/day in divided doses every 6 hours

Children ≥12 years and Adults: Heartburn, acid indigestion, sour stomach (OTC labeling): 200 mg up to twice daily; may take 30 minutes prior to eating foods or beverages expected to cause heartburn or indigestion

Adults:

Short-term treatment of active ulcers: 300 mg 4 times/day or 800 mg at bedtime or 400 mg twice daily for up to 8 weeks

Note: Higher doses of 1600 mg at bedtime for 4 weeks may be beneficial for a subpopulation of patients with larger duodenal ulcers (>1 cm defined endoscopically) who are also heavy smokers (≥1 pack/day).

Duodenal ulcer prophylaxis: 400 mg at bedtime

Gastric hypersecretory conditions: 300-600 mg every 6 hours; dosage not to exceed 2.4 g/day

Gastroesophageal reflux disease: 400 mg 4 times/day or 800 mg twice daily for 12 weeks

Helicobacter pylori eradication (off-label use): 400 mg twice daily; requires combination therapy with antibiotics

Interstitial cystitis (bladder pain syndrome) (off-label use): 600 to 800 mg daily in divided doses as 200 mg 3 times daily or as 300 to 400 mg twice daily (Dasgupta, 2001; Seshadri, 1994; Thilagarajah, 2001)

Dosing adjustment/interval in renal impairment: Children and Adults:

CrCl 10-50 mL/minute: Administer 50% of normal dose

CrCl <10 mL/minute: Administer 25% of normal dose

Hemodialysis: Slightly dialyzable (5% to 20%); administer after dialysis

Dosing adjustment/comments in hepatic impairment: Usual dose is safe in mild liver disease but use with caution and in reduced dosage in severe liver disease; increased risk of CNS toxicity in cirrhosis suggested by enhanced penetration of CNS

Additional Information Complete prescribing information should be consulted for additional detail.

Dosage Forms

Solution, Oral:

Generic: 300 mg/5 mL (237 mL, 240 mL)

Tablet, Oral:

Cimetidine Acid Reducer [OTC]: 200 mg

Tagamet HB [OTC]: 200 mg

Generic: 200 mg, 300 mg, 400 mg, 800 mg

◆ **Cimetidine Acid Reducer [OTC]** *see* Cimetidine *on page 438*

◆ **Cimzia** *see* Certolizumab Pegol *on page 409*

◆ **Cimzia Prefilled** *see* Certolizumab Pegol *on page 409*

◆ **Cimzia Starter Kit** *see* Certolizumab Pegol *on page 409*

Cinacalcet (sin a KAL cet)

Brand Names: U.S. Sensipar

Brand Names: Canada Sensipar

Index Terms AMG 073; Cinacalcet Hydrochloride

Pharmacologic Category Calcimimetic

Use

Hyperparathyroidism, primary: Treatment of severe hypercalcemia in adult patients with primary hyperparathyroidism for whom parathyroidectomy would be indicated on the basis of serum calcium levels, but who are unable to undergo parathyroidectomy

Hyperparathyroidism, secondary: Treatment of secondary hyperparathyroidism in adult patients with chronic kidney disease (CKD) on dialysis.

Limitation of use: Not indicated for use in patients with CKD who are not on dialysis (due to the increased risk of hypocalcemia)

Parathyroid carcinoma: Treatment of hypercalcemia in adult patients with parathyroid carcinoma

Pregnancy Risk Factor C

Pregnancy Considerations Adverse events have been observed in animal reproduction studies. Women who become pregnant during cinacalcet treatment are encouraged to enroll in Amgen's Pregnancy Surveillance Program (1-800-772-6436).

Breast-Feeding Considerations It is not known if cinacalcet is excreted in breast milk. Due to the potential for clinically significant adverse reactions in the nursing infant, the manufacturer recommends a decision be made whether to discontinue nursing or the drug, taking into account the importance of treatment to the mother. Women who choose to continue nursing during cinacalcet treatment are encouraged to enroll in Amgen's Lactation Surveillance Program (1-800-772-6436).

Contraindications

Serum calcium lower than the lower limit of normal range

Canadian labeling: Additional contraindications (not in U.S. labeling): Hypersensitivity to any component of the formulation

Warnings/Precautions Life-threatening and fatal events associated with hypocalcemia have occurred. Use is contraindicated if the serum calcium is less than the lower limit of the normal range. Monitor serum calcium and for symptoms of hypocalcemia (eg, muscle cramps, myalgia, paresthesia, seizure, tetany); may require treatment interruption, dose reduction, or initiation (or dose increases) of calcium-based phosphate binder and/or vitamin D to raise serum calcium depending on calcium levels or symptoms of hypocalcemia. Use with caution in patients with a seizure disorder (seizure threshold is lowered by significant serum calcium reductions); monitor calcium levels closely. Adynamic bone disease may develop if intact parathyroid hormone (iPTH) levels are suppressed <100 pg/mL; reduce dose or discontinue use of cinacalcet and/or vitamin D if iPTH levels decrease below 150 pg/mL.

Use caution in patients with moderate-to-severe hepatic impairment (Child-Pugh classes B and C); monitor serum calcium, serum phosphorus and iPTH closely. In the U.S., the long-term safety and efficacy of cinacalcet has not been evaluated in chronic kidney disease (CKD) patients with hyperparathyroidism not requiring dialysis. Not indicated for CKD patients not receiving dialysis. Although possibly related to lower baseline calcium levels, clinical studies have shown an increased incidence of hypocalcemia (<8.4 mg/dL) in patients not requiring dialysis. Cases of idiosyncratic hypotension, worsening of heart failure, and/or arrhythmia have been reported in patients with impaired cardiovascular function; may correlate with decreased serum calcium. QT prolongation and ventricular arrhythmia secondary to hypocalcemia have also been reported. Potentially significant interactions may exist, requiring dose or frequency adjustment, additional monitoring, and/or selection of alternative therapy.

Adverse Reactions

Cardiovascular: Hypertension, hypotension

Central nervous system: Depression, dizziness, fatigue, headache, noncardiac chest pain, paresthesia, seizure

Endocrine & metabolic: Dehydration, hypercalcemia, hyperkalemia, hypocalcemia, hypoparathyroidism (intact parathyroid hormone)

Gastrointestinal: Abdominal pain, anorexia, constipation, decreased appetite, diarrhea, dyspepsia, nausea, vomiting, upper abdominal pain

Hematologic & oncologic: Anemia

Neuromuscular & skeletal: Arthralgia, back pain, bone fracture, limb pain, muscle spasm, myalgia, weakness

Respiratory: Cough, dyspnea, upper respiratory tract infection

Hypersensitivity: Hypersensitivity reaction

Infection: Localized infection (dialysis access site)

Rare but important or life-threatening:Adynamic bone disease, cardiac arrhythmia, cardiac failure, hypotension (idiosyncratic), prolonged Q-T interval on ECG (secondary to hypocalcemia), ventricular arrhythmia (secondary to hypocalcemia)

Drug Interactions

Metabolism/Transport Effects Substrate of CYP1A2 (minor), CYP2D6 (minor), CYP3A4 (major); **Note:** Assignment of Major/Minor substrate status based on clinically relevant drug interaction potential; **Inhibits** CYP2D6 (strong)

Avoid Concomitant Use

Avoid concomitant use of Cinacalcet with any of the following: Conivaptan; Fusidic Acid (Systemic); Idelalisib; Pimozide; Tamoxifen; Thioridazine

Increased Effect/Toxicity

Cinacalcet may increase the levels/effects of: ARIPiprazole; AtoMOXetine; CYP2D6 Substrates; DOXOrubicin (Conventional); Eliglustat; Fesoterodine; Iloperidone; Metoprolol; Nebivolol; Pimozide; Propafenone; Tetrabenazine; Thioridazine; Tricyclic Antidepressants; Vortioxetine

The levels/effects of Cinacalcet may be increased by: Aprepitant; Ceritinib; Conivaptan; CYP3A4 Inhibitors (Moderate); CYP3A4 Inhibitors (Strong); Dasatinib; Fosaprepitant; Fusidic Acid (Systemic); Idelalisib; Ivacaftor; Luliconazole; Mifepristone; Netupitant; Simeprevir; Stiripentol

Decreased Effect

Cinacalcet may decrease the levels/effects of: Codeine; Iloperidone; Tacrolimus (Systemic); Tamoxifen; TraMADol

Food Interactions Food increases bioavailability. Management: Administer with food or shortly after a meal.

Storage/Stability Store at 25°C (77°F); excursions permitted to 15°C to 30°C (59°F to 86°F).

Mechanism of Action Increases the sensitivity of the calcium-sensing receptor on the parathyroid gland thereby, concomitantly lowering parathyroid hormone (PTH), serum calcium, and serum phosphorus levels, preventing progressive bone disease and adverse events associated with mineral metabolism disorders.

Pharmacodynamics/Kinetics

Distribution: V_d: ~1,000 L

Protein binding: ~93% to 97%

Metabolism: Hepatic (extensive) via CYP3A4, 2D6, 1A2; forms inactive metabolites

Half-life elimination: Terminal: 30 to 40 hours; moderate hepatic impairment: 65 hours; severe hepatic impairment: 84 hours

Time to peak, plasma: ~2 to 6 hours; increased with food.

Excretion: Urine ~80% (as metabolites); feces ~15%

Dosage Note: Do not titrate dose more frequently than every 2 to 4 weeks. May be used alone or in combination with vitamin D and/or phosphate binders. Dosage adjustment may be required in patients on concurrent CYP3A4 inhibitors.

Hyperparathyroidism, primary: Adults: Oral: Initial: 30 mg twice daily; increase dose incrementally (to 60 mg twice daily, 90 mg twice daily, and 90 mg 3 or 4 times daily) as necessary to normalize serum calcium levels.

Hyperparathyroidism, secondary: Adults: Oral: Initial: 30 mg once daily; increase dose incrementally (to 60 mg once daily, 90 mg once daily, 120 mg once daily, and 180 mg once daily) as necessary to maintain iPTH level between 150 to 300 pg/mL.

Parathyroid carcinoma: Adults: Oral: Initial: 30 mg twice daily; increase dose incrementally (to 60 mg twice daily, 90 mg twice daily, and 90 mg 3 or 4 times daily) as necessary to normalize serum calcium levels.

Dosage adjustment for hypocalcemia:

If serum calcium >7.5 mg/dL but <8.4 mg/dL **or** if hypocalcemia symptoms occur: Use calcium-containing phosphate binders and/or vitamin D to raise calcium levels.

If serum calcium <7.5 mg/dL **or** if hypocalcemia symptoms persist and the dose of vitamin D cannot be increased: Withhold cinacalcet until serum calcium ≥8 mg/dL and/or symptoms of hypocalcemia resolve. Reinitiate cinacalcet at the next lowest dose.

If iPTH <150 pg/mL: Reduce dose or discontinue cinacalcet and/or vitamin D.

Dosage adjustment in renal impairment: No dosage adjustment necessary.

Dosage adjustment in hepatic impairment:

Mild impairment (Child-Pugh class A): No dosage adjustment necessary.

Moderate to severe impairment (Child-Pugh class B or C); may have an increased exposure to cinacalcet and increased half-life. Dosage adjustments may be necessary based on serum calcium, serum phosphorus, and/or iPTH.

Administration Administer with food or shortly after a meal. Do not break or divide tablet; should be taken whole.

Monitoring Parameters

Monitor for signs/symptoms of hypocalcemia. Monitor serum calcium and iPTH concentrations closely in patients on concurrent CYP3A4 inhibitors, with hepatic impairment or with seizure disorders.

Hyperparathyroidism, secondary: Serum calcium and phosphorus levels prior to initiation and within a week of initiation and frequently during dose titration; iPTH should be measured 1 to 4 weeks after initiation or dosage adjustment (wait at least 12 hours after dose before drawing iPTH levels). After the maintenance dose is established, obtain serum calcium levels monthly.

Parathyroid carcinoma and hyperparathyroidism, primary: Serum calcium levels prior to initiation and within a week of initiation or dosage adjustment; once maintenance dose is established, obtain serum calcium every 2 months.

Reference Range

CKD K/DOQI guidelines definition of stages; chronic disease is kidney damage or GFR <60 mL/minute/1.73 m^2 for ≥3 months:

Stage 2: GFR 60 to 89 mL/minute/1.73 m^2 (kidney damage with mild decrease GFR)

Stage 3: GFR 30 to 59 mL/minute/1.73 m^2 (moderate decrease GFR)

Stage 4: GFR 15 to 29 mL/minute/1.73 m^2 (severe decrease GFR)

Stage 5: GFR <15 mL/minute/1.73 m^2 or dialysis (kidney failure)

Target range for iPTH: Adults:

Stage 3 CKD: 35 to 70 pg/mL

Stage 4 CKD: 70 to 110 pg/mL

Stage 5 CKD: 150 to 300 pg/mL

Serum phosphorus: Adults:

Stage 3 and 4 CKD: ≥2.7 to <4.6 mg/dL

Stage 5 CKD: 3.5 to 5.5 mg/dL

Serum calcium-phosphorus product: Adults: Stage 3 to 5 CKD: <55 mg^2/dL^2

Dosage Forms

Tablet, Oral:

Sensipar: 30 mg, 60 mg, 90 mg

◆ **Cinacalcet Hydrochloride** *see* Cinacalcet *on page 439*

Cinnarizine [INT] (si NAR i zeen)

International Brand Names Antigeron (BR); Antimet (ZA); Aplactan (JP); Aplexal (JP); Apomiterl (JP); Apotomin

(JP); Apsatan (JP); Artate (JP); Bo Rui Te (CN); Brawmicin (VN); Carecin (JP); Cebridin (UY); Celenid (MY, SG); Cerebolan (JP); Cerebrin (PK); Cerepar (CH, HN, SA); Cinabioquim (AR); Cinact (IN); Cinadil (PE, PY); Cinageron (BR); Cinar (JO); Cinaren (VE); Cinarin (LB, PH); Cinarizin (HR); Cinarizina (AR, BR, ES); Cinarizina Ratiopharm (ES, PT); Cinaziere (GB); Cinazin (CH); Cinazyn (IT); Cinedil (HR); Cinergil (CL); Cinna (DE, MY, SG, TH); Cinnabene (AT, CZ); Cinnabloc (PH); Cinnaforte (DE); Cinnageron (CH); Cinnamed (CH); Cinnar (SG); Cinnarizin AL (DE); Cinnarizin R.A.N. (DE); Cinnarizin Siegfried (DE); cinnarizin von ct (DE); Cinnarizin-ratiopharm (DE); Cinnaron (CY, SG); Cinnipirine (NL); Cinon Forte (PT); Cintigo (ID); Cisaken[tabs] (MX); Corathiem (HN, JP); Cronogeron (BR); Cysten (JP); Denapol (JP); Derozin (GR); Dismaren (AR); Dizzigo (IN); Dizzinon (PH); Eglen (JP); Fabracin (AR); Folcodal (AR); Glanyl (KR); Hilactan (JP); Hirdsyn (JP); Iroplex (AR); Katoseran (JP); Libotasin (GR); Natropas (AR); Nazin (SG); Nazine (TH); Novertigo (PK); Pericephal (AT); Pervasum (ES); Purazine (ZA); Razlin (JP); Roin (JP); Salarizine (JP); Sapratol (JP); Sepan (DK); Sinver (VE); Siptazin (JP); Spaderizine (JP); Stabin (KR); Stugeron (AR, BE, BH, BR, CH, CL, CO, CY, CZ, EE, EG, ES, GB, GR, HK, HN, HR, HU, ID, IE, IN, IT, JO, KW, LB, LT, LU, MX, MY, PE, PH, PK, PT, PY, QA, RO, SA, SG, SI, SK, TH, TR, UY, VE, VN, ZA); Stugeron Forte (EC, GB, HR); Stunarone (IL); Stutgeron (AT, DE, HU, IE); Toliman (IT); Torizin (JP); Uphageron (MY); Vasogeron (PY); Venoxil (MX); Vericin (VE); Vertigon (ID, SG); Vessel (BR)

Pharmacologic Category Antiemetic

Reported Use Management of vestibular symptoms, including vertigo, dizziness, tinnitus, nystagmus, nausea, and vomiting; prophylaxis of migraine; prophylaxis of motion sickness; adjunct therapy for symptoms of peripheral or cerebral vascular disease

Dosage Range Oral:

Children 5-12 years: 12.5 mg 3-4 times daily or 7.5-15 mg 3 times daily

Children >12 years and Adolescents: 25 mg 3-4 times daily or 30 mg 3 times daily

Adults: Usual dose range: 25-75 mg 3 times daily. Maximum daily dose: 225 mg daily

Product Availability Product available in various countries; not currently available in the U.S.

Dosage Forms

Tablet: 15 mg; 25 mg

- **Cinryze** *see* C1 Inhibitor (Human) *on page 315*
- **Cipralex (Can)** *see* Escitalopram *on page 765*
- **Cipralex MELTZ (Can)** *see* Escitalopram *on page 765*
- **Cipro** *see* Ciprofloxacin (Systemic) *on page 441*
- **Cipro XL (Can)** *see* Ciprofloxacin (Systemic) *on page 441*
- **Ciprodex** *see* Ciprofloxacin and Dexamethasone *on page 446*

Ciprofibrate [INT] (sye proe FYE brate)

International Brand Names Cetaxin (PE); Cibrato (BR); Ciprolip (BR); Dislipen (PY); Dublina (CL); Estaprol (AR, CL, UY); Fibrolip (CO, UY); Fixeril (AR, UY); Giabri (CL, CO); Hiperlipen (CO, EC, PE, PY, VE); Hyperlipen (BE, CH); Lipanor (CZ, EE, FR, HN, IL, KR, PL, PT, RU); Lipobrand (EC); Modalim (CN, CY, ID, KW, MY, NL, PH, SA, SG, TR, VN); Orodaxin (BR); Savilen (GR); Trifolget (PE)

Pharmacologic Category Antilipemic Agent, Fibric Acid

Reported Use Hypertriglyceridemia, severe; mixed hyperlipidemia

Dosage Range Adults: Oral: 100 mg/day (maximum: 100 mg daily)

Product Availability Product available in various countries; not currently available in the U.S.

Dosage Forms

Tablet, oral: 100 mg

Ciprofloxacin (Systemic) (sip roe FLOKS a sin)

Brand Names: U.S. Cipro; Cipro in D5W; Cipro XR

Brand Names: Canada ACT Ciprofloxacin; Apo-Ciproflox; Auro-Ciprofloxacin; Cipro; Cipro XL; Ciprofloxacin Injection; Ciprofloxacin Injection USP; Ciprofloxacin Intravenous Infusion; Ciprofloxacin Intravenous Infusion BP; Dom-Ciprofloxacin; JAMP-Ciprofloxacin; Mar-Ciprofloxacin; Mint-Ciproflox; Mint-Ciprofloxacin; Mylan-Ciprofloxacin; Novo-Ciprofloxacin; PHL-Ciprofloxacin; PMS-Ciprofloxacin; PMS-Ciprofloxacin XL; PRO-Ciprofloxacin; RAN-Ciproflox; ratio-Ciprofloxacin; Riva-Ciprofloxacin; Sandoz-Ciprofloxacin; Septa-Ciprofloxacin; Taro-Ciprofloxacin

Index Terms Ciprofloxacin Hydrochloride

Pharmacologic Category Antibiotic, Fluoroquinolone

Use

Children: Complicated urinary tract infections and pyelonephritis due to *E. coli*. **Note:** Although effective, ciprofloxacin is not the drug of first choice in children.

Children and Adults: To reduce incidence or progression of disease following exposure to aerolized *Bacillus anthracis*.

Adults: Treatment of the following infections when caused by susceptible bacteria: Urinary tract infections; acute uncomplicated cystitis in females; chronic bacterial prostatitis; lower respiratory tract infections (including acute exacerbations of chronic bronchitis); acute sinusitis; skin and skin structure infections; bone and joint infections; complicated intra-abdominal infections (in combination with metronidazole); infectious diarrhea; typhoid fever due to *Salmonella typhi* (eradication of chronic typhoid carrier state has not been proven); uncomplicated cervical and urethra gonorrhea (due to *N. gonorrhoeae*); nosocomial pneumonia; empirical therapy for febrile neutropenic patients (in combination with piperacillin)

Note: As of April 2007, the CDC no longer recommends the use of fluoroquinolones for the treatment of gonococcal disease.

Pregnancy Risk Factor C

Pregnancy Considerations Adverse events have been observed in some animal reproduction studies. Ciprofloxacin crosses the placenta and produces measurable concentrations in the amniotic fluid and cord serum (Ludlam 1997). Based on available data, an increased risk of teratogenic effects has not been observed following ciprofloxacin use during pregnancy (Bar-Oz 2009; Padberg 2014). Ciprofloxacin is recommended for prophylaxis and treatment of pregnant women exposed to anthrax (Meaney-Delman 2014). Serum concentrations of ciprofloxacin may be lower during pregnancy than in nonpregnant patients (Giamarellou 1989).

Breast-Feeding Considerations Ciprofloxacin is excreted in breast milk. Due to the potential for serious adverse reactions in the nursing infant, the manufacturer recommends a decision be made whether to discontinue nursing or to discontinue the drug, taking into account the importance of treatment to the mother. However infant serum levels were undetectable (<0.03 mcg/mL) in one report (Gardner 1992). There has been a single case report of perforated pseudomembranous colitis in a breast-feeding infant whose mother was taking ciprofloxacin (Harmon 1992). Ciprofloxacin is recommended for the prophylaxis and treatment of *Bacillus anthracis* in lactating women (Meaney-Delman 2014).

Contraindications Hypersensitivity to ciprofloxacin, any component of the formulation, or other quinolones; concurrent administration of tizanidine

Warnings/Precautions [U.S. Boxed Warning]: There have been reports of tendon inflammation and/or rupture with quinolone antibiotics in all ages; risk may be increased with concurrent corticosteroids, solid organ transplant recipients, and in patients >60 years of age. Rupture of the Achilles tendon sometimes requiring surgical repair has been reported most frequently; but other tendon sites (eg, rotator cuff, biceps) have also been reported. Strenuous physical activity, rheumatoid arthritis, and renal impairment may be an independent risk factor for tendonitis. Inflammation and rupture may occur bilaterally. Cases have been reported within the first 48 hours, during, and up to several months after discontinuation of therapy. Discontinue at first sign of tendon inflammation or pain. Use with caution in patients with rheumatoid arthritis; may increase risk of tendon rupture. Use with caution in patients with a history of tendon disorders.

CNS effects may occur (tremor, restlessness, confusion, and hallucinations, increased intracranial pressure [including pseudotumor cerebri] or seizures). Reactions may occur following the first dose. Use with caution in patients with known or suspected CNS disorder or consider discontinuation if CNS effects develop. Potential for seizures, although very rare, may be increased with concomitant NSAID therapy. Use with caution in individuals at risk of seizures (CNS disorders or concurrent therapy with medications which may lower seizure threshold; status epilepticus has occurred) or if clinically appropriate, consider alternative antimicrobial therapy. Discontinue if seizures occur.

Fluoroquinolones may prolong QTc interval; avoid use in patients with a history of or at risk for QTc prolongation, torsade de pointes, uncorrected hypokalemia, hypomagnesemia, cardiac disease (heart failure, myocardial infarction, bradycardia) or concurrent administration of other medications known to prolong the QT interval (including Class Ia and Class III antiarrhythmics, cisapride, erythromycin, antipsychotics, and tricyclic antidepressants). Hepatocellular, cholestatic, or mixed liver injury has been reported, including hepatic necrosis, life-threatening hepatic events, and fatalities. Acute liver injury can be rapid onset (range: 1-39 days), often associated with hypersensitivity. Most fatalities occurred in patients >55 years of age. Discontinue immediately if signs/symptoms of hepatitis (abdominal tenderness, dark urine, jaundice, pruritus) occur. Additionally, temporary increases in transaminases or alkaline phosphatase or cholestatic jaundice may occur (highest risk in patients with previous liver damage).

Prolonged use may result in fungal or bacterial superinfection, including *C. difficile*-associated diarrhea (CDAD) and pseudomembranous colitis; CDAD has been observed >2 months postantibiotic treatment. Rarely crystalluria has occurred; urine alkalinity may increase the risk. Ensure adequate hydration during therapy. Adverse effects, including those related to joints and/or surrounding tissues, are increased in pediatric patients and therefore, ciprofloxacin should not be considered as drug of choice in children (exception is anthrax treatment). Peripheral neuropathy has been reported (rare); may occur soon after initiation of therapy and may be irreversible; discontinue if symptoms of sensory or sensorimotor neuropathy occur.

Fluoroquinolones have been associated with the development of serious, and sometimes fatal, hypoglycemia, most often in elderly diabetics but also in patients without diabetes. This occurred most frequently with gatifloxacin (no longer available systemically), but may occur at a lower frequency with other quinolones.

Severe hypersensitivity reactions, including anaphylaxis, have occurred with quinolone therapy. Reactions may present as typical allergic symptoms after a single dose, or may manifest as severe idiosyncratic dermatologic, vascular, pulmonary, renal, hepatic, and/or hematologic events, usually after multiple doses. Prompt discontinuation of drug should occur if skin rash or other symptoms arise. **[U.S. Boxed Warning]: Quinolones may exacerbate myasthenia gravis; avoid use (rare, potentially life-threatening weakness of respiratory muscles may occur).** Use caution in renal impairment. Avoid excessive sunlight and take precautions to limit exposure (eg, loose fitting clothing, sunscreen); may cause moderate-to-severe photosensitivity/phototoxicity reactions. Discontinue use if photosensitivity occurs. Since ciprofloxacin is ineffective in the treatment of syphilis and may mask symptoms, all patients should be tested for syphilis at the time of gonorrheal diagnosis and 3 months later. Hemolytic reactions may (rarely) occur with quinolone use in patients with latent or actual glucose-6-phosphate dehydrogenase (G6PD) deficiency.

Potentially significant interactions may exist, requiring dose or frequency adjustment, additional monitoring, and/or selection of alternative therapy. Serious and fatal reactions including seizures, status epilepticus, cardiac arrest and respiratory failure have been reported with concomitant administration of theophylline. If concurrent use is unavoidable, monitor serum theophylline levels and adjust theophylline dose as warranted.

Adverse Reactions

Central nervous system: Fever, headache (IV administration); neurologic events (includes dizziness, insomnia, nervousness, somnolence); restlessness (IV administration)

Dermatologic: Rash

Gastrointestinal: Abdominal pain, diarrhea, dyspepsia, nausea, vomiting

Hepatic: ALT increased, AST increased

Local: Injection site reactions (IV administration)

Respiratory: Rhinitis

Rare but important or life-threatening: Abnormal gait, acute generalized exanthemous pustulosis (AGEP), acute renal failure, agitation, agranulocytosis, albuminuria, alkaline phosphatase increase, allergic reactions, anaphylactic shock, anemia, angina pectoris, angioedema, anorexia,anxiety, arthralgia, ataxia, atrial flutter, bilirubin (serum) increase, bone marrow depression (life-threatening), bronchospasm, BUN increased, candidiasis, cardiopulmonary arrest, chills, cholestatic jaundice, chromatopsia, *Clostridium difficile*-associated diarrhea (CDAD), confusion, constipation, CPK increase, crystalluria (particularly in alkaline urine), cylindruria, delirium, depression (including self-injurious behavior), dizziness, drowsiness, dyspepsia (adults), dyspnea, edema, eosinophilia, erythema multiforme/nodosum, exfoliative dermatitis, fever (adults), fixed eruption, gastrointestinal bleeding, gout flare, hallucinations, headache (oral), hematocrit decreased, hematuria, hemoglobin decreased, hemolytic anemia, hepatic failure (some fatal), hepatic necrosis, hyper-/hypoglycemia, hyper-/hypotension, hyperesthesia, hyperpigmentation, hypertonia, insomnia, interstitial nephritis, intestinal perforation, intracranial pressure increased, irritability, joint pain, laryngeal edema, LDH increased, lightheadedness, lipase increased, lymphadenopathy, malaise, manic reaction, methemoglobinemia, MI, migraine, myalgia, myasthenia gravis exacerbation, myoclonus, nephritis, nightmares, nystagmus, palpitation, pancreatitis, pancytopenia (life-threatening or fatal), paranoia, peripheral neuropathy, petechiae, photosensitivity/toxicity, pneumonitis, polyneuropathy, prolongation of PT/INR (in patients treated with vitamin K antagonists), pseudotumor cerebri, psychosis (toxic), PT decrease, pulmonary edema, renal calculi, seizure (including grand mal), serum cholesterol increased, serum creatinine increased, serum sickness-like reactions, serum triglycerides increased, status epilepticus, Stevens-Johnson syndrome, suicidal thoughts/ideation/attempts and completions, syncope, tachycardia, taste loss, tendon rupture, tendonitis, thrombocytopenia, thrombocytosis, thrombophlebitis, tinnitus, torsade de pointes, toxic epidermal necrolysis, tremor, twitching, unresponsiveness, urethral bleeding, uric acid increased, vaginitis, vasculitis, ventricular arrhythmia, visual disturbance, weakness

Drug Interactions

Metabolism/Transport Effects Substrate of OAT3, P-glycoprotein; **Inhibits** CYP1A2 (strong), CYP3A4 (weak)

Avoid Concomitant Use

Avoid concomitant use of Ciprofloxacin (Systemic) with any of the following: Agomelatine; BCG; CloZAPine; DULoxetine; Highest Risk QTc-Prolonging Agents; Ivabradine; Mifepristone; Pimozide; Pomalidomide; Strontium Ranelate; Tasimelteon; TiZANidine

Increased Effect/Toxicity

Ciprofloxacin (Systemic) may increase the levels/effects of: Agomelatine; ARIPiprazole; Bendamustine; CarBAMazepine; CloZAPine; CYP1A2 Substrates; DULoxetine; Erlotinib; Highest Risk QTc-Prolonging Agents; Hydrocodone; Lomitapide; Methotrexate; Moderate Risk QTc-Prolonging Agents; Pimozide; Pirfenidone; Pomalidomide; Porfimer; Roflumilast; ROPINIRole; Ropivacaine; Sulfonylureas; Tasimelteon; Theophylline Derivatives; TiZANidine; Varenicline; Verteporfin; Vitamin K Antagonists

The levels/effects of Ciprofloxacin (Systemic) may be increased by: Corticosteroids (Systemic); Fosphenytoin; Insulin; Ivabradine; Mifepristone; Nonsteroidal Anti-Inflammatory Agents; P-glycoprotein/ABCB1 Inhibitors; Probenecid; QTc-Prolonging Agents (Indeterminate Risk and Risk Modifying); Teriflunomide

Decreased Effect

Ciprofloxacin (Systemic) may decrease the levels/effects of: BCG; Didanosine; Fosphenytoin; Mycophenolate; Phenytoin; Sodium Picosulfate; Sulfonylureas; Thyroid Products; Typhoid Vaccine

The levels/effects of Ciprofloxacin (Systemic) may be decreased by: Antacids; Calcium Salts; Didanosine; Iron Salts; Lanthanum; Magnesium Salts; Multivitamins/Minerals (with ADEK, Folate, Iron); Multivitamins/Minerals (with AE, No Iron); P-glycoprotein/ABCB1 Inducers; Quinapril; Sevelamer; Strontium Ranelate; Sucralfate; Zinc Salts

Food Interactions Food decreases rate, but not extent, of absorption. Ciprofloxacin serum levels may be decreased if taken with divalent or trivalent cations. Rarely, crystalluria may occur. Enteral feedings may decrease plasma concentrations of ciprofloxacin probably by >30% inhibition of absorption. Management: May administer with food to minimize GI upset. Avoid or take ciprofloxacin 2 hours before or 6 hours after antacids, dairy products, or calcium-fortified juices alone or in a meal containing >800 mg calcium, oral multivitamins, or mineral supplements containing divalent and/or trivalent cations. Ensure adequate hydration during therapy. Ciprofloxacin should not be administered with enteral feedings. The feeding would need to be discontinued for 1-2 hours prior to and after ciprofloxacin administration. Nasogastric administration produces a greater loss of ciprofloxacin bioavailability than does nasoduodenal administration.

Preparation for Administration Injection, vial: May be diluted with NS, D_5W, SWFI, $D_{10}W$, $D_5$1/4NS, $D_5$1/2NS, LR.

Storage/Stability

Injection:

Premixed infusion: Store between 5°C to 25°C (41°F to 77°F); avoid freezing. Protect from light.

Vial: Store between 5°C to 30°C (41°F to 86°F); avoid freezing. Protect from light. Diluted solutions of 0.5-2 mg/mL are stable for up to 14 days refrigerated or at room temperature.

Microcapsules for oral suspension: Prior to reconstitution, store below 25°C (77°F). Protect from freezing. Following reconstitution, store below 30°C (86°F) for up to 14 days. Protect from freezing.

Tablet:

Immediate release: Store below 30°C (86°F).

Extended release: Store at room temperature of 15°C to 30°C (59°F to 86°F).

Mechanism of Action Inhibits DNA-gyrase in susceptible organisms; inhibits relaxation of supercoiled DNA and promotes breakage of double-stranded DNA

Pharmacodynamics/Kinetics

Absorption: Oral: Immediate release tablet: Rapid (~50% to 85%)

Distribution: V_d: 2.1-2.7 L/kg; tissue concentrations often exceed serum concentrations especially in kidneys, gallbladder, liver, lungs, gynecological tissue, and prostatic tissue; CSF concentrations: 10% of serum concentrations (noninflamed meninges), 14% to 37% (inflamed meninges)

Protein binding: 20% to 40%

Metabolism: Partially hepatic; forms 4 metabolites (limited activity)

Half-life elimination: Children: 2.5 hours; Adults: Normal renal function: 3-5 hours

Time to peak: Oral:

Immediate release tablet: 0.5-2 hours

Extended release tablet: Cipro XR: 1-2.5 hours

Excretion: Urine (30% to 50% as unchanged drug); feces (15% to 43%)

Dosage Note: Extended release tablets and immediate release formulations are not interchangeable. Unless otherwise specified, oral dosing reflects the use of immediate release formulations.

Usual dosage ranges:

Children (see Warnings/Precautions):

Oral: See indication-specific dosing; maximum dose: 1500 mg daily

IV: See indication-specific dosing; maximum dose: 800 mg daily

Adults:

Oral: 250-750 mg every 12 hours

IV: 200-400 mg every 12 hours

Indication-specific dosing:

Infants >3 months and Children:

Community-acquired pneumonia (CAP) (IDSA/PIDS, 2011): *H. influenzae,* moderate-to-severe infection (alternative to ampicillin, ceftriaxone, or cefotaxime): IV: 30 mg/kg/day divided every 12 hours

Children:

Anthrax:

Inhalational (postexposure prophylaxis):

Oral: 15 mg/kg/dose every 12 hours for 60 days; maximum: 500 mg dose

IV: 10 mg/kg/dose every 12 hours for 60 days; do **not** exceed 400 mg dose (800 mg daily)

Cutaneous (treatment, CDC guidelines): Oral: 10-15 mg/kg every 12 hours for 60 days (maximum: 1000 mg daily); amoxicillin 80 mg/kg/day divided every 8 hours is an option for completion of treatment after clinical improvement. **Note:** In the presence of systemic involvement, extensive edema, lesions on head/neck, refer to IV dosing for treatment of inhalational/gastrointestinal/oropharyngeal anthrax.

Inhalational/gastrointestinal/oropharyngeal (treatment, CDC guidelines): IV: Initial: 10-15 mg/kg every 12 hours for 60 days (maximum: 500 mg dose); switch to oral therapy when clinically appropriate; refer to adult dosing for notes on combined therapy and duration

Cystic fibrosis (off-label use):

Oral: 40 mg/kg/day divided every 12 hours administered following 1 week of IV therapy has been reported in a clinical trial; total duration of therapy: 10-21 days (Rubio, 1997)

IV: 30 mg/kg/day divided every 8 hours for 1 week, followed by oral therapy, has been reported in a clinical trial (Rubio, 1997)

Plague (off-label use): Children and adolescents:

Contained casualty management: IV: 15 mg/kg twice daily for 10 days (maximum: 1 g daily). Can switch to oral administration when clinically indicated (CDC [plague], 2014; Inglesby, 2000).

Mass casualty management: Oral: 20 mg/kg twice daily for 10 days (maximum: 1 g daily) (Inglesby, 2000)

Mass casualty postexposure prophylaxis: Oral: 20 mg/kg twice daily for 7 days (maximum: 1 g daily) (CDC [plague], 2014; Inglesby, 2000)

Shigella dysentery type 1 (off-label use): Oral: 30 mg/kg/day in 2 divided doses for 3 days (WHO, 2005)

Surgical (preoperative) prophylaxis (off-label use): Children ≥1 year: IV: 10 mg/kg within 120 minutes prior to surgical incision (maximum: 400 mg) (Bratzler, 2013)

Urinary tract infection (complicated) or pyelonephritis:

Oral: 20-40 mg/kg/day in 2 divided doses (every 12 hours) for 10-21 days; maximum: 1500 mg daily. **Note:** 30-40 mg/kg/day reserved for severe infections (Red Book, 2012)

IV: 6-10 mg/kg every 8 hours for 10-21 days (maximum: 400 mg dose)

Adults:

Anthrax:

Inhalational (postexposure prophylaxis):

Oral: 500 mg every 12 hours for 60 days

IV: 400 mg every 12 hours for 60 days

Cutaneous (treatment, CDC guidelines): Oral: Immediate release formulation: 500 mg every 12 hours for 60 days. **Note:** In the presence of systemic involvement, extensive edema, lesions on head/neck, refer to IV dosing for treatment of inhalational/gastrointestinal/oropharyngeal anthrax

Inhalational/gastrointestinal/oropharyngeal (treatment, CDC guidelines): IV: 400 mg every 12 hours. **Note:** Initial treatment should include two or more agents predicted to be effective (per CDC recommendations). Continue combined therapy for 60 days.

Bone/joint infections:

Oral: 500-750 mg twice daily for ≥4-6 weeks

IV: Mild-to-moderate: 400 mg every 12 hours for ≥4-6 weeks; Severe/complicated: 400 mg every 8 hours for ≥4-6 weeks

Chancroid (off-label use): Oral: 500 mg twice daily for 3 days (CDC, 2010)

Endocarditis due to HACEK organisms (off-label use) (Baddour, 2005): Note: Not first-line option; use only if intolerant of beta-lactam therapy:

Oral: 500 mg every 12 hours for 4 weeks (native valve) or 6 weeks (prosthetic valve)

IV: 400 mg every 12 hours for 4 weeks (native valve) or 6 weeks (prosthetic valve)

Epididymitis, chlamydial (off-label use): Oral: 500 mg single dose (Canadian STI Guidelines, 2008)

Febrile neutropenia: IV: 400 mg every 8 hours for 7-14 days (combination therapy with piperacillin generally recommended)

Gonococcal infections:

Urethral/cervical gonococcal infections: Oral: 250-500 mg as a single dose (CDC recommends concomitant doxycycline or azithromycin due to possible coinfection with *Chlamydia*); **Note:** As of April 2007, the CDC no longer recommends the use of fluoroquinolones for the treatment of uncomplicated gonococcal disease.

Granuloma inguinale (donovanosis) (off-label use): Oral: 750 mg twice daily for at least 3 weeks (and until lesions have healed) (CDC, 2010)

Infectious diarrhea: Oral:

Salmonella: 500 mg twice daily for 5-7 days

Shigella (including Shigella dysentery type 1) (off-label regimen): 500 mg twice daily for 3 days (IDSA, 2001)

Traveler's diarrhea (off-label regimen): Mild: 750 mg as a single dose (CDC, 2012; de la Cabada Bauch, 2011); Severe: 500 mg twice daily for 3 days (IDSA, 2001)

Vibrio cholerae (off-label regimen): 1 g as a single dose (CDC, 2011)

Intra-abdominal, complicated, community-acquired (in combination with metronidazole): Note: Avoid using in settings where *E. coli* susceptibility to fluoroquinolones is <90%:

Oral: 500 mg every 12 hours for 7-14 days

IV: 400 mg every 12 hours for 7-14 days; **Note:** 2010 IDSA guidelines recommend treatment duration of 4-7 days (provided source controlled)

Lower respiratory tract:

Oral: 500-750 mg twice daily for 7-14 days

IV: Mild-to-moderate: 400 mg every 12 hours for 7-14 days; Severe/complicated: 400 mg every 8 hours for 7-14 days

Meningococcal meningitis prophylaxis (off-label use): Oral: 500 mg as a single dose (CDC, 2005)

Nosocomial pneumonia: IV: 400 mg every 8 hours for 10-14 days

Periodontitis (off-label use): Oral: 500 mg every 12 hours for 8-10 days (Rams, 1992)

Plague (off-label use):

Contained casualty management: IV: 400 mg twice daily for 10 days. Can switch to oral administration when clinically indicated (Bossi [plague], 2004; CDC [plague], 2014; Inglesby, 2000).

Mass casualty management: Oral: 500 mg twice daily for 10 days (Inglesby, 2000)

Mass casualty postexposure prophylaxis: Oral: 500 mg twice daily for 7 days (Bossi [plague], 2004; CDC [plague], 2012; Inglesby, 2000).

Prostatitis (chronic, bacterial):

Oral: 500 mg every 12 hours for 28 days

IV: 400 mg every 12 hours for 28 days

Sinusitis (acute):

Oral: 500 mg every 12 hours for 10 days

IV: 400 mg every 12 hours for 10 days

Skin/skin structure infections:

Oral: 500-750 mg twice daily for 7-14 days

IV: Mild-to-moderate: 400 mg every 12 hours for 7-14 days; Severe/complicated: 400 mg every 8 hours for 7-14 days

Surgical (preoperative) prophylaxis (off-label use): IV: 400 mg within 120 minutes prior to surgical incision (Bratzler, 2013).

Tularemia (off-label use):

Contained casualty management: IV: 400 mg twice daily for 10 days. Can switch to oral administration when clinically indicated (Dennis, 2001).

Mass casualty management or postexposure prophylaxis: Oral: 500 or 750 mg twice daily for 14 days. At least 14 days of therapy is recommended in oral regimens (Bossi [tularemia], 2004; Dennis, 2001; Stevens, 2014).

Typhoid fever: Oral: 500 mg every 12 hours for 10 days

Urinary tract infection:

Acute uncomplicated, cystitis:

Oral:

Immediate release formulation: 250 mg every 12 hours for 3 days

Extended release formulation (Cipro XR): 500 mg every 24 hours for 3 days

IV: 200 mg every 12 hours for 7-14 days

Complicated (including pyelonephritis):

Oral:

Immediate release formulation: 500 mg every 12 hours for 7-14 days

Extended release formulation (Cipro XR): 1000 mg every 24 hours for 7-14 days

IV: 400 mg every 12 hours for 7-14 days

Elderly: No adjustment needed in patients with normal renal function

Dosage adjustment in renal impairment: Adults:

Manufacturer's recommendations:

Oral, immediate release:

CrCl >50 mL/minute: No dosage adjustment necessary

CrCl 30-50 mL/minute: 250-500 mg every 12 hours

CrCl 5-29 mL/minute: 250-500 mg every 18 hours

ESRD on intermittent hemodialysis (IHD)/peritoneal dialysis (PD) (administer after dialysis on dialysis days): 250-500 mg every 24 hours

Oral, extended release:

CrCl ≥30 mL/minute: No dosage adjustment necessary

CrCl <30 mL/minute: 500 mg every 24 hours

ESRD on intermittent hemodialysis (IHD)/peritoneal dialysis (PD) (administer after dialysis on dialysis days): 500 mg every 24 hours

IV:

CrCl ≥30 mL/minute: No dosage adjustment necessary

CrCl 5-29 mL/minute: 200-400 mg every 18-24 hours

Alternate recommendations: Oral (immediate release), IV:

CrCl >50 mL/minute: No dosage adjustment necessary (Aronoff, 2007)

CrCl 10-50 mL/minute: Administer 50% to 75% of usual dose every 12 hours (Aronoff, 2007)

CrCl <10 mL/minute: Administer 50% of usual dose every 12 hours (Aronoff, 2007)

Intermittent hemodialysis (IHD) (administer after hemodialysis on dialysis days): Minimally dialyzable (<10%): Oral: 250-500 mg every 24 hours **or** IV: 200-400 mg every 24 hours (Heintz, 2009). **Note:** Dosing dependent on the assumption of 3 times weekly, complete IHD sessions.

Continuous renal replacement therapy (CRRT) (Heintz, 2009; Trotman, 2005): Drug clearance is highly dependent on the method of renal replacement, filter type, and flow rate. Appropriate dosing requires close monitoring of pharmacologic response, signs of adverse reactions due to drug accumulation, as well as drug concentrations in relation to target trough (if appropriate). The following are general recommendations only (based on dialysate flow/ultrafiltration rates of 1-2 L/hour and minimal residual renal function) and should not supersede clinical judgment:

CVVH/CVVHD/CVVHDF: IV: 200-400 mg every 12-24 hours

Dosage adjustment in hepatic impairment: No dosage adjustment provided in manufacturer's labeling (has not been studied). No pharmacokinetic changes were noted in patients with stable chronic cirrhosis, but pharmacokinetics have not been evaluated in patients with acute impairment.

Dietary Considerations Food: Drug may cause GI upset; take without regard to meals (manufacturer prefers that immediate release tablet is taken 2 hours after meals). Extended release tablet may be taken with meals that contain dairy products (calcium content <800 mg), but not with dairy products alone.

Dairy products, calcium-fortified juices, oral multivitamins, and mineral supplements: Absorption of ciprofloxacin is decreased by divalent and trivalent cations. The manufacturer states that the usual dietary intake of calcium (including meals which include dairy products) has not been shown to interfere with ciprofloxacin absorption. Immediate release ciprofloxacin and Cipro XR may be taken 2 hours before or 6 hours after any of these products.

Caffeine: Patients consuming regular large quantities of caffeinated beverages may need to restrict caffeine intake if excessive cardiac or CNS stimulation occurs.

Administration

Oral: May administer with food to minimize GI upset; avoid antacid use; maintain proper hydration and urine output. Administer immediate release ciprofloxacin and Cipro XR at least 2 hours before or 6 hours after antacids or other products containing calcium, iron, or zinc (including dairy products or calcium-fortified juices). Separate oral administration from drugs which may impair absorption (see Drug Interactions).

Oral suspension: Should not be administered through feeding tubes (suspension is oil-based and adheres to the feeding tube). Patients should avoid chewing on the microcapsules.

Nasogastric/orogastric tube: Crush immediate-release tablet and mix with water. Flush feeding tube before and after administration. Hold tube feedings at least 1 hour before and 2 hours after administration.

Tablet, extended release: Do not crush, split, or chew. May be administered with meals containing dairy products (calcium content <800 mg), but not with dairy products alone.

Parenteral: Administer by slow IV infusion over 60 minutes into a large vein (reduces risk of venous irritation).

Monitoring Parameters CBC, renal and hepatic function during prolonged therapy

Reference Range Therapeutic: 2.6-3 mcg/mL; Toxic: >5 mcg/mL

Additional Information Although the systemic use of ciprofloxacin is only FDA-approved in children for the treatment of complicated UTI and postexposure treatment of inhalation anthrax, use of the fluoroquinolones in pediatric patients is increasing. Current recommendations by the American Academy of Pediatrics note that the systemic use of these agents in children should be restricted to infections caused by multidrug resistant pathogens with no safe or effective alternative, and when parenteral therapy is not feasible or other oral agents are not available.

Dosage Forms

Solution, Intravenous:

Cipro in D5W: 200 mg/100 mL (100 mL)

Generic: 200 mg/100 mL (100 mL); 400 mg/200 mL (200 mL); 200 mg/20 mL (20 mL); 400 mg/40 mL (40 mL)

Solution, Intravenous [preservative free]:

Cipro in D5W: 200 mg/100 mL (100 mL); 400 mg/200 mL (200 mL)

Generic: 200 mg/100 mL (100 mL); 400 mg/200 mL (200 mL); 200 mg/20 mL (20 mL); 400 mg/40 mL (40 mL)

Suspension Reconstituted, Oral:
Cipro: 250 mg/5 mL (100 mL); 500 mg/5 mL (100 mL)
Generic: 250 mg/5 mL (100 mL); 500 mg/5 mL (100 mL)
Tablet, Oral:
Cipro: 250 mg, 500 mg
Generic: 100 mg, 250 mg, 500 mg, 750 mg
Tablet Extended Release 24 Hour, Oral:
Cipro XR: 500 mg, 1000 mg
Generic: 500 mg, 1000 mg

Extemporaneous Preparations A 50 mg/mL oral suspension may be made using 2 different vehicles (a 1:1 mixture of Ora-Sweet and Ora-Plus or a 1:1 mixture of Methylcellulose 1% and Simple Syrup, NF). Crush twenty 500 mg tablets and reduce to a fine powder. Add a small amount of vehicle and mix to a uniform paste; mix while adding the vehicle in geometric proportions to **almost** 200 mL; transfer to a calibrated bottle, rinse mortar with vehicle, and add quantity of vehicle sufficient to make 200 mL. Label "shake well" and "refrigerate". Stable 91 days refrigerated and 70 days at room temperature. **Note:** Microcapsules for oral suspension available (50 mg/mL; 100 mg/mL); not for use in feeding tubes.

Nahata MC, Pai VB, and Hipple TF, *Pediatric Drug Formulations*, 5th ed, Cincinnati, OH: Harvey Whitney Books Co, 2004.

Ciprofloxacin (Ophthalmic) (sip roe FLOKS a sin)

Brand Names: U.S. Ciloxan
Brand Names: Canada Ciloxan
Index Terms Ciprofloxacin Hydrochloride
Pharmacologic Category Antibiotic, Fluoroquinolone; Antibiotic, Ophthalmic
Use Treatment of superficial ocular infections (corneal ulcers, conjunctivitis) due to susceptible strains
Pregnancy Risk Factor C
Dosage Ophthalmic:
Bacterial conjunctivitis:
Ophthalmic solution: Children ≥1 year and Adults: Instill 1-2 drops into the conjunctival sac every 2 hours while awake for 2 days and 1-2 drops every 4 hours while awake for the next 5 days
Ophthalmic ointment: Children ≥2 years and Adults: Apply a 1/2 inch ribbon into the conjunctival sac 3 times/day for the first 2 days, followed by a 1/2 inch ribbon applied twice daily for the next 5 days
Corneal ulcer: Ophthalmic solution: Children ≥1 year and Adults: Instill 2 drops into affected eye every 15 minutes for the first 6 hours, then 2 drops into the affected eye every 30 minutes for the remainder of the first day. On day 2, instill 2 drops into the affected eye hourly. On days 3-14, instill 2 drops into affected eye every 4 hours. Treatment may continue after day 14 if re-epithelialization has not occurred.

Dosage adjustment in renal impairment: No dosage adjustment provided in manufacturer's labeling.
Dosage adjustment in hepatic impairment: No dosage adjustment provided in manufacturer's labeling.

Additional Information Complete prescribing information should be consulted for additional detail.
Dosage Forms
Ointment, Ophthalmic:
Ciloxan: 0.3% (3.5 g)
Solution, Ophthalmic:
Ciloxan: 0.3% (5 mL)
Generic: 0.3% (2.5 mL, 5 mL, 10 mL)

Ciprofloxacin (Otic) (sip roe FLOKS a sin)

Brand Names: U.S. Cetraxal
Index Terms Ciprofloxacin Hydrochloride
Pharmacologic Category Antibiotic, Fluoroquinolone; Antibiotic, Otic
Use Treatment of acute otitis externa due to susceptible strains of *Pseudomonas aeruginosa* or *Staphylococcus aureus*
Pregnancy Risk Factor C
Dosage Otic: Children ≥1 year and Adults: Acute otitis externa: Instill 0.25 mL solution (contents of 1 single-dose container) into affected ear twice daily for 7 days
Additional Information Complete prescribing information should be consulted for additional detail.
Dosage Forms
Solution, Otic [preservative free]:
Cetraxal: 0.2% (1 ea)
Generic: 0.2% (1 ea)

Ciprofloxacin and Dexamethasone

(sip roe FLOKS a sin & deks a METH a sone)

Brand Names: U.S. Ciprodex
Brand Names: Canada Ciprodex
Index Terms Ciprofloxacin Hydrochloride and Dexamethasone; Dexamethasone and Ciprofloxacin
Pharmacologic Category Antibiotic, Otic; Antibiotic/Corticosteroid, Otic; Corticosteroid, Otic
Use
Acute otitis media: Treatment of acute otitis media in pediatric patients ≥6 months of age with tympanostomy tubes due to susceptible isolates of *Staphylococcus aureus*, *Streptococcus pneumoniae*, *Haemophilus influenza*, *Moraxella catarrhalis*, and *Pseudomonas aeruginosa*.
Acute otitis externa: Treatment of acute otitis externa in pediatric patients ≥6 months of age and adults due to susceptible isolates of *Staphylococcus aureus* and *Pseudomonas aeruginosa*.
Pregnancy Risk Factor C
Dosage
Acute otitis externa: Infants ≥6 months, Children, Adolescents, and Adults: Otic: Instill 4 drops into affected ear(s) twice daily for 7 days
Acute otitis media in patients with tympanostomy tubes: Infants ≥6 months, Children, and Adolescents: Otic: Instill 4 drops into affected ear(s) twice daily for 7 days

Dosage adjustment in renal impairment: There are no dosage adjustments provided in the manufacturer's labeling.
Dosage adjustment in hepatic impairment: There are no dosage adjustments provided in the manufacturer's labeling.

Additional Information Complete prescribing information should be consulted for additional detail.
Dosage Forms
Suspension, otic:
Ciprodex: Ciprofloxacin 0.3% and dexamethasone 0.1% (7.5 mL)

Ciprofloxacin and Hydrocortisone

(sip roe FLOKS a sin & hye droe KOR ti sone)

Brand Names: U.S. Cipro® HC
Brand Names: Canada Cipro® HC
Index Terms Ciprofloxacin Hydrochloride and Hydrocortisone; Hydrocortisone and Ciprofloxacin
Pharmacologic Category Antibiotic, Otic; Antibiotic/Corticosteroid, Otic; Corticosteroid, Otic
Use Treatment of acute otitis externa, sometimes known as "swimmer's ear"
Pregnancy Risk Factor C

Dosage Children >1 year of age and Adults: Otic: The recommended dosage for all patients is three drops of the suspension in the affected ear twice daily for 7 days; twice-daily dosing schedule is more convenient for patients than that of existing treatments with hydrocortisone, which are typically administered 3 or 4 times a day; a twice-daily dosage schedule may be especially helpful for parents and caregivers of young children

Dosage adjustment in renal impairment: No dosage adjustment provided in manufacturer's labeling.

Dosage adjustment in hepatic impairment: No dosage adjustment provided in manufacturer's labeling.

Additional Information Complete prescribing information should be consulted for additional detail.

Dosage Forms

Suspension, otic:

Cipro® HC: Ciprofloxacin 0.2% and hydrocortisone 1% (10 mL)

◆ **Ciprofloxacin Hydrochloride** *see* Ciprofloxacin (Ophthalmic) *on page 446*

◆ **Ciprofloxacin Hydrochloride** *see* Ciprofloxacin (Otic) *on page 446*

◆ **Ciprofloxacin Hydrochloride** *see* Ciprofloxacin (Systemic) *on page 441*

◆ **Ciprofloxacin Hydrochloride and Dexamethasone** *see* Ciprofloxacin and Dexamethasone *on page 446*

◆ **Ciprofloxacin Hydrochloride and Hydrocortisone** *see* Ciprofloxacin and Hydrocortisone *on page 446*

◆ **Ciprofloxacin Injection (Can)** *see* Ciprofloxacin (Systemic) *on page 441*

◆ **Ciprofloxacin Injection USP (Can)** *see* Ciprofloxacin (Systemic) *on page 441*

◆ **Ciprofloxacin Intravenous Infusion (Can)** *see* Ciprofloxacin (Systemic) *on page 441*

◆ **Ciprofloxacin Intravenous Infusion BP (Can)** *see* Ciprofloxacin (Systemic) *on page 441*

◆ **Cipro® HC** *see* Ciprofloxacin and Hydrocortisone *on page 446*

◆ **Cipro in D5W** *see* Ciprofloxacin (Systemic) *on page 441*

◆ **Cipro XR** *see* Ciprofloxacin (Systemic) *on page 441*

Cisatracurium (sis a tra KYOO ree um)

Brand Names: U.S. Nimbex

Brand Names: Canada Nimbex

Index Terms Cisatracurium Besylate

Pharmacologic Category Neuromuscular Blocker Agent, Nondepolarizing

Use Adjunct to general anesthesia to facilitate endotracheal intubation and to relax skeletal muscles during surgery; to facilitate mechanical ventilation in ICU patients; does not relieve pain or produce sedation

Pregnancy Risk Factor B

Pregnancy Considerations Adverse events have not been observed in animal reproduction studies.

Breast-Feeding Considerations It is not known if cisatracurium is excreted in breast milk. The manufacturer recommends that caution be exercised when administering cisatracurium to nursing women.

Contraindications Hypersensitivity to cisatracurium besylate or any component of the formulation; use of the 10 mL multiple-dose vials in premature infants (formulation contains benzyl alcohol)

Warnings/Precautions Maintenance of an adequate airway and respiratory support is critical; certain clinical conditions may result in potentiation or antagonism of neuromuscular blockade:

Potentiation: Electrolyte abnormalities, severe hyponatremia, severe hypocalcemia, severe hypokalemia, hypermagnesemia, neuromuscular diseases, acidosis, acute intermittent porphyria, renal failure, hepatic failure

Antagonism: Alkalosis, hypercalcemia, demyelinating lesions, peripheral neuropathies, diabetes mellitus

Hypothermia may slow Hoffmann elimination thereby prolonging the duration of activity (Greenberg, 2013). Increased sensitivity in patients with myasthenia gravis, Eaton-Lambert syndrome; resistance in burn patients (>30% of body) for period of 5-70 days postinjury; resistance in patients with muscle trauma, denervation, immobilization, infection. Cross-sensitivity with other neuromuscular-blocking agents may occur; use extreme caution in patients with previous anaphylactic reactions to other neuromuscular-blocking agents. Bradycardia may be more common with cisatracurium than with other neuromuscular blocking agents since it has no clinically significant effects on heart rate to counteract the bradycardia produced by anesthetics. Use caution in the elderly. Should be administered by adequately trained individuals familiar with its use.

Benzyl alcohol and derivatives: Some dosage forms may contain benzyl alcohol; large amounts of benzyl alcohol (≥99 mg/kg/day) have been associated with a potentially fatal toxicity ("gasping syndrome") in neonates; the "gasping syndrome" consists of metabolic acidosis, respiratory distress, gasping respirations, CNS dysfunction (including convulsions, intracranial hemorrhage), hypotension and cardiovascular collapse (AAP, 1997; CDC, 1982); some data suggests that benzoate displaces bilirubin from protein binding sites (Ahlfors, 2001); avoid or use dosage forms containing benzyl alcohol with caution in neonates. See manufacturer's labeling.

Adverse Reactions

Effects are minimal and transient.

Rare but important or life-threatening: Bradycardia, bronchospasm, flushing, hypotension, muscle calcification (prolonged use), myopathy (acute quadriplegic syndrome; prolonged use), pruritus, skin rash

Drug Interactions

Metabolism/Transport Effects None known.

Avoid Concomitant Use

Avoid concomitant use of Cisatracurium with any of the following: QuiNINE

Increased Effect/Toxicity

Cisatracurium may increase the levels/effects of: Cardiac Glycosides; Corticosteroids (Systemic); OnabotulinumtoxinA; RimabotulinumtoxinB

The levels/effects of Cisatracurium may be increased by: AbobotulinumtoxinA; Aminoglycosides; Calcium Channel Blockers; Capreomycin; Clindamycin (Topical); Colistimethate; CycloSPORINE (Systemic); Fosphenytoin-Phenytoin; Inhalational Anesthetics; Ketorolac (Nasal); Ketorolac (Systemic); Lincosamide Antibiotics; Lithium; Loop Diuretics; Magnesium Salts; Polymyxin B; Procainamide; QuiNIDine; QuiNINE; Spironolactone; Tetracycline Derivatives; Vancomycin

Decreased Effect

The levels/effects of Cisatracurium may be decreased by: Acetylcholinesterase Inhibitors; Fosphenytoin-Phenytoin; Loop Diuretics

Storage/Stability Refrigerate intact vials at 2°C to 8°C (36°F to 46°F). Use vials within 21 days upon removal from the refrigerator to room temperature of 25°C (77°F). Per the manufacturer, dilutions of 0.1 mg/mL in 0.9% sodium chloride (NS), dextrose 5% in water (D_5W), or

D_5NS are stable for up to 24 hours at room temperature or under refrigeration; dilutions of 0.1-0.2 mg/mL in D_5LR are stable for up to 24 hours in the refrigerator. *Additional stability data:* Dilutions of 0.1, 2, and 5 mg/mL in D_5W or NS are stable in the refrigerator for up to 30 days; at room temperature (23°C), dilutions of 0.1 and 2 mg/mL began exhibiting substantial drug loss between 7-14 days; dilutions of 5 mg/mL in D_5W or NS are stable for up to 30 days at room temperature (23°C) (Xu, 1998). Usual concentration: 0.1-0.4 mg/mL.

Mechanism of Action Blocks neural transmission at the myoneural junction by binding with cholinergic receptor sites

Pharmacodynamics/Kinetics

Onset of action: IV: 2-3 minutes

Peak effect: 3-5 minutes

Duration: Recovery begins in 20-35 minutes when anesthesia is balanced; recovery is attained in 90% of patients in 25-93 minutes

Distribution: V_{dss}: 145 mL/kg (21% larger V_{dss} when receiving inhalational anesthetics)

Protein binding: Not studied due to rapid degradation at physiologic pH

Metabolism: Undergoes rapid nonenzymatic degradation in the bloodstream (Hofmann elimination) to laudanosine and inactive metabolites; laudanosine may cause CNS stimulation (association not established in humans) and has less accumulation with prolonged use than atracurium due to lower requirements for clinical effect

Half-life elimination: 22-29 minutes

Excretion: Urine (95%; <10% as unchanged drug)

Dosage IV (not to be used IM):

Operating room administration:

Infants 1-23 months: Intubating dose: 0.15 mg/kg over 5-10 seconds

Children 2-12 years: Intubating dose: 0.1-0.15 mg/kg over 5-10 seconds. (**Note:** When given during stable opioid/nitrous oxide/oxygen anesthesia, 0.1 mg/kg produces maximum neuromuscular block in an average of 2.8 minutes and clinically effective block for 28 minutes.)

Adults: Intubating dose: 0.15-0.2 mg/kg as component of propofol/nitrous oxide/oxygen induction-intubation technique. (**Note:** May produce generally good or excellent conditions for tracheal intubation in 1.5-2 minutes with clinically effective duration of action during propofol anesthesia of 55-61 minutes.) Initial dose after succinylcholine for intubation: 0.1 mg/kg; maintenance dose: 0.03 mg/kg 40-60 minutes after initial dose, then at ~20-minute intervals based on clinical criteria

Children ≥2 years and Adults: Continuous infusion: After an initial bolus, a diluted solution can be given by continuous infusion for maintenance of neuromuscular blockade during extended surgery; adjust the rate of administration according to the patient's response as determined by peripheral nerve stimulation. An initial infusion rate of 3 **mcg**/kg/**minute** (0.18 **mg**/kg/**hour**) may be required to rapidly counteract the spontaneous recovery of neuromuscular function; thereafter, a rate of 1-2 **mcg**/kg/**minute** (0.06-0.12 **mg**/kg/**hour**) should be adequate to maintain continuous neuromuscular block in the 89% to 99% range in most pediatric and adult patients. Consider reduction of the infusion rate by 30% to 40% when administering during stable isoflurane, enflurane, sevoflurane, or desflurane anesthesia. Spontaneous recovery from neuromuscular blockade following discontinuation of infusion of cisatracurium may be expected to proceed at a rate comparable to that following single bolus administration.

Intensive care unit administration:

Manufacturer's labeling: Loading dose: 0.15-0.2 mg/kg; at initial signs of recovery from bolus dose, begin the infusion at a dose of 3 **mcg**/kg/**minute** (0.18 **mg**/kg/**hour**) and adjust rate accordingly (follow the principles for infusion in the operating room); dosage ranges of 0.5-10 **mcg**/kg/**minute** (0.03-0.6 **mg**/kg/**hour**) have been reported. If patient is allowed to recover from neuromuscular blockade, readministration of a bolus dose may be necessary to quickly re-establish neuromuscular block prior to reinstituting the infusion.

or

Loading dose: 0.1 mg/kg (additional boluses of 0.05 mg/kg until train-of-four response is 3/4 or less can be used); then initiate an infusion at 2.5-3 **mcg**/kg/**minute** (0.15-0.18 **mg**/kg/**hour**) and adjust rate accordingly (Baumann, 2004; Lagneau, 2002).

or

Loading dose: 0.1 to 0.2 mg/kg; immediately following loading dose administration, begin an infusion at 1-3 **mcg**/kg/**minute** (0.06-0.18 **mg**/kg/**hour**) and adjust rate accordingly (Greenberg, 2013).

Dosing adjustment in renal impairment: Because slower times to onset of complete neuromuscular block were observed in renal dysfunction patients, extending the interval between the administration of cisatracurium and intubation attempt may be required to achieve adequate intubation conditions.

Dosage adjustment in hepatic impairment: No dosage adjustment provided in manufacturer's labeling. The time to onset of action was ~1 minute faster in patients with end-stage liver disease, but was not associated with clinically significant changes in recovery time.

Usual Infusion Concentrations: Adult IV infusion: 100 mg in 250 mL (total volume) (concentration: 400 **mcg**/mL) of D_5W or NS

Administration Administer IV only; give undiluted as bolus injection over 5-10 seconds. Continuous infusion requires the use of an infusion pump. The use of a peripheral nerve stimulator will permit the most advantageous use of cisatracurium, minimize the possibility of overdosage or underdosage and assist in the evaluation of recovery.

Do not administer IM (excessive tissue irritation).

Monitoring Parameters Peripheral nerve stimulator measuring twitch response (when appropriate); vital signs (heart rate, blood pressure, respiratory rate)

Additional Information Cisatracurium is classified as an intermediate-duration neuromuscular-blocking agent. It does not appear to have a cumulative effect on the duration of blockade. Neuromuscular-blocking potency is 3 times that of atracurium; maximum block is up to 2 minutes longer than for equipotent doses of atracurium.

Dosage Forms

Solution, Intravenous:

Nimbex: 10 mg/5 mL (5 mL); 20 mg/10 mL (10 mL); 10 mg/mL (20 mL)

Generic: 20 mg/10 mL (10 mL)

Solution, Intravenous [preservative free]:

Generic: 10 mg/5 mL (5 mL); 10 mg/mL (20 mL)

◆ **Cisatracurium Besylate** *see* Cisatracurium *on page 447*

◆ **cis-DDP** *see* CISplatin *on page 448*

◆ **cis-Diamminedichloroplatinum** *see* CISplatin *on page 448*

CISplatin (SIS pla tin)

Brand Names: Canada Cisplatin Injection; Cisplatin Injection BP; Cisplatin Injection, Mylan STD

Index Terms CDDP; cis-DDP; cis-Diamminedichloroplatinum; Platinol; Platinol-AQ

Pharmacologic Category Antineoplastic Agent, Alkylating Agent; Antineoplastic Agent, Platinum Analog

Additional Appendix Information

Beers Criteria - Potentially Inappropriate Medications for Geriatrics *on page 2271*

Use

Bladder cancer: Treatment of advanced bladder cancer

Ovarian cancer: Treatment of metastatic ovarian cancer

Testicular cancer: Treatment of metastatic testicular cancer

Pregnancy Risk Factor D

Pregnancy Considerations Adverse effects have been observed in animal reproduction studies. Women of childbearing potential should be advised to avoid pregnancy during treatment. May case fetal harm if administered during pregnancy.

Breast-Feeding Considerations Cisplatin is excreted in breast milk. Breast-feeding is not recommended by the manufacturer.

Contraindications Hypersensitivity to cisplatin, other platinum-containing compounds, or any component of the formulation (anaphylactic-like reactions have been reported); preexisting renal impairment; myelosuppression; hearing impairment

Warnings/Precautions Hazardous agent - use appropriate precautions for handling and disposal (NIOSH 2014 [group 1]). **[U.S. Boxed Warning]: Doses >100 mg/m² once every 3 to 4 weeks are rarely used; verify with the prescriber. Exercise caution to avoid potential sound-alike/look-alike confusion between CISplatin and CARBOplatin.** Patients should receive adequate hydration, with or without diuretics, prior to and for 24 hours after cisplatin administration. **[U.S. Boxed Warning]: Cumulative renal toxicity may be severe.** Monitor serum creatinine, blood urea nitrogen, creatinine clearance, and serum electrolytes closely. According to the manufacturer's labeling, use is contraindicated in patients with preexisting renal impairment and renal function must return to normal prior to administering subsequent cycles; some literature recommends reduced doses with renal impairment. Nephrotoxicity may be potentiated by aminoglycosides.

Use caution in the elderly; may cause or exacerbate syndrome of inappropriate antidiuretic hormone secretion or hyponatremia; monitor sodium closely with initiation or dosage adjustments in older adults (Beers Criteria). Elderly patients may be more susceptible to nephrotoxicity and peripheral neuropathy; select dose cautiously and monitor closely.

[U.S. Boxed Warning]: Dose-related toxicities include myelosuppression, nausea, and vomiting. Cisplatin is associated with a high emetic potential; antiemetics are recommended to prevent nausea and vomiting (Basch, 2011; Dupuis, 2011; Roila, 2010). Nausea and vomiting are dose-related and may be immediate and/or delayed. Diarrhea may also occur. **[U.S. Boxed Warning]: Ototoxicity, which may be more pronounced in children, is manifested by tinnitus and/or loss of high frequency hearing and occasionally, deafness; may be significant.** Ototoxicity is cumulative and may be severe. Audiometric testing should be performed at baseline and prior to each dose. Certain genetic variations in the thiopurine S-methyltransferase (TPMT) gene may be associated with an increased risk of ototoxicity in children administered conventional cisplatin doses (Pussegoda, 2013). Controversy may exist regarding the role of TPMT variants in cisplatin ototoxicity (Ratain, 2013; Yang, 2013). Children without the TPMT gene variants are still at risk for ototoxicity. Cumulative dose, prior or concurrent exposure to other ototoxic agents (eg, aminoglycosides, carboplatin), prior cranial radiation, younger age, and type of cancer may also increase the risk for ototoxicity in children (Knight, 2005; Landier, 2014). Pediatric patients should receive audiometric testing at baseline, prior to each dose, and for several years after discontinuing therapy. An international grading scale (SIOP Boston scale) has been developed to assess ototoxicity in children (Brock, 2012). Severe (and possibly irreversible) neuropathies may occur with higher than recommended doses or more frequent administration; may require therapy discontinuation. Seizures, loss of motor function, loss of taste, leukoencephalopathy, and posterior reversible leukoencephalopathy syndrome (PRES [formerly RPLS]) have also been described. Serum electrolytes, particularly magnesium and potassium, should be monitored and replaced as needed during and after cisplatin therapy.

[U.S. Boxed Warning]: Anaphylactic-like reactions have been reported; may include facial edema, bronchoconstriction, tachycardia, and hypotension and may occur within minutes of administration; may be managed with epinephrine, corticosteroids, and/or antihistamines. Hyperuricemia has been reported with cisplatin use, and is more pronounced with doses >50 mg/m²; consider allopurinol therapy to reduce uric acid levels. Local infusion site reactions may occur; monitor infusion site during administration; avoid extravasation. Secondary malignancies have been reported with cisplatin in combination with other chemotherapy agents. Potentially significant drug-drug interactions may exist, requiring dose or frequency adjustment, additional monitoring, and/or selection of alternative therapy. **[U.S. Boxed Warning]: Should be administered under the supervision of an experienced cancer chemotherapy physician.** Cisplatin is a vesicant at higher concentrations, and an irritant at lower concentrations; ensure proper needle or catheter placement prior to and during infusion; avoid extravasation.

Adverse Reactions

Central nervous system: Neurotoxicity (peripheral neuropathy is dose and duration dependent)

Gastrointestinal: Nausea and vomiting

Genitourinary: Nephrotoxicity (acute renal failure and chronic renal insufficiency)

Hematologic & oncologic: Anemia, leukopenia (nadir: day 18 to 23; recovery: by day 39; dose related), thrombocytopenia (nadir: day 18 to 23; recovery: by day 39; dose related)

Hepatic: Increased liver enzymes

Local: Local irritation

Otic: Ototoxicity (as tinnitus, high frequency hearing loss; more common in children)

Rare but important or life-threatening: Alopecia (mild), ageusia, anaphylaxis, aortic thrombosis (Fernandes, 2011), autonomic neuropathy, bradycardia (Schlumbrecht, 2014), cardiac arrhythmia, cardiac failure, cerebrovascular accident, extravasation, hemolytic anemia (acute), hemolytic-uremic syndrome, hiccups, hypercholesterolemia, hyperuricemia, hypocalcemia, hypokalemia, hypomagnesemia, hyponatremia, hypophosphatemia, increased serum amylase, leukoencephalopathy, myocardial infarction, neutropenic enterocolitis (Furonaka, 2005), optic neuritis, pancreatitis (Trivedi, 2005), papilledema, peripheral ischemia (acute), phlebitis (Tokuda, 2014), SIADH, tachycardia, thrombotic thrombocytopenic purpura

Drug Interactions

Metabolism/Transport Effects None known.

Avoid Concomitant Use

Avoid concomitant use of CISplatin with any of the following: BCG; CloZAPine; Dipyrone; Natalizumab; Pimecrolimus; Tacrolimus (Topical); Tofacitinib; Vaccines (Live)

Increased Effect/Toxicity

CISplatin may increase the levels/effects of: Aminoglycosides; CloZAPine; Leflunomide; Natalizumab; Taxane Derivatives; Tofacitinib; Topotecan; Vaccines (Live); Vinorelbine

The levels/effects of CISplatin may be increased by: Denosumab; Dipyrone; Loop Diuretics; Pimecrolimus; Roflumilast; Tacrolimus (Topical); Trastuzumab

Decreased Effect

CISplatin may decrease the levels/effects of: BCG; Coccidioides immitis Skin Test; Fosphenytoin-Phenytoin; Sipuleucel-T; Vaccines (Inactivated); Vaccines (Live)

The levels/effects of CISplatin may be decreased by: Echinacea

Preparation for Administration Hazardous agent; use appropriate precautions for handling and disposal (NIOSH 2014 [group 1]). The infusion solution should have a final sodium chloride concentration ≥0.2%. Needles or IV administration sets that contain aluminum should not be used in the preparation or administration; aluminum can react with cisplatin resulting in precipitate formation and loss of potency.

Storage/Stability Store intact vials at 20°C to 25°C (68°F to 77°F). Protect from light. Do not refrigerate solution (precipitate may form). Further dilution **stability is dependent on the chloride ion concentration** and should be mixed in solutions of NS (at least 0.3% NaCl). After initial entry into the vial, solution is stable for 28 days protected from light or for at least 7 days under fluorescent room light at room temperature.

Further dilutions in NS, D_5/0.45% NaCl or D_5/NS to a concentration of 0.05 to 2 mg/mL are stable for 72 hours at 4°C to 25°C. The infusion solution should have a final sodium chloride concentration ≥0.2%.

Mechanism of Action Inhibits DNA synthesis by the formation of DNA cross-links; denatures the double helix; covalently binds to DNA bases and disrupts DNA function; may also bind to proteins; the *cis*-isomer is 14 times more cytotoxic than the *trans*-isomer; both forms cross-link DNA but cis-platinum is less easily recognized by cell enzymes and, therefore, not repaired. Cisplatin can also bind two adjacent guanines on the same strand of DNA producing intrastrand cross-linking and breakage.

Pharmacodynamics/Kinetics

Distribution: IV: Rapidly into tissue; high concentrations in kidneys, liver, ovaries, uterus, and lungs

Protein binding: >90% (O'Dwyer, 2000)

Metabolism: Nonenzymatic; inactivated (in both cell and bloodstream) by sulfhydryl groups; covalently binds to glutathione and thiosulfate

Half-life elimination: Initial: 14 to 49 minutes; Beta: 0.7 to 4.6 hours; Gamma: 24 to 127 hours (O'Dwyer, 2000)

Excretion: Urine (>90%); feces (minimal)

Dosage VERIFY ANY CISPLATIN DOSE EXCEEDING 100 mg/m² PER COURSE. Pretreatment hydration with 1 to 2 L of IV fluid is recommended. Cisplatin is associated with a high emetic potential; antiemetics are recommended to prevent nausea and vomiting (Basch, 2011; Dupuis, 2011; Roila, 2010).

Children:

Germ cell tumors (off-label use; combination chemotherapy): IV: 20 mg/m²/day on days 1 to 5 or 100 mg/m² on day 1 of a 21-day treatment cycle (Pinkerton, 1986)

Hepatoblastoma (off-label use; combination chemotherapy): IV: 80 mg/m² continuous infusion over 24 hours on day 1 of a 21-day treatment cycle (Pritchard, 2000)

Medulloblastoma (off-label use; combination chemotherapy): IV: 75 mg/m² on either day 0 or day 1 of each chemotherapy cycle (Packer, 2006)

Neuroblastoma, high-risk (off-label use; combination chemotherapy): IV: 50 mg/m²/day on days 0 to 3 of a 21-day cycle (cycles 3 and 5) (Naranjo, 2011) **or** 50 mg/m²/day on days 1 to 4 (cycles 3, 5, and 7) (Kushner, 1994)

Osteosarcoma (off-label use; combination chemotherapy): IV: 60 mg/m²/day for 2 days weeks 2, 7, 25, and 28 (neoadjuvant) or weeks 5, 10, 25, and 28 (adjuvant) (Goorin, 2003)

Adults:

Bladder cancer, advanced: IV: 50 to 70 mg/m² every 3 to 4 weeks; heavily pretreated patients: 50 mg/m² every 4 weeks

Ovarian cancer, metastatic:

Single agent: IV: 100 mg/m² every 4 weeks

Combination therapy: IV: 75 to 100 mg/m² every 4 weeks or (off-label dosing) 75 mg/m² every 3 weeks (Ozols, 2003)

Testicular cancer, metastatic: IV: 20 mg/m²/day for 5 days repeated every 3 weeks (Cushing, 2004; Saxman, 1998)

Cervical cancer (off-label use): IV: 75 mg/m² on day 1 every 3 weeks (in combination with fluorouracil and radiation) for 3 cycles (Morris, 1999) **or** 70 mg/m² on day 1 every 3 weeks for 4 cycles (in combination with fluorouracil; cycles 1 and 2 given concurrently with radiation) (Peters, 2000) **or** 50 mg/m² on day 1 every 4 weeks (in combination with radiation and fluorouracil) for 2 cycles (Whitney, 1999)

Endometrial carcinoma, recurrent, metastatic, or high-risk (off-label use): IV: 50 mg/m² on day 1 every 3 weeks (in combination with doxorubicin ± paclitaxel) for 7 cycles or until disease progression or unacceptable toxicity (Fleming, 2004)

Head and neck cancer (off-label use):

Locally advanced disease: IV: 100 mg/m² every 3 weeks for 3 doses (with concurrent radiation) (Bernier, 2004; Cooper, 2004) **or** 75 mg/m² every 3 weeks (in combination with docetaxel and fluorouracil) for 4 cycles or until disease progression or unacceptable toxicity (if no disease progression after 4 cycles, chemotherapy was followed by radiation) (Vermorken, 2007) **or** 100 mg/m² every 3 weeks (in combination with docetaxel and fluorouracil) for 3 cycles or until disease progression or unacceptable toxicity (chemotherapy was followed by chemoradiation) (Posner, 2007)

Metastatic disease: IV: 100 mg/m² every 3 weeks (in combination with fluorouracil and cetuximab) until disease progression or unacceptable toxicity or a maximum of 6 cycles (Vermorken, 2008)

Malignant pleural mesothelioma (off-label use): IV: 75 mg/m² on day 1 of each 21-day cycle (in combination with pemetrexed) (Vogelzang, 2003) **or** 100 mg/m² on day 1 of a 28-day cycle (in combination with gemcitabine) (Nowak, 2002) **or** 80 mg/m² on day 1 of a 21-day cycle (in combination with gemcitabine) (van Haarst, 2002)

Non-small cell lung cancer (NSCLC; off-label use): **Note:** There are multiple cisplatin-containing regimens for the treatment of NSCLC. Listed below are several commonly used regimens: IV:

100 mg/m² on day 1 every 4 weeks (in combination with etoposide) for 3 to 4 cycles; (Arriagada, 2007), or

100 mg/m² on day 1 every 4 weeks (in combination with vinorelbine) (Kelly, 2001; Wozniak, 1998), or

100 mg/m² on day 1 every 4 weeks (in combination with gemcitabine) (Comella, 2000), or

80 mg/m² on day 1 every 3 weeks (in combination with gemcitabine) (Ohe, 2007), or

75 mg/m² on day 1 every 3 weeks (in combination with pemetrexed) for up to 6 cycles or until disease progression or unacceptable toxicity (Scagliotti, 2008)

Ovarian cancer (off-label route): Intraperitoneal: 75 to 100 mg/m^2 on day 2 of a 21-day treatment cycle (in combination with IV and intraperitoneal paclitaxel) for 6 cycles (Armstrong, 2006; NCCN Ovarian Cancer guidelines, v.3.2014)

Small cell lung cancer (SCLC; off-label use):

Limited-stage disease: IV: 60 mg/m^2 on day 1 every 3 weeks for 4 cycles (in combination with etoposide and concurrent radiation) (Turrisi, 1999)

Extensive-stage disease: IV: 80 mg/m^2 on day 1 every 3 weeks (in combination with etoposide) for 4 cycles (Lara, 2009) or a maximum of 8 cycles (Ihde, 1994) **or** 60 mg/m^2 on day 1 every 4 weeks for 4 cycles (in combination with irinotecan) (Lara, 2009)

Testicular germ cell tumor, malignant (off-label use): IV: 25 mg/m^2 on days 2 to 5 every 3 weeks (in combination with paclitaxel and ifosfamide) for 4 cycles (Kondagunta, 2005) **or** 20 mg/m^2 on days 1 to 5 every 3 weeks (in combination with bleomycin and etoposide) for 4 cycles (Nichols, 1998) **or** 20 mg/m^2 on days 1 to 5 every 3 weeks (in combination with etoposide and ifosfamide) for 4 cycles (Nichols, 1998)

Elderly: Select dose cautiously and monitor closely in the elderly; may be more susceptible to nephrotoxicity and peripheral neuropathy.

Dosage adjustment in renal impairment: Note: The manufacturer(s) recommend that repeat courses of cisplatin should not be given until serum creatinine is <1.5 mg/dL and/or BUN is <25 mg/dL and use is contraindicated in preexisting renal impairment. The following adjustments have been recommended:

Aronoff, 2007:

CrCl 10 to 50 mL/minute: Administer 75% of dose

CrCl <10 mL/minute: Administer 50% of dose

Hemodialysis: Partially cleared by hemodialysis

Administer 50% of dose posthemodialysis

Continuous ambulatory peritoneal dialysis (CAPD): Administer 50% of dose

Continuous renal replacement therapy (CRRT): Administer 75% of dose

Janus, 2010: Hemodialysis: Reduce initial dose by 50%; administer post hemodialysis or on nondialysis days.

Kintzel, 1995:

CrCl 46 to 60 mL/minute: Administer 75% of dose

CrCl 31 to 45 mL/minute: Administer 50% of dose

CrCl <30 mL/minute: Consider use of alternative drug

Dosage adjustment in hepatic impairment: There are no dosage adjustments provided in manufacturer's labeling. However, cisplatin undergoes nonenzymatic metabolism and predominantly renal elimination; therefore, dosage adjustment is likely not necessary.

Dosing in obesity: *ASCO Guidelines for appropriate chemotherapy dosing in obese adults with cancer:* Utilize patient's actual body weight (full weight) for calculation of body surface area- or weight-based dosing, particularly when the intent of therapy is curative; manage regimen-related toxicities in the same manner as for nonobese patients; if a dose reduction is utilized due to toxicity, consider resumption of full weight-based dosing with subsequent cycles, especially if cause of toxicity (eg, hepatic or renal impairment) is resolved (Griggs, 2012).

Dietary Considerations Some products may contain sodium.

Administration Cisplatin is associated with a high emetic potential; antiemetics are recommended to prevent nausea and vomiting (Basch, 2011; Dupuis, 2011; Roila, 2010). Pretreatment hydration with 1 to 2 L of fluid is recommended prior to cisplatin administration; adequate post hydration and urinary output (>100 mL/hour) should be maintained for 24 hours after administration.

IV: Infuse over 6 to 8 hours; has also been infused (off-label rates) over 30 minutes to 3 hours, at a rate of 1 mg/minute, or as a continuous infusion; infusion rate varies by protocol (refer to specific protocol for infusion details). Avoid extravasation.

Needles or IV administration sets that contain aluminum should not be used in the preparation or administration; aluminum may react with cisplatin resulting in precipitate formation and loss of potency.

Vesicant (at higher concentrations); ensure proper needle or catheter placement prior to and during infusion; avoid extravasation.

Extravasation management: If extravasation occurs, stop infusion immediately and disconnect (leave cannula/needle in place); gently aspirate extravasated solution (do **NOT** flush the line); initiate sodium thiosulfate antidote; elevate extremity.

Sodium thiosulfate 1/6 M solution: Inject 2 mL into existing IV line for each 100 mg of cisplatin extravasated; then consider also injecting 1 mL as 0.1 mL subcutaneous injections (clockwise) around the area of extravasation, may repeat subcutaneous injections several times over the next 3 to 4 hours (Ener, 2004).

Dimethyl sulfoxide (DMSO) may also be considered an option: Apply to a region covering twice the affected area every 8 hours for 7 days; begin within 10 minutes of extravasation; do not cover with a dressing (Perez Fidalgo, 2012).

Hazardous agent; use appropriate precautions for handling and disposal (NIOSH 2014 [group 1]).

Monitoring Parameters Renal function (serum creatinine, BUN, CrCl); electrolytes (particularly magnesium, calcium, potassium [periodic]); CBC with differential and platelet count (weekly); liver function tests (periodic); audiography (baseline and prior to each subsequent dose, and following treatment in children), neurologic exam (with high dose); urine output, urinalysis

Dosage Forms

Solution, Intravenous:

Generic: 50 mg/50 mL (50 mL); 100 mg/100 mL (100 mL)

Solution, Intravenous [preservative free]:

Generic: 50 mg/50 mL (50 mL); 100 mg/100 mL (100 mL); 200 mg/200 mL (200 mL)

◆ **Cisplatin Injection (Can)** *see* CISplatin *on page 448*

◆ **Cisplatin Injection BP (Can)** *see* CISplatin *on page 448*

◆ **Cisplatin Injection, Mylan STD (Can)** *see* CISplatin *on page 448*

◆ ***Cis*-Retinoic Acid** *see* ISOtretinoin *on page 1127*

◆ **9-*cis*-Retinoic Acid** *see* Alitretinoin (Systemic) [CAN/INT] *on page 88*

◆ **13-*cis*-Retinoic Acid** *see* ISOtretinoin *on page 1127*

◆ **9-*cis*-Tretinoin** *see* Alitretinoin (Systemic) [CAN/INT] *on page 88*

◆ **13-*cis*-Vitamin A Acid** *see* ISOtretinoin *on page 1127*

Citalopram (sye TAL oh pram)

Brand Names: U.S. CeleXA

Brand Names: Canada Abbott-Citalopram; Accell-Citalopram; ACT Citalopram; AG-Citalopram; Apo-Citalopram; Auro-Citalopram; Celexa; Citalopram-Odan; CTP 30; Dom-Citalopram; ECL-Citalopram; JAMP-Citalopram; Mar-Citalopram; Mint-Citalopram; Mylan-Citalopram; Nat-Citalopram; PHL-Citalopram; PMS-Citalopram; Q-Citalopram; RAN-Citalo; Riva-Citalopram; Sandoz-Citalopram; Septa-Citalopram; Teva-Citalopram

Index Terms Citalopram Hydrobromide; Nitalapram

Pharmacologic Category Antidepressant, Selective Serotonin Reuptake Inhibitor

Use Treatment of depression

Pregnancy Risk Factor C

Pregnancy Considerations Adverse events have been observed in animal reproduction studies. Citalopram and its metabolites cross the human placenta. An increased risk of teratogenic effects, including cardiovascular defects, may be associated with maternal use of citalopram or other SSRIs; however, available information is conflicting. Nonteratogenic effects in the newborn following SSRI/SNRI exposure late in the third trimester include respiratory distress, cyanosis, apnea, seizures, temperature instability, feeding difficulty, vomiting, hypoglycemia, hypo- or hypertonia, hyper-reflexia, jitteriness, irritability, constant crying, and tremor. Symptoms may be due to the toxicity of the SSRIs/SNRIs or a discontinuation syndrome and may be consistent with serotonin syndrome associated with SSRI treatment. Persistent pulmonary hypertension of the newborn (PPHN) has also been reported with SSRI exposure. The long-term effects of *in utero* SSRI exposure on infant development and behavior are not known.

Due to pregnancy-induced physiologic changes, women who are pregnant may require adjusted doses of citalopram to achieve euthymia. The ACOG recommends that therapy with SSRIs or SNRIs during pregnancy be individualized; treatment of depression during pregnancy should incorporate the clinical expertise of the mental health clinician, obstetrician, primary healthcare provider, and pediatrician. According to the American Psychiatric Association (APA), the risks of medication treatment should be weighed against other treatment options and untreated depression. For women who discontinue antidepressant medications during pregnancy and who may be at high risk for postpartum depression, the medications can be restarted following delivery. Treatment algorithms have been developed by the ACOG and the APA for the management of depression in women prior to conception and during pregnancy.

Breast-Feeding Considerations Citalopram and its metabolites are excreted in breast milk. According to the manufacturer, the decision to continue or discontinue breast-feeding during therapy should take into account the risk of exposure to the infant and the benefits of treatment to the mother. Excessive somnolence, decreased feeding, colic, irritability, restlessness, and weight loss have been reported in breast-fed infants. The long-term effects on development and behavior have not been studied; therefore, citalopram should be prescribed to a mother who is breast-feeding only when the benefits outweigh the potential risks. Maternal use of an SSRI during pregnancy may cause delayed milk secretion.

Contraindications

Hypersensitivity to citalopram or any component of the formulation; use of MAO inhibitors intended to treat psychiatric disorders (concurrently or within 14 days of discontinuing either citalopram or the MAO inhibitor); initiation of citalopram in a patient receiving linezolid or intravenous methylene blue; concomitant use with pimozide

Canadian labeling: Additional contraindications (not in US labeling): Known QT interval prolongation or congenital long QT syndrome

Warnings/Precautions **[U.S. Boxed Warning]: Antidepressants increase the risk of suicidal thinking and behavior in children, adolescents, and young adults (18-24 years of age) with major depressive disorder (MDD) and other psychiatric disorders;** consider risk prior to prescribing. Short-term studies did not show an increased risk in patients >24 years of age and showed a decreased risk in patients ≥65 years. Closely monitor patients for clinical worsening, suicidality, or unusual changes in behavior, particularly during the initial 1-2 months of therapy or during periods of dosage adjustments (increases or decreases); the patient's family or caregiver should be instructed to closely observe the patient and communicate condition with healthcare provider. A medication guide concerning the use of antidepressants should be dispensed with each prescription. **Citalopram is not FDA approved for use in children.**

The possibility of a suicide attempt is inherent in major depression and may persist until remission occurs. Use caution in high-risk patients. Worsening depression and severe abrupt suicidality that are not part of the presenting symptoms may require discontinuation or modification of drug therapy. The patient's family or caregiver should be alerted to monitor patients for the emergence of suicidality and associated behaviors (such as agitation, irritability, hostility, impulsivity, and hypomania) and call healthcare provider.

May worsen psychosis in some patients or precipitate a shift to mania or hypomania in patients with bipolar disorder. Patients presenting with depressive symptoms should be screened for bipolar disorder. Monotherapy in patients with bipolar disorder should be avoided. **Citalopram is not FDA approved for the treatment of bipolar depression.**

Potentially life-threatening serotonin syndrome (SS) has occurred with serotonergic agents (eg, SSRIs, SNRIs), particularly when used in combination with other serotonergic agents (eg, triptans, TCAs, fentanyl, lithium, tramadol, buspirone, St. John's wort, tryptophan) or agents that impair metabolism of serotonin (eg, MAO inhibitors intended to treat psychiatric disorders, other MAO inhibitors [ie, linezolid and intravenous methylene blue]). Discontinue treatment (and any concomitant serotonergic agent) immediately if signs/symptoms arise. May increase the risks associated with electroconvulsive therapy. Has a low potential to impair cognitive or motor performance; caution operating hazardous machinery or driving. Bone fractures have been associated with antidepressant treatment. Consider the possibility of a fragility fracture if an antidepressant-treated patient presents with unexplained bone pain, point tenderness, swelling, or bruising (Rabenda, 2013; Rizzoli, 2012).

Citalopram causes dose-dependent QTc prolongation; torsade de pointes, ventricular tachycardia, and sudden death have been reported. Use is not recommended in patients with congenital long QT syndrome, bradycardia, recent MI, uncompensated heart failure, hypokalemia, and/or hypomagnesemia, or patients receiving concomitant medications which prolong the QT interval; if use is essential and cannot be avoided in these patients, ECG monitoring is recommended. Discontinue therapy in any patient with persistent QTc measurements >500 msec. Serum electrolytes, particularly potassium and magnesium, should be monitored prior to initiation and periodically during therapy in any patient at increased risk for significant electrolyte disturbances; hypokalemia and/or hypomagnesemia should be corrected prior to use. Due to the QT prolongation risk, doses >40 mg/day are not recommended. Additionally, the maximum daily dose should not exceed 20 mg/day in certain populations (eg, CYP2C19 poor metabolizers, patients with hepatic impairment, elderly patients). Potentially significant interactions may exist, requiring dose or frequency adjustment, additional monitoring, and/or selection of alternative therapy. Consult drug interactions database for more detailed information.

Use with caution in patients with a previous seizure disorder or condition predisposing to seizures such as brain damage or alcoholism. May cause or exacerbate sexual dysfunction. Use caution in elderly patients; may be potentially inappropriate in patients with a history of falls or fractures, and may cause hyponatremia/SIADH (elderly at increased risk); volume depletion and diuretics may increase risk. Monitor sodium closely with initiation or dosage adjustments in older adults (Beers Criteria). May cause mild pupillary dilation which in susceptible individuals can lead to an episode of narrow-angle glaucoma. Consider evaluating patients who have not had an iridectomy for narrow-angle glaucoma risk factors. Citalopram is not FDA-approved for use in children; however, if used, monitor weight and growth regularly during therapy due to the potential for decreased appetite and weight loss with SSRI use.

Abrupt discontinuation or interruption of antidepressant therapy has been associated with a discontinuation syndrome. Symptoms arising may vary with antidepressant however commonly include nausea, vomiting, diarrhea, headaches, light-headedness, dizziness, diminished appetite, sweating, chills, tremors, paresthesias, fatigue, somnolence, and sleep disturbances (eg, vivid dreams, insomnia). Greater risks for developing a discontinuation syndrome have been associated with antidepressants with shorter half-lives, longer durations of treatment, and abrupt discontinuation. For antidepressants of short or intermediate half-lives, symptoms may emerge within 2-5 days after treatment discontinuation and last 7-14 days (APA, 2010; Fava, 2006; Haddad, 2001; Shelton, 2001; Warner, 2006).

Adverse Reactions

Cardiovascular: Bradycardia, hypotension, orthostatic hypotension, QT prolongation, tachycardia

Central nervous system: Agitation, amnesia, anorexia, anxiety, apathy, concentration impaired, confusion, depression, fatigue (dose related), fever, insomnia (dose related), migraine, somnolence (dose related), suicide attempt, yawning (dose related)

Dermatologic: Pruritus, rash

Endocrine & metabolic: Amenorrhea, dysmenorrhea, libido decreased

Gastrointestinal: Abdominal pain, anorexia, appetite increased, diarrhea, dyspepsia, flatulence, nausea, salivation increased, taste perversion, vomiting, weight gain/loss, xerostomia

Genitourinary: Ejaculation disorder, impotence (dose related), polyuria

Neuromuscular & skeletal: Arthralgia, myalgia, paresthesia, tremor

Ocular: Abnormal accommodation

Respiratory: Cough, rhinitis, sinusitis, upper respiratory tract infection

Miscellaneous: Diaphoresis (dose related)

Rare but important or life-threatening: Allergic reaction, alopecia, anaphylaxis, anemia, angina pectoris, angioedema, arthritis, asthma, atrial fibrillation, bronchitis, bundle branch block, bursitis, cardiac arrest, cardiac failure, cataracts, catatonia, cerebrovascular accident, cholelithiasis, delirium, delusions, dependence, depersonalization, diplopia, diverticulitis, duodenal ulcer, eczema, epidermal necrolysis, erythema multiforme, extrapyramidal symptoms, extrasystoles, galactorrhea, gastric ulcer, gastrointestinal hemorrhage, glaucoma, granulocytopenia, gynecomastia, hallucinations, hemolytic anemia, hepatic necrosis, hepatitis, hyperpigmentation, hypertension, hypertrichosis, hypoglycemia, hypokalemia, hyponatremia, hypothyroidism, leukocytosis, leukopenia, lymphadenopathy, lymphocytosis, lymphopenia, muscle weakness, myocardial infarction, myocardial ischemia, neuroleptic malignant syndrome, obesity, osteoporosis, pancreatitis, phlebitis, photosensitivity, pneumonia, priapism, prolactinemia, prothrombin decreased, psoriasis, psychosis, ptosis, pulmonary embolism, renal calculi, renal failure, rhabdomyolysis, seizures, serotonin syndrome, SIADH, spontaneous abortion, syncope, thrombocytopenia, thrombosis, torsade de pointes, transient ischemic attack, urinary incontinence, urinary retention, vaginal bleeding, ventricular arrhythmia, withdrawal syndrome

Drug Interactions

Metabolism/Transport Effects Substrate of CYP2C19 (major), CYP2D6 (minor), CYP3A4 (major); **Note:** Assignment of Major/Minor substrate status based on clinically relevant drug interaction potential; **Inhibits** CYP1A2 (weak), CYP2B6 (weak), CYP2C19 (weak), CYP2D6 (weak)

Avoid Concomitant Use

Avoid concomitant use of Citalopram with any of the following: Conivaptan; Dapoxetine; Dosulepin; Fluconazole; Fusidic Acid (Systemic); Highest Risk QTc-Prolonging Agents; Idelalisib; Iobenguane I 123; Ivabradine; Linezolid; MAO Inhibitors; Methylene Blue; Mifepristone; Moderate Risk QTc-Prolonging Agents; Pimozide; Tryptophan; Urokinase

Increased Effect/Toxicity

Citalopram may increase the levels/effects of: Agents with Antiplatelet Properties; Anticoagulants; Antidepressants (Serotonin Reuptake Inhibitor/Antagonist); Antipsychotic Agents; Apixaban; Aspirin; BusPIRone; CarBAMazepine; Collagenase (Systemic); Dabigatran Etexilate; Desmopressin; Dextromethorphan; Dosulepin; Highest Risk QTc-Prolonging Agents; Hypoglycemic Agents; Ibritumomab; Methylene Blue; Mexiletine; NSAID (COX-2 Inhibitor); NSAID (Nonselective); Obinutuzumab; Pimozide; Rivaroxaban; Salicylates; Serotonin Modulators; Thiazide Diuretics; Thrombolytic Agents; Tositumomab and Iodine I 131 Tositumomab; TraMADol; Tricyclic Antidepressants; Urokinase; Vitamin K Antagonists

The levels/effects of Citalopram may be increased by: Alcohol (Ethyl); Analgesics (Opioid); Antiemetics (5HT3 Antagonists); Antipsychotic Agents; Aprepitant; BuPROPion; BusPIRone; Cimetidine; CNS Depressants; Conivaptan; CYP2C19 Inhibitors (Moderate); CYP2C19 Inhibitors (Strong); CYP3A4 Inhibitors (Moderate); CYP3A4 Inhibitors (Strong); Dapoxetine; Fluconazole; Fosaprepitant; Fusidic Acid (Systemic); Glucosamine; Herbs (Anticoagulant/Antiplatelet Properties); Ibrutinib; Idelalisib; Ivabradine; Ivacaftor; Limaprost; Linezolid; Lithium; Luliconazole; MAO Inhibitors; Metoclopramide; Metyrosine; Mifepristone; Moderate Risk QTc-Prolonging Agents; Multivitamins/Fluoride (with ADE); Multivitamins/Minerals (with ADEK, Folate, Iron); Multivitamins/Minerals (with AE, No Iron); Netupitant; Omega-3 Fatty Acids; Pentosan Polysulfate Sodium; Pentoxifylline; Prostacyclin Analogues; QTc-Prolonging Agents (Indeterminate Risk and Risk Modifying); Simeprevir; Stiripentol; Tedizolid; Tipranavir; TraMADol; Tricyclic Antidepressants; Tryptophan; Vitamin E

Decreased Effect

Citalopram may decrease the levels/effects of: Iobenguane I 123; Ioflupane I 123; Thyroid Products

The levels/effects of Citalopram may be decreased by: Bosentan; CarBAMazepine; CYP2C19 Inducers (Strong); CYP3A4 Inducers (Moderate); CYP3A4 Inducers (Strong); Cyproheptadine; Dabrafenib; Deferasirox; Mitotane; NSAID (COX-2 Inhibitor); NSAID (Nonselective); Rifampin; Siltuximab; St Johns Wort; Tocilizumab

Storage/Stability Store at 25°C (77°F); excursions permitted to 15°C to 30°C (59°F to 86°F). Protect from moisture.

Mechanism of Action A racemic bicyclic phthalane derivative, citalopram selectively inhibits serotonin reuptake in the presynaptic neurons and has minimal effects on norepinephrine or dopamine. Uptake inhibition of serotonin is primarily due to the *S*-enantiomer of citalopram. Displays little to no affinity for serotonin, dopamine, adrenergic, histamine, GABA, or muscarinic receptor subtypes.

Pharmacodynamics/Kinetics

Onset of action: Depression: The onset of action is 1-4 weeks; however, individual response varies greatly and full response may not be seen until 8-12 weeks after initiation of treatment.

Distribution: V_d: 12 L/kg

Protein binding, plasma: ~80%

Metabolism: Extensively hepatic, via CYP3A4 and 2C19 (major pathways), and 2D6 (minor pathway); metabolized to demethylcitalopram (DCT), didemethylcitalopram (DDCT), citalopram-N-oxide, and a deaminated propionic acid derivative, which are at least eight times less potent than citalopram

Bioavailability: 80%; tablets and oral solution are bioequivalent

Half-life elimination: 24-48 hours (average: 35 hours); doubled with hepatic impairment and increased by 30% (following multiple doses) to 50% (following single dose) in elderly patients (≥60 years)

Time to peak, serum: 1-6 hours, average within 4 hours

Excretion: Urine (Citalopram 10% and DCT 5%)

Note: Clearance was decreased, while half-life was significantly increased in patients with hepatic impairment. Mild-to-moderate renal impairment may reduce clearance (17%) and prolong half-life of citalopram. No pharmacokinetic information is available concerning patients with severe renal impairment. AUC and half-life were significantly increased in elderly patients (≥60 years), and in poor CYP2C19 metabolizers, steady state C_{max} and AUC was increased by 68% and 107%, respectively.

Dosage Oral:

Children and Adolescents: Obsessive-compulsive disorder (off-label use): 10-40 mg daily (Mukaddes, 2003; Thomsen, 1997; Thomsen, 2001)

Adults <60 years: Depression: Initial: 20 mg once daily; increase the dose by 20 mg at an interval of ≥1 week to a maximum dose of 40 mg daily. **Note:** Doses >40 mg daily are not recommended due to the risk of QT prolongation; additional efficacy with doses >40 mg daily has not been demonstrated in clinical trials.

Poor metabolizers of CYP2C19 or concurrent use of moderate-to-strong CYP2C19 inhibitors (eg, cimetidine, omeprazole): Maximum dose: 20 mg daily

Elderly ≥60 years: Depression: Initial: 20 mg once daily; maximum dose in adults ≥60 years: 20 mg daily due to increased exposure and the risk of QT prolongation. Refer to adult dosing.

Discontinuation of therapy: Upon discontinuation of antidepressant therapy, gradually taper the dose to minimize the incidence of withdrawal symptoms and allow for the detection of re-emerging symptoms. Evidence supporting ideal taper rates is limited. APA and NICE guidelines suggest tapering therapy over at least several weeks with consideration to the half-life of the antidepressant; antidepressants with a shorter half-life may need to be tapered more conservatively. In addition for long-term treated patients, WFSBP guidelines recommend tapering over 4-6 months. If intolerable withdrawal symptoms occur following a dose reduction, consider resuming the previously prescribed dose and/or decrease dose at a more gradual rate (APA, 2010; Bauer, 2002; Haddad, 2001; NCCMH, 2010; Schatzberg, 2006; Shelton, 2001; Warner, 2006).

MAO inhibitor recommendations:

Switching to or from an MAO inhibitor intended to treat psychiatric disorders:

Allow 14 days to elapse between discontinuing an MAO inhibitor intended to treat psychiatric disorders and initiation of citalopram.

Allow 14 days to elapse between discontinuing citalopram and initiation of an MAO inhibitor intended to treat psychiatric disorders.

Use with other MAO inhibitors (linezolid or IV methylene blue):

Do not initiate citalopram in patients receiving linezolid or IV methylene blue; consider other interventions for psychiatric condition.

If urgent treatment with linezolid or IV methylene blue is required in a patient already receiving citalopram and potential benefits outweigh potential risks, discontinue citalopram promptly and administer linezolid or IV methylene blue. Monitor for serotonin syndrome for 2 weeks or until 24 hours after the last dose of linezolid or IV methylene blue, whichever comes first. May resume citalopram 24 hours after the last dose of linezolid or IV methylene blue.

Dosage adjustment in renal impairment:

Mild-to-moderate impairment: No dosage adjustment necessary.

Severe impairment: CrCl <20 mL/minute: No dosage adjustment provided in manufacturer's labeling (has not been studied); use caution.

Dosage adjustment in hepatic impairment: Initial: 20 mg once daily; maximum recommended dose: 20 mg daily due to decreased clearance and the risk of QT prolongation

Dietary Considerations May be taken without regard to food.

Administration May be administered without regard to food.

Monitoring Parameters ECG (patients at increased risk for QT-prolonging effects due to certain conditions); electrolytes (potassium and magnesium concentrations [prior to initiation and periodically during therapy in patients at increased risk for electrolyte abnormalities]); signs/symptoms of arrhythmias (eg, dizziness, palpitations, syncope); liver function tests and CBC with continued therapy; monitor patient periodically for symptom resolution; signs/symptoms of serotonin syndrome; mental status for depression, suicidal ideation (especially at the beginning of therapy or when doses are increased or decreased), anxiety, social functioning, mania, panic attacks; akathisia

Dosage Forms

Solution, Oral:

Generic: 10 mg/5 mL (240 mL)

Tablet, Oral:

CeleXA: 10 mg, 20 mg, 40 mg

Generic: 10 mg, 20 mg, 40 mg

◆ **Citalopram Hydrobromide** *see* Citalopram *on page 451*

◆ **Citalopram-Odan (Can)** *see* Citalopram *on page 451*

◆ **Citracal Maximum [OTC]** *see* Calcium and Vitamin D *on page 326*

◆ **Citracal Petites [OTC]** *see* Calcium and Vitamin D *on page 326*

◆ **Citracal Regular [OTC]** *see* Calcium and Vitamin D *on page 326*

◆ **Citrate of Magnesia** *see* Magnesium Citrate *on page 1262*

◆ **Citric Acid and Potassium Citrate** *see* Potassium Citrate and Citric Acid *on page 1689*

◆ **Citric Acid and Sodium Citrate** *see* Sodium Citrate and Citric Acid *on page 1905*

Citric Acid, Sodium Citrate, and Potassium Citrate

(SIT rik AS id, SOW dee um SIT rate, & poe TASS ee um SIT rate)

Brand Names: U.S. Cytra-3; Virtrate-3

Index Terms Polycitra; Potassium Citrate, Citric Acid, and Sodium Citrate; Sodium Citrate, Citric Acid, and Potassium Citrate

Pharmacologic Category Alkalinizing Agent

Use Conditions where long-term maintenance of an alkaline urine is desirable as in control and dissolution of uric acid and cystine calculi of the urinary tract

Pregnancy Risk Factor Not established

Dosage Oral:

Children: 5-15 mL diluted in water after meals and at bedtime

Adults: 15-30 mL diluted in water after meals and at bedtime

Additional Information Complete prescribing information should be consulted for additional detail.

Dosage Forms

Solution, Oral:

Virtrate-3: Citric acid 334 mg, sodium citrate 500 mg, and potassium citrate 550 mg per 5 mL (473 mL)

Generic: Citric acid 334 mg, sodium citrate 500 mg, and potassium citrate 550 mg per 5 mL (473 mL)

Syrup, Oral:

Cytra-3: Citric acid 334 mg, sodium citrate 500 mg, and potassium citrate 550 mg per 5 mL (473 mL)

- ◆ **Citric Acid, Sodium Picosulfate, and Magnesium Oxide** *see* Sodium Picosulfate, Magnesium Oxide, and Citric Acid *on page 1911*
- ◆ **Citroma [OTC]** *see* Magnesium Citrate *on page 1262*
- ◆ **Citro-Mag (Can)** *see* Magnesium Citrate *on page 1262*
- ◆ **Citrovorum Factor** *see* Leucovorin Calcium *on page 1183*
- ◆ **CL-118,532** *see* Triptorelin *on page 2107*
- ◆ **CI-719** *see* Gemfibrozil *on page 956*
- ◆ **CL-184116** *see* Porfimer *on page 1682*
- ◆ **CL-232315** *see* MitoXANtrone *on page 1382*

Cladribine (KLA dri been)

Index Terms 2-CdA; 2-Chlorodeoxyadenosine; Leustatin

Pharmacologic Category Antineoplastic Agent, Antimetabolite; Antineoplastic Agent, Antimetabolite (Purine Analog)

Use Treatment of active hairy cell leukemia

Pregnancy Risk Factor D

Dosage

Children: IV:

Acute myeloid leukemia (off-label use): 8.9 mg/m²/day continuous infusion for 5 days for 1 or 2 courses (Krance, 2001) **or** 9 mg/m²/day over 30 minutes for 5 days for 1 course (in combination with cytarabine) (Crews, 2002; Rubnitz, 2009)

Langerhans cell histiocytosis, refractory (off-label use): 5 mg/m²/day over 2 hours for 5 days every 21 days for up to 6 cycles (Weitzman, 2009)

Adults: Details concerning dosing in combination regimens should also be consulted.

Hairy cell leukemia: IV: 0.09 mg/kg/day continuous infusion for 7 days for 1 cycle **or** (off-label dosing) 0.1 mg/kg/day continuous infusion for 7 days for 1 cycle (Goodman, 2003; Saven, 1998)

Acute myeloid leukemia, induction (off-label use): IV: CLAG or CLAG-M regimen: 5 mg/m²/day over 2 hours for 5 days; a second induction may be administered if needed (Robak, 2000; Wierzbowska, 2008; Wrzesień-Kuś, 2003)

Chronic lymphocytic leukemia (off-label use): IV: 0.1 mg/kg/day continuous infusion for 7 days every 4-5 weeks (Saven, 1995) **or** 0.14 mg/kg/day over 2 hours for 5 days every 28 days for 3-6 cycles (Byrd, 2003)

Mantle cell lymphoma (off-label use): IV: 5 mg/m²/day over 2 hours for 5 days every 4 weeks for 2-6 cycles (Inwards, 2008; Rummel, 1999) **or** 5 mg/m²/day over 2 hours for 5 days every 4 weeks for 2-6 cycles (in combination with rituximab) (Inwards, 2008)

Waldenström's macroglobulinemia (off-label use):

IV: 0.1 mg/kg/day continuous infusion for 7 days every 4 weeks for 2 cycles (Dimopoulos, 1994)

SubQ: 0.1 mg/kg/day for 5 consecutive days every month for 4 cycles (in combination with rituximab) (Laszlo, 2010)

Dosing adjustment in renal impairment: No dosage adjustment provided in the manufacturer's labeling (due to inadequate data); use with caution. The following adjustments have been used (Aronoff, 2007):

Children:

CrCl 10-50 mL/minute: Administer 50% of dose

CrCl <10 mL/minute: Administer 30% of dose

Hemodialysis: Administer 30% of dose

Continuous renal replacement therapy (CRRT): Administer 50% of dose

Adults:

CrCl 10-50 mL/minute: Administer 75% of dose

CrCl <10 mL/minute: Administer 50% of dose

Continuous ambulatory peritoneal dialysis (CAPD): Administer 50% of dose

Dosing adjustment in hepatic impairment: No dosage adjustment provided in the manufacturer's labeling (due to inadequate data); use with caution.

Dosing in obesity: ASCO Guidelines for appropriate chemotherapy dosing in obese adults with cancer: Utilize patient's actual body weight (full weight) for calculation of body surface area- or weight-based dosing, particularly when the intent of therapy is curative; manage regimen-related toxicities in the same manner as for nonobese patients; if a dose reduction is utilized due to toxicity, consider resumption of full weight-based dosing with subsequent cycles, especially if cause of toxicity (eg, hepatic or renal impairment) is resolved (Griggs, 2012).

Additional Information Complete prescribing information should be consulted for additional detail.

Dosage Forms

Solution, Intravenous [preservative free]:

Generic: 1 mg/mL (10 mL)

- ◆ **Claforan** *see* Cefotaxime *on page 382*
- ◆ **Claforan in D5W** *see* Cefotaxime *on page 382*
- ◆ **Claravis** *see* ISOtretinoin *on page 1127*
- ◆ **Clarifoam EF** *see* Sulfur and Sulfacetamide *on page 1953*
- ◆ **Clarinex** *see* Desloratadine *on page 594*
- ◆ **Clarinex-D® 12 Hour** *see* Desloratadine and Pseudoephedrine *on page 594*
- ◆ **Clarinex-D® 24 Hour [DSC]** *see* Desloratadine and Pseudoephedrine *on page 594*
- ◆ **Clarinex Reditabs** *see* Desloratadine *on page 594*
- ◆ **Claris** *see* Sulfur and Sulfacetamide *on page 1953*

Clarithromycin (kla RITH roe mye sin)

Brand Names: U.S. Biaxin; Biaxin XL; Biaxin XL Pac

Brand Names: Canada Accel-Clarithromycin; Apo-Clarithromycin; Apo-Clarithromycin XL; Biaxin; Biaxin BID; Biaxin XL; Dom-Clarithromycin; Mylan-Clarithromycin; PMS-Clarithromycin; RAN-Clarithromycin; Riva-Clarithromycin; Sandoz-Clarithromycin; Teva-Clarithromycin

Pharmacologic Category Antibiotic, Macrolide

Use

Infants and Children 6 months and older:

- Acute maxillary sinusitis due to susceptible *H. influenzae, S. pneumoniae,* or *Moraxella catarrhalis*
- Acute otitis media due to susceptible *H. influenzae, M. catarrhalis*, or *S. pneumoniae*
- Community-acquired pneumonia due to susceptible *Mycoplasma pneumoniae, S. pneumoniae*, or *Chlamydophila pneumoniae* (TWAR)
- Disseminated mycobacterial infections due to *M. avium* or *M. intracellulare*
- Pharyngitis/tonsillitis due to susceptible *S. pyogenes*
- Prevention of disseminated mycobacterial infections due to *M. avium* complex (MAC) disease in patients with advanced HIV infection (20 months of age and older)
- Uncomplicated skin/skin structure infection due to susceptible *S. aureus* or *S. pyogenes*

Adults:

- Pharyngitis/tonsillitis due to susceptible *S. pyogenes*
- Acute maxillary sinusitis due to susceptible *H. influenzae, M. catarrhalis,* or *S. pneumoniae*
- Acute exacerbation of chronic bronchitis due to susceptible *H. influenzae, H. parainfluenzae, M. catarrhalis*, or *S. pneumoniae*
- Community-acquired pneumonia due to susceptible *H. influenzae, H. parainfluenzae, M. catarrhalis, Mycoplasma pneumoniae, S. pneumoniae*, or *Chlamydophila pneumoniae* (TWAR)
- Uncomplicated skin/skin structure infections due to susceptible *S. aureus* or *S. pyogenes*
- Disseminated mycobacterial infections due to *M. avium* or *M. intracellulare*
- Prevention of disseminated mycobacterial infections due to MAC disease in patients with advanced HIV infection
- Duodenal ulcer disease due to *H. pylori* in regimens with other drugs including amoxicillin and lansoprazole or omeprazole, or in combination with omeprazole or ranitidine bismuth citrate (no longer marketed in the U.S.). **Note:** Regimens that contain clarithromycin as the single antimicrobial agent are more likely to be associated with the development of clarithromycin resistance.

Pregnancy Risk Factor C

Pregnancy Considerations Adverse events have been documented in some animal reproduction studies. Clarithromycin crosses the placenta (Witt, 2003). The manufacturer recommends that clarithromycin not be used in a pregnant woman unless there are no alternative therapies. Clarithromycin is generally not recommended for the treatment or prophylaxis of *Mycobacterium avium* complex (MAC) or bacterial respiratory disease in HIV-infected pregnant patients (DHHS, 2013).

Breast-Feeding Considerations Clarithromycin and its active metabolite (14-hydroxy clarithromycin) are excreted into breast milk. The manufacturer recommends that caution be used if administered to nursing women. Decreased appetite, diarrhea, rash, and somnolence have been noted in nursing infants exposed to macrolide antibiotics (Goldstein, 2009).

Contraindications Hypersensitivity to clarithromycin, erythromycin, any of the macrolide antibiotics, or any component of the formulation; history of cholestatic jaundice/hepatic dysfunction associated with prior use of clarithromycin; history of QT prolongation or ventricular cardiac arrhythmia, including torsade de pointes; concomitant use with cisapride, pimozide, ergotamine, dihydroergotamine, HMG-CoA reductase inhibitors extensively metabolized by CYP3A4 (eg, lovastatin, simvastatin), astemizole or terfenadine (not available in the U.S.); concomitant use with colchicine in patients with renal or hepatic impairment

Warnings/Precautions Use has been associated with QT prolongation and infrequent cases of arrhythmias, including torsade de pointes; use is contraindicated in patients with a history of QT prolongation and ventricular arrhythmias, including torsade de pointes. Systemic exposure is increased in the elderly; may be at increased risk of torsade de pointes, particularly if concurrent severe renal impairment. Use with caution in patients at risk of prolonged cardiac repolarization. Avoid use in patients with uncorrected hypokalemia or hypomagnesemia, clinically significant bradycardia, and patients receiving Class IA (eg, quinidine, procainamide) or Class III (eg, amiodarone, dofetilide, sotalol) antiarrhythmic agents. Use caution in patients with coronary artery disease.

Elevated liver function tests and hepatitis (hepatocellular and/or cholestatic with or without jaundice) have been reported; usually reversible after discontinuation of clarithromycin. May lead to hepatic failure or death (rarely), especially in the presence of preexisting diseases and/or concomitant use of medications. Discontinue immediately if symptoms of hepatitis occur. Dosage adjustment needed in severe renal impairment. Use with caution in patients with myasthenia gravis.

Potentially significant drug-drug interactions may exist, requiring dose or frequency adjustment, additional monitoring, and/or selection of alternative therapy. Colchicine toxicity (including fatalities) has been reported with concomitant use; concomitant use is contraindicated in patients with renal or hepatic impairment. Clarithromycin in combination with ranitidine bismuth citrate should not be used in patients with a history of acute porphyria. Prolonged use may result in fungal or bacterial superinfection, including *C. difficile*-associated diarrhea (CDAD) and pseudomembranous colitis; CDAD has been observed >2 months postantibiotic treatment. Decreased *H. pylori* eradication rates have been observed with short-term (≤7 days) combination therapy. Current guidelines recommend 10 to 14 days of therapy (triple or quadruple) for eradication of *H. pylori* in pediatric and adult patients (Chey, 2007; NASPHGAN [Koletzko 2011]).

Severe acute reactions have (rarely) been reported, including anaphylaxis, Stevens-Johnson syndrome (SJS), toxic epidermal necrolysis (TEN), drug rash with eosinophilia and systemic symptoms (DRESS), and Henoch-Schönlein purpura (IgA vasculitis); discontinue therapy and initiate treatment immediately for severe acute hypersensitivity reactions. The presence of extended release tablets in the stool has been reported, particularly in patients with anatomic (eg, ileostomy, colostomy) or functional GI disorders with decreased transit times. Consider alternative dosage forms (eg, suspension) or an alternative antimicrobial for patients with tablet residue in the stool and no signs of clinical improvement. Some dosage forms may contain propylene glycol; large amounts are potentially toxic and have been associated hyperosmolality, lactic acidosis, seizures, and respiratory depression; use caution (AAP, 1997; Zar, 2007).

Adverse Reactions

Central nervous system: Headache, insomnia

Dermatologic: Skin rash (children)

Gastrointestinal: Abdominal pain, diarrhea, dysgeusia (adults), dyspepsia (adults), nausea (adults), vomiting (children)
Hematologic & oncologic: Prolonged prothrombin time (adults)
Hepatic: Abnormal hepatic function tests
Hypersensitivity: Anaphylactoid reaction
Infection: Candidiasis (including oral)
Renal: Increased blood urea nitrogen
Rare but important or life-threatening: Acne vulgaris, ageusia, altered sense of smell, anxiety, asthma, atrial fibrillation, behavioral changes, cardiac arrest, cellulitis, cholestatic hepatitis, *Clostridium difficile* associated diarrhea, *Clostridium difficile* (colitis), dental discoloration (reversible with dental cleaning), depression, disorientation, DRESS syndrome, drowsiness, dyskinesia, epistaxis, esophagitis, extrasystoles, gastritis, gastroesophageal reflux disease, glossitis, hallucination, hearing loss (reversible), hemorrhage, hepatic failure, hyperhidrosis, hypersensitivity, hypoglycemia, IgA vasculitis, increased gamma-glutamyl transferase, increased INR, increased lactate dehydrogenase, interstitial nephritis, leukopenia, loss of consciousness, malaise, manic behavior, neck stiffness, neutropenia, pancreatitis, parasominas, paresthesia, prolonged QT interval on ECG, pruritus, pseudomembranous colitis, pulmonary embolism, renal failure, rhabdomyolysis, seizure, Stevens-Johnson syndrome, stomatitis, thrombocytopenia, tinnitus, tongue discoloration, torsades de pointes, vaginal infection, ventricular arrhythmia, ventricular tachycardia

Drug Interactions

Metabolism/Transport Effects **Substrate** of CYP3A4 (major); **Note:** Assignment of Major/Minor substrate status based on clinically relevant drug interaction potential; **Inhibits** CYP1A2 (weak), CYP3A4 (strong), P-glycoprotein

Avoid Concomitant Use

Avoid concomitant use of Clarithromycin with any of the following: Ado-Trastuzumab Emtansine; Alfuzosin; Apixaban; Astemizole; Avanafil; Axitinib; BCG; Bosutinib; Cabozantinib; Ceritinib; Cisapride; Conivaptan; Crizotinib; Dapoxetine; Dihydroergotamine; Disopyramide; Dronedarone; Eplerenone; Ergotamine; Everolimus; Fusidic Acid (Systemic); Halofantrine; Highest Risk QTc-Prolonging Agents; Ibrutinib; Idelalisib; Irinotecan; Ivabradine; Lapatinib; Lercanidipine; Lomitapide; Lovastatin; Lurasidone; Macitentan; Mifepristone; Naloxegol; Nilotinib; Nisoldipine; Olaparib; PAZOPanib; Pimozide; QuiNIDine; QuiNINE; Ranolazine; Red Yeast Rice; Regorafenib; Salmeterol; Silodosin; Simeprevir; Simvastatin; Suvorexant; Tamsulosin; Terfenadine; Ticagrelor; Tolvaptan; Topotecan; Toremifene; Trabectedin; Ulipristal; Vemurafenib; VinCRIStine (Liposomal); Vorapaxar

Increased Effect/Toxicity

Clarithromycin may increase the levels/effects of: Ado-Trastuzumab Emtansine; Afatinib; Alfentanil; Alfuzosin; Almotriptan; Alosetron; ALPRAZolam; Antifungal Agents (Azole Derivatives, Systemic); Antineoplastic Agents (Vinca Alkaloids); Apixaban; ARIPiprazole; Astemizole; AtorvaSTATin; Avanafil; Axitinib; Bedaquiline; Boceprevir; Bortezomib; Bosutinib; Brentuximab Vedotin; Brinzolamide; Budesonide (Nasal); Budesonide (Systemic, Oral Inhalation); BusPIRone; Cabazitaxel; Cabergoline; Cabozantinib; Calcium Channel Blockers; Cannabis; CarBAMazepine; Cardiac Glycosides; Ceritinib; Cilostazol; Cisapride; CloZAPine; Cobicistat; Colchicine; Conivaptan; Corticosteroids (Orally Inhaled); Corticosteroids (Systemic); Crizotinib; CYP3A4 Inducers (Strong); CYP3A4 Substrates; Dabigatran Etexilate; Dapoxetine; Dasatinib; Dienogest; Dihydroergotamine; Disopyramide; DOXOrubicin (Conventional); Dronabinol; Dronedarone; Dutasteride; Edoxaban; Eletriptan; Eplerenone; Ergot Derivatives; Ergotamine; Erlotinib; Estazolam; Etizolam; Everolimus; FentaNYL; Fesoterodine; Fluticasone (Nasal); Fluticasone (Oral Inhalation); GlipiZIDE; GlyBURIDE; GuanFACINE; Halofantrine; Highest Risk QTc-Prolonging Agents; Hydrocodone; Ibrutinib; Imatinib; Imidafenacin; Irinotecan; Ivabradine; Ivacaftor; Ixabepilone; Lacosamide; Lapatinib; Ledipasvir; Lercanidipine; Levobupivacaine; Levomilnacipran; Lomitapide; Lovastatin; Lurasidone; Macitentan; Maraviroc; MethylPREDNISolone; Midazolam; Moderate Risk QTc-Prolonging Agents; Naloxegol; Nilotinib; Nintedanib; Nisoldipine; Olaparib; Ospemifene; OxyCODONE; Paricalcitol; PAZOPanib; P-glycoprotein/ABCB1 Substrates; Pimecrolimus; Pimozide; Pitavastatin; PONATinib; Pranlukast; Pravastatin; PrednisoLONE (Systemic); PredniSONE; Protease Inhibitors; Prucalopride; QuiNIDine; QuiNINE; Ranolazine; Red Yeast Rice; Regorafenib; Repaglinide; Retapamulin; Rifaximin; Rilpivirine; Rivaroxaban; Ruxolitinib; Salmeterol; Saxagliptin; Selective Serotonin Reuptake Inhibitors; Sildenafil; Silodosin; Simeprevir; Simvastatin; Sirolimus; Suvorexant; Tacrolimus (Topical); Tadalafil; Tamsulosin; Telaprevir; Temsirolimus; Terfenadine; Tetrahydrocannabinol; Theophylline Derivatives; Ticagrelor; Tofacitinib; Tolterodine; Tolvaptan; Topotecan; Toremifene; Trabectedin; Triazolam; Ulipristal; Vardenafil; Vemurafenib; Vilazodone; VinCRIStine (Liposomal); Vitamin K Antagonists; Vorapaxar; Zidovudine; Zopiclone

The levels/effects of Clarithromycin may be increased by: Antifungal Agents (Azole Derivatives, Systemic); Boceprevir; Cobicistat; Conivaptan; CYP3A4 Inducers (Moderate); CYP3A4 Inducers (Strong); CYP3A4 Inhibitors (Moderate); CYP3A4 Inhibitors (Strong); Fusidic Acid (Systemic); Idelalisib; Ivabradine; Luliconazole; Mifepristone; Netupitant; Protease Inhibitors; QTc-Prolonging Agents (Indeterminate Risk and Risk Modifying); Stiripentol; Telaprevir

Decreased Effect

Clarithromycin may decrease the levels/effects of: BCG; Clopidogrel; Ifosfamide; Prasugrel; Sodium Picosulfate; Ticagrelor; Typhoid Vaccine; Zidovudine

The levels/effects of Clarithromycin may be decreased by: CYP3A4 Inducers (Moderate); CYP3A4 Inducers (Strong); Dabrafenib; Deferasirox; Efavirenz; Etravirine; Mitotane; Protease Inhibitors; Siltuximab; St Johns Wort; Tocilizumab

Food Interactions Immediate release: Food delays rate, but not extent of absorption; Extended release: Food increases clarithromycin AUC by ~30% relative to fasting conditions. Management: Administer immediate release products without regard to meals. Administer extended release products with food.

Storage/Stability

Extended release tablets: Store at 20°C to 25°C (68°F to 77°F); excursions are permitted between 15°C and 30°C (59°F and 86°F).
Immediate release tablets:
250 mg: Store at 15°C to 30°C (59°F to 86°F). Protect from light.
500 mg: Store at 20°C to 25°C (68°F to 77°F).
Granules for suspension: Store at 15°C to 30°C (59°F to 86°F) prior to and following reconstitution. Do not refrigerate. Use within 14 days of reconstitution.

Mechanism of Action Exerts its antibacterial action by binding to 50S ribosomal subunit resulting in inhibition of protein synthesis. The 14-OH metabolite of clarithromycin is twice as active as the parent compound against certain organisms.

Pharmacodynamics/Kinetics

Absorption:
Immediate release: Rapid; food delays rate, but not extent of absorption
Extended-release: Fasting is associated with ~30% lower AUC relative to administration with food

Distribution: Widely into most body tissues; manufacturer reports no data in regards to CNS penetration

Protein binding: 42% to 70% (Peters, 1992)

Metabolism: Partially hepatic via CYP3A4; converted to 14-OH clarithromycin (active metabolite)

Bioavailability: ~50%

Half-life elimination: Immediate release: Clarithromycin: 3-7 hours; 14-OH-clarithromycin: 5-9 hours

Time to peak: Immediate release: 2-3 hours; Extended release: 5-8 hours

Excretion: Urine (20% to 40% as unchanged drug; additional 10% to 15% as metabolite); feces (29% to 40% mostly as metabolites) (Ferrero, 1990)

Clearance: Approximates normal GFR

Dosage

Usual dosage range: Note: All pediatric dosing recommendations based on immediate release product formulations (tablet and oral suspension):

Infants ≥6 months, Children, and Adolescents: Oral: 7.5 mg/kg every 12 hours (maximum: 500 mg/dose) for 10 days

Adults: Oral: 250-500 mg every 12 hours **or** 1000 mg (two 500 mg extended release tablets) once daily for 7-14 days

Indication-specific dosing:

Children: Oral:

Acute otitis media: Infants ≥6 months, Children, and Adolescents: 7.5 mg/kg/dose (maximum: 500 mg/dose) every 12 hours for 10 days. **Note:** Due to increased *S. pneumoniae* and *H. influenzae* resistance, macrolides are not routinely recommended as a treatment option (Lieberthal, 2013).

Bartonellosis, treatment and secondary prophylaxis (excluding CNS infections and endocarditis) (off-label use): Adolescents (HIV-positive): 500 mg twice daily for at least 3 months (recommended as alternative therapy; DHHS, 2013)

Community-acquired pneumonia (CAP): Infants >3 months and Children: **Note:** A beta-lactam antibiotic should be added if typical bacterial pneumonia cannot be ruled out.

Presumed atypical *(M. pneumoniae, C. pneumoniae, C. trachomatis)* infection, mild-to-severe atypical infection or step-down therapy (alternative to azithromycin): 7.5 mg/kg/dose (maximum: 500 mg) every 12 hours (Bradley, 2011)

Lyme disease (off-label use): Children: 7.5 mg/kg/dose (maximum dose: 500 mg) twice daily for 14-21 days (Wormser, 2006)

Mycobacterial infection (prevention and treatment):

Manufacturer's recommendation: 7.5 mg/kg/dose (maximum: 500 mg/dose) twice daily; use in combination with other antimycobacterial agents for the treatment of disseminated MAC. **Note:** Safety of clarithromycin for MAC not studied in children <20 months.

Alternative recommendations:

HIV-exposed/-positive infants and children (CDC, 2009):

Primary prophylaxis: 7.5 mg/kg/dose (maximum: 500 mg/dose) twice daily

Secondary prophylaxis: 7.5 mg/kg/dose (maximum: 500 mg/dose) twice daily, plus ethambutol, with or without rifabutin

Treatment: 7.5-15 mg/kg/dose (maximum: 500 mg/dose) twice daily plus ethambutol, plus rifabutin (for severe disease)

HIV-positive adolescents (DHHS, 2013):

Primary prophylaxis: 500 mg twice daily (maximum: 1000 mg daily)

Secondary prophylaxis and treatment: 500 mg twice daily (maximum: 1000 mg daily) plus ethambutol; consider additional agents (eg, rifabutin, aminoglycoside, fluoroquinolone) for CD4 <50 cells/mm^3, high mycobacterial load, or ineffective antiretroviral therapy

Pertussis (off-label use): Infants ≥1 month, Children, and Adolescents: 7.5 mg/kg/dose (maximum: 500 mg/dose) every 12 hours for 7 days (CDC, 2005)

Pharyngitis/tonsillitis: 7.5 mg/kg/dose (maximum: 250 mg/dose) every 12 hours for 10 days. **Note:** Recommended by the Infectious Disease Society of America (IDSA) as an alternative agent for group A streptococcal pharyngitis in penicillin-allergic patients (Shulman, 2012).

Prophylaxis against infective endocarditis (off-label use): Children and Adolescents: 15 mg/kg/dose (maximum: 500 mg/dose) 30-60 minutes before procedure. **Note:** American Heart Association (AHA) guidelines now recommend prophylaxis only in patients undergoing invasive procedures and in whom underlying cardiac conditions may predispose to a higher risk of adverse outcomes should infection occur. As of April 2007, routine prophylaxis for GI/GU procedures is no longer recommended by the AHA (Wilson, 2007).

Sinusitis: Infants ≥6 months, Children, and Adolescents: 7.5 mg/kg/dose (maximum: 500 mg/dose) every 12 hours for 10 days

Skin/skin structure infections, uncomplicated: Infants ≥6 months, Children, and Adolescents: 7.5 mg/kg/dose (maximum: 250 mg dose) every 12 hours for 10 days

Adults: Oral:

Acute exacerbation of chronic bronchitis:

M. catarrhalis and *S. pneumoniae*: 250 mg every 12 hours for 7-14 days **or** 1000 mg (two 500 mg extended release tablets) once daily for 7 days

H. influenzae: 500 mg every 12 hours for 7-14 days **or** 1000 mg (two 500 mg extended release tablets) once daily for 7 days

H. parainfluenzae: 500 mg every 12 hours for 7 days **or** 1000 mg (two 500 mg extended release tablets) once daily for 7 days

Acute maxillary sinusitis: 500 mg every 12 hours for 14 days **or** 1000 mg (two 500 mg extended release tablets) once daily for 14 days

Bartonellosis, treatment and secondary prophylaxis in HIV-infected patients (excluding CNS infections and endocarditis) (off-label use): 500 mg twice daily for at least 3 months (DHHS, 2013)

Lyme disease (off-label use): 500 mg twice daily for 14-21 days (Wormser, 2006)

Mycobacterial infection (prevention and treatment):

Manufacturer recommendations: 500 mg twice daily (use with other antimycobacterial drugs, eg, ethambutol or rifampin). Continue therapy if clinical response is observed; may discontinue when patient is considered at low risk of disseminated infection.

Alternative recommendations: (DHHS, 2013):

Primary prophylaxis: 500 mg twice daily (maximum: 1 g daily)

Secondary prophylaxis and treatment: 500 mg twice daily (maximum: 1 g daily) plus ethambutol; consider additional agents (eg, rifabutin, aminoglycoside, fluoroquinolone) for CD4 <50 cells/mm^3, high mycobacterial load, or ineffective antiretroviral therapy.

Peptic ulcer disease: Eradication of *Helicobacter pylori*: Dual or triple combination regimens with bismuth subsalicylate, amoxicillin, an H_2-receptor antagonist, or proton-pump inhibitor: 500 mg every 8-12 hours for 10-14 days

Pertussis (off-label use): 500 mg twice daily for 7 days (CDC, 2005)

Pharyngitis, tonsillitis: 250 mg every 12 hours for 10 days. **Note:** Recommended by the Infectious Disease Society of America (IDSA) as an alternative agent for group A streptococcal pharyngitis in penicillin-allergic patients (Shulman, 2012).

Pneumonia:

C. pneumoniae, *M. pneumoniae*, and *S. pneumoniae*: 250 mg every 12 hours for 7-14 days **or** 1000 mg (two 500 mg extended release tablets) once daily for 7 days

H. influenzae: 250 mg every 12 hours for 7 days **or** 1000 mg (two 500 mg extended release tablets) once daily for 7 days

H. parainfluenzae and *M. catarrhalis*: 1000 mg (two 500 mg extended release tablets) once daily for 7 days

Prophylaxis against infective endocarditis (off-label use): 500 mg 30-60 minutes prior to procedure. **Note:** American Heart Association (AHA) guidelines now recommend prophylaxis only in patients undergoing invasive procedures and in whom underlying cardiac conditions may predispose to a higher risk of adverse outcomes should infection occur. As of April 2007, routine prophylaxis for GI/GU procedures is no longer recommended by the AHA (Wilson, 2007).

Skin and skin structure infection, uncomplicated: 250 mg every 12 hours for 7-14 days

Elderly: May have age-related reductions in renal function; monitor and adjust dose if necessary

Dosing adjustment in renal impairment:

CrCl <30 mL/minute: Decrease clarithromycin dose by 50%

Hemodialysis: Administer after HD session is completed (Aronoff, 2007).

In combination with atazanavir or ritonavir:

CrCl 30-60 mL/minute: Decrease clarithromycin dose by 50%

CrCl <30 mL/minute: Decrease clarithromycin dose by 75%

Dosing adjustment in hepatic impairment: No dosing adjustment is needed as long as renal function is normal

Dietary Considerations Extended release tablets should be taken with food.

Administration Immediate release tablets and granules for suspension: Administer with or without meals. Administer every 12 hours rather than twice daily to avoid peak and trough variation. Shake suspension well before each use.

Extended release tablets: Administer with food. Do not crush or chew.

Monitoring Parameters CBC with differential, BUN, creatinine; perform culture and sensitivity studies prior to initiating drug therapy as appropriate

Dosage Forms

Suspension Reconstituted, Oral:

Biaxin: 250 mg/5 mL (50 mL, 100 mL)

Generic: 125 mg/5 mL (50 mL, 100 mL); 250 mg/5 mL (50 mL, 100 mL)

Tablet, Oral:

Biaxin: 250 mg, 500 mg

Generic: 250 mg, 500 mg

Tablet Extended Release 24 Hour, Oral:

Biaxin XL: 500 mg

Biaxin XL Pac: 500 mg

Generic: 500 mg

◆ **Clarithromycin, Amoxicillin, and Omeprazole** *see* Omeprazole, Clarithromycin, and Amoxicillin *on page 1511*

◆ **Clarithromycin, Lansoprazole, and Amoxicillin** *see* Lansoprazole, Amoxicillin, and Clarithromycin *on page 1169*

◆ **Claritin [OTC]** *see* Loratadine *on page 1241*

◆ **Claritin® (Can)** *see* Loratadine *on page 1241*

◆ **Claritin-D® 12 Hour Allergy & Congestion [OTC]** *see* Loratadine and Pseudoephedrine *on page 1242*

◆ **Claritin-D® 24 Hour Allergy & Congestion [OTC]** *see* Loratadine and Pseudoephedrine *on page 1242*

◆ **Claritin® Extra (Can)** *see* Loratadine and Pseudoephedrine *on page 1242*

◆ **Claritin Eye [OTC]** *see* Ketotifen (Ophthalmic) *on page 1150*

◆ **Claritin® Kids (Can)** *see* Loratadine *on page 1241*

◆ **Claritin® Liberator (Can)** *see* Loratadine and Pseudoephedrine *on page 1242*

◆ **Claritin Reditabs [OTC]** *see* Loratadine *on page 1241*

◆ **Clarus (Can)** *see* ISOtretinoin *on page 1127*

◆ **Clasteon® (Can)** *see* Clodronate [CAN/INT] *on page 469*

◆ **Clavulanic Acid and Amoxicillin** *see* Amoxicillin and Clavulanate *on page 133*

◆ **Clavulanic Acid and Amoxycillin** *see* Amoxicillin and Clavulanate *on page 133*

◆ **Clavulin (Can)** *see* Amoxicillin and Clavulanate *on page 133*

◆ **Clear Eyes Redness Relief [OTC]** *see* Naphazoline (Ophthalmic) *on page 1426*

Clemastine (KLEM as teen)

Brand Names: U.S. Dayhist Allergy 12 Hour Relief [OTC]; Tavist Allergy [OTC]

Index Terms Clemastine Fumarate

Pharmacologic Category Ethanolamine Derivative; Histamine H_1 Antagonist; Histamine H_1 Antagonist, First Generation

Additional Appendix Information

Beers Criteria – Potentially Inappropriate Medications for Geriatrics *on page 2271*

Use Perennial and seasonal allergic rhinitis and other allergic symptoms including urticaria

Pregnancy Risk Factor B

Dosage Oral:

Infants and Children <6 years: 0.05 mg/kg/day as **clemastine base** or 0.335-0.67 mg/day clemastine fumarate (0.25-0.5 mg base/day) divided into 2 or 3 doses; maximum daily dosage: 1.34 mg (1 mg base)

Children 6-12 years: 0.67-1.34 mg clemastine fumarate (0.5-1 mg base) twice daily; do not exceed 4.02 mg/day (3 mg/day base)

Children ≥12 years and Adults:

1.34 mg clemastine fumarate (1 mg base) twice daily to 2.68 mg (2 mg base) 3 times/day; do not exceed 8.04 mg/day (6 mg base)

OTC labeling: 1.34 mg clemastine fumarate (1 mg base) twice daily; do not exceed 2 mg base/24 hours

Elderly: Lower doses should be considered in patients >60 years

Additional Information Complete prescribing information should be consulted for additional detail.

Dosage Forms

Syrup, Oral:

Generic: 0.67 mg/5 mL (120 mL)

Tablet, Oral:

Dayhist Allergy 12 Hour Relief [OTC]: 1.34 mg

Tavist Allergy [OTC]: 1.34 mg

Generic: 1.34 mg, 2.68 mg

◆ **Clemastine Fumarate** *see* Clemastine *on page 459*

Clenbuterol [INT] (klen BYOO ter ole)

International Brand Names Airum (CL); Brodilan (VE); Broncodil (IT); Broncolit (PY); Broncoterol (PT); Bronq-C (AR); Bronq-C[compr.] (AR); Brontel (PY); Buclen (VE); Cesbron (PT); Clenasma (IT); Clenbunal (VE); Contrasmina (IT); Contraspasmin (CZ, DE); Copan (KR); Crenble (KR); Mavilex (MY); Monores (IT); Oxibron (AR); Oxyflux (MX); Planipart[vet.] (FR); Prontovent (IT); Risopent (VE); Spiropent (AT, CO, CY, CZ, DE, ES, GR, HU, ID, IT, JP, MX, PE, PH, TR); Ventipulmin[vet.] (CH, DE, FR); Ventolase (ES)

Index Terms Clenbuterol Hydrochloride

Pharmacologic Category Beta$_2$-Adrenergic Agonist

Reported Use Bronchodilator in reversible airway obstruction due to asthma or COPD

Dosage Range Adults:

Oral: 20-40 mcg twice daily

Inhalation: 20 mcg 3 times/day

Product Availability Product available in various countries; not currently available in the U.S.

Dosage Forms

Tablet, as hydrochloride: 10 mcg, 20 mcg

◆ **Clenbuterol Hydrochloride** *see* Clenbuterol [INT] *on page 460*

◆ **Clenia [DSC]** *see* Sulfur and Sulfacetamide *on page 1953*

◆ **Cleocin** *see* Clindamycin (Systemic) *on page 460*

◆ **Cleocin** *see* Clindamycin (Topical) *on page 464*

◆ **Cleocin in D5W** *see* Clindamycin (Systemic) *on page 460*

◆ **Cleocin Phosphate** *see* Clindamycin (Systemic) *on page 460*

◆ **Cleocin-T** *see* Clindamycin (Topical) *on page 464*

Clevidipine (klev ID i peen)

Brand Names: U.S. Cleviprex

Index Terms Clevidipine Butyrate

Pharmacologic Category Antihypertensive; Calcium Channel Blocker; Calcium Channel Blocker, Dihydropyridine

Use Management of hypertension

Pregnancy Risk Factor C

Dosage IV:

Adults: Initial: 1-2 mg/hour

Titration: Initial: dose may be doubled at 90-second intervals toward blood pressure goal. As blood pressure approaches goal, dose may be increased by less than double every 5-10 minutes. **Note:** For every 1-2 mg/hour increase in dose, an approximate reduction of 2-4 mm Hg in systolic blood pressure may occur.

Usual maintenance: 4-6 mg/hour; maximum: 21 mg/hour (1000 mL within a 24-hour period due to lipid load restriction). There is limited short-term experience with doses up to 32 mg/hour. Data is limited beyond 72 hours.

Elderly: Initiate at the low end of the dosage range.

Dosing adjustment in renal impairment: No adjustment required with initial infusion rate

Dosing adjustment in hepatic impairment: No adjustment required with initial infusion rate

Additional Information Complete prescribing information should be consulted for additional detail.

Dosage Forms

Emulsion, Intravenous:

Cleviprex: 0.5 mg/mL (50 mL, 100 mL)

◆ **Clevidipine Butyrate** *see* Clevidipine *on page 460*

◆ **Cleviprex** *see* Clevidipine *on page 460*

Clidinium and Chlordiazepoxide
(kli DI nee um & klor dye az e POKS ide)

Brand Names: U.S. Librax

Brand Names: Canada Chlorax; Librax

Index Terms Chlordiazepoxide and Clidinium

Pharmacologic Category Antispasmodic Agent, Gastrointestinal; Benzodiazepine

Additional Appendix Information

Beers Criteria – Potentially Inappropriate Medications for Geriatrics *on page 2271*

Use Adjunct treatment of peptic ulcer; treatment of irritable bowel syndrome

Dosage Oral: 1-2 capsules 3-4 times/day, before meals or food and at bedtime

Caution: Do not abruptly discontinue after prolonged use; taper dose gradually.

Dosage adjustment in renal impairment: No dosage adjustment provided in manufacturer's labeling.

Dosage adjustment in hepatic impairment: No dosage adjustment provided in manufacturer's labeling.

Additional Information Complete prescribing information should be consulted for additional detail.

Dosage Forms

Capsule: Clidinium 2.5 mg and chlordiazepoxide 5 mg

Librax®: Clidinium 2.5 mg and chlordiazepoxide 5 mg

◆ **Climara** *see* Estradiol (Systemic) *on page 775*

◆ **ClimaraPro** *see* Estradiol and Levonorgestrel *on page 781*

◆ **Clindacin ETZ** *see* Clindamycin (Topical) *on page 464*

◆ **Clindacin-P** *see* Clindamycin (Topical) *on page 464*

◆ **Clindacin Pac** *see* Clindamycin (Topical) *on page 464*

◆ **Clindagel** *see* Clindamycin (Topical) *on page 464*

◆ **ClindaMax** *see* Clindamycin (Topical) *on page 464*

Clindamycin (Systemic) (klin da MYE sin)

Brand Names: U.S. Cleocin; Cleocin in D5W; Cleocin Phosphate

Brand Names: Canada Apo-Clindamycin; Ava-Clindamycin; Clindamycin Injection, USP; Clindamycine; Dalacin C; Mylan-Clindamycin; PMS-Clindamycin; Riva-Clindamycin; Teva-Clindamycin

Index Terms Clindamycin Hydrochloride; Clindamycin Palmitate

Pharmacologic Category Antibiotic, Lincosamide

Use

Treatment of infections: Treatment of infections due to susceptible organisms:

Bone and joint infections: Including acute hematogenous osteomyelitis caused by *Staphylococcus aureus* and as adjunctive therapy in the surgical treatment of chronic bone and joint infections caused by susceptible organisms.

Gynecological infections: Including endometritis, nongonococcal tubo-ovarian abscess, pelvic cellulitis, and postsurgical vaginal cuff infection caused by susceptible anaerobes.

Intra-abdominal infections: Including peritonitis and intra-abdominal abscess caused by susceptible anaerobic organisms.

Lower respiratory tract infections: Including pneumonia, empyema, and lung abscess caused by anaerobes, *Streptococcus pneumoniae*, other streptococci (except *Enterococcus faecalis*), and *S. aureus*.

Septicemia: Caused by *S. aureus*, streptococci (except *E. faecalis*), and susceptible anaerobes.

Serious infections: Caused by susceptible strains of streptococci, pneumococci, and staphylococci.

Skin and skin structure infections: Caused by *Streptococcus pyogenes*, *S. aureus*, and anaerobes.

Pregnancy Risk Factor B

Pregnancy Considerations Adverse events were not observed in animal reproduction studies. Clindamycin crosses the placenta and can be detected in the cord blood and fetal tissue (Philipson, 1973; Weinstein, 1976). Clindamycin pharmacokinetics are not affected by pregnancy (Philipson, 1976; Weinstein, 1976). Clindamycin therapy is recommended as an alternative treatment in certain pregnant patients for prophylaxis of group B streptococcal disease in newborns (ACOG 485, 2011); prophylaxis and treatment of *Toxoplasma gondii* encephalitis, or for the treatment of *Pneumocystis* pneumonia (PCP) (DHHS, 2013); bacterial vaginosis (CDC RR12, 2010); or malaria (CDC, 2013). Clindamycin is also one of the antibiotics recommended for prophylactic use prior to cesarean delivery and may be used in certain situations prior to vaginal delivery in women at high risk for endocarditis (ACOG 120, 2011).

Breast-Feeding Considerations Clindamycin can be detected in breast milk; reported concentrations range from 0.7 to 3.8 mcg/mL following maternal doses of 150 mg orally to 600 mg IV Due to the potential for serious adverse reactions in neonates, breast-feeding is not recommended by the manufacturer. Nondose-related effects could include modification of bowel flora. One case of bloody stools in an infant occurred after a mother received clindamycin while breast-feeding; however, a causal relationship was not confirmed (Mann, 1980).

Contraindications Hypersensitivity to preparations containing clindamycin, lincomycin, or any component of the formulation.

Warnings/Precautions Dosage adjustment may be necessary in patients with severe hepatic dysfunction. **[U.S. Boxed Warning]: Can cause severe and possibly fatal colitis.** Should be reserved for serious infections where less toxic antimicrobial agents are inappropriate. It should not be used in patients with nonbacterial infections such as most upper respiratory tract infections. Hypertoxin producing strains of *C. difficile* cause increased morbidity and mortality, as these infections can be refractory to antimicrobial therapy and may require colectomy. *C. difficile*-associated diarrhea (CDAD) must be considered in all patients who present with diarrhea following antibiotic use. CDAD has been observed >2 months postantibiotic treatment. Use with caution in patients with a history of gastrointestinal disease, particularly colitis.. Discontinue drug if significant diarrhea, abdominal cramps, or passage of blood and mucus occurs. Use may result in overgrowth of nonsusceptible organisms, particularly yeast. Should superinfection occur, appropriate measures should be taken as indicated by the clinical situation. May cause hypersensitivity. Serious anaphylactoid reactions require immediate emergency treatment with epinephrine. Oxygen and IV corticosteroids should also be administered as indicated. Severe or fatal reactions such as toxic epidermal necrolysis (TEN) have been reported. Discontinue if severe skin reaction occurs. Premature and low birth weight infants may be more likely to develop toxicity. Some products may contain tartrazine (FD&C yellow no. 5), which may cause allergic reactions in certain individuals. Allergy is frequently seen in patients who also have an aspirin hypersensitivity. Use caution in atopic patients. A subgroup of older patients with associated severe illness may tolerate diarrhea less well. Monitor carefully for changes in bowel frequency. Not appropriate for use in the treatment of meningitis due to inadequate penetration into the CSF. Do not inject IV undiluted as a bolus. Product should be diluted in compatible fluid and infused over 10 to 60 minutes. Potentially significant interactions may exist, requiring dose or frequency adjustment, additional monitoring, and/or selection of alternative therapy.

Benzyl alcohol and derivatives: Some dosage forms may contain benzyl alcohol; large amounts of benzyl alcohol (≥99 mg/kg/day) have been associated with a potentially fatal toxicity ("gasping syndrome") in neonates; the "gasping syndrome" consists of metabolic acidosis, respiratory distress, gasping respirations, CNS dysfunction (including convulsions, intracranial hemorrhage), hypotension and cardiovascular collapse (AAP, 1997; CDC, 1982); some data suggests that benzoate displaces bilirubin from protein binding sites (Ahlfors, 2001); avoid or use dosage forms containing benzyl alcohol with caution in neonates. See manufacturer's labeling.

Adverse Reactions

Cardiovascular: Cardiac arrest (rare; IV administration), hypotension (rare; IV administration), thrombophlebitis (IV)

Central nervous system: Metallic taste (IV)

Dermatologic: Acute generalized exanthematous pustulosis, erythema multiforme (rare), exfoliative dermatitis (rare), maculopapular rash, pruritus, skin rash, Stevens-Johnson syndrome (rare), toxic epidermal necrolysis, urticaria, vesiculobullous dermatitis

Gastrointestinal: Abdominal pain, antibiotic-associated colitis, *Clostridium difficile* associated diarrhea, diarrhea, esophageal ulcer, esophagitis, nausea, pseudomembranous colitis, unpleasant taste (IV), vomiting

Genitourinary: Azotemia, oliguria, proteinuria, vaginitis

Hematologic & oncologic: Agranulocytosis, eosinophilia (transient), neutropenia (transient), thrombocytopenia

Hepatic: Abnormal hepatic function tests, jaundice

Hypersensitivity: Anaphylactoid reaction (rare)

Immunologic: DRESS syndrome

Local: Abscess at injection site (IM), induration at injection site (IM), irritation at injection site (IM), pain at injection site (IM)

Neuromuscular & skeletal: Polyarthritis (rare)

Renal: Renal insufficiency (rare)

Drug Interactions

Metabolism/Transport Effects Substrate of CYP3A4 (minor); **Note:** Assignment of Major/Minor substrate status based on clinically relevant drug interaction potential

Avoid Concomitant Use

Avoid concomitant use of Clindamycin (Systemic) with any of the following: BCG; Erythromycin (Systemic)

Increased Effect/Toxicity

Clindamycin (Systemic) may increase the levels/effects of: Neuromuscular-Blocking Agents

Decreased Effect

Clindamycin (Systemic) may decrease the levels/effects of: BCG; Erythromycin (Systemic); Sodium Picosulfate; Typhoid Vaccine

The levels/effects of Clindamycin (Systemic) may be decreased by: Kaolin

Food Interactions Peak concentrations may be delayed with food. Management: May administer with food.

Preparation for Administration Never administer undiluted as bolus. For IV infusion, dilute vials with 50 to 100 mL of compatible diluent; concentration of clindamycin for IV infusion should not exceed 18 mg/mL.

Storage/Stability

Capsule: Store at room temperature of 20°C to 25°C (68°F to 77°F).

IV: Infusion solution in NS or D_5W solution is stable for 16 days at room temperature, 32 days refrigerated, or 8 weeks frozen. Prior to use, store vials and premixed bags at controlled room temperature 20°C to 25°C (68°F to 77°F). After initial use, discard any unused portion of vial after 24 hours.

Oral solution: Do not refrigerate reconstituted oral solution (it will thicken). Following reconstitution, oral solution is stable for 2 weeks at room temperature of 20°C to 25°C (68°F to 77°F).

Mechanism of Action Reversibly binds to 50S ribosomal subunits preventing peptide bond formation thus inhibiting bacterial protein synthesis; bacteriostatic or bactericidal depending on drug concentration, infection site, and organism

Pharmacodynamics/Kinetics

Absorption: Oral, hydrochloride: Rapid (90%)

Distribution: Distributed in body fluids and tissues; no significant levels in CSF, even with inflamed meninges

Metabolism: Clindamycin phosphate is converted to clindamycin HCl (active)

Half-life elimination: Children: ~2.5 hours; Adults: 3 hours; Elderly (oral) 4 hours (range: 3.4 to 5.1 hours)

Time to peak, serum: Oral: Within 60 minutes; IM: 1 to 3 hours

Excretion: Urine (10%) and feces (~4%) as active drug and metabolites

Dosage

Usual dosage ranges:

Infants and Children:

Oral: 8 to 40 mg/kg/day in 3 to 4 divided doses; Manufacturer's labeling: 8 to 20 mg/kg/day (as hydrochloride) or 8 to 25 mg/kg/day (as palmitate) in 3 to 4 divided doses; minimum dose of palmitate: 37.5 mg 3 times daily

IM, IV: Manufacturer's labeling: 20 to 40 mg/kg/day in 3 to 4 divided doses

Adults:

Oral: 150 to 450 mg/dose every 6 hours

IM, IV: 600 to 2,700 mg daily in 2 to 4 divided doses; up to 4,800 mg IV daily may be used in life-threatening infections

Indication-specific dosing:

Infants >3 months and Children:

Community-acquired pneumonia (CAP) (IDSA/PIDS, 2011): Note: In children ≥5 years, a macrolide antibiotic should be added if atypical pneumonia cannot be ruled out.

Group A *Streptococcus:*

Moderate-to-severe infection (alternative to ampicillin/penicillin): IV: 40 mg/kg/day divided every 6 to 8 hours

Mild infection, step-down therapy (alternative to amoxicillin/penicillin): Oral: 40 mg/kg/day divided every 8 hours

Presumed bacterial (in addition to recommended antibiotic therapy), *S. pneumoniae* moderate-to-severe (MICs to penicillin ≤2.0 mcg/mL) (alternative to ampicillin/penicillin): IV: 40 mg/kg/day divided every 6 to 8 hours

S. pneumoniae:

Moderate-to-severe infection (MICs to penicillin ≥4.0 mcg/mL) (alternative to ceftriaxone): IV: 40 mg/kg/day divided every 6 to 8 hours

Mild infection, step-down therapy (MICs to penicillin ≥4.0 mcg/mL) (alternative to levofloxacin or linezolid): Oral: 30 to 40 mg/kg/day divided every 8 hours

S. aureus (methicillin-susceptible):

Moderate-to-severe infection (alternative to cefazolin or oxacillin): IV: 40 mg/kg/day divided every 6 to 8 hours

Mild infection, step-down therapy (alternative to cephalexin): Oral: 30 to 40 mg/kg/day divided every 6 to 8 hours

S. aureus (methicillin-resistant/clindamycin-susceptible):

Moderate-to-severe infection (preferred): IV: 40 mg/kg/day divided every 6 to 8 hours; recommended duration: 7 to 21 days (Liu, 2011)

Mild infection, step-down therapy (preferred): Oral: 30 to 40 mg/kg/day divided every 6 to 8 hours; recommended duration: 7 to 21 days (Liu, 2011)

Children:

Acute bacterial rhinosinusitis (off-label use): Oral: 30 to 40 mg/kg/day divided every 8 hours with concomitant cefixime or cefpodoxime for 10 to 14 days. **Note:** Recommended in patients with non-type I penicillin allergy, after failure of initial therapy or in patients at risk for antibiotic resistance (eg, daycare attendance, age <2 years, recent hospitalization, antibiotic use within the past month) (Chow, 2012).

Anthrax (off-label dose): Note: For inhalational anthrax, combine with penicillin G (WHO, 2008):

Oral: 8 to 25 mg/kg/day divided every 6 to 8 hours

IV: 15 to 40 mg/kg/day divided every 6 to 8 hours

Babesiosis (off-label use): Oral: 20 to 40 mg/kg/day divided every 8 hours for 7 to 10 days *plus* quinine (*Medical Letter*, 2007)

Cellulitis due to MRSA (off-label use): Oral: 10 to 13 mg/kg/dose every 6 to 8 hours for 5 to 10 days (maximum: 40 mg/kg/day) (Liu, 2011)

Complicated skin/soft tissue infection due to MRSA (off-label use): Oral, IV: 10 to 13 mg/kg/dose every 6 to 8 hours for 7 to 14 days (maximum: 40 mg/kg/day) (Liu, 2011)

Healthcare-associated pneumonia (HAP) (methicillin-resistant/clindamycin-susceptible): Oral, IV: 30 to 40 mg/kg/day divided every 6 to 8 hours for 7 to 21 days (Liu, 2011)

Malaria, severe (off-label use): IV: Load: 10 mg/kg followed by 15 mg/kg/day divided every 8 hours *plus* IV quinidine gluconate; switch to oral therapy (clindamycin *plus* quinine) when able for total clindamycin treatment duration of 7 days (**Note:** Quinine duration is region specific, consult CDC for current recommendations) (CDC, 2009)

Malaria, uncomplicated treatment (off-label use): Oral: 20 mg/kg/day divided every 8 hours for 7 days *plus* quinine (CDC, 2009)

Osteomyelitis due to MRSA (off-label use): Oral, IV: 10 to 13 mg/kg/dose every 6 to 8 hours for a minimum of 4 to 6 weeks (maximum: 40 mg/kg/day) (Liu, 2011)

Pharyngitis, group A streptococci (IDSA recommendations): Oral:

Acute treatment in penicillin-allergic patients: 21 mg/kg/day divided every 8 hours (maximum: 300 mg per dose) for 10 days (Shulman, 2012).

Chronic carrier treatment: 20 to 30 mg/kg/day divided every 8 hours (maximum: 300 mg per dose) for 10 days (Shulman, 2012).

Prophylaxis against infective endocarditis (off-label use):

Oral: 20 mg/kg 30 to 60 minutes before procedure (Wilson, 2007)

IM, IV: 20 mg/kg 30 to 60 minutes before procedure. Intramuscular injections should be avoided in patients who are receiving anticoagulant therapy. In these circumstances, orally administered regimens should be given whenever possible. Intravenously administered antibiotics should be used for patients who are unable to tolerate or absorb oral medications (Wilson, 2007).

Note: American Heart Association (AHA) guidelines now recommend prophylaxis only in patients undergoing invasive procedures and in whom underlying cardiac conditions may predispose to a higher risk of adverse outcomes should infection occur. As of April 2007, routine prophylaxis for GI/GU procedures is no longer recommended by the AHA.

Septic arthritis due to MRSA (off-label use): Oral, IV: 10 to 13 mg/kg/dose every 6 to 8 hours for minimum of 3 to 4 weeks (maximum: 40 mg/kg/day) (Liu, 2011)

Toxoplasmosis (HIV-exposed/-positive [off-label use]):

Treatment: IV, Oral: 5 to 7.5 mg/kg (maximum dose: 600 mg) every 6 hours (plus pyrimethamine and leucovorin) (DHHS [OI Adults, 2014]; DHHS [OI Children, 2013])

Secondary prevention: Oral: 7 to 10 mg/kg (maximum dose: 600 mg) every 8 hours (plus pyrimethamine and leucovorin) (DHHS [OI Adults, 2014]; DHHS [OI Children, 2013])

Adults:

Amnionitis: IV: 450 to 900 mg every 8 hours

Anthrax (off-label dose):

Oral: 150 to 300 mg every 6 hours. **Note:** For inhalational anthrax, combine with penicillin (WHO, 2008).

IV:

Nonspecified disease: 600 to 900 mg every 6 to 8 hours. **Note:** For inhalational anthrax, combine with penicillin G (WHO, 2008)

Alternative regimens:

Inhalational, gastrointestinal, or complicated cutaneous disease with systemic involvement: 600 mg every 8 hours in combination with ciprofloxacin or doxycycline (Hicks, 2012)

Injectional: 600 mg every 8 hours in combination with ciprofloxacin and other antibiotics (eg, a 5-drug combination) (Hicks, 2012)

Babesiosis (off-label use):

Oral: 600 mg 3 times daily for 7 to 10 days with quinine (Vannier, 2012; Wormser, 2006)

IV: 300 to 600 mg every 6 hours for 7 to 10 days with quinine (Vannier, 2012; Wormser, 2006)

Note: Relapsing infection may require at least 6 weeks of therapy (Vannier, 2012)

Bacterial vaginosis (off-label use): Oral: 300 mg twice daily for 7 days (CDC, 2010)

Bite wounds (canine): Oral: 300 mg 3 times daily for 3 to 10 days (Stevens, 2005)

Cellulitis due to MRSA (off-label use): Oral: 300 to 450 mg 3 times daily for 5 to 10 days (Liu, 2011)

Complicated skin/soft tissue infection due to MRSA (off-label use): IV, Oral: 600 mg 3 times daily for 7 to 14 days (Liu, 2011)

Gangrenous pyomyositis: IV: 900 mg every 8 hours with penicillin G (Brook, 1999; Hassel, 2004; Wong, 2013)

Group B streptococcus (neonatal prophylaxis) (off-label use): IV: 900 mg every 8 hours until delivery (CDC, 2010)

Malaria, severe (off-label use): IV: Load: 10 mg/kg followed by 15 mg/kg/day divided every 8 hours *plus* IV quinidine gluconate; switch to oral therapy (clindamycin *plus* quinine) when able for total clindamycin treatment duration of 7 days (**Note:** Quinine duration is region specific, consult CDC for current recommendations) (CDC, 2009)

Malaria, uncomplicated treatment (off-label use): Oral: 20 mg/kg/day divided every 8 hours for 7 days *plus* quinine (CDC, 2009)

Osteomyelitis due to MRSA (off-label use): IV, Oral: 600 mg 3 times daily for a minimum of 8 weeks (some experts combine with rifampin) (Liu, 2011)

Pelvic inflammatory disease: IV: 900 mg every 8 hours with gentamicin (conventional or single daily dosing); 24 hours after clinical improvement may convert to oral doxycycline 100 mg twice daily **or** clindamycin 450 mg 4 times daily to complete 14 days of total therapy. Avoid doxycycline if tubo-ovarian abscess is present (CDC, 2010).

Pharyngitis, group A streptococci (IDSA recommendations):

Acute treatment in penicillin-allergic patients: 21 mg/kg/day divided every 8 hours (maximum: 300 mg per dose) for 10 days (Shulman, 2012)

Chronic carrier treatment: 20 to 30 mg/kg/day divided every 8 hours (maximum: 300 mg per dose) for 10 days (Shulman, 2012)

***Pneumocystis jirovecii* pneumonia (off-label use):**

IV: 600 to 900 mg every 6 to 8 hours with primaquine for 21 days (CDC, 2009)

Oral: 300 to 450 mg every 6 to 8 hours with primaquine for 21 days (CDC, 2009)

Pneumonia due to MRSA (off-label use): IV, Oral: 600 mg 3 times daily for 7 to 21 days (Liu, 2011)

Prophylaxis against infective endocarditis (off-label use):

Oral: 600 mg 30 to 60 minutes before procedure (Wilson, 2007)

IM, IV: 600 mg 30 to 60 minutes before procedure. Intramuscular injections should be avoided in patients who are receiving anticoagulant therapy. In these circumstances, orally administered regimens should be given whenever possible. Intravenously administered antibiotics should be used for patients who are unable to tolerate or absorb oral medications. (Wilson, 2007)

Note: American Heart Association (AHA) guidelines now recommend prophylaxis only in patients undergoing invasive procedures and in whom underlying cardiac conditions may predispose to a higher risk of adverse outcomes should infection occur. As of April 2007, routine prophylaxis for GI/GU procedures is no longer recommended by the AHA.

Prophylaxis in total joint replacement patients undergoing dental procedures which produce bacteremia (off-label use):

Oral: 600 mg 1 hour prior to procedure (ADA, 2003)

IV: 600 mg 1 hour prior to procedure (for patients unable to take oral medication) (ADA, 2003)

Prosthetic joint infection:

Chronic antimicrobial suppression, Staphylococci (oxacillin-susceptible) (alternative to cephalexin or cefadroxil) (off-label use): Oral: 300 mg every 6 hours (Osmon, 2013)

Propionibacterium acnes, treatment (alternative to penicillin G or ceftriaxone):

Oral: 300 to 450 mg every 6 hours for 4 to 6 weeks (Osmon, 2013)

IV: 600 to 900 mg every 8 hours for 4 to 6 weeks (Osmon, 2013)

Septic arthritis due to MRSA (off-label use): IV, Oral: 600 mg 3 times daily for 3 to 4 weeks (Liu, 2011)

Toxic shock syndrome: IV: 900 mg every 8 hours with additional concomitant therapy (Lappin, 2009; Wong, 2013)

Toxoplasmosis (HIV-exposed/positive [off-label use]):

Treatment: IV, Oral: 600 mg every 6 hours for ≥6 weeks (with pyrimethamine and leucovorin) (DHHS [OI Adults, 2014])

Secondary prevention: Oral: 600 mg every 8 hours (with pyrimethamine and leucovorin) (DHHS [OI Adults, 2014])

Dosage adjustment in renal impairment:

Mild to moderate impairment: No dosage adjustment necessary.

End stage renal disease (ESRD) on hemodialysis or peritoneal dialysis: Not removed from serum (eg, poorly dialyzed); no supplemental dose or dosage adjustment necessary.

Continuous renal replacement therapy (CRRT) (eg, CVVH, CVVHD, CVVHDF): No supplemental dose or dosage adjustment necessary (Heintz, 2009).

Dosage adjustment in hepatic impairment:

Mild impairment: There are no dosage adjustments provided in the manufacturer's labeling.

Moderate to severe impairment: There are no dosage adjustments provided in the manufacturer's labeling; in studies of patients with moderate or severe liver disease, half-life is prolonged, however, when administered on an every 8 hour schedule, accumulation should rarely occur. In severe liver disease, use caution and monitor liver enzymes periodically during therapy.

Dietary Considerations May be taken with food.

Administration

IM: Deep IM sites, rotate sites; do not exceed 600 mg in a single injection.

IV: **Never administer undiluted as bolus**; administer by IV intermittent infusion over at least 10-60 minutes, at a maximum rate of 30 mg/minute (do not exceed 1200 mg/hour).

Oral: Administer with a full glass of water to minimize esophageal ulceration; give around-the-clock to promote less variation in peak and trough serum levels.

Monitoring Parameters Observe for changes in bowel frequency. Monitor for colitis and resolution of symptoms. In severe liver disease monitor liver function tests periodically; during prolonged therapy monitor CBC, liver and renal function tests periodically.

Additional Information *In vitro* susceptibility rates to clindamycin are higher in community acquired versus hospital acquired MRSA, although this may vary by geographic region. The D-zone test is recommended for detection of inducible resistance to clindamycin in erythromycin-resistant but clindamycin-susceptible isolates (Liu, 2011).

Dosage Forms

Capsule, Oral:
- Cleocin: 75 mg, 150 mg, 300 mg
- Generic: 75 mg, 150 mg, 300 mg

Solution, Injection:
- Cleocin Phosphate: 300 mg/2 mL (2 mL); 600 mg/4 mL (4 mL); 900 mg/6 mL (6 mL); 9 g/60 mL (60 mL)
- Generic: 300 mg/2 mL (2 mL); 600 mg/4 mL (4 mL); 900 mg/6 mL (6 mL); 9000 mg/60 mL (60 mL); 9 g/60 mL (60 mL)

Solution, Intravenous:
- Cleocin in D5W: 300 mg/50 mL (50 mL); 600 mg/50 mL (50 mL); 900 mg/50 mL (50 mL)
- Cleocin Phosphate: 600 mg/4 mL (4 mL); 900 mg/6 mL (6 mL)
- Generic: 300 mg/50 mL (50 mL); 600 mg/50 mL (50 mL); 900 mg/50 mL (50 mL); 300 mg/2 mL (2 mL); 600 mg/4 mL (4 mL); 900 mg/6 mL (6 mL)

Solution Reconstituted, Oral:
- Cleocin: 75 mg/5 mL (100 mL)
- Generic: 75 mg/5 mL (100 mL)

Clindamycin (Topical) (klin da MYE sin)

Brand Names: U.S. Cleocin; Cleocin-T; Clindacin ETZ; Clindacin Pac; Clindacin-P; Clindagel; ClindaMax; Clindesse; Evoclin

Brand Names: Canada Clinda-T; Clindasol; Clindets; Dalacin T; Dalacin Vaginal; Taro-Clindamycin

Index Terms Clindamycin Phosphate

Pharmacologic Category Antibiotic, Lincosamide; Topical Skin Product, Acne

Use Treatment of bacterial vaginosis (vaginal cream, vaginal suppository); topically in treatment of severe acne

Pregnancy Risk Factor B

Dosage Indication-specific dosing:

Children ≥12 years and Adults: **Acne vulgaris:** Topical:

Gel (Cleocin T®, ClindaMax®), pledget, lotion, solution: Apply a thin film twice daily

Gel (Clindagel®), foam (Evoclin®): Apply once daily

Adults: **Bacterial vaginosis:** Intravaginal:

Suppositories: Insert one ovule (100 mg clindamycin) daily into vagina at bedtime for 3 days

Cream:

Cleocin®: One full applicator inserted intravaginally once daily before bedtime for 3 or 7 consecutive days in nonpregnant patients or for 7 consecutive days in pregnant patients

Clindesse®: One full applicator inserted intravaginally as a single dose at anytime during the day in nonpregnant patients

Additional Information Complete prescribing information should be consulted for additional detail.

Dosage Forms

Cream, Vaginal:
- Cleocin: 2% (40 g)
- Clindesse: 2% (5.8 g)
- Generic: 2% (40 g)

Foam, External:
- Evoclin: 1% (50 g, 100 g)
- Generic: 1% (50 g, 100 g)

Gel, External:
- Cleocin-T: 1% (30 g, 60 g)
- Clindagel: 1% (75 mL)
- ClindaMax: 1% (30 g, 60 g)
- Generic: 1% (30 g, 60 g)

Kit, External:
- Clindacin ETZ: 1%
- Clindacin Pac: 1%

Lotion, External:
- Cleocin-T: 1% (60 mL)
- ClindaMax: 1% (60 mL)
- Generic: 1% (60 mL)

Solution, External:
- Cleocin-T: 1% (30 mL, 60 mL)
- Generic: 1% (30 mL, 60 mL)

Suppository, Vaginal:
- Cleocin: 100 mg (3 ea)

Swab, External:
- Cleocin-T: 1% (60 ea)
- Clindacin ETZ: 1% (60 ea)
- Clindacin-P: 1% (69 ea)
- Generic: 1% (60 ea)

Clindamycin and Tretinoin

(klin da MYE sin & TRET i noyn)

Brand Names: U.S. Veltin™; Ziana®

Index Terms Clindamycin Phosphate and Tretinoin; Tretinoin and Clindamycin; Veltin™

Pharmacologic Category Acne Products; Retinoic Acid Derivative; Topical Skin Product; Topical Skin Product, Acne

Use Treatment of acne vulgaris

Pregnancy Risk Factor C

Dosage Topical: Children ≥12 years and Adults: Apply once daily

Additional Information Complete prescribing information should be consulted for additional detail.

Dosage Forms

Gel, topical:

Veltin™: Clindamycin phosphate 1.2% and tretinoin 0.025% (30 g, 60 g)

Ziana®: Clindamycin phosphate 1.2% and tretinoin 0.025% (30 g, 60 g)

- ◆ **Clindamycine (Can)** *see* Clindamycin (Systemic) *on page 460*
- ◆ **Clindamycin Hydrochloride** *see* Clindamycin (Systemic) *on page 460*
- ◆ **Clindamycin Injection, USP (Can)** *see* Clindamycin (Systemic) *on page 460*
- ◆ **Clindamycin Palmitate** *see* Clindamycin (Systemic) *on page 460*
- ◆ **Clindamycin Phosphate** *see* Clindamycin (Topical) *on page 464*
- ◆ **Clindamycin Phosphate and Tretinoin** *see* Clindamycin and Tretinoin *on page 464*
- ◆ **Clindasol (Can)** *see* Clindamycin (Topical) *on page 464*
- ◆ **Clinda-T (Can)** *see* Clindamycin (Topical) *on page 464*
- ◆ **Clindesse** *see* Clindamycin (Topical) *on page 464*
- ◆ **Clindets (Can)** *see* Clindamycin (Topical) *on page 464*
- ◆ **Clinolipid** *see* Fat Emulsion (Plant Based) *on page 848*
- ◆ **Clinoril** *see* Sulindac *on page 1953*
- ◆ **Clinpro 5000** *see* Fluoride *on page 895*

Clioquinol and Flumethasone [CAN/INT]

(klye ok KWIN ole & floo METH a sone)

Brand Names: Canada Locacorten® Vioform®

Index Terms Flumethasone and Clioquinol; Iodochlorhydroxyquin and Flumethasone

Pharmacologic Category Antibiotic, Topical; Antifungal Agent, Topical; Corticosteroid, Topical

Use Note: Not approved in U.S.

Otic solution: Treatment of otitis externa; otomycosis due to *Aspergillus niger*

Topical cream: Treatment of corticosteroid-responsive dermatoses complicated by infection with bacterial and/or fungal agents

Pregnancy Considerations Adverse events have been observed with corticosteroids in animal reproduction studies.

Contraindications Hypersensitivity to clioquinol, flumethasone, or any component of the formulation; viral infection of the skin; tuberculosis, syphilis, rosacea, acne vulgaris, or perioral dermatitis; suspected or verified perforation of eardrum (otic solution); application to eyes; application to ulcerated areas (topical); use in children <2 years of age

Warnings/Precautions Do not apply to large areas or denuded skin; may irritate sensitized skin. Topical application poses a potential risk of toxicity to infants and children. Known to cause serious and irreversible optic atrophy and peripheral neuropathy with muscular weakness, sensory loss, spastic paraparesis, and blindness. Use with caution in patients with iodine intolerance. Discontinue therapy if no response within 1 week. Use caution in patients with thyroid abnormalities or hepatic or renal impairment.

Systemic absorption of topical corticosteroids may cause hypothalamic-pituitary-adrenal (HPA) axis suppression (reversible) particularly in younger children. HPA axis suppression may lead to adrenal crisis. Risk is increased when used over large surface areas, for prolonged periods, or with occlusive dressings; adverse systemic effects including hyperglycemia, glycosuria, fluid and electrolyte changes, and HPA suppression may occur when used on large surface areas, for prolonged periods, or with an occlusive dressing; prolonged treatment with corticosteroids has been associated with the development of Kaposi's sarcoma (case reports); if noted, discontinuation of therapy should be considered; striae and growth suppression have been reported with use of some corticosteroids in infants and children.

Adverse Reactions

Dermatologic: Acne, burning, itching, pigmentary changes, purpura, rash, skin atrophy, skin irritation, striae, telangiectasia

Endocrine: Potentially associated with excessive/prolonged use: HPA axis suppression (rare), thyrotoxicosis

Neuromuscular & skeletal: Peripheral neuropathy

Ocular: Optic atrophy

Miscellaneous: Hypersensitivity, secondary infection

Drug Interactions

Metabolism/Transport Effects None known.

Avoid Concomitant Use There are no known interactions where it is recommended to avoid concomitant use.

Increased Effect/Toxicity There are no known significant interactions involving an increase in effect.

Decreased Effect There are no known significant interactions involving a decrease in effect.

Storage/Stability Store between 15°C and 30°C.

Mechanism of Action Topical corticosteroids have anti-inflammatory, antipruritic, and vasoconstrictive properties. May depress the formation, release, and activity of endogenous chemical mediators of inflammation (kinins, histamine, liposomal enzymes, prostaglandins) through the induction of phospholipase A_2 inhibitory proteins (lipocortins) and sequential inhibition of the release of arachidonic acid. Flumethasone is an intermediate potency fluorinated corticosteroid. Clioquinol chelates bacterial surface and trace metals needed for bacterial growth

Dosage Children >2 years and Adults:

Otic solution (drops): Instill 2-3 drops into affected ear(s) 2 times/day; generally limit duration to 10 days

Topical: Apply in a thin layer to affected area 2-3 times/day; generally limit duration to 7 days

Dosage adjustment in renal impairment: No dosage adjustment provided in manufacturer's labeling; use with caution.

Dosage adjustment in hepatic impairment: No dosage adjustment provided in manufacturer's labeling; use with caution.

Administration

Otic solution: Thorough cleaning of the external ear prior to and during therapy either by wiping or gentle syringing is essential.

Topical cream: Avoid use of occlusive dressings. Cleanse affected area before application; can stain skin and fabrics; for external use only; avoid contact with eyes and mucous membranes.

Monitoring Parameters Observe affected area for increased irritation

Product Availability Not available in U.S.

Dosage Forms: Canada

Cream, topical:

Locacorten® Vioform®: Clioquinol 3% and flumethasone 0.02% (15 g, 50 g)

Solution, otic:

Locacorten® Vioform®: Clioquinol 1% and flumethasone 0.02% (10 mL)

CloBAZam (KLOE ba zam)

Brand Names: U.S. Onfi

Brand Names: Canada Apo-Clobazam; Clobazam-10; Dom-Clobazam; Frisium; Novo-Clobazam; PMS-Clobazam

Pharmacologic Category Benzodiazepine

Use Adjunctive treatment of seizures associated with Lennox-Gastaut syndrome

Canadian labeling: Adjunctive treatment of epilepsy

Pregnancy Risk Factor C

Pregnancy Considerations Adverse events were observed in animal reproduction studies. Clobazam crosses the placenta. An increased risk of fetal malformations may be associated with first trimester exposure. The Canadian labeling contraindicates use in the first trimester. Exposure to benzodiazepines immediately prior to or during birth may result in hypothermia, hypotonia, respiratory depression, and difficulty feeding in the neonate; neonates exposed to benzodiazepines late in pregnancy may develop dependence and withdrawal. The incidence of premature birth and low birth weights may be increased following maternal use of benzodiazepines; hypoglycemia and respiratory problems in the neonate may occur following exposure late in pregnancy. Neonatal withdrawal symptoms may occur within days to weeks after birth and "floppy infant syndrome" (which also includes withdrawal symptoms) has been reported with some benzodiazepines (Bergman, 1992; Iqbal, 2002; Wikner, 2007). A combination of factors influences the potential teratogenicity of anticonvulsant therapy. When treating women with epilepsy, monotherapy with the lowest effective dose and avoidance medications known to have a high incidence of teratogenic effects is recommended (Harden, 2009; Wlodarczyk, 2012).

Patients exposed to clobazam during pregnancy are encouraged to enroll themselves into the North American Antiepileptic Drug (NAAED) Pregnancy Registry by calling 1-888-233-2334. Additional information is available at www.aedpregnancyregistry.org.

Breast-Feeding Considerations Clobazam is excreted into breast milk. Due to the potential for serious adverse reactions in the nursing infant, the U.S. manufacturer recommends a decision be made whether to discontinue nursing or to discontinue the drug, taking into account the importance of treatment to the mother. Use in nursing women is contraindicated in the Canadian labeling. Drowsiness, lethargy, or weight loss in nursing infants have been observed in case reports following maternal use of some benzodiazepines (Iqbal, 2002).

Contraindications Hypersensitivity to clobazam or any component of the formulation.

Canadian labeling (not in U.S. labeling): Hypersensitivity to clobazam or any component of the formulation (cross sensitivity with other benzodiazepines may exist); myasthenia gravis; narrow-angle glaucoma; severe hepatic or respiratory disease; sleep apnea; history of substance abuse; use in the first trimester of pregnancy; breast-feeding

Warnings/Precautions Serious reactions, including Stevens-Johnson syndrome (SJS) and toxic epidermal necrolysis (TEN), have been reported. Monitor patients closely for signs and symptoms especially during the first 8 weeks or when reintroducing therapy. Permanently discontinue if SJS/TEN suspected.

Rebound or withdrawal symptoms may occur following abrupt discontinuation or large decreases in dose (more common with prolonged treatment). Cautiously taper dose if drug discontinuation is required. Use with caution in elderly or debilitated patients, patients with mild-to-moderate hepatic impairment or with preexisting muscle weakness or ataxia (may cause muscle weakness). Concentrations of the active metabolite are 3 to 5 times higher in patients who are known CYP2C19 poor metabolizers compared to CYP2C19 extensive metabolizers; dose adjustment is needed in patients who are poor CYP2C19 metabolizers.

Causes CNS depression (dose related) resulting in sedation, dizziness, confusion, or ataxia which may impair physical and mental capabilities. Patients must be cautioned about performing tasks which require mental alertness (eg, operating machinery or driving). Use with caution in patients receiving other CNS depressants or psychoactive agents. Effects with other sedative drugs or ethanol may be potentiated. Use with caution in patients with an impaired gag reflex or respiratory disease.

Tolerance, psychological and physical dependence may occur with prolonged use. Where possible, avoid use in patients with drug abuse, alcoholism, or psychiatric disease (eg, depression, psychosis). May increase risk of suicidal thoughts/behavior.

Acute withdrawal, including seizures, may be precipitated in patients after administration of flumazenil to patients receiving long-term benzodiazepine therapy. Potentially significant interactions may exist, requiring dose or frequency adjustment, additional monitoring, and/or selection of alternative therapy.

Benzodiazepines have been associated with anterograde amnesia. Paradoxical reactions, including hyperactive or aggressive behavior, have been reported with benzodiazepines, particularly in adolescent/pediatric or psychiatric patients. Does not have analgesic, antidepressant, or antipsychotic properties.

Adverse Reactions

Central nervous system: Aggressive behavior, ataxia, drowsiness, dysarthria, fatigue, insomnia, irritability, lethargy, psychomotor agitation, sedation

Gastrointestinal: Constipation, dysphagia, increased appetite, sialorrhea, vomiting

Genitourinary: Urinary tract infection

Neuromuscular & skeletal: Dysarthria

Respiratory: Bronchitis, cough, pneumonia, upper respiratory tract infection

Miscellaneous: Fever

Postmarketing and/or case reports (Limited to important or life-threatening): Aspiration, behavioral changes, blurred vision, confusion, delirium, delusions, depression, diplopia, eosinophilia, hallucination, leukopenia, mood changes, respiratory depression, Stevens-Johnson syndrome, suicidal ideation, suicidal tendencies, thrombocytopenia, toxic epidermal necrolysis

Drug Interactions

Metabolism/Transport Effects Substrate of CYP2B6 (minor), CYP2C19 (major), CYP3A4 (minor), P-glycoprotein; **Note:** Assignment of Major/Minor substrate status based on clinically relevant drug interaction potential; **Inhibits** CYP2C9 (weak), CYP2D6 (moderate), UGT1A4, UGT1A6, UGT2B4; **Induces** CYP3A4 (weak)

Avoid Concomitant Use

Avoid concomitant use of CloBAZam with any of the following: Azelastine (Nasal); Methadone; OLANZapine; Orphenadrine; Paraldehyde; Sodium Oxybate; Thalidomide; Thioridazine

Increased Effect/Toxicity

CloBAZam may increase the levels/effects of: Azelastine (Nasal); Buprenorphine; CloZAPine; CNS Depressants; CYP2D6 Substrates; Deferiprone; DOXOrubicin (Conventional); Eliglustat; Fesoterodine; Hydrocodone; Methadone; Methotrimeprazine; Metoprolol; Metyrosine; Mirtazapine; Nebivolol; Orphenadrine; Paraldehyde; Pramipexole; ROPINIRole; Rotigotine; Selective Serotonin Reuptake Inhibitors; Sodium Oxybate; Stiripentol; Suvorexant; Thalidomide; Thioridazine; Zolpidem

The levels/effects of CloBAZam may be increased by: Alcohol (Ethyl); Brimonidine (Topical); Cannabis; CYP2C19 Inhibitors (Moderate); CYP2C19 Inhibitors (Strong); Doxylamine; Dronabinol; Droperidol; HydrOXYzine; Kava Kava; Luliconazole; Magnesium Sulfate;

Methotrimeprazine; Nabilone; OLANZapine; Perampanel; Propafenone; Rufinamide; Stiripentol; Tapentadol; Teduglutide; Tetrahydrocannabinol

Decreased Effect

CloBAZam may decrease the levels/effects of: ARIPiprazole; Codeine; Contraceptives (Estrogens); Contraceptives (Progestins); Saxagliptin; Tamoxifen; TraMADol

The levels/effects of CloBAZam may be decreased by: CYP2C19 Inducers (Strong); Dabrafenib; Theophylline Derivatives; Yohimbine

Food Interactions

Ethanol: Concomitant administration may increase bioavailability of clobazam by 50%. Management: Monitor for increased effects with coadministration.

Food: Serum concentrations may be increased by grapefruit juice. Management: Keep grapefruit consumption consistent.

Storage/Stability Tablets and suspension: Store at 20°C to 25°C (68°F to 77°F). Dispose of unused suspension 90 days after opening bottle.

Mechanism of Action Clobazam is a 1,5 benzodiazepine which binds to stereospecific benzodiazepine receptors on the postsynaptic GABA neuron at several sites within the central nervous system, including the limbic system, reticular formation. Enhancement of the inhibitory effect of GABA on neuronal excitability results by increased neuronal membrane permeability to chloride ions. This shift in chloride ions results in hyperpolarization (a less excitable state) and stabilization. Benzodiazepine receptors and effects appear to be linked to the GABA-A receptors. Benzodiazepines do not bind to GABA-B receptors.

Pharmacodynamics/Kinetics

Absorption: Rapid; ~87%

Protein binding: 80% to 90%

Metabolism: Hepatic via CYP3A4 and to a lesser extent via CYP2C19 and 2B6 (N-demethylation to active metabolite [N-desmethyl] with ~20% activity of clobazam). CYP2C19 primarily mediates subsequent hydroxylation of the N-desmethyl metabolite.

Half-life elimination: Clobazam: 36-42 hours; N-desmethyl (active): 71-82 hours

Time to peak: 30 minutes to 4 hours

Excretion: Urine (~94%), as metabolites

Dosage Oral:

Children:

Lennox-Gastaut (adjunctive): U.S. labeling: ≥2 years: Refer to adult dosing.

Epilepsy (adjunctive): Canadian labeling (not in U.S. labeling):

<2 years: Initial 0.5-1 mg/kg/day

2-16 years: Initial: 5 mg daily; may be increased (no more frequently than every 5 days) to a maximum of 40 mg daily

Epilepsy (monotherapy) (off-label use): 2-16 years: Initial: Titrate slowly over 1-3 weeks to target dose of ~0.5 mg/kg/day in 2 divided doses (Canadian Study Group, 1998)

Adults:

Lennox-Gastaut (adjunctive): U.S. labeling: **Note:** Dose should be titrated according to patient tolerability and response.

≤30 kg: Initial: 5 mg once daily for ≥1 week, then increase to 5 mg twice daily for ≥1 week, then increase to 10 mg twice daily thereafter

>30 kg: Initial: 5 mg twice daily for ≥1 week, then increase to 10 mg twice daily for ≥1 week, then increase to 20 mg twice daily thereafter

CYP2C19 poor metabolizers:

≤30 kg: Initial: 5 mg once daily for ≥2 weeks, then increase to 5 mg twice daily; after ≥1 week may increase to 10 mg twice daily

>30 kg: Initial: 5 mg once daily for ≥1 week, then increase to 5 mg twice daily for ≥1 week, then increase to 10 mg twice daily; after ≥1 week may increase to 20 mg twice daily

Epilepsy (adjunctive): Canadian labeling (not in U.S. labeling): Initial: 5-15 mg/day; dosage may be gradually adjusted (based on tolerance and seizure control) to a maximum of 80 mg/day. **Note:** Daily doses of up to 30 mg may be taken as a single dose at bedtime; higher doses should be divided.

Catamenial epilepsy (off-label use): 20-30 mg daily for 10 days during the perimenstrual period (Feely, 1984)

Elderly: Lennox-Gastaut (adjunctive):

≤30 kg: Initial: 5 mg once daily for ≥2 weeks, then increase to 5 mg twice daily; after ≥1 week may increase to 10 mg twice daily based on patient tolerability and response

>30 kg: Initial: 5 mg once daily for ≥1 week, then increase to 5 mg twice daily for ≥1 week, then increase to 10 mg twice daily; after ≥1 week may increase to 20 mg twice daily based on patient tolerability and response

Dosage adjustment in renal impairment:

U.S. labeling:

CrCl ≥30 mL/minute: No dosage adjustment necessary.

CrCl <30 mL/minute: No dosage adjustment provided in manufacturer's labeling (has not been studied); use with caution.

Canadian labeling: No dosage adjustment provided in manufacturer's labeling; however, a reduced dosage is recommended.

Dosage adjustment in hepatic impairment:

U.S. labeling:

Mild-to-moderate impairment:

≤30 kg: Initial: 5 mg once daily for ≥2 weeks, then increase to 5 mg twice daily; after ≥1 week may increase to 10 mg twice daily based on patient tolerability and response

>30 kg: Initial: 5 mg once daily for ≥1 week, then increase to 5 mg twice daily for ≥1 week, then increase to 10 mg twice daily; after ≥1 week may increase to 20 mg twice daily based on patient tolerability and response

Severe impairment: No dosage adjustment provided in manufacturer's labeling (has not been studied). Use with caution; undergoes extensive hepatic metabolism.

Canadian labeling:

Mild-to-moderate impairment: No dosage adjustment provided in manufacturer's labeling; however, a reduced dosage is recommended.

Severe impairment: Use is contraindicated.

Dietary Considerations May be taken with or without food.

Administration May be administered with or without food. Tablets can be crushed and mixed in applesauce. Shake suspension well before using; only use the oral dosing syringe supplied with the suspension. Daily doses greater than 5 mg should be divided and administered twice daily.

Monitoring Parameters Respiratory and mental status/suicidality (eg, suicidal thoughts, depression, behavioral changes). The Canadian labeling recommends periodic CBC, liver function, renal function and thyroid function tests.

Dosage Forms

Suspension, Oral:

Onfi: 2.5 mg/mL (120 mL)

Tablet, Oral:

Onfi: 10 mg, 20 mg

Dosage Forms: Canada

Tablet:

Alti-Clobazam, Apo-Clobazam, Clobazam-10, Dom-Clobazam, Frisium, Novo-Clobazam, PMS-Clobazam, ratio-Clobazam: 10 mg

◆ **Clobazam-10 (Can)** *see* CloBAZam *on page* 465

Clobetasol (kloe BAY ta sol)

Brand Names: U.S. Clobetasol Propionate E; Clobex; Clobex Spray; Clodan; Cormax Scalp Application; Olux; Olux-E; Temovate; Temovate E

Brand Names: Canada Clobex; Dermovate; Mylan-Clobetasol; Novo-Clobetasol; Olux-E; PMS-Clobetasol; ratio-Clobetasol; Taro-Clobetasol

Index Terms Clobetasol Propionate

Pharmacologic Category Corticosteroid, Topical

Additional Appendix Information

Topical Corticosteroids *on page* 2230

Use Steroid-responsive dermatoses: Short-term relief of inflammation and pruritic manifestations of moderate to severe corticosteroid-responsive dermatoses

Pregnancy Risk Factor C

Dosage Topical: Discontinue when control achieved; if improvement not seen within 2 weeks, reassessment of diagnosis may be necessary.

Children <12 years: Use is not recommended

Children ≥12 years, Adolescents, and Adults:

Oral mucosal inflammation, dental (off-label use): Cream: Apply twice daily for up to 2 weeks (maximum dose: 50 g/week); discontinue application when control is achieved; if no improvement is seen, reassessment of diagnosis may be necessary

Steroid-responsive dermatoses: Cream, emollient cream, foam, gel, ointment, solution: Apply twice daily for up to 2 weeks (maximum dose: 50 g/week or 50 mL/week)

Mild to moderate plaque-type psoriasis of nonscalp areas, and moderate to severe plaque-type psoriasis of the scalp: Foam: Apply twice daily for up to 2 weeks (maximum dose: 50 g/week)

Adolescents ≥16 years and Adults: Moderate to severe plaque-type psoriasis: Emollient cream: Apply twice daily for up to 2 weeks; may be used for up to 4 weeks when application is <10% of body surface area (maximum dose: 50 g/week). Treatment with lotion beyond 2 weeks should be limited to localized lesions (<10% body surface area) which have not improved sufficiently.

Adolescents ≥18 years and Adults:

Moderate to severe plaque-type psoriasis:

Lotion: Apply twice daily for up to 2 weeks; may be used for up to 4 weeks when application is <10% of body surface area (maximum dose: 50 g/week or 50 mL/week). Treatment with lotion beyond 2 weeks should be limited to localized lesions (<10% body surface area) which have not improved sufficiently.

Spray: Apply by spraying directly onto affected area twice daily and gently rub into skin. Limit treatment to 4 consecutive weeks; treatment beyond 2 weeks should be limited to localized lesions which have not improved sufficiently. Maximum total dose: 50 g/week or 59 mL/week. Do not use more than 26 sprays per application or 52 sprays per day.

Oral mucosal inflammation, dental (off-label use): Cream: Apply twice daily for up to 2 weeks (maximum dose: 50 g/week); discontinue application when control is achieved; if no improvement is seen, reassessment of diagnosis may be necessary

Scalp psoriasis, moderate to severe: Shampoo: Apply thin film to dry scalp once daily (maximum dose: 50 g/week or 50 mL/week); leave in place for 15 minutes, then add water, lather; rinse thoroughly. Limit treatment to 4 consecutive weeks.

Steroid-responsive dermatoses: Lotion: Apply twice daily for up to 2 weeks (maximum dose: 50 g/week or 50 mL/week)

Dosage adjustment in renal impairment: There are no dosage adjustments provided in the manufacturer's labeling.

Dosage adjustment in hepatic impairment: There are no dosage adjustments provided in the manufacturer's labeling.

Additional Information Complete prescribing information should be consulted for additional detail.

Dosage Forms

Cream, External:

Clobetasol Propionate E: 0.05% (15 g, 30 g, 60 g)

Temovate: 0.05% (30 g, 60 g)

Temovate E: 0.05% (60 g)

Generic: 0.05% (15 g, 30 g, 45 g, 60 g)

Foam, External:

Olux: 0.05% (50 g, 100 g)

Olux-E: 0.05% (50 g, 100 g)

Generic: 0.05% (50 g, 100 g)

Gel, External:

Temovate: 0.05% (60 g)

Generic: 0.05% (15 g, 30 g, 60 g)

Kit, External:

Clodan: 0.05%

Liquid, External:

Clobex Spray: 0.05% (59 mL, 125 mL)

Generic: 0.05% (59 mL, 125 mL)

Lotion, External:

Clobex: 0.05% (59 mL, 118 mL)

Generic: 0.05% (59 mL, 118 mL)

Ointment, External:

Temovate: 0.05% (15 g, 30 g)

Generic: 0.05% (15 g, 30 g, 45 g, 60 g)

Shampoo, External:

Clobex: 0.05% (118 mL)

Clodan: 0.05% (118 mL)

Generic: 0.05% (118 mL)

Solution, External:

Cormax Scalp Application: 0.05% (50 mL)

Temovate: 0.05% (50 mL)

Generic: 0.05% (25 mL, 50 mL)

◆ **Clobetasol Propionate** *see* Clobetasol *on page* 468

◆ **Clobetasol Propionate E** *see* Clobetasol *on page* 468

◆ **Clobex** *see* Clobetasol *on page* 468

◆ **Clobex Spray** *see* Clobetasol *on page* 468

Clobutinol [INT] (kloe BYOO ti nol)

International Brand Names Desketo (IT); Enantyum (ES, IT); Ketesse (CH, ES, IT, LU); Lomisat (DE, ES); mentopin Hustenstiller (DE); Nullatuss Clobutinol (DE); Quiralam (ES); Rofatuss (DE); Silomat (AR, AT, BE, BR, CZ, DE, FI, FR, IT, LU, PT); stas Hustenstiller N (DE); Sympal (DE); Tussamed (DE); Tussed (DE)

Index Terms Clobutinol Hydrochloride

Pharmacologic Category Antitussive

Reported Use Symptomatic treatment of nonproductive cough

Dosage Range Adults: Oral: 40-80 mg 3 times/day

Product Availability Product available in various countries; not currently available in the U.S.

Dosage Forms

Syrup: 40 mg/10 mL [sugar free; contains sodium benzoate]

Tablet: 40 mg

◆ **Clobutinol Hydrochloride** *see* Clobutinol [INT] *on page 468*

Clocortolone (kloe KOR toe lone)

Brand Names: U.S. Cloderm; Cloderm Pump

Brand Names: Canada Cloderm®

Index Terms Clocortolone Pivalate

Pharmacologic Category Corticosteroid, Topical

Additional Appendix Information

Topical Corticosteroids *on page 2230*

Use Inflammation of corticosteroid-responsive dermatoses (intermediate-potency topical corticosteroid)

Pregnancy Risk Factor C

Dosage Adults: Apply sparingly and gently; rub into affected area from 1-4 times/day. Therapy should be discontinued when control is achieved; if no improvement is seen, reassessment of diagnosis may be necessary.

Additional Information Complete prescribing information should be consulted for additional detail.

Dosage Forms

Cream, External:

Cloderm: 0.1% (45 g, 90 g)

Cloderm Pump: 0.1% (30 g, 75 g)

Generic: 0.1% (45 g, 75 g, 90 g)

◆ **Clocortolone Pivalate** *see* Clocortolone *on page 469*

◆ **Clodan** *see* Clobetasol *on page 468*

◆ **Cloderm** *see* Clocortolone *on page 469*

◆ **Cloderm® (Can)** *see* Clocortolone *on page 469*

◆ **Cloderm Pump** *see* Clocortolone *on page 469*

Clodronate [CAN/INT] (KLOE droh nate)

Brand Names: Canada Bonefos®; Clasteon®

Index Terms Clodronate Disodium

Pharmacologic Category Bisphosphonate Derivative

Use Note: Not approved in U.S.

Management of hypercalcemia of malignancy; management of osteolysis due to bone metastases of malignancy

Pregnancy Considerations Adverse events were observed in animal reproduction studies. It is not known if bisphosphonates cross the placenta, but fetal exposure is expected (Djokanovic, 2008; Stathopoulos, 2011). Available data have not shown that exposure to bisphosphonates during pregnancy significantly increases the risk of adverse fetal events (Djokanovic, 2008; Levy, 2009; Stathopoulos, 2011). However until additional data is available, most sources recommend discontinuing bisphosphonate therapy in women of reproductive potential as early as possible prior to a planned pregnancy; use in premenopausal women should be reserved for special circumstances when rapid bone loss is occurring (Bhalla, 2010; Pereira, 2012; Stathopoulos, 2011). Because hypocalcemia has been described following *in utero* bisphosphonate exposure, exposed infants should be monitored for hypocalcemia after birth (Djokanovic, 2008; Stathopoulos, 2011). Use of this product is contraindicated during pregnancy.

Breast-Feeding Considerations It is not known if clodronate is excreted into breast milk. Use in lactating women is contraindicated by the manufacturer.

Contraindications Hypersensitivity to clodronate, bisphosphonates, or any component of the formulation; severe GI inflammation; renal impairment (serum creatinine >5 mg/dL, SI 440 micromole/L); concomitant use with other bisphosphonates; pregnancy or breast-feeding

Warnings/Precautions Use caution in patients with renal impairment; dose reductions, as well as close monitoring of serum creatinine and BUN, are necessary. Use is contraindicated when serum creatinine >5 mg/dL (SI 440 micromole/L). May cause irritation to upper gastrointestinal mucosa. Esophagitis, dysphagia, esophageal ulcers, esophageal erosions, and esophageal stricture (rare) have been reported with bisphosphonates (oral). Use with caution in patients with dysphagia, esophageal disease, gastritis, duodenitis, or ulcers (may worsen underlying condition). Discontinue use if new or worsening symptoms develop.

Bisphosphonate therapy has been associated with osteonecrosis, primarily of the jaw; this has been observed mostly in cancer patients, but also in patients with postmenopausal osteoporosis and other diagnoses. Most reported cases occurred after IV bisphosphonate therapy; however, cases have been reported following oral therapy. Dental exams and preventive dentistry should be performed prior to placing patients with risk factors on chronic bisphosphonate therapy. Invasive dental procedures should be avoided during treatment.

Infrequently, severe (and occasionally debilitating) bone, joint, and/or muscle pain have been reported during bisphosphonate treatment. The onset of pain ranged from a single day to several months. Consider discontinuing therapy in patients who experience severe symptoms; symptoms usually resolve upon discontinuation. Some patients experienced recurrence when rechallenged with same drug or another bisphosphonate; avoid use in patients with a history of these symptoms in association with bisphosphonate therapy. May cause hypocalcemia (increased risk with intravenous administration) or transient hypophosphatemia.

For IV preparation: Dilute prior to use; adequate hydration should be ensured prior to infusion; avoid infiltration/extravasation. Do not administer as bolus injection (may precipitate acute renal failure, severe local reactions, and thrombophlebitis). Monitor renal function during and after intravenous administration. Interrupt infusion in patients experiencing deteriorating renal function during therapy.

Adverse Reactions

Endocrine & metabolic: Hypocalcemia

Gastrointestinal: GI disturbances (includes anorexia, diarrhea, gastric pain, nausea, vomiting)

Hepatic: Transaminases increased

Renal: BUN increased, serum creatinine increased

Rare but important or life-threatening: Alkaline phosphatase increased, bronchospasm (patients with aspirin-sensitive asthma), dysphagia, erythematous rash, hypersensitivity reactions (angioedema, pruritus, rash, respiratory disorder, urticaria), hypophosphatemia (transient), leukemia/myelodysplasia (rare), macropapular rash, mouth irritation, musculoskeletal pain (severe), oliguria, osteonecrosis (primarily of jaw), parathyroid hormone increased, proteinuria, renal failure, ulcerative pharyngitis

Drug Interactions

Metabolism/Transport Effects None known.

Avoid Concomitant Use There are no known interactions where it is recommended to avoid concomitant use.

Increased Effect/Toxicity

Clodronate may increase the levels/effects of: Deferasirox; Estramustine; Phosphate Supplements

The levels/effects of Clodronate may be increased by: Aminoglycosides; Nonsteroidal Anti-Inflammatory Agents; Systemic Angiogenesis Inhibitors

Decreased Effect
The levels/effects of Clodronate may be decreased by: Antacids; Calcium Salts; Iron Salts; Magnesium Salts; Multivitamins/Minerals (with ADEK, Folate, Iron); Multivitamins/Minerals (with AE, No Iron); Proton Pump Inhibitors

Food Interactions All food and beverages may interfere with absorption. Coadministration with dairy products may decrease absorption. Beverages (especially orange juice and coffee), food, and medications (eg, antacids, calcium, iron, and multivalent cations) may reduce the absorption of bisphosphonates as much as 60%. Management: Administer with a glass of plain water at least 2 hours (Bonefos®) or 1 hour (Clasteon®) before or after food.

Preparation for Administration Injection must be further diluted (in 500 mL of NS or D_5W) prior to administration.

Storage/Stability Store capsules and undiluted ampuls at room temperature (15°C to 30°C).
Clasteon®: Diluted solution should be infused within 12 hours of preparation.
Bonefos®: Diluted solution should be infused within 24 hours of preparation. Once diluted, Bonefos® may be stored up to 24 hours at room temperature.

Mechanism of Action A bisphosphonate which lowers serum calcium by inhibition of bone resorption via actions on osteoclasts or on osteoclast precursors.

Pharmacodynamics/Kinetics
Onset of calcium-lowering effects: IV: Within 48 hours
Duration of calcium-lowering effects: 5 days to 3 weeks following discontinuation
Absorption: Oral: Rapid but low absorption (~1% to 3%)
Distribution: V_d: ~20 L; 20% of absorbed clodronate is bound to bone
Protein binding: Variable (2% to 36%)
Bioavailability: Oral: 1% to 3%
Half-life elimination: Terminal: Oral: ~6 hours; IV: 13 hours (serum); prolonged in bone tissue
Time to peak, plasma: Oral: 30 minutes
Excretion: Urine (60% to 80% of absorbed dose as unchanged drug); feces (as unabsorbed drug)

Dosage Adults:
Clasteon®: Hypercalcemia of malignancy/osteolytic bone metastases:
IV:
Single infusion: 1500 mg as a single dose
Multiple infusions: 300 mg once daily; treatment duration should not exceed 10 days
Oral: Recommended daily maintenance dose following IV therapy: Range: 1600 mg (4 capsules) to 2400 mg (6 capsules) given in a single or 2 divided doses; maximum recommended daily dose: 3200 mg (8 capsules).
Bonefos®:
Hypercalcemia of malignancy:
IV: Multiple infusions: 300 mg once daily; treatment duration should not exceed 7 days
Oral: Recommended daily maintenance dose following IV therapy: Range: 1600 mg (4 capsules) to 2400 mg (6 capsules) given in single or 2 divided doses; maximum recommended daily dose: 3200 mg (8 capsules).
Osteolytic bone metastases:
IV: Multiple infusions: 300 mg once daily; treatment duration should not exceed 7 days
Oral: Initial: 1600 mg/day; may be increased to a maximum of 3200 mg/day
Note: Retreatment: Limited data suggests that patients who develop hypercalcemia following discontinuation of therapy or during oral therapy may be retreated with Bonefos® or Clasteon® at a higher oral dosage (up to 3200 mg/day) or by IV infusion with Clasteon® (1500 mg as single dose or 300 mg once daily) or Bonefos® (300 mg once daily).

Dosage adjustment in renal impairment:
Clasteon®:
Serum creatinine (S_{cr}) >5 mg/dL: Use is contraindicated
S_{cr} ≥2.5-5 mg/dL: Dosage reduction is recommended; however, there are no dosage adjustments provided in manufacturer's labeling.
Bonefos®: **Note:** S_{cr} >5 mg/dL: Use is contraindicated
IV:
CrCl: 50-80 mL/minute: Administer 75% to 100% of normal dose
CrCl: 12-49 mL/minute: Administer 50% to 75% of normal dose
CrCl: <12 mL/minute: Administer 50% of normal dose
Oral: **Note:** Daily doses >1600 mg should not be used continuously
CrCl: >50 mL/minute: No dosage reduction recommended
CrCl: 30-50 mL/minute: Administer 75% of normal dose
CrCl: <30 mL/minute: Administer 50% of normal dose

Dietary Considerations Take at least 1 hour (Clasteon®) or 2 hours (Bonefos®) before or after food.

Administration
Capsules: Administer with a glass of plain water at least 2 hours (Bonefos®) or 1 hour (Clasteon®) before or after food.
Injection: Do not administer as bolus injection; for single infusion therapy administer over at least 4 hours; for multiple-infusion therapy administered once daily, infuse over 2-6 hours. Patients should be adequately hydrated with oral or IV fluids prior to infusion.

Monitoring Parameters Serum electrolytes including calcium, phosphorous, magnesium, and potassium; monitor for hypocalcemia for at least 2 weeks after therapy; serum creatinine, BUN, CBC with differential, hepatic function

Reference Range Calcium (total): Adults: 9.0-11.0 mg/dL (SI: 2.05-2.54 mmol/L), may slightly decrease with aging; Phosphorus: 2.5-4.5 mg/dL (SI: 0.81-1.45 mmol/L)

Product Availability Not available in U.S.

Dosage Forms: Canada
Capsule, oral:
Bonefos®, Clasteon®: 400 mg
Injection, solution:
Bonefos®: 60 mg/mL (5 mL)
Clasteon®; 30 mg/mL (10 mL)

◆ **Clodronate Disodium** *see* Clodronate [CAN/INT] *on page 469*

Clofarabine (klo FARE a been)

Brand Names: U.S. Clolar
Brand Names: Canada Clolar
Index Terms CAFdA; Clofarex
Pharmacologic Category Antineoplastic Agent, Antimetabolite; Antineoplastic Agent, Antimetabolite (Purine Analog)
Use Acute lymphoblastic leukemia: Treatment of relapsed or refractory acute lymphoblastic leukemia (ALL) in patients 1 to 21 years of age (after at least 2 prior regimens)
Pregnancy Risk Factor D
Pregnancy Considerations Adverse events were observed in animal reproduction studies. May cause fetal harm if administered to a pregnant woman. Women of childbearing potential should be advised to use effective contraception and avoid becoming pregnant during therapy.
Breast-Feeding Considerations It is not known if clofarabine is excreted in breast milk. Due to the potential for serious adverse reactions in the nursing infant, breastfeeding should be avoided during clofarabine treatment.

Contraindications

There are no contraindications listed in the manufacturer's U.S. labeling.

Canadian labeling: Hypersensitivity to clofarabine or any component of the formulation; symptomatic CNS involvement; history of serious heart, liver, kidney, or pancreas disease; severe hepatic impairment (AST and/or ALT >5 x ULN, and/or bilirubin >3 x ULN); severe renal impairment (CrCl <30 mL/minute)

Warnings/Precautions Hazardous agent - use appropriate precautions for handling and disposal (NIOSH 2014 [group 1]). Cytokine release syndrome (eg, tachypnea, tachycardia, hypotension, pulmonary edema) may develop into capillary leak syndrome, systemic inflammatory response syndrome (SIRS), and organ dysfunction; discontinue with signs/symptoms of SIRS or capillary leak syndrome (rapid onset respiratory distress, hypotension, pleural/pericardial effusion, and multiorgan failure) and consider supportive treatment with diuretics, corticosteroids, and/or albumin. Prophylactic corticosteroids may prevent or diminish the signs/symptoms of cytokine release. May require dosage reduction. Monitor blood pressure during 5 days of treatment; discontinue if hypotension develops. Monitor if on concurrent medications known to affect blood pressure. Dose-dependent, reversible myelosuppression (neutropenia, thrombocytopenia, and anemia) is common; may be severe and prolonged. Monitor blood counts and platelets. May be at increased risk for infection due to neutropenia; opportunistic infection or sepsis (may be severe or fatal), is increased due to prolonged neutropenia and immunocompromised state; monitor for signs and symptoms of infection and treat promptly if infection develops. May require therapy discontinuation. Serious and fatal hemorrhages (including cerebral, gastrointestinal, and pulmonary hemorrhage) have occurred, usually associated with thrombocytopenia. Monitor and manage coagulation parameters.

Serious and fatal cases of Stevens-Johnson syndrome (SJS) and toxic epidermal necrolysis (TEN) have been reported. Discontinue clofarabine for exfoliative or bullous rash, or if SJS or TEN are suspected. Clofarabine is associated with a moderate emetic potential; antiemetics are recommended to prevent nausea and vomiting (Basch, 2011; Dupuis, 2011; Roila, 2010). Serious and fatal enterocolitis (including neutropenic colitis, cecitis, and *C. difficile* colitis) has been reported, usually occurring within 30 days of treatment, and when used in combination with other chemotherapy. May lead to complication including necrosis, perforation, hemorrhage or sepsis. Monitor for signs/symptoms of enterocolitis and manage promptly.

Has not been studied in patients with hepatic impairment; use with caution (per manufacturer's labeling). Canadian labeling contraindicates use in severe impairment or in patients with a history of serious hepatic disease. Transaminases and bilirubin may be increased during treatment; transaminase elevations generally occur within 10 days of administration and persist for ≤15 days. In some cases, hepatotoxicity was severe and fatal. The risk for hepatotoxicity, including hepatic sinusoidal obstruction syndrome (SOS; formerly called veno-occlusive disease), is increased in patients who have previously undergone a hematopoietic stem cell transplant. Monitor liver function closely; may require therapy interruption or discontinuation; discontinue if SOS is suspected. Elevated creatinine, acute renal failure, and hematuria were observed in clinical studies. Monitor renal function closely; may require dosage reduction or therapy discontinuation. A pharmacokinetic study demonstrated that systemic exposure increases as creatinine clearance decreases (CrCl <60 mL/minute) (Bonate, 2011). Dosage reduction required for moderate renal impairment (CrCl 30-60 mL/minute); use with caution in patients with CrCl <30 mL/minute (has not been studied). Canadian labeling contraindicates use in severe impairment or in patients with a history of serious kidney disease. Minimize the use of drugs known to cause renal toxicity during the 5-day treatment period; avoid concomitant hepatotoxic medications. Tumor lysis syndrome/hyperuricemia may occur as a consequence of leukemia treatment, including treatment with clofarabine, usually occurring in the first treatment cycle. May lead to life-threatening acute renal failure; adequate hydration and prophylactic antihyperuricemic therapy throughout treatment will reduce the risk/effects of tumor lysis syndrome; monitor closely. Potentially significant drug-drug interactions may exist, requiring dose or frequency adjustment, additional monitoring, and/or selection of alternative therapy.

Adverse Reactions

Cardiovascular: Edema, flushing, hyper-/hypotension, pericardial effusion, tachycardia

Central nervous system: Agitation, anxiety, chills, drowsiness, fatigue, headache, irritability, lethargy, mental status changes, pain

Dermatologic: Cellulitis, erythema, palmar-plantar erythrodysesthesia, pruritic rash, pruritus, skin rash

Gastrointestinal: Abdominal pain, anorexia, diarrhea, gingival bleeding, mouth hemorrhage, mucosal inflammation, nausea, oral candidiasis, pancreatitis, pseudomembranous colitis, rectal pain, stomatitis, typhlitis, vomiting

Genitourinary: Hematuria

Hematologic & oncologic: Anemia, febrile neutropenia, leukopenia, lymphocytopenia, neutropenia, oral mucosal petechiae, petechia, thrombocytopenia, tumor lysis syndrome

Hepatic: Hyperbilirubinemia, increased bilirubin, increased serum ALT, increased serum AST, jaundice

Hypersensitivity: Hypersensitivity

Infection: Bacteremia, candidiasis, herpes simplex infection, herpes zoster, infection (includes bacterial, fungal, and viral), sepsis (including septic shock), sepsis syndrome, staphylococcal bacteremia, staphylococcal sepsis

Local: Catheter infection

Neuromuscular & skeletal: Arthralgia, back pain, limb pain, myalgia, ostealgia, weakness

Renal: Creatinine increased

Respiratory: Dyspnea, epistaxis, pleural effusion, pneumonia, pulmonary edema, respiratory distress, respiratory tract infection, tachypnea

Miscellaneous: Fever

Rare but important or life-threatening: Bone marrow failure, enterocolitis (occurs more frequently within 30 days of treatment and with combination chemotherapy), exfoliative dermatitis, gastrointestinal hemorrhage, hallucination (Jeha, 2006), hepatomegaly (Jeha, 2006), hypokalemia (Jeha, 2006), hyponatremia, hypophosphatemia, increased right ventricular pressure (Jeha, 2006), left ventricular systolic dysfunction (Jeha, 2006), major hemorrhage (including cerebral and pulmonary; majority of cases associated with thrombocytopenia), pancytopenia, Stevens-Johnson syndrome, syncope, toxic epidermal necrolysis

Drug Interactions

Metabolism/Transport Effects None known.

Avoid Concomitant Use

Avoid concomitant use of Clofarabine with any of the following: BCG; CloZAPine; Dipyrone; Natalizumab; Pimecrolimus; Tacrolimus (Topical); Tofacitinib; Vaccines (Live)

Increased Effect/Toxicity

Clofarabine may increase the levels/effects of: CloZAPine; Leflunomide; Natalizumab; Tofacitinib; Vaccines (Live)

The levels/effects of Clofarabine may be increased by: Denosumab; Dipyrone; Pimecrolimus; Roflumilast; Tacrolimus (Topical); Trastuzumab

Decreased Effect

Clofarabine may decrease the levels/effects of: BCG; Coccidioides immitis Skin Test; Sipuleucel-T; Vaccines (Inactivated); Vaccines (Live)

The levels/effects of Clofarabine may be decreased by: Echinacea

Preparation for Administration Hazardous agent; use appropriate precautions for handling and disposal (NIOSH 2014 [group 1]). Clofarabine should be diluted with NS or D_5W to a final concentration of 0.15 to 0.4 mg/mL. Manufacturer recommends the product be filtered through a 0.2 micron filter prior to dilution.

Storage/Stability Store intact vials at room temperature of 25°C (77°F); excursions permitted to 15°C to 30°C (59°F to 86°F). Solutions diluted for infusion in D_5W or NS may be stored for 24 hours at room temperature.

Mechanism of Action Clofarabine, a purine (deoxyadenosine) nucleoside analog, is metabolized to clofarabine 5'-triphosphate. Clofarabine 5'-triphosphate decreases cell replication and repair as well as causing cell death. To decrease cell replication and repair, clofarabine 5'-triphosphate competes with deoxyadenosine triphosphate for the enzymes ribonucleotide reductase and DNA polymerase. Cell replication is decreased when clofarabine 5'-triphosphate inhibits ribonucleotide reductase from reacting with deoxyadenosine triphosphate to produce deoxynucleotide triphosphate which is needed for DNA synthesis. Cell replication is also decreased when clofarabine 5'-triphosphate competes with DNA polymerase for incorporation into the DNA chain; when done during the repair process, cell repair is affected. To cause cell death, clofarabine 5'-triphosphate alters the mitochondrial membrane by releasing proteins, an inducing factor and cytochrome C.

Pharmacodynamics/Kinetics

Distribution: V_d: Children: 172 L/m^2 or 5.8 L/kg (Bonate, 2011); Elderly: 268 L/kg (Bonate, 2011)

Protein binding: 47%, primarily to albumin

Metabolism: Intracellulary by deoxycytidine kinase and mono- and diphosphokinases to active metabolite clofarabine 5′-triphosphate; limited hepatic metabolism (0.2%)

Half-life elimination: Children: ~5 hours; Children and Adults: 7 hours (Bonate, 2011)

Excretion: Urine (49% to 60%, as unchanged drug)

Dosage Note: Consider prophylactic corticosteroids (hydrocortisone 100 mg/m^2 on days 1 to 3) to prevent signs/symptoms of capillary leak syndrome or systemic inflammatory response syndrome (SIRS), and hydration and antihyperuricemic therapy (to reduce the risk of tumor lysis syndrome/hyperuricemia). Calculate body surface area (BSA) prior to each cycle, utilizing actual body weight. Clofarabine is associated with a moderate emetic potential; antiemetics are recommended to prevent nausea and vomiting (Basch, 2011; Dupuis, 2011; Roila, 2010).

Acute lymphoblastic leukemia (ALL), relapsed or refractory: Children ≥1 year, Adolescents, and Adults ≤21 years: IV: 52 mg/m^2/day days 1 through 5; repeat every 2 to 6 weeks; subsequent cycles should begin no sooner than 14 days from day 1 of the previous cycle (subsequent cycles may be administered when ANC ≥750/mm^3)

Acute lymphoblastic leukemia, relapsed/refractory (ALL; off-label population): Adults: IV:

Monotherapy: Induction: 40 mg/m^2/day for 5 days; may repeat induction cycle once in 3 to 6 weeks (depending on marrow response and recovery) (Kantarjian, 2003)

Combination therapy:

Induction: 40 mg/m^2/day for 5 days (in combination with cytarabine); may repeat one time after day 28 (if needed) (Advani, 2010)

Consolidation: 40 mg/m^2/day for 4 days (in combination with cytarabine) for one cycle (Advani, 2010)

Acute myeloid leukemia (AML), refractory (off-label use): Adults <70 years: IV:

Induction: 25 mg/m2/day for 5 days (in combination with cytarabine and filgrastim); may repeat one time after 21 days if needed (Becker, 2011)

Consolidation: 20 mg/m2/day for 5 days (in combination with cytarabine and filgrastim) for 1 or 2 cycles (Becker, 2011)

Langerhans cell histiocytosis, refractory (off-label use): Children 1 to 18 years: IV: 25 mg/m^2/day days 1 through 5; repeat every 28 days for 2 to 8 cycles (Simko, 2014). Additional data may be necessary to further define the role of clofarabine in this condition.

Dosage adjustment for toxicity:

Hematologic toxicity: ANC <500/mm^3 lasting ≥4 weeks: Reduce dose by 25% for next cycle

Nonhematologic toxicity:

Clinically significant infection: Withhold treatment until infection is under control, then restart at full dose

Grade 3 toxicity (excluding infection, nausea and vomiting, and transient elevations in transaminases and bilirubin): Withhold treatment; may reinitiate with a 25% dose-reduction with resolution or return to baseline

Grade ≥3 increase in creatinine or bilirubin: Discontinue clofarabine; may reinitiate with 25% dosage reduction when creatinine or bilirubin return to baseline and patient is stable; administer antihyperuricemic therapy for elevated uric acid.

Grade 4 toxicity (noninfectious): Discontinue treatment

Capillary leak or SIRS early signs/symptoms (eg, hypotension, tachycardia, tachypnea, pulmonary edema): Discontinue clofarabine; institute supportive measures. May consider reinitiating with a 25% dose reduction after patient is stable and organ function recovers to baseline.

Dermatologic toxicity: Exfoliative or bullous rash, or suspected Stevens-Johnson syndrome or toxic epidermal necrolysis: Discontinue clofarabine.

Hypotension (during the 5 days of administration): Discontinue clofarabine. If hypotension is transient and resolves (without pharmacologic intervention), may reinitiate with 25% dosage reduction (Canadian labeling).

Dosage adjustment in renal impairment: Clofarabine undergoes renal elimination and exposure is increased as creatinine clearance decreases (Bonate, 2011).

Renal impairment at baseline:

U.S. labeling:

CrCl 30 to 60 mL/minute: Reduce dose by 50%

CrCl <30 mL/minute: There are no dosage adjustments provided in the manufacturer's labeling; use with caution (has not been studied).

Canadian labeling:

CrCl ≥30 mL/minute: There are no dosage adjustments provided in the manufacturer's labeling; use with caution (has not been studied).

CrCl <30 mL/minute: Use is contraindicated.

Renal toxicity during treatment: Grade 3 or higher increase in serum creatinine: Discontinue clofarabine; may reinitiate with a 25% dose reduction after patient is stable and organ function recovers to baseline.

Dosage adjustment in hepatic impairment:

Hepatic impairment at baseline: There are no dosage adjustments provided in the manufacturer's labeling; use with caution (has not been studied). Canadian labeling contraindicates use in severe impairment.

Hepatotoxicity during treatment: Grade 3 or higher increase in bilirubin: Discontinue clofarabine; may reinitiate with a 25% dose reduction after patient is stable and organ function recovers to baseline.

Dosing in obesity:

American Society of Clinical Oncology (ASCO) Guidelines for appropriate chemotherapy dosing in obese adults with cancer: Utilize patient's actual body weight (full weight) for calculation of body surface area- or weight-based dosing, particularly when the intent of therapy is curative; manage regimen-related toxicities in the same manner as for nonobese patients; if a dose reduction is utilized due to toxicity, consider resumption of full weight-based dosing with subsequent cycles, especially if cause of toxicity (eg, hepatic or renal impairment) is resolved (Griggs, 2012).

American Society for Blood and Marrow Transplantation (ASBMT) practice guideline committee position statement on chemotherapy dosing in obesity: Utilize actual body weight (full weight) for calculation of body surface area in clofarabine dosing for hematopoietic stem cell transplant conditioning regimens in pediatrics and adults (Bubalo, 2014).

Administration

Clofarabine is associated with a moderate emetic potential; antiemetics are recommended to prevent nausea and vomiting (Basch, 2011; Dupuis, 2011; Roila, 2010).

IV infusion: Infuse over 2 hours for relapsed/refractory ALL. May be infused over 1 hour for some off-label protocols (Becker, 2011; Kantarjian, 2003). Continuous IV fluids are encouraged to decrease adverse events and tumor lysis effects. Hypotension may be a sign of capillary leak syndrome or systemic inflammatory response syndrome (SIRS). Discontinue if the patient becomes hypotensive during administration; may consider therapy reinitiation with a 25% dose reduction after return to baseline. Do not administer any other medications through the same intravenous line.

Hazardous agent; use appropriate precautions for handling and disposal (NIOSH 2014 [group 1]).

Monitoring Parameters CBC with differential and platelets (daily during treatment, then 1 to 2 times weekly or as necessary); liver and kidney function (during 5 days of clofarabine administration); coagulation parameters, blood pressure, cardiac function, and respiratory status during infusion; signs and symptoms of tumor lysis syndrome, infection, hepatic sinusoidal obstruction syndrome, enterocolitis, and cytokine release syndrome (tachypnea, tachycardia, hypotension, pulmonary edema); hydration status

Dosage Forms

Solution, Intravenous [preservative free]:

Clolar: 1 mg/mL (20 mL)

◆ **Clofarex** *see* Clofarabine *on page 470*

◆ **Clofazimina** *see* Clofazimine [INT] *on page 473*

Clofazimine [INT] (kloe FAZ i meen)

International Brand Names Clofozine (IN); Hansepran (IN); Lamcoin (TH); Lampren (ES, JP, NL); Lamprene (AU, CH, CZ, EG, FR, GR, HK, IR, MY, NZ, SA); Lapren (KR); Lapren SL (KR); MB-Combi (SA)

Index Terms B-663; Clofazimina; Clofazimine; Clofaziminum; G-30320; Klofatsimiini; Klofatzimin; Klofaziminos; NSC-14106

Pharmacologic Category Antibiotic, Miscellaneous

Reported Use

Labeled: Hansen's Disease (leprosy): Treatment of severe erythema nodosum leprosum (ENL) reactions in multibacillary (MB) leprosy

Off-label/Investigational: Rarely used as treatment of multidrug resistant tuberculosis (MDR-TB) and in *Mycobacterium avium* complex (MAC) complex infections in patients with acquired immune deficiency symptoms (AIDS)

Dosage Range Oral: Leprosy:

Children: 2 mg/kg every other day (in combination with dapsone and rifampin)

Adults: 50 mg/day (in combination with dapsone and rifampin) for 24 months

Product Availability International: No longer available commercially. In nations where a national leprosy elimination program exists, the Ministries of Health make an official request to the World Health Organization (WHO) for clofazimine. In nations where no such program exists, doctors or pharmacists from individual institutions contact the WHO with a request. A request can be made to the WHO via a letter, fax, or email to verify that the drug will be used to treat a severe ENL reaction due to leprosy and how many patients need the drug. If these conditions are met, a free supply of clofazimine will then be made available. For treatment of MDR-TB, the WHO handles decisions regarding distribution on an individual case-by-case basis. For additional information: http://www.who.int/lep/mdt/clofazimine/en/.

United States: Clofazimine is distributed through the National Hansen's Disease Program (NHDP). NHDP holds the Investigational New Drug (IND) clofazimine for treatment in the United States. In order for physicians to obtain clofazimine, they will have to register as an investigator under the NHDP IND. This will require submitting a curriculum vitae and a signed FDA form 1572 to the NHDP. For further information, or to request investigator status, please call the NHDP at 1-800-642-2477. For additional information: http://www.hrsa.gov/hansens/clinical/regimens.htm.

Dosage Forms

Capsule, oral: 50 mg, 100 mg

◆ **Clofazimine** *see* Clofazimine [INT] *on page 473*

◆ **Clofaziminum** *see* Clofazimine [INT] *on page 473*

◆ **Clolar** *see* Clofarabine *on page 470*

◆ **Clomid** *see* ClomiPHENE *on page 473*

ClomiPHENE (KLOE mi feen)

Brand Names: U.S. Clomid; Serophene

Brand Names: Canada Clomid; Serophene

Index Terms Clomiphene Citrate

Pharmacologic Category Ovulation Stimulator; Selective Estrogen Receptor Modulator (SERM)

Use Treatment of ovulatory dysfunction in women desiring pregnancy

Pregnancy Risk Factor X

Pregnancy Considerations Adverse events were observed in animal reproduction studies. The incidence of adverse fetal effects following maternal use of clomiphene for ovulation induction is similar to those seen in the general population. Clomiphene is not indicated for use in women who are already pregnant.

Breast-Feeding Considerations It is not known if clomiphene is excreted into breast milk. The manufacturer recommends that caution be used if administered to nursing women. Clomiphene may decrease lactation.

Contraindications Hypersensitivity to clomiphene citrate or any of its components; liver disease or history of liver disease; abnormal uterine bleeding; enlargement or development of ovarian cyst (not due to polycystic ovarian syndrome); uncontrolled thyroid or adrenal dysfunction; presence of an organic intracranial lesion such as pituitary tumor; pregnancy

Warnings/Precautions Use with caution in patients unusually sensitive to pituitary gonadotropins (eg, polycystic ovarian syndrome [PCOS]); a lower dose may be necessary. Use caution in patients with uterine fibroids, may cause further enlargement. Blurring or other visual symptoms can occur; symptoms may increase with higher doses or duration of therapy and in some cases may be irreversible. Patients with visual disturbances should discontinue therapy and receive prompt ophthalmic evaluation. Prolonged use may increase the risk of borderline or invasive ovarian cancer. Multiple births may result from the use of this medication; advise patient of the potential risk of multiple births before starting the treatment. Use should be supervised by physicians who are thoroughly familiar with infertility problems and their management.

Ovarian enlargement may be accompanied by abdominal distention or abdominal pain and generally regresses without treatment within a few days or weeks after therapy discontinuation. If ovaries are abnormally enlarged, withhold therapy until ovaries return to pretreatment size; reduce clomiphene dose and duration of future cycles. Ovarian hyperstimulation syndrome (OHSS), an exaggerated response to ovulation induction therapy, is characterized by an increase in vascular permeability which causes a fluid shift from intravascular space to third space compartments (eg, peritoneal cavity, thoracic cavity) (ASRM 2008; SOGC-CFAS 2011). This syndrome may begin within 24 hours of treatment, but may become most severe 7 to 10 days after therapy (SOGC-CFAS 2011). OHSS is typically self-limiting with spontaneous resolution, although it may be more severe and protracted if pregnancy occurs (ASRM 2008). Symptoms of mild/moderate OHSS may include abdominal distention/discomfort, diarrhea, nausea, and/or vomiting. Severe OHSS symptoms may include abdominal pain that is severe, acute respiratory distress syndrome, anuria/oliguria, ascites, dyspnea, hypotension, nausea/vomiting (intractable), pericardial effusions, tachycardia, or thromboembolism. Decreased creatinine clearance, hemoconcentration, hypoproteinemia, elevated liver enzymes, elevated WBC, and electrolyte imbalances may also be present (ASRM 2008; Fiedler 2012; SOGC-CFAS 2011). If severe OHSS occurs, stop treatment and consider hospitalizing the patient (ASRM 2008; SOGC-CFAS 2011). Treatment is primarily symptomatic and includes fluid and electrolyte management, analgesics, and prevention of thromboembolic complications (ASRM 2008; SOGC-CFAS 2011). The ascitic, pleural, and pericardial fluids may be removed if needed to relieve symptoms (eg, pulmonary distress or cardiac tamponade) (ASRM 2008; SOGC-CFAS 2011). Women with OHSS should avoid pelvic examination and/or intercourse (ASRM 2008; SOGC-CFAS 2011).

Appropriate use: To minimize risks, use only at the lowest effective dose for the shortest duration of therapy (especially for the first course of therapy). Women with PCOS, amenorrhea-galactorrhea syndrome, psychogenic amenorrhea, post oral contraceptive amenorrhea, and some cases of secondary amenorrhea of undetermined cause may most likely benefit from clomiphene therapy.

Adverse Reactions

Central nervous system: Headache

Endocrine & metabolic: Abnormal uterine bleeding, breast discomfort, hot flashes, ovarian enlargement

Gastrointestinal: Distention/bloating/discomfort, nausea, vomiting

Ocular: Visual symptoms (includes blurred vision, diplopia, floaters, lights, phosphenes, photophobia, scotomata, waves)

Rare but important or life-threatening: Abnormal accommodation, acne, allergic reaction, arrhythmia, chest pain, depression, dizziness, dyspnea, edema, endometriosis, erythema multiforme, erythema nodosum, eye pain, fatigue, fever, hepatitis, hypertension, hypertrichosis, leukocytosis, macular edema, migraine, mood changes, neoplasms, optic neuritis, ovarian cyst, ovarian hemorrhage, palpitation, PE, phlebitis, posterior vitreous detachment, pruritus, psychosis, retinal hemorrhage, retinal thrombosis, retinal vascular spasm, seizure, stroke, syncope, tachycardia, thrombophlebitis, thyroid disorder, tinnitus, transaminase increased, tubal pregnancy, uterine hemorrhage, vision loss (temporary/prolonged)

Drug Interactions

Metabolism/Transport Effects None known.

Avoid Concomitant Use

Avoid concomitant use of ClomiPHENE with any of the following: Ospemifene

Increased Effect/Toxicity

ClomiPHENE may increase the levels/effects of: Ospemifene

Decreased Effect

ClomiPHENE may decrease the levels/effects of: Ospemifene

Storage/Stability Store at room temperature of 15°C to 30°C (59°F to 86°F). Protect from light, heat, and excessive humidity.

Mechanism of Action Clomiphene is a racemic mixture consisting of zuclomiphene (~38%) and enclomiphene (~62%), each with distinct pharmacologic properties. Clomiphene acts at the level of the hypothalamus, occupying cell surface and intracellular estrogen receptors (ERs) for longer durations than estrogen. This interferes with receptor recycling, effectively depleting hypothalamic ERs and inhibiting normal estrogenic negative feedback. Impairment of the feedback signal results in increased pulsatile GnRH secretion from the hypothalamus and subsequent pituitary gonadotropin (FSH, LH) release, causing growth of the ovarian follicle, followed by follicular rupture (ASRM 2013; Dickey, 1996).

Pharmacodynamics/Kinetics

Onset of action: Ovulation: 5 to 10 days following course of treatment

Duration: Effects are cumulative; ovulation may occur in the cycle following the last treatment (Dickey, 1996)

Absorption: Readily absorbed

Metabolism: Hepatic; undergoes enterohepatic recirculation (Goldstein 2000)

Half-life elimination: ~5 days (Goldstein 2000)

Time to peak, plasma: ~6 hours (Goldstein 2000)

Excretion: Primarily feces (42%); urine (8%); some excretion may occur for up to 6 weeks after therapy is discontinued

Dosage Oral: Adults: Ovulation induction: Females: **Note:** Intercourse should be timed to coincide with the expected time of ovulation (usually 5 to 10 days after a clomiphene course).

Initial course: 50 mg once daily for 5 days. Begin on or about the fifth day of cycle if progestin-induced bleeding is scheduled or spontaneous uterine bleeding occurs prior to therapy. Therapy may be initiated at anytime in patients with no recent uterine bleeding.

Dose adjustment: Subsequent doses may be increased to 100 mg once daily for 5 days only if ovulation does not occur at the initial dose. Lower doses (12.5 to 25 mg daily) may be used in women sensitive to clomiphene or who consistently develop large ovarian cysts (ASRM 2013).

Repeat courses: If needed, the 5-day cycle may be repeated as early as 30 days after the previous one. Exclude the presence of pregnancy. The lowest effective dose should be used.

Maximum dose: 100 mg once daily for 5 days for up to 6 cycles. Discontinue if ovulation does not occur after 3 courses of treatment; or if 3 ovulatory responses occur but pregnancy is not achieved. Long-term therapy (>6 cycles) is not recommended. Re-evaluate if menses does not occur following ovulatory response. Doses have ranged from 50 to 250 mg daily, although doses

>100 mg daily have not been shown to increase pregnancy rates (ASRM 2013). The maximum recommended dose in women with PCOS is 150 mg daily (ESHRE/ASRM 2008).

Dosage adjustment in renal impairment: There are no dosage adjustments provided in the manufacturer's labeling.

Dosage adjustment in hepatic impairment: Use is contraindicated in patients with a history of liver disease or dysfunction.

Administration The total daily dose should be taken at one time to maximize effectiveness (Dickey, 1996).

Monitoring Parameters

Prior to therapy: serum estrogen. Rule out primary pituitary or ovarian failure, endometriosis/endometrial carcinoma, adrenal disorders, thyroid disorders, hyperprolactinemia, and male infertility.

Pelvic exam prior to each course of therapy; pregnancy test prior to repeat courses; ovulation (may include serum estradiol, progesterone, urinary luteinizing hormone; ultrasound) (ASRM 2013).

OHSS: Monitoring of hospitalized patients should include abdominal circumference, albumin, cardiorespiratory status, electrolytes, fluid balance, hematocrit, hemoglobin, serum creatinine, urine output, urine specific gravity, vital signs, weight (daily or as necessary) and liver enzymes (weekly) (ASRM 2008; SOGC-CFAS 2011).

Dosage Forms

Tablet, Oral:

Clomid: 50 mg

Serophene: 50 mg

Generic: 50 mg

◆ **Clomiphene Citrate** *see* ClomiPHENE *on page 473*

ClomiPRAMINE (kloe MI pra meen)

Brand Names: U.S. Anafranil

Brand Names: Canada Anafranil®; Apo-Clomipramine®; CO Clomipramine; Dom-Clomipramine; Novo-Clomipramine

Index Terms Clomipramine Hydrochloride

Pharmacologic Category Antidepressant, Tricyclic (Tertiary Amine)

Additional Appendix Information

Beers Criteria – Potentially Inappropriate Medications for Geriatrics *on page 2271*

Use Treatment of obsessive-compulsive disorder (OCD)

Pregnancy Risk Factor C

Pregnancy Considerations Adverse events were observed in some animal reproduction studies. Clomipramine and its metabolite desmethylclomipramine cross the placenta and can be detected in cord blood and neonatal serum at birth (Loughhead, 2006; ter Horst, 2011). Data from five newborns found the half-life for clomipramine in the neonate to be 42 ± 16 hours following *in utero* exposure. Serum concentrations were not found to correlate to withdrawal symptoms (ter Horst, 2011). Withdrawal symptoms (including jitteriness, tremor, and seizures) have been observed in neonates whose mothers took clomipramine up to delivery.

The ACOG recommends that therapy for depression during pregnancy be individualized; treatment should incorporate the clinical expertise of the mental health clinician, obstetrician, primary healthcare provider, and pediatrician (ACOG, 2008). According to the American Psychiatric Association (APA), the risks of medication treatment should be weighed against other treatment options and untreated depression. For women who discontinue antidepressant medications during pregnancy and who may be at high risk for postpartum depression, the medications can be restarted following delivery (APA, 2010). Treatment algorithms have been developed by the ACOG and the APA for the management of depression in women prior to conception and during pregnancy (Yonkers, 2009).

Breast-Feeding Considerations Clomipramine is excreted in breast milk. Based on information from three mother-infant pairs, following maternal use of clomipramine 75-150 mg/day, the estimated exposure to the breast-feeding infant would be 0.4% to 4% of the weight-adjusted maternal dose. Adverse events have not been reported in nursing infants (information from seven cases). Infants should be monitored for signs of adverse events; routine monitoring of infant serum concentrations is not recommended (Fortinguerra, 2009). Due to the potential for serious adverse reactions in the nursing infant, the decision to continue or discontinue breast-feeding during therapy should take into account the risk of exposure to the infant and the benefits of treatment to the mother.

Contraindications Hypersensitivity to clomipramine, other tricyclic agents, or any component of the formulation; use of MAO inhibitors intended to treat psychiatric disorders (concurrently or within 14 days of discontinuing either clomipramine or the MAO inhibitor); initiation of clomipramine in a patient receiving linezolid or intravenous methylene blue; use in a patient during the acute recovery phase of MI

Warnings/Precautions [U.S. Boxed Warning]: Antidepressants increase the risk of suicidal thinking and behavior in children, adolescents, and young adults (18 to 24 years of age) with major depressive disorder (MDD) and other psychiatric disorders; consider risk prior to prescribing. Short-term studies did not show an increased risk in patients >24 years of age and showed a decreased risk in patients ≥65 years. Closely monitor patients for clinical worsening, suicidality, or unusual changes in behavior, particularly during the initial 1 to 2 months of therapy or during periods of dosage adjustments (increases or decreases); the patient's family or caregiver should be instructed to closely observe the patient and communicate condition with health care provider. A medication guide should be dispensed with each prescription. **Clomipramine is FDA approved for the treatment of OCD in children ≥10 years of age.**

The possibility of a suicide attempt is inherent in major depression and may persist until remission occurs. Use caution in high-risk patients. Worsening depression and severe abrupt suicidality that are not part of the presenting symptoms may require discontinuation or modification of drug therapy. The patient's family or caregiver should be alerted to monitor patients for the emergence of suicidality and associated behaviors (such as agitation, irritability, hostility, impulsivity, and hypomania) and notify the healthcare provider.

May worsen psychosis in some patients or precipitate a shift to mania or hypomania in patients with bipolar disorder. Patients presenting with depressive symptoms should be screened for bipolar disorder. Monotherapy in patients with bipolar disorder should be avoided. **Clomipramine is not FDA approved for bipolar depression.**

Potentially life-threatening serotonin syndrome (SS) has occurred with serotonergic agents (eg, SSRIs, SNRIs), particularly when used in combination with other serotonergic agents (eg, triptans, TCAs, fentanyl, lithium, tramadol, buspirone, St John's wort, tryptophan) or agents that impair metabolism of serotonin (eg, MAO inhibitors intended to treat psychiatric disorders, other MAO inhibitors [ie, linezolid and intravenous methylene blue]). Discontinue treatment (and any concomitant serotonergic agent) immediately if signs/symptoms arise. TCAs may rarely cause bone marrow suppression; monitor for any signs of infection and obtain CBC if symptoms (eg, fever, sore throat) evident. May cause seizures (relationship to dose and/or duration of therapy) - do not exceed maximum doses. Use caution in patients with a previous seizure disorder or condition predisposing to seizures such as brain damage, alcoholism, or concurrent therapy with other drugs which lower the seizure threshold. May increase the risks associated with electroconvulsive therapy. Bone fractures have been associated with antidepressant treatment. Consider the possibility of a fragility fracture if an antidepressant-treated patient presents with unexplained bone pain, point tenderness, swelling, or bruising (Rabenda, 2013; Rizzoli, 2012). Use with caution in patients with tumors of the adrenal medulla (eg, pheochromocytoma, neuroblastoma); may cause hypertensive crises. Has been associated with a high incidence of sexual dysfunction. Weight gain may occur.

May cause CNS depression, which may impair physical or mental abilities; patients must be cautioned about performing tasks that require mental alertness (eg, operating machinery or driving). The degree of sedation, anticholinergic effects, and conduction abnormalities are high relative to other antidepressants. The risk of orthostasis is moderate to high relative to other antidepressants. Use with caution in patients with a history of cardiovascular disease (including previous MI, stroke, tachycardia, or conduction abnormalities). Use with caution in patients with urinary retention, benign prostatic hyperplasia, narrow-angle glaucoma, xerostomia, visual problems, constipation, or a history of bowel obstruction. Potentially significant drug-drug interactions may exist, requiring dose or frequency adjustment, additional monitoring, and/or selection of alternative therapy.

Recommended by the manufacturer to discontinue prior to elective surgery; risks exist for drug interactions with anesthesia and for cardiac arrhythmias. However, definitive drug interactions have not been widely reported in the literature and continuation of tricyclic antidepressants is generally recommended as long as precautions are taken to reduce the significance of any adverse events that may occur (Pass, 2004). Use with caution in patients with hepatic impairment; increases in ALT/AST have occurred, including rare reports of severe hepatic injury (some fatal); monitor hepatic transaminases periodically in patients with hepatic impairment. Use with caution in patients with renal dysfunction. Avoid use in the elderly due to its potent anticholinergic and sedative properties, and potential to cause orthostatic hypotension. In addition, may also cause or exacerbate syndrome of inappropriate antidiuretic hormone secretion or hyponatremia; monitor sodium closely with initiation or dosage adjustments in older adults (Beers Criteria). May cause mild pupillary dilation which in susceptible individuals can lead to an episode of narrow-angle glaucoma. Consider evaluating patients who have not had an iridectomy for narrow-angle glaucoma risk factors.

Abrupt discontinuation or interruption of antidepressant therapy has been associated with a discontinuation syndrome. Symptoms arising may vary with antidepressant however commonly include nausea, vomiting, diarrhea, headaches, light-headedness, dizziness, diminished appetite, sweating, chills, tremors, paresthesias, fatigue, somnolence, and sleep disturbances (eg, vivid dreams, insomnia). Greater risks for developing a discontinuation syndrome have been associated with antidepressants with shorter half-lives, longer durations of treatment, and abrupt discontinuation. For antidepressants of short or intermediate half-lives, symptoms may emerge within 2-5 days after treatment discontinuation and last 7-14 days (APA, 2010; Fava, 2006; Haddad, 2001; Shelton, 2001; Warner, 2006).

Adverse Reactions

Cardiovascular: Chest pain (children & adolescents), ECG abnormality, flushing, orthostatic hypotension, palpitations, syncope (children & adolescents), tachycardia

Central nervous system: Abnormal dreams (adults), abnormality in thinking, aggressive behavior (children & adolescents), agitation (adults), anxiety (more common in adults), chills (adults), confusion (more common in adults), depersonalization, depression (adults), dizziness (more common in adults), drowsiness, emotional lability (adults), fatigue, headache (adults), hypertonia, insomnia (more common in adults), irritability (children & adolescents), lack of concentration (adults), memory impairment, migraine (adults), myasthenia, myoclonus (more common in adults), nervousness (more common in adults), pain, panic attack, paresis (children & adolescents), paresthesia (adults), psychosomatic disorder (adults), sleep disorder, speech disturbance (adults), twitching (adults), vertigo, yawning (adults)

Dermatologic: Body odor (children & adolescents), dermatitis (adults), diaphoresis (more common in adults), pruritus (adults), skin rash, urticaria (adults), xeroderma (adults)

Endocrine & metabolic: Amenorrhea (adults), change in libido (adults), hot flash, menstrual disease (adults), weight gain (more common in adults), weight loss (children & adolescents)

Gastrointestinal: Abdominal pain (adults), anorexia, aphthous stomatitis (children & adolescents), constipation (more common in adults), diarrhea, dysgeusia, dyspepsia, dysphagia (adults), esophagitis (adults), flatulence (adults), gastrointestinal disease (adults), halitosis (children & adolescents), increased appetite (adults), nausea (adults), vomiting, xerostomia (more common in adults)

Genitourinary: Breast hypertrophy (adults), cystitis (adults), difficulty in micturition (more common in adults), ejaculation failure (more common in adults), impotence (adults), lactation (nonpuerperal; adults), leukorrhea (adults), mastalgia (adults), urinary frequency (adults), urinary retention (more common in children & adolescents), urinary tract infection (adults), vaginitis (adults)

Hematologic & oncologic: Purpura (adults)

Hepatic: Increased serum ALT (>3 x ULN), increased serum AST (>3 x ULN)

Hypersensitivity: Hypersensitivity reaction (children & adolescents)

Neuromuscular & skeletal: Myalgia (adults), tremor (more common in adults), weakness (more common in children & adolescents)

Ophthalmic: Abnormal lacrimation (adults), anisocoria (children & adolescents), blepharospasm (children & adolescents), conjunctivitis (adults), mydriasis (adults), ocular allergy (children & adolescents), visual disturbance (more common in adults)

Otic: Tinnitus

Respiratory: Bronchospasm (more common in children & adolescents), dyspnea (children & adolescents), epistaxis (adults), laryngitis (children & adolescents), pharyngitis (adults), rhinitis (adults), sinusitis (adults)

Miscellaneous: Fever (adults)

Rare but important or life-threatening: Abnormal electroencephalogram, accommodation disturbance, agranulocytosis, albuminuria, alopecia, anemia, aneurysm, angle-closure glaucoma, anticholinergic syndrome, aphasia, apraxia, ataxia, atrial flutter, blepharitis, bloody stools, bone marrow depression, bradycardia, brain disease, breast fibroadenosis, bronchitis, bundle branch block, cardiac arrest, cardiac arrhythmia, cardiac failure, catalepsy, cellulitis, cerebral hemorrhage, cervical dysplasia, cheilitis, chloasma, cholinergic syndrome, choreoathetosis, chromatopsia, chronic enteritis, colitis, coma, conjunctival hemorrhage, cyanosis, deafness, dehydration, delirium, delusions, dental caries, dermal ulcer, diabetes mellitus, diplopia, duodenitis, dyskinesia, dystonia, edema, edema (oral), endometrial hyperplasia, endometriosis, enlargement of salivary glands, epididymitis, erythematous rash, exophthalmos, exostosis, extrapyramidal reaction, extrasystoles, gastric dilation, gastric ulcer, gastroesophageal reflux disease, glycosuria, goiter, gout, gynecomastia, hallucination, heart block, hematuria, hemiparesis, hemoptysis, hepatic injury (severe), hepatitis, hostility, hyperacusis, hypercholesterolemia, hyperesthesia, hyperglycemia, hyperkinesia, hyperreflexia, hyperthermia, hyperthyroidism, hyperuricemia, hyperventilation, hypnogenic hallucinations, hypoesthesia, hypokalemia, hypokinesia, hypothyroidism, hypoventilation, intestinal obstruction, irritable bowel syndrome, ischemic heart disease, keratitis, laryngismus, leukemoid reaction, leukopenia, lupus erythematous-like rash, lymphadenopathy, maculopapular rash, manic reaction, muscle spasm, mutism, myocardial infarction, myopathy, myositis, nephrolithiasis, neuralgia, neuropathy, nocturnal amblyopia, oculogyric crisis, oculomotor nerve paralysis, ovarian cyst, pancytopenia, paralytic ileus, paranoia, peptic ulcer, periarteritis nodosa, peripheral ischemia, pharyngeal edema, phobia, photophobia, pneumonia, premature ejaculation, pseudolymphoma, psoriasis, psychosis, pyelonephritis, pyuria, rectal hemorrhage, renal cyst, schizophrenic reaction, scleritis, seizure, sensory disturbance, serotonin syndrome, skin hypertrophy, skin photosensitivity, somnambulism, strabismus, stupor, suicidal ideation, thrombocytopenia, thrombophlebitis, tongue ulcer, torticollis, urinary incontinence, uterine hemorrhage, uterine inflammation, vaginal hemorrhage, vasospasm, ventricular tachycardia, visual field defect, voice disorder, withdrawal syndrome

Drug Interactions

Metabolism/Transport Effects Substrate of CYP1A2 (major), CYP2C19 (major), CYP2D6 (major), CYP3A4 (minor); **Note:** Assignment of Major/Minor substrate status based on clinically relevant drug interaction potential; **Inhibits** CYP2D6 (moderate)

Avoid Concomitant Use

Avoid concomitant use of ClomiPRAMINE with any of the following: Aclidinium; Azelastine (Nasal); Dapoxetine; Glucagon; Iobenguane I 123; Ipratropium (Oral Inhalation); Linezolid; MAO Inhibitors; Methylene Blue; Moxonidine; Orphenadrine; Paraldehyde; Potassium Chloride; Thalidomide; Thioridazine; Tiotropium; Umeclidinium

Increased Effect/Toxicity

ClomiPRAMINE may increase the levels/effects of: AbobotulinumtoxinA; Alcohol (Ethyl); Alpha-/Beta-Agonists (Direct-Acting); Alpha1-Agonists; Amphetamines; Analgesics (Opioid); Anticholinergic Agents; Antipsychotic Agents; ARIPiprazole; Aspirin; Azelastine (Nasal); Beta2-Agonists; Buprenorphine; Citalopram; CNS Depressants; CYP2D6 Substrates; Desmopressin; DOXOrubicin (Conventional); Eliglustat; Escitalopram; Fesoterodine; Glucagon; Highest Risk QTc-Prolonging Agents; Hydrocodone; Methotrimeprazine; Methylene Blue; Metoprolol; Metyrosine; Milnacipran; Mirabegron; Moderate Risk QTc-Prolonging Agents; Nebivolol; Nicorandil; NSAID (COX-2 Inhibitor); NSAID (Nonselective); OnabotulinumtoxinA; Orphenadrine; Paraldehyde; Potassium Chloride; Pramipexole; QuiNIDine; RimabotulinumtoxinB; ROPINIRole; Rotigotine; Serotonin Modulators; Sodium Phosphates; Sulfonylureas; Suvorexant; Thalidomide; Thiazide Diuretics; Thioridazine; Tiotropium; Topiramate; TraMADol; Vitamin K Antagonists; Yohimbine; Zolpidem

The levels/effects of ClomiPRAMINE may be increased by: Abiraterone Acetate; Aclidinium; Altretamine; Antiemetics (5HT3 Antagonists); Antipsychotic Agents; Brimonidine (Topical); BuPROPion; Cannabis; CarBAMazepine; Cimetidine; Cinacalcet; Citalopram; Cobicistat; CYP1A2 Inhibitors (Moderate); CYP1A2 Inhibitors (Strong); CYP2C19 Inhibitors (Moderate); CYP2C19 Inhibitors (Strong); CYP2D6 Inhibitors (Moderate); CYP2D6 Inhibitors (Strong); Dapoxetine; Darunavir; Deferasirox; Dexmethylphenidate; Doxylamine; Dronabinol; Droperidol; DULoxetine; Escitalopram; FLUoxetine; FluvoxaMINE; Grapefruit Juice; HydrOXYzine; Ipratropium (Oral Inhalation); Kava Kava; Linezolid; Lithium; Luliconazole; Magnesium Sulfate; MAO Inhibitors; Methotrimeprazine; Methylphenidate; Metoclopramide; Metyrosine; Mianserin; Mifepristone; Nabilone; PARoxetine; Peginterferon Alfa-2b; Perampanel; Pramlintide; Propafenone; Protease Inhibitors; QuiNIDine; Rufinamide; Sertraline; Sodium Oxybate; Tapentadol; Tedizolid; Terbinafine (Systemic); Tetrahydrocannabinol; Thyroid Products; TraMADol; Umeclidinium; Valproic Acid and Derivatives; Vemurafenib

Decreased Effect

ClomiPRAMINE may decrease the levels/effects of: Acetylcholinesterase Inhibitors; Alpha1-Agonists; Alpha2-Agonists; Alpha2-Agonists (Ophthalmic); Codeine; Iobenguane I 123; Itopride; Moxonidine; Secretin; Tamoxifen

The levels/effects of ClomiPRAMINE may be decreased by: Acetylcholinesterase Inhibitors; Barbiturates; Cannabis; CYP1A2 Inducers (Strong); CYP2C19 Inducers (Strong); Cyproterone; Dabrafenib; Peginterferon Alfa-2b; St Johns Wort; Teriflunomide

Food Interactions Serum concentrations/toxicity may be increased by grapefruit juice. Management: Avoid grapefruit juice.

Storage/Stability

Store at controlled room temperature at 20°C to 25°C (68°F to 77°F).

Mechanism of Action Clomipramine appears to affect serotonin uptake while its active metabolite, desmethylclomipramine, affects norepinephrine uptake

Pharmacodynamics/Kinetics

Absorption: Rapid

Protein binding: 97%, primarily to albumin

Metabolism: Hepatic to desmethylclomipramine (DMI; active); extensive first-pass effect

Half-life elimination: Clomipramine: Mean 32 hours (range: 19-37 hours); DMI: Mean 69 hours (range: 54-77 hours)

Time to peak, plasma: 2-6 hours

Excretion: Urine and feces

Dosage

Obsessive-compulsive disorder (OCD), treatment:

Children ≥10 years and Adolescents: Oral:

Initial: 25 mg daily; gradually increase as tolerated over the first 2 weeks to 3 mg/kg/day or 100 mg daily (whichever is less) in divided doses

Maintenance: May further increase over next several weeks up to maximum of 3 mg/kg/day or 200 mg daily (whichever is less); after titration, may give as a single once daily dose at bedtime

Adults: Oral:

Initial: 25 mg daily; may gradually increase as tolerated over the first 2 weeks to ~100 mg daily in divided doses

Maintenance: May further increase over next several weeks up to a maximum of 250 mg daily; after titration, may give as a single once daily dose at bedtime

Panic attacks (off-label use): Adults: Oral: Initial: 10-25 mg daily; titrate gradually (usually weekly) to an effective dose (usual dosage range: 50-150 mg daily); in some studies dose was titrated up to a maximum dose of 200-250 mg daily, if needed (Bakker, 1999; Cassano, 1988; McTavish, 1990; Modigh 1992; Stein, 2010)

Discontinuation of therapy: Upon discontinuation of antidepressant therapy, gradually taper the dose to minimize the incidence of withdrawal symptoms and allow for the detection of re-emerging symptoms. Evidence supporting ideal taper rates is limited. APA and NICE guidelines suggest tapering therapy over at least several weeks with consideration to the half-life of the antidepressant; antidepressants with a shorter half-life may need to be tapered more conservatively. In addition for long-term treated patients, WFSBP guidelines recommend tapering over 4-6 months. If intolerable withdrawal symptoms occur following a dose reduction, consider resuming the previously prescribed dose and/or decrease dose at a more gradual rate (APA, 2007; APA, 2010; Bauer, 2002; Haddad, 2001; NCCMH, 2010; Schatzberg, 2006; Shelton, 2001; Warner, 2006).

MAO inhibitor recommendations:

Switching to or from an MAO inhibitor intended to treat psychiatric disorders:

Allow 14 days to elapse between discontinuing an MAO inhibitor intended to treat psychiatric disorders and initiation of clomipramine.

Allow 14 days to elapse between discontinuing clomipramine and initiation of an MAO inhibitor intended to treat psychiatric disorders.

Use with other MAO inhibitors (linezolid or IV methylene blue):

Do not initiate clomipramine in patients receiving linezolid or IV methylene blue; consider other interventions for psychiatric condition.

If urgent treatment with linezolid or IV methylene blue is required in a patient already receiving clomipramine and potential benefits outweigh potential risks, discontinue clomipramine promptly and administer linezolid or IV methylene blue. Monitor for serotonin syndrome for 2 weeks or until 24 hours after the last dose of linezolid or IV methylene blue, whichever comes first. May resume clomipramine 24 hours after the last dose of linezolid or IV methylene blue.

Dosage adjustment in renal impairment: No dosage adjustment provided in manufacturer's labeling (has not been studied). Use with caution in patients with significantly impaired renal function.

Dosage adjustment in hepatic impairment: No dosage adjustment provided in manufacturer's labeling (has not been studied). Use with caution in patients with hepatic impairment.

Administration During titration, may divide doses and administer with meals to decrease gastrointestinal side effects. After titration, may administer total daily dose at bedtime to decrease daytime sedation.

Monitoring Parameters Pulse rate and blood pressure prior to and during therapy; ECG/cardiac status in older adults and patients with cardiac disease; suicidal ideation (especially at the beginning of therapy, after initiation, or when doses are increased or decreased); signs/symptoms of serotonin syndrome; hepatic transaminases (periodically during therapy in patients with preexisting hepatic impairment)

Dosage Forms

Capsule, Oral:

Anafranil: 25 mg, 50 mg, 75 mg

Generic: 25 mg, 50 mg, 75 mg

Dosage Forms: Canada

Tablet, Oral: 10 mg, 25 mg, 50 mg

◆ **Clomipramine Hydrochloride** *see* ClomiPRAMINE *on page 475*

◆ **Clonapam (Can)** *see* ClonazePAM *on page 478*

ClonazePAM (kloe NA ze pam)

Brand Names: U.S. KlonoPIN

Brand Names: Canada Apo-Clonazepam; Clonapam; Clonazepam-R; CO Clonazepam; Dom-Clonazepam; Dom-Clonazepam-R; Mylan-Clonazepam; PHL-Clonazepam; PHL-Clonazepam-R; PMS-Clonazepam; PMS-Clonazepam-R; PRO-Clonazepam; ratio-Clonazepam; Riva-Clonazepam; Rivotril; Sandoz-Clonazepam; Teva-Clonazepam; ZYM-Clonazepam

Pharmacologic Category Benzodiazepine

Additional Appendix Information

Beers Criteria – Potentially Inappropriate Medications for Geriatrics *on page 2271*

Use Alone or as an adjunct in the treatment of petit mal variant (Lennox-Gastaut), akinetic, and myoclonic seizures; petit mal (absence) seizures unresponsive to succimides; panic disorder with or without agoraphobia

Pregnancy Risk Factor D

Pregnancy Considerations Adverse events were observed in some animal reproduction studies. Clonazepam crosses the placenta. Teratogenic effects have been observed with some benzodiazepines; however, additional studies are needed. The incidence of premature birth and low birth weights may be increased following maternal use of benzodiazepines; hypoglycemia and respiratory problems in the neonate may occur following exposure late in pregnancy. Neonatal withdrawal symptoms may occur within days to weeks after birth and "floppy infant syndrome" (which also includes withdrawal symptoms) has been reported with some benzodiazepines, including clonazepam (Bergman, 1992; Iqbal, 2002; Wikner, 2007). A combination of factors influences the potential teratogenicity of anticonvulsant therapy. When treating women with epilepsy, monotherapy with the lowest effective dose and avoidance medications known to have a high incidence of teratogenic effects is recommended (Harden, 2009; Wlodarczyk, 2012).

Patients exposed to clonazepam during pregnancy are encouraged to enroll themselves into the AED Pregnancy Registry by calling 1-888-233-2334. Additional information is available at www.aedpregnancyregistry.org.

Breast-Feeding Considerations Clonazepam enters breast milk. Drowsiness, lethargy, or weight loss in nursing infants have been observed in case reports following maternal use of some benzodiazepines (Iqbal, 2002). The manufacturer states that women taking clonazepam should not breast-feed their infants.

Contraindications Hypersensitivity to clonazepam or any component of the formulation (cross-sensitivity with other benzodiazepines may exist); significant liver disease; acute narrow-angle glaucoma

Warnings/Precautions Hazardous agent - use appropriate precautions for handling and disposal (NIOSH 2014 [group 3]). Antiepileptics are associated with an increased risk of suicidal behavior/thoughts with use (regardless of indication); patients should be monitored for signs/symptoms of depression, suicidal tendencies, and other unusual behavior changes during therapy and instructed to inform their healthcare provider immediately if symptoms occur.

Use with caution in elderly or debilitated patients, patients with hepatic disease (including alcoholics), or renal impairment. Use with caution in patients with respiratory disease or impaired gag reflex or ability to protect the airway from secretions (salivation may be increased). Worsening of seizures may occur when added to patients with multiple seizure types. Concurrent use with valproic acid may result in absence status. Monitoring of CBC and liver function tests has been recommended during prolonged therapy.

Causes CNS depression (dose related) resulting in sedation, dizziness, confusion, or ataxia which may impair physical and mental capabilities. Patients must be cautioned about performing tasks which require mental alertness (eg, operating machinery or driving). Use with caution in patients receiving other CNS depressants or psychoactive agents. Effects with other sedative drugs or ethanol may be potentiated. Benzodiazepines have been associated with falls and traumatic injury and should be used with extreme caution in patients who are at risk of these events.

Use caution in patients with depression, particularly if suicidal risk may be present. Use with caution in patients with a history of drug dependence. Benzodiazepines have been associated with dependence and acute withdrawal symptoms, including seizures, on discontinuation or reduction in dose. Acute withdrawal, including seizures, may be precipitated in patients after administration of flumazenil to patients receiving long-term benzodiazepine therapy.

Benzodiazepines have been associated with anterograde amnesia. Paradoxical reactions, including hyperactive or aggressive behavior, have been reported with benzodiazepines, particularly in adolescent/pediatric or psychiatric patients. Does not have analgesic, antidepressant, or antipsychotic properties. Clonazepam is a long half-life benzodiazepine. Tolerance does not develop to the anxiolytic effects (Vinkers, 2012). Chronic use of this agent may increase the perioperative benzodiazepine dose needed to achieve desired effect.

In older adults, benzodiazepines increase the risk of impaired cognition, delirium, falls, fractures, and motor vehicle accidents. Due to increased sensitivity in this age group and slower metabolism of long-acting agents (such as clonazepam), avoid use for treatment of insomnia, agitation, or delirium (Beers Criteria).

Adverse Reactions Reactions reported in patients with seizure and/or panic disorder.

Cardiovascular: Edema (ankle or facial), palpitation

Central nervous system: Amnesia, ataxia, behavior problems, coma, confusion, coordination impaired, depression, dizziness, drowsiness, emotional lability, fatigue, fever, hallucinations, headache, hysteria, insomnia, intellectual ability reduced, memory disturbance, nervousness; paradoxical reactions (including aggressive behavior, agitation, anxiety, excitability, hostility, irritability, nervousness, nightmares, sleep disturbance, vivid dreams); psychosis, slurred speech, somnolence, vertigo

Dermatologic: Hair loss, hirsutism, skin rash

Endocrine & metabolic: Dysmenorrhea, libido increased/decreased

Gastrointestinal: Abdominal pain, anorexia, appetite increased/decreased, coated tongue, constipation, dehydration, diarrhea, encopresis, gastritis, gum soreness, nausea, weight changes (loss/gain), xerostomia

Genitourinary: Colpitis, dysuria, ejaculation delayed, enuresis, impotence, micturition frequency, nocturia, urinary retention, urinary tract infection

Hematologic: Anemia, eosinophilia, leukopenia, thrombocytopenia

Hepatic: Alkaline phosphatase increased (transient), hepatomegaly, transaminases increased (transient)

Neuromuscular & skeletal: Choreiform movements, coordination abnormal, dysarthria, hypotonia, muscle pain, muscle weakness, myalgia, tremor

Ocular: Blurred vision, eye movements abnormal, diplopia, nystagmus

Respiratory: Bronchitis, chest congestion, cough, hypersecretions, pharyngitis, respiratory depression, respiratory tract infection, rhinitis, rhinorrhea, shortness of breath, sinusitis

Miscellaneous: Allergic reaction, aphonia, dysdiadochokinesis, "glassy-eyed" appearance, hemiparesis, flu-like syndrome, lymphadenopathy

Rare but important or life-threatening: Apathy, burning skin, chest pain, depersonalization, dyspnea, excessive dreaming, hyperactivity, hypoesthesia, hypotension postural, infection, migraine, organic disinhibition, pain, paresthesia, paresis, periorbital edema, polyuria, suicidal attempt, suicide ideation, thick tongue, twitching, visual disturbance, xerophthalmia

Drug Interactions

Metabolism/Transport Effects **Substrate** of CYP3A4 (major); **Note:** Assignment of Major/Minor substrate status based on clinically relevant drug interaction potential

Avoid Concomitant Use

Avoid concomitant use of ClonazePAM with any of the following: Azelastine (Nasal); Conivaptan; Fusidic Acid (Systemic); Idelalisib; Methadone; OLANZapine; Orphenadrine; Paraldehyde; Sodium Oxybate; Thalidomide

Increased Effect/Toxicity

ClonazePAM may increase the levels/effects of: Alcohol (Ethyl); Azelastine (Nasal); Buprenorphine; CloZAPine; CNS Depressants; Hydrocodone; Methadone; Methotrimeprazine; Metyrosine; Mirtazapine; Orphenadrine; Paraldehyde; Pramipexole; ROPINIRole; Rotigotine; Selective Serotonin Reuptake Inhibitors; Sodium Oxybate; Suvorexant; Thalidomide; Zolpidem

The levels/effects of ClonazePAM may be increased by: Aprepitant; Brimonidine (Topical); Cannabis; Ceritinib; Cobicistat; Conivaptan; Cosyntropin; CYP3A4 Inhibitors (Moderate); CYP3A4 Inhibitors (Strong); Dasatinib; Doxylamine; Dronabinol; Droperidol; Fosaprepitant; Fusidic Acid (Systemic); HydrOXYzine; Idelalisib; Ivacaftor; Kava Kava; Luliconazole; Magnesium Sulfate; Methotrimeprazine; Mifepristone; Nabilone; Netupitant; OLANZapine; Perampanel; Rufinamide; Simeprevir; Stiripentol; Tapentadol; Teduglutide; Tetrahydrocannabinol; Vigabatrin

Decreased Effect

The levels/effects of ClonazePAM may be decreased by: Bosentan; CYP3A4 Inducers (Moderate); CYP3A4 Inducers (Strong); Dabrafenib; Deferasirox; Mitotane; Siltuximab; St Johns Wort; Theophylline Derivatives; Tocilizumab; Yohimbine

Food Interactions Clonazepam serum concentration is unlikely to be increased by grapefruit juice because of clonazepam's high oral bioavailability.

Storage/Stability Store at 25°C (77°F); excursions permitted to 15°C to 30°C (59°F to 80°F)

Mechanism of Action The exact mechanism is unknown, but believed to be related to its ability to enhance the activity of GABA; suppresses the spike-and-wave discharge in absence seizures by depressing nerve transmission in the motor cortex. Benzodiazepine receptors and effects appear to be linked to the GABA-A receptors. Benzodiazepines do not bind to GABA-B receptors.

Pharmacodynamics/Kinetics

Onset of action: ~20-40 minutes (Hanson, 1972)

Duration: Infants and young children: 6-8 hours (Hanson, 1972); Adults: ≤12 hours (Hanson, 1972)

Absorption: Rapidly and completely absorbed

Distribution: Children: V_d: 1.5-3 L/kg (Walson, 1996); Adults: V_d: 1.5-64.4 L/kg (Walson, 1996)

Protein binding: ~85%

Metabolism: Extensively hepatic via glucuronide and sulfate conjugation

Bioavailability: 90%

Half-life elimination: Children: 22-33 hours (Walson, 1996); Adults: 17-60 hours (Walson, 1996)

Time to peak, serum: 1-4 hours

Excretion: Urine (<2% as unchanged drug); metabolites excreted as glucuronide or sulfate conjugates

Dosage

Children <10 years or <30 kg: Seizure disorders: Oral:

Initial daily dose: 0.01-0.03 mg/kg/day (maximum: 0.05 mg/kg/day) given in 2-3 divided doses; increase by no more than 0.25-0.5 mg every third day until seizures are controlled or adverse effects seen

Usual maintenance dose: 0.1-0.2 mg/kg/day divided 3 times daily, not to exceed 0.2 mg/kg/day

Children >10 years or ≥30 kg, Adolescents, and Adults:

Seizure disorders: Oral:

Initial daily dose not to exceed 1.5 mg given in 3 divided doses; may increase by 0.5-1 mg every third day until seizures are controlled or adverse effects seen (maximum: 20 mg daily)

Usual maintenance dose: 2-8 mg daily in 1-2 divided doses (Brodie, 1997); do not exceed 20 mg daily

Adults:

Panic disorder: Oral: 0.25 mg twice daily; increase in increments of 0.125-0.25 mg twice daily every 3 days; target dose: 1 mg daily (maximum: 4 mg daily)

Discontinuation of treatment: To discontinue, treatment should be withdrawn gradually. Decrease dose by 0.125 mg twice daily every 3 days until medication is completely withdrawn.

Burning mouth syndrome (off-label use):

Oral: Initial: 0.25 at bedtime for 1 week; increase dose by ≤0.25 mg every week; maximum dose: 3 mg daily in 3 divided doses. **Note:** Use should be limited (Buchanan, 2008; Grushka, 1998).

Topical: May administer topically with 1 mg 3 times daily (after each meal). **Note:** Patient should be instructed to suck on the tablet, retain saliva in mouth near the pain sites without swallowing for 3 minutes, and then expectorate saliva (Gremeau-Richard, 2004).

Essential tremor (off-label use): Oral: Initial: 0.5 mg at bedtime; increase dose by 0.5 mg every 3-4 days; maximum dose: 6 mg daily (Biary, 1987; Thompson, 1984; Zesiewicz, 2005; Zesiewicz, 2011).

REM sleep behavior disorder (off-label use): 0.25-2 mg 30 minutes prior to bedtime (maximum: 4 mg 30 minutes prior to bedtime). **Note:** Use with caution in patients with dementia, gait disorders, or obstructive sleep apnea (Aurora, 2010).

Elderly: Initiate with low doses and observe closely

Dosage adjustment in renal impairment: No dosage adjustment provided in manufacturer's labeling; use with caution. Clonazepam metabolites may accumulate in patients with renal impairment.

Dosage adjustment in hepatic impairment: No dosage adjustment provided in manufacturer's labeling; use with caution.

Administration

Orally-disintegrating tablet: Open pouch and peel back foil on the blister; do not push tablet through foil. Use dry hands to remove tablet and place in mouth. May be swallowed with or without water. Use immediately after removing from package.

Tablet: Swallow whole with water.

Hazardous agent; use appropriate precautions for handling and disposal (NIOSH 2014 [group 3]).

Monitoring Parameters CBC, liver and renal function tests; observe patient for excess sedation, respiratory depression; suicidality (eg, suicidal thoughts, depression, behavioral changes)

Reference Range Relationship between serum concentration and seizure control is not well established

Timing of serum samples: Peak serum levels occur 1-3 hours after oral ingestion; the half-life is 20-40 hours; therefore, steady-state occurs in 5-7 days

Therapeutic levels: 20-80 ng/mL; Toxic concentration: >80 ng/mL

Additional Information Ethosuximide or valproic acid may be preferred for treatment of absence (petit mal) seizures. Clonazepam-induced behavioral disturbances may be more frequent in mentally handicapped patients. Abrupt discontinuation after sustained use (generally >10 days) may cause withdrawal symptoms. Flumazenil, a competitive benzodiazepine antagonist at the CNS receptor site, reverses benzodiazepine-induced CNS depression.

Dosage Forms

Tablet, Oral:

KlonoPIN: 0.5 mg, 1 mg, 2 mg

Generic: 0.5 mg, 1 mg, 2 mg

Tablet Dispersible, Oral:

Generic: 0.125 mg, 0.25 mg, 0.5 mg, 1 mg, 2 mg

Extemporaneous Preparations Hazardous agent: Use appropriate precautions for handling and disposal (NIOSH 2014 [group 3]).

A 0.1 mg/mL oral suspension may be made with tablets and one of three different vehicles (cherry syrup; a 1:1 mixture of Ora-Sweet® and Ora-Plus®; or a 1:1 mixture of Ora-Sweet® SF and Ora-Plus®). Crush six 2 mg tablets in a mortar and reduce to a fine powder. Add 10 mL of the chosen vehicle and mix to a uniform paste; mix while adding the vehicle in incremental proportions to **almost** 120 mL; transfer to a calibrated bottle, rinse mortar with vehicle, and add quantity of vehicle sufficient to make 120 mL. Label "shake well" and "protect from light". Stable for 60 days when stored in amber prescription bottles in the dark at room temperature or refrigerated.

Allen LV Jr and Erickson MA 3rd, "Stability of Acetazolamide, Allopurinol, Azathioprine, Clonazepam, and Flucytosine in Extemporaneously Compounded Oral Liquids," Am *J Health Syst Pharm*, 1996, 53(16):1944-9.

◆ **Clonazepam-R (Can)** *see* ClonazePAM *on page 478*

CloNIDine (KLON i deen)

Brand Names: U.S. Catapres; Catapres-TTS-1; Catapres-TTS-2; Catapres-TTS-3; Duraclon; Kapvay

Brand Names: Canada Apo-Clonidine®; Catapres®; Dixarit®; Dom-Clonidine; Novo-Clonidine

Index Terms Clonidine Hydrochloride

Pharmacologic Category $Alpha_2$-Adrenergic Agonist; Antihypertensive

Additional Appendix Information

Beers Criteria – Potentially Inappropriate Medications for Geriatrics *on page 2271*

Use

Oral:

Immediate release: Management of hypertension (monotherapy or as adjunctive therapy)

Extended release (Kapvay): Treatment of attention-deficit/hyperactivity disorder (ADHD) (monotherapy or as adjunctive therapy)

Epidural (Duraclon): For continuous epidural administration as adjunctive therapy with opioids for treatment of severe cancer pain in patients tolerant to or unresponsive to opioids alone; epidural clonidine is generally more effective for neuropathic pain and less effective (or possibly ineffective) for somatic or visceral pain

Transdermal patch: Management of hypertension (monotherapy or as adjunctive therapy)

Note: According to the Eighth Joint National Committee (JNC 8) guidelines, clonidine is **not** recommended for the initial treatment of hypertension (James, 2013).

Pregnancy Risk Factor C

Pregnancy Considerations Adverse events have been observed in some animal reproduction studies. Clonidine crosses the placenta; concentrations in the umbilical cord plasma are similar to those in the maternal serum and concentrations in the amniotic fluid may be 4 times those in the maternal serum. The pharmacokinetics of clonidine may be altered during pregnancy (Buchanan, 2009). Untreated chronic maternal hypertension is associated with adverse events in the fetus, infant, and mother. If treatment for hypertension during pregnancy is needed, other agents are preferred (ACOG, 2012). **[U.S. Boxed Warning]: Epidural clonidine is not recommended for obstetrical or postpartum pain** due to risk of hemodynamic instability.

Breast-Feeding Considerations Clonidine is excreted in breast milk. Concentrations have been noted as ~7% to 8% of those in the maternal plasma following oral dosing (Atkinson, 1988; Bunjes, 1993) and twice those in the maternal serum following epidural administration. The manufacturer recommends caution be used if administered to nursing women. Another source recommends avoiding use when nursing infants born <34 weeks gestation or when large maternal doses are needed (Atkinson, 1988).

Contraindications Hypersensitivity to clonidine hydrochloride or any component of the formulation

Epidural administration: Injection site infection; concurrent anticoagulant therapy; bleeding diathesis; administration above the C4 dermatome

Warnings/Precautions May cause CNS depression, which may impair physical or mental abilities; patients must be cautioned about performing tasks which require mental alertness (eg, operating machinery or driving). Sedating effects may be potentiated when used with other CNS-depressant drugs or ethanol. Use with caution in patients with severe coronary insufficiency; conduction disturbances; recent MI, CVA, or chronic renal insufficiency. The hemodynamic effects may be prolonged in those with renal impairment; elimination half-life significantly prolonged (up to 41 hours) in patients with severe renal impairment. May cause dose dependent reductions in heart rate; use with caution in patients with preexisting bradycardia or those predisposed to developing bradycardia. Caution in sinus node dysfunction. Use with caution in patients concurrently receiving agents known to reduce SA node function and/or AV nodal conduction (eg, digoxin, diltiazem, metoprolol, verapamil). May cause significant xerostomia. Clonidine may cause eye dryness in patients who wear contact lenses.

[U.S. Boxed Warning]: Must dilute concentrated epidural injectable (500 mcg/mL) solution prior to use. Epidural clonidine is not recommended for perioperative, obstetrical, or postpartum pain due to risk of hemodynamic instability. Clonidine injection should be administered via a continuous epidural infusion device. Monitor closely for catheter-related infection such as meningitis or epidural abscess. Epidural clonidine is not recommended for use in patients with severe cardiovascular disease or hemodynamic instability; may lead to cardiovascular instability (hypotension, bradycardia). Symptomatic hypotension may occur with use; in all patients, use epidural clonidine with caution due to the potential for severe hypotension especially in women and those of low body weight. Most hypotensive episodes occur within the first 4 days of initiation; however, episodes may occur throughout the duration of therapy.

Gradual withdrawal is needed (taper oral immediate release or epidural dose gradually over 2-4 days to avoid rebound hypertension) if drug needs to be stopped. Patients should be instructed about abrupt discontinuation (causes rapid increase in BP and symptoms of sympathetic overactivity). In patients on both a beta-blocker and clonidine where withdrawal of clonidine is necessary, withdraw the beta-blocker first and several days before clonidine withdrawal, then slowly decrease clonidine. In children and adolescents, extended release formulation (Kapvay™) should be tapered in decrements of no more than 0.1 mg every 3-7 days. Discontinue oral immediate release formulations within 4 hours of surgery then restart as soon as possible afterwards. Discontinue oral extended release formulations up to 28 hours prior to surgery, then restart the following day.

Oral formulations of clonidine (immediate release versus extended release) are not interchangeable on a mg:mg basis due to different pharmacokinetic profiles.

Transdermal patch may contain conducting metal (eg, aluminum); remove patch prior to MRI. Due to the potential for altered electrical conductivity, remove transdermal patch before cardioversion or defibrillation. Localized contact sensitization to the transdermal system has been reported; in these patients, allergic reactions (eg, generalized rash, urticaria, angioedema) have also occurred following subsequent substitution of oral therapy.

In the elderly, avoid use as first-line antihypertensive due to high risk of CNS adverse effects; may also cause orthostatic hypotension and bradycardia (Beers Criteria). In pediatric patients, epidural clonidine should be reserved for cancer patients with severe intractable pain, unresponsive to other analgesics or epidural or spinal opioids. Use oral formulations with caution in pediatric patients since children commonly have gastrointestinal illnesses with vomiting and are susceptible to hypertensive episodes due to abrupt inability to take oral medication.

Adverse Reactions

Oral, Transdermal: Incidence of adverse events may be less with transdermal compared to oral due to the lower peak/trough ratio.

Cardiovascular: Atrioventricular block, bradycardia, cardiac arrhythmia, cardiac failure, cerebrovascular accident, chest pain, ECG abnormality, edema, flushing, localized blanching (transdermal), orthostatic hypotension, palpitations, prolonged Q-T Interval on ECG, Raynaud's phenomenon, syncope, tachycardia

Central Nervous System: Aggressive behavior, agitation, anxiety, behavioral changes, delirium, delusions, depression, dizziness, drowsiness, emotional disturbance, fatigue, hallucination (visual and auditory), headache, insomnia, irritability, lethargy, malaise, nervousness, nightmares, numbness (localized; transdermal), paresthesia, parotid pain (oral), restlessness, sedation, throbbing (transdermal), vivid dream, withdrawal syndrome

Dermatologic: Allergic contact sensitivity (transdermal), alopecia, burning sensation of skin (transdermal), contact dermatitis (transdermal), excoriation (transdermal), hyperpigmentation (transdermal), hypopigmentation (localized; transdermal), localized vesiculation (transdermal), macular eruption, pallor, papule (transdermal), skin rash, transient skin rash (localized; characterized by pruritus and erythema; transdermal), urticaria

Endocrine & metabolic: Decreased libido, gynecomastia, hyperglycemia (transient; oral), increased thirst, weight gain

Gastrointestinal: Abdominal pain (oral), anorexia, constipation, diarrhea, gastrointestinal pseudo-obstruction (oral), nausea, parotitis (oral), sore throat, upper abdominal pain, viral gastrointestinal infection, vomiting, xerostomia

Genitourinary: Erectile dysfunction, nocturia, pollakiuria, sexual disorder, urinary incontinence, urinary retention

Hematologic & oncologic: Thrombocytopenia (oral)

Hepatic: Abnormal hepatic function tests (mild transient abnormalities), hepatitis

Hypersensitivity: Angioedema

Neuromuscular & skeletal: Arthralgia, increased creatine phosphokinase (transient; oral), leg cramps, limb pain, myalgia, tremor, weakness

Ophthalmic: Accommodation disturbance, blurred vision, burning sensation of eyes, decreased lacrimation, dry eye syndrome, increased lacrimation

Otic: Otalgia, otitis media

Respiratory: Asthma, dry nose, epistaxis, flu-like symptoms, nasal congestion, nasopharyngitis, respiratory tract infection, rhinorrhea

Miscellaneous: Crying, fever

Epidural: Note: The following adverse events occurred more often than placebo in cancer patients with intractable pain being treated with concurrent epidural morphine.

Cardiovascular: Chest pain, hypotension, orthostatic hypotension

Central nervous system: Confusion, dizziness, hallucination

Dermatologic: Diaphoresis

Gastrointestinal: Nausea and vomiting, xerostomia

Otic: Tinnitus

Drug Interactions

Metabolism/Transport Effects None known.

Avoid Concomitant Use

Avoid concomitant use of CloNIDine with any of the following: Azelastine (Nasal); Ceritinib; Iobenguane I 123; Orphenadrine; Paraldehyde; Thalidomide

Increased Effect/Toxicity

CloNIDine may increase the levels/effects of: Alcohol (Ethyl); Amifostine; Antihypertensives; Azelastine (Nasal); Beta-Blockers; Bradycardia-Causing Agents; Buprenorphine; Calcium Channel Blockers (Nondihydropyridine); Cardiac Glycosides; Ceritinib; CNS Depressants; DULoxetine; Hydrocodone; Hypotensive Agents; Lacosamide; Levodopa; Methotrimeprazine; Metyrosine; Obinutuzumab; Orphenadrine; Paraldehyde; Pramipexole; RisperiDONE; RiTUXimab; ROPINIRole; Rotigotine; Selective Serotonin Reuptake Inhibitors; Suvorexant; Thalidomide; Zolpidem

The levels/effects of CloNIDine may be increased by: Alfuzosin; Barbiturates; Beta-Blockers; Bretylium; Brimonidine (Topical); Cannabis; Diazoxide; Doxylamine; Dronabinol; Droperidol; Herbs (Hypotensive Properties); HydrOXYzine; Kava Kava; Magnesium Sulfate; MAO Inhibitors; Methotrimeprazine; Methylphenidate; Nabilone; Nicorandil; Pentoxifylline; Perampanel; Phosphodiesterase 5 Inhibitors; Prostacyclin Analogues; Rufinamide; Sodium Oxybate; Tapentadol; Tetrahydrocannabinol; Tofacitinib

Decreased Effect

CloNIDine may decrease the levels/effects of: Iobenguane I 123

The levels/effects of CloNIDine may be decreased by: Herbs (Hypertensive Properties); Mirtazapine; Serotonin/Norepinephrine Reuptake Inhibitors; Tricyclic Antidepressants; Yohimbine

Preparation for Administration Epidural formulation: Prior to administration, the 500 mcg/mL concentration must be diluted in 0.9% sodium chloride for injection (preservative-free) to a final concentration of 100 mcg/mL.

Storage/Stability

Epidural formulation: Store at 25°C (77°F); excursions permitted to 15°C to 30°C (59°F to 86°F). **Preservative free;** discard unused portion.

Tablets: Store at 25°C (77°F); excursions permitted to 15°C to 30°C (59°F to 86°F). Protect from light.

Extended release tablets: Store at 20°C to 25°C (68°F to 77°F). Protect from light.

Transdermal patches: Store below 30°C (86°F).

Mechanism of Action Stimulates alpha$_2$-adrenoceptors in the brain stem, thus activating an inhibitory neuron, resulting in reduced sympathetic outflow from the CNS, producing a decrease in peripheral resistance, renal vascular resistance, heart rate, and blood pressure; epidural clonidine may produce pain relief at spinal presynaptic and postjunctional alpha$_2$-adrenoceptors by preventing pain signal transmission; pain relief occurs only for the body regions innervated by the spinal segments where analgesic concentrations of clonidine exist. For the treatment of ADHD, the mechanism of action is unknown; it has been proposed that postsynaptic alpha$_2$-agonist stimulation regulates subcortical activity in the prefrontal cortex, the area of the brain responsible for emotions, attentions, and behaviors and causes reduced hyperactivity, impulsiveness, and distractibility.

Pharmacodynamics/Kinetics

Onset of action: Oral: Immediate release: 0.5-1 hour (maximum reduction in blood pressure: 2-4 hours); Transdermal: Initial application: 2-3 days

Duration: Oral: Immediate release: 6-10 hours

Absorption: Oral: Extended release tablets (Kapvay™) are not bioequivalent with immediate release formulations; peak plasma concentrations are 50% lower compared to immediate release formulations

Distribution: V_d: Adults: 2.9 L/kg; highly lipid soluble; distributes readily into extravascular sites

Note: Epidurally administered clonidine readily distributes into plasma via the epidural veins and attains clinically significant systemic concentrations.

Protein binding: 20% to 40%

Metabolism: Extensively hepatic to inactive metabolites; undergoes enterohepatic recirculation

Bioavailability: Oral: Immediate release: 70% to 80%; Extended release (Kapvay™): ~89% (relative to immediate release formulation); Transdermal: ~60%

Half-life elimination: Adults: Normal renal function: 12-16 hours

Epidural administration: CSF half-life elimination: 0.8-1.8 hours

Transdermal: Half-life elimination (after patch removal): ~20 hours (due to skin depot effect; increase in plasma clonidine concentrations may occur after patch removal [MacGregor, 1985])

Time to peak, plasma: Oral: Immediate release: 1-3 hours; Extended release: 7-8 hours

Excretion: Urine (40% to 60% as unchanged drug)

Dosage Note: Dosing is expressed as the salt (clonidine hydrochloride) unless otherwise noted. Formulations of clonidine (immediate release versus extended release) are not interchangeable on a mg:mg basis due to different pharmacokinetic profiles.

Children:

Oral:

Hypertension (off-label use): Children ≥12 years: Immediate release: Initial: 0.2 mg/day in 2 divided doses; increase gradually, if needed, in 0.1 mg/day increments at weekly intervals; maximum: 2.4 mg/day (rarely required) (NHBPEP, Fourth Report)

Severe hypertension (off-label use): Children: Immediate release: 0.05-0.1 mg/dose; may repeat up to a maximum total dose of 0.8 mg (NHBPEP, Fourth Report)

Clonidine tolerance test (test of growth hormone release from pituitary) (off-label use):

0.15 mg/m^2 as a single dose (Lanes, 1982)

or

5 mcg/kg as a single dose; maximum dose: 250 mcg (Richmond, 2008)

ADHD: **Note:** May be used alone or as an adjunct to stimulants.

Immediate release (off-label indication; Pliszka, 2007):

Children ≤45 kg: Initial: 0.05 mg at bedtime; sequentially increase every 3-7 days by 0.05 mg increments as twice daily, then 3 times daily, then 4 times daily; maximum daily dose: 0.2 mg/day for patients weighing 27-40.5 kg; 0.3 mg/day for patients weighing 40.5-45 kg. When discontinuing therapy, taper gradually over 1-2 weeks.

Children >45 kg: Initial: 0.1 mg at bedtime; sequentially increase every 3-7 days by 0.1 mg increments as twice daily, then 3 times daily, then 4 times daily; maximum daily dose: 0.4 mg/day. When discontinuing therapy, taper gradually over 1-2 weeks.

Extended release (Kapvay™): Children ≥6 years: Initial: 0.1 mg at bedtime; increase in 0.1 mg/day increments every 7 days until desired response, doses should be administered twice daily (either split equally or with the higher split dosage given at bedtime); maximum: 0.4 mg/day. **Note:** Maintenance treatment for >5 weeks has not been evaluated. When discontinuing therapy, taper daily dose by ≤0.1 mg every 3-7 days.

Epidural infusion: Pain management: Reserved for cancer patients with severe intractable pain, unresponsive to other opioid analgesics: Initial: 0.5 mcg/kg/**hour**; adjust with caution, based on clinical effect

Adults:

Oral:

Hypertension: Immediate release: Initial dose: 0.1 mg twice daily (maximum recommended dose: 2.4 mg/day); usual dose range (ASH/ISH [Weber, 2014]): 0.1-0.2 mg twice daily

Acute hypertension (urgency) (off-label use): Initial 0.1-0.2 mg; may be followed by additional doses of 0.1 mg every hour, if necessary, to a maximum total dose of 0.7 mg (Atkin, 1992; Jaker, 1989)

Off-label route of administration: Sublingual: Initial: 0.1-0.2 mg; followed by 0.05-0.1 mg every hour until blood pressure controlled or a cumulative dose of 0.7 mg is reached (Cunningham, 1994; Matuschka, 1999)

Nicotine withdrawal symptoms (off-label use): Initial: 0.1 mg twice daily; titrate by 0.1 mg/day every 7 days if needed; dosage range used in clinical trials: 0.15-0.75 mg/day; duration of therapy ranged from 3-10 weeks in clinical trials (Fiore, 2008)

Transdermal:

Hypertension: Initial: 0.1 mg/24 hour patch applied once every 7 days and increase by 0.1 mg at 1- to 2-week intervals (dosages >0.6 mg/24 hours do not improve efficacy); usual dose range (ASH/ISH [Weber, 2014]): 0.1-0.3 mg/24 hour patch applied once every 7 days

Nicotine withdrawal symptoms (off-label use): Initial: 0.1 mg/24 hour patch applied once every 7 days and increase by 0.1 mg at 1-week intervals if necessary; dosage range used in clinical trials: 0.1-0.2 mg/24 hour patch applied once every 7 days; duration of therapy ranged from 3-10 weeks in clinical trials (Fiore, 2008)

Epidural infusion: Pain management: Reserved for cancer patients with severe intractable pain, unresponsive to other opioid analgesics: Starting dose: 30 mcg/hour; titrate as required for relief of pain or presence of side effects; experience with doses >40 mcg/hour is limited; should be considered an adjunct to opioid therapy

Conversion from oral to transdermal: **Note:** If transitioning from oral to transdermal therapy, overlap oral regimen for 1-2 days; transdermal route takes 2-3 days to achieve therapeutic effects. An example transition is below:

Day 1: Place Catapres-TTS® 1; administer 100% of oral dose.

Day 2: Administer 50% of oral dose.

Day 3: Administer 25% of oral dose.

Day 4: Patch remains, no further oral supplement necessary.

Conversion from transdermal to oral: After transdermal patch removal, therapeutic clonidine levels persist for ~8 hours and then slowly decrease over several days. Consider starting oral clonidine no sooner than 8 hours after patch removal.

Elderly: Oral: Immediate release: Hypertension: Initial: 0.1 mg once daily at bedtime, increase gradually as needed

Dosage adjustment in renal impairment:

Children: Oral (extended release), epidural: The manufacturer recommends dosage adjustment according to degree of renal impairment; however, no specific dosage adjustment provided (has not been studied).

Adults: Oral (immediate release), transdermal, epidural: The manufacturer recommends dosage adjustment according to degree of renal impairment; however, no specific dosage adjustment provided in manufacturer's labeling. Bradycardia, sedation, and hypotension may be more likely to occur in patients with renal failure; half-life significantly prolonged in patients with severe renal failure; consider use of lower initial doses and monitor closely.

Hemodialysis: Not dialyzable (0% to 5%); supplemental dose is not necessary. Oral antihypertensive drugs given preferentially at night may reduce the nocturnal surge of blood pressure and minimize the intradialytic hypotension that may occur when taken the morning before a dialysis session (K/DOQI, 2005).

Dosage adjustment in hepatic impairment: No dosage adjustment provided in manufacturer's labeling.

Administration

Epidural: Specialized techniques are required for continuous epidural administration; administration via this route should only be performed by qualified individuals familiar with the techniques of epidural administration and patient management problems associated with this route. Familiarization of the epidural infusion device is essential. Do not discontinue clonidine abruptly; if needed, gradually reduce dose over 2-4 days to avoid withdrawal symptoms.

Oral: May be taken with or without food. Do not discontinue clonidine abruptly. If needed, gradually reduce dose over 2-4 days to avoid rebound hypertension.

Extended release tablet: Kapvay™: Swallow whole; do not crush, split, or chew.

Transdermal patch: Patches should be applied weekly at a consistent time to a clean, hairless area of the upper outer arm or chest. Rotate patch sites weekly. Redness under patch may be reduced if a topical corticosteroid spray is applied to the area before placement of the patch (Tom, 1994).

Monitoring Parameters Blood pressure, standing and sitting/supine, mental status, heart rate

When used for the treatment of ADHD, thoroughly evaluate for cardiovascular risk. Monitor heart rate, blood pressure (when started and weaned), and consider obtaining ECG prior to initiation (Vetter, 2008).

Clonidine tolerance test: In addition to growth hormone concentrations, monitor blood pressure and blood glucose (Huang, 2001).

Epidural: Carefully monitor infusion pump; inspect catheter tubing for obstruction or dislodgement to reduce risk of inadvertent abrupt withdrawal of infusion. Monitor closely for catheter-related infection (eg, meningitis or epidural abscess).

Additional Information Each 0.1 mg of clonidine hydrochloride (salt form) is equivalent to 0.087 mg of the free base.

Transdermal clonidine should only be used in patients unable to take oral medication. The transdermal product is much more expensive than oral clonidine and produces no better therapeutic effects.

When used for ADHD treatment, clonidine is recommended to be used as part of a comprehensive treatment program (eg, psychological, educational, and social) for attention-deficit disorder.

Dosage Forms

Patch Weekly, Transdermal:
- Catapres-TTS-1: 0.1 mg/24 hr (4 ea)
- Catapres-TTS-2: 0.2 mg/24 hr (4 ea)
- Catapres-TTS-3: 0.3 mg/24 hr (4 ea)
- Generic: 0.1 mg/24 hr (1 ea, 4 ea); 0.2 mg/24 hr (1 ea, 4 ea); 0.3 mg/24 hr (1 ea, 4 ea)

Solution, Epidural:
- Duraclon: 100 mcg/mL (10 mL)
- Generic: 100 mcg/mL (10 mL); 500 mcg/mL (10 mL)

Solution, Epidural [preservative free]:
- Duraclon: 100 mcg/mL (10 mL); 500 mcg/mL (10 mL)
- Generic: 100 mcg/mL (10 mL); 500 mcg/mL (10 mL)

Tablet, Oral:
- Catapres: 0.1 mg, 0.2 mg, 0.3 mg
- Generic: 0.1 mg, 0.2 mg, 0.3 mg

Tablet Extended Release 12 Hour, Oral:
- Kapvay: 0.1 mg
- Generic: 0.1 mg

Dosage Forms: Canada Note: Also refer to Dosage Forms. Epidural solution and extended-release tablets are not available in Canada.

Tablet, Oral: 0.025 mg

Extemporaneous Preparations

0.01 mg/mL concentration

A **0.01** mg/mL oral suspension may be made from tablets. Crush twenty 0.1 mg tablets in a glass mortar and reduce to a fine powder. Slowly add Ora-Blend in ~15 mL increments while mixing to form a uniform paste until approximately half of the total volume (~100 mL) is added. Transfer the suspension to a graduated cylinder. Rinse the mortar and pestle with the remaining vehicle and add quantity to fill the volume within the graduated cylinder to 200 mL. Transfer this amount to a calibrated bottle. Label "shake well". When stored in clear plastic syringes, the suspension is stable for at least 91 days at room temperature (25°C) or refrigerated (4°C).

Ma C, Decarie D, Ensom MHH. Stability of clonidine oral suspension in oral plastic syringes. *Am J Health-Syst Pharm.* 2014;71:657-661.

0.1 mg/mL concentration

A **0.1** mg/mL oral suspension may be made from tablets. Crush thirty 0.2 mg tablets in a glass mortar and reduce to a fine powder. Slowly add 2 mL Purified Water USP and mix to a uniform paste. Slowly add Simple Syrup, NF in 15 mL increments; transfer to a calibrated bottle, rinse mortar with vehicle, and add quantity of vehicle sufficient to make 60 mL. Label "shake well" and "refrigerate". Stable for 28 days when stored in amber glass bottles and refrigerated.

Levinson ML and Johnson CE. Stability of an extemporaneously compounded clonidine hydrochloride oral liquid. *Am J Hosp Pharm.* 1992;49(1):122-125.

◆ **Clonidine Hydrochloride** *see* CloNIDine *on page 480*

Clopidogrel (kloh PID oh grel)

Brand Names: U.S. Plavix

Brand Names: Canada Apo-Clopidogrel; CO Clopidogrel; Dom-Clopidogrel; JAMP-Clopidogrel; Mylan-Clopidogrel; Plavix; PMS-Clopidogrel; RAN-Clopidogrel; Sandoz-Clopidogrel; Teva-Clopidogrel

Index Terms Clopidogrel Bisulfate

Pharmacologic Category Antiplatelet Agent; Antiplatelet Agent, Thienopyridine

Additional Appendix Information

Oral Antiplatelet Comparison Chart *on page 2239*

Use

Unstable angina/non-ST-segment elevation myocardial infarction: To decrease the rate of a combined end point of cardiovascular death, MI, or stroke, as well as the rate of a combined end point of cardiovascular death, MI, stroke, or refractory ischemia in patients with non-ST-segment elevation acute coronary syndrome (unstable angina/non-ST-elevation myocardial infarction [UA/NSTEMI]), including patients who are to be managed medically and those who are to be managed with coronary revascularization.

ST-segment elevation acute myocardial infarction: To reduce the rate of death from any cause and the rate of a combined end point of death, reinfarction, or stroke in patients with ST-elevation MI (STEMI).

Recent myocardial infarction, recent stroke, or established peripheral arterial disease: To reduce the rate of a combined end point of new ischemic stroke (fatal or nonfatal), new MI (fatal or nonfatal), and other vascular death in patients with a history of recent MI, recent stroke, or established peripheral arterial disease.

Canadian labeling: Additional use (not in U.S. labeling): Prevention of atherothrombotic and thromboembolic events, including stroke, in patients with atrial fibrillation with at least 1 risk factor for vascular events who are not suitable for treatment with an anticoagulant and are at a low risk for bleeding.

Pregnancy Risk Factor B

Pregnancy Considerations Adverse events were not observed in animal reproduction studies. Information related to use during pregnancy is limited (Bauer, 2012; DeSantis, 2011; Myers, 2011).

Breast-Feeding Considerations It is not known if clopidogrel is excreted into breast milk. Due to the potential for serious adverse reactions in the nursing infant, the manufacturer recommends a decision be made whether to discontinue nursing or to discontinue the drug, taking into account the importance of treatment to the mother.

Contraindications Hypersensitivity to clopidogrel or any component of the formulation; active pathological bleeding such as peptic ulcer or intracranial hemorrhage

Canadian labeling: Additional contraindications (not in U.S. labeling): Significant liver impairment or cholestatic jaundice

Warnings/Precautions [U.S. Boxed Warning]: Patients with one or more copies of the variant *CYP2C19*2* and/or *CYP2C19*3* alleles (and potentially other reduced-function variants) may have reduced conversion of clopidogrel to its active thiol metabolite. Lower active metabolite exposure may result in reduced platelet inhibition and, thus, a higher rate of cardiovascular events following MI or stent thrombosis following PCI. Although evidence is insufficient to recommend routine genetic testing, tests are available to determine CYP2C19 genotype and may be used to determine therapeutic strategy; alternative treatment or treatment strategies may be considered if patient is identified as a CYP2C19 poor metabolizer. Genetic testing may be considered prior to initiating clopidogrel in patients at moderate or high risk for poor outcomes (eg, PCI in patients with extensive and/or very complex disease). The optimal dose for CYP2C19 poor metabolizers has yet to be determined. After initiation of clopidogrel, functional testing (eg, VerifyNow® P2Y12 assay) may also be done to determine clopidogrel responsiveness (Holmes, 2010).

Use with caution in patients who may be at risk of increased bleeding, including patients with PUD, trauma, or surgery. In patients with coronary stents, premature interruption of therapy may result in stent thrombosis with subsequent fatal and nonfatal MI. Duration of therapy, in general, is determined by the type of stent placed (bare metal or drug eluting) and whether an ACS event was ongoing at the time of placement. Consider discontinuing 5 days before elective surgery (except in patients with cardiac stents that have not completed their full course of dual antiplatelet therapy; patient-specific situations need to be discussed with cardiologist; AHA/ACC/SCAI/ACS/ADA Science Advisory provides recommendations). Discontinue at least 5 days before elective CABG; when urgent CABG is necessary, the ACCF/AHA CABG guidelines recommend discontinuation for at least 24 hours prior to surgery (ACCF/AHA [Hillis, 2011]). The ACCF/AHA STEMI guidelines recommend discontinuation for at least 24 hours prior to *on-pump* CABG if possible; *off-pump* CABG may be performed within 24 hours of clopidogrel administration if the benefits of prompt revascularization outweigh the risks of bleeding (ACCF/AHA [O'Gara, 2013]).

Because of structural similarities, cross-reactivity has been reported among the thienopyridines (clopidogrel, prasugrel, and ticlopidine); use with caution or avoid in patients with hypersensitivity or hematologic reactions to previous thienopyridine use. Use of clopidogrel is contraindicated in patients with hypersensitivity to clopidogrel, although desensitization may be considered for mild-to-moderate hypersensitivity.

Use caution in concurrent treatment with anticoagulants (eg, heparin, warfarin) or other antiplatelet drugs; bleeding risk is increased. Concurrent use with drugs known to inhibit CYP2C19 (eg, proton pump inhibitors) may reduce levels of active metabolite and subsequently reduce clinical efficacy and increase the risk of cardiovascular events; if possible, avoid concurrent use of moderate-to-strong CYP2C19 inhibitors. In patients requiring antacid therapy, consider use of an acid-reducing agent lacking (eg, ranitidine/famotidine) or with less CYP2C19 inhibition. According to the manufacturer, avoid concurrent use of omeprazole (even when scheduled 12 hours apart) or esomeprazole; if a PPI is necessary, the use of an agent with comparatively less effect on the antiplatelet activity of clopidogrel is recommended. Of the PPIs, pantoprazole has the lowest degree of CYP2C19 inhibition *in vitro* (Li, 2004) and has been shown to have has less effect on conversion of clopidogrel to its active metabolite compared to omeprazole (Angiolillo, 2011). Although lansoprazole exhibits the most potent CYP2C19 inhibition *in vitro* (Li, 2004; Ogilvie, 2012), an *in vivo* study of extensive CYP2C19 metabolizers showed less reduction of the active metabolite of clopidogrel by lansoprazole/dexlansoprazole compared to esomeprazole/omeprazole (Frelinger, 2012). Avoidance of rabeprazole appears prudent due to potent *in vitro* CYP2C19 inhibition and lack of sufficient comparative *in vivo* studies with other PPIs. In contrast to these warnings, others have recommended the continued use of PPIs, regardless of the degree of inhibition, in patients with multiple risk factors for GI bleeding who are also receiving clopidogrel since no evidence has established clinically meaningful differences in outcome; however, a clinically-significant interaction cannot be excluded in those who are poor metabolizers of clopidogrel. Staggering PPIs with clopidogrel is not recommended until further evidence is available (Abraham, 2010). Concurrent use of aspirin and clopidogrel is not recommended for secondary prevention of ischemic stroke or TIA in patients unable to take oral anticoagulants due to hemorrhagic risk (Furie, 2011).

Use with caution in patients with severe liver or renal disease (experience is limited). Cases of TTP (usually occurring within the first 2 weeks of therapy), resulting in some fatalities, have been reported; urgent plasmapheresis is required. Use in patients with severe hepatic impairment or cholestatic jaundice is contraindicated in the Canadian labeling. Cases of TTP (usually occurring within the first 2 weeks of therapy), resulting in some fatalities, have been reported; urgent plasmapheresis is required. In patients with recent lacunar stroke (within 180 days), the use of clopidogrel in addition to aspirin did not significantly reduce the incidence of the primary outcome of stroke recurrence (any ischemic stroke or intracranial hemorrhage) compared to aspirin alone; the use of clopidogrel in addition to aspirin did however increase the risk of major hemorrhage and the rate of all-cause mortality (SPS3 Investigators, 2012).

Assess bleeding risk carefully prior to initiating therapy in patients with atrial fibrillation (Canadian labeling; not an approved use in U.S. labeling); in clinical trials, a significant increase in major bleeding events (including intracranial hemorrhage and fatal bleeding events) were observed in patients receiving clopidogrel plus aspirin versus aspirin alone. Vitamin K antagonist (VKA) therapy (in suitable patients) has demonstrated a greater benefit in stroke reduction than aspirin (with or without clopidogrel).

Adverse Reactions As with all drugs which may affect hemostasis, bleeding is associated with clopidogrel. Hemorrhage may occur at virtually any site. Risk is dependent on multiple variables, including the concurrent use of multiple agents which alter hemostasis and patient susceptibility.

Dermatologic: Pruritus, skin rash

Gastrointestinal: Gastrointestinal hemorrhage

Hematologic & oncologic: Hematoma, minor hemorrhage, major hemorrhage, purpura

Respiratory: Epistaxis

Rare but important or life-threatening: Abnormal hepatic function tests, acute hepatic failure, agranulocytosis, anaphylactoid reaction, angioedema, aplastic anemia, arthralgia, arthritis, bronchospasm, bullous rash, colitis (including ulcerative or lymphocytic), confusion, diarrhea, DRESS syndrome, duodenal ulcer, eczema, eosinophilic pneumonia, erythema multiforme, erythematous rash, exfoliative rash, fever, gastric ulcer, glomerulopathy, hallucination, headache, hemophilia A (acquired), hemophthalmos (including conjunctival and retinal), hemorrhagic stroke, hepatitis, hypersensitivity reaction, hypotension, increased serum creatinine, interstitial pneumonitis, intracranial hemorrhage, lichen planus, maculopapular rash, musculoskeletal bleeding, myalgia, pancreatitis, pancytopenia, pulmonary hemorrhage, respiratory tract hemorrhage, retroperitoneal hemorrhage, serum sickness, Stevens-Johnson syndrome, stomatitis, taste disorder, thrombotic thrombocytopenic purpura, toxic epidermal necrolysis, urticaria, vasculitis, wound hemorrhage

Drug Interactions

Metabolism/Transport Effects Substrate of CYP2C19 (major), CYP3A4 (minor); **Note:** Assignment of Major/Minor substrate status based on clinically relevant drug interaction potential; **Inhibits** CYP2B6 (moderate), CYP2C8 (strong), CYP2C9 (weak), SLCO1B1

Avoid Concomitant Use

Avoid concomitant use of Clopidogrel with any of the following: Dasabuvir; Enzalutamide; Esomeprazole; Omeprazole; Urokinase

Increased Effect/Toxicity

Clopidogrel may increase the levels/effects of: Agents with Antiplatelet Properties; Anticoagulants; Apixaban; BuPROPion; Collagenase (Systemic); CYP2B6 Substrates; CYP2C8 Substrates; Dabigatran Etexilate; Dasabuvir; Enzalutamide; Ibritumomab; Obinutuzumab; Pioglitazone; Rivaroxaban; Rosuvastatin; Salicylates; Thrombolytic Agents; Tositumomab and Iodine I 131 Tositumomab; Treprostinil; Urokinase; Warfarin

The levels/effects of Clopidogrel may be increased by: Dasatinib; Glucosamine; Herbs (Anticoagulant/Antiplatelet Properties); Ibrutinib; Limaprost; Luliconazole; Multivitamins/Fluoride (with ADE); Multivitamins/Minerals (with ADEK, Folate, Iron); Multivitamins/Minerals (with AE, No Iron); Omega-3 Fatty Acids; Pentosan Polysulfate Sodium; Pentoxifylline; Prostacyclin Analogues; Rifamycin Derivatives; Tipranavir; Vitamin E

Decreased Effect

The levels/effects of Clopidogrel may be decreased by: Amiodarone; Calcium Channel Blockers; CYP2C19 Inhibitors (Moderate); CYP2C19 Inhibitors (Strong); Dexlansoprazole; Esomeprazole; Grapefruit Juice; Lansoprazole; Macrolide Antibiotics; Morphine (Liposomal); Morphine (Systemic); Omeprazole; Pantoprazole; RABEprazole

Food Interactions Consumption of three 200 mL glasses of grapefruit juice a day may substantially reduce clopidogrel antiplatelet effects. Management: Avoid or minimize the consumption of grapefruit or grapefruit juice (Holmberg, 2013).

Storage/Stability Store at 25°C (77°F); excursions permitted to 15°C to 30°C (59°F to 86°F).

Mechanism of Action Clopidogrel requires *in vivo* biotransformation to an active thiol metabolite. The active metabolite irreversibly blocks the $P2Y_{12}$ component of ADP receptors on the platelet surface, which prevents activation of the GPIIb/IIIa receptor complex, thereby reducing platelet aggregation. Platelets blocked by clopidogrel are affected for the remainder of their lifespan (~7-10 days).

Pharmacodynamics/Kinetics

Onset of action: Inhibition of platelet aggregation (IPA): Dose-dependent:

300-600 mg loading dose: Detected within 2 hours

50-100 mg/day: Detected by the second day of treatment

Peak effect: Time to maximal IPA: Dose-dependent: **Note:** Degree of IPA based on adenosine diphosphate (ADP) concentration used during light aggregometry:

300-600 mg loading dose:

ADP 5 micromole/L: 20% to 30% IPA at 6 hours post administration (Montelescot, 2006)

ADP 20 micromole/L: 30% to 37% IPA at 6 hours post administration (Montelescot, 2006)

50-100 mg/day: ADP 5 micromole/L: 50% to 60% IPA at 5-7 days (Herbert, 1993)

Absorption: Well absorbed

Protein binding: Parent drug: 98%; Inactive metabolite: 94%

Metabolism: Extensively hepatic via esterase-mediated hydrolysis to a carboxylic acid derivative (inactive) and via CYP450-mediated (CYP2C19 primarily) oxidation to a thiol metabolite (active)

Half-life elimination: Parent drug: ~6 hours; Active metabolite: ~30 minutes

Time to peak, serum: ~0.75 hours

Excretion: Following administration of a single ^{14}C-labeled clopidogrel oral dose; radioactivity measured over 5 days: Urine (50%); feces (46%)

Dosage Oral: Adults:

Recent MI, recent stroke, or established peripheral arterial disease (PAD): 75 mg once daily. **Note:** The ACCF/AHA guidelines for PAD recommend clopidogrel as an alternative to aspirin (Class Ib recommendation) or in conjunction with aspirin for those who are not at an increased risk of bleeding but are of high cardiovascular risk (Class IIb recommendation). These recommendations also pertain to those with intermittent claudication or critical limb ischemia, prior lower extremity revascularization, or prior amputation for lower extremity ischemia (Rooke, 2011).

Acute coronary syndrome (ACS):

Unstable angina, non-ST-segment elevation myocardial infarction (UA/NSTEMI): Initial: 300 mg loading dose, followed by 75 mg once daily for up to 12 months (in combination with aspirin indefinitely) (ACCF/AHA [Anderson, 2013]). The American College of Chest Physicians recommends combination aspirin dose of 75-100 mg (Guyatt, 2012).

ST-segment elevation myocardial infarction (STEMI) receiving fibrinolytic therapy (in combination with aspirin and appropriate anticoagulant) (ACCF/AHA [O'Gara, 2013]): **Note**: If patient is to undergo primary PCI, see *Percutaneous coronary intervention (PCI) for acute coronary syndrome* dosing.

Age ≤75 years: Loading dose of 300 mg followed by 75 mg once daily for at least 14 days up to 1 year (in the absence of bleeding)

Age >75 years: 75 mg once daily (no loading dose) for at least 14 days up to 1 year (in the absence of bleeding)

Percutaneous coronary intervention (PCI) for acute coronary syndrome (eg, UA/NSTEMI or STEMI) (off-label use): 600 mg (loading dose) given as early as possible before or at the time of PCI, followed by 75 mg once daily for at least 12 months (in combination with aspirin 81 mg/day) (ACCF/AHA [Anderson, 2013]; ACCF/AHA/SCAI [Levine, 2011]; ACCF/AHA [O'Gara, 2013]).

PCI after fibrinolytic therapy (ACCF/AHA [O'Gara, 2013]):

Fibrinolytic administered **with** a loading dose of clopidogrel: Continue 75 mg once daily and do not administer an additional loading dose.

Fibrinolytic administered within previous 24 hours **without** a loading dose of clopidogrel: Administer 300 mg loading dose before or at the time of PCI.

Fibrinolytic administered more than 24 hours ago without a loading dose of clopidogrel: Administer 600 mg loading dose before or at the time of PCI.

Higher versus standard maintenance dosing: May consider a maintenance dose of 150 mg once daily for 6 days, then 75 mg once daily thereafter in patients not at high risk for bleeding (ACCF/AHA [Anderson, 2013]; CURRENT-OASIS 7 Investigators, 2010); however, in another study, in patients with high on-treatment platelet reactivity, the use of 150 mg once daily for 6 months did not demonstrate a difference in 6-month incidence of death from cardiovascular causes, nonfatal MI, or stent thrombosis compared to standard dose therapy (Price, 2011).

Duration of clopidogrel (in combination with aspirin) after stent placement for ACS and non-ACS indications: **Premature interruption of therapy may result in stent thrombosis with subsequent fatal and nonfatal MI.** According to the ACCF/AHA/SCAI PCI guidelines, at least 12 months of clopidogrel is recommended for those with ACS receiving either stent type (bare metal [BMS] or drug eluting stent [DES]) or those receiving a DES for a non-ACS indication (ACCF/AHA/SCAI [Levine, 2011]). The ACCF/AHA guidelines for the management of UA/NSTEMI recommend up to 12 months of clopidogrel in patients with ACS who receive a BMS (ACCF/AHA [Anderson, 2013]). A duration >12 months may be considered in patients with DES placement. Recent data has demonstrated that continued dual antiplatelet therapy for a total of 30 months (compared to 12 months) significantly reduced the risk of stent thrombosis and major adverse cardiovascular/cerebrovascular events but was associated with a higher risk of bleeding (Mauri, 2014). Those receiving a BMS for a non-ACS indication (ie, elective PCI) should be given clopidogrel for at least 1 month and ideally up to 12 months; if patient is at increased risk of bleeding, give for a minimum of 2 weeks (ACCF/AHA/SCAI [Levine, 2011]).

CYP2C19 poor metabolizers (ie, *CYP2C19*2* or **3* carriers): Although routine genetic testing is not recommended in patients treated with clopidogrel undergoing PCI, testing may be considered to identify poor metabolizers who would be at risk for poor outcomes while receiving clopidogrel; if identified, these patients may be considered for an alternative $P2Y_{12}$ inhibitor (Levine, 2011). An appropriate regimen for this patient population has not been established in clinical outcome trials. Although a 600 mg loading dose, followed by 150 mg once daily produced greater active metabolite exposure and antiplatelet response compared to the 300 mg/75 mg regimen, it does not appear that this dosing strategy improves outcomes for this patient population (Price, 2011; Simon, 2011).

Atrial fibrillation (in patients not candidates for warfarin and at a low risk of bleeding) (Canadian labeling; ACTIVE Investigators, 2009; off-label use in U.S.): 75 mg once daily (in combination with aspirin 75-100 mg once daily). **Note:** Combination may also be used as an alternative for patients with atrial fibrillation and mitral stenosis (Guyatt, 2012).

Carotid artery stenosis, symptomatic (including recent carotid endarterectomy) (off-label use): 75 mg once daily (Guyatt, 2012)

Coronary artery disease (CAD), established (off-label use): 75 mg once daily. **Note:** Established CAD defined as patients 1-year post ACS, with prior revascularization, coronary stenosis >50% by angiogram, and/or evidence for cardiac ischemia on diagnostic testing (includes patients after the first year post-ACS and/or with prior CABG surgery) (Guyatt, 2012).

Peripheral artery percutaneous transluminal angioplasty (with or without stenting) or peripheral artery bypass graft surgery, postprocedure (off-label use): 75 mg once daily. **Note:** For below-knee bypass graft surgery with prosthetic grafts, combine with aspirin 75-100 mg/day (Guyatt, 2012).

Prevention of coronary artery bypass graft closure (saphenous vein) and postoperative adverse cardiovascular events (off-label use): Aspirin-allergic patients: 75 mg once daily (Hillis, 2011)

Secondary prevention of cardioembolic stroke (patient not candidate for oral anticoagulation) (off-label use): 75 mg once daily (in combination with aspirin) (Guyatt, 2012).

Dosing adjustment in renal impairment: No dosage adjustment necessary (Basra, 2011). **Note:** GFR stage 5 (ie, ESRD or an eGFR <15 mL/minute) is associated with higher residual platelet reactivity with maintenance dosing (Muller, 2012).

Dosing adjustment in hepatic impairment: Use with caution; experience is limited. **Note:** Inhibition of ADP-induced platelet aggregation and mean bleeding time prolongation were similar in patients with severe hepatic impairment compared to healthy subjects after repeated doses of 75 mg once daily for 10 days.

Dietary Considerations May be taken without regard to meals. Avoid grapefruit juice (Holmberg, 2013).

Administration May be administered without regard to meals.

Monitoring Parameters Signs of bleeding; hemoglobin and hematocrit periodically. May consider platelet function testing to determine platelet inhibitory response or genotyping for CYP2C19 loss of function variant if results of testing may alter management (ACCF/AHA [Anderson, 2013]).

Dosage Forms

Tablet, Oral:

Plavix: 75 mg, 300 mg

Generic: 75 mg, 300 mg

Extemporaneous Preparations A 5 mg/mL oral suspension may be made using tablets. Crush four 75 mg tablets and reduce to a fine powder. Add a small amount of a 1:1 mixture of Ora-Sweet® and Ora-Plus® and mix to a uniform paste; mix while adding the vehicle in geometric proportions to **almost** 60 mL; transfer to a calibrated bottle, rinse mortar with vehicle, and add quantity of vehicle sufficient to make 60 mL. Label "shake well". Stable 60 days at room temperature or under refrigeration.

Skillman KL, Caruthers RL, and Johnson CE, "Stability of an Extemporaneously Prepared Clopidogrel Oral Suspension," *Am J Health Syst Pharm*, 2010, 67(7):559-61.

◆ **Clopidogrel Bisulfate** *see* Clopidogrel *on page 484*

◆ **Clopixol (Can)** *see* Zuclopenthixol [CAN/INT] *on page 2219*

◆ **Clopixol-Acuphase (Can)** *see* Zuclopenthixol [CAN/INT] *on page 2219*

◆ **Clopixol Depot (Can)** *see* Zuclopenthixol [CAN/INT] *on page 2219*

Clorazepate (klor AZ e pate)

Brand Names: U.S. Tranxene-T

Brand Names: Canada Apo-Clorazepate®; Novo-Clopate

Index Terms Clorazepate Dipotassium; Tranxene T-Tab

Pharmacologic Category Benzodiazepine

Use Treatment of generalized anxiety disorder; management of ethanol withdrawal; adjunct anticonvulsant in management of partial seizures

Dosage Oral:

Children 9-12 years: Anticonvulsant: Initial: 3.75-7.5 mg/dose twice daily; increase dose by 3.75 mg at weekly intervals, not to exceed 60 mg/day in 2-3 divided doses

Children >12 years and Adults: Anticonvulsant: Initial: Up to 7.5 mg/dose 2-3 times/day; increase dose by 7.5 mg at weekly intervals, not to exceed 90 mg/day

Adults:

Anxiety: 7.5-15 mg 2-4 times/day

Ethanol withdrawal: Initial: 30 mg, then 15 mg 2-4 times/day on first day; maximum daily dose: 90 mg; gradually decrease dose over subsequent days

Dosage adjustment in renal impairment: No dosage adjustment provided in manufacturer's labeling; use with caution.

Dosage adjustment in hepatic impairment: No dosage adjustment provided in manufacturer's labeling; use with caution.

Additional Information Complete prescribing information should be consulted for additional detail.

Dosage Forms

Tablet, Oral:

Tranxene-T: 3.75 mg, 7.5 mg, 15 mg

Generic: 3.75 mg, 7.5 mg, 15 mg

◆ **Clorazepate Dipotassium** *see* Clorazepate *on page 487*

◆ **Clotrimaderm (Can)** *see* Clotrimazole (Topical) *on page 488*

◆ **Clotrimazole 3 Day [OTC]** *see* Clotrimazole (Topical) *on page 488*

Clotrimazole (Oral) (kloe TRIM a zole)

Index Terms Mycelex

Pharmacologic Category Antifungal Agent, Imidazole Derivative; Antifungal Agent, Oral Nonabsorbed

Use Treatment of susceptible fungal infections, including oropharyngeal candidiasis; limited data suggest that clotrimazole troches may be effective for prophylaxis against oropharyngeal candidiasis in neutropenic patients

Pregnancy Risk Factor C

Dosage Oral: Children >3 years and Adults:

Prophylaxis: 10 mg troche dissolved 3 times/day for the duration of chemotherapy or until steroids are reduced to maintenance levels

Treatment: 10 mg troche dissolved slowly 5 times/day for 14 consecutive days

Additional Information Complete prescribing information should be consulted for additional detail.

Dosage Forms

Lozenge, Mouth/Throat:

Generic: 10 mg (70 ea, 140 ea)

Troche, Mouth/Throat:

Generic: 10 mg

Clotrimazole (Topical) (kloe TRIM a zole)

Brand Names: U.S. Alevazol [OTC]; Clotrimazole 3 Day [OTC]; Clotrimazole Anti-Fungal [OTC]; Clotrimazole GRx [OTC]; Desenex [OTC]; Gyne-Lotrimin 3 [OTC]; Gyne-Lotrimin [OTC]; Lotrimin AF For Her [OTC]; Lotrimin AF [OTC]

Brand Names: Canada Canesten® Topical; Canesten® Vaginal; Clotrimaderm; Trivagizole-3®

Pharmacologic Category Antifungal Agent, Imidazole Derivative; Antifungal Agent, Topical; Antifungal Agent, Vaginal

Use Treatment of susceptible fungal infections, including dermatophytoses, superficial mycoses, and cutaneous candidiasis, as well as vulvovaginal candidiasis

Dosage

Children >3 years and Adults: Topical (cream, solution): Apply twice daily; if no improvement occurs after 4 weeks of therapy, re-evaluate diagnosis

Children >12 years and Adults:

Vaginal: Cream:

1%: Insert 1 applicatorful vaginal cream daily (preferably at bedtime) for 7 consecutive days

2%: Insert 1 applicatorful vaginal cream daily (preferably at bedtime) for 3 consecutive days

Topical (cream, solution): Apply to affected area twice daily (morning and evening) for 7 consecutive days

Additional Information Complete prescribing information should be consulted for additional detail.

Dosage Forms

Cream, External:

Clotrimazole Anti-Fungal [OTC]: 1% (14.17 g, 28.35 g)
Clotrimazole GRx [OTC]: 1% (14 g)
Desenex [OTC]: 1% (15 g, 30 g)
Lotrimin AF [OTC]: 1% (12 g, 24 g)
Lotrimin AF For Her [OTC]: 1% (24 g)
Generic: 1% (15 g, 30 g, 45 g)

Cream, Vaginal:

Clotrimazole 3 Day [OTC]: 2% (22.2 g)
Gyne-Lotrimin [OTC]: 1% (45 g)
Gyne-Lotrimin 3 [OTC]: 2% (21 g)
Generic: 1% (45 g)

Ointment, External:

Alevazol [OTC]: 1% (56.7 g)

Solution, External:

Generic: 1% (10 mL, 30 mL)

- **Clotrimazole and Betamethasone** *see* Betamethasone and Clotrimazole *on page 256*
- **Clotrimazole Anti-Fungal [OTC]** *see* Clotrimazole (Topical) *on page 488*
- **Clotrimazole GRx [OTC]** *see* Clotrimazole (Topical) *on page 488*

Cloxacillin [CAN/INT] (kloks a SIL in)

Brand Names: Canada Apo-Cloxi; Novo-Cloxin; Nu-Cloxi

Index Terms Cloxacillin Sodium

Pharmacologic Category Antibiotic, Penicillin

Use Note: Not approved in U.S.

Treatment of bacterial infections including endocarditis, pneumonia, bone and joint infections, skin and soft-tissue infections, and sepsis that are caused by susceptible strains of penicillinase-producing staphylococci. Exhibits good activity against *Staphylococcus aureus*; has activity against many streptococci, but is less active than penicillin and is generally not used in clinical practice to treat streptococcal infections

Pregnancy Considerations Cloxacillin crosses the placenta and distributes into fetal tissue (Prigot, 1962).

Breast-Feeding Considerations Cloxacillin is excreted into breast milk (Prigot, 1962).

Contraindications Hypersensitivity to cloxacillin, other penicillins, cephalosporins, or any component of the formulation

Warnings/Precautions Serious and occasionally severe or fatal hypersensitivity (anaphylactoid) reactions have been reported in patients on penicillin therapy, especially with a history of beta-lactam hypersensitivity, history of sensitivity to multiple allergens, or previous IgE-mediated reactions (eg, anaphylaxis, angioedema, urticaria). Use with caution in renal impairment as the rate of elimination is decreased. Use with caution in asthmatic patients. Prolonged use may result in fungal or bacterial superinfection, including *C. difficile*-associated diarrhea (CDAD) and pseudomembranous colitis; CDAD has been observed >2 months postantibiotic treatment. Use with caution in patients with a history of seizure disorders, particularly in the presence of renal impairment as increased serum levels may increase risk for seizures. Penicillin transport across the blood-brain barrier may be enhanced by inflamed meninges or during cardiopulmonary bypass increasing the risk of myoclonia, seizures, or reduced consciousness especially in patients with renal failure. Penicillin use has been associated with hematologic disorders (eg, agranulocytosis, neutropenia, thrombocytopenia) believed to be a hypersensitivity phenomena. Reactions are most often reversible upon discontinuing therapy. Renal clearance may be reduced in neonates; more frequent evaluation of clinical status and serum levels as well as more frequent dosage adjustments may be necessary with this patient population.

Adverse Reactions

Cardiovascular: Hypotension

Central nervous system: Confusion, fever, lethargy, seizure (high doses and/or renal failure)

Dermatologic: Pruritus, rash, urticaria

Gastrointestinal: Abdominal pain, black or hairy tongue, diarrhea, flatulence, nausea, oral candidiasis, pseudomembranous colitis, stomatitis, vomiting

Hematologic: Agranulocytosis, bone marrow depression, eosinophilia, granulocytopenia, hemolytic anemia, leukopenia, neutropenia, thrombocytopenia

Hepatic: Alkaline phosphatase increased, ALT increased, AST increased, hepatotoxicity

Local: Thrombophlebitis

Neuromuscular & skeletal: Arthralgia, myalgia, myoclonus

Renal: Hematuria, interstitial nephritis, proteinuria, renal insufficiency, renal tubular damage

Respiratory: Bronchospasm, laryngeal edema, laryngospasm, sneezing, wheezing

Miscellaneous: Anaphylaxis, angioedema, allergic reaction, serum sickness-like reaction

Drug Interactions

Metabolism/Transport Effects None known.

Avoid Concomitant Use

Avoid concomitant use of Cloxacillin with any of the following: BCG; Probenecid

Increased Effect/Toxicity

Cloxacillin may increase the levels/effects of: Methotrexate; Vitamin K Antagonists

The levels/effects of Cloxacillin may be increased by: Probenecid

Decreased Effect

Cloxacillin may decrease the levels/effects of: BCG; Mycophenolate; Sodium Picosulfate; Typhoid Vaccine; Vitamin K Antagonists

The levels/effects of Cloxacillin may be decreased by: Tetracycline Derivatives

Food Interactions Food decreases cloxacillin absorption; serum levels are reduced by ~50%. Management: Administer with water on an empty stomach 1 hour before or 2 hours after meals.

Preparation for Administration

IM injection: Vials should be reconstituted with appropriate volume of SWFI to make a final concentration of 125 mg/mL or 250 mg/mL

IV injection: Vials should be reconstituted with appropriate volume of SWFI to make a final concentration of 50 mg/mL or 100 mg/mL

IV infusion: Infusion is prepared in 2 stages: Initial reconstitution of powder with appropriate volume of SWFI, followed by dilution to final infusion solution.

Storage/Stability

Capsule: Store at room temperature not exceeding 25°C (77°F).

Powder for injection: Store at controlled room temperature not exceeding 25°C (77°F). Upon reconstitution the resulting solution is stable for up to 24 hours at controlled room temperature and 48 hours under refrigeration.

IV infusion: **Note:** After reconstitution of powder with appropriate volume of sterile water for injection, the manufacturer suggests further dilution to concentrations of 1-2 mg/mL in a compatible solution (eg, D_5W, NS); solutions are stable for up to 12 hours at controlled room temperature.

Powder for oral solution: Prior to mixing, store powder at room temperature not exceeding 25°C (77°F). Refrigerate oral solution after reconstitution; discard after 14 days.

Mechanism of Action Inhibits bacterial cell wall synthesis by binding to one or more of the penicillin-binding proteins (PBPs) which in turn inhibit the final transpeptidation step of peptidoglycan synthesis in bacterial cell walls, thus inhibiting cell wall biosynthesis. Bacteria eventually lyse due to ongoing activity of cell wall autolytic enzymes (autolysins and murein hydrolases) while cell wall assembly is arrested.

Pharmacodynamics/Kinetics

Absorption: Oral: ~50%; reduced by food

Distribution: Widely to most body fluids and bone; penetration into cells, into eye, and across normal meninges is poor; inflammation increases amount that crosses blood-brain barrier

Protein binding: ~94% (primarily albumin)

Metabolism: Extensively hepatic to active and inactive metabolites

Half-life elimination: 0.5-1.5 hours; prolonged with renal impairment and in neonates

Time to peak, serum: ~1 hour

Excretion: Urine and feces

Dosage Note: Dose and duration of therapy can vary depending on infecting organism, severity of infection, and clinical response of patient. Treat severe staphylococcal infections for at least 14 days; endocarditis and osteomyelitis require an extended duration of therapy for 4-6 weeks. The intravenous route should be used for severe infections.

Usual dosage range (manufacturer's labeling):

Oral:

Children ≤20 kg: 25-50 mg/kg/day in divided doses every 6 hours

Children >20 kg and Adults: 250-500 mg every 6 hours (maximum adult dose: 6 g/day)

IM, IV:

Children ≤20 kg: 25-50 mg/kg/day in divided doses every 6 hours; up to 200 mg/kg/day has been used in some studies for severe infections (Nunn, 2007; St. John, 1981)

Children >20 kg and Adults: 250-500 mg every 6 hours (maximum adult dose: 6 g/day)

Indication-specific dosing: Dosing recommendations of World Health Organization unless otherwise noted:

Arthritis (septic), methicillin-sensitive *Staphylococcus aureus* (MSSA) (off-label dosing):

Children 2 months to 5 years: IM, IV: 25-50 mg/kg (maximum: 2 g) every 4-6 hours given with ceftriaxone until clinical improvement, **followed by** oral therapy: 12.5 mg/kg (maximum: 500 mg) every 6 hours; total duration of therapy 2-3 weeks

Children >5 years: IM, IV: 25-50 mg/kg (maximum: 2 g) every 4-6 hours (maximum daily dose: 12 g/day) until clinical improvement, **followed by** oral therapy: 25 mg/kg (maximum: 500 mg) every 6 hours; total duration of therapy 2-3 weeks

Adults: IM, IV: 2 g every 6 hours for 2-3 weeks; **Note:** Oral therapy of 1 g every 6 hours may be used to complete therapy if parenteral therapy is discontinued prior to 2-3 week duration

Endocarditis (MSSA) (off-label dosing): IV:

Children: 50 mg/kg (maximum: 2 g) every 4 hours for 6 weeks; give with gentamicin for initial 7 days

Adults:

Native valve: 2 g every 4 hours for 6 weeks; may give with gentamicin for initial 5 days (Choudri, 2000)

Prosthetic valve: 2 g every 4 hours for 6 weeks; give with gentamicin for 2 weeks and rifampin for 6 weeks (Choudri, 2000)

Uncomplicated endocarditis in IV drug users: 2 g every 4 hours for 4 weeks and gentamicin for initial 5 days **or** 2 g every 4 hours and gentamicin both given for 2 weeks total (Choudri, 2000)

Osteomyelitis (MSSA) (off-label dosing):

Children 2 months to 5 years: IM, IV: 25-50 mg/kg (maximum: 2 g) every 4-6 hours given with ceftriaxone until clinical improvement, **followed by** oral therapy: 12.5 mg/kg (maximum: 500 mg) every 6 hours; total duration of therapy 3-4 weeks

Children >5 years: IM, IV: 25-50 mg/kg (maximum: 2 g) every 4-6 hours (maximum daily dose: 12 g/day) until clinical improvement, **followed by** oral therapy: 25 mg/kg (maximum: 500 mg) every 6 hours; total duration of therapy 3-4 weeks

Adults: IM, IV: 2 g every 6 hours for 4-6 weeks (preferred) **or** for a minimum of 14 days, **followed by** 1 g every 6 hours orally to complete 4-6 weeks of therapy

Pneumonia (MSSA) (off-label dosing):
Children 2 months to 5 years: Oral: 25-50 mg/kg (maximum: 2 g) every 6 hours for at least 3 weeks with gentamicin
Children >5 years: IM, IV: 50 mg/kg (maximum: 2 g) every 6 hours for 10-14 days
Adults: IM, IV: 1-2 g every 6 hours for 10-14 days

Dosage adjustment in renal impairment: No dosage adjustment necessary.
Dosage adjustment in hepatic impairment: No dosage adjustment provided in manufacturer's labeling.

Dietary Considerations Should be taken 1 hour before or 2 hours after meals with water.

Administration
Oral: Administer with water 1 hour before or 2 hours after meals
IV:
IV push: Administer slowly over 2-4 minutes
IV infusion: Administer over 30-40 minutes

Monitoring Parameters Observe for signs and symptoms of anaphylaxis during first dose; CBC with differential (prior to initiating therapy and weekly thereafter), periodic BUN, creatinine, hepatic function

Product Availability Not available in U.S.

Dosage Forms: Canada
Capsule, oral: 250 mg, 500 mg
Injection, powder for reconstitution: 250 mg, 500 mg, 1000 mg, 2000 mg
Powder for suspension, oral: 125 mg/5 mL

◆ **Cloxacillin and Amoxicillin** *see* Amoxicillin and Cloxacillin [INT] *on page 136*

◆ **Cloxacillin and Ampicillin** *see* Ampicillin and Cloxacillin [INT] *on page 144*

◆ **Cloxacillin Sodium** *see* Cloxacillin [CAN/INT] *on page 488*

CloZAPine (KLOE za peen)

Brand Names: U.S. Clozaril; FazaClo; Versacloz

Brand Names: Canada Apo-Clozapine; Clozaril; Gen-Clozapine

Pharmacologic Category Second Generation (Atypical) Antipsychotic

Additional Appendix Information
Beers Criteria – Potentially Inappropriate Medications for Geriatrics *on page 2271*

Use
Schizophrenia, treatment resistant: Treatment of severely ill patients with schizophrenia who fail to respond adequately to antipsychotic treatment.
Suicidal behavior in schizophrenia or schizoaffective disorder: To reduce the risk of suicidal behavior in patients with schizophrenia or schizoaffective disorder who are judged to be at chronic risk for reexperiencing suicidal behavior, based on history and recent clinical state.

Pregnancy Risk Factor B

Pregnancy Considerations Adverse events were not observed in animal reproduction studies. Clozapine crosses the placenta and can be detected in the fetal blood and amniotic fluid (Barnas, 1994). Antipsychotic use during the third trimester of pregnancy has a risk for abnormal muscle movements (extrapyramidal symptoms [EPS]) and/or withdrawal symptoms in newborns following delivery. Symptoms in the newborn may include agitation, feeding disorder, hypertonia, hypotonia, respiratory distress, somnolence, and tremor; these effects may be self-limiting or require hospitalization.

Clozapine may theoretically cause agranulocytosis in the fetus and should not routinely be used in pregnancy (NICE, 2007). The American College of Obstetricians and Gynecologists recommends that therapy during pregnancy be individualized; treatment with psychiatric medications during pregnancy should incorporate the clinical expertise of the mental health clinician, obstetrician, primary healthcare provider, and pediatrician. Safety data related to atypical antipsychotics during pregnancy is limited and routine use is not recommended. However, if a woman is inadvertently exposed to an atypical antipsychotic while pregnant, continuing therapy may be preferable to switching to a typical antipsychotic that the fetus has not yet been exposed to; consider risk:benefit (ACOG, 2008). An increased risk of exacerbation of psychosis should be considered when discontinuing or changing treatment during pregnancy and postpartum.

Healthcare providers are encouraged to enroll women 18 to 45 years of age exposed to clozapine during pregnancy in the Atypical Antipsychotics Pregnancy Registry (1-866-961-2388 or http://www.womensmentalhealth.org/pregnancyregistry).

Women with amenorrhea associated with use of other antipsychotic agents may return to normal menstruation when switching to clozapine therapy. Reliable contraceptive measures should be employed by women of childbearing potential switching to clozapine therapy.

Breast-Feeding Considerations Clozapine was found to accumulate in breast milk in concentrations higher than the maternal plasma (Barnas, 1994). Breast-feeding is not recommended by the manufacturer. Clozapine may theoretically cause agranulocytosis in the nursing infant and should not routinely be used in women who are breast-feeding (NICE, 2007).

Contraindications
Hypersensitivity to clozapine or any component of the formulation (eg, photosensitivity, vasculitis, erythema multiforme, or Stevens-Johnson syndrome [SJS]); history of clozapine-induced agranulocytosis or severe granulocytopenia
Canadian labeling: Additional contraindications (not in U.S. labeling): Myeloproliferative disorders; history of toxic or idiosyncratic agranulocytosis or severe granulocytopenia (unless due to previous chemotherapy); concomitant use with other agents that suppress bone marrow function; active hepatic disease associated with nausea, anorexia, or jaundice; progressive hepatic disease or hepatic failure; paralytic ileus; uncontrolled epilepsy; severe CNS depression or comatose states; severe renal impairment; severe cardiac disease (eg, myocarditis); patients unable to undergo blood testing

Warnings/Precautions [U.S. Boxed Warning]: Significant risk of potentially life-threatening agranulocytosis, defined as an ANC <500/mm³. Monitor ANC and WBC prior to and during treatment. ANC must be ≥2,000/mm³ and WBC must be ≥3,500/mm³ to begin treatment. Discontinue clozapine and do not rechallenge if ANC <1,000/mm³ or WBC is <2,000/mm³. Monitor for symptoms of agranulocytosis and infection (eg, fever, weakness, lethargy, or sore throat). Clozapine is only available through a restricted program requiring enrollment of prescribers, patients, and pharmacies to the Registry. Do not initiate in patients with a history of clozapine-induced agranulocytosis or granulocytopenia. Reported cases occurred most often in the first 2 to 3 months of therapy. Patients who have developed agranulocytosis or leukopenia are at an increased risk of subsequent episodes. Concurrent use with bone marrow suppressive agents or treatments also leads to an increased risk. The restricted distribution system ensures appropriate WBC and ANC monitoring. Eosinophilia, defined as a blood eosinophil count of

>700/mm^3, has been reported to occur with clozapine and usually occurs within the first month of treatment. If eosinophilia develops, evaluate for signs or symptoms of systemic reactions (eg, rash or other allergic symptoms), myocarditis, or organ-specific disease. If systemic disease is suspected, discontinue clozapine immediately. If an eosinophilia cause unrelated to clozapine is identified treat the underlying cause and continue clozapine. In the absence of organ involvement continue clozapine under careful monitoring. If the total eosinophil count continues to increase over several weeks in the absence of systemic disease, base interruption of treatment and rechallenge (after eosinophil count decreases) on overall clinical assessment and consultation with internist or hematologist (**Note:** The Canadian labeling recommends discontinuing therapy for eosinophil count >3,000/mm^3; may resume therapy when eosinophil count <1,000/mm^3).

[U.S. Boxed Warning]: Elderly patients with dementia-related psychosis treated with antipsychotics are at an increased risk of death compared to placebo. Most deaths appeared to be either cardiovascular (eg, heart failure, sudden death) or infectious (eg, pneumonia) in nature. Clozapine is not approved for the treatment of dementia-related psychosis. Avoid antipsychotic use for behavioral problems associated with dementia unless alternative nonpharmacologic therapies have failed and patient may harm self or others. May also be inappropriate in older adults depending on comorbidities (eg, dementia, delirium) due to its potent anticholinergic effects (Beers Criteria). The elderly are more susceptible to adverse effects (including agranulocytosis, cardiovascular, anticholinergic, and tardive dyskinesia). An increased incidence of cerebrovascular effects (eg, transient ischemic attack, stroke), including fatalities, has been reported in placebo-controlled trials of atypical antipsychotics in elderly patients with dementia-related psychosis.

May cause CNS depression, which may impair physical or mental abilities; patients must be cautioned about performing tasks that require mental alertness (eg, operating machinery or driving); use caution in patients receiving general anesthesia. **[U.S. Boxed Warning]: Seizures have been associated with clozapine use in a dose-dependent manner. Initiate treatment with no more than 12.5 mg, titrate gradually using divided dosing. Use with caution in patients at risk of seizures, including those with a history of seizures, head trauma, brain damage, alcoholism, or concurrent therapy with medications which may lower seizure threshold. Patients should be warned that a sudden loss of consciousness may occur with seizures.** Benign transient temperature elevation (>100.4°F) may occur; peaking within the first 3 weeks of treatment. May be associated with an increase or decrease in WBC count. Rule out infection, agranulocytosis, and neuroleptic malignant syndrome (NMS) in patients presenting with fever. However, clozapine may also be associated with severe febrile reactions, including neuroleptic malignant syndrome (NMS). Impaired core body temperature regulation may occur; caution with strenuous exercise, heat exposure, dehydration, and concomitant medication possessing anticholinergic effects (Kerwin, 2004; Safferman, 1991). Clozapine's potential for extrapyramidal symptoms (including tardive dyskinesia) appears to be extremely low. Risk of dystonia (and probably other EPS) may be greater with increased doses, use of conventional antipsychotics, males, and younger patients.

[U.S. Boxed Warning]: Fatalities due to myocarditis and cardiomyopathy have been reported. Upon suspicion of these reactions discontinue clozapine and obtain a cardiac evaluation. Symptoms may include chest pain, tachycardia, palpitations, dyspnea, fever, flu-like symptoms, hypotension, or ECG changes. Patients with Clozaril-related myocarditis or cardiomyopathy should generally not be rechallenged with clozapine. Myocarditis and cardiomyopathy may occur at any period during clozapine treatment, however, typically myocarditis presents within the first 2 months and cardiomyopathy after 8 weeks of treatment. Cases of thromboembolism, including pulmonary embolism and stroke resulting in fatalities, have been associated with clozapine. Clozapine is associated with QT prolongation and ventricular arrhythmias including torsade de pointes; cardiac arrest and sudden death may occur. Use caution in patients with conditions that may increase the risk of QT prolongation, including history of QT prolongation, long QT syndrome, family history of long QT syndrome or sudden cardiac death, significant cardiac arrhythmia, recent myocardial infarction, uncompensated heart failure, treatment with other medications that cause QT prolongation, treatment with medications that inhibit the metabolism of clozapine, hypokalemia, and hypomagnesemia. Consider obtaining a baseline ECG and serum chemistry panel. Correct electrolyte abnormalities prior to initiating therapy. Discontinue clozapine if QTc interval >500 msec. Undesirable changes in lipids have been observed with antipsychotic therapy; incidence varies with product. Periodically monitor total serum cholesterol, triglycerides, LDL, and HDL concentrations.

Potentially significant drug-drug interactions may exist, requiring dose or frequency adjustment, additional monitoring, and/or selection of alternative therapy. Use caution when converting from brand to generic formulation; poor tolerability, including relapse, has been reported usually soon after product switch (1 to 3 months); monitor closely during this time (Bobo, 2010).

May cause anticholinergic effects; use with caution in patients with urinary retention, benign prostatic hyperplasia, narrow-angle glaucoma, xerostomia, visual problems, constipation, or history of bowel obstruction. Because of its potential to significantly decreased GI motility, use is associated with increased risk of paralytic ileus, bowel obstruction, fecal impaction, bowel perforation, and in rare cases death. Bowel regimens and monitoring are recommended. May cause hyperglycemia; in some cases may be extreme and associated with ketoacidosis, hyperosmolar coma, or death. In some cases, hyperglycemia resolved after discontinuation of the antipsychotic; however, some patients have required continuation of antidiabetic treatment. Monitor for symptoms of hyperglycemia including polydipsia, polyuria, polyphagia, and weakness. Use with caution in patients with diabetes or other disorders of glucose regulation; monitor for worsening of glucose control. Antipsychotic use has been associated with esophageal dysmotility and aspiration; use with caution in patients at risk of aspiration pneumonia (eg, Alzheimer disease). Use with caution in patients with hepatic disease or impairment; monitor hepatic function regularly. Hepatitis has been reported as a consequence of therapy. Use with caution in patients with renal disease.

Use caution with cardiovascular or pulmonary disease; gradually increase dose. **[U.S. Boxed Warning]: Orthostatic hypotension, bradycardia, syncope, and cardiac arrest have been reported with clozapine treatment. Risk is highest during the initial titration period and with rapid dose increases. Symptoms can develop with the first dose and with doses as low as 12.5 mg per day. Initiate treatment with no more than 12.5 mg once daily or twice daily, titrate slowly, and use divided doses. Use with caution in patients at risk for these effects (eg, cerebrovascular disease, cardiovascular disease) or with predisposing conditions for hypotensive episodes (eg, hypovolemia, concurrent**

antihypertensive medication); reactions can be fatal. Consider dose reduction if hypotension occurs. May cause tachycardia; tachycardia is not limited to a reflex response to orthostatic hypotension.

The possibility of a suicide attempt is inherent in psychotic illness or bipolar disorder; use caution in high-risk patients during initiation of therapy. Prescriptions should be written for the smallest quantity consistent with good patient care. Medication should not be stopped abruptly; taper off over 1 to 2 weeks. If conditions warrant abrupt discontinuation (eg, leukopenia, myocarditis, cardiomyopathy), monitor patient for psychosis and cholinergic rebound (eg, headache, nausea, vomiting, diarrhea, profuse diaphoresis). Significant weight gain has been observed with antipsychotic therapy; incidence varies with product. Monitor waist circumference and BMI. Clozapine levels may be lower in patients who smoke. Smokers may require twice the daily dose as nonsmokers in order to obtain an equivalent clozapine concentration (Tsuda, 2014). Smoking cessation may cause toxicity in a patient stabilized on clozapine. Monitor change in smoking. Consider baseline serum clozapine levels and/or empiric dosage adjustments (30% to 40% reduction) in patients expected to have a prolonged hospital stay with forced smoking cessation. Case reports suggest symptoms from increasing clozapine concentrations may develop 2 to 4 weeks after smoking cessation (Lowe 2010). Clozapine concentrations may be increased in CYP2D6 poor metabolizers; dose reduction may be necessary. FazaClo oral disintegrating tablets contain phenylalanine.

Adverse Reactions

Cardiovascular: Angina pectoris, ECG changes, hyper-/hypotension, syncope, tachycardia

Central nervous system: Agitation, akathisia, akinesia, anxiety, ataxia, confusion, depression, dizziness, drowsiness, fatigue, headache, insomnia, lethargy, myoclonic seizures, nightmares, pain, restlessness, seizure, slurred speech

Dermatologic: Skin rash

Gastrointestinal: Abdominal discomfort, anorexia, constipation, diarrhea, heartburn, nausea, sialorrhea, sore throat, vomiting, weight gain, xerostomia

Genitourinary: Genitourinary complaint (abnormal ejaculation, retention, urgency, incontinence)

Hematologic: Leukopenia

Hepatic: Abnormal hepatic function tests

Neuromuscular & skeletal: Hyper-/hypokinesia, muscle rigidity, muscle spasm, tremor, weakness

Ocular: Visual disturbances

Respiratory: Dyspnea, nasal congestion

Miscellaneous: Diaphoresis, numbness of tongue

Rare but important or life-threatening: Abnormal electrocephalogram, agranulocytosis, amnesia, anemia, aspiration, bronchitis, cataplexy, cardiac failure, cerebrovascular accident, cholestasis, colitis, deep vein thrombosis, delirium, dermatitis, difficult micturition, edema, eosinophilia, erythema multiforme, fecal impaction, gastric ulcer, gastroenteritis, granulocytopenia, hallucinations, hematemesis, hepatotoxicity, hyperglycemia, hyperosmolar coma, hypersensitivity reaction, hyperuricemia, hypothermia, impotence, increased erythrocyte sedimentation rate, liver steatosis, mental retardation, mitral valve insufficiency, myasthenia syndrome, mydriasis, myocarditis, myoclonus, neuroleptic malignant syndrome, nocturnal enuresis, obsessive compulsive disorder, orthostatic hypotension, pancreatitis (acute), paralytic ileus, Parkinsonian-like syndrome, pericardial effusion, pericarditis, periorbital edema, phlebitis, pleural effusion, priapism, prolonged QT interval on ECG, psychosis exacerbated, pulmonary embolism, rectal hemorrhage, renal failure, respiratory arrest, rhabdomyolysis, sepsis, sialadenitis, skin photosensitivity, speech disturbance, status epilepticus, Stevens-Johnson syndrome, tardive dyskinesia, thrombocytopenia, thrombocytosis, thromboembolism, thrombophlebitis, torsade de pointes, weight loss

Drug Interactions

Metabolism/Transport Effects Substrate of CYP1A2 (major), CYP2A6 (minor), CYP2C19 (minor), CYP2C9 (minor), CYP2D6 (minor), CYP3A4 (minor); **Note:** Assignment of Major/Minor substrate status based on clinically relevant drug interaction potential; **Inhibits** CYP1A2 (weak), CYP2C19 (weak), CYP2C9 (weak), CYP2D6 (moderate), CYP2E1 (weak), CYP3A4 (weak)

Avoid Concomitant Use

Avoid concomitant use of CloZAPine with any of the following: Aclidinium; Amisulpride; Azelastine (Nasal); CarBAMazepine; Ciprofloxacin (Systemic); CYP3A4 Inducers (Strong); Glucagon; Highest Risk QTc-Prolonging Agents; Ipratropium (Oral Inhalation); Ivabradine; Metoclopramide; Mifepristone; Myelosuppressive Agents; Orphenadrine; Paraldehyde; Pimozide; Potassium Chloride; St Johns Wort; Sulpiride; Thalidomide; Thioridazine; Tiotropium; Umeclidinium

Increased Effect/Toxicity

CloZAPine may increase the levels/effects of: AbobotulinumtoxinA; Alcohol (Ethyl); Amisulpride; Analgesics (Opioid); Anticholinergic Agents; ARIPiprazole; Azelastine (Nasal); Buprenorphine; CNS Depressants; CYP2D6 Substrates; Fesoterodine; Glucagon; Highest Risk QTc-Prolonging Agents; Hydrocodone; Lomitapide; Methotrimeprazine; Methylphenidate; Metoprolol; Metyrosine; Mirabegron; Mirtazapine; Moderate Risk QTc-Prolonging Agents; Nebivolol; OnabotulinumtoxinA; Orphenadrine; Paraldehyde; Pimozide; Potassium Chloride; RimabotulinumtoxinB; Serotonin Modulators; Sulpiride; Suvorexant; Thalidomide; Thiazide Diuretics; Thioridazine; Tiotropium; Topiramate; Zolpidem

The levels/effects of CloZAPine may be increased by: Abiraterone Acetate; Acetylcholinesterase Inhibitors (Central); Aclidinium; Benzodiazepines; Brimonidine (Topical); Cannabis; CarBAMazepine; Cimetidine; Ciprofloxacin (Systemic); CYP1A2 Inhibitors (Moderate); CYP1A2 Inhibitors (Strong); Deferasirox; Doxylamine; Dronabinol; Droperidol; HydrOXYzine; Ipratropium (Oral Inhalation); Ivabradine; Kava Kava; Lithium; Macrolide Antibiotics; Magnesium Sulfate; MAO Inhibitors; Methotrimeprazine; Methylphenidate; Metoclopramide; Metyrosine; Mifepristone; Myelosuppressive Agents; Nabilone; Nefazodone; Omeprazole; Perampanel; Pramlintide; QTc-Prolonging Agents (Indeterminate Risk and Risk Modifying); Rufinamide; Selective Serotonin Reuptake Inhibitors; Serotonin Modulators; Sodium Oxybate; Tapentadol; Tetrahydrocannabinol; Umeclidinium

Decreased Effect

CloZAPine may decrease the levels/effects of: Acetylcholinesterase Inhibitors; Amphetamines; Anti-Parkinson's Agents (Dopamine Agonist); Codeine; Itopride; Quinagolide; Secretin; Tamoxifen; TraMADol

The levels/effects of CloZAPine may be decreased by: Acetylcholinesterase Inhibitors; Cannabis; CarBAMazepine; CYP3A4 Inducers (Strong); Cyproterone; Lithium; Omeprazole; St Johns Wort; Teriflunomide

Storage/Stability

Suspension: Store at ≤25°C (77°F). Protect from light. Do not refrigerate or freeze. Suspension is stable for 100 days after initial bottle opening.

Tablet: Store at ≤30°C (86°F).

Tablet, dispersible: Store at 20°C to 25°C (68°F to 77°F); excursions permitted to 15°C to 30°C (59°F to 86°F). Protect from moisture; do not remove from package until ready to use.

Mechanism of Action The therapeutic efficacy of clozapine (dibenzodiazepine antipsychotic) is proposed to be mediated through antagonism of the dopamine type 2 (D_2) and serotonin type 2A ($5\text{-}HT_{2A}$) receptors. In addition, it acts as an antagonist at alpha-adrenergic, histamine H_1, cholinergic, and other dopaminergic and serotonergic receptors.

Pharmacodynamics/Kinetics

Protein binding: 97% to serum proteins

Metabolism: Extensively hepatic; forms metabolites with limited or no activity

Bioavailability: 50% to 60% (not affected by food)

Half-life elimination: Steady state: 12 hours (range: 4-66 hours)

Time to peak: Suspension: 2.2 hours (range: 1-3.5 hours); Tablets: 2.5 hours (range: 1-6 hours)

Excretion: Urine (~50%) and feces (30%) with trace amounts of unchanged drug

Dosage Note: Prior to initiating treatment obtain a baseline WBC and ANC; the WBC must be ≥3,500/mm^3 and the ANC must be ≥2,000/mm^3 in order to initiate treatment. To continue treatment, the WBC and ANC must be monitored regularly.

Schizophrenia: Oral:

Adults: Initial: 12.5 mg once or twice daily; increase, as tolerated, in increments of 25 to 50 mg daily to a target dose of 300 to 450 mg daily (administered in divided doses) by the end of 2 weeks; may further titrate in increments not exceeding 100 mg and no more frequently than once or twice weekly. Maximum total daily dose: 900 mg. **Note:** In some efficacy studies, total daily dosage was administered in 3 divided doses.

Elderly: Experience in the elderly is limited; may initiate with 12.5 once daily for 3 days, then increase to 25 mg once daily for 3 days as tolerated; may further increase, as tolerated, in increments of 12.5 to 25 mg daily every 3 days to desired response; maximum total daily dosage: 300 mg (Howanitz, 1999). Mean recommended dosage range: 25 to 150 mg (in divided doses) (Gareri, 2003).

Suicidal behavior in schizophrenia or schizoaffective disorder: Adults: Oral: Initial: 12.5 mg once or twice daily; increase, as tolerated, in increments of 25 to 50 mg daily to a target dose of 300 to 450 mg daily (administered in divided doses) by the end of 2 weeks; may further titrate in increments not exceeding 100 mg and no more frequently than once or twice weekly. Mean dose is ~300 mg daily; maximum total daily dose: 900 mg. **Note:** If no longer a suicide risk, may resume prior antipsychotic therapy after gradually tapering off clozapine over 1 to 2 weeks (Meltzer 2003; Wagstaff 2003).

Bipolar disorder (off-label use): Adults: Oral: Initial: 25 mg daily; increased, as tolerated in increments of 25 mg daily to a maximum dose of 550 mg daily. Average daily dose ~300 mg daily (Green, 2000).

Psychosis/agitation related to Alzheimer's dementia (off-label use): Elderly: Oral: Initial: 12.5 mg once daily; if necessary, gradually increase as tolerated not to exceed 75 to 100 mg daily (Rabins, 2007).

Schizoaffective disorder (off-label use): Adults: Oral: Initial: 25 mg daily; increased, as tolerated to a maximum dose of 600 mg daily. Average daily dose: ~200 mg daily (Ciapparelli, 2003).

Dosage adjustment with concomitant therapy:

Strong CYP1A2 inhibitors (eg, fluvoxamine, ciprofloxacin):

Initiating clozapine with concomitant medication or adding a concomitant medication while taking clozapine: Use one-third of the clozapine dose.

Discontinuing concomitant medication while continuing clozapine: Increase clozapine dose based on clinical response.

Moderate or weak CYP1A2 inhibitors (eg, oral contraceptives, caffeine), CYP2D6 or CYP3A4 inhibitors (eg, cimetidine, escitalopram, erythromycin, paroxetine, bupropion, fluoxetine, quinidine, duloxetine, terbinafine, sertraline):

Initiating clozapine with concomitant medication or adding a concomitant medication while taking clozapine: Monitor for adverse reactions and if necessary, consider reducing the clozapine dose.

Discontinuing concomitant medication while continuing clozapine: Monitor for lack of effectiveness and if necessary, consider increasing the clozapine dose.

Strong CYP3A4 inducers (eg, phenytoin, carbamazepine, St John's wort, rifampin):

Initiating clozapine with concomitant medication or adding a concomitant medication while taking clozapine: Concomitant use is not recommended. However, if the CYP3A4 inducer is necessary, monitor for decreased effectiveness and if necessary, consider increasing the clozapine dose.

Discontinuing concomitant medication while continuing clozapine: Reduce clozapine dose based on clinical response.

Moderate or weak CYP1A2 (eg, tobacco smoke) or CYP3A4 inducers:

Initiating clozapine with concomitant medication or adding a concomitant medication while taking clozapine: Monitor for decreased effectiveness and if necessary, consider increasing the clozapine dose.

Discontinuing concomitant medication while continuing clozapine: Monitor for adverse reactions and if necessary, consider reducing the clozapine dose.

Reinitiation of therapy: If dosing is interrupted for ≥48 hours, therapy must be reinitiated at 12.5 to 25 mg daily to minimize the risk of hypotension, bradycardia, and syncope; if dose is well tolerated, may be increased more rapidly than with initial titration, unless cardiopulmonary arrest occurred during initial titration, then retitrate with extreme caution. Patients with clozapine discontinued for WBCs below 2,000/mm^3 or an ANC below 1,000/mm^3 must not restart clozapine.

Discontinuation of therapy: In the event of planned discontinuation of clozapine, gradual reduction in dose over a 1- to 2-week period is recommended. If conditions warrant abrupt discontinuation (eg, agranulocytosis), monitor patient for psychosis and cholinergic rebound (eg, headache, nausea, vomiting, diarrhea, profuse diaphoresis).

Dosage adjustment for toxicity:

Hematologic toxicity:

Eosinophilia: Canadian labeling: Interrupt therapy for eosinophil count >3000/mm^3; may resume therapy when eosinophil count <1000/mm^3

Leukopenia/granulocytopenia:

Mild (WBC 3000 to 3500/mm^3 and/or ANC 1500 to 2000/mm^3): Continue treatment; monitor WBC and ANC twice weekly until WBC >3500/mm^3 and ANC >2000/mm^3 then return to previous monitoring schedule.

Moderate (WBC 2000 to 3000/mm^3 and/or ANC 1000 to 1500/mm^3): Interrupt therapy and begin daily WBC/ANC monitoring until WBC >3000/mm^3 and ANC >1500/mm^3 followed by twice weekly monitoring until WBC >3500/mm^3 and ANC >2000/mm^3, then may consider restarting therapy; weekly WBC/ANC monitoring is required for 12 months in patients restarted on clozapine treatment. **Note:** Patient is at greater risk for developing agranulocytosis.

Severe (WBC <2000/mm^3 and/or ANC <1000/mm^3 [U.S. labeling] or ANC <1500/mm^3 [Canadian labeling]) or agranulocytosis (ANC <500/mm^3): Discontinue treatment and do not rechallenge patient; continue to monitor WBC/ANC daily for at least 4 weeks from day of discontinuation and until WBC >3000/mm^3 and ANC >1500/mm^3, then twice weekly until WBC >3500/mm^3 and ANC >2000/mm^3, then weekly after WBC >3500/mm^3.

Thrombocytopenia: Platelets <50,000/mm^3: Canadian labeling recommends discontinuing therapy.

Nonhematologic toxicity:

QTc interval >500 msec, cardiomyopathy/myocarditis, hepatotoxicity (clinically relevant transaminase elevations or jaundice symptoms), or neuroleptic malignant syndrome: Discontinue use. Patients with clozapine-related myocarditis or cardiomyopathy should generally not be rechallenged. If the benefit of treatment is judged to outweigh the potential risks of recurrent myocarditis or cardiomyopathy, rechallenge may be considered in consultation with a cardiologist, after a complete cardiac evaluation, and under close monitoring. If antipsychotic therapy is required following neuroleptic malignant syndrome, use with caution as symptoms can recur.

Dosage adjustment in renal impairment:

U.S. labeling: There are no dosage adjustments provided in the manufacturer's labeling; however, labeling suggests that dose reductions may be necessary with significant impairment.

Canadian labeling:

Mild to moderate impairment: Initial dose: 12.5 mg once daily

Severe impairment: Use is contraindicated

Dosage adjustment in hepatic impairment:

U.S. labeling: There are no dosage adjustments provided in the manufacturer's labeling; however, labeling suggests that dose reductions may be necessary with significant impairment.

Canadian labeling: Contraindicated in active liver disease associated with nausea, anorexia, or jaundice; progressive liver disease; or hepatic failure. There is no dosage adjustment provided in the manufacturer's labeling for stable preexisting hepatic disorders; use with caution.

Dietary Considerations Some products may contain phenylalanine.

Administration May be taken without regard to food. Total daily dose may be divided into uneven doses with larger dose administered at bedtime. The Canadian labeling suggests that maintenance doses ≤200 mg daily may be administered as single dose in the evening.

Orally disintegrating tablet: Remove from foil blister by peeling apart (do not push tablet through the foil). Remove immediately prior to use. Place tablet in mouth and chew or allow to dissolve; swallow with saliva. If dosing requires splitting tablet, throw unused portion away.

Suspension: Shake bottle prior to use. Using syringe adaptor and oral syringe provided withdrawal dose from bottle. Administer immediately after preparation using the oral syringe provided.

Monitoring Parameters Note: The Canadian labeling recommends initiating treatment in an inpatient setting or an outpatient setting with medical supervision and monitoring of vital signs for at least 6 to 8 hours after the first few doses.

Mental status; WBC (see monitoring recommendations based on WBC and ANC); vital signs (as clinically indicated); ECG (as clinically indicated); blood pressure (baseline; repeat 3 months after antipsychotic initiation, then yearly); signs and symptoms of myocarditis and cardiomyopathy; weight, height, body mass index, waist circumference (baseline; repeat at 4, 8, and 12 weeks after initiating or changing therapy, then quarterly; consider switching to a different antipsychotic for a weight gain 5% or more of initial weight); electrolytes and liver function (annually and as clinically indicated); personal and family history of obesity, diabetes, dyslipidemia, hypertension, or cardiovascular disease (baseline; repeat annually); fasting plasma glucose level/HbA_{1c} (baseline; repeat 3 months after starting antipsychotic, then yearly); lipid panel (baseline; repeat 3 months after initiation of antipsychotic; if low-density lipoprotein level is normal, repeat at 2- to 5-year intervals or more frequently if clinical indicated); changes in menstruation, libido, development of galactorrhea, and erectile and ejaculatory function (yearly); abnormal involuntary movements or parkinsonian signs (baseline; repeat weekly until dose stabilized for at least 2 weeks after introduction and for 2 weeks after any significant dose increase); tardive dyskinesia (every 12 months; high-risk patients every 6 months); ocular examination (yearly in patients older than 40 years; every 2 years in younger patients) (ADA, 2004; Lehman, 2004; Marder, 2004).

WBC and ANC should be obtained at baseline and at least weekly for the first 6 months (26 weeks) of continuous treatment. If counts remain acceptable (WBC ≥3,500/mm^3, ANC ≥2,000/mm^3) during this time period, then they may be monitored every other week for the next 6 months (26 weeks). If WBC/ANC continue to remain within these acceptable limits after the second 6 months (26 weeks) of therapy, monitoring can be decreased to every 4 weeks. If clozapine is discontinued, a weekly WBC should be conducted for an additional 4 weeks or until WBC is ≥3,500/mm^3 and ANC is ≥2,000/mm^3. **Note:** The Canadian labeling recommends weekly hematologic monitoring for an additional 6 weeks if therapy is interrupted for >3 days and for an additional 26 weeks if therapy is interrupted for ≥4 weeks.

Monitoring for hematologic toxicity:

Immature forms present: Repeat WBC and ANC.

Substantial drop in WBC or ANC (single drop or cumulative drop within 3 weeks of WBC ≥3,000/mm^3 or ANC ≥1,500/mm^3): Repeat WBC and ANC; if repeat values are WBC 3,000 to 3,500/mm^3 and ANC <2,000/mm^3, then monitor twice weekly.

Mild leukopenia/granulocytopenia (WBC 3,000 to 3,500/mm^3 and/or ANC 1,500 to 2,000/mm^3): Continue treatment; monitor WBC and ANC twice weekly until WBC >3,500/mm^3 and ANC >2,000/mm^3 then return to previous monitoring schedule.

Moderate leukopenia/granulocytopenia (WBC 2,000 to 3,000/mm^3 and/or ANC 1,000 to 1,500/mm^3):

U.S. labeling: Interrupt therapy and begin daily WBC/ANC monitoring until WBC >3,000/mm^3 and ANC >1,500/mm^3, followed by twice weekly monitoring until WBC >3,500/mm^3 and ANC >2,000/mm^3, then may consider restarting therapy; after restarting therapy, weekly WBC/ANC monitoring is required for 12 months. **Note:** Patient is at greater risk for developing agranulocytosis.

Canadian labeling: Begin twice weekly monitoring for any of the following: WBC 2,000 to 3,500 mm^3; ANC 1,500 to 2,000; single fall or sum of falls in WBC ≥3,000 mm^3 within prior 4 weeks, reaching a value <4,000 mm^3; single fall or sum of falls in ANC ≥1,500 mm^3 within prior 4 weeks, reaching a value <2,500 mm^3; flu-like symptoms or other symptoms suggesting infection.

Severe leukopenia/granulocytopenia (WBC <2,000/mm^3 and/or ANC <1,000/mm^3 [U.S. labeling] or ANC <1,500/mm^3 [Canadian labeling]) or agranulocytosis (ANC <500/mm^3): Discontinue treatment and do not rechallenge patient; continue to monitor WBC/ANC daily for at least 4 weeks from day of discontinuation and until WBC >3,000/mm^3 and ANC >1,500/mm^3, then twice weekly until WBC >3,500/mm^3 and ANC >2,000/mm^3, then weekly after WBC >3,500/mm^3.

Monitoring after interruption of therapy: If therapy is interrupted for reasons other than leukopenia/granulocytopenia and rechallenge is considered, the 6-month time period for initiation of biweekly WBCs may need to be reset. This determination depends upon the treatment duration, the length of the break in therapy, and whether or not an abnormal blood event occurred. Transitions to reduce frequency of monitoring are only permitted if all WBC ≥3,500/mm^3 and ANC ≥2,000/mm^3.

Previous therapy duration <6 months:

No abnormal blood event (WBC ≥3,500/mm^3 and ANC ≥2,000/mm^3) and interruption in therapy >3 days but ≤1 month: Do not reset clock.

No abnormal blood event (WBC ≥3,500/mm^3 and ANC ≥2,000/mm^3) and interruption in therapy >1 month: Monitor WBC and ANC weekly for 6 months.

An abnormal blood event (WBC <3,500/mm^3 or ANC <2,000/mm^3) and rechallengeable: See monitoring parameters for hematologic toxicity.

Previous therapy duration 6 to 12 months:

No abnormal blood event (WBC ≥3,500/mm^3 and ANC ≥2,000/mm^3) and interruption in therapy >3 days but ≤1 month: Monitor WBC and ANC weekly for 6 weeks, then return to every 2 weeks for 6 months.

No abnormal blood event (WBC ≥3,500/mm^3 and ANC ≥2,000/mm^3) and interruption in therapy >1 month: Monitor WBC and ANC weekly for 6 months, then return to every 2 weeks for 6 months.

An abnormal blood event (WBC <3,500/mm^3 or ANC <2,000/mm^3) and rechallengeable: See monitoring parameters for hematologic toxicity.

Previous therapy duration >12 months:

No abnormal blood event (WBC ≥3,500/mm^3 and ANC ≥2,000/mm^3) and interruption in therapy >3 days, but ≤1 month: Monitor WBC and ANC weekly for 6 weeks, then return to every 4 weeks.

No abnormal blood event (WBC ≥3,500/mm^3 and ANC ≥2,000/mm^3) and interruption in therapy >1 month: Monitor WBC and ANC weekly for 6 months, then every 2 weeks for 6 months, then return to every 4 weeks.

An abnormal blood event (WBC <3,500/mm^3 or ANC <2,000/mm^3) and rechallengeable: See monitoring parameters for hematologic toxicity.

Reference Range Clozapine levels >350 ng/mL may be associated with an increased likelihood of clinical response. However, increases of serum concentrations above this have not been shown to confer greater improvements and may increase the risk of adverse events (Remington 2013).

Dosage Forms

Suspension, Oral:

Versacloz: 50 mg/mL (100 mL)

Tablet, Oral:

Clozaril: 25 mg, 100 mg

Generic: 25 mg, 50 mg, 100 mg, 200 mg

Tablet Dispersible, Oral:

FazaClo: 12.5 mg, 25 mg, 100 mg, 150 mg, 200 mg

Generic: 12.5 mg, 25 mg, 100 mg

Dosage Forms: Canada Note: Refer to Dosage Forms. Dispersible tablet and oral suspension are not available in Canada.

- ◆ **Clozaril** *see* CloZAPine *on page 490*
- ◆ **CMA-676** *see* Gemtuzumab Ozogamicin *on page 957*
- ◆ **C-Met/Hepatocyte Growth Factor Receptor Tyrosine Kinase Inhibitor PF-02341066** *see* Crizotinib *on page 511*
- ◆ **C-Met/HGFR Tyrosine Kinase Inhibitor PF-02341066** *see* Crizotinib *on page 511*
- ◆ **CMV Hyperimmune Globulin** *see* Cytomegalovirus Immune Globulin (Intravenous-Human) *on page 541*
- ◆ **CMV-IGIV** *see* Cytomegalovirus Immune Globulin (Intravenous-Human) *on page 541*
- ◆ **CNJ-016** *see* Vaccinia Immune Globulin (Intravenous) *on page 2118*
- ◆ **CNL8 Nail** *see* Ciclopirox *on page 433*
- ◆ **CNTO-148** *see* Golimumab *on page 977*
- ◆ **CNTO 328** *see* Siltuximab *on page 1885*
- ◆ **CNTO 1275** *see* Ustekinumab *on page 2117*
- ◆ **CoActifed (Can)** *see* Triprolidine, Pseudoephedrine, and Codeine [CAN/INT] *on page 2105*
- ◆ **Coagulant Complex Inhibitor** *see* Anti-inhibitor Coagulant Complex (Human) *on page 155*
- ◆ **Coagulation Factor I** *see* Fibrinogen Concentrate (Human) *on page 874*
- ◆ **Coagulation Factor VIIa** *see* Factor VIIa (Recombinant) *on page 836*
- ◆ **CO Alendronate (Can)** *see* Alendronate *on page 79*
- ◆ **Co-Amoxiclav** *see* Amoxicillin and Clavulanate *on page 133*
- ◆ **Coartem** *see* Artemether and Lumefantrine *on page 177*
- ◆ **CO Atenolol (Can)** *see* Atenolol *on page 189*
- ◆ **CO Betahistine (Can)** *see* Betahistine [CAN/INT] *on page 252*
- ◆ **CO Bicalutamide (Can)** *see* Bicalutamide *on page 262*

Cobicistat (koe BIK i stat)

Brand Names: U.S. Tybost

Pharmacologic Category Cytochrome P-450 Inhibitor

Use

HIV-1 infection: Treatment of HIV-1 infection to increase systemic exposure of atazanavir or darunavir (once-daily dosing regimen) in combination with other antiretroviral agents

Limitations of use: Cobicistat is **not** interchangeable with ritonavir to increase systemic exposure of darunavir 600 mg twice daily, fosamprenavir, saquinavir, or tipranavir due to lack of exposure data. The use of cobicistat is not recommended with darunavir 600 mg twice daily, fosamprenavir, saquinavir, or tipranavir.

Pregnancy Risk Factor B

Pregnancy Considerations Adverse events were not observed in animal reproduction studies. The HHS Perinatal HIV Guidelines note there are insufficient data to recommend use in pregnancy.

Regardless of CD4 count or HIV RNA copy number, all HIV-infected pregnant women should receive a combination antiretroviral (ARV) drug regimen. A combination of antepartum, intrapartum, and infant ARV prophylaxis is recommended. ARV therapy should be started as soon as possible in women with symptomatic infection. Although earlier initiation may be more effective in reducing the perinatal transmission of HIV, initiation may be delayed until after 12 weeks gestation in women who do not require immediate treatment after careful consideration of maternal conditions (eg, nausea and vomiting) and the potential risks of first trimester fetal exposure for specific agents. A scheduled cesarean delivery at 38 weeks gestation is recommended for all women with HIV RNA >1000 copies/mL or unknown concentrations near delivery in order to decrease transmission. If ARV therapy must be interrupted for <24 hours during the peripartum period, stop then restart all medications simultaneously in order to decrease the chance of developing resistance. Long-term follow-up is recommended for all infants exposed to ARV medications. In couples who want to conceive, the HIV-infected partner should attain maximum viral suppression prior to conception.

Health care providers are encouraged to enroll pregnant women exposed to antiretroviral medications in the Antiretroviral Pregnancy Registry (1-800-258-4263 or www.APRegistry.com). Health care providers caring for HIV-infected women and their infants may contact the National Perinatal HIV Hotline (888-448-8765) for clinical consultation (HHS [perinatal], 2014).

Breast-Feeding Considerations It is not known if cobicistat is excreted into breast milk. Maternal or infant antiretroviral therapy does not completely eliminate the risk of postnatal HIV transmission. In addition, multiclass-resistant virus has been detected in breast-feeding infants despite maternal therapy. Therefore, in the United States, where formula is accessible, affordable, safe, and sustainable, and the risk of infant mortality due to diarrhea and respiratory infections is low, complete avoidance of breast-feeding by HIV-infected women is recommended to decrease potential transmission of HIV (HHS [perinatal], 2014).

Contraindications Concomitant use of cobicistat with atazanavir or darunavir with alfuzosin, cisapride, dronedarone, ergot derivatives (eg, dihydroergotamine, ergotamine, methylergonovine), indinavir, irinotecan, lovastatin, midazolam (oral), nevirapine, pimozide, rifampin, sildenafil (when used for pulmonary arterial hypertension), simvastatin, St John's wort, triazolam

Warnings/Precautions Patients may develop immune reconstitution syndrome resulting in the occurrence of an inflammatory response to an indolent or residual opportunistic infection during initial HIV treatment or activation of autoimmune disorders (eg, Graves' disease, polymyositis, Guillain-Barré syndrome) later in therapy; further evaluation and treatment may be required. May inhibit tubular secretion of creatinine without affecting actual renal glomerular function; use caution when interpreting serum creatinine values in patients with medical conditions or receiving drugs needing to be monitored with estimated creatinine clearance (CrCl). Patients who experience a confirmed increase in serum creatinine >0.4 mg/dL from baseline should have renal function monitored closely. Assess estimated CrCl prior to initiating therapy; consider alternative medications that do not require dosage adjustments in patients with renal impairment. When used with concomitant tenofovir, may cause renal toxicity (acute renal failure and/or Fanconi syndrome); avoid use with concurrent or recent nephrotoxic therapy. Calculate estimated creatinine clearance prior to initiation of therapy and monitor renal function (including recalculation of creatinine clearance and serum phosphorus) during therapy (DHHS [adult], 2014). In patients receiving concomitant tenofovir, urine glucose, and urine protein prior to and periodically during treatment; assess serum phosphorus in patients with or at risk for renal impairment. Do not initiate therapy in patients with CrCl <70 mL/minute.

Use with HIV-1 protease inhibitors other than atazanavir or darunavir administered once daily is not recommended; use with more than one antiretroviral that requires pharmacokinetic enhancement (eg, two protease inhibitors or elvitegravir in combination with a protease inhibitor) is not recommended. Avoid concurrent use with other cobicistat-containing products or ritonavir-containing products. Potentially significant drug-drug interactions may exist, requiring dose or frequency adjustment, additional monitoring, and/or selection of alternative therapy. Complex or unknown mechanisms of drug interactions preclude extrapolation of ritonavir drug interactions to certain cobicistat interactions. Cobicistat and ritonavir when administered with either atazanavir or darunavir may result in different drug interactions when used with concomitant medications.

Adverse Reactions All adverse reactions are from trials using cobicistat coadministered with atazanavir, emtricitabine + tenofovir unless otherwise noted.

Central nervous system: Abnormal dreams, depression, fatigue, headache, insomnia

Dermatologic: Skin rash

Endocrine & metabolic: Fanconi's syndrome, glycosuria (≥1000 mg/dL), increased gamma-glutamyl transferase (>5.0 x ULN)

Gastrointestinal: Diarrhea, increased serum amylase (>2.0 x ULN), increased serum lipase, nausea, upper abdominal pain, vomiting

Genitourinary: Hematuria (>75 RBC/HPF)

Hepatic: Hyperbilirubinemia (>2.5 x ULN), increased serum ALT (>5.0 x ULN), increased serum AST (>5.0 x ULN) jaundice

Neuromuscular & skeletal: Increased creatine phosphokinase (≥10.0 x ULN), rhabdomyolysis

Ophthalmic: Ocular icterus

Renal: Nephrolithiasis, renal disease

Rare but important or life-threatening: Hypercholesterolemia, increased HDL cholesterol, renal insufficiency

Drug Interactions

Metabolism/Transport Effects Substrate of CYP3A4 (major); **Note:** Assignment of Major/Minor substrate status based on clinically relevant drug interaction potential; **Inhibits** BCRP, CYP2D6 (weak), CYP3A4 (strong), P-glycoprotein, SLCO1B1

Avoid Concomitant Use

Avoid concomitant use of Cobicistat with any of the following: Ado-Trastuzumab Emtansine; Alfuzosin; Apixaban; Astemizole; Avanafil; Axitinib; Boceprevir; Bosutinib; Cabozantinib; Ceritinib; Cisapride; Conivaptan; Crizotinib; Dapoxetine; Dihydroergotamine; Dronedarone; Eplerenone; Ergotamine; Everolimus; Fluticasone (Oral Inhalation); Halofantrine; Ibrutinib; Irinotecan; Ivabradine; Lapatinib; Lercanidipine; Lomitapide; Lovastatin; Lurasidone; Macitentan; Methylergonovine; Midazolam; Naloxegol; Nilotinib; Nisoldipine; Olaparib; PAZOPanib; Pimozide; Ranolazine; Red Yeast Rice; Regorafenib; Rifampin; Rifapentine; Rivaroxaban; Salmeterol; Sildenafil; Silodosin; Simeprevir; Simvastatin; St Johns Wort; Suvorexant; Tamsulosin; Telaprevir; Terfenadine; Ticagrelor; Tolvaptan; Topotecan; Toremifene; Trabectedin; Triazolam; Ulipristal; Vardenafil; Vemurafenib; VinCRIStine (Liposomal); Vorapaxar

Increased Effect/Toxicity

Cobicistat may increase the levels/effects of: Ado-Trastuzumab Emtansine; Afatinib; Alfuzosin; Almotriptan; Alosetron; Apixaban; ARIPiprazole; Astemizole; AtorvaSTATin; Avanafil; Axitinib; Bedaquiline; Boceprevir; Bortezomib; Bosentan; Bosutinib; Brentuximab Vedotin; Brinzolamide; Budesonide (Nasal); Budesonide (Systemic, Oral Inhalation); Buprenorphine; Cabazitaxel; Cabozantinib; Cannabis; Ceritinib; Cisapride; Clarithromycin; ClonazePAM; Colchicine; Conivaptan; Contraceptives (Progestins); Corticosteroids (Orally Inhaled); Corticosteroids (Systemic); Crizotinib; CYP2D6 Substrates; CYP3A4 Substrates; Dabigatran Etexilate; Dapoxetine; Dasatinib; Dihydroergotamine; Dofetilide; DOXOrubicin (Conventional); Dronabinol; Dronedarone; Dutasteride; Edoxaban; Eliglustat; Eplerenone; Ergotamine; Erlotinib; Ethosuximide; Etizolam; Everolimus; FentaNYL; Fesoterodine; Fluticasone (Nasal); Fluticasone (Oral Inhalation); GuanFACINE; Halofantrine; Hydrocodone; Ibrutinib; Idelalisib; Iloperidone; Imatinib; Imidafenacin; Irinotecan; Itraconazole; Ivabradine; Ivacaftor; Ixabepilone; Ketoconazole (Systemic); Lacosamide; Lapatinib; Ledipasvir; Lercanidipine; Levobupivacaine; Levomilnacipran; Lomitapide;

Lovastatin; Lumefantrine; Lurasidone; Macitentan; Maraviroc; Methadone; Methylergonovine; MethylPREDNISolone; Midazolam; Mifepristone; Naloxegol; Nilotinib; Nintedanib; Nisoldipine; Olaparib; Ospemifene; OxyCODONE; Paricalcitol; PAZOPanib; P-glycoprotein/ABCB1 Substrates; Pimecrolimus; Pimozide; PONATinib; Pranlukast; PrednisoLONE (Systemic); PredniSONE; Propafenone; Prucalopride; QUEtiapine; Ranolazine; Red Yeast Rice; Regorafenib; Repaglinide; Retapamulin; Rifaximin; Rilpivirine; Riociguat; Rivaroxaban; RomiDEPsin; Ruxolitinib; Salmeterol; Saxagliptin; Sildenafil; Silodosin; Simeprevir; Simvastatin; SORAfenib; Suvorexant; Tadalafil; Tamsulosin; Telaprevir; Telithromycin; Tenofovir; Terfenadine; Tetrahydrocannabinol; Ticagrelor; Tofacitinib; Tolterodine; Tolvaptan; Topotecan; Toremifene; Trabectedin; Triazolam; Ulipristal; Vardenafil; Vemurafenib; Vilazodone; VinCRIStine (Liposomal); Vorapaxar; Voriconazole; Warfarin; Zopiclone; Zuclopenthixol

The levels/effects of Cobicistat may be increased by: Clarithromycin; Itraconazole; Ketoconazole (Systemic); Telithromycin; Voriconazole

Decreased Effect

Cobicistat may decrease the levels/effects of: Contraceptives (Estrogens); Ifosfamide; Prasugrel; Ticagrelor

The levels/effects of Cobicistat may be decreased by: CarBAMazepine; CYP3A4 Inducers (Moderate); CYP3A4 Inducers (Strong); Dabrafenib; Deferasirox; Dexamethasone (Systemic); Fosphenytoin-Phenytoin; Mitotane; OXcarbazepine; PHENobarbital; Rifampin; Rifapentine; Siltuximab; St Johns Wort; Tocilizumab

Storage/Stability Store at 25°C (77°F); excursions are permitted between 15°C and 30°C (59°F and 86°F). Keep tightly closed. Dispense only in original container.

Mechanism of Action Cobicistat is a mechanism-based inhibitor of cytochrome P450 3A (CYP3A). Inhibition of CYP3A-mediated metabolism by cobicistat and increases the systemic exposure of CYP3A substrates atazanavir and darunavir.

Pharmacodynamics/Kinetics

Absorption: Well absorbed with food

Protein binding: 97% to 98%

Metabolism: Via CYP3A enzymes and to a minor extent by CYP2D6 enzymes and does not undergo glucuronidation

Half-life elimination: ~3 to 4 hours

Time to peak, plasma: 3.5 hours

Excretion: Feces (~86%), urine (~8%)

Dosage HIV-1 infection in antiretroviral treatment: Adults: Oral: **Note:** Must be administered with concomitant atazanavir or darunavir and other antiretroviral drugs. See individual agents.

Treatment-naive or experienced: 150 mg once daily with concomitant atazanavir

Treatment-naive or experienced with no darunavir resistance-associated substitutions: 150 mg once daily with concomitant darunavir

Dosage adjustment in renal impairment:

When **not** used with concomitant tenofovir: No dosage adjustment necessary.

When used with concomitant tenofovir:

CrCl ≥70 mL/minute: No dosage adjustment necessary.

CrCl <70 mL/minute: Use is not recommended.

Dosage adjustment in hepatic impairment:

Mild-to-moderate hepatic impairment (Child-Pugh class A or B): No dosage adjustment necessary.

Severe hepatic impairment (Child-Pugh class C): Use is not recommended (has not been studied).

Dietary Considerations Take with food

Administration Oral: Administer with food

Monitoring Parameters CBC with differential, reticulocyte count, CD4 count, HIV RNA plasma levels, and serum creatinine at baseline and when clinically indicated during therapy; when coadministered with tenofovir, serum creatinine, urine glucose and urine protein prior to initiation and as clinically indicated during therapy; assess serum phosphorus in patients with or at risk for renal impairment. Patients who experience a confirmed increase in serum creatinine >0.4 mg/dL from baseline should have renal function monitored closely. Testing for HBV is recommended prior to the initiation of antiretroviral therapy.

Dosage Forms

Tablet, Oral:

Tybost: 150 mg

◆ **Cobicistat and Darunavir** *see* Darunavir and Cobicistat *on page 572*

◆ **Cobicistat, Emtricitabine, Tenofovir, and Elvitegravir** *see* Elvitegravir, Cobicistat, Emtricitabine, and Tenofovir *on page 718*

Cocaine (koe KANE)

Index Terms Cocaine Hydrochloride

Pharmacologic Category Local Anesthetic

Use Topical anesthesia (and vasoconstriction) for mucous membranes

Pregnancy Risk Factor C

Dosage Topical application (ear, nose, throat, bronchoscopy): Dosage depends on the area to be anesthetized, tissue vascularity, technique of anesthesia, and individual patient tolerance; the lowest dose necessary to produce adequate anesthesia should be used; concentrations of 1% to 10% may be used, with 4% being the most frequently used concentration (maximum total dose: 3 mg/kg **or** 200 mg) (Liao, 1999). Lasts for 30 minutes or longer depending on concentration and vascularity of anesthetized tissue. Use reduced dosages for children, elderly, or debilitated patients.

Additional Information Complete prescribing information should be consulted for additional detail.

Dosage Forms

Solution, External:

Generic: 4% (4 mL, 10 mL); 10% (4 mL)

◆ **Cocaine Hydrochloride** *see* Cocaine *on page 497*

◆ **CO Candesartan (Can)** *see* Candesartan *on page 335*

◆ **Co-Candesartan/HCT (Can)** *see* Candesartan and Hydrochlorothiazide *on page 338*

◆ **CO Cilazapril (Can)** *see* Cilazapril [CAN/INT] *on page 434*

◆ **CO Clomipramine (Can)** *see* ClomiPRAMINE *on page 475*

◆ **CO Clonazepam (Can)** *see* ClonazePAM *on page 478*

◆ **CO Clopidogrel (Can)** *see* Clopidogrel *on page 484*

◆ **Codar GF** *see* Guaifenesin and Codeine *on page 987*

Codeine (KOE deen)

Brand Names: Canada Codeine Contin; PMS-Codeine; ratio-Codeine

Index Terms Codeine Phosphate; Codeine Sulfate; Methylmorphine

Pharmacologic Category Analgesic, Opioid; Antitussive

Use Management of mild-to-moderately-severe pain

Pregnancy Risk Factor C

Pregnancy Considerations Adverse events have been observed in animal reproduction studies. Opioid analgesics cross the placenta. In humans, birth defects (including some heart defects) have been associated with maternal use of codeine during the first trimester of pregnancy (Broussard, 2011). If chronic opioid exposure occurs in pregnancy, adverse events in the newborn (including withdrawal) may occur; monitoring of the neonate is recommended. The minimum effective dose should be used if opioids are needed (Chou, 2009). Neonatal abstinence syndrome following opioid exposure may present with autonomic (eg, fever, temperature instability), gastrointestinal (eg, diarrhea, vomiting, poor feeding/weight gain), or neurologic (eg, high pitched crying, increased muscle tone, irritability, seizure, tremor) symptoms (Dow, 2012; Hudak, 2012).

Breast-Feeding Considerations Codeine and its metabolite (morphine) are found in breast milk and can be detected in the serum of nursing infants. The relative dose to a nursing infant has been calculated to be ~1% of the weight-adjusted maternal dose (Spigset, 2000). Higher levels of morphine may be found in the breast milk of lactating mothers who are "ultrarapid metabolizers" of codeine; patients with two or more copies of the variant CYP2D6*2 allele may have extensive conversion to morphine and thus increased opioid-mediated effects. In one case, excessively high serum concentrations of morphine were reported in a breast-fed infant following maternal use of acetaminophen with codeine. The mother was later found to be an "ultrarapid metabolizer" of codeine; symptoms in the infant included feeding difficulty and lethargy, followed by death. Caution should be used since most persons are not aware if they have the genotype resulting in "ultra-rapid metabolizer" status. When codeine is used in breast-feeding women, it is recommended to use the lowest dose for the shortest duration of time and observe the infant for increased sleepiness, difficulty in feeding or breathing, or limpness (FDA, 2007; Koren, 2006). The manufacturer recommends that caution be used if administered to a nursing woman. According to other guidelines, when treatment is needed for pain in nursing women, other agents should be used; if codeine cannot be avoided it should not be used for >4 days (Kahan, 2011; Wong, 2011).

Contraindications Hypersensitivity to codeine or any component of the formulation; respiratory depression in the absence of resuscitative equipment; acute or severe bronchial asthma or hypercarbia; presence or suspicion of paralytic ileus; postoperative pain management in children who have undergone tonsillectomy and/or adenoidectomy

Canadian labeling: Additional contraindications (not in U.S. labeling): Hypersensitivity to other opioid analgesics; cor pulmonale; acute alcoholism; delirium tremens; severe CNS depression; convulsive disorders; increased cerebrospinal or intracranial pressure; head injury; suspected surgical abdomen; use with or within 14 days of MAO inhibitors.

Warnings/Precautions [U.S. Boxed Warning]: Respiratory depression and death have occurred in children who received codeine following tonsillectomy and/or adenoidectomy and were found to have evidence of being ultra-rapid metabolizers of codeine due to a CYP2D6 polymorphism. Deaths have also occurred in nursing infants after being exposed to high concentrations of morphine because the mothers were ultra-rapid metabolizers. Use is contraindicated in the postoperative pain management of children who have undergone tonsillectomy and/or adenoidectomy. Use caution in patients with two or more copies of the variant CYP2D6*2 allele; may have extensive conversion to morphine and thus increased opioid-mediated effects. Avoid the use of codeine in these patients; consider alternative analgesics such as morphine or a nonopioid agent (Crews, 2012). The occurrence of this phenotype is seen in 0.5% to 1% of Chinese and Japanese, 0.5% to 1% of Hispanics, 1% to 10% of Caucasians, 3% of African-Americans, and 16% to 28% of North Africans, Ethiopians, and Arabs.

May cause dose-related respiratory depression. The risk is increased in elderly patients, debilitated patients, and patients with conditions associated with hypoxia, hypercapnia, or upper airway obstruction. Use with caution in patients with preexisting respiratory compromise (hypoxia and/or hypercapnia), COPD or other obstructive pulmonary disease, and kyphoscoliosis or other skeletal disorder which may alter respiratory function; critical respiratory depression may occur, even at therapeutic dosages.

After chronic maternal exposure to opioids, neonatal withdrawal syndrome may occur in the newborn; monitor neonate closely. Signs and symptoms include irritability, hyperactivity and abnormal sleep pattern, high pitched cry, tremor, vomiting, diarrhea and failure to gain weight. Onset, duration and severity depend on the drug used, duration of use, maternal dose, and rate of drug elimination by the newborn. Opioid withdrawal syndrome in the neonate, unlike in adults, may be life-threatening and should be treated according to protocols developed by neonatology experts.

Use may cause or aggravate constipation; chronic use may result in obstructive bowel disease, particularly in those with underlying intestinal motility disorders. Constipation may also be problematic in patients with unstable angina or those patients post-myocardial infarction. Avoid use in patients with gastrointestinal obstruction, particularly paralytic ileus. May cause hypotension; use with caution in patients with hypovolemia, cardiovascular disease (including acute MI), or drugs which may exaggerate hypotensive effects (including phenothiazines or general anesthetics). May cause CNS depression, which may impair physical or mental abilities; patients must be cautioned about performing tasks which require mental alertness (eg, operating machinery or driving).

Use with extreme caution in patients with head injury, intracranial lesions, or elevated intracranial pressure; exaggerated elevation of ICP may occur. Use with caution in patients with hypersensitivity reactions to other phenanthrene-derivative opioid agonists (hydrocodone, hydromorphone, levorphanol, oxycodone, oxymorphone), adrenal insufficiency (including Addison's disease), biliary tract dysfunction, pancreatitis, thyroid dysfunction, morbid obesity, prostatic hyperplasia and/or urinary stricture, or severe hepatic or renal impairment. Use may obscure diagnosis or clinical course of patients with acute abdominal conditions. May induce or aggravate seizures; use with caution in patients with seizure disorders. Avoid use in patients with CNS depression or coma as these patients are susceptible to intracranial effects of CO_2 retention.

Use with caution in patients with a history of drug abuse or acute alcoholism; potential for drug dependency exists. Tolerance, psychological and physical dependence may occur with prolonged use. Potentially significant drug interactions may exist, requiring dose or frequency adjustment, additional monitoring, and/or selection of alternative therapy. Effects may be potentiated when used with other sedative drugs or ethanol. Concurrent use of agonist/antagonist analgesics may precipitate withdrawal symptoms and/or reduced analgesic efficacy in patients following prolonged therapy with mu opioid agonists. Abrupt discontinuation following prolonged use may also lead to withdrawal symptoms.

Some preparations contain sulfites which may cause allergic reactions. Healthcare provider should be alert to the potential for abuse, misuse, and diversion.

Adverse Reactions

Cardiovascular: Bradycardia, cardiac arrest, circulatory depression, flushing, hypertension, hypotension, palpitations, shock, syncope, tachycardia

Central nervous system: Abnormal dreams, agitation, anxiety, apprehension, ataxia, chills, depression, disorientation, dizziness, drowsiness, dysphoria, euphoria, fatigue, hallucination, headache, increased intracranial pressure, insomnia, nervousness, paresthesia, sedation, shakiness, taste disorder, vertigo
Dermatologic: Diaphoresis, pruritus, skin rash, urticaria
Gastrointestinal: Abdominal cramps, abdominal pain, anorexia, biliary tract spasm, constipation, diarrhea, nausea, pancreatitis, vomiting, xerostomia
Genitourinary: Urinary hesitancy, urinary retention
Hypersensitivity: Hypersensitivity reaction
Neuromuscular & skeletal: Laryngospasm, muscle rigidity, tremor, weakness
Ophthalmic: Blurred vision, diplopia, miosis, nystagmus, visual disturbance
Respiratory: Bronchospasm, dyspnea, respiratory arrest, respiratory depression
Rare, but important or life-threatening): Hypogonadism (Brennan, 2013; Debono, 2011)

Drug Interactions

Metabolism/Transport Effects Substrate of CYP2D6 (major); **Note:** Assignment of Major/Minor substrate status based on clinically relevant drug interaction potential

Avoid Concomitant Use

Avoid concomitant use of Codeine with any of the following: Azelastine (Nasal); Orphenadrine; Paraldehyde; Thalidomide

Increased Effect/Toxicity

Codeine may increase the levels/effects of: Alcohol (Ethyl); Alvimopan; Azelastine (Nasal); Buprenorphine; CNS Depressants; Desmopressin; Diuretics; Hydrocodone; Methotrimeprazine; Metyrosine; Mirtazapine; Orphenadrine; Paraldehyde; Pramipexole; ROPINIRole; Rotigotine; Selective Serotonin Reuptake Inhibitors; Suvorexant; Thalidomide; Zolpidem

The levels/effects of Codeine may be increased by: Amphetamines; Anticholinergic Agents; Antipsychotic Agents (Phenothiazines); Brimonidine (Topical); Cannabis; Doxylamine; Dronabinol; Droperidol; HydrOXYzine; Kava Kava; Magnesium Sulfate; Methotrimeprazine; Nabilone; Perampanel; Rufinamide; Sodium Oxybate; Somatostatin Analogs; Succinylcholine; Tapentadol; Tetrahydrocannabinol

Decreased Effect

Codeine may decrease the levels/effects of: Pegvisomant

The levels/effects of Codeine may be decreased by: Ammonium Chloride; CYP2D6 Inhibitors (Moderate); CYP2D6 Inhibitors (Strong); Mixed Agonist / Antagonist Opioids; Naltrexone

Storage/Stability Oral solution, tablet: Store at controlled room temperature.

Mechanism of Action Binds to opioid receptors in the CNS, causing inhibition of ascending pain pathways, altering the perception of and response to pain; causes cough suppression by direct central action in the medulla; produces generalized CNS depression

Pharmacodynamics/Kinetics

Onset of action: Oral: Immediate release: 0.5-1 hour
Peak effect: Oral: Immediate release: 1-1.5 hours
Duration: Immediate release: 4-6 hours
Distribution: ~3-6 L/kg
Protein binding: ~7% to 25%
Metabolism: Hepatic via UGT2B7 and UGT2B4 to codeine-6-glucuronide, via CYP2D6 to morphine (active), and via CYP3A4 to norcodeine. Morphine is further metabolized via glucuronidation to morphine-3-glucuronide and morphine-6-glucuronide (active).
Bioavailability: 53%
Half-life elimination: ~3 hours
Time to peak, plasma: Immediate release: 1 hour; Controlled release [Canadian product]: 3.3 hours
Excretion: Urine (~90%, ~10% of the total dose as unchanged drug); feces

Dosage Oral:

Pain management (analgesic): **Note:** These are guidelines and do not represent the maximum doses that may be required in all patients. Doses should be titrated to pain relief/prevention.

Children (off-label use): Immediate release (tablet, oral solution): Initial: 0.5-1 mg/kg/dose every 4 hours as needed; maximum: 60 mg/dose (American Pain Society, 2008)

Adults:

Immediate release (tablet, oral solution): Initial: 15-60 mg every 4 hours as needed; maximum total daily dose: 360 mg/day; patients with prior opioid exposure may require higher initial doses. **Note:** The American Pain Society recommends an initial dose of 30-60 mg for adults with moderate pain (American Pain Society, 2008).

Controlled release: Codeine Contin [Canadian product]: **Note:** Titrate at intervals of ≥48 hours until adequate analgesia has been achieved. Daily doses >600 mg/day should not be used; patients requiring higher doses should be switched to an opioid approved for use in severe pain. In patients who receive both Codeine Contin and an immediate release or combination codeine product for breakthrough pain, the rescue dose of the immediate release codeine product should be ≤12.5% of the total daily Codeine Contin dose.

Opioid-naive patients: Initial: 50 mg every 12 hours

Conversion from immediate release codeine preparations: Immediate release codeine preparations contain ~75% codeine base. Therefore, patients who are switching from immediate release codeine preparations may be transferred to a ~25% lower total daily dose of Codeine Contin, equally divided into 2 daily doses.

Conversion from a combination codeine product (eg, codeine with acetaminophen ***or*** *aspirin):* See table:

Number of 30 mg Codeine Combination Tablets Daily	Initial Dose of Codeine Contin	Maintenance Dose of Codeine Contin
≤6	50 mg every 12 h	100 mg every 12 h
7-9	100 mg every 12 h	150 mg every 12 h
10-12	150 mg every 12 h	200 mg every 12 h
>12	200 mg every 12 h	200-300 every 12 h (maximum: 300 mg every 12 h)

Conversion from another opioid analgesic: Using the patient's current opioid dose, calculate an equivalent daily dose of immediate release codeine. A ~25% lower dose of Codeine Contin should then be initiated, equally divided into 2 daily doses.

Discontinuation of therapy: **Note:** Gradual dose reduction is recommended if clinically appropriate. Initially reduce the total daily dose by 50% and administer equally divided into 2 daily doses for 2 days followed by a 25% reduction every 2 days thereafter.

Treatment of cough (off-label use): Adults: Reported doses vary; range: 7.5-120 mg/day as a single dose or in divided doses (Bolser, 2006; Smith, 2010); **Note:** The American College of Chest Physicians does not recommend the routine use of codeine as an antitussive in patients with upper respiratory infections (Bolser, 2006).

Dosing adjustment in renal impairment:

Manufacturer's recommendations: Clearance may be reduced; active metabolites may accumulate. Initiate at lower doses or longer dosing intervals followed by careful titration.

Alternate recommendations: The following guidelines have been used by some clinicians (Aronoff, 2007):

CrCl 10-50 mL/minute: Administer 75% of dose

CrCl <10 mL/minute: Administer 50% of dose

Dosing adjustment in hepatic impairment: No dosage adjustment provided in manufacturer's labeling (has not been studied); however, initial lower doses or longer dosing intervals followed by careful titration are recommended.

Administration May administer without regard to meals. Take with food or milk to decrease adverse GI effects.

Controlled release tablets: Codeine Contin [Canadian product]: Tablets should be swallowed whole; do not chew, dissolve, or crush. All strengths may be halved, **except** the 50 mg tablets; half tablets should also be swallowed intact.

Monitoring Parameters Pain relief, respiratory and mental status, blood pressure, heart rate; signs or symptoms of hypogonadism or hypoadrenalism (Brennan, 2013)

Reference Range Therapeutic: Not established

Dosage Forms

Solution, Oral:

Generic: 30 mg/5 mL (500 mL)

Tablet, Oral:

Generic: 15 mg, 30 mg, 60 mg

Dosage Forms: Canada

Tablet, controlled release:

Codeine Contin: 50 mg, 100 mg, 150 mg, 200 mg

Extemporaneous Preparations A 3 mg/mL oral suspension may be made with codeine phosphate powder, USP. Add 600 mg of powder to a 400 mL beaker. Add 2.5 mL of Sterile Water for Irrigation, USP, and stir to dissolve the powder. Mix for 10 minutes while adding Ora-Sweet to make 200 mL; transfer to a calibrated bottle. Stable 98 days at room temperature.

Dentinger PJ and Swenson CF, "Stability of Codeine Phosphate in an Extemporaneously Compounded Syrup," *Am J Health Syst Pharm*, 2007, 64(24):2569-73.

◆ **Codeine and Acetaminophen** *see* Acetaminophen and Codeine *on page 36*

◆ **Codeine and Guaifenesin** *see* Guaifenesin and Codeine *on page 987*

◆ **Codeine and Promethazine** *see* Promethazine and Codeine *on page 1725*

◆ **Codeine, Aspirin, and Carisoprodol** *see* Carisoprodol, Aspirin, and Codeine *on page 364*

◆ **Codeine Contin (Can)** *see* Codeine *on page 497*

◆ **Codeine, Doxylamine, and Acetaminophen** *see* Acetaminophen, Codeine, and Doxylamine [CAN/INT] *on page 37*

◆ **Codeine, Guaifenesin, and Pseudoephedrine** *see* Guaifenesin, Pseudoephedrine, and Codeine *on page 989*

◆ **Codeine Phosphate** *see* Codeine *on page 497*

◆ **Codeine, Pseudoephedrine, and Triprolidine** *see* Triprolidine, Pseudoephedrine, and Codeine [CAN/INT] *on page 2105*

◆ **Codeine Sulfate** *see* Codeine *on page 497*

◆ **Codeine, Triprolidine, and Pseudoephedrine** *see* Triprolidine, Pseudoephedrine, and Codeine [CAN/INT] *on page 2105*

◆ **Co Diclo-Miso (Can)** *see* Diclofenac and Misoprostol *on page 621*

◆ **Cod Liver Oil** *see* Vitamin A and Vitamin D (Systemic) *on page 2174*

◆ **Cod Liver Oil** *see* Vitamin A and Vitamin D (Topical) *on page 2174*

◆ **Codulax [OTC] (Can)** *see* Bisacodyl *on page 265*

◆ **CO Escitalopram (Can)** *see* Escitalopram *on page 765*

◆ **CO Etidrocal (Can)** *see* Etidronate and Calcium Carbonate [CAN/INT] *on page 814*

◆ **CO Exemestane (Can)** *see* Exemestane *on page 828*

◆ **CO Famciclovir (Can)** *see* Famciclovir *on page 843*

◆ **Co-Fentanyl (Can)** *see* FentaNYL *on page 857*

◆ **CO Finasteride (Can)** *see* Finasteride *on page 878*

◆ **CO Fluconazole (Can)** *see* Fluconazole *on page 885*

◆ **CO Fluoxetine (Can)** *see* FLUoxetine *on page 899*

◆ **CO Gabapentin (Can)** *see* Gabapentin *on page 943*

◆ **Cogentin** *see* Benztropine *on page 248*

◆ **Colace [OTC]** *see* Docusate *on page 661*

◆ **Colace Clear [OTC]** *see* Docusate *on page 661*

◆ **CO Latanoprost (Can)** *see* Latanoprost *on page 1172*

◆ **Colazal** *see* Balsalazide *on page 226*

◆ **ColBenemid** *see* Colchicine and Probenecid *on page 503*

Colchicine (KOL chi seen)

Brand Names: U.S. Colcrys; Mitigare

Brand Names: Canada Jamp-Colchicine; PMS-Colchicine

Pharmacologic Category Antigout Agent

Use

Familial Mediterranean fever (Colcrys only): Treatment of familial Mediterranean fever in adults and children 4 years and older.

Gout flares: Prophylaxis and the treatment of acute gout flares when taken at the first sign of a flare. **Note:** Mitigare is only approved for prophylaxis of gout flares.

Pregnancy Risk Factor C

Pregnancy Considerations Adverse events were observed in animal reproduction studies. Colchicine crosses the human placenta. Use during pregnancy in the treatment of familial Mediterranean fever has not shown an increase in miscarriage, stillbirth, or teratogenic effects (limited data).

Breast-Feeding Considerations Colchicine enters breast milk; exclusively breast-fed infants are expected to receive <10% of the weight-adjusted maternal dose (limited data). The manufacturer recommends that caution be used if administered to a nursing woman.

Contraindications Concomitant use of a P-glycoprotein (P-gp) or strong CYP3A4 inhibitor in presence of renal or hepatic impairment

Mitigare: Patients with both renal and hepatic impairment.

Canadian labeling: Additional contraindications (not in U.S. labeling): Hypersensitivity to colchicine; serious gastrointestinal, hepatic, renal, and cardiac disease

Warnings/Precautions Hazardous agent - use appropriate precautions for handling and disposal (NIOSH 2014 [group 3]). Myelosuppression (eg, thrombocytopenia, leukopenia, granulocytopenia, pancytopenia) and aplastic anemia have been reported in patients receiving therapeutic doses. Neuromuscular toxicity (including rhabdomyolysis) has been reported in patients receiving therapeutic doses; patients with renal dysfunction and elderly patients are at increased risk. Concomitant use of cyclosporine, diltiazem, verapamil, fibrates, and statins may increase the risk of myopathy. Clearance is decreased in renal or hepatic impairment; monitor closely for adverse effects/toxicity. Dosage adjustments may be required depending on degree of impairment or indication, and may be affected by the use of concurrent medication (CYP3A4 or P-gp inhibitors). Concurrent use of P-gp or strong CYP3A4 inhibitors is contraindicated in renal impairment; fatal toxicity has been reported. Colchicine is not an analgesic and should not be used to treat pain from other causes. Potentially significant interactions may exist, requiring dose or frequency adjustment, additional monitoring, and/or selection of alternative therapy.

Adverse Reactions

Central nervous system: Fatigue, headache

Endocrine & metabolic: Gout

Gastrointestinal: Abdominal cramps, abdominal pain, diarrhea, gastrointestinal disease, nausea, vomiting

Respiratory: Pharyngolaryngeal pain

Rare but important or life-threatening: Alopecia, bone marrow depression, dermatitis, disseminated intravascular coagulation, hepatotoxicity, hypersensitivity reaction, increased creatine phosphokinase, lactose intolerance, myalgia, myasthenia, oligospermia, purpura, rhabdomyolysis, toxic neuromuscular disease

Drug Interactions

Metabolism/Transport Effects Substrate of CYP3A4 (major), P-glycoprotein; **Note:** Assignment of Major/Minor substrate status based on clinically relevant drug interaction potential

Avoid Concomitant Use

Avoid concomitant use of Colchicine with any of the following: Conivaptan; Fusidic Acid (Systemic); Idelalisib

Increased Effect/Toxicity

Colchicine may increase the levels/effects of: HMG-CoA Reductase Inhibitors

The levels/effects of Colchicine may be increased by: Cobicistat; Conivaptan; CYP3A4 Inhibitors (Moderate); CYP3A4 Inhibitors (Strong); Dasatinib; Digoxin; Fibric Acid Derivatives; Fosamprenavir; Fusidic Acid (Systemic); Idelalisib; Luliconazole; Mifepristone; P-glycoprotein/ABCB1 Inhibitors; Stiripentol; Telaprevir; Tipranavir

Decreased Effect

Colchicine may decrease the levels/effects of: Cyanocobalamin; Multivitamins/Fluoride (with ADE); Multivitamins/Minerals (with ADEK, Folate, Iron); Multivitamins/Minerals (with AE, No Iron)

The levels/effects of Colchicine may be decreased by: P-glycoprotein/ABCB1 Inducers

Food Interactions Grapefruit juice may increase colchicine serum concentrations. Management: Administer orally with water and maintain adequate fluid intake. Dose adjustment may be required based on indication if ingesting grapefruit juice. Avoid grapefruit juice with hepatic or renal impairment.

Storage/Stability Store at 20°C to 25°C (68°F to 77°F). Protect from light and moisture.

Mechanism of Action Disrupts cytoskeletal functions by inhibiting β-tubulin polymerization into microtubules, preventing activation, degranulation, and migration of neutrophils associated with mediating some gout symptoms. In familial Mediterranean fever, may interfere with intracellular assembly of the inflammasome complex present in neutrophils and monocytes that mediate activation of interleukin-1β.

Pharmacodynamics/Kinetics

Onset of action: Oral: Pain relief: ~18 to 24 hours

Distribution: Concentrates in leukocytes, kidney, spleen, and liver; does not distribute in heart, skeletal muscle, and brain

V_d: 5 to 8 L/kg

Protein binding: ~39%

Metabolism: Hepatic via CYP3A4; 3 metabolites (2 primary, 1 minor)

Bioavailability: ~45%

Half-life elimination: 27 to 31 hours (multiple oral doses; young, healthy volunteers)

Time to peak, serum: Oral: 0.5 to 3 hours

Excretion: Urine (40% to 65% as unchanged drug); enterohepatic recirculation and biliary excretion also possible

Dosage Oral:

Familial Mediterranean fever (FMF):

U.S. labeling: Colcrys only:

Children:

4 to 6 years: 0.3 to1.8 mg daily in 1 to 2 divided doses

6 to 12 years: 0.9 to 1.8 mg daily in 1 to 2 divided doses

Adolescents >12 years and Adults: 1.2 to 2.4 mg daily in 1 to 2 divided doses. Titration: Increase or decrease dose in 0.3 mg daily increments based on efficacy or adverse effects

Canadian labeling: Adolescents >12 years and Adults: 1.2 to 2.4 mg daily in 1 to 2 divided doses. Titration: Increase or decrease dose in 0.3 mg daily increments based on efficacy or adverse effects; maximum: 2.4 mg daily

Gout:

U.S. labeling:

Flare treatment: Colcrys: Adolescents >16 years and Adults: Initial: 1.2 mg at the first sign of flare, followed in 1 hour with a single dose of 0.6 mg (maximum: 1.8 mg within 1 hour). Patients receiving prophylaxis therapy may receive treatment dosing; wait 12 hours before resuming prophylaxis dose. **Note:** Current FDA-approved dose for gout flare is substantially lower than what has been historically used clinically. Doses larger than the currently recommended dosage for gout flare have not been proven to be more effective.

Prophylaxis: Colcrys (Adolescents >16 years and Adults) and Mitigare (Adults):

0.6 mg once or twice daily; maximum: 1.2 mg daily. The duration of prophylaxis is 6 months **or** 3 months (patients without tophi) to 6 months (≥1 tophi) after achieving target serum uric acid levels (ACR guidelines [Khanna, 2012]).

Canadian labeling: Adults:

Flare treatment: Initial: 1.2 mg at the first sign of flare, followed in 1 hour with a single dose of 0.6 mg (maximum: 1.8 mg within 1 hour). Do not repeat treatment for at least 3 days. Wait at least 12 hours to resume prophylactic dose.

Prophylaxis: 0.6 mg once or twice daily; maximum: 1.2 mg per 24 hours

Pericarditis (acute) (off-label use): Adults: **Note:** Use in combination with high-dose aspirin, ibuprofen, or a glucocorticoid (if intolerance or contraindications to aspirin or ibuprofen exist). Dosage strengths (0.5 mg or 1 mg tablets) are not available in the U.S.:

Patients >70 kg: 0.5 mg twice daily for 3 months (Imazio, 2013)

Patients ≤70 kg or unable to tolerate higher dosing regimen: 0.5 mg once daily for 3 months (Imazio, 2013)

Note: In patients with pericarditis after ST-elevation myocardial infarction (STEMI), the American College of Cardiology Foundation/American Heart Association recommends aspirin as first-line treatment. If unresponsive to aspirin (even with high doses), may then consider the use of colchicine (specific dose not recommended). The use of colchicine in this setting has been extrapolated from other settings. Glucocorticoids and NSAIDs should **not** be used in this setting due to risk of scar thinning and infarct expansion (ACCF/AHA [O'Gara, 2013]).

Pericarditis (recurrent) (off-label use): Adults: **Note:** Use in combination with high-dose aspirin, ibuprofen, or indomethacin. Regimens without a loading dose may improve patient compliance and reduce side effects (Imazio, 2014a). Dosage strengths (0.5 mg or 1 mg tablets) are not available in the U.S.:
Regimens with loading dose:
Patients ≥70 kg: 0.5 to 1 mg every 12 hours for 1 day, followed by 0.25 to 0.5 mg every 12 hours for 6 months (Imazio, 2005a; Imazio, 2011).
Patients <70 kg or unable to tolerate higher dosing regimen: 0.5 mg every 12 hours for 1 day followed by 0.5 mg once daily for 6 months (Imazio, 2005a; Imazio, 2011).
Regimens without loading dose:
Patients >70 kg: 0.5 mg twice daily for 6 months (Imazio, 2014a).
Patients ≤70 kg or unable to tolerate higher dosing regimen: 0.5 mg once daily for 6 months (Imazio, 2014a).

Postpericardiotomy syndrome (prevention): Note: Regimens without a loading dose may improve patient compliance and reduce side effects (Imazio, 2014b). Dosage strengths (0.5 mg or 1 mg tablets) are not available in the U.S.:
Regimens with loading dose:
Patients ≥70 kg: 1 mg twice daily given on post-operative day 3, followed by 0.5 mg twice daily for 1 month (Imazio, 2010).
Patients <70 kg or unable to tolerate higher dosing regimen: 0.5 mg twice daily given on post-operative day 3, followed by 0.5 mg once daily for 1 month (Imazio, 2010).
Regimens without loading dose:
Patients ≥70 kg: 0.5 mg twice daily initiated 48 to 72 hours prior to surgery and continued for 1 month (Imazio, 2014b).
Patients <70 kg: 0.5 mg once daily initiated 48 to 72 hours prior to surgery and continued for 1 month (Imazio, 2014b).

Elderly: Use caution; reduce prophylactic daily dose by 50% in individuals >70 years (Terkeltaub, 2009)

Dosage adjustment for concomitant therapy with CYP3A4 or P-glycoprotein (P-gp) inhibitors: Note: Colcrys labeling recommends dosage adjustments in patients receiving CYP3A4 or P-gp inhibitors up to 14 days prior to initiation of colchicine. Treatment of gout flare with colchicine is not recommended in patients receiving prophylactic colchicine and CYP3A4 inhibitors.
Coadministration of **strong** CYP3A4 inhibitor (eg, atazanavir, clarithromycin, darunavir/ritonavir, indinavir, itraconazole, ketoconazole, lopinavir/ritonavir, nefazodone, nelfinavir, ritonavir, saquinavir, telithromycin, tipranavir/ritonavir):
FMF: Maximum dose: 0.6 mg daily (0.3 mg twice daily)
Gout prophylaxis:
U.S. labeling:
Colcrys:
If original dose is 0.6 mg twice daily, adjust dose to 0.3 mg once daily
If original dose is 0.6 mg once daily, adjust dose to 0.3 mg every other day
Mitigare: Avoid concomitant use; if coadministration is necessary, reduce daily dosage or dose frequency and monitor closely.
Canadian labeling:
If original dose is 0.6 mg twice daily, adjust dose to 0.3 mg once daily
If original dose is 0.6 mg once daily, adjust dose to 0.3 mg every other day
Gout flare treatment:
U.S. labeling: Colcrys: Initial: 0.6 mg, followed in 1 hour by a single dose of 0.3 mg; do not repeat for at least 3 days
Canadian labeling: Initial: 0.6 mg, followed in 1 hour by a single dose of 0.3 mg; do not repeat for at least 3 days
Coadministration of **moderate** CYP3A4 inhibitor (eg, aprepitant, diltiazem, erythromycin, fluconazole, fosamprenavir, grapefruit juice, verapamil):
FMF: Maximum dose: 1.2 mg daily (0.6 mg twice daily)
Gout prophylaxis:
U.S. labeling:
Colcrys:
If original dose is 0.6 mg twice daily, adjust dose to 0.3 mg twice daily **or** 0.6 mg once daily
If original dose is 0.6 mg once daily, adjust dose to 0.3 mg once daily
Mitigare: Avoid concomitant use; if coadministration is necessary, reduce daily dosage or dose frequency and monitor closely.
Canadian labeling:
If original dose is 0.6 mg twice daily, adjust dose to 0.3 mg twice daily **or** 0.6 mg once daily
If original dose is 0.6 mg once daily, adjust dose to 0.3 mg once daily
Gout flare treatment: 1.2 mg as a single dose; do not repeat for at least 3 days
Coadministration of P-gp inhibitor (eg, cyclosporine, ranolazine):
FMF: Maximum dose: 0.6 mg daily (0.3 mg twice daily)
Gout prophylaxis:
U.S. labeling:
Colcrys:
If original dose is 0.6 mg twice daily, adjust dose to 0.3 mg once daily
If original dose is 0.6 mg once daily, adjust dose to 0.3 mg every other day
Mitigare: Avoid concomitant use; if coadministration is necessary, reduce daily dosage or dose frequency and monitor closely.
Canadian labeling:
If original dose is 0.6 mg twice daily, adjust dose to 0.3 mg once daily
If original dose is 0.6 mg once daily, adjust dose to 0.3 mg every other day
Gout flare treatment: Initial: 0.6 mg as a single dose; do not repeat for at least 3 days

Dosage adjustment in renal impairment: Concurrent use of colchicine and P-gp or strong CYP3A4 inhibitors is **contraindicated** in renal impairment. Fatal toxicity has been reported. Use of colchicine to treat gout flares is not recommended in patients with renal impairment receiving prophylactic colchicine.
FMF:
CrCl 30 to 80 mL/minute: Monitor closely for adverse effects; dose reduction may be necessary
CrCl <30 mL/minute: Initial dose: 0.3 mg daily; use caution if dose titrated; monitor for adverse effects
Dialysis: 0.3 mg as a single dose; use caution if dose titrated; dosing can be increased with close monitoring; monitor for adverse effects. Not removed by dialysis.
Gout prophylaxis:
CrCl 30 to 80 mL/minute:
Colcrys: Dosage adjustment not required; monitor closely for adverse effects
Mitigare: There are no dosage adjustments provided in the manufacturer's labeling (has not been studied).

CrCl <30 mL/minute:
Colcrys: Initial dose: 0.3 mg daily; use caution if dose titrated; monitor for adverse effects
Mitigare: There is no specific dosage adjustment provided in the manufacturer's labeling; dosage reduction or alternative therapy should be considered.
Dialysis:
Colcrys: 0.3 mg twice weekly; monitor closely for adverse effects
Mitigare: There are no dosage adjustments provided in the manufacturer's labeling; monitor closely.
Gout flare treatment: Colcrys: **Note:** Treatment of gout flares is not recommended in patients with renal impairment who are receiving colchicine for prophylaxis.
CrCl 30 to 80 mL/minute: Dosage adjustment not required; monitor closely for adverse effects
CrCl <30 mL/minute: Dosage reduction not required but may be considered; treatment course should not be repeated more frequently than every 14 days
Dialysis: 0.6 mg as a single dose; treatment course should not be repeated more frequently than every 14 days. Not removed by dialysis.
Hemodialysis: Avoid chronic use of colchicine.

Dosage adjustment in hepatic impairment: Concurrent use of colchicine and P-gp or strong CYP3A4 inhibitors is **contraindicated** in hepatic impairment. Fatal toxicity has been reported. Treatment of gout flare with colchicine is not recommended in patients with hepatic impairment receiving prophylactic colchicine.
FMF:
Mild to moderate impairment: Use caution; monitor closely for adverse effects
Severe impairment: There is no specific dosage adjustment provided in the manufacturer's labeling; dosage adjustment should be considered.
Gout prophylaxis:
Mild to moderate impairment:
Colcrys: Dosage adjustment not required; monitor closely for adverse effects
Mitigare: There are no dosage adjustments provided in the manufacturer's labeling (has not been studied).
Severe impairment: Colcrys and Mitigare: There is no specific dosage adjustment provided in the manufacturer's labeling; dosage adjustment should be considered.
Gout flare treatment: **Note:** Treatment of gout flares is not recommended in patients with hepatic impairment who are receiving colchicine for prophylaxis.
Mild to moderate impairment: Dosage adjustment not required; monitor closely for adverse effects
Severe impairment: Dosage reduction not required but may be considered; treatment course should not be repeated more frequently than every 14 days

Dietary Considerations May be taken without regard to meals. May need to supplement with vitamin B_{12}. Avoid grapefruit juice.

Administration Administer orally with water and maintain adequate fluid intake. May be administered without regard to meals.

Hazardous agent; use appropriate precautions for handling and disposal (NIOSH 2014 [group 3]).

Monitoring Parameters CBC, renal and hepatic function tests

Additional Information Oral colchicine had been available as an unapproved medication without FDA-approved prescribing information. In August 2009, the FDA approved prescribing information for a brand name colchicine product. The currently approved prescribing information recommends a lower than historically used dosage for the treatment of acute gout. This recommendation is based on data from the AGREE trial. In this trial, low-dose colchicine (1.8 mg total) had similar efficacy to high dose colchicine (4.8 mg total). Additionally, the low dosage regimen was associated with a lower incidence (26% vs 77%) of GI adverse events. Parenteral formulation of colchicine is no longer available in the U.S.; serious life-threatening complications (eg, neutropenia, acute renal failure, thrombocytopenia, heart failure) associated with intravenous colchicine have occurred prior to market withdrawal. The risks associated with oral colchicine are believed to be lower compared to intravenous use.

Dosage Forms
Capsule, Oral:
Mitigare: 0.6 mg
Generic: 0.6 mg
Tablet, Oral:
Colcrys: 0.6 mg
Generic: 0.6 mg

Colchicine and Probenecid
(KOL chi seen & proe BEN e sid)

Index Terms ColBenemid; Probenecid and Colchicine

Pharmacologic Category Anti-inflammatory Agent; Antigout Agent; Uricosuric Agent

Use Treatment of chronic gouty arthritis when complicated by frequent, recurrent acute attacks of gout

Dosage Oral: Adults: One tablet daily for 1 week, then 1 tablet twice daily thereafter
Note: Current prescribing information states a maximum dose of 4 tablets per day; however this exceeds the usual maximum dose of colchicine for gout prophylaxis (1.2 mg per day).

Dosage adjustment in renal impairment: CrCl <30 mL/minute: Probenecid may not be effective in patients with chronic renal insufficiency.
Dosage adjustment in hepatic impairment: No dosage adjustment provided in manufacturer's labeling; use with caution.

Additional Information Complete prescribing information should be consulted for additional detail.

Dosage Forms
Tablet: Colchicine 0.5 mg and probenecid 0.5 g

◆ **Colcrys** *see* Colchicine *on page 500*

◆ **Coldcough PD [DSC]** *see* Dihydrocodeine, Chlorpheniramine, and Phenylephrine *on page 633*

Colesevelam (koh le SEV a lam)

Brand Names: U.S. Welchol
Brand Names: Canada Lodalis
Pharmacologic Category Antilipemic Agent, Bile Acid Sequestrant
Use
Diabetes mellitus, type 2: Improve glycemic control in adults with type 2 diabetes mellitus (noninsulin dependent, NIDDM) in conjunction with diet and exercise
Heterozygous familial hypercholesterolemia: Management of heterozygous familial hypercholesterolemia (heFH) in adolescent patients (males and postmenarcheal females 10-17 years of age) used alone or in combination with a 3-hydroxy-3-methylglutaryl coenzyme A (HMG-CoA) reductase inhibitor when after an adequate trial of dietary therapy patient continues to have low-density lipoprotein-cholesterol (LDL-C) ≥190 mg/dL or LDL-C ≥160 mg/dL with positive family history of premature cardiovascular disease (CVD) or with two or more CVD risk factors.

Hyperlipidemia:

U.S. labeling: Management of elevated LDL-C in adults with primary hyperlipidemia (Fredrickson type IIa) when used alone or in combination with an HMG-CoA reductase inhibitor in conjunction with diet and exercise

Canadian labeling (Lodalis): Adjunct to diet and lifestyle modifications in the management of primary hypercholesterolemia (Fredrickson type IIa) as monotherapy or in combination with an HMG-CoA reductase inhibitor

Limitations of use: Should not be used for the treatment of type 1 diabetes or diabetic ketoacidosis. Colesevelam has not been studied in Fredrickson Type I, III, IV, and V dyslipidemias; type 2 diabetes in combination with a dipeptidyl peptidase 4 inhibitor; pediatric patients with type 2 diabetes; children <10 years of age or in premenarchal girls. No effect on cardiovascular morbidity and mortality has been established. There is no evidence of macrovascular disease risk reduction with colesevelam use.

Pregnancy Risk Factor B

Dosage Oral:

Children 10 to 17 years (males and postmenarchal females): Heterozygous familial hypercholesterolemia: 3.75 g once daily (oral suspension). **Note:** Due to large tablet size, oral suspension is recommended in pediatric patients.

Adults:

U.S. labeling: Hyperlipidemia, type 2 diabetes mellitus:

Once-daily dosing: 3.75 g (oral suspension or 6 tablets)

Twice-daily dosing: 1.875 g (3 tablets)

Canadian labeling: Hyperlipidemia:

Combination therapy: 2.5 to 3.75 g (4 to 6 tablets) daily; maximum dose: 3.75 g (6 tablets) given once daily or 1.875 g (3 tablets) given twice daily

Monotherapy: Initial: 1.875 g (3 tablets) twice daily or 3.75 g (6 tablets) once daily; maximum dose: 4.375 g (7 tablets) daily

Elderly: Refer to adult dosing.

Dosage adjustment in renal impairment: No dosage adjustments necessary; not absorbed from the gastrointestinal tract.

Dosage adjustment in hepatic impairment: No dosage adjustments necessary; not absorbed from the gastrointestinal tract.

Additional Information Complete prescribing information should be consulted for additional detail.

Dosage Forms Considerations

Welchol contains phenylalanine 27 mg per 3.75 gram packet

Dosage Forms

Packet, Oral:

Welchol: 3.75 g (30 ea)

Tablet, Oral:

Welchol: 625 mg

Dosage Forms: Canada

Tablet, oral:

Lodalis: 625 mg

◆ **Colestid** *see* Colestipol *on page 504*

◆ **Colestid Flavored** *see* Colestipol *on page 504*

Colestipol (koe LES ti pole)

Brand Names: U.S. Colestid; Colestid Flavored; Micronized Colestipol HCl

Brand Names: Canada Colestid

Index Terms Colestipol Hydrochloride

Pharmacologic Category Antilipemic Agent, Bile Acid Sequestrant

Use Primary hypercholesterolemia: Adjunctive therapy to diet in patients with primary hypercholesterolemia

Dosage Primary hypercholesterolemia: Adults: Oral:

Granules: Initial: 5 g once or twice daily; increase by 5 g per day at 1- to 2-month intervals. In patients with preexisting constipation, initiate at 5 g once daily for 5 to 7 days, then increase to 5 g twice daily. Maintenance: 5 to 30 g per day, once daily or in divided doses.

Tablets: Initial: 2 g once or twice daily; increase by 2 g once or twice daily at 1- to 2-month intervals. Maintenance: 2 to 16 g per day, once daily or in divided doses.

Dosage adjustment in renal impairment: There are no dosage adjustments provided in the manufacturer's labeling; however, dosage adjustment is unlikely because not absorbed from the gastrointestinal tract.

Dosage adjustment in hepatic impairment: There are no dosage adjustments provided in the manufacturer's labeling; however, dosage adjustment is unlikely because not absorbed from the gastrointestinal tract.

Additional Information Complete prescribing information should be consulted for additional detail.

Dosage Forms Considerations

Colestid tablets contain micronized colestipol. Generic tablets are available in micronized and non-micronized formulations.

Dosage Forms

Granules, Oral:

Colestid: 5 g (300 g, 500 g)

Colestid Flavored: 5 g (450 g)

Generic: 5 g (500 g)

Packet, Oral:

Colestid: 5 g (30 ea, 90 ea)

Colestid Flavored: 5 g (60 ea)

Generic: 5 g (30 ea, 90 ea)

Tablet, Oral:

Colestid: 1 g

Micronized Colestipol HCl: 1 g

Generic: 1 g

◆ **Colestipol Hydrochloride** *see* Colestipol *on page 504*

◆ **CO Lisinopril (Can)** *see* Lisinopril *on page 1226*

Colistimethate (koe lis ti METH ate)

Brand Names: U.S. Coly-Mycin M

Brand Names: Canada Coly-Mycin M

Index Terms Colistimethate Sodium; Colistin Methanesulfonate; Colistin Sulfomethate; Pentasodium Colistin Methanesulfonate; Polymyxin E

Pharmacologic Category Antibiotic, Miscellaneous

Use Treatment of acute or chronic infections due to sensitive strains of certain gram-negative bacilli (particularly *Pseudomonas aeruginosa*) which are resistant to other antibacterials or in patients allergic to other antibacterials

Pregnancy Risk Factor C

Pregnancy Considerations Adverse events have been observed in animal reproduction studies. Colistimethate crosses the placenta in humans.

Breast-Feeding Considerations Colistin (the active form of colistimethate sodium) and colistin sulphate (another form of colistin) are excreted in human milk. The manufacturer recommends caution if giving colistimethate sodium to a breast-feeding woman. Nondose-related effects could include modification of bowel flora.

Contraindications Hypersensitivity to colistimethate, colistin, or any component of the formulation

Warnings/Precautions Use only to prevent or treat infections strongly suspected or proven to be caused by susceptible bacteria to minimize development of bacterial drug resistance. Nephrotoxicity has been reported; use with caution in patients with preexisting renal disease; dosage adjustments may be required. Withhold treatment if signs of renal impairment occur during treatment.

Respiratory arrest has been reported with use; impaired renal function may increase the risk for neuromuscular blockade and apnea. Transient, reversible neurological disturbances (eg, dizziness, numbness, paresthesia, generalized pruritus, slurred speech, tingling, vertigo) may occur. Patients must be cautioned about performing tasks which require mental alertness (eg, operating machinery or driving). Dose reduction may reduce neurologic symptoms; monitor closely. Use of inhaled colistimethate cause bronchoconstriction. Use with caution in patients with hyperactive airways; consider administration of a bronchodilator 15 minutes prior to administration. Colistimethate solutions change to bioactive colistin, a component of which may result in severe pulmonary toxicity. Solutions for inhalation must be mixed immediately prior to administration and used within 24 hours.

Prolonged use may result in fungal or bacterial superinfection, including *C. difficile*-associated diarrhea (CDAD) and pseudomembranous colitis; CDAD has been observed >2 months postantibiotic treatment.

Potentially significant drug-drug interactions may exist, requiring dose or frequency adjustment, additional monitoring, and/or selection of alternative therapy. Use caution when prescribing or dispensing; potential for dosing errors due to lack of standardization in literature when referring to product and dose; colistimethate (inactive prodrug) and colistin base strengths are not interchangeable; verify prescribed dose is expressed in terms of colistin base prior to dispensing.

Adverse Reactions

Central nervous system: Dizziness, headache, oral paresthesia, peripheral paresthesia, slurred speech, vertigo

Dermatologic: Pruritus, skin rash, urticaria

Gastrointestinal: Gastric distress

Genitourinary: Decreased urine output, nephrotoxicity, proteinuria

Miscellaneous: Fever

Neuromuscular & skeletal: Lower extremity weakness

Renal: Increased blood urea nitrogen, increased serum creatinine

Respiratory: Apnea, respiratory distress

Rare but important or life-threatening: Pulmonary toxicity (bronchoconstriction, bronchospasm, chest tightness, respiratory distress, acute respiratory tract failure following inhalation)

Drug Interactions

Metabolism/Transport Effects None known.

Avoid Concomitant Use

Avoid concomitant use of Colistimethate with any of the following: Bacitracin (Systemic); BCG

Increased Effect/Toxicity

Colistimethate may increase the levels/effects of: Bacitracin (Systemic); Neuromuscular-Blocking Agents

The levels/effects of Colistimethate may be increased by: Aminoglycosides; Amphotericin B; Capreomycin; Polymyxin B; Vancomycin

Decreased Effect

Colistimethate may decrease the levels/effects of: BCG; Sodium Picosulfate; Typhoid Vaccine

Preparation for Administration

IV or IM use: Reconstitute each vial containing 150 mg of colistin base activity with 2 mL of SWFI resulting in a concentration of 75 mg colistin base/mL; swirl gently to avoid frothing. May further dilute in D_5W or NS for IV infusion.

Intrathecal/intraventricular use (off-label route): Reconstitute with preservative-free diluent (SWFI or NS) only; use promptly after preparation; discard unused portion of vial (Quinn, 2005).

Nebulized inhalation (off-label route): Reconstitute vial containing 150 mg of colistin base activity with 2 mL SWFI, resulting in a concentration of 75 mg colistin base activity/mL; further dilute dose to a total volume of 3-4 mL in NS (Michalopoulos, 2008); alternatively, further dilute 150 mg colistin base to a total volume of 10 mL in SWFI (concentration: 15 mg colistin base activity/mL) (Lu, 2012). Storing for >24 hours may increase the risk for potential lung toxicity; preparation immediately prior to administration is recommended (FDA, 2007; Le, 2010, Wallace, 2008).

Storage/Stability Store intact vials (prior to reconstitution) at 20°C to 25°C (68°F to 77°F); excursions permitted to 15°C to 30°C (59°F to 86°F). Reconstituted vials may be refrigerated at 2°C to 8°C (36°F to 46°F) or stored at 20°C to 25°C (68°F to 77°F) for up to 7 days. Solutions for infusion should be freshly prepared; do not use beyond 24 hours.

Mechanism of Action Colistimethate (or the sodium salt [colistimethate sodium]) is the inactive prodrug which is hydrolyzed to colistin, which acts as a cationic detergent and damages the bacterial cytoplasmic membrane causing leaking of intracellular substances and cell death

Pharmacodynamics/Kinetics

Distribution: Widely, except for CNS, synovial, pleural, and pericardial fluids

Metabolism: Colistimethate sodium (inactive prodrug) is hydrolyzed to colistin (active form)

Half-life elimination: IM, IV: 2-3 hours; Anuria: ≤2-3 days

Time to peak: IV: 10 minutes

Excretion: Primarily urine (as unchanged drug)

Dosage Note: Dosage expressed in terms of **colistin base**.

Susceptible infections: Children and Adults: IM, IV: 2.5-5 mg/kg/day in 2-4 divided doses; maximum: 5 mg/kg/day

Cystic fibrosis: Adults: IV: 3 mg/kg/day in 3 divided doses (Young, 2013)

Bronchiectasis, pulmonary colonization/infection with susceptible organisms in patients with cystic fibrosis and noncystic fibrosis (off-label use/route): Adults: Inhalation: 30-150 mg in NS (3-4 mL total) via nebulizer 1-3 times daily (maximum dose: 150 mg 2 times daily) (Le, 2010; Sabuda, 2008; Steinfort, 2007). **Note:** Lower doses have been used in noncystic fibrosis patients with bronchiectasis (Steinfort, 2007); the most commonly used dose is 150 mg twice daily (Le, 2010).

Meningitis (susceptible gram-negative organisms): Adults: Intrathecal/Intraventricular (off-label route): 10 mg/day (IDSA, 2004); **Note:** Dosage in clinical reports has ranged from 1.6-20 mg/day in 1 or 2 divided doses (maximum single dose: 10 mg) (administered with concomitant systemic antimicrobial therapy) (Guardado, 2008; Kasiakou, 2005; Katragkou, 2005)

Ventilator-associated pneumonia due to multidrug-resistant *Pseudomonas aeruginosa* or *Acinetobacter baumannii* (off-label use/route): Adults: Nebulization (via ventilator circuit): 150 mg every 8 hours delivered over 60 minutes for 14 days or until successful wean from mechanical ventilation (treatment duration range: 7-19 days) (Lu, 2012).

Dosage adjustment for toxicity:

CNS toxicity: Dose reduction may reduce neurologic symptoms.

Nephrotoxicity: Withhold treatment if signs of renal impairment occur during treatment.

Dosage adjustment in obesity: Doses should be based on ideal body weight in obese patients.

Dosage adjustment in renal impairment: IM, IV: Adults:

CrCl ≥80 mL/minute: No dosage adjustment necessary; maximum: 5 mg/kg/day

CrCl 50-79 mL/minute: 2.5-3.8 mg/kg/day in 2 divided doses

CrCl 30-49 mL/minute: 2.5 mg/kg/day once daily or in 2 divided doses

CrCl 10-29 mL/minute: 1.5 mg/kg every 36 hours

Intermittent hemodialysis (IHD) (administer after hemodialysis on dialysis days): 1.5 mg/kg every 24-48 hours (Heintz, 2009). **Note:** Dosing dependent on the assumption of 3 times/week, complete IHD sessions.

Continuous renal replacement therapy (CRRT) (Heintz, 2009; Trotman, 2005): Drug clearance is highly dependent on the method of renal replacement, filter type, and flow rate. Appropriate dosing requires close monitoring of pharmacologic response, signs of adverse reactions due to drug accumulation, as well as drug concentrations in relation to target trough (if appropriate). The following are general recommendations only (based on dialysate flow/ultrafiltration rates of 1-2 L/hour and minimal residual renal function) and should not supersede clinical judgment:

CVVH/CVVHD/CVVHDF: 2.5 mg/kg every 24-48 hours (frequency dependent upon site or severity of infection or susceptibility of pathogen)

Note: A single case report has demonstrated that the use of 2.5 mg/kg every 48 hours with a dialysate flow rate of 1 L/hour may be inadequate and that dosing every 24 hours was well-tolerated. Based on pharmacokinetic analysis, the authors recommend dosing as frequent as every 12 hours in patients receiving CVVHDF (Li, 2005).

Dosage adjustment in hepatic impairment: No dosage adjustment provided in manufacturer's labeling.

Dosing in obesity: Doses should be based on ideal body weight in obese patients.

Administration

Parenteral: Administer by IM, direct IV injection over 3-5 minutes, intermittent infusion over 30 minutes (Beringer, 2001; Conway, 1997), or by continuous IV infusion. For continuous IV infusion, one-half of the total daily dose is administered by direct IV injection over 3-5 minutes followed 1-2 hours later by the remaining one-half of the total daily dose diluted in a compatible IV solution infused over 22-23 hours. The final concentration for continuous infusion administration should be based on the patient's fluid needs; infusion should be completed within 24 hours of preparation.

Inhalation (off-label route): Administer solution via nebulizer promptly following preparation to decrease possibility of high concentrations of colistin from forming which may lead to potentially life-threatening lung toxicity. Consider use of a bronchodilator (eg, albuterol) within 15 minutes prior to administration (Le, 2010). If patient is on a ventilator, place medicine in a T-piece at the midinspiratory circuit of the ventilator. One study in adult patients with VAP administered colistimethate (150 mg colistin base/10 mL SWFI) over 60 minutes (Lu, 2012).

Note: A case report of fatal lung toxicity implicated *in vitro* colistin formation from an inhalation solution as a potential etiology, but data regarding the concentration, formulation and storage of the inhaled colistin administered to the patient were not reported (FDA, 2007; McCoy, 2007; Wallace, 2008). An acceptable limit of *in vitro* colistin formation to prevent potential toxicity is unknown. Limited stability data are available regarding the storage of colistin solution for inhaled administration (Healan, 2012; Wallace, 2008). Storing for >24 hours may increase the risk for potential lung toxicity; preparation immediately prior to administration is recommended (FDA, 2007; Le, 2010, Wallace, 2008).

Intrathecal/intraventricular (off-label route): Administer only preservative-free solutions via intrathecal/intraventricular routes. Administer promptly after preparation. Discard unused portion of vial.

Monitoring Parameters Serum creatinine, BUN; urine output; signs of neurotoxicity; signs of bronchospasm (inhalation [off-label route])

Additional Information

Colistimethate sodium 1 mg is equivalent to ~12,500 units of **colistimethate sodium**

Colistimethate sodium ~2.67 mg is equivalent to 1 mg of **colistin base**

Dosage Forms

Solution Reconstituted, Injection:

Coly-Mycin M: 150 mg (1 ea)

Generic: 150 mg (1 ea)

Solution Reconstituted, Injection [preservative free]:

Generic: 150 mg (1 ea)

◆ **Colistimethate Sodium** *see* Colistimethate *on page 504*

◆ **Colistin, Hydrocortisone, Neomycin, and Thonzonium** *see* Neomycin, Colistin, Hydrocortisone, and Thonzonium *on page 1437*

◆ **Colistin Methanesulfonate** *see* Colistimethate *on page 504*

◆ **Colistin Sulfomethate** *see* Colistimethate *on page 504*

Collagenase (Systemic) (KOL la je nase)

Brand Names: U.S. Xiaflex

Index Terms Collagenase Clostridium Histolyticum

Pharmacologic Category Enzyme

Use

Dupuytren contracture: Treatment of adults with Dupuytren contracture with a palpable cord

Peyronie disease: Treatment of adult men with Peyronie disease with a palpable plaque and curvature deformity of at least 30 degrees at the start of therapy

Pregnancy Risk Factor B

Dosage

Dupuytren contracture: Adults: Intralesional: Inject 0.58 mg per cord affecting a metacarpophalangeal (MP) joint or a proximal interphalangeal (PIP) joint. If contracture persists, finger extension procedure should be performed 24 to 72 hours following injection to facilitate cord disruption. If MP or PIP contracture remains, may reinject cord with a single dose of 0.58 mg 4 weeks following initial injection; injections and finger extension procedures may be administered up to 3 times per cord separated by ~4 week intervals. **Note:** Up to 2 injections per hand may be used during a treatment; 2 palpable cords affecting 2 joints or 1 palpable cord affecting 2 joints in the same finger may be injected at 2 locations during a treatment. Other palpable cords with contractures of MP or PIP joints may be injected at other treatment visits ~4 weeks apart.

Peyronie disease: Adults: Males: Intralesional: Inject 0.58 mg into a Peyronie plaque; repeat injection 1 to 3 days later. A penile modeling procedure should be performed 1 to 3 days after the second injection. Administer a second treatment cycle (two 0.58 mg injections 1 to 3 days apart, followed by penile modeling procedure 1 to 3 days after second injection) in ~6 weeks if needed (maximum, 4 treatment cycles [a total of 8 injection procedures and 4 penile modeling procedures]); subsequent treatment cycles should not be administered if the curvature deformity is <15 degrees after a treatment cycle or health care provider determines further treatment is not indicated. The safety of more than 1 treatment course (ie, 4 treatment cycles) is not known. **Note:** If more than 1 plaque is present, inject into the plaque causing the curvature deformity.

Dosage adjustment in renal impairment: There are no dosage adjustments provided in the manufacturer's labeling. However, dosage adjustment unlikely due to low systemic absorption.

Dosage adjustment in hepatic impairment: There are no dosage adjustments provided in the manufacturer's labeling. However, dosage adjustment unlikely due to low systemic absorption.

Additional Information Complete prescribing information should be consulted for additional detail.

Dosage Forms

Solution Reconstituted, Injection:

Xiaflex: 0.9 mg (1 ea)

Collagenase (Topical) (KOL la je nase)

Brand Names: U.S. Santyl

Brand Names: Canada Santyl®

Pharmacologic Category Enzyme, Topical Debridement

Use Promotes debridement of necrotic tissue in dermal ulcers and severe burns

Dosage Topical: Apply once daily (or more frequently if the dressing becomes soiled)

Additional Information Complete prescribing information should be consulted for additional detail.

Dosage Forms

Ointment, External:

Santyl: 250 units/g (30 g, 90 g)

- ◆ **Collagenase Clostridium Histolyticum** *see* Collagenase (Systemic) *on page 506*
- ◆ **Colocort** *see* Hydrocortisone (Topical) *on page 1014*
- ◆ **CO Lovastatin (Can)** *see* Lovastatin *on page 1252*
- ◆ **Coly-Mycin M** *see* Colistimethate *on page 504*
- ◆ **Coly-Mycin® S** *see* Neomycin, Colistin, Hydrocortisone, and Thonzonium *on page 1437*
- ◆ **Colyte** *see* Polyethylene Glycol-Electrolyte Solution *on page 1674*
- ◆ **Combantrin (Can)** *see* Pyrantel Pamoate *on page 1744*
- ◆ **Combigan** *see* Brimonidine and Timolol *on page 288*
- ◆ **CombiPatch** *see* Estradiol and Norethindrone *on page 781*
- ◆ **Combivent® [DSC]** *see* Ipratropium and Albuterol *on page 1109*
- ◆ **Combivent® Respimat®** *see* Ipratropium and Albuterol *on page 1109*
- ◆ **Combivent Respimat (Can)** *see* Ipratropium and Albuterol *on page 1109*
- ◆ **Combivent UDV (Can)** *see* Ipratropium and Albuterol *on page 1109*
- ◆ **Combivir** *see* Lamivudine and Zidovudine *on page 1160*
- ◆ **CO Meloxicam (Can)** *see* Meloxicam *on page 1283*
- ◆ **CO Metformin (Can)** *see* MetFORMIN *on page 1307*
- ◆ **Compazine** *see* Prochlorperazine *on page 1718*
- ◆ **Complera** *see* Emtricitabine, Rilpivirine, and Tenofovir *on page 722*
- ◆ **Complete Allergy Medication [OTC]** *see* DiphenhydrAMINE (Systemic) *on page 641*
- ◆ **Complete Allergy Relief [OTC]** *see* DiphenhydrAMINE (Systemic) *on page 641*
- ◆ **Compound E** *see* Cortisone *on page 510*
- ◆ **Compound F** *see* Hydrocortisone (Systemic) *on page 1013*
- ◆ **Compound F** *see* Hydrocortisone (Topical) *on page 1014*
- ◆ **Compound S** *see* Zidovudine *on page 2196*
- ◆ **Compound S, Abacavir, and Lamivudine** *see* Abacavir, Lamivudine, and Zidovudine *on page 22*
- ◆ **Compro** *see* Prochlorperazine *on page 1718*
- ◆ **Comtan** *see* Entacapone *on page 730*
- ◆ **Comvax** *see* *Haemophilus* b Conjugate and Hepatitis B Vaccine *on page 991*
- ◆ **CO Mycophenolate (Can)** *see* Mycophenolate *on page 1405*
- ◆ **Concerta** *see* Methylphenidate *on page 1336*
- ◆ **Conestat Alfa** *see* C1 Inhibitor (Recombinant) *on page 316*
- ◆ **Confidex** *see* Prothrombin Complex Concentrate (Human) [(Factors II, VII, IX, X), Protein C, and Protein S] *on page 1738*
- ◆ **Congest (Can)** *see* Estrogens (Conjugated/Equine, Systemic) *on page 787*
- ◆ **Congestac® [OTC]** *see* Guaifenesin and Pseudoephedrine *on page 989*

Conivaptan (koe NYE vap tan)

Brand Names: U.S. Vaprisol

Index Terms Conivaptan Hydrochloride; YM087

Pharmacologic Category Vasopressin Antagonist

Use Treatment of euvolemic and hypervolemic hyponatremia in hospitalized patients

Pregnancy Risk Factor C

Pregnancy Considerations Adverse events were observed in animal reproduction studies.

Breast-Feeding Considerations It is not known if conivaptan is excreted in breast milk. Due to the potential for serious adverse reactions in the nursing infant, a decision should be made whether to discontinue nursing or to discontinue the drug, taking into account the importance of treatment to the mother.

Contraindications Hypersensitivity to conivaptan, corn or corn products, or any component of the formulation; use in hypovolemic hyponatremia; concurrent use with strong CYP3A4 inhibitors (eg, ketoconazole, itraconazole, ritonavir, indinavir, and clarithromycin); anuria

Warnings/Precautions Monitor closely for rate of serum sodium increase and neurological status; overly rapid serum sodium correction (>12 mEq/L/24 hours) can lead to seizures, permanent neurological damage, coma, or death. Discontinue use if rate of serum sodium increase is undesirable; may reinitiate infusion (at reduced dose) if hyponatremia persists in the absence of neurological symptoms typically associated with rapid sodium rise. Of note, raising serum sodium concentrations with conivaptan has not demonstrated symptomatic benefit. Discontinue if hypovolemia or hypotension occurs. Safety and efficacy in patients with hypervolemic hyponatremia associated with heart failure have not been established. Use in small numbers of hypervolemic, hyponatremic heart failure patients led to increased adverse events. In other heart failure studies, conivaptan did not show significant improvements in outcomes over placebo. Coadministration with digoxin may increase digoxin concentrations; monitor digoxin concentrations. Use with caution in patients with hepatic impairment; dosage adjustment may be required. May cause injection-site reactions.

Adverse Reactions

Cardiovascular: Atrial fibrillation, ECG abnormality, hypertension, hypotension (including orthostatic), peripheral edema, phlebitis

Central nervous system: Confusion, fever, headache, insomnia, pain

Dermatologic: Erythema, pruritus

Endocrine & metabolic: Hyper-/hypoglycemia, hypokalemia, hypomagnesemia, hyponatremia

Gastrointestinal: Constipation, dehydration, diarrhea, dry mouth, nausea, oral candidiasis, vomiting

Genitourinary: Urinary tract infection

Hematologic: Anemia

Local: Injection site reactions (including pain, erythema, phlebitis, swelling)

Renal: Hematuria, polyuria

Respiratory: Pharyngolaryngeal pain, pneumonia

Miscellaneous: Thirst

Rare but important or life-threatening: Atrial arrhythmias, sepsis

Drug Interactions

Metabolism/Transport Effects Substrate of CYP3A4 (major); **Note:** Assignment of Major/Minor substrate status based on clinically relevant drug interaction potential; **Inhibits** CYP3A4 (strong)

Avoid Concomitant Use

Avoid concomitant use of Conivaptan with any of the following: Ado-Trastuzumab Emtansine; Alfuzosin; Antifungal Agents (Azole Derivatives, Systemic); Apixaban; Astemizole; Avanafil; Axitinib; Bosutinib; Cabozantinib; Ceritinib; Crizotinib; CYP3A4 Inhibitors (Strong); CYP3A4 Substrates; Dapoxetine; Dronedarone; Eplerenone; Everolimus; Fusidic Acid (Systemic); Halofantrine; Ibrutinib; Idelalisib; Irinotecan; Ivabradine; Lapatinib; Lercanidipine; Lomitapide; Lovastatin; Lurasidone; Macitentan; Naloxegol; Nilotinib; Nisoldipine; Olaparib; Pimozide; Ranolazine; Red Yeast Rice; Regorafenib; Rivaroxaban; Salmeterol; Silodosin; Simeprevir; Simvastatin; Suvorexant; Tamsulosin; Terfenadine; Ticagrelor; Tolvaptan; Toremifene; Trabectedin; Ulipristal; Vemurafenib; VinCRIStine (Liposomal); Vorapaxar

Increased Effect/Toxicity

Conivaptan may increase the levels/effects of: Ado-Trastuzumab Emtansine; Alfuzosin; Almotriptan; Alosetron; Apixaban; Astemizole; Avanafil; Axitinib; Bedaquiline; Bortezomib; Bosentan; Bosutinib; Brentuximab Vedotin; Brinzolamide; Budesonide (Nasal); Cabozantinib; Cannabis; Ceritinib; Corticosteroids (Orally Inhaled); Corticosteroids (Systemic); Crizotinib; CYP3A4 Substrates; Dapoxetine; Dienogest; Digoxin; Dofetilide; Dronabinol; Dronedarone; Dutasteride; Eplerenone; Everolimus; Fluticasone (Nasal); Halofantrine; Ibrutinib; Iloperidone; Imatinib; Imidafenacin; Irinotecan; Ivabradine; Lacosamide; Lapatinib; Lercanidipine; Levobupivacaine; Lomitapide; Lovastatin; Lumefantrine; Lurasidone; Macitentan; MethylPREDNISolone; Naloxegol; Nilotinib; Nisoldipine; Olaparib; Ospemifene; Paricalcitol; Pimecrolimus; Pimozide; PONATinib; Pranlukast; PrednisoLONE (Systemic); PredniSONE; Propafenone; Ranolazine; Red Yeast Rice; Regorafenib; Repaglinide; Retapamulin; Rilpivirine; Rivaroxaban; RomiDEPsin; Salmeterol; Silodosin; Simeprevir; Simvastatin; SORAfenib; Suvorexant; Tamsulosin; Terfenadine; Tetrahydrocannabinol; Ticagrelor; Tolvaptan; Toremifene; Trabectedin; Ulipristal; Vemurafenib; Vilazodone; VinCRIStine (Liposomal); Vorapaxar; Zuclopenthixol

The levels/effects of Conivaptan may be increased by: Antifungal Agents (Azole Derivatives, Systemic); CYP3A4 Inhibitors (Moderate); CYP3A4 Inhibitors (Strong); Fusidic Acid (Systemic); Idelalisib; Luliconazole; Netupitant

Decreased Effect

Conivaptan may decrease the levels/effects of: Ifosfamide; Prasugrel; Ticagrelor

The levels/effects of Conivaptan may be decreased by: Bosentan; CYP3A4 Inducers (Moderate); CYP3A4 Inducers (Strong); Deferasirox; Mitotane; Siltuximab; St Johns Wort; Tocilizumab

Storage/Stability Store at 25°C (77°F); brief excursions permitted up to 40°C (104°F). Protect from light and freezing. Do not remove protective overwrap until ready for use.

Mechanism of Action Conivaptan is an arginine vasopressin (AVP) receptor antagonist with affinity for AVP receptor subtypes V_{1A} and V_2. The antidiuretic action of AVP is mediated through activation of the V_2 receptor, which functions to regulate water and electrolyte balance at the level of the collecting ducts in the kidney. Serum levels of AVP are commonly elevated in euvolemic or hypervolemic hyponatremia, which results in the dilution of serum sodium and the relative hyponatremic state. Antagonism of the V_2 receptor by conivaptan promotes the excretion of free water (without loss of serum electrolytes) resulting in net fluid loss, increased urine output, decreased urine osmolality, and subsequent restoration of normal serum sodium concentrations.

Pharmacodynamics/Kinetics

Protein binding: 99%

Metabolism: Hepatic via CYP3A4 to four minimally-active metabolites

Half-life elimination: ~5-8 hours

Excretion: Feces (83%); urine (12%, primarily as metabolites)

Dosage IV: Adults: 20 mg infused over 30 minutes as a loading dose, followed by a continuous infusion of 20 mg over 24 hours (0.83 mg/hour) for 2-4 days; may increase to a maximum dose of 40 mg over 24 hours (1.7 mg/hour) if serum sodium not rising sufficiently; total duration of therapy not to exceed 4 days. **Note:** If patient requires 40 mg/24 hours, may administer two consecutive 20 mg/100 mL premixed solutions over 24 hours (ie, 20 mg over 12 hours followed by 20 mg over 12 hours).

Dosing adjustment in renal impairment:

CrCl ≥30 mL/minute: No dosage adjustment necessary.

CrCl <30 mL/minute: Use not recommended; clinical response reduced; contraindicated in anuria (no benefit expected).

Dosing adjustment in hepatic impairment:

Mild impairment: No dosage adjustment necessary.

Moderate impairment: 10 mg infused over 30 minutes as a loading dose, followed by a continuous infusion of 10 mg over 24 hours (0.42 mg/hour) for 2-4 days; may increase to a maximum dose of 20 mg over 24 hours (0.83 mg/hour) if serum sodium not rising sufficiently; total duration of therapy not to exceed 4 days.

Severe impairment: Use not recommended (not studied).

Usual Infusion Concentrations: Adult Note: Premixed solutions available.

IV infusion: 20 mg in 100 mL (concentration: 0.2 mg/mL) of D_5W

Administration For intravenous use only; infuse into large veins and change infusion site every 24 hours to minimize vascular irritation. Do not administer with any other product in the same intravenous line or container.

Monitoring Parameters Rate of serum sodium increase, blood pressure, volume status, urine output

Dosage Forms

Solution, Intravenous:

Vaprisol: 20 mg (100 mL)

◆ **Conivaptan Hydrochloride** *see* Conivaptan *on page 507*

◆ **Conjugated Estrogen** *see* Estrogens (Conjugated/Equine, Systemic) *on page 787*

◆ **Conjugated Estrogen** *see* Estrogens (Conjugated/Equine, Topical) *on page 790*

◆ **CO Norfloxacin (Can)** *see* Norfloxacin *on page 1475*

◆ **Constella (Can)** *see* Linaclotide *on page 1215*

◆ **Constulose** *see* Lactulose *on page 1156*

- ◆ **Contac® Cold 12 Hour Relief Non Drowsy (Can)** *see* Pseudoephedrine *on page 1742*
- ◆ **Contac® Cold-Chest Congestion, Non Drowsy, Regular Strength (Can)** *see* Guaifenesin and Pseudoephedrine *on page 989*
- ◆ **Continuous Renal Replacement Therapy** *see* Electrolyte Solution, Renal Replacement *on page 710*
- ◆ **Contrave** *see* Naltrexone and Bupropion *on page 1423*
- ◆ **ControlRx** *see* Fluoride *on page 895*
- ◆ **ControlRx Multi** *see* Fluoride *on page 895*
- ◆ **Conventional Amphotericin B** *see* Amphotericin B (Conventional) *on page 136*
- ◆ **Conventional Cytarabine** *see* Cytarabine (Conventional) *on page 535*
- ◆ **Conventional Daunomycin** *see* DAUNOrubicin (Conventional) *on page 577*
- ◆ **Conventional Doxorubicin** *see* DOXOrubicin (Conventional) *on page 679*
- ◆ **Conventional Paclitaxel** *see* PACLitaxel (Conventional) *on page 1550*
- ◆ **Conventional Trastuzumab** *see* Trastuzumab *on page 2085*
- ◆ **Conventional Vincristine** *see* VinCRIStine *on page 2163*
- ◆ **ConZip** *see* TraMADol *on page 2074*
- ◆ **CO Olanzapine ODT (Can)** *see* OLANZapine *on page 1491*
- ◆ **CO Olopatadine (Can)** *see* Olopatadine (Ophthalmic) *on page 1500*
- ◆ **CO Ondansetron (Can)** *see* Ondansetron *on page 1513*
- ◆ **CO Oxycodone CR (Can)** *see* OxyCODONE *on page 1538*
- ◆ **CO Paroxetine (Can)** *see* PARoxetine *on page 1579*
- ◆ **Copaxone** *see* Glatiramer Acetate *on page 963*
- ◆ **Copegus** *see* Ribavirin *on page 1797*
- ◆ **CO Pioglitazone (Can)** *see* Pioglitazone *on page 1654*
- ◆ **Copolymer-1** *see* Glatiramer Acetate *on page 963*

Copper (KOP er)

Brand Names: U.S. Coppermin [OTC]; Cu-5 [OTC]

Index Terms Cupric Chloride; Cupric Chloride Dihydrate

Pharmacologic Category Trace Element, Parenteral

Use Supplement to intravenous solutions given for total parenteral nutrition (TPN) to maintain copper serum levels and to prevent depletion of endogenous stores and subsequent deficiency symptoms

Pregnancy Risk Factor C

Dosage IV (incorporated into parenteral nutrition):

Infants and Children: 20 mcg/kg/day

Adults: 0.3-0.5 mg/day (ASPEN, 2002); 0.5-1.5 mg/day (manufacturer's product labeling)

High output intestinal fistula: Some clinicians may use twice the recommended daily allowance (ASPEN, 2002)

Elderly: Use caution. Start at the low end of dosing range.

Dosage adjustment in renal impairment: Use caution; contains aluminum

Dosage adjustment in hepatic impairment: Use caution; dosage reduction may be required

Additional Information Complete prescribing information should be consulted for additional detail.

Dosage Forms

Capsule, Oral [preservative free]:

Cu-5 [OTC]: 5 mg

Solution, Intravenous:

Generic: 0.4 mg/mL (10 mL)

Tablet, Oral:

Coppermin [OTC]: 5 mg

- ◆ **Coppermin [OTC]** *see* Copper *on page 509*
- ◆ **CO Pregabalin (Can)** *see* Pregabalin *on page 1710*
- ◆ **CO Quetiapine (Can)** *see* QUEtiapine *on page 1751*
- ◆ **Cordarone** *see* Amiodarone *on page 114*
- ◆ **Cordran** *see* Flurandrenolide *on page 906*
- ◆ **Coreg** *see* Carvedilol *on page 367*
- ◆ **Coreg CR** *see* Carvedilol *on page 367*
- ◆ **CO-Repaglinide (Can)** *see* Repaglinide *on page 1791*
- ◆ **Corfen-DM [OTC]** *see* Chlorpheniramine, Phenylephrine, and Dextromethorphan *on page 428*
- ◆ **Corgard** *see* Nadolol *on page 1411*
- ◆ **Coricidin HBP Chest Congestion and Cough [OTC]** *see* Guaifenesin and Dextromethorphan *on page 987*
- ◆ **Coricidin HBP® Cold and Flu [OTC]** *see* Chlorpheniramine and Acetaminophen *on page 426*
- ◆ **Coricidin® HBP Cough & Cold [OTC]** *see* Dextromethorphan and Chlorpheniramine *on page 610*
- ◆ **Corifact®** *see* Factor XIII Concentrate (Human) *on page 843*
- ◆ **Corifact** *see* Factor XIII Concentrate (Human) *on page 843*
- ◆ **Corlopam** *see* Fenoldopam *on page 856*
- ◆ **Cormax Scalp Application** *see* Clobetasol *on page 468*
- ◆ **CO Rosuvastatin (Can)** *see* Rosuvastatin *on page 1848*
- ◆ **Correct [OTC]** *see* Bisacodyl *on page 265*
- ◆ **Correctol Stool Softener [OTC] (Can)** *see* Docusate *on page 661*
- ◆ **Cortaid Maximum Strength [OTC]** *see* Hydrocortisone (Topical) *on page 1014*
- ◆ **CortAlo** *see* Hydrocortisone (Topical) *on page 1014*
- ◆ **Cortamed® (Can)** *see* Hydrocortisone (Topical) *on page 1014*
- ◆ **Cortef** *see* Hydrocortisone (Systemic) *on page 1013*
- ◆ **Cortenema** *see* Hydrocortisone (Topical) *on page 1014*
- ◆ **Cortenema® (Can)** *see* Hydrocortisone (Topical) *on page 1014*
- ◆ **Corticool [OTC]** *see* Hydrocortisone (Topical) *on page 1014*

Corticorelin (kor ti koe REL in)

Brand Names: U.S. Acthrel

Index Terms Corticorelin Ovine Triflutate; Human Corticotrophin-Releasing Hormone, Analogue; Ovine Corticotrophin-Releasing Hormone (oCRH)

Pharmacologic Category Diagnostic Agent

Use Diagnostic test used in adrenocorticotropic hormone (ACTH)-dependent Cushing's syndrome to differentiate between pituitary and ectopic production of ACTH

Pregnancy Risk Factor C

Dosage IV: Adults: Testing pituitary corticotrophin function: 1 mcg/kg; dosages >1 mcg/kg or >100 mcg have been associated with an increase in adverse effects and are not recommended.

Note: Venous blood samples should be drawn 15 minutes before and immediately prior to corticorelin administration to determine baseline ACTH and cortisol (baseline ACTH value is the average of the 2 samples). At 15-, 30-, and 60 minutes after administration, venous blood samples should be drawn again to determine response. **Basal**

and peak responses differ depending on AM or PM administration; therefore, any repeat evaluations on the same patient are recommended to be done at the same time of day as the initial testing.

Dosage adjustment in renal impairment: No dosage adjustment provided in manufacturer's labeling.

Dosage adjustment in hepatic impairment: No dosage adjustment provided in manufacturer's labeling.

Additional Information Complete prescribing information should be consulted for additional detail.

Dosage Forms

Solution Reconstituted, Intravenous:

Acthrel: 100 mcg (1 ea)

◆ **Corticorelin Ovine Triflutate** *see* Corticorelin *on page 509*

◆ **Cortifoam** *see* Hydrocortisone (Topical) *on page 1014*

◆ **Cortifoam™ (Can)** *see* Hydrocortisone (Topical) *on page 1014*

◆ **Cortimyxin (Can)** *see* Neomycin, Polymyxin B, and Hydrocortisone *on page 1438*

◆ **Cortisol** *see* Hydrocortisone (Systemic) *on page 1013*

◆ **Cortisol** *see* Hydrocortisone (Topical) *on page 1014*

Cortisone (KOR ti sone)

Index Terms Compound E; Cortisone Acetate

Pharmacologic Category Corticosteroid, Systemic

Additional Appendix Information

Corticosteroids Systemic Equivalencies *on page 2228*

Use Management of adrenocortical insufficiency

Dosage If possible, administer glucocorticoids before 9 AM to minimize adrenocortical suppression; dosing depends upon the condition being treated and the response of the patient. **Note:** Supplemental doses may be warranted during times of stress in the course of withdrawing therapy.

Children:

Anti-inflammatory or immunosuppressive: Oral: 2.5-10 mg/kg/day **or** 20-300 mg/m²/day in divided doses every 6-8 hours

Physiologic replacement: Oral: 0.5-0.75 mg/kg/day **or** 20-25 mg/m²/day in divided doses every 8 hours

Adults:

Anti-inflammatory or immunosuppressive: Oral: 25-300 mg/day in divided doses every 12-24 hours

Physiologic replacement: Oral: 25-35 mg/day

Hemodialysis: Supplemental dose is not necessary

Peritoneal dialysis: Supplemental dose is not necessary

Additional Information Complete prescribing information should be consulted for additional detail.

Dosage Forms

Tablet, Oral:

Generic: 25 mg

◆ **Cortisone Acetate** *see* Cortisone *on page 510*

◆ **Cortisporin** *see* Neomycin, Polymyxin B, and Hydrocortisone *on page 1438*

◆ **Cortisporin® Ointment** *see* Bacitracin, Neomycin, Polymyxin B, and Hydrocortisone *on page 223*

◆ **Cortisporin Otic (Can)** *see* Neomycin, Polymyxin B, and Hydrocortisone *on page 1438*

◆ **Cortisporin®-TC** *see* Neomycin, Colistin, Hydrocortisone, and Thonzonium *on page 1437*

◆ **Cortisporin® Topical Ointment (Can)** *see* Bacitracin, Neomycin, Polymyxin B, and Hydrocortisone *on page 223*

◆ **Cortomycin** *see* Neomycin, Polymyxin B, and Hydrocortisone *on page 1438*

◆ **Cortrosyn** *see* Cosyntropin *on page 510*

◆ **Corvert** *see* Ibutilide *on page 1036*

◆ **Cosmegen** *see* DACTINomycin *on page 551*

◆ **Cosopt®** *see* Dorzolamide and Timolol *on page 673*

◆ **Cosopt® PF** *see* Dorzolamide and Timolol *on page 673*

◆ **Cosopt® Preservative Free (Can)** *see* Dorzolamide and Timolol *on page 673*

◆ **CO Sotalol (Can)** *see* Sotalol *on page 1927*

Cosyntropin (koe sin TROE pin)

Brand Names: U.S. Cortrosyn

Brand Names: Canada Cortrosyn; Synacthen Depot

Index Terms Synacthen; Tetracosactide

Pharmacologic Category Corticosteroid, Systemic; Diagnostic Agent

Use Diagnostic test to differentiate primary adrenal from secondary (pituitary) adrenocortical insufficiency

Synacthen Depot [Canadian product]: Additional indications: Treatment of various disease states (eg, collagen, dermatologic, endocrine, ocular, hemolytic). Consult manufacturer labeling for detailed list.

Pregnancy Risk Factor C

Dosage

Diagnostic use: Screening of adrenocortical insufficiency:

Cosyntropin **powder** for injection (IM, IV) **or** cosyntropin **solution** for injection (IV only [manufacturer labeling does not recommend IM administration of solution for injection]):

Children ≤2 years: 0.125 mg

Children >2 years and Adults:

Conventional dose: 0.25 mg; **Note:** Doses in the range of 0.25-0.75 mg have been used in clinical studies; however, maximal response is seen with 0.25 mg dose. When greater cortisol stimulation is needed, an IV infusion may be used: 0.25 mg administered at 0.04 mg/hour over 6 hours

Low-dose protocol (off-label dose): 1 mcg (Abdu, 1999); **Note:** The use of the low-dose protocol has been advocated by some clinicians, particularly in mild or secondary adrenal insufficiency. The low-dose protocol is not recommended in critically-ill patients (Marik, 2008).

Synacthen Depot [Canadian product]: IM: Children >3 years and Adults: 1 mg administered as a single dose or once daily for 3 or 4 days (depending on method of testing; refer to manufacturer labeling for detailed information). **Note:** For patients with severe adrenal insufficiency, some clinicians administer dexamethasone on days that Synacthen® Depot is administered to provide steroid coverage.

Therapeutic use: Synacthen Depot [Canadian product]: IM: **Note:** Titrate to lowest effective dose at the longest effective dosing interval.

Children 3-6 years: Initial: 0.25-0.5 mg daily; maintenance: 0.25-0.5 mg every 2-8 days

Children 7-15 years: Initial: 0.25-1 mg daily; maintenance: 0.25-1 mg every 2-8 days

Children ≥16 years and Adults: Initial for acute treatment: 1 mg daily for 3 days; maintenance dose is individualized: 0.5-1 mg every 2-3 days or twice weekly or 2 mg once weekly or less frequently

Transferring from corticosteroids: Synacthen Depot [Canadian product]: Children >3 years and Adults: IM: Initial: 1 mg daily; gradually reduce steroid by 25% of original dose on successive days. Upon withdrawal from steroid adjust Synacthen® Depot dose as needed.

Transferring from animal-derived ACTH: Synacthen Depot [Canadian product]: Children >3 years and Adults: IM: Conversion varies depending on product previously used. Manufacturer suggests that patients previously receiving ACTH gel 40 units daily should receive Synacthen® Depot 0.5 mg every other day; adjust dose based on response, preferably by extending the dosing interval.

Elderly: Refer to adult dosing.

Dosage adjustment in renal impairment: No dosage adjustment provided in manufacturer's labeling (has not been studied).

Dosage adjustment in hepatic impairment: No dosage adjustment provided in manufacturer's labeling (has not been studied).

Additional Information Complete prescribing information should be consulted for additional detail.

Dosage Forms

Solution, Intravenous:
Generic: 0.25 mg/mL (1 mL)

Solution Reconstituted, Injection:
Cortrosyn: 0.25 mg (1 ea)
Generic: 0.25 mg (1 ea)

Solution Reconstituted, Injection [preservative free]:
Generic: 0.25 mg (1 ea)

Dosage Forms: Canada

Injection, suspension:
Synacthen Depot: 1 mg/mL (1 mL)

◆ **Cotazym (Can)** *see* Pancrelipase *on page 1566*
◆ **CO Temazepam (Can)** *see* Temazepam *on page 1990*
◆ **Co-Temozolomide (Can)** *see* Temozolomide *on page 1991*
◆ **CO Terbinafine (Can)** *see* Terbinafine (Systemic) *on page 2002*
◆ **Cotridin** *see* Triprolidine, Pseudoephedrine, and Codeine [CAN/INT] *on page 2105*
◆ **Co-Trimoxazole** *see* Sulfamethoxazole and Trimethoprim *on page 1946*
◆ **Cough Syrup [OTC]** *see* GuaiFENesin *on page 986*
◆ **Coumadin** *see* Warfarin *on page 2186*
◆ **CO Valacyclovir (Can)** *see* ValACYclovir *on page 2119*
◆ **Covan (Can)** *see* Triprolidine, Pseudoephedrine, and Codeine [CAN/INT] *on page 2105*
◆ **Covera (Can)** *see* Verapamil *on page 2154*
◆ **Covera-HS (Can)** *see* Verapamil *on page 2154*
◆ **Coversyl (Can)** *see* Perindopril *on page 1623*
◆ **Coversyl Plus (Can)** *see* Perindopril and Indapamide [CAN/INT] *on page 1626*
◆ **Coversyl Plus HD (Can)** *see* Perindopril and Indapamide [CAN/INT] *on page 1626*
◆ **Coversyl Plus LD (Can)** *see* Perindopril and Indapamide [CAN/INT] *on page 1626*
◆ **Co-Vidarabine** *see* Pentostatin *on page 1618*
◆ **Coviracil** *see* Emtricitabine *on page 720*
◆ **Cozaar** *see* Losartan *on page 1248*
◆ **CP-690, 550** *see* Tofacitinib *on page 2059*
◆ **CP358774** *see* Erlotinib *on page 756*
◆ **CPDG2** *see* Glucarpidase *on page 971*
◆ **CPG2** *see* Glucarpidase *on page 971*
◆ **CPM** *see* Cyclophosphamide *on page 517*
◆ **CPT-11** *see* Irinotecan *on page 1112*
◆ **CPZ** *see* ChlorproMAZINE *on page 429*
◆ **13-CRA** *see* ISOtretinoin *on page 1127*
◆ **CRA-032765** *see* Ibrutinib *on page 1030*
◆ **Creon** *see* Pancrelipase *on page 1566*
◆ **Crestor** *see* Rosuvastatin *on page 1848*
◆ **Crinone** *see* Progesterone *on page 1722*
◆ **Critic-Aid Clear AF [OTC]** *see* Miconazole (Topical) *on page 1360*
◆ **Critic-Aid Skin Care® [OTC]** *see* Zinc Oxide *on page 2200*
◆ **Crixivan** *see* Indinavir *on page 1066*

Crizotinib (kriz OH ti nib)

Brand Names: U.S. Xalkori

Brand Names: Canada Xalkori

Index Terms C-Met/Hepatocyte Growth Factor Receptor Tyrosine Kinase Inhibitor PF-02341066; C-Met/HGFR Tyrosine Kinase Inhibitor PF-02341066; MET Tyrosine Kinase Inhibitor PF-02341066; PF-02341066

Pharmacologic Category Antineoplastic Agent, Anaplastic Lymphoma Kinase Inhibitor; Antineoplastic Agent, Tyrosine Kinase Inhibitor

Use Non-small cell lung cancer: Treatment of patients with metastatic non-small cell lung cancer (NSCLC) whose tumors are anaplastic lymphoma kinase (ALK)-positive (as detected by an approved test)

Pregnancy Risk Factor D

Pregnancy Considerations Adverse events have been observed in animal reproduction studies. Based on the mechanism of action, crizotinib may cause fetal harm if administered during pregnancy. Women of childbearing potential and men of reproductive potential should use adequate contraception methods during and for at least 90 days after treatment.

Breast-Feeding Considerations It is not known if crizotinib is excreted in breast milk. Due to the potential for serious adverse reactions in the nursing infant, the decision to discontinue crizotinib or to discontinue breast-feeding should take into account the benefits of treatment to the mother.

Contraindications

U.S. labeling: There are no contraindications listed in the manufacturer's labeling.

Canadian labeling: Hypersensitivity to crizotinib or any component of the formulation; congenital long QT syndrome or with persistent Fridericia-corrected QT interval (QTcF) ≥500 msec

Warnings/Precautions Hazardous agent - use appropriate precautions for handling and disposal (NIOSH 2014 [group 1]). Approved for use only in patients with metastatic non-small cell lung cancer (NSCLC) who test positive for the abnormal anaplastic lymphoma kinase (ALK) gene. The Vysis ALK break-apart FISH probe kit is approved to test for the gene abnormality.

Fatalities due to crizotinib-induced hepatotoxicity have occurred. Grade 3 or 4 ALT increases (usually asymptomatic and reversible) have been observed in clinical trials. May require dosage interruption and/or reduction; permanent discontinuation was necessary in some cases; elevations in ALT >5 x ULN were observed; concurrent ALT elevations >3 x ULN and total bilirubin elevations >2 x ULN (without alkaline phosphatase elevations) occurred rarely. Transaminase elevation onset generally was within 2 months of treatment initiation. Monitor liver function tests, including ALT and total bilirubin every 2 weeks during the first 2 months of therapy, then monthly and as clinically necessary. Use with caution in patients with hepatic impairment (has not been studied); crizotinib is extensively metabolized in the liver and liver impairment is likely to increase crizotinib levels.

Severe, life-threatening, and potentially fatal interstitial lung disease (ILD)/pneumonitis has been associated with crizotinib. Onset was generally within 2 months of treatment initiation. Monitor for pulmonary symptoms which may indicate ILD/pneumonitis; exclude other potential causes (eg, disease progression, infection, other pulmonary disease, or radiation therapy). Permanently discontinue if treatment-related ILD/pneumonitis is confirmed.

Symptomatic bradycardia may occur; heart rate <50 beats/minute has occurred. If possible, avoid concurrent use with other agents known to cause bradycardia (eg, beta blockers, nondihydropyridine calcium channel blockers, clonidine, digoxin). Monitor heart rate and blood pressure regularly. If symptomatic bradycardia (not life-threatening) occurs, withhold treatment until recovery to asymptomatic bradycardia or to a heart rate of ≥60 beats/minute, evaluate concurrent medications, and potentially reduce crizotinib dose. Permanently discontinue for life-threatening bradycardia due to crizotinib; if life-threatening bradycardia occurs and concurrent medications associated with bradycardia can be discontinued or dose adjusted, restart crizotinib at a reduced dose (with frequent monitoring). QTc prolongation has been observed; consider periodic monitoring of ECG and electrolytes in patients with heart failure, bradyarrhythmias, electrolyte abnormalities, or who are taking medications known to prolong the QT interval. May require treatment interruption, dosage reduction, or discontinuation. Avoid use in patients with congenital long QT syndrome. Canadian labeling contraindicates use in patients with congenital long QT syndrome or persistent QTcF ≥500 msec.

Ocular toxicities (eg, blurred vision, diplopia, photophobia, photopsia, visual acuity decreased, visual brightness, visual field defect, visual impairment, and/or vitreous floaters) commonly occur. Onset is generally within 1 week of treatment initiation; the impact on daily activities is limited. Reduce initial dose in patients with severe renal impairment not requiring dialysis. Potentially significant drug-drug and drug-food interactions may exist, requiring dose or frequency adjustment, additional monitoring, and/or selection of alternative therapy. Avoid concomitant use with strong CYP3A4 inhibitors and inducers and with CYP3A4 substrates. Crizotinib is associated with a moderate emetic potential; antiemetics may be needed to prevent nausea and vomiting.

Adverse Reactions

Cardiovascular: Bradycardia, chest pain, edema, prolonged Q-T interval on ECG, pulmonary embolism, syncope

Central nervous system: Dizziness, fatigue, headache, insomnia, neuropathy (includes dysesthesia, gait disturbance, hypoesthesia, muscular weakness, neuralgia, peripheral neuropathy, parasthesia, peripheral sensory neuropathy, polyneuropathy, burning sensation in skin)

Dermatologic: Skin rash

Endocrine & metabolic: Hypokalemia, hypophosphatemia

Gastrointestinal: Abdominal pain, constipation, decreased appetite, diarrhea, disease of esophagus (includes dysphagia, epigastric burning/discomfort/pain, esophageal obstruction/pain/spasm/ulcer, esophagitis, gastroesophageal reflux, odynophagia, reflux esophagitis), dysgeusia, dyspepsia, nausea, stomatitis, vomiting

Hematologic & oncologic: Lymphocytopenia, neutropenia

Hepatic: Hepatic failure, increased serum ALT, increased serum AST

Neuromuscular & skeletal: Arthralgia (2%)

Ophthalmic: Visual disturbance (includes blurred vision, diplopia, photophobia, photopsia, visual acuity decreased, visual brightness, visual field defect, visual impairment, vitreous floaters)

Renal: Renal cyst

Respiratory: Cough, dyspnea, interstitial pulmonary disease, pneumonia, upper respiratory tract infection

Rare but important or life-threatening: Hepatotoxicity (fatal), thrombocytopenia

Drug Interactions

Metabolism/Transport Effects **Substrate** of CYP3A4 (major), P-glycoprotein; **Note:** Assignment of Major/Minor substrate status based on clinically relevant drug interaction potential; **Inhibits** CYP2B6 (moderate), CYP3A4 (moderate), OCT1, OCT2, P-glycoprotein

Avoid Concomitant Use

Avoid concomitant use of Crizotinib with any of the following: Alfentanil; Bosutinib; Ceritinib; Conivaptan; CycloSPORINE (Systemic); CYP3A4 Inducers (Strong); CYP3A4 Inhibitors (Strong); Dihydroergotamine; Ergotamine; FentaNYL; Fusidic Acid (Systemic); Grapefruit Juice; Highest Risk QTc-Prolonging Agents; Ibrutinib; Idelalisib; Ivabradine; Lomitapide; Mifepristone; Naloxegol; Olaparib; PAZOPanib; Pimozide; QuiNIDine; Silodosin; Simeprevir; Sirolimus; St Johns Wort; Tacrolimus (Systemic); Tolvaptan; Topotecan; Trabectedin; Ulipristal; VinCRIStine (Liposomal)

Increased Effect/Toxicity

Crizotinib may increase the levels/effects of: Afatinib; Alfentanil; ARIPiprazole; Avanafil; Bosentan; Bosutinib; Bradycardia-Causing Agents; Brentuximab Vedotin; Budesonide (Systemic, Oral Inhalation); BuPROPion; Cannabis; Ceritinib; Colchicine; CycloSPORINE (Systemic); CYP2B6 Substrates; CYP3A4 Substrates; Dabigatran Etexilate; Dapoxetine; Dihydroergotamine; DOXOrubicin (Conventional); Dronabinol; Edoxaban; Eplerenone; Ergotamine; Everolimus; FentaNYL; Highest Risk QTc-Prolonging Agents; Hydrocodone; Ibrutinib; Imatinib; Ivabradine; Ivacaftor; Lacosamide; Ledipasvir; Lomitapide; Lurasidone; Moderate Risk QTc-Prolonging Agents; Naloxegol; Nintedanib; Olaparib; OxyCODONE; PAZOPanib; P-glycoprotein/ABCB1 Substrates; Pimecrolimus; Pimozide; Prucalopride; QuiNIDine; Ranolazine; Rifaximin; Rivaroxaban; Salmeterol; Saxagliptin; Silodosin; Simeprevir; Sirolimus; Suvorexant; Tacrolimus (Systemic); Tetrahydrocannabinol; Tolvaptan; Topotecan; Trabectedin; Ulipristal; Vilazodone; VinCRIStine (Liposomal); Zopiclone

The levels/effects of Crizotinib may be increased by: Aprepitant; Bretylium; Conivaptan; CYP3A4 Inhibitors (Moderate); CYP3A4 Inhibitors (Strong); Dasatinib; Fosaprepitant; Fusidic Acid (Systemic); Grapefruit Juice; Idelalisib; Ivabradine; Luliconazole; Mifepristone; Netupitant; P-glycoprotein/ABCB1 Inhibitors; QTc-Prolonging Agents (Indeterminate Risk and Risk Modifying); Tofacitinib

Decreased Effect

Crizotinib may decrease the levels/effects of: Ifosfamide

The levels/effects of Crizotinib may be decreased by: Bosentan; CYP3A4 Inducers (Moderate); CYP3A4 Inducers (Strong); Dabrafenib; Deferasirox; P-glycoprotein/ABCB1 Inducers; Siltuximab; St Johns Wort; Tocilizumab

Food Interactions Grapefruit juice may increase serum crizotinib levels. Management: Avoid grapefruit and grapefruit juice.

Storage/Stability Store between 20°C and 25°C (68°F and 77°F); excursions are permitted between 15°C and 30°C (59°F and 86°F).

Mechanism of Action Tyrosine kinase receptor inhibitor, which inhibits anaplastic lymphoma kinase (ALK), Hepatocyte Growth Factor Receptor (HGFR, c-MET), and Recepteur d'Origine Nantais (RON). ALK gene abnormalities due to mutations or translocations may result in expression of oncogenic fusion proteins (eg, ALK fusion protein) which alter signaling and expression and result in increased cellular proliferation and survival in tumors which express these fusion proteins. Approximately 2% to 7% of patients with NSCLC have the abnormal echinoderm microtubule-associated protein-like 4, or EML4-ALK gene (which has a higher prevalence in never smokers or light smokers and in patients with adenocarcinoma). Crizotinib selectively inhibits ALK tyrosine kinase, which reduces proliferation of cells expressing the genetic alteration.

Pharmacodynamics/Kinetics

Distribution: V_{ss}: 1772 L

Protein binding: 91%

Metabolism: Hepatic, via CYP3A4/5

Bioavailability: 43% (range: 32% to 66%); bioavailability is reduced 14% with a high-fat meal

Half-life elimination: Terminal: 42 hours

Time to peak: 4-6 hours

Excretion: Feces (63%; 53% as unchanged drug); urine (22%; 2% as unchanged drug)

Dosage Note: Crizotinib is associated with a moderate emetic potential; antiemetics may be needed to prevent nausea and vomiting.

Non-small cell lung cancer (NSCLC), metastatic (ALK-positive): Adults: Oral: 250 mg twice daily, continue treatment until disease progression or unacceptable toxicity

Missed doses: If a dose is missed, take as soon as remembered unless it is <6 hours prior to the next scheduled dose (skip the dose if <6 hours before the next dose); do not take 2 doses at the same time to make up for a missed dose. If vomiting occurs after dose, administer the next dose at the regularly scheduled time.

Dosage adjustment for toxicity: Note: If dose reduction is necessary, reduce dose to 200 mg twice daily; if necessary, further reduce to 250 mg once daily. If unable to tolerate 250 mg once daily, permanently discontinue therapy.

Hematologic toxicity (except lymphopenia, unless lymphopenia is associated with clinical events such as opportunistic infection):

Grade 3 toxicity (WBC 1000 to 2000/mm^3, ANC 500 to 1000/mm^3, platelets 25,000 to 50,000/mm^3), grade 3 anemia: Withhold treatment until recovery to ≤ grade 2, then resume at the same dose and schedule

Grade 4 toxicity (WBC <1000/mm^3, ANC <500/mm^3, platelets <25,000/mm^3), grade 4 anemia: Withhold treatment until recovery to ≤ grade 2, then resume at 200 mg twice daily

Recurrent grade 4 toxicity on 200 mg twice daily: Withhold treatment until recovery to ≤ grade 2, then resume at 250 mg once daily

Recurrent grade 4 toxicity on 250 mg once daily: Permanently discontinue

Nonhematologic toxicities:

Cardiovascular toxicities:

QTc prolongation:

Grade 3 QTc prolongation (QTc >500 msec without life-threatening signs or symptoms) on at least 2 separate ECGs: Withhold treatment until recovery to baseline or to ≤ grade 1 (QTc ≤480 msec), then resume at 200 mg twice daily.

Recurrent grade 3 QTc prolongation at 200 mg twice daily: Withhold treatment until recovery to baseline or to ≤ grade 1, then resume at 250 mg once daily.

Recurrent grade 3 QTc prolongation at 250 mg once daily: Permanently discontinue.

Grade 4 QTc prolongation (QTc >500 msec or ≥60 msec change from baseline with life-threatening symptoms): Permanently discontinue.

Bradycardia:

Grade 2 bradycardia (symptomatic with medical intervention indicated) or grade 3 bradycardia (severe/medically significant with intervention indicated): Withhold until recovery to asymptomatic bradycardia or to a heart rate of ≥60 beats/minute and evaluate concomitant medications. If contributing concomitant medication is identified and discontinued (or dose adjusted), then resume crizotinib at the previous dose. If no contributing concomitant medication is identified (or cannot be discontinued or dose adjusted), resume crizotinib at a reduced dose.

Grade 4 bradycardia due to crizotinib (life-threatening with urgent intervention indicated): Permanently discontinue.

Grade 4 bradycardia associated with concurrent medications known to cause bradycardia or hypotension (life-threatening with urgent intervention indicated): Withhold until recovery to asymptomatic bradycardia or to a heart rate of ≥60 beats/minute, and if concurrent medication can be discontinued or dose adjusted, resume at 250 mg once daily with frequent monitoring.

Hepatotoxicity: Refer to Dosage adjustment in hepatic impairment.

Pulmonary toxicity: Interstitial lung disease (ILD)/pneumonitis (any grade; not attributable to disease progression, infection, other pulmonary disease or radiation therapy): Permanently discontinue.

Dosage adjustment in renal impairment:

Mild to moderate impairment (CrCl 30 to 89 mL/minute): No dosage adjustment necessary.

Severe impairment (CrCl <30 mL/minute) not requiring dialysis: Initial: 250 mg once daily

Dosage adjustment in hepatic impairment:

Hepatotoxicity **prior to** treatment: No dosage adjustment provided in manufacturer's labeling (has not been studied); crizotinib undergoes extensive hepatic metabolism and systemic exposure may be increased with impairment; use with caution.

Hepatotoxicity **during** treatment:

Grade 3 or 4 ALT or AST elevation (ALT or AST >5 x ULN) with ≤ grade 1 total bilirubin elevation (total bilirubin ≤1.5 x ULN): Withhold treatment until recovery to ≤ grade 1 (<3 x ULN) or baseline, then resume at 200 mg twice daily.

Recurrent grade 3 or 4 ALT or AST elevation with ≤ grade 1 total bilirubin elevation: Withhold treatment until recovery to ≤ grade 1, then resume at 250 mg once daily.

Recurrent grade 3 or 4 ALT or AST elevation on 250 mg once daily: Permanently discontinue.

Grade 2, 3, or 4 ALT or AST elevation (ALT or AST >3 x ULN) with concurrent grade 2, 3, or 4 total bilirubin elevation (>1.5 x ULN) in the absence of cholestasis or hemolysis: Permanently discontinue.

Dietary Considerations Avoid grapefruit and grapefruit juice.

Administration

Crizotinib is associated with a moderate emetic potential; antiemetics may be needed to prevent nausea and vomiting.

Swallow capsules whole (do not crush, dissolve, or open capsules). Administer with or without food. If vomiting occurs after dose, administer the next dose at the regularly scheduled time.

Hazardous agent; use appropriate precautions for handling and disposal (NIOSH 2014 [group 1]).

Monitoring Parameters ALK positivity; CBC with differential monthly and as clinically appropriate (monitor more frequently if grades 3 or 4 abnormalities observed or with fever or infection), liver function tests every 2 weeks for the first 2 months, then monthly and as clinically appropriate (monitor more frequently if grades 2, 3, or 4 abnormalities observed); renal function (baseline and periodic). Monitor pulmonary symptoms (for interstitial lung disease [ILD]/pneumonitis). Monitor heart rate and blood pressure; consider monitoring ECG and electrolytes in patients with heart failure, bradycardia, bradyarrhythmias, electrolyte abnormalities, or who are taking medications known to prolong the QT interval.

Dosage Forms

Capsule, Oral:

Xalkori: 200 mg, 250 mg

Crofelemer (kroe FEL e mer)

Brand Names: U.S. Fulyzaq

Index Terms *Croton lechleri*; Provir; SP-303

Pharmacologic Category Antidiarrheal

Use Symptomatic relief of noninfectious diarrhea in patients with HIV/AIDS on antiretroviral therapy

Pregnancy Risk Factor C

Dosage Diarrhea, noninfectious (associated with antiretroviral therapy for HIV/AIDS): Adults: Oral: 125 mg twice daily

Dosage adjustment in renal impairment: No dosage adjustment provided in the manufacturer's labeling.

Dosage adjustment in hepatic impairment: No dosage adjustment provided in the manufacturer's labeling.

Additional Information Complete prescribing information should be consulted for additional detail.

Dosage Forms

Tablet Delayed Release, Oral:

Fulyzaq: 125 mg

◆ **Crolom** *see* Cromolyn (Ophthalmic) *on page 514*
◆ **Cromoglicate** *see* Cromolyn (Nasal) *on page 514*
◆ **Cromoglicate** *see* Cromolyn (Ophthalmic) *on page 514*
◆ **Cromoglycic Acid** *see* Cromolyn (Nasal) *on page 514*
◆ **Cromoglycic Acid** *see* Cromolyn (Ophthalmic) *on page 514*

Cromolyn (Nasal) (KROE moe lin)

Brand Names: U.S. NasalCrom [OTC]

Brand Names: Canada Apo-Cromolyn Nasal Spray [OTC]; Rhinaris-CS Anti-Allergic Nasal Mist

Index Terms Cromoglicate; Cromoglycic Acid; Cromolyn Sodium; Disodium Cromoglycate; DSCG; Sodium Cromoglicate

Pharmacologic Category Mast Cell Stabilizer

Use Prevention and treatment of seasonal and perennial allergic rhinitis

Dosage Intranasal: Allergic rhinitis (treatment and prophylaxis): Children ≥2 years and Adults: 1 spray into each nostril 3-4 times/day; may be increased to 6 times/day (symptomatic relief may require 2-4 weeks)

Dosage adjustment in renal impairment: No dosage adjustment provided in manufacturer's labeling.

Dosage adjustment in hepatic impairment: No dosage adjustment provided in manufacturer's labeling.

Additional Information Complete prescribing information should be consulted for additional detail.

Dosage Forms

Aerosol Solution, Nasal:

NasalCrom [OTC]: 5.2 mg/actuation (13 mL, 26 mL)
Generic: 5.2 mg/actuation (26 mL)

Cromolyn (Ophthalmic) (KROE moe lin)

Brand Names: Canada Opticrom®

Index Terms Crolom; Cromoglicate; Cromoglycic Acid; Cromolyn Sodium; Disodium Cromoglycate; DSCG; Sodium Cromoglicate

Pharmacologic Category Mast Cell Stabilizer

Use Treatment of vernal keratoconjunctivitis, vernal conjunctivitis, and vernal keratitis

Pregnancy Risk Factor B

Dosage Ophthalmic: Children >4 years and Adults: 1-2 drops in each eye 4-6 times/day

Dosage adjustment in renal impairment: No dosage adjustment provided in manufacturer's labeling. However, dosage adjustment unlikely due to low systemic absorption.

Dosage adjustment in hepatic impairment: No dosage adjustment provided in manufacturer's labeling. However, dosage adjustment unlikely due to low systemic absorption.

Additional Information Complete prescribing information should be consulted for additional detail.

Dosage Forms

Solution, Ophthalmic:

Generic: 4% (10 mL)

◆ **Cromolyn Sodium** *see* Cromolyn (Nasal) *on page 514*
◆ **Cromolyn Sodium** *see* Cromolyn (Ophthalmic) *on page 514*

Crotamiton (kroe TAM i tonn)

Brand Names: U.S. Eurax

Brand Names: Canada Eurax Cream

Pharmacologic Category Scabicidal Agent

Use Treatment of scabies (*Sarcoptes scabiei*) and symptomatic treatment of pruritus

Pregnancy Risk Factor C

Dosage Topical:

Scabicide: Children and Adults: Wash thoroughly and scrub away loose scales, then towel dry; apply a thin layer and massage drug onto skin of the entire body from the neck to the toes (with special attention to skin folds, creases, and interdigital spaces). Repeat application in 24 hours. Take a cleansing bath 48 hours after the final application. Treatment may be repeated after 7-10 days if live mites are still present.

Pruritus: Massage into affected areas until medication is completely absorbed; repeat as necessary

Additional Information Complete prescribing information should be consulted for additional detail.

Dosage Forms

Cream, External:

Eurax: 10% (60 g)

Lotion, External:

Eurax: 10% (60 g, 454 g)

◆ ***Croton lechleri*** *see* Crofelemer *on page 514*
◆ **CRRT** *see* Electrolyte Solution, Renal Replacement *on page 710*
◆ **Cruex Prescription Strength [OTC]** *see* Miconazole (Topical) *on page 1360*
◆ **Cryselle 28** *see* Ethinyl Estradiol and Norgestrel *on page 812*
◆ **Crystalline Penicillin** *see* Penicillin G (Parenteral/Aqueous) *on page 1611*
◆ **Crystal Violet** *see* Gentian Violet *on page 962*
◆ **Crystapen® (Can)** *see* Penicillin G (Parenteral/Aqueous) *on page 1611*
◆ **Crystodigin** *see* Digitoxin [INT] *on page 627*
◆ **CS-747** *see* Prasugrel *on page 1699*
◆ **CsA** *see* CycloSPORINE (Ophthalmic) *on page 529*
◆ **CsA** *see* CycloSPORINE (Systemic) *on page 522*
◆ **C-Time [OTC]** *see* Ascorbic Acid *on page 178*
◆ **CTLA-4Ig** *see* Abatacept *on page 23*
◆ **CTP 30 (Can)** *see* Citalopram *on page 451*
◆ **CTX** *see* Cyclophosphamide *on page 517*

- **Cu-5 [OTC]** *see* Copper *on page 509*
- **Cubicin** *see* DAPTOmycin *on page 563*
- **Cupric Chloride** *see* Copper *on page 509*
- **Cupric Chloride Dihydrate** *see* Copper *on page 509*
- **Cuprimine** *see* PenicillAMINE *on page 1608*
- **Cuprimine® (Can)** *see* PenicillAMINE *on page 1608*
- **Cutivate** *see* Fluticasone (Topical) *on page 911*
- **Cutivate™ (Can)** *see* Fluticasone (Topical) *on page 911*
- **Cuvposa** *see* Glycopyrrolate *on page 975*
- **CXA 201** *see* Ceftolozane and Tazobactam *on page 394*
- **CyA** *see* CycloSPORINE (Ophthalmic) *on page 529*
- **CyA** *see* CycloSPORINE (Systemic) *on page 522*

Cyanocobalamin (sye an oh koe BAL a min)

Brand Names: U.S. Nascobal; Physicians EZ Use B-12

Index Terms Vitamin B_{12}

Pharmacologic Category Vitamin, Water Soluble

Use Treatment of pernicious anemia; vitamin B_{12} deficiency due to dietary deficiencies or malabsorption diseases, inadequate secretion of intrinsic factor, and inadequate utilization of B_{12} (eg, during neoplastic treatment); increased B_{12} requirements due to pregnancy, thyrotoxicosis, hemorrhage, malignancy, liver or kidney disease

Dosage

Adequate intake (IOM, 1998):

Children:

0-6 months: 0.4 mcg daily

7-12 months: 0.5 mcg daily

Recommended intake (IOM, 1998):

Children:

1-3 years: 0.9 mcg daily

4-8 years: 1.2 mcg daily

9-13 years: 1.8 mcg daily

Adolescents >14 years and Adults: 2.4 mcg daily

Pregnancy: 2.6 mcg daily

Lactation: 2.8 mcg daily

Vitamin B_{12} deficiency:

IM, deep SubQ:

Children (dosage not well established): 0.2 mcg/kg for 2 days, followed by 1000 mcg daily for 2-7 days, followed by 100 mcg weekly for 1 month; for malabsorptive causes of B_{12} deficiency, monthly maintenance doses of 100 mcg have been recommended **or** as an alternative 100 mcg daily for 10-15 days, then once or twice weekly for several months (Rasmussen, 2001)

Adults: May use initial treatment similar to that for pernicious anemia depending on severity of deficiency: 100 mcg daily for 6-7 days; if improvement, administer same dose on alternate days for 7 doses, then every 3-4 days for 2-3 weeks; once hematologic values have returned to normal, maintenance dosage: 100 mcg monthly.

Note: Given the lack of toxicity associated with cyanocobalamin, higher doses may be preferred, especially in cases of severe deficiency. Alternate dosing regimens exist with initial doses ranging from 100-1000 mcg every day or every other day for 1-2 weeks and maintenance doses of 100-1000 mcg every 1-3 months (Oh, 2003).

Intranasal: Adults (Nascobal): 500 mcg in one nostril once weekly

Oral: Adults: 1000-2000 mcg daily for 1-2 weeks; maintenance: 1000 mcg daily (Langan, 2011; Oh, 2003)

Pernicious anemia: IM, deep SubQ (administer concomitantly with folic acid if needed, 1 mg daily for 1 month):

Children: 30-50 mcg daily for 2 or more weeks (to a total dose of 1000-5000 mcg), then follow with 100 mcg monthly as maintenance dosage

Adults: 100 mcg daily for 6-7 days; if improvement, administer same dose on alternate days for 7 doses, then every 3-4 days for 2-3 weeks; once hematologic values have returned to normal, maintenance dosage: 100 mcg monthly.

Note: Given the lack of toxicity associated with cyanocobalamin, higher doses may be preferred, especially in cases of severe deficiency. Alternate dosing regimens exist with initial doses ranging from 100-1000 mcg every day or every other day for 1-2 weeks and maintenance doses of 100-1000 mcg every 1-3 months (Oh, 2003).

Hematologic remission (without evidence of nervous system involvement): Adults:

Intranasal (Nascobal): 500 mcg in one nostril once weekly

Oral: 1000-2000 mcg daily

IM, SubQ: 100-1000 mcg monthly

Dosage adjustment in renal impairment: There are no dosage adjustments provided in the manufacturer's labeling. Use with caution; some formulations may also contain aluminum, which may accumulate in renal impairment.

Dosage adjustment in hepatic impairment: There are no dosage adjustments provided in the manufacturer's labeling.

Additional Information Complete prescribing information should be consulted for additional detail.

Product Availability Nascobal Nasal Spray single-use device: FDA approved June 2014; availability anticipated in September 2014. The device requires no priming or assembly and will replace the currently available multi-use product.

Dosage Forms

Kit, Injection:

Physicians EZ Use B-12: 1000 mcg/mL

Liquid, Sublingual:

Generic: 3000 mcg/mL (52 mL)

Lozenge, Oral:

Generic: 50 mcg (100 ea); 100 mcg (100 ea); 250 mcg (100 ea, 250 ea); 500 mcg (100 ea, 250 ea)

Solution, Injection:

Generic: 1000 mcg/mL (1 mL, 10 mL, 30 mL)

Solution, Nasal:

Nascobal: 500 mcg/0.1 mL (1 ea, 1.3 mL)

Tablet, Oral:

Generic: 100 mcg, 250 mcg, 500 mcg, 1000 mcg

Tablet, Oral [preservative free]:

Generic: 100 mcg, 500 mcg, 1000 mcg

Tablet Extended Release, Oral:

Generic: 1000 mcg

Tablet Sublingual, Sublingual:

Generic: 2500 mcg

Tablet Sublingual, Sublingual [preservative free]:

Generic: 2500 mcg

- **Cyanocobalamin, Folic Acid, and Pyridoxine** *see* Folic Acid, Cyanocobalamin, and Pyridoxine *on page 921*
- **Cyanokit** *see* Hydroxocobalamin *on page 1020*
- **Cyclafem 1/35** *see* Ethinyl Estradiol and Norethindrone *on page 808*
- **Cyclafem 7/7/7** *see* Ethinyl Estradiol and Norethindrone *on page 808*
- **Cyclen (Can)** *see* Ethinyl Estradiol and Norgestimate *on page 810*
- **Cyclessa** *see* Ethinyl Estradiol and Desogestrel *on page 799*

Cyclobenzaprine (sye kloe BEN za preen)

Brand Names: U.S. Active-Cyclobenzaprine; Amrix; EnovaRX-Cyclobenzaprine HCl; Fexmid

Brand Names: Canada Apo-Cyclobenzaprine; Auro-Cyclobenzaprine; Ava-Cyclobenzaprine; Dom-Cyclobenzaprine; JAMP-Cyclobenzaprine; Mylan-Cyclobenzaprine; Novo-Cycloprine; PHL-Cyclobenzaprine; PMS-Cyclobenzaprine; Q-Cyclobenzaprine; ratio-Cyclobenzaprine; Riva-Cycloprine; ZYM-Cyclobenzaprine

Index Terms Cyclobenzaprine Hydrochloride; Flexeril

Pharmacologic Category Skeletal Muscle Relaxant

Additional Appendix Information

Beers Criteria - Potentially Inappropriate Medications for Geriatrics *on page 2271*

Use Short-term (2-3 weeks) treatment of muscle spasm associated with acute, painful musculoskeletal conditions

Pregnancy Risk Factor B

Pregnancy Considerations Adverse events have not been observed in animal reproduction studies. The manufacturer recommends avoiding use during pregnancy unless clearly needed.

Breast-Feeding Considerations It is not known if cyclobenzaprine is excreted in breast milk. The manufacturer recommends that caution be exercised when administering cyclobenzaprine to nursing women.

Contraindications Hypersensitivity to cyclobenzaprine or any component of the formulation; during or within 14 days of MAO inhibitors; hyperthyroidism; congestive heart failure; arrhythmias; heart block or conduction disturbances; acute recovery phase of MI

Warnings/Precautions May cause CNS depression, which may impair physical or mental abilities; ethanol and/or other CNS depressants may enhance these effects. Patients must be cautioned about performing tasks which require mental alertness (eg, operating machinery or driving). Cyclobenzaprine shares the toxic potentials of the tricyclic antidepressants (including arrhythmias, tachycardia, and conduction time prolongation) and the usual precautions of tricyclic antidepressant therapy should be observed; use with caution in patients with urinary hesitancy or retention, angle-closure glaucoma or increased intraocular pressure, hepatic impairment, or in the elderly.

Potentially life-threatening serotonin syndrome has occurred with cyclobenzaprine when used in combination with other serotonergic agents (eg, SSRIs, SNRIs, TCAs, meperidine, tramadol, buspirone, MAO inhibitors), bupropion, and verapamil. Monitor patients closely especially during initiation/dose titration for signs/symptoms of serotonin syndrome such as mental status changes (eg, agitation, hallucinations); autonomic instability (eg, tachycardia, labile blood pressure, diaphoresis); neuromuscular changes (eg, tremor, rigidity, myoclonus); GI symptoms (eg, nausea, vomiting, diarrhea); and/or seizures. Discontinue cyclobenzaprine and any concomitant serotonergic agent immediately if signs/symptoms arise. Concomitant use or use within 14 days of discontinuing an MAO inhibitor is contraindicated.

Muscle relaxants are poorly tolerated by the elderly due to potent anticholinergic effects, sedation, and risk of fracture. Efficacy is questionable at dosages tolerated by elderly patients; avoid use (Beers Criteria). Extended release capsules not recommended for use in mild-to-severe hepatic impairment or in the elderly. Potentially significant drug-drug interactions may exist, requiring dose or frequency adjustment, additional monitoring, and/or selection of alternative therapy. Effects may be potentiated when used with other CNS depressants or ethanol.

Adverse Reactions

Central nervous system: Confusion, decreased mental acuity, dizziness, drowsiness, fatigue, headache, irritability, nervousness

Gastrointestinal: Abdominal pain, acid regurgitation, constipation, diarrhea, dyspepsia, nausea, unpleasant taste, xerostomia

Neuromuscular & skeletal: Weakness

Ophthalmic: Blurred vision

Respiratory: Pharyngitis, upper respiratory tract infection

Rare but important or life-threatening: Anaphylaxis, angioedema, cardiac arrhythmia, convulsions, hepatitis (rare), hypertonia, hypotension, paresthesia, psychosis, seizure, serotonin syndrome, skin rash, syncope, tachycardia

Drug Interactions

Metabolism/Transport Effects Substrate of CYP1A2 (major), CYP2D6 (minor), CYP3A4 (minor); **Note:** Assignment of Major/Minor substrate status based on clinically relevant drug interaction potential

Avoid Concomitant Use

Avoid concomitant use of Cyclobenzaprine with any of the following: Aclidinium; Azelastine (Nasal); Dapoxetine; Glucagon; Ipratropium (Oral Inhalation); MAO Inhibitors; Orphenadrine; Paraldehyde; Potassium Chloride; Thalidomide; Tiotropium; Umeclidinium

Increased Effect/Toxicity

Cyclobenzaprine may increase the levels/effects of: AbobotulinumtoxinA; Alcohol (Ethyl); Analgesics (Opioid); Anticholinergic Agents; Antipsychotic Agents; Azelastine (Nasal); Buprenorphine; CNS Depressants; Glucagon; Hydrocodone; MAO Inhibitors; Methotrimeprazine; Metoclopramide; Metyrosine; Mirabegron; OnabotulinumtoxinA; Orphenadrine; Paraldehyde; Potassium Chloride; Pramipexole; RimabotulinumtoxinB; ROPINIRole; Rotigotine; Serotonin Modulators; Suvorexant; Thalidomide; Thiazide Diuretics; Tiotropium; Topiramate; TraMADol; Zolpidem

The levels/effects of Cyclobenzaprine may be increased by: Abiraterone Acetate; Aclidinium; Antiemetics (5HT3 Antagonists); Antipsychotic Agents; Brimonidine (Topical); Cannabis; CYP1A2 Inhibitors (Moderate); CYP1A2 Inhibitors (Strong); Dapoxetine; Deferasirox; Doxylamine; Dronabinol; Droperidol; HydrOXYzine; Ipratropium (Oral Inhalation); Kava Kava; Magnesium Sulfate; Methotrimeprazine; Mianserin; Nabilone; Peginterferon Alfa-2b; Perampanel; Pramlintide; Rufinamide; Sodium Oxybate; Tapentadol; Tetrahydrocannabinol; Umeclidinium; Vemurafenib

Decreased Effect

Cyclobenzaprine may decrease the levels/effects of: Acetylcholinesterase Inhibitors; Itopride; Secretin

The levels/effects of Cyclobenzaprine may be decreased by: Acetylcholinesterase Inhibitors

Food Interactions Food increases bioavailability (peak plasma concentrations increased by 35% and area under the curve by 20%) of the extended release capsule. Management: Monitor for increased effects if taken with food.

Storage/Stability

Amrix, Flexeril: Store at 25°C (77°F); excursions permitted to 15°C to 30°C (59°F to 86°F). Protect from light.

Fexmid: Store at 20°C to 25°C (68°F to 77°F).

Mechanism of Action Centrally-acting skeletal muscle relaxant pharmacologically related to tricyclic antidepressants; reduces tonic somatic motor activity influencing both alpha and gamma motor neurons

Pharmacodynamics/Kinetics

Metabolism: Hepatic via CYP3A4, 1A2, and 2D6; may undergo enterohepatic recirculation

Bioavailability: 33% to 55%

Half-life elimination: Immediate release tablet: 18 hours (range: 8-37 hours); Extended release capsule: 32-33 hours
Time to peak, serum: Extended release capsule: 7-8 hours
Excretion: Urine (primarily as glucuronide metabolites); feces (as unchanged drug; Hucker, 1978)

Dosage Oral: Muscle spasm: **Note:** Do not use longer than 2-3 weeks
Capsule, extended release:
Adults: Usual: 15 mg once daily; some patients may require up to 30 mg once daily
Elderly: Use not recommended
Tablet, immediate release:
Children ≥15 years and Adults: Initial: 5 mg 3 times daily; may increase up to 10 mg 3 times daily if needed
Elderly: Initial: 5 mg; titrate dose slowly and consider less frequent dosing

Dosage adjustment in renal impairment: No dosage adjustment provided in manufacturer's labeling.
Dosage adjustment in hepatic impairment:
Capsule, extended release: Mild-to-severe impairment: Use not recommended.
Tablet, immediate release:
Mild impairment: Initial: 5 mg; use with caution; titrate slowly and consider less frequent dosing
Moderate-to-severe impairment: Use not recommended

Administration Oral: Extended release capsules: Administer at the same time each day. Do not crush or chew.

Monitoring Parameters Signs/symptoms of serotonin syndrome (patients receiving other serotonergic drugs)

Dosage Forms Considerations
EnovaRX-Cyclobenzaprine and Active-Cyclobenzaprine are compounding kits. Refer to manufacturer's labeling for compounding instructions.

Dosage Forms
Capsule Extended Release 24 Hour, Oral:
Amrix: 15 mg, 30 mg
Cream, Transdermal:
Active-Cyclobenzaprine: 5% (120 g)
EnovaRX-Cyclobenzaprine HCl: 20 mg/g (120 g)
Tablet, Oral:
Fexmid: 7.5 mg
Generic: 5 mg, 7.5 mg, 10 mg

◆ **Cyclobenzaprine Hydrochloride** *see* Cyclobenzaprine *on page 516*
◆ **Cyclogyl** *see* Cyclopentolate *on page 517*
◆ **Cyclomen® (Can)** *see* Danazol *on page 558*
◆ **Cyclomydril®** *see* Cyclopentolate and Phenylephrine *on page 517*

Cyclopentolate (sye kloe PEN toe late)

Brand Names: U.S. Cyclogyl
Brand Names: Canada AK Pentolate Oph Soln; Cyclogyl; Diopentolate; Minims Cyclopentolate; PMS-Cyclopentolate
Index Terms Cyclopentolate Hydrochloride
Pharmacologic Category Anticholinergic Agent, Ophthalmic
Use Mydriasis/Cycloplegia: Produce mydriasis and cycloplegia.
Pregnancy Risk Factor C
Dosage
Mydriasis, cycloplegia: **Note:** Cyclopentolate and phenylephrine combination formulation is the preferred agent for use in infants due to lower cyclopentolate concentration and reduced risk for systemic reactions (Chew, 2005).
Infants: Ophthalmic: Instill 1 drop of 0.5% solution as a single dose.
Children and Adolescents: Ophthalmic: Instill 1 or 2 drops of 0.5%, 1%, or 2% solution; may repeat with 0.5% or 1% solution in 5 to 10 minutes.
Adults: Ophthalmic: Instill 1 or 2 drops of 0.5%, 1%, or 2% solution; may repeat in 5 to 10 minutes; heavily pigmented irides may require use of the higher strengths.
Anterior uveitis (off-label use): Adults: Ophthalmic: Instill 1 drop of 1% solution 3 times daily (AOA [Alexander, 2004]).

Dosage adjustment in renal impairment: There are no dosage adjustments provided in the manufacturer's labeling.
Dosage adjustment in hepatic impairment: There are no dosage adjustments provided in the manufacturer's labeling.

Additional Information Complete prescribing information should be consulted for additional detail.

Dosage Forms
Solution, Ophthalmic:
Cyclogyl: 0.5% (15 mL); 1% (2 mL, 5 mL, 15 mL); 2% (2 mL, 5 mL, 15 mL)
Generic: 1% (2 mL, 15 mL); 2% (2 mL, 5 mL, 15 mL)

Cyclopentolate and Phenylephrine
(sye kloe PEN toe late & fen il EF rin)

Brand Names: U.S. Cyclomydril®
Index Terms Phenylephrine and Cyclopentolate
Pharmacologic Category Ophthalmic Agent, Mydriatic
Use Mydriasis: For the production of mydriasis.
Pregnancy Risk Factor C
Dosage Diagnostic aid (mydriasis): Infants, Children, Adolescents, and Adults: Ophthalmic: Instill 1 drop into the eye every 5 to 10 minutes.
Additional Information Complete prescribing information should be consulted for additional detail.
Dosage Forms
Solution, ophthalmic:
Cyclomydril: Cyclopentolate 0.2% and phenylephrine 1% (2 mL, 5 mL)

◆ **Cyclopentolate Hydrochloride** *see* Cyclopentolate *on page 517*

Cyclophosphamide (sye kloe FOS fa mide)

Brand Names: Canada Procytox
Index Terms CPM; CTX; CYT; Cytoxan; Neosar
Pharmacologic Category Antineoplastic Agent, Alkylating Agent; Antineoplastic Agent, Alkylating Agent (Nitrogen Mustard); Antirheumatic Miscellaneous; Immunosuppressant Agent
Use
Oncology-related uses: Treatment of acute lymphoblastic leukemia (ALL), acute myelocytic leukemia (AML), breast cancer, chronic lymphocytic leukemia (CLL), chronic myeloid leukemia (CML), Hodgkin lymphoma, mycosis fungoides, multiple myeloma, neuroblastoma, non-Hodgkin lymphomas (including Burkitt lymphoma), ovarian adenocarcinoma, and retinoblastoma
Limitations of use: Although potentially effective as a single-agent in susceptible malignancies, cyclophosphamide is more frequently used in combination with other chemotherapy drugs
Canadian labeling: Additional use (not in U.S. labeling): Treatment of lung cancer
Nononcology uses: *U.S. labeling:* Nephrotic syndrome: Treatment of minimal change nephrotic syndrome (biopsy proven) in children who are unresponsive or intolerant to corticosteroid therapy

Limitations of use: The safety and efficacy for the treatment of nephrotic syndrome in adults or in other renal diseases has not been established.

Pregnancy Risk Factor D

Pregnancy Considerations Cyclophosphamide crosses the placenta and can be detected in amniotic fluid (D'Incalci, 1982). Based on the mechanism of action, cyclophosphamide may cause fetal harm if administered during pregnancy. Adverse events (including ectrodactylia) were observed in human studies following exposure to cyclophosphamide. Women of childbearing potential should avoid pregnancy while receiving cyclophosphamide and for up to 1 year after completion of treatment. Males with female partners who are or may become pregnant should use a condom during and for at least 4 months after cyclophosphamide treatment. Cyclophosphamide may cause sterility in males and females (may be irreversible) and amenorrhea in females. When treatment is needed for lupus nephritis, cyclophosphamide should be avoided in women who are pregnant or those who wish to preserve their fertility (Hahn, 2012). Chemotherapy, if indicated, may be administered to pregnant women with breast cancer as part of a combination chemotherapy regimen (common regimens administered during pregnancy include doxorubicin (or epirubicin), cyclophosphamide, and fluorouracil); chemotherapy should not be administered during the first trimester, after 35 weeks gestation, or within 3 weeks of planned delivery (Amant, 2010; Loibl, 2006).

Breast-Feeding Considerations Cyclophosphamide is excreted into breast milk. Leukopenia and thrombocytopenia were noted in an infant exposed to cyclophosphamide while nursing. The mother was treated with one course of cyclophosphamide 6 weeks prior to delivery then cyclophosphamide IV 6 mg/kg (300 mg) once daily for 3 days beginning 20 days postpartum. Complete blood counts were obtained in the breast-feeding infant on each day of therapy; WBC and platelets decreased by day 3 (Durodola, 1979). Due to the potential for serious adverse effects in the nursing infant, a decision should be made to discontinue cyclophosphamide or to discontinue breast-feeding, taking into account the importance of treatment to the mother.

Contraindications

U.S. labeling: Hypersensitivity to cyclophosphamide or any component of the formulation; urinary outflow obstruction

Canadian labeling: Hypersensitivity to cyclophosphamide or its metabolites, urinary outflow obstructions, severe myelosuppression, severe renal or hepatic impairment, active infection (especially varicella zoster), severe immunosuppression

Warnings/Precautions Hazardous agent - use appropriate precautions for handling and disposal (NIOSH 2014 [group 1]).

Cyclophosphamide is associated with the development of hemorrhagic cystitis, pyelitis, ureteritis, and hematuria. Hemorrhagic cystitis may rarely be severe or fatal. Bladder fibrosis may also occur, either with or without cystitis. Urotoxicity is due to excretion of cyclophosphamide metabolites in the urine and appears to be dose- and treatment duration-dependent, although may occur with short-term use. Increased hydration and frequent voiding is recommended to help prevent cystitis; some protocols utilize mesna to protect against hemorrhagic cystitis. Monitor urinalysis for hematuria or other signs of urotoxicity. Severe or prolonged hemorrhagic cystitis may require medical or surgical treatment. While hematuria generally resolves within a few days after treatment is withheld, it may persist in some cases. Discontinue cyclophosphamide with severe hemorrhagic cystitis. Exclude or correct any urinary tract obstructions prior to treatment initiation (use is contraindicated with bladder outlet obstruction). Use with caution (if at all) in patients with active urinary tract infection. Use with caution in patients with renal impairment; dosage adjustment may be needed. Decreased renal excretion and increased serum levels (cyclophosphamide and metabolites) may occur in patients with severe renal impairment (CrCl 10 to 24 mL/minute); monitor for signs/symptoms of toxicity. Use is contraindicated in severe impairment in the Canadian labeling. Cyclophosphamide and metabolites are dialyzable; differences in amount dialyzed may occur due to dialysis system used. If dialysis is required, maintain a consistent interval between administration and dialysis.

Leukopenia, neutropenia, thrombocytopenia, and anemia may commonly occur; may be dose related. Bone marrow failure has been reported. Bone marrow failure and severe immunosuppression may lead to serious (and fatal) infections, including sepsis and septic shock, or may reactive latent infections. Antimicrobial prophylaxis may be considered in appropriate patients. Initiate antibiotics for neutropenic fever; antifungal and antiviral medications may also be necessary. Monitor blood counts during treatment. Avoid use if neutrophils are ≤1500/mm^3 and platelets are <50,000/mm^3. Consider growth factors (primary or secondary prophylaxis) in patients at increased risk for complications due to neutropenia. Platelet and neutrophil nadirs are usually at weeks 1 and 2 of treatment and recovery is expected after ~20 days. Severe myelosuppression may be more prevalent in heavily pretreated patients or in patients receiving concomitant chemotherapy and/or radiation therapy. Monitor for infections; immunosuppression and serious infections may occur; serious infections may require dose reduction, or interruption or discontinuation of treatment.

Cardiotoxicity has been reported (some fatal), usually with high doses associated with transplant conditioning regimens, although may rarely occur with lower doses. Cardiac abnormalities do not appear to persist. Cardiotoxicities reported have included arrhythmias (supraventricular and ventricular), congestive heart failure, heart block, hemorrhagic myocarditis, hemopericardium (secondary to hemorrhagic myocarditis and myocardial necrosis), pericarditis, pericardial effusion including cardiac tamponade, and tachyarrhythmias. Cardiotoxicity is related to endothelial capillary damage; symptoms may be managed with diuretics, ACE inhibitors, beta-blockers, or inotropics (Floyd, 2005). The risk for cardiotoxicity may be increased with higher doses, advanced age, and in patients with prior radiation to the cardiac region, and in patients who have received prior or concurrent cardiotoxic medication. Use with caution in patients with preexisting cardiovascular disease or those at risk for cardiotoxicity. For patients with multiple cardiac risk factors, considering monitoring during treatment (Floyd, 2005).

Pulmonary toxicities, including pneumonitis, pulmonary fibrosis, pulmonary veno-occlusive disease, and acute respiratory distress syndrome, have been reported. Monitor for signs/symptoms of pulmonary toxicity. Consider pulmonary function testing to assess the severity of pneumonitis (Morgan, 2011). Cyclophosphamide-induced pneumonitis is rare and may present as early (within 1 to 6 months) or late onset (several months to years). Early onset may be reversible with discontinuation; late onset is associated with pleural thickening and may persist chronically (Malik, 1996). In addition, late onset pneumonitis (>6 months after therapy initiation) may be associated with increased mortality.

Hepatic sinusoidal obstruction syndrome (SOS), formerly called veno-occlusive liver disease (VOD), has been reported in patients receiving chemotherapy regimens containing cyclophosphamide. A major risk factor for SOS is cytoreductive conditioning transplantation regimens with cyclophosphamide used in combination with total body irradiation or busulfan (or other agents). Other risk factors include preexisting hepatic dysfunction, prior radiation to the abdominal area, and low performance status. Children <3 years of age are reported to be at increased risk for hepatic SOS; monitor for signs or symptoms of hepatic SOS, including bilirubin >1.4 mg/dL, unexplained weight gain, ascites, hepatomegaly, or unexplained right upper quadrant pain (Arndt, 2004). SOS has also been reported in patients receiving long-term lower doses for immunosuppressive indications. Use with caution in patients with hepatic impairment; dosage adjustment may be needed. Use is contraindicated in severe impairment in the Canadian labeling. The conversion between cyclophosphamide to the active metabolite may be reduced in patients with severe hepatic impairment, potentially reducing efficacy.

Nausea and vomiting commonly occur. Cyclophosphamide is associated with a moderate to high emetic potential (depending on dose, regimen, or administration route); antiemetics are recommended to prevent nausea and vomiting (Basch, 2011; Dupuis, 2011; Roila, 2010). Stomatitis/mucositis may also occur. Anaphylactic reactions have been reported; cross-sensitivity with other alkylating agents may occur. Hyponatremia associated with increased total body water, acute water intoxication, and a syndrome resembling SIADH (syndrome of inappropriate secretion of antidiuretic hormone) has been reported; some have been fatal. May interfere with wound healing. May impair fertility; interferes with oogenesis and spermatogenesis. Effect on fertility is generally dependent on dose and duration of treatment and may be irreversible. The age at treatment initiation and cumulative dose were determined to be risk factors for ovarian failure in cyclophosphamide use for the treatment of systemic lupus erythematosus (SLE) (Mok, 1998). Potentially significant drug-drug interactions may exist, requiring dose or frequency adjustment, additional monitoring, and/or selection of alternative therapy. Secondary malignancies (bladder cancer, myelodysplasia, acute leukemias, lymphomas, thyroid cancer, and sarcomas) have been reported with both single-agent and with combination chemotherapy regimens; onset may be delayed (up to several years after treatment). Bladder cancer usually occurs in patients previously experiencing hemorrhagic cystitis; risk may be reduced by preventing hemorrhagic cystitis.

Adverse Reactions

Dermatologic: Alopecia (reversible; onset: 3-6 weeks after start of treatment)

Endocrine & metabolic: Amenorrhea, azoospermia, gonadal suppression, oligospermia, oogenesis impaired, sterility

Gastrointestinal: Abdominal pain, anorexia, diarrhea, mucositis, nausea/vomiting (dose-related), stomatitis

Genitourinary: Hemorrhagic cystitis

Hematologic: Anemia, leukopenia (dose-related; recovery: 7-10 days after cessation), myelosuppression, neutropenia, neutropenic fever, thrombocytopenia

Miscellaneous: Infection

Rare but important or life-threatening: Acute respiratory distress syndrome, anaphylactic reactions, anaphylaxis, arrhythmias (with high-dose [HSCT] therapy), bladder/urinary fibrosis, blurred vision, cardiac tamponade (with high-dose [HSCT] therapy), cardiotoxicity, confusion, dyspnea, ejection fraction decreased, erythema multiforme, gastrointestinal hemorrhage, hearing disorders, heart block, heart failure (with high-dose [HSCT] therapy), hematuria, hemopericardium, hemorrhagic colitis, hemorrhagic myocarditis (with high-dose [HSCT] therapy), hemorrhagic ureteritis, hepatic sinusoidal obstruction syndrome (SOS; formerly called veno-occlusive liver disease), hepatitis, hepatotoxicity, hypersensitivity reactions, hyperuricemia, hypokalemia, hyponatremia, interstitial pneumonitis, interstitial pulmonary fibrosis (with high doses), jaundice, latent infection reactivation, mesenteric ischemia (acute), methemoglobinemia (with high-dose [HSCT] therapy), multiorgan failure, myocardial necrosis (with high-dose [HSCT] therapy), neurotoxicity, neutrophilic eccrine hidradenitis, ovarian fibrosis, pancreatitis, pericarditis, pigmentation changes (skin/fingernails), pneumonia, pulmonary hypertension, pulmonary infiltrates, pulmonary veno-occlusive disease, pyelonephritis, radiation recall, renal tubular necrosis, reversible posterior leukoencephalopathy syndrome (RPLS), rhabdomyolysis, secondary malignancy, septic shock, sepsis, SIADH, Stevens-Johnson syndrome, testicular atrophy, thrombocytopenia (immune mediated), thrombotic disorders (arterial and venous), toxic epidermal necrolysis, toxic megacolon, tumor lysis syndrome, wound healing impaired

Drug Interactions

Metabolism/Transport Effects **Substrate** of CYP2A6 (minor), CYP2B6 (major), CYP2C19 (minor), CYP2C9 (minor), CYP3A4 (minor); **Note:** Assignment of Major/Minor substrate status based on clinically relevant drug interaction potential; **Inhibits** CYP3A4 (weak); **Induces** CYP2B6 (moderate), CYP2C9 (moderate)

Avoid Concomitant Use

Avoid concomitant use of Cyclophosphamide with any of the following: BCG; Belimumab; CloZAPine; Dipyrone; Etanercept; Natalizumab; Pimecrolimus; Pimozide; Tacrolimus (Topical); Tofacitinib; Vaccines (Live)

Increased Effect/Toxicity

Cyclophosphamide may increase the levels/effects of: Amiodarone; Antineoplastic Agents (Anthracycline, Systemic); ARIPiprazole; CloZAPine; CycloSPORINE (Systemic); Dofetilide; Hydrocodone; Leflunomide; Lomitapide; Natalizumab; Pimozide; Sargramostim; Succinylcholine; Tofacitinib; Vaccines (Live)

The levels/effects of Cyclophosphamide may be increased by: Allopurinol; AzaTHIOprine; Belimumab; CYP2B6 Inhibitors (Moderate); Denosumab; Dipyrone; Etanercept; Filgrastim; Pentostatin; Pimecrolimus; Protease Inhibitors; Quazepam; Roflumilast; Tacrolimus (Topical); Thiazide Diuretics; Trastuzumab

Decreased Effect

Cyclophosphamide may decrease the levels/effects of: BCG; Coccidioides immitis Skin Test; CycloSPORINE (Systemic); Sipuleucel-T; Vaccines (Inactivated); Vaccines (Live)

The levels/effects of Cyclophosphamide may be decreased by: CYP2B6 Inducers (Strong); Dabrafenib; Echinacea

Preparation for Administration Hazardous agent; use appropriate precautions for handling and disposal (NIOSH 2014 [group 1]).

Injection powder for reconstitution: Reconstitute with 25 mL for a 500 mg vial, 50 mL for a 1000 mg vial, or 100 mL for a 2000 mg vial to a concentration of 20 mg/mL using NS only for direct IV push, or NS or SWFI for IV infusion; swirl gently to mix. For IV infusion, further dilute for infusion in D_5W, 1/2NS, or D_5NS, to a minimum concentration of 2 mg/mL.

Storage/Stability

Injection powder for reconstitution: Store intact vials of powder at ≤25°C (77°F). Exposure to excessive temperatures during transport or storage may cause active ingredient to melt (vials with melting may have a clear to yellow viscous liquid which may appear as droplets); do not use vials with signs of melting. Reconstituted solutions in normal saline (NS) are stable for 24 hours at room temperature and for 6 days refrigerated at 2°C to 8°C (36°F to 46°F). Solutions diluted for infusion in 1/2NS are stable for 24 hours at room temperature and for 6 days refrigerated; solutions diluted in D_5W or D_5NS are stable for 24 hours at room temperature and for 36 hours refrigerated.

Capsules: Store at 20°C to 25°C (68°F to 77°F); excursions are permitted between 15°C and 30°C (59°F and 86°F).

Tablets: Store tablets at ≤25°C (77°F); brief excursions are permitted up to 30°C (86°F); protect from temperatures >30°C (86°F).

Mechanism of Action Cyclophosphamide is an alkylating agent that prevents cell division by cross-linking DNA strands and decreasing DNA synthesis. It is a cell cycle phase nonspecific agent. Cyclophosphamide also possesses potent immunosuppressive activity. Cyclophosphamide is a prodrug that must be metabolized to active metabolites in the liver.

Pharmacodynamics/Kinetics

Absorption: Oral: Well absorbed

Distribution: V_d: 30 to 50 L (approximates total body water); crosses into CSF (not in high enough concentrations to treat meningeal leukemia)

Protein binding: ~20%; some metabolites are bound at >60%

Metabolism: Hepatic to active metabolites acrolein, 4-aldophosphamide, 4-hydroperoxycyclophosphamide, and nor-nitrogen mustard

Bioavailability: >75%

Half-life elimination: IV: 3 to 12 hours

Time to peak: Oral: ~1 hour; IV: Metabolites: 2 to 3 hours

Excretion: Urine (10% to 20% as unchanged drug); feces (4%)

Dosage Cyclophosphamide is associated with a moderate to high emetic potential (depending on dose, regimen, or administration route); antiemetics are recommended to prevent nausea and vomiting (Basch, 2011; Dupuis, 2011; Roila, 2010).

Children:

U.S. labeling:

Malignancy:

IV: 40 to 50 mg/kg in divided doses over 2 to 5 days **or** 10 to 15 mg/kg every 7 to 10 days **or** 3 to 5 mg/kg twice weekly

Oral: 1 to 5 mg/kg/day (initial and maintenance dosing)

Nephrotic syndrome, corticosteroid refractory or intolerant, or corticosteroid sparing: Oral: Initial: 2 mg/kg once daily for 8 to 12 weeks (maximum cumulative dose: 168 mg/kg); treatment beyond 90 days may increase the potential for sterility in males; treatment beyond 1 course is not recommended (Lombel, 2013)

Canadian labeling: Malignancy:

IV: Initial: 2 to 8 mg/kg (60 to 250 mg/m^2) in divided doses for 6 or more days; Maintenance: 10 to 15 mg/kg every 7 to 10 days or 30 mg/kg every 3 to 4 weeks or when bone marrow function recovers

Oral: Initial: 2 to 8 mg/kg (60 to 250 mg/m^2) in divided doses for 6 or more days; Maintenance: 2 to 5 mg/kg (50 to 150 mg/m^2) twice weekly

Indication specific and/or off-label uses/dosing:

Ewing sarcoma (off-label use): IV: VAC/IE regimen: VAC: 1200 mg/m^2 (plus mesna) on day 1 of a 21-day treatment cycle (in combination with vincristine and doxorubicin [then dactinomycin when maximum doxorubicin dose reached]), alternates with IE (ifosfamide and etoposide) for a total of 17 cycles (Grier, 2003)

Hodgkin lymphoma (off-label dosing): IV: BEACOPP escalated regimen: 1200 mg/m^2 on day 0 of a 21-day treatment cycle (in combination with bleomycin, etoposide, doxorubicin, vincristine, prednisone, and procarbazine) for 4 cycles (Kelly, 2011)

Lupus nephritis (off-label use): IV: 500 to 1000 mg/m^2 every month for 6 months, then every 3 months for a total of 2.5 to 3 years (Austin, 1986; Gourley, 1996; Lehman, 2000)

Neuroblastoma (off-label dosing): IV: CE-CAdO regimen, courses 3 and 4: 300 mg/m^2 days 1 to 5 every 21 days for 2 cycles (Rubie, 1998) **or** 10 mg/kg days 1 to 5 every 21 days for 2 cycles (Rubie, 2001). **Note:** Decreased doses may be recommended for newborns or children <10 kg.

Stem cell transplant conditioning (off-label use): Myeloablative transplant: IV: 50 mg/kg/day for 4 days beginning 5 days before transplant (with or without antithymocyte globulin [equine]) (Champlin, 2007)

Adults:

U.S. labeling: Malignancy:

IV: 40 to 50 mg/kg in divided doses over 2 to 5 days **or** 10 to 15 mg/kg every 7 to 10 days **or** 3 to 5 mg/kg twice weekly

Oral: 1 to 5 mg/kg/day (initial and maintenance dosing)

Canadian labeling: Malignancy:

IV: Initial: 40 to 50 mg/kg (1500 to 1800 mg/m^2) administered as 10 to 20 mg/kg/day over 2 to 5 days; Maintenance: 10 to 15 mg/kg (350 to 550 mg/m^2) every 7 to 10 days **or** 3 to 5 mg/kg (110 to 185 mg/m^2) twice weekly

Oral: Initial 1 to 5 mg/kg/day (depending on tolerance); Maintenance: 1 to 5 mg/kg/day

Indication specific and/or off-label uses/dosing:

Acute lymphoblastic leukemia (off-label dosing): Multiple-agent regimens:

Hyper-CVAD regimen: IV: 300 mg/m^2 over 3 hours (with mesna) every 12 hours for 6 doses on days 1, 2, and 3 during odd-numbered cycles (cycles 1, 3, 5, 7) of an 8-cycle phase (Kantarjian, 2004)

CALGB8811 regimen: IV:

Adults <60 years: Induction phase: 1200 mg/m^2 on day 1 of a 4-week cycle; Early intensification phase: 1000 mg/m^2 on day 1 of a 4-week cycle (repeat once); Late intensification phase: 1000 mg/m^2 on day 29 of an 8-week cycle (Larson, 1995)

Adults ≥60 years: Induction phase: 800 mg/m^2 on day 1 of a 4-week cycle; Early intensification phase: 1000 mg/m^2 on day 1 of a 4-week cycle (repeat once); Late intensification phase: 1000 mg/m^2 on day 29 of an 8-week cycle (Larson, 1995)

Breast cancer (off-label dosing):

AC regimen: IV: 600 mg/m^2 on day 1 every 21 days (in combination with doxorubicin) for 4 cycles (Fisher, 1990)

CEF regimen: Oral: 75 mg/m^2/day days 1 to 14 every 28 days (in combination with epirubicin and fluorouracil) for 6 cycles (Levine, 1998)

CMF regimen: Oral: 100 mg/m^2/day days 1 to 14 every 28 days (in combination with methotrexate and fluorouracil) for 6 cycles (Levine, 1998) **or** IV: 600 mg/m^2 on day 1 every 21 days (in combination with methotrexate and fluorouracil); Goldhirsch, 1998)

Chronic lymphocytic leukemia (off-label dosing): IV: R-FC regimen: 250 mg/m^2/day for 3 days every 28 days (in combination with rituximab and fludarabine) for 6 cycles (Robak, 2010)

Ewing sarcoma (off-label use): IV: VAC/IE regimen: VAC: 1200 mg/m^2 (plus mesna) on day 1 of a 21-day treatment cycle (in combination with vincristine and doxorubicin [then dactinomycin when maximum doxorubicin dose reached]), alternates with IE (ifosfamide and etoposide) for a total of 17 cycles (Grier, 2003)

Gestational trophoblastic tumors, high-risk (off-label use): IV: EMA/CO regimen: 600 mg/m^2 on day 8 of 2-week treatment cycle (in combination with etoposide, methotrexate, dactinomycin, and vincristine), continue for at least 2 treatment cycles after a normal hCG level (Escobar, 2003)

Granulomatosis with polyangiitis (GPA; Wegener granulomatosis) (off-label use; in combination with glucocorticoids):
- Low-dose: Oral: 1.5 to 2 mg/kg/day (Jayne, 2003; Stone, 2010) or 2 mg/kg/day until remission, followed by 1.5 mg/kg/day for 3 additional months (de Groot, 2009; Harper, 2012)
- Pulse: IV: 15 mg/kg (maximum dose: 1200 mg) every 2 weeks for 3 doses, followed by maintenance pulses of either 15 mg/kg IV (maximum dose: 1200 mg) every 3 weeks or 2.5 to 5 mg/kg/day orally on days 1, 2, and 3 every 3 weeks for 3 months after remission achieved (de Groot, 2009; Harper, 2012)

Hodgkin lymphoma (off-label dosing): IV:
- BEACOPP regimen: 650 mg/m^2 on day 1 every 3 weeks (in combination with bleomycin, etoposide, doxorubicin, vincristine, procarbazine, and prednisone) for 8 cycles (Diehl, 2003)
- BEACOPP escalated regimen: 1200 mg/m^2 on day 1 every 3 weeks (in combination with bleomycin, etoposide, doxorubicin, vincristine, procarbazine, and prednisone) for 8 cycles (Diehl, 2003)

Multiple myeloma (off-label dosing): Oral: CyBorD regimen: 300 mg/m^2 on days 1, 8, 15, and 22 every 4 weeks (in combination with bortezomib and dexamethasone) for 4 cycles; may continue beyond 4 cycles (Khan, 2012)

Non-Hodgkin lymphoma (off-label dosing): IV:
- R-CHOP regimen: 750 mg/m^2 on day 1 every 3 weeks (in combination with rituximab, doxorubicin, vincristine, and prednisone) for 8 cycles (Coiffier, 2002)
- R-EPOCH (dose adjusted) regimen: 750 mg/m^2 on day 5 every 3 weeks (in combination with rituximab, etoposide, prednisone, vincristine, and doxorubicin) for 6 to 8 cycles (Garcia-Suarez, 2007)
- CODOX-M/IVAC (Burkitt lymphoma): Cycles 1 and 3 (CODOX-M): 800 mg/m^2 on day 1, followed by 200 mg/m^2 on days 2 to 5 (Magrath, 1996) **or** 800 mg/m^2 on days 1 and 2 (Lacasce, 2004), in combination with vincristine, doxorubicin, and methotrexate; CODOX-M alternates with IVAC (etoposide, ifosfamide, and cytarabine) for a total of 4 cycles

Lupus nephritis (off-label use): IV: 500 mg once every 2 weeks for 6 doses or 500 to 1000 mg/m^2 once every month for 6 doses (Hahn, 2012) **or** 500 to 1000 mg/m^2 every month for 6 months, then every 3 months for a total of at least 2.5 years (Austin, 1986; Gourley, 1996)

Small cell lung cancer (SCLC), refractory (off-label use): IV: 1000 mg/m^2 (maximum: 2000 mg) on day 1 every 3 weeks (in combination with doxorubicin and vincristine) until disease progression or unacceptable toxicity (von Pawel, 1999)

Stem cell transplant conditioning (off-label use): IV:
- Nonmyeloablative transplant (allogeneic): 750 mg/m^2/day for 3 days beginning 5 days prior to transplant (in combination with fludarabine) (Khouri, 2008)
- Myeloablative transplant:
  - 100 mg/kg (based on IBW, unless actual weight <95% of IBW) as a single dose 2 days prior to transplant (in combination with total body irradiation and etoposide) (Thompson, 2008)
  - 50 mg/kg/day for 4 days beginning 5 days before transplant (with or without antithymocyte globulin [equine]) (Champlin, 2007)
  - 50 mg/kg/day for 4 days beginning 5 days prior to transplant (in combination with busulfan) (Cassileth, 1993)
  - 60 mg/kg/day for 2 days (in combination with busulfan and total body irradiation) (Anderson, 1996)
  - 1800 mg/m^2/day for 4 days beginning 7 days prior to transplant (in combination with etoposide and carmustine) (Reece, 1991)

Elderly: Refer to adult dosing. Adjust dosing for renal clearance.

Dosage adjustment for toxicity:
- *Hematologic toxicity:* May require dose reduction or treatment interruption; Canadian labeling recommends reducing initial dose by 30% to 50% if bone marrow function compromised (due to prior radiation therapy, prior chemotherapy, or tumor infiltration)
- *Hemorrhagic cystitis, severe:* Discontinue treatment.

Dosage adjustment in renal impairment:

U.S. labeling: There is no adjustment provided in the manufacturer's labeling (use with caution; elevated levels of metabolites may occur).

Canadian labeling:
- Mild impairment: There are no dosage adjustments provided in the manufacturer's labeling
- Moderate impairment: Dose reduction may be necessary; manufacturer's labeling does not provide specific dosing recommendations
- Severe impairment: Use is contraindicated.

The following adjustments have also been recommended:

Aronoff, 2007: Children and Adults:
- CrCl ≥10 mL/minute: No dosage adjustment required.
- CrCl <10 mL/minute: Administer 75% of normal dose.
- Hemodialysis: Moderately dialyzable (20% to 50%); administer 50% of normal dose; administer after hemodialysis
- Continuous ambulatory peritoneal dialysis (CAPD): Administer 75% of normal dose.
- Continuous renal replacement therapy (CRRT): Administer 100% of normal dose.

Janus, 2010: Hemodialysis: Administer 75% of normal dose; administer after hemodialysis

Dosage adjustment in hepatic impairment: The conversion between cyclophosphamide to the active metabolite may be reduced in patients with severe hepatic impairment, potentially reducing efficacy.

U.S. labeling: There are no dosage adjustments provided in the manufacturer's labeling.

Canadian labeling:
- Mild-to-moderate impairment: There are no dosage adjustments provided in the manufacturer's labeling.
- Severe impairment: Use is contraindicated.

The following adjustments have been recommended (Floyd, 2006):
- Serum bilirubin 3.1 to 5 mg/dL or transaminases >3 times ULN: Administer 75% of dose.
- Serum bilirubin >5 mg/mL: Avoid use.

Dosing in obesity:

*American Society of Clinical Oncology (ASCO) Guidelines for appropriate chemotherapy dosing in obese adults with cancer (**Note:** Excludes HSCT dosing):* Utilize patient's actual body weight (full weight) for calculation of body surface area- or weight-based dosing, particularly when the intent of therapy is curative; manage regimen-related toxicities in the same manner as for nonobese patients; if a dose reduction is utilized due to toxicity, consider resumption of full weight-based dosing with subsequent cycles, especially if cause of toxicity (eg, hepatic or renal impairment) is resolved (Griggs, 2012).

American Society for Blood and Marrow Transplantation (ASBMT) practice guideline committee position statement on chemotherapy dosing in obesity (Bubalo, 2014):
- Cy200 (cyclophosphamide total dose of 200 mg/kg): Use the lesser of IBW or actual body weight (ABW).

Cy120 (cyclophosphamide total dose of 120 mg/kg): Use either IBW or ABW for patients ≤120% IBW (preferred method for adults of all body sizes); use ABW25 for patients >120% IBW (preferred for pediatric patients).

ABW25: Adjusted wt (kg) = Ideal body weight (kg) + 0.25 [actual wt (kg) - ideal body weight (kg)]

Administration

Cyclophosphamide is associated with a moderate to high emetic potential (depending on dose, regimen, or administration route); antiemetics are recommended to prevent nausea and vomiting (Basch, 2011; Dupuis, 2011; Roila, 2010).

IV: Infusion rate may vary based on protocol (refer to specific protocol for infusion rate). Administer by direct IV injection (if reconstituted in NS), IVPB, or continuous IV infusion

Bladder toxicity: To minimize bladder toxicity, increase normal fluid intake during and for 1 to 2 days after cyclophosphamide dose. Most adult patients will require a fluid intake of at least 2 L/day. High-dose regimens should be accompanied by vigorous hydration with or without mesna therapy. Morning administration may be preferred to ensure adequate hydration throughout the day.

Hematopoietic stem cell transplant: Approaches to reduction of hemorrhagic cystitis include infusion of 0.9% NaCl 3 L/m²/24 hours, infusion of 0.9% NaCl 3 L/m²/24 hours with continuous 0.9% NaCl bladder irrigation 300 to 1000 mL/hour, and infusion of 0.9% NaCl 1.5 to 3 L/m²/24 hours with intravenous mesna. Hydration should begin at least 4 hours before cyclophosphamide and continue at least 24 hours after completion of cyclophosphamide. The dose of daily mesna used may be 67% to 100% of the daily dose of cyclophosphamide. Mesna can be administered as a continuous 24-hour intravenous infusion or be given in divided doses every 4 hours. Mesna should begin at the start of treatment, and continue at least 24 hours following the last dose of cyclophosphamide.

Oral: Tablets are not scored and should not be cut, chewed, or crushed. Swallow capsules whole; do not open, crush, or chew. To minimize bladder toxicity, increase normal fluid intake. Morning administration may be preferred to ensure adequate hydration throughout the day; do not administer tablets/capsules at bedtime.

Hazardous agent; use appropriate precautions for handling and disposal (NIOSH 2014 [group 1]). Wear gloves when handling capsules/tablets and container. Avoid exposure to broken capsules; if contact occurs, wash hands immediately and thoroughly.

Monitoring Parameters CBC with differential and platelets, BUN, UA, serum electrolytes, serum creatinine; monitor for signs/symptoms of hemorrhagic cystitis or other urinary/renal toxicity, pulmonary, cardiac, and/or hepatic toxicity

Additional Information In patients with CYP2B6 G516T variant allele, cyclophosphamide metabolism is markedly increased; metabolism is not influenced by CYP2C9 and CYP2C19 isotypes (Xie, 2006).

Dosage Forms

Capsule, Oral:

Generic: 25 mg, 50 mg

Solution Reconstituted, Injection:

Generic: 500 mg (1 ea); 1 g (1 ea); 2 g (1 ea)

Tablet, Oral:

Generic: 25 mg, 50 mg

Dosage Forms: Canada

Injection, powder for reconstitution: 200 mg

Extemporaneous Preparations Hazardous agent: Use appropriate precautions for handling and disposal (NIOSH 2014 [group 1]).

Liquid solutions for oral administration may be prepared by dissolving cyclophosphamide injection in Aromatic Elixir, N.F. Store refrigerated (in glass container) for up to 14 days.

Cyclophosphamide Prescribing Information, Baxter Healthcare Corporation, Deerfield, Il, May, 2013.

A 10 mg/mL oral suspension may be prepared by reconstituting one 2 g vial for injection with 100 mL of NaCl 0.9%, providing an initial concentration of 20 mg/mL. Mix this solution in a 1:1 ratio with either Simple Syrup, NF or Ora-Plus® to obtain a final concentration of 10 mg/mL. Label "shake well" and "refrigerate". Stable for 56 days refrigerated.

Kennedy R, Groepper D, Tagen M, et al, "Stability of Cyclophosphamide in Extemporaneous Oral Suspensions," *Ann Pharmacother*, 2010, 44(2):295-301.

◆ **Cycloset** *see* Bromocriptine *on page 291*

◆ **Cyclosporin A** *see* CycloSPORINE (Ophthalmic) *on page 529*

◆ **Cyclosporin A** *see* CycloSPORINE (Systemic) *on page 522*

CycloSPORINE (Systemic) (SYE kloe spor een)

Brand Names: U.S. Gengraf; Neoral; SandIMMUNE

Brand Names: Canada Apo-Cyclosporine; Neoral; Sandimmune I.V.; Sandoz-Cyclosporine

Index Terms Ciclosporin; CsA; CyA; Cyclosporin A

Pharmacologic Category Calcineurin Inhibitor; Immunosuppressant Agent

Use

Cyclosporine modified:

Transplant rejection prophylaxis: Prophylaxis of organ rejection in kidney, liver, and heart transplants (has been used with azathioprine and/or corticosteroids)

Rheumatoid arthritis: Treatment of severe, active rheumatoid arthritis (RA) not responsive to methotrexate alone

Psoriasis: Treatment of severe, recalcitrant plaque psoriasis in nonimmunocompromised adults unresponsive to or unable to tolerate other systemic therapy

Cyclosporine non-modified: Transplant rejection (prophylaxis/treatment): Prophylaxis of organ rejection in kidney, liver, and heart transplants (has been used with azathioprine and/or corticosteroids; treatment of chronic organ rejection)

Canadian labeling: Additional uses (not in U.S. labeling):

Cyclosporine modified: Nephrotic syndrome: Induction and maintenance of remission in steroid dependent/resistant nephrotic syndrome due to glomerular disease (eg, minimal change nephropathy, membranous glomerulonephritis, focal and segmental glomerulosclerosis); maintenance of steroid induced remission allowing for steroid dose reduction or withdrawal.

Cyclosporine modified/non-modified: Bone marrow transplant rejection (prophylaxis/treatment): Prophylaxis of graft rejection following bone marrow transplantation; prophylaxis or treatment of graft-versus-host disease (GVHD)

Pregnancy Risk Factor C

Pregnancy Considerations Adverse events were not observed following the use of oral cyclosporine in animal reproduction studies (using doses that were not maternally toxic). In humans, cyclosporine crosses the placenta; maternal concentrations do not correlate with those found in the umbilical cord. Cyclosporine may be detected in the serum of newborns for several days after birth (Claris,

1993). Based on clinical use, premature births and low birth weight were consistently observed in pregnant transplant patients (additional pregnancy complications also present). Formulations may contain alcohol; the alcohol content should be taken into consideration in pregnant women.

The pharmacokinetics of cyclosporine may be influenced by pregnancy (Grimer, 2007). Cyclosporine may be used in pregnant renal, liver, or heart transplant patients (Cowan, 2012; EBPG Expert Group on Renal Transplantation, 2002; McGuire, 2009; Parhar 2012). If therapy is needed for psoriasis, other agents are preferred; however, cyclosporine may be used as an alternative agent along with close clinical monitoring; use should be avoided during the first trimester if possible (Bae, 2012). If treatment is needed for lupus nephritis, other agents are recommended to be used in pregnant women (Hahn, 2012).

Following transplant, normal menstruation and fertility may be restored within months; however, appropriate contraception is recommended to prevent pregnancy until 1-2 years following the transplant to improve pregnancy outcomes (Cowan, 2012; EBPG Expert Group on Renal Transplantation, 2002; McGuire, 2009; Parhar 2012).

A pregnancy registry has been established for pregnant women taking immunosuppressants following any solid organ transplant (National Transplantation Pregnancy Registry, Temple University, 877-955-6877).

A pregnancy registry has also been established for pregnant women taking Neoral for psoriasis or rheumatoid arthritis (Neoral Pregnancy Registry for Psoriasis and Rheumatoid Arthritis, Thomas Jefferson University, 888-522-5581).

Breast-Feeding Considerations Cyclosporine is excreted in breast milk. Concentrations of cyclosporine in milk vary widely and breast-feeding during therapy is generally not recommended (Bae, 2012; Cowan, 2012). Due to the potential for serious adverse in the nursing infant, the decision to discontinue cyclosporine or to discontinue breast-feeding should take into account the importance of treatment to the mother. Formulations may contain alcohol which may be present in breast milk and could be absorbed orally by the nursing infant.

Contraindications

Hypersensitivity to cyclosporine or any component of the formulation. IV cyclosporine is contraindicated in hypersensitivity to polyoxyethylated castor oil (Cremophor EL).

Rheumatoid arthritis and psoriasis: Abnormal renal function, uncontrolled hypertension, malignancies. Concomitant treatment with PUVA or UVB therapy, methotrexate, other immunosuppressive agents, coal tar, or radiation therapy are also contraindications for use in patients with psoriasis.

Canadian labeling: Additional contraindications (not in U.S. labeling): Primary or secondary immunodeficiency excluding autoimmune disease; uncontrolled infection.

Warnings/Precautions Hazardous agent - use appropriate precautions for handling and disposal (NIOSH 2014 [group 2]).

[U.S. Boxed Warning]: Increased risk of lymphomas and other malignancies (including fatal outcomes), **particularly skin cancers;** risk is related to intensity/duration of therapy and the use of more than one immunosuppressive agent; all patients should avoid excessive sun/UV light exposure. **[U.S. Boxed Warning]: May cause hypertension; risk is increased with increasing doses/duration.** Use caution when changing dosage forms.

[U.S. Boxed Warning]: Renal impairment, including structural kidney damage has occurred (when used at high doses); risk is increased with increasing doses/duration; monitor renal function closely. Elevations in serum creatinine and BUN generally respond to dosage reductions. Use caution with other potentially nephrotoxic drugs (eg, acyclovir, aminoglycoside antibiotics, amphotericin B, ciprofloxacin). Elevations in serum creatinine and BUN associated with nephrotoxicity generally respond to dosage reductions. In renal transplant patients with rapidly rising BUN and creatinine, carefully evaluate to differentiate between cyclosporine-associated nephrotoxicity and renal rejection episodes. In cases of severe rejection that fail to respond to pulse steroids and monoclonal antibodies, switching to an alternative immunosuppressant agent may be preferred to increasing cyclosporine to an excessive dosage.

[U.S. Boxed Warning]: Increased risk of infection with use; serious and fatal infections have been reported. Bacterial, viral, fungal, and protozoal infections (including opportunistic infections) have occurred. Polyoma virus infections, such as the JC virus and BK virus, may result in serious and sometimes fatal outcomes. The JC virus is associated with progressive multifocal leukoencephalopathy (PML), and PML has been reported in patients receiving cyclosporine. PML may be fatal and presents with hemiparesis, apathy, confusion, cognitive deficiencies, and ataxia; consider neurologic consultation as indicated. The BK virus is associated with nephropathy, and polyoma virus-associated nephropathy (PVAN) has been reported in patients receiving cyclosporine. PVAN is associated with serious adverse effects including renal dysfunction and renal graft loss. If PML or PVAN occur in transplant patients, consider reducing immunosuppression therapy as well as the risk that reduced immunosuppression poses to grafts.

Liver injury, including cholestasis, jaundice, hepatitis, and liver failure, has been reported. These events were mainly in patients with confounding factors including infections, coadministration with other potentially hepatotoxic medications, underlying conditions, and significant comorbidities. Fatalities have also been reported rarely, primarily in transplant patients. Increased hepatic enzymes and bilirubin have occurred (when used at high doses); improvement usually seen with dosage reduction.

Should be used initially with corticosteroids in transplant patients. Significant hyperkalemia (with or without hyperchloremic metabolic acidosis) and hyperuricemia have occurred with therapy. Syndromes of microangiopathic hemolytic anemia and thrombocytopenia have occurred and may result in graft failure; it is accompanied by platelet consumption within the graft. Syndrome may occur without graft rejection. Although management of the syndrome is unclear, discontinuation or reduction of cyclosporine, in addition to streptokinase and heparin administration or plasmapheresis, has been associated with syndrome resolution. However, resolution seems to be dependent upon early detection of the syndrome via indium 111 labeled platelet scans.

May cause seizures, particularly if used with high-dose corticosteroids. Encephalopathy (including posterior reversible encephalopathy syndrome [PRES]) has also been reported; predisposing factors include hypertension, hypomagnesemia, hypocholesterolemia, high-dose corticosteroids, high cyclosporine serum concentration, and graft-versus-host disease (GVHD). Encephalopathy may be more common in patients with liver transplant compared to kidney transplant. Other neurotoxic events, such as optic disc edema (including papilloedema and potential visual impairment), have been rarely reported primarily in transplant patients.

[U.S. Boxed Warning]: The modified/non-modified formulations are not bioequivalent; cyclosporine (modified) has increased bioavailability as compared to

cyclosporine (non-modified) and the products cannot be used interchangeably without close monitoring. Cyclosporine (modified) refers to the oral solution and capsule dosage formulations of cyclosporine in an aqueous dispersion (previously referred to as "microemulsion"). Potentially significant drug-drug/drug-food interactions may exist, requiring dose or frequency adjustment, additional monitoring, and/or selection of alternative therapy. Gingival hyperplasia may occur; avoid concomitant nifedipine in patients who develop gingival hyperplasia (may increase frequency of hyperplasia). Monitor cyclosporine concentrations closely following the addition, modification, or deletion of other medication. Live, attenuated vaccines may be less effective; vaccination should be avoided. Make dose adjustments based on cyclosporine blood concentrations. **[U.S. Boxed Warning]: Cyclosporine non-modified absorption is erratic; monitor blood concentrations closely. [U.S. Boxed Warning]: Prescribing and dosage adjustment should only be under the direct supervision of an experienced physician. Adequate laboratory/medical resources and follow-up are necessary.** Anaphylaxis has been reported with IV use; reserve for patients who cannot take oral form. **[U.S. Boxed Warning]: Risk of skin cancer may be increased in transplant patients.** Due to the increased risk for nephrotoxicity in renal transplantation, avoid using standard doses of cyclosporine in combination with everolimus; reduced cyclosporine doses are recommended; monitor cyclosporine concentrations closely. Cyclosporine and everolimus combination therapy may increase the risk for proteinuria. Cyclosporine combined with either everolimus or sirolimus may increase the risk for thrombotic microangiopathy/thrombotic thrombocytopenic purpura/hemolytic uremic syndrome (TMA/TTP/HUS). Cyclosporine has extensive hepatic metabolism and exposure is increased in patients with severe hepatic impairment; may require dose reduction.

Patients with psoriasis should avoid excessive sun exposure. **[U.S. Boxed Warning]: Risk of skin cancer may be increased with a history of PUVA and possibly methotrexate or other immunosuppressants, UVB, coal tar, or radiation.**

Rheumatoid arthritis: If receiving other immunosuppressive agents, radiation or UV therapy, concurrent use of cyclosporine is not recommended.

Products may contain corn oil, ethanol (consider alcohol content in certain patient populations, including pregnant or breast feeding women, patients with liver disease, seizure disorders, alcohol dependency, or pediatrics), or propylene glycol; injection also contains the vehicle Cremophor EL (polyoxyethylated castor oil), which has been associated with hypersensitivity (anaphylactic) reactions. Some dosage forms may contain propylene glycol; large amounts are potentially toxic and have been associated hyperosmolality, lactic acidosis, seizures, and respiratory depression; use caution (AAP, 1997; Zar, 2007).

Adverse Reactions Adverse reactions reported with systemic use, including rheumatoid arthritis, psoriasis, and transplantation (kidney, liver, and heart).

Any indication:

Cardiovascular: Edema, hypertension

Central nervous system: Headache, paresthesia

Dermatologic: Hypertrichosis

Endocrine & metabolic: Female genital tract disease, hirsutism, increased serum triglycerides

Gastrointestinal: Abdominal distress, diarrhea, dyspepsia, gingival hyperplasia, nausea

Infection: Increased susceptibility to infection

Neuromuscular & skeletal: Leg cramps, tremor

Renal: Increased serum creatinine, renal insufficiency

Respiratory: Upper respiratory tract infection

Kidney, liver, and heart transplant only:

Cardiovascular: Chest pain, flushing, glomerular capillary thrombosis, myocardial infarction

Central nervous system: Anxiety, confusion, convulsions, lethargy, tingling sensation

Dermatologic: Acne vulgaris, nail disease (brittle fingernails), hair breakage, night sweats, pruritus, skin infection

Endocrine & metabolic: Gynecomastia, hyperglycemia, hypomagnesemia, weight loss

Gastrointestinal: Anorexia, aphthous stomatitis, constipation, dysphagia, gastritis, hiccups, pancreatitis, vomiting

Genitourinary: Hematuria, urinary tract infection (kidney transplant)

Hematologic & oncologic: Anemia, leukopenia, lymphoma, thrombocytopenia, upper gastrointestinal hemorrhage

Hepatic: Hepatotoxicity

Infection: Abscess, cytomegalovirus disease, fungal infection (systemic), localized fungal infection, septicemia, viral infection (kidney transplant)

Neuromuscular & skeletal: Arthralgia, myalgia, weakness

Ophthalmic: Conjunctivitis, visual disturbance

Otic: Hearing loss, tinnitus

Respiratory: Pneumonia, sinusitis

Miscellaneous: Fever

Rheumatoid arthritis only:

Cardiovascular: Abnormal heart sounds, cardiac arrhythmia, cardiac failure, chest pain, myocardial infarction, peripheral ischemia

Central nervous system: Anxiety, depression, dizziness, drowsiness, emotional lability, hypoesthesia, insomnia, lack of concentration, malaise, migraine, neuropathy, nervousness, pain, paranoia, vertigo

Dermatologic: Cellulitis, dermatological reaction, dermatitis, diaphoresis, dyschromia, eczema, enanthema, folliculitis, nail disease, pruritus, urticaria, xeroderma

Endocrine & metabolic: Decreased libido, diabetes mellitus, goiter, hot flash, hyperkalemia, hyperuricemia, hypoglycemia, increased libido, menstrual disease, weight gain, weight loss

Gastrointestinal: Constipation, dysgeusia, dysphagia, enlargement of salivary glands, eructation, esophagitis, flatulence, gastric ulcer, gastritis, gastroenteritis, gingival hemorrhage, gingivitis, glossitis, peptic ulcer, tongue disease, vomiting, xerostomia

Genitourinary: Breast fibroadenosis, hematuria, leukorrhea, mastalgia, nocturia, urine abnormality, urinary incontinence, urinary urgency, uterine hemorrhage

Hematologic & oncologic: Anemia, carcinoma, leukopenia, lymphadenopathy, purpura

Hepatic: Hyperbilirubinemia

Infection: Abscess (including renal), bacterial infection, candidiasis, fungal infection, herpes simplex infection, herpes zoster, viral infection

Neuromuscular & skeletal: Arthralgia, bone fracture, dislocation, myalgia, stiffness, synovial cyst, tendon disease, weakness

Ophthalmic: Cataract, conjunctivitis, eye pain, visual disturbance

Otic: Tinnitus, deafness, vestibular disturbance

Renal: Abscess (renal), increased blood urea nitrogen, polyuria, pyelonephritis

Respiratory: Abnormal breath sounds, bronchospasm, cough, dyspnea, epistaxis, sinusitis, tonsillitis

Psoriasis only:

Cardiovascular: Chest pain, flushing

Central nervous system: Dizziness, insomnia, nervousness, pain, psychiatric disturbance, vertigo

Dermatologic: Acne vulgaris, folliculitis, hyperkeratosis, pruritus, skin rash, xeroderma

Endocrine & metabolic: Hot flash

Gastrointestinal: Abdominal distention, constipation, gingival hemorrhage, increased appetite
Genitourinary: Urinary frequency
Hematologic & oncologic: Abnormal erythrocytes, altered platelet function, blood coagulation disorder, carcinoma, hemorrhagic diathesis
Hepatic: Hyperbilirubinemia
Neuromuscular & skeletal: Arthralgia
Ophthalmic: Visual disturbance
Respiratory: Bronchospasm, cough, dyspnea, flu-like symptoms, respiratory tract infection, rhinitis
Miscellaneous: Fever

Rare but important or life-threatening; any indication: Anaphylaxis/anaphylactoid reaction (possibly associated with Cremophor EL vehicle in injection formulation), brain disease, central nervous system toxicity, cholestasis, cholesterol increased, exacerbation of psoriasis (transformation to erythrodermic or pustular psoriasis), gout, haemolytic uremic syndrome, hepatic insufficiency, hepatitis, hyperbilirubinemia, hyperkalemia, hyperlipidemia, hypertrichosis, hyperuricemia, hypomagnesemia, impaired consciousness, increased susceptibility to infection (including JC virus and BK virus), jaundice, malignant lymphoma, migraine, myalgia, myopathy, myositis, papilledema, progressive multifocal leukoencephalopathy, pseudotumor cerebri, pulmonary edema (noncardiogenic), renal disease (polyoma virus-associated), reversible posterior leukoencephalopathy syndrome, rhabdomyolysis, thrombotic microangiopathy

Drug Interactions

Metabolism/Transport Effects **Substrate** of CYP3A4 (major), P-glycoprotein; **Note:** Assignment of Major/Minor substrate status based on clinically relevant drug interaction potential; **Inhibits** CYP2C9 (weak), CYP3A4 (moderate), P-glycoprotein

Avoid Concomitant Use

Avoid concomitant use of CycloSPORINE (Systemic) with any of the following: Aliskiren; AtorvaSTATin; BCG; Bosentan; Bosutinib; Conivaptan; Crizotinib; Dronedarone; Enzalutamide; Eplerenone; Foscarnet; Fusidic Acid (Systemic); Ibrutinib; Idelalisib; Ivabradine; Lercanidipine; Lomitapide; Lovastatin; Mifepristone; Naloxegol; Natalizumab; Olaparib; PAZOPanib; Pimecrolimus; Pimozide; Pitavastatin; Potassium-Sparing Diuretics; Silodosin; Simeprevir; Simvastatin; Sitaxentan; Tacrolimus (Systemic); Tacrolimus (Topical); Tofacitinib; Tolvaptan; Topotecan; Trabectedin; Ulipristal; Vaccines (Live); VinCRIStine (Liposomal)

Increased Effect/Toxicity

CycloSPORINE (Systemic) may increase the levels/effects of: Afatinib; Aliskiren; Ambrisentan; ARIPiprazole; AtorvaSTATin; Avanafil; Boceprevir; Bosentan; Bosutinib; Brentuximab Vedotin; Budesonide (Systemic, Oral Inhalation); Calcium Channel Blockers (Dihydropyridine); Calcium Channel Blockers (Nondihydropyridine); Cannabis; Caspofungin; Colchicine; CYP3A4 Substrates; Dabigatran Etexilate; Dapoxetine; Dexamethasone (Systemic); Digoxin; Dofetilide; DOXOrubicin (Conventional); Dronabinol; Dronedarone; Edoxaban; Eliglustat; Etoposide; Etoposide Phosphate; Everolimus; Ezetimibe; FentaNYL; Fibric Acid Derivatives; Fluvastatin; Halofantrine; Hydrocodone; Ibrutinib; Imipenem; Ivabradine; Ivacaftor; Ledipasvir; Leflunomide; Lercanidipine; Lomitapide; Loop Diuretics; Lovastatin; Lurasidone; Methotrexate; MethylPREDNISolone; Minoxidil (Systemic); Minoxidil (Topical); MitoXANtrone; Naloxegol; Natalizumab; Neuromuscular-Blocking Agents; Nintedanib; Nonsteroidal Anti-Inflammatory Agents; Olaparib; OxyCODONE; PAZOPanib; P-glycoprotein/ABCB1 Substrates; Pimozide; Pitavastatin; Pravastatin; PrednisoLONE (Systemic); PredniSONE; Propafenone; Protease Inhibitors; Prucalopride; Ranolazine; Repaglinide; Rifaximin; Rivaroxaban; Rosuvastatin; Salmeterol; Saxagliptin; Silodosin; Simeprevir; Simvastatin; Sirolimus; Sitaxentan; Suvorexant; Tacrolimus (Systemic); Tacrolimus (Topical); Tetrahydrocannabinol; Ticagrelor; Tofacitinib; Tolvaptan; Topotecan; Trabectedin; Ulipristal; Vaccines (Live); Vilazodone; VinCRIStine (Liposomal); Zopiclone; Zuclopenthixol

The levels/effects of CycloSPORINE (Systemic) may be increased by: AcetaZOLAMIDE; Aminoglycosides; Amiodarone; Amphotericin B; Androgens; Angiotensin II Receptor Blockers; Antifungal Agents (Azole Derivatives, Systemic); Aprepitant; Boceprevir; Bromocriptine; Calcium Channel Blockers (Nondihydropyridine); Carvedilol; Ceritinib; Chloramphenicol; Conivaptan; Crizotinib; Cyclophosphamide; CYP3A4 Inhibitors (Moderate); CYP3A4 Inhibitors (Strong); Dasatinib; Denosumab; Dexamethasone (Systemic); Eplerenone; Ezetimibe; Fluconazole; Fosaprepitant; Foscarnet; Fusidic Acid (Systemic); GlyBURIDE; Grapefruit Juice; Idelalisib; Imatinib; Imipenem; Lercanidipine; Luliconazole; Macrolide Antibiotics; Melphalan; Methotrexate; MethylPREDNISolone; Metoclopramide; Metreleptin; Mifepristone; Netupitant; Nonsteroidal Anti-Inflammatory Agents; Norfloxacin; Omeprazole; P-glycoprotein/ABCB1 Inhibitors; Pimecrolimus; Potassium-Sparing Diuretics; Pravastatin; PredniSoLONE (Systemic); PredniSONE; Protease Inhibitors; Pyrazinamide; Quinupristin; Ritonavir; Roflumilast; Simeprevir; Sirolimus; Stiripentol; Sulfonamide Derivatives; Tacrolimus (Systemic); Tacrolimus (Topical); Telaprevir; Temsirolimus; Trastuzumab

Decreased Effect

CycloSPORINE (Systemic) may decrease the levels/effects of: BCG; Coccidioides immitis Skin Test; GlyBURIDE; Ifosfamide; Mycophenolate; Sipuleucel-T; Vaccines (Inactivated); Vaccines (Live)

The levels/effects of CycloSPORINE (Systemic) may be decreased by: Adalimumab; Armodafinil; Ascorbic Acid; Barbiturates; Bosentan; CarBAMazepine; Colesevelam; Cyclophosphamide; CYP3A4 Inducers (Moderate); CYP3A4 Inducers (Strong); Dabrafenib; Deferasirox; Dexamethasone (Systemic); Echinacea; Efavirenz; Enzalutamide; Fibric Acid Derivatives; Fosphenytoin; Griseofulvin; Imipenem; MethylPREDNISolone; Metreleptin; Mitotane; Modafinil; Multivitamins/Fluoride (with ADE); Multivitamins/Minerals (with ADEK, Folate, Iron); Multivitamins/Minerals (with AE, No Iron); Nafcillin; Orlistat; P-glycoprotein/ABCB1 Inducers; Phenytoin; PredniSoLONE (Systemic); PredniSONE; Rifamycin Derivatives; Sevelamer; Siltuximab; Somatostatin Analogs; St Johns Wort; Sulfinpyrazone [Off Market]; Sulfonamide Derivatives; Tocilizumab; Vitamin E

Food Interactions Grapefruit juice increases cyclosporine serum concentrations. Management: Avoid grapefruit juice.

Preparation for Administration Hazardous agent - use appropriate precautions for handling and disposal (NIOSH 2014 [group 2]).

Injection: To minimize leaching of DEHP, non-PVC containers and sets should be used for preparation and administration.

Sandimmune injection: Injection should be further diluted (1 mL [50 mg] of concentrate in 20-100 mL of D_5W or NS) for administration by intravenous infusion.

Storage/Stability

Capsule: Store at controlled room temperature.

Injection: Store at controlled room temperature; do not refrigerate. Ampuls and vials should be protected from light. Stability of injection of parenteral admixture at room temperature (25°C) is 6 hours in PVC; 12-24 hours in Excel, PAB containers, or glass.

Oral solution: Store at controlled room temperature; do not refrigerate. Use within 2 months after opening; should be mixed in glass containers.

Mechanism of Action Inhibition of production and release of interleukin II and inhibits interleukin II-induced activation of resting T-lymphocytes.

Pharmacodynamics/Kinetics

Absorption: Oral:

Cyclosporine (non-modified): Erratic and incomplete; dependent on presence of food, bile acids, and GI motility; larger oral doses are needed in pediatrics due to shorter bowel length and limited intestinal absorption

Cyclosporine (modified): Erratic and incomplete; increased absorption, up to 30% when compared to cyclosporine (non-modified); less dependent on food, bile acids, or GI motility when compared to cyclosporine (non-modified)

Distribution: Widely in tissues and body fluids including the liver, pancreas, and lungs

V_{dss}: 4-6 L/kg in renal, liver, and marrow transplant recipients (slightly lower values in cardiac transplant patients; children <10 years have higher values); ESRD: 3.49 L/kg

Protein binding: 90% to 98% to lipoproteins

Metabolism: Extensively hepatic via CYP3A4; forms at least 25 metabolites; extensive first-pass effect following oral administration

Bioavailability: Oral:

Cyclosporine (non-modified): Dependent on patient population and transplant type (<10% in adult liver transplant patients and as high as 89% in renal transplant patients); bioavailability of Sandimmune capsules and oral solution are equivalent; bioavailability of oral solution is ~30% of the IV solution

Children: 28% (range: 17% to 42%); gut dysfunction common in BMT patients and oral bioavailability is further reduced

Cyclosporine (modified): Bioavailability of Neoral capsules and oral solution are equivalent:

Children: 43% (range: 30% to 68%)

Adults: 23% greater than with cyclosporine (non-modified) in renal transplant patients; 50% greater in liver transplant patients

Half-life elimination: Oral: May be prolonged in patients with hepatic impairment and shorter in pediatric patients due to the higher metabolism rate

Cyclosporine (non-modified): Biphasic: Alpha: 1.4 hours; Terminal: 19 hours (range: 10-27 hours)

Cyclosporine (modified): Biphasic: Terminal: 8.4 hours (range: 5-18 hours)

Time to peak, serum: Oral:

Cyclosporine (non-modified): 2-6 hours; some patients have a second peak at 5-6 hours

Cyclosporine (modified): Renal transplant: 1.5-2 hours

Excretion: Primarily feces; urine (6%, 0.1% as unchanged drug and metabolites)

Dosage Neoral/Gengraf and Sandimmune are not bioequivalent and cannot be used interchangeably.

Children:

Bone marrow transplantation *(Canadian labeling)*:

Note: IV administration is preferred for initial therapy.

Oral: Cyclosporine (modified): Initial: 12.5 to 15 mg/kg daily in 2 divided doses beginning 1 day prior to transplant; Maintenance: ~12.5 mg/kg daily in 2 divided doses every 12 hours for at least 3 to 6 months; decrease dose gradually to zero by 1 year following transplant. Patients who develop graft versus host disease (GVHD) after discontinuation of cyclosporine may be reinitiated on therapy with a loading dose of 10 to 12.5 mg/kg followed by the previously established maintenance dose. Patients with mild, chronic GVHD should be treated with lowest effective dose.

IV: Cyclosporine (non-modified): Initial: 3 to 5 mg/kg daily or one-third of the oral dose as a single dose (infused over 2 to 6 hours) beginning 1 day prior to transplant; Maintenance: may continue initial dose for up to 2 weeks; however, patients should be switched to an oral dosage form as soon as possible.

Nephrotic syndrome *(Canadian labeling)*: Oral: Cyclosporine (modified):

Initial: 4.2 mg/kg daily in 2 divided doses every 12 hours; titrate for induction of remission and renal function. Adjunct therapy with low-dose oral corticosteroids is recommended for patients with an inadequate response to cyclosporine (particularly if steroid-resistant).

Maintenance: Dose is individualized based on proteinuria, serum creatinine, and tolerability but should be maintained at lowest effective dose; maximum dose: 6 mg /kg daily. Discontinue if no improvement is observed after 3 months.

Solid organ transplant: Refer to adult dosing; children may require, and are able to tolerate, larger doses than adults.

Adults:

Psoriasis: Oral: Cyclosporine (modified): Initial dose: 2.5 mg/kg daily, divided twice daily

Titration:

U.S. labeling: Increase by 0.5 mg/kg daily if insufficient response is seen after 4 weeks of treatment. Additional dosage increases may be made every 2 weeks if needed (maximum dose: 4 mg/kg daily).

Canadian labeling: Increase by 0.5 to 1 mg/kg daily if insufficient response is seen after 4 weeks of treatment. Additional dosage increases may be made every 4 weeks if needed (maximum dose: 5 mg/kg daily).

Discontinue if no benefit is seen by 6 weeks of therapy at the maximum dose. Once patients are adequately controlled, the dose should be decreased to the lowest effective dose. Doses lower than 2.5 mg/kg daily may be effective. The Canadian labeling recommends attempting to wean patients off therapy if no relapse occurs within 6 months of achieving remission. Treatment longer than 1 year is not recommended.

Note: Increase the frequency of blood pressure monitoring after each alteration in dosage of cyclosporine. Cyclosporine dosage should be decreased by 25% to 50% in patients with no history of hypertension who develop sustained hypertension during therapy and, if hypertension persists, treatment with cyclosporine should be discontinued.

Rheumatoid arthritis: Oral: Cyclosporine (modified): Initial dose: 2.5 mg/kg daily, divided twice daily; salicylates, NSAIDs, and oral glucocorticoids may be continued (refer to Drug Interactions)

Titration:

U.S. labeling: Dose may be increased by 0.5 to 0.75 mg/kg daily if insufficient response is seen after 8 weeks of treatment; additional dosage increases may be made again at 12 weeks (maximum dose: 4 mg/kg daily). Discontinue if no benefit is seen by 16 weeks of therapy.

Canadian labeling: If insufficient response to initial dose after 6 weeks, may increase dose gradually as tolerated (maximum dose: 5 mg/kg daily); maintenance therapy should be individualized to the lowest effective and tolerable dose; may take up to 12 weeks before full effect is achieved.

Note: Increase the frequency of blood pressure monitoring after each alteration in dosage of cyclosporine. Cyclosporine dosage should be decreased by 25% to 50% in patients with no history of hypertension who develop sustained hypertension during therapy and, if hypertension persists, treatment with cyclosporine should be discontinued.

Solid organ transplant (newly transplanted patients): Adjunct therapy with corticosteroids is recommended. Initial dose should be given 4 to 12 hours prior to transplant or may be given postoperatively; adjust initial dose to achieve desired plasma concentration

Oral: Dose is dependent upon type of transplant and formulation:

Cyclosporine (modified):

Renal: 9 ± 3 mg/kg daily, in 2 divided doses

Liver: 8 ± 4 mg/kg daily, in 2 divided doses

Heart: 7 ± 3 mg/kg daily, in 2 divided doses

Cyclosporine (non-modified): Initial doses of 10 to 14 mg/kg daily have been used for renal transplants (the manufacturer's labeling includes dosing from initial clinical trials of 15 mg/kg daily [range: 14 to 18 mg/kg daily]; however, this higher dosing level is rarely used any longer). Continue initial dose daily for 1 to 2 weeks; taper by 5% per week to a maintenance dose of 5 to 10 mg/kg daily; some renal transplant patients may be dosed as low as 3 mg/kg daily.

Note: When using the non-modified formulation, cyclosporine levels may increase in liver transplant patients when the T-tube is closed; dose may need decreased.

IV: Cyclosporine (non-modified): Manufacturer's labeling: Initial dose: 5 to 6 mg/kg daily or one-third of the oral dose as a single dose, infused over 2 to 6 hours; use should be limited to patients unable to take capsules or oral solution; patients should be switched to an oral dosage form as soon as possible.

Note: Many transplant centers administer cyclosporine as "divided dose" infusions (in 2 to 3 doses daily) or as a continuous (24-hour) infusion; dosages range from 3 to 7.5 mg/kg daily. Specific institutional protocols should be consulted.

Conversion to cyclosporine (modified) from cyclosporine (non-modified): Start with daily dose previously used and adjust to obtain preconversion cyclosporine trough concentration. Plasma concentrations should be monitored every 4 to 7 days and dose adjusted as necessary, until desired trough level is obtained. When transferring patients with previously poor absorption of cyclosporine (non-modified), monitor trough levels at least twice weekly (especially if initial dose exceeds 10 mg/kg daily); high plasma levels are likely to occur.

Acute graft versus host disease (GVHD), prevention (off-label use in the U.S.): Adults: IV followed by oral:

Initial: IV: 3 mg/kg daily 1 day prior to transplant; may convert to oral therapy when tolerated; titrate dose to appropriate cyclosporine trough concentration (in combination with methotrexate); taper per protocol (refer to specific references for tapering and target trough details); discontinue 6 months posttransplant in the absence of acute GVHD (Ratanatharathorn, 1998; Ruutu, 2013; Storb, 1986a; Storb, 1986b)

or

Initial: IV: 5 mg/kg (continuous infusion over 20 hours) each day for 6 days (loading dose) starting 2 days prior to transplant, then 3 mg/kg over 20 hours each day for 11 days starting on posttransplant day 4, then 3.75 mg/kg over 20 hours each day for 21 days starting on day 15, then **oral** (in 2 divided daily doses): 10 mg/kg daily days 36 to 83, then 8 mg/kg daily days 84 to 97, then 6 mg/kg/day days 98 to 119, then 4 mg/kg/day days 120 to 180, then discontinue (in combination with methotrexate +/- corticosteroid) (Chao, 1993; Chao, 2000).

Bone marrow transplantation *(Canadian labeling):* **Note:** IV administration is preferred for initial therapy.

Oral: Cyclosporine (modified): Initial: 12.5 to 15 mg/kg daily in 2 divided doses beginning 1 day prior to transplant. Maintenance: ~12.5 mg/kg daily in 2 divided doses every 12 hours for at least 3 to 6 months; decrease dose gradually to zero by 1 year following transplant. Patients who develop GVHD after discontinuation of cyclosporine may be reinitiated on therapy with a loading dose of 10 to 12.5 mg/kg followed by the previously established maintenance dose. Patients with mild, chronic GVHD should be treated with lowest effective dose.

IV Cyclosporine (non-modified): Initial: 3 to 5 mg/kg daily or one-third of the oral dose as a single dose (infused over 2 to 6 hours) beginning 1 day prior to transplant; Maintenance: May continue initial dose for up to 2 weeks; however, patients should be switched to an oral dosage form as soon as possible.

Focal segmental glomerulosclerosis (off-label use in U.S.): Oral: Initial: 3.5 to 5 mg/kg/day divided every 12 hours (in combination with oral prednisone) (Braun, 2008; Cattran, 1999)

Interstitial cystitis (bladder pain syndrome) (off-label use): Oral: Initial: 2 to 3 mg/kg/day in 2 divided doses (maximum of 300 mg daily). Once symptom relief is established, the dose can be tapered as tolerated (to as low as 1 mg/kg as a single daily dose) and in some cases can be stopped with continued benefit. Treatment duration was at least 6 months to more than 1 year in some patients (Forrest, 2012; Sairanen, 2004; Sairanen, 2005; Sairanen, 2008).

Nephrotic syndrome *(Canadian labeling):* Oral: Cyclosporine (modified):

Initial: 3.5 mg/kg daily in 2 divided doses every 12 hours; titrate for induction of remission and renal function. Adjunct therapy with low-dose oral corticosteroids is recommended for patients with an inadequate response to cyclosporine (particularly if steroid-resistant).

Maintenance: Dose is individualized based on proteinuria, serum creatinine, and tolerability but should be maintained at lowest effective dose; maximum dose: 5 mg /kg daily. Discontinue if no improvement is observed after 3 months.

Lupus nephritis (off-label use): Oral: Cyclosporine (modified): Initial: 4 mg/kg daily for 1 month (reduce dose if trough concentrations >200 ng/mL); reduce dose by 0.5 mg/kg every 2 weeks to a maintenance dose of 2.5 to 3 mg/kg daily (Moroni, 2006)

Ulcerative colitis, severe (steroid-refractory) (off-label use):

IV: Cyclosporine (non-modified): 2 to 4 mg/kg daily, infused continuously over 24 hours (Lichtiger, 1994; Van Assche, 2003). **Note:** Some studies suggest no therapeutic difference between low-dose (2 mg/kg) and high-dose (4 mg/kg) cyclosporine regimens (Van Assche, 2003).

Oral: Cyclosporine (modified): 2.3 to 3 mg/kg every 12 hours (De Saussure, 2005; Weber, 2006)

Note: Patients responsive to IV therapy should be switched to oral therapy when possible.

Dosage adjustment in renal impairment:

Nephrotic syndrome: *Canadian labeling:* Initial: 2.5 mg/kg daily.

Serum creatinine levels >30% above pretreatment levels: Take another sample within 2 weeks; if the level remains >30% above pretreatment levels, decrease dosage of cyclosporine (modified) by 25% to 50%.

Psoriasis (severe):

U.S. labeling:

Serum creatinine levels ≥25% above pretreatment levels: Take another sample within 2 weeks; if the level remains ≥25% above pretreatment levels, decrease dosage of cyclosporine (modified) by 25% to 50%. If two dosage adjustments do not reverse the increase in serum creatinine levels, treatment should be discontinued.

Serum creatinine levels ≥50% above pretreatment levels: Decrease cyclosporine dosage by 25% to 50%. If two dosage adjustments do not reverse the increase in serum creatinine levels, treatment should be discontinued.

Canadian labeling: Serum creatinine levels >30% above pretreatment levels: Decrease dosage of cyclosporine (modified) by 25% to 50%. If dosage adjustment does not reverse the increase in serum creatinine levels within 30 days, discontinue treatment.

Rheumatoid arthritis: *Canadian labeling:*

Serum creatinine levels >30% above pretreatment levels: Take another sample within 2 weeks; if the level remains ≥30% above pretreatment levels, manufacturer labeling recommends reducing dose but does not provide specific dosing recommendation. If dosage adjustment does not reverse the increase in serum creatinine levels within 30 days, discontinue treatment.

Serum creatinine levels >50% above pretreatment levels: Reduce dose by 50%; if dosage adjustment does not reverse the increase in serum creatinine levels within 30 days, discontinue treatment.

Hemodialysis: Supplemental dose is not necessary.

Peritoneal dialysis: Supplemental dose is not necessary.

Dosage adjustment in hepatic impairment:

Mild to moderate impairment: No dosage adjustment provided in the manufacturer's labeling; monitor blood concentrations.

Severe impairment: No dosage adjustment provided in the manufacturer's labeling; however, metabolism is extensively hepatic (exposure is increased). Monitor blood concentrations; may require dose reduction.

Dietary Considerations Administer this medication consistently with relation to time of day and meals. Avoid grapefruit juice with oral cyclosporine use.

Administration

Oral solution: Do not administer liquid from plastic or styrofoam cup. May dilute Neoral oral solution with orange juice or apple juice. May dilute Sandimmune oral solution with milk, chocolate milk, or orange juice. Avoid changing diluents frequently. Mix thoroughly and drink at once. Use syringe provided to measure dose. Mix in a glass container and rinse container with more diluent to ensure total dose is taken. Do not rinse syringe before or after use (may cause dose variation).

Combination therapy with renal transplantation:

Everolimus: Administer cyclosporine at the same time as everolimus

Sirolimus: Administer cyclosporine 4 hours prior to sirolimus

IV: The manufacturer recommends that following dilution, intravenous admixture be administered over 2-6 hours. However, many transplant centers administer as divided doses (2-3 doses/day) or as a 24-hour continuous infusion. Discard solution after 24 hours. Anaphylaxis has been reported with IV use; reserve for patients who cannot take oral form. Patients should be under continuous observation for at least the first 30 minutes of the infusion, and should be monitored frequently thereafter. Maintain patent airway; other supportive measures and agents for treating anaphylaxis should be present when IV drug is given. To minimize leaching of DEHP, non-PVC sets should be used for administration.

Hazardous agent - use appropriate precautions for handling and disposal (NIOSH 2014 [group 2]).

Monitoring Parameters Monitor blood pressure and serum creatinine after any cyclosporine dosage changes or addition, modification, or deletion of other medications. Monitor plasma concentrations periodically.

Nephrotic syndrome (Canadian labeling): Baseline blood pressure (2 readings within 2 weeks), fasting serum creatinine (at least 3 levels within 2 weeks), creatinine clearance, urinalysis, CBC, liver function, serum uric acid, serum potassium, and malignancy screening (eg, skin, mouth, lymph nodes). Biweekly monitoring of blood pressure for initial 3 months and then monthly thereafter, frequent monitoring of renal function and periodic cyclosporine trough levels are recommended during therapy. Consider renal biopsy in patients with steroid-dependent minimal change neuropathy who have been maintained on therapy >1 year.

Transplant patients: Cyclosporine trough levels, serum electrolytes, renal function, hepatic function, blood pressure, lipid profile

Psoriasis therapy: Baseline blood pressure, serum creatinine (2 levels each), BUN, CBC, serum magnesium, potassium, uric acid, lipid profile. Biweekly monitoring of blood pressure, complete blood count, serum creatinine, and levels of BUN, uric acid, potassium, lipids, and magnesium during the first 3 months of treatment for psoriasis. Monthly monitoring is recommended after this initial period. (**Note:** The Canadian labeling recommends bimonthly monitoring of serum creatinine after the initial period if serum creatinine remains stable and cyclosporine dose is ≤2.5 mg/kg daily, and monthly monitoring for higher doses). Also evaluate any atypical skin lesions prior to therapy. Increase the frequency of blood pressure monitoring after each alteration in dosage of cyclosporine.

Rheumatoid arthritis: Baseline blood pressure, and serum creatinine (2 levels each); serum creatinine every 2 weeks for first 3 months, then monthly if patient is stable. Increase the frequency of blood pressure monitoring after each alteration in dosage of cyclosporine. Additional Canadian labeling recommendations include CBC, hepatic function, urinalysis, serum potassium and uric acid (baseline and periodic thereafter).

Reference Range Reference ranges are method dependent and specimen dependent; use the same analytical method consistently

Method-dependent and specimen-dependent: Trough levels should be obtained:

Oral: 12-18 hours after dose (chronic usage)

IV: 12 hours after dose **or** immediately prior to next dose

Therapeutic range: Not absolutely defined, dependent on organ transplanted, time after transplant, organ function and CsA toxicity:

General range of 100-400 ng/mL

Toxic level: Not well defined, nephrotoxicity may occur at any level

Recommended cyclosporine therapeutic ranges when administered in combination with everolimus for renal transplant (Zortress product labeling, 2013):

Month 1 post-transplant: 100-200 ng/mL

Months 2 and 3 post-transplant: 75-150 ng/mL

Months 4 and 5 post-transplant: 50-100 ng/mL

Months 6-12 post-transplant: 25-50 ng/mL

Additional Information Cyclosporine (modified): Refers to the capsule dosage formulation of cyclosporine in an aqueous dispersion (previously referred to as "microemulsion"). Cyclosporine (modified) has increased bioavailability as compared to cyclosporine (non-modified) and cannot be used interchangeably without close monitoring.

Dosage Forms Considerations
Cyclosporine (modified): Gengraf and Neoral
Cyclosporine (non-modified): SandIMMUNE

Dosage Forms

Capsule, Oral:
Gengraf: 25 mg, 100 mg
Neoral: 25 mg, 100 mg
SandIMMUNE: 25 mg, 100 mg
Generic: 25 mg, 50 mg, 100 mg

Solution, Intravenous:
SandIMMUNE: 50 mg/mL (5 mL)
Generic: 50 mg/mL (5 mL)

Solution, Oral:
Gengraf: 100 mg/mL (50 mL)
Neoral: 100 mg/mL (50 mL)
SandIMMUNE: 100 mg/mL (50 mL)
Generic: 100 mg/mL (50 mL)

Dosage Forms: Canada

Capsule, Oral:
Neoral: 10 mg, 25 mg, 50 mg, 100 mg

Solution, Intravenous:
SandIMMUNE IV: 50 mg/mL (1 mL, 5 mL)

Solution, Oral:
Neoral: 100 mg/mL (50 mL)

CycloSPORINE (Ophthalmic)
(SYE kloe spor een)

Brand Names: U.S. Restasis

Brand Names: Canada Restasis®

Index Terms Ciclosporin; CsA; CyA; Cyclosporin A

Pharmacologic Category Calcineurin Inhibitor; Immunosuppressant Agent

Use Increase tear production when suppressed tear production is presumed to be due to keratoconjunctivitis sicca-associated ocular inflammation (in patients not already using topical anti-inflammatory drugs or punctal plugs)

Pregnancy Risk Factor C

Dosage Ophthalmic: Adolescents ≥16 years and Adults: Keratoconjunctivitis sicca: Instill 1 drop in each eye every 12 hours

Dosage adjustment in renal impairment: No dosage adjustment provided in manufacturer's labeling. However, dosage adjustment unlikely due to low systemic absorption.

Dosage adjustment in hepatic impairment: No dosage adjustment provided in manufacturer's labeling. However, dosage adjustment unlikely due to low systemic absorption.

Additional Information Complete prescribing information should be consulted for additional detail.

Dosage Forms

Emulsion, Ophthalmic [preservative free]:
Restasis: 0.05% (1 ea)

◆ **Cyestra-35 (Can)** *see* Cyproterone and Ethinyl Estradiol [CAN/INT] *on page 532*

◆ **Cyklokapron** *see* Tranexamic Acid *on page 2081*

◆ **Cymbalta** *see* DULoxetine *on page 698*

Cyproheptadine (si proe HEP ta deen)

Brand Names: Canada Euro-Cyproheptadine; PMS-Cyproheptadine

Index Terms Cyproheptadine Hydrochloride; Periactin

Pharmacologic Category Histamine H_1 Antagonist; Histamine H_1 Antagonist, First Generation; Piperidine Derivative

Additional Appendix Information
Beers Criteria - Potentially Inappropriate Medications for Geriatrics *on page 2271*

Use Perennial and seasonal allergic rhinitis and other allergic symptoms including urticaria

Pregnancy Risk Factor B

Pregnancy Considerations Adverse events have been observed in some animal reproduction studies. Maternal antihistamine use has generally not resulted in an increased risk of birth defects; however, information specific to cyproheptadine is limited. Antihistamines are recommended for the treatment of rhinitis, urticaria, and pruritus with rash in pregnant women (although second generation antihistamines may be preferred). Antihistamines are not recommended for treatment of pruritus associated with intrahepatic cholestasis in pregnancy.

Breast-Feeding Considerations It is not known if cyproheptadine is excreted into breast milk. Premature infants and newborns have a higher risk of intolerance to antihistamines. Use while breast-feeding is contraindicated by the manufacturer. Antihistamines may decrease maternal serum prolactin concentrations when administered prior to the establishment of nursing.

Contraindications Hypersensitivity to cyproheptadine or any component of the formulation; narrow-angle glaucoma; bladder neck obstruction; pyloroduodenal obstruction; symptomatic prostatic hyperplasia; stenosing peptic ulcer; concurrent use of MAO inhibitors; use in debilitated elderly patients; use in premature and term newborns due to potential association with SIDS; breast-feeding

Warnings/Precautions May cause CNS depression, which may impair physical or mental abilities; patients must be cautioned about performing tasks which require mental alertness (eg, operating machinery or driving). Effects may be potentiated when used with other sedative drugs or ethanol. Use with caution in patients with cardiovascular disease; increased intraocular pressure; respiratory disease; or thyroid dysfunction. In the elderly, avoid use of this potent anticholinergic agent due to increased risk of confusion, dry mouth, constipation, and other anticholinergic effects; clearance decreases in patients of advanced age (Beers Criteria). Antihistamines may cause excitation in young children.

Adverse Reactions
Cardiovascular: Extrasystoles, hypotension, palpitations, tachycardia
Central nervous system: Ataxia, chills, confusion, dizziness, drowsiness, euphoria, excitement, fatigue, hallucination, headache, hysteria, insomnia, irritability, nervousness, neuritis, paresthesia, restlessness, sedation, seizure, vertigo
Dermatologic: Diaphoresis, skin photosensitivity, skin rash, urticaria
Gastrointestinal: Abdominal pain, anorexia, cholestasis, constipation, diarrhea, increased appetite, nausea, vomiting, xerostomia
Genitourinary: Difficulty in micturition, urinary frequency, urinary retention
Hematologic & oncologic: Agranulocytosis, hemolytic anemia, leukopenia, thrombocytopenia
Hepatic: Hepatic failure, hepatitis, jaundice
Hypersensitivity: Anaphylactic shock, angioedema, hypersensitivity reaction
Neuromuscular & skeletal: Tremor
Ophthalmic: Blurred vision, diplopia
Otic: Labyrinthitis (acute), tinnitus
Respiratory: Nasal congestion, pharyngitis, thickening of bronchial secretions

Drug Interactions

Metabolism/Transport Effects None known.

Avoid Concomitant Use

Avoid concomitant use of Cyproheptadine with any of the following: Aclidinium; Azelastine (Nasal); Glucagon; Ipratropium (Oral Inhalation); MAO Inhibitors; Orphenadrine; Paraldehyde; Potassium Chloride; Thalidomide; Tiotropium; Umeclidinium

Increased Effect/Toxicity

Cyproheptadine may increase the levels/effects of: AbobotulinumtoxinA; Alcohol (Ethyl); Analgesics (Opioid); Anticholinergic Agents; Azelastine (Nasal); Buprenorphine; CNS Depressants; Glucagon; Hydrocodone; Methotrimeprazine; Metyrosine; Mirabegron; Mirtazapine; OnabotulinumtoxinA; Orphenadrine; Paraldehyde; Potassium Chloride; Pramipexole; RimabotulinumtoxinB; ROPINIRole; Rotigotine; Suvorexant; Thalidomide; Thiazide Diuretics; Tiotropium; Topiramate; Zolpidem

The levels/effects of Cyproheptadine may be increased by: Aclidinium; Brimonidine (Topical); Cannabis; Doxylamine; Dronabinol; Droperidol; HydrOXYzine; Ipratropium (Oral Inhalation); Kava Kava; Magnesium Sulfate; MAO Inhibitors; Methotrimeprazine; Mianserin; Nabilone; Perampanel; Pramlintide; Rufinamide; Sodium Oxybate; Tapentadol; Tetrahydrocannabinol; Umeclidinium

Decreased Effect

Cyproheptadine may decrease the levels/effects of: Acetylcholinesterase Inhibitors; Benzylpenicilloyl Polylysine; Betahistine; Hyaluronidase; Itopride; MAO Inhibitors; Secretin; Selective Serotonin Reuptake Inhibitors

The levels/effects of Cyproheptadine may be decreased by: Acetylcholinesterase Inhibitors; Amphetamines

Storage/Stability

Oral solution: Store at 15°C to 30°C (59°F to 86°F); protect from light.

Oral syrup: Store at 20°C to 25°C (68°F to 77°F); excursions permitted to 15°C to 30°C (59°F to 86°F); protect from light.

Oral tablets: Store at 20°C to 25°C (68°F to 77°F).

Mechanism of Action A potent antihistamine and serotonin antagonist, competes with histamine for H_1-receptor sites on effector cells in the gastrointestinal tract, blood vessels, and respiratory tract

Pharmacodynamics/Kinetics

Metabolism: Primarily by hepatic glucuronidation via UGT1A (Walker, 1996)

Half-life elimination: Metabolites: ~16 hours (Paton, 1985)

Time to peak, plasma: 6-9 hours (Paton, 1985)

Excretion: Urine (~40% primarily as metabolites); feces (2% to 20%)

Dosage

Allergic conditions: Oral:

Children: 0.25 mg/kg/day or 8 mg/m^2/day in 2-3 divided doses **or**

2-6 years: 2 mg every 8-12 hours (not to exceed 12 mg daily)

7-14 years: 4 mg every 8-12 hours (not to exceed 16 mg daily)

Adults: 4-20 mg daily divided every 8 hours (not to exceed 0.5 mg/kg/day); some patients may require up to 32 mg daily for adequate control of symptoms

Migraine headache prophylaxis (off-label use): Oral:

Children: 4 mg every 8-12 hours

Adults: 2 mg every 12 hours (with or without propranolol) (Holland, 2012; Rao, 2000)

Serotonin syndrome (off-label use): Adults: Oral: Initial: 12 mg followed by 2 mg every 2 hours or 4-8 mg every 6 hours as needed for symptom control (Boyer, 2005; Sun-Edelstein, 2008)

Spasticity associated with spinal cord damage (off-label use): Adults: Oral: Initial: 2-4 mg every 8 hours; maximum: 8 mg every 8 hours (Barbeau, 1982; Wainberg, 1990)

Elderly: Initiate therapy at the lower end of the dosage range

Dosage adjustment in renal impairment: No dosage adjustment provided in manufacturer's labeling. However, elimination is diminished in renal insufficiency.

Dosage adjustment in hepatic impairment: No dosage adjustment provided in manufacturer's labeling.

Dosage Forms

Syrup, Oral:

Generic: 2 mg/5 mL (10 mL, 473 mL)

Tablet, Oral:

Generic: 4 mg

◆ **Cyproheptadine Hydrochloride** *see* Cyproheptadine *on page 529*

Cyproterone [CAN/INT] (sye PROE ter one)

Brand Names: Canada Androcur®; Androcur® Depot; Novo-Cyproterone

Index Terms Cyproterone Acetate; SH 714

Pharmacologic Category Antiandrogen; Antineoplastic Agent, Antiandrogen

Use Note: Not approved in U.S.

Palliative treatment of advanced prostate cancer

Pregnancy Considerations Not indicated for use in women. In males, sperm count and volume of ejaculate will be reduced at oral doses of 50-300 mg/day. After ~2 months of treatment, infertility may be noted. Changes are reversible upon discontinuation of therapy, usually within 3-5 months although in some patients may take up to 20 months. Production of abnormal spermatozoa has been observed although the effect on fertilization or embryo formation is unknown.

Breast-Feeding Considerations Not indicated for use in women.

Contraindications Hypersensitivity to cyproterone or any component of the formulation; liver disease or hepatic dysfunction; Dubin-Johnson syndrome; Rotor syndrome; previous or existing liver tumors (if not due to metastases from prostate cancer); presence or history of meningioma; wasting diseases (except inoperable prostate cancer); severe chronic depression; existing thromboembolic processes

Warnings/Precautions Hazardous agent - use appropriate precautions for handling and disposal (meets NIOSH 2014 criteria).

[Canadian Boxed Warning]: Use is associated with dose-dependent hepatotoxicity (jaundice, hepatitis, acute hepatic failure) including fatal case reports with doses ≥100 mg/day. Hepatotoxicity typically develops after a few weeks to several months of treatment initiation. Use in patients with prior or existing hepatic disease is contraindicated. Use caution with concurrent use of other hepatotoxic drugs. Monitor hepatic function and discontinue in patients with evidence of hepatic injury.

Use caution in patients with a history of depression (contraindicated in severe chronic depression). Cyproterone has been associated with an increased incidence of depression, particularly early in the course of therapy (initial 6-8 weeks). Use with caution in patients with diabetes or impaired glucose tolerance, may cause alterations in glucose metabolism and require dosage adjustments in diabetes medications. Use with caution in conditions that may be aggravated by fluid retention, or cardiovascular disease. May increase the risk of thromboembolism (particularly when used in combination with ethinyl estradiol) and/or alter lipid profiles.

Benign and malignant hepatic tumors have been observed (rarely) after use; rule out the presence of tumor in patients presenting with severe upper abdominal discomfort, hepatic enlargement or signs of intra-abdominal hemorrhage. Meningioma formation has been reported with chronic therapy (years) at doses ≥25 mg/day. Avoid initiation of therapy in patients with a history or presence of meningioma; discontinue treatment in patients diagnosed with meningioma. Hyperplasia of the breast has been reported; subsides usually within 1-3 months after therapy discontinuation and/or dose reduction. Risk of treatment failure should be considered prior to discontinuation or dose reduction.

Shortness of breath commonly observed in patients receiving doses of 300 mg/day; use caution in patients with existing pulmonary dysfunction. Adrenalcortical function suppression has been reported with use; monitor adrenal function periodically. Hypochromic anemia has been observed (rarely); monitor CBC regularly. May promote prostate cancer growth in some patients with metastatic prostate cancer; discontinue therapy immediately with increasing prostate specific antigen (PSA) levels and monitor 6-8 weeks for withdrawal response prior to initiating alternative treatment. Decreased PSA levels and/or clinical improvement have been reported following therapy discontinuation.

Lassitude, weakness, and fatigue are common during first few weeks of treatment; symptoms usually lessen ~3 months after therapy initiation. Patients must be cautioned about performing tasks which require mental alertness (eg, operating machinery or driving). Five-year survival rates may be lower when used concomitantly with a GnRH agonist or orchiectomy versus patients treated with castration alone. Antiandrogen effects in hypersexuality may be reduced with ethanol. Ethanol should be avoided during treatment.

[Canadian Boxed Warning]: Should be prescribed and managed by a clinician experienced with hormonal therapy in prostate cancer.

Adverse Reactions

Cardiovascular: Edema, heart failure, hypotension, MI, phlebitis, shock, stroke, syncope, tachycardia, thrombosis (DVT, embolus, superficial venous thrombosis)

Central nervous system: Aphasia, chills, coma, depression, dizziness, encephalopathy, fatigue, headache, hemiplegia, lassitude, malaise, meningioma (with chronic therapy), personality disorder, psychotic depression, pyrexia, restlessness, vascular headache, vasovagal reactions

Dermatologic: Dry skin (sebum reduction), eczema, erythema nodosum, exfoliative dermatitis, hirsutism, maculopapular rash, patchy loss of body hair, photosensitivity, pruritus, rash, scleroderma, skin discoloration, urticaria

Endocrine & metabolic: Adrenal suppression (dose related), benign nodular breast hyperplasia, diabetes mellitus, galactorrhea, gynecomastia, hot flashes, hypercalcemia, hyperglycemia, hypernatremia, impotence, inhibition of spermatogenesis, libido decreased, negative nitrogen balance

Gastrointestinal: Anorexia, constipation, diarrhea, dyspepsia, glossitis, nausea, pancreatitis, vomiting, weight gain/loss

Genitourinary: Bladder carcinoma, crystalluria, urinary frequency, uterine fibroids enlarged, uterine hemorrhage

Hematologic: Anemia, fibrinogen increased, hemolytic anemia, hemorrhage, hypochromic anemia, leukopenia, leukocytosis, normocytic anemia, PT decreased, thrombocytopenia

Hepatic: Ascites, cholestatic jaundice, cirrhosis, hepatic carcinoma, hepatic coma, hepatic dysfunction (dose related), hepatic failure, hepatic necrosis, hepatitis, hepatoma, hepatomegaly, transaminases increased

Local: Injection site reaction

Neuromuscular and skeletal: Gait abnormal, myasthenia, osteoporosis, weakness

Ocular: Abnormal accommodation, abnormal vision, blindness, optic neuritis, optic atrophy, retinal vascular disorder, retinal vein thrombosis

Renal: Hematuria, renal failure, serum creatinine increased

Respiratory: Asthma, cough, dyspnea, hyperventilation, pulmonary embolism, pulmonary fibrosis, pulmonary oil microembolism

Miscellaneous: Allergic reaction, diaphoresis

Drug Interactions

Metabolism/Transport Effects Substrate of CYP3A4 (major); **Note:** Assignment of Major/Minor substrate status based on clinically relevant drug interaction potential; **Inhibits** CYP2C19 (weak), CYP2C8 (weak), CYP2C9 (weak), CYP2D6 (weak), CYP3A4 (weak); **Induces** CYP1A2 (moderate), CYP2E1 (moderate)

Avoid Concomitant Use

Avoid concomitant use of Cyproterone with any of the following: Conivaptan; Fusidic Acid (Systemic); Idelalisib; Indium 111 Capromab Pendetide; Pimozide; Ulipristal

Increased Effect/Toxicity

Cyproterone may increase the levels/effects of: ARIPiprazole; C1 inhibitors; Dofetilide; HMG-CoA Reductase Inhibitors; Hydrocodone; Lomitapide; Pimozide

The levels/effects of Cyproterone may be increased by: Aprepitant; Ceritinib; Conivaptan; CYP3A4 Inhibitors (Moderate); CYP3A4 Inhibitors (Strong); Dasatinib; Fosaprepitant; Fusidic Acid (Systemic); Herbs (Progestogenic Properties); Idelalisib; Ivacaftor; Luliconazole; Mifepristone; Netupitant; Simeprevir; Stiripentol

Decreased Effect

Cyproterone may decrease the levels/effects of: Anticoagulants; CYP1A2 Substrates; CYP2E1 Substrates; Indium 111 Capromab Pendetide

The levels/effects of Cyproterone may be decreased by: Alcohol (Ethyl); Aminoglutethimide; Bosentan; CYP3A4 Inducers (Moderate); CYP3A4 Inducers (Strong); Dabrafenib; Deferasirox; Mitotane; Siltuximab; St Johns Wort; Tocilizumab; Ulipristal

Food Interactions Ethanol may reduce the effect of cyproterone (not established in the treatment of prostatic carcinoma). Management: Avoid concurrent use.

Storage/Stability

Injection: Store at 15°C to 30°C (59°F to 86°F).

Tablet: Store at 15°C to 30°C (59°F to 86°F). Protect from light.

Mechanism of Action Cyproterone is a steroid with antiandrogenic, antigonadotropic, and progestin-like activity. Blocks binding of dihydrotestosterone (DHT) to prostatic cancer cells and exerts negative feedback on hypothalamic-pituitary axis by inhibiting luteinizing hormone (LH) secretion leading to decreased testosterone production.

Pharmacodynamics/Kinetics

Absorption: Oral: Complete

Metabolism: Hepatic, some metabolites have activity

Half-life elimination: Oral: 38 hours (range: 33-43 hours); Depot injection: 4 days

Time to peak, plasma: Oral: 3-4 hours; Depot injection: 3 days

Excretion: Feces (60%); urine (33%)

Dosage Adults: Males:

Prostate cancer, advanced (palliative treatment):

Oral: 200-300 mg daily in 2-3 divided doses (maximum: 300 mg daily); following orchiectomy, reduce dose to 100-200 mg daily

IM: 300 mg (3 mL) once weekly; reduce dose in orchiectomized patients to 300 mg every 2 weeks

Note: May interchange between oral and IM administration during chronic therapy; dosages should remain within usual ranges (Oral: 100-300 mg daily; IM: 300 mg weekly or every 2 weeks).

Treatment of paraphilia/hypersexuality (off-label use; Guay, 2009; Reilly, 2000): **Note:** Avoid use if active pituitary pathology, hepatic failure or thromboembolic disease:

Oral: 50-600 mg daily

IM: 300-600 mg weekly or every other week

Dosage adjustment in renal impairment: Has not been studied in patients with renal impairment. Use with caution; 33% of cyproterone is excreted renally.

Dosage adjustment in hepatic impairment: Use is contraindicated with hepatic impairment or liver disease.

Dietary Considerations Tablets should be taken after meals.

Administration

IM: Administer IM injections slowly and avoid intravascular injection which can lead to pulmonary microembolism.

Oral: Administer tablets at the same time each day, after meals and with liquids. Tablets may be divided into equal halves.

Hazardous agent; use appropriate precautions for handling and disposal (meets NIOSH 2014 criteria).

Monitoring Parameters Liver function tests should be performed at baseline and periodically thereafter, or with signs or symptoms suggestive of hepatotoxicity. CBC, adrenal function, electrolytes, fasting blood glucose and glucose tolerance (diabetic patients) should be monitored periodically. In patients with PSA progression, monitor for withdrawal response syndrome (eg, decrease in PSA levels) for 6-8 weeks following therapy discontinuation.

Treatment of paraphilia/hypersexuality (Guay 2009; Reilly, 2000): ECG; hepatic function test (baseline and during treatment if suspected hepatotoxicity); CBC (baseline); serum testosterone (baseline then monthly for 4 months then every 6 months); serum luteinizing hormone and prolactin (baseline and every 6 months); follicle-stimulating hormone (baseline); glucose; bone scan (baseline then annually) if serum testosterone significantly suppressed; blood pressure; weight gain

Product Availability Not available in U.S.

Dosage Forms: Canada

Injection, solution: 100 mg/mL (3 mL)

Androcur® Depot: 100 mg/mL (3 mL)

Tablet: 50 mg

Androcur®, Apo-Cyproterone®, Gen-Cyproterone: 50 mg

◆ **Cyproterone Acetate** *see* Cyproterone [CAN/INT] *on page 530*

Cyproterone and Ethinyl Estradiol [CAN/INT] (sye PROE ter one & ETH in il es tra DYE ole)

Brand Names: Canada Cyestra-35; Diane-35®; Novo-Cyproterone/Ethinyl Estradiol

Index Terms Ethinyl Estradiol and Cyproterone Acetate

Pharmacologic Category Acne Products; Estrogen and Progestin Combination

Use Note: Not approved in U.S.

Treatment of females with severe acne, unresponsive to oral antibiotics and other therapies, with associated symptoms of androgenization (including mild hirsutism or seborrhea). **Should not be used solely for contraception;** however, will provide reliable contraception if taken as recommended for approved indications

Pregnancy Considerations Pregnancy should be ruled out prior to treatment and discontinued if pregnancy occurs. In general, the use of combination hormonal contraceptives when inadvertently taken early in pregnancy have not been associated with teratogenic effects. Upon discontinuation of therapy, women should use a nonhormonal contraceptive to delay pregnancy until at least one normal cycle has occurred. Due to increased risk of venous thromboembolism (VTE) postpartum, combination hormonal contraceptives should not be started in any woman <21 days following delivery. Women without risk factors for VTE and who are not breast-feeding may start combination hormonal contraceptives during 21-42 days postpartum. After 42 days postpartum, restrictions for use are not related to postpartum status and should be based on other medical conditions (CDC, 2011).

Breast-Feeding Considerations Jaundice and breast enlargement in the nursing infant have been reported following the use of combination hormonal contraceptives. May decrease the quality and quantity of breast milk; alternative form of contraception is recommended (per manufacturer). The theoretical concerns about decreased milk production are greatest early in the postpartum period when milk production is being established. Postpartum risk status for VTE should be considered when initiating combination hormonal contraceptives after delivery. Combined hormonal contraceptives should not be started <21 days postpartum due to increased risk of VTE. Risk of VTE is still elevated in breast-feeding women until ~42 days postpartum and is greater in women with additional risk factors. After 42 days postpartum, restrictions for use are not related to postpartum VTE risk and should be based on other medical conditions (CDC, 2011).

Contraindications Hypersensitivity to ethinyl estradiol, cyproterone, or any component of the formulation; breast cancer or other estrogen- or progestin-dependent neoplasms (current or a history of); hepatic tumors or disease; history of cholestatic jaundice; pregnancy; undiagnosed abnormal vaginal bleeding; ocular lesions arising from ophthalmic vascular disease; history of otosclerosis with deterioration during pregnancy

Use is also contraindicated in women at high risk of arterial or venous thrombotic diseases including: Cerebrovascular disease, coronary artery disease, MI, diabetes mellitus with vascular disease

Warnings/Precautions Hazardous agent - use appropriate precautions for handling and disposal (meets NIOSH 2014 criteria).

[Canadian Boxed Warning]: May increase the risk of thromboembolism; discontinue use if an arterial or venous thrombotic event occurs. Use is contraindicated in women with a history of thrombophlebitis or thromboembolic disorders. Progesterone and/or estrogen should not be taken while on this medication. [Canadian Boxed Warning]: The risk of cardiovascular side effects is increased in women who smoke cigarettes; risk increases with age (especially women >35 years of age) and the number of cigarettes smoked (≥15 cigarettes/day); women who use combination estrogen/progestin therapy should be strongly advised not to smoke.

Use with caution in patients with risk factors for coronary artery disease (eg, hypertension, hypercholesterolemia, morbid obesity, diabetes, or women who smoke); may lead to increased risk of myocardial infarction. May have a dose-related risk of vascular disease and hypertension. Women with androgen-related conditions (severe acne, hirsutism) may have an increased cardiovascular risk. Discontinue use if a significant rise in blood pressure occurs at any time during therapy.

[Canadian Boxed Warning]: Should not be prescribed solely for its contraceptive properties. Secondary nonhormonal contraception recommended in patients who may not adhere to dosing. **Should not be used in combination with other estrogen/progestin combination products.** This combination shares many of the risks of oral contraceptive agents. **Therapy should be discontinued 3-4 cycles after resolution of symptoms.** Not indicated for use after menopause or prior to menarche.

The use of combination oral contraceptive therapy has been associated with a slight increase in frequency of breast cancer; however, studies are not consistent. Use is contraindicated in women with breast cancer (current or history of). Evaluate hypothalamic-pituitary function in women with persistent (≥6 months) amenorrhea (especially associated with breast secretion) following discontinuation of therapy. Development of irregular, unresolving vaginal bleeding following previously regular cycles warrants further evaluation including endometrial sampling, if indicated, to rule out malignancy. Use with caution in patients with fibroids (leiomyomata); discontinue use with sudden enlargement, pain, or tenderness of fibroids. Discontinue at least 4 weeks prior to elective surgery. Medication should not be restarted until first menstrual period after hospital discharge following surgery.

May have adverse effects on glucose tolerance; use caution in women with diabetes. If patient has diabetes, hypertension, and obesity or if this triad of conditions develops, medication should be discontinued. Use with caution in patients with hepatic or renal impairment, cardiac disease, depression, asthma, epilepsy, or history of migraine. Estrogens may induce or exacerbate symptoms of angioedema, particularly in women with hereditary angioedema. Discontinuation of therapy may be necessary.

Combination hormonal contraceptives may affect serum triglyceride and lipoprotein levels; use with caution in patients with familial defects of lipoprotein metabolism. May have a dose-related risk of gallbladder disease; may worsen existing gallbladder disease. Risk of cholestasis may be increased with previous cholestatic jaundice of pregnancy or jaundice with prior oral contraceptive use. Hepatic adenomas and focal nodular hyperplasia have been reported with long-term oral contraceptive use. Presentation of an abdominal mass, acute abdominal pain, or intra-abdominal bleeding warrants further evaluation to rule out source.

Estrogens may cause retinal vascular thrombosis; discontinue if migraine, loss of vision, proptosis, diplopia, or other visual disturbances occur; discontinue permanently if papilledema or retinal vascular lesions are observed on examination. Use with caution in patients with myopia. Changes in contact lens tolerance or development of visual changes should be evaluated by an ophthalmologist. The use of estrogens and/or progestins may change the results of some laboratory tests (eg, coagulation factors, lipids, glucose tolerance, binding proteins). The dose, route, and the specific estrogen/progestin influences these changes. In addition, personal risk factors (eg, cardiovascular disease, smoking, diabetes, age) also contribute to adverse events; use of specific products may be contraindicated in women with certain risk factors.

Adverse Reactions Note: This listing reflects reactions reported with combination hormonal contraceptives.

Cardiovascular: Arterial thromboembolism, cerebral hemorrhage, cerebral thrombosis, edema, hypertension, mesenteric thrombosis, MI, Raynaud's phenomenon, varicosities

Central nervous system: Depression, dizziness, headache, migraine, nervousness, premenstrual syndrome, stroke

Dermatologic: Acne, angioedema, chloasma, erythema multiforme, erythema nodosum, hirsutism, loss of scalp hair, melasma (may persist), rash (allergic)

Endocrine & metabolic: Amenorrhea, breakthrough bleeding, breast changes (enlargement, secretion), breast tenderness, carbohydrate intolerance, dysmenorrhea, lactation decreased (postpartum), libido changes, menstrual flow changes, spotting, temporary infertility (following discontinuation), thyroid-binding globulin increased, triglycerides increased

Gastrointestinal: Abdominal bloating/cramps, appetite changes, cholestasis, colitis, gallbladder disease, nausea, pancreatitis, vomiting, weight gain/loss

Genitourinary: Cervical erosion changes, cervical secretion changes, cystitis-like syndrome, endocervical hyperplasia, uterine fibroids (leiomyomata) enlarged, vaginal candidiasis, vaginitis

Hematologic: Factors VII, VIII, IX, and X increased; folate levels decreased; hemolytic uremic syndrome; porphyria; prothrombin increased

Hepatic: Alkaline phosphatase increased, AST increased, benign liver tumors, Budd-Chiari syndrome, cholestatic jaundice, GGT increased, hepatic adenomas, jaundice

Local: Thrombophlebitis

Neuromuscular & skeletal: Chorea, rheumatoid arthritis exacerbation, synovitis exacerbation

Ocular: Cataracts, change in corneal curvature (steepening), contact lens intolerance, optic neuritis, retinal thrombosis

Otic: Auditory disturbances

Renal: Impaired renal function

Respiratory: Pulmonary thromboembolism, rhinitis

Miscellaneous: Hemorrhagic eruption, systemic lupus erythematosus (SLE)

Rare but important or life-threatening: Abortion, exanthema, focal nodular hyperplasia, hepatic enzymes abnormal, hepatitis, herpes zoster, hyperprolactinemia, hyperthyroidism, hypoesthesia, missed abortion, myoma, neurodermatitis, ovarian cyst, palpitations, paresthesia, photosensitivity, pigmentation, placental insufficiency, salivary gland swelling, seizures, urinary tract infection, urticaria, vision abnormal

Drug Interactions

Metabolism/Transport Effects Refer to individual components.

Avoid Concomitant Use

Avoid concomitant use of Cyproterone and Ethinyl Estradiol with any of the following: Anastrozole; Conivaptan; Dasabuvir; Dehydroepiandrosterone; Exemestane; Fusidic Acid (Systemic); Idelalisib; Indium 111 Capromab Pendetide; Ombitasvir; Ospemifene; Paritaprevir; Pimozide; Tranexamic Acid; Ulipristal

Increased Effect/Toxicity

Cyproterone and Ethinyl Estradiol may increase the levels/effects of: Agomelatine; ARIPiprazole; C1 inhibitors; Corticosteroids (Systemic); CYP1A2 Substrates; Dasabuvir; Dofetilide; HMG-CoA Reductase Inhibitors; Hydrocodone; Immune Globulin; Lenalidomide; Lomitapide; Ombitasvir; Ospemifene; Paritaprevir; Pimozide; Pirfenidone; ROPINIRole; Selegiline; Thalidomide; Tipranavir; TiZANidine; Tranexamic Acid

The levels/effects of Cyproterone and Ethinyl Estradiol may be increased by: Ascorbic Acid; Ceritinib; Conivaptan; CYP3A4 Inhibitors (Moderate); CYP3A4 Inhibitors (Strong); Dasatinib; Dehydroepiandrosterone; Fusidic Acid (Systemic); Herbs (Estrogenic Properties); Herbs (Progestogenic Properties); Idelalisib; Ivacaftor; Luliconazole; Metreleptin; Mifepristone; Netupitant; NSAID (COX-2 Inhibitor); Simeprevir; Stiripentol

Decreased Effect

Cyproterone and Ethinyl Estradiol may decrease the levels/effects of: Anastrozole; Anticoagulants; Chenodiol; CYP1A2 Substrates; CYP2E1 Substrates; Exemestane; Hyaluronidase; Indium 111 Capromab Pendetide; LamoTRIgine; Ospemifene; Thyroid Products; Ursodiol; Vitamin K Antagonists

The levels/effects of Cyproterone and Ethinyl Estradiol may be decreased by: Alcohol (Ethyl); Aminoglutethimide; Aprepitant; Armodafinil; Artemether; Barbiturates; Bexarotene (Systemic); Bile Acid Sequestrants; Boceprevir; Bosentan; CarBAMazepine; CloBAZam; Cobicistat; Colesevelam; CYP3A4 Inducers (Moderate); CYP3A4 Inducers (Strong); Dabrafenib; Deferasirox; Elvitegravir; Eslicarbazepine; Exenatide; Felbamate; Fosaprepitant; Fosphenytoin; Griseofulvin; Metreleptin; Mifepristone; Mitotane; Modafinil; Mycophenolate; Nafcillin; Nevirapine; OXcarbazepine; Phenytoin; Protease Inhibitors; Prucalopride; Retinoic Acid Derivatives; Rifamycin Derivatives; Rufinamide; Siltuximab; St Johns Wort; Telaprevir; Tipranavir; Tocilizumab; Topiramate; Ulipristal

Food Interactions CNS effects of caffeine may be enhanced if combination hormonal contraceptives are used concurrently with caffeine. Grapefruit juice increases ethinyl estradiol concentrations and would be expected to increase progesterone serum levels as well; clinical implications are unclear. Management: Monitor patients closely with concurrent use.

Storage/Stability Store at controlled room temperature of 15°C to 25°C (59°F to 77°F).

Mechanism of Action

Ethinyl estradiol: Estrogens are responsible for the development and maintenance of the female reproductive system and secondary sexual characteristics. Estrogens modulate the pituitary secretion of gonadotropins, luteinizing hormone, and follicle-stimulating hormone through a negative feedback system. Estrogen increases levels of sex hormone-binding globulin (SHBG) and may reduce unbound androgen levels. Ethinyl estradiol is a synthetic derivative of estradiol. The addition of the ethinyl group prevents rapid degradation by the liver.

Cyproterone: Steroidal compound with antiandrogenic, antigonadotropic and progestin-like activity.

Pharmacodynamics/Kinetics See individual agents.

Dosage Oral: Adults: Females: Acne: One tablet daily for 21 days, followed by 7 days off; first cycle should begin on the first day of menstrual flow. Subsequent dosing cycles should begin on the same day of the week that the first cycle was begun regardless of presence of withdrawal bleeding. Discontinue therapy 3-4 cycles after symptoms have resolved. **Note:** Retreatment may be considered with recurrence of symptoms following therapy discontinuation.

Dosage adjustment in renal impairment: Specific guidelines not available; use with caution

Dosage adjustment in hepatic impairment: Contraindicated in hepatic impairment or active liver disease

Administration Administer at the same time each day. Swallow tablet whole. A missed dose may be taken within the next 12 hours. If >12 hours, discard unused tablet and resume at usual scheduled times.

Hazardous agent; use appropriate precautions for handling and disposal (meets NIOSH 2014 criteria).

Monitoring Parameters Before starting therapy, a physical exam with reference to the breasts and pelvis are recommended, including a Papanicolaou smear. Exam may be deferred if appropriate; pregnancy should be ruled out prior to use. The first follow-up visit should be 3 months after initiation of treatment. Monitor patient closely for loss of vision, sudden onset of proptosis, diplopia, or migraine; blood pressure; signs and symptoms of thromboembolic disorders; signs and symptoms of depression; glycemic control in patients with diabetes; lipid profiles in patients being treated for hyperlipidemias; liver function tests. Adequate diagnostic measures, including endometrial sampling, if indicated, should be performed to rule out malignancy in all cases of undiagnosed abnormal vaginal bleeding.

Product Availability Not available in U.S.

Dosage Forms: Canada

Tablet, oral:

Diane-35: Cyproterone 2 mg and ethinyl estradiol 0.035 mg (21s)

- ◆ **Cyramza** *see* Ramucirumab *on page 1775*
- ◆ **Cystadane** *see* Betaine *on page 252*
- ◆ **Cystagon** *see* Cysteamine (Systemic) *on page 534*
- ◆ **Cystaran** *see* Cysteamine (Ophthalmic) *on page 535*

Cysteamine (Systemic) (sis TEE a meen)

Brand Names: U.S. Cystagon; Procysbi

Index Terms Cysteamine Bitartrate; Procysbi™

Pharmacologic Category Anticystine Agent; Urinary Tract Product

Use Treatment of nephropathic cystinosis

Pregnancy Risk Factor C

Dosage Oral:

Initial: Begin therapy as soon as the diagnosis of nephropathic cystinosis has been confirmed. Initiate therapy with 1/6 to 1/4 of maintenance dose; titrate slowly upward over 4-6 weeks.

Maintenance dose: Dosage adjustments should be made based on target WBC cystine levels (<1 nmol half-cystine/mg protein) and/or plasma cysteamine concentrations (>0.1 mg/L). If the patient is tolerating therapy, the target WBC cystine level should be <1 nmol half-cystine/mg protein; patients with poorer tolerability may still receive benefit when WBC cystine levels are kept at <2 nmol half-cystine/mg protein. If the WBC cystine level is >1 nmol half-cystine/mg protein but plasma cysteamine is >0.1 mg/L, confirm that the patient is compliant with regard to administration (including proper dosing interval and relationship between administration of medication and food).

Immediate release:

Children and Adolescents weighing ≤50 kg: 1.3 g/m^2/day or 60 mg/kg/day (off-label dose; Gahl, 2002) divided into 4 doses; maximum dose: 1.95 g/m^2/day or 90 mg/kg/day (off-label dose; Gahl, 2002).

Adolescents and Adults weighing >50 kg: 2 g daily in 4 divided doses; maximum dose: 1.95 g/m^2/day or 90 mg/kg/day (off-label dose; Gahl, 2002).

Missed doses: Administer missed dose as soon as possible. If the next scheduled dose is due in <2 hours, skip the missed dose and resume the regular dosing schedule. Do not double the dose.

Switching from cysteamine hydrochloride or phosphocysteamine solutions: Initiate immediate release cysteamine bitartrate at an equimolar dose to the cysteamine hydrochloride or phosphocysteamine dose; monitor WBC cystine levels 2 weeks after the switch, then every 3 months thereafter.

Delayed release:

Children ≥6 years, Adolescents, and Adults: 1.3 g/m^2/day divided every 12 hours; may increase as needed in 10% increments to a maximum dose of 1.95 g/m^2/day.

Missed doses: Administer missed dose as soon as possible. If the next scheduled dose is due in <4 hours, skip the missed dose and resume the regular dosing schedule. Do not double the dose.

Switching from immediate release cysteamine bitartrate to delayed release cysteamine bitartrate: Initiate delayed release cysteamine bitartrate at a total daily dose equal to the total daily dose of the immediate release formulation; monitor WBC cystine levels and/or plasma cysteamine concentration 2 weeks after the switch, then quarterly for 6 months, then two times annually thereafter.

Dosage adjustment for toxicity:

Gastrointestinal symptoms, transient skin rashes, CNS symptoms (eg, seizures, lethargy, somnolence, depression, encephalopathy):

Immediate release: Temporarily discontinue therapy. Reinitiate at a lower dose; titrate slowly.

Delayed release: Decrease dose by 10%. May temporarily discontinue therapy and reinitiate at a lower dose; titrate slowly.

Severe skin rashes (eg, erythema multiforme bullosa, toxic epidermal necrolysis): Permanently discontinue therapy.

Dosage adjustment in renal impairment: No dosage adjustment provided in manufacturer's labeling.

Dosage adjustment in hepatic impairment: No dosage adjustment provided in manufacturer's labeling.

Additional Information Complete prescribing information should be consulted for additional detail.

Dosage Forms

Capsule, Oral:

Cystagon: 50 mg, 150 mg

Capsule Delayed Release, Oral:

Procysbi: 25 mg, 75 mg

Cysteamine (Ophthalmic) (sis TEE a meen)

Brand Names: U.S. Cystaran

Index Terms Cysteamine Hydrochloride

Pharmacologic Category Anticystine Agent; Ophthalmic Agent

Use Treatment of corneal cystine crystal accumulation in patients with cystinosis

Pregnancy Risk Factor C

Dosage Ocular cystinosis: Adults: Ophthalmic: Instill 1 drop in each eye every hour while awake

Dosage adjustment in renal impairment: No dosage adjustment provided in manufacturer's labeling. However, dosage adjustment unlikely due to low systemic absorption.

Dosage adjustment in hepatic impairment: No dosage adjustment provided in manufacturer's labeling. However, dosage adjustment unlikely due to low systemic absorption.

Additional Information Complete prescribing information should be consulted for additional detail.

Dosage Forms

Solution, Ophthalmic:

Cystaran: 0.44% (15 mL)

◆ **Cysteamine Bitartrate** *see* Cysteamine (Systemic) *on page 534*

◆ **Cysteamine Hydrochloride** *see* Cysteamine (Ophthalmic) *on page 535*

◆ **Cystistat (Can)** *see* Hyaluronate and Derivatives *on page 1006*

◆ **CYT** *see* Cyclophosphamide *on page 517*

◆ **Cytarabine** *see* Cytarabine (Conventional) *on page 535*

Cytarabine (Conventional)

(sye TARE a been con VEN sha nal)

Brand Names: Canada Cytarabine Injection; Cytosar

Index Terms Ara-C; Arabinosylcytosine; Conventional Cytarabine; Cytarabine; Cytarabine Hydrochloride; Cytosar-U; Cytosine Arabinosine Hydrochloride

Pharmacologic Category Antineoplastic Agent, Antimetabolite; Antineoplastic Agent, Antimetabolite (Pyrimidine Analog)

Use

Acute myeloid leukemia: Remission induction in acute myeloid leukemia (AML)

Acute lymphocytic leukemia: Treatment of acute lymphocytic leukemia (ALL)

Chronic myeloid leukemia: Treatment of chronic myelocytic leukemia (CML; blast phase)

Meningeal leukemia: Prophylaxis and treatment of meningeal leukemia

Pregnancy Risk Factor D

Pregnancy Considerations Adverse effects were demonstrated in animal reproduction studies. Limb and ear defects have been noted in case reports of cytarabine exposure during the first trimester of pregnancy. The following have also been noted in the neonate: Pancytopenia, WBC depression, electrolyte abnormalities, prematurity, low birth weight, decreased hematocrit or platelets. Risk to the fetus is decreased if treatment can be avoided during the first trimester; however, women of childbearing potential should be advised of the potential risks.

Breast-Feeding Considerations It is not known if cytarabine is excreted in breast milk. Due to the potential for serious adverse reactions in the nursing infant, the decision to discontinue cytarabine or to discontinue breast-feeding should take into account the importance of treatment to the mother.

Contraindications Hypersensitivity to cytarabine or any component of the formulation

Warnings/Precautions Hazardous agent - use appropriate precautions for handling and disposal (NIOSH 2014 [group 1]). **[U.S. Boxed Warning]: Myelosuppression (leukopenia, thrombocytopenia and anemia) is the major toxicity of cytarabine.** Use with caution in patients with prior drug-induced bone marrow suppression. Monitor blood counts frequently; once blasts are no longer apparent in the peripheral blood, bone marrow should be monitored frequently. Monitor for signs of infection or neutropenic fever due to neutropenia or bleeding due to thrombocytopenia. **[U.S. Boxed Warning]: Toxicities (less serious) include nausea, vomiting, diarrhea, abdominal pain, oral ulcerations and hepatic dysfunction.** In adults, doses >1000 mg/m^2 are associated with a moderate emetic potential (Basch, 2011; Roila, 2010). In pediatrics, doses >200 mg/m^2 are associated with a moderate emetic potential and 3000 mg/m^2 is associated with a high emetic potential (Dupuis, 2011); antiemetics are recommended to prevent nausea and vomiting.

High-dose regimens are associated with CNS, gastrointestinal, ocular (reversible corneal toxicity and hemorrhagic conjunctivitis; prophylaxis with ophthalmic corticosteroid drops is recommended), pulmonary toxicities and cardiomyopathy. Neurotoxicity associated with high-dose treatment may present as acute cerebellar toxicity (with or without cerebral impairment), personality changes, or may be severe with seizure and/or coma; may be delayed, occurring up to 3 to 8 days after treatment has begun. Risk factors for neurotoxicity include cumulative cytarabine dose, prior CNS disease and renal impairment; high-dose therapy (>18 g/m^2 per cycle) and age >50 years also increase the risk for cerebellar toxicity (Herzig, 1987). Tumor lysis syndrome and subsequent hyperuricemia may occur; monitor, consider antihyperuricemic therapy and hydrate accordingly. Potentially significant drug-drug interactions may exist, requiring dose or frequency adjustment, additional monitoring, and/or selection of alternative therapy. There have been case reports of fatal cardiomyopathy when high dose cytarabine was used in combination with cyclophosphamide as a preparation regimen for transplantation.

Use with caution in patients with impaired renal and hepatic function; may be at higher risk for CNS toxicities; dosage adjustments may be necessary. Sudden respiratory distress, rapidly progressing to pulmonary edema and cardiomegaly has been reported with high dose cytarabine. May present as severe dyspnea with a rapid onset and refractory hypoxia with diffuse pulmonary infiltrates, leading to respiratory failure; may be fatal (Morgan, 2011). Cytarabine (ARA-C) syndrome is characterized by fever, myalgia, bone pain, chest pain (occasionally), maculopapular rash, conjunctivitis, and malaise; generally occurs 6 to 12 hours following administration; may be managed with corticosteroids. Anaphylaxis resulting in acute cardiopulmonary arrest has been reported (rare). There have been reports of acute pancreatitis in patients receiving continuous infusion cytarabine and in patients receiving cytarabine who were previously treated with L-asparaginase. **[U.S. Boxed Warning]: Should be administered under the supervision of an experienced cancer chemotherapy physician. Due to the potential toxicities, induction treatment with cytarabine should be in a facility with sufficient laboratory and supportive resources.** Some products may contain benzyl alcohol; do not use products containing benzyl alcohol or products reconstituted with bacteriostatic diluent intrathecally or for high-dose cytarabine regimens. Benzyl alcohol is associated with gasping syndrome in premature infants. Delayed progressive ascending paralysis has been reported in two children who received combination chemotherapy with IV and intrathecal cytarabine at conventional doses for the treatment of acute myeloid leukemia (was fatal in one patient). When used for intrathecal administration, should not be prepared during the preparation of any other agents; after preparation, store intrathecal medications in an isolated location or container clearly marked with a label identifying as "intrathecal" use only; delivery of intrathecal medications to the patient should only be with other medications also intended for administration into the central nervous system (Jacobson, 2009).

Adverse Reactions

Cardiovascular: Chest pain, pericarditis

Central nervous system: Dizziness, fever, headache, neural toxicity, neuritis

Dermatologic: Alopecia, pruritus, rash, skin freckling, skin ulceration, urticaria

Gastrointestinal: Abdominal pain, anal inflammation, anal ulceration, anorexia, bowel necrosis, diarrhea, esophageal ulceration, esophagitis, mucositis, nausea, pancreatitis, sore throat, vomiting

Genitourinary: Urinary retention

Hematologic: Myelosuppression, neutropenia (onset: 1 to 7 days; nadir [biphasic]: 7 to 9 days and at 15 to 24 days; recovery [biphasic]: 9 to 12 and at 24 to 34 days), thrombocytopenia (onset: 5 days; nadir: 12 to 15 days; recovery 15 to 25 days), anemia, bleeding, leukopenia, megaloblastosis, reticulocytes decreased

Hepatic: Hepatic dysfunction, jaundice, transaminases increased (acute)

Local: Injection site cellulitis, thrombophlebitis

Ocular: Conjunctivitis

Renal: Renal dysfunction

Respiratory: Dyspnea

Miscellaneous: Allergic edema, anaphylaxis, sepsis

Rare but important or life-threatening: Acute respiratory distress syndrome, amylase increased, angina, aseptic meningitis, cardiopulmonary arrest (acute), cerebral dysfunction, cytarabine syndrome (bone pain, chest pain, conjunctivitis, fever, maculopapular rash, malaise, myalgia); exanthematous pustulosis, hepatic sinusoidal obstruction syndrome (SOS; veno-occlussive disease), hyperuricemia, injection site inflammation (SubQ injection), injection site pain (SubQ injection), interstitial pneumonitis, lipase increased, paralysis (intrathecal and I.V. combination therapy), reversible posterior leukoencephalopathy syndrome (RPLS), rhabdomyolysis, toxic megacolon

Adverse events associated with high-dose cytarabine (CNS, gastrointestinal, ocular, and pulmonary toxicities are more common with high-dose regimens):

Cardiovascular: Cardiomegaly, cardiomyopathy (in combination with cyclophosphamide)

Central nervous system: Cerebellar toxicity, coma, neurotoxicity, personality change, somnolence

Dermatologic: Alopecia (complete), desquamation, rash (severe)

Gastrointestinal: Gastrointestinal ulcer, pancreatitis, peritonitis, pneumatosis cystoides intestinalis

Hepatic: Hyperbilirubinemia, liver abscess, liver damage, necrotizing colitis

Neuromuscular & skeletal: Peripheral neuropathy (motor and sensory)

Ocular: Corneal toxicity, hemorrhagic conjunctivitis

Respiratory: Pulmonary edema, syndrome of sudden respiratory distress

Miscellaneous: Sepsis

Adverse events associated with intrathecal cytarabine administration:

Central nervous system: Accessory nerve paralysis, fever, necrotizing leukoencephalopathy (with concurrent cranial irradiation, intrathecal methotrexate, and intrathecal hydrocortisone), neurotoxicity, paraplegia

Gastrointestinal: Dysphagia, nausea, vomiting

Ocular: Blindness (with concurrent systemic chemotherapy and cranial irradiation), diplopia

Respiratory: Cough, hoarseness

Miscellaneous: Aphonia

Drug Interactions

Metabolism/Transport Effects None known.

Avoid Concomitant Use

Avoid concomitant use of Cytarabine (Conventional) with any of the following: BCG; CloZAPine; Dipyrone; Natalizumab; Pimecrolimus; Tacrolimus (Topical); Tofacitinib; Vaccines (Live)

Increased Effect/Toxicity

Cytarabine (Conventional) may increase the levels/effects of: CloZAPine; Leflunomide; Natalizumab; Tofacitinib; Vaccines (Live)

The levels/effects of Cytarabine (Conventional) may be increased by: Denosumab; Dipyrone; Pimecrolimus; Roflumilast; Tacrolimus (Topical); Trastuzumab

Decreased Effect

Cytarabine (Conventional) may decrease the levels/effects of: BCG; Coccidioides immitis Skin Test; Flucytosine; Sipuleucel-T; Vaccines (Inactivated); Vaccines (Live)

The levels/effects of Cytarabine (Conventional) may be decreased by: Echinacea

Preparation for Administration Hazardous agent; use appropriate precautions for handling and disposal (NIOSH 2014 [group 1]). **Note:** Solutions containing bacteriostatic agents may be used for SubQ and standard-dose (100 to 200 mg/m^2) IV cytarabine preparations, but should not be used for the preparation of either intrathecal doses or high-dose IV therapies.

IV:

Powder for reconstitution: Reconstitute with bacteriostatic water for injection (for standard-dose).

For IV infusion: Further dilute in 250 to 1000 mL 0.9% NaCl or D_5W.

Intrathecal: Powder for reconstitution: Reconstitute with preservative free sodium chloride 0.9%; may further dilute to preferred final volume (volume generally based on institution or practitioner preference; may be up to 12 mL) with Elliott's B solution, sodium chloride 0.9% or lactated Ringer's. Intrathecal medications should not be prepared during the preparation of any other agents.

Triple intrathecal therapy (TIT): Cytarabine 30 to 50 mg with hydrocortisone sodium succinate 15 to 25 mg and methotrexate 12 mg are reported to be compatible together in a syringe (Cheung, 1984) and cytarabine 18 to 36 mg with hydrocortisone 12 to 24 mg and methotrexate 6 to 12 mg, prepared to a final volume of 6 to 12 mL, is reported compatible as well (Lin, 2008).

Intrathecal preparations should be administered as soon as possible after preparation because intrathecal preparations are preservative free.

Storage/Stability Store intact vials of powder for injection at room temperature of 20°C to 25°C (68°F to 77°F); store intact vials of solution at room temperature of 15°C to 30°C (59°F to 86°F).

IV:

Powder for reconstitution: Reconstituted solutions should be stored at room temperature and used within 48 hours.

For IV infusion: Solutions for IV infusion diluted in D_5W or NS are stable for 8 days at room temperature, although the manufacturer recommends administration as soon as possible after preparation.

Intrathecal: Administer as soon as possible after preparation. After preparation, store intrathecal medications in an isolated location or container clearly marked with a label identifying as "intrathecal" use only.

Mechanism of Action Inhibits DNA synthesis. Cytosine gains entry into cells by a carrier process, and then must be converted to its active compound, aracytidine triphosphate. Cytosine is a pyrimidine analog and is incorporated into DNA; however, the primary action is inhibition of DNA polymerase resulting in decreased DNA synthesis and repair. The degree of cytotoxicity correlates linearly with incorporation into DNA; therefore, incorporation into the DNA is responsible for drug activity and toxicity. Cytarabine is specific for the S phase of the cell cycle (blocks progression from the G_1 to the S phase).

Pharmacodynamics/Kinetics

Distribution: V_d: Total body water; widely and rapidly since it enters the cells readily; crosses blood-brain barrier with CSF levels of 40% to 50% of plasma level

Metabolism: Primarily hepatic; metabolized by deoxycytidine kinase and other nucleotide kinases to aracytidine triphosphate (active); about 86% to 96% of dose is metabolized to inactive uracil arabinoside (ARA-U); intrathecal administration results in little conversion to ARA-U due to the low levels of deaminase in the cerebral spinal fluid

Half-life elimination: IV: Initial: 7 to 20 minutes; Terminal: 1 to 3 hours; Intrathecal: 2 to 6 hours

Time to peak, plasma: SubQ: 20 to 60 minutes

Excretion: Urine (~80%; 90% as metabolite ARA-U) within 24 hours

Dosage Note: In adults, doses >1000 mg/m^2 are associated with a moderate emetic potential (Basch, 2011; Roila, 2010). In pediatrics, doses >200 mg/m^2 are associated with a moderate emetic potential and 3000 mg/m^2 is associated with a high emetic potential (Dupuis, 2011); antiemetics are recommended to prevent nausea and vomiting.

Acute myeloid leukemia (AML) remission induction: IV: Children and Adults: Standard-dose (manufacturer's labeling): 100 mg/m^2/day continuous infusion for 7 days **or** 200 mg/m^2/day continuous infusion (as 100 mg/m^2 over 12 hours every 12 hours) for 7 days

Pediatric indication-specific dosing:

AML induction: *7 + 3 regimen:* IV:

Children <3 years (off-label dosing): 3.3 mg/kg/day continuous infusion for 7 days; minimum of 2 courses (in combination with daunorubicin) (Woods, 1990)

Children ≥3 years: 100 mg/m^2/day continuous infusion for 7 days; minimum of 2 courses (in combination with daunorubicin) (Woods, 1990)

AML consolidation (off-label use): *5 + 2 + 5 regimen:* IV: Children ≥15 years: 100 mg/m^2/day continuous infusion for 5 days for 2 consolidation courses (in combination with daunorubicin and etoposide) (Bishop, 1996)

AML salvage treatment (off-label use):

Clofarabine/Cytarabine regimen: Induction: IV: Children ≥1 year and Adolescents: 1,000 mg/m^2/day over 2 hours for 5 days (in combination with clofarabine; cytarabine is administered 4 hours after initiation of clofarabine) for up to 2 induction cycles (Cooper, 2014)

FLAG regimen: IV: Children ≥11 years: 2000 mg/m^2/day over 4 hours for 5 days (in combination with fludarabine and G-CSF); may repeat once if needed (Montillo, 1998)

MEC regimen: IV:

Children ≥5 years: 1,000 mg/m^2/day over 6 hours for 6 days (in combination with etoposide and mitoxantrone) (Amadori, 1991)

Adolescents ≥15 years: 500 mg/m^2/day continuous infusion days 1, 2, and 3 and days 8, 9, and 10 (in combination with mitoxantrone and etoposide); may administer a second course if needed (Archimbaud, 1991; Archimbaud, 1995)

Acute lymphocytic leukemia (ALL; off-label dosing): *POG 8602/PVA regimen, intensification phase:* IV: Children ≥1 year: 1,000 mg/m^2 continuous infusion over 24 hours day 1 (beginning 12 hours after start of methotrexate) every 3 weeks or every 12 weeks for 6 cycles (Land, 1994)

Non-Hodgkin lymphomas (off-label use):

CODOX-M/IVAC regimen: IV: Children ≥3 years: Cycles 2 and 4 (IVAC): 2,000 mg/m^2 every 12 hours days 1 and 2 (total of 4 doses/cycle) (IVAC is combination with ifosfamide, mesna and etoposide; IVAC alternates with CODOX-M) (Magrath, 1996)

High-dose cytarabine: Children >1 year and Adolescents: IV: 3,000 mg/m^2 over 3 hours every 12 hours on days 2 and 3 (secondary phase; total of 4 doses) in combination with methotrexate and intrathecal methotrexate/ cytarabine (Bowman, 1996)

Adult indication-specific dosing:

AML induction: IV:

7 + 3 regimens (a second induction may be administered if needed; refer to specific references): 100 mg/m^2/day continuous infusion for 7 days (in combination with daunorubicin **or** idarubicin **or** mitoxantrone) (Arlin, 1990; Dillman, 1991; Fernandez, 2009; Vogler, 1992; Wiernick, 1992) **or** (Adults <60 years) 200 mg/m^2/day continuous infusion for 7 days (in combination with daunorubicin) (Dillman, 1991)

Low intensity therapy (off-label dosing): Adults ≥65 years: SubQ: 20 mg/m²/day for 14 days out of every 28-day cycle for at least 4 cycles (Fenaux, 2010) **or** 10 mg/m² every 12 hours for 21 days; if complete response not achieved, may repeat a second course after 15 days (Tilly, 1990)

AML consolidation (off-label use): IV:

5 + 2 regimens: 100 mg/m²/day continuous infusion for 5 days (in combination with daunorubicin **or** idarubicin **or** mitoxantrone) (Arlin, 1990; Wiernick, 1992)

5 + 2 + 5 regimen: 100 mg/m²/day continuous infusion for 5 days (in combination with daunorubicin **and** etoposide) (Bishop, 1996)

Single-agent: Adults ≤60 years: 3,000 mg/m² over 3 hours every 12 hours on days 1, 3, and 5 (total of 6 doses); repeat every 28-35 days for 4 courses (Mayer, 1994)

AML salvage treatment (off-label use): IV:

CLAG regimen: 2,000 mg/m²/day over 4 hours for 5 days (in combination with cladribine and G-CSF); may repeat once if needed (Wrzesień-Kuś, 2003)

CLAG-M regimen: 2,000 mg/m²/day over 4 hours for 5 days (in combination with cladribine, G-CSF, and mitoxantrone); may repeat once if needed (Wierzbowska, 2008)

FLAG regimen: 2,000 mg/m²/day over 4 hours for 5 days (in combination with fludarabine and G-CSF); may repeat once if needed (Montillo, 1998)

HiDAC (high-dose cytarabine) ± an anthracycline: 3,000 mg/m² over 1 hour every 12 hours 6 days (total of 12 doses) (Herzig, 1985)

MEC regimen: 1,000 mg/m²/day over 6 hours for 6 days (in combination with mitoxantrone and etoposide) (Amadori, 1991) **or**

Adults <60 years: 500 mg/m²/day continuous infusion days 1, 2, and 3 and days 8, 9, and 10 (in combination with mitoxantrone and etoposide); may administer a second course if needed (Archimbaud, 1991; Archimbaud, 1995)

Acute promyelocytic leukemia (APL) induction (off-label dosing): IV: 200 mg/m²/day continuous infusion for 7 days beginning on day 3 of treatment (in combination with tretinoin and daunorubicin) (Ades, 2006; Ades, 2008; Powell, 2010)

APL consolidation (off-label use): IV:

In combination with idarubicin and tretinoin: High-risk patients (WBC ≥10,000/mm³) (Sanz, 2010): Adults ≤60 years:

First consolidation course: 1000 mg/m²/day for 4 days

Third consolidation course: 150 mg/m² every 8 hours for 4 days

In combination with idarubicin, tretinoin, and thioguanine: High-risk patients (WBC >10,000/mm³) (Lo Coco, 2010): Adults ≤61 years:

First consolidation course: 1,000 mg/m²/day for 4 days

Third consolidation course: 150 mg/m² every 8 hours for 5 days

In combination with daunorubicin (Ades, 2006; Ades, 2008):

First consolidation course: 200 mg/m²/day for 7 days

Second consolidation course:

Age ≤60 years and low risk (WBC <10,000/mm³): 1,000 mg/m² every 12 hours for 4 days (8 doses)

Age <50 years and high risk (WBC ≥10,000/mm³): 2,000 mg/m² every 12 hours for 5 days (10 doses)

Age 50 to 60 years and high risk (WBC ≥10,000/mm³): 1,500 mg/m² every 12 hours for 5 days (10 doses) (Ades, 2008)

Age >60 years and high risk (WBC ≥10,000/mm³): 1,000 mg/m² every 12 hours for 4 days (8 doses)

Acute lymphocytic leukemia (ALL; off-label dosing):

Induction regimen, relapsed or refractory: IV: 3,000 mg/m² over 3 hours daily for 5 days (in combination with idarubicin [day 3]) (Weiss, 2002)

Dose-intensive regimen: IV: 3,000 mg/m² over 2 hours every 12 hours days 2 and 3 (4 doses/cycle) of even numbered cycles (in combination with methotrexate; alternates with Hyper-CVAD) (Kantarjian, 2000)

CALGB 8811 regimen (Larson, 1995): SubQ:

Early intensification phase: 75 mg/m²/dose days 1 to 4 and 8 to 11 (4-week cycle; repeat once)

Late intensification phase: 75 mg/m²/dose days 29 to 32 and 36 to 39

Linker protocol: IV: 300 mg/m²/day days 1, 4, 8, and 11 of even numbered consolidation cycles (in combination with teniposide) (Linker, 1991)

Chronic lymphocytic leukemia (CLL; off-label use):

OFAR regimen: IV: 1000 mg/m²/dose over 2 hours days 2 and 3 every 4 weeks for up to 6 cycles (in combination with oxaliplatin, fludarabine, and rituximab) (Tsimberidou, 2008)

CNS lymphoma, primary (off-label use): IV: 2,000 mg/m² over 1 hour every 12 hours days 2 and 3 (total of 4 doses) every 3 weeks (in combination with methotrexate and followed by whole brain irradiation) for a total of 4 courses (Ferreri, 2009)

Hodgkin lymphoma, relapsed or refractory (off-label use): IV:

DHAP regimen: 2,000 mg/m² over 3 hours every 12 hours day 2 (total of 2 doses/cycle) for 2 cycles (in combination with dexamethasone and cisplatin) (Josting, 2002)

ESHAP regimen: 2,000 mg/m² day 5 (in combination with etoposide, methylprednisolone, and cisplatin) every 3 to 4 weeks for 3 or 6 cycles (Aparicio, 1999)

Mini-BEAM regimen: 100 mg/m² every 12 hours days 2 through 5 (total of 8 doses) every 4 to 6 weeks (in combination with carmustine, etoposide, and melphalan) (Colwill, 1995; Martin, 2001)

BEAM regimen (transplant preparative regimen): 200 mg/m² twice daily for 4 days beginning 5 days prior to transplant (in combination with carmustine, etoposide, and melphalan) (Chopra, 1993)

Non-Hodgkin lymphomas (off-label use): IV:

CALGB 9251 regimen: Cycles 2, 4, and 6: 150 mg/m²/day continuous infusion days 4 and 5 (Lee, 2001; Rizzieri, 2004)

CODOX-M/IVAC regimen:

Adults ≤60 years: Cycles 2 and 4 (IVAC): 2,000 mg/m² every 12 hours days 1 and 2 (total of 4 doses/cycle) (IVAC is combination with ifosfamide, mesna, and etoposide; IVAC alternates with CODOX-M) (Magrath, 1996)

Adults ≤65 years: Cycles 2 and 4 (IVAC): 2,000 mg/m² over 3 hours every 12 hours days 1 and 2 (total of 4 doses/cycle) (IVAC is combination with ifosfamide, mesna, and etoposide; IVAC alternates with CODOX-M) (Mead, 2008)

Adults >65 years: Cycles 2 and 4 (IVAC): 1,000 mg/m² over 3 hours every 12 hours days 1 and 2 (total of 4 doses/cycle) (IVAC is combination with ifosfamide, mesna, and etoposide; IVAC alternates with CODOX-M) (Mead, 2008)

DHAP regimen:

Adults ≤70 years: 2,000 mg/m² over 3 hours every 12 hours day 2 (total of 2 doses/cycle) every 3-4 weeks for 6-10 cycles (in combination with dexamethasone and cisplatin) (Velasquez, 1988)

Adults >70 years: 1,000 mg/m² over 3 hours every 12 hours day 2 (total of 2 doses/cycle) every 3-4 weeks for 6-10 cycles (in combination with dexamethasone and cisplatin) (Velasquez, 1988)

ESHAP regimen: 2,000 mg/m^2 over 2 hours day 5 every 3 to 4 weeks for 6-8 cycles (in combination with etoposide, methylprednisolone, and cisplatin) (Velasquez, 1994)

BEAM regimen (transplant preparative regimen): 200 mg/m^2 twice daily for 3 days beginning 4 days prior to transplant (in combination with carmustine, etoposide, and melphalan) (Linch, 2010) **or** 100 mg/m^2 over 1 hour every 12 hours for 4 days beginning 5 days prior to transplant (in combination with carmustine, etoposide, and melphalan) (van Imhoff, 2005)

Intrathecal:

Meningeal leukemia: Note: Optimal intrathecal chemotherapy dosing should be based on age rather than on body surface area (BSA); CSF volume correlates with age and not to BSA (Bleyer, 1983; Kerr, 2001). Dosing provided in the manufacturer's labeling is BSA-based (usual dose 30 mg/m^2 every 4 days; range: 5 to 75 mg/m^2 once daily for 4 days or once every 4 days until CNS findings normalize, followed by 1 additional treatment).

Children: Age-based intrathecal dosing (off-label):

CNS prophylaxis:

<1 year: 20 mg per dose

1 to 1.99 years: 30 mg per dose

2 to 2.99 years: 50 mg per dose

≥3 years: 70 mg per dose

ALL CNS prophylaxis, age-specific doses from literature:

Administer on day 0 of induction therapy (Gaynon, 1993):

1 to <2 years: 30 mg per dose

2 to <3 years: 50 mg per dose

≥3 years: 70 mg per dose

Administer as part of triple intrathecal therapy (TIT) on days 1 and 15 of induction therapy; days 1, 15, 50, and 64 (standard risk patients) or days 1, 15, 29, and 43 (high-risk patients) during consolidation therapy; day 1 of reinduction therapy, and during maintenance therapy (very high-risk patients receive on days 1, 22, 45, and 59 of induction, days 8, 22, 36, and 50 of consolidation therapy, days 8 and 38 of reinduction therapy, and during maintenance) (Lin, 2007):

<1 year: 18 mg per dose

1 to 2 years: 24 mg per dose

2 to 3 years: 30 mg per dose

≥3 years: 36 mg per dose

Administer on day 0 of induction therapy, then as part of TIT on days 7, 14, and 21 during consolidation therapy; as part of TIT on days 0, 28, and 35 for 2 cycles of delayed intensification therapy, and then maintenance treatment as part of TIT on day 0 every 12 weeks for 38 months (boys) or 26 months (girls) from initial induction treatment (Matloub, 2006):

1 to <2 years: 16 mg per dose

2 to <3 years: 20 mg per dose

≥3 years: 24-30 mg per dose

Administer on day 15 of induction therapy, days 1 and 15 of reinduction phase; and day 1 of cycle 2 of maintenance 1A phase (Pieters, 2007):

<1 year: 15 mg per dose

≥1 year: 20 mg per dose

Treatment, CNS leukemia (ALL): Children: Administer as part of TIT weekly until CSF remission, then every 4 weeks throughout continuation treatment (Lin, 2007):

<1 year: 18 mg per dose

1 to 2 years: 24 mg per dose

2 to 3 years: 30 mg per dose

≥3 years: 36 mg per dose

Adult off-label uses or doses for intrathecal therapy:

CNS prophylaxis (ALL): 100 mg weekly for 8 doses, then every 2 weeks for 8 doses, then monthly for 6 doses (high-risk patients) **or** 100 mg on day 7 or 8 with each chemotherapy cycle for 4 doses (low risk patients) **or** 16 doses (high-risk patients) (Cortes, 1995)

or as part of TIT: 40 mg days 0 and 14 during induction, days 1, 4, 8, and 11 during CNS therapy phase, every 18 weeks during intensification and maintenance phases (Storring, 2009)

CNS prophylaxis (APL, as part of TIT): 50 mg per dose; administer 1 dose prior to consolidation and 2 doses during each of 2 consolidation phases (total of 5 doses) (Ades, 2006; Ades, 2008)

CNS leukemia treatment (ALL, as part of TIT): 40 mg twice weekly until CSF cleared (Storring, 2009)

CNS lymphoma treatment: 50 mg twice a week for 4 weeks, then weekly for 4 to 8 weeks, then every other week for 4 weeks, then every 4 weeks for 4 doses (Glantz, 1999)

Leptomeningeal metastases treatment: 25 to 100 mg twice weekly for 4 weeks, then once weekly for 4 weeks, then a maintenance regimen of once a month (Chamberlain, 2010) **or** 40 to 60 mg per dose (DeAngelis, 2005)

Dosage adjustment in renal impairment: There are no dosage adjustments provided in the manufacturers' labeling; however, the following adjustments have been recommended:

Aronoff, 2007 (Cytarabine 100 to 200 mg/m^2): Children and Adults: No adjustment necessary

Kintzel, 1995 (High-dose cytarabine 1 to 3 g/m^2):

CrCl 46 to 60 mL/minute: Administer 60% of dose

CrCl 31 to 45 mL/minute: Administer 50% of dose

CrCl <30 mL/minute: Consider use of alternative drug

Smith, 1997 (High-dose cytarabine; ≥2 g/m^2/dose):

Serum creatinine 1.5 to 1.9 mg/dL or increase (from baseline) of 0.5 to 1.2 mg/dL: Reduce dose to 1 g/m^2/dose

Serum creatinine ≥2 mg/dL or increase (from baseline) of >1.2 mg/dL: Reduce dose to 0.1 g/m^2/day as a continuous infusion

Hemodialysis: In 4 hour dialysis sessions (with high flow polysulfone membrane) 6 hours after cytarabine 1 g/m^2 over 2 hours, 63% of the metabolite ARA-U was extracted from plasma (based on a single adult case report) (based on a single adult case report) (Radeski, 2011)

Dosage adjustment in hepatic impairment: Dose may need to be adjusted in patients with liver failure since cytarabine is partially detoxified in the liver. There are no dosage adjustments provided in the manufacturers' labeling; however, the following adjustments have been recommended:

Floyd, 2006: Transaminases (any elevation): Administer 50% of dose; may increase subsequent doses in the absence of toxicities

Koren, 1992 (dose level not specified): Bilirubin >2 mg/dL: Administer 50% of dose; may increase subsequent doses in the absence of toxicities

Dosing in obesity:

American Society of Clinical Oncology (ASCO) Guidelines for appropriate chemotherapy dosing in obese adults with cancer: Utilize patient's actual body weight (full weight) for calculation of body surface area- or weight-based dosing, particularly when the intent of therapy is curative; manage regimen-related toxicities in the same manner as for nonobese patients; if a dose reduction is utilized due to toxicity, consider resumption of full weight-based dosing with subsequent cycles, especially if cause of toxicity (eg, hepatic or renal impairment) is resolved (Griggs, 2012).

American Society for Blood and Marrow Transplantation (ASBMT) practice guideline committee position statement on chemotherapy dosing in obesity: Utilize actual body weight (full weight) for calculation of body surface area in cytarabine dosing for hematopoietic stem cell transplant conditioning regimens in pediatrics and adults (Bubalo, 2014).

Administration

IV: Infuse standard dose therapy for AML (100 to 200 mg/m^2/day) as a continuous infusion. Infuse high-dose therapy (off-label) over 1 to 3 hours (usually). Other rates have been used, refer to specific reference.

In adults, doses >1000 mg/m^2 are associated with a moderate emetic potential (Basch, 2011; Roila, 2010). In pediatrics, doses >200 mg/m^2 are associated with a moderate emetic potential and 3000 mg/m^2 is associated with a high emetic potential (Dupuis, 2011); antiemetics are recommended to prevent nausea and vomiting.

Intrathecal: Intrathecal doses should be administered as soon as possible after preparation.

May also be administered SubQ.

Hazardous agent; use appropriate precautions for handling and disposal (NIOSH 2014 [group 1]).

Monitoring Parameters Liver function tests, CBC with differential and platelet count, serum creatinine, BUN, serum uric acid

Additional Information IV doses ≥1.5 g/m^2 may produce conjunctivitis which can be ameliorated with prophylactic use of corticosteroid (0.1% dexamethasone) eye drops. Dexamethasone eye drops should be administered at 1 to 2 drops every 6 hours during and for 2 to 7 days after completion of cytarabine.

Dosage Forms

Solution, Injection:
Generic: 20 mg/mL (25 mL); 100 mg/mL (20 mL)

Solution, Injection [preservative free]:
Generic: 20 mg/mL (5 mL, 50 mL); 100 mg/mL (20 mL)

Solution Reconstituted, Injection:
Generic: 100 mg (1 ea); 500 mg (1 ea); 1 g (1 ea)

◆ **Cytarabine Hydrochloride** *see* Cytarabine (Conventional) *on page 535*

◆ **Cytarabine Injection (Can)** *see* Cytarabine (Conventional) *on page 535*

◆ **Cytarabine Lipid Complex** *see* Cytarabine (Liposomal) *on page 540*

Cytarabine (Liposomal)

(sye TARE a been lye po SO mal)

Brand Names: U.S. DepoCyt

Brand Names: Canada DepoCyt®

Index Terms Cytarabine Lipid Complex; Cytarabine Liposome; DepoFoam-Encapsulated Cytarabine; DTC 101; Liposomal Cytarabine

Pharmacologic Category Antineoplastic Agent, Antimetabolite; Antineoplastic Agent, Antimetabolite (Pyrimidine Analog)

Use Treatment of lymphomatous meningitis

Pregnancy Risk Factor D

Pregnancy Considerations Reproductive studies have not been conducted with cytarabine liposomal. Cytarabine, the active component, has been associated with fetal malformations when given as a component of systemic combination chemotherapy during the first trimester. Systemic exposure following intrathecal administration of cytarabine liposomal is negligible; however, women of childbearing potential should avoid becoming pregnant during treatment.

Breast-Feeding Considerations Although the systemic exposure following intrathecal administration of cytarabine liposomal is negligible, breast-feeding is not recommended due to the potential for serious adverse reactions in the nursing infant.

Contraindications Hypersensitivity to cytarabine or any component of the formulation; active meningeal infection

Warnings/Precautions Hazardous agent - use appropriate precautions for handling and disposal (NIOSH 2014 [group 1]). **[U.S. Boxed Warning]: Chemical arachnoiditis (nausea, vomiting, headache, fever) occurs commonly; may be fatal if untreated. The incidence and severity of chemical arachnoiditis is reduced by coadministration with dexamethasone; dexamethasone should be administered concomitantly with cytarabine (liposomal) to diminish chemical arachnoid symptoms.** Hydrocephalus has been reported and may be precipitated by chemical arachnoiditis. May cause neurotoxicity (including myelopathy), which may lead to permanent neurologic deficit (rare); monitor for neurotoxicity; reduce subsequent doses; discontinue with persistent neurotoxicity. The risk of neurotoxicity is increased with concurrent radiation therapy or systemic chemotherapy. The risk for neurotoxicity is increased when administered with other antineoplastic agents or with cranial/spinal irradiation. Persistent (extreme) somnolence, hemiplegia, visual disturbances (including blindness; may be permanent), deafness, cranial nerve palsies, peripheral neuropathy, and even combined neurologic features (cauda equina syndrome) have been reported. CSF flow blockage may lead to increased free cytarabine concentrations in the CSF and increase the risk for neurotoxicity; assess CSF flow prior to administration. Infectious meningitis may be associated with intrathecal administration. **[U.S. Boxed Warning]: Should be administered under the supervision of an experienced cancer chemotherapy physician; facilities appropriate for diagnosis and management of complications should be readily available.** For intrathecal use only. Intrathecal medications should not be prepared during the preparation of any other agents; after preparation, store intrathecal medications in an isolated location or container clearly marked with a label identifying as "intrathecal" use only; delivery of intrathecal medications to the patient should only be with other medications intended for administration into the central nervous system (Jacobson, 2009).

Adverse Reactions

Cardiovascular: Edema, hyper-/hypotension, peripheral edema, syncope, tachycardia

Central nervous system: Agitation, anxiety, chemical arachnoiditis, confusion, depression, dizziness, fatigue, fever, headache, hypoesthesia, insomnia, lethargy, memory impairment, pain, seizure, sensory neuropathy

Dermatologic: Pruritus

Endocrine & metabolic: Dehydration, hyperglycemia, hypokalemia, hyponatremia

Gastrointestinal: Abdominal pain, appetite decreased, anorexia, constipation, diarrhea, dysphagia, hemorrhoids, mucosal inflammation, nausea, vomiting

Genitourinary: Incontinence, urinary retention, urinary tract infection

Hematologic: Anemia, contusion, neutropenia, thrombocytopenia

Neuromuscular & skeletal: Abnormal gait, abnormal reflexes, arthralgia, back pain, limb pain, muscle weakness, neck pain, neck stiffness, peripheral neuropathy, tremor, weakness

Ocular: Blurred vision

Otic: Hypoacusis

Respiratory: Cough, dyspnea, pneumonia

Miscellaneous: Diaphoresis

Rare but important or life-threatening: Anaphylaxis, bladder control impaired, blindness, bowel control impaired, cauda equine syndrome, cranial nerve palsies, CSF protein increased, CSF WBC increased, deafness, encephalopathy, hemiplegia, hydrocephalus, infectious meningitis, intracranial pressure increased, myelopathy, neurologic deficit, numbness, papilledema, somnolence, visual disturbance

Drug Interactions

Metabolism/Transport Effects None known.

Avoid Concomitant Use

Avoid concomitant use of Cytarabine (Liposomal) with any of the following: Tofacitinib

Increased Effect/Toxicity

Cytarabine (Liposomal) may increase the levels/effects of: Tofacitinib

Decreased Effect There are no known significant interactions involving a decrease in effect.

Preparation for Administration Hazardous agent; use appropriate precautions for handling and disposal (NIOSH 2014 [group 1]). Allow vial to warm to room temperature prior to withdrawal from vial. Particles may settle in diluent over time, and may be resuspended with gentle agitation or inversion immediately prior to withdrawing from the vial. Do not further dilute or mix with any other medications. Further reconstitution or dilution is not required. Intrathecal medications should not be prepared during the preparation of any other agents.

Storage/Stability Store under refrigeration at 2°C to 8°C (36°F to 46°F); protect from freezing. Avoid aggressive agitation. Withdraw from the vial immediately prior to administration; solutions should be used within 4 hours of withdrawal from the vial.

After preparation, store intrathecal medications in an isolated location or container clearly marked with a label identifying as "intrathecal" use only.

Mechanism of Action Cytarabine liposomal is a sustained-release formulation of the active ingredient cytarabine, an antimetabolite which acts through inhibition of DNA synthesis and is cell cycle-specific for the S phase of cell division. Cytarabine is converted intracellularly to its active metabolite cytarabine-5'-triphosphate (ara-CTP). Ara-CTP also appears to be incorporated into DNA and RNA; however, the primary action is inhibition of DNA polymerase, resulting in decreased DNA synthesis and repair. The liposomal formulation allows for gradual release, resulting in prolonged exposure.

Pharmacodynamics/Kinetics

Absorption: Systemic exposure following intrathecal administration is negligible since transfer rate from CSF to plasma is slow

Half-life elimination, CSF: 6-82 hours

Time to peak, CSF: Intrathecal: <1 hour

Dosage Note: Initiate dexamethasone 4 mg twice daily (oral or IV) for 5 days, beginning on the day of cytarabine liposomal administration.

Intrathecal: Adults:

Induction: 50 mg every 14 days for a total of 2 doses (weeks 1 and 3)

Consolidation: 50 mg every 14 days for 3 doses (weeks 5, 7, and 9), followed by an additional dose at week 13

Maintenance: 50 mg every 28 days for 4 doses (weeks 17, 21, 25, and 29)

Dosage reduction for toxicity: If drug-related neurotoxicity develops, reduce dose to 25 mg. If toxicity persists, discontinue treatment.

Dosage adjustment in renal impairment: No dosage adjustment provided in manufacturer's labeling (has not been studied).

Dosage adjustment in hepatic impairment: No dosage adjustment provided in manufacturer's labeling (has not been studied).

Administration For intrathecal use only. Dose should be removed from vial immediately before administration (must be administered within 4 hours of removal). An in-line filter should **NOT** be used. Administer directly into the CSF via an intraventricular reservoir or by direct injection into the lumbar sac. Injection should be made slowly (over 1-5 minutes). Patients should lie flat for 1 hour after lumbar puncture.

Hazardous agent; use appropriate precautions for handling and disposal (NIOSH 2014 [group 1]).

Monitoring Parameters Monitor closely for signs of an immediate reaction; neurotoxicity

Dosage Forms

Suspension, Intrathecal:

DepoCyt: 50 mg/5 mL (5 mL)

◆ **Cytarabine Liposome** *see* Cytarabine (Liposomal) *on page 540*

◆ **CytoGam®** *see* Cytomegalovirus Immune Globulin (Intravenous-Human) *on page 541*

Cytomegalovirus Immune Globulin (Intravenous-Human)

(sye toe meg a low VYE rus i MYUN GLOB yoo lin in tra VEE nus HYU man)

Brand Names: U.S. CytoGam®

Brand Names: Canada CytoGam®

Index Terms CMV Hyperimmune Globulin; CMV-IGIV

Pharmacologic Category Blood Product Derivative; Immune Globulin

Additional Appendix Information

Immunization Administration Recommendations *on page 2250*

Immunization Recommendations *on page 2255*

Use Prophylaxis of cytomegalovirus (CMV) disease associated with kidney, lung, liver, pancreas, and heart transplants; concomitant use with ganciclovir should be considered in organ transplants (other than kidney) from CMV seropositive donors to CMV seronegative recipients

Pregnancy Risk Factor C

Dosage IV: Children Adolescents, and Adults:

Prophylaxis of CMV disease in kidney transplant:

Initial dose (within 72 hours of transplant): 150 mg/kg/dose

2-, 4-, 6-, and 8 weeks after transplant: 100 mg/kg/dose

12- and 16 weeks after transplant: 50 mg/kg/dose

Prophylaxis of CMV disease in liver, lung, pancreas, or heart transplant:

Initial dose (within 72 hours of transplant): 150 mg/kg/dose

2-, 4-, 6-, and 8 weeks after transplant: 150 mg/kg/dose

12- and 16 weeks after transplant: 100 mg/kg/dose

Treatment of severe CMV pneumonitis in hematopoietic stem cell transplant (off-label use; in combination with ganciclovir): 400 mg/kg on days 1, 2, and 7, followed by 200 mg/kg on day 14; if still symptomatic, may administer an additional 200 mg/kg on day 21 (Reed, 1988) **or** 150 mg/kg twice weekly (Alexander, 2010)

Elderly: Refer to adult dosing.

Dosage adjustment in renal impairment: No dosage adjustment provided in manufacturer's labeling; use with caution. Infuse at minimum rate possible.

Dosage adjustment in hepatic impairment: No dosage adjustment provided in manufacturer's labeling.

Additional Information Complete prescribing information should be consulted for additional detail.

Dosage Forms

Injection, solution [preservative free]:

CytoGam®: 50 mg (± 10 mg)/mL (50 mL)

- ◆ **Cytomel** *see* Liothyronine *on page 1221*
- ◆ **Cytomel® (Can)** *see* Liothyronine *on page 1221*
- ◆ **Cytosar (Can)** *see* Cytarabine (Conventional) *on page 535*
- ◆ **Cytosar-U** *see* Cytarabine (Conventional) *on page 535*
- ◆ **Cytosine Arabinosine Hydrochloride** *see* Cytarabine (Conventional) *on page 535*
- ◆ **Cytostasan** *see* Bendamustine *on page 241*
- ◆ **Cytotec** *see* Misoprostol *on page 1379*
- ◆ **Cytovene** *see* Ganciclovir (Systemic) *on page 948*
- ◆ **Cytovene® (Can)** *see* Ganciclovir (Systemic) *on page 948*
- ◆ **Cytoxan** *see* Cyclophosphamide *on page 517*
- ◆ **Cytra-2** *see* Sodium Citrate and Citric Acid *on page 1905*
- ◆ **Cytra-3** *see* Citric Acid, Sodium Citrate, and Potassium Citrate *on page 455*
- ◆ **Cytra-K** *see* Potassium Citrate and Citric Acid *on page 1689*
- ◆ **D2** *see* Ergocalciferol *on page 753*
- ◆ **D2E7** *see* Adalimumab *on page 51*
- ◆ **D-3-Mercaptovaline** *see* PenicillAMINE *on page 1608*
- ◆ **d4T** *see* Stavudine *on page 1934*
- ◆ **D1694** *see* Raltitrexed [CAN/INT] *on page 1769*
- ◆ **D-23129** *see* Ezogabine *on page 835*
- ◆ **DA-1773** *see* Sodium Picosulfate, Magnesium Oxide, and Citric Acid *on page 1911*
- ◆ **DA-7157** *see* Tedizolid *on page 1981*
- ◆ **DA-7158** *see* Tedizolid *on page 1981*
- ◆ **DA-7218** *see* Tedizolid *on page 1981*

Dabigatran Etexilate (da BIG a tran ett EX ill ate)

Brand Names: U.S. Pradaxa

Brand Names: Canada Pradaxa

Index Terms Dabigatran Etexilate Mesylate

Pharmacologic Category Anticoagulant; Anticoagulant, Direct Thrombin Inhibitor

Additional Appendix Information

Beers Criteria - Potentially Inappropriate Medications for Geriatrics *on page 2271*

Oral Anticoagulant Comparison Chart *on page 2233*

Reversal of Oral Anticoagulants *on page 2235*

Use

Deep venous thrombosis and pulmonary embolism treatment and prevention: Treatment of deep venous thrombosis (DVT) and pulmonary embolism in patients who have been treated with a parenteral anticoagulant for 5 to 10 days; to reduce the risk of recurrence of DVT and pulmonary embolism in patients who have been previously treated.

Nonvalvular atrial fibrillation (to prevent stroke and systemic embolism): Prevention of stroke and systemic embolism in patients with nonvalvular atrial fibrillation (AF)

Note: The 2014 American Heart Association/American College of Cardiology/Heart Rhythm Society guidelines for the management of AF recommend oral anticoagulation for patients with nonvalvular AF or atrial flutter with prior stroke, TIA, or a CHA_2DS_2-VASc score ≥2. As an alternative to warfarin, dabigatran may also be used for 3 weeks prior and 4 weeks after cardioversion in patients with AF or atrial flutter of ≥48 hours duration or when the duration is unknown (January, 2014).

Canadian labeling: Additional uses (not in U.S. labeling): Postoperative thromboprophylaxis in patients who have undergone total hip or knee replacement procedures

Pregnancy Risk Factor C

Pregnancy Considerations Adverse events were observed in some animal reproduction studies. An *ex vivo* human placenta dual perfusion model illustrated that dabigatran crossed the placenta at term; dabigatran etexilate mesylate (prodrug) had limited placental transfer (Bapat, 2014). Data are insufficient to evaluate the safety of direct thrombin inhibitors during pregnancy; use of oral agents during pregnancy should be avoided (Guyatt, 2012). Consider the risks of bleeding and stroke if used during pregnancy.

Breast-Feeding Considerations It is not known if dabigatran etexilate is excreted into breast milk. Due to the potential for serious adverse reactions in the nursing infant, the manufacturer recommends a decision be made whether to discontinue nursing or to discontinue the drug, taking into account the importance of treatment to the mother. The use of alternative anticoagulants is preferred (Guyatt, 2012).

Contraindications

Serious hypersensitivity (eg, anaphylaxis or anaphylactic shock) to dabigatran or any component of the formulation; active pathological bleeding; patients with mechanical prosthetic heart valve(s)

Canadian labeling: Additional contraindications (not in U.S. labeling): Severe renal impairment (CrCl <30 mL/minute); bleeding diathesis or patients with spontaneous or pharmacological hemostatic impairment; lesions at risk of clinically significant bleeding (eg, hemorrhagic or ischemic cerebral infarction) within previous 6 months; concomitant therapy with oral ketoconazole; concomitant use with other anticoagulants including unfractionated heparin (except when used to maintain central venous or arterial catheter patency), low molecular weight heparins, heparin derivatives (eg, fondaparinux), antithrombin agents (eg, bivalirudin), and oral anticoagulants (eg, warfarin, rivaroxaban, apixaban) except during transitioning of therapy from or to dabigatran

Warnings/Precautions [U.S. Boxed Warning]: Upon premature discontinuation, the risk of thrombotic events is increased. If dabigatran must be discontinued for a reason other than pathological bleeding or completion of a course of therapy, consider the use of another anticoagulant during the time of interruption.

[U.S. Boxed Warning]: Spinal or epidural hematomas may occur with neuraxial anesthesia (epidural or spinal anesthesia) or spinal puncture in patients who are anticoagulated; may result in long-term or permanent paralysis. The risk of spinal/epidural hematoma is increased with the use of indwelling epidural catheters, concomitant administration of other drugs that affect hemostasis (eg, NSAIDS, platelet inhibitors, other anticoagulants), in patients with a history of traumatic or repeated epidural or spinal punctures, or a history of spinal deformity or spinal surgery. Placement or removal of an epidural catheter or lumbar puncture is best performed when the anticoagulant effect of dabigatran is low; however, the optimal timing between the administration of dabigatran and neuraxial procedures is not known. Monitor frequently for signs and symptoms of neurologic impairment (eg, midline back pain, numbness/weakness of legs, bowel/bladder dysfunction); prompt diagnosis and treatment are necessary. In patients who are anticoagulated or pharmacologic thromboprophylaxis is anticipated, assess risks versus benefits prior to

neuraxial interventions. If possible, discontinue dabigatran 1-2 days (CrCl ≥50 mL/minute) or 3-5 days (CrCl <50 mL/minute) before invasive or surgical procedures due to the increased risk of bleeding; consider longer times for patients undergoing major surgery, spinal puncture, or insertion of a spinal or epidural catheter or port. If surgery cannot be delayed, the risk of bleeding is elevated; weigh risk of bleeding with urgency of procedure. Bleeding risk can be assessed by the ecarin clotting time (ECT) if available; if ECT is not available, use of aPTT may provide an approximation of dabigatran's anticoagulant activity.

The most common complication is bleeding, and sometimes fatal bleeding. Risk factors for bleeding include concurrent use of drugs that increase the risk of bleeding (eg, antiplatelet agents, heparin), renal impairment, impairment, and elderly patients (especially if low body weight). Monitor for signs and symptoms of bleeding; discontinue in patients with active pathological bleeding. **Important:** No specific antidote exists for dabigatran reversal. Dabigatran is dialyzable (~57% removed over 4 hours); however, supporting data are limited for utilizing this method. The use of a PCC (Cofact, not available in the U.S.) has been shown to be **ineffective** for dabigatran reversal (Eerenberg, 2011); however, the manufacturer does suggest that activated PCC (eg, FEIBA NF), recombinant factor VIIa, or concentrates of factors II, IX, or X may be considered, although their use has not been evaluated in clinical trials. FEIBA NF was reported to have been effective in rapidly reversing the anticoagulant effects of dabigatran in one case study (Dager, 2013). Platelet concentrates should be considered when thrombocytopenia is present or long-acting antiplatelet drugs have been used. Use in patients with moderate hepatic impairment (Child-Pugh class B) demonstrated large inter-subject variability; however, no consistent change in exposure or pharmacodynamics was seen. Patients with active liver disease were excluded from the Randomized Evaluation of Long-term Anticoagulation Therapy (RE-LY) trial (Connolly, 2009). Use is not recommended in patients with valvular heart disease, including the presence of a bioprosthetic heart valve (has not been evaluated); use is contraindicated in patients with mechanical prosthetic heart valves. In addition to several case reports (Chu, 2012; Price, 2012; Stewart, 2012), one clinical trial reported significantly more thromboembolic events (valve thrombosis, stroke, TIA, and MI) and an excess of major bleeding (predominantly postoperative pericardial effusions requiring intervention for hemodynamic compromise) in patients with mechanical prosthetic heart valves receiving dabigatran compared with those receiving adjusted-dose warfarin.

Due to an increased risk of bleeding, avoid use, if possible, with other direct thrombin inhibitors (eg, bivalirudin), unfractionated heparin or heparin derivatives, low molecular weight heparins (eg, enoxaparin), fondaparinux, thienopyridines (eg, clopidogrel), GPIIb/IIIa antagonists (eg, eptifibatide), aspirin, coumarin derivatives, sulfinpyrazone, and ticagrelor. NSAIDs should be used cautiously. Appropriate doses of unfractionated heparin may be used to maintain catheter patency. Potentially significant interactions may exist, requiring dose or frequency adjustment, additional monitoring, and/or selection of alternative therapy.

Evaluate renal function prior to and during therapy, particularly if used in patients with any degree of preexisting renal impairment or in any condition that may result in a decline in renal function (eg, hypovolemia, dehydration, concomitant use of medications with a potential to affect renal function); dabigatran concentrations may increase in any degree of renal impairment and increase the risk of bleeding. In moderate impairment, serum concentrations may increase 3 times higher than normal compared to concentrations in patients with normal renal function. However, in patients with nonvalvular AF, U.S. labeling only requires dosage reduction in patients with severe renal impairment (CrCl 15-30 mL/minute) and dosing recommendations cannot be provided in patients with CrCl <15 mL/minute due to insufficient evidence. Per the American College of Chest Physicians, dabigatran is considered contraindicated in patients with severe renal impairment (CrCl ≤30 mL/minute) (Guyatt, 2012). The Canadian labeling also contraindicates use in severe renal impairment (CrCl <30 mL/minute) and recommends indication-specific dose reductions in patients with moderate impairment (CrCl 30-50 mL/minute). Discontinue therapy in any patient who develops acute renal failure.

In the elderly, use with extreme caution or consider other treatment options. No dosage adjustment is recommended in the U.S. labeling based on age alone (unless renal impairment coexists); however, numerous case reports of hemorrhage, including hemorrhagic stroke, have been reported in elderly patients (median age: 80 years), with a quarter of these reports occurring in patients ≥84 years of age. Some reports have resulted in fatality, particularly in those with low body weight and mild-to-moderate renal impairment; the risk is expected to be higher in patients receiving interacting drugs (eg, amiodarone) (Legrand, 2011). The RE-LY trial, although not powered to assess safety in the elderly, employed 110 mg and 150 mg twice daily regiments. The 110 mg twice daily regimen was not approved for use in the United States. The Canadian labeling recommends a dose reduction for patients ≥80 years of age with atrial fibrillation and suggests that dose reductions be considered in patients >75 years of age receiving therapy for atrial fibrillation or postoperative thromboprophylaxis. In addition, due to the frequency of renal impairment in older adults, the Canadian labeling recommends monitoring renal function at a minimum of once per year in any patient >75 years of age; use of dabigatran is contraindicated in patients with CrCl <30 mL/minute. Per the Beers Criteria, there is a greater risk of bleeding in older adults aged ≥75 years (exceeds warfarin bleeding risk) and therapy should be used with caution in patients ≥75 years of age or in patients with CrCl <30 mL/minute (Beers Criteria).

Adverse Reactions Adverse reactions listed below are reflective of both the U.S. and Canadian product information. **Important:** No specific antidote exists for dabigatran reversal; protamine and vitamin K do not reverse or impact anticoagulant effects of dabigatran. Dabigatran is dialyzable (~57% removed over 4 hours); however, supporting data are limited for utilizing this method. The use of a PCC (Cofact, not available in the U.S.) has been shown to be **ineffective** for dabigatran reversal (Eerenberg, 2011); however, the manufacturer does suggest that activated PCC (eg, FEIBA NF), recombinant factor VIIa, or concentrates of factors II, IX, or X may be considered, although their use has not been evaluated in clinical trials. FEIBA NF was reported to have been effective in rapidly reversing the anticoagulant effects of dabigatran in one case study (Dager, 2013). Platelet concentrates should be considered when thrombocytopenia is present or long-acting antiplatelet drugs have been used.

Dermatologic: Bloody discharge, postprocedural discharge, wound secretion

Gastrointestinal: Dyspepsia (includes abdominal pain, abdominal discomfort, epigatric discomfort), gastritis (includes gastroesophageal reflux disease, esophagitis, erosive gastritis, gastrointestinal hemorrhage, hemorrhagic gastritis, gastrointestinal ulcer), gastrointestinal hemorrhage, gastrointestinal symptoms (eg, dyspepsia, gastritis-like symptoms)

Genitourinary: Hematuria

Hematologic & oncologic: Anemia, hematoma, hemorrhage (includes procedural or wound), hemorrhage (life-threatening), major hemorrhage

Hepatic: Increased serum ALT

Rare but important or life-threatening: Allergic edema, anaphylactic shock, anaphylaxis, angioedema, catheter site hemorrhage, cerebrovascular accident (in patients with prosthetic heart valve), decreased hematocrit, ecchymoses, epidural hematoma (with spinal puncture or spinal/epidural anesthesia), esophageal ulcer, genitourinary tract hemorrhage, hemarthrosis, hemophthalmos, hemorrhagic death, hemorrhoidal bleeding, hepatic insufficiency, hypersensitivity reaction, incision site hemorrhage, increased serum AST, intracranial hemorrhage (includes hemorrhagic stroke, subarachnoid bleeding, subdural hematoma), muscle hemorrhage, myocardial infarction (in patients with prosthetic heart valve), rectal hemorrhage, retroperitoneal hemorrhage, severe hemorrhagic pericardial effusion (occurred postoperatively in patients with prosthetic heart valve; required intervention for hemodynamic compromise), spinal hematoma (with spinal puncture or spinal/epidural anesthesia), thrombocytopenia, thromboembolism (in patients with prosthetic heart valve), transient ischemic attacks (in patients with prosthetic heart valve)

Drug Interactions

Metabolism/Transport Effects Substrate of P-glycoprotein

Avoid Concomitant Use

Avoid concomitant use of Dabigatran Etexilate with any of the following: Anticoagulants; Apixaban; Edoxaban; Omacetaxine; P-glycoprotein/ABCB1 Inducers; Rivaroxaban; Sulfinpyrazone [Off Market]; Urokinase; Vorapaxar

Increased Effect/Toxicity

Dabigatran Etexilate may increase the levels/effects of: Anticoagulants; Collagenase (Systemic); Deferasirox; Ibritumomab; Nintedanib; Obinutuzumab; Omacetaxine; Rivaroxaban; Tositumomab and Iodine I 131 Tositumomab

The levels/effects of Dabigatran Etexilate may be increased by: Agents with Antiplatelet Properties; Amiodarone; Apixaban; Clarithromycin; Dasatinib; Dronedarone; Edoxaban; Herbs (Anticoagulant/Antiplatelet Properties); Ketoconazole (Systemic); Limaprost; Nonsteroidal Anti-Inflammatory Agents; Omega-3 Fatty Acids; Pentosan Polysulfate Sodium; P-glycoprotein/ABCB1 Inhibitors; Prostacyclin Analogues; QuiNIDine; Salicylates; Sugammadex; Sulfinpyrazone [Off Market]; Thrombolytic Agents; Tibolone; Ticagrelor; Urokinase; Verapamil; Vitamin E; Vorapaxar

Decreased Effect

The levels/effects of Dabigatran Etexilate may be decreased by: Antacids; AtorvaSTATin; Estrogen Derivatives; P-glycoprotein/ABCB1 Inducers; Progestins; Proton Pump Inhibitors

Food Interactions Food has no affect on the bioavailability of dabigatran, but delays the time to peak plasma concentrations by 2 hours. Management: Administer without regard to meals.

Storage/Stability

Blister: Store at 25°C (77°F); excursions permitted between 15°C to 30°C (59°F to 86°F). Dispense and store in original package to protect from moisture.

Bottle: Store at 25°C (77°F); excursions permitted between 15°C to 30°C (59°F to 86°F). Dispense and store in original manufacturer's bottle to protect from moisture; discard 4 months after opening original container.

Mechanism of Action Prodrug lacking anticoagulant activity that is converted *in vivo* to the active dabigatran, a specific, reversible, direct thrombin inhibitor that inhibits both free and fibrin-bound thrombin. Inhibits coagulation by preventing thrombin-mediated effects, including cleavage of fibrinogen to fibrin monomers, activation of factors V, VIII, XI, and XIII, and inhibition of thrombin-induced platelet aggregation.

Pharmacodynamics/Kinetics

Absorption: Rapid; initially slow postoperatively

Distribution: V_d: 50-70 L

Protein binding: 35%

Metabolism: Hepatic; dabigatran etexilate is rapidly and completely hydrolyzed to dabigatran (active form) by plasma and hepatic esterases; dabigatran undergoes hepatic glucuronidation to active acylglucuronide isomers (similar activity to parent compound; accounts for <10% of total dabigatran in plasma)

Bioavailability: 3% to 7%

Half-life elimination: 12-17 hours; Elderly: 14-17 hours; Mild-to-moderate renal impairment: 15-18 hours; Severe renal impairment: 28 hours (Stangier, 2010)

Time to peak, plasma: Dabigatran: 1 hour; delayed 2 hours by food (no effect on bioavailability)

Excretion: Urine (80%)

Dosage Oral:

Adults:

DVT and pulmonary embolism: 150 mg twice daily (after 5 to 10 days of parenteral anticoagulation)

Nonvalvular atrial fibrillation (to prevent stroke and systemic embolism): 150 mg twice daily.

Conversion:

Conversion from a parenteral anticoagulant: Initiate dabigatran ≤2 hours prior to the time of the next scheduled dose of the parenteral anticoagulant (eg, enoxaparin) or at the time of discontinuation for a continuously administered parenteral drug (eg, IV heparin); discontinue parenteral anticoagulant at the time of dabigatran initiation.

Conversion to a parenteral anticoagulant:

U.S. labeling: Wait 12 hours (CrCl ≥30 mL/minute) or 24 hours (CrCl <30 mL/minute) after the last dose of dabigatran before initiating a parenteral anticoagulant.

Canadian labeling: Wait 12 hours after the last dose of dabigatran before initiating a parenteral anticoagulant.

Conversion from warfarin: Discontinue warfarin and initiate dabigatran when INR <2.0

Conversion to warfarin: Since dabigatran contributes to INR elevation, warfarin's effect on the INR will be better reflected only after dabigatran has been stopped for ≥2 days. Start time must be adjusted based on CrCl:

CrCl >50 mL/minute: Initiate warfarin 3 days before discontinuation of dabigatran

CrCl 31 to 50 mL/minute: Initiate warfarin 2 days before discontinuation of dabigatran

CrCl 15 to 30 mL/minute: Initiate warfarin 1 day before discontinuation of dabigatran (dabigatran use is contraindicated in Canadian labeling when CrCl <30 mL/minute).

CrCl <15 mL/minute: There are no recommendations provided in the U.S. manufacturer's labeling.

Postoperative thromboprophylaxis (Canadian labeling):

Knee replacement: Initial: 110 mg given 1 to 4 hours after completion of surgery and establishment of hemostasis **OR** 220 mg as 1 dose in postoperative patients in whom therapy is not initiated on day of surgery regardless of reason; maintenance: 220 mg once daily (total duration of therapy: 10 days; ACCP recommendation [Guyatt, 2012]: Minimum of 10 to 14 days; extended duration of up to 35 days suggested)

Hip replacement: Initial: 110 mg given 1 to 4 hours after completion of surgery and establishment of hemostasis **OR** 220 mg as 1 dose in postoperative patients in whom therapy is not initiated on day of surgery regardless of reason; maintenance: 220 mg once daily (total duration of therapy: 28 to 35 days; ACCP recommendation [Guyatt, 2012]: Minimum of 10 to 14 days; extended duration of up to 35 days suggested)

Conversion information (Canadian labeling): When transitioning from parenteral anticoagulation therapy, initiate oral dabigatran therapy ≤2 hours prior to the time of next regularly scheduled dose of intermittent parenteral anticoagulant or at the time of discontinuation for continuously administered parenteral anticoagulation therapy. When transitioning from dabigatran to IV anticoagulation therapy following hip- or knee-replacement surgery, allow 24 hours after the last dabigatran dose before initiating IV anticoagulation therapy. When transitioning from warfarin, discontinue warfarin and initiate dabigatran when INR <2.0.

Dosing adjustment with concomitant medications:

U.S. labeling:

DVT and pulmonary embolism:

Any P-glycoprotein inducer (eg, rifampin): Avoid concurrent use.

Any P-glycoprotein inhibitor (eg, amiodarone, clarithromycin, dronedarone, quinidine, verapamil, and others) with CrCl <50 mL/minute: Avoid concurrent use.

Nonvalvular atrial fibrillation (to prevent stroke and systemic embolism):

Dronedarone or ketoconazole (oral) with CrCl 30 to 50 mL/minute: Consider dabigatran dose reduction to 75 mg twice daily.

Any P-glycoprotein inducer (eg, rifampin): Avoid concurrent use.

Any P-glycoprotein inhibitor (eg, amiodarone, clarithromycin, dronedarone, quinidine, verapamil, and others) with CrCl <30 mL/minute: Avoid concurrent use.

Canadian labeling: Postoperative thromboprophylaxis: *Strong P-gp inhibitors (eg, amiodarone, quinidine, verapamil):* Use caution and reduce dabigatran to 150 mg once daily. In patients with CrCl 30 to 50 mL/minute and receiving verapamil, consider dabigatran dose reduction to 75 mg once daily. Use with the strong P-gp inhibitor ketoconazole (oral) is contraindicated.

Elderly:

DVT and pulmonary embolism/Nonvalvular atrial fibrillation (to prevent stroke and systemic embolism):

U.S. labeling:

Patients >65 years: Refer to adult dosing. No dosage adjustment required unless renal impairment exists; however, increased risk of bleeding has been observed, particularly in elderly patients with low body weight and/or concomitant renal impairment.

Patients ≥80 years: **Use with extreme caution or consider other treatment options;** no dosage adjustment provided in manufacturer's labeling; however, numerous cases of hemorrhage, including hemorrhagic stroke, have been reported postmarketing, particularly in this age group of octogenarians. Due to a lack of available dosing options available in the U.S., consider avoiding use of dabigatran in this population.

Canadian labeling:

Patients <80 years: 150 mg twice daily; **Note:** The manufacturer labeling suggests that a dose reduction to 110 mg twice daily may be considered in patients >75 years with at least one other risk factor for bleeding (eg, moderate renal impairment [CrCl 30 to 50 mL/minute], concomitant treatment with strong P-gp inhibitors, or previous GI bleed); however, efficacy in stroke prevention may be lessened with this dose reduction.

Patients ≥80 years: 110 mg twice daily

Postoperative thromboprophylaxis (Canadian labeling): Patients >75 years: Use with caution; consider a dose of 150 mg once daily.

Dosing adjustment in renal impairment: Note: Clinical trial evaluating safety and efficacy utilized the Cockcroft-Gault formula with the use of actual body weight (data on file; Boehringer Ingelheim Pharmaceuticals Inc, 2012).

DVT and pulmonary embolism:

CrCl >30 mL/minute: No dosage adjustment necessary **unless** patient has a CrCl <50 mL/minute and is receiving concomitant P-gp inhibitors, then avoid coadministration.

CrCl ≤30 mL/minute: There are no dosage recommendations provided in the manufacturer's labeling (has not been studied). Patients with CrCl <30 mL/minute (Schulman, 2009; Schulman, 2011) or CrCl ≤30 mL/minute (Schulman, 2013) were excluded from the respective clinical trials.

Hemodialysis: There are no dosage recommendations provided in the manufacturer's labeling (has not been studied). Patients receiving hemodialysis were excluded from clinical trials (Schulman, 2009; Schulman, 2011; Schulman 2013).

Nonvalvular atrial fibrillation (to prevent stroke and systemic embolism):

U.S. labeling:

CrCl >50 mL/minute: No dosage adjustment necessary. Use with caution in mild renal impairment (CrCl 50 to 80 mL/minute) due to risk for increased dabigatran exposure (area under the curve may be increased 1.5 times higher than normal).

CrCl 30 to 50 mL/minute: No dosage adjustment necessary **unless** patient receiving concomitant dronedarone or oral ketoconazole, then consider reducing dabigatran to 75 mg twice daily. Use with caution in moderate renal impairment due to risk for increased dabigatran exposure (area under the curve may be increased 3 times higher than normal), particularly if patient is also of advanced age. In patients with moderate-to-severe chronic kidney disease, dose reduction may be considered although safety and efficacy of this approach has not been established (AHA/ACC/HRS [January, 2014]).

CrCl 15 to 30 mL/minute: 75 mg twice daily **unless** patient receiving concomitant P-gp inhibitor, then avoid concurrent use. **Note:** Patients with CrCl <30 mL/minute were excluded from the RE-LY trial (Connolly, 2009). Dose based on pharmacokinetic data; safety and efficacy has not been established. Per the American College of Chest Physicians, dabigatran is considered contraindicated in patients with severe renal impairment (CrCl ≤30 mL/minute) (Guyatt, 2012).

CrCl <15 mL/minute: There are no dosage recommendations provided in the manufacturer's labeling (has not been studied). Per the American College of Chest Physicians, dabigatran is considered contraindicated in patients with severe renal impairment (CrCl ≤30 mL/minute) (Guyatt, 2012). In addition, the AHA/ACC/HRS does not recommend dabigatran for patients with AF and end-stage chronic kidney disease (January, 2014).

Hemodialysis: There are no dosage recommendations provided in the manufacturer's labeling (has not been studied). The AHA/ACC/HRS does not recommend dabigatran for patients with AF on hemodialysis (January, 2014). **Note:** Hemodialysis removes ~57% over 4 hours

Canadian labeling:

CrCl >50 mL/minute: No dosage adjustment necessary.

CrCl 30 to 50 mL/minute: No dosage adjustment necessary. **Note:** Patients with moderate renal impairment (CrCl 30 to 50 mL/minute) are at an increased risk for bleeding; routine assessment of renal status is recommended; use recommended unadjusted dosage of 150 mg twice daily with caution in these patients. A dosage reduction to 110 mg twice daily may be considered for patients ≥75 years and/or those with other bleeding risk factors; however, efficacy in stroke prevention may be lessened with this dose.

CrCl <30 mL/minute: Use is contraindicated.

Postoperative thromboprophylaxis: Canadian labeling:

CrCl >50 mL/minute: No dosage adjustment necessary.

CrCl 30 to 50 mL/minute: Initial: 75 mg given 1 to 4 hours after completion of surgery and establishment of hemostasis; Maintenance: 150 mg once daily **unless** patient receiving concomitant verapamil, then consider reducing dabigatran to 75 mg once daily.

CrCl <30 mL/minute: Use is contraindicated.

Dosing adjustment in hepatic impairment:

U.S. labeling: There are no dosage adjustments provided in manufacturer's labeling; consistent changes in exposure or pharmacodynamics were not observed in a study of patients with moderate impairment.

Canadian labeling: Use is not recommended if hepatic enzymes >3 x ULN.

Administration Administer with a full glass of water without regard to meals. Do not break, chew, or open capsules, as this will lead to 75% increase in absorption and potentially serious adverse reactions.

Monitoring Parameters Routine monitoring of coagulation tests not required. However, the measurement of activated partial thromboplastin time (aPTT) (values >2.5 x control may indicate overanticoagulation), ecarin clotting test (ECT) if available, or thrombin time (TT; most sensitive) may be useful to determine presence of dabigatran and level of coagulopathy; CBC with differential; renal function prior to initiation and periodically as clinically indicated (ie, situations associated with a decline in renal function) and according to the AHA/ACC/HRS, at least annually in all patients (January, 2014); **Note:** Canadian labeling specifically recommends renal function be routinely assessed at least once per year in elderly patients (>75 years of age) or patients with moderate renal impairment (CrCl 30-50 mL/minute)

Reference Range

At therapeutic dabigatran doses, aPTT, ECT (ecarin clotting time), and TT (thrombin time) are prolonged. A median peak aPTT of ~2 x control and a median trough aPTT of 1.5 x control were observed in subjects taking dabigatran 150 mg twice daily in the RE-LY trial

A therapeutic range has not been established for aPTT or for other tests of anticoagulant activity

Dosage Forms

Capsule, Oral:

Pradaxa: 75 mg, 150 mg

Dosage Forms: Canada

Capsule, oral:

Pradax: 75 mg, 110 mg, 150 mg

◆ **Dabigatran Etexilate Mesylate** *see* Dabigatran Etexilate *on page 542*

Dabrafenib (da BRAF e nib)

Brand Names: U.S. Tafinlar

Brand Names: Canada Tafinlar

Index Terms GSK2118436

Pharmacologic Category Antineoplastic Agent, BRAF Kinase Inhibitor

Use Melanoma:

U.S. labeling: Treatment of unresectable or metastatic melanoma in patients with a BRAF V600E mutation (single agent therapy) or in patients with BRAF V600E or BRAF V600K mutations (in combination with trametinib); confirm BRAF V600E or BRAF V600K mutation status with an approved test prior to treatment.

Canadian labeling: Treatment of unresectable or metastatic melanoma in patients with a BRAF V600 mutation (as detected by a validated test).

Note: Not recommended in patients with wild-type BRAF melanoma.

Pregnancy Risk Factor D

Pregnancy Considerations Adverse effects were observed in animal reproduction studies. Based on its mechanism of action, dabrafenib would be expected to cause fetal harm if administered to a pregnant woman. Females of reproductive potential should use a highly effective nonhormonal contraceptive during therapy and for at least 2 weeks (single agent therapy) or 4 months (combination therapy with trametinib) after treatment is complete; hormonal contraceptives may not be effective. Spermatogenesis may be impaired in males (observed in animal studies); family planning and fertility counseling should be considered prior to therapy.

Breast-Feeding Considerations It is not known if dabrafenib is excreted into breast milk. Due to the potential for serious adverse reactions in the nursing infant, the manufacturer recommends a decision be made whether to discontinue nursing or to discontinue the drug, taking into account the importance of treatment to the mother.

Contraindications There are no contraindications listed in the manufacturer's U.S. labeling.

Canadian labeling: Hypersensitivity to dabrafenib or any component of the formulation.

Warnings/Precautions Hazardous agent – use appropriate precautions for handling and disposal (meets NIOSH 2014 criteria). Serious adverse reactions (retinal vein occlusion, interstitial lung disease), which occur with single agent trametinib, may also occur when dabrafenib is administered in combination with trametinib. Cardiomyopathy may be observed when concomitantly with trametinib. The median time to onset of cardiomyopathy was ~3 months (range: 27-253 days) when used in combination with trametinib. Assess LVEF (by echocardiogram or MUGA scan) prior to combination therapy initiation, at 1 month, and then at 2- to 3-month intervals while on combination therapy. Cardiac dysfunction may require dabrafenib treatment interruption (see Trametinib monograph for dosage modifications). Cardiomyopathy resolved in some patients following therapy adjustments. Hemorrhage, including symptomatic bleeding in a critical area/organ, may occur when dabrafenib is used in combination with trametinib. Major bleeding events (some fatal) included intracranial or gastrointestinal hemorrhage. May require treatment interruption and dosage reduction; permanently discontinue dabrafenib (and trametinib) for all grade 4 hemorrhagic events and any grade 3 event that does not improve with therapy interruption. Venous thromboembolism events (some fatal) may occur when dabrafenib is used in combination with trametinib. DVT and PE occurred at an increased incidence with combination therapy. Patients should seek immediate medical attention with symptoms of DVT or PE (shortness of breath, chest pain, arm/leg swelling). Dabrafenib therapy may be continued for uncomplicated DVT or PE; permanently discontinue dabrafenib (and trametinib) for life-threatening PE.

Serious febrile reactions and fever (any severity) complicated by hypotension, rigors or chills, dehydration, or renal failure were observed during dabrafenib single agent therapy and when used in combination with trametinib. The median time to initial fever (single agent therapy)

was 11 days (range: 1-202 days); median duration was 3 days (range: 1-129 days). In patients treated with combination therapy, the median time to onset of fever was 30 days and duration was 6 days. Interrupt dabrafenib therapy for fever ≥38.5°C (101.3°F) or for any other serious febrile reaction complicated by hypotension, rigors/chills, dehydration, or renal failure; evaluate promptly for signs/symptoms of infection. Dosage reduction may be required; when resuming therapy after a febrile reaction, may require prophylactic administration of antipyretics. Hyperglycemia may occur while on therapy (either as a single agent or in combination with trametinib); may require initiation of insulin or oral hypoglycemic agent therapy (or an increased dose if already taking). Monitor serum glucose as clinically necessary, particularly in patients with preexisting diabetes or hyperglycemia. Instruct patients to report symptoms of severe hyperglycemia (eg, polydipsia, polyuria).

Serious dermatologic toxicity (eg, rash, dermatitis, acneiform rash, palmar-plantar erythrodysesthesia syndrome, and erythema) may occur when used in combination with trametinib (known complication of single agent trametinib therapy); some patients required hospitalization for severe toxicity or for secondary skin infections. The median time to onset and resolution of skin toxicity for combination therapy was 37 days (range: 1-225 days) and 33 days (range: 3-421 days), respectively. Monitor for dermatologic toxicity and signs/symptoms of secondary infections. Treatment interruption, dose reduction, and/or therapy discontinuation may be necessary. Cutaneous squamous cell carcinoma and keratoacanthoma (cuSCC) and melanoma were observed during single agent dabrafenib therapy at an increased incidence as compared to control therapy in clinical trials. The median time to the first occurrence of cuSCC was 9 weeks (range: 1-53 weeks); approximately one-third of patients who developed cuSCC had more than one occurrence (with continued treatment). The median time between diagnosis of the first and second lesions was 6 weeks. When used in combination with trametinib, cuSCC occurred less frequently than with single agent dabrafenib therapy; time to diagnosis ranged from 136-197 days after the initiation of combination treatment. Basal cell carcinoma (BCC) occurs more frequently with combination versus single agent therapy; the incidence of BCC is 9% for combination therapy versus 2% for single agent dabrafenib. The time to BCC diagnosis ranged from 28-249 days for patients receiving combination therapy. Dermatologic evaluations should be performed prior to initiating therapy, every 2 months during therapy, and for up to 6 months post discontinuation. There are case reports of noncutaneous malignancies, including pancreatic cancer (KRAS mutation-positive), colorectal cancer (recurrent NRAS mutation-positive), hand and neck cancer, and glioblastoma, with combination therapy; monitor for signs/symptoms of noncutaneous malignancies. Dabrafenib should be permanently discontinued if RAS mutation-positive noncutaneous malignancies develop (no trametinib dosage reduction is required).

Retinal pigment epithelial detachments (RPED) were seen in clinical trials when used in combination with trametinib (known complication of trametinib single agent therapy). Detachments were typically bilateral and multifocal and occurred in the macular area of the retina. Promptly refer patients for ophthalmological evaluations if loss of vision or other visual disturbances occur; dabrafenib dosage modification is not necessary for RPED (trametinib therapy modification may be required). In clinical trials, ophthalmic exams (including retinal evaluation) were performed prior to and regularly during treatment with combination therapy. Uveitis and iritis have been reported with dabrafenib single agent therapy and when used in combination with trametinib; manage symptomatically with ophthalmic steroid and mydriatic drops. May require dabrafenib treatment interruption (does not require alteration in trametinib therapy). Monitor for signs/symptoms of uveitis (eg, eye pain, photophobia, and vision changes).

When administered at recommended doses for 15 days, a mean increase of ~12 msec in QTc interval from baseline has been observed. Use with caution in patients who may be at increased risk for arrhythmias (eg, torsade de pointes). Potentially significant drug-drug interactions may exist, requiring dose or frequency adjustment, additional monitoring, and/or selection of alternative therapy. Drugs affecting gastric pH (eg, proton pump inhibitors, H2-receptor antagonists, antacids) may alter dabrafenib solubility, resulting in decreased bioavailability. Clinical trials have not been performed to evaluate concomitant administration and its effect on dabrafenib efficacy. Patients with glucose-6-phosphate dehydrogenase (G6PD) deficiency may be at risk for hemolytic anemia when administered dabrafenib; use with caution and closely observe for signs/symptoms of hemolytic anemia. Not indicated for treatment of patients with wild-type BRAF melanoma. Exposing wild-type cells to BRAF inhibitors such as dabrafenib may result in paradoxical activation of MAP-kinase signaling and increased cell proliferation. Prior to initiating therapy, confirm BRAF V600E or BRAF V600K mutations (U.S. labeling) or BRAF V600 mutations (Canadian labeling) status with an approved test. Data regarding single agent use in patients with BRAF V600K mutation is limited; compared to BRAF V600E mutation, lower response rates have been observed with BRAF V600K mutation. Data regarding other less common BRAF V600 mutations is lacking.

Adverse Reactions

Monotherapy:

Cardiovascular: Peripheral edema, prolonged Q-T interval on ECG

Central nervous system: Chills, dizziness, fatigue, headache, insomnia

Dermatologic: Acneiform eruption, actinic keratosis, alopecia, dermatological reaction, erythema, hyperkeratosis, night sweats, palmar-plantar erythrodysesthesia, pruritus, skin rash, xeroderma

Endocrine & metabolic: Dehydration, hypercalcemia, hyperglycemia, hyperkalemia, hypoalbuminemia, hypocalcemia, hypokalemia, hypomagnesemia, hyponatremia, hypophosphatemia, increased gamma-glutamyl transferase

Gastrointestinal: Abdominal pain, constipation, decreased appetite, diarrhea, nausea, pancreatitis, vomiting, xerostomia

Genitourinary: Urinary tract infection

Hematologic & oncologic: Anemia, basal cell carcinoma, hemorrhage, leukopenia, lymphocytopenia, malignant melanoma, malignant neoplasm of skin (keratoacanthoma and squamous cell carcinoma), neutropenia, papilloma, thrombocytopenia

Hepatic: Increased serum alkaline phosphatase, increased serum ALT, increased serum AST

Hypersensitivity: Hypersensitivity (bullous rash)

Neuromuscular & skeletal: Arthralgia, back pain, limb pain, muscle spasm, myalgia

Respiratory: Cough

Ophthalmic: Uveitis (including iritis)

Renal: Increased serum creatinine, interstitial nephritis

Respiratory: Nasopharyngitis

Miscellaneous: Febrile reaction, fever

Combination therapy with trametanib:

Cardiovascular: Cardiomyopathy, hypertension, peripheral edema, prolonged Q-T interval on ECG, venous thromboembolism (deep vein thrombosis or pulmonary embolism)

Central nervous system: Chills, dizziness, fatigue, headache, insomnia

Dermatologic: Acneiform eruption, actinic keratosis, cellulitis, dermatological reaction, erythema, folliculitis, hyperhidrosis, hyperkeratosis, night sweats, palmar-plantar erythrodysesthesia, paronychia, pruritus, pustular rash, secondary skin infection, skin rash, xeroderma
Endocrine & metabolic: Dehydration, hypercalcemia, hyperglycemia, hyperkalemia, hypoalbuminemia, hypocalcemia, hypokalemia, hypomagnesemia, hyponatremia, hypophosphatemia, increased gamma-glutamyl transferase
Gastrointestinal: Abdominal pain, constipation, decreased appetite, diarrhea, nausea, pancreatitis, stomatitis, vomiting, xerostomia
Genitourinary: Urinary tract infection
Hematologic & oncologic: Anemia, basal cell carcinoma, cutaneous papilloma, hemorrhage, leukopenia, lymphocytopenia, malignant neoplasm of skin (keratoacanthoma and squamous cell carcinoma), neutropenia, thrombocytopenia
Hepatic: Hyperbilirubinemia, increased serum alkaline phosphatase, increased serum ALT, increased serum AST
Neuromuscular & skeletal: Arthralgia, back pain, limb pain, muscle spasm, myalgia, weakness
Ophthalmic: Blindness, blurred vision, retinal detachment (pigment epithelium), uveitis
Renal: Increased serum creatinine, renal failure
Respiratory: Cough, oropharyngeal pain
Miscellaneous: Febrile reaction, fever

Rare but important or life-threatening: Glioblastoma, malignant neoplasm of colon and rectum (recurrent NRAS mutation-positive), malignant neoplasm of head and neck, pancreatic adenocarcinoma (KRAS mutation-positive)

Drug Interactions

Metabolism/Transport Effects **Substrate** of BCRP, CYP2C8 (major), CYP3A4 (major), P-glycoprotein; **Note:** Assignment of Major/Minor substrate status based on clinically relevant drug interaction potential; **Inhibits** BCRP, SLCO1B1; **Induces** CYP2B6 (moderate), CYP2C19 (moderate), CYP2C8 (moderate), CYP2C9 (moderate), CYP3A4 (moderate)

Avoid Concomitant Use

Avoid concomitant use of Dabrafenib with any of the following: Axitinib; Bosutinib; Conivaptan; Enzalutamide; Fusidic Acid (Systemic); Idelalisib; Nisoldipine; Olaparib; PAZOPanib; Simeprevir

Increased Effect/Toxicity

Dabrafenib may increase the levels/effects of: Clarithromycin; Highest Risk QTc-Prolonging Agents; Moderate Risk QTc-Prolonging Agents; PAZOPanib; Topotecan

The levels/effects of Dabrafenib may be increased by: Conivaptan; CYP2C8 Inhibitors (Moderate); CYP2C8 Inhibitors (Strong); CYP3A4 Inhibitors (Moderate); CYP3A4 Inhibitors (Strong); Deferasirox; Fusidic Acid (Systemic); Idelalisib; Luliconazole; Mifepristone; Stiripentol; Trametinib

Decreased Effect

Dabrafenib may decrease the levels/effects of: ARIPiprazole; Axitinib; Bosutinib; Clarithromycin; Contraceptives (Estrogens); Contraceptives (Progestins); CYP2B6 Substrates; CYP2C19 Substrates; CYP2C8 Substrates; CYP2C9 Substrates; CYP3A4 Substrates; Enzalutamide; FentaNYL; Ibrutinib; Nisoldipine; Olaparib; Ombitasvir; Proton Pump Inhibitors; Saxagliptin; Simeprevir

The levels/effects of Dabrafenib may be decreased by: Antacids; CYP2C8 Inducers (Strong); H2-Antagonists; Proton Pump Inhibitors; St Johns Wort

Food Interactions Administration with a high-fat meal decreased C_{max} and AUC by 51% and 31%, respectively, and delayed median T_{max} by ~4 hours. Management: Administer 1 hour before or 2 hours after a meal.

Storage/Stability Store at 25°C (77°F); excursions permitted to 15°C to 30°C (59°F to 86°F).

Mechanism of Action Selectively inhibits some mutated forms of the protein kinase B-raf (BRAF). BRAF V600 mutations result in constitutive activation of the BRAF pathway; through BRAF inhibition, dabrafenib inhibits tumor cell growth. The combination of dabrafenib and trametinib allows for greater inhibition of the MAPK pathway, resulting in BRAF V600 melanoma cell death (Flaherty, 2012).

Pharmacodynamics/Kinetics

Absorption: Decreased with a high-fat meal
Distribution: 70.3 L
Protein binding: 99.7% to plasma proteins
Metabolism: Hepatic via CYP2C8 and CYP3A4 to hydroxy-dabrafenib (active) which is further metabolized via CYP3A4 oxidation to desmethyl-dabrafenib (active)
Bioavailability: 95%
Half-life elimination: Parent drug: 8 hours; Hydroxy-dabrafenib (active metabolite): 10 hours; Desmethyl-dabrafenib (active metabolite): 21-22 hours
Time to peak: 2 hours; delayed with a high-fat meal
Excretion: Feces (71%); urine (23%; metabolites only)

Dosage

U.S. labeling:

Melanoma, metastatic or unresectable (with BRAF V600E mutation): Adults: Oral: 150 mg twice daily (approximately every 12 hours) until disease progression or unacceptable toxicity (single agent therapy)

Melanoma, metastatic or unresectable (with BRAF V600E or BRAF V600K mutation): Adults: Oral: 150 mg twice daily (approximately every 12 hours) until disease progression or unacceptable toxicity (in combination with trametinib)

Canadian labeling: Melanoma, metastatic or unresectable (with BRAF V600 mutation): Adults: Oral: 150 mg twice daily (approximately every 12 hours) until disease progression or unacceptable toxicity

Missed doses: A missed dose may be administered up to 6 hours prior to the next dose; do not administer if <6 hours until the next dose.

Dosage adjustment for toxicity:

Recommended dabrafenib dose reductions for toxicity:
First dose reduction: 100 mg twice daily
Second dose reduction: 75 mg twice daily
Third dose reduction: 50 mg twice daily
Subsequent modifications (if unable to tolerate 50 mg twice daily): Permanently discontinue.

Note: If using combination therapy, refer to Trametinib monograph for recommended trametinib dose reductions.

Cardiac:

Asymptomatic, 10% or greater absolute decrease in LVEF from baseline and LVEF is below institutional lower limits of normal (LLN) from pretreatment value: No dabrafenib dosage modification is necessary.

>20% absolute decrease in LVEF from baseline and LVEF is below institutional LLN: Interrupt dabrafenib therapy; if improved, may resume at the same dose.

Symptomatic heart failure: Interrupt dabrafenib therapy; if improved, may resume at the same dose.

Dermatologic:

Intolerable grade 2 skin toxicity or grade 3 or 4 skin toxicity: Interrupt dabrafenib therapy for up to 3 weeks. If toxicity improves within 3 weeks, resume at a lower dose level. If toxicity does not improve within 3 weeks following therapy interruption, permanently discontinue dabrafenib.

New primary cutaneous malignancy: No dabrafenib dosage modification is necessary.

Fever:

Fever of 38.5°C to 40°C (101.3°F to 104°F): Interrupt dabrafenib therapy until temperature normalizes. Resume at the same or lower dose level.

Fever >40°C (104°F) and/or fever complicated by rigors, hypotension, dehydration, or renal failure: Interrupt dabrafenib therapy until temperature normalizes. Resume at a lower dose level or permanently discontinue.

Hemorrhage:

Grade 3 hemorrhage: Interrupt dabrafenib therapy. If hemorrhage improves, resume at a lower dose level. If hemorrhage does not improve following therapy interruption, permanently discontinue dabrafenib.

Grade 4 hemorrhage: Permanently discontinue dabrafenib.

Ocular:

Uveitis and iritis: Interrupt dabrafenib therapy for up to 6 weeks. If improves to ≤ grade 1 within 6 weeks following therapy interruption, resume at the same dose. If does not improve, permanently discontinue dabrafenib.

Grade 2 or 3 retinal pigment epithelial detachments (RPED): No dabrafenib dosage modification is necessary.

Retinal vein occlusion: No dabrafenib dosage modification is necessary.

Pulmonary: Interstitial lung disease or pneumonitis: No dabrafenib dosage modification is necessary.

Venous thromboembolism:

Uncomplicated DVT or PE: No dabrafenib dosage modification is necessary.

Life-threatening PE: Permanently discontinue dabrafenib.

Other toxicity:

Intolerable grade 2 or any grade 3 toxicity: Interrupt dabrafenib therapy until resolution to ≤ grade 1; resume at a lower dose level. If toxicity does not improve following therapy interruption, permanently discontinue dabrafenib.

Grade 4 toxicity (first occurrence): Interrupt dabrafenib therapy until resolution to ≤ grade 1; consider resuming at a lower dose level or permanently discontinue.

Grade 4 toxicity (recurrent after dosage reduction): Permanently discontinue dabrafenib.

New primary noncutaneous malignancy (RAS mutation-positive): Permanently discontinue dabrafenib.

Dosage adjustment for renal impairment:

Mild to moderate impairment (GFR ≥30 mL/minute/1.73 m^2): No dosage adjustment necessary.

Severe impairment (GFR <30 mL/minute/1.73 m^2): No dosage adjustment provided in manufacturer's labeling (has not been studied).

Dosage adjustment for hepatic impairment:

Mild impairment: No dosage adjustment necessary.

Moderate to severe impairment: No dosage adjustment provided in manufacturer's labeling (has not been studied); however, metabolism is primarily hepatic and exposure may be increased in patients with moderate to severe impairment.

Dietary Considerations Administer at least 1 hour before or 2 hours after a meal.

Administration Administer orally at least 1 hour before or 2 hours after a meal; doses should be ~12 hours apart. Do not open, crush, or break capsules. A missed dose may be administered up to 6 hours prior to the next dose. When administered in combination with trametinib, take the once-daily dose of trametinib at the same time each day with either the morning or evening dose of dabrafenib.

Hazardous agent; use appropriate precautions for handling and disposal (meets NIOSH 2014 criteria).

Monitoring Parameters Serum glucose (particularly in patients with preexisting diabetes mellitus or hyperglycemia); dermatologic evaluations prior to initiation, every 2 months during therapy, and for up to 6 months following discontinuation to assess for new cutaneous malignancies; monitor for febrile drug reactions and signs/symptoms of infections; signs/symptoms of uveitis (eg, eye pain, photophobia, and vision changes), RPED, or retinal vein occlusion; monitor for signs/symptoms of hemolytic anemia.

For patients receiving combination therapy with trametinib: Assess LVEF (by echocardiogram or MUGA scan) at baseline, 1 month after therapy initiation, and then at 2- to 3-month intervals; monitor for signs/symptoms of hemorrhage, venous thromboembolism, and interstitial lung disease.

Dosage Forms

Capsule, Oral:

Tafinlar: 50 mg, 75 mg

Dacarbazine (da KAR ba zeen)

Brand Names: Canada Dacarbazine for Injection

Index Terms DIC; Dimethyl Triazeno Imidazole Carboxamide; DTIC; DTIC-Dome; Imidazole Carboxamide; Imidazole Carboxamide Dimethyltriazene; WR-139007

Pharmacologic Category Antineoplastic Agent, Alkylating Agent (Triazene)

Use Treatment of malignant melanoma, Hodgkin lymphoma

Pregnancy Risk Factor C

Pregnancy Considerations **[U.S. Boxed Warning]: This agent is carcinogenic and/or teratogenic when used in animals;** adverse effects have been observed in animal studies. There are no adequate and well-controlled trials in pregnant women; use in pregnancy only if the potential benefit outweighs the potential risk to the fetus.

Breast-Feeding Considerations Due to the potential for serious adverse reactions in the nursing infant, breast-feeding is not recommended.

Contraindications Hypersensitivity to dacarbazine or any component of the formulation

Warnings/Precautions Hazardous agent - use appropriate precautions for handling and disposal (NIOSH 2014 [group 1]). **[U.S. Boxed Warnings]: Bone marrow suppression is a common toxicity;** leukopenia and thrombocytopenia may be severe; may result in treatment delays or discontinuation; monitor closely. **Hepatotoxicity with hepatocellular necrosis and hepatic vein thrombosis has been reported (rare),** usually with combination chemotherapy, but may occur with dacarbazine alone. The half-life is increased in patients with renal and/or hepatic impairment; use caution, monitor for toxicity and consider dosage reduction. Anaphylaxis may occur following dacarbazine administration. Extravasation may result in tissue damage and severe pain. **[U.S. Boxed Warnings]: May be carcinogenic and/or teratogenic. Should be administered under the supervision of an experienced cancer chemotherapy physician.** Carefully evaluate the potential benefits of therapy against the risk for toxicity. Dacarbazine is associated with a high emetic potential; antiemetics are recommended to prevent nausea and vomiting (Basch, 2011; Dupuis, 2011; Roila, 2010).

Adverse Reactions

Dermatologic: Alopecia

Gastrointestinal: Anorexia, nausea and vomiting

Hematologic: Myelosuppression (onset: 5-7 days; nadir: 7-10 days; recovery: 21-28 days), leukopenia, thrombocytopenia

Local: Pain on infusion

Infrequent, postmarketing, and/or case reports: Anaphylactic reactions, anemia, diarrhea, eosinophilia, erythema, facial flushing, facial paresthesia, flu-like syndrome (fever, myalgia, malaise), hepatic necrosis, hepatic vein occlusion, liver enzymes increased (transient), paresthesia, photosensitivity, rash, renal functions test abnormalities, taste alteration, urticaria

Drug Interactions

Metabolism/Transport Effects Substrate of CYP1A2 (major), CYP2E1 (major); **Note:** Assignment of Major/Minor substrate status based on clinically relevant drug interaction potential

Avoid Concomitant Use

Avoid concomitant use of Dacarbazine with any of the following: BCG; CloZAPine; Dipyrone; Natalizumab; Pimecrolimus; Tacrolimus (Topical); Tofacitinib; Vaccines (Live)

Increased Effect/Toxicity

Dacarbazine may increase the levels/effects of: CloZAPine; Leflunomide; Natalizumab; Tofacitinib; Vaccines (Live)

The levels/effects of Dacarbazine may be increased by: Abiraterone Acetate; CYP1A2 Inhibitors (Moderate); CYP1A2 Inhibitors (Strong); CYP2E1 Inhibitors (Moderate); CYP2E1 Inhibitors (Strong); Deferasirox; Denosumab; Dipyrone; MAO Inhibitors; Peginterferon Alfa-2b; Pimecrolimus; Roflumilast; Tacrolimus (Topical); Trastuzumab; Vemurafenib

Decreased Effect

Dacarbazine may decrease the levels/effects of: BCG; Coccidioides immitis Skin Test; Sipuleucel-T; Vaccines (Inactivated); Vaccines (Live)

The levels/effects of Dacarbazine may be decreased by: Cannabis; CYP1A2 Inducers (Strong); Cyproterone; Echinacea; SORAfenib; Teriflunomide

Preparation for Administration Hazardous agent; use appropriate precautions for handling and disposal (NIOSH 2014 [group 1]). The manufacturer recommends reconstituting 100 mg and 200 mg vials with 9.9 mL and 19.7 mL SWFI, respectively, to a concentration of 10 mg/mL; some institutions use different standard dilutions (eg, 20 mg/mL).

Standard IV dilution: Dilute in 250-1000 mL D_5W or NS.

Storage/Stability Store intact vials under refrigeration (2°C to 8°C). Protect from light. The following stability information has also been reported: Intact vials are stable for 3 months at room temperature (Cohen, 2007). Reconstituted solution is stable for 24 hours at room temperature (20°C) and 96 hours under refrigeration (4°C) when protected from light, although the manufacturer recommends use within 72 hours if refrigerated and 8 hours at room temperature. Solutions for infusion (in D_5W or NS) are stable for 24 hours at room temperature if protected from light. Decomposed drug turns pink.

Mechanism of Action Alkylating agent which is converted to the active alkylating metabolite MTIC [(methyl-triazene-1-yl)-imidazole-4-carboxamide] via the cytochrome P450 system. The cytotoxic effects of MTIC are manifested through alkylation (methylation) of DNA at the O^6, N^7 guanine positions which lead to DNA double strand breaks and apoptosis. Non-cell cycle specific.

Pharmacodynamics/Kinetics

Distribution: V_d: 0.6 L/kg, exceeding total body water; suggesting binding to some tissue (probably liver)

Protein binding: ~5%

Metabolism: Extensively hepatic to the active metabolite MTIC [(methyl-triazene-1-yl)-imidazole-4-carboxamide]

Half-life elimination: Biphasic: Initial: 20-40 minutes, Terminal: 5 hours; Patients with renal and hepatic dysfunction: Initial: 55 minutes, Terminal: 7.2 hours

Excretion: Urine (~40% as unchanged drug)

Dosage Note: Dacarbazine is associated with a high emetic potential; antiemetics are recommended to prevent nausea and vomiting (Basch, 2011; Dupuis, 2011; Roila, 2010).

Children: Hodgkin lymphoma (combination chemotherapy): IV: 375 mg/m²/dose days 1 and 15 every 4 weeks (ABVD regimen; Hutchinson, 1998)

Adults:

Hodgkin lymphoma (combination chemotherapy): IV: 375 mg/m²/dose days 1 and 15 every 4 weeks (ABVD regimen)

Metastatic melanoma: IV: 250 mg/m²/dose days 1-5 every 3 weeks

Metastatic melanoma (off-label dosing; in combination with cisplatin and vinblastine): IV: 800 mg/m² on day 1 every 3 weeks (Atkins, 2008; Eton, 2002)

Soft tissue sarcoma (off-label use; MAID regimen): IV: 250 mg/m²/day continuous infusion for 4 days every 3 weeks (total of 1000 mg/m²/cycle) (Antman, 1993; Antman, 1998)

Dosage adjustment in renal impairment: The FDA-approved labeling does not contain dosage adjustment guidelines. The following guidelines have been used by some clinicians (Kintzel, 1995):

CrCl 46-60 mL/minute: Administer 80% of dose

CrCl 31-45 mL/minute: Administer 75% of dose

CrCl <30 mL/minute: Administer 70% of dose

Dosage adjustment in hepatic impairment: The FDA-approved labeling does not contain adjustment guidelines. May cause hepatotoxicity; monitor closely for signs of toxicity.

Dosing in obesity: *ASCO Guidelines for appropriate chemotherapy dosing in obese adults with cancer:* Utilize patient's actual body weight (full weight) for calculation of body surface area- or weight-based dosing, particularly when the intent of therapy is curative; manage regimen-related toxicities in the same manner as for nonobese patients; if a dose reduction is utilized due to toxicity, consider resumption of full weight-based dosing with subsequent cycles, especially if cause of toxicity (eg, hepatic or renal impairment) is resolved (Griggs, 2012).

Administration Dacarbazine is associated with a high emetic potential; antiemetics are recommended to prevent nausea and vomiting (Basch, 2011; Dupuis, 2011; Roila, 2010).

Infuse over 30 to 60 minutes; rapid infusion may cause severe venous irritation. May also be administered as a continuous infusion (off-label administration rate) depending on the protocol.

Extravasation management: Local pain, burning sensation, and irritation at the injection site may be relieved by local application of hot packs. If extravasation occurs, apply cold packs. Protect exposed tissue from light following extravasation.

Hazardous agent; use appropriate precautions for handling and disposal (NIOSH 2014 [group 1]).

Monitoring Parameters CBC with differential, liver function

Dosage Forms

Solution Reconstituted, Intravenous:

Generic: 100 mg (1 ea); 200 mg (1 ea)

Solution Reconstituted, Intravenous [preservative free]:

Generic: 200 mg (1 ea)

◆ **Dacarbazine for Injection (Can)** *see* Dacarbazine *on page 549*

◆ **Dacogen** *see* Decitabine *on page 581*

◆ **DACT** *see* DACTINomycin *on page 551*

DACTINomycin (dak ti noe MYE sin)

Brand Names: U.S. Cosmegen

Brand Names: Canada Cosmegen

Index Terms ACT-D; Actinomycin; Actinomycin Cl; Actinomycin D; DACT

Pharmacologic Category Antineoplastic Agent, Antibiotic

Use Treatment of Wilms' tumor, childhood rhabdomyosarcoma, Ewing's sarcoma, metastatic testicular tumors (nonseminomatous), gestational trophoblastic neoplasm; regional perfusion (palliative or adjunctive) of locally recurrent or locoregional solid tumors (sarcomas, carcinomas and adenocarcinomas)

Pregnancy Risk Factor D

Dosage Note: Medication orders for dactinomycin are commonly written in MICROgrams (eg, 150 mcg) although many regimens list the dose in MILLIgrams (eg, mg/kg or mg/m²). The dose intensity per 2-week cycle should not exceed 15 mcg/kg/day for 5 days or 400-600 mcg/m²/day for 5 days. The manufacturer recommends calculation of the dosage for obese or edematous adult patients on the basis of body surface area in an effort to relate dosage to lean body mass. Dactinomycin is associated with a high emetic potential; antiemetics are recommended to prevent nausea and vomiting (Basch, 2011; Dupuis, 2011).

Wilms tumor, rhabdomyosarcoma, Ewing's sarcoma: Children >6 months and Adults: IV: 15 mcg/kg/day for 5 days (in various combination regimens and schedules)

Testicular cancer, metastatic: Adults: IV: 1000 mcg/m² on day 1 (in combination with cyclophosphamide, bleomycin, cisplatin, and vinblastine)

Gestational trophoblastic neoplasm: Adults: IV: 12 mcg/kg/day for 5 days (as a single agent) **or** 500 mcg on days 1 and 2 (in combination with etoposide, methotrexate, leucovorin, vincristine, cyclophosphamide, and cisplatin) **or** (off-label dosing for low-risk disease) 1.25 mg/m² every 2 weeks as a single agent (Osborne, 2011)

Regional perfusion: Adults (dosages and techniques may vary by institution; obese patients and patients with prior chemotherapy or radiation therapy may require lower doses): Lower extremity or pelvis: 50 mcg/kg; Upper extremity: 35 mcg/kg

Off-label dosing:

Rhabdomyosarcoma: IV:

VAC regimen:

Children <1 year: 25 mcg/kg every 3 weeks, weeks 0 to 45 (in combination with vincristine and cyclophosphamide, and mesna); dose omission required following radiation therapy (Raney, 2011)

Children ≥1 year: 45 mcg/kg (maximum dose: 2500 mcg) every 3 weeks, weeks 0 to 45 (in combination with vincristine and cyclophosphamide, and mesna); dose omission required following radiation therapy (Raney, 2011)

Wilms tumor: IV:

DD-4A regimen: Children: 45 mcg/kg on day 1 every 6 weeks for 54 weeks (in combination with doxorubicin and vincristine) (Green, 1998)

EE-4A regimen: Children: 45 mcg/kg on day 1 every 3 weeks for 18 weeks (in combination with vincristine) (Green, 1998)

VAD regimen:

Children <1 year: 750 mcg/m² every 6 weeks for 1 year (stage III disease) (in combination with vincristine and doxorubicin) (Pritchard, 1995)

Children ≥1 year: 1500 mcg/m² every 6 weeks for 1 year (stage III disease) (in combination with vincristine and doxorubicin) (Pritchard, 1995)

Osteosarcoma (off-label use): Children and Adults: IV: 600 mcg/m² on days 1, 2, and 3 of weeks 15, 31, 34, 39, and 42 (as part of a combination chemotherapy regimen) (Goorin, 2003)

Ovarian (germ cell) tumor (off-label use): Adults: IV: 500 mcg daily for 5 days every 4 weeks (in combination with vincristine and cyclophosphamide) (Gershenson, 1985) **or** 300 mcg/m²/day for 5 days every 4 weeks (in combination with vincristine and cyclophosphamide) (Slayton, 1985)

Elderly: Elderly patients are at increased risk of myelosuppression; dosing should begin at the low end of the dosing range.

Dosage adjustment in renal impairment: There are no dosage adjustments provided in the manufacturer's labeling; however, based on the amount of urinary excretion, dosage adjustments may not be necessary.

Dosage adjustment in hepatic impairment:

U.S. labeling: There are no dosage adjustments provided in manufacturer's labeling.

Canadian labeling:

Mild impairment: There are no dosage adjustments provided.

Moderate-severe impairment: Dose reduction may be considered; 33% to 50% dose reductions for patients with hyperbilirubinemia have been recommended by some clinicians.

Off-label dosing: Any transaminase increase: Reduce dose by 50%; may increase by monitoring toxicities (Floyd, 2006)

Dosing in obesity: *ASCO Guidelines for appropriate chemotherapy dosing in obese adults with cancer:* Utilize patient's actual body weight (full weight) for calculation of body surface area- or weight-based dosing, particularly when the intent of therapy is curative; manage regimen-related toxicities in the same manner as for nonobese patients; if a dose reduction is utilized due to toxicity, consider resumption of full weight-based dosing with subsequent cycles, especially if cause of toxicity (eg, hepatic or renal impairment) is resolved (Griggs, 2012).

Additional Information Complete prescribing information should be consulted for additional detail.

Dosage Forms

Solution Reconstituted, Intravenous:

Cosmegen: 0.5 mg (1 ea)

◆ **Dalacin C (Can)** *see* Clindamycin (Systemic) *on page 460*

◆ **Dalacin T (Can)** *see* Clindamycin (Topical) *on page 464*

◆ **Dalacin Vaginal (Can)** *see* Clindamycin (Topical) *on page 464*

Dalbavancin (dal ba VAN sin)

Brand Names: U.S. Dalvance

Index Terms BI 397; Zeven

Pharmacologic Category Glycopeptide

Use Acute bacterial skin and skin structure infections: Treatment of adult patients with acute bacterial skin and skin structure infections (ABSSSI) caused by susceptible isolates of the following gram-positive microorganisms: *Staphylococcus aureus* (including methicillin-susceptible and methicillin-resistant strains), *Streptococcus pyogenes*, *Streptococcus agalactiae* and *Streptococcus anginosus* group (including *S. anginosus*, *S. intermedius*, *S. constellatus*)

Pregnancy Risk Factor C

Pregnancy Considerations Adverse events were observed in some animal reproduction studies. The long half-life of dalbavancin should be considered when evaluating potential exposure to the fetus.

Breast-Feeding Considerations It is not known of dalbavancin is excreted into breast milk. The manufacturer recommends that caution be used if administered to a nursing woman.

Contraindications Hypersensitivity to dalbavancin or to any component of the formulation

Warnings/Precautions Serious hypersensitivity (anaphylactic) and skin reactions have been reported. Discontinue treatment if an allergic reaction occurs. Dalbavancin cross-sensitivity to other glycopeptides may occur; exercise caution in patients with a history of glycopeptide allergy; carefully screen for previous hypersensitivity reactions to glycopeptides prior to administration. Patients with normal baseline transaminase levels may have alanine aminotransferase (ALT) elevation >3 times the upper limit of normal (ULN) during therapy; in clinical studies, abnormalities in liver tests (ALT, AST, bilirubin) were reported with similar frequency in the dalbavancin and comparator arms. ALT elevations were reversible after discontinuation. Rapid intravenous infusions of dalbavancin (<30 minutes) may cause reactions that resemble "Red-Man Syndrome," (eg, flushing of the upper body, urticaria, pruritus, rash). Stopping or slowing the infusion may result in cessation of these reactions. Use may result in fungal or bacterial superinfection, including *Clostridium difficile*-associated diarrhea (CDAD) and pseudomembranous colitis; CDAD has been observed >2 months postantibiotic treatment.

Adverse Reactions

Cardiovascular: Flushing, phlebitis

Central nervous system: Dizziness, headache

Dermatologic: Pruritus, skin rash, urticaria

Endocrine & Metabolic: Hypoglycemia

Gastrointestinal: Abdominal pain, diarrhea, gastrointestinal hemorrhage, hematochezia, melena, nausea, oral candidiasis, pseudomembranous colitis, vomiting

Hematologic & oncologic: Acute posthemorrhagic anemia, anemia, eosinophilia, hematoma (spontaneous), increased INR, leukopenia, neutropenia, petechia, thrombocythemia, thrombocytopenia, wound hemorrhage

Hepatic: Hepatotoxicity

Hepatic: Increased serum alkaline phosphatase, increased serum transaminases

Hypersensitivity: Anaphylactoid reaction

Infection: Vulvovaginal infection (mycotic)

Respiratory: Bronchospasm

Miscellaneous: Infusion related reaction

Rare but important or life-threatening: Hypersensitivity reaction, increased serum ALT (>3 x ULN)

Drug Interactions

Metabolism/Transport Effects None known.

Avoid Concomitant Use

Avoid concomitant use of Dalbavancin with any of the following: BCG

Increased Effect/Toxicity There are no known significant interactions involving an increase in effect.

Decreased Effect

Dalbavancin may decrease the levels/effects of: BCG; Sodium Picosulfate; Typhoid Vaccine

Preparation for Administration Reconstitute with 25 mL of SWFI for each 500 mg vial. Alternate between gentle swirling and inversion of the vial until contents are completely dissolved. Do not shake. The reconstituted vial contains 20 mg/mL dalbavancin as a clear, colorless to yellow solution. Dilute for infusion in D_5W (final solution concentration 1 to 5 mg/mL).

Storage/Stability Store intact vials at 25°C (77°F); excursions are permitted between 15°C and 30°C (59°F and 86°F). Reconstituted vials and diluted solution may be stored refrigerated at 2°C to 8°C (36°F to 46°F) or at room temperature 20°C to 25°C (68°F to 77°F). Do not freeze. The total time from reconstitution to dilution to administration should be ≤48 hours.

Mechanism of Action Dalbavancin is a lipoglycopeptide which binds to the D-alanyl-D-alanine terminus of the stem pentapeptide in nascent cell wall peptidoglycan prevents cross-linking and interferes with cell wall synthesis. It is bactericidal *in vitro* against *Staphylococcus aureus* and *Streptococcus pyogenes*

Pharmacodynamics/Kinetics

Distribution: V_d: 7 to 13 L (Leighton, 2004)

Protein binding: 93% (primarily to albumin)

Metabolism: Minor metabolite (hydroxy-dalbavancin)

Half-life elimination: 346 hours

Excretion: Urine (33% as unchanged drug, 12% as hydroxy metabolite); feces (20%)

Dosage **Usual dosage range:** Adults: IV: 1000 mg as a single dose initially, followed by 500 mg as a single dose 1 week later

Indication-specific dosing: Acute bacterial skin and skin structure infections: Adults: IV: 1000 mg as a single dose initially, followed by 500 mg as a single dose 1 week later

Dosage adjustment for renal impairment:

CrCl ≥30 mL/minute: No dosage adjustment necessary

CrCl <30 mL/minute: 750 mg as a single dose initially, followed by 375 mg as a single dose 1 week later

ESRD patients receiving intermittent hemodialysis (IHD) (regularly scheduled): No dosage adjustment necessary; administer without regard to hemodialysis.

Dosage adjustment for hepatic impairment:

Mild hepatic impairment (Child-Pugh class A): No dosage adjustment necessary.

Moderate or severe hepatic impairment (Child-Pugh class B or C): There are no dosage adjustments provided in the manufacturer's labeling (has not been studied); use with caution.

Usual Infusion Concentrations: Adult *IV infusion:* 500 mg or 1000 mg in 100 to 1000 mL (concentration of 1 to 5 mg/mL) of D_5W.

Administration IV: Infuse over 30 minutes. If a common IV line is being used to administer other drugs in addition to dalbavancin, the line should be flushed before and after each infusion with D_5W.

Monitoring Parameters Baseline BUN, serum creatinine, and liver function tests (AST, ALT, bilirubin). Monitor patients for any infusion-related reactions and for superinfection during therapy.

Dosage Forms

Solution Reconstituted, Intravenous [preservative free]: Dalvance: 500 mg (1 ea)

Dalfampridine (dal FAM pri deen)

Brand Names: U.S. Ampyra

Brand Names: Canada Fampyra

Index Terms 4-aminopyridine; 4-AP; EL-970; Fampridine; Fampridine-SR

Pharmacologic Category Potassium Channel Blocker

Use Treatment to improve walking in patients with multiple sclerosis (MS)

Pregnancy Risk Factor C

Dosage Multiple sclerosis: Adults: Oral: 10 mg every 12 hours (maximum daily dose: 20 mg); no additional benefit seen with doses >20 mg daily

Missed doses: Do not administer double or extra doses if a dose is missed.

Dosing adjustment in renal impairment: Note: Creatinine clearance is estimated with Cockcroft-Gault formula.

U.S. labeling:

Mild renal impairment (CrCl 51-80 mL/minute): No dosage adjustment recommended by the manufacturer; however, use with extreme caution as risk of seizure may be increased secondary to reduced clearance.

Moderate-to-severe renal impairment (CrCl ≤50 mL/minute): Use is contraindicated.

Canadian labeling:

Mild-to-severe impairment (CrCl ≤80 mL/minute): Use is contraindicated.

Dosing adjustment in hepatic impairment: No dosage adjustment required; drug undergoes minimal metabolism and is primarily excreted unchanged in the urine.

Additional Information Complete prescribing information should be consulted for additional detail.

Dosage Forms

Tablet Extended Release 12 Hour, Oral:

Ampyra: 10 mg

Dosage Forms: Canada

Tablet, extended release, oral:

Fampyra™: 10 mg

◆ **Dalfopristin and Quinupristin** *see* Quinupristin and Dalfopristin *on page 1762*

◆ **Daliresp** *see* Roflumilast *on page 1840*

◆ **Dallergy Drops [OTC]** *see* Chlorpheniramine and Phenylephrine *on page 426*

◆ **Dalmane (Can)** *see* Flurazepam *on page 906*

◆ ***d*-Alpha Tocopherol** *see* Vitamin E *on page 2174*

Dalteparin (dal TE pa rin)

Brand Names: U.S. Fragmin

Brand Names: Canada Fragmin

Index Terms Dalteparin Sodium

Pharmacologic Category Anticoagulant; Anticoagulant, Low Molecular Weight Heparin

Use Prevention of deep vein thrombosis (DVT) which may lead to pulmonary embolism, in patients requiring abdominal surgery who are at risk for thromboembolism complications (eg, patients >40 years of age, obesity, patients with malignancy, history of DVT or pulmonary embolism, and surgical procedures requiring general anesthesia and lasting >30 minutes); prevention of DVT in patients undergoing hip-replacement surgery; patients immobile during an acute illness; prevention of ischemic complications in patients with unstable angina or non-Q-wave myocardial infarction on concurrent aspirin therapy; in patients with cancer, extended treatment (6 months) of acute symptomatic venous thromboembolism (DVT and/or PE) to reduce the recurrence of venous thromboembolism

Canadian labeling: Additional use (off-label use in U.S.): Treatment of acute DVT; prevention of venous thromboembolism (VTE) in patients at risk of VTE undergoing general surgery; anticoagulant in extracorporeal circuit during hemodialysis and hemofiltration

Pregnancy Risk Factor B

Pregnancy Considerations Adverse effects were not observed in animal reproduction studies. Low molecular weight heparin (LMWH) does not cross the placenta; increased risks of fetal bleeding or teratogenic effects have not been reported (Bates, 2012).

LMWH is recommended over unfractionated heparin for the treatment of acute venous thromboembolism (VTE) in pregnant women. LMWH is also recommended over unfractionated heparin for VTE prophylaxis in pregnant women with certain risk factors. LMWH should be discontinued at least 24 hours prior to induction of labor or a planned cesarean delivery. For women undergoing cesarean section and who have additional risk factors for developing VTE, the prophylactic use of LMWH may be considered. For women who require long-term anticoagulation with warfarin and who are considering pregnancy, LMWH substitution should be done prior to conception when possible. When choosing therapy, fetal outcomes (ie, pregnancy loss, malformations), maternal outcomes (ie, VTE, hemorrhage), burden of therapy, and maternal preference should be considered (Guyatt, 2012). LMWH may also be used in women with mechanical heart valves (consult current guidelines for details) (Bates, 2012; Nishimura, 2014).

Multiple-dose vials contain benzyl alcohol (avoid in pregnant women due to association with gasping syndrome in premature infants); use of preservative-free formulation is recommended.

Breast-Feeding Considerations In lactating women receiving prophylactic doses of dalteparin, small amounts of anti-xa activity was noted in breast milk. The milk/plasma ratio was <0.025 to 0.224. Oral absorption of low molecular weight heparin is extremely low, and is therefore unlikely to cause adverse events in a nursing infant. Use of LMWH may be continued in breast-feeding women (Guyatt, 2012).

Contraindications Hypersensitivity to dalteparin (eg, pruritus, rash, anaphylactic reactions) or any component of the formulation; history of heparin-induced thrombocytopenia (HIT) or HIT with thrombosis; hypersensitivity to heparin or pork products; active major bleeding; patients with unstable angina, non-Q-wave MI, or prolonged venous thromboembolism prophylaxis undergoing epidural/neuraxial anesthesia

Note: Use of dalteparin in patients with current HIT or HIT with thrombosis is **not** recommended and considered contraindicated due to high cross-reactivity to heparin-platelet factor-4 antibody (Guyatt [ACCP], 2012; Warkentin, 1999).

Canadian labeling: Additional contraindications (not in U.S. labeling): Septic endocarditis, major blood clotting disorders; acute gastroduodenal ulcer; cerebral hemorrhage; severe uncontrolled hypertension; diabetic or hemorrhagic retinopathy; other diseases that increase risk of hemorrhage; injuries to and operations on the CNS, eyes, and ears

Warnings/Precautions [U.S. Boxed Warning]: Spinal or epidural hematomas, including subsequent paralysis, may occur with recent or anticipated neuraxial anesthesia (epidural or spinal) or spinal puncture in patients anticoagulated with LMWH or heparinoids. Consider risk versus benefit prior to spinal procedures; risk is increased by the use of concomitant agents which may alter hemostasis, the use of indwelling epidural catheters for analgesia, a history of spinal deformity or spinal surgery, as well as traumatic or repeated epidural or spinal punctures. Optimal timing between neuraxial procedures and dalteparin administration is not known. Delay placement or removal of catheter for at least 12 hours after administration of 2,500 units once daily, at least 15 hours after the administration of 5,000 units once daily, and at least 24 hours after the administration of higher doses (200 units/kg once daily, 120 units/kg twice daily) and consider doubling these times in patients with creatinine clearance <30 mL/minute; risk of neuraxial hematoma may still exist since antifactor Xa levels are still detectable at these time points. Upon removal of catheter, consider delaying next dose of dalteparin for at least 4 hours. Patient should be observed closely for bleeding, signs and symptoms of neurological impairment, bowel and/or bladder dysfunction if therapy is administered during or immediately following diagnostic lumbar puncture, epidural anesthesia, or spinal anesthesia. If neurological compromise is noted, urgent treatment is necessary. If spinal hematoma is suspected, diagnose and treat immediately; spinal cord decompression may be considered although it may not prevent or reverse neurological sequelae. Use of dalteparin is contraindicated in patients undergoing epidural/neuraxial anesthesia. Patient should be observed closely for bleeding if dalteparin is administered during or immediately following diagnostic lumbar puncture, epidural anesthesia, or spinal anesthesia.

Use with caution in patients with preexisting thrombocytopenia, recent childbirth, subacute bacterial endocarditis, peptic ulcer disease, pericarditis or pericardial effusion, liver or renal function impairment, recent lumbar puncture, vasculitis, concurrent use of aspirin (increased bleeding risk), previous hypersensitivity to heparin, heparin-associated thrombocytopenia. Monitor platelet count closely. Cases of dalteparin-induced thrombocytopenia and thrombosis (similar to heparin-induced thrombocytopenia [HIT]), some complicated by organ infarction, limb ischemia, or death, have been observed. In patients with a history of HIT or HIT with thrombosis, dalteparin is contraindicated. Consider discontinuation of therapy in any patient developing significant thrombocytopenia (eg, <100,000/mm^3) and/or thrombosis related to initiation of dalteparin especially when associated with a positive *in vitro* test for antiplatelet antibodies. Use caution in patients with congenital or drug-induced thrombocytopenia or platelet defects.

Monitor patient closely for signs or symptoms of bleeding. Certain patients are at increased risk of bleeding. Risk factors include bacterial endocarditis; congenital or acquired bleeding disorders; active ulcerative or angiodysplastic GI diseases; severe uncontrolled hypertension; hemorrhagic stroke; or use shortly after brain, spinal, or ophthalmology surgery; in patients treated concomitantly with platelet inhibitors; recent GI bleeding; thrombocytopenia or platelet defects; hypertensive or diabetic retinopathy; or in patients undergoing invasive procedures.

Use with caution in patients with severe renal impairment or severe hepatic impairment; accumulation may occur with repeated dosing increasing the risk for bleeding. Heparin can cause hyperkalemia by affecting aldosterone. Similar reactions could occur with dalteparin. Monitor for hyperkalemia. Do **not** administer intramuscularly. Not to be used interchangeably (unit for unit) with heparin or any other low molecular weight heparins.

Benzyl alcohol and derivatives: Some dosage forms may contain benzyl alcohol and should not be used in pregnant women. In neonates, large amounts of benzyl alcohol (≥99 mg/kg/day) have been associated with a potentially fatal toxicity ("gasping syndrome"); the "gasping syndrome" consists of metabolic acidosis, respiratory distress, gasping respirations, CNS dysfunction (including convulsions, intracranial hemorrhage), hypotension, and cardiovascular collapse (AAP, 1997; CDC, 1982); some data suggests that benzoate displaces bilirubin from protein binding sites (Ahlfors, 2001); avoid or use dosage forms containing benzyl alcohol with caution in neonates. See manufacturer's labeling.

There is no consensus for adjusting/correcting the weight-based dosage of LMWH for patients who are morbidly obese (BMI ≥40 kg/m^2). The American College of Chest Physicians Practice Guidelines suggest consulting with a pharmacist regarding dosing in bariatric surgery patients and other obese patients who may require higher doses of LMWH (Gould, 2012).

Adverse Reactions Note: As with all anticoagulants, bleeding is the major adverse effect of dalteparin. Hemorrhage may occur at virtually any site. Risk is dependent on multiple variables.

Hematologic: Hemorrhage, major hemorrhage, thrombocytopenia (including heparin-induced thrombocytopenia), wound hematoma

Hepatic: Increased serum ALT (>3 x ULN), increased serum AST (>3 x ULN)

Local: Hematoma at injection site, pain at injection site

Rare but important or life-threatening: Alopecia, anaphylactoid reaction, gastrointestinal hemorrhage, hemoptysis, hypersensitivity reaction (fever, pruritus, rash, injections site reaction, bullous eruption), postoperative wound bleeding, skin necrosis, subdural hematoma, thrombosis (associated with heparin-induced thrombocytopenia). Spinal or epidural hematomas can occur following neuraxial anesthesia or spinal puncture, resulting in paralysis.

Drug Interactions

Metabolism/Transport Effects None known.

Avoid Concomitant Use

Avoid concomitant use of Dalteparin with any of the following: Apixaban; Dabigatran Etexilate; Edoxaban; Omacetaxine; Rivaroxaban; Urokinase; Vorapaxar

Increased Effect/Toxicity

Dalteparin may increase the levels/effects of: ACE Inhibitors; Aliskiren; Angiotensin II Receptor Blockers; Anticoagulants; Canagliflozin; Collagenase (Systemic); Deferasirox; Eplerenone; Ibritumomab; Nintedanib; Obinutuzumab; Omacetaxine; Palifermin; Potassium Salts; Potassium-Sparing Diuretics; Rivaroxaban; Tositumomab and Iodine I 131 Tositumomab

The levels/effects of Dalteparin may be increased by: 5-ASA Derivatives; Agents with Antiplatelet Properties; Apixaban; Dabigatran Etexilate; Dasatinib; Edoxaban; Herbs (Anticoagulant/Antiplatelet Properties); Ibrutinib; Limaprost; Nonsteroidal Anti-Inflammatory Agents; Omega-3 Fatty Acids; Pentosan Polysulfate Sodium; Pentoxifylline; Prostacyclin Analogues; Salicylates; Sugammadex; Thrombolytic Agents; Tibolone; Tipranavir; Urokinase; Vitamin E; Vorapaxar

Decreased Effect

The levels/effects of Dalteparin may be decreased by: Estrogen Derivatives; Progestins

Preparation for Administration Canadian labeling: If necessary, may dilute in isotonic sodium chloride or dextrose solutions to a concentration of 20 units/mL. Use within 24 hours of mixing.

Storage/Stability Store at 20°C to 25°C (68°F to 77°F). Multidose vials may be stored for up to 2 weeks at room temperature after entering.

Mechanism of Action Low molecular weight heparin analog with a molecular weight of 4000-6000 daltons; the commercial product contains 3% to 15% heparin with a molecular weight <3000 daltons, 65% to 78% with a molecular weight of 3000-8000 daltons and 14% to 26% with a molecular weight >8000 daltons; while dalteparin has been shown to inhibit both factor Xa and factor IIa (thrombin), the antithrombotic effect of dalteparin is characterized by a higher ratio of antifactor Xa to antifactor IIa activity (ratio = 4)

Pharmacodynamics/Kinetics

Onset of action: Anti-Xa activity: Within 1-2 hours

Duration: >12 hours

Distribution: V_d: 40-60 mL/kg

Protein binding: Low affinity for plasma proteins (Howard, 1997)

Bioavailability: SubQ: 81% to 93%

Half-life elimination (route dependent): Anti-Xa activity: 2-5 hours; prolonged in chronic renal insufficiency: 3.7-7.7 hours (following a single 5000 unit dose)

Time to peak, serum: Anti-Xa activity: ~4 hours
Excretion: Primarily renal (Howard, 1997)

Dosage Adults:

IV: Canadian labeling (not in U.S. labeling): Anticoagulant for hemodialysis and hemofiltration:

Chronic renal failure with no other bleeding risks:

Hemodialysis/filtration ≤4 hours: IV bolus: 5,000 units

Hemodialysis/filtration >4 hours: IV bolus: 30-40 units/kg, followed by an infusion of 10-15 units/kg/hour (typically produces plasma concentrations of 0.5-1 units anti-Xa/mL)

Acute renal failure and high bleeding risk: IV bolus: 5-10 units/kg, followed by an infusion of 4-5 units/kg/hour (typically produces plasma concentrations of 0.2-0.4 units anti-Xa/mL)

SubQ: **Note:** Each 2500 units of anti-Xa activity is equal to 16 mg of dalteparin.

DVT prophylaxis: **Note:** In morbidly obese patients (BMI ≥40 kg/m^2), increasing the prophylactic dose by 30% may be appropriate (Nutescu, 2009):

Abdominal surgery:

Low-to-moderate DVT risk: 2500 units 1-2 hours prior to surgery, then once daily for 5-10 days postoperatively

High DVT risk: 5000 units the evening prior to surgery and then once daily for 5-10 days postoperatively. Alternatively in patients with malignancy: 2500 units 1-2 hours prior to surgery, 2500 units 12 hours later, then 5000 units once daily for 5-10 days postoperatively.

General surgery with risk factors for VTE: Canadian labeling (not in U.S. labeling): 2500 units 1-2 hours preoperatively followed by 2500-5000 units every morning (may administer 2500 units no sooner than 4 hours after surgery and 8 hours after previous dose provided hemostasis has been achieved) or if other risk factors are present (eg, malignancy, heart failure), then may administer 5000 units the evening prior to surgery followed by 5000 units every evening postoperatively; continue treatment until patient is mobilized (approximately ≥5-7 days).

Total hip replacement surgery: **Note:** Three treatment options are currently available. Dose is given for 5-10 days, although up to 14 days of treatment have been tolerated in clinical trials. The American College of Chest Physicians (ACCP) recommends a minimum duration of at least 10-14 days; extended duration of up to 35 days is suggested (Guyatt, 2012).

Postoperative regimen:

Initial: 2500 units 4-8 hours after surgery (or later if hemostasis not achieved). The ACCP recommends initiation ≥12 hours after surgery if postoperative regimen chosen (Guyatt, 2012).

Maintenance: 5000 units once daily; allow at least 6 hours to elapse after initial postsurgical dose (adjust administration time accordingly)

Preoperative regimen (starting day of surgery):

Initial: 2500 units within 2 hours **before** surgery. The ACCP recommends initiation ≥12 hours before surgery if preoperative regimen chosen (Guyatt, 2012). At 4-8 hours **after** surgery (or later if hemostasis not achieved), administer 2500 units

Maintenance: 5000 units once daily; allow at least 6 hours to elapse after initial postsurgical dose (adjust administration time accordingly)

Preoperative regimen (starting evening prior to surgery):

Initial: 5000 units 10-14 hours **before** surgery. The ACCP recommends initiation ≥12 hours before surgery if preoperative regimen chosen (Guyatt, 2012). At 4-8 hours **after** surgery (or later if hemostasis not achieved), administer 5000 units

Maintenance: 5000 units once daily, allowing 24 hours between doses

Immobility during acute illness: 5000 units once daily

Unstable angina or non-Q-wave myocardial infarction: 120 units/kg body weight (maximum dose: 10,000 units) every 12 hours for up to 5-8 days with concurrent aspirin therapy. Discontinue dalteparin once patient is clinically stable.

Obesity: Use actual body weight to calculate dose; dose capping at 10,000 units recommended (Nutescu, 2009)

Venous thromboembolism, extended treatment in cancer patients:

Initial (month 1): 200 units/kg (maximum dose: 18,000 units) once daily for 30 days

Maintenance (months 2-6): ~150 units/kg (maximum dose: 18,000 units) once daily. If platelet count between 50,000-100,000/mm^3, reduce dose by 2,500 units until platelet count recovers to ≥100,000/mm^3. If platelet count <50,000/mm^3, discontinue dalteparin until platelet count recover to >50,000/mm^3.

Obesity: Use actual body weight to calculate dose; dose capping is not recommended (Nutescu, 2009). However, the manufacturer recommends a maximum dose of 18,000 units per day for the treatment of VTE in cancer patients.

DVT (with or without PE) treatment in noncancer patients (off-label use in U.S.): SubQ: 200 units/kg once daily (Feissinger, 1996; Jaff, 2011; Wells, 2005) **or** 100 units/kg twice daily (Jaff, 2011).

Canadian labeling: SubQ: 200 units/kg once daily (maximum dose: 18,000 units/day) **or** alternatively, may adapt dose as follows (SubQ):

46-56 kg: 10,000 units once daily
57-68 kg: 12,500 units once daily
69-82 kg: 15,000 units once daily
≥83 kg: 18,000 units once daily

Note: If increased bleeding risk, may give 100 units/kg SubQ twice daily. Concomitant treatment with a vitamin-K antagonist is usually initiated immediately.

Obesity: Use actual body weight to calculate dose; dose capping is not recommended (Nutescu, 2009). One study demonstrated similar anti-Xa levels after 3 days of therapy in obese patients (>40% above IBW; range: 82-190 kg) compared to those ≤20% above IBW or between 20% to 40% above IBW (Wilson, 2001).

Pregnant women (off-label use): 200 units/kg/dose once daily or 100 units/kg/dose every 12 hours. Discontinue ≥24 hours prior to the induction of labor or cesarean section. Dalteparin therapy may be substituted with heparin near term. Continue anticoagulation therapy for ≥6 weeks postpartum (minimum duration of therapy: 3 months). LMWH or heparin therapy is preferred over warfarin during pregnancy (Bates, 2012).

Mechanical heart valve (aortic or mitral position) to bridge anticoagulation (off-label use): 100 units/kg/dose every 12 hours (ACCP [Douketis, 2012]). **Note:** If used in pregnant patients, target anti-Xa level of 0.8 to 1.2 units/mL, 4 to 6 hours postdose (AHA/ACC [Nishimura, 2014]).

Prevention of recurrent venous thromboembolism in pregnancy (off-label use): 5000 units once daily. Therapy should continue for 6 weeks postpartum in high-risk women (Bates, 2012).

Dosing adjustment in renal impairment: Half-life is increased in patients with chronic renal failure, use with caution, accumulation can be expected; specific dosage adjustments have not been recommended. Accumulation was not observed in critically ill patients with severe renal insufficiency (CrCl <30 mL/minute) receiving prophylactic doses (5000 units) for a median of 7 days (Douketis, 2008). In cancer patients, receiving treatment for venous thromboembolism, if CrCl <30 mL/minute, manufacturer recommends monitoring anti-Xa levels to determine appropriate dose.

Dosing adjustment in hepatic impairment: No dosage adjustment provided in manufacturer's labeling; use with caution.

Administration

For deep SubQ injection; may be injected in a U-shape to the area surrounding the navel, the upper outer side of the thigh, or the upper outer quadrangle of the buttock. Use thumb and forefinger to lift a fold of skin when injecting dalteparin to the navel area or thigh. Insert needle at a 45- to 90-degree angle. The entire length of needle should be inserted. Do not expel air bubble from fixed-dose syringe prior to injection. Air bubble (and extra solution, if applicable) may be expelled from graduated syringes. In order to minimize bruising, do not rub injection site.

To convert from IV unfractionated heparin (UFH) infusion to SubQ dalteparin (Nutescu, 2007): Calculate specific dose for dalteparin based on indication, discontinue UFH and begin dalteparin within 1 hour

To convert from SubQ dalteparin to IV UFH infusion (Nutescu, 2007): Discontinue dalteparin; calculate specific dose for IV UFH infusion based on indication; omit heparin bolus/loading dose

Converting from SubQ dalteparin dosed every 12 hours: Start IV UFH infusion 10-11 hours after last dose of dalteparin

Converting from SubQ dalteparin dosed every 24 hours: Start IV UFH infusion 22-23 hours after last dose of dalteparin

IV (Canadian labeling; not an approved route in U.S. labeling): Administer as bolus IV injection or as continuous infusion. Recommended concentration for infusion: 20 units/mL.

Monitoring Parameters Periodic CBC including platelet count; stool occult blood tests; monitoring of PT and PTT is not necessary. Once patient has received 3-4 doses, anti-Xa levels, drawn 4-6 hours after dalteparin administration, may be used to monitor effect in patients with severe renal dysfunction or if abnormal coagulation parameters or bleeding should occur. For patients >190 kg, if anti-Xa monitoring is available, adjusting dose based on anti-Xa levels is recommended; if anti-Xa monitoring is unavailable, reduce dose if bleeding occurs (Nutescu, 2009).

Reference Range

Recurrent VTE prophylaxis in pregnant women: Peak anti-Xa concentrations: 0.2-0.6 units/mL (Bates, 2012)

Treatment of venous thromboembolism: Peak anti-Xa concentration target (measured 4 hours after administration): *Once-daily dosing:* 1.05 anti-Xa units/mL (Garcia, 2012); per the manufacturer, target anti-Xa range is 0.5-1.5 units/mL (measured 4-6 hours after administration and after patient received 3-4 doses)

Additional Information Neutralization of dalteparin (in overdose) with protamine 1% solution: Manufacturer's recommendations: 1 mg protamine for each 100 anti-Xa units of dalteparin; if PTT prolonged 2-4 hours after first dose (or if bleeding continues), consider additional dose of 0.5 mg for each 100 anti-Xa units of dalteparin.

Dosage Forms

Solution, Subcutaneous [preservative free]:

Fragmin: 10,000 units/mL (1 mL); 2500 units/0.2 mL (0.2 mL); 5000 units/0.2 mL (0.2 mL); 12,500 units/0.5 mL (0.5 mL); 15,000 units/0.6 mL (0.6 mL); 18,000 units/0.72 mL (0.72 mL)

◆ **Dalteparin Sodium** *see* Dalteparin *on page 553*

◆ **Dalvance** *see* Dalbavancin *on page 551*

Danaparoid [CAN/INT] (da NAP a roid)

Brand Names: Canada Orgaran®

Index Terms Danaparoid Sodium

Pharmacologic Category Anticoagulant; Anticoagulant, Heparinoid

Use Note: Not approved in U.S.

Prevention of postoperative deep vein thrombosis (DVT) following orthopedic or major abdominal and thoracic surgery; prevention of DVT in patients with confirmed diagnosis of non-hemorrhagic stroke; management of heparin-induced thrombocytopenia (HIT)

Pregnancy Considerations Teratogenic effects have not been observed in animal reproduction studies. The manufacturer labeling states that incidental observations in pregnant women during the last trimesters, gave no indication that use during pregnancy results in fetal abnormalities or exacerbation of bleeding in the mother or infant during delivery. Use in pregnant women however is generally not recommended unless deemed medically necessary and alternative therapy is unavailable. Danaparoid does not cross the placenta and is the preferred anticoagulant in pregnant women with HIT (Guyatt, 2012).

Breast-Feeding Considerations Only low amounts of anit-Xa activity have been found breast milk following maternal use of danaparoid; however, because it is not absorbed when taken orally, it is unlikely to cause adverse events in a nursing infant. Use of danaparoid may be continued in breast-feeding. The manufacturer labeling recommends that women receiving danaparoid avoid breast-feeding.

Contraindications Hypersensitivity to danaparoid, or any component of the formulation (including sulfites); history of thrombocytopenia while receiving danaparoid or when associated with a positive *in vitro* test for antiplatelet antibodies in the presence of danaparoid; hemorrhagic stroke (without systemic emboli); acute hemorrhagic stroke; patients with active major bleeding; severe hemorrhagic diathesis (hemophilia, immune thrombocytopenia [ITP]); acute or subacute bacterial endocarditis; active gastric or duodenal ulcer; surgery of CNS, eyes, or ears; diabetic or hemorrhagic retinopathy; severe uncontrolled hypertension; other conditions or diseases that increase risk of hemorrhage; not for IM use

Warnings/Precautions Hemorrhagic stroke should be ruled out by CT scan prior to initiating therapy. Do not administer intramuscularly.

Spinal or epidural hematomas, including subsequent paralysis, may occur with recent or anticipated neuraxial anesthesia (epidural or spinal anesthesia) or spinal puncture in patients anticoagulated with LMWH or heparinoids. Consider risk versus benefit prior to spinal procedures; risk is increased by the use of concomitant agents which may alter hemostasis, the use of indwelling epidural catheters for analgesia, a history of spinal deformity or spinal surgery, as well as a history of traumatic or repeated epidural or spinal punctures. Spinal procedures should be avoided for 12 hours after the last danaparoid dose; allow at least 2 hours after procedure before resuming danaparoid therapy. Patient should be observed closely for bleeding and signs and symptoms of neurological impairment if therapy is administered during or immediately following diagnostic lumbar puncture, epidural anesthesia, or spinal anesthesia.

Use with caution in patients with history of peptic ulcer disease, hepatic impairment, and severe renal impairment. Monitor patient closely for signs or symptoms of bleeding. Certain patients are at increased risk of bleeding (eg, severe hepatic disease, patients undergoing knee surgery or other invasive procedures, concomitant therapy with platelet inhibitors, elderly). Discontinue use if bleeding occurs. Danaparoid is not effectively antagonized by protamine sulfate. No other antidote is available, so extreme caution is needed in monitoring dose given and resulting Xa inhibition effect.

Use caution in patients with or with a history of thrombocytopenia (heparin-induced, congenital) or platelet defects. The manufacturer labeling recommends that patients with a history of heparin-induced thrombocytopenia be tested for cross-reactivity with danaparoid prior to initiating therapy; if test is positive, alternative therapy should be employed unless otherwise not available. If danaparoid is administered, therapy must be discontinued immediately with clinical signs of positive cross-reactivity (eg, increased reduction in platelet counts, thrombosis, skin necrosis). May resume therapy (if needed) only after laboratory confirmed negative test for danaparoid activated antiplatelet antibodies. Cutaneous allergy tests may help detect the presence of cross-reactivity between heparins and danaparoid (Grassegger, 2001).

Safety and efficacy have not been established for use as thromboprophylaxis in patients with prosthetic heart valves. Heparin can cause hyperkalemia by affecting aldosterone. A similar reaction could occur with danaparoid. Monitor for hyperkalemia. Not to be used interchangeably (unit for unit) with heparin or any other low molecular weight heparins.

This product contains sodium sulfite which may cause allergic-type reactions, including anaphylactic symptoms and life-threatening asthmatic episodes in susceptible people; this is seen more frequently in asthmatics.

Adverse Reactions As with all anticoagulants, bleeding is the major adverse effect of danaparoid. Hemorrhage may occur at virtually any site. Risk is dependent on multiple variables.

Cardiovascular: Arterial pressure decreased, atrial fibrillation, cerebral infarction, DVT, hypotension, peripheral edema

Central nervous system: Confusion, fatigue, fever, insomnia, loss of consciousness, pain, restlessness

Dermatologic: Bruising, rash

Gastrointestinal: Constipation, nausea

Genitourinary: Urinary incontinence, urinary retention

Hematologic: Cerebral hemorrhage, hematoma, hemorrhage, spinal or epidural hematomas (may occur following neuraxial anesthesia or spinal puncture, resulting in paralysis), thrombocytopenia

Hepatic: Alkaline phosphatase increased, ALT increased (transient), AST increased (transient)

Local: Injection site hematoma

Neuromuscular & skeletal: Hemiparesis, involuntary muscle contractions, tremor

Renal: Hematuria

Respiratory: Apnea, asthma

Miscellaneous: Allergic reaction, infection, sepsis

Drug Interactions

Metabolism/Transport Effects None known.

Avoid Concomitant Use

Avoid concomitant use of Danaparoid with any of the following: Apixaban; Dabigatran Etexilate; Edoxaban; Omacetaxine; Rivaroxaban; Urokinase; Vorapaxar

Increased Effect/Toxicity

Danaparoid may increase the levels/effects of: Anticoagulants; Collagenase (Systemic); Deferasirox; Ibritumomab; Nintedanib; Obinutuzumab; Omacetaxine; Rivaroxaban; Tositumomab and Iodine I 131 Tositumomab

The levels/effects of Danaparoid may be increased by: Agents with Antiplatelet Properties; Apixaban; Dabigatran Etexilate; Dasatinib; Edoxaban; Herbs (Anticoagulant/Antiplatelet Properties); Ibrutinib; Limaprost; Nonsteroidal Anti-Inflammatory Agents; Omega-3 Fatty Acids; Pentosan Polysulfate Sodium; Prostacyclin Analogues; Salicylates; Sugammadex; Thrombolytic Agents; Tibolone; Tipranavir; Urokinase; Vitamin E; Vorapaxar

Decreased Effect

The levels/effects of Danaparoid may be decreased by: Estrogen Derivatives; Progestins

Storage/Stability Store at 2°C to 30°C (36°F to 86°F). Protect from light. Stable for up to 48 hours in the following IV solutions: D_5NS, NS, Ringer's, LR, mannitol.

Mechanism of Action Inhibits factor Xa and IIa (anti-Xa effects >20 times anti-IIa effects). Prevents fibrin formation in the coagulation pathway via thrombin generation inhibition.

Pharmacodynamics/Kinetics

Onset of action: Peak effect: SubQ: Maximum antifactor Xa activities occur in 4-5 hours

Bioavailability: SubQ: ~100%

Half-life elimination: Anti-Xa activity: ~25 hours (renal impairment: 29-35 hours); Thrombin generation inhibition activity: ~7 hours

Excretion: Primarily urine

Dosage Note: Dosing recommendations per manufacturer labeling unless otherwise noted. Dose expressed as anti-Xa units.

Children: **Acute thrombosis:**

Treatment: IV: Initial: 30 units/kg as a bolus; Maintenance: 1.2-4 units/kg/hour. **Note:** Anticipated plasma anti-Xa levels after bolus: 400-700 units/L; steady-state levels: 400-600 units/L (or 500-800 units/L for higher doses).

Prophylaxis: SubQ: 10 units/kg every 12 hours

Adults:

Prevention of DVT following orthopedic, major abdominal, or thoracic surgery: SubQ: 750 units twice daily for up to 14 days; it is recommended that patients begin prophylactic therapy preoperatively and receive their last preoperative dose 1-4 hours before surgery.

Prevention of DVT in stroke (nonhemorrhagic):

Initial: IV: Up to 1000 units as single dose

Maintenance: SubQ: 750 units every 12 hours for 7-14 days

Heparin-induced thrombocytopenia (HIT):

Prevention of DVT (with current or past HIT): **Note:** May administer IV bolus of 1250 units if clinically necessary (ie, current HIT) or may initiate maintenance regimen without a bolus as follows:

SubQ:

≤90 kg: Current HIT or past HIT: 750 units every 8-12 hours for 7-10 days

>90 kg: Current HIT: 1250 units every 8-12 hours for 7-10 days; Past HIT: 1250 units every 12 hours or 750 units every 8 hours for 7-10 days

Treatment of DVT/PE (see also Linkins, 2012):

Initial IV bolus: Thrombosis <5 days old: ≤55 kg: 1250-1500 units; 55-90 kg: 2250-2500 units; >90 kg: 3750 units; followed by a maintenance IV infusion or maintenance SubQ injections. **Note:** If thrombosis is ≥5 days old, administer an IV bolus dose of 1250 units followed by maintenance SubQ injections.

Maintenance: IV infusion (after IV bolus administered): Thrombosis <5 days old: 400 units/hour for 4 hours, then 300 units/hour for 4 hours, then 150-200 units/hour for 5-7 days; adjust rate according to target anti-Xa levels

or

Maintenance: SubQ injections (after IV bolus administered):

Thrombosis <5 days old: ≤55 kg: 1500 units every 12 hours; 55-90 kg: 2000 units every 12 hours; >90 kg: 1750 units every 8 hours for 4-7 days.

Thrombosis ≥5 days old: ≤90 kg: 750 units every 8-12 hours; >90 kg: 750 units every 8 hours or 1250 units every 8-12 hours

HIT/surgical thromboprophylaxis:

Nonvascular surgery: SubQ:

≤90 kg: 750 units 1-4 hours preoperatively and at ≥6 hours postop, followed by 750 units every 12 hours beginning day 1 post-op and continued for 7-10 days

>90 kg: 750 units 1-4 hours preoperatively and at ≥6 hours postop, followed by 750 units every 8 hours or 1250 units every 12 hours beginning day 1 post-op and continued for 7-10 days

Embolectomy:

55-90 kg: IV: 2250-2500 units as a bolus preoperatively, followed by SubQ: 1250 units every 12 hours beginning ≥6 hours postop. **Note:** After several days of IV therapy, may switch to SubQ: 750 units every 8-12 hours or oral anticoagulant therapy.

>90 kg: IV: 2250-2500 units as a bolus preoperatively, followed by 150-200 units/hour beginning ≥6 hours post-op for 5-7 days. **Note:** After several days of IV therapy, may switch to SubQ: 750 units every 8-12 hours or oral anticoagulant therapy.

HIT/cardiac procedures: Note: Other therapies may be preferred (eg, bivalirudin); long half-life and irreversibility of danaparoid make it a poor choice in these settings. Refer to product labeling for dosing recommendations.

Catheter patency: Mix 750 units with 50 mL normal saline. Flush catheter with 5-10 mL of resulting solution as needed.

Conversion to oral anticoagulant therapy (OAC): Establish adequate antithrombotic effect with danaparoid prior to initiation of oral anticoagulant (OAC) therapy. PT/INR should be therapeutic before discontinuing use of danaparoid. **Note:** Laboratory values taken within 5 hours of danaparoid administration may be unreliable.

Conversion of SubQ danaparoid to OAC (based on current danaparoid dose):

Danaparoid 750 units every 12 hours: Initiate OAC and maintain danaparoid therapy until PT/INR is therapeutic; may take up to 5 days.

Danaparoid 1250 units every 12 hours: Initiate OAC and decrease danaparoid to 750 units every 12 hours; maintain danaparoid therapy until PT/INR is therapeutic; may take up to 5 days.

Conversion of IV danaparoid to OAC: Initiate OAC with concurrent danaparoid IV infusion (maximum 300 units/hour); discontinue IV infusion once INR is therapeutic (maximum INR: 3.0). If bleeding risk is present, IV infusion should be reduced to 75 units/hour and OAC initiation withheld for 24 hours **or** danaparoid IV infusion may be switched to subcutaneous route at a dose of 1250 units every 12 hours and the recommended conversion of SubQ danaparoid to OAC regimen followed (ie, subsequent reduction to 750 units every 12 hours while OAC initiated).

Dosage adjustment in renal impairment: Note: Danaparoid half-life is significantly prolonged in renal impairment; anti-Xa levels should be closely monitored. Dosage reduction, especially with maintenance doses, may be required.

Mild or moderate impairment: There are no dosage adjustments provided in manufacturer's labeling.

Severe impairment (serum creatinine ≥220 micromol/L [≥2.5 mg/dL]): Following initial dose, dose reductions or temporary discontinuation of therapy may be necessary to prevent accumulation of plasma anti-Xa (indicated by consistent, steady state-plasma anti-Xa activity >0.5 anti-Xa units).

Hemodialysis:

Children: IV:

First two dialysis sessions:

<10 years: 30 units/kg *plus* 1000 units

10-17 years: 30 units/kg *plus* 1500 units

Third and subsequent sessions (based on predialysis anti-Xa levels):

<300 units/L: Administer previous dialysis dose

300-500 units/L: Reduce total dose by 250 units

>500 units/L: No dose required with next dialysis

Adults: IV: 1500-3750 units before dialysis session. **Note:** Dose depends on frequency of dialysis regimen (eg, daily dialysis vs every-other-day or less frequently) and weight of patient with the lower dose recommended for patients <55 kg. Do not administer prior to dialysis if plasma antifactor Xa levels >400 units/L and not receiving daily dialysis; however, if fibrin threads are present in bubble chamber may administer 1500 units.

Hemofiltration: Adults: 55-90 kg: IV: 2500 units as a bolus, followed by 600 units/hour for 4 hours, then 400 units/hour for 4 hours, then 200-600 units/hour to maintain adequate anti-Xa levels. **Note:** If patient is <55 kg, reduce bolus dose to 2000 units, followed by 400 units/hour for 4 hours, then 150-400 units/hour to maintain adequate anti-Xa levels.

Dosage adjustment in hepatic impairment: There are no dosage adjustments provided in manufacturer's labeling.

Administration May administer intravenously as bolus or infusion, or by subcutaneous injection. When administered intravenously, do not mix with other drugs. For subcutaneous administration, rotate injection sites. Do **not** administer intramuscularly.

Monitoring Parameters Platelets (baseline, every other day during week 1, twice weekly during weeks 2 and 3, and once weekly thereafter); occult blood or other signs of bleeding; anti-Xa activity (if available). See manufacturer's recommendations within labeling regarding anticipated anti-Xa levels.

Product Availability Not available in U.S.

Dosage Forms: Canada

Injection, solution:

Organ®: 750 anti-Xa units/0.6 mL (0.6 mL)

◆ **Danaparoid Sodium** *see* Danaparoid [CAN/INT] *on page 556*

Danazol (DA na zole)

Brand Names: Canada Cyclomen®

Index Terms Danocrine

Pharmacologic Category Androgen

Use Treatment of endometriosis, fibrocystic breast disease, and hereditary angioedema

Pregnancy Risk Factor X

Dosage Adults: Oral:

Females: Endometriosis:

Mild disease: Initial: 200-400 mg/day in 2 divided doses

Moderate-to-severe disease: Initial: 800 mg/day in 2 divided doses

Maintenance: Mild-severe disease: Dosage should be individualized. Continue therapy uninterrupted for 3-6 months (up to 9 months).

Females: Fibrocystic breast disease: Range: 100-400 mg/day in 2 divided doses. Pain and tenderness may be eliminated in 2-3 months; elimination of nodularity may require therapy for 4-6 months.

Males/Females: Hereditary angioedema: Initial: 200 mg 2-3 times/day; after favorable response, decrease the dosage by 50% or less at intervals of 1-3 months or longer if the frequency of attacks dictates. If an attack occurs, increase the dosage by up to 200 mg/day.

Dosage adjustment in renal impairment: Use is contraindicated in patients with markedly impaired renal function.

Dosage adjustment in hepatic impairment: Use is contraindicated in patients with markedly impaired hepatic function.

Additional Information Complete prescribing information should be consulted for additional detail.

Dosage Forms

Capsule, Oral:

Generic: 50 mg, 100 mg, 200 mg

◆ **Dandrex [OTC]** *see* Selenium Sulfide *on page 1877*

◆ **Danocrine** *see* Danazol *on page 558*

◆ **Dantrium** *see* Dantrolene *on page 559*

Dantrolene (DAN troe leen)

Brand Names: U.S. Dantrium; Revonto; Ryanodex

Brand Names: Canada Dantrium

Index Terms Dantrolene Sodium

Pharmacologic Category Skeletal Muscle Relaxant

Use

IV: Management of malignant hyperthermia (MH); prevention of MH in susceptible individuals (preoperative/postoperative administration)

Oral: Treatment of spasticity associated with upper motor neuron disorders (eg, spinal cord injury, stroke, cerebral palsy, or multiple sclerosis); management of MH; prevention of MH in susceptible individuals (preoperative/postoperative administration)

Note: Dantrolene prophylaxis is not recommended for most MH-susceptible patients, provided nontriggering anesthetics are used and an adequate supply of dantrolene is available.

Pregnancy Risk Factor C

Pregnancy Considerations Adverse events have been observed in animal reproduction studies. Dantrolene crosses the human placenta. Cord blood concentrations are similar to those in the maternal plasma at term. and dantrolene can be detected in the newborn serum at delivery. Adverse events were not observed in the newborn following maternal doses of 100 mg/day administered orally prior to delivery (Shime, 1988). Uterine atony has been reported following dantrolene injection after delivery; however, this may be due in part to the mannitol contained in the IV preparation (Shin, 1995; Weingarten, 1987). Prophylactic use of dantrolene is not routinely recommended in pregnant women susceptible to MH prior to obstetric surgery, if use is needed, close monitoring of the mother and newborn is recommended (Krause, 2004; Norman, 1995).

Breast-Feeding Considerations Low amounts of dantrolene are excreted into breast milk. Due to the potential for serious adverse reactions in the nursing infant, the manufacturer recommends that a decision be made whether to discontinue nursing or to discontinue the drug, taking into account the importance of treatment to the mother. In a case report, the half-life of dantrolene in breast milk was calculated to be 9 hours; the highest milk concentration was 1.2 mcg/mL following a maternal IV dose; however, the maternal serum concentrations were not reported (Fricker, 1998).

Contraindications

IV: There are no contraindications listed within the manufacturer's labeling.

Oral: Active hepatic disease; should not be used when spasticity is used to maintain posture/balance during locomotion or to obtain/maintain increased function

Warnings/Precautions [U.S. Boxed Warning]: Oral: Has potential for hepatotoxicity. Higher doses (ie, ≥800 mg/day), even sporadic short courses, may increase the risk of severe hepatic injury although hepatic injury may occur at doses <400 mg/day. Overt hepatitis has been most frequently observed between the third and twelfth month of therapy. Hepatic injury appears to be greater in females, in patients >35 years of age, and those taking concurrent medications. A higher incidence of fatal hepatic events have been reported in the elderly, although concurrent disease states and concurrent use of hepatotoxic drugs may have contributed. Idiosyncratic and hypersensitivity reactions (sometimes fatal) of the liver have also occurred. Monitor hepatic function at baseline and as clinically indicated during treatment. Discontinue therapy if abnormal liver function tests occur or benefits are not observed within 45 days when utilized for chronic spasticity.

Loss of grip strength, weakness in the legs, dyspnea, respiratory muscle weakness, dysphagia, and decreased inspiratory capacity has occurred with IV dantrolene. Patients should not ambulate without assistance until they have normal strength and balance. Monitor patients for the adequacy of ventilation and for difficulty swallowing/choking.

Use oral therapy with caution in patients with impaired cardiac, hepatic, or pulmonary function (particularly in obstructive pulmonary disease). Oral therapy may cause photosensitivity. Lightheadedness, dizziness, somnolence, and vertigo may occur and may persist for 48-hours postdose; patients must be cautioned about performing tasks which require mental alertness (eg, operating machinery or driving). Injection may contain mannitol. In addition to IV dantrolene, supportive measures must also be utilized for management of malignant hyperthermia; administer diuretics to prevent late kidney injury due to myoglobinuria. Alkaline solution; may cause tissue necrosis if extravasated (vesicant); ensure proper needle or catheter placement prior to and during infusion; avoid extravasation. Potentially significant interactions may exist, requiring dose or frequency adjustment, additional monitoring, and/or selection of alternative therapy.

Adverse Reactions

Cardiovascular: Atrioventricular block (intravenous), cardiac failure, flushing (intravenous), phlebitis, tachycardia, variable blood pressure

Central nervous system: chills, choking sensation, confusion, depression, dizziness, drowsiness (may persist for 48 hours post dose), fatigue, feeling abnormal, headache, insomnia, malaise, myasthenia, nervousness, seizure, speech disturbance, voice disorder (intravenous)

Dermatologic: Acneiform eruption (capsules), diaphoresis, eczematous rash, erythema (intravenous), hair disease (abnormal growth), pruritus, urticaria

Gastrointestinal: Abdominal cramps, anorexia, constipation, diarrhea, dysgeusia, dysphagia (use caution at meal time on day of administration as swallowing may be difficult), gastric irritation, gastrointestinal hemorrhage, nausea, sialorrhea, vomiting

Genitourinary: Crystalluria, difficulty in micturition, erectile dysfunction, hematuria, nocturia, urinary frequency, urinary incontinence, urinary retention

Hematologic & oncologic: Anemia, aplastic anemia, leukopenia, lymphocytic lymphoma, thrombocytopenia

Hepatic: Hepatitis

Hypersensitivity: Anaphylaxis

Local: Injection site reaction (intravenous; pain, erythema, swelling), local tissue necrosis (with extravasation due to high product pH)

Neuromuscular & skeletal: Back pain, limb pain (intravenous), myalgia

Ophthalmic: Blurred vision (intravenous), diplopia, epiphora, visual disturbance

Respiratory: Dyspnea (intravenous), pleural effusion (with pericarditis), pulmonary edema (rare), respiratory depression

Miscellaneous: Fever

Rare but important or life-threatening: Decrease in forced vital capacity (intravenous), dyspnea (intravenous), hepatic disease, hepatotoxicity (oral), increased liver enzymes (oral), respiratory muscle failure (intravenous)

Drug Interactions

Metabolism/Transport Effects Substrate of CYP3A4 (major); **Note:** Assignment of Major/Minor substrate status based on clinically relevant drug interaction potential

Avoid Concomitant Use

Avoid concomitant use of Dantrolene with any of the following: Azelastine (Nasal); Calcium Channel Blockers (Nondihydropyridine); Conivaptan; Fusidic Acid (Systemic); Idelalisib; Orphenadrine; Paraldehyde; Thalidomide

Increased Effect/Toxicity

Dantrolene may increase the levels/effects of: Alcohol (Ethyl); Azelastine (Nasal); Buprenorphine; Calcium Channel Blockers (Nondihydropyridine); CNS Depressants; Hydrocodone; Methotrimeprazine; Metyrosine; Mirtazapine; Orphenadrine; Paraldehyde; Pramipexole; ROPINIRole; Rotigotine; Selective Serotonin Reuptake Inhibitors; Suvorexant; Thalidomide; Vecuronium; Zolpidem

The levels/effects of Dantrolene may be increased by: Aprepitant; Brimonidine (Topical); Cannabis; Ceritinib; Conivaptan; CYP3A4 Inhibitors (Moderate); CYP3A4 Inhibitors (Strong); Dasatinib; Dexketoprofen; Doxylamine; Dronabinol; Droperidol; Fosaprepitant; Fusidic Acid (Systemic); HydrOXYzine; Idelalisib; Ivacaftor; Kava Kava; Luliconazole; Magnesium Sulfate; Methotrimeprazine; Mifepristone; Nabilone; Netupitant; Perampanel; Rufinamide; Simeprevir; Sodium Oxybate; Stiripentol; Tapentadol; Tetrahydrocannabinol

Decreased Effect

The levels/effects of Dantrolene may be decreased by: Bosentan; CYP3A4 Inducers (Moderate); CYP3A4 Inducers (Strong); Dabrafenib; Deferasirox; Mitotane; Siltuximab; St Johns Wort; Tocilizumab

Preparation for Administration Injection, powder for reconstitution:

Dantrium, Revonto: Reconstitute vial by adding 60 mL of sterile water for injection only (**not bacteriostatic water for injection**); avoid glass bottles for IV infusion due to potential for precipitate formation.

Ryanodex: Reconstitute vial by adding 5 mL of sterile water for injection only (**not bacteriostatic water for injection**); shake well (suspension is an orange color). Do not dilute or transfer the suspension to another container to infuse the product.

Storage/Stability

Capsules: Store at 20°C to 25°C (68°F to 77°F).

Injection, powder for reconstitution: Protect from light. Use reconstituted solution within 6 hours of preparation.

Dantrium: Store unreconstituted vials and reconstituted solutions at 15°C to 30°C (59°F to 86°F).

Revonto: Store unreconstituted vials and reconstituted solutions at 20°C to 25°C (68°F to 77°F).

Ryanodex: Store unreconstituted vials at 20°C to 25°C (68°F to 77°F); excursions are permitted between 15°C and 30°C (59°F and 86°F). Store reconstituted solutions at 20°C to 25°C (68°F to 77°F).

Mechanism of Action Acts directly on skeletal muscle by interfering with release of calcium ion from the sarcoplasmic reticulum; prevents or reduces the increase in myoplasmic calcium ion concentration that activates the acute catabolic processes associated with malignant hyperthermia

Pharmacodynamics/Kinetics

Absorption: Oral: Slow and incomplete

Distribution: V_d: 24.7 to 48.1 L

Metabolism: Hepatic; major metabolites are 5-hydroxy dantrolene and an acetylamino metabolite of dantrolene.

Half-life elimination: 4 to 11 hours

Time to peak: IV: 1 minute post-dose (dantrolene); 24 hours post-dose (5-hydroxy dantrolene)

Excretion: Feces (45% to 50%); urine (25% as unchanged drug and metabolites)

Dosage

Spasticity: Oral: **Note:** Dose should be titrated and individualized for maximum effect; use the lowest dose compatible with optimal response. Some patients may not respond until a higher daily dosage is achieved; each dose level should be maintained for 7 days to determine patient response. If no further benefit observed with the higher dose level, then decrease dosage to previous dose level. Because of the potential for hepatotoxicity, stop therapy if benefits are not evident within 45 days.

Children and Adolescents: Initial: 0.5 mg/kg/dose once daily for 7 days; increase to 0.5 mg/kg/dose 3 times daily for 7 days, increase to 1 mg/kg/dose 3 times daily for 7 days, and then increase to 2 mg/kg/dose 3 times daily; some patients may require 2 mg/kg/dose 4 times daily; maximum dose: 400 mg daily

Adults: Initial: 25 mg once daily for 7 days; increase to 25 mg 3 times daily for 7 days, increase to 50 mg 3 times daily for 7 days, and then increase to 100 mg 3 times daily; some patients may require 100 mg 4 times daily; maximum dose: 400 mg daily

Malignant hyperthermia: Infants, Children, Adolescents, and Adults:

Preoperative prophylaxis: **Note:** Dantrolene prophylaxis is not recommended for most MH-susceptible patients, provided nontriggering anesthetics are used and an adequate supply of dantrolene is available.

Oral: 4 to 8 mg/kg/day in 3 to 4 divided doses, begin 1 to 2 days prior to surgery with last dose 3 to 4 hours prior to surgery

IV: 2.5 mg/kg ~1¼ hours prior to anesthesia and infused over at least 1 minute (Ryanodex) or 1 hour (Dantrium, Revonto) with additional doses as needed and individualized

Crisis: IV: 2.5 mg/kg (MHAUS recommendation, available at www.mhaus.org); continuously repeat dose until symptoms subside or a cumulative dose of 10 mg/kg is reached (rarely, some patients may require up to 30 mg/kg for initial treatment). **Note:** Manufacturer's labeling suggests an initial minimum dose of 1 mg/kg.

24-hour MH Hotline (for emergencies only):

United States: 1-800-644-9737

Outside the U.S.: 00-1-209-417-3722

Postcrisis follow-up:

MHAUS protocol suggestion: 1 mg/kg every 4 to 6 hours (route not specified) **or** a continuous IV infusion of 0.25 mg/kg/hour for at least 24 hours; further doses may be indicated

Manufacturer's recommendation: Oral: 4 to 8 mg/kg/day in 4 divided doses for 1 to 3 days; IV dantrolene may be used to prevent or attenuate recurrence of MH signs when oral therapy is not practical; individualize dosage beginning with 1 mg/kg or more as the clinical situation dictates

Neuroleptic malignant syndrome (off-label use): IV: 1 to 2.5 mg/kg, may repeat dose up to maximum cumulative dose of 10 mg/kg/day, then switch to oral dosage (Strawn, 2007; Susman, 2001)

Dosage adjustment in renal impairment: There are no dosage adjustments provided in the manufacturer's labeling.

Dosage adjustment in hepatic impairment: There are no dosage adjustments provided in the manufacturer's labeling; use of oral dantrolene in patients with active liver disease (eg, hepatitis and cirrhosis) is contraindicated.

Administration IV: Therapeutic or emergency dose can be administered with rapid continuous IV push. Follow-up doses should be administered over at least 1 minute (Ryanodex) or 1 hour (Dantrium, Revonto).

Vesicant; ensure proper needle or catheter placement prior to and during infusion; avoid extravasation.

Extravasation management: If extravasation occurs, stop infusion immediately and disconnect (leave cannula/needle in place); gently aspirate extravasated solution (do **NOT** flush the line); remove needle/cannula; elevate extremity.

Monitoring Parameters Motor performance should be monitored for therapeutic outcomes; nausea, vomiting, and liver function tests (baseline and at appropriate intervals thereafter) should be monitored for potential hepatotoxicity; intravenous administration requires cardiac, blood pressure, and respiratory monitoring.

Malignant hyperthermia: During and post-acute phase: Per MHAUS protocol, patient should be observed in an ICU for at least 24 hours since recrudescence may occur; monitor for arrhythmias; monitor vital signs (including core temperature), electrolytes, ABG, CK, end tidal CO_2 ($EtCO_2$)/capnography, urine output, urine myoglobin

Dosage Forms

Capsule, Oral:
Dantrium: 25 mg, 50 mg
Generic: 25 mg, 50 mg, 100 mg

Solution Reconstituted, Intravenous:
Dantrium: 20 mg (1 ea)
Revonto: 20 mg (1 ea)

Suspension Reconstituted, Intravenous:
Ryanodex: 250 mg (1 ea)

Extemporaneous Preparations A 5 mg/mL oral suspension may be made with dantrolene capsules, a citric acid solution, and either simple syrup or syrup BP (containing 0.15% w/v methylhydroxybenzoate). Add the contents of five 100 mg dantrolene capsules to a citric acid solution (150 mg citric acid powder in 10 mL water); mix while adding the chosen vehicle in incremental proportions to **almost** 100 mL. Transfer to a calibrated bottle and add quantity of vehicle sufficient to make 100 mL. Label "shake well" and "refrigerate". Simple syrup suspension is stable for 2 days refrigerated; syrup BP suspension is stable for 30 days refrigerated.

Nahata MC, Pai VB, and Hipple TF, *Pediatric Drug Formulations*, 5th ed, Cincinnati, OH: Harvey Whitney Books Co, 2004.

◆ **Dantrolene Sodium** *see* Dantrolene *on page 559*

Dapagliflozin and Metformin
(dap a gli FLOE zin & met FOR min)

Brand Names: U.S. Xigduo XR

Index Terms Metformin and Dapagliflozin; Metformin Hydrochloride and Dapagliflozin

Pharmacologic Category Antidiabetic Agent, Biguanide; Antidiabetic Agent, Sodium-Glucose Cotransporter 2 (SGLT2) Inhibitor; Sodium-Glucose Cotransporter 2 (SGLT2) Inhibitor

Use

Diabetes mellitus, type 2: As an adjunct to diet and exercise to improve glycemic control in adults with type 2 diabetes mellitus (noninsulin dependent, NIDDM) when treatment with both dapagliflozin and metformin is appropriate.

Limitations of use: Not indicated in patients with type 1 diabetes (insulin dependent, IDDM) or for the treatment of diabetic ketoacidosis.

Pregnancy Risk Factor C

Dosage Note: If converting from a metformin extended release product that is being taken in the evening, skip the last dose before starting the dapagliflozin/metformin combination product.

Diabetes mellitus, type 2: Oral:

Adults: Initial: Individualize based on patient's current antidiabetic regimen. May gradually increase dose based on effectiveness and tolerability; range: dapagliflozin 5 mg/metformin 500 mg once daily to dapagliflozin 10 mg/metformin 2,000 mg once daily. Maximum: dapagliflozin 10 mg/metformin 2,000 mg once daily.

Elderly: The initial and maintenance dosing should be conservative, due to the potential for decreased renal function. Generally, elderly patients should not be titrated to the maximum dose of metformin. Do not use in patients ≥80 years of age unless normal renal function has been established.

Dosage adjustment in renal impairment:

eGFR ≥60 mL/minute/1.73 m^2: No dosage adjustment necessary.

eGFR <60 mL/minute/1.73 m^2 or CrCl <60 mL/minute: Use is contraindicated.

Dosage adjustment in hepatic impairment: Avoid use; liver disease is a risk factor for the development of lactic acidosis during metformin therapy.

Additional Information Complete prescribing information should be consulted for additional detail.

Dosage Forms

Tablet Extended Release 24 Hour, Oral:
Xigduo XR: Dapagliflozin 5 mg and metformin hydrochloride 500 mg, Dapagliflozin 10 mg and metformin hydrochloride 500 mg, Dapagliflozin 5 mg and metformin hydrochloride 1000 mg, Dapagliflozin 10 mg and metformin hydrochloride 1000 mg

◆ **Dapcin** *see* DAPTOmycin *on page 563*

Dapoxetine [INT] (da POX e teen hye)

International Brand Names Dasutra (IN); Extensil (AR); Kutub (IN); Lagose (AR); Precoce (AR); Priligy (AT, BE, BG, BR, CH, CN, CO, CZ, DE, DK, EE, ES, FI, FR, GB, HK, HR, IT, KR, LB, LT, MX, MY, NL, PH, PT, RO, SE, SG, SI, SK, TH); Prolongal (AR); Xydap (IN)

Index Terms Dapoxetine HCL; Dapoxetine Hydrochloride

Pharmacologic Category Selective Serotonin Reuptake Inhibitor (SSRI)

Reported Use Premature ejaculation

Dosage Range Adults: Male patients: 30 to 60 mg as a single dose prior to sexual activity

Product Availability Product available in various countries; not currently available in the U.S.

Dosage Forms Tablet, oral: 30 mg; 60 mg

◆ **Dapoxetine HCL** *see* Dapoxetine [INT] *on page 561*

◆ **Dapoxetine Hydrochloride** *see* Dapoxetine [INT] *on page 561*

Dapsone (Systemic) (DAP sone)

Index Terms Diaminodiphenylsulfone

Pharmacologic Category Antibiotic, Miscellaneous

Use Treatment of leprosy (due to susceptible strains of *Mycobacterium leprae*) and dermatitis herpetiformis

Pregnancy Risk Factor C

Pregnancy Considerations Adverse events were observed in some animal reproduction studies. Dapsone crosses the placenta (Brabin, 2004). Per the manufacturer, dapsone has not shown an increased risk of congenital anomalies when given during all trimesters of pregnancy. Several reports have described adverse effects in the newborn after *in utero* exposure to dapsone, including neonatal hemolytic disease, methemoglobinemia, and hyperbilirubinemia (Hocking, 1968; Kabra, 1998; Thornton, 1989). Dapsone may be used in pregnant women requiring maintenance therapy of either leprosy or dermatitis herpetiformis. Dapsone may be used as an alternative agent for prophylaxis of *Pneumocystis jirovecii* pneumonia (PCP) in pregnant, HIV-infected patients (DHHS [OI], 2013).

Breast-Feeding Considerations Dapsone is excreted in breast milk and can be detected in the serum of nursing infants. Hemolytic anemia has been reported in a breast-fed infant (Sanders, 1982). Due to the potential for serious adverse reactions in the nursing infant, the manufacturer recommends a decision be made whether to discontinue nursing or to discontinue the drug, taking into account the importance of treatment to the mother.

Contraindications Hypersensitivity to dapsone or any component of the formulation

Warnings/Precautions Use with caution in patients with severe anemia, G6PD, methemoglobin reductase deficiency or hemoglobin M deficiency; hypersensitivity to other sulfonamides; aplastic anemia, agranulocytosis and other severe blood dyscrasias have resulted in death; monitor carefully; serious dermatologic reactions (including toxic epidermal necrolysis) are rare but potential occurrences; sulfone reactions may also occur as potentially fatal hypersensitivity reactions; these, but not leprosy reactional states, require drug discontinuation. Motor loss and muscle weakness have been reported with use. Prolonged use may result in fungal or bacterial superinfection, including *C. difficile*-associated diarrhea and pseudomembranous colitis.

Adverse Reactions

Cardiovascular: Tachycardia

Central nervous system: Fever, headache, insomnia, psychosis (oral/topical), vertigo

Dermatologic: Bullous and exfoliative dermatitis, erythema nodosum, exfoliative dermatitis, morbilliform and scarlatiniform reactions, phototoxicity, Stevens-Johnson syndrome, toxic epidermal necrolysis, urticaria

Endocrine & metabolic: Hypoalbuminemia (without proteinuria), male infertility

Gastrointestinal: Abdominal pain, nausea, pancreatitis, vomiting

Hematologic: Agranulocytosis, anemia, leukopenia, pure red cell aplasia (case report); hemolysis (dose related; seen in patients with and without G6PD deficiency), hemoglobin decrease (1-2 g/dL), reticulocyte increase, methemoglobinemia, red cell life span shortened

Hepatic: Cholestatic jaundice, hepatitis

Neuromuscular & skeletal: Drug-induced lupus erythematosus, lower motor neuron toxicity (prolonged therapy), peripheral neuropathy (rare, nonleprosy patients)

Ocular: Blurred vision

Otic: Tinnitus

Renal: Albuminuria, nephrotic syndrome, renal papillary necrosis

Respiratory: Interstitial pneumonitis, pulmonary eosinophilia

Miscellaneous: Infectious mononucleosis-like syndrome (rash, fever, lymphadenopathy, hepatic dysfunction)

Drug Interactions

Metabolism/Transport Effects Substrate of CYP2C19 (minor), CYP2C8 (minor), CYP2C9 (major), CYP2E1 (minor), CYP3A4 (major); **Note:** Assignment of Major/Minor substrate status based on clinically relevant drug interaction potential

Avoid Concomitant Use

Avoid concomitant use of Dapsone (Systemic) with any of the following: BCG; Conivaptan; Fusidic Acid (Systemic); Idelalisib

Increased Effect/Toxicity

Dapsone (Systemic) may increase the levels/effects of: Antimalarial Agents; Prilocaine; Sodium Nitrite; Trimethoprim

The levels/effects of Dapsone (Systemic) may be increased by: Antimalarial Agents; Ceritinib; Conivaptan; CYP2C9 Inhibitors (Moderate); CYP2C9 Inhibitors (Strong); CYP3A4 Inhibitors (Moderate); CYP3A4 Inhibitors (Strong); Dasatinib; Fosaprepitant; Fusidic Acid (Systemic); Idelalisib; Ivacaftor; Luliconazole; Mifepristone; Netupitant; Nitric Oxide; Probenecid; Simeprevir; Stiripentol; Trimethoprim

Decreased Effect

Dapsone (Systemic) may decrease the levels/effects of: BCG; Sodium Picosulfate; Typhoid Vaccine

The levels/effects of Dapsone (Systemic) may be decreased by: Bosentan; CYP2C9 Inducers (Strong); CYP3A4 Inducers (Moderate); CYP3A4 Inducers (Strong); Dabrafenib; Deferasirox; Mitotane; Rifamycin Derivatives; Siltuximab; St Johns Wort; Tocilizumab

Storage/Stability Store at 20°C to 25°C (68°F to 76°F). Protect from light.

Mechanism of Action Competitive antagonist of para-aminobenzoic acid (PABA) and prevents normal bacterial utilization of PABA for the synthesis of folic acid

Pharmacodynamics/Kinetics

Absorption: Well-absorbed

Protein binding: Dapsone: 70% to 90%; Metabolite: ~99%

Distribution: V_d: 1.5 L/kg; throughout total body water and present in all tissues, especially liver and kidney

Metabolism: Hepatic (acetylation and hydroxylation); forms multiple metabolites

Half-life elimination: 30 hours (range: 10-50 hours)

Excretion: Urine (~85%)

Dosage

Leprosy: Oral:

Children: 1-2 mg/kg/24 hours, up to a maximum of 100 mg daily, in combination with other antileprosy agents; duration of therapy is variable

Adults: 100 mg daily, in combination with other antileprosy agents; duration of therapy is variable

Dermatitis herpetiformis: Adults: Oral: Start at 50 mg daily, increase to 300 mg daily, or higher to achieve full control, reduce dosage to minimum level as soon as possible

Aphthous ulcers, severe (off-label use): Adults: Oral:

Initial: 25 mg daily for 3 days; increase dose in increments of 25 mg daily every 3 days up to 100 mg daily for 3 days, then increase by 25 mg daily every 7 days up to 150 mg daily. Administer in 2 divided doses (75 mg dose is administered in 3 divided doses).

Maintenance: 100-150 mg daily in 2 divided doses with or without concomitant colchicine (Rogers, 1982; Lynde 2009)

Bullous systemic lupus erythematosus (off-label use): Adults: Oral: 100 mg once daily with or without prednisone (Fabbri, 2003).

Pemphigus vulgaris (off-label use): Adults: Oral: 25 mg daily for 7 days, then increase dose in increments of 25 mg daily every 7 days up to 100 mg daily for 7 days (4 weeks total therapy) with concomitant prednisone. Administer in 2 divided doses (a 75 mg dose is administered in 3 divided doses) (Azizi, 2008). **Note:** If patient becomes lesion free, taper and discontinue gradually by decreasing dose 25 mg daily over 7 days. If no new lesions are seen, gradual taper is continued. If lesions recur, dose is increased by 25 mg daily at 7-day intervals until the patient develops no new lesions. Taper is usually ~4 weeks total.

Pneumocystis jirovecii pneumonia, alternative therapy (off-label use): Oral:

Prophylaxis (primary or secondary):

Infants and Children: 2 mg/kg/day once daily (maximum dose: 100 mg daily) or 4 mg/kg/dose once weekly (maximum dose: 200 mg) (CDC, 2009)

Adolescents and Adults: 100 mg daily once daily or in 2 divided doses as monotherapy or 50 mg daily in combination with weekly pyrimethamine and leucovorin **or** 200 mg weekly in combination with weekly pyrimethamine and leucovorin (DHHS, 2013)

Treatment:

Infants and Children: 2 mg/kg/day once daily (maximum dose: 100 mg daily) in combination with trimethoprim for 21 days (CDC, 2009)

Adolescents and Adults (mild-to-moderate disease): 100 mg daily once daily in combination with trimethoprim for 21 days (DHHS, 2013)

Toxoplasmosis in severely-immunocompromised patients (alternative treatment) (off-label use): Oral: Prophylaxis:

Infants and Children: 2 mg/kg or 15 mg/m^2 up to a maximum of 25 mg once daily, in combination with pyrimethamine and leucovorin (CDC, 2009)

Adolescents and Adults: Oral: 50 mg daily, in combination with pyrimethamine and leucovorin **or** 200 mg weekly in combination with pyrimethamine and leucovorin. (DHHS, 2013)

Dosing adjustment in renal impairment: No specific guidelines are available

Dietary Considerations Do not give with antacids, alkaline foods, or drugs.

Administration May administer with meals if GI upset occurs.

Monitoring Parameters Check G6PD levels (prior to initiation); CBC (weekly for first month, monthly for 6 months and semiannually thereafter); reticulocyte counts; liver function tests. Monitor patients for signs of jaundice and hemolysis.

Dosage Forms

Tablet, Oral:

Generic: 25 mg, 100 mg

Extemporaneous Preparations A 2 mg/mL oral suspension may be made with tablets and a 1:1 mixture of Ora-Sweet® and Ora-Plus®. Crush eight 25 mg tablets in a mortar and reduce to a fine powder. Add small portions of vehicle and mix to a uniform paste; mix while adding the vehicle in incremental proportions to **almost** 100 mL; transfer to a calibrated bottle, rinse mortar with vehicle, and add quantity of vehicle sufficient to make 100 mL. Label "shake well". Stable for 90 days at room temperature or refrigerated.

Jacobus Pharmaceutical Company makes a 2 mg/mL proprietary liquid formulation available under an IND for the prophylaxis of *Pneumocystis jirovecii* pneumonia.

Nahata MC, Morosco RS, and Trowbridge JM, "Stability of Dapsone in Two Oral Liquid Dosage Forms," *Ann Pharmacother*, 2000, 34 (7-8):848-50.

◆ **Daptacel** *see* Diphtheria and Tetanus Toxoids, and Acellular Pertussis Vaccine *on page 649*

DAPTOmycin (DAP toe mye sin)

Brand Names: U.S. Cubicin

Brand Names: Canada Cubicin

Index Terms Cidecin; Dapcin; LY146032

Pharmacologic Category Antibiotic, Cyclic Lipopeptide

Use

Complicated skin and skin structure infections: For the treatment of complicated skin and skin structure infections caused by susceptible isolates of the following gram-positive bacteria: *Staphylococcus aureus* (including methicillin-resistant isolates), *Streptococcus pyogenes*, *Streptococcus agalactiae*, *Streptococcus dysgalactiae* subspecies *equisimilis*, and *Enterococcus faecalis* (vancomycin-susceptible strains only).

***S. aureus* bloodstream infections:**

For the treatment of *S. aureus* bloodstream infections (bacteremia), including those with right-sided infective endocarditis, caused by methicillin-susceptible and methicillin-resistant isolates.

The efficacy of daptomycin for the treatment of left-sided infective endocarditis caused by *S. aureus* has not been demonstrated.

The clinical trial of daptomycin in patients with *S. aureus* bloodstream infections included limited data from patients with left-sided infective endocarditis; outcomes in these patients were poor.

Patients with persisting or relapsing *S. aureus* infection or poor clinical response should have repeat blood cultures. If a culture is positive for *S. aureus*, perform minimum inhibitory concentration (MIC) susceptibility testing of the isolate using a standardized procedure and diagnostic evaluation to rule out sequestered foci of infection.

General information: Daptomycin is not indicated for the treatment of pneumonia.

Pregnancy Risk Factor B

Pregnancy Considerations Adverse events were not observed in animal reproduction studies. Successful use of daptomycin during the second and third trimesters of pregnancy has been described; however, only limited information is available from case reports.

Breast-Feeding Considerations Low concentrations of daptomycin have been detected in breast milk; however, daptomycin is poorly absorbed orally. The manufacturer recommends caution if daptomycin is used during breast-feeding. Per the Canadian product labeling, daptomycin should be discontinued while breast-feeding. Nondose-related effects could include modification of bowel flora.

Contraindications Hypersensitivity to daptomycin

Warnings/Precautions May be associated with an increased incidence of myopathy; discontinue in patients with signs and symptoms of myopathy in conjunction with an increase in CPK (>5 times ULN or 1,000 units/L) or in asymptomatic patients with a CPK ≥10 times ULN. Myopathy may occur more frequently at dose and/or frequency in excess of recommended dosages. Consider temporarily interrupting therapy with other agents associated with an increased risk of myopathy (eg, HMG-CoA reductase inhibitors) during daptomycin therapy. Not indicated for the treatment of pneumonia (inactivation by pulmonary surfactant). Use caution in renal impairment (dosage adjustment required severe renal impairment [CrCl <30 mL/minute]). Limited data (eg, subgroup analysis) from cSSSI and endocarditis trials suggest possibly reduced clinical efficacy (relative to comparators) in patients with baseline moderate renal impairment (<50 mL/minute).

Symptoms suggestive of peripheral neuropathy have been observed with treatment; monitor for new-onset or worsening neuropathy. Prolonged use may result in fungal or bacterial superinfection, including *C. difficile*-associated diarrhea (CDAD) and pseudomembranous colitis; CDAD has been observed >2 months postantibiotic treatment. Repeat blood cultures in patients with persisting or relapsing *S. aureus* bacteremia/endocarditis or poor clinical response. If culture is positive for *S. aureus*, perform minimum inhibitory concentration (MIC) susceptibility testing of the isolate and diagnostic evaluation of the patient to ▶

rule out sequestered foci of infection. Appropriate surgical intervention (eg, debridement, removal of prosthetic devices, valve replacement surgery) and/or consideration of a change in antibacterial therapy may be necessary. Hypersensitivity reactions and anaphylaxis (including angioedema, and drug rash with eosinophilia and systemic symptoms [DRESS]) have been reported with use; discontinue use immediately with signs/symptoms of hypersensitivity and initiate appropriate treatment. Use has been associated with eosinophilic pneumonia; generally develops 2 to 4 weeks after therapy initiation. Monitor for signs/symptoms of eosinophilic pneumonia, including new onset or worsening fever, dyspnea, difficulty breathing, new infiltrates on chest imaging studies, and/or >25% eosinophils present in bronchoalveolar lavage. Discontinue use immediately with signs/symptoms of eosinophilic pneumonia and initiate appropriate treatment (ie, corticosteroids). May reoccur with re-exposure. Although not approved for use in children, the manufacturer recommends to avoid use in pediatric patients <12 months due to risk of potential muscular, neuromuscular, and/or nervous systems effects observed in neonatal canines.

Adverse Reactions

Cardiovascular: Chest pain, hypertension, hypotension, peripheral edema

Central nervous system: Anxiety, dizziness, headache, insomnia

Dermatologic: Diaphoresis, erythema, pruritus, skin rash

Endocrine & metabolic: Hyperkalemia, hyperphosphatemia, hypokalemia

Gastrointestinal: Abdominal pain, constipation, diarrhea, dyspepsia, gastrointestinal hemorrhage, loose stools, nausea, vomiting

Genitourinary: Urinary tract infection

Hematologic & oncologic: Anemia, eosinophilia, increased INR

Hepatic: Increased serum alkaline phosphatase, increased serum transaminases

Infection: Bacteremia, fungal infection, gram-negative organism infection, sepsis

Local: Injection site reaction

Neuromuscular & skeletal: Arthralgia, back pain, increased creatine phosphokinase, limb pain, osteomyelitis, weakness

Renal: Renal failure

Respiratory: Cough, dyspnea, pneumonia, pharyngolaryngeal pain, pleural effusion

Miscellaneous: Fever

Rare but important or life-threatening: Anaphylaxis, atrial fibrillation, atrial flutter, candidiasis, cardiac arrest, *Clostridium difficile* associated diarrhea, coma (post anaesthesia/surgery), eczema, eosinophilic pneumonitis, hallucination, hypomagnesemia, hypersensitivity, jaundice, increased lactate dehydrogenase, lymphadenopathy, mental status changes, neutropenia (Knoll, 2013), oral candidiasis, peripheral neuropathy, proteinuria, prolonged prothrombin time, renal insufficiency, rhabdomyolysis, increased serum bicarbonate, Stevens-Johnson syndrome, stomatitis, supraventricular cardiac arrhythmia, thrombocytopenia, thrombocythemia

Drug Interactions

Metabolism/Transport Effects None known.

Avoid Concomitant Use There are no known interactions where it is recommended to avoid concomitant use.

Increased Effect/Toxicity

The levels/effects of DAPTOmycin may be increased by: HMG-CoA Reductase Inhibitors

Decreased Effect There are no known significant interactions involving a decrease in effect.

Preparation for Administration Reconstitute vial with 10 mL NS to a concentration of 50 mg/mL. Add NS to vial and rotate gently to wet powder. Allow to stand for 10 minutes, then gently swirl to obtain completely reconstituted solution. Do not shake or agitate vial vigorously. If administering via IVPB, further dilute in 50 mL NS prior to administration.

Storage/Stability

Store original packages at 2°C to 8°C (36°F to 46°F); avoid excessive heat. Daptomycin vials are for single use only.

U.S. labeling: Reconstituted solution is stable in the vial for 12 hours at room temperature or up to 48 hours if refrigerated at 2°C to 8°C (36°F to 46°F). The diluted solution is stable in the infusion bag for 12 hours at room temperature or 48 hours if refrigerated. The combined time (reconstituted solution in vial and diluted solution in infusion bag) should not exceed 12 hours at room temperature or 48 hours refrigerated.

Canadian labeling: Reconstituted solution is stable in the vial or infusion solution for 12 hours at 25°C (77°F) or up to 10 days if refrigerated at 2°C to 8°C (36°F to 46°F) under normal lighting. The manufacturer recommends using reconstituted solution within 72 hours if stored under refrigeration. The combined time (reconstituted solution in vial and diluted solution in infusion bag) should not exceed 12 hours at up to 25°C (77°F) or 10 days at 2°C to 8°C (36°F to 46°F).

Mechanism of Action Daptomycin binds to components of the cell membrane of susceptible organisms and causes rapid depolarization, inhibiting intracellular synthesis of DNA, RNA, and protein. Daptomycin is bactericidal in a concentration-dependent manner.

Pharmacodynamics/Kinetics

Distribution: V_{ss}: 0.1 L/kg; Critically-ill patients: V_{ss}: 0.23 ± 0.14 L/kg (Vilay, 2010)

Protein binding: 90% to 93%; 84% to 88% in patients with CrCl <30 mL/minute

Half-life elimination: 8-9 hours (up to 28 hours in renal impairment)

Excretion: Urine (78%; primarily as unchanged drug); feces (6%)

Dosage IV: Adults:

Skin and soft tissue: 4 mg/kg once daily for 7 to 14 days

Bacteremia, right-sided native valve endocarditis caused by MSSA or MRSA:

Manufacturer labeling:

U.S. labeling: 6 mg/kg once daily for 2 to 6 weeks

Canadian labeling: 6 mg/kg once daily for 10 days to 6 weeks; may consider an additional 2 weeks of therapy

Alternate recommendation: 8 to 10 mg/kg once daily for complicated bacteremia or infective endocarditis (Liu, 2011)

Osteomyelitis (off-label use): 6 mg/kg once daily for a minimum of 8 weeks (some experts combine with rifampin) (Liu, 2011)

Prosthetic joint infection (off-label use):

Enterococcus spp (penicillin-susceptible or -resistant) (alternative treatment): 6 mg/kg every 24 hours for 4 to 6 weeks (consider adding an aminoglycoside) followed by an oral antibiotic suppressive regimen (Osmon, 2013)

Staphylococci (oxacillin-susceptible or -resistant) (alternative treatment): 6 mg/kg every 24 hours for 2 to 6 weeks used in combination with rifampin followed by oral antibiotic treatment and suppressive regimens (Osmon, 2013)

Septic arthritis (off-label use): 6 mg/kg once daily for 3 to 4 weeks (Liu, 2011)

Dosage adjustment in renal impairment:

CrCl ≥30 mL/minute: No dosage adjustment necessary.

CrCl <30 mL/minute:

Skin and soft tissue infections: 4 mg/kg every 48 hours

Staphylococcal bacteremia: 6 mg/kg every 48 hours

Intermittent hemodialysis or peritoneal dialysis (PD): Dose as in CrCl <30 mL/minute (administer after hemodialysis on dialysis days) or (off-label dosing) may administer 6 mg/kg after hemodialysis 3 times weekly (Salama, 2010)

Note: High permeability intermittent hemodialysis removes ~50% during a 4-hour session (Salama, 2010).

Continuous renal replacement therapy (CRRT) (Heintz, 2009; Trotman, 2005): Drug clearance is highly dependent on the method of renal replacement, filter type, and flow rate. Appropriate dosing requires close monitoring of pharmacologic response, signs of adverse reactions due to drug accumulation, as well as drug concentrations in relation to target trough (if appropriate). The following are general recommendations only (based on dialysate flow/ultrafiltration rates of 1 to 2 L/hour and minimal residual renal function) and should not supersede clinical judgment:

Continuous veno-venous hemodialysis (CVVHD): 8 mg/kg every 48 hours (Vilay, 2010)

Note: For other forms of CRRT (eg, CVVH or CVVHDF), dosing as with CrCl <30 mL/minute may result in low C_{max}. May consider 4-6 mg/kg every 24 hours (or 8 mg/kg every 48 hours) depending on site or severity of infection or if not responding to standard dosing; therapeutic drug monitoring and/or more frequent serum CPK levels may be necessary (Heintz, 2009).

Slow extended daily dialysis (or extended dialysis): 6 mg/kg every 24 hours (Kielstein, 2010); **Note:** Dialysis should be initiated within 8 hours of administering daptomycin dose to avoid dose accumulation.

Dosage adjustment in hepatic impairment: No dosage adjustment necessary for mild-to-moderate impairment (Child-Pugh class A or B); not evaluated in severe hepatic impairment (Child-Pugh class C)

Administration May administer IV push over 2 minutes or infuse IVPB over 30 minutes. Do not use in conjunction with ReadyMED® elastomeric infusion pumps (Cardinal Health, Inc) due to an impurity (2-mercaptobenzothiazole) leaching from the pump system into the daptomycin solution.

Monitoring Parameters Monitor signs and symptoms of infection. CPK should be monitored at least weekly during therapy; more frequent monitoring if current or prior statin therapy, unexplained CPK increases, and/or renal impairment. Monitor for muscle pain or weakness, especially if noted in distal extremities. Monitor for new onset or worsening peripheral neuropathy. Canadian labeling recommends CPK monitoring every 48 hours with unexplained muscle pain, tenderness, weakness or cramps. Monitor for signs/symptoms of eosinophilic pneumonia.

Reference Range

Trough concentrations at steady-state:

4 mg/kg once daily: 5.9 ± 1.6 mcg/mL

6 mg/kg once daily: 6.7 ± 1.6 mcg/mL

Note: Trough concentrations are not predictive of efficacy/toxicity. Drug exhibits concentration-dependent bactericidal activity, so C_{max}:MIC ratios may be a more useful parameter.

Dosage Forms

Solution Reconstituted, Intravenous [preservative free]:

Cubicin: 500 mg (1 ea)

◆ **Daraprim** *see* Pyrimethamine *on page 1749*

◆ **Daraprim [DSC] (Can)** *see* Pyrimethamine *on page 1749*

Darbepoetin Alfa (dar be POE e tin AL fa)

Brand Names: U.S. Aranesp (Albumin Free)

Brand Names: Canada Aranesp

Index Terms Erythropoiesis-Stimulating Agent (ESA); Erythropoiesis-Stimulating Protein; NESP; Novel Erythropoiesis-Stimulating Protein

Pharmacologic Category Colony Stimulating Factor; Erythropoiesis-Stimulating Agent (ESA); Hematopoietic Agent

Use Anemia: Treatment of anemia due to concurrent myelosuppressive chemotherapy in patients with cancer (nonmyeloid malignancies) receiving chemotherapy (palliative intent) for a planned minimum of 2 additional months of chemotherapy; treatment of anemia due to chronic kidney disease (including patients on dialysis and not on dialysis)

Note: Darbepoetin is **not** indicated for use under the following conditions:

- Cancer patients receiving hormonal therapy, therapeutic biologic products, or radiation therapy unless also receiving concurrent myelosuppressive chemotherapy
- Cancer patients receiving myelosuppressive chemotherapy when the expected outcome is curative
- As a substitute for RBC transfusion in patients requiring immediate correction of anemia

Note: In clinical trials, darbepoetin has not demonstrated improved quality of life, fatigue, or well-being.

Pregnancy Risk Factor C

Pregnancy Considerations Adverse events were observed in animal reproduction studies. Women who become pregnant during treatment with darbepoetin are encouraged to enroll in Amgen's Pregnancy Surveillance Program (800-772-6436).

Breast-Feeding Considerations It is not known if darbepoetin alfa is excreted in breast milk. The manufacturer recommends that caution be exercised when administering darbepoetin alfa to nursing women.

Contraindications Hypersensitivity to darbepoetin or any component of the formulation; uncontrolled hypertension; pure red cell aplasia (due to darbepoetin or other erythropoietin protein drugs)

Warnings/Precautions [U.S. Boxed Warning]: Erythropoiesis-stimulating agents (ESAs) increased the risk of serious cardiovascular events, thromboembolic events, stroke, and/or tumor progression in clinical studies when administered to target hemoglobin levels >11 g/dL (and provide no additional benefit); a rapid rise in hemoglobin (>1 g/dL over 2 weeks) may also contribute to these risks. **[U.S. Boxed Warning]: A shortened overall survival and/or increased risk of tumor progression or recurrence has been reported in studies with breast, cervical, head and neck, lymphoid, and non-small cell lung cancer patients.** It is of note that in these studies, patients received ESAs to a target hemoglobin of ≥12 g/dL; although risk has not been excluded when dosed to achieve a target hemoglobin of <12 g/dL. **[U.S. Boxed Warnings]: To decrease these risks, and risk of cardio- and thrombovascular events, use ESAs in cancer patients only for the treatment of anemia related to concurrent myelosuppressive chemotherapy and use the lowest dose needed to avoid red blood cell transfusions. Discontinue ESA following completion of the chemotherapy course. ESAs are not indicated for patients receiving myelosuppressive therapy when the anticipated outcome is curative.** A dosage modification is appropriate if hemoglobin levels rise >1 g/dL per 2-week time period during treatment (Rizzo, 2010). Use of ESAs has been associated with an increased risk of venous thromboembolism (VTE) without a reduction in transfusions in patients >65 years of age with cancer (Hershman, 2009). Improved anemia symptoms, quality of life, fatigue, or well-being have not been demonstrated in controlled clinical trials. **[U.S. Boxed Warning]: Because of the risks of decreased survival and increased risk of tumor growth or progression, all**

healthcare providers and hospitals are required to enroll and comply with the ESA APPRISE (Assisting Providers and Cancer Patients with Risk Information for the Safe use of ESAs) Oncology Program prior to prescribing or dispensing ESAs to cancer patients. Prescribers and patients will have to provide written documentation of discussed risks prior to each course.

[U.S. Boxed Warning]: An increased risk of death, serious cardiovascular events, and stroke was reported in patients with chronic kidney disease (CKD) administered ESAs to target hemoglobin levels ≥11 g/dL; use the lowest dose sufficient to reduce the need for RBC transfusions. An optimal target hemoglobin level, dose or dosing strategy to reduce these risks has not been identified in clinical trials. Hemoglobin rising >1 g/dL in a 2-week period may contribute to the risk (dosage reduction recommended). The American College of Physicians recommends against the use of ESAs in patients with mild to moderate anemia and heart failure or coronary heart disease (ACP [Qaseem, 2013]).

CKD patients who exhibit an inadequate hemoglobin response to ESA therapy may be at a higher risk for cardiovascular events and mortality compared to other patients. ESA therapy may reduce dialysis efficacy (due to increase in red blood cells and decrease in plasma volume); adjustments in dialysis parameters may be needed. Patients treated with epoetin may require increased heparinization during dialysis to prevent clotting of the extracorporeal circuit. CKD patients not requiring dialysis may have a better response to darbepoetin and may require lower doses. An increased risk of DVT has been observed in patients treated with epoetin undergoing surgical orthopedic procedures. Darbepoetin is **not** approved for reduction in allogeneic red blood cell transfusions in patients scheduled for surgical procedures. The risk for seizures is increased with darbepoetin use in patients with CKD; use with caution in patients with a history of seizures. Monitor closely for neurologic symptoms during the first several months of therapy. Use with caution in patients with hypertension; hypertensive encephalopathy has been reported. Use is contraindicated in patients with uncontrolled hypertension. If hypertension is difficult to control, reduce or hold darbepoetin alfa. Due to the delayed onset of erythropoiesis, darbepoetin alfa is **not** recommended for acute correction of severe anemia or as a substitute for emergency transfusion. Consider discontinuing in patients who receive a renal transplant.

Prior to treatment, correct or exclude deficiencies of iron, vitamin B_{12}, and/or folate, as well as other factors which may impair erythropoiesis (inflammatory conditions, infections, bleeding). Prior to and during therapy, iron stores must be evaluated. Supplemental iron is recommended if serum ferritin <100 mcg/L or serum transferrin saturation <20%; most patients with CKD will require iron supplementation. Poor response should prompt evaluation of these potential factors, as well as possible malignant processes and hematologic disease (thalassemia, refractory anemia, myelodysplastic disorder), occult blood loss, hemolysis, osteitis fibrosa cystic, and/or bone marrow fibrosis. Severe anemia and pure red cell aplasia (PRCA) with associated neutralizing antibodies to erythropoietin has been reported, predominantly in patients with CKD receiving SubQ darbepoetin (the IV route is preferred for hemodialysis patients). Cases have also been reported in patients with hepatitis C who were receiving ESAs, interferon, and ribavirin. Patients with a sudden loss of response to darbepoetin (with severe anemia and a low reticulocyte count) should be evaluated for PRCA with associated neutralizing antibodies to erythropoietin; discontinue treatment (permanently) in patients with PRCA secondary to neutralizing antibodies to erythropoietin. Antibodies may cross-react; do not switch to another ESA in patients who develop antibody-mediated anemia.

Potentially serious allergic reactions have been reported (rarely). Discontinue immediately (and permanently) in patients who experience serious allergic/anaphylactic reactions. Some products may contain albumin and the packaging of some formulations may contain latex. Some dosage forms may contain polysorbate 80 (also known as Tweens). Hypersensitivity reactions, usually a delayed reaction, have been reported following exposure to pharmaceutical products containing polysorbate 80 in certain individuals (Isaksson, 2002; Lucente 2000; Shelley, 1995). Thrombocytopenia, ascites, pulmonary deterioration, and renal and hepatic failure have been reported in premature neonates after receiving parenteral products containing polysorbate 80 (Alade, 1986; CDC, 1984). See manufacturer's labeling.

Adverse Reactions

Cardiovascular: Angina pectoris, edema, hypotension, myocardial infarction, hypertension, peripheral edema, pulmonary embolism, thromboembolism, thrombosis of vascular graft (arteriovenous), vascular injury (vascular access complications)

Central nervous system: Cerebrovascular disease

Dermatologic: Erythema, skin rash

Endocrine & metabolic: Hypervolemia

Gastrointestinal: Abdominal pain

Respiratory: Cough, dyspnea

Rare but important or life-threatening: Anaphylaxis, anemia (associated with neutralizing antibodies; severe; with or without other cytopenias), angioedema, bronchospasm, cerebrovascular accident, hypersensitivity reaction, hypertensive encephalopathy, pure red cell aplasia, seizure, tumor growth (progression/recurrence; cancer patients), urticaria

Drug Interactions

Metabolism/Transport Effects None known.

Avoid Concomitant Use There are no known interactions where it is recommended to avoid concomitant use.

Increased Effect/Toxicity

Darbepoetin Alfa may increase the levels/effects of: Lenalidomide; Thalidomide

The levels/effects of Darbepoetin Alfa may be increased by: Nandrolone

Decreased Effect There are no known significant interactions involving a decrease in effect.

Storage/Stability Store at 2°C to 8°C (36°F to 46°F); do not freeze. Do not shake. Protect from light. Store in original carton until use. The following stability information has also been reported: May be stored at room temperature for up to 7 days (Cohen, 2007).

Mechanism of Action Induces erythropoiesis by stimulating the division and differentiation of committed erythroid progenitor cells; induces the release of reticulocytes from the bone marrow into the bloodstream, where they mature to erythrocytes. There is a dose response relationship with this effect. This results in an increase in reticulocyte counts followed by a rise in hematocrit and hemoglobin levels. When administered SubQ or IV, darbepoetin's half-life is ~3 times that of epoetin alfa concentrations.

Pharmacodynamics/Kinetics

Onset of action: Increased hemoglobin levels not generally observed until 2-6 weeks after initiating treatment

Absorption: SubQ: Slow

Distribution: V_d: 0.06 L/kg

Bioavailability: CKD: SubQ: Adults: ~37% (range: 30% to 50%); Children: 54% (range: 32% to 70%)

Half-life elimination:

CKD: Adults:

IV: 21 hours

SubQ: Nondialysis patients: 70 hours (range: 35-139 hours); Dialysis patients: 46 hours (range: 12-89 hours)

Cancer: Adults: SubQ: 74 hours (range: 24-144 hours); Children: 49 hours

Note: Darbepoetin half-life is approximately threefold longer than epoetin alfa following IV administration

Time to peak: SubQ:

CKD: Adults: 48 hours (range: 12-72 hours; independent of dialysis); Children: 36 hours (range: 10-58 hours)

Cancer: Adults: 71-90 hours (range: 28-123 hours); Children: 71 hours (range: 21-143 hours)

Dosage

Anemia associated with chronic kidney disease: Individualize dosing and use the lowest dose necessary to reduce the need for RBC transfusions.

Chronic kidney disease patients ***ON dialysis*** (IV route is preferred for hemodialysis patients; initiate treatment when hemoglobin is <10 g/dL; reduce dose or interrupt treatment if hemoglobin approaches or exceeds 11 g/dL):

Children ≥1 year: Conversion from epoetin alfa: IV, SubQ: Initial dose: Epoetin alfa doses of 1500 to ≥90,000 units per week may be converted to doses ranging from 6.25-200 mcg darbepoetin alfa per week (see pediatric column in conversion table below).

Adults: IV, SubQ: Initial: 0.45 mcg/kg once weekly **or** 0.75 mcg/kg once every 2 weeks **or** epoetin alfa doses of <1500 to ≥90,000 units per week may be converted to doses ranging from 6.25-200 mcg darbepoetin alfa per week (see adult column in conversion table below).

Chronic kidney disease patients ***NOT on dialysis*** (consider initiating treatment when hemoglobin is <10 g/dL; use only if rate of hemoglobin decline would likely result in RBC transfusion and desire is to reduce risk of alloimmunization or other RBC transfusion-related risks; reduce dose or interrupt treatment if hemoglobin exceeds 10 g/dL):

Adults: IV, SubQ: Initial: 0.45 mcg/kg once every 4 weeks

Dosage adjustments for chronic kidney disease patients (either on dialysis or not on dialysis): Do not increase dose more frequently than every 4 weeks (dose decreases may occur more frequently).

If hemoglobin increases >1 g/dL in any 2-week period: Decrease dose by ≥25%

If hemoglobin does not increase by >1 g/dL after 4 weeks: Increase dose by 25%

Inadequate or lack of response: If adequate response is not achieved over 12 weeks, further increases are unlikely to be of benefit and may increase the risk for adverse events; use the minimum effective dose that will maintain a hemoglobin level sufficient to avoid red blood cell transfusions **and** evaluate patient for other causes of anemia; discontinue treatment if responsiveness does not improve

Anemia due to chemotherapy in cancer patients: Initiate treatment only if hemoglobin <10 g/dL and anticipated duration of myelosuppressive chemotherapy is ≥2 months. Titrate dosage to use the minimum effective dose that will maintain a hemoglobin level sufficient to avoid red blood cell transfusions. Discontinue darbepoetin following completion of chemotherapy. SubQ:

Adults: Initial: 2.25 mcg/kg once weekly **or** 500 mcg once every 3 weeks until completion of chemotherapy

Dosage adjustments:

Increase dose: If hemoglobin does not increase by 1 g/dL **and** remains below 10 g/dL after initial 6 weeks (for patients receiving weekly therapy only), increase dose to 4.5 mcg/kg once weekly (no dosage adjustment if using every 3 week dosing).

Reduce dose by 40% if hemoglobin increases >1 g/dL in any 2-week period **or** hemoglobin reaches a level sufficient to avoid red blood cell transfusion.

Withhold dose if hemoglobin exceeds a level needed to avoid red blood cell transfusion. Resume treatment with a 40% dose reduction when hemoglobin approaches a level where transfusions may be required.

Discontinue: On completion of chemotherapy or if after 8 weeks of therapy there is no hemoglobin response or RBC transfusions still required

Symptomatic anemia associated with MDS (off-label use): Adults: SubQ: 150-300 mcg once weekly (NCCN MDS guidelines v.2.2011)

Conversion from epoetin alfa to darbepoetin alfa: See table.

Conversion From Epoetin Alfa to Darbepoetin Alfa (Initial Dose)

Previous Dosage of Epoetin Alfa (units/week)	Children Darbepoetin Alfa Dosage (mcg/week)	Adults Darbepoetin Alfa Dosage (mcg/week)
<1500	Not established	6.25
1500-2499	6.25	6.25
2500-4999	10	12.5
5000-10,999	20	25
11,000-17,999	40	40
18,000-33,999	60	60
34,000-89,999	100	100
≥90,000	200	200

Note: In patients receiving epoetin alfa 2-3 times per week, darbepoetin alfa is administered once weekly. In patients receiving epoetin alfa once weekly, darbepoetin alfa is administered once every 2 weeks. The darbepoetin dose to be administered every 2 weeks is derived by adding together 2 weekly epoetin alfa doses and then converting to the appropriate darbepoetin dose. Titrate dose to hemoglobin response thereafter.

Dosage adjustment in renal impairment: No dosage adjustment necessary.

Dosage adjustment in hepatic impairment: No dosage adjustment provided in manufacturer's labeling.

Dietary Considerations Supplemental iron intake may be required in patients with low iron stores.

Administration May be administered by SubQ or IV injection. The IV route is recommended in hemodialysis patients. Do not shake; vigorous shaking may denature darbepoetin alfa, rendering it biologically inactive. Do not dilute or administer in conjunction with other drug solutions. Discard any unused portion of the vial; do not pool unused portions.

Monitoring Parameters Hemoglobin (at least once per week until maintenance dose established and after dosage changes; monitor less frequently once hemoglobin is stabilized); CKD patients should be also be monitored at least monthly following hemoglobin stability); iron stores (transferrin saturation and ferritin) prior to and during therapy; serum chemistry (CKD patients); blood pressure; fluid balance (CKD patients); seizures (CKD patients following initiation for first few months, includes new-onset or change in seizure frequency or premonitory symptoms)

Cancer patients: Examinations recommended by the ASCO/ASH guidelines (Rizzo, 2010) prior to treatment include peripheral blood smear (in some situations a bone marrow exam may be necessary), assessment for iron, folate, or vitamin B_{12} deficiency, reticulocyte count, renal function status, and occult blood loss; during ESA treatment, assess baseline and periodic iron, total iron-binding capacity, and transferrin saturation or ferritin levels.

Additional Information Oncology Comment: The American Society of Clinical Oncology (ASCO) and American Society of Hematology (ASH) 2010 updates to the clinical practice guidelines for the use of erythropoiesis-stimulating agents (ESAs) in patients with cancer indicate that ESAs are appropriate when used according to the parameters identified within the Food and Drug Administration (FDA) approved labeling for epoetin and darbepoetin (Rizzo, 2010). ESAs are an option for chemotherapy associated anemia when the hemoglobin has fallen to <10 g/dL to decrease the need for RBC transfusions. ESAs should only be used in conjunction with concurrent chemotherapy. Although the FDA label now limits ESA use to the palliative setting, the ASCO/ASH guidelines suggest using clinical judgment in weighing risks versus benefits as formal outcomes studies of ESA use defined by intent of chemotherapy treatment have not been conducted.

The ASCO/ASH guidelines continue to recommend following the FDA approved dosing (and dosing adjustment) guidelines as alternate dosing and schedules have not demonstrated consistent differences in effectiveness with regard to hemoglobin response. In patients who do not have a response within 6-8 weeks (hemoglobin rise <1-2 g/dL or no reduction in transfusions) ESA therapy should be discontinued.

Prior to the initiation of ESAs, other sources of anemia (in addition to chemotherapy or underlying hematologic malignancy) should be investigated. Examinations recommended prior to treatment include peripheral blood smear (in some situations a bone marrow exam may be necessary), assessment for iron, folate, or vitamin B_{12} deficiency, reticulocyte count, renal function status, and occult blood loss. During ESA treatment, assess baseline and periodic iron, total iron-binding capacity, and transferrin saturation or ferritin levels. Iron supplementation may be necessary.

The guidelines note that patients with an increased risk of thromboembolism (generally includes previous history of thrombosis, surgery, and/or prolonged periods of immobilization) and patients receiving concomitant medications that may increase thromboembolic risk, should begin ESA therapy only after careful consideration. With the exception of low-risk myelodysplasia-associated anemia (which has evidence supporting the use of ESAs without concurrent chemotherapy), the guidelines do not support the use of ESAs in the absence of concurrent chemotherapy.

Dosage Forms

Solution, Injection [preservative free]:

Aranesp (Albumin Free): 25 mcg/mL (1 mL); 40 mcg/mL (1 mL); 25 mcg/0.42 mL (0.42 mL); 60 mcg/mL (1 mL); 40 mcg/0.4 mL (0.4 mL); 100 mcg/mL (1 mL); 60 mcg/0.3 mL (0.3 mL); 100 mcg/0.5 mL (0.5 mL); 150 mcg/0.75 mL (0.75 mL); 200 mcg/mL (1 mL); 300 mcg/mL (1 mL); 150 mcg/0.3 mL (0.3 mL); 200 mcg/0.4 mL (0.4 mL); 300 mcg/0.6 mL (0.6 mL); 500 mcg/mL (1 mL)

Darifenacin (dar i FEN a sin)

Brand Names: U.S. Enablex

Brand Names: Canada Enablex®

Index Terms Darifenacin Hydrobromide; UK-88,525

Pharmacologic Category Anticholinergic Agent

Additional Appendix Information

Beers Criteria - Potentially Inappropriate Medications for Geriatrics *on page 2271*

Use Management of symptoms of bladder overactivity (urge incontinence, urgency, and frequency)

Pregnancy Risk Factor C

Pregnancy Considerations Teratogenic effects and developmental delay were observed in some animal studies. There are no adequate and well-controlled studies in pregnant women; should be used only if potential benefit outweighs possible risk to the fetus.

Breast-Feeding Considerations Although human data are not available, darifenacin is excreted in the breast milk in animals.

Contraindications Hypersensitivity to darifenacin or any component of the formulation; uncontrolled narrow-angle glaucoma; urinary retention, paralytic ileus, GI or GU obstruction

Warnings/Precautions Cases of angioedema involving the face, lips, tongue, and/or larynx have been reported during treatment; some cases have occurred after the first dose. May be life-threatening. Immediately discontinue and institute supportive care if tongue, hypopharynx, or larynx is involved. Central nervous system effects have been reported (eg, headache, confusion, hallucinations, somnolence); monitor, particularly at treatment initiation or dose increase, reduce dose or discontinue if necessary. May cause drowsiness and/or blurred vision, which may impair physical or mental abilities; patients must be cautioned about performing tasks which require mental alertness (eg, operating machinery or driving). May occur in the presence of increased environmental temperature; use caution in hot weather and/or exercise. Use with caution with hepatic impairment; dosage limitation is required in moderate hepatic impairment (Child-Pugh class B). Not recommended for use in severe hepatic impairment (Child-Pugh class C). Use with caution in patients with clinically-significant bladder outlet obstruction or prostatic hyperplasia (nonobstructive). Use caution in patients with decreased GI motility, constipation, hiatal hernia, reflux esophagitis, and ulcerative colitis. Use caution in patients with myasthenia gravis. In patients with controlled narrow-angle glaucoma, darifenacin should be used with extreme caution and only when the potential benefit outweighs risks of treatment. Use with caution in patients taking strong CYP3A4 inhibitors (see Drug Interactions); dosage limitation of darifenacin is required. This medication is associated with potent anticholinergic properties which may be inappropriate in older adults depending on comorbidities (eg, dementia, delirium) (Beers Criteria).

Adverse Reactions

Cardiovascular: Hypertension, peripheral edema

Central nervous system: Dizziness, headache, pain

Dermatological: Pruritus, skin rash, xeroderma

Endocrine & metabolic: Weight gain

Gastrointestinal: Abdominal pain, constipation, dyspepsia, nausea, vomiting, xerostomia

Genitourinary: Urinary retention (acute), urinary tract infection, vaginitis

Neuromuscular & skeletal: Arthralgia, back pain, weakness

Ophthalmic: Dry eye syndrome, visual disturbance

Respiratory: Bronchitis, flu-like symptoms, pharyngitis, rhinitis, sinusitis

Rare but important or life-threatening: Anaphylaxis, angioedema, confusion, erythema multiforme, granuloma (annulare), hallucination, hypersensitivity reaction

Drug Interactions

Metabolism/Transport Effects Substrate of CYP2D6 (minor), CYP3A4 (major); **Note:** Assignment of Major/Minor substrate status based on clinically relevant drug interaction potential; **Inhibits** CYP2D6 (moderate), CYP3A4 (weak)

Avoid Concomitant Use

Avoid concomitant use of Darifenacin with any of the following: Aclidinium; Conivaptan; Fusidic Acid (Systemic); Glucagon; Idelalisib; Ipratropium (Oral Inhalation); Pimozide; Potassium Chloride; Thioridazine; Tiotropium; Umeclidinium

Increased Effect/Toxicity

Darifenacin may increase the levels/effects of: AbobotulinumtoxinA; Analgesics (Opioid); Anticholinergic Agents; ARIPiprazole; Cannabinoid-Containing Products; CYP2D6 Substrates; Dofetilide; DOXOrubicin (Conventional); Eliglustat; Fesoterodine; Glucagon; Hydrocodone; Lomitapide; Metoprolol; Mirabegron; Nebivolol; OnabotulinumtoxinA; Pimozide; Potassium Chloride; RimabotulinumtoxinB; Thiazide Diuretics; Thioridazine; Tiotropium; Topiramate

The levels/effects of Darifenacin may be increased by: Aclidinium; Aprepitant; Ceritinib; Conivaptan; CYP3A4 Inhibitors (Moderate); CYP3A4 Inhibitors (Strong); Dasatinib; Fosaprepitant; Fusidic Acid (Systemic); Idelalisib; Ipratropium (Oral Inhalation); Ivacaftor; Luliconazole; Mianserin; Mifepristone; Netupitant; Pramlintide; Propafenone; Simeprevir; Stiripentol; Umeclidinium

Decreased Effect

Darifenacin may decrease the levels/effects of: Acetylcholinesterase Inhibitors; Codeine; Itopride; Secretin; Tamoxifen; TraMADol

The levels/effects of Darifenacin may be decreased by: Acetylcholinesterase Inhibitors; Bosentan; CYP3A4 Inducers (Moderate); CYP3A4 Inducers (Strong); Dabrafenib; Deferasirox; Mitotane; Siltuximab; St Johns Wort; Tocilizumab

Storage/Stability Store at 25°C (77°F); excursions permitted to 15°C to 30°C (59°F to 86°F). Protect from light.

Mechanism of Action Selective antagonist of the M3 muscarinic (cholinergic) receptor subtype. Blockade of the receptor limits bladder contractions, reducing the symptoms of bladder irritability/overactivity (urge incontinence, urgency and frequency).

Pharmacodynamics/Kinetics

Distribution: V_{dss}: ~163 L

Protein binding: ~98% (primarily alpha$_1$-acid glycoprotein)

Metabolism: Hepatic, via CYP3A4 (major) and CYP2D6 (minor)

Bioavailability: 15% to 19%

Half-life elimination: ~13-19 hours

Time to peak, plasma: ~7 hours

Excretion: As metabolites (inactive); urine (60%), feces (40%)

Dosage Oral: Adults: Initial: 7.5 mg once daily. If response is not adequate after a minimum of 2 weeks, dosage may be increased to 15 mg once daily.

Dosage adjustment with concomitant potent CYP3A4 inhibitors (eg, ketoconazole, itraconazole, ritonavir, nelfinavir, clarithromycin, nefazodone): Daily dosage should not exceed 7.5 mg daily

Dosage adjustment in renal impairment: No dosage adjustment necessary.

Dosage adjustment in hepatic impairment:

Mild impairment (Child-Pugh class A): No dosage adjustment necessary.

Moderate impairment (Child-Pugh class B): Daily dosage should not exceed 7.5 mg daily

Severe impairment (Child-Pugh class C): Has not been evaluated; use is not recommended

Dietary Considerations May be taken without regard to meals, with or without food.

Administration Tablet should be taken with liquid and swallowed whole; do not chew, crush, or split tablet. May be taken without regard to food.

Dosage Forms

Tablet Extended Release 24 Hour, Oral:

Enablex: 7.5 mg, 15 mg

◆ **Darifenacin Hydrobromide** *see* Darifenacin *on page 568*

Darunavir (dar OO na veer)

Brand Names: U.S. Prezista

Brand Names: Canada Prezista

Index Terms Darunavir Ethanolate; DRV; TMC-114

Pharmacologic Category Antiretroviral, Protease Inhibitor (Anti-HIV)

Use HIV infection: Treatment of HIV-1 infection, coadministered with ritonavir and other antiretroviral agents, in adults and pediatric patients 3 years and older

Pregnancy Risk Factor C

Pregnancy Considerations Teratogenic effects have not been observed in animal reproduction studies. Darunavir has a low level of transfer across the human placenta. Serum concentrations are decreased during pregnancy; therefore, once-daily dosing is not recommended; twice-daily dosing should be used. The DHHS Perinatal HIV Guidelines consider darunavir to be an alternative protease inhibitor (PI) for use in antiretroviral-naive pregnant patients when combined with low-dose ritonavir boosting. A small increased risk of preterm birth has been associated with maternal use of protease inhibitor-based combination antiretroviral (ARV) therapy during pregnancy; however, the benefits of use generally outweigh this risk and PIs should not be withheld if otherwise recommended. Hyperglycemia, new onset of diabetes mellitus, or diabetic ketoacidosis have been reported with PIs; it is not clear if pregnancy increases this risk.

Regardless of CD4 count or HIV RNA copy number, all HIV-infected pregnant women should receive an ARV drug regimen combination of antepartum, intrapartum, and infant ARV prophylaxis. ARV therapy should be started as soon as possible in women with symptomatic infection. Although earlier initiation may be more effective in reducing the perinatal transmission of HIV, initiation may be delayed until after 12 weeks gestation in women who do not require immediate treatment after careful consideration of maternal conditions (eg, nausea and vomiting) and the potential risks of first trimester fetal exposure for specific agents. A scheduled cesarean delivery at 38 weeks gestation is recommended for all women with HIV RNA >1000 copies/mL or unknown concentrations near delivery in order to decrease transmission. If ARV therapy must be interrupted for <24 hours during the peripartum period, stop then restart all medications simultaneously in order to decrease the chance of developing resistance. Long-term follow-up is recommended for all infants exposed to ARV medications. In couples who want to conceive, the HIV-infected partner should attain maximum viral suppression prior to conception.

Healthcare providers are encouraged to enroll pregnant women exposed to antiretroviral medications in the Antiretroviral Pregnancy Registry (1-800-258-4263 or www.APRegistry.com). Healthcare providers caring for HIV-infected women and their infants may contact the National Perinatal HIV Hotline (888-448-8765) for clinical consultation (HHS [perinatal], 2014).

Breast-Feeding Considerations It is not known if darunavir is excreted into breast milk. Maternal or infant antiretroviral therapy does not completely eliminate the risk of postnatal HIV transmission. In addition, multiclass-resistant virus has been detected in breast-feeding infants despite maternal therapy. Therefore, in the United States, where formula is accessible, affordable, safe, and sustainable, and the risk of infant mortality due to diarrhea and respiratory infections is low, complete avoidance of breast-feeding by HIV-infected women is recommended to decrease potential transmission of HIV (HHS [perinatal], 2014).

Contraindications Coadministration with drugs that are highly dependent on CYP3A for clearance and drugs for which elevated plasma concentrations are associated with serious and/or life-threatening events (narrow therapeutic index) (eg, alfuzosin, ergot derivatives [dihydroergotamine, ergonovine, ergotamine, methylergonovine], cisapride, pimozide, midazolam oral, triazolam, St John's wort, lovastatin, simvastatin, rifampin, sildenafil [for the treatment of pulmonary hypertension]). Must be coadministered with ritonavir; refer to individual monograph for ritonavir for additional contraindication information.

Canadian labeling: Additional contraindications: Hypersensitivity to darunavir or any component of the formulation; coadministration with amiodarone, lidocaine (systemic), quinidine; severe (Child-Pugh class C) hepatic impairment

Warnings/Precautions Darunavir has a high potential for drug interactions requiring dose or frequency adjustment, additional monitoring, and/or selection of alternative therapy.

Use with caution in patients with hepatic impairment, including active chronic hepatitis; consider interruption or discontinuation with worsening hepatic function. Not recommended in severe hepatic impairment (contraindicated in Canadian labeling). Infrequent cases of drug-induced hepatitis (including acute and cytolytic) have been reported. Liver injury has been reported with use (including some fatalities), though generally in patients on multiple medications, with advanced HIV disease, hepatitis B/C coinfection, and/or immune reconstitution syndrome. Monitor patients closely; consider interrupting or discontinuing therapy if signs/symptoms of liver impairment occur.

May cause fat redistribution (buffalo hump, increased abdominal girth, breast engorgement, facial atrophy). Patients may develop immune reconstitution syndrome resulting in the occurrence of an inflammatory response to an indolent or residual opportunistic infection during initial HIV treatment or activation of autoimmune disorders (eg, Graves disease, polymyositis, Guillain-Barré syndrome) later in therapy; further evaluation and treatment may be required. May increase cholesterol and/or triglycerides. Pancreatitis has been observed with use. Risk for pancreatitis may be increased in patients with elevated triglycerides, advanced HIV disease, or history of pancreatitis. Protease inhibitors have been associated with glucose dysregulation; use caution in patients with diabetes. Initiation or dose adjustments of antidiabetic agents may be required. Use with caution in patients with sulfonamide allergy (contains sulfa moiety) or hemophilia. Protease inhibitors have been associated with a variety of hypersensitivity events (some severe), including rash, anaphylaxis (rare), angioedema, bronchospasm, erythema multiforme, Stevens-Johnson syndrome (rare), acute generalized exanthematous pustulosis, toxic epidermal necrolysis, and/or drug rash with eosinophilia and systemic symptoms (DRESS). Discontinue treatment if severe skin reactions develop. Severe skin reactions may be accompanied by fever, malaise, fatigue, arthralgias, hepatitis, oral lesion, blisters, conjunctivitis, and/or eosinophilia. Mild-to-moderate rash may occur early in treatment and resolve with continued therapy. Treatment history and resistance data should guide use of darunavir with ritonavir. Do not administer darunavir with ritonavir in pediatric patients younger than 3 years (toxicity and mortality observed in animal studies).

Adverse Reactions As a class, protease inhibitors potentially cause dyslipidemias which includes elevated cholesterol and triglycerides and a redistribution of body fat centrally to cause increased abdominal girth, buffalo hump, facial atrophy, and breast enlargement. These agents also cause hyperglycemia. See also Ritonavir monograph.

Central nervous system: Fatigue (more common in children), headache (more common in children)

Dermatologic: Pruritus (more common in children), skin rash (more common in children)

Endocrine & metabolic: Diabetes mellitus, hypercholesterolemia (more common in adults), hyperglycemia, increased amylase (more common in adults), increased LDL cholesterol (more common in adults), increased serum triglycerides

Gastrointestinal: Abdominal distention, abdominal pain (more common in children), anorexia (more common in children), decreased appetite (more common in children), diarrhea (more common in children), dyspepsia, increased serum lipase (more common in adults), nausea (more common in children), vomiting (more common in children)

Hepatic: Increased serum ALT (more common in adults), increased serum AST (more common in adults)

Neuromuscular & skeletal: Weakness

Rare but important or life-threatening: Acute renal failure, alopecia, arthritis, bradycardia, cerebrovascular accident, depression, dermatitis (including dermatitis medicamentosa), DRESS syndrome, facial paralysis, folliculitis, gynecomastia, hematuria, hepatic failure, hepatic neoplasm (malignant), hepatitis (acute and cytolytic), hepatotoxicity, hyperlipidemia, hypersensitivity, hyperthermia, immune reconstitution syndrome, impaired consciousness, infection (including clostridium infection, parasitic infection [cryptosporidiosis], cytomegalovirus disease [encephalitis], hepatitis B, esophageal candidiasis), malignant lymphoma, myocardial infarction, nephrolithiasis, neutropenia, obesity, oropharyngeal ulcer, osteoporosis, pancreatitis, pancytopenia, peripheral neuropathy, pneumothorax, progressive multifocal leukoencephalopathy, pulmonary edema, rectal hemorrhage, redistribution of body fat (eg, buffalo hump, increased abdominal girth, breast engorgement, facial atrophy), respiratory failure, rhabdomyolysis (coadministration with HMG-CoA reductase inhibitors), seizure, sepsis, skin rash (toxic), tachycardia, uveitis

Drug Interactions

Metabolism/Transport Effects **Substrate** of CYP3A4 (major); **Note:** Assignment of Major/Minor substrate status based on clinically relevant drug interaction potential; **Inhibits** CYP2D6 (weak), CYP3A4 (strong), P-glycoprotein

Avoid Concomitant Use

Avoid concomitant use of Darunavir with any of the following: Ado-Trastuzumab Emtansine; Alfuzosin; Amiodarone; Apixaban; Astemizole; Avanafil; Axitinib; Bosutinib; Cabozantinib; Ceritinib; Cisapride; Conivaptan; Crizotinib; Dapoxetine; Dronedarone; Eplerenone; Ergot Derivatives; Everolimus; Fosphenytoin; Fusidic Acid (Systemic); Halofantrine; Ibrutinib; Idelalisib; Irinotecan; Ivabradine; Lapatinib; Lercanidipine; Lomitapide; Lopinavir; Lovastatin; Lurasidone; Macitentan; Midazolam; Naloxegol; Nilotinib; Nisoldipine; Olaparib; PAZOPanib; Pimozide; QuiNIDine; Ranolazine; Red Yeast Rice; Regorafenib; Rifampin; Rivaroxaban; Salmeterol; Saquinavir; Silodosin; Simeprevir; Simvastatin; St Johns Wort; Suvorexant; Tamsulosin; Telaprevir; Terfenadine; Ticagrelor; Tipranavir; Tolvaptan; Topotecan; Toremifene; Trabectedin; Triazolam; Ulipristal; Vemurafenib; VinCRIStine (Liposomal); Vorapaxar; Voriconazole

Increased Effect/Toxicity

Darunavir may increase the levels/effects of: Ado-Trastuzumab Emtansine; Afatinib; Alfuzosin; Almotriptan; Alosetron; ALPRAZolam; Amiodarone; Apixaban; ARIPiprazole; Astemizole; AtorvaSTATin; Avanafil; Axitinib; Bedaquiline; Bortezomib; Bosentan; Bosutinib; Brentuximab Vedotin; Brinzolamide; Budesonide (Nasal); Budesonide (Systemic, Oral Inhalation); Cabazitaxel; Cabozantinib; Calcium Channel Blockers

(Dihydropyridine); Calcium Channel Blockers (Nondihydropyridine); Cannabis; CarBAMazepine; Ceritinib; Cisapride; Clarithromycin; Colchicine; Conivaptan; Corticosteroids (Orally Inhaled); Corticosteroids (Systemic); Crizotinib; Cyclophosphamide; CycloSPORINE (Systemic); CYP2D6 Substrates; CYP3A4 Substrates; Dabigatran Etexilate; Dapoxetine; Dasatinib; Digoxin; Dofetilide; DOXOrubicin (Conventional); Dronabinol; Dronedarone; Dutasteride; Edoxaban; Efavirenz; Eliglustat; Enfuvirtide; Eplerenone; Ergot Derivatives; Erlotinib; Etizolam; Everolimus; FentaNYL; Fesoterodine; Fluticasone (Nasal); Fluticasone (Oral Inhalation); GuanFACINE; Halofantrine; Hydrocodone; Ibrutinib; Iloperidone; Imatinib; Imidafenacin; Irinotecan; Itraconazole; Ivabradine; Ivacaftor; Ixabepilone; Ketoconazole (Systemic); Lacosamide; Lapatinib; Ledipasvir; Lercanidipine; Levobupivacaine; Levomilnacipran; Lomitapide; Lovastatin; Lumefantrine; Lurasidone; Macitentan; Maraviroc; Meperidine; MethylPREDNISolone; Midazolam; Mifepristone; Naloxegol; Nefazodone; Nilotinib; Nintedanib; Nisoldipine; Olaparib; Ospemifene; OxyCODONE; Paricalcitol; PAZOPanib; P-glycoprotein/ABCB1 Substrates; Pimecrolimus; Pimozide; PONATinib; Pranlukast; Pravastatin; PrednisoLONE (Systemic); PredniSONE; Propafenone; Protease Inhibitors; Prucalopride; QUEtiapine; QuiNIDine; Ranolazine; Red Yeast Rice; Regorafenib; Repaglinide; Retapamulin; Rifabutin; Rifaximin; Rilpivirine; Riociguat; Rivaroxaban; RomiDEPsin; Rosuvastatin; Ruxolitinib; Salmeterol; Saxagliptin; Sildenafil; Silodosin; Simeprevir; Simvastatin; SORAfenib; Suvorexant; Tacrolimus (Systemic); Tacrolimus (Topical); Tadalafil; Tamsulosin; Temsirolimus; Tenofovir; Terfenadine; Tetrahydrocannabinol; Ticagrelor; Tofacitinib; Tolterodine; Tolvaptan; Topotecan; Toremifene; Trabectedin; TraZODone; Triazolam; Tricyclic Antidepressants; Ulipristal; Vardenafil; Vemurafenib; Vilazodone; VinCRIStine (Liposomal); Vorapaxar; Zopiclone; Zuclopenthixol

The levels/effects of Darunavir may be increased by: Clarithromycin; Conivaptan; CycloSPORINE (Systemic); CYP3A4 Inhibitors (Moderate); CYP3A4 Inhibitors (Strong); Delavirdine; Enfuvirtide; Etravirine; Fusidic Acid (Systemic); Idelalisib; Itraconazole; Ketoconazole (Systemic); Luliconazole; Mifepristone; Netupitant; Rifabutin; Simeprevir; Stiripentol; Tenofovir

Decreased Effect

Darunavir may decrease the levels/effects of: Abacavir; Boceprevir; Clarithromycin; Contraceptives (Estrogens); Contraceptives (Progestins); Delavirdine; Didanosine; Etravirine; Ifosfamide; Meperidine; Methadone; Norethindrone; PARoxetine; PHENobarbital; Phenytoin; Prasugrel; Sertraline; Telaprevir; Ticagrelor; Valproic Acid and Derivatives; Voriconazole; Warfarin; Zidovudine

The levels/effects of Darunavir may be decreased by: Boceprevir; Bosentan; CYP3A4 Inducers (Moderate); CYP3A4 Inducers (Strong); Dabrafenib; Deferasirox; Efavirenz; Fosphenytoin; Garlic; Lopinavir; Mitotane; Rifampin; Saquinavir; Siltuximab; St Johns Wort; Telaprevir; Tipranavir; Tocilizumab

Food Interactions Absorption and bioavailability are increased when administered with food. Management: Take with meals.

Storage/Stability

Tablets: Store at 25°C (77°F); excursions are permitted between 15°C and 30°C (59°F and 86°F).

Suspension: Store at 25°C (77°F); excursions are permitted between 15°C and 30°C (59°F and 86°F). Do not refrigerate or freeze.

Mechanism of Action Binds to the site of HIV-1 protease activity and inhibits cleavage of viral Gag-Pol polyprotein precursors into individual functional proteins required for infectious HIV. This results in the formation of immature, noninfectious viral particles.

Pharmacodynamics/Kinetics All kinetic parameters derived in the presence of ritonavir coadministration.

Absorption: Increased ~40% with food

Protein binding: ~95%; primarily to alpha$_1$ acid glycoprotein (AAG)

Metabolism: Hepatic, via CYP3A to minimally active metabolites

Bioavailability: 82%

Half-life elimination: ~15 hours

Time to peak, plasma: 2.5 to 4 hours

Excretion: Feces (~80%, 41% as unchanged drug); urine (~14%, 8% as unchanged drug)

Dosage Oral:

Children ≥3 years and Adolescents: **Note:** Coadministration with ritonavir is required; do not exceed the maximum recommended darunavir adult dose (800 mg to 1200 mg daily depending upon indication). Genotypic testing is recommended in therapy-experienced patients.

Treatment-naive patients or treatment-experienced with no darunavir resistance-associated substitutions: **Note:** Guidelines do not recommend once-daily dosing in any patient <12 years, patients 12 to 18 years who are treatment experienced with prior treatment failure, or patients ≥18 years with darunavir resistance-associated viral mutations (HHS [pediatric], 2014).

Dosing recommendations based on body weight using the oral suspension:

- ≥10 kg to <11 kg: 350 mg once daily with ritonavir 64 mg once daily
- ≥11 kg to <12 kg: 385 mg once daily with ritonavir 64 mg once daily
- ≥12 kg to <13 kg: 420 mg once daily with ritonavir 80 mg once daily
- ≥13 kg to <14 kg: 455 mg once daily with ritonavir 80 mg once daily
- ≥14 kg to <15 kg: 490 mg once daily with ritonavir 96 mg once daily

Dosing recommendations based on body weight using the oral suspension or tablets:

- ≥15 kg to <30 kg: 600 mg once daily with ritonavir 100 mg once daily
- ≥30 kg to <40 kg: 675 mg once daily with ritonavir 100 mg once daily
- ≥40 kg: 800 mg once daily with ritonavir 100 mg once daily

Treatment-experienced patients with at ≥1 darunavir resistance-associated substitution. Darunavir resistance-associated viral mutations include: V11I, V32I, L33F, I47V, I50V, I54L, I54M, T74P, L76V, I84V, and L89V. **Note:** Guidelines recommend twice-daily dosing for all patients 3 to <12 years. (HHS [pediatric], 2014).

Dosing recommendations based on body weight using the oral suspension:

- ≥10 kg to <11 kg: 200 mg twice daily with ritonavir 32 mg twice daily
- ≥11 kg to <12 kg: 220 mg twice daily with ritonavir 32 mg twice daily
- ≥12 kg to <13 kg: 240 mg twice daily with ritonavir 40 mg twice daily
- ≥13 kg to <14 kg: 260 mg twice daily with ritonavir 40 mg twice daily
- ≥14 kg to <15 kg: 280 mg twice daily with ritonavir 48 mg twice daily

Dosing recommendations based on body weight using the oral suspension or tablets:

- ≥15 kg to <30 kg: 375 mg twice daily with ritonavir 48 mg twice daily
- ≥30 kg to <40 kg: 450 mg twice daily with ritonavir 60 mg twice daily
- ≥40 kg: 600 mg twice daily with ritonavir 100 mg twice daily

Adults:

Treatment-naive: 800 mg once daily; coadministration with ritonavir 100 mg once daily is required. **Note:** Recommended (with ritonavir) as a first-line therapy with tenofovir/emtricitabine in antiretroviral naïve patients (HHS [adult], 2014).

Treatment-experienced: **Note:** Genotypic testing is recommended in therapy experienced patients.

With no darunavir resistance-associated substitutions: 800 mg once daily; coadministration with ritonavir 100 mg once daily is required

With ≥1 darunavir resistance-associated substitution: 600 mg twice daily; coadministration with ritonavir 100 mg twice daily is required

If genotypic testing is not possible: 600 mg twice daily, coadministered with ritonavir 100 mg twice daily

Dosage adjustment for toxicity:

Severe rash: Discontinue treatment

New or worsening liver dysfunction: Consider interrupting or discontinuing treatment

Dosage adjustment in renal impairment:

CrCl ≥30 mL/minute: There are no dosage adjustments provided in the manufacturer's labeling; however, need for adjustment not expected based on pharmacokinetic data.

CrCl <30 mL/minute: There are no dosage adjustments provided in the manufacturer's labeling (has not been studied).

Dosage adjustment in hepatic impairment:

Mild to moderate impairment (Child-Pugh class A or B): No dosage adjustments necessary

Severe impairment (Child-Pugh class C): Use not recommended (contraindicated in Canadian labeling).

Dietary Considerations Absorption increased with food. Take with meals.

Administration Coadministration with ritonavir and food is required (bioavailability is increased). Shake suspension prior to each dose; use provided oral dosing syringe to measure dose. In patients taking darunavir once daily, if a dose of darunavir or ritonavir is missed by >12 hours, the next dose should be taken at the regularly scheduled time. If a dose of darunavir or ritonavir is missed by <12 hours, the dose should be taken immediately, and then the next dose should be taken at the regularly scheduled time. In patients taking darunavir twice daily, if a dose of darunavir or ritonavir is missed by >6 hours, the next dose should be taken at the regularly scheduled time. If a dose of darunavir or ritonavir is missed by <6 hours, the dose should be taken immediately, and then the next dose should be taken at the regularly scheduled time.

Monitoring Parameters Viral load, CD4, baseline genotyping in treatment-experienced patients (if possible); serum glucose; transaminase levels prior to and during therapy (increase monitoring in patients at risk for liver impairment), cholesterol, triglycerides

Dosage Forms

Suspension, Oral:

Prezista: 100 mg/mL (200 mL)

Tablet, Oral:

Prezista: 75 mg, 150 mg, 600 mg, 800 mg

Darunavir and Cobicistat

(dar OO na veer & koe BIK i stat)

Brand Names: U.S. Prezcobix

Brand Names: Canada Prezcobix

Index Terms Cobicistat and Darunavir

Pharmacologic Category Antiretroviral, Protease Inhibitor (Anti-HIV); Cytochrome P-450 Inhibitor

Use

HIV infection: Treatment of HIV-1 infection, coadministered with other antiretroviral agents, in treatment-naive and in treatment-experienced patients without darunavir resistant-associated substitutions (V11I, V32I, L33F, I47V, I50V, I54L, I54M, T74P, L76V, I84V, L89V)

Note: For treatment-experienced patients, the Canadian labeling indicates use in patients without any darunavir resistant-associated substitutions

Pregnancy Considerations Refer to individual monographs. Healthcare providers are encouraged to enroll pregnant women exposed to antiretroviral medications in the Antiretroviral Pregnancy Registry (1-800-258-4263).

Breast-Feeding Considerations It is not known whether darunavir, cobicistat, or their metabolites are excreted in human milk. **To avoid the risk of postnatal transmission of HIV to an infant, women with HIV infection should not breast-feed.** Refer also to individual monographs.

Contraindications

Coadministration with alfuzosin, dronedarone, lurasidone, colchicine (in patients with renal or hepatic impairment), rifampin, ergot derivatives (eg, dihydroergotamine, ergonovine, ergotamine, methylergonovine), cisapride (not available in Canada), St John's wort, lovastatin, simvastatin, pimozide, ranolazine, sildenafil (for treatment of pulmonary arterial hypertension), oral midazolam, triazolam

Canadian labeling: Additional contraindications (not in US labeling): Hypersensitivity to darunavir, cobicistat, or any component of the formulation; severe hepatic impairment (Child-Pugh class C). Coadministration with amiodarone, bepridil (not available in Canada), lidocaine (systemic), quinidine, salmeterol, astemizole (not available in Canada), or terfenadine (not available in Canada)

Warnings/Precautions Protease inhibitors have been associated with a variety of hypersensitivity events (some severe); discontinue treatment if severe skin reactions develop. May cause redistribution of fat (eg, buffalo hump, peripheral wasting with increased abdominal girth, cushingoid appearance). Patients may develop immune reconstitution syndrome resulting in the occurrence of an inflammatory response to an indolent or residual opportunistic infection during initial HIV treatment or activation of autoimmune disorders (eg, Graves disease, polymyositis, Guillain-Barré syndrome) later in therapy; further evaluation and treatment may be required. Increases in total cholesterol and triglycerides have been reported with darunavir; screening should be done prior to therapy and periodically throughout treatment. Pancreatitis has been observed during therapy with darunavir; use caution in patients at risk for pancreatitis.

Cobicistat may inhibit tubular secretion of creatinine without affecting actual renal glomerular function; use caution when interpreting serum creatinine values. Patients who experience a confirmed increase in serum creatinine >0.4 mg/dL from baseline should have renal function monitored closely. Concomitant use of cobicistat and tenofovir may cause renal toxicity (acute renal failure and/or Fanconi syndrome); avoid use with concurrent or recent nephrotoxic therapy. Calculate estimated creatinine clearance (CrCl) prior to initiation of therapy and monitor renal function during therapy. In patients receiving concomitant tenofovir, assess urine glucose and urine protein prior to and periodically during treatment; assess serum phosphorus in patients with or at risk for renal impairment. Do not initiate therapy in patients with CrCl <70 mL/minute.

Darunavir may exacerbate preexisting hepatic dysfunction; use with caution in patients with advanced HIV disease or preexisting liver disease, hepatitis B/C coinfection, and/or immune reconstitution syndrome. Monitor LFTs closely at baseline and during treatment in all patients; in patients with baseline elevations, consider increased monitoring, especially in the first few months of therapy. Consider interrupting or discontinuing therapy if signs/symptoms of new or worsening liver impairment (eg, clinically significant LFT elevations, fatigue, anorexia, nausea, jaundice, dark urine, liver tenderness, hepatomegaly) occur. Use in severe liver impairment (Child-Pugh class C) is not recommended (US labeling) or contraindicated (Canadian labeling).

Changes in glucose tolerance, hyperglycemia, exacerbation of diabetes, DKA, and new-onset diabetes mellitus have been reported in patients receiving protease inhibitors. Initiation or dose adjustments of antidiabetic agents may be required. Use with caution in patients with hemophilia A or B; increased bleeding (eg, spontaneous skin hematomas and hemarthroses) has been reported during protease inhibitor therapy. Some patients receive additional factor VIII. In more than half of the cases, protease inhibitor treatment was continued or reintroduced if treatment was discontinued. Use with caution in patients with sulfonamide allergy (darunavir contains sulfa moiety).

Potentially significant drug-drug interactions may exist, requiring dose or frequency adjustment, additional monitoring, and/or selection of alternative therapy.

Adverse Reactions

Central nervous system: Headache
Dermatologic: Skin rash
Gastrointestinal: Abdominal pain, diarrhea, flatulence, nausea, vomiting
Hepatic: Increased liver enzymes
Hypersensitivity: Drug-induced hypersensitivity
Rare but important or life-threatening: Abnormal dreams, absence seizures, acute respiratory distress, anemia, anorexia, anxiety, arthropathy, biliary obstruction, blurred vision, breast hypertrophy, cerebral infarction, clostridium infection, conjunctivitis, convulsions, cryptosporidosis, cytomegalovirus disease, dehydration, depression, diabetes mellitus, diabetic ketoacidosis, dizziness, drug toxicity, dyspepsia, encephalitis, eosinophilia, esophageal candidiasis, exacerbation of diabetes mellitus, fanconi's syndrome, feeling of heaviness, gastritis, graves' disease, guillain-barre syndrome, hemarthrosis, hematoma, hematuria, hepatic cirrhosis, hepatic neoplasm, hepatitis, hepatomegaly, hepatotoxicity, hypercholesterolemia, hypersensitivity, hypertriglyceridemia, immune reconstitution syndrome, impaired consciousness, increased serum bilirubin, increased serum transaminases, limb pain, lipoatrophy, lipodystrophy, lipohypertrophy, liver tenderness, maculopathy, malaise, malignant lymphoma, metabolic acidosis, myocarditis, myositis, neoplasm, neuromuscular disease, obesity, oral lesion, ostealgia, osteonecrosis, pancreatitis, pancytopenia, paralysis, peripheral neuropathy, pneumothorax, polymyositis, progressive multifocal leukoencephalopathy, pulmonary edema, rectal hemorrhage, renal failure, renal insufficiency, renal tubular necrosis, respiratory failure, rhabdomyolysis, sepsis, stevens-johnson syndrome, swelling of eye, uveitis, weakness

Drug Interactions

Metabolism/Transport Effects Refer to individual components.

Avoid Concomitant Use

Avoid concomitant use of Darunavir and Cobicistat with any of the following: Ado-Trastuzumab Emtansine; Alfuzosin; Amiodarone; Apixaban; Astemizole; Avanafil; Axitinib; Boceprevir; Bosutinib; Cabozantinib; Ceritinib; Cisapride; Conivaptan; Crizotinib; Dapoxetine; Dihydroergotamine; Dronedarone; Eplerenone; Ergot Derivatives; Ergotamine; Everolimus; Fluticasone (Oral Inhalation); Fosphenytoin; Fusidic Acid (Systemic); Halofantrine; Ibrutinib; Idelalisib; Irinotecan; Ivabradine; Lapatinib; Lercanidipine; Lomitapide; Lopinavir; Lovastatin; Lurasidone; Macitentan; Methylergonovine; Midazolam; Naloxegol; Nilotinib; Nisoldipine; Olaparib; PAZOPanib; Pimozide; QuiNIDine; Ranolazine; Red Yeast Rice; Regorafenib; Rifampin; Rifapentine; Rivaroxaban; Salmeterol; Saquinavir; Sildenafil; Silodosin; Simeprevir; Simvastatin; St Johns Wort; Suvorexant; Tamsulosin; Telaprevir; Terfenadine; Ticagrelor; Tipranavir; Tolvaptan; Topotecan; Toremifene; Trabectedin; Triazolam; Ulipristal; Vardenafil; Vemurafenib; VinCRIStine (Liposomal); Vorapaxar; Voriconazole

Increased Effect/Toxicity

Darunavir and Cobicistat may increase the levels/effects of: Ado-Trastuzumab Emtansine; Afatinib; Alfuzosin; Almotriptan; Alosetron; ALPRAZolam; Amiodarone; Apixaban; ARIPiprazole; Astemizole; AtorvaSTATin; Avanafil; Axitinib; Bedaquiline; Boceprevir; Bortezomib; Bosentan; Bosutinib; Brentuximab Vedotin; Brinzolamide; Budesonide (Nasal); Budesonide (Systemic, Oral Inhalation); Cabazitaxel; Cabozantinib; Calcium Channel Blockers (Dihydropyridine); Calcium Channel Blockers (Nondihydropyridine); Cannabis; Ceritinib; Cisapride; Clarithromycin; Colchicine; Conivaptan; Contraceptives (Progestins); Corticosteroids (Orally Inhaled); Corticosteroids (Systemic); Crizotinib; Cyclophosphamide; CycloSPORINE (Systemic); CYP2D6 Substrates; CYP3A4 Substrates; Dabigatran Etexilate; Dapoxetine; Dasatinib; Digoxin; Dihydroergotamine; Dofetilide; DOXOrubicin (Conventional); Dronabinol; Dronedarone; Dutasteride; Edoxaban; Efavirenz; Eliglustat; Enfuvirtide; Eplerenone; Ergot Derivatives; Ergotamine; Erlotinib; Etizolam; Everolimus; FentaNYL; Fesoterodine; Fluticasone (Nasal); Fluticasone (Oral Inhalation); GuanFACINE; Halofantrine; Hydrocodone; Ibrutinib; Iloperidone; Imatinib; Imidafenacin; Irinotecan; Itraconazole; Ivabradine; Ivacaftor; Ixabepilone; Ketoconazole (Systemic); Lacosamide; Lapatinib; Ledipasvir; Lercanidipine; Levobupivacaine; Levomilnacipran; Lomitapide; Lovastatin; Lumefantrine; Lurasidone; Macitentan; Maraviroc; Meperidine; Methadone; Methylergonovine; MethylPREDNISolone; Midazolam; Mifepristone; Naloxegol; Nefazodone; Nilotinib; Nintedanib; Nisoldipine; Olaparib; Ospemifene; OxyCODONE; Paricalcitol; PAZOPanib; P-glycoprotein/ABCB1 Substrates; Pimecrolimus; Pimozide; PONATinib; Pranlukast; Pravastatin; PrednisoLONE (Systemic); PredniSONE; Propafenone; Protease Inhibitors; Prucalopride; QUEtiapine; QuiNIDine; Ranolazine; Red Yeast Rice; Regorafenib; Repaglinide; Retapamulin; Rifabutin; Rifaximin; Rilpivirine; Riociguat; Rivaroxaban; RomiDEPsin; Rosuvastatin; Ruxolitinib; Salmeterol; Saxagliptin; Sildenafil; Silodosin; Simeprevir; Simvastatin; SORAfenib; Suvorexant; Tacrolimus (Systemic); Tacrolimus (Topical); Tadalafil; Tamsulosin; Telaprevir; Temsirolimus; Tenofovir; Terfenadine; Tetrahydrocannabinol; Ticagrelor; Tofacitinib; Tolterodine; Tolvaptan; Topotecan; Toremifene; Trabectedin; TraZODone; Triazolam; Tricyclic Antidepressants; Ulipristal; Vardenafil; Vemurafenib; Vilazodone; VinCRIStine (Liposomal); Vorapaxar; Warfarin; Zopiclone; Zuclopenthixol

The levels/effects of Darunavir and Cobicistat may be increased by: Clarithromycin; Conivaptan; CycloSPORINE (Systemic); CYP3A4 Inhibitors (Moderate); CYP3A4 Inhibitors (Strong); Delavirdine; Enfuvirtide; Etravirine; Fusidic Acid (Systemic); Idelalisib; Itraconazole; Ketoconazole (Systemic); Luliconazole; Mifepristone; Netupitant; Rifabutin; Simeprevir; Stiripentol; Tenofovir

Decreased Effect

Darunavir and Cobicistat may decrease the levels/effects of: Abacavir; Clarithromycin; Contraceptives (Estrogens); Contraceptives (Progestins); Delavirdine; Didanosine; Etravirine; Ifosfamide; Meperidine; Methadone; Norethindrone; PARoxetine; Prasugrel; Sertraline; Telaprevir; Ticagrelor; Valproic Acid and Derivatives; Voriconazole; Warfarin; Zidovudine

The levels/effects of Darunavir and Cobicistat may be decreased by: Bosentan; CarBAMazepine; CYP3A4 Inducers (Moderate); CYP3A4 Inducers (Strong); Dabrafenib; Deferasirox; Dexamethasone (Systemic); Efavirenz; Fosphenytoin; Fosphenytoin-Phenytoin; Garlic; Lopinavir; Mitotane; OXcarbazepine; PHENobarbital; Rifampin; Rifapentine; Saquinavir; Siltuximab; St Johns Wort; Telaprevir; Tipranavir; Tocilizumab

Food Interactions Absorption and bioavailability of darunavir are increased when administered with food. Management: Take with meals.

Storage/Stability Store at 20°C to 25°C (68°F to77°F); excursions are permitted between 15°C and 30°C (59°F and 86°F).

Mechanism of Action Darunavir binds to the site of HIV-1 protease activity and inhibits cleavage of viral Gag-Pol polyprotein precursors into individual functional proteins required for infectious HIV. This results in the formation of immature, noninfectious viral particles.

Cobicistat is a mechanism-based inhibitor of cytochrome P450 3A (CYP3A). Inhibition of CYP3A-mediated metabolism by cobicistat and increases the systemic exposure of CYP3A substrates (eg, darunavir).

Pharmacodynamics/Kinetics Refer to individual monographs.

Dosage Note: Genotype testing is advised prior to therapy initiation; if testing is not feasible, use is recommended in protease-inhibitor naïve patients only. Dosage modifications are not possible with darunavir/cobicistat combination tablet.

HIV-1 infection: Adults (treatment-naive or treatment-experienced without darunavir resistance-associated substitutions; **Note:** For treatment-experienced patients, the Canadian labeling indicates use in patients without any darunavir resistant-associated substitutions): Oral: One tablet (darunavir 800 mg/cobicistat 150 mg) once daily. **Note:** Administer with other antiretroviral agents.

Missed dose: If <12 hours, take dose as soon as possible; if >12 hours resume at next regularly scheduled time.

Dosage adjustment in renal impairment:

US labeling: There are no dosage adjustments provided in the manufacturer's labeling. If CrCl <70 mL/minute, do not coadminister as part of a regimen that includes tenofovir disoproxil fumarate.

Canadian labeling: No dosage adjustment necessary. If CrCl <70 mL/minute, do not coadminister as part of regimens that include emtricitabine, lamivudine, tenofovir disoproxil fumarate, or adefovir.

Dosage adjustment in hepatic impairment:

Mild to moderate impairment (Child-Pugh class A or B): There are no dosage adjustments provided in the manufacturer's labeling (has not been studied); pharmacokinetic data with darunavir and cobicistat (as individual agents) suggest that dosage adjustment is not necessary.

Severe impairment (Child-Pugh class C):

U.S. labeling: Use is not recommended.

Canadian labeling: Use is contraindicated.

Dietary Considerations Take with meals.

Administration Administer with food. The Canadian labeling indicates that the tablet should be swallowed whole and not be crushed or broken.

Monitoring Parameters Viral load, baseline genotyping in treatment-experienced patients (if possible); serum glucose; liver function prior to and during therapy (increase monitoring in patients at risk for liver impairment), cholesterol, triglycerides; CBC with differential, reticulocyte count, CD4 count, serum creatinine at baseline and when clinically indicated during therapy; when coadministered with tenofovir, serum creatinine, urine glucose, and urine protein prior to initiation and as clinically indicated during therapy; assess serum phosphorus in patients with or at risk for renal impairment. Patients who experience a confirmed increase in serum creatinine >0.4 mg/dL from baseline should have renal function monitored closely. Testing for HBV is recommended prior to the initiation of antiretroviral therapy.

Dosage Forms

Tablet, Oral:

Prezcobix: Darunavir 800 mg and cobicistat 150 mg

◆ **Darunavir Ethanolate** *see* Darunavir *on page 569*

◆ **Dasabuvir, Ombitasvir, Paritaprevir, and Ritonavir** *see* Ombitasvir, Paritaprevir, Ritonavir, and Dasabuvir *on page 1505*

Dasatinib (da SA ti nib)

Brand Names: U.S. Sprycel

Brand Names: Canada Sprycel

Index Terms BMS-354825

Pharmacologic Category Antineoplastic Agent, BCR-ABL Tyrosine Kinase Inhibitor; Antineoplastic Agent, Tyrosine Kinase Inhibitor

Use

Acute lymphoblastic leukemia: Treatment of Philadelphia chromosome-positive (Ph+) acute lymphoblastic leukemia (ALL) with resistance or intolerance to prior therapy.

Chronic myeloid leukemia: Treatment of newly diagnosed Ph+ chronic myeloid leukemia (CML) in chronic phase; treatment of chronic, accelerated, or myeloid or lymphoid blast phase Ph+ CML with resistance or intolerance to prior therapy, including imatinib.

Pregnancy Risk Factor D

Pregnancy Considerations Animal reproduction studies have demonstrated fetal abnormalities (skeletal malformations, reduced ossification, edema, microhepatia) and fetal death. May cause fetal harm if administered to a pregnant woman. Not recommended for use during pregnancy or if contemplating pregnancy. Effective contraception is recommended for men and women of childbearing potential. Pregnant women are advised to avoid contact with crushed or broken tablets.

Breast-Feeding Considerations Due to the potential for serious adverse reactions in the nursing infant, the decision to discontinue dasatinib or to discontinue breast-feeding should take into account the benefits of treatment to the mother.

Contraindications

U.S. labeling: There are no contraindications listed within the FDA-approved manufacturer's labeling.

Canadian labeling: Hypersensitivity to dasatinib or any other component of the formulation; breast-feeding

Warnings/Precautions Hazardous agent - use appropriate precautions for handling and disposal (NIOSH 2014 [group 1]). Severe dose-related bone marrow suppression (thrombocytopenia, neutropenia, anemia) is associated with treatment (usually reversible); dosage adjustment or temporary interruption may be required for severe myelosuppression; the incidence of myelosuppression is higher in patients with advanced CML and Ph+ ALL. Monitor blood counts weekly for the first 2 months, then monthly thereafter (or as clinically necessary). Fatal intracranial and GI hemorrhage have been reported in association with dasatinib use. Severe hemorrhage (including CNS, GI) may occur due to thrombocytopenia; in addition to thrombocytopenia, dasatinib may also cause platelet dysfunction. Potentially significant drug-drug interactions may exist, requiring dose or frequency adjustment, additional monitoring, and/or selection of alternative therapy. Use caution with patients taking anticoagulants or medications interfering with platelet function; not studied in clinical trials. Avoid concomitant use with CYP3A4 inducers and inhibitors; if concomitant use cannot be avoided, consider dasatinib dosage adjustments. Elevated gastric pH may reduce dasatinib bioavailability; avoid concomitant use with proton pump inhibitors and H_2 blockers. If needed, may consider antacid administration at least 2 hours before or 2 hours after the dasatinib dose.

Cardiomyopathy, diastolic dysfunction, heart failure (congestive), left ventricular dysfunction, and MI have been reported; monitor for signs and symptoms of cardiac dysfunction. Fluid retention, including pleural and pericardial effusions, severe ascites, severe pulmonary edema, and generalized edema were reported; may be dose-related. A chest x-ray is recommended for symptoms suggestive of effusion (dyspnea or dry cough). Fluid retention may be managed with supportive care (diuretics or corticosteroids); thoracentesis and oxygen therapy may be necessary for severe fluid retention. Utilizing once-daily dosing is associated with a decreased frequency of fluid retention. The risk for pleural effusion is increased in patients with hypertension, prior cardiac history and a twice a day administration schedule; interrupt treatment for grade ≥2 effusion; may consider reinitiating at a reduced dose after resolution (Quintás-Cardama, 2007). Use caution in patients where fluid accumulation may be poorly tolerated, such as in cardiovascular disease (HF or hypertension) and pulmonary disease. Patients 65 years of age and older are more likely to experience toxicity (compared with younger patients). Pulmonary arterial hypertension (PAH) has been reported with use, sometimes after >12 months of therapy. Evaluate for underlying cardiopulmonary disease prior to therapy initiation and during therapy; evaluate and rule out alternative etiologies in patients with symptoms suggestive of PAH (eg, dyspnea, fatigue, hypoxia, fluid retention) and interrupt therapy if symptoms are severe. Discontinue permanently with confirmed PAH diagnosis.

May prolong QT interval; use caution in patients at risk for QT prolongation, including patients with long QT syndrome, patients taking antiarrhythmic medications or other medications that lead to QT prolongation or potassium-wasting diuretics, patients with cumulative high-dose anthracycline therapy, and conditions which cause hypokalemia or hypomagnesemia. Correct hypokalemia and hypomagnesemia prior to initiation of therapy. Use caution with hepatic impairment due to extensive hepatic metabolism.

Adverse Reactions

Cardiovascular: Cardiac arrhythmia, cardiac disease (includes cardiac failure, cardiomyopathy, diastolic dysfunction, ejection fraction decreased, left ventricular dysfunction, ventricular failure), chest pain, edema (generalized), flushing, hypertension, palpitations, pericardial effusion, prolonged Q-T interval on ECG, tachycardia

Central nervous system: Central nervous system toxicity (bleeding), chills, depression, dizziness, drowsiness, fatigue, headache, insomnia, myasthenia, neuropathy, pain, peripheral neuropathy

Dermatologic: Acne vulgaris, alopecia, dermatitis, eczema, hyperhidrosis, pruritus, skin rash (includes drug eruption, erythema, erythema multiforme, erythematous rash, erythrosis, exfoliative rash, follicular rash, heat rash, macular rash, maculopapular rash, milia, papular rash, pruritic rash, pustular rash, skin exfoliation, skin irritation, urticaria vesiculosa, vesicular rash), urticaria, xeroderma

Endocrine & metabolic: Fluid retention, hypocalcemia, hypokalemia, hypophosphatemia, weight gain, weight loss

Gastrointestinal: Abdominal distention, abdominal pain, anorexia, change in appetite, colitis (including neutropenic colitis), constipation, diarrhea, dysgeusia, dyspepsia, enterocolitis, gastritis, gastrointestinal hemorrhage, mucositis, nausea, stomatitis, vomiting

Hematologic & oncologic: Anemia, bruise, febrile neutropenia, hemorrhage, neutropenia, pancytopenia, thrombocytopenia

Hepatic: Ascites, increased serum ALT, increased serum AST, increased serum bilirubin

Infection: Herpes virus infection, increased susceptibility to infection (includes bacterial, fungal, viral), sepsis

Local: Localized edema (superficial)

Neuromuscular & skeletal: Arthralgia, muscle spasm, musculoskeletal pain, myalgia, myositis, stiffness, weakness

Ophthalmic: Blurred vision, decreased visual acuity, dry eye syndrome, visual disturbance

Otic: Tinnitus

Renal: Hyperuricemia, increased serum creatinine

Respiratory: Cough, pneumonia (bacterial, viral, or fungal), dyspnea, pleural effusion, pneumonitis, pulmonary edema, pulmonary hypertension, pulmonary infiltrates, upper respiratory tract infection

Miscellaneous: Fever, soft tissue injury (oral)

Rare but important or life-threatening: Abnormal platelet aggregation, acute coronary syndrome, acute respiratory distress, amnesia, anal fissure, angina pectoris, asthma, atrial fibrillation, atrial flutter, bullous skin disease, cardiomegaly, cerebrovascular accident, cholecystitis, cholestasis, conjunctivitis, cor pulmonale, cranial nerve palsy (facial), decreased libido, deep vein thrombosis, dermal ulcer, dyschromia, dysphagia, embolism, erythema nodosum, esophagitis, gynecomastia, hematoma, hematuria, hemorrhage (ocular), hepatitis, hypersensitivity, hypoalbuminemia, hypotension, increased pulmonary artery pressure, inflammation (panniculitis), interstitial pulmonary disease, intestinal obstruction, intolerance to temperature, livedo reticularis, myocardial infarction, myocarditis, optic neuritis, palmar-plantar erythrodysesthesia, pancreatitis, pericarditis, polyuria, proteinuria, pulmonary embolism, pure red cell aplasia, renal failure, rhabdomyolysis, seizure, skin photosensitivity, Sweet's syndrome, syncope, tendonitis, thrombophlebitis, thrombosis, transient ischemic attacks, tumor lysis syndrome, upper gastrointestinal tract ulcer, ventricular arrhythmia, ventricular tachycardia

Drug Interactions

Metabolism/Transport Effects **Substrate** of CYP3A4 (major); **Note:** Assignment of Major/Minor substrate status based on clinically relevant drug interaction potential; **Inhibits** CYP3A4 (weak)

Avoid Concomitant Use

Avoid concomitant use of Dasatinib with any of the following: BCG; CloZAPine; Conivaptan; Dipyrone; Fusidic Acid (Systemic); H2-Antagonists; Idelalisib; Natalizumab; Pimecrolimus; Pimozide; Proton Pump Inhibitors; St Johns Wort; Tacrolimus (Topical); Tofacitinib; Vaccines (Live)

Increased Effect/Toxicity

Dasatinib may increase the levels/effects of: Acetaminophen; Agents with Antiplatelet Properties; Anticoagulants; ARIPiprazole; CloZAPine; CYP3A4 Substrates; Highest Risk QTc-Prolonging Agents; Hydrocodone; Leflunomide; Lomitapide; Moderate Risk QTc-Prolonging Agents; Natalizumab; Pimozide; Tofacitinib; Vaccines (Live)

The levels/effects of Dasatinib may be increased by: Acetaminophen; Aprepitant; Ceritinib; Conivaptan; CYP3A4 Inhibitors (Moderate); CYP3A4 Inhibitors (Strong); Denosumab; Dipyrone; Fosaprepitant; Fusidic Acid (Systemic); Idelalisib; Ivacaftor; Luliconazole; Mifepristone; Netupitant; Pimecrolimus; Roflumilast;

Simeprevir; Stiripentol; Tacrolimus (Topical); Trastuzumab; Voriconazole

Decreased Effect

Dasatinib may decrease the levels/effects of: BCG; Coccidioides immitis Skin Test; Sipuleucel-T; Vaccines (Inactivated); Vaccines (Live)

The levels/effects of Dasatinib may be decreased by: Antacids; Bosentan; CYP3A4 Inducers (Moderate); CYP3A4 Inducers (Strong); Dabrafenib; Deferasirox; Dexamethasone (Systemic); Echinacea; H2-Antagonists; Mitotane; Proton Pump Inhibitors; Siltuximab; St Johns Wort; Tocilizumab

Food Interactions Dasatinib serum concentrations may be increased when taken with grapefruit or grapefruit juice. Management: Avoid concurrent use.

Storage/Stability Store at 20°C to 25°C (68°F to 77°F); excursions permitted to 15°C to 30°C (59°F to 86°F).

Mechanism of Action BCR-ABL tyrosine kinase inhibitor; targets most imatinib-resistant BCR-ABL mutations (except the T315I and F317V mutants) by distinctly binding to active and inactive ABL-kinase. Kinase inhibition halts proliferation of leukemia cells. Also inhibits SRC family (including SRC, LKC, YES, FYN); c-KIT, EPHA2 and platelet derived growth factor receptor (PDGFRβ)

Pharmacodynamics/Kinetics

Distribution: 2505 L

Protein binding: Dasatinib: 96%; metabolite (active): 93%

Metabolism: Hepatic (extensive); metabolized by CYP3A4 (primarily), flavin-containing mono-oxygenase-3 (FOM-3) and uridine diphosphate-glucuronosyltransferase (UGT) to an active metabolite and other inactive metabolites (the active metabolite plays only a minor role in the pharmacology of dasatinib)

Half-life elimination: Terminal: 3 to 5 hours

Time to peak, plasma: 0.5 to 6 hours

Excretion: Feces (~85%, 19% as unchanged drug); urine (~4%, 0.1% as unchanged drug)

Dosage Note: The effect of discontinuation after complete cytogenetic remission is achieved has not been studied.

Chronic myelogenous leukemia (CML), Philadelphia chromosome-positive (Ph+), newly-diagnosed in chronic phase: Adults: Oral: 100 mg once daily until disease progression or unacceptable toxicity. In clinical studies, a dose escalation to 140 mg once daily was allowed in patients not achieving hematologic or cytogenetic response at recommended initial dosage.

CML, Ph+, resistant or intolerant: Adults: Oral:

Chronic phase: 100 mg once daily until disease progression or unacceptable toxicity. In clinical studies, a dose escalation to 140 mg once daily was allowed in patients not achieving hematologic or cytogenetic response at recommended initial dosage.

Accelerated or blast phase: 140 mg once daily until disease progression or unacceptable toxicity. In clinical studies, a dose escalation to 180 mg once daily was allowed in patients not achieving hematologic or cytogenetic response at recommended initial dosage.

Acute lymphoblastic lymphoma (ALL), Ph+: Adults: Oral: 140 mg once daily until disease progression or unacceptable toxicity. In clinical studies, a dose escalation to 180 mg once daily was allowed in patients not achieving hematologic or cytogenetic response at recommended initial dosage.

Gastrointestinal stromal tumor (GIST; off-label use): Adults: Oral: 70 mg twice daily (Montemurro, 2012; Trent, 2011).

Missed doses: A missed dose should be taken at the next scheduled regular time; 2 doses should not be taken at the same time.

Dosage adjustment for concomitant CYP3A4 inhibitors: Avoid concomitant administration with strong CYP3A4 inhibitors (eg, clarithromycin, itraconazole, ketoconazole, nefazodone, protease inhibitors, telithromycin, voriconazole, grapefruit juice); if concomitant administration with a strong CYP3A4 inhibitor cannot be avoided, consider reducing dasatinib from 100 mg once daily to 20 mg once daily **or** from 140 mg once daily to 40 mg once daily, with careful monitoring. If reduced dose is not tolerated, the strong CYP3A4 inhibitor must be discontinued or dasatinib therapy temporarily held until concomitant inhibitor use has ceased. When a strong CYP3A4 inhibitor is discontinued, allow a washout period (~1 week) prior to adjusting dasatinib dose upward.

Dosage adjustment for concomitant CYP3A4 inducers: Avoid concomitant administration with strong CYP3A4 inducers (eg, carbamazepine, dexamethasone, phenobarbital, phenytoin, rifabutin, rifampin, St John's wort); if concomitant administration with a strong CYP3A4 inducer cannot be avoided, consider increasing the dasatinib dose with careful monitoring.

Dosage adjustment for toxicity:

Hematologic toxicity: Note: Growth factor support may be considered in patients with resistant myelosuppression.

Chronic phase CML (100 mg daily starting dose): For ANC <500/mm^3 or platelets <50,000/mm^3, withhold treatment until ANC ≥1000/mm^3 and platelets ≥50,000/mm^3; then resume treatment at the original starting dose if recovery occurs in ≤7 days. If platelets <25,000/mm^3 or recurrence of ANC <500/mm^3 for >7 days, withhold treatment until ANC ≥1000/mm^3 and platelets ≥50,000/mm^3; then resume treatment at 80 mg once daily (second episode). For third episode, further reduce dose to 50 mg once daily (for newly diagnosed patients) or discontinue (for patients resistant or intolerant to prior therapy)

Accelerated or blast phase CML and Ph+ ALL (140 mg once daily starting dose): For ANC <500/mm^3 or platelets <10,000/mm^3, if cytopenia unrelated to leukemia, withhold treatment until ANC ≥1000/mm^3 and platelets ≥20,000/mm^3; then resume treatment at the original starting dose. If cytopenia recurs, withhold treatment until ANC ≥1000/mm^3 and platelets ≥20,000/mm^3; then resume treatment at 100 mg once daily (second episode) or 80 mg once daily (third episode). For cytopenias related to leukemia (confirm with marrow aspirate or biopsy), consider dose escalation to 180 mg once daily.

Nonhematologic toxicity: Withhold treatment until toxicity improvement or resolution; if appropriate, resume treatment at a reduced dose based on the event severity. Fluid retention is managed with diuretics and supportive care. Effusions may require diuretics and/or dose interruption. Corticosteroids (eg, prednisone 20 mg/day for 3 days) may be considered for pleural or pericardial effusion with significant symptoms (hold dasatinib and reinitiate at a decreased dose when effusion resolves). Rash may be managed with steroids (topical or systemic), treatment interruption, dose reduction, or discontinuation (NCCN CML guidelines v.3.2014). Discontinue with confirmed pulmonary arterial hypertension.

Dosage adjustment for renal impairment: There are no dosage adjustments provided in the manufacturer's labeling. However, <4% of dasatinib and metabolites are renally excreted.

Dosage adjustment for hepatic impairment: No dosage adjustment is necessary; use with caution.

Dietary Considerations Avoid grapefruit juice.

Administration Administer once daily (morning or evening). May be taken without regard to food. Swallow whole; do not break, crush, or chew tablets. Take with a meal or with a large glass of water if GI upset occurs (NCCN CML v.3.2014).

Hazardous agent; use appropriate precautions for handling and disposal (NIOSH 2014 [group 1]).

Monitoring Parameters CBC with differential (weekly for 2 months, then monthly or as clinically necessary); bone marrow biopsy; liver function tests, electrolytes including calcium, phosphorus, magnesium; monitor for fluid retention; monitor for signs/symptoms of cardiac dysfunction; ECG monitoring if at risk for QTc prolongation; chest x-ray is recommended for symptoms suggestive of pleural effusion (eg, cough, dyspnea)

Thyroid function testing recommendations (Hamnvik, 2011):

Preexisting levothyroxine therapy: Obtain baseline TSH levels, then monitor every 4 weeks until levels and levothyroxine dose are stable, then monitor every 2 months

Without preexisting thyroid hormone replacement: TSH at baseline, then monthly for 4 months, then every 2-3 months

Dosage Forms

Tablet, Oral:

Sprycel: 20 mg, 50 mg, 70 mg, 80 mg, 100 mg, 140 mg

Extemporaneous Preparations Hazardous agent: Use appropriate precautions for handling and disposal (NIOSH 2014 [group 1]).

An oral suspension may be prepared by dissolving dasatinib tablet(s) for one dose in 30 mL chilled orange or apple juice (without preservatives). After 5 minutes, swirl the contents for 3 seconds and repeat the process every 5 minutes for a total of 20 minutes following addition of tablet(s). Minimize time between end of 20 minutes and administration since suspension will taste more bitter if allowed to stand longer. Swirl contents of container one last time, then administer immediately. To ensure the full dose is administered, rinse container with 15 mL juice and administer residue. May be administered orally (or by nasogastric tube). Discard any unused portion after 60 minutes.

Sprycel data on file, Bristol-Myers Squibb

- **Dasetta 1/35** *see* Ethinyl Estradiol and Norethindrone *on page 808*
- **Dasetta 7/7/7** *see* Ethinyl Estradiol and Norethindrone *on page 808*
- **Daunomycin** *see* DAUNOrubicin (Conventional) *on page 577*
- **DAUNOrubicin Citrate** *see* DAUNOrubicin (Liposomal) *on page 580*
- **DAUNOrubicin Citrate (Liposomal)** *see* DAUNOrubicin (Liposomal) *on page 580*
- **DAUNOrubicin Citrate Liposome** *see* DAUNOrubicin (Liposomal) *on page 580*

DAUNOrubicin (Conventional)

(daw noe ROO bi sin con VEN sha nal)

Brand Names: Canada Cerubidine; Daunorubicin Hydrochloride for Injection

Index Terms Cerubidine; Conventional Daunomycin; Daunomycin; DAUNOrubicin Hydrochloride; Rubidomycin Hydrochloride

Pharmacologic Category Antineoplastic Agent, Anthracycline; Antineoplastic Agent, Topoisomerase II Inhibitor

Use

Acute lymphocytic leukemia: Treatment (remission induction) of acute lymphocytic leukemia (ALL) in children and adults (in combination with other chemotherapy)

Acute myeloid leukemia: Treatment (remission induction) of acute myeloid leukemia (AML) in adults (in combination with other chemotherapy)

Pregnancy Risk Factor D

Pregnancy Considerations Adverse events have been observed in animal reproduction studies. Daunorubicin crosses the placenta. Women of reproductive potential should avoid pregnancy.

Breast-Feeding Considerations It is not known if daunorubicin is excreted into breast milk. Due to the potential for serious adverse reactions in the nursing infant, the manufacturer recommends a decision be made whether to discontinue nursing or to discontinue the drug, taking into account the importance of treatment to the mother.

Contraindications Hypersensitivity to daunorubicin or any component of the formulation

Warnings/Precautions Hazardous agent - use appropriate precautions for handling and disposal (NIOSH 2014 [group 1]). **[U.S. Boxed Warning]: Potent vesicant; if extravasation occurs, severe local tissue damage leading to ulceration and necrosis, and pain may occur. For IV administration only. NOT for IM or SubQ administration. Administer through a rapidly flowing IV line.** Ensure proper needle or catheter placement prior to and during infusion. Avoid extravasation. **[U.S. Boxed Warning]: Severe bone marrow suppression may occur when used at therapeutic doses; may lead to infection or hemorrhage.** Use with caution in patients with drug-induced bone marrow suppression (preexisting), unless the therapy benefit outweighs the toxicity risk. Monitor blood counts at baseline and frequently during therapy.

[U.S. Boxed Warning]: May cause cumulative, dose-related myocardial toxicity; may lead to heart failure. May occur either during treatment or may be delayed (months to years after cessations of treatment). The incidence of irreversible myocardial toxicity increases as the total cumulative (lifetime) dosages approach 550 mg/m^2 in adults, 400 mg/m^2 in adults receiving chest radiation, 300 mg/m^2 in children >2 years of age, or 10 mg/kg in children <2 years of age. Total cumulative dose should take into account prior treatment with other anthracyclines or anthracenediones, previous or concomitant treatment with cardiotoxic agents or irradiation of chest. Although the risk increases with cumulative dose, irreversible cardiotoxicity may occur at any dose level. Patients with preexisting heart disease, hypertension, concurrent administration of other antineoplastic agents, prior or concurrent chest irradiation, advanced age; and infants and children are at increased risk. Monitor left ventricular (LV) function (baseline and periodic) with ECHO or MUGA scan; monitor ECG. Cardiotoxicity may occur more frequently in elderly patients. Use with caution in patients with impaired renal function and/or poor marrow reserve due to advanced age; dosage adjustment may be necessary. Infants and children are at increased risk for developing delayed cardiotoxicity; long-term periodic cardiac function monitoring is recommended.

[U.S. Boxed Warning]: Dosage reductions are recommended in patients with renal or hepatic impairment; significant impairment may result in increased toxicities. May cause tumor lysis syndrome and hyperuricemia. Urinary alkalinization and prophylaxis with an antihyperuricemic agent may be necessary. Monitor electrolytes, renal function, and hydration status. Use with caution in patients who have received radiation therapy; reduce dosage in patients who are receiving radiation therapy simultaneously. Secondary leukemias may occur when used with combination chemotherapy or radiation therapy. **[U.S. Boxed Warning]: Should be administered under the supervision of an experienced cancer chemotherapy physician.** Use caution when selecting product for preparation and dispensing; indications, dosages, and adverse event profiles differ between conventional daunorubicin hydrochloride solution and daunorubicin liposomal.

Potentially significant drug-drug interactions may exist, requiring dose or frequency adjustment, additional monitoring, and/or selection of alternative therapy.

Adverse Reactions

Cardiovascular: Transient ECG abnormalities (supraventricular tachycardia, S-T wave changes, atrial or ventricular extrasystoles); generally asymptomatic and self-limiting. CHF, dose related, may be delayed for 7-8 years after treatment

Dermatologic: Alopecia (reversible); discoloration of saliva, sweat, or tears, radiation recall, skin "flare" at injection site

Endocrine & metabolic: Hyperuricemia

Gastrointestinal: Abdominal pain, diarrhea, GI ulceration, diarrhea, mild nausea or vomiting, stomatitis

Genitourinary: Discoloration of urine (red)

Hematologic: Myelosuppression (onset: 7 days; nadir: 10-14 days; recovery: 21-28 days), primarily leukopenia; thrombocytopenia and anemia

Rare but important or life-threatening: Anaphylactoid reaction, arrhythmia, bilirubin increased, cardiomyopathy, hepatitis, infertility; local (cellulitis, pain, thrombophlebitis at injection site); MI, myocarditis, neutropenic typhlitis, pericarditis, secondary leukemia, skin rash, sterility, systemic hypersensitivity (including urticaria, pruritus, angioedema, dysphagia, dyspnea); transaminases increased

Drug Interactions

Metabolism/Transport Effects **Substrate** of P-glycoprotein

Avoid Concomitant Use

Avoid concomitant use of DAUNOrubicin (Conventional) with any of the following: BCG; CloZAPine; Dipyrone; Natalizumab; Pimecrolimus; Tacrolimus (Topical); Tofacitinib; Vaccines (Live)

Increased Effect/Toxicity

DAUNOrubicin (Conventional) may increase the levels/effects of: CloZAPine; Leflunomide; Natalizumab; Tofacitinib; Vaccines (Live)

The levels/effects of DAUNOrubicin (Conventional) may be increased by: Bevacizumab; Cyclophosphamide; Denosumab; Dipyrone; P-glycoprotein/ABCB1 Inhibitors; Pimecrolimus; Roflumilast; Tacrolimus (Topical); Taxane Derivatives; Trastuzumab

Decreased Effect

DAUNOrubicin (Conventional) may decrease the levels/effects of: BCG; Cardiac Glycosides; Coccidioides immitis Skin Test; Sipuleucel-T; Vaccines (Inactivated); Vaccines (Live)

The levels/effects of DAUNOrubicin (Conventional) may be decreased by: Cardiac Glycosides; Echinacea; P-glycoprotein/ABCB1 Inducers

Preparation for Administration Hazardous agent; use appropriate precautions for handling and disposal (NIOSH 2014 [group 1]). Dilute vials of powder for injection [Canadian product] with 4 mL SWFI for a final concentration of 5 mg/mL. May further dilute solution or reconstituted daunorubicin solution in D_5W or NS for infusion.

Storage/Stability

Solution: Store intact vials at 2°C to 8°C (36°F to 46°F). Protect from light. Retain in carton until time of use. Solution prepared for infusion may be stored at 20°C to 25°C (68°F to 77°F) for up to 24 hours. Discard unused portion.

Lyophilized powder [Canadian product]: Store intact vials of powder at 15°C to 30°C (59°F to 86°F). Protect from light. Retain in carton until time of use. Reconstituted daunorubicin is stable for 24 hours at room temperature or 48 hours when refrigerated at 2°C to 8°C (36°F to 46°F). Protect reconstituted solution from light.

Mechanism of Action Inhibits DNA and RNA synthesis by intercalation between DNA base pairs and by steric obstruction. Daunomycin intercalates at points of local uncoiling of the double helix. Although the exact mechanism is unclear, it appears that direct binding to DNA (intercalation) and inhibition of DNA repair (topoisomerase II inhibition) result in blockade of DNA and RNA synthesis and fragmentation of DNA.

Pharmacodynamics/Kinetics

Distribution: Distributes widely into tissues, particularly the liver, kidneys, lung, spleen, and heart; does not distribute into the CNS

Metabolism: Primarily hepatic to daunorubicinol (active), then to inactive aglycones, conjugated sulfates, and glucuronides

Half-life elimination: Initial: 45 minutes; Terminal: 18.5 hours; Daunorubicinol plasma half-life: ~27 hours

Excretion: Feces (40%); urine (~25% as unchanged drug and metabolites)

Dosage Daunorubicin is associated with a moderate emetic potential; antiemetics are recommended to prevent nausea and vomiting (Basch, 2011; Dupuis, 2011; Roila, 2010).

Manufacturer's labeling:

Children: **Note:** Cumulative doses above 300 mg/m^2 in children >2 years or 10 mg/kg in children <2 years of age are associated with an increased risk of cardiomyopathy.

Acute lymphocytic leukemia (ALL):

Children <2 years or BSA <0.5 m^2: Remission induction: IV: 1 mg/kg/dose on day 1 every week for up to 4 to 6 cycles (in combination with vincristine and prednisone)

Children ≥2 years and BSA ≥0.5 m^2: Remission induction: IV: 25 mg/m^2 on day 1 every week for up to 4 to 6 cycles (in combination with vincristine and prednisone)

Adults: **Note:** Cumulative doses above 550 mg/m^2 in adults without risk factors for cardiotoxicity and above 400 mg/m^2 in adults receiving chest irradiation are associated with an increased risk of cardiomyopathy.

ALL: Adults: IV: 45 mg/m^2 on days 1, 2, and 3 (in combination with vincristine, prednisone, and asparaginase)

Acute myeloid leukemia (AML):

Adults <60 years: Induction: IV: 45 mg/m^2 on days 1, 2, and 3 of the first course of induction therapy; subsequent courses: 45 mg/m^2 on days 1 and 2 (in combination with cytarabine)

Adults ≥60 years: Induction: IV: 30 mg/m^2 on days 1, 2, and 3 of the first course of induction therapy; subsequent courses: 30 mg/m^2 on days 1 and 2 (in combination with cytarabine)

Indication-specific dosing (off-label dosing):

ALL:

CALGB 8811 regimen: Adults: IV: 45 mg/m^2 (in patients <60 years) or 30 mg/m^2 (in patients ≥60 years) on days 1, 2, and 3 of induction (Course I; 4 week cycle), in combination with cyclophosphamide, prednisone, vincristine, and asparaginase (Larson, 1995)

CCG 1961: Children ≥10 years, Adolescents, and Adults ≤21 years: IV: Induction: 25 mg/m^2 once weekly for 4 weeks (in combination with vincristine, prednisone, and asparaginase) (Nachman, 2009)

GRAALL-2003: Adolescents ≥15 years and Adults ≤60 years: IV:

Induction: 50 mg/m^2 on days 1, 2, and 3 **and** 30 mg/m^2 on days 15 and 16 (in combination with prednisone, vincristine, asparaginase, cyclophosphamide, and G-CSF support) (Huguet, 2009)

Late intensification: 30 mg/m^2 on days 1, 2, and 3 (in combination with prednisone, vincristine, asparaginase, cyclophosphamide, and G-CSF support) (Huguet, 2009)

MRC UKALLXII/ECOG E2993: Adolescents ≥15 years and Adults <60 years: IV: Induction (Phase I): 60 mg/m^2 on days 1, 8, 15, and 22 (in combination with vincristine, asparaginase, and prednisone) (Rowe, 2005)

PETHEMA ALL-96: Adolescents ≥15 years and Adults ≤30 years: IV:

Induction: 30 mg/m^2 on days 1, 8, 15, and 22 (in combination with vincristine, prednisone, asparaginase, and cyclophosphamide) (Ribera, 2008)

Consolidation-2/Reinduction: 30 mg/m^2 on days 1, 2, 8, and 9 (in combination with vincristine, dexamethasone, asparaginase, and cyclophosphamide) (Ribera, 2008)

Protocol 8707: Adults ≤60 years: IV: Induction and Consolidation 2A cycles: 60 mg/m^2 on days 1, 2, and 3 (in combination with vincristine, prednisone, and asparaginase). An additional 60 mg/m^2 daunorubicin dose may be administered on day 15 of induction if bone marrow biopsy on day 14 shows residual disease (Linker, 2002).

AML: Induction:

MRC AML 10/12: Children ≤14 years: IV: 50 mg/m^2 on days 1, 3, and 5 for 2 cycles (in combination with cytarabine and etoposide) (Gibson, 2005)

CCG 2891:

Children <3 years: IV: 0.67 mg/kg/day continuous infusion on days 0 to 4 and 10 to 14 (in combination with dexamethasone, cytarabine, thioguanine, and etoposide) (Woods, 1996)

Children ≥3 years, Adolescents and Adults <21 years: IV: 20 mg/m^2/day continuous infusion on days 0 to 4 and 10 to 14 (in combination with dexamethasone, cytarabine, thioguanine, and etoposide) (Woods, 1996)

Adults <60 years: IV: 90 mg/m^2 on days 1, 2, and 3 (in combination with cytarabine). If residual disease was observed on day 12 to day 14 bone marrow biopsy, 45 mg/m^2 for 3 days was administered (in combination with cytarabine) (Fernandez, 2009).

Adults <60 years: IV: 60 mg/m^2 on days 1, 2, and 3 (in combination with cytarabine and cladribine); may repeat if partial remission occurs (Holowiecki, 2012).

Adults ≥60 years: IV: 45 or 90 mg/m^2 on days 1, 2, and 3 (in combination with cytarabine); the escalated 90 mg/m^2 dose was associated with increased remission rates and overall survival in the subgroup of patients 60 to 65 years of age as compared to patients >65 years (Lowenberg, 2009)

Acute promyelocytic leukemia (APL):

Induction: Adults: IV: 50 mg/m^2 on days 3, 4, 5, and 6 (in combination with ATRA and cytarabine) (Powell, 2010) **or** 60 mg/m^2 on days 1, 2, and 3 (in combination with ATRA and cytarabine) (Ades, 2008)

Consolidation: Adults: IV: 50 mg/m^2 on days 1, 2, and 3 for 2 cycles (in combination with ATRA; arsenic trioxide was administered for 2 cycles prior to daunorubicin and ATRA) (Powell, 2010) **or** 60 mg/m^2 on days 1, 2, and 3 during cycle 1 of consolidation (in combination with cytarabine), followed by 45 mg/m^2 on days 1, 2, and 3 during cycle 2 of consolidation (in combination with cytarabine) (Ades, 2008)

Dosage adjustment in renal impairment:

The manufacturer's labeling recommends the following adjustment: S_{cr} >3 mg/dL: Administer 50% of normal dose

The following adjustments have also been recommended (Aronoff, 2007):

Children:

CrCl <30 mL/minute: Administer 50% of dose

Hemodialysis/continuous ambulatory peritoneal dialysis (CAPD): Administer 50% of dose

Adults: No dosage adjustment necessary.

Dosage adjustment in hepatic impairment:

The manufacturer's labeling recommends the following adjustments:

Serum bilirubin 1.2 to 3 mg/dL: Administer 75% of dose

Serum bilirubin >3 mg/dL: Administer 50% of dose

The following adjustments have also been recommended (Floyd, 2006):

Serum bilirubin 1.2 to 3 mg/dL: Administer 75% of dose

Serum bilirubin 3.1 to 5 mg/dL: Administer 50% of dose

Serum bilirubin >5 mg/dL: Avoid use

Dosing in obesity: *ASCO Guidelines for appropriate chemotherapy dosing in obese adults with cancer:* Utilize patient's actual body weight (full weight) for calculation of body surface area- or weight-based dosing, particularly when the intent of therapy is curative; manage regimen-related toxicities in the same manner as for nonobese patients; if a dose reduction is utilized due to toxicity, consider resumption of full weight-based dosing with subsequent cycles, especially if cause of toxicity (eg, hepatic or renal impairment) is resolved (Griggs, 2012).

Administration Daunorubicin is associated with a moderate emetic potential; antiemetics are recommended to prevent nausea and vomiting (Basch, 2011; Dupuis, 2011; Roila, 2010).

For IV administration only. Do not administer IM or SubQ. Administer as slow IV push over 1 to 5 minutes into the tubing of a rapidly infusing IV solution of D_5W or NS or may dilute further and infuse over 15 to 30 minutes.

Vesicant; ensure proper needle or catheter placement prior to and during infusion; avoid extravasation.

Extravasation management: If extravasation occurs, stop infusion immediately and disconnect (leave cannula/needle in place); gently aspirate extravasated solution (do **NOT** flush the line); remove needle/cannula; elevate extremity. Initiate antidote (dexrazoxane or dimethyl sulfate [DMSO]). Apply dry cold compresses for 20 minutes 4 times daily for 1 to 2 days (Perez Fidalgo, 2012); withhold cooling beginning 15 minutes before dexrazoxane infusion; continue withholding cooling until 15 minutes after infusion is completed. Topical DMSO should not be administered in combination with dexrazoxane; may lessen dexrazoxane efficacy.

Dexrazoxane: Adults: 1000 mg/m^2 (maximum dose: 2000 mg) IV (administer in a large vein remote from site of extravasation) over 1 to 2 hours days 1 and 2, then 500 mg/m^2 (maximum dose: 1000 mg) IV over 1-2 hours day 3; begin within 6 hours of extravasation. Day 2 and day 3 doses should be administered at approximately the same time (± 3 hours) as the dose on day 1 (Mouridsen, 2007; Perez Fidalgo, 2012). **Note:** Reduce dexrazoxane dose by 50% in patients with moderate to severe renal impairment (CrCl <40 mL/minute).

DMSO: Children and Adults: Apply topically to a region covering twice the affected area every 8 hours for 7 days; begin within 10 minutes of extravasation; do not cover with a dressing (Perez Fidalgo, 2012).

Hazardous agent; use appropriate precautions for handling and disposal (NIOSH 2014 [group 1]).

Monitoring Parameters CBC with differential and platelet count, liver function test, ECG, left ventricular ejection function (echocardiography [ECHO] or multigated radionuclide angiography [MUGA] scan), renal function test, signs/symptoms of extravasation

Dosage Forms

Injectable, Intravenous:

Generic: 5 mg/mL (4 mL)

Injectable, Intravenous [preservative free]:

Generic: 5 mg/mL (4 mL, 10 mL)

◆ **DAUNOrubicin Hydrochloride** *see* DAUNOrubicin (Conventional) *on page 577*

◆ **Daunorubicin Hydrochloride for Injection (Can)** *see* DAUNOrubicin (Conventional) *on page 577*

DAUNOrubicin (Liposomal)

(daw noe ROO bi sin lye po SO mal)

Brand Names: U.S. DaunoXome

Index Terms DAUNOrubicin Citrate; DAUNOrubicin Citrate (Liposomal); DAUNOrubicin Citrate Liposome; Liposomal DAUNOrubicin

Pharmacologic Category Antineoplastic Agent, Anthracycline; Antineoplastic Agent, Topoisomerase II Inhibitor

Use First-line treatment of advanced HIV-associated Kaposi's sarcoma (KS)

Pregnancy Risk Factor D

Pregnancy Considerations Adverse events were observed in animal reproduction studies. Women of childbearing potential should avoid becoming pregnant while receiving treatment.

Breast-Feeding Considerations Based on information from daunorubicin (conventional), it is not known if daunorubicin (liposomal) is excreted into breast milk. Daunorubicin (liposomal) is indicated for advanced HIV-associated Kaposi's sarcoma. In the United States, where formula is accessible, affordable, safe, and sustainable, and the risk of infant mortality due to diarrhea and respiratory infections is low, complete avoidance of breast-feeding by HIV-infected women is recommended to decrease potential transmission of HIV (DHHS [perinatal], 2012).

Contraindications Hypersensitivity to daunorubicin citrate (liposomal), daunorubicin, or any component of the formulation

Warnings/Precautions Hazardous agent - use appropriate precautions for handling and disposal (NIOSH 2014 [group 1]). **[U.S. Boxed Warning]: Monitor cardiac function regularly; especially in patients with previous therapy with high cumulative doses of anthracyclines, cyclophosphamide, or thoracic radiation, or who have preexisting cardiac disease.** Although the risk increases with cumulative dose, irreversible cardiotoxicity may occur with anthracycline treatment at any dose level. Patients with preexisting heart disease, hypertension, concurrent administration of other antineoplastic agents, prior or concurrent chest irradiation, and advanced age are at increased risk. Evaluate left ventricular ejection fraction (LVEF) prior to treatment and periodically during treatment.

[U.S. Boxed Warning]: May cause bone marrow suppression, particularly neutropenia; monitor closely for infections. **[U.S. Boxed Warning]: Use caution with hepatic impairment;** dosage reduction is recommended. Use caution with renal impairment; may require dose adjustment. **[U.S. Boxed Warning]: The lipid component is associated with infusion-related reactions (back pain, flushing, chest tightness) usually within the first 5 minutes of infusion;** monitor, interrupt infusion, and resume at reduced infusion rate. Safety and efficacy in children and the elderly have not been established. **[U.S. Boxed Warning]: Should be administered under the supervision of an experienced cancer chemotherapy physician.**

Adverse Reactions

Cardiovascular: Chest pain, CHF/cardiomyopathy, edema, hypertension, LVEF decreased, palpitation, syncope, tachycardia

Central nervous system: Abnormal thinking, amnesia, anxiety, ataxia, confusion, depression, dizziness, emotional lability, fatigue, fever, hallucination, headache, insomnia, malaise, meningitis, neutropenic fever, seizure, somnolence

Dermatologic: Alopecia, dry skin, folliculitis, pruritus, seborrhea

Endocrine & metabolic: Dehydration, hot flashes

Gastrointestinal: Abdominal pain, anorexia, appetite increased, constipation, dental caries, diarrhea, dysphagia, gastritis, gastrointestinal hemorrhage, gingival bleeding, hemorrhoids, melena, nausea, splenomegaly, stomatitis, taste perversion, tenesmus, vomiting, xerostomia

Genitourinary: Dysuria, nocturia, polyuria

Hematologic: Anemia, myelosuppression (onset: 7 days; nadir: 14 days; recovery 21 days), neutropenia, thrombocytopenia

Hepatic: Hepatomegaly

Local: Injection site inflammation

Neuromuscular & skeletal: Arthralgia, back pain, gait abnormal, hyperkinesia, hypertonia, myalgia, neuropathy, rigors, tremor

Ocular: Abnormal vision, conjunctivitis, eye pain

Otic: Deafness, earache, tinnitus

Respiratory: Cough, dyspnea, hemoptysis, pulmonary infiltrate, rhinitis, sinusitis, sputum increased

Miscellaneous: Allergic reactions, diaphoresis, flu-like syndrome, hiccups, infusion-related reactions (includes back pain, flushing, chest tightness), lymphadenopathy, opportunistic infections, thirst

Rare but important or life-threatening: Angina, atrial fibrillation, cardiac arrest, MI, pericardial effusion, pericardial tamponade, pulmonary hypertension, supraventricular tachycardia, ventricular extrasystoles

Drug Interactions

Metabolism/Transport Effects Substrate of P-glycoprotein

Avoid Concomitant Use

Avoid concomitant use of DAUNOrubicin (Liposomal) with any of the following: BCG; CloZAPine; Dipyrone; Natalizumab; Pimecrolimus; Tacrolimus (Topical); Tofacitinib; Vaccines (Live)

Increased Effect/Toxicity

DAUNOrubicin (Liposomal) may increase the levels/effects of: CloZAPine; Leflunomide; Natalizumab; Tofacitinib; Vaccines (Live)

The levels/effects of DAUNOrubicin (Liposomal) may be increased by: Bevacizumab; Cyclophosphamide; Denosumab; Dipyrone; P-glycoprotein/ABCB1 Inhibitors; Pimecrolimus; Roflumilast; Tacrolimus (Topical); Taxane Derivatives; Trastuzumab

Decreased Effect

DAUNOrubicin (Liposomal) may decrease the levels/effects of: BCG; Cardiac Glycosides; Coccidioides immitis Skin Test; Sipuleucel-T; Vaccines (Inactivated); Vaccines (Live)

The levels/effects of DAUNOrubicin (Liposomal) may be decreased by: Cardiac Glycosides; Echinacea; P-glycoprotein/ABCB1 Inducers

Preparation for Administration Hazardous agent; use appropriate precautions for handling and disposal (NIOSH 2014 [group 1]). Only fluid which may be mixed with DaunoXome® is D_5W. Dilute to a 1:1 solution (1 mg daunorubicin liposomal/mL D_5W). Must **not** be mixed with saline, bacteriostatic agents (such as benzyl alcohol), or any other solution.

Storage/Stability Store intact vials of solution under refrigeration at 2°C to 8°C (36°F to 46°F); do not freeze. Protect from light. Diluted daunorubicin liposomal for infusion may be refrigerated at 2°C to 8°C (36°F to 46°F) for a maximum of 6 hours. Do not use with in-line filters.

Mechanism of Action Liposomes have been shown to penetrate solid tumors more effectively, possibly because of their small size and longer circulation time. Once in tissues, daunorubicin is released. Daunorubicin inhibits DNA and RNA synthesis by intercalation between DNA base pairs and by steric obstruction; and intercalates at points of local uncoiling of the double helix. Although the exact mechanism is unclear, it appears that direct binding to DNA (intercalation) and inhibition of DNA repair (topoisomerase II inhibition) result in blockade of DNA and RNA synthesis and fragmentation of DNA.

Pharmacodynamics/Kinetics

Distribution: V_d: 5-8 L

Metabolism: Similar to daunorubicin, but metabolite plasma levels are low

Half-life elimination: Distribution: 4.4 hours; Terminal: 3-5 hours

Excretion: Primarily feces; some urine

Clearance, plasma: 17.3 mL/minute

Dosage Refer to individual protocols. IV:

Adults: HIV-associated KS: 40 mg/m^2 every 2 weeks

Elderly: Use with caution.

Dosage adjustment for toxicity: Withhold treatment for ANC <750/mm^3

Elderly: Use with caution.

Dosing adjustment in renal impairment: Serum creatinine >3 mg/dL: Administer 50% of normal dose

Dosing adjustment in hepatic impairment:

Bilirubin 1.2-3 mg/dL: Administer 75% of normal dose

Bilirubin >3 mg/dL: Administer 50% of normal dose

Dosing in obesity: *ASCO Guidelines for appropriate chemotherapy dosing in obese adults with cancer:* Utilize patient's actual body weight (full weight) for calculation of body surface area- or weight-based dosing, particularly when the intent of therapy is curative; manage regimen-related toxicities in the same manner as for nonobese patients; if a dose reduction is utilized due to toxicity, consider resumption of full weight-based dosing with subsequent cycles, especially if cause of toxicity (eg, hepatic or renal impairment) is resolved (Griggs, 2012).

Administration Infuse over 1 hour; do not mix with other drugs. Avoid extravasation.

Hazardous agent; use appropriate precautions for handling and disposal (NIOSH 2014 [group 1]).

Monitoring Parameters CBC with differential and platelets (prior to each dose), liver function tests, renal function tests; evaluate cardiac function (baseline left ventricular ejection fraction [LVEF] prior to treatment initiation; repeat LVEF at total cumulative doses of 320 mg/m^2, and every 160 mg/m^2 thereafter; patients with preexisting cardiac disease, history of prior chest irradiation, or history of prior anthracycline treatment should have baseline LVEF and every 160 mg/m^2 thereafter); signs and symptoms of infection or disease progression; monitor closely for infusion reactions

Dosage Forms Considerations

DaunoXome injection contains sucrose 2125 mg/25 mL

Dosage Forms

Injectable, Intravenous [preservative free]:

DaunoXome: 2 mg/mL (25 mL)

- ◆ **DaunoXome** *see* DAUNOrubicin (Liposomal) *on page 580*
- ◆ **Daxas (Can)** *see* Roflumilast *on page 1840*
- ◆ **Dayhist Allergy 12 Hour Relief [OTC]** *see* Clemastine *on page 459*
- ◆ **Daypro** *see* Oxaprozin *on page 1532*
- ◆ **Daysee** *see* Ethinyl Estradiol and Levonorgestrel *on page 803*
- ◆ **Daytrana** *see* Methylphenidate *on page 1336*
- ◆ **dCF** *see* Pentostatin *on page 1618*
- ◆ **DDAVP** *see* Desmopressin *on page 594*
- ◆ **DDAVP Melt (Can)** *see* Desmopressin *on page 594*
- ◆ **DDAVP Rhinal Tube** *see* Desmopressin *on page 594*
- ◆ **ddI** *see* Didanosine *on page 622*
- ◆ **1-Deamino-8-D-Arginine Vasopressin** *see* Desmopressin *on page 594*
- ◆ **Deblitane** *see* Norethindrone *on page 1473*
- ◆ **Debrox [OTC]** *see* Carbamide Peroxide *on page 350*
- ◆ **Decadron** *see* Dexamethasone (Systemic) *on page 599*
- ◆ **Decapeptyl (Can)** *see* Triptorelin *on page 2107*
- ◆ **De-Chlor DM [OTC]** *see* Chlorpheniramine, Phenylephrine, and Dextromethorphan *on page 428*

Decitabine (de SYE ta been)

Brand Names: U.S. Dacogen

Index Terms 5-Aza-2'-deoxycytidine; 5-Aza-dCyd; Deoxyazacytidine; Dezocitidine

Pharmacologic Category Antineoplastic Agent, Antimetabolite; Antineoplastic Agent, DNA Methylation Inhibitor

Use Treatment of myelodysplastic syndrome (MDS)

Pregnancy Risk Factor D

Pregnancy Considerations Teratogenic effects, decreased fetal weight, and increased fetal deaths were observed in animal studies. There are no adequate and well-controlled studies in pregnant women. Women of childbearing potential should be advised to avoid pregnancy during treatment and for 1 month after treatment. In addition, males should be advised to avoid fathering a child while on decitabine therapy and for 2 months after treatment.

Breast-Feeding Considerations Due to the potential for serious adverse reactions in the nursing infant, breast-feeding is not recommended.

Contraindications There are no contraindications listed within the manufacturer's labeling.

Warnings/Precautions Hazardous agent - use appropriate precautions for handling and disposal (NIOSH 2014 [group 1]). The dose-limiting toxicity is bone marrow suppression; worsening neutropenia is common in first two treatment cycles and may not correlate with progression of underlying MDS; may require dosage adjustment (after the first cycle), growth factor support and/or antimicrobial agents; monitor for infection. Not studied in hepatic and renal disease; use caution.

Adverse Reactions

Cardiovascular: Cardiac murmur, chest discomfort/pain, edema, facial edema, heart failure, hypotension, pallor, peripheral edema, tachycardia

Central nervous system: Anxiety, chills, confusion, depression, dizziness, fatigue, headache, hypoesthesia, insomnia, lethargy, malaise, pain

Dermatologic: Alopecia, bruising, cellulitis, dry skin, erythema, lesions, petechiae, pruritus, rash, urticaria

Endocrine & metabolic: Bicarbonate increased/decreased, dehydration, hyperglycemia, hyper-/hypokalemia, hyperuricemia, hypoalbuminemia, hypochloremia, hypomagnesemia, hyponatremia, hypoproteinemia, LDH increased

Gastrointestinal: Abdominal distension, abdominal pain, anorexia, appetite decreased, constipation, diarrhea, dyspepsia, dysphagia, gastroesophageal reflux, gingival bleeding, glossodynia, hemorrhoids, lip ulceration, loose stools, mucosal inflammation, nausea, oral candidiasis, oral mucosal oral pain, petechiae, stomatitis, tongue ulceration, tooth abscess, toothache, vomiting, weight loss

Genitourinary: Dysuria, polyuria, urinary tract infection

Hematologic: Anemia, bacteremia, febrile neutropenia, hematoma, leukopenia, lymphadenopathy, neutropenia, pancytopenia, thrombocytopenia

Hepatic: Alkaline phosphatase increased, ascites, AST increased, hyper-/hypobilirubinemia
Local: Catheter infection, catheter site erythema, catheter site pain, injection site swelling, tenderness
Neuromuscular & skeletal: Arthralgia, back pain, bone pain, chest wall pain, crepitation, falling, limb pain, musculoskeletal discomfort/pain, myalgia, rigors, weakness
Ocular: Blurred vision
Respiratory: Breath sounds abnormal, cough, epistaxis, hypoxia, lung crackles, pharyngitis, pharyngolaryngeal pain, pleural effusion, pneumonia, postnasal drip, pulmonary edema, rales, sinus congestion, sinusitis, upper respiratory tract infection
Miscellaneous: Candidal infection, night sweats, staphylococcal infection, transfusion reaction
Rare but important or life-threatening: Anaphylactic reaction, atrial fibrillation, bronchopulmonary aspergillosis, cardiomyopathy, cardiorespiratory arrest/failure, catheter site hemorrhage, cholecystitis, fungal infection, gastrointestinal hemorrhage, gingival pain, hemoptysis, hypersensitivity, intracranial hemorrhage, mental status change, MI, mycobacterium avium complex infection, peridiverticular abscess, pseudomonal lung infection, pulmonary embolism, pulmonary infiltrates, pulmonary mass, renal failure, respiratory arrest, sepsis, splenomegaly, supraventricular tachycardia, Sweet's syndrome (acute febrile neutrophilic dermatosis), urethral hemorrhage

Drug Interactions

Metabolism/Transport Effects None known.

Avoid Concomitant Use

Avoid concomitant use of Decitabine with any of the following: CloZAPine; Dipyrone

Increased Effect/Toxicity

Decitabine may increase the levels/effects of: CloZAPine

The levels/effects of Decitabine may be increased by: Dipyrone

Decreased Effect There are no known significant interactions involving a decrease in effect.

Preparation for Administration Hazardous agent; use appropriate precautions for handling and disposal (NIOSH 2014 [group 1]). Vials should be reconstituted with 10 mL SWFI to a concentration of 5 mg/mL. Immediately further dilute with 50-250 mL NS, D_5W, or lactated Ringer's to a final concentration of 0.1-1 mg/mL. Use appropriate precautions for handling and disposal. Solutions not administered within 15 minutes of preparation should be prepared with cold (2°C to 8°C [36°F to 46°F]) infusion solutions.

Storage/Stability Store vials at 25°C (77°F); excursions permitted to 15°C to 30°C (59°F to 86°F). Solutions diluted for infusion may be stored for up to 7 hours under refrigeration at 2°C to 8°C (36°F to 46°F) if prepared with cold infusion fluids.

Mechanism of Action After phosphorylation, decitabine is incorporated into DNA and inhibits DNA methyltransferase causing hypomethylation and subsequent cell death (within the S-phase of the cell cycle).

Pharmacodynamics/Kinetics

Distribution: 63-89 L/m^2
Protein binding: <1%
Metabolism: Possibly via deamination by cytidine deaminase
Half-life elimination: ~30-35 minutes
Time to peak: At end of infusion

Dosage IV: Adults:

MDS:

15 mg/m^2 over 3 hours every 8 hours (45 mg/m^2/day) for 3 days (135 mg/m^2/cycle) every 6 weeks (treatment is recommended for at least 4 cycles and may continue until the patient no longer continues to benefit)

Adjustment for prolonged hematologic toxicity (ANC <1000/mm^3 and platelets <50,000/mm^3):

>6 weeks but <8 weeks: Delay dose for up to 2 weeks and temporarily reduce dose to 11 mg/m^2 every 8 hours (33 mg/m^2/day) for 3 days

>8 weeks but <10 weeks: Assess for disease progression; if no disease progression, delay dose for up to 2 weeks and reduce dose to 11 mg/m^2 every 8 hours (33 mg/m^2/day) for 3 days; maintain or increase dose with subsequent cycles if clinically indicated

or

20 mg/m^2 over 1 hour daily for 5 days every 28 days (delay subsequent treatment cycles until hematologic recovery (ANC ≥1000/mm^3 and platelets ≥50,000/mm^3)

AML (off-label use): 20 mg/m^2 over 1 hour daily for 5 days every 28 days (Cashen, 2010)

Dosage adjustment for toxicity:

Hematologic toxicity (ANC <1000/mm^3 and platelets <50,000/mm^3): Delay and/or reduce dose; see recommendations specific to each MDS dosing regimen above

Nonhematologic toxicity: Temporarily hold treatment until resolution for any of the following toxicities:
Serum creatinine ≥2 mg/dL
ALT, bilirubin ≥2 times ULN
Active or uncontrolled infection

Dosage adjustment in renal impairment: No dosage adjustment provided in manufacturer's labeling (has not been studied); use with caution.

Dosage adjustment in hepatic impairment: No dosage adjustment provided in manufacturer's labeling (has not been studied); use with caution.

Dosing in obesity: *ASCO Guidelines for appropriate chemotherapy dosing in obese adults with cancer:* Utilize patient's actual body weight (full weight) for calculation of body surface area- or weight-based dosing, particularly when the intent of therapy is curative; manage regimen-related toxicities in the same manner as for nonobese patients; if a dose reduction is utilized due to toxicity, consider resumption of full weight-based dosing with subsequent cycles, especially if cause of toxicity (eg, hepatic or renal impairment) is resolved (Griggs, 2012).

Administration Infuse over 1-3 hours. Premedication with antiemetics is recommended.

Hazardous agent; use appropriate precautions for handling and disposal (NIOSH 2014 [group 1]).

Monitoring Parameters CBC with differential and platelets with each cycle, more frequently if needed; liver enzymes; serum creatinine

Dosage Forms

Solution Reconstituted, Intravenous:
Dacogen: 50 mg (1 ea)
Generic: 50 mg (1 ea)

◆ **Declomycin** *see* Demeclocycline *on page 589*

◆ **Decongestant 12Hour Max St [OTC]** *see* Pseudoephedrine *on page 1742*

◆ **Deep Sea Nasal Spray [OTC]** *see* Sodium Chloride *on page 1902*

Deferasirox (de FER a sir ox)

Brand Names: U.S. Exjade
Brand Names: Canada Exjade
Index Terms ICL670
Pharmacologic Category Chelating Agent
Use Chronic iron overload: Treatment of chronic iron overload due to blood transfusions (transfusional hemosiderosis) or due to non-transfusion-dependent thalassemia

syndromes and with a liver iron concentration (LIC) of at least 5 mg iron per gram of liver dry weight (mg Fe/g dw) and serum ferritin >300 mcg/L.

Pregnancy Risk Factor C

Pregnancy Considerations Adverse events were observed in animal reproduction studies. Information related to the use of deferasirox in pregnant women is limited (Vini 2011).

Breast-Feeding Considerations It is not known if deferasirox is excreted in breast milk. Due to the potential for serious adverse reactions in the nursing infant, the manufacturer recommends a decision be made whether to discontinue nursing or to discontinue the drug, taking into account the importance of treatment to the mother.

Contraindications

Hypersensitivity to deferasirox or any component of the formulation; platelet counts <50,000/mm^3; poor performance status; high-risk myelodysplastic syndromes; advanced malignancies; creatinine clearance <40 mL/minute or serum creatinine >2 x age-appropriate ULN

Canadian labeling: Additional contraindications (not in U.S. labeling): MDS patients with <1 year life expectancy; CrCl <60 mL/minute

Warnings/Precautions [U.S. Boxed Warning]: Acute renal failure (including fatalities and cases requiring dialysis) may occur; observed more frequently in patients with comorbid conditions and advanced hematologic malignancies. Obtain serum creatinine and calculate creatinine clearance in duplicate at baseline prior to initiation, and monitor at least monthly thereafter; in patients with underlying renal dysfunction or at risk for acute renal failure, monitor creatinine weekly during the first month then at least monthly thereafter. Dose reduction, interruption, or discontinuation should be considered for serum creatinine elevations. Monitor serum creatinine and/or creatinine clearance more frequently if creatinine levels are increasing. Use with caution in renal impairment; dosage modification or treatment discontinuation may be required; reductions in initial dose are recommended for patients with CrCl 40-60 mL/minute; use is contraindicated in patients with CrCl <40 mL/minute (U.S. labeling) or <60 mL/minute (Canadian labeling) or serum creatinine >2 times age-appropriate ULN. May cause proteinuria; monitor monthly. Renal tubular damage, including Fanconi's syndrome, has also been reported, primarily in pediatric/adolescent patients with beta-thalassemia and serum ferritin levels <1500 mcg/L.

[U.S. Boxed Warning]: Hepatic injury and failure (including fatalities) may occur. Monitor transaminases and bilirubin at baseline, every 2 weeks for 1 month, then at least monthly thereafter. Hepatitis and elevated transaminases have also been reported. Hepatotoxicity is more common in patients >55 years of age and in patients with significant comorbidities (eg, cirrhosis, multiorgan failure). Reduce dose or temporarily interrupt treatment for severe or persistent increases in transaminases/bilirubin. **[U.S. Boxed Warning]: Avoid use in patients with severe (Child-Pugh class C) hepatic impairment; a dose reduction is required in patients with moderate (Child-Pugh class B) hepatic impairment.** Monitor patients with mild (Child-Pugh class A) or moderate (Child-Pugh class B) impairment closely for efficacy and for adverse reactions requiring dosage reduction.

[U.S. Boxed Warning]: Gastrointestinal (GI) hemorrhage (including fatalities) may occur; observed more frequently in elderly patients with advanced hematologic malignancies and/or low platelet counts; discontinue treatment for suspected GI hemorrhage or ulceration. Other GI effects including irritation and ulceration have been reported. Use caution with concurrent medications that may increase risk of adverse GI effects (eg, NSAIDs, corticosteroids, anticoagulants, oral bisphosphonates). Monitor patients closely for signs/symptoms of GI ulceration/bleeding.

May cause skin rash (dose-related), including erythema multiforme; mild-to-moderate rashes may resolve without treatment interruption; for severe rash, interrupt and consider restarting at a lower dose with dose escalation and oral steroids; discontinue if erythema multiforme is suspected. Severe skin reactions, including Stevens-Johnson syndrome (SJS) and erythema multiforme, have also been reported; discontinue and evaluate if suspected. Hypersensitivity reactions, including severe reactions (anaphylaxis and angioedema) have been reported, onset is usually within the first month of treatment; discontinue if severe. Auditory (decreased hearing and high frequency hearing loss) or ocular disturbances (lens opacities, cataracts, intraocular pressure elevation, and retinal disorders) have been reported (rare); monitor and consider dose reduction or treatment interruption. Bone marrow suppression (including agranulocytosis, neutropenia, thrombocytopenia, and worsening anemia) has been reported, risk may be increased in patients with preexisting hematologic disorders; monitor blood counts regularly; interrupt treatment in patients who develop cytopenias; may reinitiate once cause of cytopenia has been determined; use contraindicated if platelet count <50,000/mm^3. Potentially significant drug-drug interactions may exist, requiring dose or frequency adjustment, additional monitoring, and/or selection of alternative therapy. Potent UGT inducers (eg, rifampin) or bile acid sequestrants (eg, cholestyramine) may decrease the efficacy of deferasirox; avoid concomitant use. If coadministration necessary, dosage modifications may be needed; monitor serum ferritin and clinical response. Not approved for use in combination with other iron chelation therapies; safety of combinations has not been established. For transfusion-related iron overload, treatment should be initiated with evidence of chronic iron overload (ie, transfusion of ≥100 mL/kg of packed RBCs [eg, ≥20 units for a 40 kg individual] and serum ferritin consistently >1000 mcg/L). For non-transfusion-dependent iron overload, initiate with liver iron concentration ≥5 mg Fe/g dry liver weight and serum ferritin >300 mcg/L. Prior to use, consider risk versus anticipated benefit with respect to individual patient's life expectancy and prognosis. Use with caution in the elderly due to the higher incidence of toxicity (eg, hepatotoxicity) and fatal events during use. Overchelation of iron may increase development of toxicity; consider temporary interruption of treatment in transfusional iron overload when serum ferritin <500 mcg/L; in non-transfusion-dependent thalassemia when serum ferritin <300 mcg/L or hepatic iron concentration <3 mg Fe/g dry weight. May contain lactose; Canadian product labeling recommends avoiding use in patients with galactose intolerance, Lapp lactase deficiency, or glucose-galactose malabsorption syndromes. Controlled studies in myelodysplastic syndromes (MDS) and chronic iron overload due to blood transfusions have not been conducted.

Adverse Reactions

Central nervous system: Fatigue, headache

Dermatologic: Skin rash (dose related), urticaria

Gastrointestinal: Abdominal pain (dose related), diarrhea (dose related), nausea (dose related), vomiting (dose related)

Genitourinary: Proteinuria

Hepatic: Increased serum ALT, increased serum transaminases

Infection: Influenza

Neuromuscular & skeletal: Arthralgia, back pain

Otic: Otic infection

Renal: Increased serum creatinine (dose related)

Respiratory: Bronchitis, cough, nasopharyngitis, pharyngitis, pharyngolaryngeal pain, respiratory tract infection, rhinitis, tonsillitis (acute)

Rare but important or life-threatening: Acute renal failure, agranulocytosis, anaphylaxis, anemia (worsening), angioedema, ascites, cataract, cholecystitis, cholelithiasis, cytopenia, drug fever, duodenal ulcer, dyschromia, edema, erythema multiforme, Fanconi's syndrome, gastric ulcer, gastritis, gastrointestinal hemorrhage, glomerulonephritis, glycosuria, hearing loss (including high frequency), hematuria, hepatic encephalopathy, hepatic failure, hepatic insufficiency, hepatitis, hyperactivity, hypersensitivity angiitis, hypersensitivity reaction, hypocalcemia, IgA vasculitis, increased intraocular pressure, interstitial nephritis, jaundice, maculopathy, neutropenia, optic neuritis, purpura, renal tubular disease, renal tubular necrosis, retinopathy, sleep disorder, Stevens-Johnson syndrome, thrombocytopenia, visual disturbance

Drug Interactions

Metabolism/Transport Effects Substrate of UGT1A1; **Inhibits** CYP1A2 (moderate), CYP2C8 (moderate); **Induces** CYP3A4 (weak)

Avoid Concomitant Use

Avoid concomitant use of Deferasirox with any of the following: Aluminum Hydroxide; Bile Acid Sequestrants; Theophylline

Increased Effect/Toxicity

Deferasirox may increase the levels/effects of: Agomelatine; CYP1A2 Substrates; CYP2C8 Substrates; Pirfenidone; Repaglinide; Theophylline

The levels/effects of Deferasirox may be increased by: Anticoagulants; Bisphosphonate Derivatives; Corticosteroids; Corticosteroids (Systemic); Nonsteroidal Anti-Inflammatory Agents

Decreased Effect

Deferasirox may decrease the levels/effects of: ARIPiprazole; CYP3A4 Substrates; Hydrocodone; Saxagliptin

The levels/effects of Deferasirox may be decreased by: Aluminum Hydroxide; Bile Acid Sequestrants; Fosphenytoin; PHENobarbital; Phenytoin; Rifampin; Ritonavir

Food Interactions Bioavailability is increased variably when taken with food. Management: Take on an empty stomach at the same time each day at least 30 minutes before food. Maintain adequate hydration, unless instructed to restrict fluid intake.

Storage/Stability Store at room temperature of 25°C (77°F); excursions permitted to 15°C and 30°C (59°F and 86°F). Protect from moisture.

Mechanism of Action Selectively binds iron, forming a complex which is excreted primarily through the feces.

Pharmacodynamics/Kinetics

Distribution: Adults: 14.4 ± 2.7L

Protein binding: ~99% to serum albumin

Metabolism: Hepatic via glucuronidation by UGT1A1(primarily) and UGT1A3; minor oxidation by CYP450; undergoes enterohepatic recirculation

Bioavailability: 70%

Half-life elimination: 8-16 hours

Time to peak, plasma: ~1.5-4 hours

Excretion: Feces (84%); urine (8%)

Dosage Note: Calculate dose to the nearest whole tablet size.

Chronic iron overload due to blood transfusion: Note: Treatment should only be initiated with evidence of chronic iron overload (ie, transfusion of ≥100 mL/kg of packed red blood cells [eg, ≥20 units for a 40 kg individual] and serum ferritin consistently >1000 mcg/L).

Children ≥2 years, Adolescents, and Adults: Oral:

U.S. labeling: Initial: 20 mg/kg once daily

Canadian labeling: Dosing based on treatment goal and patient's individual transfusion rate:

Treatment goal: Maintenance of acceptable body iron levels:

Initial: 10 mg/kg once daily if transfused packed red blood cells (pRBCs) <7 mL/kg/month (approximately <2 units per month for an adult)

Initial: 20 mg/kg once daily if transfused pRBCs ≥7 mL/kg/month (approximately >2 units per month for an adult)

Treatment goal: Iron overload reduction:

Initial: 20 mg/kg once daily if transfused pRBCs <14 mL/kg/month (approximately <4 units per month for an adult)

Initial: 30 mg/kg once daily if transfused pRBCs ≥14 mL/kg/month (approximately >4 units per month for an adult)

Maintenance: Adjust dose every 3-6 months based on serum ferritin trends; adjust by 5 or 10 mg/kg/day; titrate to individual response and treatment goals. Usual range: 20-30 mg/kg/day; doses up to 40 mg/kg/day may be considered for serum ferritin levels persistently >2500 mcg/L (doses above 40 mg/kg/day are not recommended). **Note:** Consider interrupting therapy for serum ferritin <500 mcg/L (risk of toxicity may be increased).

Chronic iron overload in non-transfusion-dependent thalassemia syndromes: Children ≥10 years, Adolescents, and Adults: Oral:

U.S. labeling: **Note:** Treatment should only be initiated with evidence of chronic iron overload (hepatic iron concentration ≥5 mg Fe/g dry weight and serum ferritin >300 mcg/L).

Initial: 10 mg/kg once daily. Consider increasing to 20 mg/kg once daily after 4 weeks if baseline hepatic iron concentration is >15 mg Fe/g dry weight.

Maintenance: Monitor serum ferritin monthly; if serum ferritin is <300 mcg/L, interrupt therapy and obtain hepatic iron concentration. Monitor hepatic iron concentration every 6 months; interrupt therapy when hepatic iron concentration <3 mg Fe/g dry weight. After 6 months of therapy, consider dose adjustment to 20 mg/kg/day if hepatic iron concentration >7 mg Fe/g dry weight. Reduce dose to ≤10 mg/kg when hepatic iron concentration is 3-7 mg Fe/g dry weight. Doses above 20 mg/kg/day are not recommended. After interruption, resume treatment when hepatic iron concentration >5 mg Fe/g dry weight.

Canadian labeling: **Note:** Treatment should only be initiated with evidence of chronic iron overload (hepatic iron concentration ≥5 mg Fe/g dry weight or serum ferritin consistently >800 mcg/L).

Initial: 10 mg/kg/day

Maintenance: Do not exceed 10 mg/kg/day in patients whose hepatic iron concentration was not evaluated and if serum ferritin ≤2000 mcg/L. Monitor serum ferritin monthly; consider dose adjustment by 5 or 10 mg/kg/day every 3-6 months if hepatic iron concentration ≥7 mg Fe/g dry weight or serum transferrin levels consistently >2000 mcg/L. Patients receiving >10 mg/kg should have their dose reduced to ≤10 mg/kg when hepatic iron concentration <7 mg Fe/g dry weight or serum ferritin <2000 mcg/L. Interrupt therapy when hepatic iron concentration <3 mg Fe/g dry weight or serum ferritin <300 mcg/L. Doses above 20 mg/kg/day are not recommended.

Dosage adjustment with concomitant bile acid sequestrants (eg, cholestyramine, colesevelam, colestipol) or potent UGT inducers (eg, rifampin, phenytoin, phenobarbital, ritonavir): Avoid concomitant use; if coadministration necessary, consider increasing the initial dose of deferasirox dose by 50%; monitor serum ferritin and clinical response.

Dosage adjustment for toxicity:

Bone marrow suppression: Interrupt treatment; may reinitiate once cause of cytopenia has been determined; use contraindicated if platelet count <50,000/mm^3

Dermatologic toxicity:

Rash (severe): Interrupt treatment; may reintroduce at a lower dose (with future dose escalation) and short-term oral corticosteroids

Severe skin reaction (Stevens-Johnson syndrome, erythema multiforme): Discontinue and evaluate.

Gastrointestinal: Discontinue treatment for suspected GI ulceration or hemorrhage.

Hearing loss or visual disturbance: Consider dose reduction or treatment interruption

Dosage adjustment in renal impairment: Creatinine clearance should be estimated using the Cockcroft-Gault formula.

Renal impairment at treatment initiation:

CrCl >60 mL/minute: No dosage adjustment necessary.

CrCl 40-60 mL/minute:

U.S. labeling: Reduce initial dose by 50%.

Canadian labeling: Use is contraindicated

CrCl <40 mL/minute or serum creatinine >2 times age-appropriate ULN: Use is contraindicated.

Renal toxicity during treatment:

U.S. labeling:

Transfusional iron overload:

Children ≥2 years and Adolescents <16 years: For increase in serum creatinine >33% above the average baseline level and above the age-appropriate ULN: Reduce daily dose by 10 mg/kg

Adolescents ≥16 years and Adults: For increase in serum creatinine ≥33% above the average baseline, repeat within 1 week; if still elevated by ≥33%: Reduce daily dose by 10 mg/kg

All patients: CrCl <40 mL/minute or serum creatinine >2 times age-appropriate ULN: Discontinue treatment.

Non-transfusion-dependent thalassemia syndromes:

Children ≥10 years and Adolescents <16 years: For increase in serum creatinine >33% above the average baseline level and above the age-appropriate ULN: Reduce daily dose by 5 mg/kg

Adolescents ≥16 years and Adults: For increase in serum creatinine ≥33% above the average baseline, repeat within 1 week; if still elevated by ≥33%: Interrupt therapy if the dose is 5 mg/kg; reduce dose by 50% if the dose is 10-20 mg/kg

All patients: CrCl <40 mL/minute or serum creatinine >2 times age-appropriate ULN: Discontinue treatment.

Canadian labeling:

Children ≥2 years and Adolescents <16 years: For increase in serum creatinine above the age-appropriate ULN for 2 consecutive levels, reduce daily dose by 10 mg/kg.

Adolescents ≥16 years and Adults: For increase in serum creatinine >33% above the average pretreatment level for 2 consecutive weekly levels, reduce daily dose by 10 mg/kg.

All patients: Progressive increase serum creatinine beyond ULN: Withhold treatment.

Dosage adjustment in hepatic impairment:

Hepatic impairment at treatment initiation:

Mild impairment (Child-Pugh class A): No dosage adjustment necessary; monitor closely for efficacy and for adverse reactions requiring dosage reduction.

Moderate impairment (Child-Pugh class B): Initial: Reduce dose by 50%; monitor closely for efficacy and for adverse reactions requiring dosage reduction.

Severe impairment (Child-Pugh class C): Avoid use.

Hepatic toxicity during treatment: Severe or persistent increases in transaminases/bilirubin: Reduce dose or temporarily interrupt treatment.

Dietary Considerations Bioavailability increased variably when taken with food; take on empty stomach 30 minutes before a meal.

Administration Oral: Administer tablets by making an oral suspension; **do not chew or swallow tablets whole.** Completely disperse tablets in water, orange juice, or apple juice (use 3.5 ounces for total doses <1 g; 7 ounces for doses ≥1 g); stir to form a fine suspension and drink entire contents. Rinse remaining residue with more fluid; drink. Avoid dispersion of tablets in milk (due to slowed dissolution) or carbonated drinks (due to foaming) (Séchaud, 2008). Administer at same time each day on an empty stomach, at least 30 minutes before food. Do not take simultaneously with aluminum-containing antacids.

Monitoring Parameters Serum ferritin (baseline, monthly thereafter), iron levels (baseline), CBC with differential, serum creatinine and creatinine clearance (2 baseline assessments then monthly thereafter; in patients who are at increased risk of complications [eg, preexisting renal conditions, elderly, comorbid conditions, or receiving other potentially nephrotoxic medications]: weekly for the first month then at least monthly thereafter); liver iron concentration (non-transfusion-dependent thalassemia; baseline, every 6 months); urine protein (monthly); monitor serum creatinine and/or creatinine clearance more frequently if creatinine levels are increasing; serum transaminases (ALT/AST) and bilirubin (baseline, every 2 weeks for the first month, then monthly); baseline and annual auditory and ophthalmic function (including slit lamp examinations and dilated fundoscopy); performance status (in patients with hematologic malignancies); signs and symptoms of GI ulcers or hemorrhage; cumulative number of RBC units received

Canadian labeling also recommends monitoring growth and body weight every 12 months in pediatric patients.

Additional Information Deferasirox has a low affinity for binding with zinc and copper, may cause variable decreases in the serum concentration of these trace minerals.

Dosage Forms

Tablet Soluble, Oral:

Exjade: 125 mg, 250 mg, 500 mg

Deferiprone (de FER i prone)

Brand Names: U.S. Ferriprox

Index Terms APO-066; Ferriprox®

Pharmacologic Category Chelating Agent

Use Treatment of transfusional iron overload due to thalassemia syndromes with inadequate response to other chelation therapy

Pregnancy Risk Factor D

Dosage Oral: **Note:** Round dose to the nearest 250 mg (or 1/2 tablet). If serum ferritin falls consistently below 500 mcg/L, consider temporary treatment interruption.

Adults: Transfusional iron overload: Initial: 25 mg/kg 3 times/day (75 mg/kg/day); individualize dose based on response and therapeutic goal; maximum dose: 33 mg/kg 3 times/day (99 mg/kg/day)

Elderly: Begin at the low end of dosing range

Dosage adjustment for toxicity:

ANC <1500/mm³: Interrupt treatment

ANC <500/mm³: In addition to treatment interruption, consider hospitalization (and other clinically-appropriate management); do not resume or rechallenge unless the potential benefits outweigh potential risks

Infection: Interrupt treatment; monitor ANC more frequently

Dosage adjustment in renal impairment: No dosage adjustments are provided in the manufacturer's labeling (has not been studied).

Dosage adjustment in hepatic impairment: No dosage adjustments are provided in the manufacturer's labeling (has not been studied).

Additional Information Complete prescribing information should be consulted for additional detail.

Dosage Forms

Tablet, Oral:

Ferriprox: 500 mg

Deferoxamine (de fer OKS a meen)

Brand Names: U.S. Desferal

Brand Names: Canada Deferoxamine Mesylate for Injection; Desferal; PMS-Deferoxamine

Index Terms Deferoxamine Mesylate; Desferrioxamine; DFM

Pharmacologic Category Antidote; Chelating Agent

Use Adjunct in the treatment of acute iron intoxication; treatment of chronic iron overload secondary to multiple transfusions

Canadian labeling (off-label use in the U.S.): Diagnosis of aluminum overload; treatment of chronic aluminum overload in patients with end-stage renal failure undergoing maintenance dialysis

Pregnancy Risk Factor C

Dosage

Acute iron toxicity: **Note:** The IV route is used when severe toxicity is evidenced by cardiovascular collapse or systemic symptoms (coma, shock, metabolic acidosis, or gastrointestinal bleeding) or potentially severe intoxications (peak serum iron level >500 mcg/dL) (Perrone, 2011). When severe symptoms are not present, the IM route may be used (per the manufacturer).

Children and Adolescents:

IM: 90 mg/kg/dose every 8 hours (maximum: 6,000 mg/24 hours)

IV: 15 mg/kg/hour (maximum: 6,000 mg/24 hours)

Canadian labeling:

IM: Initial: 90 mg/kg/dose (maximum/dose: 1,000 mg) followed by 45 mg/kg every 4 to 12 hours as needed (maximum: 6,000 mg/24 hours)

IV: 15 mg/kg/hour up to a maximum of 80 mg/kg/dose or maximum of 6000 mg/24 hours

Adults: IM, IV: Initial: 1,000 mg, may be followed by 500 mg every 4 hours for 2 doses; subsequent doses of 500 mg have been administered every 4 to 12 hours based on clinical response (maximum recommended dose: 6,000 mg/day [per manufacturer])

Canadian labeling:

IM: Initial: 90 mg/kg/dose (maximum/dose: 2,000 mg) followed by 45 mg/kg every 4 to 12 hours as needed (maximum: 6,000 mg/24 hours)

IV: 15 mg/kg/hour up to a maximum of 80 mg/kg/dose or maximum of 6,000 mg/24 hours

Chronic iron overload:

Children ≥3 years and Adolescents:

IV: 20 to 40 mg/kg/day over 8 to 12 hours for 5 to 7 days per week; dose should not exceed 40 mg/kg/day until growth has ceased

SubQ: 20 to 40 mg/kg/day over 8 to 12 hours (maximum: 1000 to 2,000 mg/day)

Off-label dosing: IV, SubQ: 25 to 30 mg/kg over 8 to 10 hours 5 to 7 days per week (Brittenham, 2011)

Adults:

IM: 500 to 1,000 mg/day (maximum: 1000 mg/day)

IV: 40 to 50 mg/kg/day (maximum: 60 mg/kg/day) over 8 to 12 hours for 5 to 7 days per week

SubQ: 1,000 to 2,000 mg/day or 20 to 40 mg/kg/day over 8 to 24 hours

Off-label dosing: IV, SubQ: 25 to 50 mg/kg over 8 to 10 hours 5 to 7 days per week (Brittenham, 2011)

Canadian labeling: IV, SubQ: 1000 to 4,000 mg/day (20 to 60 mg/kg/day) over ~12 hours (may further increase iron excretion with infusion at the same dose over 24 hours). SubQ infusions are administered 4 to 7 days per week based on the degree of iron overload.

Diagnosis of aluminum-induced toxicity with CKD (off-label use; K/DOQI guidelines, 2003): Children, Adolescents, and Adults: IV: Test dose: 5 mg/kg during the last hour of dialysis if serum aluminum levels are 60 to 200 mcg/L, or clinical signs/symptoms of toxicity, or aluminum exposure prior to parathyroid surgery. Measure aluminum just prior to deferoxamine; remeasure 2 days later (test is positive if serum aluminum is ≥50 mcg/L). Do not use if aluminum serum levels are >200 mcg/L.

Canadian labeling: **Note:** Measure serum aluminum levels prior to and after administration of deferoxamine.

Adults: IV: Test dose: 5 mg/kg/dose (infusion rate not to exceed 15 mg/kg/hour) following hemodialysis (preferred) or during the last hour of dialysis if serum aluminum levels are >60 mcg/L in association with serum ferritin levels >100 mcg/L; continuous rise in serum aluminum over the next 24 to 48 hours suggests overload. Remeasure serum aluminum levels prior to next hemodialysis, test is considered positive if serum aluminum levels increase >150 mcg/L above baseline.

Treatment of aluminum toxicity with CKD (off-label use; K/DOQI guidelines, 2003): Children, Adolescents, and Adults: IV:

Administer after diagnostic deferoxamine test dose. **Note:** The risk for deferoxamine-associated neurotoxicity is increased if aluminum serum levels are >200 mcg/L; withhold deferoxamine and administer intensive dialysis until <200 mcg/L.

Aluminum rise ≥300 mcg/L: 5 mg/kg once a week 5 hours before dialysis for 4 months

Aluminum rise <300 mcg/L: 5 mg/kg once a week during the last hour of dialysis for 2 months

Canadian labeling: Adults: Treatment should be considered for symptomatic patients with serum aluminum levels >60 mcg/L and a positive deferoxamine test dose.

Hemodialysis: IV: 5 mg/kg/dose (infusion rate not to exceed 15 mg/kg/hour) once weekly for 3 months following hemodialysis (preferred) or during the last hour of dialysis administered. Withhold treatment for 1 month then perform deferoxamine test. Further treatment is not recommended if 2 consecutive tests (performed 1 month apart) yield an increase in serum aluminum levels <75 mcg/L.

Continuous ambulatory or cyclic peritoneal dialysis: Intraperitoneal (preferred), IM, SubQ infusion (slow), or IV infusion (slow): 5 mg/kg/dose once weekly prior to final daily exchange

Dosing adjustment in renal impairment: Severe renal disease or anuria: Use is contraindicated in the manufacturer's U.S. labeling.

The following adjustments have been used by some clinicians (Aronoff, 2007): Adults:

CrCl >50 mL/minute: No adjustment required

CrCl 10 to 50 mL/minute, CRRT: Administer 25% to 50% of normal dose

CrCl<10 mL/minute, hemodialysis, peritoneal dialysis: Avoid use

Dosage adjustment in hepatic impairment: There are no dosage adjustments provided in the manufacturer's labeling (has not been studied).

Additional Information Complete prescribing information should be consulted for additional detail.

Dosage Forms

Solution Reconstituted, Injection:

Desferal: 500 mg (1 ea); 2 g (1 ea)

Generic: 500 mg (1 ea); 2 g (1 ea)

◆ **Deferoxamine Mesylate** *see* Deferoxamine *on page 586*

◆ **Deferoxamine Mesylate for Injection (Can)** *see* Deferoxamine *on page 586*

Deflazacort [INT] (de FLAZE a kort)

International Brand Names Alnacort (IN); Azacortid (AR, CL, PY, UY); Calcorrt (EC); Calcort (BB, BR, BS, CH, DE, GB, JM, KR, LU, MX, PE, TT, VE); Clobax (CO); Defas (AR); Deflan (GR, IT); Dezacor (ES); Dezartal (CL, CO); DFZ (IN); Dispercort (UY); Flacort (PE); Flamirex (AR); Flantadin (GR, IT); Flazal (BR); Flezacor (CR, GT, HN, PA, SV); Landacort (CO); Lantadin (AT); Prandin (KR); Prism (IN); Rosilan (PT); Servicor (UY); Telacort (KR); Zamene (ES)

Pharmacologic Category Corticosteroid, Systemic; Glucocorticoid

Reported Use Anti-inflammatory for use in conditions responsive to corticosteroid therapy

Dosage Range Adults: Oral: Initial: 120 mg; maintenance: 3-18 mg/day

Product Availability Product available in various countries; not currently available in the U.S.

Dosage Forms

Drops: 22.75 mg/mL [One drop = 1 mg]

Tablet: 6 mg, 30 mg

Degarelix (deg a REL ix)

Brand Names: U.S. Firmagon

Brand Names: Canada Firmagon®

Index Terms Degarelix Acetate; FE200486

Pharmacologic Category Antineoplastic Agent, Gonadotropin-Releasing Hormone Antagonist; Gonadotropin Releasing Hormone Antagonist

Use Treatment of advanced prostate cancer

Pregnancy Risk Factor X

Dosage

Prostate cancer, advanced: Adults: SubQ:

Loading dose: 240 mg administered as two 120 mg (3 mL) injections

Maintenance dose: 80 mg administered as one 4 mL injection every 28 days (beginning 28 days after initial loading dose)

Dosage adjustment in renal impairment:

CrCl 50-80 mL/minute: No dosage adjustment necessary.

CrCl <50 mL/minute: No dosage adjustment provided in manufacturer's labeling; use with caution.

Dosage adjustment in hepatic impairment:

Mild-to-moderate hepatic impairment: No dosage adjustment necessary; monitor serum testosterone levels

Severe hepatic impairment: No dosage adjustment provided in manufacturer's labeling (has not been studied); use with caution.

Additional Information Complete prescribing information should be consulted for additional detail.

Dosage Forms

Solution Reconstituted, Subcutaneous:

Firmagon: 80 mg (1 ea); 120 mg (1 ea)

◆ **Degarelix Acetate** *see* Degarelix *on page 587*

◆ **Dehydral® (Can)** *see* Methenamine *on page 1317*

◆ **Dehydrobenzperidol** *see* Droperidol *on page 695*

Delapril [INT] (DEL a pril)

International Brand Names Adecut (JP); Delaket (IT)

Index Terms Delapril Hydrochloride

Pharmacologic Category Angiotensin-Converting Enzyme (ACE) Inhibitor

Reported Use Management of hypertension

Dosage Range Adults: Oral: 15-30 mg twice daily

Product Availability Product available in various countries; not currently available in the U.S.

Dosage Forms

Tablet: 15 mg, 30 mg

◆ **Delapril Hydrochloride** *see* Delapril [INT] *on page 587*

◆ **Delatestryl (Can)** *see* Testosterone *on page 2010*

Delavirdine (de la VIR deen)

Brand Names: U.S. Rescriptor

Brand Names: Canada Rescriptor

Index Terms DLV; U-90152S

Pharmacologic Category Antiretroviral, Reverse Transcriptase Inhibitor, Non-nucleoside (Anti-HIV)

Use Treatment of HIV-1 infection in combination with at least two additional antiretroviral agents

Pregnancy Risk Factor C

Pregnancy Considerations Adverse events were observed in some animal reproduction studies. Hypersensitivity reactions (including hepatic toxicity and rash) are more common in women on NNRTI therapy; it is not known if pregnancy increases this risk.

Regardless of CD4 count or HIV RNA copy number, all HIV-infected pregnant women should receive a combination antiretroviral (ARV) drug regimen. A combination of antepartum, intrapartum, and infant ARV prophylaxis is recommended. ARV therapy should be started as soon as possible in women with symptomatic infection. Although earlier initiation may be more effective in reducing the perinatal transmission of HIV, initiation may be delayed until after 12 weeks gestation in women who do not require immediate treatment after careful consideration of maternal conditions (eg, nausea and vomiting) and the potential risks of first trimester fetal exposure for specific agents. A scheduled cesarean delivery at 38 weeks gestation is recommended for all women with HIV RNA >1000 copies/mL or unknown concentrations near delivery in order to decrease transmission. If ARV therapy must be interrupted for <24 hours during the peripartum period, stop then restart all medications simultaneously in order to decrease the chance of developing resistance. Long-term follow-up is recommended for all infants exposed to ARV medications. In couples who want to conceive, the HIV-infected partner should attain maximum viral suppression prior to conception.

Health care providers are encouraged to enroll pregnant women exposed to antiretroviral medications in the Antiretroviral Pregnancy Registry (1-800-258-4263 or www.APRegistry.com). Health care providers caring for HIV-infected women and their infants may contact the National Perinatal HIV Hotline (888-448-8765) for clinical consultation (HHS [perinatal], 2014).

Breast-Feeding Considerations It is not known if delavirdine is excreted into breast milk. Maternal or infant antiretroviral therapy does not completely eliminate the risk of postnatal HIV transmission. In addition, multiclass-resistant virus has been detected in breast-feeding infants despite maternal therapy. Therefore, in the United States, where formula is accessible, affordable, safe, and sustainable, and the risk of infant mortality due to diarrhea and respiratory infections is low, complete avoidance of breast-feeding by HIV-infected women is recommended to decrease potential transmission of HIV (HHS [perinatal], 2014).

Contraindications Hypersensitivity to delavirdine or any component of the formulation; concurrent use of alprazolam, astemizole, cisapride, ergot alkaloids, midazolam, pimozide, rifampin, terfenadine, or triazolam

Warnings/Precautions Use with caution in patients with hepatic or renal dysfunction; due to rapid emergence of resistance, delavirdine should not be used as monotherapy or as a component of an initial antiretroviral regimen; cross-resistance may be conferred to other non-nucleoside reverse transcriptase inhibitors, although potential for cross-resistance with protease inhibitors is low. Long-term effects of delavirdine are not known. May cause redistribution of fat (eg, buffalo hump, peripheral wasting with increased abdominal girth, cushingoid appearance). Patients may develop immune reconstitution syndrome resulting in the occurrence of an inflammatory response to an indolent or residual opportunistic infection during initial HIV treatment or activation of autoimmune disorders (eg, Graves' disease, polymyositis, Guillain-Barré syndrome) later in therapy; further evaluation and treatment may be required. Safety and efficacy have not been established in children. Rash, which occurs frequently, may require discontinuation of therapy; usually occurs within 1-3 weeks and lasts <2 weeks. Most patients may resume therapy following a treatment interruption. Use with caution in patients taking strong CYP3A4 inhibitors, moderate or strong CYP3A4 inducers and major CYP3A4 substrates (see Drug Interactions); consider alternative agents that avoid or lessen the potential for CYP-mediated interactions.

Adverse Reactions

Central nervous system: Anxiety, depressive symptoms, fever, headache

Dermatologic: Rash

Endocrine & metabolic: Amylase increased, bilirubin increased, transaminases increased

Gastrointestinal: Abdominal pain, diarrhea, nausea, vomiting

Hematologic: Hemoglobin decreased, prothrombin time increased

Respiratory: Bronchitis

Rare but important or life-threatening: Abscess, adenopathy, alkaline phosphatase increased, allergic reaction, angioedema, anorexia, arrhythmia, bloody stool, bone pain, bruising, cardiac insufficiency, cardiac rate abnormal, cardiomyopathy, chest congestion, cognitive impairment, colitis, confusion, conjunctivitis, dermal leukocytoclastic vasculitis, desquamation, diverticulitis, dyspnea, emotional lability, eosinophilia, erythema multiforme, fecal incontinence, fungal dermatitis, gamma glutamyl transpeptidase increased, gastroenteritis, gastrointestinal bleeding, granulocytosis, gum hemorrhage, hallucination, hematuria, hepatomegaly, hyperglycemia, hyperkalemia, hypertension, hypertriglyceridemia, hyperuricemia, hypocalcemia, hyponatremia, hypophosphatemia, infection, jaundice, kidney pain, leukopenia, lipase increased, menstrual irregularities, moniliasis (oral/vaginal), orthostatic hypotension, pancreatitis, pancytopenia, paralysis, peripheral vascular disorder, pneumonia, purpura, redistribution of body fat, renal calculi, serum creatinine increased, spleen disorder, Stevens-Johnson syndrome, tetany, thrombocytopenia, urinary tract infection, vertigo

Drug Interactions

Metabolism/Transport Effects Substrate of CYP2D6 (minor), CYP3A4 (major); **Note:** Assignment of Major/Minor substrate status based on clinically relevant drug interaction potential; **Inhibits** CYP1A2 (weak), CYP2C19 (strong), CYP2C9 (strong), CYP2D6 (strong), CYP3A4 (strong)

Avoid Concomitant Use

Avoid concomitant use of Delavirdine with any of the following: Ado-Trastuzumab Emtansine; Alfuzosin; Apixaban; Astemizole; Avanafil; Axitinib; Bosutinib; Cabozantinib; CarBAMazepine; Ceritinib; Conivaptan; Crizotinib; Dapoxetine; Dronedarone; Efavirenz; Eplerenone; Etravirine; Everolimus; Fosamprenavir; Fosphenytoin; H2-Antagonists; Halofantrine; Ibrutinib; Irinotecan; Ivabradine; Lapatinib; Lercanidipine; Lomitapide; Lovastatin; Lurasidone; Macitentan; Naloxegol; Nilotinib; Nisoldipine; Olaparib; Phenytoin; Pimozide; Proton Pump Inhibitors; Ranolazine; Red Yeast Rice; Regorafenib; Rifamycin Derivatives; Rilpivirine; Rivaroxaban; Salmeterol; Silodosin; Simeprevir; Simvastatin; St Johns Wort; Suvorexant; Tamoxifen; Tamsulosin; Terfenadine; Thioridazine; Ticagrelor; Tolvaptan; Toremifene; Trabectedin; Ulipristal; Vemurafenib; VinCRIStine (Liposomal); Vorapaxar

Increased Effect/Toxicity

Delavirdine may increase the levels/effects of: Ado-Trastuzumab Emtansine; Alfuzosin; Almotriptan; Alosetron; Apixaban; ARIPiprazole; Astemizole; AtoMOXetine; Avanafil; Axitinib; Bedaquiline; Bortezomib; Bosentan; Bosutinib; Brentuximab Vedotin; Brinzolamide; Budesonide (Nasal); Budesonide (Systemic, Oral Inhalation); Cabazitaxel; Cabozantinib; Cannabis; Ceritinib; Citalopram; Colchicine; Conivaptan; Corticosteroids (Orally Inhaled); Corticosteroids (Systemic); Crizotinib; CYP2C19 Substrates; CYP2C9 Substrates; CYP2D6 Substrates; CYP3A4 Substrates; Dapoxetine; Dasatinib; Diclofenac (Systemic); Dienogest; Dofetilide; DOXOrubicin (Conventional); Dronabinol; Dronedarone; Dutasteride; Efavirenz; Eliglustat; Eplerenone; Erlotinib; Etizolam; Etravirine; Everolimus; FentaNYL; Fesoterodine; Fluticasone (Nasal); Fluticasone (Oral Inhalation); Fosamprenavir; Fosphenytoin; GuanFACINE; Halofantrine; Hydrocodone; Ibrutinib; Idelalisib; Iloperidone; Imatinib; Imidafenacin; Irinotecan; Ivabradine; Ivacaftor; Ixabepilone; Lacosamide; Lapatinib; Lercanidipine; Levobupivacaine; Levomilnacipran; Lomitapide; Lovastatin; Lumefantrine; Lurasidone; Macitentan; Maraviroc; MethylPREDNISolone; Metoprolol; Mifepristone; Naloxegol; Nebivolol; Nilotinib; Nisoldipine; Olaparib; Ospemifene; OxyCODONE; Paricalcitol; PAZOPanib; Phenytoin; Pimecrolimus; Pimozide; PONATinib; Pranlukast; PrednisoLONE (Systemic); PredniSONE; Propafenone; Protease Inhibitors; QUEtiapine; Ranolazine; Red Yeast Rice; Regorafenib; Repaglinide; Retapamulin; Rifamycin Derivatives; Rilpivirine; Rivaroxaban; RomiDEPsin; Ruxolitinib; Salmeterol; Saxagliptin; Sildenafil; Silodosin; Simeprevir; Simvastatin; SORAfenib; Suvorexant; Tadalafil; Tamsulosin; Terfenadine; Tetrabenazine; Tetrahydrocannabinol; Thioridazine; Ticagrelor; Tofacitinib; Tolterodine; Tolvaptan; Toremifene; Trabectedin; Ulipristal; Vardenafil; Vemurafenib; Vilazodone; VinCRIStine (Liposomal); Vorapaxar; Vortioxetine; Zopiclone; Zuclopenthixol

The levels/effects of Delavirdine may be increased by: Cannabis

Decreased Effect

Delavirdine may decrease the levels/effects of: CarBAMazepine; Clopidogrel; Codeine; Efavirenz; Etravirine; Ifosfamide; Iloperidone; Prasugrel; Rilpivirine; Tamoxifen; Ticagrelor

The levels/effects of Delavirdine may be decreased by: Antacids; Bosentan; CarBAMazepine; CYP3A4 Inducers (Moderate); CYP3A4 Inducers (Strong); Dabrafenib; Deferasirox; Fosamprenavir; Fosphenytoin; H2-Antagonists; Mitotane; Phenytoin; Protease Inhibitors; Proton Pump Inhibitors; Rifamycin Derivatives; Siltuximab; St Johns Wort; Tocilizumab

Storage/Stability Store at 20°C to 25°C (68°F to 77°F). Protect from humidity.

Mechanism of Action Delavirdine binds directly to reverse transcriptase, blocking RNA-dependent and DNA-dependent DNA polymerase activities

Pharmacodynamics/Kinetics

Absorption: Rapid

Distribution: Low concentration in saliva and semen; CSF 0.4% concurrent plasma concentration

Protein binding: ~98%, primarily albumin

Metabolism: Hepatic via CYP3A4 and 2D6 (**Note:** May reduce CYP3A activity and inhibit its own metabolism.)

Bioavailability: Tablet: 85% as tablet; ~100% as oral slurry

Half-life elimination: 5.8 hours (range: 2-11 hours)

Time to peak, plasma: 1 hour

Excretion: Urine (51%, <5% as unchanged drug); feces (44%); nonlinear kinetics exhibited

Dosage Adolescents ≥16 years and Adults: Oral: 400 mg 3 times/day

Note: Only a single delavirdine mutation causes resistance; use is not recommended in initial antiretroviral regimens (HHS [adult], 2014).

Dosage adjustment in renal impairment: No dosage adjustment provided in manufacturer's labeling (has not been studied). Guidelines state that no dosage adjustment is necessary in renal impairment (HHS [adult], 2014).

Dosage adjustment in hepatic impairment: No dosage adjustment provided in manufacturer's labeling (has not been studied). However, delavirdine is primarily metabolized by the liver, use with caution.

Dietary Considerations May be taken without regard to meals.

Administration Patients with achlorhydria should take the drug with an acidic beverage; antacids and delavirdine should be separated by 1 hour. A dispersion of delavirdine may be prepared by adding four 100 mg tablets to at least 3 oz of water. Allow to stand for a few minutes and stir until uniform dispersion. Drink immediately. Rinse glass and mouth, then swallow the rinse to ensure total dose administered. The 200 mg tablets should be taken intact.

Monitoring Parameters Liver function tests if administered with saquinavir

Additional Information Potential compliance problems, frequency of administration, and adverse effects should be discussed with patients before initiating therapy to help prevent the emergence of resistance.

Dosage Forms

Tablet, Oral:

Rescriptor: 100 mg, 200 mg

Extemporaneous Preparations A dispersion of delavirdine may be made with tablets. Add four 100 mg tablets to at least 3 oz of water; allow to stand for a few minutes and stir until uniform dispersion. Administer immediately. To ensure full dose is administered, rinse glass and drink liquid; also rinse mouth and swallow following ingestion.

- **Delestrogen** *see* Estradiol (Systemic) *on page 775*
- **Delta-9-tetrahydro-cannabinol** *see* Dronabinol *on page 694*
- **Delta-9-Tetrahydrocannabinol and Cannabinol** *see* Tetrahydrocannabinol and Cannabidiol [CAN/INT] *on page 2018*
- **Delta-9 THC** *see* Dronabinol *on page 694*
- **Deltacortisone** *see* PredniSONE *on page 1706*
- **Deltadehydrocortisone** *see* PredniSONE *on page 1706*
- **Delyla** *see* Ethinyl Estradiol and Levonorgestrel *on page 803*
- **Delzicol** *see* Mesalamine *on page 1301*
- **Demadex** *see* Torsemide *on page 2071*

Demeclocycline (dem e kloe SYE kleen)

Index Terms Declomycin; Demeclocycline Hydrochloride; Demethylchlortetracycline

Pharmacologic Category Antibiotic, Tetracycline Derivative

Use Treatment of susceptible bactérial infections (eg, acne, urinary tract infections, respiratory infections) caused by both gram-negative and gram-positive organisms

Note: Use of demeclocycline as an antibacterial agent is uncommon; alternative tetracycline agents (eg, doxycycline, minocycline, tetracycline) are generally preferred.

Pregnancy Risk Factor D

Dosage

Susceptible infections: Manufacturer's labeling:

Children >8 years: Oral: 7-13 mg/kg/day (maximum: 600 mg/day) divided every 6-12 hours

Adults: Oral: 150 mg 4 times/day or 300 mg twice daily

SIADH (off-label use): Adults: Oral: 600-1200 mg/day (Goh, 2004; Gross, 2008)

Dosing adjustment in renal impairment: Use with caution; dosage adjustment and/or increase in time interval between doses recommended in manufacturer's labeling; no specific adjustment recommendations provided.

Dosing adjustment in hepatic impairment: Use with caution; dosage adjustment and/or increase in time interval between doses recommended in manufacturer's labeling; no specific adjustment recommendations provided.

Additional Information Complete prescribing information should be consulted for additional detail.

Dosage Forms

Tablet, Oral:

Generic: 150 mg, 300 mg

- **Demeclocycline Hydrochloride** *see* Demeclocycline *on page 589*
- **Demerol** *see* Meperidine *on page 1293*
- **4-Demethoxydaunorubicin** *see* IDArubicin *on page 1037*
- **Demethylchlortetracycline** *see* Demeclocycline *on page 589*
- **Demser** *see* Metyrosine *on page 1359*
- **Demulen® 30 (Can)** *see* Ethinyl Estradiol and Ethynodiol Diacetate *on page 801*
- **Denavir** *see* Penciclovir *on page 1608*

Denosumab (den OH sue mab)

Brand Names: U.S. Prolia; Xgeva

Brand Names: Canada Prolia; Xgeva

Index Terms AMG-162

Pharmacologic Category Bone-Modifying Agent; Monoclonal Antibody

Use

Hypercalcemia of malignancy (Xgeva): Treatment of hypercalcemia of malignancy refractory to bisphosphonate therapy

Osteoporosis/bone loss (Prolia): Treatment of osteoporosis in postmenopausal women at high risk of fracture; treatment of osteoporosis (to increase bone mass) in men at high risk of fracture; treatment of bone loss in men receiving androgen-deprivation therapy (ADT) for nonmetastatic prostate cancer; treatment of bone loss in women receiving aromatase inhibitor (AI) therapy for breast cancer

Tumors (Xgeva): Prevention of skeletal-related events (eg, fracture, spinal cord compression, bone pain requiring surgery/radiation therapy) in patients with bone metastases from solid tumors; treatment of giant cell tumor of the bone in adults and skeletally mature adolescents that is unresectable or where surgical resection is likely to result in severe morbidity

Limitation of use: Denosumab is NOT indicated for prevention of skeletal-related events in patients with multiple myeloma

Pregnancy Risk Factor D (Xgeva)/X (Prolia)

Pregnancy Considerations Adverse events were observed in animal reproduction studies. Specifically, increased fetal loss, stillbirths, postnatal mortality, absent lymph nodes, abnormal bone growth, and decreased neonatal growth was observed in cynomolgus monkeys exposed to denosumab throughout pregnancy. Denosumab was measurable in the offspring at one month of age. Fetal exposure to monoclonal antibodies is expected to increase as pregnancy progresses. Women of reproductive potential should be advised to use effective contraception during denosumab treatment and for at least 5 months following the last dose. If a pregnant woman is exposed, patients or their prescribers may contact the Amgen Pregnancy Surveillance Program (800-772-6436). In addition, there is potential for a fetus to be exposed to denosumab when a pregnant woman has unprotected sex with a man treated with denosumab. It is unknown the extent that denosumab is present in seminal fluid; however, the risk of harm to the fetus is expected to be low. Men receiving denosumab who have pregnant partners should be counseled regarding this potential risk.

Breast-Feeding Considerations It is not known if denosumab is excreted in breast milk. According to the manufacturer, the decision to discontinue denosumab or discontinue breast-feeding should take into account the benefits of treatment to the mother. In some animal studies, mammary gland development was impaired following exposure to denosumab during pregnancy, resulting in impaired lactation postpartum.

Contraindications Hypersensitivity to denosumab or any component of the formulation; preexisting hypocalcemia; pregnancy (Prolia only)

Warnings/Precautions Clinically significant hypersensitivity (including anaphylaxis) has been reported. May include throat tightness, facial edema, upper airway edema, lip swelling, dyspnea, pruritus, rash, urticaria, and hypotension. If anaphylaxis or clinically significant hypersensitivity occurs, initiate appropriate management and permanently discontinue. Denosumab may cause or exacerbate hypocalcemia; severe symptomatic cases (including fatalities) have been reported. An increased risk has been observed with increasing renal dysfunction, most commonly severe dysfunction (creatinine clearance <30 mL/minute and/or on dialysis), and with inadequate/no calcium supplementation. Monitor calcium levels; correct preexisting hypocalcemia prior to therapy. Monitor levels more frequently when denosumab is administered with other drugs that can also lower calcium levels. Use caution in patients with a history of hypoparathyroidism, thyroid surgery, parathyroid surgery, malabsorption syndromes, excision of small intestine, severe renal impairment/dialysis, or other conditions which would predispose the patient to hypocalcemia; monitor calcium, phosphorus, and magnesium closely during therapy. Administer calcium, vitamin D, and magnesium as necessary. Patients with severe renal impairment (CrCl <30 mL/minute) or those on dialysis may also develop marked elevations of serum parathyroid hormone (PTH). Incidence of infections may be increased, including serious skin infections, abdominal, urinary, ear, or periodontal infections. Endocarditis has also been reported following use. Patients should be advised to contact their healthcare provider if signs or symptoms of severe infection or cellulitis develop. Use with caution in patients with impaired immune systems or using concomitant immunosuppressive therapy; may be at increased risk for serious infections. Evaluate the need for continued treatment with serious infection.

Atypical femur fractures have been reported in patients receiving denosumab. The fractures may occur anywhere along the femoral shaft (may be bilateral) and commonly occur with minimal to no trauma to the area. Some patients experience prodromal pain weeks or months before the fracture occurs. Because these fractures also occur in osteoporosis patients not treated with denosumab, it is unclear if denosumab therapy is the cause for the fractures; concomitant glucocorticoids may contribute to fracture risk. Advise patients to report new/unusual hip, thigh, or groin pain; and if so, evaluate for atypical/incomplete fracture. Contralateral limb should be assessed if atypical fracture occurs. Consider interrupting therapy in patients who develop an atypical femoral fracture. Osteonecrosis of the jaw (ONJ) has been reported in patients receiving denosumab. ONJ may manifest as jaw pain, osteomyelitis, osteitis, bone erosion, tooth/periodontal infection, toothache, gingival ulceration/erosion. Risk factors include invasive dental procedures (eg, tooth extraction, dental implants, boney surgery); a diagnosis of cancer, concomitant chemotherapy or corticosteroids, poor oral hygiene, ill-fitting dentures; and comorbid disorders (anemia, coagulopathy, infection, preexisting dental disease). In studies of patients with osseous metastasis, a longer duration of denosumab exposure was associated with a higher incidence of ONJ. Patients should maintain good oral hygiene during treatment. A dental exam and preventive dentistry should be performed prior to therapy. The benefit/risk must be assessed by the treating physician and/or dentist/ surgeon prior to any invasive dental procedure; avoid invasive procedures in patients with bone metastases receiving therapy for prevention of skeletal-related events. Patients developing ONJ while on denosumab therapy should receive care by a dentist or oral surgeon; extensive dental surgery to treat ONJ may exacerbate ONJ; evaluate individually and consider discontinuing if extensive dental surgery is necessary. Severe and occasionally incapacitating bone, joint, and/or muscle pain has been reported (time to onset of symptoms has varied from one day to several months after initiating therapy). Consider discontinuing use if severe symptoms develop.

Postmenopausal osteoporosis: For use in women at high risk for fracture which is defined as a history of osteoporotic fracture or multiple risk factors for fracture. May also be used in women who failed or did not tolerate other therapies.

Bone metastases: Denosumab is not indicated for the prevention of skeletal-related events in patients with multiple myeloma. In trials of with multiple myeloma patients, denosumab was noninferior to zoledronic acid in delaying time to first skeletal-related event and mortality was increased in a subset of the denosumab-treated group.

Breast cancer: The American Society of Clinical Oncology (ASCO) updated guidelines on the role of bone-modifying agents (BMAs) in the prevention and treatment of skeletal-related events for metastatic breast cancer patients (Van Poznak, 2011). The guidelines recommend initiating a BMA (denosumab, pamidronate, zoledronic acid) in patients with metastatic breast cancer to the bone. There is currently no literature indicating the superiority of one particular BMA. Optimal duration is not defined; however, the guidelines recommend continuing therapy until substantial decline in patient's performance status. The ASCO guidelines are in alignment with package insert guidelines for dosing, renal dose adjustments, infusion times, prevention and management of osteonecrosis of the jaw, and monitoring of laboratory parameter recommendations. BMAs are not the first-line therapy for pain. BMAs are to be used as adjunctive therapy for cancer-related bone pain associated with bone metastasis, demonstrating a modest pain control benefit. BMAs should be used in conjunction with agents such as NSAIDs, opioid and nonopioid analgesics, corticosteroids, radiation/surgery, and interventional procedures.

Denosumab therapy results in significant suppression of bone turnover; the long term effects of treatment are not known but may contribute to adverse outcomes such as ONJ, atypical fractures, or delayed fracture healing; monitor. Use with caution in patients with renal impairment (CrCl <30 mL/minute) or patients on dialysis; risk of hypocalcemia is increased. Dose adjustment is not needed when administered at 60 mg every 6 months (Prolia); once-monthly dosing has not been evaluated in patients with renal impairment (Xgeva). Dermatitis, eczema, and rash (which are not necessarily specific to the injection site) have been reported; consider discontinuing if severe symptoms occur. Packaging may contain natural latex rubber. May impair bone growth in children with open growth plates or inhibit eruption of dentition. In pediatrics, indicated only for the treatment of giant cell tumor of the bone in adolescents who are skeletally mature. Do not administer Prolia and Xgeva to the same patient for different indications. Denosumab is intended for subcutaneous route only and should not be administered intravenously, intramuscularly, or intradermally.

Adverse Reactions A postmarketing safety program is available to collect information on adverse events. Prescribers may call 800-772-6436 or see http://www.proliasafety.com for more information.

Cardiovascular: Angina pectoris, peripheral edema

Central nervous system: Fatigue, headache, sciatica

Dermatologic: Dermatitis, eczema, skin rash

Endocrine & metabolic: Hypercholesterolemia, hypocalcemia (risk increased with renal dysfunction), hypophosphatemia

Gastrointestinal: Diarrhea, flatulence, nausea

Hematologic & oncologic: Malignant neoplasm (new)

Infection: Serious infection (nonfatal)

Neuromuscular & skeletal: Limb pain, myalgia, ostealgia, osteonecrosis (jaw)

Ophthalmic: Cataract

Respiratory: Nasopharyngitis, upper respiratory tract infection

Rare but important or life-threatening: Antibody development (both formulations), endocarditis, femur fracture (both formulations; diaphyseal, subtrochanteric), hypersensitivity (both formulations), hypertension, hypotension, influenza, pancreatitis

Drug Interactions

Metabolism/Transport Effects None known.

Avoid Concomitant Use

Avoid concomitant use of Denosumab with any of the following: Belimumab

Increased Effect/Toxicity

Denosumab may increase the levels/effects of: Belimumab; Immunosuppressants

Decreased Effect There are no known significant interactions involving a decrease in effect.

Storage/Stability Store in original carton under refrigeration at 2°C to 8°C (36°F to 46°F). Do not freeze. Prior to use, bring to room temperature of 25°C (77°F) in original container (usually takes 15 to 30 minutes); do not use any other methods for warming. Use within 14 days once at room temperature. Protect from direct heat and light; do not expose to temperatures >25°C (77°F). Avoid vigorous shaking.

Mechanism of Action Denosumab is a monoclonal antibody with affinity for nuclear factor-kappa ligand (RANKL). Osteoblasts secrete RANKL; RANKL activates osteoclast precursors and subsequent osteolysis which promotes release of bone-derived growth factors, such as insulin-like growth factor-1 (IGF1) and transforming growth factor-beta (TGF-beta), and increases serum calcium levels. Denosumab binds to RANKL, blocks the interaction between RANKL and RANK (a receptor located on osteoclast surfaces), and prevents osteoclast formation, leading to decreased bone resorption and increased bone mass in osteoporosis. In solid tumors with bony metastases, RANKL inhibition decreases osteoclastic activity leading to decreased skeletal related events and tumor-induced bone destruction. In giant cell tumors of the bone (which express RANK and RANKL), denosumab inhibits tumor growth by preventing RANKL from activating its receptor (RANK) on the osteoclast surface, osteoclast precursors, and osteoclast-like giant cells.

Pharmacodynamics/Kinetics

Onset of action: Decreases markers of bone resorption by ~85% within 3 days; maximal reductions observed within 1 month

Hypercalcemia of malignancy: Time to response (median): 9 days; Time to complete response (median): 23 days (Hu, 2014)

Duration: Markers of bone resorption return to baseline within 12 months of discontinuing therapy

Hypercalcemia of malignancy: Duration of response (median): 104 days; Duration of complete response (median): 34 days (Hu, 2014)

Bioavailability: SubQ: 62%

Half-life elimination: ~25 to 28 days

Time to peak, serum: 10 days (range: 3 to 21 days)

Dosage Note: Administer calcium and vitamin D as necessary to prevent or treat hypocalcemia

Hypercalcemia of malignancy (Xgeva): Adults: SubQ: 120 mg every 4 weeks; during the first month, give an additional 120 mg on days 8 and 15 (Hu, 2014)

Prevention of skeletal-related events in bone metastases from solid tumors (Xgeva): Adults: SubQ: 120 mg every 4 weeks (Fizazi, 2011; Henry, 2011; Stopeck, 2010)

Treatment of androgen deprivation-induced bone loss in men with prostate cancer (Prolia): Adults: SubQ: 60 mg as a single dose, once every 6 months (Smith, 2009)

Treatment of aromatase inhibitor-induced bone loss in women with breast cancer (Prolia): Adults: SubQ: 60 mg as a single dose, once every 6 months (Ellis, 2008)

Treatment of giant cell tumor of the bone (Xgeva): Adolescents (skeletally mature) 13 to 17 years and Adults: SubQ: 120 mg once every 4 weeks; during the first month, give an additional 120 mg on days 8 and 15 (Blay, 2011; Thomas, 2010)

Treatment of osteoporosis in men or postmenopausal women (Prolia): Adults: SubQ: 60 mg as a single dose, once every 6 months

Dosage adjustment in renal impairment: Monitor patients with severe impairment (CrCl <30 mL/minute or on dialysis) due to increased risk of hypocalcemia.

Prolia: No dosage adjustment is necessary.

Xgeva: There are no dosage adjustments provided in the manufacturer's labeling. However, in studies of patients with varying degrees of renal impairment, the degree of renal impairment had no effect on denosumab pharmacokinetics or pharmacodynamics.

Dosage adjustment in hepatic impairment: There are no dosage adjustments provided in the manufacturer's labeling (has not been studied).

Dietary Considerations Ensure adequate calcium and vitamin D intake to prevent or treat hypocalcemia. Calcium 1000 mg/day and vitamin D ≥400 units/day is recommended in product labeling (Prolia). If dietary intake is inadequate, dietary supplementation is recommended. Women and men should consume:

Calcium: 1000 mg/day (men: 50 to 70 years) **or** 1200 mg/day (women ≥51 years and men ≥71 years) (IOM, 2011; NOF, 2014)

Vitamin D: 800 to 1000 units/day (men and women ≥50 years) (NOF, 2014). Recommended Dietary Allowance (RDA): 600 units/day (men and women ≤70 years) **or** 800 units/day (men and women ≥71 years) (IOM, 2011).

Administration SubQ: Denosumab is intended for subcutaneous route only and should not be administered intravenously, intramuscularly, or intradermally. Prior to administration, bring to room temperature in original container (allow to stand ~15 to 30 minutes); do not warm by any other method. Solution may contain trace amounts of translucent to white protein particles; do not use if cloudy, discolored (normal solution should be clear and colorless to pale yellow), or contains excessive particles or foreign matter. Avoid vigorous shaking. Administer via SubQ injection in the upper arm, upper thigh, or abdomen.

Prolia: If a dose is missed, administer as soon as possible, then continue dosing every 6 months from the date of the last injection.

Monitoring Parameters Recommend monitoring of serum creatinine, serum calcium, phosphorus and magnesium, signs and symptoms of hypocalcemia, especially in patients predisposed to hypocalcemia (severe renal impairment, thyroid/parathyroid surgery, malabsorption syndromes, hypoparathyroidism); infection, or dermatologic reactions; routine oral exam (prior to treatment); dental exam if risk factors for ONJ; monitor for sings/symptoms of hypersensitivity

Osteoporosis: Bone mineral density (BMD) should be reevaluated every 2 years (or more frequently) after initiating therapy (NOF, 2014); annual measurements of height and weight, assessment of chronic back pain; serum calcium and 25(OH)D; may consider monitoring biochemical markers of bone turnover

Reference Range

Calcium (total): Adults: 9.0 to 11.0 mg/dL (2.05 to 2.54 mmol/L), may slightly decrease with aging

Phosphorus: 2.5 to 4.5 mg/dL (0.81 to 1.45 mmol/L)

Vitamin D: There is no clear consensus on a reference range for total serum 25(OH)D concentrations or the validity of this level as it relates clinically to bone health. In addition, there is significant variability in the reporting of serum 25(OH)D levels as a result of different assay types in use; however, the following ranges have been suggested:

Adults (IOM, 2011): Sufficient levels in practically all persons: ≥20 ng/mL (50 nmol/L); concern for risk of toxicity: >50 ng/mL (125 nmol/L)

Osteoporosis patients (NOF, 2014): Recommended level to reach and maintain: ~30 ng/mL (75 nmol/L)

Dosage Forms

Solution, Subcutaneous [preservative free]:

Prolia: 60 mg/mL (1 mL)

Xgeva: 120 mg/1.7 mL (1.7 mL)

- **Denta 5000 Plus** *see* Fluoride *on page 895*
- **DentaGel** *see* Fluoride *on page 895*
- **Dentapaine [OTC]** *see* Benzocaine *on page 246*
- **Denti-Care Chlorhexidine Gluconate Oral Rinse (Can)** *see* Chlorhexidine Gluconate *on page 422*
- **Dent-O-Kain/20 [OTC]** *see* Benzocaine *on page 246*
- **Deodorized Tincture of Opium (error-prone synonym)** *see* Opium Tincture *on page 1518*
- **Deoxyazacytidine** *see* Decitabine *on page 581*
- **Deoxycoformycin** *see* Pentostatin *on page 1618*
- **2'-Deoxycoformycin** *see* Pentostatin *on page 1618*
- **Depacon** *see* Valproic Acid and Derivatives *on page 2123*
- **Depakene** *see* Valproic Acid and Derivatives *on page 2123*
- **Depakote** *see* Valproic Acid and Derivatives *on page 2123*
- **Depakote ER** *see* Valproic Acid and Derivatives *on page 2123*
- **Depakote Sprinkles** *see* Valproic Acid and Derivatives *on page 2123*
- **Depen Titratabs** *see* PenicillAMINE *on page 1608*
- **DepoCyt** *see* Cytarabine (Liposomal) *on page 540*
- **DepoCyt® (Can)** *see* Cytarabine (Liposomal) *on page 540*
- **DepoDur** *see* Morphine (Liposomal) *on page 1400*
- **Depo-Estradiol** *see* Estradiol (Systemic) *on page 775*
- **DepoFoam Bupivacaine** *see* Bupivacaine (Liposomal) *on page 299*
- **DepoFoam-Encapsulated Cytarabine** *see* Cytarabine (Liposomal) *on page 540*
- **Depo-Medrol** *see* MethylPREDNISolone *on page 1340*
- **Depo-Prevera (Can)** *see* MedroxyPROGESTERone *on page 1277*
- **Depo-Provera** *see* MedroxyPROGESTERone *on page 1277*
- **Depo-SubQ Provera 104** *see* MedroxyPROGESTERone *on page 1277*
- **Depotest 100 (Can)** *see* Testosterone *on page 2010*
- **Depo-Testosterone** *see* Testosterone *on page 2010*
- **Deprenyl** *see* Selegiline *on page 1873*
- **Deprizine FusePaq** *see* Ranitidine *on page 1777*
- **Depsipeptide** *see* RomiDEPsin *on page 1841*
- **DermaFungal [OTC]** *see* Miconazole (Topical) *on page 1360*
- **Dermal Therapy Finger Care [OTC]** *see* Urea *on page 2114*
- **DermaMed [OTC]** *see* Aluminum Hydroxide *on page 103*
- **Derma-Smoothe/FS® (Can)** *see* Fluocinolone (Topical) *on page 893*
- **Derma-Smoothe/FS Body** *see* Fluocinolone (Topical) *on page 893*
- **Derma-Smoothe/FS Scalp** *see* Fluocinolone (Topical) *on page 893*
- **Dermasorb HC** *see* Hydrocortisone (Topical) *on page 1014*
- **Dermasorb TA** *see* Triamcinolone (Topical) *on page 2100*
- **Dermasorb XM** *see* Urea *on page 2114*
- **Dermatop** *see* Prednicarbate *on page 1703*
- **Dermatop® (Can)** *see* Prednicarbate *on page 1703*
- **Dermazene** *see* Iodoquinol and Hydrocortisone *on page 1105*
- **Dermazole (Can)** *see* Miconazole (Topical) *on page 1360*
- **Dermovate (Can)** *see* Clobetasol *on page 468*
- **Desenex [OTC]** *see* Clotrimazole (Topical) *on page 488*
- **Desenex [OTC]** *see* Miconazole (Topical) *on page 1360*
- **Desenex Jock Itch [OTC]** *see* Miconazole (Topical) *on page 1360*

◆ **Desenex Spray [OTC]** *see* Miconazole (Topical) *on page 1360*

◆ **Desferal** *see* Deferoxamine *on page 586*

◆ **Desferrioxamine** *see* Deferoxamine *on page 586*

◆ **Desiccated Thyroid** *see* Thyroid, Desiccated *on page 2031*

Desipramine (des IP ra meen)

Brand Names: U.S. Norpramin

Brand Names: Canada Dom-Desipramine; Novo-Desipramine; Nu-Desipramine; PMS-Desipramine

Index Terms Desipramine Hydrochloride; Desmethylimipramine Hydrochloride

Pharmacologic Category Antidepressant, Tricyclic (Secondary Amine)

Additional Appendix Information

Beers Criteria - Potentially Inappropriate Medications for Geriatrics *on page 2271*

Use Depression: Treatment of depression

Dosage

Depression: **Note:** Not FDA approved for use in pediatric patients; controlled clinical trials have not shown tricyclic antidepressants to be superior to placebo for the treatment of depression in children and adolescents (Dopheide, 2006; Wagner, 2005).

Children 6 to 12 years (off-label use): Oral: 1 to 3 mg/kg/day in divided doses; monitor carefully with doses >3 mg/kg/day; maximum dose: 5 mg/kg/day (Kliegman, 2007).

Adolescents: Oral: Initial dose: Start at a lower dosage level and increase based on tolerance and response; usual maximum of 100 mg daily; usual maintenance dose: 25 to 100 mg once daily or in divided doses; doses up to 150 mg daily may be necessary in severely depressed patients (maximum: 150 mg daily)

Adults: Oral: Initial dose: 25 to 50 mg once daily or in divided doses (APA, 2010; WFSBP 2013); increase based on tolerance and response; usual maintenance dose: 100 to 200 mg once daily or in divided doses; doses up to 300 mg daily may be necessary in severely depressed patients (maximum: 300 mg daily)

Elderly: Oral: Initial dose: Start at a lower dosage level and increase based on tolerance and response to a usual maximum of 100 mg daily; usual maintenance dose: 25 to 100 mg once daily or in divided doses; doses up to 150 mg daily may be necessary in severely depressed patients (maximum: 150 mg daily)

Neuropathic pain (off-label use): Adults: Oral: Initial: 25 mg at bedtime; increase dose in increments of 25 mg daily every 3 to 7 days as necessary until the desired effect is obtained; maximum dose: 150 mg daily (Dworkin, 2007; Max, 1992).

Discontinuation of therapy: Upon discontinuation of antidepressant therapy, gradually taper the dose to minimize the incidence of withdrawal symptoms and allow for the detection of re-emerging symptoms. Evidence supporting ideal taper rates is limited. APA and NICE guidelines suggest tapering therapy over at least several weeks with consideration to the half-life of the antidepressant; antidepressants with a shorter half-life may need to be tapered more conservatively. In addition for long-term treated patients, WFSBP guidelines recommend tapering over 4 to 6 months. If intolerable withdrawal symptoms occur following a dose reduction, consider resuming the previously prescribed dose and/or decrease dose at a more gradual rate (APA, 2010; Bauer, 2002; Haddad, 2001; NCCMH, 2010; Schatzberg, 2006; Shelton, 2001; Warner, 2006).

MAO inhibitor recommendations:

Switching to or from an MAO inhibitor intended to treat psychiatric disorders:

Allow 14 days to elapse between discontinuing an MAO inhibitor intended to treat psychiatric disorders and initiation of desipramine.

Allow 14 days to elapse between discontinuing desipramine and initiation of an MAO inhibitor intended to treat psychiatric disorders.

Use with other MAO inhibitors (linezolid or IV methylene blue):

Do not initiate desipramine in patients receiving linezolid or IV methylene blue; consider other interventions for psychiatric condition.

If urgent treatment with linezolid or IV methylene blue is required in a patient already receiving desipramine and potential benefits outweigh potential risks, discontinue desipramine promptly and administer linezolid or IV methylene blue. Monitor for serotonin syndrome for 2 weeks or until 24 hours after the last dose of linezolid or IV methylene blue, whichever comes first. May resume desipramine 24 hours after the last dose of linezolid or IV methylene blue.

Dosage adjustment in renal impairment: There are no dosage adjustments provided in the manufacturer's labeling; use with caution.

Dosage adjustment in hepatic impairment: There are no dosage adjustments provided in the manufacturer's labeling; use with caution.

Additional Information Complete prescribing information should be consulted for additional detail.

Dosage Forms

Tablet, Oral:

Norpramin: 10 mg, 25 mg, 50 mg, 75 mg, 100 mg, 150 mg

Generic: 10 mg, 25 mg, 50 mg, 75 mg, 100 mg, 150 mg

◆ **Desipramine Hydrochloride** *see* Desipramine *on page 593*

Desirudin (des i ROO din)

Brand Names: U.S. Iprivask

Index Terms CGP-39393; Desulfato-Hirudin; Desulfatohirudin; Desulphatohirudin; r-Hirudin; Recombinant Desulfatohirudin; Recombinant Hirudin

Pharmacologic Category Anticoagulant; Anticoagulant, Direct Thrombin Inhibitor

Use Deep vein thrombosis, prophylaxis: Prophylaxis of deep vein thrombosis (DVT) in patients undergoing hip-replacement surgery

Pregnancy Risk Factor C

Dosage Note: Initial dose may be given up to 5 to 15 minutes prior to surgery (after induction of regional anesthesia, if used); has been administered for up to 12 days (average: 9 to 12 days) in clinical trials

DVT prophylaxis: Adults: SubQ: 15 mg every 12 hours; interrupt therapy if aPTT exceeds 2 times control; resume at a reduced dose (based on the degree of aPTT abnormality) when aPTT is <2 times control

Dosage adjustment in renal impairment:

Moderate impairment (CrCl ≥31 to 60 mL/minute/1.73 m^2): Initial dose: 5 mg every 12 hours. Interrupt therapy if aPTT exceeds 2 times control; resume at a reduced dose (based on the degree of aPTT abnormality) when aPTT is <2 times control.

Severe impairment (CrCl <31 mL/minute/1.73 m^2): Initial dose: 1.7 mg every 12 hours. Interrupt therapy if aPTT exceeds 2 times control; resume at a reduced dose (based on the degree of aPTT abnormality) when aPTT is <2 times control.

Dosage adjustment in hepatic impairment: There are no dosage adjustments provided in the manufacturer's labeling (has not been studied); use with caution.

Additional Information Complete prescribing information should be consulted for additional detail.

Dosage Forms

Solution Reconstituted, Subcutaneous:
Iprivask: 15 mg (1 ea)

◆ **Desitin® [OTC]** *see* Zinc Oxide *on page 2200*

◆ **Desitin® Creamy [OTC]** *see* Zinc Oxide *on page 2200*

Desloratadine (des lor AT a deen)

Brand Names: U.S. Clarinex; Clarinex Reditabs

Brand Names: Canada Aerius®; Aerius® Kids; Desloratadine Allergy Control

Pharmacologic Category Histamine H_1 Antagonist; Histamine H_1 Antagonist, Second Generation; Piperidine Derivative

Use Relief of nasal and non-nasal symptoms of seasonal allergic rhinitis (SAR) and perennial allergic rhinitis (PAR); treatment of chronic idiopathic urticaria (CIU)

Pregnancy Risk Factor C

Dosage Oral:

Children:
- 6-11 months: 1 mg once daily
- 12 months to 5 years: 1.25 mg once daily
- 6-11 years: 2.5 mg once daily

Children ≥12 years and Adults: 5 mg once daily

Dosage adjustment in renal impairment:
- Children: No dosage adjustment provided in manufacturer's labeling (has not been studied).
- Adults: Mild-to-severe impairment: 5 mg every other day.

Dosage adjustment in hepatic impairment:
- Children: No dosage adjustment provided in manufacturer's labeling (has not been studied).
- Adults: Mild-to-severe impairment: 5 mg every other day.

Additional Information Complete prescribing information should be consulted for additional detail.

Dosage Forms

Syrup, Oral:
Clarinex: 0.5 mg/mL (473 mL)

Tablet, Oral:
Clarinex: 5 mg
Generic: 5 mg

Tablet Dispersible, Oral:
Clarinex Reditabs: 2.5 mg, 5 mg
Generic: 2.5 mg, 5 mg

◆ **Desloratadine Allergy Control (Can)** *see* Desloratadine *on page 594*

Desloratadine and Pseudoephedrine
(des lor AT a deen & soo doe e FED rin)

Brand Names: U.S. Clarinex-D® 12 Hour; Clarinex-D® 24 Hour [DSC]

Index Terms Pseudoephedrine and Desloratadine

Pharmacologic Category Alpha/Beta Agonist; Decongestant; Histamine H_1 Agonist; Histamine H_1 Antagonist, Second Generation; Piperidine Derivative

Use Relief of nasal and non-nasal symptoms of seasonal allergic rhinitis

Pregnancy Risk Factor C

Dosage Oral: Children ≥12 years and Adults:
- Clarinex-D® 12 Hour: One tablet twice daily
- Clarinex-D® 24 Hour: One tablet daily

Dosage adjustment in renal impairment: Use is not recommended.

Dosage adjustment in hepatic impairment: Use is not recommended.

Additional Information Complete prescribing information should be consulted for additional detail.

Dosage Forms

Tablet, variable release:
Clarinex-D® 12 Hour: Desloratadine 2.5 mg [immediate release] and pseudoephedrine 120 mg [extended release]

◆ **Desmethylimipramine Hydrochloride** *see* Desipramine *on page 593*

Desmopressin (des moe PRES in)

Brand Names: U.S. DDAVP; DDAVP Rhinal Tube; Stimate

Brand Names: Canada Apo-Desmopressin; DDAVP; DDAVP Melt; Minirin; Novo-Desmopressin; Octostim; PMS-Desmopressin

Index Terms 1-Deamino-8-D-Arginine Vasopressin; Desmopressin Acetate

Pharmacologic Category Antihemophilic Agent; Hemostatic Agent; Hormone, Posterior Pituitary; Vasopressin Analog, Synthetic

Use

Injection: Treatment of diabetes insipidus; maintenance of hemostasis and control of bleeding in hemophilia A with factor VIII coagulant activity levels >5% and mild-to-moderate classic von Willebrand's disease (type 1) with factor VIII coagulant activity levels >5%

Nasal solutions (DDAVP Nasal Spray and DDAVP Rhinal Tube): Treatment of central diabetes insipidus

Nasal spray (Stimate): Maintenance of hemostasis and control of bleeding in hemophilia A with factor VIII coagulant activity levels >5% and mild-to-moderate classic von Willebrand's disease (type 1) with factor VIII coagulant activity levels >5%

Tablet: Treatment of central diabetes insipidus, temporary polyuria and polydipsia following pituitary surgery or head trauma, primary nocturnal enuresis

Pregnancy Risk Factor B

Pregnancy Considerations Adverse events were not observed in animal reproduction studies. Anecdotal reports suggest congenital anomalies and low birth weight. However, causal relationship has not been established. Desmopressin has been used safely throughout pregnancy for the treatment of diabetes insipidus (Brewster, 2005; Schrier, 2010). The use of desmopressin is limited for the treatment of von Willebrand disease in pregnant women (NHLBI, 2007).

Breast-Feeding Considerations It is not known if desmopressin is excreted in breast milk. The manufacturer recommends that caution be exercised when administering desmopressin to nursing women.

Contraindications Hypersensitivity to desmopressin or any component of the formulation; hyponatremia or a history of hyponatremia; moderate-to-severe renal impairment (CrCl<50 mL/minute)

Canadian labeling: Additional contraindications (not in U.S. labeling): Type 2B or platelet-type (pseudo) von Willebrand's disease (injection, intranasal, oral, sublingual); known hyponatremia, habitual or psychogenic polydipsia, cardiac insufficiency or other conditions requiring diuretic therapy (intranasal, sublingual); nephrosis, severe hepatic dysfunction (sublingual); primary nocturnal enuresis (intranasal)

Warnings/Precautions Allergic reactions and anaphylaxis have been reported rarely with both the IV and intranasal formulations. Fluid intake should be adjusted downward in the elderly and very young patients to decrease the possibility of water intoxication and hyponatremia. Use may rarely lead to extreme decreases in plasma osmolality, resulting in seizures, coma, and death.

Use caution with cystic fibrosis, heart failure, renal dysfunction, polydipsia (habitual or psychogenic [contraindicated in Canadian labeling]), or other conditions associated with fluid and electrolyte imbalance due to potential hyponatremia. Use caution with coronary artery insufficiency or hypertensive cardiovascular disease; may increase or decrease blood pressure leading to changes in heart rate. Consider switching from nasal to intravenous solution if changes in the nasal mucosa (scarring, edema) occur leading to unreliable absorption. Use caution in patients predisposed to thrombus formation; thrombotic events (acute cerebrovascular thrombosis, acute myocardial infarction) have occurred (rare).

Desmopressin (intranasal and IV), when used for hemostasis in hemophilia, is not for use in hemophilia B, type 2B von Willebrand disease, severe classic von Willebrand disease (type 1), or in patients with factor VIII antibodies. In general, desmopressin is also not recommended for use in patients with ≤5% factor VIII activity level, although it may be considered in selected patients with activity levels between 2% and 5%.

Consider switching from nasal to intravenous administration if changes in the nasal mucosa (scarring, edema) occur leading to unreliable absorption. Consider alternative rout of administration (IV or intranasal) with inadequate therapeutic response at maximum recommended oral doses. Therapy should be interrupted if patient experiences an acute illness (eg, fever, recurrent vomiting or diarrhea), vigorous exercise, or any condition associated with an increase in water consumption. Some patients may demonstrate a change in response after long-term therapy (>6 months) characterized as decreased response or a shorter duration of response.

Adverse Reactions

Cardiovascular: Decreased blood pressure (IV), increased blood pressure (IV), flushing (facial)

Central nervous system: Chills (intranasal), dizziness (intranasal), headache, nostril pain (intranasal)

Dermatologic: Skin rash

Endocrine & metabolic: Hyponatremia, water intoxication

Gastrointestinal: Abdominal cramps, abdominal pain (intranasal), gastrointestinal disease (intranasal), nausea (intranasal), sore throat

Hepatic: Increased serum transaminases (transient; associated primarily with tablets)

Local: Burning sensation at injection site, erythema at injection site, swelling at injection site

Neuromuscular & skeletal: Weakness (intranasal)

Ophthalmic: Abnormal lacrimation (intranasal), conjunctivitis (intranasal), ocular edema (intranasal)

Respiratory: Cough, epistaxis (intranasal), nasal congestion, rhinitis (intranasal), upper respiratory infection

Rare but important or life-threatening: Abnormality in thinking, agitation, anaphylaxis (rare), balanitis, cerebral thrombosis (IV; acute), chest pain, coma, diarrhea, drowsiness, dyspepsia, edema, eye pruritus, hypersensitivity reaction (rare), insomnia, localized warm feeling, myocardial infarction (IV), pain, palpitations, photophobia, seizure, tachycardia, vomiting, vulvar pain

Drug Interactions

Metabolism/Transport Effects None known.

Avoid Concomitant Use There are no known interactions where it is recommended to avoid concomitant use.

Increased Effect/Toxicity

Desmopressin may increase the levels/effects of: Lithium

The levels/effects of Desmopressin may be increased by: Analgesics (Opioid); CarBAMazepine; ChlorproMAZINE; LamoTRIgine; Nonsteroidal Anti-Inflammatory Agents; Selective Serotonin Reuptake Inhibitors; Tricyclic Antidepressants

Decreased Effect

The levels/effects of Desmopressin may be decreased by: Demeclocycline; Lithium

Preparation for Administration DDAVP: Dilute solution for injection in 10 to 50 mL NS for IV infusion (10 mL for children ≤10 kg: 50 mL for adults and children >10 kg).

Storage/Stability

DDAVP:

Nasal spray: Store at controlled room temperature of 20°C to 25°C (68°F to 77°F). Keep nasal spray in upright position.

Rhinal Tube solution: Store refrigerated at 2°C to 8°C (36°F to 46°F). May store at controlled room temperature of 20°C to 25°C (68°F to 77°F) for up to 3 weeks.

Solution for injection: Store refrigerated at 2°C to 8°C (36°F to 46°F).

Tablet: Store at controlled room temperature of 20°C to 25°C (68°F to 77°F).

DDAVP Melt (CAN; not available in U.S.): Store at 15°C to 25°C (59°F to 77°F) in original container. Protect from moisture.

Stimate nasal spray: Store at room temperature not to exceed 25°C (77°F). Discard 6 months after opening bottle.

Mechanism of Action In a dose dependent manner, desmopressin increases cyclic adenosine monophosphate (cAMP) in renal tubular cells which increases water permeability resulting in decreased urine volume and increased urine osmolality; increases plasma levels of von Willebrand factor, factor VIII, and t-PA contributing to a shortened activated partial thromboplastin time (aPTT) and bleeding time.

Pharmacodynamics/Kinetics

Onset of action:

Intranasal: Antidiuretic: 15 to 30 minutes; Increased factor VIII and von Willebrand factor (vWF) activity (dose related): 30 minutes

Peak effect: Antidiuretic: 1 hour; Increased factor VIII and vWF activity: 1.5 hours

IV infusion: Increased factor VIII and vWF activity: 30 minutes (dose related)

Peak effect: 1.5 to 2 hours

Oral tablet: Antidiuretic: ~1 hour

Peak effect: 4 to 7 hours

Duration: Intranasal, IV infusion, Oral tablet: ~6 to 14 hours

Absorption: Sublingual: Rapid

Bioavailability: Intranasal: ~3.5%; Oral tablet: 5% compared to intranasal, 0.16% compared to IV

Half-life elimination: Intranasal: ~3.5 hours; IV infusion: 3 hours; Oral tablet: 2 to 3 hours

Renal impairment: ≤9 hours

Excretion: Urine

Dosage

Diabetes insipidus: Note: Fluid restriction should be observed in these patients; younger patients more susceptible to plasma osmolality shifts and possible hyponatremia. Dosing should be individualized to response.

Parenteral:

U.S. labeling: Children ≥12 years, Adolescents, and Adults: IV, SubQ: 2 to 4 mcg daily (0.5 to 1 mL) in 2 divided doses or one-tenth (1/10) of the maintenance intranasal dose. Fluid restriction should be observed.

Alternative recommendations (off-label): Infants and Children <12 years: IV, SubQ: No definitive dosing available. Adult dosing should **not** be used in this age group; adverse events such as hyponatremia-induced seizures may occur. Dose should be reduced. Some have suggested an initial dosage range of 0.1 to 1 mcg daily in 1 or 2 divided doses (Cheetham, 2002). Initiate at low dose and increase as necessary. Closely monitor serum sodium levels and urine output; fluid restriction is recommended.

Canadian labeling:

Children and Adolescents: IM, IV, SubQ: 0.4 mcg (0.1 mL) once daily or one-tenth (1/10) of the maintenance intranasal dose. Fluid restriction should be observed.

Adults: IM, IV, SubQ: 1 to 4 mcg (0.25 to 1 mL) once daily or one-tenth (1/10) of the maintenance intranasal dose. Fluid restriction should be observed.

Intranasal (using 100 mcg/mL nasal solution [eg, DDAVP]):

Infants ≥3 months and Children ≤12 years: Usual dose range: 5 to 30 mcg daily (0.05 to 0.3 mL daily) as a single dose or divided 2 times daily; adjust morning and evening doses separately for an adequate diurnal rhythm of water turnover. **Note:** The nasal spray pump can only deliver doses of 10 mcg (0.1 mL) or multiples of 10 mcg (0.1 mL); if doses other than this are needed, the rhinal tube delivery system is preferred. Fluid restriction should be observed.

Adolescents and Adults: Usual dose range: 10 to 40 mcg daily (0.1 to 0.4 mL) as a single dose or divided 2 to 3 times daily; adjust morning and evening doses separately for an adequate diurnal rhythm of water turnover. **Note:** The nasal spray pump can only deliver doses of 10 mcg (0.1 mL) or multiples of 10 mcg (0.1 mL); if doses other than this are needed, the rhinal tube delivery system is preferred. Fluid restriction should be observed.

Oral:

U.S. labeling: Children ≥4 years, Adolescents, and Adults: Initial: 0.05 mg twice daily; total daily dose should be increased or decreased as needed to obtain adequate antidiuresis (range: 0.1 to 1.2 mg divided 2 to 3 times daily). Fluid restriction should be observed.

Canadian labeling:

Children: Initial: 0.1 mg 3 times daily; total daily dose should be increased or decreased as needed to obtain adequate antidiuresis (range: 0.3 to 1.2 mg divided 3 times daily). Divide daily doses so that the evening dose is 2 times higher than the morning or afternoon dose to ensure adequate antidiuresis during the night. Fluid restriction should be observed.

Adolescents and Adults: Initial: 0.1 mg 3 times daily; total daily dose should be increased or decreased as needed to obtain adequate antidiuresis (range: 0.3 to 1.2 mg divided 3 times daily). Fluid restriction should be observed.

Sublingual formulation [Canadian product]:

Children: Initial: 60 mcg 3 times daily; total daily dose should be increased or decreased as needed to obtain adequate antidiuresis. Usual maintenance: 60 to 120 mcg 3 times daily (range: 120 to 720 mcg divided 3 times daily); divide daily doses so that the evening dose is 2 times higher than the morning or afternoon dose to ensure adequate antidiuresis during the night. Fluid restriction should be observed.

Adolescents and Adults: Initial: 60 mcg 3 times daily; total daily dose should be increased or decreased as needed to obtain adequate antidiuresis. Usual maintenance: 60 to 120 mcg 3 times daily (range: 120 to 720 mcg divided 3 times daily). Fluid restriction should be observed.

Hemophilia A and von Willebrand disease (type 1):

IV: **Note:** Adverse events such as hyponatremia-induced seizures have been reported especially in young children using this dosing regimen (Das, 2005; Molnar, 2005; Smith, 1989; Thumfart, 2005; Weinstein, 1989). Fluid restriction and careful monitoring of serum sodium levels and urine output are necessary.

Infants ≥3 months, Children, Adolescents, and Adults: 0.3 mcg/kg by slow infusion; may repeat dose if needed; if used preoperatively, administer 30 minutes before procedure

Canadian labeling (not in U.S. labeling): Maximum IV dose: 20 mcg

Intranasal (using high concentration spray [1.5 mg/mL] [eg, Stimate]): Infants ≥11 months, Children, Adolescents, and Adults: <50 kg: 150 mcg (1 spray in a single nostril); ≥50 kg: 300 mcg (1 spray each nostril); repeat use is determined by the patient's clinical condition and laboratory results. If using preoperatively, administer 2 hours before surgery.

Nocturnal enuresis:

Oral:

Children ≥6 years and Adolescents (U.S. labeling) or Children ≥5 years and Adolescents (Canadian labeling): Initial: 0.2 mg at bedtime; dose may be titrated up to 0.6 mg to achieve desired response. Fluid intake should be limited 1 hour prior to dose until the next morning, or at least 8 hours after administration.

Adults: Initial: 0.2 mg at bedtime; dose may be titrated up to 0.6 mg to achieve desired response.

Sublingual formulation [Canadian product]: Children ≥5 years and Adolescents: Initial: 120 mcg administered 1 hour before bedtime; dose may be titrated up to 360 mcg to achieve desired response. Fluid intake should be limited 1 hour prior to dose until the next morning, or at least 8 hours after administration.

Uremic bleeding associated with acute or chronic renal failure (off-label use): IV: Adults: 0.4 mcg/kg over 10 minutes (Watson, 1984)

Prevention of surgical bleeding in patients with uremia (off-label use): IV: Adults: 0.3 mcg/kg over 30 minutes (Mannucci, 1983)

Dosage adjustment in renal impairment: CrCl <50 mL/minute: Use is contraindicated according to the manufacturer; however, has been used in acute and chronic renal failure patients experiencing uremic bleeding or for prevention of surgical bleeding (off-label uses) (Mannucci, 1983; Watson, 1984)

Dosage adjustment in hepatic impairment: No dosage adjustment provided in manufacturer's labeling.

Administration

IM (Canadian labeling; not in U.S. labeling), IV push, SubQ injection: Central diabetes insipidus: Withdraw dose from ampul into appropriate syringe size (eg, insulin syringe). Further dilution is not required. Administer as direct injection.

IV infusion:

Hemophilia A, von Willebrand disease (type 1), and prevention of surgical bleeding in patients with uremia (off-label) (Mannucci, 1983): Infuse over 15 to 30 minutes

Acute uremic bleeding (off-label) (Watson, 1984): May infuse over 10 minutes

Intranasal:

DDAVP: Nasal pump spray: Delivers 0.1 mL (10 mcg); for doses <10 mcg or for other doses which are not multiples, use rhinal tube. DDAVP Nasal spray delivers fifty 10 mcg doses. For 10 mcg dose, administer in one nostril. Any solution remaining after 50 doses should be discarded. Pump must be primed prior to first use.

DDAVP Rhinal tube: Insert top of dropper into tube (arrow marked end) in downward position. Squeeze dropper until solution reaches desired calibration mark. Disconnect dropper. Grasp the tube 3/4 inch from the end and insert tube into nostril until the fingertips reach the nostril. Place opposite end of tube into the mouth (holding breath). Tilt head back and blow with a strong, short puff into the nostril (for very young patients, an adult should blow solution into the child's nose). Reseal dropper after use.

Monitoring Parameters Blood pressure and pulse should be monitored during IV infusion

Note: For all indications, fluid intake, urine volume, and signs and symptoms of hyponatremia should be closely monitored especially in high-risk patient subgroups (eg, young children, elderly, patients with heart failure).

Diabetes insipidus: Urine specific gravity, plasma and urine osmolality, serum electrolytes

Hemophilia A: Factor VIII coagulant activity, factor VIII ristocetin cofactor activity, and factor VIII antigen levels, aPTT

von Willebrand disease: Factor VIII coagulant activity, factor VIII ristocetin cofactor activity, and factor VIII von Willebrand antigen levels, bleeding time

Nocturnal enuresis: Serum electrolytes if used for >7 days

Additional Information 10 mcg of desmopressin acetate is equivalent to 40 units

Dosage Forms Considerations

DDAVP and Minirin 5 mL bottles contain 50 sprays.

Stimate 2.5 mL bottles contain 25 sprays.

Dosage Forms

Solution, Injection:

DDAVP: 4 mcg/mL (1 mL, 10 mL)

Generic: 4 mcg/mL (1 mL, 10 mL)

Solution, Nasal:

DDAVP: 0.01% (5 mL)

DDAVP Rhinal Tube: 0.01% (2.5 mL)

Stimate: 1.5 mg/mL (2.5 mL)

Generic: 0.01% (2.5 mL, 5 mL)

Tablet, Oral:

DDAVP: 0.1 mg, 0.2 mg

Generic: 0.1 mg, 0.2 mg

Dosage Forms: Canada

Tablet, sublingual:

DDAVP® Melt: 60 mcg, 120 mcg, 240 mcg

◆ **Desmopressin Acetate** *see* Desmopressin *on page 594*

◆ **Desocort (Can)** *see* Desonide *on page 597*

◆ **Desogen** *see* Ethinyl Estradiol and Desogestrel *on page 799*

Desogestrel [INT] (des oh JES trel)

International Brand Names Aizea (GB); Antigone (FR); Arlette (CL, CO, PE, PY, VE); Azalia (BG, CZ, ES, HU, PL); Babette (DE); Camelia (AR); Carmin (AR, UY); Celea (BE); Cerazet (ES, IT); Cerazette (AE, AR, AT, BE, BH, BR, CH, CL, CO, CR, CZ, DE, DK, DO, EC, EE, FI, FR, GB, GR, GT, HK, HN, HR, HU, ID, IE, IL, IN, IS, IT, JO, KW, LB, LT, MY, NI, NL, NO, NZ, PA, PE, PH, PL, PT, QA, RO, RU, SA, SE, SG, SI, SK, SV, TH, UY, VE); Cerelle (GB); Clareal (FR); Desirett (EE); Desomono (GB); Desorox (GB); Diamilla (DK, EE); Embevio (VN); Fleur (CZ); Juliet (BR); Kelly (BR); Lactafem (PE); Lueva (BE, ES); Nacrez (DK, GB); Pink (AR); Vanish (CL, PY); Zelleta (GB); Zerogen (IN)

Pharmacologic Category Contraceptive, Oral (Progestin)

Reported Use Prevention of pregnancy

Dosage Range Oral: Adults: Females: Contraception:

No previous hormonal contraceptive use: Dosage is 1 tablet daily without interruption starting on day 1 (first day of menstrual bleeding). May start later (on days 2-5), but alternative/barrier method of contraception is recommended for 7 days following the first dose.

Following first trimester abortion: Dosage is 1 tablet daily without interruption starting immediately. No additional contraceptive method necessary.

Following delivery or second trimester abortion: Dosage is 1 tablet daily without interruption. May be started prior to return of menstruation. If starting therapy >21 days postpartum/abortion, additional/barrier method of contraception is recommended for the 7 days following the first dose.

Switching from other contraceptive methods: Dosage is 1 tablet daily without interruption.

Switching from combination oral contraceptive, vaginal ring, or transdermal patch: Start therapy on the day following the last active tablet or on the day of removal of vaginal ring or transdermal patch. No additional contraceptive method necessary.

Switching from progestogen-only contraceptive: May switch any day; take first desogestrel tablet when next scheduled dose is due or on day of removal of implant/continuous release dosage form.

Missed dose <12 hours elapsed: Dose (1 tablet) can be taken immediately and then resume regular schedule

Missed dose >12 hours elapsed: Dose should be skipped and resume regular schedule. Alternate form of contraception recommended for the following 7 days.

Dosage adjustment in renal impairment: No dosage adjustment provided in manufacturer's labeling

Dosage adjustment in hepatic impairment:

Mild-to-moderate impairment: No dosage adjustment provided in manufacturer's labeling; use with caution

Severe impairment: Use is contraindicated

Product Availability Product available in various countries; not currently available in the U.S.

Dosage Forms

Tablet, oral: 75 mcg

◆ **Desogestrel and Ethinyl Estradiol** *see* Ethinyl Estradiol and Desogestrel *on page 799*

◆ **Desonate** *see* Desonide *on page 597*

Desonide (DES oh nide)

Brand Names: U.S. Desonate; DesOwen; DesOwen Cream w/Cetaphil Lot [DSC]; DesOwen Lot w/Cetaphil Cream [DSC]; DesOwen Oint w/Cetaphil Lot [DSC]; LoKara; Verdeso

Brand Names: Canada Desocort; PDP-Desonide; Tridesilon; Verdeso

Pharmacologic Category Corticosteroid, Topical

Additional Appendix Information

Topical Corticosteroids *on page 2230*

Use

Atopic dermatitis (foam and gel): Treatment of mild to moderate atopic dermatitis in patients 3 months and older

Corticosteroid-responsive dermatoses (cream, ointment, and lotion): Relief of the inflammatory and pruritic manifestations of corticosteroid-responsive dermatoses.

Pregnancy Risk Factor C

Dosage Topical:

Atopic dermatitis: Infants ≥3 months, Children, Adolescents, and Adults: Foam, gel: Apply 2 times daily sparingly. Therapy should be discontinued when control is achieved. If no improvement is seen within 4 weeks, reassessment of diagnosis may be necessary; treatment should not exceed 4 consecutive weeks.

Corticosteroid responsive dermatoses: Adults: Cream, ointment, lotion: Apply 2 to 3 times daily sparingly. Therapy should be discontinued when control is achieved. If no improvement is seen within 2 weeks, reassessment of diagnosis may be necessary.

Dosage adjustment in renal impairment: There are no dosage adjustments provided in the manufacturer's labeling.

Dosage adjustment in hepatic impairment: There are no dosage adjustments provided in the manufacturer's labeling.

Additional Information Complete prescribing information should be consulted for additional detail.

Dosage Forms

Cream, External:

DesOwen: 0.05% (60 g)

Generic: 0.05% (15 g, 60 g)

Foam, External:

Verdeso: 0.05% (100 g)

Gel, External:

Desonate: 0.05% (60 g)

Lotion, External:

DesOwen: 0.05% (59 mL, 118 mL)

LoKara: 0.05% (59 mL, 118 mL)

Generic: 0.05% (59 mL, 118 mL)

Ointment, External:

DesOwen: 0.05% (60 g)

Generic: 0.05% (15 g, 60 g)

◆ **DesOwen** *see* Desonide *on page 597*

◆ **DesOwen Cream w/Cetaphil Lot [DSC]** *see* Desonide *on page 597*

◆ **DesOwen Lot w/Cetaphil Cream [DSC]** *see* Desonide *on page 597*

◆ **DesOwen Oint w/Cetaphil Lot [DSC]** *see* Desonide *on page 597*

◆ **Desoxicream (Can)** *see* Desoximetasone *on page 598*

Desoximetasone (des oks i MET a sone)

Brand Names: U.S. Topicort; Topicort Spray

Brand Names: Canada Desoxicream; Topicort®; Topicort® Gel; Topicort® Mild; Topicort® Ointment

Index Terms Desoxymethasone

Pharmacologic Category Corticosteroid, Topical

Additional Appendix Information

Topical Corticosteroids *on page 2230*

Use

Cream, gel, ointment: Relief of inflammation and pruritic symptoms of corticosteroid-responsive dermatosis

Spray: Plaque psoriasis treatment

Pregnancy Risk Factor C

Dosage Note: Therapy should be discontinued when control is achieved; if no improvement is seen within 4 weeks, reassessment of diagnosis may be necessary.

Corticosteroid-responsive dermatoses: Children, Adolescents, and Adults: Topical: Cream, gel, ointment: Apply a thin film to affected area twice daily

Plaque psoriasis treatment: Adults: Topical: Spray: Apply a thin film to affected area twice daily

Dosage adjustment in renal impairment: No dosage adjustment provided in manufacturer's labeling.

Dosage adjustment in hepatic impairment: No dosage adjustment provided in manufacturer's labeling; use caution.

Additional Information Complete prescribing information should be consulted for additional detail.

Dosage Forms

Cream, External:

Topicort: 0.05% (15 g, 60 g, 100 g); 0.25% (15 g, 60 g, 100 g)

Generic: 0.05% (15 g, 60 g, 100 g); 0.25% (15 g, 60 g, 100 g)

Gel, External:

Topicort: 0.05% (15 g, 60 g)

Generic: 0.05% (15 g, 60 g)

Liquid, External:

Topicort Spray: 0.25% (100 mL)

Ointment, External:

Topicort: 0.05% (15 g, 60 g, 100 g); 0.25% (15 g, 60 g, 100 g)

Generic: 0.05% (60 g, 100 g); 0.25% (15 g, 60 g, 100 g)

◆ **Desoxyephedrine Hydrochloride** *see* Methamphetamine *on page 1315*

◆ **Desoxymethasone** *see* Desoximetasone *on page 598*

◆ **Desoxyn** *see* Methamphetamine *on page 1315*

◆ **Desoxyphenobarbital** *see* Primidone *on page 1714*

◆ **Desulfato-Hirudin** *see* Desirudin *on page 593*

◆ **Desulphatohirudin** *see* Desirudin *on page 593*

Desvenlafaxine (des ven la FAX een)

Brand Names: U.S. Khedezla; Pristiq

Brand Names: Canada Pristiq

Index Terms O-desmethylvenlafaxine; ODV

Pharmacologic Category Antidepressant, Serotonin/Norepinephrine Reuptake Inhibitor

Use Treatment of major depressive disorder (acute and maintenance)

Pregnancy Risk Factor C

Dosage Oral: Adults: Depression: 50 mg once daily; doses up to 400 mg once daily have been studied; however, the manufacturer states there is no evidence that doses >50 mg daily confer any additional benefit. A flat dose response curve for efficacy between 50-400 mg daily has been noted as well as an increase in adverse events.

Discontinuation of therapy: Upon discontinuation of antidepressant therapy, gradually taper the dose to minimize the incidence of withdrawal symptoms and allow for the detection of re-emerging symptoms. Evidence supporting ideal taper rates is limited. APA and NICE guidelines suggest tapering therapy over at least several weeks with consideration to the half-life of the antidepressant; antidepressants with a shorter half-life may need to be tapered more conservatively. In addition for long-term treated patients, WFSBP guidelines recommend tapering over 4-6 months. If intolerable withdrawal symptoms occur following a dose reduction, consider resuming the previously prescribed dose and/or decrease dose at a more gradual rate (APA, 2010; Bauer, 2002; Haddad, 2001; NCCMH, 2010; Schatzberg, 2006; Shelton, 2001; Warner, 2006).

MAO inhibitor recommendations:

Switching to or from an MAO inhibitor intended to treat psychiatric disorders:

Allow 14 days to elapse between discontinuing an MAO inhibitor intended to treat psychiatric disorders and initiation of desvenlafaxine.

Allow 7 days to elapse between discontinuing desvenlafaxine and initiation of an MAO inhibitor intended to treat psychiatric disorders.

Use with other MAO inhibitors (linezolid or IV methylene blue):

Do not initiate desvenlafaxine in patients receiving linezolid or IV methylene blue; consider other interventions for psychiatric condition.

If urgent treatment with linezolid or IV methylene blue is required in a patient already receiving desvenlafaxine and potential benefits outweigh potential risks, discontinue desvenlafaxine promptly and administer linezolid or IV methylene blue. Monitor for serotonin syndrome for 7 days or until 24 hours after the last dose of linezolid or IV methylene blue, whichever comes first. May resume desvenlafaxine 24 hours after the last dose of linezolid or IV methylene blue.

Dosing adjustment in renal impairment:
CrCl >50 mL/minute: No dosage adjustment necessary.
CrCl 30-50 mL/minute: 50 mg once daily (maximum)
CrCl <30 mL/minute: 50 mg every other day (maximum)
End-stage renal disease (ESRD) requiring hemodialysis (HD): 50 mg every other day (maximum). Supplemental doses should not be given after HD.

Dosing adjustment in hepatic impairment:
Mild impairment: No dosage adjustment necessary.
Moderate-to-severe impairment: Initial: 50 mg once daily; maximum dose: 100 mg daily

Additional Information Complete prescribing information should be consulted for additional detail.

Dosage Forms

Tablet Extended Release 24 Hour, Oral:
Khedezla: 50 mg, 100 mg
Pristiq: 50 mg, 100 mg
Generic: 50 mg, 100 mg

- ◆ **Desyrel** *see* TraZODone *on page 2091*
- ◆ **Detemir Insulin** *see* Insulin Detemir *on page 1085*
- ◆ **Detrol** *see* Tolterodine *on page 2063*
- ◆ **Detrol® (Can)** *see* Tolterodine *on page 2063*
- ◆ **Detrol LA** *see* Tolterodine *on page 2063*
- ◆ **Detrol® LA (Can)** *see* Tolterodine *on page 2063*
- ◆ **Detryptoreline** *see* Triptorelin *on page 2107*

Dexamethasone (Systemic)

(deks a METH a sone)

Brand Names: U.S. Baycadron; Dexamethasone Intensol; DexPak 10 Day; DexPak 13 Day; DexPak 6 Day; DoubleDex

Brand Names: Canada Apo-Dexamethasone; Dexasone; Dom-Dexamethasone; PHL-Dexamethasone; PMS-Dexamethasone; PRO-Dexamethasone; ratio-Dexamethasone

Index Terms Decadron; Dexamethasone Sodium Phosphate

Pharmacologic Category Anti-inflammatory Agent; Antiemetic; Corticosteroid, Systemic

Additional Appendix Information

Corticosteroids Systemic Equivalencies *on page 2228*

Use Primarily as an anti-inflammatory or immunosuppressant agent in the treatment of a variety of diseases including those of allergic, dermatologic, gastrointestinal, endocrine, hematologic, inflammatory, neoplastic, nervous system, ophthalmic, renal, respiratory, rheumatic, and autoimmune origin; management of cerebral edema, chronic swelling, as a diagnostic agent, diagnosis of Cushing syndrome, antiemetic

Pregnancy Risk Factor C

Pregnancy Considerations Adverse events have been observed with corticosteroids in animal reproduction studies. Betamethasone crosses the placenta (Brownfoot, 2013); and is partially metabolized by placental enzymes to an inactive metabolite (Murphy, 2007). Some studies have shown an association between first trimester systemic corticosteroid use and oral clefts (Park-Wyllie, 2000; Pradat, 2003). Systemic corticosteroids may have an effect on fetal growth (decreased birth weight); however, information is conflicting (Lunghi, 2010). Hypoadrenalism may occur in newborns following maternal use of corticosteroids during pregnancy; monitor.

Because antenatal corticosteroid administration may reduce the incidence of intraventricular hemorrhage, necrotizing enterocolitis, neonatal mortality, and respiratory distress syndrome, the injection is often used in patients with preterm premature rupture of membranes (membrane rupture between 24 0/7 weeks and 34 0/7 weeks of gestation) who are at risk of preterm delivery (ACOG, 2013). When systemic corticosteroids are needed in pregnancy, it is generally recommended to use the lowest effective dose for the shortest duration of time, avoiding high doses during the first trimester (Leachman, 2006; Lunghi, 2010; Makol, 2011; Østensen, 2009).

Women exposed to dexamethasone during pregnancy for the treatment of an autoimmune disease may contact the OTIS Autoimmune Diseases Study at 877-311-8972.

Breast-Feeding Considerations Corticosteroids are excreted in human milk; information specific to dexamethasone has not been located. The manufacturer notes that when used systemically, maternal use of corticosteroids have the potential to cause adverse events in a nursing infant (eg, growth suppression, interfere with endogenous corticosteroid production). Due to the potential for serious adverse reactions in the nursing infant, the manufacturer recommends a decision be made whether to discontinue nursing or to discontinue the drug, taking into account the importance of treatment to the mother. If there is concern about exposure to the infant, some guidelines recommend waiting 4 hours after the maternal dose of an oral systemic corticosteroid before breast feeding in order to decrease potential exposure to the nursing infant (based on a study using prednisolone) (Bae, 2011; Leachman, 2006; Makol, 2011; Ost, 1985).

Contraindications Hypersensitivity to dexamethasone or any component of the formulation, including sulfites; systemic fungal infections, cerebral malaria

Warnings/Precautions Corticosteroids are not approved for epidural injection. Serious neurologic events (eg, spinal cord infarction, paraplegia, quadriplegia, cortical blindness, stroke), some resulting in death, have been reported with epidural injection of corticosteroids, with and without use of fluoroscopy. Intra-articular injection may produce systemic as well as local effects. Appropriate examination of any joint fluid present is necessary to exclude a septic process. Avoid injection into an infected site. Do not inject into unstable joints. Patients should not overuse joints in which symptomatic benefit has been obtained as long as the inflammatory process remains active. Frequent intra-articular injection may result in damage to joint tissues.

Use with caution in patients with thyroid disease, hepatic impairment, renal impairment, cardiovascular disease, diabetes, glaucoma, cataracts, myasthenia gravis, osteoporosis, seizures, or GI diseases (diverticulitis, intestinal anastomoses, peptic ulcer, ulcerative colitis) due to perforation risk. Avoid ethanol may enhance gastric mucosal irritation. Use caution following acute MI (corticosteroids have been associated with myocardial rupture). Because of the risk of adverse effects, systemic corticosteroids should be used cautiously in the elderly in the smallest possible effective dose for the shortest duration. May affect growth velocity; growth should be routinely monitored in pediatric patients. Withdraw therapy with gradual tapering of dose.

May cause hypercorticism or suppression of hypothalamic-pituitary-adrenal (HPA) axis, particularly in younger children or in patients receiving high doses for prolonged periods. HPA axis suppression may lead to adrenal crisis. Withdrawal and discontinuation of a corticosteroid should be done slowly and carefully. Particular care is required when patients are transferred from systemic corticosteroids to inhaled products due to possible adrenal insufficiency or withdrawal from steroids, including an increase in allergic symptoms. Adult patients receiving >20 mg per day of prednisone (or equivalent) may be most susceptible. Fatalities have occurred due to adrenal insufficiency in asthmatic patients during and after transfer from systemic corticosteroids to aerosol steroids; aerosol steroids do not provide the systemic steroid needed to treat patients having trauma, surgery, or infections. ▶

Dexamethasone does not provide adequate mineralocorticoid activity in adrenal insufficiency (may be employed as a single dose while cortisol assays are performed). The lowest possible dose should be used during treatment; discontinuation and/or dose reductions should be gradual. Rare cases of anaphylactoid reactions have been observed in patients receiving corticosteroids. Patients may require higher doses when subject to stress (ie, trauma, surgery, severe infection).

Acute myopathy has been reported with high dose corticosteroids, usually in patients with neuromuscular transmission disorders; may involve ocular and/or respiratory muscles; monitor creatine kinase; recovery may be delayed. Corticosteroid use may cause psychiatric disturbances, including depression, euphoria, insomnia, mood swings, and personality changes. Preexisting psychiatric conditions may be exacerbated by corticosteroid use. Prolonged use of corticosteroids may increase the incidence of secondary infection, mask acute infection (including fungal infections), prolong or exacerbate viral infections, or limit response to vaccines. Exposure to chickenpox or measles should be avoided; corticosteroids should not be used to treat ocular herpes simplex. Corticosteroids should not be used for cerebral malaria, fungal infections, or viral hepatitis. Close observation is required in patients with latent tuberculosis and/or TB reactivity; restrict use in active TB (only fulminating or disseminated TB in conjunction with antituberculosis treatment). Amebiasis should be ruled out in any patient with recent travel to tropic climates or unexplained diarrhea prior to initiation of corticosteroids.

Prolonged treatment with corticosteroids has been associated with the development of Kaposi sarcoma (case reports); if noted, discontinuation of therapy should be considered. High-dose corticosteroids should not be used to manage acute head injury. Some products may contain sodium sulfite, a sulfite that may cause allergic-type reactions including anaphylaxis and life-threatening or less severe asthmatic episodes in susceptible patients. Potentially significant drug-drug interactions may exist, requiring dose or frequency adjustment, additional monitoring, and/or selection of alternative therapy. Some dosage forms may contain propylene glycol; large amounts are potentially toxic and have been associated hyperosmolality, lactic acidosis, seizures, and respiratory depression; use caution (AAP, 1997; Zar, 2007).

Benzyl alcohol and derivatives: Some dosage forms may contain sodium benzoate/benzoic acid; benzoic acid (benzoate) is a metabolite of benzyl alcohol; large amounts of benzyl alcohol (≥99 mg/kg/day) have been associated with a potentially fatal toxicity ("gasping syndrome") in neonates; the "gasping syndrome" consists of metabolic acidosis, respiratory distress, gasping respirations, CNS dysfunction (including convulsions, intracranial hemorrhage), hypotension, and cardiovascular collapse (AAP, 1997; CDC, 1982); some data suggests that benzoate displaces bilirubin from protein binding sites (Ahlfors, 2001); avoid or use dosage forms containing benzyl alcohol derivative with caution in neonates. See manufacturer's labeling.

Adverse Reactions

Cardiovascular: Arrhythmia, bradycardia, cardiac arrest, cardiomyopathy, CHF, circulatory collapse, edema, hypertension, myocardial rupture (post-MI), syncope, thromboembolism, vasculitis

Central nervous system: Depression, emotional instability, euphoria, headache, intracranial pressure increased, insomnia, malaise, mood swings, neuritis, personality changes, pseudotumor cerebri (usually following discontinuation), psychic disorders, seizure, vertigo

Dermatologic: Acne, allergic dermatitis, alopecia, angioedema, bruising, dry skin, erythema, fragile skin, hirsutism, hyper-/hypopigmentation, hypertrichosis, perianal pruritus (following IV injection), petechiae, rash, skin atrophy, skin test reaction impaired, striae, urticaria, wound healing impaired

Endocrine & metabolic: Adrenal suppression, carbohydrate tolerance decreased, Cushing's syndrome, diabetes mellitus, glucose intolerance decreased, growth suppression (children), hyperglycemia, hypokalemic alkalosis, menstrual irregularities, negative nitrogen balance, pituitary-adrenal axis suppression, protein catabolism, sodium retention

Gastrointestinal: Abdominal distention, appetite increased, gastrointestinal hemorrhage, gastrointestinal perforation, nausea, pancreatitis, peptic ulcer, ulcerative esophagitis, weight gain

Genitourinary: Altered (increased or decreased) spermatogenesis

Hepatic: Hepatomegaly, transaminases increased

Local: Postinjection flare (intra-articular use), thrombophlebitis

Neuromuscular & skeletal: Arthropathy, aseptic necrosis (femoral and humoral heads), fractures, muscle mass loss, myopathy (particularly in conjunction with neuromuscular disease or neuromuscular-blocking agents), neuropathy, osteoporosis, parasthesia, tendon rupture, vertebral compression fractures, weakness

Ocular: Cataracts, exophthalmos, glaucoma, intraocular pressure increased

Renal: Glucosuria

Respiratory: Pulmonary edema

Miscellaneous: Abnormal fat deposition, anaphylactoid reaction, anaphylaxis, avascular necrosis, diaphoresis, hiccups, hypersensitivity, impaired wound healing, infections, Kaposi's sarcoma, moon face, secondary malignancy

Drug Interactions

Metabolism/Transport Effects Substrate of CYP3A4 (major), P-glycoprotein; **Note:** Assignment of Major/Minor substrate status based on clinically relevant drug interaction potential; **Inhibits** P-glycoprotein; **Induces** CYP2A6 (moderate), CYP2B6 (moderate), CYP2C9 (moderate), CYP3A4 (moderate), P-glycoprotein

Avoid Concomitant Use

Avoid concomitant use of Dexamethasone (Systemic) with any of the following: Aldesleukin; Axitinib; BCG; Bosutinib; Cabozantinib; Conivaptan; Dabigatran Etexilate; Enzalutamide; Fusidic Acid (Systemic); Idelalisib; Indium 111 Capromab Pendetide; Lapatinib; Ledipasvir; Mifepristone; Natalizumab; Nilotinib; Nintedanib; Nisoldipine; Olaparib; Pimecrolimus; Rilpivirine; RomiDEPsin; Simeprevir; Sofosbuvir; Tacrolimus (Topical); Ticagrelor; Tofacitinib; VinCRIStine (Liposomal)

Increased Effect/Toxicity

Dexamethasone (Systemic) may increase the levels/effects of: Acetylcholinesterase Inhibitors; Amphotericin B; Androgens; Ceritinib; Clarithromycin; CycloSPORINE (Systemic); Deferasirox; Ifosfamide; Leflunomide; Lenalidomide; Loop Diuretics; Natalizumab; Nicorandil; NSAID (COX-2 Inhibitor); NSAID (Nonselective); Quinolone Antibiotics; Thalidomide; Thiazide Diuretics; Tofacitinib; Vaccines (Live); Warfarin

The levels/effects of Dexamethasone (Systemic) may be increased by: Aprepitant; Asparaginase (E. coli); Asparaginase (Erwinia); Ceritinib; Conivaptan; CycloSPORINE (Systemic); CYP3A4 Inhibitors (Moderate); CYP3A4 Inhibitors (Strong); Denosumab; Estrogen Derivatives; Fosaprepitant; Fusidic Acid (Systemic); Idelalisib; Indacaterol; Ivacaftor; Luliconazole; Mifepristone; Netupitant; Neuromuscular-Blocking Agents (Nondepolarizing); P-glycoprotein/ABCB1 Inhibitors; Pimecrolimus;

Roflumilast; Salicylates; Stiripentol; Tacrolimus (Topical); Telaprevir; Trastuzumab

Decreased Effect

Dexamethasone (Systemic) may decrease the levels/effects of: Afatinib; Aldesleukin; Antidiabetic Agents; ARIPiprazole; Axitinib; BCG; Bosutinib; Brentuximab Vedotin; Cabozantinib; Calcitriol; Caspofungin; Clarithromycin; Cobicistat; Coccidioides immitis Skin Test; Corticorelin; CycloSPORINE (Systemic); CYP3A4 Substrates; Dabigatran Etexilate; Dasabuvir; Dasatinib; DOXOrubicin (Conventional); Elvitegravir; Enzalutamide; FentaNYL; Hyaluronidase; Hydrocodone; Ibrutinib; Ifosfamide; Imatinib; Indium 111 Capromab Pendetide; Isoniazid; Ixabepilone; Lapatinib; Ledipasvir; Linagliptin; Nilotinib; Nintedanib; Nisoldipine; Olaparib; Ombitasvir; Paritaprevir; P-glycoprotein/ABCB1 Substrates; Rilpivirine; RomiDEPsin; Salicylates; Saxagliptin; Simeprevir; Sipuleucel-T; Sofosbuvir; SUNItinib; Telaprevir; Ticagrelor; Triazolam; Urea Cycle Disorder Agents; Vaccines (Inactivated); VinCRIStine (Liposomal)

The levels/effects of Dexamethasone (Systemic) may be decreased by: Aminoglutethimide; Antacids; Barbiturates; Bile Acid Sequestrants; Bosentan; CYP3A4 Inducers (Moderate); CYP3A4 Inducers (Strong); Dabrafenib; Deferasirox; Echinacea; Mifepristone; Mitotane; P-glycoprotein/ABCB1 Inducers; Siltuximab; St Johns Wort; Tocilizumab

Preparation for Administration

Oral: Oral administration of dexamethasone for croup may be prepared using a parenteral dexamethasone formulation and mixing it with an oral flavored syrup (Bjornson, 2004).

IV: May be given undiluted or further diluted in NS or D_5W. Use preservative-free product when used in neonates, especially premature infants.

Storage/Stability

Elixir: Store at 15°C to 30°C (59°F to 86°F); avoid freezing.

Injection: Store intact vials at 20°C to 25°C (68°F to 77°F); excursions permitted to 15°C to 30°C (59°F to 86°F). Protect from light, heat, and freezing. Diluted solutions should be used within 24 hours.

Oral concentrated solution (Intensol): Store at 20°C to 25°C (68°F to 77°F); do not freeze; do not use if precipitate is present; dispense only in original bottle and only with manufacturer-supplied calibrated dropper; discard open bottle after 90 days.

Oral solution: Store at 20°C to 25°C (68°F to 77°F).

Tablets: Store at 20°C to 25°C (68°F to 77°F); protect from moisture.

Mechanism of Action Decreases inflammation by suppression of neutrophil migration, decreased production of inflammatory mediators, and reversal of increased capillary permeability; suppresses normal immune response. Dexamethasone's mechanism of antiemetic activity is unknown.

Pharmacodynamics/Kinetics

Onset of action: IV: Prompt

Absorption: Oral: 61% to 86%

Metabolism: Hepatic

Half-life elimination: Oral: ~4 hours (Czock, 2005); IV: ~1 to 5 hours (Hochhaus, 2001; Miyabo, 1991; Rohdewald, 1987; Toth, 1999)

Time to peak, serum: Oral: 1 to 2 hours (Czock, 2005); IM: ~30 to 120 minutes (Egerman, 1997; Hochhaus, 2001); IV: 5 to 10 minutes (free dexamethasone) (Miyabo, 1991; Rohdewald, 1987)

Excretion: Urine (~10%) (Duggan 1975; Miyabo, 1991)

Dosage Refer to individual protocols.

Children:

Antiemetic (prior to chemotherapy): Refer to individual protocols and emetogenic potential: IV: 10 mg/m²/dose every 12-24 hours on days of chemotherapy for severely emetogenic chemotherapy courses

Anti-inflammatory immunosuppressant: Oral, IM, IV: 0.08-0.3 mg/kg/day **or** 2.5-10 mg/m²/day in divided doses every 6-12 hours

Extubation or airway edema: Oral, IM, IV: 0.5-2 mg/kg/day in divided doses every 6 hours beginning 24 hours prior to extubation and continuing for 4-6 doses afterwards

Cerebral edema: IV: Loading dose: 1-2 mg/kg/dose as a single dose; maintenance: 1-1.5 mg/kg/day (maximum: 16 mg/day) in divided doses every 4-6 hours, taper off over 1-6 weeks

Croup (laryngotracheobronchitis): Oral, IM, IV: 0.6 mg/kg once; usual maximum dose: 16 mg (doses as high as 20 mg have been used) (Bjornson, 2004; Hegenbarth, 2008; Rittichier, 2000); a single oral dose of 0.15 mg/kg has been shown effective in children with mild-to-moderate croup (Russell, 2004; Sparrow, 2006)

Bacterial meningitis: Infants and Children >6 weeks: IV: 0.15 mg/kg/dose every 6 hours for the first 2-4 days of antibiotic treatment; start dexamethasone 10-20 minutes before or with the first dose of antibiotic

Physiologic replacement: Oral, IM, IV: 0.03-0.15 mg/kg/day **or** 0.6-0.75 mg/m²/day in divided doses every 6-12 hours

Acute mountain sickness (AMS)/high altitude cerebral edema (HACE) (off-label use): Oral, IM, IV: 0.15 mg/kg/dose every 6 hours; consider using for high altitude pulmonary edema because of associated HACE with this condition (Luks, 2010; Pollard, 2001)

Adults:

Antiemetic:

Prophylaxis: Oral, IV: 10-20 mg 15-30 minutes before treatment on each treatment day

Continuous infusion regimen: Oral or IV: 10 mg every 12 hours on each treatment day

Mildly emetogenic therapy: Oral, IM, IV: 4 mg every 4-6 hours

Delayed nausea/vomiting: Oral: 4-10 mg 1-2 times/day for 2-4 days **or**

8 mg every 12 hours for 2 days; then
4 mg every 12 hours for 2 days **or**
20 mg 1 hour before chemotherapy; then
10 mg 12 hours after chemotherapy; then
8 mg every 12 hours for 4 doses; then
4 mg every 12 hours for 4 doses

Anti-inflammatory:

Oral, IM, IV (injections should be given as sodium phosphate): 0.75-9 mg/day in divided doses every 6-12 hours

Intra-articular, intralesional, or soft tissue (as sodium phosphate): 0.4-6 mg/day

Multiple myeloma: Oral, IV: 40 mg/day, days 1 to 4, 9 to 12, and 17 to 20, repeated every 4 weeks (alone or as part of a regimen)

Cerebral edema: IV: 10 mg stat, 4 mg IM/IV every 6 hours until response is maximized, then switch to oral regimen, then taper off if appropriate; dosage may be reduced after 2-4 days and gradually discontinued over 5-7 days

Extubation or airway edema: Oral, IM, IV (injections should be given as sodium phosphate): 0.5-2 mg/kg/day in divided doses every 6 hours beginning 24 hours prior to extubation and continuing for 4-6 doses afterwards

Dexamethasone suppression test (depression/suicide indicator) (off-label use): Oral: 1 mg at 11 PM, draw blood at 8 AM the following day for plasma cortisol determination

Cushing's syndrome, diagnostic: Oral: 1 mg at 11 PM, draw blood at 8 AM; greater accuracy for Cushing's syndrome may be achieved by the following:

Dexamethasone 0.5 mg by mouth every 6 hours for 48 hours (with 24-hour urine collection for 17-hydroxycorticosteroid excretion)

Differentiation of Cushing's syndrome due to ACTH excess from Cushing's due to other causes: Oral: Dexamethasone 2 mg every 6 hours for 48 hours (with 24-hour urine collection for 17-hydroxycorticosteroid excretion)

Multiple sclerosis (acute exacerbation): 30 mg/day for 1 week, followed by 4-12 mg/day for 1 month

Physiological replacement: Oral, IM, IV (should be given as sodium phosphate): 0.03-0.15 mg/kg/day **or** 0.6-0.75 mg/m^2/day in divided doses every 6-12 hours

Treatment of shock:

Addisonian crisis/shock (ie, adrenal insufficiency/responsive to steroid therapy): IV (given as sodium phosphate): 4-10 mg as a single dose, which may be repeated if necessary

Unresponsive shock (ie, unresponsive to steroid therapy): IV (given as sodium phosphate): 1-6 mg/kg as a single IV dose or up to 40 mg initially followed by repeat doses every 2-6 hours while shock persists

Acute mountain sickness (AMS)/high altitude cerebral edema (HACE) (off-label use):

Prevention: Oral: 2 mg every 6 hours **or** 4 mg every 12 hours starting on the day of ascent; may be discontinued after staying at the same elevation for 2-3 days or if descent is initiated; do not exceed a 10 day duration (Luks, 2010). **Note:** In situations of rapid ascent to altitudes >3500 meters (such as rescue or military operations), 4 mg every 6 hours may be considered (Luks, 2010).

Treatment: Oral, IM, IV:

AMS: 4 mg every 6 hours (Luks, 2010)

HACE: Initial: 8 mg as a single dose; Maintenance: 4 mg every 6 hours until symptoms resolve (Luks, 2010)

Antenatal fetal maturation (off-label use): IM: In women with preterm premature rupture of membranes (membrane rupture between 24 0/7 weeks and 34 0/7 weeks of gestation), a single course of corticosteroids is recommended if there is a risk of preterm delivery (ACOG, 2013). Although the optimal corticosteroid and dose have not been determined, dexamethasone 6 mg every 12 hours for a total of 4 doses has been used in most studies (Brownfoot, 2013).

Dosage adjustment in renal impairment: There are no dosage adjustments provided in the manufacturer's labeling; use with caution.

Hemodialysis: Supplemental dose is not necessary

Peritoneal dialysis: Supplemental dose is not necessary

Dosage adjustment in hepatic impairment: There are no dosage adjustments provided in the manufacturer's labeling.

Dietary Considerations May be taken with meals to decrease GI upset. May need diet with increased potassium, pyridoxine, vitamin C, vitamin D, folate, calcium, and phosphorus.

Administration

Oral: Administer with meals to decrease GI upset.

IV: Administer the 4 mg/mL or 10 mg/mL concentration intravenously as an undiluted or diluted solution.

IM: Administer the 4 mg/mL or 10 mg/mL concentration deep IM.

Intra-articular: Administer into affected joint using the 4 mg/mL concentration only.

Intralesional injection: Administer into affected area using the 4 mg/mL concentration only.

Soft tissue injection: Administer into affected tissue using the 4 mg/mL concentration only.

Monitoring Parameters Hemoglobin, occult blood loss, serum potassium, glucose, growth in children

Reference Range Dexamethasone suppression test, overnight: 8 AM cortisol <6 mcg/100 mL (dexamethasone 1 mg); plasma cortisol determination should be made on the day after giving dose

Additional Information Effects of inhaled/intranasal steroids on growth have been observed in the absence of laboratory evidence of HPA axis suppression, suggesting that growth velocity is a more sensitive indicator of systemic corticosteroid exposure in pediatric patients than some commonly used tests of HPA axis function. The long-term effects of this reduction in growth velocity associated with orally-inhaled and intranasal corticosteroids, including the impact on final adult height, are unknown. The potential for "catch up" growth following discontinuation of treatment with inhaled corticosteroids has not been adequately studied.

Withdrawal/tapering of therapy: Corticosteroid tapering following short-term use is limited primarily by the need to control the underlying disease state; tapering may be accomplished over a period of days. Following longer-term use, tapering over weeks to months may be necessary to avoid signs and symptoms of adrenal insufficiency and to allow recovery of the HPA axis. Testing of HPA axis responsiveness may be of value in selected patients. Subtle deficits in HPA response may persist for months after discontinuation of therapy, and may require supplemental dosing during periods of acute illness or surgical stress.

Dosage Forms

Concentrate, Oral:

Dexamethasone Intensol: 1 mg/mL (30 mL)

Elixir, Oral:

Baycadron: 0.5 mg/5 mL (237 mL)

Generic: 0.5 mg/5 mL (237 mL)

Kit, Injection:

DoubleDex: 10 mg/mL

Solution, Injection:

Generic: 4 mg/mL (1 mL, 5 mL, 30 mL); 20 mg/5 mL (5 mL); 120 mg/30 mL (30 mL); 10 mg/mL (1 mL, 10 mL); 100 mg/10 mL (10 mL)

Solution, Injection [preservative free]:

Generic: 10 mg/mL (1 mL)

Solution, Oral:

Generic: 0.5 mg/5 mL (240 mL, 500 mL)

Tablet, Oral:

DexPak 10 Day: 1.5 mg

DexPak 13 Day: 1.5 mg

DexPak 6 Day: 1.5 mg

Generic: 0.5 mg, 0.75 mg, 1 mg, 1.5 mg, 2 mg, 4 mg, 6 mg

Dexamethasone (Ophthalmic)

(deks a METH a sone)

Brand Names: U.S. Maxidex; Ozurdex

Brand Names: Canada Diodex; Maxidex; Ozurdex

Index Terms Dexamethasone Sodium Phosphate

Pharmacologic Category Anti-inflammatory Agent, Ophthalmic; Corticosteroid, Ophthalmic; Corticosteroid, Otic

Use

Management of steroid-responsive inflammatory conditions such as allergic conjunctivitis, iritis, or cyclitis; symptomatic treatment of corneal injury from chemical, radiation, or thermal burns, or penetration of foreign bodies. The ophthalmic solution is also indicated for otic use to treat steroid-responsive inflammatory conditions of the external auditory meatus.

Ophthalmic intravitreal implant (Ozurdex): Treatment of macular edema following branch retinal vein occlusion (BRVO) or central retinal vein occlusion (CRVO); treatment of noninfective uveitis affecting the posterior segment of the eye; treatment of diabetic macular edema

Pregnancy Risk Factor C

Dosage Adults:

Ophthalmic:

Anti-inflammatory:

Solution: Instill 1 to 2 drops into conjunctival sac every hour during the day and every other hour during the night; gradually reduce dose to 1 drop every 4 hours, then to 3 to 4 times/day

Suspension: Instill 1 to 2 drops into conjunctival sac up to 4 to 6 times/day; may use hourly in severe disease; taper prior to discontinuation

Diabetic macular edema (pseudophakic or phakic patients scheduled for cataract surgery) or macular edema (following BRVO or CRVO): Ocular implant: Intravitreal injection: 0.7 mg implant injected in affected eye

Noninfective uveitis: Ocular implant: Intravitreal injection: 0.7 mg implant injected in affected eye

Otic: Anti-inflammatory: Solution: Initial: Instill 3 to 4 drops into the aural canal 2 to 3 times a day; reduce dose gradually once a favorable response is obtained. Alternately, may pack the aural canal with a gauze wick saturated with the solution; remove from the ear after 12 to 24 hours. Repeat as necessary.

Dosage adjustment in renal impairment: There are no dosage adjustment provided in the manufacturer's labeling.

Dosage adjustment in hepatic impairment: There are no dosage adjustment provided in the manufacturer's labeling.

Additional Information Complete prescribing information should be consulted for additional detail.

Dosage Forms

Implant, Intraocular [preservative free]:

Ozurdex: 0.7 mg (1 ea)

Solution, Ophthalmic:

Generic: 0.1% (5 mL)

Suspension, Ophthalmic:

Maxidex: 0.1% (5 mL)

- ◆ **Dexamethasone and Ciprofloxacin** *see* Ciprofloxacin and Dexamethasone *on page 446*
- ◆ **Dexamethasone and Tobramycin** *see* Tobramycin and Dexamethasone *on page 2056*
- ◆ **Dexamethasone Intensol** *see* Dexamethasone (Systemic) *on page 599*
- ◆ **Dexamethasone, Neomycin, and Polymyxin B** *see* Neomycin, Polymyxin B, and Dexamethasone *on page 1437*
- ◆ **Dexamethasone Sodium Phosphate** *see* Dexamethasone (Ophthalmic) *on page 602*
- ◆ **Dexamethasone Sodium Phosphate** *see* Dexamethasone (Systemic) *on page 599*
- ◆ **Dexasone (Can)** *see* Dexamethasone (Systemic) *on page 599*

Dexchlorpheniramine (deks klor fen EER a meen)

Index Terms Dexchlorpheniramine Maleate

Pharmacologic Category Alkylamine Derivative; Histamine H_1 Antagonist; Histamine H_1 Antagonist, First Generation

Additional Appendix Information

Beers Criteria – Potentially Inappropriate Medications for Geriatrics *on page 2271*

Use Perennial and seasonal allergic rhinitis and other allergic symptoms including urticaria

Dosage Oral:

Children:

2-5 years: 0.5 mg every 4-6 hours (do not use timed release)

6-11 years: 1 mg every 4-6 hours or 4 mg timed release at bedtime

Adults: 2 mg every 4-6 hours or 4-6 mg timed release at bedtime or every 8-10 hours

Dosage adjustment in renal impairment: No dosage adjustment provided in manufacturer's labeling.

Dosage adjustment in hepatic impairment: No dosage adjustment provided in manufacturer's labeling.

Additional Information Complete prescribing information should be consulted for additional detail.

Dosage Forms

Syrup, Oral:

Generic: 2 mg/5 mL (473 mL)

- ◆ **Dexchlorpheniramine Maleate** *see* Dexchlorpheniramine *on page 603*
- ◆ **Dexchlorpheniramine Tannate, Pseudoephedrine Tannate, and Dextromethorphan Tannate** *see* Chlorpheniramine, Pseudoephedrine, and Dextromethorphan *on page 428*
- ◆ **Dexedrine** *see* Dextroamphetamine *on page 607*
- ◆ **Dexferrum** *see* Iron Dextran Complex *on page 1117*
- ◆ **Dexilant** *see* Dexlansoprazole *on page 603*
- ◆ **Dexiron (Can)** *see* Iron Dextran Complex *on page 1117*

Dexketoprofen [INT] (deks kee toe PROE fen)

International Brand Names Desketo (CL); Dexak (PL); Dexofen (BG); Dexoket (CZ); Dexomen (HR); Dolmen (EE); Enantyum (AR, AT, BE, CR, DO, GT, HN, NI, NL, PA, SE, SV); Fen Li (CN); Fendex (ID); Infen (IN); Keral (GB, IE, KR); Ketesse (AT, BE, CH, CO, CZ, DK, EC, EE, FI, FR, HK, ID, IT, KW, LB, LT, MY, PE, PH, PT, SA, SE, SG, SI, SK, TR); Kui La Lan (CN); Nor-Algifort (DO, GT, HN, SV); Simprofen (ID); Sympal (DE); Tador (RO); Tofedex (ID); Youbaifen (CN)

Pharmacologic Category Analgesic, Nonsteroidal Anti-inflammatory Drug

Reported Use Short-term treatment of mild-to-moderate pain, including dysmenorrhoea

Dosage Range Oral:

Children: Not recommended

Adults: 12.5 mg every 4-6 hours or 25 mg every 8 hours; maximum: 75 mg daily

Elderly: Maximum dose: 50 mg daily (unless well tolerated)

Product Availability Product available in various countries; not currently available in the U.S.

Dosage Forms

Tablet, scored: 25 mg

Dexlansoprazole (deks lan SOE pra zole)

Brand Names: U.S. Dexilant

Brand Names: Canada Dexilant

Index Terms Kapidex; TAK-390MR

Pharmacologic Category Proton Pump Inhibitor; Substituted Benzimidazole

Use

Erosive esophagitis: For healing of all grades of erosive esophagitis for up to 8 weeks; to maintain healing of erosive esophagitis and relief of heartburn for up to 6 months.

Gastroesophageal reflux disease: For the treatment of heartburn associated with symptomatic nonerosive gastroesophageal reflux disease (GERD) for 4 weeks.

Pregnancy Risk Factor B

Dosage Oral: Adults:

Erosive esophagitis (EE): Short-term treatment: 60 mg once daily for up to 8 weeks; maintenance of healed EE and symptomatic relief of heartburn: 30 mg once daily for up to 6 months. **Note:** Doses >30 mg do not provide additional benefit during maintenance phase.

Symptomatic GERD: Short-term treatment: 30 mg once daily for 4 weeks. **Note:** Doses >30 mg do not provide additional benefit during maintenance phase.

Dosage adjustment in renal impairment: No dosage adjustment necessary

Dosage adjustment in hepatic impairment:

Mild hepatic impairment (Child-Pugh class A): No dosage adjustment necessary

Moderate hepatic impairment (Child-Pugh class B): Consider a maximum dose of 30 mg once daily

Severe hepatic impairment (Child-Pugh class C): No dosage adjustment provided in manufacturer's labeling (has not been studied).

Additional Information Complete prescribing information should be consulted for additional detail.

Dosage Forms

Capsule Delayed Release, Oral:

Dexilant: 30 mg, 60 mg

Dexmedetomidine (deks MED e toe mi deen)

Brand Names: U.S. Precedex

Brand Names: Canada Precedex

Index Terms Dexmedetomidine Hydrochloride

Pharmacologic Category Alpha$_2$-Adrenergic Agonist; Sedative

Use

Intensive care unit sedation: Sedation of initially-intubated and mechanically-ventilated patients during treatment in an intensive care setting.

Procedural sedation: Procedural sedation prior to and/or during awake fiberoptic intubation; sedation prior to and/or during surgical or other procedures of nonintubated patients

Pregnancy Risk Factor C

Pregnancy Considerations Adverse effects were observed in some animal reproduction studies. Dexmedetomidine is expected to cross the placenta. Information related to use during pregnancy is limited (El-Tahan, 2012).

Breast-Feeding Considerations It is not known if dexmedetomidine is excreted in breast milk. The manufacturer recommends that caution be exercised when administering dexmedetomidine to nursing women.

Contraindications

There are no contraindications listed in the U.S. manufacturer's labeling.

Canadian labeling: Hypersensitivity to dexmedetomidine or any component of the formulation.

Warnings/Precautions Should be administered only by persons skilled in management of patients in intensive care setting or operating room. Patients should be continuously monitored. Episodes of bradycardia, hypotension, and sinus arrest have been associated with dexmedetomidine. Use caution in patients with heart block, severe ventricular dysfunction, hypovolemia, diabetes, chronic hypertension, and elderly. Use with caution in patients with hepatic impairment; dosage reductions recommended. Use with caution in patients receiving vasodilators or drugs which decrease heart rate. If medical intervention is required, treatment may include stopping or decreasing the infusion; increasing the rate of IV fluid administration, use of pressor agents, and elevation of the lower extremities. Transient hypertension has been primarily observed during the loading dose administration and is associated with the initial peripheral vasoconstrictive effects of dexmedetomidine. Treatment is generally unnecessary; however, reduction of infusion rate may be required. Patients may be arousable and alert when stimulated. This alone should not be considered as lack of efficacy in the absence of other clinical signs/symptoms. When withdrawn abruptly in patients who have received >24 hours of therapy, withdrawal symptoms similar to clonidine withdrawal may result (eg, hypertension, tachycardia, nervousness, nausea, vomiting, agitation, headaches). Use for >24 hours is not recommended by the manufacturer. Use of infusions >24 hours has been associated with tolerance and tachyphylaxis and dose-related increase in adverse reactions.

Adverse Reactions

Cardiovascular: Atrial fibrillation, bradycardia, edema, hypertension, hypertension (diastolic), hypotension, hypovolemia, peripheral edema, systolic hypertension, tachycardia

Central nervous system: Agitation, anxiety

Endocrine & metabolic: Hyperglycemia, hypocalcemia, hypokalemia, hypoglycemia, hypomagnesemia, increased thirst

Gastrointestinal: Constipation, nausea, xerostomia

Genitourinary: Oliguria

Hematologic & oncologic: Anemia

Renal: Acute renal failure, decreased urine output

Respiratory: Pleural effusion, respiratory depression, wheezing

Miscellaneous: Fever, withdrawal syndrome (ICU sedation)

Rare but important or life-threatening: Acidosis, apnea, atrioventricular block, bronchospasm, cardiac arrest, cardiac disease, chills, confusion, convulsions, decreased visual acuity, delirium, drug tolerance (use >24 hours), extrasystoles, hallucination, heart block, hemorrhage, hepatic insufficiency, hyperbilirubinemia, hypercapnia, hyperkalemia, hyperpyrexia, hypoxia, increased blood urea nitrogen, increased gamma-glutamyl transferase, increased serum alkaline phosphatase, increased serum ALT, increased serum AST, inversion T wave on ECG, myocardial infarction, neuralgia, neuritis, oliguria, photopsia, pulmonary congestion, respiratory acidosis, rigors, seizure, sinoatrial arrest, speech disturbance, supraventricular tachycardia, tachyphylaxis (use >24 hours), variable blood pressure, ventricular arrhythmia, ventricular tachycardia, visual disturbance

Drug Interactions

Metabolism/Transport Effects Substrate of CYP2A6 (major); **Note:** Assignment of Major/Minor substrate status based on clinically relevant drug interaction potential; **Inhibits** CYP1A2 (weak), CYP2C9 (weak), CYP3A4 (weak)

Avoid Concomitant Use

Avoid concomitant use of Dexmedetomidine with any of the following: Ceritinib; Iobenguane I 123; Pimozide

Increased Effect/Toxicity

Dexmedetomidine may increase the levels/effects of: ARIPiprazole; Beta-Blockers; Bradycardia-Causing Agents; Ceritinib; Dofetilide; DULoxetine; Hydrocodone; Hypotensive Agents; Lacosamide; Levodopa; Lomitapide; Pimozide; RisperiDONE

The levels/effects of Dexmedetomidine may be increased by: Barbiturates; Beta-Blockers; Bretylium; CYP2A6 Inhibitors (Moderate); CYP2A6 Inhibitors (Strong); MAO Inhibitors; Nicorandil; Tofacitinib

Decreased Effect

Dexmedetomidine may decrease the levels/effects of: Iobenguane I 123

The levels/effects of Dexmedetomidine may be decreased by: Mirtazapine; Serotonin/Norepinephrine Reuptake Inhibitors; Tricyclic Antidepressants

Preparation for Administration Dexmedetomidine injection concentrate (100 mcg/mL) must be diluted in 0.9% sodium chloride solution to achieve the required concentration (4 mcg/mL) prior to administration. Add 2 mL (200 mcg) of dexmedetomidine to 48 mL of 0.9% sodium chloride for a total volume of 50 mL (4 mcg/mL). Shake gently to mix.

Storage/Stability Store at controlled room temperature of 25°C (77°F); excursions permitted to 15°C to 30°C (59°F to 86°F).

Mechanism of Action Selective $alpha_2$-adrenoceptor agonist with anesthetic and sedative properties thought to be due to activation of G-proteins by $alpha_{2a}$-adrenoceptors in the brainstem resulting in inhibition of norepinephrine release; peripheral $alpha_{2b}$-adrenoceptors are activated at high doses or with rapid IV administration resulting in vasoconstriction.

Pharmacodynamics/Kinetics

Onset of action: IV Bolus: 5 to 10 minutes

Peak effect: 15 to 30 minutes

Duration (dose dependent): 60 to 120 minutes

Distribution: V_{ss}: ~118 L; rapid

Protein binding: ~94%

Metabolism: Hepatic via N-glucuronidation, N-methylation, and CYP2A6

Half-life elimination: Distribution: ~6 minutes; Terminal: ~up to 3 hours (Venn, 2002); significantly prolonged in patients with severe hepatic impairment (Cunningham, 1999)

Excretion: Urine (95%); feces (4%)

Dosage Note: Errors have occurred due to misinterpretation of dosing information. Maintenance dose expressed as mcg/kg/**hour**.

Individualized and titrated to desired clinical effect. Manufacturer recommends duration of infusion should not exceed 24 hours; however, randomized clinical trials have demonstrated efficacy and safety comparable to lorazepam and midazolam with longer-term infusions of up to ~5 days (Pandharipande, 2007; Riker, 2009).

ICU sedation:

Adults: IV: Initial: Loading infusion (optional; see **"Note"** below) of 1 mcg/kg over 10 minutes (U.S. labeling) or 20 minutes (Canadian labeling), followed by a maintenance infusion of 0.2 to 0.7 mcg/kg/**hour**; adjust rate to desired level of sedation; titration no more frequently than every 30 minutes may reduce the incidence of hypotension (Gerlach, 2009)

Note: *Loading infusion:* The loading dose may be omitted for this indication if patient is either being converted from another sedative and patient is adequately sedated or there are concerns for hemodynamic compromise. *Maintenance infusion:* Dosing ranges between 0.2 to 1.4 mcg/kg/**hour** have been reported during randomized controlled clinical trials (Pandharipande, 2007; Riker, 2009). Although infusion rates as high as 2.5 mcg/kg/**hour** have been used, it is thought that doses >1.5 mcg/kg/**hour** do not add to clinical efficacy (Venn, 2003).

Elderly (>65 years of age): Consider dosage reduction. No specific guidelines available. Dose selections should be cautious, at the low end of dosage range; titration should be slower, allowing adequate time to evaluate response.

Procedural sedation:

Adults: IV: Initial: Loading infusion of 1 mcg/kg over 10 minutes, followed by a maintenance infusion of 0.6 mcg/kg/**hour**, titrate to desired effect; usual range: 0.2 to 1 mcg/kg/**hour**

Fiberoptic intubation (awake): IV: Initial: Loading infusion of 1 mcg/kg over 10 minutes, followed by a maintenance infusion of 0.7 mcg/kg/**hour** until endotracheal tube is secured (Bergese, 2010).

Elderly (>65 years of age): IV: Initial: Loading infusion of 0.5 mcg/kg over 10 minutes; Maintenance infusion: Dosage reduction should be considered.

Craniotomy (awake) (off-label use): IV: Initial: Loading infusion of 1 mcg/kg over 10 minutes, followed by a maintenance infusion of 0.5 mcg/kg/**hour**, titrate to desired effect (Bekker, 2008); usual range: 0.1 to 0.7 mcg/kg/**hour** (Piccioni, 2008)

Dosage adjustment in renal impairment: There are no dosage adjustments provided in the manufacturer's labeling; however, dexmedetomidine pharmacokinetics were not significantly different in patients with severe renal impairment compared to those with normal renal function.

Dosage adjustment in hepatic impairment: The manufacturer's labeling recommends considering a dose reduction but does not provide specific dosing recommendations. Clearance is reduced in varying degrees based on the level of impairment.

Usual Infusion Concentrations: Pediatric IV infusion: 4 mcg/mL

Usual Infusion Concentrations: Adult IV infusion: 200 mcg in 50 mL (concentration: 4 mcg/mL) of NS

Administration Administer using a controlled infusion device. Advisable to use administration components made with synthetic or coated natural rubber gaskets. Parenteral products should be inspected visually for particulate matter and discoloration prior to administration. If loading dose used, administer over 10 minutes; may extend to 20 minutes to further reduce vasoconstrictive effects. Titration no more frequently than every 30 minutes may reduce the incidence of hypotension when used for ICU sedation (Gerlach, 2009).

Monitoring Parameters Level of sedation; heart rate, respiration, rhythm, blood pressure; pain control

Critically-ill mechanically ventilated patients: Monitor depth of sedation with either the Richmond Agitation-Sedation Scale (RASS) or Sedation-Agitation Scale (SAS) (Barr, 2013)

Dosage Forms

Solution, Intravenous [preservative free]:

Precedex: 80 mcg/20 mL (20 mL); 200 mcg/50 mL (50 mL); 400 mcg/100 mL (100 mL); 200 mcg/2 mL (2 mL)

Generic: 200 mcg/2 mL (2 mL)

◆ **Dexmedetomidine Hydrochloride** *see* Dexmedetomidine *on page 604*

Dexmethylphenidate (dex meth il FEN i date)

Brand Names: U.S. Focalin; Focalin XR

Index Terms Dexmethylphenidate Hydrochloride

Pharmacologic Category Central Nervous System Stimulant

Use Treatment of attention-deficit/hyperactivity disorder (ADHD)

Pregnancy Risk Factor C

Dosage Treatment of ADHD: Oral:

Children ≥6 years: Patients not currently taking methylphenidate:

Immediate release: Initial: 2.5 mg twice daily; dosage may be adjusted in increments of 2.5-5 mg at weekly intervals (maximum dose: 20 mg/day); doses should be taken at least 4 hours apart

Extended release: Initial: 5 mg once daily; dosage may be adjusted in increments of 5 mg/day at weekly intervals (maximum dose: 30 mg/day)

Conversion to dexmethylphenidate from methylphenidate:

Immediate release: Initial: Half the total daily dose of racemic methylphenidate (maximum dexmethylphenidate dose: 20 mg/day)

Extended release: Initial: Half the total daily dose of racemic methylphenidate (maximum dexmethylphenidate dose: 30 mg/day)

Conversion from dexmethylphenidate immediate release to dexmethylphenidate extended release: When changing from Focalin® tablets to Focalin® XR capsules, patients may be switched to the same daily dose using Focalin® XR (maximum dose: 30 mg/day)

Adults: Patients not currently taking methylphenidate:

Immediate release: Initial: 2.5 mg twice daily; dosage may be adjusted in increments of 2.5-5 mg at weekly intervals (maximum dose: 20 mg/day); doses should be taken at least 4 hours apart

Extended release: Initial: 10 mg once daily; dosage may be adjusted in increments of 10 mg/day at weekly intervals (maximum dose: 40 mg/day)

Conversion to dexmethylphenidate from methylphenidate:

Immediate release: Initial: Half the total daily dose of racemic methylphenidate (maximum dexmethylphenidate dose: 20 mg/day)

Extended release: Initial: Half the total daily dose of racemic methylphenidate (maximum dexmethylphenidate dose: 40 mg/day)

Conversion from dexmethylphenidate immediate release to dexmethylphenidate extended release: When changing from Focalin® tablets to Focalin® XR capsules, patients may be switched to the same daily dose using Focalin® XR (maximum dose: 40 mg/day)

Dose reductions and discontinuation: Children ≥6 years and Adults: Reduce dose or discontinue in patients with paradoxical aggravation of symptoms. Discontinue if no improvement is seen after one month of treatment.

Dosage adjustment in renal impairment: No data available. However, considering extensive metabolism to inactive compounds, renal insufficiency expected to have minimal effect on kinetics of dexmethylphenidate.

Dosage adjustment in hepatic impairment: No data available.

Additional Information Complete prescribing information should be consulted for additional detail.

Dosage Forms

Capsule Extended Release 24 Hour, Oral:

Focalin XR: 5 mg, 10 mg, 15 mg, 20 mg, 25 mg, 30 mg, 35 mg, 40 mg

Generic: 5 mg, 10 mg, 15 mg, 30 mg, 40 mg

Tablet, Oral:

Focalin: 2.5 mg, 5 mg, 10 mg

Generic: 2.5 mg, 5 mg, 10 mg

◆ **Dexmethylphenidate Hydrochloride** *see* Dexmethylphenidate *on page 605*

◆ **DexPak 6 Day** *see* Dexamethasone (Systemic) *on page 599*

◆ **DexPak 10 Day** *see* Dexamethasone (Systemic) *on page 599*

◆ **DexPak 13 Day** *see* Dexamethasone (Systemic) *on page 599*

Dexpanthenol (deks PAN the nole)

Index Terms Pantothenyl Alcohol

Pharmacologic Category Gastrointestinal Agent, Stimulant; Topical Skin Product

Use Prophylactic use to minimize paralytic ileus; treatment of postoperative distention; topical to relieve itching and to aid healing of minor dermatoses

Pregnancy Risk Factor C

Dosage IM: Adults:

Prevention of postoperative ileus: 250-500 mg stat, repeat in 2 hours, followed by doses every 6 hours until danger passes

Paralytic ileus: 500 mg stat, repeat in 2 hours, followed by doses every 6 hours, if needed

Dosage adjustment in renal impairment: No dosage adjustment provided in manufacturer's labeling.

Dosage adjustment in hepatic impairment: No dosage adjustment provided in manufacturer's labeling.

Additional Information Complete prescribing information should be consulted for additional detail.

Dosage Forms

Solution, Injection:

Generic: 250 mg/mL (2 mL)

Dexrazoxane (deks ray ZOKS ane)

Brand Names: U.S. Totect; Zinecard

Brand Names: Canada Zinecard

Index Terms ICRF-187

Pharmacologic Category Antidote; Antidote, Extravasation; Chemoprotective Agent

Use

Prevention of cardiomyopathy associated with doxorubicin (Zinecard, generic products): To reduce the incidence and severity of cardiomyopathy associated with doxorubicin administration in women with metastatic breast cancer who have received a cumulative doxorubicin dose of 300 mg/m^2 and will benefit from continuing doxorubicin therapy to maintain tumor control. Not recommended for use with initial doxorubicin therapy.

Extravasation of anthracyclines (Totect): Treatment of extravasation resulting from intravenous anthracycline chemotherapy.

Pregnancy Risk Factor D

Dosage

Prevention of doxorubicin cardiomyopathy: Adults: IV: A 10:1 ratio of dexrazoxane:doxorubicin (dexrazoxane 500 mg/m^2:doxorubicin 50 mg/m^2). **Note:** Cardiac monitoring should continue during dexrazoxane therapy; doxorubicin/dexrazoxane should be discontinued in patients who develop a decline in LVEF or clinical CHF.

Treatment of anthracycline extravasation: Adults: IV: 1000 mg/m^2 on days 1 and 2 (maximum dose: 2000 mg), followed by 500 mg/m^2 on day 3 (maximum dose: 1000 mg); begin treatment as soon as possible, within 6 hours of extravasation

Prevention of doxorubicin cardiomyopathy associated with acute lymphoblastic leukemia treatment (high-risk patients; off-label use): Children: IV: A 10:1 ratio of dexrazoxane:doxorubicin (eg, dexrazoxane 300 mg/m^2: doxorubicin 30 mg/m^2) was used in patients with high-risk acute lymphoblastic leukemia; dexrazoxane is administered immediately prior to the doxorubicin dose (Lipshultz, 2010; Moghrabi, 2007; Silverman, 2010).

Dosage adjustment in renal impairment: Note: Renal function may be estimated using the Cockcroft-Gault formula.

Mild (CrCl ≥40 mL/minute) impairment: No dosage adjustment necessary.

Moderate-to-severe (CrCl <40 mL/minute) impairment:

Prevention of cardiomyopathy: Reduce dose by 50%, using a 5:1 dexrazoxane:doxorubicin ratio (dexrazoxane 250 mg/m^2:doxorubicin 50 mg/m^2)

Anthracycline extravasation: Reduce dose by 50%

Dosage adjustment in hepatic impairment:

Prevention of cardiomyopathy: Since doxorubicin dosage is reduced in hyperbilirubinemia, a proportional reduction in dexrazoxane dosage is recommended (maintain a 10:1 ratio of dexrazoxane:doxorubicin)

Anthracycline extravasation: There are no dosage adjustments provided in the manufacturer's labeling (has not been studied).

Additional Information Complete prescribing information should be consulted for additional detail.

Dosage Forms

Solution Reconstituted, Intravenous:

Totect: 500 mg (1 ea)

Zinecard: 250 mg (1 ea); 500 mg (1 ea)

Generic: 250 mg (1 ea); 500 mg (1 ea)

Dextran (DEKS tran)

Brand Names: U.S. LMD in D5W; LMD in NaCl

Index Terms 10% LMD; Dextran 40; Dextran, Low Molecular Weight

Pharmacologic Category Plasma Volume Expander, Colloid

Use Blood volume expander used in treatment of shock or impending shock when blood or blood products are not available; also used as a priming fluid in pump oxygenators during cardiopulmonary bypass and for prophylaxis of venous thrombosis and pulmonary embolism in surgical procedures associated with a high risk of thromboembolic complications

Pregnancy Risk Factor C

Dosage IV: Dose and infusion rate are dependent upon the patient's fluid status and must be individualized:

Volume expansion/shock:

Children (Dextran 40): Infuse 10 mL/kg as rapidly as possible (maximum: 20 mL/kg/day for the first 24 hours; 10 mL/kg/day thereafter); therapy should not be continued beyond 5 days

Adults (Dextran 40): Infuse 500-1000 mL (~10 mL/kg) as rapidly as possible (maximum: 20 mL/kg/day for first 24 hours; 10 mL/kg/day thereafter); therapy should not be continued beyond 5 days

Pump prime (Dextran 40): Varies with the volume of the pump oxygenator; generally, the solution is added in a dose of 10-20 mL/kg (or 1-2 g/kg); usual maximum total dose: 20 mL/kg (or 2 g/kg)

Postoperative prophylaxis of venous thrombosis/pulmonary embolism (Dextran 40): Note: Current ACCP guidelines for the prevention of venous thromboembolism in surgical patients do not recommend the use of dextran; consider the use of other anticoagulants (Falck-Ytter, 2012; Gould, 2012): Per the manufacturer, begin during surgical procedure and give 500-1000 mL (~10 mL/kg); continue treatment with 500 mL once daily for 2-3 additional days. Additional 500 mL doses may be administered every 2-3 days during the period of risk (up to 2 weeks postoperatively).

Dosage adjustment in renal impairment: Use with extreme caution.

Dosage adjustment in hepatic impairment: Use with extreme caution.

Additional Information Complete prescribing information should be consulted for additional detail.

Dosage Forms

Solution, Intravenous:

LMD in D5W: 10% Dextran 40 (500 mL)

LMD in NaCl: 10% Dextran 40 (500 mL)

◆ **Dextran 40** *see* Dextran *on page 607*

◆ **Dextran, Low Molecular Weight** *see* Dextran *on page 607*

◆ **Dextrin** *see* Wheat Dextrin *on page 2190*

Dextroamphetamine (deks troe am FET a meen)

Brand Names: U.S. Dexedrine; ProCentra; Zenzedi

Brand Names: Canada Dexedrine

Index Terms Dextroamphetamine Sulfate

Pharmacologic Category Central Nervous System Stimulant

Use

Attention-deficit/hyperactivity disorder: Treatment of attention-deficit/hyperactivity disorder (ADHD) as part of a total treatment program that typically includes other remedial measures (psychological, educational, social) for a stabilizing effect in children 3 to 16 years of age.

Narcolepsy: Treatment of narcolepsy.

Pregnancy Risk Factor C

Pregnancy Considerations Adverse effects have been observed in animal reproduction studies. The majority of human data is based on illicit amphetamine/methamphetamine exposure and not from therapeutic maternal use (Golub, 2005). Use of amphetamines during pregnancy may lead to an increased risk of premature birth and low birth weight; newborns may experience symptoms of withdrawal. Behavioral problems may also occur later in childhood (LaGasse, 2012).

Breast-Feeding Considerations The majority of human data is based on illicit amphetamine/methamphetamine exposure and not from therapeutic maternal use (Golub, 2005). Amphetamines are excreted into breast milk and use may decrease milk production. Increased irritability, agitation, and crying have been reported in nursing infants (ACOG, 2011). The manufacturer recommends that mothers taking dextroamphetamine refrain from nursing.

Contraindications

Hypersensitivity or idiosyncrasy to dextroamphetamine, other sympathomimetic amines, or any component of the formulation; advanced arteriosclerosis, symptomatic cardiovascular disease, moderate-to-severe hypertension; hyperthyroidism; glaucoma; agitated states; patients with a history of drug abuse; during or within 14 days following MAO inhibitor therapy.

Documentation of allergenic cross-reactivity for amphetamines is limited. However, because of similarities in chemical structure and/or pharmacologic actions, the possibility of cross-sensitivity cannot be ruled out with certainty.

Warnings/Precautions [U.S. Boxed Warning]: Use has been associated with serious cardiovascular events including sudden death in patients with preexisting structural cardiac abnormalities or other serious heart problems (sudden death in children and adolescents; sudden death, stroke and MI in adults. These products should be avoided in the patients with known serious structural cardiac abnormalities, cardiomyopathy, serious heart rhythm abnormalities, or other serious cardiac problems that could increase the risk of sudden death that these conditions alone carry. Patients should be carefully evaluated for cardiac disease prior to initiation of therapy. Patients who develop symptoms such as exertional chest pain, unexplained syncope, or other symptoms suggestive of cardiac disease during treatment should undergo a prompt cardiac evaluation. Use with caution in patients with hypertension and other cardiovascular conditions that might be exacerbated by increases in blood pressure or heart rate. Amphetamines may impair the ability to engage in potentially hazardous activities. May cause visual disturbances. Stimulants are associated with peripheral vasculopathy, including Raynaud's phenomenon; signs/symptoms are usually mild and intermittent, and generally improve with dose reduction or discontinuation. Digital ulceration and/or soft tissue breakdown have been observed rarely; monitor for digital changes during therapy and seek further evaluation (eg, rheumatology) if necessary.

Limited information exists regarding amphetamine use in seizure disorder (Cortese, 2013). The manufacturer recommends use with caution in patients with a history of seizure disorder; may lower seizure threshold leading to new onset or breakthrough seizure activity. Use with caution in patients with preexisting psychosis or bipolar disorder. May exacerbate symptoms of behavior and thought disorder or induce mixed/manic episode, respectively. New onset psychosis or mania may also occur with stimulant use. Observe for symptoms of aggression and/or hostility. Stimulants may exacerbate tics (motor and phonic) and Tourette syndrome. Evaluate for tics and Tourette syndrome prior to therapy initiation. **[U.S. Boxed Warning]: Potential for drug dependency exists; prolonged use may lead to drug dependency.** Use is contraindicated in patients with history of ethanol or drug abuse. Prescriptions should be written for the smallest quantity consistent with good patient care to minimize possibility of overdose. Abrupt discontinuation following high doses or for prolonged periods may result in symptoms for withdrawal.

Use caution in the elderly due to CNS stimulant adverse effects. Appetite suppression may occur, particularly in children. Use of stimulants has been associated with weight loss and slowing of growth rate; monitor growth rate and weight during treatment. Treatment interruption may be necessary in patients who are not increasing in height or gaining weight as expected.

Benzyl alcohol and derivatives: Some dosage forms may contain sodium benzoate/benzoic acid; benzoic acid (benzoate) is a metabolite of benzyl alcohol; large amounts of benzyl alcohol (≥99 mg/kg/day) have been associated with a potentially fatal toxicity ("gasping syndrome") in neonates; the "gasping syndrome" consists of metabolic acidosis, respiratory distress, gasping respirations, CNS dysfunction (including convulsions, intracranial hemorrhage), hypotension, and cardiovascular collapse (AAP, 1997; CDC, 1982); some data suggests that benzoate displaces bilirubin from protein binding sites (Ahlfors, 2001); avoid or use dosage forms containing benzyl alcohol derivative with caution in neonates. See manufacturer's labeling.

Adverse Reactions Frequency not defined.

Cardiovascular: Cardiomyopathy, hypertension, palpitations, tachycardia

Central nervous system: Aggressive behavior, dizziness, dysphoria, euphoria, exacerbation of tics, Gilles de la Tourette's syndrome, headache, insomnia, mania, overstimulation, psychosis, restlessness

Dermatologic: Urticaria

Endocrine & metabolic: Change in libido, weight loss

Gastrointestinal: Anorexia, constipation, diarrhea, unpleasant taste, xerostomia

Genitourinary: Frequent erections, impotence, prolonged erection

Neuromuscular & skeletal: Dyskinesia, tremor

Ophthalmic: Accommodation disturbances, blurred vision

Drug Interactions

Metabolism/Transport Effects Substrate of CYP2D6 (minor); **Note:** Assignment of Major/Minor substrate status based on clinically relevant drug interaction potential

Avoid Concomitant Use

Avoid concomitant use of Dextroamphetamine with any of the following: Iobenguane I 123; MAO Inhibitors

Increased Effect/Toxicity

Dextroamphetamine may increase the levels/effects of: Analgesics (Opioid); Sympathomimetics

The levels/effects of Dextroamphetamine may be increased by: Alkalinizing Agents; Antacids; AtoMOXetine; Cannabinoid-Containing Products; Carbonic Anhydrase Inhibitors; Linezolid; MAO Inhibitors; Proton Pump Inhibitors; Tedizolid; Tricyclic Antidepressants

Decreased Effect

Dextroamphetamine may decrease the levels/effects of: Antihistamines; Ethosuximide; Iobenguane I 123; Ioflupane I 123; PHENobarbital; Phenytoin

The levels/effects of Dextroamphetamine may be decreased by: Ammonium Chloride; Antipsychotic Agents; Ascorbic Acid; Gastrointestinal Acidifying Agents; Lithium; Methenamine; Multivitamins/Fluoride (with ADE); Multivitamins/Minerals (with ADEK, Folate, Iron); Multivitamins/Minerals (with AE, No Iron); Urinary Acidifying Agents

Food Interactions Amphetamine serum levels may be reduced if taken with acidic food, juices, or vitamin C. Management: Monitor response when taken concurrently.

Storage/Stability Store at 20°C to 25°C (68°F to 77°F). Protect from light.

Mechanism of Action Amphetamines are noncatecholamine, sympathomimetic amines that promote release of catecholamines (primarily dopamine and norepinephrine) from their storage sites in the presynaptic nerve terminals. A less significant mechanism may include their ability to block the reuptake of catecholamines by competitive inhibition.

Pharmacodynamics/Kinetics

Half-life elimination: Adults: 10 to 12 hours

Time to peak, serum: Immediate release: ~3 hours; sustained release: ~8 hours

Excretion: Urine

Dosage

Attention-deficit/hyperactivity disorder (ADHD):

Children 3 to 5 years: Oral: Immediate release tablets or oral solution: Initial: 2.5 mg once daily; may increase in increments of 2.5 mg at weekly intervals until optimal response is obtained; maximum dose: 40 mg daily (Dopheide 2009). **Note:** Although FDA approved, current guidelines do not recommend use in children ≤5 years due to insufficient evidence (AAP, 2011).

Children ≥6 years and Adolescents: Oral:

Immediate release tablets and oral solution: Initial: 5 mg once or twice daily; may increase in increments of 5 mg at weekly intervals until optimal response is reached; maximum dose: 40 mg daily (Dopheide 2009).

Extended release capsules: Initial: 5 mg once or twice daily; may increase in increments of 5 mg at weekly intervals until optimal response is obtained. Maximum dose: 40 mg daily (Dopheide 2009); a maximum daily dose of 60 mg in divided doses has been used in children >50 kg. (Dopheide, 2009; Pliszka 2007).

Narcolepsy:

Children 6 to 12 years: Oral: Initial: 5 mg once daily; may increase in increments of 5 mg at weekly intervals until optimal response is obtained; usual dosage: 5 to 60 mg daily in divided doses.

Children >12 years, Adolescents, and Adults: Oral: Initial: 10 mg once daily; may increase in increments of 10 mg at weekly intervals until optimal response is obtained; usual dosage: 5 to 60 mg daily in divided doses.

Dosage adjustment in renal impairment: There are no dosage adjustments provided in the manufacturer's labeling.

Dosage adjustment in hepatic impairment: There are no dosage adjustments provided in the manufacturer's labeling.

Administration Administer initial dose upon awakening; do not administer doses late in the evening due to potential for insomnia.

Immediate release tablets and oral solution: If needed, 1 to 2 additional doses may be administered at intervals of 4 to 6 hours.

Extended release and sustained release capsules: Do not crush sustained release drug products. Formulations may be used for once-daily administration, if appropriate.

Monitoring Parameters Cardiac evaluation should be completed on any patient who develops exertional chest pain, unexplained syncope, and any symptom of cardiac disease during treatment with stimulants; behavioral changes; signs of peripheral vasculopathy (eg, digital changes); growth and weight in children; CNS activity in all patients; signs of misuse, abuse, or addiction.

When used for the treatment of ADHD, thoroughly evaluate for cardiovascular risk. Monitor heart rate, blood pressure, and consider obtaining ECG prior to initiation (Vetter, 2008).

Dosage Forms

Capsule Extended Release 24 Hour, Oral:

Dexedrine: 5 mg, 10 mg, 15 mg

Generic: 5 mg, 10 mg, 15 mg

Solution, Oral:

ProCentra: 5 mg/5 mL (473 mL)

Generic: 5 mg/5 mL (473 mL)

Tablet, Oral:

Dexedrine: 5 mg, 10 mg

Zenzedi: 2.5 mg, 5 mg, 7.5 mg, 10 mg, 15 mg, 20 mg, 30 mg

Generic: 5 mg, 10 mg

Dextroamphetamine and Amphetamine

(deks troe am FET a meen & am FET a meen)

Brand Names: U.S. Adderall; Adderall XR

Brand Names: Canada Adderall XR

Index Terms Amphetamine and Dextroamphetamine

Pharmacologic Category Central Nervous System Stimulant

Use Attention-deficit/hyperactivity disorder (ADHD); narcolepsy

Pregnancy Risk Factor C

Dosage Oral: **Note:** Use lowest effective individualized dose; administer first dose as soon as awake.

ADHD:

Children: <3 years: Not recommended

Children: 3-5 years (Adderall): Initial 2.5 mg once daily given every morning; increase daily dose in 2.5 mg increments at weekly intervals until optimal response is obtained (maximum dose: 40 mg daily given in 1-3 divided doses); use intervals of 4-6 hours between additional doses.

Children: 6-12 years:

Adderall: Initial: 5 mg once or twice daily; increase daily dose in 5 mg increments at weekly intervals until optimal response is obtained (usual maximum dose: 40 mg daily given in 1-3 divided doses); use intervals of 4-6 hours between additional doses

Adderall XR: 5-10 mg once daily in the morning; if needed, may increase daily dose in 5-10 mg increments at weekly intervals (maximum dose: 30 mg daily)

Conversion from immediate release to extended release formulation: Patients may be switched from the immediate release formulation to the extended release formulation using the same total daily dose once daily.

Adolescents 13-17 years:

Adderall: Initial: 5 mg once or twice daily; increase daily dose in 5 mg increments at weekly intervals until optimal response is obtained (usual maximum dose: 40 mg daily given in 1-3 divided doses); use intervals of 4-6 hours between additional doses.

Adderall XR: 10 mg once daily in the morning; maybe increased to 20 mg daily after 1 week if symptoms are not controlled; higher doses (up to 60 mg daily) have been evaluated; however, there is not adequate evidence that higher doses afford additional benefit.

Canadian labeling: Maximum dose: 30 mg daily.

Conversion from immediate release to extended release formulation: Patients may be switched from the immediate release formulation to the extended release formulation using the same total daily dose once daily.

Adults:

Adderall: Initial: 5 mg once or twice daily; increase daily dose in 5 mg increments at weekly intervals until optimal response is obtained; usual maximum dose: 40 mg daily given in 1-3 divided doses per day. Use intervals of 4-6 hours between additional doses.

Adderall XR: Initial: 20 mg once daily in the morning; higher doses (up to 60 mg once daily) have been evaluated; however, there is not adequate evidence that higher doses afforded additional benefit.

Canadian labeling: Maximum dose: 30 mg daily.

Conversion from immediate release to extended release formulation: Patients may be switched from the immediate release formulation to the extended release formulation using the same total daily dose once daily.

Narcolepsy (Adderall):

Children: 6-12 years: Initial: 5 mg daily; increase daily dose in 5 mg at weekly intervals until optimal response is obtained (maximum dose: 60 mg daily given in 1-3 divided doses with intervals of 4-6 hours between doses)

Children >12 years and Adults: Initial: 10 mg daily; increase daily dose in 10 mg increments at weekly intervals until optimal response is obtained (maximum dose: 60 mg daily given in 1-3 divided doses with intervals of 4-6 hours between doses)

Dosage adjustment in renal impairment: No dosage adjustment provided in manufacturer's labeling.

Dosage adjustment in hepatic impairment: No dosage adjustment provided in manufacturer's labeling.

Additional Information Complete prescribing information should be consulted for additional detail.

Dosage Forms

Capsule, extended release, oral:

5 mg [dextroamphetamine sulfate 1.25 mg, dextroamphetamine saccharate 1.25 mg, amphetamine aspartate monohydrate 1.25 mg, amphetamine sulfate 1.25 mg]

10 mg [dextroamphetamine sulfate 2.5 mg, dextroamphetamine saccharate 2.5 mg, amphetamine aspartate monohydrate 2.5 mg, amphetamine sulfate 2.5 mg]

15 mg [dextroamphetamine sulfate 3.75 mg, dextroamphetamine saccharate 3.75 mg, amphetamine aspartate monohydrate 3.75 mg, amphetamine sulfate 3.75 mg]

20 mg [dextroamphetamine sulfate 5 mg, dextroamphetamine saccharate 5 mg, amphetamine aspartate monohydrate 5 mg, amphetamine sulfate 5 mg]
25 mg [dextroamphetamine sulfate 6.25 mg, dextroamphetamine saccharate 6.25 mg, amphetamine aspartate monohydrate 6.25 mg, amphetamine sulfate 6.25 mg]
30 mg [dextroamphetamine sulfate 7.5 mg, dextroamphetamine saccharate 7.5 mg, amphetamine aspartate monohydrate 7.5 mg, amphetamine sulfate 7.5 mg]
Adderall XR:
5 mg [dextroamphetamine 1.25 mg, dextroamphetamine saccharate 1.25 mg, amphetamine aspartate monohydrate 1.25 mg, amphetamine sulfate 1.25 mg]
10 mg [dextroamphetamine sulfate 2.5 mg, dextroamphetamine saccharate 2.5 mg, amphetamine aspartate monohydrate 2.5 mg, amphetamine sulfate 2.5 mg]
15 mg [dextroamphetamine sulfate 3.75 mg, dextroamphetamine saccharate 3.75 mg, amphetamine aspartate monohydrate 3.75 mg, amphetamine sulfate 3.75 mg]
20 mg [dextroamphetamine sulfate 5 mg, dextroamphetamine saccharate 5 mg, amphetamine aspartate monohydrate 5 mg, amphetamine sulfate 5 mg]
25 mg [dextroamphetamine sulfate 6.25 mg, dextroamphetamine saccharate 6.25 mg, amphetamine aspartate monohydrate 6.25 mg, amphetamine sulfate 6.25 mg]
30 mg [dextroamphetamine sulfate 7.5 mg, dextroamphetamine saccharate 7.5 mg, amphetamine aspartate monohydrate 7.5 mg, amphetamine sulfate 7.5 mg]

Tablet, oral: 5 mg, 7.5 mg, 10 mg, 12.5 mg, 15 mg, 20 mg, 30 mg
5 mg [dextroamphetamine sulfate 1.25 mg, dextroamphetamine saccharate 1.25 mg, amphetamine aspartate monohydrate 1.25 mg, amphetamine sulfate 1.25 mg]
7.5 mg [dextroamphetamine sulfate 1.875 mg, dextroamphetamine saccharate 1.875 mg, amphetamine aspartate monohydrate 1.875 mg, amphetamine sulfate 1.875 mg]
10 mg [dextroamphetamine sulfate 2.5 mg, dextroamphetamine saccharate 2.5 mg, amphetamine aspartate monohydrate 2.5 mg, amphetamine sulfate 2.5 mg]
12.5 mg [dextroamphetamine sulfate 3.125 mg, dextroamphetamine saccharate 3.125 mg, amphetamine aspartate monohydrate 3.125 mg, amphetamine sulfate 3.125 mg]
15 mg [dextroamphetamine sulfate 3.75 mg, dextroamphetamine saccharate 3.75 mg, amphetamine aspartate monohydrate 3.75 mg, amphetamine sulfate 3.75 mg]
20 mg [dextroamphetamine sulfate 5 mg, dextroamphetamine saccharate 5 mg, amphetamine aspartate monohydrate 5 mg, amphetamine sulfate 5 mg]
30 mg [dextroamphetamine sulfate 7.5 mg, dextroamphetamine saccharate 7.5 mg, amphetamine aspartate monohydrate 7.5 mg, amphetamine sulfate 7.5 mg]
Adderall:
5 mg [dextroamphetamine sulfate 1.25 mg, dextroamphetamine saccharate 1.25 mg, amphetamine aspartate monohydrate 1.25 mg, amphetamine sulfate 1.25 mg]
7.5 mg [dextroamphetamine sulfate 1.875 mg, dextroamphetamine saccharate 1.875 mg, amphetamine aspartate monohydrate 1.875 mg, amphetamine sulfate 1.875 mg]
10 mg [dextroamphetamine sulfate 2.5 mg, dextroamphetamine saccharate 2.5 mg, amphetamine aspartate monohydrate 2.5 mg, amphetamine sulfate 2.5 mg]
12.5 mg [dextroamphetamine sulfate 3.125 mg, dextroamphetamine saccharate 3.125 mg, amphetamine aspartate monohydrate 3.125 mg, amphetamine sulfate 3.125 mg]
15 mg [dextroamphetamine sulfate 3.75 mg, dextroamphetamine saccharate 3.75 mg, amphetamine aspartate monohydrate 3.75 mg, amphetamine sulfate 3.75 mg]
20 mg [dextroamphetamine sulfate 5 mg, dextroamphetamine saccharate 5 mg, amphetamine aspartate monohydrate 5 mg, amphetamine sulfate 5 mg]
30 mg [dextroamphetamine sulfate 7.5 mg, dextroamphetamine saccharate 7.5 mg, amphetamine aspartate monohydrate 7.5 mg, amphetamine sulfate 7.5 mg]

◆ **Dextroamphetamine Sulfate** *see* Dextroamphetamine *on page 607*

Dextromethorphan and Chlorpheniramine

(deks troe meth OR fan & klor fen IR a meen)

Brand Names: U.S. Coricidin® HBP Cough & Cold [OTC]; Dimetapp® Children's Long Acting Cough Plus Cold [OTC]; Robitussin® Children's Cough & Cold Long-Acting [OTC]; Scot-Tussin® DM Maximum Strength [OTC]; Triaminic® Children's Softchews® Cough & Runny Nose [OTC]

Index Terms Chlorpheniramine and Dextromethorphan; Chlorpheniramine Maleate and Dextromethorphan Hydrobromide; Dextromethorphan Hydrobromide and Chlorpheniramine Maleate

Pharmacologic Category Alkylamine Derivative; Antitussive; Histamine H_1 Antagonist; Histamine H_1 Antagonist, First Generation

Use Symptomatic relief of runny nose, sneezing, itchy/watery eyes, cough, and other upper respiratory symptoms associated with hay fever, common cold, or upper respiratory allergies

Dosage General dosing guidelines; consult specific product labeling.
Antitussive/antihistamine: Oral:
Children: 6-11 years:
Liquid: Dextromethorphan 15 mg and chlorpheniramine 2 mg every 6 hours as needed (maximum: 60 mg dextromethorphan and 8 mg chlorpheniramine/24 hours)
Chewable tablet: Dextromethorphan 10 mg and chlorpheniramine 2 mg every 4-6 hours as needed (maximum: 50 mg dextromethorphan and 10 mg chlorpheniramine/24 hours)
Children ≥12 years and Adults: Dextromethorphan 30 mg and chlorpheniramine 4 mg every 6 hours as needed (maximum: 120 mg dextromethorphan and 16 mg chlorpheniramine/24 hours)

Additional Information Complete prescribing information should be consulted for additional detail.

Dosage Forms
Syrup, oral:
Dimetapp® Children's Long Acting Cough Plus Cold [OTC]: Dextromethorphan 7.5 mg and chlorpheniramine 1 mg per 5 mL (118 mL)
Robitussin® Children's Cough and Cold Long-Acting [OTC]: Dextromethorphan 7.5 mg and chlorpheniramine 1 mg per 5 mL (118 mL)
Scot-Tussin® DM Maximum Strength [OTC]: Dextromethorphan 15 mg and chlorpheniramine 2 mg per 5 mL (118 mL)

Tablet, oral:

Coricidin® HBP Cough and Cold [OTC]: Dextromethorphan 30 mg and chlorpheniramine 4 mg

Tablet, softchew, oral:

Triaminic® Children's Softchews® Cough & Runny Nose [OTC]: Dextromethorphan 5 mg and chlorpheniramine 1 mg

◆ **Dextromethorphan and Guaifenesin** *see* Guaifenesin and Dextromethorphan *on page 987*

Dextromethorphan and Phenylephrine

(deks troe meth OR fan & fen il EF rin)

Brand Names: U.S. PediaCare® Children's Multi-Symptom Cold [OTC]; Safetussin® CD [OTC]; Sudafed PE® Children's Cold & Cough [OTC]; Triaminic® Day Time Cold & Cough [OTC]

Index Terms Dextromethorphan Hydrobromide and Phenylephrine Hydrochloride; Phenylephrine and Dextromethorphan

Pharmacologic Category Antitussive; Decongestant

Use Temporary relief of symptoms of hay fever, the common cold, and upper respiratory allergies including sinus/nasal congestion, minor bronchial/throat irritation, and cough

Dosage Oral: Relief of nasal/sinus congestion and cough:

Children 4-6 years: PediaCare® Children's Multi-Symptom Cold, Sudafed PE® Children's Cold & Cough, Triaminic® Day Time Cold & Cough: 5 mL every 4 hours as needed (maximum: 30 mL/24 hours)

Children 6-12 years:

PediaCare® Children's Multi-Symptom Cold, Sudafed PE® Children's Cold & Cough, Triaminic® Day Time Cold & Cough: 10 mL every 4 hours as needed (maximum: 60 mL/24 hours)

Safetussin® CD: 5 mL every 6 hours as needed (maximum: 20 mL/24 hours)

Children ≥12 years and Adults: Safetussin® CD: 10 mL every 6 hours as needed (maximum: 40 mL/24 hours)

Additional Information Complete prescribing information should be consulted for additional detail.

Dosage Forms

Liquid, oral:

Sudafed PE® Children's Cold + Cough [OTC]: Dextromethorphan 5 mg and phenylephrine 2.5 mg per 5 mL (118 mL)

Syrup:

PediaCare® Children's Multi-Symptom Cold [OTC], Triaminic® Day Time Cold & Cough [OTC]: Dextromethorphan 5 mg and phenylephrine 2.5 mg per 5 mL

Safetussin® CD [OTC]: Dextromethorphan 15 mg and phenylephrine 2.5 mg per 5 mL

◆ **Dextromethorphan and Promethazine** *see* Promethazine and Dextromethorphan *on page 1725*

◆ **Dextromethorphan and Pseudoephedrine** *see* Pseudoephedrine and Dextromethorphan *on page 1743*

Dextromethorphan and Quinidine

(deks troe meth OR fan & KWIN i deen)

Brand Names: U.S. Nuedexta™

Brand Names: Canada Nuedexta™

Index Terms Dextromethorphan Hydrobromide and Quinidine Sulfate; Quinidine and Dextromethorphan

Pharmacologic Category N-Methyl-D-Aspartate Receptor Antagonist

Use Treatment of pseudobulbar affect (PBA)

Pregnancy Risk Factor C

Pregnancy Considerations Adverse events were observed in animal reproduction studies using this combination.

Breast-Feeding Considerations Quinidine is excreted in breast milk; excretion of dextromethorphan is not known

Contraindications Hypersensitivity to dextromethorphan, quinidine, quinine, mefloquine, or any component of the formulation; concomitant use with quinidine or other medications containing quinidine, quinine, or mefloquine; history of quinine-, mefloquine-, or quinidine-induced thrombocytopenia; hepatitis; bone marrow depression; or lupus-like syndrome; concurrent administration with or within 2 weeks of discontinuing an MAO inhibitor; patients with prolonged QT interval, congenital QT syndrome, or history of torsade de pointes; patients with heart failure; concurrent use of drugs that prolong the QT interval and are metabolized by CYP2D6 (eg, pimozide, thioridazine); patients with complete AV block without an implanted pacemaker or patients at high risk of complete AV block

Warnings/Precautions Immune-mediated thrombocytopenia (severe or fatal) may be associated with quinidine use. Unless clearly not drug related, discontinue immediately; continued use may be associated with an increase in fatal hemorrhage. Thrombocytopenia generally resolves within a few days of discontinuation. Therapy should not be restarted in sensitized patients. Agranulocytosis, angioedema, bronchospasm, lupus-like syndrome, rash or other hypersensitivity reactions may be associated with use. Quinidine has also been associated with severe hepatotoxic reactions including granulomatous hepatitis. Use is contraindicated in patients with prior history of immune-mediated thrombocytopenia associated with structurally related drugs (eg, quinine, mefloquine) and in patients with quinidine-, quinine-, or mefloquine-induced lupus-like syndrome.

Concomitant use of moderate or strong CYP3A4 inhibitors may increase quinidine levels and prolong the QTc interval. Quinidine inhibits CYP2D6; concomitant use with CYP2D6 substrates may cause an accumulation of concomitantly administered drug and/or reduce active metabolite formation, decreasing their safety and/or efficacy. Use with caution in patients who are poor metabolizers of CYP2D6 metabolized drugs. Quinidine in this combination product is used to inhibit CYP2D6 in order to increase plasma concentrations of dextromethorphan. In patients who are poor metabolizers, this effect would not be significant; however, adverse events related to quinidine may still be observed. Genotyping should be considered in patients considered to be at risk of quinidine toxicity prior to therapy. Symptoms associated with serotonin syndrome such as agitation, confusion, hallucinations, hyper-reflexia, myoclonus, shivering, and tachycardia may occur with concomitant proserotonergic drugs (ie, SSRIs/SNRIs or triptans); especially with higher dextromethorphan doses. Effects with other sedative drugs or ethanol may be potentiated.

Use caution in patients with left ventricular hypertrophy or left ventricular dysfunction which are more common in patients with chronic hypertension, coronary artery disease or history of stroke; risk of QTc prolongation may be increased. Use is contraindicated in patients with prolonged QT interval, congenital QT syndrome, or history of torsade de pointes, patients with heart failure, complete AV block without an implanted pacemaker or patients at high risk of complete AV block. Correct hypokalemia or hypomagnesemia prior to therapy. Use caution with medications which may further prolong the QT interval or cause cardiac arrhythmias. Dose dependent QTc prolongation may occur. Monitor patients at risk following the first dose. Discontinue if arrhythmia occurs.

May cause anticholinergic effects; use caution in patients with myasthenia gravis or other conditions which may be affected. May cause dizziness; use caution in patients with motor impairment or history of falls. Safety and efficacy have not been established with severe hepatic or renal impairment; increased serum concentrations may occur. Has not shown to be safe or effective in other types of commonly occurring emotional labilities (eg, Alzheimer's disease and other dementias). Patients with a history of drug abuse should be monitored closely for signs of abuse/misuse of Nuedexta™ (eg, development of tolerance, increase in dose, or drug-seeking behavior). Abuse of dextromethorphan may cause brain damage, cardiac arrhythmia, loss of consciousness, or death. Periodically reassess the need for treatment; spontaneous improvement of PBA may occur.

Adverse Reactions Also see individual agents.

Cardiovascular: Peripheral edema
Central nervous system: Dizziness
Gastrointestinal: Diarrhea, flatulence, vomiting
Genitourinary: Urinary tract infection
Hepatic: GGT increased
Neuromuscular & skeletal: Weakness
Respiratory: Cough
Miscellaneous: Influenza

Drug Interactions

Metabolism/Transport Effects Refer to individual components.

Avoid Concomitant Use

Avoid concomitant use of Dextromethorphan and Quinidine with any of the following: Amiodarone; Antifungal Agents (Azole Derivatives, Systemic); Bosutinib; Conivaptan; Crizotinib; Dapoxetine; Enzalutamide; Fingolimod; Fusidic Acid (Systemic); Haloperidol; Highest Risk QTc-Prolonging Agents; Idelalisib; Ivabradine; Macrolide Antibiotics; MAO Inhibitors; Mefloquine; Mifepristone; Moderate Risk QTc-Prolonging Agents; PAZOPanib; Pimozide; Propafenone; Protease Inhibitors; Silodosin; Tamoxifen; Thioridazine; Topotecan; VinCRIStine (Liposomal)

Increased Effect/Toxicity

Dextromethorphan and Quinidine may increase the levels/effects of: Afatinib; Antipsychotic Agents; ARIPiprazole; AtoMOXetine; Bosutinib; Brentuximab Vedotin; Calcium Channel Blockers (Dihydropyridine); Cardiac Glycosides; Colchicine; CYP2D6 Substrates; Dabigatran Etexilate; Dalfampridine; Dextromethorphan; DOXOrubicin (Conventional); Edoxaban; Everolimus; Fesoterodine; Haloperidol; Highest Risk QTc-Prolonging Agents; Ledipasvir; Lomitapide; Mefloquine; Memantine; Metoprolol; Naloxegol; Nebivolol; Neuromuscular-Blocking Agents; PAZOPanib; P-glycoprotein/ABCB1 Substrates; Pimozide; Propafenone; Propranolol; Prucalopride; Rifaximin; Rivaroxaban; Serotonin Modulators; Silodosin; Thioridazine; Topotecan; Tricyclic Antidepressants; Verapamil; VinCRIStine (Liposomal); Vitamin K Antagonists; Vortioxetine

The levels/effects of Dextromethorphan and Quinidine may be increased by: Abiraterone Acetate; Amiodarone; Antacids; Antiemetics (5HT3 Antagonists); Antifungal Agents (Azole Derivatives, Systemic); Antipsychotic Agents; Aprepitant; Boceprevir; Calcium Channel Blockers (Dihydropyridine); Carbonic Anhydrase Inhibitors; Cimetidine; Conivaptan; Crizotinib; CYP2D6 Inhibitors (Moderate); CYP2D6 Inhibitors (Strong); CYP3A4 Inhibitors (Moderate); CYP3A4 Inhibitors (Strong); Dapoxetine; Diltiazem; Fingolimod; Fosaprepitant; Fosphenytoin; Fusidic Acid (Systemic); Haloperidol; Idelalisib; Ivabradine; Ivacaftor; Luliconazole; Lurasidone; Macrolide Antibiotics; MAO Inhibitors; Mifepristone; Moderate Risk QTc-Prolonging Agents; Netupitant; Peginterferon Alfa-2b; P-glycoprotein/ABCB1 Inhibitors; PHENobarbital; Protease Inhibitors; QTc-Prolonging Agents (Indeterminate Risk and Risk Modifying); QuiNIDine; Reserpine; Selective Serotonin Reuptake Inhibitors; Simeprevir; Stiripentol; Telaprevir; Tricyclic Antidepressants; Verapamil

Decreased Effect

Dextromethorphan and Quinidine may decrease the levels/effects of: Codeine; Dihydrocodeine; Hydrocodone; Tamoxifen

The levels/effects of Dextromethorphan and Quinidine may be decreased by: Bosentan; Calcium Channel Blockers (Dihydropyridine); CYP3A4 Inducers (Moderate); CYP3A4 Inducers (Strong); Dabrafenib; Deferasirox; Enzalutamide; Etravirine; Fosphenytoin; Kaolin; Mitotane; Peginterferon Alfa-2b; P-glycoprotein/ABCB1 Inducers; PHENobarbital; Phenytoin; Potassium-Sparing Diuretics; Primidone; Rifamycin Derivatives; Siltuximab; St Johns Wort; Sucralfate; Tocilizumab

Food Interactions Grapefruit juice may increase levels of quinidine. Tonic water contains quinine. Management: Avoid grapefruit juice. Avoid tonic water.

Storage/Stability Store at controlled room temperature at 25°C (77°F); excursions permitted to 15°C to 30°C (59°F to 86°F).

Mechanism of Action Dextromethorphan may relieve the symptoms of PBA by binding to sigma-1 receptors in the brain which may be involved in behavior, however the exact mechanism of action is not known. Quinidine is used to block the rapid metabolism of dextromethorphan, thereby increasing serum concentrations. The dose of quinidine in this combination product provides serum concentrations 1% to 3% of those needed to treat cardiac arrhythmias.

Pharmacodynamics/Kinetics

Absorption: Bioavailability of dextromethorphan increased ~20-fold when administered with quinidine.
Protein binding: Dextromethorphan: 60% to 70%; Quinidine: 80% to 89%
Metabolism: Dextromethorphan: Hepatic via CYP2D6 to dextrorphan (active); Quinidine: Hepatic via CYP3A4 to 3-hydroxyquinidine (active) and other metabolites
Half-life elimination: Dextromethorphan: 13 hours in extensive metabolizers; Quinidine: 7 hours in extensive metabolizers
Time to peak: Dextromethorphan: 3-4 hours; Quinidine: 1-2 hours
Excretion: Urine

Dosage Oral: Adults: Pseudobulbar affect: One capsule once daily for 7 days, then increase to 1 capsule twice daily; reassess patient periodically to determine if continued use is necessary

Dosage adjustment in renal impairment: Dose adjustment not required for mild or moderate renal impairment; not studied with severe impairment

Dosage adjustment in hepatic impairment: Dose adjustment not required for mild or moderate hepatic impairment; however, an increase in adverse reactions is observed with moderate hepatic dysfunction; not studied with severe impairment

Dietary Considerations May be taken with or without food. Avoid grapefruit juice.

Administration May be administered with or without food. Administer twice-daily doses every 12 hours.

Monitoring Parameters QT interval 3-4 hours after the first dose in patients at risk for QTc prolongation; potassium and magnesium prior to and during therapy; CBC, liver and renal function tests; periodically assess risk factors for arrhythmias during treatment; periodically reassess the need for treatment (spontaneous improvement of PBA may occur)

Dosage Forms

Capsule, oral:

Nuedexta™: Dextromethorphan hydrobromide 20 mg and quinidine sulfate 10 mg

- **Dextromethorphan, Chlorpheniramine, and Phenylephrine** *see* Chlorpheniramine, Phenylephrine, and Dextromethorphan *on page 428*
- **Dextromethorphan, Chlorpheniramine, and Pseudoephedrine** *see* Chlorpheniramine, Pseudoephedrine, and Dextromethorphan *on page 428*
- **Dextromethorphan, Guaifenesin, and Pseudoephedrine** *see* Guaifenesin, Pseudoephedrine, and Dextromethorphan *on page 989*
- **Dextromethorphan Hydrobromide and Chlorpheniramine Maleate** *see* Dextromethorphan and Chlorpheniramine *on page 610*
- **Dextromethorphan Hydrobromide and Phenylephrine Hydrochloride** *see* Dextromethorphan and Phenylephrine *on page 611*
- **Dextromethorphan Hydrobromide and Quinidine Sulfate** *see* Dextromethorphan and Quinidine *on page 611*
- **Dex-Tuss** *see* Guaifenesin and Codeine *on page 987*
- **Dezocitidine** *see* Decitabine *on page 581*
- **dFdC** *see* Gemcitabine *on page 952*
- **dFdCyd** *see* Gemcitabine *on page 952*
- **DFM** *see* Deferoxamine *on page 586*
- **DFMO** *see* Eflornithine *on page 710*
- **D-Forte (Can)** *see* Ergocalciferol *on page 753*
- **DHAD** *see* MitoXANtrone *on page 1382*
- **DHAQ** *see* MitoXANtrone *on page 1382*
- **DHE** *see* Dihydroergotamine *on page 633*
- **D.H.E. 45** *see* Dihydroergotamine *on page 633*
- **DHPG Sodium** *see* Ganciclovir (Systemic) *on page 948*
- **Diabeta** *see* GlyBURIDE *on page 972*
- **Diabeta** *see* GlyBURIDE *on page 972*
- **DiaBeta (Can)** *see* GlyBURIDE *on page 972*
- **Diabetic Siltussin DAS-Na [OTC]** *see* GuaiFENesin *on page 986*
- **Diabetic Siltussin-DM DAS-Na [OTC]** *see* Guaifenesin and Dextromethorphan *on page 987*
- **Diabetic Siltussin-DM DAS-Na Maximum Strength [OTC]** *see* Guaifenesin and Dextromethorphan *on page 987*
- **Diabetic Tussin [OTC]** *see* GuaiFENesin *on page 986*
- **Diabetic Tussin DM [OTC]** *see* Guaifenesin and Dextromethorphan *on page 987*
- **Diabetic Tussin DM Maximum Strength [OTC]** *see* Guaifenesin and Dextromethorphan *on page 987*
- **Diabetic Tussin Mucus Relief [OTC]** *see* GuaiFENesin *on page 986*

Diacerein [INT] (dye ah CER ain)

International Brand Names Aceren (KR); Art (FR, IL); Arthrofar (GR); Artizona (CL); Artoflam (ID); Artrizan (ES); Artroda (KR); Artrodar (AR, BR, CN, CO, CZ, HK, ID, IN, MY, SK, TH, VN); Artroglobina (PE, UY); Artrolyt (AT, PT); Atrodar (TR, VE); Biojoint (IN); Bondi (ID); Cartigen (MX); Cartivix (PT); Cerhein (KR); Cominar (AR); Diatrim (IL); Distrin (KR); Duskare (IN); Dycerin (KR); Fisiodar (IT); Galaxdar (ES); Glizolan (ES); Jaizzy (IN); Myobloc (GR); Nulartrin (AR); Oacerein (MX); Ostirein (GR); Pentacrin (GR); Rumaterin (KR); Verboril (AT, GR); Zondar (FR)

Pharmacologic Category Anthraquinone

Reported Use Osteoarthritis

Dosage Range Adults: Oral: 50 mg twice daily

Dosage adjustment in renal impairment: CrCl <30 mL/minute: 25 mg twice daily

Product Availability Product available in various countries; not currently available in the U.S.

Dosage Forms

Capsule: 50 mg

- **Diacomit (Can)** *see* Stiripentol [CAN/INT] *on page 1935*
- **Dialyvite Omega-3 Concentrate [OTC]** *see* Omega-3 Fatty Acids *on page 1507*
- **Diamicron (Can)** *see* Gliclazide [CAN/INT] *on page 964*
- **Diamicron MR (Can)** *see* Gliclazide [CAN/INT] *on page 964*
- **Diaminocyclohexane Oxalatoplatinum** *see* Oxaliplatin *on page 1528*
- **Diaminodiphenylsulfone** *see* Dapsone (Systemic) *on page 561*
- **Diamode [OTC]** *see* Loperamide *on page 1236*
- **Diamox® (Can)** *see* AcetaZOLAMIDE *on page 39*
- **Diamox Sequels** *see* AcetaZOLAMIDE *on page 39*
- **Diane-35® (Can)** *see* Cyproterone and Ethinyl Estradiol [CAN/INT] *on page 532*
- **Diarr-Eze (Can)** *see* Loperamide *on page 1236*
- **Diastat® (Can)** *see* Diazepam *on page 613*
- **Diastat AcuDial** *see* Diazepam *on page 613*
- **Diastat Pediatric** *see* Diazepam *on page 613*
- **Diazemuls® (Can)** *see* Diazepam *on page 613*

Diazepam (dye AZ e pam)

Brand Names: U.S. Diastat AcuDial; Diastat Pediatric; Diazepam Intensol; Valium

Brand Names: Canada Apo-Diazepam®; Bio-Diazepam; Diastat®; Diazemuls®; Diazepam Auto Injector; Diazepam Injection USP; Novo-Dipam; PMS-Diazepam; Valium®

Pharmacologic Category Benzodiazepine

Additional Appendix Information

Beers Criteria – Potentially Inappropriate Medications for Geriatrics *on page 2271*

Use Management of anxiety disorders, ethanol withdrawal symptoms; skeletal muscle relaxant; treatment of convulsive disorders; preoperative or preprocedural sedation and amnesia

Rectal gel: Management of selected, refractory epilepsy patients on stable regimens of antiepileptic drugs requiring intermittent use of diazepam to control episodes of increased seizure activity

Pregnancy Risk Factor D

Pregnancy Considerations Teratogenic effects have been reported in animal reproduction studies. In humans, diazepam and its metabolites (N-desmethyldiazepam, temazepam, and oxazepam) cross the placenta. Teratogenic effects have been observed with diazepam; however, additional studies are needed. The incidence of premature birth and low birth weights may be increased following maternal use of benzodiazepines; hypoglycemia and respiratory problems in the neonate may occur following exposure late in pregnancy. Neonatal withdrawal symptoms may occur within days to weeks after birth and "floppy infant syndrome" (which also includes withdrawal symptoms) has been reported with some benzodiazepines (including diazepam) (Bergman, 1992; Iqbal, 2002; Wikner, 2007). A combination of factors influences the potential teratogenicity of anticonvulsant therapy. When treating women with epilepsy, monotherapy with the lowest effective dose and avoidance of medications known to have a high incidence of teratogenic effects is recommended (Harden, 2009; Wlodarczyk, 2012).

Breast-Feeding Considerations Diazepam and N-desmethyldiazepam can be found in breast milk; the oxazepam metabolite has also been detected in the urine of a nursing infant. Drowsiness, lethargy, or weight loss in nursing infants have been observed in case reports following maternal use of some benzodiazepines, including diazepam (Iqbal, 2002). Because diazepam and its metabolites may be present in breast milk for prolonged periods following administration, one manufacturer recommends discontinuing breast-feeding for an appropriate period of time.

Contraindications Hypersensitivity to diazepam or any component of the formulation (cross-sensitivity with other benzodiazepines may exist); myasthenia gravis; severe respiratory insufficiency; severe hepatic insufficiency; sleep apnea syndrome; acute narrow-angle glaucoma; not for use in infants <6 months of age (oral)

Warnings/Precautions Withdrawal has also been associated with an increase in the seizure frequency. Use with caution with drugs which may decrease diazepam metabolism. Use with caution in debilitated patients, obese patients, patients with hepatic disease (including alcoholics), or renal impairment. Active metabolites with extended half-lives may lead to delayed accumulation and adverse effects. Use with caution in patients with respiratory disease or impaired gag reflex.

Acute hypotension, muscle weakness, apnea, and cardiac arrest have occurred with parenteral administration. Acute effects may be more prevalent in patients receiving concurrent barbiturates, opioids, or ethanol. Appropriate resuscitative equipment and qualified personnel should be available during administration and monitoring. Avoid use of the injection in patients with shock, coma, or acute ethanol intoxication. Intra-arterial injection or extravasation of the parenteral formulation should be avoided. Some dosage forms may contain propylene glycol; large amounts are potentially toxic and have been associated hyperosmolality, lactic acidosis, seizures, and respiratory depression; use caution (AAP, 1997; Zar, 2007). Administration of rectal gel should only be performed by individuals trained to recognize characteristic seizure activity and monitor response.

IV administration: Vesicant; ensure proper needle or catheter placement prior to and during administration; avoid extravasation.

Benzyl alcohol and derivatives: Some dosage forms may contain benzyl alcohol and/or sodium benzoate/benzoic acid; benzoic acid (benzoate) is a metabolite of benzyl alcohol; large amounts of benzyl alcohol (≥99 mg/kg/day) have been associated with a potentially fatal toxicity ("gasping syndrome") in neonates; the "gasping syndrome" consists of metabolic acidosis, respiratory distress, gasping respirations, CNS dysfunction (including convulsions, intracranial hemorrhage), hypotension, and cardiovascular collapse (AAP, 1997; CDC, 1982); some data suggests that benzoate displaces bilirubin from protein binding sites (Ahlfors, 2001); avoid or use dosage forms containing benzyl alcohol and/or benzyl alcohol derivative with caution in neonates. See manufacturer's labeling.

Causes CNS depression (dose-related) resulting in sedation, dizziness, confusion, or ataxia which may impair physical and mental capabilities. Patients must be cautioned about performing tasks which require mental alertness (eg, operating machinery or driving). Use with caution in patients receiving other CNS depressants or psychoactive agents. Effects with other sedative drugs or ethanol may be potentiated. The dosage of opioids should be reduced by approximately one-third when diazepam is added. Benzodiazepines have been associated with falls and traumatic injury and should be used with extreme caution in patients who are at risk of these events. Benzodiazepines with long half-lives may produce prolonged sedation and increase the risk of falls and fracture. In older adults, benzodiazepines increase the risk of impaired cognition, delirium, falls, fractures, and motor vehicle accidents. Due to increased sensitivity in this age group and slower metabolism of long-acting agents (such as diazepam), avoid use for treatment of insomnia, agitation, or delirium (Beers Criteria).

Use with caution in patients taking strong CYP3A4 inhibitors, moderate or strong CYP3A4 and CYP2C19 inducers and major CYP3A4 substrates.

Use caution in patients with depression or anxiety associated with depression, particularly if suicidal risk may be present. Use with caution in patients with a history of drug dependence. Benzodiazepines have been associated with dependence and acute withdrawal symptoms on discontinuation or reduction in dose. Acute withdrawal, including seizures, may be precipitated in patients after administration of flumazenil to patients receiving long-term benzodiazepine therapy. Diazepam is a long half-life benzodiazepine. Tolerance develops to the sedative, hypnotic, and anticonvulsant effects. It does not develop to the anxiolytic or skeletal muscle relaxing effects (Vinkers, 2012). Chronic use of this agent may increase the perioperative benzodiazepine dose needed to achieve desired effect.

Diazepam has been associated with anterograde amnesia. Psychiatric and paradoxical reactions, including hyperactive or aggressive behavior, have been reported with benzodiazepines, particularly in adolescent/pediatric or elderly patients. Does not have analgesic, antidepressant, or antipsychotic properties.

Adverse Reactions Adverse reactions may vary by route of administration.

Cardiovascular: Hypotension, localized phlebitis, vasodilatation

Central nervous system: Amnesia, ataxia, confusion, depression, drowsiness, dysarthria, fatigue, headache, slurred speech, vertigo

Dermatologic: Skin rash

Endocrine & metabolic: Change in libido

Gastrointestinal: Altered salivation (dry mouth or hypersalivation), constipation, diarrhea, nausea

Genitourinary: Urinary incontinence, urinary retention

Hepatic: Jaundice

Local: Pain at injection site

Neuromuscular & skeletal: Tremor, weakness

Ophthalmic: Blurred vision, diplopia

Respiratory: Apnea, asthma, bradypnea

Miscellaneous: Paradoxical reaction (eg, aggressiveness, agitation, anxiety, delusions, hallucinations, inappropriate behavior, increased muscle spasms, insomnia, irritability, psychoses, rage, restlessness, sleep disturbances, stimulation)

Drug Interactions

Metabolism/Transport Effects Substrate of CYP1A2 (minor), CYP2B6 (minor), CYP2C19 (major), CYP2C9 (minor), CYP3A4 (major); **Note:** Assignment of Major/Minor substrate status based on clinically relevant drug interaction potential; **Inhibits** CYP2C19 (weak), CYP3A4 (weak)

Avoid Concomitant Use

Avoid concomitant use of Diazepam with any of the following: Azelastine (Nasal); Conivaptan; Fusidic Acid (Systemic); Idelalisib; Methadone; OLANZapine; Orphenadrine; Paraldehyde; Pimozide; Sodium Oxybate; Thalidomide

Increased Effect/Toxicity

Diazepam may increase the levels/effects of: Alcohol (Ethyl); Alfentanil; ARIPiprazole; Azelastine (Nasal); Buprenorphine; CloZAPine; CNS Depressants; Dofetilide; Hydrocodone; Lomitapide; Methadone; Methotrimeprazine; Metyrosine; Mirtazapine; Orphenadrine; Paraldehyde; Pimozide; Pramipexole; ROPINIRole; Rotigotine; Selective Serotonin Reuptake Inhibitors; Sodium Oxybate; Suvorexant; Thalidomide; Zolpidem

The levels/effects of Diazepam may be increased by: Aprepitant; Brimonidine (Topical); Cannabis; Ceritinib; Conivaptan; Cosyntropin; CYP2C19 Inhibitors (Moderate); CYP2C19 Inhibitors (Strong); CYP3A4 Inhibitors (Moderate); CYP3A4 Inhibitors (Strong); Dasatinib; Disulfiram; Doxylamine; Dronabinol; Droperidol; Etravirine; Fosamprenavir; Fosaprepitant; Fusidic Acid (Systemic); HydrOXYzine; Idelalisib; Ivacaftor; Kava Kava; Luliconazole; Magnesium Sulfate; Methotrimeprazine; Mifepristone; Nabilone; Netupitant; OLANZapine; Perampanel; Ritonavir; Rufinamide; Saquinavir; Simeprevir; Stiripentol; Tapentadol; Teduglutide; Tetrahydrocannabinol

Decreased Effect

The levels/effects of Diazepam may be decreased by: Bosentan; CYP2C19 Inducers (Strong); CYP3A4 Inducers (Moderate); CYP3A4 Inducers (Strong); Dabrafenib; Deferasirox; Etravirine; Mitotane; Siltuximab; St Johns Wort; Theophylline Derivatives; Tocilizumab; Yohimbine

Food Interactions Diazepam serum concentrations may be decreased if taken with food. Grapefruit juice may increase diazepam serum concentrations. Management: Avoid concurrent use of grapefruit juice. Maintain adequate hydration, unless instructed to restrict fluid intake.

Preparation for Administration Per manufacturer, do not mix IV product with other medications.

Storage/Stability

Injection: Store at 20°C to 25°C (68°F to 77°F); excursions permitted to 15°C to 30°C (59°F to 86°F). Protect from light. Potency is retained for up to 3 months when kept at room temperature. Most stable at pH 4-8; hydrolysis occurs at pH <3.

Oral solution: Store at 25°C (77°F); excursions permitted to 15°C to 30°C (59°F to 86°F).

Oral concentrated solution: Store at 25°C (77°F); excursions permitted to 15°C to 30°C (59°F to 86°F); protect from light; discard opened bottle after 90 days.

Rectal gel: Store at 25°C (77°F); excursion permitted to 15°C to 30°C (59°F to 86°F).

Tablet: Store at 15°C to 30°C (59°F to 86°F).

Mechanism of Action Binds to stereospecific benzodiazepine receptors on the postsynaptic GABA neuron at several sites within the central nervous system, including the limbic system, reticular formation. Enhancement of the inhibitory effect of GABA on neuronal excitability results by increased neuronal membrane permeability to chloride ions. This shift in chloride ions results in hyperpolarization (a less excitable state) and stabilization. Benzodiazepine receptors and effects appear to be linked to the GABA-A receptors. Benzodiazepines do not bind to GABA-B receptors.

Pharmacodynamics/Kinetics

Onset of action: IV: Almost immediate; Oral: Rapid

Duration: IV: 20-30 minutes; Oral: Variable (dose and frequency dependent)

Absorption: Oral: 85% to 100%, more reliable than IM

Distribution: V_d: Young healthy males: 0.8-1.0 L/kg

Protein binding: 98%

Metabolism: Hepatic

Half-life elimination: Parent drug: Adults: 20-50 hours; increased half-life in neonates, elderly, and those with severe hepatic disorders; Active major metabolite (desmethyldiazepam): 50-100 hours; may be prolonged in neonates

Time to peak: Oral: 15 minutes to 2 hours

Dosage Oral absorption is more reliable than IM

Children:

Conscious sedation for procedures: Oral: 0.2-0.3 mg/kg (maximum: 10 mg) 45-60 minutes prior to procedure

Muscle spasm associated with tetanus: IV, IM:

Infants >30 days and Children <5 years: 1-2 mg/dose every 3-4 hours as needed

Children ≥5 years: 5-10 mg/dose every 3-4 hours as needed

Sedation/muscle relaxant/anxiety:

Oral: 0.12-0.8 mg/kg/day in divided doses every 6-8 hours

IM, IV: 0.04-0.3 mg/kg/dose every 2-4 hours to a maximum of 0.6 mg/kg within an 8-hour period if needed

Spasticity in cerebral palsy (off-label use): Oral: Dose should be individualized:

Children ≤5 years: <8.5 kg: 0.5-1 mg at bedtime; 8.5-15 kg: 1-2 mg at bedtime (Mathew, 2005)

Children 5-16 years: 1.25 mg 3 times daily to 5 mg 4 times daily (Engle, 1966)

Status epilepticus:

IV: Infants >30 days and Children: 0.1-0.3 mg/kg (maximum dose: 10 mg) given over ≤5 mg/minute; may repeat dose after 5-10 minutes (Hegenbarth, 2008)

Manufacturer's recommendations:

Infants >30 days and Children <5 years: 0.2-0.5 mg given slowly every 2-5 minutes (maximum total dose: 5 mg); repeat in 2-4 hours if needed

Children ≥5 years: 1 mg given slowly every 2-5 minutes (maximum total dose: 10 mg); repeat in 2-4 hours if needed

Rectal gel: 0.5 mg/kg, then 0.25 mg/kg in 10 minutes if needed (maximum dose: 20 mg) (Hegenbarth, 2008).

Anticonvulsant (acute treatment): Rectal gel:

Children <2 years: Safety and efficacy have not been studied

Children 2-5 years: 0.5 mg/kg (maximum dose: 20 mg)

Children 6-11 years: 0.3 mg/kg (maximum dose: 20 mg)

Children ≥12 years: 0.2 mg/kg (maximum dose: 20 mg)

Note: Dosage should be rounded upward to the next available dose, 2.5, 5, 7.5, 10, 12.5, 15, 17.5, and 20 mg/dose; dose may be repeated in 4-12 hours if needed; do not use for more than 5 episodes per month or more than one episode every 5 days

Adolescents: Conscious sedation for procedures:

Oral: 10 mg

IV: 5 mg, may repeat with 1/2 dose if needed

Adults:

Acute ethanol withdrawal: Oral: 10 mg 3-4 times during first 24 hours, then decrease to 5 mg 3-4 times/day as needed

Anticonvulsant (acute treatment): Rectal gel: 0.2 mg/kg

Note: Dosage should be rounded upward to the next available dose, 2.5, 5, 7.5, 10, 12.5, 15, 17.5, and 20 mg/dose; dose may be repeated in 4-12 hours if needed; do not use for more than 5 episodes per month or more than one episode every 5 days.

Anxiety (symptoms/disorders): Oral, IM, IV: 2-10 mg 2-4 times/day if needed

Muscle spasm: IV, IM: Initial: 5-10 mg; then 5-10 mg in 3-4 hours, if necessary. Larger doses may be required if associated with tetanus.

Sedation in the ICU patient: IV: Loading dose: 5-10 mg; Maintenance dose: 0.03-0.1 mg/kg every 30 minutes to 6 hours (Barr, 2013)

Skeletal muscle relaxant (adjunct therapy): Oral: 2-10 mg 3-4 times/day

Status epilepticus:
IV: 5-10 mg every 5-10 minutes given over ≤5 mg/minute; maximum dose: 30 mg
Rectal gel: Premonitory/Out-of-hospital treatment: 10 mg once; may repeat once if necessary (Kälviäinen, 2007)
Rapid tranquilization of agitated patient (administer every 30-60 minutes): Oral: 5-10 mg; average total dose for tranquilization: 20-60 mg
Elderly/debilitated patients:
Oral: 2-2.5 mg 1-2 times/day initially; increase gradually as needed and tolerated
Rectal gel: Due to the increased half-life in elderly and debilitated patients, consider reducing dose.

Dosing adjustment in renal impairment: No dose adjustment recommended; decrease dose if administered for prolonged periods.
IV: Risk of propylene glycol toxicity; monitor closely if using for prolonged periods or at high doses
Hemodialysis: Not dialyzable (0% to 5%); supplemental dose is not necessary
Dosing adjustment in hepatic impairment: Decrease maintenance dose by 50%; half-life significantly prolonged.

Administration Oral solution (Intensol™) should be diluted before use.
IV: Continuous infusion is not recommended because of precipitation in IV fluids and absorption of drug into infusion bags and tubing. In children, do not exceed 1-2 mg/minute IVP; adults 5 mg/minute.
Vesicant; ensure proper needle or catheter placement prior to and during infusion; avoid extravasation.
Extravasation management: If extravasation occurs, stop IV administration immediately and disconnect (leave cannula/needle in place); gently aspirate extravasated solution (do **NOT** flush the line); remove needle/cannula; elevate extremity. Apply dry cold compresses (Hurst, 2004).
Rectal gel: Prior to administration, confirm that prescribed dose is visible and correct, and that the green "ready" band is visible. Patient should be positioned on side (facing person responsible for monitoring), with top leg bent forward. Insert rectal tip (lubricated) into rectum and push in plunger gently over 3 seconds. Remove tip of rectal syringe after 3 additional seconds. Buttocks should be held together for 3 seconds after removal. Dispose of syringe appropriately.

Monitoring Parameters Respiratory, cardiovascular, and mental status; check for orthostasis

Critically-ill mechanically-ventilated patients: Monitor depth of sedation with either the Richmond Agitation-Sedation Scale (RASS) or Sedation-Agitation Scale (SAS) (Barr, 2013)

Reference Range Therapeutic: Diazepam: 0.2-1.5 mcg/mL (SI: 0.7-5.3 micromole/L); N-desmethyldiazepam (nordiazepam): 0.1-0.5 mcg/mL (SI: 0.35-1.8 micromole/L)

Additional Information Diazepam does not have any analgesic effects.
Diastat® AcuDial™: When dispensing, consult package information for directions on setting patient's dose; confirm green "ready" band is visible prior to dispensing product.

Dosage Forms
Concentrate, Oral:
Diazepam Intensol: 5 mg/mL (30 mL)
Generic: 5 mg/mL (30 mL)
Device, Intramuscular:
Generic: 10 mg/2 mL (2 mL)
Gel, Rectal:
Diastat AcuDial: 10 mg (1 ea); 20 mg (1 ea)
Diastat Pediatric: 2.5 mg (1 ea)
Generic: 2.5 mg (1 ea); 10 mg (1 ea); 20 mg (1 ea)
Solution, Injection:
Generic: 5 mg/mL (2 mL, 10 mL)
Solution, Oral:
Generic: 1 mg/mL (5 mL, 500 mL)
Tablet, Oral:
Valium: 2 mg, 5 mg, 10 mg
Generic: 2 mg, 5 mg, 10 mg

◆ **Diazepam Auto Injector (Can)** *see* Diazepam *on page 613*
◆ **Diazepam Injection USP (Can)** *see* Diazepam *on page 613*
◆ **Diazepam Intensol** *see* Diazepam *on page 613*

Diazoxide (dye az OKS ide)

Brand Names: U.S. Proglycem
Brand Names: Canada Proglycem®
Pharmacologic Category Antidote, Hypoglycemia; Vasodilator, Direct-Acting
Use Hypoglycemia related to islet cell adenoma, carcinoma, hyperplasia, or adenomatosis; nesidioblastosis; leucine sensitivity; extrapancreatic malignancy
Pregnancy Risk Factor C
Dosage Hyperinsulinemic hypoglycemia: Oral:
Neonates and Infants: Initial dose: 10 mg/kg/day in divided doses every 8 hours; dosing range: 8-15 mg/kg/day in divided doses every 8-12 hours. Discontinue if no effect after 2-3 weeks.
Children, Adolescents, and Adults: Initial dose: 3 mg/kg/day in divided doses every 8 hours; dosing range: 3-8 mg/kg/day in divided doses every 8-12 hours. **Note:** In certain instances, patients with refractory hypoglycemia may require higher doses. Discontinue if no effect after 2-3 weeks.

Dosage adjustment in renal impairment: Half-life may be prolonged with renal impairment; a reduced dose should be considered.
Dosage adjustment in hepatic impairment: No dosage adjustment provided in manufacturer's labeling.

Additional Information Complete prescribing information should be consulted for additional detail.
Dosage Forms
Suspension, Oral:
Proglycem: 50 mg/mL (30 mL)
Dosage Forms: Canada
Capsule, oral:
Proglycem: 100 mg

Dibekacin [INT] (dye BEK a sin)

International Brand Names Debekacyl (JP, LU); Decabicin (ES); Dikacine (BE, LU); DKB-GT (JP); Ibekacin (AR); Icacine (FR); Klobamicina (ES); Nipocin (HR); Panimycin (JP)
Index Terms Dibekacine Sulfate
Pharmacologic Category Antibiotic, Aminoglycoside
Reported Use Treatment of septicemia, plurifocal infections, urinary tract infections, gyno-obstetrical infections, and bronchopulmonary infections caused by susceptible *Staphylococcus* and gram-negative organisms
Dosage Range Adults: IV: 1-3 mg/kg daily in divided doses
Product Availability Product available in various countries; not currently available in the U.S.
Dosage Forms
Injection, solution: 75 mg/1.5 mL

◆ **Dibekacine Sulfate** *see* Dibekacin [INT] *on page 616*
◆ **Dibenzyline** *see* Phenoxybenzamine *on page 1635*

- ◆ **DIC** *see* Dacarbazine *on page 549*
- ◆ **Dicel® Chewable [OTC]** *see* Chlorpheniramine and Pseudoephedrine *on page 427*
- ◆ **Dicel® DM Chewables [OTC]** *see* Chlorpheniramine, Pseudoephedrine, and Dextromethorphan *on page 428*
- ◆ **Dicetel (Can)** *see* Pinaverium [CAN/INT] *on page 1651*
- ◆ **Diclectin® (Can)** *see* Doxylamine and Pyridoxine *on page 693*
- ◆ **Diclegis®** *see* Doxylamine and Pyridoxine *on page 693*

Diclofenac (Systemic) (dye KLOE fen ak)

Brand Names: U.S. Cambia; Cataflam [DSC]; Voltaren-XR; Zipsor; Zorvolex

Brand Names: Canada Apo-Diclo; Apo-Diclo Rapide; Apo-Diclo SR; Cambia; Diclofenac EC; Diclofenac ECT; Diclofenac K; Diclofenac SR; Diclofenac-SR; Dom-Diclofenac; Dom-Diclofenac SR; PMS-Diclofenac; PMS-Diclofenac K; PMS-Diclofenac-SR; PRO-Diclo-Rapide; Sandoz-Diclofenac; Sandoz-Diclofenac Rapide; Sandoz-Diclofenac SR; Teva-Diclofenac; Teva-Diclofenac EC; Teva-Diclofenac K; Teva-Diclofenac SR; Voltaren; Voltaren Rapide; Voltaren SR

Index Terms Diclofenac Potassium; Diclofenac Sodium; Dyloject; Voltaren; Zorvolex

Pharmacologic Category Nonsteroidal Anti-inflammatory Drug (NSAID); Nonsteroidal Anti-inflammatory Drug (NSAID), Oral

Additional Appendix Information

Beers Criteria – Potentially Inappropriate Medications for Geriatrics *on page 2271*

Use

Analgesia

Capsules/immediate-release tablets only: Relief of mild to moderate acute pain

Injection only: Management of mild to moderate acute pain and moderate to severe acute pain (alone or in combination with opioid analgesics) in adults

Ankylosing spondylitis (delayed-release tablets only): Acute or long-term use in the relief of signs and symptoms of ankylosing spondylitis

Dysmenorrhea (immediate-release tablets only): Treatment of primary dysmenorrhea

Migraine (powder for oral solution only): Acute treatment of migraine attacks with or without aura in adults

Osteoarthritis (immediate-release, extended-release, and delayed-release tablets; capsules [Zorvolex]; and suppositories [Canadian product] only): Relief of signs and symptoms of osteoarthritis.

Rheumatoid arthritis (immediate-release, extended-release, and delayed-release tablets; and suppositories [Canadian product] only): Relief of signs and symptoms of rheumatoid arthritis.

Pregnancy Risk Factor C (oral, injection)/D (≥30 weeks gestation [oral, injection])

Pregnancy Considerations Adverse events were not observed in the initial animal reproduction studies; therefore, manufacturers classify most dosage forms of diclofenac as pregnancy category C (oral, injection: Category D ≥30 weeks gestation). Diclofenac crosses the placenta and can be detected in fetal tissue and amniotic fluid. NSAID exposure during the first trimester is not strongly associated with congenital malformations; however, cardiovascular anomalies and cleft palate have been observed following NSAID exposure in some studies. The use of a NSAID close to conception may be associated with an increased risk of miscarriage. Nonteratogenic effects have been observed following NSAID administration during the third trimester including: Myocardial degenerative changes, prenatal constriction of the ductus arteriosus, fetal tricuspid regurgitation, failure of the ductus arteriosus to close postnatally; renal dysfunction or failure, oligohydramnios; gastrointestinal bleeding or perforation, increased risk of necrotizing enterocolitis; intracranial bleeding (including intraventricular hemorrhage), platelet dysfunction with resultant bleeding; pulmonary hypertension. Because they may cause premature closure of the ductus arteriosus, use of NSAIDs in pregnancy (particularly late pregnancy) should be avoided. Product labeling for Cambia, Zipsor, and Zorvolex specifically notes that use at ≥30 weeks' gestation should be avoided. Use in the third trimester is contraindicated in the Canadian labeling. The chronic use of NSAIDs in women of reproductive age may be associated with infertility that is reversible upon discontinuation of the medication. A registry is available for pregnant women exposed to autoimmune medications including diclofenac. For additional information contact the Organization of Teratology Information Specialists, OTIS Autoimmune Diseases Study, at 877-311-8972

Breast-Feeding Considerations Low concentrations of diclofenac can be found in breast milk. Breast-feeding is not recommended by most manufacturers. The manufacturers of the injection recommend that caution be exercised when administering treprostinil to breast-feeding women. Use while breast-feeding is contraindicated in Canadian labeling.

Contraindications

Hypersensitivity to diclofenac (eg, anaphylactoid reactions, serious skin reactions) or bovine protein (Zipsor only) or any component of the formulation; patients who have experienced asthma, urticaria, or other allergic-type reactions after taking aspirin or other NSAIDs; treatment of perioperative pain in the setting of CABG surgery; patients with moderate to severe renal impairment in the perioperative period and who are at risk for volume depletion (injection only)

Canadian labeling: Additional contraindications (not in U.S. labeling): Severe uncontrolled heart failure, active gastric/duodenal/peptic ulcer; active GI bleed or perforation; regional ulcer, gastritis, or ulcerative colitis; cerebrovascular bleeding or other bleeding disorders; inflammatory bowel disease; severe hepatic impairment; active hepatic disease; severe renal impairment (CrCl <30 mL/minute) or deteriorating renal disease; known hyperkalemia; patients <16 years of age; breast-feeding; pregnancy (third trimester); use of diclofenac suppository if recent history of bleeding or inflammatory lesions of rectum/anus

Warnings/Precautions [U.S. Boxed Warning]: NSAIDs are associated with an increased risk of adverse cardiovascular thrombotic events, including MI and stroke. Risk may increase with dose and duration of use or preexisting cardiovascular risk factors or disease. Carefully evaluate individual cardiovascular risk profiles (eg, hypertension, ischemic heart disease, diabetes, smoking) and consider alternative agents if appropriate) prior to prescribing. May cause new-onset hypertension or worsening of existing hypertension. Monitor blood pressure closely. Use caution with fluid retention. Avoid use in heart failure (ACCF/AHA [Yancy, 2013]). Concurrent administration of ibuprofen, and potentially other nonselective NSAIDs, may interfere with aspirin's cardioprotective effect. **[U.S. Boxed Warning]: Use is contraindicated for treatment of perioperative pain in the setting of coronary artery bypass graft (CABG) surgery.** Risk of MI and stroke may be increased with use following CABG surgery.

NSAID use may compromise existing renal function; dose-dependent decreases in prostaglandin synthesis may result from NSAID use, reducing renal blood flow which may cause renal decompensation. NSAID use may increase the risk for hyperkalemia (Canadian labeling contraindicates use with known hyperkalemia). Patients ▶

with impaired renal function, dehydration, heart failure, liver dysfunction, those taking diuretics and ACEI, and the elderly are at greater risk of renal toxicity and hyperkalemia. Rehydrate patient before starting therapy; monitor renal function closely. Not recommended for use in patients with advanced renal disease. Injection is not recommended in patients with moderate to severe renal impairment and is contraindicated in patients with moderate to severe renal impairment in the perioperative period and who are at risk for volume depletion. Long-term NSAID use may result in renal papillary necrosis while persistent urinary symptoms (eg, dysuria, bladder pain), cystitis, or hematuria may occur any time after initiating NSAID therapy. Discontinue therapy with symptom onset and evaluate for origin.

[U.S. Boxed Warning]: NSAIDs may increase risk of gastrointestinal irritation, inflammation, ulceration, bleeding, and perforation. These events may occur at any time during therapy and without warning. Use caution with a history of GI disease (bleeding or ulcers), concurrent therapy with aspirin, anticoagulants and/or corticosteroids, smoking, use of alcohol, the elderly or debilitated patients. When used concomitantly with aspirin, a substantial increase in the risk of gastrointestinal complications (eg, ulcer) occurs; concomitant gastroprotective therapy (eg, proton pump inhibitors) is recommended (Bhatt, 2008).

Use the lowest effective dose for the shortest duration of time, consistent with individual patient goals, to reduce risk of cardiovascular or GI adverse events. Alternate therapies should be considered for patients at high risk. Canadian labeling contraindicates use in patients with active gastric/duodenal/peptic ulcer; active GI bleed or perforation; or regional ulcer, gastritis, or ulcerative colitis.

NSAIDs may cause photosensitivity or serious skin adverse events including exfoliative dermatitis, Stevens-Johnson syndrome (SJS), and toxic epidermal necrolysis (TEN); discontinue use at first sign of skin rash or hypersensitivity. Anaphylactoid reactions may occur, even without prior exposure; patients with "aspirin triad" (bronchial asthma, aspirin intolerance, rhinitis) may be at increased risk. Do not use in patients who experience bronchospasm, asthma, rhinitis, or urticaria with NSAID or aspirin therapy. Use caution in other forms of asthma. Platelet adhesion and aggregation may be decreased; may prolong bleeding time; patients with coagulation disorders or who are receiving anticoagulants should be monitored closely. Anemia may occur; patients on long-term NSAID therapy should be monitored for anemia. Rarely, NSAID use may cause severe blood dyscrasias (eg, agranulocytosis, aplastic anemia, thrombocytopenia).

Use with caution in patients with impaired hepatic function (Canadian labeling contraindicates use in severe hepatic impairment or active hepatic disease). Closely monitor patients with any abnormal LFT. Transaminase elevations have been observed with use, generally within the first 2 months of therapy, but may occur at any time. Risk may be higher with diclofenac than other NSAIDS (Laine, 2009; Rostom, 2005). Significant elevations in transaminases (eg, >3 x ULN) occur before patients become symptomatic; initiate monitoring 4 to 8 weeks into therapy. Rarely, severe hepatic reactions (eg, fulminant hepatitis, liver failure) have occurred; discontinue all formulations if signs or symptoms of liver disease develop, or if systemic manifestations occur. Use with caution in hepatic porphyria (may trigger attack; Jose, 2008).

NSAIDS may cause drowsiness, dizziness, blurred vision, and other neurologic effects which may impair physical or mental abilities; patients must be cautioned about performing tasks which require mental alertness (eg, operating machinery or driving). Discontinue use with blurred or diminished vision and perform ophthalmologic exam. Monitor vision with long-term therapy. May increase the risk of aseptic meningitis, especially in patients with systemic lupus erythematosus (SLE) and mixed connective tissue disorders. In the elderly, avoid chronic use (unless alternative agents ineffective and patient can receive concomitant gastroprotective agent); nonselective oral NSAID use is associated with an increased risk of GI bleeding and peptic ulcer disease in older adults in high risk category (eg, >75 years or age or receiving concomitant oral/parenteral corticosteroids, anticoagulants, or antiplatelet agents) (Beers Criteria).

Withhold for at least 4 to 6 half-lives prior to surgical or dental procedures.

Different formulations of oral diclofenac are not bioequivalent, even if the milligram strength is the same; do not interchange products. Zipsor (capsule) contains gelatin; use is contraindicated in patients with history of hypersensitivity to bovine protein. Oral solution is only indicated for the acute treatment of migraine; not indicated for migraine prophylaxis or cluster headache; contains phenylalanine. Injection is not indicated for long-term use.

Adverse Reactions

Injection:

Cardiovascular: Cerebrovascular accident, edema, hypertension, myocardial infarction, significant cardiovascular event

Central Nervous System: Dizziness, headache

Dermatologic: Exfoliative dermatitis, pruritus, skin rash, Stevens-Johnson syndrome, toxic epidermal necrolysis

Endocrine & Metabolic: Fluid retention

Gastrointestinal: Abdominal pain, constipation, diarrhea, dyspepsia, esophageal perforation, flatulence, gastrointestinal ulcer (including gastric/duodenal), heartburn, intestinal perforation, nausea, vomiting

Hematologic & Oncologic: Anemia, hemorrhage, prolonged bleeding time

Hepatic: Increased liver enzymes, increased serum ALT, increased serum AST, increased serum transaminases

Hypersensitivity: Anaphylactoid reaction

Local: Extravasation, infusion site reaction

Otic: Tinnitus

Renal: Renal insufficiency

Miscellaneous: Gastrointestinal inflammation, wound healing impairment

Rare but important or life-threatening: Abnormal Dreams, agranulocytosis, alopecia, anaphylaxis, angioedema, anxiety, aplastic anemia, asthma, auditory impairment, blurred vision, cardiac arrhythmia, change in appetite, colitis, coma, confusion, congestive heart failure, conjunctivitis, convulsions, cystitis, depression, diaphoresis, drowsiness, dyspnea, dysuria, ecchymoses, eosinophilia, eructation, erythema multiforme, esophagitis, exfoliative dermatitis, fever, fulminant hepatitis, gastritis, gastrointestinal hemorrhage, glossitis, hallucination, hematemesis, hematuria, hemolytic anemia, hepatic failure, hepatic necrosis, hepatitis, hepatotoxicity, hyperglycemia, hypertension, hypotension, infection, insomnia, interstitial nephritis, jaundice, leukopenia, lymphadenopathy, malaise, melena, meningitis, nervousness, oliguria, palpitations, pancreatitis, pancytopenia, paresthesia, pneumonia, polyuria, proteinuria, purpura, rectal hemorrhage, renal failure, respiratory depression, sepsis, skin photosensitivity, stomatitis, syncope, tachycardia, thrombocytopenia, toxic epidermal necrolysis, tremor, urticaria, vasculitis, vertigo, weakness, weight changes

Oral:

Cardiovascular: Edema, hypertension

Central nervous system: Dizziness, falling, headache, procedural pain

Dermatologic: Pruritus, skin rash

Gastrointestinal: Abdominal discomfort, abdominal pain, constipation, diarrhea, duodenal ulcer, dyspepsia, flatulence, GI adverse effects (gastric ulcer, hemorrhage, and perforation; risk increases with therapy duration), heartburn, nausea, vomiting

Genitourinary: Urinary tract infection

Hematologic & oncologic: Anemia, bruise, prolonged bleeding time,

Hepatic: Increased serum ALT, increased serum AST, increased serum transaminases

Neuromuscular & skeletal: Arthralgia, back pain, limb pain, osteoarthritis

Otic: Tinnitus

Renal: Renal function abnormality

Respiratory: Bronchitis, cough, nasopharyngitis, sinusitis, upper respiratory tract infection

Rare but important or life-threatening: Agranulocytosis, alopecia, anaphylactoid reaction, aplastic anemia, aseptic meningitis, asthma, cardiac arrhythmia, cardiac failure, cerebrovascular accident, colitis, coma, conjunctivitis, cystitis, decreased hemoglobin, depression, diplopia, eosinophilia, erythema multiforme, esophageal ulcer, esophagitis, gastritis, hearing loss, hemolytic anemia, hepatic failure, hepatitis, hyperglycemia, hypotension, interstitial nephritis, intestinal perforation, lymphadenopathy, memory impairment, meningitis, myocardial infarction, pancreatitis, pancytopenia, peptic ulcer, pneumonia, psychotic reaction, purpura, rectal hemorrhage, renal failure, respiratory depression, seizure, sepsis, skin photosensitivity, Stevens-Johnson syndrome, tachycardia, toxic epidermal necrolysis, vasculitis

Rectal suppository [Canadian product]:

Also refer to adverse reactions associated with oral formulations.

Rare but important or life-threatening: Local hemorrhage, hemorrhoids (exacerbation), proctitis

Drug Interactions

Metabolism/Transport Effects Substrate of CYP1A2 (minor), CYP2B6 (minor), CYP2C19 (minor), CYP2C8 (minor), CYP2C9 (minor), CYP2D6 (minor), CYP3A4 (minor); **Note:** Assignment of Major/Minor substrate status based on clinically relevant drug interaction potential; **Inhibits** CYP1A2 (weak), CYP2C9 (weak), CYP2E1 (weak), CYP3A4 (weak), UGT1A6

Avoid Concomitant Use

Avoid concomitant use of Diclofenac (Systemic) with any of the following: Dexketoprofen; Floctafenine; Ketorolac (Nasal); Ketorolac (Systemic); NSAID (COX-2 Inhibitor); Omacetaxine; Pimozide; Urokinase

Increased Effect/Toxicity

Diclofenac (Systemic) may increase the levels/effects of: 5-ASA Derivatives; Agents with Antiplatelet Properties; Aliskiren; Aminoglycosides; Anticoagulants; Apixaban; ARIPiprazole; Bisphosphonate Derivatives; Collagenase (Systemic); CycloSPORINE (Systemic); Dabigatran Etexilate; Deferasirox; Deferiprone; Desmopressin; Digoxin; Dofetilide; Eplerenone; Haloperidol; Hydrocodone; Ibritumomab; Lithium; Lomitapide; Methotrexate; Nonsteroidal Anti-Inflammatory Agents; NSAID (COX-2 Inhibitor); Obinutuzumab; Omacetaxine; PEMEtrexed; Pimozide; Porfimer; Potassium-Sparing Diuretics; PRALAtrexate; Quinolone Antibiotics; Rivaroxaban; Salicylates; Tacrolimus (Systemic); Tenofovir; Thrombolytic Agents; Tositumomab and Iodine I 131 Tositumomab; Urokinase; Vancomycin; Verteporfin; Vitamin K Antagonists

The levels/effects of Diclofenac (Systemic) may be increased by: ACE Inhibitors; Angiotensin II Receptor Blockers; Antidepressants (Tricyclic, Tertiary Amine); Corticosteroids (Systemic); CycloSPORINE (Systemic); CYP2C9 Inhibitors (Strong); Dasatinib; Dexketoprofen; Floctafenine; Glucosamine; Herbs (Anticoagulant/Antiplatelet Properties); Ibrutinib; Ketorolac (Nasal); Ketorolac (Systemic); Limaprost; Multivitamins/Fluoride (with ADE); Multivitamins/Minerals (with ADEK, Folate, Iron); Multivitamins/Minerals (with AE, No Iron); Omega-3 Fatty Acids; Pentosan Polysulfate Sodium; Pentoxifylline; Probenecid; Prostacyclin Analogues; Selective Serotonin Reuptake Inhibitors; Serotonin/Norepinephrine Reuptake Inhibitors; Sodium Phosphates; Tipranavir; Treprostinil; Vitamin E; Voriconazole

Decreased Effect

Diclofenac (Systemic) may decrease the levels/effects of: ACE Inhibitors; Aliskiren; Angiotensin II Receptor Blockers; Beta-Blockers; Eplerenone; HydrALAZINE; Loop Diuretics; Potassium-Sparing Diuretics; Prostaglandins (Ophthalmic); Salicylates; Selective Serotonin Reuptake Inhibitors; Thiazide Diuretics

The levels/effects of Diclofenac (Systemic) may be decreased by: Bile Acid Sequestrants; CYP2C9 Inducers (Strong); Salicylates

Preparation for Administration Oral solution: Empty contents of packet into 1-2 ounces (30-60 mL) of water (do not use other liquids); mix well and administer immediately.

Storage/Stability

Capsule, powder for oral solution: Store at 25°C (77°F); excursions permitted to 15°C to 30°C (59°F to 86°F). Protect from moisture.

Injection: Store at 20°C to 25°C (68°F to 77°F). Do not freeze. Protect from light.

Suppository [Canadian product]: Store at 15°C to 30°C (59°F to 86°F); protect from heat.

Tablet: Store immediate-release and ER tablets below 30°C (86°F); store delayed-release tablets at 20°C to 25°C (68°F to 77°F). Protect from moisture.

Mechanism of Action Reversibly inhibits cyclooxygenase-1 and 2 (COX-1 and 2) enzymes, which results in decreased formation of prostaglandin precursors; has antipyretic, analgesic, and anti-inflammatory properties

Other proposed mechanisms not fully elucidated (and possibly contributing to the anti-inflammatory effect to varying degrees), include inhibiting chemotaxis, altering lymphocyte activity, inhibiting neutrophil aggregation/activation, and decreasing proinflammatory cytokine levels.

Pharmacodynamics/Kinetics

Onset of action:

Cataflam (potassium salt) is more rapid than the sodium salt because it dissolves in the stomach instead of the duodenum

Suppository [Canadian product]: More rapid onset, but slower rate of absorption when compared to enteric coated tablet

Distribution: ~1.4 L/kg

Protein binding: >99%, primarily to albumin

Metabolism: Hepatic; undergoes first-pass metabolism; forms several metabolites (1 with weak activity)

Bioavailability: 55%

Half-life elimination: Oral: ~2 hours; Injection: ~1 to 2 hours

Time to peak, serum: **Note:** Fasted values reported for oral products; may be delayed with food

Cambia: ~0.25 hours

Cataflam, Zorvolex: ~1 hour

Voltaren XR ~5 hours

Zipsor: ~0.5 hour

Injection: ~5 minutes

Suppository [Canadian product]: ≤1 hour; **Note:** Suppository: C_{max}: Approximately two-thirds of that observed with enteric coated tablet (equivalent 50 mg dose)

Tablet, delayed release (diclofenac sodium): ~2 hours

Excretion: Urine (~65%); feces (~35%)

Dosage

Children ≥3 years and Adolescents: Juvenile idiopathic arthritis (off-label use): Oral: Delayed-release tablet (diclofenac sodium): 2 to 3 mg/kg/day in divided doses (Haapasaari, 1983; Hashkes, 2005)

Adults:

Oral:

Analgesia:

Immediate-release tablet: 50 mg 3 times daily; may administer 100 mg loading dose, followed by 50 mg every 8 hours

Canadian labeling: 50 mg every 6 to 8 hours for up to 7 days (maximum: 100 mg daily)

Immediate-release capsule:

Zipsor (diclofenac potassium): 25 mg 4 times daily

Zorvolex (diclofenac acid): 18 mg or 35 mg 3 times daily

Primary dysmenorrhea: Immediate-release tablet: 50 mg 3 times daily; may administer 100 mg loading dose, followed by 50 mg every 8 hours

Canadian labeling: Immediate release tablet: Day 1: Initial: 100 mg then 50 mg every 6 to 8 hours (maximum: 200 mg daily); Day 2 and beyond (up to 7 days): 50 mg every 6 to 8 hours (maximum: 100 mg daily)

Rheumatoid arthritis: Immediate-release tablet: 150 to 200 mg daily in 3 to 4 divided doses; Delayed-release tablet: 150 to 200 mg daily in 2 to 4 divided doses; Extended-release tablet: 100 mg daily (may increase dose to 200 mg daily in 2 divided doses)

Canadian labeling: Enteric-coated tablet: 50 mg every 8 hours (maximum: 100 mg daily); Slow-release tablet: 75 to 100 mg daily (maximum: 100 mg daily)

Osteoarthritis:

Immediate- or delayed-release tablet: 100 to 150 mg daily in 2 to 3 divided doses; Extended-release tablet: 100 mg daily

Canadian labeling: Enteric-coated tablet: 50 mg every 8 hours (maximum: 100 mg daily); Slow-release tablets: 75 to 100 mg daily (maximum: 100 mg daily)

Immediate-release capsule: Zorvolex (diclofenac acid): 35 mg 3 times daily.

Ankylosing spondylitis: Delayed-release tablet: 100 to 125 mg daily in 4 to 5 divided doses

Migraine: Oral solution: 50 mg (one packet) as a single dose at the time of migraine onset; safety and efficacy of a second dose have not been established

IV: Analgesia: 37.5 mg every 6 hours as needed (maximum: 150 mg daily).

Rectal suppository [Canadian product]:

Osteoarthritis: Insert 50 mg or 100 mg suppository rectally as single dose to substitute for final oral daily dose; maximum combined dose (rectal and oral): 100 mg daily

Rheumatoid arthritis: Insert 50 mg or 100 mg suppository rectally as single dose to substitute for final oral daily dose (maximum combined dose [rectal and oral]: 100 mg daily)

Dosage adjustment in renal impairment:

U.S. labeling: There are no dosage adjustments provided in the manufacturer's labeling; not recommended in patients with advanced renal disease or significant renal impairment; use of injection is contraindicated in patients with moderate to severe renal impairment in the perioperative period and who are at risk for volume depletion.

Canadian labeling: There are no dosage adjustments provided in the manufacturer's labeling; however, the manufacturer recommends that reduced dosages should be considered. Use in severe renal impairment (CrCl <30 mL/minute) or deteriorating renal disease is contraindicated.

Dosage adjustment in hepatic impairment:

Hepatic impairment at treatment initiation:

U.S. labeling: May require dosage adjustment due to extensive hepatic metabolism. Additional product-specific recommendations:

Cambia: Use in patients with hepatic impairment only if benefits outweigh risks

Zorvolex: Initial: Initiate treatment at the lowest dose; if efficacy is not achieved with the lowest dose, discontinue use.

Injection:

Mild impairment: No dosage adjustment necessary.

Moderate to severe impairment: Use is not recommended (has not been studied).

Canadian labeling: There are no dosage adjustments provided in the manufacturer's labeling; however, the manufacturer recommends that reduced dosages should be considered. Use is contraindicated in severe liver impairment or active liver disease.

Hepatic impairment during treatment: Persistent or worsening abnormal liver function tests, clinical signs/symptoms consistent with liver disease, or systemic manifestations of liver disease (eg, eosinophilia, rash, abdominal pain, diarrhea, dark urine): Discontinue immediately.

Elderly: Use lowest recommended dose and frequency in elderly to initiate therapy for indications listed in adult dosing

Dietary Considerations Oral formulations may be taken with food to decrease GI distress. Food may reduce effectiveness of oral solution. Some products may contain phenylalanine.

Administration

Injection: Administer as an IV bolus over 15 seconds.

Oral: Do not crush delayed- or extended-release tablets. Administer with food or milk to avoid gastric distress.

Cambia, Zorvolex: Taking with food may cause a reduction in effectiveness.

Rectal suppository [Canadian product]: Remove entire plastic wrapping prior to inserting rectally.

Monitoring Parameters

Monitor CBC, liver enzymes (periodically during chronic therapy starting 4 to 8 weeks after initiation), electrolytes, BUN/serum creatinine; monitor urine output; occult blood loss; blood pressure

Canadian labeling also recommends periodic ophthalmic evaluation during extended therapy or with onset of vision changes.

Product Availability

Dyloject injection: FDA approved December 2014; anticipated availability is currently unknown.

Dyloject is indicated as monotherapy for the management of mild to severe pain or in combination with opioid analgesics for the management of moderate to severe pain.

Dosage Forms

Capsule, Oral:

Zipsor: 25 mg

Zorvolex: 18 mg, 35 mg

Packet, Oral:

Cambia: 50 mg (1 ea, 9 ea)

Tablet, Oral:

Generic: 50 mg

Tablet Delayed Release, Oral:

Generic: 25 mg, 50 mg, 75 mg

Tablet Extended Release 24 Hour, Oral:

Voltaren-XR: 100 mg

Generic: 100 mg

Dosage Forms: Canada Note: Refer also to Dosage Forms; Zipsor and Zorvolex capsules are not currently available in Canada.

Suppository:

Voltaren: 50 mg, 100 mg

Diclofenac (Ophthalmic) (dye KLOE fen ak)

Brand Names: Canada Voltaren Ophtha

Index Terms Diclofenac Sodium

Pharmacologic Category Nonsteroidal Anti-inflammatory Drug (NSAID); Nonsteroidal Anti-inflammatory Drug (NSAID), Ophthalmic

Use Treatment of postoperative inflammation following cataract extraction; temporary relief of pain and photophobia in patients undergoing corneal refractive surgery

Pregnancy Risk Factor C

Dosage Ophthalmic: Adults:

Cataract surgery: Instill 1 drop into affected eye 4 times/day beginning 24 hours after cataract surgery and continuing for 2 weeks

Corneal refractive surgery: Instill 1-2 drops into affected eye within the hour prior to surgery, within 15 minutes following surgery, and then continue for 4 times/day, up to 3 days

Additional Information Complete prescribing information should be consulted for additional detail.

Dosage Forms

Solution, Ophthalmic:

Generic: 0.1% (2.5 mL, 5 mL)

Diclofenac and Misoprostol
(dye KLOE fen ak & mye soe PROST ole)

Brand Names: U.S. Arthrotec

Brand Names: Canada Arthrotec; Co Diclo-Miso

Index Terms Misoprostol and Diclofenac

Pharmacologic Category Nonsteroidal Anti-inflammatory Drug (NSAID), Oral; Prostaglandin

Use

Osteoarthritis: Treatment of osteoarthritis in patients at high risk for NSAID-induced gastric and duodenal ulceration

Rheumatoid arthritis: Treatment of rheumatoid arthritis in patients at high risk for NSAID-induced gastric and duodenal ulceration

Pregnancy Risk Factor X

Dosage Oral:

Adults:

U.S. labeling:

Osteoarthritis: Arthrotec 50: One tablet 3 times daily

Rheumatoid arthritis: Arthrotec 50: One tablet 3 or 4 times daily

Note: For both indications, may administer Arthrotec 50 or Arthrotec 75 one tablet twice daily if recommended dose is not tolerated; however, these options are less effective in preventing GI ulceration. May adjust dose using individual agents in combination with Arthrotec. The maximum daily dose of misoprostol is 800 mcg and the maximum single dose of misoprostol is 200 mcg. The maximum daily dose of diclofenac is 150 mg daily (osteoarthritis) or 225 mg daily (rheumatoid arthritis).

Canadian labeling: Osteoarthritis, Rheumatoid arthritis: Arthrotec 50: One tablet 2 times daily (maximum diclofenac dose: 100 mg daily)

Elderly: No specific dosage adjustment is recommended; may require reduced dosage due to lower body weight; monitor renal function

Dosage adjustment in renal impairment:

U.S. labeling: There are no dosage adjustments provided in the manufacturer's labeling; not recommended in patients with advanced renal disease.

Canadian labeling:

Mild-to-moderate impairment: Consider lowest dose and monitor closely.

Severe impairment (CrCl <30 mL/minute) or deteriorating renal disease: Use is contraindicated.

Dosage adjustment in hepatic impairment:

U.S. labeling: There are no dosage requirements in the manufacturer's labeling; however, the bioavailability of misoprostol may be increased in patients with hepatic impairment.

Canadian labeling:

Mild-to moderate impairment: There are no dosage adjustments provided in the manufacturer's labeling (monitor closely).

Significant impairment or active hepatic disease: Use is contraindicated.

Additional Information Complete prescribing information should be consulted for additional detail.

Dosage Forms

Tablet, oral: Diclofenac 50 mg and misoprostol 200 mcg; Diclofenac 75 mg and misoprostol 200 mcg

Arthrotec 50: Diclofenac 50 mg and misoprostol 200 mcg

Arthrotec 75: Diclofenac 75 mg and misoprostol 200 mcg

◆ **Diclofenac EC (Can)** *see* Diclofenac (Systemic) *on page 617*

◆ **Diclofenac ECT (Can)** *see* Diclofenac (Systemic) *on page 617*

◆ **Diclofenac K (Can)** *see* Diclofenac (Systemic) *on page 617*

◆ **Diclofenac Potassium** *see* Diclofenac (Systemic) *on page 617*

◆ **Diclofenac Sodium** *see* Diclofenac (Ophthalmic) *on page 621*

◆ **Diclofenac Sodium** *see* Diclofenac (Systemic) *on page 617*

◆ **Diclofenac SR (Can)** *see* Diclofenac (Systemic) *on page 617*

Dicloxacillin (dye kloks a SIL in)

Index Terms Dicloxacillin Sodium

Pharmacologic Category Antibiotic, Penicillin

Use Treatment of systemic infections such as pneumonia, skin and soft tissue infections, and osteomyelitis caused by penicillinase-producing staphylococci

Pregnancy Risk Factor B

Dosage

Usual dosage range:

Newborns: Use not recommended

Children <40 kg: Oral: 12.5-100 mg/kg/day divided every 6 hours

Children >40 kg: Oral: 125-250 mg every 6 hours

Adults: Oral: 125-1000 mg every 6 hours

Indication-specific dosing:

Children: Oral:

Furunculosis: 25-50 mg/kg/day divided every 6 hours

Osteomyelitis: 50-100 mg/kg/day in divided doses every 6 hours

Adults: Oral:

Erysipelas, furunculosis, mastitis, otitis externa, septic bursitis, skin abscess: 500 mg every 6 hours

Impetigo: 250 mg every 6 hours

Prosthetic joint infection: Chronic suppression therapy: Staphylococci (oxacillin-susceptible) (off-label regimen): 500 mg every 6-8 hours (Osmon, 2013)

***Staphylococcus aureus*, methicillin susceptible infection if no IV access:** 500-1000 mg every 6-8 hours

Dosage adjustment in renal impairment: No specific adjustment provided in manufacturer's labeling; a reduction in total dosage should be considered in renal impairment.

Hemodialysis: Not dialyzable (0% to 5%); supplemental dosage not necessary

Peritoneal dialysis: Supplemental dosage not necessary

Continuous arteriovenous or venovenous hemofiltration: Supplemental dosage not necessary

Dosage adjustment in hepatic impairment: No dosage adjustment provided in manufacturer's labeling.

Additional Information Complete prescribing information should be consulted for additional detail.

Dosage Forms

Capsule, Oral:

Generic: 250 mg, 500 mg

◆ **Dicloxacillin Sodium** *see* Dicloxacillin *on page 621*

◆ **Dicopanol FusePaq** *see* DiphenhydrAMINE (Systemic) *on page 641*

Dicyclomine (dye SYE kloe meen)

Brand Names: U.S. Bentyl

Brand Names: Canada Bentylol; Dicyclomine Hydrochloride Injection; Formulex; Jamp-Dicyclomine; Protylol; Riva-Dicyclomine

Index Terms Dicyclomine Hydrochloride; Dicycloverine Hydrochloride

Pharmacologic Category Anticholinergic Agent

Additional Appendix Information

Beers Criteria – Potentially Inappropriate Medications for Geriatrics *on page 2271*

Use Treatment of functional bowel/irritable bowel syndrome

Pregnancy Risk Factor B

Dosage

Adults:

Oral: Initial: 20 mg 4 times daily for 7 days; after 1 week, may increase to 40 mg 4 times daily. If efficacy not achieved in 2 weeks or if adverse effects require a dose <80 mg/day, therapy should be discontinued. Safety data are not available for doses >80 mg daily for a duration that exceeds 2 weeks.

IM **(should not be used IV)**: 10-20 mg 4 times daily for 1-2 days; convert to oral therapy as soon as possible

Elderly: Refer to adult dosing. Use caution; lower dosages may be required.

Dosage adjustment in renal impairment: No dosage adjustment provided in the manufacturer's labeling (has not been studied); use with caution.

Dosage adjustment in hepatic impairment: No dosage adjustment provided in the manufacturer's labeling (has not been studied); use with caution.

Additional Information Complete prescribing information should be consulted for additional detail.

Dosage Forms

Capsule, Oral:

Bentyl: 10 mg

Generic: 10 mg

Solution, Intramuscular:

Bentyl: 10 mg/mL (2 mL)

Solution, Oral:

Generic: 10 mg/5 mL (473 mL)

Tablet, Oral:

Bentyl: 20 mg

Generic: 20 mg

◆ **Dicyclomine Hydrochloride** *see* Dicyclomine *on page 622*

◆ **Dicyclomine Hydrochloride Injection (Can)** *see* Dicyclomine *on page 622*

◆ **Dicycloverine Hydrochloride** *see* Dicyclomine *on page 622*

◆ **Di-Dak-Sol [OTC]** *see* Sodium Hypochlorite Solution *on page 1906*

Didanosine (dye DAN oh seen)

Brand Names: U.S. Videx; Videx EC

Brand Names: Canada Videx; Videx EC

Index Terms ddI; Dideoxyinosine

Pharmacologic Category Antiretroviral, Reverse Transcriptase Inhibitor, Nucleoside (Anti-HIV)

Use HIV infection: Treatment of HIV-1 infection in combination with other antiretroviral agents.

Pregnancy Risk Factor B

Dosage Oral: Treatment of HIV infection:

Pediatric powder for oral solution (Videx): **Note:** Once-daily dosing of the oral solution is not FDA approved in children.

Infants: 2 weeks to 8 months: 100 mg/m^2 twice daily is recommended by the manufacturer; 50 mg/m^2 may be considered in infants 2 weeks to <3 months (HHS [pediatric], 2014)

Infants and Children >8 months: 120 mg/m^2 twice daily, not to exceed adult dose, is recommended by the manufacturer.

Children 3 to 21 years (off-label dose): Treatment-naive: 240 mg/m^2/dose once daily (maximum: 400 mg/dose) (HHS [pediatric], 2014)

Adolescents and Adults: Dosing based on patient weight:

<60 kg: 125 mg twice daily (preferred) or 250 mg once daily

≥60 kg: 200 mg twice daily (preferred) or 400 mg once daily

Delayed release capsule (Videx EC):

Children ≥6 years and Adults:

20 kg to <25 kg: 200 mg once daily

25 kg to <60 kg: 250 mg once daily

≥60 kg: 400 mg once daily

Children 3 to 21 years (off-label dose): Treatment-naive: 240 mg/m^2/dose once daily (maximum: 400 mg/dose) (DHHS [pediatric], 2014)

Elderly: Higher frequency of pancreatitis (10% versus 5% in younger patients); monitor renal function and dose accordingly

Dosage adjustment for concomitant therapy:

When taken with tenofovir: Adults:

<60 kg and CrCl ≥60 mL/minute: 200 mg once daily

≥60 kg and CrCl ≥60 mL/minute: 250 mg once daily

Note: Combined use of tenofovir with didanosine is no longer recommended (DHHS [adult], 2014).

Dosage adjustment in renal impairment:

Children: No specific guidelines available; consider dosage reduction using adjustments for adults.

Adults: Dosing based on patient weight, creatinine clearance, and dosage form: See table.

Recommended Dose (mg) of Didanosine by Body Weight – Adults

Creatinine Clearance (mL/min)	≥60 kg		<60 kg	
	Powder for Oral Solution	Delayed Release Capsule	Powder for Oral Solution	Delayed Release Capsule
≥60	400 mg daily or 200 mg twice daily	400 mg daily	250 mg daily or 125 mg twice daily	250 mg daily
30-59	200 mg daily or 100 mg twice daily	200 mg daily	150 mg daily or 75 mg twice daily	125 mg daily
10-29	150 mg daily	125 mg daily	100 mg daily	125 mg daily
<10	100 mg daily	125 mg daily	75 mg daily	See **Note**

Note: Per manufacturer, not suitable for use in patients <60 kg with CrCl <10 mL/minute; use alternate formulation.

Patients requiring hemodialysis or CAPD: Dose per CrCl <10 mL/minute. Didanosine is not removed via CAPD and minimal amount of dose (≤7%) is removed by hemodialysis; no supplemental dosing necessary.

Dosing adjustment in hepatic impairment: No dosage adjustment necessary.

Additional Information Complete prescribing information should be consulted for additional detail.

Dosage Forms

Capsule Delayed Release, Oral:

Videx EC: 125 mg, 200 mg, 250 mg, 400 mg

Generic: 125 mg, 200 mg, 250 mg, 400 mg

Solution Reconstituted, Oral:

Videx: 2 g (100 mL); 4 g (200 mL)

◆ **Dideoxyinosine** *see* Didanosine *on page 622*

◆ **Didrocal® (Can)** *see* Etidronate and Calcium Carbonate [CAN/INT] *on page 814*

Dienogest [CAN/INT] (dye EN oh jest)

Brand Names: Canada Visanne®

Pharmacologic Category Antiandrogen

Use Note: Not approved in U.S.

Management of pelvic pain associated with endometriosis

Pregnancy Considerations In animal studies, teratogenic effects were not observed; however, use of high dose dienogest during late pregnancy impaired fertility of female offspring. Based on limited data, inadvertent exposure in pregnancy has not shown adverse effects to the fetus, however use in known or suspected pregnancy is contraindicated. Rule out pregnancy prior to initiating therapy. Use of hormonal contraceptives is not recommended during dienogest therapy. Nonhormonal contraceptives should be employed during treatment. Ovulation is often inhibited during therapy although normal menstruation usually returns within 2 months of therapy discontinuation.

Breast-Feeding Considerations It is not known whether dienogest is excreted into human breast milk. The risk of thromboembolism may be increased immediately postpartum.

Contraindications Hypersensitivity to dienogest or any component of the formulation; undiagnosed abnormal vaginal bleeding; active venous thromboembolic disorder; history of or current arterial and cardiovascular disease (eg, MI, CVA); diabetes mellitus with vascular involvement; history of or current severe hepatic disease where liver function tests remain abnormal; history of or current hepatic neoplasia (benign or malignant); known or suspected sex-hormone-dependent malignancy; ocular lesions due to ophthalmic vascular disease, such as partial or complete vision loss or defect in visual fields; current or history of migraine with focal aura; breast-feeding; known or suspected pregnancy

Warnings/Precautions Use is associated with irregular menstrual bleeding (eg, amenorrhea, infrequent or frequent bleeding, prolonged bleeding) and may be aggravated in some women (eg, those with fibroids). Bleeding patterns generally show a reduced intensity over time. If bleeding irregularities continue with prolonged use, appropriate diagnostic measures should be taken to rule out endometrial pathology (eg, endometrial sampling, pelvic ultrasound). Consider discontinuation of therapy with prolonged heavy bleeding. Pretreatment menstrual bleeding patterns return within 2 months of therapy discontinuation. The use of combination hormonal contraceptives has been associated with a slight increase in the frequency of breast cancer however studies are not consistent. Data is insufficient to determine if progestin only contraceptives also increase this risk. Routine breast examinations are recommended during therapy. Persistent ovarian cysts which are often asymptomatic may occur during therapy. Use is associated with a moderate decrease in endogenous estrogen levels; in a small study, a reduction in mean bone mineral density was not observed 6 months after initiating therapy though long term data are not available.

Use with caution in women with diabetes. Use with caution in patients with depression; discontinue use with onset of clinically relevant depression or with aggravation of preexisting depression. Use is contraindicated in patients with a history of or current severe hepatic disease. Patients with a prior history of cholestatic jaundice during pregnancy or due to the use of sex steroids should discontinue use of dienogest if cholestatic jaundice reoccurs during therapy. Rare cases of benign and malignant hepatic tumors have been reported with use.

Progestin-only therapy has been associated with a slight but non-significant increase risk of VTE in some studies; discontinue therapy promptly with suspicion or symptoms of a thrombotic event. Discontinue use in patients with prolonged immobilization and at least 4 weeks prior to elective surgery; may resume therapy 2 weeks after complete remobilization. The risk of stroke may be increased in women with hypertension. Discontinue if clinically significant hypertension develops during therapy. The risk of cardiovascular side effects is increased in women who smoke cigarettes. Women should be advised not to smoke.

Progestin use has been associated with retinal vascular lesions; discontinue pending examination in case of sudden vision loss, complete loss of vision, sudden onset of proptosis, diplopia, or migraine. Chloasma may occur occasionally; women with a history of chloasma should avoid sun or ultraviolet radiation exposure during therapy. Patients with a prior history of pruritus during pregnancy or due to use of sex steroids should discontinue dienogest therapy if pruritus reoccurs during therapy. Not indicated for use prior to menarche or in the geriatric population. Not intended for use as a contraceptive.

Adverse Reactions

Central nervous system: Depression, headache, irritability, migraine, nervousness, sleep disturbance

Dermatologic: Acne, alopecia

Endocrine & metabolic: Breast discomfort, libido decreased, ovarian cyst

Gastrointestinal: Abdominal pain, nausea, weight gain

Genitourinary: Vaginal bleeding

Neuromuscular & skeletal: Weakness

Rare but important or life-threatening: Abdominal discomfort, anemia, anxiety, appetite increased, attention disturbance, autonomic nervous system imbalance, back pain, bone pain, breast induration, breast mass, circulatory disorder (nonspecified), constipation, dermatitis, diarrhea, dry eye, dry skin, edema, extremity pain, fibrocystic breast disease, flatulence, genital discharge, GI inflammation, glucose intolerance, heaviness in extremities, hot flashes, mood changes, muscle spasm, onychoclasis, palpitations, pelvic pain, photosensitivity, pigmentation disorder, pruritus, tinnitus, UTI, vaginal candidiasis, vomiting, vulvovaginal dryness

Drug Interactions

Metabolism/Transport Effects Substrate of CYP3A4 (major); **Note:** Assignment of Major/Minor substrate status based on clinically relevant drug interaction potential

Avoid Concomitant Use

Avoid concomitant use of Dienogest with any of the following: CYP3A4 Inducers (Strong); Griseofulvin; St Johns Wort; Tranexamic Acid; Ulipristal

Increased Effect/Toxicity

Dienogest may increase the levels/effects of: C1 inhibitors; Selegiline; Thalidomide; Tranexamic Acid; Voriconazole

The levels/effects of Dienogest may be increased by: Atazanavir; Boceprevir; Cobicistat; CYP3A4 Inhibitors (Strong); Herbs (Progestogenic Properties); Lopinavir; Metreleptin; Mifepristone; Tipranavir; Voriconazole

Decreased Effect

Dienogest may decrease the levels/effects of: Anticoagulants; Fosamprenavir; Vitamin K Antagonists

The levels/effects of Dienogest may be decreased by: Acitretin; Aminoglutethimide; Aprepitant; Artemether; Barbiturates; Bexarotene (Systemic); Bile Acid Sequestrants; Bosentan; CloBAZam; CYP3A4 Inducers (Moderate); CYP3A4 Inducers (Strong); Dabrafenib; Darunavir; Deferasirox; Efavirenz; Eslicarbazepine; Felbamate; Fosamprenavir; Fosaprepitant; Griseofulvin; LamoTRIgine; Lopinavir; Metreleptin; Mifepristone; Mycophenolate; Nelfinavir; Nevirapine; OXcarbazepine; Perampanel; Prucalopride; Retinoic Acid Derivatives; Saquinavir; Siltuximab; St Johns Wort; Sugammadex; Telaprevir; Tocilizumab; Topiramate; Ulipristal

Storage/Stability Store in original packaging at 15°C to 30°C (59°F to 86°F).

Mechanism of Action Dienogest is a steroid with antiandrogen properties that lacks androgen, mineralcorticoid or glucocorticoid activity. Exhibits strong progestogenic effects although it binds uterine progesterone receptors with an affinity much lower (about one-tenth) than that of progesterone. Decreases estradiol production and thus suppresses estradiol's trophic effects on eutopic and ectopic endometrium. Inhibits cellular proliferation via direct antiproliferative, immunologic, and antiangiogenic effects.

Pharmacodynamics/Kinetics

Absorption: Rapid and almost complete

Distribution: V_d: 40 L

Protein binding: ~90% nonspecifically to albumin

Metabolism: Hepatic via CYP3A4 to inactive metabolites

Bioavailability: ~91%

Half-life elimination: ~9-10 hours

Time to peak: ~1.5 hours

Excretion: Urine (minimal amount as unchanged drug)

Dosage Oral: Adult females: 2 mg once daily

Dosage adjustment in renal impairment: No dosage adjustment necessary.

Dosage adjustment in hepatic impairment:

Mild-to-moderate impairment: No dosage adjustment provided in manufacturer's labeling; dienogest undergoes hepatic metabolism and therefore systemic exposure may be increased.

Severe impairment: Use in patients with a history of or current severe hepatic disease is contraindicated.

Administration Administer without regard to meals. If a dose is not absorbed due to vomiting and/or diarrhea within 3-4 hours of administration, repeat dose.

Monitoring Parameters Pregnancy test prior to initiating therapy; routine physical examination that includes blood pressure and Papanicolaou smear, breast exam, mammogram; adequate diagnostic measures, including endometrial sampling, if indicated, should be performed to rule out malignancy in all cases of undiagnosed abnormal vaginal bleeding; bone mineral density (prior to therapy in patients at risk for osteoporosis); signs and symptoms of thromboembolic disorders, vision changes

Product Availability Not available in the U.S.

Dosage Forms: Canada

Tablet, oral:

Visanne®: 2 mg

◆ **Dienogest and Estradiol** *see* Estradiol and Dienogest *on page 780*

◆ **Dietary Fiber Laxative [OTC]** *see* Psyllium *on page 1744*

Diethylamine Salicylate [INT]

(dye ETH il a meen sal il si late)

International Brand Names Aciphen (HU); Algesal (BE, IT, NO); Algesal[+Myrtecaine] (AT, CH, CZ, DE, ES, FI, GB, HU, NL, SE); Algiderma (PT); Algoderm (ES); Algoflex (IT); Artrogota (ES); Gallisal (FI); Multigesic (IN); Rheumagel-Dr. Schmidgall (AT)

Pharmacologic Category Analgesic, Topical

Reported Use Topical treatment of rheumatic and muscular pain

Dosage Range Topical: Apply 2-3 times/day

Product Availability Product available in various countries; not currently available in the U.S.

Dosage Forms

Cream: 1%

Diethylpropion (dye eth il PROE pee on)

Index Terms Amfepramone; Diethylpropion Hydrochloride; Tenuate; Tenuate Dospan

Pharmacologic Category Anorexiant; Central Nervous System Stimulant; Sympathomimetic

Use Short-term (few weeks) adjunct in the management of exogenous obesity

Pharmacotherapy for weight loss is recommended only for obese patients with a body mass index ≥30 kg/m^2, or ≥27 kg/m^2 in the presence of other risk factors such as hypertension, diabetes, and/or dyslipidemia or a high waist circumference; therapy should be used in conjunction with a comprehensive weight management program.

Pregnancy Risk Factor B

Dosage Children >16 years and Adults: Oral:

Immediate release: 25 mg 3 times daily

Controlled release: 75 mg once daily at midmorning

Dosage adjustment in renal impairment: No dosage adjustment provided in manufacturer's labeling; use with caution.

Dosage adjustment in hepatic impairment: No dosage adjustment provided in manufacturer's labeling.

Additional Information Complete prescribing information should be consulted for additional detail.

Dosage Forms

Tablet, Oral:

Generic: 25 mg

Tablet Extended Release 24 Hour, Oral:

Generic: 75 mg

- **Diethylpropion Hydrochloride** *see* Diethylpropion *on page 624*
- **Differin** *see* Adapalene *on page 54*
- **Differin® (Can)** *see* Adapalene *on page 54*
- **Differin® XP (Can)** *see* Adapalene *on page 54*
- **Dificid** *see* Fidaxomicin *on page 875*
- **Dificid™ (Can)** *see* Fidaxomicin *on page 875*
- **Difimicin** *see* Fidaxomicin *on page 875*

Diflorasone (dye FLOR a sone)

Brand Names: U.S. ApexiCon; ApexiCon E

Index Terms Diflorasone Diacetate

Pharmacologic Category Corticosteroid, Topical

Additional Appendix Information

Topical Corticosteroids *on page 2230*

Use Relieves inflammation and pruritic symptoms of corticosteroid-responsive dermatosis (high to very high potency topical corticosteroid)

Pregnancy Risk Factor C

Dosage Topical: Apply ointment sparingly 1-3 times/day; apply cream sparingly 2-4 times/day. Therapy should be discontinued when control is achieved; if no improvement is seen, reassessment of diagnosis may be necessary.

Additional Information Complete prescribing information should be consulted for additional detail.

Dosage Forms

Cream, External:

ApexiCon E: 0.05% (30 g, 60 g)

Generic: 0.05% (15 g, 30 g, 60 g)

Ointment, External:

ApexiCon: 0.05% (30 g, 60 g)

Generic: 0.05% (15 g, 30 g, 60 g)

- **Diflorasone Diacetate** *see* Diflorasone *on page 625*
- **Diflucan** *see* Fluconazole *on page 885*
- **Diflucan injection (Can)** *see* Fluconazole *on page 885*
- **Diflucan One (Can)** *see* Fluconazole *on page 885*
- **Diflucan PWS (Can)** *see* Fluconazole *on page 885*

Diflucortolone [CAN/INT] (dye floo KOR toe lone)

Brand Names: Canada Nerisone Cream; Nerisone Oily Cream; Nerisone Ointment

Index Terms Diflucortolone Valerate

Pharmacologic Category Corticosteroid, Topical

Additional Appendix Information

Topical Corticosteroids *on page 2230*

Use Acute and chronic skin disease: Treatment of acute and chronic skin diseases responsive to the anti-inflammatory, antipruritic, and antiallergic effects of topical corticosteroids.

Pregnancy Considerations Adverse events have been observed with corticosteroids (including diflucortolone) in animal reproduction studies. Topical corticosteroids are preferred over systemic for treating conditions, such as psoriasis or atopic dermatitis in pregnant women; high potency corticosteroids are not recommended during the first trimester. Topical products are not recommended for extensive use, in large quantities, or for long periods of time in pregnant women (Bae, 2011; Koutroulis, 2011; Leachman, 2006).

Breast-Feeding Considerations Corticosteroids are excreted in human milk. It is not known if systemic absorption following topical administration results in detectable quantities in human milk. Do not apply topical corticosteroids to breasts; hypertension was noted in a nursing infant exposed to a topical corticosteroid while nursing (Leachman, 2006). The manufacturer notes that when used systemically, maternal use of corticosteroids have the potential to cause adverse events in a nursing infant (eg, growth suppression, interfere with endogenous corticosteroid production) and therefore recommends that caution be exercised when administering diflucortolone to nursing women.

Contraindications Hypersensitivity to diflucortolone, any component of the formulation, or other corticosteroids; infants <1 year of age; viral (eg, herpes, varicella, vaccinia) lesions of the skin, bacterial or fungal skin infections, parasitic infections, skin manifestations relating to tuberculosis or syphilis, eruptions following vaccinations; rosacea; pruritus without inflammation; perianal and genital pruritus; perioral dermatitis; acne vulgaris; ophthalmic application

Warnings/Precautions Topical corticosteroids may be absorbed percutaneously. Absorption is increased by the use of occlusive dressings, application to denuded skin, or application to large surface areas. Absorption of topical corticosteroids may cause manifestations of Cushing syndrome, hyperglycemia, or glycosuria. May cause hypercorticism or suppression of hypothalamic-pituitary-adrenal (HPA) axis, particularly in younger children or in patients receiving high doses for prolonged periods. HPA axis suppression may lead to adrenal crisis. Patients receiving large doses of potent topical steroids should be periodically evaluated for HPA axis suppression using urinary free cortisol and ACTH stimulation tests. Withdrawal and discontinuation of a corticosteroid should be done slowly and carefully by reducing the frequency of application or substitution of a less potent steroid. Recovery is usually prompt and complete upon drug discontinuation, but may require supplemental systemic corticosteroids if signs and symptoms of steroid withdrawal occur. Intracranial hypertension and Cushing syndrome have been reported in children receiving topical corticosteroids. Prolonged use in children may affect growth velocity; growth should be routinely monitored in pediatric patients.

Localized hypersensitivity reactions may occur; discontinue use if hypersensitivity occurs and treat appropriately. Prolonged use of corticosteroids may increase the incidence of secondary infection, mask acute infection (including fungal infections), prolong or exacerbate viral infections, or limit response to vaccines. Discontinue use if concomitant skin infection occurs and treat appropriately. Exposure to varicella zoster (chickenpox) should be avoided; corticosteroids should not be used to treat ocular herpes simplex. Prolonged treatment with corticosteroids has been associated with the development of Kaposi sarcoma (case reports) (Goedert, 2002); if noted, discontinuation of therapy should be considered.

Use with caution in the elderly. Use with caution in patients with psoriasis, stasis dermatitis or other skin diseases associated with impaired circulation. Application near chronic leg ulcers may increase risk of localized hypersensitivity reactions and infection. Use with caution near the eyes (do not apply to the eyes), and on the face, groin and axilla. Monitor for skin atrophy and discontinue use if observed.

Drug Interactions

Metabolism/Transport Effects None known.

Avoid Concomitant Use

Avoid concomitant use of Diflucortolone with any of the following: Aldesleukin

Increased Effect/Toxicity

Diflucortolone may increase the levels/effects of: Ceritinib; Deferasirox

The levels/effects of Diflucortolone may be increased by: Telaprevir

Decreased Effect
Diflucortolone may decrease the levels/effects of: Aldesleukin; Corticorelin; Hyaluronidase; Telaprevir

Storage/Stability Store between 15°C to 25°C (59°F to 77°F); do not freeze.

Mechanism of Action Topical corticosteroids have anti-inflammatory, antipruritic, and vasoconstrictive properties. May depress the formation, release, and activity of endogenous chemical mediators of inflammation (kinins, histamine, liposomal enzymes, prostaglandins) through the induction of phospholipase A2 inhibitory proteins (lipocortins) and sequential inhibition of the release of arachidonic acid. Diflucortolone has intermediate range potency.

Pharmacodynamics/Kinetics
Absorption: Percutaneous absorption is variable and dependent upon many factors including vehicle used, integrity and thickness of epidermis, surface area of application, and use of occlusive dressings (not recommended)
Metabolism: Hepatic
Excretion: Urine and feces

Dosage
Acute and chronic skin disease: Topical: **Note:** Lack of improvement or worsening of condition after 2 to 4 weeks of therapy may necessitate further evaluation. Maximum duration of therapy: 4 weeks
Children ≥1 year and Adolescents: Apply the least amount for the shortest duration of time needed to achieve desired therapeutic effect. May apply a thin layer using only enough to cover affected area 1 to 2 times daily.
Adults: Apply a thin layer using only enough to cover affected area 1 to 2 times daily
Elderly: Apply the least amount for the shortest duration of time needed to achieve desired therapeutic effect. Refer to adult dosing.

Dosage adjustment in renal impairment: There are no specific dosage adjustments provided in the manufacturer's labeling; however, the manufacturer recommends applying the least amount for the shortest duration of time needed to achieve desired therapeutic effect.

Dosage adjustment in hepatic impairment: There are no specific dosage adjustments provided in the manufacturer's labeling; however, the manufacturer recommends applying the least amount for the shortest duration of time needed to achieve desired therapeutic effect.

Administration For topical use only. Rub a thin layer in gently using only enough to cover affected area. Avoid use of occlusive dressings. Do not apply in or near the eye or on other mucous membranes.

Monitoring Parameters Adrenal suppression with extensive/prolonged use (ACTH stimulation test); response to treatment; growth in children

Product Availability Not available in the U.S.

Dosage Forms: Canada
Cream, External, as valerate:
Nerisone: 0.1% (30 g)
Oily Cream, External, as valerate [preservative free]:
Nerisone: 0.1% (30 g, 60 g)
Ointment, External, as valerate [preservative free]:
Nerisone: 0.1% (30 g)

◆ **Diflucortolone Valerate** *see* Diflucortolone [CAN/INT] *on page 625*

Diflunisal (dye FLOO ni sal)

Brand Names: Canada Apo-Diflunisal; Novo-Diflunisal

Index Terms Dolobid

Pharmacologic Category Nonsteroidal Anti-inflammatory Drug (NSAID), Oral

Additional Appendix Information
Beers Criteria – Potentially Inappropriate Medications for Geriatrics *on page 2271*

Use
Mild to moderate pain: For acute or long-term use for symptomatic treatment of mild to moderate pain
Osteoarthritis/Rheumatoid arthritis (RA): For acute or long-term use for symptomatic relief of osteoarthritis and RA

Pregnancy Risk Factor C

Dosage
Mild to moderate pain:
Adults: Oral: Initial: 1 g, followed by 500 mg every 12 hours; maintenance doses of 500 mg every 8 hours may be necessary in some patients; maximum daily dose: 1.5 g
Dosage adjustments: A lower dosage may be appropriate depending on pain severity, patient response, and weight: Initial: 500 mg, followed by 250 mg every 8-12 hours; maximum daily dose: 1.5 g
Elderly: Mild to moderate pain: Oral: Initial: 500 mg, followed by 250 mg every 8-12 hours; maximum daily dose: 1.5 g
Arthritis: Adults and Elderly: Oral: 500 mg to 1 g daily in 2 divided doses; maximum daily dose: 1.5 g

Dosage adjustment in renal impairment: No dosage adjustment provided in the manufacturer's labeling; however the following adjustments have been used by some clinicians (Aronoff, 2007):
CrCl <50 mL/minute: Administer 50% of normal dose
Hemodialysis: No supplement required
CAPD: No supplement required

Dosage adjustment in hepatic impairment: No dosage adjustment provided in manufacturer's labeling; use with caution.

Additional Information Complete prescribing information should be consulted for additional detail.

Dosage Forms
Tablet, Oral:
Generic: 500 mg

Dosage Forms: Canada
Tablet, Oral: 250 mg

◆ **Difluorodeoxycytidine Hydrochlorothiazide** *see* Gemcitabine *on page 952*

Difluprednate (dye floo PRED nate)

Brand Names: U.S. Durezol

Pharmacologic Category Corticosteroid, Ophthalmic

Use Treatment of inflammation and pain following ocular surgery; treatment of endogenous anterior uveitis

Pregnancy Risk Factor C

Dosage
Inflammation associated with ocular surgery: Infants, Children, Adolescents, and Adults: Ophthalmic: Instill 1 drop in conjunctival sac of the affected eye(s) 4 times daily beginning 24 hours after surgery, continue for 2 weeks, then decrease to 2 times daily for 1 week, then taper based on response
Endogenous anterior uveitis: Adults: Ophthalmic: Instill 1 drop into conjunctival sac of the affected eye(s) 4 times daily for 14 days, then taper as clinically indicated

Additional Information Complete prescribing information should be consulted for additional detail.

Dosage Forms
Emulsion, Ophthalmic:
Durezol: 0.05% (5 mL)

Difluprednate (Topical) [INT]

(dye floo PRED nate TOP i kal)

International Brand Names Epitopic (AE, FR); Myser (JP); Ribeca (KR)

Pharmacologic Category Corticosteroid, Topical

Reported Use Treatment of corticosteroid responsive dermatoses

Dosage Range Adults: Topical: Apply twice daily

Product Availability Product available in various countries; not currently available in the U.S.

Dosage Forms

Cream: 0.02% (40 g); 0.05% (15 g)

◆ **Digestive Enzyme** *see* Pancrelipase *on page 1566*

◆ **Digibind** *see* Digoxin Immune Fab *on page 630*

◆ **DigiFab** *see* Digoxin Immune Fab *on page 630*

◆ **Digitalis** *see* Digoxin *on page 627*

◆ **Digitek** *see* Digoxin *on page 627*

Digitoxin [INT] (di ji TOKS in)

International Brand Names Carditoxin (HU); Digimed (DE); Digimerck (AT, DE, HN, HU, TR); Digitalina Nativelle (IT); Digitaline (GR, PT); Digitaline Nativelle (BE, BR, CH, FR, LU); Digitossina (IT); Digitoxin Nyco (NO); Digitoxin Streuli (CH); Digitrin (NO, SE)

Index Terms Crystodigin

Pharmacologic Category Antiarrhythmic Agent, Class IV

Reported Use Treatment of congestive heart failure, atrial fibrillation, atrial flutter, paroxysmal atrial tachycardia, and cardiogenic shock

Dosage Range Adults: Oral:

Rapid loading dose: Initial: 1-1.5 mg over 24 hours in divided doses

Maintenance: 0.05-0.2 mg/day

Product Availability Product available in various countries; not currently available in the U.S.

Dosage Forms

Tablet: 0.1 mg, 0.2 mg

◆ **Digox** *see* Digoxin *on page 627*

Digoxin (di JOKS in)

Brand Names: U.S. Digitek; Digox; Lanoxin; Lanoxin Pediatric

Brand Names: Canada Apo-Digoxin; Digoxin Injection CSD; Lanoxin; Pediatric Digoxin CSD; PMS-Digoxin; Toloxin

Index Terms Digitalis

Pharmacologic Category Antiarrhythmic Agent, Miscellaneous; Cardiac Glycoside

Additional Appendix Information

Beers Criteria - Potentially Inappropriate Medications for Geriatrics *on page 2271*

Use

Atrial fibrillation: For the control of ventricular response rate in adults with chronic atrial fibrillation.

Heart failure: For the treatment of mild-to-moderate (or stage C as recommended by the ACCF/AHA) heart failure (HF) in adults; to increase myocardial contractility in pediatric patients with heart failure

Note: In treatment of atrial fibrillation (AF), use is not considered first-line in patients with AF; digoxin may be considered for rate control in patients with heart failure with reduced ejection fraction (HFrEF) without pre-excitation or in sedentary patients (AHA/ACC/HRS [January, 2014]). In the treatment of heart failure, digoxin should be considered for use only in HF with reduced ejection fraction (HFrEF) when symptoms remain despite guideline-directed medical therapy or as initial therapy in patients with severe symptoms yet to respond to guideline-directed medical therapy (ACCF/AHA [Yancy, 2013]).

Pregnancy Risk Factor C

Pregnancy Considerations Animal reproduction studies have not been conducted. Digoxin crosses the placenta and serum concentrations are similar in the mother and fetus at delivery. Digoxin is recommended as first-line in the treatment of fetal tachycardia determined to be SVT. In pregnant women with SVT, use of digoxin is recommended (Blomström-Lundqvist, 2003).

Breast-Feeding Considerations Digoxin is excreted into breast milk and similar concentrations are found within mother's serum and milk. The manufacturer recommends that caution be used when administered to nursing women.

Contraindications Hypersensitivity to digoxin (rare) or other forms of digitalis, or any component of the formulation; ventricular fibrillation

Warnings/Precautions Watch for proarrhythmic effects (especially with digoxin toxicity). Withdrawal in clinically stable patients with HF may lead to recurrence of HF symptoms. During an episode of atrial fibrillation or flutter in patients with an accessory bypass tract (eg, Wolff-Parkinson-White syndrome) or pre-excitation syndrome, use has been associated with increased anterograde conduction down the accessory pathway leading to ventricular fibrillation; avoid use in such patients (ACLS [Neumar, 2010]; AHA/ACC/HRS [January, 2014]). Because digoxin slows sinoatrial and AV conduction, the drug commonly prolongs the PR interval. Digoxin may cause severe sinus bradycardia or sinoatrial block in patients with preexisting sinus node disease. Avoid use in patients with second- or third-degree heart block (except in patients with a functioning artificial pacemaker) (Yancy, 2013); incomplete AV block (eg, Stokes-Adams attack) may progress to complete block with digoxin administration. Digoxin should be considered for use only in heart failure (HF) with reduced ejection fraction (HFrEF) when symptoms remain despite guideline-directed medical therapy. It may also be considered in patients with both HF and atrial fibrillation; however, beta blockers may offer better ventricular rate control than digoxin (ACCF/AHA [Yancy, 2013]). Avoid use in patients with hypertrophic cardiomyopathy (HCM) and outflow tract obstruction unless used to control ventricular response with atrial fibrillation; outflow obstruction may worsen due to the positive inotropic effects of digoxin. Digoxin is potentially harmful in the treatment of dyspnea in patients with HCM in the absence of atrial fibrillation (Gersh, 2011). In a murine model of viral myocarditis, digoxin in high doses was shown to be detrimental (Matsumori, 1999). If used in humans, therefore, digoxin should be used with caution and only at low doses (Frishman, 2007). The manufacturer recommends avoiding the use of digoxin in patients with myocarditis.

Use with caution in patients with hyperthyroidism (increased digoxin clearance) and hypothyroidism (reduced digoxin clearance). Atrial arrhythmias associated with hypermetabolic (eg, hyperthyroidism) or hyperdynamic (hypoxia, arteriovenous shunt) states are very difficult to treat; treat underlying condition first. Use with caution in patients with an acute MI; may increase myocardial oxygen demand. During an acute coronary syndrome, digoxin administered IV may be used to slow a rapid ventricular response and improve left ventricular (LV) function in the acute treatment of atrial fibrillation associated with severe LV function and heart failure or hemodynamic instability (AHA/ACC/HRS [January, 2014]). Reduce dose with renal impairment and when amiodarone, propafenone, quinidine, or verapamil are added to a patient on digoxin; use with caution in patients taking strong inducers or inhibitors of P-glycoprotein (eg, cyclosporine). Avoid ▶

rapid IV administration of calcium in digitalized patients; may produce serious arrhythmias.

Atrial arrhythmias associated with hypermetabolic states are very difficult to treat; treat underlying condition first; if digoxin is used, ensure digoxin toxicity does not occur. Patients with beri beri heart disease may fail to adequately respond to digoxin therapy; treat underlying thiamine deficiency concomitantly. Correct electrolyte disturbances, especially hypokalemia or hypomagnesemia, prior to use and throughout therapy; toxicity may occur despite therapeutic digoxin concentrations. Hypercalcemia may increase the risk of digoxin toxicity; maintain normocalcemia. It is not necessary to routinely reduce or hold digoxin therapy prior to elective electrical cardioversion for atrial fibrillation; however, exclusion of digoxin toxicity (eg, clinical and ECG signs) is necessary prior to cardioversion. If signs of digoxin excess exist, withhold digoxin and delay cardioversion until toxicity subsides (AHA/ACC/HRS [January, 2014]). IV administration: Vesicant; ensure proper needle or catheter placement prior to and during administration; avoid extravasation. Some dosage forms may contain propylene glycol; large amounts are potentially toxic and have been associated hyperosmolality, lactic acidosis, seizures, and respiratory depression; use caution (AAP, 1997; Zar, 2007). Use with caution in the elderly; decreases in renal clearance may result in toxic effects; in general, avoid doses >0.125 mg/day; in heart failure, higher doses may increase the risk of potential toxicity and have not been shown to provide additional benefit (Beers Criteria).

Adverse Reactions

Cardiovascular: Accelerated junctional rhythm, asystole, atrial tachycardia with or without block, AV dissociation, first-, second- (Wenckebach), or third-degree heart block, facial edema, PR prolongation, PVCs (especially bigeminy or trigeminy), ST segment depression, ventricular tachycardia or ventricular fibrillation

Central nervous system: Apathy, anxiety, confusion, delirium, depression, dizziness, fever, hallucinations, headache, mental disturbances

Dermatologic: Rash (erythematous, maculopapular [most common], papular, scarlatiniform, vesicular or bullous), pruritus, urticaria, angioneurotic edema

Gastrointestinal: Abdominal pain, anorexia, diarrhea, nausea, vomiting

Neuromuscular & skeletal: Weakness

Ocular: Visual disturbances (blurred or yellow vision)

Respiratory: Laryngeal edema

Rare but important or life-threatening: Asymmetric chorea, gynecomastia, thrombocytopenia, palpitation, intestinal ischemia, hemorrhagic necrosis of the intestines, vaginal cornification, eosinophilia, sexual dysfunction, diaphoresis

Drug Interactions

Metabolism/Transport Effects **Substrate** of CYP3A4 (minor), P-glycoprotein; **Note:** Assignment of Major/Minor substrate status based on clinically relevant drug interaction potential

Avoid Concomitant Use

Avoid concomitant use of Digoxin with any of the following: Ceritinib

Increased Effect/Toxicity

Digoxin may increase the levels/effects of: Adenosine; Bradycardia-Causing Agents; Carvedilol; Ceritinib; Colchicine; Dronedarone; Lacosamide; Midodrine

The levels/effects of Digoxin may be increased by: Aminoquinolines (Antimalarial); Amiodarone; Amphotericin B; Antithyroid Agents; AtorvaSTATin; Beta-Blockers; Boceprevir; Bretylium; Brimonidine (Topical); Calcium Channel Blockers (Nondihydropyridine); Calcium Polystyrene Sulfonate; Calcium Salts; Carvedilol; CloNIDine; Conivaptan; CycloSPORINE (Systemic); Dronedarone; Eliglustat; Epoprostenol; Etravirine; Ezogabine; Flecainide; Glycopyrrolate; Itraconazole; Lenalidomide; Licorice; Loop Diuretics; Macrolide Antibiotics; Mifepristone; Milnacipran; Mirabegron; Multivitamins/Fluoride (with ADE); Multivitamins/Minerals (with ADEK, Folate, Iron); Multivitamins/Minerals (with AE, No Iron); Nefazodone; Neuromuscular-Blocking Agents; NIFEdipine; Nonsteroidal Anti-Inflammatory Agents; Parathyroid Hormone; Paricalcitol; P-glycoprotein/ABCB1 Inhibitors; Posaconazole; Potassium-Sparing Diuretics; Propafenone; Protease Inhibitors; QuiNIDine; QuiNINE; Ranolazine; Regorafenib; Reserpine; Simeprevir; SitaGLIPtin; Sodium Polystyrene Sulfonate; Spironolactone; Telaprevir; Telmisartan; Thiazide Diuretics; Ticagrelor; Tofacitinib; Tolvaptan; Trimethoprim; Vandetanib; Vitamin D Analogs

Decreased Effect

Digoxin may decrease the levels/effects of: Antineoplastic Agents (Anthracycline, Systemic)

The levels/effects of Digoxin may be decreased by: 5-ASA Derivatives; Acarbose; Aminoglycosides; Antineoplastic Agents (Anthracycline, Systemic); Bile Acid Sequestrants; Kaolin; PenicillAMINE; P-glycoprotein/ABCB1 Inducers; Polyethylene Glycol 3350; Polyethylene Glycol 4000; Potassium-Sparing Diuretics; St Johns Wort; Sucralfate

Food Interactions Digoxin peak serum concentrations may be decreased if taken with food. Meals containing increased fiber (bran) or foods high in pectin may decrease oral absorption of digoxin.

Preparation for Administration

IM: No dilution required.

IV: May be administered undiluted or diluted fourfold in D_5W, NS, or SWFI for direct injection. Less than fourfold dilution may lead to drug precipitation.

Storage/Stability Store at 25°C (77°F); excursions permitted to 15°C to 30°C (59°F to 86°F). Protect elixir, injection, and tablets from light.

Mechanism of Action

Heart failure: Inhibition of the sodium/potassium ATPase pump in myocardial cells results in a transient increase of intracellular sodium, which in turn promotes calcium influx via the sodium-calcium exchange pump leading to increased contractility.

Supraventricular arrhythmias: Direct suppression of the AV node conduction to increase effective refractory period and decrease conduction velocity - positive inotropic effect, enhanced vagal tone, and decreased ventricular rate to fast atrial arrhythmias. Atrial fibrillation may decrease sensitivity and increase tolerance to higher serum digoxin concentrations.

Pharmacodynamics/Kinetics

Onset of action: Heart rate control: Oral: 1 to 2 hours; IV: 5 to 60 minutes

Peak effect: Heart rate control: Oral: 2 to 8 hours; IV: 1 to 6 hours; **Note:** In patients with atrial fibrillation, median time to ventricular rate control in one study was 6 hours (range: 3 to 15 hours) (Siu, 2009)

Duration: Adults: 3 to 4 days

Absorption: By passive nonsaturable diffusion in the upper small intestine; food may delay, but does not affect extent of absorption

Distribution:

Normal renal function: 6 to 7 L/kg

V_d: Extensive to peripheral tissues, with a distinct distribution phase which lasts 6 to 8 hours; concentrates in heart, liver, kidney, skeletal muscle, and intestines. Heart/serum concentration is 70:1. Pharmacologic effects are delayed and do not correlate well with serum concentrations during distribution phase.

Hyperthyroidism: Increased V_d

Hyperkalemia, hyponatremia: Decreased digoxin distribution to heart and muscle

Hypokalemia: Increased digoxin distribution to heart and muscles
Concomitant quinidine therapy: Decreased V_d
Chronic renal failure: 4 to 6 L/kg
Decreased sodium/potassium ATPase activity - decreased tissue binding
Neonates, full-term: 7.5 to 10 L/kg
Children: 16 L/kg
Adults: 7 L/kg, decreased with renal disease

Protein binding: ~25%; in uremic patients, digoxin is displaced from plasma protein binding sites

Metabolism: Via sequential sugar hydrolysis in the stomach or by reduction of lactone ring by intestinal bacteria (in ~10% of population, gut bacteria may metabolize up to 40% of digoxin dose); once absorbed, only ~16% is metabolized to 3-beta-digoxigenin, 3-keto-digoxigenin, and glucuronide and sulfate conjugates; metabolites may contribute to therapeutic and toxic effects of digoxin; metabolism is reduced with decompensated HF

Bioavailability: Oral (formulation dependent): Elixir: 70% to 85%; Tablet: 60% to 80%

Half-life elimination (age, renal and cardiac function dependent):
Neonates: Premature: 61 to 170 hours; Full-term: 35 to 45 hours
Infants: 18 to 25 hours
Children: 18 to 36 hours
Adults: 36 to 48 hours
Adults, anephric: 3.5 to 5 days

Half-life elimination: Parent drug: 38 hours; Metabolites: Digoxigenin: 4 hours; Monodigitoxoside: 3 to 12 hours

Time to peak, serum: Oral: 1 to 3 hours

Excretion: Urine (50% to 70% as unchanged drug)

Dosage

Children: When changing from oral (tablets or liquid) or IM to IV therapy, dosage should be reduced by 20% to 25%. Refer to the following: See table.

Dosage Recommendations for Digoxin[1]

Age	Total Digitalizing Dose[2,3] (mcg/kg)		Daily Maintenance Dose[3,4] (mcg/kg)	
	Oral	IV or IM[5]	Oral	IV or IM[5]
Preterm infant	20-30	15-25	5-7.5	4-6
Full-term infant	25-35	20-30	6-10	5-8
1 mo - 2 y	35-60	30-50	10-15	7.5-12
2-5 y	30-40	25-35	7.5-10	6-9
5-10 y	20-35	15-30	5-10	4-8
>10 y	10-15	8-12	2.5-5	2-3

[1]**Heart failure:** A lower serum digoxin concentration may be adequate to treat heart failure (compared to cardiac arrhythmias); consider doses at the lower end of the recommended range for treatment of heart failure; a digitalizing dose (loading dose) may not be necessary when treating heart failure (Ross, 2001).

[2]**Do not give full total digitalizing dose (TDD) at once.** Give one-half of the total digitalizing dose (TDD) in the initial dose, then give one-quarter of the TDD in each of two subsequent doses at 6- to 8-hour intervals. Obtain ECG 6 hours after each dose to assess potential toxicity.

[3]Based on lean body weight and normal renal function for age. Decrease dose in patients with decreased renal function; digitalizing dose often not recommended in infants and children.

[4]Divided every 12 hours in infants and children <10 years of age. Given once daily to children >10 years of age and adults.

[5]IM not preferred due to severe injection site pain. If IM route is necessary, administer as deep injection followed by massage of injection site.

Adults:

Atrial fibrillation (rate control) (off-label dose):

Total digitalizing dose (TDD): IV: 8 to 12 **mcg**/kg; administer half of TDD over 5 minutes with the remaining portion as 25% fractions at 4 to 8 hour intervals (ACLS [Neumar, 2010]) **or** may administer 0.25 mg with repeat dosing to a maximum of 1.5 mg over 24 hours followed by an oral maintenance regimen (AHA/ACC/HRS [January, 2014]).

Maintenance: Oral: 0.125 to 0.25 mg once daily (AHA/ACC/HRS [January, 2014])

Heart failure: Daily maintenance dose (**Note:** Loading dose not recommended): Oral: 0.125 to 0.25 mg once daily; higher daily doses (eg, 0.375 to 0.5 mg daily) are rarely necessary. If patient is >70 years of age, has impaired renal function, or has a low lean body mass, low doses (eg, 0.125 mg daily or every other day) should be used initially (ACCF/AHA [Yancy, 2013]). **Note:** IV digoxin may be used to control ventricular response in patients with atrial fibrillation and heart failure with reduced ejection fraction (HFrEF) who do not have an accessory pathway or pre-excitation syndrome (AHA/ACC/HRS [January, 2014]). The addition of a beta-blocker to digoxin is usually more effective in controlling ventricular response, particularly during exercise (ACCF/AHA [Yancy, 2013]).

Supraventricular tachyarrhythmias (rate control):

Initial: Total digitalizing dose:
Oral: 0.75 to 1.5 mg
IV, IM: 0.5 to 1 mg (**Note:** IM not preferred due to severe injection site pain.)
Give 1/2 (one-half) of the total digitalizing dose (TDD) as the initial dose, then give 1/4 (one-quarter) of the TDD in each of 2 subsequent doses at 6- to 8-hour intervals. Obtain ECG 6 hours after each dose to assess potential toxicity.

Daily maintenance dose:
Oral: 0.125 to 0.5 mg once daily
IV, IM: 0.1 to 0.4 mg once daily (**Note:** IM not preferred due to severe injection site pain.)

Elderly: Dose is based on assessment of lean body mass and renal function. Elderly patients with low lean body mass may experience higher digoxin concentrations due to reduced volume of distribution (Cheng, 2010). Decrease dose in patients with decreased renal function.
Heart failure: If patient is >70 years, low doses (eg, 0.125 mg daily or every other day) should be used (ACCF/AHA [Yancy, 2013]).

Dosage adjustment in renal impairment: Adults: No dosage adjustment provided in manufacturer's labeling; however, the following adjustments have been recommended:

Loading dose:
ESRD: If loading dose necessary, reduce dose by 50% (Aronoff, 2007)
Acute renal failure: Based on expert opinion, if patient in acute renal failure requires ventricular rate control (eg, in atrial fibrillation), consider alternative therapy. If loading digoxin becomes necessary, patient volume of distribution may be increased and reduction in loading dose may not be necessary; however, maintenance dosing will require adjustment as long as renal failure persists.

Maintenance dose (Aronoff, 2007):
CrCl >50 mL/minute: No dosage adjustment necessary.
CrCl 10 to 50 mL/minute: Administer 25% to 75% of the normal daily dose or administer normal dose every 36 hours
CrCl <10 mL/minute: Administer 10% to 25% of the normal daily dose or administer normal dose every 48 hours

Continuous renal replacement therapy (CRRT): Administer 25% to 75% of the normal daily dose or administer normal dose every 36 hours; monitor serum concentrations.

Hemodialysis: Not dialyzable; no supplemental dose necessary.

Heart failure: Initial maintenance dose (Bauman, 2006; Jusko, 1974; Koup, 1975): **Note:** The following suggested dosing recommendations are intended to achieve a target digoxin concentration of 0.7 ng/mL. Renal function estimated using Cockcroft-Gault formula.

CrCl >120 mL/minute: 0.25 mg once daily

CrCl 80 to 120 mL/minute: Alternate between doses of 0.25 mg and 0.125 mg once daily

CrCl 30 to 80 mL/minute: 0.125 mg once daily

CrCl <30 mL/minute: 0.125 mg every 48 hours

Note: A contemporary digoxin dosing nomogram using creatinine clearance and ideal body weight or height has been published for determining the initial maintenance dose in patients with heart failure to achieve a target digoxin concentration of 0.7 ng/mL (Bauman, 2006).

Dosage adjustment in hepatic impairment: No dosage adjustment provided in manufacturer's labeling.

Dietary Considerations Maintain adequate amounts of potassium in diet to decrease risk of hypokalemia (hypokalemia may increase risk of digoxin toxicity).

Administration

IM: IV route preferred. If IM injection necessary, administer by deep injection followed by massage at the injection site. Inject no more than 2 mL per injection site. May cause intense pain.

IV: May be administered undiluted or diluted. Inject slowly over ≥5 minutes.

Vesicant; ensure proper needle or catheter placement prior to and during administration; avoid extravasation.

Extravasation management: If extravasation occurs, stop IV administration immediately and disconnect (leave cannula/needle in place); gently aspirate extravasated solution (do **NOT** flush the line); remove needle/cannula; elevate extremity.

Monitoring Parameters

Heart rate and rhythm should be monitored along with periodic ECGs to assess desired effects and signs of toxicity; baseline and periodic serum creatinine. Periodically monitor serum potassium, magnesium, and calcium especially if on medications where these electrolyte disturbances can occur (eg, diuretics), or if patient has a history of hypokalemia or hypomagnesemia. Observe patients for noncardiac signs of toxicity, confusion, and depression.

When to draw serum digoxin concentrations: Digoxin serum concentrations are monitored because digoxin possesses a narrow therapeutic serum range; the therapeutic endpoint is difficult to quantify and digoxin toxicity may be life-threatening. Digoxin serum concentrations should be drawn **at least 6 to 8 hours after last dose, regardless of route of administration (optimally 12 to 24 hours after a dose). Note:** Serum digoxin concentrations may decrease in response to exercise due to increased skeletal muscle uptake; a period of rest (eg, ~2 hours) after exercise may be necessary prior to drawing serum digoxin concentrations.

Initiation of therapy:

If a loading dose is given: Digoxin serum concentration may be drawn within 12 to 24 hours after the initial loading dose administration. Concentrations drawn this early may confirm the relationship of digoxin plasma concentrations and response but are of little value in determining maintenance doses.

If a loading dose is not given: Digoxin serum concentration should be obtained after 3 to 5 days of therapy.

Maintenance therapy:

Trough concentrations should be followed just prior to the next dose or at a minimum of 6 to 8 hours after last dose.

Digoxin serum concentrations should be obtained within 5 to 7 days (approximate time to steady-state) after any dosage changes. Continue to obtain digoxin serum concentrations 7 to 14 days after any change in maintenance dose. **Note:** In patients with end-stage renal disease, it may take 15 to 20 days to reach steady-state.

Patients who are receiving electrolyte-depleting medications such as diuretics, serum potassium, magnesium, and calcium should be monitored closely.

Digoxin serum concentrations should be obtained whenever any of the following conditions occur:

Questionable patient compliance or to evaluate clinical deterioration following an initial good response

Changing renal function

Suspected digoxin toxicity

Initiation or discontinuation of therapy with drugs (eg, amiodarone, quinidine, verapamil) which potentially interact with digoxin.

Any disease changes (eg, thyroid disease)

Reference Range

Digoxin therapeutic serum concentrations:

Heart failure: 0.5 to 0.9 ng/mL (ACCF/AHA [Yancy, 2013])

Adults: <0.5 ng/mL; probably indicates underdigitalization unless there are special circumstances

Toxic: >2 ng/mL

Digoxin-like immunoreactive substance (DLIS) may cross-react with digoxin immunoassay. DLIS has been found in patients with renal and liver disease, heart failure, neonates, and pregnant women (3rd trimester).

Dosage Forms

Solution, Injection:

Lanoxin: 0.25 mg/mL (2 mL)

Lanoxin Pediatric: 0.1 mg/mL (1 mL)

Generic: 0.25 mg/mL (1 mL, 2 mL)

Solution, Oral:

Generic: 0.05 mg/mL (60 mL)

Tablet, Oral:

Digitek: 125 mcg, 250 mcg

Digox: 125 mcg, 250 mcg

Lanoxin: 62.5 mcg, 125 mcg, 187.5 mcg, 250 mcg

Generic: 125 mcg, 250 mcg

Dosage Forms: Canada

Tablet, oral:

Apo-Digoxin: 62.5 mcg, 125 mcg, 250 mcg

Digoxin Immune Fab (di JOKS in i MYUN fab)

Brand Names: U.S. DigiFab

Brand Names: Canada DigiFab

Index Terms Antidigoxin Fab Fragments, Ovine; Digibind

Pharmacologic Category Antidote

Use

Digoxin toxicity: Treatment of life-threatening or potentially life-threatening digoxin intoxication, including:

- Acute digoxin ingestion (≥10 mg in adults; 4 mg [>0.1 mg/kg] in children); resulting in serum concentration ≥10 ng/mL)
- Chronic ingestion leading to steady state digoxin concentrations >6 ng/mL in adults or >4 ng/mL in children
- Manifestations of life-threatening digoxin toxicity due to overdose (severe ventricular arrhythmias, progressive bradycardia, second or third degree heart block not responsive to atropine, serum potassium concentration >5.5 mEq/L in adults or >6 mEq/L in children)

Pregnancy Risk Factor C

Pregnancy Considerations Animal reproduction studies have not been conducted. In general, medications used as antidotes should take into consideration the health and prognosis of the mother; antidotes should be administered to pregnant women if there is a clear indication for use and should not be withheld because of fears of teratogenicity (Bailey, 2003).

Breast-Feeding Considerations It is not known if digoxin immune fab is excreted in breast milk. The manufacturer recommends caution be exercised when administering to nursing women.

Contraindications There are no contraindications listed in the manufacturer's labeling.

Warnings/Precautions Digoxin immune Fab is derived from ovine (sheep) Fab immunoglobulin fragments; hypersensitivity reactions (eg, anaphylactic or anaphylactoid reactions, delayed allergic reactions) are possible. Patients with allergies to sheep proteins and patients with prior exposure to ovine antibodies or ovine Fab may be at a higher risk for anaphylactic reactions. In patients who develop an anaphylactic reaction, discontinue the infusion immediately and administer emergency care; balance the need for epinephrine against its potential risk in the setting of digitalis toxicity. Processed with papain and may cause hypersensitivity reactions in patients allergic to papaya, other papaya extracts, papain, chymopapain, or the pineapple-enzyme bromelain. There may also be cross allergenicity with dust mite and latex allergens.

Patients experiencing acute digitalis toxicity may present with significant hyperkalemia due to shifting of potassium into the extracellular space. Upon treatment with digoxin immune Fab, potassium shifts back into the intracellular space and may result in hypokalemia. Monitor potassium closely, especially during the first few hours after administration; treat hypokalemia cautiously when clinically indicated.

In patients chronically maintained on digoxin for HF, administration of digoxin immune Fab may result in exacerbation of HF symptoms due to a reduction in digoxin serum concentration. If reinitiation is required, consider postponing until Fab fragments have been eliminated completely; elimination may take several days or longer, especially in patients with renal impairment. Use with caution in patients with renal failure (experience limited); the Fab-digoxin complex will be eliminated more slowly. Toxicity may recur; prolonged monitoring for recurrence of symptoms and evaluation of free (unbound) digoxin concentrations (if test available) may be warranted in this patient population.

Adverse Reactions

Cardiovascular: Heart failure exacerbation (due to withdrawal of digoxin), orthostatic hypotension, rapid ventricular response (patients with atrial fibrillation; due to withdrawal of digoxin)

Endocrine & metabolic: Hypokalemia

Local: Phlebitis

Miscellaneous: Allergic reactions, serum sickness

Drug Interactions

Metabolism/Transport Effects None known.

Avoid Concomitant Use There are no known interactions where it is recommended to avoid concomitant use.

Increased Effect/Toxicity There are no known significant interactions involving an increase in effect.

Decreased Effect There are no known significant interactions involving a decrease in effect.

Preparation for Administration Reconstitute each vial to a concentration of 10 mg/mL by adding 4 mL SWFI; gently mix. Add reconstituted digoxin immune fab to an appropriate volume of NS. For very small doses, the reconstituted vial can be further diluted by adding an additional 36 mL NS to achieve a final concentration of 1 mg/mL. Infants and small children who require very small doses may be administered reconstituted digoxin immune undiluted using a tuberculin syringe.

Storage/Stability Store vials at 2°C to 8°C (36°F to 46°F); do not freeze. Reconstituted solutions are stable for 4 hours when stored at 2°C to 8°C (36°F to 46°F). The following stability information has also been reported: May be stored at room temperature for up to 30 days (Cohen, 2007).

Mechanism of Action Digoxin immune antigen-binding fragments (Fab) are specific antibodies for the treatment of digitalis intoxication in carefully selected patients; binds with molecules of digoxin or DIGIToxin and is then excreted by the kidneys and removed from the body

Pharmacodynamics/Kinetics

Onset of action: IV: Digitalis toxicity: Improvement may be seen within 20 to 90 minutes (Betten, 2006)

Distribution: V_d: 0.3 L/kg

Half-life elimination: 15 to 20 hours; may be increased up to 10-fold in patient with renal impairment

Excretion: Urine

Dosage Each vial of digoxin immune Fab 40 mg will bind ~0.5 mg of digoxin or DIGIToxin.

Digoxin toxicity: Note: Estimation of the dose is based on the body burden of digitalis. This may be calculated if the amount ingested is known or the post-distribution serum drug level is known (round the dose up to the nearest whole vial). If the amount ingested is unknown, general dosing guidelines should be used.

Acute ingestion of *unknown* amount: IV: Infants, Children, Adolescents, and Adults: Initial: 10 vials; if needed, administer a second dose of 10 vials (20 vials total is adequate to treat most life-threatening ingestions).

Acute ingestion of *known* amount: IV:

Based on number of tablets or capsules ingested: Infants, Children, Adolescents, and Adults:

Step 1: Calculate total body load (mg)

*Digoxin capsules **or** DIGIToxin:*

Total body load (mg) = Amount (mg) digoxin capsules **or** DIGIToxin ingested

Digoxin tablets:

Total body load (mg) = 0.8 x (amount [mg] digoxin tablets ingested)

Step 2: Calculate number of vials needed

Digoxin Immune Fab Dose (vials) = Total body load (mg) / (0.5)

Alternatively, the following table gives an estimation of the number of vials needed based on the number of **digoxin** tablets or capsules ingested.

Approximate Dose of Digoxin Immune Fab for Reversal of a Single Large Digoxin Overdose

Number of Digoxin Tablets or Capsules Ingested[1]	Dose of Digoxin Immune Fab (# of Vials)
25	10
50	20
75	30
100	40
150	60
200	80

[1]250 mcg tablets with 80% bioavailability or 200 mcg capsules with 100% bioavailability.

Based on steady-state serum digoxin concentration:

Infants and Children <20 kg: May require smaller doses. Calculate the dose in milligrams (mg)

Digoxin Immune Fab Dose (mg) = [(serum digoxin concentration [ng/mL] x weight [kg]) / **100**] x (digoxin immune Fab amount per vial [mg/vial])

Note: Digoxin immune Fab amount per vial: 40 mg/vial.

Alternatively, the following table gives an estimation of the amount of digoxin immune Fab needed based on the steady-state serum digoxin concentration.

Infants and Small Children Dose Estimates of Digoxin Immune Fab (in mg) From Steady-State Serum Digoxin Concentration

Patient Weight (kg)	Serum Digoxin Concentration (ng/mL)						
	1	2	4	8	12	16	20
1	0.4 mg[1]	1 mg[1]	1.5 mg[1]	3 mg[1]	5 mg	6.5 mg	8 mg
3	1 mg[1]	2.5 mg[1]	5 mg	10 mg	14 mg	19 mg	24 mg
5	2 mg[1]	4 mg	8 mg	16 mg	24 mg	32 mg	40 mg
10	4 mg	8 mg	16 mg	32 mg	48 mg	64 mg	80 mg
20	8 mg	16 mg	32 mg	64 mg	96 mg	128 mg	160 mg

[1]Dilution of reconstituted vial to 1 mg/mL may be desirable.

Children >20 kg, Adolescents, and Adults:

Digoxin Immune Fab Dose (vials) = [(serum digoxin concentration [ng/mL] x weight [kg]) / **100**]

Alternatively, the following table gives an estimation of the number of vials needed based on the steady-state serum digoxin concentration.

Adult Dose Estimates of Digoxin Immune Fab (in # of Vials) From Steady-State Serum Digoxin Concentration

Patient Weight (kg)	Serum Digoxin Concentration (ng/mL)						
	1	2	4	8	12	16	20
40	0.5 vial	1 vial	2 vials	3 vials	5 vials	7 vials	8 vials
60	0.5 vial	1 vial	3 vials	5 vials	7 vials	10 vials	12 vials
70	1 vial	2 vials	3 vials	6 vials	9 vials	11 vials	14 vials
80	1 vial	2 vials	3 vials	7 vials	10 vials	13 vials	16 vials
100	1 vial	2 vials	4 vials	8 vials	12 vials	16 vials	20 vials

Based on steady-state DIGIToxin concentration: Infants, Children, Adolescents, and Adults: If the calculated dose based on the **DIGIToxin** concentration is different from the estimated dose based on the known ingested amount (if available), use the higher dose.

Digoxin Immune Fab Dose (vials) = [serum **DIGIToxin** concentration (ng/mL) x weight (kg)] / **1000**

Chronic toxicity (serum digoxin concentration unavailable): IV:

Infants and Children <20 kg: 1 vial is adequate to reverse most cases of toxicity

Children ≥20 kg, Adolescents, and Adults: 6 vials is adequate to reverse most cases of toxicity

Dosage adjustment in renal impairment: There are no dosage adjustments provided in the manufacturer's labeling; however, use with caution since digoxin-digoxin immune Fab complex is renally eliminated. Patients should undergo prolonged monitoring for recurrence of toxicity.

Dosage adjustment in hepatic impairment: There are no dosage adjustments provided in the manufacturer's labeling.

Administration Administer by slow IV infusion over at least 30 minutes. May also be given by bolus injection if cardiac arrest is imminent (infusion-related reaction may occur). Infants and small children who require very small doses can be administered reconstituted digoxin immune fab undiluted using a tuberculin syringe. Stopping the infusion and restarting at a slower rate may help if an infusion-related reaction occurs.

Monitoring Parameters Prior to the first dose of digoxin immune Fab evaluate serum potassium, serum digoxin concentration, and serum creatinine; closely monitor serum potassium (eg, hourly for 4-6 hours; at least daily thereafter), temperature, blood pressure, and electrocardiogram after administration. **Total serum digoxin concentrations will rise precipitously following administration of digoxin immune Fab due to the presence of the Fab-digoxin complex; because digoxin bound to Fab fragments cannot result in toxicity, this rise has no clinical meaning.** Therefore, avoid monitoring total serum digoxin concentrations until the Fab fragments have been eliminated completely; this may be several days to weeks in patients with renal impairment (Ujhelyi, 1995). Monitor for volume overload in children <20 kg. Monitor for signs and symptoms of a hypersensitivity reaction.

Patients with renal failure may experience a recurrence of toxicity; prolonged monitoring for recurrence of symptoms and evaluation of free (unbound) digoxin concentrations (if test available) may be warranted in this patient population.

Dosage Forms

Solution Reconstituted, Intravenous [preservative free]:

DigiFab: 40 mg (1 ea)

◆ **Digoxin Injection CSD (Can)** *see* Digoxin *on page 627*

◆ **Dihematoporphyrin Ether** *see* Porfimer *on page 1682*

◆ **Dihydroartemisinin Hemisuccinate Sodium** *see* Artesunate *on page 178*

Dihydrocodeine, Aspirin, and Caffeine

(dye hye droe KOE deen, AS pir in, & KAF een)

Brand Names: U.S. Synalgos®-DC

Index Terms Aspirin, Dihydrocodeine, and Caffeine; Caffeine, Dihydrocodeine, and Aspirin; Dihydrocodeine Compound; Dihydrocodeine, Aspirin, and Caffeine

Pharmacologic Category Analgesic, Opioid

Use Pain: Management of moderate to moderately severe pain

Dosage

Children >12 years, Adolescents, and Adults: Oral: Two capsules (aspirin 712.8 mg/caffeine 60 mg/dihydrocodeine 32 mg) every 4 hours as needed for pain

Elderly: Initial dosing should be cautious (low end of adult dosing range)

Dosage adjustment in renal impairment: There are no dosage adjustments provided in the manufacturer's labeling.

Dosage adjustment in hepatic impairment: There are no dosage adjustments provided in the manufacturer's labeling.

Additional Information Complete prescribing information should be consulted for additional detail.

Dosage Forms

Capsule, oral:

Synalgos®-DC: Dihydrocodeine 16 mg, aspirin 356.4 mg, and caffeine 30 mg

Generic: Dihydrocodeine bitartrate 16 mg, aspirin 356.4 mg, and caffeine 30 mg

◆ **Dihydrocodeine, Aspirin, and Caffeine** *see* Dihydrocodeine, Aspirin, and Caffeine *on page 632*

Dihydrocodeine, Chlorpheniramine, and Phenylephrine

(dye hye droe KOE deen, klor fen IR a meen, & fen il EF rin)

Brand Names: U.S. Coldcough PD [DSC]; Novahistine DH [DSC]; Tusscough DHC [DSC]

Index Terms Chlorpheniramine Maleate, Dihydrocodeine Bitartrate, and Phenylephrine Hydrochloride; Phenylephrine, Chlorpheniramine, and Dihydrocodeine

Pharmacologic Category Alkylamine Derivative; Alpha-Adrenergic Agonist; Analgesic, Opioid; Antitussive; Decongestant; Histamine H_1 Antagonist; Histamine H_1 Antagonist, First Generation

Use Symptomatic relief of cough and congestion associated with the upper respiratory tract

Dosage Cough and congestion: Oral:

Children 2-6 years (Novahistine DH): 1.25-2.5 mL every 4-6 hours as needed (maximum: 10 mL/24 hours)

Children 6-12 years (Novahistine DH): 2.5-5 mL every 4-6 hours as needed (maximum: 20 mL/24 hours)

Children ≥12 years and Adults (Novahistine DH): 5-10 mL every 4-6 hours as needed (maximum: 40 mL/24 hours)

Additional Information Complete prescribing information should be consulted for additional detail.

◆ **Dihydrocodeine Compound** *see* Dihydrocodeine, Aspirin, and Caffeine *on page 632*

Dihydroergotamine (dye hye droe er GOT a meen)

Brand Names: U.S. D.H.E. 45; Migranal

Brand Names: Canada Migranal®

Index Terms DHE; Dihydroergotamine Mesylate

Pharmacologic Category Antimigraine Agent; Ergot Derivative

Use Treatment of migraine headache with or without aura; injection also indicated for treatment of cluster headaches

Pregnancy Risk Factor X

Pregnancy Considerations Dihydroergotamine is oxytocic and should not be used during pregnancy.

Breast-Feeding Considerations Ergot derivatives inhibit prolactin and it is known that ergotamine is excreted in breast milk (vomiting, diarrhea, weak pulse, and unstable blood pressure have been reported in nursing infants). It is not known if dihydroergotamine would also cause these effects, however, it is likely that it is excreted in human breast milk. Do not use in nursing women.

Contraindications Hypersensitivity to dihydroergotamine or any component of the formulation; uncontrolled hypertension, ischemic heart disease, angina pectoris, history of MI, silent ischemia, or coronary artery vasospasm including Prinzmetal's angina; hemiplegic or basilar migraine; peripheral vascular disease; sepsis; severe hepatic or renal dysfunction; following vascular surgery; avoid use within 24 hours of sumatriptan, zolmitriptan, other serotonin agonists, or ergot-like agents; avoid during or within 2 weeks of discontinuing MAO inhibitors; concurrent use of peripheral and central vasoconstrictors; ergot alkaloids are contraindicated with potent inhibitors of CYP3A4 (includes protease inhibitors, azole antifungals, and some macrolide antibiotics); pregnancy, breast-feeding

Warnings/Precautions [U.S. Boxed Warning]: Ergot alkaloids are contraindicated with potent inhibitors of CYP3A4 (includes protease inhibitors, azole antifungals, and some macrolide antibiotics); concomitant use associated with an increased risk of vasospasm leading to cerebral ischemia and/or ischemia of the extremities. Do not give to patients with risk factors for CAD until a cardiovascular evaluation has been performed; if evaluation is satisfactory, the healthcare provider should administer the first dose and cardiovascular status should be periodically evaluated. May cause vasospastic reactions; persistent vasospasm may lead to gangrene or death in patients with compromised circulation. Discontinue if signs of vasoconstriction develop. Rare reports of increased blood pressure in patients without history of hypertension. Rare reports of adverse cardiac events (acute MI, life-threatening arrhythmias, death) have been reported following use of the injection. Cerebral hemorrhage, subarachnoid hemorrhage, and stroke have also occurred following use of the injection. Not for prolonged use. Pleural and peritoneal fibrosis have been reported with prolonged daily use. Cardiac valvular fibrosis has also been associated with ergot alkaloids. Use with caution in the elderly.

Migranal® Nasal Spray: Local irritation to nose and throat (usually transient and mild-moderate in severity) can occur; long-term consequences on nasal or respiratory mucosa have not been extensively evaluated.

Adverse Reactions Nasal spray:

Central nervous system: Dizziness, drowsiness, taste disorder

Endocrine & metabolic: Hot flash

Gastrointestinal: Diarrhea, nausea, vomiting

Local: Application site reaction

Neuromuscular & skeletal: Stiffness, weakness

Respiratory: Pharyngitis, rhinitis

Rare but important or life-threatening: Injection and nasal spray: Abdominal pain, anxiety, cerebral hemorrhage, cerebrovascular accident, coronary artery vasospasm, diaphoresis, diarrhea, dizziness, dyspnea, edema, fibrothorax (prolonged use), flushing, headache, hyperkinesia, hypertension, ischemic heart disease, muscle cramps, myalgia, myasthenia, myocardial infarction, palpitations, paresthesia, peripheral cyanosis, peripheral ischemia, retroperitoneal fibrosis (prolonged use), skin rash, subarachnoid hemorrhage, tremor, valvular sclerosis (associated with ergot alkaloids), ventricular fibrillation, ventricular tachycardia (transient)

Drug Interactions

Metabolism/Transport Effects Substrate of CYP3A4 (major); **Note:** Assignment of Major/Minor substrate status based on clinically relevant drug interaction potential; **Inhibits** CYP3A4 (weak)

Avoid Concomitant Use

Avoid concomitant use of Dihydroergotamine with any of the following: Alpha-/Beta-Agonists; Alpha1-Agonists; Boceprevir; Clarithromycin; Cobicistat; Conivaptan; Crizotinib; Dapoxetine; Enzalutamide; Fusidic Acid (Systemic); Idelalisib; Itraconazole; Ketoconazole (Systemic); Lorcaserin; Mifepristone; Nitroglycerin; Pimozide; Posaconazole; Protease Inhibitors; Serotonin 5-HT1D Receptor Agonists; Telaprevir; Voriconazole

Increased Effect/Toxicity

Dihydroergotamine may increase the levels/effects of: Alpha-/Beta-Agonists; Alpha1-Agonists; Antipsychotic Agents; ARIPiprazole; Dofetilide; Hydrocodone; Lomitapide; Metoclopramide; Pimozide; Serotonin 5-HT1D Receptor Agonists; Serotonin Modulators

The levels/effects of Dihydroergotamine may be increased by: Antiemetics (5HT3 Antagonists); Antipsychotic Agents; Aprepitant; Beta-Blockers; Boceprevir; Ceritinib; Clarithromycin; Cobicistat; Conivaptan; Crizotinib; CYP3A4 Inhibitors (Moderate); CYP3A4 Inhibitors (Strong); Dapoxetine; Dasatinib; Fosaprepitant; Fusidic Acid (Systemic); Idelalisib; Itraconazole; Ivacaftor; Ketoconazole (Systemic); Lorcaserin; Luliconazole; Macrolide Antibiotics; Mifepristone; Netupitant; Nitroglycerin; Posaconazole; Protease Inhibitors; Serotonin 5-HT1D Receptor Agonists; Simeprevir; Stiripentol; Tedizolid; Telaprevir; Voriconazole

Decreased Effect

Dihydroergotamine may decrease the levels/effects of: Nitroglycerin

The levels/effects of Dihydroergotamine may be decreased by: Enzalutamide

Storage/Stability

Injection: Store below 25°C (77°F); do not refrigerate or freeze; protect from heat. Protect from light.

Nasal spray: Prior to use, store below 25°C (77°F); do not refrigerate or freeze. Once spray applicator has been prepared, use within 8 hours; discard any unused solution.

Mechanism of Action Ergot alkaloid alpha-adrenergic blocker directly stimulates vascular smooth muscle to vasoconstrict peripheral and cerebral vessels; also has effects on serotonin receptors

Pharmacodynamics/Kinetics

Onset of action: IM: 15-30 minutes

Duration: IM: 3-4 hours

Distribution: V_d: ~800 L

Protein binding: 93%

Metabolism: Extensively hepatic

Half-life elimination: ~9-10 hours

Time to peak, serum: IM: 24 minutes; IV: 1-2 minutes; Intranasal: 30-60 minutes; SubQ 15-45 minutes

Excretion: Primarily feces; urine (6% to 7% as unchanged drug)

Dosage Adults:

IM, SubQ: 1 mg at first sign of headache; repeat hourly to a maximum dose of 3 mg/day; maximum dose: 6 mg/week

IV: 1 mg at first sign of headache; repeat hourly up to a maximum dose of 2 mg/day; maximum dose: 6 mg/week

Raskin protocol (off-label dosing): Initial test dose: 0.5 mg (following premedication with metoclopramide); subsequent dosing is titrated (range: 0.2-1 mg) every 8 hours for 2-3 days and administered with or without metoclopramide based on response and tolerance (Raskin, 1986; Raskin, 1990). **Note:** Some clinicians use modified versions of this protocol, with additional adjunctive medications and/or alternate antiemetic agents.

Intranasal: 1 spray (0.5 mg) of nasal spray should be administered into each nostril; if needed, repeat after 15 minutes, up to a total of 4 sprays (2 mg). **Note:** Do not exceed 6 sprays (3 mg) in a 24-hour period and no more than 8 sprays (4 mg) in a week.

Elderly: Patients >65 years of age were not included in controlled clinical studies

Dosing adjustment in renal impairment: Contraindicated in severe renal impairment

Dosing adjustment in hepatic impairment: Dosage reductions are probably necessary but specific guidelines are not available; contraindicated in severe hepatic dysfunction

Administration

Intranasal: Prior to administration of nasal spray, the nasal spray applicator must be primed (pumped 4 times); in order to let the drug be absorbed through the skin in the nose, patients should not inhale deeply through the nose while spraying or immediately after spraying; for best results, treatment should be initiated at the first symptom or sign of an attack; however, nasal spray can be used at any stage of a migraine attack.

IM, SubQ: May administer by intramuscular or subcutaneous injection.

IV: Administer slowly over 2-3 minutes (Raskin protocol)

Reference Range Minimum concentration for vasoconstriction is reportedly 0.06 ng/mL

Dosage Forms Considerations Migranal nasal solution contains caffeine 10 mg/mL

Dosage Forms

Solution, Injection:

D.H.E. 45: 1 mg/mL (1 mL)

Generic: 1 mg/mL (1 mL)

Solution, Nasal:

Migranal: 4 mg/mL (1 mL)

Generic: 4 mg/mL (1 mL)

◆ **Dihydroergotamine Mesylate** *see* Dihydroergotamine *on page 633*

◆ **Dihydrohydroxycodeinone** *see* OxyCODONE *on page 1538*

◆ **Dihydromorphinone** *see* HYDROmorphone *on page 1016*

◆ **Dihydroqinghaosu Hemisuccinate Sodium** *see* Artesunate *on page 178*

◆ **Dihydroxyanthracenedione** *see* MitoXANtrone *on page 1382*

◆ **Dihydroxyanthracenedione Dihydrochloride** *see* MitoXANtrone *on page 1382*

◆ **1,25 Dihydroxycholecalciferol** *see* Calcitriol *on page 323*

◆ **Dihydroxydeoxynorvinkaleukoblastine** *see* Vinorelbine *on page 2168*

◆ **Diiodohydroxyquin** *see* Iodoquinol *on page 1105*

◆ **Dilacor XR [DSC]** *see* Diltiazem *on page 634*

◆ **Dilantin** *see* Phenytoin *on page 1640*

◆ **Dilantin Infatabs** *see* Phenytoin *on page 1640*

◆ **Dilatrate-SR** *see* Isosorbide Dinitrate *on page 1124*

◆ **Dilaudid** *see* HYDROmorphone *on page 1016*

◆ **Dilaudid-HP** *see* HYDROmorphone *on page 1016*

◆ **Dilt-CD [DSC]** *see* Diltiazem *on page 634*

Diltiazem (dil TYE a zem)

Brand Names: U.S. Cardizem; Cardizem CD; Cardizem LA; Cartia XT; Dilacor XR [DSC]; Dilt-CD [DSC]; Dilt-XR; Diltiazem HCl CD [DSC]; Diltzac [DSC]; Matzim LA; Taztia XT; Tiazac

Brand Names: Canada ACT Diltiazem CD; ACT Diltiazem T; Apo-Diltiaz; Apo-Diltiaz CD; Apo-Diltiaz SR; Apo-Diltiaz TZ; Ava-Diltiazem; Cardizem CD; Diltiazem Hydrochloride Injection; Diltiazem TZ; Diltiazem-CD; PMS-Diltiazem CD; ratio-Diltiazem CD; Sandoz-Diltiazem CD; Sandoz-Diltiazem T; Teva-Diltiazem; Teva-Diltiazem CD; Teva-Diltiazem HCL ER Capsules; Tiazac; Tiazac XC

Index Terms Diltiazem Hydrochloride

Pharmacologic Category Antianginal Agent; Antiarrhythmic Agent, Class IV; Antihypertensive; Calcium Channel Blocker; Calcium Channel Blocker, Nondihydropyridine

Use

Oral: Primary hypertension; chronic stable angina or angina from coronary artery spasm

The 2014 guideline for the management of high blood pressure in adults (JNC 8) recommends initiation of pharmacologic treatment to lower blood pressure for the following patients (JNC8 [James, 2013]):

- Patients ≥60 years of age, with systolic blood pressure (SBP) ≥150 mm Hg or diastolic blood pressure (DBP) ≥90 mm Hg. Goal of therapy is SBP <150 mm Hg and DBP <90 mm Hg.
- Patients <60 years of age, with SBP ≥140 mm Hg or DBP ≥90 mm Hg. Goal of therapy is SBP <140 mm Hg and DBP <90 mm Hg.
- Patients ≥18 years of age with diabetes, with SBP ≥140 mm Hg or DBP ≥90 mm Hg. Goal of therapy is SBP <140 mm Hg and DBP <90 mm Hg.

- Patients ≥18 years of age with chronic kidney disease (CKD), with SBP ≥140 mm Hg or DBP ≥90 mm Hg. Goal of therapy is SBP <140 mm Hg and DBP <90 mm Hg.

In patients with chronic kidney disease (CKD), regardless of race or diabetes status, the use of an ACE inhibitor (ACEI) or angiotensin receptor blocker (ARB) as initial therapy is recommended to improve kidney outcomes. In the general nonblack population (without CKD) including those with diabetes, initial antihypertensive treatment should consist of a thiazide-type diuretic, calcium channel blocker, ACEI, or ARB. In the general black population (without CKD) including those with diabetes, initial antihypertensive treatment should consist of a thiazide-type diuretic or a calcium channel blocker **instead of** an ACEI or ARB.

Injection: Control of rapid ventricular rate in patients with atrial fibrillation or atrial flutter; conversion of paroxysmal supraventricular tachycardia (PSVT)

Pregnancy Risk Factor C

Pregnancy Considerations Adverse events have been observed in animal reproduction studies. Untreated chronic maternal hypertension is associated with adverse events in the fetus, infant, and mother. If treatment for hypertension during pregnancy is needed, other agents are preferred (ACOG, 2013). The Canadian labeling contraindicates use in pregnant women or women of childbearing potential. Women with hypertrophic cardiomyopathy who are controlled with diltiazem prior to pregnancy may continue therapy, but increased fetal monitoring is recommended (Gersh, 2011).

Breast-Feeding Considerations Diltiazem is excreted into breastmilk in concentrations similar to those in the maternal plasma (Okada, 1985). Breast-feeding is not recommended by the manufacturer.

Contraindications

Oral: Hypersensitivity to diltiazem or any component of the formulation; sick sinus syndrome (except in patients with a functioning artificial pacemaker); second- or third-degree AV block (except in patients with a functioning artificial pacemaker); severe hypotension (systolic <90 mm Hg); acute MI and pulmonary congestion

Intravenous (IV): Hypersensitivity to diltiazem or any component of the formulation; sick sinus syndrome (except in patients with a functioning artificial pacemaker); second- or third-degree AV block (except in patients with a functioning artificial pacemaker); severe hypotension (systolic <90 mm Hg); cardiogenic shock; administration concomitantly or within a few hours of the administration of IV beta-blockers; atrial fibrillation or flutter associated with accessory bypass tract (eg, Wolff-Parkinson-White syndrome); ventricular tachycardia (with wide-complex tachycardia, must determine whether origin is supraventricular or ventricular)

Canadian labeling: Additional contraindications (not in U.S. labeling): IV and Oral: Pregnancy; use in women of childbearing potential; concurrent use with intravenous dantrolene

Warnings/Precautions Can cause first-, second-, and third-degree AV block or sinus bradycardia and risk increases with agents known to slow cardiac conduction. The most common side effect is peripheral edema; occurs within 2-3 weeks of starting therapy. Symptomatic hypotension with or without syncope can rarely occur; blood pressure must be lowered at a rate appropriate for the patient's clinical condition. Ethanol may increase risk of hypotension or vasodilation. Advise patients to avoid ethanol. Use caution when using diltiazem together with a beta-blocker; may result in conduction disturbances, hypotension, and worsened LV function. Simultaneous administration of IV diltiazem and an IV beta-blocker or administration within a few hours of each other may result in asystole and is contraindicated. Use with other agents known to either reduce SA node function and/or AV nodal conduction (eg, digoxin) or reduce sympathetic outflow (eg, clonidine) may increase the risk of serious bradycardia. Use caution in left ventricular dysfunction (may exacerbate condition). The ACCF/AHA heart failure guidelines recommend to avoid use in patients with heart failure due to lack of benefit and/or worse outcomes with calcium channel blockers in general (ACCF/AHA [Yancy, 2013]). Use with caution with hypertrophic obstructive cardiomyopathy; routine use is currently not recommended due to insufficient evidence (Maron, 2003). Use with caution in hepatic or renal dysfunction. Transient dermatologic reactions have been observed with use; if reaction persists, discontinue. May (rarely) progress to erythema multiforme or exfoliative dermatitis.

Adverse Reactions

Cardiovascular: Atrioventricular block (first degree), bradycardia, edema (including lower limb), extrasystoles, flushing, hypotension, palpitations, vasodilatation

Central nervous system: Dizziness, headache, nervousness, pain

Dermatologic: Skin rash

Endocrine & metabolic: Gout

Gastrointestinal: Constipation, diarrhea, dyspepsia, vomiting

Local: Injection site reaction (itching, burning)

Neuromuscular & skeletal: Myalgia, weakness

Respiratory: Bronchitis, dyspnea, pharyngitis, rhinitis sinus congestion

Rare but important or life-threatening: amblyopia, amnesia, atrioventricular block (second or third degree), bundle branch block, cardiac arrhythmia, cardiac failure, depression, dysgeusia, extrapyramidal reaction, gingival hyperplasia, hemolytic anemia, hypersensitivity reaction, increased serum alkaline phosphatase, increased serum ALT, increased serum AST, petechiae, skin photosensitivity, Stevens-Johnson syndrome, syncope, tachycardia, thrombocytopenia, tremor, toxic epidermal necrolysis

Drug Interactions

Metabolism/Transport Effects Substrate of CYP2C9 (minor), CYP2D6 (minor), CYP3A4 (major), P-glycoprotein; **Note:** Assignment of Major/Minor substrate status based on clinically relevant drug interaction potential; **Inhibits** CYP2C9 (weak), CYP2D6 (weak), CYP3A4 (moderate)

Avoid Concomitant Use

Avoid concomitant use of Diltiazem with any of the following: Bosutinib; Ceritinib; Conivaptan; Dantrolene; Fusidic Acid (Systemic); Ibrutinib; Idelalisib; Ivabradine; Lomitapide; Naloxegol; Olaparib; Pimozide; Simeprevir; Tolvaptan; Trabectedin; Ulipristal

Increased Effect/Toxicity

Diltiazem may increase the levels/effects of: Alfentanil; Amifostine; Amiodarone; Antihypertensives; Aprepitant; ARIPiprazole; AtorvaSTATin; Atosiban; Avanafil; Beta-Blockers; Bosentan; Bosutinib; Bradycardia-Causing Agents; Budesonide (Systemic, Oral Inhalation); BusPIRone; Calcium Channel Blockers (Dihydropyridine); Cannabis; CarBAMazepine; Cardiac Glycosides; Ceritinib; Colchicine; CycloSPORINE (Systemic); CYP3A4 Substrates; Dapoxetine; Dofetilide; DOXOrubicin (Conventional); Dronabinol; Dronedarone; DULoxetine; Eletriptan; Eliglustat; Eplerenone; Everolimus; FentaNYL; Fingolimod; Fosaprepitant; Fosphenytoin; Halofantrine; Hydrocodone; Hypotensive Agents; Ibrutinib; Imatinib; Ivabradine; Ivacaftor; Lacosamide; Levodopa; Lithium; Lomitapide; Lovastatin; Lurasidone; Magnesium Salts; Midodrine; Naloxegol; Neuromuscular-Blocking Agents (Nondepolarizing); Nitroprusside; Obinutuzumab; Olaparib; OxyCODONE; Phenytoin; Pimecrolimus; Pimozide; Propafenone; QuiNIDine; Ranolazine; Red Yeast Rice; RisperiDONE; RiTUXimab; Rivaroxaban;

Salicylates; Salmeterol; Saxagliptin; Simeprevir; Simvastatin; Suvorexant; Tacrolimus (Systemic); Tacrolimus (Topical); Tetrahydrocannabinol; Tolvaptan; Trabectedin; Ulipristal; Vilazodone; Zopiclone; Zuclopenthixol

The levels/effects of Diltiazem may be increased by: Alfuzosin; Alpha1-Blockers; Anilidopiperidine Opioids; Antifungal Agents (Azole Derivatives, Systemic); Aprepitant; AtorvaSTATin; Barbiturates; Bretylium; Brimonidine (Topical); Calcium Channel Blockers (Dihydropyridine); Cimetidine; CloNIDine; Conivaptan; CycloSPORINE (Systemic); CYP3A4 Inhibitors (Moderate); CYP3A4 Inhibitors (Strong); Dantrolene; Dasatinib; Diazoxide; Dronedarone; Fluconazole; Fosaprepitant; Fusidic Acid (Systemic); Grapefruit Juice; Herbs (Hypotensive Properties); Idelalisib; Ivabradine; Lovastatin; Luliconazole; Macrolide Antibiotics; Magnesium Salts; MAO Inhibitors; Mifepristone; Netupitant; Nicorandil; Pentoxifylline; P-glycoprotein/ABCB1 Inhibitors; Phosphodiesterase 5 Inhibitors; Prostacyclin Analogues; Protease Inhibitors; Regorafenib; Simvastatin; Stiripentol; Tofacitinib

Decreased Effect

Diltiazem may decrease the levels/effects of: Clopidogrel; Ifosfamide

The levels/effects of Diltiazem may be decreased by: Barbiturates; Bosentan; Calcium Salts; CarBAMazepine; Colestipol; CYP3A4 Inducers (Moderate); CYP3A4 Inducers (Strong); Dabrafenib; Deferasirox; Efavirenz; Herbs (Hypertensive Properties); Methylphenidate; Mitotane; Nafcillin; P-glycoprotein/ABCB1 Inducers; Rifamycin Derivatives; Siltuximab; St Johns Wort; Tocilizumab; Yohimbine

Food Interactions Diltiazem serum levels may be elevated if taken with food. Serum concentrations were not altered by grapefruit juice in small clinical trials.

Storage/Stability

Capsule, tablet: Store at room temperature. Protect from light.

Solution for injection: Store in refrigerator at 2°C to 8°C (36°F to 46°F); do not freeze. May be stored at room temperature for up to 1 month. Following dilution to ≤1 mg/mL with $D_5{}^1/_2NS$, D_5W, or NS, solution is stable for 24 hours at room temperature or under refrigeration.

Mechanism of Action Nondihydropyridine calcium channel blocker which inhibits calcium ion from entering the "slow channels" or select voltage-sensitive areas of vascular smooth muscle and myocardium during depolarization, producing a relaxation of coronary vascular smooth muscle and coronary vasodilation; increases myocardial oxygen delivery in patients with vasospastic angina

Pharmacodynamics/Kinetics

Onset of action: Oral: Immediate release tablet: 30-60 minutes; IV: 3 minutes

Duration: IV: Bolus: 1-3 hours; Continuous infusion (after discontinuation): 0.5-10 hours

Absorption: Immediate release tablet: >90%; Extended release capsule: ~93%

Distribution: V_d: 3-13 L/kg

Protein binding: 70% to 80%

Metabolism: Hepatic (extensive first-pass effect); following single IV injection, plasma concentrations of N-monodesmethyldiltiazem and desacetyldiltiazem are typically undetectable; however, these metabolites accumulate to detectable concentrations following 24-hour constant rate infusion. N-monodesmethyldiltiazem appears to have 20% of the potency of diltiazem; desacetyldiltiazem is about 25% to 50% as potent as the parent compound.

Bioavailability: Oral: ~40% (undergoes extensive first-pass metabolism)

Half-life elimination: Immediate release tablet: 3-4.5 hours, may be prolonged with renal impairment; Extended release tablet: 6-9 hours; Extended release capsules: 5-10 hours; IV: single dose: ~3.4 hours; continuous infusion: 4-5 hours

Time to peak, serum: Immediate release tablet: 2-4 hours; Extended release tablet: 11-18 hours; Extended release capsule: 10-14 hours

Excretion: Urine (2% to 4% as unchanged drug; 6% to 7% as metabolites); feces

Dosage

Children (off-label use): Minimal information available; some centers use the following: Oral: Hypertension: Immediate release tablets: Initial: 1.5-2 mg/kg/day divided in 3 doses/day (maximum dose 6 mg/kg/day up to 360 mg daily) (Flynn, 2000)

Adults:

Oral:

Angina:

Capsule, extended release:

Dilacor XR, Dilt-XR, Diltia XT: Initial: 120 mg once daily; titrate over 7-14 days; usual dose range: 120-320 mg daily: maximum: 480 mg daily

Cardizem CD, Cartia XT, Dilt-CD: Initial: 120-180 mg once daily; titrate over 7-14 days; usual dose range: 120-320 mg daily; maximum: 480 mg daily

Tiazac, Taztia XT: Initial: 120-180 mg once daily; titrate over 7-14 days; usual dose range: 120-320 mg daily; maximum: 540 mg daily

Tablet, extended release (Cardizem LA, Matzim LA, Tiazac XC [CAN; not available in U.S.]): 180 mg once daily; may increase at 7- to 14-day intervals; usual dose range: 120-320 mg daily; maximum: 360 mg daily

Tablet, immediate release (Cardizem): Usual starting dose: 30 mg 4 times daily; titrate dose gradually at 1- to 2-day intervals; usual dose range: 120-320 mg daily

Hypertension:

Capsule, extended release (once-daily dosing):

Cardizem CD, Cartia XT, Dilt-CD: Initial: 180-240 mg once daily; dose adjustment may be made after 14 days; usual dose range (ASH/ISH [Weber, 2014]): 240-360 mg daily; maximum: 480 mg daily

Dilacor XR, Diltia XT, Dilt-XR: Initial: 180-240 mg once daily; dose adjustment may be made after 14 days; usual dose range (ASH/ISH [Weber, 2014]): 240-360 mg daily; maximum: 540 mg daily

Tiazac, Taztia XT: Initial: 120-240 mg once daily; dose adjustment may be made after 14 days; usual dose range (ASH/ISH [Weber, 2014]): 240-360 mg daily; maximum: 540 mg daily

Capsule, extended release (twice-daily dosing): Initial: 60-120 mg twice daily; dose adjustment may be made after 14 days; usual range: 240-360 mg daily

Note: Diltiazem is available as a generic intended for either once- or twice-daily dosing, depending on the formulation; verify appropriate extended release capsule formulation is administered.

Tablet, extended release (Cardizem LA, Matzim LA, Tiazac XC [CAN; not available in U.S.]): Initial: 180-240 mg once daily; dose adjustment may be made after 14 days; usual dose range (ASH/ISH [Weber, 2014]): 240-360 mg daily

Note: Elderly: Consider lower initial doses (eg, 120 mg once daily using extended release capsule) and titrate to response (Aronow, 2011)

Atrial fibrillation (rate control) (off-label use): Extended release (capsule or tablet): Usual maintenance dose: 120 to 360 mg once daily (AHA/ACC/HRS [January, 2014])

IV: *Atrial fibrillation, atrial flutter, PSVT:*

Initial bolus dose: 0.25 mg/kg actual body weight over 2 minutes (average adult dose: 20 mg); ACLS guideline recommends 15-20 mg

Repeat bolus dose (may be administered after 15 minutes if the response is inadequate): 0.35 mg/kg actual body weight over 2 minutes (average adult dose: 25 mg); ACLS guideline recommends 20-25 mg

Continuous infusion (infusions >24 hours or infusion rates >15 mg/hour are not recommended): Initial infusion rate of 10 mg/hour; rate may be increased in 5 mg/hour increments up to 15 mg/hour as needed; some patients may respond to an initial rate of 5 mg/hour.

If diltiazem injection is administered by continuous infusion for >24 hours, the possibility of decreased diltiazem clearance, prolonged elimination half-life, and increased diltiazem and/or diltiazem metabolite plasma concentrations should be considered.

Conversion from IV diltiazem to oral diltiazem:

Oral dose (mg daily) is approximately equal to [rate (mg/hour) x 3 + 3] x 10.

3 mg/hour = 120 mg daily
5 mg/hour = 180 mg daily
7 mg/hour = 240 mg daily
11 mg/hour = 360 mg daily

Dosing adjustment in renal impairment: Use with caution; no dosing adjustments recommended

Dialysis: Not removed by hemo- or peritoneal dialysis; supplemental dose is not necessary.

Dosing adjustment in hepatic impairment: Use with caution; no specific dosing recommendations available; extensively metabolized by the liver; half-life is increased in patients with cirrhosis

Usual Infusion Concentrations: Pediatric IV infusion: 1 mg/mL

Usual Infusion Concentrations: Adult IV infusion: 125 mg in 125 mL (total volume) (concentration: 1 mg/mL) of D_5W or NS

Administration

Oral:

Immediate release tablet (Cardizem): Administer before meals and at bedtime. Do not split, crush, or chew; swallow whole.

Long acting dosage forms: Do not open, chew, or crush; swallow whole.

Cardizem CD, Cardizem LA, Cartia XT, Dilt-CD, Matzim LA: May be administered without regards to meals.

Dilacor XR, Dilt-XR, Diltia XT: Administer on an empty stomach.

Taztia XT, Tiazac: Capsules may be opened and sprinkled on a spoonful of applesauce. Applesauce should not be hot and should be swallowed without chewing, followed by drinking a glass of water.

Tiazac XC [CAN; not available in U.S.]: Administer at bedtime

IV: Bolus doses given over 2 minutes with continuous ECG and blood pressure monitoring. Continuous infusion should be via infusion pump. Response to bolus may require several minutes to reach maximum. Response may persist for several hours after infusion is discontinued.

Monitoring Parameters Liver function tests, blood pressure, ECG, heart rate; consult individual institutional policies and procedures

Dosage Forms

Capsule Extended Release 12 Hour, Oral:
Generic: 60 mg, 90 mg, 120 mg

Capsule Extended Release 24 Hour, Oral:
Cardizem CD: 120 mg, 180 mg, 240 mg, 300 mg, 360 mg
Cartia XT: 120 mg, 180 mg, 240 mg, 300 mg
Dilt-XR: 120 mg, 180 mg, 240 mg
Taztia XT: 120 mg, 180 mg, 240 mg, 300 mg, 360 mg
Tiazac: 120 mg, 180 mg, 240 mg, 300 mg, 360 mg, 420 mg
Generic: 120 mg, 180 mg, 240 mg, 300 mg, 360 mg, 420 mg

Solution, Intravenous:
Generic: 25 mg/5 mL (5 mL, 25 mL); 50 mg/10 mL (10 mL); 125 mg/25 mL (25 mL)

Solution, Intravenous [preservative free]:
Generic: 50 mg/10 mL (10 mL); 125 mg/25 mL (25 mL)

Solution Reconstituted, Intravenous:
Generic: 100 mg (1 ea)

Tablet, Oral:
Cardizem: 30 mg, 60 mg, 120 mg
Generic: 30 mg, 60 mg, 90 mg, 120 mg

Tablet Extended Release 24 Hour, Oral:
Cardizem LA: 120 mg, 180 mg, 240 mg, 300 mg, 360 mg, 420 mg
Matzim LA: 180 mg, 240 mg, 300 mg, 360 mg, 420 mg
Generic: 180 mg, 240 mg, 300 mg, 360 mg, 420 mg

Dosage Forms: Canada Note: Also refer to Dosage Forms.

Tablet, Extended Release, Oral:
Tiazac XC: 120 mg, 180 mg, 240 mg, 300 mg, 360 mg

Extemporaneous Preparations A 12 mg/mL oral suspension may be made from tablets (regular, not extended release) and one of three different vehicles (cherry syrup, a 1:1 mixture of Ora-Sweet® and Ora-Plus®, or a 1:1 mixture of Ora-Sweet® SF and Ora-Plus®). Crush sixteen 90 mg tablets in a mortar and reduce to a fine powder. Add 10 mL of the chosen vehicle and mix to a uniform paste; mix while adding the vehicle in incremental proportions to **almost** 120 mL; transfer to a calibrated bottle, rinse mortar with vehicle, and add quantity of vehicle sufficient to make 120 mL. Label "shake well" and "protect from light". Stable for 60 days when stored in amber plastic prescription bottles in the dark at room temperature or refrigerated.

Allen LV and Erickson MA, "Stability of Baclofen, Captopril, Diltiazem Hydrochloride, Dipyridamole, and Flecainide Acetate in Extemporaneously Compounded Oral Liquids," *Am J Health Syst Pharm*, 1996, 53(18):2179-84.

◆ **Diltiazem-CD (Can)** *see* Diltiazem *on page 634*
◆ **Diltiazem HCl CD [DSC]** *see* Diltiazem *on page 634*
◆ **Diltiazem Hydrochloride** *see* Diltiazem *on page 634*
◆ **Diltiazem Hydrochloride Injection (Can)** *see* Diltiazem *on page 634*
◆ **Diltiazem TZ (Can)** *see* Diltiazem *on page 634*
◆ **Dilt-XR** *see* Diltiazem *on page 634*
◆ **Diltzac [DSC]** *see* Diltiazem *on page 634*

Dimemorfan [INT] (dye me MOR fan)

International Brand Names Astomin (JP); Dastosin (ES); Gentus (IT); Tusben (IT)

Index Terms Dimemorfan Phosphate

Pharmacologic Category Antitussive

Dosage Range Adults: Oral: 10-20 mg 3-4 times/day

Product Availability Product available in various countries; not currently available in the U.S.

Dosage Forms
Capsule: 20 mg
Solution, oral: 10 mg/5 mL (150 mL, 250 mL)

◆ **Dimemorfan Phosphate** *see* Dimemorfan [INT] *on page 637*

DimenhyDRINATE (dye men HYE dri nate)

Brand Names: U.S. Dramamine [OTC]; Driminate [OTC]; Motion Sickness [OTC]

Brand Names: Canada Apo-Dimenhydrinate [OTC]; Children's Motion Sickness Liquid [OTC]; Dimenhydrinate Injection; Dinate [OTC]; Gravol IM; Gravol [OTC]; Jamp-Dimenhydrinate [OTC]; Nauseatol [OTC]; Novo-Dimenate [OTC]; PMS-Dimenhydrinate [OTC]; Sandoz-Dimenhydrinate [OTC]; Travel Tabs [OTC]

Pharmacologic Category Ethanolamine Derivative; Histamine H_1 Antagonist; Histamine H_1 Antagonist, First Generation

Additional Appendix Information

Beers Criteria – Potentially Inappropriate Medications for Geriatrics *on page 2271*

Use

Motion sickness: Treatment and prevention of nausea, vertigo, and vomiting associated with motion sickness.

Note: In Canada, dimenhydrinate is also approved for the treatment and prevention of radiation sickness, postoperative vomiting, and drug-induced vomiting; and for the treatment of nausea, vomiting, and vertigo due to Mènière disease and other labyrinthine disturbances

Pregnancy Risk Factor B

Dosage

Motion sickness, nausea/vomiting, or vertigo:

Oral:

Children 2 to 5 years: 12.5 to 25 mg every 6 to 8 hours, maximum: 75 mg daily

Children 6 to 12 years: 25 to 50 mg every 6 to 8 hours, maximum: 150 mg daily

Adults: 50 to 100 mg every 4 to 6 hours, not to exceed 400 mg daily

IM:

Children: 1.25 mg/kg **or** 37.5 mg/m^2 4 times daily; maximum: 300 mg daily

Adults: 50 mg every 4 hours; maximum: 100 mg every 4 hours

IV: Adults: 50 mg every 4 hours; maximum: 100 mg every 4 hours

Rectal suppository [Canadian product]:

Children 6 to 8 years: 12.5 to 25 mg 2 to 3 times daily

Children 9 to 12 years: 25 to 50 mg 2 to 3 times daily

Adolescents ≥13 years: 50 mg 2 to 3 times daily

Adults: 50 to 100 mg 3 to 4 times daily

Dosage adjustment in renal impairment: There are no dosage adjustments provided in the manufacturer's labeling.

Dosage adjustment in hepatic impairment: There are no dosage adjustments provided in the manufacturer's labeling.

Additional Information Complete prescribing information should be consulted for additional detail.

Dosage Forms

Solution, Injection:

Generic: 50 mg/mL (1 mL)

Tablet, Oral:

Dramamine [OTC]: 50 mg

Driminate [OTC]: 50 mg

Motion Sickness [OTC]: 50 mg

Generic: 50 mg

Tablet Chewable, Oral:

Dramamine [OTC]: 50 mg

Dosage Forms: Canada

Suppository, Rectal:

Sandoz-Dimenhydrinate: 50 mg, 100 mg

◆ **Dimenhydrinate Injection (Can)** *see* DimenhyDRINATE *on page 637*

Dimercaprol (dye mer KAP role)

Brand Names: U.S. Bal in Oil

Index Terms 2,3-Dimercapto-1-Propanol; 2,3-Dimercaptopropan-1-Ol; 2,3-Dimercaptopropanol; BAL; British Anti-Lewisite; Dithioglycerol

Pharmacologic Category Antidote

Use Antidote to gold, arsenic (except arsine), or acute mercury poisoning (except nonalkyl mercury); adjunct to edetate CALCIUM disodium in acute lead poisoning

Pregnancy Risk Factor C

Dosage Note: Premedication with a histamine H_1 antagonist (eg, diphenhydramine) is recommended.

Children and Adults: Deep IM:

Arsenic or gold poisoning (acute, mild): 2.5 mg/kg every 6 hours for 2 days, then every 12 hours for 1 day, followed by once daily for 10 days

Arsenic or gold poisoning (acute, severe): 3 mg/kg every 4 hours for 2 days, then every 6 hours for 1 day, followed every 12 hours for 10 days

Mercury poisoning (acute): 5 mg/kg initially, followed by 2.5 mg/kg 1-2 times/day for 10 days

Lead poisoning: **Note:** For the treatment of high blood lead levels in children, the CDC recommends chelation treatment when blood lead levels are >45 mcg/dL (CDC, 2002); however, dimercaprol is only recommended for use (in combination with edetate CALCIUM disodium) in children whose blood lead levels are >70 mcg/dL or in children with lead encephalopathy (AAP, 2005; Chandran, 2010). In adults, available guidelines recommend chelation therapy with blood lead levels >50 mcg/dL and significant symptoms; chelation therapy may also be indicated with blood lead levels ≥100 mcg/dL and/or symptoms (Kosnett, 2007).

Blood lead levels ≥70 mcg/dL, symptomatic lead poisoning, or lead encephalopathy (in conjunction with edetate CALCIUM disodium): 4 mg/kg every 4 hours for 2-7 days; duration of therapy of at least 3 days is recommended by some experts (Chandran, 2010). **Note:** Begin treatment with edetate CALCIUM disodium with the second dimercaprol dose.

Dosage adjustment in renal impairment: No specific adjustment provided in manufacturer's labeling. Use with extreme caution or discontinue if acute renal insufficiency develops during therapy.

Dosage adjustment in hepatic impairment: Use is contraindicated in hepatic insufficiency (except in cases of postarsenical jaundice).

Additional Information Complete prescribing information should be consulted for additional detail.

Dosage Forms

Solution, Intramuscular:

Bal in Oil: 100 mg/mL (3 mL)

◆ **2,3-Dimercapto-1-Propanol** *see* Dimercaprol *on page 638*

◆ **2,3-Dimercaptopropan-1-Ol** *see* Dimercaprol *on page 638*

◆ **2,3-Dimercaptopropanol** *see* Dimercaprol *on page 638*

◆ **Dimetapp® Children's Long Acting Cough Plus Cold [OTC]** *see* Dextromethorphan and Chlorpheniramine *on page 610*

◆ **Dimetapp® Children's Nighttime Cold & Congestion [OTC]** *see* Diphenhydramine and Phenylephrine *on page 644*

Dimethindene [INT] (dye meth IN deen)

International Brand Names Fenistil (AT, BE, CH, DE, ES, GR, IL, IT, NL, NO, PT, TH); Foristal (IN); Neostil (PT)

Index Terms Dimethindene Maleate; Dimetindene

Pharmacologic Category Antihistamine

Reported Use Symptomatic treatment of allergic conditions; pruritus; prevention of hypersensitivity reactions; adjuvant treatment of anaphylactic reactions and serum sickness

Dosage Range Adults: Oral: 1-2 mg 3 times/day

Product Availability Product available in various countries; not currently available in the U.S.

Dosage Forms

Tablet: 1 mg

◆ **Dimethindene Maleate** *see* Dimethindene [INT] *on page 638*

Dimethyl Fumarate (dye meth il FYOO ma rate)

Brand Names: U.S. Tecfidera

Brand Names: Canada Tecfidera

Index Terms BG-12; Dimethylfumarate; DMF; FAG-201

Pharmacologic Category Fumaric Acid Derivative; Immunomodulator, Systemic

Use Multiple sclerosis, relapsing: Treatment of relapsing forms of multiple sclerosis (MS)

Pregnancy Risk Factor C

Pregnancy Considerations Adverse events were observed in animal reproduction studies.

Women exposed to dimethyl fumarate during pregnancy are encouraged to enroll in the Pregnancy Registry by calling 866-810-1462 or visiting www.tecfiderapregnancyregistry.com.

Breast-Feeding Considerations It is not known if dimethyl fumarate is excreted into breast milk. The manufacturer recommends caution be used if administered to nursing women.

Contraindications Hypersensitivity to dimethyl fumarate or any component of the formulation

Warnings/Precautions Dimethyl fumarate should only be prescribed by health care providers who are experienced in the diagnosis and management of multiple sclerosis. Anaphylaxis and angioedema may occur after the first dose or at any time during treatment. Discontinue therapy if signs and symptoms of anaphylaxis or angioedema occur. Progressive multifocal leukoencephalopathy (PML) with fatality has been reported (rare); withhold therapy immediately at the first sign or symptom suggestive of PML (eg, progressive weakness on one side of the body or clumsiness of limbs; vision disturbances; mental status changes).

Decreased lymphocyte counts may occur with use. Obtain a CBC including lymphocyte count prior to initiation of therapy, after 6 months of treatment, every 6 to 12 months thereafter, and as clinically indicated. Consider therapy interruption in patients with lymphocyte counts $<0.5 \times 10^9$/L persisting >6 months and in patients with signs and symptoms of serious infections. The Canadian labeling recommends additional CBC monitoring prior to switching patients to other therapies known to reduce lymphocyte counts and that dimethyl fumarate treatment not be initiated in patients who are immunocompromised due to other treatments (eg, antineoplastic, immunosuppressive or immune modulating therapies) or disease (eg, immunodeficiency syndrome) or in patients with signs/symptoms of a serious infection.

Use commonly causes GI events (eg, nausea, vomiting, diarrhea, abdominal pain, dyspepsia) and mild-to-moderate flushing (eg, warmth, redness, itching, burning sensation). GI events generally occur in the first month of use and decrease thereafter. To improve tolerability, administer with food or temporarily reduce the dosage. Flushing generally appears soon after initiation, and improves or resolves with subsequent dosing. Administration with food may decrease flushing incidence. Administration of aspirin (nonenteric coated ≤325 mg) 30 minutes prior to dimethyl fumarate or a temporary dose reduction may also reduce the incidence and severity of flushing. The Canadian labeling does not recommend use of aspirin >4 days for the management of flushing (has not been studied). The Canadian labeling recommends caution be exercised when administering in patients with severe active GI disease.

Transaminase elevations (usually <3 times ULN) were observed, generally occurring in the first 6 months of treatment. Use may cause rash, pruritus, or erythema. There are case reports of contact dermatitis resulting from dimethyl fumarate (DMF) exposure after use as a fungicide and desiccant in the shipping of furniture (Bruze, 2011; Giménez-Arnau, 2011; Ropper, 2012). In clinical trials, proteinuria was reported at a slightly higher incidence than that observed with placebo; significance of these findings is unknown. Potentially significant interactions may exist, requiring dose or frequency adjustment, additional monitoring, and/or selection of alternative therapy.

Adverse Reactions

Cardiovascular: Flushing

Dermatologic: Erythema, pruritus, skin rash

Gastrointestinal: Abdominal pain, diarrhea, dyspepsia, nausea, vomiting

Genitourinary: Proteinuria

Infection: Infection

Hematologic: Lymphocytopenia

Hepatic: Increased serum AST

Rare but important or life-threatening: Anaphylaxis, angioedema, eosinophilia (transient), progressive multifocal leukoencephalopathy

Drug Interactions

Metabolism/Transport Effects None known.

Avoid Concomitant Use There are no known interactions where it is recommended to avoid concomitant use.

Increased Effect/Toxicity

Dimethyl Fumarate may increase the levels/effects of: Vaccines (Live)

Decreased Effect

Dimethyl Fumarate may decrease the levels/effects of: Vaccines (Live)

Storage/Stability Store at 15°C to 30°C (50°F to 86°F). Protect capsules from light and store in the original container. Once opened, discard after 90 days.

Mechanism of Action DMF and its active metabolite, monomethyl fumarate (MMF), have been shown to activate the nuclear factor (erythroid-derived 2)-like 2 (Nrf2) pathway, which is involved in cellular response to oxidative stress. The mechanism by which dimethyl fumarate (DMF) exerts a therapeutic effect in MS is unknown, although it is believed to result from its anti-inflammatory and cytoprotective properties via activation of the Nrf2 pathway (Fox, 2012; Gold, 2012).

Pharmacodynamics/Kinetics

Distribution: V_d: MMF: 53 to 73 L

Protein binding: MMF: 27% to 45%

Metabolism: Undergoes rapid and extensive presystemic hydrolysis by esterases to its active metabolite, monomethyl fumarate (MMF); MMF is further metabolized via the tricarboxylic acid (TCA) cycle. Major serum metabolites include: MMF, fumaric acid, citric acid, and glucose.

Half-life elimination: MMF: ~1 hour

Time to peak: 2 to 2.5 hours; delayed to 5.5 hours with food

Excretion: CO_2 via exhalation (~60%); urine (16%; trace amounts as unchanged MMF), feces (1%)

Dosage Multiple sclerosis (relapsing): Adults: Oral: Initial: 120 mg twice daily for 7 days; then increase to the maintenance dose: 240 mg twice daily

Dosing adjustment for toxicity:

Flushing, GI intolerance, or intolerance to maintenance dose: Consider temporary dose reduction to 120 mg twice daily (resume recommended maintenance dose of 240 mg twice daily within 1 month). Consider discontinuation in patients who cannot tolerate return to the recommended maintenance dose.

Serious infection: Consider withholding treatment until infection resolves.

Dosage adjustment in renal impairment: No dosage adjustment necessary.

Dosage adjustment in hepatic impairment: No dosage adjustment necessary.

Dietary Considerations Taking with food may decrease the incidence or severity of flushing.

Administration Swallow capsules whole; do not crush, chew, open the capsule, or sprinkle contents on food. Administer with or without food; administering with food may decrease the incidence of flushing. Administration of aspirin (nonenteric coated ≤325 mg) 30 minutes prior to dimethyl fumarate may also reduce the incidence and severity of flushing. Canadian labeling suggests that missed doses may be taken if ≥4 hours lapse between the morning and evening doses.

Monitoring Parameters CBC including lymphocyte count (obtained prior to imitation of therapy, after 6 months of treatment, then every 6 to 12 months thereafter and as clinically necessary).

Canadian labeling recommends obtaining a CBC, hepatic transaminases, and a urinalysis within 6 months prior to use, after 6 months of therapy, then every 6 to 12 months during therapy and as clinically indicated.

Additional Information Dimethyl fumarate (DMF) has been implicated as the cause of an outbreak of contact dermatitis in Europe resulting from DMF's use as a fungicide and desiccant in the shipping of furniture (Bruze, 2011; Giménez-Arnau, 2011; Ropper, 2012); may be irritating to mucous membranes (do not crush, chew, or open capsule).

Dosage Forms

Capsule Delayed Release, Oral:

Tecfidera: 120 mg, 240 mg

Miscellaneous, Oral:

Tecfidera: Capsule, delayed release: 120 mg (14s) and Capsule, delayed release: 240 mg (46s) (60 ea)

- ◆ **Dimethylfumarate** *see* Dimethyl Fumarate *on page* 639
- ◆ **Dimethyl Triazeno Imidazole Carboxamide** *see* Dacarbazine *on page* 549
- ◆ **Dimetindene** *see* Dimethindene [INT] *on page* 638
- ◆ **Dinate [OTC] (Can)** *see* DimenhyDRINATE *on page* 637

Dinoprostone (dye noe PROST one)

Brand Names: U.S. Cervidil; Prepidil; Prostin E2

Brand Names: Canada Cervidil®; Prepidil®; Prostin E_2®

Index Terms PGE_2; Prostaglandin E_2

Pharmacologic Category Abortifacient; Prostaglandin

Use

Endocervical gel (Prepidil®): Promote cervical ripening in patients at or near term in whom there is a medical or obstetrical indication for the induction of labor

Suppositories (Prostin E_2®): Terminate pregnancy from 12th through 20th week of gestation; evacuate uterus in cases of missed abortion or intrauterine fetal death up to 28 weeks of gestation; manage benign hydatidiform mole (nonmetastatic gestational trophoblastic disease)

Tablet (oral) (Prostin E_2®; [Canadian product]): Elective induction of labor; when indications for induction of labor exist (eg, premature rupture of amniotic membranes, toxemia of pregnancy, Rh incompatibility, diabetes mellitus, hypertension, postmaturity, intrauterine death or fetal growth retardation)

Vaginal gel (Prostin E_2®; [Canadian product]): Induction of labor in patients at or near term with singleton pregnancy, vertex presentation, and favorable induction features

Vaginal insert (Cervidil®): Initiation and/or continuation of cervical ripening in patients at or near term in whom there is a medical or obstetrical indication for the induction of labor

Pregnancy Risk Factor C

Dosage Females of reproductive age:

Abortifacient: Vaginal suppository: Insert 20 mg (1 suppository) high in vagina, repeat at 3- to 5-hour intervals until abortion occurs; continued administration for longer than 2 days is not advisable

Cervical ripening:

Endocervical gel: Using catheter supplied with gel, insert 0.5 mg into the cervical canal. May repeat every 6 hours if needed. Maximum cumulative dose: 1.5 mg/24 hours

Tablet (oral) [Canadian product]:

Induction: Initial: 0.5 mg and then repeat 0.5 mg dose 1 hour later; may give additional 0.5 mg dose on an hourly basis as needed for satisfactory uterine response. Maintain patient at the lowest effective dose. **Note:** Failure to induce regular contractions after 8 hours indicates failed induction and alternative management of patient should be considered. If patient vomits an intact tablet during therapy repeat dose. If patient vomits intact tablets following 2 successive doses, withhold therapy until next scheduled dose. If patient vomits a partial tablet or if no tablet is visible, continue at next regularly scheduled dose.

Parity ≥2 times or Bishop Score of ≥6: Administer 0.5 mg hourly throughout induction (discontinue hourly dose for excessive uterine activity)

Nulliparous or multiparous and resistant to induction (Bishop Score <6): If inadequate response after 2 hours of therapy may increase dose in 0.5 mg increments at hourly intervals up to a maximum single dose of 1.5 mg.

Maintenance of labor: 0.5 mg dose hourly; may occasionally withhold hourly dose to assess need for further dosing

Vaginal gel [Canadian product]: Initial: Using prefilled syringe, insert 1 mg into the posterior fornix of the vaginal canal; may give 1 additional dose of 1-2 mg 6 hours later if needed.

Vaginal insert: Insert 10 mg transversely into the posterior fornix of the vagina (to be removed at the onset of active labor or after 12 hours)

Additional Information Complete prescribing information should be consulted for additional detail.

Dosage Forms

Gel, Vaginal:

Prepidil: 0.5 mg/3 g (3 g)

Insert, Vaginal:

Cervidil: 10 mg (1 ea)

Suppository, Vaginal:

Prostin E2: 20 mg (5 ea)

Dosage Forms: Canada

Gel, vaginal:

Prostin E_2®: 1 mg/3 g (3 g), 2 mg/3 g (3 g)

Tablet, oral:

Prostin E_2®: 0.5 mg

- ◆ **Diocaine® (Can)** *see* Proparacaine *on page* 1728
- ◆ **Diocarpine (Can)** *see* Pilocarpine (Ophthalmic) *on page* 1649
- ◆ **Diochloram® (Can)** *see* Chloramphenicol *on page* 421
- ◆ **Diocto [OTC]** *see* Docusate *on page* 661

- ◆ **Dioctyl Calcium Sulfosuccinate** *see* Docusate *on page 661*
- ◆ **Dioctyl Sodium Sulfosuccinate** *see* Docusate *on page 661*
- ◆ **Diodex (Can)** *see* Dexamethasone (Ophthalmic) *on page 602*
- ◆ **Diodoquin® (Can)** *see* Iodoquinol *on page 1105*
- ◆ **Diogent® (Can)** *see* Gentamicin (Ophthalmic) *on page 962*
- ◆ **Diomycin® (Can)** *see* Erythromycin (Ophthalmic) *on page 764*
- ◆ **Diopentolate (Can)** *see* Cyclopentolate *on page 517*
- ◆ **Dioptic's Atropine Solution (Can)** *see* Atropine *on page 200*
- ◆ **Dioptimyd® (Can)** *see* Sulfacetamide and Prednisolone *on page 1944*
- ◆ **Dioptrol® (Can)** *see* Neomycin, Polymyxin B, and Dexamethasone *on page 1437*
- ◆ **Diosulf (Can)** *see* Sulfacetamide (Ophthalmic) *on page 1943*
- ◆ **Diotame [OTC]** *see* Bismuth *on page 265*
- ◆ **Diotrope® (Can)** *see* Tropicamide *on page 2108*
- ◆ **Diovan** *see* Valsartan *on page 2127*
- ◆ **Diovan HCT** *see* Valsartan and Hydrochlorothiazide *on page 2129*
- ◆ **Diovol® (Can)** *see* Aluminum Hydroxide and Magnesium Hydroxide *on page 103*
- ◆ **Diovol® Ex (Can)** *see* Aluminum Hydroxide and Magnesium Hydroxide *on page 103*
- ◆ **Diovol Plus (Can)** *see* Aluminum Hydroxide, Magnesium Hydroxide, and Simethicone *on page 104*
- ◆ **Dipentum** *see* Olsalazine *on page 1500*
- ◆ **Dipentum® (Can)** *see* Olsalazine *on page 1500*
- ◆ **Diphen [OTC]** *see* DiphenhydrAMINE (Systemic) *on page 641*
- ◆ **Diphenhist [OTC]** *see* DiphenhydrAMINE (Systemic) *on page 641*

DiphenhydrAMINE (Systemic)

(dye fen HYE dra meen)

Brand Names: U.S. Aler-Dryl [OTC]; Allergy Relief Childrens [OTC]; Allergy Relief [OTC]; Altaryl [OTC]; Anti-Hist Allergy [OTC]; Banophen [OTC]; Benadryl Allergy Childrens [OTC]; Benadryl Allergy [OTC]; Benadryl Dye-Free Allergy [OTC]; Benadryl [OTC]; Complete Allergy Medication [OTC]; Complete Allergy Relief [OTC]; Dicopanol FusePaq; Diphen [OTC]; Diphenhist [OTC]; Genahist [OTC]; Geri-Dryl [OTC]; Naramin [OTC]; Nighttime Sleep Aid [OTC]; Nytol Maximum Strength [OTC]; Nytol [OTC]; PediaCare Childrens Allergy [OTC]; Pharbedryl; Pharbedryl [OTC]; Q-Dryl [OTC]; Quenalin [OTC]; Scot-Tussin Allergy Relief [OTC]; Siladryl Allergy [OTC]; Silphen Cough [OTC]; Simply Allergy [OTC]; Simply Sleep [OTC]; Sleep Tabs [OTC]; Sominex Maximum Strength [OTC]; Sominex [OTC]; Tetra-Formula Nighttime Sleep [OTC]; Total Allergy Medicine [OTC]; Total Allergy [OTC]; Triaminic Cough/Runny Nose [OTC]; ZzzQuil [OTC]

Brand Names: Canada Allerdryl; Allernix; Benadryl; Nytol; Nytol Extra Strength; PMS-Diphenhydramine; Simply Sleep; Sominex

Index Terms Diphenhydramine Citrate; Diphenhydramine Hydrochloride; Diphenhydramine Tannate

Pharmacologic Category Ethanolamine Derivative; Histamine H_1 Antagonist; Histamine H_1 Antagonist, First Generation

Use Symptomatic relief of allergic symptoms caused by histamine release including nasal allergies and allergic dermatosis; adjunct to epinephrine in the treatment of anaphylaxis; insomnia, occasional; prevention or treatment of motion sickness; antitussive; management of Parkinsonian syndrome including drug-induced extrapyramidal symptoms (dystonic reactions) alone or in combination with centrally acting anticholinergic agents

Pregnancy Risk Factor B

Pregnancy Considerations Adverse events have not been observed in animal reproduction studies. Diphenhydramine crosses the placenta. Maternal diphenhydramine use has generally not resulted in an increased risk of birth defects; however, adverse events (withdrawal symptoms, respiratory depression) have been reported in newborns exposed to diphenhydramine *in utero*. Antihistamines are recommended for the treatment of rhinitis, urticaria, and pruritus with rash in pregnant women (although second generation antihistamines may be preferred). Antihistamines are not recommended for treatment of pruritus associated with intrahepatic cholestasis in pregnancy.

Breast-Feeding Considerations Diphenhydramine is excreted into breast milk; drowsiness has been reported in a breast-feeding infant. Premature infants and newborns have a higher risk of intolerance to antihistamines. Breast-feeding is contraindicated by the manufacturer. Antihistamines may decrease maternal serum prolactin concentrations when administered prior to the establishment of nursing.

Contraindications Hypersensitivity to diphenhydramine, other structurally related antihistamines, or any component of the formulation; neonates or premature infants; breast-feeding

Additional contraindications: Parenteral: Use as a local anesthetic

OTC labeling: When used for self-medication, do not use in children <6 years, to make a child sleep, or with any other diphenhydramine-containing products (including topical products)

Warnings/Precautions Causes sedation, caution must be used in performing tasks which require alertness (eg, operating machinery or driving). Potentially significant drug-drug interactions may exist, requiring dose or frequency adjustment, additional monitoring, and/or selection of alternative therapy. Sedative effects of CNS depressants or ethanol are potentiated. Antihistamines may cause excitation in young children. Toxicity (overdose) in pediatric patients may result in hallucinations, convulsions, or death; neonates and young children are highly sensitive to depressive effects of diphenhydramine; use is contraindicated in neonates. Use with caution in patients with angle-closure glaucoma, pyloroduodenal obstruction (including stenotic peptic ulcer), urinary tract obstruction (including bladder neck obstruction and symptomatic prostatic hyperplasia), asthma, hyperthyroidism, increased intraocular pressure, and cardiovascular disease (including hypertension and tachycardia).

Some preparations contain soy protein; avoid use in patients with soy protein or peanut allergies. Some products may contain phenylalanine. Some products may contain alcohol. Some dosage forms may contain propylene glycol; large amounts are potentially toxic and have been associated hyperosmolality, lactic acidosis, seizures, and respiratory depression; use caution (AAP, 1997; Zar, 2007).

Benzyl alcohol and derivatives: Some dosage forms may contain sodium benzoate/benzoic acid; benzoic acid (benzoate) is a metabolite of benzyl alcohol; large amounts of benzyl alcohol (≥99 mg/kg/day) have been associated with a potentially fatal toxicity ("gasping syndrome") in neonates; the "gasping syndrome" consists of metabolic acidosis, respiratory distress, gasping respirations, CNS dysfunction (including convulsions, intracranial hemorrhage), hypotension, and cardiovascular collapse (AAP, 1997; CDC, 1982); some data suggests that benzoate displaces bilirubin from protein binding sites (Ahlfors, 2001); avoid or use dosage forms containing benzyl alcohol derivative with caution in neonates. See manufacturer's labeling.

Some dosage forms may contain polysorbate 80 (also known as Tweens). Hypersensitivity reactions, usually a delayed reaction, have been reported following exposure to pharmaceutical products containing polysorbate 80 in certain individuals (Isaksson, 2002; Lucente 2000; Shelley, 1995). Thrombocytopenia, ascites, pulmonary deterioration, and renal and hepatic failure have been reported in premature neonates after receiving parenteral products containing polysorbate 80 (Alade, 1986; CDC, 1984). See manufacturer's labeling.

Oral products: In the elderly, avoid use of this potent anticholinergic agent due to increased risk of confusion, dry mouth, constipation, and other anticholinergic effects; clearance decreases in patients of advanced age; tolerance develops to hypnotic effects; when used for severe allergic reaction, use may be appropriate (Beers Criteria). Oral solutions are available in two concentrations (ie, 12.5 mg/5 mL and 50 mg/30 mL [eg, ZzzQuil]); precautions should be taken to verify and avoid confusion between the different concentrations; dose should be clearly presented as "mg"; the 50 mg/30 mL oral solution is indicated for the occasional treatment of insomnia.

Parenteral products: Subcutaneous or intradermal use has been associated with tissue necrosis; administer IV or IM only.

Adverse Reactions

Cardiovascular: Chest tightness, extrasystoles, hypotension, palpitations, tachycardia

Central nervous system: Ataxia, chills, confusion, dizziness, drowsiness, euphoria, excitement, fatigue, headache, insomnia, irritability, nervousness, neuritis, paradoxical excitation, paresthesia, restlessness, sedation, seizure, vertigo

Dermatologic: Diaphoresis

Endocrine & metabolic: Menstrual disease (early menses)

Gastrointestinal: Anorexia, constipation, diarrhea, dry mucous membranes, epigastric distress, nausea, vomiting, xerostomia

Genitourinary: Difficulty in micturition, urinary frequency, urinary retention

Hematologic & oncologic: Agranulocytosis, hemolytic anemia, thrombocytopenia

Hypersensitivity: Anaphylactic shock

Neuromuscular & skeletal: Tremor

Ophthalmic: Blurred vision, diplopia

Otic: Labyrinthitis (acute), tinnitus

Respiratory: Constriction of the pharynx, nasal congestion, thickening of bronchial secretions, wheezing

Drug Interactions

Metabolism/Transport Effects **Inhibits** CYP2D6 (moderate)

Avoid Concomitant Use

Avoid concomitant use of DiphenhydrAMINE (Systemic) with any of the following: Aclidinium; Azelastine (Nasal); Glucagon; Ipratropium (Oral Inhalation); Orphenadrine; Paraldehyde; Potassium Chloride; Thalidomide; Thioridazine; Tiotropium; Umeclidinium

Increased Effect/Toxicity

DiphenhydrAMINE (Systemic) may increase the levels/effects of: AbobotulinumtoxinA; Alcohol (Ethyl); Analgesics (Opioid); Anticholinergic Agents; ARIPiprazole; Azelastine (Nasal); Buprenorphine; CNS Depressants; CYP2D6 Substrates; DOXOrubicin (Conventional); Eliglustat; Fesoterodine; Glucagon; Highest Risk QTc-Prolonging Agents; Hydrocodone; Methotrimeprazine; Metoprolol; Metyrosine; Mirabegron; Mirtazapine; Moderate Risk QTc-Prolonging Agents; Nebivolol; OnabotulinumtoxinA; Orphenadrine; Paraldehyde; Potassium Chloride; Pramipexole; RimabotulinumtoxinB; ROPINIRole; Rotigotine; Selective Serotonin Reuptake Inhibitors; Suvorexant; Thalidomide; Thiazide Diuretics; Thioridazine; Tiotropium; Topiramate; Zolpidem

The levels/effects of DiphenhydrAMINE (Systemic) may be increased by: Aclidinium; Brimonidine (Topical); Cannabis; Doxylamine; Dronabinol; Droperidol; HydrOXYzine; Ipratropium (Oral Inhalation); Kava Kava; Magnesium Sulfate; Methotrimeprazine; Mianserin; Mifepristone; Nabilone; Perampanel; Pramlintide; Propafenone; Rufinamide; Sodium Oxybate; Tapentadol; Tetrahydrocannabinol; Umeclidinium

Decreased Effect

DiphenhydrAMINE (Systemic) may decrease the levels/effects of: Acetylcholinesterase Inhibitors; Benzylpenicilloyl Polylysine; Betahistine; Codeine; Hyaluronidase; Itopride; Secretin; Tamoxifen; TraMADol

The levels/effects of DiphenhydrAMINE (Systemic) may be decreased by: Acetylcholinesterase Inhibitors; Amphetamines

Storage/Stability

Injection: Store at room temperature of 20°C to 25°C (68°F to 77°F); protect from light and freezing.

Oral: Store at room temperature. Protect capsules and tablets from moisture. Protect oral solution from freezing and light.

Mechanism of Action Competes with histamine for H_1-receptor sites on effector cells in the gastrointestinal tract, blood vessels, and respiratory tract; anticholinergic and sedative effects are also seen

Pharmacodynamics/Kinetics

Duration:

Histamine-induced wheal suppression: ≤10 hours (Simons, 1990)

Histamine-induced flare suppression: ≤12 hours (Simons, 1990)

Distribution: V_d: Children: 22 L/kg (range: 15 to 28 L/kg); Adults: 17 L/kg (range: 13 to 20 L/kg); Elderly: 14 L/kg (range: 7 to 20 L/kg) (Blyden, 1986; Simons, 1990)

Protein binding: 98.5% (Vozeh, 1988)

Metabolism: Extensively hepatic n-demethylation via CYP2D6; minor demethylation via CYP1A2, 2C9 and 2C19; smaller degrees in pulmonary and renal systems; significant first-pass effect (Akutsu, 2007)

Bioavailability: 42% to 62% (Paton, 1985)

Half-life elimination: Children: 5 hours (range: 4 to 7 hours); Adults: 9 hours (range: 7 to 12 hours); Elderly: 13.5 hours (range: 9 to 18 hours) (Blyden, 1986; Simons, 1990)

Time to peak, serum: ~2 hours (Blyden, 1986; Simons, 1990)

Excretion: Urine (as metabolites and unchanged drug) (Albert, 1975; Maurer, 1988)

Dosage

Pediatric:

Allergic reactions: Infants, Children, and Adolescents:

Oral, IM, IV: 5 mg/kg/day in divided doses every 6 to 8 hours; maximum: 300 mg daily

Alternate dosing by age: Oral:

2 to <6 years (off-label use): 6.25 mg every 4 to 6 hours; maximum: 37.5 mg daily (Kleigman, 2011)

6 to <12 years: 12.5 to 25 mg every 4 to 6 hours; maximum: 150 mg daily

≥12 years: 25 to 50 mg every 4 to 6 hours; maximum: 300 mg daily

Anaphylaxis (adjunct to epinephrine)/allergic reaction (off-label use): Infants, Children, and Adolescents: IM, IV, Oral: 1 to 2 mg/kg/dose; maximum: 50 mg/dose (Hegenbarth, 2008; Kliegman, 2011; Liberman, 2008; Lieberman, 2010; Simons, 2011)
Antitussive: Oral: Children ≥12 years: 25 mg every 4 hours; maximum: 150 mg daily
Dystonic reactions (off-label use): Infants, Children, and Adolescents: IM, IV: 1 to 2 mg/kg/dose; maximum single dose: 50 mg (Hegenbarth, 2008; Kliegman, 2011)
Motion sickness:
Prophylaxis: Oral:
Manufacturer recommendations: Infants, Children, and Adolescents: **Note:** Administer 30 minutes before motion
Weight-directed dosing: 5 mg/kg/day divided into 3 to 4 doses; maximum: 300 mg daily
Fixed dosing: 12.5 to 25 mg 3 to 4 times daily
Alternate dosing: Children 2 to 12 years: Limited data available: 0.5 to 1 mg/kg/dose every 6 hours; maximum single dose: 25 mg. First dose should be administered 1 hour before travel (CDC, 2014).
Treatment: Infants, Children, and Adolescents:
IM, IV: 5 mg/kg/day divided into 4 doses; maximum: 300 mg daily
Oral:
Weight-directed dosing: 5 mg/kg/day divided into 3 to 4 doses; maximum: 300 mg daily
Fixed dosing: 12.5 to 25 mg 3 to 4 times daily
Insomnia, occasional: Oral:
Children 2 to 12 years, weighing 10 to 50 kg (off-label use): Limited data available: 1 mg/kg administered 30 minutes before bedtime; maximum single dose: 50 mg (Russo, 1976)
Children ≥12 years and Adolescents: 50 mg administered 30 minutes before bedtime
Rhinitis, sneezing due to common cold: Oral:
Children 6 to <12 years: 12.5 to 25 mg every 4 to 6 hours; maximum: 150 mg daily
Children ≥12 years and Adolescents: 25 to 50 mg every 4 to 6 hours; maximum: 300 mg daily

Adults:
Allergic reactions:
Oral: 25 to 50 mg every 4 to 8 hours; maximum: 300 mg daily
IM, IV: 10 to 50 mg per dose; single doses up to 100 mg may be used if needed; maximum: 400 mg daily
Antitussive: Oral: 25 mg every 4 hours; maximum: 150 mg daily
Motion sickness: **Note:** When used for prophylaxis, administer 30 minutes before motion.
Oral (treatment or prophylaxis): 25 to 50 mg every 6 to 8 hours
IM, IV (treatment): 10 to 50 mg per dose; single doses up to 100 mg may be used if needed; maximum: 400 mg daily
Insomnia, occasional: Oral: 50 mg at bedtime
Parkinsonism:
Oral: 25 to 50 mg 3 or 4 times daily.
IM, IV: 10 to 50 mg per dose; single doses up to 100 mg may be used if needed; maximum: 400 mg daily
Rhinitis, sneezing due to common cold: Oral: 25 to 50 mg every 4 to 6 hours; maximum: 300 mg daily

Dosage adjustment in renal impairment: There are no dosage adjustments provided in the manufacturer's labeling.

Dosage adjustment in hepatic impairment: There are no dosage adjustments provided in the manufacturer's labeling.

Dietary Considerations Some products may contain sodium and/or phenylalanine.

Administration When used to prevent motion sickness, first dose should be given 30 minutes prior to exposure. When used for occasional insomnia, dose should be given 30 minutes before bedtime.
Injection solution is for IV or deep IM administration only. For IV administration, inject at a rate ≤25 mg/minute. Local necrosis may result with SubQ or intradermal use.

Monitoring Parameters Relief of symptoms, mental alertness

Dosage Forms Considerations Dicopanol FusePaq is a compounding kit for the preparation of an oral suspension. Refer to manufacturer's labeling for compounding instructions.

Dosage Forms
Capsule, Oral:
Allergy Relief [OTC]: 25 mg
Banophen [OTC]: 25 mg, 50 mg
Benadryl [OTC]: 25 mg
Benadryl Allergy [OTC]: 25 mg
Benadryl Dye-Free Allergy [OTC]: 25 mg
Genahist [OTC]: 25 mg
Geri-Dryl [OTC]: 25 mg
Pharbedryl [OTC]: 25 mg, 50 mg, 50 mg
Q-Dryl [OTC]: 25 mg
ZzzQuil [OTC]: 25 mg
Generic: 25 mg, 50 mg
Elixir, Oral:
Altaryl [OTC]: 12.5 mg/5 mL (120 mL, 480 mL, 3840 mL)
Generic: 12.5 mg/5 mL (5 mL, 10 mL)
Liquid, Oral:
Allergy Relief Childrens [OTC]: 12.5 mg/5 mL (118 mL, 480 mL)
Banophen [OTC]: 12.5 mg/5 mL (118 mL, 473 mL)
Benadryl Allergy Childrens [OTC]: 12.5 mg/5 mL (5 mL, 118 mL, 236 mL)
Diphenhist [OTC]: 12.5 mg/5 mL (118 mL, 473 mL)
Naramin [OTC]: 12.5 mg/5 mL (5 mL)
PediaCare Childrens Allergy [OTC]: 12.5 mg/5 mL (118 mL)
Q-Dryl [OTC]: 12.5 mg/5 mL (118 mL, 237 mL, 473 mL)
Scot-Tussin Allergy Relief [OTC]: 12.5 mg/5 mL (118.3 mL, 240 mL, 480 mL, 3780 mL)
Siladryl Allergy [OTC]: 12.5 mg/5 mL (118 mL, 237 mL, 473 mL)
Total Allergy Medicine [OTC]: 12.5 mg/5 mL (118 mL)
ZzzQuil [OTC]: 50 mg/30 mL (177 mL, 354 mL)
Solution, Injection:
Generic: 50 mg/mL (1 mL, 10 mL)
Solution, Injection [preservative free]:
Generic: 50 mg/mL (1 mL)
Strip, Oral:
Triaminic Cough/Runny Nose [OTC]: 12.5 mg (14 ea, 16 ea)
Suspension Reconstituted, Oral:
Dicopanol FusePaq: 5 mg/mL (150 mL)
Syrup, Oral:
Altaryl [OTC]: 12.5 mg/5 mL (120 mL, 480 mL, 3785 mL)
Quenalin [OTC]: 12.5 mg/5 mL (120 mL)
Silphen Cough [OTC]: 12.5 mg/5 mL (118 mL, 237 mL, 473 mL)
Tablet, Oral:
Aler-Dryl [OTC]: 50 mg
Allergy Relief [OTC]: 25 mg
Anti-Hist Allergy [OTC]: 25 mg
Banophen [OTC]: 25 mg
Benadryl [OTC]: 25 mg
Benadryl Allergy [OTC]: 25 mg
Complete Allergy Medication [OTC]: 25 mg
Complete Allergy Relief [OTC]: 25 mg
Diphen [OTC]: 25 mg
Diphenhist [OTC]: 25 mg
Geri-Dryl [OTC]: 25 mg
Nighttime Sleep Aid [OTC]: 25 mg

Nytol [OTC]: 25 mg
Nytol Maximum Strength [OTC]: 50 mg
Simply Allergy [OTC]: 25 mg
Simply Sleep [OTC]: 25 mg
Sleep Tabs [OTC]: 25 mg
Sominex [OTC]: 25 mg
Sominex Maximum Strength [OTC]: 50 mg
Tetra-Formula Nighttime Sleep [OTC]: 50 mg
Total Allergy [OTC]: 25 mg
Generic: 25 mg

Tablet Chewable, Oral:
Benadryl Allergy Childrens [OTC]: 12.5 mg

◆ **Diphenhydramine and Acetaminophen** *see* Acetaminophen and Diphenhydramine *on page 36*

◆ **Diphenhydramine and ASA** *see* Aspirin and Diphenhydramine *on page 185*

◆ **Diphenhydramine and Aspirin** *see* Aspirin and Diphenhydramine *on page 185*

Diphenhydramine and Phenylephrine

(dye fen HYE dra meen & fen il EF rin)

Brand Names: U.S. Aldex® CT [DSC]; Benadryl-D® Allergy & Sinus [OTC]; Benadryl-D® Children's Allergy & Sinus [OTC]; Dimetapp® Children's Nighttime Cold & Congestion [OTC]; Triaminic® Children's Night Time Cold & Cough [OTC]

Index Terms Diphenhydramine Hydrochloride and Phenylephrine Hydrochloride; Diphenhydramine Tannate and Phenylephrine Tannate; Phenylephrine and Diphenhydramine; Phenylephrine Hydrochloride and Diphenhydramine Hydrochloride; Phenylephrine Tannate and Diphenhydramine Tannate

Pharmacologic Category Alpha-Adrenergic Agonist; Decongestant; Ethanolamine Derivative; Histamine H_1 Antagonist; Histamine H_1 Antagonist, First Generation

Use Temporary relief of symptoms of allergic rhinitis, sinusitis, and other upper respiratory conditions, including sinus/nasal congestion, sneezing, stuffy/runny nose, itchy/watery eyes, and cough

Dosage Oral:
Aldex® CT:
Children 6-11 years: One-half to 1 tablet every 6 hours
Children ≥12 years and Adults: 1-2 tablets every 6 hours
OTC labeling:
Children <6 years: Use not recommended
Children 6-11 years:
Benadryl-D® Children's Allergy & Sinus: 5 mL every 4 hours as needed (maximum: 6 doses/24 hours)
Dimetapp® Children's Nighttime Cold and Congestion, Triaminic® Children's Night Time Cold & Cough: 10 mL every 4 hours as needed (maximum: 6 doses/24 hours)
Children ≥12 years and Adults: **Note:** General dosing guidelines; refer to specific product labeling:
10-20 mL every 4 hours as needed (maximum: 6 doses/24 hours) **or** 1 tablet every 4 hours as needed (maximum: 6 doses/24 hours)

Additional Information Complete prescribing information should be consulted for additional detail.

Dosage Forms

Liquid, oral:
Benadryl-D® Children's Allergy & Sinus [OTC]: Diphenhydramine 12.5 mg and phenylephrine 5 mg per 5 mL (118 mL)

Syrup, oral:
Dimetapp® Children's Nighttime Cold and Congestion [OTC]: Diphenhydramine 6.25 mg and phenylephrine 2.5 mg per 5 mL (120 mL)
Triaminic® Children's Night Time Cold & Cough [OTC]: Diphenhydramine 6.25 mg and phenylephrine 2.5 mg per 5 mL (118 mL)

Tablet, oral:
Benadryl-D® Allergy & Sinus [OTC]: Diphenhydramine 25 mg and phenylephrine 10 mg

◆ **Diphenhydramine Citrate** *see* DiphenhydrAMINE (Systemic) *on page 641*

◆ **Diphenhydramine Citrate and Aspirin** *see* Aspirin and Diphenhydramine *on page 185*

◆ **Diphenhydramine Hydrochloride** *see* DiphenhydrAMINE (Systemic) *on page 641*

◆ **Diphenhydramine Hydrochloride and Phenylephrine Hydrochloride** *see* Diphenhydramine and Phenylephrine *on page 644*

◆ **Diphenhydramine Tannate** *see* DiphenhydrAMINE (Systemic) *on page 641*

◆ **Diphenhydramine Tannate and Phenylephrine Tannate** *see* Diphenhydramine and Phenylephrine *on page 644*

Diphenoxylate and Atropine

(dye fen OKS i late & A troe peen)

Brand Names: U.S. Lomotil
Brand Names: Canada Lomotil
Index Terms Atropine and Diphenoxylate
Pharmacologic Category Antidiarrheal
Use Treatment of diarrhea
Pregnancy Risk Factor C

Pregnancy Considerations Teratogenic effects were not noted in animal studies; decreased maternal weight, fertility and litter sizes were observed. There are no adequate and well-controlled studies in pregnant women.

Breast-Feeding Considerations Atropine is excreted in breast milk (refer to Atropine monograph); the manufacturer states that diphenoxylic acid may be excreted in breast milk.

Contraindications Hypersensitivity to diphenoxylate, atropine, or any component of the formulation; obstructive jaundice; diarrhea associated with pseudomembranous enterocolitis or enterotoxin-producing bacteria; not for use in children <2 years of age

Warnings/Precautions Use in conjunction with fluid and electrolyte therapy when appropriate. In case of severe dehydration or electrolyte imbalance, withhold diphenoxylate/atropine treatment until corrective therapy has been initiated. Inhibiting peristalsis may lead to fluid retention in the intestine aggravating dehydration and electrolyte imbalance. Reduction of intestinal motility may be deleterious in diarrhea resulting from *Shigella, Salmonella*, toxigenic strains of *E. coli*, and pseudomembranous enterocolitis associated with broad-spectrum antibiotics; use is not recommended.

Use with caution in children. Younger children may be predisposed to toxicity; signs of atropinism may occur even at recommended doses, especially in patients with Down syndrome. Overdose in children may result in severe respiratory depression, coma, and possibly permanent brain damage.

Use caution with acute ulcerative colitis, hepatic or renal dysfunction. If there is no response with 48 hours, this medication is unlikely to be effective and should be discontinued; if chronic diarrhea is not improved symptomatically within 10 days at maximum dosage, control is unlikely with further use. Physical and psychological dependence have been reported with higher than recommended dosing.

Adverse Reactions

Cardiovascular: Flushing, tachycardia

Central nervous system: Confusion, depression, dizziness, drowsiness, euphoria, headache, hyperthermia, lethargy, malaise, numbness, restlessness, sedation

Dermatologic: Pruritus, urticaria, xeroderma

Gastrointestinal: Abdominal distress, anorexia, gingival swelling, nausea, pancreatitis, paralytic ileus, toxic megacolon, vomiting, xerostomia

Genitourinary: Urinary retention

Hypersensitivity: Anaphylaxis, angioedema

Drug Interactions

Metabolism/Transport Effects None known.

Avoid Concomitant Use

Avoid concomitant use of Diphenoxylate and Atropine with any of the following: Aclidinium; Azelastine (Nasal); Glucagon; Ipratropium (Oral Inhalation); Orphenadrine; Paraldehyde; Potassium Chloride; Thalidomide; Tiotropium; Umeclidinium

Increased Effect/Toxicity

Diphenoxylate and Atropine may increase the levels/effects of: AbobotulinumtoxinA; Alcohol (Ethyl); Analgesics (Opioid); Anticholinergic Agents; Azelastine (Nasal); Buprenorphine; CNS Depressants; Glucagon; Hydrocodone; Methotrimeprazine; Metyrosine; Mirabegron; Mirtazapine; OnabotulinumtoxinA; Orphenadrine; Paraldehyde; Potassium Chloride; Pramipexole; RimabotulinumtoxinB; ROPINIRole; Rotigotine; Selective Serotonin Reuptake Inhibitors; Suvorexant; Thalidomide; Thiazide Diuretics; Tiotropium; Topiramate; Zolpidem

The levels/effects of Diphenoxylate and Atropine may be increased by: Aclidinium; Brimonidine (Topical); Cannabis; Doxylamine; Dronabinol; Droperidol; HydrOXYzine; Ipratropium (Oral Inhalation); Kava Kava; Magnesium Sulfate; Methotrimeprazine; Mianserin; Nabilone; Perampanel; Pramlintide; Rufinamide; Sodium Oxybate; Tapentadol; Tetrahydrocannabinol; Umeclidinium

Decreased Effect

Diphenoxylate and Atropine may decrease the levels/effects of: Acetylcholinesterase Inhibitors; Itopride; Secretin

The levels/effects of Diphenoxylate and Atropine may be decreased by: Acetylcholinesterase Inhibitors

Storage/Stability

Oral solution: Store at 20°C to 25°C (68°F to 77°F). Discard opened bottle after 90 days.

Tablet: Store at 20°C to 25°C (68°F to 77°F); protect from light.

Mechanism of Action Diphenoxylate inhibits excessive GI motility and GI propulsion; commercial preparations contain a subtherapeutic amount of atropine to discourage abuse

Pharmacodynamics/Kinetics

Atropine: See Atropine monograph.

Diphenoxylate:

Onset of action: Antidiarrheal: 45-60 minutes

Duration: Antidiarrheal: 3-4 hours

Absorption: Well absorbed

Metabolism: Extensively hepatic via ester hydrolysis to diphenoxylic acid (active)

Half-life elimination: Diphenoxylate: 2.5 hours; Diphenoxylic acid: 12-14 hours

Time to peak, serum: 2 hours

Excretion: Primarily feces (49% as unchanged drug and metabolites); urine (~14%, <1% as unchanged drug)

Dosage Oral:

Children 2-12 years (use with caution in young children due to variable responses): Liquid: Diphenoxylate 0.3-0.4 mg/kg/day in 4 divided doses until control achieved (maximum: 10 mg/day), then reduce dose as needed; some patients may be controlled on doses as low as 25% of the initial daily dose

Adults: Diphenoxylate 5 mg 4 times/day until control achieved (maximum: 20 mg/day), then reduce dose as needed; some patients may be controlled on doses of 5 mg/day

Dosage adjustment in renal impairment: No adjustment provided in the manufacturer's labeling. Use with extreme caution in patients with advanced hepatorenal disease.

Dosage adjustment in hepatic impairment: No adjustment provided in the manufacturer's labeling. Use with extreme caution in patients with advanced hepatorenal disease or abnormal liver function tests.

Administration If there is no response within 48 hours of continuous therapy, this medication is unlikely to be effective and should be discontinued; if chronic diarrhea is not improved symptomatically within 10 days at maximum dosage, control is unlikely with further use. Use of the liquid preparation is recommended in children <13 years of age; use plastic dropper provided when measuring liquid.

Monitoring Parameters Watch for signs of atropinism (dryness of skin and mucous membranes, tachycardia, thirst, flushing); monitor number and consistency of stools; observe for signs of toxicity, fluid and electrolyte loss, hypotension, and respiratory depression

Dosage Forms

Solution, oral: Diphenoxylate 2.5 mg and atropine 0.025 mg per 5 mL

Tablet, oral: Diphenoxylate 2.5 mg and atropine 0.025 mg

◆ **Diphenylhydantoin** *see* Phenytoin *on page 1640*

Diphtheria and Tetanus Toxoid

(dif THEER ee a & TET a nus TOKS oyds)

Brand Names: U.S. Tenivac

Brand Names: Canada Td Adsorbed

Index Terms DT; Td; Tetanus and Diphtheria Toxoid

Pharmacologic Category Vaccine, Inactivated (Bacterial)

Additional Appendix Information

Immunization Recommendations *on page 2255*

Use

Diphtheria and tetanus toxoids adsorbed for pediatric use (DT): Infants and children through 6 years of age: Active immunization against diphtheria and tetanus when pertussis vaccine is contraindicated

Tetanus and diphtheria toxoids adsorbed for adult use (Td) (Tenivac): Children ≥7 years of age and Adults: Active immunization against diphtheria and tetanus; tetanus prophylaxis in wound management

The Advisory Committee on Immunization Practices (ACIP) recommends routine vaccination for the following:

- Adults and children ≥7 years should receive a booster dose of Td every 10 years; may substitute a single Td booster dose with Tdap (CDC 60[1], 2011)
- Children 7 to 10 years of age, adults, and the elderly (≥65 years) who are wounded in bombings or similar mass casualty events who have penetrating injuries or nonintact skin exposure and who cannot confirm receipt of a tetanus booster within the previous 5 years, may also receive a single dose of Td; children ≥11 years and adults may also receive Td if Tdap is unavailable (CDC [Chapman, 2008])

Pregnancy Risk Factor C

Dosage IM:

Children 6 weeks to <7 years (DT): Primary immunization:

Note: For use when a pertussis-containing vaccine is contraindicated: 0.5 mL per dose, total of 5 doses administered as follows:

Three doses, usually given at 2-, 4-, and 6 months of age; may be given as early as 6 weeks of age and repeated every 4-8 weeks

Fourth dose: Given at ~15 to 18 months of age, but at least 6 months after third dose. The fourth dose may be given as early as 12 months of age, but at least 6 months must have elapsed between the third dose and the fourth dose.

Fifth dose: Given at 4 to 6 years of age, prior to starting school or kindergarten; if the fourth dose is given at ≥4 years of age, the fifth dose may be omitted

For children who start primary immunization series ≥4 months of age, refer to current ACIP "Catch-up Immunization Schedule"

Children ≥7 years and Adults (Td):

Primary immunization:

Manufacturer labeling (Tenivac): Patients previously not immunized should receive 2 primary doses of 0.5 mL each, given at an interval of 8 weeks; third (reinforcing) dose of 0.5 mL 6 to 8 months later

ACIP recommendations: Patients previously not immunized should receive 2 primary doses of 0.5 mL each, given at an interval of 4 weeks; third (reinforcing) dose of 0.5 mL 6 to 12 months later (CDC/ACIP [Akinsanya-Beysolow, 2014]; CDC/ACIP [Bridges, 2014]).

Booster immunization: For routine booster in patients who have completed primary immunization series. The ACIP prefers Tdap for use in in some situations if no contraindications exist; refer to Diphtheria and Tetanus Toxoids, and Acellular Pertussis Vaccine monograph for additional information.

Children 11 to 12 years: A single dose when at least 5 years have elapsed since last dose of toxoid-containing vaccine. Subsequent routine doses are not recommended more often than every 10 years.

Adults: 0.5 mL every 10 years

Tetanus prophylaxis in wound management: Tetanus prophylaxis in patients with wounds should consider if the wound is clean or contaminated, the immunization status of the patient, proper use of tetanus toxoid and/or tetanus immune globulin (TIG), wound cleaning, and (if required) surgical debridement and the proper use of antibiotics. Patients with an uncertain or incomplete tetanus immunization status should have additional follow up to ensure a series is completed. Patients with a history of Arthus reaction following a previous dose of a tetanus toxoid-containing vaccine should not receive a tetanus toxoid-containing vaccine until >10 years after the most recent dose even if they have a wound that is neither clean nor minor. See table.

Tetanus Prophylaxis in Wound Management

History of Tetanus Immunization Doses	Clean, Minor Wounds		All Other Wounds[1]	
	Tetanus Toxoid[2]	TIG	Tetanus Toxoid[2]	TIG
Uncertain or <3 doses	Yes	No	Yes	Yes
3 or more doses	No[3]	No	No[4]	No

[1]Such as, but not limited to, wounds contaminated with dirt, feces, soil, and saliva; puncture wounds; wounds from crushing, tears, burns, and frostbite.

[2]Tetanus toxoid in this chart refers to a tetanus toxoid-containing vaccine. For children <7 years of age, DTaP (DT, if pertussis vaccine contraindicated) is preferred to tetanus toxoid alone. For children ≥7 years and adults, Td preferred to tetanus toxoid alone; Tdap may be preferred if the patient has not previously been vaccinated with Tdap.

[3]Yes, if ≥10 years since last dose.

[4]Yes, if ≥5 years since last dose.

Adapted from CDC "Yellow Book" (*Health Information for International Travel 2010*), "Routine Vaccine-Preventable Diseases, Tetanus" (available at http://www.cdc.gov/yellowbook) and *MMWR* 2006, 55 (RR-17).

Abbreviations: **DT** = Diphtheria and Tetanus Toxoids (formulation for age ≤6 years); **DTaP** = Diphtheria and Tetanus Toxoids, and Acellular Pertussis (formulation for age ≤6 years; Daptacel, Infanrix); **Td** = Diphtheria and Tetanus Toxoids (formulation for age ≥7 years; Tenivac); **TT**= Tetanus toxoid (adsorbed [formulation for age ≥7 years]); **Tdap** = Diphtheria and Tetanus Toxoids, and Acellular Pertussis (Adacel or Boostrix [formulations for age ≥7 years]); **TIG** = Tetanus Immune Globulin

Additional Information Complete prescribing information should be consulted for additional detail.

Dosage Forms

Injection, suspension [Td, adult; preservative free]: Diphtheria 2 Lf units and tetanus 2 Lf units per 0.5 mL (0.5 mL)

Tenivac: Diphtheria 2 Lf units and tetanus 5 Lf units per 0.5 mL (0.5 mL)

Injection, suspension [DT, pediatric; preservative free]: Diphtheria 25 Lf units and tetanus 5 Lf units per 0.5 mL (0.5 mL)

Diphtheria and Tetanus Toxoids, Acellular Pertussis, and Poliovirus Vaccine

(dif THEER ee a & TET a nus TOKS oyds, ay CEL yoo lar per TUS sis & POE lee oh VYE rus vak SEEN)

Brand Names: U.S. Kinrix®

Brand Names: Canada Adacel®-Polio

Index Terms Diphtheria and Tetanus Toxoids and Acellular Pertussis Adsorbed, and Inactivated Poliovirus Vaccine Combined; Diphtheria, Tetanus Toxoids, Acellular Pertussis (DTaP); DTaP-IPV; Poliovirus, Inactivated (IPV)

Pharmacologic Category Vaccine, Inactivated (Bacterial); Vaccine, Inactivated (Viral)

Additional Appendix Information

Immunization Administration Recommendations *on page 2250*

Immunization Recommendations *on page 2255*

Use Kinrix®: Active immunization against diphtheria, tetanus, pertussis, and poliomyelitis, used as the fifth dose in the DTaP series and the 4th dose in the IPV series

The Advisory Committee on Immunization Practices (ACIP) recommends routine vaccination for use as the fifth dose in the DTaP series and the fourth dose in the IPV series in children who received DTaP (Infanrix®) and/or DTaP-Hepatitis B-IPV (Pediarix®) as the first 3 doses and DTaP (Infanrix®) as the fourth dose. Whenever feasible, the same manufacturer should be used to provide the pertussis component; however, vaccination should not be deferred if a specific brand is not known or is not available.

Adacel®-Polio [Canadian product]: Active booster immunization against diphtheria, tetanus, pertussis, and poliomyelitis; alternative to fifth dose of DTaP-IPV; May be used for wound management when a tetanus toxoid-containing vaccine is needed for wound management [refer to current National Advisory Committee on Immunization (NACI) guidelines]

Pregnancy Risk Factor C

Dosage IM:

Kinrix®: Children 4-6 years: Immunization: 0.5 mL; **Note:** For use as the fifth dose in the DTaP series and the fourth dose in the IPV series

Adacel®-Polio [Canadian product]: Children ≥4 years and Adults: Booster immunization: 0.5 mL; **Note:** May also be used as alternative to fifth dose of DTaP-IPV in children 4-6 years.

Dosage adjustment in renal impairment: No dosage adjustment provided in manufacturer's labeling.

Dosage adjustment in hepatic impairment: No dosage adjustment provided in manufacturer's labeling.

Additional Information Complete prescribing information should be consulted for additional detail.

Dosage Forms

Injection, suspension [preservative free]:

Kinrix®: Diphtheria toxoid 25 Lf, tetanus toxoid 10 Lf, acellular pertussis antigens [inactivated pertussis toxin 25 mcg, filamentous hemagglutinin 25 mcg, pertactin 8 mcg], type 1 poliovirus 40 D-antigen units, type 2 poliovirus 8 D-antigen units, and type 3 poliovirus 32 D-antigen units per 0.5 mL (0.5 mL)

Dosage Forms: Canada

Injection, suspension [preservative free]:

Adacel®-Polio: Diphtheria toxoid 2 Lf, tetanus toxoid 5 Lf, acellular pertussis antigens [inactivated pertussis toxoid 2.5 mcg, filamentous hemagglutinin 5 mcg, pertactin 3 mcg, types 2 and 3 fimbriae 5 mcg], type 1 poliovirus 40 D-antigen units, type 2 poliovirus 8 D-antigen units, and type 3 poliovirus 32 D-antigen units per 0.5 mL (0.5 mL)

Diphtheria and Tetanus Toxoids, Acellular Pertussis, Hepatitis B (Recombinant), Poliovirus (Inactivated), and *Haemophilus influenzae* B Conjugate (Adsorbed) Vaccine [CAN/INT]

(dif THEER ee a & TET a nus TOKS oyds, ay CEL yoo lar per TUS sis, hep a TYE tis bee ree KOM be nant, POE lee oh VYE rus in ak ti VAY ted, & hem OF fi lus in floo EN za bee KON joo gate ad SORBED vak SEEN)

Brand Names: Canada Infanrix Hexa™

Index Terms Diphtheria and Tetanus Toxoids and Acellular Pertussis, Hepatitis B (Recombinant), Inactivated Poliovirus Vaccine, and *Haemophilus influenzae* Type B Combined; DTaP-HepB-IPV-Hib

Pharmacologic Category Vaccine, Inactivated (Bacterial, Viral)

Additional Appendix Information

Immunization Administration Recommendations *on page 2250*

Immunization Recommendations *on page 2255*

Use Note: Not approved in U.S.

Active primary immunization against diphtheria, tetanus, pertussis, hepatitis B, poliomyelitis and disease caused by *Haemophilus influenzae* type b in infants and children 6 weeks to 2 years of age; booster immunization (at 18 months) in infants who previously received a full primary vaccination course of each component of the vaccine

Pregnancy Considerations Not indicated for use in pregnant women.

Breast-Feeding Considerations Not indicated for use in breast-feeding women.

Contraindications Hypersensitivity to any component of vaccine or formulation; encephalopathy of unknown etiology within 1 week following prior vaccination with a pertussis-containing vaccine; moderate or severe acute febrile illness or acute infection; children >7 years of age

Warnings/Precautions

Immediate treatment (including epinephrine 1:1000) for anaphylactoid and/or hypersensitivity reactions should be available during vaccine use. Apnea has been reported following IM vaccine administration in premature infants; consider respiratory monitoring for 2-3 days following administration and/or consider risk versus benefit in infants born prematurely. Carefully consider use in patients with history of any of the following effects from previous administration of whole-cell DTP or acellular pertussis vaccine: fever ≥105°F (40.5°C) within 48 hours of unknown cause; seizures with or without fever occurring within 3 days; persistent, inconsolable crying episodes lasting ≥3 hours and occurring within 48 hours; shock or collapse within 48 hours. Syncope has been reported with use of injectable vaccines and may be accompanied by transient visual disturbances, weakness, or tonic-clonic movements. Procedures should be in place to avoid injuries from falling and to restore cerebral perfusion if syncope occurs.

Use is contraindicated in patients with moderate or severe acute illness (with or without fever); may administer to patients with mild acute illness (with or without fever). Defer administration during outbreaks of poliomyelitis. Simultaneous administration of all age-appropriate vaccines (live or inactivated) for which a person is eligible at a single clinic visit is recommended unless contraindications exist. The use of combination vaccines is generally preferred over separate injections. Use for completion of hepatitis B vaccination series in infants born to HBsAG-positive mothers and previously vaccinated with hepatitis B immune globulin or born to mothers of unknown status, has not been evaluated.

Use with caution in patients with a history of bleeding disorders (including thrombocytopenia) and/or on anticoagulant therapy. Use with caution in severely immunocompromised patients (eg, patients receiving chemo/radiation therapy or other immunosuppressive therapy (including high dose corticosteroids); may have a reduced response to vaccination. May be used in patients with HIV infection. In general, inactivated vaccines should be administered ≥2 weeks prior to planned immunosuppression when feasible (Rubin, 2014). Vaccination may not result in effective immunity in all patients. Response depends upon multiple factors (eg, type of vaccine, age of patient) and may be improved by administering the vaccine at the recommended dose, route, and interval. Vaccines may not be effective if administered during periods of altered immune competence (CDC, 2011). Use with caution in patients with personal or immediate family (parent, sibling) history of progressive neurologic disease, or conditions predisposing to seizures; consider deferring immunization until health status can be assessed and condition stabilized. Antipyretics may be considered at the time of and for 24 hours following vaccination to patients at high risk for seizures to reduce the possibility of postvaccination fever (may occur within 2-3 days). Use caution with repeat administration of any vaccine associated with the onset of Guillain-Barré syndrome within 8 weeks of immunization. Formulation may contain aluminum, neomycin, or polymyxin B.

Some dosage forms may contain polysorbate 80 (also known as Tweens). Hypersensitivity reactions, usually a delayed reaction, have been reported following exposure to pharmaceutical products containing polysorbate 80 in certain individuals (Isaksson, 2002; Lucente 2000; Shelley, 1995). Thrombocytopenia, ascites, pulmonary deterioration, and renal and hepatic failure have been reported in premature neonates after receiving parenteral products containing polysorbate 80 (Alade, 1986; CDC, 1984). See manufacturer's labeling.

Adverse Reactions All serious adverse reactions may be reported to local provincial/territorial health agencies or to the Vaccine Safety Section at Public Health Agency of Canada (1-866-844-0018).

Central nervous system: Crying abnormal, fatigue, fever ≥38°C (100.4°F), fever >39.5°C (103.1°F), irritability, nervousness, restlessness, sleeping decreased/increased

Local: Injection site: Induration, redness, pain, swelling

Gastrointestinal: Diarrhea, loss of appetite, vomiting

Rare but important or life-threatening: Allergic reaction (including anaphylactic and anaphylactoid reactions), angioedema, apnea, bronchospasm, collapse, diffuse edema of injected limb, inflammatory cellulitis (without bacterial infection), lymphadenopathy, seizure (including febrile seizure), shock-like state (hypotonic-hyporesponsiveness episode), sudden unexpected death, thrombocytopenia

Drug Interactions

Metabolism/Transport Effects None known.

Avoid Concomitant Use There are no known interactions where it is recommended to avoid concomitant use.

Increased Effect/Toxicity There are no known significant interactions involving an increase in effect.

Decreased Effect

The levels/effects of Diphtheria and Tetanus Toxoids, Acellular Pertussis, Hepatitis B (Recombinant), Poliovirus (Inactivated), and Haemophilus influenzae B Conjugate (Adsorbed) Vaccine may be decreased by: Belimumab; Immunosuppressants; Meningococcal Polysaccharide (Groups A / C / Y and W-135) Tetanus Toxoid Conjugate Vaccine

Preparation for Administration Allow vial containing the Hib pellet to stay at room temperature for at least 5 minutes. Shake Pediarix™ syringe until homogenous turbid white suspension is obtained. Add entire contents of syringe to vial containing the Hib pellet and then shake vial until pellet dissolves completely. Resulting suspension will appear slightly cloudier than suspension added from syringe.

Storage/Stability Store at 2°C to 8°C (36°F to 46°F); do not freeze (discard if frozen). Immediate use after reconstitution is recommended; however, after reconstitution vaccine may be stored for 8 hours at ~21°C (~70°F).

Mechanism of Action Promotes active immunity to diphtheria, tetanus, pertussis, hepatitis B, poliovirus (types 1, 2, and 3), and *Haemophilus influenzae* type B by inducing production of specific antibodies and antitoxins.

Pharmacodynamics/Kinetics Onset: Immune response observed to all components 1 month following the 3-dose series

Dosage IM: **Note:** Vaccinate preterm infants according to their chronological age from birth. Children 6 weeks to 2 years:

Primary immunization: 0.5 mL; repeat in 8-week intervals for a total of 3 doses. Vaccination usually begins at 2 months, but may be started at 6 weeks of age. Do not administer to infants <6 weeks of age.

Use in children previously vaccinated with one or more doses of hepatitis B vaccine: Children who received 1 dose of hepatitis B vaccine at birth may receive a 3 dose series of Infanrix Hexa™ beginning no earlier than at 6 weeks of age. Use in infants who received more than 1 dose of hepatitis B vaccine has not been studied.

Where immunization against poliovirus is desired, Infanrix Hexa™ may be administered instead to infants scheduled to receive concurrent Infanrix™ (diphtheria, tetanus and acellular pertussis vaccine) and hepatitis B vaccine.

Booster immunization: 0.5 mL administered at 18 months (in infants who have received a full primary vaccination course of each component of Infanrix Hexa™)

Note: Dosing delays should not interfere with the final immunity achieved with Infanrix Hexa™. Regardless of the time that elapses between doses, it is not necessary to restart the vaccination series.

Administration Administer by IM injection only, preferably in the anterolateral aspects of the thigh or the deltoid muscle of the upper arm. Do not administer intravenously or subcutaneously. Do not inject into the gluteal area (suboptimal hepatitis B immune response) or areas where major nerve trunks may be located. Fractional dosing (use of reduced volume) is not recommended. If more than one vaccine is to be given by IM injection use separate limbs. Rotate injection sites when completing vaccination series.

Acetaminophen may be used when needed to provide comfort; however, routine prophylactic administration of acetaminophen to prevent fever due to vaccine use is not recommended. There is evidence of a decreased immune response to some vaccines associated with acetaminophen administration; the clinical significance of this reduction in immune response has not been established.

Monitoring Parameters Signs/symptoms of hypersensitivity for 30 minutes after administration; respiratory function for 2-3 days following vaccination of infants born prematurely. Monitor for syncope for 15 minutes following administration. If seizure-like activity associated with syncope occurs, maintain patient in supine or Trendelenburg position to reestablish adequate cerebral perfusion.

Product Availability Not available in U.S.

Dosage Forms: Canada

Injection, suspension:

Infanrix Hexa™: Diphtheria toxoid 25 Lf, tetanus toxoid 10 Lf, acellular pertussis antigens [inactivated pertussis toxin 25 mcg, filamentous hemagglutinin 25 mcg, pertactin 8 mcg], HBsAg 10 mcg, type 1 poliovirus 40 D antigen units, type 2 poliovirus 8 D antigen units and type 3 poliovirus 32 D antigen units, *Haemophilus* b capsular polysaccharide 10 mcg [bound to tetanus toxoid 20-40 mcg] per 0.5 mL (0.5 mL) [contains aluminum, neomycin sulfate (trace amounts), polymyxin B (trace amounts), polysorbate 20, polysorbate 80, and yeast protein ≤5%; Pediarix™ vaccine used to reconstitute Hib forms Infanrix Hexa™]

Diphtheria and Tetanus Toxoids, Acellular Pertussis, Poliovirus and *Haemophilus* b Conjugate Vaccine

(dif THEER ee a & TET a nus TOKS oyds ay CEL yoo lar per TUS sis POE lee oh VYE rus & hem OF fi lus bee KON joo gate vak SEEN)

Brand Names: U.S. Pentacel®

Brand Names: Canada Pediacel®; Pentacel®

Index Terms *Haemophilus* B Conjugate (Hib); *Haemophilus* B Polysaccharide; Diphtheria Toxoid; Diphtheria, Tetanus Toxoids, Acellular Pertussis (DTaP); DTaP-IPV/Hib; Pertussis, Acellular (Adsorbed); Poliovirus, Inactivated (IPV); Tetanus Toxoid

Pharmacologic Category Vaccine, Inactivated (Bacterial); Vaccine, Inactivated (Viral)

Additional Appendix Information

Immunization Administration Recommendations *on page 2250*

Immunization Recommendations *on page 2255*

Use Active immunization against diphtheria, tetanus, pertussis, poliomyelitis, and invasive disease caused by *H. influenzae* type b in children 6 weeks through 4 years of age

Advisory Committee on Immunization Practices (ACIP) recommends that Pentacel® (DTaP-IPV/Hib) may be used to provide the recommended DTaP, IPV, and Hib immunization in children <5 years of age. Whenever feasible, the same manufacturer should be used to provide the pertussis component; however, vaccination should not be deferred if a specific brand is not known or is not available. The Hib component in Pentacel® contains a tetanus toxoid conjugate. A Hib vaccine containing the PRP-OMP conjugate (PedvaxHIB®) may provide a more rapid seroconversion following the first dose and may be preferable to use in certain populations (eg, American Indian or Alaska Native children).

Pregnancy Risk Factor C

Dosage IM: Children:

Primary immunization: Children 6 weeks to ≤4 years: 0.5 mL per dose administered at 2, 4, 6 and 15-18 months of age (total of 4 doses). The first dose may be administered as early as 6 weeks of age. Following completion of the 4-dose series, children should receive a dose of DTaP vaccine at 4-6 years of age (Daptacel® recommended due to same pertussis antigen used in both products).

Note: Per the ACIP, polio vaccine should not be administered more frequently than 4 weeks apart. Use of the minimum age and minimum intervals during the first 6 months of life should only be done when the vaccine recipient is at risk for imminent exposure to circulating poliovirus (shorter intervals and earlier start dates may lead to lower seroconversion. Pentacel® is not indicated for the polio booster dose given at 4-6 years of age; Kinrix® or IPV should be used.

Children previously vaccinated with ≥1 dose of Daptacel® or IPV vaccines: Pentacel® may be used to complete the first 4 doses of the DTaP or IPV series in children scheduled to receive the other components in the vaccine.

Children previously vaccinated with ≥1 dose of *Haemophilus* b conjugate vaccine: Pentacel® may be used to complete the series in children scheduled to receive the other components in the vaccine; however, if different brands of *Haemophilus* b conjugate vaccine are administered to complete the series, 3 primary immunizing doses are needed, followed by a booster dose.

Note: Completion of 3 doses of Pentacel® provides primary immunization against diphtheria, tetanus, *H. influenzae* type B, and poliomyelitis. Completion of the 4-dose series with Pentacel® provides primary immunization against pertussis. It also provides a booster vaccination against diphtheria, tetanus, *H. influenzae* type B, and poliomyelitis.

Dosage adjustment in renal impairment: No dosage adjustment provided in manufacturer's labeling.

Dosage adjustment in hepatic impairment: No dosage adjustment provided in manufacturer's labeling.

Additional Information Complete prescribing information should be consulted for additional detail.

Dosage Forms

Injection, suspension:

Pentacel®: Diphtheria toxoid 15 Lf, tetanus toxoid 5 Lf, acellular pertussis antigens, poliovirus, and *Haemophilus* b capsular polysaccharide 10 mcg per 0.5 mL (0.5 mL)

- ◆ **Diphtheria and Tetanus Toxoids and Acellular Pertussis Adsorbed, and Inactivated Poliovirus Vaccine Combined** *see* Diphtheria and Tetanus Toxoids, Acellular Pertussis, and Poliovirus Vaccine *on page 646*
- ◆ **Diphtheria and Tetanus Toxoids and Acellular Pertussis Adsorbed, Hepatitis B (Recombinant) and Inactivated Poliovirus Vaccine Combined** *see* Diphtheria, Tetanus Toxoids, Acellular Pertussis, Hepatitis B (Recombinant), and Poliovirus (Inactivated) Vaccine *on page 651*
- ◆ **Diphtheria and Tetanus Toxoids and Acellular Pertussis, Hepatitis B (Recombinant), Inactivated Poliovirus Vaccine, and *Haemophilus influenzae* Type B Combined** *see* Diphtheria and Tetanus Toxoids, Acellular Pertussis, Hepatitis B (Recombinant), Poliovirus (Inactivated), and *Haemophilus influenzae* B Conjugate (Adsorbed) Vaccine [CAN/INT] *on page 647*

Diphtheria and Tetanus Toxoids, and Acellular Pertussis Vaccine

(dif THEER ee a & TET a nus TOKS oyds & ay CEL yoo lar per TUS sis vak SEEN)

Brand Names: U.S. Adacel; Boostrix; Daptacel; Infanrix

Brand Names: Canada Adacel; Boostrix

Index Terms DTaP; Tdap; Tetanus Toxoid, Reduced Diphtheria Toxoid, and Acellular Pertussis, Adsorbed; Tripedia

Pharmacologic Category Vaccine, Inactivated (Bacterial)

Additional Appendix Information

Immunization Administration Recommendations *on page 2250*

Immunization Recommendations *on page 2255*

Use

Daptacel, Infanrix (DTaP): Active immunization against diphtheria, tetanus, and pertussis from age 6 weeks through 6 years of age (prior to seventh birthday)

Adacel, Boostrix (Tdap): Active booster immunization against diphtheria, tetanus, and pertussis in persons 10 years and older (Boostrix) or persons 10 to 64 years of age (Adacel)

The Advisory Committee on Immunization Practices (ACIP) recommends routine vaccination for the following:

Children 6 weeks to <7 years (DTaP):

- For primary immunization against diphtheria, tetanus and pertussis (Use of diphtheria toxoid [ACIP], 2000)
- Pediatric patients who are wounded in bombings or similar mass casualty events and who have penetrating injuries or nonintact skin exposure, and have an uncertain vaccination history should receive a tetanus booster with DTaP (if no contraindications exist) (CDC [Chapman, 2008]).

Children 7 to 9 years (Tdap):

- Children who did not complete a fully primary DTaP series should receive a single dose of Tdap (if no contraindications exist) (CDC 60[1], 2011)
- Children never vaccinated against diphtheria, tetanus, or pertussis, or whose vaccination status is not known should receive a series of three vaccinations containing tetanus and diphtheria toxoids and the first dose should be with Tdap (CDC 60[1], 2011)

Adolescents 10 to 18 years (Tdap):

- A single dose of Tdap as a booster dose in adolescents who have completed the recommended childhood DTaP vaccination series (preferred age of administration is 11 to 12 years) (CDC 60[1], 2011)

Adolescents ≥11 years and Adults (Tdap):

- Persons wounded in bombings or similar mass casualty events and who cannot confirm receipt of a tetanus booster within the previous 5 years and who have penetrating injuries or nonintact skin exposure should receive a single dose of Tdap (CDC 61[25], 2012; CDC [Chapman, 2008])

Pregnant patients: (Tdap): Pregnant females should receive a single dose with each pregnancy, preferably between 27-36 weeks gestation (CDC 62 [7], 2013)

Adults ≥19 years (including adults ≥65 years) (Tdap): A single dose of Tdap should be given to all patients who have not previously received Tdap or for whom their vaccine status is unknown. Following administration of Tdap, Td vaccine should be used for routine boosters (CDC/ACIP [Bridges, 2014]). The following patients, who have not yet received Tdap or for whom vaccine status is not known, should receive a single dose of Tdap as soon as feasible:

- Close contacts of children <12 months of age; Tdap should ideally be administered at least 2 weeks prior to beginning close contact (CDC/ACIP 60[41], 2011; CDC [Kretsinger, 2006]).
- Healthcare providers with direct patient contact (CDC [Kretsinger, 2006])

Note: Tdap is currently recommended for a single dose only (all age groups) (CDC 60[1], 2011; CDC/ACIP 61 [25], 2012), except pregnant females (CDC 62[7], 2013)

Pregnancy Risk Factor B/C (manufacturer specific)

Dosage Note: Tdap can be administered regardless of the interval between the last tetanus or diphtheria toxoid containing vaccine. Tdap is currently recommended for a single dose only (CDC 60[1], 2011; CDC/ACIP 61[25], 2012), except pregnant females (CDC 62 [7], 2013).

Immunization: IM:

Children 6 weeks to <7 years: Primary immunization:

Note: Whenever possible, the same product should be used for all doses. Interruption of recommended schedule does not require starting the series over; a delay between doses should not interfere with final immunity.

Daptacel, Infanrix: 0.5 mL per dose, total of 5 doses administered as follows:

Three doses, usually given at 2-, 4-, and 6 months of age; may be given as early as 6 weeks of age and repeated every 4 to 8 weeks

Fourth dose: Given at ~15 to 20 months of age, but at least 6 months after third dose. The fourth dose may be given as early as 12 months of age, but at least 6 months must have elapsed between the third dose and the fourth dose.

Fifth dose: Given at 4 to 6 years of age, prior to starting school or kindergarten; if the fourth dose is given at ≥4 years of age, the fifth dose may be omitted

For children who start primary immunization series ≥4 months of age, refer to current ACIP "Catch-up Immunization Schedule".

Children 7 to 10 years: Not fully vaccinated against pertussis, or never vaccinated against diphtheria, tetanus, or pertussis, or whose vaccination status is not known: Administer a series of 3 vaccinations containing tetanus and diphtheria toxoids; the first dose should be with Tdap (CDC 60[1], 2011).

Adolescents and Adults: Booster immunization: ACIP recommendations:

Adolescents 11 to 18 years: 0.5 mL per dose. Tdap should be given as a single booster dose at age 11 or 12 years in adolescents who have completed a childhood DTaP vaccination series, followed by booster doses of Td every 10 years. Adolescents who have not received Tdap at age 11 or 12 should receive a single dose of Tdap in place of a single Td booster dose (CDC [Broder, 2006]; CDC 60[1], 2011).

Adults ≥19 years: 0.5 mL per dose. A single dose of Tdap should be given to replace a single dose of the 10 year Td booster in patients who have not previously received Tdap or for whom vaccine status is not known. A single dose of Tdap is recommended for health care personnel who have not previously received Tdap and who have direct patient contact (CDC [Kretsinger, 2006]). Tdap should be administered regardless of interval since last tetanus- or diphtheria-containing vaccine (CDC/ACIP 61[25], 2012).

Adolescents and Adults: Booster immunization: Manufacturer's recommendations:

Children ≥10 years and Adults (Boostrix): 0.5 mL as a single dose, administered 5 years after last dose of tetanus toxoid, diphtheria toxoid, and/or pertussis-containing vaccine

Children ≥10 years and Adults ≤64 years (Adacel): 0.5 mL as a single dose, administered 5 years after last dose of tetanus toxoid, diphtheria toxoid and/or pertussis-containing vaccine

Elderly: Adults ≥65 years: Booster immunization:

ACIP recommendations: Refer to adult dosing. In adults ≥65 years Boostrix should be used if feasible; however, ACIP has concluded that either Tdap vaccine (Boostrix or Adacel) may be used (CDC 61[25], 2012).

Manufacturer's recommendations: Boostrix: 0.5 mL as a single dose, administered 5 years after last dose of tetanus toxoid, diphtheria toxoid, and/or pertussis-containing vaccine.

Wound management: IM: Children, Adolescents, Adults, and Elderly: Adacel or Boostrix may be used as an alternative to Td vaccine when a tetanus toxoid-containing vaccine is needed for wound management, and in whom the pertussis component is also indicated. Tetanus prophylaxis in patients with wounds should consider if the wound is clean or contaminated, the immunization status of the patient, proper use of tetanus toxoid and/or tetanus immune globulin (TIG), wound cleaning, and (if required) surgical debridement and the proper use of antibiotics. Patients with an uncertain or incomplete tetanus immunization status should have additional follow up to ensure a series is completed. Patients with a history of Arthus reaction following a previous dose of a tetanus toxoid-containing vaccine should not receive a tetanus toxoid-containing vaccine until >10 years after the most recent dose even if they have a wound that is neither clean nor minor. See table.

Tetanus Prophylaxis in Wound Management

History of Tetanus Immunization Doses	Clean, Minor Wounds		All Other Wounds[1]	
	Tetanus Toxoid[2]	TIG	Tetanus Toxoid[2]	TIG
Uncertain or <3 doses	Yes	No	Yes	Yes
3 or more doses	No[3]	No	No[4]	No

[1]Such as, but not limited to, wounds contaminated with dirt, feces, soil, and saliva; puncture wounds; wounds from crushing, tears, burns, and frostbite.

[2]Tetanus toxoid in this chart refers to a tetanus toxoid-containing vaccine. For children <7 years of age, DTaP (DT, if pertussis vaccine contraindicated) is preferred to tetanus toxoid alone. For children ≥7 years and adults, Td preferred to tetanus toxoid alone; Tdap may be preferred if the patient has not previously been vaccinated with Tdap.

[3]Yes, if ≥10 years since last dose.

[4]Yes, if ≥5 years since last dose.

Adapted from CDC "Yellow Book" (*Health Information for International Travel 2010*), "Routine Vaccine-Preventable Diseases, Tetanus" (available at http://www.cdc.gov/yellowbook) and *MMWR* 2006, 55 (RR-17).

Abbreviations: **DT** = Diphtheria and Tetanus Toxoids (formulation for age ≤6 years); **DTaP** = Diphtheria and Tetanus Toxoids, and Acellular Pertussis (formulation for age ≤6 years; Daptacel®, Infanrix®); **Td** = Diphtheria and Tetanus Toxoids (formulation for age ≥7 years; Decavac®,Tenivac™); **TT**= Tetanus toxoid (adsorbed [formulation for age ≥7 years]); **Tdap** = Diphtheria and Tetanus Toxoids, and Acellular Pertussis (Adacel® or Boostrix® [formulations for age ≥7 years]); **TIG** = Tetanus Immune Globulin

Additional Information Complete prescribing information should be consulted for additional detail.

Dosage Forms

Injection, suspension [Tdap, booster formulation]:

Adacel: Diphtheria 2 Lf units, tetanus 5 Lf units, and acellular pertussis antigens per 0.5 mL (0.5 mL)

Boostrix: Diphtheria 2.5 Lf units, tetanus 5 Lf units, and acellular pertussis antigens per 0.5 mL (0.5 mL)

Injection, suspension [DTaP, active immunization formulation]:

Daptacel: Diphtheria 15 Lf units, tetanus 5 Lf units, and acellular pertussis antigens per 0.5 mL (0.5 mL)

Infanrix: Diphtheria 25 Lf units, tetanus 10 Lf units, and acellular pertussis antigens per 0.5 mL (0.5 mL) [preservative free]

◆ **Diphtheria, Tetanus Toxoids, Acellular Pertussis (DTaP)** *see* Diphtheria and Tetanus Toxoids, Acellular Pertussis, and Poliovirus Vaccine *on page 646*

◆ **Diphtheria, Tetanus Toxoids, Acellular Pertussis (DTaP)** *see* Diphtheria and Tetanus Toxoids, Acellular Pertussis, Poliovirus and *Haemophilus* b Conjugate Vaccine *on page 648*

Diphtheria, Tetanus Toxoids, Acellular Pertussis, Hepatitis B (Recombinant), and Poliovirus (Inactivated) Vaccine

(dif THEER ee a, TET a nus TOKS oyds, ay CEL yoo lar per TUS sis, hep a TYE tis bee ree KOM be nant, & POE lee oh VYE rus in ak ti VAY ted vak SEEN)

Brand Names: U.S. Pediarix®

Brand Names: Canada Pediarix®

Index Terms Diphtheria and Tetanus Toxoids and Acellular Pertussis Adsorbed, Hepatitis B (Recombinant) and Inactivated Poliovirus Vaccine Combined; Diphtheria, Tetanus Toxoids, Acellular Pertussis, Hepatitis B (Recombinant), and Poliovirus (Inactivated) Vaccine; Diphtheria, Tetanus Toxoids, Acellular Pertussis, Hepatitis B (Recombinant), and Poliovirus Vaccine; DTaP-HepB-IPV

Pharmacologic Category Vaccine, Inactivated (Bacterial); Vaccine, Inactivated (Viral)

Additional Appendix Information

Immunization Administration Recommendations *on page 2250*

Immunization Recommendations *on page 2255*

Use Combination vaccine for the active immunization against diphtheria, tetanus, pertussis, hepatitis B virus (all known subtypes), and poliomyelitis (caused by poliovirus types 1, 2, and 3)

The Advisory Committee on Immunization Practices (ACIP) recommends Pediarix® for the following:

- Primary vaccination for DTaP, Hep B, and IPV in children at 2, 4, and 6 months of age.
- To complete the primary vaccination series in children who have received DTaP (Infanrix®) and who are scheduled to receive the other components of the vaccine. Whenever feasible, the same manufacturer should be used to provide the pertussis component; however, vaccination should not be deferred if a specific brand is not known or is not available. HepB and IPV from different manufacturers are interchangeable.

Pregnancy Risk Factor C

Dosage IM: Children 6 weeks to <7 years:

Primary immunization: 0.5 mL/dose; administer as a 3-dose series at 2-, 4-, and 6 months of age in 6- to 8-week intervals (preferably 8-week intervals). Vaccination usually begins at 2 months, but may be started as early as 6 weeks of age.

Note: Pediarix® is approved for the first 3 doses of polio vaccine. Per the ACIP, polio vaccine is given at 2, 4 and 6 months of age and should not be administered more frequently than 4 weeks apart. Use of the minimum age and minimum intervals during the first 6 months of life should only be done when the vaccine recipient is at risk for imminent exposure to circulating poliovirus (shorter intervals and earlier start dates may lead to lower seroconversion).

Use in children previously vaccinated with one or more component, and who are also scheduled to receive all vaccine components:

Hepatitis B vaccine: Infants previously vaccinated with 1 or 2 doses of another hepatitis B vaccine may use Pediarix® to complete the 3-dose series. Not for use as birth dose of hepatitis B vaccine. Infants born to HBsAg-positive women should begin dosing with DTaP-HepB-IPV by age 6-8 weeks after receiving the single antigen hepatitis B vaccine at birth.

Diphtheria and tetanus toxoids, and acellular pertussis vaccine (DTaP): Infants previously vaccinated with 1 or 2 doses of Infanrix® may use Pediarix® to complete the first 3 doses of the series; use of Pediarix® to complete DTaP vaccination started with products other than Infanrix® is not recommended.

Inactivated polio vaccine (IPV): Infants previously vaccinated with 1 or 2 doses of IPV may use Pediarix® to complete the first 3 doses of the series.

Dosage adjustment in renal impairment: No dosage adjustment provided in manufacturer's labeling.

Dosage adjustment in hepatic impairment: No dosage adjustment provided in manufacturer's labeling.

Additional Information Complete prescribing information should be consulted for additional detail.

Dosage Forms

Injection, suspension [preservative free]:

Pediarix®: Diphtheria toxoid 25 Lf, tetanus toxoid 10 Lf, acellular pertussis antigens per 0.5 mL (0.5 mL)

◆ **Diphtheria, Tetanus Toxoids, Acellular Pertussis, Hepatitis B (Recombinant), and Poliovirus (Inactivated) Vaccine** *see* Diphtheria, Tetanus Toxoids, Acellular Pertussis, Hepatitis B (Recombinant), and Poliovirus (Inactivated) Vaccine *on page 651*

◆ **Diphtheria, Tetanus Toxoids, Acellular Pertussis, Hepatitis B (Recombinant), and Poliovirus Vaccine** *see* Diphtheria, Tetanus Toxoids, Acellular Pertussis, Hepatitis B (Recombinant), and Poliovirus (Inactivated) Vaccine *on page 651*

◆ **Diphtheria Toxoid** *see* Diphtheria and Tetanus Toxoids, Acellular Pertussis, Poliovirus and *Haemophilus* b Conjugate Vaccine *on page 648*

◆ **Dipirona** *see* Dipyrone [INT] *on page 653*

◆ **Dipirona Sodica** *see* Dipyrone [INT] *on page 653*

◆ **Dipivalyl Epinephrine** *see* Dipivefrin *on page 651*

Dipivefrin (dye PI ve frin)

Brand Names: Canada Ophtho-Dipivefrin™; PMS-Dipivefrin; Propine®

Index Terms Dipivalyl Epinephrine; Dipivefrin Hydrochloride; DPE

Pharmacologic Category Alpha/Beta Agonist; Ophthalmic Agent, Antiglaucoma; Ophthalmic Agent, Vasoconstrictor

Use Reduces elevated intraocular pressure in chronic open-angle glaucoma; also used to treat ocular hypertension, low tension, and secondary glaucomas

Pregnancy Risk Factor B

Dosage Adults: Ophthalmic: Instill 1 drop every 12 hours into the eyes

Dosage adjustment in renal impairment: No dosage adjustment provided in manufacturer's labeling.

Dosage adjustment in hepatic impairment: No dosage adjustment provided in manufacturer's labeling.

Additional Information Complete prescribing information should be consulted for additional detail.

◆ **Dipivefrin Hydrochloride** *see* Dipivefrin *on page 651*

◆ **Diprivan** *see* Propofol *on page 1728*

◆ **Diprolene** *see* Betamethasone (Topical) *on page 255*

◆ **Diprolene AF** *see* Betamethasone (Topical) *on page 255*

◆ **Dipropylacetic Acid** *see* Valproic Acid and Derivatives *on page 2123*

◆ **Diprosone (Can)** *see* Betamethasone (Topical) *on page 255*

Dipyridamole (dye peer ID a mole)

Brand Names: U.S. Persantine

Brand Names: Canada Apo-Dipyridamole FC®; Dipyridamole For Injection; Persantine®

Pharmacologic Category Antiplatelet Agent; Vasodilator

Additional Appendix Information

Beers Criteria – Potentially Inappropriate Medications for Geriatrics *on page 2271*

Use

Oral: Used with warfarin to decrease thrombosis in patients after artificial heart valve replacement

IV: Diagnostic agent in CAD

Pregnancy Risk Factor B

Pregnancy Considerations Adverse events have not been observed in animal reproduction studies.

Breast-Feeding Considerations Dipyridamole is excreted in breast milk. The manufacturer recommends that caution be exercised when administering dipyridamole to nursing women.

Contraindications Hypersensitivity to dipyridamole or any component of the formulation

Warnings/Precautions Use with caution in patients with hypotension, unstable angina, and/or recent MI. Use with caution in hepatic impairment. Avoid use of oral dipyridamole in this age group due to risk of orthostatic hypotension and availability of more efficacious alternative agents (Beers Criteria). Use caution in patients on other antiplatelet agents or anticoagulation. Severe adverse reactions have occurred with IV administration (rarely); use the IV form with caution in patients with bronchospastic disease or unstable angina. Aminophylline should be available in case of urgency or emergency with IV use.

Adverse Reactions

Oral:

Cardiovascular: Angina pectoris, flushing

Central nervous system: Dizziness, headache

Dermatologic: Pruritus, skin rash

Gastrointestinal: Abdominal distress, diarrhea, vomiting

Hepatic: Hepatic insufficiency

Rare but important or life-threatening: Alopecia, arthritis, cholelithiasis, dyspepsia, fatigue, hepatitis, hypersensitivity reaction, hypotension, laryngeal edema, malaise, myalgia, nausea, palpitations, paresthesia, tachycardia, thrombocytopenia

IV:

Cardiovascular: Altered blood pressure, ECG abnormality (ST-T changes, extrasystoles), exacerbation of angina pectoris, flushing, hypertension, hypotension, tachycardia

Central nervous system: Dizziness, fatigue, headache, pain, paresthesia

Gastrointestinal: Nausea

Respiratory: Dyspnea

Rare but important or life-threatening: Abdominal pain, arthralgia, ataxia, back pain, bronchospasm, cardiac arrhythmia (ventricular tachycardia, bradycardia, AV block, SVT, atrial fibrillation, asystole), cardiomyopathy, cough, depersonalization, diaphoresis, dysgeusia, dyspepsia, dysphagia, ECG abnormality (unspecified), edema, eructation, flatulence, hypersensitivity reaction, hypertonia, hyperventilation, increased appetite, increased thirst, injection site reaction, leg cramps (intermittent claudication), malaise, mastalgia, muscle rigidity, myalgia, myocardial infarction, orthostatic hypotension, otalgia, palpitations, perineal pain, pharyngitis, pleuritic chest pain, pruritus, renal pain, rhinitis, skin rash, syncope, tenesmus, tinnitus, tremor, urticaria, vertigo, visual disturbance, vomiting, weakness, xerostomia

Drug Interactions

Metabolism/Transport Effects Inhibits BCRP, P-glycoprotein

Avoid Concomitant Use

Avoid concomitant use of Dipyridamole with any of the following: Bosutinib; PAZOPanib; Riociguat; Silodosin; Topotecan; Urokinase; VinCRIStine (Liposomal)

Increased Effect/Toxicity

Dipyridamole may increase the levels/effects of: Adenosine; Afatinib; Agents with Antiplatelet Properties; Anticoagulants; Apixaban; Beta-Blockers; Bosutinib; Brentuximab Vedotin; Colchicine; Collagenase (Systemic); Dabigatran Etexilate; DOXOrubicin (Conventional); DULoxetine; Edoxaban; Everolimus; Hypotensive Agents; Ibritumomab; Ledipasvir; Levodopa; Naloxegol; Obinutuzumab; PAZOPanib; P-glycoprotein/ABCB1 Substrates; Prucalopride; Regadenoson; Rifaximin; Riociguat; RisperiDONE; Rivaroxaban; Salicylates; Silodosin; Thrombolytic Agents; Topotecan; Tositumomab and Iodine I 131 Tositumomab; Urokinase; VinCRIStine (Liposomal)

The levels/effects of Dipyridamole may be increased by: Barbiturates; Dasatinib; Glucosamine; Herbs (Anticoagulant/Antiplatelet Properties); Ibrutinib; Limaprost; Multivitamins/Fluoride (with ADE); Multivitamins/Minerals (with ADEK, Folate, Iron); Multivitamins/Minerals (with AE, No Iron); Nicorandil; Omega-3 Fatty Acids; Pentosan Polysulfate Sodium; Pentoxifylline; Prostacyclin Analogues; Tipranavir; Vitamin E

Decreased Effect

Dipyridamole may decrease the levels/effects of: Acetylcholinesterase Inhibitors

Preparation for Administration Prior to administration, dilute solution for injection to a ≥1:2 ratio in NS, ½NS, or D_5W. Total volume should be ~20-50 mL.

Storage/Stability IV: Store between 15°C to 25°C (59°F to 77°F); do not freeze. Protect from light.

Mechanism of Action Inhibits the activity of adenosine deaminase and phosphodiesterase, which causes an accumulation of adenosine, adenine nucleotides, and cyclic AMP; these mediators then inhibit platelet aggregation and may cause vasodilation; may also stimulate release of prostacyclin or PGD_2; causes coronary vasodilation

Pharmacodynamics/Kinetics

Absorption: Readily, but variable

Distribution: Adults: V_d: 2-3 L/kg

Protein binding: 91% to 99%

Metabolism: Hepatic

Half-life elimination: Terminal: 10-12 hours

Time to peak, serum: 2-2.5 hours

Excretion: Feces (as glucuronide conjugates and unchanged drug)

Dosage

Oral: Children ≥12 years and Adults: Adjunctive therapy for prophylaxis of thromboembolism with cardiac valve replacement: 75-100 mg 4 times/day

IV: Adults: Evaluation of coronary artery disease: 0.14 mg/kg/minute for 4 minutes; maximum dose: 60 mg

Following dipyridamole infusion, inject thallium-201 within 5 minutes. **Note:** Aminophylline should be available for urgent/emergent use; dosing of 50-100 mg (range: 50-250 mg) IV push over 30-60 seconds.

Dosage adjustment in renal impairment: No dosage adjustment provided in manufacturer's labeling.

Dosage adjustment in hepatic impairment: No dosage adjustment provided in manufacturer's labeling.

Dietary Considerations Should be taken with water 1 hour before meals.

Administration

IV: Infuse diluted solution over 4 minutes.

Tablet: Administer with water 1 hour before meals.

Monitoring Parameters Blood pressure, heart rate, ECG (stress test)

Dosage Forms

Solution, Intravenous:

Generic: 5 mg/mL (2 mL, 10 mL)

Tablet, Oral:

Persantine: 25 mg, 50 mg, 75 mg

Generic: 25 mg, 50 mg, 75 mg

Extemporaneous Preparations A 10 mg/mL oral suspension may be made with tablets and one of three different vehicles (cherry syrup, a 1:1 mixture of Ora-Sweet® and Ora-Plus®, or a 1:1 mixture of Ora-Sweet® SF and Ora-Plus®). Crush twenty-four 50 mg tablets in a mortar and reduce to a fine powder. Add 20 mL of the chosen vehicle and mix to a uniform paste; mix while adding the vehicle in incremental proportions to **almost** 120 mL; transfer to a calibrated bottle, rinse mortar with vehicle, and add quantity of vehicle sufficient to make 120 mL. Label "shake well" and "protect from light". Stable for 60 days when stored in amber plastic prescription bottles in the dark at room temperature or refrigerated.

Allen LV and Erickson III MA, "Stability of Baclofen, Captopril, Diltiazem, Hydrochloride, Dipyridamole, and Flecainide Acetate in Extemporaneously Compounded Oral Liquids," *Am J Health Syst Pharm*, 1996, 53:2179-84.

◆ **Dipyridamole and Aspirin** *see* Aspirin and Dipyridamole *on page 185*

◆ **Dipyridamole For Injection (Can)** *see* Dipyridamole *on page 652*

Dipyrone [INT] (dye PYE rone)

International Brand Names Algimabo (ES); Algirona (BR); Algopyrin (HU); Alnex (MX); Analgin (BG, CZ, DE, EG, RU); Analgina (AR, PY); Analgine (BE); Antalgin (ID); Antalgina (PE); Causalon (UY); Conmel (CO, VE); Cornalgin (ID); Defin (MX); Di Shuang (CN); Dialgin (BG); Diprin (BR); Dolanet (PY); Dolemicin (ES); Dolgan (MX); Dolocalma (PT); Foragin (ID); Hexalgin (BG); Laper (CO); Magnopyrol (BR); Metamizol (CL); Minalgin (CH); Natralgin (GR); Nolotil (ES, PT); Novalcina (VE); Novalgin (AT, CH, CZ, DE, NL, PK); Novalgina (AR, CO, IT, PE, UY); Novalgine (BE, VN); Optalgin (HU, IL); Proalgin (BG); Promel (VE); Sinalgia (PY); Taxenil (AR); Telalgin (GR); V-Dalgin (IL)

Index Terms Dipirona; Dipirona Sodica; Metamizol Sodico; Metamizole; Metamizole Sodium; Methampyrone; Sulpyrine

Pharmacologic Category Analgesic, Nonsteroidal Anti-inflammatory Drug; Antipyretic; Nonsteroidal Anti-inflammatory Drug (NSAID), Oral; Nonsteroidal Anti-inflammatory Drug (NSAID), Parenteral; Nonsteroidal Anti-inflammatory Drug (NSAID), Suppository

Reported Use Treatment of pain or fever

Dosage Range

Children ≥3 months to Adolescents <15 years: IM, IV, Oral, Rectal: Dosing varies greatly based on weight (consult product labeling)

Adolescents ≥15 years or >53 kg and Adults:

Oral: 500 mg to 1 g up to 4 times daily; maximum: 4 g daily

IM, IV: 1 to 2.5 g up to 4 times daily; maximum: 5 g daily

Rectal (suppository): 300 mg up to 4 times daily

Product Availability Product available in various countries; not currently available in the U.S.

Dosage Forms

Solution, injection: 500 mg/mL

Solution, oral: 50 mg/mL; 500 mg/mL

Tablet, oral: 500 mg; 1 g

Suppository, rectal: 300 mg

◆ **Disalcid** *see* Salsalate *on page 1862*

◆ **Disalicylic Acid** *see* Salsalate *on page 1862*

◆ **DisCoVisc®** *see* Sodium Chondroitin Sulfate and Sodium Hyaluronate *on page 1905*

◆ **Disodium Cromoglycate** *see* Cromolyn (Nasal) *on page 514*

◆ **Disodium Cromoglycate** *see* Cromolyn (Ophthalmic) *on page 514*

◆ **Disodium Thiosulfate Pentahydrate** *see* Sodium Thiosulfate *on page 1915*

◆ ***d*-Isoephedrine Hydrochloride** *see* Pseudoephedrine *on page 1742*

Disopyramide (dye soe PEER a mide)

Brand Names: U.S. Norpace; Norpace CR

Brand Names: Canada Norpace; Rythmodan; Rythmodan-LA

Index Terms Disopyramide Phosphate

Pharmacologic Category Antiarrhythmic Agent, Class Ia

Additional Appendix Information

Beers Criteria – Potentially Inappropriate Medications for Geriatrics *on page 2271*

Use Life-threatening ventricular arrhythmias (eg, sustained ventricular tachycardia)

Pregnancy Risk Factor C

Dosage Oral:

Children: Arrhythmias: *Immediate release:*

<1 year: 10 to 30 mg/kg/24 hours in 4 divided doses

1 to 4 years: 10 to 20 mg/kg/24 hours in 4 divided doses

4 to 12 years: 10 to 15 mg/kg/24 hours in 4 divided doses

12 to 18 years: 6 to 15 mg/kg/24 hours in 4 divided doses

Adults:

Ventricular arrhythmias: **Note:** Since newer agents with less toxicity are available, the use of disopyramide for this indication has fallen out of favor. Controlled release formulation not to be used when rapid achievement of disopyramide plasma concentrations is desired. A maximum dose up to 400 mg every 6 hours (immediate release) may be required for patients with severe refractory ventricular tachycardia.

<50 kg:

Immediate release: An initial loading dose of 200 mg may be administered if rapid onset is required. Maintenance dose: 100 mg every 6 hours

Controlled release: Maintenance dose: 200 mg every 12 hours

≥50 kg:

Immediate release: An initial loading dose of 300 mg may be administered if rapid onset is required. Maintenance dose: 150 mg every 6 hours. If rapid control is necessary and no response seen within 6 hours of loading dose, may increase maintenance dose to 200 mg every 6 hours.

Controlled release: Maintenance dose: 300 mg every 12 hours

Atrial fibrillation (maintenance of sinus rhythm) (off-label use; AHA/ACC/HRS [January, 2014]): **Note:** Because of the potent anticholinergic and negative inotropic effects, may be more desirable for patients with vagally-induced AF or hypertrophic cardiomyopathy associated with dynamic outflow tract obstruction; use in combination with a beta blocker or a non-dihydropyridine calcium channel blocker.

Immediate release: Usual dose: 100 to 200 mg every 6 hours

Controlled release: Usual dose: 200 to 400 mg every 12 hours

Hypertrophic cardiomyopathy (obstructive physiology) with or without atrial fibrillation (off-label use): Initial: *Controlled release:* 200 to 250 mg twice daily. If symptoms do not improve, increase by 100 mg/day at 2-week intervals to a maximum daily dose of 600 mg (Gersh, 2011; Sherrid, 2005).

Elderly: Dose with caution, starting at the lower end of dosing range

Dosage adjustment in renal impairment:

Manufacturer recommendations:

Immediate release:

CrCl >40 mL/minute: 100 mg every 6 hours

CrCl 30 to 40 mL/minute: 100 mg every 8 hours

CrCl 15 to 30 mL/minute: 100 mg every 12 hours

CrCl <15 mL/minute: 100 mg every 24 hours

Controlled release:

CrCl >40 mL/minute: 200 mg every 12 hours

CrCl ≤40 mL/minute: Not recommended for use

Alternative recommendations (Aronoff, 2007): *Immediate release:*

CrCl >50 mL/minute: 100 to 200 mg every 8 hours

CrCl 10 to 50 mL/minute: 100 to 200 mg every 12 to 24 hours

CrCl <10 mL/minute: 100 to 200 mg every 24 to 48 hours

Dialysis: Not dialyzable (0% to 5%) by hemo- or peritoneal methods; supplemental dose is not necessary.

Dosage adjustment in hepatic impairment: Manufacturer's recommendations:

Immediate release: 100 mg every 6 hours

Controlled release: 200 mg every 12 hours

Additional Information Complete prescribing information should be consulted for additional detail.

Dosage Forms

Capsule, Oral:

Norpace: 100 mg, 150 mg

Generic: 100 mg, 150 mg

Capsule Extended Release 12 Hour, Oral:

Norpace CR: 100 mg, 150 mg

◆ **Disopyramide Phosphate** *see* Disopyramide *on page 653*

Disulfiram (dye SUL fi ram)

Brand Names: U.S. Antabuse

Pharmacologic Category Aldehyde Dehydrogenase Inhibitor

Use Management of chronic alcoholism

Dosage Adults: Oral: Do not administer until the patient has abstained from ethanol for at least 12 hours

Initial: 500 mg once daily for 1-2 weeks (maximum daily dose: 500 mg)

Average maintenance dose: 250 mg once daily (range: 125-500 mg; maximum daily dose: 500 mg); duration of therapy is to continue until the patient is fully recovered socially and a basis for permanent self-control has been established; maintenance therapy may be required for months or even years.

Dosage adjustment in renal impairment: No dosage adjustment provided in manufacturer's labeling. Use with extreme caution in chronic and acute nephritis.

Dosage adjustment in hepatic impairment: No dosage adjustment provided in manufacturer's labeling. Use with extreme caution in hepatic cirrhosis or insufficiency.

Additional Information Complete prescribing information should be consulted for additional detail.

Dosage Forms

Tablet, Oral:

Antabuse: 250 mg, 500 mg

Generic: 250 mg, 500 mg

◆ **Dithioglycerol** *see* Dimercaprol *on page 638*

◆ **Dithranol** *see* Anthralin *on page 150*

◆ **Ditropan** *see* Oxybutynin *on page 1536*

◆ **Ditropan XL** *see* Oxybutynin *on page 1536*

◆ **Diuril** *see* Chlorothiazide *on page 426*

◆ **Divalproex Sodium** *see* Valproic Acid and Derivatives *on page 2123*

◆ **Divigel** *see* Estradiol (Systemic) *on page 775*

◆ **Dixarit® (Can)** *see* CloNIDine *on page 480*

◆ **5071-1DL(6)** *see* Megestrol *on page 1281*

◆ ***dl*-Alpha Tocopherol** *see* Vitamin E *on page 2174*

◆ **DLV** *see* Delavirdine *on page 587*

◆ ***D*-Mannitol** *see* Mannitol *on page 1269*

◆ **4-DMDR** *see* IDArubicin *on page 1037*

◆ **DMF** *see* Dimethyl Fumarate *on page 639*

◆ **DMSA** *see* Succimer *on page 1939*

◆ **D-Natural-5 [OTC]** *see* Vitamin A and Vitamin D (Systemic) *on page 2174*

◆ **Doans Extra Strength [OTC]** *see* Magnesium Salicylate *on page 1265*

◆ **Doans Pills [OTC]** *see* Magnesium Salicylate *on page 1265*

DOBUTamine (doe BYOO ta meen)

Brand Names: Canada Dobutamine Injection, USP; Dobutrex

Index Terms Dobutamine Hydrochloride

Pharmacologic Category Adrenergic Agonist Agent; Inotrope

Use Short-term management of patients with cardiac decompensation

American College of Cardiology/American Heart Association heart failure (HF) guideline recommendations (ACCF/AHA [Yancy, 2013]): To maintain systemic perfusion and preserve end-organ performance in patients with cardiogenic shock; bridge therapy in stage D HF unresponsive to guideline-directed medical therapy and device therapy in patients awaiting heart transplant or mechanical circulatory support; short-term management of hospitalized patients with severe systolic dysfunction presenting with low blood pressure and significantly depressed cardiac output; long-term management (palliative therapy) in select patients with stage D HF unresponsive to guideline-directed medical therapy and device therapy who are not candidates for heart transplant or mechanical circulatory support.

Pregnancy Risk Factor B

Pregnancy Considerations Adverse events have not been observed in animal reproduction studies.

Breast-Feeding Considerations It is not known if dobutamine is excreted in breast milk. The manufacturer recommends that caution be exercised when administering dobutamine to nursing women.

Contraindications Hypersensitivity to dobutamine or sulfites (some contain sodium metabisulfate), or any component of the formulation; idiopathic hypertrophic subaortic stenosis (IHSS)

Warnings/Precautions May increase heart rate. Patients with atrial fibrillation may experience an increase in ventricular response. An increase in blood pressure is more common, but occasionally a patient may become hypotensive. May exacerbate ventricular ectopy. If needed, correct hypovolemia first to optimize hemodynamics. Ineffective therapeutically in the presence of mechanical obstruction such as severe aortic stenosis. Use caution post-MI (can increase myocardial oxygen demand). Use cautiously in the elderly starting at lower end of the dosage range. Use with extreme caution in patients taking MAO inhibitors. Dobutamine in combination with stress echo may be used diagnostically. The ACCF/AHA 2013 heart failure guidelines do not recommend long-term use of intravenous inotropic therapy except for palliative purposes in end-stage disease (ACCF/AHA [Yancy, 2013]). Product may contain sodium sulfite.

Adverse Reactions

Cardiovascular: Ventricular premature contractions (5%; dose related), angina pectoris (1% to 3%), chest pain (1% to 3%; nonspecific), palpitations (1% to 3%), hypotension, increased blood pressure, increased heart rate, localized phlebitis, ventricular ectopy (increased)

Central nervous system: Headache (1% to 3%), paresthesia

Dermatologic: Skin necrosis (isolated cases)

Endocrine & metabolic: Decreased serum potassium (slight)

Gastrointestinal: Nausea (1% to 3%)

Hematologic & oncologic: Thrombocytopenia (isolated cases)

Local: Local inflammation, local pain (from infiltration)

Neuromuscular & skeletal: Leg cramps (mild)

Respiratory: Dyspnea (1% to 3%)

Miscellaneous: Fever (1% to 3%)

Drug Interactions

Metabolism/Transport Effects Substrate of COMT

Avoid Concomitant Use

Avoid concomitant use of DOBUTamine with any of the following: Iobenguane I 123

Increased Effect/Toxicity

DOBUTamine may increase the levels/effects of: Sympathomimetics

The levels/effects of DOBUTamine may be increased by: AtoMOXetine; Cannabinoid-Containing Products; COMT Inhibitors; Linezolid; Tedizolid

Decreased Effect

DOBUTamine may decrease the levels/effects of: Iobenguane I 123

The levels/effects of DOBUTamine may be decreased by: Calcium Salts

Storage/Stability Store reconstituted solution under refrigeration for 48 hours or 6 hours at room temperature. Stability of parenteral admixture at room temperature (25°C) is 48 hours; at refrigeration (4°C) stability is 7 days. Remix solution every 24 hours. Pink discoloration of solution indicates slight oxidation but no significant loss of potency.

Mechanism of Action Stimulates beta$_1$-adrenergic receptors, causing increased contractility and heart rate, with little effect on beta$_2$- or alpha-receptors

Pharmacodynamics/Kinetics

Onset of action: IV: 1-10 minutes

Peak effect: 10-20 minutes

Metabolism: In tissues and hepatically to inactive metabolites

Half-life elimination: 2 minutes

Excretion: Urine (as metabolites)

Dosage

Cardiac decompensation: IV infusion: Children and Adults:

Initial dose: 0.5-1 mcg/kg/minute (per the manufacturer); may also initiate at higher doses (eg, 2.5 mcg/kg/minute) depending on severity of decompensation with titration to desired response (Leier, 1977).

Maintenance dose: 2-20 mcg/kg/minute. **Note:** In patients with heart failure, lower doses are preferred to minimize adverse effects (ACCF/AHA [Yancy, 2013]).

Maximum dose: 40 mcg/kg/minute. The ACCF/AHA 2013 heart failure guidelines and the Surviving Sepsis Campaign recommend a maximum dose of 20 mcg/kg/minute (ACCF/AHA [Yancy, 2013]; SCCM [Dellinger, 2013]).

Advanced life support:

Children: *Pediatric Advanced Life Support (PALS) guideline recommendation (to maintain cardiac output and for postresuscitation stabilization):* IV or I.O.: Dose range: 2-20 mcg/kg/minute (AHA [Kleinman, 2010])

Adults: *Adult Advanced Cardiovascular Life Support (ACLS) guideline recommendation (in the immediate post-cardiac arrest care setting):* IV infusion: Initial: 5-10 mcg/kg/minute; titrate to effect (AHA [Peberdy, 2010])

Dosage adjustment in renal impairment: There are no dosage adjustments provided in manufacturer's labeling.

Dosage adjustment in hepatic impairment: There are no dosage adjustments provided in manufacturer's labeling.

Usual Infusion Concentrations: Pediatric Note: Premixed solutions available.

IV infusion: 1000 **mcg**/mL, 2000 **mcg**/mL, **or** 4000 **mcg**/mL

Usual Infusion Concentrations: Adult Note: Premixed solutions available.

IV infusion: 250 mg in 500 mL (concentration: 500 **mcg**/mL), 500 mg in 250 mL (concentration: 2000 **mcg**/mL), **or** 1000 mg in 250 mL (concentration: 4000 **mcg**/mL) of D_5W or NS

Administration Use infusion device to control rate of flow; administer into large vein. Do not administer through same IV line as heparin, hydrocortisone sodium succinate, cefazolin, or penicillin.

Monitoring Parameters Blood pressure, ECG, heart rate, CVP, RAP, MAP; serum glucose, renal function; urine output; if pulmonary artery catheter is in place, monitor CI, PCWP, and SVR

Consult individual institutional policies and procedures.

Dosage Forms

Solution, Intravenous:

Generic: 1 mg/mL (250 mL); 2 mg/mL (250 mL); 4 mg/mL (250 mL); 250 mg/20 mL (20 mL); 500 mg/40 mL (40 mL)

◆ **Dobutamine Hydrochloride** *see* DOBUTamine *on page 654*

◆ **Dobutamine Injection, USP (Can)** *see* DOBUTamine *on page 654*

◆ **Dobutrex (Can)** *see* DOBUTamine *on page 654*

◆ **Docefrez** *see* DOCEtaxel *on page 656*

DOCEtaxel (doe se TAKS el)

Brand Names: U.S. Docefrez; Taxotere

Brand Names: Canada Docetaxel for Injection; Taxotere

Index Terms RP-6976

Pharmacologic Category Antineoplastic Agent, Antimicrotubular; Antineoplastic Agent, Taxane Derivative

Use

U.S. labeling:

Docefrez: Treatment of breast cancer (locally advanced/metastatic) after prior chemotherapy failure; treatment of locally advanced or metastatic non–small cell lung cancer (NSCLC); treatment of hormone-refractory metastatic prostate cancer

Taxotere: Treatment of breast cancer (locally advanced/metastatic) after prior chemotherapy failure, or adjuvant treatment of operable node-positive; locally advanced or metastatic non-small cell lung cancer (NSCLC); hormone refractory, metastatic prostate cancer; advanced gastric adenocarcinoma; locally advanced squamous cell head and neck cancer

Canadian labeling: Treatment of breast cancer (locally advanced/metastatic or adjuvant treatment of operable node-positive); locally advanced or metastatic non-small cell lung cancer (NSCLC); hormone refractory, metastatic prostate cancer; recurrent and/or metastatic squamous cell head and neck cancer; treatment of metastatic ovarian cancer following failure of first-line or subsequent chemotherapy

Pregnancy Risk Factor D

Pregnancy Considerations Adverse events have been observed in animal reproduction studies. An *ex vivo* human placenta perfusion model illustrated that docetaxel crossed the placenta at term. Placental transfer was low and affected by the presence of albumin; higher albumin concentrations resulted in lower docetaxel placental transfer (Berveiller, 2012). Women of childbearing potential should avoid becoming pregnant. A pregnancy registry is available for all cancers diagnosed during pregnancy at Cooper Health (877-635-4499).

Breast-Feeding Considerations It is not known if docetaxel is excreted into breast milk. Due to the potential for serious adverse reactions in nursing the infant, the decision to discontinue docetaxel or to discontinue breast-feeding should take into account the importance of treatment to the mother.

Contraindications

Severe hypersensitivity to docetaxel or any component of the formulation; severe hypersensitivity to other medications containing polysorbate 80; neutrophil count $<1500/mm^3$

Canadian labeling: Additional contraindications (not in U.S. labeling): Severe hepatic impairment; pregnancy; breast-feeding

Warnings/Precautions Hazardous agent - use appropriate precautions for handling and disposal (NIOSH 2014 [group 1]). **[U.S. Boxed Warning]: Avoid use in patients with bilirubin exceeding upper limit of normal (ULN) or AST and/or ALT >1.5 times ULN in conjunction with alkaline phosphatase >2.5 times ULN; patients with isolated transaminase elevations >1.5 times ULN also had a higher rate of neutropenic fever, although no increased incidence of toxic death.** Patients with abnormal liver function are also at increased risk of other treatment-related adverse events, including grade 4 neutropenia, infections, and severe thrombocytopenia, stomatitis, skin toxicity or toxic death; obtain liver function tests prior to each treatment cycle. Canadian labeling contraindicates use in severe hepatic impairment. Canadian labeling contraindicates use in severe hepatic impairment. **[U.S. Boxed Warnings]: Severe hypersensitivity reactions, characterized by generalized rash/erythema, hypotension, bronchospasms, or anaphylaxis may occur (may be fatal; has occurred in patients receiving corticosteroid premedication); minor reactions including flushing or localized skin reactions may also occur; do not administer to patients with a history of severe hypersensitivity to docetaxel or polysorbate 80 (component of formulation). Severe fluid retention, characterized by pleural effusion (requiring immediate drainage, ascites, peripheral edema (poorly tolerated), dyspnea at rest, cardiac tamponade, generalized edema, and weight gain, has been reported.** Fluid retention may begin as lower extremity peripheral edema and become generalized with a median weight gain of 2 kg. In patients with breast cancer, the median cumulative dose to onset of moderate or severe fluid retention was 819 mg/m^2; fluid retention resolves in a median of 16 weeks after discontinuation. Observe for hypersensitivity, especially with the first two infusions. Discontinue for severe reactions; do not rechallenge if severe. Patients should be premedicated with a corticosteroid (starting one day prior to administration) to reduce the incidence and severity of hypersensitivity reactions and fluid retention; severity is reduced with dexamethasone premedication starting one day prior to docetaxel administration.

[U.S. Boxed Warning]: Patients with abnormal liver function, those receiving higher doses, and patients with non–small cell lung cancer and a history of prior treatment with platinum derivatives who receive single-agent docetaxel at a dose of 100 mg/m^2 are at higher risk for treatment-related mortality.

Neutropenia is the dose-limiting toxicity. Patients with increased liver function tests experienced more episodes of neutropenia with a greater number of severe infections. **[U.S. Boxed Warning]: Patients with an absolute neutrophil count $<1500/mm^3$ should not receive docetaxel.** Platelets should recover to $>100,000/mm^3$ prior to treatment. Monitor blood counts and liver function tests frequently; dose reduction or therapy discontinuation may be necessary.

Cutaneous reactions including erythema (with edema) and desquamation have been reported; may require dose reduction. Cystoid macular edema (CME) has been reported; if vision impairment occurs, a prompt comprehensive ophthalmic exam is recommended. If CME is diagnosed, initiate appropriate CME management and discontinue docetaxel (consider non-taxane treatments). In a study of patients receiving docetaxel for the adjuvant treatment of breast cancer, a majority of patients experienced tearing, which occurred in patients with and without lacrimal duct obstruction at baseline; onset was generally after cycle 1, but subsided in most patients within 4 months after therapy completion (Chan, 2013). Dosage adjustment is recommended with severe neurosensory symptoms (paresthesia, dysesthesia, pain); persistent symptoms may require discontinuation; reversal of symptoms may be delayed after discontinuation. Some docetaxel formulations contain alcohol, which may affect the central nervous system and cause symptoms of alcohol intoxication. Consider alcohol content, particularly in patients for whom alcohol intake should be avoided or minimized. Patients should avoid driving or operating machinery immediately after the infusion. The alcohol content varies by formulation. Treatment-related acute myeloid leukemia or myelodysplasia occurred in patients receiving docetaxel in combination with anthracyclines and/or cyclophosphamide. Fatigue and weakness (may be severe) have been reported; symptoms may last a few days up to several weeks; in patients with progressive disease, weakness may be associated with a decrease in performance status. Potentially significant drug-drug interactions may exist, requiring dose or frequency adjustment, additional monitoring, and/or selection of alternative therapy. Docetaxel is an irritant with vesicant-like properties; ensure proper needle or catheter placement prior to and during infusion; avoid extravasation.

Some dosage forms may contain polysorbate 80 (also known as Tweens). Hypersensitivity reactions, usually a delayed reaction, have been reported following exposure to pharmaceutical products containing polysorbate 80 in certain individuals (Isaksson, 2002; Lucente 2000; Shelley, 1995). Thrombocytopenia, ascites, pulmonary deterioration, and renal and hepatic failure have been reported in premature neonates after receiving parenteral products containing polysorbate 80 (Alade, 1986; CDC, 1984). See manufacturer's labeling.

Adverse Reactions Frequency of adverse effects may vary depending on diagnosis, dose, liver function, prior treatment, and premedication. The incidence of adverse events was usually higher in patients with elevated liver function tests.

Cardiovascular: Decreased left ventricular ejection fraction, hypotension

Central nervous system: Central nervous system toxicity (including neuropathy), peripheral motor neuropathy (mainly distal extremity weakness)

Dermatologic: Alopecia, dermatological reaction, nail disease

Endocrine & metabolic: Fluid retention (dose dependent)

Gastrointestinal: Diarrhea, dysgeusia, nausea, stomatitis, vomiting

Hematologic & oncologic: Anemia (dose dependent), febrile neutropenia (dose dependent), leukopenia, neutropenia (nadir [median]: 7 days, duration [severe neutropenia]: 7 days; dose dependent), thrombocytopenia (dose dependent)

Hepatic: Increased serum alkaline phosphatase, increased serum bilirubin, increased serum transaminases

Hypersensitivity: Hypersensitivity

Infection: Infection (dose dependent)

Local: Infusion site reactions (including hyperpigmentation, inflammation, redness, dryness, phlebitis, extravasation, swelling of the vein)

Neuromuscular & skeletal: Arthralgia, myalgia, neuromuscular reaction, weakness

Ophthalmic: Epiphora (associated with canalicular stenosis)

Respiratory: Pulmonary reaction

Miscellaneous: Hypersensitivity (including with premedication), infection (dose dependent)

Rare but important or life-threatening: Acute myelocytic leukemia, acute respiratory distress, anaphylactic shock, anorexia, ascites, atrial fibrillation, atrial flutter, atrioventricular block, bradycardia, bronchospasm, cardiac arrhythmia, cardiac failure, cardiac tamponade, chest pain, chest tightness, colitis, confusion, conjunctivitis, constipation, cystoid macular edema, deep vein thrombosis, dehydration, disease of the lacrimal apparatus (duct obstruction), disseminated intravascular coagulation, drug fever, duodenal ulcer, dyspnea, ECG abnormality, erythema multiforme, esophagitis, gastrointestinal hemorrhage, gastrointestinal obstruction, gastrointestinal perforation, hearing loss, hemorrhagic diathesis, hepatitis, hypertension, hyponatremia, intestinal obstruction, interstitial pulmonary disease, ischemic colitis, ischemic heart disease, loss of consciousness (transient), lymphedema (peripheral), multiorgan failure, myelodysplastic syndrome, myocardial infarction, neutropenic enterocolitis, ototoxicity, palmar-plantar erythrodysesthesia, pericardial effusion, pleural effusion, pneumonia, pneumonitis, pruritus, pulmonary edema, pulmonary embolism, pulmonary fibrosis, radiation pneumonitis, radiation recall phenomenon, renal failure, renal insufficiency, respiratory failure, skin changes (scleroderma-like), seizure, sepsis, sinus tachycardia, Stevens-Johnson syndrome, subacute cutaneous lupus erythematosus, syncope, toxic epidermal necrolysis, tachycardia, thrombophlebitis, unstable angina pectoris, visual disturbance (transient)

Drug Interactions

Metabolism/Transport Effects **Substrate** of CYP3A4 (major), P-glycoprotein; **Note:** Assignment of Major/Minor substrate status based on clinically relevant drug interaction potential; **Inhibits** CYP3A4 (weak)

Avoid Concomitant Use

Avoid concomitant use of DOCEtaxel with any of the following: BCG; CloZAPine; Conivaptan; Dipyrone; Fusidic Acid (Systemic); Idelalisib; Natalizumab; Pimecrolimus; Pimozide; Tacrolimus (Topical); Tofacitinib; Vaccines (Live)

Increased Effect/Toxicity

DOCEtaxel may increase the levels/effects of: Antineoplastic Agents (Anthracycline, Systemic); ARIPiprazole; CloZAPine; Dofetilide; Hydrocodone; Leflunomide; Lomitapide; Natalizumab; Pimozide; Tofacitinib; Vaccines (Live)

The levels/effects of DOCEtaxel may be increased by: Antifungal Agents (Azole Derivatives, Systemic); Ceritinib; Conivaptan; CYP3A4 Inhibitors (Moderate); CYP3A4 Inhibitors (Strong); Dasatinib; Denosumab; Dipyrone; Dronedarone; Fusidic Acid (Systemic); Idelalisib; Ivacaftor; Luliconazole; Mifepristone; Netupitant; P-glycoprotein/ABCB1 Inhibitors; Pimecrolimus; Platinum Derivatives; Roflumilast; Simeprevir; SORAfenib; Stiripentol; Tacrolimus (Topical); Trastuzumab

Decreased Effect

DOCEtaxel may decrease the levels/effects of: BCG; Coccidioides immitis Skin Test; Sipuleucel-T; Vaccines (Inactivated); Vaccines (Live)

The levels/effects of DOCEtaxel may be decreased by: Bosentan; CYP3A4 Inducers (Moderate); CYP3A4 Inducers (Strong); Dabrafenib; Deferasirox; Echinacea; Mitotane; P-glycoprotein/ABCB1 Inducers; Siltuximab; St Johns Wort; Tocilizumab

Preparation for Administration Hazardous agent; use appropriate precautions for handling and disposal (NIOSH 2014 [group 1]).

Preparation instructions may vary by manufacturer, refer to specific prescribing information. **Note:** Some formulations contain overfill.

Note: Multiple concentrations: Docetaxel is available as a one-vial formulation at concentrations of 10 mg/mL (generic formulation) and 20 mg/mL (concentrate; Taxotere, and as a lyophilized powder (Docefrez) which is reconstituted (with provided diluent) to 20 mg/0.8 mL (20 mg vial) or 24 mg/mL (80 mg vial). Admixture errors have occurred due to the availability of various concentrations. Docetaxel was previously available as a two-vial formulation which included two vials (a concentrated docetaxel vial and a diluent vial), resulting in a reconstituted concentration of 10 mg/mL; the two-vial formulation has been discontinued by the Taxotere manufacturer (available generically).

One-vial formulations: Further dilute for infusion in 250 to 500 mL of NS or D_5W in a non-DEHP container (eg, glass, polypropylene, polyolefin) to a final concentration of 0.3 to 0.74 mg/mL. Gently rotate and invert manually to mix thoroughly; avoid shaking or vigorous agitation.

Taxotere: Use **only** a 21 gauge needle to withdraw docetaxel from the vial (larger bore needles, such as 18 gauge or 19 gauge needles, may cause stopper coring and rubber precipitates). If intact vials were stored refrigerated, allow to stand at room temperature for 5 minutes prior to dilution. Inspect vials prior to dilution; solution is supersaturated and may crystalize over time; do not use if crystalized.

Lyophilized powder: Dilute with the provided diluent (contains ethanol in polysorbate 80); add 1 mL to each 20 mg vial (resulting concentration is 20 mg/0.8 mL) and 4 mL to each 80 mg vial (resulting concentration is 24 mg/mL). Shake well to dissolve completely. Reconstituted solution is supersaturated and could crystallize over time; if crystals appear, discard the solution (should no longer be used). If air bubbles are present, allow to stand for a few minutes while air bubbles dissipate. Further dilute in 250 mL of NS or D_5W in a non-DEHP container (eg, glass, polypropylene, polyolefin) to a final concentration of 0.3 to 0.74 mg/mL (for doses >200 mg, use a larger volume of NS or D_5W, not to exceed a final concentration of 0.74 mg/mL). Mix thoroughly by manual agitation.

Two-vial formulation *(generic; concentrate plus diluent formulation):* Vials should be diluted with 13% (w/w) polyethylene glycol 400/water (provided with the drug) to a final concentration of 10 mg/mL. Do not shake. Further dilute for infusion in 250 to 500 mL of NS or D_5W in a non-DEHP container (eg, glass, polypropylene, polyolefin) to a final concentration of 0.3 to 0.74 mg/mL. Gently rotate to mix thoroughly. Do not use the two-vial formulation with the one-vial formulation for the same admixture product.

Storage/Stability Storage and stability may vary by manufacturer, refer to specific prescribing information.

Docetaxel 10 mg/mL: Store intact vials between 2°C to 25°C (36°F to 77°F) (actual recommendations may vary by generic manufacturer; consult manufacturer's labeling). Protect from bright light. Freezing does not adversely affect the product. Multi-use vials (80 mg/8 mL and 160 mg/16 mL) are stable for up to 28 days after first entry when stored between 2°C to 8°C (36°F to 46°F) and protected from light. Solutions diluted for infusion should be used within 4 hours of preparation, including infusion time.

Docetaxel 20 mg/mL concentrate:

Taxotere: Store intact vials between 2°C to 25°C (36°F to 77°F). Protect from bright light. Freezing does not adversely affect the product. Solutions diluted for infusion in non-PVC containers should be used within 6 hours of preparation, including infusion time, when stored between 2°C to 25°C (36°F to 77°F) or within 48 hours when stored between 2°C to 8°C (36°F to 46°F).

Generic formulations: Store intact vials at 25°C (77°F); excursions permitted between 15°C to 30°C (59°F to 86°F). Protect from light. Solutions diluted for infusion should be used within 4 hours of preparation, including infusion time.

Docetaxel lyophilized powder (Docefrez): Store intact vials between 2°C to 8°C (36°F to 46°F). Protect from light. Allow vials (and provided diluent) to stand at room temperature for 5 minutes prior to reconstitution. After reconstitution, may be stored refrigerated or at room temperature for up to 8 hours. Solutions diluted for infusion should be used within 6 hours of preparation, including infusion time. According to the manufacturer, physical and chemical in-use stability of the infusion solution (prepared as recommended) has been demonstrated in non-PVC bags up to 48 hours when stored between 2°C and 8°C (36°F and 46°F).

Two-vial formulation *(generic; concentrate plus diluent formulation):* Reconstituted solutions of the two-vial formulation are stable in the vial for 8 hours at room temperature or under refrigeration. Solutions diluted for infusion in polyolefin containers should be used within 4 hours of preparation, including infusion time.

Mechanism of Action Docetaxel promotes the assembly of microtubules from tubulin dimers, and inhibits the depolymerization of tubulin which stabilizes microtubules in the cell. This results in inhibition of DNA, RNA, and protein synthesis. Most activity occurs during the M phase of the cell cycle.

Pharmacodynamics/Kinetics Exhibits linear pharmacokinetics at the recommended dosage range

Distribution: Extensive extravascular distribution and/or tissue binding; V_{dss}: 113 L (mean steady state)

Protein binding: ~94% to 97%, primarily to $alpha_1$-acid glycoprotein, albumin, and lipoproteins

Metabolism: Hepatic; oxidation via CYP3A4 to metabolites

Half-life elimination: Terminal: ~11 hours

Excretion: Feces (~75%, <8% as unchanged drug); urine (~6%)

Dosage Note: Premedicate with corticosteroids for 3 days, beginning one day prior to docetaxel administration, to reduce the severity of hypersensitivity reactions and fluid retention.

U.S. labeling:

Breast cancer: Adults: IV:

Locally advanced or metastatic: 60 to 100 mg/m² every 3 weeks (as a single agent)

Operable, node-positive (adjuvant treatment): TAC regimen: 75 mg/m² every 3 weeks for 6 courses (in combination with doxorubicin and cyclophosphamide) (Mackey, 2013; Martin, 2005)

Adjuvant treatment (off-label dosing): 75 mg/m² every 21 days (in combination with cyclophosphamide) for 4 cycles (Jones, 2006) **or** 75 mg/m² every 21 days (in combination with carboplatin and trastuzumab) for 6 cycles (Slamon, 2011)

Neoadjuvant treatment (off-label dosing): 75 mg/m² (cycle 1; if tolerated, may increase to 100 mg/m² in subsequent cycles); every 21 days for a total of 4 cycles (in combination with trastuzumab and pertuzumab) (Gianni, 2012)

Metastatic treatment (off-label dosing):

Every-3-week administration: 75 mg/m² (cycle 1; may increase to 100 mg/m2 in subsequent cycles) every 21 days for at least 6 cycles (in combination with trastuzumab and pertuzumab) (Baselga, 2012; Swain, 2013) **or** 100 mg/m² every 21 days (in combination with trastuzumab) for at least 6 cycles (Marty, 2005) **or** 75 mg/m² every 21 days (in combination with capecitabine) until disease progression or unacceptable toxicity (O'Shaughnessy, 2002) **or** 60 mg/m², 75 mg/m², or 100 mg/m² every 21 days for at least 6 cycles until disease progression, unacceptable toxicity, or discontinuation (Harvey, 2006)

Weekly administration: 40 mg/m²/dose once a week (as a single agent) for 6 weeks followed by a 2-week rest, repeat until disease progression or unacceptable toxicity (Burstein, 2000) **or** 35 mg/m²/dose once weekly for 3 weeks, followed by a 1-week rest, may increase to 40 mg/m² once weekly for 3 weeks followed by a 1-week rest with cycle 2 (Rivera, 2008) **or** 35 mg/m²/dose once weekly (in combination with trastuzumab) for 3 weeks followed by a 1-week rest; repeat until disease progression or unacceptable toxicity (Esteva, 2002)

Non-small cell lung cancer: Adults: IV: 75 mg/m² every 3 weeks (as a single agent or in combination with cisplatin)

Prostate cancer: Adults: IV: 75 mg/m² every 3 weeks (in combination with prednisone)

Gastric adenocarcinoma: Adults: IV: 75 mg/m² every 3 weeks (in combination with cisplatin and fluorouracil)

Sequential chemotherapy and chemoradiation (off-label dosing): Induction: 75 mg/m^2 on days 1 and 22 (in combination with cisplatin) for 2 cycles, followed by chemoradiation: 20 mg/m^2 weekly for 5 weeks (in combination with cisplatin and radiation) (Ruhstaller, 2009)

Locally advanced or metastatic disease (off-label dosing): 50 mg/m^2 on day 1 every 2 weeks (in combination with fluorouracil, leucovorin, and oxaliplatin) until disease progression or unacceptable toxicity up to a maximum of 8 cycles (Al-Batran, 2008)

Head and neck cancer: Adults: IV: 75 mg/m^2 every 3 weeks (in combination with cisplatin and fluorouracil) for 3 or 4 cycles, followed by radiation therapy

Canadian labeling:

Breast cancer: Adults: IV:

Locally advanced or metastatic: 75 mg/m^2 (as combination therapy) **or** 100 mg/m^2 (as a single agent) every 3 weeks

Operable, node-positive (adjuvant treatment): 75 mg/m^2 every 3 weeks for 6 courses (in combination with doxorubicin and cyclophosphamide)

Non-small cell lung cancer (locally advanced or metastatic), ovarian cancer (metastatic), head and neck cancer (recurrent and/or metastatic): Adults: IV: 75 mg/m^2 (as combination therapy) **or** 100 mg/m^2 (as a single agent) every 3 weeks

Prostate cancer (hormone-refractory, metastatic): Adults: IV: 75 mg/m^2 every 3 weeks (in combination with prednisone or prednisolone)

Off-label uses:

Bladder cancer, metastatic (off-label use): Adults: IV: 100 mg/m^2 every 3 weeks (as a single agent) (McCaffrey, 1997) **or** 35 mg/m^2 on days 1 and 8 of a 21-day cycle (in combination with gemcitabine and cisplatin) for at least 6 cycles or until disease progression or unacceptable toxicity (Pectasides, 2002)

Esophageal cancer (off-label use): Adults: IV:

Sequential chemotherapy and chemoradiation: Induction: 75 mg/m^2 on days 1 and 22 (in combination with cisplatin) for 2 cycles, followed by chemoradiation: 20 mg/m^2 weekly for 5 weeks (in combination with cisplatin and radiation) (Ruhstaller, 2009)

Definitive chemoradiation: 60 mg/m^2 on days 1 and 22 (in combination with cisplatin and radiation) for 1 cycle (Li, 2010)

Locally advanced or metastatic disease: 75 mg/m^2 on day 1 every 3 weeks (in combination with cisplatin and fluorouracil) (Ajani, 2007; Van Cutsem, 2006) **or** 50 mg/m^2 on day 1 every 2 weeks (in combination with fluorouracil, leucovorin, and oxaliplatin) until disease progression or unacceptable toxicity up to a maximum of 8 cycles (Al-Batran, 2008) **or** 35 mg/m^2 on days 1, 8, 15, 29, 36, 43, 50, and 57 (in combination with cisplatin, fluorouracil, and radiotherapy; neoadjuvant setting) (Pasini, 2013)

Ewing sarcoma, osteosarcoma (recurrent or progressive; off-label uses): Children ≥8 years, Adolescents, and Adults: IV: 100 mg/m^2 on day 8 of a 21-day cycle (in combination with gemcitabine) (Navid, 2008)

Ovarian cancer (off-label use in U.S.): Adults: IV: 60 mg/m^2 every 3 weeks (in combination with carboplatin) for up to 6 cycles (Markman, 2001) **or** 75 mg/m^2 every 3 weeks (in combination with carboplatin) for 6 cycles (Vasey, 2004) **or** 35 mg/m^2 (maximum dose: 70 mg) weekly for 3 weeks followed by a 1-week rest (in combination with carboplatin) (Kushner, 2007)

Small cell lung cancer, relapsed (off-label use): Adults: IV: 100 mg/m^2 every 3 weeks (Smyth, 1994)

Soft tissue sarcoma (off-label use): Adults: IV: 100 mg/m^2 on day 8 of a 3-week treatment cycle (in combination with gemcitabine and filgrastim or pegfilgrastim) (Leu, 2004; Maki, 2007)

Unknown-primary, adenocarcinoma (off-label use): Adults: IV: 65 mg/m^2 every 3 weeks (in combination with carboplatin) (Greco, 2000) **or** 75 mg/m^2 on day 8 of a 3-week treatment cycle (in combination with gemcitabine) for up to 6 cycles (Pouessel, 2004) **or** 60 mg/m^2 on day 1 of a 3-week treatment cycle (in combination with cisplatin) (Mukai, 2010)

Dosing adjustment for concomitant CYP3A4 inhibitors: Avoid the concomitant use of strong CYP3A4 inhibitors with docetaxel. If concomitant use of a strong CYP3A4 inhibitor cannot be avoided, consider reducing the docetaxel dose by 50% (based on limited pharmacokinetic data).

Dosing adjustment for toxicity:

Note: Toxicity includes febrile neutropenia, neutrophils <500/mm^3 for >1 week, severe or cumulative cutaneous reactions; in non–small cell lung cancer, this may also include platelet nadir <25,000/mm^3 and other grade 3/4 nonhematologic toxicities.

Breast cancer (single agent): Patients dosed initially at 100 mg/m^2; reduce dose to 75 mg/m^2; **Note:** If the patient continues to experience these adverse reactions, the dosage should be reduced to 55 mg/m^2 or therapy should be discontinued; discontinue for peripheral neuropathy ≥ grade 3. Patients initiated at 60 mg/m^2 who do not develop toxicity may tolerate higher doses.

Breast cancer, adjuvant treatment (combination chemotherapy): TAC regimen should be administered when neutrophils are ≥1500/mm^3. Patients experiencing febrile neutropenia should receive G-CSF in all subsequent cycles. Patients with persistent febrile neutropenia (while on G-CSF), patients experiencing severe/cumulative cutaneous reactions, moderate neurosensory effects (signs/symptoms) or grade 3 or 4 stomatitis should receive a reduced dose (60 mg/m^2) of docetaxel. Discontinue therapy with persistent toxicities after dosage reduction.

Non-small cell lung cancer:

Monotherapy: Patients dosed initially at 75 mg/m^2 should have dose held until toxicity is resolved, then resume at 55 mg/m^2; discontinue for peripheral neuropathy ≥ grade 3.

Combination therapy (with cisplatin): Patients dosed initially at 75 mg/m^2 should have the docetaxel dosage reduced to 65 mg/m^2 in subsequent cycles; if further adjustment is required, dosage may be reduced to 50 mg/m^2.

Prostate cancer: Reduce dose to 60 mg/m^2; discontinue therapy if toxicities persist at lower dose.

Gastric cancer, head and neck cancer: **Note:** Cisplatin may require dose reductions/therapy delays for peripheral neuropathy, ototoxicity, and/or nephrotoxicity. Patients experiencing febrile neutropenia, documented infection with neutropenia or neutropenia >7 days should receive G-CSF in all subsequent cycles. For neutropenic complications despite G-CSF use, further reduce dose to 60 mg/m^2. Dosing with neutropenic complications in subsequent cycles should be further reduced to 45 mg/m^2. Patients who experience grade 4 thrombocytopenia should receive a dose reduction from 75 mg/m^2 to 60 mg/m^2. Discontinue therapy for persistent toxicities.

Gastrointestinal toxicity for docetaxel in combination with cisplatin and fluorouracil for treatment of gastric cancer or head and neck cancer:

Diarrhea, grade 3:

First episode: Reduce fluorouracil dose by 20%

Second episode: Reduce docetaxel dose by 20%

Diarrhea, grade 4:
First episode: Reduce fluorouracil and docetaxel doses by 20%
Second episode: Discontinue treatment
Stomatitis, grade 3:
First episode: Reduce fluorouracil dose by 20%
Second episode: Discontinue fluorouracil for all subsequent cycles
Third episode: Reduce docetaxel dose by 20%
Stomatitis, grade 4:
First episode: Discontinue fluorouracil for all subsequent cycles
Second episode: Reduce docetaxel dose by 20%

Canadian labeling: **Note:** Toxicity includes febrile neutropenia, neutrophils ≤500/mm^3 for >1 week, severe or cumulative cutaneous reactions, or severe neurosensory symptoms.

Patients initially dosed at 100 mg/m^2: Reduce dose to 75 mg/m^2; Patients initially dosed at 75 mg/m^2: Reduce dose to 60 mg/m^2. Discontinue therapy for persistent toxicities after dosage reduction.

Breast cancer, adjuvant treatment (combination chemotherapy): Patients experiencing febrile neutropenia should receive G-CSF in all subsequent cycles. Patients with persistent febrile neutropenia (while on G-CSF), patients experiencing severe/cumulative cutaneous reactions, severe neurosensory symptoms, or grade 3 or 4 stomatitis should receive a reduced dose (60 mg/m^2). Discontinue therapy with persistent toxicities after dosage reduction.

Concomitant use with capecitabine (treatment of metastatic breast cancer):
Grade 2 toxicities:
First episode: Interrupt therapy until resolution to < grade 2, then resume docetaxel and capecitabine at previous dose; consider prophylactic measures if appropriate and/or possible
Second episode of same toxicity: Interrupt therapy until resolution to < grade 2, then resume docetaxel at 55 mg/m^2; reduce capecitabine dose to 75% of original dose
Further episodes of same toxicity: Discontinue docetaxel; interrupt capecitabine until resolution to < grade 2, then resume at 50% of original dose (third episode) or discontinue therapy altogether (fourth episode)
Grade 3 toxicities:
First episode: Occurring at time treatment is due: Interrupt docetaxel until resolution to < grade 2 (maximum delay ≤2 weeks), then resume docetaxel at 55 mg/m^2; reduce capecitabine dose to 75% of original dose (consider prophylactic measure if appropriate); if no resolution to < grade 2 within 2 weeks, discontinue docetaxel but may resume capecitabine at 75% of original dose after resolution to < grade 2. Occurring between cycles and resolves to < grade 2 by time of next treatment: Administer docetaxel at 55 mg/m^2 and reduce capecitabine dose to 75% of original dose; consider prophylactic measures if appropriate and/or possible.
Further episodes of same toxicity: Discontinue docetaxel; interrupt capecitabine until resolution to < grade 2, then resume capecitabine at 50% of original dose (second episode) or discontinue therapy altogether (third episode)
Grade 4 toxicities: First episode: Discontinue docetaxel and capecitabine therapy or if deemed clinically necessary, capecitabine may be continued at 50% of original dose

Dosage adjustment in renal impairment: Renal excretion is minimal (~6%), therefore, the need for dosage adjustments for renal dysfunction is unlikely (Janus, 2010; Li, 2007). Not removed by hemodialysis, may be administered before or after hemodialysis (Janus, 2010).

Dosage adjustment in hepatic impairment:

U.S. labeling:
Total bilirubin greater than the ULN, or AST and/or ALT >1.5 times ULN concomitant with alkaline phosphatase >2.5 times ULN: Use is not recommended.
Hepatic impairment dosing adjustment specific for gastric or head and neck cancer:
AST/ALT >2.5 to ≤5 times ULN and alkaline phosphatase ≤2.5 times ULN: Administer 80% of dose
AST/ALT >1.5 to ≤5 times ULN and alkaline phosphatase >2.5 to ≤5 times ULN: Administer 80% of dose
AST/ALT >5 times ULN and /or alkaline phosphatase >5 times ULN: Discontinue docetaxel

Canadian labeling: **Note:** Dosing recommendations when used as a single agent; dosage adjustment when used as part of combination therapy not provided in manufacturer's labeling.
AST and/or ALT >1.5 times ULN and alkaline phosphatase >2.5 times ULN: Reduce dose from 100 mg/m^2 to 75 mg/m^2
Serum bilirubin >ULN and/or AST and ALT >3.5 times ULN associated with alkaline phosphatase >6 times ULN: Avoid use unless strictly indicated.
Severe hepatic impairment: Use is contraindicated.

The following adjustments have also been used (Floyd, 2006):
Transaminases 1.6 to 6 times ULN: Administer 75% of dose.
Transaminases >6 times ULN: Use clinical judgment.

Dosing in obesity: *ASCO Guidelines for appropriate chemotherapy dosing in obese adults with cancer:* Utilize patient's actual body weight (full weight) for calculation of body surface area- or weight-based dosing, particularly when the intent of therapy is curative; manage regimen-related toxicities in the same manner as for nonobese patients; if a dose reduction is utilized due to toxicity, consider resumption of full weight-based dosing with subsequent cycles, especially if cause of toxicity (eg, hepatic or renal impairment) is resolved (Griggs, 2012).

Administration Administer IV infusion over 1-hour through nonsorbing polyethylene lined (non-DEHP) tubing; in-line filter is not necessary (the use of a filter during administration is not recommended by the manufacturer). Infusion should be completed within 4 hours of final preparation. **Note:** Premedication with corticosteroids for 3 days, beginning the day before docetaxel administration, is recommended to reduce the incidence and severity of hypersensitivity reactions and fluid retention (see Additional Information). Some docetaxel formulations contain alcohol (content varies by formulation); use with caution in patients for whom alcohol intake should be avoided or minimized.

Irritant with vesicant-like properties; avoid extravasation. Assure proper needle or catheter position prior to administration.

Extravasation management: If extravasation occurs, stop infusion immediately and disconnect (leave cannula/needle in place); gently aspirate extravasated solution (do **NOT** flush the line); remove needle/cannula; elevate extremity. Information conflicts regarding the use of warm or cold compresses (Perez Fidalgo, 2012; Polovich, 2009).

Hazardous agent; use appropriate precautions for handling and disposal (NIOSH 2014 [group 1]).

Monitoring Parameters CBC with differential, liver function tests, bilirubin, alkaline phosphatase, renal function; monitor for hypersensitivity reactions, neurosensory symptoms, gastrointestinal toxicity (eg, diarrhea, stomatitis), cutaneous reactions, visual impairment, fluid retention, epiphora, and canalicular stenosis

Additional Information Premedication with oral corticosteroids is recommended to decrease the incidence and severity of fluid retention and severity of hypersensitivity reactions. The manufacturer recommends dexamethasone 16 mg/day (8 mg twice daily) orally for 3 days, starting the day before docetaxel administration; for prostate cancer, when prednisone is part of the antineoplastic regimen, dexamethasone 8 mg orally is administered at 12 hours, 3 hours, and 1 hour prior to docetaxel. Some docetaxel formulations contain alcohol (content varies by formulation); use with caution in patients for whom alcohol intake should be avoided or minimized.

Dosage Forms

Concentrate, Intravenous:

Taxotere: 20 mg/mL (1 mL); 80 mg/4 mL (4 mL)

Generic: 20 mg/mL (1 mL); 80 mg/4 mL (4 mL); 160 mg/8 mL (8 mL); 20 mg/0.5 mL (0.5 mL); 80 mg/2 mL (2 mL)

Concentrate, Intravenous [preservative free]:

Generic: 20 mg/mL (1 mL); 80 mg/4 mL (4 mL); 140 mg/7 mL (7 mL)

Solution, Intravenous:

Generic: 20 mg/2 mL (2 mL); 80 mg/8 mL (8 mL); 160 mg/16 mL (16 mL)

Solution Reconstituted, Intravenous:

Docefrez: 20 mg (1 ea); 80 mg (1 ea)

◆ **Docetaxel for Injection (Can)** *see* DOCEtaxel *on page 656*

◆ **Docosahexaenoic Acid** *see* Omega-3 Fatty Acids *on page 1507*

Docosanol (doe KOE san ole)

Brand Names: U.S. Abreva [OTC]

Index Terms *n*-Docosanol; Behenyl Alcohol

Pharmacologic Category Antiviral Agent, Topical

Use Treatment of herpes simplex of the face or lips

Dosage Children ≥12 years and Adults: Topical: Apply 5 times/day to affected area of face or lips. Start at first sign of cold sore or fever blister and continue until healed.

Additional Information Complete prescribing information should be consulted for additional detail.

Dosage Forms

Cream, External:

Abreva [OTC]: 10% (2 g)

◆ **DocQLace [OTC]** *see* Docusate *on page 661*

◆ **Doc-Q-Lax [OTC]** *see* Docusate and Senna *on page 662*

◆ **Docu [OTC]** *see* Docusate *on page 661*

◆ **Docuprene [OTC]** *see* Docusate *on page 661*

Docusate (DOK yoo sate)

Brand Names: U.S. Colace Clear [OTC]; Colace [OTC]; D.O.S. [OTC]; Diocto [OTC]; DocQLace [OTC]; Docu Soft [OTC]; Docu [OTC]; Docuprene [OTC]; Docusil [OTC]; DocuSol Kids [OTC]; DocuSol Mini [OTC]; DOK [OTC]; Dulcolax Stool Softener [OTC]; Enemeez Mini [OTC]; Healthy Mama Move It Along [OTC]; Kao-Tin [OTC]; KS Stool Softener [OTC]; Laxa Basic [OTC]; Pedia-Lax [OTC]; Promolaxin [OTC]; Silace [OTC]; Sof-Lax [OTC]; Stool Softener Laxative DC [OTC]; Stool Softener [OTC]; Sur-Q-Lax [OTC]; Vacuant Mini-Enema [OTC] [DSC]

Brand Names: Canada Apo-Docusate Calcium [OTC]; Apo-Docusate Sodium [OTC]; Calax [OTC]; Colace [OTC]; Correctol Stool Softener [OTC]; Docusate Sodium Odan [OTC]; Dom-Docusate Sodium [OTC]; Dosolax [OTC]; Euro-Docusate C [OTC]; Jamp-Docusate [OTC]; Novo-Docusate Calcium [OTC]; Novo-Docusate Sodium [OTC]; PHL-Docusate Sodium [OTC]; PMS-Docusate Calcium [OTC]; PMS-Docusate Sodium [OTC]; ratio-Docusate Sodium [OTC]; Selax [OTC]; Silace [OTC]; Sirop Docusate De Sodium [OTC]; Soflax C [OTC]; Soflax Pediatric Drops [OTC]; Soflax [OTC]; Taro-Docusate [OTC]; Teva-Docusate Sodium [OTC]

Index Terms Dioctyl Calcium Sulfosuccinate; Dioctyl Sodium Sulfosuccinate; Docusate Calcium; Docusate Potassium; Docusate Sodium; DOSS; DSS

Pharmacologic Category Stool Softener

Use Stool softener in patients who should avoid straining during defecation and constipation associated with hard, dry stools; prophylaxis for straining (Valsalva) following myocardial infarction. A safe agent to be used in elderly; some evidence that doses <200 mg are ineffective; stool softeners are unnecessary if stool is well hydrated or "mushy" and soft; shown to be ineffective used long-term.

Dosage Docusate salts are interchangeable; the amount of sodium or calcium per dosage unit is clinically insignificant

Infants and Children <3 years: Oral: 10-40 mg/day in 1-4 divided doses

Children: Oral:

3-6 years: 20-60 mg/day in 1-4 divided doses

6-12 years: 40-150 mg/day in 1-4 divided doses

Adolescents and Adults: Oral: 50-500 mg/day in 1-4 divided doses

Older Children and Adults: Rectal: Add 50-100 mg of docusate liquid to enema fluid (saline or water); administer as retention or flushing enema

Ceruminolytic (off-label use): Intra-aural: Administer 1 mL of docusate sodium in 2 mL syringes; if no clearance in 15 minutes, irrigate with 50-100 mL normal saline (this method is 80% effective)

Additional Information Complete prescribing information should be consulted for additional detail.

Dosage Forms

Capsule, Oral:

Colace [OTC]: 50 mg, 100 mg
Colace Clear [OTC]: 50 mg
D.O.S. [OTC]: 250 mg
DocQLace [OTC]: 100 mg
Docu Soft [OTC]: 100 mg
Docusil [OTC]: 100 mg
DOK [OTC]: 100 mg, 250 mg
Dulcolax Stool Softener [OTC]: 100 mg
Kao-Tin [OTC]: 240 mg
KS Stool Softener [OTC]: 100 mg
Laxa Basic [OTC]: 100 mg
Sof-Lax [OTC]: 100 mg
Stool Softener [OTC]: 100 mg, 250 mg
Stool Softener Laxative DC [OTC]: 240 mg
Sur-Q-Lax [OTC]: 240 mg
Generic: 100 mg, 240 mg, 250 mg

Enema, Rectal:

DocuSol Kids [OTC]: 100 mg/5 mL (5 ea)
DocuSol Mini [OTC]: 283 mg (5 ea)
Enemeez Mini [OTC]: 283 mg (5 mL)

Liquid, Oral:

Diocto [OTC]: 50 mg/5 mL (473 mL)
Docu [OTC]: 50 mg/5 mL (10 mL, 473 mL)
Pedia-Lax [OTC]: 50 mg/15 mL (118 mL)
Silace [OTC]: 150 mg/15 mL (473 mL)
Generic: 50 mg/5 mL (10 mL)

Syrup, Oral:

Diocto [OTC]: 60 mg/15 mL (473 mL)
Silace [OTC]: 60 mg/15 mL (473 mL)

Tablet, Oral:
Docuprene [OTC]: 100 mg
DOK [OTC]: 100 mg
Healthy Mama Move It Along [OTC]: 100 mg
Promolaxin [OTC]: 100 mg
Stool Softener [OTC]: 100 mg
Generic: 100 mg

Docusate and Senna (DOK yoo sate & SEN na)

Brand Names: U.S. Doc-Q-Lax [OTC]; Dok Plus [OTC]; Geri-Stool [OTC]; Peri-Colace [OTC]; Senexon-S [OTC]; Senna Plus [OTC]; SennaLax-S [OTC]; Senokot-S [OTC]; SenoSol-SS [OTC]

Index Terms Docusate and Sennosides; Senna and Docusate; Senna-S; Sennosides and Docusate

Pharmacologic Category Laxative, Stimulant; Stool Softener

Use Constipation: Relief of occasional constipation

Dosage Constipation: OTC ranges:

Children: Oral:

2 to 6 years: Initial: 4.3 mg sennosides plus 25 mg docusate (1/2 tablet) once daily (maximum: 1 tablet twice daily)

6 to 12 years: Initial: 8.6 sennosides plus 50 mg docusate (1 tablet) once daily (maximum: 2 tablets twice daily)

Children ≥12 years and Adults: Oral: Initial: Two tablets (17.2 mg sennosides plus 100 mg docusate) once daily (maximum: 4 tablets twice daily)

Elderly: Consider half the initial dose in older, debilitated patients

Additional Information Complete prescribing information should be consulted for additional detail.

Dosage Forms

Tablet: Docusate 50 mg and sennosides 8.6 mg

Doc-Q-Lax [OTC], Dok Plus [OTC], Geri-Stool [OTC], Peri-Colace [OTC], Senexon-S [OTC], SennaLax-S [OTC], Senna Plus [OTC], Senokot-S [OTC], SenoSol-SS [OTC]: Docusate 50 mg and sennosides 8.6 mg

- ◆ **Docusate and Sennosides** *see* Docusate and Senna *on page 662*
- ◆ **Docusate Calcium** *see* Docusate *on page 661*
- ◆ **Docusate Potassium** *see* Docusate *on page 661*
- ◆ **Docusate Sodium** *see* Docusate *on page 661*
- ◆ **Docusate Sodium Odan [OTC] (Can)** *see* Docusate *on page 661*
- ◆ **Docusil [OTC]** *see* Docusate *on page 661*
- ◆ **Docu Soft [OTC]** *see* Docusate *on page 661*
- ◆ **DocuSol Kids [OTC]** *see* Docusate *on page 661*
- ◆ **DocuSol Mini [OTC]** *see* Docusate *on page 661*

Dofetilide (doe FET il ide)

Brand Names: U.S. Tikosyn

Pharmacologic Category Antiarrhythmic Agent, Class III

Additional Appendix Information

Beers Criteria – Potentially Inappropriate Medications for Geriatrics *on page 2271*

Use Maintenance of normal sinus rhythm in patients with chronic atrial fibrillation/atrial flutter of longer than 1-week duration who have been converted to normal sinus rhythm; conversion of atrial fibrillation and atrial flutter to normal sinus rhythm

Pregnancy Risk Factor C

Pregnancy Considerations Adverse events have been observed in animal reproduction studies.

Breast-Feeding Considerations It is not known if dofetilide is excreted in breast milk. Breast-feeding is not recommended by the manufacturer.

Contraindications Hypersensitivity to dofetilide or any component of the formulation; patients with congenital or acquired long QT syndromes, do not use if baseline QT interval or QTc is >440 msec (500 msec in patients with ventricular conduction abnormalities); severe renal impairment (CrCl <20 mL/minute [Cockcroft-Gault method]); concurrent use with verapamil, cimetidine, hydrochlorothiazide (alone or in combinations), trimethoprim (alone or in combination with sulfamethoxazole), itraconazole (according to itraconazole prescribing information) ketoconazole, prochlorperazine, dolutegravir, or megestrol

Warnings/Precautions [U.S. Boxed Warning]: Must be initiated (or reinitiated) in a setting with continuous monitoring and staff familiar with the recognition and treatment of life-threatening arrhythmias. Patients must be monitored with continuous ECG for a minimum of 3 days, or for a minimum of 12 hours after electrical or pharmacological cardioversion to normal sinus rhythm, whichever is greater. Patients should be readmitted for continuous monitoring if dosage is later increased.

Reserve for patients who are highly symptomatic with atrial fibrillation/atrial flutter; risk of torsade de pointes (TdP) significantly increases with doses >500 mcg twice daily; hold Class I or Class III antiarrhythmics for at least three half-lives prior to starting dofetilide; use in patients previously on amiodarone therapy only if serum amiodarone level is <0.3 mg/L or if amiodarone was discontinued ≥3 months ago; correct hypokalemia or hypomagnesemia before initiating dofetilide and maintain within normal limits during treatment. The risk of TdP may be higher in certain patient subgroups (eg, patients with heart failure). Most episodes of TdP occur within the first 3 days of therapy. Risk of hypokalemia and/or hypomagnesemia may be increased by potassium-depleting diuretics, increasing the risk of TdP. Concurrent use with other drugs known to prolong QTc interval is not recommended.

In the treatment of atrial fibrillation in the elderly, avoid antiarrhythmics as first-line treatment. In older adults, data suggests rate control may provide more benefits than risks compared to rhythm control for most patients (Beers Criteria).

Patients with sick sinus syndrome or with second or third-degree heart block should not receive dofetilide unless a functional pacemaker is in place. Defibrillation threshold is reduced in patients with ventricular tachycardia or ventricular fibrillation undergoing implantation of a cardioverter-defibrillator device. Use with caution in renal impairment; **dose adjustment required for patients with CrCl ≤60 mL/minute.** Use with caution in patients with severe hepatic impairment; not studied.

Adverse Reactions Supraventricular arrhythmia patients:

Cardiovascular: AV block, bradycardia, cardiac arrest, chest pain, torsade de pointes (most frequently within the first 3 days of therapy), ventricular tachycardia

Central nervous system: CVA, dizziness, facial paralysis, flaccid paralysis, headache, insomnia, migraine, paralysis

Dermatologic: Angioedema, rash

Gastrointestinal: Abdominal pain, diarrhea, liver damage, nausea

Neuromuscular & skeletal: Back pain, paresthesia

Respiratory: Cough, dyspnea, respiratory tract infection

Miscellaneous: Flu-like syndrome

Drug Interactions

Metabolism/Transport Effects Substrate of CYP3A4 (minor); **Note:** Assignment of Major/Minor substrate status based on clinically relevant drug interaction potential

Avoid Concomitant Use

Avoid concomitant use of Dofetilide with any of the following: Antifungal Agents (Azole Derivatives, Systemic); Cimetidine; Dolutegravir; Fingolimod; Highest Risk QTc-Prolonging Agents; Ivabradine; Megestrol; Mifepristone; Moderate Risk QTc-Prolonging Agents; Prochlorperazine; Propafenone; Saquinavir; Thiazide Diuretics; Trimethoprim; Verapamil

Increased Effect/Toxicity

Dofetilide may increase the levels/effects of: Highest Risk QTc-Prolonging Agents; Lidocaine (Topical)

The levels/effects of Dofetilide may be increased by: AMILoride; Antifungal Agents (Azole Derivatives, Systemic); Cimetidine; Cobicistat; CYP3A4 Inhibitors (Moderate); CYP3A4 Inhibitors (Strong); CYP3A4 Inhibitors (Weak); Dolutegravir; Fingolimod; Ivabradine; Lidocaine (Topical); Loop Diuretics; Megestrol; MetFORMIN; Mifepristone; Moderate Risk QTc-Prolonging Agents; Prochlorperazine; Propafenone; QTc-Prolonging Agents (Indeterminate Risk and Risk Modifying); Saquinavir; Thiazide Diuretics; Triamterene; Trimethoprim; Verapamil

Decreased Effect There are no known significant interactions involving a decrease in effect.

Mechanism of Action Vaughan Williams Class III antiarrhythmic activity. Blockade of the cardiac ion channel carrying the rapid component of the delayed rectifier potassium current. Dofetilide has no effect on sodium channels, adrenergic alpha-receptors, or adrenergic beta-receptors. It increases the monophasic action potential duration due to delayed repolarization. The increase in the QT interval is a function of prolongation of both effective and functional refractory periods in the His-Purkinje system and the ventricles. Changes in cardiac conduction velocity and sinus node function have not been observed in patients with or without structural heart disease. PR and QRS width remain the same in patients with preexisting heart block and or sick sinus syndrome.

Pharmacodynamics/Kinetics

Absorption: Well absorbed

Distribution: V_d: 3 L/kg

Protein binding: 60% to 70%

Metabolism: Hepatic via CYP3A4, but low affinity for it; metabolites formed by N-dealkylation and N-oxidation

Bioavailability: >90%

Half-life elimination: ~10 hours; prolonged with renal impairment

Time to peak, serum: Fasting: 2-3 hours

Excretion: Urine (80%; 80% as unchanged drug, 20% as inactive or minimally active metabolites); renal elimination consists of glomerular filtration and active tubular secretion via cationic transport system

Dosage Atrial fibrillation/atrial flutter: Adults: Oral:

Note: QT or QTc must be determined prior to first dose. If QTc >440 msec (>500 msec in patients with ventricular conduction abnormalities), dofetilide is contraindicated.

Initial: 500 mcg twice daily. Initial dosage must be adjusted in patients with estimated CrCl <60 mL/minute (see Dosage adjustment in renal impairment). Dofetilide may be initiated at lower doses than recommended based on physician discretion.

Modification of dosage in response to **initial** dose: QTc interval should be measured 2 to 3 hours after the initial dose. If the QTc increases to more than 15% above baseline QTc or if the QTc is >500 msec (>550 msec in patients with ventricular conduction abnormalities), dofetilide dose should be reduced. If the starting dose was 500 mcg twice daily, then reduce to 250 mcg twice daily. If the starting dose was 250 mcg twice daily, then reduce to 125 mcg twice daily. If the starting dose was 125 mcg twice daily, then reduce to 125 mcg once daily. If at any time after the second dose is given the QTc is >500 msec (>550 msec in patients with ventricular conduction abnormalities), dofetilide should be discontinued.

Dosage adjustment in renal impairment: Note: Using the Modification of Diet in Renal Disease (MDRD) equation and subsequent eGFR to determine dose may lead to overestimation of creatinine clearance and overdose of medication; use only the Cockcroft-Gault equation to estimate creatinine clearance (Denetclaw, 2011). Use actual body weight when using the Cockcroft-Gault equation to calculate creatinine clearance (weight range of patients enrolled in clinical trials: 40-134 kg).

CrCl >60 mL/minute: Administer 500 mcg twice daily.

CrCl 40-60 mL/minute: Administer 250 mcg twice daily.

CrCl 20-39 mL/minute: Administer 125 mcg twice daily.

CrCl <20 mL/minute: Contraindicated.

Dosage adjustment in hepatic impairment: No dosage adjustments required in Child-Pugh class A and B. Patients with severe hepatic impairment were not studied.

Elderly: No specific dosage adjustments are recommended based on age, however, careful assessment of renal function is particularly important in this population.

Monitoring Parameters ECG monitoring with attention to QT (if heart rate <60 beats per minute) or QTc and occurrence of ventricular arrhythmias, baseline serum creatinine and changes in serum creatinine. Upon initiation (or reinitiation) continuous ECG monitoring recommended for a minimum of 3 days, or for at least 12 hours after electrical or pharmacological conversion to normal sinus rhythm, whichever is greater. Check serum potassium and magnesium levels at baseline and throughout therapy especially if on medications where these electrolyte disturbances can occur, or if patient has a history of hypokalemia or hypomagnesemia. QT or QTc must be monitored at baseline prior to the first dose and 2-3 hours afterwards. If at baseline, QTc >440 msec (>500 msec in patients with ventricular conduction abnormalities), dofetilide is contraindicated. If dofetilide initiated, QTc interval must be determined 2-3 hours after each subsequent dose of dofetilide for in-hospital doses 2-5. Thereafter, QT or QTc and creatinine clearance should be evaluated every 3 months. If at any time during therapy after the second dose the measured QTc is >500 msec (>550 msec in patients with ventricular conduction abnormalities), dofetilide should be discontinued.

Consult individual institutional policies and procedures.

Dosage Forms

Capsule, Oral:

Tikosyn: 125 mcg, 250 mcg, 500 mcg

◆ **DOK [OTC]** *see* Docusate *on page 661*

◆ **Dok Plus [OTC]** *see* Docusate and Senna *on page 662*

Dolasetron (dol A se tron)

Brand Names: U.S. Anzemet

Brand Names: Canada Anzemet

Index Terms Dolasetron Mesylate; MDL 73,147EF

Pharmacologic Category Antiemetic; Selective 5-HT_3 Receptor Antagonist

Use

U.S. labeling:

Injection: Prevention and treatment of postoperative nausea and vomiting in adults and children ≥2 years

Oral: Prevention of nausea and vomiting associated with moderately emetogenic cancer chemotherapy (initial and repeat courses) in adults and children ≥2 years

Canadian labeling: Oral: Prevention of nausea and vomiting associated with emetogenic cancer chemotherapy (initial and repeat courses)

Pregnancy Risk Factor B

Pregnancy Considerations Adverse events have not been observed in animal reproduction studies.

Breast-Feeding Considerations It is not known if dolasetron is excreted in breast milk. The manufacturer recommends that caution be exercised when administering dolasetron to nursing women.

Contraindications

U.S. labeling:

Injection: Hypersensitivity to dolasetron or any component of the formulation; intravenous administration is contraindicated when used for prevention of chemotherapy-associated nausea and vomiting

Tablet: Hypersensitivity to dolasetron or any component of the formulation

Canadian labeling: Hypersensitivity to dolasetron or any component of the formulation; use in children and adolescents <18 years of age; use for the prevention or treatment of postoperative nausea and vomiting; concomitant use with apomorphine

Warnings/Precautions Dolasetron is associated with a number of dose-dependent increases in ECG intervals (eg, PR, QRS duration, QT/QTc, JT), usually occurring 1-2 hours after IV administration and usually lasting 6-8 hours; however, may last ≥24 hours and rarely lead to heart block or arrhythmia. Clinically relevant QT-interval prolongation may occur resulting in torsade de pointes, when used in conjunction with other agents that prolong the QT interval (eg, Class I and III antiarrhythmics). Avoid use in patients at greater risk for QT prolongation (eg, patients with congenital long QT syndrome, medications known to prolong QT interval, electrolyte abnormalities, and cumulative high-dose anthracycline therapy) and/or ventricular arrhythmia. Correct potassium or magnesium abnormalities prior to initiating therapy. IV formulations of 5-HT_3 antagonists have more association with ECG interval changes, compared to oral formulations. Reduction in heart rate may also occur with the 5-HT_3 antagonists. Use with caution in children and adolescents who have or may develop QTc prolongation; rare cases of supraventricular and ventricular arrhythmias, cardiac arrest, and MI have been reported in this population. ECG monitoring is recommended in patients with renal impairment and in the elderly.

Serotonin syndrome has been reported with 5-HT_3 receptor antagonists, predominantly when used in combination with other serotonergic agents (eg, SSRIs, SNRIs, MAOIs, mirtazapine, fentanyl, lithium, tramadol, and/or methylene blue). Some of the cases have been fatal. The majority of serotonin syndrome reports due to 5-HT_3 receptor antagonist have occurred in a post-anesthesia setting or in an infusion center. Serotonin syndrome has also been reported following overdose of another 5-HT_3 receptor antagonist. Monitor patients for signs of serotonin syndrome, including mental status changes (eg, agitation, hallucinations, delirium, coma); autonomic instability (eg, tachycardia, labile blood pressure, diaphoresis, dizziness, flushing, hyperthermia); neuromuscular changes (eg, tremor, rigidity, myoclonus, hyperreflexia, incoordination); gastrointestinal symptoms (eg, nausea, vomiting, diarrhea); and/or seizures. If serotonin syndrome occurs, discontinue 5-HT_3 receptor antagonist treatment and begin supportive management.

Use with caution in patients allergic to other 5-HT_3 receptor antagonists; cross-reactivity has been reported with other 5-HT_3 receptor antagonists. **For chemotherapy-associated nausea and vomiting, should be used on a scheduled basis, not on an "as needed" (PRN) basis,** since data support the use of this drug only in the prevention of nausea and vomiting (due to antineoplastic therapy) and not in the rescue of nausea and vomiting. Not intended for treatment of nausea and vomiting or for chronic continuous therapy. If the prophylaxis dolasetron dose for postoperative nausea and vomiting has failed, a repeat dose should not be administered as rescue or treatment for postoperative nausea and vomiting. Potentially significant drug-drug interactions may exist, requiring dose or frequency adjustment, additional monitoring, and/or selection of alternative therapy.

Adverse Reactions Adverse events may vary according to indication and route of administration.

Cardiovascular: Bradycardia (may be severe after IV administration), edema, facial edema, flushing, hypotension (may be severe after IV administration), orthostatic hypotension, peripheral edema, peripheral ischemia, phlebitis, sinus arrhythmia, tachycardia, thrombophlebitis

Central nervous system: Abnormal dreams, agitation, anxiety, ataxia, chills, confusion, depersonalization, dizziness, fatigue (oral), headache (more common in oral), pain, paresthesia, shivering sleep disorder, twitching, vertigo

Dermatologic: Diaphoresis, skin rash, urticaria

Endocrine & metabolic: Increased gamma-glutamyl transferase

Gastrointestinal: Abdominal pain, anorexia, constipation, diarrhea (oral), dysgeusia, dyspepsia, pancreatitis

Genitourinary: Dysuria, hematuria

Hematologic and oncologic: Anemia, hematoma, prolonged prothrombin time, prolonged partial thromboplastin time, purpura, thrombocytopenia

Hepatic: Hyperbilirubinemia, increased serum alkaline phosphatase

Hypersensitivity: Anaphylaxis

Local: Burning sensation at injection site (IV), pain at injection site (IV)

Neuromuscular & skeletal: Arthralgia, myalgia, tremor

Ophthalmic: Photophobia, visual disturbance

Otic: Tinnitus

Renal: Acute renal failure, polyuria

Respiratory: Bronchospasm, dyspnea, epistaxis

Rare but important or life-threatening: Abnormal T waves on ECG, appearance of U waves on ECG, atrial fibrillation, atrioventricular block, bundle branch block (left and right), chest pain, extrasystoles (APCs or VPCs), increased serum ALT (transient), increased serum AST (transient), ischemic heart disease, nodal arrhythmia, prolongation P-R interval on ECG (dose-dependent), prolonged Q-T interval on ECG, serotonin syndrome, slow R wave progression, ST segment changes on ECG, supraventricular cardiac arrhythmia, syncope (may be severe after IV administration), torsades de pointes, ventricular arrhythmia (may be serious), ventricular fibrillation cardiac arrest (intravenous), wide complex tachycardia (intravenous), widened QRS complex on ECG (dose-dependent)

Drug Interactions

Metabolism/Transport Effects Substrate of CYP2C9 (minor), CYP3A4 (minor); **Note:** Assignment of Major/Minor substrate status based on clinically relevant drug interaction potential; **Inhibits** CYP2D6 (weak)

Avoid Concomitant Use

Avoid concomitant use of Dolasetron with any of the following: Apomorphine; Highest Risk QTc-Prolonging Agents; Ivabradine; Mifepristone

Increased Effect/Toxicity

Dolasetron may increase the levels/effects of: Apomorphine; ARIPiprazole; Highest Risk QTc-Prolonging Agents; Moderate Risk QTc-Prolonging Agents; Serotonin Modulators

The levels/effects of Dolasetron may be increased by: Ivabradine; Mifepristone; QTc-Prolonging Agents (Indeterminate Risk and Risk Modifying)

Decreased Effect

Dolasetron may decrease the levels/effects of: Tapentadol; TraMADol

Food Interactions Food does not affect the bioavailability of oral doses.

Preparation for Administration May be administered undiluted, or diluted in 50 mL of a compatible solution (ie, 0.9% NS, D_5W, $D_5{}^1\!/_2NS$, D_5LR, LR, and 10% mannitol injection).

Storage/Stability

Injection: Store intact vials at 20°C to 25°C (68°F to 77°F); excursions are permitted to 15°C to 30°C (59°F to 86°F). Protect from light. Solutions diluted for infusion are stable under normal lighting conditions at room temperature for 24 hours or under refrigeration for 48 hours.

Tablets: Store at 20°C to 25°C (68°F to 77°F). Protect from light.

Mechanism of Action Selective serotonin receptor ($5\text{-}HT_3$) antagonist, blocking serotonin both peripherally (primary site of action) and centrally at the chemoreceptor trigger zone

Pharmacodynamics/Kinetics

Absorption: Oral: Rapid and complete

Distribution: Hydrodolasetron: 5.8 L/kg

Protein binding: Hydrodolasetron: 69% to 77% (50% bound to $alpha_1$-acid glycoprotein)

Metabolism: Hepatic; rapid reduction by carbonyl reductase to hydrodolasetron (active metabolite); further metabolized by CYP2D6, CYP3A, and flavin monooxygenase

Bioavailability: Oral: ~75% (not affected by food)

Half-life elimination: Dolasetron: ≤10 minutes; hydrodolasetron: Adults: 6-8 hours; Children: 4-6 hours; Severe renal impairment: 11 hours; Severe hepatic impairment: 11 hours

Time to peak, plasma: Hydrodolasetron: IV: 0.6 hours; Oral: ~1 hour

Excretion: Urine ~67% (53% to 61% of the total dose as active metabolite hydrodolasetron); feces ~33%

Dosage Note: Use of intravenous dolasetron is contraindicated in the prevention of chemotherapy-associated nausea and vomiting. In Canada, use of dolasetron is also contraindicated in children and adolescents <18 years of age and in the prevention and treatment of postoperative nausea and vomiting in adults.

U.S. labeling:

Prevention of chemotherapy-associated nausea and vomiting (including initial and repeat courses):

Children 2-16 years: Oral: 1.8 mg/kg within 1 hour before chemotherapy; maximum: 100 mg/dose

Adults: Oral: 100 mg within 1 hour before chemotherapy

Prevention of postoperative nausea and vomiting:

Children 2-16 years:

Oral: 1.2 mg/kg within 2 hours before surgery; maximum: 100 mg/dose

IV: 0.35 mg/kg ~15 minutes before cessation of anesthesia; maximum: 12.5 mg/dose

Adults: IV: 12.5 mg ~15 minutes before cessation of anesthesia (do not exceed the recommended dose)

Treatment of postoperative nausea and vomiting:

Children 2-16 years: IV: 0.35 mg/kg as soon as nausea or vomiting present; maximum: 12.5 mg/dose

Adults: IV: 12.5 mg as soon as nausea or vomiting present (do not exceed the recommended dose)

Canadian labeling: **Prevention of chemotherapy-associated nausea and vomiting (including initial and repeat courses):** Adults: Oral: 100 mg within 1 hour before chemotherapy

Dosing adjustment in renal impairment: No dosage adjustment necessary; however, ECG monitoring is recommended in patients with renal impairment.

Dosing adjustment in hepatic impairment: No dosage adjustment necessary

Administration

IV injection may be given either undiluted as an IV push over 30 seconds or diluted in 50 mL of compatible fluid and infused over 15 minutes. Flush line before and after dolasetron administration.

Oral: When unable to administer in tablet form, dolasetron injection may be diluted in apple or apple-grape juice and taken orally; this dilution is stable for 2 hours at room temperature (Anzemet prescribing information, 2013).

Monitoring Parameters ECG (in patients with cardiovascular disease, elderly, renally impaired, those at risk of developing hypokalemia and/or hypomagnesemia); potassium, magnesium

Additional Information Efficacy of dolasetron, for chemotherapy treatment, is enhanced with concomitant administration of dexamethasone 20 mg (increases complete response by 10% to 20%). Oral administration of the intravenous solution is equivalent to tablets.

Dosage Forms

Solution, Intravenous:

Anzemet: 20 mg/mL (0.625 mL, 5 mL, 25 mL)

Tablet, Oral:

Anzemet: 50 mg, 100 mg

Extemporaneous Preparations Dolasetron injection may be diluted in apple or apple-grape juice and taken orally; this dilution is stable for 2 hours at room temperature (Anzemet prescribing information, 2013).

A 10 mg/mL oral suspension may be prepared with tablets and either a 1:1 mixture of Ora-Plus and Ora-Sweet SF or a 1:1 mixture of strawberry syrup and Ora-Plus. Crush twelve 50 mg tablets in a mortar and reduce to a fine powder. Slowly add chosen vehicle to **almost** 60 mL; transfer to a calibrated bottle, rinse mortar with vehicle, and add quantity of vehicle sufficient to make 60 mL. Label "shake well" and "refrigerate". Stable for 90 days refrigerated.

Anzemet® prescribing information, sanofi-aventis U.S. LLC, Bridgewater, NJ, 2013.

Johnson CE, Wagner DS, and Bussard WE, "Stability of Dolasetron in Two Oral Liquid Vehicles," *Am J Health Syst Pharm*, 2003, 60 (21):2242-4.

◆ **Dolasetron Mesylate** *see* Dolasetron *on page 663*

◆ **Dolgic Plus** *see* Butalbital, Acetaminophen, and Caffeine *on page 313*

◆ **Dolobid** *see* Diflunisal *on page 626*

◆ **Dolophine** *see* Methadone *on page 1311*

◆ **Doloral (Can)** *see* Morphine (Systemic) *on page 1394*

◆ **Dolutegravir, Lamivudine, and Abacavir** *see* Abacavir, Dolutegravir, and Lamivudine *on page 22*

◆ **Dom-Alendronate (Can)** *see* Alendronate *on page 79*

◆ **Dom-Amantadine (Can)** *see* Amantadine *on page 105*

◆ **Dom-Amiodarone (Can)** *see* Amiodarone *on page 114*

◆ **Dom-Amlodipine (Can)** *see* AmLODIPine *on page 123*

◆ **Dom-Anagrelide (Can)** *see* Anagrelide *on page 147*

◆ **Dom-Atenolol (Can)** *see* Atenolol *on page 189*

◆ **DOM-Atomoxetine (Can)** *see* AtoMOXetine *on page 191*

◆ **Dom-Atorvastatin (Can)** *see* AtorvaSTATin *on page 194*

◆ **Dom-Azithromycin (Can)** *see* Azithromycin (Systemic) *on page 216*

◆ **Dom-Baclofen (Can)** *see* Baclofen *on page 223*

◆ **Dom-Benzydamine (Can)** *see* Benzydamine [CAN/INT] *on page 249*

◆ **Dom-Bicalutamide (Can)** *see* Bicalutamide *on page 262*

◆ **Dom-Bromocriptine (Can)** *see* Bromocriptine *on page 291*

◆ **Dom-Buspirone (Can)** *see* BusPIRone *on page 311*

- ◆ **DOM-Candesartan (Can)** *see* Candesartan *on page 335*
- ◆ **Dom-Captopril (Can)** *see* Captopril *on page 342*
- ◆ **Dom-Carbamazepine (Can)** *see* CarBAMazepine *on page 346*
- ◆ **Dom-Carvedilol (Can)** *see* Carvedilol *on page 367*
- ◆ **Dom-Cephalexin (Can)** *see* Cephalexin *on page 405*
- ◆ **Dom-Cimetidine (Can)** *see* Cimetidine *on page 438*
- ◆ **Dom-Ciprofloxacin (Can)** *see* Ciprofloxacin (Systemic) *on page 441*
- ◆ **Dom-Citalopram (Can)** *see* Citalopram *on page 451*
- ◆ **Dom-Clarithromycin (Can)** *see* Clarithromycin *on page 456*
- ◆ **Dom-Clobazam (Can)** *see* CloBAZam *on page 465*
- ◆ **Dom-Clomipramine (Can)** *see* ClomiPRAMINE *on page 475*
- ◆ **Dom-Clonazepam (Can)** *see* ClonazePAM *on page 478*
- ◆ **Dom-Clonazepam-R (Can)** *see* ClonazePAM *on page 478*
- ◆ **Dom-Clonidine (Can)** *see* CloNIDine *on page 480*
- ◆ **Dom-Clopidogrel (Can)** *see* Clopidogrel *on page 484*
- ◆ **Dom-Cyclobenzaprine (Can)** *see* Cyclobenzaprine *on page 516*
- ◆ **Dom-Desipramine (Can)** *see* Desipramine *on page 593*
- ◆ **Dom-Dexamethasone (Can)** *see* Dexamethasone (Systemic) *on page 599*
- ◆ **Dom-Diclofenac (Can)** *see* Diclofenac (Systemic) *on page 617*
- ◆ **Dom-Diclofenac SR (Can)** *see* Diclofenac (Systemic) *on page 617*
- ◆ **Dom-Divalproex (Can)** *see* Valproic Acid and Derivatives *on page 2123*
- ◆ **Dom-Docusate Sodium [OTC] (Can)** *see* Docusate *on page 661*
- ◆ **Dom-Domperidone (Can)** *see* Domperidone [CAN/INT] *on page 666*
- ◆ **Dom-Doxazosin (Can)** *see* Doxazosin *on page 674*
- ◆ **Dom-Doxycycline (Can)** *see* Doxycycline *on page 689*
- ◆ **Dome Paste Bandage** *see* Zinc Gelatin *on page 2200*
- ◆ **Dom-Fenofibrate Micro (Can)** *see* Fenofibrate and Derivatives *on page 852*
- ◆ **Dom-Finasteride (Can)** *see* Finasteride *on page 878*
- ◆ **Dom-Fluconazole (Can)** *see* Fluconazole *on page 885*
- ◆ **Dom-Fluoxetine (Can)** *see* FLUoxetine *on page 899*
- ◆ **Dom-Fluvoxamine (Can)** *see* FluvoxaMINE *on page 916*
- ◆ **Dom-Furosemide (Can)** *see* Furosemide *on page 940*
- ◆ **Dom-Gabapentin (Can)** *see* Gabapentin *on page 943*
- ◆ **Dom-Glyburide (Can)** *see* GlyBURIDE *on page 972*
- ◆ **Dom-Indapamide (Can)** *see* Indapamide *on page 1065*
- ◆ **Dom-Irbesartan (Can)** *see* Irbesartan *on page 1110*
- ◆ **Dom-Isoniazid (Can)** *see* Isoniazid *on page 1120*
- ◆ **Dom-Levetiracetam (Can)** *see* LevETIRAcetam *on page 1191*
- ◆ **Dom-Levo-Carbidopa (Can)** *see* Carbidopa and Levodopa *on page 351*
- ◆ **Dom-Lisinopril (Can)** *see* Lisinopril *on page 1226*
- ◆ **Dom-Loperamide (Can)** *see* Loperamide *on page 1236*
- ◆ **Dom-Lorazepam (Can)** *see* LORazepam *on page 1243*
- ◆ **Dom-Lovastatin (Can)** *see* Lovastatin *on page 1252*
- ◆ **Dom-Loxapine (Can)** *see* Loxapine *on page 1255*
- ◆ **Dom-Medroxyprogesterone (Can)** *see* MedroxyPROGESTERone *on page 1277*
- ◆ **Dom-Mefenamic Acid (Can)** *see* Mefenamic Acid *on page 1280*
- ◆ **Dom-Meloxicam (Can)** *see* Meloxicam *on page 1283*
- ◆ **Dom-Metformin (Can)** *see* MetFORMIN *on page 1307*
- ◆ **Dom-Methimazole (Can)** *see* Methimazole *on page 1319*
- ◆ **Dom-Metoprolol-L (Can)** *see* Metoprolol *on page 1350*
- ◆ **Dom-Metoprolol-B (Can)** *see* Metoprolol *on page 1350*
- ◆ **Dom-Minocycline (Can)** *see* Minocycline *on page 1371*
- ◆ **Dom-Mirtazapine (Can)** *see* Mirtazapine *on page 1376*
- ◆ **Dom-Moclobemide (Can)** *see* Moclobemide [CAN/INT] *on page 1384*
- ◆ **Dom-Montelukast (Can)** *see* Montelukast *on page 1392*
- ◆ **Dom-Montelukast FC (Can)** *see* Montelukast *on page 1392*
- ◆ **Dom-Nortriptyline (Can)** *see* Nortriptyline *on page 1476*
- ◆ **Dom-Omeprazole DR (Can)** *see* Omeprazole *on page 1508*
- ◆ **Dom-Ondansetron (Can)** *see* Ondansetron *on page 1513*
- ◆ **Dom-Oxybutynin (Can)** *see* Oxybutynin *on page 1536*
- ◆ **Dom-Pantoprazole (Can)** *see* Pantoprazole *on page 1570*
- ◆ **Dom-Paroxetine (Can)** *see* PARoxetine *on page 1579*

Domperidone [CAN/INT] (dom PE ri done)

Brand Names: Canada Apo-Domperidone; Dom-Domperidone; Jamp-Domperidone; Mylan-Domperidone; PMS-Domperidone; RAN-Domperidone; ratio-Domperidone; Teva-Domperidone

Index Terms Domperidone Maleate

Pharmacologic Category Dopamine Antagonist; Gastrointestinal Agent, Prokinetic

Use Note: Not approved in U.S.

Symptomatic management of upper GI motility disorders associated with chronic and subacute gastritis and diabetic gastroparesis; prevention of GI symptoms associated with use of dopamine-agonist anti-Parkinson agents

Pregnancy Considerations Animal studies have not shown drug-related teratogenic or primary embryotoxic effects on animal fetuses; however, comparative studies have not been done in humans. Use only when benefit outweighs potential risk in a pregnant woman.

Breast-Feeding Considerations Domperidone is excreted in low concentrations in breast milk; however, breast-feeding is not recommended by the manufacturer.

Contraindications Hypersensitivity to domperidone or any component of the formulation; prolactin-releasing pituitary tumor (prolactinoma); patients with GI hemorrhage, mechanical obstruction, or perforation; concomitant use with ketoconazole

Warnings/Precautions Domperidone may increase prolactin levels (dose-dependent response). Elevated prolactin may be asymptomatic (clinical consequence of chronically-elevated prolactin is unknown) or may present symptomatically as galactorrhea, gynecomastia, amenorrhea, or impotence (reversible upon decreasing dose or discontinuing drug). Contraindicated in patients with prolactinomas.

[Canadian Boxed Warning]: Domperidone may be associated with an increased risk of serious ventricular arrhythmias or sudden cardiac death, particularly with doses >30 mg or when used in patients >60 years of age. QTc prolongation, life-threatening tachyarrhythmias, and cardiac arrest have been reported after domperidone use; these adverse effects may be precipitated in patients with preexisting prolonged cardiac conduction or other underlying cardiac disease, hypokalemia, or receiving other QTc-prolonging agents. Avoid use in patients with diagnosed or suspected congenital long QT syndrome. Initiate therapy at the lowest dose possible. The American College of Gastroenterology guidelines recommend baseline and follow-up ECGs and avoiding use if corrected QT is >470 msec in male patients or >450 msec in female patients (Camilleri, 2013). Use with caution in patients with severe renal impairment; dosage and/or frequency of administration may need adjusted with repeated use and/or long-term therapy. Use with caution in patients with hepatic impairment. Use caution when administering domperidone to patients with a personal or family history of breast cancer; evidence regarding an association between chronic use of dopamine-receptor antagonists and breast cancer is limited and nonconclusive. Potentially significant drug-drug interactions may exist, requiring dose or frequency adjustment, additional monitoring, and/or selection of alternative therapy.

In 2004, the Food and Drug Administration (FDA) issued a warning recommending that domperidone not be used off-label to increase milk production in breast-feeding women due to safety concerns. Several cases of cardiac arrhythmia, cardiac arrest, and sudden death have been reported in patients receiving intravenous domperidone. The risk of similar adverse events in breast-feeding women is unknown. Domperidone is not available for any use in the United States (except via severe GI disorder IND) and does not have approval for this indication in other countries.

Adverse Reactions

Central nervous system: Headache/migraine

Gastrointestinal: Xerostomia

Rare but important or life-threatening: ALT increased, AST increased, dizziness, dysuria, edema, extrapyramidal symptoms (EPS) rarely, galactorrhea, gynecomastia, hot flashes, insomnia, irritability, mastalgia, menstrual irregularities, nervousness, pruritus, rash, serum prolactin increased, sudden death, torsade de pointes

Drug Interactions

Metabolism/Transport Effects Substrate of CYP1A2 (minor), CYP2B6 (minor), CYP2C8 (minor), CYP2D6 (minor), CYP3A4 (major); **Note:** Assignment of Major/Minor substrate status based on clinically relevant drug interaction potential

Avoid Concomitant Use

Avoid concomitant use of Domperidone with any of the following: Conivaptan; Fusidic Acid (Systemic); Highest Risk QTc-Prolonging Agents; Idelalisib; Ivabradine; Ketoconazole (Systemic); Mifepristone; Moderate Risk QTc-Prolonging Agents

Increased Effect/Toxicity

Domperidone may increase the levels/effects of: Highest Risk QTc-Prolonging Agents; Ketoconazole (Systemic)

The levels/effects of Domperidone may be increased by: Aprepitant; Conivaptan; CYP3A4 Inhibitors (Moderate); CYP3A4 Inhibitors (Strong); Fosaprepitant; Fusidic Acid (Systemic); Idelalisib; Ivabradine; Ivacaftor; Ketoconazole (Systemic); Luliconazole; MAO Inhibitors; Mifepristone; Moderate Risk QTc-Prolonging Agents; Netupitant; QTc-Prolonging Agents (Indeterminate Risk and Risk Modifying); Simeprevir; Stiripentol

Decreased Effect

Domperidone may decrease the levels/effects of: MAO Inhibitors

The levels/effects of Domperidone may be decreased by: MAO Inhibitors

Storage/Stability Store at room temperature of 15°C to 30°C (59°F to 86°F). Protect from light and moisture.

Mechanism of Action Domperidone has peripheral dopamine receptor blocking properties and does not readily cross the blood-brain barrier. It increases esophageal peristalsis and increases lower esophageal sphincter pressure, increases gastric motility and peristalsis, and enhances gastroduodenal coordination, therefore, facilitating gastric emptying and decreasing small bowel transit time.

Pharmacodynamics/Kinetics

Protein binding: 93%

Metabolism: Hepatic via CYP3A4, N-dealkylation and hydroxylation

Half-life elimination: 7 hours (increases to ~21 hours in severe renal impairment)

Time to peak serum concentration: 30 minutes

Excretion: Feces (66%); urine (31%)

Dosage Oral: Adults: **Note:** Health Canada has updated dosing recommendations due to safety concerns and now recommends a maximum daily dose of 30 mg. Revisions to the manufacturer labeling are pending. Further information is available at: http://healthycanadians.gc.ca/recall-alert-rappel-avis/hc-sc/2015/43423a-eng.php.

GI motility disorders (diabetic gastroparesis, gastritis): Initiate at lowest possible dose. Usual: 10 mg 3 to 4 times daily, 15 to 30 minutes before meals and at bedtime if needed; in severe/resistant cases, may increase to maximum dose of 20 mg 3 to 4 times daily, 15 to 30 minutes before meals and at bedtime if needed. The American College of Gastroenterology recommends initiating at 10 mg 3 times daily (Camilleri, 2013).

Nausea/vomiting associated with dopamine-agonist anti-Parkinson agents: Usual: 20 mg 3 to 4 times daily (higher doses may be necessary during titration of anti-Parkinson therapy)

Dosage adjustment in renal impairment:

Mild-to-moderate impairment: No dosage adjustment necessary.

Severe impairment (serum creatinine >0.6 mmol/L or 6 mg/dL): Reduce dosing frequency to 1 to 2 times daily with prolonged therapy. Dose reduction may also be necessary.

Dosage adjustment in hepatic impairment:

Mild impairment: There are no dosage adjustments provided in the manufacturer's labeling; use with caution (undergoes hepatic metabolism).

Moderate or severe impairment: **Note:** Revisions to the manufacturer labeling are pending. Use is now contraindicated.

Administration In GI motility disorders, administer 15 to 30 minutes prior to meals and at bedtime if needed.

Monitoring Parameters Renal function; ECG

Product Availability Not available in U.S.

Dosage Forms: Canada

Tablet: 10 mg

◆ **Domperidone Maleate** *see* Domperidone [CAN/INT] *on page 666*

◆ **Dom-Pindolol (Can)** *see* Pindolol *on page 1652*

◆ **Dom-Pioglitazone (Can)** *see* Pioglitazone *on page 1654*

◆ **Dom-Piroxicam (Can)** *see* Piroxicam *on page 1662*

◆ **Dom-Pramipexole (Can)** *see* Pramipexole *on page 1695*

◆ **Dom-Pravastatin (Can)** *see* Pravastatin *on page 1700*

◆ **Dom-Pregabalin (Can)** *see* Pregabalin *on page 1710*

◆ **Dom-Propranolol (Can)** *see* Propranolol *on page 1731*

- **Dom-Quetiapine (Can)** *see* QUEtiapine *on page 1751*
- **Dom-Ramipril (Can)** *see* Ramipril *on page 1771*
- **Dom-Ranitidine (Can)** *see* Ranitidine *on page 1777*
- **Dom-Risedronate (Can)** *see* Risedronate *on page 1816*
- **Dom-Risperidone (Can)** *see* RisperiDONE *on page 1818*
- **Dom-Rizatriptan RDT (Can)** *see* Rizatriptan *on page 1836*
- **Dom-Rosuvastatin (Can)** *see* Rosuvastatin *on page 1848*
- **Dom-Salbutamol (Can)** *see* Albuterol *on page 69*
- **Dom-Sertraline (Can)** *see* Sertraline *on page 1878*
- **Dom-Simvastatin (Can)** *see* Simvastatin *on page 1890*
- **Dom-Sotalol (Can)** *see* Sotalol *on page 1927*
- **Dom-Sucralfate (Can)** *see* Sucralfate *on page 1940*
- **Dom-Sumatriptan (Can)** *see* SUMAtriptan *on page 1953*
- **Dom-Temazepam (Can)** *see* Temazepam *on page 1990*
- **Dom-Terazosin (Can)** *see* Terazosin *on page 2001*
- **Dom-Terbinafine (Can)** *see* Terbinafine (Systemic) *on page 2002*
- **Dom-Tiaprofenic (Can)** *see* Tiaprofenic Acid [CAN/INT] *on page 2034*
- **Dom-Ticlopidine (Can)** *see* Ticlopidine *on page 2040*
- **Dom-Timolol (Can)** *see* Timolol (Ophthalmic) *on page 2043*
- **Dom-Topiramate (Can)** *see* Topiramate *on page 2065*
- **Dom-Trazodone (Can)** *see* TraZODone *on page 2091*
- **Dom-Ursodiol C (Can)** *see* Ursodiol *on page 2116*
- **DOM-Valacyclovir (Can)** *see* ValACYclovir *on page 2119*
- **Dom-Valproic Acid (Can)** *see* Valproic Acid and Derivatives *on page 2123*
- **Dom-Valproic Acid E.C. (Can)** *see* Valproic Acid and Derivatives *on page 2123*
- **Dom-Venlafaxine XR (Can)** *see* Venlafaxine *on page 2150*
- **Dom-Verapamil SR (Can)** *see* Verapamil *on page 2154*
- **Dom-Zolmitriptan (Can)** *see* ZOLMitriptan *on page 2210*
- **Dom-Zopiclone (Can)** *see* Zopiclone [CAN/INT] *on page 2217*

Donepezil (doh NEP e zil)

Brand Names: U.S. Aricept; Aricept ODT

Brand Names: Canada Accel-Donepezil; ACT-Donepezil; ACT-Donepezil ODT; Apo-Donepezil; Aricept; Aricept RDT; Auro-Donepezil; Bio-Donepezil; JAMP-Donepezil; Mar-Donepezil; Mylan-Donepezil; PMS-Donepezil; RAN-Donepezil; Riva-Donepezil; Sandoz-Donepezil; Sandoz-Donepezil ODT; Teva-Donepezil

Index Terms E2020

Pharmacologic Category Acetylcholinesterase Inhibitor (Central)

Use Treatment of mild, moderate, or severe dementia of the Alzheimer's type

Pregnancy Risk Factor C

Pregnancy Considerations Adverse events have been observed in some animal reproduction studies.

Breast-Feeding Considerations It is not known if donepezil is excreted in breast milk. The manufacturer recommends that caution be used if administered to a nursing woman.

Contraindications Hypersensitivity to donepezil, piperidine derivatives, or any component of the formulation

Warnings/Precautions Cholinesterase inhibitors may have vagotonic effects which may cause bradycardia and/or heart block with or without a history of cardiac disease; syncopal episodes have been associated with donepezil. Alzheimer's treatment guidelines consider bradycardia to be a relative contraindication for use of centrally-active cholinesterase inhibitors. Use with caution with sick sinus syndrome or other supraventricular cardiac conduction abnormalities, COPD, or asthma. Use with caution in patients with a history of seizure disorder; cholinomimetics may potentially cause generalized seizures, although seizure activity may also result from Alzheimer's disease. Use with caution in patients at risk of ulcer disease (eg, previous history or NSAID use), or in patients with bladder outlet obstruction. May cause dose-related diarrhea, nausea, and/or vomiting, which usually resolves in 1 to 3 weeks. May cause anorexia and/or weight loss (dose-related). Patients weighing <55 kg may experience more nausea, vomiting, and weight loss than patients ≥55 kg. May exaggerate neuromuscular blockade effects of depolarizing neuromuscular-blocking agents (eg, succinylcholine).

Rare cases of neuroleptic malignant syndrome (NMS) have been reported (Matsumoto 2004; Warwick 2008). Discontinuation of donepezil therapy may be necessary in patients presenting with symptoms of NMS or unexplained high fever without additional symptoms. Rare cases of rhabdomyolysis (including acute renal failure) have been reported after a few months of therapy (Sahin, 2014) or in the days following therapy initiation and dose increase (Aricept Canadian product monograph, 2014). Use with caution in patients with risk factors for rhabdomyolysis. Discontinuation of therapy may be necessary for marked elevation of CPK levels and/or symptoms (eg, muscle pain, tenderness or weakness, malaise, fever, dark urine) suggesting rhabdomyolysis. Potentially significant interactions may exist, requiring dose or frequency adjustment, additional monitoring, and/or selection of alternative therapy. Consult drug interactions database for more detailed information.

Adverse Reactions

Cardiovascular: Atrial fibrillation, bradycardia, chest pain, ECG abnormal, edema, heart failure hemorrhage, hot flashes, hyper-/hypotension, peripheral edema, syncope, vasodilation

Central nervous system: Abnormal crying, abnormal dreams, aggression, agitation, anxiety, aphasia, confusion, delusions, depression, dizziness, emotional lability, fatigue, fever, hallucinations, headache, hostility, insomnia, irritability, nervousness, pain, personality disorder, restlessness, seizure, somnolence, tremor, vertigo

Dermatologic: Bruising, eczema, pruritus, rash, skin ulcer, urticaria

Endocrine & metabolic: Dehydration, hyperlipemia, libido increased

Gastrointestinal: Abdominal pain, anorexia, bloating, constipation, diarrhea (dose related), dyspepsia, epigastric pain, fecal incontinence, gastroenteritis, GI bleeding, nausea (dose related), toothache, vomiting, weight loss

Genitourinary: Cystitis, hematuria, glycosuria, nocturia, urinary frequency, urinary incontinence, UTI

Hematologic: Anemia, contusion

Hepatic: Alkaline phosphatase increased

Neuromuscular & skeletal: Arthritis, ataxia, back pain, bone fracture, CPK increased, gait abnormal, lactate dehydrogenase increased, muscle cramps, paresthesia, weakness, tremor

Ocular: Blurred vision, cataract, eye irritation

Respiratory: Bronchitis, cough increased, dyspnea, pharyngitis, pneumonia, sore throat

Miscellaneous: Accident, diaphoresis, fungal infection, flu symptoms, infection, wandering

Rare but important or life-threatening: Abscess, angina, breast fibroadenosis, cardiomegaly, cellulitis, cerebrovascular accident, cholecystitis, conjunctival hemorrhage, conjunctivitis, deep vein thrombosis, diabetes mellitus, diverticulitis, eosinophilia, fibrocystic breast, gastrointestinal ulcer, glaucoma, goiter, heart block, heart failure, hemolytic anemia, hepatitis, hyperglycemia, hypertonia, hypokalemia, hypokinesia, hyponatremia, hypoxia, intracranial hemorrhage, jaundice, LFTs increased, MI, neuroleptic malignant syndrome, pancreatitis, pleurisy, pulmonary collapse, pulmonary congestion, pyelonephritis, renal failure, retinal hemorrhage, SVT, thrombocythemia, thrombocytopenia, tongue edema, transient ischemic attack

Drug Interactions

Metabolism/Transport Effects **Substrate** of CYP2D6 (minor), CYP3A4 (minor); **Note:** Assignment of Major/Minor substrate status based on clinically relevant drug interaction potential

Avoid Concomitant Use

Avoid concomitant use of Donepezil with any of the following: Ceritinib

Increased Effect/Toxicity

Donepezil may increase the levels/effects of: Antipsychotic Agents; Beta-Blockers; Bradycardia-Causing Agents; Ceritinib; Cholinergic Agonists; Lacosamide; Succinylcholine

The levels/effects of Donepezil may be increased by: Bretylium; Corticosteroids (Systemic); Tofacitinib

Decreased Effect

Donepezil may decrease the levels/effects of: Anticholinergic Agents; Neuromuscular-Blocking Agents (Nondepolarizing)

The levels/effects of Donepezil may be decreased by: Anticholinergic Agents; Dipyridamole

Storage/Stability Store at 15°C to 30°C (59°F to 86°F).

Mechanism of Action Alzheimer's disease is characterized by cholinergic deficiency in the cortex and basal forebrain, which contributes to cognitive deficits. Donepezil reversibly and noncompetitively inhibits centrally-active acetylcholinesterase, the enzyme responsible for hydrolysis of acetylcholine. This appears to result in increased concentrations of acetylcholine available for synaptic transmission in the central nervous system.

Pharmacodynamics/Kinetics

Absorption: Well absorbed

Distribution: V_{dss}: 12-16 L/kg

Protein binding: 96%, primarily to albumin (75%) and α_1-acid glycoprotein (21%)

Metabolism: Extensively to four major metabolites (two are active) via CYP2D6 and 3A4; undergoes glucuronidation

Bioavailability: 100%

Half-life elimination: 70 hours; time to steady-state: 15 days

Time to peak, plasma: Tablet, 10 mg: 3 hours; Tablet, 23 mg: ~8 hours; **Note:** Peak plasma concentrations almost twofold higher for the 23 mg tablet compared to the 10 mg tablet

Excretion: Urine 57% (17% as unchanged drug); feces 15%

Dosage Oral:

Adults: Alzheimer's dementia:

Mild-to-moderate: Initial: 5 mg once daily; may increase to 10 mg once daily after 4-6 weeks; effective dosage range in clinical studies: 5-10 mg/day

Moderate-to-severe: Initial: 5 mg once daily; may increase to 10 mg once daily after 4-6 weeks; may increase further to 23 mg once daily after ≥3 months; effective dosage range in clinical studies: 10-23 mg/day

Elderly: Refer to adult dosing. **Note:** The Canadian labeling recommends a maximum dose of 5 mg once daily in elderly women of low body weight.

Dosage adjustment in renal impairment: No adjustment provided in manufacturer's labeling. Limited data suggest severe renal impairment does not adversely affect donepezil clearance.

Dosage adjustment in hepatic impairment: No adjustment provided in manufacturer's labeling.

Dietary Considerations May take with or without food.

Administration Administer at bedtime without regard to food.

Aricept® 5 mg or 10 mg tablet: Swallow whole with water.

Aricept® 23 mg tablet: Swallow whole with water; do **NOT** crush or chew due to an increased rate of absorption. The 23 mg strength is provided in a unique film-coated formulation different from the 5 mg or 10 mg tablet strengths, which results in an altered pharmacokinetic profile.

Aricept® ODT: Allow tablet to dissolve completely on tongue and follow with water.

Monitoring Parameters Behavior, mood, bowel function, cognitive function, general function (eg, activities of daily living)

Dosage Forms

Tablet, Oral:

Aricept: 5 mg, 10 mg, 23 mg

Generic: 5 mg, 10 mg, 23 mg

Tablet Dispersible, Oral:

Aricept ODT: 10 mg

Generic: 5 mg, 10 mg

- **Donnatal®** *see* Hyoscyamine, Atropine, Scopolamine, and Phenobarbital *on page 1027*

- **Donnatal Extentabs®** *see* Hyoscyamine, Atropine, Scopolamine, and Phenobarbital *on page 1027*

DOPamine (DOE pa meen)

Index Terms Dopamine Hydrochloride; Intropin

Pharmacologic Category Adrenergic Agonist Agent; Inotrope

Use Adjunct in the treatment of shock (eg, MI, open heart surgery, renal failure, cardiac decompensation) which persists after adequate fluid volume replacement

American College of Cardiology/American Heart Association heart failure (HF) guideline recommendations (ACCF/AHA [Yancy, 2013]): To maintain systemic perfusion and preserve end-organ performance in patients with cardiogenic shock; bridge therapy in stage D HF unresponsive to guideline-directed medical therapy and device therapy in patients awaiting heart transplant or mechanical circulatory support; short-term management of hospitalized patients with severe systolic dysfunction presenting with low blood pressure and significantly depressed cardiac output; long-term management (palliative therapy) in select patients with stage D HF unresponsive to guideline-directed medical therapy and device therapy who are not candidates for heart transplant or mechanical circulatory support.

Pregnancy Risk Factor C

Pregnancy Considerations Adverse events have been observed in some animal reproduction studies. It is not known if dopamine crosses the placenta.

Breast-Feeding Considerations It is not known if dopamine is excreted in breast milk. The manufacturer recommends that caution be exercised when administering dopamine to nursing women.

Contraindications Hypersensitivity to sulfites (commercial preparation contains sodium bisulfite); pheochromocytoma; ventricular fibrillation

Warnings/Precautions Use with caution in patients with cardiovascular disease or cardiac arrhythmias or patients with occlusive vascular disease. Correct hypovolemia and electrolytes when used in hemodynamic support. May cause increases in HR increasing the risk of tachycardia and other tachyarrhythmia. Use with caution in patients with recent myocardial infarction; may increase myocardial oxygen consumption. Use has been associated with a higher incidence of adverse events (eg, tachyarrhythmias) in adult patients with shock compared to norepinephrine. Higher 28-day mortality was also seen in patients with septic shock; the use of norepinephrine in patients with shock may be preferred. The 2012 Surviving Sepsis Campaign (SSC) guidelines suggest dopamine use as an alternative to norepinephrine only in patients with low risk of tachyarrhythmias and absolute or relative bradycardia (SCCM [Dellinger, 2013]). Use with extreme caution in patients taking MAO inhibitors.

Vesicant; ensure proper needle or catheter placement prior to and during infusion. Avoid extravasation; infuse into a large vein if possible. Avoid infusion into leg veins. Watch IV site closely. **[U.S. Boxed Warning]: If extravasation occurs, infiltrate the area with diluted phentolamine (5 to 10 mg in 10 to 15 mL of saline) with a fine hypodermic needle. Phentolamine should be administered as soon as possible after extravasation is noted to prevent sloughing/necrosis.** Product may contain sodium metabisulfite.

Adverse Reactions

Cardiovascular: Angina pectoris, atrial fibrillation, bradycardia, ectopic beats, hypertension, hypotension, palpitations, tachycardia, vasoconstriction, ventricular arrhythmia, ventricular conduction, widened QRS complex on ECG

Central nervous system: Anxiety, headache

Dermatologic: Gangrene (high dose), piloerection

Endocrine & metabolic: Increased serum glucose (usually not above normal limits)

Gastrointestinal: Nausea, vomiting

Genitourinary: Azotemia

Ophthalmic: Increased intraocular pressure, mydriasis

Renal: Polyuria

Respiratory: Dyspnea

Miscellaneous: Tissue necrosis

Drug Interactions

Metabolism/Transport Effects Substrate of COMT, OCT2

Avoid Concomitant Use

Avoid concomitant use of DOPamine with any of the following: Ergot Derivatives; Inhalational Anesthetics; Iobenguane I 123; Lurasidone

Increased Effect/Toxicity

DOPamine may increase the levels/effects of: Lurasidone; Sympathomimetics

The levels/effects of DOPamine may be increased by: AtoMOXetine; Beta-Blockers; BuPROPion; Cannabinoid-Containing Products; COMT Inhibitors; Ergot Derivatives; Hyaluronidase; Inhalational Anesthetics; Linezolid; Serotonin/Norepinephrine Reuptake Inhibitors; Tedizolid; Tricyclic Antidepressants

Decreased Effect

DOPamine may decrease the levels/effects of: Benzylpenicilloyl Polylysine; Iobenguane I 123

The levels/effects of DOPamine may be decreased by: Alpha1-Blockers; Spironolactone

Storage/Stability Protect from light. Solutions that are darker than slightly yellow should not be used.

Mechanism of Action Stimulates both adrenergic and dopaminergic receptors, lower doses are mainly dopaminergic stimulating and produce renal and mesenteric vasodilation, higher doses also are both dopaminergic and beta$_1$-adrenergic stimulating and produce cardiac stimulation and renal vasodilation; large doses stimulate alpha-adrenergic receptors

Pharmacodynamics/Kinetics

Children: Dopamine has exhibited nonlinear kinetics in children; with dose changes, may not achieve steady-state for ~1 hour rather than 20 minutes

Onset of action: Adults: Within 5 minutes

Duration: Adults: <10 minutes

Metabolism: Renal, hepatic, plasma; 75% to inactive metabolites by monoamine oxidase and 25% to norepinephrine

Half-life elimination: ~2 minutes

Excretion: Urine (as metabolites)

Clearance: Neonates: Varies and appears to be age related; clearance is more prolonged with combined hepatic and renal dysfunction

Dosage IV infusion:

Hemodynamic support:

Children: 1-20 mcg/kg/minute, maximum: 50 mcg/kg/minute continuous infusion, titrate to desired response.

Pediatric Advanced Life Support (PALS) guideline recommendation (to maintain cardiac output and for postresuscitation stabilization): IV or I.O.: Dose range: 2-20 mcg/kg/minute (AHA [Kleinman, 2010])

Adults: 1-5 mcg/kg/minute up to 20 mcg/kg/minute, titrate to desired response (maximum: 50 mcg/kg/minute; however, doses >20 mcg/kg/minute may not have a beneficial effect on blood pressure and increase the risk of tachyarrhythmias). Infusion may be increased by 1-4 mcg/kg/minute at 10- to 30-minute intervals until optimal response is obtained.

ACLS guideline recommendations (to treat hypotension especially if associated with symptomatic bradycardia in the immediate post-cardiac arrest care setting): Initial: 5-10 mcg/kg/minute; titrate to effect (AHA [Peberdy, 2010])

Note: If dosages >20-30 mcg/kg/minute are needed, a more direct-acting pressor may be more beneficial (ie, epinephrine, norepinephrine).

The hemodynamic effects of dopamine are dose dependent (however, this is relative and there is overlap of clinical effects between dosing ranges):

Low-dose: 1-3 mcg/kg/minute, increased renal blood flow and urine output

Intermediate-dose: 3-10 mcg/kg/minute, increased renal blood flow, heart rate, cardiac contractility, and cardiac output

High-dose: >10 mcg/kg/minute, alpha-adrenergic effects begin to predominate, vasoconstriction, increased blood pressure

Inotropic support in advanced heart failure: Adults: IV infusion: 5-15 mcg/kg/minute; lower doses are preferred (ACCF/AHA [Yancy, 2013]).

Usual Infusion Concentrations: Pediatric Note: Premixed solutions available.

IV infusion: 1600 **mcg**/mL **or** 3200 **mcg**/mL

Usual Infusion Concentrations: Adult Note: Premixed solutions available.

IV infusion: 400 mg in 250 mL (concentration: 1600 **mcg**/mL) **or** 800 mg in 250 mL (concentration: 3200 **mcg**/mL) of D_5W or NS

Administration Administer as a continuous infusion with the use of an infusion pump. Administer into large vein to prevent the possibility of extravasation (central line administration); monitor continuously for free flow; use infusion device to control rate of flow; administration into an umbilical arterial catheter is not recommended; when discontinuing the infusion, gradually decrease the dose of dopamine (sudden discontinuation may cause hypotension). Vials (concentrated solution) must be diluted prior to use.

Vesicant; ensure proper needle or catheter placement prior to and during infusion; avoid extravasation.

Extravasation management: If extravasation occurs, stop infusion immediately and disconnect (leave cannula/needle in place); gently aspirate extravasated solution (do **NOT** flush the line); remove needle/cannula; elevate extremity. Initiate phentolamine (or alternative) antidote. Apply dry warm compresses (Hurst, 2004).

Phentolamine: Dilute 5-10 mg in 10-15 mL NS and administer into extravasation site as soon as possible after extravasation (AHA [Peberdy, 2010])

Alternatives to phentolamine:

Nitroglycerin topical 2% ointment (based on limited case reports in neonates/infants): Apply 4 mm/kg as a thin ribbon to the affected areas; may repeat after 8 hours if needed (Wong, 1992) **or** apply a 1-inch strip on the affected site (Denkler, 1989)

Terbutaline (based on limited case reports): Infiltrate extravasation area using a solution of terbutaline 1 mg diluted to 10 mL in NS (large extravasation site; administration volume varied from 3-10 mL) **or** 1 mg diluted in 1 mL NS (small/distal extravasation site; administration volume varied from 0.5-1 mL) (Stier, 1999)

Monitoring Parameters Blood pressure, ECG, heart rate, CVP, RAP, MAP; serum glucose, renal function; urine output; if pulmonary artery catheter is in place, monitor CI, PCWP, SVR, and PVR

Consult individual institutional policies and procedures.

Additional Information Dopamine is most frequently used for treatment of hypotension because of its peripheral vasoconstrictor action. In this regard, dopamine is often used together with dobutamine and minimizes hypotension secondary to dobutamine-induced vasodilation. Thus, pressure is maintained by increased cardiac output (from dobutamine) and vasoconstriction (by dopamine). It is critical neither dopamine nor dobutamine be used in patients in the absence of correcting any hypovolemia as a cause of hypotension.

Low-dose dopamine is often used in the intensive care setting for presumed beneficial effects on renal function. However, there is no clear evidence that low-dose dopamine confers any renal or other benefit. Indeed, dopamine may act on dopamine receptors in the carotid bodies causing chemoreflex suppression. In patients with heart failure, dopamine may inhibit breathing and cause pulmonary shunting. Both these mechanisms would act to decrease minute ventilation and oxygen saturation. This could potentially be deleterious in patients with respiratory compromise and patients being weaned from ventilators.

Dosage Forms

Solution, Intravenous:

Generic: 0.8 mg/mL (250 mL, 500 mL); 1.6 mg/mL (250 mL, 500 mL); 3.2 mg/mL (250 mL); 40 mg/mL (5 mL, 10 mL); 80 mg/mL (5 mL); 160 mg/mL (5 mL)

◆ **Dopamine Hydrochloride** *see* DOPamine *on page 669*

Dopexamine [INT] (doe PEKS a meen)

International Brand Names Dopacard (CH, DE, DK, FR, GB, IE, NL, SE)

Index Terms Dopexamine Hydrochloride

Pharmacologic Category Sympathomimetic

Reported Use Inotropic support and vasodilator therapy in exacerbations of heart failure

Dosage Range Adults: IV: 0.5 mcg/kg/minute, may be increased to 1 mcg/kg/minute and further increased up to 6 mcg/kg/minute in increments of 0.5-1 mcg/kg/minute at intervals of not less than 15 minutes

Product Availability Product available in various countries; not currently available in the U.S.

Dosage Forms

Injection, solution: 10 mg/mL (5 mL)

◆ **Dopexamine Hydrochloride** *see* Dopexamine [INT] *on page 671*

◆ **Dopram** *see* Doxapram *on page 673*

◆ **Doral** *see* Quazepam *on page 1751*

◆ **Doribax** *see* Doripenem *on page 671*

Doripenem (dore i PEN em)

Brand Names: U.S. Doribax

Index Terms S-4661

Pharmacologic Category Antibiotic, Carbapenem

Use Treatment of complicated intra-abdominal infections and complicated urinary tract infections (including pyelonephritis) due to susceptible aerobic gram-positive, aerobic gram-negative (including *Pseudomonas aeruginosa*), and anaerobic bacteria

Pregnancy Risk Factor B

Pregnancy Considerations Adverse events have not been observed in animal reproduction studies. Information related to use during pregnancy has not been located.

Breast-Feeding Considerations It is not known if doripenem is excreted into breast milk. The manufacturer recommends that caution be exercised when administering doripenem to nursing women.

Contraindications Known serious hypersensitivity to doripenem or other carbapenems (eg, ertapenem, imipenem, meropenem) or any component of the formulation; anaphylactic reactions to beta-lactam antibiotics

Warnings/Precautions Serious hypersensitivity reactions, including anaphylaxis, and skin reactions have been reported in patients receiving beta-lactams. Use may result in fungal or bacterial superinfection, including *C. difficile*-associated diarrhea (CDAD) and pseudomembranous colitis; CDAD has been observed >2 months postantibiotic treatment. Not indicated for the treatment of pneumonia including ventilator-associated pneumonia; decreased efficacy and increased mortality observed in a phase 3 study using a higher dose and fixed 7-day administration (Kollef, 2012). Use with caution in patients with renal impairment; dosage adjustment required in patients with moderate-to-severe renal dysfunction. Carbapenems have been associated with CNS adverse effects, including confusional states and seizures (myoclonic); use caution with CNS disorders (eg, brain lesions, stroke, or history of seizures) and adjust dose in renal impairment to avoid drug accumulation, which may increase seizure risk. Patients receiving doses >500 mg every 8 hours may also be at increased risk of seizures. Potentially significant interactions may exist, requiring dose or frequency adjustment, additional monitoring, and/or selection of alternative therapy. Administer via intravenous infusion only. Per manufacturer's labeling, investigational experience of doripenem via inhalation resulted in pneumonitis.

Adverse Reactions

Cardiovascular: Phlebitis

Central nervous system: Headache

Dermatologic: Pruritus, skin rash (includes allergic/bullous dermatitis, erythema, macular/papular eruptions, urticaria, and erythema multiforme)

Gastrointestinal: Diarrhea, nausea, oral candidiasis, pseudomembranous colitis

Hematologic & oncologic: Anemia

Hepatic: Increased serum transaminases

Renal: Renal insufficiency

Miscellaneous: Vaginal infection

Rare but important or life-threatening: Anaphylaxis, leukopenia, neutropenia, pneumonia, seizure, Stevens-Johnson syndrome, thrombocytopenia, toxic epidermal necrolysis

Drug Interactions

Metabolism/Transport Effects None known.

Avoid Concomitant Use

Avoid concomitant use of Doripenem with any of the following: BCG; Probenecid

Increased Effect/Toxicity

The levels/effects of Doripenem may be increased by: Probenecid

Decreased Effect

Doripenem may decrease the levels/effects of: BCG; Sodium Picosulfate; Typhoid Vaccine; Valproic Acid and Derivatives

Preparation for Administration Reconstitute 250 mg vial with 10 mL of SWFI or NS; further dilute for infusion with 50 mL or 100 mL of NS or D_5W. Shake gently until clear. Reconstitute 500 mg vial with 10 mL of SWFI or NS; further dilute for infusion with 100 mL of NS or D_5W. Shake gently until clear. Reconstituted vial may be stored for up to 1 hour prior to preparation of infusion solution. To prepare a 250 mg dose using a 500 mg vial, reconstitute the 500 mg vial with 10 mL of SWFI or NS and further dilute with 100 mL of compatible solution as above, but remove and discard 55 mL from the infusion bag to leave the remaining solution containing the 250 mg dose.

Storage/Stability Store dry powder vials at 15°C to 30°C (59°F to 86°F). Stability of solution when diluted in NS is 12 hours at room temperature or 72 hours under refrigeration; stability in D_5W is 4 hours at room temperature and 24 hours under refrigeration.

Mechanism of Action Inhibits bacterial cell wall synthesis by binding to several of the penicillin-binding proteins (PBP-2, PBP-3, PBP-4), which in turn inhibits the final transpeptidation step of peptidoglycan synthesis in bacterial cell walls, thus inhibiting cell wall biosynthesis; bacteria eventually lyse due to ongoing activity of cell wall autolytic enzymes (autolysins and murein hydrolases) while cell wall assembly is arrested.

Pharmacodynamics/Kinetics Note: As with other time-dependent antibiotics, doripenem shows bacteriostatic effects at T>MIC <40% and bactericidal effects at T>MIC>40%. Of note, prolonged infusion time (over 4 hours) was more effective in increasing T>MIC over 40% to up to 81%. Pharmacokinetics are linear (AUC directly proportional to dose) at doses administered over 1 hour.

Distribution: Penetrates well into body fluids and tissues, including peritoneal and retroperitoneal fluids, gallbladder, bile, and urine

V_d: 16.8 L

Protein binding: 8% to 9%

Metabolism: Non-CYP-mediated metabolism via hydrolysis by dehydropeptidase-I to doripenem-M1 (inactive metabolite)

Half-life elimination: ~1 hour

Excretion: Urine (71% as unchanged drug; 15% as doripenem-M1 metabolite); feces (<1%)

Dialyzable with reduction in systemic levels by 48% to 62%.

Dosage Note: A switch to appropriate oral antimicrobial therapy may be considered after 3 days of parenteral therapy and demonstrated clinical improvement.

Usual dosage: Adults: IV: 500 mg every 8 hours

Indication-specific dosing: Adults: IV:

Intra-abdominal infection, complicated, severe: 500 mg every 8 hours for 5-14 days. **Note:** 2010 IDSA guidelines recommend treatment duration of 4-7 days (provided source controlled). Not recommended for mild-to-moderate, community-acquired intra-abdominal infections due to risk of toxicity and the development of resistant organisms (Solomkin, 2010).

Urinary tract infection (complicated) or pyelonephritis: 500 mg every 8 hours for 10-14 days

Intravenous catheter-related bloodstream infection (off-label use): 500 mg every 8 hours for 7-14 days (IDSA, 2009)

Dosage adjustment in renal impairment:

CrCl >50 mL/minute: No adjustment necessary

CrCl 30-50 mL/minute: 250 mg every 8 hours

CrCl 11-29 mL/minute: 250 mg every 12 hours

Hemodialysis: Dialyzable (~52% of dose removed during 4-hour session in ESRD patients)

Intermittent HD: 250 mg every 24 hours; if treating infections caused by ***Pseudomonas aeruginosa***, administer 500 mg every 12 hours on day 1, followed by 500 mg every 24 hours (Tanoue, 2011)

CVVHDF: 250 mg every 12 hours (Hidaka, 2010).

Dosage adjustment in hepatic impairment: There are no dosage adjustments provided in manufacturer's labeling (has not been studied). However, doripenem undergoes minimal hepatic metabolism.

Administration Infuse intravenously over 1 hour. Use of 4-hour infusion has been studied in the treatment of VAP (off-label use) (Chastre, 2008).

Monitoring Parameters Monitor for signs of anaphylaxis during first dose; periodic renal assessment; consider hematologic monitoring during prolonged therapy

Additional Information One mechanism of resistance to doripenem is production of the Ambler's class B metallo-beta-lactamase, a potent carbapenemase produced by *Stenotrophomonas maltophilia*.

Dosage Forms

Solution Reconstituted, Intravenous:

Doribax: 250 mg (1 ea); 500 mg (1 ea)

Dornase Alfa (DOOR nase AL fa)

Brand Names: U.S. Pulmozyme

Brand Names: Canada Pulmozyme

Index Terms Recombinant Human Deoxyribonuclease; rhDNase

Pharmacologic Category Enzyme; Mucolytic Agent

Use Cystic fibrosis: Management of cystic fibrosis patients, in conjunction with standard therapies, to improve pulmonary function; reduce the risk of respiratory tract infections requiring parenteral antibiotics in patients with a forced vital capacity (FVC) ≥40% of predicted.

Dosage

Inhalation: Cystic fibrosis:

Infants and Children ≤5 years: Not approved for use; however, studies using this therapy in small numbers of children as young as 3 months of age have reported efficacy and similar side effects.

Children >5 years and Adults: 2.5 mg daily through selected jet nebulizers in conjunction with a Pulmo-Aide, Pari-Proneb, Mobilaire, or Porta-Neb compressor system or eRapid Nebulizer System

Patients unable to inhale or exhale orally throughout the entire treatment period may use Pari-Baby nebulizer. Some patients may benefit from twice daily administration.

Intrapleural: Complicated parapneumonic effusion (off-label use): Adults: 5 mg (diluted in 30 mL sterile water) administered twice daily >2 hours after intrapleural alteplase administration (Rahman, 2011)

Dosage adjustment in renal impairment: There are no dosage adjustment provided in manufacturer's labeling.

Dosage adjustment in hepatic impairment: There are no dosage adjustment provided in manufacturer's labeling.

Additional Information Complete prescribing information should be consulted for additional detail.

Dosage Forms

Solution, Inhalation:

Pulmozyme: 1 mg/mL (2.5 mL)

- **Doryx** *see* Doxycycline *on page 689*

Dorzolamide (dor ZOLE a mide)

Brand Names: U.S. Trusopt

Brand Names: Canada Sandoz-Dorzolamide; Trusopt®

Index Terms Dorzolamide Hydrochloride

Pharmacologic Category Carbonic Anhydrase Inhibitor (Ophthalmic); Ophthalmic Agent, Antiglaucoma

Use Treatment of elevated intraocular pressure in patients with ocular hypertension or open-angle glaucoma

Pregnancy Risk Factor C

Dosage Children and Adults: Reduction of intraocular pressure: Instill 1 drop in the affected eye(s) 3 times/day

Dosage adjustment in renal impairment: CrCl <30 mL/minute: Use is not recommended (has not been studied).

Dosage adjustment in hepatic impairment: No dosage adjustment provided in manufacturer's labeling (has not been studied); use with caution.

Additional Information Complete prescribing information should be consulted for additional detail.

Dosage Forms

Solution, Ophthalmic:

Trusopt: 2% (10 mL)

Generic: 2% (10 mL)

Dosage Forms: Canada

Solution, ophthalmic [drops; preservative free]:

Trusopt®: 2% (0.2 mL)

Dorzolamide and Timolol
(dor ZOLE a mide & TYE moe lole)

Brand Names: U.S. Cosopt®; Cosopt® PF

Brand Names: Canada Apo-Dorzo-Timop; Cosopt®; Cosopt® Preservative Free; Sandoz-Dorzolamide/Timolol

Index Terms Cosopt® PF; Timolol and Dorzolamide

Pharmacologic Category Beta-Adrenergic Blocker, Nonselective; Carbonic Anhydrase Inhibitor (Ophthalmic); Ophthalmic Agent, Antiglaucoma

Use Treatment of elevated intraocular pressure in patients with ocular hypertension or open-angle glaucoma

Pregnancy Risk Factor C

Dosage Ophthalmic: Children ≥2 years and Adults: Instill 1 drop in affected eye(s) twice daily

Dosage adjustment in renal impairment: CrCl <30 mL/minute: Use is not recommended (has not been studied).

Dosage adjustment in hepatic impairment: No dosage adjustment provided in manufacturer's labeling (has not been studied): use with caution.

Additional Information Complete prescribing information should be consulted for additional detail.

Dosage Forms Considerations

Ophthalmic solution contains dorzolamide hydrochloride 2.23% [22.3 mg/mL] and timolol maleate 0.68% [6.8 mg/mL]

Dosage Forms

Solution, ophthalmic [drops]: Dorzolamide 2% [20 mg/mL] and timolol 0.5% [5 mg/mL] (10 mL)

Cosopt®: Dorzolamide 2% [20 mg/mL] and timolol 0.5% [5 mg/mL] (10 mL)

Solution, ophthalmic [drops, preservative free]:

Cosopt® PF: Dorzolamide 2% [20 mg/mL] and timolol 0.5% [5 mg/mL] (0.2 mL)

- **Dorzolamide Hydrochloride** *see* Dorzolamide *on page 673*
- **D.O.S. [OTC]** *see* Docusate *on page 661*
- **Dosolax [OTC] (Can)** *see* Docusate *on page 661*
- **DOSS** *see* Docusate *on page 661*
- **Dostinex (Can)** *see* Cabergoline *on page 319*

Dosulepin [INT] (doe SUL e pin)

International Brand Names Depropin (MY); Dopin (TH); Dopress (NZ); Dothapax (GB); Dothcin (IN); Dothep (AU, IE, MY); Dothip (IN); Espin (SG); Idom (DE); Prepadine (GB); Prothiaden (AU, BE, BH, CZ, DK, EG, ES, FR, GB, HK, IE, IN, KR, MY, NL, NZ, PK, QA, SA, SG, SK, TH, VN, ZA); Protiaden (CH, IT); Protiadene (PT); Qualiaden (HK); Thaden (ZA); Vick-Thiaden (HK); Xerenal (AT)

Index Terms Dosulepin Hydrochloride; Dosulepine; Dothiepin; Dothiepin Hydrochloride

Pharmacologic Category Antidepressant, Tricyclic

Reported Use For acute and maintenance treatment of depression

Dosage Range Adults: Oral: Depression: 75-225 mg in 1-3 divided doses (maximum single dose: 150 mg)

Dosage adjustment in elderly patients: Initial dose: 50-75 mg/day; maintenance dose: $^1/_2$ the normal dose may be adequate

Product Availability Product available in various countries; not currently available in the U.S.

Dosage Forms

Capsule, Oral, as hydrochloride: 25 mg

Tablet, Oral, as hydrochloride: 75 mg

- **Dosulepine** *see* Dosulepin [INT] *on page 673*
- **Dosulepin Hydrochloride** *see* Dosulepin [INT] *on page 673*
- **Dothiepin** *see* Dosulepin [INT] *on page 673*
- **Dothiepin Hydrochloride** *see* Dosulepin [INT] *on page 673*
- **DoubleDex** *see* Dexamethasone (Systemic) *on page 599*
- **Double Tussin DM [OTC]** *see* Guaifenesin and Dextromethorphan *on page 987*
- **Dovobet (Can)** *see* Calcipotriene and Betamethasone *on page 321*
- **Dovonex** *see* Calcipotriene *on page 321*

Doxapram (DOKS a pram)

Brand Names: U.S. Dopram

Index Terms Doxapram Hydrochloride

Pharmacologic Category Respiratory Stimulant

Use Respiratory stimulant for respiratory depression secondary to anesthesia, mild-to-moderate drug-induced respiratory and CNS depression; acute hypercapnia secondary to COPD

Note: In general, the use of doxapram as a respiratory stimulant in adults is limited; alternate therapies are preferred.

Pregnancy Risk Factor B

Dosage Note: Although manufacturer's dosing recommendations are presented for these FDA-approved indications, use of doxapram has largely been replaced by alternate preferred agents.

Respiratory depression following anesthesia: Children ≥12 years, Adolescents, and Adults: IV:

Intermittent injection: Initial: 0.5-1 mg/kg; may repeat at 5-minute intervals (only in patients who demonstrate initial response); maximum total dose: 2 mg/kg

IV infusion: Initial: 5 mg/minute until adequate response or adverse effects seen; decrease to 1-3 mg/minute; maximum total dose: 4 mg/kg

Drug-induced CNS depression: Children ≥12 years, Adolescents, and Adults:

Intermittent injection: Initial: Priming dose of 1-2 mg/kg, repeat after 5 minutes; may repeat at 1-2 hour intervals (until sustained consciousness); maximum: 3000 mg daily. May repeat in 24 hours if necessary.

IV infusion: Initial: Priming dose of 1-2 mg/kg, repeat after 5 minutes. If no response, wait 1-2 hours and repeat priming dose. If some stimulation is noted, initiate infusion at 1-3 mg/minute (depending on size of patient/depth of CNS depression); suspend infusion if patient begins to awaken. Infusion should not be continued for >2 hours. May reinstitute infusion as described above, including bolus, after rest interval of 30 minutes to 2 hours; maximum: 3000 mg daily.

Acute hypercapnia secondary to COPD: Children ≥12 years, Adolescents, and Adults: IV infusion: Initial: Initiate infusion at 1-2 mg/minute (depending on size of patient/depth of CNS depression); may increase to maximum rate of 3 mg/minute; infusion should not be continued for >2 hours. Monitor arterial blood gases prior to initiation of infusion and at 30-minute intervals during the infusion (to identify possible development of acidosis/CO_2 retention). Additional infusions are not recommended (per manufacturer).

Dosage adjustment in renal impairment: No dosage adjustment provided in manufacturer's labeling (has not been studied); however, use caution in severe impairment due to the potential for altered pharmacokinetics.

Dosage adjustment in hepatic impairment: No dosage adjustment provided in manufacturer's labeling (has not been studied); however, use caution in severe impairment due to the potential for altered pharmacokinetics.

Additional Information Complete prescribing information should be consulted for additional detail.

Dosage Forms

Solution, Intravenous:

Dopram: 20 mg/mL (20 mL)

Generic: 20 mg/mL (20 mL)

◆ **Doxapram Hydrochloride** *see* Doxapram *on page 673*

Doxazosin (doks AY zoe sin)

Brand Names: U.S. Cardura; Cardura XL

Brand Names: Canada Apo-Doxazosin; Cardura-1; Cardura-2; Cardura-4; Dom-Doxazosin; Doxazosin-1; Doxazosin-2; Doxazosin-4; Mylan-Doxazosin; PMS-Doxazosin; Teva-Doxazosin

Index Terms Doxazosin Mesylate

Pharmacologic Category Alpha$_1$ Blocker; Antihypertensive

Additional Appendix Information

Beers Criteria - Potentially Inappropriate Medications for Geriatrics *on page 2271*

Use

Immediate release formulation: Treatment of hypertension as monotherapy or in conjunction with diuretics, ACE inhibitors, beta-blockers, or calcium antagonists; treatment of urinary outflow obstruction and/or obstructive and irritative symptoms associated with benign prostatic hyperplasia (BPH)

Note: The 2014 guideline for the management of high blood pressure in adults (Eighth Joint National Committee [JNC 8]) does **not** recommend the use of doxazosin in the treatment of hypertension (JNC8 [James, 2013]).

Extended release formulation: Treatment of urinary outflow obstruction and/or obstructive and irritative symptoms associated with BPH

Pregnancy Risk Factor C

Pregnancy Considerations Adverse events were observed in some animal reproduction studies. Untreated chronic maternal hypertension is associated with adverse events in the fetus, infant, and mother. If treatment for hypertension during pregnancy is needed, other agents are generally preferred (ACOG, 2013).

Breast-Feeding Considerations Doxazosin is excreted into breast milk. Information is available from a single case report following a maternal dose of doxazosin 4 mg every 24 hours for 2 doses. Milk samples were obtained at various intervals over 24 hours, beginning ~17 hours after the first dose. Maternal serum samples were obtained at nearly the same times, beginning ~1 hour later. The highest serum and milk concentrations of doxazosin were observed ~1 hour after the dose. Using the highest milk concentration (4.15 mcg/L), the estimated dose to the nursing infant was calculated to be <1% of the weight-adjusted maternal dose (Jensen, 2013). The manufacturer recommends that caution be used if administered to nursing women.

Contraindications Hypersensitivity to quinazolines (prazosin, terazosin), doxazosin, or any component of the formulation

Warnings/Precautions Can cause significant orthostatic hypotension and syncope, especially with first dose; anticipate a similar effect if therapy is interrupted for a few days, if dosage is rapidly increased, or if another antihypertensive drug (particularly vasodilators) or a PDE-5 inhibitor is introduced. Discontinue if symptoms of angina occur or worsen. Patients should be cautioned about performing hazardous tasks when starting new therapy or adjusting dosage upward. Priapism has been associated with use (rarely). Prostate cancer should be ruled out before starting for BPH. Use with caution in mild-to-moderate hepatic impairment; not recommended in severe dysfunction. Intraoperative floppy iris syndrome has been observed in cataract surgery patients who were on or were previously treated with alpha$_1$-blockers. Causality has not been established and there appears to be no benefit in discontinuing alpha-blocker therapy prior to surgery. In the elderly, avoid use as an antihypertensive due to high risk of orthostatic hypotension; alternative agents preferred due to a more favorable risk/benefit profile (Beers Criteria).

The extended release formulation consists of drug within a nondeformable matrix; following drug release/absorption, the matrix/shell is expelled in the stool. The use of nondeformable products in patients with known stricture/narrowing of the GI tract has been associated with symptoms of obstruction. Use caution in patients with increased GI retention (eg, chronic constipation) as doxazosin exposure may be increased. Extended release formulation is not indicated for use in women or for the treatment of hypertension.

Adverse Reactions

Cardiovascular: Arrhythmia, edema, facial edema, flushing, hypotension, orthostatic hypotension

Central nervous system: Anxiety, ataxia, dizziness, fatigue, headache, hypertonia, insomnia, malaise, movement disorder, pain, somnolence, vertigo

Endocrine & metabolic: Sexual dysfunction

Gastrointestinal: Abdominal pain, dyspepsia, nausea, xerostomia

Genitourinary: Impotence, incontinence, polyuria, urinary tract infection

Neuromuscular & skeletal: Arthritis,muscle cramps, muscle weakness, myalgia

Ocular: Abnormal vision

Otic: Tinnitus

Respiratory: Dyspnea, epistaxis, respiratory disorder, rhinitis

Rare but important or life-threatening: Abnormal lacrimation, abnormal thinking, agitation, allergic reaction, alopecia, amnesia, angina, anorexia, appetite increased, arthralgia, back pain, blurred vision, bradycardia, breast pain, bronchospasm, cerebrovascular accident, chest pain, cholestasis, confusion, cough, depersonalization, diaphoresis increased, diarrhea, dry skin, dysuria, earache, eczema, emotional lability, fecal incontinence, fever, gastroenteritis, gout, gynecomastia, hematuria, hepatitis, hot flashes, hypoesthesia, hypokalemia, impaired concentration, impotence, infection, influenza-like syndrome, intraoperative floppy iris syndrome (cataract surgery), jaundice, leukopenia, liver function tests increased, libido decreased, lymphadenopathy, micturition abnormality, migraine, MI, neutropenia, nocturia, pallor, palpitation, paranoia, paresis, parosmia, peripheral ischemia, pharyngitis, photophobia, priapism, pruritus, purpura, renal calculus, rigors, sinusitis, skin rash, syncope, taste perversion, thirst, thrombocytopenia, tremor, twitching, urticaria, vomiting, weight gain/loss

Drug Interactions

Metabolism/Transport Effects Substrate of CYP2C19 (minor), CYP2D6 (minor), CYP3A4 (major); **Note:** Assignment of Major/Minor substrate status based on clinically relevant drug interaction potential

Avoid Concomitant Use

Avoid concomitant use of Doxazosin with any of the following: Alpha1-Blockers; Boceprevir; Conivaptan; Fusidic Acid (Systemic); Idelalisib

Increased Effect/Toxicity

Doxazosin may increase the levels/effects of: Alpha1-Blockers; Amifostine; Antihypertensives; Calcium Channel Blockers; DULoxetine; Hypotensive Agents; Levodopa; Obinutuzumab; RisperiDONE; RiTUXimab

The levels/effects of Doxazosin may be increased by: Aprepitant; Barbiturates; Beta-Blockers; Boceprevir; Brimonidine (Topical); Ceritinib; Conivaptan; CYP3A4 Inhibitors (Moderate); CYP3A4 Inhibitors (Strong); Dapoxetine; Dasatinib; Diazoxide; Fosaprepitant; Fusidic Acid (Systemic); Herbs (Hypotensive Properties); Idelalisib; Ivacaftor; Luliconazole; MAO Inhibitors; Mifepristone; Netupitant; Nicorandil; Pentoxifylline; Phosphodiesterase 5 Inhibitors; Prostacyclin Analogues; Simeprevir; Stiripentol

Decreased Effect

Doxazosin may decrease the levels/effects of: Alpha-/Beta-Agonists; Alpha1-Agonists

The levels/effects of Doxazosin may be decreased by: Bosentan; CYP3A4 Inducers (Moderate); CYP3A4 Inducers (Strong); Dabrafenib; Deferasirox; Herbs (Hypertensive Properties); Methylphenidate; Mitotane; Siltuximab; St Johns Wort; Tocilizumab; Yohimbine

Storage/Stability Store at 25°C (77°F); excursions permitted between 15°C to 30°C (59°F to 86°F).

Mechanism of Action

Hypertension: Competitively inhibits postsynaptic alpha$_1$-adrenergic receptors which results in vasodilation of veins and arterioles and a decrease in total peripheral resistance and blood pressure; ~50% as potent on a weight by weight basis as prazosin.

BPH: Competitively inhibits postsynaptic alpha$_1$-adrenergic receptors in prostatic stromal and bladder neck tissues. This reduces the sympathetic tone-induced urethral stricture causing BPH symptoms.

Pharmacodynamics/Kinetics Not significantly affected by increased age

Duration: >24 hours

Protein binding: ~98%

Metabolism: Extensively hepatic to active metabolites; primarily via CYP3A4; secondary pathways involve CYP2D6 and 2C19

Bioavailability: Immediate release: ~65%; Extended release relative to immediate release: 54% to 59%

Half-life elimination: Immediate release: ~22 hours; Extended release: 15-19 hours

Time to peak, serum: Immediate release: 2-3 hours; Extended release: 8-9 hours

Excretion: Feces (63%, primarily as metabolites); urine (9%, primarily as metabolites)

Dosage Oral:

Children and Adolescents 1-17 years (off-label use): Hypertension: Immediate release: Initial: 1 mg once daily; maximum: 4 mg daily (NHBPEP, 2004)

Adults:

Immediate release: 1 mg once daily in morning or evening; may be increased to 2 mg once daily. Thereafter titrate upwards, if needed, every 1-2 weeks, balancing therapeutic benefit with doxazosin-induced postural hypotension.

BPH: Goal: 4-8 mg daily; maximum dose: 8 mg daily

Hypertension: Usual dosage range (ASH/ISH [Weber, 2014]): 1-2 mg daily; Maximum dose: 16 mg daily

Ureteral calculi (distal) expulsion (off-label use): 4 mg once daily in evening (Gurbuz, 2011; Resorlu, 2011). **Note:** Patients with stones >10 mm were excluded from studies.

Reinitiation of therapy: If therapy is discontinued for several days, restart at 1 mg dose and titrate as before

Extended release: BPH: 4 mg once daily with breakfast; titrate based on response and tolerability every 3-4 weeks to maximum recommended dose of 8 mg daily

Reinitiation of therapy: If therapy is discontinued for several days, restart at 4 mg dose and titrate as before.

Conversion to extended release from immediate release: Omit final evening dose of immediate release prior to starting morning dosing with extended release product; initiate extended release product using 4 mg once daily

Elderly: Hypertension: Consider lower initial doses (eg, immediate release: 0.5 mg once daily) and titrate to response (Aronow, 2011)

Dosage adjustment in renal impairment: No dosage adjustment provided in the manufacturer's labeling (limited data suggest renal impairment does not significantly alter pharmacokinetic parameters).

Dosage adjustment in hepatic impairment: Use with caution in mild-to-moderate hepatic dysfunction. Do not use with severe impairment.

Dietary Considerations Cardura® XL: Take with morning meal.

Administration Cardura® XL: Tablets should be swallowed whole; do not crush, chew, or divide. Administer with morning meal.

Monitoring Parameters Blood pressure, standing and sitting/supine; syncope may occur usually within 90 minutes of the initial dose or dose increase

Additional Information First-dose hypotension occurs less frequently with doxazosin as compared to prazosin; this may be due to its slower onset of action.

Dosage Forms

Tablet, Oral:

Cardura: 1 mg, 2 mg, 4 mg, 8 mg

Generic: 1 mg, 2 mg, 4 mg, 8 mg

Tablet Extended Release 24 Hour, Oral:

Cardura XL: 4 mg, 8 mg

Dosage Forms: Canada Note: Refer to Dosage Forms. Extended-release capsules are not available in Canada.

◆ **Doxazosin-1 (Can)** *see* Doxazosin *on page 674*

◆ **Doxazosin-2 (Can)** *see* Doxazosin *on page 674*

◆ **Doxazosin-4 (Can)** *see* Doxazosin *on page 674*

◆ **Doxazosin Mesylate** *see* Doxazosin *on page 674*

Doxepin (Systemic) (DOKS e pin)

Brand Names: U.S. Silenor

Brand Names: Canada Apo-Doxepin; Novo-Doxepin; Silenor; Sinequan; Zonalon

Index Terms Doxepin Hydrochloride

Pharmacologic Category Antidepressant, Tricyclic (Tertiary Amine)

Additional Appendix Information

Beers Criteria – Potentially Inappropriate Medications for Geriatrics *on page 2271*

Use

Depression and/or anxiety: Treatment of psychoneurotic patients with depression and/or anxiety; depression and/or anxiety associated with alcoholism; depression and/or anxiety associated with organic disease; psychotic depressive disorders with associated anxiety, including involutional depression and manic-depressive disorders.

Insomnia (Silenor only): Treatment of insomnia characterized by difficulty with sleep maintenance.

Pregnancy Risk Factor C

Pregnancy Considerations Adverse events were observed in animal reproduction studies. Tricyclic antidepressants may be associated with irritability, jitteriness, and convulsions (rare) in the neonate (Yonkers, 2009).

The ACOG recommends that therapy for depression during pregnancy be individualized; treatment should incorporate the clinical expertise of the mental health clinician, obstetrician, primary healthcare provider, and pediatrician (ACOG, 2008). According to the American Psychiatric Association (APA), the risks of medication treatment should be weighed against other treatment options and untreated depression. For women who discontinue antidepressant medications during pregnancy and who may be at high risk for postpartum depression, the medications can be restarted following delivery (APA, 2010). Treatment algorithms have been developed by the ACOG and the APA for the management of depression in women prior to conception and during pregnancy (Yonkers, 2009).

Breast-Feeding Considerations Doxepin and N-desmethyldoxepin are excreted into breast milk (Frey, 1999; Kemp, 1985). Drowsiness, vomiting, poor feeding, and muscle hypotonia were noted in a nursing infant following maternal use of doxepin. Symptoms began to resolve 24 hours after feedings with breast milk were discontinued (Frey, 1999). In addition, product labeling notes that drowsiness and apnea have been reported in a nursing infant following maternal use of doxepin for depression. The manufacturer recommends that caution be used if administered to a nursing woman.

Contraindications

Hypersensitivity to doxepin, dibenzoxepins, or any component of the formulation; glaucoma; urinary retention; use of MAO inhibitors within 14 days

Documentation of allergenic cross-reactivity for tricyclic antidepressants is limited. However, because of similarities in chemical structure and/or pharmacologic actions, the possibility of cross-sensitivity cannot be ruled out with certainty.

Warnings/Precautions [U.S. Boxed Warning]: Antidepressants increase the risk of suicidal thinking and behavior in children, adolescents, and young adults (18-24 years of age) with major depressive disorder (MDD) and other psychiatric disorders; consider risk prior to prescribing. Short-term studies did not show an increased risk in patients >24 years of age and showed a decreased risk in patients ≥65 years. Closely monitor for clinical worsening, suicidality, or unusual changes in behavior, particularly during the initial 1 to 2 months of therapy or during periods of dosage adjustments (increases or decreases); the patient's family or caregiver should be instructed to closely observe the patient and communicate condition with healthcare provider. A medication guide should be dispensed with each prescription. **Doxepin is not approved for use in pediatric patients.**

The possibility of a suicide attempt is inherent in major depression and may persist until remission occurs. Use caution in high-risk patients. Worsening depression and severe abrupt suicidality that are not part of the presenting symptoms may require discontinuation or modification of drug therapy. The patient's family or caregiver should be alerted to monitor patients for the emergence of suicidality and associated behaviors (such as agitation, irritability, hostility, impulsivity, and hypomania) and call healthcare provider.

Risk of suicidal behavior may be increased regardless of doxepin dose; antidepressant doses of doxepin are 10- to 100-fold higher than doses for insomnia.

May precipitate a shift to mania or hypomania in patients with bipolar disorder. Patients presenting with depressive symptoms should be screened for bipolar disorder. Monotherapy in patients with bipolar disorder should be avoided. **Doxepin is not FDA approved for the treatment of bipolar depression.**

Should only be used for insomnia after evaluation of potential causes of sleep disturbance. Failure of sleep disturbance to resolve after 7 to 10 days may indicate psychiatric or medical illness. An increased risk for hazardous sleep-related activities has been noted; discontinue use with any sleep-related episodes. The risks of sedative and anticholinergic effects are high relative to other antidepressant agents. Anxiety, psychosis, and other neuropsychiatric symptoms may occur unpredictably. May cause CNS depression, which may impair physical or mental abilities; patients must be cautioned about performing tasks that require mental alertness (eg, operating machinery or driving). Also use caution in patients with benign prostatic hyperplasia, xerostomia, visual problems, constipation, or history of bowel obstruction.

May cause orthostatic hypotension or conduction disturbances (risks are moderate relative to other antidepressants). Use with caution in patients with a history of cardiovascular disease (including previous MI, stroke, tachycardia, or conduction abnormalities). Use with caution in patients with respiratory compromise or sleep apnea; use of Silenor is generally not recommended with severe sleep apnea.

Use caution in patients with a previous seizure disorder or condition predisposing to seizures such as brain damage, alcoholism, or concurrent therapy with other drugs which lower the seizure threshold (APA, 2010). Bone fractures have been associated with antidepressant treatment. Consider the possibility of a fragility fracture if an antidepressant-treated patient presents with unexplained bone pain, point tenderness, swelling, or bruising (Rabenda, 2013; Rizzoli, 2012). Use with caution in patients with hepatic dysfunction. May cause mild pupillary dilation which in susceptible individuals can lead to an episode of narrow-angle glaucoma. Consider evaluating patients who have not had an iridectomy for narrow-angle glaucoma risk factors. Potentially significant drug-drug interactions may exist, requiring dose or frequency adjustment, additional monitoring, and/or selection of alternative therapy.

May cause confusion and over sedation in the elderly. In the elderly, avoid doses >6 mg/day in this age group due to its potent anticholinergic and sedative properties, and potential to cause orthostatic hypotension; safety of doses ≤6 mg/day is comparable to placebo. In addition, may also cause or exacerbate syndrome of inappropriate antidiuretic hormone secretion or hyponatremia; monitor sodium closely with initiation or dosage adjustments in older adults (Beers Criteria).

Abrupt discontinuation or interruption of antidepressant therapy has been associated with a discontinuation syndrome. Symptoms arising may vary with antidepressant however commonly include nausea, vomiting, diarrhea, headaches, light-headedness, dizziness, diminished appetite, sweating, chills, tremors, paresthesias, fatigue, somnolence, and sleep disturbances (eg, vivid dreams, insomnia). Greater risks for developing a discontinuation syndrome have been associated with antidepressants with shorter half-lives, longer durations of treatment, and abrupt discontinuation. For antidepressants of short or intermediate half-lives, symptoms may emerge within 2-5 days after treatment discontinuation and last 7 to 14 days (APA, 2010; Fava, 2006; Haddad, 2001; Shelton, 2001; Warner, 2006).

Adverse Reactions May be dependent on diagnosis.

Cardiovascular: Edema, flushing, hypertension (chronic insomnia patients), hypotension, tachycardia

Central nervous system: Ataxia, chills, confusion, disorientation, dizziness (chronic insomnia patients), drowsiness, extrapyramidal reaction, fatigue, hallucination, headache, numbness, paresthesia, sedation (chronic insomnia patients), seizure, tardive dyskinesia

Dermatologic: Alopecia, diaphoresis (excessive), pruritus, skin photosensitivity, skin rash

Endocrine & metabolic: Altered serum glucose, change in libido, galactorrhea, gynecomastia, SIADH, weight gain

Gastrointestinal: Anorexia, aphthous stomatitis, constipation, diarrhea, dysgeusia, dyspepsia, gastroenteritis (chronic insomnia patients), nausea (chronic insomnia patients), vomiting, xerostomia

Genitourinary: Breast hypertrophy, testicular swelling, urinary retention

Hematologic & oncologic: Agranulocytosis, eosinophilia, leukopenia, purpura, thrombocytopenia

Hepatic: Jaundice

Neuromuscular & skeletal: Tremor, weakness

Ophthalmic: Blurred vision

Otic: Tinnitus

Respiratory: Exacerbation of asthma, upper respiratory tract infection (chronic insomnia patients)

Rare but important or life-threatening: Adenocarcinoma (lung, stage I), adjustment disorder, anemia, angle-closure glaucoma, atrioventricular block, bone fracture, breast cyst, cerebrovascular accident, chest pain, decreased neutrophils, decreased performance on neuropsychometrics, decreased range of motion (joints), depression, ECG abnormality (ST-T segment, QRS complex, QRS axis), eye infection, fungal infection, gastroesophageal reflux disease, hematochezia, hematoma, hemoglobinuria, hyperbilirubinemia, hyperkalemia, hypermagnesemia, hypersensitivity, hypoacusis, hypokalemia, increased serum ALT, increased serum transaminases, malignant melanoma, migraine, peripheral edema, pneumonia, sleep paralysis, somnambulism (complex sleep-related behavior [sleep-driving, cooking or eating food, making phone calls]), staphylococcal cellulitis, syncope, tenosynovitis, tooth infection, urinary incontinence, urinary tract infection, viral infection

Drug Interactions

Metabolism/Transport Effects Substrate of CYP1A2 (minor), CYP2C19 (minor), CYP2D6 (major), CYP3A4 (minor); **Note:** Assignment of Major/Minor substrate status based on clinically relevant drug interaction potential

Avoid Concomitant Use

Avoid concomitant use of Doxepin (Systemic) with any of the following: Aclidinium; Azelastine (Nasal); Dapoxetine; Glucagon; Iobenguane I 123; Ipratropium (Oral Inhalation); Linezolid; MAO Inhibitors; Methylene Blue; Moxonidine; Orphenadrine; Paraldehyde; Potassium Chloride; Thalidomide; Tiotropium; Umeclidinium

Increased Effect/Toxicity

Doxepin (Systemic) may increase the levels/effects of: AbobotulinumtoxinA; Alcohol (Ethyl); Alpha-/Beta-Agonists (Direct-Acting); Alpha1-Agonists; Amphetamines; Analgesics (Opioid); Anticholinergic Agents; Antipsychotic Agents; Aspirin; Azelastine (Nasal); Beta2-Agonists; Buprenorphine; Citalopram; CNS Depressants; Desmopressin; Escitalopram; Glucagon; Highest Risk QTc-Prolonging Agents; Hydrocodone; Methotrimeprazine; Methylene Blue; Metyrosine; Mirabegron; Moderate Risk QTc-Prolonging Agents; Nicorandil; NSAID (COX-2 Inhibitor); NSAID (Nonselective); OnabotulinumtoxinA; Orphenadrine; Paraldehyde; Potassium Chloride; Pramipexole; QuiNIDine; RimabotulinumtoxinB; ROPINIRole; Rotigotine; Serotonin Modulators; Sodium Phosphates; Sulfonylureas; Suvorexant; Thalidomide; Thiazide Diuretics; Tiotropium; Topiramate; TraMADol; Vitamin K Antagonists; Yohimbine; Zolpidem

The levels/effects of Doxepin (Systemic) may be increased by: Abiraterone Acetate; Aclidinium; Altretamine; Antiemetics (5HT3 Antagonists); Antipsychotic Agents; Brimonidine (Topical); BuPROPion; Cannabis; Cimetidine; Cinacalcet; Citalopram; Cobicistat; CYP2D6 Inhibitors (Moderate); CYP2D6 Inhibitors (Strong); Dapoxetine; Darunavir; Dexmethylphenidate; Doxylamine; Dronabinol; Droperidol; DULoxetine; Escitalopram; FLUoxetine; FluvoxaMINE; HydrOXYzine; Ipratropium (Oral Inhalation); Kava Kava; Linezolid; Lithium; Magnesium Sulfate; MAO Inhibitors; Methotrimeprazine; Methylphenidate; Metoclopramide; Metyrosine; Mianserin; Mifepristone; Nabilone; PARoxetine; Peginterferon Alfa-2b; Perampanel; Pramlintide; Protease Inhibitors; QuiNIDine; Rufinamide; Sertraline; Sodium Oxybate; Tapentadol; Tedizolid; Terbinafine (Systemic); Tetrahydrocannabinol; Thyroid Products; TraMADol; Umeclidinium; Valproic Acid and Derivatives

Decreased Effect

Doxepin (Systemic) may decrease the levels/effects of: Acetylcholinesterase Inhibitors; Alpha1-Agonists; Alpha2-Agonists; Alpha2-Agonists (Ophthalmic); Iobenguane I 123; Itopride; Moxonidine; Secretin

The levels/effects of Doxepin (Systemic) may be decreased by: Acetylcholinesterase Inhibitors; Barbiturates; CarBAMazepine; Peginterferon Alfa-2b; St Johns Wort

Food Interactions Administration with a high-fat meal increases the bioavailability of Silenor and delays the peak plasma concentration by ~3 hours. Management: Silenor should not be taken during or within 3 hours of a meal.

Preparation for Administration Concentrate, oral: Must dilute with approximately 120 mL of water, whole or skimmed milk, or orange, grapefruit, tomato, prune or pineapple juice prior to administration. Do not mix with carbonated beverages (physically incompatible). Doxepin concentrate and methadone syrup can be mixed together with Gatorade, lemon or orange juice, sugar water, Tang, or water, but not with grape juice.

Storage/Stability Store at room temperature. Protect from light.

Mechanism of Action Increases the synaptic concentration of serotonin and norepinephrine in the central nervous system by inhibition of their reuptake by the presynaptic neuronal membrane (Pinder, 1977); antagonizes the histamine (H_1) receptor for sleep maintenance

Pharmacodynamics/Kinetics
Onset of action: Individual responses may vary; 4-8 weeks of treatment are needed before determining if a patient with depression is partially or nonresponsive (APA, 2010); onset of anxiolytic effects may have a latency of 2-6 weeks (Bandelow, 2008)
Absorption: Administration with a high-fat meal increases the bioavailability of Silenor and delays the peak plasma concentration by ~3 hours
Distribution: V_d: 20.2 L/kg (Ziegler, 1978); Silenor 11,930 L
Protein binding: ~80%
Metabolism: Hepatic via CYP2C19 and 2D6; primary metabolite is N-desmethyldoxepin (active)
Half-life elimination: Adults: Doxepin: ~15 hours; N-desmethyldoxepin: 31 hours
Time to peak, serum: 3.5 hours
Excretion: Urine (<3% as unchanged drug or N-desmethyldoxepin)

Dosage
Depression or anxiety (entire daily dose may be given at bedtime): Oral:
Adults: Initial: 25-50 mg as a single dose at bedtime or in divided doses; gradually increase based on response and tolerability to a usual dose of 100-300 mg daily (APA, 2010; Bauer 2013)
Elderly: Carefully adjust the use of doxepin on a once-a-day dosage regimen in elderly patients based on the patient's condition; elderly patients generally should be started on low doses of doxepin and observed closely
Insomnia (Silenor): Oral:
Adults: 3-6 mg once daily within 30 minutes of bedtime; maximum dose: 6 mg daily
Elderly: 3 mg once daily within 30 minutes of bedtime; increase to 6 mg once daily if clinically needed; maximum dose: 6 mg daily

Discontinuation of therapy: Upon discontinuation of antidepressant therapy, gradually taper the dose to minimize the incidence of withdrawal symptoms and allow for the detection of re-emerging symptoms. Evidence supporting ideal taper rates is limited. APA and NICE guidelines suggest tapering therapy over at least several weeks with consideration to the half-life of the antidepressant; antidepressants with a shorter half-life may need to be tapered more conservatively. In addition for long-term treated patients, WFSBP guidelines recommend tapering over 4-6 months. If intolerable withdrawal symptoms occur following a dose reduction, consider resuming the previously prescribed dose and/or decrease dose at a more gradual rate (APA, 2010; Bauer, 2002; Haddad, 2001; NCCMH, 2010; Schatzberg, 2006; Shelton, 2001; Warner, 2006).

MAO inhibitor recommendations:
Switching to or from an MAO inhibitor intended to treat psychiatric disorders:
Allow 14 days to elapse between discontinuing an MAO inhibitor intended to treat psychiatric disorders and initiation of doxepin.
Allow 14 days to elapse between discontinuing doxepin and initiation of an MAO inhibitor intended to treat psychiatric disorders.
Use with other MAO inhibitors (such as linezolid or IV methylene blue):
Do not initiate doxepin in patients receiving linezolid or IV methylene blue; consider other interventions for psychiatric condition.
If urgent treatment with linezolid or IV methylene blue is required in a patient already receiving doxepin and potential benefits outweigh potential risks, discontinue doxepin promptly and administer linezolid or IV methylene blue. Monitor for serotonin syndrome for 2 weeks or until 24 hours after the last dose of linezolid or IV methylene blue, whichever comes first. May resume doxepin 24 hours after the last dose of linezolid or IV methylene blue.

Dosage adjustment in renal impairment: There are no dosage adjustments provided in manufacturer's labeling.
Dosage adjustment in hepatic impairment: Silenor: Initial: 3 mg once daily

Administration
Depression and/or anxiety: Oral: Administer the total daily dosage in divided or once a day dosage schedule. If the once a day schedule is employed the maximum recommended dose is 150 mg once daily at bedtime. The 150 mg capsule strength is intended for maintenance therapy only and is not for initiation of treatment.
Insomnia: Oral: Administer within 30 minutes prior to bedtime; do not take within 3 hours of food.

Monitoring Parameters Evaluate mental status, suicide ideation (especially at the beginning of therapy or when doses are increased or decreased); anxiety, social functioning, mania, panic attacks or other unusual changes in behavior; heart rate, blood pressure and ECG in older adults and patients with preexisting cardiac disease; blood glucose; weight and BMI; blood levels are useful for therapeutic monitoring (APA, 2010).

Insomnia: Re-evaluate diagnosis if insomnia does not remit within 7-10 days of treatment.

Reference Range Proposed therapeutic concentration (doxepin plus desmethyldoxepin): 50-250 ng/mL. Utility of serum level monitoring is controversial (Leucht, 2001).

Dosage Forms
Capsule, Oral:
Generic: 10 mg, 25 mg, 50 mg, 75 mg, 100 mg, 150 mg
Concentrate, Oral:
Generic: 10 mg/mL (118 mL, 120 mL)
Tablet, Oral:
Silenor: 3 mg, 6 mg

Dosage Forms: Canada Note: Refer to Dosage Forms. Oral concentrate is not available in Canada.

Doxepin (Topical) (DOKS e pin)

Brand Names: U.S. Prudoxin; Zonalon
Brand Names: Canada Zonalon®
Index Terms Doxepin Hydrochloride
Pharmacologic Category Topical Skin Product
Use Short-term (<8 days) management of moderate pruritus in adults with atopic dermatitis or lichen simplex chronicus
Pregnancy Risk Factor B

Dosage
Oral: Topical: Burning mouth syndrome (off-label use): Cream: Apply 3-4 times daily
Topical: Pruritus: Adults and Elderly: Apply a thin film 4 times/day with at least 3- to 4-hour interval between applications; not recommended for use >8 days. **Note:** Low-dose (25-50 mg) oral administration has also been used to treat pruritus, but systemic effects are increased.

Additional Information Complete prescribing information should be consulted for additional detail.

Dosage Forms
Cream, External:
Prudoxin: 5% (45 g)
Zonalon: 5% (30 g, 45 g)

◆ **Doxepin Hydrochloride** *see* Doxepin (Systemic) *on page 676*

◆ **Doxepin Hydrochloride** *see* Doxepin (Topical) *on page 678*

Doxercalciferol (doks er kal si fe FEER ole)

Brand Names: U.S. Hectorol

Brand Names: Canada Hectorol

Index Terms 1α-Hydroxyergocalciferol

Pharmacologic Category Vitamin D Analog

Use

Secondary hyperparathyroidism (dialysis): Injection, oral: Treatment of secondary hyperparathyroidism in patients with chronic kidney disease on dialysis

Secondary hyperparathyroidism (predialysis patients): Oral: Treatment of secondary hyperparathyroidism in patients with stage 3 or 4 chronic kidney disease

Pregnancy Risk Factor B

Dosage

Oral:

Dialysis patients:

Initial dose: iPTH >400 pg/mL: 10 mcg 3 times/week at dialysis for 8 weeks

Dose titration:

iPTH level >300 pg/mL (dose should be titrated to lower iPTH to within the range of 150 to 300 pg/mL): Increase to 12.5 mcg 3 times/week at dialysis for 8 more weeks; this titration process can continue at 8-week intervals in 2.5 mcg/dose increments (maximum: 20 mcg 3 times/week).

iPTH level 150 to 300 pg/mL: Maintain current dose

iPTH level <100 pg/mL: Suspend doxercalciferol for 1 week; resume at a reduced dose; decrease each dose (not weekly dose) by at least 2.5 mcg

Hypercalcemia, hyperphosphatemia, or serum calcium times serum phosphorus product >55 mg^2/dL^2: Decrease or suspend dose and/or adjust dose of phosphate binders; if dose is suspended, resume at a reduced dose; decrease each dose (not weekly dose) by at least 2.5 mcg.

Predialysis patients:

Initial dose: iPTH >70 pg/mL with stage 3 disease or >110 pg/mL with stage 4 disease: 1 mcg/day for 2 weeks

Dose titration:

iPTH level >70 pg/mL with stage 3 disease or >110 pg/mL with stage 4 disease (dose should be titrated to lower iPTH to 35 to 70 pg/mL with stage 3 disease or to 70 to 110 pg/mL with stage 4 disease): Increase dose by 0.5 mcg per day every 2 weeks as necessary (maximum dose: 3.5 mcg/day)

iPTH level 35 to 70 pg/mL with stage 3 disease or 70 to 110 pg/mL with stage 4 disease: Maintain current dose

iPTH level is <35 pg/mL with stage 3 disease or <70 pg/mL with stage 4 disease: Suspend doxercalciferol for 1 week, then resume at a reduced dose (at least 0.5 mcg per day lower)

Hypercalcemia, hyperphosphatemia, or serum calcium times serum phosphorus product >55 mg^2/dL^2: Decrease or suspend dose and/or adjust dose of phosphate binders; if dose is suspended, resume at a reduced dose (at least 0.5 mcg per day lower).

IV:

Dialysis patients:

Initial dose: iPTH level >400 pg/mL: 4 mcg 3 times/week after dialysis for 8 weeks

Dose titration:

iPTH level decreased by <50% and >300 pg/mL (dose should be titrated to lower iPTH to within a range of 150 to 300 pg/mL): Increase by 1 to 2 mcg at 8-week intervals, as necessary (doses >18 mcg/week have not been studied).

iPTH level decreased by >50% and >300 pg/mL: Maintain current dose

iPTH level 150 to 300 pg/mL: Maintain current dose

iPTH level <100 pg/mL: Suspend doxercalciferol for 1 week; resume at a reduced dose (at least 1 mcg lower)

Hypercalcemia, hyperphosphatemia, or serum calcium times serum phosphorus product >55 mg^2/dL^2: Decrease or suspend dose and/or adjust dose of phosphate binders; if dose is suspended, resume at a reduced dose (at least 1 mcg lower)

Dosage adjustment in renal impairment: No dosage adjustment necessary.

Dosage adjustment in hepatic impairment: There are no dosage adjustments provided in the manufacturer's labeling. Use with caution and consider more frequent monitoring of iPTH, calcium, and phosphorus levels.

Additional Information Complete prescribing information should be consulted for additional detail.

Dosage Forms

Capsule, Oral:

Hectorol: 0.5 mcg, 1 mcg, 2.5 mcg

Generic: 0.5 mcg, 1 mcg, 2.5 mcg

Solution, Intravenous:

Hectorol: 2 mcg/mL (1 mL); 4 mcg/2 mL (2 mL)

Generic: 4 mcg/2 mL (2 mL)

◆ **Doxil** *see* DOXOrubicin (Liposomal) *on page 684*

Doxofylline [INT] (doks OFF i lin)

International Brand Names Ansimar (IT, PH); Asima (KR); Axofin (MX); Coxylate (IN); Dilitair (PH); Doxfree (IN); Puroxan (CO, PH, TH); Rexifine (KR); Rexipin (KR); Roar (IN); Shuweixin (CN)

Pharmacologic Category Bronchodilator; Theophylline Derivative

Reported Use Treatment of symptoms and reversible airway obstruction due to chronic asthma, chronic bronchitis, or COPD

Dosage Range Adults: Oral: 400 mg 2-3 times/day

Product Availability Product available in various countries; not currently available in the U.S.

Dosage Forms

Capsule: 400 mg

DOXOrubicin (Conventional)

(doks oh ROO bi sin con VEN sha nal)

Brand Names: U.S. Adriamycin

Brand Names: Canada Adriamycin PFS; Doxorubicin Hydrochloride For Injection, USP; Doxorubicin Hydrochloride Injection

Index Terms ADR (error-prone abbreviation); Adria; Conventional Doxorubicin; Doxorubicin HCl; Doxorubicin Hydrochloride; Hydroxydaunomycin Hydrochloride; Hydroxyldaunorubicin Hydrochloride

Pharmacologic Category Antineoplastic Agent, Anthracycline; Antineoplastic Agent, Topoisomerase II Inhibitor

Use

Breast cancer: Treatment component of adjuvant therapy in women with evidence of axillary lymph node involvement following resection of primary breast cancer

Metastatic cancers or disseminated neoplastic conditions: Treatment of acute lymphoblastic leukemia, acute myeloid leukemia, Wilms tumor, neuroblastoma, soft tissue and bone sarcomas, breast cancer, ovarian cancer, transitional cell bladder carcinoma, thyroid carcinoma, gastric carcinoma, Hodgkin lymphoma, non-Hodgkin lymphoma, and bronchogenic carcinoma in which the small cell histologic type is the most responsive compared with other cell types

Pregnancy Risk Factor D

Pregnancy Considerations Adverse events have been observed in animal reproduction studies. Based on the mechanism of action, doxorubicin may cause fetal harm if administered during pregnancy (according to the manufacturer's labeling). Advise patients (females of reproductive potential and males with female partners of reproductive potential) to use effective nonhormonal contraception during and for 6 months following therapy. The National Comprehensive Cancer Network (NCCN) breast cancer guidelines (v3.2013) state that chemotherapy, if indicated, may be administered to pregnant women with breast cancer as part of a combination chemotherapy regimen (common regimens administered during pregnancy include doxorubicin, cyclophosphamide, and fluorouracil); chemotherapy should not be administered during the first trimester, after 35 weeks gestation, or within 3 weeks of planned delivery.

Breast-Feeding Considerations Doxorubicin and its metabolites are excreted in breast milk. Due to the potential for serious adverse reactions in the nursing infant, the manufacturer recommends a decision be made whether to discontinue nursing or to discontinue the drug, taking into account the importance of treatment to the mother. Per the NCCN guidelines (v3.2013), breast-feeding after breast-conserving treatment for breast cancer is not contraindicated; however, the quantity and quality of breast milk may not be sufficient or may be lacking some nutrients needed.

Contraindications Hypersensitivity (including anaphylaxis) to doxorubicin, any component of the formulation, or to other anthracyclines or anthracenediones; recent MI (within past 4-6 weeks), severe myocardial insufficiency, severe arrhythmia; previous therapy with high cumulative doses of doxorubicin, daunorubicin, idarubicin, or other anthracycline and anthracenediones; severe persistent drug-induced myelosuppression or baseline neutrophil count <1500/mm^3; severe hepatic impairment (Child-Pugh class C or bilirubin >5 mg/dL)

Warnings/Precautions Hazardous agent - use appropriate precautions for handling and disposal (NIOSH 2014 [group 1]). **[U.S. Boxed Warning]: May cause cumulative, dose-related, myocardial toxicity (early or delayed, including acute left ventricular failure and HF). The risk of cardiomyopathy increases with cumulative exposure and with concomitant cardiotoxic therapy; the incidence of irreversible myocardial toxicity increases as the total cumulative (lifetime) dosages approach 300-500 mg/m^2. Assess left ventricular ejection fraction (LVEF) with either an echocardiogram or MUGA scan before, during, and after therapy; increase the frequency of assessments as the cumulative dose exceeds 300 mg/m^2.** Cardiotoxicity is dose-limiting. Delayed cardiotoxicity may occur late in treatment or within months to years after completion of therapy, and is typically manifested by LVEF reduction and/or heart failure (may be life threatening). Subacute effects such as pericarditis and myocarditis may also occur. Early toxicity may consist of tachyarrhythmias, including sinus tachycardia, premature ventricular contractions, and ventricular tachycardia, as well as bradycardia. Electrocardiographic changes including ST-T wave changes, atrioventricular and bundle-branch block have also been reported. These effects are not necessarily predictive of subsequent delayed cardiotoxicity. Total cumulative dose should take into account prior treatment with other anthracyclines or anthracenediones, previous or concomitant treatment with other cardiotoxic agents or irradiation of chest. Although the risk increases with cumulative dose, irreversible cardiotoxicity may occur at any dose level. Patients with active or dominant cardiovascular disease, concurrent administration of cardiotoxic drugs, prior therapy with other anthracyclines or anthracenediones, prior or concurrent chest irradiation, advanced age, and infants and children are at increased risk. Alternative administration schedules (weekly or continuous infusions) have are associated with less cardiotoxicity.

[U.S. Boxed Warning]: Vesicant; if extravasation occurs, severe local tissue damage leading to tissue injury, blistering, ulceration, and necrosis may occur. Discontinue infusion immediately and apply ice to the affected area. For IV administration only. Do not administer IM or SubQ. Ensure proper needle or catheter placement prior to and during infusion. Avoid extravasation.

[U.S. Boxed Warning]: May cause severe myelosuppression, which may result in serious infection, septic shock, transfusion requirements, hospitalization, and death. Myelosuppression may be dose-limiting and primarily manifests as leukopenia and neutropenia; anemia and thrombocytopenia may also occur. The nadir typically occurs 10 to 14 days after administration with cell count recovery around day 21. Monitor blood counts at baseline and regularly during therapy.

[U.S. Boxed Warning]: Secondary acute myelogenous leukemia (AML) and myelodysplastic syndrome (MDS) have been reported following treatment. AML and MDS typically occur within one to three years of treatment; risk factors for development of secondary AML or MDS include treatment with anthracyclines in combination with DNA-damaging antineoplastics (eg, alkylating agents) and/or radiation therapy, heavily pretreated patients, and escalated anthracycline doses. May cause tumor lysis syndrome and hyperuricemia (in patients with rapidly growing tumors). Urinary alkalinization and prophylaxis with an antihyperuricemic agent may be necessary. Monitor electrolytes, renal function, and hydration status. **[U.S. Boxed Warning]: Dosage modification is recommended in patients with impaired hepatic function;** toxicities may be increased in patients with hepatic impairment. Use is contraindicated in patients with severe impairment (Child-Pugh class C or bilirubin >5 mg/dL). Monitor hepatic function tests (eg, transaminases, alkaline phosphatase, and bilirubin) closely. Use with caution in patients who have received radiation therapy; radiation recall may occur. May increase radiation-induced toxicity to the myocardium, mucosa, skin, and liver. Doxorubicin is associated with a moderate or high emetic potential (depending on dose or regimen); antiemetics are recommended to prevent nausea and vomiting (Basch, 2011; Dupuis, 2011; Roila, 2010). Potentially significant drug-drug interactions may exist, requiring dose or frequency adjustment, additional monitoring, and/or selection of alternative therapy.

In men, doxorubicin may damage spermatozoa and testicular tissue, resulting in possible genetic fetal abnormalities; may also result in oligospermia, azoospermia, and permanent loss of fertility (sperm counts have been reported to return to normal levels in some men, occurring several years after the end of therapy). In females of reproductive potential, doxorubicin may cause infertility and result in amenorrhea; premature menopause can occur. Children are at increased risk for developing delayed cardiotoxicity; long-term cardiac function monitoring is recommended. Doxorubicin may contribute to prepubertal growth failure in children; may also contribute to gonadal impairment (usually temporary). Radiation recall pneumonitis has been reported in children receiving concomitant dactinomycin and doxorubicin. **[U.S. Boxed Warning]: Should be administered under the supervision of an experienced cancer chemotherapy physician.** Use caution when selecting product for preparation and dispensing; indications, dosages and adverse event profiles differ between conventional doxorubicin hydrochloride solution and doxorubicin liposomal. Both formulations are the same concentration. As a result, serious errors have occurred.

Adverse Reactions

Cardiovascular:

Acute cardiotoxicity: Atrioventricular block, bradycardia, bundle branch block, ECG abnormalities, extrasystoles (atrial or ventricular), sinus tachycardia, ST-T wave changes, supraventricular tachycardia, tachyarrhythmia, ventricular tachycardia

Delayed cardiotoxicity: LVEF decreased, CHF (manifestations include ascites, cardiomegaly, dyspnea, edema, gallop rhythm, hepatomegaly, oliguria, pleural effusion, pulmonary edema, tachycardia); myocarditis, pericarditis

Central nervous system: Malaise

Dermatologic: Alopecia, itching, photosensitivity, radiation recall, rash; discoloration of saliva, sweat, or tears

Endocrine & metabolic: Amenorrhea, dehydration, infertility (may be temporary), hyperuricemia

Gastrointestinal: Abdominal pain, anorexia, colon necrosis, diarrhea, GI ulceration, mucositis, nausea, vomiting

Genitourinary: Discoloration of urine

Hematologic: Leukopenia/neutropenia (nadir: 10-14 days; recovery: by day 21); thrombocytopenia and anemia

Local: Skin "flare" at injection site, urticaria

Neuromuscular & skeletal: Weakness

Rare but important or life-threatening: Anaphylaxis, azoospermia, bilirubin increased, coma (when in combination with cisplatin or vincristine), conjunctivitis, fever, gonadal impairment (children), growth failure (prepubertal), hepatitis, hyperpigmentation (nail, skin & oral mucosa), infection, keratitis, lacrimation, myelodysplastic syndrome, neutropenic fever, neutropenic typhlitis, oligospermia, peripheral neurotoxicity (with intra-arterial doxorubicin), phlebosclerosis, radiation recall pneumonitis (children), secondary acute myelogenous leukemia, seizure (when in combination with cisplatin or vincristine), sepsis, shock, Stevens-Johnson syndrome, systemic hypersensitivity (including urticaria, pruritus, angioedema, dysphagia, and dyspnea), toxic epidermal necrolysis, transaminases increased, urticaria

Drug Interactions

Metabolism/Transport Effects **Substrate** of CYP2D6 (major), CYP3A4 (major), P-glycoprotein; **Note:** Assignment of Major/Minor substrate status based on clinically relevant drug interaction potential; **Inhibits** CYP2B6 (moderate), CYP2D6 (weak), CYP3A4 (weak); **Induces** P-glycoprotein

Avoid Concomitant Use

Avoid concomitant use of DOXOrubicin (Conventional) with any of the following: BCG; CloZAPine; Conivaptan; Dabigatran Etexilate; Dipyrone; Fusidic Acid (Systemic); Idelalisib; Ledipasvir; Natalizumab; Pimecrolimus; Pimozide; Sofosbuvir; Tacrolimus (Topical); Tofacitinib; Vaccines (Live); VinCRIStine (Liposomal)

Increased Effect/Toxicity

DOXOrubicin (Conventional) may increase the levels/effects of: ARIPiprazole; CloZAPine; CYP2B6 Substrates; Dofetilide; Hydrocodone; Leflunomide; Lomitapide; Mercaptopurine; Natalizumab; Pimozide; Tofacitinib; Vaccines (Live); Zidovudine

The levels/effects of DOXOrubicin (Conventional) may be increased by: Abiraterone Acetate; Bevacizumab; Conivaptan; Cyclophosphamide; CycloSPORINE (Systemic); CYP2D6 Inhibitors (Moderate); CYP2D6 Inhibitors (Strong); CYP3A4 Inhibitors (Moderate); CYP3A4 Inhibitors (Strong); Dasatinib; Denosumab; Dipyrone; Fusidic Acid (Systemic); Idelalisib; Luliconazole; Mifepristone; Peginterferon Alfa-2b; P-glycoprotein/ABCB1 Inhibitors; Pimecrolimus; Roflumilast; SORAfenib; Stiripentol; Tacrolimus (Topical); Taxane Derivatives; Trastuzumab

Decreased Effect

DOXOrubicin (Conventional) may decrease the levels/effects of: Afatinib; BCG; Brentuximab Vedotin; Cardiac Glycosides; Coccidioides immitis Skin Test; Dabigatran Etexilate; Ledipasvir; Linagliptin; P-glycoprotein/ABCB1 Substrates; Sipuleucel-T; Sofosbuvir; Stavudine; Vaccines (Inactivated); Vaccines (Live); VinCRIStine (Liposomal); Zidovudine

The levels/effects of DOXOrubicin (Conventional) may be decreased by: Bosentan; Cardiac Glycosides; CYP3A4 Inducers (Moderate); CYP3A4 Inducers (Strong); Dabrafenib; Deferasirox; Dexrazoxane; Echinacea; Mitotane; Peginterferon Alfa-2b; P-glycoprotein/ABCB1 Inducers; Siltuximab; St Johns Wort; Tocilizumab

Preparation for Administration Hazardous agent; use appropriate precautions for handling and disposal (NIOSH 2014 [group 1]). Reconstitute lyophilized powder with NS (using 5 mL for the 10 mg vial; 10 mL for the 20 mg vial; or 25 mL for the 50 mg vial) to a final concentration of 2 mg/mL; gently shake until contents are dissolved. May further dilute doxorubicin solution or reconstituted doxorubicin solution in 50-1000 mL D_5W or NS for infusion. Unstable in solutions with a pH <3 or >7.

Storage/Stability

Lyophilized powder: Store powder at 20°C to 25°C (68°F to 77°F). Protect from light. Retain in carton until time of use. Discard unused portion from single-dose vials. Reconstituted doxorubicin is stable for 7 days at room temperature under normal room lighting and for 15 days when refrigerated at 2°C to 8°C (36°F to 46°F). Protect reconstituted solution from light.

Solution: Store refrigerated at 2°C to 8°C (36°F to 46°F). Protect from light. Retain in carton until time of use. Discard unused portion. Storage of vials of solution under refrigeration may result in formation of a gelled product; if gelling occurs, place vials at room temperature for 2-4 hours to return the product to a slightly viscous, mobile solution.

Mechanism of Action Inhibition of DNA and RNA synthesis by intercalation between DNA base pairs by inhibition of topoisomerase II and by steric obstruction. Doxorubicin intercalates at points of local uncoiling of the double helix. Although the exact mechanism is unclear, it appears that direct binding to DNA (intercalation) and inhibition of DNA repair (topoisomerase II inhibition) result in blockade of DNA and RNA synthesis and fragmentation of DNA. Doxorubicin is also a powerful iron chelator; the iron-doxorubicin complex can bind DNA and cell membranes and produce free radicals that immediately cleave the DNA and cell membranes.

Pharmacodynamics/Kinetics

Distribution: V_d: 809-1214 L/m^2; does not cross the blood-brain barrier

Protein binding, plasma: ~75%

Metabolism: Primarily hepatic to doxorubicinol (active), then to inactive aglycones, conjugated sulfates, and glucuronides

Half-life elimination:

Distribution: ~5 minutes

Terminal: 20-48 hours

Male: 54 hours; Female: 35 hours

Excretion: Feces (~40% as unchanged drug); urine (5% to 12% as unchanged drug and metabolites)

Dosage Doxorubicin is associated with a moderate to high emetic potential (depending on dose or regimen); antiemetics are recommended to prevent nausea and vomiting (Basch, 2011; Dupuis, 2011; Roila, 2010).

Manufacturer's labeling: **Note:** Lower dosages should be considered for patients with inadequate marrow reserve (due to advanced age, prior treatment, or neoplastic marrow infiltration). Cumulative doses above 550 mg/m^2 are associated with an increased risk of cardiomyopathy.

Breast cancer: Adults: IV: 60 mg/m^2 on day 1 of a 21-day cycle (in combination with cyclophosphamide) for 4 cycles

Metastatic solid tumors, leukemia, or lymphoma: Children, Adolescents, and Adults: IV:
Single-agent therapy: 60-75 mg/m^2 every 21 days
Combination therapy: 40-75 mg/m^2 every 21-28 days

Indication-specific dosing (off-label dosing):

Acute lymphoblastic leukemia: IV:

DFCI Consortium Protocol 00-01: Children ≥1 year and Adolescents:
Induction: 30 mg/m^2/dose on days 0 and 1 of a 4-week cycle (Vrooman, 2013)
CNS therapy: High-risk patients: 30 mg/m^2 on day 1 of a 3-week cycle (with dexrazoxane) (Vrooman, 2013)
Intensification: High-risk patients: 30 mg/m^2 on day 1 of every 3-week cycle (with dexrazoxane; cumulative doxorubicin dose: 300 mg/m^2) (Vrooman, 2013)

Hyper-CVAD regimen: Adults: 50 mg/m^2 on day 4 of Courses 1, 3, 5, and 7 (in combination with cyclophosphamide, vincristine, and dexamethasone); alternating cycles with high-dose methotrexate and cytarabine (Kantarjian, 2004)

CALGB 8811 regimen: Adults: 30 mg/m^2 on days 1, 8 and 15 of late intensification (Course IV; 8-week cycle); in combination with vincristine, dexamethasone, cyclophosphamide, thioguanine, and cytarabine (Larson, 1995)

Bladder cancer, transitional cell: Adults: IV: *Dose-dense MVAC regimen:* 30 mg/m^2 on day 2 every 14 days (in combination with methotrexate, vinblastine, and cisplatin) (Sternberg, 2001)

Breast cancer: Adults: IV:

CAF regimen: 30 mg/m^2 on days 1 and 8 every 28 days for 6 cycles (in combination with cyclophosphamide and fluorouracil) (Bull, 1978)

FAC regimen: 50 mg/m^2 on day 1 (or administered as a 72-hour continuous infusion) every 21 days for 6 cycles (in combination with fluorouracil and cyclophosphamide) (Assikis, 2003)

TAC regimen: 50 mg/m^2 on day 1 every 21 days for 6 cycles (in combination with docetaxel and cyclophosphamide) (Martin, 2005)

Ewing sarcoma: IV:

VAC/IE regimen: Children, Adolescents, and Adults (≤30 years): 75 mg/m^2 on day 1 every 21 days for 5 cycles (in combination with vincristine and cyclophosphamide; after 5 cycles, dactinomycin replaced doxorubicin), alternating cycles with ifosfamide and etoposide for a total of 17 cycles (Grier, 2003)

VAIA regimen: Children, Adolescents, and Adults (<35 years): 30 mg/m^2/day on days 1 and 2 every 21 days (doxorubicin alternates with dactinomycin; in combination with vincristine and ifosfamide) for 14 cycles (Paulussen, 2008)

VIDE regimen: Children, Adolescents, and Adults: 20 mg/m^2/day over 4 hours on days 1 to 3 every 21 days for 6 cycles (in combination with vincristine, ifosfamide, and etoposide) (Juergens, 2006)

Hodgkin lymphoma: Adults: IV:

ABVD regimen: 25 mg/m^2 on days 1 and 15 every 28 days (in combination with bleomycin, vinblastine, and dacarbazine) for 2 to 4 cycles (Bonadonna, 2004; Engert, 2010)

BEACOPP and escalated BEACOPP regimens: 25 mg/m^2 (BEACOPP) or 35 mg/m^2 (escalated BEACOPP) on day 1 every 21 days (in combination with bleomycin, etoposide, cyclophosphamide, vincristine, procarbazine, and prednisone) (Engert, 2009)

Stanford V regimen: 25 mg/m^2 on weeks 1, 3, 5, 7, 9, and 11 of a 12-week cycle (in combination with mechlorethamine, vinblastine, vincristine, bleomycin, etoposide, and prednisone) (Horning, 2002)

Non-Hodgkin lymphoma: Adults: IV:

CHOP or RCHOP regimen: 50 mg/m^2 on day 1 every 21 days (in combination with cyclophosphamide, vincristine, and prednisone +/- rituximab) (Coiffier, 2010; McKelvey, 1976)

Hyper-CVAD + rituximab regimen: 50 mg/m^2 administered as a continuous infusion over 24 hours on day 4 of Courses 1, 3, 5, and 7 (21-day treatment cycles; in combination with cyclophosphamide, vincristine, dexamethasone, and rituximab); alternating cycles with high-dose methotrexate and cytarabine (Thomas, 2006)

Dose-adjusted EPOCH or REPOCH regimen: 10 mg/m^2/day administered as a continuous infusion on days 1 to 4 every 21 days (in combination with etoposide, vincristine, cyclophosphamide, and prednisone +/- rituximab) (Garcia-Suarez, 2007; Wilson, 2002)

Nordic regimen (Maxi-CHOP): 75 mg/m^2 on day 1 every 21 days (in combination with cyclophosphamide, vincristine, prednisone, and rituximab), alternating cycles with high-dose cytarabine (Geisler, 2008)

Osteosarcoma: IV:

Cisplatin/doxorubicin regimen: Children, Adolescents, and Adults (≤40 years of age): 25 mg/m^2 (bolus infusion) on days 1 to 3 every 21 days (in combination with cisplatin) (Bramwell, 1992)

High-dose methotrexate/cisplatin/doxorubicin/ifosfamide regimen: Children, Adolescents, and Adults (<40 years of age):
Preoperative: 75 mg/m^2 administered as a continuous infusion over 24 hours on day 3 of weeks 1 and 7 (in combination with methotrexate, cisplatin, and ifosfamide) (Bacci, 2003)
Postoperative: 90 mg/m^2 administered as a continuous infusion over 24 hours on weeks 13, 22, and 31 (in combination with methotrexate, cisplatin, and ifosfamide) (Bacci, 2003)

High-dose methotrexate/cisplatin/doxorubicin regimen: Children, Adolescents, and Adults (<40 years):
Preoperative: 60 mg/m^2 over 8 hours on days 9 and 36 (in combination with methotrexate and cisplatin) (Bacci, 2000)
Postoperative: 45 mg/m^2/day over 4 hours for 2 consecutive days (in combination with methotrexate, cisplatin +/- ifosfamide, +/- etoposide; refer to protocol for criteria, frequency, and other specific information) (Bacci, 2000)

Small cell lung cancer, recurrent: Adults: IV: *CAV regimen:* 45 mg/m^2 (maximum dose: 100 mg) on day 1 every 21 days (in combination with cyclophosphamide and vincristine) until disease progression or unacceptable toxicity or for at least 4 or 6 cycles past maximum response (von Pawel, 1999)

Soft tissue sarcoma: IV:

Non-specific histologies: Adults:

AD regimen: 60 mg/m^2 on day 1 every 21 days (either as a bolus infusion or administered continuously over 96 hours; in combination with dacarbazine) (Zalupski, 1991)

AIM regimen: 30 mg/m^2 on days 1 and 2 every 21 days (in combination with ifosfamide and mesna) (Edmonson, 1993)

MAID regimen: 20 mg/m²/day as a continuous infusion on days 1-3 every 21 days (in combination with ifosfamide, mesna, and dacarbazine) (Elias, 1989)

Single-agent regimen: 75 mg/m² on day 1 every 21 days until disease progression or unacceptable toxicity (Santoro, 1995)

Rhabdomyosarcoma:

VAC/IE regimen: Children, Adolescents, and Adults (<21 years of age): 37.5 mg/m² on days 1 and 2 (administered over 18 hours each day) every 6 weeks (in combination with vincristine and cyclophosphamide), alternating cycles with ifosfamide and etoposide (Arndt, 1998)

VAI regimen (based on a limited number of patients): Adults: 25 mg/m²/day on days 1-3 every 21 days (in combination with vincristine and ifosfamide) (Ogilvie, 2010)

Off-label uses:

Endometrial carcinoma, advanced: Adults: IV: 60 mg/m² on day 1 every 21 days for 8 cycles; maximum cumulative dose: 420 mg/m² (in combination with cisplatin) (Randall, 2006)

Multiple myeloma: Adults: IV:

PAD regimen: Induction: 9 mg/m²/day on days 1 to 4 for 3 cycles (in combination with bortezomib and dexamethasone) (Sonneveld, 2012)

VDT-PACE regimen: 10 mg/m²/day administered as a continuous infusion on days 1 to 4 of each cycle (in combination with bortezomib, dexamethasone, thalidomide, cisplatin, cyclophosphamide, and etoposide) (Lee, 2003; Pineda-Roman, 2008)

Thymomas and thymic malignancies: Adults: IV:

CAP regimen: 50 mg/m² on day 1 every 21 days for up to 8 cycles (in combination with cisplatin and cyclophosphamide) (Loehrer, 1994)

ADOC regimen: 40 mg/m² on day 1 every 21 days (in combination with cisplatin, vincristine, and cyclophosphamide) (Fornasiero, 1991)

Uterine sarcoma: Adults: IV: 60 mg/m² on day 1 every 21 days; maximum cumulative dose: 480 mg/m² (Omura, 1983) **or** 50 mg/m² (over 15 minutes) on day 1 every 21 days; maximum cumulative dose: 450 mg/m² (in combination with ifosfamide/mesna) (Sutton, 1996)

Waldenstrom macroglobulinemia: Adults: IV: *R-CHOP regimen:* 50 mg/m² on day 1 every 21 days for 4 to 8 cycles (in combination with cyclophosphamide, vincristine, prednisone, and rituximab) (Buske, 2009)

Dosing adjustment in toxicity: *Cardiotoxicity:* Discontinue in patients who develop signs/symptoms of cardiomyopathy.

Dosing adjustment in renal impairment:

Mild, moderate, or severe impairment: No dosage adjustment provided in the manufacturers' labeling; however, adjustments are likely not necessary given limited renal excretion.

The following adjustments have also been recommended (Aronoff, 2007):

CrCl <50 mL/minute: No dosage adjustment necessary.

Hemodialysis: Supplemental dose is not necessary.

Dosing adjustment in hepatic impairment:

The manufacturers' labeling recommends the following adjustments:

Serum bilirubin 1.2-3 mg/dL: Administer 50% of dose.

Serum bilirubin 3.1-5 mg/dL: Administer 25% of dose.

Severe hepatic impairment (Child-Pugh class C or bilirubin >5 mg/dL): Use is contraindicated.

The following adjustments have also been recommended (Floyd, 2006):

Transaminases 2-3 times ULN: Administer 75% of dose.

Transaminases >3 times ULN: Administer 50% of dose.

Dosing in obesity: *ASCO Guidelines for appropriate chemotherapy dosing in obese adults with cancer:* Utilize patient's actual body weight (full weight) for calculation of body surface area- or weight-based dosing, particularly when the intent of therapy is curative; manage regimen-related toxicities in the same manner as for nonobese patients; if a dose reduction is utilized due to toxicity, consider resumption of full weight-based dosing with subsequent cycles, especially if cause of toxicity (eg, hepatic or renal impairment) is resolved (Griggs, 2012).

Administration Doxorubicin is associated with a moderate to high emetic potential (depending on dose or regimen); antiemetics are recommended to prevent nausea and vomiting (Basch, 2011; Dupuis, 2011; Roila, 2010).

Administer IV push over at least 3-10 minutes or by continuous infusion (infusion via central venous line recommended). Do not administer IM or SubQ. Rate of administration varies by protocol, refer to individual protocol for details. Protect from light until completion of infusion. Avoid contact with alkaline solutions. Monitor for local erythematous streaking along vein and/or facial flushing (may indicate rapid infusion rate); decrease the rate if occurs.

Vesicant; ensure proper needle or catheter placement prior to and during infusion; avoid extravasation.

Extravasation management: If extravasation occurs, stop infusion immediately and disconnect (leave cannula/needle in place); gently aspirate extravasated solution (do **NOT** flush the line); remove needle/cannula; elevate extremity. Initiate antidote (dexrazoxane or dimethyl sulfate [DMSO]). Apply dry cold compresses for 20 minutes 4 times daily for 1-2 days (Perez Fidalgo, 2012); withhold cooling beginning 15 minutes before dexrazoxane infusion; continue withholding cooling until 15 minutes after infusion is completed. Topical DMSO should not be administered in combination with dexrazoxane; may lessen dexrazoxane efficacy.

Dexrazoxane: Adults: 1000 mg/m² (maximum dose: 2000 mg) IV (administer in a large vein remote from site of extravasation) over 1-2 hours days 1 and 2, then 500 mg/m² (maximum dose: 1000 mg) IV over 1-2 hours day 3; begin within 6 hours of extravasation. Day 2 and day 3 doses should be administered at approximately the same time (± 3 hours) as the dose on day 1 (Mouridsen, 2007; Perez Fidalgo, 2012). **Note:** Reduce dexrazoxane dose by 50% in patients with moderate to severe renal impairment (CrCl <40 mL/minute).

DMSO: Children and Adults: Apply topically to a region covering twice the affected area every 8 hours for 7 days; begin within 10 minutes of extravasation; do not cover with a dressing (Perez Fidalgo, 2012).

Hazardous agent; use appropriate precautions for handling and disposal (NIOSH 2014 [group 1]).

Monitoring Parameters CBC with differential and platelet count; liver function tests (bilirubin, ALT/AST, alkaline phosphatase); serum uric acid, calcium, potassium, phosphate and creatinine; hydration status; cardiac function (baseline, periodic, and followup): ECG, left ventricular ejection fraction (echocardiography [ECHO] or multigated radionuclide angiography [MUGA]); monitor infusion site

Dosage Forms

Solution, Intravenous:

Adriamycin: 2 mg/mL (5 mL, 10 mL, 25 mL, 100 mL)

Generic: 2 mg/mL (5 mL, 10 mL, 25 mL, 100 mL)

Solution, Intravenous [preservative free]:
Generic: 2 mg/mL (5 mL, 10 mL, 25 mL, 75 mL, 100 mL)
Solution Reconstituted, Intravenous:
Adriamycin: 10 mg (1 ea); 20 mg (1 ea); 50 mg (1 ea)
Generic: 50 mg (1 ea)
Solution Reconstituted, Intravenous [preservative free]:
Generic: 10 mg (1 ea)

DOXOrubicin (Liposomal)

(doks oh ROO bi sin lye po SO mal)

Brand Names: U.S. Doxil; Lipodox; Lipodox 50

Brand Names: Canada Caelyx; Myocet

Index Terms DOXOrubicin Hydrochloride (Liposomal); DOXOrubicin Hydrochloride Encapsulated Liposomes (Myocet™); DOXOrubicin Hydrochloride Liposome; DOXOrubicin Hydrochloride Liposomes (Myocet™); Lipodox; Liposomal DOXOrubicin; Pegylated DOXOrubicin Liposomal; Pegylated Liposomal DOXOrubicin; Pegylated Liposomal DOXOrubicin Hydrochloride (Doxil®, Caelyx®)

Pharmacologic Category Antineoplastic Agent, Anthracycline; Antineoplastic Agent, Topoisomerase II Inhibitor

Use

U.S. labeling: Treatment of ovarian cancer (progressive or recurrent after platinum-based treatment); multiple myeloma (in combination with bortezomib in patients who are bortezomib naïve and after failure of at least 1 prior therapy); AIDS-related Kaposi's sarcoma (after failure of or intolerance to prior systemic therapy)

Canadian labeling: Treatment of metastatic breast cancer (as monotherapy [Caelyx®] or in combination with cyclophosphamide [Myocet™]); advanced ovarian cancer (after failure of first-line treatment [Caelyx®]); AIDS-related Kaposi's sarcoma (after failure of or intolerance to prior systemic therapy [Caelyx®])

Pregnancy Risk Factor D

Pregnancy Considerations Adverse events were observed in animal reproduction studies at doses less than the equivalent human dose (based on BSA). May cause fetal harm if administered during pregnancy. Women of childbearing potential should avoid becoming pregnant during treatment.

Breast-Feeding Considerations Due to the potential for serious adverse reactions in the nursing infant, breast-feeding should be discontinued during treatment.

Contraindications Hypersensitivity to doxorubicin liposomal, conventional doxorubicin, or any component of the formulation

Canadian labeling (Caelyx®): Additional contraindications (not in U.S. labeling): Breast-feeding

Warnings/Precautions Hazardous agent - use appropriate precautions for handling and disposal (NIOSH 2014 [group 1]).

[U.S. Boxed Warning]: Doxorubicin may cause cumulative, dose-related myocardial toxicity may lead to congestive heart failure as the cumulative (lifetime) dose of pegylated doxorubicin liposomal approaches 550 mg/m^2. When calculating cumulative doses, also include prior dose of other anthracyclines and anthracenediones. Cardiotoxicity may occur at lower cumulative doses (400 mg/m^2) in patients who have received prior mediastinal irradiation or are receiving concurrent cyclophosphamide treatment. For Myocet™ [Canadian product], cardiotoxicity may occur as the cumulative (lifetime) dose approaches 750 mg/m^2. Anthracycline-induced cardiotoxicity may be delayed (after discontinuation of anthracycline treatment). Use only if potential benefits outweigh cardiovascular risk in patients with a history of cardiovascular disease. Monitor cardiac function with biopsy, echocardiography, or MUGA scan; evaluate left ventricular ejection fraction (LVEF) prior to treatment and periodically during treatment; if results indicate possible heart failure, carefully evaluate the potential effects of continued treatment.

[U.S. Boxed Warning]: Acute infusion reactions may occur, some may be serious/life-threatening (eg, allergic or anaphylactoid reactions). Reactions may include flushing, dyspnea, facial swelling, headache, chills, back pain, hypotension, and/or chest/throat tightness. Infusion reactions typically occur with the first dose and usually resolve with within several hours to a day after terminating the infusion; some have resolved with slowing the infusion rate. To minimize the risk of infusion reactions, infuse at an initial rate of 1 mg/minute. Medications for the treatment of reactions should be readily available in the event of severe reaction.

[U.S. Boxed Warning]: Use with caution in patients with hepatic impairment; dosage reduction is recommended. Use in patients with hepatic impairment has not been adequately studied; no dosing adjustment recommendations are available for multiple myeloma patients with hepatic impairment. **[U.S. Boxed Warning]: Severe myelosuppression may occur.** Monitor blood counts. Treatment delay, dosage modification, or discontinuation may be required. Leukopenia is usually transient, although persistent or severe neutropenia may result in superinfection or neutropenic fever; sepsis due to neutropenia has resulted in discontinuation (may rarely be fatal). Hemorrhage due to thrombocytopenia may occur. Hematologic toxicity may be more severe with combination chemotherapy. Palmar-plantar erythrodysesthesia (hand-foot syndrome) has been reported, more commonly in patients with ovarian cancer and multiple myeloma, and less commonly in patients with Kaposi's sarcoma. May occur early in treatment, but is usually seen after 2-3 treatment cycles. Dosage modification may be required; mild cases resolve within 1-2 weeks; in severe cases, treatment discontinuation may be required. Use of Caelyx® [Canadian product] in splenectomized patients with AIDS-related Kaposi's sarcoma is not recommended (has not been studied). **[U.S. Boxed Warning]: Liposomal formulations of doxorubicin should NOT be substituted for conventional doxorubicin hydrochloride on a mg-per-mg basis.**

Cases of secondary oral cancers (primarily squamous cell carcinoma) have been reported with long-term (>1 year) doxorubicin liposomal exposure; these secondary oral malignancies have occurred during treatment and up to 6 years after treatment. The development of oral ulceration or discomfort should be monitored and further evaluated in patients with past or present use of doxorubicin liposomal. Tissue distribution of the liposomal doxorubicin compared to free doxorubicin may play a role in the development of oral secondary malignancies associated with long-term use.

Doxorubicin may potentiate the toxicity of cyclophosphamide (hemorrhagic cystitis) and mercaptopurine (hepatotoxicity). Radiation recall reaction has been reported with doxorubicin liposomal treatment after radiation therapy. Radiation-induced toxicity (to the myocardium, mucosa, skin, and liver) may be increased by doxorubicin.

Adverse Reactions

Cardiovascular: Cardiac arrest, chest pain, deep thrombophlebitis, edema, hypotension, pallor, peripheral edema, tachycardia, vasodilation

Central nervous system: Agitation, anxiety, chills, confusion, depression, dizziness, emotional lability, fever, headache, insomnia, pain, somnolence, vertigo

Dermatologic: Acne, alopecia, bruising, dry skin, exfoliative dermatitis, fungal dermatitis, furunculosis, maculopapular rash, palmar-plantar erythrodysesthesia/hand-foot syndrome, pruritus, rash, skin discoloration, vesiculobullous rash

Endocrine & metabolic: Dehydration, hyperglycemia, hypercalcemia, hypokalemia, hyponatremia

Gastrointestinal: Abdomen enlarged, anorexia, ascites, cachexia, constipation, diarrhea, dyspepsia, dysphagia, esophagitis, flatulence, gingivitis, glossitis, ileus, intestinal obstruction, mouth ulceration, mucositis, nausea, oral moniliasis, rectal bleeding, stomatitis, taste perversion, vomiting, weight loss, xerostomia

Genitourinary: Cystitis, dysuria, leukorrhea, pelvic pain, polyuria, urinary incontinence, urinary tract infection, urinary urgency, vaginal bleeding, vaginal moniliasis

Hematologic: Anemia, hemolysis, leukopenia, myelosuppression (onset: 7 days; nadir: 10-14 days; recovery: 21-28 days), neutropenia, prothrombin time increased, thrombocytopenia

Neuromuscular & skeletal: Back pain, weakness

Respiratory: Dyspnea, pharyngitis

Hepatic: ALT increased, alkaline phosphatase increased, hyperbilirubinemia

Local: Thrombophlebitis

Neuromuscular & skeletal: Arthralgia, hypertonia, myalgia, neuralgia, neuritis (peripheral), neuropathy, paresthesia, pathological fracture,

Ocular: Conjunctivitis, dry eyes, retinitis

Otic: Ear pain

Renal: Albuminuria, hematuria

Respiratory: Apnea, cough increased, epistaxis, pleural effusion, pneumonia, rhinitis, sinusitis

Miscellaneous: Allergic reaction, diaphoresis, infection; infusion-related reactions (bronchospasm, chest tightness, chills, dyspnea, facial edema, flushing, headache, herpes simplex/zoster, hypotension, pruritus); infection, moniliasis

Rare but important or life-threatening: Abscess, acute brain syndrome, abnormal vision, acute myeloid leukemia (secondary), alkaline phosphatase increased, anaphylactic or anaphylactoid reaction, asthma, balanitis, blindness, bronchitis, BUN increased, bundle branch block, cardiomegaly, cardiomyopathy, cellulitis, CHF, colitis, creatinine increased, cryptococcosis, diabetes mellitus, erythema multiforme, erythema nodosum, eosinophilia, fecal impaction, flu-like syndrome, gastritis, glucosuria, hemiplegia, hemorrhage, hepatic failure, hepatitis, hepatosplenomegaly, hyperkalemia, hypernatremia, hyperuricemia, hyperventilation, hypoglycemia, hypolipidemia, hypomagnesemia, hypophosphatemia, hypoproteinemia, hypothermia, injection site hemorrhage, injection site pain, jaundice, ketosis, lactic dehydrogenase increased, lymphadenopathy, lymphangitis, migraine, myositis, optic neuritis, oral cancers (squamous cell; long-term use), palpitation, pancreatitis, pericardial effusion, petechia, pneumonitis, pneumothorax, pulmonary embolism, radiation injury, reddish/orange discoloration of urine/body fluids, renal failure, sclerosing cholangitis, seizure, sepsis, skin necrosis, skin ulcer, syncope, Stevens-Johnson syndrome, tenesmus, thromboplastin decreased, thrombosis, tinnitus, toxic epidermal necrolysis, urticaria, visual field defect, ventricular arrhythmia

Drug Interactions

Metabolism/Transport Effects Substrate of CYP2D6 (major), CYP3A4 (major); **Note:** Assignment of Major/Minor substrate status based on clinically relevant drug interaction potential; **Inhibits** CYP2B6 (moderate)

Avoid Concomitant Use

Avoid concomitant use of DOXOrubicin (Liposomal) with any of the following: BCG; CloZAPine; Conivaptan; Dipyrone; Fusidic Acid (Systemic); Idelalisib; Natalizumab; Pimecrolimus; Tacrolimus (Topical); Tofacitinib; Vaccines (Live)

Increased Effect/Toxicity

DOXOrubicin (Liposomal) may increase the levels/effects of: CloZAPine; CYP2B6 Substrates; Leflunomide; Natalizumab; Tofacitinib; Vaccines (Live); Zidovudine

The levels/effects of DOXOrubicin (Liposomal) may be increased by: Abiraterone Acetate; Aprepitant; Bevacizumab; Ceritinib; Conivaptan; Cyclophosphamide; CYP2D6 Inhibitors (Moderate); CYP2D6 Inhibitors (Strong); CYP3A4 Inhibitors (Moderate); CYP3A4 Inhibitors (Strong); Dasatinib; Denosumab; Dipyrone; Fosaprepitant; Fusidic Acid (Systemic); Idelalisib; Ivacaftor; Luliconazole; Mifepristone; Netupitant; Peginterferon Alfa-2b; Pimecrolimus; Roflumilast; Simeprevir; Stiripentol; Tacrolimus (Topical); Taxane Derivatives; Trastuzumab

Decreased Effect

DOXOrubicin (Liposomal) may decrease the levels/effects of: BCG; Cardiac Glycosides; Coccidioides immitis Skin Test; Sipuleucel-T; Stavudine; Vaccines (Inactivated); Vaccines (Live); Zidovudine

The levels/effects of DOXOrubicin (Liposomal) may be decreased by: Bosentan; Cardiac Glycosides; CYP3A4 Inducers (Moderate); CYP3A4 Inducers (Strong); Dabrafenib; Deferasirox; Echinacea; Mitotane; Peginterferon Alfa-2b; Siltuximab; St Johns Wort; Tocilizumab

Preparation for Administration Hazardous agent; use appropriate precautions for handling and disposal (NIOSH 2014 [group 1]).

Doxil, Caelyx: Doses ≤90 mg must be diluted in D_5W 250 mL prior to administration. Doses >90 mg should be diluted in D_5W 500 mL. Solution is not clear, but has a red, translucent appearance due to the liposomal dispersion. Dilute only in D_5W; do not use bacteriostatic agents; do not mix with other medications.

Myocet: Refer to product labeling for detailed reconstitution and preparation information.

Storage/Stability Store intact vials refrigerated at 2°C to 8°C (36°F to 46°F); avoid freezing.

Doxil®, Caelyx®: Prolonged freezing may adversely affect liposomal drug products, however, short-term freezing (<1 month) does not appear to have a deleterious effect (Doxil®). Solutions diluted for infusion should be refrigerated at 2°C to 8°C (36°F to 46°F); administer within 24 hours. **Do not infuse with in-line filters.**

Myocet™: Refer to product labeling for detailed reconstitution and preparation information. Following reconstitution, may be stored up to 8 hours at room temperature or up to 72 hours refrigerated at 2°C to 8°C (36°F to 46°F); do not freeze.

Mechanism of Action Doxorubicin inhibits DNA and RNA synthesis by intercalating between DNA base pairs causing steric obstruction and inhibits topoisomerase-II at the point of DNA cleavage. Doxorubicin is also a powerful iron chelator. The iron-doxorubicin complex can bind DNA and cell membranes, producing free hydroxyl (OH) radicals that cleave DNA and cell membranes. Active throughout entire cell cycle. Doxorubicin liposomal is a pegylated formulation which protects the liposomes, and thereby increases blood circulation time.

Pharmacodynamics/Kinetics

Distribution: V_{dss}: 2.7-2.8 L/m^2

Protein binding, plasma: Unknown; nonliposomal (conventional) doxorubicin: 70%

Half-life elimination: Terminal: Distribution: 4.7-5.2 hours, Elimination: 44-55 hours

Metabolism: Hepatic and in plasma to doxorubicinol and the sulfate and glucuronide conjugates of 4-demethyl,7-deoxyaglycones

Excretion: Urine (5% as doxorubicin or doxorubicinol)

Dosage Details concerning dosing in combination regimens should also be consulted. **Liposomal formulations of doxorubicin should NOT be substituted for conventional doxorubicin hydrochloride on a mg-per-mg basis.**

U.S. labeling:

AIDS-related Kaposi's sarcoma: IV: 20 mg/m^2 once every 3 weeks; continue as long as responding and tolerating

Multiple myeloma: IV: 30 mg/m^2 on day 4 every 3 weeks (in combination with bortezomib) for up to 8 cycles until disease progression or unacceptable toxicity

Ovarian cancer, progressive or recurrent: IV: 50 mg/m^2 once every 4 weeks (minimum of 4 cycles is recommended)

Canadian labeling:

AIDS-related Kaposi's sarcoma (Caelyx®): IV: 20 mg/m^2 once every 2-3 weeks; continue as long as responding and tolerating

Breast cancer, metastatic: IV:

Caelyx®: 50 mg/m^2 once every 4 weeks until disease progression or unacceptable toxicity

Myocet™: 60-75 mg/m^2 once every 3 weeks (in combination with cyclophosphamide)

Ovarian cancer, advanced (Caelyx®): IV: 50 mg/m^2 once every 4 weeks until disease progression or unacceptable toxicity

Off-label uses/doses:

Breast cancer, metastatic (off-label use in U.S.): IV: 50 mg/m^2 every 4 weeks (Keller, 2004)

Cutaneous T-cell lymphomas (off-label use): IV: 20 mg/m^2 days 1 and 15 every 4 weeks for 6 cycles (Dummer, 2012) **or** 20 mg/m^2 every 4 weeks (Wollina, 2003)

Hodgkin lymphoma, salvage treatment (off-label use): IV: GVD regimen: 10 mg/m^2 (post-transplant patients) or 15 mg/m^2 (transplant-naive patients) days 1 and 8 every 3 weeks (in combination with gemcitabine and vinorelbine) for 2-6 cycles (Bartlett, 2007)

Multiple myeloma (off-label dosing): IV: 40 mg/m^2 on day 1 every 4 weeks (in combination with vincristine and dexamethasone) for at least 4 cycles (Rifkin, 2006)

Soft tissue sarcoma, advanced (off-label use): IV: 50 mg/m^2 every 4 weeks for 6 cycles (Judson, 2001)

Uterine sarcoma, advanced or recurrent (off-label use): IV: 50 mg/m^2 every 4 weeks until disease progression or unacceptable toxicity (Sutton, 2005)

Dosage adjustment in renal impairment: No dosage adjustment provided in manufacturer's labeling (has not been studied).

Dosage adjustment in hepatic impairment:

U.S. labeling:

Ovarian cancer and AIDS-related Kaposi's sarcoma:

Bilirubin 1.2-3 mg/dL: Administer 50% of normal dose

Bilirubin >3 mg/dL: Administer 25% of normal dose

Multiple myeloma: Dosage adjustment information is not available.

Canadian labeling:

AIDS-related Kaposi's sarcoma (Caelyx®):

Bilirubin 1.2-3 mg/dL: Administer 50% of normal dose

Bilirubin >3 mg/dL: Administer 25% of normal dose

Breast cancer:

Caelyx®:

Bilirubin 1.2-3 mg/dL: Initial dose: Administer 75% of normal dose; if tolerated and no change in bilirubin/hepatic enzymes, may increase to full dose with cycle 2

Bilirubin >3 mg/dL: Initial dose: Administer 50% of normal dose; if tolerated and no change in bilirubin/hepatic enzymes, may increase dose to 75% of normal dose for cycle 2; if cycle 2 dose tolerated, may increase to full dose for subsequent cycles.

Myocet™:

Bilirubin 1.2-3 mg/dL: Administer 50% of normal dose

Bilirubin >3 mg/dL: Administer 25% of normal dose

Ovarian cancer (Caelyx®):

Bilirubin 1.2-3 mg/dL: Initial dose: Administer 75% of normal dose; if tolerated and no change in bilirubin/hepatic enzymes, may increase to full dose with cycle 2

Bilirubin >3 mg/dL: Initial dose: Administer 50% of normal dose; if tolerated and no change in bilirubin/hepatic enzymes, may increase dose to 75% of normal dose for cycle 2; if cycle 2 dose tolerated, may increase to full dose for subsequent cycles.

Dosing in obesity: *ASCO Guidelines for appropriate chemotherapy dosing in obese adults with cancer:* Utilize patient's actual body weight (full weight) for calculation of body surface area- or weight-based dosing, particularly when the intent of therapy is curative; manage regimen-related toxicities in the same manner as for nonobese patients; if a dose reduction is utilized due to toxicity, consider resumption of full weight-based dosing with subsequent cycles, especially if cause of toxicity (eg, hepatic or renal impairment) is resolved (Griggs, 2012).

Dosing adjustment for toxicity:

U.S. labeling: **Note:** Once a dosage reduction is implemented, the dose should not be increased at a later time.

Recommended Dose Modification Guidelines

Toxicity Grade	Dose Adjustment
HAND-FOOT SYNDROME (HFS)	
1 (Mild erythema, swelling, or desquamation not interfering with daily activities)	Redose unless patient has experienced previous Grade 3 or 4 HFS toxicity. If so, delay up to 2 weeks and decrease dose by 25%; return to original dosing interval.
2 (Erythema, desquamation, or swelling interfering with, but not precluding, normal physical activities; small blisters or ulcerations <2 cm in diameter)	Delay dosing up to 2 weeks or until resolved to Grade 0-1. If after 2 weeks there is no resolution, discontinue liposomal doxorubicin. Otherwise, if no prior Grade 3-4 HFS, continue treatment at previous dose and dosage interval. If a prior Grade 3-4 HFS has occurred, continue prior dosage interval, but decrease dose by 25%.
3 (Blistering, ulceration, or swelling interfering with walking or normal daily activities; cannot wear regular clothing)	Delay dosing up to 2 weeks or until resolved to Grade 0-1. Decrease dose by 25% and return to original dosing interval; if after 2 weeks there is no resolution, discontinue liposomal doxorubicin.
4 (Diffuse or local process causing infectious complications, or a bedridden state or hospitalization)	Delay dosing up to 2 weeks or until resolved to Grade 0-1. Decrease dose by 25% and return to original dosing interval. If after 2 weeks there is no resolution, discontinue liposomal doxorubicin.

(continued)

Recommended Dose Modification Guidelines *(continued)*

Toxicity Grade	Dose Adjustment
STOMATITIS	
1 (Painless ulcers, erythema, or mild soreness)	Redose unless patient has experienced previous Grade 3 or 4 toxicity. If so, delay up to 2 weeks and decrease by 25%. Return to original dosing interval.
2 (Painful erythema, edema, or ulcers, but can eat)	Delay dosing up to 2 weeks or until resolved to Grade 0-1. If after 2 weeks there is no resolution, discontinue liposomal doxorubicin. Otherwise, if not prior Grade 3-4 stomatitis, continue treatment at previous dose and dosage interval. If prior Grade 3-4 toxicity, continue treatment with previous dosage interval, but decrease dose by 25%.
3 (Painful erythema, edema, or ulcers, and cannot eat)	Delay dosing up to 2 weeks or until resolved to Grade 0-1. Decrease dose by 25% and return to original dosing interval. If after 2 weeks there is no resolution, discontinue liposomal doxorubicin.
4 (Requires parenteral or enteral support)	Delay dosing up to 2 weeks or until resolved to Grade 0-1. Decrease dose by 25% and return to original dosing interval. If after 2 weeks there is no resolution, discontinue liposomal doxorubicin.

See table: "Hematologic Toxicity"

Hematologic Toxicity (see below for multiple myeloma)

Grade	ANC	Platelets	Modification
1	1500-1900	75,000-150,000	Resume treatment with no dose reduction.
2	1000-<1500	50,000-<75,000	Wait until ANC ≥1500 and platelets ≥75,000; redose with no dose reduction.
3	500-999	25,000-<50,000	Wait until ANC ≥1500 and platelets ≥75,000; redose with no dose reduction.
4	<500	<25,000	Wait until ANC ≥1500 and platelets ≥75,000; redose at 25% dose reduction or continue full dose with cytokine support.

Dosing Adjustment for Toxicity in Treatment with Bortezomib (for Multiple Myeloma) (see Bortezomib monograph for bortezomib dosage reduction with toxicity guidelines):

Fever ≥38°C and ANC <1000/mm³: If prior to doxorubicin liposomal treatment (day 4), do not administer; if after doxorubicin liposomal administered, reduce dose by 25% in next cycle.

ANC <500/mm³, platelets <25,000/mm³, hemoglobin <8 g/dL: If prior to doxorubicin liposomal treatment (day 4); do not administer; if after doxorubicin liposomal administered, reduce dose by' 25% in next cycle if bortezomib dose reduction occurred for hematologic toxicity.

Grade 3 or 4 nonhematologic toxicity: Delay dose until resolved to grade <2; reduce dose by 25% for all subsequent doses.

Neuropathic pain or peripheral neuropathy: No dose reductions needed for doxorubicin liposomal, refer to Bortezomib monograph for bortezomib dosing adjustment.

Canadian labeling:

Caelyx®: Nonhematologic toxicity: Breast cancer, ovarian cancer:

Caelyx®: Recommended Dose Modification Guidelines

Toxicity Grade	Week After Prior Caelyx® Dose (Breast Cancer or Ovarian Cancer)	
	Weeks 4 and 5	Week 6
HAND-FOOT SYNDROME (HFS)		
1 (Mild erythema, swelling, or desquamation not interfering with daily activities)	Redose unless patient has experienced previous Grade 3 or 4 HFS toxicity. If so, wait an additional week	Decrease dose by 25%; return to 4-week interval
2 (Erythema, desquamation, or swelling interfering with, but not precluding, normal physical activities; small blisters or ulcerations <2 cm in diameter)	Wait an additional week	Decrease dose by 25%; return to 4-week interval
3 (Blistering, ulceration, or swelling interfering with walking or normal daily activities; cannot wear regular clothing)	Wait an additional week	Discontinue therapy
4 (Diffuse or local process causing infectious complications, or a bedridden state or hospitalization)	Wait an additional week	Discontinue therapy
STOMATITIS		
1 (Painless ulcers, erythema, or mild soreness)	Redose unless patient has experienced previous Grade 3 or 4 stomatitis. If so, wait an additional week.	Decrease dose by 25%; return to 4-week interval or if warranted, discontinue therapy
2 (Painful erythema, edema, or ulcers, but can eat)	Wait an additional week	Decrease dose by 25%; return to 4-week interval or if warranted, discontinue therapy
3 (Painful erythema, edema, or ulcers, and cannot eat)	Wait an additional week	Discontinue therapy
4 (Requires parenteral or enteral support)	Wait an additional week	Discontinue therapy

Caelyx®: Hematologic toxicity: Breast cancer, ovarian cancer: Refer to U.S. dosage adjustment for hematologic toxicity section.

Caelyx®: Nonhematologic toxicity: AIDS-related Kaposi's sarcoma:

Caelyx®: Recommended Dose Modification Guidelines: Hand-Foot Syndrome (HFS) (AIDS-related Kaposi's Sarcoma)

Toxicity Grade	Weeks Since Last Caelyx® Dose (AIDS-related Kaposi's Sarcoma)	
	3 Weeks	**4 Weeks**
HAND-FOOT SYNDROME (HFS)		
1 (Mild erythema, swelling, or desquamation not interfering with daily activities)	Redose unless patient has experienced previous Grade 3 or 4 skin toxicity. If so, wait an additional week	Decrease dose by 25%; return to 3-week interval
2 (Erythema, desquamation, or swelling interfering with, but not precluding, normal physical activities; small blisters or ulcerations <2 cm in diameter)	Wait an additional week	Decrease dose by 50%; return to 3-week interval
3 (Blistering, ulceration, or swelling interfering with walking or normal daily activities; cannot wear regular clothing)	Wait an additional week	Discontinue therapy
4 (Diffuse or local process causing infectious complications, or a bedridden state or hospitalization)	Wait an additional week	Discontinue therapy

Caelyx®: Recommended Dose Modification Guidelines: Stomatitis (AIDS-related Kaposi's Sarcoma)

STOMATITIS Toxicity grade:	Caelyx® Dosage Adjustment (AIDS-related Kaposi's Sarcoma)
1 (Painless ulcers, erythema, or mild soreness)	No dosage adjustment
2 (Painful erythema, edema, or ulcers, but can eat)	Wait 1 week and if symptoms improve, redose at 100% dose
3 (Painful erythema, edema, or ulcers, and cannot eat)	Wait 1 week and if symptoms improve, redose with a 25% dose reduction
4 (Requires parenteral or enteral support)	Wait 1 week and if symptoms improve, redose with a 50% dose reduction

Caelyx®: Hematologic toxicity: AIDS-related Kaposi's sarcoma:

Caelyx®: Hematologic Toxicity (AIDS-related Kaposi's Sarcoma)

Grade	ANC	Platelets	Modification
1	1500-1900	75,000-150,000	None
2	1000-<1500	50,000-<75,000	None
3	500-999	25,000-<50,000	Wait until ANC ≥1000 and/or platelets ≥50,000; redose with a 25% dose reduction.
4	<500	<25,000	Wait until ANC ≥1000 and/or platelets ≥50,000; redose with a 50% dose reduction.

Myocet™: Hematologic or gastrointestinal toxicity: Dosage reduction: If initial dose was 75 mg/m^2, reduce dose to 60 mg/m^2; if initial dose was 60 mg/m^2, reduce dose to 50 mg/m^2. If toxicity persists with subsequent cycles, consider reducing dose further (from 60 mg/m^2 to 50 mg/m^2 or from 50 mg/m^2 to 40 mg/m^2).

Neutropenia: If grade 4 neutropenia (ANC <500/mm^3) without fever lasting ≥7 days or grade 4 neutropenia of any duration with concurrent fever (≥38.5°C) occurs, consider reducing dose with subsequent cycles. **Note:** Prior to dose reductions, prophylactic cytokine therapy may be considered.

Thrombocytopenia or anemia: If grade 4 thrombocytopenia or anemia occurs, hold therapy until recovery to ≤ grade 2. Reduce dose with subsequent cycles or consider discontinuing treatment.

Gastrointestinal toxicity or mucositis: Grade 3 mucositis persisting ≥3 days, or grade 4 mucositis of any duration, or grade 3 or 4 gastrointestinal toxicity not responsive to interventions and/or prophylaxis: Consider dose reduction with subsequent cycles.

Administration Do not administer as a bolus injection or IM or SubQ. Avoid extravasation (irritant); monitor infusion site; extravasation may occur without stinging or burning. Monitor for infusion reaction.

Doxil, Caelyx: Administer IVPB over 60 minutes; manufacturer recommends administering at initial rate of 1 mg/minute to minimize risk of infusion reactions until the absence of a reaction has been established, then increase the infusion rate for completion over 1 hour. Do **NOT** administer undiluted. Do **NOT** infuse with in-line filters. Incompatible with heparin flushes; flush with 5-10 mL of D_5W solution before and after drug administration (do not rapidly flush through the IV line). Monitor for local erythematous streaking along vein and/or facial flushing (may indicate rapid infusion rate).

Myocet: Infuse over 1 hour.

Hazardous agent; use appropriate precautions for handling and disposal (NIOSH 2014 [group 1]).

Monitoring Parameters CBC with differential and platelet count, liver function tests (ALT/AST, bilirubin, alkaline phosphatase); monitor for infusion reactions, hand-foot syndrome, stomatitis, and oral ulceration/discomfort suggestive of secondary oral malignancy

Cardiac function (left ventricular ejection fraction [LVEF]; baseline and periodic); echocardiography, or MUGA scan may be used. Endomyocardial biopsy is the most definitive test for anthracycline myocardial injury.

Dosage Forms

Injectable, Intravenous:

Doxil: 2 mg/mL (10 mL, 25 mL)

Lipodox: 2 mg/mL (10 mL)

Lipodox 50: 2 mg/mL (25 mL)

Generic: 2 mg/mL (10 mL, 25 mL)

Dosage Forms: Canada

Injection, solution, as hydrochloride, pegylated:

Caelyx®: 2 mg/mL (10 mL, 25 mL)

Injection, encapsulated liposomes:

Myocet™: 3-vial kit (doxorubicin HCl for injection 50 mg/vial, liposomes for injection, and buffer for injection)

◆ **Doxorubicin HCl** *see* DOXOrubicin (Conventional) *on page 679*

◆ **Doxorubicin Hydrochloride** *see* DOXOrubicin (Conventional) *on page 679*

◆ **DOXOrubicin Hydrochloride Encapsulated Liposomes (Myocet™)** *see* DOXOrubicin (Liposomal) *on page 684*

◆ **Doxorubicin Hydrochloride For Injection, USP (Can)** *see* DOXOrubicin (Conventional) *on page 679*

◆ **Doxorubicin Hydrochloride Injection (Can)** *see* DOXOrubicin (Conventional) *on page 679*

◆ **DOXOrubicin Hydrochloride (Liposomal)** *see* DOXOrubicin (Liposomal) *on page 684*

◆ **DOXOrubicin Hydrochloride Liposome** *see* DOXOrubicin (Liposomal) *on page 684*

◆ **DOXOrubicin Hydrochloride Liposomes (Myocet™)** *see* DOXOrubicin (Liposomal) *on page 684*

◆ **Doxy 100** *see* Doxycycline *on page 689*

◆ **Doxycin (Can)** *see* Doxycycline *on page 689*

Doxycycline (doks i SYE kleen)

Brand Names: U.S. Acticlate; Adoxa; Adoxa Pak 1/100; Adoxa Pak 1/150; Adoxa Pak 2/100; Alodox Convenience; Avidoxy; Doryx; Doxy 100; Monodox; Morgidox; NicAzel-Doxy 30; NicAzelDoxy 60; Ocudox; Oracea; Vibramycin

Brand Names: Canada Apo-Doxy; Apo-Doxy Tabs; Apprilon; Dom-Doxycycline; Doxycin; Doxytab; Periostat; PHL-Doxycycline; PMS-Doxycycline; Teva-Doxycycline; Vibra-Tabs; Vibramycin

Index Terms Doxycycline Calcium; Doxycycline Hyclate; Doxycycline Monohydrate

Pharmacologic Category Antibiotic, Tetracycline Derivative

Use Principally in the treatment of infections caused by susceptible *Rickettsia*, *Chlamydia*, *Chlamydophila*, and *Mycoplasma*; malaria prophylaxis (areas with chloroquine-and/or pyrimethamine-sulfadoxine resistant strains) for short-term travel (<4 months); treatment for syphilis, uncomplicated *Neisseria gonorrhoeae* (alternative agent), *Listeria*, *Actinomyces israelii*, and *Clostridium* infections in penicillin-allergic patients; used for community-acquired pneumonia and other common infections due to susceptible organisms; anthrax due to *Bacillus anthracis*, including inhalational anthrax (postexposure); treatment of infections caused by uncommon susceptible gram-negative and gram-positive organisms including *Borrelia recurrentis*, *Ureaplasma urealyticum*, *Haemophilus ducreyi*, *Yersinia pestis*, *Francisella tularensis*, *Vibrio cholerae*, *Campylobacter fetus*, *Brucella* spp, *Bartonella bacilliformis*, and *Klebsiella granulomatis*, Q fever; intestinal amebiasis; severe acne

Oracea (U.S. labeling), Apprilon (Canadian labeling): Treatment of inflammatory lesions associated with rosacea

Periostat (Canadian labeling; not available in U.S.): Adjunctive periodontitis treatment to scaling and root planing to promote attachment level gain and reduce pocket depth

Pregnancy Risk Factor D

Pregnancy Considerations Tetracyclines cross the placenta and accumulate in developing teeth and long tubular bones. Therapeutic doses of doxycycline during pregnancy are unlikely to produce substantial teratogenic risk, but data are insufficient to say that there is no risk. In general, reports of exposure have been limited to short durations of therapy in the first trimester. Tetracyclines may discolor fetal teeth following maternal use during pregnancy; the specific teeth involved and the portion of the tooth affected depends on the timing and duration of exposure relative to tooth calcification. As a class, tetracyclines are generally considered second-line antibiotics in pregnant women and their use should be avoided. Tetracycline medications should be used during pregnancy only when other medications are contraindicated or ineffective (Mylonas, 2011).

Breast-Feeding Considerations Doxycycline is excreted in breast milk (Chung, 2002). According to the manufacturer, the decision to continue or discontinue breast-feeding during therapy should take into account the risk of exposure to the infant and the benefits of treatment to the mother. Although nursing is not specifically contraindicated, the effects of long-term exposure via breast milk are not known. Oral absorption of doxycycline is not markedly influenced by simultaneous ingestion of milk; therefore, oral absorption of doxycycline by the breast-feeding infant would not be expected to be diminished by the calcium in the maternal milk. Nondose-related effects could include modification of bowel flora.

Contraindications

U.S. labeling: Hypersensitivity to doxycycline, tetracycline, or any component of the formulation

Canadian labeling: Hypersensitivity to doxycycline, tetracycline, or any component of the formulation; myasthenia gravis

Periostat®, Apprilon™: Additional contraindications: Use in infants and children <8 years of age or during second or third trimester of pregnancy; breast-feeding

Warnings/Precautions Photosensitivity reaction may occur with this drug; avoid prolonged exposure to sunlight or tanning equipment. Antianabolic effects of tetracyclines can increase BUN (dose-related). Hypersensitivity syndromes have been reported, including drug rash with eosinophilia and systemic symptoms (DRESS), urticaria, angioneurotic edema, anaphylaxis, anaphylactoid purpura, serum sickness, pericarditis, and systemic lupus erythematosus exacerbation. Hepatotoxicity rarely occurs; if symptomatic, conduct LFT and discontinue drug. Intracranial hypertension (headache, blurred vision, diplopia, vision loss, and/or papilledema) has been associated with use. Women of childbearing age who are overweight or have a history of intracranial hypertension are at greater risk. Concomitant use of isotretinoin (known to cause pseudotumor cerebri) and doxycycline should be avoided. Intracranial hypertension typically resolves after discontinuation of treatment; however, permanent visual loss is possible. If visual symptoms develop during treatment, prompt ophthalmologic evaluation is warranted. Intracranial pressure can remain elevated for weeks after drug discontinuation; monitor patients until they stabilize. Prolonged use may result in fungal or bacterial superinfection, including *C. difficile*-associated diarrhea (CDAD) and pseudomembranous colitis; CDAD has been observed >2 months postantibiotic treatment. May cause tissue hyperpigmentation, tooth enamel hypoplasia, or permanent tooth discoloration; use of tetracyclines should be avoided during tooth development (last half or pregnancy, infancy, and children <8 years of age) unless other drugs are not likely to be effective or are contraindicated. However, recommended in treatment of anthrax exposure, tickborne rickettsial diseases, and Q fever. Do not use during pregnancy. In addition to affecting tooth development, tetracycline use has been associated with retardation of skeletal development and reduced bone growth. When used for malaria prophylaxis, does not completely suppress asexual blood stages of *Plasmodium* strains. ▶

Doxycycline does not suppress *Plasmodium falciparum*'s sexual blood stage gametocytes. Patients completing a regimen may still transmit the infection to mosquitoes outside endemic areas.

Oracea® (U.S. labeling) or Apprilon™ (Canadian labeling): Additional specific warnings: Should not be used for the treatment or prophylaxis of bacterial infections, since the lower dose of drug per capsule may be subefficacious and promote resistance. Syrup contains sodium metabisulfite. Effectiveness of products intended for use in periodontitis has not been established in patients with coexistent oral candidiasis; use with caution in patients with a history or predisposition to oral candidiasis.

Adverse Reactions

Central nervous system: Bulging fontanel (infants), headache, intracranial hypertension (adults), pericarditis

Dermatologic: Discoloration of thyroid gland (brown/black, no dysfunction reported), erythema multiforme, erythematous rash, exfoliative dermatitis, maculopapular rash, skin hyperpigmentation, skin photosensitivity, Stevens-Johnson syndrome, toxic epidermal necrolysis, urticaria

Endocrine & metabolic: Hypoglycemia

Gastrointestinal: Anorexia, *Clostridium difficile* associated diarrhea, dental discoloration (children), diarrhea, dysphagia, enterocolitis, esophageal ulcer, esophagitis, glossitis, nausea, upper abdominal pain, vomiting

Genitourinary: Vaginitis (bacterial, 3%), vulvovaginal disease (mycotic infection, 2%), inflammatory anogenital lesion

Hematologic & oncologic: Anaphylactoid purpura, eosinophilia, hemolytic anemia, neutropenia, thrombocytopenia

Hepatic: Hepatotoxicity (rare)

Hypersensitivity: Anaphylaxis, angioedema, serum sickness

Neuromuscular & skeletal: Exacerbation of systemic lupus erythematosus

Renal: Increased blood urea nitrogen (dose related)

Note: Additional adverse reactions not listed above that have been reported with Oracea or Periostat (Canadian availability; not available in the U.S.):

Periostat: Arthralgia (6%), dyspepsia (6%), dysmenorrhea (4%), pain (4%), bronchitis (3%)

Oracea: Nasopharyngitis (5%), hypertension (3%), sinusitis (3%), anxiety (2%), fungal infection (2%), increased blood pressure (2%), increased lactate dehydrogenase (2%), increased serum AST (2%), influenza (2%), pain (2%), abdominal pain (1% to 2%), back pain (1%), hyperglycemia (1%), sinus headache (1%), xerostomia (1%)

Drug Interactions

Metabolism/Transport Effects **Inhibits** CYP3A4 (weak)

Avoid Concomitant Use

Avoid concomitant use of Doxycycline with any of the following: BCG; Pimozide; Retinoic Acid Derivatives; Strontium Ranelate

Increased Effect/Toxicity

Doxycycline may increase the levels/effects of: ARIPiprazole; Dofetilide; Hydrocodone; Lomitapide; Mipomersen; Neuromuscular-Blocking Agents; Pimozide; Porfimer; Retinoic Acid Derivatives; Verteporfin; Vitamin K Antagonists

Decreased Effect

Doxycycline may decrease the levels/effects of: BCG; Iron Salts; Penicillins; Sodium Picosulfate; Typhoid Vaccine

The levels/effects of Doxycycline may be decreased by: Antacids; Barbiturates; Bile Acid Sequestrants; Bismuth; Bismuth Subsalicylate; Calcium Salts; CarBAMazepine; Fosphenytoin; Iron Salts; Lanthanum; Magnesium Salts; Multivitamins/Minerals (with ADEK, Folate, Iron); Multivitamins/Minerals (with AE, No Iron); Phenytoin; Quinapril; Rifampin; Strontium Ranelate; Sucralfate; Sucroferric Oxyhydroxide

Food Interactions

Ethanol: Chronic ethanol ingestion may reduce the serum concentration of doxycycline.

Food: Doxycycline serum levels may be slightly decreased if taken with food or milk. Administration with iron or calcium may decrease doxycycline absorption. May decrease absorption of calcium, iron, magnesium, zinc, and amino acids. Management: Doryx® tablets can be administered without regard to meals.

Preparation for Administration IV infusion: Following reconstitution with sterile water for injection, dilute to a final concentration of 0.1-1 mg/mL using a compatible solution.

Storage/Stability

Capsule, tablet: Store at 20°C to 25°C (68°F to 77°F); excursions are permitted between 15°C and 30°C (59°F and 86°F). Protect from light and moisture.

Syrup, oral suspension: Store below 30°C (86°F); protect from light.

IV infusion: Protect from light. Stability varies based on solution.

Mechanism of Action Inhibits protein synthesis by binding with the 30S and possibly the 50S ribosomal subunit(s) of susceptible bacteria; may also cause alterations in the cytoplasmic membrane

Periostat® capsules (Canadian availability; not available in the U.S.): Proposed mechanism: Has been shown to inhibit collagenase activity *in vitro*. Also has been noted to reduce elevated collagenase activity in the gingival crevicular fluid of patients with periodontal disease. Systemic levels do not reach inhibitory concentrations against bacteria.

Pharmacodynamics/Kinetics

Absorption: Oral: Almost complete

Distribution: Widely into body tissues and fluids including synovial, pleural, prostatic, seminal fluids, and bronchial secretions; saliva, aqueous humor, and CSF penetration is poor; Periostat® (Canadian availability; not available in the U.S.): ~53-134 L

Protein binding: 90%

Metabolism: Not hepatic; partially inactivated in GI tract by chelate formation

Bioavailability: Reduced at high pH; may be clinically significant in patients with gastrectomy, gastric bypass surgery or who are otherwise deemed achlorhydric

Half-life elimination: Single dose: 12-15 hours (usually increases to 22-24 hours with multiple doses); End-stage renal disease: 18-25 hours

Oracea® (U.S. labeling), Apprilon™ (Canadian labeling): Single dose: 21 hours

Periostat®: Single dose: 18 hours

Time to peak, serum: 1.5-4 hours

Excretion: Feces (30%); urine (23%)

Dosage

Usual dosage range:

Children >8 years (≤45 kg): Oral, IV: 2-5 mg/kg/day in 1-2 divided doses, not to exceed 200 mg/day

Children >8 years (>45 kg) and Adults: Oral, IV: 100-200 mg/day in 1-2 divided doses

Indication-specific dosing:

Children:

Anthrax: Doxycycline should be used in children if antibiotic susceptibility testing, exhaustion of drug supplies, or allergic reaction preclude use of penicillin or ciprofloxacin. For treatment, the consensus recommendation does not include a loading dose for doxycycline.

Inhalational (postexposure prophylaxis) (ACIP, 2010): Oral, IV (use oral route when possible):
≤8 years: 2.2 mg/kg every 12 hours for 60 days
>8 years and ≤45 kg: 2.2 mg/kg every 12 hours for 60 days
>8 years and >45 kg: 100 mg every 12 hours for 60 days
Cutaneous (treatment): Oral: See dosing for "Inhalational (postexposure prophylaxis)"
Note: In the presence of systemic involvement, extensive edema, and/or lesions on head/neck, doxycycline should initially be administered IV
Inhalational/gastrointestinal/oropharyngeal (treatment): IV: Refer to dosing for inhalational anthrax (postexposure prophylaxis); switch to oral therapy when clinically appropriate
Note: Initial treatment should include two or more agents predicted to be effective (CDC, 2001). Agents suggested for use in conjunction with doxycycline or ciprofloxacin include rifampin, vancomycin, imipenem, penicillin, ampicillin, chloramphenicol, clindamycin, and clarithromycin. May switch to oral antimicrobial therapy when clinically appropriate. Continue combined therapy for 60 days

Community-acquired pneumonia (CAP) (IDSA/PIDS, 2011): Oral: Children >7 years: **Note:** A beta-lactam antibiotic should be added if typical bacterial pneumonia cannot be ruled out.
Presumed atypical, mild atypical (*M. pneumoniae, C. pneumoniae, C. trachomatis*) infection or step-down therapy (alternative to azithromycin): 2-4 mg/kg/day in 2 divided doses (maximum: 200 mg/day)

Cellulitis (purulent) due to community-acquired MRSA (off-label use): Oral: Children >8 years and ≤45 kg: 2 mg/kg/dose every 12 hours for 5-10 days (Liu, 2011)

Localized juvenile periodontitis (LJP) (off-label use): Oral: 50-100 mg/day

Q fever: Oral:
Acute:
Children <8 years with high-risk criteria (eg, hospitalized or have severe illness, with preexisting heart valvulopathy, immunocompromised, or with delayed Q fever diagnosis who have experienced illness for >14 days without resolution of symptoms): 2.2 mg/kg/dose (maximum: 100 mg per dose) twice daily for 14 days (CDC, 2013).
Children <8 years with mild or uncomplicated illness: 2.2 mg/kg/dose (maximum: 100 mg per dose) twice daily for 5 days. If patient remains febrile past 5 days of treatment, switch to sulfamethoxazole and trimethoprim (CDC, 2013). **Note:** Some clinicians may recommend initial treatment with sulfamethoxazole and trimethoprim for children <8 years with mild or uncomplicated illness (Hartzell, 2008; CDC, 2013).
Children ≥8 years and Adolescents: 2.2 mg/kg/dose (maximum: 100 mg per dose) twice daily for 14 days (CDC, 2013).
Chronic: ID consult recommended for treatment of chronic Q fever (CDC, 2013)

Tickborne rickettsial disease: Oral, IV: Children ≤8 years: 2.2 mg/kg (maximum dose: 100 mg) every 12 hours for 5-7 days; severe or complicated disease may require longer treatment; human granulocytotropic anaplasmosis (HGA) should be treated for 10-14 days. **Note:** The American Academy of Pediatrics Committee on Infectious Diseases identifies doxycycline as the drug of choice in children of any age.

Tularemia: IV (may transition to oral if clinically indicated) (Dennis, 2001):
Children <45 kg: 2.2 mg/kg every 12 hours for 14-21 days
Children ≥45 kg: 100 mg every 12 hours for 14-21 days

Children ≥8 years:

Lyme disease (off-label use): Oral (Halperin, 2007; Wormser, 2006):
Prevention: 4 mg/kg (maximum: 200 mg) administered as a single dose; **Note:** Initiate within 72 hours of tick removal
Treatment (early Lyme disease without neurologic manifestations): 1-2 mg/kg twice daily for 10-21 days (maximum: 100 mg/dose)
Treatment (meningitis and other early neurologic manifestations): 4-8 mg/kg/day in 2 divided doses for 10-28 days (maximum: 200 mg/dose)

Malaria chemoprophylaxis: Oral:
Manufacturer's recommendation: 2 mg/kg/day (maximum: 100 mg daily). Start 1-2 days prior to travel to endemic area; continue daily during travel and for 4 weeks after leaving endemic area (CDC, 2012)
Alternative recommendation: 2.2 mg/kg/day (maximum: 100 mg daily). Start 1-2 days prior to travel to endemic area; continue daily during travel and for 4 weeks after leaving endemic area (CDC, 2012)

Malaria, severe, treatment (off-label use): Oral, IV:
<45 kg: 2.2 mg/kg (maximum dose: 100 mg) every 12 hours for 7 days with quinidine gluconate. **Note:** Quinidine gluconate duration is region specific; consult CDC for current recommendations (CDC, 2011).
≥45 kg: 100 mg every 12 hours for 7 days with quinidine gluconate. **Note:** Quinidine gluconate duration is region specific; consult CDC for current recommendations (CDC, 2011).

Malaria, uncomplicated, treatment (off-label use): Oral: 2.2 mg/kg (maximum dose: 100 mg) every 12 hours for 7 days with quinine sulfate. **Note:** Quinine sulfate duration is region specific; consult CDC for current recommendations (CDC, 2011).

Children >8 years (and >45 kg) and Adults:

Cellulitis (purulent) due to community-acquired MRSA (off-label use): Oral: 100 mg twice daily for 5-10 days (Liu, 2011)

Chlamydial infections, uncomplicated: Oral: *Manufacturer's recommendation:* 100 mg twice daily for 7 days; alternatively, for endocervical or urethral infections, may give 200 mg once daily for 7 days

Tickborne rickettsial disease: Oral, IV: 100 mg twice daily for 5-7 days; severe or complicated disease may require longer treatment; human granulocytotropic anaplasmosis (HGA) should be treated for 10-14 days. **Note:** The American Academy of Pediatrics Committee on Infectious Diseases identifies doxycycline as the drug of choice in children of any age.

Adults:

Acute bacterial rhinosinusitis (off-label use): Oral: 200 mg/day in 1-2 divided doses for 5-7 days (Chow, 2012)

Anthrax:
Inhalational (postexposure prophylaxis): Oral, IV (use oral route when possible): 100 mg every 12 hours for 60 days (ACIP, 2010)
Cutaneous (treatment): Oral: 100 mg every 12 hours for 60 days. **Note:** In the presence of systemic involvement, extensive edema, lesions on head/neck, refer to IV dosing for treatment of inhalational/gastrointestinal/oropharyngeal anthrax

Inhalational/gastrointestinal/oropharyngeal (treatment): IV: Initial: 100 mg every 12 hours; switch to oral therapy when clinically appropriate; some recommend initial loading dose of 200 mg, followed by 100 mg every 8-12 hours (Franz, 1997). **Note:** Initial treatment should include two or more agents predicted to be effective (CDC, 2001). Agents suggested for use in conjunction with doxycycline or ciprofloxacin include rifampin, vancomycin, imipenem, penicillin, ampicillin, chloramphenicol, clindamycin, and clarithromycin. May switch to oral antimicrobial therapy when clinically appropriate. Continue combined therapy for 60 days

Brucellosis: Oral: 100 mg twice daily for 6 weeks with rifampin or streptomycin

Community-acquired pneumonia, bronchitis: Oral, IV: 100 mg twice daily (Ailani, 1999; Mandell, 2007)

Epididymitis: Oral: 100 mg twice daily for 10 days (in combination with ceftriaxone) (CDC, 2010)

Gonococcal infection, uncomplicated: Oral: **Note:** Azithromycin is preferred over doxycycline as the second antimicrobial in combination with ceftriaxone in uncomplicated infections due to a high prevalence of tetracycline resistance in isolates (CDC, 2012).

Cervix, rectum (off-label use), urethra: 100 mg twice daily for 7 days in combination with ceftriaxone (preferred) or cefixime (only if ceftriaxone is not available and test-of-cure follow up in 7 days) (CDC, 2010; CDC, 2012).

Pharynx: 100 mg twice daily for 7 days in combination with ceftriaxone (CDC, 2012).

Alternatively, the manufacturer recommends a single-visit dose in nonanorectal infections in men: 300 mg initially, repeat dose in 1 hour (total dose: 600 mg)

Granuloma inguinale (donovanosis): Oral: 100 mg twice daily for at least 3 weeks (and until lesions have healed) (CDC, 2010)

Lyme disease (off-label use): Oral (Halperin, 2007; Wormser, 2006):

Prevention: Initiate within 72 hours of tick removal: 200 mg administered as a single dose

Treatment (early Lyme disease without neurologic manifestations): 100 mg twice daily for 10-21 days

Treatment (meningitis or other early neurologic manifestations): 100-200 mg twice daily for 14 days (range: 10-28 days)

Lymphogranuloma venereum: Oral: 100 mg twice daily for 21 days (CDC, 2010)

Malaria chemoprophylaxis: Oral: 100 mg daily. Start 1-2 days prior to travel to endemic area; continue daily during travel and for 4 weeks after leaving endemic area

Malaria, severe, treatment (off-label use): Oral, IV: 100 mg every 12 hours for 7 days with quinidine gluconate. **Note:** Quinidine gluconate duration is region specific; consult CDC for current recommendations (CDC, 2011).

Malaria, uncomplicated, treatment (off-label use): Oral: 100 mg twice daily for 7 days with quinine sulfate. **Note:** Quinine sulfate duration is region specific; consult CDC for current recommendations (CDC, 2011).

Nongonococcal urethritis: Oral: 100 mg twice daily for 7 days (CDC, 2010)

Pelvic inflammatory disease:

Treatment, inpatient: Oral, IV: 100 mg twice daily (in combination with cefoxitin or cefotetan); may transition to oral doxycycline (add clindamycin or metronidazole if tubo-ovarian abscess present) to complete 14 days of treatment (CDC, 2010)

Treatment, outpatient: Oral: 100 mg twice daily for 14 days (with or without metronidazole); preceded by a single IM dose of cefoxitin (plus oral probenecid) or ceftriaxone (CDC, 2010)

Periodontitis: Oral (Periostat® [Canadian availability; not available in the U.S.]): 20 mg twice daily as an adjunct following scaling and root planing; may treat for up to 9 months

Periodontitis, refractory (off-label use): Oral: 100-200 mg daily (Jolkovsky, 2006)

Proctitis: Oral: 100 mg twice daily for 7 days (in combination with ceftriaxone) (CDC, 2010)

Prosthetic joint infection (off-label use): Oral:

Chronic oral antimicrobial suppression:

Propionibacterium spp (alternative to penicillin or amoxicillin): 100 mg twice daily (Osmon, 2013)

Staphylococci (oxacillin-resistant): 100 mg twice daily (Osmon, 2013)

Staphylococci (oxacillin-sensitive or –resistant) oral phase treatment (after completion of pathogen-specific IV) following 1-stage exchange:

Total ankle, elbow, hip, or shoulder arthroplasty: 100 mg twice daily for 3 months; **Note:** Must be used in combination with rifampin (Osmon, 2013).

Total knee arthroplasty: 100 mg twice daily for 6 months; **Note:** Must be used in combination with rifampin (Osmon, 2013)

Q fever: Oral:

Acute: 100 mg every 12 hours for 14 days (CDC, 2013); **Note:** In patients who have valvular heart disease, consider increasing the duration of therapy to 1 year and adding hydroxychloroquine to the regimen to prevent endocarditis; consultation with an infectious disease expert is recommended (CDC, 2002; Fenollar, 2001).

Chronic (CDC, 2013):

Endocarditis or vascular infection: 100 mg every 12 hours in combination with hydroxychloroquine for ≥18 months

Noncardiac organ disease: 100 mg every 12 hours in combination with hydroxychloroquine (duration based on serologic response; ID consult recommended)

Postpartum with serologic evidence present >12 months after delivery: 100 mg every 12 hours in combination with hydroxychloroquine for 12 months

Rosacea Oral (Oracea® [U.S. labeling], Apprilon™ [Canadian labeling]): 40 mg once daily in the morning

Sclerosing agent for pleural effusion (off-label use): Intrapleural: 500 mg as a single dose in 100 mL NS (Porcel, 2006); may require a repeat dose (Kvale, 2007)

Syphilis:

Primary/secondary syphilis: Oral: 100 mg twice daily for 14 days (CDC, 2010)

Latent syphilis: Oral: 100 mg twice daily for 28 days (CDC, 2010)

Tularemia: IV (may transition to oral if clinically appropriate): Initial: 100 mg every 12 hours for 14-21 days (Dennis, 2001)

Vibrio cholerae: Oral: 300 mg as a single dose (WHO, 2004)

***Yersinia pestis* (plague):** Oral, IV: 200 mg initially then 100 mg twice daily **or** 200 mg once daily for 10 days (Daya, 2005; Inglesby, 2000)

Dosage adjustment in renal impairment: No dosage adjustment necessary.

Poorly dialyzed; no supplemental dose or dosage adjustment necessary, including patients on intermittent hemodialysis, peritoneal dialysis, or continuous renal replacement therapy (eg, CVVHD).

Dosage adjustment in hepatic impairment: There are no dosage adjustments provided in the manufacturer's labeling.

Dietary Considerations

Tetracyclines (in general): Take with food if gastric irritation occurs. While administration with food may decrease GI absorption of doxycycline by up to 20%, administration on an empty stomach is not recommended due to GI intolerance. Of currently available tetracyclines, doxycycline has the least affinity for calcium.

Doryx tablets: May be taken without regard to meals; nausea occurs more frequently when taken on an empty stomach.

Oracea (U.S. labeling), Apprilon (Canadian labeling): Take on an empty stomach 1 hour before or 2 hours after meals.

Periostat (Canadian availability; not available in the U.S.): Take at least 1 hour before morning and evening meals.

Some products may contain sodium.

Administration Oral administration is preferable unless patient has significant nausea and vomiting; IV and oral routes are bioequivalent.

Oral: May give with meals to decrease GI upset. Capsule and tablet: Administer with at least 8 ounces of water and have patient sit up for at least 30 minutes after taking to reduce the risk of esophageal irritation and ulceration.

Oracea (U.S. labeling), Apprilon (Canadian labeling): Administer on an empty stomach 1 hour before or 2 hours after meals.

Doryx: Administer without regard to meals; nausea occurs more frequently when taken on an empty stomach. May be administered by carefully breaking up the tablet and sprinkling tablet contents on a spoonful of cold applesauce. The delayed release pellets must not be crushed or damaged when breaking up tablet. Should be administered immediately after preparation and without chewing.

Periostat (Canadian availability; not available in the U.S.): Administer 1 hour before breakfast and evening meal.

IV: Infuse IV doxycycline over 1-4 hours. Avoid extravasation. Prolonged IV administration may cause thrombophlebitis. Oral administration is preferable unless patient has significant nausea and vomiting; IV and oral routes are bioequivalent.

Intrapleural (off-label route): Add to 100 mL NS and instill into chest tube (Porcel, 2006)

Monitoring Parameters Perform culture and sensitivity testing prior to initiating therapy. CBC, renal and liver function tests periodically with prolonged therapy. When used as part of alternative treatment for gonococcal infection, test of cure 7 days after dose (CDC, 2012).

Patients with no risk factors for chronic Q fever should undergo clinical and serological evaluation 6 months after diagnosis of acute Q fever to identify possible progression to chronic disease. Postpartum women treated during pregnancy for acute Q fever, others who are at high risk for progression to chronic disease or when used as part of treatment for chronic Q fever infection unrelated to endocarditis or vascular infection (eg, osteoarticular infections or chronic hepatitis), assess serologic response at 3, 6, 12, 18, and 24 months after diagnosis of acute Q fever (or after delivery in pregnant women) (CDC, 2013).

Additional Information Oracea® (U.S. labeling) or Apprilon™ (Canadian labeling) capsules are not bioequivalent to other doxycycline products.

Dosage Forms Considerations

Alodox Convenience kits contain doxycycline tablets 20 mg, plus eyelid cleanser

Morgidox kits contain doxycycline capsules 100 mg, plus AcuWash moisturizing Daily Cleanser

NizAzel Doxy kits contain doxycycline tablets 100 mg, plus NicAzel FORTE dietary supplement tablets

Ocudox kits contain doxycycline capsules 50 mg, plus eyelid cleanser and Tears Again Advanced eyelid spray

Dosage Forms

Capsule, Oral:
- Adoxa: 150 mg
- Monodox: 75 mg, 100 mg
- Morgidox: 100 mg
- Vibramycin: 100 mg
- Generic: 50 mg, 75 mg, 100 mg, 150 mg

Capsule Delayed Release, Oral:
- Oracea: 40 mg
- Generic: 40 mg

Kit, Combination:
- Alodox Convenience: 20 mg
- Morgidox: 1 x 100 mg, 2 x 100 mg
- Ocudox: 50 mg

Kit, Oral:
- NicAzelDoxy 30: 100 mg
- NicAzelDoxy 60: 100 mg

Solution Reconstituted, Intravenous [preservative free]:
- Doxy 100: 100 mg (1 ea)
- Generic: 100 mg (1 ea)

Suspension Reconstituted, Oral:
- Vibramycin: 25 mg/5 mL (60 mL)
- Generic: 25 mg/5 mL (60 mL)

Syrup, Oral:
- Vibramycin: 50 mg/5 mL (473 mL)

Tablet, Oral:
- Acticlate: 75 mg, 150 mg
- Adoxa: 50 mg, 75 mg, 100 mg
- Adoxa Pak 1/100: 100 mg
- Adoxa Pak 2/100: 100 mg
- Adoxa Pak 1/150: 150 mg
- Avidoxy: 100 mg
- Generic: 20 mg, 50 mg, 75 mg, 100 mg, 150 mg

Tablet Delayed Release, Oral:
- Doryx: 150 mg, 200 mg
- Generic: 75 mg, 100 mg, 150 mg

Dosage Forms: Canada

Capsule, oral:
- Apprilon: 40 mg [30 mg (immediate release) and 10 mg (delayed release)]
- Periostat: 20 mg

Extemporaneous Preparations If a public health emergency is declared and liquid doxycycline is unavailable for the treatment of anthrax, emergency doses may be prepared for children or adults who cannot swallow tablets.

Add 20 mL of water to one 100 mg tablet. Allow tablet to soak in the water for 5 minutes to soften. Crush into a fine powder and stir until well mixed. Appropriate dose should be taken from this mixture. To increase palatability, mix with food or drink. If mixing with drink, add 15 mL of milk, chocolate milk, chocolate pudding, or apple juice to the appropriate dose of mixture. If using apple juice, also add 4 teaspoons of sugar. Doxycycline and water mixture may be stored at room temperature for up to 24 hours.

U.S. Food and Drug Administration, Center for Drug Evaluation and Research, "Public Health Emergency Home Preparation Instructions for Doxycycline." Available at http://www.fda.gov/Drugs/EmergencyPreparedness/BioterrorismandDrugPreparedness/ucm130996.htm

◆ **Doxycycline Calcium** *see* Doxycycline *on page 689*

◆ **Doxycycline Hyclate** *see* Doxycycline *on page 689*

◆ **Doxycycline Monohydrate** *see* Doxycycline *on page 689*

Doxylamine and Pyridoxine

(dox IL a meen & peer i DOX een)

Brand Names: U.S. Diclegis®

Brand Names: Canada Diclectin®

Index Terms Doxylamine Succinate and Pyridoxine Hydrochloride; Pyridoxine and Doxylamine

Pharmacologic Category Ethanolamine Derivative; Histamine H_1 Antagonist; Histamine H_1 Antagonist, First Generation; Vitamin, Water Soluble

Use Treatment of pregnancy-associated nausea and vomiting

Pregnancy Risk Factor A

Dosage Nausea and vomiting associated with pregnancy: Adults: Oral:

U.S. labeling: Day 1: Two delayed release tablets (a total of doxylamine 20 mg and pyridoxine 20 mg) at bedtime. If symptoms are controlled the next day, continue taking 2 tablets at bedtime. If symptoms persist into the afternoon of Day 2, take 2 tablets at bedtime, then 1 tablet in the morning of Day 3 and 2 tablets at bedtime. If symptoms are controlled on Day 4, continue with 1 tablet in the morning and 2 tablets at bedtime. If symptoms are **not** controlled on Day 4, increase dose to 1 tablet in the morning, 1 tablet midafternoon, and 2 tablets in the evening. Tablets should be taken as scheduled and not on an as needed basis. Maximum dose: Four tablets daily.

Canadian labeling: Take 2 delayed release tablets (a total of doxylamine 20 mg and pyridoxine 20 mg) at bedtime. One additional tablet may be taken in the morning or midafternoon; dose should be individualized to control symptoms. Tablets should not be taken on an as needed basis. Maximum dose: Four tablets daily. A gradual tapering of the dose is recommended to prevent a sudden onset of symptoms.

Dosage adjustment in renal impairment: No dosage adjustment provided in manufacturer's labeling (has not been studied).

Dosage adjustment in hepatic impairment: No dosage adjustment provided in manufacturer's labeling (has not been studied).

Additional Information Complete prescribing information should be consulted for additional detail.

Dosage Forms

Tablet, delayed release:

Diclegis®: Doxylamine 10 mg and pyridoxine 10 mg

Dosage Forms: Canada

Tablet, delayed release:

Diclectin®: Doxylamine 10 mg and pyridoxine 10 mg

- ◆ **Doxylamine Succinate and Pyridoxine Hydrochloride** *see* Doxylamine and Pyridoxine *on page 693*
- ◆ **Doxylamine Succinate, Codeine Phosphate, and Acetaminophen** *see* Acetaminophen, Codeine, and Doxylamine [CAN/INT] *on page 37*
- ◆ **Doxytab (Can)** *see* Doxycycline *on page 689*
- ◆ **DPA** *see* Valproic Acid and Derivatives *on page 2123*
- ◆ **DPE** *see* Dipivefrin *on page 651*
- ◆ **D-Penicillamine** *see* PenicillAMINE *on page 1608*
- ◆ **DPH** *see* Phenytoin *on page 1640*
- ◆ **DPM [OTC]** *see* Urea *on page 2114*
- ◆ **Dramamine [OTC]** *see* DimenhyDRINATE *on page 637*
- ◆ **Dramamine Less Drowsy [OTC]** *see* Meclizine *on page 1277*
- ◆ **Dr Gs Clear Nail [OTC]** *see* Tolnaftate *on page 2063*
- ◆ **Driminate [OTC]** *see* DimenhyDRINATE *on page 637*
- ◆ **Drisdol** *see* Ergocalciferol *on page 753*
- ◆ **Dritho-Creme HP** *see* Anthralin *on page 150*
- ◆ **Drixoral® ND (Can)** *see* Pseudoephedrine *on page 1742*

Dronabinol (droe NAB i nol)

Brand Names: U.S. Marinol

Brand Names: Canada Marinol®

Index Terms Delta-9 THC; Delta-9-tetrahydro-cannabinol; Tetrahydrocannabinol; THC

Pharmacologic Category Antiemetic; Appetite Stimulant

Use Chemotherapy-associated nausea and vomiting refractory to other antiemetic(s); AIDS-related anorexia

Pregnancy Risk Factor C

Pregnancy Considerations Adverse events have been observed in animal reproduction studies.

Breast-Feeding Considerations Dronabinol is excreted in breast milk. Breast-feeding is not recommended by the manufacturer.

Contraindications Hypersensitivity to dronabinol, cannabinoids, sesame oil, or any component of the formulation, or marijuana; should be avoided in patients with a history of schizophrenia

Warnings/Precautions Use with caution in patients with hepatic disease or seizure disorders. Reduce dosage in patients with severe hepatic impairment. May cause additive CNS effects with sedatives, hypnotics or other psychoactive agents; patients must be cautioned about performing tasks which require mental alertness (eg, operating machinery or driving).

May have potential for abuse; drug is psychoactive substance in marijuana; use caution in patients with a history of substance abuse or potential. May cause withdrawal symptoms upon abrupt discontinuation. Use with caution in patients with mania, depression, or schizophrenia; careful psychiatric monitoring is recommended. Use caution in elderly; they are more sensitive to adverse effects.

Adverse Reactions

Cardiovascular: Palpitations, tachycardia, vasodilation/facial flushing

Central nervous system: Abnormal thinking, amnesia, anxiety, ataxia, depersonalization, dizziness, euphoria, hallucination, paranoia, somnolence

Gastrointestinal: Abdominal pain, nausea, vomiting

Neuromuscular & skeletal: Weakness

Rare but important or life-threatening: Conjunctivitis, depression, diarrhea, fatigue, fecal incontinence, flushing, hypotension, myalgia, nightmares, seizure, speech difficulties, tinnitus, vision difficulties

Drug Interactions

Metabolism/Transport Effects Substrate of CYP2C9 (minor), CYP3A4 (minor); **Note:** Assignment of Major/Minor substrate status based on clinically relevant drug interaction potential

Avoid Concomitant Use There are no known interactions where it is recommended to avoid concomitant use.

Increased Effect/Toxicity

Dronabinol may increase the levels/effects of: Alcohol (Ethyl); CNS Depressants; Sympathomimetics

The levels/effects of Dronabinol may be increased by: Anticholinergic Agents; Cocaine; CYP2C9 Inhibitors (Moderate); CYP2C9 Inhibitors (Strong); CYP3A4 Inhibitors (Moderate); CYP3A4 Inhibitors (Strong); MAO Inhibitors; Ritonavir

Decreased Effect

The levels/effects of Dronabinol may be decreased by: CYP3A4 Inducers (Strong)

Food Interactions Administration with high-lipid meals may increase absorption.

Storage/Stability Store under refrigeration (or in a cool environment) between 8°C and 15°C (46°F and 59°F); protect from freezing.

Mechanism of Action Unknown, may inhibit endorphins in the brain's emetic center, suppress prostaglandin synthesis, and/or inhibit medullary activity through an unspecified cortical action. Some pharmacologic effects appear to involve sympathimometic activity; tachyphylaxis to some effect (eg, tachycardia) may occur, but appetite-stimulating effects do not appear to wane over time. Antiemetic activity may be due to effect on cannabinoid receptors (CB1) within the central nervous system.

Pharmacodynamics/Kinetics

Onset of action: Within 1 hour

Peak effect: 2-4 hours

Duration: 24 hours (appetite stimulation)

Absorption: Oral: 90% to 95%; 10% to 20% of dose gets into systemic circulation

Distribution: V_d: 10 L/kg; dronabinol is highly lipophilic and distributes to adipose tissue

Protein binding: 97% to 99%

Metabolism: Hepatic to at least 50 metabolites, some of which are active; 11-hydroxy-delta-9-tetrahydrocannabinol (11-OH-THC) is the major metabolite; extensive first-pass effect

Half-life elimination: Dronabinol: 25-36 hours (terminal); Dronabinol metabolites: 44-59 hours

Time to peak, serum: 0.5-4 hours

Excretion: Feces (50% as unconjugated metabolites, 5% as unchanged drug); urine (10% to 15% as acid metabolites and conjugates)

Dosage Refer to individual protocols. Oral:

Antiemetic: Children and Adults: 5 mg/m^2 1-3 hours before chemotherapy, then 5 mg/m^2/dose every 2-4 hours after chemotherapy for a total of 4-6 doses/day; increase doses in increments of 2.5 mg/m^2 to a maximum of 15 mg/m^2/dose.

Appetite stimulant: Adults: Initial: 2.5 mg twice daily (before lunch and dinner); titrate up to a maximum of 20 mg/day.

Dosage adjustment in renal impairment: No dosage adjustment provided in manufacturer's labeling.

Dosage adjustment in hepatic impairment: Usual dose should be reduced in patients with severe liver failure.

Dietary Considerations Capsules contain sesame oil.

Monitoring Parameters CNS effects, heart rate, blood pressure, behavioral profile

Reference Range Antinauseant effects: 5-10 ng/mL

Dosage Forms

Capsule, Oral:

Marinol: 2.5 mg, 5 mg, 10 mg

Generic: 2.5 mg, 5 mg, 10 mg

Dronedarone (droe NE da rone)

Brand Names: U.S. Multaq

Brand Names: Canada Multaq

Index Terms Dronedarone Hydrochloride; SR33589

Pharmacologic Category Antiarrhythmic Agent, Class III

Additional Appendix Information

Beers Criteria − Potentially Inappropriate Medications for Geriatrics *on page 2271*

Use Paroxysmal or persistent atrial fibrillation: To reduce the risk of hospitalization for atrial fibrillation (AF) in patients in sinus rhythm with a history of paroxysmal or persistent AF

Pregnancy Risk Factor X

Dosage Note: Prior to initiation of dronedarone, class I or III antiarrhythmics (eg, amiodarone, flecainide, propafenone, quinidine, disopyramide, dofetilide, sotalol) or drugs that are strong inhibitors of CYP3A (eg, ketoconazole) must be stopped.

Paroxysmal or persistent atrial fibrillation: Adults: Oral: 400 mg twice daily.

Dosage adjustment in renal impairment: No dosage adjustment necessary.

Dosage adjustment in hepatic impairment:

Mild to moderate impairment: No dosage adjustment necessary.

Severe impairment: Use is contraindicated.

Additional Information Complete prescribing information should be consulted for additional detail.

Dosage Forms

Tablet, Oral:

Multaq: 400 mg

◆ **Dronedarone Hydrochloride** *see* Dronedarone *on page 695*

Droperidol (droe PER i dole)

Brand Names: Canada Droperidol Injection, USP

Index Terms Dehydrobenzperidol

Pharmacologic Category Antiemetic; First Generation (Typical) Antipsychotic

Use Prevention and/or treatment of nausea and vomiting from surgical and diagnostic procedures

Pregnancy Risk Factor C

Pregnancy Considerations Adverse events were observed in some animal reproduction studies. Although use in pregnancy has been reported, due to cases of QT prolongation and torsade de pointes (some fatal), use of other agents in pregnant women is preferred (ACOG, 2004).

Breast-Feeding Considerations It is not known if droperidol is excreted in breast milk. The manufacturer recommends that caution be exercised when administering droperidol to nursing women.

Contraindications Hypersensitivity to droperidol or any component of the formulation; known or suspected QT prolongation, including congenital long QT syndrome (prolonged QTc is defined as >440 msec in males or >450 msec in females)

Canadian labeling: Additional contraindications (not in U.S. labeling): Not for use in children ≤2 years of age

Warnings/Precautions May alter cardiac conduction. **[U.S. Boxed Warning]: Cases of QT prolongation and torsade de pointes, including some fatal cases, have been reported.** Use extreme caution in patients with bradycardia (<50 bpm), cardiac disease, concurrent MAO inhibitor therapy, Class I and Class III antiarrhythmics or other drugs known to prolong QT interval, and electrolyte disturbances (hypokalemia or hypomagnesemia), including concomitant drugs which may alter electrolytes (diuretics).

Use with caution in patients with seizures or severe liver disease. May be sedating, use with caution in disorders where CNS depression is a feature. Caution in patients with hemodynamic instability, predisposition to seizures, subcortical brain damage, pheochromocytoma or renal disease. Esophageal dysmotility and aspiration have been associated with antipsychotic use - use with caution in patients at risk of pneumonia (ie, Alzheimer's disease). Caution in breast cancer or other prolactin-dependent tumors (may elevate prolactin levels). May alter temperature regulation or mask toxicity of other drugs due to antiemetic effects. May cause orthostatic hypotension - use with caution in patients at risk of this effect or those who would tolerate transient hypotensive episodes (cerebrovascular disease, cardiovascular disease, or other medications which may predispose). Significant hypotension may occur.

May cause anticholinergic effects (confusion, agitation, constipation, xerostomia, blurred vision, urinary retention). Therefore, they should be used with caution in patients with decreased gastrointestinal motility, urinary retention, BPH, xerostomia, visual problems, or narrow-angle glaucoma (screening is recommended). Relative to other neuroleptics, droperidol has a low potency of cholinergic blockade.

May cause extrapyramidal symptoms, including pseudoparkinsonism, acute dystonic reactions, akathisia, and tardive dyskinesia. Risk of dystonia (and possibly other EPS) may be greater with increased doses, use of conventional antipsychotics, males, and younger patients. Risk of tardive dyskinesia and potential for irreversibility may be increased in elderly patients (particularly women), prolonged therapy, and higher total cumulative dose. May be associated with neuroleptic malignant syndrome (NMS). May mask toxicity of other drugs or conditions (eg, intestinal obstruction, Reye's syndrome, brain tumor) due to antiemetic effects. Use with caution in the elderly; reduce initial dose.

Adverse Reactions

Cardiovascular: Cardiac arrest, hypertension, hypotension (especially orthostatic), QTc prolongation (dose dependent), tachycardia, torsade de pointes, ventricular tachycardia

Central nervous system: Anxiety, chills, depression (postoperative, transient), dizziness, drowsiness (postoperative) increased, dysphoria, extrapyramidal symptoms (akathisia, dystonia, oculogyric crisis), hallucinations (postoperative), hyperactivity, neuroleptic malignant syndrome (NMS) (rare), restlessness

Respiratory: Bronchospasm, laryngospasm

Miscellaneous: Anaphylaxis, shivering

Drug Interactions

Metabolism/Transport Effects None known.

Avoid Concomitant Use

Avoid concomitant use of Droperidol with any of the following: Aclidinium; Amisulpride; Azelastine (Nasal); Glucagon; Highest Risk QTc-Prolonging Agents; Ipratropium (Oral Inhalation); Ivabradine; Metoclopramide; Mifepristone; Orphenadrine; Paraldehyde; Potassium Chloride; Sulpiride; Thalidomide; Tiotropium; Umeclidinium

Increased Effect/Toxicity

Droperidol may increase the levels/effects of: AbobotulinumtoxinA; Alcohol (Ethyl); Amisulpride; Anticholinergic Agents; Azelastine (Nasal); Buprenorphine; CNS Depressants; Glucagon; Highest Risk QTc-Prolonging Agents; Hydrocodone; Methotrimeprazine; Methylphenidate; Metoclopramide; Mirabegron; Moderate Risk QTc-Prolonging Agents; OnabotulinumtoxinA; Orphenadrine; Paraldehyde; Potassium Chloride; RimabotulinumtoxinB; Selective Serotonin Reuptake Inhibitors; Serotonin Modulators; Sulpiride; Suvorexant; Thalidomide; Thiazide Diuretics; Tiotropium; Zolpidem

The levels/effects of Droperidol may be increased by: Acetylcholinesterase Inhibitors (Central); Aclidinium; Brimonidine (Topical); Cannabis; Dronabinol; Ipratropium (Oral Inhalation); Ivabradine; Kava Kava; Lithium; Magnesium Sulfate; MAO Inhibitors; Methotrimeprazine; Methylphenidate; Metyrosine; Mifepristone; Nabilone; Perampanel; Pramlintide; QTc-Prolonging Agents (Indeterminate Risk and Risk Modifying); Rufinamide; Serotonin Modulators; Sodium Oxybate; Tapentadol; Tetrahydrocannabinol; Umeclidinium

Decreased Effect

Droperidol may decrease the levels/effects of: Acetylcholinesterase Inhibitors; Amphetamines; Anti-Parkinson's Agents (Dopamine Agonist); Itopride; Quinagolide; Secretin

The levels/effects of Droperidol may be decreased by: Acetylcholinesterase Inhibitors; Anti-Parkinson's Agents (Dopamine Agonist); Lithium

Preparation for Administration IV infusion: Dilute in 50-100 mL NS or D_5W.

Storage/Stability Store at 20°C to 25°C (68°F to 77°F); excursions permitted to 15°C to 30°C (59°F to 86°F). Protect from light. Solutions diluted in NS or D_5W are stable at room temperature for up to 7 days in PVC bags or glass bottles. Solutions diluted in LR are stable at room temperature for 24 hours in PVC bags and up to 7 days in glass bottles.

Mechanism of Action Droperidol is a butyrophenone antipsychotic; antiemetic effect is a result of blockade of dopamine stimulation of the chemoreceptor trigger zone. Other effects include alpha-adrenergic blockade, peripheral vascular dilation, and reduction of the pressor effect of epinephrine resulting in hypotension and decreased peripheral vascular resistance; may also reduce pulmonary artery pressure

Pharmacodynamics/Kinetics

Onset of action: 3-10 minutes

Peak effect: ~30 minutes

Duration: 2-4 hours, may extend to 12 hours

Absorption: IM: Rapid

Distribution: Crosses blood-brain barrier and placenta

V_d: Children: ~0.6 L/kg; Adults: ~1.5 L/kg

Protein binding: 85% to 90%

Metabolism: Hepatic, to *p*-fluorophenylacetic acid, benzimidazolone, *p*-hydroxypiperidine

Half-life elimination: ~2.3 hours

Excretion: Urine (75%, <1% as unchanged drug); feces (22%, 11% as unchanged drug)

Dosage Note: Titrate carefully to desired effect

IM, IV:

Children 2-12 years: Prevention of postoperative nausea and vomiting (PONV):

Manufacturer labeling: Maximum dose: 0.1 mg/kg; additional doses may be repeated with caution to achieve desired effect

Consensus guideline recommendations: 0.01-0.015 mg/kg (maximum: 1.25 mg) IV administered at the end of surgery (Gan, 2007)

Adults: Prevention of PONV:

Manufacturer labeling: Maximum initial dose: 2.5 mg; additional doses of 1.25 mg may be administered with caution to achieve desired effect

Consensus guideline recommendations: 0.625-1.25 mg IV administered at the end of surgery (Gan, 2007)

Canadian labeling: IV: Prevention and treatment of PONV:

Children >2 years and Adolescents: 0.02-0.05 mg/kg (maximum dose: 1.25 mg) 30 minutes prior to anticipated end of surgery, and then every 6 hours as needed for breakthrough PONV

Adults: 0.625-1.25 mg 30 minutes prior to anticipated end of surgery, and then every 6 hours as needed for breakthrough PONV

Elderly: PONV: 0.625 mg 30 minutes prior to anticipated end of surgery and then every 6 hours as needed for breakthrough PONV; additional dosing should be administered with caution

Dosage adjustment in renal impairment:

U.S. labeling: Specific dosing recommendations are not provided; use with caution

Canadian labeling: IV: 0.625 mg; additional dosing should be administered with caution

Dosage adjustment in hepatic impairment:

U.S. labeling: Specific dosing recommendations are not provided; use with caution

Canadian labeling: IV: 0.625 mg; additional dosing should be administered with caution

Administration Administer IM or IV; according to the manufacturer, IV push administration should be slow. For IV infusion, further dilute.

Monitoring Parameters To identify QT prolongation, a 12-lead ECG prior to use is recommended; continued ECG monitoring for 2-3 hours following administration is recommended. Vital signs; serum magnesium and potassium; mental status, abnormal involuntary movement scale (AIMS); observe for dystonias, extrapyramidal side effects, and temperature changes

Dosage Forms

Solution, Injection:

Generic: 2.5 mg/mL (2 mL)

- **Droperidol Injection, USP (Can)** *see* Droperidol *on page 695*
- **Drospirenone and Ethinyl Estradiol** *see* Ethinyl Estradiol and Drospirenone *on page 801*
- **Drospirenone, Ethinyl Estradiol, and Levomefolate Calcium** *see* Ethinyl Estradiol, Drospirenone, and Levomefolate *on page 812*
- **Droxia** *see* Hydroxyurea *on page 1021*
- **DRV** *see* Darunavir *on page 569*
- **Drymira (Can)** *see* Ciclesonide (Nasal) *on page 432*
- **DSCG** *see* Cromolyn (Nasal) *on page 514*
- **DSCG** *see* Cromolyn (Ophthalmic) *on page 514*
- **DSS** *see* Docusate *on page 661*
- **DT** *see* Diphtheria and Tetanus Toxoid *on page 645*
- **DTaP** *see* Diphtheria and Tetanus Toxoids, and Acellular Pertussis Vaccine *on page 649*
- **DTaP-HepB-IPV** *see* Diphtheria, Tetanus Toxoids, Acellular Pertussis, Hepatitis B (Recombinant), and Poliovirus (Inactivated) Vaccine *on page 651*
- **DTaP-HepB-IPV-Hib** *see* Diphtheria and Tetanus Toxoids, Acellular Pertussis, Hepatitis B (Recombinant), Poliovirus (Inactivated), and *Haemophilus influenzae* B Conjugate (Adsorbed) Vaccine [CAN/INT] *on page 647*
- **DTaP-IPV** *see* Diphtheria and Tetanus Toxoids, Acellular Pertussis, and Poliovirus Vaccine *on page 646*
- **DTaP-IPV/Hib** *see* Diphtheria and Tetanus Toxoids, Acellular Pertussis, Poliovirus and *Haemophilus* b Conjugate Vaccine *on page 648*
- **DTC 101** *see* Cytarabine (Liposomal) *on page 540*
- **DTIC** *see* Dacarbazine *on page 549*
- **DTIC-Dome** *see* Dacarbazine *on page 549*
- **DTO (error-prone abbreviation)** *see* Opium Tincture *on page 1518*
- **D-Trp(6)-LHRH** *see* Triptorelin *on page 2107*
- **Duavee** *see* Estrogens (Conjugated/Equine) and Bazedoxifene *on page 782*
- **Ducodyl [OTC]** *see* Bisacodyl *on page 265*
- **Duetact™** *see* Pioglitazone and Glimepiride *on page 1654*
- **Dukoral® (Can)** *see* Travelers' Diarrhea and Cholera Vaccine [CAN/INT] *on page 2088*

Dulaglutide (doo la GLOO tide)

Brand Names: U.S. Trulicity

Index Terms LY2189265

Pharmacologic Category Antidiabetic Agent, Glucagon-Like Peptide-1 (GLP-1) Receptor Agonist

Use Type 2 diabetes mellitus: Adjunct to diet and exercise to improve glycemic control in adults with type 2 diabetes mellitus (noninsulin dependent, NIDDM)

Pregnancy Risk Factor C

Pregnancy Considerations Adverse events have been observed in some animal reproduction studies.

In women with diabetes, maternal hyperglycemia can be associated with congenital malformations as well as adverse effects in the fetus, neonate, and the mother (ACOG, 2005; ADA, 2014; Kitzmiller, 2008; Metzger, 2007). To prevent adverse outcomes, prior to conception and throughout pregnancy maternal blood glucose and HbA_{1c} should be kept as close to normal as possible but without causing significant hypoglycemia (ACOG, 2013; ADA, 2014; Blumer, 2013; Kitzmiller, 2008). Prior to pregnancy, effective contraception should be used until glycemic control is achieved (ADA, 2014; Kitzmiller, 2008). Other agents are currently recommended to treat diabetes in pregnant women (ACOG, 2013; Blumer, 2013).

Breast-Feeding Considerations It is not known if dulaglutide is excreted in breast milk. Due to the potential for serious adverse reactions in the nursing infant, the manufacturer recommends a decision be made whether to discontinue nursing or to discontinue the drug, taking into account the importance of treatment to the mother.

Contraindications Serious hypersensitivity to dulaglutide or any component of the formulation; personal or family history of medullary thyroid carcinoma (MTC); patients with multiple endocrine neoplasia syndrome type 2 (MEN2)

Warnings/Precautions [U.S. Boxed Warning] Thyroid C-cell tumors have developed in animal studies with glucagon-like peptide-1 (GLP-1) receptor agonists; it is not known if dulaglutide causes thyroid C-cell tumor, including medullary thyroid carcinoma (MTC) in humans. Routine serum calcitonin or thyroid ultrasound monitoring is of uncertain value. Patients should be counseled on the risk and symptoms (eg, neck mass, dysphagia, dyspnea, persistent hoarseness) of thyroid tumors. Use is contraindicated in patients with or a family history of MTC and in patients with multiple endocrine neoplasia syndrome type 2 (MEN2). Consultation with an endocrinologist is recommended in patients with thyroid nodules on physical examination or neck imaging and in patients who develop elevated calcitonin concentrations.

Use is not recommended in patients with preexisting severe gastrointestinal disease. Hypersensitivity reactions have been reported; discontinue therapy in the event of a hypersensitivity reaction. Cases of pancreatitis have been reported; monitor for signs and symptoms of pancreatitis (eg, persistent severe abdominal pain). If pancreatitis is suspected, discontinue use. Do not resume therapy if pancreatitis is confirmed. Consider antidiabetic therapies other than dulaglutide in patients with a history of pancreatitis.

Use with caution in patients with renal impairment, particularly during initiation of therapy and dose escalation. Acute renal failure and chronic renal failure exacerbation (sometimes requiring hemodialysis) have been reported; some cases have been reported in patients with no known preexisting renal disease. A majority of reported cases occurred in patients with nausea/vomiting/diarrhea or dehydration. Use with caution in patients with hepatic impairment.

Not recommended for first-line therapy in patients inadequately controlled on diet and exercise alone. Do not use in patients with type 1 diabetes mellitus or for the treatment of diabetic ketoacidosis; not a substitute for insulin. Diabetes self-management education (DSME) is essential to maximize the effectiveness of therapy. Potentially significant drug-drug interactions may exist, requiring dose or frequency adjustment, additional monitoring, and/or selection of alternative therapy.

Adverse Reactions

Cardiovascular: Sinus tachycardia, prolongation P-R interval on ECG, first degree atrioventricular block

Central nervous system: Fatigue

Endocrine & metabolic: Hypoglycemia
Gastrointestinal: Abdominal distension, abdominal pain, constipation, decreased appetite, diarrhea, dyspepsia, eructation, flatulence, gastroesophageal reflux disease, nausea, vomiting
Immunologic: Antibody development
Rare but important or life-threatening: Acute renal failure, chronic renal failure, hypersensitivity reaction, increased serum amylase, increased serum lipase, injection site reaction, pancreatitis

Drug Interactions

Metabolism/Transport Effects None known.

Avoid Concomitant Use There are no known interactions where it is recommended to avoid concomitant use.

Increased Effect/Toxicity

Dulaglutide may increase the levels/effects of: Insulin; Sulfonylureas

The levels/effects of Dulaglutide may be increased by: Androgens; Pegvisomant

Decreased Effect

The levels/effects of Dulaglutide may be decreased by: Corticosteroids (Orally Inhaled); Corticosteroids (Systemic); Danazol; Luteinizing Hormone-Releasing Hormone Analogs; Somatropin; Thiazide Diuretics

Storage/Stability Store at 36°F to 46°F (2°C to 8°C). Do not freeze. Protect from light. If needed, each single-dose pen or prefilled syringe can be kept at room temperature, not to exceed 86°F (30°C) for a total of 14 days.

Mechanism of Action Dulaglutide is an agonist of human glucagon-like peptide-1 (GLP-1) receptor and augments glucose dependent insulin secretion and slows gastric emptying.

Pharmacodynamics/Kinetics

Bioavailability: 47% to 65%
Distribution: V_d: ~17 to 19 L
Metabolism: Degradation to amino acids by protein catabolism pathways.
Half-life elimination: ~5 days
Time to peak, plasma: 24 to 72 hours

Dosage Type 2 diabetes mellitus: Adults: SubQ: 0.75 mg once weekly; may increase to 1.5 mg once weekly if inadequate glycemic response; maximum: 1.5 mg once weekly

Missed doses: If a dose is missed, administer as soon as possible within 3 days after the missed dose; dosing can then be resumed on the usual day of administration. If there are less than 3 days until next scheduled dose, omit the missed dose and resume administration at the next regularly scheduled weekly dose.

Dosage adjustment in renal impairment: No dosage adjustment necessary; use caution when initiating or escalating doses.

Dosage adjustment in hepatic impairment: There are no dosage adjustments provided in the manufacturer's labeling; use with caution.

Dietary Considerations Individualized medical nutrition therapy (MNT) based on ADA recommendations is an integral part of therapy.

Administration Do not inject intravenously or intramuscularly. Inject subcutaneously into the upper arm, thigh, or abdomen; when administering within the same body region, use a different injection site each week. Administer once weekly on the same day each week, without regard to meals or time of day. The day of weekly administration may be changed, as long as the last dose was administered ≥3 days before. If using concomitantly with insulin, administer as separate injections (do not mix); may inject in the same body region as insulin, but not adjacent to one another.

Monitoring Parameters Plasma glucose, HbA_{1c}, renal function, signs/symptoms of pancreatitis

Reference Range

Recommendations for glycemic control in nonpregnant adults with diabetes (ADA, 2015):
HbA_{1c}: <7% (a more aggressive [<6.5%] or less aggressive [<8%] HbA_{1c} goal may be targeted based on patient-specific characteristics)
Preprandial capillary plasma glucose: 80 to 130 mg/dL
Peak postprandial capillary blood glucose: <180 mg/dL

Recommendations for glycemic control in pediatric (all age groups) patients with type 1 diabetes (ADA, 2015):
HbA_{1c}: <7.5% (individualization may be appropriate based on patient-specific characteristics; <7% is reasonable if it can be achieved without excessive hypoglycemia)
Preprandial capillary plasma glucose: 90 to 130 mg/dL
Bedtime and overnight capillary blood glucose: 90 to 150 mg/dL

Dosage Forms

Solution Pen-injector, Subcutaneous:

Trulicity: 0.75 mg/0.5 mL (0.5 mL); 1.5 mg/0.5 mL (0.5 mL)

◆ **Dulcolax [OTC]** *see* Bisacodyl *on page 265*

◆ **Dulcolax For Women [OTC] (Can)** *see* Bisacodyl *on page 265*

◆ **Dulcolax Milk of Magnesia [OTC]** *see* Magnesium Hydroxide *on page 1263*

◆ **Dulcolax Stool Softener [OTC]** *see* Docusate *on page 661*

◆ **Dulera** *see* Mometasone and Formoterol *on page 1392*

DULoxetine (doo LOX e teen)

Brand Names: U.S. Cymbalta

Brand Names: Canada Cymbalta

Index Terms (+)-(*S*)-*N*-Methyl-γ-(1-naphthyloxy)-2-thiophenepropylamine Hydrochloride; Duloxetine Hydrochloride; LY248686

Pharmacologic Category Antidepressant, Serotonin/Norepinephrine Reuptake Inhibitor

Use

Chronic musculoskeletal pain: Management of chronic musculoskeletal pain.

Diabetic peripheral neuropathic pain: Management of diabetic peripheral neuropathy.

Fibromyalgia: Management of fibromyalgia.

Generalized anxiety disorder: Treatment of generalized anxiety disorder (GAD).

Major depressive disorder: Treatment of major depressive disorder (MDD).

Pregnancy Risk Factor C

Pregnancy Considerations Adverse events were observed in animal reproduction studies. Nonteratogenic effects in the newborn following SSRI/SNRI exposure late in the third trimester include respiratory distress, cyanosis, apnea, seizures, temperature instability, feeding difficulty, vomiting, hypoglycemia, hyper- or hypotonia, hyperreflexia, jitteriness, irritability, constant crying, and tremor. Symptoms may be due to the toxicity of the SNRIs/SSRIs or a discontinuation syndrome and may be consistent with serotonin syndrome associated with SSRI treatment. The long-term effects of *in utero* SNRI/SSRI exposure on infant development and behavior are not known.

The ACOG recommends that therapy with SSRIs or SNRIs during pregnancy be individualized; treatment of depression during pregnancy should incorporate the clinical expertise of the mental health clinician, obstetrician, primary healthc are provider, and pediatrician. According to the American Psychiatric Association (APA), the risks of medication treatment should be weighed against other treatment options and untreated depression. For women who discontinue antidepressant medications during pregnancy and who may be at high risk for postpartum depression, the medications can be restarted following delivery. Treatment algorithms have been developed by the ACOG and the APA for the management of depression in women prior to conception and during pregnancy.

Health care providers are encouraged to enroll women exposed to duloxetine during pregnancy in the Cymbalta Pregnancy Registry (866-814-6975 or http://cymbaltapregnancyregistry.com).

Breast-Feeding Considerations Duloxetine is excreted in human milk and has been detected in the serum of a nursing infant. The manufacturer recommends that caution be exercised when administering duloxetine to nursing women. The long-term effects on neurobehavior have not been studied, thus one should prescribe duloxetine to a mother who is breast-feeding only when the benefits outweigh the potential risks.

Contraindications Use of monoamine oxidase (MAO) inhibitors intended to treat psychiatric disorders (concurrently or within 14 days of discontinuing the MAO inhibitor); initiation of MAO inhibitor intended to treat psychiatric disorders within 5 days of discontinuing duloxetine; initiation of duloxetine in a patient receiving linezolid or intravenous methylene blue.

Canadian labeling: Additional contraindications (not in U.S. labeling): Hypersensitivity to duloxetine or any component of the formulation; hepatic impairment; severe renal impairment (eg, CrCl <30 mL/minute) or end-stage renal disease (ESRD); concomitant use with thioridazine or with CYP1A2 inhibitors.

Warnings/Precautions [U.S. Boxed Warning]: Antidepressants increase the risk of suicidal thinking and behavior in children, adolescents, and young adults (18 to 24 years of age) with major depressive disorder (MDD) and other psychiatric disorders; consider risk prior to prescribing. Short-term studies did not show an increased risk in patients >24 years of age and showed a decreased risk in patients ≥65 years. Closely monitor for clinical worsening, suicidality, or unusual changes in behavior, particularly during the initial 1 to 2 months of therapy or during periods of dosage adjustments (increases or decreases); the patient's family or caregiver should be instructed to closely observe the patient and communicate condition with healthcare provider. A medication guide concerning the use of antidepressants in children and teenagers should be dispensed with each prescription. **Duloxetine is not FDA approved for use in children.**

The possibility of a suicide attempt is inherent in major depression and may persist until remission occurs. Use caution in high-risk patients. Worsening depression and severe abrupt suicidality that are not part of the presenting symptoms may require discontinuation or modification of drug therapy. The patient's family or caregiver should be alerted to monitor patients for the emergence of suicidality and associated behaviors (such as agitation, irritability, hostility, impulsivity, and hypomania) and call healthcare provider.

May worsen psychosis in some patients or precipitate a shift to mania or hypomania in patients with bipolar disorder. Patients presenting with depressive symptoms should be screened for bipolar disorder. Monotherapy in patients with bipolar disorder should be avoided. **Duloxetine is not FDA approved for the treatment of bipolar depression.**

May cause orthostatic hypotension/syncope at therapeutic doses especially within the first week of therapy and after dose increases. Consider dose reduction or discontinuation of duloxetine if orthostatic hypotension or syncope occurs. Monitor blood pressure with initiation of therapy, dose increases (especially in patients receiving >60 mg/day), or with concomitant use of vasodilators, CYP2D6 inhibitors/substrates, or CYP1A2 inhibitors. Use caution in patients with hypertension. May increase blood pressure. Rare cases of hypertensive crisis have been reported; evaluate blood pressure prior to initiating therapy and periodically thereafter; consider dose reduction or gradual discontinuation of therapy in individuals with sustained hypertension during therapy. Falls with serious consequences including bone fractures and hospitalization have been reported in patients receiving therapeutic doses of duloxetine. The risk of falling appears related to the degree of orthostatic decrease in blood pressure. Risks may also be greater in elderly patients, patients taking concomitant medications that induce orthostatic hypotension or are potent CYP1A2 inhibitors, and in patients taking doses >60 mg/day. Consider dose reduction or discontinuation of duloxetine if falls occur.

Modest increases in serum glucose and hemoglobin A_{1c} (HbA_{1c}) levels have been observed in some diabetic patients receiving duloxetine therapy for diabetic peripheral neuropathic pain (DPNP). Duloxetine may cause increased urinary resistance; advise patient to report symptoms of urinary hesitation/difficulty. Has a low potential to impair cognitive or motor performance. Use caution in patients with a previous seizure disorder or condition predisposing to seizures such as brain damage or alcoholism (Montgomery, 2005). Avoid use in patients with substantial ethanol intake, evidence of liver disease, or hepatic impairment (contraindicated in Canadian labeling). Rare cases of hepatic failure (including fatalities) have been reported with use. Hepatitis with abdominal pain, hepatomegaly, elevated transaminase levels >20 times the upper limit of normal (ULN) with and without jaundice have all been observed. Discontinue therapy with the presentation of jaundice or other signs of hepatic dysfunction and do not reinitiate therapy unless another source or cause is identified. Use caution in patients with impaired gastric motility (eg, some diabetics) may affect stability of the capsule's enteric coating.

Severe skin reactions (including Stevens-Johnson syndrome and erythema multiforme) have been reported; discontinue immediately if hypersensitivity reaction suspected. May cause hyponatremia/SIADH (elderly at increased risk); volume depletion (diuretics may increase risk). May cause mild pupillary dilation which in susceptible individuals can lead to an episode of narrow-angle glaucoma. Consider evaluating patients who have not had an iridectomy for narrow-angle glaucoma risk factors. May cause or exacerbate sexual dysfunction. Use caution with renal impairment (contraindicated in Canadian labeling for severe renal impairment or ESRD). May impair platelet aggregation; use caution with concomitant use of NSAIDs, ASA, or other drugs that affect coagulation; the risk of bleeding may be potentiated. Bone fractures have been associated with antidepressant treatment. Consider the possibility of a fragility fracture if an antidepressant-treated patient presents with unexplained bone pain, point tenderness, swelling, or bruising (Rabenda, 2013; Rizzoli, 2012).

Potentially life-threatening serotonin syndrome (SS) has occurred with serotonergic agents (eg, SSRIs, SNRIs), particularly when used in combination with other serotonergic agents (eg, triptans, tricyclic antidepressants, fentanyl, lithium, tramadol, tryptophan, buspirone, and St John's wort) or drugs that impair serotonin metabolism (eg, MAO inhibitors, specifically linezolid, methylene blue, and others used for psychiatric disorders). Monitor patients closely for signs/symptoms of SS which may include mental status changes (eg, agitation, hallucinations, delirium), seizures, autonomic instability (eg, tachycardia, dizziness, diaphoresis), neuromuscular symptoms (eg, tremor, rigidity, myoclonus), or gastrointestinal symptoms (eg, nausea, vomiting, diarrhea). Discontinue treatment (and any concomitant serotonergic agents) immediately if signs/symptoms of SS arise.

Use caution in elderly patients; may cause or exacerbate syndrome of inappropriate antidiuretic hormone secretion or hyponatremia; monitor sodium closely with initiation or dosage adjustments in older adults (Beers Criteria). Formulation contains sucrose; patients with fructose intolerance, glucose-galactose malabsorption, or sucrase-isomaltase deficiency should avoid use.

Abrupt discontinuation or interruption of antidepressant therapy has been associated with a discontinuation syndrome. Symptoms arising may vary with antidepressant however commonly include nausea, vomiting, diarrhea, headaches, lightheadedness, dizziness, diminished appetite, sweating, chills, tremors, paresthesias, fatigue, somnolence, and sleep disturbances (eg, vivid dreams, insomnia). Greater risks for developing a discontinuation syndrome have been associated with antidepressants with shorter half-lives, longer durations of treatment, and abrupt discontinuation. For antidepressants of short or intermediate half-lives, symptoms may emerge within 2 to 5 days after treatment discontinuation and last 7 to 14 days (APA, 2010; Fava, 2006; Haddad, 2001; Shelton, 2001; Warner, 2006).

Adverse Reactions

Cardiovascular: Flushing, increased blood pressure, palpitations

Central nervous system: Abnormal dreams, agitation, anorgasmia, anxiety, chills, delayed ejaculation, dizziness, drowsiness, fatigue, headache, hypoesthesia, insomnia, lethargy, paresthesia, rigors, sleep disorder, vertigo, yawning

Dermatologic: Diaphoresis, pruritus

Endocrine & metabolic: Decreased libido, hot flash, orgasm abnormal, weight gain, weight loss (more common in pediatric)

Gastrointestinal: Abdominal pain, constipation, decreased appetite, diarrhea dysgeusia, dyspepsia, flatulence, nausea, vomiting, xerostomia

Genitourinary: Ejaculatory disorder, erectile dysfunction, urinary frequency

Hepatic: Increased serum ALT

Neuromuscular & skeletal: Musculoskeletal pain, tremor

Ophthalmic: Blurred vision

Respiratory: Cough, oropharyngeal pain

Rare but important or life-threatening: Angle-closure glaucoma, apathy, bruxism, cholestatic jaundice, disorientation, dysarthria, dysphagia, dysuria, emotional lability, epistaxis, erythema multiforme, extrapyramidal reaction, falling, gastroenteritis, gastrointestinal hemorrhage, hallucination, hematoma, hepatic failure, hostility, hyperglycemia, hyperkalemia, hyperlipidemia, hypersensitivity, hypokalemia, hypothyroidism, impulsivity, increased serum bicarbonate, menopausal symptoms, menstrual disease, muscle spasm, myocardial infarction, night sweats, oropharyngeal pain, orthostatic hypotension, otalgia, outbursts of anger (particularly early in treatment or after treatment discontinuation), panic attack, restless leg syndrome, seizure, sensation of cold, serotonin syndrome, SIADH, skin photosensitivity, Stevens-Johnson syndrome, supraventricular cardiac arrhythmia, syncope, tachycardia, testicular pain, trismus, urinary retention, urinary urgency, weakness

Drug Interactions

Metabolism/Transport Effects **Substrate** of CYP1A2 (major), CYP2D6 (major); **Note:** Assignment of Major/Minor substrate status based on clinically relevant drug interaction potential; **Inhibits** CYP2D6 (moderate)

Avoid Concomitant Use

Avoid concomitant use of DULoxetine with any of the following: CYP1A2 Inhibitors (Strong); Dapoxetine; Iobenguane I 123; Linezolid; MAO Inhibitors; Methylene Blue; Thioridazine; Urokinase

Increased Effect/Toxicity

DULoxetine may increase the levels/effects of: Agents with Antiplatelet Properties; Alpha-/Beta-Agonists; Anticoagulants; Antipsychotic Agents; Apixaban; ARIPiprazole; Aspirin; Collagenase (Systemic); CYP2D6 Substrates; Dabigatran Etexilate; DOXOrubicin (Conventional); Eliglustat; Fesoterodine; Ibritumomab; Methylene Blue; Metoclopramide; Metoprolol; Nebivolol; NSAID (Nonselective); Obinutuzumab; PARoxetine; Rivaroxaban; Salicylates; Serotonin Modulators; Thioridazine; Thrombolytic Agents; Tositumomab and Iodine I 131 Tositumomab; Tricyclic Antidepressants; Urokinase

The levels/effects of DULoxetine may be increased by: Abiraterone Acetate; Alcohol (Ethyl); Antiemetics (5HT3 Antagonists); Antipsychotic Agents; ARIPiprazole; Cobicistat; CYP1A2 Inhibitors (Moderate); CYP1A2 Inhibitors (Strong); CYP2D6 Inhibitors (Moderate); CYP2D6 Inhibitors (Strong); Dapoxetine; Darunavir; Dasatinib; Deferasirox; Glucosamine; Herbs (Anticoagulant/Antiplatelet Properties); Hypotensive Agents; Ibrutinib; Limaprost; Linezolid; MAO Inhibitors; Multivitamins/Fluoride (with ADE); Multivitamins/Minerals (with ADEK, Folate, Iron); Multivitamins/Minerals (with AE, No Iron); Omega-3 Fatty Acids; PARoxetine; Peginterferon Alfa-2b; Pentosan Polysulfate Sodium; Pentoxifylline; Propafenone; Prostacyclin Analogues; Tedizolid; Vemurafenib; Vitamin E

Decreased Effect

DULoxetine may decrease the levels/effects of: Codeine; Iobenguane I 123; Ioflupane I 123; Tamoxifen

The levels/effects of DULoxetine may be decreased by: Cannabis; CYP1A2 Inducers (Strong); Cyproterone; Peginterferon Alfa-2b; Teriflunomide

Storage/Stability Store at 25°C (77°F); excursions are permitted between 15°C and 30°C (59°F and 86°F).

Mechanism of Action Duloxetine is a potent inhibitor of neuronal serotonin and norepinephrine reuptake and a weak inhibitor of dopamine reuptake. Duloxetine has no significant activity for muscarinic cholinergic, H_1-histaminergic, or alpha$_2$-adrenergic receptors. Duloxetine does not possess MAO-inhibitory activity.

Pharmacodynamics/Kinetics

Absorption: Well absorbed, 2-hour delay in absorption after ingestion; food decreases extent of absorption ~10% (no effect on C_{max})

Distribution: 1,640 L

Protein binding: >90%; primarily to albumin and alpha$_1$-acid glycoprotein

Metabolism: Hepatic, via CYP1A2 and CYP2D6; forms multiple metabolites (inactive)

Half-life elimination: 12 hours (range: 8 to 17 hours)

Time to peak: 6 hours; 10 hours when ingested with food

Excretion: Urine (~70%; <1% of total dose as unchanged drug); feces (~20%)

Dosage Oral:

Children and Adolescents 7 to 17 years: Generalized anxiety disorder: Initial: 30 mg once daily; after 2 weeks may increase based on response and tolerability to 60 mg once daily; titrate doses >60 mg daily in increments of 30 mg daily; maximum dose: 120 mg daily.

Adults:

Major depressive disorder: Initial: 40 to 60 mg daily; dose may be divided (ie, 20 or 30 mg twice daily) or given as a single daily dose of 60 mg. For some patients it may be desirable to start at 30 mg once daily for 1 week (to allow patients to adjust to the medication) before increasing to 60 mg once daily. Maintenance: 60 mg once daily; maximum dose: 120 mg daily. **Note:** Doses >60 mg daily have not been demonstrated to be more effective than 60 mg daily.

Diabetic neuropathy: 60 mg once daily; lower initial doses may be considered in patients where tolerability is a concern and/or renal impairment is present; maximum dose: 60 mg daily. **Note:** Doses >60 mg daily administered in clinical trials offered no additional benefit and were less well tolerated than dose of 60 mg daily.

Fibromyalgia: 30 mg once daily for 1 week, then increase to 60 mg once daily as tolerated; maximum dose: 60 mg daily. **Note:** Doses >60 mg daily administered in clinical trials offered no additional benefit and were less well tolerated than dose of 60 mg daily.

Generalized anxiety disorder: Initial: 60 mg daily as a single daily dose; for some patients it may be desirable to start at 30 mg once daily for 1 week (to allow patients to adjust to the medication) before increasing to 60 mg once daily. For doses >60 mg daily, titrate dose in increments of 30 mg daily over 1 week as tolerated; maximum dose: 120 mg daily. **Note:** Doses >60 mg daily have not been demonstrated to be more effective than 60 mg daily.

Chronic musculoskeletal pain: Initial: 30 mg once daily for 1 week, then increase to 60 mg once daily as tolerated; maximum dose: 60 mg daily. **Note:** Doses >60 mg daily administered in clinical trials offered no additional benefit and were less well tolerated than dose of 60 mg daily.

Stress urinary incontinence (off-label use): 80 mg once daily or in 2 divided doses (range: 20 to 120 mg) for 12 weeks (Mariappan, 2005).

Elderly:

Major depressive disorder: Refer to adult dosing.

Generalized anxiety disorder: Initial: 30 mg once daily; after 2 weeks may increase to 60 mg once daily; titrate doses >60 mg daily in increments of 30 mg daily; maximum dose: 120 mg daily.

Other indications: Refer to adult dosing

Discontinuation of therapy: Upon discontinuation of antidepressant therapy, gradually taper the dose to minimize the incidence of withdrawal symptoms and allow for the detection of re-emerging symptoms. Evidence supporting ideal taper rates is limited. APA and NICE guidelines suggest tapering therapy over at least several weeks with consideration to the half-life of the antidepressant; antidepressants with a shorter half-life may need to be tapered more conservatively. In addition for long-term treated patients, WFSBP guidelines recommend tapering over 4-6 months. If intolerable withdrawal symptoms occur following a dose reduction, consider resuming the previously prescribed dose and/or decrease dose at a more gradual rate (APA, 2010; Bauer, 2002; Haddad, 2001; NCCMH, 2010; Schatzberg, 2006; Shelton, 2001; Warner, 2006).

MAO inhibitor recommendations:

Switching to or from an MAO inhibitor intended to treat psychiatric disorders:

Allow 14 days to elapse between discontinuing an MAO inhibitor intended to treat psychiatric disorders and initiation of duloxetine.

Allow ≥5 to 14 days to elapse between discontinuing duloxetine and initiation of an MAO inhibitor intended to treat psychiatric disorders.

Use with other MAO inhibitors (such as linezolid or IV methylene blue):

Do not initiate duloxetine in patients receiving linezolid or IV methylene blue; consider other interventions for psychiatric condition.

If urgent treatment with linezolid or IV methylene blue is required in a patient already receiving duloxetine and potential benefits outweigh potential risks, discontinue duloxetine promptly and administer linezolid or IV methylene blue. Monitor for serotonin syndrome for 5 days or until 24 hours after the last dose of linezolid or IV methylene blue, whichever comes first. May resume duloxetine 24 hours after the last dose of linezolid or IV methylene blue.

Dosage adjustment in renal impairment:

CrCl <30 mL/minute: Avoid use

End-stage renal disease (ESRD): Avoid use (contraindicated in Canadian labeling)

Dosage adjustment in hepatic impairment: Avoid use in hepatic impairment (contraindicated in Canadian labeling)

Dietary Considerations May be taken without regard to meals.

Administration Capsule should be swallowed whole; do not crush or chew. Although the manufacturer does not recommend opening the capsule to facilitate administration, the contents of capsule may be sprinkled on applesauce or in apple juice and swallowed (without chewing) immediately; do not sprinkle contents on chocolate pudding (Wells, 2008). Administer without regard to meals.

Monitoring Parameters Blood pressure should be checked prior to initiating therapy and then regularly monitored, especially in patients with a high baseline blood pressure; mental status for depression, suicidal ideation (especially at the beginning of therapy or when doses are increased or decreased), anxiety, social functioning, mania, panic attacks or other unusual changes in behavior; glucose levels and HbA_{1c} levels in diabetic patients, creatinine, BUN, transaminases

Dosage Forms

Capsule Delayed Release Particles, Oral:

Cymbalta: 20 mg, 30 mg, 60 mg

Generic: 20 mg, 30 mg, 60 mg

- **Duloxetine Hydrochloride** *see* DULoxetine *on page 698*
- **Duodopa (Can)** *see* Carbidopa and Levodopa *on page 351*
- **Duodote** *see* Atropine and Pralidoxime *on page 203*
- **DuoNeb®** *see* Ipratropium and Albuterol *on page 1109*
- **Duopa** *see* Carbidopa and Levodopa *on page 351*
- **DuoTrav PQ (Can)** *see* Travoprost and Timolol [CAN/INT] *on page 2090*
- **Duovent® UDV (Can)** *see* Ipratropium and Fenoterol [CAN/INT] *on page 1109*
- **DuP 753** *see* Losartan *on page 1248*
- **Duraclon** *see* CloNIDine *on page 480*
- **Duragesic** *see* FentaNYL *on page 857*
- **Duragesic MAT (Can)** *see* FentaNYL *on page 857*
- **Duramorph** *see* Morphine (Systemic) *on page 1394*
- **Duratocin™ (Can)** *see* Carbetocin [CAN/INT] *on page 350*
- **Durela (Can)** *see* TraMADol *on page 2074*
- **Durezol** *see* Difluprednate *on page 626*
- **Duricef** *see* Cefadroxil *on page 372*
- **Durolane (Can)** *see* Hyaluronate and Derivatives *on page 1006*

Dutasteride (doo TAS teer ide)

Brand Names: U.S. Avodart

Brand Names: Canada ACT-Dutasteride; Apo-Dutasteride; Avodart; Med-Dutasteride; Mint-Dutasteride; PMS-Dutasteride; Riva-Dutasteride; Sandoz-Dutasteride; Teva-Dutasteride

Pharmacologic Category 5 Alpha-Reductase Inhibitor

Use Treatment of symptomatic benign prostatic hyperplasia (BPH) as monotherapy or combination therapy with tamsulosin

Pregnancy Risk Factor X

Dosage Oral: Adults: Males: BPH: 0.5 mg once daily alone or in combination with tamsulosin

Dosage adjustment in renal impairment: No adjustment required

Dosage adjustment in hepatic impairment: Use caution; no specific adjustments recommended

Additional Information Complete prescribing information should be consulted for additional detail.

Dosage Forms

Capsule, Oral:

Avodart: 0.5 mg

Dutasteride and Tamsulosin
(doo TAS teer ide & tam SOO loe sin)

Brand Names: U.S. Jalyn

Brand Names: Canada Jalyn

Index Terms Tamsulosin and Dutasteride; Tamsulosin Hydrochloride and Dutasteride

Pharmacologic Category 5 Alpha-Reductase Inhibitor; Alpha$_1$ Blocker

Use Benign prostatic hyperplasia: Treatment of symptomatic benign prostatic hyperplasia (BPH) in men with an enlarged prostate

Pregnancy Risk Factor X

Dosage Benign prostatic hypertrophy (BPH): Adults: Males: Oral: One capsule (0.5 mg dutasteride/0.4 mg tamsulosin) once daily ~30 minutes after the same meal each day

Dosage adjustment in renal impairment:

CrCl 10-30 mL/minute/1.73 m^2: No dosage adjustment necessary.

CrCl <10 mL/minute/1.73 m^2: No dosage adjustment provided in the manufacturer's labeling (has not been studied).

Dosage adjustment in hepatic impairment: No dosage adjustment provided in the manufacturer's labeling.

Additional Information Complete prescribing information should be consulted for additional detail.

Dosage Forms

Capsule, oral:

Jalyn™: Dutasteride 0.5 mg and tamsulosin hydrochloride 0.4 mg

- ◆ **Duvoid® (Can)** *see* Bethanechol *on page 257*
- ◆ **DW286** *see* Gemifloxacin *on page 957*
- ◆ **DX-88** *see* Ecallantide *on page 703*
- ◆ **Dyazide** *see* Hydrochlorothiazide and Triamterene *on page 1012*

Dyclonine (DYE kloe neen)

Brand Names: U.S. Sucrets® Children's [OTC]; Sucrets® Maximum Strength [OTC]; Sucrets® Regular Strength [OTC]

Index Terms Dyclonine Hydrochloride

Pharmacologic Category Local Anesthetic, Oral

Use Temporary relief of pain associated with oral mucosa

Dosage Oral: Children ≥2 years and Adults: Lozenge: One lozenge every 2 hours as needed (maximum: 10 lozenges/day)

Additional Information Complete prescribing information should be consulted for additional detail.

Dosage Forms

Lozenge, oral:

Sucrets® Children's [OTC]: 1.2 mg (18s)
Sucrets® Maximum Strength [OTC]: 3 mg (18s)
Sucrets® Regular Strength [OTC]: 2 mg (18s)

- ◆ **Dyclonine Hydrochloride** *see* Dyclonine *on page 702*

Dydrogesterone [INT] (dye droe JES ter one)

International Brand Names Dabroston (HR); Dufaston (IT); Duphaston (AE, AT, AU, BE, BH, BR, CH, CL, CO, CY, CZ, DE, EC, EE, EG, ES, FR, GB, GR, HK, HN, HR, HU, ID, IE, IL, IN, JO, KR, KW, LB, LT, LU, MY, NL, PH, PK, PL, PT, PY, QA, RO, RU, SA, SE, SG, SK, TH, TR, TW, VE, VN, ZA); Terolut (DK, FI, NO)

Pharmacologic Category Progestin

Reported Use Treatment of progesterone deficiencies; counteract unopposed estrogen in hormone replacement therapy

Dosage Range Adults: Oral: 5-40 mg/day

Product Availability Product available in various countries; not currently available in the U.S.

Dosage Forms

Tablet: 10 mg

- ◆ **Dyloject** *see* Diclofenac (Systemic) *on page 617*
- ◆ **Dymista™** *see* Azelastine and Fluticasone *on page 214*
- ◆ **Dyrenium** *see* Triamterene *on page 2101*
- ◆ **Dyspel [OTC]** *see* Ibuprofen *on page 1032*
- ◆ **Dysport** *see* AbobotulinumtoxinA *on page 28*
- ◆ **Dysport (Glabellar Lines)** *see* AbobotulinumtoxinA *on page 28*
- ◆ **7E3** *see* Abciximab *on page 24*
- ◆ **E-400 [OTC]** *see* Vitamin E *on page 2174*
- ◆ **E-400-Clear [OTC]** *see* Vitamin E *on page 2174*
- ◆ **E-400-Mixed [OTC]** *see* Vitamin E *on page 2174*
- ◆ **E2020** *see* Donepezil *on page 668*
- ◆ **E 2080** *see* Rufinamide *on page 1854*
- ◆ **E7389** *see* Eribulin *on page 755*
- ◆ **EACA** *see* Aminocaproic Acid *on page 113*
- ◆ **Ear Drops Earwax Aid [OTC]** *see* Carbamide Peroxide *on page 350*
- ◆ **Ear Wax Remover [OTC] [DSC]** *see* Carbamide Peroxide *on page 350*
- ◆ **Earwax Treatment Drops [OTC]** *see* Carbamide Peroxide *on page 350*

Ebastine [INT] (EB as teen)

International Brand Names Alastina (ES); Aleva (PH); Bactil (ES); Bromselon (ES); Busidril (ES); Clever (IT); Ebasitin (VN); Ebast (IN, PK); Ebastel (AE, AR, BR, CL, CY, DE, EC, ES, JP, KR, KW, LB, SA, TR, TW, VE); Ebastin (TW); Ebatis (KR); Ebost (VN); Erostin (IN); Estel (KR); Estimin (TW); Estivan (BE); Evastel (MX); Evastel Z (MX); Histagone (PH); Kestin (FR); Kestine (AT, DK, EE, FI, GR, HK, IE, IS, IT, LT, NL, NO, PK, PT, RU, SE, SG, TR, ZA); Kestinlyo (FR); Pinavalt (CO, MX); Si Jin (CN)

Pharmacologic Category Antihistamine, Nonsedating

Reported Use Symptomatic treatment of idiopathic chronic urticaria and seasonal and perennial allergic rhinitis

Dosage Range Adults: Oral: Allergic rhinitis (seasonal and perennial) and urticaria (chronic idiopathic): 10-20 mg/day

Product Availability Product available in various countries; not currently available in the U.S.

Dosage Forms

Solution, oral: 5 mg/5 mL

Tablet: 10 mg

◆ **Ebixa (Can)** *see* Memantine *on page 1286*

Ecallantide (e KAL lan tide)

Brand Names: U.S. Kalbitor

Index Terms DX-88

Pharmacologic Category Kallikrein Inhibitor

Use Hereditary angioedema: Treatment of acute attacks of hereditary angioedema (HAE) in patients 12 years and older

Pregnancy Risk Factor C

Dosage Hereditary angioedema (HAE) treatment: Children ≥12 years, Adolescents, and Adults: SubQ: 30 mg (as three 10 mg [1 mL] injections); if attack persists, may repeat an additional 30 mg within 24 hours

Dosage adjustment in renal impairment: There are no dosage adjustments provided in the manufacturer's labeling (has not been studied).

Dosage adjustment in hepatic impairment: There are no dosage adjustments provided in the manufacturer's labeling (has not been studied).

Additional Information Complete prescribing information should be consulted for additional detail.

Dosage Forms

Solution, Subcutaneous [preservative free]:

Kalbitor: 10 mg/mL (1 mL)

Echothiophate Iodide
(ek oh THYE oh fate EYE oh dide)

Brand Names: U.S. Phospholine Iodide

Index Terms Ecostigmine Iodide

Pharmacologic Category Acetylcholinesterase Inhibitor; Ophthalmic Agent, Antiglaucoma; Ophthalmic Agent, Miotic

Use Used as miotic in treatment of chronic, open-angle glaucoma; may be useful in specific cases of angle-closure glaucoma (postiridectomy or where surgery refused/contraindicated); postcataract surgery-related glaucoma; accommodative esotropia

Pregnancy Risk Factor C

Dosage Ophthalmic:

Children: Accommodative esotropia:

Diagnosis: Instill 1 drop (0.125%) once daily into both eyes at bedtime for 2-3 weeks

Treatment: Usual dose: Instill 1 drop of 0.06% once daily or 0.125% every other day (maximum: 0.125% daily). **Note:** Use lowest concentration and frequency which gives satisfactory response; if necessary, doses >0.125% daily may be used for short periods of time.

Adults: Open-angle or secondary glaucoma:

Initial: Instill 1 drop (0.03%) twice daily into eyes with 1 dose just prior to bedtime

Maintenance: Some patients have been treated with 1 dose daily or every other day

Conversion from other ophthalmic agents: If IOP control was unsatisfactory, patients may be expected to require higher doses of echothiophate (eg, ≥0.06%); however, patients should be initially started on the 0.03% strength for a short period to better tolerance.

Dosage adjustment in renal impairment: No dosage adjustment provided in manufacturer's labeling.

Dosage adjustment in hepatic impairment: No dosage adjustment provided in manufacturer's labeling.

Additional Information Complete prescribing information should be consulted for additional detail.

Dosage Forms

Solution Reconstituted, Ophthalmic:

Phospholine Iodide: 0.125% (5 mL)

◆ **ECL-Citalopram (Can)** *see* Citalopram *on page 451*

◆ **EC-Naprosyn** *see* Naproxen *on page 1427*

◆ ***E. coli* Asparaginase** *see* Asparaginase (*E. coli*) *on page 179*

Econazole (e KONE a zole)

Brand Names: U.S. Ecoza

Index Terms Econazole Nitrate; Ecoza

Pharmacologic Category Antifungal Agent, Imidazole Derivative; Antifungal Agent, Topical

Use Fungal infection:

Cream: Treatment of tinea pedis, tinea cruris, and tinea corporis caused by *Trichophyton rubrum*, *Trichophyton mentagrophytes*, *Trichophyton tonsurans*, *Microsporum canis*, *Microsporum audouini*, *Microsporum gypseum*, and *Epidermophyton floccosum* in the treatment of cutaneous candidiasis, and in the treatment of tinea versicolor.

Foam: Treatment of interdigital tinea pedis caused by *Trichophyton rubrum*, *Trichophyton mentagrophytes*, and *Epidermophyton floccosum* in patients 12 years and older

Pregnancy Risk Factor C

Dosage

Children ≥12 years, Adolescents, and Adults: Topical:

Foam: Tinea pedis: Apply sufficient amount to cover affected area once daily for 4 weeks

Adults: Topical: Cream:

Tinea pedis: Apply sufficient amount to cover affected areas once daily for 4 weeks

Tinea cruris, tinea corporis, tinea versicolor: Apply sufficient amount to cover affected areas once daily for 2 weeks

Cutaneous candidiasis: Apply sufficient quantity twice daily (morning and evening) for 2 weeks

Additional Information Complete prescribing information should be consulted for additional detail.

Product Availability Ecoza topical foam: FDA approved October 2013; anticipated availability currently unknown

Dosage Forms

Cream, External:

Generic: 1% (15 g, 30 g, 85 g)

Foam, External:

Ecoza: 1% (70 g)

◆ **Econazole Nitrate** *see* Econazole *on page 703*

◆ **Econopred** *see* PrednisoLONE (Ophthalmic) *on page 1706*

◆ **Ecostigmine Iodide** *see* Echothiophate Iodide *on page 703*

◆ **Ecotrin [OTC]** *see* Aspirin *on page 180*

◆ **Ecotrin Arthritis Strength [OTC]** *see* Aspirin *on page 180*

◆ **Ecotrin Low Strength [OTC]** *see* Aspirin *on page 180*

◆ **Ecoza** *see* Econazole *on page 703*

Eculizumab (e kue LIZ oo mab)

Brand Names: U.S. Soliris

Brand Names: Canada Soliris

Index Terms h5G1.1; Monoclonal Antibody 5G1.1; Monoclonal Antibody Anti-C5

Pharmacologic Category Monoclonal Antibody; Monoclonal Antibody, Complement Inhibitor

Use

Atypical hemolytic uremic syndrome: Treatment of atypical hemolytic uremic syndrome (aHUS) to inhibit complement-mediated thrombotic microangiopathy.

Limitation of use: Eculizumab is not indicated for the treatment of patients with Shiga toxin *Escherichia coli*-related hemolytic uremic syndrome.

Paroxysmal nocturnal hemoglobinuria: Treatment of paroxysmal nocturnal hemoglobinuria (PNH) to reduce hemolysis.

Pregnancy Risk Factor C

Pregnancy Considerations Adverse events were observed in animal reproduction studies. Eculizumab is a recombinant IgG molecule with IgG2 and IgG4 sequences; human IgG is known to cross the placenta, however IgG2 may have reduced placental transfer compared to other IgG subclasses. Pregnant women with PNH and their fetuses have high rates of morbidity and mortality during pregnancy and the postpartum period. Limited information is available related to use during pregnancy. Use during pregnancy only if clearly needed.

Breast-Feeding Considerations It is not known if eculizumab is excreted in human milk. However, human IgG is excreted in breast milk, and therefore, eculizumab may also be excreted in milk. Although antibodies in human milk do not enter neonatal or infant circulation in substantial amounts, the risks to the infant from gastrointestinal or limited systemic exposure are unknown.

Contraindications Unresolved serious *Neisseria meningitidis* infection; patients not currently vaccinated against *Neisseria meningitidis* (unless risks of treatment delay outweigh risk of developing a meningococcal infection)

Warnings/Precautions [U.S. Boxed Warning]: Meningococcal *(Neisseria meningitides)* infections have occurred in patients receiving eculizumab; may be fatal or life-threatening if not detected and treated promptly. Monitor closely for early signs of meningococcal infection; evaluate and treat promptly if suspected. Follow current meningococcal immunization recommendations for patients with complement deficiencies. Vaccinate with meningococcal vaccine at least 2 weeks prior to initiation of treatment (unless the risks of delaying eculizumab outweigh the risk of developing meningococcal infection); revaccinate according to current guidelines. Polyvalent meningococcal vaccines are recommended. If urgent treatment is necessary in an unvaccinated patient, administer meningococcal vaccine as soon as possible. Although the risk/benefits of prophylactic meningococcal antibiotic therapy have not been determined, prophylactic antibiotics were administered in clinical studies until at least 2 weeks after vaccination. Meningococcal infections developed in some patients despite vaccination. Discontinue eculizumab during the treatment of serious meningococcal infections. In addition to meningitis, the risk of other infections, especially encapsulated bacteria (eg, *Streptococcus pneumoniae, H. influenzae*) is increased with eculizumab treatment (because eculizumab blocks terminal complement activation). Aspergillus infections have occurred in immunocompromised and neutropenic patients. Children should receive vaccination for prevention of *S. pneumoniae, H. influenzae* according to current ACIP guidelines. Use caution in patients with concurrent systemic infection. Patients should be up to date with all immunizations before initiating therapy. **[U.S. Boxed Warning]: Access is restricted through a REMS program. Prescribers must be enrolled in the program; enrollment and additional information is available at 1-888-765-4747.** Counsel patients on the risk of meningococcal infection; ensure patients are vaccinated and provide educational materials.

Infusion reactions, including anaphylaxis or hypersensitivity, may occur; interrupt infusion for severe reaction (eg, cardiovascular instability, respiratory compromise). Continue monitoring for 1 hour after completion of infusion. Patients with PNH who discontinue treatment may be at increased risk for serious hemolysis; monitor closely for at least 8 weeks after treatment discontinuation. When used for aHUS, monitor for at least 12 weeks after treatment discontinuation for signs/symptoms of thrombotic microangiopathy (TMA) complications (angina, dyspnea, mental status changes, seizure, or thrombosis; occurrence of two or repeated measurement of any one of the following: Serum creatinine elevation (≥25% from baseline or nadir), serum LDH elevation (≥25% from baseline or nadir), thrombocytopenia (platelet decrease by ≥25% compared to baseline or peak). If TMA complications occur after stopping eculizumab, consider reinitiation of treatment, plasmapheresis, plasma exchange, fresh frozen plasma infusion, and/or appropriate organ-specific measures. In clinical trials, anticoagulant therapy was continued in patients who were receiving these agents (due to history of or risk for thromboembolism) prior to initiation of eculizumab. Potentially significant drug-drug interactions may exist, requiring dose or frequency adjustment, additional monitoring, and/or selection of alternative therapy. The effect of anticoagulant therapy withdrawal is unknown; treatment with eculizumab should not alter anticoagulation management

Adverse Reactions

Cardiovascular: Hypertension (more common in aHUS patients), hypotension, peripheral edema, tachycardia

Central nervous system: Fatigue, headache, insomnia

Dermatologic: Pruritus, skin rash

Endocrine & metabolic: Hypokalemia

Gastrointestinal: Abdominal pain, constipation, diarrhea (more common in adults), dyspepsia, gastroenteritis, nausea, vomiting (more common in adults)

Genitourinary: Proteinuria, urinary tract infection (more common in adults), uropathy

Hematologic & oncologic: Anemia, leukopenia, neoplasm

Immunologic: Antibody development

Infection: Herpes virus infection, viral infection, meningococcal infection

Local: Catheter infection

Neuromuscular & skeletal: Arthralgia, back pain, limb pain, muscle spasm, myalgia, weakness

Ophthalmic: Eye disease

Renal: Renal insufficiency

Respiratory: Bronchitis, cough, flu-like symptoms, nasal congestion, nasopharyngitis (more common in adults), oropharyngeal pain, respiratory tract infection, rhinitis, sinusitis, upper respiratory tract infection

Miscellaneous: Fever (more common in infants, children, and adolescents 2 months through 17 years)

Rare but important or life-threatening: Aspergillosis, cholangitis, endometritis, hematoma (mild), infusion related reaction, pyelonephritis

Drug Interactions

Metabolism/Transport Effects None known.

Avoid Concomitant Use

Avoid concomitant use of Eculizumab with any of the following: BCG; Belimumab; Natalizumab; Pimecrolimus; Tacrolimus (Topical); Tofacitinib; Vaccines (Live)

Increased Effect/Toxicity

Eculizumab may increase the levels/effects of: Belimumab; Leflunomide; Natalizumab; Tofacitinib; Vaccines (Live)

The levels/effects of Eculizumab may be increased by: Denosumab; Pimecrolimus; Roflumilast; Tacrolimus (Topical); Trastuzumab

Decreased Effect

Eculizumab may decrease the levels/effects of: BCG; Coccidioides immitis Skin Test; Sipuleucel-T; Vaccines (Inactivated); Vaccines (Live)

The levels/effects of Eculizumab may be decreased by: Echinacea

Preparation for Administration Add eculizumab to an infusion bag and dilute with an equal volume of D_5W, sodium chloride 0.9%, sodium chloride 0.45%, or Ringer's injection to a final concentration of 5 mg/mL (eg, 300 mg to a total volume of 60 mL, 600 mg in a total volume of 120 mL, 900 mg in a total volume of 180 mL, or 1200 mg to a total volume of 240 mL). Gently invert bag to mix thoroughly; do not shake.

Storage/Stability Prior to dilution, store intact vials at 2°C to 8°C (36°F to 46°F); do not freeze. Protect from light; do not shake. Following dilution, store at room temperature or refrigerate; protect from light; use within 24 hours. If refrigerated, allow admixture to reach room temperature prior to administration (do not use a heat source or warming).

Mechanism of Action Terminal complement-mediated intravascular hemolysis is a key clinical feature of paroxysmal nocturnal hemoglobinuria (PNH); blocking the formation of membrane attack complex (MAC) results in stabilization of hemoglobin and a reduction in the need for RBC transfusions. Impairment of complement activity regulation leads to uncontrolled complement activation in atypical hemolytic uremic syndrome (aHUS). Eculizumab is a humanized monoclonal IgG antibody that binds to complement protein C5, preventing cleavage into C5a and C5b. Blocking the formation of C5b inhibits the subsequent formation of terminal complex C5b-9 or MAC.

Pharmacodynamics/Kinetics

Onset of action: PNH: Reduced hemolysis: ≤1 week

Distribution: PNH: 7.7 L; aHUS: 6.14 L

Half-life elimination: PNH: ~11 days (range: ~8-15 days); aHUS: ~12 days (during plasma exchange the half-life is reduced to 1.26 hours)

Dosage Note: Patients must receive meningococcal vaccine at least 2 weeks prior to treatment initiation; revaccinate according to current guidelines. Treatment should be administered at the recommended time interval although administration may be varied by ±2 days.

Atypical hemolytic uremic syndrome (aHUS): IV:

Children 5 kg to <10 kg: Induction: 300 mg weekly for 1 dose; Maintenance: 300 mg at week 2, then 300 mg every 3 weeks

Children 10 kg to <20 kg: Induction: 600 mg weekly for 1 dose; Maintenance: 300 mg at week 2, then 300 mg every 2 weeks

Children 20 kg to <30 kg: Induction: 600 mg weekly for 2 doses; Maintenance: 600 mg at week 3, then 600 mg every 2 weeks

Children 30 kg to <40 kg: Induction: 600 mg weekly for 2 doses; Maintenance: 900 mg at week 3, then 900 mg every 2 weeks

Children ≥40 kg and Adults: Induction: 900 mg weekly for 4 doses; Maintenance: 1200 mg at week 5, then 1200 mg every 2 weeks

Supplemental dosing for patients receiving plasmapheresis or plasma exchange:

If most recent dose was 300 mg, administer 300 mg within 60 minutes after each plasmapheresis or plasma exchange

If most recent dose was ≥600 mg, administer 600 mg within 60 minutes after each plasmapheresis or plasma exchange

Supplemental dosing for patients receiving fresh frozen plasma infusion: If most recent dose was ≥300 mg, administer 300 mg within 60 minutes prior to each infusion of fresh frozen plasma

Paroxysmal nocturnal hemoglobinuria (PNH): IV: Adults: 600 mg weekly for 4 doses, followed by 900 mg 1 week later, then 900 mg every 2 weeks

Dosage adjustment in renal impairment: There are no dosage adjustments provided in the manufacturer's labeling (has not been studied).

Dosage adjustment in hepatic impairment: There are no dosage adjustments provided in the manufacturer's labeling (has not been studied).

Administration IV: Allow to reach room temperature prior to administration. Infuse over 35 minutes in adults and over 1 to 4 hours in pediatric patients; do not administer as an IV push or bolus. Decrease infusion rate or discontinue for infusion reactions; do not exceed a maximum 2-hour duration of infusion in adults. Monitor for at least 1 hour following completion of infusion (for signs/symptoms of infusion reaction).

Monitoring Parameters CBC with differential, lactic dehydrogenase (LDH), serum creatinine, AST, urinalysis; early signs/symptoms of meningococcal infection; signs and symptoms of infusion reaction (during infusion and for 1 hour after infusion complete).

After discontinuation:

aHUS: Signs/symptoms of thrombotic microangiopathy (TMA) complications (monitor for at least 12 weeks after treatment discontinuation), including angina, dyspnea, mental status changes, seizure, or thrombosis; occurrence of two or repeated measurement of any one of the following: Serum creatinine elevation (≥25% from baseline or nadir), serum LDH elevation (≥25% from baseline or nadir), thrombocytopenia (platelet decrease by ≥25% compared to baseline or peak).

PNH: Signs and symptoms of intravascular hemolysis (monitor for at least 8 weeks after discontinuation), including anemia, fatigue, pain, dark urine, dyspnea, or thrombosis.

Dosage Forms

Solution, Intravenous [preservative free]:

Soliris: 10 mg/mL (30 mL)

- ◆ **Ed-A-Hist™ [OTC]** *see* Chlorpheniramine and Phenylephrine *on page 426*
- ◆ **Ed A-Hist DM [OTC]** *see* Chlorpheniramine, Phenylephrine, and Dextromethorphan *on page 428*
- ◆ **Ed A-Hist PSE [OTC]** *see* Triprolidine and Pseudoephedrine *on page 2105*
- ◆ **Edarbi** *see* Azilsartan *on page 214*
- ◆ **Edarbyclor** *see* Azilsartan and Chlorthalidone *on page 215*
- ◆ **Edarbyclor™ (Can)** *see* Azilsartan and Chlorthalidone *on page 215*
- ◆ **Ed Bron GP [OTC]** *see* Guaifenesin and Phenylephrine *on page 988*
- ◆ **Ed ChlorPed D [OTC]** *see* Chlorpheniramine and Phenylephrine *on page 426*
- ◆ **Edecrin** *see* Ethacrynic Acid *on page 797*

Edetate CALCIUM Disodium

(ED e tate KAL see um dye SOW dee um)

Index Terms CaEDTA; Calcium Disodium Edetate; Calcium Disodiumethylenediaminetetraacetic Acid; Edetate Disodium CALCIUM; EDTA (CALCIUM Disodium) (error-prone abbreviation)

Pharmacologic Category Chelating Agent

Use Treatment of symptomatic acute and chronic lead poisoning

Pregnancy Risk Factor B

Dosage IM, IV:

Lead poisoning: **Note:** For the treatment of high blood lead levels in children, the CDC recommends chelation treatment when blood lead levels are >45 mcg/dL (CDC, 2002). The AAP recommends succimer as the drug used for initial management in asymptomatic children when blood lead levels are >45 mcg/dL and <70 mcg/dL. Edetate CALCIUM disodium can be used in children allergic to succimer (AAP, 2005; Chandran, 2010). Combination therapy with edetate CALCIUM disodium and dimercaprol is recommended for use in children whose blood lead levels are ≥70 mcg/dL or in children with lead encephalopathy (AAP, 2005; Chandran, 2010). In adults, available guidelines recommend chelation therapy with blood lead levels >50 mcg/dL and significant symptoms; chelation therapy may also be indicated with blood lead levels ≥100 mcg/dL and/or symptoms (Kosnett, 2007). Depending upon the blood lead level, additional courses may be necessary; at least 2-4 days should elapse before repeat treatment is initiated.

Blood lead levels <70 mcg/dL and asymptomatic:

Children: 1000 mg/m²/day for 5 days or 50 mg/kg/day (maximum: 1000 mg/day) for 5 days (Chandran, 2010)

Adults: 1000 mg/m²/day for 5 days

Blood lead levels ≥70 mcg/dL or symptomatic lead poisoning (in conjunction with dimercaprol): **Note:** Begin treatment with edetate CALCIUM disodium with the second dimercaprol dose:

Children: 1000 mg/m²/day **or** 25-50 mg/kg/day (maximum: 1000 mg/day) for 5 days (Chandran, 2010; Howland, 2011)

Adults: 1000 mg/m²/day **or** 25-50 mg/kg/day for 5 days; a maximum dose of 3000 mg has been suggested (Howland, 2011)

Lead encephalopathy (in conjunction with dimercaprol): **Note:** Begin treatment with edetate CALCIUM disodium with the second dimercaprol dose:

Children: 1500 mg/m²/day **or** 50-75 mg/kg/day (maximum: 1000 mg/day) for 5 days (Chandran, 2010; Howland, 2011)

Adults: 1500 mg/m²/day **or** 50-75 mg/kg/day for 5 days; a maximum dose of 3000 mg has been suggested (Howland, 2011)

Lead nephropathy: Adults: An alternative dosing regimen reflecting the reduction in renal clearance is based upon the serum creatinine; **Note:** Repeat regimen monthly until lead levels are reduced to an acceptable level:

S_{cr} 2-3 mg/dL: 500 mg/m² every 24 hours for 5 days

S_{cr} 3-4 mg/dL: 500 mg/m² every 48 hours for 3 doses

S_{cr} >4 mg/dL: 500 mg/m² once weekly

Dosage adjustment in renal impairment: Dose should be reduced with preexisting mild renal disease. Limiting the daily dose to 1 g in children and 2 g in adults may decrease risk of nephrotoxicity, although larger doses may be needed in the treatment of lead encephalopathy (Howland, 2011).

Additional Information Complete prescribing information should be consulted for additional detail.

Dosage Forms

Solution, Injection:

Generic: 1 g/5 mL (5 mL)

◆ **Edetate Disodium CALCIUM** *see* Edetate CALCIUM Disodium *on page 705*

◆ **Edex** *see* Alprostadil *on page 96*

◆ **Edluar** *see* Zolpidem *on page 2212*

Edrophonium (ed roe FOE nee um)

Brand Names: U.S. Enlon

Brand Names: Canada Enlon®; Tensilon®

Index Terms Edrophonium Chloride

Pharmacologic Category Acetylcholinesterase Inhibitor; Antidote; Diagnostic Agent

Use Diagnosis of myasthenia gravis; differentiation of cholinergic crises from myasthenia crises; reversal of nondepolarizing neuromuscular blockers

Dosage Usually administered IV, however, if not possible, IM or SubQ may be used:

Infants:

IM: 0.5-1 mg

IV: Initial: 0.1 mg, followed by 0.4 mg if no response; total dose = 0.5 mg

Children:

Diagnosis: Initial: 0.04 mg/kg over 1 minute followed by 0.16 mg/kg if no response, to a maximum total dose of 5 mg for children <34 kg, or 10 mg for children >34 kg **or**

Alternative dosing (manufacturer's recommendation):

≤34 kg: 1 mg; if no response after 45 seconds, repeat dosage in 1 mg increments every 30-45 seconds, up to a total of 5 mg

>34 kg: 2 mg; if no response after 45 seconds, repeat dosage in 1 mg increments every 30-45 seconds, up to a total of 10 mg

IM:

<34 kg: 1 mg

>34 kg: 5 mg

Titration of oral anticholinesterase therapy: 0.04 mg/kg once given 1 hour after oral intake of the drug being used in treatment; if strength improves, an increase in neostigmine or pyridostigmine dose is indicated

Adults:

Diagnosis:

IV: 2 mg test dose administered over 15-30 seconds; 8 mg given 45 seconds later if no response is seen; test dose may be repeated after 30 minutes

IM: Initial: 10 mg; if no cholinergic reaction occurs, administer 2 mg 30 minutes later to rule out false-negative reaction

Titration of oral anticholinesterase therapy: 1-2 mg given 1 hour after oral dose of anticholinesterase; if strength improves, an increase in neostigmine or pyridostigmine dose is indicated

Reversal of nondepolarizing neuromuscular blocking agents (neostigmine with atropine usually preferred): IV: 10 mg over 30-45 seconds; may repeat every 5-10 minutes up to 40 mg

Termination of paroxysmal atrial tachycardia: IV rapid injection: 5-10 mg

Differentiation of cholinergic from myasthenic crisis: IV: 1 mg; may repeat after 1 minute. **Note:** Intubation and controlled ventilation may be required if patient has cholinergic crisis

Dosage adjustment in renal impairment: Dose may need to be reduced in patients with chronic renal failure

Dosage adjustment in hepatic impairment: No dosage adjustment provided in manufacturer's labeling.

Additional Information Complete prescribing information should be consulted for additional detail.

Dosage Forms

Solution, Injection:

Enlon: 10 mg/mL (15 mL)

Edrophonium and Atropine

(ed roe FOE nee um & A troe peen)

Brand Names: U.S. Enlon-Plus®

Index Terms Atropine Sulfate and Edrophonium Chloride; Edrophonium Chloride and Atropine Sulfate

Pharmacologic Category Acetylcholinesterase Inhibitor; Anticholinergic Agent; Antidote

Use Reversal of nondepolarizing neuromuscular blockers; adjunct treatment of respiratory depression caused by curare overdose

Pregnancy Risk Factor C

Dosage IV: Adults: Reversal of neuromuscular blockade: 0.05-0.1 mL/kg given over 45-60 seconds. The dose delivered is 0.5-1 mg/kg of edrophonium and 0.007-0.014 mg/kg of atropine. An edrophonium dose of 1 mg/kg should rarely be exceeded. **Note:** Monitor closely for bradyarrhythmias.

Dosage adjustment in renal impairment: Adjustment not required.

Dosage adjustment in hepatic impairment: Adjustment not required.

Additional Information Complete prescribing information should be consulted for additional detail.

Dosage Forms

Injection, solution:

Enlon-Plus®: Edrophonium 10 mg/mL and atropine 0.14 mg/mL (5 mL, 15 mL)

- ◆ **Edrophonium Chloride** *see* Edrophonium *on page 706*
- ◆ **Edrophonium Chloride and Atropine Sulfate** *see* Edrophonium and Atropine *on page 706*
- ◆ **Ed-Spaz** *see* Hyoscyamine *on page 1026*
- ◆ **EDTA (CALCIUM Disodium) (error-prone abbreviation)** *see* Edetate CALCIUM Disodium *on page 705*
- ◆ **Edurant** *see* Rilpivirine *on page 1810*
- ◆ **Edurant® (Can)** *see* Rilpivirine *on page 1810*
- ◆ **EES (Can)** *see* Erythromycin (Systemic) *on page 762*
- ◆ **E.E.S. 400** *see* Erythromycin (Systemic) *on page 762*
- ◆ **E.E.S. Granules** *see* Erythromycin (Systemic) *on page 762*

Efavirenz (e FAV e renz)

Brand Names: U.S. Sustiva

Brand Names: Canada Mylan-Efavirenz; Sustiva; Teva-Efavirenz

Pharmacologic Category Antiretroviral, Reverse Transcriptase Inhibitor, Non-nucleoside (Anti-HIV)

Use HIV-1 infection: Treatment of HIV-1 infection in combination with other antiretroviral agents in adults and pediatric patients at least 3 months old and weighing at least 3.5 kg

Pregnancy Risk Factor D

Pregnancy Considerations Teratogenic effects have been observed in primates receiving efavirenz. Efavirenz has a moderate level of transfer across the human placenta. Based on data from the Antiretroviral Pregnancy Registry, an increased risk of overall birth defects has not been observed following first trimester exposure to efavirenz; however, neural tube and other CNS defects have been reported. Due to the low number of first trimester exposures and the low incidence of neural tube defects in the general population, available data are insufficient to evaluate risk. Other antiretroviral agents should strongly be considered for use in women of childbearing potential who are planning to become pregnant or who are sexually active and not using effective contraception. Nonpregnant women of reproductive age should undergo pregnancy testing prior to initiation of efavirenz. Barrier contraception should be used in combination with other (hormonal) methods of contraception during therapy and for 12 weeks after efavirenz is discontinued. Neural tube defects would occur following exposure during the first 5 to 6 weeks of gestation (most pregnancies are not detected before 4 to 6 weeks gestation). For women who present in the first trimester already on an efavirenz-containing regimen and who have adequate viral suppression, efavirenz may be continued; changing regimens may lead to loss of viral control and increase the risk of perinatal transmission. Pharmacokinetic data from available studies do not suggest dose alterations are needed during pregnancy. The DHHS Perinatal HIV Guidelines consider efavirenz to be a preferred NNRTI for use in antiretroviral-naive pregnant women after 8 weeks gestation. Hypersensitivity reactions (including hepatic toxicity and rash) are more common in women on NNRTI therapy; it is not known if pregnancy increases this risk.

Regardless of CD4 count or HIV RNA copy number, all HIV-infected pregnant women should receive a combination antiretroviral (ARV) drug regimen. A combination of antepartum, intrapartum, and infant ARV prophylaxis is recommended. ARV therapy should be started as soon as possible in women with symptomatic infection. Although earlier initiation may be more effective in reducing the perinatal transmission of HIV, initiation may be delayed until after 12 weeks gestation in women who do no require immediate treatment after careful consideration of maternal conditions (eg, nausea and vomiting) and the potential risks of first trimester fetal exposure for specific agents. A scheduled cesarean delivery at 38 weeks gestation is recommended for all women with HIV RNA >1000 copies/mL or unknown concentration near delivery in order to decrease transmission. If ARV therapy must be interrupted for <24 hours during the peripartum period, stop then restart all medications simultaneously in order to decrease the chance of developing resistance. Long-term follow-up is recommended for all infants exposed to ARV medications. In couples who want to conceive, the HIV-infected partner should attain maximum viral suppression prior to conception.

Health care providers are encouraged to enroll pregnant women exposed to antiretroviral medications in the Antiretroviral Pregnancy Registry (1-800-258-4263 or www.APRegistry.com). Health care providers caring for HIV-infected women and their infants may contact the National Perinatal HIV Hotline (888-448-8765) for clinical consultation (HHS [perinatal], 2014).

Breast-Feeding Considerations Efavirenz is excreted into breast milk. Although breast-feeding is not recommended, plasma concentrations of efavirenz in nursing infants have been reported as ~13% of maternal plasma concentrations.

Maternal or infant antiretroviral therapy does not completely eliminate the risk of postnatal HIV transmission. In addition, multiclass-resistant virus has been detected in breast-feeding infants despite maternal therapy. Therefore, in the United States, where formula is accessible, affordable, safe, and sustainable, and the risk of infant mortality due to diarrhea and respiratory infections is low, complete avoidance of breast-feeding by HIV-infected women is recommended to decrease potential transmission of HIV (HHS [perinatal], 2014).

Contraindications Hypersensitivity (eg, Stevens-Johnson syndrome, erythema multiforme, toxic skin eruptions) to efavirenz or any component of the formulation

Warnings/Precautions Do not use as single-agent therapy. Avoid pregnancy; women of childbearing potential should undergo pregnancy testing prior to initiation of therapy. Use caution with other agents metabolized by cytochrome P450 isoenzyme 3A4 (see Contraindications); concomitant use of other efavirenz-containing products should be avoided (unless needed for dosage adjustment with concomitant rifampin treatment). Use caution with history of mental illness/drug abuse (predisposition to psychological reactions); may cause CNS and psychiatric symptoms, which include impaired concentration, dizziness or drowsiness (avoid potentially hazardous tasks such as driving or operating machinery if these effects are noted); CNS effects may be potentiated when used with other psychoactive drugs or ethanol. Serious psychiatric side effects have been associated with efavirenz, including severe depression, suicidal ideation, nonfatal suicide attempts, paranoia, and mania; instruct patients to contact healthcare provider if serious psychiatric effects occur. May cause mild-to-moderate maculopapular rash; usually occurs within 2 weeks of starting therapy; discontinue if severe rash (involving blistering, desquamation, mucosal involvement, or fever) develops; contraindicated in patients with a history of a severe cutaneous reaction (eg, Stevens-Johnson syndrome). Children are more susceptible.

Caution in patients with known or suspected hepatitis B or C infection or Child-Pugh class A hepatic impairment; not recommended in Child-Pugh class B or C hepatic impairment. Persistent elevations of serum transaminases >5 times the upper limit of normal should prompt evaluation - benefit of continued therapy should be weighed against possible risk of hepatotoxicity. Hepatic failure has been reported, including patients with no preexisting hepatic disease or other identifiable risk factors. Monitor liver function tests in patients with underlying hepatic disease (eg, hepatitis B or C, marked transaminase elevations or taking concomitant medications that may cause hepatotoxicity). Ethanol may increase hepatotoxic potential; instruct patients to limit or avoid alcohol. Increases in total cholesterol and triglycerides have been reported; screening should be done prior to therapy and periodically throughout treatment. May cause redistribution of fat (eg, buffalo hump, peripheral wasting with increased abdominal girth, cushingoid appearance). Patients may develop immune reconstitution syndrome resulting in the occurrence of an inflammatory response to an indolent or residual opportunistic infection during initial HIV treatment or activation of autoimmune disorders (eg, Graves' disease, polymyositis, Guillain-Barré syndrome) later in therapy; further evaluation and treatment may be required. Use with caution in patients with a history of seizure disorder; seizures have been associated with use. Efavirenz administered as monotherapy or added on to a failing regimen may result in rapid viral resistance to efavirenz. Consider cross-resistance when adding antiretroviral agents on to efavirenz therapy.

Adverse Reactions

Central nervous system: Abnormal dreams, anxiety, depression, dizziness, fatigue, fever, hallucinations, headache, impaired concentration, insomnia, nervousness, pain, severe depression, somnolence

Dermatologic: Pruritus, rash

Endocrine & metabolic: HDL increased, hyperglycemia, total cholesterol increased, triglycerides increased

Gastrointestinal: Abdominal pain, amylase increased, anorexia, diarrhea, dyspepsia, nausea, vomiting

Hematologic: Neutropenia

Hepatic: ALT increased, AST increased

Respiratory: Cough

Rare but important or life-threatening: Allergic reaction, ataxia, body fat accumulation/redistribution, cerebellar coordination disturbances, delusions, dermatitis (photoallergic), erythema multiforme, gynecomastia, hepatic failure, hepatitis, immune reconstitution syndrome, malabsorption, mania, neuropathy, neurosis, palpitations, pancreatitis, paranoia, psychosis, seizures, Stevens-Johnson syndrome, suicide attempts, suicidal ideation, visual abnormalities

Drug Interactions

Metabolism/Transport Effects **Substrate** of CYP2B6 (major), CYP3A4 (major); **Note:** Assignment of Major/Minor substrate status based on clinically relevant drug interaction potential; **Inhibits** CYP2C19 (moderate), CYP2C9 (moderate); **Induces** CYP2B6 (moderate), CYP3A4 (moderate)

Avoid Concomitant Use

Avoid concomitant use of Efavirenz with any of the following: Atovaquone; Axitinib; Azelastine (Nasal); Boceprevir; Bosutinib; CarBAMazepine; Dasabuvir; Elvitegravir; Enzalutamide; Etravirine; Itraconazole; Ketoconazole (Systemic); Nevirapine; Nisoldipine; Olaparib; Orphenadrine; Paraldehyde; Paritaprevir; Posaconazole; Reverse Transcriptase Inhibitors (Non-Nucleoside); Rilpivirine; Simeprevir; St Johns Wort; Thalidomide; Ulipristal

Increased Effect/Toxicity

Efavirenz may increase the levels/effects of: Alcohol (Ethyl); Azelastine (Nasal); Bosentan; Cannabis; Carvedilol; Citalopram; CNS Depressants; CYP2C19 Substrates; CYP2C9 Substrates; Dasabuvir; Dronabinol; Etravirine; Fosphenytoin; Hydrocodone; Ifosfamide; Methotrimeprazine; Metyrosine; Mirtazapine; Nevirapine; Orphenadrine; Paraldehyde; Paritaprevir; Phenytoin; Pramipexole; Rilpivirine; Ritonavir; ROPINIRole; Rotigotine; Selective Serotonin Reuptake Inhibitors; Suvorexant; Tetrahydrocannabinol; Thalidomide; Vitamin K Antagonists; Zolpidem

The levels/effects of Efavirenz may be increased by: Boceprevir; Brimonidine (Topical); Cannabis; CYP2B6 Inhibitors (Moderate); Darunavir; Doxylamine; Dronabinol; Droperidol; HydrOXYzine; Kava Kava; Magnesium Sulfate; Methotrimeprazine; Mifepristone; Nabilone; Nevirapine; Perampanel; Quazepam; Reverse Transcriptase Inhibitors (Non-Nucleoside); Ritonavir; Rufinamide; Saquinavir; Sodium Oxybate; Tapentadol; Tetrahydrocannabinol; Voriconazole

Decreased Effect

Efavirenz may decrease the levels/effects of: Alcohol (Ethyl); ARIPiprazole; Artemether; Atazanavir; AtorvaSTATin; Atovaquone; Axitinib; Boceprevir; Bosutinib; Buprenorphine; BuPROPion; Calcium Channel Blockers; Canagliflozin; CarBAMazepine; Caspofungin; Clarithromycin; Clopidogrel; Contraceptives (Progestins); CycloSPORINE (Systemic); CYP3A4 Substrates; Darunavir; Dasabuvir; Diltiazem; Dolutegravir; Elvitegravir; Enzalutamide; Etonogestrel; Etravirine; Everolimus; FentaNYL; Fosamprenavir; Ibrutinib; Ifosfamide; Indinavir; Itraconazole; Ketoconazole (Systemic); Lopinavir; Lovastatin; Maraviroc; Methadone; Nisoldipine; Norgestimate; Olaparib; Ombitasvir; Paritaprevir; Posaconazole; Pravastatin; Proguanil; Raltegravir; Rifabutin; Rilpivirine; Saquinavir; Saxagliptin; Sertraline; Simeprevir; Simvastatin; Sirolimus; Tacrolimus (Systemic); Telaprevir; Ulipristal; Vitamin K Antagonists; Voriconazole

The levels/effects of Efavirenz may be decreased by: Bosentan; CarBAMazepine; CYP2B6 Inducers (Strong); CYP3A4 Inducers (Moderate); CYP3A4 Inducers (Strong); Dabrafenib; Deferasirox; Fosphenytoin; Ginkgo Biloba; Mitotane; Nevirapine; Phenytoin; Reverse Transcriptase Inhibitors (Non-Nucleoside); Rifabutin; Rifampin; Siltuximab; St Johns Wort; Telaprevir; Tocilizumab

Food Interactions High-fat meals increase the absorption of efavirenz. CNS effects are possible. Management: Avoid high-fat meals. Administer at or before bedtime on an empty stomach unless using capsule sprinkle method in patients unable to swallow capsules or tablets. If capsule sprinkle method is used, patient should not consume additional food for 2 hours after administration.

Storage/Stability Store at 25°C (77°F); excursion permitted to 15°C to 30°C (59°F to 86°F).

Mechanism of Action As a non-nucleoside reverse transcriptase inhibitor, efavirenz has activity against HIV-1 by binding to reverse transcriptase. It consequently blocks the RNA-dependent and DNA-dependent DNA polymerase activities including HIV-1 replication. It does not require intracellular phosphorylation for antiviral activity.

Pharmacodynamics/Kinetics

Absorption: Increased by fatty meals

Distribution: CSF concentrations exceed free fraction in serum

Protein binding: >99%, primarily to albumin

Metabolism: Hepatic via CYP3A4 and 2B6 to inactive hydroxylated metabolites; may induce its own metabolism

Half-life elimination: Single dose: 52 to 76 hours; Multiple doses: 40 to 55 hours

Time to peak: 3 to 5 hours

Excretion: Feces (16% to 61% primarily as unchanged drug); urine (14% to 34% as metabolites)

Dosage Oral: HIV infection (as part of combination therapy):

Children ≥3 months and ≥3.5 kg: Dosage is based on body weight:

3.5 kg to <5 kg: 100 mg once daily
5 kg to <7.5 kg: 150 mg once daily
7.5 kg to <15 kg: 200 mg once daily
15 kg to <20 kg: 250 mg once daily
20 kg to <25 kg: 300 mg once daily
25 kg to <32.5 kg: 350 mg once daily
32.5 kg to <40 kg: 400 mg once daily
≥40 kg: 600 mg once daily; **Note:** Dosage adjustments may be necessary if patient receives certain concomitant medications. Refer to adult dosing.

Adults: 600 mg once daily; **Note:** Efavirenz is a component of a recommended regimen (with tenofovir and emtrictabine) for all therapy-naive patients and a component of a recommended regimen (with abacavir and lamivudine) for therapy-naïve patients with a pre-ART plasma HIV RNA <100,000 copies/mL who are HLA-B*5701 negative (HHS, [adult] 2014).

Dosage adjustment for concomitant rifampin (only if patient weighs ≥50 kg): Increase efavirenz dose to 800 mg once daily

Dosage adjustment for concomitant voriconazole: Reduce efavirenz dose to 300 mg once daily and increase voriconazole to 400 mg every 12 hours

Dosing adjustment in renal impairment: There are no dosage adjustments provided in manufacturer's labeling (has not been studied); however, undergoes minimal renal excretion.

Dosing comments in hepatic impairment:

Mild impairment (Child-Pugh class A): No dosage adjustment necessary; use with caution.

Moderate-to-severe impairment (Child-Pugh class B or C): No dosage adjustment provided in manufacturer's labeling (has not been adequately studied); use not recommended.

Dietary Considerations Should be taken on an empty stomach unless using capsule sprinkle method in patients unable to swallow capsules or tablets. If capsule sprinkle method is used, do not consume additional food for 2 hours after administration.

Administration Administer on an empty stomach. Dosing at or before bedtime is recommended to limit central nervous system effects (HHS, [adult] 2014). Tablets should not be broken.

Capsule contents may be sprinkled onto a small amount of soft food (eg, applesauce, grape jelly, yogurt) for pediatric or adult patients who cannot swallow capsules. Place 1-2 teaspoonfuls of food in a small container. Hold capsule horizontally over container and carefully twist in opposite directions to open, sprinkling contents over food. If more than 1 capsule is needed for a dose, add contents of all capsules needed to 1-2 teaspoonfuls of food; do not add more food. Use a small spoon to gently mix capsule contents with food and administer all of mixture to patient. To ensure entire capsule contents are administered, add another 2 teaspoonfuls of food to the container, mix to incorporate any drug residue, and administer.

Capsule contents may also be mixed with infant formula only for pediatric patients who cannot reliably consume solid foods. Combine entire contents of capsule(s) with 10 mL of reconstituted, room temperature infant formula in a 30 mL medicine cup, stir carefully, then draw up mixture in a 10 mL oral syringe for administration. If more than 1 capsule is needed for a dose, add contents of all capsules needed to 10 mL of formula; do not add more formula. To ensure entire capsule contents are administered, add another 10 mL of formula to the cup, stir to incorporate any drug residue, draw up in oral syringe and administer.

Administer within 30 minutes of mixing. Patient should not consume any additional food or administer additional formula for 2 hours after administration.

Monitoring Parameters Serum transaminases (discontinuation of treatment should be considered for persistent elevations >5 times the upper limit of normal); cholesterol and triglycerides (prior to therapy and periodically during); signs and symptoms of infection; psychiatric effects

Additional Information Early virologic failure was observed with tenofovir and didanosine delayed release capsules, plus either efavirenz or nevirapine; use caution in treatment-naive patients with high baseline viral loads.

Dosage Forms

Capsule, Oral:

Sustiva: 50 mg, 200 mg

Tablet, Oral:

Sustiva: 600 mg

Efavirenz, Emtricitabine, and Tenofovir

(e FAV e renz, em trye SYE ta been, & ten OF oh vir)

Brand Names: U.S. Atripla

Brand Names: Canada Atripla

Index Terms Emtricitabine, Efavirenz, and Tenofovir; FTC, TDF, and EFV; Tenofovir Disoproxil Fumarate, Efavirenz, and Emtricitabine

Pharmacologic Category Antiretroviral, Reverse Transcriptase Inhibitor, Non-nucleoside (Anti-HIV); Antiretroviral, Reverse Transcriptase Inhibitor, Nucleoside (Anti-HIV); Antiretroviral, Reverse Transcriptase Inhibitor, Nucleotide (Anti-HIV)

Use Treatment of HIV-1 infection

Pregnancy Risk Factor D

Dosage Note: Prior to initiation, patients should be tested for hepatitis B infection, and baseline estimated creatinine clearance, serum phosphorus, urine glucose, and urine protein should be assessed in all patients.

Oral: Children ≥12 years and ≥40 kg, Adolescents, and Adults: One tablet once daily. **Note:** Recommended as an initial regimen for antiretroviral-naive patients (HHS [adult], 2014).

Dosage adjustment in renal impairment: Moderate-to-severe renal impairment (CrCl <50 mL/minute): Use not recommended

Dosage adjustment in hepatic impairment:

Mild hepatic impairment (Child-Pugh class A): Use with caution

Moderate or severe hepatic impairment (Child-Pugh class B, C): Not recommended

Additional Information Complete prescribing information should be consulted for additional detail.

Dosage Forms

Tablet, oral:

Atripla: Efavirenz 600 mg, emtricitabine 200 mg, and tenofovir disoproxil fumarate 300 mg

◆ **Effer-K** *see* Potassium Bicarbonate and Potassium Citrate *on page 1687*

◆ **Effexor XR** *see* Venlafaxine *on page 2150*

◆ **Effient** *see* Prasugrel *on page 1699*

Efinaconazole (ef in a KON a zole)

Brand Names: U.S. Jublia

Brand Names: Canada Jublia

Pharmacologic Category Antifungal Agent, Topical

Use Onychomycosis: Topical treatment of onychomycosis of the toenail(s) due to *Trichophyton rubrum* and *Trichophyton mentagrophytes*

Pregnancy Risk Factor C

Dosage Onychomycosis: Adults: Topical: Apply to affected toenail(s) once daily for 48 weeks.

Dosage adjustment in renal impairment: There are no dosage adjustments provided in the manufacturer's labeling.

Dosage adjustment in hepatic impairment: There are no dosage adjustments provided in the manufacturer's labeling.

Additional Information Complete prescribing information should be consulted for additional detail.

Dosage Forms

Solution, External:

Jublia: 10% (4 mL)

Eflornithine (ee FLOR ni theen)

Brand Names: U.S. Vaniqa

Brand Names: Canada Vaniqa®

Index Terms DFMO; Eflornithine Hydrochloride

Pharmacologic Category Antiprotozoal; Topical Skin Product

Use Reduce unwanted hair from face and adjacent areas under the chin

Pregnancy Risk Factor C

Dosage

Children ≥12 years and Adults: Females: Topical: Unwanted facial hair: Apply thin layer of cream to affected areas of face and areas under the chin twice daily, at least 8 hours apart

Adults: IV infusion: Treatment of infections caused by *Trypanosoma brucei gambiense* infection (sleeping sickness) (off-label use): 100 mg/kg/dose given every 6 hours for 14 days (Kappagoda, 2011)

Dosing adjustment in renal impairment: Injection: Dose should be adjusted although no specific guidelines are available.

Additional Information Complete prescribing information should be consulted for additional detail.

Dosage Forms

Cream, External:

Vaniqa: 13.9% (45 g)

◆ **Eflornithine Hydrochloride** *see* Eflornithine *on page 710*

◆ **Eformoterol** *see* Formoterol *on page 926*

◆ **Eformoterol and Budesonide** *see* Budesonide and Formoterol *on page 297*

◆ **Eformoterol and Mometasone** *see* Mometasone and Formoterol *on page 1392*

◆ **Efraloctocog Alfa** *see* Antihemophilic Factor (Recombinant) *on page 152*

◆ **Efudex** *see* Fluorouracil (Topical) *on page 899*

◆ **Efudex® (Can)** *see* Fluorouracil (Topical) *on page 899*

◆ **Egaten** *see* Triclabendazole [INT] *on page 2102*

◆ **Egrifta** *see* Tesamorelin *on page 2010*

◆ **EHDP** *see* Etidronate *on page 813*

◆ **Eicosapentaenoic Acid** *see* Omega-3 Fatty Acids *on page 1507*

◆ **EL-970** *see* Dalfampridine *on page 552*

◆ **Elaprase** *see* Idursulfase *on page 1040*

◆ **Elavil** *see* Amitriptyline *on page 119*

◆ **Eldepryl** *see* Selegiline *on page 1873*

◆ **Eldopaque [OTC] [DSC]** *see* Hydroquinone *on page 1020*

◆ **Eldopaque® (Can)** *see* Hydroquinone *on page 1020*

◆ **Eldopaque Forte [DSC]** *see* Hydroquinone *on page 1020*

◆ **Eldoquin [OTC] [DSC]** *see* Hydroquinone *on page 1020*

◆ **Eldoquin® (Can)** *see* Hydroquinone *on page 1020*

◆ **Eldoquin Forte [DSC]** *see* Hydroquinone *on page 1020*

◆ **Electrolyte Lavage Solution** *see* Polyethylene Glycol-Electrolyte Solution *on page 1674*

Electrolyte Solution, Renal Replacement

(ee LEK trow lite soe LOO shun REE nil ree PLASE ment)

Brand Names: U.S. Normocarb HF® 25; Normocarb HF® 35; PrismaSol

Index Terms Continuous Renal Replacement Therapy; CRRT; Renal Replacement Solution

Pharmacologic Category Alkalinizing Agent; Electrolyte Supplement

Use Used as a replacement solution to replenish water, correct electrolytes, and adjust acid-base balance depleted by hemofiltration or hemodiafiltration (continuous renal replacement therapy [CRRT]); drug poisoning when CRRT is used to remove filterable substances

Dosage Note: If using PrismaSol™, ensure that compartment A and B are mixed.

Continuous renal replacement circuit: Children and Adults:

Pre- or post-filter: Volume of solution administered depends upon the patient's fluid balance, target fluid balance, body weight, and amount of fluid removed during hemofiltration process.

Post-filter replacement: Volume infused/hour should not be greater than 1/3 of blood flow rate (eg, blood flow rate 100 mL/minute [6000 mL/hour], post-filter replacement rate ≤2000 mL/hour)

Dosage adjustment in hepatic impairment: Ability to convert lactate to bicarbonate may be impaired; use solutions containing lactate cautiously.

Additional Information Complete prescribing information should be consulted for additional detail.

Dosage Forms

Injection, solution [concentrate; preservative free]:

Normocarb HF® 25: Bicarbonate 25 mEq/L, chloride 116.5 mEq/L, magnesium 1.5 mEq/L, sodium 140 mEq/L (240 mL) [strength represents final solution after mixing; when diluted as directed, makes 3240 mL of infusate]

Normocarb HF® 35: Bicarbonate 35 mEq/L, chloride 106.5 mEq/L, magnesium 1.5 mEq/L, sodium 140 mEq/L (240 mL) [strength represents final solution after mixing; when diluted as directed, makes 3240 mL of infusate]

Injection, solution [preservative free]:

PrismaSol B22GK 2/0: Bicarbonate 22 mEq/L, chloride 118.5 mEq/L, dextrose 100 mg/dL, lactate 3 mEq/L, magnesium 1.5 mEq/L, potassium 2 mEq/L, sodium 140 mEq/L (5000 mL) [strength represents final solution after mixing]

PrismaSol B22GK 4/0: Bicarbonate 22 mEq/L, chloride 120.5 mEq/L, dextrose 100 mg/dL, lactate 3 mEq/L, magnesium 1.5 mEq/L, potassium 4 mEq/L, sodium 140 mEq/L (5000 mL) [strength represents final solution after mixing]

PrismaSol BGK 0/2.5: Bicarbonate 32 mEq/L, calcium 2.5 mEq/L, chloride 109 mEq/L, dextrose 100 mg/dL, lactate 3 mEq/L, magnesium 1.5 mEq/L, sodium 140 mEq/L (5000 mL) [strength represents final solution after mixing]

PrismaSol BGK 2/0: Bicarbonate 32 mEq/L, chloride 108 mEq/L, dextrose 100 mg/dL, lactate 3 mEq/L, magnesium 1 mEq/L, potassium 2 mEq/L, sodium 140 mEq/L (5000 mL) [strength represents final solution after mixing]

PrismaSol BGK 2/3.5: Bicarbonate 32 mEq/L, calcium 3.5 mEq/L, chloride 111.5 mEq/L, dextrose 100 mg/dL, lactate 3 mEq/L, magnesium 1 mEq/L, potassium 2 mEq/L, sodium 140 mEq/L (5000 mL) [strength represents final solution after mixing]

PrismaSol BGK 4/0/1.2: Bicarbonate 32 mEq/L, chloride 110.2 mEq/L, dextrose 100 mg/dL, lactate 3 mEq/L, magnesium 1.2 mEq/L, potassium 4 mEq/L, sodium 140 mEq/L (5000 mL) [strength represents final solution after mixing]

PrismaSol BGK 4/2.5: Bicarbonate 32 mEq/L, calcium 2.5 mEq/L, chloride 113 mEq/L, dextrose 100 mg/dL, lactate 3 mEq/L, magnesium 1.5 mEq/L, potassium 4 mEq/L, sodium 140 mEq/L (5000 mL) [strength represents final solution after mixing]

PrismaSol BK 0/0/1.2: Bicarbonate 32 mEq/L, chloride 106.2 mEq/L, lactate 3 mEq/L, magnesium 1.2 mEq/L, sodium 140 mEq/L (5000 mL) [strength represents final solution after mixing]

◆ **Elelyso** *see* Taliglucerase Alfa *on page 1971*

◆ **Elestrin** *see* Estradiol (Systemic) *on page 775*

Eletriptan (el e TRIP tan)

Brand Names: U.S. Relpax

Brand Names: Canada Relpax®

Index Terms Eletriptan Hydrobromide

Pharmacologic Category Antimigraine Agent; Serotonin 5-$HT_{1B,\ 1D}$ Receptor Agonist

Use Migraines: Acute treatment of migraine, with or without aura in adults

Pregnancy Risk Factor C

Pregnancy Considerations Adverse events were observed in animal reproduction studies. Information related to eletriptan use in pregnancy is limited (Källén, 2011; Nezvalová-Henriksen, 2010; Nezvalová-Henriksen, 2012). Until additional information is available, other agents are preferred for the initial treatment of migraine in pregnancy (Da Silva, 2012; MacGregor, 2012; Williams, 2012).

Breast-Feeding Considerations Eletriptan is excreted in breast milk. Eight women were given a single dose of eletriptan 80 mg. The amount of drug detected in breast milk over 24 hours was ~0.02% of the maternal dose and the milk-to-plasma ratio was variable. The presence of the active metabolite was not measured. The manufacturer recommends that caution be exercised when administering eletriptan to nursing women.

Contraindications

Ischemic coronary artery disease (eg, angina pectoris, history of myocardial infarction, documented silent ischemia); coronary artery vasospasm, including Prinzmetal's angina; Wolff-Parkinson-White syndrome or arrhythmias associated with other cardiac accessory conduction pathway disorders; history of stroke, transient ischemic attack, or history or current evidence of hemiplegic or basilar migraine; peripheral vascular disease; ischemic bowel disease; uncontrolled hypertension; recent use (within 24 hours) of treatment with another 5-HT_1 agonist, or an ergotamine-containing or ergot-type medication (eg, dihydroergotamine or methysergide); recent use (within at least 72 hours) of the following potent CYP3A4 inhibitors: ketoconazole, itraconazole, nefazodone, troleandomycin, clarithromycin, ritonavir, or nelfinavir; known hypersensitivity to eletriptan or any component of the formulation.

Canadian labeling: Additional contraindications (not in U.S. labeling): Cardiac arrhythmias (especially tachycardias), valvular heart disease, congenital heart disease, atherosclerotic disease; ophthalmoplegic migraine; Raynaud's syndrome; severe hepatic impairment.

Documentation of allergenic cross-reactivity for serotonin 5-HT_1 receptor agonists (triptans) in this class is limited. However, because of similarities in chemical structure and/or pharmacologic actions, the possibility of cross-sensitivity cannot be ruled out with certainty.

Warnings/Precautions Only indicated for treatment of acute migraine; not indicated for migraine prophylaxis, or for the treatment of cluster headache, hemiplegic or basilar migraine. If a patient does not respond to the first dose, the diagnosis of migraine should be reconsidered. Acute migraine agents (eg, triptans, opioids, ergotamine, or a combination of the agents) used for 10 or more days per month may lead to worsening of headaches (medication overuse headache); withdrawal treatment may be necessary in the setting of overuse. Do not give to patients with risk factors for CAD until a cardiovascular evaluation has been performed; if evaluation is satisfactory, the health care provider should administer the first dose (consider ECG monitoring) and cardiovascular status should be periodically evaluated. Cardiac events (coronary artery vasospasm, transient ischemia, MI, ventricular tachycardia/fibrillation, cardiac arrest, and death), cerebral/subarachnoid hemorrhage, stroke (some fatal), peripheral vascular ischemia, gastrointestinal vascular ischemia/infarction, and Raynaud's syndrome have been reported with 5-HT_1 agonist administration. Patients who experience sensations of chest pain/pressure/tightness or symptoms suggestive of angina following dosing should be evaluated for coronary artery disease or Prinzmetal's angina before receiving additional doses; if dosing is resumed and similar symptoms recur, monitor with ECG. Significant elevation in blood pressure, including hypertensive crisis with acute impairment of organ systems, has been reported on rare occasions in patients with and without a history of hypertension; monitor blood pressure.

Not recommended for use in patients with severe hepatic impairment; the Canadian labeling contraindicates use in patients with severe impairment. Symptoms of agitation, confusion, hallucinations, hyper-reflexia, myoclonus, shivering, and tachycardia (serotonin syndrome) may occur with concomitant proserotonergic drugs (ie, SSRIs/SNRIs or triptans) or agents which reduce eletriptan's metabolism. Concurrent use of serotonin precursors (eg, tryptophan) is not recommended. If concomitant administration with SSRIs is warranted, monitor closely, especially at initiation and with dose increases. Discontinue eletriptan if serotonin syndrome is suspected. Potentially significant drug-drug interactions may exist, requiring dose or frequency adjustment, additional monitoring, and/or selection of alternative therapy. Use is contraindicated within 72 hours of patients taking strong CYP3A4 inhibitors. Anaphylaxis, anaphylactoid, and hypersensitivity reactions (including angioedema) have occurred; may be life-threatening or fatal.

Adverse Reactions

Cardiovascular: Chest pain (chest tightness, pain, and pressure), palpitations

Central nervous system: Chills, dizziness, drowsiness, headache, hypertonia, hypoesthesia, pain, paresthesia, vertigo

Dermatologic: Diaphoresis

Gastrointestinal: Abdominal pain (pain, discomfort, stomach pain, cramps, and pressure), dyspepsia, dysphagia, nausea, xerostomia

Neuromuscular & skeletal: Back pain, weakness

Respiratory: Pharyngitis

Rare but important or life-threatening: Abnormal hepatic function tests, anaphylactoid reaction, anaphylaxis, angina pectoris, angioedema, cardiac arrhythmia, confusion, depersonalization, depression, edema, emotional lability, hyperesthesia, hyperkinesia, hypersensitivity reaction, hypertension, impotence, increased creatine phosphokinase, insomnia, ischemic colitis, lacrimation, myalgia, myasthenia, myocardial infarction, peripheral vascular disorder, photophobia, polyuria, Prinzmetal angina, seizure, skin rash, speech disturbance, stupor, tachycardia, thrombophlebitis, vasospasm, ventricular fibrillation, visual disturbance

Drug Interactions

Metabolism/Transport Effects Substrate of CYP3A4 (major); **Note:** Assignment of Major/Minor substrate status based on clinically relevant drug interaction potential

Avoid Concomitant Use

Avoid concomitant use of Eletriptan with any of the following: Conivaptan; Dapoxetine; Ergot Derivatives; Fusidic Acid (Systemic); Idelalisib; Itraconazole; Ketoconazole (Systemic); Posaconazole; Voriconazole

Increased Effect/Toxicity

Eletriptan may increase the levels/effects of: Antipsychotic Agents; Droxidopa; Ergot Derivatives; Metoclopramide; Serotonin Modulators

The levels/effects of Eletriptan may be increased by: Antiemetics (5HT3 Antagonists); Antipsychotic Agents; Aprepitant; Calcium Channel Blockers (Nondihydropyridine); Ceritinib; Conivaptan; CYP3A4 Inhibitors (Moderate); CYP3A4 Inhibitors (Strong); Dapoxetine; Dasatinib; Ergot Derivatives; Fluconazole; Fosaprepitant; Fusidic Acid (Systemic); Idelalisib; Itraconazole; Ivacaftor; Ketoconazole (Systemic); Luliconazole; Macrolide Antibiotics; Mifepristone; Netupitant; Posaconazole; Simeprevir; Stiripentol; Tedizolid; Voriconazole

Decreased Effect There are no known significant interactions involving a decrease in effect.

Food Interactions A high-fat meal increases bioavailability. Management: Administer without regard to meals.

Storage/Stability Store at 20°C to 25°C (68°F to 77°F); excursions are permitted between 15°C and 30°C (59°F and 86°F).

Mechanism of Action Selective agonist for serotonin (5-HT_{1B}, 5-HT_{1D}, and 5-HT_{1F} receptors) in cranial arteries; causes vasoconstriction and reduces sterile inflammation associated with antidromic neuronal transmission correlating with relief of migraine

Pharmacodynamics/Kinetics

Absorption: Well absorbed

Distribution: V_d: 138 L

Protein binding: ~85%

Metabolism: Hepatic via CYP3A4; forms one metabolite (active)

Bioavailability: ~50%, increased with high-fat meal

Half-life elimination: ~4 hours (Elderly: 4.4-5.7 hours); Metabolite: ~13 hours

Time to peak, plasma: 1.5-2 hours

Dosage Note: If the first dose is ineffective, diagnosis needs to be re-evaluated. Safety of treating >3 headaches/month has not been established.

U.S. labeling: Acute migraine: Adults: Oral: Initial: 20-40 mg as a single dose (maximum: 40 mg/dose); if the headache improves but returns, dose may be repeated after 2 hours have elapsed since first dose (maximum: 80 mg daily)

Canadian labeling: Acute migraine: Adults: Oral: Initial: 20-40 mg as a single dose (maximum: 40 mg/dose). If after an initial dose of 20 mg, the headache improves but returns a repeat 20 mg dose may be administered after 2 hours have elapsed since first dose. If an initial dose of 40 mg was administered, a repeat dose is not recommended (maximum: 40 mg daily).

Dosage adjustment in renal impairment: No dosing adjustment provided in manufacturer's labeling, however, dosage adjustment likely not needed based on pharmacokinetic analysis; monitor for increased blood pressure.

Dosage adjustment in hepatic impairment:

Mild-to-moderate impairment: No dosage adjustment necessary

Severe impairment:

U.S. labeling: Use is not recommended.

Canadian labeling: Use is contraindicated.

Administration Administer orally as soon as symptoms appear. May take with or without food.

Monitoring Parameters Headache severity; signs/symptoms suggestive of angina; blood pressure, heart rate, and/or ECG with first dose in patients with likelihood of unrecognized coronary disease, such as patients with significant hypertension, hypercholesterolemia, obese patients, patients with diabetes, smokers with other risk factors or strong family history of coronary artery disease; signs/symptoms of serotonin syndrome and hypersensitivity reactions

Dosage Forms

Tablet, Oral:

Relpax: 20 mg, 40 mg

◆ **Eletriptan Hydrobromide** *see* Eletriptan *on page 711*

◆ **Elidel** *see* Pimecrolimus *on page 1650*

◆ **Eligard** *see* Leuprolide *on page 1186*

Eliglustat (el i GLOO stat)

Brand Names: U.S. Cerdelga

Index Terms Genz-112638

Pharmacologic Category Enzyme Inhibitor; Glucosylceramide Synthase Inhibitor

Use

Gaucher disease: Treatment of adult patients with Gaucher disease type 1 (GD1) who are CYP2D6 extensive metabolizers (EMs), intermediate metabolizers (IMs), or poor metabolizers (PMs).

Limitations of use: Patients who are CYP2D6 ultra-rapid metabolizers (URMs) may not achieve adequate concentrations of eliglustat to achieve a therapeutic effect. A specific dosage cannot be recommended for those patients whose CYP2D6 genotype cannot be determined (IMs).

Pregnancy Risk Factor C

Pregnancy Considerations

Adverse events were observed in some animal reproduction studies.

Uncontrolled type 1 Gaucher disease is associated an increased risk of spontaneous abortion; maternal hepatosplenomegaly and thrombocytopenia may also occur and lead to adverse pregnancy outcomes.

Breast-Feeding Considerations It is not known if eliglustat is excreted into breast milk. Due to the potential for serious adverse reactions in the nursing infant, the manufacturer recommends a decision be made whether to discontinue nursing or to discontinue the drug, taking into account the importance of treatment to the mother.

Contraindications Concomitant use of a moderate or strong CYP2D6 inhibitor with a moderate or strong CYP3A inhibitor in extensive metabolizers (EMs) or intermediate metabolizers (IMs); concomitant use of a strong CYP3A inhibitor in poor metabolizers (PMs) or IMs

Warnings/Precautions May cause increases in ECG intervals (PR, QTc, and QRS) at substantially elevated plasma concentrations; use is not recommended in patients with preexisting cardiac disease (CHF, recent acute MI, eliglustat bradycardia, heart block, ventricular arrhythmia), long QT syndrome, and in combination with Class IA (eg, quinidine, procainamide) and Class III (eg, amiodarone, sotalol) antiarrhythmic medications (has not been studied). Not recommended in hepatic impairment or cirrhosis (has not been studied). Not recommended in patients with moderate-to-severe renal impairment or end-stage renal disease; use with caution in patients with mild renal impairment. Dosing has not been studied in poor metabolizers (PMs); monitor these patients for adverse reactions. Potentially significant drug-drug interactions may exist, requiring dose or frequency adjustment, additional monitoring, and/or selection of alternative therapy. A registry has been established and all patients with Gaucher disease, and health care providers who treat Gaucher disease are encouraged to participate. Information on the International Collaborative Gaucher Group (ICGG) Gaucher Registry may be obtained at https://www.-registrynxt.com or by calling 1-800-745-4447 (ext.15500).

Adverse Reactions

Cardiovascular: Palpitations

Central nervous system: Dizziness, fatigue, headache, migraine

Dermatologic: Skin rash

Gastrointestinal: Constipation, diarrhea, dyspepsia, flatulence, gastroesophageal reflux disease, nausea, upper abdominal pain

Neuromuscular & skeletal: Arthralgia, back pain, limb pain, weakness

Respiratory: Cough, oropharyngeal pain

Drug Interactions

Metabolism/Transport Effects **Substrate** of CYP2D6 (major), CYP3A4 (major); **Note:** Assignment of Major/Minor substrate status based on clinically relevant drug interaction potential; **Inhibits** CYP2D6 (moderate), CYP3A4 (weak), P-glycoprotein

Avoid Concomitant Use

Avoid concomitant use of Eliglustat with any of the following: Bosutinib; Conivaptan; CYP3A4 Inducers (Strong); Fusidic Acid (Systemic); Grapefruit Juice; Highest Risk QTc-Prolonging Agents; Idelalisib; Ivabradine; Mifepristone; Moderate Risk QTc-Prolonging Agents; PAZOPanib; Pimozide; Silodosin; St Johns Wort; Thioridazine; Topotecan; VinCRIStine (Liposomal)

Increased Effect/Toxicity

Eliglustat may increase the levels/effects of: Afatinib; Bosutinib; Brentuximab Vedotin; Colchicine; CYP2D6 Substrates; Dabigatran Etexilate; Digoxin; DOXOrubicin (Conventional); Edoxaban; Everolimus; Fesoterodine; Highest Risk QTc-Prolonging Agents; Hydrocodone; Ledipasvir; Lomitapide; Metoprolol; Naloxegol; Nebivolol; PAZOPanib; P-glycoprotein/ABCB1 Substrates; Pimozide; Prucalopride; Rifaximin; Rivaroxaban; Silodosin; Thioridazine; Topotecan; VinCRIStine (Liposomal)

The levels/effects of Eliglustat may be increased by: Abiraterone Acetate; Conivaptan; CYP2D6 Inhibitors (Moderate); CYP2D6 Inhibitors (Strong); CYP3A4 Inhibitors (Moderate); CYP3A4 Inhibitors (Strong); Fusidic Acid (Systemic); Grapefruit Juice; Idelalisib; Ivabradine; Ivacaftor; Luliconazole; Mifepristone; Moderate Risk QTc-Prolonging Agents; Peginterferon Alfa-2b; QTc-Prolonging Agents (Indeterminate Risk and Risk Modifying); Simeprevir; Stiripentol

Decreased Effect

Eliglustat may decrease the levels/effects of: Codeine; Tamoxifen; TraMADol

The levels/effects of Eliglustat may be decreased by: Bosentan; CYP3A4 Inducers (Moderate); CYP3A4 Inducers (Strong); Dabrafenib; Deferasirox; Peginterferon Alfa-2b; Siltuximab; St Johns Wort; Tocilizumab

Storage/Stability Store at 20°C to 25°C (68°F to 77°F); excursions are permitted between 15°C and 30°C (59°F and 86°F).

Mechanism of Action Eliglustat inhibits the enzyme needed to produce glycosphingolipids and decreases the rate of glycosphingolipid glucosylceramide formation. Glucosylceramide accumulates in type 1 Gaucher disease, causing complications specific to this disease.

Pharmacodynamics/Kinetics

Absorption: Systemic exposure depends upon the patient's CYP2D6 phenotype; systemic exposure is up to 9-fold higher in poor metabolizers (PMs).

Distribution: V_d: 835 L

Protein binding: 76% to 83%

Metabolism: Extensive by CYP2D6 (major) and CYP3A4

Bioavailability: Extensive metabolizers (EMs): <5%

Half-life elimination: EMs: 6.5 hours; PMs: 8.9 hours

Time to peak: EMs: 1.5 to 2 hours; PMs: 3 hours

Excretion: Urine (41.8%) and feces (51.4%) as inactive metabolites

Dosage

Gaucher disease: Adults: Oral: **Note:** Dosage is based on patient CYP2D6 metabolizer status (extensive metabolizers [EMs], intermediate metabolizers [IMs], or poor metabolizers [PMs]) determined by an FDA-cleared test.

EMs and IMs: 84 mg twice daily

PMs: 84 mg once daily. **Note:** Dosage has not been studied; however the predicted systemic exposures in these patients are within the range of those observed in clinical studies.

Missed dose: If a dose is missed, take the prescribed dose at the next scheduled time; do not double the next dose.

Dosage adjustment for concomitant therapy with strong or moderate CYP2D6 or CYP3A4 inhibitors:

EMs and IMs taking strong or moderate CYP2D6 inhibitors: 84 mg once daily

EMs taking strong or moderate CYP3A inhibitors: 84 mg once daily

Dosage adjustment in renal impairment:

Mild renal impairment: No dosage adjustment necessary.

Moderate to severe renal impairment: Use is not recommended (has not been studied).

End-stage renal disease (ESRD): Use is not recommended (has not been studied).

Dosage adjustment in hepatic impairment: Use is not recommended (has not been studied).

Dietary Considerations Avoid grapefruit or grapefruit juice.

Administration Oral: Administer with or without food. Swallow capsules whole with water; do not crush, dissolve, or open. Avoid grapefruit or grapefruit juice.

Monitoring Parameters Adverse reactions (especially in PMs)

Dosage Forms

Capsule, Oral:

Cerdelga: 84 mg

◆ **Elimite** *see* Permethrin *on page* 1627

- ◆ **Elimite** *see* Permethrin *on page 1627*
- ◆ **Eliphos** *see* Calcium Acetate *on page 326*
- ◆ **Eliquis** *see* Apixaban *on page 158*
- ◆ **Elitek** *see* Rasburicase *on page 1783*
- ◆ **Elixophyllin** *see* Theophylline *on page 2026*
- ◆ **ElixSure Congestion [OTC]** *see* Pseudoephedrine *on page 1742*
- ◆ **Ella** *see* Ulipristal *on page 2113*
- ◆ **Ellence** *see* Epirubicin *on page 739*
- ◆ **Ellence® (Can)** *see* Epirubicin *on page 739*
- ◆ **Elmiron** *see* Pentosan Polysulfate Sodium *on page 1617*
- ◆ **Elmiron® (Can)** *see* Pentosan Polysulfate Sodium *on page 1617*
- ◆ **Elocom (Can)** *see* Mometasone (Topical) *on page 1391*
- ◆ **Elocon** *see* Mometasone (Topical) *on page 1391*
- ◆ **Eloctate** *see* Antihemophilic Factor (Recombinant) *on page 152*

Elosulfase Alfa (el oh SUL fase AL fa)

Brand Names: U.S. Vimizim

Index Terms Elosulfase alfa; N-acetylgalactosamine-6-sulfatase

Pharmacologic Category Enzyme

Use Mucopolysaccharidosis type IVA: Treatment of mucopolysaccharidosis type IVA (MPS IVA; Morquio A syndrome)

Pregnancy Risk Factor C

Dosage Note: Premedicate with antihistamines with or without antipyretics 30 to 60 minutes prior to infusion.

MPS IVA: Children ≥5 years, Adolescents, and Adults: IV: 2 mg/kg once weekly

Dosage adjustment in renal impairment: There are no dosage adjustments provided in manufacturer's labeling.

Dosage adjustment in hepatic impairment: There are no dosage adjustments provided in manufacturer's labeling.

Additional Information Complete prescribing information should be consulted for additional detail.

Dosage Forms

Solution, Intravenous [preservative free]:

Vimizim: 5 mg/5 mL (5 mL)

- ◆ **Elosulfase alfa** *see* Elosulfase Alfa *on page 714*
- ◆ **Eloxatin** *see* Oxaliplatin *on page 1528*
- ◆ **Elspar [DSC]** *see* Asparaginase (*E. coli*) *on page 179*
- ◆ **Eltor® (Can)** *see* Pseudoephedrine *on page 1742*

Eltrombopag (el TROM boe pag)

Brand Names: U.S. Promacta

Brand Names: Canada Revolade

Index Terms Eltrombopag Olamine; Revolade; SB-497115; SB-497115-GR

Pharmacologic Category Colony Stimulating Factor; Hematopoietic Agent; Thrombopoietic Agent

Use

Chronic immune (idiopathic) thrombocytopenia: Treatment of thrombocytopenia in patients with chronic immune (idiopathic) thrombocytopenia (ITP) who have had insufficient response to corticosteroids, immune globulin, or splenectomy.

Chronic hepatitis C infection-associated thrombocytopenia: Treatment of thrombocytopenia in patients with chronic hepatitis C (CHC) to allow the initiation and maintenance of interferon-based therapy.

Severe aplastic anemia: Treatment of severe aplastic anemia in patients who have had an insufficient response to immunosuppressive therapy.

Limitations of use: For ITP, use eltrombopag only if the degree of thrombocytopenia and clinical condition increase the risk for bleeding. For chronic hepatitis C (CHC), use eltrombopag only if the degree of thrombocytopenia prevents initiation of or limits the ability to maintain interferon-based therapy. For CHC, safety and efficacy have not been established when used in combination with direct-acting antiviral agents used without interferon for treatment of CHC infection.

Pregnancy Risk Factor C

Pregnancy Considerations Adverse effects were observed in animal reproduction studies. Use during pregnancy only if the potential benefit to the mother outweighs the potential risk to the fetus. A Promacta pregnancy registry has been established to monitor outcomes of women exposed to eltrombopag during pregnancy (1-888-825-5249).

Breast-Feeding Considerations It is not known if eltrombopag is excreted in breast milk. Due to the potential for serious adverse effects in the nursing infant, the decision to discontinue therapy or to discontinue breastfeeding should take into account the importance of treatment to the mother.

Contraindications There are no contraindications listed in the manufacturer's labeling.

Warnings/Precautions Liver enzyme elevations may occur; obtain ALT, AST, and bilirubin prior to treatment initiation, every 2 weeks during adjustment phase, then monthly (after stable dose established); obtain fractionation for elevated bilirubin levels. Repeat abnormal liver function tests within 3 to 5 days; if confirmed abnormal, monitor weekly until resolves, stabilizes, or returns to baseline. Discontinue treatment for ALT levels ≥3 times the upper limit of normal (ULN) in patients with normal hepatic function, or ≥3 times baseline in those with preexisting transaminase elevations and which are progressive, or persistent (≥4 weeks), or accompanied by increased direct bilirubin, or accompanied by clinical signs of liver injury or evidence of hepatic decompensation. Hepatotoxicity may reoccur with retreatment after therapy interruption; however, if the benefit of treatment outweighs the hepatotoxicity risk, initiate carefully, and monitor liver function tests weekly during the dose adjustment phase; permanently discontinue if liver abnormalities persist, worsen, or recur with rechallenge. Use with caution in patients with preexisting hepatic impairment (clearance may be reduced); dosage reductions are recommended in patients with ITP and severe aplastic anemia who have hepatic dysfunction (no initial dose reductions are necessary in patients with chronic hepatitis C-related thrombocytopenia); monitor closely.

[U.S. Boxed Warning]: May increase risk of hepatic decompensation when used in combination with interferon and ribavirin in patients with chronic hepatitis C. In clinical trials, patients with low albumin (<3.5 g/dL) or a Model for End-Stage Liver Disease (MELD) score ≥10 at baseline had an increased risk of hepatic decompensation; closely monitor these patients during therapy. If antiviral therapy is discontinued for hepatic decompensation according to interferon/ribavirin recommendations, eltrombopag should also be discontinued. Indirect hyperbilirubinemia is commonly observed with eltrombopag when used in combination with peginterferon and ribavirin. In addition, ascites, encephalopathy, and thrombotic events were reported more frequently than placebo in chronic hepatitis C trials.

May increase the risk for bone marrow reticulin formation or progression (Canadian labeling). Monitor peripheral blood smear for cellular morphologic abnormalities;

analyze CBC monthly; discontinue treatment with onset of new or worsening abnormalities (eg, teardrop and nucleated RBC, immature WBC) or cytopenias and consider bone marrow biopsy (with staining for fibrosis).

Thromboembolism may occur with excess increases in platelet levels. Use with caution in patients with known risk factors for thromboembolism (eg, Factor V Leiden, ATIII deficiency, antiphospholipid syndrome, chronic liver disease). Thrombotic events, primarily involving the portal venous system, were more commonly seen in eltrombopag-treated chronic hepatitis C patients with thrombocytopenia (when compared to placebo). Thrombotic events (including portal venous thrombosis) were also reported in a study of non-ITP thrombocytopenic patients with chronic liver disease undergoing elective invasive procedures receiving eltrombopag 75 mg once daily. Symptoms of portal vein thrombosis include abdominal pain, nausea, vomiting, and diarrhea. The risk for portal venous thrombosis is increased in thrombocytopenic patients with chronic liver disease receiving 75 mg once daily for 2 weeks as preparation for invasive procedures. Stimulation of cell surface thrombopoietin (TPO) receptors may increase the risk for hematologic malignancies (Canadian labeling).

Cataract formation or worsening was observed in clinical trials. Monitor regularly for signs and symptoms of cataracts; obtain ophthalmic exam at baseline and during therapy. Use with caution in patients at risk for cataracts (eg, advanced age, long-term glucocorticoid use). Potentially significant drug-drug interactions may exist, requiring dose or frequency adjustment, additional monitoring, and/or selection of alternative therapy. Allow at least 4 hours between dosing of eltrombopag and antacids, minerals (eg, iron, calcium, aluminum, magnesium, selenium, zinc), or foods high in calcium; may reduce eltrombopag levels. Patients of East-Asian ethnicity (eg, Chinese, Japanese, Korean, Taiwanese) may have greater drug exposure (compared to non-East Asians); therapy should be initiated with lower starting doses in ITP and severe aplastic anemia patients. Use with caution in renal impairment (any degree) and monitor closely; initial dosage adjustment is not necessary.

Do not use to normalize platelet counts. *ITP:* Indicated only when the degree of thrombocytopenia and clinical conditions increase the risk for bleeding in patients with chronic immune ITP; use the lowest dose necessary to achieve and maintain platelet count ≥50,000/mm^3. Discontinue if platelet count does not respond to a level to avoid clinically important bleeding after 4 weeks at the maximum recommended dose. *Chronic hepatitis C-associated thrombocytopenia:* Use only when thrombocytopenia prevents the initiation and maintenance of interferon-based therapy; discontinue if antiviral therapy is discontinued. Safety and efficacy have not been established when combined with direct acting antiviral medications approved for chronic hepatitis C genotype 1 infection therapy. *Severe aplastic anemia:* Use the lowest dose to achieve and maintain hematologic response. Discontinue if no hematologic response has occurred after 16 weeks of therapy, excessive platelet count responses or important liver test abnormalities. Consider discontinuation if new cytogenetic abnormalities are observed.

Adverse Reactions Adverse reactions reported are associated with ITP unless otherwise indicated.

Cardiovascular: Peripheral edema (chronic hepatitis C), thrombosis (chronic hepatitis C)

Central nervous system: Brain disease, chills (chronic hepatitis C), dizziness (aplastic anemia), fatigue (incidence similar in chronic hepatitis C as in aplastic anemia), headache (incidence similar in chronic hepatitis C as in aplastic anemia), insomnia (chronic hepatitis C)

Dermatologic: Alopecia (more common in chronic hepatitis C), ecchymosis (aplastic anemia), pruritus (chronic hepatitis C), skin rash

Gastrointestinal: Abdominal pain (aplastic anemia), appetite decreased (chronic hepatitis C), diarrhea (more common in aplastic anemia), nausea (more common in aplastic anemia), vomiting, xerostomia

Genitourinary: Urinary tract infection

Hematologic: Anemia (chronic hepatitis C), myelofibrosis (bone marrow biopsy)

Hepatic: Abnormal hepatic function, alkaline phosphatase increased, ascites (chronic hepatitis C), hyperbilirubinemia (≥1.5 x ULN), increased serum ALT, increased serum AST, increased serum transaminases (aplastic anemia)

Neuromuscular & skeletal: Arm pain (aplastic anemia), arthralgia (aplastic anemia), back pain, leg pain (aplastic anemia), muscle spasm (aplastic anemia), musculoskeletal pain, myalgia, paresthesia, weakness (chronic hepatitis C)

Ophthalmic: Cataract

Respiratory: Cough (more common in aplastic anemia), dyspnea (aplastic anemia), oropharyngeal pain (more common in aplastic anemia), pharyngitis, rhinorrhea (aplastic anemia), upper respiratory infection

Miscellaneous: Fever (more common in chronic hepatitis C), flu-like syndrome (more common in chronic hepatitis C)

Rare but important or life-threatening: Abdominal distension, deep vein thrombosis, drowsiness, dysgeusia, dyspepsia, facial swelling, fecal discoloration, hemorrhage (due to thrombocytopenia or rebound thrombocytopenia), hepatic lesions, hypokalemia, increased hemoglobin, increased serum albumin, increased serum creatinine, increased serum total protein, malignant neoplasm (rectosigmoid), non-Hodgkin lymphoma, oropharyngeal blistering, ostealgia, portal vein thrombosis, pulmonary embolism, retinal hemorrhage, sinus tachycardia, superficial thrombophlebitis, tachycardia, thrombocytopenia (rebound), upper abdominal pain, visual acuity decreased

Drug Interactions

Metabolism/Transport Effects **Substrate** of CYP1A2 (minor), CYP2C8 (minor), UGT1A1, UGT1A3; **Note:** Assignment of Major/Minor substrate status based on clinically relevant drug interaction potential; **Inhibits** CYP2C8 (moderate), SLCO1B1, UGT1A1, UGT1A3, UGT1A4, UGT1A6, UGT1A9, UGT2B15, UGT2B7

Avoid Concomitant Use There are no known interactions where it is recommended to avoid concomitant use.

Increased Effect/Toxicity

Eltrombopag may increase the levels/effects of: CYP2C8 Substrates; Deferiprone; OATP1B1/SLCO1B1 Substrates; Rosuvastatin

Decreased Effect

The levels/effects of Eltrombopag may be decreased by: Aluminum Hydroxide; Calcium Salts; Iron Salts; Magnesium Salts; Multivitamins/Minerals (with ADEK, Folate, Iron); Multivitamins/Minerals (with AE, No Iron); Selenium; Sucralfate; Zinc Salts

Food Interactions Food, especially dairy products, may decrease the absorption of eltrombopag. Management: Take on an empty stomach at least 1 hour before or 2 hours after a meal. Separate intake from antacids, foods high in calcium, or minerals (eg, iron, calcium, aluminum, magnesium, selenium, zinc) by at least 4 hours.

Storage/Stability Store at 20°C to 25°C (68°F to 77°F); excursions are permitted between 15°C and 30°C (59°F and 86°F). If present, do not remove desiccant. Dispense in original bottle.

Mechanism of Action Thrombopoietin (TPO) nonpeptide agonist which increases platelet counts by binding to and activating the human TPO receptor. Activates intracellular signal transduction pathways to increase proliferation and differentiation of marrow progenitor cells. Does not induce platelet aggregation or activation.

Pharmacodynamics/Kinetics

Onset of action: Platelet count increase: Within 1 to 2 weeks

Peak platelet count increase: 14 to 16 days

Duration: Platelets return to baseline: 1 to 2 weeks after last dose

Protein binding: >99%

Metabolism: Extensive hepatic metabolism; via CYP 1A2, 2C8 oxidation and UGT 1A1, 1A3 glucuronidation

Bioavailability: ~52%

Half-life elimination: ~21 to 32 hours in healthy individuals; ~26 to 35 hours in patients with ITP

Time to peak, plasma: 2 to 6 hours

Excretion: Feces (~59%, 20% as unchanged drug, 21% glutathione-related conjugates); urine (31%, 20% glucuronide of the phenylpyrazole moiety)

Dosage Note: Do not use eltrombopag to normalize platelet counts.

Chronic immune (idiopathic) thrombocytopenia (ITP): Adults: Oral: **Note:** Use the lowest dose to achieve and maintain platelet count ≥50,000/mm^3 as needed to reduce the risk of bleeding. Discontinue if platelet count does not respond to a level that avoids clinically important bleeding after 4 weeks at the maximum daily dose of 75 mg.

Initial: 50 mg once daily (25 mg once daily for patients of East-Asian ethnicity [eg, Chinese, Japanese, Korean, Taiwanese]); dose should be titrated based on platelet response. Maximum dose: 75 mg once daily.

Dosage adjustment based on platelet response:

Platelet count <50,000/mm^3 (≥2 weeks after treatment initiation or a dose increase): Increase daily dose by 25 mg (if taking 12.5 mg once daily, increase dose to 25 mg once daily prior to increasing the dose amount by 25 mg daily); maximum: 75 mg once daily

Platelet count ≥200,000/mm^3 and ≤400,000/mm^3 (at any time): Reduce daily dose by 25 mg; reassess in 2 weeks

Platelet count >400,000/mm^3: Withhold dose; assess platelet count twice weekly; when platelet count <150,000/mm^3, resume with the daily dose reduced by 25 mg (if taking 25 mg once daily, resume with 12.5 mg once daily)

Platelet count >400,000/mm^3 after 2 weeks at the lowest dose: Discontinue treatment

Chronic hepatitis C-associated thrombocytopenia: Adults: Oral: **Note:** Use the lowest dose to achieve the target platelet count necessary to initiate antiviral therapy (peginterferon and ribavirin) or to avoid dose reductions of peginterferon during antiviral therapy. Discontinue when antiviral therapy is stopped.

Initial: 25 mg once daily; dose should be titrated based on platelet response. Maximum dose: 100 mg once daily

Dosage adjustment based on platelet response:

Platelet count <50,000/mm^3 (after at least 2 weeks): Increase daily dose by 25 mg every 2 weeks; maximum dose: 100 mg once daily

Platelet count ≥200,000/mm^3 and ≤400,000/mm^3 (at any time): Reduce daily dose by 25 mg; reassess in 2 weeks

Platelet count >400,000/mm^3: Withhold dose; assess platelet count twice weekly; when platelet count <150,000/mm^3, resume with the daily dose reduced by 25 mg (if taking 25 mg once daily, resume with 12.5 mg once daily)

Platelet count >400,000/mm^3 after 2 weeks at the lowest dose: Discontinue treatment

Severe aplastic anemia: Adults: Oral: **Note:** Use the lowest dose to achieve and maintain hematologic response. Hematologic response may take up to 16 weeks and requires dose titration. Discontinue therapy if hematologic response is not achieved after 16 weeks of treatment, for excessive platelet responses or for liver function abnormalities. Consider discontinuing if new cytogenetic abnormalities are observed.

Initial: 50 mg once daily (25 mg once daily for patients of East-Asian ethnicity); dose should be titrated based on platelet response. Maximum dose: 150 mg once daily.

Dosage adjustment based on platelet response:

Platelet count <50,000/mm^3 (≥2 weeks after treatment initiation or a dose increase): Increase daily dose by 50 mg (if taking 25 mg once daily, increase dose to 50 mg once daily prior to increasing the dose amount by 50 mg daily); maximum: 150 mg once daily

Platelet count ≥200,000/mm^3 and ≤400,000/mm^3 (at any time): Reduce daily dose by 50 mg; reassess in 2 weeks

Platelet count >400,000/mm^3: Withhold dose for 1 week; when platelet count <150,000/mm^3, resume with the daily dose reduced by 50 mg

Platelet count >400,000/mm^3 after 2 weeks at the lowest dose: Discontinue treatment

For patients who achieve tri-lineage response, including transfusion independence, lasting 8 weeks, may reduce the dose by 50%. If counts remain stable after 8 weeks at the reduced dose, discontinue and monitor blood counts. If platelets counts drop to <30,000/mm^3, hemoglobin to <9 g/dL, or ANC to <500/ mm^3, may reinitiate at the prior effective dose.

Dosage adjustment in renal impairment: There are no dosage adjustments necessary.

Dosage adjustment in hepatic impairment:

Adjustment for hepatic impairment prior to initiating treatment:

Chronic ITP: **Note:** In patients with ITP and hepatic impairment, wait 3 weeks (instead of 2 weeks) after therapy initiation or subsequent dosage changes prior to increasing dose.

Mild, moderate, or severe impairment (Child-Pugh classes A, B, or C): Initial: 25 mg once daily

Patients of East-Asian ethnicity with hepatic impairment (Child-Pugh classes A, B, or C): Initial: 12.5 mg once daily

Chronic hepatitis C-associated thrombocytopenia: Initial: No dosage adjustment is necessary.

Severe aplastic anemia: Mild, moderate, or severe impairment (Child-Pugh classes A, B, or C): Initial: 25 mg once daily

Adjustment for hepatic impairment during treatment:

ALT levels ≥3 times the upper limit of normal (ULN) in patients with normal hepatic function or ≥3 times baseline in those with preexisting transaminase elevations **and** which are progressive, persistent (≥4 weeks), accompanied by increased direct bilirubin, or accompanied by clinical signs of liver injury or evidence of hepatic decompensation: Discontinue treatment. Hepatotoxicity may recur with retreatment after therapy interruption, but if determined to be clinically beneficial, may cautiously resume treatment; monitor ALT weekly during dosage titration; permanently discontinue if liver function test elevations persist, worsen, or recur.

Dietary Considerations Food, especially dairy products, may decrease the absorption of eltrombopag; allow at least 4 hours between dosing of eltrombopag and polyvalent cation intake (eg, dairy products, calcium-rich foods, multivitamins with minerals).

Administration Administer on an empty stomach, 1 hour before or 2 hours after a meal. Do not administer concurrently with antacids, foods high in calcium, or minerals (eg, iron, calcium, aluminum, magnesium, selenium, zinc); separate by at least 4 hours. Do not administer more than one dose within 24 hours.

Monitoring Parameters Thrombocytopenia due to CHC and chronic ITP: Liver function tests, including ALT, AST, and bilirubin (baseline, every 2 weeks during dosage titration, then monthly; evaluate abnormal liver function tests within 3-5 days; monitor weekly until abnormalities resolve, stabilize, or return to baseline or if retreating [not recommended] after therapy interruption for hepatotoxicity); bilirubin fractionation (for elevated bilirubin); CBC with differential and platelet count (weekly at initiation and during dosage titration, then monthly when stable; after cessation, monitor weekly for ≥4 weeks); peripheral blood smear (baseline and monthly when stable), bone marrow biopsy with staining for fibrosis (if peripheral blood smear reveals abnormality); ophthalmic exam (baseline and during treatment)

Severe aplastic anemia: CBC with differential and platelets (regularly throughout therapy), liver function tests (regularly throughout therapy); ophthalmic exam (baseline and during treatment)

Reference Range Target platelet count (with treatment) of 50,000 to 200,000/mm^3; platelet life span: 8 to 11 days

Additional Information Restricted access to Promacta was previously a REMS requirement via the Promacta® Cares™ program. Patients, prescribers, and pharmacies were required to be enrolled in this program. However, the FDA eliminated this REMS requirement in December 2011. There is currently no restricted access to obtaining Promacta®.

Dosage Forms

Tablet, Oral:

Promacta: 12.5 mg, 25 mg, 50 mg, 75 mg

◆ **Eltrombopag Olamine** *see* Eltrombopag *on page 714*

◆ **Eltroxin (Can)** *see* Levothyroxine *on page 1205*

Elvitegravir (el vi TEG ra vir)

Brand Names: U.S. Vitekta

Index Terms Vitekta

Pharmacologic Category Antiretroviral, Integrase Inhibitor (Anti-HIV)

Use HIV-1 infection: In combination with an HIV protease inhibitor coadministered with ritonavir and with other antiretroviral drug(s) for the treatment of HIV-1 infection in antiretroviral treatment-experienced adults

Pregnancy Risk Factor B

Pregnancy Considerations Adverse events were not observed in animal reproduction studies. The DHHS Perinatal HIV Guidelines note there are insufficient data to recommend use in pregnancy.

Regardless of CD4 count or HIV RNA copy number, all HIV-infected pregnant women should receive a combination antiretroviral (ARV) drug regimen. A combination of antepartum, intrapartum, and infant ARV prophylaxis is recommended. ARV therapy should be started as soon as possible in women with symptomatic infection. Although earlier initiation may be more effective in reducing the perinatal transmission of HIV, initiation may be delayed until after 12 weeks gestation in women who do not require immediate treatment after careful consideration of maternal conditions (eg, nausea and vomiting) and the potential risks of first trimester fetal exposure for specific agents. A scheduled cesarean delivery at 38 weeks gestation is recommended for all women with HIV RNA >1,000 copies/mL or unknown concentrations near delivery in order to decrease transmission. If ARV therapy must be interrupted for <24 hours during the peripartum period, stop then restart all medications simultaneously in order to decrease the chance of developing resistance. Long-term follow-up is recommended for all infants exposed to ARV medications. In couples who want to conceive, the HIV-infected partner should attain maximum viral suppression prior to conception.

Health care providers are encouraged to enroll pregnant women exposed to antiretroviral medications in the Antiretroviral Pregnancy Registry (1-800-258-4263 or www.APRegistry.com). Health care providers caring for HIV-infected women and their infants may contact the National Perinatal HIV Hotline (888-448-8765) for clinical consultation (DHHS [perinatal], 2014).

Breast-Feeding Considerations It is not known of elvitegravir is excreted in breast milk. Maternal or infant antiretroviral therapy does not completely eliminate the risk of postnatal HIV transmission. In addition, multiclass-resistant virus has been detected in breast-feeding infants despite maternal therapy. Therefore, in the United States, where formula is accessible, affordable, safe, and sustainable, and the risk of infant mortality due to diarrhea and respiratory infections is low, complete avoidance of breast-feeding by HIV-infected women is recommended to decrease potential transmission of HIV (DHHS [perinatal], 2014).

Contraindications There are no contraindications listed in the manufacturer's labeling.

Warnings/Precautions Patients may develop immune reconstitution syndrome resulting in the occurrence of an inflammatory response to an indolent or residual opportunistic infection during initial HIV treatment or activation of autoimmune disorders (eg, Graves' disease, polymyositis, Guillain-Barré syndrome) later in therapy; further evaluation and treatment may be required. Use is not recommended in severe hepatic impairment (Child-Pugh class C); has not been studied in this population. Not recommended in combination with a protease inhibitor and cobicistat due to lack of dosing recommendations, potential suboptimal plasma concentrations, loss of therapeutic effect, or development of resistance. Avoid concurrent use with other elvitegravir-containing products. Potentially significant interactions may exist, requiring dose or frequency adjustment, additional monitoring, and/or selection of alternative therapy.

Adverse Reactions

Central nervous system: Depression, fatigue, headache, insomnia, suicidal ideation

Dermatologic: Skin rash

Gastrointestinal: Abdominal pain, diarrhea, dyspepsia, nausea, vomiting

Immunologic: Immune reconstitution syndrome

Drug Interactions

Metabolism/Transport Effects Substrate of CYP3A4 (major); **Note:** Assignment of Major/Minor substrate status based on clinically relevant drug interaction potential; **Induces** CYP2C9 (moderate)

Avoid Concomitant Use

Avoid concomitant use of Elvitegravir with any of the following: Efavirenz; Nevirapine; Rifabutin; Rifampin; Rifapentine; St Johns Wort

Increased Effect/Toxicity

The levels/effects of Elvitegravir may be increased by: Itraconazole; Ketoconazole (Systemic); Voriconazole

Decreased Effect

Elvitegravir may decrease the levels/effects of: Contraceptives (Estrogens); Warfarin

The levels/effects of Elvitegravir may be decreased by: Antacids; Bosentan; CarBAMazepine; CYP3A4 Inducers (Moderate); CYP3A4 Inducers (Strong); Dabrafenib; Deferasirox; Dexamethasone (Systemic); Efavirenz; Fosphenytoin-Phenytoin; Mitotane; Nevirapine; OXcarbazepine; PHENobarbital; Rifabutin; Rifampin; Rifapentine; Siltuximab; St Johns Wort; Tocilizumab

Storage/Stability Store below 30°C (86°F). Dispense only in original container.

Mechanism of Action Integrase is an HIV-1 encoded enzyme that is required for viral replication. Inhibition of integrase prevents the integration of HIV-1 DNA into host genomic DNA, blocking the formation of the HIV-1 provirus and propagation of the viral infection. Elvitegravir does not inhibit human topoisomerases I or II.

Pharmacodynamics/Kinetics

Absorption: AUC increases with food

Protein binding: 99%

Metabolism: Hepatic via CYP3A enzymes and also hepatic glucuronidation mediated by UGT1A1/3

Half-life elimination: Terminal: ~9 hours

Time to peak, plasma: ~4 hours

Excretion: Feces (~95%); urine (~7%)

Dosage

HIV-1 infection in antiretroviral treatment-experienced patients: Note: Must be administered in combination with a protease inhibitor, ritonavir, and another antiretroviral drug. See individual agents.

Adults: Oral:

Administered with concomitant atazanavir and ritonavir or lopinavir and ritonavir: 85 mg once daily

Administered with concomitant darunavir and ritonavir, fosamprenavir and ritonavir, or tipranavir and ritonavir: 150 mg once daily

Dosage adjustment in renal impairment: No dosage adjustment necessary.

Dosage adjustment in hepatic impairment:

Mild-to-moderate hepatic impairment (Child-Pugh class A or B): No dosage adjustment necessary.

Severe hepatic impairment (Child-Pugh class C): Use is not recommended (has not been studied).

Dietary Considerations Take with food.

Administration Oral: Administer once daily with food.

Monitoring Parameters CBC with differential, reticulocyte count, CD4 count, HIV RNA plasma levels, hepatic function tests, testing for HBV is recommended prior to the initiation of antiretroviral therapy.

Product Availability Vitekta; FDA approved September 2014; anticipated availability is currently undetermined.

Dosage Forms

Tablet, Oral:

Vitekta: 85 mg, 150 mg

Elvitegravir, Cobicistat, Emtricitabine, and Tenofovir

(el vi TEG ra vir, koe BIK i stat, em trye SYE ta been, & ten OF oh vir)

Brand Names: U.S. Stribild

Brand Names: Canada Stribild

Index Terms Cobicistat, Emtricitabine, Tenofovir, and Elvitegravir; Elvitegravir, Cobicistat, Emtricitabine, and Tenofovir Disoproxil Fumarate; Emtricitabine, Tenofovir, Elvitegravir, and Cobicistat; EVG/COBI/FTC/TDF; Quad Pill; Tenofovir, Elvitegravir, Cobicistat, and Emtricitabine

Pharmacologic Category Antiretroviral, Integrase Inhibitor (Anti-HIV); Antiretroviral, Reverse Transcriptase Inhibitor, Nucleoside (Anti-HIV); Antiretroviral, Reverse Transcriptase Inhibitor, Nucleotide (Anti-HIV); Cytochrome P-450 Inhibitor

Use HIV infection: Treatment of HIV-1 infection in adults who are antiretroviral treatment-naïve; as a replacement for the current antiretroviral regimen in adults who are virologically-suppressed (HIV-1 RNA <50 copies/mL) on a stable antiretroviral regimen for ≥6 months with no history of treatment failure and no known substitutions associated with resistance to elvitegravir, cobicistat, emtricitabine, or tenofovir.

Pregnancy Risk Factor B

Dosage Note: Prior to initiation, patients should be tested for hepatitis B infection, and baseline estimated creatinine clearance, urine glucose, and urine protein should be assessed in all patients.

Oral: Adults: HIV-1: One tablet once daily. **Note:** This combination is a recommended regimen for antiretroviral-naive patients with CrCl >70 mL/minute (DHHS [INSTI], 2013; DHHS [adult], 2014).

Dosing adjustment in renal impairment:

CrCl ≥70 mL/minute: No dosage adjustment necessary.

CrCl <70 mL/minute at initiation of therapy: Initial use is not recommended.

CrCl <50 mL/minute during therapy: Continued use is not recommended.

ESRD requiring dialysis: Use is not recommended.

Dosing adjustment in hepatic impairment:

Mild-to-moderate hepatic impairment (Child-Pugh class A or B): No dosage adjustment necessary.

Severe hepatic impairment (Child-Pugh class C): Use is not recommended (has not been studied).

Additional Information Complete prescribing information should be consulted for additional detail.

Dosage Forms

Tablet, oral:

Stribild: Elvitegravir 150 mg, cobicistat 150 mg, emtricitabine 200 mg, and tenofovir disoproxil fumarate 300 mg

◆ **Elvitegravir, Cobicistat, Emtricitabine, and Tenofovir Disoproxil Fumarate** *see* Elvitegravir, Cobicistat, Emtricitabine, and Tenofovir *on page* 718

◆ **E-Max-1000 [OTC]** *see* Vitamin E *on page* 2174

◆ **Emcyt** *see* Estramustine *on page* 782

◆ **EMD 68843** *see* Vilazodone *on page* 2158

◆ **Emend** *see* Aprepitant *on page* 166

◆ **Emend** *see* Fosaprepitant *on page* 929

◆ **Emend® IV (Can)** *see* Fosaprepitant *on page* 929

◆ **EMLA®** *see* Lidocaine and Prilocaine *on page* 1213

◆ **Emo-Cort® (Can)** *see* Hydrocortisone (Topical) *on page* 1014

◆ **Emoquette** *see* Ethinyl Estradiol and Desogestrel *on page* 799

Empagliflozin (em pa gli FLOE zin)

Brand Names: U.S. Jardiance

Index Terms BI10773

Pharmacologic Category Antidiabetic Agent, Sodium-Glucose Cotransporter 2 (SGLT2) Inhibitor; Sodium-Glucose Cotransporter 2 (SGLT2) Inhibitor

Use Diabetes mellitus, type 2: Treatment of type 2 diabetes mellitus (noninsulin dependent, NIDDM) as an adjunct to diet and exercise to improve glycemic control

Pregnancy Risk Factor C

Pregnancy Considerations Adverse events were observed in some animal reproduction studies. The manufacturer recommends the use of alternative therapies in pregnant women, especially during the second and third trimesters.

In women with diabetes, maternal hyperglycemia can be associated with congenital malformations as well as adverse effects in the fetus, neonate, and the mother (ACOG, 2005; ADA, 2014; Kitzmiller, 2008; Metzger, 2007). To prevent adverse outcomes, prior to conception and throughout pregnancy maternal blood glucose and HbA_{1c} should be kept as close to normal as possible but without causing significant hypoglycemia (ACOG, 2013; ADA, 2014; Blumer, 2013; Kitzmiller, 2008). Prior to pregnancy, effective contraception should be used until glycemic control is achieved (ADA, 2014; Kitzmiller, 2008). Other agents are currently recommended to treat diabetes in pregnant women (ACOG, 2013; Blumer, 2013).

Breast-Feeding Considerations It is not known if empagliflozin is excreted into breast milk. Due to the potential for serious adverse reactions in the nursing infant, the manufacturer recommends a decision be made whether to discontinue nursing or to discontinue the drug, taking into account the importance of treatment to the mother.

Contraindications Hypersensitivity to empagliflozin or any component of the formulation; severe renal impairment (eGFR <30 mL/minute/1.73 m^2), end-stage renal disease (ESRD), or dialysis

Warnings/Precautions May cause symptomatic hypotension due to intravascular volume depletion especially in patients with renal impairment, the elderly, patients on diuretics, or those with low systolic blood pressure. Assess volume status prior to initiation in patients at risk of hypotension and correct if depleted; monitor signs and symptoms of hypotension after initiation. Abnormalities in renal function (decreased eGFR, increased serum creatinine) may occur; elderly patients and patients with preexisting renal impairment may be at greater risk. Glycemic efficacy may be decreased and risk of adverse reactions (eg, adverse reaction related to volume depletion, renal impairment, UTI) may be increased with worsening renal function. Assess renal function prior to initiation and periodically during treatment; empagliflozin should not be initiated if initial eGFR is <45 mL/minute/1.73 m^2 and should be discontinued when eGFR is persistently <45 mL/minute/1.73 m^2. Use is contraindicated in severe renal impairment (eGFR <30 mL/minute/1.73 m^2), ESRD, and dialysis patients. May increase the risk of genital mycotic infections (eg, vulvovaginal mycotic infection, vulvovaginal candidiasis, vulvovaginitis, candida balanitis, balanoposthitis). Patients with a history of these infections or uncircumcised males are at greater risk. Risk for UTI may be increased; monitor for signs and symptoms of UTI and treat as needed. May cause low-density lipoprotein cholesterol (LDL-C) elevation; monitor LDL-C and treat as needed. Risk of intravascular volume depletion, renal impairment, and UTI may be increased in elderly patients. Should not be used in patients with type 1 diabetes mellitus (insulin-dependent, IDDM) or DKA. Potentially significant drug-drug interactions may exist, requiring dose or frequency adjustment, additional monitoring, and/or selection of alternative therapy.

Adverse Reactions

Endocrine & metabolic: Dyslipidemia, hypoglycemia, Increased LDL cholesterol, increased thirst (including polydipsia)

Gastrointestinal: Nausea

Genitourinary: Increased urine output (includes polyuria, pollakiuria, nocturia), urinary tract infection (includes bacteriuria [asymptomatic], cystitis)

Hematologic & oncologic: Increased hematocrit

Infection: Genitourinary fungal infection (females: includes bacterial vaginosis, cervicitis, vulvitis, vulvovaginal candidiasis, vulvovaginal infection, vulvovaginitis; males: includes balanitis, balanoposthitis, genitourinary fungal infection, penile infection, scrotal abscess)

Rare but important or life-threatening: Decreased estimated GFR (eGFR), hypotension, hypovolemia, increased serum creatinine, phimosis

Drug Interactions

Metabolism/Transport Effects Substrate of BCRP, OAT3, P-glycoprotein, SLCO1B1, UGT1A3, UGT1A8, UGT1A9, UGT2B7

Avoid Concomitant Use There are no known interactions where it is recommended to avoid concomitant use.

Increased Effect/Toxicity

Empagliflozin may increase the levels/effects of: DULoxetine; Hypoglycemic Agents; Hypotensive Agents; Levodopa; RisperiDONE

The levels/effects of Empagliflozin may be increased by: Androgens; Barbiturates; Nicorandil; Pegvisomant; Teriflunomide

Decreased Effect

The levels/effects of Empagliflozin may be decreased by: Corticosteroids (Orally Inhaled); Corticosteroids (Systemic); Danazol; Luteinizing Hormone-Releasing Hormone Analogs; Somatropin; Thiazide Diuretics

Storage/Stability Store at 25°C (77°F); excursions are permitted between 15°C and 30°C (59°F and 86°F).

Mechanism of Action By inhibiting sodium-glucose cotransporter 2 (SGLT2) in the proximal renal tubules, empagliflozin reduces reabsorption of filtered glucose from the tubular lumen and lowers the renal threshold for glucose (RT_G). SGLT2 is the main site of filtered glucose reabsorption; reduction of filtered glucose reabsorption and lowering of RT_G result in increased urinary excretion of glucose, thereby reducing plasma glucose concentrations.

Pharmacodynamics/Kinetics

Distribution: V_d: 73.8 L

Protein binding: 86.2%

Metabolism: Primarily through glucuronidation by UGT2B7, UGT1A3, UGT1A8, and UGT1A9 to minor metabolites

Half-life Elimination: 12.4 hours

Time to Peak: 1.5 hours

Excretion: Urine (54.4%; 50% as unchanged drug); feces (41.2%; majority as unchanged drug)

Dosage Note: If present, correct volume depletion prior to initiation.

Diabetes mellitus, type 2: Adults: Oral: Initial: 10 mg once daily; may increase to 25 mg once daily

Dosage adjustment in renal impairment:

eGFR ≥45 mL/minute/1.73 m^2: No dosage adjustment necessary.

eGFR <45 mL/minute/1.73 m^2: Do not initiate therapy; in patients already taking empagliflozin, discontinue therapy when eGFR is persistently <45 mL/minute/1.73 m^2

eGFR <30 mL/minute/1.73 m^2: Use is contraindicated.

ESRD, dialysis: Use is contraindicated.

Dosage adjustment in hepatic impairment: There are no dosage adjustments provided in the manufacturer's labeling; may be used in patients with hepatic impairment.

Dietary Considerations Individualized medical nutrition therapy (MNT) based on ADA recommendations is an integral part of therapy

Administration Administer once daily in the morning, with or without food.

Monitoring Parameters Blood glucose, HbA_{1c}; renal function (baseline and periodically during treatment); LDL-C; monitor for genital mycotic infections and UTI; monitor blood pressure

Reference Range

Recommendations for glycemic control in nonpregnant adults with diabetes (ADA, 2015):

HbA_{1c}: <7% (a more aggressive [<6.5%] or less aggressive [<8%] HbA_{1c} goal may be targeted based on patient-specific characteristics)

Preprandial capillary plasma glucose: 80 to 130 mg/dL

Peak postprandial capillary blood glucose: <180 mg/dL

Recommendations for glycemic control in pediatric (all age groups) patients with type 1 diabetes (ADA, 2015):

HbA_{1c}: <7.5% (individualization may be appropriate based on patient-specific characteristics; <7% is reasonable if it can be achieved without excessive hypoglycemia)

Preprandial capillary plasma glucose: 90 to 130 mg/dL

Bedtime and overnight capillary blood glucose: 90 to 150 mg/dL

Dosage Forms

Tablet, Oral:

Jardiance: 10 mg, 25 mg

◆ **Emsam** *see* Selegiline *on page 1873*

◆ **Emtec** *see* Acetaminophen and Codeine *on page 36*

Emtricitabine (em trye SYE ta been)

Brand Names: U.S. Emtriva

Brand Names: Canada Emtriva®

Index Terms BW524W91; Coviracil; FTC

Pharmacologic Category Antiretroviral, Reverse Transcriptase Inhibitor, Nucleoside (Anti-HIV)

Use Treatment of HIV infection in combination with at least two other antiretroviral agents

Pregnancy Risk Factor B

Pregnancy Considerations Adverse events were not observed in animal studies. Emtricitabine has a high level of transfer across the human placenta; no increased risk of overall birth defects has been observed according to data collected by the antiretroviral pregnancy registry. Cases of lactic acidosis/hepatic steatosis syndrome related to mitochondrial toxicity have been reported in pregnant women with prolonged use of nucleoside analogues. It is not known if pregnancy itself potentiates this known side effect; however, women may be at increased risk of lactic acidosis and liver damage. In addition, these adverse events are similar to other rare but life-threatening syndromes which occur during pregnancy (eg, HELLP syndrome). Hepatic enzymes and electrolytes should be monitored in women receiving nucleoside analogues and clinicians should watch for early signs of the syndrome. In addition, mitochondrial dysfunction may develop in infants following in utero exposure. A pharmacokinetic study shows a slight decrease in emtricitabine serum levels during the third trimester and immediately postpartum; however, there is no clear need to adjust the dose. The DHHS Perinatal HIV Guidelines consider emtricitabine with tenofovir to be a preferred NRTI backbone in antiretroviral-naive pregnant women. The DHHS Perinatal HIV Guidelines consider emtricitabine plus tenofovir a recommended dual NRTI/NtRTI backbone for HIV/HBV coinfected pregnant women.

Regardless of CD4 count or HIV RNA copy number, all HIV-infected pregnant women should receive a combination antiretroviral (ARV) drug regimen. A combination of antepartum, intrapartum, and infant ARV prophylaxis is recommended. ARV therapy should be started as soon as possible in women with symptomatic infection. Although earlier initiation may be more effective in reducing the perinatal transmission of HIV, initiation may be delayed until after 12 weeks gestation in women who do not require immediate treatment after careful consideration of maternal conditions (eg, nausea and vomiting) and the potential risks of first trimester fetal exposure for specific agents. A scheduled cesarean delivery at 38 weeks gestation is recommended for all women with HIV RNA >1,000 copies/mL or unknown concentrations near delivery in order to decrease transmission. If ARV therapy must be interrupted for <24 hours during the peripartum period, stop then restart all medications simultaneously in order to decrease the chance of developing resistance. Long-term follow-up is recommended for all infants exposed to ARV medications. In couples who want to conceive, the HIV-infected partner should attain maximum viral suppression prior to conception.

Health care providers are encouraged to enroll pregnant women exposed to antiretroviral medications in the Antiretroviral Pregnancy Registry (1-800-258-4263 or www.-APRegistry.com). Healthcare providers caring for HIV-infected women and their infants may contact the National Perinatal HIV Hotline (888-448-8765) for clinical consultation (HHS [perinatal], 2014).

Breast-Feeding Considerations Emtricitabine is excreted into breast milk. Maternal or infant antiretroviral therapy does not completely eliminate the risk of postnatal HIV transmission. In addition, multiclass-resistant virus has been detected in breast-feeding infants despite maternal therapy. Therefore, in the United States, where formula is accessible, affordable, safe, and sustainable, and the risk of infant mortality due to diarrhea and respiratory infections is low, complete avoidance of breast-feeding by HIV-infected women is recommended to decrease potential transmission of HIV (HHS [perinatal], 2014).

Contraindications Hypersensitivity to emtricitabine or any component of the formulation

Warnings/Precautions **[U.S. Boxed Warning]: Lactic acidosis, severe hepatomegaly with steatosis, and hepatic failure have occurred rarely with emtricitabine (similar to other nucleoside analogues).** Some cases have been fatal; stop treatment if lactic acidosis or hepatotoxicity occur. Prior liver disease, obesity, extended duration of therapy, and female gender may represent risk factors for severe hepatic reactions. Testing for hepatitis B is recommended prior to the initiation of therapy; **[U.S. Boxed Warnings]: Hepatitis B may be exacerbated following discontinuation of emtricitabine; not indicated for treatment of chronic hepatitis B; safety and efficacy in HIV/HBV coinfected patients not established.** May be associated with fat redistribution (buffalo hump, increased abdominal girth, breast engorgement, facial atrophy, and dyslipidemia). Immune reconstitution syndrome may develop resulting in the occurrence of an inflammatory response to an indolent or residual opportunistic infection during initial HIV treatment or activation of autoimmune disorders (eg, Graves' disease, polymyositis, Guillain-Barré syndrome) later in therapy; further evaluation and treatment may be required. Use caution in patients with renal impairment (dosage adjustment required). Concomitant use of other emtricitabine-containing products should be avoided. Concomitant use of lamivudine or lamivudine-containing products should be avoided; cross-resistance may develop.

Adverse Reactions

Central nervous system: Abnormal dreams, depression, dizziness, headache, insomnia, neuropathy/neuritis

Dermatologic: Hyperpigmentation (primarily of palms and/or soles but may include tongue, arms, lip and nails; generally mild and nonprogressive without associated local reactions such as pruritus or rash), rash (includes pruritus, maculopapular rash, vesiculobullous rash, pustular rash, and allergic reaction)

Endocrine & metabolic: Disordered glucose homeostasis, serum amylase increased, serum triglycerides increased

Gastrointestinal: Abdominal pain, diarrhea, dyspepsia, nausea, serum amylase increased, vomiting
Genitourinary: Hematuria
Hematologic: Anemia, neutropenia
Hepatic: Alkaline phosphatase increased, bilirubin increased, transaminases increased
Neuromuscular & skeletal: Arthralgia, CPK increased, creatinine kinase increased, myalgia, paresthesia, weakness
Respiratory: Cough, respiratory tract infection (upper), pharyngitis, rhinitis, sinusitis
Rare but important or life-threatening: Immune reconstitution syndrome

Drug Interactions

Metabolism/Transport Effects None known.

Avoid Concomitant Use

Avoid concomitant use of Emtricitabine with any of the following: LamiVUDine

Increased Effect/Toxicity

The levels/effects of Emtricitabine may be increased by: Ganciclovir-Valganciclovir; LamiVUDine; Ribavirin

Decreased Effect There are no known significant interactions involving a decrease in effect.

Food Interactions Food decreases peak plasma concentrations, but does not alter the extent of absorption or overall systemic exposure. Management: Administer without regard to meals.

Storage/Stability

Capsules: Store at 25°C (77°F); excursions permitted to 15°C to 30°C (59°F to 86°F).

Oral solution: Store at 2°C to 8°C (36°F to 46°F). Use within 3 months if stored at 25°C (77°F) with excursions permitted to 15°C to 30°C (59°F to 86°F).

Mechanism of Action Nucleoside reverse transcriptase inhibitor; emtricitabine is a cytosine analogue which is phosphorylated intracellularly to emtricitabine 5'-triphosphate which interferes with HIV viral RNA dependent DNA polymerase resulting in inhibition of viral replication.

Pharmacodynamics/Kinetics

Absorption: Rapid, extensive
Protein binding: <4%
Metabolism: Limited, via oxidation and conjugation (not via CYP isoenzymes)
Bioavailability: Capsule: 93%; solution: 75%
Half-life elimination: Normal renal function: Adults: 10 hours; children: 5-18 hours
Time to peak, plasma: 1-2 hours
Excretion: Urine (86% primarily as unchanged drug, 13% as metabolites); feces (14%)

Dosage Oral:

Children:
0 to 3 months: Solution: 3 mg/kg/day
3 months to 17 years:
Capsule: Children >33 kg: 200 mg once daily
Solution: 6 mg/kg once daily; maximum: 240 mg/day

Adults: **Note:** Emtricitabine in combination with tenofovir is a component of recommended regimens (with atazanavir/ritonavir, with darunavir/ritonavir, with dolutegravir, with efavirenz, or with raltegravir) in all treatment-naive patients and a component of a recommended regimen (with rilpivirine) for treatment-naive patients with CD4 count >200 cells/mm^3 (HHS [adult], 2014).
Capsule: 200 mg once daily
Solution: 240 mg once daily

Dosage adjustment in renal impairment: Adults (consider similar adjustments in children):
CrCl 30 to 49 mL/minute: Capsule: 200 mg every 48 hours; solution: 120 mg every 24 hours
CrCl 15 to 29 mL/minute: Capsule: 200 mg every 72 hours; solution: 80 mg every 24 hours
CrCl <15 mL/minute (including hemodialysis patients): Capsule: 200 mg every 96 hours; solution: 60 mg every 24 hours; administer after dialysis

Dosage adjustment in hepatic impairment: No dosage adjustment required.

Dietary Considerations May be taken with or without food.

Administration May be administered with or without food.

Monitoring Parameters Viral load, CD4, liver function tests; hepatitis B testing is recommended prior to initiation of therapy

Dosage Forms

Capsule, Oral:
Emtriva: 200 mg

Solution, Oral:
Emtriva: 10 mg/mL (170 mL)

Emtricitabine and Tenofovir

(em trye SYE ta been & ten OF oh vir)

Brand Names: U.S. Truvada

Brand Names: Canada Truvada

Index Terms Tenofovir and Emtricitabine

Pharmacologic Category Antiretroviral, Reverse Transcriptase Inhibitor, Nucleoside (Anti-HIV); Antiretroviral, Reverse Transcriptase Inhibitor, Nucleotide (Anti-HIV)

Use

Treatment of HIV-1 infection in combination with other antiretroviral agents in adults and pediatric patients ≥12 years of age

Pre-exposure prophylaxis (PrEP) for prevention of HIV-1 infection in adults who are at high risk for acquiring HIV

High risk individuals include those with partners known to be HIV-1 infected or who engage in sexual activity within a high prevalence area or social network, and one or more of the following:
- Inconsistent or no condom use
- Diagnosis of sexually-transmitted infections
- Exchange of sex for commodities
- Use of illicit drugs or alcohol dependence
- Incarceration
- Partner of unknown HIV-1 status with any of the above risk factors

When prescribing PrEP healthcare providers **MUST**:
- Include PrEP as part of a comprehensive prevention strategy because PrEP alone is not always effective in preventing HIV-1 infection
- Counsel all uninfected patients to strictly adhere to the dosing schedule, because adherence was strongly correlated with effectiveness in clinical trials
- Confirm a negative HIV-1 test prior to starting PrEP; if a candidate has acute viral infection symptoms and unprotected exposure events <1 month prior, delay PrEP for at least 1 month and retest HIV-1 status or use an Food and Drug Administration (FDA) test approved for HIV-1 diagnosis, including acute or primary HIV-1 infection
- Retest for HIV-1 infection at least every 3 months while the patient receives PrEP

Pregnancy Risk Factor B

Dosage Note: Avoid concurrent use with adefovir or lamivudine-containing products or other emtricitabine- and/or tenofovir-containing products.

HIV-1 infection: Children ≥12 (and ≥35 kg), Adolescents (≥35 kg), and Adults: Oral: One tablet (emtricitabine 200 mg and tenofovir 300 mg) once daily. **Note:** Emtricitabine plus tenofovir is a component of recommended regimens (in combination with atazanavir/ritonavir or darunavir/ritonavir or efavirenz or raltegravir) in antiretroviral-naive patients and a component of a recommended regimen (with rilpivirine) in antiretroviral-naive patients with CD4 count >200 cells/mm^3 (HHS [adult], 2014).

Preexposure prophylaxis (PrEP) for prevention of HIV infection in uninfected high-risk individuals: Adults: Oral: One tablet (emtricitabine 200 mg and tenofovir 300 mg) once daily

Hepatitis B treatment in patients with antiviral-resistant HBV or coinfection with HIV (off-label use): Adults: Oral: One tablet (emtricitabine 200 mg and tenofovir 300 mg) once daily (Lok, 2009)

Occupational HIV postexposure, prophylaxis (PEP) (off-label use): Adults: Oral: One tablet (emtricitabine 200 mg and tenofovir 300 mg) once daily for 4 weeks with concomitant raltegravir. Recommended as preferred therapy (Kuhar, 2013)

PrEP for prevention of HIV infection in injecting drug users (IDU) who are at risk for parenteral acquisition of HIV but not at risk for sexual acquisition of HIV (off-label use): Adults: Oral: One tablet (emtricitabine 200 mg and tenofovir 300 mg) once daily (CDC, 2013)

Dosage adjustment in renal impairment: Adults:

HIV-1 infection:

CrCl ≥50 mL/minute: No dosage adjustment necessary

CrCl 30 to 49 mL/minute: Increase interval to every 48 hours.

CrCl <30 mL/minute or hemodialysis: Not recommended.

PrEP:

CrCl ≥60 mL/minute: No dosage adjustment necessary

CrCl <60 mL/minute: Not recommended.

Dosage adjustment in hepatic impairment: No dosing adjustment necessary for tenofovir in moderate-to-severe hepatic compromise; no specific data available on emtricitabine in hepatic impairment, but given limited hepatic metabolism, dose adjustments are unlikely.

Additional Information Complete prescribing information should be consulted for additional detail.

Dosage Forms

Tablet:

Truvada: Emtricitabine 200 mg and tenofovir 300 mg

◆ **Emtricitabine, Efavirenz, and Tenofovir** *see* Efavirenz, Emtricitabine, and Tenofovir *on page 709*

Emtricitabine, Rilpivirine, and Tenofovir

(em trye SYE ta been, ril pi VIR een, & ten OF oh vir)

Brand Names: U.S. Complera

Brand Names: Canada Complera

Index Terms FTC/RPV/TDF; Rilpivirine, Emtricitabine, and Tenofovir; Tenofovir Disoproxil Fumarate, Rilpivirine, and Emtricitabine; Tenofovir, Emtricitabine, and Rilpivirine

Pharmacologic Category Antiretroviral, Reverse Transcriptase Inhibitor, Non-nucleoside (Anti-HIV); Antiretroviral, Reverse Transcriptase Inhibitor, Nucleoside (Anti-HIV); Antiretroviral, Reverse Transcriptase Inhibitor, Nucleotide (Anti-HIV)

Use HIV infection: For use as a complete regimen for the treatment of HIV-1 infection in antiretroviral treatment-naive adult patients with HIV-1 RNA ≤100,000 copies/mL at the start of therapy, and in certain virologically suppressed (HIV-1 RNA <50 copies/mL) adult patients on a stable antiretroviral regimen at start of therapy in order to replace their current antiretroviral treatment regimen.

Pregnancy Risk Factor B

Dosage HIV: Adults: Oral: One tablet once daily

Dosage adjustment for concomitant therapy with rifabutin: One tablet once daily plus rilpivirine 25 mg

Dosage adjustment in renal impairment:

CrCl ≥50 mL/minute: No dosage adjustments necessary.

CrCl <50 mL/minute: Use is not recommended

ESRD requiring dialysis: Use is not recommended

Dosage adjustment in hepatic impairment:

Mild-to-moderate impairment (Child-Pugh class A or B): No dosage adjustments necessary.

Severe impairment (Child-Pugh class C): There are no dosage adjustments provided in the manufacturer's labeling (has not been studied).

Additional Information Complete prescribing information should be consulted for additional detail.

Dosage Forms

Tablet, oral:

Complera: Emtricitabine 200 mg, rilpivirine 25 mg, and tenofovir 300 mg

◆ **Emtricitabine, Tenofovir, Elvitegravir, and Cobicistat** *see* Elvitegravir, Cobicistat, Emtricitabine, and Tenofovir *on page 718*

◆ **Emtriva** *see* Emtricitabine *on page 720*

◆ **Emtriva® (Can)** *see* Emtricitabine *on page 720*

◆ **ENA 713** *see* Rivastigmine *on page 1833*

◆ **Enablex** *see* Darifenacin *on page 568*

◆ **Enablex® (Can)** *see* Darifenacin *on page 568*

Enalapril

(e NAL a pril)

Brand Names: U.S. Epaned; Vasotec

Brand Names: Canada ACT-Enalapril; Apo-Enalapril; Mylan-Enalapril; PMS-Enalapril; PRO-Enalapril; RAN-Enalapril; Riva-Enalapril; Sandoz-Enalapril; Sig-Enalapril; Taro-Enalapril; Teva-Enalapril; Vasotec

Index Terms Enalapril Maleate

Pharmacologic Category Angiotensin-Converting Enzyme (ACE) Inhibitor; Antihypertensive

Use

Asymptomatic left ventricular dysfunction: Treatment of asymptomatic left ventricular dysfunction

Heart failure: Treatment of symptomatic heart failure (HF)

Note: The ACCF/AHA 2013 heart failure guidelines recommend the use of ACE inhibitors, along with other guideline directed medical therapies, to prevent heart failure in patients with a reduced ejection fraction who have a history of MI (Stage B HF), to prevent heart failure in any patient with a reduced ejection fraction (Stage B HF), or to treat those with heart failure and reduced ejection fraction (Stage C HFrEF) (ACCF/AHA [Yancy, 2013]).

Hypertension: Treatment of hypertension

The 2014 guideline for the management of high blood pressure in adults (Eighth Joint National Committee [JNC 8]) recommends initiation of pharmacologic treatment to lower blood pressure for the following patients:

- Patients ≥60 years of age with systolic blood pressure (SBP) ≥150 mm Hg or diastolic blood pressure (DBP) ≥90 mm Hg. Goal of therapy is SBP <150 mm Hg and DBP <90 mm Hg.
- Patients <60 years of age with SBP ≥140 mm Hg or DBP is ≥90 mm Hg. Goal of therapy is SBP <140 mm Hg and DBP <90 mm Hg.
- Patients ≥18 years of age with diabetes and SBP ≥140 mm Hg or DBP ≥90 mm Hg. Goal of therapy is SBP <140 mm Hg and DBP <90 mm Hg.
- Patients ≥18 years of age with chronic kidney disease (CKD) and SBP ≥140 mm Hg or DBP ≥90 mm Hg. Goal of therapy is SBP <140 mm Hg and DBP <90 mm Hg.

In patients with CKD, regardless of race or diabetes status, the use of an ACE inhibitor (ACEI) or angiotensin receptor blocker (ARB) as initial therapy is recommended to improve kidney outcomes. In the general nonblack population (without CKD) including those with diabetes, initial antihypertensive treatment should consist of a thiazide-type diuretic, calcium channel blocker, ACEI, or ARB. In the general black population (without CKD) including those with diabetes, initial antihypertensive treatment should consist of a thiazide-type diuretic or a calcium channel blocker **instead of** an ACEI or ARB.

Pregnancy Risk Factor D

Pregnancy Considerations [U.S. Boxed Warning]: Drugs that act on the renin-angiotensin system can cause injury and death to the developing fetus. Discontinue as soon as possible once pregnancy is detected. Enalaprilat, the active metabolite of enalapril, crosses the placenta; teratogenic effects may occur following maternal use during pregnancy. Drugs that act on the renin-angiotensin system are associated with oligohydramnios. Oligohydramnios, due to decreased fetal renal function, may lead to fetal lung hypoplasia and skeletal malformations. The use of these drugs in pregnancy is also associated with anuria, hypotension, renal failure, skull hypoplasia, and death in the fetus/neonate. Chronic maternal hypertension itself is also associated with adverse events in the fetus/infant. ACE inhibitors are not recommended during pregnancy to treat maternal hypertension or heart failure. Use of an ACE inhibitor should also be avoided in any woman of reproductive age. Women who are planning a pregnancy should be considered for other medication options if an ACE inhibitor is currently prescribed or the ACE inhibitor should be discontinued as soon as possible once pregnancy is detected. The exposed fetus should be monitored for fetal growth, amniotic fluid volume, and organ formation. Infants exposed to an ACE inhibitor *in utero* should be monitored for hyperkalemia, hypotension, and oliguria (exchange transfusions or dialysis may be needed). These adverse events are generally associated with maternal use in the second and third trimesters.

Untreated chronic maternal hypertension is also associated with adverse events in the fetus, infant, and mother. The use of ACE inhibitors is not recommended to treat chronic uncomplicated hypertension in pregnant women and should generally be avoided in women of reproductive potential (ACOG, 2013).

Breast-Feeding Considerations Enalapril and enalaprilat are excreted in breast milk. Breast-feeding is not recommended by the manufacturer.

Contraindications

Hypersensitivity to enalapril or any component of the formulation; angioedema related to previous treatment with an ACE inhibitor; patients with idiopathic or hereditary angioedema; concomitant use with aliskiren in patients with diabetes mellitus

Documentation of allergenic cross-reactivity for ACE inhibitors is limited. However, because of similarities in chemical structure and/or pharmacologic actions, the possibility of cross-sensitivity cannot be ruled out with certainty.

Canadian labeling: Additional contraindications (not in U.S. labeling): Concomitant use with aliskiren-containing drugs in patients with moderate-to-severe renal impairment (GFR <60 mL/minute/1.73 m^2)

Warnings/Precautions Anaphylactic reactions may occur rarely with ACE inhibitors. At any time during treatment (especially following first dose) angioedema may occur rarely with ACE inhibitors; it may involve the head and neck (potentially compromising airway) or the intestine (presenting with abdominal pain). African-Americans may be at an increased risk. Prolonged frequent monitoring may be required especially if tongue, glottis, or larynx are involved as they are associated with airway obstruction. Patients with a history of airway surgery may have a higher risk of airway obstruction. Aggressive early and appropriate management is critical. Use in patients with idiopathic or hereditary angioedema or previous angioedema associated with ACE inhibitor therapy is contraindicated. Severe anaphylactoid reactions may be seen during hemodialysis (eg, CVVHD) with high-flux dialysis membranes (eg, AN69), and rarely, during low density lipoprotein apheresis with dextran sulfate cellulose. Rare cases of anaphylactoid reactions have been reported in patients undergoing sensitization treatment with hymenoptera (bee, wasp) venom while receiving ACE inhibitors.

Symptomatic hypotension with or without syncope can occur with ACE inhibitors (usually with the first several doses); effects are most often observed in volume depleted patients; correct volume depletion prior to initiation; close monitoring of patient is required especially with initial dosing and dosing increases; blood pressure must be lowered at a rate appropriate for the patient's clinical condition. Initiation of therapy in patients with ischemic heart disease or cerebrovascular disease warrants close observation due to the potential consequences posed by falling blood pressure (eg, MI, stroke). Use with caution in hypertrophic cardiomyopathy with outflow tract obstruction, severe aortic stenosis, or before, during, or immediately after major surgery. **[U.S. Boxed Warning]: Drugs that act on the renin-angiotensin system can cause injury and death to the developing fetus. Discontinue as soon as possible once pregnancy is detected.**

Hyperkalemia may occur with ACE inhibitors; risk factors include renal dysfunction, diabetes mellitus, concomitant use of potassium-sparing diuretics, potassium supplements, and/or potassium-containing salts. Use cautiously, if at all, with these agents and monitor potassium closely. Cough may occur with ACE inhibitors. Other causes of cough should be considered (eg, pulmonary congestion in patients with heart failure) and excluded prior to discontinuation.

May be associated with deterioration of renal function and/or increases in serum creatinine, particularly in patients with low renal blood flow (eg, renal artery stenosis, heart failure) whose glomerular filtration rate (GFR) is dependent on efferent arteriolar vasoconstriction by angiotensin II; deterioration may result in oliguria, acute renal failure, and progressive azotemia. Small increases in serum creatinine may occur following initiation; consider discontinuation only in patients with progressive and/or significant deterioration in renal function. Use with caution in patients with unstented unilateral/bilateral renal artery stenosis. When unstented bilateral renal artery stenosis is present, use is generally avoided due to the elevated risk of deterioration in renal function unless possible benefits outweigh risks. Potentially significant drug-drug interactions may exist, requiring dose or frequency adjustment, additional monitoring, and/or selection of alternative therapy.

Rare toxicities associated with ACE inhibitors include cholestatic jaundice (which may progress to fulminant hepatic necrosis), agranulocytosis, neutropenia or leukopenia with myeloid hypoplasia. Patients with collagen vascular diseases (especially with concomitant renal impairment) or renal impairment alone may be at increased risk for hematologic toxicity; periodically monitor CBC with differential in these patients.

Adverse Reactions

Cardiovascular: Chest pain, hypotension, orthostatic effect, orthostatic hypotension, syncope

Central nervous system: Dizziness, fatigue, headache

Dermatologic: Skin rash

Gastrointestinal: Abdominal pain, anorexia, constipation, diarrhea, dysgeusia, nausea, vomiting

Neuromuscular & skeletal: Weakness

Renal: Increased serum creatinine, renal insufficiency (in patients with bilateral renal artery stenosis or hypovolemia)

Respiratory: Bronchitis, cough, dyspnea

Rare but important or life-threatening: Acute generalized exanthematous pustulosis, agranulocytosis, alopecia, anaphylactoid reaction, angina pectoris, angioedema, anosmia, arthritis, asthma, ataxia, atrial fibrillation, atrial tachycardia, bone marrow depression, bradycardia, cardiac arrest, cardiac arrhythmia, cerebrovascular accident, cholestatic jaundice, confusion, conjunctivitis, depression, eosinophilia, eosinophilic pneumonitis, erythema multiforme, exfoliative dermatitis, giant-cell arteritis, gynecomastia, hallucination, hemolysis (with G6PD), herpes zoster, IgA vasculitis, increased erythrocyte sedimentation rate, intestinal obstruction, insomnia, interstitial nephritis, leukocytosis, lichenoid eruption, melena, myocardial infarction, myositis, neutropenia, ototoxicity, pancreatitis, pemphigus, pemphigus foliaceus, peripheral neuropathy, positive ANA titer, psychosis, pulmonary edema, pulmonary embolism, pulmonary infarct, pulmonary infiltrates, Raynaud's phenomenon, serositis, Sjogren's syndrome, skin photosensitivity, Stevens-Johnson syndrome, stomatitis, systemic lupus erythematosus, thrombocytopenia, toxic epidermal necrolysis, upper respiratory tract infection, vasculitis, visual hallucination (Doane, 2013)

Drug Interactions

Metabolism/Transport Effects None known.

Avoid Concomitant Use There are no known interactions where it is recommended to avoid concomitant use.

Increased Effect/Toxicity

Enalapril may increase the levels/effects of: Allopurinol; Amifostine; Antihypertensives; AzaTHIOprine; DULoxetine; Ferric Gluconate; Gold Sodium Thiomalate; Grass Pollen Allergen Extract (5 Grass Extract); Hypotensive Agents; Iron Dextran Complex; Levodopa; Lithium; Nonsteroidal Anti-Inflammatory Agents; Obinutuzumab; RisperiDONE; RiTUXimab; Sodium Phosphates

The levels/effects of Enalapril may be increased by: Alfuzosin; Aliskiren; Angiotensin II Receptor Blockers; Barbiturates; Brimonidine (Topical); Canagliflozin; Dapoxetine; Diazoxide; DPP-IV Inhibitors; Eplerenone; Everolimus; Heparin; Heparin (Low Molecular Weight); Herbs (Hypotensive Properties); Loop Diuretics; MAO Inhibitors; Nicorandil; Pentoxifylline; Phosphodiesterase 5 Inhibitors; Potassium Salts; Potassium-Sparing Diuretics; Prostacyclin Analogues; Sirolimus; Temsirolimus; Thiazide Diuretics; TiZANidine; Tolvaptan; Trimethoprim

Decreased Effect

The levels/effects of Enalapril may be decreased by: Aprotinin; Herbs (Hypertensive Properties); Icatibant; Lanthanum; Methylphenidate; Nonsteroidal Anti-Inflammatory Agents; Salicylates; Yohimbine

Preparation for Administration Epaned: Solution kit (for 150 mL, enalapril solution 1 mg/mL): Kit contains 1 bottle of enalapril powder and 1 bottle of Ora-Sweet SF dilution to be added to the enalapril powder prior to dispensing. Firmly tap the enalapril powder for oral solution bottle on a hard surface 5 times. Add approximately one-half (75 mL) of the Ora-Sweet SF diluent to the enalapril 150 mL oral solution bottle and shake well for 30 seconds. Add the remainder of the Ora-Sweet SF diluent and shake well for an additional 30 seconds. May be used for 60 days after reconstitution.

Storage/Stability

Solution kit: Store at 25°C (77°F); excursions are permitted between 15°C and 30°C (59°F and 86°F). Do not freeze. Protect from moisture. Once reconstituted, the solution should be stored at 15°C to 30°C (59°F to 86°F) and may be stored for up to 60 days.

Tablet: Store at 25°C (77°F); excursions permitted to 15°C to 30°C (59°F to 86°F). Protect from moisture.

Mechanism of Action Competitive inhibitor of angiotensin-converting enzyme (ACE); prevents conversion of angiotensin I to angiotensin II, a potent vasoconstrictor; results in lower levels of angiotensin II which causes an increase in plasma renin activity and a reduction in aldosterone secretion

Pharmacodynamics/Kinetics

Onset of action: ~1 hour

Peak effect: 4 to 6 hours

Duration: 12 to 24 hours

Absorption: 55% to 75%

Protein binding: ~50% (Davies, 1984)

Metabolism: Prodrug, undergoes hepatic biotransformation to enalaprilat

Half-life elimination:

Enalapril: Adults: Healthy: 2 hours; Congestive heart failure: 3.4 to 5.8 hours

Enalaprilat: Infants 6 weeks to 8 months of age: 6 to 10 hours (Lloyd, 1989); Adults: ~35 hours (Till, 1984; Ulm, 1982)

Time to peak, serum: Oral: Enalapril: 0.5 to 1.5 hours; Enalaprilat (active metabolite): 3 to 4.5 hours

Excretion: Urine (61%; 18% of which was enalapril, 43% was enalaprilat); feces (33%; 6% of which was enalapril, 27% was enalaprilat) (Ulm, 1982)

Dosage Use lower listed initial dose in patients with hyponatremia, hypovolemia, severe congestive heart failure, decreased renal function, or in those receiving diuretics.

Oral:

Children ≥1 month and Adolescents: Hypertension: Initial: 0.08 mg/kg (up to 5 mg) once daily; adjust dosage based on patient response; doses >0.58 mg/kg (40 mg) have not been evaluated in pediatric patients

Infants and Children: Heart failure (off-label dosing): Initial: 0.1 mg/kg/day in 1 to 2 divided doses; increase as required over 2 weeks to maximum of 0.5 mg/kg/day. **Note:** Mean dose required for CHF improvement in 39 children (9 days to 17 years) was 0.36 mg/kg/day; select individuals have been treated with doses up to 0.94 mg/kg/day (Leversha, 1994).

Adults:

Asymptomatic left ventricular dysfunction: 2.5 mg twice daily, titrated as tolerated to 20 mg daily

Heart failure with reduced ejection fraction (HFrEF): Initial: 2.5 mg twice daily (usual range: 5 to 40 mg daily in 2 divided doses); titrate slowly at 1- to 2-week intervals. Target dose: 10 to 20 mg twice daily (ACCF/AHA [Yancy, 2013])

Hypertension: 2.5to 5 mg daily then increase as required, usually at 1- to 2-week intervals; usual dose range (ASH/ISH [Weber, 2014]): 10 to 40 mg daily. Target dose (JNC 8 [James, 2013]): 20 mg daily in 1 or 2 divided doses. **Note:** Initiate with 2.5 mg if patient is taking a diuretic which cannot be discontinued. May add a diuretic if blood pressure cannot be controlled with enalapril alone.

Conversion from IV **enalaprilat** to oral **enalapril** therapy: If not concurrently receiving diuretics, initiate enalapril 5 mg once daily; if concurrently receiving diuretics and responding to enalaprilat 0.625 mg IV every 6 hours, initiate with enalapril 2.5 mg once daily; subsequent titration as needed.

Dosage adjustment in renal impairment: Note: Use in infants and children ≤16 years of age with GFR <30 mL/minute/1.73 m^2 is not recommended (no dosing data exists).

Manufacturer's recommendations:

CrCl >30 mL/minute: No dosage adjustment necessary

CrCl ≤30 mL/minute: Administer 2.5 mg day; titrated upward until blood pressure is controlled.

Heart failure patients with sodium <130 mEq/L or serum creatinine >1.6 mg/dL: Initiate dosage with 2.5 mg daily, increasing to twice daily as needed. Increase further in increments of 2.5 mg/dose at >4-day intervals to a maximum daily dose of 40 mg.

Intermittent hemodialysis (IHD): Moderately dialyzable (20% to 50%): Initial: 2.5 mg on dialysis days; adjust dose on nondialysis days depending on blood pressure response.

Conversion from IV **enalaprilat** to oral **enalapril** therapy:

CrCl >30 mL/minute: May initiate enalapril 5 mg once daily.

CrCl ≤30 mL/minute: May initiate enalapril 2.5 mg once daily.

Alternate recommendations (Aronoff, 2007):

CrCl >50 mL/minute: No dosage adjustment necessary

CrCl 10 to 50 mL/minute: Administer 75% to 100% of usual dose

CrCl <10 mL/minute: Administer 50% of usual dose

Peritoneal dialysis: Supplemental dose is not necessary, although some removal of drug occurs.

Dosage adjustment in hepatic impairment: No dosage adjustment is necessary. Hydrolysis of enalapril to enalaprilat may be delayed and/or impaired in patients with severe hepatic impairment, but the pharmacodynamic effects of the drug do not appear to be significantly altered.

Dietary Considerations Limit salt substitutes or potassium-rich diet.

Monitoring Parameters Blood pressure; serum creatinine and potassium; if patient has collagen vascular disease and/or renal impairment, periodically monitor CBC with differential

2013 ACCF/AHA Heart Failure guideline recommendations: Within 1-2 weeks after initiation and periodically thereafter, reassess renal function and serum potassium especially in patients with preexisting hypotension, hyponatremia, diabetes mellitus, azotemia, or those taking potassium supplements (ACCF/AHA [Yancy, 2013]).

Dosage Forms

Solution Reconstituted, Oral:

Epaned: 1 mg/mL (150 mL)

Tablet, Oral:

Vasotec: 2.5 mg, 5 mg, 10 mg, 20 mg

Generic: 2.5 mg, 5 mg, 10 mg, 20 mg

Dosage Forms: Canada Note: Refer to Dosage Forms. Oral powder for reconstitution is not available in Canada.

Extemporaneous Preparations Note: Commercial oral solution kit is available (1 mg/mL).

A 1 mg/mL oral suspension may be made with tablets, Bicitra [discontinued] or equivalent, and Ora-Sweet SF. Place ten 20 mg tablets in a 200 mL polyethylene terephthalate bottle; add 50 mL of Bicitra [discontinued] or equivalent and shake well for at least 2 minutes. Let stand for 1 hour then shake for 1 additional minute; add 150 mL of Ora-Sweet SF and shake well. Label "shake well" and "refrigerate". Stable for 30 days when stored in a polyethylene terephthalate bottle and refrigerated (Vasotec prescribing information, 2011).

A 1 mg/mL oral suspension may be made with tablets and one of three different vehicles (cherry syrup, a 1:1 mixture of Ora-Sweet and Ora-Plus, or a 1:1 mixture of Ora-Sweet SF and Ora-Plus). Crush six 20 mg tablets in a mortar and reduce to a fine powder. Add 15 mL of the chosen vehicle and mix to a uniform paste; mix while adding the vehicle in incremental proportions to **almost** 120 mL; transfer to a calibrated bottle, rinse mortar with vehicle, and add quantity of vehicle sufficient to make 120 mL. Label "shake well" and "protect from light". Stable for 60 days when stored in amber plastic prescription bottles in the dark at room temperature or refrigerated (Allen, 1998).

A 1 mg/mL oral suspension may be made with tablets and one of three different vehicles (deionized water, citrate buffer solution at pH 5.0, or a 1:1 mixture of Ora-Sweet and Ora-Plus). Crush twenty 10 mg tablets in a mortar and reduce to a fine powder. Add small portions of the chosen vehicle and mix to a uniform paste; mix while adding vehicle in incremental proportions to **almost** 200 mL; transfer to a graduated cylinder, rinse mortar with vehicle, and add quantity of vehicle sufficient to make 200 mL. Label "shake well" and "protect from light". Preparations made in citrate buffer solution at pH 5.0 and the 1:1 mixture of Ora-Sweet and Ora-Plus are stable for 91 days when stored in plastic prescription bottles in the dark at room temperature or refrigerated. Preparation made in deionized water is stable for 91 days refrigerated or 56 days at room temperature when stored in plastic prescription bottles in the dark. **Note:** To prepare the isotonic citrate buffer solution (pH 5.0), see reference (Nahata, 1998).

A more dilute, 0.1 mg/mL oral suspension may be made with tablets and an isotonic buffer solution at pH 5.0. Grind one 20 mg tablet in a glass mortar and reduce to a fine powder; mix with isotonic citrate buffer (pH 5.0) and filter; add quantity of buffer solution sufficient to make 200 mL. Label "shake well", "protect from light", and "refrigerate". Stable for 90 days (Boulton, 1994).

Allen LV Jr and Erickson MA 3rd, "Stability of Alprazolam, Chloroquine Phosphate, Cisapride, Enalapril Maleate, and Hydralazine Hydrochloride in Extemporaneously Compounded Oral Liquids," *Am J Health Syst Pharm*, 1998, 55(18):1915-20.

Boulton DW, Woods DJ, Fawcett JP, et al, "The Stability of an Enalapril Maleate Oral Solution Prepared From Tablets," *Aust J Hosp Pharm*, 1994, 24(2):151-6.

Nahata MC, Morosco RS, and Hipple TF, "Stability of Enalapril Maleate in Three Extemporaneously Prepared Oral Liquids," *Am J Health Syst Pharm*, 1998, 55(11):1155-7.

Vasotec® prescribing information, Valeant Pharmaceuticals North America LLC, Bridgewater, NJ; 2011.

Enalapril and Hydrochlorothiazide

(e NAL a pril & hye droe klor oh THYE a zide)

Brand Names: U.S. Vaseretic

Brand Names: Canada Apo-Enalapril Maleate/Hctz; Novo-Enalapril/Hctz; Vaseretic

Index Terms Enalapril Maleate and Hydrochlorothiazide; Hydrochlorothiazide and Enalapril

Pharmacologic Category Angiotensin-Converting Enzyme (ACE) Inhibitor; Antihypertensive; Diuretic, Thiazide

Use Treatment of hypertension

Pregnancy Risk Factor D

Dosage Oral: Adults: Enalapril 5-10 mg and hydrochlorothiazide 12.5-25 mg once daily (maximum: 40 mg/day [enalapril]; 50 mg/day [hydrochlorothiazide])

Dosage adjustment in renal impairment:

CrCl >30 mL/minute: No dosage adjustment required.

Severe renal failure: Avoid; loop diuretics are recommended.

Dosage adjustment in hepatic impairment: No dosage adjustment provided in manufacturer's labeling; use with caution.

Additional Information Complete prescribing information should be consulted for additional detail.

Dosage Forms

Tablet: 5/12.5: Enalapril 5 mg and hydrochlorothiazide 12.5 mg; 10/25: Enalapril 10 mg and hydrochlorothiazide 25 mg

Vaseretic: 10/25: Enalapril 10 mg and hydrochlorothiazide 25 mg

◆ **Enalapril Maleate** *see* Enalapril *on page 722*

◆ **Enalapril Maleate and Hydrochlorothiazide** *see* Enalapril and Hydrochlorothiazide *on page 725*

◆ **Enbrel** *see* Etanercept *on page 795*

◆ **Enbrel SureClick** *see* Etanercept *on page 795*

◆ **Endocet** *see* Oxycodone and Acetaminophen *on page 1541*

◆ **Endodan®** *see* Oxycodone and Aspirin *on page 1542*
◆ **Endometrin** *see* Progesterone *on page 1722*
◆ **Enduron** *see* Methyclothiazide *on page 1331*
◆ **Enemeez Mini [OTC]** *see* Docusate *on page 661*
◆ **Enerjets [OTC]** *see* Caffeine *on page 319*

Enfuvirtide (en FYOO vir tide)

Brand Names: U.S. Fuzeon
Brand Names: Canada Fuzeon
Index Terms T-20
Pharmacologic Category Antiretroviral, Fusion Protein Inhibitor (Anti-HIV)
Use HIV-1 infection: Treatment of HIV-1 infection in combination with other antiretroviral agents in treatment-experienced patients with evidence of HIV-1 replication despite ongoing antiretroviral therapy
Pregnancy Risk Factor B
Dosage HIV treatment:
Children and Adolescents 6 to 16 years: SubQ: 2 mg/kg twice daily (maximum dose: 90 mg twice daily)
Adolescents >16 years and Adults: SubQ: 90 mg twice daily

Dosage adjustment in renal impairment: No dosage adjustment necessary.
Dosage adjustment in hepatic impairment: No dosage adjustment necessary (has not been studied).

Additional Information Complete prescribing information should be consulted for additional detail.
Dosage Forms
Solution Reconstituted, Subcutaneous:
Fuzeon: 90 mg (1 ea)

◆ **Engerix-B** *see* Hepatitis B Vaccine (Recombinant) *on page 1002*
◆ **Engerix-B® and Havrix®** *see* Hepatitis A and Hepatitis B Recombinant Vaccine *on page 1000*
◆ **Enhanced-Potency Inactivated Poliovirus Vaccine** *see* Poliovirus Vaccine (Inactivated) *on page 1673*
◆ **Enjuvia** *see* Estrogens (Conjugated B/Synthetic) *on page 785*
◆ **Enlon** *see* Edrophonium *on page 706*
◆ **Enlon® (Can)** *see* Edrophonium *on page 706*
◆ **Enlon-Plus®** *see* Edrophonium and Atropine *on page 706*
◆ **EnovaRX-Baclofen** *see* Baclofen *on page 223*
◆ **EnovaRX-Cyclobenzaprine HCl** *see* Cyclobenzaprine *on page 516*
◆ **EnovaRX-Ibuprofen** *see* Ibuprofen *on page 1032*
◆ **EnovaRX-Lidocaine HCl** *see* Lidocaine (Topical) *on page 1211*
◆ **EnovaRX-Naproxen** *see* Naproxen *on page 1427*
◆ **EnovaRX-Tramadol** *see* TraMADol *on page 2074*

Enoxaparin (ee noks a PA rin)

Brand Names: U.S. Lovenox
Brand Names: Canada Lovenox; Lovenox HP; Lovenox With Preservative
Index Terms Enoxaparin Sodium
Pharmacologic Category Anticoagulant; Anticoagulant, Low Molecular Weight Heparin
Use
Acute coronary syndromes: Unstable angina (UA), non-ST-elevation (NSTEMI), and ST-elevation myocardial infarction (STEMI)
DVT prophylaxis: Following hip or knee replacement surgery, abdominal surgery, or in medical patients with severely-restricted mobility during acute illness who are at risk for thromboembolic complications. **Note:** Patients at risk of thromboembolic complications who undergo abdominal surgery include those with one or more of the following risk factors: >40 years of age, obesity, general anesthesia lasting >30 minutes, malignancy, history of deep vein thrombosis or pulmonary embolism
DVT treatment (acute): Inpatient treatment (patients with or without pulmonary embolism) and outpatient treatment (patients without pulmonary embolism)

Pregnancy Risk Factor B
Pregnancy Considerations Adverse events were not observed in animal reproduction studies. Low molecular weight heparin (LMWH) does not cross the placenta; increased risks of fetal bleeding or teratogenic effects have not been reported (Bates, 2012).

LMWH is recommended over unfractionated heparin for the treatment of acute venous thromboembolism (VTE) in pregnant women. LMWH is also recommended over unfractionated heparin for VTE prophylaxis in pregnant women with certain risk factors (eg, homozygous factor V Leiden, antiphospholipid antibody syndrome with ≥3 previous pregnancy losses). Prophylaxis is not routinely recommended for women undergoing assisted reproduction therapy; however, LMWH therapy is recommended for women who develop severe ovarian hyperstimulation syndrome. LMWH should be discontinued at least 24 hours prior to induction of labor or a planned cesarean delivery. For women undergoing cesarean section and who have additional risk factors for developing VTE, the prophylactic use of LMWH may be considered (Bates, 2012).

LMWH may also be used in women with mechanical heart valves (consult current guidelines for details) (Bates, 2012; Nishimura, 2014). Women who require long-term anticoagulation with warfarin and who are considering pregnancy, LMWH substitution should be done prior to conception when possible. When choosing therapy, fetal outcomes (ie, pregnancy loss, malformations), maternal outcomes (ie, VTE, hemorrhage), burden of therapy, and maternal preference should be considered (Bates, 2012). Monitoring antifactor Xa levels is recommended (Bates, 2012; Nishimura, 2014).

Multiple-dose vials contain benzyl alcohol (avoid in pregnant women due to association with gasping syndrome in premature infants); use of preservative-free formulations is recommended.

Breast-Feeding Considerations Small amounts of LMWH have been detected in breast milk; however, because it has a low oral bioavailability, it is unlikely to cause adverse events in a nursing infant. Enoxaparin product labeling does not recommend use in nursing women; however, antithrombotic guidelines state that use of LMWH may be continued in breast-feeding women (Guyatt, 2012).

Contraindications
Hypersensitivity to enoxaparin, heparin, pork products, or any component of the formulation (including benzyl alcohol in multiple-dose vials); thrombocytopenia associated with a positive *in vitro* test for antiplatelet antibodies in the presence of enoxaparin; active major bleeding
Canadian labeling: Additional contraindications (not in U.S. labeling): Use of multiple-dose vials in newborns or premature neonates; history of confirmed or suspected immunologically-mediated heparin-induced thrombocytopenia; acute or subacute bacterial endocarditis; major blood clotting disorders; active gastric or duodenal ulcer; hemorrhagic cerebrovascular accident (except if there are systemic emboli); severe uncontrolled hypertension; diabetic or hemorrhagic retinopathy; other conditions or

diseases involving an increased risk of hemorrhage; injuries to and operations on the brain, spinal cord, eyes, and ears; spinal/epidural anesthesia when repeated dosing of enoxaparin (1 mg/kg every 12 hours or 1.5 mg/kg daily) is required, due to increased risk of bleeding.

Note: Use of enoxaparin in patients with current heparin-induced thrombocytopenia (HIT) or HIT with thrombosis is **not** recommended and considered contraindicated due to high cross-reactivity to heparin-platelet factor-4 antibody (Guyatt [ACCP], 2012; Warkentin, 1999).

Warnings/Precautions [U.S. Boxed Warning]: Spinal or epidural hematomas, including subsequent long-term or permanent paralysis, may occur with recent or anticipated neuraxial anesthesia (epidural or spinal anesthesia) or spinal puncture in patients anticoagulated with LMWH or heparinoids. Consider risk versus benefit prior to spinal procedures; risk is increased by the use of concomitant agents which may alter hemostasis, the use of indwelling epidural catheters, a history of spinal deformity or spinal surgery, as well as a history of traumatic or repeated epidural or spinal punctures. Optimal timing between neuraxial procedures and enoxaparin administration is not known. Delay placement or removal of catheter for at least 12 hours after administration of low-dose enoxaparin (eg, 30 to 60 mg/day) and at least 24 hours after high-dose enoxaparin (eg, 0.75 to 1 mg/kg twice daily or 1.5 mg/kg once daily) and consider doubling these times in patients with creatinine clearance <30 mL/minute; risk of neuraxial hematoma may still exist since antifactor Xa levels are still detectable at these time points. Patients receiving twice daily high-dose enoxaparin should have the second dose withheld to allow a longer time period prior to catheter placement or removal. Upon removal of catheter, consider withholding enoxaparin for at least 4 hours. **Patient should be observed closely for bleeding and signs and symptoms of neurological impairment if therapy is administered during or immediately following diagnostic lumbar puncture, epidural anesthesia, or spinal anesthesia. If neurological compromise is noted, urgent treatment is necessary.** If spinal hematoma is suspected, diagnose and treat immediately; spinal cord decompression may be considered although it may not prevent or reverse neurological sequelae.

Do not administer intramuscularly. Discontinue use 12 to 24 hours prior to CABG and dose with unfractionated heparin per institutional practice (ACCF/AHA [Anderson, 2013]). Not recommended for thromboprophylaxis in patients with prosthetic heart valves (especially pregnant women). Not to be used interchangeably (unit for unit) with heparin or any other low molecular weight heparins. Monitor patient closely for signs or symptoms of bleeding. Certain patients are at increased risk of bleeding. Risk factors include bacterial endocarditis; congenital or acquired bleeding disorders; active ulcerative or angiodysplastic GI diseases; severe uncontrolled hypertension; hemorrhagic stroke; use shortly after brain, spinal, or ophthalmic surgery; patients treated concomitantly with platelet inhibitors; recent GI bleeding or ulceration; renal dysfunction and hemorrhage; thrombocytopenia or platelet defects or history of heparin-induced thrombocytopenia; severe liver disease; hypertensive or diabetic retinopathy; or in patients undergoing invasive procedures. To minimize risk of bleeding following PCI, achieve hemostasis at the puncture site after PCI. If a closure device is used, sheath can be removed immediately. If manual compression is used, remove sheath 6 hours after the last IV/SubQ dose of enoxaparin. Do not administer further doses until 6 to 8 hours after sheath removal; observe for signs of bleeding/hematoma formation. Cases of enoxaparin-induced thrombocytopenia and thrombosis (similar to heparin-induced thrombocytopenia [HIT]), some complicated by organ infarction, limb ischemia, or death, have been observed. Use with extreme caution or avoid in patients with history of HIT, especially if administered within 100 days of HIT episode (Warkentin, 2001); monitor platelet count closely. Use is contraindicated in patients with thrombocytopenia associated with a positive *in vitro* test for antiplatelet antibodies in the presence of enoxaparin. Discontinue therapy and consider alternative treatment if platelets are <100,000/mm^3 and/or thrombosis develops. Use caution in patients with congenital or drug-induced thrombocytopenia or platelet defects. Risk of bleeding may be increased in women <45 kg and in men <57 kg. Use caution in patients with renal failure; dosage adjustment needed if CrCl <30 mL/minute. Use with caution in the elderly (delayed elimination may occur); dosage alteration/adjustment may be required (eg, omission of IV bolus in acute STEMI in patients ≥75 years of age). Monitor for hyperkalemia; can cause hyperkalemia possibly by suppressing aldosterone production.

Benzyl alcohol and derivatives: Some dosage forms may contain benzyl alcohol and should not be used in pregnant women. In neonates, large amounts of benzyl alcohol (≥99 mg/kg/day) have been associated with a potentially fatal toxicity ("gasping syndrome"); the "gasping syndrome" consists of metabolic acidosis, respiratory distress, gasping respirations, CNS dysfunction (including convulsions, intracranial hemorrhage), hypotension, and cardiovascular collapse (AAP, 1997; CDC, 1982); some data suggests that benzoate displaces bilirubin from protein binding sites (Ahlfors, 2001); avoid or use dosage forms containing benzyl alcohol with caution in neonates. See manufacturer's labeling.

Safety and efficacy of prophylactic dosing of enoxaparin has not been established in patients who are obese (>30 kg/m^2) nor is there a consensus regarding dosage adjustments. The American College of Chest Physicians Practice Guidelines suggest consulting with a pharmacist regarding dosing in bariatric surgery patients and other obese patients who may require higher doses of LMWH (ACCP [Gould, 2012]).

Adverse Reactions As with all anticoagulants, bleeding is the major adverse effect of enoxaparin. Hemorrhage may occur at virtually any site. Risk is dependent on multiple variables. At the recommended doses, single injections of enoxaparin do not significantly influence platelet aggregation or affect global clotting time (ie, PT or aPTT).

Central nervous system: Confusion, pain
Gastrointestinal: Diarrhea, nausea
Hematologic & oncologic: Anemia, bruise, major hemorrhage (includes cases of intracranial, retroperitoneal, or intraocular hemorrhage; incidence varies with indication/population), thrombocytopenia
Hepatic: Increased serum ALT, increased serum AST
Local: Bruising at injection site, erythema at injection site, hematoma at injection site, irritation at injection site, pain at injection site
Renal: Hematuria
Miscellaneous: Fever
Rare but important or life-threatening: Alopecia, anaphylaxis, anaphylactoid reaction, eczematous rash (plaques), eosinophilia, epidural hematoma (spinal; after neuroaxial anesthesia or spinal puncture; risk may be increased with indwelling epidural catheter or concomitant use of other drugs affecting hemostasis), headache, hepatic injury (hepatocellular and cholestatic), hyperkalemia, hyperlipidemia (very rare), hypersensitivity angiitis, hypersensitivity reaction, hypertriglyceridemia, intracranial hemorrhage (up to 0.8%), osteoporosis (following long-term therapy), pruritic erythematous rash (patches), pruritus, purpura, retroperitoneal hemorrhage, severe anemia (hemorrhagic), shock, skin necrosis,

thrombocythemia, thrombocytopenia, thrombosis (prosthetic value [in pregnant females] or associated with enoxaparin-induced thrombocytopenia; can cause limb ischemia or organ infarction), urticaria, vesicobullous rash

Drug Interactions

Metabolism/Transport Effects None known.

Avoid Concomitant Use

Avoid concomitant use of Enoxaparin with any of the following: Apixaban; Dabigatran Etexilate; Edoxaban; Omacetaxine; Rivaroxaban; Urokinase; Vorapaxar

Increased Effect/Toxicity

Enoxaparin may increase the levels/effects of: ACE Inhibitors; Aliskiren; Angiotensin II Receptor Blockers; Anticoagulants; Canagliflozin; Collagenase (Systemic); Deferasirox; Eplerenone; Ibritumomab; Nintedanib; Obinutuzumab; Omacetaxine; Palifermin; Potassium Salts; Potassium-Sparing Diuretics; Rivaroxaban; Tositumomab and Iodine I 131 Tositumomab

The levels/effects of Enoxaparin may be increased by: 5-ASA Derivatives; Agents with Antiplatelet Properties; Apixaban; Dabigatran Etexilate; Dasatinib; Edoxaban; Herbs (Anticoagulant/Antiplatelet Properties); Ibrutinib; Limaprost; Nonsteroidal Anti-Inflammatory Agents; Omega-3 Fatty Acids; Pentosan Polysulfate Sodium; Pentoxifylline; Prostacyclin Analogues; Salicylates; Sugammadex; Thrombolytic Agents; Tibolone; Tipranavir; Urokinase; Vitamin E; Vorapaxar

Decreased Effect

The levels/effects of Enoxaparin may be decreased by: Estrogen Derivatives; Progestins

Storage/Stability Store at 25°C (77°F); excursions permitted to 15°C to 30°C (59°F to 86°F); do not freeze. Do not store multiple-dose vials for >28 days after first use.

Mechanism of Action Standard heparin consists of components with molecular weights ranging from 4000 to 30,000 daltons with a mean of 16,000 daltons. Heparin acts as an anticoagulant by enhancing the inhibition rate of clotting proteases by antithrombin III impairing normal hemostasis and inhibition of factor Xa. Low molecular weight heparins have a small effect on the activated partial thromboplastin time and strongly inhibit factor Xa. Enoxaparin is derived from porcine heparin that undergoes benzylation followed by alkaline depolymerization. The average molecular weight of enoxaparin is 4500 daltons which is distributed as (≤20%) 2000 daltons (≥68%) 2000 to 8000 daltons, and (≤15%) >8000 daltons. Enoxaparin has a higher ratio of antifactor Xa to antifactor IIa activity than unfractionated heparin.

Pharmacodynamics/Kinetics

Onset of action: Peak effect: SubQ: Antifactor Xa and antithrombin (antifactor IIa): 3 to 5 hours

Duration: 40 mg dose: Antifactor Xa activity: ~12 hours

Distribution: 4.3 L (based on antifactor Xa activity)

Protein binding: Does not bind to heparin binding proteins

Metabolism: Hepatic, to lower molecular weight fragments (little activity)

Half-life elimination, plasma: 2 to 4 times longer than standard heparin, independent of dose; based on anti-Xa activity: 4.5 to 7 hours

Excretion: Urine (40% of dose; 10% as active fragments)

Dosage Note: One mg of enoxaparin is equal to 100 units of anti-Xa activity (World Health Organization First International Low Molecular Weight Heparin Reference Standard).

Infants and Children (off-label use; Monagle, 2012): SubQ:

Infants <2 months: Initial:

Prophylaxis: 0.75 mg/kg every 12 hours

Treatment: 1.5 mg/kg every 12 hours

Infants >2 months and Children ≤18 years: Initial:

Prophylaxis: 0.5 mg/kg every 12 hours

Treatment: 1 mg/kg every 12 hours

Maintenance: See **Dosage Titration** table:

Enoxaparin Pediatric Dosage Titration[1]

Anti-Xa Result	Dose Titration	Time to Repeat Anti-Xa Measurement
<0.35 units/mL	Increase dose by 25%	4 h after next dose
0.35-0.49 units/mL	Increase dose by 10%	4 h after next dose
0.5-1 unit/mL	Keep same dosage	Next day, then 1 wk later, then monthly (4 h after dose)
1.1-1.5 units/mL	Decrease dose by 20%	Before next dose
1.6-2 units/mL	Hold dose for 3 h and decrease dose by 30%	Before next dose, then 4 h after next dose
>2 units/mL	Hold all doses until anti-Xa is 0.5 units/mL, then decrease dose by 40%	Before next dose and every 12 h until anti-Xa <0.5 units/mL

[1]Nomogram to be used for treatment dosing.

Modified from Duplaga BA, et al, "Dosing and Monitoring of Low-Molecular-Weight Heparins in Special Populations," *Pharmacotherapy*, 2001, 21(2):218-34.

Adults: Note: Weight-based doses (eg, 1 mg/kg) are commonly rounded to the nearest 10 mg; also see institution-specific rounding protocols if available. Most available prefilled syringes are graduated in 10 mg increments.

DVT prophylaxis: SubQ:

Obesity: **Note:** In morbidly-obese patients (BMI ≥40 kg/m^2), increasing the prophylactic dose by 30% may be appropriate for some indications (Nutescu, 2009). For bariatric surgery, dose increases may be >30% based on clinical trial data.

Abdominal surgery: 40 mg once daily, with initial dose given 2 hours prior to surgery; continue until risk of DVT has diminished (usually 7 to 10 days).

Hip replacement surgery:

Twice-daily dosing: 30 mg every 12 hours, with initial dose within 12 to 24 hours after surgery, and every 12 hours for at least 10 days or until risk of DVT has diminished or the patient is adequately anticoagulated on warfarin. The American College of Chest Physicians recommends initiation ≥12 hours preoperatively **or** ≥12 hours postoperatively; extended duration of up to 35 days suggested (Guyatt, 2012).

Once-daily dosing: 40 mg once daily, with initial dose within 9 to 15 hours before surgery, and daily for at least 10 days (or up to 35 days postoperatively) or until risk of DVT has diminished or the patient is adequately anticoagulated on warfarin. The American College of Chest Physicians recommends initiation ≥12 hours preoperatively **or** ≥12 hours postoperatively; extended duration of up to 35 days suggested (Guyatt, 2012).

Knee replacement surgery: 30 mg every 12 hours, with initial dose within 12 to 24 hours after surgery, and every 12 hours for at least 10 days or until risk of DVT has diminished or the patient is adequately anticoagulated on warfarin. The American College of Chest Physicians recommends initiation ≥12 hours preoperatively **or** ≥12 hours postoperatively; extended duration of up to 35 days suggested (Guyatt, 2012).

Medical patients with severely-restricted mobility during acute illness: 40 mg once daily; continue until risk of DVT has diminished (usually 6 to 11 days).

Bariatric surgery (off-label use): Roux-en-Y gastric bypass: Appropriate dosing strategies have not been clearly defined (Borkgren-Okonek, 2008):

BMI ≤50 kg/m^2: 40 mg every 12 hours

BMI >50 kg/m^2: 60 mg every 12 hours

Note: The 2013 AACE/TOS/ASMBS bariatric surgery guidelines recommend, along with early ambulation, both sequential compression devices and subcutaneous LMWH or unfractionated heparin administered within 24 hours after surgery with consideration of extended prophylaxis for those who are at high risk for VTE (eg, history of DVT) (AACE/TOS/ASMBS [Mechanick, 2013]).

Prevention of recurrent venous thromboembolism in pregnancy (off-label use): 40 mg once daily. Therapy should continue for 6 weeks postpartum in high-risk women (Bates, 2012).

DVT treatment (acute): SubQ: **Note:** Start warfarin on the first or second treatment day and continue enoxaparin until INR is ≥2 for at least 24 hours (usually 5 to 7 days) (Guyatt, 2012).

Inpatient treatment (with or without pulmonary embolism): 1 mg/kg/dose every 12 hours or 1.5 mg/kg once daily.

Outpatient treatment (without pulmonary embolism): 1 mg/kg/dose every 12 hours.

Obesity: Use actual body weight to calculate dose; dose capping not recommended; use of twice daily dosing preferred (Nutescu, 2009).

Pregnant women (off-label use): 1 mg/kg/dose every 12 hours. Discontinue ≥24 hours prior to the induction of labor or cesarean section. Enoxaparin therapy may be substituted with heparin near term. Continue anticoagulation therapy for ≥6 weeks postpartum (minimum duration of therapy: 3 months). LMWH or heparin therapy is preferred over warfarin during pregnancy (Bates, 2012).

Mechanical heart valve (aortic or mitral position) to bridge anticoagulation (off-label use): SubQ: 1 mg/kg every 12 hours (ACCP [Douketis, 2012]). **Note:** If used in pregnant patients, target anti-Xa level of 0.8 to 1.2 units/mL, 4 to 6 hours postdose (AHA/ACC [Nishimura, 2014]).

ST-elevation myocardial infarction (STEMI):

Patients <75 years of age: Initial: 30 mg IV single bolus plus 1 mg/kg (maximum: 100 mg for the first 2 doses only) SubQ every 12 hours. The first SubQ dose should be administered with the IV bolus. Maintenance: After first 2 doses, administer 1 mg/kg SubQ every 12 hours.

Patients ≥75 years of age: Initial: SubQ: 0.75 mg/kg every 12 hours (**Note:** No IV bolus is administered in this population); a maximum dose of 75 mg is recommended for the first 2 doses. Maintenance: After first 2 doses, administer 0.75 mg/kg SubQ every 12 hours

Obesity: Use weight-based dosing; a maximum dose of 100 mg is recommended for the first 2 doses (Nutescu, 2009)

Additional notes on STEMI treatment: Therapy may be continued for up to 8 days or until revascularization. Unless contraindicated, all patients should receive aspirin (indefinitely) and clopidogrel (ACCF/AHA [O'Gara, 2013]). In patients with STEMI receiving thrombolytics, initiate enoxaparin dosing between 15 minutes before and 30 minutes after fibrinolytic therapy.

Unstable angina or non-ST-elevation myocardial infarction (NSTEMI): SubQ: 1 mg/kg every 12 hours in conjunction with oral aspirin therapy; continue for the duration of hospitalization (a minimum of at least 2 days) or up to 8 days (ACCF/AHA [Anderson, 2013])

Obesity: Use actual body weight to calculate dose; dose capping not recommended (Nutescu, 2009)

Percutaneous coronary intervention (PCI), adjunctive therapy (off-label dosing) (ACCF/AHA/SCAI [Levine, 2011]): IV:

If patient undergoing PCI has been treated with multiple doses of enoxaparin and PCI occurs within 8 hours after the last SubQ enoxaparin dose: No additional enoxaparin is needed.

If PCI occurs 8 to 12 hours after the last SubQ enoxaparin dose or the patient received only 1 therapeutic SubQ dose (eg, 1 mg/kg): Administer a single IV dose of 0.3 mg/kg.

If PCI occurs >12 hours after the last SubQ dose: May use an established anticoagulation regimen (eg, full-dose unfractionated heparin or bivalirudin).

If patient has not received prior anticoagulant therapy: 0.5 to 0.75 mg/kg IV bolus dose

Conversion from IV unfractionated heparin (UFH) infusion to SubQ enoxaparin (Nutescu, 2007): Calculate specific dose for enoxaparin based on indication, discontinue UFH and begin enoxaparin within 1 hour.

Conversion from SubQ enoxaparin to IV UFH infusion (Nutescu, 2007): Discontinue enoxaparin, calculate specific dose for IV UFH infusion based on indication, omit heparin bolus/loading dose:

Converting from SubQ enoxaparin dosed every 12 hours: Start IV UFH infusion 10 to 11 hours after last dose of enoxaparin

Converting from SubQ enoxaparin dosed every 24 hours: Start IV UFH infusion 22 to 23 hours after last dose of enoxaparin

Elderly: Refer to adult dosing. Increased incidence of bleeding with doses of 1.5 mg/kg/day or 1 mg/kg every 12 hours; injection-associated bleeding and serious adverse reactions are also increased in the elderly. Careful attention should be paid to elderly patients, particularly those <45 kg. **Note:** Dosage alteration/adjustment may be required.

Dosage adjustment in renal impairment:

CrCl ≥30 mL/minute: No specific adjustment recommended (per manufacturer); monitor closely for bleeding

CrCl <30 mL/minute:

DVT prophylaxis in abdominal surgery, hip replacement, knee replacement, or in medical patients during acute illness: SubQ: 30 mg once daily. **Note:** The Canadian labeling recommends 20 to 30 mg once daily (based on risk/benefit assessment) for prophylaxis in abdominal or colorectal surgery or in medical patients during acute illness.

DVT treatment (inpatient or outpatient treatment in conjunction with warfarin): SubQ: 1 mg/kg once daily

STEMI:

<75 years: Initial: IV: 30 mg as a single dose with the first dose of the SubQ maintenance regimen administered at the same time as the IV bolus; Maintenance: SubQ: 1 mg/kg once daily. **Note:** Canadian labeling recommends a maximum dose of 100 mg for the first SubQ dose.

≥75 years of age: Omit IV bolus; Maintenance: SubQ: 1 mg/kg once daily. **Note:** Canadian labeling recommends a maximum dose of 100 mg for the first SubQ dose.

Unstable angina, NSTEMI: SubQ: 1 mg/kg once daily

Dialysis: Enoxaparin has not been FDA approved for use in dialysis patients. Its elimination is primarily via the renal route. Serious bleeding complications have been reported with use in patients who are dialysis dependent or have severe renal failure. LMWH administration at fixed doses without monitoring has greater unpredictable anticoagulant effects in patients with chronic kidney disease. If used, dosages should be reduced and anti-Xa levels frequently monitored, as accumulation may occur with repeated doses. Many clinicians would not use enoxaparin in this population especially without timely anti-Xa levels.

Hemodialysis: Supplemental dose is not necessary.

Peritoneal dialysis: Significant drug removal is unlikely based on physiochemical characteristics.

Dosage adjustment in hepatic impairment: There are no dosage adjustments provided in the manufacturer's labeling (has not been studied); use with caution.

Administration Note: Enoxaparin is available in 100 mg/mL and 150 mg/mL concentrations.

SubQ: Administer by deep SubQ injection alternating between the left or right anterolateral and left or right posterolateral abdominal wall. Do not mix with other infusions or injections. In order to minimize bruising, do not rub injection site. To avoid loss of drug from the 30 mg and 40 mg prefilled syringes, do not expel the air bubble from the syringe prior to injection.

IV: STEMI and PCI only: The U.S. labeling recommends using the multiple-dose vial to prepare IV doses. The Canadian labeling recommends either the multiple-dose vial or a prefilled syringe. Do not mix or coadminister with other medications; may be administered with NS or D_5W. Flush IV access site with a sufficient amount of NS or D_5W prior to and following IV bolus administration. When used prior to percutaneous coronary intervention or as part of treatment for ST-elevation myocardial infarction (STEMI), a single dose may be administered IV except when the patient is ≥75 years of age and is experiencing STEMI then only administer by SubQ injection.

Monitoring Parameters Platelets, occult blood, anti-Xa levels, serum creatinine; monitoring of PT and/or aPTT is not necessary. Routine monitoring of anti-Xa levels is not required, but has been utilized in patients with obesity and/ or renal insufficiency. Monitoring anti-Xa levels is recommended in pregnant women receiving therapeutic doses of enoxaparin or when receiving enoxaparin for the prevention of thromboembolism with mechanical heart valves (Guyatt, 2012). For patients >190 kg, if anti-Xa monitoring is available, adjusting dose based on anti-Xa levels is recommended; if anti-Xa monitoring is unavailable, reduce dose if bleeding occurs (Nutescu, 2009). Monitor obese patients closely for signs/symptoms of thromboembolism.

Reference Range The following therapeutic ranges for anti-Xa levels have been suggested, but have not been validated in a controlled trial. Anti-Xa level measured 4 hours postdose.

Treatment of venous thromboembolism: Anti-Xa concentration target (Garcia, 2012):

Once-daily dosing: >1 anti-Xa units/mL; the manufacturer recommends a range of 1 to 2 anti-Xa units/mL

Twice-daily dosing: 0.6 to 1 anti-Xa units/mL

Recurrent VTE prophylaxis in pregnant women: Peak anti-Xa concentrations: 0.2 to 0.6 units/mL (Bates, 2012)

Additional Information Neutralization of enoxaparin (in overdose) with protamine 1% solution: Manufacturer's recommendations:

Enoxaparin administered in ≤8 hours: Dose of protamine should equal the dose of enoxaparin administered. Therefore, 1 mg of protamine sulfate neutralizes 1 mg of enoxaparin

Enoxaparin administered in >8 hours or if it has been determined that a second dose is required (eg, if aPTT measured 2-4 hours after the first dose remains prolonged or if bleeding continues): 0.5 mg of protamine sulfate for every 1 mg of enoxaparin administered

Dosage Forms

Solution, Injection:

Lovenox: 300 mg/3 mL (3 mL)

Generic: 300 mg/3 mL (3 mL)

Solution, Subcutaneous:

Lovenox: 30 mg/0.3 mL (0.3 mL); 40 mg/0.4 mL (0.4 mL); 60 mg/0.6 mL (0.6 mL); 80 mg/0.8 mL (0.8 mL); 100 mg/mL (1 mL); 120 mg/0.8 mL (0.8 mL); 150 mg/mL (1 mL)

Generic: 30 mg/0.3 mL (0.3 mL); 40 mg/0.4 mL (0.4 mL); 60 mg/0.6 mL (0.6 mL); 80 mg/0.8 mL (0.8 mL); 100 mg/mL (1 mL); 120 mg/0.8 mL (0.8 mL); 150 mg/mL (1 mL)

Solution, Subcutaneous [preservative free]:

Lovenox: 30 mg/0.3 mL (0.3 mL); 40 mg/0.4 mL (0.4 mL); 60 mg/0.6 mL (0.6 mL); 80 mg/0.8 mL (0.8 mL); 100 mg/mL (1 mL); 120 mg/0.8 mL (0.8 mL); 150 mg/mL (1 mL)

Generic: 30 mg/0.3 mL (0.3 mL); 40 mg/0.4 mL (0.4 mL); 60 mg/0.6 mL (0.6 mL); 80 mg/0.8 mL (0.8 mL); 100 mg/mL (1 mL); 120 mg/0.8 mL (0.8 mL); 150 mg/mL (1 mL)

◆ **Enoxaparin Sodium** *see* Enoxaparin *on page 726*

Enoximone [INT] (EN oks i mone)

International Brand Names Cardomel (ES); Perfan (BE, DE, GB, IE, IT, NL); Perfane (FR, IT, LU)

Pharmacologic Category Phosphodiesterase Enzyme Inhibitor

Reported Use Treatment of congestive heart failure

Dosage Range Adults:

Slow IV infusion:

Initial: 0.5-1 mg/kg, then 500 mcg/kg every 30 minutes until satisfactory response or total of 3 mg/kg given

Maintenance: Initial dose of up to 3 mg/kg may be repeated every 3-6 hours as needed

IV infusion: Initial: 90 mcg/kg/minute over 10-30 minutes, followed by continuous or intermittent infusion of 5-20 mcg/kg/minute; maximum dose: 24 mg/kg/24 hours

Product Availability Product available in various countries; not currently available in the U.S.

Dosage Forms

Injection, solution: 5 mg/mL (20 mL)

◆ **Enpresse** *see* Ethinyl Estradiol and Levonorgestrel *on page 803*

◆ **Enskyce** *see* Ethinyl Estradiol and Desogestrel *on page 799*

Entacapone (en TA ka pone)

Brand Names: U.S. Comtan

Brand Names: Canada Comtan; Mylan-Entacapone; Sandoz-Entacapone; Teva-Entacapone

Pharmacologic Category Anti-Parkinson's Agent, COMT Inhibitor

Use Parkinson disease: Adjunct to levodopa/carbidopa therapy in patients with idiopathic Parkinson disease who experience "wearing-off" symptoms at the end of a dosing interval

Pregnancy Risk Factor C

Dosage Parkinson disease: Adults: Oral: 200 mg with each dose of levodopa/carbidopa, up to a maximum of 8 times daily (maximum daily dose: 1600 mg daily).

Note: To optimize therapy, the dosage of levodopa may need to be reduced or the dosing interval may need to be extended. Patients taking levodopa ≥800 mg daily or who had moderate-to-severe dyskinesias prior to therapy required an average decrease of 25% in the daily levodopa dose.

Dosage adjustment in renal impairment: There are no dosage adjustments provided in the manufacturer's labeling; however, renal function was not found to significantly affect the pharmacokinetics of entacapone.

Dosage adjustment in hepatic impairment:

U.S. labeling: There are no dosage adjustments provided in the manufacturer's labeling. Treat with caution and monitor carefully; AUC and C_{max} may possibly be doubled.

Canadian labeling: Use is contraindicated.

Additional Information Complete prescribing information should be consulted for additional detail.

Dosage Forms

Tablet, Oral:

Comtan: 200 mg

Generic: 200 mg

◆ **Entacapone, Carbidopa, and Levodopa** *see* Levodopa, Carbidopa, and Entacapone *on page 1196*

Entecavir (en TE ka veer)

Brand Names: U.S. Baraclude

Brand Names: Canada Apo-Entecavir; Baraclude; PMS-Entecavir

Pharmacologic Category Antihepadnaviral, Reverse Transcriptase Inhibitor, Nucleoside (Anti-HBV)

Use

U.S. labeling: Treatment of chronic hepatitis B virus (HBV) infection in adults and pediatric patients 2 years and older with evidence of active viral replication and either evidence of persistent transaminase elevations or histologically-active disease. **Note:** In adults, indication is based on data in patients with compensated and decompensated liver disease; in children, indication is based on data in patients with compensated liver disease.

Canadian labeling: Treatment of chronic hepatitis B virus (HBV) infection in adults with compensated liver disease and evidence of active viral replication and either evidence of persistent transaminase elevations or histologically-active disease.

Pregnancy Risk Factor C

Pregnancy Considerations Teratogenic effects have been observed in animal studies. Information related to use in pregnancy is limited; use only if other options are inappropriate (DHHS [OI], 2013). Pregnant women taking entecavir should enroll in the pregnancy registry by calling 1-800-258-4263.

Breast-Feeding Considerations It is not known if entecavir is excreted in breast milk. Due to the potential for serious adverse reactions in the nursing infant, the manufacturer recommends a decision be made whether to discontinue nursing or to discontinue the drug, taking into account the importance of treatment to the mother.

Contraindications There are no contraindications listed in the manufacturer's U.S. labeling.

Canadian labeling: Hypersensitivity to entecavir or any component of the formulation

Warnings/Precautions Hazardous agent - use appropriate precautions for handling and disposal (NIOSH 2014 [group 2]).

[U.S. Boxed Warning]: Lactic acidosis and severe hepatomegaly with steatosis (including fatal cases) have been reported with nucleoside analogue inhibitors; use with caution in patients with risk factors for liver disease (risk may be increased with female gender, decompensated liver disease, obesity, or prolonged nucleoside inhibitor exposure) and suspend treatment in any patient who develops clinical or laboratory findings suggestive of lactic acidosis or hepatotoxicity (transaminase elevation may/may not accompany hepatomegaly and steatosis)

[U.S. Boxed Warning]: Severe, acute exacerbation of hepatitis B may occur upon discontinuation of antihepatitis B therapy, including entecavir. Monitor liver function for at least several months after stopping treatment; reinitiation of antihepatitis B therapy may be required. Use caution in patients with renal impairment or in patients receiving concomitant therapy which may reduce renal function; dose adjustment recommended for CrCl <50 mL/minute. Cross-resistance may develop in patients failing previous therapy with lamivudine. There are limited data available on the use of entecavir in lamivudine-experienced pediatric patients; use in these patients only if the potential benefit justifies the potential risk to the child.

HIV: **[U.S. Boxed Warning]: May cause the development of HIV resistance in chronic hepatitis B patients with unrecognized or untreated HIV infection.** Determine HIV status prior to initiating treatment with entecavir. **Not recommended for HIV/HBV coinfected patients unless also receiving highly active antiretroviral therapy (HAART).** The manufacturer's labeling states that entecavir does not exhibit any clinically-relevant activity against human immunodeficiency virus (HIV type 1). However, a small number of case reports have indicated declines in virus levels during entecavir therapy. HIV resistance to a common HIV drug has been reported in an HIV/HBV-infected patient receiving entecavir as monotherapy for HBV.

Dose adjustment not required in patients with hepatic impairment. Limited data supporting treatment of chronic hepatitis B in patients with decompensated liver disease; observe for increased adverse reactions, including hepatorenal dysfunction.

Some dosage forms may contain polysorbate 80 (also known as Tweens). Hypersensitivity reactions, usually a delayed reaction, have been reported following exposure to pharmaceutical products containing polysorbate 80 in certain individuals (Isaksson, 2002; Lucente 2000; Shelley, 1995). Thrombocytopenia, ascites, pulmonary deterioration, and renal and hepatic failure have been reported in premature neonates after receiving parenteral products containing polysorbate 80 (Alade, 1986; CDC, 1984). See manufacturer's labeling.

Adverse Reactions Adverse reactions are generally similar in adult and pediatric patients.

Cardiovascular: Peripheral edema (with decompensated liver disease)

Central nervous system: Dizziness, fatigue, headache

Dermatologic: Skin rash

Endocrine & metabolic: Decreased serum bicarbonate (with decompensated liver disease), glycosuria, hyperglycemia

Gastrointestinal: Abdominal pain, diarrhea, dyspepsia, increased serum amylase, increased serum lipase, nausea, unpleasant taste, vomiting

Genitourinary: Hematuria

Hepatic: Ascites (with decompensated liver disease), increased serum ALT, increased serum bilirubin, hepatic encephalopathy

Hematologic & oncologic: Hepatic carcinoma (with decompensated liver disease)

Renal: Increased serum creatinine

Respiratory: Upper respiratory tract infection (with decompensated liver disease)

Miscellaneous: Fever (with decompensated liver disease)

Rare but important or life-threatening: Alopecia, anaphylactoid reaction, hepatomegaly, insomnia, lactic acidosis, macular edema (Muqit, 2011), renal failure, thrombocytopenia

Drug Interactions

Metabolism/Transport Effects None known.

Avoid Concomitant Use There are no known interactions where it is recommended to avoid concomitant use.

Increased Effect/Toxicity

The levels/effects of Entecavir may be increased by: Ganciclovir-Valganciclovir; Ribavirin

Decreased Effect There are no known significant interactions involving a decrease in effect.

Food Interactions Food delays absorption and reduces AUC by 18% to 20%. Management: Administer on an empty stomach 2 hours before or after a meal.

Storage/Stability Store at 25°C (77°F); excursions permitted to 15°C to 30°C (59°F to 86°F). Protect from light. After opening, oral solution can be used up to expiration date on the bottle.

Mechanism of Action Entecavir is intracellularly phosphorylated to guanosine triphosphate which competes with natural substrates to effectively inhibit hepatitis B viral polymerase; enzyme inhibition blocks reverse transcriptase activity thereby reducing viral DNA synthesis.

Pharmacodynamics/Kinetics

Absorption: Delayed with food; C_{max} decreased 44% to 46%, AUC decreased 18% to 20%

Distribution: Extensive (V_d in excess of body water)

Protein binding: ~13%

Metabolism: Minor hepatic glucuronide/sulfate conjugation

Half-life elimination: Terminal: ~5-6 days; accumulation: ~24 hours

Time to peak, plasma: 0.5-1.5 hours

Excretion: Urine (60% to 73% as unchanged drug)

Dosage

Hepatitis B virus (HBV) infection, treatment: Oral:

U.S. labeling:

Children ≥2 years and Adolescents: **Note:** Oral solution should be used for patients weighing ≤30 kg.

Treatment-naive:
- 10 to 11 kg: 0.15 mg once daily (oral solution)
- >11 to 14 kg: 0.2 mg once daily (oral solution)
- >14 to 17 kg: 0.25 mg once daily (oral solution)
- >17 to 20 kg: 0.3 mg once daily (oral solution)
- >20 to 23 kg: 0.35 mg once daily (oral solution)
- >23 to 26 kg: 0.4 mg once daily (oral solution)
- >26 to 30 kg: 0.45 mg once daily (oral solution)
- >30 kg: 0.5 mg once daily (oral solution or tablet)

Lamivudine-experienced:
- 10 to 11 kg: 0.3 mg once daily (oral solution)
- >11 to 14 kg: 0.4 mg once daily (oral solution)
- >14 to 17 kg: 0.5 mg once daily (oral solution)
- >17 to 20 kg: 0.6 mg once daily (oral solution)
- >20 to 23 kg: 0.7 mg once daily (oral solution)
- >23 to 26 kg: 0.8 mg once daily (oral solution)
- >26 to 30 kg: 0.9 mg once daily (oral solution)
- >30 kg: 1 mg once daily (oral solution or tablet)

Adults:

Nucleoside treatment-naive: 0.5 mg once daily

Lamivudine-refractory or -resistant viremia (or known lamivudine- or telbivudine-resistance mutations): 1 mg once daily

Decompensated liver disease: 1 mg once daily

Canadian labeling: Adolescents ≥16 years and Adults:

Nucleoside treatment-naive: 0.5 mg once daily

Lamivudine-refractory or known lamivudine-resistance mutations: 1 mg once daily

HBV reinfection prophylaxis, post liver transplant (with or without HBIG) (off-label use): Adults: Oral: 0.5 mg once daily (Fung, 2011) or 1 mg once daily (Perrillo, 2012)

HIV/HBV coinfection (off-label use): Adults: Oral:

Nucleoside treatment naive: 0.5 mg once daily

Lamivudine refractory or resistant: 1 mg once daily

Note: Only recommended in patients who cannot take tenofovir; must be used in addition to a fully suppressive antiretroviral therapy regimen (DHHS, 2013).

Treatment duration (AASLD Practice Guidelines, 2009):

Hepatitis Be antigen (HBeAg) positive chronic hepatitis: Treat ≥1 year until HBeAg seroconversion and undetectable serum HBV DNA; continue therapy for ≥6 months after HBeAg seroconversion

HBeAg negative chronic hepatitis: Treat >1 year until hepatitis B surface antigen (HBsAg) clearance

Decompensated liver disease: Lifelong treatment is recommended

Note: Patients not achieving a primary response (<2 log decrease in serum HBV DNA) after at least 6 months of therapy should either receive additional treatment or be switched to an alternative therapy.

Dosage adjustment in renal impairment:

Children >2 years and Adolescents: Insufficient data to recommend a specific dose adjustment in pediatric patients with renal impairment; consider a reduction in the dose or an increase in the dosing interval similar to adjustments for adults.

Adults (Canadian labeling: Adolescents ≥16 years and Adults): Daily-dosage regimen preferred:
- CrCl ≥50 mL/minute: No dosage adjustment necessary.
- CrCl 30-49 mL/minute: Administer 50% of usual dose daily or administer the normal dose every 48 hours
- CrCl 10-29 mL/minute: Administer 30% of usual dose daily or administer the normal dose every 72 hours
- CrCl <10 mL/minute (including hemodialysis and CAPD): Administer 10% of usual dose daily or administer the normal dose every 7 days; administer after hemodialysis

Dosage adjustment in hepatic impairment:

Children >2 years and Adolescents: There are no dosage adjustments provided in the manufacturer's labeling (has not been studied).

Adults (Canadian labeling: Adolescents ≥16 years and Adults): No dosage adjustment necessary.

Dietary Considerations Take on an empty stomach (2 hours before or after a meal).

Administration Administer on an empty stomach (2 hours before or after a meal). Do not dilute or mix oral solution with water or other beverages; use calibrated oral dosing syringe. Oral solution and tablet are bioequivalent on a mg-to-mg basis.

Hazardous agent - use appropriate precautions for handling and disposal (NIOSH 2014 [group 2]).

Monitoring Parameters HIV status (prior to initiation of therapy); liver function tests, renal function; in HBV/HIV-coinfected patients, monitor HIV viral load and CD4 count; HBeAg, HBV DNA; in patients with lamivudine-refractory or -resistant viremia (or known lamivudine- or telbivudine-resistance mutations) entecavir resistance can develop rapidly. Monitor HBV DNA every 3 months (DHHS, 2013)

Dosage Forms

Solution, Oral:

Baraclude: 0.05 mg/mL (210 mL)

Tablet, Oral:

Baraclude: 0.5 mg, 1 mg

Generic: 0.5 mg, 1 mg

- ◆ **Entereg** *see* Alvimopan *on page* 104
- ◆ **Enterotoxigenic *Escherichia coli* and *Vibrio cholera* Vaccine** *see* Travelers' Diarrhea and Cholera Vaccine [CAN/INT] *on page* 2088
- ◆ **Entex® LA (Can)** *see* Guaifenesin and Pseudoephedrine *on page* 989
- ◆ **Entex PAC [OTC]** *see* Guaifenesin, Pseudoephedrine, and Dextromethorphan *on page* 989
- ◆ **Entocort (Can)** *see* Budesonide (Systemic) *on page* 293
- ◆ **Entocort EC** *see* Budesonide (Systemic) *on page* 293

- ◆ **Entre-Cough [OTC]** *see* Guaifenesin, Pseudoephedrine, and Dextromethorphan *on page 989*
- ◆ **Entre-Hist PSE** *see* Triprolidine and Pseudoephedrine *on page 2105*
- ◆ **Entrophen (Can)** *see* Aspirin *on page 180*
- ◆ **Entsol [OTC]** *see* Sodium Chloride *on page 1902*
- ◆ **Entsol Nasal [OTC]** *see* Sodium Chloride *on page 1902*
- ◆ **Entsol Nasal Wash [OTC]** *see* Sodium Chloride *on page 1902*
- ◆ **Entyvio** *see* Vedolizumab *on page 2146*
- ◆ **Enulose** *see* Lactulose *on page 1156*

Enzalutamide (en za LOO ta mide)

Brand Names: U.S. Xtandi

Brand Names: Canada Xtandi

Index Terms MDV3100

Pharmacologic Category Antineoplastic Agent, Antiandrogen

Use Prostate cancer: Treatment of metastatic, castration-resistant prostate cancer

Pregnancy Risk Factor X

Pregnancy Considerations Adverse effects were observed in animal reproduction studies. Enzalutamide is an androgen receptor inhibitor and would be expected to cause fetal harm based on its mechanism of action. Enzalutamide is not indicated for use in women and is specifically contraindicated for use in women who are or may become pregnant. Men using this medication should use a condom if having intercourse with a pregnant woman. A condom plus another effective method of birth control is recommended during therapy and for 3 months after treatment for men using this medication and who are having intercourse with a woman of reproductive potential.

Breast-Feeding Considerations Enzalutamide is not indicated for use in women.

Contraindications Women who are or may become pregnant

Canadian labeling: Additional contraindications (not in U.S. labeling): Hypersensitivity to enzalutamide or any component of the formulation; women who are lactating

Warnings/Precautions Hazardous agent - use appropriate precautions for handling and disposal (meets NIOSH 2014 criteria). Seizures were observed in clinical trials (onset: ~1-20 months after treatment initiation). Therapy was permanently discontinued and patients were not rechallenged; seizures resolved upon therapy cessation. Patients with predisposing factors for seizure were excluded from the trials; factors include seizure history, underlying brain injury with loss of consciousness, transient ischemic attack within the past 12 months, cerebral vascular accident, brain metastases, brain arteriovenous malformation, or (in one study) the use of concomitant medications which may lower the seizure threshold. Enzalutamide should be used with caution in patients with a history of seizure disorders or other predisposing factors. Discontinue permanently if seizures develop during treatment. Enzalutamide may cause hypospermatogenesis and may impair male fertility. Androgen-deprivation therapy may increase the risk of cardiovascular disease (Levine, 2010). An increase in systolic and diastolic blood pressures has been observed (Scher, 2012); may worsen preexisting hypertension.

Potentially significant drug-drug interactions may exist, requiring dose or frequency adjustment, additional monitoring, and/or selection of alternative therapy. May contain sorbitol; Canadian product labeling recommends avoiding use in patients with fructose intolerance.

Adverse Reactions

Cardiovascular: Hypertension, peripheral edema

Central nervous system: Altered mental status, anxiety, cauda equina syndrome, dizziness, falling, fatigue, hallucination, headache, hypoesthesia, insomnia, myasthenia, paresthesia, restless leg syndrome, spinal cord compression

Dermatologic: Pruritus, xeroderma

Endocrine & metabolic: Gynecomastia, hot flash, weight loss

Gastrointestinal: Constipation, decreased appetite, diarrhea, dysgeusia

Genitourinary: Hematuria, pollakiuria

Hematologic & oncologic: Neutropenia, thrombocytopenia

Hepatic: Increased serum bilirubin

Infection: Infection (including sepsis)

Neuromuscular & skeletal: Arthralgia, back pain, bone fracture, musculoskeletal pain, stiffness, weakness

Respiratory: Dyspnea, epistaxis, lower respiratory tract infection, upper respiratory tract infection

Rare but important or life-threatening: Seizure

Drug Interactions

Metabolism/Transport Effects Substrate of CYP2C8 (major), CYP3A4 (major); **Note:** Assignment of Major/Minor substrate status based on clinically relevant drug interaction potential; **Inhibits** P-glycoprotein; **Induces** CYP2C19 (moderate), CYP2C9 (moderate), CYP3A4 (strong)

Avoid Concomitant Use

Avoid concomitant use of Enzalutamide with any of the following: Abiraterone Acetate; Alfentanil; Apixaban; Apremilast; Artemether; Axitinib; Bedaquiline; Boceprevir; Bortezomib; Bosutinib; Cabozantinib; Ceritinib; CloZAPine; Crizotinib; CycloSPORINE (Systemic); CYP2C8 Inducers (Strong); CYP2C8 Inhibitors (Strong); CYP3A4 Inducers (Moderate); CYP3A4 Inducers (Strong); Dasabuvir; Dienogest; Dihydroergotamine; Dronedarone; Eliglustat; Ergotamine; Everolimus; FentaNYL; Fosphenytoin-Phenytoin; Ibrutinib; Idelalisib; Indium 111 Capromab Pendetide; Irinotecan; Itraconazole; Ivacaftor; Lapatinib; Lumefantrine; Lurasidone; Macitentan; Mifepristone; Naloxegol; Netupitant; NIFEdipine; Nilotinib; Nisoldipine; Olaparib; Ombitasvir; Paritaprevir; PAZOPanib; Perampanel; Pimozide; PONATinib; Praziquantel; QuiNIDine; Ranolazine; Regorafenib; Rivaroxaban; Roflumilast; RomiDEPsin; Simeprevir; Sirolimus; SORAfenib; St Johns Wort; Suvorexant; Tacrolimus (Systemic); Tasimelteon; Telaprevir; Ticagrelor; Tofacitinib; Tolvaptan; Toremifene; Trabectedin; Ulipristal; Vandetanib; Vemurafenib; VinCRIStine (Liposomal); Vorapaxar; Warfarin

Increased Effect/Toxicity

Enzalutamide may increase the levels/effects of: Clarithromycin; Ifosfamide

The levels/effects of Enzalutamide may be increased by: Clarithromycin; CYP2C8 Inhibitors (Moderate); CYP2C8 Inhibitors (Strong); CYP3A4 Inhibitors (Strong); Deferasirox

Decreased Effect

Enzalutamide may decrease the levels/effects of: Abiraterone Acetate; Alfentanil; Apixaban; Apremilast; ARIPiprazole; Artemether; Axitinib; Bedaquiline; Boceprevir; Bortezomib; Bosutinib; Brentuximab Vedotin; Cabozantinib; Cannabidiol; Cannabis; Ceritinib; Clarithromycin; CloZAPine; Crizotinib; CycloSPORINE (Systemic); CYP3A4 Substrates; Dasabuvir; Dasatinib; Dienogest; Dihydroergotamine; DOXOrubicin (Conventional); Dronabinol; Dronedarone; Eliglustat; Ergotamine; Erlotinib; Everolimus; Exemestane; FentaNYL; Fosphenytoin-Phenytoin; Gefitinib; GuanFACINE; Hydrocodone; Ibrutinib; Idelalisib; Ifosfamide; Imatinib; Indium 111 Capromab Pendetide; Irinotecan; Itraconazole; Ivacaftor; Ixabepilone; Lapatinib; Linagliptin; Lumefantrine; Lurasidone;

Macitentan; Maraviroc; Mifepristone; Naloxegol; Netupitant; NIFEdipine; Nilotinib; Nisoldipine; Olaparib; Ombitasvir; Paritaprevir; PAZOPanib; Perampanel; Pimozide; PONATinib; Praziquantel; QUEtiapine; QuiNIDine; Ranolazine; Regorafenib; Rivaroxaban; Roflumilast; RomiDEPsin; Saxagliptin; Simeprevir; Sirolimus; SORAfenib; SUNItinib; Suvorexant; Tacrolimus (Systemic); Tadalafil; Tasimelteon; Telaprevir; Tetrahydrocannabinol; Ticagrelor; Tofacitinib; Tolvaptan; Toremifene; Trabectedin; Ulipristal; Vandetanib; Vemurafenib; Vilazodone; VinCRIStine (Liposomal); Vorapaxar; Vortioxetine; Warfarin; Zuclopenthixol

The levels/effects of Enzalutamide may be decreased by: CYP2C8 Inducers (Strong); CYP3A4 Inducers (Moderate); CYP3A4 Inducers (Strong); Deferasirox; Siltuximab; St Johns Wort; Tocilizumab

Storage/Stability Store at 20°C to 25°C (68°F to 77°F); excursions permitted to 15°C to 30°C (59°F to 86°F). Protect from moisture; keep bottle tightly closed.

Mechanism of Action Enzalutamide is a pure androgen receptor signaling inhibitor; unlike other antiandrogen therapies, it has no known agonistic properties. It inhibits androgen receptor nuclear translocation, DNA binding, and coactivator mobilization, leading to cellular apoptosis and decreased prostate tumor volume.

Pharmacodynamics/Kinetics

Absorption: Rapid

Distribution: 110 L

Protein binding: Parent drug: 97% to 98% to primarily albumin; active metabolite: 95% to plasma proteins

Metabolism: Primarily hepatic via CYP2C8 (responsible for formation of active metabolite N-desmethyl enzalutamide) and CYP3A4

Half-life elimination: 5.8 days (range: 2.8 to 10.2 days)

Time to peak: 1 hour (range: 0.5 to 3 hours)

Excretion: Urine (71%); feces (14%); primarily as inactive metabolite

Dosage Prostate cancer, metastatic, castration-resistant: Adults: Oral: 160 mg once daily

Dosage adjustment for concomitant strong CYP2C8 inhibitors: Avoid concomitant use if possible. If coadministration is necessary, reduce enzalutamide dose to 80 mg once daily. If the strong CYP2C8 inhibitor is discontinued, adjust the enzalutamide dose back up to the dose used prior to the initiation of the strong CYP2C8 inhibitor.

Dosage adjustment for toxicity: If ≥ grade 3 toxicity or intolerable side effects occur, withhold treatment for 1 week or until symptom(s) improve to ≤ grade 2, then resume at same dose, or reduce dose to 120 mg or 80 mg once daily, if necessary.

Seizures: Permanently discontinue treatment.

Dosage adjustment in renal impairment:

Preexisting mild-to-moderate impairment (CrCl 30 to 89 mL/minute): No initial dosage adjustment necessary.

Preexisting severe impairment (CrCl <30 mL/minute), including end-stage renal disease: There are no dosage adjustments provided in the manufacturer's labeling (has not been studied).

Dosage adjustment in hepatic impairment:

Preexisting mild to moderate impairment (Child-Pugh class A or B): No dosage adjustment necessary.

Preexisting severe impairment (Child-Pugh class C): There are no dosage adjustments provided in the manufacturer's U.S. labeling (has not been studied). Canadian labeling recommends to avoid use in severe impairment.

Administration May be administered with or without food; take at the same time each day. Swallow capsules whole; do not chew, dissolve, or open the capsules. Hazardous agent; use appropriate precautions for handling and disposal (meets NIOSH 2014 criteria).

Monitoring Parameters Monitor for signs/symptoms of seizure, loss of consciousness, dizziness, and hallucinations; CBC with differential and liver function tests (baseline and periodic); additional INR monitoring (if on warfarin); blood pressure (baseline and periodic)

Dosage Forms

Capsule, Oral:

Xtandi: 40 mg

◆ **Epaned** *see* Enalapril *on page 722*

◆ **EPEG** *see* Etoposide *on page 816*

EPHEDrine (Systemic) (e FED rin)

Index Terms Ephedrine Sulfate

Pharmacologic Category Alpha/Beta Agonist

Use Treatment of anesthesia-induced hypotension

Note: The use of ephedrine for the treatment of acute bronchospasm, Stokes-Adams syndrome (ie, presyncope/syncope) with complete heart block, narcolepsy, or depression has fallen out of favor given the availability of more effective agents for these conditions.

Pregnancy Risk Factor C

Dosage

Infants, Children, and Adolescents ≤15 years: Hypotension induced by anesthesia (off-label dose): IV: 0.1 to 0.2 mg/kg/dose slow IV push; administer as needed to maintain blood pressure; maximum: 25 mg (Taguchi, 1996)

Adolescents >15 years and Adults:

Hypotension induced by anesthesia: IV: 5 to 25 mg/dose slow IV push repeated after 5 to 10 minutes as needed to maintain blood pressure

Idiopathic orthostatic hypotension (off-label use): Oral: 25 to 50 mg 3 times daily; maximum: 150 mg daily. **Note:** Not considered first-line for this indication.

Postoperative nausea and vomiting (PONV) refractory to traditional antiemetics (off-label use): IM: 0.5 mg/kg at the end of surgery (Gan, 2007; Hagemann, 2000)

Additional Information Complete prescribing information should be consulted for additional detail.

Dosage Forms

Solution, Injection:

Generic: 50 mg/mL (1 mL)

Solution, Injection [preservative free]:

Generic: 50 mg/mL (1 mL)

Ephedrine and Theophylline [INT]

(e FED rin & thee OFF i lin)

International Brand Names Asmadex (ID); Asmano (ID); Asmasolon (ID); Asthma (MY); Asthma Soho (ID); Franol (BR); Multimix (IN); Tedral (CO); Theocodil (ID)

Index Terms Theophylline and Ephedrine

Pharmacologic Category Theophylline Derivative

Reported Use Symptomatic relief of chronic bronchial asthma, asthmatic bronchitis, and other bronchospastic disorders; prophylactically use to stop or decrease asthmatic attacks

Dosage Range Oral:

Children: 1/2-1 regular-release tablet (containing ephedrine 24 mg and theophylline 130 mg) 4 times/day or at first sign of an asthma attack

Adults: 1-2 regular-release tablets (containing ephedrine 24 mg and theophylline 130 mg) 4 times/day or at first sign of an asthma attack

Product Availability Product available in various countries; not currently available in the U.S.

Dosage Forms

Tablet (Tedral®): Ephedrine hydrochloride 24 mg and theophylline monohydrate 130 mg

Tablet, sustained action (Tedral® SA): Ephedrine hydrochloride 48 mg and theophylline monohydrate 198 mg

◆ **Ephedrine Sulfate** *see* EPHEDrine (Systemic) *on page 734*

◆ **E-Pherol [OTC]** *see* Vitamin E *on page 2174*

◆ **Epidoxorubicin** *see* Epirubicin *on page 739*

◆ **Epiduo®** *see* Adapalene and Benzoyl Peroxide *on page 54*

◆ **Epifoam®** *see* Pramoxine and Hydrocortisone *on page 1698*

EPINEPHrine (Systemic, Oral Inhalation)

(ep i NEF rin)

Brand Names: U.S. Adrenaclick; Adrenalin; Asthmanefrin Refill [OTC]; Asthmanefrin Starter Kit [OTC]; Auvi-Q; EpiPen 2-Pak; EpiPen Jr 2-Pak; Micronefrin [OTC] [DSC]; S2 [OTC]

Brand Names: Canada Adrenalin; Allerject; Anapen; Anapen Junior; EpiPen; EpiPen Jr; S2; Twinject

Index Terms Adrenaline; Adrenaline Bitartrate; Adrenaline Hydrochloride; Epinephrine Bitartrate; Epinephrine Hydrochloride; Racemic Epinephrine; Racepinephrine

Pharmacologic Category Alpha/Beta Agonist

Use

Hypersensitivity: Treatment of type I allergic reactions including anaphylactic reactions

Hypotension/shock: Treatment of hypotension associated with septic shock (increase mean arterial blood pressure)

Mydriasis during intraocular surgery: Induction and maintenance of mydriasis during intraocular surgery

OTC labeling: Treatment of bronchospasm associated with bronchial asthma

Pregnancy Risk Factor C

Pregnancy Considerations Teratogenic effects have been observed in animal reproduction studies. Epinephrine crosses the placenta and may cause fetal anoxia. Use during pregnancy when the potential benefit to the mother outweighs the possible risk to the fetus.

Breast-Feeding Considerations It is not known if epinephrine is excreted in breast milk. The manufacturer recommends that caution be exercised when administering epinephrine to nursing women.

Contraindications

There are no absolute contraindications to the use of injectable epinephrine (including Adrenaclick, Auvi-Q, EpiPen, EpiPen Jr, Allerject [Canadian product], and Twinject [Canadian product]) in a life-threatening situation. Some products include the following contraindications: Hypersensitivity to sympathomimetic amines; general anesthesia with halogenated hydrocarbons (eg, halothane) or cyclopropane; narrow angle glaucoma; nonanaphylactic shock; in combination with local anesthesia of certain areas such as fingers, toes, and ears; use in situations where vasopressors may be contraindicated (eg, thyrotoxicosis, diabetes, in obstetrics when maternal blood pressure is in excess of 130/80 mm Hg and in hypertension and other cardiovascular disorders)

Injectable solution (Adrenalin, Epinephrine injection, USP): There are no contraindications listed in the manufacturer's labeling.

Oral inhalation (OTC labeling): Concurrent use or within 2 weeks of MAO inhibitors

Warnings/Precautions Use with caution in elderly patients, patients with diabetes mellitus, cardiovascular diseases (eg, coronary artery disease, hypertension), thyroid disease, cerebrovascular disease, in patients with prostate enlargement or urinary retention, or Parkinson's disease. May induce cardiac arrhythmias; use with caution especially in patients with cardiac disease or those receiving drugs that sensitize the myocardium. Due to peripheral constriction and cardiac stimulation, pulmonary edema may occur. Due to renal blood vessel constriction, decreased urine output may occur. In hypovolemic patients, correct blood volume depletion before administering any vasopressor. Some products contain sulfites as preservatives; the presence of sulfites in some products should not deter administration during a serious allergic or other emergency situation even if the patient is sulfite-sensitive. Potentially significant drug-drug interactions may exist, requiring dose or frequency adjustment, additional monitoring, and/or selection of alternative therapy.

IV administration: Rapid IV administration may cause death from cerebrovascular hemorrhage or cardiac arrhythmias. However, rapid IV administration during pulseless arrest is necessary. Vesicant; ensure proper needle or catheter placement prior to and during infusion; avoid extravasation. Accidental injection into digits, hands, or feet may result in local reactions, including injection site pallor, coldness and hypoesthesia or injury, resulting in bruising, bleeding, discoloration, erythema or skeletal injury; patient should seek immediate medical attention if this occurs. Rapid IV administration may cause death from cerebrovascular hemorrhage or cardiac arrhythmias; however, rapid IV administration during pulseless arrest is necessary. Prior to intraocular use, must dilute 1:**1000** (1 mg/mL) solution to a concentration of 1:**100,000** to 1:**1,000,000** (10 **mcg**/mL to 1 **mcg**/mL) prior to intraocular use. When used undiluted, has been associated with corneal endothelial damage.

Self medication (OTC use): Oral inhalation: Prior to self-medication, patients should contact healthcare provider. The product should only be used in persons with a diagnosis of asthma. If symptoms are not relieved in 20 minutes or become worse do not continue to use the product - seek immediate medical assistance. The product should not be used more frequently or at higher doses than recommended unless directed by a healthcare provider. This product should not be used in patients who have required hospitalization for asthma or if a patient is taking prescription medication for asthma. Use with caution in patients with prostate enlargement or urinary retention. Do not use if you have taken a MAO inhibitor (certain drugs used for depression, Parkinson's disease, or other conditions) within 2 weeks.

Adverse Reactions

Cardiovascular: Angina, cardiac arrhythmia, chest pain, flushing, hypertension, pallor, palpitation, sudden death, tachycardia (parenteral), vasoconstriction, ventricular ectopy, ventricular fibrillation

Central nervous system: Anxiety (transient), apprehensiveness, cerebral hemorrhage, dizziness, headache, insomnia, lightheadedness, nervousness, restlessness

Gastrointestinal: Dry throat, loss of appetite, nausea, vomiting, xerostomia

Genitourinary: Acute urinary retention in patients with bladder outflow obstruction

Neuromuscular & skeletal: Tremor, weakness

Ocular: Allergic lid reaction, burning, corneal endothelial damage (intraocular use), eye pain, ocular irritation, precipitation of or exacerbation of narrow-angle glaucoma, transient stinging

Respiratory: Dyspnea, pulmonary edema

Miscellaneous: Diaphoresis

Drug Interactions

Metabolism/Transport Effects Substrate of COMT

Avoid Concomitant Use

Avoid concomitant use of EPINEPHrine (Systemic, Oral Inhalation) with any of the following: Ergot Derivatives; Iobenguane I 123; Lurasidone

Increased Effect/Toxicity

EPINEPHrine (Systemic, Oral Inhalation) may increase the levels/effects of: Lurasidone; Sympathomimetics

The levels/effects of EPINEPHrine (Systemic, Oral Inhalation) may be increased by: AtoMOXetine; Beta-Blockers; Cannabinoid-Containing Products; COMT Inhibitors; Ergot Derivatives; Hyaluronidase; Inhalational Anesthetics; Linezolid; MAO Inhibitors; Serotonin/Norepinephrine Reuptake Inhibitors; Tedizolid; Tricyclic Antidepressants

Decreased Effect

EPINEPHrine (Systemic, Oral Inhalation) may decrease the levels/effects of: Benzylpenicilloyl Polylysine; Iobenguane I 123

The levels/effects of EPINEPHrine (Systemic, Oral Inhalation) may be decreased by: Alpha1-Blockers; Promethazine; Spironolactone

Preparation for Administration

Endotracheal (off-label route): Dilute in NS or sterile water.

Intraocular: Dilute 1 mL of 1 mg/mL (1:**1000**) solution in 100 mL to 1000 mL of an ophthalmic irrigation fluid for a final concentration of 1:**100,000** to 1:**1,000,000** (10 **mcg**/mL to 1 **mcg**/mL); may use this solution as an irrigation as needed during the procedure. May also prepare a dilution of 1:**100,000** to 1:**400,000** (10 **mcg**/mL to 2.5 **mcg**/mL) for intracameral administration.

Intravenous: Although the manufacturer recommends dilution in dextrose containing solutions (provides protection against significant loss of potency by oxidation) and does not recommend dilution in NS alone, dilution in NS has been reported to be physically compatible (Trissel, 2014).

Oral inhalation: S2, Asthmanefrin: If using jet nebulizer, must be diluted with 3-5 mL NS. If using handheld rubber bulb nebulizer, dilution is not required.

Storage/Stability Epinephrine is sensitive to light and air. Protection from light is recommended. Oxidation turns drug pink, then a brown color. **Solutions should not be used if they are discolored or contain a precipitate.**

Adrenaclick: Store between 20°C to 25°C (68°F to 77°F); excursions permitted to 15°C to 30°C (59°F to 86°F); do not freeze or refrigerate. Protect from light.

Adrenalin: Store between 20°C to 25°C (68°F to 77°F); do not freeze. Protect from light.

Allerject [Canadian product]: Store between 15°C to 30°C (59°F to 86°F); do not refrigerate. Protect from light.

Asthmanefrin: Store between 20°C to 25°C (68°F to 77°F); protect from light and excessive heat.

Auvi-Q: Store between 20°C to 25°C (68°F to 77°F); excursions permitted to 15°C to 30°C (59°F to 86°F); do not refrigerate. Protect from light by storing in outer case provided.

Epinephrine injection, USP: Store between 20°C to 25°C (68°F to 77°F); do not refrigerate; protect from freezing. Protect from light until ready for use.

EpiPen and EpiPen Jr: Store at 25°C (77°F); excursions permitted to 15°C to 30°C (59°F to 86°F); do not freeze or refrigerate. Protect from light by storing in carrier tube provided.

Twinject [Canadian product]: Store between 20°C to 25°C (68°F to 77°F); excursions permitted to 15°C to 30°C (59°F to 86°F); do not freeze or refrigerate. Protect from light.

S2, Asthmanefrin: Store between 2°C to 20°C (36°F to 68°F). Protect from light.

Stability of injection of parenteral admixture at room temperature (25°C) or refrigeration (4°C) is 24 hours.

Mechanism of Action Stimulates alpha-, beta$_1$-, and beta$_2$-adrenergic receptors resulting in relaxation of smooth muscle of the bronchial tree, cardiac stimulation (increasing myocardial oxygen consumption), and dilation of skeletal muscle vasculature; small doses can cause vasodilation via beta$_2$-vascular receptors; large doses may produce constriction of skeletal and vascular smooth muscle

Pharmacodynamics/Kinetics

Onset of action: Bronchodilation: SubQ: ~5 to 10 minutes; Inhalation: ~1 minute

Metabolism: Taken up into the adrenergic neuron and metabolized by monoamine oxidase and catechol-o-methyltransferase; circulating drug hepatically metabolized

Half-life elimination: IV: <5 minutes

Excretion: Urine (as inactive metabolites, metanephrine, and sulfate and hydroxy derivatives of mandelic acid, small amounts as unchanged drug)

Dosage

Infants, Children, and Adolescents:

Asystole/pulseless arrest, pulseless VT/VF (after failed defibrillation attempts) (PALS [Kleinman, 2010]):

IV, I.O.: 0.01 mg/kg (0.1 mL/kg of **1:10,000** [0.1 mg/mL] solution) (maximum single dose: 1 mg) every 3 to 5 minutes until return of spontaneous circulation

Endotracheal: 0.1 mg/kg (0.1 mL/kg of **1:1000** [1 mg/mL] solution) (maximum single dose: 2.5 mg) every 3 to 5 minutes until IV/I.O. access established or return of spontaneous circulation. Flush with 5 mL of NS immediately after administration. May cause false-negative reading with exhaled CO_2 detectors; use second method to confirm tube placement if CO_2 is not detected (ACLS [Neumar, 2010]).

Postresuscitation infusion to maintain cardiac output or stabilize: IV, I.O.: 0.1 to 1 mcg/kg/minute; doses <0.3 mcg/kg/minute generally produce beta-adrenergic effects and higher doses (>0.3 mcg/kg/minute) generally produce alpha-adrenergic vasoconstriction; titrate dosage to desired effect

Bradycardia (symptomatic; unresponsive to atropine or pacing) (PALS [Kleinman, 2010]):

IV, I.O.: 0.01 mg/kg (0.1 mL/kg of **1:10,000** [0.1 mg/mL] solution) (maximum single dose: 1 mg) every 3 to 5 minutes as needed

Endotracheal: 0.1 mg/kg or (0.1 mL/kg of **1:1000** [1 mg/mL] solution) (maximum single dose: 2.5 mg) every 3 to 5 minutes as needed until IV/I.O. access established. Flush with 5 mL of NS immediately after administration. May cause false-negative reading with exhaled CO_2 detectors; use second method to confirm tube placement if CO_2 is not detected (ACLS [Neumar, 2010]).

Continuous infusion: IV, I.O.: 0.1 to 1 mcg/kg/minute; doses <0.3 mcg/kg/minute generally produce beta-adrenergic effects and higher doses (>0.3 mcg/kg/minute) generally produce alpha-adrenergic vasoconstriction; titrate dosage to desired effect

Bronchodilator: Nebulization: Racemic epinephrine (2.25% solution): OTC labeling: Children ≥4 years and Adolescents:

Hand-bulb nebulizer: Add 0.5 mL (~10 drops) to nebulizer; 1 to 3 inhalations up to every 3 hours if needed

Jet nebulizer: Add 0.5 mL (~10 drops) to nebulizer and dilute with 3 to 5 mL of NS; administer over ~15 minutes every 3 to 4 hours as needed

Croup (laryngotracheobronchitis), airway edema (off-label use): Nebulization: **Note:** Typically relief of symptoms occurs within 10 to 30 minutes and lasts 2 to 3 hours; patients should be observed for rapid symptom recurrence and possible repeat treatment.

Racemic epinephrine (2.25% solution): 0.05 to 0.1 mL/kg (maximum dose: 0.5 mL) diluted in 2 mL NS, may repeat dose every 20 minutes; others have reported use of 0.5 mL as a fixed dose for all patients; use lower end of dosing range for younger infants (Hegenbarth, 2008; Rosekrans, 1998; Rotta, 2003; Wright, 2002)

L-epinephrine: 0.5 mL/kg of **1:1000** solution (maximum dose: 5 mL) diluted in NS, may repeat dose every 20 minutes; **Note:** Racemic epinephrine 10 mg = 5 mg L-epinephrine (Hegenbarth, 2008)

Hypersensitivity reaction (eg, anaphylaxis): **Note:** SubQ administration results in slower absorption and is less reliable. IM administration in the anterolateral aspect of the middle third of the thigh is preferred in the setting of anaphylaxis (AHA [Vanden Hoek, 2010]; Kemp, 2008).

IM, SubQ: Larger IM or SubQ doses, use of IV route, or continuous IV infusion may be needed for severe anaphylactic reactions (Kemp, 2008; Lieberman, 2010). If clinician deems appropriate, the 5-minute interval between injections may be shortened to allow for more frequent administration (Lieberman, 2010).

Children <30 kg: 0.01 mg/kg (0.01 mL/kg of 1:**1000** [1 mg/mL] solution) (maximum single dose: 0.3 mg) every 5 to 10 minutes

Children ≥30 kg: 0.3 to 0.5 mg (0.3 to 0.5 mL of 1:**1000** [1 mg/mL] solution) every 5 to 10 minutes

Self-administration following severe allergic reactions (eg, insect stings, food): **Note:** World Health Organization (WHO) and Anaphylaxis Canada recommend the availability of 1 dose for every 10 to 20 minutes of travel time to a medical emergency facility. If anaphylactic symptoms persist after first dose, may repeat dose in 5 to 15 minutes (AHA [Vanden Hoek, 2010]); more than 2 sequential doses should only be administered under direct medical supervision.

Adrenaclick: IM, SubQ:

Children 15 to 29 kg: 0.15 mg

Children ≥30 kg: 0.3 mg

Allerject [Canadian product]: IM

Children 15 to 29 kg: 0.15 mg

Children ≥30 kg: 0.3 mg

Auvi-Q: IM, SubQ:

Children 15 to 29 kg: 0.15 mg; if anaphylactic symptoms persist, dose may be repeated

Children ≥30 kg: 0.3 mg; if anaphylactic symptoms persist, dose may be repeated

EpiPen Jr: IM, SubQ: Children 15 to 29 kg: 0.15 mg; if anaphylactic symptoms persist, dose may be repeated using an additional EpiPen

EpiPen: IM, SubQ: Children ≥30 kg: 0.3 mg; if anaphylactic symptoms persist, dose may be repeated using an additional EpiPen

Twinject [Canadian product]: IM SubQ:

Children 15 to 29 kg: 0.15 mg; if anaphylactic symptoms persist, dose may be repeated in 5 to 15 minutes using the same device after partial disassembly

Children ≥30 kg: 0.3 mg; if anaphylactic symptoms persist, dose may be repeated in 5 to 15 minutes using the same device after partial disassembly

Alternate auto-injector dose: IM (Sicherer, 2007):

Children 10 to 25 kg: 0.15 mg

Children >25 kg: 0.3 mg

Hypotension/shock, fluid-resistant (off-label use): Continuous IV infusion: 0.1 to 1 mcg/kg/minute; doses up to 5 mcg/kg/minute may rarely be necessary (Hegenbarth, 2008)

Mydriasis during intraocular surgery, induction and maintenance: Intraocular: Must dilute 1:**1000** (1 mg/mL) solution to a concentration of 1:**100,000** to 1:**1,000,000** (10 **mcg**/mL to 1 **mcg**/mL) prior to intraocular use: May use as an irrigation solution as needed during the procedure or may administer intracamerally (ie, directly into the anterior chamber of the eye) with a bolus dose of 0.1 mL of a 1:**100,000** to 1:**400,000** (10 **mcg**/mL to 2.5 **mcg**/mL) dilution.

Adults:

Asystole/pulseless arrest, pulseless VT/VF (ACLS [Neumar, 2010]):

IV, I.O.: 1 mg every 3 to 5 minutes until return of spontaneous circulation; if this approach fails, higher doses of epinephrine (up to 0.2 mg/kg) have been used for treatment of specific problems (eg, beta-blocker or calcium channel blocker overdose)

Endotracheal: 2 to 2.5 mg every 3 to 5 minutes until IV/I.O. access established or return of spontaneous circulation; dilute in 5 to 10 mL NS or sterile water. **Note:** Absorption may be greater with sterile water (Naganobu, 2000). May cause false-negative reading with exhaled CO_2 detectors; use second method to confirm tube placement if CO_2 is not detected (ACLS [Neumar, 2010]).

Bradycardia (symptomatic; unresponsive to atropine or pacing): IV infusion: 2 to 10 mcg/minute **or** 0.1 to 0.5 mcg/kg/minute (7 to 35 mcg/minute in a 70 kg patient); titrate to desired effect (ACLS [Neumar, 2010]):

Bronchodilator:

SubQ: Acute severe asthma unresponsive to inhaled beta-agonist (off-label use): 0.01 mg/kg divided into 3 doses of approximately 0.3 mg every 20 minutes. **Note:** The **1:1000** (1 mg/mL) concentration is recommended (AHA [Vanden Hoek, 2010]).

Nebulization: Racemic epinephrine (2.25% solution): OTC labeling:

Hand-bulb nebulizer: Add 0.5 mL (~10 drops) to nebulizer; 1 to 3 inhalations up to every 3 hours if needed

Jet nebulizer: Add 0.5 mL (~10 drops) to nebulizer and dilute with 3 to 5 mL of NS; administer over ~15 minutes every 3 to 4 hours as needed

Hypersensitivity reaction (eg, anaphylaxis):**Note:** SubQ administration results in slower absorption and is less reliable. IM administration in the anterolateral aspect of the middle third of the thigh is preferred in the setting of anaphylaxis (AHA [Vanden Hoek, 2010]; Kemp, 2008).

IM, SubQ: 0.2 to 0.5 mg (**1:1000** [1 mg/mL] solution) every 5 to 15 minutes in the absence of clinical improvement (AHA [Vanden Hoek, 2010]; Kemp, 2008; Lieberman, 2010). If clinician deems appropriate, the 5-minute interval between injections may be shortened to allow for more frequent administration (Lieberman, 2010).

IV: 0.1 mg (**1:10,000** [0.1 mg/mL] solution) over 5 minutes; may infuse at 1 to 4 mcg/minute to prevent the need to repeat injections frequently **or** may initiate with an infusion at 5 to 15 mcg/minute (with crystalloid administration) (AHA [Vanden Hoek, 2010]; Brown, 2004). In general, IV administration should only be done in patients who are profoundly hypotensive or are in cardiopulmonary arrest refractory to volume resuscitation and several epinephrine injections (Lieberman, 2010).

Self-administration following severe allergic reactions (eg, insect stings, food): **Note:** The World Health Organization (WHO) and Anaphylaxis Canada recommend the availability of one dose for every 10 to 20 minutes of travel time to a medical emergency facility. If anaphylactic symptoms persist after first dose, may repeat dose in 5 to 15 minutes (AHA [Vanden Hoek, 2010]); more than 2 sequential doses should only be administered under direct medical supervision.

Adrenaclick: IM, SubQ: 0.3 mg

Allerject [Canadian product]: IM: 0.3 mg

Auvi-Q: IM, SubQ: 0.3 mg; if anaphylactic symptoms persist, dose may be repeated

EpiPen: IM, SubQ: 0.3 mg; if anaphylactic symptoms persist, dose may be repeated using an additional EpiPen

Twinject [Canadian product]: IM, SubQ: 0.3 mg; if anaphylactic symptoms persist, dose may be repeated in 5 to 15 minutes using the same device after partial disassembly

Hypotension/septic shock:

Manufacturer recommendation: Septic shock: IV infusion: Initial: 0.05 to 2 mcg/kg/minute (3.5 to 140 mcg/minute in a 70 kg patient); titrate to desired mean arterial pressure (MAP). May adjust dose every 10 to 15 minutes by 0.05 to 0.2 mcg/kg/minute to achieve desired blood pressure goal. After hemodynamic stabilization, may wean incrementally every 30 minutes over 12 to 24 hours.

American Heart Association recommendation: Severe and fluid resistant (off-label dosing): IV infusion: Initial: 0.1 to 0.5 mcg/kg/minute (7 to 35 mcg/minute in a 70 kg patient); titrate to desired response (AHA [Peberdy, 2010]).

Mydriasis during intraocular surgery, induction and maintenance: Intraocular: Must dilute 1:**1000** (1 mg/mL) solution to a concentration of 1:**100,000** to 1:**1,000,000** (10 **mcg**/mL to 1 **mcg**/mL) prior to intraocular use: May use as an irrigation solution as needed during the procedure or may administer intracamerally (ie, directly into the anterior chamber of the eye) with a bolus dose of 0.1 mL of a 1:**100,000** to 1:**400,000** (10 **mcg**/mL to 2.5 **mcg**/mL) dilution.

Dosage adjustment in renal impairment: There are no dosage adjustments provided in the manufacturer's labeling.

Dosage adjustment in hepatic impairment: There are no dosage adjustments provided in the manufacturer's labeling.

Usual Infusion Concentrations: Pediatric IV infusion: 16 **mcg**/mL, 32 **mcg**/mL, or 64 **mcg**/mL

Usual Infusion Concentrations: Adult IV infusion: 1 mg in 250 mL (concentration: 4 **mcg**/mL) **or** 4 mg in 250 mL (concentration: 16 **mcg**/mL) of D_5W or NS; 1 mg in 1,000 mL (concentration: 1 **mcg**/mL) in D_5W or D_5NS

Administration Epinephrine solutions for injection can be administered IM, I.O., endotracheally, IV, or SubQ. **Note:** Adrenaclick, Allerject [Canadian product], Auvi-Q, EpiPen and EpiPen Jr Auto-Injectors contain a single, fixed-dose of epinephrine and may only be administered IM (preferred) or SubQ. Twinject Auto-Injectors [Canadian product] contain two doses; the first fixed-dose is available for auto-injection; the second dose is available for manual injection following partial disassembly of device.

IV: When administering as a continuous infusion, central line administration is preferred. IV infusions require an infusion pump. If central line not available, as a temporary measure, may administer through a large vein. Avoid use of ankle veins (due to potential for gangrene), leg veins in elderly patients, or leg veins in those suffering from occlusive vascular diseases (eg, diabetic endarteritis, Buerger's disease, arteriosclerosis, atherosclerosis). Vesicant; ensure proper needle or catheter placement prior to and during infusion; avoid extravasation.

Extravasation management: If extravasation occurs, stop infusion immediately and disconnect (leave cannula/needle in place); gently aspirate extravasated solution (do **NOT** flush the line); remove needle/cannula; elevate extremity. Initiate phentolamine (or alternative antidote). Apply dry warm compresses (Hurst, 2004).

Phentolamine: Dilute 5 to 10 mg in 10 to 15 mL NS and administer into extravasation site as soon as possible after extravasation (Peberdy, 2010).

Alternatives to phentolamine (due to shortage):

Nitroglycerin topical 2% ointment (based on limited case reports in neonates/infants): Apply 4 mm/kg as a thin ribbon to the affected areas; may repeat after 8 hours if needed (Wong, 1992) **or** apply a 1-inch strip on the affected site (Denkler, 1989).

Terbutaline (based on limited case reports): Infiltrate extravasation area using a solution of terbutaline 1 mg diluted to 10 mL in NS (large extravasation site; administration volume varied from 3 to 10 mL) **or** 1 mg diluted in 1 mL NS (small/distal extravasation site; administration volume varied from 0.5 to 1 mL) (Stier, 1999).

Subcutaneous: SubQ administration results in slower absorption and is less reliable.

IM: IM administration in the anterolateral aspect of the middle third of the thigh is preferred in the setting of anaphylaxis (AHA [Vanden Hoek, 2010]; Kemp, 2008). IM administration into the buttocks should be avoided. Adrenaclick, Allerject [Canadian product], Auvi-Q, EpiPen, EpiPen Jr, and Twinject Auto-Injectors [Canadian product] should only be injected into the anterolateral aspect of the thigh, through clothing if necessary.

Obesity: In overweight or obese children, because skin surface to muscle depth is greater in the upper half of the thigh, administration into the lower half of the thigh may be preferred. In very obese children, injection into the calf will provide an even greater chance of intramuscular administration (Arkwright, 2013).

Endotracheal (cardiac arrest): Dilute in NS or sterile water. Absorption may be greater with sterile water (Naganobu, 2000). Stop compressions, spray drug quickly down tube. Follow immediately with several quick insufflations and continue chest compressions. May cause false-negative reading with exhaled CO_2 detectors; use second method to confirm tube placement if CO_2 is not detected (ACLS [Neumar, 2010]).

Oral inhalation: S2, Asthmanefrin: If using jet nebulizer: Administer diluted over ~15 minutes. If using handheld rubber bulb nebulizer, dilution is not required.

Monitoring Parameters Heart rate, blood pressure (invasive blood pressure monitoring and central venous pressure monitoring recommended while receiving continuous infusion); monitor site of infusion for blanching/extravasation; continuous cardiac monitoring required during continuous infusion. If using to treat hypotension, assess intravascular volume prior to and during therapy; support as needed.

Consult individual institutional policies and procedures.

Dosage Forms

Device, Injection:

Auvi-Q: 0.15 mg/0.15 mL (2 ea); 0.3 mg/0.3 mL (2 ea)

EpiPen 2-Pak: 0.3 mg/0.3 mL (2 ea)

EpiPen Jr 2-Pak: 0.15 mg/0.3 mL (2 ea)

Nebulization Solution, Inhalation:

Asthmanefrin Refill [OTC]: 2.25% (1 ea)

Asthmanefrin Starter Kit [OTC]: 2.25% (1 ea)

Nebulization Solution, Inhalation [preservative free]:

S2 [OTC]: 2.25% (1 ea)

Solution, Injection:

Adrenalin: 1 mg/mL (1 mL); 30 mg/30 mL (30 mL)

Generic: 0.1 mg/mL (10 mL); 1 mg/mL (1 mL, 30 mL)

Solution, Intravenous [preservative free]:

Generic: 1 mg/mL (1 mL)

Solution Auto-injector, Injection:

Adrenaclick: 0.15 mg/0.15 mL (2 ea); 0.3 mg/0.3 mL (2 ea)

Generic: 0.15 mg/0.15 mL (1 ea, 2 ea); 0.3 mg/0.3 mL (1 ea, 2 ea)

Solution Prefilled Syringe, Injection:

Generic: 0.1 mg/mL (10 mL)

- **Epinephrine and Lidocaine** *see* Lidocaine and Epinephrine *on page 1212*
- **Epinephrine Bitartrate** *see* EPINEPHrine (Systemic, Oral Inhalation) *on page 735*
- **Epinephrine Hydrochloride** *see* EPINEPHrine (Systemic, Oral Inhalation) *on page 735*
- **EpiPen (Can)** *see* EPINEPHrine (Systemic, Oral Inhalation) *on page 735*
- **EpiPen 2-Pak** *see* EPINEPHrine (Systemic, Oral Inhalation) *on page 735*
- **EpiPen Jr (Can)** *see* EPINEPHrine (Systemic, Oral Inhalation) *on page 735*
- **EpiPen Jr 2-Pak** *see* EPINEPHrine (Systemic, Oral Inhalation) *on page 735*
- **Epipodophyllotoxin** *see* Etoposide *on page 816*
- **Epipodophyllotoxin** *see* Etoposide Phosphate *on page 820*
- **EpiQuin Micro** *see* Hydroquinone *on page 1020*

Epirubicin (ep i ROO bi sin)

Brand Names: U.S. Ellence

Brand Names: Canada Ellence®; Epirubicin for Injection; Epirubicin Hydrochloride Injection; Pharmorubicin®

Index Terms Epidoxorubicin; Epirubicin Hydrochloride; Pidorubicin; Pidorubicin Hydrochloride

Pharmacologic Category Antineoplastic Agent, Anthracycline; Antineoplastic Agent, Topoisomerase II Inhibitor

Use Adjuvant therapy component for primary breast cancer

Pregnancy Risk Factor D

Dosage Note: Patients receiving 120 mg/m^2/cycle as part of combination therapy (CEF-120 regimen) should also receive prophylactic therapy with sulfamethoxazole/trimethoprim or a fluoroquinolone. Lower starting doses may be necessary for heavily pretreated patients, patients with preexisting myelosuppression, or with bone marrow involvement. Epirubicin is associated with a moderate to high emetic potential (depending on dose or regimen); antiemetics are recommended to prevent nausea and vomiting (Basch, 2011; Dupuis, 2011; Roila, 2010).

Breast cancer, adjuvant treatment: Adults: IV: Usual dose: 100-120 mg/m^2 per 3- or 4-week treatment cycle as follows:

60 mg/m^2 on days 1 and 8 every 28 days for 6 cycles in combination with cyclophosphamide and fluorouracil (CEF-120 regimen; Levine, 2005) **or**

100 mg/m^2 on day 1 every 21 days for 6 cycles in combination with cyclophosphamide and fluorouracil (FEC-100 regimen; Bonneterre, 2005) **or**

Breast cancer (off-label regimens; as a part of combination chemotherapy): Adults: IV:

60 mg/m^2 on day 1 every 21 days for 8 cycles (EC regimen; Piccart, 2001) **or**

75 mg/m^2 on day 1 every 21 days for 4 cycles (FEC regimen; Buzdar, 2005) **or**

75 mg/m^2 on day 1 every 21 days for 6 cycles (EP or EC regimen; Langley, 2005) **or**

90 mg/m^2 on day 1 every 21 days for 4 or 6 cycles (FEC regimen ± paclitaxel; Martin, 2008) **or**

50 mg/m^2 on days 1 and 8 every 21-28 days for 6-9 cycles (CEF regimen; Ackland, 2001)

Esophageal cancer (off-label use; as part of combination chemotherapy): Adults: IV:

50 mg/m^2 on day 1 every 21 days for up to 8 cycles (ECF, ECX, EOF, and EOX regimens; Cunningham, 2008) **or**

50 mg/m^2 on day 1 every 21 days for 3 preoperative and 3 postoperative cycles (ECF regimen; Cunningham, 2006)

Gastric cancer (off-label use; as part of combination chemotherapy): Adults: IV:

50 mg/m^2 on day 1 every 21 days for up to 8 cycles (ECF, ECX, EOF, and EOX regimens [Cunningham, 2008]; ECF regimen [Waters, 1999]) **or**

50 mg/m^2 on day 1 every 21 days for 3 preoperative and 3 postoperative cycles (ECF regimen; Cunningham, 2006)

Dosage modifications (breast cancer; labeled dosing):

Delay day 1 dose until platelets are ≥100,000/mm^3, ANC ≥1500/mm^3, and nonhematologic toxicities have recovered to ≤ grade 1

Reduce day 1 dose in subsequent cycles to 75% of previous day 1 dose if patient experiences nadir platelet counts <50,000/mm^3, ANC <250/mm^3, neutropenic fever, or grade 3/4 nonhematologic toxicity during the previous cycle

For CEF-120 regimen, reduce day 8 dose to 75% of day 1 dose if platelet counts are 75,000-100,000/mm^3 and ANC is 1000-1499/mm^3; omit day 8 dose if platelets are <75,000/mm^3, ANC <1000/mm^3, or grade 3/4 nonhematologic toxicity

Elderly: Plasma clearance of epirubicin in elderly female patients was noted to be reduced by 35%. Although no initial dosage reduction is specifically recommended, particular care should be exercised in monitoring toxicity and adjusting subsequent dosage in elderly patients (particularly females >70 years of age).

Dosage adjustment in bone marrow dysfunction: Heavily-treated patients, patients with preexisting bone marrow depression or neoplastic bone marrow infiltration: Lower starting doses (75-90 mg/m^2) should be considered.

Dosage adjustment in renal impairment: The manufacturer's labeling recommends lower doses (dose not specified) in patients with severe renal impairment (serum creatinine >5 mg/dL). Other sources (Aronoff, 2007) suggest no dosage adjustment is needed for CrCl <50 mL/minute.

Dosage adjustment in hepatic impairment: The manufacturer's labeling recommends the following adjustments (based on clinical trial information):

Bilirubin 1.2-3 mg/dL or AST 2-4 times the upper limit of normal: Administer 50% of recommended starting dose

Bilirubin >3 mg/dL or AST >4 times the upper limit of normal: Administer 25% of recommended starting dose

Severe hepatic impairment: Use is not recommended (has not been studied)

Dosing in obesity: *ASCO Guidelines for appropriate chemotherapy dosing in obese adults with cancer:* Utilize patient's actual body weight (full weight) for calculation of body surface area- or weight-based dosing, particularly when the intent of therapy is curative; manage regimen-related toxicities in the same manner as for nonobese patients; if a dose reduction is utilized due to toxicity, consider resumption of full weight-based dosing with subsequent cycles, especially if cause of toxicity (eg, hepatic or renal impairment) is resolved (Griggs, 2012).

Additional Information Complete prescribing information should be consulted for additional detail.

Dosage Forms

Solution, Intravenous [preservative free]:

Ellence: 50 mg/25 mL (25 mL); 200 mg/100 mL (100 mL)

Generic: 50 mg/25 mL (25 mL); 200 mg/100 mL (100 mL)

Solution Reconstituted, Intravenous:

Generic: 50 mg (1 ea)

- **Epirubicin for Injection (Can)** *see* Epirubicin *on page 739*
- **Epirubicin Hydrochloride** *see* Epirubicin *on page 739*

◆ **Epirubicin Hydrochloride Injection (Can)** *see* Epirubicin *on page 739*

◆ **Epitol** *see* CarBAMazepine *on page 346*

◆ **Epival (Can)** *see* Valproic Acid and Derivatives *on page 2123*

◆ **Epival ECT (Can)** *see* Valproic Acid and Derivatives *on page 2123*

◆ **Epivir** *see* LamiVUDine *on page 1157*

◆ **Epivir HBV** *see* LamiVUDine *on page 1157*

Eplerenone (e PLER en one)

Brand Names: U.S. Inspra

Brand Names: Canada Inspra

Pharmacologic Category Antihypertensive; Diuretic, Potassium-Sparing; Selective Aldosterone Blocker

Use

Heart failure post-myocardial infarction (MI): Treatment of heart failure (HF) (LVEF ≤40%) following acute MI

Note: According to the Eighth Joint National Committee (JNC 8) guidelines, aldosterone antagonists are **not** recommended for the initial treatment of hypertension (James, 2013).

The ACCF/AHA 2013 heart failure guidelines recommend the use of aldosterone antagonists, along with other guideline directed medical therapies, to reduce morbidity and mortality in patients with an LVEF ≤40% following acute MI who develop symptoms of HF or have a history of diabetes mellitus (Yancy, 2013).

According to the 2013 ACCF/AHA guidelines for the management of ST-elevation myocardial infarction (STEMI) and the guidelines for the management of unstable angina/non-STEMI, an aldosterone antagonist should be given to patients who are already on an ACE inhibitor and beta-blocker, who have an LVEF ≤40% and either symptomatic HF or diabetes mellitus (ACCF/AHA [Anderson, 2013]; ACCF/AHA [O'Gara, 2013]).

Hypertension: Treatment of hypertension (may be used alone or in combination with other antihypertensive agents)

Note: According to the Eighth Joint National Committee (JNC 8) guidelines, aldosterone antagonists are **not** recommended for the initial treatment of hypertension (James, 2013).

Canadian labeling: Additional use (not in U.S. labeling): **Heart failure:** Treatment of NYHA class II chronic heart failure (HF) with left ventricular systolic dysfunction

Pregnancy Risk Factor B

Pregnancy Considerations Adverse events were observed in some animal reproduction studies. Information related to eplerenone use in pregnancy is limited (Cabassi, 2012; Morton, 2011). The use of mineralocorticoid receptor antagonists is not recommended to treat chronic uncomplicated hypertension in pregnant women and should generally be avoided in women of reproductive potential (ACOG, 2013).

Breast-Feeding Considerations It is not known if eplerenone is excreted in breast milk. Due to the potential for serious adverse reactions in the nursing infant, the manufacturer recommends a decision be made whether to discontinue nursing or to discontinue the drug, taking into account the importance of treatment to the mother.

Contraindications

U.S. labeling: Serum potassium >5.5 mEq/L at initiation; CrCl ≤30 mL/minute; concomitant use of strong CYP3A4 inhibitors (see Drug Interactions for details)

The following additional contraindications apply to patients with hypertension: Type 2 diabetes mellitus (noninsulin dependent, NIDDM) with microalbuminuria; serum creatinine >2.0 mg/dL in males or >1.8 mg/dL in females; CrCl <50 mL/minute; concomitant use with potassium supplements or potassium-sparing diuretics

Canadian labeling: Hypersensitivity to eplerenone or any component of the formulation; serum potassium >5 mEq/L at initiation; severe hepatic impairment (Child-Pugh class C); severe renal impairment (eGFR <30 mL/minute/1.73 m^2); clinically significant hyperkalemia; concomitant use with potassium supplements, potassium-sparing diuretics or strong CYP3A4 inhibitors

The following additional contraindications apply to patients with hypertension: Type 2 diabetes mellitus (noninsulin dependent, NIDDM) with microalbuminuria; serum creatinine >1.5 mg/dL [132 micromole/L] in males or >1.3 mg/dL [115 micromole/L] in females; eGFR <50 mL/minute/1.73 m^2

Warnings/Precautions Monitor closely for hyperkalemia; increases in serum potassium were dose related during clinical trials and rates of hyperkalemia also increased with declining renal function. The concurrent use of larger doses of ACE inhibitors (eg, ≥ lisinopril 10 mg daily) also increases the risk of hyperkalemia (ACCF/AHA [Yancy, 2013]). Dose reduction or interruption of therapy may be necessary with development of hyperkalemia. Use is contraindicated in patients with potassium >5.5 mEq/L (U.S. labeling) or >5 mEq/L (Canadian labeling) at initiation of therapy. Safety and efficacy have not been established in patients with severe hepatic impairment (Canadian labeling contraindicates use in severe hepatic impairment). Use with caution in HF patients post-MI with diabetes (especially if patient has proteinuria); risk of hyperkalemia is increased. Risk of hyperkalemia is increased with declining renal function. Based on indication and degree of renal impairment, use may be contraindicated (refer to Contraindications field). Use with caution in patients with mild renal impairment; contraindicated with moderate-severe impairment. Potentially significant drug-drug interactions may exist, requiring dose or frequency adjustment, additional monitoring, and/or selection of alternative therapy. Avoid potassium supplements, potassium-containing salt substitutes, a diet rich in potassium, or other drugs that can cause hyperkalemia (eg, other potassium-sparing diuretics, NSAIDS). Concomitant use of potassium supplements or potassium-sparing diuretics is contraindicated in the treatment of hypertension (U.S. labeling) or in all patients regardless of indication (Canadian labeling).

When evaluating a heart failure patient for eplerenone treatment, eGFR should be >30 mL/minute/1.73 m^2 or creatinine should be ≤2.5 mg/dL (men) or ≤2 mg/dL (women) with no recent worsening and potassium <5 mEq/L with no history of severe hyperkalemia (ACCF/AHA [Yancy, 2013]). Serum potassium levels require close monitoring and management if elevated. The manufacturer recommends to withhold therapy if serum potassium >6 mEq/L. The ACCF/AHA recommends considering discontinuation upon the development of serum potassium >5.5 mEq/L or worsening renal function with careful evaluation of the entire medical regimen. Avoid routine triple therapy with the combined use of an ACE inhibitor, ARB, and eplerenone. Instruct patients with heart failure to discontinue use during an episode of diarrhea or dehydration or when loop diuretic therapy is interrupted (ACCF/AHA [Yancy, 2013]).

Adverse Reactions

Central nervous system: Dizziness, fatigue

Endocrine & metabolic: Breast pain, creatinine increased, gynecomastia, hypercholesterolemia, hyperkalemia, hypertriglyceridemia (dose related), hyponatremia (dose related)

Gastrointestinal: Abdominal pain, diarrhea

Genitourinary: Abnormal vaginal bleeding

Renal: Albuminuria, creatinine increased

Respiratory: Cough

Miscellaneous: Flu-like syndrome

Rare but important or life-threatening: Angioneurotic edema, BUN increased, liver function tests increased, rash, uric acid increased

Drug Interactions

Metabolism/Transport Effects Substrate of CYP3A4 (major); **Note:** Assignment of Major/Minor substrate status based on clinically relevant drug interaction potential

Avoid Concomitant Use

Avoid concomitant use of Eplerenone with any of the following: Conivaptan; CycloSPORINE (Systemic); CYP3A4 Inhibitors (Strong); Fusidic Acid (Systemic); Idelalisib; Itraconazole; Ketoconazole (Systemic); Posaconazole; Tacrolimus (Systemic); Voriconazole

Increased Effect/Toxicity

Eplerenone may increase the levels/effects of: ACE Inhibitors; Amifostine; Ammonium Chloride; Angiotensin II Receptor Blockers; Antihypertensives; Cardiac Glycosides; CycloSPORINE (Systemic); DULoxetine; Hypotensive Agents; Levodopa; Lithium; Obinutuzumab; Potassium Salts; Potassium-Sparing Diuretics; RisperiDONE; RiTUXimab; Sodium Phosphates; Tacrolimus (Systemic)

The levels/effects of Eplerenone may be increased by: Alfuzosin; Analgesics (Opioid); Barbiturates; Brimonidine (Topical); Canagliflozin; Conivaptan; CYP3A4 Inhibitors (Moderate); CYP3A4 Inhibitors (Strong); Dasatinib; Diazoxide; Fluconazole; Fusidic Acid (Systemic); Heparin; Heparin (Low Molecular Weight); Herbs (Hypotensive Properties); Idelalisib; Itraconazole; Ivacaftor; Ketoconazole (Systemic); Luliconazole; MAO Inhibitors; Mifepristone; Nicorandil; Nitrofurantoin; Nonsteroidal Anti-Inflammatory Agents; Pentoxifylline; Phosphodiesterase 5 Inhibitors; Posaconazole; Prostacyclin Analogues; Simeprevir; Tolvaptan; Trimethoprim; Voriconazole

Decreased Effect

Eplerenone may decrease the levels/effects of: Cardiac Glycosides; QuiNIDine

The levels/effects of Eplerenone may be decreased by: Bosentan; CYP3A4 Inducers (Moderate); CYP3A4 Inducers (Strong); Dabrafenib; Deferasirox; Herbs (Hypertensive Properties); Methylphenidate; Mitotane; Nonsteroidal Anti-Inflammatory Agents; Siltuximab; St Johns Wort; Tocilizumab; Yohimbine

Food Interactions Grapefruit juice increases eplerenone AUC ~25%. Management: Dosage adjustments of eplerenone may be needed.

Storage/Stability Store at controlled room temperature of 25°C (77°F); excursions permitted to 15°C to 30°C (59°F to 86°F).

Mechanism of Action Aldosterone, a mineralocorticoid, increases blood pressure primarily by inducing sodium and water retention. Overexpression of aldosterone is thought to contribute to myocardial fibrosis (especially following myocardial infarction) and vascular fibrosis. Mineralocorticoid receptors are located in the kidney, heart, blood vessels, and brain. Eplerenone selectively blocks mineralocorticoid receptors reducing blood pressure in a dose-dependent manner and appears to prevent myocardial and vascular fibrosis.

Pharmacodynamics/Kinetics

Distribution: V_d: 43-90 L

Protein binding: ~50%; primarily to alpha$_1$-acid glycoproteins

Metabolism: Primarily hepatic via CYP3A4; metabolites inactive

Bioavailability: 69%

Half-life elimination: 4-6 hours

Time to peak, plasma: ~1.5 hours; may take up to 4 weeks for full antihypertensive effect

Excretion: Urine (~67%); feces (32%); <5% as unchanged drug in urine and feces

Dosage Oral: Adults:

Hypertension: Initial: 50 mg once daily; may increase to 50 mg twice daily if response is not adequate; may take up to 4 weeks for full therapeutic response. Doses >100 mg/day are associated with increased risk of hyperkalemia and no greater therapeutic effect.

Concurrent use with **moderate** CYP3A4 inhibitors: Initial: 25 mg once daily

Heart failure (HF):

U.S. labeling:

Heart failure (HF) (post-MI): Initial: 25 mg once daily; dosage goal: Titrate to 50 mg once daily within 4 weeks, as tolerated

Dosage adjustment per serum potassium concentrations for HF (post-MI):

<5 mEq/L:

Increase dose from 25 mg every other day to 25 mg daily **or**

Increase dose from 25 mg daily to 50 mg daily

5 to 5.4 mEq/L: No adjustment needed

5.5 to 5.9 mEq/L:

Decrease dose from 50 mg daily to 25 mg daily **or**

Decrease dose from 25 mg daily to 25 mg every other day **or**

Modify dose from 25 mg every other day to withhold medication

≥6 mEq/L: Withhold medication until potassium <5.5 mEq/L, then restart at 25 mg every other day

Alternatively, the ACCF/AHA 2013 HF guidelines recommend withholding treatment if potassium >5.5 mEq/L or renal function worsens; hold doses until potassium is <5 mEq/L and consider restarting with a reduced dose after confirming resolution of hyperkalemia/renal insufficiency for at least 72 hours (ACCF/AHA [Yancy, 2013]).

Heart failure (NYHA class II-IV with LVEF ≤35%) (off-label dose): Initial: 25 mg once daily; may increase to a maximum dose of 50 mg once daily (ACCF/AHA [Yancy, 2013])

Canadian labeling:

Chronic HF (NYHA class II) or HF (post-MI):

eGFR ≥50 mL/minute/1.73 m^2 and potassium ≤5 mEq/L: Initial: 25 mg once daily; may increase within 4 weeks as tolerated to a target dose of 50 mg once daily (maximum dose). **Note:** Treatment following MI should be initiated 3 to 14 days after MI.

Concurrent use with **mild-to-moderate** CYP3A4 inhibitors: Maximum dose: 25 mg once daily

eGFR 30 to 49 mL/minute/1.73 m^2 and potassium ≤5 mEq/L: Initial: 25 mg every other day; may increase within 4 weeks as tolerated to a target dose of 25 mg once daily (maximum dose). **Note:** Treatment following MI should be initiated 3 to 14 days after MI.

Concurrent use with **mild-to-moderate** CYP3A4 inhibitors: Avoid concurrent use (target dose <25 mg once daily has not been studied).

Dosage adjustment (after initiation) per serum potassium concentrations:

<5 mEq/L:

Current dose is 25 mg every other day: Increase to 25 mg daily

Current dose is 25 mg daily and eGFR ≥50 mL/minute/1.73 m^2 or **not taking** concurrent mild-to-moderate CYP3A4 inhibitor: Increase to 50 mg daily

Current dose is 25 mg daily and eGFR 30-49 mL/minute/1.73 m^2 or **if taking** concurrent mild-to-moderate CYP3A4 inhibitor: Do not increase dose.

5 to 5.4 mEq/L: No adjustment needed

5.5 to 5.9 mEq/L:
Current dose is 50 mg daily: Decrease to 25 mg daily
Current dose is 25 mg daily: Decrease to 25 mg every other day
Decrease dose is 25 mg every other day: Withhold further doses; reinitiate only if potassium <5 mEq/L
≥6 mEq/L: Withhold further doses until potassium <5 mEq/L, then may temporarily resume therapy at 25 mg every other day (dose efficacy has not been established); reassess potassium levels in 1 week and if within acceptable limits, increase dose to 25 mg once daily; reassess potassium levels again in 1 week to determine whether therapy should be continued or interrupted.

Dosage adjustment in renal impairment:

U.S. labeling:

Hypertension:
CrCl ≥50 mL/minute: There are no dosage adjustments provided in the manufacturer's labeling.
CrCl <50 mL/minute or serum creatinine >2 mg/dL (males) or >1.8 mg/dL (females): Use is contraindicated; risk of hyperkalemia increases with declining renal function.

Heart failure (post-MI):
CrCl ≥50 mL/minute: There are no dosage adjustments provided in the manufacturer's labeling.
CrCl 31 to 50 mL/minute or serum creatinine >2 mg/dL (males) or >1.8 mg/dL (females): There are no dosage adjustments provided in the manufacturer's labeling; use with caution.There are no dosage adjustments provided in the manufacturer's labeling; use with caution..
CrCl ≤30 mL/minute: Use is contraindicated.

Heart failure (including post-MI) (ACCF/AHA [Yancy, 2013]):
eGFR ≥50 mL/minute/1.73 m^2: Initial dose: 25 mg once daily, Maintenance dose (after 4 weeks of treatment and potassium ≤5 mEq/L): 50 mg once daily
eGFR 30 to 49 mL/minute/1.73 m^2: Initial dose: 25 mg once every other day; Maintenance dose (after 4 weeks of treatment and potassium ≤5 mEq/L): 25 mg once daily
eGFR <30 mL/minute/1.73 m^2: Not recommended

Canadian labeling:

Hypertension:
eGFR ≥50 mL/minute/1.73 m^2: There are no dosage adjustments provided in the manufacturer's labeling; monitor serum potassium closely.
eGFR <50 mL/minute/1.73 m^2 or serum creatinine >1.5 mg/dL [132 micromol/L] in males or >1.3 mg/dL [115 micromol/L] in females: Use is contraindicated.

Chronic HF (NYHA class II) or HF (post-MI):
eGFR ≥50 mL/minute/1.73 m^2: No dosage adjustment necessary unless receiving concurrent mild-to-moderate CYP3A4 inhibitor, then maximum dose is 25 mg once daily.
eGFR 30 to 49 mL/minute/1.73 m^2: Initial: 25 mg every other day; titrate to 25 mg once daily (maximum dose) within 4 weeks, as tolerated. Avoid concurrent use with mild-to-moderate CYP3A4 inhibitors.
eGFR ≤30 mL/minute/1.73 m^2: Use is contraindicated.

Dosage adjustment in hepatic impairment:

U.S. labeling:

Mild-to-moderate impairment: No dosage adjustment necessary.
Severe impairment: No dosage adjustment provided in manufacturer's labeling (has not been studied).

Canadian labeling:

Mild-to-moderate impairment: No dosage adjustment necessary.
Severe impairment: Use is contraindicated.

Dietary Considerations May be taken with or without food. Do not use salt substitutes containing potassium.

Administration May be administered with or without food.

Monitoring Parameters Blood pressure; serum potassium (prior to therapy, within the first week, 1 month after start of treatment or dose adjustment, then periodically as clinically indicated); additionally, check serum potassium in 3-7 days after initiating concurrent therapy with moderate CYP3A4 inhibitor; serum creatinine

ACCF/AHA heart failure guideline recommendations (ACCF/AHA [Yancy, 2013]): Serum potassium and renal function should be checked in 3 days after initiation, at 1 week after initiation, at least monthly for the first 3 months of therapy, and every 3 months thereafter. If adding or increasing the dose of concomitant ACE inhibitors or ARBs, a new cycle of monitoring should be done. If serum potassium increases to >5.5 mEq/L or renal function worsens, hold doses until potassium is <5 mEq/L and consider restarting with a reduced dose after confirming resolution of hyperkalemia/renal insufficiency for at least 72 hours.

Dosage Forms

Tablet, Oral:
Inspra: 25 mg, 50 mg
Generic: 25 mg, 50 mg

◆ **EPO** *see* Epoetin Alfa *on page 742*

Epoetin Alfa (e POE e tin AL fa)

Brand Names: U.S. Epogen; Procrit

Brand Names: Canada Eprex

Index Terms *r*HuEPO; *r*HuEPO-α; EPO; Erythropoiesis-Stimulating Agent (ESA); Erythropoietin

Pharmacologic Category Colony Stimulating Factor; Erythropoiesis-Stimulating Agent (ESA); Hematopoietic Agent

Use Treatment of anemia due to concurrent myelosuppressive chemotherapy in patients with cancer (nonmyeloid malignancies) receiving chemotherapy (palliative intent) for a planned minimum of 2 additional months of chemotherapy; treatment of anemia due to chronic kidney disease (including patients on dialysis and not on dialysis) to decrease the need for RBC transfusion; treatment of anemia associated with HIV (zidovudine) therapy when endogenous erythropoietin levels ≤500 mUnits/mL; reduction of allogeneic RBC transfusion for elective, noncardiac, nonvascular surgery when perioperative hemoglobin is >10 to ≤13 g/dL and there is a high risk for blood loss

Note: Epoetin is **not** indicated for use under the following conditions:

- Cancer patients receiving hormonal therapy, therapeutic biologic products, or radiation therapy unless also receiving concurrent myelosuppressive chemotherapy
- Cancer patients receiving myelosuppressive chemotherapy when the expected outcome is curative
- Surgery patients who are willing to donate autologous blood
- Surgery patients undergoing cardiac or vascular surgery
- As a substitute for RBC transfusion in patients requiring immediate correction of anemia

Note: In clinical trials (and one meta-analysis), epoetin has not demonstrated improved quality of life, fatigue, or well-being.

Pregnancy Risk Factor C

Pregnancy Considerations Adverse events were observed in animal reproduction studies. In vitro studies suggest that recombinant erythropoietin does not cross the human placenta (Reisenberger, 1997). Polyhydramnios and intrauterine growth retardation have been reported with use in women with chronic kidney disease (adverse effects also associated with maternal disease). Hypospadias and pectus excavatum have been reported with first trimester exposure (case report).

Recombinant erythropoietin alfa has been evaluated as adjunctive treatment for severe pregnancy associated iron deficiency anemia (Breymann, 2001; Krafft, 2009) and has been used in pregnant women with iron-deficiency anemia associated with chronic kidney disease (CKD) (Furaz-Czerpak 2012; Josephson, 2007).

Amenorrheic premenopausal women should be cautioned that menstruation may resume following treatment with recombinant erythropoietin (Furaz-Czerpak, 2012). Multidose formulations containing benzyl alcohol are contraindicated for use in pregnant women; if treatment during pregnancy is needed, single dose preparations should be used.

Women who become pregnant during treatment with epoetin are encouraged to enroll in Amgen's Pregnancy Surveillance Program (1-800-772-6436).

Breast-Feeding Considerations Endogenous erythropoietin is found in breast milk (Semba, 2002). It is not known if recombinant erythropoietin alfa is excreted into breast milk. The manufacturer recommends caution be used if the single dose vial preparation is administered to nursing women; use of the multiple dose vials containing benzyl alcohol is contraindicated in breast-feeding women. When administered enterally to neonates (mixed with human milk or infant formula), recombinant erythropoietin did not significantly increase serum EPO concentrations. If passage via breast milk does occur, risk to a nursing infant appears low (Juul, 2003).

Contraindications Hypersensitivity to epoetin or any component of the formulation; uncontrolled hypertension; pure red cell aplasia (due to epoetin or other epoetin protein drugs); multidose vials contain benzyl alcohol and are contraindicated in neonates, infants, pregnant women, and nursing women

Warnings/Precautions **[U.S. Boxed Warning]: Erythropoiesis-stimulating agents (ESAs) increased the risk of serious cardiovascular events, thromboembolic events, stroke, mortality, and/or tumor progression in clinical studies when administered to target hemoglobin levels >11 g/dL** (and provide no additional benefit); a rapid rise in hemoglobin (>1 g/dL over 2 weeks) may also contribute to these risks. **[U.S. Boxed Warning]: A shortened overall survival and/or increased risk of tumor progression or recurrence has been reported in studies with breast, cervical, head and neck, lymphoid, and non-small cell lung cancer patients.** It is of note that in these studies, patients received ESAs to a target hemoglobin of ≥12 g/dL; although risk has not been excluded when dosed to achieve a target hemoglobin of <12 g/dL. **[U.S. Boxed Warnings]: To decrease these risks, and risk of cardio- and thrombovascular events, use the lowest dose needed to avoid red blood cell transfusions. Use ESAs in cancer patients only for the treatment of anemia related to concurrent myelosuppressive chemotherapy; discontinue ESA following completion of the chemotherapy course. ESAs are not indicated for patients receiving myelosuppressive therapy when the anticipated outcome is curative.** A dosage modification is appropriate if hemoglobin levels rise >1 g/dL per 2-week time period during treatment (Rizzo, 2010). Use of ESAs has been associated with an increased risk of venous thromboembolism (VTE) without a reduction in transfusions in patients with cancer (Hershman, 2009). Improved anemia symptoms, quality of life, fatigue, or well-being have not been demonstrated in controlled clinical trials. **[U.S. Boxed Warning]: Because of the risks of decreased survival and increased risk of tumor growth or progression, all healthcare providers and hospitals are required to enroll and comply with the ESA APPRISE (Assisting Providers and Cancer Patients with Risk Information for the Safe use of ESAs) Oncology Program prior to prescribing or dispensing ESAs to cancer patients.** Prescribers and patients will have to provide written documentation of discussed risks prior to each new course.

[U.S. Boxed Warning]: An increased risk of death, serious cardiovascular events, and stroke was reported in chronic kidney disease (CKD) patients administered ESAs to target hemoglobin levels ≥11 g/dL; use the lowest dose sufficient to reduce the need for RBC transfusions. An optimal target hemoglobin level, dose or dosing strategy to reduce these risks has not been identified in clinical trials. Hemoglobin rising >1 g/dL in a 2-week period may contribute to the risk (dosage reduction recommended). The American College of Physicians recommends against the use of ESAs in patients with mild to moderate anemia and heart failure or coronary heart disease (ACP [Qaseem, 2013]).

Chronic kidney disease patients who exhibit an inadequate hemoglobin response to ESA therapy may be at a higher risk for cardiovascular events and mortality compared to other patients. ESA therapy may reduce dialysis efficacy (due to increase in red blood cells and decrease in plasma volume); adjustments in dialysis parameters may be needed. Patients treated with epoetin may require increased heparinization during dialysis to prevent clotting of the extracorporeal circuit. **[U.S. Boxed Warning]: DVT prophylaxis is recommended in perisurgery patients due to the risk of DVT.** Increased mortality was also observed in patients undergoing coronary artery bypass surgery who received epoetin alfa; these deaths were associated with thrombotic events. Epoetin is **not** approved for reduction of red blood cell transfusion in patients undergoing cardiac or vascular surgery and is **not** indicated for surgical patients willing to donate autologous blood.

Use with caution in patients with hypertension (contraindicated in uncontrolled hypertension) or with a history of seizures; hypertensive encephalopathy and seizures have been reported. If hypertension is difficult to control, reduce or hold epoetin alfa. An excessive rate of rise of hemoglobin is associated with hypertension or exacerbation of hypertension; decrease the epoetin dose if the hemoglobin increase exceeds 1 g/dL in any 2-week period. Blood pressure should be controlled prior to start of therapy and monitored closely throughout treatment. The risk for seizures is increased with epoetin use in patients with CKD; monitor closely for neurologic symptoms during the first several months of therapy. Due to the delayed onset of erythropoiesis, epoetin alfa is **not** recommended for acute correction of severe anemia or as a substitute for emergency transfusion.

Prior to treatment, correct or exclude deficiencies of iron, vitamin B_{12}, and/or folate, as well as other factors which may impair erythropoiesis (inflammatory conditions, infections). Prior to and periodically during therapy, iron stores must be evaluated. Supplemental iron is recommended if serum ferritin <100 mcg/L or serum transferrin saturation <20%; most patients with chronic kidney disease will require iron supplementation. Poor response should prompt evaluation of these potential factors, as well as possible malignant processes and hematologic disease (thalassemia, refractory anemia, myelodysplastic disorder), occult blood loss, hemolysis, ostetis fibrosa cystic, and/or bone marrow fibrosis. Severe anemia and pure red cell aplasia (PRCA) with associated neutralizing antibodies to erythropoietin has been reported, predominantly in patients with CKD receiving SubQ epoetin (the IV route is preferred for hemodialysis patients). Cases have also been reported in patients with hepatitis C who were receiving ESAs, interferon, and ribavirin. Patients with a sudden loss of response to epoetin alfa (with severe anemia and a low reticulocyte count) should be evaluated for PRCA with associated neutralizing antibodies to erythropoietin; discontinue treatment (permanently) in patients with PRCA secondary to neutralizing antibodies to epoetin.

Potentially serious allergic reactions have been reported (rarely). Discontinue immediately (and permanently) in patients who experience serious allergic/anaphylactic reactions.

Some dosage forms may contain polysorbate 80 (also known as Tweens). Hypersensitivity reactions, usually a delayed reaction, have been reported following exposure to pharmaceutical products containing polysorbate 80 in certain individuals (Isaksson, 2002; Lucente 2000; Shelley, 1995). Thrombocytopenia, ascites, pulmonary deterioration, and renal and hepatic failure have been reported in premature neonates after receiving parenteral products containing polysorbate 80 (Alade, 1986; CDC, 1984). See manufacturer's labeling.

Some products may contain albumin.

Benzyl alcohol and derivatives: Some dosage forms may contain benzyl alcohol; large amounts of benzyl alcohol (≥99 mg/kg/day) have been associated with a potentially fatal toxicity ("gasping syndrome") in neonates; the "gasping syndrome" consists of metabolic acidosis, respiratory distress, gasping respirations, CNS dysfunction (including convulsions, intracranial hemorrhage), hypotension and cardiovascular collapse (AAP, 1997; CDC, 1982); some data suggests that benzoate displaces bilirubin from protein binding sites (Ahlfors, 2001); avoid or use dosage forms containing benzyl alcohol with caution in neonates. See manufacturer's labeling.

Adverse Reactions

Cardiovascular: Deep vein thrombosis, edema, hypertension, thrombosis

Central nervous system: Chills, depression, dizziness, fever, headache, insomnia

Dermatologic: Pruritus, rash,urticaria

Endocrine & metabolic: Hyperglycemia, hypokalemia

Gastrointestinal: Dysphagia, nausea, stomatitis, vomiting, weight loss

Hematologic: Leukopenia

Local: Clotted vascular access, injection site reaction

Neuromuscular & skeletal: Arthralgia, bone pain, muscle spasm, myalgia

Respiratory: Cough, pulmonary embolism, respiratory congestion, upper respiratory infection

Rare but important or life-threatening: Allergic reaction, anaphylactic reaction, angioedema, bronchospasm, erythema, hypersensitivity reactions, hypertensive encephalopathy, microvascular thrombosis, MI, neutralizing antibodies, porphyria, pure red cell aplasia (PRCA), renal vein thrombosis, retinal artery thrombosis, seizure, stroke, tachycardia, temporal vein thrombosis, thrombophlebitis, TIA, tumor progression

Drug Interactions

Metabolism/Transport Effects None known.

Avoid Concomitant Use There are no known interactions where it is recommended to avoid concomitant use.

Increased Effect/Toxicity

Epoetin Alfa may increase the levels/effects of: Lenalidomide; Thalidomide

The levels/effects of Epoetin Alfa may be increased by: Nandrolone

Decreased Effect There are no known significant interactions involving a decrease in effect.

Preparation for Administration Prior to SubQ administration, preservative free solutions may be mixed with bacteriostatic NS containing benzyl alcohol 0.9% in a 1:1 ratio.

Storage/Stability Vials should be stored at 2°C to 8°C (36°F to 46°F); **do not freeze or shake**. Protect from light.

Single-dose 1 mL vial contains no preservative: Use one dose per vial. Do not re-enter vial; discard unused portions.

Single-dose vials (except 40,000 units/mL vial) are stable for 2 weeks at room temperature (Cohen, 2007). Single-dose 40,000 units/mL vial is stable for 1 week at room temperature.

Multidose 1 mL or 2 mL vial contains preservative. Store at 2°C to 8°C after initial entry and between doses. Discard 21 days after initial entry.

Multidose vials (with preservative) are stable for 1 week at room temperature (Cohen, 2007).

Prefilled syringes containing the 20,000 units/mL formulation with preservative are stable for 6 weeks refrigerated (2°C to 8°C) (Naughton, 2003).

Dilutions of 1:10 and 1:20 (1 part epoetin:19 parts sodium chloride) are stable for 18 hours at room temperature (Ohls, 1996).

Prior to SubQ administration, preservative free solutions may be mixed with bacteriostatic NS containing benzyl alcohol 0.9% in a 1:1 ratio (Corbo, 1992).

Dilutions of 1:10 in $D_{10}W$ with human albumin 0.05% or 0.1% are stable for 24 hours.

Mechanism of Action Induces erythropoiesis by stimulating the division and differentiation of committed erythroid progenitor cells; induces the release of reticulocytes from the bone marrow into the bloodstream, where they mature to erythrocytes. There is a dose response relationship with this effect. This results in an increase in reticulocyte counts followed by a rise in hematocrit and hemoglobin levels.

Pharmacodynamics/Kinetics

Onset of action: Several days

Peak effect: Hemoglobin level: 2-6 weeks

Distribution: V_d: 9 L; rapid in the plasma compartment; concentrated in liver, kidneys, and bone marrow

Metabolism: Some degradation does occur

Bioavailability: SubQ: ~21% to 31%; intraperitoneal epoetin: 3% (Macdougall, 1989)

Half-life elimination: Cancer: SubQ: 16-67 hours; Chronic kidney disease: IV: 4-13 hours

Time to peak, serum: Chronic kidney disease: SubQ: 5-24 hours

Excretion: Feces (majority); urine (small amounts, 10% unchanged in normal volunteers)

Dosage

Anemia associated with chronic kidney disease: Individualize dosing and use the lowest dose necessary to reduce the need for RBC transfusions.

Chronic kidney disease patients ***ON dialysis*** (IV route is preferred for hemodialysis patients; initiate treatment when hemoglobin is <10 g/dL; reduce dose or interrupt treatment if hemoglobin approaches or exceeds 11 g/dL):

Children 1 month to 16 years: IV, SubQ: Initial dose: 50 units/kg 3 times/week

Adults: IV, SubQ: Initial dose: 50-100 units/kg 3 times/week

*Chronic kidney disease patients **NOT on dialysis*** (consider initiating treatment when hemoglobin is <10 g/dL; use only if rate of hemoglobin decline would likely result in RBC transfusion and desire is to reduce risk of alloimmunization or other RBC transfusion-related risks; reduce dose or interrupt treatment if hemoglobin exceeds 10 g/dL):

Adults: IV, SubQ: Initial dose: 50-100 units/kg 3 times/week

Dosage adjustments for chronic kidney disease patients (either on dialysis or not on dialysis):

If hemoglobin does not increase by >1 g/dL after 4 weeks: Increase dose by 25%; do not increase the dose more frequently than once every 4 weeks

If hemoglobin increases >1 g/dL in any 2-week period: Reduce dose by ≥25%; dose reductions can occur more frequently than once every 4 weeks; avoid frequent dosage adjustments

Inadequate or lack of response over a 12-week escalation period: Further increases are unlikely to improve response and may increase risks; use the minimum effective dose that will maintain a Hgb level sufficient to avoid RBC transfusions and evaluate patient for other causes of anemia. Discontinue therapy if responsiveness does not improve.

Anemia due to chemotherapy in cancer patients: Initiate treatment only if hemoglobin <10 g/dL and anticipated duration of myelosuppressive chemotherapy is ≥2 months. Titrate dosage to use the minimum effective dose that will maintain a hemoglobin level sufficient to avoid red blood cell transfusions. Discontinue erythropoietin following completion of chemotherapy.

Children ≥5 years: IV: Initial dose: 600 units/kg once weekly until completion of chemotherapy.

Dosage adjustments:

If hemoglobin does not increase by >1 g/dL **and** remains <10 g/dL after initial 4 weeks: Increase to 900 units/kg (maximum dose: 60,000 units); discontinue after 8 weeks of treatment if RBC transfusions are still required or there is no hemoglobin response.

If hemoglobin exceeds a level needed to avoid red blood cell transfusion: Withhold dose; resume treatment with a 25% dose reduction when hemoglobin approaches a level where transfusions may be required.

If hemoglobin increases >1 g/dL in any 2-week period **or** hemoglobin reaches a level sufficient to avoid red blood cell transfusion: Reduce dose by 25%.

Adults: SubQ: Initial dose: 150 units/kg 3 times/week or 40,000 units once weekly until completion of chemotherapy

Dosage adjustments:

If hemoglobin does not increase by >1 g/dL **and** remains below 10 g/dL after initial 4 weeks: Increase to 300 units/kg 3 times/week or 60,000 units weekly; discontinue after 8 weeks of treatment if RBC transfusions are still required or there is no hemoglobin response

If hemoglobin exceeds a level needed to avoid red blood cell transfusion: Withhold dose; resume treatment with a 25% dose reduction when hemoglobin approaches a level where transfusions may be required.

If hemoglobin increases >1 g/dL in any 2-week period **or** hemoglobin reaches a level sufficient to avoid red blood cell transfusion: Reduce dose by 25%.

Anemia due to zidovudine in HIV-infected patients: Titrate dosage to use the minimum effective dose that will maintain a hemoglobin level sufficient to avoid red blood cell transfusions. Hemoglobin levels should not exceed 12 g/dL.

Children 8 months to 17 years (based on limited data): IV, SubQ: Reported dosing range: 50-400 units/kg 2-3 times/week

Adults (with serum erythropoietin levels ≤500 mUnits/mL and zidovudine doses ≤4200 mg/week): IV, SubQ: Initial: 100 units/kg 3 times/week; if hemoglobin does not increase after 8 weeks, increase dose by ~50-100 units/kg at 4-8 week intervals until hemoglobin reaches a level sufficient to avoid RBC transfusion; maximum dose: 300 units/kg. Withhold dose if hemoglobin exceeds 12 g/dL, may resume treatment with a 25% dose reduction once hemoglobin <11 g/dL. Discontinue if hemoglobin increase is not achieved with 300 units/kg for 8 weeks.

Surgery patients (perioperative hemoglobin should be >10 g/dL and ≤13 g/dL; DVT prophylactic anticoagulation is recommended): Adults: SubQ: Initial dose:

300 units/kg/day beginning 10 days before surgery, on the day of surgery, and for 4 days after surgery **or**

600 units/kg once weekly for 4 doses, given 21-, 14-, and 7 days before surgery, and on the day of surgery

Symptomatic anemia associated with MDS (off-label use): Adults: SubQ: 40,000-60,000 units 1-3 times/week (NCCN MDS guidelines v.2.2011)

Dosage adjustment in renal impairment: No dosage adjustment necessary.

Dosage adjustment in hepatic impairment: No dosage adjustment provided in manufacturer's labeling.

Administration

SubQ is the preferred route of administration **except** in patients with CKD on hemodialysis; 1:1 dilution with bacteriostatic NS (containing benzyl alcohol) acts as a local anesthetic to reduce pain at the injection site

Patients with CKD on hemodialysis: IV route preferred; it may be administered into the venous line at the end of the dialysis procedure

Monitoring Parameters Transferrin saturation and serum ferritin (prior to and during treatment); hemoglobin (weekly after initiation and following dose adjustments until stable and sufficient to minimize need for RBC transfusion, CKD patients should be also be monitored at least monthly following hemoglobin stability); blood pressure; seizures (CKD patients following initiation for first few months, includes new-onset or change in seizure frequency or premonitory symptoms)

Cancer patients: Examinations recommended by the ASCO/ASH guidelines (Rizzo, 2010) prior to treatment include: peripheral blood smear (in some situations a bone marrow exam may be necessary), assessment for iron, folate, or vitamin B_{12} deficiency, reticulocyte count, renal function status, and occult blood loss; during ESA treatment, assess baseline and periodic iron, total iron-binding capacity, and transferrin saturation or ferritin levels.

Reference Range Zidovudine-treated HIV patients: Available evidence indicates patients with endogenous serum erythropoietin levels >500 mU/mL are unlikely to respond

Additional Information Oncology Comment: The American Society of Clinical Oncology (ASCO) and American Society of Hematology (ASH) 2010 updates to the clinical practice guidelines for the use of erythropoiesis-stimulating agents (ESAs) in patients with cancer indicate that ESAs are most appropriate when used according to the parameters identified within the Food and Drug Administration (FDA) approved labeling for epoetin and darbepoetin (Rizzo, 2010). ESAs are an option for chemotherapy associated anemia when the hemoglobin has fallen to <10 g/dL to decrease the need for RBC transfusions. ESAs should only be used in conjunction with concurrent chemotherapy. Although the FDA label now limits ESA use to the palliative setting, the ASCO/ASH guidelines suggest using clinical judgment in weighing risks versus benefits as formal outcomes studies of ESA use defined by intent of chemotherapy treatment have not been conducted.

The ASCO/ASH guidelines continue to recommend following the FDA approved dosing (and dosing adjustment) guidelines as alternate dosing and schedules have not demonstrated consistent differences in effectiveness with regard to hemoglobin response. In patients who do not have a response within 6-8 weeks (hemoglobin rise <1-2 g/dL or no reduction in transfusions) ESA therapy should be discontinued.

Prior to the initiation of ESAs, other sources of anemia (in addition to chemotherapy or underlying hematologic malignancy) should be investigated. Examinations recommended prior to treatment include peripheral blood smear (in some situations a bone marrow exam may be necessary), assessment for iron, folate, or vitamin B_{12} deficiency, reticulocyte count, renal function status, and occult blood loss. During ESA treatment, assess baseline and periodic iron, total iron-binding capacity, and transferrin saturation or ferritin levels. Iron supplementation may be necessary

The guidelines note that patients with an increased risk of thromboembolism (generally includes previous history of thrombosis, surgery, and/or prolonged periods of immobilization) and patients receiving concomitant medications that may increase thromboembolic risk, should begin ESA therapy only after careful consideration. With the exception of low-risk myelodysplasia-associated anemia (which has evidence supporting the use of ESAs without concurrent chemotherapy), the guidelines do not support the use of ESAs in the absence of concurrent chemotherapy.

Dosage Forms

Solution, Injection:

Epogen: 10,000 units/mL (2 mL); 20,000 units/mL (1 mL)

Procrit: 10,000 units/mL (2 mL); 20,000 units/mL (1 mL)

Solution, Injection [preservative free]:

Epogen: 2000 units/mL (1 mL); 3000 units/mL (1 mL); 4000 units/mL (1 mL); 10,000 units/mL (1 mL)

Procrit: 2000 units/mL (1 mL); 3000 units/mL (1 mL); 4000 units/mL (1 mL); 10,000 units/mL (1 mL); 40,000 units/mL (1 mL)

Dosage Forms: Canada

Injection, solution [preservative free]:

Eprex®: 1000 units/0.5 mL (0.5 mL), 2000 units/0.5 mL (0.5 mL), 3000 units/0.3 mL (0.3 mL), 4000 units/0.4 mL (0.4 mL), 5000 units/0.5 mL (0.5 mL), 6000 units/0.6 mL (0.6 mL), 8000 units/0.8 mL (0.8 mL), 10,000 units/mL (1 mL), 20,000 units/0.5 mL (0.5 mL), 30,000 units/0.75 mL (0.75 mL), 40,000 units/mL (1 mL) [contains polysorbate 80; prefilled syringe, free of human serum albumin]

◆ **Epogen** *see* Epoetin Alfa *on page* 742

Epoprostenol (e poe PROST en ole)

Brand Names: U.S. Flolan; Veletri

Brand Names: Canada Caripul; Flolan

Index Terms Epoprostenol Sodium; PGI_2; PGX; Prostacyclin

Pharmacologic Category Prostacyclin; Prostaglandin; Vasodilator

Use Treatment of pulmonary arterial hypertension (PAH) (WHO Group I) in patients with NYHA Class III or IV symptoms to improve exercise capacity

Pregnancy Risk Factor B

Pregnancy Considerations Adverse events were not observed in animal reproduction studies. Women with PAH are encouraged to avoid pregnancy (McLaughlin, 2009).

Breast-Feeding Considerations It is not known if epoprostenol is excreted in breast milk. The manufacturer recommends that caution be exercised when administering epoprostenol to nursing women.

Contraindications Hypersensitivity to epoprostenol or to structurally-related compounds; chronic use in patients with heart failure due to severe left ventricular systolic dysfunction; patients who develop pulmonary edema during dose initiation

Warnings/Precautions Initiation or transition to epoprostenol requires specialized cardiopulmonary monitoring in a critical care setting where clinicians are experienced in advanced management of pulmonary arterial hypertension. Abrupt interruptions or large sudden reductions in dosage may result in rebound pulmonary hypertension; some patients with PAH have developed pulmonary edema during dosing adjustment and acute vasodilator testing (not an approved use), which may be associated with concomitant heart failure (LV systolic dysfunction with significantly elevated left heart filling pressures) or pulmonary veno-occlusive disease/pulmonary capillary hemangiomatosis. During chronic use, unless contraindicated, anticoagulants should be coadministered to reduce the risk of thromboembolism. Use cautiously in patients who have conditions that increase bleeding risk (inhibits platelet aggregation). Use with caution in patients receiving anticoagulants and antiplatelet agents. Chronic continuous IV infusion of epoprostenol via a chronic indwelling central venous catheter (CVC) has been associated with local infections and serious blood stream infections. Clinical studies of epoprostenol in pulmonary hypertension did not include sufficient numbers of patients ≥65 years of age to substantiate its safety and efficacy in the geriatric population. As a result, in general, dose selection for an elderly patient should be cautious usually starting at the low end of the dosing range.

Adverse Reactions Note: Adverse events reported during dose initiation and escalation include flushing, headache, nausea/vomiting, hypotension, anxiety/nervousness/agitation, chest pain; dizziness, abdominal pain, bradycardia, musculoskeletal pain, dyspnea, back pain, diaphoresis, dyspepsia, hypoesthesia/paresthesia, and tachycardia are also reported. Although some adverse reactions may be related to the underlying disease state, abdominal pain, anxiety/nervousness/agitation, arthralgia, bleeding, bradycardia, diarrhea, diaphoresis, flu-like syndrome, flushing, headache, hypotension, jaw pain, nausea, pain, pulmonary edema, rash, tachycardia, thrombocytopenia, and vomiting are clearly contributed to epoprostenol. The following adverse events have been reported during chronic administration for idiopathic or heritable PAH:

Cardiovascular: Flushing, hypotension, tachycardia

Central nervous system: Agitation, anxiety, chills, dizziness, fever, flu-like syndrome, headache, nervousness, sepsis, tremor

Dermatologic: Dermal ulcer, eczema, skin rash, urticaria

Gastrointestinal: Anorexia, diarrhea, nausea, vomiting

Local: Injection site reactions: Infection, pain

Neuromuscular & skeletal: Arthralgia, hyperesthesia, hypoesthesia, jaw pain, musculoskeletal pain, myalgia, neck pain, pain, paresthesia

Rare but important or life-threatening: Abdominal pain, anemia, ascites, dyspnea, fatigue, hemorrhage, hepatic failure, hyperthyroidism, pancytopenia, pulmonary edema, pulmonary embolism, splenomegaly, thrombocytopenia

Drug Interactions

Metabolism/Transport Effects None known.

Avoid Concomitant Use There are no known interactions where it is recommended to avoid concomitant use.

Increased Effect/Toxicity

Epoprostenol may increase the levels/effects of: Agents with Antiplatelet Properties; Anticoagulants; Antihypertensives; Digoxin

The levels/effects of Epoprostenol may be increased by: Thrombolytic Agents

Decreased Effect There are no known significant interactions involving a decrease in effect.

Preparation for Administration

Preparation of Epoprostenol Infusion

To make solution with concentration:	Flolan Instructions	Veletri or Caripul Instructions
	Note: Flolan may only be prepared with sterile diluent provided.	**Note:** Veletri or Caripul may only be prepared with sterile water for injection (SWFI) or NS.
3000 ng/mL	Dissolve one 0.5 mg vial with 5 mL supplied diluent, withdraw 3 mL, and add to a sufficient volume of supplied diluent to make a total of 100 mL.	Dissolve one 0.5 mg vial with 5 mL of SWFI or NS, withdraw 3 mL, and add to a sufficient volume of the identical diluent to make a total of 100 mL.
5000 ng/mL	Dissolve one 0.5 mg vial with 5 mL supplied diluent, withdraw entire vial contents, and add to a sufficient volume of supplied diluent to make a total of 100 mL.	Dissolve one 0.5 mg vial with 5 mL of SWFI or NS, withdraw entire vial contents, and add to a sufficient volume of the identical diluent to make a total of 100 mL.
10,000 ng/mL	Dissolve two 0.5 mg vials each with 5 mL supplied diluent, withdraw entire vial contents, and add to a sufficient volume of supplied diluent to make a total of 100 mL.	Dissolve two 0.5 mg vials each with 5 mL of SWFI or NS, withdraw entire vial contents, and add to a sufficient volume of the identical diluent to make a total of 100 mL.
15,000 ng/mL	Dissolve one 1.5 mg vial with 5 mL supplied diluent, withdraw entire vial contents, and add to a sufficient volume of supplied diluent to make a total of 100 mL.	Dissolve one 1.5 mg vial with 5 mL of SWFI or NS, withdraw entire vial contents, and add to a sufficient volume of the identical diluent to make a total of 100 mL.
20,000 ng/mL	Dissolve two 0.5 mg vials each with 5 mL supplied diluent, withdraw entire vial contents, and add to a sufficient volume of supplied diluent to make a total of **50 mL** (DeWet, 2004).	
30,000 ng/mL		Dissolve two 1.5 mg vials each with 5 mL of SWFI or NS, withdraw entire vial contents, and add to a sufficient volume of the identical diluent to make a total of 100 mL.

Storage/Stability

Flolan: Prior to use, store vials at 15°C to 25°C (59°F to 77°F); do not freeze. Protect from light. Following reconstitution, solution must be stored under refrigeration at 2°C to 8°C (36°F to 46°F) if not used immediately; do not freeze. Protect from light. Total storage and infusion time must not exceed 48 hours for reconstituted solutions. Each reservoir of solution may be refrigerated for ≤40 hours and infused at room temperature over ≤8 hours; alternatively, each reservoir may be refrigerated for ≤24 hours and infused with the use of a cold pouch over ≤24 hours (gel packs must be changed every 12 hours).

Veletri: Prior to use, store vials at 20°C to 25°C (68°F to 77°F); do not freeze. Protect from light. Reconstituted vials must be further diluted prior to use.

Caripul [Canadian product]: Prior to use, store vials at 15°C to 30°C (59°F to 86°F); do not freeze. Reconstituted vials must be further diluted prior to use.

Reconstituted solutions of Veletri or Caripul immediately diluted to a final concentration within a drug delivery reservoir may be administered immediately or stored at 2°C to 8°C (36°F to 46°F) for up to 8 days; do not freeze. Protect from light.

If administered immediately, the following maximum durations of administration at room temperature (25°C [77°F]) according to solution concentration are recommended:

U.S. labeling (Veletri):

3000 to <15,000 ng/mL: 48 hours

15,000 to <60,000 ng/mL: 48 hours

≥60,000 ng/mL: 72 hours

Canadian labeling (Caripul):

3000 to <15,000 ng/mL: 48 hours

≥15,000: 48 hours

If stored at 2°C to 8°C (36°F to 46°F) for up to 8 days, the following maximum durations of administration at room temperature (25°C [77°F]) according to solution concentration are recommended:

3000 to <15,000 ng/mL: 24 hours

15,000 to <60,000 ng/mL: 48 hours

≥60,000 ng/mL: 48 hours

Short excursions at 40°C (104°F) are permitted as follows:

Solution concentration <15,000 ng/mL: Up to 2 hours

Solution concentration 15,000 to <60,000 ng/mL: Up to 4 hours

Solution concentration ≥60,000 ng/mL: Up to 8 hours

The following maximum durations of administration at temperatures >25°C to 40°C (>77°F up to 104°F) administered either immediately or after up to 8 days storage at 2°C to 8°C (36°F to 46°F) according to solution concentration are recommended:

Use at temperature >25°C to 30°C (>77°F up to 86°F):

U.S. labeling (Veletri):

<60,000 ng/mL: 24 hours

≥60,000 ng/mL: 48 hours

Canadian labeling (Caripul): All concentrations: 24 hours

Use at temperature up to 40°C (104°F):

U.S. labeling (Veletri): ≥60,000 ng/mL: 24 hours (immediately administered after preparation)

Mechanism of Action Epoprostenol is also known as prostacyclin and PGI_2. It is a strong vasodilator of all vascular beds. In addition, it is a potent endogenous inhibitor of platelet aggregation. The reduction in platelet aggregation results from epoprostenol's activation of intracellular adenylate cyclase and the resultant increase in cyclic adenosine monophosphate concentrations within the platelets. Additionally, it is capable of decreasing thrombogenesis and platelet clumping in the lungs by inhibiting platelet aggregation.

Pharmacodynamics/Kinetics

Metabolism: Rapidly hydrolyzed; subject to some enzymatic degradation; forms two active metabolites (6-keto-prostaglandin $F_1\alpha$ and 6,15-diketo-13,14-dihydro-prostaglandin $F_1\alpha$) with minimal activity and 14 inactive metabolites

Half-life elimination: ~6 minutes

Excretion: Urine (84%); feces (4%)

Dosage

IV:

Pulmonary arterial hypertension (PAH): Children (off-label use), Adolescents (off-label use), and Adults: Initial: 2 ng/kg/minute; a lower initial dose may be used if patient is intolerant of starting dose. Increase dose in increments of 2 ng/kg/minute at intervals of ≥15 minutes until dose-limiting side effects (eg, flushing, jaw pain, headache, hypotension, nausea) are noted or response to epoprostenol plateaus. Usual optimal dose (monotherapy): 25-40 ng/kg/minute (McLaughlin, 2009); significant patient variability in optimal dose exists. Maximum dose with chronic therapy has not been defined; however, doses as high as 195 ng/kg/minute have been described in children (Rosenzweig, 1999).

Dose adjustment during chronic phase of treatment:

If PAH symptoms persist or recur following improvement, increase dose in 1-2 ng/kg/minute increments at intervals of ≥15 minutes. May also increase dose at intervals of 24-48 hours or longer (eg, every 1-2 weeks). **Note:** The need for increased doses should be expected with chronic use; incremental increases occur more frequently during the first few months after the drug is initiated.

In case of dose-limiting pharmacologic events (eg, hypotension, severe nausea, vomiting), decrease dose in 2 ng/kg/minute decrements at intervals of ≥15 minutes. Avoid abrupt withdrawal or sudden large dose reductions. **Note:** Adverse event may resolve without dosage adjustment.

Lung transplant: In patients receiving lung transplants, epoprostenol may be tapered after sequential lung transplantation once the allografts have been reperfused. If cardiopulmonary bypass utilized, epoprostenol may be tapered after pump perfusion has been initiated.

Acute vasodilator testing in patients with PAH (off-label use; McLaughlin, 2009): Adults: **Note:** Acute vasodilator testing should only be done in patients who might be considered candidates for calcium channel blocker therapy.

Initial: 2 ng/kg/minute; increase dose in increments of 2 ng/kg/minute every 10-15 minutes; dosing range during testing: 2-10 ng/kg/minute

Inhalation (off-label route): Adults:

Intraoperative pulmonary hypertension during cardiac surgery with cardiopulmonary bypass (CPB) (off-label use): **Note:** Institution-specific protocols vary.

Administration after induction of anesthesia before incision: Flolan: 60 mcg (4 mL of 15,000 ng/mL concentration) via jet nebulizer; effect persists for ~25 minutes (Hache, 2003)

or

Intraoperative administration: Nebulization via ventilator circuit: Flolan: Using a 15,000 ng/mL concentration and an oxygen flow of 8 L/minute, begin administration via jet nebulizer 5 minutes prior to weaning from CPB; discontinue at least 60 minutes after CPB weaned (Fattouch, 2006)

Post-cardiothoracic surgery pulmonary hypertension, right ventricular dysfunction, or refractory hypoxemia (off-label use) (DeWet, 2004): Flolan: **Note:** May need to change ventilator filter every 2 hours due to glycine buffer diluent; may cause ventilator valve malfunction. Tidal volume delivered by ventilator may require adjustment.

Nebulization via ventilator circuit: Flolan: Using a 20,000 ng/mL concentration, prime nebulizer chamber with 15 mL; administer remainder at a constant rate of 8 mL/hour; delivers ~38 ng/kg/minute (based on a 70 kg patient); set oxygen flow at 2-3 L/minute; wean as tolerated. **Note:** Although not achieved with this regimen, in general, doses >50 ng/kg/minute do not provide additional benefit and may increase the risk of hypotension.

or

Nebulization via facemask with Venturi attachment: Flolan: Using a 20,000 ng/mL concentration, prime nebulizer chamber with 15 mL; set oxygen flow at 2-3 L/minute; 8 mL/hour will be nebulized; wean as tolerated.

Weaning procedure: Reduce dose by 50% every 2-4 hours (ie, 20,000 ng/mL to 10,000 ng/mL to 5000 ng/mL) until a concentration of 2500 ng/mL is reached; carefully discontinue once patient remains stable on this concentration for at least 4 hours.

Dosage adjustment in renal impairment: There are no dosage adjustments provided in the manufacturer's labeling.

Dosage adjustment in hepatic impairment: There are no dosage adjustments provided in the manufacturer's labeling.

Administration

IV: Use infusion sets with an in-line 0.22 micron filter for Veletri or Caripul infusions. Flolan labeling does not specifically recommend filtering; however, the use of an in-line 0.22 micron filter was used during clinical trials. The ambulatory infusion pump should be small and lightweight, be able to adjust infusion rates in 2 ng/kg/minute increments, have occlusion, end of infusion, and low battery alarms, have ± 6% accuracy of the programmed rate, and have positive continuous or pulsatile pressure with intervals ≤3 minutes between pulses. The reservoir should be made of polyvinyl chloride, polypropylene, or glass. Immediate access to back up pump, infusion sets and medication is essential to prevent treatment interruptions.

When administered on an ongoing basis, must be infused through a central venous catheter. Peripheral infusion may be used temporarily until central line is established. Infuse using an infusion pump. Avoid abrupt withdrawal (including interruptions in delivery) or sudden large reductions in dosing.

Inhalation (off-label route):

Intraoperative administration: Administer via jet nebulizer connected to the inspiratory limb of the ventilator near the endotracheal tube with a bypass oxygen flow of 8 L/minute to achieve administration of a high proportion of small particles (Fattouch, 2006; Hache, 2003).

Post-cardiothoracic surgery: May also be administered via jet nebulizer connected to the inspiratory limb of the ventilator near the endotracheal tube or via face mask with a Venturi attachment for aerosolization with a bypass oxygen flow of 2-3 L/minute (De Wet, 2004). **Note:** Glycine buffer diluent may cause ventilator valve malfunction; it has been recommended that filters be changed on the ventilator every 2 hours; may also use a ventilator heating coil (De Wet, 2004).

Monitoring Parameters Monitor for improvements in pulmonary function, decreased exertional dyspnea, fatigue, syncope and chest pain, pulmonary vascular resistance, pulmonary arterial pressure and quality of life. In addition, the pump device and catheters should be monitored frequently to avoid "system" related failure. Monitor arterial pressure; assess all vital functions. Hypoxia, flushing, and tachycardia may indicate overdose.

Dosage Forms

Solution Reconstituted, Intravenous:

Flolan: 0.5 mg (1 ea); 1.5 mg (1 ea)

Veletri: 0.5 mg (1 ea); 1.5 mg (1 ea)

Generic: 0.5 mg (1 ea); 1.5 mg (1 ea)

Dosage Forms: Canada

Solution Reconstituted, Intravenous:

Caripul: 0.5 mg (1 ea); 1.5 mg (1 ea)

Flolan: 0.5 mg (1 ea); 1.5 mg (1 ea)

◆ **Epoprostenol Sodium** *see* Epoprostenol *on page 746*

◆ **Epothilone B Lactam** *see* Ixabepilone *on page 1138*

◆ **Eprex (Can)** *see* Epoetin Alfa *on page 742*

Eprosartan (ep roe SAR tan)

Brand Names: U.S. Teveten

Brand Names: Canada Teveten

Pharmacologic Category Angiotensin II Receptor Blocker; Antihypertensive

Use Hypertension: Treatment of hypertension; may be used alone or in combination with other antihypertensives

The 2014 guideline for the management of high blood pressure in adults (Eighth Joint National Committee [JNC 8; James, 2013]) recommends initiation of pharmacologic treatment to lower blood pressure for the following patients:

- Patients ≥60 years of age with systolic blood pressure (SBP) ≥150 mm Hg or diastolic blood pressure (DBP) ≥90 mm Hg. Goal of therapy is SBP <150 mm Hg and DBP <90 mm Hg.
- Patients <60 years of age with SBP ≥140 mm Hg or DBP ≥90 mm Hg. Goal of therapy is SBP <140 mm Hg and DBP <90 mm Hg.
- Patients ≥18 years of age with diabetes and SBP ≥140 mm Hg or DBP ≥90 mm Hg. Goal of therapy is SBP <140 mm Hg and DBP <90 mm Hg.
- Patients ≥18 years of age with chronic kidney disease (CKD) and SBP ≥140 mm Hg or DBP ≥90 mm Hg. Goal of therapy is SBP <140 mm Hg and DBP <90 mm Hg.

In patients with CKD, regardless of race or diabetes status, the use of an ACE inhibitor (ACEI) or angiotensin receptor blocker (ARB) as initial therapy is recommended to improve kidney outcomes. In the general nonblack population (without CKD), including those with diabetes, initial antihypertensive treatment should consist of a thiazide-type diuretic, calcium channel blocker, ACEI, or ARB. In the general black population (without CKD), including those with diabetes, initial antihypertensive treatment should consist of a thiazide-type diuretic or a calcium channel blocker instead of an ACEI or ARB.

Pregnancy Risk Factor D

Pregnancy Considerations **[U.S. Boxed Warning]: Drugs that act on the renin-angiotensin system can cause injury and death to the developing fetus. Discontinue as soon as possible once pregnancy is detected.** The use of drugs which act on the renin-angiotensin system are associated with oligohydramnios. Oligohydramnios, due to decreased fetal renal function, may lead to fetal lung hypoplasia and skeletal malformations. Use is also associated with anuria, hypotension, renal failure, skull hypoplasia, and death in the fetus/neonate. The exposed fetus should be monitored for fetal growth, amniotic fluid volume, and organ formation. Infants exposed *in utero* should be monitored for hyperkalemia, hypotension, and oliguria (exchange transfusions or dialysis may be needed). These adverse events are generally associated with maternal use in the second and third trimesters.

Untreated chronic maternal hypertension is also associated with adverse events in the fetus, infant, and mother. The use of angiotensin II receptor blockers is not recommended to treat chronic uncomplicated hypertension in pregnant women and should generally be avoided in women of reproductive potential (ACOG, 2013).

Breast-Feeding Considerations It is not known if eprosartan is excreted into breast milk. Due to the potential for serious adverse reactions in the nursing infant, the US manufacturer recommends a decision be made whether to discontinue nursing or to discontinue the drug, taking into account the importance of treatment to the mother. Canadian labeling contraindicates use in breast-feeding women.

Contraindications

Hypersensitivity to eprosartan or any component of the formulation; coadministration with aliskiren in patients with diabetes

Documentation of allergenic cross-reactivity for angiotensin II receptor blockers is limited. However, because of similarities in chemical structure and/or pharmacologic actions, the possibility of cross-sensitivity cannot be ruled out with certainty.

Canadian labeling: Additional contraindications (not in US labeling): Hemodynamically significant bilateral renovascular disease or severe stenosis of a solitary functioning kidney; hereditary problems of galactose intolerance, the Lapp lactase deficiency, or glucose-galactose malabsorption; concomitant use with aliskiren in patients with moderate to severe renal impairment (GFR <60 mL/minute/1.73 m^2); pregnancy; breast-feeding

Warnings/Precautions **[U.S. Boxed Warning]: Drugs that act on the renin-angiotensin system can cause injury and death to the developing fetus. Discontinue as soon as possible once pregnancy is detected.** May cause hyperkalemia; risk factors include renal dysfunction, diabetes mellitus, concomitant use of ACE inhibitors, aliskiren, potassium-sparing diuretics, potassium supplements and/or potassium containing salts. Use cautiously, if at all, with these agents and monitor potassium closely. Avoid ace inhibitors, aliskiren, and potassium supplementation unless specifically required by health care provider. Avoid use or use a smaller dose in patients who are volume depleted; correct depletion first. May be associated with deterioration of renal function and/or increases in serum creatinine, particularly in patients with low renal blood flow (eg, renal artery stenosis, heart failure) whose glomerular filtration rate (GFR) is dependent on efferent arteriolar vasoconstriction by angiotensin II. Use with caution in unstented unilateral/bilateral renal artery stenosis. When unstented bilateral renal artery stenosis is present, use is generally avoided due to the elevated risk of deterioration in renal function unless possible benefits outweigh risks. Use with caution in preexisting renal insufficiency; significant aortic/mitral stenosis. Potentially significant drug-drug interactions may exist, requiring dose or frequency adjustment, additional monitoring, and/or selection of alternative therapy. Concomitant use of an angiotensin-converting enzyme (ACE) inhibitor or renin inhibitor (eg, aliskiren) is associated with an increased risk of hypotension, hyperkalemia, and renal dysfunction; concomitant use with aliskiren should be avoided in patients with GFR <60 mL/minute and is contraindicated in patients with diabetes mellitus (regardless of GFR). In surgical patients on chronic angiotensin receptor blocker (ARB) therapy, intraoperative hypotension may occur with induction and maintenance of general anesthesia.

Angioedema has been reported rarely with some angiotensin II receptor antagonists (ARBs) and may occur at any time during treatment (especially following first dose). It may involve the head and neck (potentially compromising airway) or the intestine (presenting with abdominal pain). Patients with idiopathic or hereditary angioedema or previous angioedema associated with ACE-inhibitor therapy may be at an increased risk. Prolonged frequent monitoring may be required, especially if tongue, glottis, or larynx are involved, as they are associated with airway obstruction. Patients with a history of airway surgery may have a higher risk of airway obstruction. Discontinue therapy immediately if angioedema occurs. Aggressive early management is critical. Intramuscular (IM) administration of epinephrine may be necessary. Do not readminister to patients who have had angioedema with ARBs.

Adverse Reactions

Central nervous system: Depression, fatigue

Endocrine & metabolic: Hypertriglyceridemia

Gastrointestinal: Abdominal pain

Genitourinary: Urinary tract infection

Respiratory: Cough, pharyngitis, rhinitis, upper respiratory tract infection

Miscellaneous: Injury, viral infection

Rare but important or life-threatening: Abnormal ECG, angina, arthritis, asthma, ataxia, bradycardia, BUN increased, creatinine increased,eczema, edema, esophagitis, ethanol intolerance, gingivitis, gout, hypotension, influenza-like symptoms, leg cramps, leukopenia, maculopapular rash, migraine, neuritis, neutropenia, orthostasis, palpitation, paresthesia, peripheral ischemia, purpura, renal calculus, somnolence, tachycardia, tendonitis, thrombocytopenia, tinnitus, tremor, urinary incontinence, vertigo; rhabdomyolysis has been reported (rarely) with angiotensin-receptor antagonists.

Drug Interactions

Metabolism/Transport Effects **Inhibits** CYP2C9 (weak)

Avoid Concomitant Use There are no known interactions where it is recommended to avoid concomitant use.

Increased Effect/Toxicity

Eprosartan may increase the levels/effects of: ACE Inhibitors; Amifostine; Antihypertensives; CycloSPORINE (Systemic); DULoxetine; Hypotensive Agents; Levodopa; Lithium; Nonsteroidal Anti-Inflammatory Agents; Obinutuzumab; Potassium-Sparing Diuretics; RisperiDONE; RiTUXimab; Sodium Phosphates

The levels/effects of Eprosartan may be increased by: Alfuzosin; Aliskiren; Barbiturates; Brimonidine (Topical); Canagliflozin; Dapoxetine; Diazoxide; Eplerenone; Heparin; Heparin (Low Molecular Weight); Herbs (Hypotensive Properties); MAO Inhibitors; Nicorandil; Pentoxifylline; Phosphodiesterase 5 Inhibitors; Potassium Salts; Prostacyclin Analogues; Tolvaptan; Trimethoprim

Decreased Effect

The levels/effects of Eprosartan may be decreased by: Herbs (Hypertensive Properties); Methylphenidate; Nonsteroidal Anti-Inflammatory Agents; Yohimbine

Storage/Stability Store at 20°C to 25°C (68°F to 77°F).

Mechanism of Action Angiotensin II is formed from angiotensin I in a reaction catalyzed by angiotensin-converting enzyme (ACE, kininase II). Angiotensin II is the principal pressor agent of the renin-angiotensin system, with effects that include vasoconstriction, stimulation of synthesis and release of aldosterone, cardiac stimulation, and renal reabsorption of sodium. Eprosartan blocks the vasoconstrictor and aldosterone-secreting effects of angiotensin II by selectively blocking the binding of angiotensin II to the AT1 receptor in many tissues, such as vascular smooth muscle and the adrenal gland. Its action is therefore independent of the pathways for angiotensin II synthesis. Blockade of the renin-angiotensin system with ACE inhibitors, which inhibit the biosynthesis of angiotensin II from angiotensin I, is widely used in the treatment of hypertension. ACE inhibitors also inhibit the degradation of bradykinin, a reaction also catalyzed by ACE. Because eprosartan does not inhibit ACE (kininase II), it does not affect the response to bradykinin. Whether this difference has clinical relevance is not yet known. Eprosartan does not bind to or block other hormone receptors or ion channels known to be important in cardiovascular regulation.

Pharmacodynamics/Kinetics

Protein binding: 98%

Metabolism: Minimally hepatic

Bioavailability: 300 mg dose: 13%

Half-life elimination: Terminal: 5 to 9 hours (Bottorff, 1999)

Time to peak, serum: Fasting: 1 to 2 hours

Excretion: Feces (90%); urine (7%, mostly as unchanged drug)

Dosage Hypertension:

Adults: Oral: Dosage must be individualized; can administer once or twice daily with total daily doses of 400 to 800 mg. Usual starting dose is 600 mg once daily as monotherapy in patients who are euvolemic. Target dose (JNC 8 [James, 2013]): 600 to 800 mg daily in 1 or 2 divided doses. Limited clinical experience with doses >800 mg.

Elderly:

U.S. labeling: No initial dosage adjustment is necessary.

Canadian labeling: Consider decreasing initial dose to 400 mg once daily.

Dosage adjustment in renal impairment:

U.S. labeling:

Mild impairment: No initial dosage adjustment necessary.

Moderate to severe impairment: No initial dosage adjustment necessary; maximum dose: 600 mg daily

Hemodialysis: There are no dosage adjustments provided in the manufacturer's labeling; eprosartan is poorly removed by hemodialysis (Cl_{HD} <1 L/hour)

Canadian labeling:

CrCl ≥60 mL/minute: No dosage adjustment necessary.

CrCl 30 to 59 mL/minute: No initial dosage adjustment necessary; monitor closely. Maximum dose: 600 mg daily.

CrCl 5 to 29 mL/minute: Initial dose: Consider decreasing to 400 mg once daily; monitor closely. Maximum dose: 600 mg daily.

Hemodialysis: There are no dosage adjustments provided in manufacturer's labeling; eprosartan is poorly removed by hemodialysis (Cl_{HD} <1 L/hour)

Dosage adjustment in hepatic impairment:

U.S. labeling: No dosage adjustment necessary.

Canadian labeling: Consider decreasing initial dose to 400 mg once daily

Administration May be administered with or without food.

Monitoring Parameters Serum potassium, serum creatinine, BUN, urinalysis, blood pressure

Product Availability Teveten 400 mg tablets have been discontinued in the U.S. more than 1 year.

Dosage Forms

Tablet, Oral:

Teveten: 600 mg

Generic: 600 mg

Eprosartan and Hydrochlorothiazide

(ep roe SAR tan & hye droe klor oh THYE a zide)

Brand Names: U.S. Teveten HCT

Brand Names: Canada Teveten Plus

Index Terms Eprosartan Mesylate and Hydrochlorothiazide; Hydrochlorothiazide and Eprosartan

Pharmacologic Category Angiotensin II Receptor Blocker; Antihypertensive; Diuretic, Thiazide

Use Hypertension: Treatment of hypertension

Limitations of use: Not indicated for initial treatment.

Pregnancy Risk Factor D

Dosage Hypertension: Oral:

Adults: Dose is individualized (combination substituted for individual components): Usual recommended dose:

U.S. labeling: Eprosartan 600 mg/hydrochlorothiazide 12.5 mg once daily; may titrate to eprosartan 600 mg/hydrochlorothiazide 25 mg once daily if response is inadequate. If additional blood pressure control is needed or to maintain a twice-daily schedule of monotherapy, eprosartan 300 mg may be added as an evening dose.

Canadian labeling: Eprosartan 600 mg/hydrochlorothiazide 12.5 mg once daily. **Note:** Combination product is only available in one strength and may be used after successful titration of individual agents to corresponding dose. Dose titration is not possible with available dosage form.

Elderly:

U.S. labeling: No initial dosage adjustment necessary.

Canadian labeling: Consider decreasing initial dose of eprosartan (monotherapy) to 400 mg once daily

Dosage adjustment in renal impairment:

U.S. labeling:

Mild impairment: No initial dosage adjustment necessary.

Moderate-to-severe impairment: No initial dosage adjustments necessary. Maximum dose of eprosartan: 600 mg daily. Hydrochlorothiazide is ineffective in patients with CrCl <30 mL/minute.

Hemodialysis: There are no dosage adjustments provided in the manufacturer's labeling; eprosartan is poorly removed by hemodialysis (Cl_{HD} <1 L/hour)

Canadian labeling:

CrCl ≥30 mL/minute: No dosage adjustment necessary.

CrCl <30 mL/minute: Use is contraindicated.

Dosage adjustment in hepatic impairment:

US labeling: No dosage adjustments necessary; use with caution

Canadian labeling: Use is not recommended (contraindicated in severe impairment).

Additional Information Complete prescribing information should be consulted for additional detail.

Dosage Forms

Tablet:

Teveten® HCT: 600 mg/12.5 mg: Eprosartan 600 mg and hydrochlorothiazide 12.5 mg; 600 mg/25 mg: Eprosartan 600 mg and hydrochlorothiazide 25 mg

- ◆ **Eprosartan Mesylate and Hydrochlorothiazide** *see* Eprosartan and Hydrochlorothiazide *on page 750*
- ◆ **Epsilon Aminocaproic Acid** *see* Aminocaproic Acid *on page 113*
- ◆ **Epsom Salt [OTC]** *see* Magnesium Sulfate *on page 1265*
- ◆ **Epsom Salts** *see* Magnesium Sulfate *on page 1265*
- ◆ **EPT** *see* Teniposide *on page 1997*
- ◆ **Eptacog Alfa (Activated)** *see* Factor VIIa (Recombinant) *on page 836*

Eptaplatin [INT] (ep ta PLA tin)

International Brand Names Sunpla (KR)

Index Terms Heptaplatin; SKI-2053R

Pharmacologic Category Antineoplastic Agent, Alkylating Agent

Reported Use Small cell lung cancer; stomach, cervical, and colon cancer

Dosage Range Adults: IV: Refer to individual protocols: 360 mg/m^2 (range: 320-400 mg/m^2); schedule varies by protocol/indication

Product Availability Product available in various countries; not currently available in the U.S.

Dosage Forms

Vial: 50 mg

Eptifibatide (ep TIF i ba tide)

Brand Names: U.S. Integrilin

Brand Names: Canada Eptifibatide Injection; Integrilin

Index Terms Intrifiban

Pharmacologic Category Antiplatelet Agent, Glycoprotein IIb/IIIa Inhibitor

Use

Acute coronary syndrome: Treatment of patients with acute coronary syndrome (unstable angina/non-ST-segment elevation myocardial infarction [UA/NSTEMI]), including patients who are to be managed medically and those undergoing percutaneous coronary intervention (PCI)

Percutaneous coronary intervention: Treatment of patients undergoing PCI, including those undergoing intracoronary stenting.

Pregnancy Risk Factor B

Pregnancy Considerations Adverse events have not been observed in animal reproduction studies.

Breast-Feeding Considerations It is not known if eptifibatide is excreted in breast milk. The manufacturer recommends that caution be exercised when administering eptifibatide to nursing women.

Contraindications

Hypersensitivity to eptifibatide or any component of the formulation; active abnormal bleeding within the previous 30 days or a history of bleeding diathesis; history of stroke within 30 days or a history of hemorrhagic stroke; severe hypertension (systolic blood pressure >200 mm Hg or diastolic blood pressure >110 mm Hg) not adequately controlled on antihypertensive therapy; major surgery within the preceding 6 weeks; current or planned administration of another parenteral GP IIb/IIIa inhibitor; dependency on hemodialysis

Canadian labeling: Additional contraindications (not in U.S. labeling): PT >1.2 times control or INR ≥2.0; known history of intracranial disease (eg, neoplasm, arteriovenous malformation, aneurysm); severe renal impairment (CrCl <30 mL/minute); thrombocytopenia (<100,000 cells/mm^3); clinically significant liver disease

Warnings/Precautions The most common complication is bleeding, including retroperitoneal, pulmonary, and spontaneous GI and/or GU bleeding; monitor closely for bleeding, especially the arterial access site for the cardiac catheterization. Risk factors for bleeding include older age, a history of bleeding disorders, and concomitant use of drugs that increase the risk of bleeding (thrombolytics, oral anticoagulants, NSAIDs, and/or P2Y12 inhibitors). Patients caution with administration of other drugs affecting hemostasis. Minimize invasive procedures, including arterial and venous punctures, IM injections, and the use of urinary catheters, nasotracheal intubation and nasogastric tubes. Discontinue ≥2 to 4 hours prior to coronary artery bypass graft surgery (Hillis, 2011). Acute, profound thrombocytopenia (immune-mediated and nonimmune mediated) has occurred. Use with extreme caution in patients with platelet counts <100,000/mm^3 (contraindicated in the Canadian labeling). If platelet count decreases to <100,000/mm^3 during therapy, discontinue eptifibatide and heparin if administered concurrently.

Prior to sheath removal, heparin should be discontinued for 3 to 4 hours and the aPTT or ACT should be checked (do not remove unless aPTT is <50 seconds or the ACT <180 seconds). Of note, full dose anticoagulation is no longer used after successful PCI procedures (ACCF/AHA/SCAI [Levine, 2011]). Use caution in renal dysfunction (estimated CrCl <50 mL/minute, using Cockcroft-Gault equation); dosage adjustment required. Use is contraindicated in patients dependent upon hemodialysis. Hypersensitivity reactions have occurred, including anaphylaxis and urticaria. Potentially significant drug-drug interactions may exist, requiring dose or frequency adjustment, additional monitoring, and/or selection of alternative therapy.

Adverse Reactions Bleeding is the major drug-related adverse effect. Incidence of bleeding is also related to heparin intensity (aPTT goal 50-70 seconds). Patients weighing <70 kg may have an increased risk of major bleeding.

Cardiovascular: Hypotension

Hematologic: Bleeding, thrombocytopenia

Local: Injection site reaction

Rare but important or life-threatening: Acute profound thrombocytopenia (including immune-mediated thrombocytopenia), fatal bleeding events, GI hemorrhage, pulmonary hemorrhage

Drug Interactions

Metabolism/Transport Effects None known.

Avoid Concomitant Use

Avoid concomitant use of Eptifibatide with any of the following: Urokinase

Increased Effect/Toxicity

Eptifibatide may increase the levels/effects of: Agents with Antiplatelet Properties; Anticoagulants; Apixaban; Collagenase (Systemic); Dabigatran Etexilate; Ibritumomab; Obinutuzumab; Rivaroxaban; Salicylates; Thrombolytic Agents; Tositumomab and Iodine I 131 Tositumomab; Urokinase

The levels/effects of Eptifibatide may be increased by: Dasatinib; Glucosamine; Herbs (Anticoagulant/Antiplatelet Properties); Ibrutinib; Limaprost; Multivitamins/Fluoride (with ADE); Multivitamins/Minerals (with ADEK, Folate, Iron); Multivitamins/Minerals (with AE, No Iron); Omega-3 Fatty Acids; Pentosan Polysulfate Sodium; Pentoxifylline; Prostacyclin Analogues; Tipranavir; Vitamin E

Decreased Effect There are no known significant interactions involving a decrease in effect.

Storage/Stability Vials should be stored refrigerated at 2°C to 8°C (36°F to 46°F). Vials can be kept at room temperature for 2 months, after which they must be discarded. Protect from light until administration. Do not use beyond the expiration date. Discard any unused portion left in the vial.

Mechanism of Action Eptifibatide is a cyclic heptapeptide which blocks the platelet glycoprotein IIb/IIIa receptor, the binding site for fibrinogen, von Willebrand factor, and other ligands. Inhibition of binding at this final common receptor reversibly blocks platelet aggregation and prevents thrombosis.

Pharmacodynamics/Kinetics

Onset of action: Immediate after initial bolus (>80% inhibition of ADP-induced aggregation achieved 5 minutes after bolus dose); maximal effect achieved within 1 hour (Gilchrist, 2001; Tardiff, 2001)

Duration: Platelet function restored ~4 to 8 hours following discontinuation (Tardiff, 2001)

Protein binding: ~25%

Half-life elimination: ~2.5 hours

Excretion: Primarily urine (as eptifibatide and metabolites)

Clearance: Total body: ~55 mL/kg/hour; Renal: ~50% of total body clearance in healthy subjects

Dosage IV: Adults:

Acute coronary syndrome: 180 mcg/kg bolus (maximum: 22.6 mg) administered as soon as possible following diagnosis, followed by a continuous infusion of 2 mcg/kg/minute (maximum: 15 mg/hour) until hospital discharge or initiation of CABG surgery (discontinue ≥2 to 4 hours before surgery (ACCF/AHA [Hillis, 2011]), up to 72 hours. If PCI performed during initial 72 hours, maintain continuous infusion at the time of PCI and continue until hospital discharge or for up to 18 to 24 hours, whichever comes first (total infusion time ≤96 hours). Concurrent aspirin and heparin therapy (target aPTT 50 to 70 seconds) are recommended. **Note:** If UA/NSTEMI, administration ≥12 hours before angiography was shown not to be superior to provisional use at the time of PCI and has a higher incidence of bleeding (Giugliano, 2009).

Percutaneous coronary intervention (PCI) with or without stenting: 180 mcg/kg bolus (maximum: 22.6 mg) administered immediately before the initiation of PCI, followed by a continuous infusion of 2 mcg/kg/minute (maximum: 15 mg/hour). A second 180 mcg/kg bolus (maximum: 22.6 mg) should be administered 10 minutes after the first bolus. Infusion should be continued until hospital discharge or for up to 18 to 24 hours, whichever comes first; shorter infusion durations (ie, <2 hours) may be considered for nonemergent uncomplicated PCI in patients adequately pretreated with clopidogrel (Fung, 2007). Preprocedural aspirin and heparin therapy (ACT 200 to 250 seconds during PCI) and daily aspirin are recommended. Heparin infusion after PCI is discouraged. In patients who undergo CABG surgery, discontinue infusion ≥2 to 4 hours prior to surgery (ACCF/AHA [Hillis, 2011]).

Primary percutaneous coronary intervention (PCI) during ST-elevation myocardial infarction with or without stenting or pretreatment with clopidogrel (off-label use): Bolus of 180 mcg/kg (maximum: 22.6 mg) administered at the time of PCI, followed by a continuous infusion of 2 mcg/kg/minute (maximum: 15 mg/hour) in combination with heparin or bivalirudin. A second 180 mcg/kg bolus (maximum: 22.6 mg) should be administered 10 minutes after the first bolus (ACCF/AHA [O'Gara, 2013]). Infusion was continued for 24 hours in one study (Zeymer, 2010).

Elderly: No dosing adjustment for the elderly appears to be necessary; adjust carefully to renal function.

Dosage adjustment in renal impairment:

Note: The Cockcroft-Gault equation using actual body weight should be used to estimate renal function.

Acute coronary syndrome:

CrCl ≥50 mL/minute: No dosage adjustment necessary.

CrCl <50 mL/minute: 180 mcg/kg bolus (maximum: 22.6 mg) administered as soon as possible following diagnosis, followed by a continuous infusion of 1 mcg/kg/minute (maximum: 7.5 mg/hour)

End-stage renal disease (ie, dialysis dependent): Use is contraindicated.

Percutaneous coronary intervention (PCI) with or without stenting:

CrCl ≥50 mL/minute: No dosage adjustment necessary.

CrCl <50 mL/minute: 180 mcg/kg bolus (maximum: 22.6 mg) administered immediately before the initiation of PCI and followed by a continuous infusion of 1 mcg/kg/minute (maximum: 7.5 mg/hour). Administer a second 180 mcg/kg (maximum: 22.6 mg) bolus 10 minutes after the first bolus

End-stage renal disease (ie, dialysis dependent): Use is contraindicated.

Dosage adjustment in hepatic impairment: There are no dosage adjustments provided in the manufacturer's labeling (has not been studied).

Administration Bolus dose should be withdrawn from the 10 mL vial into a syringe and administered by IV push. Begin continuous infusion (using an IV infusion pump) immediately following bolus administration, administered undiluted directly from the 100 mL vial. The 100 mL vial should be spiked with a vented infusion set.

Monitoring Parameters Coagulation parameters, signs/symptoms of excessive bleeding. Laboratory tests at baseline and monitoring during therapy: hematocrit and hemoglobin, platelet count, serum creatinine, PT/aPTT (maintain aPTT between 50-70 seconds unless PCI is to be performed), and ACT with PCI (maintain ACT between 200-300 seconds during PCI).

Assess sheath insertion site and distal pulses of affected leg every 15 minutes for the first hour and then every 1 hour for the next 6 hours. Arterial access site care is important to prevent bleeding. Care should be taken when attempting vascular access that only the anterior wall of the femoral artery is punctured, avoiding a Seldinger (through and through) technique for obtaining sheath access. Femoral vein sheath placement should be avoided unless needed. While the vascular sheath is in place, patients should be maintained on complete bedrest with the head of the bed at a 30° angle and the affected limb restrained in a straight position.

Observe patient for mental status changes, hemorrhage, assess nose and mouth mucous membranes, puncture sites for oozing, ecchymosis and hematoma formation, and examine urine, stool and emesis for presence of occult or frank blood; gentle care should be provided when removing dressings.

Dosage Forms

Solution, Intravenous:

Integrilin: 0.75 mg/mL (100 mL); 2 mg/mL (10 mL, 100 mL)

- ◆ **Eptifibatide Injection (Can)** *see* Eptifibatide *on page 751*
- ◆ **Epuris (Can)** *see* ISOtretinoin *on page 1127*
- ◆ **Epzicom** *see* Abacavir and Lamivudine *on page 22*
- ◆ **Equanil** *see* Meprobamate *on page 1296*
- ◆ **Equetro** *see* CarBAMazepine *on page 346*
- ◆ **ER-086526** *see* Eribulin *on page 755*
- ◆ **Eraxis** *see* Anidulafungin *on page 150*
- ◆ **Erbitux** *see* Cetuximab *on page 413*
- ◆ **Erdol (Can)** *see* Ergocalciferol *on page 753*

Erdosteine [INT] (ER do stine)

International Brand Names A Duo Ting (CN); Biopulmin (CL); Dostin (PK); Dostol (EC); Ectrin (PH); Edopect (ID); Eldostam (KR); Erdine (KR); Erdobat (ID); Erdoce (KR); Erdomac (IN); Erdomed (AT, BG, CZ, HN, PL, RO, SK); Erdopect (FI); Erdos (KR, TH); Erdotin (DK, GB, IE, IL, IT, PT); Erdozets (IN); Ertusin (ID); Fluidasa (AR); Lactrin (ID); Mucodox (BE); Mucofor (CH); Mucotec (QA); SP Edonal (VN); Theovix (GR); Vectrine (FR, ID, VN); Vestein (ID); Zertin (PH)

Pharmacologic Category Mucolytic Agent

Reported Use Acute and chronic airway diseases such as bronchitis, rhinitis, sinusitis, laryngopharyngitis, and exacerbations of chronic bronchitis; preventive treatment of stable and chronic bronchitis in smokers; recurrent infectious episodes and related conditions; co-treatment with antibiotics in cases of bacterial exacerbations

Dosage Range Adults: Oral: 300 mg twice daily

Product Availability Product available in various countries; not currently available in the U.S.

Dosage Forms

Capsule: 300 mg

Ergocalciferol (er goe kal SIF e role)

Brand Names: U.S. Calcidol [OTC]; Calciferol [OTC]; Drisdol; Drisdol [OTC]

Brand Names: Canada D-Forte; Erdol

Index Terms Activated Ergosterol; D2; Viosterol; Vitamin D2

Pharmacologic Category Vitamin D Analog

Use

Dietary supplement: For use as a vitamin D supplement.

Familial hypophosphatemia: Treatment of familial hypophosphatemia.

Hypoparathyroidism: Treatment of hypoparathyroidism.

Rickets: Treatment of refractory rickets, also known as vitamin D-resistant rickets.

Pregnancy Risk Factor C

Dosage Oral: **Note:** 1 mcg = 40 units

Dietary Reference Intake for Vitamin D:

Infants 0 to 12 months: Adequate intake: 400 units/day (IOM, 2011)

Breast-fed (fully or partially) Infants: Oral: 10 mcg/day (400 units/day) beginning in the first few days of life; continue supplementation until infant is weaned to ≥1 L/day or 1 quart/day of vitamin D-fortified formula or whole milk (after 12 months of age) (Wagner, 2008)

Nonbreast-fed Infants, Older Children ingesting <1000 mL of vitamin D-fortified formula or milk: Oral: 10 mcg/day (400 units/day) (Wagner, 2008)

Children with increased risk of vitamin D deficiency (chronic fat malabsorption, maintained on chronic antiseizure medications): Oral: Higher doses may be required; use laboratory testing [25 (OH)D, PTH, bone mineral status] to evaluate (Wagner, 2008)

Children and Adolescents 1 to 18 years: RDA: 600 units/day (IOM, 2011)

Adults:

19 to 70 years: RDA: 600 units/day (IOM, 2011)

Pregnancy/Lactating: RDA: 600 units/day (IOM, 2011)

Elderly >70 years: RDA: 800 units/day (IOM, 2011)

Osteoporosis prevention (off-label use): Adults ≥50 years: 800 to 1000 units/day (NOF guidelines, 2014)

Vitamin D deficiency treatment (off-label dose) (Holick, 2011):

Infants 0 to 1 year: 2000 units daily or 50,000 units once weekly for 6 weeks to achieve a 25(OH)D level >30 ng/mL; then maintenance dose of 400 to 1000 units daily.

Children and Adolescents 1 to 18 years: 2000 units daily or 50,000 units once weekly for at least 6 weeks to achieve a 25(OH)D level >30 ng/mL; then maintenance dose of 600 to 1000 units daily.

Adults: 6000 units daily or 50,000 units once weekly for at least 8 weeks to achieve a 25(OH)D level >30 ng/mL; then maintenance dose of 1500 to 2000 units daily.

Special populations (obese patients, patients on medications known to affect vitamin D metabolism, patients with malabsorption syndromes): 6000 to 10,000 units daily to achieve a 25(OH)D level >30 ng/mL; then maintenance dose of 3000 to 6000 units daily

Vitamin D deficiency/insufficiency in patients with CKD stages 3 to 4 (K/DOQI guidelines): **Note:** Dose is based on 25-hydroxyvitamin D serum level (25[OH]D):

Children (treatment duration should be a total of 3 months) (K/DOQI, 2005):

Serum 25(OH)D <5 ng/mL:

8000 units/day for 4 weeks, then 4000 units/day for 2 months **or**

50,000 units/week for 4 weeks, then 50,000 units twice a month for 2 months

Serum 25(OH)D 5 to 15 ng/mL:

4000 int units/day **or**

50,000 int units every other week

Serum 25(OH)D 16 to 30 ng/mL:

2000 units/day **or**

50,000 units every 4 weeks

Adults (treatment duration should be a total of 6 months) (K/DOQI, 2003):

Serum 25(OH)D <5 ng/mL:

50,000 units/week for 12 weeks, then 50,000 units/month

Serum 25(OH)D 5 to 15 ng/mL:

50,000 units/week for 4 weeks, then 50,000 units/month

Serum 25(OH)D 16 to 30 ng/mL:

50,000 units/month

Hypoparathyroidism: Children, Adolescents, and Adults: 1.25 to 5 mg/day (50,000 to 200,000 units) with calcium supplements

Vitamin D-*resistant* rickets: Children, Adolescents, and Adults: 12,000 to 500,000 units/day

Dosage adjustment in renal impairment: There are no dosage adjustments provided in the manufacturer's labeling.

Dosage adjustment in hepatic impairment: There are no dosage adjustments provided in manufacturer's labeling.

Additional Information Complete prescribing information should be consulted for additional detail.

Dosage Forms

Capsule, Oral:

Drisdol: 50,000 units

Generic: 50,000 units

Solution, Oral:

Calcidol [OTC]: 8000 units/mL (60 mL)

Calciferol [OTC]: 8000 units/mL (60 mL)

Drisdol [OTC]: 8000 units/mL (60 mL)

Generic: 8000 units/mL (60 mL)

Tablet, Oral:

Generic: 400 units, 2000 units

◆ **Ergomar** *see* Ergotamine *on page 754*

◆ **Ergometrine Maleate** *see* Ergonovine [CAN/INT] *on page 754*

Ergonovine [CAN/INT] (er goe NOE veen)

Brand Names: Canada Ergonovine Maleate Injection

Index Terms Ergometrine Maleate; Ergonovine Maleate

Pharmacologic Category Ergot Derivative

Use Note: Not approved in U.S.

Prevention and treatment of postpartum and postabortion hemorrhage caused by uterine atony

Pregnancy Considerations Ergonovine is used in the third stage of labor for the prevention or treatment of postpartum hemorrhage and should not be used prior to delivery of the placenta. Prior to administration, the placenta should be delivered and the possibility of twin pregnancy ruled out. Administration causes hyperstimulation of the uterus and may cause uterine tetany, decreased uteroplacental blood flow, uterine rupture, cervical and perineal lacerations, amniotic fluid embolism, and possible trauma to the infant.

Breast-Feeding Considerations May cause ergotism in breast-feeding infants. The manufacturer labeling states that breast-feeding is contraindicated when more than a single dose of ergonovine is administered to the postpartum mother. Administration of a single dose of ergonovine does not preclude a mother from nursing.

Contraindications Hypersensitivity to ergonovine, other ergot preparations, or any component of the formulation; ergot alkaloids are contraindicated with potent inhibitors of CYP3A4 (includes protease inhibitors, azole antifungals, and some macrolide antibiotics); induction of labor, threatened spontaneous abortion, pregnancy, toxemia; hypertension; breast-feeding (if >1 dose is administered)

Warnings/Precautions Hazardous agent - use appropriate precautions for handling and disposal (NIOSH 2014 [group 3]). Use caution in patients with sepsis, obliterative vascular disease, cardiovascular disease, hepatic or renal involvement, or second stage of labor; administer with extreme caution if using intravenously. Pleural and peritoneal fibrosis have been reported with prolonged daily use. Cardiac valvular fibrosis has also been associated with ergot alkaloids. Ergot alkaloid use may result in ergotism (intense vasoconstriction) resulting in peripheral vascular ischemia and possible gangrene. Concomitant use with potent inhibitors of CYP3A4 (includes protease inhibitors, azole antifungals, and some macrolide antibiotics) and ergot alkaloids has been associated with acute ergot toxicity (ergotism); the product labeling for various potent CYP3A4 inhibitors (eg, ritonavir, clarithromycin, itraconazole) contraindicates concomitant use with ergot derivatives. Use with caution in the elderly. Restore uterine responsiveness in calcium-deficient patients who do not respond to ergonovine by IV calcium administration.

Adverse Reactions

Cardiovascular: Angina (transient), bradycardia, hypertension, MI, palpitation, shock, thrombophlebitis

Central nervous system: Dizziness, hallucination, headache, vertigo

Endocrine & metabolic: Water intoxication

Gastrointestinal: Abdominal pain, diarrhea, nausea, vomiting

Renal: Hematuria

Respiratory: Dyspnea

Miscellaneous: Allergic reactions, diaphoresis, ergotism

Drug Interactions

Metabolism/Transport Effects Substrate of CYP3A4 (major); **Note:** Assignment of Major/Minor substrate status based on clinically relevant drug interaction potential

Avoid Concomitant Use

Avoid concomitant use of Ergonovine with any of the following: Alpha-/Beta-Agonists; Alpha1-Agonists; Boceprevir; Conivaptan; Dapoxetine; Fusidic Acid (Systemic); Idelalisib; Itraconazole; Ketoconazole (Systemic); Lorcaserin; Nitroglycerin; Posaconazole; Protease Inhibitors; Serotonin 5-HT1D Receptor Agonists; Telaprevir; Voriconazole

Increased Effect/Toxicity

Ergonovine may increase the levels/effects of: Alpha-/Beta-Agonists; Alpha1-Agonists; Antipsychotic Agents; Metoclopramide; Serotonin 5-HT1D Receptor Agonists; Serotonin Modulators

The levels/effects of Ergonovine may be increased by: Antiemetics (5HT3 Antagonists); Antipsychotic Agents; Aprepitant; Beta-Blockers; Boceprevir; Ceritinib; Conivaptan; CYP3A4 Inhibitors (Moderate); CYP3A4 Inhibitors (Strong); Dapoxetine; Dasatinib; Fosaprepitant; Fusidic Acid (Systemic); Idelalisib; Itraconazole; Ivacaftor; Ketoconazole (Systemic); Lorcaserin; Luliconazole; Macrolide Antibiotics; Mifepristone; Netupitant; Nitroglycerin; Posaconazole; Protease Inhibitors; Serotonin 5-HT1D Receptor Agonists; Simeprevir; Stiripentol; Tedizolid; Telaprevir; Voriconazole

Decreased Effect

Ergonovine may decrease the levels/effects of: Nitroglycerin

Storage/Stability Store at 2°C to 8°C (36°F to 46°F). Protect from light.

Mechanism of Action Similar smooth muscle actions as seen with ergotamine; however, it affects primarily uterine smooth muscles producing sustained contractions and thereby shortens the third stage of labor.

Pharmacodynamics/Kinetics

Onset of action: IM: 2-3 minutes; IV: 1 minute

Duration: IM: Uterine effect: 3 hours; IV: ~45 minutes

Dosage Adults: IM, IV (IV should be reserved for emergency use only): 0.2 mg, may repeat dose in 2-4 hours if needed, up to maximum of 5 total doses

Administration May be administered by IV or IM injection. IV use should be limited to patients with severe uterine bleeding or other life-threatening emergency situations. IV doses should be administered over a period of not <1 minute.

Hazardous agent; use appropriate precautions for handling and disposal (NIOSH 2014 [group 3]).

Monitoring Parameters Blood pressure, pulse, uterine response; cramping

Product Availability Not available in the U.S.

Dosage Forms: Canada

Injection, solution: 0.25 mg/mL (1 mL)

◆ **Ergonovine Maleate** *see* Ergonovine [CAN/INT] *on page 754*

◆ **Ergonovine Maleate Injection (Can)** *see* Ergonovine [CAN/INT] *on page 754*

Ergotamine (er GOT a meen)

Brand Names: U.S. Ergomar

Index Terms Ergotamine Tartrate

Pharmacologic Category Antimigraine Agent; Ergot Derivative

Use Abort or prevent vascular headaches, such as migraine, migraine variants, or so-called "histaminic cephalalgia"

Pregnancy Risk Factor X

Dosage Migraine: Adults: Sublingual: 2 mg (1 tablet) under tongue at first sign of migraine, then 2 mg every 30 minutes if needed; maximum dose: 6 mg per 24 hours, 10 mg per week

Dosage adjustment in renal impairment: Use is contraindicated in patients with impaired renal function.

Dosage adjustment in hepatic impairment: Use is contraindicated in patients with impaired hepatic function.

Additional Information Complete prescribing information should be consulted for additional detail.

Dosage Forms

Tablet Sublingual, Sublingual:

Ergomar: 2 mg

◆ **Ergotamine Tartrate** *see* Ergotamine *on page 754*

Eribulin (er i BUE lin)

Brand Names: U.S. Halaven

Brand Names: Canada Halaven

Index Terms B1939; E7389; ER-086526; Eribulin Mesylate; Halichondrin B Analog

Pharmacologic Category Antineoplastic Agent, Antimicrotubular

Use Breast cancer, metastatic: Treatment of metastatic breast cancer in patients who have received at least 2 prior chemotherapy regimens for the treatment of metastatic disease (prior treatment should have included an anthracycline and a taxane in either the adjuvant or metastatic setting)

Pregnancy Risk Factor D

Pregnancy Considerations Adverse effects were observed in animal reproduction studies. Based on its mechanism of action, eribulin would be expected to cause fetal harm if administered during pregnancy. Women of childbearing potential should use effective contraception to avoid pregnancy during eribulin treatment; the Canadian labeling recommends continuing effective contraception for at least 3 months after treatment.

Breast-Feeding Considerations It is not known if eribulin is excreted in breast milk. Due to the potential for serious adverse reactions in the nursing infant, a decision should be made to discontinue eribulin or to discontinue breast-feeding, taking into account the importance of treatment to the mother.

Contraindications There are no contraindications listed in the manufacturer's labeling.

Canadian labeling (not in U.S. labeling): Hypersensitivity to eribulin mesylate, halichondrin B, or its chemical derivatives.

Warnings/Precautions Hazardous agent - use appropriate precautions for handling and disposal (NIOSH 2014 [group 1]). Hematologic toxicity, including severe neutropenia, has occurred; may require treatment delay and dosage reduction. A higher incidence of grade 4 neutropenia and neutropenic fever occurred in patients with ALT or AST >3 x ULN or bilirubin >1.5 x ULN. Monitor complete blood counts prior to each dose; more frequently if severe cytopenias develop. Patients with baseline neutrophils <1,500/mm^3 were not included in clinical studies.

Peripheral neuropathy commonly occurs and is the most frequent toxicity leading to discontinuation. Peripheral neuropathy may be prolonged (>1 year in 5% of patients); may require treatment delay. Monitor for signs of peripheral motor or sensory neuropathy. Some patients may have preexisting neuropathy because of prior chemotherapy; monitor closely for worsening.

QT prolongation was observed on day 8 of eribulin therapy (in an uncontrolled study); monitor ECG in patients with heart failure, bradyarrhythmia, with concomitant medication known to prolong the QT interval, or with electrolyte imbalance; correct hypokalemia and hypomagnesemia prior to treatment; monitor electrolytes periodically during treatment. Avoid use in patients with congenital long QT syndrome.

Dosage reduction required in patients with mild to moderate (Child-Pugh class A or B) hepatic impairment; use has not been studied in patients with severe hepatic impairment; transaminase or bilirubin elevations are associated with a higher incidence of grade 4 neutropenia and neutropenic fever. Dosage reduction required in patients with moderate or severe renal impairment (CrCl 15 to 49 mL/minute). Potentially significant drug-drug interactions may exist, requiring dose or frequency adjustment, additional monitoring, and/or selection of alternative therapy. Some products available internationally may have vial strength and dosing expressed as the base (instead of as the salt); refer to prescribing information for specific dosing information.

Adverse Reactions

Cardiovascular: Peripheral edema

Central nervous system: Depression, dizziness, fatigue, headache, insomnia, myasthenia, peripheral neuropathy

Dermatologic: Alopecia, skin rash

Endocrine & metabolic: Hypokalemia, weight loss

Gastrointestinal: Abdominal pain, anorexia, constipation, diarrhea, dysgeusia, dyspepsia, mucosal inflammation, nausea, stomatitis, vomiting, xerostomia

Genitourinary: Urinary tract infection

Hematologic & oncologic: Anemia, febrile neutropenia, neutropenia, thrombocytopenia

Hepatic: Increased serum ALT

Neuromuscular & skeletal: Arthralgia, back pain, limb pain, muscle spasm, myalgia, ostealgia, weakness

Ophthalmic: Increased lacrimation

Respiratory: Cough, dyspnea, upper respiratory tract infection

Miscellaneous: Fever

Rare but important or life-threatening: Dehydration, drug-induced hypersensitivity, hepatotoxicity, hypomagnesemia, interstitial pulmonary disease, lymphocytopenia, pancreatitis, pneumonia, prolonged Q-T interval on ECG, sepsis

Drug Interactions

Metabolism/Transport Effects Substrate of CYP3A4 (minor); **Note:** Assignment of Major/Minor substrate status based on clinically relevant drug interaction potential; **Inhibits** CYP3A4 (weak)

Avoid Concomitant Use

Avoid concomitant use of EriBULin with any of the following: CloZAPine; Dipyrone; Highest Risk QTc-Prolonging Agents; Ivabradine; Mifepristone; Pimozide

Increased Effect/Toxicity

EriBULin may increase the levels/effects of: ARIPiprazole; CloZAPine; Highest Risk QTc-Prolonging Agents; Hydrocodone; Lomitapide; Moderate Risk QTc-Prolonging Agents; Pimozide

The levels/effects of EriBULin may be increased by: Dipyrone; Ivabradine; Mifepristone; QTc-Prolonging Agents (Indeterminate Risk and Risk Modifying)

Decreased Effect There are no known significant interactions involving a decrease in effect.

Preparation for Administration Hazardous agent; use appropriate precautions for handling and disposal (NIOSH 2014 [group 1]). No dilution required. May prepare by drawing into a syringe for administration or may dilute in 100 mL normal saline. Discard unused portion of vial.

Storage/Stability Store intact vials at 25°C (77°F); excursions permitted between 15°C and 30°C (59°F and 86°F); do not freeze. Store in original carton. Undiluted solutions in a syringe and solutions diluted in normal saline for infusion are stable for up to 4 hours at room temperature or up to 24 hours refrigerated at 4°C (40°F).

Mechanism of Action Eribulin is a non-taxane microtubule inhibitor which is a halichondrin B analog. It inhibits the growth phase of the microtubule by inhibiting formation of mitotic spindles causing mitotic blockage and arresting the cell cycle at the G_2/M phase; suppresses microtubule polymerization yet does not affect depolymerization.

Pharmacodynamics/Kinetics

Distribution: V_d: 43 to 114 L/m^2

Protein binding: 49% to 65%

Metabolism: Negligible

Half-life, elimination: ~40 hours

Excretion: Feces (82%, predominantly as unchanged drug); urine (9%, primarily as unchanged drug)

Dosage Note: *International Considerations:* Some products available internationally may have vial strength and dosing expressed as the base (instead of as the salt). Refer to prescribing information for specific dosing information.

Breast cancer, metastatic: Adults: IV: Eribulin mesylate: 1.4 mg/m^2/dose on days 1 and 8 of a 21-day treatment cycle

Dosing adjustment in toxicity:

ANC <1,000/mm^3 or platelets <75,000/mm^3 or grade 3 or 4 nonhematologic toxicity on day 1 or 8: Withhold dose; may delay day 8 dose up to 1 week. If toxicity resolves to ≤ grade 2 by day 15, administer a reduced dose and wait at least 2 weeks before beginning the next cycle. Omit dose if not resolved to ≤ grade 2 by day 15. Do not re-escalate dose after reduction.

Permanently reduce dose from eribulin mesylate 1.4 mg/m^2 to 1.1 mg/m^2 for the following:

ANC <500/mm^3 for >7 days

ANC <1,000/mm^3 with fever or infection

Platelets <25,000/mm^3

Platelets <50,000/mm^3 requiring transfusion

Nonhematologic toxicity of grade 3 or 4

Dose omission or delay due to toxicity on day 8 of prior cycle

Permanently reduce dose from eribulin mesylate 1.1 mg/m^2 to 0.7 mg/m^2 for occurrence of any of the above events; discontinue treatment if the above toxicities occur at the 0.7 mg/m^2 dose level.

Dosage adjustment in renal impairment:

Mild impairment (CrCl ≥50 mL/minute): No dosage adjustment required.

Moderate impairment (CrCl 30 to 49 mL/minute): Reduce to eribulin mesylate 1.1 mg/m^2/dose

Severe impairment (CrCl 15 to 29 mL/minute): Reduce to eribulin mesylate 1.1 mg/m^2/dose

ESRD (*Canadian labeling*): Use is not recommended.

Dosage adjustment in hepatic impairment:

Mild hepatic impairment (Child-Pugh class A): Reduce to eribulin mesylate 1.1 mg/m^2/dose

Moderate hepatic impairment (Child-Pugh class B): Reduce to eribulin mesylate 0.7 mg/m^2/dose

Severe hepatic impairment (Child-Pugh class C): There are no dosage adjustments provided in the manufacturer's U.S. labeling (has not been studied); use is not recommended in the Canadian labeling.

Dosing in obesity: *ASCO Guidelines for appropriate chemotherapy dosing in obese adults with cancer:* Utilize patient's actual body weight (full weight) for calculation of body surface area- or weight-based dosing, particularly when the intent of therapy is curative; manage regimen-related toxicities in the same manner as for nonobese patients; if a dose reduction is utilized due to toxicity, consider resumption of full weight-based dosing with subsequent cycles, especially if cause of toxicity (eg, hepatic or renal impairment) is resolved (Griggs, 2012).

Administration IV: Infuse over 2 to 5 minutes. May be administered undiluted or diluted. Do not administer other medications through the same IV line, or through a line containing dextrose.

Hazardous agent; use appropriate precautions for handling and disposal (NIOSH 2014 [group 1]).

Monitoring Parameters CBC with differential prior to each dose; renal and liver function tests; serum electrolytes, including potassium and magnesium. Assess for peripheral neuropathy prior to each dose. Monitor ECG in patients with heart failure, bradyarrhythmia, with concomitant medication known to prolong the QT interval, and electrolyte abnormalities (eg, hypokalemia, hypomagnesemia).

Additional Information *International considerations:* Eribulin mesylate 1.4 mg is equivalent to eribulin (base) 1.23 mg.

Dosage Forms

Solution, Intravenous:

Halaven: 1 mg/2 mL (2 mL)

- **Eribulin Mesylate** *see* Eribulin *on page 755*
- **Erivedge** *see* Vismodegib *on page 2171*

Erlotinib (er LOE tye nib)

Brand Names: U.S. Tarceva

Brand Names: Canada Tarceva

Index Terms CP358774; Erlotinib Hydrochloride; OSI-774

Pharmacologic Category Antineoplastic Agent, Epidermal Growth Factor Receptor (EGFR) Inhibitor; Antineoplastic Agent, Tyrosine Kinase Inhibitor

Use

Non-small cell lung cancer (NSCLC): First-line treatment of metastatic non-small cell lung cancer (NSCLC) in tumors with epidermal growth factor receptor (EGFR) exon 19 deletions or exon 21 (L858R) substitution mutations as detected by an approved test; treatment of locally advanced or metastatic NSCLC after failure of at least 1 prior chemotherapy regimen; maintenance treatment of locally advanced or metastatic NSCLC which has not progressed after 4 cycles of first-line platinum-based chemotherapy

Limitations of use: Use in combination with platinum-based chemotherapy is not recommended. First-line treatment in patients with metastatic NSCLC with EGFR mutations other than exon 19 deletion or exon 21 (L858R) substitution has not been evaluated.

Pancreatic cancer (not an approved use in Canada): First-line treatment of locally advanced, unresectable, or metastatic pancreatic cancer (in combination with gemcitabine)

Pregnancy Risk Factor D

Pregnancy Considerations Adverse events were observed in animal reproduction studies. Based on the mechanism of action, may cause fetal harm if administered in pregnancy. Females of reproductive potential should be advised to avoid pregnancy; highly effective contraception is recommended during treatment and for at least 2 weeks after treatment has been completed.

Breast-Feeding Considerations It is not known if erlotinib is excreted in breast milk. Due to the potential for serious adverse reactions in the nursing infant, the decision to discontinue breast-feeding or discontinue erlotinib should take into account the benefits of treatment to the mother.

Contraindications

There are no contraindications listed in the manufacturer's U.S. labeling.

Canadian labeling: Hypersensitivity to erlotinib or any component of the formulation

Warnings/Precautions Hazardous agent - use appropriate precautions for handling and disposal (NIOSH 2014 [group 1]). Rare, sometimes fatal, interstitial lung disease (ILD) has occurred; symptoms include acute respiratory distress syndrome, interstitial pneumonia, obliterative bronchiolitis, pneumonitis (including radiation and hypersensitivity), pulmonary fibrosis, and pulmonary infiltrates. The onset of symptoms has been within 5 days to more than 9 months after treatment initiation (median: 39 days). Interrupt treatment for unexplained new or worsening pulmonary symptoms (dyspnea, cough, and fever); permanently discontinue for confirmed ILD.

Hepatic failure and hepatorenal syndrome have been reported, particularly in patients with baseline hepatic impairment (although have also been observed in patients with normal hepatic function). Monitor liver function (transaminases, bilirubin, and alkaline phosphatase); patients with any hepatic impairment (total bilirubin >ULN; Child-Pugh class A, B, or C) should be closely monitored, including those with hepatic disease due to tumor burden. Dosage reduction, interruption, or discontinuation may be recommended for changes in hepatic function. Use with extreme caution in patients with total bilirubin >3 times ULN. Interrupt therapy if total bilirubin is >3 times ULN or transaminases are >5 times ULN in patients without preexisting hepatic impairment. In patients with baseline hepatic dysfunction or biliary obstruction, interrupt therapy if bilirubin doubles or transaminases triple from baseline values. Increased monitoring of liver function is required in patients with preexisting hepatic impairment or biliary obstruction. Acute renal failure, renal insufficiency, and hepatorenal syndrome have been reported, either secondary to hepatic impairment at baseline or due to severe dehydration; use with caution in patients with or at risk for renal impairment. Monitor closely for dehydration; monitor renal function and electrolytes in patients at risk for dehydration. If severe renal impairment develops, interrupt therapy until toxicity resolves. Gastrointestinal perforation has been reported with use; risk for perforation is increased with concurrent anti-angiogenic agents, corticosteroids, NSAIDs, and/or taxane based-therapy, and patients with history of peptic ulcers or diverticular disease; permanently discontinue in patients who develop perforation.

Bullous, blistering, or exfoliating skin conditions, some suggestive of Stevens-Johnson or toxic epidermal necrolysis (TEN) have been reported. An acne-like rash commonly appears on the face, back, and upper chest. Generalized or severe acneiform, erythematous or maculopapular rash may occur. Skin rash may correlate with treatment response and prolonged survival (Saif, 2008); management of skin rashes that are not serious should include alcohol-free lotions, topical antibiotics, or topical corticosteroids, or if necessary, oral antibiotics and systemic corticosteroids; avoid sunlight. Reduce dose or temporarily interrupt treatment for severe skin reactions; discontinue treatment for bullous, blistering or exfoliative skin toxicity. Corneal perforation and ulceration have been reported with use; decreased tear production, abnormal eyelash growth, keratoconjunctivitis sicca, or keratitis have also been reported and are known risk factors for corneal ulceration/perforation. Interrupt or discontinue treatment in patients presenting with eye pain or other acute or worsening ocular symptoms. Consider a baseline ophthalmologic exam and reassess for ocular toxicities at 4 to 8 weeks after treatment initiation (Renouf, 2012).

MI, CVA, and microangiopathic hemolytic anemia with thrombocytopenia have been reported (rarely) with erlotinib in combination with gemcitabine. Elevated INR and bleeding events (including fatal hemorrhage) have been reported; monitor prothrombin time and INR closely. Erlotinib levels may be lower in patients who smoke; advise patients to stop smoking. Smokers treated with 300 mg/day exhibited steady-state erlotinib levels comparable to former- and never-smokers receiving 150 mg/day (Hughes, 2009). Potentially significant drug-drug interactions may exist, requiring dose or frequency adjustment, additional monitoring, and/or selection of alternative therapy. Avoid concomitant use with proton pump inhibitors. If taken with an H_2-receptor antagonist (eg, ranitidine), administer erlotinib 10 hours after the H_2-receptor antagonist dose and at least 2 hours prior to the next H_2-receptor dose. If an antacid is necessary, separate dosing by several hours. In patients with NSCLC, EGFR mutations, specifically exon 19 deletions and exon 21 mutation (L858R), are associated with better response to erlotinib (Riely, 2006); erlotinib treatment is not recommended in patients with *K-ras* mutations; they are not likely to benefit from erlotinib treatment (Eberhard, 2005; Miller, 2008). Concurrent erlotinib plus platinum-based chemotherapy is not recommended for first line treatment of locally advanced or metastatic NSCLC due to a lack of clinical benefit. The cobas EGFR mutation test has been approved to detect EGFR mutation for first-line NSCLC treatment. Product may contain lactose; avoid use in patients with Lapp lactase deficiency, glucose-galactose malabsorption, or glucose intolerance.

Adverse Reactions

Adverse reactions reported with monotherapy:

Cardiovascular: Chest pain, peripheral edema

Central nervous system: Anxiety, dizziness, fatigue, headache, insomnia, neurotoxicity, pain, paresthesia, voice disorder

Dermatologic: Acne vulgaris, acneiform eruption, alopecia, bullous dermatitis, dermatitis, erythema, erythematous rash, exfoliative dermatitis, folliculitis, hypertrichosis, nail disease, palmar-plantar erythrodysesthesia, paronychia, pruritus, skin fissure, skin rash, xeroderma

Endocrine & metabolic: Weight loss

Gastrointestinal: Abdominal pain, anorexia, constipation, decreased appetite, diarrhea, dyspepsia, mucositis, nausea, stomatitis, taste disorder, vomiting, xerostomia

Genitourinary: Urinary tract infection

Hematologic & oncologic: Anemia, leukopenia, lymphocytopenia, thrombocytopenia

Hepatic: Hepatic failure, hyperbilirubinemia, increased gamma-glutamyl transferase, increased serum ALT

Infection: Increased susceptibility to infection

Miscellaneous: Fever

Neuromuscular and skeletal: Arthralgia, back pain, muscle spasm, musculoskeletal pain (including chest), ostealgia, weakness

Ophthalmic: Conjunctivitis, keratoconjunctivitis sicca, ophthalmic signs and symptoms

Otic: Tinnitus

Renal: Increased serum creatinine, renal failure

Respiratory: Cough, dyspnea, epistaxis, nasopharyngitis, pneumonitis, pulmonary embolism, pulmonary fibrosis, respiratory tract infection

Rare but important or life-threatening: Interstitial pulmonary disease

Adverse reactions reported with combination (erlotinib plus gemcitabine) therapy:

Cardiovascular: Cardiac arrhythmia, cerebrovascular accident (including cerebral hemorrhage), deep vein thrombosis, edema, myocardial infarction, syncope, thrombosis

Central nervous system: Anxiety, depression, dizziness, fatigue, headache

Dermatologic: Alopecia, skin rash

Gastrointestinal: Abdominal pain, anorexia, diarrhea, dyspepsia, flatulence, intestinal obstruction, nausea, pancreatitis, stomatitis, vomiting, weight loss

Hematologic & oncologic: Hemolytic anemia, microangiopathic hemolytic anemia with thrombocytopenia

Hepatic: Hyperbilirubinemia, increased serum ALT, increased serum AST

Infection: Increased susceptibility to infection

Miscellaneous: Fever

Neuromuscular & skeletal: Myalgia, neuropathy, ostealgia, rigors

Renal: Renal failure, renal insufficiency

Respiratory: Cough, dyspnea, interstitial pulmonary disease

Rare but important or life-threatening: Bullous dermatitis, exfoliative dermatitis, hepatic failure

Mono- or combination therapy: Rare but important or life-threatening: Acute peptic ulcer with hemorrhage, bronchiolitis, corneal perforation, corneal ulcer, episcleritis, gastritis, gastrointestinal hemorrhage, gastrointestinal perforation, hearing loss, hematemesis, hematochezia, hepatorenal syndrome, hepatotoxicity, hirsutism, hyperpigmentation, hypokalemia, keratitis, melena, myopathy (in combination with statin therapy), peptic ulcer, rhabdomyolysis (in combination with statin therapy), skin photosensitivity, skin rash (acneiform; sparing prior radiation field), Stevens-Johnson syndrome, toxic epidermal necrolysis, tympanic membrane perforation

Drug Interactions

Metabolism/Transport Effects **Substrate** of CYP1A2 (minor), CYP3A4 (major); **Note:** Assignment of Major/Minor substrate status based on clinically relevant drug interaction potential

Avoid Concomitant Use

Avoid concomitant use of Erlotinib with any of the following: Conivaptan; Fusidic Acid (Systemic); Idelalisib; Proton Pump Inhibitors

Increased Effect/Toxicity

Erlotinib may increase the levels/effects of: Warfarin

The levels/effects of Erlotinib may be increased by: Aprepitant; Ceritinib; Ciprofloxacin (Systemic); Conivaptan; CYP3A4 Inhibitors (Moderate); CYP3A4 Inhibitors (Strong); Dasatinib; FluvoxaMINE; Fosaprepitant; Fusidic Acid (Systemic); Grapefruit Juice; Idelalisib; Ivacaftor; Luliconazole; Mifepristone; Netupitant; Simeprevir; Stiripentol

Decreased Effect

The levels/effects of Erlotinib may be decreased by: Antacids; Bosentan; CYP3A4 Inducers (Moderate); CYP3A4 Inducers (Strong); Dabrafenib; Deferasirox; H2-Antagonists; Mitotane; Proton Pump Inhibitors; Siltuximab; St Johns Wort; Tocilizumab

Food Interactions Erlotinib bioavailability is increased with food. Grapefruit or grapefruit juice may decrease metabolism and increase erlotinib plasma concentrations. Management: Take on an empty stomach at least 1 hour before or 2 hours after the ingestion of food. Avoid grapefruit and grapefruit juice. Maintain adequate nutrition and hydration, unless instructed to restrict fluid intake.

Storage/Stability Store at 25°C (77°F); excursions are permitted between 15°C and 30°C (59°F and 86°F).

Mechanism of Action Reversibly inhibits overall epidermal growth factor receptor (HER1/EGFR) - tyrosine kinase activity. Intracellular phosphorylation is inhibited which prevents further downstream signaling, resulting in cell death. Erlotinib has higher binding affinity for EGFR exon 19 deletion or exon 21 L858R mutations than for the wild type receptor.

Pharmacodynamics/Kinetics

Absorption: Oral: 60% on an empty stomach; almost 100% on a full stomach

Distribution: 232 L

Protein binding: ~93% to albumin and alpha$_1$-acid glycoprotein

Metabolism: Hepatic, via CYP3A4 (major), CYP1A1 (minor), CYP1A2 (minor), and CYP1C (minor)

Bioavailability: Almost 100% when given with food; 60% without food

Half-life elimination: 36 hours

Time to peak, plasma: 4 hours

Excretion: Primarily as metabolites: Feces (83%; 1% as unchanged drug); urine (8%; <1% as unchanged drug)

Dosage

Non-small cell lung cancer (NSCLC), metastatic, first-line therapy in patients with EGFR exon 19 deletions or exon 21 (L858R) substitution mutations: Adults: Oral: 150 mg once daily until disease progression or unacceptable toxicity (Rosell, 2012; Zhou, 2011).

NSCLC, refractory: Adults: Oral: 150 mg once daily until disease progression or unacceptable toxicity (Shepherd, 2005)

NSCLC, maintenance therapy: Adults: Oral: 150 mg once daily until disease progression or unacceptable toxicity (Capuzzo, 2010)

Pancreatic cancer: Adults: Oral: 100 mg once daily until disease progression or unacceptable toxicity (in combination with gemcitabine) (Moore, 2007)

Dosage adjustment for concomitant CYP3A4 inhibitors/inducers:

CYP3A4 inhibitors: Avoid concurrent use if possible; consider dose reductions for severe adverse reactions if erlotinib is administered concomitantly with strong CYP3A4 inhibitors (eg, azole antifungals, clarithromycin, erythromycin, nefazodone, protease inhibitors, telithromycin, grapefruit, or grapefruit juice). Dose reduction (if required) should be done in decrements of 50 mg (after toxicity has resolved to baseline or ≤ grade 1).

Concomitant CYP3A4 and CYP1A2 inhibitor (eg, ciprofloxacin): Avoid concurrent use if possible; consider dose reductions in decrements of 50 mg if severe adverse reactions occur (after toxicity has resolved to baseline or ≤ grade 1).

CYP3A4 inducers: Alternatives to the enzyme-inducing agent should be utilized first. Concomitant administration with CYP3A4 inducers (eg, carbamazepine, phenobarbital, phenytoin, rifamycins, and St John's wort) may require increased erlotinib doses (increase as tolerated at 2-week intervals in 50 mg increments to a maximum of 450 mg); doses >150 mg daily should be considered with rifampin (the maximum erlotinib dose studied in combination with rifampin was 450 mg). Immediately reduce erlotinib dose to recommended starting dose when CYP3A4 inducer is discontinued.

Dosage adjustment for concomitant smoking: Increase dose at 2-week intervals in 50 mg increments to a maximum dose of 300 mg (with careful monitoring) in patients who continue to smoke; immediately reduce erlotinib dose to recommended starting dose upon smoking cessation.

Dosage adjustment for toxicity:

Dermatologic toxicity:

Bullous, blistering or exfoliative skin toxicity (severe): Discontinue treatment.

Severe rash (unresponsive to medical management): Withhold treatment; may reinitiate with a 50 mg dose reduction after toxicity has resolved to baseline or ≤ grade 1.

Gastrointestinal toxicity:

Diarrhea: Manage with loperamide; in severe diarrhea (unresponsive to loperamide) or dehydration due to diarrhea, withhold treatment; may reinitiate with a 50 mg dose reduction after toxicity has resolved to baseline or ≤ grade 1.

Gastrointestinal perforation: Discontinue treatment.

Ocular toxicities:

Acute or worsening ocular toxicities (eg, eye pain): Interrupt and consider discontinuing treatment. If therapy is resumed, reinitiate with a 50 mg dose reduction after toxicity has resolved to baseline or ≤ grade 1.

Corneal perforation or severe ulceration: Discontinue treatment.

Keratitis (grade 3 or 4 or grade 2 persisting >2 weeks): Withhold treatment; may reinitiate with a 50 mg dose reduction after toxicity has resolved to baseline or ≤ grade 1.

Pulmonary symptoms: Acute onset (or worsening) of pulmonary symptoms (eg, dyspnea, cough, fever): Interrupt treatment and evaluate for drug-induced interstitial lung disease; discontinue permanently with development of interstitial lung disease

Dosage adjustment in renal impairment:

Renal impairment at treatment initiation: There are no dosage adjustments provided in the manufacturer's labeling (has not been studied), although <9% of a single dose is excreted in the urine.

Renal toxicity during treatment: Withhold treatment for grades 3/4 renal toxicity (consider discontinuing) and for risk of renal failure due to dehydration; may resume after euvolemia re-established (at previous dose). If treatment withheld due to toxicity and therapy is resumed, reinitiate with a 50 mg dose reduction after toxicity has resolved to baseline or ≤ grade 1.

Dosage adjustment in hepatic impairment:

Hepatic impairment at treatment initiation:

U.S. labeling:

Total bilirubin > ULN or Child-Pugh classes A, B, and C: There are no dosage adjustments provided in the manufacturer's labeling; use with caution and monitor closely during treatment.

Total bilirubin >3 times ULN: Use extreme caution.

Canadian labeling:

Moderate impairment: There are no dosage adjustments provided in the manufacturer's labeling; however, a reduced dose should be considered.

Severe impairment (including total bilirubin >3 times ULN and/or transaminases >5 times ULN): Use is not recommended.

The following adjustments have also been studied: A reduced starting dose (75 mg once daily) has been recommended in patients with hepatic dysfunction (AST ≥3 times ULN or direct bilirubin 1-7 mg/dL), with individualized dosage escalation if tolerated (Miller, 2007); another study determined that pharmacokinetic and safety profiles were similar between patients with normal hepatic function and moderate hepatic impairment (O'Bryant, 2012).

Hepatotoxicity during treatment: U.S. labeling:

Patients with normal hepatic function at baseline: If total bilirubin >3 times ULN and/or transaminases >5 times ULN during use: Interrupt therapy (consider discontinuing); if treatment is resumed, reinitiate with a 50 mg dose reduction after bilirubin and transaminases return to baseline; discontinue treatment if there is no significant improvement or resolution within 3 weeks.

Patients with baseline hepatic impairment or biliary obstruction: If bilirubin doubles or transaminases triple over baseline during use: Interrupt therapy (consider discontinuing); if treatment is resumed, reinitiate with a 50 mg dose reduction after bilirubin and transaminases return to baseline; discontinue treatment if there is no significant improvement or resolution of hepatotoxicity within 3 weeks.

Dietary Considerations Take this medicine an empty stomach, 1 hour before or 2 hours after a meal. Avoid grapefruit juice.

Administration The manufacturer recommends administration on an empty stomach (at least 1 hour before or 2 hours after the ingestion of food). Avoid concomitant use with proton pump inhibitors. If taken with an H_2-receptor antagonist (eg, ranitidine), administer erlotinib 10 hours after the H_2-receptor antagonist dose and at least 2 hours prior to the next H_2-receptor dose. If an antacid is necessary, separate dosing by several hours.

For patients unable to swallow whole, tablets may be dissolved in 100 mL water and administered orally or via feeding tube (silicone-based); to ensure full dose is received, rinse container with 40 mL water, administer residue and repeat rinse (data on file, Genentech [contact product manufacturer to obtain current information]; Siu, 2007; Soulieres, 2004).

Hazardous agent; use appropriate precautions for handling and disposal (NIOSH 2014 [group 1]).

Monitoring Parameters Periodic liver function tests (transaminases, bilirubin, and alkaline phosphatase); monitor more frequently with worsening liver function; periodic renal function tests and serum electrolytes (in patients at risk for dehydration); hydration status; signs/symptoms of pulmonary toxicity; prothrombin time and INR (in patients on concomitant warfarin therapy); consider a baseline ophthalmologic exam and reassess for ocular toxicities at 4 to 8 weeks after treatment initiation (Renouf, 2012); EGFR mutation status in patients with NSCLC adenocarcinoma (Keedy, 2011); the cobas EGFR mutation test has been approved to detect EGFR mutation for first-line NSCLC treatment

Additional Information In patients with NSCLC, some factors which correlate positively with response to EGFR-tyrosine kinase inhibitor (TKI) therapy include patients who have never smoked, EGFR mutation, and patients of Asian origin. EGFR mutations, specifically exon 19 deletions and exon 21 mutation (L858R) correlate with response to tyrosine kinase inhibitors (Riely, 2006). *K-ras* mutations correlated with poorer outcome with EGFR-TKI therapy in patients with NSCLC (Cooley, 2008; Jackman, 2008; Masarelli, 2007; Shepherd, 2005).

Dosage Forms

Tablet, Oral:

Tarceva: 25 mg, 100 mg, 150 mg

Extemporaneous Preparations Hazardous agent; use appropriate precautions for handling and disposal (NIOSH 2014 [group 1]).

A suspension for oral or feeding tube (silicone-based) administration may be prepared by dissolving tablets needed for dose in 100 mL water. To ensure full dose is received, rinse container with 40 mL water, administer residue and repeat rinse. Administer immediately after preparation; stability of solution is unknown (Data on file from Genentech [contact product manufacturer to obtain current information]).

Siu LL, Soulieres D, Chen EX, et al, "Phase I/II Trial of Erlotinib and Cisplatin in Patients With Recurrent or Metastatic Squamous Cell Carcinoma of the Head and Neck: A Princess Margaret Hospital Phase II Consortium and National Cancer Institute of Canada Clinical Trials Group Study," *J Clin Oncol*, 2007, 25(16):2178-83. [PubMed 17538162]

Soulieres D, Senzer NN, Vokes EE, et al, "Multicenter Phase II Study of Erlotinib, an Oral Epidermal Growth Factor Receptor Tyrosine Kinase Inhibitor, in Patients With Recurrent or Metastatic Squamous Cell Cancer of the Head and Neck," *J Clin Oncol*, 2004, 22(1):77-85. [PubMed 14701768]

◆ **Erlotinib Hydrochloride** *see* Erlotinib *on page 756*

◆ **E-R-O Ear Drops [OTC]** *see* Carbamide Peroxide *on page 350*

◆ **E-R-O Ear Wax Removal System [OTC]** *see* Carbamide Peroxide *on page 350*

◆ **Errin** *see* Norethindrone *on page 1473*

◆ **Ertaczo** *see* Sertaconazole *on page 1877*

Ertapenem (er ta PEN em)

Brand Names: U.S. INVanz

Brand Names: Canada Invanz

Index Terms Ertapenem Sodium; L-749,345; MK0826

Pharmacologic Category Antibiotic, Carbapenem

Use Moderate-to-severe infections:

Acute pelvic infections: For the treatment of acute pelvic infections, including postpartum endomyometritis, septic abortion, and postsurgical gynecologic infections caused by *Streptococcus agalactiae*, *Escherichia coli*, *Bacteroides fragilis*, *Porphyromonas asaccharolytica*, *Peptostreptococcus* spp, or *Prevotella bivia*.

Community-acquired pneumonia: For the treatment of community-acquired pneumonia (CAP) caused by *Streptococcus pneumoniae* (penicillin-susceptible isolates only), including cases with concurrent bacteremia; *Haemophilus influenzae* (beta-lactamase-negative isolates only); or *Moraxella catarrhalis*.

Complicated intra-abdominal infections: For the treatment of complicated intra-abdominal infections caused by *E. coli*, *Clostridium clostridioforme*, *Eubacterium lentum*, *Peptostreptococcus* spp, *B. fragilis*, *Bacteroides distasonis*, *Bacteroides ovatus*, *Bacteroides thetaiotaomicron*, or *Bacteroides uniformis*.

Complicated skin and skin structure infections: For the treatment of complicated skin and skin structure infections, including diabetic foot infections without osteomyelitis caused by *Staphylococcus aureus* (methicillin-susceptible isolates only), *S. agalactiae*, *Streptococcus pyogenes*, *E. coli*, *Klebsiella pneumoniae*, *Proteus mirabilis*, *B. fragilis*, *Peptostreptococcus* spp, *P. asaccharolytica*, or *P. bivia*. Ertapenem has not been studied in diabetic foot infections with concomitant osteomyelitis.

Complicated urinary tract infections: For the treatment of complicated urinary tract infections (UTIs), including pyelonephritis caused by *E. coli*, including cases with concurrent bacteremia or *K. pneumoniae*.

Prophylaxis of surgical-site infection in colorectal surgery: For the prophylaxis of surgical-site infection in adults following elective colorectal surgery.

Note: Methicillin-resistant *Staphylococcus aureus*, *Enterococcus* spp, penicillin-resistant strains of *Streptococcus pneumoniae*, *Acinetobacter*, and *Pseudomonas aeruginosa*, are **resistant** to ertapenem while most extended-spectrum beta-lactamase (ESBL)-producing bacteria remain sensitive to ertapenem.

Pregnancy Risk Factor B

Pregnancy Considerations Teratogenic effects were not observed in animal reproduction studies. Ertapenem is approved for the treatment of postpartum endomyometritis, septic abortion, and postsurgical infections. Information related to use during pregnancy has not been located.

Breast-Feeding Considerations Ertapenem is excreted in breast milk. The low concentrations in milk and low oral bioavailability suggest minimal exposure risk to the infant. The manufacturer recommends that caution be exercised when administering ertapenem to nursing women. Non-dose-related effects could include modification of bowel flora.

Contraindications Known hypersensitivity to any component of this product or to other drugs in the same class or in patients who have demonstrated anaphylactic reactions to beta-lactams; known hypersensitivity to local anesthetics of the amide type due to the use of lidocaine as a diluent (IM use only).

Warnings/Precautions Use caution with renal impairment. Dosage adjustment required in patients with moderate to severe renal dysfunction; elderly patients often require lower doses (based upon renal function). Use may result in fungal or bacterial superinfection, including *C. difficile*-associated diarrhea (CDAD) and pseudomembranous colitis; CDAD has been observed >2 months postantibiotic treatment. Carbapenems have been associated with CNS adverse effects, including confusional states and seizures (myoclonic); use caution with CNS disorders (eg, brain lesions and history of seizures) and adjust dose in renal impairment to avoid drug accumulation, which may increase seizure risk. Serious hypersensitivity reactions, including anaphylaxis, have been reported (some without a history of previous allergic reactions to beta-lactams). Doses for IM administration are mixed with lidocaine; consult Lidocaine (Systemic) information for associated Warnings/Precautions. May decrease divalproex sodium/valproic acid concentrations leading to breakthrough seizures; concomitant use not recommended.

Adverse Reactions

Cardiovascular: Chest pain, edema, hypotension, phlebitis, thrombophlebitis

Central nervous system: Altered mental status (ie, agitation, confusion, disorientation, mental acuity decreased, somnolence, stupor), dizziness, headache, hypothermia (infants, children, and adolescents), insomnia

Dermatologic: Diaper rash (infants and children), genital rash (infants, children, and adolescents), pruritus, skin lesion (infants, children, and adolescents), skin rash

Gastrointestinal: Abdominal pain, constipation, decreased appetite (infants, children, and adolescents), diarrhea, nausea, vomiting

Genitourinary: Erythrocyturia, vaginitis

Hematologic & oncologic: Decreased hematocrit, decreased hemoglobin, decreased neutrophils, eosinophilia, leukocyturia, leukopenia, thrombocythemia

Hepatic: Increased serum alkaline, increased serum ALT, increased serum AST

Infection: Herpes simplex infection (infants, children, and adolescents)

Local: Infused vein complication

Neuromuscular & skeletal: Arthralgia (infants, children, and adolescents)

Otic: Otic infection (infants, children, and adolescents)

Respiratory: Cough, dyspnea, nasopharyngitis (infants, children, and adolescents), rhinitis (infants, children, and adolescents), rhinorrhea (infants, children, and adolescents), upper respiratory tract infection (infants, children, and adolescents), wheezing (infants, children, and adolescents)

Miscellaneous: Fever

Rare but important or life-threatening: Anaphylactoid reaction, anaphylaxis, anuria, asthma, asystole, atrial fibrillation, bradycardia, bronchoconstriction, cardiac arrest, cardiac arrhythmia, cardiac failure, cholelithiasis, *Clostridium difficile* associated diarrhea, delirium, DRESS syndrome, extravasation, gastrointestinal hemorrhage, gout, heart murmur, hemoptysis, hyperglycemia, hyperkalemia, hypertension, hypoxemia, impaired consciousness, intestinal obstruction, jaundice, oral candidiasis, oliguria, pancreatitis, pleural effusion, prolonged prothrombin time, renal insufficiency, seizure, septicemia, septic shock, subdural hematoma, tachycardia, thrombocytopenia, tissue necrosis, ventricular tachycardia

Drug Interactions

Metabolism/Transport Effects None known.

Avoid Concomitant Use

Avoid concomitant use of Ertapenem with any of the following: BCG

Increased Effect/Toxicity

Ertapenem may increase the levels/effects of: Tacrolimus (Systemic)

The levels/effects of Ertapenem may be increased by: Probenecid

Decreased Effect

Ertapenem may decrease the levels/effects of: BCG; Sodium Picosulfate; Typhoid Vaccine; Valproic Acid and Derivatives

Preparation for Administration

IM: Reconstitute 1 g vial with 3.2 mL of 1% lidocaine HCl injection (without epinephrine). Shake well.

IV: Reconstitute 1 g vial with 10 mL of sterile water for injection, 0.9% sodium chloride injection, or bacteriostatic water for injection. Shake well. For adults, transfer dose to 50 mL of 0.9% sodium chloride injection; for children, dilute dose with NS to a final concentration ≤20 mg/mL.

Storage/Stability Prior to reconstitution, store vials at ≤25°C (77°F). The reconstituted IM solution should be used within 1 hour after preparation. The reconstituted IV solution may be stored at room temperature (25°C [77°F]) and used within 6 hours, or stored for 24 hours under refrigeration (5°C [41°F]) and used within 4 hours after removal from refrigeration. Do not freeze.

Mechanism of Action Inhibits bacterial cell wall synthesis by binding to one or more of the penicillin-binding proteins; which in turn inhibits the final transpeptidation step of peptidoglycan synthesis in bacterial cell walls, thus inhibiting cell wall biosynthesis. Bacteria eventually lyse due to ongoing activity of cell wall autolytic enzymes (autolysins and murein hydrolases) while cell wall assembly is arrested.

Pharmacodynamics/Kinetics

Absorption: IM: Almost complete

Distribution: V_{dss}:

- Children 3 months to 12 years: ~0.2 L/kg
- Children 13-17 years: ~0.16 L/kg
- Adults: ~0.12 L/kg

Protein binding (concentration dependent, primarily to albumin): 85% at 300 mcg/mL, 95% at <100 mcg/mL

Metabolism: Non-CYP-mediated hydrolysis to inactive metabolite

Bioavailability: IM: ~90%

Half-life elimination:

- Children 3 months to 12 years: ~2.5 hours
- Children ≥13 years and Adults: ~4 hours

Time to peak: IM: ~2.3 hours

Excretion: Urine (~80% as unchanged drug and metabolite); feces (~10%)

Dosage Note: IV therapy may be administered for up to 14 days; IM therapy for up to 7 days

Usual dosage ranges:

Infants ≥3 months and Children: IM, IV: 15 **mg**/kg twice daily (maximum: 1 g daily)

Adolescents and Adults: IM, IV: 1 g once daily

Indication-specific dosing:

Infants ≥3 months and Children: IM, IV:

Community-acquired pneumonia, complicated urinary tract infections (including pyelonephritis): 15 **mg**/kg twice daily (maximum: 1 g daily); duration of total antibiotic treatment: 10-14 days (**Note:** Duration includes possible switch to appropriate oral therapy after at least 3 days of parenteral treatment, once clinical improvement demonstrated.)

Intra-abdominal infection: 15 **mg**/kg twice daily (maximum: 1 g daily) for 5-14 days

Pelvic infections (acute): 15 **mg**/kg twice daily (maximum: 1 g daily) for 3-10 days

Skin and skin structure infections: 15 **mg**/kg twice daily (maximum: 1 g daily) for 7-14 days

Adolescents and Adults: IM, IV:

Community-acquired pneumonia, complicated urinary tract infections (including pyelonephritis): 1 g once daily; duration of total antibiotic treatment: 10-14 days; duration includes possible switch to appropriate oral therapy after at least 3 days of parenteral treatment, once clinical improvement demonstrated. **Note:** The carbapenems, including ertapenem, are preferred agents for *Enterobacter* spp and *Burkholderia pseudomallei*, and are considered alternative agents for anaerobes in aspiration pneumonia (IDSA, 2007).

Intra-abdominal infection: 1 g once daily for 5-14 days; **Note:** 2010 IDSA guidelines recommend a treatment duration of 4-7 days (provided source controlled) for community-acquired, mild-to-moderate intra-abdominal infections (Solomkin, 2010)

Pelvic infections (acute): 1 g once daily for 3-10 days

Skin and skin structure infections (excluding diabetic foot infections with osteomyelitis): 1 g once daily for 7-14 days. **Note:** For diabetic foot infections, recommended treatment duration is up to 4 weeks depending on severity of infection and response to therapy (Lipsky, 2012); guidelines recommend ertapenem as a preferred agent for animal bites. (IDSA, 2005).

Adults: IV:

Prophylaxis of surgical site following colorectal surgery: 1 g as a single dose given 1 hour preoperatively

Intravenous catheter-related bloodstream infection (off-label use): 1 g once daily (**Note:** Carbapenems, including ertapenem, are preferred agents for extended-spectrum β-lactamase [ESBL]-positive *Escherichia coli* and *Klebsiella, Enterobacter,* and *Serratia* [IDSA, 2009].)

Prosthetic joint infection, *Enterobacter* spp (off-label use): 1 g every 24 hours for 4-6 weeks (Osmon, 2013)

Dosage adjustment in renal impairment:

Children: No data available for pediatric patients with renal insufficiency.

Adults:

- CrCl >30 mL/minute/1.73 m^2: No dosage adjustment necessary.
- CrCl ≤30 mL/minute/1.73 m^2 and ESRD: 500 mg daily

Hemodialysis: Adults: When the daily dose is given within 6 hours prior to hemodialysis, a supplementary dose of 150 mg is required following hemodialysis. If ertapenem is given at least 6 hours prior to hemodialysis, no supplementary dose is needed.

CAPD: IV: 500 mg daily (Cardone, 2011)

Dosage adjustment in hepatic impairment: Adjustments cannot be recommended (lack of experience and research in this patient population).

Dietary Considerations Some products may contain sodium.

Administration

IM: Avoid injection into a blood vessel. Make sure patient does not have an allergy to lidocaine or another anesthetic of the amide type. Administer by deep IM injection into a large muscle mass (eg, gluteal muscle or lateral part of the thigh). Do not administer IM preparation or drug reconstituted for IM administration intravenously.

IV: Infuse over 30 minutes

Monitoring Parameters Periodic renal, hepatic, and hematopoietic assessment during prolonged therapy; neurological assessment

Dosage Forms

Solution Reconstituted, Injection:

INVanz: 1 g (1 ea)

Solution Reconstituted, Intravenous:

INVanz: 1 g (1 ea)

◆ **Ertapenem Sodium** *see* Ertapenem *on page 760*

◆ **Erwinase (Can)** *see* Asparaginase (*Erwinia*) *on page 180*

◆ **Erwinaze** *see* Asparaginase (*Erwinia*) *on page 180*

◆ ***Erwinia chrysanthemi*** *see* Asparaginase (*Erwinia*) *on page 180*

◆ **Ery** *see* Erythromycin (Topical) *on page 765*

◆ **Erybid (Can)** *see* Erythromycin (Systemic) *on page 762*

◆ **Eryc (Can)** *see* Erythromycin (Systemic) *on page 762*

◆ **Erygel** *see* Erythromycin (Topical) *on page 765*

◆ **EryPed 200** *see* Erythromycin (Systemic) *on page 762*

◆ **EryPed 400** *see* Erythromycin (Systemic) *on page 762*

◆ **Erysol (Can)** *see* Erythromycin (Topical) *on page 765*

◆ **Ery-Tab** *see* Erythromycin (Systemic) *on page 762*

◆ **Erythrocin Lactobionate** *see* Erythromycin (Systemic) *on page 762*

◆ **Erythrocin Stearate** *see* Erythromycin (Systemic) *on page 762*

Erythromycin (Systemic) (er ith roe MYE sin)

Brand Names: U.S. E.E.S. 400; E.E.S. Granules; Ery-Tab; EryPed 200; EryPed 400; Erythrocin Lactobionate; Erythrocin Stearate; PCE

Brand Names: Canada Apo-Erythro Base; Apo-Erythro E-C; Apo-Erythro-ES; Apo-Erythro-S; EES; Erybid; Eryc; Novo-Rythro Estolate; Novo-Rythro Ethylsuccinate; Nu-Erythromycin-S; PCE

Index Terms Erythromycin Base; Erythromycin Ethylsuccinate; Erythromycin Lactobionate; Erythromycin Stearate

Pharmacologic Category Antibiotic, Macrolide

Use Treatment of susceptible bacterial infections including *S. pyogenes*, some *S. pneumoniae*, some *S. aureus*, *M. pneumoniae*, *Legionella pneumophila*, diphtheria, pertussis, *Chlamydia*, erythrasma, *N. gonorrhoeae*, *E. histolytica*, syphilis and nongonococcal urethritis, and *Campylobacter* gastroenteritis; used in conjunction with neomycin for decontaminating the bowel

Pregnancy Risk Factor B

Pregnancy Considerations Adverse events were not observed in animal reproduction studies. Erythromycin crosses the placenta and low concentrations are found in the fetal serum. Cardiovascular anomalies following exposure in early pregnancy have been reported in some observational studies. Serum concentrations of erythromycin may be variable in pregnant women (Kiefer, 1955; Philipson, 1976).

In patients with acute infections during pregnancy, erythromycin may be given if an antibiotic is required and appropriate based on bacterial sensitivity (ACOG No. 120, 2011). Erythromycin is the antibiotic of choice for preterm premature rupture of membranes (with membrane rupture between 24 0/7 to 33 6/7 weeks gestation) (ACOG 2013), the treatment of granuloma inguinale, and lymphogranuloma venereum in pregnancy (CDC [RR-12], 2010), and the treatment of or long-term suppression of *Bartonella* infection in HIV-infected pregnant patients [DHHS, 2013]. Erythromycin may be appropriate as an alternative agent for the treatment of chlamydial infections in pregnant women (consult current guidelines) (CDC [RR-12], 2010).

Breast-Feeding Considerations Erythromycin is excreted in breast milk; therefore, the manufacturer recommends that caution be exercised when administering erythromycin to breast-feeding women. Decreased appetite, diarrhea, rash, and somnolence have been reported in nursing infants exposed to macrolide antibiotics (Goldstein, 2009).

One case report and a cohort study raise the possibility for a connection with pyloric stenosis in neonates exposed to erythromycin via breast milk and an alternative antibiotic may be preferred for breast-feeding mothers of infants in this age group (Sorensen, 2003; Stang, 1986).

Contraindications Hypersensitivity to erythromycin, any macrolide antibiotics, or any component of the formulation

Concomitant use with pimozide, cisapride, ergotamine or dihydroergotamine, terfenadine, astemizole, lovastatin, or simvastatin

Warnings/Precautions Use caution with hepatic impairment with or without jaundice has occurred, it may be accompanied by malaise, nausea, vomiting, abdominal colic, and fever; discontinue use if these occur. Use caution with other medication relying on CYP3A4 metabolism; high potential for drug interactions exists. Prolonged use may result in fungal or bacterial superinfection, including *C. difficile*-associated diarrhea (CDAD) and pseudomembranous colitis; CDAD has been observed >2 months postantibiotic treatment. Use in infants has been associated with infantile hypertrophic pyloric stenosis (IHPS). Macrolides have been associated with rare QTc prolongation and ventricular arrhythmias, including torsade de pointes; avoid use in patients with prolonged QT interval, uncorrected hypokalemia or hypomagnesemia, clinically significant bradycardia, or concurrent use of Class IA (eg, quinidine, procainamide) or Class III (eg, amiodarone, dofetilide, sotalol) antiarrhythmic agents. Avoid concurrent use with strong CYP3A inhibitors; may increase the risk of sudden cardiac death (Ray, 2004). Use caution in elderly patients, as risk of adverse events may be increased. Use caution in myasthenia gravis patients; erythromycin may aggravate muscular weakness.

Benzyl alcohol and derivatives: Some dosage forms may contain benzyl alcohol; large amounts of benzyl alcohol (≥99 mg/kg/day) have been associated with a potentially fatal toxicity ("gasping syndrome") in neonates; the "gasping syndrome" consists of metabolic acidosis, respiratory distress, gasping respirations, CNS dysfunction (including convulsions, intracranial hemorrhage), hypotension and cardiovascular collapse (AAP, 1997; CDC, 1982); some data suggests that benzoate displaces bilirubin from protein binding sites (Ahlfors, 2001); avoid or use dosage forms containing benzyl alcohol with caution in neonates. See manufacturer's labeling.

Adverse Reactions

Cardiovascular: QTc prolongation, torsade de pointes, ventricular arrhythmia, ventricular tachycardia

Central nervous system: Seizure

Dermatologic: Erythema multiforme, pruritus, rash, Stevens-Johnson syndrome, toxic epidermal necrolysis

Gastrointestinal: Abdominal pain, anorexia, diarrhea, infantile hypertrophic pyloric stenosis, nausea, oral candidiasis, pancreatitis, pseudomembranous colitis, vomiting

Hepatic: Cholestatic jaundice (most common with estolate), hepatitis, liver function tests abnormal

Local: Phlebitis at the injection site, thrombophlebitis

Neuromuscular & skeletal: Weakness

Otic: Hearing loss

Miscellaneous: Allergic reactions, anaphylaxis, hypersensitivity reactions, interstitial nephritis, urticaria

Drug Interactions

Metabolism/Transport Effects Substrate of CYP2B6 (minor), CYP3A4 (major), P-glycoprotein; **Note:** Assignment of Major/Minor substrate status based on clinically relevant drug interaction potential; **Inhibits** CYP3A4 (moderate), P-glycoprotein

Avoid Concomitant Use

Avoid concomitant use of Erythromycin (Systemic) with any of the following: BCG; Bosutinib; Cisapride; Clindamycin (Topical); Conivaptan; Disopyramide; Fluconazole; Fusidic Acid (Systemic); Highest Risk QTc-Prolonging Agents; Ibrutinib; Idelalisib; Ivabradine; Lincosamide Antibiotics; Lomitapide; Lovastatin; Mifepristone; Naloxegol; Olaparib; PAZOPanib; Pimozide; QuiNIDine; QuiNINE; Silodosin; Simeprevir; Simvastatin; Terfenadine; Tolvaptan; Topotecan; Trabectedin; Ulipristal; VinCRIStine (Liposomal)

Increased Effect/Toxicity

Erythromycin (Systemic) may increase the levels/effects of: Afatinib; Alfentanil; ALPRAZolam; Antifungal Agents (Azole Derivatives, Systemic); Antineoplastic Agents (Vinca Alkaloids); ARIPiprazole; AtorvaSTATin; Avanafil; Bosentan; Bosutinib; Brentuximab Vedotin; Budesonide (Systemic, Oral Inhalation); BusPIRone; Calcium Channel Blockers; Cannabis; CarBAMazepine; Cardiac Glycosides; Cilostazol; Cisapride; CloZAPine; Colchicine; CycloSPORINE (Systemic); CYP3A4 Substrates; Dabigatran Etexilate; Dapoxetine; Disopyramide; DOXOrubicin (Conventional); Dronabinol; Edoxaban; Eletriptan; Eplerenone; Ergot Derivatives; Estazolam; Everolimus; FentaNYL; Fexofenadine; Highest Risk QTc-Prolonging Agents; Hydrocodone; Ibrutinib; Imatinib; Ivabradine; Ivacaftor; Ledipasvir; Lomitapide; Lovastatin; Lurasidone; Midazolam; Moderate Risk QTc-Prolonging Agents; Naloxegol; Nintedanib; Olaparib; OxyCODONE; PAZOPanib; P-glycoprotein/ABCB1 Substrates; Pimecrolimus; Pimozide; Pitavastatin; Pravastatin; QuiNIDine; QuiNINE; Ranolazine; Repaglinide; Rifamycin Derivatives; Rifaximin; Rilpivirine; Rivaroxaban; Salmeterol; Saxagliptin; Selective Serotonin Reuptake Inhibitors; Sildenafil; Silodosin; Simeprevir; Simvastatin; Sirolimus; Suvorexant; Tacrolimus (Systemic); Tacrolimus (Topical); Telaprevir; Temsirolimus; Terfenadine; Tetrahydrocannabinol; Theophylline Derivatives; Tolvaptan; Topotecan; Trabectedin; Triazolam; Ulipristal; Vardenafil; Vilazodone; VinCRIStine (Liposomal); Vitamin K Antagonists; Zopiclone

The levels/effects of Erythromycin (Systemic) may be increased by: Antifungal Agents (Azole Derivatives, Systemic); Aprepitant; Conivaptan; CYP3A4 Inhibitors (Moderate); CYP3A4 Inhibitors (Strong); Dasatinib; Fluconazole; Fosaprepitant; Fusidic Acid (Systemic); Idelalisib; Ivabradine; Luliconazole; Mifepristone; Netupitant; P-glycoprotein/ABCB1 Inhibitors; QTc-Prolonging Agents (Indeterminate Risk and Risk Modifying); Stiripentol; Telaprevir

Decreased Effect

Erythromycin (Systemic) may decrease the levels/effects of: BCG; Clindamycin (Topical); Clopidogrel; Ifosfamide; Sodium Picosulfate; Typhoid Vaccine; Zafirlukast

The levels/effects of Erythromycin (Systemic) may be decreased by: Bosentan; CYP3A4 Inducers (Moderate); CYP3A4 Inducers (Strong); Dabrafenib; Deferasirox; Etravirine; Lincosamide Antibiotics; Mitotane; P-glycoprotein/ABCB1 Inducers; Siltuximab; St Johns Wort; Tocilizumab

Food Interactions

Ethanol: Ethanol may decrease absorption of erythromycin or enhance effects of ethanol. Management: Avoid ethanol.

Food: Erythromycin serum levels may be altered if taken with food (formulation-dependent). GI upset, including diarrhea, is common. Management: May be taken with food to decrease GI upset, otherwise take around-the-clock with a full glass of water. Do not give with milk or acidic beverages (eg, soda, juice).

Preparation for Administration Erythromycin lactobionate should be reconstituted with sterile water for injection without preservatives to avoid gel formation. IV form has the longest stability in NS and should be prepared in this base solution whenever possible. Do not use D_5W as a diluent unless sodium bicarbonate is added to solution. If IV must be prepared in D_5W, 0.5 mL of the 8.4% sodium bicarbonate solution should be added per each 100 mL of D_5W.

Standard diluent: 500 mg/250 mL D_5W/NS; 750 mg/250 mL D_5W/NS; 1 g/250 mL D_5W/NS.

Storage/Stability

Injection: Store unreconstituted vials at 15°C to 30°C (59°F to 86°F). Reconstituted solution is stable for 2 weeks when refrigerated or for 8 hours at room temperature. Erythromycin IV infusion solution is stable at pH 6-8; stability of lactobionate is pH dependent; IV form has longest stability in NS. Stability of parenteral admixture at room temperature (25°C) and at refrigeration temperature (4°C) is 24 hours.

Oral suspension:

Granules: Prior to mixing, store at <30°C (86°F). After mixing, store under refrigeration and use within 10 days.

Powder: Prior to mixing, store at <30°C (86°F). After mixing, store at ≤25°C (77°F) and use within 35 days.

Tablet and capsule formulations: Store at <30°C (86°F).

Mechanism of Action Inhibits RNA-dependent protein synthesis at the chain elongation step; binds to the 50S ribosomal subunit resulting in blockage of transpeptidation

Pharmacodynamics/Kinetics

Absorption: Oral: Variable but better with salt forms than with base form; 18% to 45%; ethylsuccinate may be better absorbed with food

Distribution:

Relative diffusion from blood into CSF: Minimal even with inflammation

CSF:blood level ratio: Normal meninges: 2% to 13%; Inflamed meninges: 7% to 25%

Protein binding: Base: 73% to 81%

Metabolism: Demethylation primarily via hepatic CYP3A4

Half-life elimination: Peak: 1.5-2 hours; End-stage renal disease: 5-6 hours

Time to peak, serum: Base: 4 hours; Ethylsuccinate: 0.5-2.5 hours; delayed with food due to differences in absorption

Excretion: Primarily feces; urine (2% to 15% as unchanged drug)

Dosage Note: Due to differences in absorption, 400 mg erythromycin ethylsuccinate produces the same serum levels as 250 mg erythromycin base or stearate.

Usual dosage range:

Infants and Children:

Oral:

Base: 30-50 mg/kg/day in 2-4 divided doses; maximum: 2 g daily

Ethylsuccinate: 30-50 mg/kg/day in 2-4 divided doses; maximum: 3.2 g daily

Stearate: 30-50 mg/kg/day in 2-4 divided doses; maximum: 2 g daily

IV: Lactobionate: 15-50 mg/kg/day divided every 6 hours, not to exceed 4 g daily

Adults:

Oral:

Base: 250-500 mg every 6-12 hours; maximum: 4 g daily

Ethylsuccinate: 400-800 mg every 6-12 hours; maximum: 4 g daily

IV: Lactobionate: 15-20 mg/kg/day divided every 6 hours or 500 mg to 1 g every 6 hours, or given as a continuous infusion over 24 hours; maximum: 4 g daily

Indication-specific dosing:

Infants and Children:

***Bartonella* spp infections (bacillary angiomatosis [BA], peliosis hepatis [PH]) (off-label use):** Oral: 40 mg/kg/day (ethylsuccinate) in 4 divided doses (maximum: 2 g daily) for 3 months (BA) or 4 months (PH) (Rolain, 2004)

Chlamydial infection *(C. trachomatis):* Children <45 kg: Oral: 50 mg/kg/day (base or ethylsuccinate) in 4 divided doses for 14 days (CDC, 2010)

Community-acquired pneumonia (CAP) (IDSA/PIDS, 2011): Infants >3 months and Children: **Note:** A beta-lactam antibiotic should be added if typical bacterial pneumonia cannot be ruled out.

Presumed atypical *(M. pneumoniae, C. pneumoniae, C. trachomatis)* infection, mild atypical infection or step-down therapy (alternative to azithromycin): Oral: 10 mg/kg/dose every 6 hours

Moderate-to-severe atypical infection (alternative to azithromycin): IV: 5 mg/kg/dose every 6 hours

Mild/moderate infection: Oral: 30-50 mg/kg/day in divided doses every 6-12 hours

Pertussis: Oral: 40-50 mg/kg/day in 4 divided doses for 14 days; maximum: 2 g daily (not preferred agent for infants <1 month due to IHPS)

Pharyngitis, tonsillitis (streptococcal): Oral: 20 mg (base)/kg/day or 40 mg (ethylsuccinate)/kg/day in 2 divided doses for 10 days. **Note:** No longer preferred therapy due to increased organism resistance.

Surgical (preoperative) prophylaxis (colorectal) (off-label use): Children ≥1 year: Oral: 20 mg (base)/kg (maximum dose: 1000 mg) at 1 PM, 2 PM, and 11 PM on the day before 8 AM surgery combined with mechanical cleansing of the large intestine, oral neomycin. Perioperative IV antibiotics are also given on the day of surgery (Bratzler, 2013).

Severe infection: IV: 15-50 mg/kg/day; maximum: 4 g daily

Adults:

***Bartonella* spp infections (bacillary angiomatosis [BA], peliosis hepatis [PH]) (off-label use):** Oral: 500 mg (base) 4 times daily for 3 months (BA) or 4 months (PH) (Koehler, 1992; Rolain, 2004; Stevens, 2005; Tappero, 1993)

Chancroid (off-label use): Oral: 500 mg (base) 3 times daily for 7 days; **Note:** Not a preferred agent; isolates with intermediate resistance have been documented (CDC, 2010)

Gastroparesis (off-label use):

IV: 3 mg/kg administered over 45 minutes every 8 hours (Camilleri, 2013)

Oral: Patients refractory/intolerant to other prokinetic agents (eg, metoclopramide, domperidone): 250-500 mg (base) 3 times daily before meals. Limit duration of therapy, tachyphylaxis may occur after 4 weeks (Camilleri, 2013).

Granuloma inguinale (donovanosis) (off-label use): Oral: 500 mg (base) 4 times daily for 21 days (CDC, 2010)

Legionnaires' disease: Oral: 1.6-4 g (ethylsuccinate) daily or 1-4 g (base) daily in divided doses for 21 days. **Note:** No longer preferred therapy and only used in nonhospitalized patients.

Lymphogranuloma venereum: Oral: 500 mg (base) 4 times daily for 21 days; **Note:** Preferred therapy for pregnant or lactating women (CDC, 2010)

Nongonococcal urethritis (including coinfection with *C. trachomatis):* Oral: 500 mg (base) 4 times daily for 7 days or 800 mg (ethylsuccinate) 4 times daily for 7 days. **Note:** May use 250 mg (base) or 400 mg (ethylsuccinate) 4 times daily for 14 days if gastrointestinal intolerance.

Pertussis: Oral: 500 mg (base) every 6 hours for 14 days

Surgical (preoperative) prophylaxis (colorectal) (off-label dose): Oral: 1 g erythromycin base per dose at 1 PM, 2 PM, and 11 PM on the day before 8 AM surgery combined with mechanical cleansing of the large intestine, oral neomycin. Perioperative IV antibiotics are also given on the day of surgery (Bratzler, 2013).

Dosage adjustment in renal impairment: Dialysis: Slightly dialyzable (5% to 20%); no supplemental dosage necessary in hemo- or peritoneal dialysis or in continuous arteriovenous or venovenous hemofiltration

Dosage adjustment in hepatic impairment: No dosage adjustment provided in manufacturer's labeling; use with caution.

Dietary Considerations Drug may cause GI upset; may take with food. Some products may contain sodium.

Administration

Oral: Do not crush enteric coated drug product. GI upset, including diarrhea, is common. May be administered with food to decrease GI upset. Do not give with milk or acidic beverages.

IV: Infuse 1 g over 20-60 minutes. IV infusion may be very irritating to the vein. If phlebitis/pain occurs, consider diluting further (eg, 1:5) if fluid status of the patient will tolerate, or consider administering in larger available vein. The addition of lidocaine or bicarbonate does not decrease the irritation of erythromycin infusions.

Dosage Forms

Capsule Delayed Release Particles, Oral:

Generic: 250 mg

Solution Reconstituted, Intravenous:

Erythrocin Lactobionate: 500 mg (1 ea); 1000 mg (1 ea)

Suspension Reconstituted, Oral:

E.E.S. Granules: 200 mg/5 mL (100 mL, 200 mL)

EryPed 200: 200 mg/5 mL (100 mL)

EryPed 400: 400 mg/5 mL (100 mL)

Tablet, Oral:

E.E.S. 400: 400 mg

Erythrocin Stearate: 250 mg

Generic: 250 mg, 400 mg, 500 mg

Tablet Delayed Release, Oral:

Ery-Tab: 250 mg, 333 mg, 500 mg

PCE: 333 mg, 500 mg

Erythromycin (Ophthalmic) (er ith roe MYE sin)

Brand Names: U.S. Ilotycin; Romycin

Brand Names: Canada Diomycin®; PMS-Erythromycin

Index Terms Erythromycin Base

Pharmacologic Category Antibiotic, Macrolide; Antibiotic, Ophthalmic

Use Treatment of superficial eye infections involving the conjunctiva or cornea

Pregnancy Risk Factor B

Dosage Ophthalmic: Children and Adults: Usual dosage range: Instill 1/2" (1.25 cm) 2-6 times/day depending on the severity of the infection

Additional Information Complete prescribing information should be consulted for additional detail.

Dosage Forms

Ointment, Ophthalmic:

Ilotycin: 5 mg/g (1 g)

Romycin: 5 mg/g (3.5 g)

Generic: 5 mg/g (1 g, 3.5 g)

Erythromycin (Topical) (er ith roe MYE sin)

Brand Names: U.S. Akne-Mycin [DSC]; Ery; Erygel

Brand Names: Canada Erysol

Pharmacologic Category Acne Products; Antibiotic, Macrolide; Antibiotic, Topical; Topical Skin Product; Topical Skin Product, Acne

Use Acne: Treatment of acne vulgaris

Pregnancy Risk Factor B

Dosage Acne: Topical:

Children ≥12 years, Adolescents, and Adults: Erysol gel [Canadian product]: Apply thin film to affected area twice daily (morning and evening); may decrease to once daily if irritation develops at application site. Therapeutic response may take up to 6-8 weeks; discontinue use if no improvement after 6-8 weeks or if condition worsens. Maximum therapy duration: 3 months.

Adults:

Gel: Apply sparingly as a thin film over the affected area once or twice daily. Therapeutic response may take up to 6-8 weeks; discontinue use if no improvement after 6-8 weeks or if condition worsens.

Ointment, solution: Apply to affected area twice daily (morning and evening); drying and peeling may be controlled by reducing the frequency of application.

Pads: Rub pads over affected areas twice daily (morning and evening); additional pads may be used, if needed.

Dosage adjustment in renal impairment: There are no dosage adjustments provided in manufacturer's labeling.

Dosage adjustment in hepatic impairment: There are no dosage adjustments provided in manufacturer's labeling.

Additional Information Complete prescribing information should be consulted for additional detail.

Dosage Forms

Gel, External:

Erygel: 2% (30 g, 60 g)

Generic: 2% (30 g, 60 g)

Pad, External:

Ery: 2% (60 ea)

Generic: 2% (60 ea)

Solution, External:

Generic: 2% (60 mL)

Dosage Forms: Canada

Gel, topical:

Erysol: 2% (25 g)

Erythromycin and Benzoyl Peroxide

(er ith roe MYE sin & BEN zoe il per OKS ide)

Brand Names: U.S. Benzamycin®; Benzamycin® Pak

Brand Names: Canada Benzamycin®

Index Terms Benzoyl Peroxide and Erythromycin

Pharmacologic Category Acne Products; Topical Skin Product, Acne

Use Topical control of acne vulgaris

Pregnancy Risk Factor C

Dosage Adolescents ≥12 years and Adults: Apply twice daily, morning and evening

Additional Information Complete prescribing information should be consulted for additional detail.

Dosage Forms

Gel, topical: Erythromycin 30 mg and benzoyl peroxide 50 mg per g (23 g, 47g)

Benzamycin®: Erythromycin 30 mg and benzoyl peroxide 50 mg per g (47 g)

Benzamycin® Pak: Erythromycin 30 mg and benzoyl peroxide 50 mg per 0.8 g packet (60s)

Erythromycin and Sulfisoxazole

(er ith roe MYE sin & sul fi SOKS a zole)

Brand Names: U.S. E.S.P.®

Brand Names: Canada Pediazole®

Index Terms Sulfisoxazole and Erythromycin

Pharmacologic Category Antibiotic, Macrolide; Antibiotic, Macrolide Combination; Antibiotic, Sulfonamide Derivative

Use Treatment of otitis media caused by susceptible strains of *Haemophilus influenzae*

Pregnancy Risk Factor C

Dosage Oral: Otitis media: Infants ≥2 months and Children: Erythromycin 50 mg/kg/day and sulfisoxazole 150 mg/kg/day in divided doses every 6-8 hours for 10 days; maximum: Erythromycin 2 g/day or sulfisoxazole 6 g/day

Dosage adjustment in renal impairment: No dosage adjustment provided in the manufacturer's labeling.

Dosage adjustment in hepatic impairment: No dosage adjustment provided in manufacturer's labeling; use with caution.

Additional Information Complete prescribing information should be consulted for additional detail.

Dosage Forms

Powder for oral suspension: Erythromycin 200 mg and sulfisoxazole 600 mg per 5 mL

E.S.P.®: Erythromycin 200 mg and sulfisoxazole 600 mg per 5 mL

◆ **Erythromycin Base** *see* Erythromycin (Ophthalmic) *on page 764*

◆ **Erythromycin Base** *see* Erythromycin (Systemic) *on page 762*

◆ **Erythromycin Ethylsuccinate** *see* Erythromycin (Systemic) *on page 762*

◆ **Erythromycin Lactobionate** *see* Erythromycin (Systemic) *on page 762*

◆ **Erythromycin Stearate** *see* Erythromycin (Systemic) *on page 762*

◆ **Erythropoiesis-Stimulating Agent (ESA)** *see* Darbepoetin Alfa *on page 565*

◆ **Erythropoiesis-Stimulating Agent (ESA)** *see* Epoetin Alfa *on page 742*

◆ **Erythropoiesis-Stimulating Protein** *see* Darbepoetin Alfa *on page 565*

◆ **Erythropoietin** *see* Epoetin Alfa *on page 742*

Escitalopram (es sye TAL oh pram)

Brand Names: U.S. Lexapro

Brand Names: Canada Apo-Escitalopram; Cipralex; Cipralex MELTZ; CO Escitalopram; JAMP-Escitalopram; Mar-Escitalopram; Mylan-Escitalopram; PMS-Escitalopram; Priva-Escitalopram; RAN-Escitalopram; Riva-Escitalopram; Sandoz Escitalopram; Teva-Escitalopram

Index Terms Escitalopram Oxalate; Lu-26-054; S-Citalopram

Pharmacologic Category Antidepressant, Selective Serotonin Reuptake Inhibitor

Use Treatment of major depressive disorder; generalized anxiety disorders (GAD)

Canadian labeling: Additional use (not in U.S. labeling): Treatment of obsessive-compulsive disorder (OCD)

Pregnancy Risk Factor C

Pregnancy Considerations Adverse events have been observed in animal reproduction studies. Escitalopram crosses the placenta and is distributed into the amniotic fluid. An increased risk of teratogenic effects, including cardiovascular defects, may be associated with maternal use of escitalopram or other SSRIs; however, available information is conflicting. Nonteratogenic effects in the newborn following SSRI/SNRI exposure late in the third trimester include respiratory distress, cyanosis, apnea, seizures, temperature instability, feeding difficulty, vomiting, hypoglycemia, hypo- or hypertonia, hyper-reflexia, jitteriness, irritability, constant crying, and tremor. Symptoms may be due to the toxicity of the SSRIs/SNRIs or a discontinuation syndrome and may be consistent with serotonin syndrome associated with SSRI treatment. Persistent pulmonary hypertension of the newborn (PPHN) has also been reported with SSRI exposure. The long-term effects of *in utero* SSRI exposure on infant development and behavior are not known. Escitalopram is the S-enantiomer of the racemic derivative citalopram; also refer to the Citalopram monograph.

Due to pregnancy-induced physiologic changes, some pharmacokinetic parameters of escitalopram may be altered. The ACOG recommends that therapy with SSRIs or SNRIs during pregnancy be individualized; treatment of depression during pregnancy should incorporate the clinical expertise of the mental health clinician, obstetrician, primary healthcare provider, and pediatrician. According to the American Psychiatric Association (APA), the risks of medication treatment should be weighed against other treatment options and untreated depression. For women who discontinue antidepressant medications during pregnancy and who may be at high risk for postpartum depression, the medications can be restarted following delivery. Treatment algorithms have been developed by the ACOG and the APA for the management of depression in women prior to conception and during pregnancy.

Breast-Feeding Considerations Escitalopram and its metabolite are excreted into breast milk. Limited data is available concerning the effects escitalopram may have in the nursing infant and the long-term effects on development and behavior have not been studied. Adverse effects have been reported in nursing infants exposed to some SSRIs. According to the manufacturer, the decision to continue or discontinue breast-feeding during therapy should take into account the risk of exposure to the infant and the benefits of treatment to the mother. Maternal use of an SSRI during pregnancy may cause delayed milk secretion. Escitalopram is the S-enantiomer of the racemic derivative citalopram; also refer to the Citalopram monograph.

Contraindications Hypersensitivity to escitalopram, citalopram, or any component of the formulation; use of MAO inhibitors intended to treat psychiatric disorders (concurrently or within 14 days of discontinuing either escitalopram or the MAO inhibitor); initiation of escitalopram in a patient receiving linezolid or intravenous methylene blue; concurrent use of pimozide

Canadian labeling: Additional contraindications (not in U.S. labeling): Known QT-interval prolongation or congenital long QT syndrome

Warnings/Precautions [U.S. Boxed Warning]: Antidepressants increase the risk of suicidal thinking and behavior in children, adolescents, and young adults (18-24 years of age) with major depressive disorder (MDD) and other psychiatric disorders; consider risk prior to prescribing. Short-term studies did not show an increased risk in patients >24 years of age and showed a decreased risk in patients ≥65 years. Closely monitor patients for clinical worsening, suicidality, or unusual changes in behavior, particularly during the initial 1-2 months of therapy or during periods of dosage adjustments (increases or decreases); the patient's family or caregiver should be instructed to closely observe the patient and communicate condition with healthcare provider. A medication guide concerning the use of antidepressants should be dispensed with each prescription. **Escitalopram is not FDA approved for use in children <12 years of age.**

The possibility of a suicide attempt is inherent in major depression and may persist until remission occurs. Use caution in high-risk patients. Worsening depression and severe abrupt suicidality that are not part of the presenting symptoms may require discontinuation or modification of drug therapy. The patient's family or caregiver should be alerted to monitor patients for the emergence of suicidality and associated behaviors (such as agitation, irritability, hostility, impulsivity, and hypomania) and call healthcare provider.

May precipitate a shift to mania or hypomania in patients with bipolar disorder. Patients presenting with depressive symptoms should be screened for bipolar disorder. Monotherapy in patients with bipolar disorder should be avoided. Escitalopram is not FDA approved for the treatment of bipolar depression.

Potentially life-threatening serotonin syndrome (SS) has occurred with serotonergic agents (eg, SSRIs, SNRIs), particularly when used in combination with other serotonergic agents (eg, triptans, TCAs, fentanyl, lithium, tramadol, buspirone, St John's wort, tryptophan) or agents that impair metabolism of serotonin (eg, MAO inhibitors intended to treat psychiatric disorders, other MAO inhibitors [ie, linezolid and intravenous methylene blue]). Discontinue treatment (and any concomitant serotonergic agent) immediately if signs/symptoms arise. May increase the risks associated with electroconvulsive therapy. Has a low potential to impair cognitive or motor performance; caution operating hazardous machinery or driving. Bone fractures have been associated with antidepressant treatment. Consider the possibility of a fragility fracture if an antidepressant-treated patient presents with unexplained bone pain, point tenderness, swelling, or bruising (Rabenda, 2013; Rizzoli, 2012).

Use with caution in patients with a recent history of MI or unstable heart disease. Use has been associated with dose-dependent QT-interval prolongation with doses of 10 mg and 30 mg/day in healthy subjects (mean change from baseline: 4.3 msec and 10.7 msec, respectively); prolongation of QT interval and ventricular arrhythmia (including torsade de pointes) have been reported, particularly in females with preexisting QT prolongation or other risk factors (eg, hypokalemia, other cardiac disease).

Use caution with a previous seizure disorder or condition predisposing to seizures such as brain damage, alcoholism, or concurrent therapy with other drugs which lower the seizure threshold. May cause hyponatremia/SIADH (elderly at increased risk); volume depletion (diuretics may increase risk) may occur. Use caution in patients with metabolic disease. May cause or exacerbate sexual dysfunction. Use caution in elderly patients; may be potentially inappropriate in patients with a history of falls or fractures, and may cause or exacerbate syndrome of inappropriate antidiuretic hormone secretion or hyponatremia; monitor sodium closely with initiation or dosage adjustments in older adults (Beers Criteria). Bioavailability and half-life are increased by 50% in the elderly. Use caution with severe renal impairment or liver impairment; concomitant CNS depressants. May cause mild pupillary dilation which in susceptible individuals can lead to an episode of narrow-angle glaucoma. Consider evaluating patients who have not had an iridectomy for narrow-angle glaucoma risk factors. Use with caution in patients who are hemodynamically unstable. Potentially significant drug-drug interactions may exist, requiring dose or frequency adjustment, additional monitoring, and/or selection of alternative therapy. Escitalopram systemic exposure may be increased in CYP2C19 poor metabolizers; Canadian labeling recommends a dosage adjustment in this patient population.

Abrupt discontinuation or interruption of antidepressant therapy has been associated with a discontinuation syndrome. Symptoms arising may vary with antidepressant however commonly include nausea, vomiting, diarrhea, headaches, light-headedness, dizziness, diminished appetite, sweating, chills, tremors, paresthesias, fatigue, somnolence, and sleep disturbances (eg, vivid dreams, insomnia). Greater risks for developing a discontinuation syndrome have been associated with antidepressants with shorter half-lives, longer durations of treatment, and abrupt discontinuation. For antidepressants of short or intermediate half-lives, symptoms may emerge within 2-5 days after treatment discontinuation and last 7-14 days (APA, 2010; Fava, 2006; Haddad, 2001; Shelton, 2001; Warner, 2006).

Some dosage forms may contain propylene glycol; large amounts are potentially toxic and have been associated hyperosmolality, lactic acidosis, seizures, and respiratory depression; use caution (AAP, 1997; Zar, 2007).

Adverse Reactions

Central nervous system: Abnormal dreams, anorgasmia, dizziness, drowsiness, fatigue, headache, insomnia, lethargy, paresthesia, yawning

Dermatologic: Diaphoresis

Endocrine & metabolic: Decreased libido, menstrual disease

Gastrointestinal: Abdominal pain, constipation, decreased appetite, diarrhea, dyspepsia, flatulence, nausea, toothache, vomiting, xerostomia

Genitourinary: Ejaculatory disorder, impotence, urinary tract infection (children)

Neuromuscular & skeletal: Back pain (children), neck pain, shoulder pain

Respiratory: Flu-like symptoms, nasal congestion (children), rhinitis, sinusitis

Rare but important or life-threatening: Abdominal cramps, abnormal gait, acute renal failure, aggressive behavior, agitated depression, agitation, agranulocytosis, akathisia, alopecia, amnesia, anaphylaxis, anemia, angioedema, angle-closure glaucoma, anxiety, apathy, aplastic anemia, arthralgia, ataxia, atrial fibrillation, blurred vision, bradycardia, bronchitis, cardiac failure, cerebrovascular accident, chest pain, choreoathetosis, deep vein thrombosis, delirium, delusions, depersonalization, dermatitis, diabetes mellitus, diplopia, dyskinesia, dysmenorrhea, dysphagia, dyspnea, dystonia, dysuria, ecchymoses, edema, epistaxis, erythema multiforme, extrapyramidal reaction, fever, flushing, gastroenteritis, gastroesophageal reflux disease, gastrointestinal hemorrhage, hallucination, heartburn, hemolytic anemia, hepatic failure, hepatic necrosis, hepatitis, hot flash, hypercholesterolemia, hyperglycemia, hypermenorrhea, hyperprolactinemia, hypersensitivity reaction, hypertension, hypertensive crisis, hypoesthesia, hypoglycemia, hypokalemia, hyponatremia, hypoprothrombinemia, hypotension, immune thrombocytopenia, increased appetite, increased INR, increased liver enzymes, increased serum bilirubin, irritability, jaw tightness, lack of concentration, leukopenia, limb pain, migraine, myalgia, myasthenia, mydriasis, myocardial infarction, myoclonus, neuroleptic malignant syndrome (Stevens, 2008), nightmares, nystagmus, orthostatic hypotension, palpitations, pancreatitis, panic, paranoia, Parkinsonian-like syndrome, phlebitis, priapism, prolonged Q-T interval on ECG, psychosis, pulmonary embolism, rectal hemorrhage, rhabdomyolysis, seizure, serotonin syndrome, SIADH, sinus congestion, sinus headache, skin photosensitivity, skin rash, spontaneous abortion, Stevens-Johnson syndrome, suicidal ideation, suicidal tendencies, syncope, tachycardia, tardive dyskinesia, thrombocytopenia, thrombosis, tinnitus, torsades de pointes, toxic epidermal necrolysis, tremor, urinary frequency, urinary retention, urticaria, ventricular arrhythmia, ventricular tachycardia, vertigo, visual disturbance, withdrawal syndrome

Drug Interactions

Metabolism/Transport Effects Substrate of CYP2C19 (major), CYP3A4 (major); **Note:** Assignment of Major/Minor substrate status based on clinically relevant drug interaction potential; **Inhibits** CYP2D6 (weak)

Avoid Concomitant Use

Avoid concomitant use of Escitalopram with any of the following: Conivaptan; Dapoxetine; Dosulepin; Fusidic Acid (Systemic); Highest Risk QTc-Prolonging Agents; Idelalisib; Iobenguane I 123; Ivabradine; Linezolid; MAO Inhibitors; Methylene Blue; Mifepristone; Moderate Risk QTc-Prolonging Agents; Pimozide; Tryptophan; Urokinase

Increased Effect/Toxicity

Escitalopram may increase the levels/effects of: Agents with Antiplatelet Properties; Anticoagulants; Antidepressants (Serotonin Reuptake Inhibitor/Antagonist); Antipsychotic Agents; Apixaban; Aspirin; BusPIRone; CarBAMazepine; Collagenase (Systemic); Dabigatran Etexilate; Desmopressin; Dextromethorphan; Dosulepin; Highest Risk QTc-Prolonging Agents; Hypoglycemic Agents; Ibritumomab; Methylene Blue; Mexiletine; NSAID (COX-2 Inhibitor); NSAID (Nonselective); Obinutuzumab; Pimozide; Rivaroxaban; Salicylates; Serotonin Modulators; Thiazide Diuretics; Thrombolytic Agents; Tositumomab and Iodine I 131 Tositumomab; TraMADol; Tricyclic Antidepressants; Urokinase; Vitamin K Antagonists

The levels/effects of Escitalopram may be increased by: Alcohol (Ethyl); Analgesics (Opioid); Antiemetics (5HT3 Antagonists); Antipsychotic Agents; Aprepitant; BusPIRone; Cimetidine; CNS Depressants; Conivaptan; CYP2C19 Inhibitors (Moderate); CYP2C19 Inhibitors (Strong); CYP3A4 Inhibitors (Moderate); CYP3A4 Inhibitors (Strong); Dapoxetine; Fosaprepitant; Fusidic Acid (Systemic); Glucosamine; Herbs (Anticoagulant/Antiplatelet Properties); Ibrutinib; Idelalisib; Ivabradine; Ivacaftor; Limaprost; Linezolid; Lithium; Luliconazole; MAO Inhibitors; Metoclopramide; Metyrosine; Mifepristone; Moderate Risk QTc-Prolonging Agents; Multivitamins/Fluoride (with ADE); Multivitamins/Minerals (with ADEK, Folate, Iron); Multivitamins/Minerals (with AE, No Iron); Netupitant; Omega-3 Fatty Acids; Omeprazole; Pentosan Polysulfate Sodium; Pentoxifylline; Prostacyclin Analogues; QTc-Prolonging Agents (Indeterminate Risk and Risk Modifying); Stiripentol; Tedizolid; Tipranavir; TraMADol; Tricyclic Antidepressants; Tryptophan; Vitamin E

Decreased Effect

Escitalopram may decrease the levels/effects of: Iobenguane I 123; Ioflupane I 123; Simeprevir; Thyroid Products

The levels/effects of Escitalopram may be decreased by: Boceprevir; Bosentan; CarBAMazepine; CYP2C19 Inducers (Strong); CYP3A4 Inducers (Moderate); CYP3A4 Inducers (Strong); Cyproheptadine; Dabrafenib; Deferasirox; Mitotane; NSAID (COX-2 Inhibitor); NSAID (Nonselective); Siltuximab; St Johns Wort; Telaprevir; Tocilizumab

Storage/Stability Store at 25°C (77°F); excursions permitted to 15°C to 30°C (59°F to 86°F). Cipralex MELTZ [Canadian product] should be stored in original package and protected from light.

Mechanism of Action Escitalopram is the S-enantiomer of the racemic derivative citalopram, which selectively inhibits the reuptake of serotonin with little to no effect on norepinephrine or dopamine reuptake. It has no or very low affinity for 5-HT_{1-7}, alpha- and beta-adrenergic, D_{1-5}, H_{1-3}, M_{1-5}, and benzodiazepine receptors. Escitalopram does not bind to or has low affinity for Na^+, K^+, Cl^-, and Ca^{++} ion channels.

Pharmacodynamics/Kinetics

Onset of action: Depression: The onset of action is within a week; however, individual response varies greatly and full response may not be seen until 8-12 weeks after initiation of treatment.

Distribution: V_d: ~20 L/kg (Søgaard, 2005)

Protein binding: ~56% to plasma proteins

Metabolism: Hepatic via CYP2C19 and 3A4 to S-desmethylcitalopram (S-DCT); S-DCT is metabolized to S-didesmethylcitalopram (S-DDCT) via CYP2D6; *in vitro* data suggest metabolites do not contribute significantly to the antidepressant effects of escitalopram

Half-life elimination: ~27-32 hours (increased ~50% in the elderly and doubled in patients with hepatic impairment)

Time to peak: Escitalopram: ~5 hours

Excretion: Urine (8% as unchanged drug; S-DCT 10%)

Dosage Oral:

U.S. labeling:

Children ≥12 years: Major depressive disorder: Initial: 10 mg once daily; dose may be increased to a maximum of 20 mg once daily after at least 3 weeks

Adults: Major depressive disorder, generalized anxiety disorder: Initial: 10 mg once daily; dose may be increased to a maximum of 20 mg once daily after at least 1 week

Elderly: 10 mg once daily

Canadian labeling: **Note:** Orodispersible tablets should only be used for doses that can be accommodated with whole tablets (ie, 10 mg or multiples of that).

Adults: Major depressive disorder, generalized anxiety disorder (GAD), obsessive compulsive disorder (OCD): Initial: 10 mg once daily (may consider 5 mg once daily where sensitivity is a concern); dose may be increased as tolerated to a maximum of 20 mg once daily. In poor CYP2C19 metabolizers, initiate at a dose of 5 mg once daily; may increase dose to a maximum of 10 mg once daily. Patients with GAD or OCD who require extended therapy should be maintained at the lowest effective dose and assessed periodically to determine the need for continued therapy.

Elderly: Initial: 5 mg once daily; dose may be increased as tolerated to a maximum of 10 mg once daily

Adults: Hot flashes (off-label use): Initial: 10 mg once daily, increase to 20 mg once daily after 4 weeks if symptoms not adequately controlled (Carpenter, 2012; Freeman, 2011).

Discontinuation of therapy: Upon discontinuation of antidepressant therapy, gradually taper the dose to minimize the incidence of withdrawal symptoms and allow for the detection of re-emerging symptoms. Evidence supporting ideal taper rates is limited. APA and NICE guidelines suggest tapering therapy over at least several weeks with consideration to the half-life of the antidepressant; antidepressants with a shorter half-life may need to be tapered more conservatively. In addition for long-term treated patients, WFSBP guidelines recommend tapering over 4-6 months. If intolerable withdrawal symptoms occur following a dose reduction, consider resuming the previously prescribed dose and/or decrease dose at a more gradual rate (APA, 2010; Bauer, 2002; Haddad, 2001; NCCMH, 2010; Schatzberg, 2006; Shelton, 2001; Warner, 2006).

MAO inhibitor recommendations: *U.S. labeling:*

Switching to or from an MAO inhibitor intended to treat psychiatric disorders:

Allow 14 days to elapse between discontinuing an MAO inhibitor intended to treat psychiatric disorders and initiation of escitalopram.

Allow 14 days to elapse between discontinuing escitalopram and initiation of an MAO inhibitor intended to treat psychiatric disorders.

Use with other MAO inhibitors (linezolid or IV methylene blue):

Do not initiate escitalopram in patients receiving linezolid or IV methylene blue; consider other interventions for psychiatric condition.

If urgent treatment with linezolid or IV methylene blue is required in a patient already receiving escitalopram and potential benefits outweigh potential risks, discontinue escitalopram promptly and administer linezolid or IV methylene blue. Monitor for serotonin syndrome for 2 weeks or until 24 hours after the last dose of linezolid or IV methylene blue, whichever comes first. May resume escitalopram 24 hours after the last dose of linezolid or IV methylene blue.

Dosage adjustment with concomitant medications: *Canadian labeling:* Escitalopram dose should not exceed 10 mg once daily in patients taking omeprazole or cimetidine.

Dosage adjustment in renal impairment:

Mild-to-moderate impairment: No dosage adjustment is necessary

Severe impairment: CrCl <20 mL/minute (U.S. labeling) or CrCl <30 mL/minute (Canadian labeling): Use with caution.

Dosage adjustment in hepatic impairment:

U.S. labeling: 10 mg once daily

Canadian labeling:

Mild or moderate impairment (Child-Pugh class A or B): Initial: 5 mg once daily; dose may be increased as tolerated to 10 mg once daily (maximum dose)

Severe Impairment (Child-Pugh class C): No dosage adjustment provided in manufacturer's labeling; has not been studied. Use with caution.

Dietary Considerations May be taken with or without food.

Administration Administer once daily (morning or evening), with or without food.

Cipralex MELTZ [Canadian product] should be dissolved on the tongue and swallowed without water.

Monitoring Parameters Administer once daily (morning or evening), with or without food.

Cipralex MELTZ [Canadian product] should be dissolved on the tongue and swallowed without water.

Additional Information The tablet and oral solution dosage forms are bioequivalent. Cipralex MELTZ orodispersible tablets [Canadian product] are considered bioequivalent to Cipralex tablets [Canadian product].

Clinically, escitalopram 20 mg is equipotent to citalopram 40 mg. Do not coadminister with citalopram.

Dosage Forms

Solution, Oral:

Lexapro: 5 mg/5 mL (240 mL)

Generic: 5 mg/5 mL (240 mL)

Tablet, Oral:

Lexapro: 5 mg, 10 mg, 20 mg

Generic: 5 mg, 10 mg, 20 mg

Dosage Forms: Canada

Tablet:

Cipralex: 10 mg, 20 mg

Tablet, Orodispersible, as base:

Cipralex MELTZ: 10 mg, 20 mg [mint flavor]

◆ **Escitalopram Oxalate** *see* Escitalopram *on page 765*

- **Eserine Salicylate** *see* Physostigmine *on page 1647*
- **Esgic** *see* Butalbital, Acetaminophen, and Caffeine *on page 313*
- **Esgic-Plus** *see* Butalbital, Acetaminophen, and Caffeine *on page 313*
- **Eskalith** *see* Lithium *on page 1230*

Esmolol (ES moe lol)

Brand Names: U.S. Brevibloc; Brevibloc in NaCl

Brand Names: Canada Brevibloc; Brevibloc Premixed

Index Terms Esmolol Hydrochloride

Pharmacologic Category Antiarrhythmic Agent, Class II; Antihypertensive; Beta-Blocker, Beta-1 Selective

Use Treatment of supraventricular tachycardia (SVT) and atrial fibrillation/flutter (control ventricular rate); treatment of intraoperative and postoperative tachycardia and/or hypertension; treatment of noncompensatory sinus tachycardia

Pregnancy Risk Factor C

Pregnancy Considerations Adverse events were observed in some animal reproduction studies. Esmolol has been shown to decrease fetal heart rate. Adverse fetal/neonatal events have also been observed with the chronic use of beta-blockers during pregnancy. Esmolol is a short-acting beta-blocker and not indicated for the chronic treatment of hypertension. Esmolol has been evaluated for use during intubation as an agent to offset the exaggerated pressor response observed in pregnant women with hypertension undergoing surgery (Bansal, 2002).

Breast-Feeding Considerations It is not known if esmolol is excreted into breast milk. Due to the potential for serious adverse reactions in the nursing infant, the manufacturer recommends a decision be made whether to discontinue nursing or to discontinue the drug, taking into account the importance of treatment to the mother. The short half-life and the fact that it is not intended for chronic use should limit any potential exposure to the nursing infant.

Contraindications Hypersensitivity to esmolol or any component of the formulation; severe sinus bradycardia; heart block greater than first degree (except in patients with a functioning artificial ventricular pacemaker); sick sinus syndrome; cardiogenic shock; decompensated heart failure; IV administration of calcium channel blockers (eg, verapamil) in close proximity to esmolol (ie, while effects of other drug are still present); pulmonary hypertension

Canadian labeling: Additional contraindications (not in U.S. labeling): Patients requiring inotropic agents and/or vasopressors to maintain cardiac output and systolic blood pressure; hypotension; right ventricular failure secondary to pulmonary hypertension; untreated pheochromocytoma

Warnings/Precautions Can cause bradycardia including sinus pause, heart block, severe bradycardia, and cardiac arrest. Consider preexisting conditions such as first degree AV block, sick sinus syndrome, or other conduction disorders before initiating; use is contraindicated in patients with sick sinus syndrome or second- or third-degree AV block (except in patients with a functioning artificial ventricular pacemaker). Bradycardia may be observed more frequently in elderly patients (>65 years of age); dosage reductions may be necessary. Hypotension is common; patients need close blood pressure monitoring. If an unacceptable drop in blood pressure occurs, reduction in dose or discontinuation may reverse hypotension (usually within 30 minutes). Avoid use in patients with hypovolemia; treat hypovolemia first, otherwise, use of esmolol may attenuate reflex tachycardia and further increase the risk of hypotension. Administer cautiously in compensated heart failure and monitor for a worsening of the condition; use is contraindicated in patients with decompensated heart failure.

Esmolol has been associated with elevations in serum potassium and development of hyperkalemia especially in patients with risk factors (eg, renal impairment); monitor serum potassium during therapy. Use with caution in patients with myasthenia gravis. Use caution in patients with renal dysfunction (active metabolite retained). Adequate alpha-blockade is required prior to use of any beta-blocker for patients with untreated pheochromocytoma; Canadian labeling contraindicates use in this patient population. Use beta-blockers cautiously in patients with bronchospastic disease; monitor pulmonary status closely. Use cautiously in patients with diabetes because it can mask prominent hypoglycemic symptoms. May mask signs of hyperthyroidism (eg, tachycardia); if hyperthyroidism is suspected, carefully manage and monitor; abrupt withdrawal may exacerbate symptoms of hyperthyroidism or precipitate thyroid storm. Use esmolol with caution in patients with hypertension associated with hypothermia; monitor vital signs closely and titrate esmolol slowly. Use caution with history of severe anaphylaxis to allergens; patients taking beta-blockers may become more sensitive to repeated challenges. Treatment of anaphylaxis (eg, epinephrine) in patients taking beta-blockers may be ineffective or promote undesirable effects. Can precipitate or aggravate symptoms of arterial insufficiency in patients with PVD and Raynaud's disease; use with caution and monitor for progression of arterial obstruction.

Use caution with concurrent use of digoxin, verapamil or diltiazem; bradycardia or heart block can occur (may be fatal). Use is contraindicated when IV calcium channel blockers have been administered in close proximity to esmolol (ie, while effects of other drug are still present). Beta-blocker therapy should not be withdrawn abruptly (particularly in patients with CAD), but gradually tapered to avoid acute tachycardia, hypertension, and/or ischemia. Vesicant; ensure proper needle or catheter placement prior to and during infusion; avoid extravasation. Extravasation can lead to skin necrosis and sloughing; avoid infusions into small veins or through a butterfly catheter.

Adverse Reactions

Cardiovascular: Asymptomatic hypotension, blood pressure decreased, peripheral ischemia, symptomatic hypotension

Central nervous system: Agitation, confusion, dizziness, headache, somnolence

Gastrointestinal: Nausea, vomiting

Local: Infusion site reaction (including irritation, inflammation, and severe reactions associated with extravasation [eg, thrombophlebitis, necrosis, and blistering])

Rare but important or life-threatening: Abdominal discomfort, abnormal thinking, angioedema, anorexia, anxiety, bradycardia, bronchospasm, cardiac arrest, constipation, coronary arteriospasm, decompensated heart failure, depression, dyspepsia, flushing, heart block, hyperkalemia, lightheadedness, pallor, paresthesia, psoriasis, renal tubular acidosis, seizure, severe bradycardia/asystole (rare), syncope, urinary retention, urticaria, xerostomia

Drug Interactions

Metabolism/Transport Effects None known.

Avoid Concomitant Use

Avoid concomitant use of Esmolol with any of the following: Ceritinib; Floctafenine; Methacholine

Increased Effect/Toxicity

Esmolol may increase the levels/effects of: Alpha-/Beta-Agonists (Direct-Acting); Alpha1-Blockers; Alpha2-Agonists; Amifostine; Antihypertensives; Antipsychotic Agents (Phenothiazines); Bradycardia-Causing Agents; Bupivacaine; Cardiac Glycosides; Ceritinib; Cholinergic

Agonists; Disopyramide; DULoxetine; Ergot Derivatives; Fingolimod; Grass Pollen Allergen Extract (5 Grass Extract); Hypotensive Agents; Insulin; Lacosamide; Levodopa; Lidocaine (Systemic); Lidocaine (Topical); Mepivacaine; Methacholine; Midodrine; Obinutuzumab; RisperiDONE; RiTUXimab; Sulfonylureas

The levels/effects of Esmolol may be increased by: Acetylcholinesterase Inhibitors; Alpha2-Agonists; Aminoquinolines (Antimalarial); Amiodarone; Anilidopiperidine Opioids; Antipsychotic Agents (Phenothiazines); Barbiturates; Bretylium; Brimonidine (Topical); Calcium Channel Blockers (Dihydropyridine); Calcium Channel Blockers (Nondihydropyridine); Diazoxide; Dipyridamole; Disopyramide; Dronedarone; Floctafenine; Herbs (Hypotensive Properties); MAO Inhibitors; Nicorandil; Pentoxifylline; Phosphodiesterase 5 Inhibitors; Propafenone; Prostacyclin Analogues; Regorafenib; Reserpine; Tofacitinib

Decreased Effect

Esmolol may decrease the levels/effects of: Beta2-Agonists; Theophylline Derivatives

The levels/effects of Esmolol may be decreased by: Barbiturates; Herbs (Hypertensive Properties); Methylphenidate; Nonsteroidal Anti-Inflammatory Agents; Rifamycin Derivatives; Yohimbine

Storage/Stability Clear, colorless to light yellow solution which should be stored at 25°C (77°F); excursions permitted to 15°C to 30°C (59°F to 86°F); do not freeze. Protect from excessive heat. Stable for at least 24 hours (under refrigeration or at controlled room temperature) at a final concentration of 10 mg/mL.

Mechanism of Action Class II antiarrhythmic: Competitively blocks response to beta$_1$-adrenergic stimulation with little or no effect of beta$_2$-receptors except at high doses, no intrinsic sympathomimetic activity, no membrane stabilizing activity

Pharmacodynamics/Kinetics

Onset of action: Beta-blockade: IV: 2-10 minutes (quickest when loading doses are administered)

Duration of hemodynamic effects: 10-30 minutes; prolonged following higher cumulative doses, extended duration of use

Distribution: V_d: Esmolol: ~3.4 L/kg; Acid metabolite: ~0.4 L/kg

Protein binding: Esmolol: 55%; Acid metabolite: 10%

Metabolism: In blood by red blood cell esterases; forms acid metabolite (negligible activity; produces no clinically important effects) and methanol (does not achieve concentrations associated with methanol toxicity)

Half-life elimination: Adults: Esmolol: 9 minutes; Acid metabolite: 3.7 hours; elimination of metabolite decreases with end-stage renal disease

Excretion: Urine (~73% to 88% as acid metabolite, <2% unchanged drug)

Dosage IV: Adults:

U.S. labeling:

Intraoperative and postoperative tachycardia and/or hypertension:

Immediate control: Initial bolus: 1 **mg**/kg over 30 seconds, followed by a 150 mcg/kg/minute infusion, if necessary. Adjust infusion rate as needed to maintain desired heart rate and/or blood pressure (up to 300 mcg/kg/minute)

Gradual control: Initial bolus: 0.5 **mg**/kg over 1 minute, followed by a 50 mcg/kg/minute infusion for 4 minutes. Infusion may be continued at 50 mcg/kg/minute or, if the response is inadequate, titrated upward in 50 mcg/kg/minute increments (increased no more frequently than every 4 minutes) to a maximum of 300 mcg/kg/minute; may administer an optional loading dose equal to the initial bolus (0.5 **mg**/kg over 1 minute) prior to each increase in infusion rate.

For control of tachycardia, doses >200 mcg/kg/minute provide minimal additional effect. *For control of postoperative hypertension,* as many as one-third of patients may require higher doses (250-300 mcg/kg/minute) to control blood pressure; the safety of doses >300 mcg/kg/minute has not been studied.

Supraventricular tachycardia (SVT) or noncompensatory sinus tachycardia: Loading dose (optional): 0.5 **mg**/kg over 1 minute; follow with a 50 mcg/kg/minute infusion for 4 minutes; response to this initial infusion rate may be a rough indication of the responsiveness of the ventricular rate.

Infusion may be continued at 50 mcg/kg/minute or, if the response is inadequate, titrated upward in 50 mcg/kg/minute increments (increased no more frequently than every 4 minutes) to a maximum of 200 mcg/kg/minute.

To achieve more rapid response, following the initial loading dose and 50 mcg/kg/minute infusion, rebolus with a second 0.5 **mg**/kg loading dose over 1 minute, and increase the maintenance infusion to 100 mcg/kg/minute for 4 minutes. If necessary, a third (and final) 0.5 **mg**/kg loading dose may be administered, prior to increasing to an infusion rate of 150 mcg/kg/minute. After 4 minutes of the 150 mcg/kg/minute infusion, the infusion rate may be increased to a maximum rate of 200 mcg/kg/minute (without a bolus dose).

Note: If a loading dose is not administered, a continuous infusion at a fixed dose reaches steady-state in ~30 minutes. In general, the usual effective dose is 50-200 mcg/kg/minute; doses as low as 25 mcg/kg/minute may be adequate. Maintenance infusions may be continued for up to 48 hours.

Acute coronary syndromes (when relative contraindications to beta-blockade exist; off-label use): 0.5 **mg**/kg over 1 minute; follow with a 50 mcg/kg/minute infusion; if tolerated and response inadequate, may titrate upward in 50 mcg/kg/minute increments every 5-15 minutes to a maximum of 300 mcg/kg/minute (Mitchell, 2002); an additional bolus (0.5 **mg**/kg over 1 minute) may be administered prior to each increase in infusion rate (Mooss, 1994)

Electroconvulsive therapy (off-label use): 1 **mg**/kg administered 1 minute prior to induction of anesthesia (Weinger, 1991)

Intubation (off-label use): 1-2 **mg**/kg given 1.5-3 minutes prior to intubation (Kindler, 1996)

Thyrotoxicosis or thyroid storm (off-label use): 50-100 mcg/kg/minute (Bahn, 2011)

Canadian labeling: **Note:** Not recommended for use >24 hours.

Perioperative tachycardia and/or hypertension:

Associated with intubation (off-label use): Bolus: 1.5 **mg**/kg (maximum dose: 100 **mg**) over 30 seconds given 1-2 minutes prior to intubation.

Intraoperative/postoperative tachycardia and/or hypertension: Initial bolus: 1.5 **mg**/kg (maximum dose: 100 **mg**) over 30 seconds, followed by 150 mcg/kg/minute infusion. Adjust infusion rate as needed to maintain desired heart rate or blood pressure (up to 300 mcg/kg/minute).

Atrial fibrillation/atrial flutter:

Loading dose: 0.5 **mg**/kg over 1 minute; follow with a 50 mcg/kg/minute infusion for 4 minutes; response to this initial infusion rate may be a rough indication of the responsiveness of the ventricular rate.

Infusion may be continued at 50 mcg/kg/minute or, if the response is inadequate, rebolus with a second 0.5 **mg**/kg loading dose over 1 minute, and increase the maintenance infusion to 100 mcg/kg/minute for 4 minutes. If necessary, repeat same procedure (ie, 0.5 **mg**/kg loading dose and increase maintenance infusion by 50 mcg/kg/minute for 4 minutes) until target heart rate or safety end point (eg, hypotension) begins to occur then omit subsequent loading dose and decrease dosing increment of maintenance infusion to ≤25 mcg/kg/minute or alternatively, the manufacturer labeling suggests that the titration interval may be extended from 5 minutes to 10 minutes. If safety endpoints are exceeded discontinue infusion and when appropriate, resume infusion at reduced dose.

Note: In general, the usual effective dose is 50-200 mcg/kg/minute; doses as low as 25 mcg/kg/minute may be adequate.

Guidelines for transfer to oral therapy (beta-blocker, calcium channel blocker):

Infusion should be reduced by 50% thirty minutes following the first dose of the alternative agent

Manufacturer suggests following the second dose of the alternative drug, patient's response should be monitored and if control is adequate for the first hour, esmolol may be discontinued.

Dosage adjustment in renal impairment: No dosage adjustment necessary. Dialysis: Not removed by hemo- or peritoneal dialysis; supplemental dose is not necessary.

Dosage adjustment in hepatic impairment: No dosage adjustment necessary

Usual Infusion Concentrations: Pediatric Note: Premixed solutions available.

IV infusion: 10,000 **mcg**/mL or 20,000 **mcg**/mL

Usual Infusion Concentrations: Adult Note: Premixed solutions available.

IV infusion: 2500 mg in 250 mL (concentration: 10,000 **mcg**/mL) **or** 2000 mg in 100 mL (concentration: 20,000 **mcg**/mL) of D_5W or NS

Administration IV: Loading doses (eg, 0.5 **mg**/kg) may be administered over 30 seconds to 1 minute depending on how urgent the need for effect. Infusion into small veins or through a butterfly catheter should be avoided (can cause thrombophlebitis). Medication port of premixed bags should be used to withdraw only the initial bolus, if necessary (not to be used for withdrawal of additional bolus doses).

Vesicant; ensure proper needle or catheter placement prior to and during infusion; avoid extravasation.

Extravasation management: If extravasation occurs, stop infusion immediately and disconnect (leave cannula/needle in place); gently aspirate extravasated solution (do **NOT** flush the line); remove needle/cannula; elevate extremity.

Monitoring Parameters Blood pressure, MAP, heart rate, continuous ECG, respiratory rate, IV site; serum potassium (especially with renal impairment); consult individual institutional policies and procedures

Dosage Forms

Solution, Intravenous:

Brevibloc: 10 mg/mL (10 mL)

Brevibloc in NaCl: 2000 mg (100 mL); 2500 mg (250 mL)

Generic: 10 mg/mL (10 mL)

Solution, Intravenous [preservative free]:

Generic: 10 mg/mL (10 mL); 100 mg/10 mL (10 mL)

◆ **Esmolol Hydrochloride** *see* Esmolol *on page* 769

Esomeprazole (es oh ME pray zol)

Brand Names: U.S. NexIUM; NexIUM I.V.

Brand Names: Canada Apo-Esomeprazole; Mylan-Esomeprazole; Nexium; PMS-Esomeprazole DR

Index Terms Esomeprazole Magnesium; Esomeprazole Sodium; Esomeprazole Strontium; Nexium 24HR

Pharmacologic Category Proton Pump Inhibitor; Substituted Benzimidazole

Use

Oral:

Esomeprazole magnesium and esomeprazole strontium:

Gastroesophageal reflux disease (Rx only):

Healing of erosive esophagitis: Short-term (4 to 8 weeks) treatment of erosive esophagitis

Maintenance of healing of erosive esophagitis: Maintaining symptom resolution and healing of erosive esophagitis

Symptomatic gastroesophageal reflux disease: Short-term (4 to 8 weeks) treatment of symptomatic gastroesophageal reflux disease (GERD)

***Helicobacter pylori* eradication (Rx only):** As part of a multidrug regimen for *Helicobacter pylori* eradication in patients with duodenal ulcer disease (active or history of within the past 5 years)

Risk reduction of nonsteroidal anti-inflammatory drug-associated gastric ulcer (Rx only): Prevention of gastric ulcers associated with continuous NSAID therapy in patients at risk (age ≥60 years and/or history of gastric ulcer)

Pathological hypersecretory conditions, including Zollinger-Ellison syndrome (Rx only): Treatment (long-term) of pathological hypersecretory conditions including Zollinger-Ellison syndrome

Canadian labeling: Additional use (not in U.S. labeling): Oral: Treatment of nonerosive reflux disease (NERD); treatment of NSAID-induced gastric ulcers

Esomeprazole magnesium:

Heartburn (OTC labeling): Treatment of frequent heartburn (≥2 days per week).

IV: Esomeprazole sodium:

Gastroesophageal reflux disease (Rx only): Short-term (≤10 days) treatment of gastroesophageal reflux disease (GERD) when oral therapy is not possible or appropriate

Risk reduction of ulcer rebleeding postprocedure (Rx only): Decrease the risk of rebleeding postendoscopy for acute gastric or duodenal ulcers

Pregnancy Risk Factor C

Pregnancy Considerations Adverse events were observed in some animal reproduction studies. An increased risk of hypospadias was reported following maternal use of proton pump inhibitors (PPIs) during pregnancy (Anderka, 2012), but this was based on a small number of exposures and the same association was not found in another study (Erichsen, 2012). An increased risk of major birth defects following maternal use of PPIs during pregnancy was not observed in an additional study (Pasternak, 2010). Esomeprazole is the s-isomer of omeprazole; refer to the Omeprazole monograph for additional information. When treating GERD in pregnancy, PPIs may be used when clinically indicated (Katz, 2013).

Breast-Feeding Considerations Esomeprazole and strontium (limited data) are excreted in breast milk. The manufacturer of esomeprazole recommends that caution be exercised when administering to nursing women. The manufacturer of esomeprazole strontium recommends a decision be made whether to discontinue nursing or to discontinue the drug, taking into account the importance of treatment to the mother. Esomeprazole is the s-isomer of omeprazole and omeprazole is excreted in breast milk; refer to Omeprazole monograph for additional information.

Contraindications Hypersensitivity to esomeprazole, other substituted benzimidazole proton pump inhibitors, or any component of the formulation

Warnings/Precautions Use of proton pump inhibitors (PPIs) may increase the risk of gastrointestinal infections (eg, *Salmonella, Campylobacter*). Relief of symptoms does not preclude the presence of a gastric malignancy. ▶

Atrophic gastritis (by biopsy) has been noted with long-term omeprazole therapy; this may also occur with esomeprazole. No reports of enterochromaffin-like (ECL) cell carcinoids, dysplasia, or neoplasia have occurred. Use of PPIs may increase risk of CDAD, especially in hospitalized patients; consider CDAD diagnosis in patients with persistent diarrhea that does not improve. Use the lowest dose and shortest duration of PPI therapy appropriate for the condition being treated. Safety and efficacy of IV therapy for GERD >10 days have not been established; transition from IV to oral therapy as soon possible. Bioavailability may be increased in Asian populations, the elderly, and patients with hepatic dysfunction. Decreased *H. pylori* eradication rates have been observed with short-term (≤7 days) combination therapy. The American College of Gastroenterology recommends 10-14 days of therapy (triple or quadruple) for eradication of *H. pylori* (Chey, 2007).

PPIs may diminish the therapeutic effect of clopidogrel, thought to be due to reduced formation of the active metabolite of clopidogrel. The manufacturer of clopidogrel recommends either avoidance of both omeprazole (even when scheduled 12 hours apart) and esomeprazole or use of a PPI with comparatively less effect on the active metabolite of clopidogrel (eg, pantoprazole). In contrast to these warnings, others have recommended the continued use of PPIs, regardless of the degree of inhibition, in patients with a history of GI bleeding or multiple risk factors for GI bleeding who are also receiving clopidogrel since no evidence has established clinically meaningful differences in outcome; however, a clinically-significant interaction cannot be excluded in those who are poor metabolizers of clopidogrel (Abraham, 2010; Levine, 2011). Additionally, potentially significant drug-drug interactions may exist, requiring dose or frequency adjustment, additional monitoring, and/or selection of alternative therapy.

Increased incidence of osteoporosis-related bone fractures of the hip, spine, or wrist may occur with PPI therapy. Patients on high-dose or long-term therapy should be monitored. Use the lowest effective dose for the shortest duration of time, use vitamin D and calcium supplementation, and follow appropriate guidelines to reduce risk of fractures in patients at risk.

Hypomagnesemia, reported rarely, usually with prolonged PPI use of >3 months (most cases >1 year of therapy); may be symptomatic or asymptomatic; severe cases may cause tetany, seizures, and cardiac arrhythmias. Consider obtaining serum magnesium concentrations prior to beginning long-term therapy, especially if taking concomitant digoxin, diuretics, or other drugs known to cause hypomagnesemia; and periodically thereafter. Hypomagnesemia may be corrected by magnesium supplementation, although discontinuation of esomeprazole may be necessary; magnesium levels typically return to normal within 1 week of stopping.

Prolonged treatment (≥2 years) may lead to vitamin B_{12} malabsorption and subsequent vitamin B_{12} deficiency. The magnitude of the deficiency is dose-related and the association is stronger in females and those younger in age (<30 years); prevalence is decreased after discontinuation of therapy (Lam, 2013).

Severe liver dysfunction may require dosage reductions. Dosage adjustments are not necessary for any degree of renal impairment when using esomeprazole magnesium or esomeprazole sodium; however, since pharmacokinetics of the strontium may be reduced in mild to moderate renal impairment, esomeprazole strontium is not recommended for use in severe impairment (has not been studied). Esomeprazole strontium competes with calcium for intestinal absorption and is incorporated into bone; use of esomeprazole strontium in pediatric patients is not recommended. When used for self-medication (OTC), do not use for >14 days.

Serum chromogranin A (CgA) levels increase secondary to drug-induced decreases in gastric acid. May cause false positive results in diagnostic investigations for neuroendocrine tumors. Temporarily stop omeprazole treatment ≥14 days before CgA test; if CgA level high, repeat test to confirm. Use same commercial lab for testing to prevent variable results.

Adverse Reactions

Central nervous system: Dizziness, drowsiness, headache

Dermatologic: Pruritus

Gastrointestinal: Abdominal pain, constipation, diarrhea, flatulence, nausea, xerostomia

Local: Injection site reaction (IV)

Rare but important or life-threatening: Aggression, agranulocytosis, alopecia, anaphylaxis, anemia, angioedema, anorexia, benign polyps/nodules, blurred vision, bone fracture, cervical lymphadenopathy, chest pain, *Clostridium difficile*-associated diarrhea (CDAD), conjunctivitis, cyanocobalamin deficiency, cystitis, depression, dermatitis, dysgeusia, dysmenorrhea, epistaxis, erythema multiforme, exacerbation of arthritis, exacerbation of asthma, fibromyalgia syndrome, fungal infection, gastric carcinoid tumor, gastroenteritis, GI dysplasia, GI moniliasis, goiter, gynecomastia, hallucinations, hematuria, hepatic encephalopathy, hepatic failure, hepatitis, hernia, hyperhidrosis, hyperparathyroidism, hypersensitivity reactions, hypertension, hypertonia, hyperuricemia, hypoesthesia, hypokalemia, hypomagnesemia (with or without hypocalcemia and/or hypokalemia), hyponatremia, impotence, increased gastrin, increased serum alkaline phosphatase, increased serum ALT, increased serum AST, increased serum creatinine, increased thyroid-stimulating hormone, insomnia, interstitial nephritis, jaundice, laryngeal edema, leukocytosis, leukopenia, microscopic colitis, migraine, moniliasis, myasthenia, otitis media, pancreatitis, pancytopenia, parosmia, pathological fracture due to osteoporosis, phlebitis, photosensitivity, pneumonia, polymyalgia rheumatica, proteinuria, pruritus ani, rigors, skin rash (erythematous and maculopapular), Stevens-Johnson syndrome, stomatitis, tachycardia, thrombocytopenia, thrombophlebitis, toxic epidermal necrolysis, vaginitis, visual field defect, weight changes

Drug Interactions

Metabolism/Transport Effects Substrate of CYP2C19 (major), CYP3A4 (minor); **Note:** Assignment of Major/Minor substrate status based on clinically relevant drug interaction potential; **Inhibits** CYP2C19 (moderate)

Avoid Concomitant Use

Avoid concomitant use of Esomeprazole with any of the following: Clopidogrel; Dasatinib; Delavirdine; Erlotinib; Nelfinavir; PAZOPanib; Rifampin; Rilpivirine; Risedronate; St Johns Wort

Increased Effect/Toxicity

Esomeprazole may increase the levels/effects of: Amphetamine; Cilostazol; Citalopram; CYP2C19 Substrates; Dexmethylphenidate; Dextroamphetamine; Methotrexate; Methylphenidate; Raltegravir; Risedronate; Saquinavir; Tacrolimus (Systemic); Vitamin K Antagonists; Voriconazole

The levels/effects of Esomeprazole may be increased by: Fluconazole; Ketoconazole (Systemic); Voriconazole

Decreased Effect

Esomeprazole may decrease the levels/effects of: Atazanavir; Bisphosphonate Derivatives; Bosutinib; Cefditoren; Clopidogrel; Dabigatran Etexilate; Dabrafenib; Dasatinib; Delavirdine; Erlotinib; Gefitinib; Indinavir; Iron Salts; Itraconazole; Ketoconazole (Systemic); Ledipasvir; Mesalamine; Multivitamins/Minerals (with ADEK, Folate, Iron); Mycophenolate; Nelfinavir; Nilotinib; PAZOPanib;

Posaconazole; Rilpivirine; Riociguat; Risedronate; Vismodegib

The levels/effects of Esomeprazole may be decreased by: CYP2C19 Inducers (Strong); Dabrafenib; Rifampin; St Johns Wort; Tipranavir

Food Interactions Prolonged treatment (≥2 years) may lead to malabsorption of dietary vitamin B_{12} and subsequent vitamin B_{12} deficiency (Lam, 2013).

Preparation for Administration

Granules for oral administration: Empty the 2.5 mg or 5 mg packet into a container with 5 mL of water or empty the 10 mg, 20 mg, or 40 mg packet into a container with 15 mL of water and stir; leave 2-3 minutes to thicken.

Powder for injection:

For IV injection (≥3 minutes): Adults: Reconstitute powder with 5 mL NS.

For IV infusion (10 to 30 minutes):

Children: Initially reconstitute powder (20 mg or 40 mg) with 5 mL of NS, LR, or D_5W, then further dilute to a final volume of 50 mL; withdraw the appropriate amount of the final solution to administer the intended dose.

Adults: Initially reconstitute powder with 5 mL of NS, LR, or D_5W, then further dilute to a final volume of 50 mL.

For IV infusion (loading dose and continuous infusion): Prepare the 80 mg loading dose by reconstituting two 40 mg vials with NS (5 mL each); the contents of the two vials should then be further diluted in NS 100 mL. To prepare the continuous infusion, also reconstitute two 40 mg vials with NS (5 mL each); the contents of the two vials should then be further diluted in NS 100 mL.

Storage/Stability

Capsules: Keep container tightly closed.

Esomeprazole magnesium: Store at 25°C (77°F); excursions permitted to 15°C to 30°C (59°F to 86°F).

Esomeprazole strontium: Store at 20°C to 25°C (68°F to 77°F); excursions permitted to 15°C to 30°C (59°F to 86°F).

Granules: Store at 25°C (77°F); excursions permitted to 15°C to 30°C (59°F to 86°F).

Powder for injection: Store at 25°C (77°F); excursions permitted to 15°C to 30°C (59°F to 86°F). Protect from light. Per the manufacturer, following reconstitution, solution for injection prepared in NS, and solution for infusion prepared in NS or LR should be used within 12 hours. Following reconstitution, solution for infusion prepared in D_5W should be used within 6 hours. Refrigeration is not required following reconstitution.

Additional stability data: Following reconstitution, solutions for infusion prepared in D_5W, NS, or LR in PVC bags are chemically and physically stable for 48 hours at room temperature (25°C) and for at least 120 hours under refrigeration (4°C) (Kupiec, 2008).

Mechanism of Action Proton pump inhibitor suppresses gastric acid secretion by inhibition of the H^+/K^+-ATPase in the gastric parietal cell. Esomeprazole is the S-isomer of omeprazole.

Pharmacodynamics/Kinetics

Distribution: V_{dss}: 16 L

Protein binding: 97%

Metabolism: Hepatic via CYP2C19 primarily and (to a lesser extent) via 3A4 to hydroxy, desmethyl, and sulfone metabolites (all inactive)

Bioavailability: Oral: 90% with repeat dosing

Half-life elimination: ~1 to 1.5 hours

Time to peak: Oral: 1.5 to 2 hours

Excretion: Urine (80%, primarily as inactive metabolites; <1% as active drug); feces (20%)

Dosage Note: All dosing is expressed in terms of esomeprazole base, regardless of the salt associated with the dosing information. Esomeprazole strontium 24.65 mg is equivalent to 20 mg of esomeprazole base; esomeprazole strontium 49.3 mg is equivalent to 40 mg of esomeprazole base. Esomeprazole strontium is not recommended for use in pediatrics.

Oral:

Children 1 month to <1 year: Erosive esophagitis (healing): Esomeprazole magnesium: **Note:** Safety and efficacy of doses >1.33 mg/kg/day and/or therapy beyond 6 weeks have not been established.

3 to 5 kg: 2.5 mg once daily for up to 6 weeks

>5 to 7.5 kg: 5 mg once daily for up to 6 weeks

>7.5 to 12 kg: 10 mg once daily for up to 6 weeks

Children 1 to 11 years: **Note:** Safety and efficacy of doses >1 mg/kg/day and/or therapy beyond 8 weeks have not been established.

Symptomatic GERD: Esomeprazole magnesium: 10 mg once daily for up to 8 weeks

Erosive esophagitis (healing): Esomeprazole magnesium:

<20 kg: 10 mg once daily for 8 weeks

≥20 kg: 10 to 20 mg once daily for 8 weeks

Nonerosive reflux disease (NERD) (Canadian labeling): Esomeprazole magnesium: 10 mg once daily for up to 8 weeks

Adolescents 12 to 17 years:

Erosive esophagitis (healing): Esomeprazole magnesium: 20 to 40 mg once daily for 4 to 8 weeks

Symptomatic GERD: Esomeprazole magnesium: 20 mg once daily for up to 4 weeks

NERD (Canadian labeling): Esomeprazole magnesium: 20 mg once daily for 2 to 4 weeks; lack of symptom control after 4 weeks warrants further evaluation

Adults:

Erosive esophagitis (healing): Esomeprazole magnesium, esomeprazole strontium: Initial: 20 to 40 mg once daily for 4 to 8 weeks; if incomplete healing, may continue for an additional 4 to 8 weeks; maintenance: 20 mg once daily (controlled studies did not extend beyond 6 months)

NERD (Canadian labeling): Esomeprazole magnesium: Initial: 20 mg once daily for 2 to 4 weeks; lack of symptom control after 4 weeks warrants further evaluation; maintenance (in patients with successful initial therapy): 20 mg once daily as needed

Symptomatic GERD: Esomeprazole magnesium, esomeprazole strontium: 20 mg once daily for 4 weeks; may continue an additional 4 weeks if symptoms persist

Heartburn (OTC labeling): 20 mg once daily for 14 days (maximum: 20 mg/day); treatment may be repeated after 4 months if needed

Helicobacter pylori eradication:

Manufacturer labeling: Esomeprazole magnesium, esomeprazole strontium: 40 mg once daily administered with amoxicillin 1,000 mg *and* clarithromycin 500 mg twice daily for 10 days

American College of Gastroenterology guidelines (Chey, 2007):

Nonpenicillin allergy: 40 mg once daily administered with amoxicillin 1,000 mg *and* clarithromycin 500 mg twice daily for 10 to 14 days

Penicillin allergy: 40 mg once daily administered with clarithromycin 500 mg *and* metronidazole 500 mg twice daily for 10 to 14 days **or** 40 mg once daily administered with bismuth subsalicylate 525 mg *and* metronidazole 250 mg *plus* tetracycline 500 mg 4 times daily for 10 to 14 days

Canadian labeling: Esomeprazole magnesium: 20 mg twice daily for 7 days; requires combination therapy

Prevention of NSAID-induced gastric ulcers:

U.S. labeling: Esomeprazole magnesium, esomeprazole strontium: 20 to 40 mg once daily for up to 6 months

Canadian labeling: Esomeprazole magnesium: 20 mg once daily for up to 6 months

Note: 40 mg daily did not show additional benefit over 20 mg daily in clinical trials.

Treatment of NSAID-induced gastric ulcers (Canadian labeling; off-label in U.S.): Esomeprazole magnesium: 20 mg once daily for 4 to 8 weeks (Goldstein, 2007)

Pathological hypersecretory conditions (Zollinger-Ellison syndrome): Esomeprazole magnesium, esomeprazole strontium: 40 mg twice daily; adjust regimen to individual patient needs; doses up to 240 mg daily have been administered

IV:

Treatment of GERD (short-term): **Note:** Indicated only in cases where oral therapy is inappropriate or not possible; safety/efficacy ≥10 days has not been established.

Children 1 month to <1 year: 0.5 mg/kg once daily

Children 1 to 17 years: <55 kg: 10 mg once daily; ≥55 kg: 20 mg once daily

Adults: 20 mg or 40 mg once daily

Prevention of recurrent gastric or duodenal ulcer bleeding postendoscopy: Adults: 80 mg over 30 minutes, followed by 8 mg/hour continuous infusion for a total of 72 hours, then 40 mg *orally* once daily for 27 additional days (Sung, 2009) or may follow continuous infusion with any single daily-dose oral proton pump inhibitor (PPI) for a duration dictated by the underlying etiology (Barkun, 2010). **Note:** The use of intermittent PPIs was found to be comparable with the use of continuous infusion PPIs in patients with high-risk endoscopic findings and may be preferred (Sachar, 2014).

Dosage adjustment in renal impairment:

Oral:

Esomeprazole magnesium: Mild to severe impairment: No dosage adjustment necessary.

Esomeprazole strontium:

Mild to moderate impairment: No dosage adjustment necessary.

Severe impairment: Use is not recommended (has not been studied).

IV: Mild to severe impairment: No dosage adjustment necessary.

Dosage adjustment in hepatic impairment: Oral, IV:

Safety and efficacy not established in children with hepatic impairment.

Mild to moderate impairment (Child-Pugh class A or B):

Treatment of GERD (short-term): No dosage adjustment necessary

Prevention of recurrent gastric or duodenal ulcer bleeding postendoscopy: 80 mg over 30 minutes, followed by a continuous infusion of ≤6 mg/hour

Severe impairment (Child-Pugh class C):

Treatment of GERD (short-term): Dose should not exceed 20 mg (esomeprazole base) daily.

Prevention of recurrent gastric or duodenal ulcer bleeding postendoscopy: 80 mg over 30 minutes, followed by a continuous infusion of ≤4 mg/hour

Dietary Considerations Take at least 1 hour before meals; best if taken before breakfast.

Usual Infusion Concentrations: Pediatric IV infusion: 0.4 mg/mL **or** 0.8 mg/mL

Usual Infusion Concentrations: Adult IV infusion: 20 mg in 50 mL (concentration: 0.4 mg/mL) **or** 40 mg in 50 mL (concentration: 0.8 mg/mL) of D_5W, LR, or NS

Administration

Oral:

Capsule: Should be swallowed whole and taken at least 1 hour before eating (best if taken before breakfast). Capsule can be opened and contents mixed with 1 tablespoon of applesauce. Swallow immediately; mixture should not be chewed or warmed. For patients with difficulty swallowing, use of granules may be more appropriate.

Granules: Empty the 2.5 mg or 5 mg packet into a container with 5 mL of water or the 10 mg, 20 mg, or 40 mg packet into a container with 15 mL of water and stir; leave 2 to 3 minutes to thicken. Stir and drink within 30 minutes. If any medicine remains after drinking, add more water, stir and drink immediately.

Tablet (Canadian formulation, not available in U.S.): Swallow whole or may be dispersed in a half a glass of noncarbonated water. Stir until tablets disintegrate, leaving a liquid containing pellets. Drink contents within 30 minutes. Do not chew or crush pellets. After drinking, rinse glass with water and drink.

IV: Flush line prior to and after administration with NS, LR, or D_5W.

Children: Administer by intermittent infusion (10 to 30 minutes); the manufacturer recommends that children receive intravenous esomeprazole by intermittent infusion only.

Adults:

Treatment of GERD: May be administered by injection (≥3 minutes), or intermittent infusion (10 to 30 minutes)

Prevention of recurrent gastric or duodenal ulcer bleeding postendoscopy: Administer the loading dose over 30 minutes, followed by the continuous infusion over 71.5 hours (adjust rate of continuous infusion in patients with hepatic dysfunction)

Nasogastric tube:

Capsule: Open capsule and place intact granules into a 60 mL catheter-tip syringe; mix with 50 mL of water. Replace plunger and shake vigorously for 15 seconds. Ensure that no granules remain in syringe tip. Do not administer if pellets dissolve or disintegrate. Use immediately after preparation. After administration, flush nasogastric tube with additional water.

Granules: Delayed release oral suspension granules can also be given by nasogastric or gastric tube. If using a 2.5 mg or 5 mg packet, first add 5 mL of water to a catheter-tipped syringe, then add granules from packet. If using a 10 mg, 20 mg, or 40 mg packet, first add 15 mL of water to a catheter-tipped syringe, then add granules from packet. Shake the syringe, leave 2 to 3 minutes to thicken. Shake the syringe and administer through nasogastric or gastric tube (size 6 French or greater) within 30 minutes. Refill the syringe with equal amount (5 mL or 15 mL) of water, shake and flush nasogastric/gastric tube.

Tablet (Canadian formulation, not available in U.S.): Disperse tablets in 50 mL of noncarbonated water. Stir until tablets disintegrate leaving a liquid containing pellets. After administration, flush with additional 25 to 50 mL of water to clear the syringe and tube.

Monitoring Parameters Susceptibility testing recommended in patients who fail *H. pylori* eradication regimen. Monitor for rebleeding in patients with peptic ulcer bleed. For patients expected to be on prolonged therapy or who take PPIs with medications such as digoxin or drugs that may cause hypomagnesemia (eg, diuretics), consider monitoring magnesium levels prior to initiation of treatment and periodically thereafter.

Product Availability Esomeprazole strontium 24.65 mg capsules have been discontinued for more than 1 year.

Dosage Forms Considerations Esomeprazole strontium 49.3 mg is equivalent to 40 mg of esomeprazole base.

Dosage Forms

Capsule Delayed Release, Oral:

NexIUM: 20 mg, 40 mg

Generic: 49.3 mg

Packet, Oral:

NexIUM: 2.5 mg (30 ea); 5 mg (30 ea); 10 mg (30 ea); 20 mg (30 ea); 40 mg (30 ea)

Solution Reconstituted, Intravenous:

NexIUM I.V.: 40 mg (1 ea)

Generic: 20 mg (1 ea); 40 mg (1 ea)

Dosage Forms: Canada Note: Strength expressed as base.

Granules, for oral suspension, delayed release, as magnesium:

Nexium®: 10 mg/packet (28s)

Tablet, extended release, as magnesium:

Nexium®: 20 mg, 40 mg

◆ **Esomeprazole Magnesium** *see* Esomeprazole *on page 771*

◆ **Esomeprazole Sodium** *see* Esomeprazole *on page 771*

◆ **Esomeprazole Strontium** *see* Esomeprazole *on page 771*

◆ **Esoterica Daytime [OTC]** *see* Hydroquinone *on page 1020*

◆ **Esoterica Facial [OTC]** *see* Hydroquinone *on page 1020*

◆ **Esoterica Fade Nighttime [OTC]** *see* Hydroquinone *on page 1020*

◆ **Esoterica Sensitive Skin [OTC]** *see* Hydroquinone *on page 1020*

◆ **E.S.P.®** *see* Erythromycin and Sulfisoxazole *on page 765*

◆ **Estalis (Can)** *see* Estradiol and Norethindrone *on page 781*

◆ **Estarylla** *see* Ethinyl Estradiol and Norgestimate *on page 810*

Estazolam (es TA zoe lam)

Index Terms ProSom

Pharmacologic Category Benzodiazepine

Additional Appendix Information

Beers Criteria – Potentially Inappropriate Medications for Geriatrics *on page 2271*

Use Short-term management of insomnia

Pregnancy Risk Factor X

Dosage Insomnia:

Adults: Oral: 1 mg at bedtime, some patients may require 2 mg

Elderly: Oral: Initial: 0.5-1 mg at bedtime; initiate at lower dose in debilitated or small elderly patients

Dosage adjustment in renal impairment: No dosage adjustment provided in manufacturer's labeling (has not been studied); use with caution.

Dosage adjustment in hepatic impairment: No dosage adjustment provided in manufacturer's labeling (has not been studied); use with caution.

Additional Information Complete prescribing information should be consulted for additional detail.

Dosage Forms

Tablet, Oral:

Generic: 1 mg, 2 mg

◆ **Esterified Estrogens** *see* Estrogens (Esterified) *on page 790*

◆ **Estiripentol** *see* Stiripentol [CAN/INT] *on page 1935*

◆ **Estrace** *see* Estradiol (Systemic) *on page 775*

◆ **Estrace** *see* Estradiol (Topical) *on page 780*

◆ **Estradiol** *see* Estradiol (Systemic) *on page 775*

◆ **17β-estradiol** *see* Estradiol (Topical) *on page 780*

Estradiol (Systemic) (es tra DYE ole)

Brand Names: U.S. Alora; Climara; Delestrogen; Depo-Estradiol; Divigel; Elestrin; Estrace; Estrasorb [DSC]; Estrogel; Evamist; Femring; Menostar; Minivelle; Vivelle-Dot

Brand Names: Canada Climara; Depo-Estradiol; Divigel; Estradot; EstroGel; Menostar; Oesclim; Sandoz-Estradiol Derm 100; Sandoz-Estradiol Derm 50; Sandoz-Estradiol Derm 75

Index Terms Estradiol; Estradiol Acetate; Estradiol Transdermal; Estradiol Valerate

Pharmacologic Category Estrogen Derivative

Additional Appendix Information

Beers Criteria – Potentially Inappropriate Medications for Geriatrics *on page 2271*

Use Treatment of moderate-to-severe vasomotor symptoms associated with menopause; treatment of moderate-to-severe vulvar and vaginal atrophy associated with menopause; hypoestrogenism (due to hypogonadism, castration, or primary ovarian failure); advanced prostatic cancer (palliation); metastatic breast cancer (palliation) in men and postmenopausal women; postmenopausal osteoporosis (prophylaxis)

Pregnancy Risk Factor X

Pregnancy Considerations In general, the use of estrogen and progestin as in combination hormonal contraceptives has not been associated with teratogenic effects when inadvertently taken early in pregnancy. These products are contraindicated for use during pregnancy.

Breast-Feeding Considerations Estrogens are excreted in breast milk and have been shown to decrease the quantity and quality of human milk. The manufacturer recommends that caution be used if administered to breast-feeding women. Monitor the growth of the infant closely.

Contraindications Angioedema, anaphylactic reaction, or hypersensitivity to estradiol or any component of the formulation; undiagnosed abnormal vaginal bleeding; DVT or PE (current or history of); active or history of arterial thromboembolic disease (eg, stroke, MI); carcinoma of the breast (known, suspected or history of), except in appropriately selected patients being treated for metastatic disease; estrogen-dependent tumor; liver impairment or disease; known protein C, protein S, antithrombin deficiency or other known thrombophilic disorders; pregnancy

Warnings/Precautions Hazardous agent - use appropriate precautions for handling and disposal (NIOSH 2014 [group 2]). Anaphylaxis requiring emergency medical management has been reported and may develop at any time during therapy. Angioedema involving the face, feet, hands, larynx, and tongue has also been reported. Exogenous estrogens may exacerbate symptoms in women with hereditary angioedema.

[U.S. Boxed Warning]: The use of unopposed estrogen in women with an intact uterus is associated with an increased risk of endometrial cancer. The addition of a progestin to estrogen therapy may decrease the risk of endometrial hyperplasia, a precursor to endometrial cancer. The use of a progestin is not generally required when low doses of estrogen are used locally for vaginal atrophy (NAMS, 2012). **Adequate diagnostic measures, including endometrial sampling if indicated, should be performed to rule out malignancy in postmenopausal women with undiagnosed abnormal vaginal bleeding.** Estrogens may exacerbate endometriosis. Malignant transformation of residual endometrial implants has been reported posthysterectomy with unopposed estrogen therapy. Consider adding a progestin in women with residual endometriosis posthysterectomy. Postmenopausal estrogen therapy and combined estrogen/progesterone therapy may increase the risk of ovarian cancer; however, the absolute risk to an individual woman is small. Although results from various studies are not consistent, risk does not appear to be significantly associated with the duration, route, or dose of therapy. In one study, the risk decreased after 2 years following discontinuation of therapy (Mørch, 2009). Although the risk of ovarian cancer is rare, women who are at an increased risk (eg, family history) should be counseled about the association (NAMS, 2012). **[U.S. Boxed Warning]: Based on data from the Women's Health Initiative (WHI) studies, an increased risk of invasive breast cancer was observed in postmenopausal women using conjugated estrogens (CE) in combination with medroxyprogesterone acetate (MPA).** This risk may be associated with duration of use and declines once combined therapy is discontinued (Chlebowski, 2009). The risk of invasive breast cancer was decreased in postmenopausal women with a hysterectomy using CE only, regardless of weight. However, the risk was not significantly decreased in women at high risk for breast cancer (family history of breast cancer, personal history of benign breast disease) (Anderson, 2012). An increase in abnormal mammogram findings has also been reported with estrogen alone or in combination with progestin therapy. Estrogen use may lead to severe hypercalcemia in patients with breast cancer and bone metastases; discontinue estrogen if hypercalcemia occurs.

[U.S. Boxed Warning]: Estrogens with or without progestin should not be used to prevent coronary heart disease. Using data from the Women's Health Initiative (WHI) studies, an increased risk of deep vein thrombosis (DVT) and stroke has been reported with CE and an increased risk of DVT, stroke, pulmonary emboli (PE) and myocardial infarction (MI) has been reported with CE with MPA in postmenopausal women. Additional risk factors include diabetes mellitus, hypercholesterolemia, hypertension, SLE, obesity, tobacco use, and/or history of venous thromboembolism (VTE). Adverse cardiovascular events have also been reported in males taking estrogens for prostate cancer. Risk factors should be managed appropriately; discontinue use if adverse cardiovascular events occur or are suspected. Women with inherited thrombophilias (eg, protein C or S deficiency) may have increased risk of venous thromboembolism (DeSancho, 2010; van Vlijmen, 2011). Use is contraindicated in women with protein C, protein S, antithrombin deficiency or other known thrombophilic disorders.

[U.S. Boxed Warning]: Estrogens with or without progestin should not be used to prevent dementia. In the Women's Health Initiative Memory Study (WHIMS), an increased incidence of dementia was observed in women ≥65 years of age taking CE alone or in combination with MPA.

[U.S. Boxed Warning]: Estrogens with or without progestin should be used for the shortest duration possible at the lowest effective dose consistent with treatment goals. Before prescribing estrogen therapy to postmenopausal women, the risks and benefits must be weighed for each patient. Women should be informed of these risks and benefits, as well as possible effects of progestin when added to estrogen therapy. Patients should be reevaluated as clinically appropriate to determine if treatment is still necessary. Available data related to treatment risks are from Women's Health Initiative (WHI) studies, which evaluated oral CE 0.625 mg with or without MPA 2.5 mg relative to placebo in postmenopausal women. Other combinations and dosage forms of estrogens and progestins were not studied. **Outcomes reported from clinical trials using CE with or without MPA should be assumed to be similar for other doses and other dosage forms of estrogens and progestins until comparable data becomes available.**

Estrogen compounds are generally associated with lipid effects such as increased HDL-cholesterol and decreased LDL-cholesterol. Triglycerides may also be increased; discontinue if pancreatitis occurs. Estrogens may increase thyroid-binding globulin (TBG) levels leading to increased circulating total thyroid hormone levels. Women on thyroid replacement therapy may require higher doses of thyroid hormone while receiving estrogens.

Estrogens may cause retinal vascular thrombosis; discontinue if migraine, loss of vision, proptosis, diplopia, or other visual disturbances occur; discontinue permanently if papilledema or retinal vascular lesions are observed on examination. Estrogens are poorly metabolized in patients with hepatic dysfunction. Use caution with a history of cholestatic jaundice associated with prior estrogen use or pregnancy. Discontinue if jaundice develops or if acute or chronic hepatic disturbances occur. Use is contraindicated with hepatic disease. Use caution with asthma, epilepsy, hepatic hemangiomas, migraine, porphyria, or SLE; may exacerbate disease. May have adverse effects on glucose tolerance; use caution in women with diabetes. Use caution with diseases which may be exacerbated by fluid retention, including cardiac or renal dysfunction. Use of postmenopausal estrogen may be associated with an increased risk of gallbladder disease requiring surgery. Use caution with hypoparathyroidism; estrogen-induced hypocalcemia may occur. In the elderly, avoid oral and transdermal patch estrogen products (with or without progestins) due to potential of increased risk of breast and endometrial cancers, and lack of proven cardioprotection and cognitive protection (Beers Criteria). Prior to puberty, estrogens may cause premature closure of the epiphyses, premature breast development in girls or gynecomastia in boys. Vaginal bleeding and vaginal cornification may also be induced in girls. Whenever possible, estrogens should be discontinued at least 4-6 weeks prior to elective surgery associated with an increased risk of thromboembolism or during periods of prolonged immobilization. The use of estrogens and/or progestins may change the results of some laboratory tests (eg, coagulation factors, lipids, glucose tolerance, binding proteins). The dose, route, and the specific estrogen/progestin influences these changes. In addition, personal risk factors (eg, cardiovascular disease, smoking, diabetes, age) also contribute to adverse events; use of specific products may be contraindicated in women with certain risk factors.

Estradiol may be transferred to another person following skin-to-skin contact with the application site. **[U.S. Boxed Warning]: Breast budding and breast masses in prepubertal females and gynecomastia and breast masses in prepubertal males have been reported following unintentional contact with application sites of women using topical estradiol (Evamist). Patients should strictly adhere to instructions for use in order to prevent secondary exposure. In most cases, conditions resolved with removal of estradiol exposure.** If unexpected changes in sexual development occur in prepubertal children, the possibility of unintentional estradiol exposure should be evaluated by a healthcare provider. Discontinue if conditions for the safe use of the topical spray cannot be met.

Some products may contain chlorobutanol (a chloral derivative) as a preservative, which may be habit forming; some products may contain tartrazine.

Benzyl alcohol and derivatives: Some dosage forms may contain benzyl alcohol; large amounts of benzyl alcohol (≥99 mg/kg/day) have been associated with a potentially fatal toxicity ("gasping syndrome") in neonates; the "gasping syndrome" consists of metabolic acidosis, respiratory distress, gasping respirations, CNS dysfunction (including convulsions, intracranial hemorrhage), hypotension and cardiovascular collapse (AAP, 1997; CDC, 1982); some data suggests that benzoate displaces bilirubin from protein binding sites (Ahlfors, 2001); avoid or use dosage forms containing benzyl alcohol with caution in neonates. See manufacturer's labeling.

Topical emulsion, gel, spray: Absorption of the topical emulsion (Estrasorb) and topical gel (Elestrin) is increased by application of sunscreen; do not apply sunscreen within close proximity of estradiol. When sunscreen is applied ~1 hour prior to the topical spray (Evamist), no change in absorption was observed (estradiol absorption was decreased when sunscreen is applied 1 hour after Evamist). Application of Divigel or EstroGel with sunscreen has not been evaluated.

Transdermal patch: May contain conducting metal (eg, aluminum); remove patch prior to MRI.

Vaginal ring: Use may not be appropriate in women with narrow vagina, vaginal stenosis, vaginal infections, cervical prolapse, rectoceles, cystoceles, or other conditions which may increase the risk of vaginal irritation, ulceration, or increase the risk of expulsion. Ring should be removed in case of ulceration, erosion, or adherence to vaginal wall; do not reinsert until healing is complete. Ensure proper vaginal placement of the ring to avoid inadvertent urinary bladder insertion.

Osteoporosis: For use only in women at significant risk of osteoporosis and for who other nonestrogen medications are not considered appropriate.

Vulvar and vaginal atrophy: When used solely for the treatment of vulvar and vaginal atrophy, topical vaginal products should be considered. Use caution applying topical products to severely atrophic vaginal mucosa. Use of a progestin is normally not required when low-dose estrogen is applied locally and only for this purpose (NAMS, 2013).

Adverse Reactions Some adverse reactions observed with estrogen and/or progestin combination therapy.

Cardiovascular: Cerebrovascular accident, deep vein thrombosis, edema, hypertension, local thrombophlebitis, myocardial infarction, pulmonary thromboembolism, retinal thrombosis, thrombophlebitis, venous thromboembolism

Central nervous system: Anxiety, chorea, dementia, depression, dizziness, exacerbation of epilepsy, headache, hypoesthesia, irritability, migraine, mood disorder, nervousness, nipple pain, pain

Dermatologic: Chloasma, erythema multiforme, erythema nodosum, localized erythema (transdermal patch), loss of scalp hair, pruritus, skin discoloration (melasma), skin rash, urticaria

Endocrine & metabolic: Change in libido, change in menstrual flow (alterations in frequency and flow of bleeding patterns), exacerbation of diabetes mellitus, exacerbation of porphyria, fibrocystic breast changes, fluid retention, galactorrhea, hirsutism, hot flash, hypocalcemia, increased serum triglycerides, weight gain, weight loss

Gastrointestinal: Abdominal cramps, abdominal pain, bloating, carbohydrate intolerance, constipation, diarrhea, dyspepsia, flatulence, gallbladder disease, gastroenteritis, nausea, pancreatitis, vomiting

Genitourinary: Abnormal uterine bleeding, breakthrough bleeding, breast hypertrophy, breast tenderness, cervical polyp, change in cervical ectropion, change in cervical secretions, dysmenorrhea, endometrial hyperplasia, endometrium disease, leukorrhea, mastalgia, nipple discharge, spotting, urinary tract infection, uterine fibroids (size increased), uterine pain, vaginal discomfort (vaginal ring; burning, irritation, itching), vaginal hemorrhage, vaginitis, vulvovaginal candidiasis

Hematologic & oncologic: Hemorrhagic eruption, hypercoagulability state, malignant neoplasm of breast, ovarian cancer

Hepatic: Cholestatic jaundice, exacerbation of hepatic hemangioma

Hypersensitivity: Anaphylactoid reaction, anaphylaxis, angioedema, hypersensitivity reaction

Infection: Fungal infection, infection

Local: Application site reaction (gel, spray, transdermal patch)

Neuromuscular & skeletal: Arthralgia, arthropathy, back pain, exacerbation of systemic lupus erythematosus, leg cramps, limb pain, myalgia, neck pain, weakness

Ophthalmic: Change in corneal curvature (steepening), conjunctivitis, contact lens intolerance

Otic: Otitis media

Respiratory: asthma, bronchitis, cough, exacerbation of asthma, flu-like symptoms, nasopharyngitis, pharyngitis, rhinitis, sinus congestion, sinus headache, sinusitis, upper respiratory tract infection

Miscellaneous: Accidental injury, cyst

Rare but important or life-threatening: Bowel obstruction (vaginal ring), genitourinary complaint (inadvertent ring insertion into the bladder should be considered with unexplained urinary complaints), hemorrhage, mechanical complication of genitourinary device (ring adherence to vaginal or bladder wall), portal vein thrombosis, toxic shock syndrome (vaginal ring), unstable angina pectoris

Drug Interactions

Metabolism/Transport Effects **Substrate** of CYP1A2 (major), CYP2A6 (minor), CYP2B6 (minor), CYP2C19 (minor), CYP2C9 (minor), CYP2D6 (minor), CYP2E1 (minor), CYP3A4 (major), P-glycoprotein; **Note:** Assignment of Major/Minor substrate status based on clinically relevant drug interaction potential; **Inhibits** CYP1A2 (weak), CYP2C8 (weak); **Induces** CYP3A4 (weak)

Avoid Concomitant Use

Avoid concomitant use of Estradiol (Systemic) with any of the following: Anastrozole; Dehydroepiandrosterone; Exemestane; Indium 111 Capromab Pendetide; Ospemifene

Increased Effect/Toxicity

Estradiol (Systemic) may increase the levels/effects of: C1 inhibitors; Corticosteroids (Systemic); Immune Globulin; Lenalidomide; Ospemifene; ROPINIRole; Thalidomide; Theophylline Derivatives; Tipranavir

The levels/effects of Estradiol (Systemic) may be increased by: Ascorbic Acid; Dehydroepiandrosterone; Herbs (Estrogenic Properties); NSAID (COX-2 Inhibitor); P-glycoprotein/ABCB1 Inhibitors

Decreased Effect

Estradiol (Systemic) may decrease the levels/effects of: Anastrozole; Anticoagulants; ARIPiprazole; Chenodiol; Exemestane; Hyaluronidase; Hydrocodone; Indium 111 Capromab Pendetide; Ospemifene; Saxagliptin; Somatropin; Thyroid Products; Ursodiol

The levels/effects of Estradiol (Systemic) may be decreased by: Bosentan; Cannabis; CYP1A2 Inducers (Strong); CYP3A4 Inducers (Moderate); CYP3A4 Inducers (Strong); Cyproterone; Dabrafenib; Deferasirox; Mitotane; P-glycoprotein/ABCB1 Inducers; Siltuximab; St Johns Wort; Teriflunomide; Tipranavir; Tocilizumab

Food Interactions Folic acid absorption may be decreased. Routine use of ethanol increases estrogen level and risk of breast cancer; may also increase the risk of osteoporosis. Management: Avoid ethanol.

Storage/Stability Store all products at controlled room temperature. In addition:

Climara, Menostar: Do not store >30°C (>86°F); store in protective pouch.

Femring: Store in pouch. Insert immediately upon removal from the protective pouch.

Mechanism of Action Estrogens are responsible for the development and maintenance of the female reproductive system and secondary sexual characteristics. Estradiol is the principle intracellular human estrogen and is more potent than estrone and estriol at the receptor level; it is the primary estrogen secreted prior to menopause. Following menopause, estrone and estrone sulfate are more highly produced. Estrogens modulate the pituitary secretion of gonadotropins, luteinizing hormone, and follicle-stimulating hormone through a negative feedback system; estrogen replacement reduces elevated levels of these hormones in postmenopausal women.

Pharmacodynamics/Kinetics

Absorption: Well absorbed from the gastrointestinal tract, mucous membranes, and the skin. Average serum estradiol concentrations (C_{avg}) vary by product

Injection: Estradiol valerate and estradiol cypionate are absorbed over several weeks following IM injection

Topical:

Alora: C_{avg}: 41-98 pg/mL

Climara: C_{avg}: 22-106 pg/mL

Divigel: C_{avg}: 9.8-30.5 pg/mL

Elestrin: C_{avg}: 15.4-39.2 pg/mL; Exposure increased by 55% with application of sunscreen 10 minutes prior to dose

Estrasorb: Mean serum concentration on day 22 of therapy: ~35-65 pg/mL; Exposure increased by 35% with application of sunscreen 10 minutes prior to dose

Estrogel: C_{avg} on day 14 of therapy: 28.3 pg/mL

Evamist: C_{avg}: 19.6-30.9 pg/mL

Menostar: C_{avg}: 13.7 pg/mL

Vivelle-Dot: C_{avg}: 34-104 pg/mL

Vaginal: Femring: Rapid during the first hour following application, then declines to a steady rate over 3 months; C_{avg}: 40.6-76 pg/mL

Distribution: Widely distributed; high concentrations in the sex hormone target organs

Protein binding: Bound to sex hormone-binding globulin and albumin

Metabolism: Hepatic; partial metabolism via CYP3A4 enzymes; estradiol is reversibly converted to estrone and estriol; oral estradiol also undergoes enterohepatic recirculation by conjugation in the liver, followed by excretion of sulfate and glucuronide conjugates into the bile, then hydrolysis in the intestine and estrogen reabsorption. Sulfate conjugates are the primary form found in postmenopausal women. With transdermal application, less estradiol is metabolized leading to higher circulating concentrations of estradiol and lower concentrations of estrone and conjugates.

Excretion: Primarily urine (as estradiol, estrone, estriol and their glucuronide and sulfate conjugates)

Dosage All dosage needs to be adjusted based upon the patient's response

Oral:

Prostate cancer, advanced (androgen-dependent) (Estrace): 1-2 mg 3 times/day

Breast cancer, metastatic (appropriately selected patients): Males and postmenopausal females (Estrace): 10 mg 3 times/day **or** (off-label dosing) postmenopausal women: 2 mg 3 times/day (Ellis, 2009)

Osteoporosis prophylaxis in postmenopausal females (Estrace): Lowest effective dose has not been determined; doses of 0.5 mg/day in a cyclic regimen for 23 days of a 28-week cycle were used in clinical studies

Female hypoestrogenism (due to hypogonadism, castration, or primary ovarian failure) (Estrace): 1-2 mg/day; titrate as necessary to control symptoms using minimal effective dose for maintenance therapy

Vasomotor symptoms associated with menopause (Estrace): 1-2 mg/day, adjusted as necessary to limit symptoms; administration should be cyclic (3 weeks on, 1 week off)

Vulvar and vaginal atrophy associated with menopause (Estrace): 1-2 mg/day, adjusted as necessary to limit symptoms; administration should be cyclic (3 weeks on, 1 week off)

IM:

Prostate cancer, advanced (androgen-dependent): Valerate (Delestrogen): 30 mg or more every 1-2 weeks

Vasomotor symptoms associated with menopause:

Cypionate (Depo-Estradiol): 1-5 mg every 3-4 weeks

Valerate (Delestrogen): 10-20 mg every 4 weeks

Female hypoestrogenism (due to hypogonadism): Cypionate (Depo-Estradiol): 1.5-2 mg monthly

Female hypoestrogenism (due to hypogonadism, castration, or primary ovarian failure): Valerate (Delestrogen): 10-20 mg every 4 weeks

Vulvar and vaginal atrophy associated with menopause: Valerate (Delestrogen): 10-20 mg every 4 weeks

Topical:

Emulsion: Vasomotor symptoms associated with menopause (Estrasorb): 3.48 g applied once daily in the morning

Gel:

Vasomotor symptoms associated with menopause:

Divigel: 0.25 g/day; adjust dose based on patient response. Dosing range: 0.25-1 g/day

Elestrin: 0.87 g/day applied at the same time each day; adjust dose based on patient response. Dosing range: 0.87-1.7 g/day.

EstroGel: 1.25 g/day applied at the same time each day

Vulvar and vaginal atrophy associated with menopause (EstroGel): 1.25 g/day applied at the same time each day

Spray: Vasomotor symptoms associated with menopause (Evamist): Initial: One spray (1.53 mg) per day. Adjust dose based on patient response. Dosing range: 1-3 sprays per day.

Transdermal patch: **Note:** Indicated dose may be used continuously in patients without an intact uterus. Some product labeling states they may be given continuously or cyclically (3 weeks on, 1 week off) in patients with an intact uterus (**exception - Menostar, see specific dosing instructions**). When changing patients from oral to transdermal therapy, start transdermal patch 1 week after discontinuing oral hormone (may begin sooner if symptoms reappear within 1 week):

Once-weekly patch:

Vasomotor symptoms associated with menopause, vulvar and vaginal atrophy associated with menopause, female hypoestrogenism (due to hypogonadism, castration, or primary ovarian failure) (Climara): Apply 0.025 mg/day patch once weekly. Adjust dose as necessary to control symptoms.

Osteoporosis prophylaxis in postmenopausal women:

Climara: Apply patch once weekly; minimum effective dose: 0.025 mg/day; adjust dosage based on response to therapy as indicated by biochemical markers and bone mineral density

Menostar: Apply patch once weekly (0.014 mg/day). In women with a uterus, also administer a progestin for 14 days every 6-12 months

Twice-weekly patch:

Vasomotor symptoms associated with menopause, vulvar/vaginal atrophy associated with menopause, female hypoestrogenism (due to hypogonadism, castration, or primary ovarian failure): Titrate to lowest dose possible to control symptoms, adjusting initial dose after the first month of therapy:

Alora: Apply 0.05 mg patch twice weekly

Vivelle-Dot: Apply 0.0375 mg patch twice weekly

Vasomotor symptoms associated with menopause: Titrate to lowest dose possible to control symptoms:

Minivelle: Apply 0.0375 mg patch twice weekly

Prevention of osteoporosis in postmenopausal women:

Alora, Minivelle, Vivelle-Dot: Apply 0.025 mg patch twice weekly, increase dose as necessary

Vaginal ring: Vasomotor symptoms associated with menopause; vulvar and vaginal atrophy associated with menopause (Femring): Initial: 0.05 mg intravaginally; following insertion, ring should remain in place for 3 months; dose may be increased to 0.1 mg if needed

Dosage adjustment in renal impairment: For most products, there are no dosage adjustments provided in the manufacturer's labeling; (has not been studied).

Dosage adjustment in hepatic impairment: For most products, there are no dosage adjustments provided in the manufacturer's labeling (has not been studied); use is contraindicated with hepatic dysfunction or disease

Dietary Considerations Ensure adequate calcium and vitamin D intake when used for the prevention of osteoporosis.

Administration The use of a progestin should be considered when administering estrogens to postmenopausal women with an intact uterus.

Injection formulation: Intramuscular use only. Estradiol valerate should be injected into the upper outer quadrant of the gluteal muscle; administer with a dry needle (solution may become cloudy with wet needle).

Emulsion (Estrasorb): Apply to clean, dry skin while in a sitting position. Contents of two pouches (total 3.48 g) are to be applied individually, once daily in the morning. Apply contents of first pouch to left thigh; massage into skin of left thigh and calf until thoroughly absorbed (~3 minutes). Apply excess from both hands to the buttocks. Apply contents of second pouch to the right thigh; massage into skin of right thigh and calf until thoroughly absorbed (~3 minutes). Apply excess from both hands to buttocks. Wash hands with soap and water. Allow skin to dry before covering legs with clothing. Do not apply to other areas of body. Do not apply to red or irritated skin.

Gel: Apply to clean, dry, unbroken skin at the same time each day. Allow to dry for 5 minutes prior to dressing. Gel is flammable; avoid fire or flame until dry. After application, wash hands with soap and water. Prior to the first use, pump must be primed. Do not apply gel to breast.

Divigel: Apply entire contents of packet to right or left upper thigh each day (alternate sites). Do not apply to face, breasts, vaginal area or irritated skin. Apply over an area ~5x7 inches. Do not wash application site for 1 hour. Allow gel to dry before dressing

Elestrin: Apply to upper arm and shoulder area using two fingers to spread gel. Apply after bath or shower; allow at least 2 hours between applying gel and going swimming. Wait at least 25 minutes before applying sunscreen to application area. Do not apply sunscreen to application area for ≥7 days (may increase absorption of gel).

EstroGel: Apply gel to the arm, from the wrist to the shoulder. Spread gel as thinly as possible over one arm.

Spray: Evamist: Prior to first use, prime pump by spraying 3 sprays with the cover on. To administer dose, hold container upright and vertical and rest the plastic cone flat against the skin while spraying. Spray to the inner surface of the forearm, starting near the elbow. If more than one spray is needed, apply to adjacent but not overlapping areas. Apply at the same time each day. Allow spray to dry for ~2 minutes; do not rub into skin; do not cover with clothing until dry. Do not wash application site for at least 60 minutes. Apply to clean, dry, unbroken skin. Do not apply to skin other than that of the forearm. Make sure that children do not come in contact with any skin area where the drug was applied. If contact with children is unavoidable, wear a garment with long sleeves that covers the site of application. If direct exposure should occur, wash the child in the area of exposure with soap and water as soon as possible. Solution contained in the spray is flammable; avoid fire, flame, or smoking until spray has dried. If needed, sunscreen should be applied ~1 hour prior to application of Evamist.

Transdermal patch: Do not apply transdermal system to breasts, but place on trunk of body (preferably abdomen). Rotate application sites allowing a 1-week interval between applications at a particular site. Do not apply to oily, damaged or irritated skin; avoid waistline or other areas where tight clothing may rub the patch off. Apply patch immediately after removing from protective pouch. In general, if patch falls off, the same patch may be reapplied or a new system may be used for the remainder of the dosing interval (not recommended with all products). When replacing patch, reapply to a new site. Swimming, bathing or showering are not expected to affect use of the patch. Note the following exceptions:

Climara, Menostar, Minivelle: Swimming, bathing, or wearing patch while in a sauna have not been studied; adhesion of patch may be decreased or delivery of estradiol may be affected. Showering is not expected to cause the Minivelle patch to fall off. Remove patch slowly after use to avoid skin irritation. If any adhesive remains on the skin after removal, first allow skin to dry for 15 minutes, then gently rub area with an oil-based cream or lotion. If patch falls off, a new patch should be applied for the remainder of the dosing interval.

Vaginal ring: Exact positioning is not critical for efficacy; however, patient should not feel anything once inserted. In case of discomfort, ring should be pushed further into vagina. If ring is expelled prior to 90 days, it may be rinsed off with warm water and reinserted. Ensure proper vaginal placement of the ring to avoid inadvertent urinary bladder insertion. If vaginal infection develops, Femring may remain in place during local treatment of a vaginal infection.

Hazardous agent; use appropriate precautions for handling and disposal (NIOSH 2014 [group 2]).

Monitoring Parameters Routine physical examination that includes blood pressure and Papanicolaou smear, breast exam, mammogram. Monitor for signs of endometrial cancer in female patients with uterus. Adequate diagnostic measures, including endometrial sampling, if indicated, should be performed to rule out malignancy in all cases of undiagnosed abnormal vaginal bleeding. Monitor for loss of vision, sudden onset of proptosis, diplopia, migraine; signs and symptoms of thromboembolic disorders; glycemic control in patients with diabetes; lipid profiles in patients being treated for hyperlipidemias; thyroid function in patients on thyroid hormone replacement therapy.

Menostar: When used in a woman with a uterus, endometrial sampling is recommended at yearly intervals or when clinically indicated.

Menopausal symptoms, vulvar and vaginal atrophy: Assess need for therapy at 3- to 6-month intervals

Prevention of osteoporosis: Bone density measurement

Reference Range
Children 6 months to 10 years: <15 pg/mL (SI: <55 pmol/L)
Males: 10-50 pg/mL (SI: 37-184 pmol/L)
Females:
Premenopausal: 30-400 pg/mL (SI: 110-1468 pmol/L) (depending on phase of menstrual cycle)
Postmenopausal: 0-30 pg/mL (SI: 0-110 pmol/L)

Dosage Forms
Gel, Transdermal:
Divigel: 0.25 mg/0.25 g (1 ea); 0.5 mg/0.5 g (1 ea); 1 mg/g (1 g)
Elestrin: 0.06% (26 g)
Estrogel: 0.06% (50 g)
Oil, Intramuscular:
Delestrogen: 10 mg/mL (5 mL); 20 mg/mL (5 mL); 40 mg/mL (5 mL)
Depo-Estradiol: 5 mg/mL (5 mL)
Generic: 20 mg/mL (5 mL); 40 mg/mL (5 mL)
Patch Twice Weekly, Transdermal:
Alora: 0.025 mg/24 hr (1 ea, 8 ea); 0.05 mg/24 hr (1 ea, 8 ea); 0.075 mg/24 hr (1 ea, 8 ea); 0.1 mg/24 hr (1 ea, 8 ea)
Minivelle: 0.025 mg/24 hr (8 ea); 0.0375 mg/24 hr (8 ea); 0.05 mg/24 hr (8 ea); 0.075 mg/24 hr (8 ea); 0.1 mg/24 hr (8 ea)
Vivelle-Dot: 0.025 mg/24 hr (8 ea); 0.0375 mg/24 hr (1 ea, 8 ea); 0.05 mg/24 hr (1 ea, 8 ea); 0.075 mg/24 hr (1 ea, 8 ea); 0.1 mg/24 hr (1 ea, 8 ea)
Generic: 0.025 mg/24 hr (8 ea); 0.0375 mg/24 hr (8 ea); 0.05 mg/24 hr (8 ea); 0.075 mg/24 hr (8 ea); 0.1 mg/24 hr (8 ea)
Patch Weekly, Transdermal:
Climara: 0.025 mg/24 hr (4 ea); 0.0375 mg/24 hr (4 ea); 0.05 mg/24 hr (1 ea, 4 ea); 0.06 mg/24 hr (4 ea); 0.075 mg/24 hr (4 ea); 0.1 mg/24 hr (1 ea, 4 ea)
Menostar: 14 mcg/24 hr (4 ea)
Generic: 0.025 mg/24 hr (4 ea); 0.0375 mg/24 hr (4 ea); 0.05 mg/24 hr (4 ea); 0.06 mg/24 hr (4 ea); 0.075 mg/24 hr (4 ea); 0.1 mg/24 hr (4 ea)
Ring, Vaginal:
Femring: 0.05 mg/24 hr (1 ea); 0.1 mg/24 hr (1 ea)
Solution, Transdermal:
Evamist: 1.53 mg/spray (8.1 mL)
Tablet, Oral:
Estrace: 0.5 mg, 1 mg, 2 mg
Generic: 0.5 mg, 1 mg, 2 mg

Estradiol (Topical) (es tra DYE ole)

Brand Names: U.S. Estrace; Estring; Vagifem
Brand Names: Canada Estrace; Estring; Vagifem; Vagifem10
Index Terms 17β-estradiol
Pharmacologic Category Estrogen Derivative
Additional Appendix Information
Beers Criteria - Potentially Inappropriate Medications for Geriatrics *on page 2271*
Use Vulvar and vaginal atrophy associated with menopause: Treatment of moderate-to-severe vulvar and vaginal atrophy associated with menopause
Dosage All dosage needs to be adjusted based upon the patient's response.
Vulvar and vaginal atrophy associated with menopause:
Adults: Intravaginal:
Vaginal cream (Estrace): Insert 2 to 4 g daily intravaginally for 1 to 2 weeks, then gradually reduce to 1/2 the initial dose for 1 to 2 weeks, followed by a maintenance dose of 1 g 1 to 3 times per week
Vaginal ring (Estring): 2 mg intravaginally; following insertion, ring should remain in place for 90 days
Vaginal tablet (Vagifem): Initial: Insert 1 tablet (10 mcg) once daily for 2 weeks; Maintenance: Insert 1 tablet twice weekly
Dosage adjustment in renal impairment: There are no dosage adjustments provided in the manufacturer's labeling (has not been studied).
Dosage adjustment in hepatic impairment: There are no dosage adjustments provided in the manufacturer's labeling (has not been studied); use is contraindicated with hepatic impairment or disease
Additional Information Complete prescribing information should be consulted for additional detail.
Dosage Forms
Cream, Vaginal:
Estrace: 0.1 mg/g (42.5 g)
Ring, Vaginal:
Estring: 2 mg (1 ea)
Tablet, Vaginal:
Vagifem: 10 mcg

◆ **Estradiol Acetate** *see* Estradiol (Systemic) *on page 775*

Estradiol and Dienogest
(es tra DYE ole & dye EN oh jest)

Brand Names: U.S. Natazia®
Index Terms Dienogest and Estradiol; Estradiol Valerate and Dienogest
Pharmacologic Category Contraceptive; Estrogen and Progestin Combination
Use Prevention of pregnancy; treatment of heavy menstrual bleeding
Dosage Oral: Adults: Females: Contraception or treatment of heavy menstrual bleeding: Take 1 tablet daily in the order presented in the blister pack
Initial dosing: Start on day 1 of menstrual period (first day of bleeding). A nonhormonal contraceptive should be used for the first 9 days.
Switching from another combination oral contraceptive tablet: Take the first dark yellow tablet on the first day of withdrawal bleeding; do not continue taking tablets from previous contraceptive pack. If withdrawal bleeding does not occur, rule-out pregnancy before starting therapy. A non-hormonal contraceptive should be used for the first 9 days.
Switching from a vaginal ring or patch: Take the first dark yellow tablet on the day the ring or patch is removed. A nonhormonal contraceptive should be used for the first 9 days.
Switching from a progestin-only contraceptive: Take the first dark yellow tablet on the day the next progestin-only tablet would have been given, or the day the progestin implant or IUD is removed, or on the day the next injection would have been given. A nonhormonal contraceptive should be used for the first 9 days.

Missed doses: If ≤12 hours late, take tablet as soon as remembering and take the next tablet at the usual time. If >12 hours late, instructions vary by day of cycle and number of tablets missed:
If missed ONE dose:
Days 1-17: Take missed tablet immediately; take next tablet at usual time; use back-up (nonhormonal) contraception for the next 9 days; continue taking 1 tablet each day for the rest of the cycle
Days 18-24: Do not continue using current blister pack (throw away); take day 1 of new blister pack; use back-up (nonhormonal) contraception for the next 9 days; continue taking 1 tablet each day for the rest of the cycle

Days 25-28: Take missed tablet immediately; take next tablet at usual time; continue taking 1 tablet each day for the rest of the cycle; no backup method of contraception is needed.

If missed TWO doses in a row:

Days 1-17: Do not take missed tablets; start by taking the tablet for the day it was first noticed that the tablet was missed; use back-up (nonhormonal) contraception for the next 9 days; continue taking 1 tablet each day for the rest of the cycle. If tablets were missed on days 17 and 18, follow directions for missed tablets on days 17-25.

Days 17-25: Do not continue using current blister pack (throw away); take day 3 of new blister pack; use back-up (nonhormonal) contraception for the next 9 days; continue taking 1 tablet each day for the rest of the cycle. If tablets were missed on days 25 and 26, follow directions for missed tablets on days 25-28.

Days 25-28: Do not continue using current blister pack (throw away); start a new pack on the same day, or start a new pack the day it would normally be started; continue taking 1 tablet each day for the rest of the cycle; no backup method of contraception is needed.

Dosage adjustment in renal impairment: Safety and efficacy have not been evaluated; dose adjustment not expected to be required

Dosage adjustment in hepatic impairment: Use is contraindicated with hepatic disease. Discontinue if hepatic dysfunction occurs.

Additional Information Complete prescribing information should be consulted for additional detail.

Dosage Forms

Tablet, oral [four-phasic formulation]:

Natazia®:

Days 1-2: Estradiol valerate 3 mg [2 dark yellow tablets]

Days 3-7: Estradiol valerate 2 mg and dienogest 2 mg [5 medium red tablets]

Days 8-24: Estradiol valerate 2 mg and dienogest 3 mg [17 light yellow tablets]

Days 25-26: Estradiol valerate 1 mg [2 dark red tablets]

Days 27-28: 2 white inactive tablets (28s)

Estradiol and Levonorgestrel

(es tra DYE ole & LEE voe nor jes trel)

Brand Names: U.S. ClimaraPro

Index Terms Levonorgestrel and Estradiol

Pharmacologic Category Estrogen and Progestin Combination

Use

Moderate to severe vasomotor symptoms: Treatment of moderate to severe vasomotor symptoms associated with menopause in women with an intact uterus

Osteoporosis prevention: Prevention of postmenopausal osteoporosis in women with an intact uterus

Limitations of use: Osteoporosis: For use only in women at significant risk of osteoporosis and for whom other nonestrogen medications are not considered appropriate

Dosage Note: Patients should be treated with the lowest effective dose and for the shortest duration, consistent with treatment goals.

Transdermal: Adult females with an intact uterus: Treatment of moderate to severe vasomotor symptoms associated with menopause or prevention of postmenopausal osteoporosis: Estradiol 0.045 mg/levonorgestrel 0.015 mg: Apply one patch weekly. When used for the treatment of vasomotor symptoms associated with menopause, evaluate to see if therapy is still needed/attempt to discontinue every 3-6 months.

Dosage adjustment in renal impairment: No dosage adjustment provided in manufacturer's labeling. Total estradiol serum concentrations may be excessive in women with end stage renal disease receiving hemodialysis.

Dosage adjustment in hepatic impairment: Use is contraindicated in women with known hepatic impairment or disease.

Additional Information Complete prescribing information should be consulted for additional detail.

Dosage Forms

Patch, transdermal:

ClimaraPro: Estradiol 0.045 mg and levonorgestrel 0.015 mg per 24 hours (4s)

Estradiol and Norethindrone

(es tra DYE ole & nor eth IN drone)

Brand Names: U.S. Activella; CombiPatch; Lopreeza; Mimvey; Mimvey Lo

Brand Names: Canada Estalis

Index Terms Norethindrone and Estradiol

Pharmacologic Category Estrogen and Progestin Combination

Use Women with an intact uterus:

Tablet: Treatment of moderate-to-severe vasomotor symptoms associated with menopause; treatment of moderate-to-severe symptoms of vulvar and vaginal atrophy associated with menopause; prophylaxis for postmenopausal osteoporosis

Transdermal patch: Treatment of moderate-to-severe vasomotor symptoms associated with menopause; treatment of moderate-to-severe symptoms of vulvar and vaginal atrophy associated with menopause; treatment of hypoestrogenism due to hypogonadism, castration, or primary ovarian failure

Dosage Note: Patients should be treated with the lowest effective dose and for the shortest duration, consistent with treatment goals. Adults: Females:

Oral:

Moderate-to-severe vasomotor symptoms of menopause, postmenopausal osteoporosis prophylaxis:

Activella: Estradiol 1 mg/norethindrone 0.5 mg or estradiol 0.5 mg/norethindrone 0.1 mg: One tablet daily

Mimvey: Estradiol 1 mg/ norethindrone 0.5 mg: One tablet daily

Vulvar and vaginal atrophy associated with menopause:

Activella, Mimvey: Estradiol 1 mg/norethindrone 0.5 mg: One tablet daily

Transdermal patch:

CombiPatch: Hypoestrogenism, menopause (moderate-to-severe vasomotor symptoms; vulvar and vaginal atrophy):

Continuous combined regimen: Apply 1 patch twice weekly

Continuous sequential regimen: Apply estradiol-only patch for first 14 days of cycle, followed by one CombiPatch® applied twice weekly for the remaining 14 days of a 28-day cycle

Estalis [Canadian product]: Menopause (moderate-to-severe vasomotor symptoms; vulvar and vaginal atrophy): Continuous combined regimen: Apply a new patch twice weekly during a 28-day cycle

Dosage adjustment in renal impairment: No dosage adjustment provided in manufacturer's labeling (has not been studied); use with caution.

Dosage adjustment in hepatic impairment: No dosage adjustment provided in manufacturer's labeling (has not been studied). Use is contraindicated with hepatic dysfunction or disease.

Additional Information Complete prescribing information should be consulted for additional detail.

Dosage Forms

Patch, transdermal:

CombiPatch:

0.05/0.14: Estradiol 0.05 mg and norethindrone 0.14 mg per day (8s) [9 sq cm]

0.05/0.25: Estradiol 0.05 mg and norethindrone 0.25 mg per day (8s) [16 sq cm]

Tablet, oral: 0.5/0.1: Estradiol 0.5 mg and norethindrone acetate 0.1 mg (28s); Estradiol 1 mg and norethindrone acetate 0.5 mg (28s)

Activella, Lopreeza, Mimvey Lo: 0.5/0.1: Estradiol 0.5 mg and norethindrone acetate 0.1 mg (28s)

Activella, Lopreeza, Mimvey: 1/0.5: Estradiol 1 mg and norethindrone acetate 0.5 mg (28s)

Dosage Forms: Canada

Patch, transdermal:

Estalis:

140/50: Norethindrone 140 mcg and estradiol 50 mcg per day (8s) [9 sq cm; total norethindrone 2.7 mg, total estradiol 0.62 mg]

250/50 Norethindrone 250 mcg and estradiol 50 mcg per day (8s) [16 sq cm; total norethindrone 4.8 mg, total estradiol 0.51 mg]

◆ **Estradiol Transdermal** *see* Estradiol (Systemic) *on page 775*

◆ **Estradiol Valerate** *see* Estradiol (Systemic) *on page 775*

◆ **Estradiol Valerate and Dienogest** *see* Estradiol and Dienogest *on page 780*

◆ **Estradot (Can)** *see* Estradiol (Systemic) *on page 775*

◆ **Estragyn (Can)** *see* Estrogens (Esterified) *on page 790*

Estramustine (es tra MUS teen)

Brand Names: U.S. Emcyt

Brand Names: Canada Emcyt

Index Terms Estramustine Phosphate; Estramustine Phosphate Sodium

Pharmacologic Category Antineoplastic Agent, Alkylating Agent; Antineoplastic Agent, Antimicrotubular; Antineoplastic Agent, Hormone (Estrogen/Nitrogen Mustard)

Use

Prostate cancer: Treatment (palliative) of progressive or metastatic prostate cancer

Limitation of use: A clinical practice guideline from the American Society of Clinical Oncology (ASCO) and Cancer Care Ontario recommends that estramustine not be offered to men with metastatic castration-resistant prostate cancer due to a lack of benefit in survival or quality of life (Basch, 2014).

Dosage Note: Estramustine is associated with a moderate emetic potential; antiemetics are recommended to prevent nausea and vomiting.

Prostate cancer, progressive or metastatic: Adults: Males: Oral: 14 mg/kg/day (range: 10-16 mg/kg/day) in 3 or 4 divided doses

Dosage adjustment in renal impairment: There are no dosage adjustments provided in the manufacturer's labeling; use with caution.

Dosage adjustment in hepatic impairment: There are no dosage adjustments provided in the manufacturer's labeling; use with caution (may be poorly metabolized).

Dosing in obesity: *ASCO Guidelines for appropriate chemotherapy dosing in obese adults with cancer:* Utilize patient's actual body weight (full weight) for calculation of body surface area- or weight-based dosing, particularly when the intent of therapy is curative; manage regimen-related toxicities in the same manner as for nonobese patients; if a dose reduction is utilized due to toxicity, consider resumption of full weight-based dosing with subsequent cycles, especially if cause of toxicity (eg, hepatic or renal impairment) is resolved (Griggs, 2012).

Additional Information Complete prescribing information should be consulted for additional detail.

Dosage Forms

Capsule, Oral:

Emcyt: 140 mg

◆ **Estramustine Phosphate** *see* Estramustine *on page 782*

◆ **Estramustine Phosphate Sodium** *see* Estramustine *on page 782*

◆ **Estrasorb [DSC]** *see* Estradiol (Systemic) *on page 775*

◆ **Estratab® (Can)** *see* Estrogens (Esterified) *on page 790*

◆ **Estring** *see* Estradiol (Topical) *on page 780*

◆ **Estrogel** *see* Estradiol (Systemic) *on page 775*

◆ **EstroGel (Can)** *see* Estradiol (Systemic) *on page 775*

◆ **Estrogenic Substances, Conjugated** *see* Estrogens (Conjugated/Equine, Systemic) *on page 787*

◆ **Estrogenic Substances, Conjugated** *see* Estrogens (Conjugated/Equine, Topical) *on page 790*

Estrogens (Conjugated/Equine) and Bazedoxifene

(ES troe jenz, KON joo gate ed/EE kwine & ba ze DOX i feen)

Brand Names: U.S. Duavee

Index Terms Bazedoxifene and Estrogens (Conjugated/Equine); Estrogens (Conjugated/Equine) and Bazedoxifene Acetate

Pharmacologic Category Estrogen Derivative; Selective Estrogen Receptor Modulator (SERM); Tissue-Selective Estrogen Complex (TSEC)

Use

Postmenopausal osteoporosis prophylaxis: Prevention of postmenopausal osteoporosis in women with a uterus

Vasomotor symptoms: Treatment of moderate-to-severe vasomotor symptoms associated with menopause in women with a uterus

Pregnancy Risk Factor X

Dosage Menopause (moderate-to-severe vasomotor symptoms), prevention of postmenopausal osteoporosis: Adults: Females: Oral: One tablet daily

Dosage adjustment in renal impairment: No dosage adjustment provided in manufacturer's labeling (has not been studied). Use is not recommended.

Dosage adjustment in hepatic impairment: Use is contraindicated with hepatic dysfunction or disease.

Additional Information Complete prescribing information should be consulted for additional detail.

Dosage Forms

Tablet, oral:

Duavee: Conjugated estrogens 0.45 mg and bazedoxifene 20 mg

Estrogens (Conjugated A/Synthetic)

(ES troe jenz, KON joo gate ed, aye, sin THET ik)

Brand Names: U.S. Cenestin [DSC]

Brand Names: Canada Cenestin

Pharmacologic Category Estrogen Derivative

Additional Appendix Information

Beers Criteria – Potentially Inappropriate Medications for Geriatrics *on page 2271*

Use Treatment of moderate-to-severe vasomotor symptoms of menopause; treatment of vulvar and vaginal atrophy

Pregnancy Considerations Estrogens are not indicated for use during pregnancy or immediately postpartum. In general, the use of estrogen and progestin as in combination hormonal contraceptives have not been associated with teratogenic effects when inadvertently taken early in pregnancy. This product is contraindicated for use during pregnancy.

Breast-Feeding Considerations Estrogens can be detected in breast milk and have been shown to decrease the quantity and quality of human milk. The manufacturer recommends that caution be used if administered to nursing women.

Contraindications Hypersensitivity to estrogens or any component of the formulation; undiagnosed abnormal vaginal bleeding; history of or current thrombophlebitis or venous thromboembolic disorders (including DVT, PE); active or recent (within 1 year) arterial thromboembolic disease (eg, stroke, MI); carcinoma of the breast; estrogen-dependent tumor; hepatic dysfunction or disease; pregnancy

Warnings/Precautions Hazardous agent - use appropriate precautions for handling and disposal (NIOSH 2014 [group 2]).

Cardiovascular-related considerations: **[U.S. Boxed Warning]: Estrogens with or without progestin should not be used to prevent cardiovascular disease.** Using data from the Women's Health Initiative (WHI) studies, an increased risk of deep vein thrombosis (DVT) and stroke has been reported with conjugated estrogens [CE] and an increased risk of DVT, stroke, pulmonary emboli (PE) and myocardial infarction (MI) has been reported with CE with medroxyprogesterone acetate [MPA] in postmenopausal women. Additional risk factors include diabetes mellitus, hypercholesterolemia, hypertension, SLE, obesity, tobacco use, and/or history of venous thromboembolism (VTE). Adverse cardiovascular events have also been reported in males taking estrogens for prostate cancer. Risk factors should be managed appropriately; discontinue use if adverse cardiovascular events occur or are suspected. Estrogen compounds are generally associated with lipid effects such as increased HDL-cholesterol and decreased LDL-cholesterol. Triglycerides may also be increased; use with caution in patients with familial defects of lipoprotein metabolism. Whenever possible, estrogens should be discontinued at least 4-6 weeks prior to elective surgery associated with an increased risk of thromboembolism or during periods of prolonged immobilization. Women with inherited thrombophilias (eg, protein C or S deficiency) may have increased risk of venous thromboembolism (DeSancho, 2010; van Vlijmen, 2011).

Neurological considerations: **[U.S. Boxed Warning]: Estrogens with or without progestin should not be used to prevent dementia. In the Women's Health Initiative Memory Study (WHIMS), an increased incidence of dementia was observed in women ≥65 years of age taking CE alone or in combination with MPA.**

Cancer-related considerations: **[U.S. Boxed Warning]: Based on data from the Women's Health Initiative (WHI) studies, an increased risk of invasive breast cancer was observed in postmenopausal women using conjugated estrogens (CE) in combination with medroxyprogesterone acetate (MPA).** This risk may be associated with duration of use and declines once combined therapy is discontinued (Chlebowski, 2009). The risk of invasive breast cancer was decreased in postmenopausal women with a hysterectomy using CE only, regardless of weight. However, the risk was not significantly decreased in women at high risk for breast cancer (family history of breast cancer, personal history of benign breast disease) (Anderson, 2012). An increase in abnormal mammogram findings has also been reported with estrogen alone or in combination with progestin therapy. Estrogen use may also lead to severe hypercalcemia in patients with breast cancer and bone metastases; discontinue estrogen if hypercalcemia occurs. Use is contraindicated in patients with known or suspected breast cancer. **[U.S. Boxed Warning]: The use of unopposed estrogen in women with an intact uterus is associated with an increased risk of endometrial cancer. The addition of a progestin to estrogen therapy may decrease the risk of endometrial hyperplasia, a precursor to endometrial cancer. Adequate diagnostic measures, including endometrial sampling if indicated, should be performed to rule out malignancy in postmenopausal women with undiagnosed abnormal vaginal bleeding.** Estrogens may exacerbate endometriosis. Malignant transformation of residual endometrial implants has been reported posthysterectomy with unopposed estrogen therapy. Consider adding a progestin in women with residual endometriosis posthysterectomy. Postmenopausal estrogen therapy and combined estrogen/progesterone therapy may increase the risk of ovarian cancer; however, the absolute risk to an individual woman is small. Although results from various studies are not consistent, risk does not appear to be significantly associated with the duration, route, or dose of therapy. In one study, the risk decreased after 2 years following discontinuation of therapy (Mørch, 2009). Although the risk of ovarian cancer is rare, women who are at an increased risk (eg, family history) should be counseled about the association (NAMS, 2012).

Estrogens may cause retinal vascular thrombosis; discontinue if migraine, loss of vision, proptosis, diplopia, or other visual disturbances occur; discontinue permanently if papilledema or retinal vascular lesions are observed on examination. Use caution in patients with asthma, epilepsy, hepatic hemangiomas, hereditary angioedema, migraine, porphyria, or SLE; may exacerbate disease. May have adverse effects on glucose tolerance; use caution in women with diabetes. Use with caution in patients with diseases which may be exacerbated by fluid retention, including cardiac or renal dysfunction. Use of postmenopausal estrogen may be associated with an increased risk of gallbladder disease requiring surgery. Estrogens are poorly metabolized in patients with hepatic dysfunction. Use caution with a history of cholestatic jaundice associated with prior estrogen use or pregnancy. Discontinue if jaundice develops or if acute or chronic hepatic disturbances occur. Use is contraindicated with hepatic disease. Use with caution in patients with severe hypocalcemia. Estrogens may increase thyroid-binding globulin (TBG) levels leading to increased circulating total thyroid hormone levels. Women on thyroid replacement therapy may require higher doses of thyroid hormone while receiving estrogens.

Avoid use of oral estrogen (with or without progestins) in the elderly due to potential of increased risk of breast and endometrial cancers, and lack of proven cardioprotection and cognitive protection (Beers Criteria). Safety and efficacy have not been established in children. Prior to puberty, estrogens may cause premature closure of the epiphyses, premature breast development in girls or gynecomastia in boys. Vaginal bleeding and vaginal cornification may also be induced in girls. Whenever possible, estrogens should be discontinued at least 4-6 weeks prior to elective surgery associated with an increased risk of thromboembolism or during periods of prolonged immobilization. The use of estrogens and/or progestins may change the results of some laboratory tests (eg, coagulation factors, lipids, glucose tolerance, binding proteins). The dose, route, and the specific estrogen/progestin influences these changes. In addition, personal risk factors (eg, cardiovascular disease, smoking, diabetes, age) also contribute to adverse events; use of specific products may be contraindicated in women with certain risk factors.

[U.S. Boxed Warning]: Estrogens with or without progestin should be used for the shortest duration possible at the lowest effective dose consistent with treatment goals. Before prescribing estrogen therapy to postmenopausal women, the risks and benefits must be weighed for each patient. Women should be informed of these risks and benefits, as well as possible effects of progestin when added to estrogen therapy. Patients should be reevaluated as clinically appropriate to determine if treatment is still necessary. Available data related to treatment risks are from Women's Health Initiative (WHI) studies, which evaluated oral CE 0.625 mg with or without MPA 2.5 mg relative to placebo in postmenopausal women. Other combinations and dosage forms of estrogens and progestins were not studied. **Outcomes reported from clinical trials using CE with or without MPA should be assumed to be similar for other doses and other dosage forms of estrogens and progestins until comparable data becomes available.**

Vulvar and vaginal atrophy use: When used solely for the treatment of vulvar and vaginal atrophy, topical vaginal products should be considered.

Adverse Reactions

Central nervous system: Anxiety, dizziness, fever, headache, pain

Endocrine & metabolic: Breast pain, endometrial thickening, metrorrhagia

Gastrointestinal: Abdominal pain, constipation, diarrhea, dyspepsia, nausea, vomiting, weight gain

Genitourinary: Vaginitis

Neuromuscular & skeletal: Back pain, hypertonia, leg cramps, paresthesia

Respiratory: Cough, rhinitis, upper respiratory tract infection

Miscellaneous: Infection

In addition, the following have been reported with estrogen and/or progestin therapy:

Cardiovascular: Edema, hypertension, MI, stroke, venous thromboembolism

Central nervous system: Epilepsy exacerbation, irritability, mental depression, migraine, mood disturbances, nervousness

Dermatologic: Angioedema, chloasma, erythema multiforme, erythema nodosum, hemorrhagic eruption, hirsutism, melasma, pruritus, rash, scalp hair loss, urticaria

Endocrine & metabolic: Breast cancer, breast enlargement, breast tenderness, HDL-cholesterol increased, hyper-/hypocalcemia, impaired glucose tolerance, LDL-cholesterol decreased, libido changes, serum triglycerides/phospholipids increased, thyroid-binding globulin increased, total thyroid hormone (T_4) increased

Gastrointestinal: Abdominal cramps, bloating, cholecystitis, cholelithiasis, gallbladder disease, pancreatitis, weight gain/loss

Genitourinary: Alterations in frequency and flow of menses, cervical secretion changes, endometrial cancer, endometrial hyperplasia, uterine leiomyomata size increased, vaginal candidiasis

Hematologic: Aggravation of porphyria, antithrombin III and antifactor Xa decreased, fibrinogen levels increased, platelet aggregability and platelet count increased; prothrombin and factors VII, VIII, IX, X increased

Hepatic: Cholestatic jaundice, hepatic hemangiomas enlarged

Neuromuscular & skeletal: Arthralgias, chorea, leg cramps

Local: Thrombophlebitis

Ocular: Contact lens intolerance, corneal curvature steepening, retinal vascular thrombosis

Respiratory: Asthma exacerbation, pulmonary thromboembolism

Miscellaneous: Anaphylactoid/anaphylactic reactions, carbohydrate intolerance

Drug Interactions

Metabolism/Transport Effects Substrate of CYP1A2 (major), CYP2A6 (minor), CYP2B6 (minor), CYP2C19 (minor), CYP2C9 (minor), CYP2D6 (minor), CYP2E1 (minor), CYP3A4 (major); **Note:** Assignment of Major/Minor substrate status based on clinically relevant drug interaction potential; **Inhibits** CYP1A2 (weak); **Induces** CYP3A4 (weak)

Avoid Concomitant Use

Avoid concomitant use of Estrogens (Conjugated A/Synthetic) with any of the following: Anastrozole; Dehydroepiandrosterone; Exemestane; Indium 111 Capromab Pendetide; Ospemifene

Increased Effect/Toxicity

Estrogens (Conjugated A/Synthetic) may increase the levels/effects of: C1 inhibitors; Corticosteroids (Systemic); Immune Globulin; Lenalidomide; Ospemifene; ROPINIRole; Thalidomide; Theophylline Derivatives; Tipranavir

The levels/effects of Estrogens (Conjugated A/Synthetic) may be increased by: Ascorbic Acid; Dehydroepiandrosterone; Herbs (Estrogenic Properties); NSAID (COX-2 Inhibitor)

Decreased Effect

Estrogens (Conjugated A/Synthetic) may decrease the levels/effects of: Anastrozole; Anticoagulants; ARIPiprazole; Chenodiol; Exemestane; Hyaluronidase; Hydrocodone; Indium 111 Capromab Pendetide; Ospemifene; Saxagliptin; Somatropin; Thyroid Products; Ursodiol

The levels/effects of Estrogens (Conjugated A/Synthetic) may be decreased by: Bosentan; Cannabis; CYP1A2 Inducers (Strong); CYP3A4 Inducers (Moderate); CYP3A4 Inducers (Strong); Cyproterone; Dabrafenib; Deferasirox; Mitotane; Siltuximab; St Johns Wort; Teriflunomide; Tipranavir; Tocilizumab

Food Interactions Routine use of ethanol increases estrogen level and risk of breast cancer. Management: Avoid ethanol.

Storage/Stability Store at room temperature of 25°C (77°F).

Mechanism of Action Conjugated A/synthetic estrogens contain a mixture of 9 synthetic estrogen substances, including sodium estrone sulfate, sodium equilin sulfate, sodium 17 alpha-dihydroequilin, sodium 17 alpha-estradiol and sodium 17 beta-dihydroequilin. Estrogens are responsible for the development and maintenance of the female reproductive system and secondary sexual characteristics. Estradiol is the principle intracellular human estrogen and is more potent than estrone and estriol at the receptor level; it is the primary estrogen secreted prior to menopause. Following menopause, estrone and estrone sulfate are more highly produced. Estrogens modulate the pituitary secretion of gonadotropins, luteinizing hormone, and follicle-stimulating hormone through a negative feedback system; estrogen replacement reduces elevated levels of these hormones in postmenopausal women.

Pharmacodynamics/Kinetics

Absorption: Well absorbed over a period of several hours

Protein-binding: Sex hormone-binding globulin (SHBG) and albumin

Metabolism: Hepatic via CYP3A4; estradiol is converted to estrone and estriol; also undergoes enterohepatic recirculation; estrone sulfate is the main metabolite in postmenopausal women

Excretion: Urine (primarily estriol, also as estradiol, estrone, and conjugates)

Dosage The lowest dose that will control symptoms should be used; medication should be discontinued as soon as possible. Oral:

Adults:

Moderate-to-severe vasomotor symptoms: 0.45 mg/day; may be titrated up to 1.25 mg/day. Attempts to discontinue medication should be made at 3- to 6-month intervals.

Vulvar and vaginal atrophy: 0.3 mg/day

Elderly: Refer to adult dosing. A higher incidence of stroke and invasive breast cancer were observed in women >75 years in a WHI substudy using conjugated equine estrogen.

Dosage adjustment in renal impairment: No dosage adjustment provided in manufacturer's labeling (has not been studied); use with caution.

Dosage adjustment in hepatic impairment: No dosage adjustment provided in manufacturer's labeling (has not been studied); use with caution.

Administration Administer at the same time each day. Hazardous agent; use appropriate precautions for handling and disposal (NIOSH 2014 [group 2]).

Monitoring Parameters Yearly physical examination that includes blood pressure and Papanicolaou smear, breast exam, mammogram. Monitor for signs of endometrial cancer in female patients with uterus. Adequate diagnostic measures, including endometrial sampling, if indicated, should be performed to rule out malignancy in all cases of undiagnosed abnormal vaginal bleeding. Monitor for loss of vision, sudden onset of proptosis, diplopia, migraine; signs and symptoms of thromboembolic disorders; glycemic control in patients with diabetes; lipid profiles in patients being treated for hyperlipidemias; thyroid function in patients on thyroid hormone replacement therapy.

Menopausal symptoms: Assess need for therapy at 3- to 6-month intervals

Additional Information Not biologically equivalent to conjugated estrogens from equine source. Contains 9 unique estrogenic compounds (equine source contains at least 10 active estrogenic compounds).

Estrogens (Conjugated B/Synthetic)

(ES troe jenz, KON joo gate ed, bee, sin THET ik)

Brand Names: U.S. Enjuvia

Pharmacologic Category Estrogen Derivative

Additional Appendix Information

Beers Criteria – Potentially Inappropriate Medications for Geriatrics *on page 2271*

Use Treatment of moderate-to-severe vasomotor symptoms of menopause; treatment of vulvar and vaginal atrophy associated with menopause; treatment of moderate-to-severe vaginal dryness and pain with intercourse associated with menopause

Pregnancy Considerations Estrogens are not indicated for use during pregnancy or immediately postpartum. In general, the use of estrogen and progestin as in combination hormonal contraceptives have not been associated with teratogenic effects when inadvertently taken early in pregnancy. This product is contraindicated for use during pregnancy.

Breast-Feeding Considerations Estrogens can be detected in breast milk and have been shown to decrease the quantity and quality of human milk. The manufacturer recommends that caution be used if administered to nursing women.

Contraindications Hypersensitivity to estrogens or any component of the formulation; undiagnosed abnormal vaginal bleeding; history of or current thrombophlebitis or venous thromboembolic disorders (including DVT, PE); active or recent (within 1 year) arterial thromboembolic disease (eg, stroke, MI); carcinoma of the breast; estrogen-dependent tumor; hepatic dysfunction or disease; pregnancy

Warnings/Precautions Hazardous agent - use appropriate precautions for handling and disposal (NIOSH 2014 [group 2]).

Cardiovascular-related considerations: **[U.S. Boxed Warning]: Estrogens with or without progestin should not be used to prevent cardiovascular disease.** Using data from the Women's Health Initiative (WHI) studies, an increased risk of deep vein thrombosis (DVT) and stroke has been reported with CE and an increased risk of DVT, stroke, pulmonary emboli (PE), and myocardial infarction (MI) has been reported with CE with MPA in postmenopausal women. Additional risk factors include diabetes mellitus, hypercholesterolemia, hypertension, SLE, obesity, tobacco use, and/or history of venous thromboembolism (VTE). Risk factors should be managed appropriately; discontinue use if adverse cardiovascular events occur or are suspected. Estrogen compounds are generally associated with lipid effects such as increased HDL-cholesterol and decreased LDL-cholesterol. Triglycerides may also be increased; use with caution in patients with familial defects of lipoprotein metabolism. Whenever possible, estrogens should be discontinued at least 4-6 weeks prior to elective surgery associated with an increased risk of thromboembolism or during periods of prolonged immobilization. Women with inherited thrombophilias (eg, protein C or S deficiency) may have increased risk of venous thromboembolism (DeSancho, 2010; van Vlijmen, 2011).

Neurological considerations: **[U.S. Boxed Warning]: Estrogens with or without progestin should not be used to prevent dementia.** In the Women's Health Initiative Memory Study (WHIMS), an increased incidence of dementia was observed in women ≥65 years of age taking CE alone or in combination with MPA.

Cancer-related considerations: **[U.S. Boxed Warning]: Based on data from the Women's Health Initiative (WHI) studies, an increased risk of invasive breast cancer was observed in postmenopausal women using conjugated estrogens (CE) in combination with medroxyprogesterone acetate (MPA).** This risk may be associated with duration of use and declines once combined therapy is discontinued (Chlebowski, 2009). The risk of invasive breast cancer was decreased in postmenopausal women with a hysterectomy using CE only, regardless of weight. However, the risk was not significantly decreased in women at high risk for breast cancer (family history of breast cancer, personal history of benign breast disease) (Anderson, 2012). An increase in abnormal mammogram findings has also been reported with estrogen alone or in combination with progestin therapy. Estrogen use may also lead to severe hypercalcemia in patients with breast cancer and bone metastases; discontinue estrogen if hypercalcemia occurs. Use is contraindicated in patients with known or suspected breast cancer. **[U.S. Boxed Warning]: The use of unopposed estrogen in women with an intact uterus is associated with an increased risk of endometrial cancer. The addition of a progestin to estrogen therapy may decrease the risk of endometrial hyperplasia, a precursor to endometrial cancer. Adequate diagnostic measures, including endometrial sampling if indicated, should be performed to rule out malignancy in postmenopausal women with undiagnosed abnormal vaginal bleeding.** Estrogens may exacerbate endometriosis. Malignant transformation of residual endometrial implants has been reported posthysterectomy with unopposed estrogen therapy. Consider adding a progestin in women with residual endometriosis posthysterectomy. Postmenopausal estrogen therapy and combined estrogen/progesterone therapy may increase the risk of ovarian cancer; however, the absolute risk to an individual woman is small. Although results from various studies are not consistent, risk does not appear to be significantly associated with the duration, route, or dose of therapy. In one study, the risk decreased after 2 years following discontinuation of therapy (Mørch, 2009). Although the risk of ovarian cancer is rare, women who are at an increased risk (eg, family history) should be counseled about the association (NAMS, 2012).

Estrogens may cause retinal vascular thrombosis; discontinue if migraine, loss of vision, proptosis, diplopia, or other visual disturbances occur; discontinue permanently if papilledema or retinal vascular lesions are observed on examination. Use caution in patients with asthma, epilepsy, hepatic hemangiomas, hereditary angioedema, migraine, porphyria, or SLE; may exacerbate disease. May have adverse effects on glucose tolerance; use caution in women with diabetes. Use with caution in patients with diseases which may be exacerbated by fluid retention, including cardiac or renal dysfunction. Use of postmenopausal estrogen may be associated with an increased risk of gallbladder disease requiring surgery. Estrogens are poorly metabolized in patients with hepatic dysfunction. Use caution with a history of cholestatic jaundice associated with prior estrogen use or pregnancy. Discontinue if jaundice develops or if acute or chronic hepatic disturbances occur. Use is contraindicated with hepatic disease. Use with caution in patients with severe hypocalcemia. Estrogens may increase thyroid-binding globulin (TBG) levels leading to increased circulating total thyroid hormone levels. Women on thyroid replacement therapy may require higher doses of thyroid hormone while receiving estrogens. Avoid use of oral estrogen (with or without progestins) in the elderly due to potential of increased risk of breast and endometrial cancers, and lack of proven cardioprotection and cognitive protection (Beers Criteria). Safety and efficacy have not been established in children. Prior to puberty, estrogens may cause premature closure of the epiphyses, premature breast development in girls or gynecomastia in boys. Vaginal bleeding and vaginal cornification may also be induced in girls. Whenever possible, estrogens should be discontinued at least 4-6 weeks prior to elective surgery associated with an increased risk of thromboembolism or during periods of prolonged immobilization. The use of estrogens and/or progestins may change the results of some laboratory tests (eg, coagulation factors, lipids, glucose tolerance, binding proteins). The dose, route, and the specific estrogen/progestin influences these changes. In addition, personal risk factors (eg, cardiovascular disease, smoking, diabetes, age) also contribute to adverse events; use of specific products may be contraindicated in women with certain risk factors.

[U.S. Boxed Warning]: Estrogens with or without progestin should be used for the shortest duration possible at the lowest effective dose consistent with treatment goals. Before prescribing estrogen therapy to postmenopausal women, the risks and benefits must be weighed for each patient. Women should be informed of these risks and benefits, as well as possible effects of progestin when added to estrogen therapy. Patients should be reevaluated as clinically appropriate to determine if treatment is still necessary. Available data related to treatment risks are from Women's Health Initiative (WHI) studies, which evaluated oral CE 0.625 mg with or without MPA 2.5 mg relative to placebo in postmenopausal women. Other combinations and dosage forms of estrogens and progestins were not studied. **Outcomes reported from clinical trials using CE with or without MPA should be assumed to be similar for other doses and other dosage forms of estrogens and progestins until comparable data becomes available.** When used solely for the treatment of vaginal dryness and pain with intercourse, or vulvar and vaginal atrophy, topical vaginal products should be considered.

Adverse Reactions

Central nervous system: Dizziness, headache, pain

Endocrine & metabolic: Breast pain, dysmenorrhea

Gastrointestinal: Abdominal pain, flatulence, nausea

Genitourinary: Vaginitis

Neuromuscular & skeletal: Paresthesia

Respiratory: Bronchitis, rhinitis, sinusitis

Miscellaneous: Flu-like syndrome

In addition, the following have been reported with estrogen and/or progestin therapy:

Cardiovascular: Edema, hypertension, MI, stroke, venous thromboembolism

Central nervous system: Epilepsy exacerbation, irritability, mental depression, migraine, mood disturbances, nervousness

Dermatologic: Angioedema, chloasma, erythema multiforme, erythema nodosum, hemorrhagic eruption, hirsutism, loss of scalp hair, melasma, pruritus, rash, urticaria

Endocrine & metabolic: Breast cancer, breast enlargement, breast tenderness, HDL-cholesterol increased, hyper-/hypocalcemia, impaired glucose tolerance, LDL-cholesterol decreased, libido (changes in), serum triglycerides/phospholipids increased, thyroid-binding globulin increased, total thyroid hormone (T_4) increased

Gastrointestinal: Abdominal cramps, bloating, cholecystitis, cholelithiasis, gallbladder disease, pancreatitis, weight gain/loss

Genitourinary: Alterations in frequency and flow of menses, changes in cervical secretions, endometrial cancer, endometrial hyperplasia, increased size of uterine leiomyomata, vaginal candidiasis

Hematologic: Aggravation of porphyria; antithrombin III and antifactor Xa decreased; fibrinogen levels increased; platelet aggregability and platelet count increased; prothrombin and factors VII, VIII, IX, X increased

Hepatic: Cholestatic jaundice, hepatic hemangiomas enlarged

Local: Thrombophlebitis

Neuromuscular & skeletal: Arthralgias, chorea, leg cramps

Ocular: Contact lens intolerance, corneal curvature steepening, retinal vascular thrombosis

Respiratory: Asthma exacerbation, pulmonary thromboembolism

Miscellaneous: Anaphylactoid/anaphylactic reactions, carbohydrate intolerance

Drug Interactions

Metabolism/Transport Effects Substrate of CYP3A4 (major); **Note:** Assignment of Major/Minor substrate status based on clinically relevant drug interaction potential

Avoid Concomitant Use

Avoid concomitant use of Estrogens (Conjugated B/Synthetic) with any of the following: Anastrozole; Dehydroepiandrosterone; Exemestane; Indium 111 Capromab Pendetide; Ospemifene

Increased Effect/Toxicity

Estrogens (Conjugated B/Synthetic) may increase the levels/effects of: C1 inhibitors; Corticosteroids (Systemic); Immune Globulin; Lenalidomide; Ospemifene; ROPINIRole; Thalidomide; Theophylline Derivatives; Tipranavir

The levels/effects of Estrogens (Conjugated B/Synthetic) may be increased by: Ascorbic Acid; Dehydroepiandrosterone; Herbs (Estrogenic Properties); NSAID (COX-2 Inhibitor)

Decreased Effect

Estrogens (Conjugated B/Synthetic) may decrease the levels/effects of: Anastrozole; Anticoagulants; Chenodiol; Exemestane; Hyaluronidase; Indium 111 Capromab Pendetide; Ospemifene; Somatropin; Thyroid Products; Ursodiol

The levels/effects of Estrogens (Conjugated B/Synthetic) may be decreased by: Bosentan; CYP3A4 Inducers (Moderate); CYP3A4 Inducers (Strong); Dabrafenib; Deferasirox; Mitotane; Siltuximab; St Johns Wort; Tipranavir; Tocilizumab

Food Interactions Routine use of ethanol increases estrogen level and risk of breast cancer. Management: Avoid ethanol.

Storage/Stability Store at room temperature of 25°C (77°F).

Mechanism of Action Conjugated B/synthetic estrogens contain a mixture of 10 synthetic estrogen substances, including sodium estrone sulfate, sodium equilin sulfate, sodium 17-alpha-dihydroequilin, sodium 17-alpha-estradiol, and sodium 17-beta-dihydroequilin. Estrogens are responsible for the development and maintenance of the female reproductive system and secondary sexual characteristics. Estradiol is the principle intracellular human estrogen and is more potent than estrone and estriol at the receptor level; it is the primary estrogen secreted prior to menopause. Following menopause, estrone and estrone sulfate are more highly produced. Estrogens modulate the pituitary secretion of gonadotropins, luteinizing hormone, and follicle-stimulating hormone through a negative feedback system; estrogen replacement reduces elevated levels of these hormones in postmenopausal women.

Pharmacodynamics/Kinetics

Absorption: Well absorbed over a period of several hours

Protein-binding: Sex hormone-binding globulin (SHBG) and albumin

Metabolism: Hepatic via CYP3A4; estradiol is converted to estrone and estriol; also undergoes enterohepatic recirculation; estrone sulfate is the main metabolite in postmenopausal women

Half-life elimination: Conjugated estrone: 8-20 hours; conjugated equilin: 5-17 hours

Excretion: Urine (primarily estriol, also as estradiol, estrone, and conjugates)

Dosage The lowest dose that will control symptoms should be used; medication should be discontinued as soon as possible. Oral:

Adults:

Moderate-to-severe vasomotor symptoms associated with menopause: 0.3 mg/day; may be titrated up to 1.25 mg/day. Attempts to discontinue medication should be made at 3- to 6-month intervals.

Vaginal dryness/vulvar and vaginal atrophy associated with menopause: 0.3 mg/day. Attempts to discontinue medication should be made at 3- to 6-month intervals.

Elderly: A higher incidence of stroke and invasive breast cancer were observed in women >75 years in a WHI substudy using conjugated equine estrogen.

Administration Administer at the same time each day. May be taken with or without food. Hazardous agent; use appropriate precautions for handling and disposal (NIOSH 2014 [group 2]).

Monitoring Parameters Yearly physical examination that may include blood pressure and Papanicolaou smear, breast exam, mammogram. Monitor for signs of endometrial cancer in female patients with uterus. Adequate diagnostic measures, including endometrial sampling, if indicated, should be performed to rule out malignancy in all cases of undiagnosed abnormal vaginal bleeding. Monitor for loss of vision, sudden onset of proptosis, diplopia, migraine; signs and symptoms of thromboembolic disorders; glycemic control in patients with diabetes; lipid profiles in patients being treated for hyperlipidemias; thyroid function in patients on thyroid hormone replacement therapy.

Additional Information Not biologically equivalent to conjugated estrogens from equine source. Contains 10 unique estrogenic compounds (equine source contains at least 10 active estrogenic compounds).

Dosage Forms

Tablet, Oral:

Enjuvia: 0.3 mg, 0.45 mg, 0.625 mg, 0.9 mg, 1.25 mg

Estrogens (Conjugated/Equine, Systemic) (ES troe jenz KON joo gate ed, EE kwine)

Brand Names: U.S. Premarin

Brand Names: Canada C.E.S.®; Congest; PMS-Conjugated Estrogens C.S.D.; Premarin®

Index Terms C.E.S.; CE; CEE; Conjugated Estrogen; Estrogenic Substances, Conjugated

Pharmacologic Category Estrogen Derivative

Additional Appendix Information

Beers Criteria – Potentially Inappropriate Medications for Geriatrics *on page 2271*

Use Treatment of moderate-to-severe vasomotor symptoms associated with menopause; treatment of vulvar and vaginal atrophy due to menopause; hypoestrogenism (due to hypogonadism, castration, or primary ovarian failure); prostatic cancer (palliation); breast cancer (palliation); postmenopausal osteoporosis (prophylaxis); abnormal uterine bleeding

Pregnancy Considerations Estrogens are not indicated for use during pregnancy or immediately postpartum. In general, the use of estrogen and progestin as in combination hormonal contraceptives have not been associated with teratogenic effects when inadvertently taken early in pregnancy. These products are contraindicated for use during pregnancy.

Breast-Feeding Considerations Estrogen has been shown to decrease the quantity and quality of human milk. Use only if clearly needed. Monitor the growth of the infant closely.

Contraindications Angioedema or anaphylactic reaction to estrogens or any component of the formulation; undiagnosed abnormal vaginal bleeding; history of or current thrombophlebitis or venous thromboembolic disorders (including DVT, PE); active or history of arterial thromboembolic disease (eg, stroke, MI); carcinoma of the breast (except in appropriately selected patients being treated for metastatic disease); estrogen-dependent tumor; hepatic dysfunction or disease; known protein C, protein S, antithrombin deficiency or other known thrombophilic disorders; pregnancy

Canadian labeling: Additional contraindications (not in U.S. labeling): Endometrial hyperplasia; partial or complete vision loss due to ophthalmic vascular disease; migraine with aura

Warnings/Precautions Hazardous agent - use appropriate precautions for handling and disposal (NIOSH 2014 [group 2]).

Anaphylaxis requiring emergency medical management has been reported within minutes to hours of taking conjugated estrogen (CE) tablets. Angioedema involving the face, feet, hands, larynx, and tongue has also been reported. Exogenous estrogens may exacerbate symptoms in women with hereditary angioedema.

[U.S. Boxed Warning]: Based on data from the Women's Health Initiative (WHI) studies, an increased risk of invasive breast cancer was observed in postmenopausal women using conjugated estrogens (CE) in

combination with medroxyprogesterone acetate (MPA). This risk may be associated with duration of use and declines once combined therapy is discontinued (Chlebowski, 2009). The risk of invasive breast cancer was decreased in postmenopausal women with a hysterectomy using CE only, regardless of weight. However, the risk was not significantly decreased in women at high risk for breast cancer (family history of breast cancer, personal history of benign breast disease) (Anderson, 2012). An increase in abnormal mammogram findings has also been reported with estrogen alone or in combination with progestin therapy. Estrogen use may lead to severe hypercalcemia in patients with breast cancer and bone metastases; discontinue estrogen if hypercalcemia occurs. **[U.S. Boxed Warning]: The use of unopposed estrogen in women with an intact uterus is associated with an increased risk of endometrial cancer. The addition of a progestin to estrogen therapy may decrease the risk of endometrial hyperplasia, a precursor to endometrial cancer. Adequate diagnostic measures, including endometrial sampling if indicated, should be performed to rule out malignancy in postmenopausal women with undiagnosed abnormal vaginal bleeding.** Estrogens may exacerbate endometriosis. Malignant transformation of residual endometrial implants has been reported posthysterectomy with unopposed estrogen therapy. Consider adding a progestin in women with residual endometriosis posthysterectomy. Postmenopausal estrogen therapy and combined estrogen/progesterone therapy may increase the risk of ovarian cancer; however, the absolute risk to an individual woman is small. Although results from various studies are not consistent, risk does not appear to be significantly associated with the duration, route, or dose of therapy. In one study, the risk decreased after 2 years following discontinuation of therapy (Mørch, 2009). Although the risk of ovarian cancer is rare, women who are at an increased risk (eg, family history) should be counseled about the association (NAMS, 2012).

[U.S. Boxed Warning]: Estrogens with or without progestin should not be used to prevent cardiovascular disease. Using data from the Women's Health Initiative (WHI) studies, an increased risk of deep vein thrombosis (DVT) and stroke has been reported with CE and an increased risk of DVT, stroke, pulmonary emboli (PE) and myocardial infarction (MI) has been reported with CE with MPA in postmenopausal women. Additional risk factors include diabetes mellitus, hypercholesterolemia, hypertension, SLE, obesity, tobacco use, and/or history of venous thromboembolism (VTE). Adverse cardiovascular events have also been reported in males taking estrogens for prostate cancer. Risk factors should be managed appropriately; discontinue use if adverse cardiovascular events occur or are suspected. Women with inherited thrombophilias (eg, protein C or S deficiency) may have increased risk of venous thromboembolism (DeSancho, 2010; van Vlijmen, 2011). Use is contraindicated in women with protein C, protein S, antithrombin deficiency, or other known thrombophilic disorders.

[U.S. Boxed Warning]: Estrogens with or without progestin should not be used to prevent dementia. In the Women's Health Initiative Memory Study (WHIMS), an increased incidence of dementia was observed in women ≥65 years of age taking CE alone or in combination with MPA.

Estrogen compounds are generally associated with lipid effects such as increased HDL-cholesterol and decreased LDL-cholesterol. Triglycerides may also be increased; discontinue if pancreatitis occurs. Use with caution in patients with familial defects of lipoprotein metabolism. Estrogens may increase thyroid-binding globulin (TBG) levels leading to increased circulating total thyroid hormone levels. Women on thyroid replacement therapy may require higher doses of thyroid hormone while receiving estrogens. Use caution in patients with hypoparathyroidism; estrogen-induced hypocalcemia may occur. May have adverse effects on glucose tolerance; use caution in women with diabetes. Use caution in patients with asthma, epilepsy, hepatic hemangiomas, porphyria, or SLE; may exacerbate disease. Use with caution in patients with diseases which may be exacerbated by fluid retention, including cardiac or renal dysfunction. Use of postmenopausal estrogen may be associated with an increased risk of gallbladder disease requiring surgery. Use caution with migraine; may exacerbate disease. Canadian labeling contraindicates use in migraine with aura. Estrogens may cause retinal vascular thrombosis; discontinue if migraine, loss of vision, proptosis, diplopia, or other visual disturbances occur; discontinue permanently if papilledema or retinal vascular lesions are observed on examination.

Estrogens are poorly metabolized in patients with hepatic dysfunction. Use caution with a history of cholestatic jaundice associated with prior estrogen use or pregnancy. Discontinue if jaundice develops or if acute or chronic hepatic disturbances occur. Use is contraindicated with hepatic disease.

Whenever possible, estrogens should be discontinued at least 4-6 weeks prior to elective surgery associated with an increased risk of thromboembolism or during periods of prolonged immobilization. Avoid use of oral estrogen (with or without progestins) in the elderly due to potential of increased risk of breast and endometrial cancers, and lack of proven cardioprotection and cognitive protection (Beers Criteria). Prior to puberty, estrogens may cause premature closure of the epiphyses, premature breast development in girls or gynecomastia in boys. Vaginal bleeding and vaginal cornification may also be induced in girls. The use of estrogens and/or progestins may change the results of some laboratory tests (eg, coagulation factors, lipids, glucose tolerance, binding proteins). The dose, route, and the specific estrogen/progestin influences these changes. In addition, personal risk factors (eg, cardiovascular disease, smoking, diabetes, age) also contribute to adverse events; use of specific products may be contraindicated in women with certain risk factors.

[U.S. Boxed Warning]: Estrogens with or without progestin should be used for the shortest duration possible at the lowest effective dose consistent with treatment goals. Before prescribing estrogen therapy to postmenopausal women, the risks and benefits must be weighed for each patient. Women should be informed of these risks and benefits, as well as possible effects of progestin when added to estrogen therapy. Patients should be reevaluated as clinically appropriate to determine if treatment is still necessary. Available data related to treatment risks are from Women's Health Initiative (WHI) studies, which evaluated oral CE 0.625 mg with or without MPA 2.5 mg relative to placebo in postmenopausal women. Other combinations and dosage forms of estrogens and progestins were not studied. **Outcomes reported from clinical trials using CE with or without MPA should be assumed to be similar for other doses and other dosage forms of estrogens and progestins until comparable data becomes available.**

Benzyl alcohol and derivatives: Some dosage forms may contain benzyl alcohol; large amounts of benzyl alcohol (≥99 mg/kg/day) have been associated with a potentially fatal toxicity ("gasping syndrome") in neonates; the "gasping syndrome" consists of metabolic acidosis, respiratory distress, gasping respirations, CNS dysfunction (including convulsions, intracranial hemorrhage), hypotension and cardiovascular collapse (AAP, 1997; CDC, 1982); some data suggests that benzoate displaces bilirubin from protein binding sites (Ahlfors, 2001); avoid or use dosage forms containing benzyl alcohol with caution in neonates. See manufacturer's labeling.

Vulvar and vaginal atrophy use: Moderate-to-severe symptoms of vulvar and vaginal atrophy include vaginal dryness, dyspareunia, and atrophic vaginitis. When used solely for the treatment of vulvar and vaginal atrophy, topical vaginal products should be considered (NAMS, 2007).

Osteoporosis use: For use only in women at significant risk of osteoporosis and for who other nonestrogen medications are not considered appropriate.

Adverse Reactions

Central nervous system: Depression, dizziness, headache, nervousness, pain
Dermatologic: Pruritus
Endocrine & metabolic: Breast pain
Gastrointestinal: Abdominal pain, diarrhea, flatulence
Genitourinary: Leukorrhea, vaginal hemorrhage, vaginal moniliasis, vaginitis
Neuromuscular & skeletal: Arthralgia, back pain, leg cramps, weakness
Respiratory: Cough increased, pharyngitis, sinusitis
Additional adverse reactions reported with injection; frequency not defined: Local: injection site: Edema, pain, phlebitis
Rare but important or life-threatening: Alopecia, anaphylaxis, angioedema, asthma exacerbation, benign meningioma (possible growth), bloating, breast cancer, breast discharge/enlargement/tenderness, cervical secretion changes, chloasma, cholestatic jaundice, contact lens intolerance, dementia, deep vein thrombosis (DVT), dysmenorrhea, edema, endometrial cancer, endometrial hyperplasia, epilepsy exacerbation, erythema multiforme, erythema nodosum, fibrocystic breast changes, galactorrhea, gallbladder disease, glucose intolerance, gynecomastia (males), hepatic hemangiomas (enlargement), hirsutism, hypersensitivity reactions, hypertension, irritability, ischemic colitis, libido changes, melasma, MI, migraine, mood disturbances, nausea, ovarian cancer, pancreatitis, pulmonary emboli (PE), pelvic pain, porphyria exacerbation, rash, retinal vascular thrombosis, stroke, superficial venous thrombosis, thrombophlebitis, triglyceride increase, urticaria, uterine bleeding (abnormal), uterine leiomyomata (increase in size), vaginal candidiasis, vomiting, weight changes

Drug Interactions

Metabolism/Transport Effects Substrate of CYP1A2 (major), CYP2A6 (minor), CYP2B6 (minor), CYP2C19 (minor), CYP2C9 (minor), CYP2D6 (minor), CYP2E1 (minor), CYP3A4 (major); **Note:** Assignment of Major/Minor substrate status based on clinically relevant drug interaction potential; **Inhibits** CYP1A2 (weak); **Induces** CYP3A4 (weak)

Avoid Concomitant Use

Avoid concomitant use of Estrogens (Conjugated/Equine, Systemic) with any of the following: Anastrozole; Dehydroepiandrosterone; Exemestane; Indium 111 Capromab Pendetide; Ospemifene

Increased Effect/Toxicity

Estrogens (Conjugated/Equine, Systemic) may increase the levels/effects of: C1 inhibitors; Corticosteroids (Systemic); Immune Globulin; Lenalidomide; Ospemifene; ROPINIRole; Thalidomide; Theophylline Derivatives; Tipranavir

The levels/effects of Estrogens (Conjugated/Equine, Systemic) may be increased by: Ascorbic Acid; Dehydroepiandrosterone; Herbs (Estrogenic Properties); NSAID (COX-2 Inhibitor)

Decreased Effect

Estrogens (Conjugated/Equine, Systemic) may decrease the levels/effects of: Anastrozole; Anticoagulants; ARIPiprazole; Chenodiol; Exemestane; Hyaluronidase; Hydrocodone; Indium 111 Capromab Pendetide; Ospemifene; Saxagliptin; Somatropin; Thyroid Products; Ursodiol

The levels/effects of Estrogens (Conjugated/Equine, Systemic) may be decreased by: Bosentan; Cannabis; CYP1A2 Inducers (Strong); CYP3A4 Inducers (Moderate); CYP3A4 Inducers (Strong); Cyproterone; Dabrafenib; Deferasirox; Mitotane; Siltuximab; St Johns Wort; Teriflunomide; Tipranavir; Tocilizumab

Food Interactions Folic acid absorption may be decreased. Routine use of ethanol increases estrogen level and risk of breast cancer; may also increase the risk of osteoporosis. Management: Avoid ethanol.

Preparation for Administration Injection: Reconstitute with sterile water for injection; slowly inject diluent against side wall of the vial. Agitate gently; do not shake violently.

Hazardous agent; use appropriate precautions for handling and disposal (NIOSH 2014 [group 2]).

Storage/Stability

Injection: Refrigerate at 2°C to 8°C (36°F to 46°F) prior to reconstitution. Use immediately following reconstitution.
Tablets: Store at room temperature 20°C to 25°C (68°F to 77°F).

Mechanism of Action Conjugated estrogens contain a mixture of estrone sulfate, equilin sulfate, 17 alpha-dihydroequilin, 17 alpha-estradiol and 17 beta-dihydroequilin. Estrogens are responsible for the development and maintenance of the female reproductive system and secondary sexual characteristics. Estradiol is the principle intracellular human estrogen and is more potent than estrone and estriol at the receptor level; it is the primary estrogen secreted prior to menopause. Following menopause, estrone and estrone sulfate are more highly produced. Estrogens modulate the pituitary secretion of gonadotropins, luteinizing hormone, and follicle-stimulating hormone through a negative feedback system; estrogen replacement reduces elevated levels of these hormones in postmenopausal women.

Pharmacodynamics/Kinetics

Absorption: Well absorbed
Protein binding: Binds to sex-hormone-binding globulin and albumin
Metabolism: Hepatic via CYP3A4; estradiol is converted to estrone and estriol; also undergoes enterohepatic recirculation (avoided with vaginal administration); estrone sulfate is the main metabolite in postmenopausal women
Half-life elimination: Total estrone: 27 hours
Time to peak, plasma: Total estrone: 7 hours
Excretion: Urine (primarily estriol, also as estradiol, estrone, and conjugates

Dosage Adults:

Males: Androgen-dependent prostate cancer palliation: Oral: 1.25-2.5 mg 3 times/day

Females:

Prevention of postmenopausal osteoporosis: Oral:
U.S. labeling: Initial: 0.3 mg/day cyclically* or daily, depending on medical assessment of patient. Dose may be adjusted based on bone mineral density and clinical response. The lowest effective dose should be used.
Canadian labeling: 0.625 mg once daily
Moderate-to-severe vasomotor symptoms associated with menopause: Oral: Initial: 0.3 mg/day, cyclically* or daily, depending on medical assessment of patient. Adjust dose based on patient's response. The lowest dose that will control symptoms should be used.
Vulvar and vaginal atrophy: Oral: Initial: 0.3 mg/day; the lowest dose that will control symptoms should be used.

May be given cyclically* or daily, depending on medical assessment of patient. Adjust dose based on patient's response.

Abnormal uterine bleeding: Acute/heavy bleeding:

Oral (off-label route): 10-20 mg/day in 4 divided doses has been used in place of IM/IV doses (ACOG, 2000)

IM, IV: 25 mg, may repeat in 6-12 hours if needed (manufacturer's labeling) **or** 25 mg IV repeated every 4 hours for 24 hours (ACOG, 2000). Patients who do not respond to 1-2 doses should be re-evaluated (ACOG, 2000).

Note: Treatment should be followed by a low-dose oral contraceptive; medroxyprogesterone acetate along with or following estrogen therapy can also be given

Female hypogonadism: Oral: 0.3-0.625 mg/day given cyclically*; dose may be titrated in 6- to 12-month intervals; progestin treatment should be added to maintain bone mineral density once skeletal maturity is achieved.

Female castration, primary ovarian failure: Oral: 1.25 mg/day given cyclically*; adjust according to severity of symptoms and patient response. For maintenance, adjust to the lowest effective dose.

***Cyclic administration:** Either 3 weeks on, 1 week off **or** 25 days on, 5 days off

Males and Females:

Breast cancer palliation, metastatic disease in selected patients: Oral: 10 mg 3 times/day for at least 3 months

Uremic bleeding (off-label use): IV: 0.6 mg/kg/day for 5 days (Livio, 1986)

Elderly: Refer to adult dosing; a higher incidence of stroke and invasive breast cancer was observed in women >75 years in a WHI substudy.

Dosage adjustment in renal impairment: No dosage adjustment provided in manufacturer's labeling (has not been studied). Use with caution; may increase risk of fluid retention.

Dosage adjustment in hepatic impairment: Use is contraindicated with hepatic dysfunction or disease.

Dietary Considerations Ensure adequate calcium and vitamin D intake when used for the prevention of osteoporosis. Powder for reconstitution for injection (25 mg) contains lactose 200 mg.

Administration

Injection: May also be administered intramuscularly; when administered IV, drug should be administered slowly to avoid the occurrence of a flushing reaction

Oral tablet: Administer at bedtime to minimize adverse effects. May be administered without regard to meals.

Abnormal uterine bleeding: High-dose therapy (eg, 10-20 mg/day) may cause nausea; consider concomitant use of an antiemetic

Hazardous agent; use appropriate precautions for handling and disposal (NIOSH 2014 [group 2]).

Monitoring Parameters Routine physical examination that includes blood pressure and Papanicolaou smear, breast exam, mammogram. Monitor for signs of endometrial cancer in female patients with uterus. Adequate diagnostic measures, including endometrial sampling, if indicated, should be performed to rule out malignancy in all cases of undiagnosed abnormal vaginal bleeding. Monitor for loss of vision, sudden onset of proptosis, diplopia, migraine; signs and symptoms of thromboembolic disorders; glycemic control in patients with diabetes; lipid profiles in patients being treated for hyperlipidemias; thyroid function in patients on thyroid hormone replacement therapy.

Menopausal symptoms: Assess need for therapy at 3- to 6-month intervals

Prevention of osteoporosis: Bone density measurement

Uremic bleeding: Bleeding time

Reference Range

Children: <10 mcg/24 hours (SI: <35 µmol/day) (values at Mayo Medical Laboratories)

Adults:

Males: 15-40 mcg/24 hours (SI: 52-139 micromole/day)

Females:

Menstruating: 15-80 mcg/24 hours (SI: 52-277 micromole/day)

Postmenopausal: <20 mcg/24 hours (SI: <69 micromole/day)

Dosage Forms

Solution Reconstituted, Injection:

Premarin: 25 mg (1 ea)

Tablet, Oral:

Premarin: 0.3 mg, 0.45 mg, 0.625 mg, 0.9 mg, 1.25 mg

Estrogens (Conjugated/Equine, Topical)

(ES troe jenz KON joo gate ed, EE kwine)

Brand Names: U.S. Premarin

Brand Names: Canada Premarin®

Index Terms C.E.S.; CE; CEE; Conjugated Estrogen; Estrogenic Substances, Conjugated

Pharmacologic Category Estrogen Derivative

Additional Appendix Information

Beers Criteria – Potentially Inappropriate Medications for Geriatrics *on page 2271*

Use Treatment of atrophic vaginitis and kraurosis vulvae; moderate-to-severe dyspareunia (pain during intercourse) due to vaginal/vulvar atrophy of menopause

Dosage Adults: Females:

Atrophic vaginitis, kraurosis vulvae: Intravaginal: 0.5 g/day (range 0.5-2 g/day) administered cyclically (21 days on, 7 days off). Adjust dose based on patient response. **Note:** Canadian labeling recommends oral estrogen therapy (~1.25 mg/day for 10 days) prior to initiating topical estrogen in severe atrophic vaginitis.

Moderate-to-severe dyspareunia due to menopause: Intravaginal: 0.5 g twice weekly (eg, Monday and Thursday) **or** once daily cyclically (21 days on, 7 days off)

Dosage adjustment in renal impairment: No dosage adjustment provided in manufacturer's labeling (has not been studied). Use with caution; may increase risk of fluid retention.

Dosage adjustment in hepatic impairment: Use is contraindicated with hepatic dysfunction or disease.

Additional Information Complete prescribing information should be consulted for additional detail.

Dosage Forms

Cream, Vaginal:

Premarin: 0.625 mg/g (30 g)

◆ **Estrogens (Conjugated/Equine) and Bazedoxifene Acetate** *see* Estrogens (Conjugated/Equine) and Bazedoxifene *on page 782*

Estrogens (Esterified) (ES troe jenz, es TER i fied)

Brand Names: U.S. Menest

Brand Names: Canada Estragyn; Estratab®; Menest®

Index Terms Esterified Estrogens

Pharmacologic Category Estrogen Derivative

Additional Appendix Information

Beers Criteria – Potentially Inappropriate Medications for Geriatrics *on page 2271*

Use Treatment of moderate-to-severe vasomotor symptoms associated with menopause; treatment of moderate-to-severe vulvar and vaginal atrophy associated with menopause; hypoestrogenism (due to hypogonadism, castration, or primary ovarian failure); advanced prostatic cancer (palliation), metastatic breast cancer (palliation) in men and postmenopausal women

Pregnancy Considerations In general, the use of estrogen and progestin as in combination hormonal contraceptives have not been associated with teratogenic effects when inadvertently taken early in pregnancy. This product is contraindicated for use during pregnancy.

Breast-Feeding Considerations Estrogen has been shown to decrease the quantity and quality of human milk; use only if clearly needed; monitor the growth of the infant closely.

Contraindications Hypersensitivity to estrogens or any component of the formulation; undiagnosed abnormal vaginal bleeding; DVT or PE (current or history of); active or recent (within 1 year) arterial thromboembolic disease (eg, stroke, MI); carcinoma of the breast (known, suspected or history of), except in appropriately selected patients being treated for metastatic disease; estrogen-dependent tumor; hepatic dysfunction or disease; pregnancy

Warnings/Precautions Hazardous agent - use appropriate precautions for handling and disposal (NIOSH 2014 [group 2]).

[U.S. Boxed Warning]: Based on data from the Women's Health Initiative (WHI) studies, an increased risk of invasive breast cancer was observed in postmenopausal women using conjugated estrogens (CE) in combination with medroxyprogesterone acetate (MPA). This risk may be associated with duration of use and declines once combined therapy is discontinued (Chlebowski, 2009). The risk of invasive breast cancer was decreased in postmenopausal women with a hysterectomy using CE only, regardless of weight. However, the risk was not significantly decreased in women at high risk for breast cancer (family history of breast cancer, personal history of benign breast disease) (Anderson, 2012). An increase in abnormal mammogram findings has also been reported with estrogen alone or in combination with progestin therapy. Estrogen use may also lead to severe hypercalcemia in patients with breast cancer and bone metastases; discontinue estrogen if hypercalcemia occurs. **[U.S. Boxed Warning]: The use of unopposed estrogen in women with an intact uterus is associated with an increased risk of endometrial cancer. The addition of a progestin to estrogen therapy may decrease the risk of endometrial hyperplasia, a precursor to endometrial cancer. Adequate diagnostic measures, including endometrial sampling if indicated, should be performed to rule out malignancy in postmenopausal women with undiagnosed abnormal vaginal bleeding.** Estrogens may exacerbate endometriosis. Malignant transformation of residual endometrial implants has been reported posthysterectomy with unopposed estrogen therapy. Consider adding a progestin in women with residual endometriosis posthysterectomy. Postmenopausal estrogen therapy and combined estrogen/progesterone therapy may increase the risk of ovarian cancer; however, the absolute risk to an individual woman is small. Although results from various studies are not consistent, risk does not appear to be significantly associated with the duration, route, or dose of therapy. In one study, the risk decreased after 2 years following discontinuation of therapy (Mørch, 2009). Although the risk of ovarian cancer is rare, women who are at an increased risk (eg, family history) should be counseled about the association (NAMS, 2012).

[U.S. Boxed Warning]: Estrogens with or without progestin should not be used to prevent cardiovascular disease. Using data from the Women's Health Initiative (WHI) studies, an increased risk of deep vein thrombosis (DVT) and stroke has been reported with CE and an increased risk of DVT, stroke, pulmonary emboli (PE) and myocardial infarction (MI) has been reported with CE with MPA in postmenopausal women. Additional risk factors include diabetes mellitus, hypercholesterolemia, hypertension, SLE, obesity, tobacco use, and/or history of venous thromboembolism (VTE). Adverse cardiovascular events have also been reported in males taking estrogens for prostate cancer. Risk factors should be managed appropriately; discontinue use if adverse cardiovascular events occur or are suspected. Women with inherited thrombophilias (eg, protein C or S deficiency) may have increased risk of venous thromboembolism (DeSancho, 2010; van Vlijmen, 2011).

[U.S. Boxed Warning]: Estrogens with or without progestin should not be used to prevent dementia. In the Women's Health Initiative Memory Study (WHIMS), an increased incidence of dementia was observed in women ≥65 years of age taking CE alone or in combination with MPA.

[U.S. Boxed Warning]: Estrogens with or without progestin should be used for the shortest duration possible at the lowest effective dose consistent with treatment goals. Before prescribing estrogen therapy to postmenopausal women, the risks and benefits must be weighed for each patient. Women should be informed of these risks and benefits, as well as possible effects of progestin when added to estrogen therapy. Patients should be reevaluated as clinically appropriate to determine if treatment is still necessary. Available data related to treatment risks are from Women's Health Initiative (WHI) studies, which evaluated oral CE 0.625 mg with or without MPA 2.5 mg relative to placebo in postmenopausal women. Other combinations and dosage forms of estrogens and progestins were not studied. **Outcomes reported from clinical trials using CE with or without MPA should be assumed to be similar for other doses and other dosage forms of estrogens and progestins until comparable data becomes available.**

Estrogen compounds are generally associated with lipid effects such as increased HDL-cholesterol and decreased LDL-cholesterol. Triglycerides may also be increased; use with caution in patients with familial defects of lipoprotein metabolism. Estrogens may increase thyroid-binding globulin (TBG) levels leading to increased circulating total thyroid hormone levels. Women on thyroid replacement therapy may require higher doses of thyroid hormone while receiving estrogens.

Estrogens may cause retinal vascular thrombosis; discontinue if migraine, loss of vision, proptosis, diplopia or other visual disturbances occur; discontinue permanently if papilledema or retinal vascular lesions are observed on examination. Estrogens are poorly metabolized in patients with hepatic dysfunction. Use caution with a history of cholestatic jaundice associated with prior estrogen use or pregnancy. Discontinue if jaundice develops or if acute or chronic hepatic disturbances occur. Use is contraindicated with hepatic disease. Use caution in patients with asthma, epilepsy, hepatic hemangiomas, migraine, porphyria, or SLE; may exacerbate disease. May have adverse effects on glucose tolerance; use caution in women with diabetes. Use with caution in patients with diseases which may be exacerbated by fluid retention, including cardiac or renal dysfunction. Use of postmenopausal estrogen may be associated with an increased risk of gallbladder disease requiring surgery. Use with caution in patients with severe hypocalcemia. Avoid use of oral estrogen (with or without ▶

progestins) in the elderly due to potential of increased risk of breast and endometrial cancers, and lack of proven cardioprotection and cognitive protection (Beers Criteria). Prior to puberty, estrogens may cause premature closure of the epiphyses, premature breast development in girls or gynecomastia in boys. Vaginal bleeding and vaginal cornification may also be induced in girls. Whenever possible, estrogens should be discontinued at least 4-6 weeks prior to elective surgery associated with an increased risk of thromboembolism or during periods of prolonged immobilization. The use of estrogens and/or progestins may change the results of some laboratory tests (eg, coagulation factors, lipids, glucose tolerance, binding proteins). The dose, route, and the specific estrogen/progestin influences these changes. In addition, personal risk factors (eg, cardiovascular disease, smoking, diabetes, age) also contribute to adverse events; use of specific products may be contraindicated in women with certain risk factors.

Adverse Reactions

Cardiovascular: Edema, hypertension, MI, stroke, venous thromboembolism

Central nervous system: Dementia exacerbation, dizziness, epilepsy exacerbation, headache, irritability, mental depression, migraine, mood disturbances, nervousness

Dermatologic: Angioedema, chloasma, erythema multiforme, erythema nodosum, hemorrhagic eruption, hirsutism, pruritus, loss of scalp hair, melasma, rash, urticaria

Endocrine & metabolic: Breast cancer, breast enlargement, breast tenderness, carbohydrate intolerance, fibrocystic breast changes, galactorrhea, hypocalcemia, libido (changes in), nipple discharge, premenstrual like syndrome

Gastrointestinal: Abdominal cramps, bloating, gallbladder disease, nausea, pancreatitis, vomiting, weight gain/loss

Genitourinary: Alterations in frequency and flow of menstrual patterns, breakthrough bleeding, changes in cervical secretions, cervical ectropion changes, cystitis-like syndrome, dysmenorrhea, endometrial hyperplasia, endometrial cancer, increased size of uterine leiomyomata, ovarian cancer, vaginal candidiasis, vaginitis

Hematologic: Aggravation of porphyria

Hepatic: Cholestatic jaundice, hemangioma enlargement

Local: Thrombophlebitis

Neuromuscular & skeletal: Arthralgia, chorea, leg cramps

Ocular: Contact lens intolerance, corneal curvature steepening, retinal vascular thrombosis

Respiratory: Asthma exacerbation, pulmonary embolism

Miscellaneous: Anaphylactoid/anaphylactic reactions

Drug Interactions

Metabolism/Transport Effects Substrate of CYP1A2 (major), CYP2B6 (minor), CYP2C9 (minor), CYP2E1 (minor), CYP3A4 (major); **Note:** Assignment of Major/Minor substrate status based on clinically relevant drug interaction potential

Avoid Concomitant Use

Avoid concomitant use of Estrogens (Esterified) with any of the following: Anastrozole; Dehydroepiandrosterone; Exemestane; Indium 111 Capromab Pendetide; Ospemifene

Increased Effect/Toxicity

Estrogens (Esterified) may increase the levels/effects of: C1 inhibitors; Corticosteroids (Systemic); Immune Globulin; Lenalidomide; Ospemifene; ROPINIRole; Thalidomide; Theophylline Derivatives; Tipranavir

The levels/effects of Estrogens (Esterified) may be increased by: Ascorbic Acid; Dehydroepiandrosterone; Herbs (Estrogenic Properties); NSAID (COX-2 Inhibitor)

Decreased Effect

Estrogens (Esterified) may decrease the levels/effects of: Anastrozole; Anticoagulants; Chenodiol; Exemestane; Hyaluronidase; Indium 111 Capromab Pendetide; Ospemifene; Somatropin; Thyroid Products; Ursodiol

The levels/effects of Estrogens (Esterified) may be decreased by: Bosentan; Cannabis; CYP1A2 Inducers (Strong); CYP3A4 Inducers (Moderate); CYP3A4 Inducers (Strong); Cyproterone; Dabrafenib; Deferasirox; Mitotane; Siltuximab; St Johns Wort; Teriflunomide; Tipranavir; Tocilizumab

Food Interactions Folic acid absorption may be decreased. Routine use of ethanol increases estrogen level and risk of breast cancer; may also increase the risk of osteoporosis. Management: Avoid ethanol.

Mechanism of Action Esterified estrogens contain a mixture of estrogenic substances; the principle component is estrone. Preparations contain 75% to 85% sodium estrone sulfate and 6% to 15% sodium equilin sulfate such that the total is not <90%. Estrogens are responsible for the development and maintenance of the female reproductive system and secondary sexual characteristics. Estradiol is the principle intracellular human estrogen and is more potent than estrone and estriol at the receptor level; it is the primary estrogen secreted prior to menopause. In males and following menopause in females, estrone and estrone sulfate are more highly produced. Estrogens modulate the pituitary secretion of gonadotropins, luteinizing hormone, and follicle-stimulating hormone through a negative feedback system; estrogen replacement reduces elevated levels of these hormones.

Pharmacodynamics/Kinetics

Absorption: Readily

Distribution: Widely distributed; high concentrations in the sex hormone target organs

Protein binding: Bound to sex hormone-binding globulin and albumin

Metabolism: Hepatic; partial metabolism via CYP3A4 enzymes; estradiol is reversibly converted to estrone and estriol; oral estradiol also undergoes enterohepatic recirculation by conjugation in the liver, followed by excretion of sulfate and glucuronide conjugates into the bile, then hydrolysis in the intestine and estrogen reabsorption. Sulfate conjugates are the primary form found in postmenopausal women.

Excretion: Primarily urine (as estradiol, estrone, estriol, and their glucuronide and sulfate conjugates)

Dosage Oral: Adults:

Prostate cancer, advanced: 1.25-2.5 mg 3 times/day

Female hypoestrogenism due to hypogonadism: 2.5-7.5 mg/day in divided doses for 20 days followed by a 10-day rest period. Administer cyclically (3 weeks on and 1 week off). If bleeding does not occur by the end of the 10-day period, repeat the same dosing schedule; the number of courses is dependent upon the responsiveness of the endometrium. If bleeding occurs before the end of the 10-day period, begin an estrogen-progestin cyclic regimen of 2.5-7.5 mg/day in divided doses for 20 days; during the last 5 days of estrogen therapy, give an oral progestin. If bleeding occurs before regimen is concluded, discontinue therapy and resume on the fifth day of bleeding.

Female hypoestrogenism due to castration and primary ovarian failure: 1.25 mg/day, cyclically. Adjust dosage upward or downward, according to the severity of symptoms and patient response. For maintenance, adjust dosage to lowest level that will provide effective control.

Vasomotor symptoms associated with menopause: 1.25 mg/day administered cyclically (3 weeks on and 1 week off). If patient has not menstruated within the last 2 months or more, cyclic administration is started arbitrary. If the patient is menstruating, cyclical administration is started on day 5 of the bleeding. For short-term use only and should be discontinued as soon as possible. Re-evaluate at 3- to 6-month intervals for tapering or discontinuation of therapy.

Vulvar and vaginal atrophy associated with menopause: 0.3 to ≥1.25 mg/day, depending on the tissue response of the individual patient. Administer cyclically. For short-term use only and should be discontinued as soon as possible. Re-evaluate at 3- to 6-month intervals for tapering or discontinuation of therapy.

Breast cancer, metastatic (appropriately selected patients): Males and postmenopausal females: 10 mg 3 times/day for at least 3 months

Elderly: Refer to adult dosing.

Dosage adjustment in renal impairment: No dosage adjustment provided in manufacturer's labeling; use with caution.

Dosage adjustment in hepatic impairment: No dosage adjustment provided in manufacturer's labeling; use with caution.

Dietary Considerations Should be taken with food at same time each day.

Administration Administer with food at same time each day.

Hazardous agent; use appropriate precautions for handling and disposal (NIOSH 2014 [group 2]).

Monitoring Parameters Routine physical examination that includes blood pressure and Papanicolaou smear, breast exam, mammogram. Monitor for signs of endometrial cancer in female patients with uterus. Adequate diagnostic measures, including endometrial sampling, if indicated, should be performed to rule out malignancy in all cases of undiagnosed abnormal vaginal bleeding. Monitor for loss of vision, sudden onset of proptosis, diplopia, migraine; signs and symptoms of thromboembolic disorders; glycemic control in patients with diabetes; lipid profiles in patients being treated for hyperlipidemias; thyroid function in patients on thyroid hormone replacement therapy.

Menopausal symptoms; vulvar and vaginal atrophy: Assess need for therapy at 3- to 6-month intervals

Dosage Forms

Tablet, Oral:

Menest: 0.3 mg, 0.625 mg, 1.25 mg, 2.5 mg

Estropipate (ES troe pih pate)

Brand Names: U.S. Ortho-Est 0.625; Ortho-Est 1.25

Brand Names: Canada Ogen

Index Terms Ortho Est; Piperazine Estrone Sulfate

Pharmacologic Category Estrogen Derivative

Use

Hypoestrogenism, female: Treatment of hypoestrogenism due to hypogonadism, castration, or primary ovarian failure.

Postmenopausal osteoporosis: Prevention of postmenopausal osteoporosis.

Vasomotor symptoms associated with menopause: Treatment of moderate to severe vasomotor symptoms associated with menopause.

Vulval and vaginal atrophy associated with menopause: Treatment of moderate to severe symptoms of vulval and vaginal atrophy associated with menopause.

Pregnancy Risk Factor X

Dosage Oral:

Adults:

Moderate-to-severe vasomotor symptoms associated with menopause: Usual dosage range: 0.75 to 6 mg estropipate daily; use the lowest dose and regimen that will control symptoms, and discontinue as soon as possible. Attempt to discontinue or taper medication at 3- to 6-month intervals. If a patient with vasomotor symptoms has not menstruated within the last ≥2 months, start the cyclic administration arbitrarily. If the patient has menstruated, start cyclic administration on day 5 of bleeding.

Female hypogonadism: 1.5 to 9 mg estropipate daily for the first 3 weeks, followed by a rest period of 8 to 10 days; use the lowest dose and regimen that will control symptoms. Repeat if bleeding does not occur by the end of the rest period. The duration of therapy necessary to product the withdrawal bleeding will vary according to the responsiveness of the endometrium. If satisfactory withdrawal bleeding does not occur, give an oral progestin in addition to estrogen during the third week of the cycle.

Female castration or primary ovarian failure: 1.5 to 9 mg estropipate daily for the first 3 weeks of a theoretical cycle, followed by a rest period of 8 to 10 days; use the lowest dose and regimen that will control symptoms

Osteoporosis prophylaxis: 0.75 mg estropipate daily for 25 days of a 31-day cycle

Atrophic vaginitis or kraurosis vulvae: 0.75 to 6 mg estropipate daily; administer cyclically. Use the lowest dose and regimen that will control symptoms; discontinue as soon as possible.

Elderly: Refer to adult dosing. A higher incidence of stroke and invasive breast cancer were observed in women >75 years in a WHI substudy using conjugated equine estrogen.

Dosage adjustment in renal impairment: There are no dosage adjustments provided in the manufacturer's labeling (has not been studied).

Dosage adjustment in hepatic impairment: There are no dosage adjustments provided in the manufacturer's labeling (has not been studied); use is contraindicated with hepatic dysfunction or disease.

Additional Information Complete prescribing information should be consulted for additional detail.

Dosage Forms

Tablet, Oral:

Ortho-Est 0.625: 0.75 mg

Ortho-Est 1.25: 1.5 mg

Generic: 0.75 mg, 1.5 mg, 3 mg

◆ **Estrostep Fe** *see* Ethinyl Estradiol and Norethindrone *on page 808*

Eszopiclone (es zoe PIK lone)

Brand Names: U.S. Lunesta

Pharmacologic Category Hypnotic, Miscellaneous

Additional Appendix Information

Beers Criteria – Potentially Inappropriate Medications for Geriatrics *on page 2271*

Use Insomnia: Treatment of insomnia

Pregnancy Risk Factor C

Pregnancy Considerations Adverse effects were observed in animal reproduction studies. Eszopiclone is the S-isomer of the racemic derivative zopiclone. Refer to Zopiclone monograph for related information.

Breast-Feeding Considerations It is not known if eszopiclone is excreted in breast milk. Eszopiclone is the S-isomer of the racemic derivative zopiclone. Zopiclone is excreted in human milk and is not recommended for use while breast-feeding. Refer to Zopiclone monograph for related information.

Contraindications Hypersensitivity to eszopiclone or any component of the formulation.

Warnings/Precautions Symptomatic treatment of insomnia should be initiated only after careful evaluation of potential causes of sleep disturbance. Failure of sleep disturbance to resolve after 7 to 10 days may indicate psychiatric and/or medical illness. Tolerance did not develop over 6 months of use. Daytime function may be impaired in patients taking higher doses (2 mg or 3 mg) even if used as prescribed; patients taking 3 mg must be cautioned about performing tasks which require mental alertness (operating machinery or driving) the day after use. An increased risk of next-day psychomotor impairment may occur if taken with less than a full night of sleep (7 to 8 hours); if higher than recommended dose is taken; if co-administered with other CNS depressants or other drugs that increase blood concentrations of eszopiclone. Dose adjustment may be necessary if taking concomitant CNS depressants; the use of concomitant sedative-hypnotics at bedtime or in the middle of the night is not recommended. Potentially significant drug-drug interactions may exist, requiring dose or frequency adjustment, additional monitoring, and/or selection of alternative therapy.

Use with caution in patients with depression; worsening of depression, including suicidal ideation has been reported with the use of hypnotics. Intentional overdose may be an issue with this population. The minimum dose that will effectively treat the individual patient should be used. Prescriptions should be written for the smallest quantity consistent with good patient care. Use caution in patients with a history of drug dependence. Hypnotics/sedatives have been associated with abnormal thinking and behavior changes including decreased inhibition, aggression, bizarre behavior, agitation, hallucinations, and depersonalization. These changes may occur unpredictably and may indicate previously unrecognized psychiatric disorders; evaluate appropriately. An increased risk for hazardous sleep-related activities such as sleep-driving, cooking and eating food, and making phone calls while asleep has also been noted; amnesia may also occur. The use of alcohol, other CNS depressants, and exceeding the recommended maximum dose may increase the risk of these activities. Discontinue treatment in patients who report any sleep-related episodes. Use caution in patients with respiratory compromise, COPD, sleep apnea, and hepatic dysfunction (dose adjustment recommended with severe impairment). Because of the rapid onset of action, administer immediately prior to bedtime or after the patient has gone to bed and is having difficulty falling asleep. Abrupt discontinuance or rapid dose decreases may lead to withdrawal symptoms. Hypersensitivity reactions including anaphylaxis as well as angioedema have been reported, in some cases following initial dosing. Patients who develop severe reactions should not be rechallenged.

Use with caution in debilitated and elderly patients; dosage adjustment recommended. Closely monitor elderly or debilitated patients for impaired cognitive and/or motor performance, confusion, and potential for falling. Avoid chronic use (>90 days) in older adults; adverse events, including delirium, falls, fractures, have been observed with nonbenzodiazepine hypnotic use in the elderly similar to events observed with benzodiazepines. Data suggests improvements in sleep duration and latency are minimal (Beers Criteria).

Adverse Reactions

Cardiovascular: Chest pain, peripheral edema

Central nervous system: Abnormal dreams, anxiety, confusion, depression, dizziness, hallucinations, headache, migraine, nervousness, pain, somnolence,

Dermatologic: Pruritus, rash

Endocrine & metabolic: Dysmenorrhea, gynecomastia, libido decreased

Gastrointestinal: Diarrhea, dyspepsia, nausea, unpleasant taste, vomiting, xerostomia

Genitourinary: Urinary tract infection

Neuromuscular & skeletal: Neuralgia

Miscellaneous: Accidental injury, infection, viral infection

Rare but important or life-threatening: Abnormal thinking, alopecia, amenorrhea, anaphylaxis, anemia, anorexia, ataxia, breast enlargement, breast neoplasm, breast pain, bursitis, cholelithiasis, colitis, complex sleep-related behavior (sleep-driving, cooking or eating food, making phone calls), conjunctivitis, contact dermatitis, cystitis, dehydration, dysphagia, emotional lability, epistaxis, gastritis, gout, halitosis, heat stroke, hepatitis, hepatomegaly, herpes zoster, hypercholesterolemia, hypertension, hypokalemia, insomnia, kidney calculus, laryngitis, lymphadenopathy, memory impairment, menorrhagia, myasthenia, mydriasis, myopathy, neck rigidity, neuritis, neuropathy, nystagmus, oliguria, photosensitivity, ptosis, pyelonephritis, rectal hemorrhage, reflexes decreased, skin discoloration, stomach ulcer, thrombophlebitis, ulcerative stomatitis, urethritis, urinary incontinence, vaginal hemorrhage, vaginitis, vestibular disorder, vesiculobullous rash

Drug Interactions

Metabolism/Transport Effects Substrate of CYP2E1 (minor), CYP3A4 (major); **Note:** Assignment of Major/Minor substrate status based on clinically relevant drug interaction potential

Avoid Concomitant Use

Avoid concomitant use of Eszopiclone with any of the following: Azelastine (Nasal); Conivaptan; Fusidic Acid (Systemic); Idelalisib; Orphenadrine; Paraldehyde; Sodium Oxybate; Thalidomide

Increased Effect/Toxicity

Eszopiclone may increase the levels/effects of: Alcohol (Ethyl); Azelastine (Nasal); Buprenorphine; CNS Depressants; Hydrocodone; Methotrimeprazine; Metyrosine; Mirtazapine; Orphenadrine; Paraldehyde; Pramipexole; ROPINIRole; Rotigotine; Selective Serotonin Reuptake Inhibitors; Sodium Oxybate; Suvorexant; Thalidomide; Zolpidem

The levels/effects of Eszopiclone may be increased by: Aprepitant; Brimonidine (Topical); Cannabis; Ceritinib; Conivaptan; CYP3A4 Inhibitors (Moderate); CYP3A4 Inhibitors (Strong); Dasatinib; Doxylamine; Dronabinol; Droperidol; Fosaprepitant; Fusidic Acid (Systemic); HydrOXYzine; Idelalisib; Ivacaftor; Kava Kava; Luliconazole; Magnesium Sulfate; Methotrimeprazine; Mifepristone; Nabilone; Netupitant; Perampanel; Rufinamide; Simeprevir; Stiripentol; Tapentadol; Tetrahydrocannabinol

Decreased Effect

The levels/effects of Eszopiclone may be decreased by: Bosentan; CYP3A4 Inducers (Moderate); CYP3A4 Inducers (Strong); Dabrafenib; Deferasirox; Flumazenil; Mitotane; Siltuximab; St Johns Wort; Tocilizumab

Food Interactions Onset of action may be reduced if taken with or immediately after a heavy meal. Management: Take immediately prior to bedtime, not with or immediately after a heavy or high-fat meal.

Storage/Stability Store at 25°C (77°F); excursions permitted to 15°C to 30°C (59°F to 86°F).

Mechanism of Action May interact with GABA-receptor complexes at binding domains located close to or allosterically coupled to benzodiazepine receptors.

Pharmacodynamics/Kinetics

Absorption: Rapid; high-fat/heavy meal may delay absorption

Protein binding: 52% to 59%

Metabolism: Hepatic via oxidation and demethylation (CYP2E1, 3A4); (S)-N-desmethyl zopiclone metabolite has less activity than parent compound

Half-life elimination: ~6 hours; Elderly (≥65 years): ~9 hours

Time to peak, plasma: ~1 hour

Excretion: Urine (up to 75%, primarily as metabolites; <10% as parent drug)

Dosage Oral: **Note:** The lowest effective dose should be used.

Adults: Insomnia: Initial: 1 mg immediately before bedtime; dosing may be increased to 2 mg or 3 mg if clinically necessary (maximum dose: 3 mg daily)

Debilitated patients: Initial: 1 mg immediately before bedtime (maximum dose: 2 mg)

Concurrent use with strong CYP3A4 inhibitor: Initial: 1 mg immediately before bedtime (maximum dose: 2 mg)

Elderly: Initial: 1 mg immediately before bedtime (maximum dose: 2 mg)

Dosage adjustment in renal impairment: No dosage adjustment necessary.

Dosage adjustment in hepatic impairment:

Mild to moderate impairment: No dosage adjustment necessary.

Severe impairment: Initial: 1 mg immediately before bedtime (maximum dose: 2 mg); use with caution; systemic exposure is doubled in severe impairment.

Dietary Considerations Avoid taking after a heavy meal; may delay onset.

Administration Because of the rapid onset of action, eszopiclone should be administered immediately prior to bedtime or after the patient has gone to bed and is having difficulty falling asleep. Do not take with, or immediately following, a high-fat meal (may delay onset).

Dosage Forms

Tablet, Oral:

Lunesta: 1 mg, 2 mg, 3 mg

Generic: 1 mg, 2 mg, 3 mg

Etamsylate [INT] (e TAM si late)

International Brand Names Altodor (DE); Dicinone (BR, CH, ES); Dicynene (CH, GB, IE); Dicynone (BE, CH, FR, HR, HU, IT, LU); Eselin (IT); Ethamsyl (IN); Hemo 141 (ES); Hemoced (FR); Impedil (AR)

Index Terms Ethamsylate

Pharmacologic Category Hemostatic Agent

Reported Use Prevention and treatment of capillary hemorrhages; treatment of menorrhagia or metrorrhagia

Dosage Range Adults:

Oral:

Preoperative: 250-500 mg 1 hour before surgery

Postoperative: 250-500 mg every 4-6 hours as risk of bleeding persists

Menorrhagia: 500 mg 4 times/day

IM, IV:

Preoperative: 250-500 mg 1 hour before surgery

During and after surgery: 250-500 mg repeating every 4-6 hours as risk of bleeding persists

Product Availability Product available in various countries; not currently available in the U.S.

Dosage Forms

Injection, solution: 125 mg/mL (2 mL) [contains sodium bisulphite]

Tablet: 250 mg, 500 mg

Etanercept (et a NER sept)

Brand Names: U.S. Enbrel; Enbrel SureClick

Brand Names: Canada Enbrel

Pharmacologic Category Antirheumatic, Disease Modifying; Tumor Necrosis Factor (TNF) Blocking Agent

Use

Ankylosing spondylitis: For reducing signs and symptoms in patients with active ankylosing spondylitis.

Plaque psoriasis: For treatment of adults ≥18 years of age with chronic moderate to severe plaque psoriasis who are candidates for systemic therapy or phototherapy.

Polyarticular juvenile idiopathic arthritis: For reducing signs and symptoms of moderately to severely active polyarticular juvenile idiopathic arthritis in patients ≥2 years of age.

Psoriatic arthritis: For reducing signs and symptoms, inhibiting the progression of structural damage of active arthritis, and improving physical function in patients with psoriatic arthritis. Etanercept can be used in combination with methotrexate in patients who do not respond adequately to methotrexate alone.

Rheumatoid arthritis: For reducing signs and symptoms, inducing major clinical response, inhibiting the progression of structural damage, and improving physical function in patients with moderately to severely active rheumatoid arthritis (RA). Etanercept can be initiated in combination with methotrexate or used alone.

Pregnancy Risk Factor B

Pregnancy Considerations Adverse events were not observed in animal reproduction studies. Etanercept crosses the placenta. Following in utero exposure, concentrations in the newborn at delivery are 3% to 32% of the maternal serum concentration.

A pregnancy registry has been established to monitor outcomes of women exposed to etanercept during pregnancy (800-772-6436).

Breast-Feeding Considerations Etanercept is excreted into breast milk in low concentrations and is minimally absorbed by a nursing infant (limited data). The manufacturer recommends that caution be used if administered to a nursing woman, taking into account the importance of the drug to the mother and potential effects to the nursing infant. A lactation surveillance program has been established to monitor outcomes of breastfed infants exposed to etanercept (800-772-6436).

Contraindications Sepsis

Warnings/Precautions [U.S. Boxed Warning]: Patients receiving etanercept are at increased risk for serious infections which may result in hospitalization and/or fatality; infections usually developed in patients receiving concomitant immunosuppressive agents (eg, methotrexate or corticosteroids) and may present as disseminated (rather than local) disease. Active tuberculosis (or reactivation of latent tuberculosis), invasive fungal (including aspergillosis, blastomycosis, candidiasis, coccidioidomycosis, histoplasmosis, and pneumocystosis) and bacterial, viral or other opportunistic infections (including legionellosis and listeriosis) have been reported in patients receiving TNF-blocking agents, including etanercept. Monitor closely for signs/symptoms of infection. Discontinue for serious infection or sepsis. Consider risks versus benefits prior to use in patients with a history of chronic or recurrent infection. Consider empiric antifungal therapy in patients who are at risk for invasive fungal infection and develop severe systemic illness. Caution should be exercised when considering use in the elderly or in patients with conditions that predispose them to infections (eg, diabetes) or residence/travel from areas of endemic mycoses (blastomycosis, coccidioidomycosis, histoplasmosis), or with latent or localized infections. Do not initiate etanercept therapy with clinically important active infection. Patients who develop a new infection while undergoing treatment should be monitored closely. **[U.S. Boxed Warning]: Tuberculosis (disseminated or extrapulmonary) has been reported in patients receiving etanercept; both reactivation of latent infection and new infections have been reported.** Patients should be evaluated for tuberculosis risk factors and for latent tuberculosis infection with a tuberculin skin test prior to starting therapy. Treatment of latent tuberculosis should be initiated before etanercept therapy; consider antituberculosis treatment if adequate course of treatment cannot be confirmed in patients with a history of latent or active tuberculosis or with risk factors despite negative skin test. Some patients who tested negative prior to therapy have developed active infection; tests for latent tuberculosis infection may be falsely negative while on etanercept therapy. Monitor for signs and symptoms of tuberculosis in all patients. Rare reactivation of hepatitis B virus (HBV) has occurred in chronic virus carriers, usually in patients receiving concomitant immunosuppressants; evaluate for HBV prior to initiation in all patients. Monitor during and for several months following discontinuation of treatment in HBV carriers; interrupt therapy if reactivation occurs and treat appropriately with antiviral therapy; if resumption of therapy is deemed necessary, exercise caution and monitor patient closely. Patients should be brought up to date with all immunizations before initiating therapy. Live vaccines should not be given concurrently with etanercept; there is no data available concerning secondary transmission of live vaccines in patients receiving therapy. Patients with a significant exposure to varicella virus should temporarily discontinue etanercept. Treatment with varicella zoster immune globulin should be considered.

[U.S. Boxed Warning]: Lymphoma and other malignancies have been reported in children and adolescent patients receiving TNF-blocking agents, including etanercept. Half of the malignancies reported in children were lymphomas (Hodgkin and non-Hodgkin) while other cases varied and included malignancies not typically observed in this population. The impact of etanercept on the development and course of malignancy is not fully defined. Compared to the general population, an increased risk of lymphoma has been noted in clinical trials; however, rheumatoid arthritis alone has been previously associated with an increased rate of lymphoma. Lymphomas and other malignancies were also observed (at rates higher than expected for the general population) in adult patients receiving etanercept. Etanercept is not recommended for use in patients with Wegener's granulomatosis who are receiving immunosuppressive therapy due to higher incidence of noncutaneous solid malignancies. Hepatosplenic T-cell lymphoma (HSTCL), a rare T-cell lymphoma, has also been associated with TNF-blocking agents, primarily reported in adolescent and young adult males with Crohn disease or ulcerative colitis. Melanoma, nonmelanoma skin cancer, and Merkel cell carcinoma have been reported in patients receiving TNF-blocking agents, including etanercept. Perform periodic skin examinations in all patients during therapy, particularly those at increased risk of skin cancer. Positive antinuclear antibody titers have been detected in patients (with negative baselines). Rare cases of autoimmune disorder, including lupus-like syndrome or autoimmune hepatitis, have been reported; monitor and discontinue if symptoms develop.

Allergic reactions may occur; if an anaphylactic reaction or other serious allergic reaction occurs, administration should be discontinued immediately and appropriate therapy initiated. Use with caution in patients with preexisting or recent onset CNS demyelinating disorders; rare cases of new-onset or exacerbation of CNS demyelinating disorders have occurred; may present with mental status changes and some may be associated with permanent disability. Optic neuritis, transverse myelitis, multiple sclerosis, Guillain-Barré syndrome, other peripheral demyelinating neuropathies, and new-onset or exacerbation of seizures have been reported. Use with caution in patients with heart failure or decreased left ventricular function; worsening and new-onset heart failure has been reported, including in patients without known preexisting cardiovascular disease. Use caution in patients with a history of significant hematologic abnormalities; has been associated with pancytopenia and aplastic anemia (rare). Patients must be advised to seek medical attention if they develop signs and symptoms suggestive of blood dyscrasias; discontinue if significant hematologic abnormalities are confirmed. Use with caution in patients with moderate to severe alcoholic hepatitis. Compared to placebo, the mortality rate in patients treated with etanercept was similar at one month but significantly higher after 6 months.

Due to a higher incidence of serious infections, concomitant use with anakinra is not recommended. Hypoglycemia has been reported in patients receiving concomitant therapy with etanercept and antidiabetic medications; dose reduction of antidiabetic medication may be necessary. Use with caution in patient with diabetes; monitor blood glucose as clinically necessary. Some dosage forms may contain dry natural rubber (latex).

Benzyl alcohol and derivatives: Diluent for injection may contain benzyl alcohol; large amounts of benzyl alcohol (≥99 mg/kg/day) have been associated with a potentially fatal toxicity ("gasping syndrome") in neonates; the "gasping syndrome" consists of metabolic acidosis, respiratory distress, gasping respirations, CNS dysfunction (including convulsions, intracranial hemorrhage), hypotension and cardiovascular collapse (AAP, 1997; CDC, 1982); some data suggests that benzoate displaces bilirubin from protein binding sites (Ahlfors, 2001); avoid or use dosage forms containing benzyl alcohol with caution in neonates. See manufacturer's labeling.

Adverse Reactions

Central nervous system: Dizziness, headache

Dermatologic: Pruritus, skin rash

Gastrointestinal: Abdominal pain (more common in children), diarrhea, nausea (children), vomiting

Infection: Infection

Local: Injection site reaction (bleeding, bruising, erythema, itching, pain, or swelling)

Neuromuscular & skeletal: Weakness

Respiratory: Cough, pharyngitis, respiratory distress, respiratory tract infection, rhinitis, sinusitis, upper respiratory tract infection

Miscellaneous: Antibody development (positive antidouble-stranded DNA antibodies), fever, positive ANA titer

Rare but important or life-threatening: Abscess, adenopathy, anemia, angioedema, anorexia, aplastic anemia, appendicitis, aseptic meningitis, aspergillosis, autoimmune hepatitis, blood coagulation disorder, bursitis, cardiac failure, cerebral ischemia, cerebrovascular accident, cholecystitis, cutaneous lupus erythematous, deep vein thrombosis, demyelinating disease of the central nervous system (suggestive of multiple sclerosis, transverse myelitis, or optic neuritis), depression, dermal ulcer, erythema multiforme, gastritis, gastroenteritis, gastrointestinal hemorrhage, glomerulopathy (membranous), herpes zoster, hydrocephalus (with normal pressure), hypersensitivity, hypersensitivity reaction, hypertension, hypotension, inflammatory bowel disease, interstitial pulmonary disease, intestinal perforation, ischemic heart disease, leukemia, leukopenia, lupus-like syndrome, lymphadenopathy, malignant lymphoma, malignant melanoma, malignant neoplasm, Merkel cell carcinoma, myocardial infarction, multiple sclerosis, nephrolithiasis, neutropenia, optic neuritis, oral mucosa ulcer, pancreatitis, pancytopenia, pneumonia due to *Pneumocystis carinii*, polymyositis, psoriasis (including new onset, palmoplantar, pustular, or exacerbation), pulmonary disease, pulmonary embolism, reactivation of HBV, sarcoidosis, scleritis, seizure, skin carcinoma, Stevens-Johnson syndrome, subcutaneous nodule, thrombocytopenia, thrombophlebitis, toxic epidermal necrolysis, tuberculosis, tuberculous arthritis, urinary tract infection, uveitis, varicella zoster infection, vasculitis (cutaneous and systemic), weight gain

Drug Interactions

Metabolism/Transport Effects None known.

Avoid Concomitant Use

Avoid concomitant use of Etanercept with any of the following: Abatacept; Anakinra; BCG; Belimumab; Canakinumab; Certolizumab Pegol; Cyclophosphamide; InFLIXimab; Natalizumab; Pimecrolimus; Rilonacept; Tacrolimus (Topical); Tocilizumab; Tofacitinib; Vaccines (Live); Vedolizumab

Increased Effect/Toxicity

Etanercept may increase the levels/effects of: Abatacept; Anakinra; Belimumab; Canakinumab; Certolizumab Pegol; Cyclophosphamide; InFLIXimab; Leflunomide; Natalizumab; Rilonacept; Tofacitinib; Vaccines (Live); Vedolizumab

The levels/effects of Etanercept may be increased by: Denosumab; Pimecrolimus; Roflumilast; Tacrolimus (Topical); Tocilizumab; Trastuzumab

Decreased Effect

Etanercept may decrease the levels/effects of: BCG; Coccidioides immitis Skin Test; Sipuleucel-T; Vaccines (Inactivated); Vaccines (Live)

The levels/effects of Etanercept may be decreased by: Echinacea

Preparation for Administration Reconstitute lyophilized powder aseptically with 1 mL sterile bacteriostatic water for injection, USP (supplied); swirl gently, do not shake. Do not filter reconstituted solution during preparation or administration.

Storage/Stability

Refrigerate at 2°C to 8°C (36°F to 46°F). Do not freeze. Do not store in extreme heat or cold. Store in the original carton to protect from light or physical damage until the time of use.

For convenience and a more comfortable injection, autoinjectors, prefilled syringes, or individual dose trays (containing multi-use vials and diluent syringes) may be stored at room temperature for a maximum single period of 14 days with protection from light and sources of heat, and humidity. Once an autoinjector, prefilled syringe or dose tray has been stored at room temperature, it should not be placed back into the refrigerator; discard after 14 days.

Once the multi-use vial has been reconstituted, use the reconstituted solution immediately or refrigerate at 2°C to 8°C (36°F to 46°F). Reconstituted solution must be used within 14 days; discard after 14 days.

Mechanism of Action Etanercept is a recombinant DNA-derived protein composed of tumor necrosis factor receptor (TNFR) linked to the Fc portion of human IgG1. Etanercept binds tumor necrosis factor (TNF) and blocks its interaction with cell surface receptors. TNF plays an important role in the inflammatory processes and the resulting joint pathology of rheumatoid arthritis (RA), polyarticular-course juvenile idiopathic arthritis (JIA), ankylosing spondylitis (AS), and plaque psoriasis.

Pharmacodynamics/Kinetics

Onset of action: ~2-3 weeks; RA: 1-2 weeks

Half-life elimination: RA: SubQ: 72-132 hours

Time to peak: RA: SubQ: 35-103 hours

Dosage SubQ:

Ankylosing spondylitis, psoriatic arthritis, rheumatoid arthritis: Adults: **Note:** Methotrexate, glucocorticoids, salicylates, NSAIDs, or analgesics may be continued during etanercept therapy: 50 mg once weekly **or** 25 mg given twice weekly (off-label dose; Bathon, 2000; Calin, 2004; Davis, 2003; Genovese, 2002; Mease, 2000; Mease, 2002); maximum dose (rheumatoid arthritis): 50 mg weekly

Juvenile idiopathic arthritis: Children ≥2 years: **Note:** Glucocorticoids, NSAIDs, or analgesics may be continued during etanercept therapy: 0.8 mg/kg (maximum: 50 mg/dose) once weekly **or** 0.4 mg/kg (maximum: 25 mg/dose) twice weekly (off-label dose; Lovell, 2000; Lovell, 2006; Lovell, 2008)

Plaque psoriasis: Adults:

Initial: 50 mg twice weekly; maintain initial dose for 3 months (starting doses of 25 or 50 mg once weekly have also been used successfully)

Maintenance dose: 50 mg once weekly

Acute graft-versus-host disease (GVHD), treatment (off-label use): Children ≥1 year, Adolescents, and Adults: 0.4 mg/kg (maximum: 25 mg/dose) twice weekly for 8 weeks (in combination with methylprednisolone) (Levine, 2008)

Elderly: Refer to adult dosing. Although greater sensitivity of some elderly patients cannot be ruled out, no overall differences in safety or effectiveness were observed.

Dosage adjustment in renal impairment: No dosage adjustment provided in manufacturer's labeling (has not been studied).

Dosage adjustment in hepatic impairment: No dosage adjustment provided in manufacturer's labeling (has not been studied).

Administration Administer subcutaneously. Rotate injection sites; may inject into the thigh (preferred), abdomen (avoiding the 2-inch area around the navel), or upper arm. New injections should be given at least one inch from an old site and never into areas where the skin is tender, bruised, red, or hard or into any raised thick, red or scaly skin patches or lesions. For a more comfortable injection, autoinjectors, prefilled syringes, and dose trays may be allowed to reach room temperature by removing from the refrigerator 15-30 minutes prior to injection. **Note:** If the physician determines that it is appropriate, patients may self-inject after proper training in injection technique.

Monitoring Parameters Monitor improvement of symptoms and physical function assessments. Latent TB screening prior to initiating and during therapy; signs/symptoms of infection (prior to, during, and following therapy); CBC with differential; signs/symptoms/worsening of heart failure; HBV screening prior to initiating (all patients), HBV carriers (during and for several months following therapy); signs and symptoms of hypersensitivity reaction; symptoms of lupus-like syndrome; signs/symptoms of malignancy (eg, splenomegaly, hepatomegaly, abdominal pain, persistent fever, night sweats, weight loss).

Dosage Forms

Kit, Subcutaneous [preservative free]:

Enbrel: 25 mg

Solution Auto-injector, Subcutaneous [preservative free]:

Enbrel SureClick: 50 mg/mL (0.98 mL)

Solution Prefilled Syringe, Subcutaneous [preservative free]:

Enbrel: 25 mg/0.5 mL (0.51 mL); 50 mg/mL (0.98 mL)

◆ **Ethacrynate Sodium** *see* Ethacrynic Acid *on page 797*

Ethacrynic Acid (eth a KRIN ik AS id)

Brand Names: U.S. Edecrin; Sodium Edecrin

Brand Names: Canada Edecrin; Sodium Edecrin

Index Terms Ethacrynate Sodium

Pharmacologic Category Diuretic, Loop

Use Management of edema associated with congestive heart failure; hepatic cirrhosis or renal disease; short-term management of ascites due to malignancy, idiopathic edema, and lymphedema

Pregnancy Risk Factor B

Dosage IV formulation should be diluted in D_5W or NS (1 mg/mL) and infused over several minutes.

Children: Oral: 1 mg/kg/dose once daily; increase at intervals of 2-3 days as needed, to a maximum of 3 mg/kg/day.

Adults:

Oral: 50-200 mg/day in 1-2 divided doses; may increase in increments of 25-50 mg at intervals of several days; doses up to 200 mg twice daily may be required with severe, refractory edema.

IV: 0.5-1 mg/kg/dose (maximum: 100 mg/dose); repeat doses not routinely recommended; however, if indicated, repeat doses every 8-12 hours.

Dosage adjustment in renal impairment: CrCl <10 mL/minute: Avoid use.

Dialysis: Not removed by hemo- or peritoneal dialysis; supplemental dose is not necessary.

Dosage adjustment in hepatic impairment: No dosage adjustment provided in manufacturer's labeling, use with caution.

Additional Information Complete prescribing information should be consulted for additional detail.

Dosage Forms

Solution Reconstituted, Intravenous:

Sodium Edecrin: 50 mg (1 ea)

Tablet, Oral:

Edecrin: 25 mg

Ethambutol (e THAM byoo tole)

Brand Names: U.S. Myambutol

Brand Names: Canada Etibi®

Index Terms Ethambutol Hydrochloride

Pharmacologic Category Antitubercular Agent

Use Treatment of pulmonary tuberculosis in conjunction with other antituberculosis agents

Pregnancy Risk Factor C

Pregnancy Considerations Teratogenic effects have been seen in animals. There are no adequate and well-controlled studies in pregnant women; there have been reports of ophthalmic abnormalities in infants born to women receiving ethambutol as a component of antitubercular therapy. Use only during pregnancy if benefits outweigh risks.

Breast-Feeding Considerations The manufacturer suggests use during breast-feeding only if benefits to the mother outweigh the possible risk to the infant. Some references suggest that exposure to the infant is low and does not produce toxicity, and breast-feeding should not be discouraged. Other references recommend if breast-feeding, monitor the infant for rash, malaise, nausea, or vomiting.

Contraindications Hypersensitivity to ethambutol or any component of the formulation; optic neuritis (risk vs benefit decision); use in young children, unconscious patients, or any other patient who may be unable to discern and report visual changes

Warnings/Precautions May cause optic neuritis (unilateral or bilateral), resulting in decreased visual acuity or other vision changes. Discontinue promptly in patients with changes in vision, color blindness, or visual defects (effects normally reversible, but reversal may require up to a year). Irreversible blindness has been reported. Monitor visual acuity prior to and during therapy. Evaluation of visual acuity changes may be more difficult in patients with cataracts, optic neuritis, diabetic retinopathy, and inflammatory conditions of the eye; consideration should be given to whether or not visual changes are related to disease progression or effects of therapy. Use only in children whose visual acuity can accurately be determined and monitored (not recommended for use in children <13 years of age unless the benefit outweighs the risk). Dosage modification is required in patients with renal insufficiency; monitor renal function prior to and during treatment. Hepatic toxicity has been reported, possibly due to concurrent therapy; monitor liver function prior to and during treatment.

Adverse Reactions

Cardiovascular: Myocarditis, pericarditis

Central nervous system: Confusion, disorientation, dizziness, fever, hallucinations, headache, malaise

Dermatologic: Dermatitis, erythema multiforme, exfoliative dermatitis, pruritus, rash

Endocrine & metabolic: Acute gout or hyperuricemia

Gastrointestinal: Abdominal pain, anorexia, GI upset, nausea, vomiting

Hematologic: Eosinophilia, leukopenia, lymphadenopathy, neutropenia, thrombocytopenia

Hepatic: Hepatitis, hepatotoxicity (possibly related to concurrent therapy), LFTs abnormal

Neuromuscular & skeletal: Arthralgia, peripheral neuritis

Ocular: Optic neuritis; symptoms may include decreased acuity, scotoma, color blindness, or visual defects (usually reversible with discontinuation, irreversible blindness has been described)

Renal: Nephritis

Respiratory: Infiltrates (with or without eosinophilia), pneumonitis

Miscellaneous: Anaphylaxis, anaphylactoid reaction; hypersensitivity syndrome (cutaneous reactions, eosinophilia, and organ-specific inflammation)

Drug Interactions

Metabolism/Transport Effects None known.

Avoid Concomitant Use There are no known interactions where it is recommended to avoid concomitant use.

Increased Effect/Toxicity There are no known significant interactions involving an increase in effect.

Decreased Effect

The levels/effects of Ethambutol may be decreased by: Aluminum Hydroxide

Storage/Stability Store at controlled room temperature of 20°C to 25°C (68°F to 77°F).

Mechanism of Action Inhibits arabinosyl transferase resulting in impaired mycobacterial cell wall synthesis

Pharmacodynamics/Kinetics

Absorption: ~80%

Distribution: Widely throughout body; concentrated in kidneys, lungs, saliva, and red blood cells

Relative diffusion from blood into CSF: Adequate with or without inflammation (exceeds usual MICs)

CSF:blood level ratio: Normal meninges: 0%; Inflamed meninges: 25%

Protein binding: 20% to 30%

Metabolism: Hepatic (20%) to inactive metabolite

Half-life elimination: 2.5-3.6 hours; End-stage renal disease: 7-15 hours

Time to peak, serum: 2-4 hours

Excretion: Urine (~50% as unchanged drug, 8% to 15% as metabolites); feces (~20% as unchanged drug)

Dosage

Usual dosage range: Oral:

Children: 15-20 mg/kg/day (maximum: 1 g/day) **or** 50 mg/kg/dose twice weekly (maximum: 2.5 g/dose)

Adults: 15-25 mg/kg daily (maximum dose: 1.5-2.5 g) **or** 25-30 mg/kg/dose 3 times/week (maximum: 2.4 g/dose) **or** 50 mg/kg/dose twice weekly (maximum: 4 g/dose)

Indication-specific dosing: Oral:

Infants and Children:

***Mycobacterium avium* (MAC), secondary prophylaxis or treatment: HIV-exposed/-infected (off-label):** 15-25 mg/kg/day once daily (maximum: 2.5 g/day) with clarithromycin (or azithromycin) with or without rifabutin (CDC, 2009)

Children:

Tuberculosis, active: Note: Used as part of a multidrug regimen; treatment regimens consist of an initial 2-month phase, followed by a continuation phase of 4 or 7 additional months; frequency of dosing may differ depending on phase of therapy.

HIV negative: Daily therapy: 15-20 mg/kg/day (maximum: 1 g/day); Twice weekly directly observed therapy (DOT): 50 mg/kg (maximum: 2.5 g/dose) (*MMWR*, 2003)

HIV-exposed/-infected: Daily therapy: 15-25 mg/kg/day (maximum: 2.5 g/day) (CDC, 2009)

Adolescents ≥13 years:

Tuberculosis, active: Refer to adult dosing.

Adults:

Disseminated *Mycobacterium avium* (MAC) treatment in patients with advanced HIV infection (off-label use; ATS/IDSA guidelines, 2007): 15 mg/kg ethambutol in combination with clarithromycin or azithromycin with/without rifabutin

Nontuberculous mycobacterium *(M. kansasii)* (off-label use; ATS/IDSA guidelines, 2007): 15 mg/kg/day ethambutol for duration to include 12 months of culture-negative sputum; typically used in combination with rifampin and isoniazid; **Note:** Previous recommendations stated to use 25 mg/kg/day for the initial 2 months of therapy; however, IDSA guidelines state this may be unnecessary given the success of rifampin-based regimens with ethambutol 15 mg/kg/day or omitted altogether.

Tuberculosis, active: Note: Used as part of a multidrug regimen; treatment regimens consist of an initial 2-month phase, followed by a continuation phase of 4 or 7 additional months; frequency of dosing may differ depending on phase of therapy.

FDA-approved labeling: Adolescents ≥13 years and Adults: Initial: 15 mg/kg once daily (maximum dose: 1.5 g); Retreatment (previous antituberculosis therapy): 25 mg/kg once daily (maximum dose: 2.5 g) for 60 days or until bacteriologic smears and cultures become negative, followed by 15 mg/kg daily.

Suggested doses by lean body weight (CDC, 2003)

Daily therapy: 15-25 mg/kg (maximum dose: 1.6 g)
- 40-55 kg: 800 mg
- 56-75 kg: 1200 mg
- 76-90 kg: 1600 mg

Twice weekly directly observed therapy (DOT): 50 mg/kg (maximum dose: 4 g)
- 40-55 kg: 2000 mg
- 56-75 kg: 2800 mg
- 76-90 kg: 4000 mg

Three times/week DOT: 25-30 mg/kg (maximum dose: 2.4 g)
- 40-55 kg: 1200 mg
- 56-75 kg: 2000 mg
- 76-90 kg: 2400 mg

Dosage adjustment in renal impairment:

MMWR, 2003: CrCl <30 mL/minute and hemodialysis: 15-25 mg/kg/dose 3 times weekly

Aronoff, 2007

CrCl 10-50 mL/minute: Administer every 24-36 hours

CrCl <10 mL/minute: Administer every 48 hours

Hemodialysis: Slightly dialyzable (5% to 20%); Administer dose postdialysis

Peritoneal dialysis: Dose for CrCl <10 mL/minute: Administer every 48 hours

Continuous arteriovenous or venovenous hemofiltration: Dose for CrCl 10-50 mL/minute: Administer every 24-36 hours

Dosage adjustment in hepatic impairment: No dosage adjustment provided in manufacturer's labeling; use with caution.

Dietary Considerations May be taken with food as absorption is not affected, may cause gastric irritation.

Monitoring Parameters Baseline and periodic (monthly) visual testing (each eye individually, as well as both eyes tested together) in patients receiving >15 mg/kg/day; baseline and periodic renal, hepatic, and hematopoietic tests

Dosage Forms

Tablet, Oral:

Myambutol: 100 mg, 400 mg

Generic: 100 mg, 400 mg

◆ **Ethambutol Hydrochloride** *see* Ethambutol *on page 798*

◆ **Ethamolin** *see* Ethanolamine Oleate *on page 799*

◆ **Ethamsylate** *see* Etamsylate [INT] *on page 795*

◆ **Ethanoic Acid** *see* Acetic Acid *on page 39*

Ethanolamine Oleate (ETH a nol a meen OH lee ate)

Brand Names: U.S. Ethamolin

Index Terms Monoethanolamine

Pharmacologic Category Sclerosing Agent

Use Sclerosing agent used for bleeding esophageal varices

Pregnancy Risk Factor C

Dosage Adults: 1.5-5 mL per varix, up to 20 mL total or 0.4 mL/kg for a 50 kg patient; doses should be decreased in patients with severe hepatic dysfunction and should receive less than recommended maximum dose

Dosage adjustment in renal impairment: No dosage adjustment provided in manufacturer's labeling.

Dosage adjustment in hepatic impairment: No dosage adjustment provided in manufacturer's labeling.

Additional Information Complete prescribing information should be consulted for additional detail.

Dosage Forms

Solution, Intravenous:

Ethamolin: 5% (2 mL)

◆ **Etherified Starch** *see* Tetrastarch *on page 2019*

◆ **Ethinyl Estradiol and Cyproterone Acetate** *see* Cyproterone and Ethinyl Estradiol [CAN/INT] *on page 532*

Ethinyl Estradiol and Desogestrel

(ETH in il es tra DYE ole & des oh JES trel)

Brand Names: U.S. Apri; Azurette; Caziant; Cyclessa; Desogen; Emoquette; Enskyce; Kariva; Mircette; Ortho-Cept; Pimtrea; Reclipsen; Velivet; Viorele

Brand Names: Canada Cyclessa; Linessa; Marvelon; Ortho-Cept

Index Terms Desogestrel and Ethinyl Estradiol; Ortho Cept

Pharmacologic Category Contraceptive; Estrogen and Progestin Combination

Use Contraception: Prevention of pregnancy.

Pregnancy Risk Factor X

Dosage Oral: Adults: Females: Contraception:

Schedule 1 (Sunday starter): Dose begins on first Sunday after onset of menstruation; if the menstrual period starts on Sunday, take first tablet that very same day. **With a Sunday start, an additional method of contraception should be used until after the first 7 days of consecutive administration.**

For 21-tablet package: Dosage is 1 tablet daily for 21 consecutive days, followed by 7 days off of the medication; a new course begins on the 8th day after the last tablet is taken.

For 28-tablet package: Dosage is 1 tablet daily without interruption.

Schedule 2 (Day 1 starter): Dose starts on first day of menstrual cycle taking 1 tablet daily.

For 21-tablet package: Dosage is 1 tablet daily for 21 consecutive days, followed by 7 days off of the medication; a new course begins on the 8th day after the last tablet is taken.

For 28-tablet package: Dosage is 1 tablet daily without interruption.

If all doses have not been taken on schedule and one menstrual period is missed, the possibility of pregnancy should be considered. If two consecutive menstrual periods are missed, pregnancy test is required before new dosing cycle is started.

Missed doses **monophasic formulations** (refer to package insert for complete information):

One dose missed: Take as soon as remembered or take 2 tablets next day

Two consecutive doses missed in the first 2 weeks: Take 2 tablets as soon as remembered or 2 tablets next 2 days. **An additional method of contraception should be used for 7 days after missed dose.**

Two consecutive doses missed in week 3 or three consecutive doses missed at any time:

Schedule 1 (Sunday starter): Continue to take 1 tablet daily until Sunday, then discard the rest of the pack, and a new pack is started that same day. **An additional method of contraception should be used for 7 days after missed dose.**

Schedule 2 (Day 1 starter): Current pack should be discarded, and a new pack started that same day. **An additional method of contraception should be used for 7 days after missed dose.**

Missed doses **biphasic/triphasic formulations** (refer to package insert for complete information):

One dose missed: Take as soon as remembered.

Two consecutive doses missed in week 1 or week 2 of the pack: Take 2 tablets as soon as remembered and 2 tablets the next day. Resume taking 1 tablet daily until the pack is empty. **An additional method of contraception should be used for 7 days after a missed dose.**

Two consecutive doses missed in week 3 of the pack; **an additional method of contraception must be used for 7 days after a missed dose**:

Schedule 1 (Sunday starter): Take 1 tablet every day until Sunday. Discard the remaining pack and start a new pack of pills on the same day.

Schedule 2 (Day 1 starter): Discard the remaining pack and start a new pack the same day.

Three or more consecutive doses missed; **an additional method of contraception must be used for 7 days after a missed dose**:

Schedule 1 (Sunday starter): Take 1 tablet every day until Sunday; on Sunday, discard the pack and start a new pack.

Schedule 2 (Day 1 starter): Discard the remaining pack and begin new pack of tablets starting on the same day.

Dosage adjustment in renal impairment: No dosage adjustment provided in manufacturer's labeling; use with caution and monitor blood pressure closely. Consider other forms of contraception.

Dosage adjustment in hepatic impairment: Contraindicated in patients with hepatic impairment

Additional Information Complete prescribing information should be consulted for additional detail.

Dosage Forms

Tablet, oral [low dose formulation]:

Azurette:

Day 1-21: Ethinyl estradiol 0.02 mg and desogestrel 0.15 mg [21 white tablets]

Day 22-23: 2 inactive green tablets

Day 24-28: Ethinyl estradiol 0.01 mg [5 blue tablets] (28s)

Kariva:

Day 1-21: Ethinyl estradiol 0.02 mg and desogestrel 0.15 mg [21 white tablets]

Day 22-23: 2 inactive light green tablets

Day 24-28: Ethinyl estradiol 0.01 mg [5 light blue tablets] (28s)

Mircette:

Day 1-21: Ethinyl estradiol 0.02 mg and desogestrel 0.15 mg [21 white tablets]

Day 22-23: 2 inactive green tablets

Day 24-28: Ethinyl estradiol 0.01 mg [5 yellow tablets] (28s)

Pimtrea:

Day 1-21: Ethinyl estradiol 0.02 mg and desogestrel 0.15 mg [21 dark blue tablets]

Day 22-23: 2 inactive white tablets

Day 24-28: Ethinyl estradiol 0.01 mg [5 green tablets] (28s)

Viorele:

Day 1-21: Ethinyl estradiol 0.02 mg and desogestrel 0.15 mg [21 white tablets]

Day 22-23: 2 inactive green tablets

Day 24-28: Ethinyl estradiol 0.01 mg [5 yellow tablets] (28s)

Tablet, oral [monophasic formulation]:

Apri 28: Ethinyl estradiol 0.03 mg and desogestrel 0.15 mg [21 rose tablets and 7 white inactive tablets] (28s)

Desogen, Reclipsen: Ethinyl estradiol 0.03 mg and desogestrel 0.15 mg [21 white tablets and 7 green inactive tablets] (28s)

Emoquette: Ethinyl estradiol 0.03 mg and desogestrel 0.15 mg [21 white tablets and 7 light green inactive tablets] (28s)

Enskyce: Ethinyl estradiol 0.03 mg and desogestrel 0.15 mg [21 light orange tablets and 7 green inactive tablets] (28s)

Ortho-Cept 28: Ethinyl estradiol 0.03 mg and desogestrel 0.15 mg [21 light orange tablets and 7 green inactive tablets] (28s)

Tablet, oral [triphasic formulation]:

Caziant:

Day 1-7: Ethinyl estradiol 0.025 mg and desogestrel 0.1 mg [7 white tablets]

Day 8-14: Ethinyl estradiol 0.025 mg and desogestrel 0.125 mg [7 light blue tablets]

Day 15-21: Ethinyl estradiol 0.025 mg and desogestrel 0.15 mg [7 blue tablets]

Day 22-28: 7 green inactive tablets (28s)

Cyclessa:

Day 1-7: Ethinyl estradiol 0.025 mg and desogestrel 0.1 mg [7 light yellow tablets]

Day 8-14: Ethinyl estradiol 0.025 mg and desogestrel 0.125 mg [7 orange tablets]

Day 15-21: Ethinyl estradiol 0.025 mg and desogestrel 0.15 mg [7 red tablets]
Day 22-28: 7 green inactive tablets (28s)
Velivet:
Day 1-7: Ethinyl estradiol 0.025 mg and desogestrel 0.1 mg [7 beige tablets]
Day 8-14: Ethinyl estradiol 0.025 mg and desogestrel 0.125 mg [7 orange tablets]
Day 15-21: Ethinyl estradiol 0.025 mg and desogestrel 0.15 mg [7 pink tablets]
Day 22-28: 7 white inactive tablets (28s)

Ethinyl Estradiol and Drospirenone

(ETH in il es tra DYE ole & droh SPYE re none)

Brand Names: U.S. Gianvi; Loryna; Nikki; Ocella; Syeda; Vestura; Yasmin; Yaz; Zarah

Brand Names: Canada Mya; Yasmin; Yaz; Zamine; Zarah

Index Terms Drospirenone and Ethinyl Estradiol

Pharmacologic Category Contraceptive; Estrogen and Progestin Combination

Use

Acne vulgaris (Gianvi, Loryna, Nikki, Vestura, Yaz): Treatment of moderate acne vulgaris in women 14 years and older only if the patient desires an oral contraceptive for birth control

Contraception: Prevention of pregnancy

Premenstrual dysphoric disorder (Gianvi, Yaz): Treatment of premenstrual dysphoric disorder (PMDD) for women who choose to use an oral contraceptive for contraception

Dosage Oral: **Note:** Not to be used prior to menarche.

Adolescents ≥14 years and Adults: Females: Acne (Gianvi, Loryna, Nikki, Vestura, Yaz): Refer to dosing for contraception

Adults: Females: PMDD (Gianvi, Yaz): Refer to dosing for contraception

Adults: Females: Contraception: Dosage is 1 tablet daily for 28 consecutive days. Dosing may be started on the first day of menstrual period (Day 1 starter) or on the first Sunday after the onset of the menstrual period (Sunday starter). **An additional method of contraception should be used until after the first 7 days of consecutive administration.**

Day 1 starter: Dose starts on first day of menstrual cycle taking 1 tablet daily.

Sunday starter: Dose begins on first Sunday after onset of menstruation; if the menstrual period starts on Sunday, take first tablet that very same day.

Switching from a different contraceptive:

Oral contraceptive: Start on the same day that a new pack of the previous oral contraceptive would have been taken

Transdermal patch, vaginal ring, injection: Start on the day the next dose would have been due

IUD or implant: Start on the day of removal

Use after childbirth (in women who are not breast-feeding) or after second trimester abortion: Therapy may be started ≥4 weeks postpartum. Pregnancy should be ruled out prior to treatment if menstrual periods have not restarted and an additional method of contraception (nonhormonal) should be used until after the first 7 days of consecutive administration.

Missed doses:

If all doses have been taken on schedule and one menstrual period is missed, continue dosing cycle. If two consecutive menstrual periods are missed, pregnancy test is required before new dosing cycle is started.

If doses have been missed during the first 3 weeks and the menstrual period is missed, pregnancy should be ruled out prior to continuing treatment.

Missed doses (monophasic formulations) (refer to package insert for complete information):

One dose missed: Take as soon as remembered or take 2 tablets next day

Two consecutive doses missed in the first 2 weeks: Take 2 tablets as soon as remembered or 2 tablets next 2 days. **An additional method of contraception should be used for 7 days after missed dose.**

Two consecutive doses missed in week 3 or three consecutive doses missed at any time: **An additional method of contraception must be used for 7 days after a missed dose.**

Day 1 starter: Current pack should be discarded, and a new pack should be started that same day.

Sunday starter: Continue dose of 1 tablet daily until Sunday, then discard the rest of the pack, and a new pack should be started that same day.

Any number of doses missed in week 4: Continue taking one pill each day until pack is empty; no back-up method of contraception is needed

Dosage adjustment in renal impairment: Contraindicated in patients with renal dysfunction

Dosage adjustment in hepatic impairment: Contraindicated in patients with hepatic dysfunction

Additional Information Complete prescribing information should be consulted for additional detail.

Dosage Forms

Tablet, oral: Ethinyl estradiol 0.03 mg and drospirenone 3 mg [21 active tablets and 7 inactive tablets] (28s)

Gianvi: Ethinyl estradiol 0.03 mg and drospirenone 3 mg [24 light pink active tablets and 4 white inactive tablets] (28s)

Loryna: Ethinyl estradiol 0.02 mg and drospirenone 3 mg [24 peach active tablets and 4 white inactive tablets] (28s)

Nikki: Ethinyl estradiol 0.02 mg and drospirenone 3 mg [24 pink active tablets and 4 white inactive tablets] (28s)

Ocella, Syeda, Yasmin: Ethinyl estradiol 0.03 mg and drospirenone 3 mg [21 yellow active tablets and 7 white inactive tablets] (28s)

Vestura: Ethinyl estradiol 0.02 mg and drospirenone 3 mg [24 pink active tablets and 4 peach inactive tablets] (28s)

Yaz: Ethinyl estradiol 0.02 mg and drospirenone 3 mg [24 light pink active tablets and 4 white inactive tablets] (28s)

Zarah: Ethinyl estradiol 0.03 mg and drospirenone 3 mg [21 blue active tablets and 7 peach inactive tablets] (28s)

Ethinyl Estradiol and Ethynodiol Diacetate

(ETH in il es tra DYE ole & e thye noe DYE ole dye AS e tate)

Brand Names: U.S. Kelnor™; Zovia®

Brand Names: Canada Demulen® 30

Index Terms Ethynodiol Diacetate and Ethinyl Estradiol

Pharmacologic Category Contraceptive; Estrogen and Progestin Combination

Use Prevention of pregnancy

Pregnancy Risk Factor X

Dosage Oral: Adults: Females: Contraception:

Schedule 1 (Sunday starter): Dose begins on first Sunday after onset of menstruation; if the menstrual period starts on Sunday, take first tablet that very same day. **With a Sunday start, an additional method of contraception should be used until after the first 7 days of consecutive administration.**

For 21-tablet package: 1 tablet/day for 21 consecutive days, followed by 7 days off of the medication; a new course begins on the 8th day after the last tablet is taken.

For 28-tablet package: 1 tablet/day without interruption.

Schedule 2 (Day 1 starter): Dose starts on first day of menstrual cycle taking 1 tablet daily.

For 21-tablet package: 1 tablet/day for 21 consecutive days, followed by 7 days off of the medication; a new course begins on the 8th day after the last tablet is taken.

For 28-tablet package: 1 tablet/day without interruption.

If all doses have been taken on schedule and one menstrual period is missed, continue dosing cycle. If two consecutive menstrual periods are missed, pregnancy test is required before new dosing cycle is started.

Missed doses **monophasic formulations** (refer to package insert for complete information):

One dose missed: Take as soon as remembered or take 2 tablets next day

Two consecutive doses missed in the first 2 weeks: Take 2 tablets as soon as remembered or 2 tablets next 2 days. **An additional method of contraception should be used for 7 days after missed dose.**

Two consecutive doses missed in week 3 or three consecutive doses missed at any time: **An additional method of contraception should be used for 7 days after missed dose:**

Schedule 1 (Sunday starter): Continue dose of 1 tablet daily until Sunday, then discard the rest of the pack, and a new pack should be started that same day.

Schedule 2 (Day 1 starter): Current package should be discarded, and a new pack should be started that same day.

Dosage adjustment in renal impairment: Specific guidelines not available; use with caution and monitor blood pressure closely. Consider other forms of contraception.

Dosage adjustment in hepatic impairment: Contraindicated in patients with hepatic impairment

Additional Information Complete prescribing information should be consulted for additional detail.

Dosage Forms

Tablet, oral [monophasic formulation]:

Kelnor™ 1/35: Ethinyl estradiol 0.035 mg and ethynodiol diacetate 1 mg [21 light yellow tablets and 7 white inactive tablets] (28s)

Zovia® 1/35-28: Ethinyl estradiol 0.035 mg and ethynodiol diacetate 1 mg [21 light pink tablets and 7 white inactive tablets] (28s)

Zovia® 1/50-28: Ethinyl estradiol 0.05 mg and ethynodiol diacetate 1 mg [21 pink tablets and 7 white inactive tablets] (28s)

Ethinyl Estradiol and Etonogestrel

(ETH in il es tra DYE ole & et oh noe JES trel)

Brand Names: U.S. NuvaRing®

Brand Names: Canada NuvaRing®

Index Terms Etonogestrel and Ethinyl Estradiol

Pharmacologic Category Contraceptive; Estrogen and Progestin Combination

Use Contraception: For the prevention of pregnancy

Dosage Vaginal: Adults: Females: Contraception: One ring, inserted vaginally and left in place for 3 consecutive weeks, then removed for 1 week. A new ring is inserted 7 days after the last was removed (even if bleeding is not complete) and should be inserted at approximately the same time of day the ring was removed the previous week.

Initial treatment should begin as follows (pregnancy should always be ruled out first):

No hormonal contraceptive use in the past month: Insert ring on the first day of menstrual cycle ("Day 1"). May also insert on days 2-5 even if bleeding is not complete, however, **a spermicide or barrier method of contraception should be used for the following 7 days.***

Switching from combination oral contraceptive: Ring can be inserted on any day within 7 days after the last **active** tablet in the cycle was taken and no later than the first day a new cycle of tablets would begin. Additional forms of contraception are not needed.

Switching from progestin-only contraceptive: **A spermicide or barrier method of contraception should be used for the following 7 days with any of the following.***

If previously using a progestin-only mini-pill, insert the ring on any day of the month; insert the vaginal ring on the day after the last mini-pill; do not skip days between the last pill and insertion of the ring.

If previously using an implant, insert the ring on the same day of implant removal.

If previously using a progestin-containing IUD, insert the ring on day of IUD removal.

If previously using a progestin injection, insert the ring on the day the next injection would be given.

Following complete 1st trimester abortion or miscarriage: Insert ring within the first 5 days of abortion or miscarriage. If not inserted within 5 days, follow instructions for "No hormonal contraceptive use within the past month" and instruct patient to use a nonhormonal contraceptive in the interim.

Following delivery or 2nd trimester abortion or miscarriage: Insert ring no sooner than 4 weeks postpartum (in women who are not breast-feeding) or following 2nd trimester abortion or miscarriage. **A spermicide or barrier method of contraception should be used for the following 7 days.***

If the ring is accidentally removed from the vagina at any time during the 3-week period of use, it may be rinsed with cool or lukewarm water (not hot) and reinserted as soon as possible. If the ring is not reinserted within 3 hours, contraceptive effectiveness will be decreased. If the ring is accidently removed from the vagina for >3 hours during weeks 1 and 2, the ring should be reinserted as soon as the woman remembers and **a spermicide or barrier method of contraception should be used until the ring has been in place for 7 consecutive days.*** If the ring is accidently removed from the vagina for >3 hours during week 3, the ring should be discarded. A new ring may be inserted immediately, restarting a new 3-week cycle, OR a new ring may be inserted ≤7 days from the time the previous ring was removed or expelled (the second option should only be done if a vaginal ring was in continuous use for ≥7 days prior to the inadvertent expulsion/removal). With either option, a **spermicide or barrier method of contraception should be used until the ring has been in place for 7 consecutive days.*** Additional guidelines are available (CDC, 2013).

If the ring has been removed for longer than 1 week, pregnancy must be ruled out prior to restarting therapy. **A spermicide or barrier method of contraception should be used for the following 7 days.***

If the ring has been left in place for >3 weeks, a new ring should be inserted following a 1-week (ring-free) interval. Protection continues during week 4, however, if the ring is left in place >4 weeks, pregnancy must be ruled out prior to insertion and **a spermicide or barrier method of contraception should be used for the following 7 days.***

Disconnected ring: In the event the ring disconnects at the weld joint, discard and replace with a new ring.

*Note: Diaphragms may interfere with proper ring placement, and therefore, are not recommended for use as an additional form of contraception.

Dosage adjustment in renal impairment: No dosage adjustment provided in manufacturer's labeling (has not been studied).

Dosage adjustment in hepatic impairment: No dosage adjustment provided in manufacturer's labeling (has not been studied). Use is contraindicated in patients with hepatic impairment.

Additional Information Complete prescribing information should be consulted for additional detail.

Dosage Forms

Ring, vaginal:

NuvaRing®: Ethinyl estradiol 0.015 mg/day and etonogestrel 0.12 mg/day (3s) [3-week duration]

Ethinyl Estradiol and Levonorgestrel

(ETH in il es tra DYE ole & LEE voe nor jes trel)

Brand Names: U.S. Altavera; Amethia; Amethia Lo; Amethyst; Aubra; Aviane; camrese; Chateal; Daysee; Delyla; Enpresse; FaLessa Kit; Falmina; Introvale; Jolessa; Kurvelo; Lessina; Levonest; Levora; LoSeasonique; Lutera; Lybrel; Marlissa; Myzilra; Orsythia; Portia; Quartette; Quasense; Seasonique; Sronyx; Trivora

Brand Names: Canada Alesse; Aviane; Min-Ovral; Seasonale; Triphasil; Triquilar

Index Terms Levonorgestrel and Ethinyl Estradiol

Pharmacologic Category Contraceptive; Estrogen and Progestin Combination

Use Prevention of pregnancy; postcoital contraception

Pregnancy Risk Factor X

Pregnancy Considerations Pregnancy should be ruled out prior to treatment and discontinued if pregnancy occurs. In general, the use of combination hormonal contraceptives when inadvertently taken early in pregnancy have not been associated with teratogenic effects. Hormonal contraceptives may be less effective in obese patients. An increase in oral contraceptive failure was noted in women with a BMI >27.3 kg/m^2. Similar findings were noted in patients weighing ≥90 kg (198 lb) using the contraceptive patch.

Due to increased risk of venous thromboembolism (VTE) postpartum, combination hormonal contraceptives should not be started in any woman <21 days following delivery. Women without risk factors for VTE and who are not breast-feeding may start combination hormonal contraceptives during 21-42 days postpartum. After 42 days postpartum, restrictions for use are not related to postpartum status and should be based on other medical conditions (CDC, 2011). Some manufacturers recommend waiting ≥4 weeks postpartum before starting this combination.

Breast-Feeding Considerations Jaundice and breast enlargement in the nursing infant have been reported following the use of combination hormonal contraceptives. May decrease the quality and quantity of breast milk; alternative form of contraception is recommended (per manufacturer). The theoretical concerns about decreased milk production are greatest early in the postpartum period when milk production is being established. Postpartum risk status for VTE should be considered when initiating combination hormonal contraceptives after delivery. Combined hormonal contraceptives should not be started <21 days postpartum due to increased risk of VTE. Risk of VTE is still elevated in breast-feeding women until ~42 days postpartum and is greater in women with additional risk factors. After 42 days postpartum, restrictions for use are not related to postpartum VTE risk and should be based on other medical conditions (CDC, 2011). Some manufacturers recommend waiting ≥4 weeks postpartum before starting this combination.

Contraindications Breast cancer or other estrogen- or progestin-dependent neoplasms (current or a history of), hepatic tumors or disease, pregnancy, undiagnosed abnormal uterine bleeding

Use is also contraindicated in women at high risk of arterial or venous thrombotic diseases including: Cerebrovascular disease, coronary artery disease, diabetes mellitus with vascular disease, DVT or PE (current or history of), hypercoagulopathies (inherited or acquired), headaches with focal neurological symptoms, hypertension (uncontrolled), migraine headaches if >35 years of age, thrombogenic valvular or rhythm diseases of the heart (eg, subacute bacterial endocarditis with valvular disease or atrial fibrillation), women >35 years of age who smoke.

Canadian-labeling: Additional contraindication: Ocular lesions due to ophthalmic vascular disease including partial or complete loss of vision or defect in visual fields; severe dyslipoproteinemia; hereditary or acquired predisposition for venous or arterial thrombosis

Warnings/Precautions Hazardous agent - use appropriate precautions for handling and disposal (NIOSH 2014 [group 2]).

Combination hormonal contraceptives do not protect against HIV infection or other sexually-transmitted diseases. **[U.S. Boxed Warning]: The risk of cardiovascular side effects is increased in women who smoke cigarettes; risk increases with age (especially women >35 years of age) and the number of cigarettes smoked; women who use combination hormonal contraceptives should be strongly advised not to smoke. Use is contraindicated in patients >35 years of age who smoke.** Use with caution in patients with risk factors for coronary artery disease (eg, hypertension, hypercholesterolemia, morbid obesity, diabetes, or women who smoke); may lead to increased risk of myocardial infarction. May have a dose-related risk of vascular disease and hypertension; women with hypertension should be encouraged to use a nonhormonal form of contraception. Use is contraindicated with uncontrolled hypertension. May increase the risk of thromboembolism; discontinue use of combination hormonal contraceptives if an arterial or venous thrombotic event occurs. Women with inherited thrombophilias (eg, protein C or S deficiency) may have increased risk of venous thromboembolism (DeSancho, 2010; van Vlijmen, 2011). Use is contraindicated in women with hypercoagulopathies (inherited or acquired). Whenever possible, combination hormonal contraceptives should be discontinued at least 4 weeks prior to and for 2 weeks following elective surgery associated with an increased risk of thromboembolism or during periods of prolonged immobilization. Combination hormonal contraceptives may have a dose-related risk of gallbladder disease and may worsen existing gallbladder disease. Women with renal disease should be encouraged to use another form of contraception. May have adverse effects on glucose tolerance; use caution in women with diabetes.

Combination hormonal contraceptives may affect serum triglyceride and lipoprotein levels. Triglycerides may also be increased; use with caution in patients with familial defects of lipoprotein metabolism. The use of combination hormonal contraceptives has been associated with a slight increase in frequency of breast cancer; however, studies are not consistent. Use is contraindicated in women with (or history of) breast cancer. Use caution with conditions that may be aggravated by fluid retention, depression, or history of migraine. Evaluate new, recurrent, severe or persistent headaches. Use with migraine headaches with or without aura if >35 years of age is contraindicated. Not for use prior to menarche. Estrogens may cause retinal vascular thrombosis; discontinue if migraine, loss of vision, proptosis, diplopia or other visual disturbances occur; discontinue permanently if papilledema or retinal vascular lesions are observed on examination. Risk of chloasma may be increased with history of chloasma gravidarum. Women with history of chloasma should avoid exposure to sun or ultraviolet radiation during therapy. May induce or exacerbate symptoms of hereditary angioedema.

Presentation of irregular, unresolving vaginal bleeding warrants further evaluation including endometrial sampling, if indicated, to rule out malignancy; evaluate hypothalamic-pituitary-function in women with persistent (≥6 months) amenorrhea (especially associated with breast secretion) following discontinuation of therapy. Discontinue use with the onset of sudden enlargement, pain, or tenderness of fibroids (leiomyomata). Extremely rare adenomas and focal nodular hyperplasia resulting in fatal intra-abdominal hemorrhage have been reported in association with long-term oral contraceptive use. Presentation of an abdominal mass, acute abdominal pain, or intra-abdominal bleeding warrants further evaluation to rule out source. Combination hormonal contraceptives may be poorly metabolized in women with hepatic impairment. Discontinue if jaundice develops during therapy or if liver function becomes abnormal. Use is contraindicated with preexisting hepatic tumors or disease. Risk of cholestasis may be increased with previous cholestatic jaundice of pregnancy or jaundice with prior oral contraceptive use. Estrogens may increase thyroid-binding globulin (TBG) levels leading to increased circulating total thyroid hormone levels. Women on thyroid replacement therapy may require higher doses of thyroid hormone while receiving estrogens. The use of estrogens and/or progestins may change the results of some laboratory tests (eg, coagulation factors, lipids, glucose tolerance, binding proteins). The dose, route, and the specific estrogen/progestin influences these changes. In addition, personal risk factors (eg, cardiovascular disease, smoking, diabetes, age) also contribute to adverse events; use of specific products may be contraindicated in women with certain risk factors. Some products may contain tartrazine, which may cause allergic reactions in certain individuals.

The minimum dosage combination of estrogen/progestin that will effectively treat the individual patient should be used. New patients should be started on products containing ≤0.035 mg of estrogen per tablet. Extended cycle regimen contraceptives provide more hormonal exposure per year than conventional monthly contraceptives.

Adverse Reactions The following reactions have been associated with oral contraceptive use:

Increased risk or evidence of association with use:

Cardiovascular: Arterial thromboembolism, cerebral hemorrhage, cerebral thrombosis, hypertension, mesenteric thrombosis, MI, venous thrombosis (with or without embolism)

Gastrointestinal: Gallbladder disease

Hepatic: Hepatic adenomas, liver tumors (benign)

Local: Thrombophlebitis

Ocular: Retinal thrombosis

Respiratory: Pulmonary embolism

Adverse reactions considered drug related:

Cardiovascular: Edema, varicose vein aggravation

Central nervous system: Depression, migraine, mood changes

Dermatologic: Chloasma, melasma, rash (allergic)

Endocrine & metabolic: Amenorrhea, breakthrough bleeding, breast changes (enlargement, pain, secretion, tenderness), carbohydrate tolerance decreased, fluid retention, infertility (temporary), lactation decreased (with use immediately postpartum), menstrual flow changes, spotting

Gastrointestinal: Abdominal bloating, abdominal cramps, abdominal pain, appetite changes, nausea, weight changes, vomiting

Genitourinary: Cervical ectropion, cervical secretion/erosion, endocervical hyperplasia, fibroid enlargement, vaginal candidiasis, vaginitis

Hematologic: Folate decreased, porphyria exacerbation

Hepatic: Cholestatic jaundice, focal nodular hyperplasia

Neuromuscular & skeletal: Chorea exacerbation

Ocular: Contact lens intolerance, corneal curvature changes (steepening)

Respiratory: Rhinitis

Miscellaneous: Anaphylactic/anaphylactoid reactions (including angioedema, circulatory collapse, respiratory collapse, urticaria), SLE exacerbation

Adverse reactions in which association is not confirmed or denied: Acne, auditory disturbances, Budd-Chiari syndrome, cataracts, cervical smear abnormal, colitis, cystitis-like syndrome, dizziness, dysmenorrhea, erythema multiforme, erythema nodosum, headache, hemolytic uremic syndrome, hemorrhagic eruption, hirsutism, libido changes, nervousness, optic neuritis (with or without partial or complete loss of vision), pancreatitis, premenstrual syndrome, renal function impaired, scalp hair loss

Drug Interactions

Metabolism/Transport Effects Refer to individual components.

Avoid Concomitant Use

Avoid concomitant use of Ethinyl Estradiol and Levonorgestrel with any of the following: Anastrozole; Dasabuvir; Dehydroepiandrosterone; Exemestane; Griseofulvin; Indium 111 Capromab Pendetide; Ombitasvir; Ospemifene; Paritaprevir; Pimozide; Tranexamic Acid; Ulipristal

Increased Effect/Toxicity

Ethinyl Estradiol and Levonorgestrel may increase the levels/effects of: Agomelatine; ARIPiprazole; C1 inhibitors; Corticosteroids (Systemic); CYP1A2 Substrates; Dasabuvir; Dofetilide; Hydrocodone; Immune Globulin; Lenalidomide; Lomitapide; Ombitasvir; Ospemifene; Paritaprevir; Pimozide; Pirfenidone; ROPINIRole; Selegiline; Thalidomide; Theophylline Derivatives; Tipranavir; TiZANidine; Tranexamic Acid; Voriconazole

The levels/effects of Ethinyl Estradiol and Levonorgestrel may be increased by: Ascorbic Acid; Atazanavir; Boceprevir; Cobicistat; Dehydroepiandrosterone; Herbs (Estrogenic Properties); Herbs (Progestogenic Properties); Lopinavir; Metreleptin; Mifepristone; NSAID (COX-2 Inhibitor); Tipranavir; Voriconazole

Decreased Effect

Ethinyl Estradiol and Levonorgestrel may decrease the levels/effects of: Anastrozole; Anticoagulants; Chenodiol; Exemestane; Fosamprenavir; Hyaluronidase; Indium 111 Capromab Pendetide; LamoTRIgine; Ospemifene; Thyroid Products; Ursodiol; Vitamin K Antagonists

The levels/effects of Ethinyl Estradiol and Levonorgestrel may be decreased by: Acitretin; Aminoglutethimide; Aprepitant; Armodafinil; Artemether; Barbiturates; Bexarotene (Systemic); Bile Acid Sequestrants; Boceprevir; Bosentan; CarBAMazepine; CloBAZam; Cobicistat; Colesevelam; CYP3A4 Inducers (Moderate); CYP3A4 Inducers (Strong); Dabrafenib; Darunavir; Deferasirox; Efavirenz; Elvitegravir; Eslicarbazepine; Exenatide; Felbamate; Fosamprenavir; Fosaprepitant; Fosphenytoin; Griseofulvin; LamoTRIgine; Lopinavir; Metreleptin; Mifepristone; Mitotane; Modafinil; Mycophenolate; Nafcillin; Nelfinavir; Nevirapine; OXcarbazepine; Perampanel; Phenytoin; Primidone; Protease Inhibitors; Prucalopride; Retinoic Acid Derivatives; Rifamycin Derivatives; Rufinamide; Saquinavir; Siltuximab; St Johns Wort; Sugammadex; Telaprevir; Tipranavir; Tocilizumab; Topiramate; Ulipristal

Storage/Stability Store at controlled room temperature of 20°C to 25°C (68°F to 77°F).

Mechanism of Action Combination hormonal contraceptives inhibit ovulation via a negative feedback mechanism on the hypothalamus, which alters the normal pattern of gonadotropin secretion of a follicle-stimulating hormone (FSH) and luteinizing hormone by the anterior pituitary. The follicular phase FSH and midcycle surge of gonadotropins are inhibited. In addition, combination hormonal contraceptives produce alterations in the genital tract, including changes in the cervical mucus, rendering it unfavorable for sperm penetration even if ovulation occurs. Changes in the endometrium may also occur, producing an unfavorable environment for nidation. Combination hormonal contraceptive drugs may alter the tubal transport of the ova through the fallopian tubes. Progestational agents may also alter sperm fertility.

Pharmacodynamics/Kinetics

Absorption: Rapid

Distribution: Ethinyl estradiol: 4.3 L/kg; Levonorgestrel: 1.8 L/kg

Protein binding:

Ethinyl estradiol: 95% to 97% to albumin

Levonorgestrel: 97% to 99% primarily to sex hormone binding globulin (SHBG), lesser amounts to albumin

Metabolism:

Ethinyl estradiol: Hepatic via CYP3A4; undergoes first-pass metabolism; forms metabolites

Levonorgestrel: Forms conjugated in unconjugated metabolites

Bioavailability: Ethinyl estradiol: 38% to 48%; Levonorgestrel: 100%

Half-life elimination: Ethinyl estradiol: 12-23 hours; Levonorgestrel: 22-49 hours

Excretion:

Ethinyl estradiol: Urine and feces

Levonorgestrel: Urine (40% to 68%, parent drug and metabolites); feces (16% to 48% as metabolites)

Dosage Oral: Adults: Females:

Contraception, 28-day cycle:

Schedule 1 (Sunday starter): Dose begins on first Sunday after onset of menstruation; if the menstrual period starts on Sunday, take first tablet that very same day. With a Sunday start, an additional method of contraception should be used until after the first 7 days of consecutive administration:

For 21-tablet package: 1 tablet/day for 21 consecutive days, followed by 7 days off of the medication; a new course begins on the 8th day after the last tablet is taken

For 28-tablet package: 1 tablet/day without interruption

Schedule 2 (Day 1 starter): Dose starts on first day of menstrual cycle taking 1 tablet/day:

For 21-tablet package: 1 tablet/day for 21 consecutive days, followed by 7 days off of the medication; a new course begins on the 8th day after the last tablet is taken

For 28-tablet package: 1 tablet/day without interruption

If all doses have been taken on schedule and one menstrual period is missed, continue dosing cycle. If two consecutive menstrual periods are missed, pregnancy test is required before new dosing cycle is started.

Missed doses **monophasic formulations** (refer to package insert for complete information):

One dose missed: Take as soon as remembered or take 2 tablets next day

Two consecutive doses missed in the first 2 weeks: Take 2 tablets as soon as remembered or 2 tablets next 2 days. An additional method of contraception should be used for 7 days after missed dose.

Two consecutive doses missed in week 3 or three consecutive doses missed at any time: An additional method of contraception must be used for 7 days after a missed dose:

Schedule 1 (Sunday starter): Continue dose of 1 tablet daily until Sunday, then discard the rest of the pack, and a new pack should be started that same day.

Schedule 2 (Day 1 starter): Current pack should be discarded, and a new pack should be started that same day.

Missed doses **biphasic/triphasic formulations** (refer to package insert for complete information):

One dose missed: Take as soon as remembered or take 2 tablets next day.

Two consecutive doses missed in week 1 or week 2 of the pack: Take 2 tablets as soon as remembered and 2 tablets the next day. Resume taking 1 tablet daily until the pack is empty. An additional method of contraception should be used for 7 days after a missed dose.

Two consecutive doses missed in week 3 of the pack: An additional method of contraception must be used for 7 days after a missed dose.

Schedule 1 (Sunday starter): Take 1 tablet every day until Sunday. Discard the remaining pack and start a new pack of pills on the same day.

Schedule 2 (Day 1 starter): Discard the remaining pack and start a new pack the same day.

Three or more consecutive doses missed: An additional method of contraception must be used for 7 days after a missed dose.

Schedule 1 (Sunday starter): Take 1 tablet every day until Sunday; on Sunday, discard the pack and start a new pack.

Schedule 2 (Day 1 starter): Discard the remaining pack and begin new pack of tablets starting on the same day.

Contraception, 91-day cycle (extended cycle regimen): Dose begins on first Sunday after onset of menstruation; if the menstrual period starts on Sunday, take first tablet that very same day. An additional method of contraception should be used until after the first 7 days of consecutive administration:

Introvale, Jolessa, Quasense, Seasonale [Canadian product]: One active tablet/day for 84 consecutive days, followed by 1 inactive tablet/day for 7 days; if all doses have been taken on schedule and one menstrual period is missed, pregnancy should be ruled out prior to continuing therapy.

Seasonique, LoSeasonique, Quartette: One active tablet/day for 84 consecutive days, followed by 1 low dose estrogen tablet/day for 7 days; if all doses have been taken on schedule and one menstrual period is missed, pregnancy should be ruled out prior to continuing therapy.

Missed doses:

One dose missed: Take as soon as remembered or take 2 tablets the next day

Two consecutive doses missed: Take 2 tablets as soon as remembered or 2 tablets the next 2 days. An additional nonhormonal method of contraception should be used for 7 consecutive days after the missed dose.

Three or more consecutive doses missed: Do not take the missed doses; continue taking 1 tablet/day until pack is complete. Bleeding may occur during the following week. An additional nonhormonal method of contraception should be used for 7 consecutive days after the missed dose.

Any number of pills during week 13: Throw away the missed pills and keep taking scheduled pills until the pack is finished. A back-up method of contraception is not needed

Contraception, continuous use (extended cycle regimen):

Lybrel: Take one tablet daily, at the same time each day, without a tablet-free interval. Therapy should be initiated as follows:

No previous contraception: Begin on the first day of menstrual cycle. Back-up contraception is not needed.

Previously taking a 21-day or 28-day combination hormonal contraceptive: Begin on day 1 of the withdrawal bleed (at the latest, 7 days after the last active tablet). Back-up contraception is not needed.

Previously using a progestin-only pill: Begin the day after taking a progestin only pill. Back-up contraception is needed for the first 7 days of therapy.

Previously using contraceptive implant: Begin the day of implant removal. Back-up contraception is needed for the first 7 days of therapy.

Previously using contraceptive injection: Begin when the next injection is due. Back-up contraception is needed for the first 7 days of therapy.

Missed doses:

One dose missed: Take as soon as remembered then take the next tablet at the regular time (2 tablets in 1 day). An additional nonhormonal method of contraception should also be used for 7 consecutive days.

Two consecutive doses missed: If remembered the day of the second missed tablet, take 2 tablets as soon as remembered, then 1 tablet the next day. If remembered the day after the second tablet is missed, take 2 tablets the day remembered, then 2 tablets the next day. An additional nonhormonal method of contraception should also be used for 7 consecutive days.

Three or more consecutive doses missed: Take 1 tablet daily and contact healthcare provider; do not take the missed pills. An additional nonhormonal method of contraception should also be used for 7 consecutive days.

Dosage adjustment in renal impairment: Specific guidelines not available; use with caution and monitor blood pressure closely. Consider other forms of contraception.

Dosage adjustment in hepatic impairment: Contraindicated in patients with hepatic impairment

Dietary Considerations Should be taken at the same time each day.

Administration Administer at the same time each day.

Quartette: If severe diarrhea or vomiting occur within 3-4 hours after taking a light pink, pink, or purple tablet, it should be considered a missed dose; additional contraceptive measures are recommended.

Hazardous agent; use appropriate precautions for handling and disposal (NIOSH 2014 [group 2]).

Monitoring Parameters Before starting therapy, a physical exam with reference to the breasts and pelvis are recommended, including a Papanicolaou smear. Exam may be deferred if appropriate; pregnancy should be ruled out prior to use. Monitor patient closely for loss of vision, sudden onset of proptosis, diplopia, migraine; blood pressure; signs and symptoms of thromboembolic disorders; signs or symptoms of depression; glycemic control in patients with diabetes; lipid profiles in patients being treated for hyperlipidemias. Adequate diagnostic measures, including endometrial sampling, if indicated, should be performed to rule out malignancy in all cases of undiagnosed abnormal vaginal bleeding.

Dosage Forms

Tablet, oral [low-dose formulation]: Ethinyl estradiol 0.02 mg and levonorgestrel 0.1 mg [21 tablets and 7 inactive tablets] (28s)

Aubra: Ethinyl estradiol 0.02 mg and levonorgestrel 0.1 mg [21 light yellow tablets and 7 brown inactive tablets] (28s)

Aviane: Ethinyl estradiol 0.02 mg and levonorgestrel 0.1 mg [21 orange tablets and 7 light green inactive tablets] (28s)

Delyla: Ethinyl estradiol 0.02 mg and levonorgestrel 0.1 mg [21 white tablets and 7 yellow inactive tablets] (28s)

FaLessa Kit: Ethinyl estradiol 0.02 mg and levonorgestrel 0.1 mg [21 orange tablets and 7 white inactive tablets] (28s) [packaged with Quatrefolic folate tablets]

Falmina: Ethinyl estradiol 0.02 mg and levonorgestrel 0.1 mg [21 orange tablets and 7 white inactive tablets] (28s)

Lessina: Ethinyl estradiol 0.02 mg and levonorgestrel 0.1 mg [21 pink tablets and 7 white inactive tablets] (28s)

Lutera, Sronyx: Ethinyl estradiol 0.02 mg and levonorgestrel 0.1 mg [21 white tablets and 7 peach inactive tablets] (28s)

Orsythia: Ethinyl estradiol 0.02 mg and levonorgestrel 0.1 mg [21 pink tablets and 7 light green inactive tablets] (28s)

Tablet, oral [monophasic formulation]: Ethinyl estradiol 0.03 mg and levonorgestrel 0.15 mg [21 tablets and 7 inactive tablets] (28s)

Altavera: Ethinyl estradiol 0.03 mg and levonorgestrel 0.15 mg [21 peach tablets and 7 white inactive tablets] (28s)

Chateal: Ethinyl estradiol 0.03 mg and levonorgestrel 0.15 mg [21 white tablets and 7 green inactive tablets] (28s)

Kurvelo: Ethinyl estradiol 0.03 mg and levonorgestrel 0.15 mg [21 light orange tablets and 7 pink inactive tablets] (28s)

Levora: Ethinyl estradiol 0.03 mg and levonorgestrel 0.15 mg [21 white tablets and 7 peach inactive tablets] (28s)

Marlissa: Ethinyl estradiol 0.03 mg and levonorgestrel 0.15 mg [21 light orange tablets and 7 pink inactive tablets] (28s)

Portia 28: Ethinyl estradiol 0.03 mg and levonorgestrel 0.15 mg [21 pink tablets and 7 white inactive tablets] (28s)

Tablet, oral [extended cycle regimen]: Ethinyl estradiol 0.02 mg and levonorgestrel 0.1 mg [84 tablets] and ethinyl estradiol 0.01 mg [7 tablets] (91s); Ethinyl estradiol 0.03 mg and levonorgestrel 0.15 mg [84 tablets and 7 inactive tablets] (91s)

Amethia: Ethinyl estradiol 0.03 mg and levonorgestrel 0.15 mg [84 white tablets] and ethinyl estradiol 0.01 mg [7 light blue tablets] (91s)

Amethia Lo: Ethinyl estradiol 0.02 mg and levonorgestrel 0.1 mg [84 white tablets] and ethinyl estradiol 0.01 mg [7 blue tablets] (91s)

camrese: Ethinyl estradiol 0.03 mg and levonorgestrel 0.15 mg [84 light blue-green tablets] and ethinyl estradiol 0.01 mg [7 yellow tablets] (91s)

Daysee: Ethinyl estradiol 0.03 mg and levonorgestrel 0.15 mg [84 light blue tablets] and ethinyl estradiol 0.01 mg [7 mustard tablets] (91s)

Introvale: Ethinyl estradiol 0.03 mg and levonorgestrel 0.15 mg [84 peach tablets and 7 white inactive tablets] (91s)

Jolessa: Ethinyl estradiol 0.03 mg and levonorgestrel 0.15 mg [84 pink tablets and 7 white inactive tablets] (91s)

LoSeasonique: Ethinyl estradiol 0.02 mg and levonorgestrel 0.1 mg [84 orange tablets] and ethinyl estradiol 0.01 mg [7 yellow tablets] (91s)

Quartette:
Day 1-42: Ethinyl estradiol 0.02 mg and levonorgestrel 0.15 mg [42 light pink tablets]
Day 43-63: Ethinyl estradiol 0.025 mg and levonorgestrel 0.15 mg [21 pink tablets]
Day 64-84: Ethinyl estradiol 0.03 mg and levonorgestrel 0.15 mg [21 purple tablets]
Day 85-91: Ethinyl estradiol 0.01 mg [7 yellow tablets] (91s)
Quasense: Ethinyl estradiol 0.03 mg and levonorgestrel 0.15 mg] [84 white tablets and 7 peach inactive tablets] (91s)
Seasonique: Ethinyl estradiol 0.03 mg and levonorgestrel 0.15 mg [84 light blue-green tablets] and ethinyl estradiol 0.01 mg [7 yellow tablets] (91s)

Tablet, oral [noncyclic regimen]:
Amethyst: Ethinyl estradiol 0.02 mg and levonorgestrel 0.09 mg [28 white tablets] (28s)
Lybrel: Ethinyl estradiol 0.02 mg and levonorgestrel 0.09 mg [28 yellow tablets] (28s)

Tablet, oral [triphasic formulation]:
Enpresse:
Day 1-6: Ethinyl estradiol 0.03 mg and levonorgestrel 0.05 mg [6 pink tablets]
Day 7-11: Ethinyl estradiol 0.04 mg and levonorgestrel 0.075 mg [5 white tablets]
Day 12-21: Ethinyl estradiol 0.03 mg and levonorgestrel 0.125 mg [10 orange tablets]
Day 22-28: 7 light green inactive tablets (28s)
Levonest:
Day 1-6: Ethinyl estradiol 0.03 mg and levonorgestrel 0.05 mg [6 yellow tablets]
Day 7-11: Ethinyl estradiol 0.04 mg and levonorgestrel 0.075 mg [5 green tablets]
Day 12-21: Ethinyl estradiol 0.03 mg and levonorgestrel 0.125 mg [10 light brown tablets]
Day 22-28: 7 white inactive tablets (28s)
Myzilra:
Day 1-6: Ethinyl estradiol 0.03 mg and levonorgestrel 0.05 mg [6 beige tablets]
Day 7-11: Ethinyl estradiol 0.04 mg and levonorgestrel 0.075 mg [5 white tablets]
Day 12-21: Ethinyl estradiol 0.03 mg and levonorgestrel 0.125 mg [10 light yellow tablets]
Day 22-28: 7 light green inactive tablets (28s)
Trivora:
Day 1-6: Ethinyl estradiol 0.03 mg and levonorgestrel 0.05 mg [6 blue tablets]
Day 7-11: Ethinyl estradiol 0.04 mg and levonorgestrel 0.075 mg [5 white tablets]
Day 12-21: Ethinyl estradiol 0.03 mg and levonorgestrel 0.125 mg [10 pink tablets]
Day 22-28: 7 peach inactive tablets (28s)

◆ **Ethinyl Estradiol and NGM** *see* Ethinyl Estradiol and Norgestimate *on page 810*

Ethinyl Estradiol and Norelgestromin

(ETH in il es tra DYE ole & nor el JES troe min)

Brand Names: U.S. Ortho Evra®; Xulane
Brand Names: Canada Evra®
Index Terms Norelgestromin and Ethinyl Estradiol; Ortho-Evra
Pharmacologic Category Contraceptive; Estrogen and Progestin Combination
Use Prevention of pregnancy
Pregnancy Risk Factor X
Dosage Topical: Adults: Females:
Contraception: Apply one patch each week for 3 weeks (21 total days); followed by one week that is patch-free. Each patch should be applied on the same day each week ("patch change day") and only one patch should be worn at a time. No more than 7 days should pass during the patch-free interval.
Schedule 1 (Sunday starter): Dose begins on first Sunday after onset of menstruation; if the menstrual period starts on Sunday, apply one patch that very same day. **With a Sunday start, an additional method of contraception (nonhormonal) must be used until after the first 7 days of consecutive administration.** Each patch change will then occur on Sunday.
Schedule 2 (Day 1 starter): Dose starts on first day of menstrual cycle, applying one patch during the first 24 hours of menstrual cycle. No back-up method of contraception is needed as long as the patch is applied on the first day of cycle. Each patch change will then occur on that same day of the week.

Additional dosing considerations:
No bleeding during patch-free week/missed menstrual period: If patch has been applied as directed, continue treatment on usual "patch change day". If used correctly, no bleeding during patch-free week does not necessarily indicate pregnancy. However, if no withdrawal bleeding occurs for 2 consecutive cycles, pregnancy should be ruled out. If patch has not been applied as directed, and one menstrual period is missed, pregnancy should be ruled out prior to continuing treatment.
If a patch becomes partially or completely detached for <24 hours: Try to reapply to same place, or replace with a new patch immediately. Do not reapply if patch is no longer sticky, if it is sticking to itself or another surface, or if it has material sticking to it.
If a patch becomes partially or completely detached for >24 hours (or time period is unknown): Apply a new patch and use this day of the week as the new "patch change day" from this point on. **An additional method of contraception (nonhormonal) must be used until after the first 7 days of consecutive administration.**
Switching from oral contraceptives or vaginal ring: Complete current cycle and apply the first patch on the day the next pill cycle would be started or ring would be inserted. If there is no menstrual bleeding within 7 days of taking the last active tablet, the patient can initiate the first patch application; however, pregnancy must be ruled out. If patch is applied later than 7 days after the last active pill or removal of the vaginal ring, **an additional method of contraception (nonhormonal) should be used until after the first 7 days of consecutive administration**
Use after childbirth: Therapy should not be started <4 weeks after childbirth. Pregnancy should be ruled out prior to treatment if menstrual periods have not restarted. **An additional method of contraception (nonhormonal) should be used until after the first 7 days of consecutive administration.**
Use after abortion or miscarriage: Therapy may be started immediately if abortion/miscarriage occurs within the first trimester. If therapy is not started within 5 days, follow instructions for first time use. An additional method of contraception (nonhormonal) should be used until after the first 7 days of consecutive administration. If abortion/miscarriage occurs during the second trimester, therapy should not be started for at least 4 weeks. Follow directions for use after childbirth.

Dosage adjustment in renal impairment: Specific guidelines not available; use with caution and monitor blood pressure closely. Consider other forms of contraception.
Dosage adjustment in hepatic impairment: Contraindicated in patients with hepatic impairment
Additional Information Complete prescribing information should be consulted for additional detail.

Dosage Forms

Patch, transdermal:

Ortho Evra®: Ethinyl estradiol 0.75 mg and norelgestromin 6 mg [releases ethinyl estradiol 35 mcg and norelgestromin 150 mcg per day] (1s, 3s)

Xulane: Ethinyl estradiol 0.53 mg and norelgestromin 4.86 mg [releases ethinyl estradiol 35 mcg and norelgestromin 150 mcg per day] (3s)

Dosage Forms: Canada

Patch, transdermal:

Evra®: Ethinyl estradiol 0.6 mg and norelgestromin 6 mg (1s, 3s)

Ethinyl Estradiol and Norethindrone

(ETH in il es tra DYE ole & nor eth IN drone)

Brand Names: U.S. Alyacen 1/35; Alyacen 7/7/7; Aranelle; Balziva; Brevicon; Briellyn; Cyclafem 1/35; Cyclafem 7/7/7; Dasetta 1/35; Dasetta 7/7/7; Estrostep Fe; Femcon Fe; femhrt; Generess Fe; Gildagia; Gildess 24 Fe; Gildess FE 1.5/30; Gildess FE 1/20; Jinteli; Junel 1.5/30; Junel 1/20; Junel Fe 1.5/30; Junel Fe 1/20; Larin 1.5/30; Larin 1/20; Larin Fe 1.5/30; Larin Fe 1/20; Leena; Lo Loestrin Fe; Lo Minastrin Fe [DSC]; Loestrin 21 1.5/30; Loestrin 21 1/20; Loestrin 24 Fe; Loestrin Fe 1.5/30; Loestrin Fe 1/20; Lomedia 24 Fe; Microgestin 1.5/30; Microgestin 1/20; Microgestin Fe 1.5/30; Microgestin Fe 1/20; Minastrin 24 Fe; Modicon; Necon 0.5/35; Necon 1/35; Necon 10/11; Necon 7/7/7; Norinyl 1+35; Nortrel 0.5/35; Nortrel 1/35; Nortrel 7/7/7; Ortho-Novum 1/35; Ortho-Novum 7/7/7; Ovcon 35; Philith; Pirmella 1/35; Pirmella 7/7/7; Tarina FE 1/20; Tilia Fe; Tri-Legest Fe; Tri-Norinyl; Vyfemla; Wera; Wymzya Fe; Zenchent; Zenchent Fe

Brand Names: Canada Brevicon 0.5/35; Brevicon 1/35; FemHRT; Loestrin 1.5/30; Minestrin 1/20; Ortho 0.5/35; Ortho 1/35; Ortho 7/7/7; Select 1/35; Synphasic

Index Terms Norethindrone Acetate and Ethinyl Estradiol; Ortho Novum

Pharmacologic Category Contraceptive; Estrogen and Progestin Combination

Use

Acne vulgaris: For the treatment of moderate acne vulgaris in females at least 15 years of age.

Limitations of Use: When used for acne, use only in females ≥15 years of age who have achieved menarche, who also desire combination hormonal contraceptive therapy, are unresponsive to topical treatments, have no contraindications to combination hormonal contraceptive use, and plan to stay on therapy for ≥6 months.

Contraception: For the prevention of pregnancy.

Moderate to severe vasomotor symptoms: Treatment of moderate to severe vasomotor symptoms associated with menopause.

Osteoporosis prevention: For prevention of postmenopausal osteoporosis.

Limitations of use: For use only in women at significant risk of osteoporosis and for whom other nonestrogen medications are not considered appropriate.

Pregnancy Risk Factor X

Dosage Oral:

Adolescents ≥15 years and Adults: Females: Acne: Estrostep Fe: Refer to dosing for contraception

Adults: Females:

Moderate-to-severe vasomotor symptoms associated with menopause: Initial: femhrt 0.5/2.5: 1 tablet daily; patient should be re-evaluated at 3- to 6-month intervals to determine if treatment is still necessary; patient should be maintained at the lowest effective dose

Prevention of osteoporosis: Initial: femhrt 0.5/2.5: 1 tablet daily; patient should be maintained on the lowest effective dose

Contraception:

Schedule 1 (Sunday starter): Dose begins on first Sunday after onset of menstruation; if the menstrual period starts on Sunday, take first tablet that very same day. (This schedule is not preferred for all products [eg, Generess Fe, Lo Loestrin Fe, Lo Minastrin Fe]). With a Sunday start, an additional method of contraception should be used until after the first 7 days of consecutive administration (all products).

For 21-tablet package: Dosage is 1 tablet daily for 21 consecutive days, followed by 7 days off of the medication; a new course begins on the 8th day after the last tablet is taken.

For 28-tablet package: Dosage is 1 tablet daily without interruption.

Schedule 2 (Day 1 starter): Dose starts on first day of menstrual cycle taking 1 tablet daily.

For 21-tablet package: Dosage is 1 tablet daily for 21 consecutive days, followed by 7 days off of the medication; a new course begins on the 8th day after the last tablet is taken.

For 28-tablet package: Dosage is 1 tablet daily without interruption.

If all doses have not been taken on schedule and one menstrual period is missed, the possibility of pregnancy should be considered. If two consecutive menstrual periods are missed, pregnancy test is required before new dosing cycle is started.

Missed doses **monophasic formulations** (refer to package insert for complete information):

One dose missed: Take as soon as remembered. Take the next tablet at your regular time. You may take 2 tablets in 1 day.

Two consecutive doses missed in the first 2 weeks: Take 2 tablets as soon as remembered and 2 tablets the next day. An additional method of contraception should be used for 7 days after missed dose.

Two consecutive doses missed in week 3 (all products) or in week 4 (some products), or three consecutive doses missed at any time (all products): An additional method of contraception must be used for 7 days after a missed dose.

Schedule 1 (Sunday starter): Continue dose of 1 tablet daily until Sunday, then discard the rest of the pack, and a new pack should be started that same day.

Schedule 2 (Day 1 starter): Current pack should be discarded, and a new pack should be started that same day.

Missed doses **biphasic/triphasic formulations** (refer to package insert for complete information):

One dose missed: Take the next tablet at your regular time. You may take 2 tablets in 1 day.

Two consecutive doses missed in week 1 or week 2 of the pack: Take 2 tablets as soon as remembered and 2 tablets the next day. Resume taking 1 tablet daily until the pack is empty. An additional method of contraception should be used for 7 days after a missed dose.

Two consecutive doses missed in week 3 of the pack: An additional method of contraception must be used for 7 days after a missed dose.

Schedule 1 (Sunday Starter): Take 1 tablet every day until Sunday. Discard the remaining pack and start a new pack of pills on the same day.

Schedule 2 (Day 1 starter): Discard the remaining pack and start a new pack the same day.

Three or more consecutive doses missed: An additional method of contraception must be used for 7 days after a missed dose.

Schedule 1 (Sunday Starter): Take 1 tablet every day until Sunday; on Sunday, discard the pack and start a new pack.

Schedule 2 (Day 1 Starter): Discard the remaining pack and begin new pack of tablets starting on the same day.

Switching from a different contraceptive:

Oral contraceptive: Start on the same day that a new pack of the previous oral contraceptive would have been taken.

Transdermal patch, vaginal ring, injection: Start on the day the next dose would have been due.

IUD or implant: Start on the day of removal. A backup method of contraception may be required following IUD removal.

Use after childbirth (in women who are not breastfeeding) or after second trimester abortion: Therapy may be started ≥4 weeks postpartum. Pregnancy should be ruled out prior to treatment if menstrual periods have not restarted and an additional method of contraception (nonhormonal) should be used until after the first 7 days of consecutive administration.

Dosage adjustment in renal impairment: No dosage adjustment provided in manufacturer's labeling; use with caution and monitor blood pressure closely. Consider other forms of contraception.

Dosage adjustment in hepatic impairment: Contraindicated in patients with hepatic impairment.

Additional Information Complete prescribing information should be consulted for additional detail.

Dosage Forms

Tablet, oral:

femhrt 0.5/2.5: Ethinyl estradiol 0.0025 mg and norethindrone acetate 0.5 mg [white tablets] (28s)

Jinteli: Ethinyl estradiol 0.005 mg and norethindrone acetate 1 mg [white tablets] (28s, 90s)

Tablet, oral [monophasic formulation]:

Alyacen 1/35: Ethinyl estradiol 0.035 mg and norethindrone 1 mg [21 peach tablets and 7 light green inactive tablets] (28s)

Balziva: Ethinyl estradiol 0.035 mg and norethindrone 0.4 mg [21 light peach tablets and 7 white inactive tablets] (28s)

Brevicon: Ethinyl estradiol 0.035 mg and norethindrone 0.5 mg [21 blue tablets and 7 orange inactive tablets] (28s)

Briellyn: Ethinyl estradiol 0.035 mg and norethindrone 0.4 mg [21 light peach tablets and 7 white-off-white inactive tablets] (28s)

Cyclafem 1/35: Ethinyl estradiol 0.035 mg and norethindrone 1 mg [21 pink tablets and 7 light green inactive tablets] (28s)

Dasetta 1/35: Ethinyl estradiol 0.035 mg and norethindrone 1 mg [21 orange tablets and 7 white inactive tablets] (28s)

Gildagia: Ethinyl estradiol 0.035 mg and norethindrone 0.4 mg [21 peach tablets and 7 light green inactive tablets] (28s)

Gildess FE 1/20: Ethinyl estradiol 0.02 mg and norethindrone acetate 1 mg [21 white tablets] and ferrous fumarate 75 mg [7 white-speckled brown tablets] (28s)

Gildess FE 1.5/30: Ethinyl estradiol 0.03 mg and norethindrone acetate 1.5 mg [21 light green tablets] and ferrous fumarate 75 mg [7 white-speckled brown tablets] (28s)

Gildess 24 Fe: Ethinyl estradiol 0.02 mg and norethindrone acetate 1 mg [21 white tablets] and ferrous fumarate 75 mg [7 white-speckled brown tablets] (28s)

Junel 1/20: Ethinyl estradiol 0.02 mg and norethindrone acetate 1 mg [yellow tablets] (21s)

Junel 1.5/30, Loestrin 21 1.5/30: Ethinyl estradiol 0.03 mg and norethindrone acetate 1.5 mg [pink tablets] (21s)

Junel Fe 1/20: Ethinyl estradiol 0.02 mg and norethindrone acetate 1 mg [21 yellow tablets] and ferrous fumarate 75 mg [7 brown tablets] (28s)

Junel Fe 1.5/30, Loestrin Fe 21 1.5/30: Ethinyl estradiol 0.03 mg and norethindrone acetate 1.5 mg [21 pink tablets] and ferrous fumarate 75 mg [7 brown tablets] (28s)

Larin 1/20: Ethinyl estradiol 0.02 mg and norethindrone acetate 1 mg [21 pale yellow tablets] (21s)

Larin 1.5/30: Ethinyl estradiol 0.03 mg and norethindrone acetate 1.5 mg [21 green tablets] (21s)

Larin Fe 1/20: Ethinyl estradiol 0.02 mg and norethindrone acetate 1 mg [21 pale yellow tablets] and ferrous fumarate 75 mg [7 brown tablets] (28s)

Larin Fe 1.5/30: Ethinyl estradiol 0.03 mg and norethindrone acetate 1.5 mg [21 green tablets] and ferrous fumarate 75 mg [7 brown tablets] (28s) [contains soya lecithin]

Loestrin 21 1/20: Ethinyl estradiol 0.02 mg and norethindrone acetate 1 mg [light yellow tablets] (21s)

Loestrin 24 Fe: Ethinyl estradiol 0.02 mg and norethindrone acetate 1 mg [24 white tablets] and ferrous fumarate 75 mg [4 brown tablets] (28s)

Loestrin Fe 1/20: Ethinyl estradiol 0.02 mg and norethindrone acetate 1 mg [21 light yellow tablets] and ferrous fumarate 75 mg [7 brown tablets] (28s)

Loestrin Fe 1.5/30: Ethinyl estradiol 0.03 mg and norethindrone acetate 1.5 mg [21 pink tablets] and ferrous fumarate 75 mg [7 brown tablets] (28s)

Lomedia 24 Fe: Ethinyl estradiol 0.02 mg and norethindrone acetate 1 mg [24 white tablets] and ferrous fumarate 75 mg [4 brown tablets] (28s)

Microgestin 1/20: Ethinyl estradiol 0.02 mg and norethindrone acetate 1 mg [white tablets] (21s)

Microgestin 1.5/30: Ethinyl estradiol 0.03 mg and norethindrone acetate 1.5 mg [green tablets] (21s)

Microgestin Fe 1/20: Ethinyl estradiol 0.02 mg and norethindrone acetate 1 mg [21 white tablets] and ferrous fumarate 75 mg [7 brown tablets] (28s)

Microgestin Fe 1.5/30: Ethinyl estradiol 0.03 mg and norethindrone acetate 1.5 mg [21 green tablets] and ferrous fumarate 75 mg [7 brown tablets] (28s)

Modicon: Ethinyl estradiol 0.035 mg and norethindrone 0.5 mg [21 white tablets and 7 green inactive tablets] (28s)

Necon 0.5/35, Nortrel 0.5/35: Ethinyl estradiol 0.035 mg and norethindrone 0.5 mg [21 light yellow tablets and 7 white inactive tablets] (28s)

Necon 1/35: Ethinyl estradiol 0.035 mg and norethindrone 1 mg [21 dark yellow tablets and 7 white inactive tablets] (28s)

Norinyl 1+35: Ethinyl estradiol 0.035 mg and norethindrone 1 mg [21 yellow-green tablets and 7 orange inactive tablets] (28s)

Nortrel 1/35:

Ethinyl estradiol 0.035 mg and norethindrone 1 mg [yellow tablets] (21s)

Ethinyl estradiol 0.035 mg and norethindrone 1 mg [21 yellow tablets and 7 white inactive tablets] (28s)

Ortho-Novum 1/35: Ethinyl estradiol 0.035 mg and norethindrone 1 mg [21 peach tablets and 7 green inactive tablets] (28s)

Ovcon 35: Ethinyl estradiol 0.035 mg and norethindrone 0.4 mg [21 light peach tablets and 7 green inactive tablets] (28s)

Philith: Ethinyl estradiol 0.035 mg and norethindrone 0.4 mg [21 tan tablets and 7 white inactive tablets] (28s)

Pirmella 1/35: Ethinyl estradiol 0.035 mg and norethindrone 1 mg [21 peach tablets and 7 green inactive tablets] (28s)

Tarina FE 1/20: Ethinyl estradiol 0.02 mg and norethindrone acetate 1 mg [21 white tablets] and ferrous fumarate 75 mg [7 brown tablets] (28s)

Vyfemla: Ethinyl estradiol 0.035 mg and norethindrone 0.4 mg [21 light peach tablets and 7 white inactive tablets] (28s)
Wera: Ethinyl estradiol 0.035 mg and norethindrone 0.5 mg [21 light peach tablets and 7 white inactive tablets] (28s)
Zenchent: Ethinyl estradiol 0.035 mg and norethindrone 0.4 mg [21 orange tablets and 7 white inactive tablets] (28s)

Tablet, chewable, oral [monophasic formulation]: Ethinyl estradiol 0.035 mg and norethindrone 0.4 mg [21 tablets] and ferrous fumarate 75 mg [7 tablets] (28s)
Femcon Fe, Wymzya Fe: Ethinyl estradiol 0.035 mg and norethindrone 0.4 mg [21 white tablets] and ferrous fumarate 75 mg [7 brown tablets] (28s)
Generess Fe: Ethinyl estradiol 0.025 mg and norethindrone 0.8 mg [24 light green tablets] and ferrous fumarate 75 mg [4 brown tablets] (28s)
Minastrin 24 Fe: Ethinyl estradiol 0.02 mg and norethindrone 1 mg [24 white tablets] and ferrous fumarate 75 mg [4 brown tablets] (28s)
Zenchent Fe: Ethinyl estradiol 0.035 mg and norethindrone 0.4 mg [21 light yellow tablets] and ferrous fumarate 75 mg [7 brown tablets] (28s)

Tablet, oral [biphasic formulation]:
Lo Loestrin Fe:
Day 1-24: Ethinyl estradiol 0.01 mg and norethindrone acetate 1 mg [24 blue tablets]
Day 25-26: Ethinyl estradiol 0.01 mg [2 white tablets]
Day 27-28: Ferrous fumarate 75 mg [2 brown tablets] (28s)
Necon 10/11:
Day 1-10: Ethinyl estradiol 0.035 mg and norethindrone 0.5 mg [10 light yellow tablets]
Day 11-21: Ethinyl estradiol 0.035 mg and norethindrone 1 mg [11 dark yellow tablets]
Day 22-28: 7 white inactive tablets (28s)

Tablet, oral [triphasic formulation]:
Alyacen 7/7/7:
Day 1-7: Ethinyl estradiol 0.035 mg and norethindrone 0.5 mg [7 white-off-white tablets]
Day 8-14: Ethinyl estradiol 0.035 mg and norethindrone 0.75 mg [7 light peach tablets]
Day 15-21: Ethinyl estradiol 0.035 mg and norethindrone 1 mg [7 peach tablets]
Day 22-28: 7 light green inactive tablets (28s)
Aranelle:
Day 1-7: Ethinyl estradiol 0.035 mg and norethindrone 0.5 mg [7 light yellow tablets]
Day 8-16: Ethinyl estradiol 0.035 mg and norethindrone 1 mg [9 white tablets]
Day 17-21: Ethinyl estradiol 0.035 mg and norethindrone 0.5 mg [5 light yellow tablets]
Day 22-28: 7 peach inactive tablets (28s)
Cyclafem 7/7/7:
Day 1-7: Ethinyl estradiol 0.035 mg and norethindrone 0.5 mg [7 white tablets]
Day 8-14: Ethinyl estradiol 0.035 mg and norethindrone 0.75 mg [7 light pink tablets]
Day 15-21: Ethinyl estradiol 0.035 mg and norethindrone 1 mg [7 pink tablets]
Day 22-28: 7 light green inactive tablets (28s)
Dasetta 7/7/7:
Day 1-7: Ethinyl estradiol 0.035 mg and norethindrone 0.5 mg [7 light peach tablets]
Day 8-14: Ethinyl estradiol 0.035 mg and norethindrone 0.75 mg [7 peach tablets]
Day 15-21: Ethinyl estradiol 0.035 mg and norethindrone 1 mg [7 orange tablets]
Day 22-28: 7 white inactive tablets (28s)
Estrostep Fe, Tilia Fe:
Day 1-5: Ethinyl estradiol 0.02 mg and norethindrone acetate 1 mg [5 white triangular tablets]
Day 6-12: Ethinyl estradiol 0.03 mg and norethindrone acetate 1 mg [7 white square tablets]
Day 13-21: Ethinyl estradiol 0.035 mg and norethindrone acetate 1 mg [9 white round tablets]
Day 22-28: Ferrous fumarate 75 mg [7 brown tablets] (28s)
Leena:
Day 1-7: Ethinyl estradiol 0.035 mg and norethindrone 0.5 mg [7 light blue tablets]
Day 8-16: Ethinyl estradiol 0.035 mg and norethindrone 1 mg [9 light yellow-green tablets]
Day 17-21: Ethinyl estradiol 0.035 mg and norethindrone 0.5 mg [5 light blue tablets]
Day 22-28: 7 orange inactive tablets (28s)
Necon 7/7/7, Ortho-Novum 7/7/7:
Day 1-7: Ethinyl estradiol 0.035 mg and norethindrone 0.5 mg [7 white tablets]
Day 8-14: Ethinyl estradiol 0.035 mg and norethindrone 0.75 mg [7 light peach tablets]
Day 15-21: Ethinyl estradiol 0.035 mg and norethindrone 1 mg [7 peach tablets]
Day 22-28: 7 green inactive tablets (28s)
Nortrel 7/7/7:
Day 1-7: Ethinyl estradiol 0.035 mg and norethindrone 0.5 mg [7 light yellow tablets]
Day 8-14: Ethinyl estradiol 0.035 mg and norethindrone 0.75 mg [7 blue tablets]
Day 15-21: Ethinyl estradiol 0.035 mg and norethindrone 1 mg [7 peach tablets]
Day 22-28: 7 white inactive tablets (28s)
Pirmella 7/7/7:
Day 1-7: Ethinyl estradiol 0.035 mg and norethindrone 0.5 mg [7 white tablets]
Day 8-14: Ethinyl estradiol 0.035 mg and norethindrone 0.75 mg [7 light peach tablets]
Day 15-21: Ethinyl estradiol 0.035 mg and norethindrone 1 mg [7 peach tablets]
Day 22-28: 7 green inactive tablets (28s)
Tri-Legest Fe:
Day 1-5: Ethinyl estradiol 0.02 mg and norethindrone acetate 1 mg [5 light pink tablets]
Day 6-12: Ethinyl estradiol 0.03 mg and norethindrone acetate 1 mg [7 light yellow tablets]
Day 13-21: Ethinyl estradiol 0.035 mg and norethindrone acetate 1 mg [9 light blue tablets]
Day 22-28: Ferrous fumarate 75 mg [7 brown tablets] (28s)
Tri-Norinyl:
Day 1-7: Ethinyl estradiol 0.035 mg and norethindrone 0.5 mg [7 blue tablets]
Day 8-16: Ethinyl estradiol 0.035 mg and norethindrone 1 mg [9 yellow-green tablets]
Day 17-21: Ethinyl estradiol 0.035 mg and norethindrone 0.5 mg [5 blue tablets]
Day 22-28: 7 orange inactive tablets (28s)

Ethinyl Estradiol and Norgestimate

(ETH in il es tra DYE ole & nor JES ti mate)

Brand Names: U.S. Estarylla; MonoNessa; Ortho Tri-Cyclen; Ortho Tri-Cyclen Lo; Ortho-Cyclen; Previfem; Sprintec; Tri-Estarylla; Tri-Previfem; Tri-Sprintec; TriNessa

Brand Names: Canada Cyclen; Tri-Cyclen; Tri-Cyclen Lo

Index Terms Ethinyl Estradiol and NGM; Norgestimate and Ethinyl Estradiol; Ortho Cyclen; Ortho Tri Cyclen

Pharmacologic Category Contraceptive; Estrogen and Progestin Combination

Use

Acne vulgaris: For the treatment of moderate acne vulgaris in females at least 15 years of age

Limitations of use: When used for acne, use only in females ≥15 years of age who achieved menarche, who also desire combination hormonal contraceptive therapy, are unresponsive to topical treatments, have no contraindications to combination hormonal contraceptive use, and plan to stay on therapy for ≥6 months

Contraception: For the prevention of pregnancy.

Pregnancy Risk Factor X

Dosage Oral:

Children ≥15 years and Adults: Females: Acne (Ortho Tri-Cyclen): Refer to dosing for contraception

Adults: Females:

Contraception:

Schedule 1 (Sunday starter): Dose begins on first Sunday after onset of menstruation; if the menstrual period starts on Sunday, take first tablet that very same day. **With a Sunday start, an additional method of contraception should be used until after the first 7 days of consecutive administration.**

For 21-tablet package: Dosage is 1 tablet daily for 21 consecutive days, followed by 7 days off of the medication; a new course begins on the 8th day after the last tablet is taken.

For 28-tablet package: Dosage is 1 tablet daily without interruption.

Schedule 2 (Day 1 starter): Dose starts on first day of menstrual cycle taking 1 tablet daily.

For 21-tablet package: Dosage is 1 tablet daily for 21 consecutive days, followed by 7 days off of the medication; a new course begins on the 8th day after the last tablet is taken.

For 28-tablet package: Dosage is 1 tablet daily without interruption.

If all doses have not been taken on schedule and one menstrual period is missed, the possibility of pregnancy should be considered. If two consecutive menstrual periods are missed, pregnancy test is required before new dosing cycle is started.

Missed doses **monophasic formulations** (refer to package insert for complete information):

One dose missed: Take as soon as remembered or take 2 tablets next day

Two consecutive doses missed in the first 2 weeks: Take 2 tablets as soon as remembered or 2 tablets next 2 days. **An additional method of contraception should be used for 7 days after missed dose.**

Two consecutive doses missed in week 3 or three consecutive doses missed at any time: **An additional method of contraception must be used for 7 days after a missed dose:**

Schedule 1 (Sunday starter): Continue dose of 1 tablet daily until Sunday, then discard the rest of the pack, and a new pack should be started that same day.

Schedule 2 (Day 1 starter): Current pack should be discarded, and a new pack should be started that same day.

Missed doses **biphasic/triphasic formulations** (refer to package insert for complete information):

One dose missed: Take as soon as remembered.

Two consecutive doses missed in week 1 or week 2 of the pack: Take 2 tablets as soon as remembered and 2 tablets the next day. Resume taking 1 tablet daily until the pack is empty. **An additional method of contraception must be used for 7 days after a missed dose.**

Two consecutive doses missed in week 3 of the pack. **An additional method of contraception must be used for 7 days after a missed dose.**

Schedule 1 (Sunday starter): Take 1 tablet every day until Sunday. Discard the remaining pack and start a new pack of pills on the same day.

Schedule 2 (Day 1 starter): Discard the remaining pack and start a new pack the same day.

Three or more consecutive doses missed. **An additional method of contraception must be used for 7 days after a missed dose.**

Schedule 1 (Sunday starter): Take 1 tablet every day until Sunday; on Sunday, discard the pack and start a new pack.

Schedule 2 (Day 1 starter): Discard the remaining pack and begin new pack of tablets starting on the same day.

Dosage adjustment in renal impairment: No dosage adjustment provided in manufacturer's labeling (has not been studied); use with caution and monitor blood pressure closely. Consider other forms of contraception.

Dosage adjustment in hepatic impairment: Contraindicated in patients with hepatic impairment.

Additional Information Complete prescribing information should be consulted for additional detail.

Dosage Forms

Tablet, oral [monophasic formulation]:

Estarylla: Ethinyl estradiol 0.035 mg and norgestimate 0.25 mg [21 blue tablets and 7 green inactive tablets] (28s)

MonoNessa, Ortho-Cyclen: Ethinyl estradiol 0.035 mg and norgestimate 0.25 mg [21 blue tablets and 7 dark green inactive tablets] (28s)

Previfem: Ethinyl estradiol 0.035 mg and norgestimate 0.25 mg [21 blue tablets and 7 light green inactive tablets] (28s)

Sprintec: Ethinyl estradiol 0.035 mg and norgestimate 0.25 mg [21 blue tablets and 7 white inactive tablets] (28s)

Tablet, oral [triphasic formulation]:

Ortho Tri-Cyclen, TriNessa:

Day 1-7: Ethinyl estradiol 0.035 mg and norgestimate 0.18 mg [7 white tablets]

Day 8-14: Ethinyl estradiol 0.035 mg and norgestimate 0.215 mg [7 light blue tablets]

Day 15-21: Ethinyl estradiol 0.035 mg and norgestimate 0.25 mg [7 blue tablets]

Day 22-28: 7 dark green inactive tablets (28s)

Tri-Estarylla

Day 1-7: Ethinyl estradiol 0.035 mg and norgestimate 0.18 mg [7 white tablets]

Day 8-14: Ethinyl estradiol 0.035 mg and norgestimate 0.215 mg [7 light blue tablets]

Day 15-21: Ethinyl estradiol 0.035 mg and norgestimate 0.25 mg [7 blue tablets]

Day 22-28: 7 green inactive tablets (28s)

Tri-Previfem::

Day 1-7: Ethinyl estradiol 0.035 mg and norgestimate 0.18 mg [7 white tablets]

Day 8-14: Ethinyl estradiol 0.035 mg and norgestimate 0.215 mg [7 light blue tablets]

Day 15-21: Ethinyl estradiol 0.035 mg and norgestimate 0.25 mg [7 blue tablets]

Day 22-28: 7 light green inactive tablets (28s)

Tri-Sprintec:

Day 1-7: Ethinyl estradiol 0.035 mg and norgestimate 0.18 mg [7 gray tablets]

Day 8-14: Ethinyl estradiol 0.035 mg and norgestimate 0.215 mg [7 light blue tablets]

Day 15-21: Ethinyl estradiol 0.035 mg and norgestimate 0.25 mg [7 blue tablets]

Day 22-28: 7 white inactive tablets (28s)

Ortho Tri-Cyclen Lo:
Day 1-7: Ethinyl estradiol 0.025 mg and norgestimate 0.18 mg [7 white tablets]
Day 8-14: Ethinyl estradiol 0.025 mg and norgestimate 0.215 mg [7 light blue tablets]
Day 15-21: Ethinyl estradiol 0.025 mg and norgestimate 0.25 mg [7 dark blue tablets]
Day 22-28: 7 dark green inactive tablets (28s)

Ethinyl Estradiol and Norgestrel

(ETH in il es tra DYE ole & nor JES trel)

Brand Names: U.S. Cryselle 28; Low-Ogestrel; Ogestrel
Brand Names: Canada Lo-Femenal 21; Ovral®
Index Terms Lo Ovral; Morning After Pill; Norgestrel and Ethinyl Estradiol
Pharmacologic Category Contraceptive; Estrogen and Progestin Combination
Use Prevention of pregnancy; postcoital contraceptive or "morning after" pill
Pregnancy Risk Factor X
Dosage Oral: Adults: Females:
Contraception:
Schedule 1 (Sunday starter): Dose begins on first Sunday after onset of menstruation; if the menstrual period starts on Sunday, take first tablet that very same day. **With a Sunday start, an additional method of contraception should be used until after the first 7 days of consecutive administration.**
For 21-tablet package: Dosage is 1 tablet daily for 21 consecutive days, followed by 7 days off of the medication; a new course begins on the 8th day after the last tablet is taken.
For 28-tablet package: Dosage is 1 tablet daily without interruption.
Schedule 2 (Day 1 starter): Dose starts on first day of menstrual cycle taking 1 tablet daily.
For 21-tablet package: Dosage is 1 tablet daily for 21 consecutive days, followed by 7 days off of the medication; a new course begins on the 8th day after the last tablet is taken.
For 28-tablet package: Dosage is 1 tablet daily without interruption.
If all doses have been taken on schedule and one menstrual period is missed, continue dosing cycle. If two consecutive menstrual periods are missed, pregnancy test is required before new dosing cycle is started.
Missed doses **monophasic formulations** (refer to package insert for complete information):
One dose missed: Take as soon as remembered or take 2 tablets next day
Two consecutive doses missed in the first 2 weeks: Take 2 tablets as soon as remembered or 2 tablets next 2 days. **An additional method of contraception should be used for 7 days after missed dose.**
Two consecutive doses missed in week 3 or three consecutive doses missed at any time:
Schedule 1 (Sunday starter): Continue to take 1 tablet daily until Sunday, then discard the rest of the pack, and a new pack is started that same day.
Schedule 2 (Day 1 starter): Current pack should be discarded, and a new pack started that same day. **An additional method of contraception should be used for 7 days after missed dose.**

Postcoital contraception:
Ethinyl estradiol 0.03 mg and norgestrel 0.3 mg formulation: 4 tablets within 72 hours of unprotected intercourse and 4 tablets 12 hours after first dose
Ethinyl estradiol 0.05 mg and norgestrel 0.5 mg formulation: 2 tablets within 72 hours of unprotected intercourse and 2 tablets 12 hours after first dose

Dosage adjustment in renal impairment: Specific guidelines not available; use with caution and monitor blood pressure closely. Consider other forms of contraception.
Dosage adjustment in hepatic impairment: Contraindicated in patients with hepatic impairment.
Additional Information Complete prescribing information should be consulted for additional detail.
Dosage Forms
Tablet, oral [monophasic formulation]: Ethinyl estradiol 0.03 mg and norgestrel 0.3 mg [21 tablets and 7 inactive tablets] (28s)
Cryselle 28: Ethinyl estradiol 0.03 mg and norgestrel 0.3 mg [21 white tablets and 7 light green inactive tablets] (28s)
Low-Ogestrel: Ethinyl estradiol 0.03 mg and norgestrel 0.3 mg [21 white tablets and 7 peach inactive tablets] (28s)
Ogestrel: Ethinyl estradiol 0.05 mg and norgestrel 0.5 mg [21 white tablets and 7 peach inactive tablets] (28s)

Ethinyl Estradiol, Drospirenone, and Levomefolate

(ETH in il es tra DYE ole, droh SPYE re none, & lee voe me FOE late)

Brand Names: U.S. Beyaz; Safyral
Brand Names: Canada Yaz Plus
Index Terms Drospirenone, Ethinyl Estradiol, and Levomefolate Calcium; Ethinyl Estradiol, Drospirenone, and Levomefolate Calcium; Levomefolate Calcium, Drospirenone, and Ethinyl Estradiol; Levomefolate, Drospirenone, and Ethinyl Estradiol
Pharmacologic Category Contraceptive; Estrogen and Progestin Combination
Use Prevention of pregnancy; treatment of premenstrual dysphoric disorder (PMDD); treatment of acne; folate supplementation
Dosage Oral:
Children ≥14 years and Adults: Females: Acne (Beyaz): Refer to dosing for contraception
Adults: Females: PMDD (Beyaz): Refer to dosing for contraception
Adults: Females: Contraception (Beyaz, Safyral): Dosage is 1 tablet daily
Beyaz: One pink tablet daily for 24 consecutive days, then one light orange tablet daily on days 25-28
Safyral: One orange tablet daily for 21 consecutive days, then one light orange tablet daily on days 22-28
Dose should be taken at the same time each day, either after the evening meal or at bedtime. Dosing may be started on the first day of menstrual period (Day 1 starter) or on the first Sunday after the onset of the menstrual period (Sunday starter).

Day 1 starter: Dose starts on first day of menstrual cycle taking 1 tablet daily. If first dose is taken later than the first day of the menstrual cycle, **an additional method of contraception should be used until after the first 7 days of consecutive administration.**
Sunday starter: Dose begins on first Sunday after onset of menstruation; if the menstrual period starts on Sunday, take first tablet that very same day. **With a Sunday start, an additional method of contraception should be used until after the first 7 days of consecutive administration.**

Switching from a different contraceptive:
Oral contraceptive: Start on the same day that a new pack of the previous oral contraceptive would have been taken
Transdermal patch, vaginal ring, injection: Start on the day the next dose would have been due
IUD or implant: Start on the day of removal

Use after childbirth (in women who are not breast-feeding) or after second trimester abortion: Therapy may be started ≥4 weeks postpartum. Pregnancy should be ruled out prior to treatment if menstrual periods have not restarted and an additional method of contraception (non-hormonal) should be used until after the first 7 days of consecutive administration.

Missed doses:

If all doses have been taken on schedule and one menstrual period is missed, continue dosing cycle. If two consecutive menstrual periods are missed, rule out pregnancy and discontinue if pregnancy is confirmed.

If doses have been missed during the first 3 weeks or if active tablets (pink tablets) were started later than as directed and the menstrual period is missed, pregnancy should be ruled out prior to continuing treatment.

Missed doses (monophasic formulations) (refer to package insert for complete information):

One dose missed: Take as soon as remembered or take 2 tablets next day

Two consecutive doses missed in the first 2 weeks: Take 2 tablets as soon as remembered or 2 tablets next 2 days. **An additional method of contraception should be used for 7 days after missed dose.**

Two consecutive doses missed in week 3 or three consecutive doses missed at any time: **An additional method of contraception must be used for 7 days after a missed dose.**

Day 1 starter: Current pack should be discarded, and a new pack should be started that same day.

Sunday starter: Continue dose of 1 tablet daily until Sunday, then discard the rest of the pack, and a new pack should be started that same day.

Any number of doses missed in week 4: Throw away the pills that were missed. Continue taking one pill each day until pack is empty; no back-up method of contraception is needed

Dosage adjustment in renal impairment: Contraindicated in patients with renal dysfunction

Dosage adjustment in hepatic impairment: Contraindicated in patients with hepatic disease. Exposure to drospirenone is ~3 times higher with moderate liver impairment; information not available for severe impairment.

Additional Information Complete prescribing information should be consulted for additional detail.

Dosage Forms

Tablet, oral:

Beyaz: Ethinyl estradiol 0.02 mg, drospirenone 3 mg, and levomefolate calcium 0.451 mg [24 pink tablets] and levomefolate calcium 0.451 mg [4 light orange tablets] (28s)

Safyral: Ethinyl estradiol 0.03 mg, drospirenone 3 mg, and levomefolate calcium 0.451 mg [21 orange tablets] and levomefolate calcium 0.451 mg [7 light orange tablets] (28s)

- ◆ **Ethinyl Estradiol, Drospirenone, and Levomefolate Calcium** *see* Ethinyl Estradiol, Drospirenone, and Levomefolate *on page 812*
- ◆ **Ethiofos** *see* Amifostine *on page 109*

Ethosuximide (eth oh SUKS i mide)

Brand Names: U.S. Zarontin

Brand Names: Canada Zarontin®

Pharmacologic Category Anticonvulsant, Succinimide

Use Management of absence (petit mal) seizures

Dosage Oral:

Children 3-6 years: Initial: 250 mg/day; increase every 4-7 days; usual maintenance dose: 20 mg/kg/day; maximum dose: 1.5 g/day in divided doses

Children ≥6 years and Adults: Initial: 500 mg/day; increase by 250 mg as needed every 4-7 days, up to 1.5 g/day in divided doses; usual maintenance dose for most pediatric patients is 20 mg/kg/day.

Dosing comment in renal impairment: No dosage adjustment provided in manufacturer's labeling; use with caution.

Dosing comment in hepatic impairment: No dosage adjustment provided in manufacturer's labeling; use with caution.

Additional Information Complete prescribing information should be consulted for additional detail.

Dosage Forms

Capsule, Oral:

Zarontin: 250 mg

Generic: 250 mg

Solution, Oral:

Zarontin: 250 mg/5 mL (474 mL)

Generic: 250 mg/5 mL (473 mL, 474 mL)

- ◆ **Ethoxynaphthamido Penicillin Sodium** *see* Nafcillin *on page 1414*
- ◆ **Ethyl Aminobenzoate** *see* Benzocaine *on page 246*
- ◆ **Ethyl Eicosapentaenoate** *see* Omega-3 Fatty Acids *on page 1507*
- ◆ **Ethyl-Eicosapentaenoic Acid** *see* Omega-3 Fatty Acids *on page 1507*
- ◆ **Ethyl-EPA** *see* Omega-3 Fatty Acids *on page 1507*
- ◆ **Ethyl Esters of Omega-3 Fatty Acids** *see* Omega-3 Fatty Acids *on page 1507*
- ◆ **Ethyl Icosapentate** *see* Omega-3 Fatty Acids *on page 1507*
- ◆ **Ethynodiol Diacetate and Ethinyl Estradiol** *see* Ethinyl Estradiol and Ethynodiol Diacetate *on page 801*
- ◆ **Ethyol** *see* Amifostine *on page 109*
- ◆ **Etibi® (Can)** *see* Ethambutol *on page 798*

Etidronate (e ti DROE nate)

Brand Names: Canada ACT Etidronate; Mylan-Etidronate

Index Terms EHDP; Etidronate Disodium; Sodium Etidronate

Pharmacologic Category Bisphosphonate Derivative

Use Symptomatic treatment of Paget's disease; prevention and treatment of heterotopic ossification due to spinal cord injury or after total hip replacement

Pregnancy Risk Factor C

Dosage Note: Patients should receive supplemental calcium and vitamin D if dietary intake is inadequate.

Paget's disease: Adults: Oral:

Initial: 5-10 mg/kg/day (not to exceed 6 months) or 11-20 mg/kg/day (not to exceed 3 months). The recommended initial dose is 5 mg/kg/day (not to exceed 6 months). Higher doses should be used only when lower doses are ineffective or there is a need to suppress rapid bone turnover (ie, potential for irreversible neurologic damage) or reduce elevated cardiac output. Doses >20 mg/kg/day are **not** recommended.

Retreatment: Initiate only after etidronate-free period ≥90 days. Monitor patients every 3-6 months. Retreatment regimens are the same as for initial treatment.

Heterotopic ossification: Adults: Oral:

Caused by spinal cord injury: 20 mg/kg/day for 2 weeks, then 10 mg/kg/day for 10 weeks; total treatment period: 12 weeks

Complicating total hip replacement: 20 mg/kg/day for 1 month preoperatively then 20 mg/kg/day for 3 months postoperatively; total treatment period is 4 months

Dosage adjustment in renal impairment: Manufacturer's labeling recommends decreasing the dose when GFR is reduced; however, no specific dosage adjustments are provided. Use with caution and monitor closely; etidronate is eliminated intact via the kidneys.

Dosage adjustment in hepatic impairment: No dosage adjustment provided in manufacturer's labeling.

Additional Information Complete prescribing information should be consulted for additional detail.

Dosage Forms

Tablet, Oral:

Generic: 200 mg, 400 mg

Etidronate and Calcium Carbonate [CAN/INT] (e ti DROE nate & KAL see um KAR bun ate)

Brand Names: Canada CO Etidrocal; Didrocal®; Mylan-Eti-Cal Carepac; Novo-Etidronatecal

Index Terms Calcium Carbonate and Etidronate Disodium; Etidronate Disodium and Calcium

Pharmacologic Category Bisphosphonate Derivative; Calcium Salt

Use Note: Not approved in U.S.

Treatment and prevention of postmenopausal osteoporosis; prevention of corticosteroid-induced osteoporosis

Pregnancy Considerations Adverse events were observed in some animal reproduction studies. Refer to individual agents. According to the manufacturer, this product is not intended for use in pregnant women.

Breast-Feeding Considerations Calcium is excreted into breast milk (refer to Calcium Carbonate monograph for additional information); excretion of etidronate is not known. Due to the potential for serious adverse reactions in the nursing infant, the manufacturer recommends a decision be made whether to discontinue nursing or to discontinue the drug, taking into account the importance of treatment to the mother. This product is not intended for use in nursing women.

Contraindications Hypersensitivity to etidronate disodium, bisphosphonates, or any component of the formulation; clinically-overt osteomalacia (appropriate treatment to resolve osteomalacia should be initiated before prescribing Didrocal™ therapy).

Warnings/Precautions Use with caution in patients with restricted calcium and vitamin D intake; IV form of etidronate has been noted to be nephrotoxic; therefore, this drug should be used with caution, if at all, in patients with impaired renal function or a history of kidney stones. There is no specific experience to guide cyclic therapy in patients with renal impairment or a history of renal calculi; monitor urine calcium and other relevant parameters if therapy is implemented.

Bisphosphonate therapy has been associated with osteonecrosis, primarily of the jaw; this has been observed mostly in cancer patients, but also in patients with postmenopausal osteoporosis and other diagnoses. Most reported cases occurred after IV bisphosphonate therapy; however, cases have been reported following oral therapy. Dental exams and preventive dentistry should be performed prior to placing patients with risk factors on chronic bisphosphonate therapy. Invasive dental procedures should be avoided during treatment. Esophagitis, dysphagia, esophageal ulcers, esophageal erosions, and esophageal stricture (rare) have been reported with oral bisphosphonates; use with caution in patients with dysphagia, esophageal disease, gastritis, duodenitis, or ulcers (may worsen underlying condition). Discontinue use if new or worsening symptoms develop.

Atypical femur fractures have been reported in patients receiving bisphosphonates for treatment/prevention of osteoporosis. The fractures include subtrochanteric femur (bone just below the hip joint) and diaphyseal femur (long segment of the thigh bone). Some patients experience prodromal pain weeks or months before the fracture occurs. It is unclear if bisphosphonate therapy is the cause for these fractures, although the majority have been reported in patients taking bisphosphonates. Patients receiving long-term (>3-5 years) therapy may be at an increased risk. Discontinue bisphosphonate therapy in patients who develop a femoral shaft fracture.

Infrequently, severe (and occasionally debilitating) bone, joint, and/or muscle pain have been reported during bisphosphonate treatment. The onset of pain ranged from a single day to several months. Consider discontinuing therapy in patients who experience severe symptoms; symptoms usually resolve upon discontinuation. Some patients experienced recurrence when rechallenged with same drug or another bisphosphonate; avoid use in patients with a history of these symptoms in association with bisphosphonate therapy.

Calcium carbonate absorption is impaired in achlorhydria (common in elderly); administer calcium component with food; while hypercalcemia and hypercalciuria may result when therapeutic replacement amounts are given for prolonged periods, they are most likely to occur in hypoparathyroid patients receiving high doses of vitamin D.

Safety and efficacy have not been established in pediatric patients.

Adverse Reactions

Central nervous system: Dizziness, headache

Gastrointestinal: Constipation, diarrhea, dyspepsia, flatulence, nausea, vomiting

Rare but important or life-threatening: Agranulocytosis, alopecia, amnesia, angioedema, arthropathies, asthma exacerbation, bone fracture, burning tongue, confusion, depression, diaphyseal femur fracture, erythema multiforme, esophageal cancer, esophagitis, follicular eruption, glossitis, hallucinations, leukopenia, leukemia (1 in 100,000 patients), musculoskeletal pain, pancytopenia, paresthesia, peptic ulcer disease (exacerbation), rash (maculopapular), Stevens-Johnson syndrome, subtrochanteric femur fracture, urticaria

Drug Interactions

Avoid Concomitant Use There are no known interactions where it is recommended to avoid concomitant use.

Increased Effect/Toxicity There are no known significant interactions involving an increase in effect.

Decreased Effect There are no known significant interactions involving a decrease in effect.

Food Interactions Food decreases the absorption and bioavailability of the etidronate. Management: Administer on an empty stomach with a full glass of plain water or fruit juice (6-8 oz) 2 hours before food.

Storage/Stability Store at 15°C to 30°C (59°F to 86°F).

Mechanism of Action See individual agents.

Pharmacodynamics/Kinetics See individual agents.

Dosage Note: 90-day treatment regimen involves sequential administration of two products within the packaging; not to be taken concurrently. The first blister card contains white tablets containing etidronate disodium, while the remaining four blister cards contains blue, capsule-shaped tablets containing calcium carbonate.

Oral: Adults: Etidronate disodium 400 mg once daily for 14 days, followed by calcium carbonate 1250 mg (500 mg elemental calcium) once daily for 76 days

Dosage adjustment in renal impairment: Not recommended for treatment in renally-impaired patients.

Dietary Considerations

Etidronate: Administer tablet with water on an empty stomach; avoid administering foods/supplements with calcium, iron, or magnesium within 2 hours of drug; maintain adequate intake of calcium and vitamin D.

Calcium: As a dietary supplement, should be given with meals to increase absorption. May decrease iron absorption, so should be administered 1-2 hours before or after iron supplementation; limit intake of with bran, foods high in oxalates, or whole grain cereals which may decrease calcium absorption. Dietary calcium should be adjusted to supply at least 1500 mg/day (Didrocal™ supplies 500 mg/day), and dietary vitamin D intake should provide 400 units/day.

Administration Administer etidronate tablets with a full glass of water on an empty stomach 2 hours before meals. The calcium carbonate tablets may be administered with food.

Monitoring Parameters Bone mass should be monitored; if not stabilized within 4 cycles (1 year) of therapy, consider discontinuation of treatment

Product Availability Not available in U.S.

Dosage Forms: Canada

Combination package [each package contains 5 blister cards (90-day supply)]:

Didrocal®:

Tablet, etidronate: 400 mg (14s) [first card (white tablets)]

Tablet, calcium: 1250 mg (76s) [remaining cards (blue tablets)]

◆ **Etidronate Disodium** *see* Etidronate *on page 813*

◆ **Etidronate Disodium and Calcium** *see* Etidronate and Calcium Carbonate [CAN/INT] *on page 814*

Etilefrine [INT] (e TIL e frine)

International Brand Names Adrenam (DE); Bioflutin-N (DE); Cardanat (DE); Cardialgine (DE); Circupon (AT, CH, DE); Circuvit E (DE); Confidol (DE); Corcanfol (AR); Effortil (AR, AT, BE, CH, CY, DE, FI, FR, HR, IT, LU, NO, PT, SE); Effortil PL (BE, LU); Efortil (BR, ES); Ethyfron (JP); Eti-Puren (DE); etil von ct (DE); Etilefrin (DE); Etilefrin AL (DE); Etilefrin-Neosan (DE); Etilefrin-ratiopharm (DE); Etilefrina (AR); Etilefrina Denver Farma (AR); Etilefrina Fabra (AR); Etilefrina Larjan (AR); Hishiherin-S (JP); Kertasin (AR); Kreislauf Katovit (DE); Logomed Kreislauf-Tabletten (DE); Mandroton (DE); Menegradil (AR); Pulsamin (JP); Theoral (JP); Thomasin (DE); Tonus-Forte (DE); Tonustab (DE); Tulupressin (DE)

Index Terms Etilefrine Hydrochloride

Pharmacologic Category Alpha/Beta Agonist

Reported Use Treatment of symptomatic or orthostatic hypotension

Dosage Range Adults: Oral: 5-10 mg 3 times/day or 25 mg long-acting capsule once or twice daily

Product Availability Product available in various countries; not currently available in the U.S.

Dosage Forms

Capsule, long acting: 25 mg

Tablet: 5 mg

◆ **Etilefrine Hydrochloride** *see* Etilefrine [INT] *on page 815*

Etodolac (ee toe DOE lak)

Brand Names: Canada Apo-Etodolac; Utradol

Index Terms Etodolic Acid; Lodine

Pharmacologic Category Nonsteroidal Anti-inflammatory Drug (NSAID), Oral

Additional Appendix Information

Beers Criteria – Potentially Inappropriate Medications for Geriatrics *on page 2271*

Use Acute and long-term use in the management of signs and symptoms of osteoarthritis; rheumatoid arthritis and juvenile idiopathic arthritis (JIA); management of acute pain

Pregnancy Risk Factor C

Dosage Note: For chronic conditions, response is usually observed within 2 weeks.

Children 6-16 years: Oral: Juvenile idiopathic arthritis (JIA):

Extended release formulation:

20-30 kg: 400 mg once daily

31-45 kg: 600 mg once daily

46-60 kg: 800 mg once daily

>60 kg: 1000 mg once daily

Adults: Oral:

Acute pain: Immediate release formulation: 200-400 mg every 6-8 hours, as needed, not to exceed total daily doses of 1000 mg

Rheumatoid arthritis, osteoarthritis:

Immediate release formulation: 400 mg 2 times/day **or** 300 mg 2-3 times/day **or** 500 mg 2 times/day (doses >1000 mg/day have not been evaluated)

Extended release formulation: 400-1000 mg once daily

Elderly: Refer to adult dosing; in patients ≥65 years, no dosage adjustment required based on pharmacokinetics. The elderly are more sensitive to antiprostaglandin effects and may need dosage adjustments.

Dosage adjustment in renal impairment:

Mild-to-moderate: No adjustment required

Severe: Use not recommended; use with caution

Hemodialysis: Not removed

Dosage adjustment in hepatic impairment: No adjustment required.

Additional Information Complete prescribing information should be consulted for additional detail.

Dosage Forms

Capsule, Oral:

Generic: 200 mg, 300 mg

Tablet, Oral:

Generic: 400 mg, 500 mg

Tablet Extended Release 24 Hour, Oral:

Generic: 400 mg, 500 mg, 600 mg

Dosage Forms: Canada Refer to Dosage Forms. **Note:** Tablets and Extended Release tablets are not available in Canada.

◆ **Etodolic Acid** *see* Etodolac *on page 815*

Etofenamate [INT] (E toe fen a mate)

International Brand Names Activon (CH); Afrolate (ES); Algesalona E (DE); Bayro (IT, MX); Bayrogel (AR, BR); Deiron (ES); Etofen (CH); Etogel (CZ); F-525 (GR); Fenax (CH); Fenogel (PT); Flexium (BE); Flogol (AR); Flogoprofen (ES); Irifone (GR); Pazergicel (GR); Reumon (PT); Rheuma-Gel-ratiopharm (DE); Rheumon (AT, CH, DE, LU, PT); Riscom (CH); Traumalix (CH); Traumon (AT, DE, LU); Zenavan (ES)

Pharmacologic Category Anti-inflammatory Agent

Reported Use Treatment of rheumatic diseases of soft tissues of the musculoskeletal system (eg, muscular rheumatism, lumbago, sciatica, tenosynovitis, bursitis, blunt traumas such as those caused by a sporting injury [contusions, sprains, and strains])

Dosage Range Adults: Topical: Apply to affected area 3-4 times/day

Product Availability Product available in various countries; not currently available in the U.S.

Dosage Forms

Gel: 50 mg/g (40 g)

Etomidate (e TOM i date)

Brand Names: U.S. Amidate

Pharmacologic Category General Anesthetic

Use Induction and maintenance of general anesthesia

Pregnancy Risk Factor C

Pregnancy Considerations Adverse events have been observed in animal reproduction studies.

Breast-Feeding Considerations It is not known if etomidate is excreted in breast milk. The manufacturer recommends that caution be exercised when administering etomidate to nursing women.

Contraindications Hypersensitivity to etomidate or any component of the formulation

Warnings/Precautions Etomidate inhibits 11-B-hydroxylase, an enzyme important in adrenal steroid production. A single induction dose blocks the normal stress-induced increase in adrenal cortisol production for 4-8 hours, up to 24 hours in elderly and debilitated patients. Continuous infusion of etomidate for sedation in the ICU may increase mortality because patients may not be able to respond to stress. No increase in mortality has been identified with a single dose for induction of anesthesia. Consider exogenous corticosteroid replacement in patients undergoing severe stress.

Adverse Reactions

Gastrointestinal: Hiccups, nausea, vomiting on emergence from anesthesia

Local: Pain at injection site

Neuromuscular & skeletal: Myoclonus, transient skeletal movements, uncontrolled eye movements

Rare but important or life-threatening: Apnea, arrhythmia, bradycardia, decreased cortisol synthesis, hyper-/hypotension, hyper-/hypoventilation, laryngospasm, tachycardia

Drug Interactions

Metabolism/Transport Effects None known.

Avoid Concomitant Use There are no known interactions where it is recommended to avoid concomitant use.

Increased Effect/Toxicity There are no known significant interactions involving an increase in effect.

Decreased Effect There are no known significant interactions involving a decrease in effect.

Storage/Stability Store at room temperature.

Mechanism of Action Ultrashort-acting nonbarbiturate hypnotic (benzylimidazole) used for the induction of anesthesia; chemically, it is a carboxylated imidazole which produces a rapid induction of anesthesia with minimal cardiovascular effects; produces EEG burst suppression at high doses

Pharmacodynamics/Kinetics

Onset of action: 30 to 60 seconds

Peak effect: 1 minute

Duration: 3 to 5 minutes; terminated by redistribution

Distribution: V_d: 2 to 4.5 L/kg

Protein binding: 76%

Metabolism: Hepatic and plasma esterases

Half-life elimination: Terminal: 2.6 hours

Dosage IV: Children >10 years, Adolescents, and Adults:

Anesthesia: Initial: 0.2 to 0.6 mg/kg over 30 to 60 seconds for induction of anesthesia; maintenance: 5 to 20 mcg/kg/minute

Procedural sedation (off-label use): Initial: 0.1 to 0.2 mg/kg, followed by 0.05 mg/kg every 3-5 minutes as needed (Bahn, 2005; Miner, 2007; Vinson, 2002)

Dosage adjustment in renal impairment: There are no dosage adjustments provided in the manufacturer's labeling.

Dosage adjustment in hepatic impairment: There are no dosage adjustments provided in the manufacturer's labeling; use with caution.

Administration Administer IV push over 30-60 seconds. Solution is highly irritating; avoid administration into small vessels; in some cases, preadministration of lidocaine may be considered.

Monitoring Parameters Cardiac monitoring and blood pressure required

Additional Information Etomidate decreases cerebral metabolism and cerebral blood flow while maintaining perfusion pressure. Premedication with opioids or benzodiazepines can decrease myoclonus. Etomidate can enhance somatosensory evoked potential recordings.

Dosage Forms

Solution, Intravenous:

Amidate: 2 mg/mL (10 mL, 20 mL)

Generic: 2 mg/mL (10 mL, 20 mL)

Solution, Intravenous [preservative free]:

Generic: 2 mg/mL (10 mL, 20 mL)

◆ **Etonogestrel and Ethinyl Estradiol** *see* Ethinyl Estradiol and Etonogestrel *on page 802*

◆ **ETOP** *see* Etoposide Phosphate *on page 820*

◆ **Etopophos** *see* Etoposide Phosphate *on page 820*

Etoposide (e toe POE side)

Brand Names: U.S. Toposar

Brand Names: Canada Etoposide Injection; Etoposide Injection USP; Vepesid

Index Terms EPEG; Epipodophyllotoxin; VePesid; VP-16; VP-16-213; VP16

Pharmacologic Category Antineoplastic Agent, Podophyllotoxin Derivative; Antineoplastic Agent, Topoisomerase II Inhibitor

Use

Small cell lung cancer (oral and IV): Treatment (first-line) of small cell lung cancer (SCLC)

Testicular cancer (IV): Treatment of refractory testicular tumors (injectable formulation)

Canadian labeling: Treatment of small cell lung cancer (SCLC; first- and second-line); treatment of non-small cell lung cancer (NSCLC); treatment of non-Hodgkin lymphomas (first-line); treatment of testicular cancer (first-line [injectable formulation] and refractory)

Pregnancy Risk Factor D

Pregnancy Considerations Adverse events were observed in animal reproduction studies. Etoposide may cause fetal harm if administered during pregnancy. Women of childbearing potential should be advised to avoid pregnancy.

Breast-Feeding Considerations It is not known if etoposide is excreted in breast milk. Due to the potential for serious adverse reactions in the nursing infant, the decision to discontinue etoposide or to discontinue breastfeeding during treatment should take into account the benefits of treatment to the mother.

Contraindications Hypersensitivity to etoposide or any component of the formulation

Canadian labeling: Additional contraindications (not in U.S. labeling): Severe leukopenia or thrombocytopenia; severe hepatic impairment; severe renal impairment

Warnings/Precautions Hazardous agent - use appropriate precautions for handling and disposal (NIOSH 2014 [group 1]). **[U.S. Boxed Warning]: Severe dose-limiting and dose-related myelosuppression with resulting infection or bleeding may occur.** Treatment should be withheld for platelets <50,000/mm^3 or absolute neutrophil count (ANC) <500/mm^3. May cause anaphylactic-like reactions manifested by chills, fever, tachycardia, bronchospasm, dyspnea, and hypotension. In addition, facial/tongue swelling, coughing, chest tightness, cyanosis, laryngospasm, diaphoresis, hypertension, back pain, loss of consciousness, and flushing have also been reported less commonly. Incidence is primarily associated with intravenous administration (up to 2%) compared to oral administration (<1%). Infusion should be interrupted and medications for the treatment of anaphylaxis should be available for immediate use. High drug concentration and rate of infusion, as well as presence of polysorbate 80 and benzyl alcohol in the etoposide intravenous formulation have been suggested as contributing factors to the development of hypersensitivity reactions. Etoposide intravenous formulations may contain polysorbate 80 and/or benzyl alcohol, while etoposide phosphate (the water soluble prodrug of etoposide) intravenous formulation does not contain either vehicle. Case reports have suggested that etoposide phosphate has been used successfully in patients with previous hypersensitivity reactions to etoposide (Collier, 2008; Siderov, 2002). The use of concentrations higher than recommended were associated with higher rates of anaphylactic-like reactions in children.

Secondary acute leukemias have been reported with etoposide, either as monotherapy or in combination with other chemotherapy agents. Must be diluted; do not give IV push, infuse over at least 30 to 60 minutes; hypotension is associated with rapid infusion. If hypotension occurs, interrupt infusion and administer IV hydration and supportive care; decrease infusion upon reinitiation. Etoposide is an irritant; tissue irritation and inflammation have occurred following extravasation. Do not administer IM or SubQ. Dosage should be adjusted in patients with hepatic or renal impairment (Canadian labeling contraindicates use in severe hepatic and/or renal impairment). Use with caution in patients with low serum albumin; may increase risk for toxicities. Use with caution in elderly patients; may be more likely to develop severe myelosuppression and/or GI effects (eg, nausea/vomiting). **[U.S. Boxed Warning]: Should be administered under the supervision of an experienced cancer chemotherapy physician.**

Oral etoposide is associated with a low (adults) or moderate (children) emetic potential; antiemetics may be recommended to prevent nausea and vomiting (Dupuis, 2011; Roila, 2010). Potentially significant drug-drug interactions may exist, requiring dose or frequency adjustment, additional monitoring, and/or selection of alternative therapy.

Injectable formulation contains polysorbate 80; do not use in premature infants. Injectable formulation contains alcohol (~33% v/v); may contribute to adverse reactions, especially with higher etoposide doses.

Benzyl alcohol and derivatives: Some dosage forms may contain benzyl alcohol; large amounts of benzyl alcohol (≥99 mg/kg/day) have been associated with a potentially fatal toxicity ("gasping syndrome") in neonates; the "gasping syndrome" consists of metabolic acidosis, respiratory distress, gasping respirations, CNS dysfunction (including convulsions, intracranial hemorrhage), hypotension, and cardiovascular collapse (AAP, 1997; CDC, 1982); some data suggests that benzoate displaces bilirubin from protein binding sites (Ahlfors, 2001); avoid or use dosage forms containing benzyl alcohol with caution in neonates. See manufacturer's labeling.

Adverse Reactions Note: The following may occur with higher doses used in stem cell transplantation: Alopecia, ethanol intoxication, hepatitis, hypotension (infusion-related), metabolic acidosis, mucositis, nausea and vomiting (severe), secondary malignancy, skin lesions (resembling Stevens-Johnson syndrome).

Cardiovascular: Hypotension (due to rapid infusion)

Dermatologic: Alopecia

Gastrointestinal: Abdominal pain, anorexia, diarrhea, nausea/vomiting, stomatitis

Hematologic: Anemia, leukopenia (nadir: 7-14 days; recovery: By day 20), thrombocytopenia (nadir: 9-16 days; recovery: By day 20)

Hepatic: Hepatic toxicity

Neuromuscular & skeletal: Peripheral neuropathy

Miscellaneous: Anaphylactic-like reaction (including chills, fever, tachycardia, bronchospasm, dyspnea)

Rare but important or life-threatening: Amenorrhea, blindness (transient/cortical), cyanosis, extravasation (induration/necrosis), facial swelling, hypersensitivity, hypersensitivity-associated apnea, interstitial pneumonitis, laryngospasm, maculopapular rash, metabolic acidosis, MI, mucositis, myocardial ischemia, optic neuritis, perivasculitis, pruritus, pulmonary fibrosis, radiation-recall dermatitis, rash, reversible posterior leukoencephalopathy syndrome (RPLS), seizure, Stevens-Johnson syndrome, tongue swelling, toxic epidermal necrolysis, toxic megacolon, vasospasm

Drug Interactions

Metabolism/Transport Effects Substrate of CYP1A2 (minor), CYP2E1 (minor), CYP3A4 (major), P-glycoprotein; **Note:** Assignment of Major/Minor substrate status based on clinically relevant drug interaction potential; **Inhibits** CYP2C9 (weak), CYP3A4 (weak)

Avoid Concomitant Use

Avoid concomitant use of Etoposide with any of the following: BCG; CloZAPine; Conivaptan; Dipyrone; Fusidic Acid (Systemic); Idelalisib; Natalizumab; Pimecrolimus; Pimozide; Tacrolimus (Topical); Tofacitinib; Vaccines (Live)

Increased Effect/Toxicity

Etoposide may increase the levels/effects of: ARIPiprazole; CloZAPine; Dofetilide; Hydrocodone; Leflunomide; Lomitapide; Natalizumab; Pimozide; Tofacitinib; Vaccines (Live); Vitamin K Antagonists

The levels/effects of Etoposide may be increased by: Aprepitant; Atovaquone; Ceritinib; Conivaptan; CycloSPORINE (Systemic); CYP3A4 Inhibitors (Moderate); CYP3A4 Inhibitors (Strong); Dasatinib; Denosumab; Dipyrone; Fosaprepitant; Fusidic Acid (Systemic); Idelalisib; Ivacaftor; Luliconazole; Mifepristone; Netupitant; P-glycoprotein/ABCB1 Inhibitors; Pimecrolimus; Roflumilast; Simeprevir; Stiripentol; Tacrolimus (Topical); Trastuzumab

Decreased Effect

Etoposide may decrease the levels/effects of: BCG; Coccidioides immitis Skin Test; Sipuleucel-T; Vaccines (Inactivated); Vaccines (Live)

The levels/effects of Etoposide may be decreased by: Barbiturates; Bosentan; CYP3A4 Inducers (Moderate); CYP3A4 Inducers (Strong); Dabrafenib; Deferasirox; Fosphenytoin; Mitotane; P-glycoprotein/ABCB1 Inducers; Phenytoin; Siltuximab; St Johns Wort; Tocilizumab

Preparation for Administration Hazardous agent; use appropriate precautions for handling and disposal (NIOSH 2014 [group 1]). Etoposide should be diluted to a concentration of 0.2 to 0.4 mg/mL in D_5W or NS for administration. Diluted solutions have concentration-dependent stability: More concentrated solutions have shorter stability times. Precipitation may occur with concentrations >0.4 mg/mL.

Storage/Stability

Capsules: Store oral capsules at 2°C to 8°C (36°F to 46°F); do not freeze. Dispense in a light-resistant container.

Injection: Store intact vials of injection at 20°C to 25°C (68°F to 77°F; do not freeze. According to the manufacturer's labeling, stability for solutions diluted for infusion in D_5W or NS (in glass or plastic containers) varies based on concentration; 0.2 mg/mL solutions are stable for 96 hours at room temperature and 0.4 mg/mL solutions are stable for 24 hours at room temperature (precipitation may occur at concentrations above 0.4 mg/mL).

Etoposide injection contains polysorbate 80 which may cause leaching of diethylhexyl phthalate (DEHP), a plasticizer contained in polyvinyl chloride (PVC) bags and tubing. Higher concentrations and longer storage time after preparation in PVC bags may increase DEHP leaching. Preparation in glass or polyolefin containers will minimize patient exposure to DEHP. When undiluted etoposide injection is stored in acrylic or ABS (acrylonitrile, butadiene and styrene) plastic containers, the containers may crack and leak.

Mechanism of Action Etoposide has been shown to delay transit of cells through the S phase and arrest cells in late S or early G_2 phase. The drug may inhibit mitochondrial transport at the NADH dehydrogenase level or inhibit uptake of nucleosides into HeLa cells. It is a topoisomerase II inhibitor and appears to cause DNA strand breaks. Etoposide does not inhibit microtubular assembly.

Pharmacodynamics/Kinetics

Absorption: Oral: Significant inter- and intrapatient variation

Distribution: Average V_d: 7 to 17 L/m²; poor penetration across the blood-brain barrier; CSF concentrations <5% of plasma concentrations

Protein binding: 94% to 98%

Metabolism: Hepatic, via CYP3A4 and 3A5, to various metabolites; in addition, conversion of etoposide to the O-demethylated metabolites (catechol and quinine) via prostaglandin synthases or myeloperoxidase occurs, as well as glutathione and glucuronide conjugation via GSTT1/GSTP1 and UGT1A1 (Yang, 2009)

Bioavailability: Oral: ~50% (range: 25% to 75%)

Half-life elimination: Terminal: IV: 4 to 11 hours; Children: Normal renal/hepatic function: 6 to 8 hours

Excretion:

Children: IV: Urine (~55% as unchanged drug) in 24 hours

Adults: IV: Urine (56%; 45% as unchanged drug) within 120 hours; feces (44%) within 120 hours

Dosage Note: Oral etoposide is associated with a low (adults) or moderate (children) emetic potential; antiemetics may be recommended to prevent nausea and vomiting (Dupuis, 2011; Roila, 2010).

Children (off-label uses):

Acute myeloid leukemia (AML) induction (combination chemotherapy; Woods, 1996): IV:

<3 years: 3.3 mg/kg/day continuous infusion for 4 days

≥3 years: 100 mg/m²/day continuous infusion for 4 days

Central nervous system tumors (combination chemotherapy): IV:

<3 years: 6.5 mg/kg/dose days 3 and 4 of each 28-day "B" treatment cycle (Duffner, 1993)

≥3 years: 100 mg/m²/day on days 1, 2, and 3 of a 3-week treatment cycle (Taylor, 2003)

≥6 years: 150 mg/m²/day on days 3 and 4 of a 3-week treatment course (Kovnar, 1990)

Hematopoietic stem cell transplant conditioning regimen: IV: 60 mg/kg/dose over 4 hours as a single dose 3 or 4 days prior to transplantation (Horning, 1994; Snyder, 1993)

Hodgkin lymphoma: IV: 200 mg/m²/day on days 1, 2, and 3 every 3 weeks (Kelly, 2002)

Neuroblastoma: IV:

Induction: 100 mg/m²/day on days 1-5 of each cycle (Kaneko, 2002)

Hematopoietic stem cell transplant conditioning regimen: 200 mg/m²/day for 4 days beginning 8 or 9 days prior to transplantation (Kaneko, 2002)

Sarcoma, refractory: IV: 100 mg/m²/day on days 1-5 of cycle; repeat cycle every 21 days (Van Winkle, 2005)

Adults:

U.S. labeling:

Small cell lung cancer (combination chemotherapy):

IV: 35 mg/m²/day for 4 days, up to 50 mg/m²/day for 5 days every 3 to 4 weeks

Oral: Due to poor bioavailability, oral doses should be twice the IV dose (and rounded to the nearest 50 mg)

Testicular cancer (combination chemotherapy): IV: 50 to 100 mg/m²/day for days 1 to 5 **or** 100 mg/m²/day on days 1, 3, and 5 repeated every 3 to 4 weeks

Canadian labeling: Non-Hodgkin lymphoma (in combination with other agents), non-small cell lung cancer (alone or in combination), small cell lung cancer (first-line in combination; second-line alone or in combination), testicular cancer (in combination; oral therapy for refractory disease):

IV: 50 to 100 mg/m²/day for 5 days

Oral: 100 to 200 mg/m²/day for 5 days; administer daily doses >200 mg in 2 divided doses.

Adult off-label uses and/or dosing:

Hematopoietic stem cell transplant conditioning regimen, lymphoid malignancies: IV: 60 mg/kg over 4 hours as a single dose 3 or 4 days prior to transplantation (Horning, 1994; Snyder, 1993; Weaver, 1994)

Non-small cell lung cancer: IV: 100 mg/m² days 1, 2, and 3 every 3 weeks for 4 cycles or every 4 weeks for 3 to 4 cycles (in combination with cisplatin) (Arriagada, 2004) **or** 50 mg/m² days 1 to 5 and days 29 to 33 (in combination with cisplatin and radiation therapy) (Albain, 2009)

Ovarian cancer, refractory: Oral: 50 mg/m² once daily for 21 days every 4 weeks until disease progression or unacceptable toxicity (Rose, 1998)

Small cell lung cancer, limited stage (combination chemotherapy): IV: 120 mg/m²/day on days 1, 2, and 3 every 3 weeks for 4 courses (Turrisi, 1999) **or** 100 mg/m²/day on days 1, 2, and 3 for induction therapy, followed by consolidation chemotherapy (Saito, 2006) **or** 100 mg/m²/day on days 1, 2, and 3 every 3 weeks up to a maximum of 6 cycles (Skarlos, 2001) **or** 100 mg/m²/day IV on day 1, followed by 200 mg/m²/day **orally** on days 2 through 4 every 3 weeks for a maximum of 5 courses (Sundstrom, 2002)

Small cell lung cancer, extensive stage (combination chemotherapy): 100 mg/m²/day IV on days 1, 2, and 3 every 3 weeks for 4 cycles (Lara, 2009) **or** 100 mg/m²/day IV on day 1, followed by 200 mg/m²/day **orally** on days 2 through 4 every 3 weeks for a maximum of 5 courses (Sundstrom, 2002) **or** IV: 80 mg/m²/day on days 1, 2, and 3 every 3 weeks up to 8 cycles (Ihede, 1994)

Testicular cancer (combination chemotherapy):

Nonseminoma: IV: 100 mg/m²/day on days 1 through 5 every 21 days for 3 to 4 courses (Saxman, 1998)

Nonseminoma, metastatic (high-dose regimens): IV: 750 mg/m²/day administered 5, 4, and 3 days before peripheral blood stem cell infusion, repeat for a second cycle after recovery of granulocyte and platelet counts (Einhorn, 2007) **or** 400 mg/m²/day (beginning on cycle 3) on days 1, 2, and 3, with peripheral blood stem cell support, administered at 14- to 21-day intervals for 3 cycles (Kondagunta, 2007)

Thymoma, locally advanced or metastatic: IV: 120 mg/m² days 1, 2, and 3 every 3 weeks (in combination with cisplatin) for up to 8 cycles (Giaccone, 1996)

Unknown primary adenocarcinoma: Oral: 50 mg once daily on days 1, 3, 5, 7, and 9 alternating with 100 mg once daily on days 2, 4, 6, 8, and 10 every 3 weeks (in combination with paclitaxel and carboplatin) (Greco, 2000; Hainsworth, 2006)

Dosage adjustment for toxicity: Oral, IV:

Infusion (hypersensitivity) reactions: Interrupt infusion.

ANC <500/mm^3 or platelets <50,000/mm^3: Withhold treatment until recovery.

Severe adverse reactions (nonhematologic): Reduce dose or discontinue treatment.

WBC 2000-3000/mm^3 or platelets 75,000 to 100,000/mm^3: Canadian labeling (not in U.S. labeling): Reduce dose by 50%.

Dosage adjustment in renal impairment: Oral, IV:

The manufacturer's U.S. labeling recommends the following adjustments:

CrCl >50 mL/minute: No adjustment required.

CrCl 15 to 50 mL/minute: Administer 75% of dose.

CrCl <15 mL minute: Data not available; consider further dose reductions.

The following adjustments have also been recommended:

Aronoff, 2007:

Children:

CrCl 10 to 50 mL/minute/1.73 m^2: Administer 75% of dose.

CrCl <10 mL minute/1.73 m^2: Administer 50% of dose.

Hemodialysis: Administer 50% of dose.

Peritoneal dialysis: Administer 50% of dose.

Continuous renal replacement therapy (CRRT): Administer 75% of dose and reduce for hyperbilirubinemia.

Adults:

CrCl 10 to 50 mL/minute: Administer 75% of dose.

CrCl <10 mL minute: Administer 50% of dose.

Hemodialysis: Administer 50% of dose; supplemental posthemodialysis dose is not necessary.

Peritoneal dialysis: Administer 50% of dose; supplemental dose is not necessary.

Continuous renal replacement therapy (CRRT): Administer 75% of dose.

Janus, 2010: Hemodialysis: Reduce dose by 50%; not removed by hemodialysis so may be administered before or after dialysis.

Kintzel, 1995:

CrCl 46 to 60 mL/minute: Administer 85% of dose.

CrCl 31 to 45 mL/minute: Administer 80% of dose.

CrCl ≤30 mL/minute: Administer 75% of dose.

Dosage adjustment in hepatic impairment:

Manufacturer's U.S. labeling: There are no dosage adjustments provided in the manufacturer's labeling.

Canadian labeling:

Mild-to-moderate impairment: There are no dosage adjustments provided in the manufacturer's labeling.

Severe impairment: Use is contraindicated.

The following adjustments have also been recommended:

Donelli, 1998: Liver dysfunction may reduce the metabolism and increase the toxicity of etoposide. Normal doses of IV etoposide should be given to patients with liver dysfunction (dose reductions may result in subtherapeutic concentrations); however, use caution with concomitant liver dysfunction (severe) and renal dysfunction as the decreased metabolic clearance cannot be compensated by increased renal clearance.

Floyd, 2006: Bilirubin 1.5 to 3 mg/dL or AST >3 times ULN: Administer 50% of dose

King, 2001; Koren, 1992: Bilirubin 1.5 to 3 mg/dL or AST >180 units/L: Administer 50% of dose

Dosing in obesity:

*American Society of Clinical Oncology (ASCO) Guidelines for appropriate chemotherapy dosing in obese adults with cancer (**Note:** Excludes HSCT dosing):* Utilize patient's actual body weight (full weight) for calculation of body surface area- or weight-based dosing, particularly when the intent of therapy is curative; manage regimen-related toxicities in the same manner as for nonobese patients; if a dose reduction is utilized due to toxicity, consider resumption of full weight-based dosing with subsequent cycles, especially if cause of toxicity (eg, hepatic or renal impairment) is resolved (Griggs, 2012).

American Society for Blood and Marrow Transplantation (ASBMT) practice guideline committee position statement on chemotherapy dosing in obesity: Utilize actual body weight (full weight) for calculation of body surface area (BSA) for BSA-based dosing and utilize adjusted body weight 25% (ABW25) for mg/kg dosing for hematopoietic stem cell transplant conditioning regimens in adults (Bubalo, 2014).

ABW25: Adjusted wt (kg) = Ideal body weight (kg) + 0.25 [actual wt (kg) - ideal body weight (kg)]

Administration

Oral etoposide is associated with a low (adults) or moderate (children) emetic potential; antiemetics may be recommended to prevent nausea and vomiting (Dupuis, 2011; Roila, 2010).

Oral: Doses ≤200 mg/day as a single once daily dose; doses >200 mg should be given in 2 divided doses. If necessary, the injection may be used for oral administration (see Extemporaneous Preparations). Canadian labeling recommends administering capsule on an empty stomach.

IV: Administer standard doses over at least 30 to 60 minutes to minimize the risk of hypotension. Higher (off-label) doses used in transplantation may be infused over longer time periods depending on the protocol. Etoposide injection contains polysorbate 80 which may cause leaching of diethylhexyl phthalate (DEHP), a plasticizer contained in polyvinyl chloride (PVC) tubing. Administration through non-PVC (low sorbing) tubing will minimize patient exposure to DEHP. Etoposide is an irritant; tissue irritation and inflammation have occurred following extravasation; avoid extravasation.

Concentrations >0.4 mg/mL are very unstable and may precipitate within a few minutes. For large doses, where dilution to ≤0.4 mg/mL is not feasible, consideration should be given to slow infusion of the undiluted drug through a running normal saline, dextrose or saline/dextrose infusion; or use of etoposide phosphate. Due to the risk for precipitation, an inline filter may be used; etoposide solutions of 0.1 to 0.4 mg/mL may be filtered through a 0.22 micron filter without damage to the filter; etoposide solutions of 0.2 mg/mL may be filtered through a 0.22 micron filter without significant loss of drug.

Hazardous agent; use appropriate precautions for handling and disposal (NIOSH 2014 [group 1]).

Monitoring Parameters CBC with differential; liver function (bilirubin, ALT, AST), albumin, renal function tests; vital signs (blood pressure); signs of an infusion reaction

Dosage Forms

Capsule, Oral:

Generic: 50 mg

Solution, Intravenous:

Toposar: 100 mg/5 mL (5 mL); 500 mg/25 mL (25 mL); 1 g/50 mL (50 mL)

Generic: 100 mg/5 mL (5 mL); 500 mg/25 mL (25 mL); 1 g/50 mL (50 mL)

Extemporaneous Preparations Hazardous agent: Use appropriate precautions for handling and disposal (NIOSH 2014 [group 1]).

Etoposide 10 mg/mL oral solution: Dilute etoposide for injection 1:1 with normal saline to a concentration of 10 mg/mL. This solution is stable in plastic oral syringes for 22 days at room temperature. Prior to oral administration, further mix with fruit juice (orange, apple, or lemon; **NOT** grapefruit juice) to a concentration of <0.4 mg/mL; once mixed with fruit juice, use within 3 hours.

McLeod HL and Relling MV, "Stability of Etoposide Solution for Oral Use," *Am J Hosp Pharm*, 1992, 49(11):2784-5.

◆ **Etoposide Injection (Can)** *see* Etoposide *on page 816*

◆ **Etoposide Injection USP (Can)** *see* Etoposide *on page 816*

Etoposide Phosphate (e toe POE side FOS fate)

Brand Names: U.S. Etopophos

Index Terms Epipodophyllotoxin; ETOP

Pharmacologic Category Antineoplastic Agent, Podophyllotoxin Derivative; Antineoplastic Agent, Topoisomerase II Inhibitor

Use Treatment of refractory testicular tumors; treatment of small cell lung cancer

Pregnancy Risk Factor D

Pregnancy Considerations Animal studies have demonstrated teratogenicity and fetal loss. There are no adequate and well-controlled studies in pregnant women. Women of childbearing potential should be advised to avoid pregnancy.

Breast-Feeding Considerations Due to the potential for serious adverse reactions in the nursing infant, breast feeding is not recommended.

Contraindications Hypersensitivity to etoposide, etoposide phosphate, or any component of the formulation

Warnings/Precautions Hazardous agent - use appropriate precautions for handling and disposal (NIOSH 2014 [group 1]). **[U.S. Boxed Warning]: Severe dose-limiting and dose-related myelosuppression with resulting infection or bleeding may occur.** Treatment should be withheld for platelets <50,000/mm^3 or absolute neutrophil count (ANC) <500/mm^3. May cause anaphylactic-like reactions manifested by chills, fever, tachycardia, bronchospasm, dyspnea, and hypotension. In addition, facial/tongue swelling, coughing, throat tightness, cyanosis, laryngospasm, diaphoresis, back pain, hypertension, flushing, apnea and loss of consciousness have also been reported less commonly. Anaphylactic-type reactions have occurred with the first infusion. Infusion should be interrupted and medications for the treatment of anaphylaxis should be available for immediate use. Underlying mechanisms behind the development of hypersensitivity reactions is unknown, but have been attributed to high drug concentration and rate of infusion. Another possible mechanism may be due to the differences between available etoposide intravenous formulations. Etoposide intravenous formulation contains polysorbate 80 and benzyl alcohol, while etoposide phosphate (the water soluble prodrug of etoposide) intravenous formulation does not contain either vehicle. Case reports have suggested that etoposide phosphate has been used successfully in patients with previous hypersensitivity reactions to etoposide (Collier, 2008; Siderov, 2002).

Secondary acute leukemias have been reported with etoposide, either as monotherapy or in combination with other chemotherapy agents. Dosage should be adjusted in patients with hepatic or renal impairment. Use with caution in patients with low serum albumin; may increase risk for toxicities. Doses of etoposide phosphate >175 mg/m^2 have not been evaluated. Use caution in elderly patients (may be more likely to develop severe myelosuppression and/or GI effects. Administer by slow IV infusion; hypotension has been reported with etoposide phosphate administration, generally associated with rapid IV infusion. Injection site reactions may occur; monitor infusion site closely. **[U.S. Boxed Warning]: Should be administered under the supervision of an experienced cancer chemotherapy physician.**

Adverse Reactions Note: Also see adverse reactions for **etoposide;** etoposide phosphate is converted to etoposide, adverse reactions experienced with etoposide would also be expected with etoposide phosphate.

Cardiovascular: Facial flushing, hyper-/hypotension

Central nervous system: Chills/fever, dizziness

Dermatologic: Alopecia, skin rash

Gastrointestinal: Abdominal pain, anorexia, constipation, diarrhea (6%), mucositis, nausea/vomiting, taste perversion (6%)

Hematologic: Anemia, leukopenia, neutropenia, thrombocytopenia

Local: Extravasation/phlebitis (including swelling, pain, cellulitis, necrosis, and/or skin necrosis at site of infiltration)

Neuromuscular & skeletal: Weakness/malaise

Miscellaneous: Anaphylactic-type reactions (including chills, diaphoresis, fever, rigor, tachycardia, bronchospasm, dyspnea, pruritus)

Rare but important or life-threatening: Acute leukemia (with/without preleukemia phase), anaphylactic-like reactions, blindness (transient, cortical), cyanosis, dysphagia, erythema, facial swelling, hepatic toxicity, hyperpigmentation, hypersensitivity-associated apnea, infection, interstitial pneumonitis, laryngospasm, maculopapular rash, neutropenic fever, optic neuritis, perivasculitis, pruritus, pulmonary fibrosis, radiation recall dermatitis, seizure, Stevens-Johnson syndrome, tongue swelling, toxic epidermal necrolysis, urticaria

Drug Interactions

Metabolism/Transport Effects Substrate of CYP1A2 (minor), CYP2E1 (minor), CYP3A4 (major), P-glycoprotein; **Note:** Assignment of Major/Minor substrate status based on clinically relevant drug interaction potential; **Inhibits** CYP2C9 (weak), CYP3A4 (weak)

Avoid Concomitant Use

Avoid concomitant use of Etoposide Phosphate with any of the following: BCG; CloZAPine; Conivaptan; Dipyrone; Fusidic Acid (Systemic); Idelalisib; Natalizumab; Pimecrolimus; Pimozide; Tacrolimus (Topical); Tofacitinib; Vaccines (Live)

Increased Effect/Toxicity

Etoposide Phosphate may increase the levels/effects of: ARIPiprazole; CloZAPine; Dofetilide; Hydrocodone; Leflunomide; Lomitapide; Natalizumab; Pimozide; Tofacitinib; Vaccines (Live)

The levels/effects of Etoposide Phosphate may be increased by: Aprepitant; Ceritinib; Conivaptan; CycloSPORINE (Systemic); CYP3A4 Inhibitors (Moderate); CYP3A4 Inhibitors (Strong); Dasatinib; Denosumab; Dipyrone; Fosaprepitant; Fusidic Acid (Systemic); Idelalisib; Ivacaftor; Luliconazole; Mifepristone; Netupitant; P-glycoprotein/ABCB1 Inhibitors; Pimecrolimus; Roflumilast; Simeprevir; Stiripentol; Tacrolimus (Topical); Trastuzumab

Decreased Effect

Etoposide Phosphate may decrease the levels/effects of: BCG; Coccidioides immitis Skin Test; Sipuleucel-T; Vaccines (Inactivated); Vaccines (Live)

The levels/effects of Etoposide Phosphate may be decreased by: Barbiturates; Bosentan; CYP3A4 Inducers (Moderate); CYP3A4 Inducers (Strong); Dabrafenib; Deferasirox; Echinacea; Fosphenytoin; Mitotane; P-glycoprotein/ABCB1 Inducers; Phenytoin; Siltuximab; St Johns Wort; Tocilizumab

Preparation for Administration Hazardous agent; use appropriate precautions for handling and disposal (NIOSH 2014 [group 1]). Reconstitute vials with 5 mL or 10 mL SWFI, D_5W, NS, bacteriostatic SWFI, or bacteriostatic NS to a concentration of 20 mg/mL or 10 mg/mL etoposide equivalent. These solutions may be administered without further dilution or may be diluted in 50-500 mL of D_5W or NS to a concentration as low as 0.1 mg/mL.

Storage/Stability Store intact vials under refrigeration at 2°C to 8°C (36°F to 46°F). Protect from light. Reconstituted solution is stable refrigerated at 2°C to 8°C (36°F to 46°F) for 7 days. At room temperature of 20°C to 25°C (68°F to 77°F), reconstituted solutions are stable for 24 hours when reconstituted with SWFI, D_5W, or NS, or for 48 hours when reconstituted with bacteriostatic SWFI or bacteriostatic NS. Further diluted solutions for infusion are stable at room temperature 20°C to 25°C (68°F to 77°F) or under refrigeration 2°C to 8°C (36°F to 46°F) for up to 24 hours.

Mechanism of Action Etoposide phosphate is converted *in vivo* to the active moiety, etoposide, by dephosphorylation. Etoposide inhibits mitotic activity; inhibits cells from entering prophase; inhibits DNA synthesis. Initially thought to be mitotic inhibitors similar to podophyllotoxin, but actually have no effect on microtubule assembly. However, later shown to induce DNA strand breakage and inhibition of topoisomerase II (an enzyme which breaks and repairs DNA); etoposide acts in late S or early G2 phases.

Pharmacodynamics/Kinetics

Distribution: Average V_d: 7-17 L/m^2; poor penetration across blood-brain barrier; concentrations in CSF being <10% that of plasma

Protein binding: 97%

Metabolism:

Etoposide phosphate: Rapidly and completely converted to etoposide in plasma

Etoposide: Hepatic, via CYP3A4 and 3A5 to various metabolites; in addition, conversion of etoposide to the O-demethylated metabolites (catechol and quinine) via prostaglandin synthases or myeloperoxidase occurs, as well as glutathione and glucuronide conjugation via GSTT1/GSTP1 and UGT1A1 (Yang, 2009)

Half-life elimination: Terminal: 4-11 hours; Children: Normal renal/hepatic function: 6-8 hours

Excretion: Urine (56%; 45% as etoposide) within 120 hours; feces (44%) within 120 hours

Children: Urine (~55% as etoposide) in 24 hours

Dosage Adults: **Note:** Etoposide phosphate is a prodrug of etoposide; equivalent doses should be used when converting from etoposide to etoposide phosphate. Each 100 mg vial of etoposide phosphate is equivalent to 100 mg of etoposide.

Small cell lung cancer (in combination with other approved chemotherapeutic drugs): IV: Etoposide 35 mg/m^2/day for 4 days up to 50 mg/m^2/day for 5 days. Courses are repeated at 3- to 4-week intervals after adequate recovery from toxicity.

Testicular cancer (in combination with other approved chemotherapeutic agents): IV: Etoposide 50-100 mg/m^2/day on days 1-5 to 100 mg/m^2/day on days 1, 3, and 5. Courses are repeated at 3- to 4-week intervals after adequate recovery from toxicity.

Indication-specific off-label dosing: Refer to Etoposide monograph.

Dosage adjustment in renal impairment:

Manufacturer recommended guidelines:

CrCl >50 mL/minute: No adjustment required

CrCl 15-50 mL/minute: Administer 75% of dose

CrCl <15 mL minute: Data are not available; consider further dose reductions

Etoposide phosphate is rapidly and completely converted to etoposide in plasma, please refer to Etoposide monograph for additional renal dosing adjustments (for etoposide).

Dosage adjustment in hepatic impairment: The FDA-approved labeling does not contain dosing adjustment guidelines. Etoposide phosphate is rapidly and completely converted to etoposide in plasma; please refer to Etoposide monograph for etoposide hepatic dosing adjustments.

Dosing in obesity: *ASCO Guidelines for appropriate chemotherapy dosing in obese adults with cancer (**Note:** Excludes HSCT dosing):* Utilize patient's actual body weight (full weight) for calculation of body surface area- or weight-based dosing, particularly when the intent of therapy is curative; manage regimen-related toxicities in the same manner as for nonobese patients; if a dose reduction is utilized due to toxicity, consider resumption of full weight-based dosing with subsequent cycles, especially if cause of toxicity (eg, hepatic or renal impairment) is resolved (Griggs, 2012).

Administration Infuse by slow IV infusion over 5 to 210 minutes; risk of hypotension may increase with rate of infusion. Do not administer as a bolus injection.

Hazardous agent; use appropriate precautions for handling and disposal (NIOSH 2014 [group 1]).

Monitoring Parameters CBC with differential and platelets (prior to initial treatment and each cycle), vital signs (blood pressure), bilirubin, AST/ALT, renal function

Additional Information Each 100 mg vial of etoposide phosphate is equivalent to 100 mg of etoposide. Equivalent doses should be used when converting from etoposide to etoposide phosphate.

Dosage Forms

Solution Reconstituted, Intravenous:

Etopophos: 100 mg (1 ea)

Etoricoxib [INT] (e toe ri KOKS ib)

International Brand Names Acoxxel (RU); Arcoxia (AE, AR, AT, AU, BE, BG, BH, BR, CH, CL, CN, CO, CY, CZ, DE, DK, EC, EE, FI, FR, GB, GR, HK, HN, HR, ID, IE, IL, IS, IT, KW, LB, LT, MY, NL, NO, NZ, PE, PH, PT, QA, RO, RU, SA, SE, SG, SI, SK, TH, TR, TW, UY, VE, VN, ZA); Arcoxib (PH); Cox (IN); Doricox (IN); Eoxy (TW); Exinef (DE); Exxiv (PT, RU); Goutix (VN); Novlen (PY); Ranacox (BE); Tauxib (SE); Turox (GR, PT, SE); Xibra-90 (PH)

Pharmacologic Category Analgesic, Nonsteroidal Anti-inflammatory Drug; Nonsteroidal Anti-inflammatory Drug (NSAID), COX-2 Selective

Reported Use Treatment of pain and inflammation in osteoarthritis, dental surgery (postoperative), rheumatoid arthritis, ankylosing spondylitis, and acute gouty arthritis

Dosage Range Adolescents >16 years and Adults: Oral:

Osteoarthritis: 30-60 mg once daily

Rheumatoid arthritis: 90 mg once daily

Acute gouty arthritis: 120 mg once daily

Ankylosing spondylitis: 90 mg once daily

Postoperative dental surgery pain: 90 mg once daily

Product Availability Product available in various countries; not currently available in the U.S.

Dosage Forms

Tablet: 60 mg, 90 mg, 120 mg

◆ **ETR** *see* Etravirine *on page* *821*

Etravirine (et ra VIR een)

Brand Names: U.S. Intelence

Brand Names: Canada Intelence®

Index Terms ETR; TMC125

Pharmacologic Category Antiretroviral, Reverse Transcriptase Inhibitor, Non-nucleoside (Anti-HIV)

Use Treatment of HIV-1 infection in combination with at least two additional antiretroviral agents in treatment-experienced patients exhibiting viral replication with documented non-nucleoside reverse transcriptase inhibitor (NNRTI) resistance

Pregnancy Risk Factor B

Dosage Oral:

Children 6 to <18 years:
- ≥16 kg to <20 kg: 100 mg twice daily
- ≥20 kg to <25 kg: 125 mg twice daily
- ≥25 kg to <30 kg: 150 mg twice daily
- ≥30 kg: 200 mg twice daily

Adults: 200 mg twice daily

Dosage adjustment in renal impairment: No dosage adjustment necessary

Due to extensive protein binding, significant removal by hemodialysis or peritoneal dialysis is unlikely.

Dosage adjustment in hepatic impairment:

Mild-to-moderate impairment (Child-Pugh class A or B): No dosage adjustment necessary.

Severe impairment (Child-Pugh class C): There are no dosage adjustments provided in the manufacturer's labeling (has not been studied).

Additional Information Complete prescribing information should be consulted for additional detail.

Dosage Forms

Tablet, Oral:

Intelence: 25 mg, 100 mg, 200 mg

- ◆ **Euflex (Can)** *see* Flutamide *on page 907*
- ◆ **Euflexxa** *see* Hyaluronate and Derivatives *on page 1006*
- ◆ **Euglucon (Can)** *see* GlyBURIDE *on page 972*
- ◆ **Eulexin** *see* Flutamide *on page 907*
- ◆ ***Euphorbia peplus* Derivative** *see* Ingenol Mebutate *on page 1083*
- ◆ **Eurax** *see* Crotamiton *on page 514*
- ◆ **Eurax Cream (Can)** *see* Crotamiton *on page 514*
- ◆ **Euro-Cyproheptadine (Can)** *see* Cyproheptadine *on page 529*
- ◆ **Euro-Docusate C [OTC] (Can)** *see* Docusate *on page 661*
- ◆ **Euro-Lac (Can)** *see* Lactulose *on page 1156*
- ◆ **Eutectic Mixture of Lidocaine and Tetracaine** *see* Lidocaine and Tetracaine *on page 1214*
- ◆ **Evac [OTC]** *see* Psyllium *on page 1744*
- ◆ **Evamist** *see* Estradiol (Systemic) *on page 775*

Everolimus (e ver OH li mus)

Brand Names: U.S. Afinitor; Afinitor Disperz; Zortress

Brand Names: Canada Afinitor

Index Terms RAD001

Pharmacologic Category Antineoplastic Agent, mTOR Kinase Inhibitor; Immunosuppressant Agent; mTOR Kinase Inhibitor

Use

Breast cancer, advanced (Afinitor only): Treatment of advanced hormone receptor-positive, HER2-negative breast cancer in postmenopausal women (in combination with exemestane and after letrozole or anastrozole failure)

Pancreatic neuroendocrine tumors (Afinitor only): Treatment of advanced, metastatic or unresectable pancreatic neuroendocrine tumors (PNET)

Limitations of use: Not indicated for the treatment of functional carcinoid tumors.

Renal angiomyolipoma with tuberous sclerosis complex (Afinitor only): Treatment of renal angiomyolipoma with tuberous sclerosis complex (TSC) not requiring immediate surgery

Renal cell carcinoma, advanced (Afinitor only): Treatment of advanced renal cell cancer (RCC) after sunitinib or sorafenib failure

Subependymal giant cell astrocytoma (Afinitor or Afinitor Disperz only): Treatment of subependymal giant cell astrocytoma (SEGA) associated with TSC which requires intervention, but cannot be curatively resected

Liver transplantation (Zortress only): Prophylaxis of organ rejection in liver transplantation (in combination with corticosteroids and reduced doses of tacrolimus)

Renal transplantation (Zortress only): Prophylaxis of organ rejection in renal transplant patients at low to moderate immunologic risk (in combination with basiliximab induction and concurrent with corticosteroids and reduced doses of cyclosporine)

Pregnancy Risk Factor D (Afinitor) / C (Zortress)

Pregnancy Considerations Adverse events were observed in animal reproduction studies with exposures lower than expected with human doses. Based on the mechanism of action, may cause fetal harm if administered during pregnancy. Women of reproductive potential should be advised to avoid pregnancy and use highly effective birth control during treatment and for up to 8 weeks after everolimus discontinuation.

The National Transplantation Pregnancy Registry (NTPR) (Temple University) is a registry for pregnant women taking immunosuppressants following any solid organ transplant. The NTPR encourages reporting of all immunosuppressant exposures during pregnancy in transplant recipients at 877-955-6877.

Breast-Feeding Considerations It is not known if everolimus is excreted in breast milk. Due to the potential for serious adverse reactions in the nursing infant, breastfeeding should be avoided.

Contraindications Hypersensitivity to everolimus, sirolimus, other rapamycin derivatives, or any component of the formulation.

Warnings/Precautions Hazardous agent - use appropriate precautions for handling and disposal (NIOSH 2014 [group 1]). To avoid potential contact with everolimus, caregivers should wear gloves when preparing suspension from tablets for oral suspension. Noninfectious pneumonitis (sometimes fatal) has been observed with mTOR inhibitors including everolimus; symptoms include dyspnea, cough, hypoxia and/or pleural effusion; promptly evaluate worsening respiratory symptoms. Consider opportunistic infections such as *Pneumocystis jiroveci* pneumonia (PCP) when evaluating clinical symptoms. May require treatment interruption followed by dose reduction (pneumonitis has developed even with reduced doses) and/or corticosteroid therapy; discontinue for grade 4 pneumonitis. Consider discontinuation for recurrence of grade 3 toxicity after dosage reduction. In patients who require steroid therapy for symptom management, consider PCP prophylaxis. Imaging may overestimate the incidence of clinical pneumonitis. **[U.S. Boxed Warning]: Everolimus has immunosuppressant properties which may result in infection;** the risk of developing bacterial (including mycobacterial), viral, fungal and protozoal infections and for local, opportunistic (including polyomavirus infection), and/or systemic infections is increased; may lead to sepsis, respiratory failure, hepatic failure, or fatality. Polyomavirus infection in transplant patients may be serious and/or fatal. Polyoma virus-associated nephropathy (due to BK virus), which may result in serious cases of deteriorating renal function and renal graft loss, has been observed with use. JC virus-associated progressive multiple leukoencephalopathy (PML) may also be associated with everolimus use in transplantation. Reduced immunosuppression (taking into account the risks of rejection) should be considered with evidence of polyoma virus infection or PML. Reactivation of hepatitis B has been observed in patients receiving everolimus. Resolve preexisting invasive fungal infections prior to treatment initiation. Cases (some fatal) of *Pneumocystis jiroveci* pneumonia (PCP) have been reported with everolimus use. Consider PCP prophylaxis in patients receiving concomitant corticosteroid or other immunosuppressant therapy. In addition, transplant recipient patients should receive prophylactic therapy for PCP and for cytomegalovirus (CMV). Monitor for signs and symptoms of infection during treatment. Discontinue if invasive systemic fungal infection is diagnosed (and manage with appropriate antifungal therapy).

[U.S. Boxed Warning]: Immunosuppressant use may result in the development of malignancy, including lymphoma and skin cancer. The risk is associated with treatment intensity and the duration of therapy. To minimize the risk for skin cancer, limit exposure to sunlight and ultraviolet light; wear protective clothing and use effective sunscreen.

[U.S. Boxed Warning]: Due to the increased risk for nephrotoxicity in renal transplantation, avoid standard doses of cyclosporine in combination with everolimus; reduced cyclosporine doses are recommended when everolimus is used in combination with cyclosporine. Therapeutic monitoring of cyclosporine and everolimus concentrations is recommended. Monitor for proteinuria; the risk of proteinuria is increased when everolimus is used in combination with cyclosporine, and with higher serum everolimus concentrations. Everolimus and cyclosporine combination therapy may increase the risk for thrombotic microangiopathy/thrombotic thrombocytopenic purpura/hemolytic uremic syndrome (TMA/TTP/HUS); monitor blood counts. Elevations in serum creatinine (generally mild), renal failure, and proteinuria have been also observed with everolimus use; monitor renal function (BUN, creatinine, and/or urinary protein). Risk of nephrotoxicity may be increased when administered with calcineurin inhibitors (eg, cyclosporine, tacrolimus); dosage adjustment of calcineurin inhibitor is necessary. An increased incidence of rash, infection and dose interruptions have been reported in patients with renal insufficiency (CrCl ≤60 mL/minute) who received mTOR inhibitors for the treatment of renal cell cancer (Gupta, 2011); serum creatinine elevations and proteinuria have been reported. Monitor renal function (BUN, serum creatinine, urinary protein) at baseline and periodically, especially if risk factors for further impairment exist; pharmacokinetic studies have not been conducted; dosage adjustments are not required based on renal impairment. **[U.S. Boxed Warning]: An increased risk of renal arterial and venous thrombosis has been reported with use in renal transplantation, generally within the first 30 days after transplant; may result in graft loss.** MTOR inhibitors are associated with an increase in hepatic artery thrombosis, most cases have been reported within 30 days after transplant and usually proceeded to graft loss or death; do not use everolimus prior to 30 days post liver transplant.

Potentially significant drug-drug/drug-food interactions may exist, requiring dose or frequency adjustment, additional monitoring, and/or selection of alternative therapy. In transplant patients, avoid the use of certain HMG-CoA reductase inhibitors (eg, simvastatin, lovastatin); may increase the risk for rhabdomyolysis due to the potential interaction with cyclosporine (which may be given in combination with everolimus for transplantation).

Use is associated with mouth ulcers, mucositis and stomatitis; manage with topical therapy; avoid the use of alcohol-, hydrogen peroxide-, iodine-, or thyme-based mouthwashes (due to the high potential for drug interactions, avoid the use of systemic antifungals unless fungal infection has been diagnosed). Everolimus is associated with the development of angioedema; concomitant use with other agents known to cause angioedema (eg, ACE inhibitors) may increase the risk. Everolimus use may delay wound healing and increase the occurrence of wound-related complications (eg, wound dehiscence, infection, incisional hernia, lymphocele, seroma); may require surgical intervention; use with caution in the perisurgical period. Generalized edema, including peripheral edema and lymphedema, and local fluid accumulation (eg, pericardial effusion, pleural effusion, ascites) may also occur.

Everolimus exposure is increased in patients with hepatic impairment. For patients with breast cancer, PNET, RCC, or renal angiomyolipoma with mild and moderate hepatic impairment, reduced doses are recommended; in patients with severe hepatic impairment, use is recommended (at reduced doses) if the potential benefit outweighs risks. Reduced doses are recommended in transplant patients with hepatic impairment; pharmacokinetic information does not exist for renal transplant patients with severe impairment (Child-Pugh class B or C); monitor whole blood trough levels closely for patients with SEGA, reduced doses may be needed for mild and moderate hepatic impairment (based on therapeutic drug monitoring), and are recommended in severe hepatic impairment; monitor whole blood trough levels. The Canadian labeling recommends against the use of everolimus in patients <18 years of age with SEGA and hepatic impairment.

[U.S. Boxed Warning]: Increased mortality (usually associated with infections) within the first 3 months after transplant was noted in a study of patients with *de novo* heart transplant receiving immunosuppressive regimens containing everolimus (with or without induction therapy). Use in heart transplantation is not recommended. Hyperglycemia, hyperlipidemia, and hypertriglyceridemia have been reported. Higher serum everolimus concentrations are associated with an increased risk for hyperlipidemia. Use has not been studied in patients with baseline cholesterol >350 mg/dL. Monitor fasting glucose and lipid profile prior to treatment initiation and periodically thereafter; monitor more frequently in patients with concomitant medications affecting glucose. Manage with appropriate medical therapy (if possible, optimize glucose control and lipids prior to treatment initiation). Antihyperlipidemic therapy may not normalize levels. May alter insulin and/or oral hypoglycemic therapy requirements in patients with diabetes; the risk for new onset diabetes is increased with everolimus use after transplantation. Decreases in hemoglobin, neutrophils, platelets, and lymphocytes have been reported; monitor blood counts at baseline and periodically. Patients should not be immunized with live viral vaccines during or shortly after treatment and should avoid close contact with recently vaccinated (live vaccine) individuals; consider the timing of routine immunizations prior to the start of therapy in pediatric patients treated for SEGA. Continue treatment with everolimus for renal cell cancer as long as clinical benefit is demonstrated or until occurrence of unacceptable toxicity. Safety and efficacy have not been established for the use of everolimus in the treatment of carcinoid tumors. Decreases in hemoglobin, neutrophils, platelets, and lymphocytes have been reported with use. Increases in serum glucose are common; may alter insulin and/or oral hypoglycemic therapy requirements in patients with diabetes; the risk for new onset diabetes is increased with everolimus use after transplantation. Patients should not be immunized with live viral vaccines during or shortly after treatment and should avoid close contact with recently vaccinated (live vaccine) individuals. In pediatric patients treated for SEGA, complete recommended series of live virus childhood vaccinations prior to treatment (if immediate everolimus treatment is not indicated); an accelerated vaccination schedule may be appropriate. Continue treatment with everolimus for renal cell cancer as long as clinical benefit is demonstrated or until occurrence of unacceptable toxicity.

Tablets (Afinitor, Zortress) and tablets for oral suspension (Afinitor Disperz) are not interchangeable; Afinitor Disperz is only indicated in conjunction with therapeutic monitoring for the treatment of SEGA. Do not combine formulations to achieve total desired dose. May cause infertility; in females, menstrual irregularities, secondary amenorrhea, and increases in luteinizing hormone and follicle-stimulating hormone have occurred; azoospermia and oligospermia have been observed in males. Avoid use in patients with hereditary galactose intolerance, Lapp lactase deficiency, or glucose-galactose malabsorption; may result in diarrhea and malabsorption. The safety and efficacy of everolimus in renal transplantation patients with high-immunologic risk or in solid organ transplant other than renal or liver have not been established. **[U.S. Boxed Warning]: In transplantation, everolimus should only be used by physicians experienced in immunosuppressive therapy and management of transplant patients. Adequate laboratory and supportive medical resources must be readily available.** For indications requiring whole blood trough concentrations to determine dosage adjustments, a consistent method should be used; concentration values from different assay methods may not be interchangeable.

Adverse Reactions

Cardiovascular: Angina pectoris, atrial fibrillation, cardiac failure, chest discomfort, chest pain, deep vein thrombosis, edema (generalized), hypertension (including hypertensive crisis), hypotension, palpitations, peripheral edema, pulmonary embolism, renal artery thrombosis, syncope, tachycardia, venous thromboembolism

Central nervous system: Agitation, behavioral changes (anxiety/aggression/behavioral disturbance; SEGA), chills, depression, dizziness, drowsiness, fatigue, hallucination, headache, hemiparesis, hypoesthesia, insomnia, lethargy, malaise, migraine, neuralgia, paresthesia, seizure

Dermatologic: Acneiform eruption, acne vulgaris, alopecia, cellulitis (SEGA), contact dermatitis, eczema, erythema, excoriation, hyperhidrosis, hypertrichosis, nail disease (including onychoclasis), night sweats, palmar-plantar erythrodysesthesia (hand-foot syndrome), papule, pityriasis rosea, pruritus, skin lesion, skin rash, xeroderma

Endocrine & metabolic: Amenorrhea, cushingoid appearance, cyanocobalamin deficiency, decreased serum albumin, decreased serum bicarbonate, dehydration, diabetes mellitus (new onset; more common in liver transplant), exacerbation of diabetes mellitus, gout, hirsutism, hypercalcemia, hypercholesterolemia, hyperglycemia, hyperkalemia (renal transplant), hyperlipidemia (renal, liver transplant), hypermenorrhea, hyperparathyroidism, hyperphosphatemia, hypertriglyceridemia, hyperuricemia, hypocalcemia, hypoglycemia, hypokalemia, hypomagnesemia (renal transplant), hyponatremia, hypophosphatemia, increased follicle-stimulating hormone, increased luteinizing hormone, iron deficiency, irregular menses, lipid metabolism disorder (renal transplant), menstrual disease, ovarian cyst

Gastrointestinal: Abdominal distention, abdominal pain, ageusia, anorexia, constipation, decreased appetite, diarrhea, dysgeusia, dyspepsia, dysphagia, epigastric distress, flatulence, gastritis, gastroenteritis, gastroesophageal reflux disease, gingival hyperplasia, hematemesis, hemorrhoids, intestinal obstruction, mucositis, nausea, oral herpes, peritonitis, stomatitis (more common in oncology uses), vomiting, weight loss, xerostomia

Genitourinary: Bladder spasm, dysmenorrhea, dysuria (renal transplant), erectile dysfunction, hematuria (renal transplant), irregular menses, pollakiuria, proteinuria, pyuria, scrotal edema, urinary retention, urinary tract infection, urinary urgency, vaginal hemorrhage

Hematologic & oncologic: Anemia, hemorrhage, leukocytosis, leukopenia (more common in oncology uses), lymphadenopathy, lymphocytopenia, neoplasm (liver transplant), neutropenia, pancytopenia (renal, liver transplant), prolonged partial thromboplastin time (SEGA), thrombocytopenia (more common in oncology uses)

Hepatic: Abnormal hepatic function tests (liver transplant), ascites (liver transplant), increased serum alkaline phosphatase (more common in oncology uses), increased serum ALT, increased serum AST, increased serum bilirubin, increased serum transaminases

Hypersensitivity: Hypersensitivity (including anaphylaxis, dyspnea, flushing, chest pain, angioedema)

Infection: BK virus, candidiasis, herpes virus infection, infection, sepsis

Neuromuscular & skeletal: Arthralgia, back pain, jaw pain, joint swelling, limb pain, muscle spasm, musculoskeletal pain, myalgia, osteonecrosis, osteopenia, osteoporosis, spondylitis, tremor, weakness

Ophthalmic: Blurred vision, cataract, conjunctivitis, eyelid edema, ocular hyperemia

Otic: Otitis

Renal: Hydronephrosis, increased blood urea nitrogen, increased serum creatinine, interstitial nephritis, polyuria, renal failure, renal insufficiency

Respiratory: Atelectasis, bronchitis, cough, dyspnea, epistaxis, lower respiratory tract infection, nasal congestion, nasopharyngitis, oropharyngeal pain, pharyngolaryngeal pain, pharyngitis, pleural effusion, pneumonia, pneumonitis (including alveolitis, interstitial lung disease, lung infiltrate, pulmonary alveolar hemorrhage, pulmonary toxicity), pulmonary edema, rhinitis, rhinorrhea, sinus congestion, sinusitis, upper respiratory tract infection, wheezing

Miscellaneous: Fever, postoperative wound complication (including incisional hernia), wound healing impairment (more common in renal and liver transplant)

Rare but important or life-threatening: Aspergillosis, azoospermia, cardiac arrest, cholecystitis, cholelithiasis, decreased plasma testosterone, fluid retention, hemolytic uremic syndrome, hepatic artery thrombosis, influenza, intrahepatic cholestasis, malignant lymphoma, oligospermia, pancreatitis, pneumonia due to *pneumocystis jiroveci*, progressive multifocal leukoencephalopathy, reactivation of HBV, respiratory distress, skin neoplasm, synovitis (severe), thrombosis of vascular graft, thrombotic thrombocytopenic purpura

Drug Interactions

Metabolism/Transport Effects Substrate of CYP3A4 (major), P-glycoprotein; **Note:** Assignment of Major/Minor substrate status based on clinically relevant drug interaction potential

Avoid Concomitant Use

Avoid concomitant use of Everolimus with any of the following: BCG; CloZAPine; Conivaptan; CYP3A4 Inducers (Strong); CYP3A4 Inhibitors (Strong); Dipyrone; Fusidic Acid (Systemic); Grapefruit Juice; Idelalisib; Natalizumab; Pimecrolimus; St Johns Wort; Tacrolimus (Topical); Tofacitinib; Vaccines (Live); Voriconazole

Increased Effect/Toxicity

Everolimus may increase the levels/effects of: ACE Inhibitors; CloZAPine; Leflunomide; Natalizumab; Tofacitinib; Vaccines (Live)

The levels/effects of Everolimus may be increased by: Conivaptan; CycloSPORINE (Systemic); CYP3A4 Inhibitors (Moderate); CYP3A4 Inhibitors (Strong); Dasatinib; Denosumab; Dipyrone; Fusidic Acid (Systemic); Grapefruit Juice; Idelalisib; Luliconazole; Mifepristone; P-glycoprotein/ABCB1 Inhibitors; Pimecrolimus; Roflumilast; Tacrolimus (Topical); Trastuzumab; Voriconazole

Decreased Effect

Everolimus may decrease the levels/effects of: BCG; Coccidioides immitis Skin Test; Sipuleucel-T; Vaccines (Inactivated); Vaccines (Live)

The levels/effects of Everolimus may be decreased by: Bosentan; CYP3A4 Inducers (Moderate); CYP3A4 Inducers (Strong); Dabrafenib; Deferasirox; Echinacea; Efavirenz; P-glycoprotein/ABCB1 Inducers; Siltuximab; St Johns Wort; Tocilizumab

Food Interactions Grapefruit juice may increase levels of everolimus. Absorption with food may be variable. Management: Avoid grapefruit juice. Take with or without food, but be consistent with regard to food.

Storage/Stability Tablets and tablets for suspension: Store at room temperature of 25°C (77°F); excursions permitted to 15°C to 30°C (59°F to 86°F). Protect from light; protect from moisture.

Mechanism of Action Everolimus is a macrolide immunosuppressant and a mechanistic target of rapamycin (mTOR) inhibitor which has antiproliferative and antiangiogenic properties, and also reduces lipoma volume in patients with angiomyolipoma. Reduces protein synthesis and cell proliferation by binding to the FK binding protein-12 (FKBP-12), an intracellular protein, to form a complex that inhibits activation of mTOR (mechanistic target of rapamycin) serine-threonine kinase activity. Also reduces angiogenesis by inhibiting vascular endothelial growth factor (VEGF) and hypoxia-inducible factor (HIF-1) expression. Angiomyolipomas may occur due to unregulated mTOR activity in TSC-associated renal angiomyolipoma (Budde, 2012); everolimus reduces lipoma volume (Bissler, 2012).

Pharmacodynamics/Kinetics

Absorption: Rapid, but moderate

Protein binding: ~74%

Metabolism: Extensively metabolized in the liver via CYP3A4; forms 6 weak metabolites

Bioavailability:

Tablets: ~30%; systemic exposure reduced by 22% with a high-fat meal and by 32% with a light-fat meal

Tablets for suspension: AUC equivalent to tablets although peak concentrations are 20% to 36% lower; steady state concentrations are similar

Half-life elimination: ~30 hours

Time to peak, plasma: 1-2 hours

Excretion: Feces (80%, based on solid organ transplant studies); Urine (~5%, based on solid organ transplant studies)

Dosage Note: Tablets (Afinitor, Zortress) and tablets for oral suspension (Afinitor Disperz) are not interchangeable; Afinitor Disperz is only indicated for the treatment of subependymal giant cell astrocytoma (SEGA), in conjunction with therapeutic monitoring. Do not combine formulations to achieve total desired dose.

Breast cancer, advanced, hormone receptor-positive, HER2-negative: Adults: Oral: 10 mg once daily (in combination with exemestane), continue treatment until no longer clinically beneficial or until unacceptable toxicity

Liver transplantation, rejection prophylaxis (begin at least 30 days post-transplant): Adults: Oral: Initial: 1 mg twice daily; adjust maintenance dose if needed at a 4- to 5-day interval (from prior dose adjustment) based on serum concentrations, tolerability, and response; goal serum concentration is between 3 and 8 ng/mL (based on an LC/MS/MS assay method); administer in combination with tacrolimus (reduced dose required) and corticosteroids

Pancreatic neuroendocrine tumors (PNET), advanced: Adults: Oral: 10 mg once daily, continue treatment until no longer clinically beneficial or until unacceptable toxicity

Renal angiomyolipoma: Adults: Oral: 10 mg once daily, continue treatment until no longer clinically beneficial or until unacceptable toxicity

Renal cell cancer (RCC), advanced: Adults: Oral: 10 mg once daily, continue treatment until no longer clinically beneficial or until unacceptable toxicity

Renal transplantation, rejection prophylaxis: Adults: Oral: Initial: 0.75 mg twice daily; adjust maintenance dose if needed at a 4- to 5-day interval (from prior dose adjustment) based on serum concentrations, tolerability, and response; goal serum concentration is between 3 and 8 ng/mL (based on an LC/MS/MS assay method); administer in combination with basiliximab induction and concurrently with cyclosporine (dose adjustment required) and corticosteroids

Subependymal giant cell astrocytoma (SEGA; dosing based on body surface area [BSA]): Children ≥1 year and Adults: Oral: **Note:** Continue until disease progression or unacceptable toxicity.

Initial dose: 4.5 mg/m^2 once daily; round to nearest tablet (tablet or tablet for oral suspension) size.

If trough <5 ng/mL: Increase dose by 2.5 mg daily (tablets) or 2 mg daily (tablets for oral suspension).

If trough >15 ng/mL: Reduce dose by 2.5 mg daily (tablets) or 2 mg daily (tablets for oral suspension). If dose reduction necessary in patients receiving the lowest strength available, administer every other day.

Therapeutic drug monitoring: Assess trough concentration ~2 weeks after initiation or with dosage modifications, initiation or changes to concurrent CYP3A4/P-glycoprotein (P-gp) inhibitor/inducer therapy, changes in hepatic impairment, or when changing dosage forms between tablets and tablets for oral suspension; adjust maintenance dose if needed at 2-week intervals to achieve and maintain trough concentrations between 5 and 15 ng/mL; once stable dose is attained and if BSA is stable throughout treatment, monitor trough concentrations every 6 to 12 months (monitor every 3 to 6 months if BSA is changing).

Carcinoid tumors, advanced (off-label use): Adults: Oral:10 mg once daily (in combination with octreotide LAR) until disease progression or toxicity (Pavel, 2011)

Waldenström's macroglobulinemia, relapsed or refractory (off-label use): Adults: Oral: 10 mg once daily until disease progression or toxicity (Ghobrial, 2010)

Dosage adjustment for toxicity:

Breast cancer (adjustments apply to everolimus), PNET, RCC, renal angiomyolipoma; Toxicities may require temporary dose interruption (with or without a subsequent dose reduction) or discontinuation; reduce everolimus dose by ~50% if dosage adjustment is necessary:

Noninfectious pneumonitis:

Grade 1 (asymptomatic radiological changes suggestive of pneumonitis): No dosage adjustment is necessary; monitor appropriately.

Grade 2 (symptomatic but not interfering with activities of daily living [ADL]): Consider interrupting treatment, rule out infection, and consider corticosteroids until symptoms improve to ≤ grade 1; reinitiate at a lower dose. Discontinue if recovery does not occur within 4 weeks.
Grade 3 (symptomatic, interferes with ADL; oxygen indicated): Interrupt treatment until symptoms improve to ≤ grade 1; rule out infection and consider corticosteroid treatment; may reinitiate at a lower dose. If grade 3 toxicity recurs, consider discontinuing.
Grade 4 (life-threatening; ventilatory support indicated): Discontinue treatment; rule out infection; consider corticosteroid treatment.

Stomatitis (avoid the use of products containing alcohol, hydrogen peroxide, iodine, or thyme derivatives):
Grade 1 (minimal symptoms, normal diet): No dosage adjustment is necessary; manage with mouth wash (nonalcoholic or isotonic salt water) several times a day
Grade 2 (symptomatic but can eat and swallow modified diet): Interrupt treatment until symptoms improve to ≤ grade 1; reinitiate at same dose; if stomatitis recurs at grade 2, interrupt treatment until symptoms improve to ≤ grade 1 and then reinitiate at a lower dose. Also manage with topical (oral) analgesics (eg, benzocaine, butyl aminobenzoate, tetracaine, menthol, or phenol) ± topical (oral) corticosteroids (eg, triamcinolone).
Grade 3 (symptomatic and unable to orally aliment or hydrate adequately): Interrupt treatment until symptoms improve to ≤ grade 1; then reinitiate at a lower dose. Also manage with topical (oral) analgesics (eg, benzocaine, butyl aminobenzoate, tetracaine, menthol, or phenol) ± topical (oral) corticosteroids (eg, triamcinolone).
Grade 4 (life-threatening symptoms): Discontinue treatment; initiate appropriate medical intervention.

Metabolic toxicity (eg, hyperglycemia, dyslipidemia):
Grade 1: No dosage adjustment is necessary; initiate appropriate medical intervention and monitor.
Grade 2: No dosage adjustment is necessary; manage with appropriate medical intervention and monitor.
Grade 3: Temporarily interrupt treatment; reinitiate at a lower dose; manage with appropriate medical intervention and monitor.
Grade 4: Discontinue treatment; manage with appropriate medical intervention.

Nonhematologic toxicities (excluding pneumonitis, stomatitis, or metabolic toxicity):
Grade 1: If toxicity is tolerable, no dosage adjustment is necessary; initiate appropriate medical intervention and monitor.
Grade 2: If toxicity is tolerable, no dosage adjustment is necessary; initiate appropriate medical intervention and monitor. If toxicity becomes intolerable, temporarily interrupt treatment until improvement to ≤ grade 1 and reinitiate at the same dose; if toxicity recurs at grade 2, temporarily interrupt treatment until improvement to ≤ grade 1 and then reinitiate at a lower dose.
Grade 3: Temporarily interrupt treatment until improvement to ≤ grade 1; initiate appropriate medical intervention and monitor. May reinitiate at a lower dose; if toxicity recurs at grade 3, consider discontinuing.
Grade 4 (life-threatening symptoms): Discontinue treatment; initiate appropriate medical intervention.

Liver or renal transplantation:
Evidence of polyoma virus infection or PML: Consider reduced immunosuppression (taking into account the allograft risks associated with decreased immunosuppression)
Pneumonitis (grade 4 symptoms) or invasive systemic fungal infection: Discontinue

SEGA: *Severe/intolerable adverse reactions:* Temporarily interrupt or permanently discontinue treatment; if dose reduction is required upon reinitiation, reduce dose by ~50%; if dose reduction is required for patients receiving the lowest available strength, consider alternate-day dosing.

Dosage adjustment for concomitant CYP3A4 inhibitors/inducers and/or P-gp inhibitors:

Breast cancer, PNET, RCC, renal angiomyolipoma:
CYP3A4/P-gp inducers: Strong inducers: Avoid coadministration with strong CYP3A4/P-gp inducers (eg, carbamazepine, phenobarbital, phenytoin, rifabutin, rifampin, rifapentine, St John's wort); if concomitant use cannot be avoided, consider doubling the everolimus dose, using increments of 5 mg or less, with careful monitoring (Canadian labeling recommends a maximum daily dose of 20 mg in patients with renal angiomyolipoma). If the strong CYP3A4/P-gp enzyme inducer is discontinued, consider allowing 3 to 5 days to elapse prior to reducing everolimus to the dose used prior to initiation of the CYP3A4/P-gp inducer.
CYP3A4/P-gp inhibitors:
Strong inhibitors: Avoid concomitant administration with strong CYP3A4/P-gp inhibitors (eg, atazanavir, clarithromycin, indinavir, itraconazole, ketoconazole, nefazodone, nelfinavir, ritonavir, saquinavir, telithromycin, voriconazole).
Moderate CYP3A4/P-gp inhibitors (eg, amprenavir, aprepitant, diltiazem, erythromycin, fluconazole, fosamprenavir, verapamil):
U.S. labeling: Reduce everolimus dose to 2.5 mg once daily; may consider increasing from 2.5 mg to 5 mg once daily based on patient tolerance. When the moderate inhibitor is discontinued, allow ~2 to 3 days to elapse prior to adjusting the everolimus upward to the recommended starting dose or to the dose used prior to initiation of the moderate inhibitor.
Canadian labeling: Reduce everolimus dose by 50%; further reductions may be necessary for adverse reactions. If dose reduction is required for patients receiving the lowest available strength, consider alternate day dosing. When the moderate inhibitor is discontinued, allow at least 3 days or 4 elimination half-lives to elapse prior to adjusting the everolimus to the dose used prior to initiation of the moderate inhibitor.

Renal transplantation: Dosage adjustments may be necessary based on everolimus serum concentrations

SEGA:
CYP3A4/P-gp inducers: Strong inducers:
U.S. labeling: Avoid concomitant administration with strong CYP3A4/P-gp inducers (eg, carbamazepine, phenobarbital, phenytoin, rifabutin, rifampin, rifapentine, St John's wort); if concomitant use cannot be avoided, an initial starting everolimus dose of 9 mg/m^2 once daily is recommended, or, double the everolimus dose and assess tolerability; assess trough concentration after ~2 weeks; adjust dose as necessary based on therapeutic drug monitoring to maintain target trough concentrations of 5 to 15 ng/mL. If the strong CYP3A4/P-gp enzyme inducer is discontinued, reduce the everolimus dose by ~50% or to the dose used prior to initiation of the CYP3A4/P-gp inducer; reassess trough concentration after ~2 weeks.
Canadian labeling: Avoid concomitant administration with strong CYP3A4 inducers (eg, carbamazepine, oxcarbazepine, phenobarbital, phenytoin, rifampin, rifabutin, rifapentine, St John's wort); if concomitant use cannot be avoided and everolimus level <5 ng/mL, may increase daily dose by 2.5 mg every 2 weeks (tablets) or 2 mg every 2 weeks (tablets for oral

suspension) until target everolimus trough concentration is 5 to 15 ng/mL. If the strong CYP3A4/P-gp inducer is discontinued, reduce everolimus to the dose used prior to initiation of the CYP3A4/P-gp inducer. Assess trough concentrations ~2 weeks after any change in dose or after any initiation or change in CYP3A4/P-gp inducer therapy.

CYP3A4/P-gp inhibitors:

Strong inhibitors: Avoid concomitant administration with strong CYP3A4/P-gp inhibitors (eg, atazanavir, clarithromycin, indinavir, itraconazole, ketoconazole, nefazodone, nelfinavir, ritonavir, saquinavir, telithromycin, voriconazole).

Moderate CYP3A4/P-gp inhibitors (eg, amprenavir, aprepitant, diltiazem, erythromycin, fluconazole, fosamprenavir, verapamil):

U.S. labeling: Currently taking a moderate CYP3A4/P-gp inhibitor and starting everolimus: Initial: 2.5 mg/m^2 once daily.

Currently taking everolimus and starting a moderate CYP3A4/P-gp inhibitor: Initial: Reduce everolimus dose by ~50%; if dose reduction is required for patients receiving the lowest strength available, administer every other day.

Discontinuing a moderate CYP3A4/P-gp inhibitor after concomitant use with everolimus: Discontinue moderate inhibitor and allow 2 to 3 days to elapse prior to resuming the everolimus dose used prior to initiation of the moderate inhibitor.

Therapeutic drug monitoring: Assess trough concentration ~2 weeks after everolimus initiation or dosage modifications, or initiation or changes to concurrent CYP3A4/P-gp inhibitor therapy; adjust maintenance dose if needed at 2-week intervals to achieve and maintain trough concentrations between 5 and 15 ng/mL.

Canadian labeling: Reduce everolimus dose by ~50% (if dose reduction is required for patients receiving the lowest strength available, consider alternate-day dosing). If the moderate inhibitor is discontinued, the everolimus dose should be returned to the dose used prior to initiation of the inhibitor.

Therapeutic drug monitoring: Assess trough concentration ~2 weeks after everolimus initiation or dosage modifications, or initiation or changes to concurrent CYP3A4/P-gp inhibitor therapy. Maintain trough concentrations between 5 and 15 ng/mL; may increase dose within the target range to achieve higher concentrations as tolerated.

Dosage adjustment in renal impairment: No dosage adjustment is necessary.

Dosage adjustment in hepatic impairment:

Mild impairment (Child-Pugh class A):

Breast cancer, PNET, RCC, renal angiomyolipoma: Reduce dose to 7.5 mg once daily; if not tolerated, may further reduce to 5 mg once daily.

Liver or renal transplantation: Reduce initial dose by ~33%; individualize subsequent dosing based on therapeutic drug monitoring (target trough concentration: 3 to 8 ng/mL).

SEGA:

U.S. labeling: Adjustment to initial dose may not be necessary; subsequent dosing is based on therapeutic drug monitoring (monitor ~2 weeks after initiation, dosage modifications, or after any change in hepatic status; target trough concentration: 5 to 15 ng/mL).

Canadian labeling: Initial:

Patients ≥18 years of age: 75% of usual dose based on calculated BSA (rounded to the nearest strength). Assess trough concentrations ~2 weeks after initiation, dosage modifications, or after any change in hepatic status. Target trough concentration: 5 and 15 ng/mL; may increase dose within the target range to achieve higher concentrations as tolerated.

Patients <18 years of age: Use is not recommended.

Moderate impairment (Child-Pugh class B):

Breast cancer, PNET, RCC, renal angiomyolipoma: Reduce dose to 5 mg once daily; if not tolerated, may further reduce to 2.5 mg once daily.

Liver or renal transplantation: Reduce initial dose by ~50%; individualize subsequent dosing based on therapeutic drug monitoring (target trough concentration: 3 to 8 ng/mL).

SEGA:

U.S. labeling: Adjustment to initial dose may not be necessary; subsequent dosing is based on therapeutic drug monitoring (monitor ~2 weeks after initiation, dosage modifications, or after any change in hepatic status; target trough concentration: 5 to 15 ng/mL).

Canadian labeling: Initial:

Patients ≥18 years of age: 50% of usual dose based on calculated BSA (rounded to the nearest strength). Assess trough concentrations ~2 weeks after initiation, dosage modifications, or after any change in hepatic status. Target trough concentration: 5 to 15 ng/mL; may increase dose within the target range to achieve higher concentrations as tolerated.

Patients <18 years of age: Use is not recommended

Severe impairment (Child-Pugh class C):

Breast cancer, PNET, RCC, renal angiomyolipoma: If potential benefit outweighs risks, a maximum dose of 2.5 mg once daily may be used.

Liver or renal transplantation: Reduce initial dose by ~50%; individualize subsequent dosing based on therapeutic drug monitoring (target trough concentration: 3 to 8 ng/mL).

SEGA:

U.S. labeling: Reduce initial dose to 2.5 mg/m^2 once daily (or current dose by ~50%); subsequent dosing is based on therapeutic drug monitoring (monitor ~2 weeks after initiation, dosage modifications, or after any change in hepatic status; target trough concentration: 5 to 15 ng/mL).

Canadian labeling: Use is not recommended.

Dietary Considerations Avoid grapefruit juice.

Administration May be taken with or without food; to reduce variability, take consistently with regard to food. Afinitor missed doses may be taken up to 6 hours after regularly scheduled time; if >6 hours, resume at next regularly scheduled time.

Tablets: Swallow whole with a glass of water. Do not break, chew, or crush (do not administer tablets that are crushed or broken). Avoid contact with or exposure to crushed or broken tablets.

Tablets for oral suspension: Administer as a suspension only. Administer immediately after preparation; discard if not administered within 60 minutes after preparation. Prepare suspension in water only. Do not break or crush tablets.

Preparation in an oral syringe: Place dose into 10 mL oral syringe (maximum: 10 mg/syringe; use an additional syringe for doses >10 mg). Draw ~5 mL of water and ~4 mL of air into oral syringe; allow to sit (tip up) in a container until tablets are in suspension (3 minutes). Gently invert syringe 5 times immediately prior to administration; administer contents, then add ~5 mL water and ~4 mL of air to same syringe, swirl to suspend remaining particles and administer entire contents.

Preparation in a small glass: Place dose into a small glass (≤100 mL) containing ~25 mL water (maximum: 10 mg/glass; use and additional glass for doses >10 mg); allow to sit until tablets are in suspension (3 minutes). Stir gently with spoon immediately prior to administration; administer contents, then add ~25 mL water to same glass, swirl with same spoon to suspend remaining particles and administer entire contents.

Breast cancer, pancreatic neuroendocrine tumors, renal cell cancer, renal angiolipoma, SEGA: Administer at the same time each day.

Liver transplantation: Administer consistently ~12 hours apart; administer at the same time as tacrolimus.

Renal transplantation: Administer consistently ~12 hours apart; administer at the same time as cyclosporine.

Hazardous agent; use appropriate precautions for handling and disposal (NIOSH 2014 [group 1]). To avoid potential contact with everolimus, caregivers should wear gloves when preparing suspension from tablets for oral suspension.

Monitoring Parameters CBC with differential (baseline and periodic), liver function; serum creatinine, urinary protein, and BUN (baseline and periodic); fasting serum glucose and lipid profile (baseline and periodic); monitor for signs and symptoms of infection, noninfectious pneumonitis, or malignancy

For liver or renal transplantation, monitor everolimus whole blood trough concentrations (based on an LC/MS/MS assay method), especially in patients with hepatic impairment, with concomitant CYP3A4 inhibitors and inducers, and when cyclosporine formulations or doses are changed; dosage adjustments should be made on trough concentrations obtained 4 to 5 days after a previous dosage adjustment; monitor cyclosporine concentrations; monitor for proteinuria

For SEGA, monitor everolimus whole blood trough concentrations ~2 weeks after treatment initiation or with dosage modifications, initiation or changes to concurrent CYP3A4/P-glycoprotein (P-gp) inhibitor/inducer therapy, changes in hepatic function and when changing dosage forms between Afinitor tablets and Afinitor Disperz. Maintain trough concentrations between 5 and 15 ng/mL; once stable dose is attained and if BSA is stable throughout treatment, monitor trough concentrations every 6 to 12 months (monitor every 3 to 6 months if BSA is changing).

Reference Range Recommended range for everolimus whole blood trough concentrations:

Liver and renal transplantation: 3-8 ng/mL (based on an LCMSMS assay method)

Subependymal giant cell astrocytoma (SEGA): 5-15 ng/mL (high concentrations may be associated with larger reductions in SEGA volumes, responses have been observed at concentrations as low as 5 ng/mL)

Dosage Forms

Tablet, Oral:

Afinitor: 2.5 mg, 5 mg, 7.5 mg, 10 mg

Zortress: 0.25 mg, 0.5 mg, 0.75 mg

Tablet Soluble, Oral:

Afinitor Disperz: 2 mg, 3 mg, 5 mg

Extemporaneous Preparations Hazardous agent: Use appropriate precautions for handling and disposal (NIOSH 2014 [group 1]).

Tablets: An oral liquid may be prepared using tablets. Disperse tablet in ~30 mL (1 oz) of water; gently stir. Administer and rinse container with additional 30 mL (1 oz) water and administer to ensure entire dose is administered. Administer immediately after preparation.

Afinitor (everolimus) [prescribing information]. East Hanover, NJ: Novartis Pharmaceuticals Corporation; July 2012.

Tablets for oral suspension: Administer as a suspension only. Administer immediately after preparation; discard if not administered within 60 minutes after preparation. Prepare suspension in water only. Do not break or crush tablets.

Preparation in an oral syringe: Place dose into 10 mL oral syringe (maximum 10 mg/syringe; use an additional syringe for doses >10 mg). Draw ~5 mL of water and ~4 mL of air into oral syringe; allow to sit (tip up) in a container until tablets are in suspension (3 minutes). Gently invert syringe 5 times immediately prior to administration; administer contents, then add ~5 mL water and ~4 mL of air to same syringe, swirl to suspend remaining particles and administer entire contents.

Preparation in a small glass: Place dose into a small glass (≤100 mL) containing ~25 mL water (maximum 10 mg/glass; use an additional glass for doses >10 mg); allow to sit until tablets are in suspension (3 minutes). Stir gently with spoon immediately prior to administration; administer contents, then add ~25 mL water to same glass, swirl with same spoon to suspend remaining particles and administer entire contents.

Administer immediately after preparation; discard if not administered within 60 minutes after preparation.

Afinitor and Afinitor Disperz (everolimus) [prescribing information]. East Hanover, NJ: Novartis Pharmaceuticals Corporation; August 2012.

- ◆ **Everone 200 (Can)** *see* Testosterone *on page 2010*
- ◆ **EVG/COBI/FTC/TDF** *see* Elvitegravir, Cobicistat, Emtricitabine, and Tenofovir *on page 718*
- ◆ **Evista** *see* Raloxifene *on page 1765*
- ◆ **Evoclin** *see* Clindamycin (Topical) *on page 464*
- ◆ **Evoxac** *see* Cevimeline *on page 415*
- ◆ **Evoxac® (Can)** *see* Cevimeline *on page 415*
- ◆ **Evra® (Can)** *see* Ethinyl Estradiol and Norelgestromin *on page 807*
- ◆ **Evzio** *see* Naloxone *on page 1419*
- ◆ **Exactacain** *see* Benzocaine, Butamben, and Tetracaine *on page 247*
- ◆ **Exalgo** *see* HYDROmorphone *on page 1016*
- ◆ **Excedrin Extra Strength [OTC]** *see* Acetaminophen, Aspirin, and Caffeine *on page 37*
- ◆ **Excedrin Migraine [OTC]** *see* Acetaminophen, Aspirin, and Caffeine *on page 37*
- ◆ **Excedrin PM® [OTC]** *see* Acetaminophen and Diphenhydramine *on page 36*
- ◆ **Excedrin Tension Headache [OTC]** *see* Acetaminophen *on page 32*
- ◆ **ExeFen-IR** *see* Guaifenesin and Pseudoephedrine *on page 989*
- ◆ **Exelderm** *see* Sulconazole *on page 1943*
- ◆ **Exelderm® (Can)** *see* Sulconazole *on page 1943*
- ◆ **Exelon** *see* Rivastigmine *on page 1833*

Exemestane (ex e MES tane)

Brand Names: U.S. Aromasin

Brand Names: Canada Aromasin; CO Exemestane

Pharmacologic Category Antineoplastic Agent, Aromatase Inhibitor

Use Breast cancer: Treatment of advanced breast cancer in postmenopausal women whose disease has progressed following tamoxifen therapy; adjuvant treatment of postmenopausal women with estrogen receptor-positive early breast cancer following 2-3 years of tamoxifen (for a total of 5 consecutive years of adjuvant therapy).

Pregnancy Risk Factor X

Pregnancy Considerations Adverse events were observed in animal reproduction studies. Exemestane is not indicated for use in premenopausal women and use during pregnancy is contraindicated. Based on the mechanism of action, exemestane is expected to cause fetal harm if administered to a pregnant woman.

Breast-Feeding Considerations Exemestane is indicated for use only in postmenopausal women. Due to the potential for serious adverse reactions in the nursing infant, the manufacturer recommends a decision be made whether to discontinue nursing or to discontinue the drug, taking into account the importance of treatment to the mother.

Contraindications Hypersensitivity to exemestane or any component of the formulation; women who are or may become pregnant; premenopausal women

Warnings/Precautions Hazardous agent - use appropriate precautions for handling and disposal (NIOSH 2014 [group 1]). Due to decreased circulating estrogen levels, exemestane is associated with a reduction in bone mineral density over time; decreases (from baseline) in lumbar spine and femoral neck density have been observed; assess bone mineral density at baseline in patients with, or at risk for osteoporosis; monitor exemestane therapy and initiate osteoporosis treatment if indicated. Due to high prevalence of vitamin D deficiency in women with breast cancer, assess 25-hydroxy vitamin D levels at baseline and supplement accordingly. Grade 3 or 4 lymphopenia has been observed with exemestane, although most patients had preexisting lower grade lymphopenia; some patients improved or recovered while continuing exemestane; lymphopenia did not result in a significant increase in viral infections, and no opportunistic infections were observed. Elevations of AST, ALT, alkaline phosphatase, and gamma glutamyl transferase >5 times ULN have been observed (rarely) in patients with advanced breast cancer; may be attributable to underlying liver and/or bone metastases. In patients with early breast cancer, elevations of bilirubin, alkaline phosphatase, and serum creatinine were more common with exemestane treatment than with tamoxifen or placebo. Potentially significant drug-drug interactions may exist, requiring dose or frequency adjustment, additional monitoring, and/or selection of alternative therapy. Not to be given with estrogen-containing agents. Dose adjustment recommended with concomitant strong CYP3A4 inducers.

Adverse Reactions

Cardiovascular: Cardiac ischemic events (MI, angina, myocardial ischemia), chest pain, edema, hypertension

Central nervous system: Anxiety, confusion, depression, dizziness, fatigue, fever, headache, hypoesthesia, insomnia, pain

Dermatologic: Alopecia, dermatitis, hyperhidrosis, itching, rash

Endocrine & metabolic: Hot flashes, weight gain

Gastrointestinal: Abdominal pain, anorexia, appetite increased, constipation, diarrhea, dyspepsia, nausea, vomiting

Genitourinary: Urinary tract infection

Hepatic: Alkaline phosphatase increased, bilirubin increased

Neuromuscular & skeletal: Arthralgia, back pain, carpal tunnel syndrome, cramps, limb pain, myalgia, osteoarthritis, osteoporosis, paresthesia, pathological fracture, weakness

Ocular: Visual disturbances

Renal: Creatinine increased

Respiratory: Bronchitis, cough, dyspnea, pharyngitis, rhinitis, sinusitis, upper respiratory infection

Miscellaneous: Flu-like syndrome, infection, lymphedema

Rare but important or life-threatening: Acute generalized exanthematous pustulosis, cardiac failure, cholestatic hepatitis, endometrial hyperplasia, gastric ulcer, GGT increased, hepatitis, hypersensitivity, neuropathy, osteochondrosis, pruritus, thromboembolism, transaminases increased, trigger finger, urticaria, uterine polyps

A dose-dependent decrease in sex hormone-binding globulin has been observed with daily doses of ≥2.5 mg. Serum luteinizing hormone and follicle-stimulating hormone levels have increased with this medicine.

Drug Interactions

Metabolism/Transport Effects **Substrate** of CYP3A4 (major); **Note:** Assignment of Major/Minor substrate status based on clinically relevant drug interaction potential; **Induces** CYP3A4 (weak)

Avoid Concomitant Use

Avoid concomitant use of Exemestane with any of the following: Estrogen Derivatives

Increased Effect/Toxicity

Exemestane may increase the levels/effects of: Methadone

Decreased Effect

Exemestane may decrease the levels/effects of: ARIPiprazole; Hydrocodone; Saxagliptin

The levels/effects of Exemestane may be decreased by: Bosentan; CYP3A4 Inducers (Moderate); CYP3A4 Inducers (Strong); Dabrafenib; Deferasirox; Estrogen Derivatives; Mitotane; Siltuximab; St Johns Wort; Tocilizumab

Food Interactions Plasma levels increased by 40% when exemestane was taken with a fatty meal. Management: Administer after a meal.

Storage/Stability Store at 25°C (77°F); excursions permitted to 15°C to 30°C (59°F to 86°F).

Mechanism of Action Exemestane is an irreversible, steroidal aromatase inactivator. It is structurally related to androstenedione, and is converted to an intermediate that irreversibly blocks the active site of the aromatase enzyme, leading to inactivation ("suicide inhibition") and thus preventing conversion of androgens to estrogens in peripheral tissues. Significantly lowers circulating estrogens in postmenopausal breast cancers where growth is estrogen-dependent.

Pharmacodynamics/Kinetics

Absorption: Rapid and moderate (~42%) following oral administration; AUC and C_{max} increased by 59% and 39%, respectively, following a high-fat breakfast (compared to fasted state)

Distribution: Extensive into tissues

Protein binding: 90%, primarily to albumin and α_1-acid glycoprotein

Metabolism: Extensively hepatic; oxidation (CYP3A4) of methylene group, reduction of 17-keto group with formation of many secondary metabolites; metabolites are inactive

Half-life elimination: ~24 hours

Time to peak: Women with breast cancer: 1.2 hours

Excretion: Urine (<1% as unchanged drug, 39% to 45% as metabolites); feces (36% to 48%)

Dosage

Breast cancer, advanced: Adults: Postmenopausal females: Oral: 25 mg once daily; continue until tumor progression

Breast cancer, early (adjuvant treatment): Adults: Postmenopausal females: Oral: 25 mg once daily (following 2-3 years of tamoxifen therapy) for a total duration of 5 consecutive years of endocrine therapy (in the absence of recurrence or contralateral breast cancer)

Breast cancer, early (first-line adjuvant treatment; off-label use): Adults: Postmenopausal females: Oral: 25 mg once daily for 5 years (Burstein, 2010; van de Velde, 2011)

Breast cancer, risk reduction (off-label use): Adults: Postmenopausal females ≥35 years: Oral: 25 mg once daily for 5 years (Goss, 2011; Visvanathan, 2013)

Dosage adjustment with strong CYP3A4 inducers: U.S. labeling: 50 mg once daily when used with potent inducers (eg, rifampin, phenytoin)

Dosing adjustment in renal impairment: No adjustment necessary (although the safety of chronic doses in patients with moderate-to-severe renal impairment has not been studied, dosage adjustment does not appear necessary).

Dosing adjustment in hepatic impairment: No adjustment necessary (although the safety of chronic doses in patients with moderate-to-severe hepatic impairment has not been studied, dosage adjustment does not appear necessary).

Dietary Considerations Patients on aromatase inhibitor therapy should receive vitamin D and calcium supplements.

Administration Administer after a meal. Hazardous agent; use appropriate precautions for handling and disposal (NIOSH 2014 [group 1]).

Monitoring Parameters 25-hydroxy vitamin D levels (at baseline); bone mineral density

Dosage Forms

Tablet, Oral:

Aromasin: 25 mg

Generic: 25 mg

Exenatide (ex EN a tide)

Brand Names: U.S. Bydureon; Byetta 10 MCG Pen; Byetta 5 MCG Pen

Brand Names: Canada Byetta

Index Terms AC 2993; AC002993; Exendin-4; LY2148568

Pharmacologic Category Antidiabetic Agent, Glucagon-Like Peptide-1 (GLP-1) Receptor Agonist

Use

Type 2 diabetes mellitus: Treatment of type 2 diabetes mellitus (noninsulin dependent, NIDDM) to improve glycemic control as an adjunct to diet and exercise.

Limitations of use: Because of the uncertain relevance of the rat thyroid C-cell tumor findings to humans, prescribe exenatide ER only to patients for whom the potential benefits are considered to outweigh the potential risks. Exenatide ER is not recommended as first-line therapy for patients who have inadequate glycemic control on diet and exercise.

Pregnancy Risk Factor C

Pregnancy Considerations Adverse events were observed in some animal reproduction studies. Based on *in vitro* data, exenatide has a low potential to cross the placenta (Hiles, 2003).

In women with diabetes, maternal hyperglycemia can be associated with congenital malformations as well as adverse effects in the fetus, neonate, and the mother (ACOG, 2005; ADA, 2014; Kitzmiller, 2008; Metzger, 2007). To prevent adverse outcomes, prior to conception and throughout pregnancy maternal blood glucose and HbA_{1c} should be kept as close to normal as possible but without causing significant hypoglycemia (ACOG, 2013; ADA, 2014; Blumer, 2013; Kitzmiller, 2008). Prior to pregnancy, effective contraception should be used until glycemic control is achieved (ADA, 2014; Kitzmiller, 2008). Other agents are currently recommended to treat diabetes in pregnant women (ACOG, 2013; Blumer, 2013).

Health care providers are encouraged to enroll women exposed to exenatide during pregnancy in the pregnancy registry (800-633-9081).

Breast-Feeding Considerations It is not known if exenatide is excreted in breast milk. According to the manufacturer, the decision to continue or discontinue breast-feeding during therapy should take into account the risk of exposure to the infant and the benefits of treatment to the mother; use caution if administering exenatide to nursing women.

Contraindications

History of or family history of medullary thyroid carcinoma (exenatide ER only); patients with multiple endocrine neoplasia syndrome type 2 (exenatide ER only); hypersensitivity to exenatide or any component of the formulation.

Byetta: Canadian labeling: Additional contraindications (not in U.S. labeling): End-stage renal disease (ESRD) or severe renal impairment (CrCl <30 mL/minute) including dialysis patients; diabetic ketoacidosis, diabetic coma/precoma or type 1 diabetes mellitus

Warnings/Precautions Bydureon: **[U.S. Boxed Warning] Dose- and duration-dependent thyroid C-cell tumors have developed in animal studies with exenatide extended release therapy; relevance in humans unknown. Patients should be counseled on the risk and symptoms (eg, neck mass, dysphagia, dyspnea, persistent hoarseness) of thyroid tumors. Use is contraindicated in patients with a personal or a family history of medullary thyroid cancer and in patients with multiple endocrine neoplasia syndrome type 2 (MEN2).** Consultation with an endocrinologist is recommended in patients who develop elevated calcitonin concentrations or have thyroid nodules detected during imaging studies or physical exam. All cases of MTC should be reported to the applicable state cancer registry.

Mechanism requires the presence of insulin, therefore use in type 1 diabetes (insulin dependent, IDDM) or diabetic ketoacidosis is not recommended (use is contraindicated in the Canadian labeling); it is not a substitute for insulin in insulin-requiring patients. Bydureon is not recommended for first-line therapy in patients inadequately controlled on diet and exercise alone.

Exenatide is frequently associated with gastrointestinal adverse effects and is not recommended for use in patients with gastroparesis or severe gastrointestinal disease. Gastrointestinal effects may be dose-related and may decrease in frequency/severity with gradual titration and continued use. Cases of acute pancreatitis (including hemorrhagic and necrotizing with some fatalities) have been reported; monitor for signs and symptoms of pancreatitis, (eg, persistent severe abdominal pain which may radiate to the back, and which may or may not be accompanied by vomiting). If pancreatitis is suspected, discontinue use. Do not resume unless an alternative etiology of pancreatitis is confirmed. Consider alternative antidiabetic therapy in patients with a history of pancreatitis. Use may be associated with the development of anti-exenatide antibodies. Low titers are not associated with a loss of efficacy; however, high titers (observed in 6% to 12% of patients in clinical studies) may result in an attenuation of response. May be associated with weight loss (due to reduced intake) independent of the change in hemoglobin A_{1c}. Serious hypersensitivity reactions (eg, anaphylaxis, angioedema) have been reported discontinue therapy in the event of a hypersensitivity reaction. Serious injection-site reactions (eg, abscess, cellulitis, and necrosis), with or without subcutaneous nodules have been reported with use. Isolated cases required surgical intervention. Potentially significant drug-drug interactions may exist, requiring dose or frequency adjustment, additional monitoring, and/or selection of alternative therapy.

Not recommended in severe renal impairment (CrCl <30 mL/minute) or end-stage renal disease (ESRD) (use in these patients and in dialysis patients is contraindicated in the Canadian labeling). Patients with ESRD receiving dialysis may be more susceptible to GI effects (eg, nausea, vomiting) which may result in hypovolemia and further reductions in renal function. Use with caution in patients with renal transplantation or in patients with moderate renal impairment (CrCl 30-50 mL/minute). Cases of acute renal failure and chronic renal failure exacerbation, including severe cases requiring hemodialysis, have been reported, predominately in patients with nausea/vomiting/diarrhea or dehydration; renal dysfunction was usually reversible with appropriate corrective measures, including discontinuation of exenatide. Risk may be increased in patients receiving concomitant medications affecting renal function and/or hydration status.

According to the Centers for Disease Control and Prevention (CDC), pen-shaped injection devices should never be used for more than one person (even when the needle is changed) because of the risk of infection. The injection device should be clearly labeled with individual patient information to ensure that the correct pen is used (CDC, 2012).

Adverse Reactions **Note:** Combination therapy may include a sulfonylurea, a thiazolidinedione, insulin glargine, or a combination of oral agents unless otherwise specified.

Central nervous system: Dizziness, fatigue, headache, jitteriness

Dermatologic: Hyperhidrosis

Endocrine & metabolic: Hypoglycemia (occurs more frequently with combination therapy), severe hypoglycemia

Gastrointestinal: Abdominal distension, constipation, decreased appetite, diarrhea, dyspepsia, flatulence, gastroesophageal reflux disease, nausea (dose-dependent and usually decreases over time), viral gastroenteritis, vomiting

Immunologic: Antibody development to exenatide (associated with attenuated glycemic response)

Local: Injection site nodule, injection site reaction, itching at injection site

Neuromuscular & skeletal: Weakness

Rare but important or life-threatening: Abscess at injection site, acute pancreatitis, acute renal failure, alopecia, anaphylaxis, angioedema, cellulitis at injection site, chest pain, drowsiness, exacerbation of renal failure, hemorrhagic pancreatitis, hypersensitivity pneumonitis (chronic), influenza, kidney transplant dysfunction, necrotizing pancreatitis (sometimes resulting in death), pain (stomach, side, or abdominal pain possibly radiating to the back), renal insufficiency, severe diarrhea, severe nausea, severe vomiting, tissue necrosis at injection site, upper respiratory tract infection, urticaria

Drug Interactions

Metabolism/Transport Effects None known.

Avoid Concomitant Use There are no known interactions where it is recommended to avoid concomitant use.

Increased Effect/Toxicity

Exenatide may increase the levels/effects of: Insulin; Sulfonylureas; Vitamin K Antagonists

The levels/effects of Exenatide may be increased by: Androgens; Pegvisomant

Decreased Effect

Exenatide may decrease the levels/effects of: Contraceptives (Estrogens); Oral Contraceptive (Progestins)

The levels/effects of Exenatide may be decreased by: Corticosteroids (Orally Inhaled); Corticosteroids (Systemic); Danazol; Luteinizing Hormone-Releasing Hormone Analogs; Somatropin; Thiazide Diuretics

Preparation for Administration Bydureon: Reconstitute vial using provided diluent; use immediately.

Storage/Stability

Bydureon: Store under refrigeration at 2°C to 8°C (36°F to 46°F); vials may be stored at ≤25°C (≤77°F) for up to 4 weeks. Do not freeze (discard if freezing occurs). Protect from light.

Byetta: Prior to initial use, store under refrigeration at 2°C to 8°C (36°F to 46°F); after initial use, may store at ≤25°C (≤77°F). Do not freeze (discard if freezing occurs). Protect from light. Pen should be discarded 30 days after initial use.

Mechanism of Action Exenatide is an analog of the hormone incretin (glucagon-like peptide 1 or GLP-1) which increases glucose-dependent insulin secretion, decreases inappropriate glucagon secretion, increases B-cell growth/replication, slows gastric emptying, and decreases food intake. Exenatide administration results in decreases in hemoglobin A_{1c} by approximately 0.5% to 1% (immediate release) or 1.5% to 1.9% (extended release).

Pharmacodynamics/Kinetics

Distribution: V_d: 28.3 L

Metabolism: Minimal systemic metabolism; proteolytic degradation may occur following glomerular filtration

Half-life elimination:

Immediate release (daily) formulation: 2.4 hours

Extended release (weekly) formulation: ~2 weeks

Time to peak, plasma: SubQ:

Immediate release (daily) formulation: 2.1 hours

Extended release (weekly) formulation: Triphasic: Phase 1: 2-5 hours; Phase 2: ~2 weeks; Phase 3: ~7 weeks

Excretion: Urine (majority of dose)

Dosage SubQ: Adults:

Immediate release: Initial: 5 mcg twice daily within 60 minutes prior to a meal; after 1 month, may be increased to 10 mcg twice daily (based on response)

Extended release: 2 mg once weekly

Note: May administer a missed dose as soon as noticed if the next regularly scheduled dose is due in ≥3 days; resume normal schedule thereafter. To establish a new day of the week administration schedule, wait ≥3 days after last dose given, then administer next dose on new desired day of the week.

Conversion from immediate release to extended release: Initiate weekly administration of exenatide extended release the day after discontinuing exenatide immediate release. **Note:** May experience increased blood glucose levels for ~2 weeks after conversion. Pretreatment with immediate release exenatide is not required when initiating extended release exenatide.

Dosage adjustment in renal impairment:

Mild impairment (CrCl ≥50 mL/minute): No dosage adjustment necessary

Moderate impairment (CrCl 30-50 mL/minute): There are no dosage adjustments provided in manufacturer's labeling; use caution.

Severe impairment (CrCl <30 mL/minute) or end-stage renal disease (ESRD):

U.S. labeling: Use is not recommended

Canadian labeling: Use is contraindicated.

Renal transplantation: Use with caution

Dosage adjustment in hepatic impairment: There are no dosage adjustments provided in manufacturer's labeling (has not been studied); however, hepatic dysfunction is not expected to affect exenatide pharmacokinetics.

Administration SubQ:

Immediate release: Use only if clear, colorless, and free of particulate matter. Administer via injection in the upper arm, thigh, or abdomen. Administer within 60 minutes prior to morning and evening meal (or prior to the 2 main meals of the day, approximately ≥6 hours apart). Set up each new pen before the first use by priming it. See pen user manual for further details. Dial the dose into the dose window before each administration.

Extended release: Administer subcutaneously in the upper arm, thigh, or abdomen; rotate injection sites weekly. Administer immediately after reconstitution in diluent, the mixture should be white to off-white and cloudy. Do not substitute needles or any other components provided with the single-dose tray. May administer without regard to meals or time of day.

Monitoring Parameters Serum glucose, hemoglobin A_{1c}, renal function, signs/symptoms of pancreatitis

Reference Range

Recommendations for glycemic control in nonpregnant adults with diabetes (ADA, 2015):

HbA_{1c}: <7% (a more aggressive [<6.5%] or less aggressive [<8%] HbA_{1c} goal may be targeted based on patient-specific characteristics)

Preprandial capillary plasma glucose: 80 to 130 mg/dL

Peak postprandial capillary blood glucose: <180 mg/dL

Recommendations for glycemic control in pediatric (all age groups) patients with type 1 diabetes (ADA, 2015):

HbA_{1c}: <7.5% (individualization may be appropriate based on patient-specific characteristics; <7% is reasonable if it can be achieved without excessive hypoglycemia)

Preprandial capillary plasma glucose: 90 to 130 mg/dL

Bedtime and overnight capillary blood glucose: 90 to 150 mg/dL

Additional Information A dosing strategy which employs progressive dose escalation of exenatide (initiating at 0.02 mcg/kg 3 times daily and increasing in increments of 0.02 mcg/kg every 3 days) has been described, limiting the frequency and severity of gastrointestinal adverse effects. The complexity of this regimen may limit its clinical application.

In animal models, exenatide has been a useful adjunctive therapy when added to immunotherapy protocols, resulting in recovery of beta cell function and sustained remission.

Dosage Forms

Pen-injector, Subcutaneous:

Bydureon: 2 mg (1 ea)

Solution Pen-injector, Subcutaneous:

Byetta 10 MCG Pen: 10 mcg/0.04 mL (2.4 mL)

Byetta 5 MCG Pen: 5 mcg/0.02 mL (1.2 mL)

Suspension Reconstituted, Subcutaneous:

Bydureon: 2 mg (1 ea)

- ◆ **Exendin-4** *see* Exenatide *on page* 830
- ◆ **Exforge®** *see* Amlodipine and Valsartan *on page* 126
- ◆ **Exforge HCT®** *see* Amlodipine, Valsartan, and Hydrochlorothiazide *on page* 127
- ◆ **Exjade** *see* Deferasirox *on page* 582
- ◆ **Ex-Lax Ultra [OTC]** *see* Bisacodyl *on page* 265
- ◆ **Exparel** *see* Bupivacaine (Liposomal) *on page* 299
- ◆ **Extavia** *see* Interferon Beta-1b *on page* 1103
- ◆ **Extended Release Epidural Morphine** *see* Morphine (Liposomal) *on page* 1400
- ◆ **Extina** *see* Ketoconazole (Topical) *on page* 1145
- ◆ **Extraneal** *see* Icodextrin *on page* 1037
- ◆ **Extra Strength Allergy Relief [OTC] (Can)** *see* Cetirizine *on page* 411
- ◆ **Exuviance Lightening Complex [OTC]** *see* Hydroquinone *on page* 1020
- ◆ **EYE001** *see* Pegaptanib *on page* 1588
- ◆ **EyeFlur** *see* Fluorescein and Benoxinate *on page* 895
- ◆ **Eye-Sed [OTC]** *see* Zinc Sulfate *on page* 2200
- ◆ **Eylea** *see* Aflibercept (Ophthalmic) *on page* 63
- ◆ **EZ Char [OTC]** *see* Charcoal, Activated *on page* 416

Ezetimibe (ez ET i mibe)

Brand Names: U.S. Zetia

Brand Names: Canada ACH-Ezetimibe; ACT Ezetimibe; Apo-Ezetimibe; Bio-Ezetimibe; Ezetrol; JAMP-Ezetimibe; Mar-Ezetimibe; Mint-Ezetimibe; Mylan-Ezetimibe; PMS-Ezetimibe; Priva-Ezetimibe; RAN-Ezetimibe; Riva-Ezetimibe; Sandoz Ezetimibe; Teva-Ezetimibe

Pharmacologic Category Antilipemic Agent, 2-Azetidinone

Use

Homozygous familial hypercholesterolemia: In combination with atorvastatin or simvastatin for the reduction of elevated total cholesterol (total-C) and low-density lipoprotein cholesterol (LDL-C) levels in patients with homozygous familial hypercholesterolemia as an adjunct to other lipid-lowering treatments (eg, LDL apheresis) or if such treatments are unavailable.

Homozygous sitosterolemia: As adjunctive therapy to diet for the reduction of elevated sitosterol and campesterol levels in patients with homozygous familial sitosterolemia.

Primary hyperlipidemia:

Combination therapy with HMG-CoA reductase inhibitors: In combination with a 3-hydroxy-3-methylglutaryl-coenzyme A (HMG-CoA) reductase inhibitor (statin) as adjunctive therapy to diet for the reduction of elevated total-C, LDL-C, apolipoprotein B (apo B), and non-high-density lipoprotein cholesterol (non-HDL-C) in patients with primary (heterozygous familial and nonfamilial) hyperlipidemia.

Combination therapy with fenofibrate: In combination with fenofibrate as adjunctive therapy to diet for the reduction of elevated total-C, LDL-C, apo B, and non-HDL-C in adult patients with mixed hyperlipidemia.

Monotherapy: As adjunctive therapy to diet for the reduction of elevated total-C, LDL-C, apo B, and non-HDL-C in patients with primary (heterozygous familial and non-familial) hyperlipidemia.

Pregnancy Risk Factor C

Pregnancy Considerations Use is contraindicated in women who are or who may become pregnant.

Breast-Feeding Considerations It is not known if ezetimibe is excreted in breast milk. According to the manufacturer, the decision to continue or discontinue breast-feeding during therapy should take into account the risk of exposure to the infant and the benefits of treatment to the mother. Use is contraindicated in nursing women who require combination therapy with an HMG-CoA reductase inhibitor.

Contraindications Hypersensitivity to ezetimibe or any component of the formulation; concomitant use with an HMG-CoA reductase inhibitor (statin) in patients with active hepatic disease or unexplained persistent elevations in serum transaminases; pregnancy and breast-feeding (when used concomitantly with a statin)

Warnings/Precautions Secondary causes of hyperlipidemia should be ruled out prior to therapy. Use caution with severe renal (CrCl ≤30 mL/minute/1.73 m^2); systemic exposure is increased ~1.5-fold. If using concurrent simvastatin in patients with moderate to severe renal impairment (CrCl <60 mL/minute/1.73m^2), the manufacturer of ezetimibe recommends that simvastatin doses exceeding 20 mg be used with caution and close monitoring for adverse events (eg, myopathy). Myopathy, including rhabdomyolysis, has been reported (rarely) with ezetimibe monotherapy; risk may be increased with concomitant use of a statin or fibrate. Discontinue ezetimibe and statin or fibrate immediately if myopathy is suspected or confirmed (symptomatic patient with CPK >10 x ULN).

A higher incidence of elevated transaminases (≥3 x ULN) has been observed with concomitant use of ezetimibe and statins compared to statin monotherapy; transaminase changes were generally not associated with symptoms or cholestasis and returned to baseline with or without discontinuation of therapy. Consider discontinuation of ezetimibe and/or the statin for persistently elevated transaminases (ALT or AST ≥3 x ULN). Systemic exposure is increased in hepatic impairment. Use caution with mild hepatic impairment (Child-Pugh class A); use is not recommended in patients with moderate or severe hepatic impairment (Child-Pugh classes B and C). Potentially significant drug-drug interactions may exist, requiring dose or frequency adjustment, additional monitoring, and/or selection of alternative therapy.

Adverse Reactions

Central nervous system: Fatigue

Gastrointestinal: Diarrhea

Hepatic: Transaminases increased (with HMG-CoA reductase inhibitors) (≥3 x ULN)

Neuromuscular & skeletal: Arthralgia, pain in extremity

Respiratory: Sinusitis, upper respiratory tract infection

Miscellaneous: Influenza

Rare but important or life-threatening: Abdominal pain, anaphylaxis, angioedema, autoimmune hepatitis (Stolk, 2006), cholecystitis, cholelithiasis, cholestatic hepatitis (Stolk, 2006), CPK increased, depression, dizziness, erythema multiforme, headache, hepatitis, hypersensitivity reactions, myalgia, myopathy, nausea, pancreatitis, paresthesia, rash, rhabdomyolysis, thrombocytopenia, urticaria

Drug Interactions

Metabolism/Transport Effects Substrate of SLCO1B1

Avoid Concomitant Use

Avoid concomitant use of Ezetimibe with any of the following: Bezafibrate; Gemfibrozil

Increased Effect/Toxicity

Ezetimibe may increase the levels/effects of: CycloSPORINE (Systemic)

The levels/effects of Ezetimibe may be increased by: Bezafibrate; CycloSPORINE (Systemic); Eltrombopag; Fenofibrate and Derivatives; Gemfibrozil; Teriflunomide

Decreased Effect

The levels/effects of Ezetimibe may be decreased by: Bile Acid Sequestrants

Storage/Stability Store at 25°C (77°F); excursions are permitted between 15°C and 30°C (59°F and 86°F). Protect from moisture.

Mechanism of Action Inhibits absorption of cholesterol at the brush border of the small intestine via the sterol transporter, Niemann-Pick C1-Like1 (NPC1L1). This leads to a decreased delivery of cholesterol to the liver, reduction of hepatic cholesterol stores and an increased clearance of cholesterol from the blood; decreases total C, LDL-cholesterol (LDL-C), ApoB, and triglycerides (TG) while increasing HDL-cholesterol (HDL-C).

Pharmacodynamics/Kinetics

Protein binding: >90% to plasma proteins

Metabolism: Undergoes glucuronide conjugation in the small intestine and liver; forms metabolite (active); may undergo enterohepatic recycling

Half-life elimination: 22 hours (ezetimibe and metabolite)

Time to peak, plasma: 4-12 hours

Excretion: Feces (78%, 69% as ezetimibe); urine (11%, 9% as metabolite)

Dosage Homozygous familial hypercholesterolemia, primary hyperlipidemia, homozygous sitosterolemia: Children ≥10 years, Adolescents, and Adults: Oral: 10 mg daily

Elderly: Refer to adult dosing

Dosage adjustment in renal impairment: No dosage adjustment necessary.

Dosage adjustment in hepatic impairment:

Mild impairment (Child-Pugh class A): No dosage adjustment necessary.

Moderate to severe impairment (Child-Pugh class B or C): Use of ezetimibe not recommended

Dietary Considerations Before initiation of therapy, patients should be placed on a standard cholesterol-lowering diet for 6 weeks and the diet should be continued during drug therapy.

Administration May be administered without regard to meals. May be taken at the same time as a statin or fenofibrate. Administer ≥2 hours before or ≥4 hours after bile acid sequestrants.

Monitoring Parameters Total cholesterol profile prior to therapy, and when clinically indicated and/or periodically thereafter. When used in combination with fenofibrate, monitor LFTs and signs and symptoms of cholelithiasis.

2013 ACC/AHA Blood Cholesterol Guideline recommendations (Stone, 2013): Baseline LFTs (reasonable); when used in combination with statin therapy, monitor LFTs when clinically indicated; discontinue use of ezetimibe if ALT elevations >3 times upper limit of normal persist.

Dosage Forms

Tablet, Oral:

Zetia: 10 mg

Dosage Forms: Canada

Tablet, Oral:

Ezetrol: 10 mg

Ezetimibe and Atorvastatin

(ez ET i mibe & a TORE va sta tin)

Brand Names: U.S. Liptruzet

Index Terms Atorvastatin and Ezetimibe

Pharmacologic Category Antilipemic Agent, 2-Azetidinone; Antilipemic Agent, HMG-CoA Reductase Inhibitor

Use

Homozygous familial hypercholesterolemia: As an adjunct to diet for the reduction of elevated total cholesterol, and low-density lipoprotein cholesterol (LDL-C) in patients with homozygous familial hypercholesterolemia, as an adjunct to other lipid-lowering treatments (eg, LDL apheresis) or if such treatments are unavailable.

Primary hyperlipidemia: As an adjunct to diet for the reduction of elevated total cholesterol, LDL-C, apolipoprotein B (apo B), triglycerides, and non-high-density lipoprotein cholesterol (non-HDL-C), and to increase HDL-C in patients with primary (heterozygous familial and nonfamilial) hyperlipidemia or mixed hyperlipidemia.

Atorvastatin: Primary and secondary prevention of atherosclerotic cardiovascular disease (ASCVD) according to the American College of Cardiology/American Heart Association: To reduce the risk of ASCVD in patients with clinical ASCVD (eg, coronary heart disease, stroke/TIA, or peripheral arterial disease presumed to be of atherosclerotic origin); in patients without clinical ASCVD if LDL-C is 190 mg/dL or greater; in patients without clinical ASCVD who have type 1 or type 2 diabetes and are between 40 and 75 years of age; in patients with an estimated 10-year ASCVD risk 7.5% or greater and who are between 40 and 75 years of age (Stone, 2013). Specific recommendations from the Kidney Disease: Improving Global Outcomes (KDIGO) organization have also been released for patients with chronic kidney disease (KDIGO [Tonelli, 2013]).

Pregnancy Risk Factor X

Dosage

Homozygous familial hypercholesterolemia: Adults: Oral: Ezetimibe 10 mg and atorvastatin 40 or 80 mg once daily

Primary hyperlipidemia: Adults: Oral: Initial: Ezetimibe 10 mg and atorvastatin 10 or 20 mg once daily; dosing range: Ezetimibe 10 mg and atorvastatin 10 to 80 mg once daily

Patients requiring >55% reduction in LDL-C: Initial: Ezetimibe 10 mg and atorvastatin 40 mg once daily

Dosage adjustment with concomitant medications:

Clarithromycin, itraconazole, saquinavir plus ritonavir, darunavir plus ritonavir, fosamprenavir, or fosamprenavir plus ritonavir: Use lowest effective dose; atorvastatin dose should not exceed 20 mg once daily.

Lopinavir plus ritonavir: Use lowest effective dose.

Nelfinavir or boceprevir: Use lowest effective dose; atorvastatin dose should not exceed 40 mg once daily.

Dosage adjustment in renal impairment: No dosage adjustment necessary.

Dosage adjustment in hepatic impairment: There are no dosage adjustments provided in the manufacturer's labeling; however, use is contraindicated in active liver disease or in patients with unexplained persistent elevations of serum transaminases.

Additional Information Complete prescribing information should be consulted for additional detail.

Dosage Forms

Tablet, oral:

Liptruzet10/10: Ezetimibe 10 mg and atorvastatin 10 mg
Liptruzet 10/20: Ezetimibe 10 mg and atorvastatin 20 mg
Liptruzet 10/40: Ezetimibe 10 mg and atorvastatin 40 mg
Liptruzet 10/80: Ezetimibe 10 mg and atorvastatin 80 mg

Ezetimibe and Simvastatin

(ez ET i mibe & SIM va stat in)

Brand Names: U.S. Vytorin

Index Terms Simvastatin and Ezetimibe

Pharmacologic Category Antilipemic Agent, 2-Azetidinone; Antilipemic Agent, HMG-CoA Reductase Inhibitor

Use

Homozygous familial hypercholesterolemia: As an adjunct to diet for the reduction of elevated total cholesterol (total-C) and low-density lipoprotein cholesterol (LDL-C) in patients with homozygous familial hypercholesterolemia, as an adjunct to other lipid-lowering treatments (eg, LDL apheresis), or if such treatments are unavailable

Primary hyperlipidemia: As an adjunct to diet for the reduction of elevated total-C, LDL-C, apolipoprotein B (apo B), triglycerides, and non-high-density lipoprotein cholesterol (HDL-C), and to increase HDL-C in patients with primary (heterozygous familial and nonfamilial) hyperlipidemia or mixed hyperlipidemia

Simvastatin: Primary and secondary prevention of atherosclerotic cardiovascular disease (ASCVD) according to the American College of Cardiology/ American Heart Association: To reduce the risk of ASCVD in patients with clinical ASCVD (eg, coronary heart disease, stroke/TIA, or peripheral arterial disease presumed to be of atherosclerotic origin) who are greater than 75 years of age or not a candidate for high-intensity statin therapy; in patients without clinical ASCVD if LDL-C is 190 mg/dL or greater and not a candidate for high-intensity statin therapy; in patients without clinical ASCVD who have type 1 or type 2 diabetes and are between 40 and 75 years of age; in patients with an estimated 10-year ASCVD risk 7.5% or greater and who are between 40 and 75 years of age (Stone, 2013). Specific recommendations from the Kidney Disease: Improving Global Outcomes (KDIGO) organization have also been released for patients with chronic kidney disease (KDIGO [Tonelli, 2013]).

Limitations of use: No incremental benefit of ezetimibe/simvastatin on cardiovascular morbidity and mortality over and above that demonstrated for simvastatin has been established. Ezetimibe/simvastatin has not been studied in Fredrickson type I, III, IV, and V dyslipidemias.

Pregnancy Risk Factor X

Dosage Note: Dosing limitation: Simvastatin 80 mg is limited to patients that have been taking this dose for >12 consecutive months without evidence of myopathy and are not currently taking or beginning a simvastatin dose-limiting or contraindicated interacting medication. If patient is unable to achieve low-density lipoprotein-cholesterol (LDL-C) goal using the 40 mg dose of simvastatin, increasing to 80 mg dose is not recommended. Instead, switch patient to an alternative LDL-C-lowering treatment providing greater LDL-C reduction. After initiation or titration, monitor lipid response after ≥2 weeks and adjust dose as necessary.

Homozygous familial hypercholesterolemia: Adults: Oral: Ezetimibe 10 mg and simvastatin 40 mg once daily in the evening.

Primary hyperlipidemia:

Children and Adolescents 10 to 17 years (males and postmenarchal females) (off-label use): Heterozygous familial hypercholesterolemia (HeFH): Oral: Initial: Ezetimibe 10 mg and simvastatin 10 to 20 mg once daily in the evening (van der Graaf, 2008). Dosing range: Ezetimibe 10 mg and simvastatin 10 to 40 mg once daily; maximum dose: Ezetimibe 10 mg and simvastatin 40 mg once daily.

Adults: Oral: Initial: Ezetimibe 10 mg and simvastatin 10 to 20 mg once daily in the evening. Start patients who require >55% reduction in LDL-C at ezetimibe 10 mg and simvastatin 40 mg once daily in the evening. Dosing range: Ezetimibe 10 mg and simvastatin 10 to 40 mg once daily

Dosage adjustment with concomitant medications: Note: Patients currently tolerating and requiring a dose of simvastatin 80 mg who require initiation of an interacting drug with a dose cap for simvastatin should be switched to an alternative statin with less potential for drug-drug interaction.

Amiodarone, amlodipine, or ranolazine: Simvastatin dose should **not** exceed 20 mg once daily

Diltiazem, dronedarone, or verapamil: Simvastatin dose should **not** exceed 10 mg once daily

Lomitapide: Reduce simvastatin dose by 50% when initiating lomitapide. Simvastatin dose should **not** exceed 20 mg once daily (or 40 mg once daily for those who previously tolerated simvastatin 80 mg daily for ≥1 year without evidence of muscle toxicity).

Dosage adjustment in Chinese patients on niacin doses ≥1 g daily: Use caution with simvastatin doses exceeding 20 mg daily; because of an increased risk of myopathy, do not administer simvastatin 80 mg

Dosage adjustment in renal impairment:

GFR ≥60 mL/minute/1.73 m^2: No dosage adjustment necessary.

GFR <60 mL/minute/1.73 m^2: Ezetimibe 10 mg and simvastatin 20 mg once daily in the evening (higher doses should be used with caution).

Dosage adjustment in hepatic impairment: Use is contraindicated in patients with active liver disease or with unexplained transaminase elevations.

Additional Information Complete prescribing information should be consulted for additional detail.

Dosage Forms

Tablet:

Vytorin:

10/10: Ezetimibe 10 mg and simvastatin 10 mg
10/20: Ezetimibe 10 mg and simvastatin 20 mg
10/40: Ezetimibe 10 mg and simvastatin 40 mg
10/80: Ezetimibe 10 mg and simvastatin 80 mg

◆ **Ezetrol (Can)** *see* Ezetimibe *on page* 832

◆ **EZFE 200 [OTC]** *see* Polysaccharide-Iron Complex *on page* 1677

◆ **EZG** *see* Ezogabine *on page* 835

Ezogabine (e ZOG a been)

Brand Names: U.S. Potiga

Index Terms D-23129; EZG; Retigabine; RTG

Pharmacologic Category Anticonvulsant, Neuronal Potassium Channel Opener

Use Adjuvant treatment of partial-onset seizures in patients ≥18 years of age who have responded inadequately to several alternative treatments and for whom the benefits outweigh the risk of retinal abnormalities and potential decline in visual acuity.

Pregnancy Risk Factor C

Pregnancy Considerations Adverse events were observed in animal reproduction studies. Patients exposed to ezogabine during pregnancy are encouraged to enroll themselves into the North American Antiepileptic Drug (NAAED) Pregnancy Registry by calling 1-888-233-2334. Additional information is available at www.aedpregnancyregistry.org.

Breast-Feeding Considerations According to the manufacturer, due to the potential for serious adverse reactions in the nursing infant, the decision to continue or discontinue breast-feeding during therapy should take into account the risk of exposure to the infant and the benefits to the mother.

Contraindications There are no contraindications listed in the manufacturer's labeling.

Warnings/Precautions [U.S. Boxed Warning]: Retinal abnormalities that may progress to vision loss have been reported and were seen in about one-third of patients after approximately 4 years of treatment. These retinal abnormalities exhibited fundoscopic features similar to those of retinal pigment dystrophies. The rate of progression and reversibility of these retinal abnormalities is unknown. Limit use to patients who have responded inadequately to other treatments and in whom the benefits of therapy exceed the risk of vision loss. Visual monitoring (at least visual acuity and dilated fundus photography) by an ophthalmic professional is recommended at baseline and at 6-month intervals. Other visual tests may include fluorescein angiograms, ocular coherence tomography, perimetry, and electroretinograms. Discontinue use if there is no substantial benefit after adequate titration or if retinal pigmentary abnormalities or vision changes are detected. If no other treatment options are available and the benefits of treatment outweigh the potential risk of vision loss, then may cautiously continue treatment with ezogabine.

Skin discoloration has been reported; typically blue in color (but may also be grey-blue or brown) and is predominantly located on or around the lips, nail beds of the fingers or toes, face and legs; and discoloration of the palate, sclera, and conjunctiva may also occur. Skin discoloration developed in ~10% of patients, generally after ≥2 years of treatment and at higher doses (≥900 mg). If detected, consider other treatment options or discontinue use.

Urinary retention, including retention requiring catheterization, has been reported, generally within the first 6 months of treatment. All patients should be monitored for urologic symptoms; close monitoring is recommended in patients with other risk factors for urinary retention (eg, benign prostatic hyperplasia), patients unable to communicate clinical symptoms, or patients who use concomitant medications that may affect voiding (eg, anticholinergics). Dose-related neuropsychiatric disorders, including confusion, psychotic symptoms, and hallucinations, have been reported, generally within the first 8 weeks of treatment; some patients required hospitalization. Symptoms resolved in most patients within 7 days of discontinuation of ezogabine. The risk appears to be greatest with rapid titration at greater than the recommended doses. Dose-related dizziness and somnolence (generally mild-to-moderate) have been reported; effects generally occur during dose titration and appear to diminish with continued use. Patients must be cautioned about performing tasks which require mental alertness (eg, operating machinery or driving). QT prolongation has been observed; monitor ECG in patients with electrolyte abnormalities (eg, hypokalemia, hypomagnesemia), hypothyroidism, familial long QT syndrome, concomitant medications which may augment QT prolongation, or any underlying cardiac abnormality which may also potentiate risk (eg, heart failure, ventricular hypertrophy). Pooled analysis of trials involving various antiepileptics (regardless of indication) showed an increased risk of suicidal thoughts/behavior (incidence rate: 0.43% treated patients compared to 0.24% of patients receiving placebo); risk observed as early as 1 week after initiation and continued through duration of trials (most trials ≤24 weeks). Monitor all patients for notable changes in behavior that might indicate suicidal thoughts or depression; notify healthcare provider immediately if symptoms occur.

Dosage adjustment recommended in hepatic impairment; ezogabine exposure increases in moderate-to-severe impairment. Dosage adjustment recommended in renal impairment; ezogabine undergoes significant renal elimination. Use caution in elderly due to potential for urinary retention, particularly in older men with symptomatic BPH. Systemic exposure is increased in the elderly; dosage adjustment is recommended in patients ≥65 years of age.

Anticonvulsants should not be discontinued abruptly because of the possibility of increasing seizure frequency; therapy should be withdrawn gradually over a period of ≥3 weeks to minimize the potential of increased seizure frequency, unless safety concerns require a more rapid withdrawal.

Adverse Reactions

Central nervous system: Abnormal gait (dose related), amnesia, anxiety, aphasia (dose related), confusion (dose related), coordination impaired (dose related), disorientation, dizziness (dose related), drowsiness (dose related), dysarthria, dysphasia, equilibrium disturbance (dose related), fatigue, hallucination, lack of concentration, memory impairment (dose related), paresthesia, vertigo

Endocrine & metabolic: Weight gain (dose related)

Gastrointestinal: Constipation (dose related), dysphagia, nausea

Genitourinary: Dysuria (dose related), hematuria, urinary hesitancy, urinary retention, urine discoloration (dose related)

Infection: Influenza

Ophthalmic: Blurred vision (dose related), diplopia

Neuromuscular & skeletal: Tremor (dose related), weakness

Rare but important or life-threatening: Alopecia, brain disease, coma, euphoria, hydronephrosis, hyperhidrosis, hypokinesia, increased appetite, increased liver enzymes, leukopenia, muscle spasm, nephrolithiasis, neutropenia, nystagmus, peripheral edema, prolonged Q-T Interval on ECG (mean: 7.7 msec), psychotic symptoms, renal colic, skin rash, syncope, thrombocytopenia

Drug Interactions

Metabolism/Transport Effects None known.

Avoid Concomitant Use

Avoid concomitant use of Ezogabine with any of the following: Azelastine (Nasal); Highest Risk QTc-Prolonging Agents; Ivabradine; Mifepristone; Orphenadrine; Paraldehyde; Thalidomide

Increased Effect/Toxicity

Ezogabine may increase the levels/effects of: Azelastine (Nasal); Buprenorphine; CNS Depressants; Digoxin; Highest Risk QTc-Prolonging Agents; Hydrocodone; Methotrimeprazine; Metyrosine; Mirtazapine; Moderate Risk QTc-Prolonging Agents; Orphenadrine; Paraldehyde; Pramipexole; ROPINIRole; Rotigotine; Selective Serotonin Reuptake Inhibitors; Suvorexant; Thalidomide; Zolpidem

The levels/effects of Ezogabine may be increased by: Alcohol (Ethyl); Brimonidine (Topical); Cannabis; Doxylamine; Dronabinol; Droperidol; HydrOXYzine; Ivabradine; Kava Kava; Magnesium Sulfate; Methotrimeprazine; Mifepristone; Nabilone; Perampanel; QTc-Prolonging Agents (Indeterminate Risk and Risk Modifying); Rufinamide; Sodium Oxybate; Tapentadol; Tetrahydrocannabinol

Decreased Effect

Ezogabine may decrease the levels/effects of: LamoTRIgine

The levels/effects of Ezogabine may be decreased by: CarBAMazepine; Mefloquine; Orlistat; Phenytoin

Storage/Stability Store at 25°C (77°F); excursions permitted to 15°C to 30°C (59°F to 86°F).

Mechanism of Action Ezogabine binds the KCNQ (Kv7.2-7.5) voltage-gated potassium channels, thereby stabilizing the channels in the open formation and enhancing the M-current. As a result, neuronal excitability is regulated and epileptiform activity is suppressed. In addition, ezogabine may also exert therapeutic effects through augmentation of GABA-mediated currents.

Pharmacodynamics/Kinetics

Absorption: Rapid

Distribution: V_{dss}: 2-3 L/kg

Protein binding: Ezogabine: 80%; N-acetyl active metabolite (NAMR): 45%

Metabolism: Glucuronidation via UGT1A4, UGT1A1, UGT1A3, and UGT1A9 and acetylation via NAT2 to an N-acetyl active metabolite (NAMR) and other inactive metabolites (eg, N-glucuronides, N-glucoside)

Bioavailability: Oral: ~60%

Half-life elimination: Ezogabine and NAMR: 7-11 hours; increased by ~30% in elderly patients

Time to peak, plasma: 0.5-2 hours; delayed by 0.75 hours when administered with high-fat food

Excretion: Urine (85%, 36% of total dose as unchanged drug, 18% of total dose as NAMR); feces (14%, 3% of total dose as unchanged drug)

Dosage Partial-onset seizures, adjunct: Oral:

Adults: Initial: 100 mg 3 times daily; may increase at weekly intervals in increments of ≤150 mg daily to a maintenance dose of 200-400 mg 3 times daily based on tolerability (maximum: 1200 mg daily). In clinical trials, no additional benefit and an increase in adverse effects was observed with doses >900 mg daily. **Note:** If there is no substantial benefit after adequate titration, then discontinue use and consider other treatment options.

Elderly: Initial: 50 mg 3 times daily; may increase at weekly intervals in increments of ≤150 mg daily to a maximum daily dose of 750 mg daily

Dosage adjustment in renal impairment:

CrCl ≥50 mL/minute: No dosage adjustment necessary.

CrCl <50 mL/minute: Initial: 50 mg 3 times daily; may increase at weekly intervals in increments of ≤150 mg daily to a maximum daily dose of 600 mg daily

ESRD requiring hemodialysis: Initial: 50 mg 3 times daily; may increase at weekly intervals in increments of ≤150 mg daily to a maximum daily dose of 600 mg daily

Dosage adjustment in hepatic impairment:

Mild impairment (Child-Pugh ≤7): No dosage adjustment necessary.

Moderate impairment (Child-Pugh 7-9): Initial: 50 mg 3 times daily; may increase at weekly intervals in increments of ≤150 mg daily to a maximum daily dose of 750 mg daily

Severe impairment (Child-Pugh >9): Initial: 50 mg 3 times daily; may increase at weekly intervals in increment of ≤150 mg daily to a maximum daily dose of 600 mg daily

Administration Oral: Swallow tablets whole. If therapy is discontinued, gradually reduce dose over ≥3 weeks unless safety concerns require abrupt withdrawal.

Monitoring Parameters Seizures; electrolytes, bilirubin, ALT, AST, serum creatinine, QT interval; urinary retention; observe patient for excessive sedation, confusion, psychotic symptoms, and hallucinations; suicidality (eg, suicidal thoughts, depression, behavioral changes); evaluate for signs/symptoms of ezogabine toxicity, including skin discoloration (blue, or grey-blue or brown in color) around the lips, nail beds of fingers or toes, face and legs.

Ophthalmic exams (at least visual acuity testing and dilated fundus photography) at baseline and 6-month intervals; fluorescein angiograms, ocular coherence tomography, perimetry, and electroretinograms may also be considered.

Dosage Forms

Tablet, Oral:

Potiga: 50 mg, 200 mg, 300 mg, 400 mg

- ◆ **F_3T** *see* Trifluridine *on page* 2103
- ◆ **FA-8 [OTC]** *see* Folic Acid *on page* 919
- ◆ **FaBB** *see* Folic Acid, Cyanocobalamin, and Pyridoxine *on page* 921
- ◆ **Fabior** *see* Tazarotene *on page* 1980
- ◆ **Fabrazyme** *see* Agalsidase Beta *on page* 64
- ◆ **Fabrazyme® (Can)** *see* Agalsidase Beta *on page* 64
- ◆ **Factive** *see* Gemifloxacin *on page* 957
- ◆ **Factive® (Can)** *see* Gemifloxacin *on page* 957
- ◆ **3 Factor PCC** *see* Factor IX Complex (Human) [(Factors II, IX, X)] *on page* 838
- ◆ **4 Factor PCC** *see* Prothrombin Complex Concentrate (Human) [(Factors II, VII, IX, X), Protein C, and Protein S] *on page* 1738

Factor VIIa (Recombinant)

(FAK ter SEV en aye ree KOM be nant)

Brand Names: U.S. NovoSeven RT

Brand Names: Canada Niastase; Niastase RT

Index Terms Coagulation Factor VIIa; Eptacog Alfa (Activated); rFVIIa

Pharmacologic Category Antihemophilic Agent

Use Bleeding episodes and perioperative management: Treatment of bleeding episodes and perioperative management in adults and children with hemophilia A or B with inhibitors, congenital factor VII (FVII) deficiency, and Glanzmann's thrombasthenia with refractoriness to platelet transfusions, with or without antibodies to platelets; treatment of bleeding episodes and perioperative management in adults with acquired hemophilia.

Pregnancy Risk Factor C

Pregnancy Considerations Adverse events were observed in animal reproduction studies.

Breast-Feeding Considerations It is not known if factor VIIa (recombinant) is excreted in breast milk. Due to the potential for serious adverse reactions in the nursing infant, a decision should be made whether to discontinue nursing or to discontinue the drug, taking into account the importance of treatment to the mother.

Contraindications There are no contraindications listed in the manufacturer's labeling.

Warnings/Precautions [U.S. Boxed Warning]: Serious thrombotic events are associated with the use of factor VIIa outside labeled indications. Arterial and venous thrombotic and thromboembolic events, some fatal, following administration of factor VIIa have been reported during postmarketing surveillance. All patients receiving factor VIIa should be monitored for signs and symptoms of activation of the coagulation system or thrombosis; thrombotic events due to circulating tissue factor or predisposing coagulopathy may be increased in patients with disseminated intravascular coagulation (DIC), advanced atherosclerotic disease, sepsis, crush injury, concomitant treatment with activated or non-activated prothrombin complex concentrates, or uncontrolled post-partum hemorrhage. Use with caution in patients with an increased risk of thromboembolic complications (eg, coronary heart disease, liver disease, DIC, postoperative immobilization, elderly patients, and neonates). Decreased dosage or discontinuation is warranted with confirmed intravascular coagulation or presence of clinical thrombosis.

Hypersensitivity reactions, including anaphylaxis, have been reported with use. Use with caution in patients with known hypersensitivity to mouse, hamster, or bovine proteins, or factor VIIa, or any components of the product. If hypersensitivity reaction occurs, discontinue use and administer appropriate treatment; carefully consider the benefits versus the risk of continued treatment with factor VIIa. Efficacy with prolonged infusions and data evaluating this agent's long-term adverse effects are limited. In patients with factor VII deficiency, if factor VIIa activity does not reach the expected level, prothrombin time is not corrected, or bleeding is uncontrolled (with recommended doses), suspect antibody formation and perform antibody analysis. Prothrombin time and factor VII coagulant activity should be measured before and after administration in patients with factor VII deficiency.

Adverse Reactions

Cardiovascular: Bradycardia, edema, hypertension, hypotension, thrombosis

Central nervous system: Cerebrovascular disease, headache, pain

Dermatologic: Pruritus, skin rash

Endocrine & metabolic: Decreased serum fibrinogen

Gastrointestinal: Vomiting

Hematologic & oncologic: Decreased prothrombin time, disseminated intravascular coagulation, increased fibrinolysis, purpura

Hepatic: Abnormal hepatic function tests

Hypersensitivity: Hypersensitivity reaction

Local: Injection site reaction

Neuromuscular & skeletal: Osteoarthrosis

Renal: Renal function abnormality

Respiratory: Pneumonia

Miscellaneous: Decreased therapeutic response, fever

Rare but important or life-threatening: Anaphylactic shock, anaphylaxis, angina pectoris, angioedema, antibody development, arterial embolism (retinal), arterial thrombosis, arterial thrombosis (limb, retinal), bowel infarction, cerebral infarction, cerebral ischemia, cerebrovascular accident, deep vein thrombosis, hepatic artery thrombosis, hypersensitivity, immunogenicity, increased fibrin degradation products (including D-dimer elevation), intracardiac thrombus, local phlebitis, myocardial infarction, myocardial ischemia, nausea, occlusion of cerebral arteries, peripheral ischemia, portal vein thrombosis, pulmonary embolism, renal artery thrombosis, thrombophlebitis, venous thrombosis at injection site

Drug Interactions

Metabolism/Transport Effects None known.

Avoid Concomitant Use There are no known interactions where it is recommended to avoid concomitant use.

Increased Effect/Toxicity

The levels/effects of Factor VIIa (Recombinant) may be increased by: Factor XIII A-Subunit (Recombinant)

Decreased Effect There are no known significant interactions involving a decrease in effect.

Preparation for Administration Prior to reconstitution, bring vials to room temperature. Add recommended diluent along wall of vial; do not inject directly onto powder. Gently swirl until dissolved.

NovoSeven RT: Reconstitute each vial to a final concentration of 1 mg/mL using the provided histidine diluent as follows:

1 mg vial: 1.1 mL histidine diluent vial or 1 mL prefilled histidine diluent syringe

2 mg vial: 2.1 mL histidine diluent vial or 2 mL prefilled histidine diluent syringe

5 mg vial: 5.2 mL histidine diluent vial or 5 mL prefilled histidine diluent syringe

8 mg vial: 8.1 mL histidine diluent vial or 8 mL prefilled histidine diluent syringe

Storage/Stability NovoSeven RT: Prior to reconstitution, store under refrigeration or between 2°C to 25°C (36°F to 77°F); do not freeze. Protect from light. Reconstituted solutions may be stored at room temperature or under refrigeration, but must be infused within 3 hours of reconstitution. Do not freeze reconstituted solutions. Do not store reconstituted solutions in syringes.

Mechanism of Action Recombinant factor VIIa, a vitamin K-dependent glycoprotein, promotes hemostasis by activating the extrinsic pathway of the coagulation cascade. It replaces deficient activated coagulation factor VII, which complexes with tissue factor and may activate coagulation factor X to Xa and factor IX to IXa. When complexed with other factors, coagulation factor Xa converts prothrombin to thrombin, a key step in the formation of a fibrin-platelet hemostatic plug.

Pharmacodynamics/Kinetics

Distribution: V_d: 103 mL/kg (range: 78 to 139)

Half-life elimination: 2.3 hours (range: 1.7 to 2.7)

Excretion: Clearance: 33 mL/kg/hour (range: 27 to 49)

Dosage

Children and Adults: IV:

Hemophilia A or B with inhibitors:

Bleeding episodes: 90 mcg/kg every 2 hours until hemostasis is achieved or until the treatment is judged ineffective. Doses between 35 to 120 mcg/kg have been used successfully in clinical trials. The dose, interval, and duration of therapy may be adjusted based upon the severity of bleeding and the degree of hemostasis achieved. For patients experiencing severe bleeds, dosing should be continued at 3- to 6-hour intervals after hemostasis has been achieved and the duration of dosing should be minimized.

Surgical interventions: 90 mcg/kg immediately before surgery; repeat at 2-hour intervals for the duration of surgery. For minor surgery, continue 90 mcg/kg every 2 hours for 48 hours, then every 2 to 6 hours until healed. For major surgery, continue 90 mcg/kg every 2 hours for 5 days, then every 4 hours until healed.

Congenital factor VII deficiency:

Bleeding episodes: 15 to 30 mcg/kg every 4 to 6 hours until hemostasis is achieved. Doses as low as 10 mcg/kg have been effective.

Surgical interventions: 15 to 30 mcg/kg immediately before surgery; repeat every 4 to 6 hours for the duration of surgery and until hemostasis achieved. Doses as low as 10 mcg/kg have been effective.

Glanzmann's thrombasthenia:

Bleeding episodes (refractory to platelet transfusions): 90 mcg/kg every 2 to 6 hours until hemostasis is achieved

Surgical interventions: 90 mcg/kg immediately before surgery; repeat at 2-hour intervals for the duration of surgery. Continue 90 mcg/kg every 2 to 6 hours to prevent post-operative bleeding.

Adults: IV:

Acquired hemophilia:

Bleeding episodes: 70 to 90 mcg/kg every 2 to 3 hours until hemostasis is achieved.

Surgical interventions: 70 to 90 mcg/kg immediately before surgery; repeat every 2 to 3 hours for the duration of surgery and until hemostasis achieved.

Intracerebral hemorrhage (ICH) (warfarin-related) (off-label use; Freeman, 2004; Ilyas, 2008): 10 to 100 mcg/kg (see **"Note"** below) administered concurrently with IV vitamin K (to correct the nonfactor VII coagulation factors).

Note: Lower doses (10 to 20 mcg/kg) are generally preferred given the higher risk of thromboembolic complications with higher doses; response is highly variable; monitor INR frequently after administration since rebound increases in INR occur quickly given the short half-life of rFVIIa; duration of INR correction is dose dependent. Routine use as a sole agent is not recommended for warfarin-related ICH (Morgenstern, 2010).

Treatment of refractory bleeding after cardiac surgery in nonhemophiliac patients: Dosing not established; doses in the range of 35 to 70 mcg/kg have been recommended based on low-quality evidence (case series, observational studies) (Chapman, 2011; Ferraris, 2011; Karkouti, 2007); in patients with a left ventricular assist device, lower doses (ie, 10 to 20 mcg/kg) may be preferred to reduce thromboembolic events (Bruckner, 2009).

Dosage adjustment in renal impairment: There are no dosage adjustments provided in the manufacturer's labeling.

Dosage adjustment in hepatic impairment: There are no dosage adjustments provided in the manufacturer's labeling; use with caution.

Dietary Considerations Some products may contain sodium.

Administration IV administration only; bolus over 2 to 5 minutes (depending on the dose administered). Use NS to flush line (if necessary) before and after administration. Administer within 3 hours after reconstitution.

Monitoring Parameters Monitor for evidence of hemostasis; although the prothrombin time/INR, aPTT, and factor VII clotting activity have no correlation with achieving hemostasis, these parameters may be useful as adjunct tests to evaluate efficacy and guide dose or interval adjustments

Additional Information The Hemophilia and Thrombosis Research Society (HTRS) Registry surveillance program is designed to collect data on the treatment of congenital and acquired bleeding disorders. All prescribers can obtain information regarding contribution of patient data to this program by calling 1-877-362-7355 or at www.novosevensurveillance.com.

Dosage Forms

Solution Reconstituted, Intravenous [preservative free]:

NovoSeven RT: 1 mg (1 ea); 2 mg (1 ea); 5 mg (1 ea); 8 mg (1 ea)

- ◆ **Factor VIII** *see* Antihemophilic Factor (Recombinant [Porcine Sequence]) *on page 153*
- ◆ **Factor VIII Concentrate** *see* Antihemophilic Factor/von Willebrand Factor Complex (Human) *on page 154*
- ◆ **Factor VIII (Human)** *see* Antihemophilic Factor (Human) *on page 152*
- ◆ **Factor VIII (Human)/von Willebrand Factor** *see* Antihemophilic Factor/von Willebrand Factor Complex (Human) *on page 154*
- ◆ **Factor VIII Inhibitor Bypassing Activity** *see* Anti-inhibitor Coagulant Complex (Human) *on page 155*
- ◆ **Factor Eight Inhibitor Bypassing Activity** *see* Anti-inhibitor Coagulant Complex (Human) *on page 155*
- ◆ **Factor VIII (Recombinant)** *see* Antihemophilic Factor (Recombinant) *on page 152*
- ◆ **Factor VIII (Recombinant)** *see* Antihemophilic Factor (Recombinant [Porcine Sequence]) *on page 153*

Factor IX Complex (Human) [(Factors II, IX, X)] (FAK ter nyne KOM pleks HYU man FAKter too nyne ten)

Brand Names: U.S. Bebulin; Bebulin VH; Profilnine SD

Index Terms 3 Factor PCC; 3-Factor PCC; PCC (Caution: Confusion-prone synonym); Prothrombin Complex Concentrate (Caution: Confusion-prone synonym); Three-Factor PCC

Pharmacologic Category Antihemophilic Agent; Blood Product Derivative; Prothrombin Complex Concentrate (PCC)

Additional Appendix Information

Reversal of Oral Anticoagulants *on page 2235*

Use Prevention and control of bleeding in patients with factor IX deficiency (hemophilia B or Christmas disease)

Pregnancy Risk Factor C

Pregnancy Considerations Animal reproduction studies have not been conducted. Factor IX concentrations do not change significantly in pregnant women with coagulation disorders and women with factor IX deficiency may be at increased risk of postpartum hemorrhage. Pregnant women should have clotting factors monitored, particularly at 28 and 34 weeks gestation and prior to invasive procedures. Prophylaxis may be needed if factor IX concentrations are <50 units/mL at term and treatment should continue for 3-5 days postpartum depending on route of delivery. Because parvovirus infection may cause hydrops fetalis or fetal death, a recombinant product is preferred if prophylaxis or treatment is needed. The neonate may also be at an increased risk of bleeding following delivery and should be tested for the coagulation disorder (Chi, 2012; Kadir, 2009; Lee, 2006).

Contraindications There are no contraindications listed in the manufacturer's labeling.

Warnings/Precautions **Factor IX Complex (Human) [Factors II, IX, X] (Bebulin, Profilnine) contains low or nontherapeutic levels of factor VII component** and should not be confused with Prothrombin complex concentrate (Human) [(Factors II, VII, IX, X), Protein C, Protein S] (Kcentra, Octaplex) which contains therapeutic levels of factor VII. Factor IX Complex (Human) [Factors II, IX, X] (Bebulin, Profilnine) should not be used for the treatment of factor VII deficiency. When treating warfarin associated hemorrhage (off-label use), administration of additional fresh frozen plasma (FFP) or factor VIIa should be considered. Hypersensitivity and anaphylactic reactions have been reported with use. Delayed reactions (up to 20 days after infusion) in previously untreated patients may also occur. Due to potential for allergic reactions, the initial ~10-20 administrations should be performed under appropriate medical supervision. The development of factor IX antibodies (or inhibitors) has been reported with factor IX therapy (usually occurs within the first 10-20 exposure days); the risk of severe hypersensitivity reactions occurring may be greater in these patients. Patients experiencing allergic reactions should be evaluated for factor IX inhibitors. When clinical response is suboptimal or patient is to undergo surgical procedure, screen for inhibitors. Patients with severe gene defects (eg, gene deletion or inversion) are more likely to develop inhibitors (WFH [Srivastava 2005]).

Observe closely for signs or symptoms of intravascular coagulation or thrombosis. Use with caution when administering to patients with liver disease, postoperatively, neonates, or patients at risk of thromboembolic phenomena, disseminated intravascular coagulation or patients with signs of fibrinolysis due to the potential risk of thromboembolic complications. Use with caution in patients with liver dysfunction; may be at increased risk of developing thrombosis or DIC. Product of human plasma; may potentially contain infectious agents which could transmit disease. Screening of donors, as well as testing and/or inactivation or removal of certain viruses, reduces the risk. Infections thought to be transmitted by this product should be reported to the manufacturer. Some products may contain heparin. Use with caution in patients with a history of heparin-induced thrombocytopenia. Some product packaging may contain natural rubber latex.

Adverse Reactions

Cardiovascular: Flushing, thrombosis (sometimes fatal)

Central nervous system: Chills, fever, headache, lethargy, somnolence

Dermatologic: Rash, urticaria

Gastrointestinal: Nausea, vomiting

Hematologic: DIC

Neuromuscular & skeletal: Paresthesia

Respiratory: Dyspnea

Miscellaneous: Anaphylactic shock, clotting factor antibodies (development of), heparin-induced thrombocytopenia (with products containing heparin)

Drug Interactions

Metabolism/Transport Effects None known.

Avoid Concomitant Use

Avoid concomitant use of Factor IX Complex (Human) [(Factors II, IX, X)] with any of the following: Aminocaproic Acid

Increased Effect/Toxicity

The levels/effects of Factor IX Complex (Human) [(Factors II, IX, X)] may be increased by: Aminocaproic Acid

Decreased Effect There are no known significant interactions involving a decrease in effect.

Preparation for Administration Bring diluent and concentrate to room temperature; gently rotate or agitate to dissolve.

Storage/Stability

Bebulin® VH: Prior to use, store under refrigeration at 2°C to 8°C (36°F to 46°F); avoid freezing. Following reconstitution, do not refrigerate and use within 3 hours.

Profilnine® SD: Prior to use, store under refrigeration at 2°C to 8°C (36°F to 46°F); avoid freezing; may also stored at room temperature (not to exceed 30°C) for up to 3 months. Following reconstitution, do not refrigerate and use within 3 hours.

Mechanism of Action Replaces deficient clotting factor including factor X; hemophilia B, or Christmas disease, is an X-linked recessively inherited disorder of blood coagulation characterized by insufficient or abnormal synthesis of the clotting protein factor IX. Factor IX is a vitamin K-dependent coagulation factor which is synthesized in the liver. Factor IX is activated by factor XIa in the intrinsic coagulation pathway. Activated factor IX (IXa), in combination with factor VII:C, activates factor X to Xa, resulting ultimately in the conversion of prothrombin to thrombin and the formation of a fibrin clot. The infusion of exogenous factor IX to replace the deficiency present in hemophilia B temporarily restores hemostasis.

Pharmacodynamics/Kinetics Half-life elimination: IX component: ~24 hours

Dosage Note: Factor IX complex (Human) [Factors II, IX, X] (Bebulin, Profilnine) contains low or nontherapeutic levels of factor VII component and should not be confused with Prothrombin Complex Concentrate (Human) [(Factors II, VII, IX, X), Protein C, Protein S] (Kcentra, Octaplex)) which contains therapeutic levels of factor VII.

Children and Adults: Dosage is expressed in units of factor IX activity and must be individualized based on severity of factor IX deficiency, extent and location of bleeding, and clinical status of patient. When multiple doses are required, administer at 24-hour intervals unless otherwise specified. Administer IV only:

Formula for units required to raise blood level %:

Bebulin® VH: In general, factor IX 1 unit/kg will increase the plasma factor IX level by 0.8%

Number of Factor IX units required = body weight (kg) x desired factor IX increase (as %) x 1.2 units/kg

Profilnine® SD: In general, factor IX 1 unit/kg will increase the plasma factor IX level by 1%:

Number of factor IX units required = bodyweight (kg) x desired factor IX increase (as %) x 1 unit/kg

For example, to increase factor IX level to 25% of normal in a 70 kg patient: Number of factor IX units needed = 70 kg x 25 x 1 unit/kg = 1750 units

As a general rule, the level of factor IX required for treatment of different conditions is listed below:

Hemorrhage: IV:

Minor bleeding (early hemarthrosis, minor epistaxis, gingival bleeding, mild hematuria):

Bebulin® VH: Raise factor IX level to 20% of normal [typical initial dose: 25-35 units/kg]; generally a single dose is sufficient.

Profilnine® SD: Mild-to-moderate bleeding: Raise factor IX level to 20% to 30% of normal.

Moderate bleeding (severe joint bleeding, early hematoma, major open bleeding, minor trauma, minor hemoptysis, hematemesis, melena, major hematuria):

Bebulin® VH: Raise factor IX level to 40% of normal [typical initial dose: 40-55 units/kg]; average duration of treatment is 2 days or until adequate wound healing.

Profilnine® SD: Mild-to-moderate bleeding: raise factor IX level to 20% to 30% of normal.

Major bleeding (severe hematoma, major trauma, severe hemoptysis, hematemesis, melena):

Bebulin® VH: Raise factor IX level to ≥60% of normal [typical initial dose: 60-70 units/kg]; average duration of treatment is 2-3 days or until adequate wound healing. Do not raise >60% in patients who may be predisposed to thrombosis.

Profilnine® SD: Raise factor IX level to 30% to 50% of normal.

Surgical procedures: IV:

Dental surgery:

Bebulin® VH: Raise factor IX level to 40% to 60% of normal on day of surgery [typical dose: 50-60 units/kg]. One infusion, administered 1 hour prior to surgery, is generally sufficient for the extraction of one tooth; for the extraction of multiple teeth, replacement therapy may be required for up to 1 week (See dosing guidelines for *Minor Surgery*).

Profilnine® SD: Raise factor IX level to 50% of normal immediately prior to procedure.

Minor surgery:

Bebulin® VH: Raise factor IX level to 40% to 60% of normal on day of surgery [typical initial dose: 50-60 units/kg]. Decrease factor IX level from 40% of normal to 20% of normal during initial postoperative period (1-2 weeks or until adequate wound healing) [typical dose: 55 units/kg decreasing to 25 units/kg]. The preoperative dose should be given 1 hour prior to surgery. The average dosing interval may be every 12 hours initially, then every 24 hours later in the postoperative period.

Profilnine® SD: Raise factor IX level to 30% to 50% of normal for at least 1 week following surgery.

Major surgery:

Bebulin® VH: Raise factor IX level to ≥60% of normal on day of surgery [typical initial dose: 70-95 units/kg]; do not raise >60% in patients who may be predisposed to thrombosis. Decrease factor IX level from 60% of normal to 20% of normal during initial postoperative period (1-2 weeks) [typical dose: 70 units/kg decreasing to 35 units/kg]; further decrease to maintain a factor IX level of 20% of normal during late postoperative period (≥3 weeks) and continuing until adequate wound healing is achieved [typical dose: 35 units/kg decreasing to 25 units/kg]. The preoperative dose should be given 1 hour prior to surgery. The average dosing interval may be every 12 hours initially, then every 24 hours later in the postoperative period.

Profilnine® SD: Raise Factor IX level to 30% to 50% of normal for at least 1 week following surgery.

Hemorrhage: IV:

Long-term prophylactic treatment: Bebulin® VH: 20-30 units/kg once or twice a week may reduce frequency of spontaneous hemorrhage; dosing regimen should be individualized.

Warfarin associated hemorrhage (off-label use): IV:

Note: Products contain low or nontherapeutic levels of factor VII component; therefore, additional fresh frozen plasma (FFP) or factor VIIa may be considered (Masotti, 2011). When immediate INR reversal is required, concomitant use of 1-2 units of FFP should be considered to ensure acute INR reversal (Baker, 2004; Chong, 2010; Holland, 2009). Administer vitamin K (phytonadione) 5-10 mg by slow IV infusion (Guyatt, 2012); vitamin K may be repeated every 12 hours if INR is persistently elevated.

Adjusted-dose regimen, weight based (Chong, 2010):

Profilnine® SD:

INR <5: 30 units/kg

INR >5 (emergent): 50 units/kg

Note: If after administration, INR remains >1.2 consider repeating dose and administering more FFP until INR <1.2

The following 2 methods have also been suggested, but are not product specific:

Adjusted-dose regimen, weight based (Liumbruno, 2009):

INR <2.0: 20 units/kg

INR 2.0-4.0: 30 units/kg

INR >4.0: 50 units/kg

Note: If after administration, INR remains >1.5 consider repeating dose appropriate for INR.

May also determine dose based on presenting INR and estimated functional prothrombin complex (PC) expressed as percentage of normal plasma levels (see table; Masotti, 2011):

Units needed to be infused = (**target** % of functional PC to be reached – **current** estimated % of functional PC) x kg of body weight

Example:

Patient (weight: 70 kg) presents with INR of 4.5 which corresponds to an **estimated % functional PC** of 10% (see table). Target INR of 1.4 corresponds to an **estimated target % functional PC** of 40%.

Units needed to be infused = (40 - 10) x 70 kg = 2100 units

Conversion of the INR to Estimated Functional Prothrombin Complex (PC)

INR Value	Estimated Functional PC
≥5.0	5%
4-4.9	10%
2.6-3.2	15%
2.2-2.5	20%
1.9-2.1	25%
1.7-1.8	30%
1.4-1.6	40%
1.0-1.3	100%

Dosage adjustment in renal impairment: No dosage adjustment provided in manufacturer's labeling.

Dosage adjustment in hepatic impairment: No dosage adjustment provided in manufacturer's labeling; use with caution.

Administration IV administration only; should be infused **slowly**. Rate should not exceed 2 mL/minute for Bebulin® VH or 10 mL/minute for Profilnine® SD. Slowing the rate of infusion, changing the lot of medication, or administering antihistamines may relieve some adverse reactions

Monitoring Parameters Levels of factor IX; PT, PTT; INR (when used for warfarin reversal); signs and symptoms of hypersensitivity reactions, DIC, thrombosis

Reference Range Average normal factor IX levels are 50% to 150%; patients with severe hemophilia B will have factor IX levels <1%, often undetectable. Moderate forms of the disease have levels of 1% to 5% while some mild cases may have 5% to 49% of normal factor IX.

Additional Information Vaccination with hepatitis A and hepatitis B vaccines are recommended at diagnosis for patients with hemophilia.

Factor IX concentrate containing only factor IX is also available and preferable for hemophilia B (or Christmas disease). Prothrombin complex concentrates also contain factor II, factor VII, and factor X and are of intermediate purity. Heparin may be present in some products to decrease thrombotic effects.

Dosage Forms Considerations

Strengths expressed as an approximate value. Consult individual vial labels for exact potency within each vial.

Bebulin VH packaged contents may contain natural rubber latex.

Dosage Forms

Solution Reconstituted, Intravenous:

Bebulin: 200-1200 UNIT (1 ea)

Bebulin VH: 200-1200 UNIT (1 ea)

Profilnine SD: 500 units (1 ea); 1000 units (1 ea); 1500 units (1 ea)

◆ **Factor IX Concentrate** *see* Factor IX (Human) *on page 840*

◆ **Factor IX Concentrate** *see* Factor IX (Recombinant) *on page 841*

Factor IX (Human) (FAK ter nyne HYU man)

Brand Names: U.S. AlphaNine SD; Mononine

Brand Names: Canada Immunine VH

Index Terms Factor IX Concentrate

Pharmacologic Category Antihemophilic Agent; Blood Product Derivative

Use Prevention and control of bleeding in patients with hemophilia B (congenital factor IX deficiency or Christmas disease)

NOTE: Contains **nondetectable levels of factors II, VII, and X**. Therefore, **NOT INDICATED** for replacement therapy of any other clotting factor besides factor IX or for reversal of anticoagulation due to either vitamin K antagonists or other anticoagulants (eg, dabigatran), for hemophilia A patients with factor VIII inhibitors, or for patients in a hemorrhagic state caused by reduced production of liver-dependent coagulation factors (eg, hepatitis, cirrhosis).

Pregnancy Risk Factor C

Dosage NOTE: Contains **nondetectable levels of factors II, VII, and X**. Therefore, **NOT INDICATED** for replacement therapy of any other clotting factor besides factor IX or for reversal of anticoagulation due to either vitamin K antagonists or other anticoagulants (eg, dabigatran), for hemophilia A patients with factor VIII inhibitors, or for patients in a hemorrhagic state caused by reduced production of liver-dependent coagulation factors (eg, hepatitis, cirrhosis).

Control or prevention of bleeding in patients with factor IX deficiency (hemophilia B or Christmas disease): Infants, Children, Adolescents, and Adults: IV: *AlphaNine SD, Mononine:* Dosage is expressed in units of factor IX activity; dosing must be individualized based on severity of factor IX deficiency, extent and location of bleeding, and clinical status of patient. Refer to product information for specific manufacturer recommended dosing. Alternatively, the World Federation of Hemophilia (WFH) has recommended general dosing for factor IX products.

Formula to determine units required to obtain desired factor IX level: **Note:** If patient has severe hemophilia (ie, baseline factor IX level is or presumed to be <1%), then may just use "desired factor IX level" instead of "desired factor IX level increase".

Number of factor IX units required = patient weight (in kg) x desired factor IX level increase (as % or units/dL) x 1 unit/kg

For example, to attain an 80% level in a 70 kg patient who has a baseline level of 20%: Number of factor IX units needed = 70 kg x 60% x 1 unit/kg = 4200 units

Alternative dosing (off-label): Infants, Children, Adolescents, and Adults: **Note:** The following recommendations may vary from those found within prescribing information or practitioner preference.

Prophylaxis: 15 to 30 units/kg/dose twice weekly weekly (Utrecht protocol; WFH [Srivastava 2013]) **or** 25 to 40 units/kg/dose twice weekly (Malmö protocol; WFH [Srivastava 2013]) **or** 40 to 100 units/kg/dose 2 to 3 times weekly (National Hemophilia Foundation, MASAC recommendation, 2007); optimum regimen has yet to be defined.

Treatment:

2013 World Federation of Hemophilia Treatment Recommendations (When No Significant Resource Constraint Exists):

Site of Hemorrhage/ Clinical Situation	Desired Factor IX Level to Maintain	Duration
Joint	40 to 60 units/dL	1 to 2 days, may be longer if response is inadequate
Superficial muscle/ no neurovascular compromise	40 to 60 units/dL	2 to 3 days, sometimes longer if response is inadequate
Iliopsoas and deep muscle with neurovascular injury, or substantial blood loss	*Initial:* 60 to 80 units/dL *Maintenance:* 30 to 60 units/dL	*Initial:* 1 to 2 days *Maintenance:* 3 to 5 days, sometimes longer as secondary prophylaxis during physiotherapy
CNS/head	*Initial:* 60 to 80 units/dL *Maintenance:* 30 units/dL	*Initial:* 1 to 7 days *Maintenance:* 8 to 21 days
Throat and neck	*Initial:* 60 to 80 units/dL *Maintenance:* 30 units/dL	*Initial:* 1 to 7 days *Maintenance:* 8 to 14 days
Gastrointestinal	*Initial:* 60 to 80 units/dL *Maintenance:* 30 units/dL	*Initial:* 7 to 14 days *Maintenance:* Not specified
Renal	40 units/dL	3 to 5 days
Deep laceration	40 units/dL	5 to 7 days
Surgery (major)	*Preop:* 60 to 80 units/dL	
	Postop: 40 to 60 units/dL 30 to 50 units/dL 20 to 40 units/dL	*Postop:* 1 to 3 days 4 to 6 days 7 to 14 days
Surgery (minor)	*Preop:* 50 to 80 units/dL	
	Postop: 30 to 80 units/dL	*Postop:* 1 to 5 days depending on procedure type

Note: Factor IX level may either be expressed as units/dL or as %. Dosing frequency most commonly corresponds to the half-life of factor IX but should be determined based on an assessment of factor IX levels before the next dose.

Continuous infusion (for patients who require prolonged periods of treatment [eg, intracranial hemorrhage or surgery] to avoid peaks and troughs associated with intermittent infusions) (Batorova, 2002; Poon, 2012; Rickard, 1995; WFH [Srivastava 2013]): Following initial bolus to achieve the desired factor IX level: Initiate 4 to 6 units/kg/hour; adjust dose based on frequent factor assays and calculation of factor IX clearance at steady-state using the following equations:

Factor IX clearance (mL/kg/hour) = (current infusion rate in units/kg/hour) divided by (plasma level in units/mL)

New infusion rate (units/kg/hour) = (factor IX clearance in mL/kg/hour) x (desired plasma level in units/mL)

Additional Information Complete prescribing information should be consulted for additional detail.

Dosage Forms Considerations

Strengths expressed with approximate values. Consult individual vial labels for exact potency within each vial.

Dosage Forms

Solution Reconstituted, Intravenous [preservative free]:

AlphaNine SD: 500 units (1 ea); 1000 units (1 ea); 1500 units (1 ea)

Mononine: 250 units (1 ea); 500 units (1 ea)

Factor IX (Recombinant)

(FAK ter nyne ree KOM be nant)

Brand Names: U.S. Alprolix; BeneFIX; Rixubis

Brand Names: Canada BeneFix

Index Terms Alprolix; Factor IX Concentrate

Pharmacologic Category Antihemophilic Agent

Use Factor IX deficiency: Prevention and control of bleeding in patients with factor IX deficiency (hemophilia B [Christmas disease]); perioperative management in patients with hemophilia B; routine prophylaxis to prevent or reduce the frequency of bleeding episodes in patients with hemophilia B (Alprolix and Rixubis).

NOTE: Contains **only factor IX**. Therefore, **NOT INDICATED** for replacement therapy of any other clotting factor besides factor IX or for reversal of anticoagulation due to either vitamin K antagonists or other anticoagulants (eg, dabigatran), for hemophilia A patients with factor VIII inhibitors, or for patients in a hemorrhagic state caused by reduced production of liver-dependent coagulation factors (eg, hepatitis, cirrhosis).

Pregnancy Risk Factor C

Dosage NOTE: Contains **only factor IX**. Therefore, **NOT INDICATED** for replacement therapy of any other clotting factor besides factor IX or for reversal of anticoagulation due to either vitamin K antagonists or other anticoagulants (eg, dabigatran), for hemophilia A patients with factor VIII inhibitors, or for patients in a hemorrhagic state caused by reduced production of liver-dependent coagulation factors (eg, hepatitis, cirrhosis).

Control or prevention of bleeding in patients with factor IX deficiency (hemophilia B or Christmas disease): IV: Dosage is expressed in units of factor IX activity; dosing must be individualized based on severity of factor IX deficiency, extent and location of bleeding, clinical status of patient, and recovery of factor IX. As compared to Benefix and Rixubis, Alprolix displays a longer half-life. Therefore, Alprolix dosing and frequency may differ. Patients <12 years of age receiving Alprolix may have a higher factor IX bodyweight-adjusted clearance, shorter half-life, and lower recovery; higher dose per kilogram or more frequent dosing may be necessary. **Refer to product information for specific manufacturer recommended dosing.** Alternatively, the World Federation of Hemophilia (WFH) has recommended general dosing for factor IX products.

Formula for units required to raise blood level %: **Note:** If patient has severe hemophilia (ie, baseline factor IX level is or presumed to be <1%), then may just use "desired factor IX level" instead of "desired factor IX level *increase*". On average, the observed recovery for BeneFix is 0.7 units/dL per units/kg in children <15 years of age and 0.8 units/dL per units/kg in adults.

Infants, Children, Adolescents, and Adults: Number of factor IX units required = patient weight (in kg) x desired factor IX level increase (as % or units/dL) x reciprocal of observed recovery (as units/kg per units/dL).

Alternative dosing (off-label): Infants, Children, Adolescents, and Adults: **Note:** The following recommendations may vary from those found within prescribing information or practitioner preference.

Prophylaxis: 15 to 30 units/kg/dose twice weekly (Utrecht protocol; WFH [Srivastava 2013]) **or** 25 to 40 units/kg/dose twice weekly (Malmö protocol; WFH [Srivastava 2013]) **or** 40 to 100 units/kg/dose 2 to 3 times weekly (National Hemophilia Foundation, MASAC recommendation, 2007); optimum regimen has yet to be defined.

Treatment:

2013 World Federation of Hemophilia Treatment Recommendations (When No Significant Resource Constraint Exists):

Site of Hemorrhage/ Clinical Situation	Desired Factor IX Level to Maintain	Duration
Joint	40-60 units/dL	1-2 days, may be longer if response is inadequate
Superficial muscle/ no neurovascular compromise	40-60 units/dL	2-3 days, sometimes longer if response is inadequate
Iliopsoas and deep muscle with neurovascular injury, or substantial blood loss	*Initial:* 60-80 units/dL *Maintenance:* 30-60 units/dL	*Initial:* 1-2 days *Maintenance:* 3-5 days, sometimes longer as secondary prophylaxis during physiotherapy
CNS/head	*Initial:* 60-80 units/dL *Maintenance:* 30 units/dL	*Initial:* 1-7 days *Maintenance:* 8-21 days
Throat and neck	*Initial:* 60-80 units/dL *Maintenance:* 30 units/dL	*Initial:* 1-7 days *Maintenance:* 8-14 days
Gastrointestinal	*Initial:* 60-80 units/dL *Maintenance:* 30 units/dL	*Initial:* 7-14 days *Maintenance:* Not specified
Renal	40 units/dL	3-5 days
Deep laceration	40 units/dL	5-7 days
Surgery (major)	*Preop:* 60-80 units/dL	
	Postop: 40-60 units/dL 30-50 units/dL 20-40 units/dL	*Postop:* 1-3 days 4-6 days 7-14 days
Surgery (minor)	*Preop:* 50-80 units/dL	
	Postop: 30-80 units/dL	*Postop:* 1-5 days depending on procedure type

Note: Factor IX level may either be expressed as units/dL or as %. Dosing frequency most commonly corresponds to the half-life of factor IX but should be determined based on an assessment of factor IX levels before the next dose.

Continuous infusion (For patients who require prolonged periods of treatment [eg, intracranial hemorrhage or surgery] to avoid peaks and troughs associated with intermittent infusions) (Batorova, 2002; Poon, 2012; Rickard, 1995; WFH [Srivastava 2013]): **Note:** Evidence supporting the use of continuous infusion is primarily with BeneFix (Chowdary, 2001): Following initial bolus to achieve the desired factor IX level, initiate 4 to 6 units/kg/hour; adjust dose based on frequent factor assays and calculation of factor IX clearance at steady-state using the following equations:

Factor IX clearance (mL/kg/hour) = (current infusion rate in units/kg/hour)/(plasma level in units/**m**L)

New infusion rate (units/kg/hour) = (factor IX clearance in mL/kg/hour) x (desired plasma level in units/**m**L)

Routine prophylaxis to prevent bleeding episodes in patients with factor IX deficiency (hemophilia B or Christmas disease): IV:

Alprolix: Children, Adolescents, and Adults: 50 units/kg once weekly or 100 units/kg once every 10 days; adjust dose based on individual response

Rixubis:

Children <12 years: 60 to 80 units/kg twice weekly; may titrate dose depending upon age, bleeding pattern, and physical activity.

Children ≥12 years, Adolescents and Adults: 40 to 60 units/kg twice weekly; may titrate dose depending upon age, bleeding pattern, and physical activity.

Dosage adjustment in renal impairment: There are no dosage adjustments provided in the manufacturer's labeling; monitor factor IX levels.

Dosage adjustment in hepatic impairment: There are no dosage adjustments provided in the manufacturer's labeling; monitor factor IX levels. Use with caution due to the risk of thromboembolic complications.

Additional Information Complete prescribing information should be consulted for additional detail.

Product Availability Alprolix: FDA approved March 2014; availability anticipated in May 2014.

Dosage Forms Considerations Strengths expressed with approximate values. Consult individual vial labels for exact potency within each vial.

Dosage Forms

Solution Reconstituted, Intravenous [preservative free]:

Alprolix: 500 units (1 ea); 1000 units (1 ea); 2000 units (1 ea); 3000 units (1 ea)

BeneFIX: 250 units (1 ea); 500 units (1 ea); 1000 units (1 ea); 2000 units (1 ea)

Rixubis: 250 units (1 ea); 500 units (1 ea); 1000 units (1 ea); 2000 units (1 ea); 3000 units (1 ea)

◆ **Factor 13** *see* Factor XIII Concentrate (Human) *on page 843*

Factor XIII Concentrate (Human)

(FAK ter THIR teen KON cen trate HYU man)

Brand Names: U.S. Corifact

Index Terms Activated Factor XIII; Corifact®; Factor 13; FXIII

Pharmacologic Category Antihemophilic Agent; Blood Product Derivative

Use Prophylaxis against bleeding episodes and management of perioperative surgical bleeding in patients with congenital factor XIII deficiency

Pregnancy Risk Factor C

Dosage Congenital factor XIII deficiency: Infants, Children, Adolescents, and Adults: IV:

Prophylaxis:

Initial: 40 units/kg

Maintenance: Dose adjustment should be based on factor XIII activity trough levels (target level of 5% to 20% using Berichrom® activity assay) and clinical response; repeat every 28 days

One trough level of <5%: Increase dosage by 5 units/kg

Trough level of 5% to 20%: No dosage change

Two trough levels of >20%: Decrease dosage by 5 units/kg

One trough level of >25%: Decrease dosage by 5 units/kg

Perioperative management of surgical bleeding: Individualize dosing based on factor XIII activity level, type of surgery, and clinical response; monitor factor XIII activity levels during and after surgery:

If time since last prophylactic dose ≤7 days: Additional dose may not be needed.

If time since last prophylactic dose 8-21 days: Additional partial or full dose may be necessary based on factor XIII activity level

If time since last prophylactic dose 21-28 days: Administer full prophylactic dose

Dosage adjustment in renal impairment: No dosage adjustment provided in the manufacturer's labeling.

Dosage adjustment in hepatic impairment: No dosage adjustment provided in the manufacturer's labeling.

Additional Information Complete prescribing information should be consulted for additional detail.

Dosage Forms

Kit, Intravenous [preservative free]:

Corifact: 1000 - 1600 units

◆ **FAG-201** *see* Dimethyl Fumarate *on page 639*

◆ **FaLessa Kit** *see* Ethinyl Estradiol and Levonorgestrel *on page 803*

◆ **Falmina** *see* Ethinyl Estradiol and Levonorgestrel *on page 803*

Famciclovir (fam SYE kloe veer)

Brand Names: U.S. Famvir

Brand Names: Canada Apo-Famciclovir®; Ava-Famciclovir; CO Famciclovir; Famvir®; PMS-Famciclovir; Sandoz-Famciclovir

Pharmacologic Category Antiviral Agent

Use Treatment of acute herpes zoster (shingles) in immunocompetent patients; treatment and suppression of recurrent episodes of genital herpes in immunocompetent patients; treatment of herpes labialis (cold sores) in immunocompetent patients; treatment of recurrent orolabial/genital (mucocutaneous) herpes simplex in HIV-infected patients

Pregnancy Risk Factor B

Pregnancy Considerations Teratogenic effects were not observed in animal reproduction studies. Data in pregnant women is limited. A registry has been established for women exposed to famciclovir during pregnancy (888-669-6682).

Breast-Feeding Considerations There is no specific data describing the excretion of famciclovir in breast milk. Breast-feeding is not recommended by the manufacturer unless the potential benefits outweigh any possible risk. If herpes lesions are on breast, breast-feeding should be avoided in order to avoid transmission to infant.

Contraindications Hypersensitivity to famciclovir, penciclovir, or any component of the formulation

Warnings/Precautions Has not been established for use in immunocompromised patients (except HIV-infected patients with orolabial or genital herpes, patients with ophthalmic or disseminated zoster or with initial episode of genital herpes, and in Black and African American patients with recurrent episodes of genital herpes. Acute renal failure has been reported with use of inappropriate high doses in patients with underlying renal disease. Dosage adjustment is required in patients with renal insufficiency. Tablets contain lactose; do not use with galactose intolerance, severe lactase deficiency, or glucose-galactose malabsorption syndromes.

Adverse Reactions

Central nervous system: Fatigue, headache, migraine

Dermatologic: Pruritus, rash

Endocrine & metabolic: Dysmenorrhea

Gastrointestinal: Abdominal pain, diarrhea, flatulence, nausea, vomiting

Hematologic: Neutropenia

Hepatic: Bilirubin increased, transaminases increased

Neuromuscular & skeletal: Paresthesia

Rare but important or life-threatening: Anemia, angioedema (eyelid, face, periorbital, pharyngeal edema), cholestatic jaundice, confusion, delirium, disorientation, dizziness, erythema multiforme, hallucinations, leukocytoclastic vasculitis, palpitations, somnolence, Stevens-Johnson syndrome, thrombocytopenia, toxic epidermal necrolysis, urticaria

Drug Interactions

Metabolism/Transport Effects None known.

Avoid Concomitant Use

Avoid concomitant use of Famciclovir with any of the following: Zoster Vaccine

Increased Effect/Toxicity There are no known significant interactions involving an increase in effect.

Decreased Effect

Famciclovir may decrease the levels/effects of: Zoster Vaccine

Food Interactions Rate of absorption and/or conversion to penciclovir and peak concentration are reduced with food, but bioavailability is not affected. Management: Administer without regard to meals.

Storage/Stability Store at 25°C (77°F); excursions permitted to 15°C to 30°C (59°F to 86°F).

Mechanism of Action Famciclovir undergoes rapid biotransformation to the active compound, penciclovir (prodrug), which is phosphorylated by viral thymidine kinase in HSV-1, HSV-2, and VZV-infected cells to a monophosphate form; this is then converted to penciclovir triphosphate and competes with deoxyguanosine triphosphate to inhibit HSV-2 polymerase, therefore, herpes viral DNA synthesis/replication is selectively inhibited.

Pharmacodynamics/Kinetics

Absorption: Food decreases maximum peak penciclovir concentration and delays time to penciclovir peak; AUC remains the same

Distribution: V_d: Penciclovir: 0.91-1.25 L/kg

Protein binding: Penciclovir: <20%

Metabolism: Famciclovir is rapidly deacetylated and oxidized to penciclovir (active prodrug); *in vitro* data demonstrate that metabolism does not occur via CYP isoenzymes

Bioavailability: Penciclovir: 69% to 85%

Half-life elimination: Penciclovir: 2-4 hours; Prolonged in renal impairment: CrCl 20-39 mL/minute: 5-8 hours, CrCl <20 mL/minute: 3-24 hours

Time to peak: Penciclovir: ~1 hour

Excretion: Urine (73% primarily as penciclovir); feces (27%)

Dosage Adults: Oral:

Immunocompetent patients:

Acute herpes zoster: 500 mg every 8 hours for 7 days (**Note:** Initiate therapy as soon as possible after diagnosis and within 72 hours of rash onset)

Genital herpes simplex virus (HSV) infection:

Initial episode: 250 mg 3 times/day for 7-10 days (CDC, 2010)

Recurrence: 1000 mg twice daily for 1 day (**Note:** Initiate therapy as soon as possible and within 6 hours of symptoms/lesions onset)

Alternatively, the following regimens are also recommended: 125 mg twice daily for 5 days or 500 mg as a single dose, followed by 250 mg twice daily for 2 days (CDC, 2010). **Note:** Canadian labeling recommends 125 mg twice daily for 5 days.

Suppressive therapy: 250 mg twice daily for up to 1 year; **Note:** Duration not established, but efficacy/safety have been demonstrated for 1 year (CDC, 2010)

Recurrent herpes labialis (cold sores): 1500 mg as a single dose; initiate therapy at first sign or symptom such as tingling, burning, or itching (initiated within 1 hour in clinical studies)

HIV patients (**Note:** Initiate therapy as soon as possible and within 48 hours of symptoms/lesions onset):

Recurrent orolabial/genital (mucocutaneous) HSV infection: 500 mg twice daily for 7 days or 5-10 days (CDC, 2010).

Prevention of HSV reactivation: 500 mg twice daily (CDC, 2010)

Dosing adjustment in renal impairment:

Herpes zoster:

CrCl ≥60 mL/minute: No dosage adjustment necessary

CrCl 40-59 mL/minute: Administer 500 mg every 12 hours

CrCl 20-39 mL/minute: Administer 500 mg every 24 hours

CrCl <20 mL/minute: Administer 250 mg every 24 hours

Hemodialysis: Administer 250 mg after each dialysis session.

Recurrent genital herpes: Treatment:

U.S. labeling (single-day regimen):

CrCl ≥60 mL/minute: No dosage adjustment necessary

CrCl 40-59 mL/minute: Administer 500 mg every 12 hours for 1 day

CrCl 20-39 mL/minute: Administer 500 mg as a single dose

CrCl <20 mL/minute: Administer 250 mg as a single dose

Hemodialysis: Administer 250 mg as a single dose after a dialysis session.

Canadian labeling:

CrCl >20 mL/minute/1.73 m^2: No dosage adjustment necessary

CrCl <20 mL/minute/1.73 m^2: Administer 125 mg every 24 hours

Hemodialysis: Administer 125 mg after each dialysis session.

Recurrent genital herpes: Suppression:

CrCl ≥40 mL/minute: No dosage adjustment necessary

CrCl 20-39 mL/minute: Administer 125 mg every 12 hours

CrCl <20 mL/minute: Administer 125 mg every 24 hours

Hemodialysis: Administer 125 mg after each dialysis session.

Recurrent herpes labialis: Treatment (single-dose regimen):

CrCl ≥60 mL/minute: No dosage adjustment necessary

CrCl 40-59 mL/minute: Administer 750 mg as a single dose

CrCl 20-39 mL/minute: Administer 500 mg as a single dose

CrCl <20 mL/minute: Administer 250 mg as a single dose

Hemodialysis: Administer 250 mg as a single dose after a dialysis session.

Recurrent orolabial/genital (mucocutaneous) herpes in HIV-infected patients:

CrCl ≥40 mL/minute: No dosage adjustment necessary

CrCl 20-39 mL/minute: Administer 500 mg every 24 hours

CrCl <20 mL/minute: Administer 250 mg every 24 hours

Hemodialysis: Administer 250 mg after each dialysis session.

Dosage adjustment in hepatic impairment:

Mild-to-moderate impairment: No dosage adjustment is necessary

Severe impairment: No dosage adjustment provided in manufacturer's labeling; has not been studied. However, a 44% decrease in the C_{max} of penciclovir (active metabolite) was noted in patients with mild-to-moderate impairment; impaired conversion of famciclovir to penciclovir may affect efficacy.

Dietary Considerations May be taken without regard to meals.

Administration May be administered without regard to meals.

Monitoring Parameters Periodic CBC during long-term therapy

Additional Information Most effective for herpes zoster if therapy is initiated within 48 hours of initial lesion. Resistance may occur by alteration of thymidine kinase, resulting in loss of or reduced penciclovir phosphorylation (cross-resistance occurs between acyclovir and famciclovir). When treatment for herpes labialis is initiated within 1 hour of symptom onset, healing time is reduced by ~2 days.

Dosage Forms

Tablet, Oral:

Famvir: 125 mg, 250 mg, 500 mg

Generic: 125 mg, 250 mg, 500 mg

Famotidine (fa MOE ti deen)

Brand Names: U.S. Acid Reducer Maximum Strength [OTC]; Acid Reducer [OTC]; Heartburn Relief Max St [OTC]; Heartburn Relief [OTC]; Pepcid

Brand Names: Canada Acid Control; Apo-Famotidine; Famotidine Omega; Maximum Strength Pepcid AC; Mylan-Famotidine; Pepcid AC; Pepcid Complete; Peptic guard; Teva-Famotidine; Ulcidine

Pharmacologic Category Histamine H_2 Antagonist

Use Maintenance therapy and treatment of duodenal ulcer; treatment of gastroesophageal reflux disease (GERD), active benign gastric ulcer; pathological hypersecretory conditions

OTC labeling: Relief of heartburn, acid indigestion, and sour stomach

Pregnancy Risk Factor B

Pregnancy Considerations Adverse events have not been observed in animal reproduction studies; therefore, famotidine is classified as pregnancy category B. Famotidine crosses the placenta. An increased risk of congenital malformations or adverse events in the newborn has generally not been observed following maternal use of famotidine during pregnancy. Histamine H_2 antagonists have been evaluated for the treatment of gastroesophageal reflux disease (GERD), as well as gastric and duodenal ulcers, during pregnancy. Although if needed, famotidine is not the agent of choice. Histamine H_2 antagonists may be used for aspiration prophylaxis prior to cesarean delivery.

Breast-Feeding Considerations Famotidine is excreted into breast milk with peak concentrations occurring ~6 hours after the maternal dose. According to the manufacturer, the decision to continue or discontinue breast-feeding during therapy should take into account the risk of exposure to the infant and the benefits of treatment to the mother.

Contraindications Hypersensitivity to famotidine, other H_2 antagonists, or any component of the formulation

Warnings/Precautions Modify dose in patients with moderate-to-severe renal impairment. Prolonged QT interval has been reported in patients with renal dysfunction. The FDA has received reports of torsade de pointes occurring with famotidine (Poluzzi, 2009). Relief of symptoms does not preclude the presence of a gastric malignancy. Reversible confusional states, usually clearing within 3-4 days after discontinuation, have been linked to use. Prolonged treatment (≥2 years) may lead to vitamin B_{12} malabsorption and subsequent vitamin B_{12} deficiency. The magnitude of the deficiency is dose-related and the association is stronger in females and those younger in age (<30 years); prevalence is decreased after discontinuation of therapy (Lam, 2013). Increased age (>50 years) and renal or hepatic impairment are thought to be associated.

Benzyl alcohol and derivatives: Some dosage forms may contain benzyl alcohol and/or sodium benzoate/benzoic acid; benzoic acid (benzoate) is a metabolite of benzyl alcohol; large amounts of benzyl alcohol (≥99 mg/kg/day) have been associated with a potentially fatal toxicity ("gasping syndrome") in neonates; the "gasping syndrome" consists of metabolic acidosis, respiratory distress, gasping respirations, CNS dysfunction (including convulsions, intracranial hemorrhage), hypotension, and cardiovascular collapse (AAP, 1997; CDC, 1982); some data suggests that benzoate displaces bilirubin from protein binding sites (Ahlfors, 2001); avoid or use dosage forms containing benzyl alcohol and/or benzyl alcohol derivative with caution in neonates. See manufacturer's labeling.

OTC labeling: When used for self-medication, patients should be instructed not to use if they have difficulty swallowing, are vomiting blood, or have bloody or black stools. Not for use with other acid reducers.

Adverse Reactions

Central nervous system: Dizziness, headache

Gastrointestinal: Constipation, diarrhea, necrotizing enterocolitis (VLBW neonates; Guillet, 2006)

Rare but important or life-threatening: Abdominal discomfort, acne, agitation, agranulocytosis, allergic reaction, alopecia, anaphylaxis, angioedema, anorexia, anxiety, arrhythmia, arthralgia, AV block, bronchospasm, cholestatic jaundice, confusion, conjunctival injection, depression, dry skin, facial edema, fatigue, fever, flushing, hallucinations, hepatitis, injection site reactions, insomnia, interstitial pneumonia, leukopenia, libido decreased, liver function tests increased, muscle cramps, nausea, palpitation, pancytopenia, paresthesia, pruritus, QT-interval prolongation, rash, rhabdomyolysis, seizure, somnolence, Stevens-Johnson syndrome, taste disorder, tinnitus, thrombocytopenia, torsade de pointes, toxic epidermal necrolysis, urticaria, vomiting, weakness, xerostomia

Drug Interactions

Metabolism/Transport Effects Substrate of OCT2

Avoid Concomitant Use

Avoid concomitant use of Famotidine with any of the following: Dasatinib; Delavirdine; PAZOPanib; Risedronate

Increased Effect/Toxicity

Famotidine may increase the levels/effects of: Dexmethylphenidate; Highest Risk QTc-Prolonging Agents; Methylphenidate; Moderate Risk QTc-Prolonging Agents; Risedronate; Saquinavir; Varenicline

The levels/effects of Famotidine may be increased by: BuPROPion; Mifepristone

Decreased Effect

Famotidine may decrease the levels/effects of: Atazanavir; Bosutinib; Cefditoren; Cefpodoxime; Cefuroxime; Dabrafenib; Dasatinib; Delavirdine; Erlotinib; Fosamprenavir; Gefitinib; Indinavir; Iron Salts; Itraconazole; Ketoconazole (Systemic); Ledipasvir; Mesalamine; Multivitamins/Minerals (with ADEK, Folate, Iron); Nelfinavir; Nilotinib; PAZOPanib; Posaconazole; Rilpivirine; Vismodegib

Food Interactions Prolonged treatment (≥2 years) may lead to malabsorption of dietary vitamin B_{12} and subsequent vitamin B_{12} deficiency (Lam, 2013).

Preparation for Administration Solution for injection:

IV push: Dilute famotidine with NS (or another compatible solution) to a total of 5-10 mL (may also administer undiluted [Lipsy, 1995])

Infusion: Dilute with D_5W 100 mL or another compatible solution.

Storage/Stability

Oral:

Powder for oral suspension: Prior to mixing, dry powder should be stored at controlled room temperature of 25°C (77°F). Reconstituted oral suspension is stable for 30 days at room temperature; do not freeze.

Tablet: Store controlled room temperature. Protect from moisture.

IV:

Solution for injection: Prior to use, store at 2°C to 8°C (36°F to 46°F). If solution freezes, allow to solubilize at controlled room temperature. May be stored at room temperature for up to 3 months (data on file [Bedford Laboratories, 2011]).

IV push: Following preparation, solutions for IV push should be used immediately, or may be stored in refrigerator and used within 48 hours.

Infusion: Following preparation, the manufacturer states may be stored for up to 48 hours under refrigeration; however, solutions for infusion have been found to be physically and chemically stable for 7 days at room temperature.

Solution for injection, premixed bags: Store at controlled room temperature of 25°C (77°F); avoid excessive heat.

Mechanism of Action Competitive inhibition of histamine at H_2 receptors of the gastric parietal cells, which inhibits gastric acid secretion

Pharmacodynamics/Kinetics

Onset of action: Antisecretory effect: Oral: Within 1 hour; IV: Within 30 minutes

Peak effect: Antisecretory effect: Oral: Within 1-3 hours (dose-dependent)

Duration: Antisecretory effect: IV, Oral: 10-12 hours

Absorption: Oral: Incompletely absorbed

Distribution: V_d:

Infants: 0-3 months: ~1.4-1.8 L/kg; >3-12 months: ~2.3 L/kg

Children: ~2 L/kg

Adults: ~1 L/kg

Protein binding: 15% to 20%

Metabolism: Minimal first-pass metabolism; forms one metabolite (S-oxide)

Bioavailability: Oral: 40% to 45%

Half-life elimination:

Infants: 0-3 months: ~8-10.5 hours; >3-12 months: ~4.5 hours

Children: 3.4 hours

Adults: 2.5-3.5 hours; prolonged with renal impairment; Oliguria: >20 hours

Time to peak, serum: Oral: ~1-3 hours

Excretion: Urine (25% to 30% [oral], 65% to 70% [IV] as unchanged drug)

Dosage

Children: Treatment duration and dose should be individualized

Peptic ulcer: 1-16 years:

Oral: 0.5 mg/kg/day at bedtime or divided twice daily (maximum dose: 40 mg/day); doses of up to 1 mg/kg/day have been used in clinical studies

IV: 0.25 mg/kg every 12 hours (maximum dose: 40 mg/day); doses of up to 0.5 mg/kg have been used in clinical studies

GERD: Oral:

<3 months: 0.5 mg/kg once daily

3-12 months: 0.5 mg/kg twice daily

1-16 years: 1 mg/kg/day divided twice daily (maximum dose: 40 mg twice daily); doses of up to 2 mg/kg/day have been used in clinical studies

Children ≥12 years and Adults: Heartburn, indigestion, sour stomach: OTC labeling: Oral: 10-20 mg every 12 hours; dose may be taken 15-60 minutes before eating foods known to cause heartburn

Adults:

Duodenal ulcer: Oral: Acute therapy: 40 mg/day at bedtime (or 20 mg twice daily) for 4-8 weeks; maintenance therapy: 20 mg/day at bedtime

Helicobacter pylori eradication (off-label use): Oral: 40 mg once daily; requires combination therapy with antibiotics

Gastric ulcer: Oral: Acute therapy: 40 mg/day at bedtime

GERD: Oral: 20 mg twice daily for 6 weeks

Hypersecretory conditions: Oral: Initial: 20 mg every 6 hours, may increase in increments up to 160 mg every 6 hours

Esophagitis and accompanying symptoms due to GERD: Oral: 20 mg or 40 mg twice daily for up to 12 weeks

Stress ulcer prophylaxis, ICU patients (off-label use): Oral, IV, or nasogastric (NG) tube: 20 mg twice daily (ASHP, 1999; Baghaie, 1995); **Note:** Intended for patients with associated risk factors (eg, coagulopathy, mechanical ventilation for >48 hours, severe sepsis); discontinue use once risk factors have resolved. The Surviving Sepsis Campaign guidelines suggest the use of proton pump inhibitors rather than H_2 antagonist therapy (Dellinger, 2013).

Patients unable to take oral medication: IV: 20 mg every 12 hours

Dosage adjustment in renal impairment: CrCl <50 mL/minute: Manufacturer recommendation: Administer 50% of dose **or** increase the dosing interval to every 36-48 hours (to limit potential CNS adverse effects).

Dietary Considerations May be taken without regard to meals.

Administration

Oral: May administer with antacids.

Suspension: Shake vigorously before use. May be taken without regard to meals.

Tablet: May be taken without regard to meals.

IV:

IV push: Inject over at least 2 minutes.

Solution for infusion: Administer over 15-30 minutes.

Dosage Forms

Solution, Intravenous:

Generic: 20 mg (50 mL); 20 mg/2 mL (2 mL); 40 mg/4 mL (4 mL); 200 mg/20 mL (20 mL); 500 mg/50 mL (50 mL)

Solution, Intravenous [preservative free]:

Generic: 20 mg/2 mL (2 mL)

Suspension Reconstituted, Oral:

Pepcid: 40 mg/5 mL (50 mL)

Generic: 40 mg/5 mL (50 mL)

Tablet, Oral:

Acid Reducer [OTC]: 10 mg

Acid Reducer Maximum Strength [OTC]: 20 mg

Heartburn Relief [OTC]: 10 mg

Heartburn Relief Max St [OTC]: 20 mg

Pepcid: 20 mg, 40 mg

Generic: 10 mg, 20 mg, 40 mg

Extemporaneous Preparations An 8 mg/mL oral suspension may be made with tablets. Crush seventy 40 mg tablets in a mortar and reduce to a fine powder. Add small portions of sterile water and mix to a uniform paste. Mix while adding a 1:1 mixture of Ora-Plus® and Ora-Sweet® in incremental proportions to **almost** 350 mL; transfer to a calibrated bottle, rinse mortar with vehicle, and add quantity of vehicle sufficient to make 350 mL. Label "shake well". Stable for 95 days at room temperature.

Dentinger PJ, Swenson CF, and Anaizi NH, "Stability of Famotidine in an Extemporaneously Compounded Oral Liquid," *Am J Health Syst Pharm*, 2000, 57(14):1340-2.

- **Famotidine Omega (Can)** *see* Famotidine *on page* 845
- **Fampridine** *see* Dalfampridine *on page* 552
- **Fampridine-SR** *see* Dalfampridine *on page* 552
- **Fampyra (Can)** *see* Dalfampridine *on page* 552
- **Famvir** *see* Famciclovir *on page* 843
- **Famvir® (Can)** *see* Famciclovir *on page* 843
- **Fanapt** *see* Iloperidone *on page* 1044
- **Fanapt Titration Pack** *see* Iloperidone *on page* 1044
- **2F-ara-AMP** *see* Fludarabine *on page* 890
- **Fareston** *see* Toremifene *on page* 2071
- **Fareston® (Can)** *see* Toremifene *on page* 2071
- **Faslodex** *see* Fulvestrant *on page* 939
- **Faslodex® (Can)** *see* Fulvestrant *on page* 939
- **Fasturtec® (Can)** *see* Rasburicase *on page* 1783

Fat Emulsion (Fish Oil Based) [CAN/INT]

(fat e MUL shun fish oyl baste)

Brand Names: Canada SMOFlipid

Index Terms Intravenous Fat Emulsion (Fish-Oil Based)

Pharmacologic Category Caloric Agent

Use Note: Not approved in U.S.

Caloric/fatty acid source: Source of calories, essential fatty acids, and omega-3 fatty acids for patients requiring parenteral nutrition

Pregnancy Considerations Has not been studied in pregnant women. The manufacturer recommends careful consideration be given when considering administration in pregnant women.

Breast-Feeding Considerations Has not been studied in nursing women. The manufacturer recommends careful consideration be given when considering administration in nursing women.

Contraindications Hypersensitivity to fish-, egg-, or soybean or peanut protein or any other component of the formulation; severe hyperlipidemia; severe hepatic insufficiency; severe blood coagulation disorders; severe renal insufficiency without access to hemofiltration or dialysis; acute shock; acute pulmonary edema; hyperhydration; decompensated cardiac insufficiency; unstable conditions (eg, severe post-traumatic conditions, uncompensated diabetes mellitus, acute MI, CVA, embolism, metabolic acidosis, severe sepsis, hypotonic dehydration)

Warnings/Precautions Contains soybean oil, fish oil, and egg phospholipids; hypersensitivity reactions may occur (rare). Cross-sensitivity has been observed between soybean and peanut. Discontinue use immediately if a reaction occurs and treat appropriately. Fat overload syndrome may occur with intravenous fat emulsion in patients with impaired ability to eliminate triglycerides, severe hypertriglyceridemia and/or sudden change in clinical status (eg, renal impairment, infection). Monitor for signs of fat overload syndrome (eg, hyperlipidemia, fever, hepatomegaly with/without jaundice, anemia, hepatic impairment, splenomegaly, coagulation disorder, leukopenia, thrombocytopenia) and interrupt infusion if they occur; usually reversible upon discontinuation. Hypertriglyceridemia may occur with intravenous fat emulsion; monitor triglycerides closely during therapy. Consider dose reduction or discontinuation of lipid infusion if plasma triglyceride concentrations exceed 3 mmol/L (265 mg/dL) during or after the infusion.

Use with caution in patients with anemia and bleeding disorders (contraindicated with severe blood coagulation disorders). Use with caution in patients with diabetes mellitus (limited data); use is contraindicated in uncompensated diabetes mellitus. Use with caution in patients with pancreatitis without hyperlipidemia or hepatic or renal impairment (contraindicated in severe hepatic impairment and severe renal impairment when hemofiltration or dialysis are not available). Use with caution in patients with respiratory disease, hypothyroidism, sepsis (contraindicated in severe sepsis), or patients who may be at danger for fat embolism.

Simultaneous infusion of a carbohydrate/amino acid solution is recommended to minimize the risk of metabolic acidosis. Lipid emulsion in a three-in-one mixture may obscure the presence of a precipitate; follow compounding guidelines, especially for calcium and phosphate additions.

Adverse Reactions

Cardiovascular: Thrombophlebitis

Central nervous system: Headache, hypoesthesia, increased body temperature, paresthesia

Endocrine & metabolic: Hyperglycemia, increased serum triglycerides

Gastrointestinal: Flatulence, nausea, vomiting

Hepatic: Hyperbilirubinemia

Respiratory: Pneumonia

Rare but important or life-threatening: Anaphylaxis, cyanosis, decreased appetite, edema, flank pain, glycosuria, hepatitis, hyperchloremia, hypernatremia, hypersensitivity reaction, hypertension, hypotension, ostealgia, priapism

Storage/Stability Store up to 25°C (77°F). Keep in overwrap just prior to use; once removed from overwrap use immediately. If not used immediately, the manufacturer suggests storing at 2°C to 8°C (35.6°F to 46.4°F) for no longer than 24 hours. Do not freeze.

Mechanism of Action SMOFlipid is composed of 4 different lipid types (soybean oil, medium-chain triglycerides [MCT], olive oil, and fish-oil). The fat emulsion provides energy, essential fatty acids and omega-3 fatty acids. MCT and olive oil mainly provide energy. Essential fatty acids (obtained mainly from soybean oil) are important for cell membrane structure and function. Fish-oil provides omega-3 fatty acids docosahexaenoic acid (DHA) and eicosapentaenoic acid (EPA), both of which are important structural components of cell membranes. EPA is metabolized to eicosanoids (eg, prostaglandins, thromboxanes, leukotrienes) with lower inflammatory potential than those derived from arachidonic acid. The formulation also contains vitamin E which protects against lipid peroxidation of unsaturated fatty acids.

Pharmacodynamics/Kinetics Half-life elimination: Serum triglycerides: A shorter half-life observed with SMOFlipid when compared to soybean oil emulsion.

Dosage Caloric source: Adults: IV: 1-2 g lipid/kg daily or 5-10 mL/kg daily; maximum rate of infusion is 0.15 g lipid/kg/hour or 0.75 mL/kg/hour. **Note:** At the onset of therapy, observe patient for any immediate allergic reactions (eg, dyspnea, cyanosis, and fever).

Dosage adjustment for toxicity:

Hypersensitivity: Discontinue infusion immediately.

Triglycerides >3 mmol/L (>265 mg/dL): Interrupt therapy or consider dose reduction if it is necessary to continue therapy.

Dosage adjustment in renal impairment:

Mild-to moderate impairment: No dosage adjustment provided in manufacturer's labeling.

Severe impairment: Use is contraindicated unless hemofiltration or dialysis is available (no dosage adjustment provided in manufacturer's labeling).

Dosage adjustment in hepatic impairment:

Mild-to moderate impairment: No dosage adjustment provided in manufacturer's labeling.

Severe impairment: Use is contraindicated.

Dietary Considerations Caloric content: 2 kcal/mL

Fat content of parenteral nutrition formulation should not exceed 2.5 g/kg daily (Mirtallo, 2004).

Administration IV: Gently invert bag prior to use. Do not use if discolored or if the emulsion contains a precipitate, phase separation, or there are leaks in the bag. Infuse IV through peripheral or central venous line using DEHP-free administration sets and lines. Do not exceed a rate of 0.15 g lipid/kg/hour (equivalent to 0.75 mL/kg/hour). Change tubing after each infusion. May be simultaneously infused with amino acid dextrose mixtures by means of Y-connector located near infusion site. Peripheral administration of parenteral nutrition is dependent upon osmolality of solution (ie, should not exceed 900 mOsm/L; Mirtallo, 2004).

Monitoring Parameters At the onset of therapy, the patient should be observed for any immediate allergic reactions such as dyspnea, cyanosis, and fever. Monitor line site for signs and symptoms of infection.

Monitor triglycerides before initiation of lipid therapy and closely thereafter during therapy (some recommend until triglycerides are stable and when changes are made in the amount of fat administered; ASPEN Guidelines, 2002); signs/symptoms of fat overload; electrolytes, glucose, hepatic function, acid/base metabolism, CBC, fluid status.

Additional Information Lipid emulsions have been used to reverse local anesthetic toxicity; lipid emulsion probably extracts lipophilic local anesthesia from cardiac muscle. Exogenous lipids provide an alternative source of binding of lipid-soluble local anesthetics (Rowlingson, 2008), commonly known as the "lipid sink" effect. This is more relevant to bupivacaine, levobupivacaine, and ropivacaine than mepivacaine and prilocaine. High lipid partition constant and large volumes of distribution are good predictors of success when using lipid therapy (French, 2011). Lipid administration may also affect the heart in a metabolically advantageous way by improving fatty acid transport (Weinberg, 2006). The use of SMOFlipid in reversing anesthetic toxicity has been studied in animals (Melo, 2012); however, human data appear to be lacking.

Product Availability Not available in the U.S.

Dosage Forms: Canada

Emulsion, Intravenous:

SMOFlipid 20%: Soybean oil 6%, medium chain triglycerides 6%, olive oil 5%, and fish oil 3% (100 mL, 250 mL, 500 mL)

Fat Emulsion (Plant Based)

(fat e MUL shun plant baste)

Brand Names: U.S. Intralipid; Liposyn III; Nutrilipid

Brand Names: Canada Intralipid

Index Terms Clinolipid; Intravenous Fat Emulsion

Pharmacologic Category Caloric Agent

Use Caloric/fatty acid source: Source of calories and essential fatty acids for patients requiring parenteral nutrition for extended periods of time (usually for longer than 5 days) or when oral or enteral nutrition is not possible, insufficient, or contraindicated; to prevent and treat essential fatty acid deficiency (except Clinolipid and Nutrilipid)

Pregnancy Risk Factor C

Dosage IV: **Note:** At the onset of therapy, the patient should be observed for any immediate allergic reactions (eg, dyspnea, cyanosis, and fever).

Caloric source: **Note:** Fat emulsion should not exceed 60% of the total daily calories.

Infants: Initial dose: 1-2 g/kg/day, increase by 0.5-1 g/kg/day to a maximum of 3 g/kg/day depending on needs/nutritional goals; daily dose may be infused over 24 hours (ASPEN Guidelines, 2002; ASPEN Pediatric Nutrition Support Core Curriculum, 2010)

Children 1-10 years: Initial dose: 1-2 g/kg/day, increase by 0.5-1 g/kg/day to a maximum of 2-3 g/kg/day depending upon the needs/nutritional goals; daily dose may be infused over 24 hours (ASPEN Guidelines, 2002; ASPEN Pediatric Nutrition Support Core Curriculum, 2010)

Adolescents: Initial dose: 1 g/kg/day (not to exceed 500 mL Intralipid 10% or 20% or 330 mL Intralipid 30% [over 4-6 hours] on the first day of therapy); increase by 1 g/kg/day to a maximum of 2.5 g/kg/day depending upon the needs/nutritional goals; daily dose may be infused over 12-24 hours (ASPEN Guidelines, 2002; ASPEN Pediatric Nutrition Support Core Curriculum, 2010)

Adults: Initial dose: 1 to 1.5 g/kg/day (not to exceed 500 mL Intralipid 10% or 20% or 330 mL Intralipid 30% [over 4-6 hours] on the first day of therapy); daily dose may be infused over 12-24 hours; maximum daily dose: 2.5 g/kg/day

Essential fatty acid deficiency (EFAD), prevention: Children, Adolescents, and Adults: Administer at least 2% to 4% of total caloric intake as linoleic acid and 0.25% to 0.5% as alpha linolenic acid (Mirtallo, 2004; Mirtallo, 2010)

Essential fatty acid deficiency (EFAD), treatment: Children, Adolescents, and Adults: Intralipid, Liposyn III: Administer 8% to 10% of total caloric intake as fat emulsion; may infuse up to once daily (Riella, 1975). If EFAD occurs with stress, the dosage needed to correct EFAD may be increased.

Local anesthetic toxicity (off-label use): Adults: 20%: 1.5 **mL**/kg administered over 1 minute, followed immediately by an infusion of 0.25 **mL**/kg/minute. Continue chest compressions (lipid must circulate). Repeat the bolus 1-2 times as needed for persistent asystole, pulseless electrical activity, or re-emergence of hemodynamic instability. Increase the infusion rate to 0.5 **mL**/kg/minute if hemodynamic instability persists or recurs. Continue the infusion for at least 10 minutes after hemodynamic stability is restored; discontinue within 1 hour, if possible (ACMT, 2010; Neal, 2012).

Dosage adjustment in renal impairment: There are no dosage adjustments provided in manufacturer's labeling; use with caution.

Dosage adjustment in hepatic impairment: There are no dosage adjustments provided in manufacturer's labeling; use with caution.

Additional Information Complete prescribing information should be consulted for additional detail.

Product Availability Clinolipid: FDA approved October 2013; anticipated availability is currently unknown. Refer to the prescribing information for additional information.

Dosage Forms Considerations

Product oil source for Intralipid, Liposyn III, and Nutrilipid: soybean

Dosage Forms

Emulsion, Intravenous:

Intralipid: 20% (100 mL, 250 mL, 500 mL, 1000 mL); 30% (500 mL)

Liposyn III: 10% (200 mL, 250 mL, 500 mL); 20% (200 mL, 250 mL, 500 mL)

Nutrilipid: 20% (250 mL, 500 mL, 1000 mL)

◆ **Father John's® Plus [OTC]** *see* Chlorpheniramine, Phenylephrine, and Dextromethorphan *on page* 428

◆ **FazaClo** *see* CloZAPine *on page* 490

◆ **5-FC** *see* Flucytosine *on page* 889

◆ **FC1157a** *see* Toremifene *on page* 2071

◆ **FC1271a** *see* Ospemifene *on page* 1527

◆ **FE200486** *see* Degarelix *on page* 587

Febuxostat (feb UX oh stat)

Brand Names: U.S. Uloric

Brand Names: Canada Uloric

Index Terms TEI-6720; TMX-67

Pharmacologic Category Antigout Agent; Xanthine Oxidase Inhibitor

Use Hyperuricemia: Chronic management of hyperuricemia in patients with gout. **Note:** Not recommended for treatment of asymptomatic hyperuricemia.

Pregnancy Risk Factor C

Pregnancy Considerations Animal studies have demonstrated increased neonatal mortality and reduction in weight gain, but not teratogenic effects. Use during pregnancy only if potential benefit to the mother outweighs potential risk to the fetus.

Breast-Feeding Considerations It is not known if febuxostat is excreted in breast milk. The U.S. manufacturer labeling recommends that caution be exercised when administering febuxostat to nursing women. Canadian labeling recommends avoiding use in nursing women.

Contraindications Concurrent use with azathioprine or mercaptopurine

Canadian labeling: Additional contraindications (not in U.S. labeling): Hypersensitivity to febuxostat or any component of the formulation.

Warnings/Precautions Hypersensitivity and serious skin reactions (eg, Stevens-Johnson syndrome) have been reported, particularly in patients with prior skin reactions to allopurinol; use with caution if a patient has a history of hypersensitivity reaction to allopurinol. Administer concurrently with an NSAID or colchicine (up to 6 months) to prevent gout flare which may occur upon initiation of therapy. Do not use to treat asymptomatic or secondary hyperuricemia. Use in secondary hyperuricemia has not been studied; avoid use in patients at increased risk of urate formation (eg, malignancy and its treatment; Lesch-Nyhan syndrome). Postmarketing cases of hepatic failure (both fatal and nonfatal) have been reported (causal relationship has not been established). Significant hepatic transaminase elevations (>3 x ULN), MI, stroke and cardiovascular deaths have been reported in controlled trials (causal relationship not established). Monitor patients for signs/symptoms of MI and stroke. Liver function tests should be evaluated at baseline and periodically thereafter; evaluate liver function tests promptly in patients experiencing signs and symptoms of hepatic injury (eg, fatigue, anorexia, right upper quadrant pain, dark urine, jaundice). Interrupt therapy in patients who develop abnormal liver function tests (eg, ALT >3 x ULN); permanently discontinue use if no other explanation for the abnormalities is elucidated and in patients who develop ALT >3 x ULT **and** serum total bilirubin >2 x ULN. All other patients may be cautiously restarted on febuxostat. Use with caution in patients with severe hepatic impairment (Child-Pugh class C); has not been studied. Canadian labeling recommends avoiding use in severe impairment.

Use with caution in patients with severe renal impairment (CrCl <30 mL/minute); insufficient data. Canadian labeling recommends avoiding use in severe impairment or end-stage renal disease (ESRD) requiring dialysis. Formulation contains lactose; Canadian labeling recommends avoiding use in patients with hereditary conditions of galactose intolerance, Lapp lactase deficiency, or glucose-galactose malabsorption.

Adverse Reactions

Dermatologic: Rash

Gastrointestinal: Nausea

Hepatic: Liver function abnormalities

Neuromuscular & skeletal: Arthralgia

Rare but important or life-threatening: Aggression, agitation, alkaline phosphatase increased, alopecia, amylase increased, anaphylactic reaction, anaphylaxis, anemia, angina, angioedema, anorexia, anxiety, aPTT prolonged, atrial fibrillation/flutter, bicarbonate decreased, blurred vision, bruising, BUN increased, cardiac murmur, cerebrovascular accident, cholecystitis, cholelithiasis, constipation, CPK increased, creatinine increased, deafness, dehydration, depression, dermatitis, dermographism, diabetes mellitus, dyspepsia, dyspnea, ECG abnormal, eczema, edema, EEG abnormal, epistaxis, erectile dysfunction, flushing, gait disturbance, gastritis, gastroesophageal reflux, gingival pain, Guillain-Barré syndrome, gynecomastia, hair color change, hair growth abnormal, hematemesis, hematochezia, hematocrit decreased, hematuria, hemiparesis, hepatic failure (fatal and nonfatal), hepatic steatosis, hepatitis, hepatomegaly, herpes zoster, hot flashes, hyperchlorhydria, hypercholesterolemia, hyperglycemia, hyperhidrosis, hyperkalemia, hyperlipidemia, hypernatremia, hypersensitivity, hyper/hypotension, hypertriglyceridemia, hypokalemia, immune thrombocytopenia (ITP), incontinence, influenza-like syndrome, jaundice, joint swelling, lacunar infarction, LDH increased, lethargy, leukocytosis, leukopenia, libido decreased, lymphocytopenia, MCV increased, MI, migraine, mouth ulceration, muscle spasm/twitching, myalgia, nephrolithiasis, neutropenia, pain, palpitation, pancreatitis, pancytopenia, panic attack, paresthesia, peptic ulcer, personality change, petechiae, pharyngeal edema, photosensitivity, pollakiuria, proteinuria, PSA increased, psychotic behavior, PT prolonged, renal failure, respiratory infection, rhabdomyolysis, sinus bradycardia, skin/pigmentation discoloration, splenomegaly, Stevens-Johnson syndrome, stroke, tachycardia, taste altered, thrombocytopenia, TIA, tinnitus, tremor, TSH increased, tubulointerstitial nephritis, urinary tract infection, urine output decreased/increased, urticaria, vertigo, vomiting, weakness, weight gain/loss

Drug Interactions

Metabolism/Transport Effects None known.

Avoid Concomitant Use

Avoid concomitant use of Febuxostat with any of the following: AzaTHIOprine; Didanosine; Mercaptopurine; Pegloticase

Increased Effect/Toxicity

Febuxostat may increase the levels/effects of: AzaTHIOprine; Didanosine; Mercaptopurine; Pegloticase; Theophylline Derivatives

Decreased Effect There are no known significant interactions involving a decrease in effect.

Storage/Stability Store at 25°C (77°F); excursions permitted to 15°C to 30°C (59°F to 86°F). Protect from light.

Mechanism of Action Selectively inhibits xanthine oxidase, the enzyme responsible for the conversion of hypoxanthine to xanthine to uric acid thereby decreasing uric acid. At therapeutic concentration does not inhibit other enzymes involved in purine and pyrimidine synthesis.

Pharmacodynamics/Kinetics

Absorption: ≥49%

Distribution: V_{ss}: ~50 L

Protein binding: ~99%, primarily to albumin

Metabolism: Extensive conjugation via uridine diphosphate glucuronosyltransferases (UGTs) 1A1, 1A3, 1A9, and 2B7 and oxidation via cytochrome P450 (CYP) 1A2, 2C8, and 2C9 as well as non-P450 enzymes. Oxidation leads to formation of active metabolites (67M-1, 67M-2, 67M-4)

Half-life elimination: ~5 to 8 hours

Time to peak, plasma: 1 to 1.5 hours

Excretion: Urine (~49% mostly as metabolites, 3% as unchanged drug); feces (~45% mostly as metabolites, 12% as unchanged drug)

Dosage Note: It is recommended to take an NSAID or colchicine with initiation of therapy and may continue for up to 6 months to help prevent gout flares. If a gout flare occurs, febuxostat does not need to be discontinued.

Hyperuricemia: Adults: Oral:

U.S. labeling: Initial: 40 mg once daily; may increase to 80 mg once daily in patients who do not achieve a serum uric acid level <6 mg/dL after 2 weeks. The dose may be increased further to 120 mg once daily if clinically indicated (ACR guidelines [Khanna, 2012]).

Canadian labeling: 80 mg once daily

Dosing adjustment in renal impairment:

Mild-to-moderate impairment (CrCl 30 to 89 mL/minute): No dosage adjustment necessary

Severe impairment (CrCl <30 mL/minute): There are no dosage adjustments provided in the manufacturer's labeling (insufficient data); use caution (use not recommended in the Canadian labeling)

Dialysis: There are no dosage adjustments provided in the manufacturer's labeling; has not been studied (use not recommended in the Canadian labeling)

Dosing adjustment in hepatic impairment:

Mild-to-moderate impairment (Child-Pugh class A or B): No dosage adjustment necessary

Severe impairment (Child-Pugh class C): There are no dosage adjustments provided in the manufacturer's labeling (has not been studied); use caution (use not recommended in the Canadian labeling)

Dietary Considerations Take with or without meals or antacids.

Administration Administer with or without meals or antacids.

Monitoring Parameters Liver function tests at baseline and then periodically, serum uric acid levels (as early as 2 weeks after initiation); signs/symptoms of MI or stroke, signs/symptoms of hypersensitivity or severe skin reactions

Reference Range Uric acid, serum: An increase occurs during childhood

Adults:

Males: 3.4 to 7 mg/dL or slightly more

Females: 2.4 to 6 mg/dL or slightly more

Target: <6 mg/dL

Values >7 mg/dL are sometimes arbitrarily regarded as hyperuricemia, but there is no sharp line between normals on the one hand, and the serum uric acid of those with clinical gout. Normal ranges cannot be adjusted for purine ingestion, but high purine diet increases uric acid. Uric acid may be increased with body size, exercise, and stress.

Dosage Forms

Tablet, Oral:

Uloric: 40 mg, 80 mg

◆ **Feiba** *see* Anti-inhibitor Coagulant Complex (Human) *on page 155*

◆ **FEIBA NF** *see* Anti-inhibitor Coagulant Complex (Human) *on page 155*

◆ **FEIBA VH** *see* Anti-inhibitor Coagulant Complex (Human) *on page 155*

Felbamate (FEL ba mate)

Brand Names: U.S. Felbatol

Pharmacologic Category Anticonvulsant, Miscellaneous

Use Monotherapy or adjunctive therapy in the treatment of partial seizures (with and without generalization); adjunctive therapy in the treatment of partial and generalized seizures associated with Lennox-Gastaut syndrome; not indicated for use as first-line treatment

Pregnancy Risk Factor C

Dosage Anticonvulsant:

Monotherapy: Children >14 years and Adults:

Initial: 1200 mg/day in divided doses 3 or 4 times/day; titrate previously untreated patients under close clinical supervision, increasing the dosage in 600 mg increments every 2 weeks to 2400 mg/day based on clinical response and thereafter to 3600 mg/day if clinically indicated

Conversion to monotherapy: Initiate at 1200 mg/day in divided doses 3 or 4 times/day, reduce the dosage of the concomitant anticonvulsant(s) by 33% at the initiation of felbamate therapy; at week 2, increase the felbamate dosage to 2400 mg/day while reducing the dosage of the other anticonvulsant(s) up to an additional 33% of their original dosage; at week 3, increase the felbamate dosage up to 3600 mg/day and continue to reduce the dosage of the other anticonvulsant(s) as clinically indicated

Adjunctive therapy: **Note:** Dose of concomitant carbamazepine, phenobarbital, phenytoin, or valproic acid should be decreased by 20% when initiating felbamate therapy. Further dosage reductions may be necessary as dose of felbamate is increased.

Children 2-14 years with Lennox-Gastaut syndrome: Initial: 15 mg/kg/day in divided doses 3 or 4 times/day; increase once per week by 15 mg/kg/day increments up to 45 mg/kg/day in divided doses 3 or 4 times/day.

Children >14 years and Adults: Initial: 1200 mg/day in divided doses 3 or 4 times/day; increase once per week by 1200 mg/day increments up to 3600 mg/day in divided doses 3 or 4 times/day.

Dosage adjustment in renal impairment: Use caution; reduce initial and maintenance doses by 50%.

Dosage adjustment in hepatic impairment: Use is contraindicated.

Additional Information Complete prescribing information should be consulted for additional detail.

Dosage Forms

Suspension, Oral:

Felbatol: 600 mg/5 mL (237 mL, 946 mL)

Generic: 600 mg/5 mL (237 mL, 240 mL, 473 mL, 946 mL)

Tablet, Oral:

Felbatol: 400 mg, 600 mg

Generic: 400 mg, 600 mg

◆ **Felbatol** *see* Felbamate *on page 850*

Felbinac [INT] (FEL bi nak)

International Brand Names Dolinac (IT); Dolo Target (CH); Flexfree (BE, LU); Napageln (JP); Seltouch (JP); Traxam (GB, IE, IT)

Pharmacologic Category Anti-inflammatory Agent

Reported Use Anti-inflammatory and analgesic product given for the relief of symptoms associated with soft tissue injuries, rheumatic pain, and nonserious arthritic conditions

Dosage Range Adults: Topical: Apply 2-4 times/day; therapy should be reviewed after 14 days

Product Availability Product available in various countries; not currently available in the U.S.

Dosage Forms

Foam: 3% (100 g)

Gel: 3% (75 g, 100 g)

◆ **Feldene** *see* Piroxicam *on page 1662*

Felodipine (fe LOE di peen)

Brand Names: Canada Plendil; Sandoz-Felodipine

Index Terms Plendil

Pharmacologic Category Antihypertensive; Calcium Channel Blocker; Calcium Channel Blocker, Dihydropyridine

Use

Hypertension: Treatment of hypertension

The 2014 guideline for the management of high blood pressure in adults (JNC 8) recommends initiation of pharmacologic treatment to lower blood pressure for the following patients (JNC8 [James, 2013]):

- Patients ≥ 60 years of age, with systolic blood pressure (SBP) ≥150 mm Hg or diastolic blood pressure (DBP) ≥90 mm Hg. Goal of therapy is SBP <150 mm Hg and DBP <90 mm Hg.

- Patients <60 years of age, with SBP ≥140 mm Hg or DBP ≥90 mm Hg. Goal of therapy is SBP <140 mm Hg and DBP <90 mm Hg.
- Patients ≥18 years of age with diabetes, with SBP ≥140 mm Hg or DBP ≥90 mm Hg. Goal of therapy is SBP <140 mm Hg and DBP <90 mm Hg.
- Patients ≥18 years of age with chronic kidney disease (CKD), with SBP ≥140 mm Hg or DBP ≥90 mm Hg. Goal of therapy is SBP <140 mm Hg and DBP <90 mm Hg.

In patients with chronic kidney disease (CKD), regardless of race or diabetes status, the use of an ACE inhibitor (ACEI) or angiotensin receptor blocker (ARB) as initial therapy is recommended to improve kidney outcomes. In the general nonblack population (without CKD) including those with diabetes, initial antihypertensive treatment should consist of a thiazide-type diuretic, calcium channel blocker, ACEI, or ARB. In the general black population (without CKD) including those with diabetes, initial antihypertensive treatment should consist of a thiazide-type diuretic or a calcium channel blocker **instead of** an ACEI or ARB.

Pregnancy Risk Factor C

Pregnancy Considerations Adverse events were observed in animal reproduction studies. Untreated chronic maternal hypertension is associated with adverse events in the fetus, infant, and mother. If treatment for hypertension during pregnancy is needed, other agents are preferred (ACOG, 2013). The Canadian labeling contraindicates use in women of childbearing potential and during pregnancy.

Breast-Feeding Considerations It is not known if felodipine is excreted in breast milk. Due to the potential for serious adverse reactions in the nursing infant, the U.S. labeling recommends a decision be made whether to discontinue nursing or to discontinue the drug, taking into account the importance of treatment to the mother. The Canadian labeling contraindicates use in nursing women.

Contraindications

Hypersensitivity to felodipine or any component of the formulation.

Canadian labeling: Additional contraindications (not in U.S. labeling): Hypersensitivity to other dihydropyridines; women of childbearing potential, in pregnancy, and during lactation.

Warnings/Precautions Increased angina and/or MI has occurred with initiation or dosage titration of dihydropyridine calcium channel blockers, reflex tachycardia may occur resulting in angina and/or MI in patients with obstructive coronary disease especially in the absence of concurrent beta-blockade. Use with extreme caution in patients with severe aortic stenosis. Use caution in patients with hypertrophic cardiomyopathy with outflow tract obstruction. The ACCF/AHA heart failure guidelines recommend to avoid use in patients with heart failure due to lack of benefit and/or worse outcomes with calcium channel blockers in general (Yancy, 2013). Elderly patients and patients with hepatic impairment should start off with a lower dose. Peripheral edema (dose dependent) is the most common side effect (occurs within 2 to 3 weeks of starting therapy). Symptomatic hypotension with or without syncope can rarely occur; blood pressure must be lowered at a rate appropriate for the patient's clinical condition. Potentially significant drug-drug interactions may exist, requiring dose or frequency adjustment, additional monitoring, and/or selection of alternative therapy. May contain lactose; if necessary, consider alternative agents in patients intolerant of lactose.

Adverse Reactions

Cardiovascular: Flushing, peripheral edema, tachycardia

Central nervous system: Headache

Rare but important or life-threatening: Angina, angioedema, anxiety, arrhythmia, CHF, CVA, decreased libido, depression, dizziness, gingival hyperplasia, dyspnea, dysuria, gynecomastia, hypotension, impotence, insomnia, irritability, leukocytoclastic vasculitis, MI, nervousness, paresthesia, somnolence, syncope, urticaria, vomiting

Drug Interactions

Metabolism/Transport Effects Substrate of CYP3A4 (major); **Note:** Assignment of Major/Minor substrate status based on clinically relevant drug interaction potential; **Inhibits** CYP2C8 (moderate), CYP2C9 (weak), CYP2D6 (weak), CYP3A4 (weak)

Avoid Concomitant Use

Avoid concomitant use of Felodipine with any of the following: Conivaptan; Fusidic Acid (Systemic); Idelalisib; Itraconazole; Ketoconazole (Systemic); Pimozide

Increased Effect/Toxicity

Felodipine may increase the levels/effects of: Amifostine; Antihypertensives; ARIPiprazole; Atosiban; Beta-Blockers; Calcium Channel Blockers (Nondihydropyridine); CYP2C8 Substrates; Dofetilide; DULoxetine; Fosphenytoin; Hydrocodone; Hypotensive Agents; Levodopa; Lomitapide; Magnesium Salts; Neuromuscular-Blocking Agents (Nondepolarizing); Nitroprusside; Obinutuzumab; Phenytoin; Pimozide; RisperiDONE; RiTUXimab; Tacrolimus (Systemic)

The levels/effects of Felodipine may be increased by: Alfuzosin; Alpha1-Blockers; Antifungal Agents (Azole Derivatives, Systemic); Aprepitant; Barbiturates; Brimonidine (Topical); Calcium Channel Blockers (Nondihydropyridine); Ceritinib; Cimetidine; Conivaptan; CycloSPORINE (Systemic); CYP3A4 Inhibitors (Moderate); CYP3A4 Inhibitors (Strong); Dapoxetine; Dasatinib; Diazoxide; Fluconazole; Fosaprepitant; Fusidic Acid (Systemic); Grapefruit Juice; Herbs (Hypotensive Properties); Idelalisib; Itraconazole; Ivacaftor; Ketoconazole (Systemic); Luliconazole; Macrolide Antibiotics; Magnesium Salts; MAO Inhibitors; Mifepristone; Netupitant; Nicorandil; Pentoxifylline; Phosphodiesterase 5 Inhibitors; Prostacyclin Analogues; Protease Inhibitors; Simeprevir; Stiripentol

Decreased Effect

Felodipine may decrease the levels/effects of: Clopidogrel

The levels/effects of Felodipine may be decreased by: Barbiturates; Bosentan; Calcium Salts; CarBAMazepine; CYP3A4 Inducers (Moderate); CYP3A4 Inducers (Strong); Dabrafenib; Deferasirox; Efavirenz; Herbs (Hypertensive Properties); Melatonin; Methylphenidate; Mitotane; Nafcillin; Rifamycin Derivatives; Siltuximab; St Johns Wort; Tocilizumab; Yohimbine

Food Interactions

Ethanol: Ethanol increases felodipine absorption. Management: Monitor for a greater hypotensive effect if ethanol is consumed.

Food: Compared to a fasted state, felodipine peak plasma concentrations are increased up to twofold when taken after a meal high in fat or carbohydrates. Grapefruit juice similarly increases felodipine C_{max} by twofold. Increased therapeutic and vasodilator side effects, including severe hypotension and myocardial ischemia, may occur. Management: May be taken with a small meal that is low in fat and carbohydrates; avoid grapefruit juice during therapy.

Storage/Stability Store below 30°C (86°F); protect from light.

Mechanism of Action Inhibits calcium ions from entering the "slow channels" or select voltage-sensitive areas of vascular smooth muscle and myocardium during depolarization, producing a relaxation of coronary vascular smooth muscle and coronary vasodilation; increases myocardial oxygen delivery in patients with vasospastic angina

Pharmacodynamics/Kinetics

Onset of action: Antihypertensive: 2 to 5 hours

Duration of antihypertensive effect: 24 hours

Absorption: 100%; Absolute: 20% due to first-pass effect

Protein binding: >99%

Metabolism: Hepatic; CYP3A4 substrate (major); extensive first-pass effect

Half-life elimination: Immediate release: 11 to 16 hours

Excretion: Urine (70% as metabolites); feces 10%

Dosage Hypertension:

Children ≥6 years and Adolescents (off-label use): Oral: Initial: 2.5 mg once daily; may increase as needed at no less than 2-week intervals to a maximum of 10 mg once daily (NHLBI, 2011)

Adults: Oral: Initial: 5 mg once daily; adjust dose as needed at no less than 2-week intervals. Usual dose range: 5 to10 mg once daily (ASH/ISH [Weber, 2014]) although some patients may benefit from 2.5 mg once daily. Doses >10 mg daily are associated with greater antihypertensive effects but also a large increase in the incidence of peripheral edema and other vasodilatory adverse effects.

Elderly: Oral: Consider lower initial doses (eg, 2.5 mg once daily) and titrate at no less than 2-week intervals to response (Aronow, 2011). The Canadian labeling recommends a maximum dose of 10 mg daily.

Dosage adjustment in renal impairment: No dosage adjustment necessary.

Dosage adjustment in hepatic impairment: Initial: 2.5 mg once daily; monitor blood pressure closely during titration. The Canadian labeling recommends a maximum dose of 10 mg daily.

Dietary Considerations May be taken with a small meal that is low in fat and carbohydrates.

Administration Swallow tablet whole; tablet should not be divided, crushed, or chewed. May be administered without food or with a small meal that is low in fat and carbohydrates.

Dosage Forms

Tablet Extended Release 24 Hour, Oral:

Generic: 2.5 mg, 5 mg, 10 mg

- **Femara** *see* Letrozole *on page 1181*
- **Femcon Fe** *see* Ethinyl Estradiol and Norethindrone *on page 808*
- **femhrt** *see* Ethinyl Estradiol and Norethindrone *on page 808*
- **FemHRT (Can)** *see* Ethinyl Estradiol and Norethindrone *on page 808*
- **Fem-Prin [OTC]** *see* Acetaminophen, Aspirin, and Caffeine *on page 37*
- **Femring** *see* Estradiol (Systemic) *on page 775*
- **Femstat® One (Can)** *see* Butoconazole *on page 314*

Fenbufen [INT] (fen BYOO fen)

International Brand Names Afiancen (AR); Bifene (PT); Cincopal (ES); Cinopal (DK); Lederfen (AT, GB, LU); Reugast (PT)

Pharmacologic Category Analgesic, Nonsteroidal Anti-inflammatory Drug

Reported Use Treatment of pain and inflammation in rheumatic disease and other musculoskeletal disorders

Dosage Range Oral:

Children <14 years: Not recommended

Adults: 300 mg in the morning and 600 mg at bedtime or 450 mg twice daily

Product Availability Product available in various countries; not currently available in the U.S.

Dosage Forms

Capsule: 300 mg

Tablet: 300 mg, 450 mg

- **Fenesin DM IR [OTC]** *see* Guaifenesin and Dextromethorphan *on page 987*
- **Fenesin IR [OTC]** *see* GuaiFENesin *on page 986*
- **Fenesin PE IR** *see* Guaifenesin and Phenylephrine *on page 988*

Fenofibrate and Derivatives

(fen oh FYE brate & dah RIV ah tives)

Brand Names: U.S. Antara; Fenoglide; Fibricor; Lipofen; Lofibra; Tricor; Triglide; Trilipix

Brand Names: Canada Apo-Feno-Micro; Apo-Feno-Super; Apo-Fenofibrate; Ava-Fenofibrate Micro; Dom-Fenofibrate Micro; Feno-Micro-200; Fenofibrate Micro; Fenofibrate-S; Lipidil EZ; Lipidil Micro; Lipidil Supra; Mylan-Fenofibrate Micro; Novo-Fenofibrate Micronized; PHL-Fenofibrate Micro; PMS-Fenofibrate Micro; PRO-Feno-Super; Q-Fenofibrate Micro; ratio-Fenofibrate MC; Riva-Fenofibrate Micro; Sandoz-Fenofibrate E; Sandoz-Fenofibrate S; Teva-Fenofibrate S

Index Terms ABT-335; Choline Fenofibrate; Fenofibric Acid; Procetofene; Proctofene

Pharmacologic Category Antilipemic Agent, Fibric Acid

Use

Hypercholesterolemia or mixed dyslipidemia: Adjunctive therapy to diet for the reduction of low-density lipoprotein cholesterol (LDL-C), total cholesterol (total-C), triglycerides, and apolipoprotein B (apo B), and to increase high-density lipoprotein cholesterol (HDL-C) in adults with primary hypercholesterolemia or mixed dyslipidemia (Fredrickson types IIa and IIb). Use lipid-altering agents in addition to a diet restricted in saturated fat and cholesterol when response to diet and nonpharmacological interventions alone has been inadequate.

Trilipix is also indicated as an adjunct to diet in combination with a statin to reduce triglycerides and increase HDL-C in patients with mixed dyslipidemia and coronary heart disease (CHD) or a CHD risk equivalent who are on optimal statin therapy.

Hypertriglyceridemia: Adjunctive therapy to diet for treatment of adult patients with severe hypertriglyceridemia (Fredrickson types IV and V hyperlipidemia).

Pregnancy Risk Factor C

Pregnancy Considerations Maternal toxicity was observed in pregnant rats at doses approximately equivalent to the human dose; adverse events were not observed in reproduction studies done in rabbits. Reports of using fenofibrate during pregnancy are limited (Goldberg, 2012; Sunman, 2012; Whitten, 2011). Other agents are generally preferred if treatment for hypertriglyceridemia during pregnancy (Berglund, 2012) or treatment of lipid disorders in women of reproductive age (NCEP, 2001) is required. Use during pregnancy is specifically contraindicated in Canadian product labeling; some products recommend using effective birth control when treating women of reproductive age and discontinuing therapy several months prior to conception if planning a pregnancy.

Breast-Feeding Considerations It is not known if fenofibrate is excreted into breast milk. Use is contraindicated in nursing women. The manufacturer recommends a decision be made whether to discontinue nursing or to discontinue the drug, taking into account the importance of treatment to the mother.

Contraindications

Active liver disease, including primary biliary cirrhosis and unexplained, persistent liver function abnormality; severe renal dysfunction, including those receiving dialysis;

preexisting gallbladder disease; breast-feeding; hypersensitivity to fenofibrate or fenofibric acid.

Documentation of allergenic cross-reactivity for fibrates is limited. However, because of similarities in chemical structure and/or pharmacologic actions, the possibility of cross-sensitivity cannot be ruled out with certainty.

Canadian labeling: Additional contraindications (not in U.S. labeling): Pregnancy; known photoallergy or phototoxic reaction during treatment with fibrates or ketoprofen

Lipidil EZ, Lipidil Micro, Lipidil Supra: Additional contraindications: Allergy to soya lecithin or peanut or arachis oil; chronic or acute pancreatitis; patients <18 years of age; coadministration with HMG-CoA reductase inhibitors in patients with a predisposition for myopathy.

Warnings/Precautions Secondary causes of hyperlipidemia should be ruled out prior to therapy. Hepatic transaminases can become significantly elevated (dose-related); hepatocellular, chronic active, and cholestatic hepatitis have been reported. Regular monitoring of liver function tests is required; discontinue therapy in patients whose enzyme levels persist above 3 times the upper limit of normal. Use with caution in patients with mild-to-moderate renal impairment; dosage adjustment may be required. Contraindicated with severe renal impairment including those receiving dialysis. Contraindicated active liver disease, including primary biliary cirrhosis and unexplained persistent liver function abnormalities. Increases in serum creatinine (>2 mg/dL) have been observed with use; clinical significance unknown. Fenofibrate has been shown to increase creatinine production (unknown mechanism) resulting in an equal increase of creatinuria thereby demonstrating that the increase does not reflect a reduction in creatinine clearance (Hottelart, 2002). Monitor renal function in patients with renal impairment and consider monitoring patients with increased risk for developing renal impairment. May cause cholelithiasis.

Therapy should be discontinued in patients who develop markedly elevated CPK concentrations or if myopathy/myositis is suspected or diagnosed. No incremental benefit of combination therapy on cardiovascular morbidity and mortality over statin monotherapy has been established. In patients with type 2 diabetes mellitus, neither fenofibrate monotherapy nor the addition of fenofibrate to simvastatin compared to placebo has been shown to reduce cardiovascular disease morbidity and mortality in patients with type 2 diabetes. Potentially significant drug-drug interactions may exist, requiring dose or frequency adjustment, additional monitoring, and/or selection of alternative therapy. In combination with HMG-CoA reductase inhibitors, fenofibrate is generally regarded as safer than gemfibrozil due to limited pharmacokinetic interaction with statins. According to the 2013 ACC/AHA Blood Cholesterol Guidelines, fenofibrate may be considered in patients on low- or moderate-intensity statin therapy (ie, statin therapy intended to lower LDL-C by <30% or ~30% to 50%, respectively) only if the benefits from atherosclerotic cardiovascular disease (ASCVD) risk reduction or triglyceride lowering when triglycerides are >500 mg/dL, outweigh the potential risk for adverse effects (Stone, 2013). Therapy should be withdrawn if an adequate response is not obtained after 2-3 months of therapy at the maximal daily dose. In patients with severe hypertriglyceridemia, the occurrence of pancreatitis may represent a failure of efficacy, a direct effect of the drug, or obstruction of the common bile duct due to biliary tract stone or sludge formation. A paradoxical, severe, and reversible decrease in HDL-C (as low as 2 mg/dL) with a simultaneous decrease in apolipoprotein A1 has been reported within 2 weeks to years after initiation of fibrate therapy; clinical significance unknown. Monitor HDL-C within a few months of initiation of therapy and discontinue if HDL-C becomes severely depressed; do not restart therapy. The occurrence of pancreatitis may represent a failure of efficacy in patients with severely elevated triglycerides. May cause mild-to-moderate decreases in hemoglobin, hematocrit, and WBC upon initiation of therapy which usually stabilizes with long-term therapy. Agranulocytosis and thrombocytopenia have been reported (rare). Periodic monitoring of blood counts is recommended during the first year of therapy.

Rare hypersensitivity reactions may occur. Use has been associated with pulmonary embolism (PE) and deep vein thrombosis (DVT). Use with caution in patients with risk factors for VTE. Dose adjustment may be required for elderly patients.

Some products may contain soya lecithin or peanut or arachis oil; use is contraindicated in patients with a soya lecithin allergy or a peanut or arachis allergy for applicable formulations.

Adverse Reactions Adverse reactions reported as observed during fenofibrate and fenofibric acid monotherapy and concurrent administration with a statin (HMG-CoA reductase inhibitor).

Cardiovascular: Hypertension

Central nervous system: Dizziness, fatigue, headache, insomnia, pain

Hepatic: Increased serum transaminases (dose related)

Dermatologic: Urticaria

Gastrointestinal: Constipation, diarrhea, dyspepsia, nausea

Genitourinary: Urinary tract infection

Hepatic: Increased serum ALT, increased serum AST

Infection: Influenza

Neuromuscular & skeletal: Arthralgia, back pain, increased creatine phosphokinase, limb pain, myalgia, muscle spasm, musculoskeletal pain

Renal: Increased serum creatinine

Respiratory: Bronchitis, cough, nasopharyngitis, pharyngolaryngeal pain, rhinitis, sinusitis, upper respiratory tract infection

Rare but important or life-threatening: Acute renal failure, agranulocytosis, anemia, angina pectoris, anorexia, arthritis, asthma, atrial fibrillation, cardiac arrhythmia, cataract, cholecystitis, cholelithiasis, cholestatic hepatitis, colitis, conjunctivitis, cyst, cystitis, decreased HDL-C (paradoxical), deep vein thrombosis, dermal ulcer, diabetes mellitus, duodenal ulcer, ECG abnormality, eosinophilia, error of refraction, esophagitis, extrasystoles, gastritis, gastroenteritis, gout, gynecomastia, hepatic cirrhosis, hepatitis (including hepatocellular and chronic active), hernia, herpes simplex infection, herpes zoster, homocysteinemia, hypersensitivity pneumonitis, hypersensitivity reaction, hypertonia, hyperuricemia, hypoglycemia, hypotension, infection, leukopenia, liver steatosis, lymphadenopathy, maculopapular rash, migraine, myopathy, myocardial infarction, myositis, neuralgia, osteoarthritis, pancreatitis, peptic ulcer, pneumonia, prostatic disease, pulmonary embolism, rectal hemorrhage, rhabdomyolysis, skin photosensitivity, Stevens-Johnson syndrome, tachycardia, thrombocytopenia, toxic epidermal necrolysis, urolithiasis, vulvovaginal candidiasis

Drug Interactions

Metabolism/Transport Effects **Inhibits** CYP2A6 (weak), CYP2C8 (weak), CYP2C9 (weak)

Avoid Concomitant Use

Avoid concomitant use of Fenofibrate and Derivatives with any of the following: Ciprofibrate

Increased Effect/Toxicity

Fenofibrate and Derivatives may increase the levels/effects of: Colchicine; Ezetimibe; HMG-CoA Reductase Inhibitors; Sulfonylureas; Vitamin K Antagonists; Warfarin

The levels/effects of Fenofibrate and Derivatives may be increased by: Acipimox; Ciprofibrate; CycloSPORINE (Systemic); Raltegravir; Tacrolimus (Systemic)

Decreased Effect

Fenofibrate and Derivatives may decrease the levels/ effects of: Chenodiol; CycloSPORINE (Systemic); Ursodiol

The levels/effects of Fenofibrate and Derivatives may be decreased by: Bile Acid Sequestrants

Food Interactions

Antara (micronized): When administered under fasted conditions or with a low-fat meal, the extent of absorption and the time to peak did not change; however peak concentrations were increased in the presence of a low-fat meal. When administered with a high fat meal, a 26% increase in the AUC and 108% increase in the peak concentration were seen in comparison to the fasted state. Management: Administer with or without food.

Fenoglide: When administered with a high-fat meal, the peak concentration was increased by 44% as compared to fasting conditions. Management: Administer with meals.

Fibricor: When administered with a high-fat meal, the peak concentration was decreased by ~35% while AUC remained unchanged as compared to fasting conditions. Management: Administer with or without food.

Lipidil EZ [Canadian product]: Bioavailability was not significantly different when administered under fasting and nonfasting conditions. Management: Administer with or without food.

Lipidil Micro [Canadian product]: In comparison with nonmicronized fenofibrate formulations, micronized fenofibrate is better absorbed when administered with a low-fat meal; absorption is less influenced by a higher fat content meal. Management: Administer with meals.

Lipidil Supra [Canadian product]: In general, fenofibrate absorption is low and variable when administered under fasting conditions; absorption is increased when administered with food. Management: Administer with meals.

Lipofen: When administered with a low-fat and high-fat meal, the extent of absorption is increased by ~25% and ~58%, respectively, as compared to fasting conditions. Management: Administer with meals.

Lofibra (micronized) capsules: Absorption is increased by ~35% under fed as compared to fasting conditions. Management: Administer with meals.

Lofibra tablets: Peak concentrations and AUC were not significantly different when a single dose was administered under fasting and nonfasting conditions. Management: Administer with or without food.

TriCor: Peak concentrations and AUC were not significantly different when a single dose was administered under fasting and nonfasting conditions. Management: Administer with or without food.

Triglide: When administered with food, the rate of absorption was increased ~55% as compared to fasting conditions; the AUC remained unchanged. Management: Administer with or without food.

Trilipix: Peak concentrations and AUC were not significantly different when a single dose was administered under fasting and nonfasting conditions. Management: Administer with or without food.

Storage/Stability Store at 25°C (77°F); excursions are permitted between 15°C and 30°C (59°F and 86°F). Protect Fibricor, Lipofen, Lofibra, TriCor, Triglide, and Trilipix from moisture. Protect Fibricor, Lofibra tablets, Lipofen, and Triglide from light.

Canadian products: Lipidil EZ, Lipidil Micro, Lipidil Supra: Store at 15°C to 25°C (59°F to 77°F). Protect Lipidil EZ, Lipidil Micro, and Lipidil Supra from moisture. Protect Lipidil EZ and Lipidil Supra from light.

Mechanism of Action Fenofibric acid, an agonist for the nuclear transcription factor peroxisome proliferator-activated receptor-alpha (PPAR-alpha), downregulates apoprotein C-III (an inhibitor of lipoprotein lipase) and upregulates the synthesis of apolipoprotein A-I, fatty acid transport protein, and lipoprotein lipase resulting in an increase in VLDL catabolism, fatty acid oxidation, and elimination of triglyceride-rich particles; as a result of a decrease in VLDL levels, total plasma triglycerides are reduced by 30% to 60%; modest increase in HDL occurs in some hypertriglyceridemic patients.

Pharmacodynamics/Kinetics

Absorption: Increased when taken with meals

Distribution: Widely to most tissues

Protein binding: ~99%

Metabolism: Fenofibrate is metabolized in the tissue and plasma via esterases to the active form, fenofibric acid; fenofibric acid then undergoes inactivation by glucuronidation hepatically or renally

Bioavailability: Fenofibric acid: ~81%

Half-life elimination: Fenofibric acid: Mean: 20 hours (range: 10-35 hours); half-life prolonged in patients with renal impairment

Time to peak: 2-8 hours

Excretion: Urine (60% as metabolites); feces (25%); hemodialysis has no effect on removal of fenofibric acid from plasma

Dosage Oral: **Note:** At least 2-3 months of therapy is required to determine efficacy.

Adults:

Hypertriglyceridemia: Initial:

Antara (micronized): 43-130 mg once daily; maximum dose: 130 mg once daily

Fenoglide: 40-120 mg once daily; maximum dose: 120 mg once daily

Fibricor: 35-105 mg once daily; maximum dose: 105 mg once daily

Lipidil EZ [Canadian product]: 145 mg once daily; maximum dose: 145 mg once daily

Lipidil Micro [Canadian product]: 200 mg once daily; maximum dose: 200 mg once daily

Lipidil Supra [Canadian product]: 160 mg once daily; maximum dose: 200 mg once daily

Lipofen: 50-150 mg once daily; maximum dose: 150 mg once daily

Lofibra (micronized): 67-200 mg once daily; maximum dose: 200 mg once daily

Lofibra (tablets): 54-160 mg once daily; maximum dose: 160 mg once daily

TriCor: 48-145 mg once daily; maximum dose: 145 mg once daily

Triglide: 50-160 mg once daily; maximum dose: 160 mg once daily

Trilipix: 45-135 mg once daily; maximum dose: 135 mg once daily

Hypercholesterolemia or mixed hyperlipidemia:

Antara (micronized): 130 mg once daily

Fenoglide: 120 mg once daily

Fibricor: 105 mg once daily

Lipidil EZ [Canadian product]: 145 mg once daily; maximum dose: 145 mg once daily

Lipidil Micro [Canadian product]: 200 mg once daily; maximum dose: 200 mg once daily

Lipidil Supra [Canadian product]: 160 mg once daily; maximum dose: 200 mg once daily

Lipofen: 150 mg once daily

Lofibra (micronized): 200 mg once daily

Lofibra (tablets): 160 mg once daily

TriCor: 145 mg once daily

Triglide: 160 mg once daily

Trilipix: 135 mg once daily; **Note:** Trilipix is approved for use with a statin in patients with mixed dyslipidemia; may be administered at the same time. Avoid coadministration with the maximum dose of a statin unless the benefits are expected to outweigh the risks

Elderly: Initial:

Antara (micronized): Adjust dosage based on renal function.

Fenoglide: Adjust dosage based on renal function.

Fibricor: Adjust dosage based on renal function.

Lipidil EZ [Canadian product]: 48 mg once daily

Lipidil Micro [Canadian product]: Adjust dosage based on creatinine clearance

Lipidil Supra [Canadian product]: Adjust dosage based on creatinine clearance

Lipofen: Adjust dosage based on renal function.

Lofibra (micronized): 67 mg once daily

Lofibra (tablets): 54 mg once daily

TriCor: Adjust dosage based on renal function.

Triglide: Adjust dosage based on renal function.

Trilipix: Adjust dosage based on renal function.

Dosage adjustment for toxicity:

Cholelithiasis: Discontinue if gallstones are found upon gallbladder studies.

CPK elevation, myopathy, and/or myositis: Discontinue therapy if the patient develops markedly elevated CPK concentrations or if myopathy/myositis is suspected or diagnosed.

HDL-C reductions: Permanently discontinue therapy if HDL-C becomes severely depressed; monitor HDL-C concentrations until returned to baseline.

Dosage adjustment in renal impairment: Monitor renal function and lipid panel before adjusting. **Note:** Use in severe renal impairment (including patients on dialysis) is contraindicated (see specific product labeling):

Antara (micronized):

CrCl >80 mL/minute or eGFR ≥60 mL/minute/1.73 m^2: No dosage adjustment necessary.

CrCl >30-80 mL/minute or eGFR 30-59 mL/minute/1.73 m^2: Initiate at 43 mg once daily

CrCl ≤30 mL/minute or eGFR <30 mL/minute/1.73 m^2: Use is contraindicated.

Dialysis: Use is contraindicated.

Fenoglide:

CrCl >80 mL/minute or eGFR ≥60 mL/minute/1.73 m^2: No dosage adjustment necessary.

CrCl >30-80 mL/minute or eGFR 30-59 mL/minute/1.73 m^2: Initiate at 40 mg once daily

CrCl ≤30 mL/minute or eGFR <30 mL/minute/1.73 m^2: Use is contraindicated.

Dialysis: Use is contraindicated.

Fibricor:

CrCl >80 mL/minute: No dosage adjustment necessary.

CrCl >30-80 mL/minute: Initiate at 35 mg once daily

CrCl ≤30 mL/minute: Use is contraindicated.

Dialysis: Use is contraindicated.

Lipidil EZ [Canadian product]: **Note:** Interrupt treatment in patients with an increase in creatinine concentrations >50% the upper limit of normal (ULN).

CrCl >50 mL/minute: No dosage adjustment necessary.

CrCl 20-50 mL/minute: Initiate at 48 mg once daily

CrCl <20 mL/minute: Use is contraindicated.

Dialysis: Use is contraindicated.

Lipidil Micro [Canadian product]: **Note:** Interrupt treatment in patients with an increase in creatinine concentrations >50% the upper limit of normal (ULN).

CrCl >85 mL/minute (women) or >95 mL/minute (men): No dosage adjustment necessary.

CrCl 20-85 mL/minute (women) or 20-95 mL/minute (men): Initiate therapy with Lipidil EZ formulation with a dose of 48 mg once daily.

CrCl <20 mL/minute: Use is contraindicated.

Dialysis: Use is contraindicated.

Lipidil Supra [Canadian product]: **Note:** Interrupt treatment in patients with an increase in creatinine concentrations >50% the upper limit of normal (ULN).

CrCl >100 mL/minute: No dosage adjustment necessary.

CrCl 20-100 mL/minute: Initiate at 100 mg once daily

CrCl <20 mL/minute: Use is contraindicated.

Dialysis: Use is contraindicated.

Lipofen:

eGFR ≥90 mL/minute/1.73 m^2: No dosage adjustment necessary.

eGFR 30-89 mL/minute/1.73 m^2: Initiate at 50 mg once daily

eGFR <30 mL/minute/1.73 m^2: Use is contraindicated.

Dialysis: Use is contraindicated.

Lofibra (micronized):

CrCl >80 mL/minute: No dosage adjustment necessary.

CrCl >30-80 mL/minute: Initiate at 67 mg once daily

CrCl ≤30 mL/minute: Use is contraindicated.

Dialysis: Use is contraindicated.

Lofibra (tablets):

eGFR ≥60 mL/minute/1.73 m^2: No dosage adjustment necessary.

eGFR 30-59 mL/minute/1.73 m^2: Initiate at 54 mg once daily

eGFR <30 mL/minute/1.73 m^2: Use is contraindicated.

Dialysis: Use is contraindicated.

TriCor:

eGFR ≥60 mL/minute/1.73 m^2: No dosage adjustment necessary.

eGFR 30-59 mL/minute/1.73 m^2: Initiate at 48 mg once daily

eGFR <30 mL/minute/1.73 m^2: Use is contraindicated.

Dialysis: Use is contraindicated.

Triglide:

CrCl >80 mL/minute or eGFR ≥60 mL/minute/1.73 m^2: No dosage adjustment necessary.

CrCl >30-80 mL/minute or eGFR 30-59 mL/minute/1.73 m^2: Initiate at 50 mg once daily

CrCl ≤30 mL/minute or eGFR <30 mL/minute/1.73 m^2: Use is contraindicated.

Dialysis: Use is contraindicated.

Trilipix:

eGFR ≥60 mL/minute/1.73 m^2: No dosage adjustment necessary.

eGFR 30-59 mL/minute/1.73 m^2: Initiate at 45 mg once daily

eGFR <30 mL/minute/1.73 m^2: Use is contraindicated.

Dialysis: Use is contraindicated.

Dosage adjustment in hepatic impairment: Use is contraindicated. Regular monitoring of liver function tests is required; discontinue therapy in patients whose enzyme levels persist above 3 times the upper limit of normal.

Dietary Considerations

Antara, Fibricor, Lipidil EZ [Canadian product], Lofibra tablets, TriCor, Triglide, Trilipix: May be taken with or without food.

Fenoglide, Lipidil Micro [Canadian product], Lipidil Supra [Canadian product], Lipofen, Lofibra (micronized capsules): Take with meals.

Administration

Antara, Fibricor, Lipidil EZ [Canadian product], Lofibra tablets, TriCor, Triglide, Trilipix: Administer with or without food. Swallow whole; do not open (capsules), crush, dissolve, or chew.

Lipidil Micro [Canadian product]; Lofibra (micronized) capsules: Administer with meals.

Fenoglide, Lipofen, Lipidil Supra [Canadian product]: Administer with meals. Swallow whole; do not open (capsules), crush, dissolve, or chew.

Monitoring Parameters Periodic blood counts during first year of therapy. Monitor lipid profile periodically. Monitor LFTs regularly and discontinue therapy if levels remain >3 times normal limits. Monitor renal function in patients with renal impairment or in those at increased risk for developing renal impairment.

2013 ACC/AHA Blood Cholesterol Guideline recommendations (Stone, 2013): Evaluate renal status at baseline, within 3 months after initiation, and every 6 months thereafter.

Dosage Forms Considerations

Micronized formulations: Antara, Lofibra capsules

Strength of choline fenofibrate products are expressed in terms of fenofibric acid.

Dosage Forms

Capsule, Oral:

Antara: 30 mg, 90 mg

Lipofen: 50 mg, 150 mg

Lofibra: 67 mg, 134 mg, 200 mg

Generic: 43 mg, 50 mg, 67 mg, 130 mg, 134 mg, 150 mg, 200 mg

Capsule Delayed Release, Oral:

Trilipix: 45 mg, 135 mg

Generic: 45 mg, 135 mg

Tablet, Oral:

Fenoglide: 40 mg, 120 mg

Fibricor: 35 mg, 105 mg

Lofibra: 54 mg, 160 mg

Tricor: 48 mg, 145 mg

Triglide: 160 mg

Generic: 35 mg, 48 mg, 54 mg, 105 mg, 145 mg, 160 mg

◆ **Fenofibrate Micro (Can)** *see* Fenofibrate and Derivatives *on page 852*

◆ **Fenofibrate-S (Can)** *see* Fenofibrate and Derivatives *on page 852*

◆ **Fenofibric Acid** *see* Fenofibrate and Derivatives *on page 852*

◆ **Fenoglide** *see* Fenofibrate and Derivatives *on page 852*

Fenoldopam (fe NOL doe pam)

Brand Names: U.S. Corlopam

Index Terms Fenoldopam Mesylate

Pharmacologic Category Antihypertensive; Dopamine Agonist

Use Treatment of severe hypertension (up to 48 hours in adults), including in patients with renal compromise; short-term (up to 4 hours) blood pressure reduction in pediatric patients

Pregnancy Risk Factor B

Pregnancy Considerations Fetal harm was not observed in animal studies; however, safety and efficacy have not been established for use during pregnancy. Use during pregnancy only if clearly needed.

Breast-Feeding Considerations It is not known if fenoldopam is excreted in breast milk. The manufacturer recommends that caution be exercised when administering fenoldopam to nursing women.

Contraindications There are no contraindications listed within the manufacturer's approved labeling.

Warnings/Precautions Use with caution in patients with open-angle glaucoma or intraocular hypertension; fenoldopam causes a dose-dependent increase in intraocular pressure. Dose-related tachycardia can occur, especially at infusion rates >0.1 mcg/kg/minute. Use with extreme caution in patients with obstructive coronary disease or ongoing angina pectoris; can increase myocardial oxygen demand due to tachycardia leading to angina pectoris. Serum potassium concentrations <3 mEq/L were observed within 6 hours of fenoldopam initiation; monitor potassium concentrations appropriately. Use with caution in patients with increased intracranial pressure; use has not been studied in this population. For continuous infusion only (no bolus doses). Some dosage forms may contain propylene glycol; large amounts are potentially toxic and have been associated hyperosmolality, lactic acidosis, seizures, and respiratory depression; use caution (AAP, 1997; Zar, 2007). Contains sulfites; may cause allergic reaction in susceptible individuals.

Adverse Reactions

Cardiovascular: Angina, bradycardia, chest pain, cutaneous flushing, extrasystoles, heart failure, hypotension, MI, orthostatic hypotension, palpitation, ST-T abnormalities, T-wave inversion, tachycardia

Central nervous system: Anxiety, dizziness, fever, headache, insomnia

Endocrine & metabolic: Hyperglycemia, hypokalemia, LDH increased

Gastrointestinal: Abdominal pain/fullness, constipation, diarrhea, nausea, vomiting

Genitourinary: Urinary tract infection

Hematologic: Bleeding, leukocytosis

Hepatic: Transaminases increased

Local: Injection site reactions

Neuromuscular & skeletal: Back pain, limb cramps

Ocular: Intraocular pressure increased

Renal: BUN increased, creatinine increased, oliguria

Respiratory: Dyspnea, nasal congestion

Miscellaneous: Diaphoresis

Drug Interactions

Metabolism/Transport Effects None known.

Avoid Concomitant Use There are no known interactions where it is recommended to avoid concomitant use.

Increased Effect/Toxicity There are no known significant interactions involving an increase in effect.

Decreased Effect There are no known significant interactions involving a decrease in effect.

Storage/Stability Store undiluted product at 2°C to 30°C (35°F to 86°F). Following dilution, store at room temperature and use solution within 24 hours.

Mechanism of Action A selective postsynaptic dopamine agonist (D_1-receptors) which exerts hypotensive effects by decreasing peripheral vasculature resistance with increased renal blood flow, diuresis, and natriuresis; 6 times as potent as dopamine in producing renal vasodilatation; has minimal adrenergic effects

Pharmacodynamics/Kinetics

Onset of action: IV: 10 minutes

Duration: IV: 1 hour

Distribution: V_d: 0.6 L/kg

Half-life elimination: IV: Children: 3-5 minutes; Adults: ~5 minutes

Metabolism: Hepatic via methylation, glucuronidation, and sulfation; the 8-sulfate metabolite may have some activity; extensive first-pass effect

Excretion: Urine (90%); feces (10%)

Dosage IV: Hypertension, severe:

Children: Initial: 0.2 mcg/kg/minute; may be increased to dosages of 0.3-0.5 mcg/kg/minute every 20-30 minutes (maximum dose: 0.8 mcg/kg/minute); limited to short-term (4 hours) use

Adults: Initial: 0.03-0.1 mcg/kg/minute (associated with less reflex tachycardia); may be increased in increments of 0.05-0.1 mcg/kg/minute every 15 minutes until target blood pressure is reached; the maximal infusion rate reported in clinical studies was 1.6 mcg/kg/minute

Dosing adjustment in renal impairment: No dosage adjustment required; the effects of hemodialysis on fenoldopam have not been evaluated.

Dosing adjustment in hepatic impairment: No dosage adjustment required.

Usual Infusion Concentrations: Pediatric IV infusion: 60 **mcg**/mL

Usual Infusion Concentrations: Adult IV infusion: 10 mg in 250 mL (concentration: 40 **mcg**/mL) of D_5W or NS

Administration For continuous IV infusion only.

Monitoring Parameters Blood pressure, heart rate, ECG; serum potassium concentrations (eg, every 6 hours)

Dosage Forms

Solution, Intravenous:

Corlopam: 10 mg/mL (1 mL); 20 mg/2 mL (2 mL)

Generic: 10 mg/mL (1 mL); 20 mg/2 mL (2 mL)

◆ **Fenoldopam Mesylate** *see* Fenoldopam *on page 856*

◆ **Feno-Micro-200 (Can)** *see* Fenofibrate and Derivatives *on page 852*

Fenoprofen (fen oh PROE fen)

Brand Names: U.S. Nalfon

Brand Names: Canada Nalfon

Index Terms Fenoprofen Calcium

Pharmacologic Category Nonsteroidal Anti-inflammatory Drug (NSAID), Oral

Additional Appendix Information

Beers Criteria – Potentially Inappropriate Medications for Geriatrics *on page 2271*

Use Symptomatic treatment of acute and chronic rheumatoid arthritis and osteoarthritis; relief of mild-to-moderate pain

Pregnancy Risk Factor C

Dosage Adults: Oral:

Rheumatoid arthritis, osteoarthritis: 300-600 mg 3-4 times/day; maximum dose: 3.2 g/day

Mild-to-moderate pain: 200 mg every 4-6 hours as needed; maximum dose: 3.2 g/day

Dosage adjustment in renal impairment: Not recommended in patients with advanced renal disease

Dosage adjustment in hepatic impairment: No dosage adjustment provided in manufacturer's labeling.

Additional Information Complete prescribing information should be consulted for additional detail.

Dosage Forms

Capsule, Oral:

Nalfon: 400 mg

Generic: 400 mg

Tablet, Oral:

Generic: 600 mg

◆ **Fenoprofen Calcium** *see* Fenoprofen *on page 857*

Fenoterol [INT] (fen oh TER ole)

International Brand Names Berotec (AE, AR, AT, AU, BE, BH, BR, CH, CZ, DE, DK, EC, EG, ES, FI, FR, GB, HR, HU, IE, KW, LU, NL, NO, NZ, PL, PT, QA, SA, SE, SI, VN); Berotec N (LT, PL, RO, SK); Dosberotec (DE, IT); Fenostad (AT); Fenoterol (PL); Fensol (ZA); Partusisten (CH, CZ, DE, HR, HU, NL, PL); Partusisten intrapartal (PL)

Pharmacologic Category Beta2 Agonist

Reported Use Bronchodilator used for symptomatic relief of asthma and other conditions such as chronic bronchitis or emphysema

Dosage Range Adults: Bronchospasm:

Metered-dose inhaler: 1 or 2 inhalations up to 3-4 times/day as needed; maximum dose: 8 inhalations/day

Solution for nebulization: 0.5-1 mg every 6 hours as needed; in refractory cases, up to 2.5 mg every 6 hours as needed

Oral: 2.5-5 mg 3 times/day; maximum daily dose: 15 mg

Product Availability Product available in various countries; not currently available in the U.S.

Dosage Forms

Aerosol for inhalation: 100 mcg/inhalation (10 mL)

Solution for inhalation: 0.1% (20 mL, 50 mL)

Tablet: 2.5 mg

◆ **Fenoterol and Ipratropium** *see* Ipratropium and Fenoterol [CAN/INT] *on page 1109*

◆ **Fenoterol Hydrobromide and Ipratropium Bromide** *see* Ipratropium and Fenoterol [CAN/INT] *on page 1109*

Fenoverine [INT] (fen oh VER een)

International Brand Names Noven (KR); Ranspa (KR); Spasmopriv (CO, IN, MX, PH, PK, SG, TH, TW, VN); Syncrospas (IN); Tavidan (TH)

Pharmacologic Category Antispasmodic Agent, Gastrointestinal

Reported Use Symptomatic treatment of gastrointestinal spasm, gastric and duodenal ulcer, monorrhagia, biliary duct and urinary tract spasm

Dosage Range Oral:

Adults: 100 mg 3 times/day or 200 mg twice daily with meals for up to 6 weeks

Elderly: Do not exceed maximum dose: 300 mg/day

Product Availability Product available in various countries; not currently available in the U.S.

Dosage Forms

Capsule: 100 mg, 200 mg

◆ **Fenprocumone** *see* Phenprocoumon [INT] *on page 1635*

FentaNYL (FEN ta nil)

Brand Names: U.S. Abstral; Actiq; Duragesic; Fentora; Lazanda; Onsolis; Subsys

Brand Names: Canada Abstral; Apo-Fentanyl Matrix; Co-Fentanyl; Duragesic MAT; Fentanyl Citrate Injection, USP; Fentora; Mylan-Fentanyl Matrix Patch; PMS-Fentanyl MTX; RAN-Fentanyl Matrix Patch; Sandoz Fentanyl Patch; Teva-Fentanyl

Index Terms Fentanyl Citrate; Fentanyl Hydrochloride; Fentanyl Patch; OTFC (Oral Transmucosal Fentanyl Citrate)

Pharmacologic Category Analgesic, Opioid; Anilidopiperidine Opioid; General Anesthetic

Additional Appendix Information

Opioid Conversion Table *on page 2232*

Use

Injection:

Pain management: Relief of pain, preoperative medication.

Surgery: Adjunct to general or regional anesthesia.

Transdermal patch (eg, Duragesic): **Chronic pain:** Management of pain in opioid-tolerant patients, severe enough to require daily, around-the-clock, long-term opioid treatment and for which alternative treatment options are inadequate.

Limitations of use: Because of the risks of addiction, abuse, and misuse with opioids, even at recommended doses, and because of the greater risks of overdose and death with extended-release opioid formulations, reserve fentanyl transdermal patch for use in patients ▶

for whom alternative treatment options (eg, nonopioid analgesics, immediate-release opioids) are ineffective, not tolerated, or would be otherwise inadequate to provide sufficient management of pain.

Transmucosal lozenge (eg, Actiq), buccal tablet (Fentora), buccal film (Onsolis), nasal spray (Lazanda), sublingual tablet (Abstral), sublingual spray (Subsys): **Cancer pain:** Management of breakthrough cancer pain in opioid-tolerant patients who are already receiving and who are tolerant to around-the-clock opioid therapy for their underlying persistent cancer pain.

Note: "Opioid-tolerant" patients are defined as patients who are taking at least:

Oral morphine 60 mg/day, **or**
Transdermal fentanyl 25 mcg/hour, **or**
Oral oxycodone 30 mg/day, **or**
Oral hydromorphone 8 mg/day, **or**
Oral oxymorphone 25 mg/day, **or**
Equianalgesic dose of another opioid for at least 1 week

Pregnancy Risk Factor C

Pregnancy Considerations Adverse events were observed in some animal reproduction studies. Fentanyl crosses the placenta.

Fentanyl injection may be used for the management of pain during labor (ACOG, 2002). When used for pain relief during labor, opioids may temporarily affect the heart rate of the fetus (ACOG, 2002). Transient muscular rigidity has been observed in the neonate with fentanyl; symptoms of respiratory or neurological depression were not different than those observed in infants of untreated mothers.

[U.S. Boxed Warning]: Prolonged maternal use of opioids during pregnancy can cause neonatal withdrawal syndrome in the newborn which may be life-threatening if not recognized and treated according to protocols developed by neonatology experts. If prolonged opioid therapy is required in a pregnant woman, ensure treatment is available and warn patient of risk to the neonate. If chronic opioid exposure occurs in pregnancy, adverse events in the newborn (including withdrawal) may occur; monitoring of the neonate is recommended. The minimum effective dose should be used if opioids are needed (Chou, 2009). Symptoms characteristic of neonatal abstinence syndrome have been observed following chronic fentanyl use in pregnant women. Neonatal abstinence syndrome following opioid exposure may present with autonomic (eg, fever, temperature instability), gastrointestinal (eg, diarrhea, vomiting, poor feeding/weight gain), or neurologic (eg, high pitched crying, increased muscle tone, irritability, seizure, tremor) symptoms (Dow, 2012; Hudak, 2012).

Long-term opioid use may cause secondary hypogonadism, which may lead to sexual dysfunction or infertility (Brennan, 2013).

Transdermal patch, transmucosal lozenge, nasal spray (Lazanda), sublingual tablet, sublingual spray (Subsys), buccal tablet (Fentora), and buccal film (Onsolis) are not recommended for analgesia during labor and delivery. Transdermal patch Canadian labeling contraindicates use in pregnant women and during labor and delivery.

Breast-Feeding Considerations Fentanyl is excreted in low concentrations into breast milk and breast-feeding is not recommended by the manufacturers.

Parenteral opioids used during labor have the potential to interfere with a newborn's natural reflex to nurse within the first few hours after birth. When needed, a short-acting opioid, such as fentanyl, is preferred for women who will be nursing (Montgomery, 2012)

Breast-feeding is considered acceptable following single doses to the mother; however, limited information is available when used long-term (Spigset, 2000). Nursing infants exposed to large doses of opioids should be monitored for apnea and sedation (Montgomery, 2012).

Note: Transdermal patch, transmucosal lozenge, sublingual tablet, sublingual spray (Subsys), buccal tablet (Fentora), and buccal film (Onsolis) are not recommended in nursing women due to potential for sedation and/or respiratory depression. Transdermal patch Canadian labeling contraindicates use in nursing women.

Contraindications Hypersensitivity to fentanyl or any component of the formulation

Additional contraindications for transdermal patches (eg, Duragesic): Severe respiratory disease or depression including acute asthma (unless patient is mechanically ventilated); paralytic ileus; patients requiring short-term therapy, management of acute or intermittent pain, postoperative or mild pain, and in patients who are **not** opioid tolerant

Additional contraindications for transmucosal buccal tablets (Fentora), buccal films (Onsolis), lozenges (eg, Actiq), sublingual tablets (Abstral), sublingual spray (Subsys), nasal spray (Lazanda): Contraindicated in the management of acute or postoperative pain (including headache, migraine, or dental pain), and in patients who are **not** opioid tolerant. Abstral and Onsolis also are contraindicated for acute pain management in the emergency room.

Canadian labeling: Additional contraindication (not in U.S. labeling):

Injection: Septicemia; severe hemorrhage or shock; local infection at proposed injection site; disturbances in blood morphology and/or anticoagulant therapy or other concomitant drug therapy or medical conditions which could contraindicate the technique of epidural administration

Sublingual tablets (Abstral): Severe respiratory depression or severe obstructive lung disease.

Transdermal patch: Hypersensitivity to other opioids; suspected surgical abdomen (eg, acute appendicitis, pancreatitis); known or suspected mechanical GI obstruction (eg, bowel obstruction, strictures); acute alcoholism, delirium tremens, and convulsive disorders; severe CNS depression, increased cerebrospinal or intracranial pressure and head injury; concurrent use of monoamine oxidase (MAO) inhibitors or within 14 days of therapy; women who are nursing, pregnant, or during labor and delivery

Warnings/Precautions An opioid-containing analgesic regimen should be tailored to each patient's needs and based upon the type of pain being treated (acute versus chronic), the route of administration, degree of tolerance for opioids (naive versus chronic user), age, weight, and medical condition. The optimal analgesic dose varies widely among patients. Doses should be titrated to pain relief/prevention. May cause CNS depression, which may impair physical or mental abilities; patients must be cautioned about performing tasks which require mental alertness (eg, operating machinery or driving). Effects may be potentiated when used with other sedative drugs or ethanol. Fentanyl shares the toxic potentials of opioid agonists, and precautions of opioid agonist therapy should be observed; use with caution in patients with bradycardia or bradyarrhythmias; rapid IV infusion may result in skeletal muscle and chest wall rigidity leading to respiratory distress and/or apnea, bronchoconstriction, laryngospasm; inject slowly over 3 to 5 minutes. Monitor for respiratory depression in patients with significant chronic obstructive pulmonary disease or cor pulmonale, and patients having a substantially decreased respiratory reserve, hypoxia, hypercarbia, or preexisting respiratory depression, particularly when initiating therapy and titrating with fentanyl; even therapeutic doses may decrease respiratory drive to the point of apnea. Consider the use of alternative nonopioid analgesics in these patients. **[U.S. Boxed Warning]: Users are exposed to the risks of addiction, abuse, and misuse, potentially leading to overdose and death. Assess each patient's risk prior to prescribing; monitor all patients for development of these behaviors or conditions.** Tolerance or drug dependence may result from extended use. The elderly may be particularly susceptible to the CNS depressant and constipating effects of opioids. Use extreme caution in patients with COPD or other chronic respiratory conditions (some products may be contraindicated). Use caution with biliary tract impairment, pancreatitis, head injuries (some products may be contraindicated), morbid obesity, renal impairment, or hepatic dysfunction. **[U.S. Boxed Warning]: Use with strong or moderate CYP3A4 inhibitors may result in increased effects and potentially fatal respiratory depression. In addition, discontinuation of a concomitant CYP 3A4 inducer may result in increased fentanyl concentrations. Monitor patients receiving any CYP 3A4 inhibitor or inducer.** Concurrent use of mixed agonist/antagonist analgesics (eg, pentazocine, nalbuphine, butorphanol) or partial agonist (eg, buprenorphine) analgesics may precipitate withdrawal symptoms and/or reduced analgesic efficacy in patients following prolonged therapy with mu opioid agonists. Abrupt discontinuation following prolonged use may also lead to withdrawal symptoms. Potentially significant interactions may exist, requiring dose or frequency adjustment, additional monitoring, and/or selection of alternative therapy.

Pediatric patients: **[U.S. Boxed Warning]: Buccal film, buccal tablet, nasal spray, sublingual tablet, sublingual spray, and lozenge preparations contain an amount of medication that can be fatal to children. Keep all used and unused products out of the reach of children at all times and discard products properly.** Patients and caregivers should be counseled on the dangers to children including the risk of exposure to partially-consumed products.

[U.S. Boxed Warning] Abstral, Actiq, Duragesic, Fentora, Lazanda, Onsolis, Subsys: May cause serious, life-threatening, or fatal respiratory depression, even when used as recommended. Monitor closely for respiratory depression, especially during initiation or dose escalation. Abstral, Actiq, Duragesic, Fentora, Lazanda, Onsolis, or Subsys should only be prescribed for opioid-tolerant patients. Risk of respiratory depression increased in elderly patients, debilitated patients, and patients with conditions associated with hypoxia or hypercapnia; usually occurs after administration of initial dose in nontolerant patients or when given with other drugs that depress respiratory function.

Transmucosal (buccal film/tablet, sublingual spray/tablet, lozenge) and nasal spray: **[U.S. Boxed Warning]: Transmucosal and nasal fentanyl formulations are contraindicated in the management of acute or postoperative pain and in opioid nontolerant patients.** Should be used only for the care of opioid-tolerant cancer patients with breakthrough pain and is intended for use by specialists who are knowledgeable in treating cancer pain. **[U.S. Boxed Warning]: Substantial differences exist in the pharmacokinetic profile of fentanyl products. Do not convert patients on a mcg-per-mcg basis from one fentanyl product to another fentanyl product; the substitution of one fentanyl product for another fentanyl product may result in a fatal overdose. [U.S. Boxed Warning]: Available only through the TIRF REMS ACCESS program, a restricted distribution program with outpatients, prescribers who prescribe to outpatients, pharmacies (inpatient and outpatient), and distributor-required enrollment.** Avoid use of topical nasal decongestants (eg, oxymetazoline) during episodes of rhinitis when using fentanyl nasal spray; response to fentanyl may be delayed or reduced. Avoid use of sublingual spray in cancer patients with grade 2 or higher mucositis (fentanyl exposure increased); use with caution in patients with grade 1 mucositis, and closely monitor for respiratory and CNS depression.

Transdermal patch (Duragesic): **[U.S. Boxed Warning]: Transdermal patch is contraindicated for use as an as-needed analgesic, in the management of acute or postoperative pain, or in patients who are opioid nontolerant. Monitor closely for respiratory depression during use, particularly during initiation of therapy or after dose increases.** Should only be prescribed by health care professionals who are knowledgeable in the use of potent opioids in the management of chronic pain. For patients undergoing cordotomy or other pain-relieving procedures, the Canadian labeling recommends withholding transdermal fentanyl within 72 hours prior to the procedure and in the immediate postoperative period; dose adjustment may be necessary upon resuming therapy. **[U.S. Boxed Warning]: Exposure of application site and surrounding area to direct external heat sources (eg, heating pads, electric blankets, heat or tanning lamps, sunbathing, hot tubs) may increase fentanyl absorption and has resulted in fatalities. Patients who experience fever or increase in core body temperature should be monitored closely.** Serum fentanyl concentrations may increase by approximately one-third for patients with a body temperature of 40°C (104°F) secondary to a temperature-dependent increase in fentanyl release from the patch and increased skin permeability. **[U.S. Boxed Warning]: Accidental exposure to fentanyl transdermal patch has resulted in fatal overdose in children and adults. Strict adherence to recommended handling and disposal instructions is necessary to prevent accidental exposures.** Avoid unclothed/unwashed application site exposure, inadvertent person-to-person patch transfer (eg, while hugging), incidental exposure (eg, sharing same bed, sitting on patch), intentional exposure (eg, chewing), or accidental exposure by caregivers when applying/removing patch. **[U.S. Boxed Warning]: Prolonged maternal use of opioids during pregnancy can cause neonatal withdrawal syndrome in the newborn which may be life-threatening if not recognized and treated according to protocols developed by neonatology experts. If prolonged opioid therapy is required in a pregnant woman, patient should be warned of risk to the neonate and ensure treatment is available.** Should be applied only to intact skin. Use of a patch that has been cut, damaged, or altered in any way may result in overdosage. Patients who experience adverse reactions should be monitored for at least 24 hours after removal of the patch. Drug continues to be absorbed from the skin for 24 hours or more following removal of the patch. May contain conducting metal (eg, aluminum); remove patch prior to MRI.

Adverse Reactions

Cardiovascular: Bradycardia, cardiac arrhythmia, cardiorespiratory arrest, chest pain, chest wall rigidity (high dose IV), deep vein thrombosis, edema, flushing, hypertension, hypotension, orthostatic hypotension, palpitations, peripheral edema, pulmonary embolism (nasal spray), sinus tachycardia, syncope, tachycardia, vasodilatation

Central nervous system: Abnormal dreams, abnormal gait, abnormality in thinking, agitation, altered sense of smell, amnesia, anxiety, ataxia, central nervous system depression, chills, confusion, depression, disorientation, dizziness, drowsiness, dysphoria, euphoria, fatigue, hallucination, headache, hypoesthesia, insomnia, irritability, lack of concentration, lethargy, malaise, mental status changes, migraine, nervousness, neuropathy, paranoia, paresthesia, restlessness, rigors, sedation, speech disturbance, stupor, vertigo, withdrawal syndrome

Dermatologic: Alopecia, cellulitis, decubitus ulcer, diaphoresis, erythema, hyperhidrosis, night sweats, pallor, papule, pruritus, skin rash

Endocrine & metabolic: Dehydration, hot flash, hypercalcemia, hyperglycemia, hypoalbuminemia, hypocalcemia, hypoglycemia, hypokalemia, hypomagnesemia, hyponatremia, weight loss

Gastrointestinal: Abdominal distention, abdominal pain, anorexia, biliary tract spasm, constipation, decreased appetite, diarrhea, dysgeusia, dyspepsia, dysphagia (buccal tablet/film/sublingual spray), flatulence, gastritis, gastroenteritis, gastroesophageal reflux disease, gastrointestinal hemorrhage, gastrointestinal ulcer (gingival, lip, mouth; transmucosal use/nasal spray), gingival pain (buccal tablet), gingivitis (lozenge), glossitis (lozenge), hematemesis, hiccups, intestinal obstruction, nausea, periodontal abscess (lozenge/buccal tablet), rectal pain, stomatitis (lozenge/buccal tablet/sublingual tablet/sublingual spray), tongue disease (sublingual tablet), vomiting, xerostomia

Genitourinary: Dysuria, erectile dysfunction, mastalgia, urinary incontinence, urinary retention, urinary tract infection, vaginal hemorrhage, vaginitis

Hematologic & oncologic: Anemia, bruise, leukopenia, lymphadenopathy, neutropenia, thrombocytopenia

Hepatic: Ascites, increased serum alkaline phosphatase, increased serum AST, jaundice

Hypersensitivity: Hypersensitivity

Local: Application site erythema, application site irritation, application site pain

Neuromuscular & skeletal: Arthralgia, back pain, limb pain, muscle rigidity, myalgia, tremor, weakness

Ophthalmic: Blepharoptosis, blurred vision, diplopia, dry eye syndrome, miosis, strabismus, swelling of eye

Renal: Renal failure

Respiratory: Apnea, asthma, bronchitis, cough, dyspnea, dyspnea (exertional), epistaxis, flu-like symptoms, hemoptysis, hypoventilation, hypoxia, laryngitis, nasal congestion (nasal spray), nasal discomfort (nasal spray), nasopharyngitis, pharyngitis, pharyngolaryngeal pain, pneumonia, postnasal drip (nasal spray), respiratory depression, rhinitis, rhinorrhea (nasal spray), sinusitis, upper respiratory tract infection, wheezing

Miscellaneous: Fever

Rare but important or life-threatening: Amblyopia, anaphylaxis, angina pectoris, aphasia, bladder pain, bronchospasm, central nervous system stimulation, delirium, depersonalization, dizziness (paradoxical), drug dependence (physical and psychological; with prolonged use), dysesthesia, emotional lability, esophageal stenosis, exfoliative dermatitis, fecal impaction, genitourinary tract spasm, gingival hemorrhage (lozenge), gum line erosion (lozenge), hematuria, hostility, hypertonia, hypogonadism (Brennan, 2013; Debono, 2011), hypotonia, laryngospasm, myasthenia, nocturia, oliguria, pancytopenia, pleural effusion, polyuria, pustules, seizure, stertorous breathing, tooth loss (lozenge), urticaria, vertigo

Drug Interactions

Metabolism/Transport Effects Substrate of CYP3A4 (major); **Note:** Assignment of Major/Minor substrate status based on clinically relevant drug interaction potential; **Inhibits** CYP3A4 (weak)

Avoid Concomitant Use

Avoid concomitant use of FentaNYL with any of the following: Azelastine (Nasal); Conivaptan; Crizotinib; Dapoxetine; Enzalutamide; Fusidic Acid (Systemic); Idelalisib; MAO Inhibitors; Mifepristone; Orphenadrine; Paraldehyde; Pimozide; Thalidomide

Increased Effect/Toxicity

FentaNYL may increase the levels/effects of: Alcohol (Ethyl); Alvimopan; Antipsychotic Agents; ARIPiprazole; Azelastine (Nasal); Beta-Blockers; Buprenorphine; Calcium Channel Blockers (Nondihydropyridine); CNS Depressants; Desmopressin; Diuretics; Dofetilide; Hydrocodone; Lomitapide; MAO Inhibitors; Methotrimeprazine; Metoclopramide; Metyrosine; Orphenadrine; Paraldehyde; Pimozide; Pramipexole; ROPINIRole; Rotigotine; Serotonin Modulators; Suvorexant; Thalidomide; Zolpidem

The levels/effects of FentaNYL may be increased by: Amphetamines; Anticholinergic Agents; Antiemetics (5HT3 Antagonists); Antipsychotic Agents; Antipsychotic Agents (Phenothiazines); Brimonidine (Topical); Cannabis; Conivaptan; Crizotinib; CYP3A4 Inhibitors (Moderate); CYP3A4 Inhibitors (Strong); Dapoxetine; Dasatinib; Doxylamine; Dronabinol; Droperidol; Fusidic Acid (Systemic); HydrOXYzine; Idelalisib; Ivacaftor; Kava Kava; Luliconazole; Magnesium Sulfate; Methotrimeprazine; Mifepristone; Nabilone; Perampanel; Rufinamide; Simeprevir; Sodium Oxybate; Stiripentol; Succinylcholine; Tapentadol; Tetrahydrocannabinol

Decreased Effect

FentaNYL may decrease the levels/effects of: Ioflupane I 123; Pegvisomant

The levels/effects of FentaNYL may be decreased by: Alpha-/Beta-Agonists (Indirect-Acting); Alpha1-Agonists; Ammonium Chloride; CYP3A4 Inducers (Moderate); CYP3A4 Inducers (Strong); Enzalutamide; Mixed Agonist/ Antagonist Opioids; Naltrexone; St Johns Wort

Food Interactions Fentanyl concentrations may be increased by grapefruit juice. Management: Avoid concurrent intake of large quantities (>1 quart/day) of grapefruit juice.

Storage/Stability

Injection formulation: Store intact vials/ampules at controlled room temperature of 20°C to 25°C (68°F to 77°F). Protect from light. Canadian labeling (not in U.S. labeling) recommends that when admixing injection formulation in NS for epidural administration, the resulting solution be used within 24 hours.

Nasal spray: Do not store above 25°C (77°F); do not freeze. Protect from light. Bottle should be stored in the provided child-resistant container when not in use and kept out of the reach of children at all times.

Transdermal patch: Do not store above 25°C (77°F). Keep out of the reach of children.

Transmucosal (buccal film, buccal tablet, lozenge, sublingual spray, sublingual tablet): Store at controlled room temperature of 20°C to 25°C (68°F to 77°F). Protect from freezing and moisture. Keep out of the reach of children.

Mechanism of Action Binds with stereospecific receptors at many sites within the CNS, increases pain threshold, alters pain reception, inhibits ascending pain pathways

Pharmacodynamics/Kinetics

Onset of action: Analgesic: IM: 7-8 minutes; IV: Almost immediate (maximal analgesic and respiratory depressant effects may not be seen for several minutes); Transdermal (initial placement): 6 hours; Transmucosal: 5-15 minutes

Duration: IM: 1-2 hours; IV: 0.5-1 hour; Transdermal (removal of patch/no replacement): Related to blood level; some effects may last 72-96 hours due to extended half-life and absorption from the skin, fentanyl concentrations decrease by ~50% in 20-27 hours; Transmucosal: Related to blood level; respiratory depressant effect may last longer than analgesic effect

Absorption:

Transdermal: Initial application: Drug is released at a nearly constant rate from the transdermal matrix system into the skin, where it accumulates; this results in a depot of fentanyl in the outer layer of skin. Fentanyl is absorbed into systemic circulation from the depot. This results in a gradual increase in serum concentration over the first 12-24 hours, followed by fairly constant concentrations for the remainder of the dosing interval. Absorption is decreased in cachectic patients (compared to normal size patients). Exposure to external heat increases drug absorption from patch.

Transmucosal, buccal tablet and buccal film: Rapid, ~50% from the buccal mucosa; remaining 50% swallowed with saliva and slowly absorbed from GI tract.

Transmucosal, lozenge: Rapid, ~25% from the buccal mucosa; 75% swallowed with saliva and slowly absorbed from GI tract

Distribution: 4-6 L/kg; Highly lipophilic, redistributes into muscle and fat

Protein binding: 80% to 85%

Metabolism: Hepatic, primarily via CYP3A4

Bioavailability:

Buccal film: 71% (mucositis did not have a clinically significant effect on C_{max} and AUC; however, bioavailability is expected to decrease if film is inappropriately chewed and swallowed)

Buccal tablet: 65%

Lozenge: ~50%

Sublingual spray: 76%

Sublingual tablet: 54%

Half-life elimination:

IV: 2-4 hours; when administered as a continuous infusion, the half-life prolongs with infusion duration due to the large volume of distribution (Sessler, 2008)

Transdermal patch: 20-27 hours (apparent half-life is influenced by continued fentanyl absorption from skin)

Transmucosal products: 3-14 hours (dose dependent); Nasal spray: 15-25 hours (based on a multiple-dose pharmacokinetic study when doses are administered in the same nostril and separated by a 1-, 2-, or 4-hour time lapse)

Time to peak:

Buccal film: 0.75-4 hours (median: 1 hour)

Buccal tablet: 20-240 minutes (median: 47 minutes)

Lozenge: 20-480 minutes (median: 20-40 minutes)

Nasal spray: Median: 15-21 minutes

Sublingual spray: 10-120 minutes (median: 90 minutes)

Sublingual tablet: 15-240 minutes (median: 30-60 minutes)

Transdermal patch: 20-72 hours; steady state serum concentrations are reached after two sequential 72-hour applications

Excretion: Urine 75% (primarily as metabolites, <7% to 10% as unchanged drug); feces ~9%

Dosage Note: Ranges listed may not represent the maximum doses that may be required in some patients. Doses and dosage intervals should be titrated to pain relief/prevention. Monitor vital signs routinely. Single IM doses have duration of 1 to 2 hours, single IV doses last 0.5 to 1 hour.

Surgery:

Children ≥2 years and Adolescents: Adjunct to anesthesia (induction and maintenance): Slow IV: 2 to 3 mcg/**kg**/dose every 1 to 2 hours as needed

Adults:

Premedication: IM: 50 to 100 mcg administered 30 to 60 minutes prior to surgery **or** slow IV: 25 to 50 mcg given shortly before induction (Barash, 2009)

Adjunct to general anesthesia: Slow IV:

Low dose: 1 to 2 mcg/**kg** depending on the indication (Miller, 2010); additional maintenance doses are generally not needed

Moderate dose (fentanyl plus a sedative/hypnotic): Initial: 2 to 4 mcg/**kg**; Maintenance (bolus or infusion): 25 to 50 mcg every 15 to 30 minutes or 0.5 to 2 mcg/kg/**hour**. Discontinuing fentanyl infusion 30 to 60 minutes prior to the end of surgery will usually allow adequate ventilation upon emergence from anesthesia.

High dose (opioid anesthesia): 4 to 20 mcg/**kg** bolus then 2 to 10 mcg/kg/**hour** (Miller, 2010); **Note:** High-dose fentanyl (ie, 20 to 50 mcg/kg) is rarely used, but is still described in the manufacturer's labeling. The concept of fast-tracking and early extubation following cardiac surgery has essentially replaced high-dose fentanyl anesthesia.

Adjunct to regional anesthesia: 50 to 100 mcg IM or slow IV over 1 to 2 minutes. **Note:** An IV should be in place with regional anesthesia so the IM route is rarely used but still maintained as an option in the manufacturer's labeling.

Postoperative recovery: IM, slow IV: 50 to 100 mcg every 1 to 2 hours as needed.

Postoperative pain: Epidural (Canadian labeling; not in U.S. labeling): Initial: 100 mcg (diluted in 8 mL of preservative free NS to final concentration of 10 mcg/mL); may repeat with additional 100 mcg boluses on demand or alternatively may administer by continuous infusion at a rate of 1 mcg/kg/hour.

Pain management:

Children <50 kg: Patient-controlled analgesia (PCA) (off-label use; American Pain Society, 2008): Opioid-naive: IV:

Usual concentration: 10 to 50 mcg/mL (varies by patient weight and institution)

Demand dose: 0.5 to 1 mcg/kg/dose

Lockout interval: 6 to 8 minutes

Usual basal rate (optional): ≤0.5 mcg/kg/**hour**. **Note:** Due to safety concerns, continuous basal infusions are not recommended for initial programming and should rarely be used (Grass, 2005).

Adults: ***Severe pain:***

IM, IV:

Intermittent dosing (off-label dose): Slow IV: 25 to 35 mcg (based on ~70 kg patient) **or** 0.35 to 0.5 mcg/kg every 30 to 60 minutes as needed (SCCM [Barr, 2013]). **Note:** After the first dose, if severe pain persists and adverse effects are minimal at the time of expected peak effect (eg, ~5 minutes after IV administration), may repeat dose (APS, 2008). In addition, since the duration of activity with IV administration is 30 to 60 minutes, more frequent administration may be necessary when administered by this route.

Patient-controlled analgesia (PCA) (off-label use; American Pain Society, 2008; Miller, 2010): Opioid-naive: IV:

Usual concentration: 10 mcg/mL

Demand dose: Usual: 10 to 20 mcg

Lockout interval: 4 to 10 minutes

Usual basal rate: ≤50 mcg/hour. **Note:** Due to safety concerns, continuous basal infusions are not recommended for initial programming and should rarely be used; consider limiting infusion rate to 10 mcg/hour if used (Grass, 2005).

Critically-ill patients (off-label dose): Slow IV: 25 to 35 mcg (based on ~70 kg patient) **or** 0.3 to 0.5 mcg/kg every 30 to 60 minutes as needed (SCCM [Barr, 2013]). **Note:** More frequent dosing may be needed (eg, mechanically-ventilated patients).

Continuous infusion: 50 to 700 mcg/hour (based on ~70 kg patient) **or** 0.7 to 10 mcg/kg/**hour** (SCCM [Barr, 2013])

Alternative continuous infusion dosing: 1 to 2 mcg/kg bolus followed by an initial rate of 1 to 2 mcg/**kg**/hour (Peng, 1999) **or** 25 to 100 mcg bolus followed by an initial rate of 25 to 200 mcg/**hour** (Liu, 2003). **Note:** When pain is not controlled, may administer an additional small bolus dose (eg, 25 to 50 mcg) prior to increasing the infusion rate (Loper 1990; Peng, 1999; Salomaki, 1991).

Intrathecal (off-label use; American Pain Society, 2008): **Must be preservative-free.** Doses must be adjusted for age, injection site, and patient's medical condition and degree of opioid tolerance.

Single dose: 5 to 25 mcg; may provide adequate relief for up to 6 hours

Continuous infusion: Not recommended in acute pain management due to risk of excessive accumulation. For chronic cancer pain, infusion of very small doses may be practical (American Pain Society, 2008).

Epidural (off-label use; American Pain Society, 2008): **Must be preservative-free.** Doses must be adjusted for age, injection site, and patient's medical condition and degree of opioid tolerance

Single dose: 25 to 100 mcg; may provide adequate relief for up to 8 hours

Continuous infusion: 25 to 100 mcg/hour (fentanyl alone). When combined with a local anesthetic (eg, bupivacaine or ropivacaine), fentanyl requirements are less (Manion, 2011)

Breakthrough cancer pain: For patients who are tolerant to and currently receiving opioid therapy for persistent cancer pain; dosing should be individually titrated to provide adequate analgesia with minimal side effects. Dose titration should be done if patient requires more than 1 dose/breakthrough pain episode for several consecutive episodes. Patients experiencing >4 breakthrough pain episodes per day should have the dose of their long-term opioid re-evaluated. **Patients must remain on around-the-clock opioids during use.**

Adolescents ≥16 years and Adults: Transmucosal: Lozenge (Actiq): **Note:** Do **not** convert patients from any other fentanyl product to Actiq on a mcg-per-mcg basis. Patients previously using another fentanyl product should be initiated at a dose of 200 mcg; individually titrate to provide adequate analgesia while minimizing adverse effects.

Initial dose: 200 mcg (consumed over 15 minutes) for all patients; if after 30 minutes from the start of the lozenge (ie, 15 minutes following the completion of the lozenge) the pain is unrelieved, a second 200 mcg dose may be given over 15 minutes. A maximum of 1 additional dose can be given per pain episode; **must wait at least 4 hours before treating another episode**. To limit the number of units in the home during titration, only prescribe an initial titration supply of six 200 mcg lozenges.

Dose titration: From the initial dose, closely follow patients and modify the dose until patient reaches a dose providing adequate analgesia using a single dosage unit per breakthrough cancer pain episode. If signs/symptoms of excessive opioid effects (eg, respiratory depression) occur, immediately remove the dosage unit from the patient's mouth, dispose of properly, and reduce subsequent doses. If adequate relief is not achieved 15 minutes after completion of the first dose (ie, 30 minutes after the start of the lozenge), only 1 additional lozenge of the same strength may be given for that episode; **must wait at least 4 hours before treating another episode.**

Maintenance dose: Once titrated to an effective dose, patients should generally use a single dosage unit per breakthrough pain episode. During any pain episode, if adequate relief is not achieved 15 minutes after completion of the first dose (ie, 30 minutes after the start of the lozenge), only 1 additional lozenge of the same strength may be given over 15 minutes for that episode; **must wait at least 4 hours before treating another episode**. Consumption should be limited to ≤4 units per day (once an effective breakthrough dose is found). If adequate analgesia is **not** provided after treating several episodes of breakthrough pain using the same dose, increase dose to next highest lozenge strength (initially dispense no more than 6 units of the new strength). Consider increasing the around-the-clock opioid therapy in patients experiencing >4 breakthrough pain episodes per day. If signs/symptoms of excessive opioid effects (eg, respiratory depression) occur, immediately remove the dosage unit from the patient's mouth, dispose of properly, and reduce subsequent doses.

Adults: Transmucosal:

Buccal film (Onsolis): **Note:** Do **not** convert patients from any other fentanyl product to Onsolis on a mcg-per-mcg basis. Patients previously using another fentanyl product should be initiated at a dose of 200 mcg; individually titrate to provide adequate analgesia while minimizing adverse effects.

Initial dose: 200 mcg for all patients; if after 30 minutes pain is unrelieved, the patient may use an alternative rescue medication as directed by their health care provider. Do **not** redose with Onsolis within an episode; buccal film should only be used once per breakthrough cancer pain episode. **Must wait at least 2 hours before treating another episode with buccal film.**

Dose titration: If titration required, increase dose in 200 mcg increments once per episode using multiples of the 200 mcg film (for doses up to 800 mcg); do not redose within a single episode of breakthrough pain and separate single doses by ≥2 hours. During titration, do not exceed 4 simultaneous applications of the 200 mcg films (800 mcg) (when using multiple films, do not place on top of each other; film may be placed on both sides of mouth); if >800 mcg required, treat next episode with one 1200 mcg film (maximum dose: 1200 mcg). Once maintenance dose is determined, all other unused films should be disposed of and that strength (using a single film) should be used. During any pain episode, if adequate relief is not achieved after 30 minutes following buccal film application, a rescue medication (as determined by health care provider) may be used.

Maintenance dose: Determined dose applied as a single film once per episode and separated by ≥2 hours (dose range: 200 to 1200 mcg); limit to 4 applications per day. Consider increasing the around-the-clock opioid therapy in patients experiencing >4 breakthrough pain episodes per day.

Buccal tablet (Fentora): **Note:** Do **not** convert patients from any other fentanyl product to Fentora on a mcg-per-mcg basis. Patients previously using another fentanyl product should be initiated at a dose of 100 mcg; individually titrate to provide adequate analgesia while minimizing adverse effects. For patients previously using the transmucosal lozenge (Actiq), the initial dose should be selected using the conversions listed; see *Conversion from lozenge (Actiq) to buccal tablet (Fentora)*.

Initial dose: 100 mcg for all patients unless patient already using Actiq; see *Conversion from lozenge (Actiq) to buccal tablet (Fentora)*; if after 30 minutes pain is unrelieved, the U.S. labeling suggests that a second 100 mcg dose may be administered (maximum of 2 doses per breakthrough pain episode). The Canadian labeling recommends only a single dose per breakthrough pain episode; patients experiencing breakthrough pain after administration may take an alternative analgesic as rescue medication after 30 minutes. **Must wait at least 4 hours before treating another episode with Fentora buccal tablet.**

Dose titration: If titration required, 100 mcg dose may be increased to 200 mcg using two 100 mcg tablets (one on each side of mouth) with the next breakthrough pain episode. If 200 mcg dose is not successful, patient can use four 100 mcg tablets (two on each side of mouth) with the next breakthrough pain episode. If titration requires >400 mcg per dose, titrate using 200 mcg tablets; do not use more than 4 tablets simultaneously (maximum single dose: 800 mcg). During any pain episode, if adequate relief is not achieved after 30 minutes following buccal tablet application, a second dose of same strength per breakthrough pain episode may be used. The Canadian labeling recommends only a single dose per breakthrough pain episode; patients experiencing breakthrough pain after administration may take an alternative analgesic as rescue medication after 30 minutes. **Must wait at least 4 hours before treating another episode with Fentora buccal tablet.**

Maintenance dose: Following titration, the effective maintenance dose using 1 tablet of the appropriate strength should be administered once per episode; if after 30 minutes pain is unrelieved, may administer a second dose of the same strength. The Canadian labeling recommends only a single dose per breakthrough pain episode; patients experiencing breakthrough pain after administration may take an alternative analgesic as rescue medication after 30 minutes. **Must wait at least 4 hours before treating another episode with Fentora buccal tablet.** Limit to 4 applications per day. Consider increasing the around-the-clock opioid therapy in patients experiencing >4 breakthrough pain episodes per day. Once an effective maintenance dose has been established, the buccal tablet may be administered sublingually (alternate route). To prevent confusion, patient should only have one strength available at a time. Once maintenance dose is determined, all other unused tablets should be disposed of and that strength (using a single tablet) should be used. Using more than four buccal tablets at a time has not been studied.

Conversion from lozenge (Actiq) to buccal tablet (Fentora):

Lozenge dose 200 to 400 mcg: Initial buccal tablet dose is 100 mcg; may titrate using multiples of 100 mcg

Lozenge dose 600 to 800 mcg: Initial buccal tablet dose is 200 mcg; may titrate using multiples of 200 mcg

Lozenge dose 1200 to 1600 mcg: Initial buccal tablet dose is 400 mcg (using two 200 mcg tablets); may titrate using multiples of 200 mcg

Nasal spray (Lazanda): **Note:** Do **not** convert patients from any other fentanyl product to Lazanda on a mcg-per-mcg basis. Patients previously using another fentanyl product should be initiated at a dose of 100 mcg; individually titrate to provide adequate analgesia while minimizing adverse effects.

Initial dose: 100 mcg (one 100 mcg spray in one nostril) for all patients; if after 30 minutes pain is unrelieved, an alternative rescue medication may be used as directed by their health care provider. **Must wait at least 2 hours before treating another episode with Lazanda nasal spray.** However, for the next pain episode, increase to a higher dose using the recommended dose titration steps.

Dose titration: If titration required, increase to a higher dose for the next pain episode using these titration steps **(Note: Must wait at least 2 hours before treating another episode with Lazanda nasal spray)**: If no relief with 100 mcg dose, increase to 200 mcg dose per episode (one 100 mcg spray in each nostril); if no relief with 200 mcg dose, increase to 400 mcg per episode (one 400 mcg spray in one nostril or two 100 mcg sprays in each nostril); if no relief with 400 mcg dose, increase to 800 mcg dose per episode (one 400 mcg spray in each nostril). **Note:** Single doses >800 mcg have not been evaluated. There are no data supporting the use of a combination of dose strengths.

Maintenance dose: Once maintenance dose for breakthrough pain episode has been determined, use that dose for subsequent episodes. For pain that is not relieved after 30 minutes of Lazanda administration or if a separate breakthrough pain episode occurs within the 2 hour window before the next Lazanda dose is permitted, a rescue medication may be used. Limit Lazanda use to ≤4 episodes of breakthrough pain per day. If patient is experiencing >4 breakthrough pain episodes per day, consider increasing the around-the-clock, long-acting opioid therapy; if long-acting opioid therapy dose is altered, re-evaluate and retitrate Lazanda dose as needed. If response to maintenance dose changes (increase in adverse reactions or alterations in pain relief), dose readjustment may be necessary.

Sublingual spray (Subsys): **Note:** Do **not** convert patients from any other fentanyl product to Subsys on a mcg-per-mcg basis. Patients previously using another fentanyl product should be initiated at a dose of 100 mcg; individually titrate to provide adequate analgesia while minimizing adverse effects. For patients previously using the transmucosal lozenge (Actiq), the initial dose should be selected using the conversions listed; see *Conversion from lozenge (Actiq) to sublingual spray (Subsys)*.

Initial dose: 100 mcg for all patients unless patient already using Actiq; see *Conversion from lozenge (Actiq) to sublingual spray (Subsys)*. If pain is unrelieved, 1 additional 100 mcg dose may be given 30 minutes after administration of the first dose. A maximum of 2 doses can be given per breakthrough pain episode. **Must wait at least 4 hours before treating another episode with sublingual spray.**

Dose titration: If titration required, titrate to a dose that provides adequate analgesia (with tolerable side effects) using the following titration steps: If no relief with 100 mcg dose, increase to 200 mcg dose (using one 200 mcg unit); if no relief with 200 mcg dose, increase to 400 mcg dose (using one 400 mcg unit); if no relief with 400 mcg dose, increase to 600 mcg dose (using one 600 mcg unit); if no relief with 600 mcg dose, increase to 800 mcg dose (using one 800 mcg unit); if no relief with 800 mcg dose, increase to 1200 mcg dose (using two 600 mcg units); if no relief with 1200 mcg dose, increase to 1600 mcg dose (using two 800 mcg units). During dose titration, if breakthrough pain unrelieved 30 minutes after Subsys administration, 1 additional dose using the same strength may be administered (maximum: 2 doses per breakthrough pain episode); **patient must wait 4 hours before treating another breakthrough pain episode with sublingual spray.**

Maintenance dose: Once maintenance dose for breakthrough pain episode has been determined, use that dose for subsequent episodes. If occasional episodes of unrelieved breakthrough pain occur following 30 minutes of Subsys administration, 1 additional dose using the same strength may be administered (maximum: 2 doses per breakthrough pain episode); **patient must wait 4 hours before treating another breakthrough pain episode with Subsys**. Once maintenance dose is determined, limit Subsys use to ≤4 episodes of breakthrough pain per day. If response to maintenance dose changes (increase in adverse reactions or alterations in pain relief), dose readjustment may be necessary. If patient is experiencing >4 breakthrough pain episodes per day, consider increasing the around-the-clock, long-acting opioid therapy.

Conversion from lozenge (Actiq) to sublingual spray (Subsys):

Lozenge dose 200 to 400 mcg: Initial sublingual spray dose is 100 mcg; may titrate using multiples of 100 mcg

Lozenge dose 600 to 800 mcg: Initial sublingual spray dose is 200 mcg; may titrate using multiples of 200 mcg

Lozenge dose 1,200 to 1,600 mcg: Initial sublingual spray dose is 400 mcg; may titrate using multiples of 400 mcg

Sublingual tablet (Abstral): **Note:** Do **not** convert patients from any other fentanyl product to Abstral on a mcg-per-mcg basis. Patients previously using another fentanyl product should be initiated at a dose of 100 mcg; individually titrate to provide adequate analgesia while minimizing adverse effects.

Initial dose:

U.S. labeling: 100 mcg for all patients; if pain is unrelieved, a second 100 mcg dose may be given 30 minutes after administration of the first dose. A maximum of 2 doses can be given per breakthrough pain episode. **Must wait at least 2 hours before treating another episode with sublingual tablet.**

Canadian labeling: 100 mcg for all patients; if pain is unrelieved 30 minutes after administration of Abstral, an alternative rescue medication (other than Abstral) may be given. Administer only 1 dose of Abstral per breakthrough pain episode. **Must wait at least 2 hours before treating another episode with sublingual tablet.**

Dose titration: If titration required, increase in 100 mcg increments (up to 400 mcg) over consecutive breakthrough episodes. If titration requires >400 mcg per dose, increase in increments of 200 mcg, starting with 600 mcg dose and titrating up to 800 mcg. During titration, patients may use multiples of 100 mcg and/or 200 mcg tablets for any single dose; do not exceed 4 tablets at one time; safety and efficacy of doses >800 mcg have not been evaluated. During dose titration, if breakthrough pain unrelieved 30 minutes after sublingual tablet administration, the U.S. labeling suggests that 1 additional dose using the same strength may be administered (maximum: 2 doses per breakthrough pain episode); the Canadian labeling recommends use of an alternative rescue medication and limits use of Abstral to 1 dose per breakthrough pain episode. **Patient must wait 2 hours before treating another breakthrough pain episode with sublingual tablet.**

Maintenance dose: Once maintenance dose for breakthrough pain episode has been determined, use only 1 tablet in the appropriate strength per episode; if pain is unrelieved with maintenance dose:

U.S. labeling: A second dose may be given after 30 minutes; maximum of 2 doses/episode of breakthrough pain; separate treatment of subsequent episodes by ≥2 hours; limit treatment to ≤4 breakthrough episodes per day.

Canadian labeling: Administer alternative rescue medication after 30 minutes; maximum of 1 Abstral dose/episode of breakthrough pain; separate treatment of subsequent episodes by ≥2 hours; limit treatment to ≤4 breakthrough episodes per day.

Consider increasing the around-the-clock long-acting opioid therapy in patients experiencing >4 breakthrough pain episodes per day; if long-acting opioid therapy dose altered, re-evaluate and retitrate Abstral dose as needed.

Conversion from lozenge (Actiq) to sublingual tablet (Abstral):

Lozenge dose 200 mcg: Initial sublingual tablet dose is 100 mcg; may titrate using multiples of 100 mcg

Lozenge dose 400 mcg: Initial sublingual tablet dose is 200 mcg; may titrate using multiples of 100 mcg

Lozenge dose 600 to 1,200 mcg: Initial sublingual tablet dose is 200 mcg; may titrate using multiples of 200 mcg

Lozenge dose 1,600 mcg: Initial sublingual tablet dose is 400 mcg; may titrate using multiples of 400 mcg

Elderly >65 years: Transmucosal lozenge (eg, Actiq): In clinical trials, patients who were >65 years of age were titrated to a mean dose that was 200 mcg less than that of younger patients.

Chronic pain management (opioid-tolerant patients only): Children ≥2 years, Adolescents, and Adults (U.S. labeling) or Adults (Canadian labeling): Transdermal patch: Discontinue or taper all other around-the-clock or extended release opioids when initiating therapy with fentanyl transdermal patch.

Initial: To convert patients from oral or parenteral opioids to transdermal patch, a 24-hour analgesic requirement should be calculated (based on prior opioid use). Using the tables, the appropriate initial dose can be determined. The initial fentanyl dosage may be approximated from the 24-hour morphine dosage equivalent and titrated to minimize adverse effects and provide analgesia. Substantial interpatient variability exists in relative potency. Therefore, it is safer to underestimate a patient's daily fentanyl requirement and provide breakthrough pain relief with rescue medication (eg, immediate release opioid) than to overestimate requirements. With the initial application, the absorption of transdermal fentanyl requires several hours to reach plateau; therefore transdermal fentanyl is inappropriate for management of acute pain. Change patch every 72 hours.

Conversion from continuous infusion of fentanyl: In patients who have adequate pain relief with a fentanyl infusion, fentanyl may be converted to transdermal dosing at a rate equivalent to the intravenous rate. A two-step taper of the infusion to be completed over 12 hours has been recommended (Kornick, 2001) after the patch is applied. The infusion is decreased to 50% of the original rate six hours after the application of the first patch, and subsequently discontinued twelve hours after application.

Titration: Short-acting agents may be required until analgesic efficacy is established and/or as supplements for "breakthrough" pain. The amount of supplemental doses should be closely monitored. Appropriate dosage increases may be based on daily supplemental dosage using the ratio of 45 mg/24 hours of oral morphine to a 12.5 mcg/hour increase in fentanyl dosage (U.S. labeling) or using the ratio of 45 to 59 mg/24 hours of oral morphine to a 12 mcg/hour increase in fentanyl dosage (Canadian labeling).

Frequency of adjustment: The dosage should not be titrated more frequently than every 3 days after the initial dose or every 6 days thereafter. Titrate dose based on the daily dose of supplemental opioids required by the patient on the second or third day of the initial application. **Note:** Upon discontinuation, ~17 hours are required for a 50% decrease in fentanyl levels.

Frequency of application: The majority of patients may be controlled on every 72-hour administration; however, a small number of adult patients require every 48-hour administration.

Discontinuation: When discontinuing transdermal fentanyl and not converting to another opioid, use a gradual downward titration, such as decreasing the dose by 50% every 6 days, to reduce the possibility of withdrawal symptoms.

Dose conversion guidelines for transdermal fentanyl (see tables below and on next page).

Note: U.S. and Canadian dose conversion guidelines differ; consult appropriate table. The conversion factors in these tables are only to be used for the conversion from current opioid therapy to Duragesic. Conversion factors in this table cannot be used to convert from Duragesic to another opioid (doing so may lead to fatal overdose due to overestimation of the new opioid). This is not a table of equianalgesic doses.

U.S. Labeling: Dose Conversion Guidelines (Children ≥2 years, Adolescents, and Adults): Recommended Initial Duragesic Dose Based Upon Daily Oral Morphine Dose[1,2]

Oral 24-Hour Morphine (mg/day)	Duragesic Dose[3] (mcg/h)
60 to 134	25
135 to 224	50
225 to 314	75
315 to 404	100
405 to 494	125
495 to 584	150
585 to 674	175
675 to 764	200
765 to 854	225
855 to 944	250
945 to 1034	275
1035 to 1124	300

[1]The table should NOT be used to convert from transdermal fentanyl (Duragesic) to other opioid analgesics. Rather, following removal of the patch, titrate the dose of the new opioid until adequate analgesia is achieved.

[2]Recommendations are based on U.S. product labeling for Duragesic.

[3]Pediatric patients initiating therapy on a 25 mcg/hour Duragesic system should be opioid-tolerant and receiving at least 60 mg oral morphine equivalents per day.

U.S. Labeling: Dose Conversion Guidelines (Children ≥2 years, Adolescents, and Adults)[1,2]

Current Analgesic	Daily Dosage (mg/day)			
Morphine (IM/IV)	10 to 22	23 to 37	38 to 52	53 to 67
Oxycodone (oral)	30 to 67	67.5 to 112	112.5 to 157	157.5 to 202
Codeine (oral)	150 to 447	-	-	-
Hydromorphone (oral)	8 to 17	17.1 to 28	28.1 to 39	39.1 to 51
Hydromorphone (IV)	1.5 to 3.4	3.5 to 5.6	5.7 to 7.9	8 to 10
Meperidine (IM)	75 to 165	166 to 278	279 to 390	391 to 503
Methadone (oral)	20 to 44	45 to 74	75 to 104	105 to 134
Fentanyl transdermal recommended dose (mcg/h)	**25 mcg/h**	**50 mcg/h**	**75 mcg/h**	**100 mcg/h**

[1]The table should NOT be used to convert from transdermal fentanyl (Duragesic) to other opioid analgesics. Rather, following removal of the patch, titrate the dose of the new opioid until adequate analgesia is achieved.

[2]Recommendations are based on U.S. product labeling for Duragesic.

Transdermal patch (Duragesic MAT [Canadian product]):

Adults:

Canadian Labeling: Dose Conversion Guidelines (Adults): Recommended Initial Duragesic MAT Dose Based Upon Daily Oral Morphine Dose[1,2]

Oral 24-Hour Morphine (Current Dose in mg/day)	Duragesic MAT Dose (Initial Dose in mcg/h)
45 to 59	12
60 to 134	25
135 to 179	37
180 to 224	50
225 to 269	62
270 to 314	75
315 to 359	87
360 to 404	100
405 to 494	125
495 to 584	150
585 to 674	175
675 to 764	200
765 to 854	225
855 to 944	250
945 to 1034	275
1035 to 1124	300

[1]The table should NOT be used to convert from transdermal fentanyl (Duragesic MAT) to other opioid analgesics. Rather, following removal of the patch, titrate the dose of the new opioid until adequate analgesia is achieved.

[2]Recommendations are based on Canadian product labeling for Duragesic MAT.

Note: The 12 mcg/hour dose included in this table is to be used for incremental dose adjustment and is generally not recommended for initial dosing, except for patients in whom lower starting doses are deemed clinically appropriate.

Canadian Labeling: Dose Conversion Guidelines (Adults)[1,2]

Current Analgesic	Daily Dosage (mg/day)						
Morphine[3] (IM/IV)	20 to 44	45 to 60	61 to 75	76 to 90	n/a[4]	n/a[4]	n/a[4]
Oxycodone (oral)	30 to 66	67 to 90	91 to 112	113 to 134	135 to 157	158 to 179	180 to 202
Codeine (oral)	150 to 447	448 to 597	598 to 747	748 to 897	898 to 1047	1048 to 1197	1198 to 1347
Hydromorphone (oral)	8 to 16	17 to 22	23 to 28	29 to 33	34 to 39	40 to 45	46 to 51
Hydromorphone (IV)	4 to 8.4	8.5 to 11.4	11.5 to 14.4	14.5 to 16.5	16.6 to 19.5	19.6 to 22.5	22.6 to 25.5
Fentanyl transdermal recommended dose (mcg/h)	**25 mcg/h**	**37 mcg/h**	**50 mcg/h**	**62 mcg/h**	**75 mcg/h**	**87 mcg/h**	**100 mcg/h**

[1]The table should NOT be used to convert from transdermal fentanyl (Duragesic MAT) to other opioid analgesics. Rather, following removal of the patch, titrate the dose of the new opioid until adequate analgesia is achieved.

[2]Recommendations are based on Canadian product labeling for Duragesic MAT.

[3]Morphine dose conversion based upon I.M to oral dose ratio of 1:3.

[4]Insufficient data available to provide specific dosing recommendations. Use caution; adjust dose conservatively.

Dosage adjustment in renal impairment:

Injection: There are no dosage adjustments provided in the manufacturer's labeling; use with caution.

Transdermal (patch): Degree of impairment (ie, CrCl) not defined in manufacturer's labeling.

U.S. labeling:

Mild-to-moderate impairment: Initial: Reduce dose by 50%.

Severe impairment: Use not recommended.

Canadian labeling: There are no specific dosage adjustments provided in the manufacturer's labeling; monitor closely for toxicity and reduce dose if necessary.

Transmucosal (buccal film/tablet, sublingual spray/tablet, lozenge) and nasal spray: There are no dosage adjustments provided in the manufacturer's labeling. Although fentanyl pharmacokinetics may be altered in renal disease, fentanyl can be used successfully in the management of breakthrough cancer pain. Doses should be titrated to reach clinical effect with careful monitoring of patients with severe renal disease.

Dosage adjustment in hepatic impairment:

Injection: There are no dosage adjustments provided in the manufacturer's labeling; use with caution.

Transdermal (patch):

U.S. labeling:

Mild-to-moderate impairment: Initial: Reduce dose by 50%.

Severe impairment: Use not recommended.

Canadian labeling: There are no specific dosage adjustments provided in the manufacturer's labeling; monitor closely for toxicity and reduce dose if necessary.

Transmucosal (buccal film/tablet, sublingual spray/tablet, lozenge) and nasal spray: There are no dosage adjustments provided in the manufacturer's labeling. Although fentanyl pharmacokinetics may be altered in hepatic disease, fentanyl can be used successfully in the management of breakthrough cancer pain. Doses should be titrated to reach clinical effect with careful monitoring of patients with severe hepatic disease.

Dietary Considerations Transmucosal lozenge contains 2 g sugar per unit.

Usual Infusion Concentrations: Pediatric IV infusion: 10 **mcg**/mL

Usual Infusion Concentrations: Adult IV infusion: 10 **mcg**/mL

Administration

Epidural (Canadian labeling; not in U.S. labeling): For postoperative pain management may administer as bolus dose (diluted in preservative free NS to a final concentration of 10 mcg/mL) or by continuous infusion at a rate of 1 mcg/kg/hour. Use within 24 hours.

IV: Administer as slow IV infusion over 1 to 2 minutes. May also be administered as continuous infusion or PCA (off-label use) routes. Muscular rigidity may occur with rapid IV administration.

Transdermal patch (eg, Duragesic): Apply to nonirritated and nonirradiated skin, such as chest, back, flank, or upper arm. Do not shave skin; hair at application site should be clipped. Prior to application, clean site with clear water and allow to dry completely. Do not use damaged, cut or leaking patches; patch may be less effective. Skin exposure from fentanyl gel leaking from patch may lead to serious adverse effects; thoroughly wash affected skin surfaces with water (do not use soap). Firmly press in place and hold for 30 seconds. Change patch every 72 hours. Do **not** use soap, alcohol, or other solvents to remove transdermal gel if it accidentally touches skin; use copious amounts of water. Avoid exposing application site to external heat sources (eg, heating pad, electric blanket, heat lamp, hot tub). If there is difficulty with patch adhesion, the edges of the system may be taped in place with first-aid tape. If there is continued difficulty with adhesion, an adhesive film dressing (eg, Bioclusive, Tegaderm) may be applied over the system.

Lozenge: Foil overwrap should be removed just prior to administration. Place the unit in mouth between the cheek and gum and allow it to dissolve. Do not chew. Lozenge may be moved from one side of the mouth to the other. The unit should be consumed over a period of 15 minutes. Handle should be removed after the lozenge is consumed; early removal should be considered if the patient has achieved an adequate response and/or shows signs of respiratory depression.

Buccal film: Foil overwrap should be removed just prior to administration. Prior to placing film, wet inside of cheek using tongue or by rinsing with water. Place film inside mouth with the pink side of the unit against the inside of the moistened cheek. With finger, press the film against cheek and hold for 5 seconds. The film should stick to the inside of cheek after 5 seconds. The film should be left in place until it dissolves (usually within 15-30 minutes after application). Liquids may be consumed after 5 minutes of application. Food can be eaten after film dissolves. If using more than 1 film simultaneously (during titration period), apply films on either side of mouth (do not apply on top of each other). Do not chew or swallow film. Do not cut or tear the film. All patients must initiate therapy using the 200 mcg film.

Buccal tablet: Patient should not open blister until ready to administer. The blister backing should be peeled back to expose the tablet; tablet should not be pushed out through the blister. Immediately use tablet once removed from blister. Place entire tablet in the buccal cavity (above a rear molar, between the upper cheek and gum) or under the tongue (U.S. labeling recommends for maintenance dosing only; Canadian labeling does not restrict sublingual use to maintenance dosing only); should dissolve in about 14 to 25 minutes. If remnants remain after 30 minutes, they may be swallowed with water. Tablet should not be split, crushed, sucked, chewed, or swallowed whole. When possible, alternate sides of mouth with each dose.

Nasal spray: Prior to initial use, prime device by spraying 4 sprays into the provided pouch (the counting window will show a green bar when the bottle is ready for use). Insert nozzle a short distance into the nose (~1/2 inch or 1 cm) and point towards the bridge of the nose (while closing off the other nostril using 1 finger). Press on finger grips until a "click" sound is heard and the number in the counting window advances by one. The "click" sound and dose counter are the only reliable methods for ensuring a dose has been administered (spray is not always felt on the nasal mucosa). Patient should remain seated for at least 1 minute following administration. Do not blow nose for ≥30 minutes after administration. Wash hands before and after use. If not used within 5 days, re-prime by spraying once. There are 8 full therapeutic sprays in each bottle; do not continue to use bottle after "8" sprays have been used. Dispose of bottle and contents if it has been ≥60 days since first use. Spray the remaining contents into the provided pouch, seal in the child-resistant container, and dispose of in the trash.

Sublingual spray: Open sealed blister unit with scissors immediately prior to administration. Contents of unit should be sprayed into mouth under the tongue.

Sublingual tablet: Remove from the blister unit immediately prior to administration. Place tablet directly under the tongue on the floor of the mouth and allow to completely dissolve; do not chew, suck, or swallow. Do not eat or drink anything until tablet is completely dissolved. In patients with a dry mouth, water may be used to moisten the buccal mucosa just before administration. All patients must initiate therapy using the 100 mcg tablet.

Monitoring Parameters

Respiratory and cardiovascular status, blood pressure, heart rate; signs of misuse, abuse, or addiction; signs or symptoms of hypogonadism or hypoadrenalism (Brennan, 2013)

Transdermal patch: Monitor for 24 hours after application of first dose

Additional Information Fentanyl is 50 to 100 times as potent as morphine; morphine 10 mg IM is equivalent to fentanyl 0.1 to 0.2 mg IM; fentanyl has less hypotensive effects than morphine due to lack of histamine release. However, fentanyl may cause rigidity with high doses. If the patient has required high-dose analgesia or has used for a prolonged period (~7 days), taper dose to prevent withdrawal; monitor for signs and symptoms of withdrawal.

Transmucosal (nasal spray, Lazanda): Disposal of nasal spray: Before disposal, all unopened or partially used bottles must be completely emptied by spraying the contents into the provided pouch. After "8" therapeutic sprays has been reached on the counter, patients should continue to spray an additional four sprays into the pouch to ensure that any residual fentanyl has been expelled (an audible click will no longer be heard and the counter will not advance beyond "8"). The empty bottle and the sealed pouch must be put into the child-resistant container before placing in the trash. Wash hands with soap and water immediately after handling the pouch. If the pouch is lost, another one can be ordered by the patient or caregiver by calling 1-866-458-6389.

Transmucosal (oral lozenge, Actiq): Disposal of lozenge units: After consumption of a complete unit, the handle may be disposed of in a trash container that is out of the reach of children. For a partially consumed unit, or a unit that still has any drug matrix remaining on the handle, the handle should be placed under hot running tap water until the drug matrix has dissolved. Special child-resistant containers are available to temporarily store partially consumed units that cannot be disposed of immediately.

Transmucosal (buccal film, Onsolis): Disposal of film: Remove foil overwrap from any unused, unneeded films and dispose by flushing in the toilet.

Transmucosal (sublingual spray, Subsys): Disposal of spray: Dispose of each unit dose immediately after use; place used unit into one of the provided white disposal bags. After sealing appropriately, discard in the trash. Dispose of any unused units as soon as no longer needed. Prior to disposal, empty all the medicine into the provided charcoal-lined disposal pouch. The disposal pouch should then be placed into the white disposal bag, sealed appropriately, and discarded in the trash.

Transmucosal (sublingual tablet, Abstral): Disposal of tablets: Remove any unused tablets from the blister cards and dispose by flushing in the toilet.

Transdermal patch (Duragesic): Upon removal of the patch, ~17 hours are required before serum concentrations fall to 50% of their original values. Opioid withdrawal symptoms are possible. Gradual downward titration (potentially by the sequential use of lower-dose patches) is recommended. Keep transdermal patch (both used and unused) out of the reach of children. Do **not** use soap, alcohol, or other solvents to remove transdermal gel if it accidentally touches skin as they may increase transdermal absorption, use copious amounts of water. Avoid exposure of direct external heat sources (eg, heating pads, electric blankets, heat lamps, saunas, hot tubs, heated water beds) to application site.

Dosage Forms

Film, for buccal application:

Onsolis: 200 mcg (30s); 400 mcg (30s); 600 mcg (30s); 800 mcg (30s); 1200 mcg (30s)

Injection, solution [preservative free]: 0.05 mg/mL (2 mL, 5 mL, 10 mL, 20 mL, 30 mL, 50 mL)

Liquid, sublingual, [spray]:

Subsys: 100 mcg (30s); 200 mcg (30s); 400 mcg (30s); 600 mcg (30s); 800 mcg (30s)

Lozenge, oral: 200 mcg (30s); 400 mcg (30s); 600 mcg (30s); 800 mcg (30s); 1200 mcg (30s); 1600 mcg (30s)

Actiq: 200 mcg (30s); 400 mcg (30s); 600 mcg (30s); 800 mcg (30s); 1200 mcg (30s); 1600 mcg (30s)

Patch, transdermal: 12 [delivers 12.5 mcg/hr] (5s); 25 [delivers 25 mcg/hr] (5s); 50 [delivers 50 mcg/hr] (5s); 75 [delivers 75 mcg/hr] (5s); 100 [delivers 100 mcg/hr] (5s)

Duragesic: 12 [delivers 12.5 mcg/hr] (5s); 25 [delivers 25 mcg/hr] (5s); 50 [delivers 50 mcg/hr] (5s); 75 [delivers 75 mcg/hr] (5s); 100 [delivers 100 mcg/hr] (5s)

Powder, for prescription compounding: USP: 100% (1 g)

Solution, intranasal, as citrate [spray]:

Lazanda: 100 mcg/spray (5 mL); 400 mcg/spray (5 mL) [delivers 8 metered sprays]

Tablet, for buccal application:

Fentora: 100 mcg (28s); 200 mcg (28s); 400 mcg (28s); 600 mcg (28s); 800 mcg (28s)

Tablet, sublingual:

Abstral: 100 mcg (12s, 32s); 200 mcg (12s, 32s); 300 mcg (12s, 32s); 400 mcg (12s, 32s); 600 mcg (32s); 800 mcg (32s)

Dosage Forms: Canada

Patch, transdermal, as base: 12 mcg/hr (5s); 25 mcg/hr (5s); 50 mcg/hr (5s); 75 mcg/hr (5s); 100 mcg/hr (5s)

Duragesic MAT: 12 mcg/hr (5s); 25 mcg/hr (5s); 50 mcg/hr (5s); 75 mcg/hr (5s); 100 mcg/hr (5s)

◆ **Fentanyl Citrate** *see* FentaNYL *on page 857*

◆ **Fentanyl Citrate Injection, USP (Can)** *see* FentaNYL *on page 857*

◆ **Fentanyl Hydrochloride** *see* FentaNYL *on page 857*

◆ **Fentanyl Patch** *see* FentaNYL *on page 857*

Fenticonazole [INT] (fen ti KOE na zole)

International Brand Names Derma-Lomexin (SA); Falvin (IT); Fenizolan (DE); Fentiderm (IT); Fentigyn (IT); Fentizol (BR); Fenzol (PK); Gyno-Lomexin (SA); Gynoxin (BE, GB, HU, NL, PL); Laurimic (ES); Lomexin (AE, AR, AT, BG, BH, BR, CO, CY, CZ, DE, ES, FR, GR, IT, KR, KW, LB, LT, MX, PK, PT, QA, RO, RU, SG, SK, TR, TW, ZA); Lomexin T (AE, BH, KW, LB); Micofulvin (ES); Mycodermil (CH); Mycofentin (VE); Terlomexin (FR)

Index Terms Fenticonazole Nitrate

Pharmacologic Category Antifungal Agent

Reported Use Treatment of fungal infections including dermatomycoses, pityriasis versicolor, or vaginal candidiasis

Dosage Range Adults:

Cream, gel, spray: Skin infections: Apply to skin daily

Vaginal ovule: Vaginal candidiasis (thrush): Insert 1-600 mg ovule intravaginally at bedtime for 1 day or 200 mg ovule intravaginally at bedtime for 3 days

Product Availability Product available in various countries; not currently available in the U.S.

Dosage Forms

Cream 2%: 30 g

Gel: 30 g

Spray: 30 mL

Vaginal ovule: 200 mg, 600 mg

◆ **Fenticonazole Nitrate** *see* Fenticonazole [INT] *on page 868*

◆ **Fentora** *see* FentaNYL *on page 857*

◆ **Feosol Original** *see* Ferrous Sulfate *on page 871*

◆ **Feraheme** *see* Ferumoxytol *on page 871*

◆ **Ferate [OTC]** *see* Ferrous Gluconate *on page 870*

◆ **Fergon [OTC]** *see* Ferrous Gluconate *on page 870*

◆ **Ferinject** *see* Ferric Carboxymaltose *on page 868*

◆ **Fer-In-Sol [OTC]** *see* Ferrous Sulfate *on page 871*

◆ **Fer-In-Sol® (Can)** *see* Ferrous Sulfate *on page 871*

◆ **Fer-Iron [OTC]** *see* Ferrous Sulfate *on page 871*

◆ **Ferodan™ (Can)** *see* Ferrous Sulfate *on page 871*

◆ **FeroSul [OTC]** *see* Ferrous Sulfate *on page 871*

◆ **Ferretts [OTC]** *see* Ferrous Fumarate *on page 870*

◆ **Ferrex 150 [OTC]** *see* Polysaccharide-Iron Complex *on page 1677*

◆ **Ferric (III) Hexacyanoferrate (II)** *see* Ferric Hexacyanoferrate *on page 870*

Ferric Carboxymaltose

(FER ik kar box ee MAWL tose)

Brand Names: U.S. Injectafer

Index Terms Ferinject; Iron Carboxymaltose; Iron Dextri-Maltose; VIT 45

Pharmacologic Category Iron Salt

Use Iron-deficiency anemia (IDA): Treatment of IDA in adults with intolerance to oral iron or unsatisfactory response to oral iron; treatment of IDA in adults with nondialysis-dependent chronic kidney disease (ND-CKD)

Pregnancy Risk Factor C

Pregnancy Considerations Adverse events were observed in some animal reproduction studies.

Breast-Feeding Considerations Ferric carboxymaltose is excreted into breast milk. Iron concentrations are higher than those following oral ferrous sulfate administration.

Contraindications Hypersensitivity to ferric carboxymaltose or any component of the formulation

Warnings/Precautions Serious hypersensitivity reactions, including anaphylactic-type reactions (some life-threatening and fatal) have been reported. Monitor during and for ≥30 minutes after administration and until clinically stable. Signs/symptoms of serious hypersensitivity reaction include shock, hypotension, loss of consciousness, and/or collapse. Equipment for resuscitation, medication, and trained personnel experienced in handling emergencies should be immediately available during infusion. Transient elevations in systolic blood pressure, (sometimes with facial flushing, dizziness, or nausea) were observed in studies; generally occurred immediately after dosing and resolved within 30 minutes. Monitor blood pressure following infusion. Lab assays may overestimate serum iron and transferrin bound irons for ~24 hours after infusion.

Adverse Reactions

Cardiovascular: Flushing, hypertension, hypotension, increased blood pressure (transient, systolic)

Central nervous system: Dizziness, headache

Dermatologic: Skin discoloration at injection site

Endocrine & metabolic: Decreased serum phosphate (<2 mg/dL [0.65 mmol/L]; transient)

Gastrointestinal: Constipation, dysgeusia, nausea, vomiting

Hepatic: Increased serum ALT

Rare but important or life-threatening): Anaphylaxis, angioedema, hypersensitivity, syncope, tachycardia

Drug Interactions

Metabolism/Transport Effects None known.

Avoid Concomitant Use

Avoid concomitant use of Ferric Carboxymaltose with any of the following: Dimercaprol

Increased Effect/Toxicity
The levels/effects of Ferric Carboxymaltose may be increased by: Dimercaprol

Decreased Effect There are no known significant interactions involving a decrease in effect.

Preparation for Administration May administer undiluted (for IV push) or diluted (for infusion). When administering as an IV infusion, dilute up to 750 mg in a maximum of 250 mL of 0.9% sodium chloride injection to a concentration of 2-4 mg/mL; concentration should be ≥2 mg/mL. Discard unused portion of vial (single-use).

Storage/Stability Store intact vials at 20°C to 25°C (68°F to 77°F); excursions permitted between 15°C to 30°C (59°F to 86°F); do not freeze. Solutions diluted in 0.9% sodium chloride at concentrations of 2-4 mg/mL are stable for 72 hours at room temperature.

Mechanism of Action Ferric carboxymaltose is a colloidal iron (III) hydroxide in complex with carboxymaltose, a carbohydrate polymer that releases iron necessary to the function of hemoglobin, myoglobin, and specific enzyme systems; allows transport of oxygen via hemoglobin. Ferric carboxymaltose is a non-dextran formulation that allows for iron uptake (into reticuloendothelial system) without the release of free iron (Szczech, 2010).

Pharmacodynamics/Kinetics

Onset of action: Maximum iron levels (37-333 mcg/mL): 0.25-1.2 hours

Distribution: V_d: ~3 L

Half-life elimination: 7-12 hours

Excretion: Urine (negligible)

Dosage Note: Dose expressed as elemental iron.

Iron-deficiency anemia (IDA): Adults: IV:

<50 kg: 15 mg/kg on day 1; repeat dose after at least 7 days (maximum: 1500 mg per course). May repeat course if anemia reoccurs.

≥50 kg: 750 mg on day 1; repeat dose after at least 7 days (maximum: 1500 mg per course). May repeat course if anemia reoccurs.

Dosage adjustment in renal impairment: Chronic kidney disease (CKD), nondialysis dependent: No dosage adjustment necessary (indicated for use in nondialysis CKD)

Dosage adjustment in hepatic impairment: No dosage adjustment provided in manufacturer's labeling.

Administration

Administer as slow IV push (undiluted) at a rate of ~100 mg/minute or by IV infusion (diluted to ≥ 2 mg/mL) over at least 15 minutes.

Avoid extravasation (may cause persistent discoloration). Monitor; if extravasation occurs, discontinue administration at that site.

Monitoring Parameters Hemoglobin and hematocrit, serum ferritin, iron saturation; vital signs (including blood pressure); signs and symptoms of hypersensitivity (monitor for ≥30 minutes following the end of administration and until clinically stable); monitor infusion site for extravasation.

NKF KDOQI guidelines (2006) recommend monitoring iron status every 1-3 months, with more frequent monitoring after course of IV iron therapy.

Reference Range CKD patients should have sufficient iron to achieve and maintain hemoglobin of 11-12 g/dL; to achieve and maintain this target Hgb for patients with nondialysis dependent CKD, sufficient iron should be administered to maintain a transferrin saturation (TSAT) of 20%, and a serum ferritin level ≥100 ng/mL (NKF KDOQI, 2006)

Dosage Forms Considerations Each mL of Injectafer contains 50 mg of elemental iron

Dosage Forms

Solution, Intravenous:

Injectafer: 750 mg/15 mL (15 mL)

Ferric Citrate (FER ik SIT rate)

Brand Names: U.S. Auryxia

Index Terms Auryxia; Tetraferric Tricitrate Decahydrate

Pharmacologic Category Phosphate Binder

Use Hyperphosphatemia: For the control of serum phosphorus levels in patients with chronic kidney disease (CKD) receiving dialysis

Pregnancy Risk Factor B

Dosage Note: Each tablet contains 210 mg of ferric iron equivalent to 1 g ferric citrate.

Hyperphosphatemia: Adults: Oral:

Initial: 2 tablets (420 mg ferric iron) 3 times daily

Maintenance: Increase or decrease dose by 1 tablet or 2 tablets (420 mg to 840 mg ferric iron) as needed at 1 week or longer intervals to achieve target serum phosphorus levels (maximum dose: 12 tablets [2,520 mg ferric iron] daily).

Dosage adjustment in renal impairment: There are no dosage adjustments provided in the manufacturer's labeling.

Dosage adjustment in hepatic impairment: There are no dosage adjustments provided in the manufacturer's labeling.

Additional Information Complete prescribing information should be consulted for additional detail.

Product Availability Auryxia: FDA approved September 2014; anticipated availability is late 2014

Dosage Forms

Tablet, Oral:

Auryxia: Ferric iron 210 mg (ferric citrate 1 g)

◆ **Ferric Ferrocyanide** *see* Ferric Hexacyanoferrate *on page 870*

Ferric Gluconate (FER ik GLOO koe nate)

Brand Names: U.S. Ferrlecit

Brand Names: Canada Ferrlecit

Index Terms Sodium Ferric Gluconate; Sodium Ferric Gluconate Complex

Pharmacologic Category Iron Salt

Use Iron deficiency anemia: Treatment of iron-deficiency anemia in patients undergoing hemodialysis in conjunction with erythropoietin therapy

Pregnancy Risk Factor B

Dosage

Iron-deficiency anemia, hemodialysis patients:

Children ≥6 years: IV: 1.5 mg/kg of elemental iron (maximum: 125 mg/dose) per dialysis session. Doses >1.5 mg/kg are associated with increased adverse events.

Adults: IV: 125 mg elemental iron per dialysis session. Most patients will require a cumulative dose of 1 g elemental iron over approximately 8 sequential dialysis treatments to achieve a favorable response.

Note: A test dose of 2 mL diluted in NS 50 mL administered over 60 minutes was previously recommended (not in current manufacturer labeling). Doses >125 mg are associated with increased adverse events.

Chemotherapy-associated anemia (off-label use): Adults: IV infusion: 125 mg once every week for 6 doses (Pedrazzoli, 2008) or for 8 doses (Henry, 2007).

Dosage adjustment in renal impairment: No dosage adjustment necessary. The ferric gluconate iron complex is not dialyzable.

Dosage adjustment in hepatic impairment: No dosage adjustment necessary.

Additional Information Complete prescribing information should be consulted for additional detail.

Dosage Forms Considerations Strength of ferric gluconate injection is expressed as elemental iron.

Dosage Forms

Solution, Intravenous:

Ferrlecit: 12.5 mg/mL (5 mL)

Generic: 12.5 mg/mL (5 mL)

Ferric Hexacyanoferrate

(FER ik hex a SYE an oh fer ate)

Brand Names: U.S. Radiogardase

Index Terms Ferric (III) Hexacyanoferrate (II); Ferric Ferrocyanide; Insoluble Prussian Blue; Prussian Blue

Pharmacologic Category Antidote

Use Internal contamination: Treatment of patients with known or suspected internal contamination with radioactive cesium and/or radioactive or nonradioactive thallium to increase their rates of elimination.

Pregnancy Risk Factor C

Dosage Internal contamination with radioactive cesium and/or radioactive or nonradioactive thallium: **Note:** Treatment should begin as soon as possible following exposure, but is also effective if therapy is delayed. Treatment typically continues for ≥30 days.

Children 2 to 12 years: Oral: 1 g 3 times daily

Adolescents and Adults: Oral:

Manufacturer recommendations: 3 g 3 times daily

Alternative recommendations: Cesium exposure: 1 to 3 g 3 times daily (REMM, 2014)

Elderly: Refer to adult dosing

Dosage adjustment in renal impairment: There are no dosage adjustments provided in the manufacturer's labeling; however, ferric hexacyanoferrate is not renally eliminated.

Dosage adjustment in hepatic impairment: There are no dosage adjustments provided in the manufacturer's labeling; however, effectiveness may be decreased due to decreased biliary excretion of cesium and thallium.

Additional Information Complete prescribing information should be consulted for additional detail.

Dosage Forms

Capsule, Oral:

Radiogardase: 0.5 g

◆ **Ferric x-150 [OTC]** *see* Polysaccharide-Iron Complex *on page* 1677

◆ **Ferrimin 150 [OTC]** *see* Ferrous Fumarate *on page* 870

◆ **Ferriprox®** *see* Deferiprone *on page* 585

◆ **Ferriprox** *see* Deferiprone *on page* 585

◆ **Ferrlecit** *see* Ferric Gluconate *on page* 869

◆ **Ferro-Bob [OTC]** *see* Ferrous Sulfate *on page* 871

◆ **Ferrocite [OTC]** *see* Ferrous Fumarate *on page* 870

Ferrous Fumarate (FER us FYOO ma rate)

Brand Names: U.S. Ferretts [OTC]; Ferrimin 150 [OTC]; Ferrocite [OTC]; Hemocyte [OTC]

Brand Names: Canada Palafer®

Index Terms Iron Fumarate

Pharmacologic Category Iron Salt

Use Prevention and treatment of iron-deficiency anemias

Dosage

Dietary Reference Intake: Dose is RDA presented as elemental iron unless otherwise noted:

0-6 months: 0.27 mg/day (adequate intake)

7-12 months: 11 mg/day

1-3 years: 7 mg/day

4-8 years: 10 mg/day

9-13 years: 8 mg/day

14-18 years: Males: 11 mg/day; Females: 15 mg/day; Pregnant females: 27 mg/day; Lactating females: 10 mg/day

19-50 years: Males: 8 mg/day; Females: 18 mg/day; Pregnant females: 27 mg/day; Lactating females: 9 mg/day

≥50 years: 8 mg/day

Doses expressed in terms of elemental iron; elemental iron content of ferrous fumarate is 33%. Oral:

Children:

Severe iron-deficiency anemia: 4-6 mg elemental iron/kg/day in 3 divided doses

Mild-to-moderate iron-deficiency anemia: 3 mg elemental iron/kg/day in 1-2 divided doses

Prophylaxis: 1-2 mg elemental iron/kg/day

Adults:

Iron deficiency: Usual range: 150-200 mg elemental iron/day in divided doses; 60-100 mg elemental iron twice daily, up to 60 mg elemental iron 4 times/day

Prophylaxis: 60-100 mg elemental iron/day

To avoid GI upset, start with a single daily dose and increase by 1 tablet/day each week or as tolerated until desired daily dose is achieved

Elderly: Lower doses (15-50 mg elemental iron/day) may have similar efficacy and less GI adverse events (eg, nausea,constipation) as compared to higher doses (eg, 150 mg elemental iron/day) (Rimon, 2005).

Additional Information Complete prescribing information should be consulted for additional detail.

Dosage Forms

Tablet, Oral:

Ferretts [OTC]: 325 mg (106 mg elemental iron)

Ferrimin 150 [OTC]: Elemental iron 150 mg

Ferrocite [OTC]: 324 mg (106 mg elemental iron)

Hemocyte [OTC]: 324 mg (106 mg elemental iron)

Generic: 90 mg (29.5 mg elemental iron), 324 mg (106 mg elemental iron), Elemental iron 29 mg

Ferrous Gluconate (FER us GLOO koe nate)

Brand Names: U.S. Ferate [OTC]; Fergon [OTC]

Brand Names: Canada Apo-Ferrous Gluconate®; Novo-Ferrogluc

Index Terms Iron Gluconate

Pharmacologic Category Iron Salt

Use Prevention and treatment of iron-deficiency anemias

Dosage Oral:

Dietary Reference Intake: Dose is RDA presented as elemental iron unless otherwise noted:

0-6 months: 0.27 mg/day (adequate intake)

7-12 months: 11 mg/day

1-3 years: 7 mg/day

4-8 years: 10 mg/day

9-13 years: 8 mg/day

14-18 years: Males: 11 mg/day; Females: 15 mg/day; Pregnant females: 27 mg/day; Lactating females: 10 mg/day

19-50 years: Males: 8 mg/day; Females: 18 mg/day; Pregnant females: 27 mg/day; Lactating females: 9 mg/day

≥50 years: 8 mg/day

Dose expressed in terms of elemental iron:

Children:

Severe iron-deficiency anemia: 4-6 mg Fe/kg/day in 3 divided doses

Mild to moderate iron deficiency anemia: 3 mg Fe/kg/day in 1-2 divided doses

Prophylaxis: 1-2 mg Fe/kg/day

Adults:
Iron deficiency: 60 mg twice daily up to 60 mg 4 times/day
Prophylaxis: 60 mg/day
Elderly: Lower doses (15-50 mg elemental iron/day) may have similar efficacy and less GI adverse events (eg, nausea, constipation) as compared to higher doses (eg, 150 mg elemental iron/day) (Rimon, 2005).

Additional Information Complete prescribing information should be consulted for additional detail.

Dosage Forms

Tablet, Oral:
Fergon [OTC]: 240 (27 Fe) mg
Generic: 240 (27 Fe) mg, 324 (37.5 Fe) mg 324 (38 Fe) mg, 325 (36 Fe) mg

Tablet, Oral [preservative free]:
Ferate [OTC]: 240 (27 Fe) mg

Ferrous Sulfate (FER us SUL fate)

Brand Names: U.S. BProtected Pedia Iron [OTC]; Fer-In-Sol [OTC]; Fer-Iron [OTC]; FeroSul [OTC]; Ferro-Bob [OTC]; FerrouSul [OTC]; Iron Supplement Childrens [OTC]; Slow Fe [OTC]; Slow Iron [OTC]; Slow Release Iron [OTC] [DSC]

Brand Names: Canada Apo-Ferrous Sulfate®; Fer-In-Sol®; Ferodan™

Index Terms Feosol Original; $FeSO_4$; Iron Sulfate

Pharmacologic Category Iron Salt

Use Prevention and treatment of iron-deficiency anemias

Dosage Oral: **Note:** Multiple concentrations of ferrous sulfate oral liquid exist; close attention must be paid to the concentration when ordering and administering ferrous sulfate; incorrect selection or substitution of one ferrous sulfate liquid for another without proper dosage volume adjustment may result in serious over- or underdosing.

Dietary Reference Intake: Dose is RDA presented as elemental iron unless otherwise noted:
0-6 months: 0.27 mg/day (adequate intake)
7-12 months: 11 mg/day
1-3 years: 7 mg/day
4-8 years: 10 mg/day
9-13 years: 8 mg/day
14-18 years: Males: 11 mg/day; Females: 15 mg/day; Pregnant females: 27 mg/day; Lactating females: 10 mg/day
19-50 years: Males: 8 mg/day; Females: 18 mg/day; Pregnant females: 27 mg/day; Lactating females: 9 mg/day
≥50 years: 8 mg/day

Children **(dose expressed in terms of elemental iron)**:
Severe iron-deficiency anemia: 4-6 mg Fe/kg/day in 3 divided doses
Mild-to-moderate iron deficiency anemia: 3 mg Fe/kg/day in 1-2 divided doses
Prophylaxis: 1-2 mg Fe/kg/day up to a maximum of 15 mg/day

Adults **(dose expressed in terms of ferrous sulfate)**:
Iron deficiency: 300 mg twice daily up to 300 mg 4 times/day or 250 mg (extended release) 1-2 times/day
Prophylaxis: 300 mg/day

Elderly: Lower doses (15-50 mg elemental iron/day) may have similar efficacy and less GI adverse events (eg, nausea, constipation) as compared to higher doses (eg, 150 mg elemental iron/day) (Rimon, 2005).

Additional Information Complete prescribing information should be consulted for additional detail.

Dosage Forms

Elixir, Oral:
FeroSul [OTC]: 220 (44 Fe) mg/5 mL (473 mL)
Generic: 220 (44 Fe) mg/5 mL (5 mL, 473 mL)

Liquid, Oral:
Generic: 220 (44 Fe) mg/5 mL (473 mL)

Solution, Oral:
BProtected Pedia Iron [OTC]: 75 (15 Fe) mg/mL (50 mL)
Fer-In-Sol [OTC]: 75 (15 Fe) mg/mL (50 mL)
Fer-Iron [OTC]: 75 (15 Fe) mg/mL (50 mL)
Iron Supplement Childrens [OTC]: 75 (15 Fe) mg/mL (50 mL)
Generic: 75 (15 Fe) mg/mL (50 mL)

Syrup, Oral:
Generic: 300 (60 Fe) mg/5 mL (5 mL)

Tablet, Oral:
Ferro-Bob [OTC]: 325 (65 Fe) mg
Generic: 325 (65 Fe) mg

Tablet, Oral [preservative free]:
FerrouSul [OTC]: 325 (65 Fe) mg
Generic: 325 (65 Fe) mg

Tablet Delayed Release, Oral:
Generic: 324 (65 Fe) mg, 325 (65 Fe) mg

Tablet Extended Release, Oral:
Slow Fe [OTC]: 142 (45 Fe) mg, 160 (50 Fe) mg

Tablet Extended Release, Oral [preservative free]:
Slow Iron [OTC]: 160 (50 Fe) mg
Generic: 140 (45 Fe) mg

◆ **FerrouSul [OTC]** *see* Ferrous Sulfate *on page* 871

Ferumoxytol (fer ue MOX i tol)

Brand Names: U.S. Feraheme

Brand Names: Canada Feraheme

Pharmacologic Category Iron Salt

Use Iron-deficiency anemia in chronic kidney disease: Treatment of iron-deficiency anemia in adults with chronic kidney disease

Pregnancy Risk Factor C

Dosage Doses expressed in mg of **elemental** iron. **Note:** Test dose: Product labeling does not indicate need for a test dose.

IV: Adults: Iron-deficiency anemia in chronic kidney disease: 510 mg (17 mL) as a single dose, followed by a second 510 mg dose 3 to 8 days (U.S. labeling) or 2 to 8 days (Canadian labeling) after initial dose. Assess response at least 30 days following the second dose. U.S. manufacturer labeling states the recommended dose may be readministered in patients with persistent or recurrent iron-deficiency anemia.

Dosage adjustment in renal impairment: No dosage adjustment necessary.

Hemodialysis: Not removed by hemodialysis; however, administer dose after at least 1 hour of hemodialysis has been completed and once blood pressure has stabilized.

Dosage adjustment in hepatic impairment: There are no dosage adjustment provided in the manufacturer's labeling.

Additional Information Complete prescribing information should be consulted for additional detail.

Dosage Forms Considerations

Strength of ferumoxytol is expressed as elemental iron

Dosage Forms

Solution, Intravenous [preservative free]:
Feraheme: 510 mg/17 mL (17 mL)

◆ **FerUS [OTC] [DSC]** *see* Polysaccharide-Iron Complex *on page* 1677

◆ **FESO** *see* Fesoterodine *on page* 872

◆ **$FeSO_4$** *see* Ferrous Sulfate *on page* 871

Fesoterodine (fes oh TER oh deen)

Brand Names: U.S. Toviaz

Index Terms FESO; Fesoterodine Fumarate

Pharmacologic Category Anticholinergic Agent

Additional Appendix Information

Beers Criteria – Potentially Inappropriate Medications for Geriatrics *on page 2271*

Use Treatment of patients with an overactive bladder with symptoms of urinary frequency, urgency, or urge incontinence.

Pregnancy Risk Factor C

Pregnancy Considerations Teratogenic effects were observed in some animal reproduction studies.

Breast-Feeding Considerations It is not known if fesoterodine is excreted in breast milk. Breast-feeding is not recommended by the manufacturer.

Contraindications Hypersensitivity to fesoterodine or tolterodine (both are metabolized to 5-hydroxymethyl tolterodine) or any component of the formulation; urinary retention; gastric retention; uncontrolled narrow-angle glaucoma

Warnings/Precautions Cases of angioedema involving the face, lips, tongue, and/or larynx have been reported. Immediately discontinue if tongue, hypopharynx, or larynx are involved. May cause drowsiness and/or blurred vision, which may impair physical or mental abilities; patients must be cautioned about performing tasks which require mental alertness (eg, operating machinery or driving). CNS effects may be potentiated when used with other sedative drugs or ethanol. Consider dose reduction or discontinuation if CNS effects occur. Patients may experience decreased sweating; caution use in hot weather or during exercise. Use is not recommended in patients with severe hepatic impairment (Child-Pugh class C). Doses >4 mg are not recommended for patients with severe renal impairment (CrCl <30 mL/minute) or patients receiving concurrent therapy with strong CYP3A4 inhibitors (no dosing adjustments are recommended in patients receiving moderate CYP3A4 inhibitors). Use caution in patients with bladder flow obstruction, gastrointestinal obstructive disorders, myasthenia gravis, and treated narrow-angle glaucoma. This medication is associated with potent anticholinergic properties which may be inappropriate in older adults depending on comorbidities (eg, dementia, delirium) (Beers Criteria). In addition, risk of adverse effects may be increased in elderly patients.

Adverse Reactions

Central nervous system: Insomnia

Dermatological: Rash

Gastrointestinal: Abdominal pain, constipation, dyspepsia, nausea, xerostomia (dose related)

Genitourinary: Dysuria, urinary retention, urinary tract infection

Hepatic: ALT increased, GGT increased

Neuromuscular & skeletal: Back pain

Ocular: Dry eyes

Respiratory: Cough, dry throat, upper respiratory tract infection

Miscellaneous: Peripheral edema

Rare but important or life-threatening: Angina, angioedema, diverticulitis, gastroenteritis, heat prostration, hypersensitivity reactions, irritable bowel syndrome, QTc prolongation

Drug Interactions

Metabolism/Transport Effects Substrate of CYP2D6 (minor), CYP3A4 (major); **Note:** Assignment of Major/Minor substrate status based on clinically relevant drug interaction potential

Avoid Concomitant Use

Avoid concomitant use of Fesoterodine with any of the following: Aclidinium; Conivaptan; Fusidic Acid (Systemic); Glucagon; Idelalisib; Ipratropium (Oral Inhalation); Potassium Chloride; Tiotropium; Umeclidinium

Increased Effect/Toxicity

Fesoterodine may increase the levels/effects of: AbobotulinumtoxinA; Analgesics (Opioid); Anticholinergic Agents; Cannabinoid-Containing Products; Glucagon; Mirabegron; OnabotulinumtoxinA; Potassium Chloride; RimabotulinumtoxinB; Thiazide Diuretics; Tiotropium; Topiramate

The levels/effects of Fesoterodine may be increased by: Aclidinium; Alcohol (Ethyl); Aprepitant; Ceritinib; Conivaptan; CYP2D6 Inhibitors; CYP3A4 Inhibitors (Moderate); CYP3A4 Inhibitors (Strong); Dasatinib; Fosaprepitant; Fusidic Acid (Systemic); Idelalisib; Ipratropium (Oral Inhalation); Ivacaftor; Luliconazole; Mianserin; Mifepristone; Netupitant; Pramlintide; Simeprevir; Stiripentol; Umeclidinium

Decreased Effect

Fesoterodine may decrease the levels/effects of: Acetylcholinesterase Inhibitors; Itopride; Secretin

The levels/effects of Fesoterodine may be decreased by: Acetylcholinesterase Inhibitors; Bosentan; CYP3A4 Inducers (Moderate); CYP3A4 Inducers (Strong); Dabrafenib; Deferasirox; Mitotane; Siltuximab; St Johns Wort; Tocilizumab

Storage/Stability Store at 20°C to 25°C (68°F to 77°F); excursions permitted between 15°C to 30°C (59°F to 86°F). Protect from moisture.

Mechanism of Action Fesoterodine acts as a prodrug and is converted to an active metabolite, 5-hydroxymethyl tolterodine (5-HMT); 5-HMT is responsible for fesoterodine's antimuscarinic activity and acts as a competitive antagonist of muscarinic receptors.

Urinary bladder contractions are mediated by muscarinic receptors; fesoterodine inhibits the receptors in the bladder preventing symptoms of urgency and frequency.

Pharmacodynamics/Kinetics

Absorption: Well absorbed

Distribution: IV: 5-HMT: V_d: 169 L

Protein binding: 5-HMT: ~50% (primarily to albumin and alpha$_1$-acid glycoprotein)

Metabolism: Fesoterodine is rapidly and extensively metabolized to its active metabolite (5-hydroxymethyl tolterodine; 5-HMT) by nonspecific esterases; 5-HMT is further metabolized via CYP2D6 and CYP3A4 to inactive metabolites.

Bioavailability: 5-HMT: 52%

Half-life elimination: ~7 hours

Time to peak, plasma: 5-HMT: ~5 hours; C_{max} higher in poor CYP2D6 metabolizers

Excretion: Urine (~70%; 16% as 5-HMT, ~53% as inactive metabolites); feces (7%)

Dosage Oral: Adults: Overactive bladder: 4 mg once daily; may be increased to 8 mg once daily based on individual response and tolerability

Dosing adjustment for concomitant strong CYP3A4 inhibitors (eg, ketoconazole, itraconazole, clarithromycin): 4 mg once daily; maximum dose: 4 mg once daily

Dosing adjustment in renal impairment:

CrCl ≥30 mL/minute: No dosage adjustment necessary

CrCl <30 mL/minute: 4 mg once daily; maximum dose: 4 mg once daily

Dosing adjustment in hepatic impairment:

Mild-to-moderate impairment (Child-Pugh class A or B): No dosage adjustment necessary

Severe impairment (Child-Pugh class C): Use is not recommended; has not been studied

Dietary Considerations May be taken with or without food.

Administration May be administered with or without food. Swallow whole; do not chew, crush, or divide.

Dosage Forms

Tablet Extended Release 24 Hour, Oral:

Toviaz: 4 mg, 8 mg

- ◆ **Fesoterodine Fumarate** *see* Fesoterodine *on page 872*
- ◆ **FeverAll Adult [OTC]** *see* Acetaminophen *on page 32*
- ◆ **FeverAll Childrens [OTC]** *see* Acetaminophen *on page 32*
- ◆ **FeverAll Infants [OTC]** *see* Acetaminophen *on page 32*
- ◆ **FeverAll Junior Strength [OTC]** *see* Acetaminophen *on page 32*
- ◆ **Fexmid** *see* Cyclobenzaprine *on page 516*

Fexofenadine (feks oh FEN a deen)

Brand Names: U.S. Allegra Allergy Childrens [OTC]; Allegra Allergy [OTC]; Fexofenadine HCl Childrens [OTC]; Mucinex Allergy [OTC]

Brand Names: Canada Allegra 12 Hour (OTC); Allegra 24 Hour (OTC)

Index Terms Fexofenadine Hydrochloride

Pharmacologic Category Histamine H_1 Antagonist; Histamine H_1 Antagonist, Second Generation; Piperidine Derivative

Use

Chronic idiopathic urticaria: Treatment of chronic idiopathic urticaria

OTC labeling: Relief of symptoms associated with allergic rhinitis

Pregnancy Risk Factor C

Pregnancy Considerations Adverse events have been observed in animal reproduction studies; therefore, the manufacturer classifies fexofenadine as pregnancy category C. The use of antihistamines for the treatment of rhinitis during pregnancy is generally considered to be safe at recommended doses. Information related to the use of fexofenadine during pregnancy is limited; therefore, other agents are preferred.

Breast-Feeding Considerations Following administration of terfenadine to nursing mothers, fexofenadine (active metabolite of terfenadine) was found to cross into human breast milk (Allegra Canadian product monograph, 2006). The U.S. manufacturer recommends that caution be exercised when administering fexofenadine to nursing women. The Canadian labeling recommends avoiding use in nursing women.

Contraindications Hypersensitivity to fexofenadine or any component of the formulation

Warnings/Precautions Use with caution in patients with renal impairment; dosage adjustment recommended. Orally disintegrating tablet contains phenylalanine. Effects may be potentiated when used with other sedative drugs or ethanol.

Adverse Reactions

Central nervous system: Dizziness, drowsiness, fatigue, fever, headache, pain, somnolence

Endocrine & metabolic: Dysmenorrhea

Gastrointestinal: Diarrhea, dyspepsia, nausea, vomiting

Neuromuscular & skeletal: Back pain, myalgia, pain in extremities

Otic: Otitis media

Respiratory: Cough, rhinorrhea, sinusitis, upper respiratory tract infection

Miscellaneous: Viral infection

Rare but important or life-threatening: Hypersensitivity reactions (anaphylaxis, angioedema, chest tightness, dyspnea, flushing, pruritus, rash, urticaria); insomnia, nervousness, sleep disorders, paroniria (terrifying dreams)

Drug Interactions

Metabolism/Transport Effects Substrate of CYP3A4 (minor), P-glycoprotein, SLCO1B1; **Note:** Assignment of Major/Minor substrate status based on clinically relevant drug interaction potential; **Inhibits** CYP2D6 (weak)

Avoid Concomitant Use

Avoid concomitant use of Fexofenadine with any of the following: Aclidinium; Azelastine (Nasal); Glucagon; Ipratropium (Oral Inhalation); Orphenadrine; Paraldehyde; Potassium Chloride; Thalidomide; Tiotropium; Umeclidinium

Increased Effect/Toxicity

Fexofenadine may increase the levels/effects of: AbobotulinumtoxinA; Alcohol (Ethyl); Analgesics (Opioid); Anticholinergic Agents; ARIPiprazole; Azelastine (Nasal); Buprenorphine; CNS Depressants; Glucagon; Hydrocodone; Methotrimeprazine; Metyrosine; Mirabegron; Mirtazapine; OnabotulinumtoxinA; Orphenadrine; Paraldehyde; Potassium Chloride; Pramipexole; RimabotulinumtoxinB; ROPINIRole; Rotigotine; Selective Serotonin Reuptake Inhibitors; Suvorexant; Thalidomide; Thiazide Diuretics; Tiotropium; Topiramate; Zolpidem

The levels/effects of Fexofenadine may be increased by: Aclidinium; Brimonidine (Topical); Cannabis; Doxylamine; Dronabinol; Droperidol; Eltrombopag; Erythromycin (Systemic); HydrOXYzine; Ipratropium (Oral Inhalation); Itraconazole; Kava Kava; Ketoconazole (Systemic); Magnesium Sulfate; Methotrimeprazine; Mianserin; Nabilone; Perampanel; P-glycoprotein/ABCB1 Inhibitors; Pramlintide; Rifampin; Rufinamide; Sodium Oxybate; Tapentadol; Teriflunomide; Tetrahydrocannabinol; Umeclidinium; Verapamil

Decreased Effect

Fexofenadine may decrease the levels/effects of: Acetylcholinesterase Inhibitors; Benzylpenicilloyl Polylysine; Betahistine; Hyaluronidase; Itopride; Secretin

The levels/effects of Fexofenadine may be decreased by: Acetylcholinesterase Inhibitors; Amphetamines; Antacids; Grapefruit Juice; P-glycoprotein/ABCB1 Inducers; Rifampin

Food Interactions High-fat meals decrease the bioavailability of fexofenadine by ~50%. Fruit juice (apple, grapefruit, orange) may decrease bioavailability of fexofenadine by ~36%. Management: Administer with water only, avoid fruit juice.

Storage/Stability

U.S. labeling: Store at controlled room temperature of 20°C to 25°C (68°F to 77°F). Protect from excessive moisture.

Canadian labeling: Store at 15°C to 30°C (59°F to 86°F). Protect from moisture.

Mechanism of Action Fexofenadine is an active metabolite of terfenadine and like terfenadine it competes with histamine for H_1-receptor sites on effector cells in the gastrointestinal tract, blood vessels and respiratory tract; it appears that fexofenadine does not cross the blood-brain barrier to any appreciable degree, resulting in a reduced potential for sedation

Pharmacodynamics/Kinetics

Onset of action: 60 minutes

Duration: Antihistaminic effect: ≥12 hours

Absorption: Rapid

Protein binding: 60% to 70%, primarily albumin and alpha$_1$-acid glycoprotein

Metabolism: Minimal (Hepatic ~5%)

Half-life elimination: 14.4 hours (31% to 72% longer in renal impairment)

Time to peak, serum: ODT: 2 hours (4 hours with high-fat meal); Tablet: ~2.6 hours; Suspension: ~1 hour

Excretion: Feces (~80%) and urine (~11%) as unchanged drug

Dosage

Chronic idiopathic urticaria: Oral:

U.S. labeling:

Children 6 months to <2 years: 15 mg twice daily

Children 2 to 11 years: 30 mg twice daily

Children ≥12 years, Adolescents, and Adults: 60 mg twice daily **or** 180 mg once daily

Elderly: Starting dose: Use caution; adjust dose for renal impairment

Canadian labeling: Children ≥12 years, Adolescents, and Adults: 60 mg every 12 hours

Allergic rhinitis (OTC labeling): Oral:

U.S. labeling:

Children 2 to 11 years: 30 mg twice daily

Children ≥12 years, Adolescents, and Adults: 60 mg twice daily **or** 180 mg once daily

Canadian labeling: Children ≥12 years, Adolescents, and Adults: 60 mg every 12 hours **or** 120 mg once daily.

Dosage adjustment in renal impairment: Note: Canadian labeling does not approve of use in children <12 years.

CrCl <80 mL/minute:

Children 6 months to <2 years: Initial: 15 mg once daily

Children 2 to 11 years: Initial: 30 mg once daily

Children ≥12 years, Adolescents, and Adults: Initial: 60 mg once daily

Hemodialysis: Not effectively removed by hemodialysis

Dosage adjustment in hepatic impairment: There are no dosage adjustment provided in the manufacturer's labeling; however, need for adjustment not likely since undergoes minimal hepatic metabolism.

Dietary Considerations Some products may contain phenylalanine and/or sodium. Take suspension and tablets with water only; do not administer with fruit juices.

Administration

Suspension, tablet: Administer with water only; do not administer with fruit juices. Shake suspension well before use.

Orally disintegrating tablet: Take on an empty stomach. Do not remove from blister pack until administered. Using dry hands, place immediately on tongue. Tablet will dissolve within seconds, and may be swallowed with or without liquid (do not administer with fruit juices). Do not split or chew.

Monitoring Parameters Relief of symptoms

Dosage Forms

Suspension, Oral:

Allegra Allergy Childrens [OTC]: 30 mg/5 mL (120 mL, 240 mL)

Fexofenadine HCl Childrens [OTC]: 30 mg/5 mL (118 mL)

Tablet, Oral:

Allegra Allergy [OTC]: 60 mg, 180 mg

Allegra Allergy Childrens [OTC]: 30 mg

Mucinex Allergy [OTC]: 180 mg

Generic: 60 mg, 180 mg

Tablet Dispersible, Oral:

Allegra Allergy Childrens [OTC]: 30 mg

Dosage Forms: Canada

Tablet, Oral:

Allegra 12 Hour: 60 mg

Allegra 24 Hour: 120 mg

Fexofenadine and Pseudoephedrine

(feks oh FEN a deen & soo doe e FED rin)

Brand Names: U.S. Allegra-D® 12 Hour; Allegra-D® 24 Hour

Brand Names: Canada Allegra-D®

Index Terms Pseudoephedrine and Fexofenadine

Pharmacologic Category Alpha/Beta Agonist; Decongestant; Histamine H_1 Antagonist; Histamine H_1 Antagonist, Second Generation; Piperidine Derivative

Use Relief of symptoms associated with seasonal allergic rhinitis in adults and children ≥12 years of age

Pregnancy Risk Factor C

Dosage Oral: Children ≥12 years and Adults:

Allegra-D® 12 Hour: One tablet twice daily

Allegra-D® 24 Hour: One tablet once daily

Dosage adjustment in renal impairment:

Allegra-D® 12 Hour: CrCl <80 mL/minute (based on fexofenadine component): One tablet once daily

Allegra-D® 24 Hour: Avoid use.

Dosage adjustment in hepatic impairment: No dosage adjustment provided in manufacturer's labeling; however, need for adjustment not likely since fexofenadine undergoes minimal hepatic metabolism; impact of hepatic impairment on pseudoephedrine pharmacokinetics are unknown.

Additional Information Complete prescribing information should be consulted for additional detail.

Dosage Forms

Tablet, extended release: Fexofenadine 60 mg [immediate release] and pseudoephedrine 120 mg [extended release]; fexofenadine 180 mg [immediate release] and pseudoephedrine 240 mg [extended release]

Allegra-D® 12 Hour: Fexofenadine 60 mg [immediate release] and pseudoephedrine 120 mg [extended release]

Allegra-D® 24 Hour: Fexofenadine 180 mg [immediate release] and pseudoephedrine 240 mg [extended release]

◆ **Fexofenadine HCl Childrens [OTC]** *see* Fexofenadine *on page 873*

◆ **Fexofenadine Hydrochloride** *see* Fexofenadine *on page 873*

◆ **Fiber Therapy [OTC]** *see* Psyllium *on page 1744*

◆ **Fibricor** *see* Fenofibrate and Derivatives *on page 852*

Fibrinogen Concentrate (Human)

(fi BRIN o gin KON suhn trate HYU man)

Brand Names: U.S. RiaSTAP®

Index Terms Coagulation Factor I

Pharmacologic Category Blood Product Derivative

Use Treatment of acute bleeding episodes in patients with congenital fibrinogen deficiency (afibrinogenemia and hypofibrinogenemia)

Pregnancy Risk Factor C

Dosage IV: Children and Adults: Congenital fibrinogen deficiency: **Note:** Adjust dose based on laboratory values and condition of patient. Maintain a target fibrinogen level of 100 mg/dL until hemostasis is achieved.

When baseline fibrinogen level is known:

Dose (mg/kg) = [Target level (mg/dL) - measured level (mg/dL)] **divided by** 1.7 (mg/dL per mg/kg body weight)

When baseline fibrinogen level is not known: 70 mg/kg

Dosage adjustment in renal impairment: No dosage adjustment provided in manufacturer's labeling.

Dosage adjustment in hepatic impairment: No dosage adjustment provided in manufacturer's labeling.

Additional Information Complete prescribing information should be consulted for additional detail.

Dosage Forms

Injection, powder for reconstitution:

RiaSTAP®: 900-1300 mg [contains albumin (human); exact potency labeled on vial]

◆ **Fibristal (Can)** *see* Ulipristal *on page 2113*

Fidaxomicin (fye DAX oh mye sin)

Brand Names: U.S. Dificid

Brand Names: Canada Dificid™

Index Terms Difimicin; Lipiarrmycin; OPT-80; PAR-101; Tiacumicin B

Pharmacologic Category Antibiotic, Macrolide

Use Treatment of *Clostridium difficile*-associated diarrhea (CDAD)

Pregnancy Risk Factor B

Pregnancy Considerations Adverse events were not observed in animal reproduction studies. Due to the limited systemic absorption of fidaxomicin, exposure to the fetus is expected to be low.

Breast-Feeding Considerations It is not known if fidaxomicin is excreted in breast milk. The manufacturer recommends that caution be exercised when administering fidaxomicin to nursing women.

Contraindications Hypersensitivity to fidaxomicin

Warnings/Precautions Do not use for systemic infections; fidaxomicin systemic absorption is negligible. Hypersensitivity reactions (angioedema [mouth, face, throat], dyspnea, pruritus, and rash) to fidaxomicin have been reported. Patients with a history of macrolide allergy may be at increased risk. If a severe reaction occurs, discontinue drug and institute supportive care. Use only in patients with proven or strongly suspected *Clostridium difficile (C. difficile)* infections.

Adverse Reactions

Gastrointestinal: Abdominal pain, gastrointestinal hemorrhage, nausea, vomiting

Hematologic: Anemia, neutropenia

Drug Interactions

Metabolism/Transport Effects None known.

Avoid Concomitant Use There are no known interactions where it is recommended to avoid concomitant use.

Increased Effect/Toxicity

Fidaxomicin may increase the levels/effects of: Rilpivirine

Decreased Effect

Fidaxomicin may decrease the levels/effects of: Sodium Picosulfate

Storage/Stability Store at 20°C to 25°C (68°F to 77°F); excursions permitted to 15°C to 30°C (59°F to 86°F).

Mechanism of Action Inhibits RNA polymerase sigma subunit resulting in inhibition of protein synthesis and cell death in susceptible organisms including *C. difficile*; bactericidal

Pharmacodynamics/Kinetics

Absorption: Oral: Minimal systemic absorption

Distribution: Largely confined to the gastrointestinal tract; in single- and multiple-dose studies, fecal concentrations of fidaxomicin and its active metabolite (OP-1118) are very high while serum concentrations are minimally detectable to undetectable

Metabolism: Intestinal hydrolysis to less active metabolite (OP-1118)

Excretion: Feces (>92% as unchanged drug and metabolites); urine (<1% as metabolite)

Dosage Oral: Adults: Diarrhea due to *Clostridium difficile* (CDAD): 200 mg twice daily for 10 days

Dosing adjustment in renal impairment: No dosage adjustment necessary (minimal systemic absorption).

Dosing adjustment in hepatic impairment: No dosage adjustment provided in manufacturer's label (has not been studied); However, due to minimal systemic absorption no dosage adjustment predicted.

Administration May be administered with or without food.

Additional Information Fidaxomicin is bactericidal against gram-positive anaerobes (including *C. difficile* NAP1/B1/027 strain) and gram-positive aerobes. Fidaxomicin spectrum does **not** include gram-negative aerobes or gram-negative anaerobes (eg, *Bacteroides spp*). At the approved dose, concentrations in feces substantially exceed the 90% MIC of *C. difficile*. Postantibiotic effects against *C. difficile* in clinical studies range from 6-10 hours. Clinical studies excluded patients with a history of >1 recurrent *C. difficile*-associated diarrhea (CDAD) episode within 3 months.

Dosage Forms

Tablet, Oral:

Dificid: 200 mg

Filgrastim (fil GRA stim)

Brand Names: U.S. Granix; Neupogen

Brand Names: Canada Neupogen

Index Terms G-CSF; Granulocyte Colony Stimulating Factor; Tbo-Filgrastim; Tevagrastim

Pharmacologic Category Colony Stimulating Factor; Hematopoietic Agent

Use

Myelosuppressive chemotherapy recipients with nonmyeloid malignancies:

Neupogen: To decrease the incidence of infection (neutropenic fever) in patients with nonmyeloid malignancies receiving myelosuppressive chemotherapy associated with a significant incidence of neutropenia with fever.

Granix: To decrease the duration of severe neutropenia in patients with nonmyeloid malignancies receiving myelosuppressive chemotherapy associated with a clinically significant incidence of neutropenic fever.

Acute myeloid leukemia (AML) patients following induction or consolidation chemotherapy (Neupogen): To reduce the time to neutrophil recovery and reduce the duration of fever following induction or consolidation chemotherapy in adults with AML.

Bone marrow transplantation (Neupogen): To reduce the duration of neutropenia and neutropenia-related events (eg, neutropenic fever) in patients with nonmyeloid malignancies receiving myeloablative chemotherapy followed by marrow transplantation.

Peripheral blood progenitor cell collection and therapy (Neupogen): Mobilization of hematopoietic progenitor cells into peripheral blood for apheresis collection (mobilization allows for collection of increased numbers of progenitor cells capable of engraftment, which may lead to more rapid engraftment).

Severe chronic neutropenia (Neupogen): Long-term administration to reduce the incidence and duration of neutropenic complications (eg, fever, infections, oropharyngeal ulcers) in symptomatic patients with congenital, cyclic, or idiopathic neutropenia.

Pregnancy Risk Factor C

Pregnancy Considerations Adverse events have been observed in animal reproduction studies. Filgrastim has been shown to cross the placenta in humans.

Women who become pregnant during Neupogen treatment are encouraged to enroll in the manufacturer's Pregnancy Surveillance Program (1-800-772-6436).

Breast-Feeding Considerations It is not known if filgrastim or tbo-filgrastim is excreted in breast milk. The manufacturers recommend that caution be exercised when administering filgrastim or tbo-filgrastim to nursing women.

Women who are nursing during Neupogen treatment are encouraged to enroll in the manufacturer's Lactation Surveillance program (1-800-772-6436).

Contraindications

Neupogen: Hypersensitivity to filgrastim, *E. coli*-derived proteins, or any component of the formulation

Granix: There are no contraindications listed in the manufacturer's labeling

Warnings/Precautions Anaphylaxis, rash, urticaria, facial edema, wheezing, dyspnea, tachycardia, and/or hypotension have occurred with first or subsequent doses. Reactions tended to involve two or more body systems and occur more frequently with intravenous administration and generally within 30 minutes of administration. Symptoms recurred in >50% of patients when rechallenged. Management may include administration of antihistamines, steroids, bronchodilators, and/or epinephrine. Do not administer tbo-filgrastim to patients who experienced serious allergic reaction to filgrastim or pegfilgrastim. Permanently discontinue tbo-filgrastim in patients with serious allergic reactions. Rare cases of splenic rupture have been reported (may be fatal); in patients with upper abdominal pain, left upper quadrant pain, or shoulder tip pain, withhold treatment and evaluate for enlarged spleen or splenic rupture. Cutaneous vasculitis has been reported with filgrastim, generally occurring in patients with severe chronic neutropenia on chronic therapy; symptoms generally developed with increasing absolute neutrophil count (ANC) and subsided when the ANC decreased; dose reductions may improve symptoms to allow for continued therapy. Capillary leak syndrome (CLS), characterized by hypotension, hypoalbuminemia, edema, and hemoconcentration, may occur in patients receiving human granulocyte colony-stimulating factors (G-CSF). CLS episode may vary in frequency and severity. If CLS develops, monitor closely and manage symptomatically (may require intensive care). CLS may be life-threatening if treatment is delayed.

White blood cell counts of ≥100,000/mm^3 have been reported with filgrastim doses >5 mcg/kg/day. Monitor CBC twice weekly during therapy. Thrombocytopenia has also been reported with filgrastim; monitor platelet counts. Although the incidence of antibody development has not been determined, there is a potential for immunogenicity, which may result in cytopenias. Filgrastim should not be routinely used in the treatment of established neutropenic fever. Colony-stimulating factors may be considered in cancer patients with febrile neutropenia who are at high risk for infection-associated complications or who have prognostic factors indicative of a poor clinical outcome (eg, prolonged and severe neutropenia, age >65 years, hypotension, pneumonia, sepsis syndrome, presence of invasive fungal infection, uncontrolled primary disease, hospitalization at the time of fever development) (Freifeld, 2011; Smith, 2006). Do not use filgrastim in the period 24 hours before to 24 hours after administration of cytotoxic chemotherapy because of the potential sensitivity of rapidly dividing myeloid cells to cytotoxic chemotherapy. Transient increase in neutrophil count is seen 1-2 days after filgrastim initiation; however, for sustained neutrophil response, continue until post-nadir ANC reaches 10,000/mm^3. Avoid simultaneous use of filgrastim with chemotherapy and radiation therapy. Safety and efficacy have not been established with patients receiving chemotherapy associated with delayed myelosuppression (eg, nitrosoureas, mitomycin). Avoid concurrent radiation therapy with filgrastim; safety and efficacy have not been established with patients receiving radiation therapy. May potentially act as a growth factor for any tumor type; caution should be exercised when using in any malignancy with myeloid characteristics. When used for stem cell mobilization, may release tumor cells from marrow which could be collected in leukapheresis product; potential effect of tumor cell reinfusion is unknown.

May precipitate severe sickle cell crises, sometimes resulting in fatalities, in patients with sickle cell disorders; carefully evaluate potential risks and benefits. Discontinue in patients undergoing sickle cell crisis. Cytogenic abnormalities and transformation to AML or myelodysplastic syndrome (MDS) have been reported in patients with severe chronic neutropenia (SCN), including patients receiving cytokine therapy; carefully consider the risks of continued filgrastim treatment if abnormal cytogenetics or myelodysplasia develop. Establish diagnosis prior to filgrastim initiation; use prior to appropriate diagnosis of SCN may impair or delay proper evaluation and treatment for neutropenia due to conditions other than SCN. Acute respiratory distress syndrome (ARDS) has been reported (possibly due to influx of neutrophils to sites of lung inflammation); patients must be instructed to report respiratory distress; monitor for fever, pulmonary infiltrates, or respiratory distress; discontinue in patients with ARDS. Reports of alveolar hemorrhage, manifested as pulmonary infiltrates and hemoptysis, have occurred in healthy donors undergoing PBPC mobilization (off-label for use in healthy donors); hemoptysis resolved upon discontinuation. The packaging of some dosage forms may contain latex. Some products available internationally may have vial strength and dosing expressed as units (instead of as micrograms). Refer to prescribing information for specific strength and dosing information.

Adverse Reactions

Cardiovascular: Cardiac arrhythmia, hypertension, myocardial infarction

Central nervous system: Headache

Dermatologic: Skin rash

Endocrine & metabolic: Increased lactate dehydrogenase, increased uric acid

Gastrointestinal: Nausea, peritonitis, vomiting

Hematologic & oncologic: Leukocytosis, petechiae, splenomegaly, thrombocytopenia

Hepatic: Increased serum alkaline phosphatase

Neuromuscular & skeletal: Ostealgia (commonly in the lower back, posterior iliac crest, and sternum)

Respiratory: Epistaxis

Hypersensitivity: Transfusion reaction

Miscellaneous: Fever

Rare but important or life-threatening: Alopecia, capillary leak syndrome, cerebral hemorrhage, decreased bone mineral density, erythema nodosum, exacerbation of psoriasis, hematuria, hepatomegaly, hemoptysis, hypersensitivity angiitis, hypersensitivity reaction, osteoporosis, pericarditis, proteinuria, pulmonary hemorrhage, pulmonary infiltrates, renal insufficiency, respiratory distress syndrome, severe sickle cell crisis, splenic rupture, supraventricular cardiac arrhythmia, Sweet's syndrome, tachycardia, thrombophlebitis

Drug Interactions

Metabolism/Transport Effects None known.

Avoid Concomitant Use There are no known interactions where it is recommended to avoid concomitant use.

Increased Effect/Toxicity

Filgrastim may increase the levels/effects of: Bleomycin; Cyclophosphamide; Topotecan

Decreased Effect There are no known significant interactions involving a decrease in effect.

Preparation for Administration Visually inspect prior to use; discard if discolored or if particulates are present.

Neupogen: **Do not dilute with saline at any time; product may precipitate.** Filgrastim may be diluted with D_5W to a concentration of 5 to 15 mcg/mL for IV infusion administration (minimum concentration: 5 mcg/mL). Concentrations of 5 to 15 mcg/mL require addition of albumin (final albumin concentration of 2 mg/mL) to prevent adsorption to plastics. Dilution to <5 mcg/mL is not recommended. Do not shake. Discard unused portion of vial/prefilled syringe.

Granix: Remove needle shield and expel extra volume if needed (depending on dose). Prefilled syringe is single use; discard unused portion.

Storage/Stability

Neupogen: Store intact vials/prefilled syringes at 2°C to 8°C (36°F to 46°F). Do not shake. Protect from direct sunlight. Prior to injection, allow to reach room temperature for a maximum of 24 hours. Discard any vial or prefilled syringe left at room temperature for more than 24 hours.

Extended storage information may be available for undiluted filgrastim; contact product manufacturer to obtain current recommendations. Sterility has been assessed and maintained for up to 7 days when prepared under strict aseptic conditions (Jacobson, 1996; Singh, 1994). The manufacturer recommends using syringes within 24 hours due to the potential for bacterial contamination.

Granix: Store prefilled syringes at 2°C to 8°C (36°F to 46°F). Protect from light. Do not shake. May be removed from 2°C to 8°C (36°F to 46°F) storage for a single period of up to 5 days between 23°C to 27°C (73°F to 81°F). If not used within 5 days, the product may be returned to 2°C to 8°C (36°F to 46°F) up to the expiration date. Exposure to -1°C to -5°C (23°F to 30°F) for up to 72 hours and temperatures as low as -15°C to -25°C (5°F to -13°F) for up to 24 hours do not adversely affect stability. Discard unused product.

Mechanism of Action Filgrastim and tbo-filgrastim are granulocyte colony stimulating factors (G-CSF) produced by recombinant DNA technology. G-CSFs stimulate the production, maturation, and activation of neutrophils to increase both their migration and cytotoxicity.

Pharmacodynamics/Kinetics

Onset of action:

Filgrastim: ~24 hours; plateaus in 3 to 5 days

Tbo-filgrastim: Time to maximum ANC: 3 to 5 days

Duration:

Filgrastim: Neutrophil counts generally return to baseline within 4 days

Tbo-filgrastim: ANC returned to baseline by 21 days after completion of chemotherapy

Absorption: SubQ: 100%

Distribution: V_d: 150 mL/kg; no evidence of drug accumulation over a 11- to 20-day period

Metabolism: Systemically degraded

Bioavailability: Tbo-filgrastim: SubQ: 33%

Half-life elimination: Filgrastim: ~3.5 hours; Tbo-filgrastim: 3 to 4 hours

Time to peak, serum: SubQ: Filgrastim: 2 to 8 hours; Tbo-filgrastim: 4 to 6 hours

Dosage Note: Do not administer in the period 24 hours before to 24 hours after cytotoxic chemotherapy. May round the dose to the nearest vial size in adults for convenience and cost minimization (Ozer, 2000). **International considerations:** Dosages below expressed as micrograms; 1 mcg = 100,000 units (Hoglund, 1998).

Myelosuppressive chemotherapy recipients with nonmyeloid malignancies (Neupogen): Infants, Children, Adolescents, and Adults: SubQ, IV: 5 mcg/kg/day; doses may be increased by 5 mcg/kg (for each chemotherapy cycle) according to the duration and severity of the neutropenia; continue for up to 14 days until the ANC reaches 10,000/mm^3. Discontinue if the ANC surpasses 10,000/mm^3 after the expected chemotherapy-induced neutrophil nadir. In clinical studies, efficacy was observed at doses of 4 to 8 mcg/kg/day.

Myelosuppressive chemotherapy recipients with nonmyeloid malignancies (Granix): Adults: SubQ: 5 mcg/kg/day; continue until anticipated nadir has passed and neutrophil count has recovered to normal range

Acute myeloid leukemia (AML) following induction or consolidation chemotherapy (Neupogen): Adults: SubQ, IV: 5 mcg/kg/day; doses may be increased by 5 mcg/kg (for each chemotherapy cycle) according to the duration and severity of the neutropenia; continue for up to 14 days until the ANC reaches 10,000/mm^3. Discontinue if the ANC surpasses 10,000/mm^3 after the expected chemotherapy-induced neutrophil nadir. In clinical studies, efficacy was observed at doses of 4 to 8 mcg/kg/day.

Bone marrow transplantation (Neupogen): Infants, Children, Adolescents, and Adults: SubQ, IV: 10 mcg/kg/day (administer ≥24 hours after chemotherapy and ≥24 hours after bone marrow infusion); adjust the dose according to the duration and severity of neutropenia; recommended steps based on neutrophil response:

When ANC >1000/mm^3 for 3 consecutive days: Reduce filgrastim dose to 5 mcg/kg/day

If ANC remains >1000/mm^3 for 3 more consecutive days: Discontinue filgrastim

If ANC decreases to <1000/mm^3: Resume at 5 mcg/kg/day

If ANC decreases to <1000/mm^3 during the 5 mcg/kg/day dose, increase filgrastim to 10 mcg/kg/day and follow the above steps

Peripheral blood progenitor cell collection and therapy (Neupogen): Infants, Children, Adolescents, and Adults: SubQ: 10 mcg/kg daily, usually for 6 to 7 days. Begin at least 4 days before the first apheresis and continue until the last apheresis; consider dose adjustment for WBC >100,000/mm^3

Severe chronic neutropenia (Neupogen): Infants ≥1 month, Children, Adolescents, and Adults: SubQ:

Congenital: Initial: 6 mcg/kg twice daily; adjust the dose based on ANC and clinical response; mean dose: 6 mcg/kg/day

Idiopathic: Initial: 5 mcg/kg/day; adjust the dose based on ANC and clinical response; mean dose: 1.2 mcg/kg/day

Cyclic: Initial: 5 mcg/kg/day; adjust the dose based on ANC and clinical response; mean dose: 2.1 mcg/kg/day

Anemia in myelodysplastic syndrome (off-label use; in combination with epoetin): Adults: SubQ: 300 mcg weekly in 2-3 divided doses (Malcovati, 2013) **or** 1 mcg/kg once daily (Greenberg, 2009) **or** 75 mcg, 150 mcg, or 300 mcg per dose 3 times weekly (Hellstrom-Lindberg, 2003)

Hematopoietic stem cell mobilization in autologous transplantation in patients with non-Hodgkin's lymphoma or multiple myeloma (in combination with plerixafor; off-label use): Adults: SubQ: 10 mcg/kg once daily; begin 4 days before initiation of plerixafor; continue G-CSF on each day prior to apheresis for up to 8 days (DiPersio, 2009a; DiPersio, 2009b)

Hepatitis C treatment-associated neutropenia (off-label use): Adults: SubQ: 150 mcg once weekly to 300 mcg 3 times weekly; titrate to maintain ANC between 750 to 10,000/mm^3 (Younossi, 2008)

Treatment of radiation-induced myelosuppression of the bone marrow (off-label use): Infants, Children, Adolescents, and Adults: SubQ: 5 mcg/kg/day; continue until ANC >1000/mm^3 (Smith, 2006; Waselenko, 2004).

Dosage adjustment in renal impairment:

Neupogen: There are no dosage adjustments provided in the manufacturer's labeling.

Granix:

Mild impairment: No dosage adjustment necessary.

Moderate to severe impairment: There are no dosage adjustments provided in the manufacturer's labeling (has not been studied).

Dosage adjustment in hepatic impairment: There are no dosage adjustments provided in the manufacturer's labeling.

Dietary Considerations Some products may contain sodium.

Administration Do not administer earlier than 24 hours after or in the 24 hours prior to cytotoxic chemotherapy.

IV (Neupogen): May be administered IV as a short infusion over 15 to 30 minutes (chemotherapy-induced neutropenia) or by continuous infusion (chemotherapy-induced neutropenia) or as a 4- or 24-hour infusion (bone marrow transplantation).

SubQ: May be administered by SubQ, either as a bolus injection (chemotherapy-induced neutropenia, peripheral blood progenitor cell collection, severe chronic neutropenia) or as a continuous infusion (chemotherapy-induced neutropenia, bone marrow transplantation, and peripheral blood progenitor cell collection). Administer into the outer upper arm, abdomen (except within 2 inches of navel), front middle thigh, or the upper outer buttocks area. Rotate injection site; do not inject into areas that are tender, red, bruised, hardened, or scarred, or sites with stretch marks.

Some patients (or caregivers) may be appropriate for subQ self-administration with proper training; patients/caregivers should follow the manufacturer instructions for preparation and administration. Granix is available in prefilled syringes with and without a needle guard; the prefilled syringe without a safety needle guard is intended for patient/caregiver self-administration.

Monitoring Parameters

Chemotherapy-induced neutropenia: CBC with differential and platelets prior to chemotherapy and twice weekly during growth factor treatment.

Bone marrow transplantation: CBC with differential and platelets at least 3 times a week.

Peripheral progenitor cell collection: Neutrophil counts after 4 days of filgrastim treatment.

Severe chronic neutropenia: CBC with differential and platelets twice weekly during the first month of therapy and for 2 weeks following dose adjustments; once clinically stable, monthly for 1 year and quarterly thereafter. Monitor bone marrow and karyotype prior to treatment; and monitor marrow and cytogenetics annually throughout treatment.

Reference Range No additional clinical benefit seen when filgrastim is used with ANC >10,000/mm^3

Dosage Forms Considerations

Prefilled syringes: Granix, Neupogen: 300 mcg/0.5 mL (0.5 mL); 480 mcg/0.8 mL (0.8 mL)

Vials: Neupogen: 300 mcg/mL (1 mL); 480 mcg/1.6 mL (1.6 mL)

Dosage Forms

Solution, Injection:

Neupogen: 300 mcg/mL (1 mL); 480 mcg/1.6 mL (1.6 mL)

Solution, Injection [preservative free]:

Neupogen: 300 mcg/0.5 mL (0.5 mL); 480 mcg/0.8 mL (0.8 mL)

Solution Prefilled Syringe, Subcutaneous [preservative free]:

Granix: 300 mcg/0.5 mL (0.5 mL); 480 mcg/0.8 mL (0.8 mL)

◆ **Finacea** *see* Azelaic Acid *on page* 213

Finasteride (fi NAS teer ide)

Brand Names: U.S. Propecia; Proscar

Brand Names: Canada Apo-Finasteride; Auro-Finasteride; CO Finasteride; Dom-Finasteride; JAMP-Finasteride; Mint-Finasteride; Mylan-Finasteride; PMS-Finasteride; Propecia; Proscar; RAN-Finasteride; ratio-Finasteride; Sandoz-Finasteride; Sandoz-Finasteride A; Teva-Finasteride

Pharmacologic Category 5 Alpha-Reductase Inhibitor

Use

Propecia®: Treatment of male pattern hair loss in **men only**. Safety and efficacy were demonstrated in men between 18-41 years of age.

Proscar®: Treatment of symptomatic benign prostatic hyperplasia (BPH); can be used in combination with an alpha-blocker, doxazosin

Pregnancy Risk Factor X

Pregnancy Considerations Abnormalities of external male genitalia were reported in animal reproduction studies. Use is not indicated in women. Pregnant women are advised to avoid contact with crushed or broken tablets and the semen from a male partner exposed to finasteride.

Breast-Feeding Considerations It is not known if finasteride is excreted in breast milk. Use is contraindicated in women of childbearing potential.

Contraindications Hypersensitivity to finasteride or any component of the formulation; women of childbearing potential

Warnings/Precautions Hazardous agent - use appropriate precautions for handling and disposal (NIOSH 2014 [group 3]). Other urological diseases (including prostate cancer) should be ruled out before initiating. For BPH, a minimum of 6 months of treatment may be necessary to determine whether an individual will respond to finasteride; for male pattern hair loss, daily use for 3 months or longer may be required before benefit is observed. Reduces prostate specific antigen (PSA) by ~50%; in patients treated for ≥6 months the PSA value should be doubled when comparing to normal ranges in untreated patients (for interpretation of serial PSAs, a new PSA baseline should be established ≥6 months after treatment initiation and PSA monitored periodically thereafter). Failure to demonstrate a meaningful PSA decrease (<50%) or a PSA increase while on this medication may be associated with an increased risk for prostate cancer (NCCN prostate cancer early detection guidelines, v.1.2011). Patients on a 5-alpha-reductase inhibitor (5-ARI) with any increase in PSA levels, even if within normal limits, should be evaluated; may indicate presence of prostate cancer. Use with caution in patients with hepatic dysfunction; finasteride is extensively metabolized in the liver. When compared to placebo, 5-ARIs have been shown to reduce the overall incidence of prostate cancer, although an increase in the incidence of high-grade prostate cancers has been observed; 5-ARIs are not approved in the U.S. or Canada for the prevention of prostate cancer. Carefully monitor patients with a large residual urinary volume or severely diminished urinary flow for obstructive uropathy; these patients may not be candidates for finasteride therapy. Rare reports of male breast cancer have been observed with finasteride use. Patients should promptly report any breast changes, including breast enlargement, lumps, tenderness, pain, or nipple discharge to their healthcare provider. Active ingredient of crushed or broken tablets can be absorbed through the skin; unbroken tablets are coated which prevents contact with the active ingredient during normal handling. Women should avoid contact with crushed or broken tablets and the semen from a male partner exposed to finasteride; finasteride may negatively impact fetal development.

Adverse Reactions

Cardiovascular: Edema, orthostatic hypotension

Central nervous system: Dizziness, drowsiness

Dermatologic: Skin rash

Endocrine & metabolic: Decreased libido, gynecomastia

Genitourinary: Breast tenderness, decreased ejaculate volume, ejaculatory disorder, impotence

Neuromuscular & skeletal: Weakness

Respiratory: Dyspnea, rhinitis

Rare but important or life-threatening: Altered mental status, decreased testicular size, depression, disturbed sleep, hypersensitivity (angioedema, facial swelling, pharyngeal edema, pruritus, skin rash, swelling of the lips, swollen tongue, urticaria), male infertility (temporary), malignant neoplasm of the male breast, prostate cancer - high grade, prostatitis, reduction in penile curvature, reduction in penile size, sexual disorder (may not be reversible with discontinuation), testicular pain

Drug Interactions

Metabolism/Transport Effects Substrate of CYP3A4 (minor); **Note:** Assignment of Major/Minor substrate status based on clinically relevant drug interaction potential

Avoid Concomitant Use There are no known interactions where it is recommended to avoid concomitant use.

Increased Effect/Toxicity There are no known significant interactions involving an increase in effect.

Decreased Effect There are no known significant interactions involving a decrease in effect.

Storage/Stability

Propecia: Store at 15°C to 30°C (59°F to 86°F). Protect from moisture.

Proscar: Store below 30°C (86°F). Protect from light.

Mechanism of Action Finasteride is a competitive inhibitor of both tissue and hepatic 5-alpha reductase. This results in inhibition of the conversion of testosterone to dihydrotestosterone and markedly suppresses serum dihydrotestosterone levels

Pharmacodynamics/Kinetics

Onset of action: BPH: 6 months; Male pattern hair loss: ≥3 months of daily use

Duration:

After a single oral dose as small as 0.5 mg: 65% depression of plasma dihydrotestosterone levels persists 5-7 days

After 6 months of treatment with 5 mg/day: Circulating dihydrotestosterone levels are reduced to castrate levels without significant effects on circulating testosterone; levels return to normal within 14 days of discontinuation of treatment

Distribution: V_{dss}: 76 L

Protein binding: ~90%

Metabolism: Hepatic via CYP3A4; two active metabolites (<20% activity of finasteride)

Bioavailability: Mean: 65%

Half-life elimination, serum: 6 hours (range: 3-16 hours); Elderly: 8 hours (range: 6-15 hours)

Time to peak, serum: 1-2 hours

Excretion: Feces (57%) and urine (39%) as metabolites

Dosage Oral: Adults:

Males:

Benign prostatic hyperplasia (Proscar®): 5 mg once daily as a single dose; clinical responses occur within 12 weeks to 6 months of initiation of therapy; long-term administration is recommended for maximal response

Male pattern baldness (Propecia®): 1 mg daily

Female hirsutism (off-label use): 5 mg/day (Moghetti, 2000)

Dosing adjustment in renal impairment: No dosage adjustment is necessary

Dosing adjustment in hepatic impairment: Use with caution in patients with liver function abnormalities because finasteride is metabolized extensively in the liver

Dietary Considerations May be taken without regard to meals.

Administration May be administered without regard to meals. Women of childbearing age should not touch or handle broken tablets.

Hazardous agent; use appropriate precautions for handling and disposal (NIOSH 2014 [group 3]).

Monitoring Parameters Objective and subjective signs of relief of benign prostatic hyperplasia, including improvement in urinary flow, reduction in symptoms of urgency, and relief of difficulty in micturition; for interpretation of serial PSAs, establish a new PSA baseline ≥6 months after treatment initiation and monitor PSA periodically thereafter. Finasteride does not interfere with free PSA levels.

Dosage Forms

Tablet, Oral:

Propecia: 1 mg

Proscar: 5 mg

Generic: 1 mg, 5 mg

Fingolimod (fin GOL i mod)

Brand Names: U.S. Gilenya

Brand Names: Canada Gilenya

Index Terms FTY720

Pharmacologic Category Sphingosine 1-Phosphate (S1P) Receptor Modulator

Use Multiple sclerosis: Treatment of relapsing forms of multiple sclerosis (MS) to reduce the frequency of clinical exacerbations and to delay the accumulation of physical disability.

Pregnancy Risk Factor C

Pregnancy Considerations Adverse events have been observed in animal reproduction studies. Elimination of fingolimod takes approximately 2 months; to avoid potential fetal harm, women of childbearing potential should use effective contraception to avoid pregnancy during and for 2 months after discontinuing treatment. Health care providers are encouraged to enroll pregnant women, or pregnant women may enroll themselves, in the Gilenya™ Pregnancy Registry (1-877-598-7237 or https://www.-gilenyapregnancyregistry.com).

Breast-Feeding Considerations It is not known if fingolimod is excreted in breast milk. Due to the potential for serious adverse reactions in the nursing infant, the manufacturer recommends a decision be made whether to discontinue nursing or to discontinue the drug, taking into account the importance of treatment to the mother.

Contraindications

MI, unstable angina, stroke, transient ischemic attack, decompensated heart failure requiring hospitalization, or New York Heart Association (NYHA) class III/IV heart failure in the past 6 months; Mobitz Type II second- or third-degree atrioventricular (AV) block or sick sinus syndrome (unless patient has a functioning pacemaker); baseline QTc interval ≥500 msec; concurrent use of a class Ia or III antiarrhythmic.

Canadian labeling: Additional contraindications (not in U.S. labeling): Hypersensitivity to fingolimod or any component of the formulation; patients at increased risk for opportunistic infections, including those who are immunocompromised; severe active infections; known active malignancy (excluding basal cell carcinoma); severe hepatic impairment (Child-Pugh class C)

Warnings/Precautions Hazardous agent - use appropriate precautions for handling and disposal (NIOSH 2014 [group 2]).

Increased blood pressure may occur ~1 month after initiation of therapy; monitor blood pressure throughout treatment. Therapy may result in transient and asymptomatic atrioventricular (AV) conduction delays; recurrence may be observed following discontinuation (>2 weeks) and subsequent reinitiation of therapy. Decreased heart rate may occur with initiation of therapy. Initiation must occur in a setting with resources and personnel capable of appropriately managing symptomatic bradycardia. Following the first dose, heart rate may decrease as soon as 1 hour postdose, with the maximal decrease usually occurring ~6 hours postdose. Heart rate typically returns to baseline after 1 month of therapy. Due to the risk of bradycardia and AV conduction delays, electrocardiogram (ECG) is required prior to initiation of therapy and after the initial observation period (6 hours) in all patients. Patients receiving concomitant therapy with drugs that slow heart rate or AV conduction (eg, beta blockers, heart rate-lowering calcium channel blockers, digoxin) or with other cardiac risk factors (eg, AV block, sick sinus syndrome, prolonged QT interval, ischemic cardiac disease, history of myocardial infarction [MI], symptomatic bradycardia, and/or cardiac arrest, heart failure, cerebrovascular disease, uncontrolled hypertension, recurrent syncope, severe sleep apnea [untreated]) require continuous overnight ECG monitoring in a medical facility after the first dose. May cause QT prolongation; patients with a prolonged QT interval at baseline (males: >450 msec; females: >470 msec) or during the first 6 hours of treatment initiation, or are at an increased risk of QT prolongation (eg, hypokalemia, hypomagnesemia, concomitant QT-prolonging drugs, congenital long-QT syndrome, concomitant QT-prolonging drugs, congenital long-QT syndrome) require continuous overnight ECG monitoring in a medical facility after the initial dose.

Posterior reversible encephalopathy syndrome (PRES) has been observed. Monitor for signs/symptoms of PRES (eg, sudden onset of severe headache, altered mental status, visual disturbances, seizure); symptoms are usually reversible, but may evolve into ischemic stroke or cerebral hemorrhage. Discontinue use if PRES is suspected. May increase risk of infection due to dose-dependent reduction of lymphocytes; lymphocyte counts may be decreased for up to 2 months following discontinuation of therapy. Do not initiate treatment in patients with acute or chronic infections until the infection has resolved. Use with caution in patients receiving concomitant immunosuppressant, immune modulating, or antineoplastic medications or when switching from other immunosuppressants (consider the duration and mode of action for each substance to avoid additive effects).

Use with caution and closely monitor patients with severe hepatic impairment (contraindicated in the Canadian labeling). Elevated liver enzymes may occur; recurrence of liver transaminase elevations may occur with rechallenge. Obtain baseline liver enzymes in all patients prior to therapy initiation; monitor liver enzymes in patients who develop symptoms of hepatic dysfunction (eg, nausea, vomiting, abdominal pain, fatigue, anorexia, jaundice, dark urine). Use caution in patients with preexisting liver disease; may be at increased risk of increased liver enzymes. Discontinue treatment with confirmation of liver injury; transaminases tend to return to normal within 2 months of discontinuation. Macular edema may occur; use with caution in patients with a history of diabetes mellitus or uveitis. Ophthalmologic exams should be performed prior to therapy and 3-4 months after treatment initiation; more frequent examination is warranted in patients with diabetes or a history of uveitis. Reductions of forced expiratory volume in the first second of expiration (FEV_1) and diffusion lung capacity for carbon monoxide (DLCO) are dose-dependent and may occur within the first month of therapy or when switching from other immunosuppressants (consider the duration and mode of action for each substance to avoid additive effects). FEV_1 changes may be reversible with drug discontinuation.

Consider varicella zoster virus (VZV) vaccination prior to initiation of treatment in VZV antibody negative patients; postpone fingolimod treatment for 1 month after varicella zoster vaccination. Potentially significant drug-drug interactions may exist, requiring dose or frequency adjustment, additional monitoring, and/or selection of alternative therapy.

Adverse Reactions

Cardiovascular: Bradycardia, hypertension

Central nervous system: Depression, dizziness, headache, migraine

Dermatologic: Alopecia, eczema, pruritus

Endocrine & metabolic: Increased triglycerides

Gastrointestinal: Diarrhea, gastroenteritis, weight loss

Hematologic: Leukopenia, lymphopenia

Hepatic: Increased ALT, increased AST, increased GGT

Neuromuscular & skeletal: Back pain, paresthesia, weakness

Ocular: Blurred vision, eye pain

Respiratory: Bronchitis, cough, dyspnea, sinusitis

Miscellaneous: Flu-like syndrome, herpes infection, tinea infection

Rare but important or life-threatening: Asystole, AV block, death, lymphoma, macular edema (incidence increased in patients with uveitis or diabetes mellitus), QT prolongation, syncope

Drug Interactions

Metabolism/Transport Effects Substrate of CYP2D6 (minor), CYP2E1 (minor), CYP3A4 (minor); **Note:** Assignment of Major/Minor substrate status based on clinically relevant drug interaction potential

Avoid Concomitant Use

Avoid concomitant use of Fingolimod with any of the following: Antiarrhythmic Agents (Class Ia); Antiarrhythmic Agents (Class III); BCG; Ceritinib; Highest Risk QTc-Prolonging Agents; Ivabradine; Mifepristone; Natalizumab; Pimecrolimus; Tacrolimus (Topical); Tofacitinib; Vaccines (Live)

Increased Effect/Toxicity

Fingolimod may increase the levels/effects of: Antiarrhythmic Agents (Class Ia); Antiarrhythmic Agents (Class III); Bradycardia-Causing Agents; Ceritinib; Highest Risk QTc-Prolonging Agents; Lacosamide; Leflunomide; Moderate Risk QTc-Prolonging Agents; Natalizumab; Tofacitinib; Vaccines (Live)

The levels/effects of Fingolimod may be increased by: Beta-Blockers; Bretylium; Denosumab; Diltiazem; Ivabradine; Ketoconazole (Systemic); Mifepristone; Pimecrolimus; QTc-Prolonging Agents (Indeterminate Risk and Risk Modifying); Roflumilast; Tacrolimus (Topical); Trastuzumab; Verapamil

Decreased Effect

Fingolimod may decrease the levels/effects of: BCG; Coccidioides immitis Skin Test; Sipuleucel-T; Vaccines (Inactivated); Vaccines (Live)

The levels/effects of Fingolimod may be decreased by: CarBAMazepine; Echinacea

Storage/Stability Store at 25°C (77°F); excursions are permitted between 15°C and 30°C (59°F and 86°F). Protect from moisture.

Mechanism of Action Fingolimod-phosphate, active metabolite of fingolimod, binds to sphingosine 1-phosphate receptors 1, 3, 4, and 5. Fingolimod-phosphate blocks the lymphocytes' ability to emerge from lymph nodes; therefore, the amount of lymphocytes available to the central nervous system is decreased, which reduces central inflammation.

Pharmacodynamics/Kinetics

Distribution: V_d: 940 to1460 L: distributes into red blood cells (86%)

Protein binding: >99.7% (fingolimod and fingolimod-phosphate)

Metabolism: Hepatic via CYP4F2 to fingolimod-phosphate (active) and other metabolites (inactive); CYP2D6, 2E1, 3A4, and 4F12 also contribute to metabolism
Bioavailability: 93%
Half-life elimination: 6 to 9 days
Time to peak, plasma: 12 to 16 hours
Excretion: Urine (~81% as inactive metabolites); feces (fingolimod and fingolimod phosphate: <2.5% of dose)

Dosage Multiple sclerosis: Adults: Oral: 0.5 mg once daily; doses >0.5 mg daily associated with increased adverse events and no additional benefit. **Note:** The first dose and doses following therapy interruption should be administered in a setting in which resources to appropriately manage symptomatic bradycardia are available.

Dosage adjustment in renal impairment: There are no dosage adjustments provided in the manufacturer's labeling; use with caution in severe renal impairment (exposure is increased).

Dosage adjustment in hepatic impairment:
Mild to moderate impairment: No dosage adjustment necessary.
Severe impairment: There are no dosage adjustments provided in the manufacturer's labeling; use with caution and closely monitor; exposure is doubled in severe hepatic impairment. Use is contraindicated in the Canadian labeling.

Administration Administer with or without food.

Hazardous agent; use appropriate precautions for handling and disposal (NIOSH 2014 [group 2]).

Monitoring Parameters CBC (baseline and periodically thereafter); ECG (baseline; repeat after initial dose observation period); heart rate, blood pressure and signs and symptoms of bradycardia (hourly for 6 hours following first dose; continued observation (until resolved) required if 6-hour postdose heart rate is either <45 bpm, is lowest post-baseline measurement, or new-onset second degree or higher AV block occurs on repeat ECG); continuous (until symptoms resolved) ECG monitoring if postdose symptomatic bradycardia occurs (overnight continuous ECG in a medical facility and repeat observation period for second dose if pharmacologic intervention for bradycardia necessary)

Initial monitoring procedures (ECG, heart rate, blood pressure) must be repeated for
- treatment interruption of ≥1 day during the first 2 weeks after treatment initiation, or
- treatment interruption of >7 days during weeks 3-4 after treatment initiation, or
- treatment interruption of >14 days after ≥1 month of treatment initiation

Ophthalmologic exam at baseline and 3-4 months after initiation of treatment (continue periodic examinations for duration of therapy in patients with diabetes or history of uveitis); baseline transaminase and bilirubin (obtained ≤6 months prior to treatment initiation), repeat if clinically indicated; respiratory function (FEV_1, DLCO) if clinically indicated; VZV antibodies (patients with no history of chickenpox or previous VZV vaccination); signs and symptoms of infection and/or PRES

Dosage Forms
Capsule, Oral:
Gilenya: 0.5 mg

- **Fioricet** *see* Butalbital, Acetaminophen, and Caffeine *on page 313*
- **Fiorinal®** *see* Butalbital, Aspirin, and Caffeine *on page 314*
- **Firazyr** *see* Icatibant *on page 1037*
- **Firmagon** *see* Degarelix *on page 587*
- **Firmagon® (Can)** *see* Degarelix *on page 587*
- **First-Hydrocortisone** *see* Hydrocortisone (Topical) *on page 1014*
- **First-Lansoprazole** *see* Lansoprazole *on page 1166*
- **First-Omeprazole** *see* Omeprazole *on page 1508*
- **First-Progesterone VGS 25** *see* Progesterone *on page 1722*
- **First-Progesterone VGS 50** *see* Progesterone *on page 1722*
- **First-Progesterone VGS 100** *see* Progesterone *on page 1722*
- **First-Progesterone VGS 200** *see* Progesterone *on page 1722*
- **First-Progesterone VGS 400** *see* Progesterone *on page 1722*
- **First-Testosterone** *see* Testosterone *on page 2010*
- **First-Testosterone MC** *see* Testosterone *on page 2010*
- **First-Vancomycin 25** *see* Vancomycin *on page 2130*
- **First-Vancomycin 50** *see* Vancomycin *on page 2130*
- **Fisalamine** *see* Mesalamine *on page 1301*
- **Fish Oil** *see* Omega-3 Fatty Acids *on page 1507*
- **Fish Oil Ultra [OTC]** *see* Omega-3 Fatty Acids *on page 1507*
- **FK228** *see* RomiDEPsin *on page 1841*
- **FK506** *see* Tacrolimus (Systemic) *on page 1962*
- **Flagyl** *see* MetroNIDAZOLE (Systemic) *on page 1353*
- **Flagyl ER** *see* MetroNIDAZOLE (Systemic) *on page 1353*
- **Flagystatin (Can)** *see* Metronidazole and Nystatin [CAN/INT] *on page 1358*
- **Flamazine® (Can)** *see* Silver Sulfadiazine *on page 1887*
- **Flanax Pain Relief [OTC]** *see* Naproxen *on page 1427*
- **Flarex** *see* Fluorometholone *on page 896*
- **Flarex® (Can)** *see* Fluorometholone *on page 896*

FlavoxATE (fla VOKS ate)

Brand Names: Canada Apo-Flavoxate®; Urispas®
Index Terms Flavoxate Hydrochloride; Urispas
Pharmacologic Category Antispasmodic Agent, Urinary
Additional Appendix Information
Beers Criteria – Potentially Inappropriate Medications for Geriatrics *on page 2271*

Use Antispasmodic to provide symptomatic relief of dysuria, nocturia, suprapubic pain, urgency, and incontinence in patients with cystitis, urethritis, urethrocystitis, urethrotrigonitis, and prostatitis

Pregnancy Risk Factor B

Dosage Children >12 years and Adults: Oral: 100-200 mg 3-4 times daily; reduce the dose when symptoms improve
Dosage adjustment in renal impairment: No dosage adjustment provided in manufacturer's labeling.
Dosage adjustment in hepatic impairment: No dosage adjustment provided in manufacturer's labeling.

Additional Information Complete prescribing information should be consulted for additional detail.

Dosage Forms
Tablet, Oral:
Generic: 100 mg

- **Flavoxate Hydrochloride** *see* FlavoxATE *on page 881*
- **Flebogamma** *see* Immune Globulin *on page 1056*
- **Flebogamma DIF** *see* Immune Globulin *on page 1056*

Flecainide (fle KAY nide)

Brand Names: U.S. Tambocor [DSC]

Brand Names: Canada Apo-Flecainide®; Tambocor™

Index Terms Flecainide Acetate

Pharmacologic Category Antiarrhythmic Agent, Class Ic

Additional Appendix Information

Beers Criteria - Potentially Inappropriate Medications for Geriatrics *on page 2271*

Use Prevention and suppression of documented life-threatening ventricular arrhythmias (eg, sustained ventricular tachycardia); controlling symptomatic, disabling paroxysmal supraventricular tachycardias (including atrial fibrillation) in patients without structural heart disease in whom other agents fail

Pregnancy Risk Factor C

Pregnancy Considerations Adverse events have been observed in some animal reproduction studies.

Breast-Feeding Considerations Flecainide is excreted in human breast milk at concentrations as high as 4 times corresponding plasma levels.

Contraindications Hypersensitivity to flecainide or any component of the formulation; preexisting second- or third-degree AV block or with right bundle branch block when associated with a left hemiblock (bifascicular block) (except in patients with a functioning artificial pacemaker); cardiogenic shock; coronary artery disease (based on CAST study results); concurrent use of ritonavir or amprenavir

Warnings/Precautions [U.S. Boxed Warning]: In the Cardiac Arrhythmia Suppression Trial (CAST), recent (>6 days but <2 years ago) myocardial infarction patients with asymptomatic, non-life-threatening ventricular arrhythmias did not benefit and may have been harmed by attempts to suppress the arrhythmia with flecainide or encainide. An increased mortality or non-fatal cardiac arrest rate (7.7%) was seen in the active treatment group compared with patients in the placebo group (3%). The applicability of the CAST results to other populations is unknown. The risks of class 1C agents and the lack of improved survival make use in patients without life-threatening arrhythmias generally unacceptable. **[U.S. Boxed Warning]: Watch for proarrhythmic effects;** monitor and adjust dose to prevent QTc prolongation. Not recommended for patients with chronic atrial fibrillation. In the treatment of atrial fibrillation in the elderly, avoid antiarrhythmics as first-line treatment. In older adults, data suggests rate control may provide more benefits than risks compared to rhythm control for most patients (Beers Criteria). **[U.S. Boxed Warning]: When treating atrial flutter, 1:1 atrioventricular conduction may occur; pre-emptive negative chronotropic therapy (eg, digoxin, beta-blockers) may lower the risk.** Preexisting hypokalemia or hyperkalemia should be corrected before initiation (can alter drug's effect). A worsening or new arrhythmia may occur (proarrhythmic effect). Use caution in heart failure (may precipitate or exacerbate HF). Dose-related increases in PR, QRS, and QT intervals occur. Use with caution in sick sinus syndrome or with permanent pacemakers or temporary pacing wires (can increase endocardial pacing thresholds). Cautious use in significant hepatic impairment.

Adverse Reactions

Cardiovascular: Chest pain, edema, palpitation, proarrhythmic, sinus node dysfunction, syncope, tachycardia

Central nervous system: Anxiety, ataxia, depression, dizziness, fatigue, fever, headache, hypoesthesia, insomnia, malaise, nervousness, paresis, somnolence, tinnitus, vertigo

Dermatologic: Rash

Gastrointestinal: Abdominal pain, anorexia, constipation, diarrhea, nausea

Neuromuscular & skeletal: Paresthesias, tremor, weakness

Ocular: Blurred vision, diplopia, visual disturbances

Respiratory: Dyspnea

Rare but important or life-threatening: Alopecia, alters pacing threshold, amnesia, angina, AV block, bradycardia, bronchospasm, CHF, corneal deposits, depersonalization, euphoria, exfoliative dermatitis, granulocytopenia, heart block, increased P-R, leukopenia, metallic taste, neuropathy, paradoxical increase in ventricular rate in atrial fibrillation/flutter, paresthesia, photophobia, pneumonitis, pruritus, QRS duration, swollen lips/tongue/mouth, tardive dyskinesia, thrombocytopenia, urinary retention, urticaria, ventricular arrhythmia

Drug Interactions

Metabolism/Transport Effects Substrate of CYP1A2 (minor), CYP2D6 (major); **Note:** Assignment of Major/Minor substrate status based on clinically relevant drug interaction potential; **Inhibits** CYP2D6 (weak)

Avoid Concomitant Use

Avoid concomitant use of Flecainide with any of the following: Fosamprenavir; Highest Risk QTc-Prolonging Agents; Ivabradine; Mifepristone; Ritonavir; Saquinavir; Tipranavir

Increased Effect/Toxicity

Flecainide may increase the levels/effects of: ARIPiprazole; Digoxin; Highest Risk QTc-Prolonging Agents; Moderate Risk QTc-Prolonging Agents

The levels/effects of Flecainide may be increased by: Abiraterone Acetate; Amiodarone; Boceprevir; Carbonic Anhydrase Inhibitors; Cobicistat; CYP2D6 Inhibitors (Moderate); CYP2D6 Inhibitors (Strong); Darunavir; Fosamprenavir; Ivabradine; Mifepristone; Mirabegron; Peginterferon Alfa-2b; QTc-Prolonging Agents (Indeterminate Risk and Risk Modifying); Ritonavir; Saquinavir; Sodium Bicarbonate; Sodium Lactate; Telaprevir; Tipranavir; Tromethamine; Verapamil

Decreased Effect

The levels/effects of Flecainide may be decreased by: Etravirine; Peginterferon Alfa-2b; Sodium Bicarbonate

Food Interactions Clearance may be decreased in patients following strict vegetarian diets due to urinary pH ≥8. Dairy products (milk, infant formula, yogurt) may interfere with the absorption of flecainide in infants; there is one case report of a neonate (GA 34 weeks PNA >6 days) who required extremely large doses of oral flecainide when administered every 8 hours with feedings ("milk feeds"); changing the feedings from "milk feeds" to 5% glucose feeds alone resulted in a doubling of the flecainide serum concentration and toxicity.

Mechanism of Action Class Ic antiarrhythmic; slows conduction in cardiac tissue by altering transport of ions across cell membranes; causes slight prolongation of refractory periods; decreases the rate of rise of the action potential without affecting its duration; increases electrical stimulation threshold of ventricle, His-Purkinje system; possesses local anesthetic and moderate negative inotropic effects

Pharmacodynamics/Kinetics

Absorption: Oral: Rapid

Distribution: Adults: V_d: 5-13.4 L/kg

Protein binding: $Alpha_1$ acid glycoprotein: 40% to 50%

Metabolism: Hepatic

Bioavailability: 85% to 90%

Half-life elimination: Infants: 11-12 hours; Children: 8 hours; Adults: 7-22 hours, increased with congestive heart failure or renal dysfunction; End-stage renal disease: 19-26 hours

Time to peak, serum: ~1.5-3 hours

Excretion: Urine (80% to 90%, 10% to 50% as unchanged drug and metabolites)

Dosage Oral:

Children:

Initial: 3 mg/kg/day or 50 to 100 mg/m²/day in 3 divided doses

Usual: 3-6 mg/kg/day or 100 to 150 mg/m²/day in 3 divided doses; up to 11 mg/kg/day or 200 mg/m²/day for uncontrolled patients with subtherapeutic levels

Adults:

Life-threatening ventricular arrhythmias:

Initial: 100 mg every 12 hours

Increase by 50 to 100 mg/day (given in 2 doses/day) every 4 days; maximum: 400 mg/day.

Use of higher initial doses and more rapid dosage adjustments have resulted in an increased incidence of proarrhythmic events and congestive heart failure, particularly during the first few days. Do not use a loading dose. Use very cautiously in patients with history of congestive heart failure or myocardial infarction.

Paroxysmal supraventricular arrhythmias (eg, PSVT, atrial fibrillation) without structural heart disease (maintenance of sinus rhythm): Initial: 50 mg every 12 hours; increase by 50 mg twice daily at 4-day intervals; maximum: 300 mg per day. The AHA/ACC/HRS atrial fibrillation guidelines recommend a maximum dose of 400 mg per day (January, 2014).

Atrial fibrillation or flutter (pharmacological cardioversion) (off-label dose): Outpatient: "Pill-in-the-pocket" dose: 200 mg (weight <70 kg), 300 mg (weight ≥70 kg). May not repeat in ≤24 hours (Alboni, 2004; AHA/ACC/HRS [January, 2014]). **Note:** An initial inpatient cardioversion trial should have been successful before sending patient home on this approach. Patient must be taking an AV nodal-blocking agent (eg, beta-blocker, nondihydropyridine calcium channel blocker) prior to initiation of antiarrhythmic.

Dosing adjustment in severe renal impairment: GFR ≤50 mL/minute: Decrease dose by 50%; dose increases should be made cautiously at intervals >4 days and serum levels monitored frequently.

Hemodialysis: No supplemental dose recommended.

Peritoneal dialysis: No supplemental dose recommended.

Dosing adjustment/comments in hepatic impairment: Monitoring of plasma levels is recommended because of significantly increased half-life.

When transferring from another antiarrhythmic agent, allow for 2 to 4 half-lives of the agent to pass before initiating flecainide therapy.

Administration Administer around-the-clock to promote less variation in peak and trough serum levels

Monitoring Parameters ECG, blood pressure, pulse, periodic serum concentrations, especially in patients with renal or hepatic impairment

Reference Range Therapeutic: 0.2-1 mcg/mL; pediatric patients may respond at the lower end of the recommended therapeutic range

Dosage Forms

Tablet, Oral:

Generic: 50 mg, 100 mg, 150 mg

Extemporaneous Preparations A 20 mg/mL oral liquid suspension may be made from tablets and one of three different vehicles (cherry syrup, a 1:1 mixture of Ora-Sweet® and Ora-Plus®, or a 1:1 mixture of Ora-Sweet® SF and Ora-Plus®). Crush twenty-four 100 mg tablets in a mortar and reduce to a fine powder. Add 20 mL of the chosen vehicle and mix to a uniform paste; mix while adding the vehicle in incremental proportions to **almost** 120 mL; transfer to a calibrated bottle, rinse mortar with vehicle, and add quantity of vehicle sufficient to make 120 mL. Label "shake well" and "protect from light". Stable for 60 days when stored in amber plastic prescription bottles in the dark at room temperature or refrigerated.

Allen LV and Erickson III MA, "Stability of Baclofen, Captopril, Diltiazem, Hydrochloride, Dipyridamole, and Flecainide Acetate in Extemporaneously Compounded Oral Liquids," *Am J Health Syst Pharm*, 1996, 53:2179-84.

- **Flecainide Acetate** *see* Flecainide *on page 882*
- **Fleet Bisacodyl [OTC]** *see* Bisacodyl *on page 265*
- **Fleet Enema [OTC]** *see* Sodium Phosphates *on page 1909*
- **Fleet Enema (Can)** *see* Sodium Phosphates *on page 1909*
- **Fleet Enema Extra [OTC]** *see* Sodium Phosphates *on page 1909*
- **Fleet Laxative [OTC]** *see* Bisacodyl *on page 265*
- **Fleet Pedia-Lax Enema [OTC]** *see* Sodium Phosphates *on page 1909*
- **Flexbumin** *see* Albumin *on page 67*
- **Flexeril** *see* Cyclobenzaprine *on page 516*
- **Floctafenina** *see* Floctafenine [CAN/INT] *on page 883*

Floctafenine [CAN/INT] (flok ta FEN een)

Index Terms Floctafenina; Floctafeninum

Pharmacologic Category Nonsteroidal Anti-inflammatory Drug (NSAID), Oral

Use Note: Not approved in U.S.

Short-term management of acute, mild-to-moderate pain

Pregnancy Considerations Floctafenic acid (active metabolite) crosses the placenta; therefore, the benefits of use must be weighed against risk to mother and fetus. In late pregnancy, NSAIDs may cause premature closure of the ductus arteriosus.

Breast-Feeding Considerations Floctafenic acid, the active metabolite of floctafenine, is excreted into breast milk. Breast-feeding is not recommended by the manufacturer.

Contraindications Hypersensitivity to floctafenine, aspirin, other NSAIDS, or any component of the formulation; active peptic ulcer or a history of ulcerative disease; inflammatory gastrointestinal disease; severe cardiac insufficiency or ischemic cardiomyopathy; significant hepatic impairment or active liver disease; severely impaired (CrCl <30 mL/minute) or deteriorating renal function; concurrent use with other NSAIDS; severe heart failure, coronary heart disease; concurrent use with beta-blockers; nasal polyp syndrome (complete or partial); patients who experience "aspirin triad" (bronchial asthma, rhinitis complicated by polyps, aspirin intolerance) with aspirin or NSAID therapy

Warnings/Precautions NSAIDs are associated with an increased risk of adverse cardiovascular events, including MI, stroke, and new onset or worsening of preexisting hypertension. Risk may be increased with duration of use or preexisting cardiovascular risk factors or disease. Carefully evaluate individual cardiovascular risk profiles prior to prescribing. Use caution with fluid retention. Avoid use in heart failure. Use is contraindicated with severe cardiac insufficiency. Use of NSAIDs is not recommended for treatment of perioperative pain in the setting of coronary artery bypass graft (CABG) surgery. Risk of MI and stroke may be increased with use following CABG surgery.

NSAIDS may increase risk of gastrointestinal irritation, inflammation, ulceration, perforation, and bleeding. These events can sometimes be severe and occasionally fatal, and can occur at any time during therapy and without warning. If ulceration is suspected or confirmed, or if bleeding occurs, discontinue use. Elderly and debilitated patients are more susceptible to adverse GI effects of

NSAIDS. Lower dosing and close monitoring of these patients may be required. Use caution with excessive alcohol intake, smoking, concurrent therapy with aspirin, anticoagulants, and/or corticosteroids. Use is contraindicated in patients with active peptic ulcer, history of ulcer disease, or inflammatory GI disease. When used concomitantly with ≤325 mg of aspirin, a substantial increase in the risk of gastrointestinal complications (eg, ulcer) occurs; concomitant gastroprotective therapy (eg, proton pump inhibitors) is recommended (Bhatt, 2008).

Use of lowest effective dose and for shortest duration of time, consistent with individual patient goals, to reduce risk of cardiovascular or GI adverse events. Alternate therapies should be considered for patients at high risk.

Platelet adhesion and aggregation may be decreased; may prolong bleeding time; patients with coagulation disorders or who are receiving anticoagulants should be monitored closely. Anemia may occur; patients on long-term NSAID therapy should be monitored for anemia. Rarely, NSAID use may cause severe blood dyscrasias (eg, agranulocytosis, aplastic anemia, thrombocytopenia).

NSAID use may compromise existing renal function; dose-dependent decreases in prostaglandin synthesis may result from NSAID use, reducing renal blood flow which may cause renal decompensation. NSAID use may increase the risk for hyperkalemia. Patients with impaired renal function, dehydration, heart failure, liver dysfunction, those taking diuretics, and ACE inhibitors, and the elderly are at greater risk of renal toxicity and hyperkalemia. Rehydrate patient before starting therapy; monitor renal function closely. Contraindicated in patients with deteriorating function or severe impairment (CrCl <30 mL/minute). Long-term NSAID use may result in renal papillary necrosis.

Use caution in hepatic disease; contraindicated in patients with severe or active impairment. Although rare, severe reactions including jaundice and reports of fatal hepatitis have been associated with NSAID use. Closely monitor patients with any abnormal LFT. Discontinue use if signs or symptoms of liver disease develop, or if systemic manifestations occur.

NSAIDS may cause drowsiness, dizziness, blurred vision and other neurologic effects which may impair physical or mental abilities; patients must be cautioned about performing tasks which require mental alertness (eg, operating machinery or driving). Discontinue use with blurred or diminished vision and perform ophthalmologic exam. Monitor vision with long-term therapy.

Symptoms of aseptic meningitis have been observed with NSAID therapy. Patients with autoimmune disorders may be more predisposed. NSAIDS may cause serious skin adverse events including exfoliative dermatitis, Stevens-Johnson syndrome (SJS), and toxic epidermal necrolysis (TEN); discontinue use at first sign of skin rash or hypersensitivity. Anaphylactoid reactions may occur even without prior exposure; patients with "aspirin triad" (bronchial asthma, aspirin intolerance, rhinitis) may be at increased risk. Do not use in patients who experience bronchospasm, asthma, rhinitis, or urticaria with NSAID or aspirin therapy. Use caution in other forms of asthma.

Safety and efficacy in children have not been established.

Withhold for at least 4-6 half-lives prior to surgical or dental procedures.

Adverse Reactions

Cardiovascular: Edema, flushing, tachycardia

Central nervous system: Depression, dizziness, drowsiness, fatigue, headache, insomnia, irritability, malaise, nervousness, vertigo

Dermatologic: Angioedema, pruritus, rash, urticaria

Endocrine & metabolic: Fluid retention, hyperkalemia

Gastrointestinal: Abdominal pain, bitter taste, constipation, diarrhea, dyspepsia, flatulence, gastrointestinal bleeding, gastrointestinal ulcer, gross bleeding with perforation, heartburn, nausea, vomiting, xerostomia

Hematologic: Agranulocytosis, aplastic anemia, bleeding, leukopenia, neutropenia, thrombocytopenia

Hepatic: Hepatotoxicity, liver enzymes increased

Ocular: Blurred and/or diminished vision

Otic: Tinnitus

Renal: Burning micturition, cystitis, dysuria, hematuria, interstitial nephritis, polyuria, reversible acute renal insufficiency with or without oliguria/anuria, strong smelling urine, urethritis

Respiratory: Asthmatic-type dyspnea

Miscellaneous: Anaphylaxis, diaphoresis, thirst

Drug Interactions

Metabolism/Transport Effects None known.

Avoid Concomitant Use

Avoid concomitant use of Floctafenine with any of the following: Aspirin; Beta-Blockers; Dexketoprofen; Ketorolac (Nasal); Ketorolac (Systemic); Nonsteroidal Anti-Inflammatory Agents; Omacetaxine; Urokinase

Increased Effect/Toxicity

Floctafenine may increase the levels/effects of: 5-ASA Derivatives; Agents with Antiplatelet Properties; Aliskiren; Aminoglycosides; Anticoagulants; Apixaban; Aspirin; Beta-Blockers; Bisphosphonate Derivatives; Collagenase (Systemic); CycloSPORINE (Systemic); Dabigatran Etexilate; Deferasirox; Desmopressin; Digoxin; Eplerenone; Haloperidol; Ibritumomab; Lithium; Methotrexate; Nonsteroidal Anti-Inflammatory Agents; Obinutuzumab; Omacetaxine; PEMEtrexed; Porfimer; Potassium-Sparing Diuretics; PRALAtrexate; Quinolone Antibiotics; Rivaroxaban; Salicylates; Tacrolimus (Systemic); Tenofovir; Thrombolytic Agents; Tositumomab and Iodine I 131 Tositumomab; Urokinase; Vancomycin; Verteporfin; Vitamin K Antagonists

The levels/effects of Floctafenine may be increased by: ACE Inhibitors; Angiotensin II Receptor Blockers; Antidepressants (Tricyclic, Tertiary Amine); Corticosteroids (Systemic); CycloSPORINE (Systemic); Dasatinib; Dexketoprofen; Glucosamine; Herbs (Anticoagulant/Antiplatelet Properties); Ibrutinib; Ketorolac (Nasal); Ketorolac (Systemic); Limaprost; Multivitamins/Fluoride (with ADE); Multivitamins/Minerals (with ADEK, Folate, Iron); Multivitamins/Minerals (with AE, No Iron); Omega-3 Fatty Acids; Pentosan Polysulfate Sodium; Pentoxifylline; Probenecid; Prostacyclin Analogues; Selective Serotonin Reuptake Inhibitors; Serotonin/Norepinephrine Reuptake Inhibitors; Sodium Phosphates; Tipranavir; Treprostinil; Vitamin E

Decreased Effect

Floctafenine may decrease the levels/effects of: ACE Inhibitors; Aliskiren; Angiotensin II Receptor Blockers; Aspirin; Eplerenone; HydrALAZINE; Loop Diuretics; Potassium-Sparing Diuretics; Prostaglandins (Ophthalmic); Salicylates; Selective Serotonin Reuptake Inhibitors; Thiazide Diuretics

The levels/effects of Floctafenine may be decreased by: Bile Acid Sequestrants; Salicylates

Storage/Stability Store at 15°C to 30°C (59°F to 86°F). Protect from light.

Mechanism of Action Reversibly inhibits cyclooxygenase-1 and 2 (COX-1 and 2) enzymes, which results in decreased formation of prostaglandin precursors; has antipyretic, analgesic, and anti-inflammatory properties

Other proposed mechanisms not fully elucidated (and possibly contributing to the anti-inflammatory effect to varying degrees), include inhibiting chemotaxis, altering lymphocyte activity, inhibiting neutrophil aggregation/activation, and decreasing proinflammatory cytokine levels.

Pharmacodynamics/Kinetics

Duration: 6-8 hours

Absorption: Rapid, well absorbed

Metabolism: Hepatic

Half-life elimination: Initial phase (distribution): 1 hour; second phase (elimination): 8 hours

Time to peak, plasma: 1-2 hours

Excretion: Feces and bile (60%); urine (40%)

Dosage Oral:

Children: Dosage not established; use not recommended

Adults: 200-400 mg every 6-8 hours as needed, up to a maximum of 1200 mg/day

Elderly/debilitated: Initiate therapy with lower than usual adult starting dose; adjust dose when necessary and under close observation

Dosage adjustment in renal impairment: Although no specific recommendations are given, initial doses should be lower than usual adult starting doses; individual adjustments to dose should be made when necessary and under close supervision.

Dosage adjustment in hepatic impairment: Use with caution and under close supervision.

Dietary Considerations Should be taken with food with a glass of water.

Administration Administer after food or meal with glass of water.

Monitoring Parameters CBC, liver function tests, renal function (including bun and creatinine); edema; GI effects (eg, abdominal pain, dyspepsia, bleeding); vision

Additional Information No interactions have been noted with concomitant administration of antacids.

Product Availability Not available in U.S.

Dosage Forms: Canada

Tablet, Oral: 200 mg, 400 mg

- **Floctafeninum** *see* Floctafenine [CAN/INT] *on page 883*
- **Flolan** *see* Epoprostenol *on page 746*
- **Flomax** *see* Tamsulosin *on page 1974*
- **Flomax CR (Can)** *see* Tamsulosin *on page 1974*
- **Flonase [DSC]** *see* Fluticasone (Nasal) *on page 910*
- **Flonase (Can)** *see* Fluticasone (Nasal) *on page 910*
- **Flonase Allergy Relief** *see* Fluticasone (Nasal) *on page 910*
- **Flonase Allergy Relief [OTC]** *see* Fluticasone (Nasal) *on page 910*
- **Flo-Pred** *see* PrednisoLONE (Systemic) *on page 1703*
- **Florical [OTC]** *see* Calcium Carbonate *on page 327*
- **Florinef** *see* Fludrocortisone *on page 891*
- **Florinef® (Can)** *see* Fludrocortisone *on page 891*
- **Flovent** *see* Fluticasone (Oral Inhalation) *on page 907*
- **Flovent Diskus** *see* Fluticasone (Oral Inhalation) *on page 907*
- **Flovent HFA** *see* Fluticasone (Oral Inhalation) *on page 907*
- **Floxin Otic Singles** *see* Ofloxacin (Otic) *on page 1491*
- **Fluad (Can)** *see* Influenza Virus Vaccine (Inactivated) *on page 1075*
- **Fluanxol® (Can)** *see* Flupentixol [CAN/INT] *on page 903*
- **Fluanxol® Depot (Can)** *see* Flupentixol [CAN/INT] *on page 903*
- **Fluarix** *see* Influenza Virus Vaccine (Inactivated) *on page 1075*
- **Fluarix Quadrivalent** *see* Influenza Virus Vaccine (Inactivated) *on page 1075*
- **Flubenisolone** *see* Betamethasone (Systemic) *on page 253*
- **Flucaine** *see* Proparacaine and Fluorescein *on page 1728*
- **Flucelvax** *see* Influenza Virus Vaccine (Inactivated) *on page 1075*
- **Flucinom** *see* Flutamide *on page 907*

Flucloxacillin [INT] (flu cloks a SIL in)

International Brand Names Aofolin (CN); Flopen (AU); Floxapen (AE, AT, AU, BE, CH, GB, GR, KW, MX, NL, PT, SA, VE, ZA); Floxin (KR); Flucil (NZ); Fluclox (DE, PH); Flucloxil (MY); Flucloxin (NZ); Genaflox (VN); Geriflox (IE); Heracillin (DK, SE); Kun Te (CN); Neoflox (IN); Ramaxir (TR); Staphlex (NZ); Staphycid (BE); Staphylex (AU, DE); Yifen (CN)

Index Terms Flucloxacillin Sodium

Pharmacologic Category Antibiotic, Penicillin

Reported Use Treatment of susceptible infections due to gram-positive organisms, including Beta-lactamase-producing Staphylococci

Dosage Range

Oral: **Note:** Take at least 30 minutes before food:

Children <2 years: 62.5 mg every 6 hours

Children 2-10 years: 125 mg every 6 hours

Adults: 250-500 mg every 6 hours

IM: Adults: 250 mg every 6 hours

IV: Adults: 250 mg-2 g every 6 hours

Product Availability Product available in various countries; not currently available in the U.S.

Dosage Forms

Capsule: 250 mg, 500 mg

Injection, powder for reconstitution: 250 mg, 500 mg

Solution, oral: 125 mg/5 mL (100 mL)

- **Flucloxacillin Sodium** *see* Flucloxacillin [INT] *on page 885*

Fluconazole (floo KOE na zole)

Brand Names: U.S. Diflucan

Brand Names: Canada ACT Fluconazole; Apo-Fluconazole; CanesOral; CO Fluconazole; Diflucan; Diflucan injection; Diflucan One; Diflucan PWS; Dom-Fluconazole; Fluconazole Injection; Fluconazole Injection SDZ; Fluconazole Omega; Monicure; Mylan-Fluconazole; Novo-Fluconazole; PHL-Fluconazole; PMS-Fluconazole; PRO-Fluconazole; Riva-Fluconazole; Taro-Fluconazole

Pharmacologic Category Antifungal Agent, Oral; Antifungal Agent, Parenteral

Use Treatment of candidiasis (esophageal, oropharyngeal, peritoneal, urinary tract, vaginal); systemic candida infections (eg, candidemia, disseminated candidiasis, and pneumonia); cryptococcal meningitis; antifungal prophylaxis in allogeneic bone marrow transplant recipients

Pregnancy Risk Factor C (single dose for vaginal candidiasis)/D (all other indications)

Pregnancy Considerations Adverse events have been observed in some animal reproduction studies. When used in high doses, fluconazole is teratogenic in animal studies. Following exposure during the first trimester, case reports have noted similar malformations in humans when used in higher doses (400 mg/day) over extended periods of time (Aleck, 1997). Abnormalities reported include abnormal facies, abnormal calvarial development, arthrogryposis, brachycephaly, cleft palate, congenital heart disease, femoral bowing, thin ribs and long bones. Use of lower doses (150 mg as a single dose) does not suggest an increase risk to the fetus. Most azole antifungals, including fluconazole, are recommended to be avoided during pregnancy (Pappas, 2009).

Breast-Feeding Considerations Fluconazole is excreted in breast milk. The manufacturer recommends that caution be exercised when administering fluconazole to nursing women. Fluconazole is found in breast milk at concentrations similar to maternal plasma.

Contraindications Hypersensitivity to fluconazole or any component of the formulation (cross-reaction with other azole antifungal agents may occur, but has not been established; use caution); coadministration of terfenadine in adult patients receiving multiple doses of 400 mg or higher or with CYP3A4 substrates which may lead to QTc prolongation (eg, astemizole, cisapride, erythromycin, pimozide, or quinidine)

Warnings/Precautions Hazardous agent; use appropriate precautions for handling and disposal (NIOSH 2014 [group 3]). Serious (and sometimes fatal) hepatic toxicity (eg, hepatitis, cholestasis, fulminant hepatic failure) has been observed. Use with caution in patients with renal and hepatic dysfunction or previous hepatotoxicity from other azole derivatives. Patients who develop abnormal liver function tests during fluconazole therapy should be monitored closely and discontinued if symptoms consistent with liver disease develop. Rare exfoliative skin disorders have been observed; fatal outcomes have been reported in patients with serious concomitant diseases. Monitor patients with deep seated fungal infections closely for rash development and discontinue if lesions progress. In patients with superficial fungal infections who develop a rash attributable to fluconazole, treatment should also be discontinued. Cases of QTc prolongation and torsade de pointes associated with fluconazole use have been reported (usually high dose or in combination with agents known to prolong the QT interval); use caution in patients with concomitant medications or conditions which are arrhythmogenic. Potentially significant drug-drug interactions may exist, requiring dose or frequency adjustment, additional monitoring, and/or selection of alternative therapy. May occasionally cause dizziness or seizures; use caution driving or operating machines.

Powder for oral suspension contains sucrose; use caution with fructose intolerance, sucrose-isomaltase deficiency, or glucose-galactose malabsorption.

Benzyl alcohol and derivatives: Some dosage forms may contain sodium benzoate/benzoic acid; benzoic acid (benzoate) is a metabolite of benzyl alcohol; large amounts of benzyl alcohol (≥99 mg/kg/day) have been associated with a potentially fatal toxicity ("gasping syndrome") in neonates; the "gasping syndrome" consists of metabolic acidosis, respiratory distress, gasping respirations, CNS dysfunction (including convulsions, intracranial hemorrhage), hypotension, and cardiovascular collapse (AAP, 1997; CDC, 1982); some data suggests that benzoate displaces bilirubin from protein binding sites (Ahlfors, 2001); avoid or use dosage forms containing benzyl alcohol derivative with caution in neonates. See manufacturer's labeling.

Adverse Reactions

Cardiovascular: Angioedema (rare)

Central nervous system: Dizziness, headache

Dermatologic: Rash

Gastrointestinal: Abdominal pain, diarrhea, dysgeusia, dyspepsia, nausea, vomiting

Hepatic: Alkaline phosphatase increased, ALT increased, AST increased, hepatic failure (rare), hepatitis, jaundice

Miscellaneous: Anaphylactic reactions (rare)

Rare but important or life-threatening: Agranulocytosis, alopecia, cholestasis, diaphoresis, drug eruption, exanthematous pustulosis, fatigue, fever, hypercholesterolemia, hypertriglyceridemia, hypokalemia, insomnia, leukopenia, malaise, myalgia, neutropenia, paresthesia, QT prolongation, seizure, somnolence, Stevens-Johnson syndrome, thrombocytopenia, torsade de pointes, toxic epidermal necrolysis, tremor, vertigo, weakness, xerostomia

Drug Interactions

Metabolism/Transport Effects Inhibits CYP1A2 (weak), CYP2C19 (strong), CYP2C9 (moderate), CYP3A4 (moderate)

Avoid Concomitant Use

Avoid concomitant use of Fluconazole with any of the following: Bosutinib; Cisapride; Citalopram; Conivaptan; Erythromycin (Systemic); Highest Risk QTc-Prolonging Agents; Ibrutinib; Ivabradine; Lomitapide; Mifepristone; Naloxegol; Olaparib; Ospemifene; Pimozide; QuiNIDine; Ranolazine; Saccharomyces boulardii; Simeprevir; Tolvaptan; Trabectedin; Ulipristal; Voriconazole

Increased Effect/Toxicity

Fluconazole may increase the levels/effects of: Alfentanil; Amitriptyline; ARIPiprazole; AtorvaSTATin; Avanafil; Bosentan; Bosutinib; Budesonide (Systemic, Oral Inhalation); BusPIRone; Busulfan; Calcium Channel Blockers; Cannabis; CarBAMazepine; Carvedilol; Cilostazol; Cisapride; Citalopram; Colchicine; Conivaptan; CycloSPORINE (Systemic); CYP2C19 Substrates; CYP2C9 Substrates; CYP3A4 Substrates; Dapoxetine; DOCEtaxel; DOXOrubicin (Conventional); Dronabinol; Eletriptan; Eplerenone; Erythromycin (Systemic); Etravirine; Everolimus; FentaNYL; Fluvastatin; Fosphenytoin; Highest Risk QTc-Prolonging Agents; Hydrocodone; Ibrutinib; Imatinib; Ivabradine; Ivacaftor; Lomitapide; Lovastatin; Lurasidone; Macrolide Antibiotics; Methadone; Moderate Risk QTc-Prolonging Agents; Naloxegol; Nevirapine; Olaparib; Ospemifene; OxyCODONE; Phenytoin; Pimecrolimus; Pimozide; PredniSONE; Proton Pump Inhibitors; QuiNIDine; Ramelteon; Ranolazine; Red Yeast Rice; Rifamycin Derivatives; Rivaroxaban; Ruxolitinib; Salmeterol; Saxagliptin; Sildenafil; Simeprevir; Simvastatin; Sirolimus; Solifenacin; Sulfonylureas; SUNItinib; Suvorexant; Tacrolimus (Systemic); Tadalafil; Temsirolimus; Tetrahydrocannabinol; Tipranavir; Tofacitinib; Tolvaptan; Trabectedin; Ulipristal; Vardenafil; Vilazodone; Vitamin K Antagonists; Voriconazole; Zidovudine; Zolpidem; Zopiclone

The levels/effects of Fluconazole may be increased by: Amitriptyline; Etravirine; Ivabradine; Macrolide Antibiotics; Mifepristone; QTc-Prolonging Agents (Indeterminate Risk and Risk Modifying)

Decreased Effect

Fluconazole may decrease the levels/effects of: Amphotericin B; Clopidogrel; Ifosfamide; Losartan; Saccharomyces boulardii

The levels/effects of Fluconazole may be decreased by: Didanosine; Etravirine; Rifamycin Derivatives

Storage/Stability

Tablet: Store at <30°C (86°F).

Powder for oral suspension: Store dry powder at <30°C (86°F). Following reconstitution, store at 5°C to 30°C (41°F to 86°F). Discard unused portion after 2 weeks. Do not freeze.

Injection: Store injection in glass at 5°C to 30°C (41°F to 86°F). Store injection in plastic flexible containers at 5°C to 25°C (41°F to 77°F). Brief exposure of up to 40°C (104°F) does not adversely affect the product. Do not freeze. Do not unwrap unit until ready for use.

Mechanism of Action Interferes with fungal cytochrome P450 activity (lanosterol 14-α-demethylase), decreasing ergosterol synthesis (principal sterol in fungal cell membrane) and inhibiting cell membrane formation

Pharmacodynamics/Kinetics

Distribution: V_d: ~0.6 L/kg; widely throughout body with good penetration into CSF, eye, peritoneal fluid, sputum, skin, and urine

Relative diffusion blood into CSF: Adequate with or without inflammation (exceeds usual MICs)

CSF:blood level ratio: Normal meninges: 50% to 90%; Inflamed meninges: ~80%

Protein binding, plasma: 11% to 12%

Bioavailability: Oral: >90%

Half-life elimination: Normal renal function: ~30 hours (range: 20-50 hours); Elderly: ~46 hours

Time to peak, serum: Oral: 1-2 hours

Excretion: Urine (80% as unchanged drug)

Dosage The daily dose of fluconazole is the same for oral and IV administration

Usual dosage ranges: Oral, IV:

Children: Loading dose: 6 to 12 mg/kg/dose; maintenance: 3 to 12 mg/kg/dose once daily; duration and dosage depend on location and severity of infection

Adults: 150 mg once **or** Loading dose: 200 to 800 mg; maintenance: 200 to 800 mg once daily; duration and dosage depend on location and severity of infection

Indication-specific dosing:

Children:

Candidiasis: Oral, IV:

Esophageal:

Manufacturer's recommendation: Loading dose: 6 mg/kg/dose; maintenance: 3 to 12 mg/kg/dose once daily for 21 days and for at least 2 weeks following resolution of symptoms (maximum: 600 mg/day)

HIV-exposed/-infected: Loading dose: 6 mg/kg/dose once on day 1; maintenance: 3 to 6 mg/kg/dose once daily for 4 to 21 days (maximum: 400 mg/day) (CDC, 2009)

Relapse suppression (HIV-exposed/-infected): 3 to 6 mg/kg/dose once daily (maximum: 200 mg/day) (CDC, 2009)

Invasive disease (alternative therapy): 5 to 6 mg/kg/dose every 12 hours for ≥28 days (maximum: 600 mg/day) (CDC, 2009)

Oropharyngeal:

Manufacturer's recommendation: Loading dose: 6 mg/kg/dose; maintenance: 3 mg/kg/dose once daily for ≥2 weeks (maximum: 600 mg/day)

HIV-exposed/-infected: 3 to 6 mg/kg/dose once daily for 7 to 14 days (maximum: 400 mg/day) (CDC, 2009)

Surgical (perioperative) prophylaxis in high-risk patients undergoing liver, pancreas, kidney, or pancreas-kidney transplantation (off-label use): IV: 6 mg/kg given in the perioperative period and continued in the postoperative period for ≤28 days (maximum dose 400 mg). Time of initiation and duration varies with transplant type and operative protocol (Bratzler, 2013).

Coccidioidomycosis: Oral, IV: *Meningeal infection, or in a stable patient with diffuse pulmonary or disseminated disease* (HIV-exposed/-infected):

Treatment: 5 to 6 mg/kg/dose twice daily (maximum daily dose: 800 mg/**day**) (CDC, 2009), followed by chronic suppressive therapy (see below)

Relapse suppression: 6 mg/kg/dose once daily (maximum daily dose: 400 mg/**day**) (CDC, 2009)

Cryptococcosis: Oral, IV:

Manufacturer's recommendation: Meningitis: 12 mg/kg/dose for 1 dose, then 6 to 12 mg/kg/day for 10 to 12 weeks following negative CSF culture

HIV-exposed/-infected:

CNS disease (alternative therapy in patients intolerant of amphotericin B): Induction: 12 mg/kg/dose for 1 dose, then 6-12 mg/kg/day (maximum: 800 mg/day) for ≥2 weeks (in combination with flucytosine) (CDC, 2009)

Consolidation: 10 to 12 mg/kg/day for 8 weeks (Perfect, 2010) **or** 12 mg/kg/dose for 1 dose, then 6 to 12 mg/kg/day (maximum: 800 mg/day) for 8 weeks (CDC, 2009)

Maintenance (suppression): 6 mg/kg/day (maximum: 200 mg/day) (CDC, 2009; Perfect, 2010)

Non-CNS disease, disseminated (including severe pulmonary disease) (alternative therapy; off-label use): Induction: 12 mg/kg/dose for 1 dose, then 6 to 12 mg/kg/day (maximum: 600 mg/day) (CDC, 2009)

Non-CNS disease, localized (including isolated pulmonary disease) (off-label use): 12 mg/kg/dose for 1 dose, then 6 to 12 mg/kg/day (maximum: 600 mg/day). **Note:** Duration depends upon infection site and severity (CDC, 2009). For patients with pulmonary disease (not delineated by severity), the IDSA recommends a duration of 6 to 12 months (Perfect, 2010).

Primary antifungal prophylaxis in pediatric oncology patients (guideline recommendations; Science, 2014): Oral, IV:

Allogeneic hematopoietic stem cell transplant (HSCT): Infants ≥1 month, Children, and Adolescents <19 years: 6 to 12 mg/kg/day (maximum: 400 mg/day), begin at the start of conditioning; continue until engraftment

Allogeneic HSCT with grades 2 to 4 acute graft-versus-host-disease (GVHD) or chronic extensive GVHD: Begin with GVHD diagnosis, continue until GVHD resolves:

Infants ≥1 month and Children <13 years: 6 to 12 mg/kg/day (maximum: 400 mg/day)

Adolescents ≥13 years (where posaconazole is contraindicated): 6 to 12 mg/kg/day (maximum: 400 mg/day)

Autologous HSCT with neutropenia anticipated >7 days: Infants ≥1 month, Children, and Adolescents <19 years: 6 to 12 mg/kg/day (maximum: 400 mg/day), begin at the start of conditioning; continue until engraftment

Acute myeloid leukemia (AML) or myelodysplastic syndromes (MDS): Infants ≥1 month, Children, and Adolescents <19 years: 6 to 12 mg/kg/day (maximum: 400 mg/day) during chemotherapy associated neutropenia; alternative antifungals may be suggested for children ≥13 years in centers with a high local incidence of mold infections or if fluconazole is not available

Adults:

Blastomycosis (off-label use): Oral: *CNS disease:* Consolidation: 800 mg daily for ≥12 months and until resolution of CSF abnormalities (Chapman, 2008)

Candidiasis: Oral, IV:

Candidemia (neutropenic and non-neutropenic): Loading dose: 800 mg (12 mg/kg) on day 1, then 400 mg daily (6 mg/kg/day) for 14 days after first negative blood culture and resolution of signs/symptoms. **Note:** Not recommended for patients with recent azole exposure, critical illness, or if *C. krusei* or *C. glabrata* are suspected (Pappas, 2009).

Chronic, disseminated: 400 mg daily (6 mg/kg/day) until calcification or lesion resolution (Pappas, 2009)

CNS candidiasis (alternative therapy): 400 to 800 mg daily (6 to 12 mg/kg/day) until CSF/radiological abnormalities resolved. **Note:** Recommended as alternative therapy in patients intolerant of amphotericin B (Pappas, 2009).

Endocarditis, prosthetic valve (off to label use): 400 to 800 mg daily (6 to 12 mg/kg/day) for 6 weeks after valve replacement (as step-down in stable, culture-negative patients); long-term suppression in absence of valve replacement: 400 to 800 mg daily (Pappas, 2009)

Endophthalmitis (off-label use): 400 to 800 mg daily (6 to 12 mg/kg/day) for 4-6 weeks until examination indicates resolution (Pappas, 2009)

Esophageal:

Manufacturer's recommendation: Loading dose: 200 mg on day 1, then maintenance dose of 100 to 400 mg daily for 21 days and for at least 2 weeks following resolution of symptoms

Alternative dosing: 200 to 400 mg daily for 14 to 21 days; suppressive therapy of 100 to 200 mg 3 times weekly may be used for recurrent infections (Pappas, 2009)

Intertrigo (off-label use): 50 mg daily or 150 mg once weekly (Coldiron, 1991; Nozickova, 1998; Stengel, 1994)

Oropharyngeal:

Manufacturer's recommendation: Loading dose: 200 mg on day 1; maintenance dose 100 mg daily for ≥2 weeks. **Note:** Therapy with 100 mg daily is associated with resistance development (Rex, 1995).

Alternative dosing: 100 to 200 mg daily for 7 to 14 days for uncomplicated, moderate-to-severe disease; chronic therapy of 100 mg 3 times weekly is recommended in immunocompromised patients with history of oropharyngeal candidiasis (OPC) (Pappas, 2009)

Osteoarticular: 400 mg daily for 6 to 12 months (osteomyelitis) or 6 weeks (septic arthritis) (Pappas, 2009)

Pacemaker (or ICD, VAD) infection (off-label use): 400 to 800 mg daily (6 to 12 mg/kg/day) for 4 to 6 weeks after device removal (as step-down in stable, culture-negative patients); long-term suppression when VAD cannot be removed: 400 to 800 mg daily (Pappas, 2009)

Pericarditis or myocarditis: 400 to 800 mg daily for several months (Pappas, 2009)

Peritonitis: 50-200 mg/day. **Note:** Some clinicians do not recommend using <200 mg daily (Chen, 2004).

Prophylaxis:

Bone marrow transplant: 400 mg once daily. Patients anticipated to have severe granulocytopenia should start therapy several days prior to the anticipated onset of neutropenia and continue for 7 days after the neutrophil count is >1000 mm^3.

High-risk ICU patients in units with high incidence of invasive candidiasis: 400 mg once daily (Pappas, 2009)

Neutropenic patients: 400 mg once daily for duration of neutropenia (Pappas, 2009)

Peritoneal dialysis associated infection (concurrently treated with antibiotics), prevention of secondary fungal infection: 200 mg every 48 hours (Restrepo, 2010)

Solid organ transplant: 200 to 400 mg once daily for at least 7 to 14 days (Pappas, 2009)

Surgical (perioperative) prophylaxis in high-risk patients undergoing liver, pancreas, kidney, or pancreas-kidney transplantation (off-label use): IV: 400 mg given in the perioperative period and continued in the postoperative period for ≤28 days. Time of initiation and duration varies with transplant type and operative protocol (Bratzler, 2013).

Thrombophlebitis, suppurative (off-label use): 400 to 800 mg daily (6 to 12 mg/kg/day) and as step-down in stable patients for ≥ 2 weeks (Pappas, 2009)

Urinary tract:

Cystitis:

Manufacturer's recommendation: UTI: 50 to 200 mg once daily

Asymptomatic, patient undergoing urologic procedure: 200 to 400 mg once daily several days before and after the procedure (Pappas, 2009)

Symptomatic: 200 mg once daily for 2 weeks (Pappas, 2009)

Fungus balls: 200 to 400 mg once daily (Pappas, 2009)

Pyelonephritis: 200 to 400 mg once daily for 2 weeks (Pappas, 2009)

Vaginal:

Uncomplicated: Manufacturer's recommendation: 150 mg as a single oral dose

Complicated: 150 mg every 72 hours for 3 doses (Pappas, 2009)

Recurrent: 150 mg once daily for 10 to 14 days, followed by 150 mg once weekly for 6 months (Pappas, 2009), **or** fluconazole (oral) 100 mg, 150 mg, or 200 mg every third day for a total of 3 doses (day 1, 4, and 7), then 100 mg, 150 mg, or 200 mg dose weekly for 6 months (CDC, 2010)

Coccidioidomycosis, treatment: Oral, IV:

HIV-infected (off-label use):

Meningitis: 400 to 800 mg once daily continued indefinitely (CDC, 2009)

Pneumonia, focal, mild or positive serology alone: 400 mg once daily continued indefinitely (CDC, 2009)

Pneumonia, diffuse or severe extrathoracic disseminated disease (after clinical improvement noted with amphotericin B): 400 mg once daily (CDC, 2009)

Non-HIV infected (off-label use):

Disseminated, extrapulmonary: 400 mg once daily (some experts use 2000 mg daily [Galgiani, 2005])

Meningitis: 400 mg once daily (some experts use initial doses of 800 to 1000 mg daily), lifelong duration (Galgiani, 2005)

Pneumonia, acute, uncomplicated: 200 to 400 mg daily for 3 to 6 months (Catanzaro, 1995; Galgiani, 2000)

Pneumonia, chronic progressive, fibrocavitary: 200 to 400 mg daily for 12 months (Catanzaro, 1995; Galgiani, 2000)

Pneumonia, diffuse: Consolidation after amphotericin B induction: 400 mg daily for 12 months (lifelong in chronically immunosuppressed) (Galgiani, 2005)

Coccidioidomycosis, prophylaxis: Oral:

HIV-infected, positive serology, CD4+ count <250 cells/microL (off-label use): 400 mg once daily (CDC, 2009)

Solid organ transplant (off-label use): **Note:** Prophylaxis regimens in this setting have not been established; the following regimen has been proposed for transplant recipients who maintain residence in a *Coccidioides* spp endemic area.

Previous history >12 months prior to transplant: 200 mg once daily for 6 to 12 months (Vikram, 2009; Vucicevic, 2011)

Previous history ≤12 months prior to transplant: 400 mg once daily, lifelong treatment (Vikram, 2009; Vucicevic, 2011)

Positive serology before or at transplant: 400 mg once daily, lifelong treatment; if serology is negative at 12 months, consider a dose reduction to 200 mg daily (Vikram, 2009; Vucicevic, 2011)

No history (at risk for *de novo* post-transplant disease): some clinicians treat with 200 mg daily for 6 to 12 months (Vucicevic, 2011)

Cryptococcosis: Oral, IV:

Meningitis: Manufacturer's recommendation: 400 mg for 1 dose, then 200 to 400 mg once daily for 10 to 12 weeks following negative CSF culture

HIV-infected:

Meningitis (in patients amphotericin B resistant or intolerant): Induction: 400 to 800 mg once daily for 4 to 6 weeks with concomitant flucytosine (CDC, 2009) **or** 800 to 1200 mg once daily with concomitant flucytosine for 6 weeks (Perfect, 2010)

Consolidation: 400 mg once daily for 8 weeks (CDC, 2009)

Maintenance (suppression): 200 mg once daily lifelong or until CD4+ count >200 (CDC, 2009)

Pulmonary (immunocompetent) (off-label use): 400 mg once daily for 6 to 12 months (Perfect, 2010)

Dosage adjustment in renal impairment:

Manufacturer's recommendation: **Note:** Renal function estimated using the Cockcroft-Gault formula

No adjustment for vaginal candidiasis single-dose therapy

For multiple dosing in adults, administer loading dose of 50 to 400 mg, then adjust daily doses as follows (dosage reduction in children should parallel adult recommendations):

CrCl >50 mL/minute: No dosage adjustment necessary

CrCl ≤50 mL/minute (no dialysis): Reduce dose by 50%

End-stage renal disease on intermittent hemodialysis (IHD):

Manufacturer's recommendations: 100% of daily dose (according to indication) after each dialysis session; on non-dialysis days, patient should receive a reduced dose according to their CrCl.

Alternate recommendations: Doses of 200 to 400 mg every 48 to 72 hours **or** 100 to 200 mg every 24 hours have been recommended. **Note:** Dosing dependent on the assumption of 3 times/week, complete IHD sessions (Heintz, 2009).

Continuous renal replacement therapy (CRRT) (Heintz, 2009; Trotman, 2005): Drug clearance is highly dependent on the method of renal replacement, filter type, and flow rate. Appropriate dosing requires close monitoring of pharmacologic response, signs of adverse reactions due to drug accumulation, as well as drug concentrations in relation to target trough (if appropriate). The following are general recommendations only (based on dialysate flow/ultrafiltration rates of 1 to 2 L/hour and minimal residual renal function) and should not supersede clinical judgment:

CVVH: Loading dose of 400 to 800 mg followed by 200 to 400 mg every 24 hours

CVVHD/CVVHDF: Loading dose of 400 to 800 mg followed by 400 to 800 mg every 24 hours (CVVHD or CVVHDF) **or** 800 mg every 24 hours (CVVHDF)

Note: Higher maintenance doses of 400 mg every 24 hours (CVVH), 800 mg every 24 hours (CVVHD), and 500 to 600 mg every 12 hours (CVVHDF) may be considered when treating resistant organisms and/or when employing combined ultrafiltration and dialysis flow rates of ≥2 L/hour for CVVHD/CVVHDF (Heintz, 2009; Trotman, 2005).

Dosage adjustment in hepatic impairment: There are no dosage adjustments provided in the manufacturer's labeling; use with caution.

Administration

IV: Do not use if cloudy or precipitated. Infuse over ~1 to 2 hours; do not exceed 200 mg/hour.

Oral: May be administered without regard to meals.

Hazardous agent; use appropriate precautions for handling and disposal (NIOSH 2014 [group 3]).

Monitoring Parameters Periodic liver function tests (AST, ALT, alkaline phosphatase) and renal function tests, potassium

Dosage Forms

Solution, Intravenous:

Generic: 100 mg (50 mL); 200 mg (100 mL); 400 mg (200 mL)

Solution, Intravenous [preservative free]:

Generic: 200 mg (100 mL); 400 mg (200 mL)

Suspension Reconstituted, Oral:

Diflucan: 10 mg/mL (35 mL); 40 mg/mL (35 mL)

Generic: 10 mg/mL (35 mL); 40 mg/mL (35 mL)

Tablet, Oral:

Diflucan: 50 mg, 100 mg, 150 mg, 200 mg

Generic: 50 mg, 100 mg, 150 mg, 200 mg

◆ **Fluconazole Injection (Can)** *see* Fluconazole *on page 885*

◆ **Fluconazole Injection SDZ (Can)** *see* Fluconazole *on page 885*

◆ **Fluconazole Omega (Can)** *see* Fluconazole *on page 885*

Flucytosine (floo SYE toe seen)

Brand Names: U.S. Ancobon

Index Terms 5-FC; 5-Fluorocytosine; 5-Flurocytosine

Pharmacologic Category Antifungal Agent, Oral

Use Adjunctive treatment of systemic fungal infections (eg, septicemia, endocarditis, UTI, meningitis, or pulmonary) caused by susceptible strains of *Candida* or *Cryptococcus*

Pregnancy Risk Factor C

Dosage

Usual dosage ranges: Children (off-label use) and Adults: Oral: 50 to 150 mg/kg/day in divided doses every 6 hours

Indication-specific dosing:

Children (off-label use) and Adults: Oral: **Meningoencephalitis, cryptococcal:** Induction: 25 mg/kg/dose (with amphotericin B) every 6 hours for at least 4 weeks, or if HIV-infected at least 2 weeks; if clinical improvement, may discontinue both amphotericin and flucytosine and follow with an extended course of fluconazole (Perfect, 2010)

Adults: Oral: **Endocarditis:** 100 mg/kg daily in 3 or 4 divided doses (with amphotericin B) for at least 4 to 6 weeks after valve replacement (Gould, 2012; Pappas, 2009)

Dosage adjustment in renal impairment: No dosage adjustment provided in manufacturer's labeling (**Note:** Manufacturer recommends dose reduction); however, the following adjustments have been recommended:

Adults (based upon dosing of 25 mg/kg every 6 hours):

CrCl >40 mL/minute: No dosage adjustment recommended (Perfect, 2010)

CrCl 20 to 40 mL/minute: 50% of standard dose every 6 hours (Perfect, 2010)

CrCl 10 to 20 mL/minute: 25% of standard dose every 6 hours (Perfect, 2010)

ESRD on intermittent hemodialysis (IHD): 25 to 50 mg/kg every 48 to 72 hours; administer dose after hemodialysis (Drew, 1999; DHHS, 2013)

Adults and Adolescents (HIV positive patients) (based upon dosing of 25 mg/kg every 6 hours) (DHHS, 2013):

CrCl >40 mL/minute: No dosage adjustment recommended

CrCl 20 to 40 mL/minute: 25 mg/kg every 12 hours

CrCl 10 to ≤20 mL/minute: 25 mg/kg every 24 hours

CrCl <10 mL/minute: 25 mg/kg every 48 hours

ESRD on intermittent hemodialysis (IHD): 25 to 50 mg/kg every 48 to 72 hours; administer dose after hemodialysis

Infants, Children, and non-HIV positive Adolescents (based upon dosing of 100 to 150 mg/kg/day divided every 6 hours) (Aronoff, 2007): **Note:** Flucytosine should be avoided in children with severe renal impairment (DHHS [pediatric], 2013):

CrCl 30 to 50 mL/minute: 25 to 37.5 mg/kg every 8 hours

CrCl 10 to 29 mL/minute: 25 to 37.5 mg/kg every 12 hours

CrCl <10 mL/minute: 25 to 37.5 mg/kg every 24 hours

Hemodialysis: 25 to 37.5 mg/kg every 24 hours

Peritoneal dialysis: 25 to 37.5 mg/kg every 24 hours

Continuous renal replacement therapy: 25 to 37.5 mg/kg every 8 hours (monitor serum concentrations)

Dosage adjustment in hepatic impairment: No dosage adjustment provided in manufacturer's labeling; use with caution.

Additional Information Complete prescribing information should be consulted for additional detail.

Dosage Forms

Capsule, Oral:

Ancobon: 250 mg, 500 mg

Generic: 250 mg, 500 mg

◆ **Fludara** *see* Fludarabine *on page 890*

Fludarabine (floo DARE a been)

Brand Names: U.S. Fludara

Brand Names: Canada Fludara; Fludarabine Phosphate for Injection; Fludarabine Phosphate for Injection, USP; Fludarabine Phosphate Injection, PPC STD.

Index Terms 2F-ara-AMP; Fludarabine Phosphate

Pharmacologic Category Antineoplastic Agent, Antimetabolite; Antineoplastic Agent, Antimetabolite (Purine Analog)

Use

Chronic lymphocytic leukemia: Treatment of progressive or refractory B-cell chronic lymphocytic leukemia (CLL)

Canadian labeling: Second-line treatment of chronic lymphocytic leukemia (CLL); second-line treatment of low-grade, refractory non-Hodgkin lymphoma (NHL)

Pregnancy Risk Factor D

Dosage Details concerning dosing in combination regimens should also be consulted.

Children (off-label use): IV:

AML: 10.5 mg/m^2 bolus over 15 minutes followed by a continuous infusion of 30.5 mg/m^2/day for 48 hours (Lange, 2008)

ALL or AML, relapsed: 10.5 mg/m^2 bolus over 15 minutes followed by a continuous infusion of 30.5 mg/m^2/day for 48 hours (Avramis, 1998)

Stem cell transplant (allogeneic) conditioning regimen, reduced-intensity: 30 mg/m^2/dose for 6 doses beginning 7 to 10 days prior to transplant (in combination with busulfan and antithymocyte globulin) (Pulsipher, 2009)

Adults: IV:

CLL: 25 mg/m^2/day for 5 days every 28 days

CLL combination regimens (off-label dosing):

CFAR: 20 mg/m^2/day for 3 days every 28 days for 6 cycles (in combination with cyclophosphamide, rituximab and alemtuzumab) (Wierda, 2008)

FC: 30 mg/m^2/day for 3 days every 28 days for 6 cycles (in combination with cyclophosphamide) (Eichhorst, 2006) **or** 20 mg/m^2/day for 5 days every 28 days for 6 cycles (in combination with cyclophosphamide) (Flinn, 2007)

FCR: 25 mg/m^2/day for 3 days every 28 days for 6 cycles (in combination with cyclophosphamide and rituximab) (Keating, 2005; Robak, 2010; Wierda, 2005)

FluCam: 30 mg/m^2/day for 3 days every 28 days for 4-6 cycles (in combination with alemtuzumab) (Elter, 2005)

FR: 25 mg/m^2/day for 5 days every 28 days for 6 cycles (in combination with rituximab) (Byrd, 2003)

OFAR: 30 mg/m^2/day for 2 days every 28 days for 6 cycles (in combination with oxaliplatin, cytarabine, and rituximab) (Tsimberidou, 2008)

AML, high-risk patients (off-label use): 30 mg/m^2/day for 5 days induction therapy, followed by post remission therapy of 30 mg/m^2/day for 4 days every other cycle (in combination with cytarabine with or without filgrastim) (Borthakur, 2008)

AML, refractory (off-label use): 30 mg/m^2/day for 5 days (in combination with cytarabine and filgrastim), may repeat once for partial remission (Montillo, 1998) **or** 30 mg/m^2/day for 5 days for 1 or 2 cycles (in combination with cytarabine, idarubicin, and filgrastim) (Virchis, 2004)

Non-Hodgkin lymphomas:

Canadian labeling: IV: 25 mg/m^2 for 5 days every 28 days; dosage adjustment may be necessary for hematologic or nonhematologic toxicity.

Follicular lymphoma (off-label use):

FCR: 25 mg/m^2/day for 3 days every 21 days for 4 cycles (in combination with cyclophosphamide and rituximab) (Sacchi, 2007)

FCMR: 25 mg/m^2/day for 3 days every 28 days for 4 cycles (in combination with cyclophosphamide, mitoxantrone, and rituximab) (Forstpointner, 2004; Forstpointner, 2006)

FND: 25 mg/m^2/day for 3 days every 28 days for up to 8 cycles (in combination with mitoxantrone and dexamethasone) (McLaughlin, 1996; Tsimberidou, 2002)

FNDR: 25 mg/m^2/day for 3 days every 28 days for up to 8 cycles (in combination with mitoxantrone, dexamethasone, and rituximab) (McLaughlin, 2000)

FR: 25 mg/m^2/day for 5 days every 28 days for 6 cycles (in combination with rituximab) (Czuczman, 2005)

Mantle cell lymphoma (off-label use):

FC: 20 mg/m^2/day for 4 to 5 days or 25 mg/m^2/day for 3 to 5 days (in combination with cyclophosphamide) (Cohen, 2001)

FCMR: 25 mg/m^2/day for 3 days every 28 days for 4 cycles (in combination with cyclophosphamide, mitoxantrone, and rituximab) (Forstpointner, 2004; Forstpointner, 2006)

Waldenstron's macroglobulinemia (off-label use): 25 mg/m^2/day for 5 days every 28 days (Foran, 1999) **or** 25 mg/m^2/day for 5 days every 28 days for 6 cycles (in combination with rituximab) (Treon, 2009)

Stem cell transplant (allogeneic) conditioning regimen, reduced-intensity, (off-label use): 30 mg/m^2/dose for 6 doses beginning 10 days prior to transplant **or** 30 mg/m^2/dose for 5 days beginning 6 days prior to transplant (in combination with busulfan with or without antithymocyte globulin) (Schetelig, 2003)

Stem cell transplant (allogeneic) nonmyeloablative conditioning regimen (off-label use): 30 mg/m^2/dose for 3 doses beginning 5 days prior to transplant (in combination with cyclophosphamide and rituximab) (Khouri, 2008) **or** 30 mg/m^2/dose for 3 doses beginning 4 days prior to transplant (in combination with total body irradiation) (Rezvani, 2008)

Oral (Canadian labeling; not available in U.S.): Adults: CLL: 40 mg/m^2 once daily for 5 days every 28 days

Dosage adjustment for toxicity:

Hematologic or nonhematologic toxicity (other than neurotoxicity): Consider treatment delay or dosage reduction

Hemolysis: Discontinue treatment

Neurotoxicity: Consider treatment delay or discontinuation

Dosage adjustment in renal impairment:

U.S. labeling: Adults: CLL: IV:

CrCl 50 to 79 mL/minute: Decrease dose to 20 mg/m^2

CrCl 30 to 49 mL/minute: Decrease dose to 15 mg/m^2

CrCl <30 mL/minute: Avoid use

Canadian labeling: CLL (Oral, IV), NHL (IV):

CrCl 30 to 70 mL/minute: Reduce dose by up to 50%

CrCl <30 mL/minute: Use is contraindicated

The following guidelines have been used by some clinicians: Aronoff, 2007: IV:

Children:

CrCl 30 to 50 mL/minute: Administer 80% of dose

CrCl <30 mL/minute: Not recommended

Hemodialysis: Administer 25% of dose

Continuous ambulatory peritoneal dialysis (CAPD): Not recommended

Continuous renal replacement therapy (CRRT): Administer 80% of dose

Adults:

CrCl 10 to 50 mL/minute: Administer 75% of dose

CrCl <10 mL/minute: Administer 50% of dose

Hemodialysis: Administer after dialysis

Continuous ambulatory peritoneal dialysis (CAPD): Administer 50% of dose

Continuous renal replacement therapy (CRRT): Administer 75% of dose

Dosage adjustment in hepatic impairment: There are no dosage adjustments provided in the manufacturer's labeling.

Dosing in obesity:

*American Society of Clinical Oncology (ASCO) Guidelines for appropriate chemotherapy dosing in obese adults with cancer (**Note:** Excludes HSCT dosing):* Utilize patient's actual body weight (full weight) for calculation of body surface area- or weight-based dosing, particularly when the intent of therapy is curative; manage regimen-related toxicities in the same manner as for nonobese patients; if a dose reduction is utilized due to toxicity, consider resumption of full weight-based dosing with subsequent cycles, especially if cause of toxicity (eg, hepatic or renal impairment) is resolved (Griggs, 2012).

American Society for Blood and Marrow Transplantation (ASBMT) practice guideline committee position statement on chemotherapy dosing in obesity: Utilize actual body weight (full weight) for calculation of body surface area in fludarabine dosing for hematopoietic stem cell transplant conditioning regimens in adults (Bubalo, 2014).

Additional Information Complete prescribing information should be consulted for additional detail.

Dosage Forms

Solution, Intravenous:

Generic: 50 mg/2 mL (2 mL)

Solution Reconstituted, Intravenous:

Fludara: 50 mg (1 ea)

Generic: 50 mg (1 ea)

Solution Reconstituted, Intravenous [preservative free]:

Generic: 50 mg (1 ea)

Dosage Forms: Canada

Tablet, oral:

Fludara: 10 mg

- ◆ **Fludarabine Phosphate** *see* Fludarabine *on page 890*
- ◆ **Fludarabine Phosphate for Injection (Can)** *see* Fludarabine *on page 890*
- ◆ **Fludarabine Phosphate for Injection, USP (Can)** *see* Fludarabine *on page 890*
- ◆ **Fludarabine Phosphate Injection, PPC STD. (Can)** *see* Fludarabine *on page 890*

Fludrocortisone (floo droe KOR ti sone)

Brand Names: Canada Florinef®

Index Terms 9α-Fluorohydrocortisone Acetate; Florinef; Fludrocortisone Acetate; Fluohydrisone Acetate; Fluohydrocortisone Acetate

Pharmacologic Category Corticosteroid, Systemic

Additional Appendix Information

Corticosteroids Systemic Equivalencies *on page 2228*

Use Partial replacement therapy for primary and secondary adrenocortical insufficiency in Addison's disease; treatment of salt-losing adrenogenital syndrome (or congenital adrenal hyperplasia)

Pregnancy Risk Factor C

Dosage Oral:

Infants, Children, and Adolescents: Congenital adrenal hyperplasia due to 21-hydroxylase deficiency (Endocrine Society guidelines): 0.05-0.2 mg daily in 1-2 divided doses in combination with sodium chloride supplementation (Speiser, 2010).

Adults:

Addison's disease: Initial: 0.1 mg daily; if transient hypertension develops, reduce dose to 0.05 mg daily; maintenance dosage range: 0.1 mg 3 times weekly to 0.2 mg daily. Preferred administration with cortisone (10-37.5 mg daily) or hydrocortisone (10-30 mg daily).

Salt-losing adrenogenital syndrome (or congenital adrenal hyperplasia): 0.1-0.2 mg daily

The Endocrine Society recommends a maintenance dose range of 0.05-0.2 mg once daily (in combination with hydrocortisone) for patients with congenital adrenal hyperplasia due to 21-hydroxylase deficiency (Speiser, 2010).

Orthostatic hypotension (off-label use; Kearney, 2009; Lahrmann, 2006; Lanier, 2011): Initial: 0.1 mg daily in conjunction with a high-salt diet and adequate fluid intake; may be increased in increments of 0.1 mg per week; maximum dose: 1 mg daily. **Note:** Doses exceeding 0.3 mg daily may not be beneficial and predispose patient to unwanted side effects (eg, hypertension, hypokalemia).

Dosage adjustment in renal impairment: No dosage adjustment provided in manufacturer's labeling; use with caution.

Dosage adjustment in hepatic impairment: No dosage adjustment provided in manufacturer's labeling.

Additional Information Complete prescribing information should be consulted for additional detail.

Dosage Forms

Tablet, Oral:

Generic: 0.1 mg

- ◆ **Fludrocortisone Acetate** *see* Fludrocortisone *on page 891*

◆ **Flugerel** *see* Flutamide *on page 907*

Fluindione [INT] (flu in DY one)

International Brand Names Previscan (FR)
Pharmacologic Category Anticoagulant, Indanedione
Reported Use Prophylaxis and treatment of venous thrombosis, pulmonary embolism, and thromboembolic disorders in connection with certain fibrillations, mitral valvulopathies, valvular prosthesis, myocardial infarctions, hip surgery, or catheter placement
Dosage Range Adults: Oral: Initial: 20 mg once daily; maintenance: Adjust according to coagulation (INR) monitoring
Product Availability Product available in various countries; not currently available in the U.S.
Dosage Forms
Tablet: 20 mg

◆ **Flulaval** *see* Influenza Virus Vaccine (Inactivated) *on page 1075*
◆ **Flulaval Quadrivalent** *see* Influenza Virus Vaccine (Inactivated) *on page 1075*
◆ **Flumadine** *see* Rimantadine *on page 1813*
◆ **Flumadine® (Can)** *see* Rimantadine *on page 1813*

Flumazenil (FLOO may ze nil)

Brand Names: Canada Anexate; Flumazenil Injection; Flumazenil Injection, USP; Romazicon
Pharmacologic Category Antidote
Use Benzodiazepine antagonist; reverses sedative effects of benzodiazepines used in conscious sedation and general anesthesia; treatment of benzodiazepine overdose
Pregnancy Risk Factor C
Dosage
IV:
Children ≥1 year: Reversal of conscious sedation:
Initial dose: 0.01 mg/kg over 15 seconds (maximum: 0.2 mg)
Repeat doses (maximum: 4 doses): If desired level of consciousness is not obtained, 0.01 mg/kg (maximum: 0.2 mg) repeated at 1-minute intervals
Maximum total cumulative dose: 1 mg or 0.05 mg/kg (whichever is lower)
Mean total dose: 0.65 mg (range: 0.08-1 mg)
Adults:
Reversal of conscious sedation and general anesthesia:
Initial dose: 0.2 mg over 15 seconds
Repeat doses (maximum: 4 doses): If desired level of consciousness is not obtained, 0.2 mg may be repeated at 1-minute intervals.
Maximum total cumulative dose: 1 mg (usual total dose: 0.6-1 mg). In the event of resedation: Repeat doses may be given at 20-minute intervals as needed at 0.2 mg per minute to a maximum of 1 mg total dose and 3 mg in 1 hour.
Suspected benzodiazepine overdose:
Initial dose: 0.2 mg over 30 seconds; if the desired level of consciousness is not obtained 30 seconds after the dose, 0.3 mg can be given over 30 seconds
Repeat doses: 0.5 mg over 30 seconds repeated at 1-minute intervals
Maximum total cumulative dose: 3 mg (usual total dose: 1-3 mg). Patients with a partial response at 3 mg may require (rare) additional titration up to a total dose of 5 mg (although doses >3 mg do not reliably produce additional effects). If a patient has not responded 5 minutes after cumulative dose of 5 mg, the major cause of sedation is not likely due to benzodiazepines. In the event of resedation, repeat doses may be given at 20-minute intervals if needed, at 0.5 mg per minute to a maximum of 1 mg total dose and 3 mg in 1 hour.
Elderly: No differences in safety or efficacy have been reported; however, increased sensitivity may occur in some elderly patients.
Dosing in renal impairment: No dosage adjustment provided in manufacturer's labeling; however, pharmacokinetics are not significantly affected by renal failure (CrCl <10 mL/minute) or hemodialysis.
Dosing in hepatic impairment: Initial reversal: No dosage adjustment necessary. Repeat doses: Reduce dose or frequency.
Additional Information Complete prescribing information should be consulted for additional detail.
Dosage Forms
Solution, Intravenous:
Generic: 0.5 mg/5 mL (5 mL); 1 mg/10 mL (10 mL)

◆ **Flumazenil Injection (Can)** *see* Flumazenil *on page 892*
◆ **Flumazenil Injection, USP (Can)** *see* Flumazenil *on page 892*
◆ **Flumethasone and Clioquinol** *see* Clioquinol and Flumethasone [CAN/INT] *on page 465*
◆ **FluMist** *see* Influenza Virus Vaccine (Live/Attenuated) *on page 1080*
◆ **FluMist Quadrivalent** *see* Influenza Virus Vaccine (Live/Attenuated) *on page 1080*

Flunarizine [CAN/INT] (floo NAR i zeen)

Brand Names: Canada Novo-Flunarizine
Index Terms Flunarizine Hydrochloride
Pharmacologic Category Calcium Channel Blocker
Use Note: Not approved in U.S.
Prophylaxis of migraine (with and without aura)
Pregnancy Considerations Teratogenic events have not been observed in animal reproduction studies.
Breast-Feeding Considerations It is not known if flunarizine is excreted into breast milk. Breast-feeding is not recommended by the manufacturer.
Contraindications Hypersensitivity to flunarizine or any component of the formulation; history of depression; preexisting symptoms of Parkinson's disease, or other extrapyramidal disorders
Warnings/Precautions Not indicated for treatment of acute migraine attacks. May produce extrapyramidal symptoms in individuals with no prior history of neurological deficits; risk is increased in elderly patients. May precipitate depression (greater risk in younger patients). Use may be associated with sedation and/or drowsiness; use caution in performing tasks requiring alertness (eg, operating machinery or driving). Effects may be potentiated when used with other sedative drugs or ethanol. Monitor for extrapyramidal, depressive, and/or fatigue symptoms and discontinue use if observed. Galactorrhea has been reported rarely in female patients during the first 2 months of therapy; usually resolves with discontinuation of therapy. Mild but significant increase in serum prolactin levels have been observed with use. Discontinue use if inadequate response after 3 months of therapy. Closely monitor for adverse effects (eg, CNS effects) in patients treated for >6 months; discontinue therapy with onset of adverse effects. Risk for adverse effects may be decreased by allowing 2 consecutive drug-free days per week.
Adverse Reactions
Central nervous system: Anxiety, depression, dizziness, drowsiness, fatigue, insomnia, sedation, vertigo
Dermatologic: Rash
Endocrine & metabolic: Galactorrhea, menstrual irregularities, prolactin levels increased

Gastrointestinal: Appetite increased, epigastric pain, heartburn, nausea, vomiting, weight gain, xerostomia

Neuromuscular & skeletal: Extrapyramidal symptoms, muscle ache, weakness

Drug Interactions

Metabolism/Transport Effects Substrate of CYP2D6 (minor); **Note:** Assignment of Major/Minor substrate status based on clinically relevant drug interaction potential

Avoid Concomitant Use

Avoid concomitant use of Flunarizine with any of the following: Azelastine (Nasal); Orphenadrine; Paraldehyde; Thalidomide

Increased Effect/Toxicity

Flunarizine may increase the levels/effects of: Alcohol (Ethyl); Azelastine (Nasal); Buprenorphine; CNS Depressants; Hydrocodone; Methotrimeprazine; Metyrosine; Mirtazapine; Orphenadrine; Paraldehyde; Pramipexole; ROPINIRole; Rotigotine; Selective Serotonin Reuptake Inhibitors; Suvorexant; Thalidomide; Zolpidem

The levels/effects of Flunarizine may be increased by: Brimonidine (Topical); Cannabis; Doxylamine; Dronabinol; Droperidol; HydrOXYzine; Kava Kava; Magnesium Sulfate; Methotrimeprazine; Nabilone; Perampanel; Rufinamide; Sodium Oxybate; Tapentadol; Tetrahydrocannabinol

Decreased Effect

The levels/effects of Flunarizine may be decreased by: CarBAMazepine; Fosphenytoin; Phenytoin

Storage/Stability Store at 15°C to 30°C (59°F to 86°F). Protect from light and moisture.

Mechanism of Action Flunarizine is a selective calcium channel blocker that prevents cellular calcium overload by reducing transmembrane calcium influx; also has antihistamine properties. Has greater effect on decreasing the frequency of migraine attacks than on decreasing the severity or duration of attacks.

Pharmacodynamics/Kinetics

Absorption: Well absorbed

Distribution: V_d: Mean: 43.2 L/kg

Protein binding: 99%

Metabolism: Hepatic: N-oxidation, aromatic hydroxylation

Half-life elimination: ~19 days

Time to peak, plasma: 2-4 hours

Excretion: Feces (<6%); urine (minimal)

Dosage Oral: Adults <65 years: Migraine prophylaxis: 5-10 mg once daily (Pryse-Phillips, 1997); incidence of adverse effects may be decreased by allowing 2 consecutive medication-free days each week. If no significant improvement is seen after 3 months of therapy, discontinue use.

Dosage adjustment in renal impairment: There are no dosage adjustments provided in manufacturer's labeling. Drug accumulation does not appear to be likely as flunarizine primarily undergoes hepatic metabolism and minimal urinary excretion.

Dosage adjustment in hepatic impairment: There are no dosage adjustments provided in manufacturer's labeling. Flunarizine is hepatically metabolized; use with caution.

Administration Administer at bedtime.

Monitoring Parameters Monitor for extrapyramidal, depressive, and/or fatigue symptoms

Product Availability Not available in U.S.

Dosage Forms: Canada

Capsule, oral: 5 mg

◆ **Flunarizine Hydrochloride** *see* Flunarizine [CAN/INT] *on page 892*

Flunisolide (Nasal) (floo NISS oh lide)

Brand Names: Canada Apo-Flunisolide®; Nasalide®; Rhinalar®

Pharmacologic Category Corticosteroid, Nasal

Use Seasonal or perennial rhinitis

Pregnancy Risk Factor C

Dosage Intranasal: Rhinitis:

Children 6-14 years: 1 spray each nostril 3 times daily **or** 2 sprays in each nostril twice daily; not to exceed 4 sprays/day in each nostril

Children ≥15 years and Adults: 2 sprays each nostril twice daily (morning and evening); may increase to 2 sprays 3 times daily; maximum dose: 8 sprays/day in each nostril

Dosage adjustment in renal impairment: No dosage adjustment provided in manufacturer's labeling.

Dosage adjustment in hepatic impairment: No dosage adjustment provided in manufacturer's labeling.

Additional Information Complete prescribing information should be consulted for additional detail.

Dosage Forms

Solution, Nasal:

Generic: 25 mcg/actuation (0.025%) (25 mL)

Fluocinolone (Topical) (floo oh SIN oh lone)

Brand Names: U.S. Capex; Derma-Smoothe/FS Body; Derma-Smoothe/FS Scalp; Fluocinolone Acetonide Body; Fluocinolone Acetonide Scalp; Synalar; Synalar (Cream); Synalar (Ointment); Synalar TS

Brand Names: Canada Capex®; Derma-Smoothe/FS®; Synalar®

Index Terms Fluocinolone Acetonide

Pharmacologic Category Corticosteroid, Topical

Additional Appendix Information

Topical Corticosteroids *on page 2230*

Use Relief of susceptible inflammatory dermatosis (low, medium corticosteroid); dermatitis or psoriasis of the scalp; atopic dermatitis in adults and children ≥3 months of age

Pregnancy Risk Factor C

Dosage Topical:

Atopic dermatitis (Derma-Smoothe/FS® body oil):

Children ≥3 months: Moisten skin; apply a thin film to affected area twice daily; do not use for longer than 4 weeks

Adults: Apply a thin film to affected area 3 times/day

Corticosteroid-responsive dermatoses: Children and Adults: Cream, ointment, solution: Apply a thin layer to affected area 2-4 times/day; may use occlusive dressings to manage psoriasis or recalcitrant conditions

Inflammatory and pruritic manifestations (dental use): Adults: Apply to oral lesion 4 times/day, after meals and at bedtime

Scalp psoriasis (Derma-Smoothe/FS® scalp oil): Adults: Massage thoroughly into wet or dampened hair/scalp; cover with shower cap. Leave on overnight (or for at least 4 hours). Remove by washing hair with shampoo and rinsing thoroughly.

Seborrheic dermatitis of the scalp (Capex®): Adults: Apply no more than 1 ounce to scalp once daily; work into lather and allow to remain on scalp for ~5 minutes. Remove from hair and scalp by rinsing thoroughly with water.

Additional Information Complete prescribing information should be consulted for additional detail.

Dosage Forms

Cream, External:

Synalar: 0.025% (120 g)

Generic: 0.01% (15 g, 60 g); 0.025% (15 g, 60 g)

Kit, External:
Synalar (Cream): 0.025%
Synalar (Ointment): 0.025%
Synalar TS: 0.01%

Oil, External:
Derma-Smoothe/FS Body: 0.01% (118.28 mL)
Derma-Smoothe/FS Scalp: 0.01% (118.28 mL)
Fluocinolone Acetonide Body: 0.01% (118.28 mL)
Fluocinolone Acetonide Scalp: 0.01% (118.28 mL)

Ointment, External:
Synalar: 0.025% (120 g)
Generic: 0.025% (15 g, 60 g)

Shampoo, External:
Capex: 0.01% (120 mL)

Solution, External:
Synalar: 0.01% (60 mL, 90 mL)
Generic: 0.01% (60 mL)

◆ **Fluocinolone Acetonide** *see* Fluocinolone (Topical) *on page 893*

◆ **Fluocinolone Acetonide Body** *see* Fluocinolone (Topical) *on page 893*

◆ **Fluocinolone Acetonide Scalp** *see* Fluocinolone (Topical) *on page 893*

Fluocinolone, Hydroquinone, and Tretinoin

(floo oh SIN oh lone, HYE droe kwin one, & TRET i noyn)

Brand Names: U.S. Tri-Luma®

Index Terms Hydroquinone, Fluocinolone Acetonide, and Tretinoin; Tretinoin, Fluocinolone Acetonide, and Hydroquinone

Pharmacologic Category Corticosteroid, Topical; Depigmenting Agent; Retinoic Acid Derivative

Use Short-term treatment of moderate-to-severe melasma of the face

Pregnancy Risk Factor C

Dosage Topical: Adults: Melasma: Apply a thin film once daily to affected areas; not indicated for use beyond 8 weeks

Additional Information Complete prescribing information should be consulted for additional detail.

Dosage Forms

Cream, topical:
Tri-Luma®: Fluocinolone acetonide 0.01%, hydroquinone 4%, and tretinoin 0.05% (30 g)

Fluocinonide (floo oh SIN oh nide)

Brand Names: U.S. Vanos

Brand Names: Canada Lidemol®; Lidex®; Lyderm®; Tiamol®; Topactin; Topsyn®

Index Terms Lidex

Pharmacologic Category Corticosteroid, Topical

Additional Appendix Information

Topical Corticosteroids *on page 2230*

Use Anti-inflammatory, antipruritic; treatment of plaque-type psoriasis (up to 10% of body surface area) [high-potency topical corticosteroid]

Pregnancy Risk Factor C

Dosage

Children and Adults: Pruritus and inflammation: Topical (0.05% cream): Apply thin layer to affected area 2-4 times/day depending on the severity of the condition. Therapy should be discontinued when control is achieved; if no improvement is seen, reassessment of diagnosis may be necessary.

Children ≥12 years and Adults: Plaque-type psoriasis (Vanos™): Topical (0.1% cream): Apply a thin layer once or twice daily to affected areas (limited to <10% of body surface area). **Note:** Not recommended for use >2 consecutive weeks or >60 g/week total exposure. Discontinue when control is achieved.

Additional Information Complete prescribing information should be consulted for additional detail.

Dosage Forms

Cream, External:
Vanos: 0.1% (30 g, 60 g, 120 g)
Generic: 0.05% (15 g, 30 g, 60 g, 120 g); 0.1% (30 g, 60 g, 120 g)

Gel, External:
Generic: 0.05% (15 g, 30 g, 60 g)

Ointment, External:
Generic: 0.05% (15 g, 30 g, 60 g)

Solution, External:
Generic: 0.05% (20 mL, 60 mL)

◆ **Fluohydrisone Acetate** *see* Fludrocortisone *on page 891*

◆ **Fluohydrocortisone Acetate** *see* Fludrocortisone *on page 891*

◆ **Fluor-I-Strips A.T.** *see* Fluorescein *on page 894*

◆ **Fluorabon** *see* Fluoride *on page 895*

◆ **Fluor-A-Day** *see* Fluoride *on page 895*

Fluorescein (FLURE e seen)

Brand Names: U.S. AK-Fluor; Bio Glo; Fluor-I-Strips A.T.; Fluorescite; Fluorets [DSC]; Ful-Glo

Brand Names: Canada Fluorescite®

Index Terms Fluorescein Sodium; Sodium Fluorescein; Soluble Fluorescein

Pharmacologic Category Diagnostic Agent

Use

Injection: Diagnostic aid in ophthalmic angiography and angioscopy

Ophthalmic: To stain the anterior segment of the eye for procedures (such as fitting contact lenses), disclosing corneal injury, and in applanation tonometry

Pregnancy Risk Factor C

Dosage

Diagnostic staining: Ophthalmic: Strips: Children and Adults: Moisten strip with sterile water, saline or ophthalmic fluid. Touch conjunctiva or fornix with tip of strip until adequately stained.

Ophthalmic angiography: Solution for injection: **Note:** Prior to use, an intradermal test dose of 0.05 mL may be used if an allergy is suspected. Evaluate 30-60 minutes following intradermal injection. A negative skin test does not exclude the potential for a reaction to occur.

IV:

Children: 3.5 mg/lb (7.7 mg/kg) as a single dose into antecubital vein; maximum: 500 mg

Adults: 500 mg as a single dose into antecubital vein; a dose of 200 mg may be appropriate in cases when a highly sensitive imaging system (eg, scanning laser ophthalmoscope) is used.

Oral (off-label route): Adults: 1 g of injection solution has been administered orally; clarity of photographs, particularly during early arterial phase, is reportedly poorer than photographs obtained following IV administration (Hara, 1998)

Dosage adjustment in renal impairment: No dosage adjustment provided in manufacturer's labeling.

Dosage adjustment in hepatic impairment: No dosage adjustment provided in manufacturer's labeling.

Additional Information Complete prescribing information should be consulted for additional detail.

Dosage Forms

Solution, Injection:

AK-Fluor: 10% (5 mL); 25% (2 mL)

Fluorescite: 10% (5 mL)

Strip, Ophthalmic:

Bio Glo: 1 mg (100 ea, 300 ea)

Fluor-I-Strips A.T.: 1 mg (300 ea)

Ful-Glo: 0.6 mg (300 ea); 1 mg (100 ea)

Fluorescein and Benoxinate

(FLURE e seen & ben OX i nate)

Brand Names: U.S. EyeFlur; Fluress® [DSC]; Flurox™

Index Terms Benoxinate Hydrochloride and Fluorescein Sodium

Pharmacologic Category Anesthetic, Topical; Diagnostic Agent; Ophthalmic Agent

Use For use in ophthalmic procedures when a topical disclosing agent is needed along with an anesthetic

Pregnancy Risk Factor C

Dosage Ophthalmic: Adults:

Removal of foreign bodies, sutures, or tonometry: Instill 1 or 2 drops (single instillations) into each eye before operating

Deep ophthalmic anesthesia: Instill 2 drops into each eye every 90 seconds up to 3 doses

Dosage adjustment in renal impairment: No dosage adjustment provided in manufacturer's labeling.

Dosage adjustment in hepatic impairment: No dosage adjustment provided in manufacturer's labeling.

Additional Information Complete prescribing information should be consulted for additional detail.

Dosage Forms

Solution, ophthalmic: Fluorescein 0.25% and benoxinate 0.4% (5 mL)

EyeFlur, Flurox™: Fluorescein 0.25% and benoxinate 0.4% (5 mL)

◆ **Fluorescein and Proparacaine** *see* Proparacaine and Fluorescein *on page 1728*

◆ **Fluorescein Sodium** *see* Fluorescein *on page 894*

◆ **Fluorescite** *see* Fluorescein *on page 894*

◆ **Fluorescite® (Can)** *see* Fluorescein *on page 894*

◆ **Fluorets [DSC]** *see* Fluorescein *on page 894*

Fluoride (FLOR ide)

Brand Names: U.S. Act Kids [OTC]; Act Restoring [OTC]; Act Total Care [OTC]; Act [OTC]; CaviRinse; Clinpro 5000; ControlRx; ControlRx Multi; Denta 5000 Plus; DentaGel; Fluor-A-Day; Fluorabon; Fluorinse; Fluoritab; Flura-Drops; Gel-Kam Rinse; Gel-Kam [OTC]; Just For Kids [OTC]; Lozi-Flur; NeutraCare; NeutraGard Advanced; Omni Gel [OTC]; OrthoWash; PerioMed; Phos-Flur; Phos-Flur Rinse [OTC]; PreviDent; PreviDent 5000 Booster; PreviDent 5000 Booster Plus; PreviDent 5000 Dry Mouth; PreviDent 5000 Plus; StanGard Perio; Stop

Brand Names: Canada Fluor-A-Day

Index Terms Acidulated Phosphate Fluoride; Sodium Fluoride; Stannous Fluoride

Pharmacologic Category Nutritional Supplement

Use Prevention of dental caries

Pregnancy Risk Factor B

Dosage Oral: Children 6 months to 16 years (Fluor-A-Day, Fluorabon, Fluoritab drops, Flura-Drops, Lozi-Flur):

The recommended daily dose of oral fluoride supplement (mg), based on fluoride ion content (ppm) in drinking water (2.2 mg of sodium fluoride is equivalent to 1 mg of fluoride ion): See table.

Fluoride Ion

Fluoride Content of Drinking Water	Daily Dose, Oral (mg)
<0.3 ppm	
Birth - 6 mo	None
6 mo - 3 y	0.25
3-6 y	0.5
6-16 y	1
0.3-0.6 ppm	
Birth - 6 mo	None
6 mo - 3 y	None
3-6 y	0.25
6-16 y	0.5

Adapted from Recommended Dosage Schedule of The American Dental Association, The American Academy of Pediatric Dentistry, and The American Academy of Pediatrics.

Dental cream or paste:

Clinpro 5000 paste, Control Rx 1.1%, Denta 5000 Plus: Children ≥6 years, Adolescents, and Adults: Once daily, in place of conventional toothpaste, brush teeth with a thin ribbon or pea-sized amount of paste for at least 2 minutes. May be used in areas with fluoridated drinking water.

Prevident 5000 Sensitive: Children ≥12 years, Adolescents, and Adults: Twice daily, brush teeth with a 1 inch strip of toothpaste for at least 1 minute. After brushing, expectorate and rinse mouth thoroughly. May be used in areas with fluoridated drinking water.

Dental rinse or gel:

ACT Restoring 0.02% rinse, ACT Total Care 0.02% rinse: Children ≥6 years, Adolescents, and Adults: Twice daily after brushing, rinse 10 mL around and between teeth for 1 minute, then spit. Do not eat, drink, or rinse mouth for at least 30 minutes after treatment; do not swallow

ACT 0.05% rinse, Phos-Flur Rinse: Children ≥6 years, Adolescents, and Adults: Once daily after brushing, rinse 10 mL around and between teeth for 1 minute, then spit. Do not eat, drink, or rinse mouth for at least 30 minutes after treatment; do not swallow

Cavirinse, PreviDent rinse: Children >6 years, Adolescents, and Adults: Once weekly, rinse 10 mL vigorously around and between teeth for 1 minute, then spit; this should be done preferably at bedtime, after thoroughly brushing teeth; do not swallow. For maximum benefit with PreviDent rinse, do not eat, drink, or rinse mouth for at least 30 minutes after treatment. Children 6 to 16 years of age should rinse mouth thoroughly with water following Cavirinse.

Gel-Kam rinse: Children ≥12 years, Adolescents, and Adults: After diluting solution as directed, rinse with 15 mL for 1 minute at least daily, then spit. Repeat with remaining solution.

Just for Kids gel: Children ≥6 years: Once daily after brushing, apply a pea sized amount of gel to teeth and brush thoroughly. Allow gel to remain on teeth for 1 minute prior to spitting out. Do not eat or drink for 30 minutes after using

Lozenge: Lozi-Flur: Adults: One lozenge daily regardless of fluoride content of drinking water

Additional Information Complete prescribing information should be consulted for additional detail.

Dosage Forms

Cream, oral: 1.1% (51 g)

Denta 5000 Plus: 1.1% (51 g)

PreviDent 5000 Plus: 1.1% (51 g)

Gel, oral:
PreviDent 5000 Booster: 1.1% (100 mL, 106 mL)
PreviDent 5000 Booster Plus: 1.1% (100 mL)
PreviDent 5000 Dry Mouth: 1.1% (100 mL)
Gel, topical: 1.1% (56 g)
DentaGel: 1.1% (56 g)
Gel-Kam [OTC]: 0.4% (129 g)
Just For Kids [OTC]: 0.4% (122 g)
NeutraCare: 1.1% (60 g)
NeutraGard Advanced: 1.1% (60 g)
Omni Gel [OTC]: 0.4% (122 g); 0.4% (122 g)
Phos-Flur: 1.1% (51 g)
PreviDent: 1.1% (56 g)
Stop: 0.4% (120 g)
Liquid, oral:
Fluoritab: 0.125 mg/drop
Lozenge, oral:
Lozi-Flur: 2.21 mg (90s)
Paste, oral:
Clinpro 5000: 1.1% (113 g)
ControlRx: 1.1% (57 g)
ControlRx Multi: 1.1% (57 g)
Solution, oral: 1.1 mg/mL (50 mL); 0.2% (473 mL); 0.63% (300 mL)
Act [OTC]: 0.05% (532 mL)
Act Kids [OTC]: 0.05% (500 mL, 532 mL)
Act Restoring [OTC]: 0.02% (1000 mL); 0.05% (532 mL)
Act Total Care [OTC]: 0.02% (1000 mL); 0.05% (88 mL, 532 mL)
CaviRinse: 0.2% (240 mL)
Fluor-A-Day: 0.278 mg/drop (30 mL)
Fluorabon: 0.55 mg/0.6 mL (60 mL)
Fluorinse: 0.2% (480 mL)
Flura-Drops: 0.55 mg/drop (24 mL)
Gel-Kam Rinse: 0.63% (300 mL)
OrthoWash: 0.044% (480 mL)
PerioMed: 0.63% (284 mL)
Phos-Flur Rinse [OTC]: 0.044% (473 mL, 500 mL)
PreviDent: 0.2% (473 mL)
StanGard Perio: 0.63% (284 mL)
Tablet, chewable, oral: 0.55 mg, 1.1 mg, 2.2 mg
Fluor-A-Day: 0.55 mg, 1.1 mg, 2.2 mg
Fluoritab: 1.1 mg, 2.2 mg

◆ **Fluorinse** *see* Fluoride *on page 895*

◆ **Fluoritab** *see* Fluoride *on page 895*

◆ **5-Fluorocytosine** *see* Flucytosine *on page 889*

◆ **9α-Fluorohydrocortisone Acetate** *see* Fludrocortisone *on page 891*

Fluorometholone (flure oh METH oh lone)

Brand Names: U.S. Flarex; FML; FML Forte; FML Liquifilm

Brand Names: Canada Flarex®; FML Forte®; FML®; PMS-Fluorometholone

Pharmacologic Category Corticosteroid, Ophthalmic

Use Treatment of steroid-responsive inflammatory conditions of the eye

Pregnancy Risk Factor C

Dosage Ophthalmic:

Children ≥2 years, Adolescents, and Adults: Re-evaluate therapy if improvement is not seen within 2 days; use care not to discontinue prematurely; in chronic conditions, gradually decrease dosing frequency prior to discontinuing treatment

Ointment (FML®): Apply small amount (~1/2 inch ribbon) to conjunctival sac 1-3 times daily; may increase application to every 4 hours during the initial 24-48 hours

Suspension (FML®, FML® Forte): Instill 1 drop into conjunctival sac 2-4 times daily; may instill 1 drop every 4 hours during initial 24-48 hours

Adults: Suspension (Flarex®): Instill 1-2 drops into conjunctival sac 4 times daily; may increase application to 2 drops every 2 hours during initial 24-48 hours

Dosage adjustment in renal impairment: No dosage adjustment provided in manufacturer's labeling.

Dosage adjustment in hepatic impairment: No dosage adjustment provided in manufacturer's labeling.

Additional Information Complete prescribing information should be consulted for additional detail.

Dosage Forms

Ointment, Ophthalmic:
FML: 0.1% (3.5 g)
Suspension, Ophthalmic:
Flarex: 0.1% (5 mL)
FML Forte: 0.25% (5 mL, 10 mL)
FML Liquifilm: 0.1% (5 mL, 10 mL)
Generic: 0.1% (5 mL, 10 mL, 15 mL)

◆ **Fluoroplex** *see* Fluorouracil (Topical) *on page 899*

◆ **Fluoroplex® (Can)** *see* Fluorouracil (Topical) *on page 899*

◆ **Fluoro Uracil** *see* Fluorouracil (Systemic) *on page 896*

◆ **5-Fluorouracil** *see* Fluorouracil (Systemic) *on page 896*

◆ **5-Fluorouracil** *see* Fluorouracil (Topical) *on page 899*

Fluorouracil (Systemic) (flure oh YOOR a sil)

Brand Names: U.S. Adrucil

Brand Names: Canada Fluorouracil Injection

Index Terms 5-Fluorouracil; 5-Fluracil; 5-FU; Fluoro Uracil; Fluouracil; FU

Pharmacologic Category Antineoplastic Agent, Antimetabolite; Antineoplastic Agent, Antimetabolite (Pyrimidine Analog)

Use Treatment of breast cancer, colon cancer, rectal cancer, pancreatic cancer, and stomach (gastric) cancer

Pregnancy Risk Factor D

Pregnancy Considerations Adverse effects (increased resorptions, embryolethality, and teratogenicity) have been observed in animal reproduction studies. Based on the mechanism of action, fluorouracil may cause fetal harm if administered during pregnancy (according to the manufacturer's labeling). The National Comprehensive Cancer Network (NCCN) breast cancer guidelines (v.3.2012) state that chemotherapy, if indicated, may be administered to pregnant women with breast cancer as part of a combination chemotherapy regimen (common regimens administered during pregnancy include doxorubicin, cyclophosphamide, and fluorouracil); chemotherapy should not be administered during the first trimester, after 35 weeks gestation, or within 3 weeks of planned delivery.

Breast-Feeding Considerations Based on the mechanism of action, the manufacturer's labeling recommends against breast-feeding if receiving fluorouracil.

Contraindications Hypersensitivity to fluorouracil or any component of the formulation; poor nutritional states; depressed bone marrow function; potentially serious infections

Warnings/Precautions Hazardous agent - use appropriate precautions for handling and disposal (NIOSH 2014 [group 1]). Use with caution in patients with impaired kidney or liver function. Discontinue if intractable vomiting or diarrhea, precipitous falls in leukocyte or platelet counts, gastrointestinal ulcer or bleeding, stomatitis, or esophagopharyngitis, hemorrhage, or myocardial ischemia occurs. Use with caution in poor-risk patients who have had high-dose pelvic radiation or previous use of alkylating agents and in patients with widespread metastatic marrow involvement. Palmar-plantar erythrodysesthesia (hand-foot) syndrome has been associated with use (symptoms include a tingling sensation, which may progress to pain, and then to symmetrical swelling and erythema with tenderness; desquamation may occur; with treatment interruption, generally resolves over 5-7 days).

Administration to patients with a genetic deficiency of dihydropyrimidine dehydrogenase (DPD) has been associated with prolonged clearance and increased toxicity (diarrhea, neutropenia, and neurotoxicity) following administration; rechallenge has resulted in recurrent toxicity (despite dose reduction). **[U.S. Boxed Warning]: Should be administered under the supervision of an experienced cancer chemotherapy physician; the manufacturer's labeling recommends hospitalizing patients during the first treatment course due to the potential for severe toxicity.**

Adverse Reactions Toxicity depends on duration of treatment and/or rate of administration

Cardiovascular: Angina, arrhythmia, heart failure, MI, myocardial ischemia, vasospasm, ventricular ectopy

Central nervous system: Acute cerebellar syndrome, confusion, disorientation, euphoria, headache, nystagmus, stroke

Dermatologic: Alopecia, dermatitis, dry skin, fissuring, nail changes (nail loss), palmar-plantar erythrodysesthesia syndrome, pruritic maculopapular rash, photosensitivity, Stevens-Johnson syndrome, toxic epidermal necrolysis, vein pigmentation

Gastrointestinal: Anorexia, bleeding, diarrhea, esophagopharyngitis, mesenteric ischemia (acute), nausea, sloughing, stomatitis, ulceration, vomiting

Hematologic: Agranulocytosis, anemia, leukopenia (nadir: days 9-14; recovery by day 30), pancytopenia, thrombocytopenia

Local: Thrombophlebitis

Ocular: Lacrimation, lacrimal duct stenosis, photophobia, visual changes

Respiratory: Epistaxis

Miscellaneous: Anaphylaxis, generalized allergic reactions

Drug Interactions

Metabolism/Transport Effects **Inhibits** CYP2C9 (strong)

Avoid Concomitant Use

Avoid concomitant use of Fluorouracil (Systemic) with any of the following: BCG; CloZAPine; Dipyrone; Gimeracil; Natalizumab; Pimecrolimus; Tacrolimus (Topical); Tofacitinib; Vaccines (Live)

Increased Effect/Toxicity

Fluorouracil (Systemic) may increase the levels/effects of: Bosentan; Carvedilol; CloZAPine; CYP2C9 Substrates; Diclofenac (Systemic); Dronabinol; Fosphenytoin; Lacosamide; Leflunomide; Natalizumab; Ospemifene; Phenytoin; Tetrahydrocannabinol; Tofacitinib; Vaccines (Live); Vitamin K Antagonists

The levels/effects of Fluorouracil (Systemic) may be increased by: Cannabis; Cimetidine; Denosumab; Dipyrone; Gemcitabine; Gimeracil; Leucovorin Calcium-Levoleucovorin; MetroNIDAZOLE (Systemic); Pimecrolimus; Roflumilast; SORAfenib; Tacrolimus (Topical); Trastuzumab

Decreased Effect

Fluorouracil (Systemic) may decrease the levels/effects of: BCG; Coccidioides immitis Skin Test; Sipuleucel-T; Vaccines (Inactivated); Vaccines (Live)

The levels/effects of Fluorouracil (Systemic) may be decreased by: Echinacea; SORAfenib

Preparation for Administration Hazardous agent; use appropriate precautions for handling and disposal (NIOSH 2014 [group 1]). May dispense in a syringe or dilute in 50-1000 mL NS or D_5W for infusion.

Storage/Stability Store intact vials at room temperature. Do not refrigerate or freeze. Protect from light. Slight discoloration may occur during storage; does not usually denote decomposition. If exposed to cold, a precipitate may form; **gentle** heating to 60°C (140°F) will dissolve the precipitate without impairing the potency. According to the manufacturer, pharmacy bulk vials should be used within 4 hours of initial entry. Solutions for infusion should be used promptly. Fluorouracil 50 mg/mL in NS was stable in polypropylene infusion pump syringes for 7 days when stored at 30°C (86°F) (Stiles, 1996). Stability of fluorouracil 1 mg/mL or 10 mg/mL in NS or D_5W in PVC bags was demonstrated for up to 14 days at 4°C (39.2°F) and 21°C (69.8°F) (Martel, 1996). Stability of undiluted fluorouracil (50 mg/mL) in ethylene-vinyl acetate ambulatory pump reservoirs was demonstrated for 3 days at 4°C (39.2°F) (precipitate formed after 3 days) and for 14 days at 33°C (91.4°F) (Martel, 1996). Stability of undiluted fluorouracil (50 mg/mL) in PVC ambulatory pump reservoirs was demonstrated for 5 days at 4°C (39.2°F) (precipitate formed after 5 days) and for 14 days at 33°C (91.4°F) (Martel, 1996).

Mechanism of Action A pyrimidine analog antimetabolite that interferes with DNA and RNA synthesis; after activation, F-UMP (an active metabolite) is incorporated into RNA to replace uracil and inhibit cell growth; the active metabolite F-dUMP, inhibits thymidylate synthetase, depleting thymidine triphosphate (a necessary component of DNA synthesis).

Pharmacodynamics/Kinetics

Distribution: Penetrates extracellular fluid, CSF, and third space fluids (eg, pleural effusions and ascitic fluid), marrow, intestinal mucosa, liver and other tissues

Metabolism: Hepatic (90%); via a dehydrogenase enzyme; FU must be metabolized to be active metabolites, 5-fluoroxyuridine monophosphate (F-UMP) and 5-5-fluoro-2'-deoxyuridine-5'-O-monophosphate (F-dUMP)

Half-life elimination: 16 minutes (range: 8-20 minutes); two metabolites, F-dUMP and F-UMP, have prolonged half-lives depending on the type of tissue

Excretion: Primarily metabolized in the liver; excreted in lung (as expired CO_2) and urine (7% to 20% as unchanged drug within 6 hours; also as metabolites within 9-10 hours)

Dosage Details concerning dosing in combination regimens should be consulted: Adults:

Breast cancer (off-label dosing): IV:

CEF regimen: 500 mg/m^2 on days 1 and 8 every 28 days (in combination with cyclophosphamide and epirubicin) for 6 cycles (Levine, 1998)

CMF regimen: 600 mg/m^2 on days 1 and 8 every 28 days (in combination with cyclophosphamide and methotrexate) for 6 cycles (Goldhirsch, 1998; Levine, 1998)

FAC regimen: 500 mg/m^2 on days 1 and 8 every 21-28 days (in combination with cyclophosphamide and doxorubicin) for 6 cycles (Assikis, 2003)

Colorectal cancer (off-label dosing): IV:

FLOX regimen: 500 mg/m^2 bolus on days 1, 8, 15, 22, 29, and 36 (1 hour after leucovorin) every 8 weeks (in combination with leucovorin and oxaliplatin) for 3 cycles (Kuebler, 2007)

FOLFOX6 and mFOLFOX6 regimen: 400 mg/m^2 bolus on day 1, followed by 1200 mg/m^2/day continuous infusion for 2 days (over 46 hours) every 2 weeks (in combination with leucovorin and oxaliplatin) until disease progression or unacceptable toxicity (Cheeseman, 2002)

FOLFIRI regimens: 400 mg/m^2 bolus on day 1, followed by 1200 mg/m^2/day continuous infusion for 2 days (over 46 hours) every 2 weeks (in combination with leucovorin and irinotecan) until disease progression or unacceptable toxicity; after 2 cycles, may increase

continuous infusion fluorouracil dose to 1500 mg/m²/day (over 46 hours) (Andre, 1999)
Roswell Park regimen: 500 mg/m² (bolus) on days 1, 8, 15, 22, 29, and 36 (1 hour after leucovorin) every 8 weeks (in combination with leucovorin) for 4 cycles (Haller, 2005)

Gastric cancer (off-label dosing): IV:
CF regimen: 750-1000 mg/m²/day continuous infusion days 1-4 and 29-32 of a 35-day treatment cycle (preoperative chemoradiation; in combination with cisplatin) (Tepper, 2008; NCCN Gastric Cancer Guidelines v2.2012)
ECF regimen (resectable disease): 200 mg/m²/day continuous infusion days 1-21 every 3 weeks (in combination with epirubicin and cisplatin) for 6 cycles (3 cycles preoperatively and 3 cycles postoperatively) (Cunningham, 2006)
ECF or EOF regimen (advanced disease): 200 mg/m²/day continuous infusion days 1-21 every 3 weeks (in combination with epirubicin and either cisplatin or oxaliplatin) for a planned duration of 24 weeks (Sumpter, 2005)
TCF or DCF regimen: 750 mg/m²/day continuous infusion days 1-5 every 3 weeks or 1000 mg/m²/day continuous infusion days 1-5 every 4 weeks (in combination with docetaxel and cisplatin) until disease progression or unacceptable toxicity (Ajani, 2007; Van Cutsem, 2006; NCCN Gastric Cancer Guidelines v2.2012)
ToGA regimen (HER2-positive): 800 mg/m²/day continuous infusion days 1-5 every 3 weeks (in combination with cisplatin and trastuzumab) until disease progression or unacceptable toxicity (Bang, 2010)

Pancreatic cancer (off-label dosing): IV:
Chemoradiation therapy: 250 mg/m²/day continuous infusion for 3 weeks prior to and then throughout radiation therapy (Regine, 2008)
Fluorouracil-Leucovorin: 425 mg/m²/day (bolus) days 1-5 every 28 days (in combination with leucovorin) for 6 cycles (Neoptolemos, 2010)
FOLFIRINOX regimen: 400 mg/m² bolus on day 1, followed by 1200 mg/m²/day continuous infusion for 2 days (over 46 hours) every 14 days (in combination with leucovorin, irinotecan, and oxaliplatin) until disease progression or unacceptable toxicity for a recommended 12 cycles (Conroy, 2011)

Anal carcinoma (off-label use): IV: 1000 mg/m²/day continuous infusion days 1-4 and days 29-32 (in combination with mitomycin and radiation therapy) (Ajani, 2008)

Bladder cancer (off-label use): IV: 500 mg/m²/day continuous infusion days 1-5 and days 16-20 (in combination with mitomycin and radiation therapy) (James, 2012)

Cervical cancer (off-label use): IV: 1000 mg/m²/day continuous infusion days 1-4 (in combination with cisplatin and radiation therapy) every 3 weeks for 3 cycles (Eifel, 2004)

Esophageal cancer (off-label use): IV:
CF regimen: 750-1000 mg/m²/day continuous infusion days 1-4 and 29-32 of a 35-day treatment cycle (preoperative chemoradiation; in combination with cisplatin) (Tepper, 2008; NCCN Esophageal and Esophagogastric Junction Cancers Guidelines v2.2012)
ECF regimen (resectable disease): 200 mg/m²/day continuous infusion days 1-21 every 3 weeks (in combination with epirubicin and cisplatin) for 6 cycles (3 cycles preoperatively and 3 cycles postoperatively) (Cunningham, 2006)
ECF or EOF regimen (advanced disease): 200 mg/m²/day continuous infusion days 1-21 every 3 weeks (in combination with epirubicin and either cisplatin or oxaliplatin) for a planned duration of 24 weeks (Sumpter, 2005)
TCF or DCF regimen: 750 mg/m²/day continuous infusion days 1-5 every 3 weeks or 1000 mg/m²/day continuous infusion days 1-5 every 4 weeks (in combination with docetaxel and cisplatin) until disease progression or unacceptable toxicity (Ajani, 2007; Van Cutsem, 2006; NCCN Esophageal and Esophagogastric Junction Cancers Guidelines v2.2012)

Head and neck cancer, squamous cell (off-label use): IV:
Platinum-Fluorouracil regimen: 1000 mg/m²/day continuous infusion days 1-4 every 3 weeks (in combination with cisplatin) for at least 6 cycles (Gibson, 2005) **or** 600 mg/m²/day continuous infusion days 1-4, 22-25, and 43-46 (in combination with carboplatin and radiation) (Denis, 2004; Bourhis, 2012)
TPF regimen: 1000 mg/m²/day continuous infusion days 1-4 every 3 weeks (in combination with docetaxel and cisplatin) for 3 cycles, and followed by chemoradiotherapy (Posner, 2007) **or** 750 mg/m²/day continuous infusion days 1-5 every 3 weeks (in combination with docetaxel and cisplatin) for up to 4 cycles (Vermorken, 2007)
Platinum, 5-FU, and cetuximab regimen: 1000 mg/m²/day continuous infusion days 1-4 every 3 weeks (in combination with either cisplatin or carboplatin and cetuximab) for a total of up to 6 cycles (Vermorken, 2008)

Hepatobiliary cancer (off-label use): IV: 600 mg/m² (bolus) on days 1, 8, and 15 every 4 weeks (in combination with gemcitabine and leucovorin) (Alberts, 2005)

Dosage adjustment for toxicity: *According to the manufacturer, treatment should be discontinued for the following:* Stomatitis or esophagopharyngitis, leukopenia (WBC <3500/mm³), rapidly falling white blood cell count, intractable vomiting, diarrhea, frequent bowel movements, watery stools, gastrointestinal ulcer or bleeding, thrombocytopenia (platelets <100,000/mm³), hemorrhage

Dosage adjustment for renal impairment: No dosage adjustment provided in the manufacturer's labeling; however, extreme caution should be used in patients with renal impairment. The following adjustments have been recommended:
CrCl <50 mL/minute and continuous renal replacement therapy (CRRT): No dosage adjustment necessary (Aronoff, 2007).
Hemodialysis:
Administer standard dose following hemodialysis on dialysis days (Janus, 2010).
Administer 50% of standard dose following hemodialysis (Aronoff, 2007).

Dosage adjustment for hepatic impairment: No dosage adjustment provided in the manufacturer's labeling; however, extreme caution should be used in patients with hepatic impairment. The following adjustments have been recommended:
Floyd, 2006: Bilirubin >5 mg/dL: Avoid use.
Koren, 1992: Hepatic impairment (degree not specified): Administer <50% of dose, then increase if toxicity does not occur.

Dosing in obesity: *ASCO Guidelines for appropriate chemotherapy dosing in obese adults with cancer:* Utilize patient's actual body weight (full weight) for calculation of body surface area- or weight-based dosing, particularly when the intent of therapy is curative; manage regimen-related toxicities in the same manner as for nonobese patients; if a dose reduction is utilized due to toxicity, consider resumption of full weight-based dosing with subsequent cycles, especially if cause of toxicity (eg, hepatic or renal impairment) is resolved (Griggs, 2012).

Dietary Considerations Increase dietary intake of thiamine.

Administration IV: Administration rate varies by protocol; refer to specific reference for protocol. May be administered by IV push, IV bolus, or as a continuous infusion. Avoid extravasation (may be an irritant).

Hazardous agent; use appropriate precautions for handling and disposal (NIOSH 2014 [group 1]).

Monitoring Parameters CBC with differential and platelet count, renal function tests, liver function tests, signs of palmar-plantar erythrodysesthesia syndrome, stomatitis, diarrhea, hemorrhage, or gastrointestinal ulcers or bleeding

Additional Information Oncology Comment: An investigational uridine prodrug, uridine triacetate (formerly called vistonuridine), has been studied in a limited number of cases of fluorouracil overdose. Of 17 patients receiving uridine triacetate beginning within 8-96 hours after fluorouracil overdose, all patients fully recovered (von Borstel, 2009). Updated data has described a total of 28 patients treated with uridine triacetate for fluorouracil overdose (including overdoses related to continuous infusions delivering fluorouracil at rates faster than prescribed), all of whom recovered fully (Bamat, 2010). Refer to Uridine Triacetate monograph.

Dosage Forms

Solution, Intravenous:

Adrucil: 500 mg/10 mL (10 mL); 2.5 g/50 mL (50 mL); 5 g/100 mL (100 mL)

Generic: 500 mg/10 mL (10 mL); 1 g/20 mL (20 mL); 2.5 g/50 mL (50 mL); 5 g/100 mL (100 mL)

Fluorouracil (Topical) (flure oh YOOR a sil)

Brand Names: U.S. Carac; Efudex; Fluoroplex

Brand Names: Canada Efudex®; Fluoroplex®

Index Terms 5-Fluorouracil; 5-FU; FU

Pharmacologic Category Antineoplastic Agent, Antimetabolite; Antineoplastic Agent, Antimetabolite (Pyrimidine Analog); Topical Skin Product

Use Management of actinic or solar keratoses and superficial basal cell carcinomas

Pregnancy Risk Factor X

Dosage Topical: Refer to individual protocols: Adults:

Actinic keratoses:

Carac™: Apply thin film to lesions once daily for up to 4 weeks, as tolerated

Efudex®: Apply to lesions twice daily for 2-4 weeks; complete healing may not be evident for 1-2 months following treatment

Fluoroplex®: Apply to lesions twice daily for 2-6 weeks

Superficial basal cell carcinoma: Efudex® 5%: Apply to affected lesions twice daily for 3-6 weeks; treatment may be continued for up to 10-12 weeks

Additional Information Complete prescribing information should be consulted for additional detail.

Dosage Forms

Cream, External:

Carac: 0.5% (30 g)

Efudex: 5% (40 g)

Fluoroplex: 1% (30 g)

Generic: 0.5% (30 g); 5% (40 g)

Solution, External:

Generic: 2% (10 mL); 5% (10 mL)

◆ **Fluorouracil Injection (Can)** *see* Fluorouracil (Systemic) *on page 896*

◆ **Fluouracil** *see* Fluorouracil (Systemic) *on page 896*

FLUoxetine (floo OKS e teen)

Brand Names: U.S. PROzac; PROzac Weekly; Sarafem

Brand Names: Canada Apo-Fluoxetine; Ava-Fluoxetine; CO Fluoxetine; Dom-Fluoxetine; Fluoxetine Capsules BP; FXT 40; Gen-Fluoxetine; JAMP-Fluoxetine; Mint-Fluoxetine; Mylan-Fluoxetine; Novo-Fluoxetine; Nu-Fluoxetine; PHL-Fluoxetine; PMS-Fluoxetine; PRO-Fluoxetine; Prozac; Q-Fluoxetine; ratio-Fluoxetine; Riva-Fluoxetine; Sandoz-Fluoxetine; Teva-Fluoxetine; ZYM-Fluoxetine

Index Terms Fluoxetine Hydrochloride

Pharmacologic Category Antidepressant, Selective Serotonin Reuptake Inhibitor

Use Treatment of major depressive disorder (MDD); treatment of binge-eating and vomiting in patients with moderate-to-severe bulimia nervosa; obsessive-compulsive disorder (OCD); premenstrual dysphoric disorder (PMDD); panic disorder with or without agoraphobia; in combination with olanzapine for treatment-resistant or bipolar I depression

Pregnancy Risk Factor C

Pregnancy Considerations Adverse events have been observed in animal reproduction studies. Fluoxetine and its metabolite cross the human placenta. An increased risk of teratogenic effects, including cardiovascular defects, may be associated with maternal use of fluoxetine or other SSRIs; however, available information is conflicting. Nonteratogenic effects in the newborn following SSRI/SNRI exposure late in the third trimester include respiratory distress, cyanosis, apnea, seizures, temperature instability, feeding difficulty, vomiting, hypoglycemia, hypo- or hypertonia, hyper-reflexia, jitteriness, irritability, constant crying, and tremor. Symptoms may be due to the toxicity of the SSRIs/SNRIs or a discontinuation syndrome and may be consistent with serotonin syndrome associated with SSRI treatment. Persistent pulmonary hypertension of the newborn (PPHN) has also been reported with SSRI exposure. The long-term effects of *in utero* SSRI exposure on infant development and behavior are not known.

Due to pregnancy-induced physiologic changes, women who are pregnant may require dose adjustments of fluoxetine to achieve euthymia. The ACOG recommends that therapy with SSRIs or SNRIs during pregnancy be individualized; treatment of depression during pregnancy should incorporate the clinical expertise of the mental health clinician, obstetrician, primary healthcare provider, and pediatrician. According to the American Psychiatric Association (APA), the risks of medication treatment should be weighed against other treatment options and untreated depression. For women who discontinue antidepressant medications during pregnancy and who may be at high risk for postpartum depression, the medications can be restarted following delivery. Treatment algorithms have been developed by the ACOG and the APA for the management of depression in women prior to conception and during pregnancy.

Breast-Feeding Considerations Fluoxetine and its metabolite are excreted into breast milk and can be detected in the serum of breast-feeding infants. Concentrations in breast milk are variable. In comparison to other SSRIs, fluoxetine concentrations in breast milk are higher and adverse events have been observed in nursing infants. Maternal use of an SSRI during pregnancy may cause delayed milk secretion. Breast-feeding is not recommended by the manufacturer. Long-term effects on development and behavior have not been studied.

Contraindications Hypersensitivity to fluoxetine or any component of the formulation; use of MAO inhibitors intended to treat psychiatric disorders (concurrently, within 5 weeks of discontinuing fluoxetine, or within 2 weeks of discontinuing the MAO inhibitor); initiation of fluoxetine in a patient receiving linezolid or intravenous methylene blue; use with pimozide or thioridazine (**Note:** Thioridazine should not be initiated until 5 weeks after the discontinuation of fluoxetine)

Warnings/Precautions [U.S. Boxed Warning]: Antidepressants increase the risk of suicidal thinking and behavior in children, adolescents, and young adults (18-24 years of age) with major depressive disorder (MDD) and other psychiatric disorders; consider risk prior to prescribing. Short-term studies did not show an increased risk in patients >24 years of age and showed a decreased risk in patients ≥65 years. Closely monitor all patients for clinical worsening, suicidality, or unusual changes in behavior, particularly during the initial 1-2 months of therapy or during periods of dosage adjustments (increases or decreases); the patient's family or caregiver should be instructed to closely observe the patient and communicate condition with healthcare provider. A medication guide concerning the use of antidepressants should be dispensed with each prescription. **Fluoxetine is FDA approved for the treatment of OCD in children ≥7 years of age and MDD in children ≥8 years of age.**

The possibility of a suicide attempt is inherent in major depression and may persist until remission occurs. Use caution in high-risk patients. Worsening depression and severe abrupt suicidality that are not part of the presenting symptoms may require discontinuation or modification of drug therapy. Prescriptions should be written for the smallest quantity consistent with good patient care. The patient's family or caregiver should be alerted to monitor patients for the emergence of suicidality and associated behaviors (such as agitation, irritability, hostility, impulsivity, and hypomania) and call healthcare provider.

May worsen psychosis in some patients or precipitate a shift to mania or hypomania in patients with bipolar disorder. Patients presenting with depressive symptoms should be screened for bipolar disorder. Monotherapy in patients with bipolar disorder should be avoided. **Fluoxetine monotherapy is not FDA approved for the treatment of bipolar depression.** May cause insomnia, anxiety, nervousness, or anorexia. Use with caution in patients where weight loss is undesirable. May impair cognitive or motor performance; caution operating hazardous machinery or driving.

QT prolongation and ventricular arrhythmia including torsade de pointes has occurred. Use with caution in patients with risk factors for QT prolongation, under conditions that predispose to arrhythmias, or increased fluoxetine exposure. Consider discontinuation of fluoxetine if ventricular arrhythmia suspected and initiate cardiac evaluation. Avoid concurrent use with other medications that increase QT interval.

Potentially life-threatening serotonin syndrome (SS) has occurred with serotonergic agents (eg, SSRIs, SNRIs), particularly when used in combination with other serotonergic agents (eg, triptans, TCAs, fentanyl, lithium, tramadol, buspirone, St John's wort, tryptophan) or agents that impair metabolism of serotonin (eg, MAO inhibitors intended to treat psychiatric disorders, other MAO inhibitors [ie, linezolid and intravenous methylene blue]). Discontinue treatment (and any concomitant serotonergic agent) immediately if signs/symptoms arise. Fluoxetine use has been associated with occurrences of significant rash and allergic events, including vasculitis, lupus-like syndrome, laryngospasm, anaphylactoid reactions, and pulmonary inflammatory disease. Discontinue if underlying cause of rash cannot be identified.

Use caution in patients with a previous seizure disorder or condition predisposing to seizures such as brain damage or alcoholism. Use with caution in patients with hepatic or severe renal dysfunction and in elderly patients. Use caution in elderly patients; may be potentially inappropriate in patients with a history of falls or fractures, and may cause or exacerbate syndrome of inappropriate antidiuretic hormone secretion or hyponatremia; monitor sodium closely with initiation or dosage adjustments in older adults (Beers Criteria). May also cause agitation, sleep disturbances, and excessive CNS stimulation. May cause hyponatremia/SIADH (elderly at increased risk); volume depletion (diuretics may increase risk). May increase the risks associated with electroconvulsive treatment. Use caution with history of MI or unstable heart disease; use in these patients is limited. May alter glycemic control in patients with diabetes. Due to the long half-life of fluoxetine and its metabolites, the effects and interactions noted may persist for prolonged periods following discontinuation. May cause or exacerbate sexual dysfunction. May cause mild pupillary dilation, which in susceptible individuals can lead to an episode of narrow-angle glaucoma. Consider evaluating patients who have not had an iridectomy for narrow-angle glaucoma risk factors. Bone fractures have been associated with antidepressant treatment. Consider the possibility of a fragility fracture if an antidepressant-treated patient presents with unexplained bone pain, point tenderness, swelling, or bruising (Rabenda, 2013; Rizzoli, 2012). Potentially significant drug-drug interactions may exist, requiring dose or frequency adjustment, additional monitoring, and/or selection of alternative therapy.

Abrupt discontinuation or interruption of antidepressant therapy has been associated with a discontinuation syndrome. Symptoms arising may vary with antidepressant however commonly include nausea, vomiting, diarrhea, headaches, light-headedness, dizziness, diminished appetite, sweating, chills, tremors, paresthesias, fatigue, somnolence, and sleep disturbances (eg, vivid dreams, insomnia). Greater risks for developing a discontinuation syndrome have been associated with antidepressants with shorter half-lives, longer durations of treatment, and abrupt discontinuation. For antidepressants of short or intermediate half-lives, symptoms may emerge within 2-5 days after treatment discontinuation and last 7-14 days (APA, 2010; Fava, 2006; Haddad, 2001; Shelton, 2001; Warner, 2006).

Benzyl alcohol and derivatives: Some dosage forms may contain sodium benzoate/benzoic acid; benzoic acid (benzoate) is a metabolite of benzyl alcohol; large amounts of benzyl alcohol (≥99 mg/kg/day) have been associated with a potentially fatal toxicity ("gasping syndrome") in neonates; the "gasping syndrome" consists of metabolic acidosis, respiratory distress, gasping respirations, CNS dysfunction (including convulsions, intracranial hemorrhage), hypotension, and cardiovascular collapse (AAP, 1997; CDC, 1982); some data suggests that benzoate displaces bilirubin from protein binding sites (Ahlfors, 2001); avoid or use dosage forms containing benzyl alcohol derivative with caution in neonates. See manufacturer's labeling.

Adverse Reactions

Cardiovascular: Chest pain, hemorrhage, hypertension, palpitation, vasodilation

Central nervous system: Abnormal dreams, abnormal thinking, agitation, amnesia, anxiety, chills, confusion, dizziness, emotional lability, headache, insomnia, nervousness, sleep disorder, somnolence

Dermatologic: Pruritus, rash

Endocrine & metabolic: Ejaculation abnormal, impotence, libido decreased, menorrhagia

Gastrointestinal: Anorexia, appetite decreased, constipation, diarrhea, dyspepsia, flatulence, nausea, taste perversion, thirst, vomiting, weight gain, weight loss, xerostomia

Genitourinary: Urinary frequency

Neuromuscular & skeletal: Hyperkinesia, tremor, weakness

Ocular: Vision abnormal

Otic: Ear pain, tinnitus

Respiratory: Pharyngitis, sinusitis, yawn

Miscellaneous: Diaphoresis, epistaxis, flu-like syndrome

Rare but important or life-threatening: Acne, acute abdominal syndrome, akathisia, albuminuria, allergies, alopecia, amenorrhea, anaphylactoid reactions, anemia, angina, aphthous stomatitis, aplastic anemia, arrhythmia, arthritis, asthma, ataxia, atrial fibrillation, balance disorder, bone pain, bruising, bruxism, bursitis, cardiac arrest, cataract, cerebrovascular accident, CHF, cholelithiasis, cholestatic jaundice, colitis, dehydration, delusions, depersonalization, dyskinesia, dysphagia, dysuria, ecchymosis, edema, eosinophilic pneumonia, erythema multiforme, erythema nodosum, esophagitis, euphoria, exfoliative dermatitis, extrapyramidal symptoms (rare), gastritis, gastroenteritis, GI ulcer, glossitis, gout, gynecological bleeding, gynecomastia, hallucinations, hepatic failure/necrosis, hepatitis, hiccup, hostility, hypercholesteremia, hyperprolactinemia, hypertonia, hyperventilation, hypoglycemia, hypokalemia, hyponatremia (possibly in association with SIADH), hypotension, hypothyroidism, immune-related hemolytic anemia, kidney failure, laryngospasm, laryngeal edema, leg cramps, liver function test abnormalities, lupus-like syndrome, malaise, melena, migraine, misuse/abuse, MI, mydriasis, myoclonus, neuroleptic malignant syndrome (NMS), optic neuritis, orthostatic hypotension, pancreatitis, pancytopenia, paranoid reaction, petechia, photosensitivity reaction, priapism, pulmonary embolism, pulmonary fibrosis, pulmonary hypertension, purpuric rash, QT prolongation, serotonin syndrome, Stevens-Johnson syndrome, suicidal ideation, syncope, tachycardia, thrombocytopenia, thrombocytopenic purpura, toxic epidermal necrolysis, vasculitis, ventricular tachycardia (including torsade de pointes), violent behavior

Drug Interactions

Metabolism/Transport Effects Substrate of CYP1A2 (minor), CYP2B6 (minor), CYP2C19 (minor), CYP2C9 (major), CYP2D6 (major), CYP2E1 (minor), CYP3A4 (minor); **Note:** Assignment of Major/Minor substrate status based on clinically relevant drug interaction potential; **Inhibits** CYP1A2 (weak), CYP2B6 (weak), CYP2C19 (moderate), CYP2C9 (weak), CYP2D6 (strong)

Avoid Concomitant Use

Avoid concomitant use of FLUoxetine with any of the following: Dapoxetine; Dosulepin; Haloperidol; Highest Risk QTc-Prolonging Agents; Iobenguane I 123; Ivabradine; Linezolid; MAO Inhibitors; Methylene Blue; Mifepristone; Moderate Risk QTc-Prolonging Agents; Pimozide; Propafenone; Tamoxifen; Thioridazine; Tryptophan; Urokinase; Ziprasidone

Increased Effect/Toxicity

FLUoxetine may increase the levels/effects of: Agents with Antiplatelet Properties; Anticoagulants; Antidepressants (Serotonin Reuptake Inhibitor/Antagonist); Antipsychotic Agents; Apixaban; ARIPiprazole; Aspirin; AtoMOXetine; Beta-Blockers; BusPIRone; CarBAMazepine; Collagenase (Systemic); CYP2C19 Substrates; CYP2D6 Substrates; Dabigatran Etexilate; Desmopressin; Dextromethorphan; Dosulepin; DOXOrubicin (Conventional); Fesoterodine; Fosphenytoin; Haloperidol; Highest Risk QTc-Prolonging Agents; Hypoglycemic Agents; Ibritumomab; Methylene Blue; Metoprolol; Mexiletine; Nebivolol; NIFEdipine; NiMODipine; NSAID (COX-2 Inhibitor); NSAID (Nonselective); Obinutuzumab; Phenytoin; Pimozide; Propafenone; Rivaroxaban; Salicylates; Serotonin Modulators; Thiazide Diuretics; Thioridazine; Thrombolytic Agents; Tositumomab and Iodine I 131 Tositumomab; TraMADol; Tricyclic Antidepressants; Urokinase; Vitamin K Antagonists; Vortioxetine; Ziprasidone

The levels/effects of FLUoxetine may be increased by: Abiraterone Acetate; Alcohol (Ethyl); Analgesics (Opioid); Antiemetics (5HT3 Antagonists); Antipsychotic Agents; ARIPiprazole; BuPROPion; BusPIRone; Cimetidine; CNS Depressants; Cobicistat; CYP2C9 Inhibitors (Moderate); CYP2C9 Inhibitors (Strong); CYP2D6 Inhibitors (Moderate); CYP2D6 Inhibitors (Strong); Dapoxetine; Darunavir; Fosphenytoin; Glucosamine; Herbs (Anticoagulant/Antiplatelet Properties); Ibrutinib; Ivabradine; Limaprost; Linezolid; Lithium; MAO Inhibitors; Metoclopramide; Metyrosine; Mifepristone; Moderate Risk QTc-Prolonging Agents; Multivitamins/Fluoride (with ADE); Multivitamins/Minerals (with ADEK, Folate, Iron); Multivitamins/Minerals (with AE, No Iron); Omega-3 Fatty Acids; Pentosan Polysulfate Sodium; Pentoxifylline; Propafenone; Prostacyclin Analogues; QTc-Prolonging Agents (Indeterminate Risk and Risk Modifying); Tedizolid; TraMADol; Tryptophan; Vitamin E; Ziprasidone

Decreased Effect

FLUoxetine may decrease the levels/effects of: Clopidogrel; Codeine; Iobenguane I 123; Ioflupane I 123; Tamoxifen; Thyroid Products

The levels/effects of FLUoxetine may be decreased by: CarBAMazepine; CYP2C9 Inducers (Strong); Cyproheptadine; Dabrafenib; NSAID (COX-2 Inhibitor); NSAID (Nonselective); Peginterferon Alfa-2b

Storage/Stability All dosage forms should be stored at controlled room temperature. Protect from light.

Mechanism of Action Inhibits CNS neuron serotonin reuptake; minimal or no effect on reuptake of norepinephrine or dopamine; does not significantly bind to alpha-adrenergic, histamine, or cholinergic receptors

Pharmacodynamics/Kinetics

Onset of action: Depression: The onset of action is within a week; however, individual response varies greatly and full response may not be seen until 8-12 weeks after initiation of treatment.

Absorption: Well absorbed; delayed 1-2 hours with weekly formulation

Distribution: V_d: 12-43 L/kg

Protein binding: 95% to albumin and $alpha_1$ glycoprotein

Metabolism: Hepatic, via CYP2C19 and 2D6, to norfluoxetine (activity equal to fluoxetine)

Half-life elimination: Adults:

Parent drug: 1-3 days (acute), 4-6 days (chronic), 7.6 days (cirrhosis)

Metabolite (norfluoxetine): 9.3 days (range: 4-16 days), 12 days (cirrhosis)

Time to peak, serum: 6-8 hours

Excretion: Urine (10% as norfluoxetine, 2.5% to 5% as fluoxetine)

Note: Weekly formulation results in greater fluctuations between peak and trough concentrations of fluoxetine and norfluoxetine compared to once-daily dosing (24% daily/164% weekly; 17% daily/43% weekly, respectively). Trough concentrations are 76% lower for fluoxetine and 47% lower for norfluoxetine than the concentrations maintained by 20 mg once-daily dosing. Steady-state fluoxetine concentrations are ~50% lower following the once-weekly regimen compared to 20 mg once daily. Average steady-state concentrations of once-daily dosing were highest in children ages 6 to <13 (fluoxetine 171 ng/mL; norfluoxetine 195 ng/mL), followed by adolescents ages 13 to <18 (fluoxetine 86 ng/mL; norfluoxetine 113 ng/mL); concentrations were considered to be within the ranges reported in adults (fluoxetine 91-302 ng/mL; norfluoxetine 72-258 ng/mL).

Dosage Oral:

Children:

Depression: 8-18 years: 10-20 mg/day; lower-weight children can be started at 10 mg/day, may increase to 20 mg/day after 1 week if needed

Depression associated with bipolar I disorder (in combination with olanzapine): 10-17 years: Initial: 20 mg in the evening; adjust dose, if needed, as tolerated; safety of fluoxetine doses >50 mg in combination with doses >12 mg of olanzapine has not been studied in pediatrics. See **"Note"** below.

Obsessive-compulsive disorder: 7-17 years: Initial: 10 mg/day; may increase after 2 weeks if inadequate clinical response to 20 mg/day; further increases may be considered after several weeks to recommended range of 20-30 mg/day (lower weight children) or 20-60 mg/day (adolescents and higher weight children)

Selective mutism (off-label use): 5-18 years: Initial: 5-10 mg/day; titrate upwards as needed (usual maximum dose: 60 mg/day)

Adults: Depression, obessive-compulsive disorder: 20 mg/day in the morning; may increase after several weeks by 20 mg/day increments; maximum: 80 mg/day; doses >20 mg may be given once daily or divided twice daily. **Note:** Lower doses of 5-10 mg/day have been used for initial treatment.

Indication-specific dosing:

Bulimia nervosa: 60 mg/day; may titrate dose to 60 mg over several days

Depression: Initial: 20 mg/day; may increase after several weeks if inadequate response (maximum: 80 mg/day). Patients maintained on Prozac 20 mg/day may be changed to Prozac Weekly 90 mg/week, starting dose 7 days after the last 20 mg/day dose

Depression associated with bipolar I disorder (in combination with olanzapine): Initial: 20 mg in the evening; adjust as tolerated to usual range of 20-50 mg/day. See **"Note"** below.

Fibromyalgia (off-label use): Range: 20-80 mg/day (Arnold, 2002)

Obsessive-compulsive disorder: Initial: 20 mg/day; may increase after several weeks if inadequate response; recommended range: 20-60 mg/day (maximum: 80 mg/day)

Panic disorder: Initial: 10 mg/day; after 1 week, increase to 20 mg/day; may increase after several weeks; doses >60 mg/day have not been evaluated

Post-traumatic stress disorder (PTSD) (off-label use): 20-40 mg/day

Premenstrual dysphoric disorder (Sarafem): 20 mg/day continuously, **or** 20 mg/day starting 14 days prior to menstruation and through first full day of menses (repeat with each cycle)

Raynaud's phenomena (off-label use): 20 mg/day (Coleiro, 2001)

Social anxiety disorder (off-label use): Target dose: 40 mg/day; range 30-60 mg/day (Davidson, 2004)

Treatment-resistant depression (in combination with olanzapine): Initial: 20 mg in the evening; adjust as tolerated to usual range of 20-50 mg/day. See **"Note."**

Note: When using individual components of fluoxetine with olanzapine rather than fixed-dose combination product (Symbyax), approximate dosage correspondence is as follows:

Olanzapine 2.5 mg + fluoxetine 20 mg = Symbyax 3/25

Olanzapine 5 mg + fluoxetine 20 mg = Symbyax 6/25

Olanzapine 12.5 mg + fluoxetine 20 mg = Symbyax 12/25

Olanzapine 5 mg + fluoxetine 50 mg = Symbyax 6/50

Olanzapine 12.5 mg + fluoxetine 50 mg = Symbyax 12/50

Elderly: Depression: Some patients may require an initial dose of 10 mg/day with dosage increases of 10 and 20 mg every several weeks as tolerated; should not be taken at night unless patient experiences sedation

Discontinuation of therapy: Upon discontinuation of antidepressant therapy, gradually taper the dose to minimize the incidence of withdrawal symptoms and allow for the detection of re-emerging symptoms. Evidence supporting ideal taper rates is limited. APA and NICE guidelines suggest tapering therapy over at least several weeks with consideration to the half-life of the antidepressant; antidepressants with a shorter half-life may need to be tapered more conservatively. In addition for long-term treated patients, WFSBP guidelines recommend tapering over 4-6 months. If intolerable withdrawal symptoms occur following a dose reduction, consider resuming the previously prescribed dose and/or decrease dose at a more gradual rate (APA, 2010; Bauer, 2002; Haddad, 2001; NCCMH, 2010; Schatzberg, 2006; Shelton, 2001; Warner, 2006).

MAO inhibitor recommendations:

Switching to or from an MAO inhibitor intended to treat psychiatric disorders:

Allow 14 days to elapse between discontinuing an MAO inhibitor intended to treat psychiatric disorders and initiation of fluoxetine.

Allow 5 weeks to elapse between discontinuing fluoxetine and initiation of an MAO inhibitor intended to treat psychiatric disorders.

Use with other MAO inhibitors (linezolid or IV methylene blue):

Do not initiate fluoxetine in patients receiving linezolid or IV methylene blue; consider other interventions for psychiatric condition.

If urgent treatment with linezolid or IV methylene blue is required in a patient already receiving fluoxetine and potential benefits outweigh potential risks, discontinue fluoxetine promptly and administer linezolid or IV methylene blue. Monitor for serotonin syndrome for 5 weeks or until 24 hours after the last dose of linezolid or IV methylene blue, whichever comes first. May resume fluoxetine 24 hours after the last dose of linezolid or IV methylene blue.

Dosing adjustment in renal impairment:

Single dose studies: Pharmacokinetics of fluoxetine and norfluoxetine were similar among subjects with all levels of impaired renal function, including anephric patients on chronic hemodialysis

Chronic administration: Additional accumulation of fluoxetine or norfluoxetine may occur in patients with severely impaired renal function

Hemodialysis: Not removed by hemodialysis; use of lower dose or less frequent dosing is not usually necessary.

Dosing adjustment in hepatic impairment: Elimination half-life of fluoxetine is prolonged in patients with hepatic impairment; a lower or less frequent dose of fluoxetine should be used in these patients

Cirrhosis patients: Administer a lower dose or less frequent dosing interval

Compensated cirrhosis without ascites: Administer 50% of normal dose

Dietary Considerations May be taken without regard to meals.

Administration Administer without regard to meals.

Bipolar I disorder and treatment-resistant depression: Take once daily in the evening.

Major depressive disorder and obsessive compulsive disorder: Once daily doses should be taken in the morning, or twice daily (morning and noon).

Bulimia: Take once daily in the morning.

Monitoring Parameters Mental status for depression, suicidal ideation (especially at the beginning of therapy or when doses are increased or decreased), anxiety, social functioning, mania, panic attacks; signs/symptoms of serotonin syndrome; akathisia, sleep status; blood glucose (for diabetic patients), baseline liver function; ECG assessment and periodic monitoring in patients with risk factors for QT prolongation and ventricular arrhythmia

Reference Range Therapeutic levels have not been well established

Therapeutic: Fluoxetine: 100-800 ng/mL (SI: 289-2314 nmol/L); Norfluoxetine: 100-600 ng/mL (SI: 289-1735 nmol/L)

Toxic: Fluoxetine plus norfluoxetine: >2000 ng/mL

Additional Information ECG may reveal S-T segment depression. Not shown to be teratogenic in rodents; 15-60 mg/day, buspirone and cyproheptadine, may be useful in treatment of sexual dysfunction during treatment with a selective serotonin reuptake inhibitor.

Weekly capsules are a delayed release formulation containing enteric-coated pellets of fluoxetine hydrochloride, equivalent to 90 mg fluoxetine. Therapeutic equivalence of weekly formulation with daily formulation for delaying time to relapse has not been established.

Dosage Forms

Capsule, Oral:

PROzac: 10 mg, 20 mg, 40 mg

Generic: 10 mg, 20 mg, 40 mg

Capsule Delayed Release, Oral:

PROzac Weekly: 90 mg

Generic: 90 mg

Solution, Oral:

Generic: 20 mg/5 mL (5 mL, 120 mL)

Tablet, Oral:

Sarafem: 10 mg, 20 mg

Generic: 10 mg, 20 mg, 60 mg

Dosage Forms: Canada Note: Refer to Dosage Forms. Delayed release capsules and tablets are not available in Canada.

Extemporaneous Preparations Note: Commercial oral solution is available (4 mg/mL)

A 1 mg/mL fluoxetine oral solution may be prepared using the commercially available preparation (4 mg/mL). In separate graduated cylinders, measure 5 mL of the commercially available fluoxetine preparation and 15 mL of Simple Syrup, NF. Mix thoroughly in incremental proportions. For a 2 mg/mL solution, mix equal proportions of both the commercially available fluoxetine preparation and Simple Syrup, NF. Label "refrigerate". Both concentrations are stable for up to 56 days.

Nahata MC, Pai VB, and Hipple TF, *Pediatric Drug Formulations*, 5th ed, Cincinnati, OH: Harvey Whitney Books Co, 2004.

◆ **Fluoxetine Capsules BP (Can)** *see* FLUoxetine *on page 899*

◆ **Fluoxetine Hydrochloride** *see* FLUoxetine *on page 899*

Fluoxymesterone (floo oks i MES te rone)

Brand Names: U.S. Androxy [DSC]

Pharmacologic Category Androgen

Use Replacement therapy in the treatment of delayed male puberty; male hypogonadism (primary or hypogonadotropic); inoperable metastatic female breast cancer

Pregnancy Risk Factor X

Dosage Adults: Oral:

Male:

Hypogonadism: 5-20 mg daily

Delayed puberty: 2.5-20 mg daily for 4-6 months

Female: Inoperable breast carcinoma: 10-40 mg daily in divided doses for ≥3 months

Dosage adjustment in renal impairment: No dosage adjustment provided in manufacturer's labeling; use with caution.

Dosage adjustment in hepatic impairment: No dosage adjustment provided in manufacturer's labeling; use with caution.

Additional Information Complete prescribing information should be consulted for additional detail.

◆ **Flupenthixol Decanoate** *see* Flupentixol [CAN/INT] *on page 903*

◆ **Flupenthixol Dihydrochloride** *see* Flupentixol [CAN/INT] *on page 903*

Flupentixol [CAN/INT] (floo pen TIKS ol)

Brand Names: Canada Fluanxol®; Fluanxol® Depot

Index Terms Flupenthixol Decanoate; Flupenthixol Dihydrochloride; Flupentixol Decanoate; Flupentixol Dihydrochloride

Pharmacologic Category First Generation (Typical) Antipsychotic

Use Note: Not approved in U.S.

Maintenance therapy of chronic schizophrenic patients whose main manifestations do **not** include excitement, agitation, or hyperactivity

Pregnancy Considerations There are no adequate and well-controlled studies in pregnant women. Antipsychotic use during the third trimester of pregnancy has a risk for abnormal muscle movements (extrapyramidal symptoms [EPS]) and withdrawal symptoms in newborns following delivery. Symptoms in the newborn may include agitation, feeding disorder, hypertonia, hypotonia, respiratory distress, somnolence, and tremor; these effects may be self-limiting or require hospitalization.

Breast-Feeding Considerations At therapeutic doses, flupentixol is found at low concentrations in human breast milk. Adverse effects are not likely in a nursing infant when used within the therapeutic dosing range.

Contraindications Hypersensitivity to flupentixol, thioxanthenes, or any component of the formulation; acute intoxication (ethanol, barbiturate, or opioid); CNS depression due to any cause; coma; severely-agitated psychotic patients, psychoneurotic patients, or geriatric patients with confusion and/or agitation; suspected or established subcortical brain damage; cerebrovascular or renal insufficiency; severe cardiovascular disease/circulatory collapse; liver damage; concomitant use with large doses of hypnotics

Warnings/Precautions [Canadian Boxed Warning]: Neuroleptic malignant syndrome (NMS) has been associated with use of antipsychotic agents, including flupentixol; monitor for mental status changes, fever, muscle rigidity, and/or autonomic instability (risk may be increased in patients with Parkinson's disease or Lewy body dementia). Discontinue treatment immediately with onset of NMS; recurrence has been reported in patients rechallenged with antipsychotic therapy.

May alter cardiac conduction; life-threatening arrhythmias have occurred with therapeutic doses of antipsychotics. Avoid use in patients with underlying QT prolongation, in those taking medicines that prolong the QT interval, or cause polymorphic ventricular tachycardia; monitor ECG closely for dose-related QT effects. May cause orthostatic hypotension; use with caution in patients at risk of this effect or in those who would not tolerate transient hypotensive episodes (cerebrovascular disease, cardiovascular disease, hypovolemia, or concurrent medication use which may predispose to hypotension/bradycardia). VTE has been reported with antipsychotics; evaluate VTE risk prior to and during therapy.

Use is contraindicated in patients with severe cardiovascular disease, liver damage, or renal insufficiency. Use with caution in patients with known or suspected glaucoma (avoid use in patients with known or suspected narrow-angle glaucoma), hepatic impairment, Parkinson's disease, breast cancer or other prolactin-dependent tumors, renal impairment, or seizure disorder. Leukopenia, neutropenia, and agranulocytosis (sometimes fatal) have been reported in clinical trials and postmarketing reports with antipsychotic use.

Antipsychotic use has been associated with esophageal dysmotility and aspiration; use with caution in patients at risk of pneumonia (ie, Alzheimer's disease). May cause extrapyramidal symptoms, including pseudoparkinsonism, acute dystonic reactions, akathisia, and tardive dyskinesia. Risk of dystonia (and possibly other EPS) may be greater with increased doses, use of conventional antipsychotics, males, and younger patients. Risk of tardive dyskinesia and potential for irreversibility may be increased in elderly patients (particularly women), prolonged therapy, and higher total cumulative dose.

Elderly patients with dementia-related psychosis who are treated with antipsychotics are at an increased risk of death compared to placebo. Most deaths appeared to be either cardiovascular (eg, heart failure, sudden death) or infectious (eg, pneumonia) in nature. An increased incidence of cerebrovascular adverse events (including fatalities) has been reported in elderly patients with dementia-related psychosis. Flupentixol is not approved for use in elderly patients with dementia or dementia-related psychosis.

May be sedating, use with caution in disorders where CNS depression is a feature; patients must be cautioned about performing tasks which require mental alertness (eg, operating machinery or driving). May cause anticholinergic effects (constipation, xerostomia, blurred vision, urinary retention); use with caution in patients with decreased gastrointestinal motility, paralytic ileus, urinary retention, BPH, xerostomia, or visual problems. Impaired core body temperature regulation may occur; caution with strenuous exercise, heat exposure, dehydration, and concomitant medication possessing anticholinergic effects. Relative to other neuroleptics, flupentixol has a low potency of cholinergic blockade. May mask toxicity of other drugs or conditions (eg, intestinal obstruction, Reye's syndrome, brain tumor) due to antiemetic effects.

Lens opacity has been reported rarely with use. Similar drugs have been associated with pigmentary retinopathy, corneal and lenticular deposits, and photosensitivity. Not recommended for use in excitable, overactive, or manic patients. Avoid abrupt withdrawal in patients receiving maintenance therapy; withdrawal symptoms (eg, n/v, insomnia, restlessness, agitation) may appear 1-4 days after discontinuing therapy and subside within 7-14 days. Surgical patients receiving high-dose flupentixol should be monitored closely for hypotension; dose reduction of anesthetic or CNS depressants may be necessary. Adverse effects of decanoate may be prolonged.

Adverse Reactions

Cardiovascular: Palpitation

Central nervous system: Extrapyramidal effects (up to 30%; including akathisia, dystonia, pseudoparkinsonism, tardive dyskinesia), depression, dizziness, drowsiness, fainting, fatigue, headache, hypomania, insomnia, oculogyric crises, opisthotonos, psychomotor agitation, restlessness, seizure, somnolence

Dermatologic: Contact dermatitis, eczema, erythema, exfoliative dermatitis, pruritus, rash, seborrhea, urticaria

Endocrine & metabolic: Amenorrhea, galactorrhea, gynecomastia, hyperprolactinemia, impotence, libido decreased/increased

Gastrointestinal: Constipation, nausea, paralytic ileus, salivation increased, weight changes, xerostomia

Genitourinary: Micturition disorder

Hematologic: Eosinophilia

Hepatic: Alkaline phosphatase increased, ALT increased, AST increased, jaundice

Neuromuscular & skeletal: Hyperreflexia, hypertonia, tremor

Ocular: Blurred vision, lens opacity

Miscellaneous: Diaphoresis increased

Rare but important or life-threatening: Abdominal pain, accommodation abnormal, amenorrhea, dyspepsia, dyspnea, erectile dysfunction, glucose tolerance impaired, granulocytopenia, hot flashes, hyperglycemia, muscle rigidity, myalgia, neuroleptic malignant syndrome (NMS), neutropenia, priapism, QT prolongation, thrombocytopenia, torsade de pointes, ventricular arrhythmias, ventricular fibrillation, ventricular tachycardia, vomiting, weakness

Additional adverse events associated with antipsychotics include agranulocytosis, arrhythmias, angioedema, asthma, cerebral edema, corneal deposits, CSF proteins altered, CVA, ECG changes, EEG changes, glaucoma, glycosuria, gynecomastia, hemolytic anemia, hepatotoxicity, hypoglycemia, hypo/hypertension, laryngeal edema, lenticular deposits, leukopenia, menstrual abnormalities, miosis, mydriasis, nonthrombocytopenic purpura, pancytopenia, peripheral edema, photosensitivity, pigmentary retinopathy, skin pigmentation, SLE, sudden death, syncope, tachycardia, VTE

Drug Interactions

Metabolism/Transport Effects None known.

Avoid Concomitant Use

Avoid concomitant use of Flupentixol with any of the following: Aclidinium; Amisulpride; Azelastine (Nasal); Glucagon; Highest Risk QTc-Prolonging Agents; Ipratropium (Oral Inhalation); Ivabradine; Metoclopramide; Mifepristone; Moderate Risk QTc-Prolonging Agents; Orphenadrine; Paraldehyde; Potassium Chloride; Sulpiride; Thalidomide; Tiotropium; Umeclidinium

Increased Effect/Toxicity

Flupentixol may increase the levels/effects of: AbobotulinumtoxinA; Alcohol (Ethyl); Amisulpride; Analgesics (Opioid); Anticholinergic Agents; Azelastine (Nasal); Buprenorphine; CNS Depressants; Glucagon; Highest Risk QTc-Prolonging Agents; Hydrocodone; Methotrimeprazine; Methylphenidate; Metyrosine; OnabotulinumtoxinA; Orphenadrine; Paraldehyde; Potassium Chloride; RimabotulinumtoxinB; Selective Serotonin Reuptake Inhibitors; Serotonin Modulators; Sulpiride; Suvorexant; Thalidomide; Thiazide Diuretics; Tiotropium; Topiramate; Zolpidem

The levels/effects of Flupentixol may be increased by: Acetylcholinesterase Inhibitors (Central); Aclidinium; Brimonidine (Topical); Cannabis; Doxylamine; Dronabinol; Ipratropium (Oral Inhalation); Ivabradine; Kava Kava; Magnesium Sulfate; Methotrimeprazine; Methylphenidate; Metoclopramide; Metyrosine; Mifepristone; Moderate Risk QTc-Prolonging Agents; Nabilone; Perampanel; Pramlintide; QTc-Prolonging Agents (Indeterminate Risk and Risk Modifying); Rufinamide; Serotonin Modulators; Sodium Oxybate; Tapentadol; Tetrahydrocannabinol; Umeclidinium

Decreased Effect

Flupentixol may decrease the levels/effects of: Acetylcholinesterase Inhibitors; Amphetamines; Anti-Parkinson's Agents (Dopamine Agonist); Itopride; Quinagolide; Secretin

The levels/effects of Flupentixol may be decreased by: Acetylcholinesterase Inhibitors; Anti-Parkinson's Agents (Dopamine Agonist)

Storage/Stability

Ampules for injection: Store at 15°C to 25°C (59°F to 77°F). Protect from light.

Tablets: Store at 15°C to 30°C (59°F to 86°F). Protect from light.

Mechanism of Action Flupentixol is a thioxanthene-derivative antipsychotic which blocks postsynaptic dopamine receptors in the CNS, resulting in inhibition of dopamine-mediated effects.

Pharmacodynamics/Kinetics

Onset: IM depot: 24-72 hours following injection

Duration: IM depot: 2-4 weeks

Distribution: V_d: ~14 L/kg

Protein binding: ~99%

Metabolism: Hepatic via sulfoxidation and dealkylation; also undergoes glucuronidation; metabolites are inactive

Bioavailability: Oral: ~40%

Half-life elimination: Oral: ~35 hours; IM depot: 3 weeks

Time to peak: Oral: 3-8 hours; IM depot: 4-7 days

Excretion: Mostly feces (as metabolites); urine (small amounts)

Dosage

IM (depot): Adults:

Initial:

Patients naive to treatment with long-acting depot antipsychotics: Administer test dose of 5-20 mg (5 mg dose is recommended in elderly, frail, cachectic patients or patients with predisposition to extrapyramidal reactions). Closely monitor therapeutic response and for the appearance of extrapyramidal symptoms over the following 5-10 days. Oral antipsychotic drugs may be continued, but dosage should be reduced during this overlapping period and eventually discontinued.

Patients with prior exposure and good tolerance of long-acting depot antipsychotics: 20-40 mg

Maintenance: 20-40 mg may be given 4-10 days after initial injection (if well tolerated), followed by usual maintenance dose of 20-40 mg every 2-3 weeks. Dose is individualized and titrated in maximum increments of ≤20 mg (doses >80 mg are not usually necessary but have been used in some patients). Dose should be maintained at the lowest effective dose.

Oral: Adults: Initial: 1 mg 3 times/day; dose must be individualized. May be increased by 1 mg every 2-3 days based on tolerance and control of symptoms. Usual maintenance dosage: 3-6 mg/day in divided doses (doses ≥12 mg/day have been used in some patients).

Conversion from oral tablets to maintenance dosing with IM injection (decanoate): Note: When transitioning to the depot injection, continue oral therapy at decreasing dosages for the first week following the initial injection.

If IM administration every 2 weeks: Use decanoate dose equal to 4 times the total daily oral dose

If IM administration every 4 weeks: Use decanoate dose equal to 8 times the total daily oral dose

Conversion from other antipsychotic depot formulations to IM flupentixol decanoate: Conversion ratios to calculate the equivalent dose:

Flupentixol decanoate 40 mg = fluphenazine decanoate 25 mg

Flupentixol decanoate 40 mg = zuclopenthixol decanoate 200 mg

Flupentixol decanoate 40 mg = haloperidol decanoate 50 mg

Dosage adjustment in renal impairment: The manufacturer's product labeling recommendations are unclear. Use in renal insufficiency is contraindicated however the labeling also suggests that dosage adjustments are not required in renal impairment; flupentixol systemic exposure is not likely to be influenced by renal impairment as the drug undergoes extensive hepatic metabolism and is primarily excreted in the feces.

Dosage adjustment in hepatic impairment: There are no dosage adjustments provided in manufacturer's labeling; flupentixol undergoes extensive hepatic metabolism. Use caution.

Administration

IM: Administer by deep IM injection, preferably in the gluteus maximus; doses requiring more than 2 mL should be administered as divided doses between 2 injection sites. **Do not administer IV**

Oral: Tablets may be taken with or without food. During initial therapy, may consider reducing evening dose in patients with sleep disturbance. Maintenance dose may be given as single morning dose. Missed doses should be taken at the next regularly scheduled time.

Monitoring Parameters Vital signs; hepatic function tests, lipid profile, CBC, fasting blood glucose/HbA_{1c}; BMI; mental status, abnormal involuntary movement scale (AIMS), extrapyramidal symptoms (EPS)

Additional Information Lundbeck Canada Inc changed the generic name of flupenthixol to flupentixol in the product monograph for Fluanxol® and Fluanxol® Depot in February 2011. Per Lundbeck, the name was changed to align with nomenclature used internationally for flupentixol.

Product Availability Not available in U.S.

Dosage Forms: Canada

Injection, Solution [depot]:

Fluanxol: 20 mg/mL (1 mL); 100 mg/mL (1 mL)

Tablet, Oral:

Fluanxol: 0.5 mg, 3 mg

◆ **Flupentixol Decanoate** *see* Flupentixol [CAN/INT] *on page 903*

◆ **Flupentixol Dihydrochloride** *see* Flupentixol [CAN/INT] *on page 903*

FluPHENAZine (floo FEN a zeen)

Brand Names: Canada Apo-Fluphenazine Decanoate®; Apo-Fluphenazine®; Modecate®; Modecate® Concentrate; PMS-Fluphenazine Decanoate

Index Terms Fluphenazine Decanoate; Fluphenazine Hydrochloride

Pharmacologic Category First Generation (Typical) Antipsychotic

Additional Appendix Information

Beers Criteria – Potentially Inappropriate Medications for Geriatrics *on page 2271*

Use Management of manifestations of psychotic disorders and schizophrenia; depot formulation may offer improved outcome in individuals with psychosis who are nonadherent with oral antipsychotics

Dosage

Adults: Psychoses:

Oral: Initial: 2.5 to 10 mg/day in divided doses at 6- to 8-hour intervals; Maintenance: 1 to 5 mg/day; **Note:** Some patients may require up to 40 mg/day for symptom control (long-term safety of higher doses not established)

PORT guidelines: Acute therapy: 6 to 20 mg/day for up to 6 weeks; Maintenance: 6 to 12 mg/day (Buchanan, 2009)

IM (hydrochloride): Initial: 1.25 mg as a single dose; depending on severity and duration, may need 2.5 to 10 mg/day in divided doses at 6- to 8-hour intervals (4 mg IM fluphenazine HCl is approximately equivalent to 10 mg oral fluphenazine HCl); use caution with doses >10 mg/day; once symptoms stabilized, transition to oral maintenance therapy

Long-acting maintenance injections (decanoate):

IM, SubQ (decanoate): Initial: 12.5 to 25 mg every 2 to 4 weeks; response may last up to 6 weeks in some patients; titrate dose cautiously, if doses >50 mg are needed, increase in 12.5 mg increments (maximum dose: 100 mg)

Conversion from hydrochloride dosage forms to decanoate IM: 12.5 mg of decanoate every 2 to 4 weeks is approximately equivalent to 10 mg of oral hydrochloride/day; **Note:** Clinically, an every-2-week interval is frequently utilized

PORT guidelines: 6.25 to 25 mg every 2 weeks (Buchanan, 2009)

Note: Decrease the oral fluphenazine (or current antipsychotic) dose by half after the initial injection; consider discontinuation of oral therapy after second injection (McEvoy, 2006).

Elderly: Oral: Initial: 1 to 2.5 mg daily; titrated gradually based on patient response

Hemodialysis: Not dialyzable (0% to 5%)

Additional Information Complete prescribing information should be consulted for additional detail.

Dosage Forms

Concentrate, Oral:
Generic: 5 mg/mL (120 mL)

Elixir, Oral:
Generic: 2.5 mg/5 mL (60 mL, 473 mL)

Solution, Injection:
Generic: 2.5 mg/mL (10 mL); 25 mg/mL (5 mL)

Tablet, Oral:
Generic: 1 mg, 2.5 mg, 5 mg, 10 mg

Dosage Forms: Canada Note: Refer also to Dosage Forms. Oral concentrate, oral elixir, and solution for injection (as hydrochloride) are not available in Canada.

Solution, Injection, as decanoate: 100 mg/mL (1 mL)

- **Fluphenazine Decanoate** *see* FluPHENAZine *on page 905*
- **Fluphenazine Hydrochloride** *see* FluPHENAZine *on page 905*
- **5-Fluracil** *see* Fluorouracil (Systemic) *on page 896*
- **Flura-Drops** *see* Fluoride *on page 895*

Flurandrenolide (flure an DREN oh lide)

Brand Names: U.S. Cordran

Index Terms Flurandrenolone

Pharmacologic Category Corticosteroid, Topical

Additional Appendix Information

Topical Corticosteroids *on page 2230*

Use Corticosteroid-responsive dermatoses: Relief of inflammatory and pruritic manifestations of corticosteroid-responsive dermatoses

Pregnancy Risk Factor C

Dosage Topical: Therapy should be discontinued when control is achieved; if no improvement is seen within 2 weeks, reassessment of diagnosis may be necessary.

Children, Adolescents, and Adults:

Cream, lotion, ointment: Apply thin film to affected area 2 to 3 times per day

Tape: Apply 1 to 2 times per day

Dosage adjustment in renal impairment: There are no dosage adjustments provided in the manufacturer's labeling.

Dosage adjustment in hepatic impairment: There are no dosage adjustments provided in the manufacturer's labeling.

Additional Information Complete prescribing information should be consulted for additional detail.

Dosage Forms

Cream, External:
Cordran: 0.05% (15 g, 30 g, 60 g, 120 g)

Lotion, External:
Cordran: 0.05% (15 mL, 60 mL, 120 mL)

Ointment, External:
Cordran: 0.05% (60 g)

Tape, External:
Cordran: 4 mcg/cm^2 (1 ea)

- **Flurandrenolone** *see* Flurandrenolide *on page 906*

Flurazepam (flure AZ e pam)

Brand Names: Canada Apo-Flurazepam; Bio-Flurazepam; Dalmane; PMS-Flurazepam; Som Pam

Index Terms Flurazepam Hydrochloride

Pharmacologic Category Hypnotic, Benzodiazepine

Additional Appendix Information

Beers Criteria – Potentially Inappropriate Medications for Geriatrics *on page 2271*

Use Insomnia: For the treatment of insomnia characterized by difficulty in falling asleep, frequent nocturnal awakenings, and/or early-morning awakenings.

Pregnancy Risk Factor C

Dosage Insomnia:

Adults: Oral: Initial: 15 mg at bedtime for women, and 15 to 30 mg at bedtime for men; may increase dose to 30 mg at bedtime as needed based on response

Elderly/Debilitated: Oral: 15 mg at bedtime

Dosage adjustment in renal impairment: There are no dosage adjustments provided in the manufacturer's labeling; use with caution.

Dosage adjustment in hepatic impairment: There are no dosage adjustments provided in the manufacturer's labeling; use with caution.

Additional Information Complete prescribing information should be consulted for additional detail.

Dosage Forms

Capsule, Oral:
Generic: 15 mg, 30 mg

- **Flurazepam Hydrochloride** *see* Flurazepam *on page 906*

Flurbiprofen (Systemic) (flure BI proe fen)

Brand Names: Canada Alti-Flurbiprofen; Ansaid; Apo-Flurbiprofen; Froben; Froben-SR; Novo-Flurprofen; Nu-Flurprofen

Index Terms Flurbiprofen Sodium

Pharmacologic Category Nonsteroidal Anti-inflammatory Drug (NSAID), Oral

Use Treatment of rheumatoid arthritis and osteoarthritis

Pregnancy Risk Factor C

Dosage Oral:

Rheumatoid arthritis and osteoarthritis: 200-300 mg/day in 2, 3, or 4 divided doses; do not administer more than 100 mg for any single dose; maximum: 300 mg/day

Dental: Management of postoperative pain (off-label use): 100 mg every 12 hours

Dosage adjustment in renal impairment: Not recommended in patients with advanced renal disease.

Dosage adjustment in hepatic impairment: No dosage adjustment provided in manufacturer's labeling; patients with hepatic insufficiency may require reduced doses due to extensive hepatic metabolism.

Additional Information Complete prescribing information should be consulted for additional detail.

Dosage Forms

Tablet, Oral:
Generic: 50 mg, 100 mg

Flurbiprofen (Ophthalmic) (flure BI proe fen)

Brand Names: U.S. Ocufen

Index Terms Flurbiprofen Sodium

Pharmacologic Category Nonsteroidal Anti-inflammatory Drug (NSAID), Ophthalmic

Use Inhibition of intraoperative miosis

Pregnancy Risk Factor C

Dosage Ophthalmic: Instill 1 drop every 30 minutes, beginning 2 hours prior to surgery for a total of 4 drops in each affected eye.

Dosage adjustment in renal impairment: No dosage adjustment provided in manufacturer's labeling.

Dosage adjustment in hepatic impairment: No dosage adjustment provided in manufacturer's labeling.

Additional Information Complete prescribing information should be consulted for additional detail.

Dosage Forms

Solution, Ophthalmic:

Ocufen: 0.03% (2.5 mL)

Generic: 0.03% (2.5 mL)

- ◆ **Flurbiprofen Sodium** *see* Flurbiprofen (Ophthalmic) *on page 906*
- ◆ **Flurbiprofen Sodium** *see* Flurbiprofen (Systemic) *on page 906*
- ◆ **Fluress® [DSC]** *see* Fluorescein and Benoxinate *on page 895*
- ◆ **5-Flurocytosine** *see* Flucytosine *on page 889*
- ◆ **Flurox™** *see* Fluorescein and Benoxinate *on page 895*

Flutamide (FLOO ta mide)

Brand Names: Canada Apo-Flutamide; Euflex; PMS-Flutamide; Teva-Flutamide

Index Terms Eulexin; Flucinom; Flugerel; Niftolid; SCH 13521

Pharmacologic Category Antineoplastic Agent, Antiandrogen

Use Prostate cancer: Management of locally confined Stage B_2 to C and Stage D_2 metastatic prostate cancer (in combination with a luteinizing hormone-releasing hormone [LHRH] agonist). For Stage B_2 to C prostate cancer, flutamide treatment (and goserelin) should start 8 weeks prior to initiating radiation therapy and continue during radiation therapy. To achieve treatment benefit in Stage D_2 metastatic prostate cancer, initiate flutamide with the LHRH agonist and continue until disease progression.

Pregnancy Risk Factor D

Dosage

Prostate cancer, metastatic: Adults (males): Oral: 250 mg 3 times daily (every 8 hours)

Dosage adjustment in renal impairment: No dosage adjustment is necessary in patients with chronic renal insufficiency.

Dosage adjustment in hepatic impairment:

Mild to moderate impairment: There are no dosage adjustments provided in the manufacturer's labeling.

Severe impairment: Use is contraindicated.

Additional Information Complete prescribing information should be consulted for additional detail.

Dosage Forms

Capsule, Oral:

Generic: 125 mg

Dosage Forms: Canada

Tablet, Oral: 250 mg

Fluticasone (Oral Inhalation) (floo TIK a sone)

Brand Names: U.S. Arnuity Ellipta; Flovent Diskus; Flovent HFA

Brand Names: Canada Flovent Diskus; Flovent HFA

Index Terms Flovent; Fluticasone Propionate

Pharmacologic Category Corticosteroid, Inhalant (Oral)

Additional Appendix Information

Inhaled Corticosteroids *on page 2229*

Use

Asthma:

Arnuity Ellipta: Maintenance treatment of asthma as prophylactic therapy in patients 12 years and older

Flovent Diskus and Flovent HFA: Maintenance treatment of asthma as prophylactic therapy in patients 4 years and older; for patients requiring oral corticosteroid therapy for asthma to assist in total discontinuation or reduction of total oral dose

Limitations of use: Not indicated for relief of acute bronchospasm

Pregnancy Risk Factor C

Pregnancy Considerations Adverse events were observed in some animal reproduction studies. Hypoadrenalism may occur in infants born to mothers receiving corticosteroids during pregnancy. Based on available data, an overall increased risk of congenital malformations or a decrease in fetal growth has not been associated with maternal use of inhaled corticosteroids during pregnancy (Bakhireva, 2005; NAEPP, 2005; Namazy, 2004). Uncontrolled asthma is associated with adverse events in pregnancy (increased risk of perinatal mortality, pre-eclampsia, preterm birth, low birth weight infants). Inhaled corticosteroids are recommended for the treatment of asthma during pregnancy (most information available using budesonide) (ACOG, 2008; NAEPP, 2005).

Breast-Feeding Considerations Systemic corticosteroids are excreted in human milk. It is not known if sufficient quantities of fluticasone are absorbed following inhalation to produce detectable amounts in breast milk. The manufacturer recommends that caution be exercised when administering fluticasone to nursing women. The use of inhaled corticosteroids is not considered a contraindication to breast-feeding (NAEPP, 2005).

Contraindications

Hypersensitivity to fluticasone or any component of the formulation; severe hypersensitivity to milk proteins or lactose (Arnuity Ellipta and Flovent Diskus); primary treatment of status asthmaticus or other acute episodes of asthma requiring intensive measures

Documentation of allergenic cross-reactivity for corticosteroids in this class is limited. However, because of similarities in chemical structure and/or pharmacologic actions, the possibility of cross-sensitivity cannot be ruled out with certainty.

Canadian labeling: Additional contraindications (not in U.S. labeling): Moderate-to-severe bronchiectasis; untreated fungal, bacterial or tubercular infections of the respiratory tract

Warnings/Precautions May cause hypercorticism or suppression of hypothalamic-pituitary-adrenal (HPA) axis. HPA axis suppression may lead to adrenal crisis. Withdrawal and discontinuation of a corticosteroid should be done slowly and carefully. Particular care is required when patients are transferred from systemic corticosteroids to inhaled corticosteroids due to possible adrenal insufficiency or withdrawal from steroids, including an increase in allergic symptoms. Patients receiving ≥20 mg per day of prednisone (or equivalent) may be most susceptible. Fatalities have occurred due to adrenal insufficiency in asthmatic patients during and after transfer from systemic corticosteroids to aerosol steroids; aerosol steroids do **not** provide the systemic steroid needed to treat patients having trauma, surgery, or infections.

Bronchospasm may occur with wheezing after inhalation; if this occurs, stop steroid and treat with a fast-acting bronchodilator. Hypersensitivity reactions including, allergic dermatitis, anaphylaxis, angioedema, bronchospasm, ▶

flushing, hypotension, urticaria, and rash have been reported. Supplemental steroids (oral or parenteral) may be needed during stress or severe asthma attacks. Corticosteroid use may cause psychiatric disturbances, including depression, euphoria, insomnia, mood swings, and personality changes. Preexisting psychiatric conditions may be exacerbated by corticosteroid use. Prolonged use of corticosteroids may also increase the incidence of secondary infection, mask acute infection (including fungal infections), prolong or exacerbate viral infections, or limit response to vaccines. Avoid use if possible in patients with ocular herpes; active or quiescent tuberculosis infections of the respiratory tract; or untreated viral, fungal, parasitic or bacterial systemic infections (Canadian labeling contraindicates use with untreated respiratory infections). Exposure to chickenpox and measles should be avoided; if the patient is exposed, prophylaxis with varicella zoster immune globulin or pooled intramuscular immunoglobulin, respectively, may be indicated; if chickenpox develops, treatment with antiviral agents may be considered. Rare cases of vasculitis (Churg-Strauss syndrome) or other systemic eosinophilic conditions can occur. Prolonged treatment with corticosteroids has been associated with the development of Kaposi's sarcoma (case reports); if noted, discontinuation of therapy should be considered.

Use with caution in patients with thyroid disease, hepatic impairment, renal impairment, cardiovascular disease, diabetes, glaucoma, cataracts, myasthenia gravis, patients at risk for osteoporosis, patients at risk for seizures, or GI diseases (diverticulitis, peptic ulcer, ulcerative colitis) due to perforation risk. Use caution following acute MI (corticosteroids have been associated with myocardial rupture). When transferring to oral inhaler, previously-suppressed allergic conditions (rhinitis, conjunctivitis, eczema) may be unmasked.

Orally-inhaled corticosteroids may cause a reduction in growth velocity in pediatric patients (~1 centimeter per year [range: 0.3-1.8 cm per year] and related to dose and duration of exposure). To minimize the systemic effects of orally-inhaled corticosteroids, each patient should be titrated to the lowest effective dose. Growth should be routinely monitored in pediatric patients.

Potentially significant drug-drug interactions may exist, requiring dose or frequency adjustment, additional monitoring, and/or selection of alternative therapy. Not to be used in status asthmaticus or for the relief of acute bronchospasm. Flovent Diskus and Arnuity Ellipta contain lactose; very rare anaphylactic reactions have been reported in patients with severe milk protein allergy. Withdraw systemic corticosteroid therapy with gradual tapering of dose; consider reducing the daily prednisone dose by 2.5 to 5 mg on a weekly basis beginning at least 1 week after inhalation therapy. Monitor lung function, beta-agonist use, asthma symptoms, and for signs and symptoms of adrenal insufficiency (fatigue, lassitude, weakness, nausea and vomiting, hypotension) during withdrawal. Local yeast infections (eg, oropharyngeal candidiasis) may occur.

Adverse Reactions

Cardiovascular: Hypertension, subarachnoid hemorrhage

Central nervous system: Fatigue, headache, herniated disk, malaise, pain, procedural pain, voice disorder

Dermatologic: Skin rash, pruritus

Gastrointestinal: Abdominal pain, gastrointestinal distress, gastrointestinal pain, nausea and vomiting, oral candidiasis, oropharyngeal candidiasis, toothache, viral gastroenteritis, viral gastrointestinal infection

Hematologic & oncologic: Malignant neoplasm of breast

Infection: Abscess, influenza, viral infection

Neuromuscular & skeletal: Arthralgia, arthritis, back pain, muscle injury, musculoskeletal pain

Respiratory: Allergic rhinitis, bronchitis, cough, hoarseness, nasal congestion, nasopharyngitis, oropharyngeal pain, pharyngitis, rhinitis, sinus infection, sinusitis, throat irritation, upper respiratory tract infection, upper respiratory tract inflammation, viral respiratory infection

Miscellaneous: Accidental injury, amputation, fever

Rare but important or life-threatening: Adrenocortical insufficiency, aggressive behavior, agitation, allergic skin reaction, anxiety, aphonia, bacterial infection, bacterial reproductive infection, behavioral changes (very rare: includes hyperactivity and irritability in children), blepharoconjunctivitis, bronchospasm (immediate and delayed), bruise, burn, cataract (long-term use), change in appetite, chest tightness, cholecystitis, Churg-Strauss syndrome, conjunctivitis, cranial nerve palsy, Cushingoid appearance, decreased bone mineral density (long-term use) decreased linear skeletal growth rate (children/adolescents), dental caries, dental discoloration, depression, dermatitis, diarrhea, disturbance in fluid balance, dizziness, drug toxicity, dyspnea, ecchymoses, edema, eosinophilia, epistaxis, esophageal candidiasis, exacerbation of asthma, facial edema, folliculitis, fungal infection, gastrointestinal disease, glaucoma (long-term use), hematoma, HPA-axis suppression, hypercorticoidism, hyperglycemia, hypersensitivity reaction (immediate and delayed; includes ear, nose, and throat allergic disorders, anaphylaxis, angioedema, bronchospasm, hypotension, skin rash, urticaria), increased intraocular pressure (long-term use), inflammation (musculoskeletal), keratitis, laceration, laryngitis, migraine, mobility disorder, mood disorder, mouth disease (and tongue disease), muscle cramps, muscle rigidity (stiffness, tightness), muscle spasm, oral discomfort (and pain), oral mucosa ulcer, oral rash (and erythema), oropharyngeal edema, palpitations, paradoxical bronchospasm, paranasal sinus disease, photodermatitis, pneumonia, polyp (ear, nose, throat), pressure-induced disorder, reduced salivation, restlessness, rhinorrhea, sleep disorder, soft tissue injury, urinary tract infection, vasculitis, viral skin infection, wheezing, wound

Drug Interactions

Metabolism/Transport Effects Substrate of CYP3A4 (major); **Note:** Assignment of Major/Minor substrate status based on clinically relevant drug interaction potential

Avoid Concomitant Use

Avoid concomitant use of Fluticasone (Oral Inhalation) with any of the following: Aldesleukin; BCG; Cobicistat; Conivaptan; Fusidic Acid (Systemic); Idelalisib; Natalizumab; Pimecrolimus; Tacrolimus (Topical); Tipranavir; Tofacitinib

Increased Effect/Toxicity

Fluticasone (Oral Inhalation) may increase the levels/effects of: Amphotericin B; Ceritinib; Deferasirox; Leflunomide; Loop Diuretics; Natalizumab; Thiazide Diuretics; Tofacitinib

The levels/effects of Fluticasone (Oral Inhalation) may be increased by: Aprepitant; Ceritinib; Cobicistat; Conivaptan; CYP3A4 Inhibitors (Moderate); CYP3A4 Inhibitors (Strong); Dasatinib; Denosumab; Fosaprepitant; Fusidic Acid (Systemic); Idelalisib; Ivacaftor; Luliconazole; Mifepristone; Netupitant; Pimecrolimus; Simeprevir; Stiripentol; Tacrolimus (Topical); Telaprevir; Tipranavir; Trastuzumab

Decreased Effect

Fluticasone (Oral Inhalation) may decrease the levels/effects of: Aldesleukin; Antidiabetic Agents; BCG; Coccidioides immitis Skin Test; Corticorelin; Hyaluronidase; Sipuleucel-T; Telaprevir; Vaccines (Inactivated)

The levels/effects of Fluticasone (Oral Inhalation) may be decreased by: Echinacea

Storage/Stability

Arnuity Ellipta and Flovent Diskus: Store at 20°C to 25°C (68°F to 77°F); excursions are permitted from 15°C to 30°C (59°F to 86°F). Store in a dry place away from direct heat or sunlight. Discard after 6 weeks (Arnuity Ellipta and 50 mcg diskus) or after 2 months (100 mcg and 250 mcg diskus) from removal from protective foil pouch or when the dose counter reads "0" (whichever comes first); device is not reusable.

Flovent HFA: Store between 20°C and 25°C (68°F and 77°F); excursions are permitted from 15°C to 30°C (59°F to 86°F). Discard device when the dose counter reads "000". Store with mouthpiece down. Do not expose to temperatures >120°F. Do not puncture or incinerate.

Mechanism of Action Fluticasone belongs to a group of corticosteroids which utilizes a fluorocarbothioate ester linkage at the 17 carbon position; extremely potent vasoconstrictive and anti-inflammatory activity. The effectiveness of inhaled fluticasone is due to its direct local effect.

Pharmacodynamics/Kinetics

Onset of action: Maximal benefit may take 1 to 2 weeks or longer

Absorption: Absorbed systemically primarily via lungs, minimal GI absorption (<1%) due to presystemic metabolism

Distribution: 4.2 L/kg

Protein binding: >99%

Metabolism: Hepatic via CYP3A4 to 17β-carboxylic acid (negligible activity)

Bioavailability: Oral inhalation: 13.9%; Flovent Diskus: ~8%

Half-life elimination: IV: ~8 hours; Oral inhalation (plasma elimination phase following repeat dosing): 24 hours

Time to peak, plasma: 0.5 to 1 hour

Excretion: Feces (as parent drug and metabolites); urine (<5% as metabolites)

Dosage

Asthma: Inhalation, oral: **Note:** Titrate to lowest effective dose once asthma stability achieved.

Arnuity Ellipta (fluticasone furoate): Adolescents ≥12 years and Adults: Dosing based on previous asthma therapy: **Note:** May increase dose after 2 weeks of therapy in patients who are not adequately controlled.

No prior treatment with inhaled corticosteroids: Initial: 100 mcg once daily; maximum: 200 mcg once daily

Prior treatment with inhaled corticosteroids: Initial: 100 to 200 mcg once daily; maximum: 200 mcg once daily

Flovent HFA (fluticasone propionate):

U.S. labeling:

Children 4 to 11 years: Initial: 88 mcg twice daily; maximum: 88 mcg twice daily

Adolescents ≥12 years and Adults: Dosing based on previous asthma therapy: **Note:** May increase dose after 2 weeks of therapy in patients who are not adequately controlled.

Bronchodilator alone: Initial: 88 mcg twice daily; maximum: 440 mcg twice daily

Inhaled corticosteroids: Initial: 88 to 220 mcg twice daily (initial dose >88 mcg twice daily may be considered in patients previously requiring higher doses of inhaled corticosteroids); maximum: 440 mcg twice daily

Oral corticosteroids (OCS): Initial: 440 mcg twice daily; maximum: 880 mcg twice daily

Asthma Guidelines (NAEPP, 2007) (administer in divided doses twice daily):

"Low" dose:

0 to 4 years: 176 mcg/day

5 to 11 years: 88 to 176 mcg/day

≥12 years: 88 to 264 mcg/day

"Medium" dose:

0 to 4 years: >176 to 352 mcg/day

5 to 11 years: >176 to 352 mcg/day

≥12 years: >264 to 440 mcg/day

"High" dose:

0 to 4 years: >352 mcg/day

5 to 11 years: >352 mcg/day

≥12 years: >440 mcg/day

Canadian labeling:

Children 1 to 3 years: 100 mcg twice daily

Children 4 to 15 years: 100 mcg twice daily. **Note:** Canadian labeling recommends Flovent HFA be administered as a minimum of 2 inhalations twice daily; therefore, patients requiring lower or higher dosages than 100 mcg twice daily should use Flovent Diskus.

Adolescents ≥16 years and Adults: **Note:** May increase dose after ~1 week of therapy in patients who are not adequately controlled.

Mild asthma: 100 to 250 mcg twice daily

Moderate asthma: 250 to 500 mcg twice daily

Severe asthma: 500 mcg twice daily; may increase up to 1000 mcg twice daily in very severe patients (eg, patients using oral corticosteroids [OCS])

Flovent Diskus (fluticasone propionate):

U.S. labeling:

Children 4 to 11 years: Initial: 50 mcg twice daily; may increase to maximum dose of 100 mcg twice daily in patients not adequately controlled after 2 weeks of therapy. Initial dose >50 mcg twice daily may be considered in patients with poorer asthma control or those previously requiring high ranges of inhaled corticosteroids

Adolescents ≥12 years and Adults: **Note:** May increase dose after 2 weeks of therapy in patients who are not adequately controlled.

Dosing based on previous asthma therapy:

Bronchodilator alone: Initial: 100 mcg twice daily; maximum: 500 mcg twice daily

Inhaled corticosteroids: Initial: 100 to 250 mcg twice daily; maximum: 500 mcg twice daily; initial dose >100 mcg twice daily may be considered in patients with poorer asthma control or those previously requiring high ranges of inhaled corticosteroids

Oral corticosteroids (OCS): Initial: 500 to 1000 mcg twice daily; maximum: 1000 mcg twice daily

Asthma Guidelines (NAEPP, 2007) (administer in divided doses twice daily):

"Low" dose:

5 to 11 years: 100 to 200 mcg/day

≥12 years: 100 to 300 mcg/day

"Medium" dose:

5 to 11 years: >200 to 400 mcg/day

≥12 years: >300 to 500 mcg/day

"High" dose:

5 to 11 years: >400 mcg/day

≥12 years: >500 mcg/day

Canadian labeling:

Children 4 to 16 years: Initial: 50 to 100 mcg twice daily; may increase up to 200 mcg twice daily after ~1 week of therapy in patients not adequately controlled

Adolescents ≥16 years and Adults: **Note:** May increase dose after ~1 week of therapy in patients who are not adequately controlled.

Mild asthma: 100 to 250 mcg twice daily

Moderate asthma: 250 to 500 mcg twice daily

Severe asthma: 500 mcg twice daily; may increase up to 1000 mcg twice daily in very severe patients (eg, patients using oral corticosteroids [OCS])

Conversion from oral systemic corticosteroids to orally inhaled corticosteroids: When converting from oral corticosteroids (OCS) to orally inhaled corticosteroids, initiate oral inhalation therapy in patients whose asthma is previously stabilized on OCS. Gradual OCS dose reductions should begin ~7 days after starting inhaled therapy. U.S. labeling recommends reducing prednisone dose no more rapidly than 2.5 to 5 mg/day (or equivalent of other OCS) weekly in children ≥12 years but does not provide a recommendation for children <12 years. A similar approach to OCS dose reduction would however seem advisable. The Canadian labeling recommends decreasing the daily dose of prednisone by 1 mg (or equivalent of other OCS) no more rapidly than weekly (adults) or every 8 days (children) if closely monitored or every 10 days (adults) and 20 days (children) if not closely monitored. If adrenal insufficiency occurs, resume OCS therapy; initiate a more gradual withdrawal. When transitioning from systemic to inhaled corticosteroids, supplemental systemic corticosteroid therapy may be necessary during periods of stress or during severe asthma attacks.

Chronic obstructive pulmonary disease (stable) (off-label use): Inhalation, oral: 50 to 500 mcg/day in combination with a long-acting bronchodilator (GOLD 2014)

Elderly: Refer to adult dosing.

Dosage adjustment in renal impairment:

Arnuity Ellipta: No dosage adjustment necessary.

Flovent HFA and Flovent Diskus: There are no dosage adjustments provided in the manufacturer's labeling (has not been studied).

Dosage adjustment in hepatic impairment: There are no dosage adjustments provided in the manufacturer's labeling (has not been studied); however, fluticasone is primarily cleared in the liver and plasma levels may be increased in patients with hepatic impairment. Use with caution and closely monitor.

Dietary Considerations Arnuity Ellipta and Flovent Diskus contains lactose; very rare anaphylactic reactions have been reported in patients with severe milk protein allergy.

Administration

Aerosol inhalation: Flovent HFA: Shake container thoroughly before using. Take 3-5 deep breaths. Use inhaler on inspiration. Allow 1 full minute between inhalations. Rinse mouth with water after use to reduce aftertaste and incidence of candidiasis; do not swallow. Inhaler must be primed before first use, when not used for 7 days, or if dropped. To prime the first time, release 4 sprays into air; shake well before each spray and spray away from face. If dropped or not used for 7 days, prime by releasing a single test spray. Patient should contact pharmacy for refill when the dose counter reads "020". Discard device when the dose counter reads "000". Do not use "float" test to determine contents.

Powder for oral inhalation:

Arnuity Ellipta: Administer the dose at the same time every day. Do not shake inhaler. When ready to use, open and prepare mouthpiece of the inhaler and slide the cover down to activate the first dose. Exhale fully (not into mouthpiece), take one deep breath through mouth without blocking air vents and hold breath for about 3 to 4 seconds. If the cover is opened and closed without inhaling the medicine, the dose will be lost. The lost dose will be held in the inhaler, but it will no longer be available to be inhaled. It is not possible to accidentally take a double dose or an extra dose in one inhalation. Following administration, rinse mouth with water after use (do not swallow). Routine cleaning of the inhaler is not required; may clean the mouthpiece if needed, using a dry tissue, before the cover is closed. Discard inhaler after 30 sprays or when the counter reads "0".

Flovent Diskus: Do not use with a spacer device. Do not exhale into Diskus. Do not wash or take apart. Use in horizontal position. Mouth should be rinsed with water after use (do not swallow). Discard after 6 weeks (50 mcg diskus) or after 2 months (100 mcg and 250 mcg diskus) once removed from protective pouch or when the dose counter reads "0", whichever comes first (device is not reusable).

Monitoring Parameters Growth (adolescents and children via stadiometry); signs/symptoms of HPA axis suppression/adrenal insufficiency; possible eosinophilic conditions (including Churg-Strauss syndrome); FEV_1, peak flow, and/or other pulmonary function tests; asthma symptoms; bone mineral density; hepatic impairment

Additional Information Effects of inhaled steroids on growth have been observed in the absence of laboratory evidence of HPA axis suppression, suggesting that growth velocity is a more sensitive indicator of systemic corticosteroid exposure in pediatric patients than some commonly used tests of HPA axis function. The long-term effects of this reduction in growth velocity associated with orally-inhaled corticosteroids, including the impact on final adult height, are unknown. The potential for "catch up" growth following discontinuation of treatment with inhaled corticosteroids has not been adequately studied.

In the United States, dosage for the metered dose inhaler (Flovent HFA) is expressed as the amount of drug which leaves the actuater and is delivered to the patient. This differs from other countries, which express the dosage as the amount of drug which leaves the valve.

Dosage Forms Considerations Flovent HFA 10.6 g and 12 g canisters contain 120 inhalations.

Dosage Forms

Aerosol, Inhalation:

Flovent HFA: 44 mcg/actuation (10.6 g); 110 mcg/actuation (12 g); 220 mcg/actuation (12 g)

Aerosol Powder Breath Activated, Inhalation:

Arnuity Ellipta: 100 mcg/actuation (14 ea, 30 ea); 200 mcg/actuation (14 ea, 30 ea)

Flovent Diskus: 50 mcg/blister (60 ea); 100 mcg/blister (28 ea, 60 ea); 250 mcg/blister (28 ea, 60 ea)

Dosage Forms: Canada

Aerosol, for oral inhalation:

Flovent HFA: 50 mcg/inhalation (120 actuations); 125 mcg/inhalation (60 or 120 actuations); 250 mcg/inhalation (60 or 120 actuations)

Powder, for oral inhalation

Flovent Diskus: 50 mcg (60s); 100 mcg (60s); 250 mcg (60s); 500 mcg (60s)

Fluticasone (Nasal) (floo TIK a sone)

Brand Names: U.S. Flonase Allergy Relief [OTC]; Flonase [DSC]; Veramyst

Brand Names: Canada Apo-Fluticasone; Avamys; Flonase; ratio-Fluticasone

Index Terms Flonase Allergy Relief; Fluticasone Furoate; Fluticasone Propionate

Pharmacologic Category Corticosteroid, Nasal

Additional Appendix Information

Inhaled Corticosteroids *on page 2229*

Use

Flonase: **Allergic and nonallergic rhinitis**: Management of the nasal symptoms of seasonal and perennial allergic and nonallergic rhinitis in adults and pediatric patients ≥4 years.

Veramyst, Avamys (Canadian availability; not available in the US): Management of seasonal and perennial allergic rhinitis

OTC labeling: Relief of hay fever or other upper respiratory allergies (eg, nasal congestion, runny nose, sneezing, itchy nose) in adults and children ≥4 years.

Pregnancy Risk Factor C

Dosage Intranasal: Rhinitis:

Children and Adolescents:

Flonase (fluticasone propionate): Children ≥4 years and Adolescents: Initial: 1 spray (50 mcg/spray) per nostril once daily (100 mcg/day); patients not adequately responding or patients with more severe symptoms may use 2 sprays per nostril once daily (200 mcg/day); once symptoms are controlled, dosage should be reduced to 1 spray per nostril once daily (100 mcg/day). Total daily dosage should not exceed 2 sprays in each nostril (200 mcg)/day. Dosing should be at regular intervals.

Flonase OTC (fluticasone propionate):

Children 4 to 11 years: 1 spray (50 mcg/spray) per nostril once daily (100 mcg/day). Do not use for more than 2 months per year unless instructed by health care provider.

Children ≥12 years and Adolescents: Initial: 2 sprays (50 mcg/spray) per nostril once daily (200 mcg/day); after 1 week, may adjust to 1 or 2 sprays per nostril once daily (100 to 200 mcg/day). Do not use for more than 6 months unless instructed by health care provider.

Veramyst (fluticasone furoate):

Children 2 to 11 years: Initial: 1 spray (27.5 mcg/spray) per nostril once daily (55 mcg/day); patients not adequately responding may use 2 sprays per nostril once daily (110 mcg/day); once symptoms are controlled, dosage may be reduced to 55 mcg once daily. Total daily dosage should not exceed 2 sprays in each nostril (110 mcg)/day; once symptoms are controlled, dosage may be reduced to 1 spray per nostril once daily (55 mcg/day). Total daily dosage should not exceed 2 sprays in each nostril (110 mcg)/day.

Children ≥12 years and Adolescents: Initial: 2 sprays (27.5 mcg/spray) per nostril once daily (110 mcg/day). Once symptoms are controlled, dosage may be reduced to 1 spray per nostril once daily (55 mcg/day) for maintenance therapy.

Avamys (fluticasone furoate) (Canadian availability; not available in the US):

Children 2 to 11 years: Initial: 1 spray (27.5 mcg/spray) per nostril once daily (55 mcg/day); patients not adequately responding may use 2 sprays per nostril once daily (110 mcg/day); once symptoms are controlled, dosage should be reduced to 1 spray per nostril once daily (55 mcg/day). Total daily dosage should not exceed 2 sprays in each nostril (110 mcg)/day.

Children ≥12 years and Adolescents: Initial: 2 sprays (27.5 mcg/spray) per nostril once daily (110 mcg/day). Total daily dosage should not exceed 2 sprays in each nostril (110 mcg)/day.

Adults:

Flonase (fluticasone propionate): Initial: 2 sprays (50 mcg/spray) per nostril once daily (200 mcg/day); alternatively, the same total daily dosage may be divided and given as 1 spray per nostril twice daily (200 mcg/day). After the first few days, dosage may be reduced to 1 spray per nostril once daily for maintenance therapy (100 mcg/day).

Flonase OTC (fluticasone propionate): Initial: 2 sprays (50 mcg/spray) per nostril once daily (200 mcg/day); after 1 week, may adjust to 1 or 2 sprays per nostril once daily (100 to 200 mcg/day). Do not use for more than 6 months unless instructed by health care provider.

Veramyst (fluticasone furoate): Initial: 2 sprays (27.5 mcg/spray) per nostril once daily (110 mcg/day); once symptoms are controlled, may reduce dosage to 1 spray per nostril once daily (55 mcg/day) for maintenance therapy.

Avamys (fluticasone furoate) (Canadian availability; not available in the US): 2 sprays (27.5 mcg/spray) in each nostril once daily (110 mcg/day). Total daily dosage should not exceed 2 sprays in each nostril (110 mcg)/day.

Dosing adjustment in renal impairment: No dosage adjustment necessary.

Dosing adjustment in hepatic impairment: There are no dosage adjustments provided in the manufacturer's labeling; use caution with severe impairment.

Additional Information Complete prescribing information should be consulted for additional detail.

Product Availability

Flonase Allergy Relief: FDA approved July 2014; availability anticipated in early 2015.

Flonase Allergy Relief is an over-the-counter (OTC) treatment for hay fever symptoms including nasal congestion, runny nose, sneezing, itchy nose and itchy, watery eyes.

Dosage Forms Considerations Flonase 16 g bottles and Veramyst 10 g bottles contain 120 sprays each.

Dosage Forms

Suspension, Nasal:

Flonase Allergy Relief [OTC]: 50 mcg/actuation (9.9 mL, 15.8 mL)

Veramyst: 27.5 mcg/spray (10 g)

Generic: 50 mcg/actuation (16 g); 50 mcg/actuation (16 g)

Dosage Forms: Canada

Suspension, intranasal, as furoate [spray]:

Avamys®: 27.5 mcg/inhalation (4.5 g, 10 g)

Fluticasone (Topical) (floo TIK a sone)

Brand Names: U.S. Cutivate

Brand Names: Canada Cutivate™

Index Terms Fluticasone Propionate

Pharmacologic Category Corticosteroid, Topical

Additional Appendix Information

Topical Corticosteroids *on page 2230*

Use Relief of inflammation and pruritus associated with corticosteroid-responsive dermatoses; atopic dermatitis

Pregnancy Risk Factor C

Dosage Topical:

Children:

Corticosteroid-responsive dermatoses: Children ≥3 months: Cream: Apply sparingly to affected area twice daily. If no improvement is seen within 2 weeks, reassessment of diagnosis may be necessary.

Atopic dermatitis

Children ≥3 months: Cream: Apply sparingly to affected area 1-2 times/day. If no improvement is seen within 2 weeks, reassessment of diagnosis may be necessary.

Children ≥1 year: Lotion: Apply sparingly to affected area once daily

Adults:

Corticosteroid-responsive dermatoses: Cream, lotion, ointment: Apply sparingly to affected area twice daily. If no improvement is seen within 2 weeks, reassessment of diagnosis may be necessary.

Atopic dermatitis: Cream, lotion: Apply sparingly to affected area once or twice daily. If no improvement is seen within 2 weeks, reassessment of diagnosis may be necessary.

Additional Information Complete prescribing information should be consulted for additional detail.

Dosage Forms
Cream, External:
Cutivate: 0.05% (30 g, 60 g)
Generic: 0.05% (15 g, 30 g, 60 g)
Lotion, External:
Cutivate: 0.05% (120 mL)
Generic: 0.05% (60 mL, 120 mL)
Ointment, External:
Cutivate: 0.005% (30 g, 60 g)
Generic: 0.005% (15 g, 30 g, 60 g)

Fluticasone and Salmeterol

(floo TIK a sone & sal ME te role)

Brand Names: U.S. Advair Diskus; Advair HFA
Brand Names: Canada Advair; Advair Diskus
Index Terms Fluticasone Propionate and Salmeterol Xinafoate; Salmeterol and Fluticasone
Pharmacologic Category $Beta_2$ Agonist; $Beta_2$-Adrenergic Agonist, Long-Acting; Corticosteroid, Inhalant (Oral)
Use
Asthma: Treatment of asthma in patients 4 years and older (Diskus) and in patients 12 years and older (HFA).
Chronic obstructive pulmonary disease (Diskus only): Twice-daily maintenance treatment of airflow obstruction in patients with chronic obstructive pulmonary disease (COPD), including chronic bronchitis and/or emphysema. Fluticasone 250 mcg/salmeterol 50 mcg Diskus is also indicated to reduce exacerbations of COPD in patients with a history of exacerbations.
Fluticasone 250 mcg/salmeterol 50 mcg Diskus twice daily is the only approved dosage for the treatment of COPD because an efficacy advantage of the higher strength fluticasone 500 mcg/salmeterol 50 mcg Diskus over fluticasone 250 mcg/salmeterol 50 mcg Diskus has not been demonstrated.

General information: Fluticasone/salmeterol is not indicated for the relief of acute bronchospasm.
Pregnancy Risk Factor C
Pregnancy Considerations Adverse events were observed in animal reproduction studies using this combination. Refer to individual agents.
Breast-Feeding Considerations It is not known if fluticasone or salmeterol are excreted into breast milk. The manufacturer recommends that caution be used if administering this combination to breast-feeding women. Refer to individual agents.
Contraindications
Hypersensitivity to fluticasone, salmeterol, or any component of the formulation; status asthmaticus; acute episodes of asthma or COPD; severe hypersensitivity to milk proteins (Advair Diskus)
Documentation of allergenic cross-reactivity for corticosteroids and sympathomimetics are limited. However, because of similarities in chemical structure and/or pharmacologic actions, the possibility of cross-sensitivity cannot be ruled out with certainty.
Warnings/Precautions See individual agents.
Adverse Reactions
Cardiovascular: Cardiac arrhythmia, chest symptoms, edema, myocardial infarction, palpitations, syncope, tachycardia
Central nervous system: Dizziness, headache, migraine, mouth pain, pain, sleep disorder
Dermatologic: Dermatitis, diaphoresis, eczema, exfoliation of skin, urticaria, viral skin infection
Endocrine & metabolic: Fluid retention, hypothyroidism, weight gain
Gastrointestinal: Constipation, diarrhea, dysgeusia, gastrointestinal infection (including viral), nausea, oral candidiasis, oral mucosa ulcer, vomiting
Genitourinary: Urinary tract infection
Hematologic & oncologic: Hematoma
Hepatic: Abnormal hepatic function tests
Hypersensitivity: Hypersensitivity reaction
Infection: Bacterial infection, candidiasis, viral infection
Neuromuscular & skeletal: Arthralgia, bone disease, bone fracture, muscle cramps, muscle injury, muscle rigidity, muscle spasm, musculoskeletal pain, myalgia, ostealgia, rheumatoid arthritis, tremor
Ophthalmic: Conjunctivitis, eye redness, keratitis, xerophthalmia
Respiratory: Bronchitis, chest congestion, cough, ENT infection, epistaxis, hoarseness, laryngitis, lower respiratory signs and symptoms (hemorrhage), lower respiratory tract infection (COPD diagnosis and age >65 years increase risk), nasal signs and symptoms (irritation), pharyngitis, rhinitis, rhinorrhea, sinusitis, sneezing, throat irritation, upper respiratory tract infection, upper respiratory tract inflammation, viral respiratory tract infection
Miscellaneous: Burn, laceration, wound
Rare but important or life-threatening: Aggressive behavior, atrial fibrillation, cataract, Churg-Strauss syndrome, Cushing's syndrome, decreased linear skeletal growth rate, depression, dysmenorrhea, ecchymoses, esophageal candidiasis, exacerbation of asthma (serious and some fatal), glaucoma, hyperactivity, hyperglycemia, hypersensitivity reaction (immediate and delayed), hypertension, hypokalemia, hypothyroidism, influenza, irritability, lassitude, myositis, osteoporosis, pallor, paranasal sinus disease, paresthesia, pelvic inflammatory disease, photodermatitis, skin rash, supraventricular tachycardia, syncope, tracheitis, ventricular tachycardia, vulvovaginitis
Drug Interactions
Metabolism/Transport Effects Refer to individual components.
Avoid Concomitant Use
Avoid concomitant use of Fluticasone and Salmeterol with any of the following: Aldesleukin; BCG; Beta-Blockers (Nonselective); Cobicistat; Conivaptan; CYP3A4 Inhibitors (Strong); Fusidic Acid (Systemic); Idelalisib; Iobenguane I 123; Long-Acting Beta2-Agonists; Natalizumab; Pimecrolimus; Tacrolimus (Topical); Telaprevir; Tipranavir; Tofacitinib
Increased Effect/Toxicity
Fluticasone and Salmeterol may increase the levels/effects of: Amphotericin B; Atosiban; Ceritinib; Deferasirox; Highest Risk QTc-Prolonging Agents; Leflunomide; Long-Acting Beta2-Agonists; Loop Diuretics; Moderate Risk QTc-Prolonging Agents; Natalizumab; Sympathomimetics; Thiazide Diuretics; Tofacitinib

The levels/effects of Fluticasone and Salmeterol may be increased by: Aprepitant; AtoMOXetine; Cannabinoid-Containing Products; Ceritinib; Cobicistat; Conivaptan; CYP3A4 Inhibitors (Moderate); CYP3A4 Inhibitors (Strong); Dasatinib; Denosumab; Fosaprepitant; Fusidic Acid (Systemic); Idelalisib; Ivacaftor; Linezolid; Luliconazole; MAO Inhibitors; Mifepristone; Netupitant; Pimecrolimus; Simeprevir; Tacrolimus (Topical); Tedizolid; Telaprevir; Tipranavir; Trastuzumab; Tricyclic Antidepressants
Decreased Effect
Fluticasone and Salmeterol may decrease the levels/effects of: Aldesleukin; Antidiabetic Agents; BCG; Coccidioides immitis Skin Test; Corticorelin; Hyaluronidase; Iobenguane I 123; Sipuleucel-T; Vaccines (Inactivated)

The levels/effects of Fluticasone and Salmeterol may be decreased by: Beta-Blockers (Beta1 Selective); Beta-Blockers (Nonselective); Betahistine; Echinacea

Storage/Stability

Advair Diskus: Store at 20°C to 25°C (68°F to 77°F). Store in a dry place out of direct heat or sunlight. Diskus device should be discarded 1 month after removal from foil pouch, or when dosing indicator reads "0" (whichever comes first); device is not reusable.

Advair HFA: Store at 20°C to 25°C (68°F to 77°F), excursions permitted from 15°C to 30°C (59°F to 86°F). Store with mouthpiece down. Discard after 120 inhalations. Discard device when the dose counter reads "000". Device is not reusable.

Mechanism of Action Combination of fluticasone (corticosteroid) and salmeterol (long-acting beta$_2$-agonist) designed to improve pulmonary function and control over what is produced by either agent when used alone. Because fluticasone and salmeterol act locally in the lung, plasma levels do not predict therapeutic effect.

Fluticasone: The mechanism of action for all topical corticosteroids is believed to be a combination of three important properties: Anti-inflammatory activity, immunosuppressive properties, and antiproliferative actions. Fluticasone has extremely potent vasoconstrictive and anti-inflammatory activity.

Salmeterol: Relaxes bronchial smooth muscle by selective action on beta$_2$-receptors with little effect on heart rate

Pharmacodynamics/Kinetics See individual agents.

Dosage Oral inhalation: **Note:** Do not use to transfer patients from systemic corticosteroid therapy. Patients receiving fluticasone/salmeterol should not use additional salmeterol or other inhaled, long-acting beta$_2$-agonists (eg, formoterol, arformoterol) for any other reason.

COPD: Adults:

Advair Diskus: Fluticasone 250 mcg/salmeterol 50 mcg twice daily, 12 hours apart. **Note:** This is the maximum dose.

Advair Diskus [Canadian labeling; not in approved U.S. labeling]: Fluticasone 250 mcg/salmeterol 50 mcg **or** fluticasone 500 mcg/salmeterol 50 mcg twice daily, 12 hours apart.

Maximum dose: Fluticasone 500 mcg/salmeterol 50 mcg per inhalation (2 inhalations/day)

Asthma:

Children 4-11 years: Advair Diskus: Fluticasone 100 mcg/salmeterol 50 mcg twice daily, 12 hours apart. **Note:** This is the maximum dose.

Children ≥12 years and Adults:

Advair Diskus: One inhalation twice daily, morning and evening, 12 hours apart

Maximum dose: Fluticasone 500 mcg/salmeterol 50 mcg per inhalation (2 inhalations/day)

Advair HFA: Two inhalations twice daily, morning and evening, 12 hours apart

Maximum dose: Fluticasone 230 mcg/salmeterol 21 mcg per inhalation (4 inhalations/day)

Advair 125 or Advair 250 [Canadian labeling; not in approved U.S. labeling]: Two inhalations twice daily, morning and evening, 12 hours apart

Maximum dose: Fluticasone 250 mcg/salmeterol 25 mcg per inhalation (4 inhalations/day)

Note: Initial dose prescribed should be based upon asthma severity. Dose should be increased after 2 weeks if adequate response is not achieved. Patients should be titrated to lowest effective dose once stable.

Elderly: Refer to adult dosing.

Dosage adjustment in renal impairment: There are no dosage adjustments provided in the manufacturer's labeling (has not been studied).

Dosage adjustment in hepatic impairment: No dosage adjustment required; manufacturer suggests close monitoring of patients with hepatic impairment.

Dietary Considerations Advair Diskus powder for oral inhalation contains lactose; very rare anaphylactic reactions have been reported in patients with severe milk protein allergy.

Administration

Advair Diskus: After removing from box and foil pouch, write the "Pouch opened" and "Use by" dates on the label on top of the Diskus. The "Use by" date is 1 month from date of opening the pouch. Every time the lever is pushed back, a dose is ready to be inhaled. Do not close or tilt the Diskus after the lever is pushed back. Do not play with the lever or move the lever more than once. The dose indicator tells you how many doses are left. When the numbers 5 to 0 appear in red, only a few doses remain. Discard device 1 month after you remove it from the foil pouch or when the dose counter reads "0" (whichever comes first). Rinse mouth with water after use and spit to reduce risk of oral candidiasis.

Advair HFA: Shake well for 5 seconds before each spray. Prime with 4 test sprays (into air and away from face) before using for the first time. If canister is dropped or not used for >4 weeks, prime with 2 sprays. Patient should contact pharmacy for refill when the dose counter reads "020". Discard device when the dose counter reads "000". Do not spray in eyes. Rinse mouth with water after use and spit to reduce risk of oral candidiasis.

Monitoring Parameters FEV$_1$, peak flow, and/or other pulmonary function tests; blood pressure, heart rate; CNS stimulation; glaucoma and cataracts. Monitor for increased use of short-acting beta$_2$-agonist inhalers; may be marker of a deteriorating asthma condition. The growth of pediatric patients receiving inhaled corticosteroids should be monitored routinely (eg, via stadiometry).

Additional Information Effects of inhaled/intranasal steroids on growth have been observed in the absence of laboratory evidence of HPA axis suppression, suggesting that growth velocity is a more sensitive indicator of systemic corticosteroid exposure in pediatric patients than some commonly used tests of HPA axis function. The long-term effects of this reduction in growth velocity associated with orally-inhaled and intranasal corticosteroids, including the impact on final adult height, are unknown. The potential for "catch up" growth following discontinuation of treatment with inhaled corticosteroids has not been adequately studied.

Advair HFA: Salmeterol (base) 21 mcg is equivalent to 30.45 mcg of salmeterol xinafoate.

Dosage Forms

Aerosol, for oral inhalation:

Advair HFA:

45/21: Fluticasone propionate 45 mcg and salmeterol 21 mcg (8 g, 12 g) [chlorofluorocarbon free]

115/21: Fluticasone propionate 115 mcg and salmeterol 21 mcg (8 g, 12 g) [chlorofluorocarbon free]

230/21: Fluticasone propionate 230 mcg and salmeterol 21 mcg (8 g, 12 g) [chlorofluorocarbon free]

Powder, for oral inhalation:

Advair Diskus:

100/50: Fluticasone propionate 100 mcg and salmeterol 50 mcg (14s, 60s)

250/50: Fluticasone propionate 250 mcg and salmeterol 50 mcg (14s, 60s)

500/50: Fluticasone propionate 500 mcg and salmeterol 50 mcg (14s, 60s)

Dosage Forms: Canada

Aerosol, for oral inhalation:

Advair: 125/25: Fluticasone propionate 125 mcg and salmeterol 25 mcg (12 g); 250/25: Fluticasone propionate 250 mcg and salmeterol 25 mcg (12 g)

Fluticasone and Vilanterol

(floo TIK a sone & VYE lan ter ol)

Brand Names: U.S. Breo Ellipta

Brand Names: Canada Breo Ellipta

Index Terms Fluticasone Furoate and Vilanterol; Vilanterol and Fluticasone; Vilanterol and Fluticasone Furoate

Pharmacologic Category $Beta_2$ Agonist; $Beta_2$-Adrenergic Agonist, Long-Acting; Corticosteroid, Inhalant (Oral)

Use

Chronic obstructive pulmonary disease: Maintenance treatment of airflow obstruction in patients with chronic obstructive pulmonary disease (COPD), including chronic bronchitis and/or emphysema; to reduce exacerbations of COPD in patients with a history of exacerbations

Limitations of use: Not indicated for the relief of acute bronchospasm or for the treatment of asthma.

Pregnancy Risk Factor C

Pregnancy Considerations Adverse events have not been observed in animal reproduction studies. Hypoadrenalism may occur in infants born to mothers receiving corticosteroids during pregnancy (refer to the Fluticasone [Oral Inhalation] monograph for additional details). Beta-agonists have the potential to affect uterine contractility if administered during labor.

Breast-Feeding Considerations It is not known if sufficient quantities of fluticasone or vilanterol are absorbed following inhalation to produce detectable amounts in breast milk. The manufacturer recommends that caution be exercised when administering fluticasone/vilanterol to breast-feeding women.

Contraindications Hypersensitivity to fluticasone, vilanterol or any component of the formulation; severe hypersensitivity to milk proteins

Warnings/Precautions [U.S. Boxed Warning]: Long-acting $beta_2$-agonists (LABAs) increase the risk of asthma-related deaths. Data from a placebo-controlled trial that compared the safety of another LABA (salmeterol) with placebo added to asthma therapy showed an increase in asthma-related deaths in subjects receiving salmeterol; this finding is considered a class effect of LABAs, including vilanterol. Data are not available to determine whether the rate of death in patients with COPD is increased by LABAs. **The safety and efficacy of fluticasone/vilanterol in patients with asthma have not been established; fluticasone/vilanterol is not indicated for the treatment of asthma.**

Do **not** use for acute bronchospasm or acute symptomatic COPD. Short-acting $beta_2$-agonist (eg, albuterol) should be used for acute symptoms and symptoms occurring between treatments. Do **not** initiate in patients with significantly worsening or acutely deteriorating COPD. Therapy should not be used more than once daily; do not exceed recommended dose. Do not use with other long-acting $beta_2$-agonists; clinically significant cardiovascular effects and fatalities have been reported in association with excessive use of inhaled sympathomimetic drugs. Patients must be instructed to use short-acting $beta_2$-agonist (eg, albuterol) for acute COPD symptoms and to seek medical attention in cases where acute symptoms are not relieved or a previous level of response is diminished. The need to increase frequency of use of inhaled short-acting $beta_2$-agonist may indicate deterioration of COPD, and medical evaluation must not be delayed.

Severe hypersensitivity reactions have been reported. Contains lactose; anaphylactic reactions have been reported in patients with severe milk protein allergy using other lactose-containing powder products. Can produce paradoxical bronchospasm, which may be life threatening. If paradoxical bronchospasm occurs following, fluticasone/vilanterol should be discontinued immediately and alternative therapy should be instituted. An increase in the incidence of pneumonia and other lower respiratory tract infections (some fatal) have been reported in patients with COPD following use; monitor COPD patients closely since pneumonia symptoms may overlap symptoms of exacerbations.

Use caution in patients with cardiovascular disease, especially coronary insufficiency (arrhythmia, hypertension), seizure disorders, diabetes, ocular disease, osteoporosis, hepatic impairment (moderate to severe), thyrotoxicosis, or hypokalemia. Long-term use may affect bone mineral density in adults. Infections with *Candida albicans* in the mouth and throat (thrush) have been reported with use. Potentially significant drug-drug interactions may exist, requiring dose or frequency adjustment, additional monitoring, and/or selection of alternative therapy.

Fluticasone may cause hypercorticism or suppression of hypothalamic-pituitary-adrenal (HPA) axis, including adrenal crisis, in patients sensitive to these effects. Withdrawal and discontinuation of a corticosteroid should be done slowly and carefully. Particular care is required when patients are transferred from systemic corticosteroids to inhaled corticosteroids; deaths due to adrenal insufficiency have occurred in patients with asthma during and after transfer from systemic steroids to a less systemically available inhaled corticosteroid. Patients receiving ≥20 mg per day of prednisone (or equivalent) may be most susceptible. Fluticasone/vilanterol does not provide the systemic steroid dose needed to treat patients having trauma, surgery, or infections. Do not use this product to transfer patients from oral corticosteroid therapy. Observe patients carefully for any evidence of systemic corticosteroid effects; particular care should be taken in observing patients postoperatively or during periods of stress for evidence of inadequate adrenal response. If systemic corticosteroid withdrawal effects occur (eg, fatigue, lassitude, weakness, nausea, vomiting, hypotension), taper fluticasone/vilanterol slowly and other treatments for management of COPD symptoms should be considered.

Use increases susceptibility to infections (eg, chickenpox and measles, sometimes more serious or even fatal, in susceptible children or adults using corticosteroids). Avoid exposure in such patients who have not had these diseases or been properly immunized. Use with caution (if at all) in patients with active or quiescent tuberculosis infections of the respiratory tract; systemic fungal, bacterial, viral, or parasitic infections; or ocular herpes simplex.

Adverse Reactions

Cardiovascular: Hypertension, peripheral edema

Central nervous system: Headache

Gastrointestinal: Diarrhea, oropharyngeal candidiasis

Infection: Influenza

Neuromuscular & skeletal: Arthralgia, back pain, bone fracture

Respiratory: Bronchitis, chronic obstructive pulmonary disease, cough, nasopharyngitis, oropharyngeal pain, pharyngitis, pneumonia, sinusitis, upper respiratory tract infection

Miscellaneous: Fever

Rare but important or life-threatening: Cataract, glaucoma, hypersensitivity reaction, paradoxical bronchospasm

Drug Interactions

Metabolism/Transport Effects Refer to individual components.

Avoid Concomitant Use

Avoid concomitant use of Fluticasone and Vilanterol with any of the following: Aldesleukin; BCG; Beta-Blockers (Nonselective); Cobicistat; Conivaptan; Fusidic Acid (Systemic); Idelalisib; Iobenguane I 123; Long-Acting Beta2-Agonists; Natalizumab; Pimecrolimus; Tacrolimus (Topical); Tipranavir; Tofacitinib

Increased Effect/Toxicity

Fluticasone and Vilanterol may increase the levels/effects of: Amphotericin B; Atosiban; Ceritinib; Deferasirox; Highest Risk QTc-Prolonging Agents; Leflunomide; Long-Acting Beta2-Agonists; Loop Diuretics; Moderate Risk QTc-Prolonging Agents; Natalizumab; Sympathomimetics; Thiazide Diuretics; Tofacitinib

The levels/effects of Fluticasone and Vilanterol may be increased by: Aprepitant; AtoMOXetine; Cannabinoid-Containing Products; Ceritinib; Cobicistat; Conivaptan; CYP3A4 Inhibitors (Moderate); CYP3A4 Inhibitors (Strong); Dasatinib; Denosumab; Fosaprepitant; Fusidic Acid (Systemic); Idelalisib; Ivacaftor; Linezolid; Luliconazole; MAO Inhibitors; Mifepristone; Netupitant; Pimecrolimus; Simeprevir; Stiripentol; Tacrolimus (Topical); Tedizolid; Telaprevir; Tipranavir; Trastuzumab; Tricyclic Antidepressants

Decreased Effect

Fluticasone and Vilanterol may decrease the levels/effects of: Aldesleukin; Antidiabetic Agents; BCG; Coccidioides immitis Skin Test; Corticorelin; Hyaluronidase; Iobenguane I 123; Sipuleucel-T; Telaprevir; Vaccines (Inactivated)

The levels/effects of Fluticasone and Vilanterol may be decreased by: Beta-Blockers (Beta1 Selective); Beta-Blockers (Nonselective); Betahistine; Echinacea

Storage/Stability Store between 20°C and 25°C (68°F and 77°F); excursions permitted from 15°C to 30°C (59°F to 86°F). Store in a dry place away from heat and sunlight. Store inside the unopened foil tray prior to initial use. Discard 6 weeks after opening the foil tray or after the labeled number of inhalations have been used, whichever comes first.

Mechanism of Action

Fluticasone is a corticosteroid with anti-inflammatory activity, immunosuppressive properties, and antiproliferative actions.

Vilanterol, a long-acting beta$_2$-agonist, relaxes bronchial smooth muscle by selective action on beta$_2$-receptors with little effect on heart rate.

Pharmacodynamics/Kinetics See individual agents.

Dosage Chronic obstructive pulmonary disease (COPD): Adults: Oral inhalation: One inhalation (fluticasone 100 mcg/vilanterol 25 mcg) once daily (maximum: 1 inhalation [fluticasone 100 mcg/vilanterol 25 mcg] once daily)

Dosage adjustment in renal impairment: No dosage adjustment necessary.

Dosage adjustment in hepatic impairment:

Mild impairment: No dosage adjustment necessary.

Moderate-to-severe impairment: No dosage adjustment necessary. However, use with caution; systemic fluticasone exposure may be increased up to threefold.

Administration Oral inhalation: Administer at the same time each day. Do not use more than one inhalation in 24 hours. Discard device 6 weeks after it is removed from the foil tray or when the dose counter reads "0" (whichever comes first). Rinse mouth with water after inhalation and spit.

Monitoring Parameters FEV$_1$, peak flow, and/or other pulmonary function tests; bone mineral density (at baseline and periodically thereafter); blood pressure, heart rate; ocular changes (intraocular pressure, cataracts); signs/symptoms of oral or systemic infection, hypercorticism, or adrenal suppression

Dosage Forms Powder, for oral inhalation:

Breo Ellipta: Fluticasone furoate 100 mcg and vilanterol 25 mcg per actuation [contains lactose; blister pack]

◆ **Fluticasone Furoate** *see* Fluticasone (Nasal) *on page 910*

◆ **Fluticasone Furoate and Vilanterol** *see* Fluticasone and Vilanterol *on page 914*

◆ **Fluticasone Propionate** *see* Fluticasone (Nasal) *on page 910*

◆ **Fluticasone Propionate** *see* Fluticasone (Oral Inhalation) *on page 907*

◆ **Fluticasone Propionate** *see* Fluticasone (Topical) *on page 911*

◆ **Fluticasone Propionate and Azelastine Hydrochloride** *see* Azelastine and Fluticasone *on page 214*

◆ **Fluticasone Propionate and Salmeterol Xinafoate** *see* Fluticasone and Salmeterol *on page 912*

Fluvastatin (FLOO va sta tin)

Brand Names: U.S. Lescol; Lescol XL

Brand Names: Canada Lescol; Lescol XL; Teva-Fluvastatin

Pharmacologic Category Antilipemic Agent, HMG-CoA Reductase Inhibitor

Use To be used as a component of multiple risk factor intervention in patients at risk for atherosclerosis vascular disease due to hypercholesterolemia

Adjunct to dietary therapy to reduce elevated total cholesterol (total-C), LDL-C, triglyceride, and apolipoprotein B (apo-B) levels and to increase HDL-C in primary hypercholesterolemia and mixed dyslipidemia (Fredrickson types IIa and IIb); to slow the progression of coronary atherosclerosis in patients with coronary heart disease; reduce risk of coronary revascularization procedures in patients with coronary heart disease

Primary and secondary prevention of atherosclerotic cardiovascular disease (ASCVD) according to the American College of Cardiology/American Heart Association: To reduce the risk of ASCVD in patients with clinical ASCVD (eg, coronary heart disease, stroke/TIA, or peripheral arterial disease presumed to be of atherosclerotic origin) who are greater than 75 years of age or not a candidate for high-intensity statin therapy; in patients without clinical ASCVD if LDL-C is 190 mg/dL or greater and not a candidate for high-intensity statin therapy; in patients without clinical ASCVD who have type 1 or type 2 diabetes and are between 40 and 75 years of age; in patients with an estimated 10-year ASCVD risk 7.5% or greater and who are between 40 and 75 years of age (Stone, 2013). Specific recommendations from the Kidney Disease: Improving Global Outcomes (KDIGO) organization have also been released for patients with chronic kidney disease (KDIGO [Tonelli, 2013]).

Pregnancy Risk Factor X

Dosage Oral:

Adolescents 10-16 years: Heterozygous familial hypercholesterolemia: Initial: 20 mg once daily; may increase every 6 weeks based on tolerability and response to a maximum recommended dose of 80 mg/day, given in 2 divided doses (immediate release capsule) or as a single daily dose (extended release tablet)

Note: Indicated only for adjunctive therapy when diet alone cannot reduce LDL-C below 190 mg/dL, or 160 mg/dL (with cardiovascular risk factors). Female patients must be 1 year postmenarche.

Concomitant use with cyclosporine or fluconazole: Refer to adult dosing.

Adults:

Patients requiring ≥25% decrease in LDL-C: 40 mg capsule once daily in the evening, 80 mg extended release tablet once daily (anytime), or 40 mg capsule twice daily

Patients requiring <25% decrease in LDL-C: Initial: 20 mg capsule once daily in the evening; may increase based on tolerability and response to a maximum recommended dose of 80 mg/day, given in 2 divided doses (immediate release capsule) or as a single daily dose (extended release tablet)

Concomitant use with cyclosporine or fluconazole: Immediate release: Do not exceed fluvastatin 20 mg twice daily

ACC/AHA Blood Cholesterol Guideline recommendations to reduce the risk of atherosclerotic cardiovascular disease (ASCVD) (Stone, 2013): Adults ≥21 years:

Primary prevention:

LDL-C ≥190 mg/dL: High-intensity therapy necessary; use alternate statin therapy (eg, atorvastatin, rosuvastatin)

Type 1 or 2 diabetes and age 40-75 years: Moderate intensity therapy:

Immediate release: 40 mg twice daily.

Extended release: 80 mg once daily.

Type 1 or 2 diabetes, age 40-75 years, and an estimated 10-year ASCVD risk ≥7.5%: High-intensity therapy necessary; use alternate statin therapy (eg, atorvastatin, rosuvastatin).

Age 40-75 years and an estimated 10-year ASCVD risk ≥7.5%: Moderate- to high-intensity therapy:

Immediate release: 40 mg twice daily or consider using high-intensity statin therapy (eg, atorvastatin, rosuvastatin).

Extended release: 80 mg once daily or consider using high-intensity statin therapy (eg, atorvastatin, rosuvastatin).

Secondary prevention:

Patient has clinical ASCVD (eg, coronary heart disease, stroke/TIA, or peripheral arterial disease presumed to be of atherosclerotic origin) **and**:

Age ≤75 years: High-intensity therapy necessary; use alternate statin therapy (eg, atorvastatin, rosuvastatin).

Age >75 years or not a candidate for high-intensity therapy: Moderate-intensity therapy:

Immediate release: 40 mg twice daily.

Extended release: 80 mg once daily.

Dosage adjustment for toxicity:

Severe muscle symptoms or fatigue: Promptly discontinue use; evaluate CPK, creatinine, and urinalysis for myoglobinuria (Stone, 2013).

Mild to moderate muscle symptoms: Discontinue use until symptoms can be evaluated; evaluate patient for conditions that may increase the risk for muscle symptoms (eg, hypothyroidism, reduced renal or hepatic function, rheumatologic disorders such as polymyalgia rheumatica, steroid myopathy, vitamin D deficiency, or primary muscle diseases). Upon resolution, resume the original or lower dose of fluvastatin. If muscle symptoms recur, discontinue fluvastatin use. After muscle symptom resolution, may then use a low dose of a different statin; gradually increase if tolerated. In the absence of continued statin use, if muscle symptoms or elevated CPK continues after 2 months, consider other causes of muscle symptoms. If determined to be due to another condition aside from statin use, may resume statin therapy at the original dose (Stone, 2013).

Dosage adjustment in renal impairment: Note: Less than 6% excreted renally

Mild-to-moderate renal impairment: No dosage adjustment necessary

Severe renal impairment: Use with caution (particularly at doses >40 mg/day; has not been studied)

Dosage adjustment in hepatic impairment: Manufacturer labeling does not provide specific dosing recommendations; however, systemic exposure may be increased in patients with liver disease (increased AUC and C_{max}); use is contraindicated in active liver disease or unexplained transaminase elevations.

Elderly: No dosage adjustment necessary based on age

Additional Information Complete prescribing information should be consulted for additional detail.

Dosage Forms

Capsule, Oral:

Lescol: 20 mg, 40 mg

Generic: 20 mg, 40 mg

Tablet Extended Release 24 Hour, Oral:

Lescol XL: 80 mg

- **Fluviral (Can)** *see* Influenza Virus Vaccine (Inactivated) *on page 1075*
- **Fluvirin** *see* Influenza Virus Vaccine (Inactivated) *on page 1075*
- **Fluvirin Preservative Free** *see* Influenza Virus Vaccine (Inactivated) *on page 1075*

FluvoxaMINE (floo VOKS a meen)

Brand Names: U.S. Luvox CR [DSC]

Brand Names: Canada ACT-Fluvoxamine; Apo-Fluvoxamine; Ava-Fluvoxamine; Dom-Fluvoxamine; Luvox; Novo-Fluvoxamine; PHL-Fluvoxamine; PMS-Fluvoxamine; ratio-Fluvoxamine; Riva-Fluvox; Sandoz-Fluvoxamine

Index Terms Luvox

Pharmacologic Category Antidepressant, Selective Serotonin Reuptake Inhibitor

Use Treatment of obsessive-compulsive disorder (OCD)

Pregnancy Risk Factor C

Pregnancy Considerations Adverse events have been observed in animal reproduction studies. Fluvoxamine crosses the human placenta. An increased risk of teratogenic effects, including cardiovascular defects, may be associated with maternal use of fluvoxamine or other SSRIs; however, available information is conflicting. Nonteratogenic effects in the newborn following SSRI/SNRI exposure late in the third trimester include respiratory distress, cyanosis, apnea, seizures, temperature instability, feeding difficulty, vomiting, hypoglycemia, hypo- or hypertonia, hyper-reflexia, jitteriness, irritability, constant crying, and tremor. Symptoms may be due to the toxicity of the SSRIs/SNRIs or a discontinuation syndrome and may be consistent with serotonin syndrome associated with SSRI treatment. Persistent pulmonary hypertension of the newborn (PPHN) has also been reported with SSRI exposure. The long-term effects of *in utero* SSRI exposure on infant development and behavior are not known.

The ACOG recommends that therapy with SSRIs or SNRIs during pregnancy be individualized; treatment of depression during pregnancy should incorporate the clinical expertise of the mental health clinician, obstetrician, primary healthcare provider, and pediatrician. According to the American Psychiatric Association (APA), the risks of medication treatment should be weighed against other treatment options and untreated depression. For women who discontinue antidepressant medications during pregnancy and who may be at high risk for postpartum depression, the medications can be restarted following delivery. Treatment algorithms have been developed by the ACOG and the APA for the management of depression in women prior to conception and during pregnancy.

Breast-Feeding Considerations Fluvoxamine is excreted in breast milk. Based on case reports, the dose the infant receives is relatively small and adverse events have not been observed. Adverse events have been reported in nursing infants exposed to some SSRIs. According to the manufacturer, the decision to continue or discontinue breast-feeding during therapy should take into account the risk of exposure to the infant and the benefits of treatment to the mother.

The long-term effects on development and behavior have not been studied; therefore, fluvoxamine should be prescribed to a mother who is breast-feeding only when the benefits outweigh the potential risks. Maternal use of an SSRI during pregnancy may cause delayed milk secretion.

Contraindications Concurrent use with alosetron, pimozide, ramelteon, thioridazine, or tizanidine; use of MAO inhibitors intended to treat psychiatric disorders (concurrently or within 14 days of discontinuing either fluvoxamine or the MAO inhibitor); initiation of fluvoxamine in a patient receiving linezolid or intravenous methylene blue

Warnings/Precautions [U.S. Boxed Warning]: Antidepressants increase the risk of suicidal thinking and behavior in children, adolescents, and young adults (18 to 24 years of age) with major depressive disorder (MDD) and other psychiatric disorders; consider risk prior to prescribing. Short-term studies did not show an increased risk in patients >24 years of age and showed a decreased risk in patients ≥65 years. Closely monitor patients for clinical worsening, suicidality, or unusual changes in behavior, particularly during the initial 1 to 2 months of therapy or during periods of dosage adjustments (increases or decreases); the patient's family or caregiver should be instructed to closely observe the patient and communicate condition with healthcare provider. A medication guide concerning the use of antidepressants should be dispensed with each prescription. **Fluvoxamine is FDA approved for the treatment of OCD in children ≥8 years of age.**

The possibility of a suicide attempt is inherent in major depression and may persist until remission occurs. Use caution in high-risk patients. Worsening depression and severe abrupt suicidality that are not part of the presenting symptoms may require discontinuation or modification of drug therapy. The patient's family or caregiver should be alerted to monitor patients for the emergence of suicidality and associated behaviors (such as agitation, irritability, hostility, impulsivity, and hypomania) and call healthcare provider.

May worsen psychosis in some patients or precipitate a shift to mania or hypomania in patients with bipolar disorder. Patients presenting with depressive symptoms should be screened for bipolar disorder. Monotherapy in patients with bipolar disorder should be avoided. **Fluvoxamine is not FDA approved for the treatment of bipolar depression.**

Potentially life-threatening serotonin syndrome (SS) has occurred with serotonergic agents (eg, SSRIs, SNRIs), particularly when used in combination with other serotonergic agents (eg, triptans, TCAs, fentanyl, lithium, tramadol, buspirone, St John's wort, tryptophan) or agents that impair metabolism of serotonin (eg, MAO inhibitors intended to treat psychiatric disorders, other MAO inhibitors [ie, linezolid and intravenous methylene blue]). Discontinue treatment (and any concomitant serotonergic agent) immediately if signs/symptoms arise. Fluvoxamine has a low potential to impair cognitive or motor performance; caution operating hazardous machinery or driving. Use caution in patients with a previous seizure disorder or condition predisposing to seizures such as brain damage or alcoholism. Potentially significant drug-drug interactions may exist, requiring dose or frequency adjustment, additional monitoring, and/or selection of alternative therapy. Fluvoxamine levels may be lower in patients who smoke.

May increase the risks associated with electroconvulsive therapy. Bone fractures have been associated with antidepressant treatment. Consider the possibility of a fragility fracture if an antidepressant-treated patient presents with unexplained bone pain, point tenderness, swelling, or bruising (Rabenda, 2013; Rizzoli, 2012). Use with caution in patients with hepatic dysfunction and in elderly patients. May cause hyponatremia/SIADH (elderly at increased risk); volume depletion (diuretics may increase risk). Use with caution in patients at risk of bleeding or receiving concurrent anticoagulant therapy, although not consistently noted, fluvoxamine may cause impairment in platelet function. May cause or exacerbate sexual dysfunction. Use caution in elderly patients; may be potentially inappropriate in patients with a history of falls or fractures, and may cause or exacerbate SIADH or hyponatremia; monitor sodium closely with initiation or dosage adjustments in older adults (Beers Criteria). May cause mild pupillary dilation which in susceptible individuals can lead to an episode of narrow-angle glaucoma. Consider evaluating patients who have not had an iridectomy for narrow-angle glaucoma risk factors.

Abrupt discontinuation or interruption of antidepressant therapy has been associated with a discontinuation syndrome. Symptoms arising may vary with antidepressant however commonly include nausea, vomiting, diarrhea, headaches, light-headedness, dizziness, diminished appetite, sweating, chills, tremors, paresthesias, fatigue, somnolence, and sleep disturbances (eg, vivid dreams, insomnia). Greater risks for developing a discontinuation syndrome have been associated with antidepressants with shorter half-lives, longer durations of treatment, and abrupt discontinuation. For antidepressants of short or intermediate half-lives, symptoms may emerge within 2 to 5 days after treatment discontinuation and last 7 to 14 days (APA, 2010; Fava, 2006; Haddad, 2001; Shelton, 2001; Warner, 2006).

Adverse Reactions

Cardiovascular: Chest pain, edema, hypertension, hypotension, palpitations, syncope, vasodilation

Central nervous system: Abnormal dreams, abnormality in thinking, agitation, amnesia, anorgasmia, anxiety, apathy, central nervous system stimulation, chills, depression, dizziness, drowsiness, headache, hypertonia, insomnia, malaise, manic reaction, myoclonus, nervousness, pain, paresthesia, psychoneurosis, psychotic reaction, twitching, yawning

Dermatologic: Acne vulgaris, diaphoresis, ecchymoses

Endocrine & metabolic: Decreased libido (incidence higher in males), hypermenorrhea, weight gain, weight loss

Gastrointestinal: Abdominal pain, anorexia, constipation, diarrhea, dysgeusia, dyspepsia, dysphagia, flatulence, gingivitis, nausea, vomiting, xerostomia

Genitourinary: Ejaculatory disorder, impotence, sexual disorder, urinary frequency, urinary retention, urinary tract infection

Hepatic: Abnormal hepatic function tests

Infection: Viral infection

Neuromuscular & skeletal: Hyperkinesia, hypokinesia, myalgia, tremor, weakness

Ophthalmic: Amblyopia

Renal: Polyuria

Respiratory: Bronchitis, dyspnea, epistaxis, flu-like symptoms, increased cough, laryngitis, pharyngitis, sinusitis, upper respiratory tract infection

Rare but important or life-threatening: Acute renal failure, agranulocytosis, akinesia, anaphylaxis, anemia, angina, angioedema, angle-closure glaucoma, anuria, aplastic anemia, apnea, asthma, ataxia, bradycardia, bullous skin disease, cardiac conduction delay, cardiac failure, cardiomyopathy, cardiorespiratory arrest, cerebrovascular accident, cholecystitis, cholelithiasis, colitis, coronary artery disease, decreased white blood cell count, dental caries, dental extraction, diplopia, dyskinesia, dystonia, extrapyramidal reaction, first degree atrioventricular block, gastrointestinal hemorrhage, goiter, hallucination, hematemesis, hematuria, hemoptysis, hepatitis, homicidal ideation, hypercholesterolemia, hyperglycemia, hypersensitivity reaction, hypoglycemia, hypokalemia, hyponatremia, hypothyroidism, IgA vasculitis, interstitial pulmonary disease, intestinal obstruction, jaundice, leukocytosis, leukopenia, loss of consciousness, lymphadenopathy, myasthenia, myocardial infarction, myopathy, neuroleptic malignant syndrome (Stevens, 2008), pancreatitis, paralysis, pericarditis, porphyria, prolonged Q-T interval on ECG, purpura, rhabdomyolysis, seizure, serotonin syndrome, ST segment changes on ECG, Stevens-Johnson syndrome, suicidal tendencies, supraventricular extrasystole, tachycardia, tardive dyskinesia, thrombocytopenia, thromboembolism, tooth abscess, toothache, toxic epidermal necrolysis, vasculitis, ventricular arrhythmia, ventricular tachycardia (including torsades de pointes)

Drug Interactions

Metabolism/Transport Effects Substrate of CYP1A2 (major), CYP2D6 (major); **Note:** Assignment of Major/Minor substrate status based on clinically relevant drug interaction potential; **Inhibits** CYP1A2 (strong), CYP2B6 (weak), CYP2C19 (strong), CYP2C9 (weak), CYP2D6 (weak), CYP3A4 (weak)

Avoid Concomitant Use

Avoid concomitant use of FluvoxaMINE with any of the following: Agomelatine; Alosetron; Dapoxetine; Dosulepin; DULoxetine; Iobenguane I 123; Linezolid; MAO Inhibitors; Methylene Blue; Pimozide; Pomalidomide; Ramelteon; Tasimelteon; Thioridazine; TiZANidine; Tryptophan; Urokinase

Increased Effect/Toxicity

FluvoxaMINE may increase the levels/effects of: Agents with Antiplatelet Properties; Agomelatine; Alosetron; ALPRAZolam; Anticoagulants; Antidepressants (Serotonin Reuptake Inhibitor/Antagonist); Antipsychotic Agents; Apixaban; ARIPiprazole; Asenapine; Aspirin; Bendamustine; Bromazepam; BusPIRone; CarBAMazepine; Citalopram; CloZAPine; Collagenase (Systemic); CYP1A2 Substrates; CYP2C19 Substrates; Dabigatran Etexilate; Desmopressin; Dofetilide; Dosulepin; DULoxetine; Erlotinib; Etizolam; Fosphenytoin; Haloperidol; Hydrocodone; Hypoglycemic Agents; Ibritumomab; Lomitapide; Methadone; Methylene Blue; Mexiletine; NSAID (COX-2 Inhibitor); NSAID (Nonselective); Obinutuzumab; OLANZapine; Phenytoin; Pimozide; Pirfenidone; Pomalidomide; Propafenone; Propranolol; QuiNIDine; Ramelteon; Rivaroxaban; Roflumilast; Ropivacaine; Salicylates; Serotonin Modulators; Tasimelteon; Theophylline Derivatives; Thiazide Diuretics; Thioridazine; Thrombolytic Agents; TiZANidine; Tositumomab and Iodine I 131 Tositumomab; TraMADol; Tricyclic Antidepressants; Urokinase; Vitamin K Antagonists; Zolpidem

The levels/effects of FluvoxaMINE may be increased by: Abiraterone Acetate; Alcohol (Ethyl); Analgesics (Opioid); Antiemetics (5HT3 Antagonists); Antipsychotic Agents; BuPROPion; BusPIRone; Cimetidine; CNS Depressants; Cobicistat; CYP1A2 Inhibitors (Moderate); CYP1A2 Inhibitors (Strong); CYP2D6 Inhibitors (Moderate); CYP2D6 Inhibitors (Strong); Dapoxetine; Darunavir; Dasatinib; Deferasirox; Glucosamine; Grapefruit Juice; Herbs (Anticoagulant/Antiplatelet Properties); Ibrutinib; Limaprost; Linezolid; Lithium; MAO Inhibitors; Metoclopramide; Metyrosine; Multivitamins/Fluoride (with ADE); Multivitamins/Minerals (with ADEK, Folate, Iron); Multivitamins/Minerals (with AE, No Iron); Omega-3 Fatty Acids; Peginterferon Alfa-2b; Pentosan Polysulfate Sodium; Pentoxifylline; Prostacyclin Analogues; QuiNIDine; Tedizolid; TraMADol; Tryptophan; Vemurafenib; Vitamin E

Decreased Effect

FluvoxaMINE may decrease the levels/effects of: Clopidogrel; Iobenguane I 123; Ioflupane I 123; Thyroid Products

The levels/effects of FluvoxaMINE may be decreased by: Cannabis; CarBAMazepine; CYP1A2 Inducers (Strong); Cyproheptadine; Cyproterone; NSAID (COX-2 Inhibitor); NSAID (Nonselective); Peginterferon Alfa-2b; Teriflunomide

Storage/Stability Protect from high humidity and store at controlled room temperature 25°C (77°F).

Mechanism of Action Inhibits CNS neuron serotonin uptake; minimal or no effect on reuptake of norepinephrine or dopamine; does not significantly bind to alpha-adrenergic, histamine or cholinergic receptors

Pharmacodynamics/Kinetics

Onset of action: Depression: The onset of action is within a week; however, individual response varies greatly and full response may not be seen until 8-12 weeks after initiation of treatment.

Absorption: Steady-state plasma concentrations have been noted to be 2-3 times higher in children than those in adolescents; female children demonstrated a significantly higher AUC than males

Distribution: V_d: ~25 L/kg

Protein binding: ~80%, primarily to albumin

Metabolism: Extensively hepatic via oxidative demethylation and deamination

Bioavailability: Immediate release: 53%; not significantly affected by food

Half-life elimination: 15-16 hours; 17-26 hours in the elderly

Time to peak, plasma: 3-8 hours

Excretion: Urine (~85% as metabolites; ~2% as unchanged drug)

Dosage Oral:

Obsessive-compulsive disorder:

Children 8-17 years: Immediate release: Initial: 25 mg once daily at bedtime; may be increased in 25 mg increments at 4- to 7-day intervals, as tolerated, to maximum therapeutic benefit; usual dose range: 50-200 mg/day. **Note:** When total daily dose exceeds 50 mg, the dose should be given in 2 divided doses with larger portion administered at bedtime.

Maximum: Children: 8-11 years: 200 mg/day, adolescents: 300 mg/day; lower doses may be effective in female versus male patients

Adults:

Immediate release: Initial: 50 mg once daily at bedtime; may be increased in 50 mg increments at 4- to 7-day intervals, as tolerated; usual dose range: 100-300 mg/day; maximum dose: 300 mg/day. **Note:** When total daily dose exceeds 100 mg, the dose should be given in 2 divided doses with larger portion administered at bedtime.

Extended release: Initial: 100 mg once daily at bedtime; may be increased in 50 mg increments at intervals of at least 1 week; usual dosage range: 100-300 mg/day; maximum dose: 300 mg/day

Social anxiety disorder (off-label use): Adults: Extended release: Initial: 100 mg once daily at bedtime; may be increased in 50 mg increments at intervals of at least 1 week; usual dosage range: 100-300 mg/day; maximum dose: 300 mg/day (Davidson, 2004; Stein, 2003; Westenberg, 2004)

Post-traumatic stress disorder (PTSD) (off-label use): Adults: Immediate release: 75 mg twice daily (Spivak, 2006)

Elderly: Reduce dose, titrate slowly

Discontinuation of therapy: Upon discontinuation of antidepressant therapy, gradually taper the dose to minimize the incidence of withdrawal symptoms and allow for the detection of re-emerging symptoms. Evidence supporting ideal taper rates is limited. APA and NICE guidelines suggest tapering therapy over at least several weeks with consideration to the half-life of the antidepressant; antidepressants with a shorter half-life may need to be tapered more conservatively. In addition for long-term treated patients, WFSBP guidelines recommend tapering over 4-6 months. If intolerable withdrawal symptoms occur following a dose reduction, consider resuming the previously prescribed dose and/or decrease dose at a more gradual rate (APA, 2007; APA, 2010; Bauer, 2002; Haddad, 2001; NCCMH, 2010; Schatzberg, 2006; Shelton, 2001; Warner, 2006).

MAO inhibitor recommendations:

Switching to or from an MAO inhibitor intended to treat psychiatric disorders:

Allow 14 days to elapse between discontinuing an MAO inhibitor intended to treat psychiatric disorders and initiation of fluvoxamine.

Allow 14 days to elapse between discontinuing fluvoxamine and initiation of an MAO inhibitor intended to treat psychiatric disorders.

Use with other MAO inhibitors (linezolid or IV methylene blue):

Do not initiate fluvoxamine in patients receiving linezolid or IV methylene blue; consider other interventions for psychiatric condition.

If urgent treatment with linezolid or IV methylene blue is required in a patient already receiving fluvoxamine and potential benefits outweigh potential risks, discontinue fluvoxamine promptly and administer linezolid or IV methylene blue. Monitor for serotonin syndrome for 2 weeks or until 24 hours after the last dose of linezolid or IV methylene blue, whichever comes first. May resume fluvoxamine 24 hours after the last dose of linezolid or IV methylene blue.

Dosage adjustment in renal impairment: No dosage adjustment provided in manufacturer's labeling. Limited data suggest fluvoxamine does not accumulate in patients with renal impairment.

Dosage adjustment in hepatic impairment: No dosage adjustment provided in manufacturer's labeling. Limited data suggest fluvoxamine clearance is reduced in patients with hepatic impairment. Reduced initial dose and slow titration may be required.

Dietary Considerations May be taken with or without food.

Administration May be administered with or without food. Do not crush, open, or chew extended release capsules.

Monitoring Parameters Mental status for depression, suicide ideation (especially at the beginning of therapy or when doses are increased or decreased), anxiety, social functioning, mania, panic attacks; signs/symptoms of serotonin syndrome; akathisia; weight gain or loss, nutritional intake, sleep; liver function assessment prior to beginning drug therapy

Dosage Forms

Capsule Extended Release 24 Hour, Oral:

Generic: 100 mg, 150 mg

Tablet, Oral:

Generic: 25 mg, 50 mg, 100 mg

Dosage Forms: Canada Note: Refer to Dosage Forms. Extended release capsules are not available in Canada.

- ◆ **Fluzone** *see* Influenza Virus Vaccine (Inactivated) *on page 1075*
- ◆ **Fluzone High-Dose** *see* Influenza Virus Vaccine (Inactivated) *on page 1075*
- ◆ **Fluzone Pediatric PF [DSC]** *see* Influenza Virus Vaccine (Inactivated) *on page 1075*
- ◆ **Fluzone Preservative Free** *see* Influenza Virus Vaccine (Inactivated) *on page 1075*
- ◆ **Fluzone Quadrivalent** *see* Influenza Virus Vaccine (Inactivated) *on page 1075*
- ◆ **FML** *see* Fluorometholone *on page 896*
- ◆ **FML® (Can)** *see* Fluorometholone *on page 896*
- ◆ **FML Forte** *see* Fluorometholone *on page 896*
- ◆ **FML Forte® (Can)** *see* Fluorometholone *on page 896*
- ◆ **FML Liquifilm** *see* Fluorometholone *on page 896*
- ◆ **Focalin** *see* Dexmethylphenidate *on page 605*
- ◆ **Focalin XR** *see* Dexmethylphenidate *on page 605*
- ◆ **Foille [OTC]** *see* Benzocaine *on page 246*
- ◆ **Folacin** *see* Folic Acid *on page 919*
- ◆ **Folacin, Vitamin B_{12}, and Vitamin B_6** *see* Folic Acid, Cyanocobalamin, and Pyridoxine *on page 921*
- ◆ **Folastin [DSC]** *see* Folic Acid, Cyanocobalamin, and Pyridoxine *on page 921*
- ◆ **Folate** *see* Folic Acid *on page 919*
- ◆ **Folbee®** *see* Folic Acid, Cyanocobalamin, and Pyridoxine *on page 921*
- ◆ **Folbic™** *see* Folic Acid, Cyanocobalamin, and Pyridoxine *on page 921*
- ◆ **Folcaps™ [DSC]** *see* Folic Acid, Cyanocobalamin, and Pyridoxine *on page 921*
- ◆ **Folgard RX®** *see* Folic Acid, Cyanocobalamin, and Pyridoxine *on page 921*

Folic Acid (FOE lik AS id)

Brand Names: U.S. FA-8 [OTC]

Brand Names: Canada Apo-Folic®

Index Terms Folacin; Folate; Pteroylglutamic Acid

Pharmacologic Category Vitamin, Water Soluble

Use Treatment of megaloblastic and macrocytic anemias due to folate deficiency

Pregnancy Risk Factor A

Pregnancy Considerations Water soluble vitamins cross the placenta. Folate requirements increase during pregnancy. Folate supplementation during the periconceptual period decreases the risk of neural tube defects. Folate supplementation (doses larger than the RDA) is recommended for women who may become pregnant (IOM, 1998).

Breast-Feeding Considerations Folate is found in breast milk; concentrations are not affected by dietary intake unless the mother has a severe deficiency (IOM, 1998).

Contraindications Hypersensitivity to folic acid or any component of the formulation

Warnings/Precautions Not appropriate for monotherapy with pernicious, aplastic, or normocytic anemias when anemia is present with vitamin B_{12} deficiency. Doses >0.1 mg/day may obscure pernicious anemia with continuing irreversible nerve damage progression. Resistance to treatment may occur with depressed hematopoiesis, alcoholism, and deficiencies of other vitamins. Injection contains benzyl alcohol (1.5%) as preservative (use care in administration to neonates).

Aluminum: The parenteral product may contain aluminum; toxic aluminum concentrations may be seen with high doses, prolonged use, or renal dysfunction. Premature neonates are at higher risk due to immature renal function and aluminum intake from other parenteral sources. Parenteral aluminum exposure of >4 to 5 mcg/kg/day is associated with CNS and bone toxicity; tissue loading may occur at lower doses (Federal Register, 2002). See manufacturer's labeling.

Benzyl alcohol and derivatives: Some dosage forms may contain benzyl alcohol; large amounts of benzyl alcohol (≥99 mg/kg/day) have been associated with a potentially fatal toxicity ("gasping syndrome") in neonates; the "gasping syndrome" consists of metabolic acidosis, respiratory distress, gasping respirations, CNS dysfunction (including convulsions, intracranial hemorrhage), hypotension and cardiovascular collapse (AAP, 1997; CDC, 1982); some data suggests that benzoate displaces bilirubin from protein binding sites (Ahlfors, 2001); avoid or use dosage forms containing benzyl alcohol with caution in neonates. See manufacturer's labeling.

Adverse Reactions

Cardiovascular: Flushing (slight)
Central nervous system: Malaise (general)
Dermatologic: Erythema, pruritus, rash
Respiratory: Bronchospasm
Miscellaneous: Allergic reaction

Drug Interactions

Metabolism/Transport Effects None known.

Avoid Concomitant Use

Avoid concomitant use of Folic Acid with any of the following: Raltitrexed

Increased Effect/Toxicity There are no known significant interactions involving an increase in effect.

Decreased Effect

Folic Acid may decrease the levels/effects of: Fosphenytoin; PHENobarbital; Phenytoin; Primidone; Raltitrexed

The levels/effects of Folic Acid may be decreased by: Green Tea; SulfaSALAzine

Storage/Stability Store at 20°C to 25°C (68°F to 77°F); protect from light.

Mechanism of Action Folic acid is necessary for formation of a number of coenzymes in many metabolic systems, particularly for purine and pyrimidine synthesis; required for nucleoprotein synthesis and maintenance in erythropoiesis; stimulates WBC and platelet production in folate deficiency anemia. Folic acid enhances the metabolism of formic acid, the toxic metabolite of methanol, to nontoxic metabolites (off-label use).

Pharmacodynamics/Kinetics

Onset of action: Peak effect: Oral: 0.5-1 hour
Absorption: Proximal part of small intestine
Metabolism: Hepatic
Excretion: Urine

Dosage

Oral, IM, IV, SubQ: Anemia:
- Infants: 0.1 mg/day
- Children <4 years: Up to 0.3 mg/day
- Children >4 years and Adults: 0.4 mg/day
- Pregnant and lactating women: 0.8 mg/day

Oral:

Adequate intake (AI) (IOM, 1998): Expressed as folate equivalents: Infants:
- 1-6 months: 65 mcg/day
- 7-12 months: 80 mcg/day

Recommended daily allowance (RDA) (IOM, 1998):
Expressed as dietary folate equivalents:
Children:
- 1-3 years: 150 mcg/day
- 4-8 years: 200 mcg/day
- 9-13 years: 300 mcg/day

Children ≥14 years and Adults: 400 mcg/day
- Pregnancy: 600 mcg/day
- Lactation: 500 mcg/day

Elderly: Vitamin B_{12} deficiency must be ruled out before initiating folate therapy due to frequency of combined nutritional deficiencies: RDA requirements (1999): 400 mcg/day (0.4 mg) minimum

Prevention of neural tube defects (off-label use):
- Females of childbearing potential: 400-800 mcg/day (USPSTF, 2009)
- Females at high risk or with family history of neural tube defects: 4 mg/day (ACOG, 2003)

Dietary Considerations As of January 1998, the FDA has required manufacturers of enriched flour, bread, corn meal, pasta, rice, and other grain products to add folic acid to their products. The intent is to help decrease the risk of neural tube defects by increasing folic acid intake. Other foods which contain folic acid include dark green leafy vegetables, citrus fruits and juices, and lentils.

Administration Oral preferred, but may also be administered by deep IM, SubQ, or IV injection.

IV administration: May administer ≤5 mg dose undiluted over ≥1 minute **or** may dilute ≤5 mg in 50 mL of NS or D_5W and infuse over 30 minutes. May also be added to IV maintenance solutions and given as an infusion.

Reference Range Therapeutic: 0.005-0.015 mcg/mL

Additional Information The RDA for folic acid is presented as dietary folate equivalents (DFE). DFE adjusts for the difference in bioavailability of folic acid from food as compared to dietary supplements.

Dosage Forms

Capsule, Oral [preservative free]:
- FA-8 [OTC]: 0.8 mg
- Generic: 5 mg, 20 mg

Solution, Injection:
- Generic: 5 mg/mL (10 mL)

Tablet, Oral:
- Generic: 400 mcg, 800 mcg, 1 mg

Tablet, Oral [preservative free]:
- FA-8 [OTC]: 800 mcg
- Generic: 400 mcg, 800 mcg

Extemporaneous Preparations A 1 mg/mL folic acid oral solution may be made with tablets. Heat 90 mL of purified water almost to boiling. Dissolve parabens (methylparaben 200 mg and propylparaben 20 mg) in the heated water; cool to room temperature. Crush one-hundred 1 mg tablets, then dissolve folic acid in the solution. Adjust pH to 8-8.5 with sodium hydroxide 10%; add sufficient quantity of purified water to make 100 mL; mix well. Stable for 30 days at room temperature (Allen, 2007).

A 0.05 mg/mL folic acid oral solution may be prepared using the injectable formulation (5 mg/mL). Mix 1 mL of injectable folic acid with 90 mL of purified water. Adjust pH to 8-8.5 with sodium hydroxide 10%; add sufficient quantity of purified water to make 100 mL; mix well. Stable for 30 days at room temperature (Nahata, 2004).

Allen LV Jr, "Folic Acid 1-mg/mL Oral Liquid," *Int J Pharm Compound*, 2007, 11(3):244.

Nahata MC, Pai VB, and Hipple TF, *Pediatric Drug Formulations*, 5th ed, Cincinnati, OH: Harvey Whitney Books Co, 2004.

Folic Acid, Cyanocobalamin, and Pyridoxine

(FOE lik AS id, sye an oh koe BAL a min, & peer i DOKS een)

Brand Names: U.S. FaBB; Folastin [DSC]; Folbee®; Folbic™; Folcaps™ [DSC]; Folgard RX®; Folplex 2.2; Foltabs™ 800 [OTC]; Homocysteine Guard [OTC]; Lev-Tov [OTC]; Tri-B® [OTC]; Tricardio B; Virt-Vite; Virt-Vite Forte; Vita-Respa®

Index Terms Cyanocobalamin, Folic Acid, and Pyridoxine; Folacin, Vitamin B_{12}, and Vitamin B_6; Pyridoxine, Folic Acid, and Cyanocobalamin

Pharmacologic Category Vitamin

Use Nutritional supplement in end-stage renal failure, dialysis, hyperhomocysteinemia, homocystinuria, malabsorption syndromes, dietary deficiencies

Dosage Oral: Adults: One tablet daily

Additional Information Complete prescribing information should be consulted for additional detail.

Dosage Forms

Tablet: Folic acid 0.8 mg, cyanocobalamin 1000 mcg, and pyridoxine 50 mg

FaBB, Folgard RX®: Folic acid 2.2 mg, cyanocobalamin 1000 mcg, and pyridoxine 25 mg

Folbee®, Virt-Vite: Folic acid 2.5 mg, cyanocobalamin 1000 mcg, and pyridoxine 25 mg

Folbic™, Virt-Vite Forte: Folic acid 2.5 mg, cyanocobalamin 2000 mcg, and pyridoxine 25 mg

Folplex 2.2: Folic acid 2.2 mg, cyanocobalamin 500 mcg, and pyridoxine 25 mg

Foltabs™ 800 [OTC]: Folic acid 0.8 mg, cyanocobalamin 115 mcg, and pyridoxine 10 mg

Homocysteine Guard [OTC], Tri-B® [OTC]: Folic acid 0.8 mg, cyanocobalamin 400 mcg, and pyridoxine 25 mg

Lev-Tov [OTC]: Folic acid 0.8 mg, cyanocobalamin 250 mcg, and pyridoxine 25 mg

Tricardio B: Folic acid 0.4 mg, cyanocobalamin 250 mcg, and pyridoxine 25 mg

Vita-Respa®: Folic acid 2.2 mg, cyanocobalamin 1300 mcg, and pyridoxine 25 mg

- **Folinate Calcium** *see* Leucovorin Calcium *on page 1183*
- **Folinic Acid (error prone synonym)** *see* Leucovorin Calcium *on page 1183*
- **Follicle-Stimulating Hormone, Human** *see* Urofollitropin *on page 2116*
- **Follicle Stimulating Hormone, Recombinant** *see* Follitropin Alfa *on page 921*
- **Follicle Stimulating Hormone, Recombinant** *see* Follitropin Beta *on page 921*
- **Follistim AQ** *see* Follitropin Beta *on page 921*

Follitropin Alfa (foe li TRO pin AL fa)

Brand Names: U.S. Gonal-f; Gonal-f RFF; Gonal-f RFF Pen; Gonal-f RFF Rediject

Brand Names: Canada Gonal-f; Gonal-f Pen

Index Terms Follicle Stimulating Hormone, Recombinant; FSH; rFSH-alpha; rhFSH-alpha

Pharmacologic Category Gonadotropin; Ovulation Stimulator

Use

Multifollicular development during Assisted Reproductive Technology (ART): To stimulate the development of multiple follicles with ART

Ovulation induction: Induction of ovulation in oligo-anovulatory infertile patients in whom the cause of infertility is functional and not caused by primary ovarian failure

Spermatogenesis induction (Gonal-f only): Induction of spermatogenesis in men with primary and secondary hypogonadotropic hypogonadism in whom the cause of infertility is not due to primary testicular failure

Pregnancy Risk Factor X

Dosage Adults: **Note:** Dose should be individualized. Use the lowest dose consistent with the expectation of good results. Over the course of treatment, doses may vary depending on individual patient response.

Females:

Ovulation induction: SubQ: Initial: 75 units daily; incremental dose adjustments of up to 37.5 units may be considered after 14 days; further dose increases of the same magnitude can be made, if necessary, every 7 days (maximum dose: 300 units daily). If response to follitropin is appropriate, hCG is given 1 day following the last dose. Withhold hCG if serum estradiol is >2000 pg/mL; discontinue if the ovaries are abnormally enlarged, or if abdominal pain occurs. In general, therapy should not exceed 35 days.

Multifollicular development during ART: SubQ: Initiate therapy with follitropin alfa in the early follicular phase (cycle day 2 or day 3) at a dose of 150 units daily, until sufficient follicular development is attained. In most cases, therapy should not exceed 10 days. In patients ≥35 years whose endogenous gonadotropin levels are suppressed, initiate follitropin alfa at a dose of 225 units daily. Continue treatment until adequate follicular development is indicated as determined by ultrasound in combination with measurement of serum estradiol levels. Consider adjustments to dose after 5 days based on the patient's response; adjust subsequent dosage every 3-5 days by ≤75-150 units additionally at each adjustment. Doses >450 units daily are not recommended. Once adequate follicular development is evident, administer hCG to induce final follicular maturation in preparation for oocyte retrieval. Withhold hCG if the ovaries are abnormally enlarged.

Males: Spermatogenesis induction: Gonal-f: SubQ: Therapy should begin with hCG pretreatment until serum testosterone is in normal range, then initiate Gonal-f at 150 units 3 times weekly with hCG 3 times weekly; continue with lowest dose needed to induce spermatogenesis (maximum dose: 300 units 3 times weekly); may be given for up to 18 months

Dosage adjustment in renal impairment: No dosage adjustment provided in manufacturer's labeling (has not been studied).

Dosage adjustment in hepatic impairment: No dosage adjustment provided in manufacturer's labeling (has not been studied).

Additional Information Complete prescribing information should be consulted for additional detail.

Dosage Forms

Solution, Subcutaneous:

Gonal-f RFF Pen: 300 units/0.5 mL (0.5 mL); 450 units/0.75 mL (0.75 mL); 900 units/1.5 mL (1.5 mL)

Gonal-f RFF Rediject: 300 units/0.5 mL (0.5 mL); 450 units/0.75 mL (0.75 mL); 900 units/1.5 mL (1.5 mL)

Solution Reconstituted, Injection:

Gonal-f: 450 units (1 ea); 1050 units (1 ea)

Solution Reconstituted, Subcutaneous:

Gonal-f RFF: 75 units (1 ea)

Follitropin Beta (foe li TRO pin BAY ta)

Brand Names: U.S. Follistim AQ

Brand Names: Canada Puregon

Index Terms Follicle Stimulating Hormone, Recombinant; FSH; rFSH-beta; rhFSH-beta

Pharmacologic Category Gonadotropin; Ovulation Stimulator

Use

Females: Induction of ovulation and pregnancy in anovulatory infertile patients in whom the cause of infertility is functional and not caused by primary ovarian failure; induction of pregnancy in normal ovulatory women undergoing Assisted Reproductive Technology (ART) (eg, *in vitro* fertilization [IVF], intracytoplasmic sperm injection [ICSI])

Males: Induction of spermatogenesis in men with primary and secondary hypogonadotropic hypogonadism in whom the cause of infertility is not due to primary testicular failure.

Pregnancy Risk Factor X

Dosage Adults: **Note:** Dose should be individualized. Use the lowest dose consistent with the expectation of good results. Over the course of treatment, doses may vary depending on individual patient response.

Females:

Ovulation induction:

Follistim® AQ: IM, SubQ: Stepwise approach: Initiate therapy with 75 units/day for at least the first 7 days. Increase by 25 or 50 units at weekly intervals until follicular growth or serum estradiol levels indicate an adequate response. The maximum (individualized) daily dose that has been safely used for ovulation induction in patients during clinical trials is 300 units. If response to follitropin is appropriate, hCG is given 1 day following the last dose. Withhold hCG if the ovaries are abnormally enlarged, or if abdominal pain occurs.

Follistim® AQ Cartridge: SubQ: Stepwise approach: Initiate therapy with 50 units/day for at least the first 7 days. Increase by 25 or 50 units at weekly intervals until follicular growth or serum estradiol levels indicate an adequate response. The maximum (individualized) daily dose that has been safely used for ovulation induction in patients during clinical trials is 250 units. If response to follitropin is appropriate, hCG is given 1 day following the last dose. Withhold hCG if the ovaries are abnormally enlarged, or if abdominal pain occurs. See **"Note"** for dosage adjustment for this product.

ART:

Follistim® AQ: IM, SubQ: Stepwise approach: A starting dose of 150-225 units is recommended for at least the first 4 days of treatment. The dose may be adjusted for the individual patient based upon their ovarian response. The maximum daily dose used in clinical studies is 600 units. When a sufficient number of follicles of adequate size are present, the final maturation of the follicles is induced by administering hCG. Oocyte retrieval is performed 34-36 hours later. Withhold hCG in cases where the ovaries are abnormally enlarged on the last day of follitropin beta therapy.

Follistim® AQ Cartridge: SubQ: Stepwise approach: A starting dose of 200 units is recommended for at least the first 7 days of treatment. The dose may be adjusted for the individual patient based upon their ovarian response. The maximum daily dose used in clinical studies is 500 units. When a sufficient number of follicles of adequate size are present, the final maturation of the follicles is induced by administering hCG. Oocyte retrieval is performed 34-36 hours later. Withhold hCG in cases where the ovaries are abnormally enlarged on the last day of follitropin beta therapy. See **"Note"** for dosage adjustment for this product.

Males: Spermatogenesis induction (Follistim® AQ, Follistim® AQ Cartridge): **Note:** Pretreatment with hCG monotherapy is required prior to concomitant therapy with follitropin beta and hCG. Follitropin beta therapy may be initiated after normal serum testosterone levels have been reached. SubQ: 450 units/week (administered as 225 units twice weekly or 150 units 3 times/weekly). A lower dose of Follistim® AQ Cartridge may be considered. See **"Note"** for dosage adjustment for this product.

Note: Dose adjustment for Follistim® AQ Cartridge: When administered using the Follistim Pen®, the Follistim® AQ Cartridge delivers 18% more follitropin beta when compared to dissolved lyophilized follitropin beta administered by a conventional syringe. If the above starting doses were previously used when administering a recombinant lyophilized gonadotropin product via a conventional syringe, lower starting and maintenance doses should be considered when switching to Follistim® AQ Cartridge. The following dose conversion may be used:

Follistim® AQ Dosing Conversion[1]

Dose Administered Using Powder for Solution/Conventional Syringe	Follistim® AQ Dose Administered Using Follistim Pen®
75 units	50 units
150 units	125 units
225 units	175 units
300 units	250 units
375 units	300 units
450 units	375 units

[1]Values listed are rounded to the nearest 25 unit increment.

Dosage adjustment in renal impairment: No dosage adjustment provided in manufacturer's labeling (has not been studied).

Dosage adjustment in hepatic impairment: No dosage adjustment provided in manufacturer's labeling (has not been studied).

Additional Information Complete prescribing information should be consulted for additional detail.

Dosage Forms

Solution, Injection:

Follistim AQ: 75 units/0.5 mL (0.5 mL); 150 units/0.5 mL (0.5 mL)

Solution, Subcutaneous:

Follistim AQ: 300 units/0.36 mL (0.42 mL); 600 units/0.72 mL (0.78 mL); 900 units/1.08 mL (1.17 mL)

◆ **Folotyn** *see* PRALAtrexate *on page 1693*

◆ **Folplex 2.2** *see* Folic Acid, Cyanocobalamin, and Pyridoxine *on page 921*

◆ **Foltabs™ 800 [OTC]** *see* Folic Acid, Cyanocobalamin, and Pyridoxine *on page 921*

Fomepizole (foe ME pi zole)

Brand Names: U.S. Antizol

Brand Names: Canada Antizol

Index Terms 4-Methylpyrazole; 4-MP

Pharmacologic Category Antidote

Use Treatment of methanol or ethylene glycol poisoning alone or in combination with hemodialysis

Pregnancy Risk Factor C

Pregnancy Considerations Animal reproduction studies have not been conducted. In general, medications used as antidotes should take into consideration the health and prognosis of the mother; antidotes should be administered to pregnant women if there is a clear indication for use and should not be withheld because of fears of teratogenicity (Bailey, 2003).

Breast-Feeding Considerations It is not known if fomepizole is excreted in breast milk. The manufacturer recommends that caution be exercised when administering fomepizole to nursing women.

Contraindications Hypersensitivity to fomepizole, other pyrazoles, or any component of the formulation

Warnings/Precautions Should not be given undiluted or by bolus injection. Fomepizole is metabolized in the liver and excreted in the urine; use caution with hepatic or renal impairment. Hemodialysis should be considered as an adjunct to fomepizole in patients with renal failure, significant acidosis (pH <7.25-7.3), worsening metabolic acidosis, or ethylene glycol or methanol concentrations ≥50 mg/dL. Pediatric administration is not FDA approved; however, safe and efficacious use in this patient population for ethylene glycol and methanol intoxication has been reported (Baum, 2000; Benitez, 2000; Boyer, 2001; Brown, 2001; De Brabander, 2005; Detaille, 2004; Fisher, 1998); consider consultation with a clinical toxicologist or poison control center.

Adverse Reactions

Cardiovascular: Bradycardia, facial flush, hypotension, shock, tachycardia

Central nervous system: Agitation, anxiety, dizziness, drowsiness increased, fever, headache, lightheadedness, seizure, vertigo

Dermatologic: Rash

Endocrine & metabolic: Liver function tests increased

Gastrointestinal: Abdominal pain, appetite decreased, bad/metallic taste, diarrhea, heartburn, nausea, vomiting

Hematologic: Anemia, disseminated intravascular coagulation (DIC), eosinophilia, lymphangitis

Local: Application site reaction, injection site inflammation, pain during injection, phlebitis

Neuromuscular & skeletal: Backache

Ocular: Nystagmus, transient blurred vision, visual disturbances

Renal: Anuria

Respiratory: Abnormal smell, hiccups, pharyngitis

Miscellaneous: Multiorgan failure, speech disturbances

Rare but important or life-threatening: Mild allergic reactions (mild rash, eosinophilia)

Drug Interactions

Metabolism/Transport Effects None known.

Avoid Concomitant Use There are no known interactions where it is recommended to avoid concomitant use.

Increased Effect/Toxicity There are no known significant interactions involving an increase in effect.

Decreased Effect There are no known significant interactions involving a decrease in effect.

Food Interactions Ethanol decreases the rate of fomepizole elimination by ~50%; conversely, fomepizole decreases the rate of elimination of ethanol by ~40%.

Preparation for Administration Prior to administration, dilute in at least 100 mL 0.9% sodium chloride or dextrose 5% water for injection. Although, it is chemically and physically stable when diluted as recommended, sterile precautions should be observed because diluents generally do not contain preservatives.

Storage/Stability Store at controlled room temperature, 20°C to 25°C (68°F to 77°F); fomepizole solidifies at temperatures <25°C (77°F). If solution becomes solid in the vial, it be should be carefully warmed by running the vial under warm water or by holding in the hand. Solidification does not affect the efficacy, safety, or stability of the drug. Diluted solution should be used within 24 hours and may be stored at room temperature or under refrigeration.

Mechanism of Action Fomepizole competitively inhibits alcohol dehydrogenase, an enzyme which catalyzes the metabolism of ethanol, ethylene glycol, and methanol to their toxic metabolites. Ethylene glycol is metabolized to glycoaldehyde, then oxidized to glycolate, glyoxylate, and oxalate. Glycolate and oxalate are responsible for metabolic acidosis and renal damage. Methanol is metabolized to formaldehyde, then oxidized to formic acid. Formic acid is responsible for metabolic acidosis and visual disturbances.

Pharmacodynamics/Kinetics

Onset of effect: Peak effect: Maximum: 1.5-2 hours

Absorption: Oral: Readily absorbed

Distribution: V_d: 0.6-1.02 L/kg; rapidly into total body water

Protein binding: Negligible

Metabolism: Hepatic to 4-carboxypyrazole (80% to 85% of dose), 4-hydroxymethylpyrazole, and their N-glucuronide conjugates; following multiple doses, induces its own metabolism via CYP oxidases after 30-40 hours

Half-life elimination: Has not been calculated; varies with dose

Excretion: Urine (1% to 3.5% as unchanged drug and metabolites)

Dosage Note: Fomepizole therapy should begin immediately upon suspicion of ethylene glycol or methanol ingestion.

Children, Adolescents (off-label use; Baum, 2000; Benitez, 2000; Boyer, 2001; Brown, 2001; De Brabander, 2005; Detaille, 2004; Fisher, 1998), and Adults: Ethylene glycol and methanol toxicity: IV: A loading dose of 15 mg/kg should be administered, followed by doses of 10 mg/kg every 12 hours for 4 doses, then 15 mg/kg every 12 hours thereafter until ethylene glycol or methanol concentrations have been reduced to <20 mg/dL and patient is asymptomatic with normal pH. **Note:** For severe toxicity requiring concomitant hemodialysis, see Dosage adjustment in renal impairment.

Dosage adjustment in renal impairment: Note: Hemodialysis should be considered as an adjunct to fomepizole in patients with renal failure, significant or worsening metabolic acidosis, or ethylene glycol or methanol concentrations ≥50 mg/dL. The following dosing adjustments should be used for any patient receiving hemodialysis regardless of renal function.

Prior to the start of hemodialysis:

To determine if the patient requires a dose of fomepizole at the start of hemodialysis, determine when the last dose was administered.

If the last dose of fomepizole was given <6 hours ago, do not administer another dose upon beginning hemodialysis.

If the last dose of fomepizole was given ≥6 hours ago, administer next scheduled dose upon beginning hemodialysis.

During hemodialysis: During hemodialysis, administer fomepizole every 4 hours. Alternatively, a loading dose of 10-20 mg/kg followed by 1-1.5 mg/kg/hour continuous infusion during hemodialysis has been described in case reports (Jobard, 1996).

Upon completion of hemodialysis:

To determine if the patient requires a dose of fomepizole at the time of completion of hemodialysis, determine when the last dose was administered.

If the last dose of fomepizole was given <1 hour ago, do not administer a dose at the end of hemodialysis.

If the last dose of fomepizole was given 1-3 hours ago, administer one-half of the next scheduled dose at the end of hemodialysis.

If the last dose of fomepizole was given >3 hours ago, administer the next scheduled dose at the end of hemodialysis.

Maintenance dose when off hemodialysis: Administer fomepizole every 12 hours (starting 12 hours from last dose administered).

Dosage adjustment in hepatic impairment: Fomepizole is metabolized in the liver; specific dosage adjustments have not been determined in patients with hepatic impairment

Administration The appropriate dose of fomepizole should be drawn from the vial with a syringe and injected into at least 100 mL of sterile 0.9% sodium chloride injection or dextrose 5% injection. All doses should be administered as a slow intravenous infusion (IVPB) over 30 minutes.

Monitoring Parameters Fomepizole plasma levels should be monitored; response to fomepizole; monitor plasma/urinary ethylene glycol or methanol levels, urinary oxalate (ethylene glycol), plasma/urinary osmolality, renal/hepatic function, serum electrolytes, arterial blood gases; anion and osmolar gaps, resolution of clinical signs and symptoms of ethylene glycol or methanol intoxication

Reference Range The manufacturer recommends concentrations 100-300 micromole/L (8.2-24.6 mg/L) to achieve enzyme inhibition of alcohol dehydrogenase; according to practice guidelines, serum fomepizole concentrations of ≥0.8 mg/L provide constant inhibition of alcohol dehydrogenase

Dosage Forms

Solution, Intravenous [preservative free]:

Antizol: 1 g/mL (1.5 mL)

Generic: 1 g/mL (1.5 mL); 1.5 g/1.5 mL (1.5 mL)

Fondaparinux (fon da PARE i nuks)

Brand Names: U.S. Arixtra

Brand Names: Canada Arixtra

Index Terms Fondaparinux Sodium

Pharmacologic Category Anticoagulant; Anticoagulant, Factor Xa Inhibitor

Use Prophylaxis of deep vein thrombosis (DVT) in patients undergoing surgery for hip replacement, knee replacement, hip fracture (including extended prophylaxis following hip fracture surgery), or abdominal surgery (in patients at risk for thromboembolic complications); treatment of acute pulmonary embolism (PE); treatment of acute DVT without PE

Canadian labeling: Additional uses (not approved in U.S.): Unstable angina or non-ST segment elevation myocardial infarction (UA/NSTEMI) for the prevention of death and subsequent MI; ST segment elevation MI (STEMI) for the prevention of death and myocardial reinfarction

Pregnancy Risk Factor B

Pregnancy Considerations Adverse events were not observed in animal reproduction studies. Based on case reports, small amounts of fondaparinux have been detected in the umbilical cord following multiple doses during pregnancy (Dempfle, 2004). Use of fondaparinux in pregnancy should be limited to those women who have severe allergic reactions to heparin, including heparin-induced thrombocytopenia, and who cannot receive danaparoid (Guyatt, 2012).

Breast-Feeding Considerations It is not known if fondaparinux is excreted into breast milk. The manufacturer recommends caution be used if administered to nursing women. The use of alternative anticoagulants is preferred (Guyatt, 2012).

Contraindications Serious hypersensitivity (eg, angioedema, anaphylactoid/anaphylactic reactions) to fondaparinux or any component of the formulation; severe renal impairment (CrCl <30 mL/minute); body weight <50 kg (prophylaxis); active major bleeding; bacterial endocarditis; thrombocytopenia associated with a positive *in vitro* test for antiplatelet antibody in the presence of fondaparinux

Warnings/Precautions **[U.S. Boxed Warning]: Spinal or epidural hematomas, including subsequent paralysis, may occur with recent or anticipated neuraxial anesthesia (epidural or spinal anesthesia) or spinal puncture in patients anticoagulated with LMWH, heparinoids, or fondaparinux.** Consider risk versus benefit prior to spinal procedures; risk is increased by the use of concomitant agents which may alter hemostasis, the use of indwelling epidural catheters for analgesia, a history of spinal deformity or spinal surgery, as well as a history of traumatic or repeated epidural or spinal punctures. Patient should be observed closely for bleeding and signs and symptoms of neurological impairment (eg, midline back pain, sensory and motor deficits [numbness, tingling, weakness in lower limbs], bowel or bladder dysfunction) if therapy is administered during or immediately following diagnostic lumbar puncture, epidural anesthesia, or spinal anesthesia. Optimal timing between administration of fondaparinux and neuraxial procedures is unknown.

Discontinue use 24 hours prior to CABG and dose with unfractionated heparin per institutional practice (ACCF/AHA [Anderson, 2013]). Use caution in patients with moderate renal dysfunction (CrCl 30-50 mL/minute); contraindicated in patients with CrCl <30 mL/minute. Discontinue if severe dysfunction or labile function develops.

Use caution in congenital or acquired bleeding disorders; bacterial endocarditis; renal impairment; hepatic impairment; active ulcerative or angiodysplastic gastrointestinal disease; hemorrhagic stroke; shortly after brain, spinal, or ophthalmologic surgery; or in patients taking platelet inhibitors. Risk of major bleeding may be increased if initial dose is administered earlier than recommended (initiation recommended at 6 to 8 hours following surgery). Discontinue agents that may enhance the risk of hemorrhage if possible. Although considered an insensitive measure of fondaparinux activity, there have been postmarketing reports of bleeding associated with elevated aPTT. Has occurred with administration, including very rare reports of thrombocytopenia with thrombosis similar to heparin-induced thrombocytopenia (HIT); however, has been used in patients with current or history of HIT due to a lack of an immune-mediated effect on platelets (ACCP [Guyatt, 2012]; Savi, 2005). Use is contraindicated in patients with thrombocytopenia associated with a positive *in vitro* test for antiplatelet antibodies in the presence of fondaparinux. Monitor patients closely and discontinue therapy if platelets fall to <100,000/mm^3 and/or thrombosis develops.

For subcutaneous administration; not for IM administration. Do not use interchangeably (unit for unit) with low molecular weight heparins, heparin, or heparinoids. Use caution in patients <50 kg who are being treated for DVT/PE; dosage reduction recommended. Contraindicated in patients <50 kg when used for prophylactic therapy. Use with caution in the elderly. The needle guard contains natural latex rubber.

The administration of fondaparinux as the sole anticoagulant is **not recommended** during PCI due to an increased risk for guiding-catheter thrombosis. Use of an anticoagulant with antithrombin activity (eg, unfractionated heparin) is recommended as adjunctive therapy to PCI even if prior treatment with fondaparinux (must take into account whether GP IIb/IIIa antagonists have been administered) (ACCF/AHA [Anderson, 2013]; Levine, 2011). Do not administer with other agents that increase the risk of hemorrhage unless they are essential for the management of the underlying condition (eg, warfarin for treatment of VTE).

Adverse Reactions As with all anticoagulants, bleeding is the major adverse effect. Hemorrhage may occur at any site. Risk appears increased by a number of factors including renal dysfunction, age (>75 years), and weight (<50 kg).

Cardiovascular: Hypotension
Central nervous system: Confusion, dizziness, insomnia
Dermatologic: Increased wound secretion, skin blister
Endocrine & metabolic: Hypokalemia
Hematologic & oncologic: Anemia, hematoma, major hemorrhage (risk of major hemorrhage increased as high as 5% in patients receiving initial dose <6 hours following surgery), minor hemorrhage, postoperative hemorrhage, purpura, thrombocytopenia (50,000 to 100,000/mm^3)
Hepatic: Increased serum ALT (>3 × ULN), increased serum AST (>3 × ULN)
Infection: Post-operative wound infection (abdominal surgery)
Respiratory: Epistaxis (VTE)
Rare but important or life-threatening: Anaphylactoid reaction, anaphylaxis, angioedema, catheter site thrombosis (during PCI; without heparin), elevated aPTT associated with bleeding, epidural hematoma, hemorrhagic death, injection site reaction (bleeding at injection site, skin rash, pruritus), intracranial hemorrhage, re-operation due to bleeding, severe thrombocytopenia (<50,000/mm^3), spinal hematoma, thrombocytopenia (with thrombosis)

Drug Interactions

Metabolism/Transport Effects None known.

Avoid Concomitant Use

Avoid concomitant use of Fondaparinux with any of the following: Apixaban; Dabigatran Etexilate; Edoxaban; Omacetaxine; Rivaroxaban; Urokinase; Vorapaxar

Increased Effect/Toxicity

Fondaparinux may increase the levels/effects of: Anticoagulants; Collagenase (Systemic); Deferasirox; Ibritumomab; Nintedanib; Obinutuzumab; Omacetaxine; Rivaroxaban; Tositumomab and Iodine I 131 Tositumomab

The levels/effects of Fondaparinux may be increased by: Agents with Antiplatelet Properties; Apixaban; Dabigatran Etexilate; Dasatinib; Edoxaban; Herbs (Anticoagulant/Antiplatelet Properties); Ibrutinib; Limaprost; Nonsteroidal Anti-Inflammatory Agents; Omega-3 Fatty Acids; Pentosan Polysulfate Sodium; Prostacyclin Analogues; Salicylates; Sugammadex; Thrombolytic Agents; Tibolone; Tipranavir; Urokinase; Vitamin E; Vorapaxar

Decreased Effect

The levels/effects of Fondaparinux may be decreased by: Estrogen Derivatives; Progestins

Preparation for Administration Canadian labeling: For IV administration: May mix with 25 mL or 50 mL NS

Storage/Stability Store at 25°C (77°F); excursions permitted to 15°C to 30°C (59°F to 86°F).

Canadian labeling: For IV administration: Manufacturer recommends immediate use once diluted in NS, but is stable for up to 24 hours at 15°C to 30°C (59°F to 86°F).

Mechanism of Action Fondaparinux is a synthetic pentasaccharide that causes an antithrombin III-mediated selective inhibition of factor Xa. Neutralization of factor Xa interrupts the blood coagulation cascade and inhibits thrombin formation and thrombus development.

Pharmacodynamics/Kinetics

Absorption: SubQ: Rapid and complete
Distribution: V_d: 7 to 11 L; mainly in blood
Protein binding: ≥94% to antithrombin III
Bioavailability: SubQ: 100%
Half-life elimination: 17 to 21 hours; prolonged with renal impairment
Time to peak: SubQ: 2 to 3 hours
Excretion: Urine (~77%, unchanged drug)

Dosage SubQ: Adults:

DVT prophylaxis: Adults ≥50 kg: 2.5 mg once daily. **Note:** Prophylactic use contraindicated in patients <50 kg. Initiate dose after hemostasis has been established, 6 to 8 hours postoperatively.

DVT prophylaxis with history of HIT (off-label use): 2.5 mg once daily (Blackmer, 2009; Harenberg, 2004; Parody, 2003)

Usual duration: 5 to 9 days (up to 10 days following abdominal surgery or up to 11 days following hip replacement or knee replacement). The American College of Chest Physicians recommends a minimum of 10 to 14 days for patients undergoing total hip arthroplasty, total knee arthroplasty, or hip fracture surgery; extended duration of up to 35 days suggested (Guyatt, 2012).

Acute DVT/PE treatment: **Note:** Start warfarin on the first or second treatment day and continue fondaparinux until INR is ≥2 for at least 24 hours (usually 5 to 7 days) (Guyatt, 2012):
<50 kg: 5 mg once daily
50 to 100 kg: 7.5 mg once daily
>100 kg: 10 mg once daily
Usual duration: 5 to 9 days (has been administered up to 26 days)

Acute coronary syndrome (Canadian labeling; off-label use in U.S.):
UA/NSTEMI: SubQ: 2.5 mg once daily; initiate as soon as possible after presentation; treat for the duration of hospitalization, up to 8 days (ACCF/AHA [Anderson, 2013]; Yusuf 2006a)
STEMI: IV: 2.5 mg once; subsequent doses (starting the following day): SubQ: 2.5 mg once daily; treat for the duration of the hospitalization, up to 8 days, or until revascularization (ACCF/AHA [O'Gara, 2013]; Yusuf, 2006b)
Note: Discontinue fondaparinux 24 hours prior to coronary artery bypass graft (CABG) surgery; instead, administer unfractionated heparin per institutional practice (ACCF/AHA [Anderson, 2013]).

Acute symptomatic superficial vein thrombosis (≥5 cm in length) of the legs (off-label use): 2.5 mg once daily for 45 days (Decousus, 2010; Guyatt, 2012)

Acute thrombosis (unrelated to HIT) in patients with a past history of HIT (off-label use; Guyatt, 2012; Warkentin, 2011):
<50 kg: 5 mg once daily
50 to 100 kg: 7.5 mg once daily
>100 kg: 10 mg once daily

Dosage adjustment in renal impairment:

CrCl 30 to 50 mL/minute: Use caution; total clearance ~40% lower compared to patients with normal renal function. When used for thromboprophylaxis, the American College of Chest Physicians suggests a 50% reduction in dose or use of low-dose heparin instead of fondaparinux (Garcia, 2012).
CrCl <30 mL/minute: Use is contraindicated.

Dosage adjustment in hepatic impairment:

Mild-to-moderate impairment: Dosage adjustment not required; monitor for signs of bleeding.
Severe impairment: There are no dosage adjustment provided in the manufacturer's labeling (has not been studied).

Administration Do **not** administer IM; intended for SubQ administration. Do not mix with other injections or infusions. Do not expel air bubble from syringe before injection. Administer according to recommended regimen; when used for DVT prophylaxis, early initiation (before 6 hours after orthopedic surgery) has been associated with increased bleeding. For STEMI patients (Canadian labeling; off-label use in U.S.) may administer initial dose as IV push or mix in 25 to 50 mL of NS (do not mix with other agents) and infuse over 2 minutes; flush tubing with NS after infusion to ensure complete administration for fondaparinux.

To convert from IV unfractionated heparin (UFH) infusion to SubQ fondaparinux (Nutescu, 2007): Calculate specific dose for fondaparinux based on indication, discontinue UFH, and begin fondaparinux within 1 hour

To convert from SubQ fondaparinux to IV UFH infusion (Nutescu, 2007): Discontinue fondaparinux; calculate specific dose for IV UFH infusion based on indication; omit heparin bolus/loading dose

For subQ fondaparinux dosed every 24 hours: Start IV UFH infusion 22 to 23 hours after last dose of fondaparinux

Monitoring Parameters Periodic monitoring of CBC, platelet count, serum creatinine, occult blood testing of stools recommended. Anti-Xa activity of fondaparinux can be measured by the assay if fondaparinux is used as the calibrator. PT and aPTT are insensitive measures of fondaparinux activity. If unexpected changes in coagulation parameters or major bleeding occur, discontinue fondaparinux (elevated aPTT associated with bleeding events have been reported in postmarketing data).

Reference Range Note: Routine monitoring is not recommended; the following fondaparinux-specific anti-Xa concentrations have been reported (Garcia, 2012):

Thromboprophylaxis dose: Anti-Xa activity at 3 hours post dose: ~0.39 to 0.5 mg/L

Therapeutic dosing (eg, 7.5 mg once daily): Anti-Xa activity at 3 hours post dose: 1.2 to 1.26 mg/L

Dosage Forms

Solution, Subcutaneous:

Generic: 2.5 mg/0.5 mL (0.5 mL); 5 mg/0.4 mL (0.4 mL); 7.5 mg/0.6 mL (0.6 mL); 10 mg/0.8 mL (0.8 mL)

Solution, Subcutaneous [preservative free]:

Arixtra: 2.5 mg/0.5 mL (0.5 mL); 5 mg/0.4 mL (0.4 mL); 7.5 mg/0.6 mL (0.6 mL); 10 mg/0.8 mL (0.8 mL)

Generic: 2.5 mg/0.5 mL (0.5 mL); 5 mg/0.4 mL (0.4 mL); 7.5 mg/0.6 mL (0.6 mL); 10 mg/0.8 mL (0.8 mL)

- ◆ **Fondaparinux Sodium** *see* Fondaparinux *on page 924*
- ◆ **Foradil (Can)** *see* Formoterol *on page 926*
- ◆ **Foradil Aerolizer** *see* Formoterol *on page 926*
- ◆ **Forfivo XL** *see* BuPROPion *on page 305*

Formestane [INT] (FOR mes tane)

International Brand Names Lentaron (AR, AT, BE, CH, DE, DK, ES, HU, IT, LU, NL, PT)

Pharmacologic Category Aromatase Inhibitor

Reported Use Treatment of advanced breast cancer in postmenopausal women

Dosage Range IM: Adults: 250 mg every 14 days

Product Availability Product available in various countries; not currently available in the U.S.

Dosage Forms

Injection, suspension: 250 mg/2 mL

Formoterol (for MOH te rol)

Brand Names: U.S. Foradil Aerolizer; Perforomist

Brand Names: Canada Foradil; Oxeze Turbuhaler

Index Terms Eformoterol; Formoterol Fumarate; Formoterol Fumarate Dihydrate

Pharmacologic Category $Beta_2$ Agonist; $Beta_2$-Adrenergic Agonist, Long-Acting

Use

U.S. labeling: Treatment of asthma (only as concomitant therapy with an inhaled corticosteroid) in patients with reversible obstructive airway disease, including patients with symptoms of nocturnal asthma (Foradil Aerolizer); maintenance treatment of bronchoconstriction in patients with COPD (Foradil Aerolizer, Perforomist); prevention of exercise-induced bronchospasm when administered on an as-needed basis (monotherapy may be indicated in patients without persistent asthma) (Foradil Aerolizer)

Canadian labeling: Treatment of asthma (only as concomitant therapy with an inhaled corticosteroid) in patients with reversible obstructive airway disease, including patients with symptoms of nocturnal asthma (Foradil, Oxeze Turbuhaler); maintenance treatment of COPD (Foradil); prevention of exercise-induced bronchospasm when administered on an as-needed basis (monotherapy may be indicated in patients without persistent asthma) (Oxeze Turbuhaler)

Pregnancy Risk Factor C

Pregnancy Considerations Adverse events were observed in some animal reproduction studies. Formoterol has the potential to affect uterine contractility if administered during labor.

Uncontrolled asthma is associated with adverse events on pregnancy (increased risk of perinatal mortality, preeclampsia, preterm birth, low birth weight infants). Although data related to its use in pregnancy is limited, formoterol may be used as an alternative agent when a long-acting beta agonist is needed to treat moderate persistent or severe persistent asthma in pregnant women (NAEPP, 2005).

Breast-Feeding Considerations It is not known if formoterol is excreted into breast milk. The manufacturer recommends that caution be exercised when administering formoterol to nursing women. The use of $beta_2$-receptor agonists are not considered a contraindication to breast-feeding (NAEPP, 2005).

Contraindications

Hypersensitivity to formoterol or any component of the formulation (Foradil Aerolizer only); treatment of status asthmaticus or other acute episodes of asthma or COPD (Foradil Aerolizer only); monotherapy in the treatment of asthma (ie, use without a concomitant long-term asthma control medication, such as an inhaled corticosteroid)

Canadian labeling: Additional contraindications (not in U.S. labeling): Presence of tachyarrhythmias

Warnings/Precautions [U.S. Boxed Warning]: Long-acting $beta_2$-agonists (LABAs) increase the risk of asthma-related deaths. Formoterol should only be used in asthma patients as adjuvant therapy in patients who are currently receiving but are not adequately controlled on a long-term asthma control medication (ie, an inhaled corticosteroid). Monotherapy with an LABA is contraindicated in the treatment of asthma. In a large, randomized, placebo-controlled U.S. clinical trial (SMART, 2006), salmeterol was associated with an increase in asthma-related deaths (when added to usual asthma therapy); risk is considered a class effect among all LABAs. Data are not available to determine if the addition of an inhaled corticosteroid lessens this increased risk of death associated with LABA use. Assess patients at regular intervals once asthma control is maintained on combination therapy to determine if step-down therapy is appropriate and the LABA can be discontinued (without loss of asthma control), and the patient can be maintained on an inhaled corticosteroid. LABAs are not appropriate in patients whose asthma is adequately controlled on low- or medium-dose inhaled corticosteroids. Do **not** use for acute bronchospasm. Short-acting $beta_2$-agonist (eg, albuterol) should be used for acute symptoms and symptoms occurring between treatments. Do **not** initiate in patients with significantly worsening or acutely deteriorating asthma; reports of severe (sometimes fatal) respiratory events have been reported when formoterol has been initiated in this situation. Corticosteroids should not be stopped or reduced when formoterol is initiated. Formoterol is not a substitute for inhaled or systemic corticosteroids and should not be used as monotherapy. During initiation, watch for signs of worsening asthma. **[U.S. Boxed Warning] (Foradil Aerolizer): LABAs may increase the risk of asthma-related hospitalization in pediatric and adolescent patients.** In general, a combination product containing a LABA and an inhaled corticosteroid is preferred in patients <18 years of age to ensure compliance.

Because LABAs may disguise poorly controlled persistent asthma, frequent or chronic use of LABAs for exercise-induced bronchospasm is discouraged by the NIH Asthma Guidelines (NIH, 2007). The safety and efficacy of Perforomist in asthma patients have not been established and is not FDA approved for the treatment of asthma.

Do **not** use for acute episodes of COPD. Do **not** initiate in patients with significantly worsening or acutely deteriorating COPD. Data are not available to determine if LABA use increases the risk of death in patients with COPD. Increased use and/or ineffectiveness of short-acting beta$_2$-agonists may indicate rapidly deteriorating disease and should prompt re-evaluation of the patient's condition.

Immediate hypersensitivity reactions (urticaria, angioedema, rash, bronchospasm) have been reported. Do not exceed recommended dose or frequency; serious adverse events (including serious asthma exacerbations and fatalities) have been associated with excessive use of inhaled sympathomimetics. Beta$_2$-agonists may increase risk of arrhythmias, decrease serum potassium, prolong QTc interval, or increase serum glucose. These effects may be exacerbated in hypoxemia. Use caution in patients with cardiovascular disease (arrhythmia, coronary insufficiency, hypertension, HF, or aneurysm), seizures, diabetes, hyperthyroidism, pheochromocytoma, or hypokalemia. Beta-agonists may cause elevation in blood pressure and heart rate, and result in CNS stimulation/excitation. Tolerance to the bronchodilator effect, measured by FEV$_1$, has been observed in studies.

Powder for oral inhalation contains lactose; very rare anaphylactic reactions have been reported in patients with severe milk protein allergy. The contents of the Foradil Aerolizer capsules are for inhalation only via the Aerolizer device. There have been reports of incorrect administration (swallowing of the capsules).

Adverse Reactions

Cardiovascular: Chest pain, palpitation

Central nervous system: Anxiety, dizziness, dysphonia, fever, headache, insomnia

Dermatologic: Pruritus, rash

Gastrointestinal: Abdominal pain, diarrhea, dyspepsia, gastroenteritis, nausea, vomiting, xerostomia

Neuromuscular & skeletal: Muscle cramps, tremor

Respiratory: Asthma exacerbation, bronchitis, dyspnea, infection, pharyngitis, sinusitis, tonsillitis

Miscellaneous: Viral infection

Rare but important or life-threatening: Acute asthma deterioration, anaphylactic reactions (severe hypotension/ angioedema), agitation, angina, arrhythmia, atrial fibrillation, bronchospasm (paradoxical), cough, fatigue, hyperglycemia, hypertension, hypokalemia, glucose intolerance, malaise, metabolic acidosis, nervousness, QTc prolongation, tachycardia, ventricular extrasystoles

Drug Interactions

Metabolism/Transport Effects

Substrate of CYP2C9 (minor); **Note:** Assignment of Major/Minor substrate status based on clinically relevant drug interaction potential

Avoid Concomitant Use

Avoid concomitant use of Formoterol with any of the following: Beta-Blockers (Nonselective); Highest Risk QTc-Prolonging Agents; Iobenguane I 123; Ivabradine; Long-Acting Beta2-Agonists; Mifepristone

Increased Effect/Toxicity

Formoterol may increase the levels/effects of: Atosiban; Highest Risk QTc-Prolonging Agents; Long-Acting Beta2-Agonists; Loop Diuretics; Moderate Risk QTc-Prolonging Agents; Sympathomimetics; Thiazide Diuretics

The levels/effects of Formoterol may be increased by: AtoMOXetine; Caffeine and Caffeine Containing Products; Cannabinoid-Containing Products; Inhalational Anesthetics; Ivabradine; Linezolid; MAO Inhibitors; Mifepristone; QTc-Prolonging Agents (Indeterminate Risk and Risk Modifying); Tedizolid; Theophylline Derivatives; Tricyclic Antidepressants

Decreased Effect

Formoterol may decrease the levels/effects of: Iobenguane I 123

The levels/effects of Formoterol may be decreased by: Beta-Blockers (Beta1 Selective); Beta-Blockers (Nonselective); Betahistine

Storage/Stability

Foradil Aerolizer: Prior to dispensing, store in refrigerator at 2°C to 8°C (36°F to 46°F). After dispensing, store at room temperature at 20°C to 25°C (68°F to 77°F). Protect from heat and moisture. Capsules should always be stored in the blister and only removed immediately before use.

Perforomist: Prior to dispensing, store in refrigerator at 2°C to 8°C (36°F to 46°F). After dispensing, store at 2°C to 25°C (36°F to 77°F) for up to 3 months. Protect from heat. Unit-dose vials should always be stored in the foil pouch and only removed immediately before use.

Mechanism of Action Relaxes bronchial smooth muscle by selective action on beta$_2$ receptors with little effect on heart rate. Formoterol has a long-acting effect.

Pharmacodynamics/Kinetics

Onset of action: Powder for inhalation: Within 3 minutes

Peak effect: Powder for inhalation: 80% of peak effect within 15 minutes; Solution for nebulization: 2 hours

Duration: Improvement in FEV$_1$ observed for 12 hours in most patients

Absorption: Rapidly into plasma

Protein binding: 61% to 64% *in vitro* at higher concentrations than achieved with usual dosing

Metabolism: Hepatic via direct glucuronidation and O-demethylation; CYP2D6, CYP2C8/9, CYP2C19, CYP2A6 involved in O-demethylation

Half-life elimination: Powder: ~10-14 hours; Nebulized solution: ~7 hours

Time to peak: Maximum improvement in FEV$_1$ in 1-3 hours

Excretion:

Children 5-12 years: Urine (7% to 9% as direct glucuronide metabolites, 6% as unchanged drug)

Adults: Urine (15% to 18% as direct glucuronide metabolites, 2% to 10% as unchanged drug)

Dosage

Asthma treatment: **Note:** For asthma control, long-acting beta$_2$-agonists (LABAs) should be used in combination with inhaled corticosteroids and not as monotherapy.

U.S. labeling: Foradil Aerolizer: Inhalation: Children ≥5 years, Adolescents, and Adults: 12 mcg every 12 hours (maximum: 24 mcg daily)

Canadian labeling:

Foradil:

Children 6 to 16 years: Inhalation: 12 mcg every 12 hours (maximum: 24 mcg daily)

Adolescents ≥17 years and Adults: Inhalation: 12 mcg every 12 hours; in severe cases, 24 mcg every 12 hours may be given (maximum: 48 mcg daily)

Oxeze Turbuhaler:

Children 6 to 16 years: Inhalation: 6 mcg or 12 mcg every 12 hours (maximum: 24 mcg daily)

Adolescents ≥17 years and Adults: Inhalation: 6 mcg or 12 mcg every 12 hours (maximum: 48 mcg daily)

Prevention of exercise-induced bronchospasm: **Note:** If already using for asthma maintenance, then should not use additional doses for exercise-induced bronchospasm. Because LABAs may disguise poorly controlled persistent asthma, frequent or chronic use of LABAs for exercise-induced bronchospasm is discouraged by the Asthma Guidelines (NAEPP, 2007).

U.S. labeling: Foradil Aerolizer: Children ≥5 years, Adolescents, and Adults: Inhalation: 12 mcg at least 15 minutes before exercise on an occasional "as needed" basis; additional doses should not be used for another 12 hours

Canadian labeling: Oxeze Turbuhaler: Children ≥6 years, Adolescents, and Adults: Inhalation: 6 mcg or 12 mcg at least 15 minutes before exercise on an occasional "as needed" basis (maximum: Children and Adolescents: 24 mcg/24-hour period; Adults: 48 mcg/24-hour period)

COPD maintenance treatment: Adults: Inhalation:

U.S. labeling:

Foradil Aerolizer: 12 mcg every 12 hours (maximum: 24 mcg daily)

Perforomist: 20 mcg twice daily (maximum dose: 40 mcg daily)

Canadian labeling: Foradil: 12 mcg or 24 mcg twice daily (maximum dose: 48 mcg daily)

Dosage adjustment in renal impairment: No dosage adjustment provided in manufacturer's labeling (has not been studied).

Dosage adjustment in hepatic impairment: No dosage adjustment provided in manufacturer's labeling (has not been studied).

Administration

Foradil Aerolizer: Remove capsule from foil blister **immediately** before use. Place capsule in the capsule-chamber in the base of the Aerolizer Inhaler. Capsules must not be swallowed whole; must only use the Aerolizer Inhaler. Press both buttons **once only** and then release. Keep inhaler in a level, horizontal position. Exhale fully. Do not exhale into inhaler. Tilt head slightly back and inhale (rapidly, steadily, and deeply). Hold breath as long as possible. If any powder remains in capsule, exhale and inhale again. Repeat until capsule is empty. Throw away empty capsule; do not leave in inhaler. Do not use a spacer with the Aerolizer Inhaler. Always keep capsules and inhaler dry.

Perforomist: Remove unit-dose vial from foil pouch **immediately** before use. Solution does not require dilution prior to administration; do not mix other medications with formoterol solution. Place contents of unit-dose vial into the reservoir of a standard jet nebulizer connected to an air compressor; assemble nebulizer based on the manufacturer's instructions and turn nebulizer on; breathe deeply and evenly until all of the medication has been inhaled. Discard any unused medication immediately; do not ingest contents of vial. Clean nebulizer after use.

Oxeze Turbuhaler (Canadian availability): Hold inhaler upright. Turn colored grip as far as it will go in one direction and then turn back to original position; a clicking sound should be heard which means the inhaler is ready for use. Exhale fully. Do not exhale into mouthpiece of inhaler. Place mouthpiece to lips and inhale forcefully and deeply. Do not chew or bite on mouthpiece. Clean outside of mouthpiece once weekly with a dry tissue. Avoid getting inhaler wet. If the inhaler is accidently dropped or shaken, or if the patient exhales into the inhaler, the dose will be lost and a new dose should be loaded.

Monitoring Parameters FEV_1, peak flow, and/or other pulmonary function tests; blood pressure, heart rate; CNS stimulation; serum glucose, serum potassium

Dosage Forms

Capsule, Inhalation:

Foradil Aerolizer: 12 mcg

Nebulization Solution, Inhalation:

Perforomist: 20 mcg/2 mL (2 mL)

Dosage Forms: Canada

Powder for oral inhalation:

Oxeze Turbuhaler: 6 mcg/inhalation, 12 mcg/inhalation

- ◆ **Formoterol and Budesonide** *see* Budesonide and Formoterol *on page 297*
- ◆ **Formoterol and Mometasone** *see* Mometasone and Formoterol *on page 1392*
- ◆ **Formoterol and Mometasone Furoate** *see* Mometasone and Formoterol *on page 1392*
- ◆ **Formoterol Fumarate** *see* Formoterol *on page 926*
- ◆ **Formoterol Fumarate Dihydrate** *see* Formoterol *on page 926*
- ◆ **Formoterol Fumarate Dihydrate and Budesonide** *see* Budesonide and Formoterol *on page 297*
- ◆ **Formoterol Fumarate Dihydrate and Mometasone** *see* Mometasone and Formoterol *on page 1392*
- ◆ **Formula E 400 [OTC]** *see* Vitamin E *on page 2174*
- ◆ **Formulex (Can)** *see* Dicyclomine *on page 622*
- ◆ **5-Formyl Tetrahydrofolate** *see* Leucovorin Calcium *on page 1183*
- ◆ **Fortamet** *see* MetFORMIN *on page 1307*
- ◆ **Fortaz** *see* CefTAZidime *on page 392*
- ◆ **Fortaz in D5W** *see* CefTAZidime *on page 392*
- ◆ **Forteo** *see* Teriparatide *on page 2008*
- ◆ **Forteo® (Can)** *see* Teriparatide *on page 2008*
- ◆ **Fortesta** *see* Testosterone *on page 2010*
- ◆ **Fortical** *see* Calcitonin *on page 322*
- ◆ **Fosamax** *see* Alendronate *on page 79*
- ◆ **Fosamax Plus D®** *see* Alendronate and Cholecalciferol *on page 81*

Fosamprenavir (FOS am pren a veer)

Brand Names: U.S. Lexiva

Brand Names: Canada Telzir

Index Terms Fosamprenavir Calcium; GW433908G

Pharmacologic Category Antiretroviral, Protease Inhibitor (Anti-HIV)

Use Treatment of HIV infections in combination with at least two other antiretroviral agents

Pregnancy Risk Factor C

Dosage Oral: HIV infection:

Children:

U.S. labeling: Infants ≥4 weeks to Children <18 years: **Note:** Twice-daily dosing is recommended; once-daily dosing (without or without ritonavir) is **not** recommended in any pediatric patient.

Protease inhibitor (PI)-naive patients:

Ritonavir-boosted regimen: Infants ≥4 weeks: **Note:** Should not be administered to infants born <38 weeks gestation and who have not attained a postnatal age of 28 days.

<11 kg: Fosamprenavir 45 mg/kg/dose twice daily **plus** ritonavir 7 mg/kg/dose twice daily (maximum: Fosamprenavir 700 mg/ritonavir 100 mg twice daily)

11 to <15 kg: Fosamprenavir 30 mg/kg/dose twice daily **plus** ritonavir 3 mg/kg/dose twice daily (maximum: Fosamprenavir 700 mg/ritonavir 100 mg twice daily)

15 to <20 kg: Fosamprenavir 23 mg/kg/dose twice daily **plus** ritonavir 3 mg/kg/dose twice daily (maximum: Fosamprenavir 700 mg/ritonavir 100 mg twice daily)

≥20 kg: Fosamprenavir 18 mg/kg/dose twice daily **plus** ritonavir 3 mg/kg/dose twice daily (maximum: Fosamprenavir 700 mg/ritonavir 100 mg twice daily)

Note: When combined with ritonavir, the adult regimen of fosamprenavir 700 mg plus ritonavir 100 mg twice daily can be used in children who weigh ≥39 kg while ritonavir capsules may be used for children who weigh ≥33 kg.

Unboosted regimen:

Children <2 years: Fosamprenavir without ritonavir is not recommended

Children ≥2 years and <47 kg: Fosamprenavir 30 mg/kg/dose twice daily (not to exceed adult dosage of 1400 mg twice daily)

Children ≥2 years and ≥47 kg: The adult regimen of fosamprenavir 1400 mg twice daily may be used

Protease inhibitor (PI)-experienced patients:

Ritonavir-boosted regimen:

Infants <6 months: Not recommended in PI-experienced patients

Infants ≥6 months:

<11 kg: Fosamprenavir 45 mg/kg/dose twice daily **plus** ritonavir 7 mg/kg/dose twice daily (maximum: Fosamprenavir 700 mg/ritonavir 100 mg twice daily)

11 to <15 kg: Fosamprenavir 30 mg/kg/dose twice daily **plus** ritonavir 3 mg/kg/dose twice daily (maximum: Fosamprenavir 700 mg/ritonavir 100 mg twice daily)

15 to <20 kg: Fosamprenavir 23 mg/kg/dose twice daily **plus** ritonavir 3 mg/kg/dose twice daily (maximum: Fosamprenavir 700 mg/ritonavir 100 mg twice daily)

≥20 kg: Fosamprenavir 18 mg/kg/dose twice daily **plus** ritonavir 3 mg/kg/dose twice daily (maximum: Fosamprenavir 700 mg/ritonavir 100 mg twice daily)

Note: When combined with ritonavir, the adult regimen of fosamprenavir 700 mg plus ritonavir 100 mg twice daily can be used in children who weigh ≥39 kg while ritonavir capsules may be used for children who weigh ≥33 kg.

Unboosted regimen: **Note:** No information provided in manufacturer's labeling regarding unboosted fosamprenavir in PI-experienced pediatric patients except that fosamprenavir without ritonavir is not recommended in children <2 years of age and the adult unboosted regimen of 1400 mg twice daily may be used for pediatric patients who weigh ≥47 kg.

Canadian labeling: **Note:** Use of fosamprenavir without ritonavir (unboosted regimen) is not an approved use in the Canadian labeling.

PI-naive and PI-experienced patients: *Ritonavir boosted regimen:* Children ≥6 years: 18 mg/kg/dose **plus** ritonavir 3 mg/kg/dose twice daily; maximum dose: Fosamprenavir 700 mg/ritonavir 100 mg twice daily; adult regimen of fosamprenavir 700 mg/ritonavir 100 mg twice daily can be used in children who weigh ≥39 kg while ritonavir tablets may be used for children who weigh ≥33 kg and can swallow tablets whole.

Adults:

Antiretroviral therapy-naive patients:

Unboosted regimen (per manufacturer's labeling): 1400 mg twice daily (without ritonavir); **Note:** This regimen is not recommended in adults due to inferior potency compared to other protease inhibitor based regimens and the potential for cross-resistance to darunavir (HHS [adults], 2014).

Ritonavir-boosted regimens:

Once-daily regimen: Fosamprenavir 1400 mg plus ritonavir 100-200 mg once daily

Twice-daily regimen: Fosamprenavir 700 mg plus ritonavir 100 mg twice daily

Protease inhibitor (PI)-experienced patients: Fosamprenavir 700 mg plus ritonavir 100 mg twice daily. **Note:** Once-daily administration is not recommended in protease inhibitor-experienced patients.

Dosage adjustments for concomitant therapy: Adults:

Combination therapy with efavirenz (ritonavir-boosted regimen):

Once-daily regimen (PI-naive patients only): Fosamprenavir 1400 mg plus ritonavir 300 mg plus efavirenz 600 mg once daily

Twice-daily regimen: Fosamprenavir 700 mg plus ritonavir 100 mg twice daily plus efavirenz 600 mg once daily

Combination therapy with maraviroc: Fosamprenavir 700 mg plus ritonavir 100 mg plus maraviroc 150 mg twice daily

Dosage adjustment in renal impairment: No dosage adjustment necessary.

Dosage adjustment in hepatic impairment: Adults (not established in pediatric patients):

Mild impairment (Child-Pugh score 5-6): Reduce dosage of fosamprenavir to 700 mg twice daily without concurrent ritonavir (therapy naive) **or** fosamprenavir 700 mg twice daily plus ritonavir 100 mg once daily (therapy naive or PI experienced)

Moderate impairment (Child-Pugh score 7-9): Reduce dosage of fosamprenavir to 700 mg twice daily without concurrent ritonavir (therapy naive) **or** fosamprenavir 450 mg twice daily plus ritonavir 100 mg once daily (therapy naive or PI experienced)

Severe impairment (Child-Pugh score 10-15): Reduce dosage of fosamprenavir to 350 mg twice daily without concurrent ritonavir (therapy naive) **or** fosamprenavir 300 mg twice daily plus ritonavir 100 mg once daily (therapy naive or PI experienced).

Additional Information Complete prescribing information should be consulted for additional detail.

Dosage Forms

Suspension, Oral:

Lexiva: 50 mg/mL (225 mL)

Tablet, Oral:

Lexiva: 700 mg

Dosage Forms: Canada

Tablet:

Telzir: 700 mg

Suspension, oral:

Telzir: 50 mg/mL

◆ **Fosamprenavir Calcium** *see* Fosamprenavir *on page 928*

Fosaprepitant (fos a PRE pi tant)

Brand Names: U.S. Emend

Brand Names: Canada Emend® IV

Index Terms Aprepitant Injection; Fosaprepitant Dimeglumine; L-758,298; MK 0517

Pharmacologic Category Antiemetic; Substance P/Neurokinin 1 Receptor Antagonist

Use Prevention of acute and delayed nausea and vomiting associated with moderately- and highly-emetogenic chemotherapy (in combination with other antiemetics)

Pregnancy Risk Factor B

Pregnancy Considerations Teratogenic effects were not observed in animal reproduction studies for aprepitant. Use during pregnancy only if clearly needed. Efficacy of hormonal contraceptive may be reduced; alternative or additional methods of contraception should be used both during treatment with fosaprepitant or aprepitant and for at least 1 month following the last fosaprepitant/aprepitant dose.

Breast-Feeding Considerations It is not known if fosaprepitant is excreted in breast milk. Due to the potential for serious adverse reactions in the nursing infant, a decision should be made whether to discontinue nursing or to discontinue the drug, taking into account the importance of treatment to the mother.

Contraindications Hypersensitivity to fosaprepitant, aprepitant, polysorbate 80, or any component of the formulation; concurrent use with pimozide or cisapride

Canadian labeling: Additional contraindications (not in U.S. labeling): Concurrent use with astemizole or terfenadine

Warnings/Precautions Fosaprepitant is rapidly converted to aprepitant, which has a high potential for drug interactions. Potentially significant drug-drug interactions may exist, requiring dose or frequency adjustment, additional monitoring, and/or selection of alternative therapy. Immediate hypersensitivity has been reported (rarely) with fosaprepitant; stop infusion with hypersensitivity symptoms (dyspnea, erythema, flushing, or anaphylaxis); do not reinitiate. Contains polysorbate 80, which is associated with hypersensitivity reactions. Use caution with hepatic impairment; has not been studied in patients with severe hepatic impairment (Child-Pugh class C). Not studied for treatment of existing nausea and vomiting. Chronic continuous administration of fosaprepitant is not recommended.

Adverse Reactions Adverse reactions reported with aprepitant and fosaprepitant (as part of a combination chemotherapy regimen) occurring at a higher frequency than standard antiemetic therapy:

Central nervous system: Fatigue, headache

Gastrointestinal: Anorexia, constipation, diarrhea, dyspepsia, eructation

Hepatic: ALT increased, AST increased

Local: Injection site reactions (includes erythema, induration, pain, pruritus, or thrombophlebitis)

Neuromuscular & skeletal: Weakness

Miscellaneous: Hiccups

Rare but important or life-threatening: Abdominal pain, alkaline phosphatase increased, anaphylactic reaction, anemia, angioedema, bradycardia, candidiasis, cardiovascular disorder, chest discomfort, chills, cognitive disorder, conjunctivitis, cough, disorientation, dizziness, duodenal ulcer (perforating), dyspnea, edema, erythema, flushing, gait disturbance, hematuria (microscopic), hyperglycemia, hyperhydrosis, hypersensitivity reaction, hypertension, hyponatremia, miosis, nausea, neutropenia, neutropenic colitis, neutropenic fever, palpitation, photosensitivity, pollakiuria, polyuria, pruritus, rash, sensory disturbance, somnolence, staphylococcal infection, Stevens-Johnson syndrome, stomatitis, subileus, tinnitus, toxic epidermal necrolysis, urticaria, visual acuity decreased, vomiting, wheezing

Drug Interactions

Metabolism/Transport Effects Substrate of CYP1A2 (minor), CYP2C19 (minor), CYP3A4 (major); **Note:** Assignment of Major/Minor substrate status based on clinically relevant drug interaction potential; **Inhibits** CYP2C19 (weak), CYP2C9 (weak), CYP3A4 (moderate); **Induces** CYP2C9 (moderate), CYP3A4 (weak)

Avoid Concomitant Use

Avoid concomitant use of Fosaprepitant with any of the following: Astemizole; Bosutinib; Cisapride; Conivaptan; Fusidic Acid (Systemic); Ibrutinib; Idelalisib; Ivabradine; Lomitapide; Naloxegol; Olaparib; Pimozide; Simeprevir; Terfenadine; Tolvaptan; Trabectedin; Ulipristal

Increased Effect/Toxicity

Fosaprepitant may increase the levels/effects of: Astemizole; Avanafil; Bosentan; Bosutinib; Budesonide (Systemic, Oral Inhalation); Cannabis; Cisapride; Colchicine; Corticosteroids (Systemic); CYP3A4 Substrates; Dapoxetine; Diltiazem; Dofetilide; DOXOrubicin (Conventional); Dronabinol; Eliglustat; Eplerenone; Everolimus; FentaNYL; Halofantrine; Hydrocodone; Ibrutinib; Ifosfamide; Imatinib; Ivabradine; Ivacaftor; Lomitapide; Lurasidone; Naloxegol; Olaparib; OxyCODONE; Pimecrolimus; Pimozide; Propafenone; Ranolazine; Rivaroxaban; Salmeterol; Saxagliptin; Simeprevir; Sirolimus; Suvorexant; Terfenadine; Tetrahydrocannabinol; Tolvaptan; Trabectedin; Ulipristal; Vilazodone; Zopiclone; Zuclopenthixol

The levels/effects of Fosaprepitant may be increased by: Aprepitant; Ceritinib; Conivaptan; CYP3A4 Inhibitors (Moderate); CYP3A4 Inhibitors (Strong); Dasatinib; Diltiazem; Fusidic Acid (Systemic); Idelalisib; Luliconazole; Mifepristone; Netupitant; Stiripentol

Decreased Effect

Fosaprepitant may decrease the levels/effects of: ARIPiprazole; Contraceptives (Estrogens); Contraceptives (Progestins); Hydrocodone; PARoxetine; Saxagliptin; TOLBUTamide; Warfarin

The levels/effects of Fosaprepitant may be decreased by: Bosentan; CYP3A4 Inducers (Moderate); CYP3A4 Inducers (Strong); Dabrafenib; Deferasirox; Mitotane; PARoxetine; Rifampin; Siltuximab; St Johns Wort; Tocilizumab

Food Interactions Aprepitant serum concentration may be increased when taken with grapefruit juice. Management: Avoid concurrent use.

Preparation for Administration Reconstitute vial with 5 mL of sodium chloride 0.9%, directing diluent down side of vial to avoid foaming; swirl gently. Add reconstituted contents of the 150 mg vial to 145 mL sodium chloride 0.9%, resulting in a final concentration of 1 mg/mL; gently invert bag to mix. Solutions may be diluted to a final volume of 250 mL (0.6 mg/mL) (data on file [Merck, 2013]).

Storage/Stability Store intact vials at 2°C to 8°C (36°F to 46°F). Solutions diluted to 1 mg/mL for infusion are stable for 24 hours at room temperature or at ≤25°C (≤77°F). Solutions diluted to a final volume of 250 mL (0.6 mg/mL) should be administered within 24 hours (data on file [Merck, 2013]).

Mechanism of Action Fosaprepitant is a prodrug of aprepitant, a substance P/neurokinin 1 (NK1) receptor antagonist. It is rapidly converted to aprepitant which prevents acute and delayed vomiting by inhibiting the substance P/neurokinin 1 (NK1) receptor; augments the antiemetic activity of the 5-HT_3 receptor antagonist and corticosteroid activity and inhibits chemotherapy-induced emesis.

Pharmacodynamics/Kinetics

Distribution: Fosaprepitant: ~5 L; Aprepitant: V_d: ~70 L; crosses the blood-brain barrier

Protein binding: Aprepitant: >95%

Metabolism:

Fosaprepitant: Hepatic and extrahepatic; rapidly (within 30 minutes after the end of infusion) converted to aprepitant (nearly complete conversion)

Aprepitant: Hepatic via CYP3A4 (major); CYP1A2 and CYP2C19 (minor); forms 7 weakly-active metabolites

Half-life elimination: Fosaprepitant: ~2 minutes; Aprepitant: ~9-13 hours

Time to peak, plasma: Fosaprepitant is converted to aprepitant within 30 minutes after the end of infusion

Excretion: Urine (57%); feces (45%)

Dosage Prevention of chemotherapy-induced nausea/ vomiting: Adults: IV:

Single-dose regimen for highly-emetogenic chemotherapy: 150 mg ~30 minutes prior to chemotherapy on day 1 only (in combination with a 5-HT_3 antagonist on day 1 and dexamethasone on days 1 to 4)

Single-dose regimen for moderately-emetogenic chemotherapy: 150 mg ~30 minutes prior to chemotherapy on day 1 only (in combination with a 5-HT_3 antagonist and dexamethasone on day 1, and either a 5-HT_3 antagonist or dexamethasone on days 2 and 3) (NCCN Antiemesis guidelines v.1.2013)

Dosage adjustment in renal impairment:

Mild, moderate, or severe impairment: No dosage adjustment necessary.

Dialysis-dependent end-stage renal disease (ESRD): No dosage adjustment necessary.

Dosage adjustment in hepatic impairment:

Mild or moderate impairment (Child-Pugh class A or B): No dosage adjustment necessary.

Severe impairment (Child-Pugh class C): Has not been evaluated; use with caution.

Administration 150 mg: Infuse over 20-30 minutes ~30 minutes prior to chemotherapy

Dosage Forms

Solution Reconstituted, Intravenous:

Emend: 150 mg (1 ea)

◆ **Fosaprepitant Dimeglumine** *see* Fosaprepitant *on page 929*

◆ **Fosavance (Can)** *see* Alendronate and Cholecalciferol *on page 81*

Foscarnet (fos KAR net)

Brand Names: U.S. Foscavir

Brand Names: Canada Foscavir®

Index Terms PFA; Phosphonoformate; Phosphonoformic Acid

Pharmacologic Category Antiviral Agent

Use Treatment of acyclovir-resistant mucocutaneous herpes simplex virus (HSV) infections in immunocompromised persons (eg, with advanced AIDS); treatment of CMV retinitis in persons with AIDS.

Pregnancy Risk Factor C

Dosage

CMV retinitis: Adults: IV:

Induction treatment: 60 mg/kg/dose every 8 hours **or** 90 mg/kg every 12 hours for 14 to 21 days

Maintenance therapy: 90 to 120 mg/kg/day as a single daily infusion

Herpes simplex infections (acyclovir-resistant): Adults: Induction: IV: 40 mg/kg/dose every 8 to 12 hours for 14 to 21 days

Therapy of CMV infection in cancer patients (off-label use): Adults: IV:

Prophylaxis: 60 mg/kg every 8 to 12 hours for 7 days, followed by 90 to 120 mg/kg daily until day 100 after HSCT

Pre-emptive treatment: 60 mg/kg every 12 hours for 14 days; if CMV still detectable, continue with 90 mg/kg daily for 5 days/week for 2 additional weeks

Treatment: 90 mg/kg every 12 hours for 2 weeks, followed by 120 mg/kg daily for ≥2 weeks

Dosage adjustment in renal impairment: Induction and maintenance dosing schedules based on creatinine clearance (mL/minute/kg): See tables.

Induction Dosing of Foscarnet in Patients With Abnormal Renal Function

CrCl (mL/min/kg)	HSV Equivalent to 40 mg/kg every 12 hours	HSV Equivalent to 40 mg/kg every 8 hours	CMV Equivalent to 60 mg/kg every 8 hours	CMV Equivalent to 90 mg/kg every 12 hours
<0.4	Not recommended	Not recommended	Not recommended	Not recommended
≥0.4-0.5	20 mg/kg every 24 hours	35 mg/kg every 24 hours	50 mg/kg every 24 hours	50 mg/kg every 24 hours
>0.5-0.6	25 mg/kg every 24 hours	40 mg/kg every 24 hours	60 mg/kg every 24 hours	60 mg/kg every 24 hours
>0.6-0.8	35 mg/kg every 24 hours	25 mg/kg every 12 hours	40 mg/kg every 12 hours	80 mg/kg every 24 hours
>0.8-1	20 mg/kg every 12 hours	35 mg/kg every 12 hours	50 mg/kg every 12 hours	50 mg/kg every 12 hours
>1-1.4	30 mg/kg every 12 hours	30 mg/kg every 8 hours	45 mg/kg every 8 hours	70 mg/kg every 12 hours
>1.4	40 mg/kg every 12 hours	40 mg/kg every 8 hours	60 mg/kg every 8 hours	90 mg/kg every 12 hours

Maintenance Dosing of Foscarnet in Patients With Abnormal Renal Function

CrCl (mL/min/kg)	CMV Equivalent to 90 mg/kg every 24 hours	CMV Equivalent to 120 mg/kg every 24 hours
<0.4	Not recommended	Not recommended
≥0.4-0.5	50 mg/kg every 48 hours	65 mg/kg every 48 hours
>0.5-0.6	60 mg/kg every 48 hours	80 mg/kg every 48 hours
>0.6-0.8	80 mg/kg every 48 hours	105 mg/kg every 48 hours
>0.8-1	50 mg/kg every 24 hours	65 mg/kg every 24 hours
>1-1.4	70 mg/kg every 24 hours	90 mg/kg every 24 hours
>1.4	90 mg/kg every 24 hours	120 mg/kg every 24 hours

Hemodialysis:

Foscarnet is highly removed by hemodialysis (up to ~38% in 2.5 hours HD with high-flux membrane)

Doses of 50 mg/kg/dose posthemodialysis have been found to produce similar serum concentrations as doses of 90 mg/kg twice daily in patients with normal renal function

Doses of 60-90 mg/kg/dose loading dose (posthemodialysis) followed by 45-60 mg/kg/dose posthemodialysis (3 times/week) with the monitoring of weekly plasma concentrations to maintain peak plasma concentrations in the range of 400-800 µMolar have been recommended by some clinicians

Continuous arteriovenous or venovenous hemodiafiltration effects: Dose as for CrCl 10-50 mL/minute

Dosage adjustment in hepatic impairment: There are no dosage adjustments provided in the manufacturer's labeling.

Additional Information Complete prescribing information should be consulted for additional detail.

Dosage Forms

Solution, Intravenous:

Foscavir: 24 mg/mL (250 mL)

Generic: 24 mg/mL (500 mL)

◆ **Foscavir** *see* Foscarnet *on page 931*

◆ **Foscavir® (Can)** *see* Foscarnet *on page 931*

Fosfomycin (fos foe MYE sin)

Brand Names: U.S. Monurol

Brand Names: Canada Monurol®

Index Terms Fosfomycin Tromethamine

Pharmacologic Category Antibiotic, Miscellaneous

Use Single oral dose in the treatment of uncomplicated urinary tract infections in women due to susceptible strains of *E. coli* and *Enterococcus faecalis*

Pregnancy Risk Factor B

Dosage Adults: Oral:

Females: Uncomplicated UTI: Single dose of 3 g in 3-4 oz (90-120 mL) of water

Males:

Complicated UTI (off-label): 3 g every 2-3 days for 3 doses

Prostatitis (off-label): 3 g every 3 days for a total of 21 days (Shrestha, 2000)

Dosage adjustment in renal impairment: No dosage adjustment provided in manufacturer's labeling.

Dosage adjustment in hepatic impairment: No dosage adjustment provided in manufacturer's labeling.

Additional Information Complete prescribing information should be consulted for additional detail.

Dosage Forms

Packet, Oral:

Monurol: 3 g (1 ea)

◆ **Fosfomycin Tromethamine** *see* Fosfomycin *on page 932*

Fosinopril (foe SIN oh pril)

Brand Names: Canada Apo-Fosinopril; Ava-Fosinopril; Jamp-Fosinopril; Mylan-Fosinopril; PMS-Fosinopril; RAN-Fosinopril; Riva-Fosinopril; Teva-Fosinopril

Index Terms Fosinopril Sodium; Monopril

Pharmacologic Category Angiotensin-Converting Enzyme (ACE) Inhibitor; Antihypertensive

Use

Hypertension: Treatment of hypertension, either alone or in combination with other antihypertensive agents

The 2014 guideline for the management of high blood pressure in adults (Eighth Joint National Committee [JNC 8]) recommends initiation of pharmacologic treatment to lower blood pressure for the following patients:

- Patients ≥60 years of age with systolic blood pressure (SBP) ≥150 mm Hg or diastolic blood pressure (DBP) ≥90 mm Hg. Goal of therapy is SBP <150 mm Hg and DBP <90 mm Hg.
- Patients <60 years of age with SBP ≥140 mm Hg or DBP is ≥90 mm Hg. Goal of therapy is SBP <140 mm Hg and DBP <90 mm Hg.
- Patients ≥18 years of age with diabetes and SBP ≥140 mm Hg or DBP ≥90 mm Hg. Goal of therapy is SBP <140 mm Hg and DBP <90 mm Hg.
- Patients ≥18 years of age with chronic kidney disease (CKD) and SBP ≥140 mm Hg or DBP ≥90 mm Hg. Goal of therapy is SBP <140 mm Hg and DBP <90 mm Hg.

In patients with CKD, regardless of race or diabetes status, the use of an ACE inhibitor (ACEI) or angiotensin receptor blocker (ARB) as initial therapy is recommended to improve kidney outcomes. In the general nonblack population (without CKD) including those with diabetes, initial antihypertensive treatment should consist of a thiazide-type diuretic, calcium channel blocker, ACEI, or ARB. In the general black population (without CKD) including those with diabetes, initial antihypertensive treatment should consist of a thiazide-type diuretic or a calcium channel blocker **instead of** an ACEI or ARB.

Heart failure: Adjunctive treatment of heart failure (HF)

The ACCF/AHA 2013 heart failure guidelines recommend the use of ACE inhibitors, along with other guideline directed medical therapies, to prevent heart failure in patients with a reduced ejection fraction who have a history of MI (Stage B HF), to prevent HF in any patient with a reduced ejection fraction (Stage B HF), or to treat those with HF and reduced ejection fraction (Stage C HFrEF) (ACCF/AHA [Yancy, 2013]).

Pregnancy Risk Factor D

Pregnancy Considerations **[U.S. Boxed Warning]: Drugs that act on the renin-angiotensin system can cause injuy and death to the developing fetus. Discontinue as soon as possible once pregnancy is detected.** Drugs that act on the renin-angiotensin system are associated with oligohydramnios. Oligohydramnios, due to decreased fetal renal function, may lead to fetal lung hypoplasia and skeletal malformations. Their use in pregnancy is also associated with anuria, hypotension, renal failure, skull hypoplasia, and death in the fetus/neonate. The exposed fetus should be monitored for fetal growth, amniotic fluid volume, and organ formation. Infants exposed *in utero* should be monitored for hyperkalemia, hypotension, and oliguria (exchange transfusions or dialysis may be needed). These adverse events are generally associated with maternal use in the second and third trimesters.

Untreated chronic maternal hypertension is associated with adverse events in the fetus, infant, and mother. The of use angiotensin-converting enzyme inhibitors is not recommended to treat chronic uncomplicated hypertension or heart failure in pregnant women and should generally be avoided in women of reproductive potential (ACOG, 2013; Yancy, 2013).

Breast-Feeding Considerations Fosinoprilat is excreted in breast milk. Breast-feeding is not recommended by the manufacturer.

Contraindications Hypersensitivity to fosinopril, any other ACE inhibitor, or any component of the formulation; angioedema related to previous treatment with an ACE inhibitor; concomitant use with aliskiren in patients with diabetes mellitus

Warnings/Precautions Anaphylactic reactions may occur rarely with ACE inhibitors. At any time during treatment (especially following first dose), angioedema may occur rarely with ACE inhibitors; it may involve the head and neck (potentially compromising airway) or the intestine (presenting with abdominal pain). African-Americans may be at an increased risk and patients with idiopathic or hereditary angioedema may be at an increased risk. Prolonged frequent monitoring may be required especially if tongue, glottis, or larynx are involved as they are associated with airway obstruction. Patients with a history of airway surgery may have a higher risk of airway obstruction. Aggressive early and appropriate management is critical. Use in patients with previous angioedema associated with ACE inhibitor therapy is contraindicated. Severe anaphylactoid reactions may be seen during hemodialysis (eg, CVVHD) with high-flux dialysis membranes (eg, AN69), and rarely, during low density lipoprotein apheresis with dextran sulfate cellulose. Rare cases of anaphylactoid reactions have been reported in patients undergoing sensitization treatment with hymenoptera (bee, wasp) venom while receiving ACE inhibitors.

Symptomatic hypotension with or without syncope can occur with ACE inhibitors (usually with the first several doses); effects are most often observed in volume-depleted patients; correct volume depletion prior to initiation; close monitoring of patient is required especially with initial dosing and dosing increases; blood pressure must be lowered at a rate appropriate for the patient's clinical condition. Initiation of therapy in patients with ischemic heart disease or cerebrovascular disease warrants close observation due to the potential consequences posed by falling blood pressure (eg, MI, stroke). Use with caution in hypertrophic cardiomyopathy with outflow tract obstruction, severe aortic stenosis, or before, during, or immediately after major surgery. **[U.S. Boxed Warning]: Drugs that act on the renin-angiotensin system can cause injury and death to the developing fetus. Discontinue as soon as possible once pregnancy is detected.**

Hyperkalemia may occur with ACE inhibitors; risk factors include renal dysfunction, diabetes mellitus, concomitant use of potassium-sparing diuretics, potassium supplements, and/or potassium-containing salts. Use cautiously, if at all, with these agents and monitor potassium closely. Cough may occur with ACE inhibitors. Other causes of cough should be considered (eg, pulmonary congestion in patients with heart failure) and excluded prior to discontinuation. Use with caution in hepatic impairment; fosinopril undergoes hepatic and gut wall metabolism to its active form (fosinoprilat) and may accumulate in hepatic impairment. In patients with alcoholic or biliary cirrhosis, the rate of fosinoprilat formation was slowed, its total body clearance decreased and its AUC ~doubled.

May be associated with deterioration of renal function and/or increases in serum creatinine, particularly in patients with low renal blood flow (eg, renal artery stenosis, heart failure) whose glomerular filtration rate (GFR) is dependent on efferent arteriolar vasoconstriction by angiotensin II; deterioration may result in oliguria, acute renal failure, and progressive azotemia. Small increases in serum creatinine may occur following initiation; consider discontinuation only in patients with progressive and/or significant deterioration in renal function. Use with caution in patients with unstented unilateral/bilateral renal artery stenosis. When unstented bilateral renal artery stenosis is present, use is generally avoided due to the elevated risk of deterioration in renal function unless possible benefits outweigh risks. Potentially significant drug-drug interactions may exist, requiring dose or frequency adjustment, additional monitoring, and/or selection of alternative therapy.

Rare toxicities associated with ACE inhibitors include cholestatic jaundice (which may progress to fulminant hepatic necrosis), agranulocytosis, neutropenia or leukopenia with myeloid hypoplasia. Patients with collagen vascular diseases (especially with concomitant renal impairment) or renal impairment alone may be at increased risk for hematologic toxicity; periodically monitor CBC with differential in these patients.

Adverse Reactions Higher rates of adverse reactions have generally been noted in patients with CHF. However, the frequency of adverse effects associated with placebo is also increased in this population.

Cardiovascular: Orthostatic hypotension, palpitation
Central nervous system: Dizziness, fatigue, headache
Endocrine & metabolic: Hyperkalemia
Gastrointestinal: Diarrhea, nausea, vomiting
Hepatic: Transaminases increased
Neuromuscular & skeletal: Musculoskeletal pain, noncardiac chest pain, weakness
Renal: Renal function worsening (in patients with bilateral renal artery stenosis or hypovolemia), serum creatinine increased
Respiratory: Cough
Miscellaneous: Upper respiratory infection
Rare but important or life-threatening: Anaphylactoid reaction, angina, angioedema, arthralgia, bronchospasm, cerebral infarction, cerebrovascular accident, gout, hepatitis, hepatomegaly, myalgia, MI, pancreatitis, paresthesia, photosensitivity, pleuritic chest pain, pruritus, rash, renal insufficiency, shock, sudden death, syncope, TIA, tinnitus, urticaria, vertigo. In a small number of patients, a symptom complex of cough, bronchospasm, and eosinophilia has been observed with fosinopril.
Other events reported with ACE inhibitors: Acute renal failure, agranulocytosis, anemia, aplastic anemia, bullous pemphigus, cardiac arrest, eosinophilic pneumonitis, exfoliative dermatitis, gynecomastia, hemolytic anemia, hepatic failure, jaundice, neutropenia, pancytopenia, Stevens-Johnson syndrome, symptomatic hyponatremia, thrombocytopenia. In addition, a syndrome which may include arthralgia, elevated ESR, eosinophilia and positive ANA, fever, interstitial nephritis, myalgia, rash, and vasculitis has been reported for other ACE inhibitors.

Drug Interactions

Metabolism/Transport Effects None known.

Avoid Concomitant Use There are no known interactions where it is recommended to avoid concomitant use.

Increased Effect/Toxicity

Fosinopril may increase the levels/effects of: Allopurinol; Amifostine; Antihypertensives; AzaTHIOprine; DULoxetine; Ferric Gluconate; Gold Sodium Thiomalate; Grass Pollen Allergen Extract (5 Grass Extract); Hypotensive Agents; Iron Dextran Complex; Levodopa; Lithium; Nonsteroidal Anti-Inflammatory Agents; Obinutuzumab; RisperiDONE; RiTUXimab; Sodium Phosphates

The levels/effects of Fosinopril may be increased by: Alfuzosin; Aliskiren; Angiotensin II Receptor Blockers; Barbiturates; Brimonidine (Topical); Canagliflozin; Dapoxetine; Diazoxide; DPP-IV Inhibitors; Eplerenone; Everolimus; Heparin; Heparin (Low Molecular Weight); Herbs (Hypotensive Properties); Loop Diuretics; MAO Inhibitors; Nicorandil; Pentoxifylline; Phosphodiesterase 5 Inhibitors; Potassium Salts; Potassium-Sparing Diuretics; Prostacyclin Analogues; Sirolimus; Temsirolimus; Thiazide Diuretics; TiZANidine; Tolvaptan; Trimethoprim

Decreased Effect

The levels/effects of Fosinopril may be decreased by: Antacids; Aprotinin; Herbs (Hypertensive Properties); Icatibant; Lanthanum; Methylphenidate; Nonsteroidal Anti-Inflammatory Agents; Salicylates; Yohimbine

Storage/Stability Store at 25°C (77°F); excursions permitted to 15°C to 30°C (59°F to 86°F). Protect from moisture.

Mechanism of Action Competitive inhibitor of angiotensin-converting enzyme (ACE); prevents conversion of angiotensin I to angiotensin II, a potent vasoconstrictor; results in lower levels of angiotensin II which causes an increase in plasma renin activity and a reduction in aldosterone secretion; a CNS mechanism may also be involved in hypotensive effect as angiotensin II increases adrenergic outflow from CNS; vasoactive kallikreins may be decreased in conversion to active hormones by ACE inhibitors, thus reducing blood pressure

Pharmacodynamics/Kinetics

Onset of action: 1 hour
Duration: 24 hours
Absorption: 36%
Protein binding: >99%
Metabolism: Prodrug, hydrolyzed to its active metabolite fosinoprilat by intestinal wall and hepatic esterases
Bioavailability: 36%
Half-life elimination, serum (fosinoprilat): 12 hours
Time to peak, serum: ~3 hours
Excretion: Urine and feces (as fosinoprilat and other metabolites in roughly equal proportions)

Dosage Oral:

Children ≥6 years and Adolescents >50 kg: Hypertension: Initial: 5 to 10 mg once daily (maximum: 40 mg once daily)

Adults:

Heart failure: Per the manufacturer: Initial: 10 mg once daily (5 mg once daily if moderate to severe renal dysfunction is present or if aggressively diuresed);

increase dose as needed and as tolerated over several weeks. Usual dosage range: 20 to 40 mg once daily (maximum dose: 40 mg once daily) If hypotension, orthostasis, or azotemia occur during titration, consider decreasing concomitant diuretic dose, if any.

ACCF/AHA 2013 heart failure guidelines: Initial: 5 to 10 mg once daily. Target dose: 40 mg once daily (Yancy, 2013).

Hypertension: Initial: 10 mg once daily; maximum dose: 80 mg once daily. May need to divide the dose into two if trough effect is inadequate. If patient is receiving a diuretic prior to initiation, consider discontinuation of the diuretic to reduce likelihood of hypotension, if possible 2 to 3 days before initiation of therapy. If blood pressure response is inadequate, resume diuretic therapy carefully. Usual dose range (ASH/ISH [Weber, 2014]): 10 to 40 mg daily.

Dosage adjustment in renal impairment:

Moderate to severe impairment: Initial dose reduction to 5 mg once daily recommended for heart failure patients. No other dose adjustments are required; hepatobiliary elimination partially compensates for diminished renal elimination.

Hemodialysis: Poorly dialyzed; supplemental dose not required (Gehr, 1993)

Peritoneal dialysis: Poorly dialyzed; supplemental dose not required (Gehr, 1991).

Dosage adjustment in hepatic impairment: No dosage adjustment provided in manufacturer's labeling.

Dietary Considerations Should not take a potassium salt supplement without the advice of healthcare provider.

Monitoring Parameters Blood pressure; BUN, serum creatinine and potassium; if patient has collagen vascular disease and/or renal impairment, periodically monitor CBC with differential

2013 ACCF/AHA Heart Failure guideline recommendations: Within 1 to 2 weeks after initiation and periodically thereafter, reassess renal function and serum potassium especially in patients with preexisting hypotension, hyponatremia, diabetes mellitus, azotemia, or those taking potassium supplements (ACCF/AHA [Yancy, 2013]).

Dosage Forms

Tablet, Oral:

Generic: 10 mg, 20 mg, 40 mg

◆ **Fosinopril Sodium** *see* Fosinopril *on page 932*

Fosphenytoin (FOS fen i toyn)

Brand Names: U.S. Cerebyx

Brand Names: Canada Cerebyx

Index Terms Cerebyx; Fosphenytoin Sodium

Pharmacologic Category Anticonvulsant, Hydantoin

Use Used for the control of generalized convulsive status epilepticus and prevention and treatment of seizures occurring during neurosurgery; indicated for short-term parenteral administration when other means of phenytoin administration are unavailable, inappropriate, or deemed less advantageous (the safety and effectiveness of fosphenytoin use for more than 5 days has not been systematically evaluated)

Pregnancy Risk Factor D

Pregnancy Considerations Fosphenytoin is the prodrug of phenytoin. Refer to Phenytoin on page 1640 for additional information.

Breast-Feeding Considerations Fosphenytoin is the prodrug of phenytoin. It is not known if fosphenytoin is excreted in breast milk prior to conversion to phenytoin. Refer to Phenytoin monograph for additional information.

Contraindications Hypersensitivity to phenytoin, other hydantoins, or any component of the formulation; patients with sinus bradycardia, sinoatrial block, second- and third-degree AV block, or Adams-Stokes syndrome; occurrence of rash during treatment (should not be resumed if rash is exfoliative, purpuric, or bullous); treatment of absence seizures; concurrent use of delavirdine (due to loss of virologic response and possible resistance to delavirdine or other non-nucleoside reverse transcriptase inhibitors [NNRTIs])

Warnings/Precautions Hazardous agent - use appropriate precautions for handling and disposal (NIOSH 2014 [group 2]).

[U.S. Boxed Warning]: Fosphenytoin administration should not exceed 150 mg phenytoin equivalents (PE)/minute in adult patients. Hypotension and severe cardiac arrhythmias (eg, heart block, ventricular tachycardia, ventricular fibrillation) may occur with rapid administration; adverse cardiac events have been reported at or below the recommended infusion rate. In the treatment of status epilepticus, the rate of administration is 150 mg PE/minute. In a nonemergent situation, administer more slowly or use oral phenytoin. Cardiac monitoring is necessary during and after administration of intravenous fosphenytoin; reduction in rate of administration or discontinuation of infusion may be necessary.

Doses of fosphenytoin are always expressed as their phenytoin sodium equivalent (PE). 1 mg PE is equivalent to 1 mg phenytoin sodium. Do not change the recommended doses when substituting fosphenytoin for phenytoin or vice versa as they are not equivalent on a mg to mg basis. Dosing errors have also occurred due to misinterpretation of vial concentrations resulting in two- or tenfold overdoses (some fatal); ensure correct volume of fosphenytoin is withdrawn from vial. Severe burning or itching, and/or paresthesias, mostly perineal, may occur upon administration, usually at the maximum administration rate and last from minutes to hours; occurrence and intensity may be lessened by slowing or temporarily stopping the infusion. Antiepileptic drugs should not be abruptly discontinued. Acute hepatotoxicity associated with a hypersensitivity syndrome characterized by fever, skin eruptions, and lymphadenopathy has been reported to occur within the first 2 months of treatment. Discontinue if skin rash or lymphadenopathy occurs. A spectrum of hematologic effects have been reported with use (eg, neutropenia, leukopenia, thrombocytopenia, pancytopenia, and anemias). Use with caution in patients with hypotension, severe myocardial insufficiency, diabetes mellitus, porphyria, hypoalbuminemia, hypothyroidism, fever, or hepatic dysfunction. Use with caution in patients with renal impairment; also consider the phosphate load of fosphenytoin (0.0037 mmol phosphate/mg PE fosphenytoin). Effects with other sedative drugs or ethanol may be potentiated. Severe reactions, including toxic epidermal necrolysis (TEN) and Stevens-Johnson syndromes, although rarely reported, have resulted in fatalities; drug should be discontinued if there are any signs of rash and patient should be evaluated for signs and symptoms of drug reaction with eosinophilia and systemic symptoms (DRESS). Patients of Asian descent with the variant *HLA-B*1502* may be at an increased risk of developing Stevens-Johnson syndrome and/or TEN.

The "purple glove syndrome" (ie, discoloration with edema and pain of distal limb) may occur following peripheral IV administration of fosphenytoin. This syndrome may or may not be associated with drug extravasation. Symptoms may resolve spontaneously; however, skin necrosis and limb ischemia may occur. In general, fosphenytoin has significantly less venous irritation and phlebitis compared with an equimolar dose of phenytoin (Jamerson, 1994). Sedation, confusional states, or cerebellar dysfunction (loss of motor coordination) may occur at higher total serum concentrations or at lower total serum concentrations when the free fraction of phenytoin is increased.

Adverse Reactions The more important adverse clinical events caused by the IV use of fosphenytoin or phenytoin are cardiovascular collapse and/or central nervous system depression. Hypotension can occur when either drug is administered rapidly by the IV route.

The adverse clinical events most commonly observed with the use of fosphenytoin in clinical trials were nystagmus, dizziness, pruritus, paresthesia, headache, somnolence, and ataxia. Paresthesia and pruritus were seen more often following fosphenytoin (versus phenytoin) administration and occurred more often with IV fosphenytoin than with IM administration. These events were dose and rate related (adult doses ≥15 mg/kg at a rate of 150 mg PE/minute). These sensations, generally described as itching, burning, or tingling are usually not at the infusion site. The location of the discomfort varied with the groin mentioned most frequently. The paresthesia and pruritus were transient events that occurred within several minutes of the start of infusion and generally resolved within 10 minutes after completion of infusion.

Transient pruritus, tinnitus, nystagmus, somnolence, and ataxia occurred 2-3 times more often at adult doses ≥15 mg/kg and rates ≥150 mg PE/minute.

IV and IM administration (as reported in clinical trials):

Cardiovascular: Facial edema, hypertension

Central nervous system: Chills, fever, intracranial hypertension, nervousness

Endocrine & metabolic: Hypokalemia

Neuromuscular & skeletal: Hyperreflexia, myasthenia

IV administration (maximum dose/rate):

Central nervous system: Ataxia, dizziness, nystagmus, somnolence

Dermatologic: Pruritus

Cardiovascular: Hypotension, tachycardia, vasodilation

Central nervous system: Agitation, brain edema, dysarthria, extrapyramidal syndrome, headache, hypoesthesia, incoordination, paresthesia, stupor, tremor, vertigo

Gastrointestinal: Dry mouth, nausea, tongue disorder, vomiting

Neuromuscular & skeletal: Back pain, muscle weakness, pelvic pain

Ocular: Amblyopia, diplopia

Otic: Deafness, tinnitus

Miscellaneous: Taste perversion

IM administration (substitute for oral phenytoin):

Central nervous system: Ataxia, dizziness, headache, incoordination, nystagmus, paresthesia, reflexes decreased, somnolence, tremor

Dermatologic: Pruritus

Gastrointestinal: Nausea, vomiting

Hematologic/lymphatic: Ecchymosis

Neuromuscular & skeletal: Muscle weakness

IV and IM administration: Rare but important or life-threatening: Acidosis, acute hepatic failure, acute hepatotoxicity, alkalosis, akathisia, amnesia, anemia, anorexia, aphasia, apnea, arthralgia, asthma, atrial flutter, Babinski sign positive, bundle branch block, cachexia, cardiac arrest, cardiomegaly, cerebral hemorrhage, cerebral infarct, CHF, circumoral paresthesia, CNS depression, cyanosis, dehydration, diabetes insipidus, dyskinesia, dysphagia, dyspnea, edema, emotional lability, encephalopathy, epistaxis, extrapyramidal symptoms, GI hemorrhage, hemiplegia, hemoptysis, hostility, hyperacusis, hyperesthesia, hyper-/hypokinesia, hyperkalemia, hyperventilation, hypochromic anemia, hypophosphatemia, hypotonia, hypoxia, ileus, injection site (edema, hemorrhage, inflammation), ketosis, leg cramps, leukocytosis, leukopenia, LFTs abnormal, malaise, migraine, myalgia, mydriasis, myopathy, neurosis, orthostatic hypotension, palpitation, paralysis, parosmia, petechia, photophobia, photosensitivity reaction, psychosis, pulmonary embolus, QT interval prolongation, rash (maculopapular or pustular), renal failure, sinus bradycardia, shock, subdural hematoma, syncope, Stevens-Johnson syndrome, tenesmus, thrombocytopenia, thrombophlebitis, tongue edema, toxic epidermal necrolysis, urticaria, ventricular extrasystoles, visual field defect

Drug Interactions

Metabolism/Transport Effects Substrate of CYP2C19 (major), CYP2C9 (major), CYP3A4 (minor); **Note:** Assignment of Major/Minor substrate status based on clinically relevant drug interaction potential; **Induces** CYP2B6 (strong), CYP2C19 (strong), CYP2C8 (strong), CYP2C9 (strong), CYP3A4 (strong), P-glycoprotein

Avoid Concomitant Use

Avoid concomitant use of Fosphenytoin with any of the following: Abiraterone Acetate; Apixaban; Apremilast; Artemether; Axitinib; Azelastine (Nasal); Bedaquiline; Boceprevir; Bortezomib; Bosutinib; Cabozantinib; Ceritinib; CloZAPine; Crizotinib; Dabigatran Etexilate; Darunavir; Dasabuvir; Delavirdine; Dienogest; Dolutegravir; Dronedarone; Eliglustat; Enzalutamide; Etravirine; Everolimus; Ibrutinib; Idelalisib; Irinotecan; Itraconazole; Ivacaftor; Lapatinib; Ledipasvir; Lumefantrine; Lurasidone; Macitentan; Mifepristone; Naloxegol; Netupitant; NIFEdipine; Nilotinib; Nintedanib; Nisoldipine; Olaparib; Ombitasvir; Orphenadrine; Paraldehyde; Paritaprevir; PAZOPanib; PONATinib; Praziquantel; Ranolazine; Regorafenib; Rilpivirine; Rivaroxaban; Roflumilast; RomiDEPsin; Simeprevir; Sofosbuvir; SORAfenib; Suvorexant; Tasimelteon; Telaprevir; Thalidomide; Ticagrelor; Tofacitinib; Tolvaptan; Toremifene; Trabectedin; Ulipristal; Vandetanib; Vemurafenib; VinCRIStine (Liposomal); Vorapaxar

Increased Effect/Toxicity

Fosphenytoin may increase the levels/effects of: Amiodarone; Azelastine (Nasal); Buprenorphine; Ciprofloxacin (Systemic); Clarithromycin; CNS Depressants; FLUoxetine; Fosamprenavir; Highest Risk QTc-Prolonging Agents; Hydrocodone; Lithium; Methotrexate; Methotrimeprazine; Metyrosine; Moderate Risk QTc-Prolonging Agents; Neuromuscular-Blocking Agents (Nondepolarizing); Orphenadrine; Paraldehyde; PHENobarbital; Pramipexole; QuiNIDine; ROPINIRole; Rotigotine; Selective Serotonin Reuptake Inhibitors; Thalidomide; Vitamin K Antagonists; Zolpidem

The levels/effects of Fosphenytoin may be increased by: Alcohol (Ethyl); Amiodarone; Antifungal Agents (Azole Derivatives, Systemic); Benzodiazepines; Brimonidine (Topical); Calcium Channel Blockers; Cannabis; Capecitabine; CarBAMazepine; Carbonic Anhydrase Inhibitors; CeFAZolin; Cimetidine; Clarithromycin; CYP2C19 Inhibitors (Moderate); CYP2C19 Inhibitors (Strong); CYP2C9 Inhibitors (Moderate); CYP2C9 Inhibitors (Strong); Delavirdine; Dexketoprofen; Dexmethylphenidate; Disopyramide; Disulfiram; Doxylamine; Dronabinol; Droperidol; Efavirenz; Eslicarbazepine; Ethosuximide; Felbamate; Floxuridine; Fluconazole; Fluorouracil (Systemic); Fluorouracil (Topical); FLUoxetine; FluvoxaMINE; Halothane; HydrOXYzine; Isoniazid; Kava Kava; Luliconazole; Magnesium Sulfate; Methotrimeprazine; Methylphenidate; MetroNIDAZOLE (Systemic); Miconazole (Oral); Nabilone; Omeprazole; OXcarbazepine; Rufinamide; Sertraline; Sodium Oxybate; Tacrolimus (Systemic); Tapentadol; Tegafur; Telaprevir; Tetrahydrocannabinol; Ticlopidine; Topiramate; TraZODone; Trimethoprim; Vitamin K Antagonists

Decreased Effect

Fosphenytoin may decrease the levels/effects of: Abiraterone Acetate; Acetaminophen; Afatinib; Amiodarone; Antifungal Agents (Azole Derivatives, Systemic); Apixaban; Apremilast; ARIPiprazole; Artemether; Axitinib; Bazedoxifene; Bedaquiline; Boceprevir; Bortezomib; Bosutinib; Brentuximab Vedotin; Busulfan; Cabozantinib; Canagliflozin; Cannabidiol; Cannabis; CarBAMazepine; Ceritinib; Clarithromycin; CloZAPine; Cobicistat; Contraceptives (Estrogens); Contraceptives (Progestins); Crizotinib; CycloSPORINE (Systemic); CYP2B6 Substrates; CYP2C19 Substrates; CYP2C8 Substrates; CYP2C9 Substrates; CYP3A4 Substrates; Dabigatran Etexilate; Darunavir; Dasabuvir; Dasatinib; Deferasirox; Delavirdine; Diclofenac (Systemic); Dienogest; Disopyramide; Dolutegravir; DOXOrubicin (Conventional); Doxycycline; Dronabinol; Dronedarone; Efavirenz; Eliglustat; Elvitegravir; Enzalutamide; Erlotinib; Eslicarbazepine; Ethosuximide; Etoposide; Etoposide Phosphate; Etravirine; Everolimus; Exemestane; Felbamate; FentaNYL; Flunarizine; Gefitinib; GuanFACINE; HMG-CoA Reductase Inhibitors; Ibrutinib; Idelalisib; Imatinib; Irinotecan; Itraconazole; Ivacaftor; Ixabepilone; Lacosamide; LamoTRIgine; Lapatinib; Ledipasvir; Levodopa; Linagliptin; Loop Diuretics; Lopinavir; Lumefantrine; Lurasidone; Macitentan; Maraviroc; Mebendazole; Meperidine; Methadone; MethylPREDNISolone; MetroNIDAZOLE (Systemic); Metyrapone; Mexiletine; Mianserin; Mifepristone; Naloxegol; Nelfinavir; Netupitant; Neuromuscular-Blocking Agents (Nondepolarizing); NIFEdipine; Nilotinib; Nintedanib; Nisoldipine; Olaparib; Ombitasvir; Omeprazole; OXcarbazepine; Paritaprevir; PAZOPanib; Perampanel; P-glycoprotein/ABCB1 Substrates; PONATinib; Praziquantel; PrednisoLONE (Systemic); PredniSONE; Primidone; QUEtiapine; QuiNIDine; QuiNINE; Ranolazine; Regorafenib; Rilpivirine; Ritonavir; Rivaroxaban; Roflumilast; RomiDEPsin; Rufinamide; Saxagliptin; Sertraline; Simeprevir; Sirolimus; Sofosbuvir; SORAfenib; SUNItinib; Suvorexant; Tacrolimus (Systemic); Tadalafil; Tasimelteon; Telaprevir; Temsirolimus; Teniposide; Tetrahydrocannabinol; Theophylline Derivatives; Thyroid Products; Ticagrelor; Tipranavir; Tofacitinib; Tolvaptan; Topiramate; Topotecan; Toremifene; Trabectedin; TraZODone; Treprostinil; Trimethoprim; Ulipristal; Valproic Acid and Derivatives; Vandetanib; Vemurafenib; Vilazodone; VinCRIStine; VinCRIStine (Liposomal); Vorapaxar; Vortioxetine; Zonisamide

The levels/effects of Fosphenytoin may be decreased by: Alcohol (Ethyl); CarBAMazepine; Ciprofloxacin (Systemic); CYP2C19 Inducers (Strong); CYP2C9 Inducers (Strong); Dabrafenib; Diazoxide; Enzalutamide; Folic Acid; Fosamprenavir; Leucovorin Calcium-Levoleucovorin; Levomefolate; Lopinavir; Mefloquine; Methotrexate; Methylfolate; Mianserin; Multivitamins/Minerals (with ADEK, Folate, Iron); Nelfinavir; PHENobarbital; Platinum Derivatives; Pyridoxine; Rifampin; Ritonavir; Theophylline Derivatives; Tipranavir; Valproic Acid and Derivatives; Vigabatrin; VinCRIStine

Food Interactions

Acute use: Ethanol inhibits metabolism of phenytoin. Management: Monitor patients.

Chronic use: Ethanol stimulates metabolism of phenytoin. Management: Monitor patients.

Preparation for Administration Hazardous agent; use appropriate precautions for handling and disposal (NIOSH 2014 [group 2]).

Must be diluted to concentrations of 1.5-25 mg PE/mL, in normal saline or D_5W, for IV infusion.

Storage/Stability Refrigerate at 2°C to 8°C (36°F to 46°F). Do not store at room temperature for more than 48 hours. Do not use vials that develop particulate matter. Has been shown to be stable at 1, 8, and 20 mg PE/mL in normal saline or D_5W at 25°C (77°F) for 30 days in glass container and at 4°C to 20°C (39°F to 68°F) for 30 days in PVC bag. Undiluted fosphenytoin injection (50 mg PE/mL) is stable in polypropylene syringes for 30 days at 25°C, 4°C, or frozen at -20°C. Fosphenytoin at concentrations of 1, 8, and 20 mg PE/mL prepared in $D_5{}^1/_2$NS, $D_5{}^1/_2$NS with KCl 20 mEq/L, $D_5{}^1/_2$NS with 40 mEq/L, LR, D_5LR, D_{10}W, amino acid 10%, mannitol 20%, hetastarch 6% in NS or Plasma-Lyte® A injection is stable in polyvinyl chloride bags for 7 days when stored at 25°C (room temperature) (Fischer, 1997).

Mechanism of Action Diphosphate ester salt of phenytoin which acts as a water soluble prodrug of phenytoin; after administration, plasma esterases convert fosphenytoin to phosphate, formaldehyde, and phenytoin as the active moiety; phenytoin works by stabilizing neuronal membranes and decreasing seizure activity by increasing efflux or decreasing influx of sodium ions across cell membranes in the motor cortex during generation of nerve impulses

Pharmacodynamics/Kinetics Also refer to Phenytoin monograph for additional information.

Distribution: Fosphenytoin: V_d: 4.3-10.8 L

Protein binding: Fosphenytoin: 95% to 99% to albumin; can displace phenytoin and increase free fraction (up to 30% unbound) during the period required for conversion of fosphenytoin to phenytoin. **Note:** In patients with renal and/or hepatic impairment or hypoalbuminemia, the fraction of unbound phenytoin may be increased.

Metabolism: Fosphenytoin is rapidly converted via hydrolysis to phenytoin; phenytoin is metabolized in the liver and forms metabolites

Bioavailability: IM: Fosphenytoin: 100%

Half-life elimination:

Fosphenytoin: Conversion half-life: 15 minutes

Phenytoin: Variable (mean: 12-29 hours); kinetics of phenytoin are saturable

Time to peak: Conversion to phenytoin: Following IV administration (maximum rate of administration): 15 minutes; following IM administration, peak phenytoin levels are reached in 3 hours; therapeutic phenytoin concentrations may be achieved as early as 5-20 minutes following IM (gluteal) administration (Pryor, 2001)

Excretion: Phenytoin: Urine (as inactive metabolites)

Dosage The dose, concentration in solutions, and infusion rates for fosphenytoin are expressed as phenytoin sodium equivalents (PE); fosphenytoin should always be prescribed and dispensed in phenytoin sodium equivalents (PE)

Infants and Children (off-label use): IV: **Note:** A limited number of clinical studies have been conducted in pediatric patients; based on pharmacokinetic studies, experts recommend the following (Fischer, 2003): Use the pediatric IV phenytoin dosing guidelines to dose fosphenytoin using doses in **PE** equal to the phenytoin doses (ie, phenytoin 1 mg = fosphenytoin 1 mg **PE**). Further pediatric studies are needed.

Adults:

Status epilepticus: IV: Loading dose: 15-20 mg PE/kg administered at 100-150 mg PE/minute

Nonemergent loading and maintenance dosing: IV or IM:

Loading dose: 10-20 mg PE/kg (IV rate: Infuse more slowly [eg, over 30 minutes]; maximum rate: 150 mg PE/minute)

Initial daily maintenance dose: 4-6 mg PE/kg/day in divided doses

IM or IV substitution for oral phenytoin therapy: May be substituted for oral phenytoin sodium at the same total daily dose; however, Dilantin® capsules are ~90% bioavailable by the oral route; phenytoin, supplied as fosphenytoin, is 100% bioavailable by both the IM and IV routes; for this reason, plasma phenytoin concentrations may increase when IM or IV fosphenytoin is substituted for oral phenytoin sodium therapy; in clinical trials, IM fosphenytoin was administered as a single daily dose utilizing either 1 or 2 injection sites; some patients may require more frequent dosing

Dosage adjustment in renal impairment: No initial dosage adjustment necessary. Free (unbound) phenytoin concentrations should be monitored closely in patients with renal disease or in those with hypoalbuminemia; furthermore, fosphenytoin clearance to phenytoin may be increased without a similar increase in phenytoin clearance in these patients leading to increase frequency and severity of adverse events.

Dosage adjustment in hepatic impairment: No initial dosage adjustment necessary. Phenytoin clearance may be substantially reduced in cirrhosis and plasma level monitoring with dose adjustment advisable. Free (unbound) phenytoin concentrations should be monitored closely in patients with hepatic disease or in those with hypoalbuminemia; furthermore, fosphenytoin clearance to phenytoin may be increased without a similar increase in phenytoin clearance in these patients leading to increased frequency and severity of adverse events.

Dietary Considerations Provides phosphate 0.0037 mmol/mg PE fosphenytoin

Administration

IM: May be administered as a single daily dose using 1-4 injection sites (up to 20 mL per site well tolerated in adults) (Meek, 1999; Pryor, 2001).

IV: Rates of infusion:

Children: 1-3 mg PE/kg/minute (**maximum rate: 150 mg PE/minute**) (Pellock, 1996)

Adults: **Do not exceed 150 mg PE/minute.** Slower administration reduces incidence of cardiovascular events (eg, hypotension, arrhythmia) as well as severity of paresthesias and pruritus. For nonemergent situations, may administer loading dose more slowly (eg, over 30 minutes [~33 mg PE/minute for 1000 mg PE] **or** 50-100 mg PE/minute [Fischer, 2003]). Highly-sensitive patients (eg, elderly, patients with preexisting cardiovascular conditions) should receive fosphenytoin more slowly (eg, 25-50 mg PE/minute) (Meek, 1999).

Hazardous agent; use appropriate precautions for handling and disposal (NIOSH 2014 [group 2]).

Monitoring Parameters Continuous blood pressure, ECG, and respiratory function monitoring with loading dose and for 10-20 minutes following infusion; vital signs, CBC, hepatic function tests, plasma phenytoin concentration monitoring (plasma concentrations should not be measured until conversion to phenytoin is complete, ~2 hours after an IV infusion or ~4 hours after an IM injection). **Note:** If available, free (unbound) phenytoin concentrations should be obtained in patients with renal impairment and/or hypoalbuminemia; if free phenytoin concentrations are unavailable, the adjusted total concentration may be determined based upon equations in adult patients. Trough concentrations are generally recommended for routine monitoring.

Consult individual institutional policies and procedures.

Reference Range

Therapeutic: 10-20 mcg/mL (SI: 40-79 micromole/L); toxicity is measured clinically, and some patients require levels outside the suggested therapeutic range

Toxic: >30 mcg/mL (SI: 120 micromole/L)

Lethal: >100 mcg/mL (SI: >400 micromole/L)

Manifestations of toxicity:

Nystagmus: 20 mcg/mL (SI: 79 micromole/L)

Ataxia: 30 mcg/mL (SI: 118.9 micromole/L)

Decreased mental status: 40 mcg/mL (SI: 159 micromole/L)

Coma: 50 mcg/mL (SI: 200 micromole/L)

Peak serum phenytoin level after a 375 mg IM fosphenytoin dose in healthy males: 5.7 mcg/mL

Peak serum fosphenytoin levels and phenytoin levels after a 1.2 g infusion (IV) in healthy subjects over 30 minutes were 129 mcg/mL and 17.2 mcg/mL, respectively

Additional Information 1.5 mg fosphenytoin is approximately equivalent to 1 mg phenytoin. Equimolar fosphenytoin dose is 375 mg (75 mg/mL solution) to phenytoin 250 mg (50 mg/mL). **However, doses of fosphenytoin are always expressed as their phenytoin sodium equivalent (PE). Thus, 1 mg PE is equivalent to 1 mg phenytoin sodium. Do not change the recommended doses when substituting fosphenytoin for phenytoin or vice versa as they are not equivalent on a mg to mg basis.**

Dosage Forms

Solution, Injection:

Cerebyx: 100 mg PE/2 mL (2 mL); 500 MG PE/10ML (2 mL, 10 mL); 500 mg PE/10 mL (10 mL)

Generic: 100 mg PE/2 mL (2 mL); 500 mg PE/10 mL (10 mL)

◆ **Fosphenytoin Sodium** *see* Fosphenytoin *on page 934*

◆ **Fosrenol** *see* Lanthanum *on page 1169*

Fotemustine [INT] (foe te MUS teen)

International Brand Names Muphoran (AT, AU, BE, BR, CN, FR, GR, IL, IT, PT, SI, TR); Mustoforan (ES); Mustophoran (BG, CZ, HU, PL, RO, RU, SK)

Pharmacologic Category Antineoplastic Agent; Antineoplastic Agent, Alkylating Agent (Nitrosourea)

Reported Use To treat malignant melanoma

Dosage Range Adults: IV: 100 mg/m²/week for 3 weeks, follow up 4-5 weeks after first dose (blood counts permitting): 100 mg/m² every 3 weeks

Product Availability Product available in various countries; not currently available in the U.S.

Dosage Forms

Injection, powder for reconstitution: 208 mg

◆ **Four-Factor PCC** *see* Prothrombin Complex Concentrate (Human) [(Factors II, VII, IX, X), Protein C, and Protein S] *on page 1738*

◆ **FR901228** *see* RomiDEPsin *on page 1841*

◆ **Fragmin** *see* Dalteparin *on page 553*

Framycetin [INT] (fra mye SEE tin)

International Brand Names Daryant-Tulle (ID); Fracitin (SG); Frade (IN); Framycin (PK); Isofra (RU); Leukase N (DE); Sofra-Tulle (IN, SA, TH, ZA); Soframycin (IN, ZA); Soframycin Ear/Eye Drops (AU, NZ); Soframycine (BE)

Index Terms Framycetin Sulfate; Framycetin Sulphate

Pharmacologic Category Antibiotic, Ophthalmic; Antibiotic, Otic

Reported Use Conjunctivitis, blepharitis, styes, corneal abrasions, and burns; prophylactically following foreign body removal from the eye; corneal ulcers; otitis externa

Dosage Range Adults:

Ophthalmic:

Drops: Initial: 1-2 drops into affected eye(s) every 1-2 hours for 2-3 days, decreasing to 2-3 drops 3 times/day

Ointment: 3 times/day into affected eye(s), or at bedtime, if drops are used during the day

Otic:

Drops: 2-3 drops or a saturated wick into external auditory meatus 3 times/day

Ointment: Apply 3 times/day

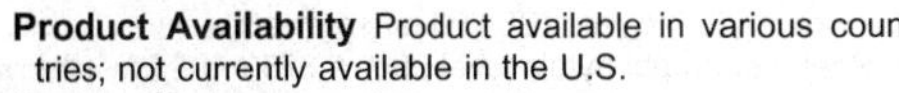

Product Availability Product available in various countries; not currently available in the U.S.

Dosage Forms

Ointment, ophthalmic/otic: 5 g

Solution, ophthalmic/otic drops: 8 mL

- ◆ **Framycetin Sulfate** *see* Framycetin [INT] *on page 937*
- ◆ **Framycetin Sulphate** *see* Framycetin [INT] *on page 937*
- ◆ **Fraxiparine (Can)** *see* Nadroparin [CAN/INT] *on page 1412*
- ◆ **Fraxiparine Forte (Can)** *see* Nadroparin [CAN/INT] *on page 1412*
- ◆ **Fresenius Propoven** *see* Propofol *on page 1728*
- ◆ **Frisium (Can)** *see* CloBAZam *on page 465*
- ◆ **Froben (Can)** *see* Flurbiprofen (Systemic) *on page 906*
- ◆ **Froben-SR (Can)** *see* Flurbiprofen (Systemic) *on page 906*
- ◆ **Frova** *see* Frovatriptan *on page 938*

Frovatriptan (froe va TRIP tan)

Brand Names: U.S. Frova

Brand Names: Canada Frova

Index Terms Frovatriptan Succinate

Pharmacologic Category Antimigraine Agent; Serotonin $5\text{-HT}_{1B,\ 1D}$ Receptor Agonist

Use Migraines: Acute treatment of migraine with or without aura in adults.

Pregnancy Risk Factor C

Pregnancy Considerations Adverse events were observed in animal reproduction studies. Information related to the use of frovatriptan in pregnancy has not been located. Until additional information is available, other agents are preferred for the initial treatment of migraine in pregnancy (Da Silva, 2012; MacGregor, 2012; Williams, 2012).

Breast-Feeding Considerations It is not known if frovatriptan is excreted in breast milk. Due to the potential for serious adverse reactions in the nursing infant, the manufacturer recommends a decision be made whether to discontinue nursing or to discontinue the drug, taking into account the importance of treatment to the mother.

Contraindications

Ischemic coronary artery disease (eg, angina pectoris, history of MI, documented silent ischemia); coronary artery vasospasm, including Prinzmetal's angina; Wolff-Parkinson-White syndrome or arrhythmias associated with other cardiac accessory conduction pathway disorders; history of stroke, transient ischemic attack, or history of hemiplegic or basilar migraine; peripheral vascular disease; ischemic bowel disease; uncontrolled hypertension; recent use (within 24 hours) of another 5-HT_1 agonist, an ergotamine containing or ergot-type medication (eg, dihydroergotamine, methysergide); hypersensitivity to frovatriptan or any component of the formulation.

Canadian labeling: Additional contraindications (not in U.S. labeling): Cardiac arrhythmias, valvular heart disease (especially tachycardia), congenital heart disease, atherosclerotic disease; management of ophthalmoplegic migraine; severe hepatic impairment; Raynaud's syndrome

Documentation of allergenic cross-reactivity for triptans is limited. However, because of similarities in chemical structure and/or pharmacologic actions, the possibility of cross-sensitivity cannot be ruled out with certainty.

Warnings/Precautions Not intended for migraine prophylaxis, or treatment of cluster headaches, hemiplegic or basilar migraines. Rule out underlying neurologic disease in patients with atypical headache, migraine (with no prior history of migraine) or inadequate clinical response to initial dosing. Cardiac events (coronary artery vasospasm, transient ischemia, MI, ventricular tachycardia/fibrillation, cardiac arrest, and death), cerebral/subarachnoid hemorrhage, stroke (some fatal), peripheral vascular ischemia, gastrointestinal vascular ischemia and infarction, splenic infarction, and Raynaud's syndrome have been reported with 5-HT_1 agonist administration. Partial vision loss and blindness (transient and permanent) have been reported with use of 5-HT_1 agonists; a causal relationship between these events and 5-HT_1 agonist administration has not been clearly determined. Patients who experience sensations of chest pain/pressure/tightness or symptoms suggestive of angina following dosing should be evaluated for coronary artery disease or Prinzmetal's angina before receiving additional doses; if dosing is resumed and similar symptoms recur, monitor with ECG. Do not give to patients with risk factors for CAD until a cardiovascular evaluation has been performed; if evaluation is satisfactory, the healthcare provider should administer the first dose (consider ECG monitoring) and cardiovascular status should be periodically evaluated. Significant elevation in blood pressure, including hypertensive crisis with acute impairment of organ systems, has been reported on rare occasions in patients using other 5-HT_{1D} agonists with and without a history of hypertension; monitor blood pressure. Blood pressure was increased to a greater extent in elderly.

Use with caution in severe hepatic impairment (has not been studied) (Canadian labeling contraindicates use in severe impairment). Potentially significant drug-drug interactions may exist, requiring dose or frequency adjustment, additional monitoring, and/or selection of alternative therapy. Symptoms of agitation, confusion, hallucinations, hyper-reflexia, myoclonus, shivering, and tachycardia (serotonin syndrome) may occur with concomitant proserotonergic drugs (ie, SSRIs/SNRIs or triptans) or agents which reduce frovatriptan's metabolism. Concurrent use of serotonin precursors (eg, tryptophan) is not recommended. If concomitant administration with SSRIs is warranted, monitor closely, especially at initiation and with dose increases. Discontinue frovatriptan if serotonin syndrome is suspected. Anaphylaxis, anaphylactoid, and hypersensitivity reactions (including angioedema) have occurred; may be life-threatening or fatal.

Adverse Reactions

Cardiovascular: Chest pain, flushing, hot or cold flashes, palpitations

Central nervous system: Anxiety, dizziness, drowsiness, dysesthesia, fatigue, headache, hypoesthesia, insomnia, pain, paresthesia

Dermatologic: Diaphoresis

Gastrointestinal: Abdominal pain, diarrhea, dyspepsia, nausea, vomiting, xerostomia

Neuromuscular & skeletal: Musculoskeletal pain

Ophthalmic: Visual disturbance

Otic: Tinnitus

Respiratory: Rhinitis, sinusitis

Rare but important or life-threatening: Abnormal gait, abnormal lacrimation, abnormal reflexes, amnesia, anaphylactoid reactions, anaphylaxis, anorexia, ataxia, bradycardia, bullous rash, cheilitis, chest tightness, confusion, conjunctivitis, dehydration, depersonalization, depression, dysgeusia, ECG changes, emotional lability, epistaxis, esophageal spasm, euphoria, eye pain, gastroesophageal reflux disease, hyperacusis, hyperesthesia, hypersensitivity reaction (including angioedema), hypertonia, hyperventilation, hypocalcemia, hypoglycemia, hypotonia, involuntary muscle movements, jaw tightness, lack of concentration, laryngitis, myocardial infarction, nocturia, osteoarthritis, peptic ulcer, personality disorder, pharyngitis, polyuria, purpura, renal pain, rigors, salivary gland pain, seizure, sialorrhea, significant cardiovascular event, speech disturbance, stomatitis, syncope, tachycardia, tightness in chest and throat, tongue paralysis

Drug Interactions

Metabolism/Transport Effects Substrate of CYP1A2 (minor); **Note:** Assignment of Major/Minor substrate status based on clinically relevant drug interaction potential

Avoid Concomitant Use

Avoid concomitant use of Frovatriptan with any of the following: Dapoxetine; Ergot Derivatives

Increased Effect/Toxicity

Frovatriptan may increase the levels/effects of: Antipsychotic Agents; Droxidopa; Ergot Derivatives; Metoclopramide; Serotonin Modulators

The levels/effects of Frovatriptan may be increased by: Antiemetics (5HT3 Antagonists); Antipsychotic Agents; Dapoxetine; Ergot Derivatives; Tedizolid

Decreased Effect There are no known significant interactions involving a decrease in effect.

Food Interactions Food does not affect frovatriptan bioavailability.

Storage/Stability Store at 25°C (77°F); excursions are permitted between 15°C and 30°C (59°F and 86°F). Protect from moisture.

Mechanism of Action Selective agonist for serotonin (5-HT_{1B} and 5-HT_{1D} receptors) in cranial arteries; causes vasoconstriction and reduces sterile inflammation associated with antidromic neuronal transmission correlating with relief of migraine.

Pharmacodynamics/Kinetics

Distribution: Male: 4.2 L/kg; Female: 3 L/kg
Protein binding: ~15%
Metabolism: Primarily hepatic via CYP1A2
Bioavailability: Male: ~20%; Female: ~30%
Half-life elimination: ~26 hours
Time to peak: 2-4 hours
Excretion: Feces (62%); urine (32%)

Dosage Note: If the first dose is ineffective, diagnosis needs to be re-evaluated. The safety of treating >4 migraines/month has not been established.

Migraine: Adults: Oral:

U.S. labeling: Initial: 2.5 mg; if headache recurs, a second dose may be administered after 2 hours have elapsed since the first dose (maximum: 7.5 mg daily)

Canadian labeling: Initial: 2.5 mg; if headache recurs, a second dose may be administered after 4 hours have elapsed since the first dose (maximum: 5 mg daily)

Dosage adjustment in renal impairment: No dosage adjustment necessary

Dosage adjustment in hepatic impairment:

Mild-to-moderate impairment: No dosage adjustment necessary.

Severe impairment:

U.S. labeling: Use with caution (has not been studied).

Canadian labeling: Use is contraindicated.

Administration Administer orally with fluids as soon as symptoms appear.

Monitoring Parameters Headache severity, blood pressure, signs/symptoms suggestive of angina; perform a cardiovascular evaluation in triptan-naïve patients who have multiple cardiovascular risk factors (eg, increased age, diabetes, hypertension, smoking, obesity, strong family history of CAD), monitor ECG with first dose in patients with multiple cardiovascular risk factors who have a negative cardiovascular evaluation and consider periodic cardiovascular evaluation in such patients if they are intermittent long-term users; signs/symptoms of serotonin syndrome and hypersensitivity reactions.

Dosage Forms

Tablet, Oral:

Frova: 2.5 mg

- ◆ **Frovatriptan Succinate** *see* Frovatriptan *on page 938*
- ◆ **Fruit C [OTC]** *see* Ascorbic Acid *on page 178*
- ◆ **Fruit C 500 [OTC]** *see* Ascorbic Acid *on page 178*
- ◆ **Fruity C [OTC]** *see* Ascorbic Acid *on page 178*
- ◆ **Frusemide** *see* Furosemide *on page 940*
- ◆ **FSH** *see* Follitropin Alfa *on page 921*
- ◆ **FSH** *see* Follitropin Beta *on page 921*
- ◆ **FSH** *see* Urofollitropin *on page 2116*
- ◆ **FTC** *see* Emtricitabine *on page 720*
- ◆ **FTC/RPV/TDF** *see* Emtricitabine, Rilpivirine, and Tenofovir *on page 722*
- ◆ **FTC, TDF, and EFV** *see* Efavirenz, Emtricitabine, and Tenofovir *on page 709*
- ◆ **FTY720** *see* Fingolimod *on page 879*
- ◆ **FU** *see* Fluorouracil (Systemic) *on page 896*
- ◆ **FU** *see* Fluorouracil (Topical) *on page 899*
- ◆ **5-FU** *see* Fluorouracil (Systemic) *on page 896*
- ◆ **5-FU** *see* Fluorouracil (Topical) *on page 899*
- ◆ **Fucidin (Can)** *see* Fusidic Acid (Topical) [CAN/INT] *on page 943*
- ◆ **Fucithalmic (Can)** *see* Fusidic Acid (Ophthalmic) [CAN/INT] *on page 942*
- ◆ **Ful-Glo** *see* Fluorescein *on page 894*

Fulvestrant (fool VES trant)

Brand Names: U.S. Faslodex

Brand Names: Canada Faslodex®

Index Terms ICI-182,780; ZD9238

Pharmacologic Category Antineoplastic Agent, Estrogen Receptor Antagonist

Use Treatment of hormone receptor positive metastatic breast cancer in postmenopausal women with disease progression following antiestrogen therapy

Pregnancy Risk Factor D

Dosage IM: Adults (postmenopausal women): Breast cancer, metastatic: Initial: 500 mg on days 1, 15, and 29; Maintenance: 500 mg once monthly

Dosage adjustment in renal impairment: No dosage adjustment provided in manufacturer's labeling (has not been studied). However, renal elimination of fulvestrant is negligible.

Dosage adjustment in hepatic impairment:

Moderate impairment (Child-Pugh class B): Decrease initial and maintenance dose to 250 mg

Severe impairment (Child-Pugh class C): Use has not been evaluated.

Additional Information Complete prescribing information should be consulted for additional detail.

Dosage Forms

Solution, Intramuscular:

Faslodex: 250 mg/5 mL (5 mL)

- ◆ **Fulyzaq** *see* Crofelemer *on page 514*
- ◆ **Fungi-Guard [OTC]** *see* Tolnaftate *on page 2063*
- ◆ **Fungizone (Can)** *see* Amphotericin B (Conventional) *on page 136*
- ◆ **Fungoid-D [OTC]** *see* Tolnaftate *on page 2063*
- ◆ **Fungoid Tincture [OTC]** *see* Miconazole (Topical) *on page 1360*
- ◆ **Furadantin** *see* Nitrofurantoin *on page 1463*

Furazolidone [INT] (fyoor a ZOE li done)

International Brand Names Diapectolin (PH); Diralox (ID); Furidona (AR); Furopine (VN); Furoxona (CL, CO, MX, PE, VE); Furoxone (IN, PH, PK); Fuxol (MX); Giardil (AR); Giarlam (BR); Neo Prodiar (ID)

Pharmacologic Category Antiprotozoal

Reported Use Treatment of bacterial or protozoal diarrhea and enteritis caused by susceptible organisms *Giardia lamblia* and *Vibrio cholerae*

Dosage Range Adults: Diarrhea/enteritis: Oral: 100 mg 4 times/day

Product Availability Product available in various countries; not currently available in the U.S.

Dosage Forms

Tablet: 100 mg

◆ **Furazosin** *see* Prazosin *on page 1703*

Furosemide (fyoor OH se mide)

Brand Names: U.S. Lasix

Brand Names: Canada Apo-Furosemide; AVA-Furosemide; Bio-Furosemide; Dom-Furosemide; Furosemide Injection Sandoz Standard; Furosemide Injection, USP; Furosemide Special; Furosemide Special Injection; Lasix; Lasix Special; Novo-Semide; NTP-Furosemide; Nu-Furosemide; PMS-Furosemide; Teva-Furosemide

Index Terms Frusemide

Pharmacologic Category Antihypertensive; Diuretic, Loop

Use

Management of edema associated with heart failure and hepatic or renal disease; acute pulmonary edema; treatment of hypertension (alone or in combination with other antihypertensives)

Note: According to the Eighth Joint National Committee (JNC 8) guidelines, loop diuretics are **not** recommended for the initial treatment of hypertension (James, 2013). In patients with chronic kidney disease (ie, eGFR <30 mL/minute/1.73 m^2), the American Society of Hypertension/International Society of Hypertension (ASH/ISH) suggests that the use of a loop diuretic may be necessary (Weber, 2014).

Canadian labeling: Additional use: Furosemide Special Injection and Lasix Special (products not available in the U.S.): Adjunctive treatment of oliguria in patients with severe renal impairment

Pregnancy Risk Factor C

Pregnancy Considerations Adverse events have been observed in animal reproduction studies. Furosemide crosses the placenta (Riva 1978). Furosemide has been used to treat heart failure in pregnant women (ESC 2011; Johnson-Coyle 2012). Monitor fetal growth if used during pregnancy; may increase birth weight.

Breast-Feeding Considerations Furosemide is excreted into breast milk; maternal use may suppress lactation. The U.S. manufacturer recommends that caution be used if administered to a nursing woman. Canadian labeling contraindicates use while breast-feeding.

Contraindications Hypersensitivity to furosemide or any component of the formulation; anuria

Canadian labeling: Additional contraindications (not in U.S. labeling): Hypersensitivity to sulfonamide-derived drugs; complete renal shutdown; hepatic coma and precoma; uncorrected states of electrolyte depletion, hypovolemia, or hypotension; jaundiced newborn infants or infants with disease(s) capable of causing hyperbilirubinemia and possibly kernicterus; breast-feeding. **Note:** Manufacturer labeling for Lasix® Special and Furosemide Special Injection also includes: GFR <5 mL/minute or GFR >20 mL/minute; hepatic cirrhosis; renal failure accompanied by hepatic coma and precoma; renal failure due to poisoning with nephrotoxic or hepatotoxic substances.

Warnings/Precautions [U.S. Boxed Warning]: If given in excessive amounts, furosemide, similar to other loop diuretics, can lead to profound diuresis, resulting in fluid and electrolyte depletion; close medical supervision and dose evaluation are required. Watch for and correct electrolyte disturbances; adjust dose to avoid dehydration. When electrolyte depletion is present, therapy should not be initiated unless serum electrolytes, especially potassium, are normalized. In cirrhosis, avoid electrolyte and acid/base imbalances that might lead to hepatic encephalopathy; correct electrolyte and acid/base imbalances prior to initiation when hepatic coma is present. Coadministration of antihypertensives may increase the risk of hypotension.

Monitor fluid status and renal function in an attempt to prevent oliguria, azotemia, and reversible increases in BUN and creatinine; close medical supervision of aggressive diuresis is required. May increase risk of contrast-induced nephropathy. Rapid IV administration, renal impairment, excessive doses, hypoproteinemia, and concurrent use of other ototoxins is associated with ototoxicity. Asymptomatic hyperuricemia has been reported with use; rarely, gout may precipitate. Photosensitization may occur.

Use with caution in patients with prediabetes or diabetes mellitus; may see a change in glucose control. Use with caution in patients with systemic lupus erythematosus (SLE); may cause SLE exacerbation or activation. Use with caution in patients with prostatic hyperplasia/urinary stricture; may cause urinary retention. May lead to nephrocalcinosis or nephrolithiasis in premature infants or in children <4 years of age with chronic use. May prevent closure of patent ductus arteriosus in premature infants. Chemical similarities are present among sulfonamides, sulfonylureas, carbonic anhydrase inhibitors, thiazides, and loop diuretics (except ethacrynic acid). A risk of cross-reaction exists in patients with allergy to any of these compounds; avoid use when previous reaction has been severe. Discontinue if signs of hypersensitivity are noted. Some dosage forms may contain propylene glycol; large amounts are potentially toxic and have been associated hyperosmolality, lactic acidosis, seizures, and respiratory depression; use caution (AAP, 1997; Zar, 2007).

Adverse Reactions

Cardiovascular: Acute hypotension, chronic aortitis, necrotizing angiitis, orthostatic hypotension, vasculitis

Central nervous system: Dizziness, fever, headache, hepatic encephalopathy, lightheadedness, restlessness, vertigo

Dermatologic: Bullous pemphigoid, cutaneous vasculitis, drug rash with eosinophilia and systemic symptoms (DRESS), erythema multiforme, exanthematous pustulosis (generalized), exfoliative dermatitis, photosensitivity, pruritus, purpura, rash, Stevens-Johnson syndrome, toxic epidermal necrolysis, urticaria

Endocrine & metabolic: Cholesterol and triglycerides increased, glucose tolerance test altered, gout, hyperglycemia, hyperuricemia, hypocalcemia, hypochloremia, hypokalemia, hypomagnesemia, hyponatremia, metabolic alkalosis

Gastrointestinal: Anorexia, constipation, cramping, diarrhea, nausea, oral and gastric irritation, pancreatitis, vomiting

Genitourinary: Urinary bladder spasm, urinary frequency

Hematological: Agranulocytosis (rare), anemia, aplastic anemia (rare), eosinophilia, hemolytic anemia, leukopenia, thrombocytopenia

Hepatic: Intrahepatic cholestatic jaundice, ischemic hepatitis, liver enzymes increased

Local: Injection site pain (following IM injection), thrombophlebitis
Neuromuscular & skeletal: Muscle spasm, paresthesia, weakness
Ocular: Blurred vision, xanthopsia
Otic: Hearing impairment (reversible or permanent with rapid IV or IM administration), tinnitus
Renal: Allergic interstitial nephritis, fall in glomerular filtration rate and renal blood flow (due to overdiuresis), glycosuria, transient rise in BUN
Miscellaneous: Anaphylaxis (rare), exacerbate or activate systemic lupus erythematosus

Drug Interactions

Metabolism/Transport Effects **Substrate** of OAT3

Avoid Concomitant Use

Avoid concomitant use of Furosemide with any of the following: Chloral Hydrate; Ethacrynic Acid

Increased Effect/Toxicity

Furosemide may increase the levels/effects of: ACE Inhibitors; Allopurinol; Amifostine; Aminoglycosides; Antihypertensives; Cardiac Glycosides; Chloral Hydrate; CISplatin; Dofetilide; DULoxetine; Ethacrynic Acid; Foscarnet; Hypotensive Agents; Ivabradine; Levodopa; Lithium; Methotrexate; Neuromuscular-Blocking Agents; Obinutuzumab; RisperiDONE; RiTUXimab; Salicylates; Sodium Phosphates; Topiramate

The levels/effects of Furosemide may be increased by: Alfuzosin; Analgesics (Opioid); Barbiturates; Beta2-Agonists; Brimonidine (Topical); Canagliflozin; Corticosteroids (Orally Inhaled); Corticosteroids (Systemic); CycloSPORINE (Systemic); Diazoxide; Herbs (Hypotensive Properties); Licorice; MAO Inhibitors; Methotrexate; Nicorandil; Pentoxifylline; Phosphodiesterase 5 Inhibitors; Probenecid; Prostacyclin Analogues; Teriflunomide

Decreased Effect

Furosemide may decrease the levels/effects of: Hypoglycemic Agents; Lithium; Neuromuscular-Blocking Agents

The levels/effects of Furosemide may be decreased by: Aliskiren; Bile Acid Sequestrants; Fosphenytoin; Herbs (Hypertensive Properties); Methotrexate; Methylphenidate; Nonsteroidal Anti-Inflammatory Agents; Phenytoin; Probenecid; Salicylates; Sucralfate; Yohimbine

Food Interactions Furosemide serum levels may be decreased if taken with food. Management: Administer on an empty stomach.

Preparation for Administration IV infusion solution may be mixed in NS or D_5W solution. May also be diluted for infusion to 1-2 mg/mL (maximum: 10 mg/mL).

Storage/Stability

Injection: Store at room temperature of 15°C to 30°C (59°F to 86°F). Protect from light. Exposure to light may cause discoloration; do not use furosemide solutions if they have a yellow color. Furosemide solutions are unstable in acidic media, but very stable in basic media. Refrigeration may result in precipitation or crystallization; however, resolubilization at room temperature or warming may be performed without affecting the drug's stability. Infusion solution is stable for 24 hours at room temperature.

Tablet: Store at 25°C (77°F); excursions permitted to 15°C to 30°C (59°F to 89°F). Protect from light.

Mechanism of Action Inhibits reabsorption of sodium and chloride in the ascending loop of Henle and distal renal tubule, interfering with the chloride-binding cotransport system, thus causing increased excretion of water, sodium, chloride, magnesium, and calcium

Pharmacodynamics/Kinetics

Onset of action: Diuresis: Oral, S.L: 30-60 minutes; IM: 30 minutes; IV: ~5 minutes
Symptomatic improvement with acute pulmonary edema: Within 15-20 minutes; occurs prior to diuretic effect
Peak effect: Oral, S.L.: 1-2 hours
Duration: Oral, S.L.: 6-8 hours; IV: 2 hours
Protein binding: 91% to 99%; primarily to albumin
Metabolism: Minimally hepatic
Bioavailability: Oral tablet: 47% to 64%; Oral solution: 50%; S.L. administration of oral tablet: ~60%; results of a small comparative study (n=11) showed bioavailability of S.L. administration of tablet was ~12% higher than oral administration of tablet (Haegeli, 2007)
Half-life elimination: Normal renal function: 0.5-2 hours; End-stage renal disease: 9 hours
Excretion: Urine (Oral: 50%, IV: 80%) within 24 hours; feces (as unchanged drug); nonrenal clearance prolonged in renal impairment

Dosage

Infants and Children: Edema, heart failure:
Oral: Initial: 2 mg/kg/dose increased in increments of 1-2 mg/kg/dose with each succeeding dose at intervals of 6-8 hours until a satisfactory response is achieved; maximum dose: 6 mg/kg/dose
IM, IV: Initial: 1 mg/kg/dose; if response not adequate, may increase dose in increments of 1 mg/kg/dose and administer not sooner than 2 hours after previous dose, until a satisfactory response is achieved; may administer maintenance dose at intervals of every 6-12 hours; maximum dose: 6 mg/kg/dose

Children 1-17 years: Hypertension, resistant (off-label; AAP, 2004): Oral: Initial: 0.5-2 mg/kg/dose once or twice daily; maximum dose: 6 mg/kg/dose

Adults:
Edema, heart failure:
Oral: Initial: 20-80 mg/dose; if response is not adequate, may repeat the same dose or increase dose in increments of 20-40 mg/dose at intervals of 6-8 hours; may be titrated up to 600 mg daily with severe edematous states; usual maintenance dose interval is once or twice daily. ACCF/AHA 2013 heart failure guidelines recommend initial dosing of 20-40 mg once or twice daily and a maximum total daily dose of 600 mg (Yancy, 2013). **Note:** Dosing frequency may be adjusted based on patient-specific diuretic needs.
IM, IV: Initial: 20-40 mg/dose; if response is not adequate, may repeat the same dose or increase dose in increments of 20 mg/dose and administer 1-2 hours after previous dose (maximum dose: 200 mg/dose). Individually determined dose should then be given once or twice daily although some patients may initially require dosing as frequent as every 6 hours.
Continuous IV infusion (ACCF/AHA [Yancy, 2013]); Brater, 1998; Howard, 2001): Initial: IV bolus dose 40-100 mg, followed by continuous IV infusion rate of 10-40 mg/hour; repeat loading dose before increasing infusion rate. **Note:** With lower baseline CrCl (eg, CrCl <25 mL/minute), the upper end of the initial infusion dosage range should be considered. If urine output is <1 mL/kg/hour, double as necessary to a maximum of 80-160 mg/hour (Howard, 2001; Schuller, 1997). The risk associated with higher infusion rates (80-160 mg/hour) must be weighed against alternative strategies.

Acute pulmonary edema: IV: 40 mg over 1-2 minutes. If response not adequate within 1 hour, may increase dose to 80 mg. **Note:** Minimal additional response is gained by single doses over 160-200 mg; maximum dose: 200 mg (Brater, 1998).

Hypertension:

Oral: Initial: 40 mg twice daily; individualize according to patient response and use minimal dose necessary to maintain therapeutic response. If response inadequate, may add another antihypertensive. Usual dosage (ASH/ISH [Weber, 2014]): 40 mg twice daily.

Elderly: Oral, IM, IV: Initial: 20 mg/day; increase slowly to desired response.

Dosing adjustment/comments in renal impairment: Acute renal failure: High doses (up to 1-3 g daily - oral/IV) have been used to initiate desired response; avoid use in oliguric states.

Dialysis: Not removed by hemo- or peritoneal dialysis; supplemental dose is not necessary.

Dosing adjustment/comments in hepatic disease: Diminished natriuretic effect with increased sensitivity to hypokalemia and volume depletion in cirrhosis; monitor effects, particularly with high doses.

Dietary Considerations May cause potassium loss; potassium supplement or dietary changes may be required.

Usual Infusion Concentrations: Pediatric IV infusion: 1 mg/mL **or** 2 mg/mL **or** undiluted as 10 mg/mL

Usual Infusion Concentrations: Adult IV infusion: 1 mg/mL **or** 2 mg/mL **or** undiluted as 10 mg/mL

Administration

IV: IV injections should be given slowly. In adults, undiluted direct IV injections may be administered at a rate of 20-40 mg per minute; maximum rate of administration for short-term intermittent infusion is 4 mg/minute; exceeding this rate increases the risk of ototoxicity. In children, a maximum rate of 0.5 mg/kg/minute has been recommended.

Oral: Administer on an empty stomach (Bard, 2004). May be administered with food or milk if GI distress occurs; however, this may reduce diuretic efficacy.

Note: When IV or oral administration is not possible, the sublingual route may be used. Place 1 tablet under tongue for at least 5 minutes to allow for maximal absorption. Patients should be advised not to swallow during disintegration time (Haegeli, 2007).

Monitoring Parameters Monitor weight and I & O daily; blood pressure, orthostasis; serum electrolytes, renal function; monitor hearing with high doses or rapid IV administration

Dosage Forms

Solution, Injection:

Generic: 10 mg/mL (2 mL, 4 mL, 10 mL)

Solution, Injection [preservative free]:

Generic: 10 mg/mL (2 mL, 4 mL, 10 mL)

Solution, Oral:

Generic: 8 mg/mL (5 mL, 500 mL); 10 mg/mL (60 mL, 120 mL)

Tablet, Oral:

Lasix: 20 mg, 40 mg, 80 mg

Generic: 20 mg, 40 mg, 80 mg

Dosage Forms: Canada

Injection, solution [preservative free]:

Furosemide Special Injection: 10 mg/mL (25 mL)

Tablet, oral:

Lasix Special: 500 mg [scored]

- ◆ **Furosemide Injection Sandoz Standard (Can)** *see* Furosemide *on page 940*
- ◆ **Furosemide Injection, USP (Can)** *see* Furosemide *on page 940*
- ◆ **Furosemide Special (Can)** *see* Furosemide *on page 940*
- ◆ **Furosemide Special Injection (Can)** *see* Furosemide *on page 940*
- ◆ **Fusidate Sodium** *see* Fusidic Acid (Ophthalmic) [CAN/INT] *on page 942*
- ◆ **Fusidate Sodium** *see* Fusidic Acid (Systemic) [INT] *on page 942*
- ◆ **Fusidate Sodium** *see* Fusidic Acid (Topical) [CAN/INT] *on page 943*

Fusidic Acid (Systemic) [INT] (fyoo SI dik AS id)

International Brand Names Fucidin (AE, AU, CH, EG, FI, HK, IL, KR, KW, MY, NZ, PH, RO, SA, SG, SI, TH, UY); Fucidin IV (ZA); Fucidine (DK, ES, FR, PT, SE)

Index Terms Fusidate Sodium; Sodium Fusidate

Pharmacologic Category Antibiotic, Miscellaneous

Reported Use Treatment of infections caused by susceptible organisms, including staphylococci

Dosage Range Oral:

Infants: Suspension: 50 mg/kg/day administered in 3 divided doses

Children 1-5 years: Suspension: 250 mg 3 times daily

Children 5-12 years:

Suspension: 500-1000 mg 3 times daily

Tablets: 250-500 mg 3 times daily

Adolescents, Adults, and Elderly:

Suspension: 750-1500 mg 3 times daily

Tablets: 250 mg twice daily or 500-1000 mg 3 times daily

Product Availability Product available in various countries; not currently available in the U.S.

Dosage Forms

Suspension, Oral, as fusidic acid hemihydrate: 250 mg/5 mL

Tablet, Oral, as sodium fusidate: 250 mg

Fusidic Acid (Ophthalmic) [CAN/INT]

(fyoo SI dik AS id)

Brand Names: Canada Fucithalmic

Index Terms Fusidate Sodium; Fusidic Acid Hemihydrate; Sodium Fusidate

Pharmacologic Category Antibiotic, Miscellaneous; Antibiotic, Ophthalmic

Use Note: Not approved in U.S.

Treatment of superficial infections of the eye and conjunctiva caused by susceptible organisms (*Staphylococcus aureus*, *Streptococcus pneumoniae*, and *Haemophilus* influenzae)

Pregnancy Considerations Adverse effects were not observed in animal reproduction studies. Fusidic acid crosses the placenta during systemic administration. According to the Canadian labeling, the decision to use fusidic acid during pregnancy should take into account the risk of exposure to the fetus.

Breast-Feeding Considerations Fusidic acid is excreted in breast milk following systemic administration. According to the Canadian labeling, the decision to use ophthalmic fusidic acid in nursing women should take into account the risk of exposure to the infant.

Contraindications Hypersensitivity to fusidic acid or any component of the formulation

Warnings/Precautions For topical use only; do not inject into the eye. Prolonged use may result in superinfection (including fungal infections). Discontinue use if superinfection occurs; evaluate and treat appropriately. Discontinue use if irritation (other than transient stinging upon administration) develops. Contact lenses should not be worn during therapy. Multidose vials contain benzalkonium chloride; may be absorbed by contact lenses. Not indicated for use in neonatal conjunctivitis.

Adverse Reactions

Ophthalmic: Eye irritation (transient)

Rare but important or life-threatening: Abscess (eyelid), chest infection, conjunctival abnormalities (cobblestone appearance of the conjunctival sulcus), exacerbation of eye infection (conjunctivitis), local hypersensitivity reaction, oral candidiasis, skin rash, tonsillitis, urinary incontinence, urticaria, vomiting

Drug Interactions

Metabolism/Transport Effects None known.

Avoid Concomitant Use There are no known interactions where it is recommended to avoid concomitant use.

Increased Effect/Toxicity There are no known significant interactions involving an increase in effect.

Decreased Effect There are no known significant interactions involving a decrease in effect.

Storage/Stability Store at 2°C to 25°C (36°F to 77°F). Discard multidose tube 1 month after opening.

Mechanism of Action Inhibits protein synthesis by blocking aminoacyl-tRNA transfer to protein in susceptible bacteria.

Pharmacodynamics/Kinetics Absorption: Good; lacrimal fluid concentrations range 15.7-40 mcg/mL and 1.4 mcg-5.6 mcg/mL at 1 hour and 12 hours respectively after administration. Median concentrations of 0.3 mcg/mL (single dose) and 0.8 mcg/mL (repeated dosing) were maintained in aqueous humor over 12 hours (Hansen, 1985).

Dosage Ophthalmic infections/conjunctivitis: Children ≥2 years, Adolescents, and Adults: Ophthalmic: Instill 1 drop into the conjunctival sac of each eye every 12 hours for 7 days; reassess if infection has not resolved after 7 days

Administration For ophthalmic use only. Tilt head back, pull down lower eyelid and instill drop into eye. Wash hands before and after instillation; avoid touching tip of applicator to eye or other surfaces. Contact lenses should not be worn during therapy.

Product Availability Not available in U.S.

Dosage Forms: Canada

Suspension, ophthalmic, as fusidic acid:

Fucithalmic: 10 mg/g (1%)

Fusidic Acid (Topical) [CAN/INT]

(fyoo SI dik AS id)

Brand Names: Canada Fucidin

Index Terms Fusidate Sodium; Fusidic Acid Hemihydrate; Sodium Fusidate

Pharmacologic Category Antibiotic, Miscellaneous; Antibiotic, Topical

Use Note: Not approved in U.S.

Treatment of primary and secondary skin infections caused by susceptible organisms; active against *staphylococcus aureus*, *streptococcus spp*, *corynebacterium spp*, *clostridium spp*, *neisseria spp*, and *bacteroides spp*

Pregnancy Considerations Adverse effects were not observed in animal reproduction studies. Fusidic acid crosses the placenta during systemic administration. According to the Canadian labeling, the decision to use fusidic acid during pregnancy should take into account the risk of exposure to the fetus.

Breast-Feeding Considerations Fusidic acid is excreted in breast milk following systemic administration. The Canadian product labeling recommends weighing benefits to the mother versus potential risks to the nursing infants prior to use of topical fusidic acid.

Contraindications Hypersensitivity to fusidic acid or any component of the formulation

Warnings/Precautions Prolonged use may result in superinfection (including fungal infections). Discontinue use if superinfection occurs; evaluate and treat appropriately. Do not use near the eye; conjunctival irritation may occur. Supplemental systemic therapy may be necessary for severe or refractory lesions.

Adverse Reactions

Central nervous system: Pain (with treatment of deep leg ulcers)

Dermatologic: Skin irritation (mild)

Hypersensitivity: Hypersensitivity reaction (rare)

Rare but important or life-threatening: Anaphylaxis (Park, 2013)

Drug Interactions

Metabolism/Transport Effects None known.

Avoid Concomitant Use

Avoid concomitant use of Fusidic Acid (Topical) with any of the following: BCG

Increased Effect/Toxicity There are no known significant interactions involving an increase in effect.

Decreased Effect

Fusidic Acid (Topical) may decrease the levels/effects of: BCG; Sodium Picosulfate

Storage/Stability

Cream: Store at 15°C to 25°C (59°F to 77°F). Use within 3 months of first opening the tube.

Ointment: Store at 15°C to 30°C (59°F to 86°F). Use within 3 months of first opening the tube.

Mechanism of Action Inhibits protein synthesis by blocking aminoacyl-tRNA transfer to protein in susceptible bacteria.

Dosage Topical: Children, Adolescents and Adults: Superficial dermatologic infections: Apply small amount to affected area 3-4 times daily until favorable results are achieved. If a gauze dressing is used, frequency of application may be reduced to 1-2 times daily.

Administration For topical use only; do not use near the eyes. Crust of impetigo contagiosa does not need to be removed prior to use.

Product Availability Not available in U.S.

Dosage Forms: Canada

Cream, Topical, as fusidic acid:

Fucidin: 2% (15 g, 30 g)

Ointment, Topical, as sodium fusidate:

Fucidin: 2% (15 g, 30 g)

- ◆ **Fusidic Acid Hemihydrate** *see* Fusidic Acid (Ophthalmic) [CAN/INT] *on page 942*
- ◆ **Fusidic Acid Hemihydrate** *see* Fusidic Acid (Topical) [CAN/INT] *on page 943*
- ◆ **Fusilev** *see* LEVOleucovorin *on page 1200*
- ◆ **Fuzeon** *see* Enfuvirtide *on page 726*
- ◆ **FVIII/vWF** *see* Antihemophilic Factor/von Willebrand Factor Complex (Human) *on page 154*
- ◆ **FXIII** *see* Factor XIII Concentrate (Human) *on page 843*
- ◆ **FXT 40 (Can)** *see* FLUoxetine *on page 899*
- ◆ **Fycompa** *see* Perampanel *on page 1620*
- ◆ **G-30320** *see* Clofazimine [INT] *on page 473*
- ◆ **GA101** *see* Obinutuzumab *on page 1482*
- ◆ **GAA** *see* Alglucosidase Alfa *on page 85*

Gabapentin (GA ba pen tin)

Brand Names: U.S. Gralise; Gralise Starter; Neurontin

Brand Names: Canada Apo-Gabapentin; Auro-Gabapentin; CO Gabapentin; Dom-Gabapentin; Gabapentin Tablets USP; GD-Gabapentin; JAMP-Gabapentin; Mylan-Gabapentin; Neurontin; PHL-Gabapentin; PMS-Gabapentin; PRO-Gabapentin; RAN-Gabapentin; ratio-Gabapentin; Riva-Gabapentin; Teva-Gabapentin

Pharmacologic Category Anticonvulsant, Miscellaneous; GABA Analog

Use

Postherpetic neuralgia: Management of postherpetic neuralgia (PHN) in adults.

Seizures, partial onset (excluding Gralise): As adjunctive therapy in the treatment of partial seizures with and without secondary generalization in adults and pediatric patients 3 years and older with epilepsy.

Pregnancy Risk Factor C

Pregnancy Considerations Adverse events have been observed in animal reproduction studies. Gabapentin crosses the placenta. In a small study (n=6), the umbilical/maternal plasma concentration ratio was ~1.74. Neonatal concentrations declined quickly after delivery and at 24 hours of life were ~27% of the cord blood concentrations at birth (gabapentin neonatal half-life ~14 hours) (Ohman, 2005). Outcome data following maternal use of gabapentin during pregnancy is limited (Holmes, 2012).

Patients exposed to gabapentin during pregnancy are encouraged to enroll in the North American Antiepileptic Drug (NAAED) Pregnancy Registry by calling 1-888-233-2334. Additional information is available at www.aedpregnancyregistry.org.

Breast-Feeding Considerations Gabapentin is excreted in human breast milk. Per the manufacturer, a nursed infant could be exposed to ~1 mg/kg/day of gabapentin; the effect on the child is not known. Use in breast-feeding women only if the benefits to the mother outweigh the potential risk to the infant.

In a small study of breast-feeding women (n=6), the estimated exposure of gabapentin to the nursing infants was ~1% to 4% of the weight-adjusted maternal dose (sampling occurred from 12-97 days after delivery and maternal doses ranged from 600-2100 mg daily). Gabapentin was detected in the serum of 2 nursing infants 2-3 weeks after delivery and in 1 infant after 3 months of breast-feeding. Serum concentrations were <12% of the maternal plasma concentrations and <5% of those measured in the umbilical cord. Adverse events were not reported in the breast-fed infants (Ohman, 2005).

Contraindications Hypersensitivity to gabapentin or any component of the formulation

Warnings/Precautions Antiepileptics are associated with an increased risk of suicidal behavior/thoughts with use (regardless of indication); patients should be monitored for signs/symptoms of depression, suicidal tendencies, and other unusual behavior changes during therapy and instructed to inform their healthcare provider immediately if symptoms occur. Avoid abrupt withdrawal, may precipitate seizures; Gralise should be withdrawn over ≥1 week. Use cautiously in patients with severe renal dysfunction; male rat studies demonstrated an association with pancreatic adenocarcinoma (clinical implication unknown). May cause CNS depression including somnolence and dizziness, which may impair physical or mental abilities. Patients must be cautioned about performing tasks which require mental alertness (eg, operating machinery or driving). Pediatric patients have shown increased incidence of CNS-related adverse effects, including emotional lability, hostility, thought disorder, and hyperkinesia. Gabapentin immediate release and Gralise products are not interchangeable with each other **or** with gabapentin enacarbil (Horizant). The safety and efficacy of Gralise has not been studied in patients with epilepsy. Potentially serious, sometimes fatal multiorgan hypersensitivity (also known as drug reaction with eosinophilia and systemic symptoms [DRESS]) has been reported with some antiepileptic drugs, including gabapentin; may affect lymphatic, hepatic, renal, cardiac, and/or hematologic systems; fever, rash, and eosinophilia may also be present. Discontinue immediately if suspected.

Adverse Reactions

Cardiovascular: Peripheral edema, vasodilatation

Central nervous system: Abnormal gait, abnormality in thinking, amnesia, ataxia, depression, dizziness (more common in adults), drowsiness (more common in adults), emotional lability (children), fatigue (more common in adults), headache, hostility (children), hyperesthesia, hyperkinesia (children), lethargy, nervousness, pain, tremor, twitching, vertigo

Dermatologic: Pruritus, skin rash

Endocrine & metabolic: Hyperglycemia, weight gain

Gastrointestinal: Abdominal pain, constipation, dental disease, diarrhea, dry throat, dyspepsia, flatulence, increased appetite, nausea and vomiting (more common in children), xerostomia

Genitourinary: Impotence, urinary tract infection

Hematologic & oncologic: Decreased white blood cell count, leukopenia

Infection: Infection, viral infection (children)

Neuromuscular & skeletal: Back pain, bone fracture, dysarthria, limb pain, myalgia, weakness

Ophthalmic: Blurred vision, conjunctivitis, diplopia, nystagmus

Otic: Otitis media

Respiratory: Bronchitis (children), cough, nasopharyngitis, pharyngitis, respiratory tract infection (children), rhinitis

Miscellaneous: Fever (children)

Rare but important or life-threatening: Acute renal failure, altered serum glucose, anemia, angina pectoris, angioedema, aphasia, aspiration pneumonia, blindness, blood coagulation disorder, bradycardia, brain disease, breast hypertrophy, cardiac arrhythmia (various), cardiac failure, cerebrovascular accident, CNS neoplasm, colitis, confusion, Cushingoid appearance, DRESS syndrome, drug abuse, drug dependence, erythema multiforme, facial paralysis, fecal incontinence, gastroenteritis, glaucoma, glycosuria, hearing loss, heart block, hematemesis, hematuria, hemiplegia, hemorrhage, hepatitis, hepatomegaly, herpes zoster, hyperlipidemia, hypertension, hyperthyroidism, hyperventilation, hyponatremia, hypotension, hypothyroidism, hypoventilation, increased creatine phosphokinase, increased liver enzymes, increased serum creatinine, jaundice, joint swelling, leukocytosis, lymphadenopathy, lymphocytosis, memory impairment, meningism, migraine, movement disorder, myocardial infarction, myoclonus (local), nephrolithiasis, nephrosis, nerve palsy, non-Hodgkin's lymphoma, ovarian failure, pancreatitis, peptic ulcer, pericardial effusion, pericardial rub, pericarditis, peripheral vascular disease, pneumonia, psychosis, pulmonary thromboembolism, purpura, retinopathy, rhabdomyolysis, seasonal allergy, skin necrosis, status epilepticus, Stevens-Johnson syndrome, subdural hematoma, suicidal ideation, suicidal tendencies, syncope, tachycardia, thrombocytopenia, thrombophlebitis, tumor growth, withdrawal syndrome

Drug Interactions

Metabolism/Transport Effects None known.

Avoid Concomitant Use

Avoid concomitant use of Gabapentin with any of the following: Azelastine (Nasal); Orphenadrine; Paraldehyde; Thalidomide

Increased Effect/Toxicity

Gabapentin may increase the levels/effects of: Alcohol (Ethyl); Azelastine (Nasal); Buprenorphine; CNS Depressants; Hydrocodone; Methotrimeprazine; Metyrosine; Mirtazapine; Orphenadrine; Paraldehyde; Pramipexole; ROPINIRole; Rotigotine; Selective Serotonin Reuptake Inhibitors; Suvorexant; Thalidomide; Zolpidem

The levels/effects of Gabapentin may be increased by: Brimonidine (Topical); Cannabis; Doxylamine; Dronabinol; Droperidol; HydrOXYzine; Kava Kava; Magnesium Salts; Methotrimeprazine; Nabilone; Perampanel; Rufinamide; Sodium Oxybate; Tapentadol; Tetrahydrocannabinol

Decreased Effect

The levels/effects of Gabapentin may be decreased by: Antacids; Magnesium Salts; Mefloquine; Mianserin; Orlistat

Food Interactions Tablet, solution (immediate release): No significant effect on rate or extent of absorption; tablet (Gralise): Increases rate and extent of absorption. Management: Administer immediate release products without regard to food. Administer Gralise with food.

Storage/Stability

Capsules and tablets: Store at 25°C (77°F); excursions permitted to 15°C to 30°C (59°F to 86°F). Use scored 600 or 800 mg tablets that are broken in half within 28 days of breaking the tablet.

Oral solution: Store refrigerated at 2°C to 8°C (36°F to 46°F).

Mechanism of Action Gabapentin is structurally related to GABA. However, it does not bind to $GABA_A$ or $GABA_B$ receptors, and it does not appear to influence synthesis or uptake of GABA. High affinity gabapentin binding sites have been located throughout the brain; these sites correspond to the presence of voltage-gated calcium channels specifically possessing the alpha-2-delta-1 subunit. This channel appears to be located presynaptically, and may modulate the release of excitatory neurotransmitters which participate in epileptogenesis and nociception.

Pharmacodynamics/Kinetics

Absorption: Variable, from proximal small bowel by L-amino transport system

Distribution: V_d: 58 ± 6 L

Protein binding: <3%

Bioavailability: Inversely proportional to dose due to saturable absorption:

Immediate release:

900 mg/day: 60%

1,200 mg/day: 47%

2,400 mg/day: 34%

3,600 mg/day: 33%

4,800 mg/day: 27%

Gralise: Variable; increased with higher fat content meal

Half-life elimination: 5 to 7 hours

Time to peak: Immediate release: 2 to 4 hours; Gralise: 8 hours

Excretion: Proportional to renal function; urine (as unchanged drug)

Dosage

Postherpetic neuralgia: Adults: Oral:

Day 1: 300 mg, Day 2: 300 mg twice daily, Day 3: 300 mg 3 times daily; dose may be titrated as needed for pain relief (range: 1,800 to 3,600 mg/day in divided doses, daily doses >1,800 mg do not generally show greater benefit)

Gralise only: Day 1: 300 mg, Day 2: 600 mg, Days 3 to 6: 900 mg once daily, Days 7 to 10: 1,200 mg once daily, Days 11 to 14: 1,500 mg once daily, Days ≥15: 1,800 mg once daily

Seizures, partial onset: Oral (excluding Gralise):

Children 3 to 4 years: Initial: 10 to 15 mg/kg/day in 3 divided doses; titrate to effective dose over ~3 days; increase dosage based on response and tolerability; usual dosage: 40 mg/kg/day in 3 divided doses; dosages of up to 50 mg/kg/day have been tolerated in clinical studies

Children 5 to 11 years: Initial: 10 to15 mg/kg/day in 3 divided doses; titrate to effective dose over ~3 days; increase dosage based on response and tolerability; usual dosage: 25 to 35 mg/kg/day in 3 divided doses; dosages of up to 50 mg/kg/day have been tolerated in clinical studies

Children ≥12 years and Adults: Initial: 300 mg 3 times daily; increase dosage based on response and tolerability; usual dosage 900 to 1,800 mg/day administered in 3 divided doses; doses of up to 2400 mg/day have been tolerated in long-term clinical studies; up to 3,600 mg/day has been tolerated in short-term studies.

Note: If gabapentin is discontinued or if another anticonvulsant is added to therapy, it should be done slowly over a minimum of 1 week

Diabetic neuropathy (off-label use): Adults: Oral: Immediate release: 900 to 3,600 mg/day (Bril, 2011)

Neuropathic pain (off-label use): Adults: Oral: Immediate release: 300 to 3,600 mg/day (Attal, 2010; Dworkin, 2010)

Neuropathic pain, critically-ill patients (off-label use): Adults: Oral: Immediate release: Initial: 100 mg 3 times daily in combination with IV opioids; Maintenance: 300 to 1,200 mg 3 times daily; maximum dose: 3,600 mg daily (Barr, 2013)

Postoperative pain (adjunct) (off-label use): Adults: Oral: Immediate release: Usual dose: 300 to 1,200 mg given the night before or 1 to 2 hours prior to surgery (Dauri, 2009)

Restless legs syndrome (RLS) (off-label use): Adults: Oral: Immediate release: Initial: 300 mg once daily 2 hours before bedtime. Doses ≥600 mg/day have been given in 2 divided doses (late afternoon and 2 hours before bedtime). Dose may be titrated every 2 weeks until symptom relief achieved (range: 300 to 1,800 mg/day). Suggested maintenance dosing schedule: One-third of total daily dose given at 12 pm, remaining two-thirds total daily dose given at 8 pm. (Garcia-Borreguero, 2002; Happe, 2003; Saletu, 2010; Vignatelli, 2006)

Hot flashes (off-label use): Adults: Oral: Immediate release: Day 1: 300 mg at bedtime, Day 2: 300 mg twice daily, followed by 300 mg 3 times daily for 4 weeks and then tapered off (Butt, 2008)

Dosing adjustment in renal impairment: Children ≥12 years and Adults:

All products, excluding Gralise:

CrCl ≥60 mL/minute: 300 to 1,200 mg 3 times daily

CrCl >30 to 59 mL/minute: 200 to 700 mg twice daily

CrCl >15 to 29 mL/minute: 200 to 700 mg once daily

CrCl 15 mL/minute: 100 to 300 mg once daily

CrCl <15 mL/minute: Reduce daily dose in proportion to creatinine clearance based on dose for creatinine clearance of 15 mL/minute (eg, reduce dose by one-half [range: 50 to 150 mg/day] for CrCl 7.5 mL/minute)

ESRD requiring hemodialysis: Dose based on CrCl plus a single supplemental dose of 125 to 350 mg (given after each 4 hours of hemodialysis)

Gralise only: **Note:** Follow initial dose titration schedule if treatment-naive.

CrCl ≥60 mL/minute: 1,800 mg once daily

CrCl >30 to 59 mL/minute: 600 to 1,800 mg once daily; dependent on tolerability and clinical response

CrCl <30 mL/minute: Use is not recommended.

ESRD requiring hemodialysis: Use is not recommended.

Dosing adjustment in hepatic impairment: There are no dosage adjustments provided in the manufacturer's labeling; however, gabapentin is not hepatically metabolized.

Dietary Considerations Tablet (excluding Gralise) and solution may be taken without regard to meals; Gralise should be taken with food.

Administration

Tablet (excluding Gralise), solution: Administer first dose on first day at bedtime to avoid somnolence and dizziness. Dosage must be adjusted for renal function; when given 3 times daily, the maximum time between doses should not exceed 12 hours.

Gralise: Take with evening meal. Swallow whole; do not chew, crush, or split.

Monitoring Parameters Monitor serum levels of concomitant anticonvulsant therapy; suicidality (eg, suicidal thoughts, depression, behavioral changes)

Dosage Forms

Capsule, Oral:

Neurontin: 100 mg, 300 mg, 400 mg

Generic: 100 mg, 300 mg, 400 mg

Miscellaneous, Oral:

Gralise Starter: 300 & 600 mg (78 ea)

Solution, Oral:

Neurontin: 250 mg/5 mL (470 mL)

Generic: 250 mg/5 mL (5 mL, 6 mL, 470 mL, 473 mL)

Tablet, Oral:

Gralise: 300 mg, 600 mg

Neurontin: 600 mg, 800 mg

Generic: 600 mg, 800 mg

Extemporaneous Preparations Note: Commercial oral solution is available (50 mg/mL)

A 100 mg/mL suspension may be made with tablets (immediate release) and either a 1:1 mixture of Ora-Sweet® (100 mL) and Ora-Plus® (100 mL) or 1:1 mixture of methylcellulose 1% (100 mL) and Simple Syrup N.F. (100 mL). Crush sixty-seven 300 mg tablets in a mortar and reduce to a fine powder. Add small portions of the chosen vehicle and mix to a uniform paste; mix while adding the vehicle in incremental proportions to **almost** 200 mL; transfer to a calibrated bottle, rinse mortar with vehicle, and add sufficient quantity of vehicle to make 200 mL. Label "shake well" and "refrigerate". Stable for 91 days refrigerated (preferred) or 56 days at room temperature.

Nahata MC, Pai VB, and Hipple TF, *Pediatric Drug Formulations*, 5th ed, Cincinnati, OH: Harvey Whitney Books Co, 2004.

Gabapentin Enacarbil (gab a PEN tin en a KAR bil)

Brand Names: U.S. Horizant

Index Terms GSK 1838262; Solzira; XP13512

Pharmacologic Category Anticonvulsant, Miscellaneous

Use Treatment of moderate-to-severe restless leg syndrome (RLS); management of postherpetic neuralgia (PHN)

Pregnancy Risk Factor C

Dosage Oral: Adults:

Postherpetic neuralgia (PHN): Initial: 600 mg once daily in the morning for 3 days, then increase to 600 mg twice daily; increasing to >1200 mg daily provided no additional benefit and increased side effects

Restless legs syndrome (RLS): 600 mg once daily (at ~5:00 pm); increasing to 1200 mg daily provided no additional benefit and increased side effects

Dosage adjustment in renal impairment: Note: Estimation of renal function for the purpose of drug dosing should be done using the Cockcroft-Gault formula.

PHN:

CrCl 30-59 mL/minute: Initial: 300 mg every morning for 3 days, then increase to 300 mg twice daily. May increase to 600 mg twice daily as needed based on tolerability and efficacy. When discontinuing, reduce current dose to once daily in the morning for 1 week.

CrCl 15-29 mL/minute: Initial: 300 mg in the morning on day 1 and on day 3; then increase to 300 mg once daily. May increase to 300 mg twice daily if needed based on tolerability and efficacy. When discontinuing, if current dose is 300 mg twice daily, reduce to 300 mg once daily for 1 week. If current dose is 300 mg once daily, no taper is needed.

CrCl <15 mL/minute: 300 mg every other day in the morning; may increase dose to 300 mg once daily if needed based on tolerability and efficacy. When discontinuing, no taper is needed.

CrCl <15 mL/minute and on hemodialysis: 300 mg following every dialysis. May increase to 600 mg following every dialysis if needed based on tolerability and efficacy. When discontinuing, no taper is needed.

RLS:

CrCl 30-59 mL/minute: Initial dose: 300 mg daily; increase to 600 mg daily as needed

CrCl 15-29 mL/minute: 300 mg daily

CrCl <15 mL/minute: 300 mg every other day

CrCl <15 mL/minute and on hemodialysis: Use is not recommended.

Dosage adjustment in hepatic impairment: No dosage adjustment provided in manufacturer's labeling.

Additional Information Complete prescribing information should be consulted for additional detail.

Dosage Forms

Tablet Extended Release, Oral:

Horizant: 300 mg, 600 mg

◆ **Gabapentin Tablets USP (Can)** *see* Gabapentin *on page 943*

◆ **Gabitril** *see* TiaGABine *on page 2032*

◆ **Gablofen** *see* Baclofen *on page 223*

Galantamine (ga LAN ta meen)

Brand Names: U.S. Razadyne; Razadyne ER

Brand Names: Canada Auro-Galantamine ER; Galantamine ER; Mylan-Galantamine ER; PAT-Galantamine ER; PMS-Galantamine ER; Reminyl ER; Teva-Galantamine ER

Index Terms Galantamine Hydrobromide

Pharmacologic Category Acetylcholinesterase Inhibitor (Central)

Use Treatment of mild-to-moderate dementia of Alzheimer's disease

Pregnancy Risk Factor C

Pregnancy Considerations Adverse events have been observed in animal reproduction studies.

Breast-Feeding Considerations It is not known if galantamine is excreted in breast milk. The manufacturer recommends that caution be exercised when administering galantamine to nursing women.

Contraindications Hypersensitivity to galantamine or any component of the formulation

Canadian labeling: Additional contraindications (not in U.S. labeling): Hypersensitivity to other tertiary alkaloids

Warnings/Precautions Use caution in patients with supraventricular conduction delays (without a functional pacemaker in place); Alzheimer's treatment guidelines consider bradycardia to be a relative contraindication for use of centrally active cholinesterase inhibitors. Use caution in patients taking medicines that slow conduction through SA or AV node. Use caution in peptic ulcer disease (or in patients at risk); seizure disorder; asthma; COPD; mild to moderate liver dysfunction; moderate renal dysfunction. May cause bladder outflow obstruction. May cause CNS depression, which may impair physical or mental abilities; patients must be cautioned about performing tasks that require mental alertness (eg, operating machinery or driving). Skin reactions including Stevens-Johnson syndrome, acute generalized exanthematous pustulosis and erythema multiforme have been reported (Reminyl ER Canadian product monograph, 2014); treatment discontinuation may be necessary if skin reaction occurs. Weight loss has been observed; monitor body weight. Limited safety data in patients ≥85 years of age. Use with caution particularly in elderly patients with low body weight and/or serious comorbidities; adjust dose with caution. Potentially significant drug-drug interactions may exist, requiring dose or frequency adjustment, additional monitoring, and/or selection of alternative therapy.

Adverse Reactions

Cardiovascular: Bradycardia, chest pain, hypertension, peripheral edema, syncope (dose related)

Central nervous system: Agitation, anxiety, confusion, depression, dizziness, fatigue, fever, hallucination, headache, insomnia, malaise, somnolence

Dermatologic: Purpura

Gastrointestinal: Abdominal pain, anorexia, constipation, diarrhea, dyspepsia, flatulence, nausea, vomiting, weight loss

Genitourinary: Hematuria, incontinence, urinary tract infection

Hematologic: Anemia

Neuromuscular & skeletal: Back pain, fall, tremor, weakness

Respiratory: Bronchitis, cough, rhinitis, upper respiratory infection

Rare but important or life-threatening): Aphasia, apraxia, ataxia, atrial fibrillation, AV block, bundle branch block, cystitis, dehydration, delirium, diverticulitis, dysphagia, epistaxis, esophageal perforation, gastrointestinal bleeding, heart failure, hepatitis, hyperglycemia, hyper-/hypokinesia, hypersensitivity reactions, hypertonia, hypokalemia, hypotension, libido increased, liver enzymes increased, MI, nightmares, nocturia, orthostatic hypotension, QT prolongation, rectal hemorrhage, renal calculi, renal failure (due to dehydration), seizure, stroke, suicide, supraventricular tachycardia, T-wave inversion, thrombocytopenia, TIA, urinary retention, ventricular tachycardia

Drug Interactions

Metabolism/Transport Effects Substrate of CYP2D6 (minor), CYP3A4 (minor); **Note:** Assignment of Major/Minor substrate status based on clinically relevant drug interaction potential

Avoid Concomitant Use

Avoid concomitant use of Galantamine with any of the following: Ceritinib

Increased Effect/Toxicity

Galantamine may increase the levels/effects of: Antipsychotic Agents; Beta-Blockers; Bradycardia-Causing Agents; Ceritinib; Cholinergic Agonists; Highest Risk QTc-Prolonging Agents; Lacosamide; Moderate Risk QTc-Prolonging Agents; Succinylcholine

The levels/effects of Galantamine may be increased by: Bretylium; Corticosteroids (Systemic); Mifepristone; Selective Serotonin Reuptake Inhibitors; Tofacitinib

Decreased Effect

Galantamine may decrease the levels/effects of: Anticholinergic Agents; Neuromuscular-Blocking Agents (Nondepolarizing)

The levels/effects of Galantamine may be decreased by: Anticholinergic Agents; Dipyridamole

Storage/Stability Store at 25°C (77°F); excursions permitted to 15°C to 30°C (59°F to 86°F). Do not freeze oral solution.

Mechanism of Action Centrally-acting cholinesterase inhibitor (competitive and reversible). It elevates acetylcholine in cerebral cortex by slowing the degradation of acetylcholine. Modulates nicotinic acetylcholine receptor to increase acetylcholine from surviving presynaptic nerve terminals. May increase glutamate and serotonin levels.

Pharmacodynamics/Kinetics

Duration: 3 hours; maximum inhibition of erythrocyte acetylcholinesterase ~40% at 1 hour post 8 mg oral dose; levels return to baseline at 30 hours

Absorption: Rapid and complete

Distribution: 175 L; levels in the brain are 2-3 times higher than in plasma

Protein binding: 18%

Metabolism: Hepatic; linear, CYP2D6 and 3A4; metabolized to epigalanthaminone and galanthaminone both of which have acetylcholinesterase inhibitory activity 130 times less than galantamine

Bioavailability: ~90%

Half-life elimination: ~7 hours

Time to peak: Immediate release: 1 hour (2.5 hours with food); extended release: 4.5-5 hours

Excretion: Urine (20%)

Dosage Oral: Adults: **Note:** If therapy is interrupted for ≥3 days, restart at the lowest dose and increase to current dose.

Alzheimer's dementia (mild-to-moderate):

Immediate release tablet or solution: Initial: 4 mg twice a day for 4 weeks; if tolerated, increase to 8 mg twice daily for ≥4 weeks; if tolerated, increase to 12 mg twice daily. Range: 16-24 mg/day in 2 divided doses

Extended-release capsule: Initial: 8 mg once daily for 4 weeks; if tolerated, increase to 16 mg once daily for ≥4 weeks; if tolerated, increase to 24 mg once daily. Range: 16-24 mg once daily

Conversion from immediate release to extended release formulation: Patients may be switched from the immediate release formulation to the extended release formulation by taking the last immediate release dose in the evening and beginning the extended release dose the following morning; the same total daily dose should be used.

Conversion to galantamine from other cholinesterase inhibitors: Patients experiencing poor tolerability with donepezil or rivastigmine should wait until side effects subside or allow a 7-day washout period prior to beginning galantamine. Patients not experiencing side effects with donepezil or rivastigmine may begin galantamine therapy the day immediately following discontinuation of previous therapy (Morris, 2001).

Elderly: Refer to adult dosing; adjust dose with caution in patients with low body weight and/or serious comorbidities.

Dosage adjustment in renal impairment:

Mild impairment: There are no dosage adjustments provided in the manufacturer's labeling.

Moderate impairment: Maximum dose: 16 mg/day.

Severe impairment (CrCl <9 mL/minute): Use is not recommended

Dosage adjustment in hepatic impairment:

U.S. labeling:

Mild impairment (Child-Pugh score 5 to 6): There are no dosage adjustments provided in the manufacturer's labeling; however, single-dose galantamine pharmacokinetics were similar to that observed in healthy subjects.

Moderate impairment (Child-Pugh score 7 to 9): Maximum dose: 16 mg/day

Severe impairment (Child-Pugh score 10 to 15): Use is not recommended

Canadian labeling:

Mild impairment: (Child-Pugh score 5 to 6): There are no dosage adjustments provided in the manufacturer's labeling; however, single-dose galantamine pharmacokinetics were similar to that observed in healthy subjects.

Moderate impairment: (Child-Pugh score 7 to 9): Initial: 8 mg every other day for at least 1 week, then increase to 8 mg once daily for at least 4 weeks (maximum dose: 16 mg daily)

Severe impairment (Child-Pugh score 10 to 15): Use is not recommended

Dietary Considerations Administration with food is preferred, but not required; should be taken with breakfast and dinner (tablet or solution) or with breakfast (capsule).

Administration Oral: Administer solution or tablet with breakfast and dinner; administer extended release capsule with breakfast. If therapy is interrupted for ≥3 days, restart at the lowest dose and increase to current dose. If using oral solution, mix dose with 3-4 ounces of any nonalcoholic beverage; mix well and drink immediately.

Monitoring Parameters Mental status; body weight

Dosage Forms

Capsule Extended Release 24 Hour, Oral:

Razadyne ER: 8 mg, 16 mg, 24 mg

Generic: 8 mg, 16 mg, 24 mg

Solution, Oral:

Generic: 4 mg/mL (100 mL)

Tablet, Oral:

Razadyne: 4 mg, 8 mg, 12 mg

Generic: 4 mg, 8 mg, 12 mg

- ◆ **Galantamine ER (Can)** *see* Galantamine *on page 946*
- ◆ **Galantamine Hydrobromide** *see* Galantamine *on page 946*
- ◆ **Galexos (Can)** *see* Simeprevir *on page 1887*

Gallamine Triethiodide [INT]

(GAL a meen trye eth EYE oh dide)

International Brand Names Flaxedil (AR, AU, GB, HR, NL); Flaxedyl (HU); Galaflax (AR); Gallasin (KR); Galonin (KR); Miowas G (ES); Relaxan (DK)

Pharmacologic Category Skeletal Muscle Relaxant

Reported Use Produce skeletal muscle relaxation during surgery after general anesthesia has been induced; aid controlled ventilation

Dosage Range IV: 80-120 mg for prolonged procedures; an additional dose of 20-40 mg may be used

Product Availability Product available in various countries; not currently available in the U.S.

Dosage Forms Injection: 20 mg/mL (10 mL)

- ◆ **Galzin** *see* Zinc Acetate *on page 2199*
- ◆ **GamaSTAN S/D** *see* Immune Globulin *on page 1056*
- ◆ **Gamastan S/D (Can)** *see* Immune Globulin *on page 1056*
- ◆ **Gamma Benzene Hexachloride** *see* Lindane *on page 1217*
- ◆ **Gammagard** *see* Immune Globulin *on page 1056*
- ◆ **Gammagard Liquid (Can)** *see* Immune Globulin *on page 1056*
- ◆ **Gammagard S/D** *see* Immune Globulin *on page 1056*
- ◆ **Gammagard S/D Less IgA** *see* Immune Globulin *on page 1056*
- ◆ **Gamma Globulin** *see* Immune Globulin *on page 1056*
- ◆ **Gamma Hydroxybutyric Acid** *see* Sodium Oxybate *on page 1908*
- ◆ **Gammaked** *see* Immune Globulin *on page 1056*
- ◆ **Gammaphos** *see* Amifostine *on page 109*
- ◆ **Gammaplex** *see* Immune Globulin *on page 1056*
- ◆ **Gamunex (Can)** *see* Immune Globulin *on page 1056*
- ◆ **Gamunex-C** *see* Immune Globulin *on page 1056*

Ganciclovir (Systemic) (gan SYE kloe veer)

Brand Names: U.S. Cytovene

Brand Names: Canada Cytovene®

Index Terms DHPG Sodium; GCV Sodium; Nordeoxyguanosine

Pharmacologic Category Antiviral Agent

Use Treatment of CMV retinitis in immunocompromised individuals, including patients with acquired immunodeficiency syndrome; prophylaxis of CMV infection in transplant patients

Pregnancy Risk Factor C

Pregnancy Considerations [U.S. Boxed Warning]: Animal studies have demonstrated carcinogenic and teratogenic effects, and inhibition of spermatogenesis. Female patients should use effective contraception during therapy; male patients should use a barrier contraceptive during and for at least 90 days after therapy.

Breast-Feeding Considerations Due to the carcinogenic and teratogenic effects observed in animal studies, the possibility of adverse events in a nursing infant is considered likely. Therefore, nursing should be discontinued during therapy. In addition, the CDC recommends **not** to breast-feed if diagnosed with HIV to avoid postnatal transmission of the virus.

Contraindications Hypersensitivity to ganciclovir, acyclovir, or any component of the formulation

Warnings/Precautions Hazardous agent - use appropriate precautions for handling and disposal (NIOSH 2014 [group 2]).

[U.S. Boxed Warning]: Granulocytopenia (neutropenia), anemia, and thrombocytopenia may occur. Dosage adjustment or interruption of ganciclovir therapy may be necessary in patients with neutropenia and/or thrombocytopenia and patients with impaired renal function. **[U.S. Boxed Warning]: Animal studies have demonstrated carcinogenic and teratogenic effects, and inhibition of spermatogenesis;** contraceptive precautions for female and male patients need to be followed during and for at least 90 days after therapy with the drug; take care to administer only into veins with good blood flow. **[U.S. Boxed Warning]: Indicated only for treatment of CMV retinitis in the immunocompromised patient and CMV prevention in transplant patients at risk.**

Adverse Reactions

Central nervous system: Chills, fever, neuropathy

Dermatologic: Pruritus

Gastrointestinal: Anorexia, diarrhea, vomiting

Hematologic: Anemia, leukopenia, neutropenia with ANC $<500/mm^3$, thrombocytopenia

Ocular: Retinal detachment (relationship to ganciclovir not established)

Renal: Serum creatinine increased

Miscellaneous: Diaphoresis, sepsis

Rare but important or life-threatening: Allergic reaction (including anaphylaxis), alopecia, arrhythmia, bronchospasm, cardiac arrest, cataracts, cholestasis, coma, dyspnea, edema, encephalopathy, exfoliative dermatitis, extrapyramidal symptoms, hepatitis, hepatic failure, pancreatitis, pancytopenia, pulmonary fibrosis, psychosis, rhabdomyolysis, seizure, alopecia, urticaria, eosinophilia, hemorrhage, Stevens-Johnson syndrome, torsade de pointes, renal failure, SIADH, visual loss

Drug Interactions

Metabolism/Transport Effects None known.

Avoid Concomitant Use

Avoid concomitant use of Ganciclovir (Systemic) with any of the following: Imipenem

Increased Effect/Toxicity

Ganciclovir (Systemic) may increase the levels/effects of: Imipenem; Mycophenolate; Reverse Transcriptase Inhibitors (Nucleoside); Tenofovir

The levels/effects of Ganciclovir (Systemic) may be increased by: Mycophenolate; Probenecid; Tenofovir

Decreased Effect There are no known significant interactions involving a decrease in effect.

Preparation for Administration Hazardous agent; use appropriate precautions for handling and disposal (NIOSH 2014 [group 2]).

Reconstitute 500 mg vial with 10 mL unpreserved sterile water **not** bacteriostatic water because parabens may cause precipitation. Typically, dilute in 100 mL D_5W or NS to a concentration ≤10 mg/mL for infusion.

Storage/Stability Store intact vials at temperatures below 40°C (104°F). Reconstituted solution is stable for 12 hours at room temperature, however, conflicting data indicates that reconstituted solution is stable for 60 days under refrigeration (4°C). Stability of parenteral admixture at room temperature (25°C) and at refrigeration temperature (4°C) for 35 days has been reported. However, the manufacturer recommends use within 24 hours of preparation.

Mechanism of Action Ganciclovir is phosphorylated to a substrate which competitively inhibits the binding of deoxyguanosine triphosphate to DNA polymerase resulting in inhibition of viral DNA synthesis

Pharmacodynamics/Kinetics

Distribution: V_d: 15.26 L/1.73 m^2; widely to all tissues including CSF and ocular tissue

Protein binding: 1% to 2%

Half-life elimination: 1.7-5.8 hours; prolonged with renal impairment; End-stage renal disease: 5-28 hours

Excretion: Urine (80% to 99% as unchanged drug)

Dosage

CMV CNS infection in HIV-exposed/-infected patients (off-label use; CDC, 2009): Infants, Children, and Adults: IV: 5 mg/kg/dose every 12 hours plus foscarnet until symptoms improve followed by chronic suppression

CMV retinitis:

Children and Adults: IV (slow infusion):

Induction therapy: 5 mg/kg/dose every 12 hours for 14-21 days followed by maintenance therapy

Maintenance therapy: 5 mg/kg/day as a single daily dose for 7 days/week or 6 mg/kg/day for 5 days/week

Prevention (secondary) of CMV disease in HIV-exposed/-infected patients (off-label use; CDC, 2009): Infants, Children, and Adults: IV: 5 mg/kg/dose daily

Prevention (secondary) of CMV disease in transplant patients: Children and Adults: IV (slow infusion): 5 mg/kg/dose every 12 hours for 7-14 days; duration of maintenance therapy is dependent on clinical condition and degree of immunosuppression

Varicella zoster: Progressive outer retinal necrosis in HIV-exposed/-infected patients (off-label use; CDC, 2009): Infants, Children, and Adults: IV: 5 mg/kg/dose every 12 hours plus systemic foscarnet and intravitreal ganciclovir or intravitreal foscarnet

Elderly: Refer to adult dosing; in general, dose selection should be cautious, reflecting greater frequency of organ impairment

Dosage adjustment in renal impairment:

IV (Induction):

CrCl 50-69 mL/minute: Administer 2.5 mg/kg/dose every 12 hours

CrCl 25-49 mL/minute: Administer 2.5 mg/kg/dose every 24 hours

CrCl 10-24 mL/minute: Administer 1.25 mg/kg/dose every 24 hours

CrCl <10 mL/minute: Administer 1.25 mg/kg/dose 3 times/week following hemodialysis

IV (Maintenance):

CrCl 50-69 mL/minute: Administer 2.5 mg/kg/dose every 24 hours

CrCl 25-49 mL/minute: Administer 1.25 mg/kg/dose every 24 hours

CrCl 10-24 mL/minute: Administer 0.625 mg/kg/dose every 24 hours

CrCl <10 mL/minute: Administer 0.625 mg/kg/dose 3 times/week following hemodialysis

Intermittent hemodialysis (IHD) (administer after hemodialysis on dialysis days): Dialyzable (50%): CMV Infection: IV: Induction: 1.25 mg/kg every 48-72 hours; Maintenance: 0.625 mg/kg every 48-72 hours. **Note:** Dosing dependent on the assumption of 3 times/week, complete IHD sessions.

Peritoneal dialysis (PD): Dose as for CrCl <10 mL/minute.

Continuous renal replacement therapy (CRRT) (Heintz, 2009; Trotman, 2005): Drug clearance is highly dependent on the method of renal replacement, filter type, and flow rate. Appropriate dosing requires close monitoring of pharmacologic response, signs of adverse reactions due to drug accumulation, as well as drug concentrations in relation to target trough (if appropriate). The following are general recommendations only (based on dialysate flow/ultrafiltration rates of 1-2 L/hour and minimal residual renal function) and should not supersede clinical judgment: CMV Infection:

CVVH: IV: Induction: 2.5 mg/kg every 24 hours; Maintenance: 1.25 mg/kg every 24 hours

CVVHD/CVVHDF: IV: Induction: 2.5 mg/kg every 12 hours; Maintenance: 2.5 mg/kg every 24 hours

Dosage adjustment in hepatic impairment: No dosage adjustment provided in manufacturer's labeling.

Dietary Considerations Some products may contain sodium.

Administration Should not be administered by IM, SubQ, or rapid IVP; administer by slow IV infusion over at least 1 hour. Too rapid infusion can cause increased toxicity and excessive plasma levels. Flush line well with NS before and after administration.

Hazardous agent; use appropriate precautions for handling and disposal (NIOSH 2014 [group 2]).

Monitoring Parameters CBC with differential and platelet count, serum creatinine

Dosage Forms

Solution Reconstituted, Intravenous:

Cytovene: 500 mg (1 ea)

Generic: 500 mg (1 ea)

Ganirelix (ga ni REL ix)

Brand Names: Canada Orgalutran®

Index Terms Antagon; Ganirelix Acetate

Pharmacologic Category Gonadotropin Releasing Hormone Antagonist

Use Inhibits premature luteinizing hormone (LH) surges in women undergoing controlled ovarian hyperstimulation

Pregnancy Risk Factor X

Dosage Adult: SubQ: 250 mcg/day during the mid-to-late phase after initiating follicle-stimulating hormone on day 2 or 3 of cycle. Treatment should be continued daily until the day of chorionic gonadotropin administration.

Dosage adjustment in renal impairment: No dosage adjustment provided in manufacturer's labeling (has not been studied).

Dosage adjustment in hepatic impairment: No dosage adjustment provided in manufacturer's labeling (has not been studied).

Additional Information Complete prescribing information should be consulted for additional detail.

Dosage Forms

Solution, Subcutaneous:

Generic: 250 mcg/0.5 mL (0.5 mL)

◆ **Ganirelix Acetate** *see* Ganirelix *on page 949*

◆ **GAR-936** *see* Tigecycline *on page 2040*

◆ **Garamycin** *see* Gentamicin (Ophthalmic) *on page 962*

◆ **Garamycin® (Can)** *see* Gentamicin (Ophthalmic) *on page 962*

◆ **Gardasil** *see* Papillomavirus (Types 6, 11, 16, 18) Vaccine (Human, Recombinant) *on page 1574*

Gatifloxacin (gat i FLOKS a sin)

Brand Names: U.S. Zymaxid

Brand Names: Canada Zymar

Pharmacologic Category Antibiotic, Fluoroquinolone; Antibiotic, Ophthalmic

Use Treatment of bacterial conjunctivitis

Pregnancy Risk Factor C

Dosage Ophthalmic: Children ≥1 year and Adults: Bacterial conjunctivitis:

Zymar:

Days 1 and 2: Instill 1 drop into affected eye(s) every 2 hours while awake (maximum: 8 times/day)

Days 3-7: Instill 1 drop into affected eye(s) 4 times/day while awake

Zymaxid:

Day 1: Instill 1 drop into affected eye(s) every 2 hours while awake (maximum: 8 times/day)

Days 2-7: Instill 1 drop into affected eye(s) 2-4 times/day while awake

Dosage adjustment in renal impairment: No dosage adjustment provided in manufacturer's labeling. However, dosage adjustment unlikely due to low systemic absorption.

Dosage adjustment in hepatic impairment: No dosage adjustment provided in manufacturer's labeling. However, dosage adjustment unlikely due to low systemic absorption.

Additional Information Complete prescribing information should be consulted for additional detail.

Dosage Forms

Solution, Ophthalmic:

Zymaxid: 0.5% (2.5 mL)

Generic: 0.5% (2.5 mL)

Dosage Forms: Canada

Solution, ophthalmic [drops]:

Zymar: 0.3% (1 mL, 2.5 mL, 5 mL)

- ◆ **Gattex** *see* Teduglutide *on page* 1982
- ◆ **GaviLAX [OTC]** *see* Polyethylene Glycol 3350 *on page* 1674
- ◆ **GaviLyte-C** *see* Polyethylene Glycol-Electrolyte Solution *on page* 1674
- ◆ **GaviLyte-G** *see* Polyethylene Glycol-Electrolyte Solution *on page* 1674
- ◆ **GaviLyte-N** *see* Polyethylene Glycol-Electrolyte Solution *on page* 1674
- ◆ **Gaviscon® Extra Strength [OTC]** *see* Aluminum Hydroxide and Magnesium Carbonate *on page* 103
- ◆ **Gaviscon® Liquid [OTC]** *see* Aluminum Hydroxide and Magnesium Carbonate *on page* 103
- ◆ **Gaviscon® Tablet [OTC]** *see* Aluminum Hydroxide and Magnesium Trisilicate *on page* 103
- ◆ **Gazyva** *see* Obinutuzumab *on page* 1482
- ◆ **G-CSF** *see* Filgrastim *on page* 875
- ◆ **G-CSF (PEG Conjugate)** *see* Pegfilgrastim *on page* 1589
- ◆ **GCV Sodium** *see* Ganciclovir (Systemic) *on page* 948
- ◆ **GD-Amlodipine (Can)** *see* AmLODIPine *on page* 123
- ◆ **GD-Atorvastatin (Can)** *see* AtorvaSTATin *on page* 194
- ◆ **GD-Azithromycin (Can)** *see* Azithromycin (Systemic) *on page* 216
- ◆ **GDC-0449** *see* Vismodegib *on page* 2171
- ◆ **GD-Gabapentin (Can)** *see* Gabapentin *on page* 943
- ◆ **GD-Latanoprost (Can)** *see* Latanoprost *on page* 1172
- ◆ **GD-Mirtazapine OD (Can)** *see* Mirtazapine *on page* 1376
- ◆ **GD-Pregabalin (Can)** *see* Pregabalin *on page* 1710
- ◆ **GD-Quinapril (Can)** *see* Quinapril *on page* 1756
- ◆ **GD-Sertraline (Can)** *see* Sertraline *on page* 1878
- ◆ **GD-Sildenafil (Can)** *see* Sildenafil *on page* 1882
- ◆ **GD-Terbinafine (Can)** *see* Terbinafine (Systemic) *on page* 2002
- ◆ **GD-Topiramate (Can)** *see* Topiramate *on page* 2065
- ◆ **GD-Venlafaxine XR (Can)** *see* Venlafaxine *on page* 2150

Gefitinib [CAN/INT] (ge FI tye nib)

Brand Names: Canada IRESSA

Index Terms ZD1839

Pharmacologic Category Antineoplastic Agent, Epidermal Growth Factor Receptor (EGFR) Inhibitor; Antineoplastic Agent, Tyrosine Kinase Inhibitor

Use Note: Not approved in U.S.

Non-small cell lung cancer: First-line treatment of locally advanced (nonresponsive to curative therapy) or metastatic non-small cell lung cancer (NSCLC) with activating mutations of the epidermal growth factor receptor tyrosine kinase (EGFR-TK)

Pregnancy Considerations Adverse events have been observed in animal reproduction studies. Gefitinib may cause fetal harm when administered to a pregnant woman.

Breast-Feeding Considerations It is not known if gefitinib is excreted in breast milk. Due to the potential for serious adverse reactions in the nursing infant, breast-feeding is not recommended by the manufacturer.

Contraindications Hypersensitivity to gefitinib or any component of the formulation

Warnings/Precautions Hazardous agent - use appropriate precautions for handling and disposal (meets NIOSH 2014 criteria). **[Canadian Boxed Warning]: Should be administered under the supervision of an experienced cancer chemotherapy healthcare professional. [Canadian Boxed Warning]: Not to be used in patients with EGFR mutation-negative tumors.** EGFR mutation-positive status must be established prior to initiating therapy. Incidence of positive mutation is higher in Asian patients (~40%) than non-Asian patients (~10%). In all patients, independent predictors of positive mutation include female gender, never smoker, and adenocarcinoma histology. EGFR mutations, specifically exon 19 deletions and exon 21 mutation (L858R), are associated with better response to gefitinib in patients with NSCLC (Riely, 2006).

[Canadian Boxed Warning]: Gastrointestinal perforation has been observed, including some fatalities; cases have been rare and mostly associated with other risk factors (eg, concomitant steroids or NSAIDS, increased age, history of GI ulceration, smoking). If perforation is confirmed, interrupt or discontinue use. Diarrhea, nausea/vomiting, anorexia, and stomatitis have been observed. Advise patients to consult health care provider for severe or persistent symptoms.

[Canadian Boxed Warning]: Hepatic failure and fulminant hepatitis have been reported rarely (with some fatalities). Asymptomatic increases in transaminases have also been reported; monitor liver function periodically. Use caution with mild to moderate changes in hepatic function. Consider discontinuing therapy if changes are severe. Gefitinib exposure may be increased in patients with moderate to severe hepatic impairment due to cirrhosis. Some data suggest systemic exposure in moderate or severe impairment secondary to hepatic metastases was similar to that with normal hepatic function. Monitor closely; dosage adjustments are not recommended for moderate to severe impairment. **[Canadian Boxed Warning]: Use in severe renal impairment has not been studied.** Renal failure secondary to dehydration has been observed. Interrupt therapy for severe/persistent diarrhea or cases leading to dehydration, particularly in the presence of other risk factors (eg, renal disease, concurrent use of diuretics or NSAIDS); rehydrate as clinically indicated. Monitor renal function and electrolytes in patients at high risk of dehydration.

Rare, sometimes fatal, interstitial lung disease (ILD) has occurred; may be acute in onset. Therapy should be interrupted in patients with worsening pulmonary symptoms (dyspnea, cough, fever); discontinue if ILD is confirmed. Epistaxis and hematuria have been commonly reported. Ophthalmic infections (eg, conjunctivitis, blepharitis) and dry eye are commonly observed, although symptoms are typically mild. Corneal erosion has been reported (rarely); corneal erosion is reversible and occasionally associated with abnormal eyelash growth. Keratoconjunctivitis sicca or keratitis have also been reported; recent corneal surgery and contact lens wearing are risk factors for ocular toxicity. Advise patients to promptly report developing eye symptoms and promptly refer for ophthalmic evaluation if signs of keratitis. Interrupt therapy if ulcerative keratitis is confirmed, and manage symptoms as clinically indicated. Consider permanent discontinuation if symptoms do not resolve or recur upon rechallenge. Safety of contact lens use during therapy has not been studied.

Skin rash is commonly observed; toxic epidermal necrolysis, Stevens-Johnson syndrome, and erythema multiforme have been observed (rarely) with some fatalities. Cutaneous vasculitis and skin fissures (including rhagades) have also been reported. Gefitinib may also have photosensitivity potential. Weakness has been reported; advise patients who experience weakness to use caution when driving or operating machinery. Potentially significant drug-drug interactions may exist, requiring dose or frequency adjustment, additional monitoring, and/or selection of alternative therapy. Systemic exposure of gefitinib may be increased in CYP2D6 poor metabolizers. May contain lactose; consider intolerance risk in patients with galactose intolerance, Lapp lactase deficiency, or glucose-galactose malabsorption.

Adverse Reactions

Central nervous system: Fatigue, hypoesthesia, insomnia, peripheral neuropathy, peripheral sensory neuropathy

Dermatologic: Acneiform eruption, acne vulgaris, alopecia, dermatological reaction (including pustular rash, itching, dry skin, skin fissures on an erythematous base), nail disease, paronychia, pruritus, skin rash, xeroderma

Endocrine & metabolic: Dehydration (secondary to diarrhea, nausea, vomiting, or anorexia)

Gastrointestinal: Anorexia, constipation, diarrhea, nausea, stomatitis, vomiting, xerostomia

Genitourinary: Cystitis, proteinuria

Hematologic & oncologic: Anemia, hemorrhage (including epistaxis, hematuria), leukopenia, neutropenia, pulmonary hemorrhage, thrombocytopenia

Hepatic: Increased serum ALT, increased serum AST, increased serum bilirubin

Neuromuscular & skeletal: Arthralgia, myalgia, weakness

Ophthalmic: Eye disease (including conjunctivitis, blepharitis, and dry eye)

Renal: Increased serum creatinine

Respiratory: Cough, interstitial pulmonary disease

Miscellaneous: Fever

Rare but important or life-threatening: Corneal erosion (reversible; may be associated with aberrant eyelash growth), erythema multiforme, gastrointestinal perforation, hemorrhagic cystitis, hepatic failure, hepatitis, hypersensitivity angiitis, hypersensitivity reaction, keratitis, keratoconjunctivitis sicca, pancreatitis, renal failure, Stevens-Johnson syndrome

Drug Interactions

Metabolism/Transport Effects **Substrate** of BCRP, CYP2D6 (major), CYP3A4 (major); **Note:** Assignment of Major/Minor substrate status based on clinically relevant drug interaction potential; **Inhibits** BCRP, CYP2C19 (weak), CYP2D6 (weak)

Avoid Concomitant Use

Avoid concomitant use of Gefitinib with any of the following: Conivaptan; Fusidic Acid (Systemic); Idelalisib; PAZOPanib

Increased Effect/Toxicity

Gefitinib may increase the levels/effects of: ARIPiprazole; PAZOPanib; Topotecan; Vinorelbine; Vitamin K Antagonists

The levels/effects of Gefitinib may be increased by: Abiraterone Acetate; Aprepitant; Ceritinib; Conivaptan; CYP2D6 Inhibitors (Moderate); CYP2D6 Inhibitors (Strong); CYP3A4 Inhibitors (Moderate); CYP3A4 Inhibitors (Strong); Dasatinib; Fosaprepitant; Fusidic Acid (Systemic); Idelalisib; Ivacaftor; Luliconazole; Mifepristone; Netupitant; Peginterferon Alfa-2b; Simeprevir; Stiripentol; Teriflunomide

Decreased Effect

The levels/effects of Gefitinib may be decreased by: Bosentan; CYP3A4 Inducers (Moderate); CYP3A4 Inducers (Strong); Dabrafenib; Deferasirox; H2-Antagonists; Mitotane; Peginterferon Alfa-2b; Proton Pump Inhibitors; Siltuximab; St Johns Wort; Tocilizumab

Food Interactions Grapefruit juice may increase serum gefitinib concentrations. Management: Avoid concurrent use.

Storage/Stability Store tablets at 15°C to 30°C (59°F to 86°F). Protect from moisture.

Mechanism of Action Gefitinib is a tyrosine kinase inhibitor (TKI) which inhibits numerous tyrosine kinases associated with transmembrane cell surface receptors found on both normal and cancer cells, including the tyrosine kinase associated with the epidermal growth factor receptor, EGFR. Tyrosine kinase activity appears to be vitally important to cell proliferation and survival.

Pharmacodynamics/Kinetics

Absorption: Oral: Slow

Distribution: 1400 L

Protein binding: 90%, albumin and alpha$_1$-acid glycoprotein

Metabolism: Hepatic, primarily via CYP3A4; forms metabolites

Bioavailability: 60%

Half-life elimination: Oral: 41 hours

Time to peak, plasma: Oral: 3 to 7 hours

Excretion: Feces (86%); urine (<4%)

Dosage Non-small cell lung cancer (NSCLC), first-line therapy in patients with EGFR mutations:

Adolescents ≥17 years and Adults: Oral: 250 mg once daily

Elderly: Refer to adult dosing.

Dosage adjustment for toxicity:

Worsening pulmonary symptoms (cough, dyspnea, fever): Interrupt treatment and evaluate promptly; discontinue if interstitial lung disease is confirmed

Diarrhea (poorly tolerated or associated with dehydration) or skin toxicity: Interrupt treatment for up to 14 days; may reinitiate at 250 mg once daily. Discontinue gefitinib if patient is unable to tolerate rechallenge following treatment interruption.

Ocular symptoms: Evaluate and interrupt treatment based on symptoms; once symptoms or eye changes have resolved, may consider reinitiating at 250 mg once daily. Discontinue gefitinib if patient is unable to tolerate rechallenge following treatment interruption.

Dosage adjustment in renal impairment: No dosage adjustment necessary. Use caution in severe impairment (CrCl ≤20 mL/minute).

Dosage adjustment in hepatic impairment: No dosage adjustment necessary. Use caution in moderate to severe impairment (Child-Pugh class B or C) (systemic exposure may be increased); monitor closely.

Administration Oral: Administer with or without food. For missed doses, administer as soon as possible if at least 12 hours until next scheduled dose. If <12 hours, skip missed dose and take next dose at regularly scheduled time.

Hazardous agent; use appropriate precautions for handling and disposal (meets NIOSH 2014 criteria).

Monitoring Parameters EGFR mutation status prior to initiating therapy; liver function tests (ALT, AST, bilirubin at baseline and periodically thereafter); BUN, creatinine, and electrolytes (baseline and periodically thereafter); INR or prothrombin time (with concurrent warfarin treatment), pulmonary symptoms

Additional Information Oncology Comment: Recent studies have demonstrated a subset of patients who are more likely to respond to treatment with gefitinib. This subset includes: patients of Asian origin, never-smokers, women, patients with bronchoalveolar adenocarcinoma, and patients with EGFR-mutated tumors. Deletion in exon 19 and mutation in exon 21 are the two most commonly found EGFR mutations; both mutations correlate with clinical response, resulting in increased response rates in patients with the mutation (Riely, 2006). Studies have compared gefitinib in treatment naïve patients to combination chemotherapy in the subsets of patients described above, resulting in a longer progression free survival in the gefitinib arm (Mok, 2009). Based on these data, the ASCO guidelines state that the first-line use of gefitinib may be recommended in stage IV disease with activating EGFR mutations (Azzoli, 2009; Azzoli, 2011). In patients with a *KRAS* mutation, however, EGFR-TKI therapy is not recommended.

Product Availability Not available in U.S.

Dosage Forms: Canada

Tablet, oral:

Iressa: 250 mg

- ◆ **Gel-Kam [OTC]** *see* Fluoride *on page 895*
- ◆ **Gel-Kam Rinse** *see* Fluoride *on page 895*
- ◆ **Gelnique** *see* Oxybutynin *on page 1536*
- ◆ **Gel-One** *see* Hyaluronate and Derivatives *on page 1006*
- ◆ **Gelucast®** *see* Zinc Gelatin *on page 2200*
- ◆ **Gelusil [OTC]** *see* Aluminum Hydroxide, Magnesium Hydroxide, and Simethicone *on page 104*
- ◆ **Gelusil (Can)** *see* Aluminum Hydroxide, Magnesium Hydroxide, and Simethicone *on page 104*
- ◆ **Gelusil® Extra Strength (Can)** *see* Aluminum Hydroxide and Magnesium Hydroxide *on page 103*

Gemcitabine (jem SITE a been)

Brand Names: U.S. Gemzar

Brand Names: Canada Gemcitabine For Injection; Gemcitabine For Injection Concentrate; Gemcitabine For Injection, USP; Gemcitabine Hydrochloride For Injection; Gemcitabine Injection; Gemcitabine Sun For Injection; Gemzar

Index Terms dFdC; dFdCyd; Difluorodeoxycytidine Hydrochlorothiazide; Gemcitabine Hydrochloride; LY-188011

Pharmacologic Category Antineoplastic Agent, Antimetabolite; Antineoplastic Agent, Antimetabolite (Pyrimidine Analog)

Use

Breast cancer: First-line treatment of metastatic breast cancer (in combination with paclitaxel) after failure of adjuvant chemotherapy which contained an anthracycline (unless contraindicated)

Non-small cell lung cancer (NSCLC): First-line treatment of inoperable, locally-advanced (stage IIIA or IIIB) or metastatic (stage IV) NSCLC (in combination with cisplatin)

Ovarian cancer: Treatment of advanced ovarian cancer (in combination with carboplatin) that has relapsed at least 6 months following completion of platinum-based chemotherapy

Pancreatic cancer: First-line treatment of locally-advanced (nonresectable stage II or III) or metastatic (stage IV) pancreatic adenocarcinoma

Pregnancy Risk Factor D

Pregnancy Considerations Adverse events were observed in animal reproduction studies. May cause fetal harm if administered during pregnancy; adverse effects in reproduction are anticipated based on the mechanism of action.

Breast-Feeding Considerations It is not known if gemcitabine is excreted in breast milk. Due to the potential for serious adverse reactions in the nursing infant, the decision to discontinue gemcitabine or to discontinue breast-feeding should take into account the benefits of treatment to the mother.

Contraindications Hypersensitivity to gemcitabine or any component of the formulation

Warnings/Precautions Hazardous agent - use appropriate precautions for handling and disposal (NIOSH 2014 [group 1]). Gemcitabine may suppress bone marrow function (neutropenia, thrombocytopenia, and anemia); myelosuppression is usually the dose-limiting toxicity; toxicity is increased when used in combination with other chemotherapy; monitor blood counts; dosage adjustments are frequently required.

Hemolytic uremic syndrome (HUS) has been reported; may lead to renal failure and dialysis (including fatalities); monitor for evidence of anemia with microangiopathic hemolysis (elevation of bilirubin or LDH, reticulocytosis, severe thrombocytopenia, and/or renal failure) and monitor renal function at baseline and periodically during treatment. Permanently discontinue if HUS or severe renal impairment occurs; renal failure may not be reversible despite discontinuation. Serious hepatotoxicity (including liver failure and death) has been reported (when used alone or in combination with other hepatotoxic medications); use in patients with hepatic impairment (history of cirrhosis, hepatitis, or alcoholism) or in patients with hepatic metastases may lead to exacerbation of hepatic impairment. Monitor hepatic function at baseline and periodically during treatment; consider dose adjustments with elevated bilirubin; discontinue if severe liver injury develops. Capillary leak syndrome (CLS) with serious consequences has been reported, both with single-agent gemcitabine and with combination chemotherapy; discontinue if CLS develops.

Pulmonary toxicity, including adult respiratory distress syndrome, interstitial pneumonitis, pulmonary edema, and pulmonary fibrosis, has been observed; may lead to respiratory failure (some fatal) despite discontinuation. Onset for symptoms of pulmonary toxicity may be delayed up to 2 weeks beyond the last dose. Discontinue for unexplained dyspnea (with or without bronchospasm) or other evidence or pulmonary toxicity. Posterior reversible encephalopathy syndrome (PRES) has been reported, both with single-agent therapy and with combination chemotherapy. PRES may manifest with blindness, confusion, headache, hypertension, lethargy, seizure, and other visual and neurologic disturbances. If PRES diagnosis is confirmed, discontinue therapy. Not indicated for use with concurrent radiation therapy; radiation toxicity, including tissue injury, severe mucositis, esophagitis, or pneumonitis, has been reported with concurrent and nonconcurrent administration; may have radiosensitizing activity when gemcitabine and radiation therapy are given ≤7 days apart; radiation recall may occur when gemcitabine and radiation therapy are given >7 days apart. Potentially significant drug-drug interactions may exist, requiring dose or frequency adjustment, additional monitoring, and/or selection of alternative therapy.

Prolongation of the infusion duration >60 minutes or more frequent than weekly dosing have been shown to alter the half-life and increase toxicity (hypotension, flu-like symptoms, myelosuppression, weakness); a fixed-dose rate (FDR) infusion rate of 10 mg/m^2/minute has been studied in adults in order to optimize the pharmacokinetics (off-label); prolonged infusion times increase the intracellular accumulation of the active metabolite, gemcitabine triphosphate (Ko, 2006; Tempero, 2003); patients who receive gemcitabine FDR experience more grade 3/4 hematologic toxicity (Ko, 2006; Poplin, 2009).

Adverse Reactions Adverse reactions reported for single-agent use of gemcitabine only; bone marrow depression is the dose-limiting toxicity.

Cardiovascular: Edema, peripheral edema

Central nervous system: Drowsiness, paresthesia

Dermatologic: Alopecia, skin rash

Gastrointestinal: Diarrhea, nausea and vomiting, stomatitis

Genitourinary: Hematuria, proteinuria

Hematologic & oncologic: Anemia, hemorrhage, neutropenia, thrombocytopenia

Hepatic: Increased serum alkaline phosphatase, increased serum ALT, increased serum AST, increased serum bilirubin

Infection: Infection

Local: Injection site reaction

Renal: Increased blood urea nitrogen, increased serum creatinine

Respiratory: Bronchospasm, dyspnea, flu-like symptoms

Miscellaneous: Fever

Rare but important or life-threatening (reported with single-agent use or with combination therapy): Adult respiratory distress syndrome (acute), anaphylactoid reaction, Budd-Chiari syndrome, bullous pemphigoid, capillary leak syndrome, cardiac arrhythmia, cardiac failure, cellulitis, cerebrovascular accident, desquamation, digital vasculitis, gangrene of skin or other tissue, hemolytic-uremic syndrome, hepatic cirrhosis, hepatic necrosis, hepatic veno-occlusive disease, hepatotoxicity (rare), hypertension, hypotension, increased gamma-glutamyl transferase, interstitial pneumonitis, myocardial infarction, neuropathy, petechiae, pulmonary edema, pulmonary fibrosis, radiation recall phenomenon, renal failure, respiratory failure, reversible posterior leukoencephalopathy syndrome, sepsis, supraventricular cardiac arrhythmia, thrombotic thrombocytopenic purpura

Drug Interactions

Metabolism/Transport Effects None known.

Avoid Concomitant Use

Avoid concomitant use of Gemcitabine with any of the following: BCG; CloZAPine; Dipyrone; Natalizumab; Pimecrolimus; Tacrolimus (Topical); Tofacitinib; Vaccines (Live)

Increased Effect/Toxicity

Gemcitabine may increase the levels/effects of: Bleomycin; CloZAPine; Fluorouracil (Systemic); Fluorouracil (Topical); Leflunomide; Natalizumab; Tofacitinib; Vaccines (Live); Warfarin

The levels/effects of Gemcitabine may be increased by: Denosumab; Dipyrone; Pimecrolimus; Roflumilast; Tacrolimus (Topical); Trastuzumab

Decreased Effect

Gemcitabine may decrease the levels/effects of: BCG; Coccidioides immitis Skin Test; Sipuleucel-T; Vaccines (Inactivated); Vaccines (Live)

The levels/effects of Gemcitabine may be decreased by: Echinacea

Preparation for Administration

Hazardous agent; use appropriate precautions for handling and disposal (NIOSH 2014 [group 1]).

Reconstitute lyophilized powder with preservative free NS; add 5 mL to the 200 mg vial, add 25 mL to the 1000 mg vial, or add 50 mL to the 2000 mg vial, resulting in a reconstituted concentration of 38 mg/mL (solutions must be reconstituted to ≤40 mg/mL to completely dissolve). Gemcitabine is also supplied as a concentrated solution for injection in different concentrations (40 mg/mL [Canada only] and 38 mg/mL); verify product concentration prior to preparation for administration.

Further dilute reconstituted lyophilized powder or concentrated solution for injection in NS for infusion; to concentrations as low as 0.1 mg/mL.

Storage/Stability

Lyophilized powder: Store intact vials at room temperature of 20°C to 25°C (68°F to 77°F); excursions permitted to 15°C to 30°C (59°F to 86°F). Reconstituted vials are stable for 24 hours at room temperature. Do not refrigerate (may form crystals).

Solution for injection: Store intact vials refrigerated at 2°C to 8°C (36°F to 46°F); do not freeze.

Solutions diluted for infusion in NS are stable for 24 hours at room temperature. Do not refrigerate.

Mechanism of Action A pyrimidine antimetabolite that inhibits DNA synthesis by inhibition of DNA polymerase and ribonucleotide reductase, cell cycle-specific for the S-phase of the cycle (also blocks cellular progression at G1/S-phase). Gemcitabine is phosphorylated intracellularly by deoxycytidine kinase to gemcitabine monophosphate, which is further phosphorylated to active metabolites gemcitabine diphosphate and gemcitabine triphosphate. Gemcitabine diphosphate inhibits DNA synthesis by inhibiting ribonucleotide reductase; gemcitabine triphosphate incorporates into DNA and inhibits DNA polymerase.

Pharmacodynamics/Kinetics

Distribution: Infusions <70 minutes: 50 L/m^2; Long infusion times (70-285 minutes): 370 L/m^2

Protein binding: Negligible

Metabolism: Metabolized intracellularly by nucleoside kinases to the active diphosphate (dFdCDP) and triphosphate (dFdCTP) nucleoside metabolites

Half-life elimination:

Gemcitabine: Infusion time ≤70 minutes: 42 to 94 minutes; infusion time 3 to 4 hours: 4 to 10.5 hours (affected by age and gender)

Metabolite (gemcitabine triphosphate), terminal phase: 1.7 to 19.4 hours

Time to peak, plasma: 30 minutes after completion of infusion

Excretion: Urine (92% to 98%; primarily as inactive uracil metabolite); feces (<1%)

Dosage Note: Prolongation of the infusion duration >60 minutes and administration more frequently than once weekly have been shown to increase toxicity.

Pediatrics (refer to specific references for ages of populations studied):

Germ cell tumor, refractory (off-label use): IV: 1000 mg/m^2 over 30 minutes days 1, 8, and 15 every 28 days (in combination with paclitaxel) for up to 6 cycles (Hinton, 2002)

Hodgkin lymphoma, relapsed (off-label use): IV: 1000 mg/m^2 over 100 minutes days 1 and 8; repeat cycle every 21 days (in combination with vinorelbine) (Cole; 2009) **or** 800 mg/m^2 days 1 and 4; repeat cycle every 21 days (in combination with ifosfamide, mesna, vinorelbine, and prednisolone) (Santoro, 2007)

Sarcomas (off-label use): IV:

Ewing's sarcoma, refractory: 675 mg/m^2 over 90 minutes days 1 and 8; repeat cycle every 21 days (in combination with docetaxel) (Navid, 2008)

Osteosarcoma, refractory: 675 mg/m^2 over 90 minutes days 1 and 8; repeat cycle every 21 days (in combination with docetaxel) (Navid, 2008) **or** 1000 mg/m^2 weekly for 7 weeks followed by 1 week rest; then weekly for 3 weeks out of every 4 weeks (Merimsky, 2000)

Adults:

Breast cancer, metastatic: IV: 1250 mg/m^2 over 30 minutes days 1 and 8; repeat cycle every 21 days (in combination with paclitaxel) **or** (off-label dosing; as a single agent) 800 mg/m^2 over 30 minutes days 1, 8, and 15 of a 28-day treatment cycle (Carmichael, 1995)

Non-small cell lung cancer, locally-advanced or metastatic: IV: 1000 mg/m^2 over 30 minutes days 1, 8, and 15; repeat cycle every 28 days (in combination with cisplatin) **or** 1250 mg/m^2 over 30 minutes days 1 and 8; repeat cycle every 21 days (in combination with cisplatin) **or** (off-label combination) 1000 mg/m^2 over 30 minutes days 1 and 8; repeat cycle every 21 days (in combination with carboplatin) for up to 4 cycles (Grønberg, 2009) **or** (off-label combination) 1000 mg/m^2 over 30 minutes days 1, 8, and 15; repeat cycle every 28 days (in combination with carboplatin) for up to 4 cycles (Danson, 2003) **or** (off-label combination) 1000 mg/m^2 over 30 minutes days 1 and 8; repeat cycle every 21 days (in combination with docetaxel) for 8 cycles (Pujol, 2005) **or** (off-label combination) 1000 mg/m^2 days 1, 8, and 15; repeat cycle every 28 days (in combination with vinorelbine) for 6 cycles (Greco, 2007)

Ovarian cancer, advanced: IV: 1000 mg/m^2 over 30 minutes days 1 and 8; repeat cycle every 21 days (in combination with carboplatin) **or** (off-label dosing; as a single agent) 1000 mg/m^2 over 30-60 minutes days 1 and 8; repeat cycle every 21 days (Mutch, 2007) **or** (off-label combination) 1000 mg/m^2 over 30 minutes days 1, 8, and 15; repeat cycle every 28 days (in combination with paclitaxel) for up to 6 cycles (Hinton, 2002)

Pancreatic cancer, locally advanced or metastatic: IV: Initial: 1000 mg/m^2 over 30 minutes once weekly for 7 weeks followed by 1 week rest; then once weekly for 3 weeks out of every 4 weeks **or** (off-label combinations) 1000 mg/m^2 over 30 minutes weekly for up to 7 weeks followed by 1 week rest; then weekly for 3 weeks out of every 4 weeks (in combination with erlotinib) (Moore, 2007) **or** 1000 mg/m^2 over 30 minutes days 1, 8, and 15 every 28 days (in combination with capecitabine) (Cunningham, 2009) **or** 1000 mg/m^2 over 30 minutes days 1 and 15 every 28 days (in combination with cisplatin) (Heinemann, 2006) **or** 1000 mg/m^2 infused at 10 mg/m^2/minute every 14 days (in combination with oxaliplatin) (Louvet, 2005) **or** 1000 mg/m^2 days 1, 8, and 15 every 28 days (in combination with paclitaxel [protein bound]) (Von Hoff, 2013)

Bladder cancer (off-label use):

Advanced or metastatic: IV: 1000 mg/m^2 over 30-60 minutes days 1, 8, and 15; repeat cycle every 28 days (in combination with cisplatin) (von der Maase, 2000) **or** 1000 mg/m^2 over 30 minutes days 1 and 8; repeat cycle every 21 days (in combination with carboplatin) until disease progression or unacceptable toxicity (De Santis, 2012)

Transitional cell carcinoma: Intravesicular instillation: 2000 mg (in 100 mL NS; retain for 1 hour) twice weekly for 3 weeks; repeat cycle every 4 weeks for at least 2 cycles (Dalbagni, 2006)

Cervical cancer, recurrent or persistent (off-label use): IV: 1000 mg/m^2 days 1 and 8; repeat cycle every 21 days (in combination with cisplatin) (Monk, 2009) **or** 1250 mg/m^2 over 30 minutes days 1 and 8; repeat cycle every 21 days (in combination with cisplatin) (Burnett, 2000) **or** 800 mg/m^2 over 30 minutes days 1, 8, and 15; repeat cycle every 28 days (as a single-agent) (Schilder, 2005) **or** 800 mg/m^2 days 1 and 8; repeat cycle every 28 days (in combination with cisplatin) (Brewer, 2006)

Head and neck cancer, nasopharyngeal (off-label use): IV: 1000 mg/m^2 over 30 minutes days 1, 8, and 15 every 28 days (Zhang, 2008) **or** 1000 mg/m^2 over 30 minutes days 1 and 8 every 21 days (in combination with vinorelbine) (Chen, 2012)

Hepatobiliary cancer, advanced (off-label use): IV: 1000 mg/m^2 over 30 minutes days 1 and 8; repeat cycle every 21 days (in combination with cisplatin) (Valle, 2010) **or** 1000 mg/m^2 over 30 minutes days 1 and 8; repeat cycle every 21 days (in combination with capecitabine) (Knox, 2005) **or** 1000 mg/m^2 infused at 10 mg/m^2/minute every 2 weeks (in combination with oxaliplatin) (Andre, 2004)

Hodgkin lymphoma, relapsed (off-label use): IV: 1000 mg/m^2 (800 mg/m^2 for post-transplant patients) over 30 minutes days 1 and 8; repeat cycle every 21 days (in combination with vinorelbine and doxorubicin liposomal) (Bartlett, 2007) **or** 800 mg/m^2 days 1 and 4; repeat cycle every 21 days (in combination with ifosfamide, mesna, vinorelbine, and prednisolone) (Santoro, 2007)

Malignant pleural mesothelioma (off-label use; in combination with cisplatin): IV: 1000 mg/m^2 over 30 minutes days 1, 8 and 15 every 28 days for up to 6 cycles (Nowak, 2002) **or** 1250 mg/m^2 over 30 minutes days 1 and 8 every 21 days for up to 6 cycles (van Haarst, 2002)

Non-Hodgkin lymphoma, refractory (off-label use): IV: 1000 mg/m^2 over 30 minutes days 1 and 8; repeat cycle every 21 days (in combination with cisplatin and dexamethasone) (Crump, 2004) **or** 1000 mg/m^2 every 15-21days (in combination with oxaliplatin and rituximab) (Lopez, 2008)

Sarcoma (off-label uses): IV:

Ewing's sarcoma, refractory: 675 mg/m^2 over 90 minutes days 1 and 8; repeat cycle every 21 days (in combination with docetaxel) (Navid, 2008)

Osteosarcoma, refractory: 675 mg/m^2 over 90 minutes days 1 and 8; repeat cycle every 21 days (in combination with docetaxel) (Navid, 2008) **or** 1000 mg/m^2 weekly for 7 weeks followed by 1 week rest; then weekly for 3 weeks out of every 4 weeks (Merimsky, 2000)

Soft tissue sarcoma, advanced: 800 mg/m^2 over 90 minutes days 1 and 8; repeat cycle every 21 days (in combination with vinorelbine) (Dileo, 2007) **or** 675 mg/m^2 over 90 minutes days 1 and 8; repeat cycle every 21 days (in combination with docetaxel) (Leu, 2004) **or** 900 mg/m^2 over 90 minutes days 1 and 8; repeat cycle every 21 days (in combination with docetaxel) (Maki, 2007)

Small cell lung cancer, refractory or relapsed (off-label use): IV: 1000-1250 mg/m^2 over 30 minutes days 1, 8, and 15 every 28 days (as a single agent) (Masters, 2003)

Testicular cancer, refractory germ cell (off-label use): IV: 1000-1250 mg/m^2 over 30 minutes days 1 and 8 every 21 days (in combination with oxaliplatin) (DeGiorgi, 2006; Kohllmannsberger, 2004; Pectasides, 2004) **or** 1000 mg/m^2 over 30 minutes days 1, 8, and 15 every 28 days for up to 6 cycles (in combination with paclitaxel) (Hinton, 2002) **or** 800 mg/m^2 over 30 minutes days 1 and 8 every 21 days (in combination with oxaliplatin and paclitaxel) (Bokemeyer, 2008)

Unknown-primary, adenocarcinoma (off-label use): IV: 1250 mg/m^2 days 1 and 8 every 21 days (in combination with cisplatin) (Culine, 2003) **or** 1000 mg/m^2 over 30 minutes days 1 and 8 every 21 days for up to 6 cycles (in combination with docetaxel) (Pouessel, 2004)

Uterine cancer (off-label use): IV: 900 mg/m^2 over 90 minutes days 1 and 8 every 21 days (in combination with docetaxel) (Hensley, 2008) **or** 1000 mg/m^2 over 30 minutes days 1, 8, and 15 every 28 days (Look, 2004)

Dosing adjustment for toxicity:

Nonhematologic toxicity (all indications):

Hold or decrease gemcitabine dose by 50% for the following: Severe (grade 3 or 4) nonhematologic toxicity until resolved (excludes nausea, vomiting, or alopecia [no dose modifications recommended])

Permanently discontinue gemcitabine for any of the following: Unexplained dyspnea (or other evidence of severe pulmonary toxicity), severe hepatotoxicity, hemolytic uremic syndrome (HUS), capillary leak syndrome (CLS), posterior reversible encephalopathy syndrome (PRES)

Hematologic toxicity:

Breast cancer:

Day 1:

Absolute granulocyte count (AGC) ≥1500/mm^3 and platelet count ≥100,000/mm^3: Administer 100% of full dose

AGC <1500/mm^3 or platelet count <100,000/mm^3: Hold dose

Day 8:

AGC ≥1200/mm^3 and platelet count >75,000/mm^3: Administer 100% of full dose

AGC 1000-1199/mm^3 or platelet count 50,000-75,000/mm^3: Administer 75% of full dose

AGC 700-999/mm^3 and platelet count ≥50,000/mm^3: Administer 50% of full dose

AGC <700/mm^3 or platelet count <50,000/mm^3: Hold dose

Non-small cell lung cancer (cisplatin dosage may also require adjustment):

AGC ≥1000/mm^3 and platelet count ≥100,000/mm^3: Administer 100% of full dose

AGC 500-999/mm^3 or platelet count 50,000-99,999/mm^3: Administer 75% of full dose

AGC <500/mm^3 or platelet count <50,000/mm^3: Hold dose

Ovarian cancer:

Day 1:

AGC ≥1500/mm^3 and platelet count ≥100,000/mm^3: Administer 100% of full dose

AGC <1500/mm^3 or platelet count <100,000/mm^3: Delay treatment cycle

Day 8:

AGC ≥1500/mm^3 and platelet count ≥100,000/mm^3: Administer 100% of full dose

AGC 1000-1499/mm^3 or platelet count 75,000-99,999/mm^3: Administer 50% of full dose

AGC <1000/mm^3 or platelet count <75,000/mm^3: Hold dose

Hematologic toxicity in previous cycle (dosing adjustment for subsequent cycles):

Initial occurrence: AGC <500/mm^3 for >5 days, AGC <100/mm^3 for >3 days, febrile neutropenia, platelet count <25,000/mm^3, or cycle delay >1 week due to toxicity: Permanently reduce gemcitabine to 800 mg/m^2 on days 1 and 8.

Subsequent occurrence: AGC <500/mm^3 for >5 days, AGC <100/mm^3 for >3 days, neutropenic fever, platelet count <25,000/mm^3, or cycle delay >1 week due to toxicity: Permanently reduce gemcitabine to 800 mg/m^2 and administer on day 1 only.

Pancreatic cancer:

AGC ≥1000/mm^3 and platelet count ≥100,000/mm^3: Administer 100% of full dose

AGC 500-999/mm^3 or platelet count 50,000-99,999/mm^3: Administer 75% of full dose

AGC <500/mm^3 or platelet count <50,000/mm^3: Hold dose

Dosing adjustment in renal impairment: There are no dosage adjustments provided in the manufacturer's labeling; use with caution in patients with preexisting renal dysfunction. Discontinue if severe renal toxicity or hemolytic uremic syndrome (HUS) occur during gemcitabine treatment.

Mild-to-severe renal impairment: No dosage adjustment necessary (Janus, 2010; Li, 2007)

ESRD (on hemodialysis): Hemodialysis should begin 6-12 hours after gemcitabine infusion (Janus 2010; Li, 2007)

Dosing adjustment in hepatic impairment: There are no dosage adjustments provided in the manufacturer's labeling; use with caution. Discontinue if severe hepatotoxicity occurs during gemcitabine treatment. The following adjustments have been reported:

Transaminases elevated (with normal bilirubin): No dosage adjustment necessary (Venook, 2000)

Serum bilirubin >1.6 mg/dL: Use initial dose of 800 mg/m^2; may escalate if tolerated (Ecklund, 2005; Floyd, 2006; Venook, 2000)

Dosing in obesity: *ASCO Guidelines for appropriate chemotherapy dosing in obese adults with cancer:* Utilize patient's actual body weight (full weight) for calculation of body surface area- or weight-based dosing, particularly when the intent of therapy is curative; manage regimen-related toxicities in the same manner as for nonobese patients; if a dose reduction is utilized due to toxicity, consider resumption of full weight-based dosing with subsequent cycles, especially if cause of toxicity (eg, hepatic or renal impairment) is resolved (Griggs, 2012).

Administration Infuse over 30 minutes; for off-label uses, infusion times may vary (refer to specific references). **Note:** Prolongation of the infusion time >60 minutes has been shown to increase toxicity. Gemcitabine has been administered at a fixed-dose rate (FDR) infusion rate of 10 mg/m^2/minute to optimize the pharmacokinetics (off-label); prolonged infusion times increase the intracellular accumulation of the active metabolite, gemcitabine triphosphate (Ko, 2006; Tempero, 2003). Patients who receive gemcitabine FDR experience more grade 3/4 hematologic toxicity (Ko, 2006; Poplin, 2009).

For intravesicular (bladder) instillation (off-label route), gemcitabine was diluted in 50 to 100 mL normal saline; patients were instructed to retain in the bladder for 1 hour (Addeo, 2010; Dalbaghi, 2006)

Hazardous agent; use appropriate precautions for handling and disposal (NIOSH 2014 [group 1]).

Monitoring Parameters CBC with differential and platelet count (prior to each dose); hepatic and renal function (prior to initiation of therapy and periodically, thereafter); monitor

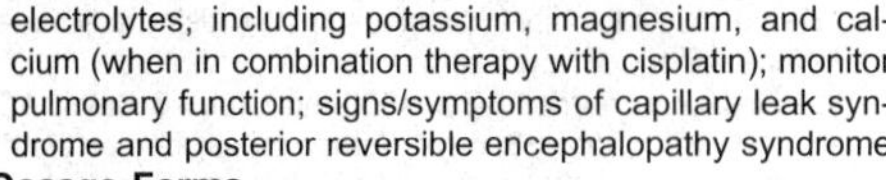

electrolytes, including potassium, magnesium, and calcium (when in combination therapy with cisplatin); monitor pulmonary function; signs/symptoms of capillary leak syndrome and posterior reversible encephalopathy syndrome

Dosage Forms

Solution, Intravenous:

Generic: 200 mg/5.26 mL (5.26 mL); 1 g/26.3 mL (26.3 mL); 2 g/52.6 mL (52.6 mL)

Solution Reconstituted, Intravenous:

Gemzar: 200 mg (1 ea); 1 g (1 ea)

Generic: 200 mg (1 ea); 1 g (1 ea); 2 g (1 ea)

Solution Reconstituted, Intravenous [preservative free]:

Generic: 200 mg (1 ea); 1 g (1 ea)

Dosage Forms: Canada

Solution, Intravenous: 200 mg/5mL, 1 g/25 mL, 2 g/50 mL [40 mg/mL]

Solution, Intravenous: 200 mg/5.3 mL, 1 g/26.3 mL, 2 g/52.6 mL [38 mg/mL]

Solution Reconstituted, Intravenous: 200 mg, 1 g, 2 g

- ◆ **Gemcitabine For Injection (Can)** *see* Gemcitabine *on page 952*
- ◆ **Gemcitabine For Injection Concentrate (Can)** *see* Gemcitabine *on page 952*
- ◆ **Gemcitabine For Injection, USP (Can)** *see* Gemcitabine *on page 952*
- ◆ **Gemcitabine Hydrochloride** *see* Gemcitabine *on page 952*
- ◆ **Gemcitabine Hydrochloride For Injection (Can)** *see* Gemcitabine *on page 952*
- ◆ **Gemcitabine Injection (Can)** *see* Gemcitabine *on page 952*
- ◆ **Gemcitabine Sun For Injection (Can)** *see* Gemcitabine *on page 952*

Gemfibrozil (jem FI broe zil)

Brand Names: U.S. Lopid

Brand Names: Canada Apo-Gemfibrozil; Gen-Gemfibrozil; GMD-Gemfibrozil; Lopid; Mylan-Gemfibrozil; Novo-Gemfibrozil; Nu-Gemfibrozil; PMS-Gemfibrozil

Index Terms CI-719

Pharmacologic Category Antilipemic Agent, Fibric Acid

Use Treatment of hypertriglyceridemia in Fredrickson types IV and V hyperlipidemia for patients who are at greater risk for pancreatitis and who have not responded to dietary intervention; to reduce the risk of CHD development in Fredrickson type IIb patients without a history or symptoms of existing CHD who have not responded to dietary and other interventions (including pharmacologic treatment) and who have decreased HDL, increased LDL, and increased triglycerides

Pregnancy Risk Factor C

Pregnancy Considerations Adverse events have been observed in animal reproduction studies. The Canadian product labeling specifically contraindicates use during pregnancy and recommends gemfibrozil be discontinued several months prior to conception.

Breast-Feeding Considerations It is not known if gemfibrozil is excreted in breast milk. Due to the potential for serious adverse reactions in the nursing infant, a decision should be made whether to discontinue nursing or to discontinue the drug, taking into account the importance of treatment to the mother. The Canadian product labeling specifically contraindicates use during breast-feeding.

Contraindications

Hypersensitivity to gemfibrozil or any component of the formulation; hepatic or severe renal dysfunction; primary biliary cirrhosis; preexisting gallbladder disease; concurrent use with repaglinide or simvastatin.

Documentation of allergenic cross-reactivity for fibrates is limited. However, because of similarities in chemical structure and/or pharmacologic actions, the possibility of cross-sensitivity cannot be ruled out with certainty.

Warnings/Precautions Secondary causes of hyperlipidemia should be ruled out prior to therapy. Possible increased risk of malignancy and cholelithiasis. Anemia, leukopenia, thrombocytopenia, and bone marrow hypoplasia have rarely been reported. Periodic monitoring recommended during the first year of therapy. Elevations in serum transaminases can be seen. Discontinue if lipid response not seen. Be careful in patient selection; this is not a first- or second-line choice. Other agents may be more suitable. Has been associated with rare myositis or rhabdomyolysis; patients should be monitored closely. Patients should be instructed to report unexplained muscle pain, tenderness, weakness, or brown urine. Potentially significant drug-drug interactions may exist, requiring dose or frequency adjustment, additional monitoring, and/or selection of alternative therapy. Use with caution in patients with mild-to-moderate renal impairment; contraindicated in patients with severe impairment. Renal function deterioration has been seen when used in patients with a serum creatinine >2 mg/dL.

Adverse Reactions

Central nervous system: Fatigue, vertigo

Dermatologic: Eczema, rash

Gastrointestinal: Dyspepsia

Gastrointestinal: Abdominal pain, nausea, vomiting

Rare but important or life-threatening (including case reports with probable causation): Alkaline phosphatase increased, anemia, angioedema, arthralgia, bilirubin increased, blurred vision, bone marrow hypoplasia, cholelithiasis, cholecystitis, cholestatic jaundice, creatine phosphokinase increased, depression, dermatitis, dermatomyositis/polymyositis, dizziness, eosinophilia, exfoliative dermatitis, headache, hypoesthesia, hypokalemia, impotence, laryngeal edema, leukopenia, libido decreased, myalgia, myasthenia, myopathy, nephrotoxicity, painful extremities, paresthesia, peripheral neuritis, pruritus, Raynaud's phenomenon, rhabdomyolysis, somnolence, synovitis, taste perversion, transaminases increased, urticaria

Reports where causal relationship has not been established: Alopecia, anaphylaxis, cataracts, colitis, confusion, decreased fertility (male), drug-induced lupus-like syndrome, extrasystoles, hepatoma, intracranial hemorrhage, pancreatitis, peripheral vascular disease, photosensitivity, positive ANA, renal dysfunction, retinal edema, seizure, syncope, thrombocytopenia, vasculitis, weight loss

Drug Interactions

Metabolism/Transport Effects **Substrate** of CYP3A4 (minor); **Note:** Assignment of Major/Minor substrate status based on clinically relevant drug interaction potential; **Inhibits** CYP1A2 (moderate), CYP2C19 (strong), CYP2C8 (strong), CYP2C9 (strong)

Avoid Concomitant Use

Avoid concomitant use of Gemfibrozil with any of the following: AtorvaSTATin; Bexarotene (Systemic); Ciprofibrate; Dasabuvir; Enzalutamide; Ezetimibe; Fluvastatin; Irinotecan; Lovastatin; Pitavastatin; Pravastatin; Repaglinide; Rosuvastatin; Simvastatin

Increased Effect/Toxicity

Gemfibrozil may increase the levels/effects of: Agomelatine; Antidiabetic Agents (Thiazolidinedione); AtorvaSTATin; Bexarotene (Systemic); Bosentan; Carvedilol; Citalopram; Colchicine; CYP1A2 Substrates; CYP2C19 Substrates; CYP2C8 Substrates; CYP2C9 Substrates; Dasabuvir; Diclofenac (Systemic); Dronabinol; Enzalutamide; Ezetimibe; Fluvastatin; Irinotecan; Lacosamide; Lovastatin; Ospemifene; Pioglitazone; Pirfenidone; Pitavastatin; Pravastatin; Repaglinide; Rosuvastatin;

Simvastatin; Sulfonylureas; Tetrahydrocannabinol; Treprostinil; Vitamin K Antagonists

The levels/effects of Gemfibrozil may be increased by: Acipimox; Cannabis; Ciprofibrate; CycloSPORINE (Systemic); Raltegravir

Decreased Effect

Gemfibrozil may decrease the levels/effects of: Chenodiol; Clopidogrel; CycloSPORINE (Systemic); Imatinib; Ursodiol

The levels/effects of Gemfibrozil may be decreased by: Bile Acid Sequestrants

Food Interactions When given after meals, the AUC of gemfibrozil is decreased. Management: Administer 30 minutes prior to breakfast and dinner.

Storage/Stability Store at 20°C to 25°C (68°F to 77°F). Protect from light and moisture.

Mechanism of Action The exact mechanism of action of gemfibrozil is unknown, however, several theories exist regarding the VLDL effect; it can inhibit lipolysis and decrease subsequent hepatic fatty acid uptake as well as inhibit hepatic secretion of VLDL; together these actions decrease serum VLDL levels; increases HDL-cholesterol; the mechanism behind HDL elevation is currently unknown

Pharmacodynamics/Kinetics

Onset of action: May require several days

Absorption: Well absorbed

Protein binding: 99%

Metabolism: Hepatic via oxidation to two inactive metabolites; undergoes enterohepatic recycling

Half-life elimination: 1.5 hours

Time to peak, serum: 1 to 2 hours

Excretion: Urine (~70% primarily as conjugated drug); feces (6%)

Dosage Adults: Oral: 600 mg twice daily 30 minutes before breakfast and dinner. **Note:** Discontinue if lipid response is inadequate after 3 months of therapy.

Dosage adjustment in renal impairment:

Manufacturer's recommendations:

Mild-to-moderate impairment: There are no dosage adjustments provided in the manufacturer's labeling; use with caution; deterioration of renal function has been reported in patients with baseline serum creatinine >2 mg/dL

Severe impairment: There are no dosage adjustments provided in the manufacturer's labeling; use is contraindicated

Alternate recommendations (Aronoff, 2007):

GFR >50 mL/minute: No dosage adjustment necessary.

GFR 10 to 50 mL/minute: Administer 75% of dose.

GFR <10 mL/minute: Administer 50% of dose.

Intermittent hemodialysis: Supplemental dose not necessary.

Peritoneal dialysis: Administer 50% of dose as supplement for dialysis.

Dosage adjustment in hepatic impairment: There are no dosage adjustments provided in the manufacturer's labeling; use is contraindicated

Dietary Considerations Before initiation of therapy, patients should be placed on a standard cholesterol-lowering diet for 3 to 6 months and the diet should be continued during drug therapy. Administer 30 minutes prior to breakfast and dinner

Administration Administer 30 minutes prior to breakfast and dinner.

Monitoring Parameters Serum cholesterol, LFTs periodically, CBC periodically (first year)

Dosage Forms

Tablet, Oral:

Lopid: 600 mg

Generic: 600 mg

Dosage Forms: Canada

Capsule, Oral: 300 mg

Gemifloxacin (je mi FLOKS a sin)

Brand Names: U.S. Factive

Brand Names: Canada Factive®

Index Terms DW286; Gemifloxacin Mesylate; LA 20304a; SB-265805

Pharmacologic Category Antibiotic, Fluoroquinolone; Antibiotic, Respiratory Fluoroquinolone

Use Treatment of acute exacerbation of chronic bronchitis; treatment of community-acquired pneumonia (CAP), including pneumonia caused by multidrug-resistant strains of *S. pneumoniae* (MDRSP)

Pregnancy Risk Factor C

Dosage

Usual dosage range:

Adults: Oral: 320 mg once daily

Indication-specific dosing:

Adults: Oral:

Acute exacerbations of chronic bronchitis: 320 mg once daily for 5 days

Community-acquired pneumonia (mild-to-moderate): 320 mg once daily for 5 or 7 days (decision to use 5- or 7-day regimen should be guided by initial sputum culture; 7 days are recommended for MDRSP, *Klebsiella*, or *M. catarrhalis* infection)

Sinusitis (off-label use): 320 mg once daily for 10 days

Elderly: Refer to adult dosing.

Dosage adjustment in renal impairment:

CrCl >40 mL/minute: No adjustment required

CrCl ≤40 mL/minute (or patients on hemodialysis/CAPD): 160 mg once daily (administer dose following hemodialysis)

Dosage adjustment in hepatic impairment: No adjustment required

Additional Information Complete prescribing information should be consulted for additional detail.

Dosage Forms

Tablet, Oral:

Factive: 320 mg

◆ **Gemifloxacin Mesylate** *see* Gemifloxacin *on page 957*

Gemtuzumab Ozogamicin

(gem TOO zoo mab oh zog a MY sin)

Index Terms CMA-676; Mylotarg

Pharmacologic Category Antineoplastic Agent, Anti-CD33; Antineoplastic Agent, Antibody Drug Conjugate; Antineoplastic Agent, Monoclonal Antibody

Use Due to safety concerns, as well as lack of clinical benefit demonstrated in a post-approval clinical trial, gemtuzumab was withdrawn from the U.S. commercial market in 2010.

Pregnancy Considerations Teratogenic effects have been observed in animal reproduction studies. May cause fetal harm when administered to a pregnant woman. Women of childbearing potential should avoid becoming pregnant while receiving treatment.

Breast-Feeding Considerations It is not known if gemtuzumab ozogamicin is excreted in breast milk. Because human IgG is secreted in breast milk and the potential for serious adverse reactions in the nursing infant exists, a decision should be made whether to discontinue nursing or to discontinue the drug, taking into account the importance of treatment to the mother.

Contraindications Hypersensitivity to gemtuzumab ozogamicin, calicheamicin derivatives, or any component of the formulation; patients with anti-CD33 antibody

Warnings/Precautions Hazardous agent - use appropriate precautions for handling and disposal (NIOSH 2014 [group 1]).

Gemtuzumab has been associated with hepatotoxicity, including severe hepatic sinusoidal obstruction syndrome (SOS; formerly called veno-occlusive disease [VOD]). Symptoms of SOS include right upper quadrant pain, rapid weight gain, ascites, hepatomegaly, and bilirubin/transaminase elevations. Risk may be increased by combination chemotherapy, underlying hepatic disease, or hematopoietic stem cell transplant.

Severe hypersensitivity reactions (including anaphylaxis) and other infusion-related reactions may occur. Infusion-related events are common, generally reported to occur with the first dose after the end of the 2-hour intravenous infusion. These symptoms usually resolved after 2-4 hours with a supportive therapy of acetaminophen, diphenhydramine, and intravenous fluids. Other severe and potentially fatal infusion related pulmonary events (including dyspnea and hypoxia) have been reported infrequently. Symptomatic intrinsic lung disease or high peripheral blast counts may increase the risk of severe reactions. Fewer infusion-related events were observed after the second dose. Postinfusion reactions (may include fever, chills, hypotension, or dyspnea) may occur during the first 24 hours after administration. Consider discontinuation in patients who develop severe infusion-related reactions. In addition to infusion-related pulmonary events, gemtuzumab therapy is also associated with acute respiratory distress syndrome, pulmonary infiltrates, pleural effusion, noncardiogenic pulmonary edema, and pulmonary insufficiency.

Severe myelosuppression occurs in all patients at recommended dosages. Tumor lysis syndrome may occur as a consequence of leukemia treatment, adequate hydration and prophylactic allopurinol must be instituted prior to use. Other methods to lower WBC <30,000 cells/mm^3 may be considered (hydroxyurea or leukapheresis) to minimize the risk of tumor lysis syndrome, and/or severe infusion reactions. An increased number of deaths have been reported in patients receiving gemtuzumab in combination with chemotherapy, compared to those receiving chemotherapy alone.

Adverse Reactions

Cardiovascular: Cerebral hemorrhage, hyper-/hypotension, peripheral edema, tachycardia

Central nervous system: Anxiety, chills, depression, dizziness, fever, headache, insomnia, intracranial hemorrhage, pain

Dermatologic: Bruising, petechiae, pruritus, rash

Endocrine & metabolic: Hyperglycemia, hypocalcemia, hypokalemia, hypomagnesemia, hypophosphatemia

Gastrointestinal: Abdominal pain, anorexia, diarrhea, dyspepsia, gingival hemorrhage, melena, mucositis, nausea, stomatitis, vomiting

Genitourinary: Vaginal bleeding, vaginal hemorrhage

Hematologic: Anemia, disseminated intravascular coagulation (DIC), hemorrhage, leukopenia, lymphopenia, neutropenia (median recovery 40-51 days), neutropenic fever, thrombocytopenia (median recovery 36-51 days)

Hepatic: Alkaline phosphatase increased, ALT increased, ascites, AST increased, hyperbilirubinemia, LDH increased, prothrombin time increased, PTT increased, sinusoidal obstruction syndrome (SOS; veno-occlusive disease; higher frequency in patients with prior history of or subsequent hematopoietic stem cell transplant)

Local: Local reaction

Neuromuscular & skeletal: Arthralgia, back pain, myalgia, weakness

Renal: Creatinine increased, hematuria

Respiratory: Cough, dyspnea, epistaxis, hypoxia, pharyngitis, pneumonia, rhinitis

Miscellaneous: Cutaneous herpes simplex, infection, infusion reaction, sepsis

Rare but important or life-threatening: Acute respiratory distress syndrome, anaphylaxis, bradycardia, Budd-Chiari syndrome, gastrointestinal hemorrhage, hepatic failure, hepatosplenomegaly, hypersensitivity reactions, jaundice, neutropenic sepsis, noncardiogenic pulmonary edema, portal vain thrombosis, pulmonary hemorrhage, renal impairment, renal failure (including renal failure secondary to tumor lysis syndrome)

Drug Interactions

Metabolism/Transport Effects None known.

Avoid Concomitant Use

Avoid concomitant use of Gemtuzumab Ozogamicin with any of the following: BCG; Belimumab; CloZAPine; Dipyrone; Natalizumab; Pimecrolimus; Tacrolimus (Topical); Tofacitinib; Vaccines (Live)

Increased Effect/Toxicity

Gemtuzumab Ozogamicin may increase the levels/effects of: Belimumab; CloZAPine; Leflunomide; Natalizumab; Tofacitinib; Vaccines (Live)

The levels/effects of Gemtuzumab Ozogamicin may be increased by: Denosumab; Dipyrone; Pimecrolimus; Roflumilast; Tacrolimus (Topical); Trastuzumab

Decreased Effect

Gemtuzumab Ozogamicin may decrease the levels/effects of: BCG; Coccidioides immitis Skin Test; Sipuleucel-T; Vaccines (Inactivated); Vaccines (Live)

The levels/effects of Gemtuzumab Ozogamicin may be decreased by: Echinacea

Preparation for Administration Hazardous agent; use appropriate precautions for handling and disposal (NIOSH 2014 [group 1]). Protect from light during preparation (and administration). Prepare in biologic safety hood with shielded fluorescent light; (some institutions prepare in a darkened room with the lights in the biologic safety cabinet turned off). Allow to warm to room temperature prior to reconstitution. Reconstitute each 5 mg vial with sterile water for injection to a concentration of 1 mg/mL. Dilute in 100 mL of 0.9% sodium chloride injection.

Storage/Stability Light sensitive; protect from light (including direct and indirect sunlight, and unshielded fluorescent light). The infusion container should be placed in a UV protectant bag immediately after preparation. Store intact vials under refrigeration at 2°C to 8°C (36°F to 46°F). Reconstituted solutions may be stored for up to 2 hours at room temperature or under refrigeration. Following dilution for infusion, solutions are stable for up to 16 hours at room temperature. Administration requires 2 hours; therefore, the maximum elapsed time from initial reconstitution to completion of infusion should be 20 hours.

Mechanism of Action Antibody to CD33 antigen, which is expressed on leukemic blasts in 80% of AML patients. Binds to the CD33 antigen, resulting in internalization of the antibody-antigen complex. Following internalization, the calicheamicin derivative is released inside the myeloid cell. The calicheamicin derivative binds to DNA resulting in double strand breaks and cell death. Pluripotent stem cells and nonhematopoietic cells are not affected.

Pharmacodynamics/Kinetics

Distribution: V_{ss}: Adults: Initial dose: 21 L; Repeat dose: 10 L

Half-life elimination: Total calicheamicin: Initial: 41-45 hours, Repeat dose: 60-64 hours; Unconjugated: 100-143 hours (no change noted in repeat dosing)

Dosage IV: Adults: **Note:** Patients should receive diphenhydramine 50 mg orally and acetaminophen 650-1000 mg orally 1 hour prior to administration of each dose. Acetaminophen dosage should be repeated as needed every 4 hours for 2 additional doses. Pretreatment with methylprednisolone may ameliorate infusion-related symptoms.

AML (off-label/investigational use):

<60 years: 9 mg/m^2 infused over 2 hours. A full treatment course is a total of 2 doses administered with 14-28 days between doses (Larson, 2005).

≥60 years: 9 mg/m^2 infused over 2 hours. A full treatment course is a total of 2 doses administered with 14-28 days between doses (Larson, 2002; Larson, 2005).

APL (off-label/investigational use):

Single-agent therapy: 6 mg/m^2 infused over 2 hours on days 1 and 15; for patients testing PCR negative after 2 doses, a third dose was administered (LoCoco, 2004).

Combination therapy (high-risk patients; Ravandi, 2009):

Induction: 9 mg/m^2 as a single dose on day 1 (in combination with arsenic trioxide and tretinoin)

Post remission therapy (if arsenic trioxide or tretinoin discontinued due to toxicity): 9 mg/m^2 once every 4-5 weeks until 28 weeks after complete remission

Dosage adjustment for toxicity:

Dyspnea or significant hypotension: Interrupt infusion; monitor

Anaphylaxis, pulmonary edema, acute respiratory distress syndrome: Strongly consider discontinuing treatment

Dosage adjustment in renal impairment: No dosage adjustment provided in manufacturer's labeling (has not been studied).

Dosage adjustment in hepatic impairment: No dosage adjustment provided in manufacturer's labeling (has not been studied); use with caution.

Administration Do not administer as IV push or bolus. Administer via IV infusion, over at least 2 hours through a low protein-binding (0.2 to 1.2 micron) in-line filter. Protect from light during infusion. Premedicate with acetaminophen and diphenhydramine prior to each infusion.

Hazardous agent; use appropriate precautions for handling and disposal (NIOSH 2014 [group 1]).

Monitoring Parameters Monitor vital signs during the infusion and for 4 hours following the infusion. Monitor for signs/symptoms of postinfusion reaction. Monitor electrolytes, liver function, CBC with differential and platelets frequently. Monitor for signs and symptoms of hepatic sinusoidal obstruction syndrome (SOS; veno-occlusive disease; weight gain, right upper quadrant abdominal pain, hepatomegaly, ascites).

Product Availability No longer commercially available in the U.S. market for new patients. Available in Canada through a special access program.

- **Gemzar** *see* Gemcitabine *on page 952*
- **Genahist [OTC]** *see* DiphenhydrAMINE (Systemic) *on page 641*
- **Genaphed [OTC]** *see* Pseudoephedrine *on page 1742*
- **Gen-Clozapine (Can)** *see* CloZAPine *on page 490*
- **Gene-Activated Human Acid-Beta-Glucosidase** *see* Velaglucerase Alfa *on page 2147*
- **Generess Fe** *see* Ethinyl Estradiol and Norethindrone *on page 808*
- **Generlac** *see* Lactulose *on page 1156*
- **Gen-Fluoxetine (Can)** *see* FLUoxetine *on page 899*
- **Gen-Gemfibrozil (Can)** *see* Gemfibrozil *on page 956*
- **Gengraf** *see* CycloSPORINE (Systemic) *on page 522*
- **Gen-Hydroxychloroquine (Can)** *see* Hydroxychloroquine *on page 1021*
- **Gen-Hydroxyurea (Can)** *see* Hydroxyurea *on page 1021*
- **Gen-Ipratropium (Can)** *see* Ipratropium (Systemic) *on page 1108*
- **Gen-Medroxy (Can)** *see* MedroxyPROGESTERone *on page 1277*
- **Gen-Nabumetone (Can)** *see* Nabumetone *on page 1411*
- **Gen-Nizatidine (Can)** *see* Nizatidine *on page 1471*
- **Genotropin** *see* Somatropin *on page 1918*
- **Genotropin GoQuick (Can)** *see* Somatropin *on page 1918*
- **Genotropin MiniQuick** *see* Somatropin *on page 1918*
- **Genpril [OTC]** *see* Ibuprofen *on page 1032*
- **Gen-Selegiline (Can)** *see* Selegiline *on page 1873*
- **Gentak** *see* Gentamicin (Ophthalmic) *on page 962*
- **Gentak® (Can)** *see* Gentamicin (Ophthalmic) *on page 962*

Gentamicin (Systemic) (jen ta MYE sin)

Brand Names: Canada Gentamicin Injection, USP

Index Terms Gentamicin Sulfate

Pharmacologic Category Antibiotic, Aminoglycoside

Use Treatment of susceptible bacterial infections, normally gram-negative organisms, including *Pseudomonas*, *Proteus*, *Serratia*, and gram-positive *Staphylococcus*; treatment of bone infections, respiratory tract infections, skin and soft tissue infections, as well as abdominal and urinary tract infections, and septicemia; treatment of infective endocarditis

Pregnancy Risk Factor D

Pregnancy Considerations Gentamicin crosses the placenta and produces detectable serum levels in the fetus. Renal toxicity has been described in two case reports following first trimester exposure. There are several reports of total irreversible bilateral congenital deafness in children whose mothers received streptomycin during pregnancy; therefore, the manufacturer classifies gentamicin as pregnancy category D. Although ototoxicity has not been reported following maternal use of gentamicin, a potential for harm exists. **[U.S. Boxed Warning]: Aminoglycosides may cause fetal harm if administered to a pregnant woman.**

Due to pregnancy induced physiologic changes, some pharmacokinetic parameters of gentamicin may be altered. Pregnant women have an average-to-larger volume of distribution which may result in lower serum peak levels than for the same dose in nonpregnant women. Serum half-life is also shorter.

Breast-Feeding Considerations Gentamicin is excreted into breast milk; however, it is not well absorbed when taken orally. This limited oral absorption may minimize exposure to the nursing infant. Nondose-related effects could include modification of bowel flora.

Contraindications Hypersensitivity to gentamicin or other aminoglycosides

Warnings/Precautions [U.S. Boxed Warning]: Aminoglycosides may cause neurotoxicity and/or nephrotoxicity; usual risk factors include preexisting renal impairment, concomitant neuro-/nephrotoxic medications, advanced age and dehydration. Ototoxicity may be directly proportional to the amount of drug given and the duration of treatment; tinnitus or vertigo are indications of vestibular injury and impending hearing loss; renal damage is usually reversible. May cause neuromuscular blockade and respiratory paralysis; especially when given soon after anesthesia or muscle relaxants.

Not intended for long-term therapy due to toxic hazards associated with extended administration; use caution in preexisting renal insufficiency, vestibular or cochlear impairment, myasthenia gravis, hypocalcemia, conditions which depress neuromuscular transmission. Dosage modification required in patients with impaired renal function. Prolonged use may result in fungal or bacterial superinfection, including *C. difficile*-associated diarrhea (CDAD) and pseudomembranous colitis; CDAD has been observed >2 months postantibiotic treatment.

Adverse Reactions

Cardiovascular: Edema, hyper/hypotension

Central nervous system: Ataxia, confusion, depression, dizziness, drowsiness, encephalopathy, fever, headache, lethargy, pseudomotor cerebri, seizures, vertigo

Dermatologic: Alopecia, erythema, itching, purpura, rash, urticaria

Endocrine & metabolic: Hypocalcemia, hypokalemia, hypomagnesemia, hyponatremia

Gastrointestinal: Anorexia, appetite decreased, *C. difficile*-associated diarrhea, enterocolitis, nausea, salivation increased, splenomegaly, stomatitis, vomiting, weight loss

Hematologic: Agranulocytosis, anemia, eosinophilia, granulocytopenia, leukopenia, reticulocytes increased/decreased, thrombocytopenia

Hepatic: Hepatomegaly, LFTs increased

Local: Injection site reactions, pain at injection site, phlebitis/thrombophlebitis

Neuromuscular & skeletal: Arthralgia, gait instability, muscle cramps, muscle twitching, muscle weakness, myasthenia gravis-like syndrome, numbness, paresthesia, peripheral neuropathy, tremor, weakness

Ocular: Visual disturbances

Otic: Hearing impairment, hearing loss (associated with persistently increased serum concentrations; early toxicity usually affects high-pitched sound), tinnitus

Renal: BUN increased, casts (hyaline, granular) in urine, creatinine clearance decreased, distal tubular dysfunction, Fanconi-like syndrome (high dose, prolonged course) (infants and adults), oliguria, renal failure (high trough serum concentrations), polyuria, proteinuria, serum creatinine increased, tubular necrosis, urine specific gravity decreased

Respiratory: Dyspnea, laryngeal edema, pulmonary fibrosis, respiratory depression

Miscellaneous: Allergic reaction, anaphylaxis, anaphylactoid reactions

Drug Interactions

Metabolism/Transport Effects None known.

Avoid Concomitant Use

Avoid concomitant use of Gentamicin (Systemic) with any of the following: Agalsidase Alfa; Agalsidase Beta; BCG; Foscarnet; Mannitol

Increased Effect/Toxicity

Gentamicin (Systemic) may increase the levels/effects of: AbobotulinumtoxinA; Bisphosphonate Derivatives; CARBOplatin; Colistimethate; CycloSPORINE (Systemic); Neuromuscular-Blocking Agents; OnabotulinumtoxinA; RimabotulinumtoxinB; Tenofovir

The levels/effects of Gentamicin (Systemic) may be increased by: Amphotericin B; Capreomycin; Cephalosporins (2nd Generation); Cephalosporins (3rd Generation); Cephalosporins (4th Generation); CISplatin; Foscarnet; Loop Diuretics; Mannitol; Nonsteroidal Anti-Inflammatory Agents; Tenofovir; Vancomycin

Decreased Effect

Gentamicin (Systemic) may decrease the levels/effects of: Agalsidase Alfa; Agalsidase Beta; BCG; Sodium Picosulfate; Typhoid Vaccine

The levels/effects of Gentamicin (Systemic) may be decreased by: Penicillins

Storage/Stability Gentamicin is a colorless to slightly yellow solution which should be stored between 2°C to 30°C, but refrigeration is not recommended. IV infusion solutions mixed in NS or D_5W solution are stable for 48 hours at room temperature and refrigeration (Goodwin, 1991). Premixed bag: Manufacturer expiration date; remove from overwrap stability: 30 days.

Mechanism of Action Interferes with bacterial protein synthesis by binding to 30S and 50S ribosomal subunits resulting in a defective bacterial cell membrane

Pharmacodynamics/Kinetics

Absorption:

Intramuscular: Rapid and complete

Oral: None

Distribution: Primarily into extracellular fluid (highly hydrophilic); high concentration in the renal cortex; minimal penetration to ocular tissues via IV route

V_d: Increased by edema, ascites, fluid overload; decreased with dehydration

Neonates: 0.4-0.6 L/kg

Children: 0.3-0.35 L/kg

Adults: 0.2-0.3 L/kg

Relative diffusion from blood into CSF: Minimal even with inflammation

CSF:blood level ratio: Normal meninges: Nil; Inflamed meninges: 10% to 30%

Protein binding: <30%

Half-life elimination:

Infants: <1 week: 3-11.5 hours; 1 week to 6 months: 3-3.5 hours

Adults: 1.5-3 hours; End-stage renal disease: 36-70 hours

Time to peak, serum: IM: 30-90 minutes; IV: 30 minutes after 30-minute infusion

Excretion: Urine (as unchanged drug)

Clearance: Directly related to renal function

Dosage Note: Dosage Individualization is **critical** because of the low therapeutic index.

In underweight and nonobese patients, use of total body weight (TBW) instead of ideal body weight for determining the initial mg/kg/dose is widely accepted (Nicolau, 1995). Ideal body weight (IBW) also may be used to determine doses for patients who are neither underweight nor obese (Gilbert, 2009).

Initial and periodic plasma drug levels (eg, peak and trough with conventional dosing, post dose level at a prespecified time with extended-interval dosing) should be determined, particularly in critically-ill patients with serious infections or in disease states known to significantly alter aminoglycoside pharmacokinetics (eg, cystic fibrosis, burns, or major surgery).

Usual dosage ranges:

Infants and Children <5 years: IM, IV: 2.5 mg/kg/dose every 8 hours*

Children ≥5 years: IM, IV: 2-2.5 mg/kg/dose every 8 hours*

***Note:** Higher individual doses and/or more frequent intervals (eg, every 6 hours) may be required in selected clinical situations (cystic fibrosis) or serum levels document the need.

Adults:

IM, IV:

Conventional: 1-2.5 mg/kg/dose every 8-12 hours; to ensure adequate peak concentrations early in therapy, higher initial dosage may be considered in selected patients when extracellular water is increased (edema, septic shock, postsurgical, or trauma)

Once daily: 4-7 mg/kg/dose once daily; some clinicians recommend this approach for all patients with normal renal function; this dose is at least as efficacious with similar, if not less, toxicity than conventional dosing

Intrathecal: 4-8 mg/day

Indication-specific dosing:

Children ≥1 year: IV:

Surgical (preoperative) prophylaxis (off-label use): 2.5 mg/kg within 60 minutes prior to surgical incision with or without other antibiotics (procedure dependent). **Note:** Dose is based on actual body weight unless >20% above ideal body weight, then dosage requirement may best be estimated using a dosing weight of IBW + 0.4 (TBW - IBW) (Bratzler, 2013).

Children and Adults: IM, IV:

Brucellosis: 240 mg (IM) daily or 5 mg/kg (IV) daily for 7 days; either regimen recommended in combination with doxycycline

Cholangitis: 4-6 mg/kg once daily with ampicillin

Diverticulitis (complicated): 1.5-2 mg/kg every 8 hours (with ampicillin and metronidazole)

Endocarditis: Treatment: 3 mg/kg/day in 1-3 divided doses

Meningitis: *Enterococcus* sp or *Pseudomonas aeruginosa*: Loading dose 2 mg/kg, then 1.7 mg/kg/dose every 8 hours (administered with another bacteriocidal drug)

Pelvic inflammatory disease: Loading dose: 2 mg/kg, then 1.5 mg/kg every 8 hours

Alternate therapy: 4.5 mg/kg once daily

Plague *(Yersinia pestis)*: Treatment: 5 mg/kg/day, followed by postexposure prophylaxis with doxycycline

Pneumonia, hospital- or ventilator-associated: 7 mg/kg/day (with antipseudomonal beta-lactam or carbapenem)

Synergy (for gram-positive infections): 3 mg/kg/day in 1-3 divided doses (with ampicillin)

Tularemia: 5 mg/kg/day divided every 8 hours for 1-2 weeks

Urinary tract infection: 1.5 mg/kg/dose every 8 hours

Adults: IV:

Surgical (preoperative) prophylaxis (off-label use): 5 mg/kg within 60 minutes prior to surgical incision with or without other antibiotics (procedure dependent). **Note:** Dose is based on actual body weight unless >20% above ideal body weight, then dosage requirement may best be estimated using a dosing weight of IBW + 0.4 (TBW - IBW) (Bratzler, 2013).

Dosing interval in renal impairment:

Conventional dosing:

CrCl ≥60 mL/minute: Administer every 8 hours

CrCl 40-60 mL/minute: Administer every 12 hours

CrCl 20-40 mL/minute: Administer every 24 hours

CrCl <20 mL/minute: Loading dose, then monitor levels

High-dose therapy: Interval may be extended (eg, every 48 hours) in patients with moderate renal impairment (CrCl 30-59 mL/minute) and/or adjusted based on serum level determinations.

Intermittent hemodialysis (IHD) (administer after hemodialysis on dialysis days) (Heintz, 2009): Dialyzable (~50%; variable; dependent on filter, duration, and type of IHD):

Loading dose of 2-3 mg/kg loading dose followed by:

Mild UTI or synergy: 1 mg/kg every 48-72 hours; consider redosing for pre-HD or post-HD concentrations <1 mg/L

Moderate-to-severe UTI: 1-1.5 mg/kg every 48-72 hours; consider redosing for pre-HD concentrations <1.5-2 mg/L or post-HD concentrations <1 mg/L

Systemic gram-negative rod infection: 1.5-2 mg/kg every 48-72 hours; consider redosing for pre-HD concentrations <3-5 mg/L or post-HD concentrations <2 mg/L

Note: Dosing dependent on the assumption of 3 times/week, complete IHD sessions.

Peritoneal dialysis (PD):

Administration via PD fluid:

Gram-positive infection (eg, synergy): 3-4 mg/L (3-4 mcg/mL) of PD fluid

Gram-negative infection: 4-8 mg/L (4-8 mcg/mL) of PD fluid

Administration via IV, IM route during PD: Dose as for CrCl <10 mL/minute and follow levels

Continuous renal replacement therapy (CRRT) (Heintz, 2009; Trotman, 2005): Drug clearance is highly dependent on the method of renal replacement, filter type, and flow rate. Appropriate dosing requires close monitoring of pharmacologic response, signs of adverse reactions due to drug accumulation, as well as drug concentrations in relation to target trough (if appropriate). The following are general recommendations only (based on dialysate flow/ultrafiltration rates of 1-2 L/hour and minimal residual renal function) and should not supersede clinical judgment:

CVVH/CVVHD/CVVHDF: Loading dose of 2-3 mg/kg followed by:

Mild UTI or synergy: 1 mg/kg every 24-36 hours (redose when concentration <1 mg/L)

Moderate-to-severe UTI: 1-1.5 mg/kg every 24-36 hours (redose when concentration <1.5-2 mg/L)

Systemic gram-negative infection: 1.5-2.5 mg/kg every 24-48 hours (redose when concentration <3-5 mg/L)

Dosing adjustment/comments in hepatic disease: Monitor plasma concentrations

Dosing in obesity: In moderate obesity (TBW/IBW ≥1.25) or greater (eg, morbid obesity [TBW/IBW >2]), initial dosage requirement may be estimated using a dosing weight of IBW + 0.4 (TBW - IBW) (Traynor, 1995).

Dietary Considerations Calcium, magnesium, potassium: Renal wasting may cause hypocalcemia, hypomagnesemia, and/or hypokalemia.

Administration

IM: Administer by deep IM route if possible. Slower absorption and lower peak concentrations, probably due to poor circulation in the atrophic muscle, may occur following IM injection; in paralyzed patients, suggest IV route.

IV: Infuse over 30-120 minutes.

Some penicillins (eg, carbenicillin, ticarcillin, and piperacillin) have been shown to inactivate aminoglycosides *in vitro*. This has been observed to a greater extent with tobramycin and gentamicin, while amikacin has shown greater stability against inactivation. Concurrent use of these agents may pose a risk of reduced antibacterial efficacy *in vivo*, particularly in the setting of profound renal impairment. However, definitive clinical evidence is lacking. If combination penicillin/aminoglycoside therapy is desired in a patient with renal dysfunction, separation of doses (if feasible), and routine monitoring of aminoglycoside levels, CBC, and clinical response should be considered.

Monitoring Parameters Urinalysis, urine output, BUN, serum creatinine, plasma gentamicin levels (as appropriate to dosing method). Levels are typically obtained after the third dose in conventional dosing. Hearing should be tested before, during, and after treatment; particularly in those at risk for ototoxicity or who will be receiving prolonged therapy (>2 weeks)

Some penicillin derivatives may accelerate the degradation of aminoglycosides *in vitro*. This may be clinically-significant for certain penicillin (ticarcillin, piperacillin, carbenicillin) and aminoglycoside (gentamicin, tobramycin) combination therapy in patients with significant renal impairment. Close monitoring of aminoglycoside levels is warranted.

Reference Range

Timing of serum samples: Draw peak 30 minutes after 30-minute infusion has been completed or 1 hour after IM injection; draw trough immediately before next dose

Therapeutic levels:

Peak:

Serious infections: 6-8 mcg/mL (12-17 micromole/L)

Life-threatening infections: 8-10 mcg/mL (17-21 micromole/L)

Urinary tract infections: 4-6 mcg/mL

Synergy against gram-positive organisms: 3-5 mcg/mL

Trough:

Serious infections: 0.5-1 mcg/mL

Life-threatening infections: 1-2 mcg/mL

The American Thoracic Society (ATS) recommends trough levels of <1 mcg/mL for patients with hospital-acquired pneumonia.

Obtain drug levels after the third dose unless renal dysfunction/toxicity suspected

Dosage Forms

Solution, Injection:

Generic: 10 mg/mL (2 mL); 40 mg/mL (2 mL, 20 mL)

Solution, Injection [preservative free]:

Generic: 10 mg/mL (2 mL)

Solution, Intravenous:

Generic: 60 mg (50 mL); 70 mg (50 mL); 80 mg (50 mL, 100 mL); 90 mg (100 mL); 100 mg (50 mL, 100 mL); 120 mg (100 mL); 10 mg/mL (6 mL, 8 mL, 10 mL)

Gentamicin (Ophthalmic) (jen ta MYE sin)

Brand Names: U.S. Garamycin; Gentak

Brand Names: Canada Diogent®; Garamycin®; Gentak®; Gentocin; PMS-Gentamicin

Index Terms Gentamicin Sulfate

Pharmacologic Category Antibiotic, Aminoglycoside; Antibiotic, Ophthalmic

Use Treatment of ophthalmic infections caused by susceptible bacteria

Pregnancy Risk Factor C

Dosage Ophthalmic: Children and Adults:

Ointment: Instill 1/2" (1.25 cm) 2-3 times/day to every 3-4 hours

Solution: Instill 1-2 drops every 4 hours, up to 2 drops every hour for severe infections

Additional Information Complete prescribing information should be consulted for additional detail.

Dosage Forms

Ointment, Ophthalmic:

Gentak: 0.3% (3.5 g)

Generic: 0.3% (3.5 g)

Solution, Ophthalmic:

Garamycin: 0.3% (5 mL)

Generic: 0.3% (5 mL, 15 mL)

- ◆ **Gentamicin and Prednisolone** *see* Prednisolone and Gentamicin *on page* 1706
- ◆ **Gentamicin Injection, USP (Can)** *see* Gentamicin (Systemic) *on page* 959
- ◆ **Gentamicin Sulfate** *see* Gentamicin (Ophthalmic) *on page* 962
- ◆ **Gentamicin Sulfate** *see* Gentamicin (Systemic) *on page* 959

Gentian Violet (JEN shun VYE oh let)

Index Terms Crystal Violet; Methylrosaniline Chloride

Pharmacologic Category Antibiotic, Topical; Antifungal Agent, Topical

Use Treatment of cutaneous or mucocutaneous infections caused by *Candida albicans* and other superficial skin infections; external treatment of minor abrasions or cuts

Dosage Children and Adults: Topical: Apply to affected area once or twice daily. Solutions diluted to 0.25% to 0.5% may be less irritating. Solutions diluted to 0.01% have been recommended for use in closed cavities.

Additional Information Complete prescribing information should be consulted for additional detail.

Dosage Forms

Solution, External:

Generic: 1% (59 mL); 2% (59 mL, 59.14 mL)

- ◆ **Gen-Ticlopidine (Can)** *see* Ticlopidine *on page* 2040
- ◆ **Gen-Tizanidine (Can)** *see* TiZANidine *on page* 2051
- ◆ **Gentle Laxative [OTC]** *see* Bisacodyl *on page* 265
- ◆ **Gentocin (Can)** *see* Gentamicin (Ophthalmic) *on page* 962
- ◆ **Genz-112638** *see* Eliglustat *on page* 712
- ◆ **Geodon** *see* Ziprasidone *on page* 2201
- ◆ **Geri-Dryl [OTC]** *see* DiphenhydrAMINE (Systemic) *on page* 641
- ◆ **Geri-Mox [OTC]** *see* Aluminum Hydroxide, Magnesium Hydroxide, and Simethicone *on page* 104
- ◆ **Geri-Mucil [OTC]** *see* Psyllium *on page* 1744
- ◆ **Geri-Pectate [OTC]** *see* Bismuth *on page* 265
- ◆ **Geri-Stool [OTC]** *see* Docusate and Senna *on page* 662
- ◆ **Geri-Tussin [OTC]** *see* GuaiFENesin *on page* 986

Gestrinone [INT] (JES tri none)

International Brand Names Dimetriose (AU, IE, PT); Dimetrose (BE, BR, IT, LU); Florizel (GB); Nemestran (AR, CH, CZ, ES, MX, NL)

Pharmacologic Category Antigonadotropic Agent

Reported Use Treatment of endometriosis

Dosage Range Adults: Oral: 2.5 mg twice weekly starting on first day of cycle with second dose 3 days later, repeated on same two days preferably at same time each week; duration of treatment usually 6 months

Product Availability Product available in various countries; not currently available in the U.S.

Dosage Forms

Capsule: 2.5 mg

- ◆ **GF196960** *see* Tadalafil *on page* 1968
- ◆ **GG** *see* GuaiFENesin *on page* 986
- ◆ **GHB** *see* Sodium Oxybate *on page* 1908
- ◆ **GI87084B** *see* Remifentanil *on page* 1789
- ◆ **Gianvi** *see* Ethinyl Estradiol and Drospirenone *on page* 801
- ◆ **Giazo** *see* Balsalazide *on page* 226
- ◆ **Gildagia** *see* Ethinyl Estradiol and Norethindrone *on page* 808
- ◆ **Gildess 24 Fe** *see* Ethinyl Estradiol and Norethindrone *on page* 808
- ◆ **Gildess FE 1.5/30** *see* Ethinyl Estradiol and Norethindrone *on page* 808
- ◆ **Gildess FE 1/20** *see* Ethinyl Estradiol and Norethindrone *on page* 808
- ◆ **Gilenya** *see* Fingolimod *on page* 879
- ◆ **Gilotrif** *see* Afatinib *on page* 61
- ◆ **Giotrif (Can)** *see* Afatinib *on page* 61
- ◆ **Glargine Insulin** *see* Insulin Glargine *on page* 1086

Glatiramer Acetate (gla TIR a mer AS e tate)

Brand Names: U.S. Copaxone

Brand Names: Canada Copaxone

Index Terms Copolymer-1

Pharmacologic Category Biological, Miscellaneous

Use Multiple sclerosis: Treatment of relapsing forms of multiple sclerosis

Pregnancy Risk Factor B

Pregnancy Considerations Adverse events were not observed in animal studies.

Breast-Feeding Considerations It is not known if glatiramer acetate is excreted in breast milk. The manufacturer recommends that caution be exercised when administering glatiramer acetate to nursing women.

Contraindications Hypersensitivity to glatiramer acetate, mannitol, or any component of the formulation

Warnings/Precautions Glatiramer acetate is antigenic, and may interfere with recognition of foreign antigens affecting tumor surveillance and infection defense systems. Immediate postinjection systemic reactions occur in a substantial percentage of patients (~16% [20 mg/mL] and ~2% [40 mg/mL] in studies); symptoms (anxiety, chest pain, dyspnea, dysphagia, flushing, palpitations, urticaria) are usually self-limited and transient. These symptoms generally occur several months after initiation of glatiramer. Chest pain may or may not occur with the immediate postinjection reaction; described as a transient pain usually resolving in a few minutes; often unassociated with other symptoms. Episodes usually begin ≥1 month after initiation of glatiramer. Lipoatrophy may occur locally at injection site at various times after treatment and may not resolve; advise patient to follow proper injection technique and rotate site daily. Skin necrosis has been observed rarely.

Adverse Reactions

Cardiovascular: Chest pain, edema, facial edema, hypertension, palpitations, peripheral edema, syncope, tachycardia, vasodilatation

Central nervous system: Abnormal dreams, anxiety, chills, emotional lability, migraine, nervousness, pain, speech disturbance, stupor

Dermatologic: Diaphoresis, eczema, erythema, hyperhidrosis, pruritus, pustular rash, skin atrophy, skin rash, urticaria, warts

Endocrine & metabolic: Weight gain, amenorrhea, hypermenorrhea

Gastrointestinal: Aphthous stomatitis, bowel urgency, dental caries, dysphagia, enlargement of salivary glands, gastroenteritis, nausea, oral candidiasis, vomiting

Genitourinary: Abnormal Pap smear, hematuria, impotence, urinary urgency, vaginal hemorrhage, volvovaginal candidiasis

Hematologic & oncologic: Benign skin neoplasm, bruise, lymphadenopathy

Hypersensitivity: Hypersensitivity, immediate hypersensitivity (postinjection, including flushing, chest pain, palpitations, anxiety, dyspnea, throat constriction, and/or urticaria)

Immunologic: Development of IgG antibodies

Infection: Abscess, herpes zoster, infection

Local: Injection site reactions: Abscess, bleeding, erythema, fibrosis, hypersensitivity reaction, inflammation, itching, lipoatrophy, pain, residual mass, swelling

Neuromuscular & skeletal: Back pain, laryngospasm, neck pain, tremor, weakness

Ophthalmic: Diplopia, visual field defect

Respiratory: Bronchitis, cough, dyspnea, flu-like symptoms, hyperventilation, laryngismus, nasopharyngitis, rhinitis, viral respiratory tract infection

Miscellaneous: Fever

Rare but important or life-threatening: Amyotrophy, anaphylactoid reaction, anemia, angina pectoris, angioedema, aphasia, arthritis, asthma, ataxia, atrial fibrillation, blepharoptosis, blindness, bradycardia, bursitis, carcinoma (breast, bladder, lung, ovarian), cardiac arrhythmia, cardiac failure, cardiomegaly, cardiomyopathy, cataract, cerebral edema, cerebrovascular accident, cholecystitis, cholelithiasis, CNS neoplasm, colitis, coma, corneal ulcer, coronary occlusion, Cushing's syndrome, cyanosis, decreased libido, deep vein thrombophlebitis, depersonalization, dermatitis, dry eye syndrome, duodenal ulcer, eosinophilia, erythema nodosum, esophageal ulcer, esophagitis, facial paralysis, fibrocystic breast disease, fourth heart sound, fungal dermatitis, furunculosis, gastrointestinal carcinoma, gastrointestinal hemorrhage, gastrointestinal ulcer, genitourinary neoplasm, glaucoma, gout, hallucination, hematemesis, hepatic cirrhosis, hepatitis, hepatomegaly, hernia, hydrocephalus, hypercholesterolemia, hyperthyroidism, hypokinesia, hypotension, hypothyroidism, hypoventilation, increased appetite, leukemia, leukopenia, lupus erythematosus, lymphedema, maculopapular rash, malignant neoplasm of cervix, malignant neoplasm of skin, mania, memory impairment, meningitis, mitral valve prolapse syndrome, moon face, muscle spasm, mydriasis, myelitis, myocardial infarction, myoclonus, nephrolithiasis, nephrosis, neuralgia, optic neuritis, oral mucosa ulcer, orthostatic hypotension, osteomyelitis, otitis externa, ovarian cyst, pancreatitis, pancytopenia, paraplegia, pericardial effusion, peripheral vascular disease, photophobia, pneumonia, priapism, pseudolymphoma, psoriasis, psychotic depression, pulmonary embolism, pyelonephritis, rectal hemorrhage, renal failure, seizures, sepsis, serum sickness, skin hypertrophy, skin photosensitivity, skin pigmentation, splenomegaly, stomatitis, suicidal tendencies, systemic lupus erythematosus, systolic heart murmur, tenosynovitis, thrombocytopenia, thrombophlebitis, thrombosis, tissue necrosis at injection site, urethritis, vesicobullous rash, weight loss, xeroderma

Drug Interactions

Metabolism/Transport Effects None known.

Avoid Concomitant Use

Avoid concomitant use of Glatiramer Acetate with any of the following: BCG; Natalizumab; Pimecrolimus; Tacrolimus (Topical); Tofacitinib; Vaccines (Live)

Increased Effect/Toxicity

Glatiramer Acetate may increase the levels/effects of: Leflunomide; Natalizumab; Tofacitinib; Vaccines (Live)

The levels/effects of Glatiramer Acetate may be increased by: Denosumab; Pimecrolimus; Roflumilast; Tacrolimus (Topical); Trastuzumab

Decreased Effect

Glatiramer Acetate may decrease the levels/effects of: BCG; Coccidioides immitis Skin Test; Sipuleucel-T; Vaccines (Inactivated); Vaccines (Live)

The levels/effects of Glatiramer Acetate may be decreased by: Echinacea

Storage/Stability Store refrigerated at 2°C to 8°C (36°F to 46°F). If needed, may store at 15°C to 30°C (59°F to 86°F) for up to 1 month (refrigeration is preferred). Avoid exposure to high temperatures; protect from intense light. Do not freeze. Discard if syringe freezes.

Mechanism of Action Glatiramer is a mixture of random polymers of four amino acids; L-alanine, L-glutamic acid, L-lysine, and L-tyrosine, the resulting mixture is antigenically similar to myelin basic protein, which is an important component of the myelin sheath of nerves; glatiramer is thought to induce and activate T-lymphocyte suppressor cells specific for a myelin antigen, it is also proposed that glatiramer interferes with the antigen-presenting function of certain immune cells opposing pathogenic T-cell function

Pharmacodynamics/Kinetics

Distribution: Small amounts of intact and partial hydrolyzed drug enter lymphatic circulation

Metabolism: SubQ: Large percentage hydrolyzed locally

Dosage Adults: SubQ: 20 mg daily or 40 mg 3 times per week administered at least 48 hours apart.

Note: Glatiramer 20 mg/mL and 40 mg/mL formulations are not interchangeable.

Dosage adjustment in renal impairment: No dosage adjustment provided in manufacturer's labeling (has not been studied).

Dosage adjustment in hepatic impairment: No dosage adjustment provided in manufacturer's labeling.

Administration For SubQ administration in the arms, abdomen, hips, or thighs; rotate injection sites to prevent lipoatrophy. Administer the 40 mg dose on the same 3 days each week (eg, Monday, Wednesday, Friday) at least 48 hours apart. Allow syringe to stand at room temperature for 20 minutes prior to injection. Solution in the syringe should appear clear and colorless to slightly yellow; discard if solution is cloudy or contains any particulate matter. Discard unused portions.

Dosage Forms

Kit, Subcutaneous:

Copaxone: 20 mg/mL

Solution Prefilled Syringe, Subcutaneous:

Copaxone: 40 mg/mL (1 mL)

- **GlcCerase** *see* Velaglucerase Alfa *on page 2147*
- **Gleevec** *see* Imatinib *on page 1047*
- **Gleostine** *see* Lomustine *on page 1235*
- **Gliadel Wafer** *see* Carmustine *on page 364*
- **Glibenclamide** *see* GlyBURIDE *on page 972*

Gliclazide [CAN/INT] (GLYE kla zide)

Brand Names: Canada Apo-Gliclazide; AVA-Gliclazide; Diamicron; Diamicron MR; Gliclazide MR; Gliclazide-80; Mint-Gliclazide MR; Mylan-Gliclazide; PMS-Gliclazide; Teva-Gliclazide

Pharmacologic Category Antidiabetic Agent, Sulfonylurea

Use Note: Not approved in U.S.

Management of type 2 diabetes mellitus (noninsulin dependent, NIDDM)

Pregnancy Considerations Use during pregnancy is contraindicated. Maternal hyperglycemia can be associated with adverse effects in the fetus, including macrosomia, neonatal hyperglycemia, and hyperbilirubinemia; the risk of congenital malformations is increased when the Hb A_{1c} is above the normal range. Diabetes can also be associated with adverse effects in the mother. Poorly-treated diabetes may cause end-organ damage that may in turn negatively affect obstetric outcomes. Physiologic glucose levels should be maintained prior to and during pregnancy to decrease the risk of adverse events in the mother and the fetus. Insulin is the drug of choice for the control of diabetes mellitus during pregnancy.

Breast-Feeding Considerations Potential for neonatal hypoglycemia in a nursing infant contraindicates use.

Contraindications Hypersensitivity to gliclazide, other sulfonylureas or sulfonamides, or any component of the formulation; unstable and/or type 1 diabetes mellitus (insulin dependent, IDDM); diabetic ketoacidosis; diabetic precoma and coma; severe renal or hepatic impairment; stress conditions (eg, serious infection, trauma, surgery); concurrent use with miconazole (systemic or oromucosal gel); pregnancy; breast-feeding

Warnings/Precautions All sulfonylurea drugs are capable of producing severe hypoglycemia. The incidence of hypoglycemia is least with gliclazide compared to other sulfonylureas (eg, glimepiride or glyburide) (Canadian Diabetes Association [CDA], 2013). Hypoglycemia is more likely to occur when caloric intake is deficient, after severe or prolonged exercise, when ethanol is ingested, or when more than one glucose-lowering drug is used. Hypoglycemia is also more likely in elderly patients, malnourished patients or in patients with endocrine disorders, severe vascular disease or impaired renal or hepatic function. Hypoglycemic effects (eg, dizziness, weakness) may impair physical or mental abilities; patients must be cautioned about performing tasks which require mental alertness (eg, operating machinery or driving).

Loss of efficacy may be observed following prolonged use as a result of the progression of type 2 diabetes mellitus which results in continued beta cell destruction. In patients who were previously responding to sulfonylurea therapy, consider additional factors which may be contributing to decreased efficacy (eg, inappropriate dose, nonadherence to diet and exercise regimen). If no contributing factors can be identified, consider discontinuing use of the sulfonylurea due to secondary failure of treatment. Additional antidiabetic therapy (eg, insulin) will be required. Diabetes self-management education (DSME) is essential to maximize the effectiveness of therapy.

Chemical similarities are present among sulfonamides, sulfonylureas, carbonic anhydrase inhibitors, thiazides, and loop diuretics (except ethacrynic acid). Use in patients with sulfonamide allergy is contraindicated in the product labeling due to the risk of cross-reaction that exists in patients with an allergy to any of these compounds especially when the previous reaction has been severe. Use with caution in hepatic or renal impairment as metabolism and/or excretion may be impaired; dose reductions may be necessary. Discontinue use if cholestatic jaundice occurs during therapy. Use in severe hepatic or renal impairment or during periods of stress (eg, trauma, infection, surgery) is contraindicated. Patients with glucose-6-phosphate dehydrogenase (G6PD) deficiency may be at an increased risk of sulfonylurea-induced hemolytic anemia; however, cases have also been described in patients without G6PD deficiency during postmarketing surveillance. Use with caution and consider a nonsulfonylurea alternative in patients with G6PD deficiency

U.S. product labeling of sulfonylureas states oral hypoglycemic drugs may be associated with an increased cardiovascular mortality as compared to treatment with diet alone or diet plus insulin. Data to support this association are limited, and several studies, including a large prospective trial (UKPDS), have not supported an association. Formulation may contain lactose; avoid use in patients with galactose intolerance, glucose-galactose malabsorption or Lapp lactose deficiency.

Adverse Reactions

Cardiovascular: Angina, hypertension, peripheral edema

Central nervous system: Depression, dizziness, headache, insomnia

Dermatologic: Dermatitis, pruritus, rash (including maculopapular, morbilliform), skin disorder

Endocrine & metabolic: Hyperlipidemia, hypoglycemia, lipid metabolism disorder

Gastrointestinal: Abdominal pain, constipation, diarrhea, gastritis, gastroenteritis, nausea

Genitourinary: Urinary tract infection

Neuromuscular & skeletal: Arthralgia, arthritis, arthrosis, back pain, myalgia, neuralgia, tendonitis,weakness

Ocular: Conjunctivitis

Otic: Otitis media

Respiratory: Bronchitis, cough, pharyngitis, pneumonia, rhinitis, sinusitis, upper respiratory infection

Miscellaneous: Viral infection

Rare but important or life-threatening: Agranulocytosis, albuminuria, allergic vasculitis, allergy, anal fissure, anemia, appetite increased, arteritis, arthropathy, asthma, balanitis, breast neoplasm (female; benign), bursitis, bullous reactions, cardiac failure, carpal tunnel syndrome, cataracts, cholestatic jaundice, colitis, coma (hypoglycemic), conjunctival hemorrhage, diplopia, disulfiram-like reaction, duodenal ulcer, eczema, erythrocytopenia, esophagitis, fecal incontinence, fungal dermatitis, fungal infection, gastroesophageal reflux, GI neoplasm (benign), glaucoma, glycosuria, gout, hearing decreased, hemolytic anemia, hepatitis, hepatomegaly, hernia (congenital), hypercholesterolemia, hyperkeratosis, hypertriglyceridemia, hyponatremia, hypotension, hypothyroidism, impotence, leukopenia, mastitis, melena, MI, neuropathy, nocturia, onychomycosis, palpitation, pancreatitis, pancytopenia, prostatic disorder, renal calculus, renal cyst, retinal disorder, skin ulceration, spine malformation, tachycardia, thrombocytopenia, thrombophlebitis, tracheitis, vaginitis, vitreous disorder, weight gain

Drug Interactions

Metabolism/Transport Effects Substrate of CYP2C9 (major); **Note:** Assignment of Major/Minor substrate status based on clinically relevant drug interaction potential

Avoid Concomitant Use There are no known interactions where it is recommended to avoid concomitant use.

Increased Effect/Toxicity

Gliclazide may increase the levels/effects of: Alcohol (Ethyl); Carbocisteine; Hypoglycemic Agents; Porfimer; Verteporfin; Vitamin K Antagonists

The levels/effects of Gliclazide may be increased by: Androgens; Beta-Blockers; Ceritinib; Chloramphenicol; Cimetidine; Cyclic Antidepressants; CYP2C9 Inhibitors (Moderate); CYP2C9 Inhibitors (Strong); Dexketoprofen; Fibric Acid Derivatives; Fluconazole; GLP-1 Agonists; Herbs (Hypoglycemic Properties); MAO Inhibitors; Metreleptin; Miconazole (Oral); Mifepristone; Pegvisomant; Probenecid; Quinolone Antibiotics; Ranitidine; Salicylates; Selective Serotonin Reuptake Inhibitors; SGLT2 Inhibitors; Sulfonamide Derivatives; Vitamin K Antagonists; Voriconazole

Decreased Effect

The levels/effects of Gliclazide may be decreased by: Corticosteroids (Orally Inhaled); Corticosteroids (Systemic); CYP2C9 Inducers (Strong); Dabrafenib; Danazol; Loop Diuretics; Luteinizing Hormone-Releasing Hormone Analogs; Quinolone Antibiotics; Rifampin; Somatropin; Thiazide Diuretics

Food Interactions Ethanol may cause rare disulfiram reactions. Management: Monitor patients.

Storage/Stability Store at 15°C to 30°C (59°F to 86°F).

Mechanism of Action Stimulates insulin release from the pancreatic beta cells; reduces insulin uptake and glucose output by the liver; insulin sensitivity is increased at peripheral target sites. Reduces microthrombosis by decreasing platelet aggregation and adhesion, and by restoring fibrinolysis with an increase in tissue plasminogen activator (t-PA) activity. Antioxidant effects include a decrease in plasma levels of peroxidized lipids and increased erythrocyte superoxide dismutase activity.

Pharmacodynamics/Kinetics

Duration of action: Modified release tablet: 24 hours

Absorption: Immediate release formulation: Rapid; Modified release formulation: Slow and complete

Bioavailability: 97%

Protein binding: ~94% to 95%

Metabolism: Hepatic (via CYP2C9 and CYP2C19; Elliot, 2007) to inactive metabolites

Half-life elimination: Immediate release tablet: 10 hours; Modified release tablet: 16 hours (range: 12-20 hours)

Time to peak: Immediate release tablet: 4-6 hours; Modified release tablet: ~6 hours

Excretion: Urine (60% to 70%; <1% as unchanged drug); feces (10% to 20%) as metabolites

Dosage Oral: Adults:

Type 2 diabetes: **Note:** There is no fixed-dosage regimen for the management of diabetes mellitus with gliclazide. Dose must be individualized based on frequent determinations of blood glucose during dose titration and throughout maintenance.

Immediate release tablet: Recommended initial: 80 mg twice daily; titrate based on blood glucose levels. Usual dosage range: 80-320 mg/day (maximum dose: 320 mg/day); dosage of ≥160 mg should be divided into 2 equal parts for twice-daily administration

Modified release tablet: Initial: 30 mg once daily; titrate in 30 mg increments every 2 weeks based on blood glucose levels. Maximum dose: 120 mg once daily

Maturity-onset diabetes: May consider conversion from insulin to gliclazide therapy in patients receiving <40 units/day insulin. Prior to conversion, discontinue insulin for 48-72 hours with close monitoring (≥3 times/day) of urine for glucose and ketones. Patients with ketonuria and glycosuria 12-24 hours after discontinuing insulin should not be converted to gliclazide therapy and should remain on insulin therapy.

Elderly: Refer to adult dosing.

Dosage adjustment in renal impairment:

Mild-to-moderate impairment: Initial dosage adjustments are not required; however, as gliclazide is primarily excreted in the urine, dose reductions may be necessary.

Severe impairment: Use is contraindicated.

Dosage adjustment in hepatic impairment:

Mild-to-moderate impairment: Initial dosage adjustments are not required; dose reductions may be necessary; however, as gliclazide is primarily excreted in the urine.

Severe impairment: Use is contraindicated.

Dietary Considerations Should be taken with meals. Individualized medical nutrition therapy (MNT) based on CDA recommendations is an integral part of therapy.

Administration Patients that are NPO or require decreased caloric intake may need doses held to avoid hypoglycemia. Administer with meals (modified release tablet should be administered with breakfast). May split the 60 mg modified release tablets in half; however, the 30 mg modified release tablets must be swallowed whole. Modified release tablets should not be crushed or chewed.

Monitoring Parameters Signs and symptoms of hypoglycemia, fasting blood glucose, hemoglobin A_{1c}; renal and hepatic function (baseline [all patients] then periodically thereafter in patients with mild-moderate dysfunction)

Reference Range

Recommendations for glycemic control in nonpregnant adults with diabetes (ADA, 2015):

HbA_{1c}: <7% (a more aggressive [<6.5%] or less aggressive [<8%] HbA_{1c} goal may be targeted based on patient-specific characteristics)

Preprandial capillary plasma glucose: 80 to 130 mg/dL

Peak postprandial capillary blood glucose: <180 mg/dL

Recommendations for glycemic control in pediatric (all age groups) patients with type 1 diabetes (ADA, 2015):

HbA_{1c}: <7.5% (individualization may be appropriate based on patient-specific characteristics; <7% is reasonable if it can be achieved without excessive hypoglycemia)

Preprandial capillary plasma glucose: 90 to 130 mg/dL

Bedtime and overnight capillary blood glucose: 90 to 150 mg/dL

Additional Information Note: 30 mg modified release tablet equals 80 mg immediate release tablet

Product Availability Not available in U.S.

Dosage Forms: Canada

Tablet, oral:

Diamicron®: 80 mg

Tablet, modified release, oral:

Diamicron® MR: 30 mg, 60 mg

◆ **Gliclazide-80 (Can)** *see* Gliclazide [CAN/INT] *on page 964*

◆ **Gliclazide MR (Can)** *see* Gliclazide [CAN/INT] *on page 964*

Glimepiride (GLYE me pye ride)

Brand Names: U.S. Amaryl

Brand Names: Canada Amaryl; Apo-Glimepiride; Novo-Glimepiride; PMS-Glimepiride; ratio-Glimepiride; Sandoz-Glimepiride

Pharmacologic Category Antidiabetic Agent, Sulfonylurea

Use Type 2 diabetes mellitus: As an adjunct to diet and exercise to improve glycemic control in adults with type 2 diabetes mellitus

Pregnancy Risk Factor C

Pregnancy Considerations Adverse events have been observed in some animal reproduction studies. Severe hypoglycemia lasting 4 to 10 days has been noted in infants born to mothers taking a sulfonylurea at the time of delivery.

In women with diabetes, maternal hyperglycemia can be associated with congenital malformations as well as adverse effects in the fetus, neonate, and the mother (ACOG, 2005; ADA, 2014; Kitzmiller, 2008; Metzger, 2007). To prevent adverse outcomes, prior to conception and throughout pregnancy maternal blood glucose and HbA_{1c} should be kept as close to normal as possible but without causing significant hypoglycemia (ACOG, 2013; ADA, 2014; Blumer, 2013; Kitzmiller, 2008). Prior to pregnancy, effective contraception should be used until glycemic control is achieved (ADA, 2014; Kitzmiller, 2008). Other agents are currently recommended to treat diabetes in pregnant women (ACOG, 2013; Blumer, 2013).

Breast-Feeding Considerations It is not known if glimepiride is excreted in breast milk. According to the manufacturer, due to the potential for hypoglycemia in the nursing infant, a decision should be made whether to discontinue nursing or to discontinue the drug, taking into account the importance of treatment to the mother.

Contraindications

Hypersensitivity to glimepiride, any component of the formulation, or sulfonamides; diabetic ketoacidosis (with or without coma)

Documentation of allergenic cross-reactivity for drugs in this class is limited. However, because of similarities in chemical structure and/or pharmacologic actions, the possibility of cross-sensitivity cannot be ruled out with certainty.

Canadian labeling: Additional contraindications (not in U.S. labeling): Pregnancy; breast-feeding; type 1 diabetes; severe renal or hepatic impairment

Warnings/Precautions All sulfonylurea drugs are capable of producing severe hypoglycemia. Hypoglycemia is more likely to occur when caloric intake is deficient, after severe or prolonged exercise, when ethanol is ingested, or when more than one glucose-lowering drug is used. It is also more likely in elderly patients, malnourished patients and in patients with impaired renal or hepatic function; use with caution. Reduce dosage in patients with renal impairment.

Loss of efficacy may be observed following prolonged use as a result of the progression of type 2 diabetes mellitus which results in continued beta cell destruction. In patients who were previously responding to sulfonylurea therapy, consider additional factors which may be contributing to decreased efficacy (eg, inappropriate dose, nonadherence to diet and exercise regimen). If no contributing factors can be identified, consider discontinuing use of the sulfonylurea due to secondary failure of treatment. Additional antidiabetic therapy (eg, insulin) will be required. It may be necessary to discontinue therapy and administer insulin if the patient is exposed to stress (fever, trauma, infection, surgery).

Chemical similarities are present among sulfonamides, sulfonylureas, carbonic anhydrase inhibitors, thiazides, and loop diuretics (except ethacrynic acid); a risk of cross-reaction exists in patients with allergy to any of these compounds. Use in patients with sulfonamide allergy is contraindicated. Patients with G6PD deficiency may be at an increased risk of sulfonylurea-induced hemolytic anemia; however, cases have also been described in patients without G6PD deficiency during postmarketing surveillance. Use with caution and consider a nonsulfonylurea alternative in patients with G6PD deficiency. Systemic exposure of glimepiride is increased in patients with CYP2C9*3 allele; dose reductions may be necessary (Niemi, 2002).

Product labeling states oral hypoglycemic drugs may be associated with an increased cardiovascular mortality as compared to treatment with diet alone or diet plus insulin. Data to support this association are limited, and several studies, including a large prospective trial (UKPDS) have not supported an association.

Adverse Reactions

Central nervous system: Dizziness, headache

Endocrine & metabolic: Hypoglycemia

Gastrointestinal: Nausea

Hepatic: Increased serum ALT

Respiratory: Flu-like symptoms

Miscellaneous: Accidental injury

Rare but important or life-threatening: Abnormal hepatic function tests, accommodation disturbance (early treatment), agranulocytosis, anaphylaxis, angioedema, anorexia, aplastic anemia, cholestatic jaundice, disulfiram-like reaction, epigastric fullness, hemolytic anemia, hepatic failure, hepatic porphyria, hepatitis, hypersensitivity, hypersensitivity angiitis, hyponatremia, hypotension, leukopenia, maculopapular rash, morbilliform rash, pancytopenia, porphyria cutanea tarda, shock, SIADH, skin photosensitivity, Stevens-Johnson syndrome, thrombocytopenia, weight gain

Drug Interactions

Metabolism/Transport Effects Substrate of CYP2C9 (major); **Note:** Assignment of Major/Minor substrate status based on clinically relevant drug interaction potential

Avoid Concomitant Use There are no known interactions where it is recommended to avoid concomitant use.

Increased Effect/Toxicity

Glimepiride may increase the levels/effects of: Alcohol (Ethyl); Carbocisteine; Hypoglycemic Agents; Porfimer; Verteporfin; Vitamin K Antagonists

The levels/effects of Glimepiride may be increased by: Androgens; Beta-Blockers; Ceritinib; Chloramphenicol; Cimetidine; Cyclic Antidepressants; CYP2C9 Inhibitors (Moderate); CYP2C9 Inhibitors (Strong); Dexketoprofen; Fibric Acid Derivatives; Fluconazole; GLP-1 Agonists; Herbs (Hypoglycemic Properties); MAO Inhibitors; Metreleptin; Miconazole (Oral); Mifepristone; Pegvisomant; Probenecid; Quinolone Antibiotics; Ranitidine; Salicylates; Selective Serotonin Reuptake Inhibitors; SGLT2 Inhibitors; Sulfonamide Derivatives; Vitamin K Antagonists; Voriconazole

Decreased Effect
The levels/effects of Glimepiride may be decreased by: Colesevelam; Corticosteroids (Orally Inhaled); Corticosteroids (Systemic); CYP2C9 Inducers (Strong); Dabrafenib; Danazol; Loop Diuretics; Luteinizing Hormone-Releasing Hormone Analogs; Quinolone Antibiotics; Rifampin; Somatropin; Thiazide Diuretics

Food Interactions Ethanol may cause rare disulfiram reactions. Management: Monitor patients.

Storage/Stability Store at 25°C (77°F); excursions permitted between 20°C and 25°C (68°F and 77°F)

Mechanism of Action Stimulates insulin release from the pancreatic beta cells; reduces glucose output from the liver; insulin sensitivity is increased at peripheral target sites

Pharmacodynamics/Kinetics
Onset of action: Peak effect: Blood glucose reductions: 2-3 hours
Duration: 24 hours
Absorption: 100%; delayed when given with food
Distribution: V_d: 8.8 L
Protein binding: >99.5%
Metabolism: Hepatic oxidation via CYP2C9 to M1 metabolite (~33% activity of parent compound); further oxidative metabolism to inactive M2 metabolite
Half-life elimination: 5-9 hours
Time to peak, plasma: 2-3 hours
Excretion: Urine (60%, 80% to 90% as M1 and M2 metabolites); feces (40%, 70% as M1 and M2 metabolites)

Dosage Type 2 diabetes:
Adults: Oral: Initial: 1-2 mg once daily, administered with breakfast or the first main meal; based on response, may increase dose by 1-2 mg every 1-2 weeks up to maximum of 8 mg once daily. If inadequate response to maximal dose, combination therapy with other agents (eg, metformin, insulin) may be considered. Combination therapy is individualized based on glycemic response.
Conversion from therapy with long half-life agents: Observe patient carefully for 1-2 weeks when converting from a longer half-life agent (eg, chlorpropamide) to glimepiride due to overlapping hypoglycemic effects.
Elderly: Initial: 1 mg once daily; dose titration and maintenance dosing should be conservative to avoid hypoglycemia

Dosage adjustment in renal impairment:
U.S. labeling: Initial: 1 mg once daily; titrate carefully based on fasting blood glucose levels
Canadian labeling:
Mild-to-moderate impairment: Initial: 1 mg once daily; titrate carefully based on fasting blood glucose levels
Severe impairment: Use is contraindicated

Dosage adjustment in hepatic impairment:
U.S. labeling: No dosage adjustment provided in manufacturer's labeling (has not been studied).
Canadian labeling:
Mild-to-moderate impairment: No dosage adjustment provided in manufacturer's labeling (has not been studied).
Severe impairment: Use is contraindicated.

Dietary Considerations Take with breakfast or the first main meal of the day. Individualized medical nutrition therapy (MNT) based on ADA recommendations is an integral part of therapy.

Administration Administer once daily with breakfast or first main meal of the day. Patients that are NPO or require decreased caloric intake may need doses held to avoid hypoglycemia.

Monitoring Parameters Monitor for signs and symptoms of hypoglycemia (fatigue, excessive hunger, profuse sweating, numbness of extremities), fasting blood glucose, hemoglobin A_{1c}

Reference Range
Recommendations for glycemic control in nonpregnant adults with diabetes (ADA, 2015):
HbA_{1c}: <7% (a more aggressive [<6.5%] or less aggressive [<8%] HbA_{1c} goal may be targeted based on patient-specific characteristics)
Preprandial capillary plasma glucose: 80 to 130 mg/dL
Peak postprandial capillary blood glucose: <180 mg/dL

Recommendations for glycemic control in pediatric (all age groups) patients with type 1 diabetes (ADA, 2015):
HbA_{1c}: <7.5% (individualization may be appropriate based on patient-specific characteristics; <7% is reasonable if it can be achieved without excessive hypoglycemia)
Preprandial capillary plasma glucose: 90 to 130 mg/dL
Bedtime and overnight capillary blood glucose: 90 to 150 mg/dL

Dosage Forms
Tablet, Oral:
Amaryl: 1 mg, 2 mg, 4 mg
Generic: 1 mg, 2 mg, 4 mg

- ◆ **Glimepiride and Pioglitazone** *see* Pioglitazone and Glimepiride *on page 1654*
- ◆ **Glimepiride and Pioglitazone Hydrochloride** *see* Pioglitazone and Glimepiride *on page 1654*
- ◆ **Glimepiride and Rosiglitazone Maleate** *see* Rosiglitazone and Glimepiride *on page 1847*

GlipiZIDE (GLIP i zide)

Brand Names: U.S. GlipiZIDE XL; Glucotrol; Glucotrol XL

Index Terms Glydiazinamide

Pharmacologic Category Antidiabetic Agent, Sulfonylurea

Use Management of type 2 diabetes mellitus (noninsulin dependent, NIDDM) as an adjunct to diet and exercise to lower blood glucose; may be used in combination with metformin or insulin in patients whose hyperglycemia cannot be controlled by diet and exercise in conjunction with a single oral hypoglycemic agent

Pregnancy Risk Factor C

Pregnancy Considerations Adverse events have been observed in some animal reproduction studies. Glipizide was found to cross the placenta in vitro (Elliott, 1994). Severe hypoglycemia lasting 4 to 10 days has been noted in infants born to mothers taking a sulfonylurea at the time of delivery.

In women with diabetes, maternal hyperglycemia can be associated with congenital malformations as well as adverse effects in the fetus, neonate, and the mother (ACOG, 2005; ADA, 2014; Kitzmiller, 2008; Metzger, 2007). To prevent adverse outcomes, prior to conception and throughout pregnancy maternal blood glucose and HbA_{1c} should be kept as close to normal as possible but without causing significant hypoglycemia (ACOG, 2013; ADA, 2014; Blumer, 2013; Kitzmiller, 2008). Prior to pregnancy, effective contraception should be used until glycemic control is achieved (ADA, 2014; Kitzmiller, 2008). Other agents are currently recommended to treat diabetes in pregnant women (ACOG, 2013; Blumer, 2013).

The manufacturer recommends if glipizide is used during pregnancy, it should be discontinued at least 1 month before the expected delivery date.

Breast-Feeding Considerations Data from two mother-infant pairs note that glipizide was not detected in breast milk (Feig, 2005). According to the manufacturer, due to the potential for hypoglycemia in the nursing infant, a decision should be made whether to discontinue nursing or to discontinue the drug, taking into account the ▶

importance of treatment to the mother. Breast-feeding is encouraged for all women, including those with diabetes (ACOG, 2005; Blumer, 2013; Metzger, 2007). Small snacks before feeds may help decrease the risk of hypoglycemia in women with pregestational diabetes (ACOG, 2005; Reader, 2004). All types of insulin may be used while breast-feeding and some oral agents, including glipizide, may be acceptable for use as well (Metzger, 2007).

Contraindications Hypersensitivity to glipizide or any component of the formulation; type 1 diabetes mellitus (insulin dependent, IDDM); diabetic ketoacidosis (with or without coma)

Warnings/Precautions All sulfonylurea drugs are capable of producing severe hypoglycemia. Hypoglycemia is more likely to occur when caloric intake is deficient, after severe or prolonged exercise, when ethanol is ingested, or when more than one glucose-lowering drug is used. It is also more likely in elderly patients, malnourished patients and in patients with impaired renal or hepatic function; use with caution. Autonomic neuropathy, advanced age, and concomitant use of beta-blockers or other sympatholytic agents may impair the patient's ability to recognize the signs and symptoms of hypoglycemia; use with caution.

Use with caution in patients with hepatic or renal impairment. It may be necessary to discontinue therapy and administer insulin if the patient is exposed to stress (fever, trauma, infection, surgery). Loss of efficacy may be observed following prolonged use as a result of the progression of type 2 diabetes mellitus which results in continued beta cell destruction. In patients who were previously responding to sulfonylurea therapy, consider additional factors which may be contributing to decreased efficacy (eg, inappropriate dose, nonadherence to diet and exercise regimen). If no contributing factors can be identified, consider discontinuing use of the sulfonylurea due to secondary failure of treatment. Additional antidiabetic therapy (eg, insulin) will be required.

Chemical similarities are present among sulfonamides, sulfonylureas, carbonic anhydrase inhibitors, thiazides, and loop diuretics (except ethacrynic acid). Use in patients with sulfonamide allergy is not specifically contraindicated in product labeling; however, a risk of cross-reaction exists in patients with allergy to any of these compounds; avoid use when previous reaction has been severe. Patients with G6PD deficiency may be at an increased risk of sulfonylurea-induced hemolytic anemia; however, cases have also been described in patients without G6PD deficiency during postmarketing surveillance. Use with caution and consider a nonsulfonylurea alternative in patients with G6PD deficiency.

Product labeling states oral hypoglycemic drugs may be associated with an increased cardiovascular mortality as compared to treatment with diet alone or diet plus insulin. Data to support this association are limited, and several studies, including a large prospective trial (UKPDS) have not supported an association. Avoid use of extended release tablets (Glucotrol XL®) in patients with known stricture/narrowing of the GI tract.

Adverse Reactions

Cardiovascular: Syncope

Central nervous system: Anxiety, depression, dizziness, drowsiness, headache, hypoesthesia, insomnia, nervousness, pain

Dermatologic: Eczema, erythema, maculopapular eruptions, morbilliform eruptions, pruritus, rash, urticaria

Endocrine & metabolic: Hypoglycemia

Gastrointestinal: Abdominal pain, constipation, diarrhea, dyspepsia, flatulence, nausea, vomiting

Hepatic: Alkaline phosphatase increased, AST increased, LDH increased

Neuromuscular & skeletal: Arthralgia, leg cramps, myalgia, paresthesia, tremor

Ocular: Blurred vision

Renal: Blood urea nitrogen increased, creatinine increased

Respiratory: Rhinitis

Miscellaneous: Diaphoresis

Rare but important or life-threatening: Agranulocytosis, anorexia, aplastic anemia, arrhythmia, blood in stool, cholestatic jaundice, conjunctivitis, disulfiram-like reaction, edema, gait instability, hemolytic anemia, hypertension, hypertonia, hyponatremia, jaundice, leukopenia, liver injury, migraine, pancytopenia, photosensitivity, porphyria, retinal hemorrhage, SIADH, thrombocytopenia, vertigo

Drug Interactions

Metabolism/Transport Effects **Substrate** of CYP2C9 (major); **Note:** Assignment of Major/Minor substrate status based on clinically relevant drug interaction potential

Avoid Concomitant Use There are no known interactions where it is recommended to avoid concomitant use.

Increased Effect/Toxicity

GlipiZIDE may increase the levels/effects of: Alcohol (Ethyl); Carbocisteine; Hypoglycemic Agents; Porfimer; Verteporfin; Vitamin K Antagonists

The levels/effects of GlipiZIDE may be increased by: Androgens; Beta-Blockers; Ceritinib; Chloramphenicol; Cimetidine; Clarithromycin; Cyclic Antidepressants; CYP2C9 Inhibitors (Moderate); CYP2C9 Inhibitors (Strong); Dexketoprofen; Fibric Acid Derivatives; Fluconazole; GLP-1 Agonists; Herbs (Hypoglycemic Properties); MAO Inhibitors; Metreleptin; Miconazole (Oral); Mifepristone; Pegvisomant; Posaconazole; Probenecid; Quinolone Antibiotics; Ranitidine; Salicylates; Selective Serotonin Reuptake Inhibitors; SGLT2 Inhibitors; Sulfonamide Derivatives; Vitamin K Antagonists; Voriconazole

Decreased Effect

The levels/effects of GlipiZIDE may be decreased by: Colesevelam; Corticosteroids (Orally Inhaled); Corticosteroids (Systemic); CYP2C9 Inducers (Strong); Dabrafenib; Danazol; Loop Diuretics; Luteinizing Hormone-Releasing Hormone Analogs; Quinolone Antibiotics; Rifampin; Somatropin; Thiazide Diuretics

Food Interactions

Ethanol: May cause rare disulfiram reactions. Management: Monitor patients.

Food: A delayed release of insulin may occur if glipizide is taken with food. Management: Immediate release tablets should be administered 30 minutes before meals to avoid erratic absorption.

Storage/Stability Store below 30°C (86°F)

Mechanism of Action Stimulates insulin release from the pancreatic beta cells; reduces glucose output from the liver; insulin sensitivity is increased at peripheral target sites

Pharmacodynamics/Kinetics

Duration: 12-24 hours

Absorption: Immediate release: Rapid and complete; delayed with food

Distribution: 10-11 L

Protein binding: 98% to 99%; primarily to albumin

Bioavailability: 90% to 100%

Metabolism: Hepatic via CYP2C9; forms metabolites (inactive)

Half-life elimination: 2-5 hours

Time to peak: 1-3 hours; extended release tablets: 6-12 hours

Excretion: Urine (<10% as unchanged drug; 80% as metabolites); feces (10%)

Dosage

Oral: Adults:

Immediate release tablet: Initial: 5 mg once daily; titrate in 2.5-5 mg increments no more frequently than every few days based on blood glucose response; if once-daily dose is ineffective, may divide the dose; doses >15 mg/day should be administered in divided doses. Maximum recommended once-daily dose: 15 mg; maximum recommended total daily dose: 40 mg (some clinicians recommend a maximum total daily dose of 20 mg [Defronzo, 1999]).

Extended release tablet (Glucotrol XL®): Initial: 5 mg once daily; usual dose: 5-10 mg once daily; maximum recommended dose: 20 mg/day; dosage adjustments based on blood glucose monitoring should be made no more frequently than every 7 days

When transferring from immediate release to extended release glipizide: May switch the total daily dose of immediate release to the nearest equivalent daily dose of the extended release tablet and administer once daily; alternatively, may initiate extended release at 5 mg once daily and titrate accordingly.

When transferring from insulin to glipizide immediate release or extended release tablet:

Current insulin requirement ≤20 units: Discontinue insulin and initiate glipizide at usual dose

Current insulin requirement >20 units: Decrease insulin by 50% and initiate glipizide at usual dose; gradually decrease insulin dose based on patient response

Conversion from therapy with long half-life agents: Observe patient carefully for 1-2 weeks when converting from a longer half-life agent (eg, chlorpropamide) to glipizide due to overlapping hypoglycemic effects.

Elderly:

Immediate release tablet: Initial: 2.5 mg once daily; consider titrating by 2.5-5 mg/day at 1- to 2-week intervals

Extended release tablet: Initial and maintenance dosing should be on the lower end of the recommended range.

Dosing adjustment in renal impairment: No dosage adjustment provided in manufacturer's labeling although caution is recommended.

The following guidelines have been used by some clinicians (Aronoff, 2007): GFR ≤50 mL/minute: Decrease dose by 50%

Dosing adjustment in hepatic impairment:

Immediate release tablet: Initial: 2.5 mg once daily

Extended release tablet: There are no dosage adjustments provided in manufacturer's labeling; however, drug undergoes hepatic metabolism and use of a lower initial and maintenance dose should be considered.

Dietary Considerations Take immediate release tablets 30 minutes before meals (preferably before breakfast if once-daily dosing); extended release tablets should be taken with breakfast. Individualized medical nutrition therapy (MNT) based on ADA recommendations is an integral part of therapy.

Administration Administer immediate release tablets 30 minutes before a meal (preferably before breakfast if once-daily dosing) to achieve greatest reduction in postprandial hyperglycemia. Extended release tablets should be given with breakfast. Patients that are NPO or require decreased caloric intake may need doses held to avoid hypoglycemia.

Monitoring Parameters Signs and symptoms of hypoglycemia (fatigue, excessive hunger, profuse sweating, numbness of extremities), blood glucose, hemoglobin A_{1c} every 3 months for unstable patients and twice yearly for stable patients

Reference Range

Recommendations for glycemic control in nonpregnant adults with diabetes (ADA, 2015):

HbA_{1c}: <7% (a more aggressive [<6.5%] or less aggressive [<8%] HbA_{1c} goal may be targeted based on patient-specific characteristics)

Preprandial capillary plasma glucose: 80 to 130 mg/dL

Peak postprandial capillary blood glucose: <180 mg/dL

Recommendations for glycemic control in pediatric (all age groups) patients with type 1 diabetes (ADA, 2015):

HbA_{1c}: <7.5% (individualization may be appropriate based on patient-specific characteristics; <7% is reasonable if it can be achieved without excessive hypoglycemia)

Preprandial capillary plasma glucose: 90 to 130 mg/dL

Bedtime and overnight capillary blood glucose: 90 to 150 mg/dL

Dosage Forms

Tablet, Oral:

Glucotrol: 5 mg, 10 mg

Generic: 5 mg, 10 mg

Tablet Extended Release 24 Hour, Oral:

GlipiZIDE XL: 2.5 mg, 5 mg, 10 mg

Glucotrol XL: 2.5 mg, 5 mg, 10 mg

Generic: 2.5 mg, 5 mg, 10 mg

◆ **GlipiZIDE XL** *see* GlipiZIDE *on page 967*

Glipizide and Metformin

(GLIP i zide & met FOR min)

Index Terms Glipizide and Metformin Hydrochloride; Metformin and Glipizide

Pharmacologic Category Antidiabetic Agent, Biguanide; Antidiabetic Agent, Sulfonylurea

Use Indicated as an adjunct to diet and exercise to improve glycemic control in adults with type 2 diabetes mellitus (noninsulin dependent, NIDDM)

Pregnancy Risk Factor C

Dosage Oral: Type 2 diabetes:

Adults:

Patients inadequately controlled on diet and exercise alone: Initial dose: Glipizide 2.5 mg/metformin 250 mg once daily with a meal. In patients with fasting plasma glucose (FPG) 280-320 mg/dL, initiate therapy with glipizide 2.5 mg/metformin 500 mg twice daily.

Note: Increase dose by 1 tablet/day every 2 weeks (maximum daily dose: Glipizide 10 mg/metformin 2000 mg in divided doses)

Patients inadequately controlled on a sulfonylurea and/or metformin: Initial dose: Glipizide 2.5 mg/metformin 500 mg or glipizide 5 mg/metformin 500 mg twice daily with morning and evening meals; starting dose should not exceed current daily dose of glipizide (or sulfonylurea equivalent) and/or metformin.

Note: Increase dose in increments of no more than glipizide 5 mg/metformin 500 mg (maximum daily dose: Glipizide 20 mg/metformin 2000 mg)

Elderly: Conservative doses are recommended in the elderly due to potentially decreased renal function; **do not titrate to maximum dose**; should not be used in patients ≥80 years unless renal function is verified as normal

Dosage adjustment in renal impairment: Contraindicated in the presence of renal disease or renal dysfunction (serum creatinine ≥1.5 mg/dL [males], ≥1.4 mg/dL [females], or abnormal creatinine clearance)

Dosage adjustment in hepatic impairment: Avoid use in patients with impaired liver function

Additional Information Complete prescribing information should be consulted for additional detail.

Dosage Forms

Tablet, oral: 2.5/250: Glipizide 2.5 mg and metformin 250 mg; 2.5/500: Glipizide 2.5 mg and metformin 500 mg; 5/500: Glipizide 5 mg and metformin 500 mg

◆ **Glipizide and Metformin Hydrochloride** *see* Glipizide and Metformin *on page 969*

Gliquidone [INT] (GLI kwi done)

International Brand Names Glurenor (DE, IT); Glurenorm (AT, BE, CZ, DE, HR, HU)

Pharmacologic Category Antidiabetic Agent, Sulfonylurea

Reported Use Treatment of type 2 (noninsulin-dependent) diabetes mellitus

Dosage Range Adults: Oral: Initial: 15 mg daily before breakfast; range: 45-60 mg daily in 2-3 divided doses; maximum single dose: 60 mg; maximum daily dose: 180 mg

Product Availability Product available in various countries; not currently available in the U.S.

Dosage Forms

Tablet: 30 mg

◆ **Glivec** *see* Imatinib *on page 1047*

◆ **Gln** *see* Glutamine *on page 971*

◆ **GlucaGen** *see* Glucagon *on page 970*

◆ **GlucaGen HypoKit** *see* Glucagon *on page 970*

Glucagon (GLOO ka gon)

Brand Names: U.S. GlucaGen; GlucaGen HypoKit; Glucagon Emergency

Brand Names: Canada GlucaGen; GlucaGen HypoKit

Index Terms Glucagon Hydrochloride

Pharmacologic Category Antidote; Antidote, Hypoglycemia; Diagnostic Agent

Use

Diagnostic aid: As a diagnostic aid during radiologic examinations to temporarily inhibit movement of the GI tract in adults.

Hypoglycemia: Treatment of severe hypoglycemia in pediatric and adult patients.

Pregnancy Risk Factor B

Pregnancy Considerations Adverse events have not been observed in animal reproduction studies.

Breast-Feeding Considerations Glucagon is not absorbed from the GI tract and therefore, it is unlikely adverse effects would occur in a breast-feeding infant.

Contraindications Known hypersensitivity to glucagon, lactose, or any component of the formulation; patients with pheochromocytoma or insulinoma

Warnings/Precautions Use of glucagon is contraindicated in insulinoma; exogenous glucagon may cause an initial rise in blood glucose followed by rebound hypoglycemia. Use of glucagon is contraindicated in pheochromocytoma; exogenous glucagon may cause the release of catecholamines, resulting in an increase in blood pressure. Use caution with prolonged fasting, starvation, adrenal insufficiency, glucagonoma, or chronic hypoglycemia; levels of glucose stores in liver may be decreased. Allergic reactions including skin rash and anaphylactic shock (with hypotension and respiratory difficulties) have been reported; reactions have generally been associated with endoscopic patients. Use with caution in patients with cardiac disease undergoing endoscopic or radiographic procedures. Use caution if using as diagnostic aid in patients with diabetes on insulin; may cause hyperglycemia. Supplemental carbohydrates should be given to patients who respond to glucagon for severe hypoglycemia to prevent secondary hypoglycemia. Monitor blood glucose levels closely.

In patients with hypoglycemia secondary to insulin or sulfonylurea overdose, dextrose should be immediately administered; if IV access cannot be established or if dextrose is not available, glucagon may be considered as alternative acute treatment until dextrose can be administered.

May contain lactose; avoid administration in hereditary galactose intolerance, Lapp lactase deficiency, or glucose-galactose malabsorption.

Adverse Reactions Frequency not defined.

Cardiovascular: Hypertension, hypotension (up to 2 hours after GI procedures), increased blood pressure, increased pulse, tachycardia

Gastrointestinal: Nausea, vomiting (high incidence with rapid administration of high doses)

Miscellaneous: Anaphylaxis, hypersensitivity reaction

Rare but important or life-threatening: Hypoglycemia, hypoglycemic coma, respiratory distress, urticaria

Drug Interactions

Metabolism/Transport Effects None known.

Avoid Concomitant Use

Avoid concomitant use of Glucagon with any of the following: Anticholinergic Agents

Increased Effect/Toxicity

Glucagon may increase the levels/effects of: Vitamin K Antagonists

The levels/effects of Glucagon may be increased by: Anticholinergic Agents

Decreased Effect

The levels/effects of Glucagon may be decreased by: Indomethacin

Food Interactions Glucagon depletes glycogen stores.

Preparation for Administration Reconstitute powder for injection by adding 1 mL of manufacturer-supplied sterile diluent or sterile water for injection to a vial containing 1 unit of the drug, to provide solutions containing 1 mg of glucagon/mL. Gently roll vial to dissolve. Solution for infusion may be prepared by reconstitution with and further dilution in NS or D_5W (Love, 1998).

Storage/Stability Prior to reconstitution, store at controlled room temperature of 20°C to 25°C (69°F to 77°F) up to 24 months; excursions are permitted between 15°C and 30°C (59°F and 86°F). Do not freeze. Protect from light. Use reconstituted solution immediately; discard unused portion.

Mechanism of Action Stimulates adenylate cyclase to produce increased cyclic AMP, which promotes hepatic glycogenolysis and gluconeogenesis, causing a raise in blood glucose levels; antihypoglycemic effect requires preexisting hepatic glycogen stores. Extra hepatic effects of glucagon include relaxation of the smooth muscle of the stomach, duodenum, small bowel, and colon.

Pharmacodynamics/Kinetics

Onset of action:

Blood glucose levels: Peak effect: IV: 5 to 20 minutes; IM: 30 minutes; SubQ: 30 to 45 minutes

GI relaxation: IV: 1 minute; IM: 4 to 10 minutes

Duration:

Glucose elevation: IV, IM, SubQ: 60 to 90 minutes

GI relaxation: IV: 9 to 25 minutes; IM: 12 to 32 minutes

Distribution: V_d: ~0.25 L/kg

Metabolism: Primarily hepatic; some inactivation occurring renally and in plasma

Half-life elimination, plasma: IV: 8 to 18 minutes; IM (apparent): ~45 minutes

Time to peak: IM: 13 minutes; SubQ: 20 minutes

Dosage

Diagnostic aid: Adults:

Relaxation of stomach, duodenal bulb, duodenum, and small bowel:

IM: 1 mg

IV: 0.2 to 0.5 mg

Relaxation of colon:

IM: 1 to 2 mg

IV: 0.5 to 0.75 mg

Hypoglycemia: **Note:** IV dextrose should be administered as soon as it is available; if patient fails to respond to glucagon, IV dextrose must be given.

Infants, Children, and Adolescents: IM, IV, SubQ:

Glucagon Emergency Kit:

<20 kg: 0.5 mg or 0.02 to 0.03 mg/kg/dose; may repeat in 15 minutes as needed

≥20 kg: 1 mg; may repeat in 15 minutes as needed

GlucaGen:

Age-based dosing (if weight is unknown):

Infants and Children <6 years: 0.5 mg; may repeat in 15 minutes if needed

Children and Adolescents ≥6 years: 1 mg; may repeat in 15 minutes if needed

Weight-based dosing:

<25 kg: 0.5 mg; may repeat in 15 minutes if needed

≥25 kg: 1 mg; may repeat in 15 minutes if needed

Adults: IM, IV, SubQ: *Glucagon Emergency Kit or GlucaGen:* 1 mg; may repeat in 15 minutes as needed

Anaphylactic reaction (refractory) in patients on beta-blocker therapy (off-label use; Lieberman, 2010):

Children: IV: Initial: 20 to 30 **mcg/kg** (maximum: 1 mg); followed by an infusion of 5 to 15 **mcg/minute**; titrate the infusion rate to achieve an adequate clinical response.

Adults: IV: Initial: 1 to 5 mg; followed by an infusion of 5 to 15 **mcg/minute**; titrate the infusion rate to achieve an adequate clinical response.

Beta-blocker- or calcium channel blocker-induced myocardial depression (with or without hypotension) unresponsive to standard measures (off-label use; AHA [Vanden Hoek, 2010]; Bailey, 2003; PALS [Kleinman, 2010]): IV:

Children: Initial bolus of 30 to 150 **mcg**/kg followed by an infusion of 70 **mcg**/kg/hour (maximum: 5 mg/hour) (Hegenbarth, 2008)

Adolescents: Initial: 5 to 10 mg over several minutes followed by infusion of 1 to 5 mg/hour (Hegenbarth, 2008; PALS [Kleinman, 2010])

Adults: 3 to 10 mg (or 0.05 to 0.15 mg/kg) bolus followed by an infusion of 3 to 5 mg/hour (or 0.05 to 0.1 mg/kg/hour); titrate infusion rate to achieve adequate hemodynamic response (AHA [Vanden Hoek, 2010])

Dosage adjustment in renal impairment: There are no dosage adjustments provided in the manufacturer's labeling.

Dosage adjustment in hepatic impairment: There are no dosage adjustment provided in the manufacturer's labeling.

Dietary Considerations Administer carbohydrates to patient as soon as possible after response to treatment.

Usual Infusion Concentrations: Adult IV infusion: 4 mg in 50 mL (concentration: 0.08 mg/mL) of D_5W

Administration IV: Rapid injection may be associated with increased nausea and vomiting; place patient in lateral recumbent position to protect airway (Liberman, 2010) and to prevent choking when consciousness returns.

Anaphylactic reaction (refractory) in patients on beta-blocker therapy: Administer bolus over 5 minutes (Lieberman, 2010).

Beta-blocker/calcium channel blocker toxicity: Administer bolus over 3 to 5 minutes; continuous infusions may be used. Ensure adequate supply available to continue therapy (AHA [Vanden Hoek], 2010).

Monitoring Parameters Blood pressure, blood glucose, ECG, heart rate, mentation

Additional Information 1 unit = 1 mg

The American Diabetes Association (ADA) recommends that glucagon be prescribed for all patients at significant risk of severe hypoglycemia; caregivers or family members of these patients should be trained on how to administer glucagon (ADA, 2013).

Dosage Forms

Kit, Injection:

Glucagon Emergency: 1 mg

Solution Reconstituted, Injection:

GlucaGen: 1 mg (1 ea)

GlucaGen HypoKit: 1 mg (1 ea)

◆ **Glucagon Emergency** *see* Glucagon *on page 970*

◆ **Glucagon Hydrochloride** *see* Glucagon *on page 970*

Glucarpidase (gloo KAR pid ase)

Brand Names: U.S. Voraxaze

Index Terms Carboxypeptidase-G2; CPDG2; CPG2; Voraxaze

Pharmacologic Category Antidote; Enzyme

Use Treatment of toxic plasma methotrexate concentrations (>1 micromole/L) in patients with delayed clearance due to renal impairment

Note: Due to the risk of subtherapeutic methotrexate exposure, glucarpidase is **NOT** indicated when methotrexate clearance is within expected range (plasma methotrexate concentration ≤2 standard deviations of mean methotrexate excretion curve specific for dose administered) **or** with normal renal function or mild renal impairment.

Pregnancy Risk Factor C

Dosage Children, Adolescents, and Adults:

IV: Methotrexate toxicity: 50 units/kg (Buchen, 2005; Widemann, 1997; Widemann, 2010)

Intrathecal: Intrathecal methotrexate overdose (off-label route/use): 2000 units as soon as possible after accidental methotrexate overdose (Widemann, 2004)

Dosage adjustment in renal impairment: No dosage adjustment necessary

Dosage adjustment in hepatic impairment: There are no dosage adjustments provided in the manufacturer's labeling (has not been studied).

Additional Information Complete prescribing information should be consulted for additional detail.

Dosage Forms

Solution Reconstituted, Intravenous [preservative free]:

Voraxaze: 1000 units (1 ea)

◆ **Glucobay (Can)** *see* Acarbose *on page 29*

◆ **GlucoNorm® (Can)** *see* Repaglinide *on page 1791*

◆ **Glucophage** *see* MetFORMIN *on page 1307*

◆ **Glucophage XR** *see* MetFORMIN *on page 1307*

◆ **Glucotrol** *see* GlipiZIDE *on page 967*

◆ **Glucotrol XL** *see* GlipiZIDE *on page 967*

◆ **Glucovance** *see* Glyburide and Metformin *on page 974*

◆ **Glulisine Insulin** *see* Insulin Glulisine *on page 1086*

◆ **Glumetza** *see* MetFORMIN *on page 1307*

Glutamine (GLOO ta meen)

Brand Names: U.S. NutreStore; Sympt-X G.I. [OTC]; Sympt-X [OTC]

Index Terms Gln; L-Glutamine

Pharmacologic Category Amino Acid; Gastrointestinal Agent, Miscellaneous

Use

NutreStore™: Treatment of short bowel syndrome (SBS) when used in combination with specialized nutritional support and growth hormone therapy

OTC products: Medical food used to promote GI tract healing and nutritional supplementation with GI disorders, HIV/AIDS, cancer, and other critical illnesses

Pregnancy Risk Factor C

Dosage Oral: Adults:

Nutritional supplement (Enterex® Glutapak-10®, Resource® GlutaSolve®, Sympt-X, Sympt-X G.I.): Average dose: 10 g 3 times/day; dosing range: 5-30 g/day

Short bowel syndrome (NutreStore™): 30 g/day administered as 5 g 6 times/day (every 2-3 hours while awake) for up to 16 weeks; to be used in combination with growth hormone and nutritional support

Dosage adjustment in renal impairment: No dosage adjustment provided in manufacturer's labeling.

Dosage adjustment in hepatic impairment: No dosage adjustment provided in manufacturer's labeling; use with caution.

Additional Information Complete prescribing information should be consulted for additional detail.

Dosage Forms

Capsule, Oral:

Generic: 500 mg

Packet, Oral:

NutreStore: 5 g (84 ea)

Sympt-X G.I. [OTC]: 10 g (60 ea)

Powder, Oral:

Sympt-X [OTC]: (480 g)

Tablet, Oral:

Generic: 500 mg

◆ **Glybenclamide** *see* GlyBURIDE *on page 972*

◆ **Glybenzcyclamide** *see* GlyBURIDE *on page 972*

GlyBURIDE (GLYE byoor ide)

Brand Names: U.S. Diabeta; Glynase

Brand Names: Canada Apo-Glyburide; Ava-Glyburide; DiaBeta; Dom-Glyburide; Euglucon; Mylan-Glybe; PMS-Glyburide; PRO-Glyburide; ratio-Glyburide; Riva-Glyburide; Sandoz-Glyburide; Teva-Glyburide

Index Terms Diabeta; Glibenclamide; Glybenclamide; Glybenzcyclamide; Micronase

Pharmacologic Category Antidiabetic Agent, Sulfonylurea

Additional Appendix Information

Beers Criteria – Potentially Inappropriate Medications for Geriatrics *on page 2271*

Use Type 2 diabetes mellitus: Adjunct to diet and exercise to improve glycemic control in adults with type 2 diabetes mellitus (noninsulin dependent, NIDDM)

Pregnancy Risk Factor B/C (manufacturer dependent)

Pregnancy Considerations Outcomes of animal reproduction studies differ by manufacturer labeling. Glyburide crosses the placenta. Some pharmacokinetic properties of glyburide may change during pregnancy (Hebert, 2009).

Severe hypoglycemia lasting 4 to 10 days has been noted in infants born to mothers taking a sulfonylurea at the time of delivery. Additional adverse maternal and fetal events have been noted in some studies and may be influenced by maternal glycemic control and/or differences in study design (Bertini, 2005; Ekpebegh, 2007; Joy, 2012; Langer, 2000; Langer, 2005).

In women with diabetes, maternal hyperglycemia can be associated with congenital malformations as well as adverse effects in the fetus, neonate, and the mother (ACOG, 2005; ADA, 2014; Kitzmiller, 2008; Metzger, 2007). To prevent adverse outcomes, prior to conception and throughout pregnancy maternal blood glucose and HbA_{1c} should be kept as close to normal as possible but without causing significant hypoglycemia (ACOG, 2013; ADA, 2014; Blumer, 2013; Kitzmiller, 2008). Prior to pregnancy, effective contraception should be used until glycemic control is achieved (ADA, 2014; Kitzmiller, 2008).

Glyburide may be used to treat GDM when nonpharmacologic therapy is not effective in maintaining glucose control (ACOG, 2013; Blumer, 2013). Women with type 2 diabetes are usually treated with insulin prior to and during pregnancy (Blumer, 2013). According to the manufacturer, if glyburide is used during pregnancy, it should be discontinued at least 2 weeks before the expected delivery date.

Breast-Feeding Considerations Data from initial studies note that glyburide was not detected in breast milk (Feig, 2005). According to the manufacturer, due to the potential for hypoglycemia in the nursing infant, a decision should be made whether to discontinue nursing or to discontinue the drug, taking into account the importance of treatment to the mother. Current guidelines note that breast-feeding is encouraged for all women, including those with diabetes (ACOG, 2005; Blumer, 2013; Metzger, 2007). Small snacks before feeds may help decrease the risk of hypoglycemia in women with pregestational diabetes (ACOG, 2005; Reader, 2004). Glyburide may be used in breast-feeding women (Blumer, 2013; Metzger, 2007).

Contraindications

Hypersensitivity to glyburide or any component of the formulation; type 1 diabetes mellitus or diabetic ketoacidosis, with or without coma; concomitant use with bosentan.

Canadian labeling: Additional contraindications (not in U.S. labeling): Diabetic precoma or coma, stress conditions (eg, severe infections, trauma, surgery); liver disease or frank jaundice; renal impairment; pregnancy; breast-feeding.

Documentation of allergenic cross-reactivity for sulfonylureas is limited. However, because of similarities in chemical structure and/or pharmacologic actions, the possibility of cross-sensitivity cannot be ruled out with certainty.

Warnings/Precautions All sulfonylurea drugs are capable of producing severe hypoglycemia. Hypoglycemia is more likely to occur when caloric intake is deficient, after severe or prolonged exercise, when ethanol is ingested, or when more than one glucose-lowering drug is used. It is also more likely in elderly patients, malnourished, or debilitated patients and in patients with severe renal or hepatic impairment; adrenal and/or pituitary insufficiency; use with caution.

It may be necessary to discontinue therapy and administer insulin if the patient is exposed to stress (fever, trauma, infection, surgery). Loss of efficacy may be observed following prolonged use as a result of the progression of type 2 diabetes mellitus which results in continued beta cell destruction. In patients who were previously responding to sulfonylurea therapy, consider additional factors which may be contributing to decreased efficacy (eg, inappropriate dose, nonadherence to diet and exercise regimen). If no contributing factors can be identified, consider discontinuing use of the sulfonylurea due to secondary failure of treatment. Additional antidiabetic therapy (eg, insulin) will be required.

Avoid use in elderly patients due to increased risk of prolonged hypoglycemia (Beers Criteria). If therapy is initiated, dosing should be conservative; monitor closely for hypoglycemia.

Chemical similarities are present among sulfonamides, sulfonylureas, carbonic anhydrase inhibitors, thiazides, and loop diuretics (except ethacrynic acid). Use in patients with sulfonamide allergy is not specifically contraindicated in product labeling, however, a risk of cross-reaction exists in patients with allergy to any of these compounds; avoid use when previous reaction has been severe.

Product labeling states oral hypoglycemic drugs may be associated with an increased cardiovascular mortality as compared to treatment with diet alone or diet plus insulin. Data to support this association are limited, and several studies, including a large prospective trial (UKPDS) have not supported an association.

Patients with G6PD deficiency may be at an increased risk of sulfonylurea-induced hemolytic anemia; however, cases have also been described in patients without G6PD deficiency during postmarketing surveillance. Use with caution and consider a nonsulfonylurea alternative in patients with G6PD deficiency.

Micronized glyburide tablets are **not** bioequivalent to *conventional* glyburide tablets; retitration should occur if patients are being transferred to a different glyburide formulation (eg, micronized-to-conventional or vice versa) or from other hypoglycemic agents.

Adverse Reactions

Cardiovascular: Vasculitis

Central nervous system: Dizziness, headache

Dermatologic: Angioedema, erythema, maculopapular eruptions, morbilliform eruptions, photosensitivity reaction, pruritus, purpura, rash, urticaria

Endocrine & metabolic: Disulfiram-like reaction, hypoglycemia, hyponatremia (SIADH reported with other sulfonylureas)

Gastrointestinal: Anorexia, constipation, diarrhea, epigastric fullness, heartburn, nausea

Genitourinary: Nocturia

Hematologic: Agranulocytosis, aplastic anemia, hemolytic anemia, leukopenia, pancytopenia, porphyria cutanea tarda, thrombocytopenia

Hepatic: Cholestatic jaundice, hepatitis, liver failure, transaminase increased

Neuromuscular & skeletal: Arthralgia, myalgia, paresthesia

Ocular: Blurred vision

Renal: Diuretic effect (minor)

Miscellaneous: Allergic reaction

Drug Interactions

Metabolism/Transport Effects Substrate of CYP2C9 (major); **Note:** Assignment of Major/Minor substrate status based on clinically relevant drug interaction potential; **Inhibits** CYP2C8 (weak), CYP3A4 (weak)

Avoid Concomitant Use

Avoid concomitant use of GlyBURIDE with any of the following: Bosentan; Pimozide

Increased Effect/Toxicity

GlyBURIDE may increase the levels/effects of: Alcohol (Ethyl); ARIPiprazole; Bosentan; Carbocisteine; CycloSPORINE (Systemic); Dofetilide; Hydrocodone; Hypoglycemic Agents; Lomitapide; Pimozide; Porfimer; Verteporfin; Vitamin K Antagonists

The levels/effects of GlyBURIDE may be increased by: Androgens; Beta-Blockers; Ceritinib; Chloramphenicol; Cimetidine; Clarithromycin; Cyclic Antidepressants; CYP2C9 Inhibitors (Moderate); CYP2C9 Inhibitors (Strong); Dexketoprofen; Fibric Acid Derivatives; Fluconazole; GLP-1 Agonists; Herbs (Hypoglycemic Properties); MAO Inhibitors; Metreleptin; Miconazole (Oral); Mifepristone; Pegvisomant; Probenecid; Quinolone Antibiotics; Ranitidine; Salicylates; Selective Serotonin Reuptake Inhibitors; SGLT2 Inhibitors; Sulfonamide Derivatives; Vitamin K Antagonists; Voriconazole

Decreased Effect

GlyBURIDE may decrease the levels/effects of: Bosentan

The levels/effects of GlyBURIDE may be decreased by: Bosentan; Colesevelam; Corticosteroids (Orally Inhaled); Corticosteroids (Systemic); CycloSPORINE (Systemic); CYP2C9 Inducers (Strong); Dabrafenib; Danazol; Loop Diuretics; Luteinizing Hormone-Releasing Hormone Analogs; Quinolone Antibiotics; Rifampin; Somatropin; Thiazide Diuretics

Food Interactions Ethanol may cause rare disulfiram reactions. Management: Monitor patients.

Storage/Stability

Conventional tablets (Diaβeta): Store at 25°C (77°F); excursions are permitted between 15°C and 30°C (59°F and 86°F).

Micronized tablets (Glynase PresTab): Store at 20°C to 25°C (68°F to 77°F).

Mechanism of Action Stimulates insulin release from the pancreatic beta cells; reduces glucose output from the liver; insulin sensitivity is increased at peripheral target sites

Pharmacodynamics/Kinetics

Onset of action: Serum insulin levels begin to increase 15-60 minutes after a single dose

Duration: ≤24 hours

Absorption: Significant within 1 hour

Protein binding, plasma: Extensive, primarily to albumin

Metabolism: Hepatic; forms metabolites (weakly active)

Bioavailability: Variable among oral dosage forms

Half-life elimination: Diaβeta: 10 hours; Glynase PresTab: ~4 hours; may be prolonged with renal or hepatic impairment

Time to peak, serum: Adults: 2-4 hours

Excretion: Feces (50%) and urine (50%) as metabolites

Dosage Oral: **Note:** Micronized glyburide tablets are **not** bioequivalent to conventional glyburide tablets; retitration should occur if patients are being transferred to a different glyburide formulation (eg, micronized-to-conventional or vice versa) or from other hypoglycemic agents. When converting to glyburide from other oral hypoglycemic agents with a long half-life (eg, chlorpropamide), observe patient carefully for 2 weeks due to overlapping hypoglycemic effects.

Conventional tablets (Diaβeta): Adults:

Initial: 2.5-5 mg daily, administered with breakfast or the first main meal of the day. In patients who are more sensitive to hypoglycemic drugs, start at 1.25 mg daily.

Increase in increments of no more than 2.5 mg daily at weekly intervals based on the patient's blood glucose response

Maintenance: 1.25-20 mg daily given as single or divided doses. Some patients (especially those receiving >10 mg daily) may have a more satisfactory response with twice-daily dosing. Maximum: 20 mg daily

Elderly: Initial: 1.25 mg daily. Conservative initial and maintenance doses are recommended to avoid hypoglycemic reactions

Debilitated or malnourished patients or patients with adrenal or pituitary insufficiency: Initial: 1.25 mg daily. Conservative initial and maintenance doses are recommended to avoid hypoglycemic reactions.

Micronized tablets (Glynase PresTab): Adults:

Initial: 1.5-3 mg daily, administered with breakfast or the first main meal of the day. In patients who are more sensitive to hypoglycemic drugs, start at 0.75 mg daily. Increase in increments of no more than 1.5 mg daily in weekly intervals based on the patient's blood glucose response.

Maintenance: 0.75-12 mg daily given as a single dose or in divided doses. Some patients (especially those receiving >6 mg daily) may have a more satisfactory response with twice-daily dosing. Maximum: 12 mg daily

Elderly: Initial: 0.75 mg daily. Conservative initial and maintenance doses are recommended to avoid hypoglycemic reactions.

Debilitated or malnourished patients or patients with adrenal or pituitary insufficiency: 0.75 mg daily. Conservative initial and maintenance doses are recommended to avoid hypoglycemic reactions.

Management of noninsulin-dependent diabetes mellitus in patients previously maintained on insulin: Initial dosage dependent upon current insulin dosage, see table.

Dose Conversion: Insulin to Glyburide

Current Daily Insulin Dosage (units daily)	Initial Glyburide Dosage *Conventional Formulation* (mg daily)	Initial Glyburide Dosage *Micronized Formulation* (mg daily)	Insulin Dosage Change (after glyburide started)
<20	2.5-5	1.5-3	Discontinue
20-40	5	3	Discontinue
>40	5 (increase in increments of 1.25-2.5 mg every 2-10 days)	3 (increase in increments of 0.75-1.5 mg every 2-10 days)	Reduce insulin dosage by 50% (gradually taper off insulin as glyburide dosage increased)

Dosing adjustment/comments in renal impairment: There are no dosage adjustments provided in manufacturer's labeling; however, use conservative initial and maintenance doses.

Dosing adjustment in hepatic impairment: There are no dosage adjustments provided in manufacturer's labeling; however, use conservative initial and maintenance doses.

Dietary Considerations Should be taken with meals at the same time each day (twice-daily dosing may be beneficial if conventional glyburide doses are >10 mg or micronized glyburide doses are >6 mg). Individualized medical nutrition therapy (MNT) based on ADA recommendations is an integral part of therapy.

Administration Administer with meals at the same time each day (twice-daily dosing may be beneficial if conventional glyburide doses are >10 mg or micronized glyburide doses are >6 mg). Patients that are NPO or require decreased caloric intake may need doses held to avoid hypoglycemia.

Monitoring Parameters Signs and symptoms of hypoglycemia, urine glucose test, fasting blood glucose, hemoglobin A_{1c}

Reference Range Recommendations for glycemic control in nonpregnant adults with diabetes (ADA, 2013):

HbA_{1c}: <7% (a more aggressive [<6.5%] or less aggressive [<8%] HbA_{1c} goal may be targeted based on patient-specific characteristics)

Preprandial capillary plasma glucose: 70-130 mg/dL

Peak postprandial capillary blood glucose: <180 mg/dL

Dosage Forms Considerations Micronized formulation: Glynase

Dosage Forms

Tablet, Oral:

Diabeta: 1.25 mg, 2.5 mg, 5 mg

Glynase: 1.5 mg, 3 mg, 6 mg

Generic: 1.25 mg, 1.5 mg, 2.5 mg, 3 mg, 5 mg, 6 mg

Glyburide and Metformin

(GLYE byoor ide & met FOR min)

Brand Names: U.S. Glucovance

Index Terms Glyburide and Metformin Hydrochloride; Metformin and Glyburide

Pharmacologic Category Antidiabetic Agent, Biguanide; Antidiabetic Agent, Sulfonylurea

Use Type 2 diabetes mellitus: As an adjunct to diet and exercise, to improve glycemic control in adults with type 2 diabetes (noninsulin dependent, NIDDM)

Pregnancy Risk Factor B

Dosage Note: Dose must be individualized. Dosages expressed as glyburide/metformin components.

Type 2 diabetes: Adults: Oral:

Patients with inadequate glycemic control on diet and exercise alone: Initial: 1.25 mg/250 mg once daily with a meal; patients with HbA_{1c} >9% or fasting plasma glucose (FPG) >200 mg/dL may start with 1.25 mg/250 mg twice daily with meals.

Adjustment: Dosage may be increased in increments of 1.25 mg/250 mg per day at intervals of not less than 2 weeks; maximum daily dose: 10 mg/2000 mg (limited experience with higher doses). **Note:** Doses of 5 mg/500 mg should not be used as initial therapy, due to risk of hypoglycemia.

Patients with inadequate glycemic control on a sulfonylurea and/or metformin: Initial: 2.5 mg/500 mg or 5 mg/500 mg twice daily with meals.

Adjustment: Dosage may be increased in increments no greater than 5 mg/500 mg; maximum daily dose: 20 mg/2000 mg. **Note:** When switching patients previously on a sulfonylurea and metformin together, do not exceed the daily dose of glyburide (or glyburide equivalent) or metformin.

Combination with thiazolidinedione: May be combined with a thiazolidinedione in patients with an inadequate response to glyburide/metformin therapy; however, the risk of hypoglycemia may be increased. When adding a thiazolidinedione, continue glyburide and metformin at current dose and initiate thiazolidinedione at recommended starting dose; may increase based on the thiazolidinedione suggested titration schedule.

Elderly: Oral: Conservative doses are recommended in the elderly due to potentially decreased renal function; **do not titrate to maximum dose**; should not be used in patients ≥80 years of age unless renal function is verified as normal

Dosage adjustment in renal impairment: Use is contraindicated in the presence of renal disease or renal dysfunction (serum creatinine ≥1.5 mg/dL in males, or ≥1.4 mg/dL in females, or abnormal creatinine clearance).

Dosage adjustment in hepatic impairment: No dosage adjustment provided in manufacturer's labeling (has not been studied). However, hepatic dysfunction has been associated with some cases of lactic acidosis; generally avoid use in patients with hepatic disease.

Additional Information Complete prescribing information should be consulted for additional detail.

Dosage Forms

Tablet, oral: Glyburide 1.25 mg and metformin 250 mg; glyburide 2.5 mg and metformin 500 mg; glyburide 5 mg and metformin 500 mg

Glucovance®: 2.5 mg/500 mg: Glyburide 2.5 mg and metformin 500 mg; 5 mg/500 mg: Glyburide 5 mg and metformin 500 mg

◆ **Glyburide and Metformin Hydrochloride** *see* Glyburide and Metformin *on page 974*

◆ **Glycate** *see* Glycopyrrolate *on page 975*

- ◆ **Glycerol Guaiacolate** *see* GuaiFENesin *on page 986*
- ◆ **Glyceryl Trinitrate** *see* Nitroglycerin *on page 1465*
- ◆ **GlycoLax [OTC]** *see* Polyethylene Glycol 3350 *on page 1674*
- ◆ **Glycon (Can)** *see* MetFORMIN *on page 1307*
- ◆ **Glycophos** *see* Sodium Glycerophosphate Pentahydrate *on page 1906*

Glycopyrrolate (glye koe PYE roe late)

Brand Names: U.S. Cuvposa; Glycate; Robinul; Robinul-Forte

Brand Names: Canada Glycopyrrolate Injection, USP; Seebri Breezhaler

Index Terms Glycopyrronium Bromide; NVA237

Pharmacologic Category Anticholinergic Agent

Use Inhibit salivation and excessive secretions of the respiratory tract preoperatively; control of upper airway secretions; intraoperatively to counteract drug-induced or vagal mediated bradyarrhythmias; adjunct in treatment of peptic ulcer (indication listed in product labeling but currently has no place in management of peptic ulcer disease)

Cuvposa: Reduce chronic, severe drooling in those with neurologic conditions (eg, cerebral palsy) associated with drooling

Seebri Breezhaler [Canadian product]: Maintenance treatment of chronic obstructive pulmonary disease (COPD) including chronic bronchitis and emphysema

Pregnancy Risk Factor B (injection) / C (oral solution)

Pregnancy Considerations Teratogenic effects were not observed in animal studies. Small amounts of glycopyrrolate cross the human placenta.

Breast-Feeding Considerations May suppress lactation

Contraindications Hypersensitivity to glycopyrrolate or any component of the formulation; medical conditions that preclude use of anticholinergic medication; severe ulcerative colitis, toxic megacolon complicating ulcerative colitis, paralytic ileus, obstructive disease of GI tract (eg, pyloric stenosis), intestinal atony in the elderly or debilitated patient; unstable cardiovascular status in acute hemorrhage; narrow-angle glaucoma; acute hemorrhage; tachycardia; obstructive uropathy; myasthenia gravis

Oral solution: Additional contraindication: Concomitant use of potassium chloride in a solid oral dosage form

Seebri Breezhaler [Canadian product]: Hypersensitivity to glycopyrronium bromide or any component of the formulation

Warnings/Precautions Diarrhea may be a sign of incomplete intestinal obstruction, treatment should be discontinued if this occurs. Use caution in elderly and in patients with autonomic neuropathy, narrow-angle glaucoma, renal disease, or ulcerative colitis; may precipitate/aggravate ileus or toxic megacolon, hyperthyroidism, CAD, CHF, arrhythmias, tachycardia, BPH, bladder neck obstruction, or hiatal hernia with reflux. Use of anticholinergics in gastric ulcer treatment may cause a delay in gastric emptying. Caution should be used in individuals demonstrating decreased pigmentation (skin and iris coloration, dark versus light) since there has been some evidence that these individuals have an enhanced sensitivity to the anticholinergic response. May cause drowsiness, eye sensitivity to light, or blurred vision; caution should be used when performing tasks which require mental alertness, such as driving. The risk of heat stroke with this medication may be increased during exercise or hot weather. Seebri® Breezhaler® [Canadian product] is not indicated for the initial (rescue) treatment of acute episodes of bronchospasm or with acutely deteriorating COPD; after initiation of therapy, patients should use short-acting bronchodilators only on an as needed basis for acute symptoms. Rarely, paradoxical bronchospasm may occur with use of inhaled bronchodilating agents; discontinue use of inhaler and consider other therapy if bronchospasm occurs. Patients using Seebri® Breezhaler® should avoid getting the powder into their eyes.

Benzyl alcohol and derivatives: Some dosage forms may contain benzyl alcohol; large amounts of benzyl alcohol (≥99 mg/kg/day) have been associated with a potentially fatal toxicity ("gasping syndrome") in neonates; the "gasping syndrome" consists of metabolic acidosis, respiratory distress, gasping respirations, CNS dysfunction (including convulsions, intracranial hemorrhage), hypotension and cardiovascular collapse (AAP, 1997; CDC, 1982); some data suggests that benzoate displaces bilirubin from protein binding sites (Ahlfors, 2001); avoid or use dosage forms containing benzyl alcohol with caution in neonates. See manufacturer's labeling. Some dosage forms may contain propylene glycol; large amounts are potentially toxic and have been associated hyperosmolality, lactic acidosis, seizures, and respiratory depression; use caution (AAP, 1997; Zar, 2007).

Adverse Reactions

Cardiovascular: Arrhythmias, cardiac arrest, flushing, heart block, hyper-/hypotension, malignant hyperthermia, pallor, palpitation, QTc-interval prolongation, tachycardia

Central nervous system: Aggressiveness, agitation, confusion, crying (abnormal), dizziness, drowsiness, excitement, headache, insomnia, irritability, mood changes, pain, restlessness, nervousness, seizure

Dermatologic: Dry skin, pruritus, rash, urticaria

Endocrine & metabolic: Dehydration, lactation suppression

Gastrointestinal: Abdominal distention, abdominal pain, constipation, flatulence, retching, bloated feeling, intestinal obstruction, loss of taste, nausea, pseudo-obstructio, vomiting, xerostomia

Genitourinary: Impotence, urinary hesitancy, urinary retention, urinary tract infection

Local: Injection site reactions (edema, erythema, pain)

Neuromuscular & skeletal: Weakness

Ocular: Blurred vision, cycloplegia, mydriasis, nystagmus, ocular tension increased, photophobia, sensitivity to light increased

Respiratory: Bronchial secretion (thickening), nasal congestion, nasal dryness, pneumonia, respiratory depression, sinusitis, upper respiratory tract infection

Miscellaneous: Anaphylactoid reactions, diaphoresis decreased, hypersensitivity reactions

As reported with Seebri® Breezhaler® [Canadian product]:

Central nervous system: Headache

Gastrointestinal: Dyspepsia, gastroenteritis, vomiting, xerostomia

Genitourinary: Dysuria, urinary tract infection

Neuromuscular & skeletal: Musculoskeletal pain

Respiratory: Nasopharyngitis, rhinitis

Rare but important or life-threatening: Cough, cystitis, dental caries, diabetes mellitus, epistaxis, fatigue, hypoesthesia, palpitations, rash, throat irritation, urinary retention, weakness

Drug Interactions

Metabolism/Transport Effects None known.

Avoid Concomitant Use

Avoid concomitant use of Glycopyrrolate with any of the following: Aclidinium; Glucagon; Ipratropium (Oral Inhalation); Potassium Chloride; Tiotropium; Umeclidinium

Increased Effect/Toxicity

Glycopyrrolate may increase the levels/effects of: AbobotulinumtoxinA; Analgesics (Opioid); Anticholinergic Agents; Atenolol; Cannabinoid-Containing Products; Digoxin; Glucagon; MetFORMIN; Mirabegron;

OnabotulinumtoxinA; Potassium Chloride; RimabotulinumtoxinB; Thiazide Diuretics; Tiotropium; Topiramate

The levels/effects of Glycopyrrolate may be increased by: Aclidinium; Amantadine; Ipratropium (Oral Inhalation); MAO Inhibitors; Mianserin; Pramlintide; Umeclidinium

Decreased Effect

Glycopyrrolate may decrease the levels/effects of: Acetylcholinesterase Inhibitors; Haloperidol; Itopride; Levodopa; Secretin

The levels/effects of Glycopyrrolate may be decreased by: Acetylcholinesterase Inhibitors

Food Interactions Administration with a high-fat meal significantly reduced absorption. Management: Administer on an empty stomach.

Storage/Stability Store at 20°C to 25°C (68°F to 77°F).

Oral capsules for inhalation [Canadian product]: Store at 15°C to 25°C (59°F to 77°F) in blister. Capsules should be stored in the blister pack and only removed immediately before use. Once protective foil is peeled back and/or removed the capsule should be used immediately; if capsule is not used immediately, it should be discarded. Do not store capsules in Seebri® Breezhaler®. Protect from moisture.

Mechanism of Action Blocks the action of acetylcholine at parasympathetic sites in smooth muscle, secretory glands, and the CNS; indirectly reduces the rate of salivation by preventing the stimulation of acetylcholine receptors

In COPD, competitively and reversibly inhibits the action of acetylcholine at muscarinic receptor subtypes 1-3 (greater affinity for subtypes 1 and 3) in bronchial smooth muscle thereby causing bronchodilation

Pharmacodynamics/Kinetics Note: Oral powder for inhalation is not available in the U.S.

Onset of action: Oral: 50 minutes; IM: 15-30 minutes; IV: ~1 minute

Peak effect: Oral: ~1 hour; IM: 30-45 minutes

Duration: Vagal effect: 2-3 hours; Inhibition of salivation: Up to 7 hours; Anticholinergic: Oral: 8-12 hours

Absorption: Oral tablet: Poor and erratic; Oral solution: 23% lower compared to tablet; Oral powder for inhalation: Rapid

Distribution: V_d: Children: 1.3-1.8 L/kg; Adults: 0.2-0.62 L/kg

Metabolism: Hepatic (minimal)

Bioavailability: Tablet: ~1% to 13%; Oral powder for inhalation: ~40%

Half-life elimination: Infants: 22-130 minutes; Children 19-99 minutes; Adults: ~60-75 minutes; Oral solution: Adults: 3 hours; Oral powder for inhalation: 13-22 hours (Sechaud, 2012)

Time to peak, plasma: Oral powder for inhalation: 5 minutes

Excretion: Urine (as unchanged drug, IM: 80%, IV: 85%); bile (as unchanged drug)

Dosage

Children:

Reduction of secretions (preanesthetic):

Oral (off-label): 40-100 mcg/kg/dose 3-4 times/day

IM, IV (off-label): 4-10 mcg/kg/dose every 3-4 hours; maximum: 0.2 mg/dose or 0.8 mg/24 hours

Intraoperative: IV: 4 mcg/kg not to exceed 0.1 mg; repeat at 2- to 3-minute intervals as needed

Preoperative: IM:

<2 years: 4-9 mcg/kg 30-60 minutes before procedure

>2 years: 4 mcg/kg 30-60 minutes before procedure

Drooling, chronic: Children 3-16 years: Oral solution (Cuvposa™): Initial: 0.02 mg/kg 3 times/day; titrate in increments of 0.02 mg/kg every 5-7 days as tolerated, up to a maximum dose of 0.1 mg/kg 3 times/day, not to exceed 1.5-3 mg/dose

Children and Adults: Reverse neuromuscular blockade: IV: 0.2 mg for each 1 mg of neostigmine or 5 mg of pyridostigmine administered or 5-15 mcg/kg glycopyrrolate with 25-70 mcg/kg of neostigmine or 0.1-0.3 mg/kg of pyridostigmine (agents usually administered simultaneously, but glycopyrrolate may be administered first if bradycardia is present)

Adults:

COPD: Oral powder for inhalation: Seebri® Breezhaler® [Canadian product]: 50 mcg (contents of one capsule) once daily

Reduction of secretions:

Intraoperative: IV: 0.1 mg repeated as needed at 2- to 3-minute intervals

Preoperative: IM: 4 mcg/kg 30-60 minutes before procedure

Dosage adjustment in renal impairment: No dosage adjustment provided in manufacturer's labeling. However, data suggest renal impairment reduces glycopyrrolate elimination; use with caution.

Dosage adjustment in hepatic impairment: No dosage adjustment provided in manufacturer's labeling (has not been studied).

Administration

IV: Administer IV at a rate of 0.2 mg over 1-2 minutes. May be administered IM or IV without dilution. May also be administered via the tubing of a running IV infusion of a compatible solution. May be administered IV in the same syringe with neostigmine or pyridostigmine.

Oral: Administer oral solution on an empty stomach, 1 hour before or 2 hours after meals

Oral inhalation [Canadian product]: Administer once daily preferably at the same time each day using the Seebri® Breezhaler® only. Remove capsule from foil blister immediately before use. Do not swallow capsule. Avoid getting powder into eyes. Place capsule in the capsule-chamber in the base of the Seebri® Breezhaler®. A click is heard as it fully closes. Hold inhaler with mouthpiece in upright position and pierce capsule within chamber by simultaneously pressing piercing buttons on base of inhaler (click is heard as capsule is pierced). Release buttons. Exhale fully. Do not exhale into inhaler. Tilt head slightly back and place mouthpiece in mouth with piercing buttons on base of inhaler in horizontal position and not up and down. Do not press piercing buttons. Inhale (rapidly, steadily and deeply); the capsule vibration should be heard within the device. Hold breath for at least 5-10 seconds or as long as possible. Remove mouthpiece prior to exhalation. Patient should not breathe out through the mouthpiece. If any powder remains in capsule, exhale and inhale again. Repeat until capsule is empty. Throw away empty capsule; do not leave in inhaler. Always keep capsules and inhaler dry. **Note:** If a dose is missed, take as soon as possible on that day; do not take 2 doses on the same day.

Monitoring Parameters Heart rate; anticholinergic effects; bowel sounds; bowel movements; effects on drooling

Oral inhalation: FEV_1, peak flow (or other pulmonary function studies)

Dosage Forms

Solution, Injection:

Robinul: 0.2 mg/mL (1 mL); 0.4 mg/2 mL (2 mL); 1 mg/5 mL (5 mL); 4 mg/20 mL (20 mL)

Generic: 0.2 mg/mL (1 mL); 0.4 mg/2 mL (2 mL); 1 mg/5 mL (5 mL); 4 mg/20 mL (20 mL)

Solution, Oral:

Cuvposa: 1 mg/5 mL (473 mL)

Tablet, Oral:
Glycate: 1.5 mg
Robinul: 1 mg
Robinul-Forte: 2 mg
Generic: 1 mg, 2 mg

Dosage Forms: Canada

Powder, for oral inhalation:
Seebri® Breezhaler®: 50 mcg/capsule (30s)

Extemporaneous Preparations A 0.5 mg/mL oral suspension may be made with 1 mg tablets and a 1:1 mixture of Ora-Plus® and either Ora-Sweet® or Ora-Sweet® SF. Crush thirty 1 mg tablets in a mortar and reduce to a fine powder. Prepare diluent by mixing 30 mL of Ora-Plus® with 30 mL of either Ora-Sweet® or Ora-Sweet® SF and stir vigorously. Add 30 mL of diluent (via geometric dilution) to powder until smooth suspension is obtained. Transfer suspension to 60 mL amber bottle. Rinse contents of mortar into bottle with sufficient quantity of remaining diluent to obtain 60 mL (final volume). Label "shake well". Stable at room temperature for 90 days. Due to bitter aftertaste, chocolate syrup may be administered prior to or mixed (1:1 v/v) with suspension immediately before administration (Cober, 2011).

A 0.5 mg/mL oral solution can be made from tablets. Crush fifty 1 mg tablets in a mortar and reduce to a fine powder. Add enough distilled water to make about 90 mL, mix well. Transfer to a bottle, rinse mortar with water, and add a quantity of water sufficient to make 100 mL. Label "shake well" and "protect from light". Stable at room temperature for 25 days (Gupta, 2001).

A 0.1 mg/mL oral solution may be made using glycopyrrolate 0.2 mg/mL injection without preservatives. Withdraw 50 mL from vials with a needle and syringe, add to 50 mL of a 1:1 mixture of Ora-Sweet® and Ora-Plus® in a bottle. Label "shake well", "protect from light," and "refrigerate". Stable refrigerated for 35 days (Landry, 2005).

Cober MP, Johnson CE, Sudekum D, et al, "Stability of Extemporaneously Prepared Glycopyrrolate Oral Suspensions," *Am J Health Syst Phar,*. 2011, 68(9):843-5.
Gupta VD, "Stability of an Oral Liquid Dosage Form of Glycopyrrolate Prepared from Tablets," *IJPC* 2001, 5(6):480-1.
Landry C, "Stability and Subjective Taste Acceptability of Four Glycopyrrolate Solutions for Oral Administration," *IJPC*, 2005, 9(5):396-98.

◆ **Glycopyrrolate Injection, USP (Can)** *see* Glycopyrrolate *on page 975*
◆ **Glycopyrronium and Indacaterol** *see* Indacaterol and Glycopyrronium [CAN/INT] *on page 1063*
◆ **Glycopyrronium Bromide** *see* Glycopyrrolate *on page 975*
◆ **Glycopyrronium Bromide and Indacaterol Maleate** *see* Indacaterol and Glycopyrronium [CAN/INT] *on page 1063*
◆ **Glydiazinamide** *see* GlipiZIDE *on page 967*
◆ **Glydo** *see* Lidocaine (Topical) *on page 1211*
◆ **Glynase** *see* GlyBURIDE *on page 972*
◆ **Gly-Oxide [OTC]** *see* Carbamide Peroxide *on page 350*
◆ **Glyquin® XM (Can)** *see* Hydroquinone *on page 1020*
◆ **Glyset** *see* Miglitol *on page 1367*
◆ **GM-CSF** *see* Sargramostim *on page 1865*
◆ **GMD-Gemfibrozil (Can)** *see* Gemfibrozil *on page 956*
◆ **GnRH** *see* Gonadorelin [CAN/INT] *on page 980*
◆ **GnRH Agonist** *see* Histrelin *on page 1005*

Golimumab (goe LIM ue mab)

Brand Names: U.S. Simponi; Simponi Aria
Brand Names: Canada Simponi; Simponi I.V.
Index Terms CNTO-148

Pharmacologic Category Antipsoriatic Agent; Antirheumatic, Disease Modifying; Monoclonal Antibody; Tumor Necrosis Factor (TNF) Blocking Agent

Use

Ankylosing spondylitis (Simponi): Treatment of adults with active ankylosing spondylitis

Psoriatic arthritis (Simponi): Treatment of adults with active psoriatic arthritis (alone or in combination with methotrexate)

Rheumatoid arthritis (Simponi, Simponi Aria): Treatment of adults with moderately-to-severely active rheumatoid arthritis (in combination with methotrexate)

Ulcerative colitis (Simponi): Treatment of adults with moderately-to-severely active ulcerative colitis in patients with corticosteroid dependence or who are refractory or intolerant to oral aminosalicylates, oral corticosteroids, azathioprine, or 6-mercaptopurine (to induce and maintain clinical response, improve mucosal appearance during induction, induce clinical remission, and achieve and sustain remission in induction responders)

Pregnancy Risk Factor B

Pregnancy Considerations Adverse events have not been observed in animal reproduction studies. Golimumab crosses the placenta. Based on data from other TNF-blockers, antibodies may be present in the newborn serum for up to 6 months and infants exposed to golimumab *in utero* may be at risk of increased infection. Administration of live vaccines to newborns is not recommended until 6 months after the last maternal dose. Canadian labeling recommends that women of childbearing potential use reliable contraception during and for at least 6 months after discontinuation of golimumab therapy.

Breast-Feeding Considerations It is not known whether golimumab is excreted in breast milk. Because many immunoglobulins are excreted in milk and the potential for serious adverse reactions exists, the manufacturer recommends a decision should be made whether to discontinue breast-feeding or discontinue the drug, taking into account the importance of the drug to the mother.

Contraindications

There are no contraindications listed in the manufacturer's U.S labeling.

Canadian labeling: Additional contraindications (not in U.S. labeling): Hypersensitivity to golimumab, latex, or any other component of formulation or packaging; patients with severe infections (eg, sepsis, tuberculosis, opportunistic infections); moderate or severe heart failure (NYHA class III/IV)

Warnings/Precautions [U.S. Boxed Warning]: Patients receiving golimumab are at increased risk for serious infections which may result in hospitalization and/or fatality; infections usually developed in patients receiving concomitant immunosuppressive agents (eg, methotrexate or corticosteroids). Active tuberculosis (or reactivation of latent tuberculosis), invasive fungal (including aspergillosis, blastomycosis, candidiasis, coccidioidomycosis, histoplasmosis, and pneumocystosis) and bacterial, viral or other opportunistic infections (including legionellosis and listeriosis) have been reported in patients receiving TNF-blocking agents, including golimumab. May present as disseminated (rather than local) disease. Histoplasmosis testing (antigen or antibody) may be negative in some patients with active infection. Monitor closely for signs/symptoms of infection. Discontinue for serious infection or sepsis. Consider risks versus benefits prior to use in patients with a history of chronic or recurrent infection. Consider empiric antifungal therapy in patients who are at risk for invasive fungal infection and develop severe systemic illness. Caution should be exercised when considering use in the elderly, patients taking concomitant immunosuppressants, patients with chronic or recurrent infection, patients who have been exposed to tuberculosis, patients with a history of opportunistic infection, patients with comorbid conditions that predispose them to infections (eg, diabetes), or residence/travel from areas of endemic mycoses (blastomycosis, coccidioidomycosis, histoplasmosis). Do not initiate golimumab therapy in patients with with active infection, including localized infection which is clinically important. Patients who develop a new infection while undergoing treatment should be monitored closely.

[U.S. Boxed Warning]: Tuberculosis (disseminated or extrapulmonary) has been reported in patients receiving golimumab; both reactivation of latent infection and new infections have been reported. Patients should be evaluated for tuberculosis risk factors and latent tuberculosis infection (with a tuberculin skin test) prior to and during therapy. Treatment of latent tuberculosis should be initiated before use. Patients with initial negative tuberculin skin tests should receive continued monitoring for tuberculosis throughout treatment; active tuberculosis has developed in this population during treatment with TNF-blocking agents. Use with caution in patients who have resided in regions where tuberculosis is endemic. Consider antituberculosis therapy if an adequate course of treatment cannot be confirmed in patients with a history of latent or active tuberculosis or for patients with risk factors despite negative skin test.

Rare reactivation of hepatitis B virus (HBV), sometimes fatal, has occurred in chronic virus carriers (usually in patients receiving concomitant immunosuppressants); evaluate prior to initiation in all patients. Patients who test positive for HBV surface antigen should be referred for hepatitis B evaluation/treatment prior to golimumab initiation. Monitor during and for several months following discontinuation of treatment in HBV carriers; interrupt therapy if reactivation occurs and treat appropriately with antiviral therapy; if resumption of therapy is deemed necessary, exercise caution and monitor patient closely. Patients should be brought up to date with all immunizations before initiating therapy. Live vaccines should not be given concurrently; there is no data available concerning secondary transmission of infection by live vaccines in patients receiving therapy. In clinical trials, humoral response to pneumococcal vaccine was not suppressed in psoriatic arthritis patients.

[U.S. Boxed Warning]: Lymphoma and other malignancies (some fatal) have been reported in children and adolescent patients receiving TNF-blocking agents. Half of the malignancies reported in children were lymphomas (Hodgkin's and non-Hodgkin's) while other cases varied and included malignancies not typically observed in this population. The onset of malignancy was after a median of 30 months (range: 1 to 84 months) after the initiation of the TNF-blocking agent; most patients were receiving concomitant immunosuppressants. The impact of golimumab on the development and course of malignancy is not fully defined. Compared to the general population, an increased risk of lymphoma has been noted in clinical trials; however, rheumatoid arthritis alone has been previously associated with an increased rate of lymphoma. Lymphomas and other malignancies were also observed (at rates higher than expected for the general population) in adult patients receiving TNF-blocking agents. Hepatosplenic T-cell lymphoma (HSTCL), a rare T-cell lymphoma, has also been associated with TNF-blocking agents, primarily reported in adolescent and young adult males with Crohn disease or ulcerative colitis treated with a TNF-blocking agent and concurrent or prior azathioprine or mercaptopurine. Melanoma and Merkel cell carcinoma have been reported in patients receiving TNF-blocking agents including golimumab. Perform periodic skin examinations in all patients during therapy, particularly those at increased risk for skin cancer. Consider risks versus benefits in patients with a known malignancy (other than a successfully treated nonmelanoma skin cancer) and if considering continuing treatment in a patient who develops a malignancy. Cases of pancytopenia and other significant cytopenias, including aplastic anemia, have been reported with TNF-blocking agents. Pancytopenia, leukopenia, neutropenia and thrombocytopenia have occurred with golimumab; use with caution in patients with underlying hematologic disorders. Consider discontinuing therapy with significant hematologic abnormalities. Treatment may result in the formation of autoimmune antibodies; cases of autoimmune disease have not been described.

Use with caution in patients with preexisting or recent onset central or peripheral nervous system demyelinating disorders; rare cases of new-onset or exacerbation of demyelinating disorders (eg, multiple sclerosis, optic neuritis, Guillain-Barré syndrome, polyneuropathy) have been reported. Consider discontinuing use in patients who develop peripheral or central nervous system demyelinating disorders during treatment. Use with caution in patients with heart failure or decreased left ventricular function; monitor closely and discontinue with new-onset or worsening of symptoms. Canadian labeling contraindicates use in moderate or severe heart failure (NYHA class III/IV). Severe systemic hypersensitivity reactions (including anaphylaxis), have been reported (some have occurred with the first dose) following subcutaneous administration; discontinue immediately if signs develop and initiate appropriate treatment.

Avoid concomitant use with abatacept (increased incidence of serious infections) or anakinra (increased incidence of neutropenia and serious infection). Potentially significant drug-drug interactions may exist, requiring dose or frequency adjustment, additional monitoring, and/or selection of alternative therapy. Use caution when switching between biological disease-modifying antirheumatic drugs (DMARDs); overlapping of biological activity may increase the risk for infection. Use with caution in the elderly (general incidence of infection is higher). Packaging (prefilled syringe and needle cover) contains dry natural rubber (latex). Some dosage forms may contain dry natural rubber (latex) and/or polysorbate 80. The safety and efficacy of switching between the IV and SubQ formulations and routes have not been studied.

Adverse Reactions

Cardiovascular: Hypertension

Central nervous system: Dizziness, paresthesia

Dermatologic: Skin rash

Gastrointestinal: Constipation

Hematologic & oncologic: Leukopenia, Positive ANA titer (≥1:160 titer, newly positive)

Hepatic: Increased serum ALT, increased serum AST

Immunologic: Antibody development

Infection: Bacterial infection, fungal infection (superficial), viral infection (includes herpes and influenza)

Local: Injection site reaction

Respiratory: Bronchitis, sinusitis, upper respiratory tract infection (includes laryngitis, nasopharyngitis, pharyngitis, and rhinitis)

Miscellaneous: Fever, infection, infusion related reaction

Rare but important or life-threatening: Anaphylaxis, aspergillosis, atypical mycobacterial infection (subcutaneous), blastomycosis, candidiasis, cellulitis, coccidioidomycosis, congestive heart failure, exacerbation of existing heart failure, histoplasmosis, Hodgkin lymphoma (initiation of therapy ≤18 years old), hypersensitivity reaction, infective bursitis (subcutaneous), interstitial pulmonary disease (subcutaneous), leukemia, lupus-like syndrome, malignant lymphoma, malignant melanoma, malignant neoplasm (other than nonmelanoma skin cancer), Merkel cell carcinoma, multiple sclerosis, non-Hodgkin lymphoma (initiation of therapy ≤18 years old), neutropenia, optic neuritis, pancytopenia, peripheral demyelinating polyneuropathy, pneumocystosis, pneumonia, psoriasis (subcutaneous) including new onset, palmoplantar, pustular, or exacerbation), pyelonephritis, reactivation of HBV, sarcoidosis, sepsis, septic arthritis (subcutaneous), septic shock (subcutaneous), serious infection, thrombocytopenia, tuberculosis (including reactivation of latent and new infection), vasculitis (subcutaneous)

Drug Interactions

Metabolism/Transport Effects None known.

Avoid Concomitant Use

Avoid concomitant use of Golimumab with any of the following: Abatacept; Anakinra; BCG; Belimumab; Canakinumab; Certolizumab Pegol; InFLIXimab; Natalizumab; Pimecrolimus; Rilonacept; Tacrolimus (Topical); Tocilizumab; Tofacitinib; Vaccines (Live); Vedolizumab

Increased Effect/Toxicity

Golimumab may increase the levels/effects of: Abatacept; Anakinra; Belimumab; Canakinumab; Certolizumab Pegol; InFLIXimab; Leflunomide; Natalizumab; Rilonacept; Tofacitinib; Vaccines (Live); Vedolizumab

The levels/effects of Golimumab may be increased by: Denosumab; Pimecrolimus; Roflumilast; Tacrolimus (Topical); Tocilizumab; Trastuzumab

Decreased Effect

Golimumab may decrease the levels/effects of: BCG; Coccidioides immitis Skin Test; Sipuleucel-T; Vaccines (Inactivated); Vaccines (Live)

The levels/effects of Golimumab may be decreased by: Echinacea

Preparation for Administration Intact solution should be colorless to light yellow; solution may develop a few fine, translucent particles.

SubQ: Bring to room temperature by allowing syringe/autoinjector to sit at room temperature outside the carton for 30 minutes prior to administration (do not warm in any other way). Do not use if discolored, cloudy, or if foreign particles are present.

IV: Do not use if solution is discolored, or contains opaque or foreign particles. Dilute for infusion by slowly adding calculated dose/volume to sodium chloride 0.9% to a total volume of 100 mL. Gently mix.

Discard unused portion of vial/syringe/autoinjector.

Storage/Stability Store intact vials and syringes refrigerated at 2°C to 8°C (36°F to 46°F); do not freeze. Do not shake. Protect from light.

IV: Solutions diluted for infusion may be stored at room temperature for 4 hours.

Mechanism of Action Human monoclonal antibody that binds to human tumor necrosis factor alpha (TNFα), thereby interfering with endogenous TNFα activity. Biological activities of TNFα include the induction of proinflammatory cytokines (interleukin [IL]-6, IL-8, Granulocyte-colony stimulating factor, granulocyte-macrophage colony stimulating factor), expression of adhesion molecules (E-selectin, vascular cell adhesion molecule [VCAM]-1, intercellular adhesion molecule [ICAM]-1) necessary for leukocyte infiltration, activation of neutrophils and eosinophils.

Pharmacodynamics/Kinetics

Distribution: V_d: IV: 151 ± 61 mL/kg (distributed primarily to circulatory system with limited extravascular distribution)

Bioavailability: SubQ: ~53%

Metabolism: Pathway unknown

Half-life elimination: ~2 weeks

Time to peak, serum: SubQ: 2-6 days

Dosage Note: Corticosteroids, *nonbiologic* disease-modifying antirheumatic drugs (DMARDs), and/or NSAIDs may be continued for the treatment of rheumatoid arthritis, psoriatic arthritis, or ankylosing spondylitis. Golimumab should not be used in combination with *biologic* DMARDs.

Ankylosing spondylitis: Adults: SubQ: 50 mg once a month (either alone or in combination with methotrexate or other nonbiologic DMARDs)

Psoriatic arthritis: Adults: SubQ: 50 mg once a month (either alone or in combination with methotrexate or other nonbiologic DMARDs)

Rheumatoid arthritis: Adults:

IV: 2 mg/kg at weeks 0, 4, and then every 8 weeks thereafter (in combination with methotrexate)

SubQ: 50 mg once a month (in combination with methotrexate)

Ulcerative colitis: Adults:

U.S. labeling: SubQ: Induction: 200 mg at week 0, then 100 mg at week 2, followed by maintenance therapy of 100 mg every 4 weeks

Canadian labeling: SubQ: Induction: 200 mg at week 0, then 100 mg at week 2, followed by maintenance therapy of 50 mg every 4 weeks (maintenance dose may be increased to 100 mg every 4 weeks if needed)

Dosage adjustment in renal impairment: There are no dosage adjustments provided in manufacturer's labeling (has not been studied).

Dosage adjustment in hepatic impairment: There are no dosage adjustments provided in manufacturer's labeling (has not been studied).

Administration

IV: Dilute prior to use. Infuse over 30 minutes, using an infusion set with an in-line low protein-binding 0.22 micron filter. Do not infuse in the same line with other medications.

Subcutaneous injection: Hold autoinjector firmly against skin and inject subcutaneously into thigh, lower abdomen (below navel), or upper arm. A loud click is heard when injection has begun. Continue to hold autoinjector against skin until second click is heard (may take 3-15 seconds). Following second click, lift autoinjector from injection site. Rotate injection sites and avoid injecting into tender, red, scaly, hard, or bruised skin, or areas with scars or stretch marks. If multiple injections are required for a single dose, administer at different sites on body.

Monitoring Parameters CBC with differential; latent TB screening (prior to initiating and periodically during therapy); HBV screening (prior to initiating [all patients]; during and for several months following therapy [HBV carriers]); monitor improvement of symptoms and physical function assessments; signs/symptoms of infection (prior to, during, and following therapy); signs/symptoms/worsening of heart failure signs and symptoms of hypersensitivity reaction; symptoms of lupus-like syndrome; signs/symptoms of malignancy (eg, splenomegaly, hepatomegaly, abdominal pain, persistent fever, night sweats, weight loss) including periodic skin examination

Dosage Forms

Solution, Intravenous [preservative free]:

Simponi Aria: 50 mg/4 mL (4 mL)

Solution Auto-injector, Subcutaneous [preservative free]:

Simponi: 50 mg/0.5 mL (0.5 mL); 100 mg/mL (1 mL)

Solution Prefilled Syringe, Subcutaneous [preservative free]:

Simponi: 50 mg/0.5 mL (0.5 mL); 100 mg/mL (1 mL)

◆ **GoLYTELY** *see* Polyethylene Glycol-Electrolyte Solution *on page 1674*

Gonadorelin [CAN/INT] (goe nad oh RELL in)

Brand Names: Canada Lutrepulse

Index Terms GnRH; Gonadorelin Acetate; Gonadotropin Releasing Hormone; LHRH; LRH; Luteinizing Hormone Releasing Hormone

Pharmacologic Category Gonadotropin

Use Note: Not approved in U.S.

Induction of ovulation in females with hypothalamic amenorrhea

Pregnancy Considerations The risk of fetal harm appears remote if gonadorelin is used during pregnancy. Clinical studies of pregnant women have not demonstrated an increased risk of fetal abnormalities during the first trimester. Follow-up reports of infants born to exposed mothers revealed no adverse effects or complications attributed to gonadorelin therapy. Based on its indicated use, gonadorelin treatment is continued for 2 weeks following ovulation to maintain the corpus luteum; initiation of treatment is not appropriate if pregnancy has been established.

Breast-Feeding Considerations It is not known if gonadorelin is excreted into breast milk. Not indicated for use in nursing women.

Contraindications Hypersensitivity to gonadorelin or any component of the formulation; women with any condition (eg, pituitary prolactinoma) that could be exacerbated by pregnancy; patients who have ovarian cysts; any condition (eg, hormone-dependent tumor) that may be worsened by reproductive hormones

Warnings/Precautions

Ovarian cancer: **[Canadian Boxed Warning]: Ovarian cancer has been reported in a very small number of infertile women treated with fertility drugs. A causal relationship has not been established.**

Ovarian hyperstimulation syndrome (OHSS): **[Canadian Boxed Warning]: OHSS is a risk of ovulation induction therapy although it is rare with pulsatile gonadotropin releasing hormone (GnRH) therapy. Clinicians should be alert for evidence of ascites, pleural effusion, fluid/electrolyte imbalance, hemoconcentration, cyst rupture, sepsis. Discontinue therapy if OHSS occurs; spontaneous resolution may be expected.** OHSS, an exaggerated response to ovulation induction therapy, is characterized by an increase in vascular permeability, which causes a fluid shift from intravascular space to third-space compartments (eg, peritoneal cavity, thoracic cavity) (ASRM, 2008; SOGC-CFAS, 2011). This syndrome may begin within 24 hours of treatment, but may become most severe 7 to 10 days after therapy (SOGC-CFAS, 2011). OHSS is typically self-limiting with spontaneous resolution, although it may be more severe and protracted if pregnancy occurs (ASRM, 2008). Symptoms of mild/moderate OHSS may include abdominal distention/discomfort, diarrhea, nausea, and/or vomiting. Severe OHSS symptoms may include abdominal pain that is severe, acute respiratory distress syndrome, anuria/oliguria, ascites, dyspnea, hypotension, nausea/vomiting (intractable), pericardial effusions, tachycardia, or thromboembolism. Decreased creatinine clearance, hemoconcentration, hypoproteinemia, elevated liver enzymes, elevated WBC, and electrolyte imbalances may also be present (ASRM, 2008; Fiedler, 2012; SOGC-CFAS, 2011). If severe OHSS occurs, stop treatment and consider hospitalizing the patient. (ASRM, 2008; SOGC-CFAS, 2011). Treatment is primarily symptomatic and includes fluid and electrolyte management, analgesics, and prevention of thromboembolic complications (ASRM, 2008; SOGC-CFAS, 2011). The ascitic, pleural, and pericardial fluids may be removed if needed to relieve symptoms (eg, pulmonary distress or cardiac tamponade) (ASRM, 2008; SOGC-CFAS, 2011). Women with OHSS should avoid pelvic examination and/or intercourse (ASRM, 2008; SOGC-CFAS, 2011).

Hypersensitivity and anaphylactic reactions have been reported rarely. Therapy should only be conducted by clinicians familiar with infertility problems and their management. Multiple births may result from the use of these medications; advise patients of the potential risk of multiple births before starting treatment.

Adverse Reactions Local: Injection site irritation, superficial thrombophlebitis

Rare but important or life-threatening: Abdominal pain, anaphylactic reaction, anaphylactic shock, antibody formation (with long term therapy resulting in therapy failure), fever, headache, injection site reddening, injection site thrombophlebitis (mild and severe), menstrual bleeding increased, ovarian hyperstimulation (moderate)

Drug Interactions

Metabolism/Transport Effects None known.

Avoid Concomitant Use There are no known interactions where it is recommended to avoid concomitant use.

Increased Effect/Toxicity There are no known significant interactions involving an increase in effect.

Decreased Effect There are no known significant interactions involving a decrease in effect.

Preparation for Administration Lutrepulse vials for IV or SubQ use: Reconstitute gonadorelin vial with 8 mL of supplied diluent immediately prior to use. Shake vial until solution is clear and particulate-free. Transfer to a polypropylene plastic reservoir. Following dilution of the 0.8 mg vial with 8 mL of diluent, the pump can be set to deliver a dose/pulse of 2.5 mcg or 5 mcg. Following dilution of the 3.2 mg vial with 8 mL of diluent, the pump can be set to deliver a dose/pulse of 10 mcg or 20 mcg.

Storage/Stability Store gonadorelin acetate and diluent (0.9% sodium chloride) at 15°C to 30°C (59°F to 86°F).

Mechanism of Action Stimulates the release of luteinizing hormone (LH) from the anterior pituitary gland

Pharmacodynamics/Kinetics

Onset of action: Response to therapy usually observed within 2-3 weeks

Distribution: V_d: ~10-15 L

Metabolism: Primarily renal

Half-life elimination: Terminal: ~10-40 minutes; increased in patients with renal impairment

Excretion: Urine (as inactive metabolites)

Dosage Primary hypothalamic amenorrhea: Adults (females): IV, SubQ.: Initial dose: 5 mcg every 90 minutes via suitable pulsatile pump. Dosage adjustments may be made every 21 days if necessary. An increase in dosage may be necessary if no response after 3 treatment intervals. In clinical trials, doses of 1-20 mcg were successfully administered. Treatment should be continued for 2 weeks after ovulation to maintain the corpus luteum.

Note: Appropriate vial should be selected for individualized treatment. Typical dose (5 mcg) is delivered with use of 0.8 mg vial.

Administration Lutrepulse vials for IV or SubQ use: Following reconstitution, administer IV or SubQ using a suitable pulsatile pump. Set the pump to deliver 25 or 50 mcL of solution, based upon the dose required and vial strength used. When using the 0.8 mg vial, the pump can be set to deliver a dose of 2.5 mcg (25 mcL) per pulse or 5 mcg (50 mcL) per pulse. When using the 3.2 mg vial, the pump can be set to deliver a dose of 10 mcg (25 mcL) per pulse or 20 mcg (50 mcL) per pulse. Pump should deliver dose over a pulse period of 1 minute and a pulse frequency of 90 minutes.

Monitoring Parameters

Ovarian ultrasound at baseline and at least weekly while on therapy or until ovulation is confirmed; LH, FSH, estradiol, progesterone (midluteal phase); basal body temperature; pelvic exam; injection site

OHSS: Monitoring of hospitalized patients should include abdominal circumference, albumin, cardiorespiratory status, electrolytes, fluid balance, hematocrit, hemoglobin, serum creatinine, urine output, urine specific gravity, vital signs, weight (all daily or as necessary) and liver enzymes (weekly) (ASRM, 2008; SOGC-CFAS, 2011)

Product Availability Not available in U.S.

Dosage Forms: Canada

Injection, powder for reconstitution:

Lutrepulse: 0.8 mg, 3.2 mg

◆ **Gonadorelin Acetate** *see* Gonadorelin [CAN/INT] *on page 980*

◆ **Gonadotropin Releasing Hormone** *see* Gonadorelin [CAN/INT] *on page 980*

◆ **Gonal-f** *see* Follitropin Alfa *on page 921*

◆ **Gonal-f Pen (Can)** *see* Follitropin Alfa *on page 921*

◆ **Gonal-f RFF** *see* Follitropin Alfa *on page 921*

◆ **Gonal-f RFF Pen** *see* Follitropin Alfa *on page 921*

◆ **Gonal-f RFF Redijectt** *see* Follitropin Alfa *on page 921*

◆ **GoodSense Acid Reducer [OTC]** *see* Ranitidine *on page 1777*

◆ **GoodSense Mucus Relief [OTC]** *see* GuaiFENesin *on page 986*

◆ **Goody's Extra Strength Headache Powder [OTC]** *see* Acetaminophen, Aspirin, and Caffeine *on page 37*

◆ **Goody's Extra Strength Pain Relief [OTC]** *see* Acetaminophen, Aspirin, and Caffeine *on page 37*

◆ **Goody's PM® [OTC]** *see* Acetaminophen and Diphenhydramine *on page 36*

◆ **Gordons Urea** *see* Urea *on page 2114*

◆ **Gordons-Vite A [OTC]** *see* Vitamin A *on page 2173*

◆ **Gordons-Vite E [OTC]** *see* Vitamin E *on page 2174*

◆ **Gormel [OTC]** *see* Urea *on page 2114*

◆ **Gormel 10 [OTC]** *see* Urea *on page 2114*

Goserelin (GOE se rel in)

Brand Names: U.S. Zoladex

Brand Names: Canada Zoladex; Zoladex LA

Index Terms Goserelin Acetate; ICI-118630; ZDX

Pharmacologic Category Antineoplastic Agent, Gonadotropin-Releasing Hormone Agonist; Gonadotropin Releasing Hormone Agonist

Use

Breast cancer, advanced (3.6 mg only): Palliative treatment of advanced breast cancer in pre- and perimenopausal women (estrogen and progesterone receptor values may help to predict if goserelin is likely to be beneficial).

Endometrial thinning (3.6 mg only): Endometrial-thinning agent prior to endometrial ablation for dysfunctional uterine bleeding.

Endometriosis (3.6 mg only): Management of endometriosis, including pain relief and reduction of endometriotic lesions for the duration of therapy (goserelin experience for endometriosis has been limited to women 18 years and older treated for 6 months).

Prostate cancer, advanced: Palliative treatment of advanced carcinoma of the prostate.

Prostate cancer, stage B2 to C: Management of locally confined stage T2b to T4 (stage B2 to C) prostate cancer (in combination with flutamide); begin goserelin and flutamide 8 weeks prior to initiating radiation therapy and continue during radiation therapy.

Pregnancy Risk Factor X (endometriosis, endometrial thinning); D (advanced breast cancer)

Pregnancy Considerations Adverse events were observed in animal reproduction studies. Goserelin induces hormonal changes which increase the risk for fetal loss and use is contraindicated in pregnancy unless being used for palliative treatment of advanced breast cancer.

Breast cancer: If used for the palliative treatment of breast cancer during pregnancy, the potential for increased fetal loss should be discussed with the patient.

Endometriosis, endometrial thinning: Use is contraindicated during pregnancy. Women of childbearing potential should not receive therapy until pregnancy has been excluded. Nonhormonal contraception is recommended for premenopausal women during therapy and for 12 weeks after therapy is discontinued. Although ovulation is usually inhibited and menstruation may stop, pregnancy prevention is not ensured during goserelin therapy. Changes in reproductive function may occur following chronic administration.

Breast-Feeding Considerations It is not known if goserelin is excreted in breast milk, although goserelin is inactivated when used orally. Due to the potential for serious adverse reactions in the breast-feeding infant, a decision should be made to discontinue breast-feeding or to discontinue the drug, taking into account the importance of treatment to the mother.

Contraindications Hypersensitivity to goserelin, GnRH, GnRH agonist analogues, or any component of the formulation; pregnancy (except if using for palliative treatment of advanced breast cancer)

Warnings/Precautions Hazardous agent - use appropriate precautions for handling and disposal (NIOSH 2014 [group 1]). Transient increases in serum testosterone (in men with prostate cancer) and estrogen (in women with breast cancer) may result in a worsening of disease signs and symptoms (tumor flare) during the first few weeks of treatment. Some patients experienced a temporary worsening of bone pain, which may be managed symptomatically. Spinal cord compression and urinary tract obstruction have been reported when used for prostate cancer; closely observe patients for symptoms (eg, ureteral obstruction, weakness, paresthesias) in first few weeks of therapy. Manage with standard treatment; consider orchiectomy for extreme cases.

Androgen deprivation therapy may increase the risk for cardiovascular disease (Levine, 2010). An increased risk for MI, sudden cardiac death, and stroke has been observed. Monitor for signs/symptoms of cardiovascular disease; manage according to current clinical practice. Androgen deprivation therapy may cause prolongation of the QT/QTc interval; evaluate risk versus benefit in patients with congenital long QT syndrome, heart failure, frequent electrolyte abnormalities, and in patients taking medication known to prolong the QT interval. Correct electrolytes prior to initiation and consider periodic electrolyte and ECG monitoring. Hyperglycemia has been reported in males and may manifest as diabetes or worsening of preexisting diabetes (worsening glycemic control); monitor blood glucose and HbA_{1c} and manage diabetes appropriately.

Hypersensitivity reactions (including acute anaphylactic reactions) and antibody formation may occur; monitor. Hypercalcemia has been reported in prostate and breast cancer patients with bone metastases; initiate appropriate management if hypercalcemia occurs. Rare cases of pituitary apoplexy (frequently secondary to pituitary adenoma) have been observed with GnRH agonist administration (onset from 1 hour to usually <2 weeks); may present as sudden headache, vomiting, visual or mental status changes, and infrequently cardiovascular collapse; immediate medical attention required. A decreased AUC may be observed when using the 3-month implant in obese patients; monitor testosterone levels if desired clinical response is not observed. If implant removal is necessary, implant may be located by ultrasound.

Decreased bone density has been reported in women and may be irreversible; use caution if other risk factors are present; evaluate and institute preventive treatment if necessary. Cervical resistance may be increased; use caution when dilating the cervix for endometrial ablation. Women of childbearing potential should not receive therapy until pregnancy has been excluded. Nonhormonal contraception is recommended during therapy and for 12 weeks after therapy is discontinued. The 3-month implant currently has no approved indications for use in women. Chronic administration may result in effects on reproductive function due to antigonadotropic properties.

Adverse Reactions

Cardiovascular: Cardiac arrhythmia (males), cardiac failure (males), cerebrovascular accident (males), chest pain, edema (more common in males), hypertension, myocardial infarction (males), palpitations, peripheral edema (females), peripheral vascular disease (males), tachycardia (females), varicose veins (males), vasodilatation (females)

Central nervous system: Abnormality in thinking, anxiety, chills (males), depression (more common in females), dizziness (more common in females), drowsiness, dyspareunia (females), emotional lability (female), headache (more common in females),insomnia, lethargy (females), malaise (females), migraine (females), nervousness (females), pain, paresthesia, voice disorder (females)

Dermatologic: Acne vulgaris (females; usually within 1 month after starting treatment), alopecia, diaphoresis (more common in females), hair disease (females), pruritus (females), seborrhea (females), skin discoloration, skin rash (males), xeroderma

Endocrine & metabolic: Decreased libido (females), gout (males), gynecomastia (males), hot flash (more common in females), hirsutism, hyperglycemia (males), increased libido (females), weight gain

Gastrointestinal: Abdominal pain (females), anorexia, constipation, diarrhea, dyspepsia, flatulence, gastric ulcer (males), increased appetite (females), nausea, vomiting, xerostomia

Genitourinary: Breast atrophy (females), breast hypertrophy (females), breast swelling (males), decrease in erectile frequency, genitourinary signs and symptoms (lower; males), mastalgia, pelvic pain (more common in females), pelvic symptoms (females), sexual disorder (males), urinary frequency, urinary tract infection, urinary tract obstruction (males), uterine hemorrhage, vaginal hemorrhage, vaginitis, vulvovaginitis

Hematologic & oncologic: Anemia (males), bruise, hemorrhage, tumor flare (more common in females)

Hypersensitivity: Hypersensitivity reaction

Infection: Infection (more common in females), sepsis (males)

Local: Application site reaction (females)

Neuromuscular & skeletal: Arthralgia, arthropathy, decreased bone mineral density (more common in females), hypertonia (more common in females), leg cramps (more common in females), myalgia (more common in females), weakness (females)

Ophthalmic: Amblyopia, dry eye syndrome

Renal: Renal insufficiency

Respiratory: Bronchitis, chronic obstructive pulmonary disease (males), cough, epistaxis, flu-like symptoms (more common in females), pharyngitis (females), rhinitis, sinusitis (more common in females), upper respiratory tract infection (males)

Miscellaneous: Fever

Rare but important or life-threatening: Anaphylaxis, convulsions, deep vein thrombosis, diabetes mellitus, hypercalcemia, hypercholesterolemia, increased HDL cholesterol, increased serum ALT, increased serum AST, osteoporosis, ovarian cyst, ovarian hyperstimulation syndrome, pituitary apoplexy, pituitary neoplasm (including adenoma), pulmonary embolism, psychotic reaction, transient ischemic attacks

Drug Interactions

Metabolism/Transport Effects None known.

Avoid Concomitant Use

Avoid concomitant use of Goserelin with any of the following: Corifollitropin Alfa; Highest Risk QTc-Prolonging Agents; Indium 111 Capromab Pendetide; Ivabradine; Mifepristone

Increased Effect/Toxicity

Goserelin may increase the levels/effects of: Corifollitropin Alfa; Highest Risk QTc-Prolonging Agents; Moderate Risk QTc-Prolonging Agents

The levels/effects of Goserelin may be increased by: Ivabradine; Mifepristone; QTc-Prolonging Agents (Indeterminate Risk and Risk Modifying)

Decreased Effect

Goserelin may decrease the levels/effects of: Antidiabetic Agents; Indium 111 Capromab Pendetide

Storage/Stability Store at room temperature not to exceed 25°C (77°F).

Mechanism of Action Goserelin (a gonadotropin-releasing hormone [GnRH] analog) causes an initial increase in luteinizing hormone (LH) and follicle stimulating hormone (FSH), chronic administration of goserelin results in a sustained suppression of pituitary gonadotropins. Serum testosterone falls to levels comparable to surgical castration. The exact mechanism of this effect is unknown, but may be related to changes in the control of LH or down-regulation of LH receptors.

Pharmacodynamics/Kinetics

Onset:

Females: Estradiol suppression reaches postmenopausal levels within 3 weeks and FSH and LH are suppressed to follicular phase levels within 4 weeks of initiation

Males: Testosterone suppression reaches castrate levels within 2 to 4 weeks after initiation

Duration:

Females: Estradiol, LH and FSH generally return to baseline levels within 12 weeks following the last monthly implant.

Males: Testosterone levels maintained at castrate levels throughout the duration of therapy.

Absorption: SubQ: Rapid and can be detected in serum in 30 to 60 minutes; 3.6 mg: released slowly in first 8 days, then rapid and continuous release for 28 days

Distribution: V_d: Male: 44.1 L; Female: 20.3 L

Protein binding: ~27%

Metabolism: Hepatic hydrolysis of the C-terminal amino acids

Time to peak, serum: SubQ: Male: 12 to 15 days, Female: 8 to 22 days

Excretion: Urine (>90%; 20% as unchanged drug)

Dosage

Prostate cancer, advanced: Adult males: SubQ:

28-day implant: 3.6 mg every 28 days

12-week implant: 10.8 mg every 12 weeks

Prostate cancer, stage B2 to C (in combination with an antiandrogen and radiotherapy; begin 8 weeks prior to radiotherapy): Adult males: SubQ:

Combination 28-day/12-week implant: 3.6 mg implant, followed in 28 days by 10.8 mg implant

28-day implant (alternate dosing): 3.6 mg; repeated every 28 days for a total of 4 doses

Breast cancer, advanced: Adult females: SubQ: 3.6 mg every 28 days

Endometriosis: Adult females: SubQ: 3.6 mg every 28 days for 6 months

Endometrial thinning: Adult females: SubQ: 3.6 mg every 28 days for 1 or 2 doses

Prevention of early menopause during chemotherapy for early stage hormone receptor negative breast cancer (off-label use): Adult females: SubQ: 3.6 mg every 28 days starting 1 week prior to the first chemotherapy dose; continue until disease progression or unacceptable toxicity (Moore, 2014)

Dosing adjustment in renal impairment: No dosage adjustment necessary

Dosing adjustment in hepatic impairment: No dosage adjustment necessary

Administration SubQ: Administer implant by inserting needle at a 30 to 45 degree angle into the anterior abdominal wall below the navel line. Goserelin is an implant; therefore, do not attempt to eliminate air bubbles prior to injection (may displace implant). Do not attempt to aspirate prior to injection; if a large vessel is penetrated, blood will be visualized in the syringe chamber (if vessel is penetrated, withdraw needle and inject elsewhere with a new syringe). Do not penetrate into muscle or peritoneum. Implant may be detected by ultrasound if removal is required.

Hazardous agent; use appropriate precautions for handling and disposal (NIOSH 2014 [group 1]).

Monitoring Parameters Monitor blood glucose and HbA_{1c} (periodically), bone mineral density, serum calcium, cholesterol/lipids

Prostate cancer: Consider periodic ECG and electrolyte monitoring. Monitor for weakness, paresthesias, tumor flare, urinary tract obstruction, and spinal cord compression in first few weeks of therapy.

Dosage Forms

Implant, Subcutaneous:

Zoladex: 3.6 mg (1 ea); 10.8 mg (1 ea)

- ◆ **Goserelin Acetate** *see* Goserelin *on page 981*
- ◆ **GP 47680** *see* OXcarbazepine *on page 1532*
- ◆ **GR38032R** *see* Ondansetron *on page 1513*
- ◆ **Gralise** *see* Gabapentin *on page 943*
- ◆ **Gralise Starter** *see* Gabapentin *on page 943*
- ◆ **Gramicidin, Neomycin, and Polymyxin B** *see* Neomycin, Polymyxin B, and Gramicidin *on page 1437*

Granisetron (gra NI se tron)

Brand Names: U.S. Granisol [DSC]; Sancuso

Brand Names: Canada Granisetron Hydrochloride Injection; Kytril

Index Terms BRL 43694; Kytril

Pharmacologic Category Antiemetic; Selective $5\text{-}HT_3$ Receptor Antagonist

Use

Chemotherapy-associated nausea and vomiting: Prevention of nausea and vomiting associated with initial and repeat courses of emetogenic chemotherapy, including high-dose cisplatin (injection and tablets); prevention of nausea and vomiting associated with moderately and/or highly emetogenic chemotherapy regimens of up to 5 consecutive days of duration (transdermal).

Radiation-associated nausea and vomiting: Prevention of nausea and vomiting associated with radiation therapy, including total body radiation and fractionated abdominal radiation (tablets).

Pregnancy Risk Factor B

Pregnancy Considerations Adverse events were not observed in animal reproduction studies. Injection (1 mg/mL strength) contains benzyl alcohol which may cross the placenta. The Canadian labeling does not recommend use during pregnancy.

Breast-Feeding Considerations It is not known if granisetron is excreted in breast milk. The U.S. labeling recommends that caution be exercised when administering granisetron to nursing women. The Canadian labeling does not recommend use in nursing women.

Contraindications

Hypersensitivity to granisetron or any component of the formulation

Canadian labeling: Additional contraindications (not in U.S. labeling): Concomitant use with apomorphine

Warnings/Precautions Use with caution in patients with congenital long QT syndrome or other risk factors for QT prolongation (eg, medications known to prolong QT interval, electrolyte abnormalities, and cumulative high-dose anthracycline therapy). $5\text{-}HT_3$ antagonists have been associated with a number of dose-dependent increases in ECG intervals (eg, PR, QRS duration, QT/QTc, JT), usually occurring 1 to 2 hours after IV administration. In general, these changes are not clinically relevant, however, when used in conjunction with other agents that prolong these intervals, arrhythmia may occur. When used with agents that prolong the QT interval (eg, Class I and III antiarrhythmics), clinically relevant QT interval prolongation may occur resulting in torsade de pointes. IV formulations of $5\text{-}HT_3$ antagonists have more association with ECG interval changes, compared to oral formulations.

Antiemetics are most effective when used prophylactically (Roila, 2010). If emesis occurs despite optimal antiemetic prophylaxis, re-evaluate emetic risk, disease, concurrent morbidities and medications to assure antiemetic regimen is optimized (Basch, 2011).

Serotonin syndrome has been reported with $5\text{-}HT_3$ receptor antagonists, predominantly when used in combination with other serotonergic agents (eg, SSRIs, SNRIs, MAOIs, mirtazapine, fentanyl, lithium, tramadol, and/or methylene blue). Some of the cases have been fatal. The majority of serotonin syndrome reports due to $5\text{-}HT_3$ receptor antagonist have occurred in a postanesthesia setting or in an infusion center. Serotonin syndrome has also been reported following overdose of another $5\text{-}HT_3$ receptor antagonist. Monitor patients for signs of serotonin syndrome, including mental status changes (eg, agitation, hallucinations, delirium, coma); autonomic instability (eg, tachycardia, labile blood pressure, diaphoresis, dizziness, flushing, hyperthermia); neuromuscular changes (eg, tremor, rigidity, myoclonus, hyperreflexia, incoordination); gastrointestinal symptoms (eg, nausea, vomiting, diarrhea); and/or seizures. If serotonin syndrome occurs, discontinue $5\text{-}HT_3$ receptor antagonist treatment and begin supportive management. Use with caution in patients allergic to other $5\text{-}HT_3$ receptor antagonists; cross-reactivity has been reported. Does not stimulate gastric or intestinal peristalsis (should not be used instead of nasogastric suction); may mask progressive ileus and/or gastric distension. Application site reactions, generally mild, have occurred with transdermal patch use; if skin reaction is severe or generalized, remove patch. Cover patch application site with clothing to protect from natural or artificial sunlight exposure while patch is applied and for 10 days following removal; granisetron may potentially be affected by natural or artificial sunlight. Do not apply patch to red, irritated, or damaged skin. Potentially significant drug-drug interactions may exist, requiring dose or frequency adjustment, additional monitoring, and/or selection of alternative therapy

Benzyl alcohol and derivatives: Some dosage forms may contain benzyl alcohol; large amounts of benzyl alcohol (≥99 mg/kg/day) have been associated with a potentially fatal toxicity ("gasping syndrome") in neonates; the "gasping syndrome" consists of metabolic acidosis, respiratory distress, gasping respirations, CNS dysfunction (including ▶

convulsions, intracranial hemorrhage), hypotension and cardiovascular collapse (AAP, 1997; CDC, 1982); some data suggests that benzoate displaces bilirubin from protein binding sites (Ahlfors, 2001); avoid or use dosage forms containing benzyl alcohol with caution in neonates. See manufacturer's labeling.

Adverse Reactions

Cardiovascular: Hypertension, prolonged Q-T interval on ECG (>450 milliseconds, not associated with any arrhythmias)

Central nervous system: Agitation, anxiety, central nervous system stimulation, dizziness, drowsiness, headache (more common in oral and IV), insomnia

Dermatologic: Alopecia, skin rash

Gastrointestinal: Abdominal pain, constipation (more common in oral and IV), decreased appetite, diarrhea, dysgeusia, dyspepsia, nausea, vomiting

Hematologic and oncologic: Anemia, leukopenia, thrombocytopenia

Hepatic: Increased serum ALT (>2 x ULN), increased serum AST (>2 x ULN)

Neuromuscular & skeletal: Weakness (more common in oral)

Miscellaneous: Fever

Rare but important or life-threatening: Angina pectoris, application site reactions (transdermal: allergic rash including erythematous, macular, popular rash, or pruritus), atrial fibrillation, atrioventricular block (IV), cardiac arrhythmia, ECG abnormality (IV), extrapyramidal reaction (oral), hypersensitivity reaction (includes anaphylaxis, dyspnea, hypotension, urticaria), hypotension, serotonin syndrome, sinus bradycardia (IV), ventricular ectopy (IV; includes non-sustained tachycardia)

Drug Interactions

Metabolism/Transport Effects Substrate of CYP3A4 (minor); **Note:** Assignment of Major/Minor substrate status based on clinically relevant drug interaction potential

Avoid Concomitant Use

Avoid concomitant use of Granisetron with any of the following: Apomorphine; Highest Risk QTc-Prolonging Agents; Ivabradine; Mifepristone

Increased Effect/Toxicity

Granisetron may increase the levels/effects of: Apomorphine; Highest Risk QTc-Prolonging Agents; Moderate Risk QTc-Prolonging Agents; Serotonin Modulators

The levels/effects of Granisetron may be increased by: Ivabradine; Mifepristone; QTc-Prolonging Agents (Indeterminate Risk and Risk Modifying)

Decreased Effect

Granisetron may decrease the levels/effects of: Tapentadol; TraMADol

Storage/Stability

IV: Store at 15°C to 30°C (59°F to 86°F). Protect from light. Do not freeze vials. Stable when mixed in NS or D_5W for 7 days under refrigeration and for 3 days at room temperature.

Oral: Store tablet or oral solution at 15°C to 30°C (59°F to 86°F). Protect from light.

Transdermal patch: Store at 20°C to 25°C (68°F to 77°F). Keep patch in original packaging until immediately prior to use.

Mechanism of Action Selective 5-HT_3-receptor antagonist, blocking serotonin, both peripherally on vagal nerve terminals and centrally in the chemoreceptor trigger zone

Pharmacodynamics/Kinetics

Duration: Oral, IV: Generally up to 24 hours

Absorption: Oral: Tablets and oral solution are bioequivalent; Transdermal patch: ~66% over 7 days

Distribution: V_d: 2 to 4 L/kg; widely throughout body

Protein binding: ~65%

Metabolism: Hepatic via N-demethylation, oxidation, and conjugation; some metabolites may have 5-HT_3 antagonist activity

Half-life elimination: Oral: 6 hours; IV: ~9 hours

Time to peak, plasma: Transdermal patch: Maximum systemic concentrations: ~48 hours after application (range: 24 to 168 hours)

Excretion: Urine (12% as unchanged drug, 48% to 49% as metabolites); feces (34% to 38% as metabolites)

Dosage

Prevention of chemotherapy-associated nausea and vomiting:

IV: Children ≥2 years, Adolescents, and Adults: 10 mcg/kg 30 minutes prior to chemotherapy; only on the day(s) chemotherapy is given.

Oral: Adults: 2 mg once daily up to 1 hour before chemotherapy or 1 mg twice daily; the first 1 mg dose should be given up to 1 hour before chemotherapy. Administer only on the day(s) chemotherapy is given.

Transdermal patch: Adults: Prophylaxis of chemotherapy-related emesis: Apply 1 patch at least 24 hours prior to chemotherapy; may be applied up to 48 hours before chemotherapy. Remove patch a minimum of 24 hours after chemotherapy completion. Maximum duration: Patch may be worn up to 7 days, depending on chemotherapy regimen duration.

Adult guideline recommendations:

American Society of Clinical Oncology (ASCO; Basch, 2011): High emetic risk:

IV: 1 mg or 10 mcg/kg on the day(s) chemotherapy is administered (antiemetic regimen also includes dexamethasone and aprepitant or fosaprepitant)

Oral: 2 mg on the day(s) chemotherapy is administered (antiemetic regimen also includes dexamethasone and aprepitant or fosaprepitant)

Multinational Association of Supportive Care in Cancer (MASCC) and European Society of Medical Oncology (ESMO) (Roila, 2010):

Highly emetic chemotherapy:

IV: 1 mg or 10 mcg/kg (antiemetic regimen includes dexamethasone and aprepitant/fosaprepitant) prior to chemotherapy on day 1

Oral: 2 mg (antiemetic regimen includes dexamethasone and aprepitant/fosaprepitant) prior to chemotherapy on day 1

Moderately emetic chemotherapy:

IV: 1 mg or 10 mcg/kg (antiemetic regimen includes dexamethasone [and aprepitant/fosaprepitant for AC chemotherapy regimen]) prior to chemotherapy on day 1

Oral: 2 mg (antiemetic regimen includes dexamethasone [and aprepitant/fosaprepitant for AC chemotherapy regimen]) prior to chemotherapy on day 1

Low emetic risk:

IV: 1 mg or 10 mcg/kg prior to chemotherapy on day 1

Oral: 2 mg prior to chemotherapy on day 1

Pediatric guideline recommendations:

Prevention of chemotherapy-induced nausea and vomiting (off-label dosing; Dupuis, 2013):

Highly emetogenic chemotherapy: Infants ≥1 month and Children <12 years: IV: 40 mcg/kg as a single daily dose prior to chemotherapy. Antiemetic regimen also includes dexamethasone.

Highly emetogenic chemotherapy: Children ≥12 years and Adolescents: IV: 40 mcg/kg as a single daily dose prior to chemotherapy. Antiemetic regimen includes dexamethasone and (if no known or suspected drug interactions) aprepitant.

Moderately emetogenic chemotherapy: Infants ≥1 month, Children, and Adolescents:

IV: 40 mcg/kg as a single daily dose. Antiemetic regimen also includes dexamethasone

Oral: 40 mcg/kg every 12 hours. Antiemetic regimen also includes dexamethasone

Low emetogenic chemotherapy: Infants ≥1 month, Children, and Adolescents:

IV: 40 mcg/kg as a single daily dose.

Oral: 40 mcg/kg every 12 hours.

Prevention of radiation-associated nausea and vomiting: Adults: Oral: 2 mg once daily within 1 hour of radiation therapy.

Prevention of postoperative nausea and vomiting (off-label use): Adults: IV: 0.35 to 3 mg (5 to 20 **mcg**/kg) administered at the end of surgery (Gan, 2014).

Dosage adjustment in renal impairment: No dosage adjustment necessary.

Dosage adjustment in hepatic impairment: Kinetic studies in patients with hepatic impairment showed that total clearance was approximately halved; however, standard doses were very well tolerated, and dose adjustments are not necessary.

Administration

Oral: Doses should be given up to 1 hour prior to initiation of chemotherapy/radiation

IV: Administer IV push over 30 seconds or as a 5- to 10-minute infusion

Transdermal (Sancuso): Apply patch to clean, dry, intact skin on upper outer arm. Do not use on red, irritated, or damaged skin. Remove patch from pouch immediately before application. Do not cut patch.

Dosage Forms

Patch, Transdermal:

Sancuso: 3.1 mg/24 hr (1 ea)

Solution, Intravenous:

Generic: 0.1 mg/mL (1 mL); 1 mg/mL (1 mL); 4 mg/4 mL (4 mL)

Solution, Intravenous [preservative free]:

Generic: 0.1 mg/mL (1 mL); 1 mg/mL (1 mL)

Tablet, Oral:

Generic: 1 mg

Dosage Forms: Canada Refer to Dosage Forms. **Note:** Transdermal patch is not available in Canada

Extemporaneous Preparations Note: Commercial oral solution is available (0.2 mg/mL)

A 0.2 mg/mL oral suspension may be made with tablets. Crush twelve 1 mg tablets in a mortar and reduce to a fine powder. Add 30 mL distilled water, mix well, and transfer to a bottle. Rinse the mortar with 10 mL cherry syrup and add to bottle. Add sufficient quantity of cherry syrup to make a final volume of 60 mL. Label "shake well". Stable 14 days at room temperature or refrigerated (Quercia, 1997).

A 50 mcg/mL oral suspension may be made with tablets and one of three different vehicles (Ora-Sweet®, Ora-Plus®, or a mixture of methylcellulose 1% and Simple Syrup, N.F.). Crush one 1 mg tablet in a mortar and reduce to a fine powder. Add 20 mL of the chosen vehicle and mix to a uniform paste; transfer to a calibrated bottle. Label "shake well" and "refrigerate". Stable for 91 days refrigerated (Nahata, 1998).

Nahata MC, Morosco RS, and Hipple TF, "Stability of Granisetron Hydrochloride in Two Oral Suspensions," *Am J Health Syst Pharm*, 1998, 55(23):2511-3.

Quercia RA, Zhang J, Fan C, et al, "Stability of Granisetron Hydrochloride in an Extemporaneously Prepared Oral Liquid," *Am J Health Syst Pharm*, 1997, 54(12):1404-6.

◆ **Granisetron Hydrochloride Injection (Can)** *see* Granisetron *on page 983*

◆ **Granisol [DSC]** *see* Granisetron *on page 983*

◆ **Granix** *see* Filgrastim *on page 875*

◆ **Granulex®** *see* Trypsin, Balsam Peru, and Castor Oil *on page 2109*

◆ **Granulocyte Colony Stimulating Factor** *see* Filgrastim *on page 875*

◆ **Granulocyte Colony Stimulating Factor (PEG Conjugate)** *see* Pegfilgrastim *on page 1589*

◆ **Granulocyte-Macrophage Colony Stimulating Factor** *see* Sargramostim *on page 1865*

Grass Pollen Allergen Extract (Timothy Grass) (GRAS POL uhn al er juhn EK strakt TIM oh thee GRAS)

Brand Names: U.S. Grastek

Brand Names: Canada Grastek

Pharmacologic Category Allergen-Specific Immunotherapy

Use

Grass pollen-induced allergic rhinitis: Immunotherapy for the treatment of grass pollen-induced allergic rhinitis with or without conjunctivitis confirmed by positive skin test or *in vitro* testing for pollen-specific IgE antibodies for timothy grass or cross-reactive grass pollens in patients 5 through 65 years of age. Not indicated for the immediate relief of allergy symptoms.

Canadian labeling: Treatment of signs and symptoms of moderate to severe seasonal timothy and related grass pollen induced allergic rhinitis with or without conjunctivitis in patients ≥5 years of age who have a positive skin test and/or positive titer to *Phleum pretense* specific IgE; symptoms for ≥2 pollen seasons; and patients who are not tolerant or responsive to conventional therapy.

Pregnancy Risk Factor B

Dosage Dosage strength expressed in Bioequivalent Allergy Units (BAU). **Note:** Initiate treatment ≥12 weeks (U.S. labeling) or ≥8 weeks (Canadian labeling) before expected onset of each grass pollen season and continue throughout pollen season. May be taken daily for 3 consecutive years (including intervals between grass pollen seasons). Safety and efficacy of initiating treatment during grass pollen season or restarting treatment after missing a dose have not been established. In clinical trials, treatment interruptions ≤7 days were allowed.

Grass pollen-induced allergic rhinitis: Sublingual: Children ≥5 years, Adolescents, and Adults ≤65 years: One tablet (2800 BAU) once daily

Dosage adjustment in renal impairment: There are no dosage adjustments provided in the manufacturer's labeling.

Dosage adjustment in hepatic impairment: There are no dosage adjustments provided in the manufacturer's labeling.

Additional Information Complete prescribing information should be consulted for additional detail.

Dosage Forms

Tablet Sublingual, Sublingual:

Grastek: 2800 bau

◆ **Grastek** *see* Grass Pollen Allergen Extract (Timothy Grass) *on page 985*

◆ **Gravol [OTC] (Can)** *see* DimenhyDRINATE *on page 637*

◆ **Gravol IM (Can)** *see* DimenhyDRINATE *on page 637*

◆ **Grifulvin V** *see* Griseofulvin *on page 985*

Griseofulvin (gri see oh FUL vin)

Brand Names: U.S. Grifulvin V; Gris-PEG

Index Terms Griseofulvin Microsize; Griseofulvin Ultramicrosize

Pharmacologic Category Antifungal Agent, Oral

Use Treatment of tinea infections of the skin, hair, and nails caused by susceptible species of *Microsporum, Epidermophyton,* or *Trichophyton*

Pregnancy Risk Factor X

Dosage Oral:

Children >2 years:

Microsize: 10-20 mg/kg/day in single or 2 divided doses (maximum: 1000 mg daily) (*Red Book*, 2012)

Tinea capitis: Higher dosages (20-25 mg/kg/day) have been recommended (Ali, 2007; Lipozenic, 2002; Sethi, 2006)

Ultramicrosize: 5-15 mg/kg/day in single dose or 2 divided doses (maximum: 750 mg daily) (*Red Book*, 2012)

Adults:

Microsize:

Tinea corporis, tinea cruris, tinea capitis: 500 mg daily in single or divided doses

Tinea pedis, tinea unguium: 1000 mg daily in single or divided doses

Ultramicrosize: 375 mg daily in single or divided doses; doses up to 750 mg daily in divided doses have been used for infections more difficult to eradicate such as tinea unguium and tinea pedis

Duration of therapy depends on the site of infection:

Children and Adults:

Tinea corporis: 2-4 weeks

Tinea cruris: 2-6 weeks (*Red Book*, 2012)

Tinea capitis:

Manufacturer's labeling: 4-6 weeks

Alternate recommendations: Children: 6-12 weeks; use up to 16 weeks may be required (AAP *Red Book®* recommends continuing treatment for 2 weeks after clinical resolution of symptoms) (Ali, 2007; Lipozenic, 2002; Sethi, 2006)

Tinea pedis: 4-8 weeks

Tinea unguium: 4-6 months or longer

Additional Information Complete prescribing information should be consulted for additional detail.

Dosage Forms Considerations

Microsized formulations: Suspensions, Grifulvin V tablets

Ultramicrosize formulation: Gris-PEG tablets

Dosage Forms

Suspension, Oral:

Generic: 125 mg/5 mL (118 mL, 120 mL)

Tablet, Oral:

Grifulvin V: 500 mg

Gris-PEG: 125 mg, 250 mg

Generic: 125 mg, 250 mg, 500 mg

- ◆ **Griseofulvin Microsize** *see* Griseofulvin *on page 985*
- ◆ **Griseofulvin Ultramicrosize** *see* Griseofulvin *on page 985*
- ◆ **Gris-PEG** *see* Griseofulvin *on page 985*
- ◆ **Growth Hormone, Human** *see* Somatropin *on page 1918*
- ◆ **GRx HiCort 25** *see* Hydrocortisone (Topical) *on page 1014*
- ◆ **GS-1101** *see* Idelalisib *on page 1038*
- ◆ **GS-5885** *see* Ledipasvir and Sofosbuvir *on page 1173*
- ◆ **GSK-580299** *see* Papillomavirus (Types 16, 18) Vaccine (Human, Recombinant) *on page 1574*
- ◆ **GSK1120212** *see* Trametinib *on page 2077*
- ◆ **GSK 1838262** *see* Gabapentin Enacarbil *on page 946*
- ◆ **GSK2118436** *see* Dabrafenib *on page 546*
- ◆ **GTN** *see* Nitroglycerin *on page 1465*
- ◆ **Guaiatussin AC** *see* Guaifenesin and Codeine *on page 987*
- ◆ **Guaicon DMS [OTC]** *see* Guaifenesin and Dextromethorphan *on page 987*

GuaiFENesin (gwye FEN e sin)

Brand Names: U.S. Altarussin [OTC]; Bidex [OTC]; Buckleys Chest Congestion [OTC]; Cough Syrup [OTC]; Diabetic Siltussin DAS-Na [OTC]; Diabetic Tussin Mucus Relief [OTC]; Diabetic Tussin [OTC]; Fenesin IR [OTC]; Geri-Tussin [OTC]; GoodSense Mucus Relief [OTC]; Iophen-NR [OTC]; Liquibid [OTC]; Liquituss GG [OTC]; Mucinex Chest Congestion Child [OTC]; Mucinex For Kids [OTC]; Mucinex Maximum Strength [OTC]; Mucinex [OTC]; Mucosa [OTC]; Mucus Relief Childrens [OTC]; Mucus Relief [OTC]; Mucus-ER [OTC]; Organ-I NR [OTC]; Q-Tussin [OTC]; Refenesen 400 [OTC]; Refenesen [OTC]; Robafen [OTC]; Robitussin Chest Congestion [OTC]; Robitussin Mucus+Chest Congest [OTC]; Scot-Tussin Expectorant [OTC]; Siltussin DAS [OTC]; Siltussin SA [OTC]; Tussin [OTC]; Xpect [OTC]

Brand Names: Canada Balminil Expectorant; Benylin® E Extra Strength; Koffex Expectorant; Robitussin®

Index Terms Cheratussin; GG; Glycerol Guaiacolate

Pharmacologic Category Expectorant

Use Help loosen phlegm and thin bronchial secretions to make coughs more productive

Dosage Oral:

Children:

6 months to 2 years: 25-50 mg every 4 hours, not to exceed 300 mg/day

2-5 years: 50-100 mg every 4 hours, not to exceed 600 mg/day

6-11 years: 100-200 mg every 4 hours, not to exceed 1.2 g/day

Children >12 years and Adults: 200-400 mg every 4 hours to a maximum of 2.4 g/day

Extended release tablet: 600-1200 mg every 12 hours, not to exceed 2.4 g/day

Additional Information Complete prescribing information should be consulted for additional detail.

Dosage Forms

Liquid, Oral:

Buckleys Chest Congestion [OTC]: 100 mg/5 mL (118 mL)

Diabetic Siltussin DAS-Na [OTC]: 100 mg/5 mL (118 mL)

Diabetic Tussin [OTC]: 100 mg/5 mL (118 mL)

Diabetic Tussin Mucus Relief [OTC]: 200 mg/5 mL (118 mL)

Iophen-NR [OTC]: 100 mg/5 mL (473 mL)

Liquituss GG [OTC]: 200 mg/5 mL (118 mL, 473 mL)

Mucinex Chest Congestion Child [OTC]: 100 mg/5 mL (118 mL)

Mucus Relief Childrens [OTC]: 100 mg/5 mL (118 mL)

Robitussin Mucus+Chest Congest [OTC]: 100 mg/5 mL (118 mL)

Scot-Tussin Expectorant [OTC]: 100 mg/5 mL (30 mL, 118 mL, 240 mL, 480 mL, 3780 mL)

Siltussin DAS [OTC]: 100 mg/5 mL (118 mL)

Packet, Oral:

Mucinex For Kids [OTC]: 50 mg (12 ea); 100 mg (12 ea)

Solution, Oral:

Generic: 100 mg/5 mL (5 mL, 10 mL, 15 mL); 200 mg/10 mL (10 mL); 300 mg/15 mL (15 mL)

Syrup, Oral:

Altarussin [OTC]: 100 mg/5 mL (120 mL, 236 mL, 240 mL, 473 mL, 480 mL, 3840 mL)

Cough Syrup [OTC]: 100 mg/5 mL (118 mL, 473 mL)

Geri-Tussin [OTC]: 100 mg/5 mL (473 mL)

Q-Tussin [OTC]: 100 mg/5 mL (118 mL, 240 mL, 473 mL)

Robafen [OTC]: 100 mg/5 mL (118 mL, 473 mL)

Robitussin Chest Congestion [OTC]: 100 mg/5 mL (118 mL, 237 mL)
Siltussin SA [OTC]: 100 mg/5 mL (118 mL, 237 mL, 473 mL)
Tussin [OTC]: 100 mg/5 mL (118 mL, 237 mL)
Generic: 100 mg/5 mL (480 mL)

Tablet, Oral:
Bidex [OTC]: 400 mg
Diabetic Tussin Mucus Relief [OTC]: 400 mg
Fenesin IR [OTC]: 400 mg
GoodSense Mucus Relief [OTC]: 400 mg
Liquibid [OTC]: 400 mg
Mucosa [OTC]: 400 mg
Mucus Relief [OTC]: 400 mg
Organ-I NR [OTC]: 200 mg
Refenesen [OTC]: 200 mg
Refenesen 400 [OTC]: 400 mg
Xpect [OTC]: 400 mg
Generic: 200 mg, 400 mg

Tablet Extended Release 12 Hour, Oral:
Mucinex [OTC]: 600 mg
Mucinex Maximum Strength [OTC]: 1200 mg
Mucus-ER [OTC]: 600 mg
Generic: 600 mg

◆ **Guaifenesin AC Liquid** *see* Guaifenesin and Codeine *on page 987*

Guaifenesin and Codeine
(gwye FEN e sin & KOE deen)

Brand Names: U.S. Allfen CD; Allfen CDX; Codar GF; Dex-Tuss; Guaiatussin AC; Guaifenesin AC Liquid; Iophen C-NR; M-Clear; M-Clear WC; Mar-Cof CG; Robafen AC; Virtussin A/C

Index Terms Codeine and Guaifenesin; Robitussin AC

Pharmacologic Category Antitussive; Cough Preparation; Expectorant

Use Temporary control of cough due to minor throat and bronchial irritation

Dosage Oral:
Children 6-11 years:
Capsule: Guaifenesin 200 mg and codeine 9 mg: One capsule every 4 hours (maximum: 6 capsules/24 hours)
Liquid:
Guaifenesin 100 mg and codeine 6.33 mg per 5 mL: 7.5 mL every 4-6 hours (maximum: 45 mL/24 hours)
Guaifenesin 100-200 mg and codeine 8-10 mg per 5 mL: 5 mL every 4 hours (maximum: 30 mL/24 hours)
Guaifenesin 300 mg and codeine 10 mg per 5 mL: 2.5 mL every 4-6 hours (maximum: 20 mL/24 hours)
Tablet: Guaifenesin 400 mg and codeine 10-20 mg: One-half tablet every 4-6 hours (maximum: 3 tablets/24 hours)
Children ≥12 years and Adults:
Capsule: Guaifenesin 200 mg and codeine 9 mg: Two capsules every 4 hours (maximum: 12 capsules/24 hours)
Liquid:
Guaifenesin 100 mg and codeine 6.33 mg per 5 mL: 15 mL every 4-6 hours (maximum: 45 mL/24 hours)
Guaifenesin 100-200 mg and codeine 8-10 mg per 5 mL: 10 mL every 4 hours (maximum: 60 mL/24 hours)
Guaifenesin 300 mg and codeine 10 mg per 5 mL: 5 mL every 4-6 hours (maximum: 40 mL/24 hours)
Tablet: Guaifenesin 400 mg and codeine 10-20 mg: One tablet every 4-6 hours (maximum: 6 tablets/24 hours)

Additional Information Complete prescribing information should be consulted for additional detail.

Dosage Forms
Capsule, oral:
M-Clear: Guaifenesin 200 mg and codeine 9 mg
Liquid, oral:
Codar GF: Guaifenesin 200 mg and codeine 8 mg per 5 mL
Dex-Tuss: Guaifenesin 300 mg and codeine 10 mg per 5 mL
Iophen C-NR: Guaifenesin 100 mg and codeine 10 mg per 5 mL
M-Clear WC: Guaifenesin 100 mg and codeine 6.33 mg per 5 mL
Solution, oral: Guaifenesin 100 mg and codeine 10 mg per 5 mL
Mar-Cof CG: Guaifenesin 225 mg and codeine 7.5 mg per 5 mL
Virtussin A/C: Guaifenesin 100 mg and codeine phosphate 10 mg per 5 mL
Syrup, oral: Guaifenesin 100 mg and codeine 10 mg per 5 mL
Guaiatussin AC, Robafen AC: Guaifenesin 100 mg and codeine 10 mg per 5 mL
Tablet, oral:
Allfen CD: Guaifenesin 400 mg and codeine 10 mg
Allfen CDX: Guaifenesin 400 mg and codeine 20 mg

Guaifenesin and Dextromethorphan
(gwye FEN e sin & deks troe meth OR fan)

Brand Names: U.S. Cheracol D [OTC]; Cheracol Plus [OTC]; Coricidin HBP Chest Congestion and Cough [OTC]; Diabetic Siltussin-DM DAS-Na Maximum Strength [OTC]; Diabetic Siltussin-DM DAS-Na [OTC]; Diabetic Tussin DM Maximum Strength [OTC]; Diabetic Tussin DM [OTC]; Double Tussin DM [OTC]; Fenesin DM IR [OTC]; Guaicon DMS [OTC]; Iophen DM-NR [OTC]; Kolephrin GG/DM [OTC]; Mucinex DM Maximum Strength [OTC]; Mucinex DM [OTC]; Mucinex Fast-Max DM Max [OTC]; Mucinex Kid's Cough Mini-Melts [OTC]; Mucinex Kid's Cough [OTC]; Q-Tussin DM [OTC]; Refenesen DM [OTC]; Robafen DM [OTC]; Robitussin Peak Cold Cough + Chest Congestion DM [OTC]; Robitussin Peak Cold Maximum Strength Cough + Chest Congestion DM [OTC]; Robitussin Peak Cold Sugar-Free Cough + Chest Congestion DM [OTC]; Safe Tussin DM [OTC]; Scot-Tussin Senior [OTC]; Silexin [OTC]; Siltussin DM DAS [OTC]; Siltussin DM [OTC]; Vicks 44E [OTC]; Vicks DayQuil Mucus Control DM [OTC]; Vicks Nature Fusion Cough & Chest Congestion [OTC]; Vicks Pediatric Formula 44E [OTC]; Zyncof [OTC]

Brand Names: Canada Balminil DM E; Benylin DM-E

Index Terms Dextromethorphan and Guaifenesin

Pharmacologic Category Antitussive; Cough Preparation; Expectorant

Use Temporary control of cough due to minor throat and bronchial irritation

Dosage Oral:
Children 2-6 years:
General dosing guidelines: Guaifenesin 50-100 mg and dextromethorphan 2.5-5 mg every 4 hours (maximum dose: Guaifenesin 600 mg and dextromethorphan 30 mg per day)
Product-specific labeling: Vicks Pediatric Formula 44E: 7.5 mL every 4 hours (maximum: 6 doses/24 hours)
Children: 6-12 years:
General dosing guidelines: Guaifenesin 100-200 mg and dextromethorphan 5-10 mg every 4 hours (maximum dose: Guaifenesin 1200 mg and dextromethorphan 60 mg per day)
Product-specific labeling:
Vicks 44E: 7.5 mL every 4 hours (maximum: 6 doses/24 hours)
Vicks Pediatric Formula 44E: 15 mL every 4 hours (maximum: 6 doses/24 hours)

Children ≥12 years and Adults:

General dosing guidelines: Guaifenesin 200-400 mg and dextromethorphan 10-20 mg every 4 hours (maximum dose: Guaifenesin 2400 mg and dextromethorphan 120 mg per day)

Product-specific labeling:

Mucinex DM: 1-2 tablets every 12 hours (maximum: 4 tablets/24 hours)

Vicks 44E: 15 mL every 4 hours (maximum: 6 doses/24 hours)

Vicks Pediatric Formula 44E: 30 mL every 4 hours (maximum: 6 doses/24 hours)

Additional Information Complete prescribing information should be consulted for additional detail.

Dosage Forms

Caplet, oral:

Fenesin DM IR [OTC]: Guaifenesin 400 mg and dextromethorphan 15 mg

Refenesen DM [OTC]: Guaifenesin 400 mg and dextromethorphan 20 mg

Capsule, softgel, oral:

Coricidin HBP Chest Congestion and Cough [OTC]: Guaifenesin 200 mg and dextromethorphan 10 mg

Granules, oral:

Mucinex Kid's Cough Mini-Melts: Guaifenesin 100 mg and dextromethorphan 5 mg per packet (12s)

Liquid, oral: Guaifenesin 100 mg and dextromethorphan 10 mg per 5 mL

Diabetic Tussin DM [OTC], Iophen DM-NR [OTC]: Guaifenesin 100 mg and dextromethorphan 10 mg per 5 mL

Iophen DM-NR: Guaifenesin 100 mg and dextromethorphan hydrobromide 10 mg per 5 mL (480 mL)

Diabetic Tussin DM Maximum Strength [OTC]: Guaifenesin 200 mg and dextromethorphan 10 mg per 5 mL

Double Tussin DM [OTC]: Guaifenesin 300 mg and dextromethorphan 20 mg per 5 mL

Kolephrin GG/DM [OTC]: Guaifenesin 150 mg and dextromethorphan 10 mg per 5 mL

Mucinex Fast-Max DM Max [OTC]: Guaifenesin 400 mg and dextromethorphan 20 mg per 20 mL

Mucinex Kid's Cough [OTC]: Guaifenesin 100 mg and dextromethorphan 5 mg per 5 mL

Safe Tussin DM [OTC]: Guaifenesin 100 mg and dextromethorphan 15 mg per 5 mL

Scot-Tussin Senior [OTC]: Guaifenesin 200 mg and dextromethorphan 15 mg per 5 mL

Vicks 44E [OTC]: Guaifenesin 200 mg and dextromethorphan 20 mg per 15 mL

Vicks DayQuil Mucus Control DM [OTC]: Guaifenesin 200 mg and dextromethorphan 10 mg per 15 mL

Vicks Nature Fusion Cough & Chest Congestion [OTC]: Guaifenesin 200 mg and dextromethorphan 20 mg per 30 mL

Vicks Pediatric Formula 44E [OTC]: Guaifenesin 100 mg and dextromethorphan 10 mg per 15 mL

Syrup, oral: Guaifenesin 100 mg and dextromethorphan 10 mg per 5 mL

Cheracol D [OTC], Cheracol Plus [OTC], Diabetic Siltussin-DM DAS-Na [OTC], Diabetic Siltussin-DM DAS-Na Maximum Strength [OTC], Guaicon DMS [OTC], Robafen DM [OTC], Robitussin Peak Cold Cough + Chest Congestion DM [OTC], Robitussin Peak Cold Sugar-Free Cough + Chest Congestion DM [OTC], Silexin [OTC], Siltussin DM [OTC], Siltussin DM DAS [OTC]: Guaifenesin 100 mg and dextromethorphan 10 mg per 5 mL

Q-Tussin DM [OTC]: Guaifenesin 100 mg and dextromethorphan 10 mg per 5 mL

Robitussin Peak Cold Maximum Strength Cough + Chest Congestion DM [OTC]: Guaifenesin 200 mg and dextromethorphan 10 mg per 5 mL

Zyncof [OTC]: Guaifenesin 400 mg and dextromethorphan hydrobromide 20 mg per 5 mL

Tablet, oral: Guaifenesin 1000 mg and dextromethorphan 60 mg; guaifenesin 1200 mg and dextromethorphan 60 mg

Silexin [OTC]: Guaifenesin 100 mg and dextromethorphan 10 mg

Tablet, extended release, oral:

Mucinex DM [OTC]: Guaifenesin 600 mg and dextromethorphan 30 mg

Mucinex DM Maximum Strength [OTC]: Guaifenesin 1200 mg and dextromethorphan 60 mg

Tablet, timed release, oral [scored]: Guaifenesin 1200 mg and dextromethorphan 60 mg

Guaifenesin and Phenylephrine

(gwye FEN e sin & fen il EF rin)

Brand Names: U.S. Ambi 10PEH/400GFN [OTC]; Ed Bron GP [OTC]; Fenesin PE IR; J-Max [OTC]; Liquibid® D-R [OTC]; Liquibid® PD-R [OTC]; Medent®-PEI [OTC]; MucaphEd [OTC]; Mucinex® Cold [OTC]; Mucus Relief Sinus [OTC]; Nu-COPD [OTC]; OneTab™ Congestion & Cold [OTC]; Refenesen™ PE [OTC]; Rescon GG [OTC]; Sudafed PE® Non-Drying Sinus [OTC]; Triaminic® Children's Chest & Nasal Congestion [OTC]

Index Terms Guaifenesin and Phenylephrine Tannate; Phenylephrine Hydrochloride and Guaifenesin

Pharmacologic Category Decongestant; Expectorant

Use Temporary relief of nasal congestion, sinusitis, rhinitis, and hay fever; temporary relief of cough associated with upper respiratory tract conditions, especially when associated with dry, nonproductive cough

Dosage Oral:

Children 2-5 years (Rescon GG): 2.5 mL every 4-6 hours; maximum: 10 mL/24 hours

Children 6-11 years (Rescon GG): 5 mL every 4-6 hours; maximum: 20 mL/24 hours

Children ≥12 years and Adults (Rescon GG): 10 mL every 4-6 hours; maximum: 40 mL/24 hours

Additional Information Complete prescribing information should be consulted for additional detail.

Dosage Forms

Caplet, oral:

Fenesin PE IR, OneTab™ Congestion & Cold [OTC], Refenesen™ PE [OTC]: Guaifenesin 400 mg and phenylephrine 10 mg

Sudafed PE® Non-Drying Sinus [OTC]: Guaifenesin 200 mg and phenylephrine 5 mg

Liquid, oral:

Ed Bron GP [OTC]: Guaifenesin 100 mg and phenylephrine 5 mg per 5 mL (480 mL)

Mucinex® Cold [OTC]: Guaifenesin 100 mg and phenylephrine 2.5 mg per 5 mL (480 mL)

Nu-COPD [OTC]: Guaifenesin 200 mg and phenylephrine 10 mg per 5 mL (480 mL)

Rescon GG [OTC]: Guaifenesin 100 mg and phenylephrine 5 mg per 5 mL (120 mL, 480 mL)

Syrup, oral:

J-Max [OTC]: Guaifenesin 200 mg and phenylephrine hydrochloride 5 mg per 5 mL (473 mL)

Triaminic® Children's Chest & Nasal Congestion [OTC]: Guaifenesin 50 mg and phenylephrine 2.5 mg per 5 mL (118 mL)

Tablet, oral:

Ambi 10PEH/400GFN [OTC], Liquibid® D-R [OTC], Medent®-PEI [OTC], MucaphEd [OTC], Mucus Relief Sinus [OTC], Nu-COPD [OTC]: Guaifenesin 400 mg and phenylephrine 10 mg

Liquibid® PD-R [OTC]: Guaifenesin 200 mg and phenylephrine 5 mg

◆ **Guaifenesin and Phenylephrine Tannate** *see* Guaifenesin and Phenylephrine *on page* 988

Guaifenesin and Pseudoephedrine
(gwye FEN e sin & soo doe e FED rin)

Brand Names: U.S. Ambifed-G [OTC]; Congestac® [OTC]; ExeFen-IR; Maxifed [OTC]; Maxifed-G [OTC] [DSC]; Mucinex® D Maximum Strength [OTC]; Mucinex® D [OTC]; Refenesen Plus [OTC]

Brand Names: Canada Contac® Cold-Chest Congestion, Non Drowsy, Regular Strength; Entex® LA; Novahistex® Expectorant with Decongestant

Index Terms Pseudoephedrine and Guaifenesin

Pharmacologic Category Alpha/Beta Agonist; Expectorant

Use Temporary relief of nasal congestion and to help loosen phlegm and thin bronchial secretions in the treatment of cough

Dosage Oral:

Children 2-6 years (Maxifed-G®): One-third to 1/2 tablet every 12 hours (maximum: 1 tablet/12 hours)

Children 6-12 years:

Ambifed-G, Maxifed®: One-half caplet or tablet every 12 hours (maximum: 1 tablet/24 hours)

Congestac®: One-half caplet every 4-6 hours (maximum: 2 caplets/24 hours)

Maxifed-G®: One-half to 1 tablet every 12 hours (maximum: 2 tablets/24 hours)

Children >12 years and Adults:

Ambifed-G, Mucinex® D Maximum Strength: One tablet every 12 hours (maximum: 2 tablets/24 hours)

Congestac®: One caplet every 4-6 hours (maximum: 4 caplets in 24 hours)

Maxifed-G®, Mucinex® D: 1-2 tablets every 12 hours (maximum: 4 tablets/24 hours)

Maxifed®: One to 1 1/2 tablets every 12 hours (maximum: 3 tablets/24 hours)

Additional Information Complete prescribing information should be consulted for additional detail.

Dosage Forms

Caplet, oral:

Congestac® [OTC], Refenesen Plus [OTC]: Guaifenesin 400 mg and pseudoephedrine 60 mg

Tablet, oral:

Ambifed-G [OTC]: Guaifenesin 400 mg and pseudoephedrine 20 mg

ExeFen-IR: Guaifenesin 400 mg and pseudoephedrine 30 mg

Maxifed [OTC]: Guaifenesin 400 mg and pseudoephedrine 60 mg

Tablet, extended release, oral:

Mucinex® D [OTC]: Guaifenesin 600 mg and pseudoephedrine 60 mg

Mucinex® D Maximum Strength [OTC]: Guaifenesin 1200 mg and pseudoephedrine 120 mg

Guaifenesin, Pseudoephedrine, and Codeine
(gwye FEN e sin, soo doe e FED rin, & KOE deen)

Brand Names: U.S. Cheratussin® DAC; Lortuss EX; Mytussin® DAC; Tricode® GF

Brand Names: Canada Benylin® 3.3 mg-D-E; Calmylin with Codeine

Index Terms Codeine, Guaifenesin, and Pseudoephedrine; Pseudoephedrine, Guaifenesin, and Codeine

Pharmacologic Category Antitussive/Decongestant/Expectorant

Use Temporarily relieves nasal congestion and controls cough associated with upper respiratory infections and related conditions (common cold, sinusitis, bronchitis, influenza)

Pregnancy Risk Factor C

Dosage Oral: **Note:** Products listed in dosage forms may contain differing amounts of active ingredients; however, the dosing volume and frequency are the same.

Children 6-12 years: 5 mL every 4 hours (maximum: 20 mL/24 hours)

Children >12 years and Adults: 10 mL every 4 hours (maximum: 40 mL/24 hours)

Additional Information Complete prescribing information should be consulted for additional detail.

Dosage Forms

Liquid, oral:

Lortuss EX: Guaifenesin 100 mg, pseudoephedrine 30 mg and codeine 10 mg per 5 mL (473 mL)

Tricode® GF: Guaifenesin 200 mg, pseudoephedrine 30 mg, and codeine 8 mg per 5 mL (473 mL)

Syrup, oral: Guaifenesin 100 mg, pseudoephedrine 30 mg, and codeine 10 mg per 5 mL (473 mL)

Cheratussin® DAC: Guaifenesin 100 mg, pseudoephedrine 30 mg and codeine 10 mg per 5 mL (473 mL)

Mytussin® DAC: Guaifenesin 100 mg, pseudoephedrine 30 mg, and codeine 10 mg per 5 mL (118 mL, 473 mL)

Guaifenesin, Pseudoephedrine, and Dextromethorphan
(gwye FEN e sin, soo doe e FED rin, & deks troe meth OR fan)

Brand Names: U.S. Aldex GS DM; AMBI 60PSE/400GFN/20DM; BP 8 Cough [OTC]; Capmist DM [OTC]; Entex PAC [OTC]; Entre-Cough [OTC]; Tusnel Pediatric [OTC]; Tusnel [OTC]; Tusnel-DM Pediatric [OTC]; Z-Cof 1 [OTC] [DSC]; Z-Cof 12 DM [OTC] [DSC]

Brand Names: Canada Balminil DM + Decongestant + Expectorant; Balminil DM + Decongestant + Expectorant Extra Strength; Benylin Cough and Chest Congestion; Benylin Cough Plus Cold Relief; Robitussin Cough & Cold Extra Strength

Index Terms Dextromethorphan, Guaifenesin, and Pseudoephedrine; Pseudoephedrine, Dextromethorphan, and Guaifenesin

Pharmacologic Category Antitussive/Decongestant/Expectorant

Use Cough and upper respiratory tract symptoms: Temporarily relieves nasal congestion and controls cough due to minor throat and bronchial irritation; helps loosen phlegm and thin bronchial secretions to make coughs more productive

Dosage Cough and upper respiratory tract symptoms:

Oral: Note: Dosing may vary by product. Consult specific product labeling.

Drops (dextromethorphan 2.5 mg/guaifenesin 25 mg/pseudoephedrine 7.5 mg per mL):

Children 2 to 5 years: 2 mL every 4 to 6 hours, up to 8 mL per day

Liquid (dextromethorphan 5 mg/guaifenesin 50 mg/pseudoephedrine 15 mg per 5 mL):

Children 2 to 5 years: 5 mL every 4 to 6 hours, up to 20 mL per day

Children 6 to 11 years: 10 mL every 4 to 6 hours, up to 40 mL per day

Liquid (dextromethorphan 15 mg/guaifenesin 175 mg/pseudoephedrine 30 mg per 5 mL):

Children 6 to 11 years: 5 mL every 8 hours, up to 15 mL per day

Children ≥12 years, Adolescents, and Adults: 10 mL every 8 hours, up to 30 mL per day

Liquid (dextromethorphan 15 mg/guaifenesin 200 mg/pseudoephedrine 30 mg per 5 mL):

Children 6 to <12 years: 5 mL every 6 hours, up to 20 mL per day

Children >12 years, Adolescents, and Adults: 10 mL every 6 hours, up to 40 mL per day

Liquid (dextromethorphan 20 mg per 5 mL) and tablets (guaifenesin 375 mg/pseudoephedrine 60 mg):

Children 6 to 11 years:

Liquid: 2.5 mL every 4 hours, up to 10 mL per day

Tablets: One-half tablet every 4 to 6 hours, up to 2 tablets per day

Children ≥12 years, Adolescents, and Adults:

Liquid: 5 mL every 4 hours, up to 20 mL per day

Tablets: One tablet every 4 to 6 hours, up to 4 tablets per day

Suspension (dextromethorphan 15 mg/guaifenesin 211 mg/pseudoephedrine 30 mg per 5 mL):

Children 6 to 11 years: 5 mL every 8 hours, up to 15 mL per day

Children ≥12 years, Adolescents, and Adults: 10 mL every 8 hours, up to 30 mL per day

Tablets (dextromethorphan 15 mg/guaifenesin 190 mg/ pseudoephedrine 30 mg):

Children 6 to 11 years: One tablet every 6 hours, up to 4 tablets per day

Children ≥12 years, Adolescents, and Adults: Two tablets every 6 hours, up to 8 tablets per day

Tablets (dextromethorphan 15 mg/guaifenesin 400 mg/ pseudoephedrine 60 mg):

Children 6 to 11 years: One-half tablet every 4 hours, up to 2 tablets per day

Children ≥12 years, Adolescents, and Adults: One tablet every 4 hours, up to 4 tablets per day

Tablets (dextromethorphan 20 mg/guaifenesin 400 mg/ pseudoephedrine 60 mg):

Children 6 to <12 years: One-half tablet every 4 to 6 hours, up to 2 tablets per day

Children >12 years, Adolescents, and Adults: One tablet every 4 to 6 hours, up to 4 tablets per day

Dosage adjustment in renal impairment: There are no dosage adjustments provided in the manufacturer's labeling.

Dosage adjustment in hepatic impairment: There are no dosage adjustments provided in the manufacturer's labeling.

Additional Information Complete prescribing information should be consulted for additional detail.

Dosage Forms

Combination Package, Oral:

Entex PAC:

Liquid (Entex S): Dextromethorphan hydrobromide 20 mg per 5 mL

Tablet (Entex T): Guaifenesin 375 mg and pseudoephedrine hydrochloride 60 mg

Liquid, Oral:

BP 8 Cough: Guaifenesin 175 mg, pseudoephedrine hydrochloride 30 mg, and dextromethorphan hydrobromide 15 mg per 5 mL

Entre-Cough: Guaifenesin 175 mg, pseudoephedrine hydrochloride 30 mg, and dextromethorphan hydrobromide 15 mg per 5 mL

Tusnel: Guaifenesin 200 mg, pseudoephedrine hydrochloride 30 mg, and dextromethorphan hydrobromide 15 mg per 5 mL

Tusnel-DM Pediatric: Guaifenesin 25 mg, pseudoephedrine hydrochloride 7.5 mg, and dextromethorphan hydrobromide 2.5 mg per 1 mL

Tusnel Pediatric: Guaifenesin 50 mg, pseudoephedrine hydrochloride 15 mg, and dextromethorphan hydrobromide 5 mg per 5 mL

Tablet, Oral:

Aldex GS DM: Guaifenesin 190 mg, pseudoephedrine hydrochloride 30 mg, and dextromethorphan hydrobromide 15 mg

AMBI 60PSE/400GFN/20DM: Guaifenesin 400 mg, pseudoephedrine hydrochloride 60 mg, and dextromethorphan hydrobromide 20 mg

Capmist DM: Guaifenesin 400 mg, pseudoephedrine hydrochloride 60 mg, and dextromethorphan hydrobromide 15 mg

GuanFACINE (GWAHN fa seen)

Brand Names: U.S. Intuniv; Tenex

Brand Names: Canada Intuniv XR

Index Terms Guanfacine Hydrochloride

Pharmacologic Category $Alpha_2$-Adrenergic Agonist; Antihypertensive

Additional Appendix Information

Beers Criteria - Potentially Inappropriate Medications for Geriatrics *on page 2271*

Use

Tablet, immediate release: Management of hypertension

Tablet, extended release: Treatment of attention-deficit/ hyperactivity disorder (ADHD) as monotherapy or adjunctive therapy to stimulants

Pregnancy Risk Factor B

Dosage Oral:

Extended release (Intuniv): Children ≥6 years and Adolescents (U.S. labeling) or Children 6 to 12 years (Canadian labeling): ADHD, monotherapy or adjunct to stimulants: Initial: 1 mg once daily; may adjust by increments no larger than 1 mg/week as tolerated, based on clinical response; maximum dose: 4 mg/day.

Note: Clinical response is associated with doses of 0.05 to 0.08 mg/kg/day. Doses up to 0.12 mg/kg/day may provide additional benefit; however, doses >4 mg/day have not been evaluated.

Dosage adjustment for concomitant CYP3A4 inhibitors/inducers: Extended release:

Strong CYP3A4 inhibitors: If initiating guanfacine while taking a strong CYP3A4 inhibitor, do not exceed a maximum guanfacine dose of 2 mg/day. If continuing guanfacine and adding a strong CYP3A4 inhibitor, decrease guanfacine dose by 50%. If the strong CYP3A4 inhibitor is discontinued, double the guanfacine dose (maximum dose: 4 mg/day).

Strong CYP3A4 inducers: If initiating guanfacine while taking a strong CYP3A4 inducer, may titrate guanfacine up to 8 mg/day; consider faster titration (eg, 2 mg/week). If continuing guanfacine and adding a strong CYP3A4 inducer, consider increasing guanfacine gradually over 1 to 2 weeks to double the original dose. If the strong CYP3A4 inducer is discontinued, decrease guanfacine dose by 50% over 1 to 2 weeks (maximum dose: 4 mg/day).

Conversion from immediate release to extended release: Discontinue the immediate release formulation, and titrate according to extended release recommendations.

Missed doses of extended release: If ≥2 consecutive doses are missed, consider repeating dosage titration based on patient tolerability.

Discontinuation of extended release: Gradually discontinue by tapering dose in decrements of ≤1 mg every 3 to 7 days.

Immediate release:

Children ≥12 years and Adults: Hypertension: 1 mg usually at bedtime, may increase if needed at 3- to 4-week intervals; usual dose range (JNC 7): 0.5-2 mg once daily

Elderly: Hypertension: Consider lower initial doses and titrate to response (Aronow, 2011)

Dosage adjustment in renal impairment:

Extended release (Intuniv): Children ≥6 years and Adolescents (U.S. labeling) or Children 6 to 12 years (Canadian labeling): There are no dosage adjustments provided in the manufacturer's labeling (has not been studied); however, dosage adjustments may be necessary in patients with significant renal impairment.

Immediate release: Children ≥12 years and Adults: There are no specific dosage adjustments provided in the manufacturer's labeling; however, the lower end of the dosing range is recommended in patients with renal impairment.

Hemodialysis: Immediate release or extended release: Dialysis clearance is low (~15% of total clearance).

Dosage adjustment in hepatic impairment:

Extended release (Intuniv): Children ≥6 years and Adolescents (U.S. labeling) or Children 6 to 12 years (Canadian labeling): There are no dosage adjustments provided in the manufacturer's labeling (has not been studied); however, dosage adjustments may be necessary in patients with significant hepatic impairment.

Immediate release: Children ≥12 years and Adults: There are no dosage adjustments provided in the manufacturer's labeling; however, use with caution in chronic hepatic impairment.

Additional Information Complete prescribing information should be consulted for additional detail.

Dosage Forms

Tablet, Oral:

Tenex: 1 mg, 2 mg

Generic: 1 mg, 2 mg

Tablet Extended Release 24 Hour, Oral:

Intuniv: 1 mg, 2 mg, 3 mg, 4 mg

Generic: 1 mg, 2 mg, 3 mg, 4 mg

- ◆ **Guanfacine Hydrochloride** *see* GuanFACINE *on page 990*
- ◆ **GUM Paroex (Can)** *see* Chlorhexidine Gluconate *on page 422*
- ◆ **GW506U78** *see* Nelarabine *on page 1435*
- ◆ **GW-1000-02** *see* Tetrahydrocannabinol and Cannabidiol [CAN/INT] *on page 2018*
- ◆ **GW433908G** *see* Fosamprenavir *on page 928*
- ◆ **GW572016** *see* Lapatinib *on page 1169*
- ◆ **GW786034** *see* PAZOPanib *on page 1584*
- ◆ **Gynazole-1** *see* Butoconazole *on page 314*
- ◆ **Gynazole-1® (Can)** *see* Butoconazole *on page 314*
- ◆ **Gyne-Lotrimin [OTC]** *see* Clotrimazole (Topical) *on page 488*
- ◆ **Gyne-Lotrimin 3 [OTC]** *see* Clotrimazole (Topical) *on page 488*
- ◆ **H1N1 Influenza Vaccine** *see* Influenza Virus Vaccine (Inactivated) *on page 1075*
- ◆ **H1N1 Influenza Vaccine** *see* Influenza Virus Vaccine (Live/Attenuated) *on page 1080*
- ◆ **h5G1.1** *see* Eculizumab *on page 703*
- ◆ **H5N1 Influenza Vaccine** *see* Influenza A Virus Vaccine (H5N1) *on page 1074*
- ◆ **HA** *see* Typhoid and Hepatitis A Vaccine [CAN/INT] *on page 2111*
- ◆ **Habitrol** *see* Nicotine *on page 1449*

Haemophilus b Conjugate and Hepatitis B Vaccine

(he MOF i lus bee KON joo gate & hep a TYE tis bee vak SEEN)

Brand Names: U.S. Comvax

Index Terms *Haemophilus* b (meningococcal protein conjugate) Conjugate Vaccine; Hepatitis B Vaccine (Recombinant); Hib Conjugate Vaccine; Hib-HepB

Pharmacologic Category Vaccine, Inactivated (Bacterial); Vaccine, Inactivated (Viral)

Additional Appendix Information

Immunization Administration Recommendations *on page 2250*

Immunization Recommendations *on page 2255*

Use

Immunization against invasive disease caused by *H. influenzae* type b and against infection caused by all known subtypes of hepatitis B virus in infants 6 weeks to 15 months of age born of hepatitis B surface antigen (HBsAg)-negative mothers

Infants born of HBsAg-positive mothers or mothers of unknown HBsAg status should receive hepatitis B vaccine (recombinant) at birth and should complete the hepatitis B vaccination series given according to a particular schedule (refer to current ACIP recommendations).

Pregnancy Risk Factor C

Dosage Infants: IM: 0.5 mL/dose; one dose at 2, 4, and 12-15 months of age (total of 3 doses)

If the recommended schedule cannot be followed, the interval between the first two doses should be at least 6 weeks and the interval between the second and third dose should be as close as possible to 8-11 months. Minimum age for first dose is 6 weeks.

Modified Schedule: Children who receive one dose of hepatitis B vaccine at or shortly after birth may receive Comvax® on a schedule of 2, 4, and 12-15 months of age

Dosage adjustment in renal impairment: No dosage adjustment provided in manufacturer's labeling.

Dosage adjustment in hepatic impairment: No dosage adjustment provided in manufacturer's labeling.

Additional Information Complete prescribing information should be consulted for additional detail.

Product Availability Production of Comvax has been discontinued by the manufacturer (Merck). As of December 31, 2014, Comvax is no longer available for direct purchase from Merck. Product may still be available from wholesalers and physician distributors. Refer to the following for additional information https://www.merckvaccines.com/is-bin/intershop.static/WFS/Merck-MerckVaccines-Site/Merck-MerckVaccines/en_US/Professional-Resources/Documents/announcements/VACC-1114028-0000.pdf.

Dosage Forms

Injection, suspension [preservative free]:

Comvax®: *Haemophilus* b capsular polysaccharide 7.5 mcg and hepatitis B surface antigen 5 mcg per 0.5 mL (0.5 mL)

◆ ***Haemophilus* B Conjugate (Hib)** *see* Diphtheria and Tetanus Toxoids, Acellular Pertussis, Poliovirus and *Haemophilus* b Conjugate Vaccine *on page 648*

Haemophilus b Conjugate Vaccine

(he MOF fi lus bee KON joo gate vak SEEN)

Brand Names: U.S. ActHIB; Hiberix; PedvaxHIB

Brand Names: Canada ActHIB; PedvaxHIB

Index Terms *Haemophilus influenzae* Type b; Hib; PRP-OMP (PedvaxHIB); PRP-T (ActHIB); PRP-T (Hiberix)

Pharmacologic Category Vaccine, Inactivated (Bacterial)

Additional Appendix Information

Immunization Administration Recommendations *on page 2250*

Immunization Recommendations *on page 2255*

Use

Active immunization for the prevention of invasive disease caused by *Haemophilus influenzae* type b (Hib):

ActHIB: Immunization of infants and children 2 months to 5 years of age.

Hiberix: Booster dose in children 15 months to 4 years of age (prior to fifth birthday).

PedvaxHIB: Routine vaccination of infants and children 2 to 71 months of age.

The Advisory Committee on Immunization Practices (ACIP) recommends vaccination for the following (CDC/ACIP [Akinsanya-Beysolow, 2014]; CDC/ACIP [Bridges, 2014]); CDC/ACIP [Briere, 2014]):

- Routine immunization of all infants and children through age 59 months
- Unimmunized (defined as those who have not received a primary series and booster dose or at least 1 dose of a Hib vaccine after 14 months of age) children 12 to 59 months including chemotherapy recipients, anatomic or functional aspleina (including sickle cell disease), HIV infection, immuneoglobulin deficiency or early component complement deficiency

Efficacy data are not available for use in older children and adults with chronic conditions associated with an increased risk of Hib disease. However, use may be considered for:

- Unimmunized (defined as those who have not received a primary series and booster dose or at least 1 dose of a Hib vaccine after 14 months of age) children ≥5 years, adolescents and adults with functional or anatomic asplenia, (including sickle cell disease)
- Unimmunized (defined as those who have not received a primary series and booster dose or at least 1 dose of a Hib vaccine after 14 months of age) children ≥5 years and adolescents with HIV infection
- Children <5 years undergoing chemotherapy or radiation treatment
- Successful hematopoietic stem cell transplant recipients
- Children ≥15 months and adolescents undergoing elective splenectomy

Pregnancy Risk Factor C

Dosage IM:

Children: 0.5 mL as a single dose should be administered to previously unvaccinated children according to one of the following "brand-specific" schedules; number of doses in series is dependent upon age at first dose. ActHIB and PedvaxHIB are approved for a complete vaccine series; Hiberix is approved only as a booster (final) dose in children who have received primary immunization.

ActHIB: *Age at first dose:*

2 months: Immunization consists of 3 doses (0.5 mL/dose) administered at 2, 4, and 6 months of age. A booster dose is given at 15-18 months.

7-11 months: Two doses (0.5 mL/dose) administered 8 weeks apart, with a booster dose at 15-18 months

12-14 months: One dose (0.5 mL) followed by a booster dose 8 weeks later

15 months to 5 years: One dose (0.5 mL)

PedvaxHIB: *Age at first dose:*

2-10 months: Two doses (0.5 mL/dose) administered 2 months apart; booster dose at 12-15 months

11-14 months: Two doses (0.5 mL/dose) administered 2 months apart

15-71 months: One 0.5 mL dose

Hiberix: 15-59 months: One 0.5 mL booster dose (per manufacturer). The ACIP recommends booster dose administration at 12-15 months (CDC/ACIP [Briere, 2013])

Children, Adolescents, and Adults who are recipients of a successful hematopoietic stem cell transplant: Revaccinate with a 3-dose regimen beginning 6-12 months after the transplant, regardless of vaccination history. Doses should be administered ≥4 weeks apart (CDC/ACIP [Briere, 2013])

Children ≥5 years and Adolescents who have not received the childhood Hib series **and** are at increased risk for invasive Hib disease due to HIV infection, anatomic/functional asplenia or splenectomy, immunoglobulin deficiency, early component complement deficiency, or chemotherapy or radiation therapy. ACIP recommendations: One dose (0.5 mL); may use any of the Hib conjugate vaccines (CDC/ACIP [Briere, 2013])

Adults who have not received the childhood Hib series **and** are at increased risk for invasive Hib disease due to sickle cell disease, anatomic/functional asplenia or splenectomy. ACIP recommendations: One dose (0.5 mL); may use any of the Hib conjugate vaccines (CDC/ACIP [Briere, 2013)

Dosage adjustment in renal impairment: There are no dosage adjustments provided in the manufacturer's labeling.

Dosage adjustment in hepatic impairment: There are no dosage adjustments provided in the manufacturer's labeling.

Additional Information Complete prescribing information should be consulted for additional detail.

Dosage Forms

Injection, powder for reconstitution [preservative free]:

ActHIB: *Haemophilus* b capsular polysaccharide 10 mcg per 0.5 mL

Hiberix: *Haemophilus* b capsular polysaccharide 10 mcg per 0.5 mL

Injection, suspension:

PedvaxHIB: *Haemophilus* b capsular polysaccharide 7.5 mcg

◆ ***Haemophilus* b (meningococcal protein conjugate) Conjugate Vaccine** *see Haemophilus* b Conjugate and Hepatitis B Vaccine *on page 991*

◆ ***Haemophilus* B Polysaccharide** *see* Diphtheria and Tetanus Toxoids, Acellular Pertussis, Poliovirus and *Haemophilus* b Conjugate Vaccine *on page 648*

◆ ***Haemophilus influenzae* Type b** *see Haemophilus* b Conjugate Vaccine *on page 991*

◆ **Hair Regrowth Treatment Men [OTC]** *see* Minoxidil (Topical) *on page 1374*

◆ **Halaven** *see* Eribulin *on page 755*

Halcinonide (hal SIN oh nide)

Brand Names: U.S. Halog

Pharmacologic Category Corticosteroid, Topical

Additional Appendix Information

Topical Corticosteroids *on page 2230*

Use Relief of inflammatory and pruritic effects of corticosteroid-responsive dermatoses [high potency topical corticosteroid]

Pregnancy Risk Factor C

Dosage Children and Adults: Topical: Steroid-responsive dermatoses: Apply sparingly 2-3 times daily, occlusive dressing may be used for severe or resistant dermatoses; a thin film is effective; avoid excessive application. Therapy should be discontinued when control is achieved; if no improvement is seen, reassessment of diagnosis may be necessary.

Additional Information Complete prescribing information should be consulted for additional detail.

Dosage Forms

Cream, External:

Halog: 0.1% (30 g, 60 g, 216 g)

Ointment, External:

Halog: 0.1% (30 g, 60 g)

- **Halcion** *see* Triazolam *on page 2101*
- **Haldol** *see* Haloperidol *on page 993*
- **Haldol Decanoate** *see* Haloperidol *on page 993*
- **Haley's M-O** *see* Magnesium Hydroxide and Mineral Oil *on page 1264*
- **Halfprin [OTC]** *see* Aspirin *on page 180*
- **Halichondrin B Analog** *see* Eribulin *on page 755*

Halobetasol (hal oh BAY ta sol)

Brand Names: U.S. Halonate; Ultravate

Brand Names: Canada Ultravate®

Index Terms Halobetasol Propionate

Pharmacologic Category Corticosteroid, Topical

Additional Appendix Information

Topical Corticosteroids *on page 2230*

Use Relief of inflammatory and pruritic manifestations of corticosteroid-response dermatoses [super high potency topical corticosteroid]

Pregnancy Risk Factor C

Dosage Topical: Children ≥12 years and Adults: Steroid-responsive dermatoses: Apply sparingly to skin once or twice daily, rub in gently and completely; treatment should not exceed 2 consecutive weeks and total dosage should not exceed 50 g/week. Therapy should be discontinued when control is achieved; if no improvement is seen, reassessment of diagnosis may be necessary.

Additional Information Complete prescribing information should be consulted for additional detail.

Dosage Forms

Cream, External:

Ultravate: 0.05% (50 g)

Generic: 0.05% (15 g, 50 g)

Kit, External:

Halonate: 0.05 & 12% (Foam)

Ointment, External:

Ultravate: 0.05% (50 g)

Generic: 0.05% (15 g, 50 g)

- **Halobetasol Propionate** *see* Halobetasol *on page 993*

Halofantrine [INT] (ha loe FAN trin)

International Brand Names Halfan (AE, AT, BE, BF, BH, BJ, CI, CO, CY, DE, EG, ES, ET, FR, GB, GH, GM, GN, IL, IQ, IR, JO, KE, KW, LB, LR, LU, LY, MA, ML, MR, MU, MW, NE, NG, NL, OM, PK, PT, QA, SA, SC, SD, SL, SN, SY, TN, TZ, UG, YE, ZA, ZM, ZW)

Index Terms Halofantrine Hydrochloride

Pharmacologic Category Antimalarial Agent

Reported Use Treatment of mild-to-moderate acute malaria caused by susceptible strains of *Plasmodium falciparum* and *Plasmodium vivax*

Dosage Range Oral:

Children:

<37 kg: 8 mg/kg every 6 hours for 3 doses; repeat in 1 week

≥37 kg: 500 mg every 6 hours for 3 doses; repeat in 1 week

Adults: 500 mg every 6 hours for 3 doses; repeat in 1 week

Product Availability Product available in various countries; not currently available in the U.S.

Dosage Forms

Tablet, as hydrochloride: 250 mg

- **Halofantrine Hydrochloride** *see* Halofantrine [INT] *on page 993*
- **Halog** *see* Halcinonide *on page 992*

Halometasone [INT] (ha loe MET a sone)

International Brand Names Sicorten (AT, BE, CH, CZ, DE, ES, HU, LU, NL)

Pharmacologic Category Corticosteroid, Topical

Reported Use Treatment of steroid responsive skin disorders

Dosage Range Topical: Apply once or twice daily

Product Availability Product available in various countries; not currently available in the U.S.

Dosage Forms

Cream: 0.05% (10 g, 30 g)

Ointment, topical: 0.05% (30 g)

- **Halonate** *see* Halobetasol *on page 993*

Haloperidol (ha loe PER i dole)

Brand Names: U.S. Haldol; Haldol Decanoate

Brand Names: Canada Apo-Haloperidol; Apo-Haloperidol LA; Haloperidol Injection, USP; Haloperidol Long Acting; Haloperidol-LA; Haloperidol-LA Omega; Novo-Peridol; PMS-Haloperidol; PMS-Haloperidol LA

Index Terms Haloperidol Decanoate; Haloperidol Lactate

Pharmacologic Category First Generation (Typical) Antipsychotic

Additional Appendix Information

Beers Criteria - Potentially Inappropriate Medications for Geriatrics *on page 2271*

Use Management of schizophrenia; control of tics and vocal utterances of Tourette's disorder in children and adults; severe behavioral problems in children

Pregnancy Risk Factor C

Pregnancy Considerations Adverse events were observed in animal reproduction studies. Haloperidol crosses the placenta in humans (Newport, 2007). Although haloperidol has not been found to be a major human teratogen, an association with limb malformations following first trimester exposure in humans cannot be ruled out (ACOG, 2008; Diav-Citrin, 2005). Antipsychotic use during the third trimester of pregnancy has a risk for abnormal muscle movements (extrapyramidal symptoms [EPS]) and withdrawal symptoms in newborns following delivery. Symptoms in the newborn may include agitation, feeding disorder, hypertonia, hypotonia, respiratory distress, somnolence, and tremor; these effects may be selflimiting or require hospitalization. If needed, the minimum effective maternal dose should be used in order to decrease the risk of EPS (ACOG, 2008).

Breast-Feeding Considerations Haloperidol is found in breast milk and has been detected in the plasma and urine of nursing infants (Whalley, 1981; Yoshida, 1999). Breast engorgement, gynecomastia, and lactation are known side effects with the use of haloperidol. Breast-feeding is not recommended by the manufacturer.

Contraindications Hypersensitivity to haloperidol or any component of the formulation; Parkinson's disease; severe CNS depression; coma

Warnings/Precautions [U.S. Boxed Warning]: Elderly patients with dementia-related psychosis treated with antipsychotics are at an increased risk of death compared to placebo. Most deaths appeared to be either cardiovascular (eg, heart failure, sudden death) or infectious (eg, pneumonia) in nature. Haloperidol is not approved for the treatment of dementia-related psychosis.

Hypotension may occur, particularly with parenteral administration. Although the short-acting form (lactate) is used clinically, the IV use of the injection is not an FDA-approved route of administration; the decanoate form should never be administered intravenously.

May alter cardiac conduction and prolong QT interval; life-threatening arrhythmias have occurred with therapeutic doses of antipsychotics but risk may be increased with doses exceeding recommendations and/or intravenous administration (off-label route). Use caution or avoid use in patients with electrolyte abnormalities (eg, hypokalemia, hypomagnesemia), hypothyroidism, familial long QT syndrome, concomitant medications which may augment QT prolongation, or any underlying cardiac abnormality which may also potentiate risk. Monitor ECG closely for dose-related QT effects. Adverse effects of decanoate may be prolonged. Avoid in thyrotoxicosis.

Leukopenia, neutropenia, and agranulocytosis (sometimes fatal) have been reported in clinical trials and postmarketing reports with antipsychotic use; presence of risk factors (eg, preexisting low WBC or history of drug-induced leuko-/neutropenia) should prompt periodic blood count assessment. Discontinue therapy at first signs of blood dyscrasias or if absolute neutrophil count <1000/mm^3.

May be sedating, use with caution in disorders where CNS depression is a feature. Effects may be potentiated when used with other sedative drugs or ethanol. Caution in patients with severe cardiovascular disease, predisposition to seizures, subcortical brain damage, or renal disease. Esophageal dysmotility and aspiration have been associated with antipsychotic use - use with caution in patients at risk of pneumonia (eg, Alzheimer's disease). Use associated with increased prolactin levels; clinical significance of hyperprolactinemia in patients with breast cancer or other prolactin-dependent tumors is unknown. May alter temperature regulation or mask toxicity of other drugs due to antiemetic effects. May cause orthostatic hypotension; use with caution in patients at risk of this effect or those who would tolerate transient hypotensive episodes (cerebrovascular disease, cardiovascular disease, or other medications which may predispose). Some tablets contain tartrazine. Antipsychotics have been associated with pigmentary retinopathy.

May cause anticholinergic effects (confusion, agitation, constipation, xerostomia, blurred vision, urinary retention). Therefore, they should be used with caution in patients with decreased gastrointestinal motility, urinary retention, BPH, xerostomia, visual problems, or narrow-angle glaucoma (screening is recommended). Relative to other neuroleptics, haloperidol has a low potency of cholinergic blockade.

May cause extrapyramidal symptoms, including pseudoparkinsonism, acute dystonic reactions, akathisia, and tardive dyskinesia. Risk of dystonia (and possibly other EPS) may be greater with increased doses, use of conventional antipsychotics, males, and younger patients. Risk of tardive dyskinesia and potential for irreversibility may be increased in elderly patients (particularly women), prolonged therapy, and higher total cumulative dose; antipsychotics may also mask signs/symptoms of tardive dyskinesia. May be associated with neuroleptic malignant syndrome (NMS). Use in elderly patients with dementia is associated with an increased risk of mortality and cerebrovascular accidents; avoid antipsychotic use for behavioral problems associated with dementia unless alternative nonpharmacologic therapies have failed and patient may harm self or others. In addition, use may cause or exacerbate syndrome of inappropriate antidiuretic hormone secretion or hyponatremia; monitor sodium closely with initiation or dosage adjustments in older adults (Beers Criteria). Increased risk for developing tardive dyskinesia, particularly elderly women.

Benzyl alcohol and derivatives: Some dosage forms may contain benzyl alcohol; large amounts of benzyl alcohol (≥99 mg/kg/day) have been associated with a potentially fatal toxicity ("gasping syndrome") in neonates; the "gasping syndrome" consists of metabolic acidosis, respiratory distress, gasping respirations, CNS dysfunction (including convulsions, intracranial hemorrhage), hypotension and cardiovascular collapse (AAP, 1997; CDC, 1982); some data suggests that benzoate displaces bilirubin from protein binding sites (Ahlfors, 2001); avoid or use dosage forms containing benzyl alcohol with caution in neonates. See manufacturer's labeling.

Adverse Reactions

Cardiovascular: Abnormal T waves with prolonged ventricular repolarization, arrhythmia, hyper-/hypotension, QT prolongation, sudden death, tachycardia, torsade de pointes

Central nervous system: Agitation, akathisia, altered central temperature regulation, anxiety, confusion, depression, drowsiness, dystonic reactions, euphoria, extrapyramidal reactions, headache, insomnia, lethargy, neuroleptic malignant syndrome (NMS), pseudoparkinsonian signs and symptoms, restlessness, seizure, tardive dyskinesia, tardive dystonia, vertigo

Dermatologic: Alopecia, contact dermatitis, hyperpigmentation, photosensitivity (rare), pruritus, rash

Endocrine & metabolic: Amenorrhea, breast engorgement, galactorrhea, gynecomastia, hyper-/hypoglycemia, hyponatremia, lactation, mastalgia, menstrual irregularities, sexual dysfunction

Gastrointestinal: Anorexia, constipation, diarrhea, dyspepsia, hypersalivation, nausea, vomiting, xerostomia

Genitourinary: Priapism, urinary retention

Hematologic: Agranulocytosis (rare), leukopenia, leukocytosis, neutropenia, anemia, lymphomonocytosis

Hepatic: Cholestatic jaundice, obstructive jaundice

Ocular: Blurred vision

Respiratory: Bronchospasm, laryngospasm

Miscellaneous: Diaphoresis, heat stroke

Drug Interactions

Metabolism/Transport Effects Substrate of CYP1A2 (minor), CYP2D6 (major), CYP3A4 (major); **Note:** Assignment of Major/Minor substrate status based on clinically relevant drug interaction potential; **Inhibits** CYP2D6 (moderate), CYP3A4 (moderate)

Avoid Concomitant Use

Avoid concomitant use of Haloperidol with any of the following: Aclidinium; Amisulpride; Azelastine (Nasal); Bosutinib; Conivaptan; FLUoxetine; Fusidic Acid (Systemic); Glucagon; Highest Risk QTc-Prolonging Agents; Ibrutinib; Idelalisib; Ipratropium (Oral Inhalation); Ivabradine; Lomitapide; Metoclopramide; Mifepristone; Naloxegol; Olaparib; Orphenadrine; Paraldehyde; Pimozide; Potassium Chloride; QuiNIDine; Simeprevir; Sulpiride; Thalidomide; Thioridazine; Tiotropium; Tolvaptan; Trabectedin; Ulipristal; Umeclidinium

Increased Effect/Toxicity

Haloperidol may increase the levels/effects of: AbobotulinumtoxinA; Alcohol (Ethyl); Amisulpride; Analgesics (Opioid); Anticholinergic Agents; ARIPiprazole; Avanafil; Azelastine (Nasal); Bosentan; Bosutinib; Budesonide (Systemic, Oral Inhalation); Buprenorphine; Cannabis; ChlorproMAZINE; CNS Depressants; Colchicine; CYP2D6 Substrates; CYP3A4 Substrates; Dapoxetine; DOXOrubicin (Conventional); Dronabinol; Eplerenone; Everolimus; FentaNYL; Fesoterodine; Glucagon; Highest Risk QTc-Prolonging Agents; Hydrocodone; Ibrutinib; Imatinib; Ivabradine; Ivacaftor; Lomitapide; Lurasidone;

Methotrimeprazine; Methylphenidate; Metoprolol; Metyrosine; Mirabegron; Mirtazapine; Moderate Risk QTc-Prolonging Agents; Naloxegol; Nebivolol; Olaparib; OnabotulinumtoxinA; Orphenadrine; OxyCODONE; Paraldehyde; Pimecrolimus; Pimozide; Potassium Chloride; QuiNIDine; Ranolazine; RimabotulinumtoxinB; Rivaroxaban; Salmeterol; Saxagliptin; Selective Serotonin Reuptake Inhibitors; Serotonin Modulators; Simeprevir; Sulpiride; Suvorexant; Tetrahydrocannabinol; Thalidomide; Thiazide Diuretics; Thioridazine; Tiotropium; Tolvaptan; Topiramate; Trabectedin; Ulipristal; Vilazodone; Zolpidem; Zopiclone

The levels/effects of Haloperidol may be increased by: Abiraterone Acetate; Acetylcholinesterase Inhibitors (Central); Aclidinium; Aprepitant; ARIPiprazole; Brimonidine (Topical); Cannabis; ChlorproMAZINE; Conivaptan; CYP2D6 Inhibitors (Moderate); CYP2D6 Inhibitors (Strong); CYP3A4 Inhibitors (Moderate); CYP3A4 Inhibitors (Strong); Dasatinib; Doxylamine; Dronabinol; Droperidol; FLUoxetine; FluvoxaMINE; Fosaprepitant; Fusidic Acid (Systemic); HydrOXYzine; Idelalisib; Ipratropium (Oral Inhalation); Ivabradine; Kava Kava; Lithium; Luliconazole; Magnesium Sulfate; Methotrimeprazine; Methylphenidate; Metoclopramide; Metyrosine; Mifepristone; Nabilone; Netupitant; Nonsteroidal Anti-Inflammatory Agents; Peginterferon Alfa-2b; Perampanel; Pramlintide; QTc-Prolonging Agents (Indeterminate Risk and Risk Modifying); QuiNIDine; Rufinamide; Serotonin Modulators; Sodium Oxybate; Stiripentol; Tapentadol; Tetrahydrocannabinol; Umeclidinium

Decreased Effect

Haloperidol may decrease the levels/effects of: Acetylcholinesterase Inhibitors; Amphetamines; Anti-Parkinson's Agents (Dopamine Agonist); Codeine; Ifosfamide; Itopride; Quinagolide; Secretin; Tamoxifen; TraMADol; Urea Cycle Disorder Agents

The levels/effects of Haloperidol may be decreased by: Acetylcholinesterase Inhibitors; Anti-Parkinson's Agents (Dopamine Agonist); ARIPiprazole; Bosentan; CarBAMazepine; CYP3A4 Inducers (Moderate); CYP3A4 Inducers (Strong); Dabrafenib; Deferasirox; Glycopyrrolate; Lithium; Mitotane; Peginterferon Alfa-2b; Siltuximab; St Johns Wort; Tocilizumab

Preparation for Administration Haloperidol lactate may be administered IVPB or IV infusion in D_5W solutions. NS solutions should not be used due to reports of decreased stability and incompatibility.

Usual concentration range: 0.5 to 100 mg/50 to 100 mL D_5W.

Storage/Stability Protect oral dosage forms from light. Haloperidol lactate injection should be stored at controlled room temperature; do not freeze or expose to temperatures >40°C. Protect from light; exposure to light may cause discoloration and the development of a grayish-red precipitate over several weeks. Stability of standardized solutions is 38 days at room temperature (24°C).

Mechanism of Action Haloperidol is a butyrophenone antipsychotic which blocks postsynaptic mesolimbic dopaminergic D_1 and D_2 receptors in the brain; depresses the release of hypothalamic and hypophyseal hormones; believed to depress the reticular activating system thus affecting basal metabolism, body temperature, wakefulness, vasomotor tone, and emesis

Pharmacodynamics/Kinetics

Onset of action: Sedation: IM, IV: 30 to 60 minutes
Duration: Decanoate: 2 to 4 weeks
Distribution: V_d: 8 to 18 L/kg
Protein binding: 90%
Metabolism: Hepatic: 50% to 60% glucuronidation (inactive); 23% CYP3A4-mediated reduction to inactive metabolites (some back-oxidation to haloperidol); and 20% to 30% CYP3A4-mediated N-dealkylation, including minor oxidation pathway to toxic pyridinium derivative (Kudo, 1999)
Bioavailability: Oral: 60% to 70%
Half-life elimination: 18 hours; Decanoate: 21 days
Time to peak, serum: Oral: 2 to 6 hours; IM: 20 minutes; Decanoate: 7 days
Excretion: Urine (30%, 1% as unchanged drug); feces (15%)

Dosage

Children: 3 to 12 years (15 to 40 kg): Oral:
Initial: 0.5 mg/day given in 2 to 3 divided doses; increase by 0.5 mg every 5 to 7 days; maximum: 0.15 mg/kg/day
Usual maintenance:
Nonpsychotic disorders, Tourette's disorder: 0.05 to 0.075 mg/kg/day in 2 to 3 divided doses
Psychotic disorders: 0.05 to 0.15 mg/kg/day in 2 to 3 divided doses

Children 6 to 12 years: Sedation/psychotic disorders: IM (as lactate): 1 to 3 mg/dose every 4 to 8 hours to a maximum of 0.15 mg/kg/day; convert to oral therapy as soon as able

Adults:
Psychosis:
Oral: 0.5 to 5 mg 2 to 3 times daily; usual maximum: 30 mg daily
IM (as lactate): 2 to 5 mg every 4 to 8 hours as needed
IM (as decanoate):
Initial: 10 to 20 times the daily oral dose administered at 4-week intervals. The initial dose should not exceed 100 mg regardless of previous antipsychotic requirements. If the initial dose conversion requires >100 mg, administer the dose in 2 injections (maximum of 100 mg for first injection) separated by 3 to 7 days.
Maintenance dose: 10 to 15 times the previous daily oral dose or 50 to 200 mg administered at 4-week intervals (Buchanan, 2009; Hasan, 2013)

Delirium in the intensive care unit, treatment (off-label use, off-label route): **Note:** The optimal dose and regimen of haloperidol for the treatment of severe agitation and/or delirium has not been established. Currently, there are no studies evaluating the role of haloperidol on duration or severity of delirium. Haloperidol has been used for symptomatic treatment (severe agitation) of delirious patients. Current guidelines do not advocate use of haloperidol for the treatment or prevention of delirium due to insufficient evidence (Barr, 2013).

IV: Initial: 0.5 to 10 mg depending on degree of agitation; if inadequate response, may repeat bolus dose (with sequential doubling of initial bolus dose) every 15 to 30 minutes until calm achieved, then administer 25% of the last bolus dose every 6 hours; monitor ECG and QTc interval. After the patient is controlled, haloperidol therapy should be tapered over several days. This strategy is based upon expert opinion; efficacy and safety have not been formally evaluated (Tesar, 1988).

Note: QTc prolongation may occur with cumulative doses ≥35 mg per day and the risk of torsade de pointes is greater if ≥35 mg is received within <6 hours (Sharma, 1998). Continuous infusions have also been used with doses in the range of 0.5 to 2 mg/hour with an optional loading dose of 2.5 mg (Reade, 2009).

Delirium in the intensive care unit (patients at high risk of delirium), prevention (off-label use, off-label route): **Note:** The optimal dose and regimen of haloperidol for prevention of ICU delirium has not been established. Current guidelines do not advocate use of haloperidol for the treatment or prevention of delirium due to insufficient evidence (Barr, 2013). Haloperidol may decrease the incidence of delirium (Van den Boogaard, 2013; Wang, 2012).

IV: 0.5 mg followed by a continuous infusion of 0.1 mg/hour for 12 hours (Wang, 2012) **or** 0.5 to 1 mg every 8 hours (Van den Boogaard, 2013)

Rapid tranquilization of severely-agitated patient (off-label use): Administer every 30 to 60 minutes:

Oral: 5 to 10 mg

IM (as lactate): 5 mg

Average total dose (oral or IM) for tranquilization: 10 to 20 mg

Postoperative nausea and vomiting (PONV) (off-label use): IM, IV: 0.5 to 2 mg (Gan, 2007)

Elderly: Nonpsychotic patient, dementia behavior (off-label use): Initial: Oral: 0.25 to 0.5 mg 1 to 2 times daily; increase dose at 4- to 7-day intervals by 0.25 to 0.5 mg/day; increase dosing intervals (twice daily, 3 times/day, etc) as necessary to control response or side effects

Dosage adjustment in renal impairment:

There are no dosage adjustments provided in the manufacturer's labeling.

Hemodialysis/peritoneal dialysis: Supplemental dose is not necessary

Dosage adjustment in hepatic impairment: There are no dosage adjustments provided in the manufacturer's labeling.

Administration

Injection oil (decanoate): The decanoate injectable formulation should be administered IM only, **do not administer decanoate IV.** A 21-guage needle is recommended. The maximum volume per injection site should not exceed 3 mL. Administer in the gluteal muscle by deep IM injection; Z-track injection techniques are recommended to limit leakage after injections (Baweja, 2012; Gillespie, 2013; McEvoy, 2006).

Injection solution (lactate): The lactate injectable formulation may be administered IM or IV (off-label route). Rate of IV administration not well defined; rates of a maximum of 5 mg/minute (Lerner, 1979) and 0.125 mg/kg (in 10 mL NS) over 1 to 2 minutes (Magliozzi, 1985) have been reported. **Note:** IV administration has been associated with QT prolongation and the manufacturer recommends ECG monitoring for QT prolongation and arrhythmias. Consult individual institutional policies and procedures prior to administration.

Oral solution (lactate): Dilute the oral concentrate with water or juice before administration. Avoid skin contact with oral solution; may cause contact dermatitis.

Monitoring Parameters Mental status; vital signs (as clinically indicated); ECG (as clinically indicated and with off-label intravenous administration); weight, height, BMI, waist circumference (baseline; at every visit for the first 6 months; quarterly with stable antipsychotic dose); CBC (as clinically indicated; monitor frequently during the first few months of therapy in patients with preexisting low WBC or history of drug-induced leukopenia/neutropenia); electrolytes and liver function (annually and as clinically indicated); fasting plasma glucose level/ HbA_{1c} (baseline, then yearly; in patients with diabetes risk factors or if gaining weight repeat 4 months after starting antipsychotic, then yearly); lipid panel (baseline; repeat every 2 years if LDL level is normal; repeat every 6 months if LDL level is >130 mg/dL); changes in menstruation, libido, development of galactorrhea, erectile and ejaculatory function (at each visit for the first 12 weeks after the antipsychotic is initiated or until the dose is stable, then yearly); abnormal involuntary movements or parkinsonian signs (baseline; repeat weekly until dose stabilized for at least 2 weeks after introduction and for 2 weeks after any significant dose increase); tardive dyskinesia (every 6 months; high-risk patients every 3 months); visual changes (inquire yearly); ocular examination (yearly in patients >40 years; every 2 years in younger patients) (ADA, 2004; Lehman, 2004; Marder, 2004).

ICU delirium: Monitor either the Confusion Assessment Method for the ICU (CAM-ICU) or the Intensive Care Delirium Screening Checklist (ICDSC)

Reference Range

Therapeutic: 5 to 20 ng/mL (SI: 10 to 40 nmol/L) (psychotic disorders - less for Tourette's and mania)

Toxic: >42 ng/mL (SI: >84 nmol/L)

Dosage Forms

Concentrate, Oral:

Generic: 2 mg/mL (5 mL, 15 mL, 120 mL)

Solution, Injection:

Haldol: 5 mg/mL (1 mL)

Generic: 5 mg/mL (1 mL, 10 mL)

Solution, Injection [preservative free]:

Generic: 5 mg/mL (1 mL)

Solution, Intramuscular:

Haldol Decanoate: 50 mg/mL (1 mL); 100 mg/mL (1 mL)

Generic: 50 mg/mL (1 mL, 5 mL); 100 mg/mL (1 mL, 5 mL)

Tablet, Oral:

Generic: 0.5 mg, 1 mg, 2 mg, 5 mg, 10 mg, 20 mg

- ◆ **Haloperidol Decanoate** *see* Haloperidol *on page 993*
- ◆ **Haloperidol Injection, USP (Can)** *see* Haloperidol *on page 993*
- ◆ **Haloperidol-LA (Can)** *see* Haloperidol *on page 993*
- ◆ **Haloperidol Lactate** *see* Haloperidol *on page 993*
- ◆ **Haloperidol-LA Omega (Can)** *see* Haloperidol *on page 993*
- ◆ **Haloperidol Long Acting (Can)** *see* Haloperidol *on page 993*
- ◆ **Harkoseride** *see* Lacosamide *on page 1154*
- ◆ **Harvoni** *see* Ledipasvir and Sofosbuvir *on page 1173*
- ◆ **Havrix** *see* Hepatitis A Vaccine *on page 1001*
- ◆ **HAVRIX (Can)** *see* Hepatitis A Vaccine *on page 1001*
- ◆ **Havrix® and Engerix-B®** *see* Hepatitis A and Hepatitis B Recombinant Vaccine *on page 1000*
- ◆ **HBIG** *see* Hepatitis B Immune Globulin (Human) *on page 1002*
- ◆ **hBNP** *see* Nesiritide *on page 1439*
- ◆ **hCG** *see* Chorionic Gonadotropin (Human) *on page 431*
- ◆ **H-Chlor 12 [OTC]** *see* Sodium Hypochlorite Solution *on page 1906*
- ◆ **HCTZ (error-prone abbreviation)** *see* Hydrochlorothiazide *on page 1009*
- ◆ **HDCV** *see* Rabies Vaccine *on page 1764*
- ◆ **HealthyLax [OTC]** *see* Polyethylene Glycol 3350 *on page 1674*
- ◆ **Healthy Mama Move It Along [OTC]** *see* Docusate *on page 661*
- ◆ **Heartburn Relief [OTC]** *see* Famotidine *on page 845*
- ◆ **Heartburn Relief 24 Hour [OTC] [DSC]** *see* Lansoprazole *on page 1166*
- ◆ **Heartburn Relief Max St [OTC]** *see* Famotidine *on page 845*
- ◆ **Heartburn Treatment 24 Hour [OTC]** *see* Lansoprazole *on page 1166*
- ◆ **Heather** *see* Norethindrone *on page 1473*
- ◆ **Hecoria** *see* Tacrolimus (Systemic) *on page 1962*
- ◆ **Hectorol** *see* Doxercalciferol *on page 679*

◆ **Hedgehog Antagonist GDC-0449** *see* Vismodegib *on page 2171*

◆ **Helixate FS** *see* Antihemophilic Factor (Recombinant) *on page 152*

◆ **Hemabate** *see* Carboprost Tromethamine *on page 360*

◆ **Hemangeol** *see* Propranolol *on page 1731*

◆ **Hemocyte [OTC]** *see* Ferrous Fumarate *on page 870*

◆ **Hemofil M** *see* Antihemophilic Factor (Human) *on page 152*

◆ **Hemorrhoidal HC** *see* Hydrocortisone (Topical) *on page 1014*

◆ **Hemril-30 [DSC]** *see* Hydrocortisone (Topical) *on page 1014*

◆ **HepA** *see* Hepatitis A Vaccine *on page 1001*

◆ **HepaGam B** *see* Hepatitis B Immune Globulin (Human) *on page 1002*

◆ **HepA-HepB** *see* Hepatitis A and Hepatitis B Recombinant Vaccine *on page 1000*

Heparin (HEP a rin)

Brand Names: U.S. Hep Flush-10

Brand Names: Canada Heparin Leo; Heparin Lock Flush; Heparin Sodium Injection, USP

Index Terms Heparin Calcium; Heparin Lock Flush; Heparin Sodium; Heparinized Saline

Pharmacologic Category Anticoagulant; Anticoagulant, Heparin

Additional Appendix Information

Reversal of Oral Anticoagulants *on page 2235*

Use Anticoagulation: Prophylaxis and treatment of thromboembolic disorders. As an anticoagulant for extracorporeal and dialysis procedures

Note: Heparin lock flush solution is intended only to maintain patency of IV devices and is **not** to be used for systemic anticoagulant therapy.

Pregnancy Risk Factor C

Pregnancy Considerations Increased resorptions were observed in some animal reproduction studies. Heparin does not cross the placenta. Heparin may be used for the prevention and treatment of thromboembolism in pregnant women; however the use of low molecular weight heparin (LMWH) is preferred. Twice-daily heparin should be discontinued prior to induction of labor or a planned cesarean delivery. In pregnant women with mechanical heart valves, adjusted-dose LMWH or adjusted-dose heparin may be used throughout pregnancy or until week 13 of gestation when therapy can be changed to warfarin. LMWH or heparin should be resumed close to delivery. In women who are at a very high risk for thromboembolism (older generation prosthesis in mitral position or history of thromboembolism), warfarin can be used throughout pregnancy and replaced with LMWH or heparin near term; the use of low-dose aspirin is also recommended. When choosing therapy, fetal outcomes (ie, pregnancy loss, malformations), maternal outcomes (ie, VTE, hemorrhage), burden of therapy, and maternal preference should be considered (Guyatt, 2012).

Some products contain benzyl alcohol as a preservative; their use in pregnant women is contraindicated by some manufacturers; use of a preservative free formulation is recommended.

Breast-Feeding Considerations Heparin is not excreted into breast milk and can be used in breast-feeding women (Guyatt, 2012). Some products contain benzyl alcohol as a preservative; their use in breast-feeding women is contraindicated by some manufacturers due to the association of gasping syndrome in premature infants.

Contraindications Hypersensitivity to heparin or any component of the formulation (unless a life-threatening situation necessitates use and use of an alternative anticoagulant is not possible); severe thrombocytopenia; uncontrolled active bleeding except when due to disseminated intravascular coagulation (DIC); not for use when appropriate blood coagulation tests cannot be obtained at appropriate intervals (applies to full-dose heparin only)

Note: Some products contain benzyl alcohol as a preservative; their use in neonates, infants, or pregnant or nursing mothers is contraindicated by some manufacturers.

Warnings/Precautions Hypersensitivity reactions can occur. Only in life-threatening situations when use of an alternative anticoagulant is not possible should heparin be cautiously used in patients with a documented hypersensitivity reaction. Hemorrhage is the most common complication. Monitor for signs and symptoms of bleeding. Certain patients are at increased risk of bleeding. Risk factors for bleeding include bacterial endocarditis; congenital or acquired bleeding disorders; active ulcerative or angiodysplastic GI diseases; continuous GI tube drainage; severe uncontrolled hypertension; history of hemorrhagic stroke; or use shortly after brain, spinal, or ophthalmology surgery; patient treated concomitantly with platelet inhibitors; conditions associated with increased bleeding tendencies (hemophilia, vascular purpura); recent GI bleeding; thrombocytopenia or platelet defects; severe liver disease; hypertensive or diabetic retinopathy; renal failure; or in patients undergoing invasive procedures including spinal tap or spinal anesthesia. Many concentrations of heparin are available ranging from 1 unit/mL to 20,000 units/mL. Clinicians **must** carefully examine each prefilled syringe or vial prior to use ensuring that the correct concentration is chosen; fatal hemorrhages have occurred related to heparin overdose especially in pediatric patients. A higher incidence of bleeding has been reported in patients >60 years of age, particularly women. They are also more sensitive to the dose. Discontinue heparin if hemorrhage occurs; severe hemorrhage or overdosage may require protamine.

May cause thrombocytopenia; monitor platelet count closely. Patients who develop HIT may be at risk of developing a new thrombus (heparin-induced thrombocytopenia and thrombosis [HITT]). Discontinue therapy and consider alternatives if platelets are <100,000/mm^3 and/or thrombosis develops. HIT or HITT may be delayed and can occur up to several weeks after discontinuation of heparin. Use with extreme caution (for a limited duration) or avoid in patients with history of HIT, especially if administered within 100 days of HIT episode (Dager, 2007; Warkentin, 2001); monitor platelet count closely. Osteoporosis may occur with prolonged use (>6 months) due to a reduction in bone mineral density. Monitor for hyperkalemia; can cause hyperkalemia by suppressing aldosterone production. Patients >60 years of age may require lower doses of heparin.

Benzyl alcohol and derivatives: Some dosage forms may contain benzyl alcohol as a preservative. In neonates, large amounts of benzyl alcohol (≥99 mg/kg/day) have been associated with a potentially fatal toxicity ("gasping syndrome"); the "gasping syndrome" consists of metabolic acidosis, respiratory distress, gasping respirations, CNS dysfunction (including convulsions, intracranial hemorrhage), hypotension, and cardiovascular collapse (AAP, 1997; CDC, 1982); some data suggests that benzoate displaces bilirubin from protein binding sites (Ahlfors, 2001); avoid or use dosage forms containing benzyl alcohol with caution in neonates. See manufacturer's labeling. Use in neonates, infants, or pregnant or nursing mothers is contraindicated by some manufacturers; the use of ▶

preservative-free heparin is, therefore, recommended in these populations. Some preparations contain sulfite which may cause allergic reactions.

Heparin resistance may occur in patients with antithrombin deficiency, increased heparin clearance, elevations in heparin-binding proteins, elevations in factor VIII and/or fibrinogen; frequently encountered in patients with fever, thrombosis, thrombophlebitis, infections with thrombosing tendencies, MI, cancer, and in postsurgical patients; measurement of anticoagulant effects using antifactor Xa levels may be of benefit.

Adverse Reactions Note: Immunologically mediated heparin-induced thrombocytopenia (HIT) occurs in a small percentage of patients and is and is marked by a progressive fall in platelet counts and, in some cases, thromboembolic complications (skin necrosis, pulmonary embolism, gangrene of the extremities, stroke, or MI).

Cardiovascular: Allergic vasospastic reaction (possibly related to thrombosis), chest pain, hemorrhagic shock, shock, thrombosis

Central nervous system: Chills, fever, headache

Dermatologic: Alopecia (delayed, transient), bruising (unexplained), cutaneous necrosis, dysesthesia pedis, erythematous plaques (case reports), eczema, urticaria, purpura

Endocrine & metabolic: Adrenal hemorrhage, hyperkalemia (suppression of aldosterone synthesis), ovarian hemorrhage, rebound hyperlipidemia on discontinuation

Gastrointestinal: Constipation, hematemesis, nausea, tarry stools, vomiting

Genitourinary: Frequent or persistent erection

Hematologic: Bleeding from gums, epistaxis, hemorrhage, ovarian hemorrhage, retroperitoneal hemorrhage, thrombocytopenia (see **"Note"**)

Hepatic: Liver enzymes increased

Local: Irritation, erythema, pain, hematoma, and ulceration have been rarely reported with deep SubQ injections; IM injection (not recommended) is associated with a high incidence of these effects

Neuromuscular & skeletal: Peripheral neuropathy, osteoporosis (chronic therapy effect)

Ocular: Conjunctivitis (allergic reaction), lacrimation

Renal: Hematuria

Respiratory: Asthma, bronchospasm (case reports), hemoptysis, pulmonary hemorrhage, rhinitis

Miscellaneous: Allergic reactions, anaphylactoid reactions, heparin resistance, hypersensitivity (including chills, fever, and urticaria)

Drug Interactions

Metabolism/Transport Effects None known.

Avoid Concomitant Use

Avoid concomitant use of Heparin with any of the following: Apixaban; Corticorelin; Dabigatran Etexilate; Edoxaban; Omacetaxine; Oritavancin; Palifermin; Rivaroxaban; Streptokinase; Telavancin; Urokinase; Vorapaxar

Increased Effect/Toxicity

Heparin may increase the levels/effects of: ACE Inhibitors; Aliskiren; Angiotensin II Receptor Blockers; Anticoagulants; Canagliflozin; Collagenase (Systemic); Corticorelin; Deferasirox; Eplerenone; Ibritumomab; Nintedanib; Obinutuzumab; Omacetaxine; Palifermin; Potassium Salts; Potassium-Sparing Diuretics; Rivaroxaban; Tositumomab and Iodine I 131 Tositumomab

The levels/effects of Heparin may be increased by: 5-ASA Derivatives; Agents with Antiplatelet Properties; Apixaban; Aspirin; Dabigatran Etexilate; Dasatinib; Edoxaban; Herbs (Anticoagulant/Antiplatelet Properties); Ibrutinib; Limaprost; Nonsteroidal Anti-Inflammatory Agents; Omega-3 Fatty Acids; Pentosan Polysulfate Sodium; Pentoxifylline; Prostacyclin Analogues; Salicylates; Streptokinase; Sugammadex; Thrombolytic Agents; Tibolone; Tipranavir; Urokinase; Vitamin E; Vorapaxar

Decreased Effect

The levels/effects of Heparin may be decreased by: Estrogen Derivatives; Nitroglycerin; Oritavancin; Progestins; Telavancin

Storage/Stability Heparin solutions are colorless to slightly yellow. Minor color variations do not affect therapeutic efficacy. Heparin should be stored at controlled room temperature. Protect from freezing and temperatures >40°C.

Stability at room temperature and refrigeration:

Prepared bag: 24-72 hours (specific to solution, concentration, and/or study conditions)

Premixed bag: After seal is broken, 4 days.

Out of overwrap stability: 30 days.

Mechanism of Action Potentiates the action of antithrombin III and thereby inactivates thrombin (as well as activated coagulation factors IX, X, XI, XII, and plasmin) and prevents the conversion of fibrinogen to fibrin; heparin also stimulates release of lipoprotein lipase (lipoprotein lipase hydrolyzes triglycerides to glycerol and free fatty acids)

Pharmacodynamics/Kinetics

Onset of action: Anticoagulation: IV: Immediate; SubQ: ~20-30 minutes

Absorption: Oral, rectal: Erratic at best from these routes of administration; SubQ absorption is also erratic, but considered acceptable for prophylactic use

Metabolism: Hepatic; may be partially metabolized in the reticuloendothelial system

Half-life elimination:

Dose-dependent: IV bolus: 25 units/kg: 30 minutes (Bjornsson, 1982); 100 units/kg: 60 minutes (de Swart, 1982); 400 units/kg: 150 minutes (Olsson, 1963)

Mean: 1.5 hours; Range: 1 to 2 hours; affected by obesity, renal function, malignancy, presence of pulmonary embolism, and infections

Note: At therapeutic doses, elimination occurs rapidly via nonrenal mechanisms. With very high doses, renal elimination may play more of a role; however, dosage adjustment remains unnecessary for patients with renal impairment (Kandrotas, 1992).

Excretion: Urine (small amounts as unchanged drug)

Dosage Note: Many concentrations of heparin are available ranging from 1 unit/mL to 20,000 units/mL. Carefully examine each prefilled syringe or vial prior to use ensuring that the correct concentration is chosen. Heparin lock flush solution is intended only to maintain patency of IV devices and is not to be used for anticoagulant therapy.

Children >1 year:

Prophylaxis for cardiac catheterization (arterial approach): IV: Bolus: 100 units/kg (Freed, 1974; Monagle, 2012)

Systemic heparinization:

Intermittent IV: Initial: 50 to 100 units/kg, then 50 to 100 units/kg every 4 hours (**Note:** Continuous IV infusion is preferred)

IV infusion: Initial loading dose: 75 units/kg given over 10 minutes, then initial maintenance dose: 20 units/kg/hour; adjust dose to maintain aPTT of 60 to 85 seconds (assuming this reflects an antifactor Xa level of 0.35 to 0.7 units/mL); see table on next page.

Pediatric Protocol For Systemic Heparin Adjustment

To be used after initial loading dose and maintenance IV infusion dose (see usual dosage listed above) to maintain aPTT of 60 to 85 seconds (assuming this reflects antifactor Xa level of 0.35 to 0.7 units/mL).

Obtain blood for aPTT 4 hours after heparin loading dose and 4 hours after every infusion rate change.
Obtain daily CBC and aPTT after aPTT is therapeutic.

aPTT (seconds)	Dosage Adjustment	Time to Repeat aPTT
<50	Give 50 units/kg bolus and increase infusion rate by 10%	4 h after rate change
50-59	Increase infusion rate by 10%	4 h after rate change
60-85	Keep rate the same	Next day
86-95	Decrease infusion rate by 10%	4 h after rate change
96-120	Hold infusion for 30 minutes and decrease infusion rate by 10%	4 h after rate change
>120	Hold infusion for 60 minutes and decrease infusion rate by 15%	4 h after rate change

Modified from Andrew M, et al, "Heparin Therapy in Pediatric Patients: A Prospective Cohort Study," *Pediatr Research*, 1994, 35(1):78-83.
Note: The aPTT range of 60 to 85 seconds corresponds to an anti-Xa level of 0.35 to 0.7 units/mL.

Adults:

Thromboprophylaxis (low-dose heparin): SubQ: 5000 units every 8 to 12 hours. **Note:** The American College of Chest Physicians recommends a minimum of 10 to 14 days for patients undergoing total hip arthroplasty, total knee arthroplasty, or hip fracture surgery (Guyatt, 2012).

Intermittent administration (anticoagulation): IV: Initial: 10,000 units, then 50 to 70 units/kg (5000 to 10,000 units) every 4 to 6 hours

Percutaneous coronary intervention (off-label use; Levine, 2011):

No prior anticoagulant therapy:

If no GPIIb/IIIa inhibitor use planned: Initial bolus of 70 to 100 units/kg (target ACT 250 to 300 seconds for HemoTec®, 300 to 350 seconds for Hemochron®)

or

If planning GPIIb/IIIa inhibitor use: Initial bolus of 50 to 70 units/kg (target ACT 200 to 250 seconds regardless of device)

Prior anticoagulant therapy:

If no GPIIb/IIIa inhibitor use planned: Additional heparin as needed (eg, 2000 to 5000 units) (target ACT 250 to 300 seconds for HemoTec®, 300 to 350 seconds for Hemochron®)

or

If planning GPIIb/IIIa inhibitor use: Additional heparin as needed (eg, 2000 to 5000 units) (target ACT 200 to 250 seconds regardless of device)

IV infusion (weight-based dosing per institutional nomogram recommended):

Acute coronary syndromes (off-label use):

STEMI: Adjunct to fibrinolysis (full-dose alteplase, reteplase, or tenecteplase): Initial bolus of 60 units/kg (maximum: 4000 units), then 12 units/kg/hour (maximum: 1000 units/hour) as continuous infusion. Check aPTT every 4 to 6 hours; adjust to target of 1.5 to 2 times the upper limit of control (50 to 70 seconds). Continue for a minimum of 48 hours, and preferably for the duration of hospitalization (up to 8 days) or until revascularization (if performed) (ACCF/AHA [O'Gara, 2013]).

Unstable angina (UA)/non-ST-elevation myocardial infarction (NSTEMI): Initial bolus of 60 units/kg (maximum: 4000 units), followed by an initial infusion of 12 units/kg/hour (maximum: 1000 units/hour). Check aPTT every 4 to 6 hours; adjust to target of 1.5 to 2 times the upper limit of control (50 to 70 seconds). Optimal duration of therapy is unknown; however, most trials continued therapy for 2 to 5 days. Recommended duration is 48 hours or until percutaneous coronary intervention is performed (AHA/ACC [Amsterdam, 2014]).

Treatment of venous thromboembolism: **Note:** Start warfarin on the first or second treatment day and continue heparin until INR is ≥2 for at least 24 hours (usually 5 to 7 days) (Guyatt, 2012).

DVT/PE (off-label dosing): IV: 80 units/kg (or alternatively 5000 units) IV push followed by continuous infusion of 18 units/kg/hour (or alternatively 1000 units/hour) (Guyatt, 2012)

or

DVT/PE (off-label dosing): SubQ: *Unmonitored dosing regimen:* Initial: 333 units/kg then 250 units/kg every 12 hours (Guyatt, 2012; Kearon, 2006)

Interstitial cystitis (bladder pain syndrome) (off-label use): Intravesical: **Note:** Various dosage regimens of heparin (20,000 to 50,000 units) alone or with alkalinized lidocaine (1% to 4%) have been used. When lidocaine and heparin are mixed, there is a risk of precipitation if proper alkalinization does not occur. Lidocaine stability and pH should be determined after the components have been mixed, prior to administration.

Single-dose regimen: Instill the combination of 50,000 units of heparin, lidocaine 200 mg, and sodium bicarbonate 420 mg in 15 mL of sterile water into the bladder via catheter and allow to dwell for 30 minutes before draining (Parsons, 2012).

Once-weekly dosing regimen: Instill the combination of 20,000 units of heparin, lidocaine 4% (5 mL), and sodium bicarbonate 7% (25 mL) into an empty bladder via catheter once weekly for 12 weeks and allow to dwell for 30 minutes before draining (Nomiya, 2013).

Twice-weekly dosing regimen: Instill 25,000 units of heparin (diluted with 5 mL of sterile water) into bladder via catheter twice weekly for 3 months (Kuo, 2001).

Maintenance of line patency (line flushing): When using daily flushes of heparin to maintain patency of single and double lumen central catheters, 10 units/mL is commonly used for younger infants (eg, <10 kg) while 100 units/mL is used for older infants, children, and adults. Capped PVC catheters and peripheral heparin locks require flushing more frequently (eg, every 6 to 8 hours). Volume of heparin flush is usually similar to volume of catheter (or slightly greater). Additional flushes should be given when stagnant blood is observed in catheter, after catheter is used for drug or blood administration, and after blood withdrawal from catheter.

Parenteral nutrition: Addition of heparin (0.5 to 3 unit/mL) to peripheral and central parenteral nutrition has not been shown to decrease catheter-related thrombosis. The final concentration of heparin used for TPN solutions may need to be decreased to 0.5 units/mL in small infants receiving larger amounts of volume in order to avoid approaching therapeutic amounts. Arterial lines are heparinized with a final concentration of 1 unit/mL.

Dosing adjustments in the elderly: Patients >60 years of age may have higher serum levels and clinical response (longer aPTTs) as compared to younger patients receiving similar dosages; lower dosages may be required

Dosage adjustment in renal impairment: No dosage adjustment required; adjust therapeutic heparin according to aPTT or anti-Xa activity.

Dosage adjustment in hepatic impairment: No dosage adjustment required; adjust therapeutic heparin according to aPTT or anti-Xa activity.

Usual Infusion Concentrations: Pediatric Note: Premixed solutions available

IV infusion: 100 units/mL

Usual Infusion Concentrations: Adult Note: Premixed solutions available

IV infusion: 25,000 units in 250 mL (concentration: 100 units/mL) of D_5W, 1/2NS, or NS

Administration

SubQ: Inject in subcutaneous tissue only (not muscle tissue). Injection sites should be rotated (usually left and right portions of the abdomen, above iliac crest).

IM: Do not administer IM due to pain, irritation, and hematoma formation.

Continuous IV infusion: Infuse via infusion pump. If preparing solution, mix thoroughly prior to administration.

Heparin lock: Inject via injection cap using positive pressure flushing technique. Heparin lock flush solution is intended only to maintain patency of IV devices and is **not** to be used for anticoagulant therapy.

Central venous catheters: Must be flushed with heparin solution when newly inserted, daily (at the time of tubing change), after blood withdrawal or transfusion, and after an intermittent infusion through an injectable cap. A volume of at least 10 mL of blood should be removed and discarded from a heparinized line before blood samples are sent for coagulation testing.

Intravesical (off-label use): Various dosage regimens of heparin (20,000 to 50,000 units) alone or with alkalinized lidocaine (1% to 4%) have been instilled into the bladder.

Monitoring Parameters Hemoglobin, hematocrit, signs of bleeding; fecal occult blood test; aPTT (or antifactor Xa activity levels) or ACT depending upon indication

Platelet counts should be routinely monitored (eg, every 2-3 days on days 4-14 of heparin therapy) when the risk of HIT is >1% (eg, receiving therapeutic dose heparin, postoperative antithrombotic prophylaxis), if the patient has received heparin or low molecular weight heparin (eg, enoxaparin) within the past 100 days, if pre-exposure history is uncertain, or if anaphylactoid reaction to heparin occurs. When the risk of HIT is <1% (eg, medical/obstetrical patients receiving heparin flushes), routine platelet count monitoring is not recommended (Guyatt, 2012).

For intermittent IV injections, aPTT is measured 3.5-4 hours after IV injection.

Note: Continuous IV infusion is preferred over IV intermittent injections. For full-dose heparin (ie, nonlow-dose), the dose should be titrated according to aPTT results. For anticoagulation, an aPTT 1.5-2.5 times normal is usually desired. Because of variation among hospitals in the control aPTT values, nomograms should be established at each institution, designed to achieve aPTT values in the target range (eg, for a control aPTT of 30 seconds, the target range [1.5-2.5 times control] would be 45-75 seconds). Measurements should be made prior to heparin therapy, 6 hours (pediatric: 4 hours) after initiation, and 6 hours (pediatric: 4 hours) after any dosage change, and should be used to adjust the heparin infusion until the aPTT exhibits a therapeutic level. When two consecutive aPTT values are therapeutic, subsequent measurements may be made every 24 hours, and if necessary, dose adjustment carried out. In addition, a significant change in the patient's clinical condition (eg, recurrent ischemia, bleeding, hypotension) should prompt an immediate aPTT determination, followed by dose adjustment if necessary. In general, may increase or decrease infusion by 2-4 units/kg/hour dependent upon aPTT.

Heparin infusion dose adjustment: A number of dose-adjustment nomograms have been developed which target an aPTT range of 1.5-2.5 times control (Cruickshank, 1991; Flaker, 1994; Hull, 1992; Raschke, 1993). However, institution-specific and indication-specific nomograms should be consulted for dose adjustment. **Note:** aPTT values vary throughout the day with maximum values occurring during the night (Decousus, 1985).

Reference Range Venous thromboembolism: Heparin: 0.3 to 0.7 unit/mL (children: 0.35 to 0.7 unit/mL) anti-Xa activity (by chromogenic assay) or 0.2 to 0.4 unit/mL (by protamine titration); aPTT: 1.5 to 2.5 times control (usually reflects an aPTT of 60 to 85 seconds) (Garcia, 2012; Monagle, 2012)

When used with thrombolytic therapy in patients with acute MI, a lower therapeutic range corresponding to an aPTT of 1.5 to 2 times control (or approximately an aPTT of 50 to 70 seconds) is recommended (ACCF/AHA [O'Gara, 2013).

Dosage Forms

Solution, Injection:

Generic: 1000 units (500 mL); 2000 units (1000 mL); 25,000 units (250 mL, 500 mL); 1000 units/mL (1 mL, 10 mL, 30 mL); 2500 units/mL (10 mL); 5000 units/mL (1 mL, 10 mL); 10,000 units/mL (1 mL, 4 mL, 5 mL); 20,000 units/mL (1 mL)

Solution, Injection [preservative free]:

Generic: 1000 units/mL (2 mL); 5000 units/0.5 mL (0.5 mL)

Solution, Intravenous:

Hep Flush-10: 10 units/mL (10 mL)

Generic: 10,000 units (250 mL); 12,500 units (250 mL); 20,000 units (500 mL); 25,000 units (250 mL, 500 mL); 1 units/mL (1 mL, 2 mL, 2.5 mL, 3 mL, 5 mL, 10 mL); 2 units/mL (3 mL); 10 units/mL (1 mL, 2 mL, 2.5 mL, 3 mL, 5 mL, 10 mL, 30 mL); 100 units/mL (1 mL, 2 mL, 2.5 mL, 3 mL, 5 mL, 10 mL, 30 mL); 2000 units/mL (5 mL)

Solution, Intravenous [preservative free]:

Generic: 1 units/mL (3 mL); 10 units/mL (1 mL, 3 mL, 5 mL); 100 units/mL (1 mL, 3 mL, 5 mL)

- ◆ **Heparin Calcium** *see* Heparin *on page 997*
- ◆ **Heparinized Saline** *see* Heparin *on page 997*
- ◆ **Heparin Leo (Can)** *see* Heparin *on page 997*
- ◆ **Heparin Lock Flush** *see* Heparin *on page 997*
- ◆ **Heparin Sodium** *see* Heparin *on page 997*
- ◆ **Heparin Sodium Injection, USP (Can)** *see* Heparin *on page 997*

Hepatitis A and Hepatitis B Recombinant Vaccine

(hep a TYE tis aye & hep a TYE tis bee ree KOM be nant vak SEEN)

Brand Names: U.S. Twinrix®

Brand Names: Canada Twinrix®; Twinrix® Junior

Index Terms Engerix-B® and Havrix®; Havrix® and Engerix-B®; HepA-HepB; Hepatitis B and Hepatitis A Vaccine

Pharmacologic Category Vaccine, Inactivated (Viral)

Additional Appendix Information

Immunization Administration Recommendations *on page 2250*

Immunization Recommendations *on page 2255*

Use Active immunization against disease caused by hepatitis A virus and hepatitis B virus (all known subtypes) in populations desiring protection against or at high risk of exposure to these viruses.

Populations include travelers or people living in or relocating to areas of intermediate/high endemicity for **both** HAV and HBV and are at increased risk of HBV infection due to behavioral or occupational factors; patients with chronic liver disease; laboratory workers who handle live HAV and HBV; healthcare workers, police, and other personnel who render first-aid or medical assistance; workers who come in contact with sewage; employees of day care centers and correctional facilities; patients/staff of hemodialysis units; men who have sex with men; patients frequently receiving blood products; military personnel; users of injectable illicit drugs; close household contacts of patients with hepatitis A and hepatitis B infection; residents of drug and alcohol treatment centers

Pregnancy Risk Factor C

Dosage Primary immunization: IM:

U.S. labeling: Adults: Three doses (1 mL each) given on a 0-, 1-, and 6-month schedule

Alternative regimen: Accelerated regimen: Four doses (1 mL each) on day 0, 7, and 21-30, followed by a booster at 12 months

Canadian labeling:

Children ≥1 year and Adolescents (Twinrix Junior): Three doses (0.5 mL each) given on a 0-, 1-, and 6-month schedule

Alternative regimen: Children ≥1 year and Adolescents ≤15 years (Twinrix): One dose (1 mL) given on elected date followed by second dose (1 mL) 6-12 months later

Adults (Twinrix): Three doses (1 mL each) given on a 0-, 1-, and 6-month schedule

Alternative regimen: Accelerated regimen: Four doses (1 mL each) on day 0, 7, and 21, followed by a booster at 12 months

Dosage adjustment in renal impairment: No dosage adjustment provided in manufacturer's labeling.

Dosage adjustment in hepatic impairment: No dosage adjustment provided in manufacturer's labeling.

Additional Information Complete prescribing information should be consulted for additional detail.

Dosage Forms

Injection, suspension [preservative free]:

Twinrix®: Hepatitis A virus antigen 720 ELISA units and hepatitis B surface antigen 20 mcg per mL (1 mL)

Dosage Forms: Canada

Injection, suspension [preservative free]:

Twinrix® Junior: Hepatitis A virus antigen 360 ELISA units and hepatitis B surface antigen 10 mcg per 0.5 mL (0.5 mL)

◆ **Hepatitis A and Typhoid Vaccine** *see* Typhoid and Hepatitis A Vaccine [CAN/INT] *on page 2111*

Hepatitis A Vaccine (hep a TYE tis aye vak SEEN)

Brand Names: U.S. Havrix; VAQTA

Brand Names: Canada Avaxim; Avaxim-Pediatric; HAVRIX; VAQTA

Index Terms HepA

Pharmacologic Category Vaccine, Inactivated (Viral)

Additional Appendix Information

Immunization Administration Recommendations *on page 2250*

Immunization Recommendations *on page 2255*

Use Hepatitis A virus vaccination:

For active immunization of persons 12 months and older against disease caused by hepatitis A virus (HAV).

The Advisory Committee on Immunization Practices (ACIP) recommends routine vaccination for:

- All children ≥12 months of age (CDC/ACIP [Fiore, 2006])
- All unvaccinated adults requesting protection from HAV infection (CDC/ACIP [Fiore, 2006])
- Unvaccinated persons with any of the following conditions: Men who have sex with men; injection and noninjection illicit drug users; persons who work with HAV-infected primates or with HAV in a research laboratory setting; persons with chronic liver disease; patients who receive clotting-factor concentrates; persons traveling to or working in countries with high or intermediate levels of endemic HAV infection (CDC/ACIP [Fiore, 2006])
- Unvaccinated persons who anticipate close personal contact with international adoptee from a country of intermediate to high endemicity of HAV, during their first 60 days of arrival into the United States (eg, household contacts, babysitters) (CDC 58[36], 2009)
- Vaccination can be a component of hepatitis A outbreak response or as postexposure prophylaxis, as determined by local public health authorities (CDC 56[41], 2007; CDC/ACIP [Fiore, 2006])

Pregnancy Risk Factor C

Dosage IM: **Note:** When used for primary immunization, the vaccine should be given at least 2 weeks prior to expected HAV exposure. When used prior to an international adoption, the vaccination series should begin when adoption is being planned, but ideally ≥2 weeks prior to expected arrival of adoptee (CDC, 58[36], 2009). When used for postexposure prophylaxis, the vaccine should be given as soon as possible (CDC, 56[41], 2007).

Primary immunization: Advisory Committee on Immunization Practices (ACIP): Children ≥12 months: All children should receive primary immunization with a two-dose series. The series should be initiated at 12 to 23 months; the two doses should be separated by 6-18 months (CDC/ACIP [Fiore, 2006]).

Manufacturer's labeling:

Avaxim [Canadian product]: Children ≥12 years, Adolescents, and Adults: 160 units (0.5 mL) with a booster dose of 160 units (0.5 mL) to be given 6-36 months following primary immunization

Avaxim-Pediatric [Canadian product]: Children ≥12 months and Adolescents ≤15 years: 80 units (0.5 mL) with a booster dose of 80 units (0.5 mL) to be given 6 to 12 months following primary immunization

Havrix:

Children ≥12 months and Adolescents: 720 ELISA units (0.5 mL) with a booster dose of 720 ELISA units (0.5 mL) to be given 6 t 12 months following primary immunization

Adults: 1440 ELISA units (1 mL) with a booster dose of 1440 ELISA units (1 mL) to be given 6 to 12 months following primary immunization

VAQTA:

Children ≥12 months and Adolescents: 25 units (0.5 mL) with a booster dose of 25 units (0.5 mL) to be given 6 to 18 months after primary immunization (6-12 months if initial dose was with Havrix).

Adults: 50 units (1 mL) with a booster dose of 50 units (1 mL) to be given 6 to 18 months after primary immunization (6 to 12 months if initial dose was with Havrix). **Note:** Canadian labeling recommends that adults with HIV receive a booster dose 6 months after primary immunization.

Postexposure prophylaxis: Children, Adolescents, and Adults without immunity: IM: 0.5 mL once as soon as possible following recent exposure to hepatitis A virus (during last 2 weeks) (CDC 56[41], 2007).

Dosage adjustment in renal impairment: There are no dosage adjustments provided in the manufacturer's labeling.

Dosage adjustment in hepatic impairment: There are no specific recommendations provided in manufacturer's labeling. However, data suggest patients with chronic liver disease have a lower antibody response to HAVRIX than healthy subjects.

Additional Information Complete prescribing information should be consulted for additional detail.

Dosage Forms

Injection, suspension [preservative free]:

Havrix: Hepatitis A virus antigen 720 ELISA units/0.5 mL (0.5 mL); Hepatitis A virus antigen 1440 ELISA units/mL (1 mL)

VAQTA: Hepatitis A virus antigen 25 units/0.5 mL (0.5 mL); Hepatitis A virus antigen 50 units/mL (1 mL)

Dosage Forms: Canada Also refer to Dosage Forms.

Injection, suspension [pediatric/adolescent]:

Avaxim-Pediatric: Hepatitis A virus antigen 80 units/0.5 mL [contains aluminum, polysorbate 80, neomycin (may have trace amounts)]

Injection, suspension [adolescent/adult]:

Avaxim: Hepatitis A virus antigen 160 units/0.5 mL [contains aluminum, polysorbate 80, neomycin (may have trace amounts)]

◆ **Hepatitis B and Hepatitis A Vaccine** *see* Hepatitis A and Hepatitis B Recombinant Vaccine *on page 1000*

Hepatitis B Immune Globulin (Human)

(hep a TYE tis bee i MYUN GLOB yoo lin YU man)

Brand Names: U.S. HepaGam B; HyperHEP B S/D; Nabi-HB

Brand Names: Canada HepaGam B; HyperHEP B S/D

Index Terms HBIG

Pharmacologic Category Blood Product Derivative; Immune Globulin

Additional Appendix Information

Immunization Recommendations *on page 2255*

Use

Passive prophylactic immunity to hepatitis B following: Acute exposure to blood containing hepatitis B surface antigen (HBsAg); perinatal exposure of infants born to HBsAg-positive mothers; sexual exposure to HBsAg-positive persons; household exposure to persons with acute HBV infection

Prevention of hepatitis B virus recurrence after liver transplantation in HBsAg-positive transplant patients

Note: Hepatitis B immune globulin is not indicated for treatment of active hepatitis B infection and is ineffective in the treatment of chronic active hepatitis B infection.

Pregnancy Risk Factor C

Dosage

IM:

Infants born to HBsAg-positive mothers: 0.5 mL as soon after birth as possible (within 12 hours); active vaccination with hepatitis B vaccine may begin at the same time in a different site (if not contraindicated). If first dose of hepatitis B vaccine is delayed for as long as 3 months, dose may be repeated. If hepatitis B vaccine is refused, dose may be repeated at 3 and 6 months.

Infants born to mothers with unknown HBsAg status at birth (CDC, 2005):

Birth weight <2 kg: 0.5 mL within 12 hours of birth (along with hepatitis B vaccine) if unable to determine maternal HBsAg status within that time

Birth weight ≥2 kg: If the mother is determined to be HBsAg positive, administer 0.5 mL as soon as possible, but within 7 days of birth

Infants <12 months: Household exposure prophylaxis: 0.5 mL (to be administered if mother or primary caregiver has acute HBV infection)

Children ≥12 months and Adults: Postexposure prophylaxis: 0.06 mL/kg as soon as possible after exposure (ie, within 24 hours of needlestick, ocular, or mucosal exposure or within 14 days of sexual exposure); repeat at 28-30 days after exposure in nonresponders to hepatitis B vaccine or in patients who refuse vaccination

Adults: Postexposure management of health care personnel (HCP) (CDC 62 [10], 2013): 0.06 mL/kg

If the HCP has prior documentation of ≥3 doses of a hepatitis B vaccine and a postvaccination anti-HBs ≥10 mIU/mL, then HBIG is not needed, regardless of the patients HBsAg status.

If the HCP is unvaccinated or incompletely vaccinated, and if the source patient is HBsAG positive or their status is unknown, one dose HBIG should be administered. If the source patient is HBsAG negative, then HBIG is not needed.

If the HCP is vaccinated with 3 doses of hepatitis B vaccine but postvaccination anti-HBs status is unknown, test HCP for anti-HBs. If anti-HBs ≥10 mIU/mL then HBIG is not needed. If anti-HBs <10 mIU/mL, and if the source patient is HBsAG positive or their status is unknown, 1 dose of HBIG should be administered. If anti-HBs <10 mIU/mL, and if the source patient is HBsAG negative, then HBIG is not needed.

If the HCP is vaccinated with 6 doses of hepatitis B vaccine but documented as a nonresponder to the vaccine, and if the source patient is HBsAG negative, then HBIG is not needed. If the source patient is HBsAG positive or unknown, administer 2 doses of HBIG separated by 1 month.

IV: Adults: Prevention of hepatitis B virus recurrence after liver transplantation (HepaGam B): 20,000 units/dose according to the following schedule:

Anhepatic phase (Initial dose): One dose given with the liver transplant

Week 1 postop: One dose daily for 7 days (days 1-7)

Weeks 2-12 postop: One dose every 2 weeks starting day 14

Month 4 onward: One dose monthly starting on month 4

Dose adjustment: Adjust dose to reach anti-HBs levels of 500 units/L within the first week after transplantation. In patients with surgical bleeding, abdominal fluid drainage >500 mL or those undergoing plasmapheresis, administer 10,000 units/dose every 6 hours until target anti-HBs levels are reached.

Dosage adjustment in renal impairment: No dosage adjustment provided in manufacturer's labeling.

Dosage adjustment in hepatic impairment: No dosage adjustment provided in manufacturer's labeling.

Additional Information Complete prescribing information should be consulted for additional detail.

Dosage Forms

Solution, Injection [preservative free]:

HepaGam B: (1 mL, 5 mL)

Solution, Intramuscular:

HyperHEP B S/D: (0.5 mL, 1 mL, 5 mL)

Nabi-HB: (1 mL, 5 mL)

◆ **Hepatitis B Inactivated Virus Vaccine (recombinant DNA)** *see* Hepatitis B Vaccine (Recombinant) *on page 1002*

Hepatitis B Vaccine (Recombinant)

(hep a TYE tis bee vak SEEN ree KOM be nant)

Brand Names: U.S. Engerix-B; Recombivax HB

Brand Names: Canada Engerix-B; Recombivax HB

Index Terms Hepatitis B Inactivated Virus Vaccine (recombinant DNA); HepB

Pharmacologic Category Vaccine, Inactivated (Viral)

Additional Appendix Information

Immunization Administration Recommendations *on page 2250*

Immunization Recommendations *on page 2255*

Use Immunization against infection caused by all known subtypes of hepatitis B virus (HBV)

The Advisory Committee on Immunization Practices (ACIP) recommends routine vaccination for the following:
- All infants at birth (CDC/ACIP [Mast, 2005])
- All infants and children not previously vaccinated (CDC/ACIP [Mast, 2005]) (post-birth dose; refer to recommended vaccination schedule)
- All unvaccinated adults requesting protection from HBV infection (CDC/ACIP [Mast, 2006])
- All unvaccinated adults at risk for HBV infection such as those with:

Behavioral risks: Sexually-active persons with >1 partner in a 6-month period; persons seeking evaluation or treatment for a sexually-transmitted disease; men who have sex with men; injection drug users (CDC/ACIP [Mast, 2006])

Occupational risks: Healthcare personnel (HCP) and public safety workers with reasonably anticipated risk for exposure to blood or blood contaminated body fluids (CDC/ACIP [Mast, 2006])

Medical risks: Persons with end-stage renal disease (including predialysis, hemodialysis, peritoneal dialysis, and home dialysis); persons with HIV infection; persons with chronic liver disease (CDC/ACIP [Mast, 2006]). Adults (19 through 59 years of age) with diabetes mellitus type 1 or type 2 should be vaccinated as soon as possible following diagnosis. Adults ≥60 years with diabetes mellitus may also be vaccinated at the discretion of their treating clinician (CDC/ACIP 60[50], 2011).

Other risks: Household contacts and sex partners of persons with chronic HBV infection; residents and staff of facilities for developmentally disabled persons; international travelers to regions with high or intermediate levels of endemic HBV infection (CDC/ACIP [Mast, 2006])

In addition, the ACIP recommends vaccination for any persons who are wounded in bombings or similar mass casualty events who have penetrating injuries or nonintact skin exposure, or who have contact with mucous membranes (exception - superficial contact with intact skin), and who cannot confirm receipt of a hepatitis B vaccination (CDC [Chapman, 2008]).

Pregnancy Risk Factor C

Dosage IM:

Primary immunization:

Infants: 0.5 mL/dose (pediatric/adolescent formulation) for 3 total doses administered at 0, 1, and 6 months. Alternate dosing regimens are also available for children who begin vaccination ≥1 year of age.

Note: Doses are presented using the pediatric/adolescent formulations. Pediatric/adolescent formulations of hepatitis B vaccine products differ by concentration (mcg/mL). However, when dosed in terms of volume (mL), the dose of Engerix-B and Recombivax HB are the same (both 0.5 mL).

Note: Combination vaccines (eg, vaccines containing HepB with DTaP, HIB) should not be used for the "birth" dose but may be used to complete the course beginning after the infant is ≥6 weeks of age (CDC/ACIP [Mast, 2005]). Please see combination vaccine monographs for dose and schedule details.

Infants (HBsAg-**negative** mothers):

First dose: 0.5 mL at birth or before discharge (may be delayed in certain cases)

Second dose: 0.5 mL at 1 to 2 months of age

Third dose: 0.5 mL at 6 to 18 months of age, but no sooner than 24 weeks of age

Note: Premature neonates <2 kg may have the initial dose deferred up to 30 days of chronological age or at hospital discharge (CDC/ACIP [Mast, 2005]).

Infants (HBsAg-**positive** mothers):

First dose: 0.5 mL within first 12 hours of life, even if premature and regardless of birth weight (hepatitis immune globulin should also be administered at the same time at a different site)

Second dose: 0.5 mL at 1 to 2 months of age

Third dose: 0.5 mL at 6 months of age but no sooner than 24 weeks of age

Note: Anti-HBs and HBsAg levels should be checked at 9 to 18 months of age (ie, next well-child visit after series completion). If HBsAg negative and anti-HBs levels <10 mIU/mL, reimmunize with 3 doses and reassess 1 to 2 months after the third dose.

Note: In premature neonates <2 kg, the birth dose should not be counted as part of the 3-dose vaccine series (CDC/ACIP [Mast, 2005]).

Infants (mother's HBsAg status **unknown**):

First dose: 0.5 mL within 12 hours of birth even if premature and regardless of birth weight

Second dose: 0.5 mL at 1 to 2 months of age

Third dose: 0.5 mL at 6 months of age but no sooner than 24 weeks of age

Note: If mother is later determined to be HBsAg-positive, the infant should receive hepatitis immune globulin as soon as possible (no later than age 1 week).

Note: In premature neonates <2 kg, the birth dose should not be counted as part of the 3-dose vaccine series (CDC/ACIP [Mast, 2005]).

Children: 0.5 mL/dose (pediatric/adolescent formulation) administered at 0, 1, and 6 months (for 3 total doses). Alternate dosing regimens are also available for children who begin vaccination ≥1 year of age.

Alternate dosing schedules (selection of schedule should optimize compliance with vaccination):

Children 1 to 10 years: 0.5 mL (pediatric/adolescent formulation) at the following intervals (two schedules presented):

0, 2, and 4 months (CDC/ACIP [Mast, 2005])

0, 1, 2, and 12 months (Engerix-B)

Children 5 to 10 years: 0.5 mL (pediatric/adolescent formulation) at 0, 12, and 24 months (Engerix-B)

Children 11 to 15 years: 1 mL (adult formulation) at 0 and 4 to 6 months (Recombivax HB)

Children 11 to 16 years: 0.5 mL (pediatric/adolescent formulation) at 0, 12, and 24 months (Engerix-B)

Children 11 to 18 years: 0.5 mL (pediatric/adolescent formulation) at the following intervals (three schedules presented):

0, 1, and 4 months (CDC/ACIP [Mast, 2005])

0, 2, and 4 months (CDC/ACIP [Mast, 2005])

0, 12, and 24 months (CDC/ACIP [Mast, 2005])

Children 11 to 18 years: 1 mL (adult formulation) at 0, 1, 2, and 12 months (Engerix-B)

Adults: 1 mL/dose (adult formulation) for 3 total doses administered at 0, 1, and 6 months

Note: Adult formulations of hepatitis B vaccine products differ by concentration (mcg/mL) but when dosed in terms of volume (mL), the dose of Engerix-B and Recombivax HB are the same (both 1 mL).

Alternate dosing schedules (selection of schedule should optimize compliance with vaccination): All regimens use the adult formulation administered as one dose at the following intervals (three schedules presented):

0, 1, and 4 months (CDC/ACIP [Mast, 2006)

0, 2, and 4 months (CDC/ACIP [Mast, 2006)

0, 1, 2, and 12 months (Engerix-B) (CDC/ACIP [Mast, 2006])

Bombings or similar mass casualty events: In persons without a reliable history of vaccination against HepB and who have no known contraindications to the vaccine, vaccination should begin within 24 hours (but no later than 7 days) following the event (CDC [Chapman, 2008]).

Postexposure management of health care personnel (HCP) (CDC [Schillie, 2013]): IM:

Documented vaccine responder: If the HCP has prior documentation of ≥3 doses of a hepatitis B vaccine and a postvaccination anti-HBs ≥10 mIU/mL, then additional hepatitis B vaccine is not needed, regardless of the patients HBsAg status. HCP is considered seroprotected.

Unvaccinated or incompletely vaccinated: The primary vaccination series should be completed regardless of the source patients HBsAg status. If the source patient is HBsAg positive or their status is unknown, 1 dose of hepatitis B vaccine and 1 dose of hepatitis B immunoglobulin (HBIG) should be administered as soon as possible.

Vaccinated with 3 doses of hepatitis B vaccine but postvaccination anti-HBs status is unknown: Test HCP for anti-HBs. If anti-HBs ≥10 mIU/mL additional hepatitis B vaccine is not needed. If anti-HBs <10 mIU/mL, initiate revaccination by administering a single dose of the vaccine and retesting for anti-HBs in 1 to 2 months; if needed 2 additional doses may be given and then retest anti-HBs level. Alternately, administer 3 consecutive doses of the vaccine and then retest anti-HBs level. Minimum dosing intervals are 4 weeks between doses 1 and 2, and 8 weeks between doses 2 and 3; maximum total 6 doses of hepatitis B vaccine (including the original series). If the source patient is HBsAg positive or their status is unknown, 1 dose of HBIG should also be administered.

Vaccinated with 6 doses of hepatitis B vaccine but documented as a nonresponder to the vaccine: No postexposure vaccination is recommended. If the source patient is HBsAg positive or unknown, administer two doses of HBIG separated by 1 month.

Dosage adjustment for renal impairment: Adults on dialysis:

Engerix-B 20 mcg/mL: Administer 2 mL per dose at 0, 1, 2, and 6 months

Recombivax HB 40 mcg/mL: Administer 1 mL per dose at 0, 1, and 6 months

Note: Serologic testing is recommended 1 to 2 months after the final dose of the primary vaccine series and annually to determine the need for booster doses. Persons with anti-HBs concentrations of <10 mIU/mL should be revaccinated with 3 doses of the vaccine (CDC/ACIP [Mast, 2006]).

Dosage adjustment in hepatic impairment: There are no dosage adjustments provided in the manufacturer's labeling.

Additional Information Complete prescribing information should be consulted for additional detail.

Dosage Forms

Injection, suspension [preservative free]:

Engerix-B: Hepatitis B surface antigen 10 mcg/0.5 mL (0.5 mL); Hepatitis B surface antigen 20 mcg/mL (1 mL)

Recombivax HB: Hepatitis B surface antigen 5 mcg/0.5 mL (0.5 mL); Hepatitis B surface antigen 10 mcg/mL (1 mL); Hepatitis B surface antigen 40 mcg/mL (1 mL)

◆ **Hepatitis B Vaccine (Recombinant)** *see Haemophilus* b Conjugate and Hepatitis B Vaccine *on page 991*

◆ **HepB** *see* Hepatitis B Vaccine (Recombinant) *on page 1002*

◆ **Hep Flush-10** *see* Heparin *on page 997*

◆ **Hepsera** *see* Adefovir *on page 54*

◆ **Heptaplatin** *see* Eptaplatin [INT] *on page 751*

◆ **Heptovir (Can)** *see* LamiVUDine *on page 1157*

◆ **Herceptin** *see* Trastuzumab *on page 2085*

◆ **Herpes Zoster Vaccine** *see* Zoster Vaccine *on page 2218*

◆ **HES** *see* Hetastarch *on page 1004*

◆ **HES** *see* Tetrastarch *on page 2019*

◆ **HES 130/0.4** *see* Tetrastarch *on page 2019*

◆ **HES 450/0.7** *see* Hetastarch *on page 1004*

◆ **Hespan** *see* Hetastarch *on page 1004*

Hetastarch (HET a starch)

Brand Names: U.S. Hespan; Hextend

Brand Names: Canada Hextend

Index Terms HES; HES 450/0.7; Hydroxyethyl Starch

Pharmacologic Category Plasma Volume Expander, Colloid

Use

Granulocyte yield increase (Hespan): Used as an adjunct in leukapheresis to improve harvesting and increase the yield of granulocytes by centrifugation

Hypovolemia: Blood volume expander used in treatment of hypovolemia

Pregnancy Risk Factor C

Dosage

Plasma volume expansion: Adults: IV: 500-1000 mL (up to 1500 mL daily) or 20 mL/kg/day (up to 1500 mL daily). **Note:** With severe dehydration, administer crystalloid first. Daily dose and rate of infusion dependent on amount of blood lost, on maintenance or restoration of hemodynamics, and on amount of hemodilution. Titrate to individual colloid needs, hemodynamics, and hydration status. Do not use in the critically ill, those undergoing open heart surgery and cardiopulmonary bypass, or those with preexisting renal dysfunction.

Leukapheresis (Hespan): Adults: 250-700 mL; **Note:** Citrate anticoagulant is added before use and then mixture is administered to the input line of the centrifuge apparatus.

Dosage adjustment in renal impairment: Avoid use in patients with preexisting renal dysfunction. Use is contraindicated in renal failure with oliguria or anuria (not related to hypovolemia). Discontinue use at the first sign of renal injury.

Dosage adjustment in hepatic impairment: No dosage adjustment provided in manufacturer's labeling; use with caution.

Additional Information Complete prescribing information should be consulted for additional detail.

Dosage Forms

Solution, Intravenous:

Hespan: 6% (500 mL)

Hextend: 6% (500 mL)

Generic: 6% (500 mL)

◆ **Hetlioz** *see* Tasimelteon *on page 1979*

◆ **Hexachlorocyclohexane** *see* Lindane *on page 1217*

◆ **Hexamethylenetetramine** *see* Methenamine *on page 1317*

◆ **Hextend** *see* Hetastarch *on page 1004*

◆ **hFSH** *see* Urofollitropin *on page 2116*

◆ **hGH** *see* Somatropin *on page 1918*

◆ **HHT** *see* Omacetaxine *on page 1501*

◆ **Hib** *see Haemophilus* b Conjugate Vaccine *on page 991*

◆ **Hib Conjugate Vaccine** *see Haemophilus* b Conjugate and Hepatitis B Vaccine *on page 991*

- **Hiberix** *see Haemophilus* b Conjugate Vaccine *on page 991*
- **Hib-HepB** *see Haemophilus* b Conjugate and Hepatitis B Vaccine *on page 991*
- **Hibiclens [OTC]** *see* Chlorhexidine Gluconate *on page 422*
- **Hibistat [OTC]** *see* Chlorhexidine Gluconate *on page 422*
- **Hib-MenCY-TT** *see* Meningococcal Polysaccharide (Groups C and Y) and *Haemophilus* b Tetanus Toxoid Conjugate Vaccine *on page 1291*
- **Highly Pathogenic Avian Influenza (HPAI) A (H5N1) Virus Vaccine** *see* Influenza A Virus Vaccine (H5N1) *on page 1074*
- **High-Molecular-Weight Iron Dextran (DexFerrum)** *see* Iron Dextran Complex *on page 1117*
- **High Potency Fish Oil [OTC] [DSC]** *see* Omega-3 Fatty Acids *on page 1507*
- **Hiprex** *see* Methenamine *on page 1317*
- **Hiprex® (Can)** *see* Methenamine *on page 1317*
- **Hirulog** *see* Bivalirudin *on page 268*
- **Histantil (Can)** *see* Promethazine *on page 1723*

Histrelin (his TREL in)

Brand Names: U.S. Supprelin LA; Vantas
Brand Names: Canada Vantas
Index Terms GnRH Agonist; Histrelin Acetate; LH-RH Agonist
Pharmacologic Category Antineoplastic Agent, Gonadotropin-Releasing Hormone Agonist; Gonadotropin Releasing Hormone Agonist
Use
Central precocious puberty: Treatment of central precocious puberty (CPP) in children
Prostate cancer, advanced: Palliative treatment of advanced prostate cancer
Pregnancy Risk Factor X
Dosage
Central precocious puberty (CPP) (Supprelin LA): Children ≥2 years: SubQ: 50 mg implant surgically inserted every 12 months. Discontinue at the appropriate time for the onset of puberty.
Prostate cancer, advanced (Vantas): Adults: SubQ: 50 mg implant surgically inserted every 12 months
Elderly: Refer to adult dosing

Dosage adjustment in renal impairment:
Vantas: CrCl ≥15 mL/minute: No dosage adjustment necessary.
Supprelin LA: There are no dosage adjustments provided in the manufacturer's labeling.
Dosage adjustment in hepatic impairment: There are no dosage adjustments provided in the manufacturers' labeling (has not been studied).
Additional Information Complete prescribing information should be consulted for additional detail.
Dosage Forms
Kit, Subcutaneous:
Supprelin LA: 50 mg
Vantas: 50 mg

- **Histrelin Acetate** *see* Histrelin *on page 1005*
- **Hizentra** *see* Immune Globulin *on page 1056*
- **Hizentra 20%** *see* Immune Globulin *on page 1056*
- **hMG** *see* Menotropins *on page 1292*
- **HMR1726** *see* Teriflunomide *on page 2006*
- **HMR 3647** *see* Telithromycin *on page 1987*
- **HN_2** *see* Mechlorethamine (Systemic) *on page 1276*
- **HOE 140** *see* Icatibant *on page 1037*
- **Holkira Pak (Can)** *see* Ombitasvir, Paritaprevir, Ritonavir, and Dasabuvir *on page 1505*
- **Homatropaire** *see* Homatropine *on page 1005*

Homatropine (hoe MA troe peen)

Brand Names: U.S. Homatropaire; Isopto Homatropine
Index Terms Homatropine Hydrobromide
Pharmacologic Category Anticholinergic Agent, Ophthalmic; Ophthalmic Agent, Mydriatic
Additional Appendix Information
Beers Criteria – Potentially Inappropriate Medications for Geriatrics *on page 2271*
Use
Ciliary spasm: Relief of ciliary spasm.
Iritis/iridocyclitis: Treatment of iritis and iridocyclitis.
Mydriasis and cycloplegia for refraction: Producing cycloplegia and mydriasis for refraction; for pre- and postoperative states when cycloplegic and mydriasis is required.
Optical aid: Use as an optical aid in some cases of axial lens opacities.
Uveitis: Treatment of inflammatory conditions of the uveal tract.
Pregnancy Risk Factor C
Dosage
Children >3 months and Adults: Ophthalmic: **Note:** Children (>3 months of age) should only use the 2% strength solution; patients with heavily pigmented irides may require increased dose.
Ciliary spasm/iritis/iridocyclitis/uveitis: 2% or 5% solution: 1-2 drops 2-3 times daily, up to every 4 hours for severe uveitis (Alexander, 2004)
Refraction:
2% solution: 1-2 drops into eye(s); repeat every 10-15 minutes if necessary; maximum: 5 doses
5% solution: 1-2 drops into eye(s); repeat dose in 15 minutes.

Dosage adjustment in renal impairment: No dosage adjustment provided in manufacturer's labeling.
Dosage adjustment in hepatic impairment: No dosage adjustment provided in manufacturer's labeling.
Additional Information Complete prescribing information should be consulted for additional detail.
Dosage Forms
Solution, Ophthalmic:
Homatropaire: 5% (5 mL)
Isopto Homatropine: 2% (5 mL); 5% (5 mL)
Generic: 5% (5 mL)

- **Homatropine and Hydrocodone** *see* Hydrocodone and Homatropine *on page 1013*
- **Homatropine Hydrobromide** *see* Homatropine *on page 1005*
- **Homocysteine Guard [OTC]** *see* Folic Acid, Cyanocobalamin, and Pyridoxine *on page 921*
- **Homoharringtonine** *see* Omacetaxine *on page 1501*
- **Horizant** *see* Gabapentin Enacarbil *on page 946*
- **Horse Antihuman Thymocyte Gamma Globulin** *see* Antithymocyte Globulin (Equine) *on page 157*
- **hpAT** *see* Antithrombin *on page 156*
- **Hp-PAC® (Can)** *see* Lansoprazole, Amoxicillin, and Clarithromycin *on page 1169*
- **HPV2** *see* Papillomavirus (Types 16, 18) Vaccine (Human, Recombinant) *on page 1574*
- **HPV4** *see* Papillomavirus (Types 6, 11, 16, 18) Vaccine (Human, Recombinant) *on page 1574*

- ◆ **HPV 16/18 L1 VLP/AS04 VAC** *see* Papillomavirus (Types 16, 18) Vaccine (Human, Recombinant) *on page 1574*
- ◆ **HPV Vaccine (Bivalent)** *see* Papillomavirus (Types 16, 18) Vaccine (Human, Recombinant) *on page 1574*
- ◆ **HPV Vaccine (Quadrivalent)** *see* Papillomavirus (Types 6, 11, 16, 18) Vaccine (Human, Recombinant) *on page 1574*
- ◆ **HRIG** *see* Rabies Immune Globulin (Human) *on page 1764*
- ◆ **HU** *see* Hydroxyurea *on page 1021*
- ◆ **HuIFN-alpha-Le** *see* Interferon Alpha, Multi-Subtype [INT] *on page 1100*
- ◆ **HumaLOG** *see* Insulin Lispro *on page 1087*
- ◆ **Humalog® (Can)** *see* Insulin Lispro *on page 1087*
- ◆ **HumaLOG KwikPen** *see* Insulin Lispro *on page 1087*
- ◆ **Humalog® Mix 25 (Can)** *see* Insulin Lispro Protamine and Insulin Lispro *on page 1088*
- ◆ **HumaLOG® Mix 50/50™** *see* Insulin Lispro Protamine and Insulin Lispro *on page 1088*
- ◆ **HumaLOG® Mix 50/50™ KwikPen™** *see* Insulin Lispro Protamine and Insulin Lispro *on page 1088*
- ◆ **HumaLOG® Mix 75/25™** *see* Insulin Lispro Protamine and Insulin Lispro *on page 1088*
- ◆ **HumaLOG® Mix 75/25™ KwikPen™** *see* Insulin Lispro Protamine and Insulin Lispro *on page 1088*
- ◆ **Human Albumin Grifols** *see* Albumin *on page 67*
- ◆ **Human Antitumor Necrosis Factor Alpha** *see* Adalimumab *on page 51*
- ◆ **Human C1 Inhibitor** *see* C1 Inhibitor (Human) *on page 315*
- ◆ **Human Corticotrophin-Releasing Hormone, Analogue** *see* Corticorelin *on page 509*
- ◆ **Human Diploid Cell Cultures Rabies Vaccine** *see* Rabies Vaccine *on page 1764*
- ◆ **Human Growth Hormone** *see* Somatropin *on page 1918*
- ◆ **Humanized IgG1 Anti-CD52 Monoclonal Antibody** *see* Alemtuzumab *on page 75*
- ◆ **Human Menopausal Gonadotropin** *see* Menotropins *on page 1292*
- ◆ **Human Normal Immunoglobulin** *see* Immune Globulin *on page 1056*
- ◆ **Human Papillomavirus Vaccine (Bivalent)** *see* Papillomavirus (Types 16, 18) Vaccine (Human, Recombinant) *on page 1574*
- ◆ **Human Papillomavirus Vaccine (Quadrivalent)** *see* Papillomavirus (Types 6, 11, 16, 18) Vaccine (Human, Recombinant) *on page 1574*
- ◆ **Human Rotavirus Vaccine, Attenuated (HRV)** *see* Rotavirus Vaccine *on page 1851*
- ◆ **Human Thyroid Stimulating Hormone** *see* Thyrotropin Alfa *on page 2031*
- ◆ **Humate-P** *see* Antihemophilic Factor/von Willebrand Factor Complex (Human) *on page 154*
- ◆ **Humatin (Can)** *see* Paromomycin *on page 1579*
- ◆ **Humatrope** *see* Somatropin *on page 1918*
- ◆ **HuMax-CD20** *see* Ofatumumab *on page 1488*
- ◆ **Humira** *see* Adalimumab *on page 51*
- ◆ **Humira Pediatric Crohns Start** *see* Adalimumab *on page 51*
- ◆ **Humira Pen** *see* Adalimumab *on page 51*
- ◆ **Humira Pen-Crohns Starter** *see* Adalimumab *on page 51*
- ◆ **Humira Pen-Psoriasis Starter** *see* Adalimumab *on page 51*
- ◆ **Humist [OTC]** *see* Sodium Chloride *on page 1902*
- ◆ **Humulin® 20/80 (Can)** *see* Insulin NPH and Insulin Regular *on page 1090*
- ◆ **HumuLIN® 70/30** *see* Insulin NPH and Insulin Regular *on page 1090*
- ◆ **Humulin® 70/30 (Can)** *see* Insulin NPH and Insulin Regular *on page 1090*
- ◆ **HumuLIN® 70/30 KwikPen** *see* Insulin NPH and Insulin Regular *on page 1090*
- ◆ **HumuLIN N [OTC]** *see* Insulin NPH *on page 1089*
- ◆ **Humulin® N (Can)** *see* Insulin NPH *on page 1089*
- ◆ **HumuLIN N KwikPen [OTC]** *see* Insulin NPH *on page 1089*
- ◆ **HumuLIN N Pen [OTC] [DSC]** *see* Insulin NPH *on page 1089*
- ◆ **HumuLIN R [OTC]** *see* Insulin Regular *on page 1091*
- ◆ **Humulin R (Can)** *see* Insulin Regular *on page 1091*
- ◆ **HumuLIN R U-500 (CONCENTRATED)** *see* Insulin Regular *on page 1091*
- ◆ **Hurricaine [OTC]** *see* Benzocaine *on page 246*
- ◆ **HurriCaine One [OTC]** *see* Benzocaine *on page 246*
- ◆ **Hyalgan** *see* Hyaluronate and Derivatives *on page 1006*
- ◆ **Hyaluronan** *see* Hyaluronate and Derivatives *on page 1006*

Hyaluronate and Derivatives

(hye al yoor ON ate & dah RIV ah tives)

Brand Names: U.S. Amvisc; Amvisc Plus; Bionect; Euflexxa; Gel-One; Hyalgan; Hylase Wound; Juvederm Ultra; Juvederm Ultra Plus; Juvederm Ultra Plus XC; Juvederm Ultra XC; Juvederm Voluma XC; Monovisc; Orthovisc; Perlane; Perlane-L; Provisc; Restylane; Restylane-L; Supartz; Synvisc; Synvisc-One

Brand Names: Canada Cystistat; Durolane; OrthoVisc; Suplasyn

Index Terms Hyaluronan; Hyaluronic Acid; Hylan G-F 20; Hylan Polymers; Restylane Silk; Sodium Hyaluronate

Pharmacologic Category Antirheumatic Miscellaneous; Ophthalmic Agent, Viscoelastic; Skin and Mucous Membrane Agent, Miscellaneous

Use

Intra-articular injection: Treatment of pain in osteoarthritis in knee in patients who have failed nonpharmacologic treatment or simple analgesics (Euflexxa, Gel-One, Hyalgan, Monovisc, OrthoVisc, Supartz, Synvisc, Synvisc-One) or nonsteroidal anti-inflammatory drugs (NSAIDS) (Gel-One)

Intradermal:

Juvederm (all formulations except Voluma XC), Perlane, Perlane-L, Restylane, Restylane-L: Correction of moderate to severe facial wrinkles or folds

Restylane Silk: Correction of perioral rhytids in adults >21 years.

Subcutaneous/supraperiosteal: Juvederm Voluma XC: Correction of age-related volume deficit (deep [subcutaneous and/or supraperiosteal] injection) for cheek augmentation in the mid-face in adults >21 years

Ophthalmic: Surgical aid in cataract extraction (Amvisc, Amvisc Plus, Provisc); intraocular lens implantation (Amvisc, Amvisc Plus, Provisc); corneal transplant (Amvisc, Amvisc Plus); glaucoma filtration (Amvisc, Amvisc Plus); and retinal attachment surgery (Amvisc, Amvisc Plus)

Submucosal: Lip augmentation in adults >21 years (Restylane, Restylane-L, Restylane Silk)

Topical cream, gel: Management of skin ulcers and wounds (Bionect, Hylase Wound)

Dosage Adults:

Osteoarthritis of the knee: Intra-articular:

Euflexxa: Inject 20 mg (2 mL) once weekly for 3 weeks (total of 3 injections)

Gel-One: Inject 30 mg (3 mL) once

Hyalgan: Inject 20 mg (2 mL) once weekly for 5 weeks (total of 5 injections); some patients may benefit with a total of 3 injections

Monovisc: Inject 88 mg (4 mL) once

Orthovisc: Inject 30 mg (2 mL) once weekly for 3-4 weeks (total of 3-4 injections)

Supartz: Inject 25 mg (2.5 mL) once weekly for 5 weeks (total of 5 injections); some patients may benefit with a total of 3 injections

Synvisc: Inject 16 mg (2 mL) once weekly for 3 weeks (total of 3 injections)

Synvisc-One: Inject 48 mg (6 mL) once

Facial wrinkles/folds: Intradermal:

Note: Formulations differ in terms of recommended injection depth: Juvederm (all formulations except Voluma XC), Restylane, and Restylane-L are intended for mid to deep intradermal injection; Perlane and Perlane-L are intended for injection into the deep dermis to superficial subcutis

Juvederm (all formulations except Voluma XC): Inject as required for cosmetic result; typical treatment regimen requires 1.6 mL/treatment site typical volume for repeat treatment is 0.7 mL/treatment site; maximum: 20 mL/60 kg/year

Perlane, Perlane-L: Inject as required into deep dermis/superficial subcutis for cosmetic result; median total dose: 3 mL; maximum: 6 mL per treatment

Restylane, Restylane-L: Inject as required for cosmetic result; median total dose: 3 mL; maximum: 6 mL per treatment

Cheek augmentation: Subcutaneous/Supraperiosteal (Juvederm Voluma XC): Adults >21 years: Inject as required for cosmetic result; typical treatment regimen requires small boluses of 0.1-0.2 mL over a large area to volumize and contour the cheek; an additional treatment may be needed to achieve the desired level of correction; maximum: 20 mL/60 kg/year

Lip augmentation: Submucosal (Restylane, Restylane-L, Restylane Silk): Adults ≥ 21 years: Maximum: 1.5 mL per lip (upper or lower) per treatment session

Perioral rhytids: Intradermal (Restylane Silk): Adults >21 years: Maximum: 1 mL per correction per treatment session

Surgical aid: Ophthalmic (Amvisc, Amvisc Plus, Provisc): Intraocular: Depends upon procedure (slowly introduce a sufficient quantity into eye)

Topical:

Bionect cream, gel: Apply a thin layer to clean and disinfected wound or ulcer 2-3 times daily

Hylase Wound gel: Apply liberally to ulcer cavity or wound and to surrounding areas once daily

Interstitial cystitis, refractory (off-label use): Intravesical (off-label route): 40 mg (as hyaluronic acid) in 50 mL saline intravesically (retain in bladder for at least 30 minutes) once weekly for 4 weeks, then monthly for up to 1 year in patients showing an initial response (Morales, 1996)

Additional Information Complete prescribing information should be consulted for additional detail.

Product Availability Restylane Silk: FDA approved June 2014; anticipated availability is currently unknown.

Dosage Forms

Cream, topical:

Bionect: 0.2% (25 g)

Foam, topical:

Bionect: 0.2% (113.4 g)

Gel, topical:

Bionect: 0.2% (30 g, 60 g)

Hylase Wound: 2.5% (75 g)

Injection, gel, intra-articular [cross-linked hyaluronate]:

Gel-One: 10 mg/mL (3 mL)

Injection, gel, intradermal [hyaluronic acid]:

Juvederm Ultra: 24 mg/mL (0.4 mL, 0.8 mL)

Juvederm Ultra Plus: 24 mg/mL (0.4 mL, 0.8 mL)

Juvederm Ultra Plus XC: Hyaluronic acid 24 mg/mL and lidocaine 0.3% (0.4 mL, 0.8 mL)

Juvederm Ultra XC: Hyaluronic acid 24 mg/mL and lidocaine 0.3% (0.4 mL, 0.8 mL)

Perlane-L: Hyaluronic acid 20 mg/mL and lidocaine 0.3% (1 mL, 2 mL)

Restylane-L: Hyaluronic acid 20 mg/mL and lidocaine 0.3% (0.5 mL, 1 mL, 2 mL)

Injection, gel, intradermal [sodium hyaluronate]:

Perlane: 20 mg/mL (1 mL)

Restylane: 20 mg/mL (0.4 mL, 1 mL, 2 mL)

Injection, gel, subcutaneous/supraperiosteal [cross-linked hyaluronic acid]:

Juvederm Voluma XC: Hyaluronic acid 20 mg/mL and lidocaine 0.3%

Injection, solution, intra-articular:

Euflexxa: 10 mg/mL (2 mL)

Hyalgan: 10 mg/mL (2 mL)

Monovisc: 88 mg/4 mL (4 mL)

Orthovisc: 15 mg/mL (2 mL)

Supartz: 10 mg/mL (2.5 mL)

Synvisc-One: 8 mg/mL (6 mL)

Synvisc: 8 mg/mL (2 mL)

Injection, solution, intraocular:

Amvisc: 12 mg/mL (0.5 mL, 0.8 mL)

Amvisc Plus: 16 mg/mL (0.5 mL, 0.8 mL)

Provisc: 10 mg/mL (0.4 mL, 0.55 mL, 0.85 mL)

◆ **Hyaluronic Acid** *see* Hyaluronate and Derivatives *on page 1006*

◆ **Hycamptamine** *see* Topotecan *on page 2069*

◆ **Hycamtin** *see* Topotecan *on page 2069*

◆ **hycet®** *see* Hydrocodone and Acetaminophen *on page 1012*

◆ **Hycodan** *see* Hydrocodone and Homatropine *on page 1013*

◆ **Hycort™ (Can)** *see* Hydrocortisone (Topical) *on page 1014*

◆ **Hydeltra T.B.A. (Can)** *see* PrednisoLONE (Systemic) *on page 1703*

◆ **Hyderm (Can)** *see* Hydrocortisone (Topical) *on page 1014*

HydrALAZINE (hye DRAL a zeen)

Brand Names: Canada Apo-Hydralazine; Apresoline; Novo-Hylazin; Nu-Hydral

Index Terms Apresoline; Hydralazine Hydrochloride

Pharmacologic Category Antihypertensive; Vasodilator

Use

Hypertension: Management of moderate to severe hypertension

Note: According to the Eighth Joint National Committee (JNC 8) guidelines, hydralazine is **not** recommended for the initial treatment of hypertension (James, 2013).

Pregnancy Risk Factor C

Pregnancy Considerations Adverse events were observed in some animal reproduction studies. Hydralazine crosses the placenta (Liedholm, 1982). Intravenous hydralazine is recommended for use in the management of acute onset, severe hypertension (systolic BP ≥160 mm Hg or diastolic BP ≥110 mm Hg) with preeclampsia or eclampsia in pregnant and postpartum women. Untreated chronic maternal hypertension is associated with adverse events in the fetus, infant, and mother. If treatment for chronic hypertension in pregnancy is needed, other oral agents are preferred as initial therapy (ACOG, 2013; Magee, 2014).

Breast-Feeding Considerations Hydralazine is excreted into breast milk. In a case report, following a maternal dose of hydralazine 50 mg three times daily, exposure to the infant was calculated to be 0.013 mg per 75 mL breast milk (Liedholm, 1982). The manufacturer recommends that caution be used if administered to a nursing woman.

Contraindications Hypersensitivity to hydralazine or any component of the formulation; mitral valve rheumatic heart disease

Warnings/Precautions May cause peripheral neuritis or a drug-induced lupus-like syndrome (more likely on larger doses, longer duration). Discontinue hydralazine in patients who develop SLE-like syndrome or positive ANA. Use with caution in patients with severe renal disease or cerebral vascular accidents or with known or suspected coronary artery disease; monitor blood pressure closely with IV use. Slow acetylators, patients with decreased renal function, and patients receiving >200 mg/day (chronically) are at higher risk for SLE. Titrate dosage cautiously to patient's response. Hypotensive effect after IV administration may be delayed and unpredictable in some patients. Usually administered with diuretic and a beta-blocker to counteract side effects of sodium and water retention and reflex tachycardia.

Adjust dose in severe renal dysfunction. Use with caution in CAD (increase in tachycardia may increase myocardial oxygen demand). Use with caution in pulmonary hypertension (may cause hypotension). Patients may be poorly compliant because of frequent dosing. Hydralazine-induced fluid and sodium retention may require addition or increased dosage of a diuretic.

Adverse Reactions

Cardiovascular: Angina pectoris, flushing, orthostatic hypotension, palpitations, paradoxical hypertension, peripheral edema, tachycardia, vascular collapse

Central nervous system: Anxiety, chills, depression, disorientation, dizziness, fever, headache, increased intracranial pressure (IV; in patient with preexisting increased intracranial pressure), psychotic reaction

Dermatologic: Pruritus, rash, urticaria

Gastrointestinal: Anorexia, constipation, diarrhea, nausea, paralytic ileus, vomiting

Genitourinary: Dysuria, impotence

Hematologic: Agranulocytosis, eosinophilia, erythrocyte count reduced, hemoglobin decreased, hemolytic anemia, leukopenia, thrombocytopenia (rare)

Neuromuscular & skeletal: Muscle cramps, peripheral neuritis, rheumatoid arthritis, tremor, weakness

Ocular: Conjunctivitis, lacrimation

Respiratory: Dyspnea, nasal congestion

Miscellaneous: Diaphoresis, drug-induced lupus-like syndrome (dose related; fever, arthralgia, splenomegaly, lymphadenopathy, asthenia, myalgia, malaise, pleuritic chest pain, edema, positive ANA, positive LE cells, maculopapular facial rash, positive direct Coombs' test, pericarditis, pericardial tamponade)

Drug Interactions

Metabolism/Transport Effects Inhibits CYP3A4 (weak)

Avoid Concomitant Use

Avoid concomitant use of HydrALAZINE with any of the following: Pimozide

Increased Effect/Toxicity

HydrALAZINE may increase the levels/effects of: Amifostine; Antihypertensives; ARIPiprazole; Dofetilide; DULOxetine; Hydrocodone; Hypotensive Agents; Levodopa; Lomitapide; Obinutuzumab; Pimozide; RisperiDONE; RiTUXimab

The levels/effects of HydrALAZINE may be increased by: Alfuzosin; Barbiturates; Brimonidine (Topical); Dapoxetine; Diazoxide; Herbs (Hypotensive Properties); MAO Inhibitors; Nicorandil; Pentoxifylline; Phosphodiesterase 5 Inhibitors; Prostacyclin Analogues

Decreased Effect

The levels/effects of HydrALAZINE may be decreased by: Herbs (Hypertensive Properties); Methylphenidate; Nonsteroidal Anti-Inflammatory Agents; Yohimbine

Food Interactions Food enhances bioavailability of hydralazine. Management: Administer without regard to food, but keep consistent.

Preparation for Administration Hydralazine should be diluted in NS for IVPB administration due to decreased stability in D_5W. Stability of IVPB solution in NS is 4 days at room temperature.

Storage/Stability Intact ampuls/vials of hydralazine should not be stored under refrigeration because of possible precipitation or crystallization.

Mechanism of Action Direct vasodilation of arterioles (with little effect on veins) with decreased systemic resistance

Pharmacodynamics/Kinetics

Onset of action: Oral: 20-30 minutes; IV: 5-20 minutes

Duration: Oral: Up to 8 hours; IV: 1-4 hours; **Note:** May vary depending on acetylator status of patient

Protein binding: 85% to 90%

Metabolism: Hepatically acetylated; extensive first-pass effect (oral)

Bioavailability: 30% to 50%; increased with food

Half-life elimination: Normal renal function: 2-8 hours; End-stage renal disease: 7-16 hours

Excretion: Urine (14% as unchanged drug)

Dosage

Children:

Oral: Initial: 0.75 to 1 mg/kg/day in 2 to 4 divided doses; increase over 3 to 4 weeks to maximum of 7.5 mg/kg/day in 2 to 4 divided doses; maximum daily dose: 200 mg/day

IM, IV: 0.1 to 0.2 mg/kg/dose (not to exceed 20 mg) every 4 to 6 hours as needed, up to 1.7 to 3.5 mg/kg/day in 4 to 6 divided doses

Adults:

Oral:

Hypertension: Initial dose: 10 mg 4 times daily for the first 2 to 4 days; increase to 25 mg 4 times daily for the balance of the first week; further increase by 10 to 25 mg/dose gradually (every 2 to 5 days) to 50 mg 4 times daily (maximum: 300 mg daily in divided doses).

Heart failure (off-label use): Initial dose: 25 to 50 mg 3 or 4 times daily; use in combination with isosorbide dinitrate; maximum dose: 300 mg daily in divided doses (ACCF/AHA [Yancy, 2013])

IM, IV:

Hypertensive emergency (off-label dose): **Note:** Use is generally not recommended due to unpredictable and prolonged antihypertensive effects (Marik, 2007): IM, IV: 10 to 20 mg every 4 to 6 hours as needed (Rhoney, 2009)

Hypertensive emergency in pregnancy (systolic BP ≥160 mm Hg or diastolic BP ≥110 mm Hg) (off-label dose): IM, IV: Initial: 5 or 10 mg; may repeat dose in 20 to 40 minutes with 5 to 10 mg if blood pressure continues to exceed thresholds (ACOG, 2015; Magee, 2014; Too, 2013). Also refer to administration protocols developed by the American College of

Obstetricians and Gynecologists (ACOG, 2015). A maximum total cumulative dose of 20 mg (IV) or 30 mg (IM) is recommended (Magee, 2014). **Note:** After the initial dose, may initiate a continuous infusion of 0.5 to 10 mg/hour instead of intermittent dosing (Magee, 2014).

Perioperative hypertension (off-label dose): IV: 3 to 20 mg every 20 to 60 minutes as needed (Varon, 2008). **Note:** The lower end of the dosage range is preferred in the immediate perioperative period and in patients with renal failure. The use of hydralazine in this setting especially in patients with ischemic heart disease, aortic dissection, or an intracranial process is best avoided due to unpredictable and prolonged antihypertensive effects (Lien, 2012; Varon, 2008).

Dosage interval in renal impairment:

CrCl 10 to 50 mL/minute: Administer every 8 hours.

CrCl <10 mL/minute: Administer every 8 to 16 hours in fast acetylators and every 12 to 24 hours in slow acetylators.

Hemodialysis: Supplemental dose is not necessary.

Peritoneal dialysis: Supplemental dose is not necessary.

Dosage adjustment in hepatic impairment: No dosage adjustment provided in manufacturer's labeling. However, hydralazine undergoes extensive hepatic metabolism.

Dietary Considerations Administer tablet with meals.

Administration Solution for injection: Administer as a slow IV push; maximum rate: 5 mg/minute

Monitoring Parameters Blood pressure (monitor closely with IV use), standing and sitting/supine, heart rate, ANA titer

Dosage Forms

Solution, Injection:

Generic: 20 mg/mL (1 mL)

Tablet, Oral:

Generic: 10 mg, 25 mg, 50 mg, 100 mg

Extemporaneous Preparations A 4 mg/mL oral suspension may be made with tablets and a 1:1 mixture of Ora-Sweet SF and Ora-Plus. Crush four 100 mg tablets in a mortar and reduce to a fine powder. Add 15 mL of the vehicle and mix to a uniform paste; mix while adding the vehicle in incremental proportions to **almost** 100 mL; transfer to a calibrated bottle, rinse mortar with vehicle, and add quantity of vehicle sufficient to make 100 mL. Label "Shake Well", "Protect From Light", "Store in a Refrigerator". Stable for 2 days when stored in amber plastic prescription bottles in the dark and refrigerated (Allen, 1998).

Note: Stability reduced to 24 hours if Ora-Sweet is substituted for Ora-Sweet SF.

Allen LV Jr, Erickson MA 3rd. Stability of alprazolam, chloroquine phosphate, cisapride, enalapril maleate, and hydralazine hydrochloride in extemporaneously compounded oral liquids. *Am J Health-Syst Pharm.* 1998;55(18):1915-1920.

◆ **Hydralazine and Isosorbide Dinitrate** *see* Isosorbide Dinitrate and Hydralazine *on page 1126*

◆ **Hydralazine Hydrochloride** *see* HydrALAZINE *on page 1007*

◆ **Hydrated Chloral** *see* Chloral Hydrate [CAN/INT] *on page 418*

◆ **Hydrea** *see* Hydroxyurea *on page 1021*

◆ **Hydrea® (Can)** *see* Hydroxyurea *on page 1021*

◆ **Hydro 35** *see* Urea *on page 2114*

◆ **Hydro 40** *see* Urea *on page 2114*

Hydrochlorothiazide (hye droe klor oh THYE a zide)

Brand Names: U.S. Microzide

Brand Names: Canada Apo-Hydro; Ava-Hydrochlorothiazide; Bio-Hydrochlorothiazide; PMS-Hydrochlorothiazide; Teva-Hydrochlorothiazide; Urozide

Index Terms HCTZ (error-prone abbreviation); Hydrodiuril

Pharmacologic Category Antihypertensive; Diuretic, Thiazide

Use

Edema: Treatment of edema due to heart failure, hepatic cirrhosis (see **"Note"**), various forms of renal dysfunction (eg, nephrotic syndrome, acute glomerulosclerosis, chronic renal failure) (see **"Note"**), corticosteroid and estrogen therapy

Note: The use of hydrochlorothiazide in the treatment of edema for hepatic cirrhosis has largely been replaced by spironolactone. The use of hydrochlorothiazide in the management of edema in patients with renal dysfunction has largely been replaced by the use of loop diuretics (eg, furosemide).

Hypertension: Management of mild-to-moderate hypertension

The 2014 guideline for the management of high blood pressure in adults (Eighth Joint National Committee [JNC 8]) recommends initiation of pharmacologic treatment to lower blood pressure for the following patients:

- Patients ≥60 years of age with systolic blood pressure (SBP) ≥150 mm Hg or diastolic blood pressure (DBP) ≥90 mm Hg. Goal of therapy is SBP <150 mm Hg and DBP <90 mm Hg.
- Patients <60 years of age with SBP ≥140 mm Hg or DBP is ≥90 mm Hg. Goal of therapy is SBP <140 mm Hg and DBP <90 mm Hg.
- Patients ≥18 years of age with diabetes and SBP ≥140 mm Hg or DBP ≥90 mm Hg. Goal of therapy is SBP <140 mm Hg and DBP <90 mm Hg.
- Patients ≥18 years of age with chronic kidney disease (CKD) and SBP ≥140 mm Hg or DBP ≥90 mm Hg. Goal of therapy is SBP <140 mm Hg and DBP <90 mm Hg.

In patients with CKD, regardless of race or diabetes status, the use of an ACE inhibitor (ACEI) or angiotensin receptor blocker (ARB) as initial therapy is recommended to improve kidney outcomes. In the general nonblack population (without CKD) including those with diabetes, initial antihypertensive treatment should consist of a thiazide-type diuretic, calcium channel blocker, ACEI, or ARB. In the general black population (without CKD), including those with diabetes, initial antihypertensive treatment should consist of a thiazide-type diuretic or a calcium channel blocker **instead of** an ACEI or ARB.

Canadian labeling: Additional uses (not in U.S. labeling):

Premenstrual tension with edema: Management of premenstrual tension with edema

Toxemia of pregnancy: Management of toxemia of pregnancy (including eclampsia). **Note:** Guidelines recommend alternative agents (Magee, 2008)

Pregnancy Risk Factor B

Pregnancy Considerations Adverse events were not observed in animal reproduction studies. Thiazide diuretics cross the placenta and are found in cord blood. Maternal use may cause may cause fetal or neonatal jaundice, thrombocytopenia, or other adverse events observed in adults. Use of thiazide diuretics to treat edema during normal pregnancies is not appropriate; use may be considered when edema is due to pathologic causes (as in the nonpregnant patient); monitor. Untreated chronic maternal hypertension is associated with adverse events in the fetus, infant, and mother (ACOG, 2013). Women who required thiazide diuretics for the treatment of hypertension prior to pregnancy may continue their use (ACOG, 2013).

Breast-Feeding Considerations Thiazide diuretics are found in breast milk. Following a single oral maternal dose of hydrochlorothiazide 50 mg, the mean breast milk concentration was 80 ng/mL (samples collected over 24 hours) and hydrochlorothiazide was not detected in the blood of the breast feeding infant (limit of detection 20 ng/mL) (Miller, 1982). Peak plasma concentrations reported in adults following hydrochlorothiazide 12.5-100 mg are 70-490 ng/mL. Due to the potential for serious adverse reactions in the nursing infant, the manufacturer recommends a decision be made whether to discontinue nursing or to discontinue the drug, taking into account the importance of treatment to the mother (Canadian labeling contraindicates use in nursing women). Diuretics have the potential to decrease milk volume and suppress lactation.

Contraindications Hypersensitivity to hydrochlorothiazide, any component of the formulation, or sulfonamide-derived drugs; anuria

Canadian labeling: Additional contraindications (not in U.S. labeling): Increasing azotemia and oliguria during treatment of severe progressive renal disease; breast-feeding

Warnings/Precautions Hypersensitivity reactions may occur with hydrochlorothiazide. Risk is increased in patients with a history of allergy or bronchial asthma. Avoid in severe renal disease (ineffective as a diuretic). Electrolyte disturbances (hypokalemia, hypochloremic alkalosis, hypomagnesemia, hyponatremia) can occur. Development of electrolyte disturbances can be minimized when used in combination with other electrolyte sparing antihypertensives (eg, ACE inhibitors or angiotensin receptor blockers). (Sica, 2011) Use with caution in severe hepatic dysfunction; hepatic encephalopathy can be caused by electrolyte disturbances. Gout may be precipitated in certain patients with a history of gout, a familial predisposition to gout, or chronic renal failure. Thiazide diuretics reduce calcium excretion; pathologic changes in the parathyroid glands with hypercalcemia and hypophosphatemia have been observed with prolonged use. Should be discontinued prior to testing for parathyroid function. Use with caution in patients with prediabetes and diabetes; may alter glucose control. May cause SLE exacerbation or activation. Use with caution in patients with moderate or high cholesterol concentrations. Photosensitization may occur. Correct hypokalemia before initiating therapy. Thiazide diuretics may decrease renal calcium excretion; consider avoiding use in patients with hypercalcemia. May cause acute transient myopia and acute angle-closure glaucoma, typically occurring within hours to weeks following initiation; discontinue therapy immediately in patients with acute decreases in visual acuity or ocular pain. Risk factors may include a history of sulfonamide or penicillin allergy. Cumulative effects may develop, including azotemia, in patients with impaired renal function.

Chemical similarities are present among sulfonamides, sulfonylureas, carbonic anhydrase inhibitors, thiazides, and loop diuretics (except ethacrynic acid). Use in patients with sulfonamide allergy is specifically contraindicated in product labeling, however, a risk of cross-reaction exists in patients with allergy to any of these compounds; avoid use when previous reaction has been severe. Discontinue if signs of hypersensitivity are noted.

Adverse Reactions The occurrence of adverse events are dose related, with the majority occurring with doses ≥25 mg.

Cardiovascular: Hypotension, necrotizing angiitis, orthostatic hypotension

Central nervous system: Dizziness, headache, paresthesia, restlessness, vertigo

Dermatologic: Alopecia, erythema multiforme, exfoliative dermatitis, skin photosensitivity, skin rash, Stevens-Johnson syndrome, toxic epidermal necrolysis, urticaria

Endocrine & metabolic: Glycosuria, hypercalcemia, hyperglycemia, hyperuricemia, hypochloremic alkalosis, hypokalemia, hypomagnesemia, hyponatremia

Gastrointestinal: Abdominal cramps, anorexia, constipation, diarrhea, gastric irritation, nausea, pancreatitis, sialadenitis, vomiting

Genitourinary: Impotence

Hematologic & oncologic: Agranulocytosis, aplastic anemia, hemolytic anemia, leukopenia, purpura, thrombocytopenia

Hepatic: Jaundice

Hypersensitivity: Anaphylaxis

Neuromuscular & skeletal: Muscle spasm, weakness

Ophthalmic: Blurred vision (transient), xanthopsia

Renal: Interstitial nephritis, renal failure, renal insufficiency

Respiratory: Respiratory distress, pneumonitis, pulmonary edema

Miscellaneous: Fever

Rare but important or life-threatening: Allergic myocarditis, eosinophilic pneumonitis, hepatic insufficiency, lip cancer (Friedman, 2012), systemic lupus erythematosus

Drug Interactions

Metabolism/Transport Effects None known.

Avoid Concomitant Use

Avoid concomitant use of Hydrochlorothiazide with any of the following: Dofetilide

Increased Effect/Toxicity

Hydrochlorothiazide may increase the levels/effects of: ACE Inhibitors; Allopurinol; Amifostine; Antihypertensives; Benazepril; Calcium Salts; CarBAMazepine; Cardiac Glycosides; Cyclophosphamide; Diazoxide; Dofetilide; DULoxetine; Hypotensive Agents; Ivabradine; Levodopa; Lithium; Multivitamins/Minerals (with ADEK, Folate, Iron); Multivitamins/Minerals (with AE, No Iron); Obinutuzumab; OXcarbazepine; Porfimer; RisperiDONE; RiTUXimab; Sodium Phosphates; Topiramate; Toremifene; Valsartan; Verteporfin; Vitamin D Analogs

The levels/effects of Hydrochlorothiazide may be increased by: Alcohol (Ethyl); Alfuzosin; Analgesics (Opioid); Anticholinergic Agents; Barbiturates; Beta2-Agonists; Brimonidine (Topical); Corticosteroids (Orally Inhaled); Corticosteroids (Systemic); Dexketoprofen; Diazoxide; Herbs (Hypotensive Properties); Licorice; MAO Inhibitors; Multivitamins/Fluoride (with ADE); Nicorandil; Pentoxifylline; Phosphodiesterase 5 Inhibitors; Prostacyclin Analogues; Selective Serotonin Reuptake Inhibitors; Valsartan

Decreased Effect

Hydrochlorothiazide may decrease the levels/effects of: Antidiabetic Agents

The levels/effects of Hydrochlorothiazide may be decreased by: Benazepril; Bile Acid Sequestrants; Herbs (Hypertensive Properties); Methylphenidate; Nonsteroidal Anti-Inflammatory Agents; Yohimbine

Storage/Stability Store at 20°C to 25°C (68°F to 77°F) (USP Controlled Room Temperature). Protect from light and moisture.

Mechanism of Action Inhibits sodium reabsorption in the distal tubules causing increased excretion of sodium and water as well as potassium and hydrogen ions

Pharmacodynamics/Kinetics

Onset of action: Diuresis: ~2 hours

Peak effect: 4 to 6 hours

Duration: 6 to 12 hours

Absorption: Well absorbed; when administered with food, time to maximum concentration increases from 1.6 to 2.9 hours. Absorption is reduced in patients with CHF.

Distribution: 3.6 to 7.8 L/kg (correlates with dose administered and concentration achieved)

Protein binding: ~40% to 68%

Metabolism: Not metabolized

Bioavailability: 65% to 75% (reduced by 10% when administered with food)
Half-life elimination: 6 to 15 hours
Time to peak: ~1 to 5 hours
Excretion: Urine (as unchanged drug)

Dosage

Infants and Children: Edema, hypertension (in pediatric patients, chlorothiazide may be preferred over hydrochlorothiazide as there are more dosage formulations [eg, suspension] available): Oral (effect of drug may be decreased when used every day):

Manufacturer's labeling: Usual dose:

<6 months: 1 to 3 mg/kg/day in 1 to 2 divided doses; maximum: 37.5 mg daily

>6 months to 2 years: 1 to 2 mg/kg/day in a single or 2 divided doses; maximum: 37.5 mg daily

>2 to 12 years: 1 to 2 mg/kg/day in a single or 2 divided doses; maximum: 100 mg daily

Alternate recommendations: Children and Adolescents: Oral: Initial: 1 mg/kg/day in a single dose once daily; maximum: 3 mg/kg/day not to exceed 50 mg daily (NHBPEP, 2005)

Adults:

Manufacturer recommendations:

Edema: Oral: 25 to 100 mg daily in 1 to 2 divided doses; may administer intermittently on alternate days or on 3 to 5 days each week.

Hypertension: Oral:

U.S. labeling: Initial: 12.5 to 25 mg once daily administered alone or in combination with other antihypertensives; may increase up to 50 mg daily in 1 to 2 divided doses; minimal increase in response and more electrolyte disturbances are seen with doses >50 mg daily.

Canadian labeling: Initial: 12.5 to 100 mg daily as a single dose or in divided doses; titrate for effect. Up to 200 mg daily (in divided doses) may be necessary. If used concomitantly with other antihypertensive agents, reduce the dose of the concomitant antihypertensive by 50%.

Premenstrual tension with edema: Canadian labeling (not in U.S. labeling): Oral: 25 to 50 mg daily once or twice daily (initiate at onset of symptoms and continue through the start of menses).

Toxemia of pregnancy (Canadian labeling; not in U.S. labeling): Oral: 100 mg daily; may temporarily increase to 200 mg daily in divided doses for severe cases. May administer daily or intermittently once every 4 days. **Note:** Guidelines recommend use of alternative agents (Magee, 2008).

Alternate recommendations:

Fluid retention (mild) in heart failure: Oral: Initial: 25 mg once or twice daily; maximum daily dose: 200 mg (ACCF/AHA [Yancy, 2013])

Hypertension: Oral: Initial: 12.5 to 25 mg once daily; may increase dose to a target dose range of 25 to 50 mg once daily in 1 to 2 divided doses (JNC 8 [James, 2014]); usual dosage range (ASH/ISH [Weber, 2013]): 12.5 to 50 mg daily

Off-label use:

Calcium nephrolithiasis: 50 mg daily in 1 or 2 divided doses (AUA Guidelines [Pearle, 2014])

Elderly: Oral: Initial: 12.5 to 25 mg once daily; titrate as necessary in increments of 12.5 mg. Minimal increase in response and more electrolyte disturbances are seen with doses >50 mg daily.

Dosage adjustment in renal impairment: There are no dosage adjustments provided in the manufacturer's labeling; however, the following adjustments have been recommended (Aronoff, 2007):

CrCl ≥10 mL/minute: No dosage adjustment necessary. Usually ineffective with CrCl <30 mL/minute unless in combination with a loop diuretic

CrCl <10 mL/minute: Use not recommended; use is contraindicated with anuria.

Dosage adjustment in hepatic impairment: There are no dosage adjustments provided in the manufacturer's labeling. Use with caution and monitor for precipitation of hepatic coma.

Administration May be administered with or without food. Take early in day to avoid nocturia. Take the last dose of multiple doses no later than 6 PM unless instructed otherwise.

Monitoring Parameters Assess weight, I & O reports daily to determine fluid loss; blood pressure, serum electrolytes, BUN, creatinine

Dosage Forms

Capsule, Oral:
Microzide: 12.5 mg
Generic: 12.5 mg

Tablet, Oral:
Generic: 12.5 mg, 25 mg, 50 mg

◆ **Hydrochlorothiazide, Aliskiren, and Amlodipine** *see* Aliskiren, Amlodipine, and Hydrochlorothiazide *on page 87*

◆ **Hydrochlorothiazide, Amlodipine, and Aliskiren** *see* Aliskiren, Amlodipine, and Hydrochlorothiazide *on page 87*

◆ **Hydrochlorothiazide, Amlodipine, and Valsartan** *see* Amlodipine, Valsartan, and Hydrochlorothiazide *on page 127*

◆ **Hydrochlorothiazide and Aliskiren** *see* Aliskiren and Hydrochlorothiazide *on page 87*

◆ **Hydrochlorothiazide and Benazepril** *see* Benazepril and Hydrochlorothiazide *on page 240*

◆ **Hydrochlorothiazide and Bisoprolol** *see* Bisoprolol and Hydrochlorothiazide *on page 267*

◆ **Hydrochlorothiazide and Candesartan** *see* Candesartan and Hydrochlorothiazide *on page 338*

◆ **Hydrochlorothiazide and Captopril** *see* Captopril and Hydrochlorothiazide *on page 345*

◆ **Hydrochlorothiazide and Cilazapril** *see* Cilazapril and Hydrochlorothiazide [CAN/INT] *on page 436*

◆ **Hydrochlorothiazide and Enalapril** *see* Enalapril and Hydrochlorothiazide *on page 725*

◆ **Hydrochlorothiazide and Eprosartan** *see* Eprosartan and Hydrochlorothiazide *on page 750*

◆ **Hydrochlorothiazide and Irbesartan** *see* Irbesartan and Hydrochlorothiazide *on page 1112*

◆ **Hydrochlorothiazide and Lisinopril** *see* Lisinopril and Hydrochlorothiazide *on page 1229*

◆ **Hydrochlorothiazide and Losartan** *see* Losartan and Hydrochlorothiazide *on page 1250*

◆ **Hydrochlorothiazide and Moexipril** *see* Moexipril and Hydrochlorothiazide *on page 1388*

◆ **Hydrochlorothiazide and Olmesartan Medoxomil** *see* Olmesartan and Hydrochlorothiazide *on page 1498*

◆ **Hydrochlorothiazide and Pindolol** *see* Pindolol and Hydrochlorothiazide [CAN/INT] *on page 1653*

◆ **Hydrochlorothiazide and Ramipril** *see* Ramipril and Hydrochlorothiazide [CAN/INT] *on page 1773*

◆ **Hydrochlorothiazide and Telmisartan** *see* Telmisartan and Hydrochlorothiazide *on page 1990*

Hydrochlorothiazide and Triamterene

(hye droe klor oh THYE a zide & trye AM ter een)

Brand Names: U.S. Dyazide; Maxzide; Maxzide-25

Brand Names: Canada Apo-Triazide; Pro-Triazide; Teva-Triamterene HCTZ

Index Terms Triamterene and Hydrochlorothiazide

Pharmacologic Category Antihypertensive; Diuretic, Potassium-Sparing; Diuretic, Thiazide

Use Treatment of hypertension or edema (not recommended for initial treatment) when hypokalemia has developed on hydrochlorothiazide alone or when the development of hypokalemia must be avoided

Pregnancy Risk Factor C

Dosage Oral: Adults:

Hydrochlorothiazide 25 mg and triamterene 37.5 mg: 1-2 tablets/capsules once daily

Hydrochlorothiazide 50 mg and triamterene 75 mg: 1/2-1 tablet daily

Dosage adjustment in renal impairment: Efficacy of hydrochlorothiazide is limited in patients with CrCl <30 mL/minute, contraindicated in patients with anuria, acute and chronic renal insufficiency, or significant renal impairment.

Dosage adjustment in hepatic impairment: No dosage adjustment provided in manufacturer's labeling; use with caution. Use with caution and monitor for precipitation of hepatic coma.

Additional Information Complete prescribing information should be consulted for additional detail.

Dosage Forms

Capsule: Hydrochlorothiazide 25 mg and triamterene 37.5 mg; hydrochlorothiazide 25 mg and triamterene 50 mg

Dyazide: Hydrochlorothiazide 25 mg and triamterene 37.5 mg

Tablet: Hydrochlorothiazide 25 mg and triamterene 37.5 mg; hydrochlorothiazide 50 mg and triamterene 75 mg

Maxzide: Hydrochlorothiazide 50 mg and triamterene 75 mg [scored]

Maxzide-25: Hydrochlorothiazide 25 mg and triamterene 37.5 mg [scored]

- ◆ **Hydrochlorothiazide and Valsartan** *see* Valsartan and Hydrochlorothiazide *on page 2129*
- ◆ **Hydrochlorothiazide, Olmesartan, and Amlodipine** *see* Olmesartan, Amlodipine, and Hydrochlorothiazide *on page 1498*

Hydrocodone and Acetaminophen

(hye droe KOE done & a seet a MIN oh fen)

Brand Names: U.S. hycet®; Lorcet® 10/650 [DSC]; Lorcet® Plus [DSC]; Lortab®; Maxidone [DSC]; Norco; Stagesic [DSC]; Verdrocet; Vicodin ES; Vicodin HP; Vicodin®; Xodol 10/300; Xodol 5/300; Xodol 7.5/300; Zamicet [DSC]; Zolvit [DSC]; Zydone [DSC]

Index Terms Acetaminophen and Hydrocodone

Pharmacologic Category Analgesic Combination (Opioid); Analgesic, Opioid

Use Pain: Reief of moderate-to-severe pain

Pregnancy Risk Factor C

Dosage Oral (doses should be titrated to appropriate analgesic effect): Analgesic:

Children 2-13 years or <50 kg: Hydrocodone 0.1-0.2 mg/kg/dose every 4-6 hours; do not exceed 6 doses/day or the maximum recommended dose of acetaminophen

Children and Adults ≥50 kg: Average starting dose in opioid naive patients: Hydrocodone 5-10 mg 4 times/day; the dosage of acetaminophen should be limited to ≤4 g/day (and possibly less in patients with hepatic impairment or ethanol use).

Dosage ranges (based on specific product labeling): Hydrocodone 2.5-10 mg every 4-6 hours (maximum dose of hydrocodone may be limited by the acetaminophen content of specific product)

Elderly: Doses should be titrated to appropriate analgesic effect; 2.5-5 mg of the hydrocodone component every 4-6 hours. Do not exceed 4 g/day of acetaminophen.

Dosage adjustment in renal impairment: No dosage adjustment provided in manufacturer's labeling; use with caution.

Dosage adjustment in hepatic impairment: Use with caution. Limited, low-dose therapy usually well tolerated in hepatic disease/cirrhosis; however, cases of hepatotoxicity at daily acetaminophen dosages <4 g/day have been reported. Avoid chronic use in hepatic impairment.

Additional Information Complete prescribing information should be consulted for additional detail.

Dosage Forms

Solution, oral: Hydrocodone 7.5 mg and acetaminophen 325 mg per 15 mL

hycet®: Hydrocodone 7.5 mg and acetaminophen 325 mg per 15 mL

Tablet, oral:

Generics:

Hydrocodone 2.5 mg and acetaminophen 325 mg
Hydrocodone 5 mg and acetaminophen 300 mg
Hydrocodone 5 mg and acetaminophen 325 mg
Hydrocodone 7.5 mg and acetaminophen 300 mg
Hydrocodone 7.5 mg and acetaminophen 325 mg
Hydrocodone 10 mg and acetaminophen 300 mg
Hydrocodone 10 mg and acetaminophen 325 mg

Brands:

Norco®: Hydrocodone 5 mg and acetaminophen 325 mg; hydrocodone 7.5 mg and acetaminophen 325 mg; hydrocodone 10 mg and acetaminophen 325 mg

Verdrocet: Hydrocodone 2.5 mg and acetaminophen 325 mg

Vicodin®: Hydrocodone 5 mg and acetaminophen 300 mg

Vicodin ES®: Hydrocodone 7.5 mg and acetaminophen 300 mg

Vicodin HP®: Hydrocodone 10 mg and acetaminophen 300 mg

Xodol®: 5/300: Hydrocodone 5 mg and acetaminophen 300 mg; 7.5/300: Hydrocodone 7.5 mg and acetaminophen 300 mg; 10/300: Hydrocodone 10 mg and acetaminophen 300 mg

Hydrocodone and Chlorpheniramine

(hye droe KOE done & klor fen IR a meen)

Brand Names: U.S. TussiCaps; Tussionex Pennkinetic; Vituz

Index Terms Chlorpheniramine Maleate and Hydrocodone Bitartrate; Hydrocodone Polistirex and Chlorpheniramine Polistirex; Tussionex

Pharmacologic Category Alkylamine Derivative; Analgesic, Opioid; Antitussive; Histamine H_1 Antagonist; Histamine H_1 Antagonist, First Generation

Use Symptomatic relief of cough and upper respiratory symptoms associated with cold and allergy

Pregnancy Risk Factor C

Dosage Oral:

Children 6 to <12 years:

Capsules: Extended release: Hydrocodone 5 mg and chlorpheniramine 4 mg: One capsule every 12 hours (maximum: 2 capsules daily)

Suspension: Extended release: 2.5 mL every 12 hours; do not exceed 5 mL daily

Children ≥12 years, Adolescents, and Adults:

Capsules: Extended release: Hydrocodone 10 mg and chlorpheniramine 8 mg: One capsule every 12 hours (maximum: 2 capsules daily)

Suspension: Extended release: 5 mL every 12 hours; do not exceed 10 mL daily

Adults: Immediate release: Solution: 5 mL every 4-6 hours as needed; do not exceed 20 mL daily

Additional Information Complete prescribing information should be consulted for additional detail.

Dosage Forms

Capsule, extended release:

TussiCaps® 5/4: Hydrocodone bitartrate 5 mg and chlorpheniramine maleate 4 mg

TussiCaps® 10/8: Hydrocodone bitartrate 10 mg and chlorpheniramine maleate 8 mg

Solution, oral:

Vituz®: Hydrocodone bitartrate 5 mg and chlorpheniramine maleate 4 mg per 5 mL

Suspension, extended release: Hydrocodone bitartrate 10 mg and chlorpheniramine maleate 8 mg per 5 mL

Tussionex® Pennkinetic® Hydrocodone bitartrate 10 mg and chlorpheniramine maleate 8 mg per 5 mL

Hydrocodone and Homatropine

(hye droe KOE done & hoe MA troe peen)

Brand Names: U.S. Hydromet; Tussigon

Index Terms Homatropine and Hydrocodone; Hycodan; Hydrocodone Bitartrate and Homatropine Methylbromide

Pharmacologic Category Antitussive

Use Cough: Symptomatic relief of cough

Pregnancy Risk Factor C

Dosage Oral:

Children 6 to 12 years: 1/2 tablet or 2.5 mL every 4 to 6 hours as needed (maximum: 3 tablets or 15 mL/24 hours)

Children >12 years, Adolescents, and Adults: One tablet or 5 mL every 4 to 6 hours as needed (maximum: 6 tablets/24 hours or 30 mL/24 hours)

Dosage adjustment in renal impairment: There are no dosage adjustments provided in manufacturer's labeling; use with caution.

Dosage adjustment in hepatic impairment: There are no dosage adjustments provided in manufacturer's labeling; use with caution.

Additional Information Complete prescribing information should be consulted for additional detail.

Dosage Forms

Syrup:

Hydromet: Hydrocodone 5 mg and homatropine 1.5 mg per 5 mL

Generic: Hydrocodone 5 mg and homatropine 1.5 mg per 5 mL

Tablet:

Tussigon: Hydrocodone 5 mg and homatropine 1.5 mg

Generic: Hydrocodone 5 mg and homatropine 1.5 mg

Hydrocodone and Ibuprofen

(hye droe KOE done & eye byoo PROE fen)

Brand Names: U.S. Ibudone; Reprexain; Vicoprofen

Brand Names: Canada Vicoprofen

Index Terms Hydrocodone Bitartrate and Ibuprofen; Ibuprofen and Hydrocodone

Pharmacologic Category Analgesic Combination (Opioid); Nonsteroidal Anti-inflammatory Drug (NSAID), Oral

Use Pain: Short-term (generally less than 10 days) management of acute pain (not indicated for treatment of chronic conditions [eg, osteoarthritis or rheumatoid arthritis]).

Pregnancy Risk Factor C

Dosage

Pain: Oral:

Adolescents ≥16 years and Adults: One tablet (hydrocodone 2.5 mg to 10 mg/ibuprofen 200 mg) every 4 to 6 hours as needed (maximum dose: 5 tablets/24 hours). **Note:** Short-term use is recommended (<10 days total therapy).

Elderly: Use with caution and at reduced doses. Refer to adult dosing.

Dosage adjustment in renal impairment: There are no dosage adjustments provided in the manufacturer's labeling (has not been studied). Not recommended in advanced renal disease.

Dosage adjustment in hepatic impairment: There are no dosage adjustments provided in the manufacturer's labeling (has not been studied); use with caution in severe impairment.

Additional Information Complete prescribing information should be consulted for additional detail.

Dosage Forms

Tablet: Hydrocodone 2.5 mg and ibuprofen 200 mg; Hydrocodone 5 mg and ibuprofen 200 mg; Hydrocodone 7.5 mg and ibuprofen 200 mg; Hydrocodone bitartrate 10 mg and ibuprofen 200 mg

Ibudone: 5/200: Hydrocodone 5 mg and ibuprofen 200 mg; 10/200: Hydrocodone 10 mg and ibuprofen 200 mg

Reprexain: 2.5/200: Hydrocodone 2.5 mg and ibuprofen 200 mg; 5/200: Hydrocodone 5 mg and ibuprofen 200 mg; 10/200: Hydrocodone 10 mg and ibuprofen 200 mg

Vicoprofen: 7.5/200: Hydrocodone 7.5 mg and ibuprofen 200 mg

Xylon: 10/200: Hydrocodone 10 mg and ibuprofen 200 mg

◆ **Hydrocodone Bitartrate and Homatropine Methylbromide** *see* Hydrocodone and Homatropine *on page 1013*

◆ **Hydrocodone Bitartrate and Ibuprofen** *see* Hydrocodone and Ibuprofen *on page 1013*

◆ **Hydrocodone Polistirex and Chlorpheniramine Polistirex** *see* Hydrocodone and Chlorpheniramine *on page 1012*

Hydrocortisone (Systemic)

(hye droe KOR ti sone)

Brand Names: U.S. A-Hydrocort; Cortef; Solu-CORTEF

Brand Names: Canada Cortef; Solu-Cortef

Index Terms A-hydroCort; Compound F; Cortisol; Hydrocortisone Sodium Succinate

Pharmacologic Category Corticosteroid, Systemic

Additional Appendix Information

Corticosteroids Systemic Equivalencies *on page 2228*

Use Primarily as an anti-inflammatory or immunosuppressant agent in the treatment of a variety of diseases including those of dermatologic, endocrine, GI, hematologic, allergic, inflammatory, neoplastic, neurologic, ophthalmic, renal, respiratory, and autoimmune origin.

Pregnancy Risk Factor C

Dosage Dose should be based on severity of disease and patient response

Adrenal insufficiency (acute): IM, IV:
Infants and Young Children: 1-2 mg/kg/dose bolus, then 25-150 mg/day in divided doses every 6-8 hours
Older Children: 1-2 mg/kg bolus then 150-250 mg/day in divided doses every 6-8 hours
Adults (off-label dosing): 100 mg IV bolus, then 50-75 mg every 6 hours for 24 hours then slowly taper over the next 72 hours administering every 4-6 hours during taper. Alternatively, after the bolus dose, may administer as a continuous infusion at a rate of 10 mg/hour for the first 24 hours followed by a gradual reduction in dose over the next 72 hours. Once patient is stable, may change to an oral maintenance regimen. **Note:** Patients with primary adrenal insufficiency may require mineralocorticoid supplementation (eg, fludrocortisone) when shifting to an oral maintenance regimen (Gardner, 2011).

Adrenal insufficiency (chronic), physiologic replacement (off-label dosing): Adults: Oral: 15-25 mg/day in 2-3 divided doses. **Note:** Studies suggest administering one-half to two-thirds of the daily dose in the morning in order to mimic the physiological cortisol secretion pattern. If the twice-daily regimen is utilized, the second dose should be administered 6-8 hours following the first dose (Arlt, 2003).

Anti-inflammatory or immunosuppressive:
Infants and Children:
Oral: 2.5-10 mg/kg/day **or** 75-300 mg/m^2/day every 6-8 hours
IM, IV: 1-5 mg/kg/day **or** 30-150 mg/m^2/day divided every 12-24 hours
Adolescents and Adults: Oral, IM, IV: 15-240 mg every 12 hours

Congenital adrenal hyperplasia (off-label dosing): Oral: **Note:** Doses must be individualized by monitoring growth, bone age, and hormonal levels.
Children: 10-15 mg/m^2/day in 3 divided doses; higher initial doses may be required to achieve initial target hormone serum concentrations in infancy (Speiser, 2010)
Adolescents and Adults: 15-25 mg/day in 2-3 divided doses (Speiser, 2010)

Physiologic replacement: Children: Oral: 8-10 mg/m^2/day divided every 8 hours; up to 12 mg/m^2/day in some patients (Ahmet, 2011; Gupta, 2008; Maguire, 2007)

Status asthmaticus: Children and Adults: IV: 1-2 mg/kg/dose every 6 hours for 24 hours, then maintenance of 0.5-1 mg/kg every 6 hours

Stress dosing (surgery) in patients known to be adrenally-suppressed or on chronic systemic steroids: IV: Adults:
Minor stress (ie, inguinal herniorrhaphy): 25 mg/day for 1 day
Moderate stress (ie, joint replacement, cholecystectomy): 50-75 mg/day (25 mg every 8-12 hours) for 1-2 days
Major stress (pancreatoduodenectomy, esophagogastrectomy, cardiac surgery): 100-150 mg/day (50 mg every 8-12 hours) for 2-3 days

Septic shock (off-label use): IV:
Children: Initial: 1-2 mg/kg/day (intermittent or as continuous infusion); may titrate up to 50 mg/kg/day for shock reversal (Brierley, 2009); alternative dosing suggests 50 mg/m^2/day (Dellinger, 2013). **Note:** Use recommended only in fluid refractory, catecholamine-resistant shock, and suspected or proven absolute (classic) adrenal insufficiency.
Adults: 50 mg every 6 hours (Annane, 2002; COIITSS Study Investigators, 2010). Practice guidelines suggest administering 200 mg daily as a continuous infusion over 24 hours to prevent adverse effects (eg, hyperglycemia) (Dellinger, 2013; Weber-Carstens, 2007); however, the impact of continuous infusion on patient outcomes has not been formally evaluated. Taper slowly (over several days) when vasopressors are no longer required; do not stop abruptly. **Note:** Hydrocortisone should be used alone (ie, without fludrocortisone) (Dellinger, 2013).

Thyroid storm (off-label use): IV: 300 mg loading dose, followed by 100 mg every 8 hours (Bahn, 2011)

Dosage adjustment in renal impairment: There are no dosage adjustments provided in the manufacturer's labeling; use with caution.

Dosage adjustment in hepatic impairment: There are no dosage adjustments provided in the manufacturer's labeling.

Additional Information Complete prescribing information should be consulted for additional detail.

Dosage Forms

Solution Reconstituted, Injection:
A-Hydrocort: 100 mg (1 ea)
Solu-CORTEF: 100 mg (1 ea)

Solution Reconstituted, Injection [preservative free]:
Solu-CORTEF: 100 mg (1 ea); 250 mg (1 ea); 500 mg (1 ea); 1000 mg (1 ea)

Tablet, Oral:
Cortef: 5 mg, 10 mg, 20 mg
Generic: 5 mg, 10 mg, 20 mg

Hydrocortisone (Topical) (hye droe KOR ti sone)

Brand Names: U.S. Ala Cort; Ala Scalp; Anti-Itch Maximum Strength [OTC]; Anucort-HC; Anusol-HC; Aquanil HC [OTC]; Beta HC [OTC]; Colocort; Cortaid Maximum Strength [OTC]; CortAlo; Cortenema; Corticool [OTC]; Cortifoam; Dermasorb HC; First-Hydrocortisone; GRx HiCort 25; Hemril-30 [DSC]; Hydro Skin Maximum Strength [OTC]; Hydrocortisone Max St [OTC]; Hydrocortisone Max St/12 Moist [OTC]; HydroSKIN [OTC]; Instacort 10 [OTC]; Instacort 5 [OTC]; Locoid; Locoid Lipocream; Med-Derm Hydrocortisone [OTC]; Medi-First Hydrocortisone [OTC]; NuCort; NuZon [DSC]; Pandel; Pediaderm HC; Preparation H Hydrocortisone [OTC]; Procto-Pak; Proctocort; Proctosol HC; Proctozone-HC; Recort Plus [OTC]; Rectacort-HC; Rederm [OTC]; Sarnol-HC [OTC]; Scalacort; Scalacort DK; Scalpicin Maximum Strength [OTC]; Texacort; TheraCort [OTC]; Westcort

Brand Names: Canada Aquacort®; Cortamed®; Cortenema®; Cortifoam™; Emo-Cort®; Hycort™; Hyderm; HydroVal®; Locoid®; Prevex® HC; Sarna® HC; Westcort®

Index Terms A-hydroCort; Compound F; Cortisol; Hemorrhoidal HC; Hydrocortisone Acetate; Hydrocortisone Butyrate; Hydrocortisone Probutate; Hydrocortisone Valerate; Nutracort

Pharmacologic Category Antihemorrhoidal Agent; Corticosteroid, Rectal; Corticosteroid, Topical

Use Relief of inflammation of corticosteroid-responsive dermatoses (low and medium potency topical corticosteroid); adjunctive treatment of ulcerative colitis; mild-to-moderate atopic dermatitis; inflamed hemorrhoids, postirradiation (factitial) proctitis, and other inflammatory conditions of anorectum and pruritus ani

Pregnancy Risk Factor C

Dosage

Topical:
Children 3 months to 18 years: Atopic dermatitis: Hydrocortisone butyrate (Locoid Lipocream®): Apply thin film to affected area twice daily
Children and Adults: Dermatosis: Apply thin film to affected area 2-4 times/day. Products labeled for OTC use (self-medication) should not be used in children <2 years of age.
Children ≥12 years and Adults: External anal and genital itching: (OTC labeling): Apply to clean dry skin up to 3-4 times/day

Adults: Dermatosis:
Hydrocortisone probutate (Pandel®): Apply thin film to affected area 1-2 times/day
Hydrocortisone valerate (Westcort®): Apply thin film to affected area 2-3 times/day
Rectal: Adults:
Hemorrhoids: Suppository: One suppository (30 mg) twice daily for 2 weeks. For severe cases of proctitis, 1 suppository 3 times/day or 2 suppositories twice daily may be needed. For factitial proctitis, duration of treatment may be up to 6-8 weeks.
Ulcerative colitis:
Foam: One applicatorful (80 mg) 1-2 times/day for 2-3 weeks, and then every other day thereafter; use lowest dose to maintain clinical response; taper dose to discontinue long-term therapy
Suspension: One enema (100 mg) every night for 21 days or until remission (clinical improvement may precede improvement of mucosal integrity); 2-3 months of therapy may be required; taper dose to discontinue long-term therapy

Additional Information Complete prescribing information should be consulted for additional detail.

Dosage Forms

Cream, External:
Ala Cort: 1% (28.4 g, 85.2 g)
Anti-Itch Maximum Strength [OTC]: 1% (28 g)
Cortaid Maximum Strength [OTC]: 1% (14 g, 28 g)
Hydrocortisone Max St [OTC]: 1% (28.4 g)
Hydrocortisone Max St/12 Moist [OTC]: 1% (28.4 g)
HydroSKIN [OTC]: 1% (28 g)
Instacort 5 [OTC]: 0.5% (28.4 g)
Locoid: 0.1% (15 g, 45 g)
Locoid Lipocream: 0.1% (45 g, 60 g)
Med-Derm Hydrocortisone [OTC]: 0.5% (30 g); 1% (30 g)
Medi-First Hydrocortisone [OTC]: 1% (1 ea)
Pandel: 0.1% (15 g, 45 g, 80 g)
Preparation H Hydrocortisone [OTC]: 1% (26 g)
Recort Plus [OTC]: 1% (30 g)
Generic: 0.1% (15 g, 45 g, 60 g); 0.2% (15 g, 45 g, 60 g); 0.5% (15 g, 28.35 g, 28.4 g, 30 g); 1% (1 g, 1.5 g, 14.2 g, 20 g, 28 g, 28.35 g, 28.4 g, 30 g, 120 g, 453.6 g, 454 g); 2.5% (20 g, 28 g, 28.35 g, 30 g, 453.6 g)

Cream, Rectal:
Anusol-HC: 2.5% (30 g)
Procto-Pak: 1% (28.4 g)
Proctocort: 1% (28.35 g)
Proctosol HC: 2.5% (28.35 g)
Proctozone-HC: 2.5% (30 g)

Enema, Rectal:
Colocort: 100 mg/60 mL (60 mL)
Cortenema: 100 mg/60 mL (60 mL)
Generic: 100 mg/60 mL (60 mL)

Foam, Rectal:
Cortifoam: 90 mg (15 g)

Gel, External:
CortAlo: 2% (43 g)
Corticool [OTC]: 1% (42.53 g)
First-Hydrocortisone: 10% (60 g)
Instacort 10 [OTC]: 1% (30 g)

Kit, External:
Dermasorb HC: 2%
Pediaderm HC: 2%
Scalacort DK: Hydrocortisone lotion 2% and Sal Acid 2% and sulfur 2%

Lotion, External:
Ala Scalp: 2% (29.6 mL)
Aquanil HC [OTC]: 1% (120 mL)
Beta HC [OTC]: 1% (60 mL)
Hydro Skin Maximum Strength [OTC]: 1% (118 mL)
Locoid: 0.1% (59 mL, 118 mL)
NuCort: 2% (60 g)
Rederm [OTC]: 1% (120 mL)
Sarnol-HC [OTC]: 1% (59 mL)
Scalacort: 2% (29.6 mL)
TheraCort [OTC]: 1% (118 mL)
Generic: 1% (114 g); 2.5% (59 mL, 118 mL)

Ointment, External:
Locoid: 0.1% (15 g, 45 g)
Westcort: 0.2% (15 g, 45 g, 60 g)
Generic: 0.1% (15 g, 45 g); 0.2% (15 g, 45 g, 60 g); 0.5% (28.35 g, 30 g); 1% (25 g, 28 g, 28.35 g, 28.4 g, 30 g, 110 g, 430 g, 453.6 g); 2.5% (20 g, 28.35 g, 453.6 g, 454 g)

Solution, External:
Locoid: 0.1% (60 mL)
Scalpicin Maximum Strength [OTC]: 1% (44 mL)
Texacort: 2.5% (30 mL)
Generic: 0.1% (20 mL, 60 mL)

Suppository, Rectal:
Anucort-HC: 25 mg (12 ea, 24 ea, 100 ea)
Anusol-HC: 25 mg (12 ea, 24 ea)
GRx HiCort 25: 25 mg (12 ea)
Proctocort: 30 mg (12 ea)
Rectacort-HC: 25 mg (12 ea, 24 ea)
Generic: 25 mg (12 ea, 24 ea); 30 mg (12 ea)

- ◆ **Hydrocortisone Acetate** *see* Hydrocortisone (Topical) *on page 1014*
- ◆ **Hydrocortisone, Acetic Acid, and Propylene Glycol Diacetate** *see* Acetic Acid, Propylene Glycol Diacetate, and Hydrocortisone *on page 40*
- ◆ **Hydrocortisone and Benzoyl Peroxide** *see* Benzoyl Peroxide and Hydrocortisone *on page 248*
- ◆ **Hydrocortisone and Ciprofloxacin** *see* Ciprofloxacin and Hydrocortisone *on page 446*
- ◆ **Hydrocortisone and Iodoquinol** *see* Iodoquinol and Hydrocortisone *on page 1105*
- ◆ **Hydrocortisone and Pramoxine** *see* Pramoxine and Hydrocortisone *on page 1698*
- ◆ **Hydrocortisone and Urea** *see* Urea and Hydrocortisone *on page 2115*
- ◆ **Hydrocortisone, Bacitracin, Neomycin, and Polymyxin B** *see* Bacitracin, Neomycin, Polymyxin B, and Hydrocortisone *on page 223*
- ◆ **Hydrocortisone Butyrate** *see* Hydrocortisone (Topical) *on page 1014*
- ◆ **Hydrocortisone Max St [OTC]** *see* Hydrocortisone (Topical) *on page 1014*
- ◆ **Hydrocortisone Max St/12 Moist [OTC]** *see* Hydrocortisone (Topical) *on page 1014*
- ◆ **Hydrocortisone, Neomycin, and Polymyxin B** *see* Neomycin, Polymyxin B, and Hydrocortisone *on page 1438*
- ◆ **Hydrocortisone, Neomycin, Colistin, and Thonzonium** *see* Neomycin, Colistin, Hydrocortisone, and Thonzonium *on page 1437*
- ◆ **Hydrocortisone Probutate** *see* Hydrocortisone (Topical) *on page 1014*
- ◆ **Hydrocortisone Sodium Succinate** *see* Hydrocortisone (Systemic) *on page 1013*
- ◆ **Hydrocortisone Valerate** *see* Hydrocortisone (Topical) *on page 1014*
- ◆ **Hydrodiuril** *see* Hydrochlorothiazide *on page 1009*
- ◆ **Hydromet** *see* Hydrocodone and Homatropine *on page 1013*
- ◆ **Hydromorph Contin (Can)** *see* HYDROmorphone *on page 1016*

HYDROmorphone (hye droe MOR fone)

Brand Names: U.S. Dilaudid; Dilaudid-HP; Exalgo

Brand Names: Canada Apo-Hydromorphone; Dilaudid; Dilaudid-HP; Hydromorph Contin; Hydromorphone HP; Hydromorphone HP 10; Hydromorphone HP 20; Hydromorphone HP 50; Hydromorphone HP Forte; Hydromorphone Hydrochloride Injection, USP; Jurnista; PMS-Hydromorphone; Teva-Hydromorphone

Index Terms Dihydromorphinone; Hydromorphone Hydrochloride

Pharmacologic Category Analgesic, Opioid

Additional Appendix Information

Opioid Conversion Table *on page 2232*

Use

Pain:

Immediate release formulation, injection, suppository: Management of moderate-to-severe pain

Extended release tablets: Management of pain in opioid tolerant patients severe enough to require daily, around-the-clock, long-term opioid treatment and for which alternative treatment options are inadequate

Limitations of use:

Because of the risks of addiction, abuse, and misuse with opioids, even at recommended doses, and because of the greater risks of overdose and death with extended-release opioid formulations, reserve for use in patients for whom alternative treatment options (eg, nonopioid analgesics, immediate-release opioids) are ineffective, not tolerated, or would be otherwise inadequate to provide sufficient management of pain

Not indicated as an as-needed analgesic

Pregnancy Risk Factor C

Pregnancy Considerations Adverse events were observed in some animal reproduction studies. Hydromorphone crosses the placenta. Some dosage forms are specifically contraindicated for use in obstetrical analgesia.

When used for pain relief during labor, opioids may temporarily affect the heart rate of the fetus (ACOG, 2002). Monitor the neonate for respiratory depression if hydromorphone is used during labor.

[U.S. Boxed Warning]: Prolonged maternal use of opioids during pregnancy can cause neonatal withdrawal syndrome in the newborn which may be life-threatening if not recognized and treated according to protocols developed by neonatology experts. If prolonged opioid therapy is required in a pregnant woman, ensure treatment is available and warn patient of risk to the neonate. If chronic opioid exposure occurs in pregnancy, adverse events in the newborn (including withdrawal) may occur; monitoring of the neonate is recommended. The minimum effective dose should be used if opioids are needed (Chou, 2009). Neonatal abstinence syndrome following opioid exposure may present with autonomic (eg, fever, temperature instability), gastrointestinal (eg, diarrhea, vomiting, poor feeding/weight gain), or neurologic (eg, high pitched crying, increased muscle tone, irritability, seizure, tremor) symptoms (Dow, 2012; Hudak, 2012).

Long-term opioid use may cause secondary hypogonadism, which may lead to sexual dysfunction or infertility (Brennan, 2013).

Breast-Feeding Considerations Low concentrations of hydromorphone can be found in breast milk. Withdrawal symptoms may be observed in breast-feeding infants when opioid analgesics are discontinued. Breast-feeding is not recommended by the manufacturer. Parenteral opioids used during labor have the potential to interfere with a newborn's natural reflex to nurse within the first few hours after birth. Nursing infants exposed to large doses of opioids should be monitored for apnea and sedation (Montgomery, 2012).

Contraindications Hypersensitivity to hydromorphone, any component of the formulation; acute or severe asthma, severe respiratory depression (in absence of resuscitative equipment or ventilatory support)

Additional product-specific contraindications:

Dilaudid liquid and tablets: Obstetrical analgesia

Dilaudid injection, Dilaudid-HP injection: Opioid nontolerant patients (Dilaudid-HP injection only); patients with risk of developing GI obstruction, especially paralytic ileus

Exalgo: Opioid nontolerant patients, paralytic ileus (known or suspected), preexisting GI surgery or diseases resulting in narrowing of GI tract, loops in the GI tract or GI obstruction

Suppository: Intracranial lesion associated with increased intracranial pressure; whenever ventilatory function is depressed (COPD, cor pulmonale, emphysema, kyphoscoliosis, status asthmaticus)

Warnings/Precautions Use with caution in patients with hypersensitivity reactions to other phenanthrene derivative opioid agonists (codeine, hydrocodone, levorphanol, oxycodone, oxymorphone). Hydromorphone shares toxic potential of opioid agonists, including CNS depression and respiratory depression. Precautions associated with opioid agonist therapy should be observed. May cause CNS depression, which may impair physical or mental abilities; patients must be cautioned about performing tasks which require mental alertness (eg, operating machinery or driving). Myoclonus and seizures have been reported with high doses; use with caution in patients with a history of seizure disorder. Use with caution in patients with cardiovascular disease, morbid obesity, adrenocortical insufficiency, hypothyroidism, acute alcoholism, delirium tremens, toxic psychoses, prostatic hyperplasia and/or urinary stricture, or severe liver or renal failure. Use with caution and monitor for respiratory depression in patients with significant chronic obstructive pulmonary disease or cor pulmonale, and patients having a substantially decreased respiratory reserve, hypoxia, hypercarbia, or preexisting respiratory depression, particularly when initiating therapy and titrating with hydromorphone; even therapeutic doses may decrease respiratory drive to the point of apnea. Consider the use of alternative nonopioid analgesics in these patients. Avoid use in patients with CNS depression or coma as these patients are susceptible to intracranial effects of CO_2 retention. Use with caution in patients with biliary tract dysfunction. Hydromorphone may increase biliary tract pressure following spasm in sphincter of Oddi. Use caution in patients with inflammatory or obstructive bowel disorder, acute pancreatitis secondary to biliary tract disease, and patients undergoing biliary surgery. Use extreme caution in patients with head injury, intracranial lesions, or elevated intracranial pressure; exaggerated elevation of ICP may occur (in addition, hydromorphone may complicate neurologic evaluation due to pupillary dilation and CNS depressant effects). Use with caution in patients with depleted blood volume or drugs which may exaggerate hypotensive effects (including phenothiazines or general anesthetics). May obscure diagnosis or clinical course of patients with acute abdominal conditions. Effects may be potentiated when used with other CNS depressants (eg, sedatives, anxiolytics, hypnotics, neuroleptics, other opioids). Potentially significant interactions may exist, requiring dose or frequency adjustment, additional monitoring, and/or selection of alternative therapy.

An opioid-containing analgesic regimen should be tailored to each patient's needs and based upon the type of pain being treated (acute versus chronic), the route of administration, degree of tolerance for opioids (naive versus chronic user), age, weight, and medical condition. The optimal analgesic dose varies widely among patients. Doses should be titrated to pain relief/prevention. IM use may result in variable absorption and a lag time to peak effect. Concurrent use of mixed agonist/antagonist analgesics (eg, pentazocine, nalbuphine, butorphanol) or partial agonist (eg, buprenorphine) analgesics may precipitate withdrawal symptoms and/or reduced analgesic efficacy in patients following prolonged therapy with mu opioid agonists. Abrupt discontinuation following prolonged use may also lead to withdrawal symptoms.

Dosage form specific warnings:

Some dosage forms contain trace amounts of sodium metabisulfite which may cause allergic reactions in susceptible individuals.

Immediate release formulations: **[U.S. Boxed Warning]: High potential for abuse and risk of producing respiratory depression. Alcohol, other opioids, and CNS depressants potentiate the respiratory depressant effects of hydromorphone, increasing the risk of respiratory depression that might result in death.**

Injection: Vial stoppers of single-dose injectable vials may contain latex. **[U.S. Boxed Warning]: Dilaudid-HP: Extreme caution should be taken to avoid confusing the highly-concentrated (Dilaudid-HP) injection with the less-concentrated (Dilaudid) injectable product.** Dilaudid-HP should only be used in patients who are opioid-tolerant.

Controlled release capsules (Canadian labeling): Capsules should only be used when continuous analgesia is required over an extended period of time. Controlled release products are not to be used on an "as needed" (PRN) basis.

Extended release tablets: **[U.S. Boxed Warning]: May cause serious, life-threatening, or fatal respiratory depression. Monitor closely for respiratory depression, especially during initiation or dose escalation. Patients should swallow tablets whole; crushing, chewing, or dissolving can cause rapid release and a potentially fatal dose.** Carbon dioxide retention from opioid-induced respiratory depression can exacerbate the sedating effects of opioids. **[U.S. Boxed Warning]: Users are exposed to the risks of addiction, abuse, and misuse, potentially leading to overdose and death. Assess each patient's risk prior to prescribing; monitor all patients regularly for development of these behaviors or conditions.** Risk of opioid abuse is increased in patients with a history or family history of alcohol or drug abuse or mental illness. Tolerance or drug dependence may result from extended use; however, concerns for abuse should not prevent effective management of pain. In general, abrupt discontinuation of therapy in dependent patients should be avoided. **[U.S. Boxed Warning]: Prolonged maternal use of opioids during pregnancy can cause neonatal withdrawal syndrome in the newborn which may be life-threatening if not recognized and treated according to protocols developed by neonatology experts. If prolonged opioid therapy is required in a pregnant woman, ensure treatment is available and warn patient of risk to the neonate.** Signs and symptoms include irritability, hyperactivity and abnormal sleep pattern, high pitched cry, tremor, vomiting, diarrhea and failure to gain weight. Onset, duration and severity depend on the drug used, duration of use, maternal dose, and rate of drug elimination by the newborn. Therapy should only be prescribed by healthcare professionals familiar with the use of potent opioids for chronic pain. Exalgo tablets are nondeformable; do not administer to patients with preexisting severe gastrointestinal narrowing (eg, esophageal motility, small bowel inflammatory disease, short gut syndrome, history of peritonitis, cystic fibrosis, chronic intestinal pseudo-obstruction, Meckel's diverticulum); obstruction may occur. Tablets may be visible on abdominal x-rays, especially when digital enhancing techniques are used.

Adverse Reactions

Cardiovascular: Bradycardia, extrasystoles, flushing (facial), hypertension, hypotension, palpitations, peripheral edema, peripheral vasodilation, syncope, tachycardia

Central nervous system: Abnormal dreams, abnormal gait, abnormality in thinking, aggressive behavior, agitation, apprehension, ataxia, brain disease, burning sensation of skin (Exalgo), central nervous system depression, chills, cognitive dysfunction, confusion, decreased body temperature (Exalgo), depression, disruption of body temperature regulation (Exalgo), dizziness, drowsiness, drug dependence, dysarthria, dysphoria, equilibrium disturbance, euphoria, fatigue, hallucination, headache, hyperesthesia, hyperreflexia, hypoesthesia, hypothermia, increased intracranial pressure, insomnia, lack of concentration, lethargy, malaise, memory impairment, mood changes, myoclonus, nervousness, painful defecation, panic attack, paranoia, paresthesia, psychomotor agitation, restlessness, sedation, seizure, sleep disorder (Exalgo), suicidal ideation, uncontrolled crying, vertigo

Dermatologic: Diaphoresis, erythema (Exalgo), hyperhidrosis, pruritus, skin rash, urticaria

Endocrine & metabolic: Antidiuretic effect, decreased amylase, decreased libido, decreased plasma testosterone, dehydration, fluid retention, hyperuricemia, hypokalemia, weight loss

Gastrointestinal: Abdominal distention, anal fissure, anorexia, bezoar formation (Exalgo), biliary tract spasm, constipation, decreased appetite, decreased gastrointestinal motility (Exalgo), delayed gastric emptying, diarrhea, diverticulitis, diverticulosis, duodenitis, dysgeusia, dysphagia, eructation, flatulence, gastroenteritis, gastroesophageal reflux disease (aggravated; Exalgo), hematochezia, increased appetite, intestinal perforation (large intestine; Exalgo), nausea, paralytic ileus, stomach cramps, vomiting, xerostomia

Genitourinary: Bladder spasm, decreased urine output, difficulty in micturition, dysuria, erectile dysfunction, hypogonadism, sexual disorder, ureteral spasm, urinary frequency, urinary hesitancy, urinary retention

Hematologic & oncologic: Oxygen desaturation

Hepatic: Increased liver enzymes

Hypersensitivity: Histamine release

Local: Pain at injection site, post-injection flare

Neuromuscular & skeletal: Arthralgia, dyskinesia, laryngospasm, muscle rigidity, muscle spasm, myalgia, tremor, weakness

Ophthalmic: Blurred vision, diplopia, dry eye syndrome, miosis, nystagmus

Otic: Tinnitus

Respiratory: Apnea, bronchospasm, dyspnea, flu-like symptoms (Exalgo), hyperventilation, hypoxia, respiratory depression, respiratory distress, rhinorrhea

Rare but important or life-threatening: Angioedema, hypersensitivity

Drug Interactions

Metabolism/Transport Effects None known.

Avoid Concomitant Use

Avoid concomitant use of HYDROmorphone with any of the following: Azelastine (Nasal); MAO Inhibitors; Orphenadrine; Paraldehyde; Thalidomide

Increased Effect/Toxicity

HYDROmorphone may increase the levels/effects of: Alcohol (Ethyl); Alvimopan; Azelastine (Nasal); Buprenorphine; CNS Depressants; Desmopressin; Diuretics;

Hydrocodone; Methotrimeprazine; Metyrosine; Mirtazapine; Orphenadrine; Paraldehyde; Pramipexole; ROPINIRole; Rotigotine; Selective Serotonin Reuptake Inhibitors; Suvorexant; Thalidomide; Zolpidem

The levels/effects of HYDROmorphone may be increased by: Amphetamines; Anticholinergic Agents; Antipsychotic Agents (Phenothiazines); Brimonidine (Topical); Cannabis; Doxylamine; Dronabinol; Droperidol; HydrOXYzine; Kava Kava; Magnesium Sulfate; MAO Inhibitors; Methotrimeprazine; Nabilone; Perampanel; Rufinamide; Sodium Oxybate; Succinylcholine; Tapentadol; Tetrahydrocannabinol

Decreased Effect

HYDROmorphone may decrease the levels/effects of: Pegvisomant

The levels/effects of HYDROmorphone may be decreased by: Ammonium Chloride; Mixed Agonist / Antagonist Opioids; Naltrexone

Storage/Stability

Injection: Store at 15°C to 30°C (59°F to 86°F). A slightly yellowish discoloration has not been associated with a loss of potency. Stable for at least 24 hours when protected from light and stored at 25°C in most common large volume parenteral solutions.

Oral dosage forms: Store at 15°C to 30°C (59°F to 86°F). Protect tablets from light.

Suppository: Store in refrigerator. Protect from light.

Mechanism of Action Binds to opioid receptors in the CNS, causing inhibition of ascending pain pathways, altering the perception of and response to pain; causes cough supression by direct central action in the medulla; produces generalized CNS depression

Pharmacodynamics/Kinetics

Onset of action: Analgesic:
- Immediate release formulations:
  - Oral: 15 to 30 minutes; Peak effect: 30 to 60 minutes
  - IV: 5 minutes; Peak effect: 10 to 20 minutes
- Extended release tablet: 6 hours; Peak effect: ~9 hours (Angst, 2001)

Duration:
- Immediate release formulations: Oral, IV: 3 to 4 hours
- Extended release tablet: ~13 hours (Angst, 2001)

Absorption: Extended release tablet: Delayed; IM: Variable and delayed

Distribution: V_d: 4 L/kg

Protein binding: ~8% to 19%

Metabolism: Hepatic via glucuronidation; to inactive metabolites

Bioavailability: 62%

Half-life elimination:
- Immediate release formulations: 2 to 3 hours
- Extended release tablets: Apparent half-life: ~11 hours (range: 8 to 15 hours)

Time to peak, plasma:
- Immediate release tablet: ≤1 hour
- Extended release tablet: 12 to 16 hours

Excretion: Urine (primarily as glucuronide conjugates)

Dosage

Acute pain (moderate-to-severe): Note: These are guidelines and do not represent the maximum doses that may be required in all patients. Doses should be titrated to provide adequate pain relief. When changing routes of administration, oral doses and parenteral doses are **NOT** equivalent; parenteral doses are up to 5 times more potent. Therefore, when administered parenterally, one-fifth of the oral dose will provide similar analgesia.

Children >50 kg and Adults:

Oral: Immediate release: Initial: Opioid-naive: 2 to 4 mg every 4 to 6 hours as needed; elderly/debilitated patients may require lower doses; patients with prior opioid exposure may require higher initial doses. **Note:** In adults with severe pain, the American Pain Society recommends an initial dose of 4 to 8 mg.

IV: Initial: Opioid-naive: 0.2 to 1 mg every 2 to 3 hours as needed; patients with prior opioid exposure may require higher initial doses

Critically ill patients (off-label dosing): 0.2 to 0.6 mg every 1 to 2 hours as needed **or** 0.5 mg every 3 hours as needed (Barr, 2013)

Continuous infusion: Usual dosage range: 0.5 to 3 mg/hour (Barr, 2013)

Patient-controlled analgesia (PCA) (off-label dosing) (American Pain Society, 2008): **Note:** Opioid-naive: Consider lower end of dosing range. A continuous (basal) infusion is not recommended in opioid-naive patients (ISMP, 2009):
- Usual concentration: 0.2 mg/mL
- Demand dose: Usual initial dose: 0.2 mg; range: 0.05 to 0.4 mg
- Lockout interval: 5 to 10 minutes

Epidural PCA (off-label dosing) (de Leon-Casasola, 1996; Liu, 2010; Smith, 2009):
- Usual concentration: 0.01 mg/mL
- Bolus dose: 0.4 to 1 mg
- Infusion rate: 0.03 to 0.3 mg/**hour**
- Demand dose: 0.02 to 0.05 mg
- Lockout interval: 10 to 15 minutes

IM, SubQ: **Note:** IM use may result in variable absorption and lag time to peak effect; IM route not recommended for use (American Pain Society, 2008)

Initial: Opioid-naive: 0.8 to 1 mg every 3 to 4 hours as needed; patients with prior opioid exposure may require higher initial doses

Rectal: 3 mg every 6 to 8 hours as needed

Elderly: Acute pain, opioid-naive:

Oral: Use with caution; initiation at the low end of dosage range is recommended. For patients >70 years, The American Pain Society recommends consideration to lowering initial doses by 25% to 50% followed by upward or downward titration (APS, 2008).

IV: Reduce initial dose to 0.2 mg

Chronic pain: Adults: Oral: **Note:** Patients taking opioids chronically may become tolerant and require doses higher than the usual dosage range to maintain the desired effect. Tolerance can be managed by appropriate dose titration. There is no optimal or maximal dose for hydromorphone in chronic pain. The appropriate dose is one that relieves pain throughout its dosing interval without causing unmanageable side effects.

Controlled release capsule (Hydromorph Contin, not available in U.S.): 3 to 30 mg every 12 hours. **Note:** A patient's hydromorphone requirement should be established using prompt release formulations; conversion to long acting products may be considered when chronic, continuous treatment is required. Higher dosages should be reserved for use only in opioid-tolerant patients.

Extended release tablet (Exalgo): **Note:** For use in opioid-tolerant patients only. Patients considered opioid tolerant are those who are receiving, for one week or longer, at least 60 mg oral morphine daily, 25 mcg transdermal fentanyl per hour, 30 mg oral oxycodone daily, 8 mg oral hydromorphone daily, 25 mg oral oxymorphone daily, or an equianalgesic dose of another opioid.

Opioid-tolerant patients: Discontinue or taper all other extended release opioids when starting therapy.

Individualization of dose: Suggested recommendations for converting to Exalgo from other analgesics are presented, but when selecting the initial dose, other characteristics (eg, patient status, degree of opioid tolerance, concurrent medications, type of pain, risk factors for addiction, abuse, and misuse) should also be considered. Pain relief and adverse events should be assessed frequently.

Conversion from other oral hydromorphone formulations to Exalgo: Start with the equivalent total daily dose of immediate-release hydromorphone administered once daily.

Conversion from other opioids to Exalgo: Discontinue all other around-the-clock opioids when therapy is initiated. Substantial interpatient variability exists in relative potency. Therefore, it is safer to underestimate a patient's daily oral hydromorphone requirement and provide breakthrough pain relief with rescue medication (eg, immediate release opioid) than to overestimate requirements. In general, start Exalgo at 50% of the calculated total daily dose every 24 hours (see Conversion Factors to Exalgo). The following conversion ratios may be used to convert from **oral** opioid therapy to Exalgo.

Conversion factors to Exalgo (see table): Select the opioid, sum the current total daily dose, multiply by the conversion factor on the table to calculate the *approximate* oral hydromorphone daily dose, then calculate the approximate starting dose for Exalgo at 50% of the calculated oral hydromorphone daily dose; administer every 24 hours. Round down, if necessary, to the nearest strength available. For patients on a regimen of more than one opioid, calculate the approximate oral hydromorphone dose for each opioid and sum the totals to obtain the approximate total hydromorphone daily dose. For patients on a regimen of fixed-ratio opioid/nonopioid analgesic medications, only the opioid component of these medications should be used in the conversion. **Note:** The conversion factors in this conversion table are only to be used for the conversion from current oral opioid therapy to Exalgo. Conversion factors in this table cannot be used to convert from Exalgo to another oral opioid (doing so may lead to fatal overdose due to overestimation of the new opioid). This is not a table of equianalgesic doses.

Conversion Factors to Exalgo[1]

Previous Oral Opioid	Oral Conversion Factor
Hydromorphone	1
Codeine	0.06
Hydrocodone	0.4
Methadone[2]	0.6
Morphine	0.2
Oxycodone	0.4
Oxymorphone	0.6

[1]Conversion factors for the conversion from one of the listed current oral opioid agents to Exalgo.

[2]Monitor closely; ratio between methadone and other opioid agonists may vary widely as a function of previous drug exposure. Methadone has a long half-life and may accumulate in the plasma.

Conversion from transdermal fentanyl to Exalgo: Treatment with Exalgo can be started 18 hours after the removal of the transdermal fentanyl patch. For every fentanyl 25 mcg/hour transdermal dose, the equianalgesic dose of Exalgo is 12 mg every 24 hours. An appropriate starting dose is 50% of the calculated total daily dose given every 24 hours. If necessary, round down to the appropriate Exalgo tablet strength available.

Titration and maintenance: Dose adjustments in 4 to 8 mg increments may occur every 3 to 4 days. In patients experiencing breakthrough pain, consider increasing the dose of Exalgo or providing rescue medication of an immediate-release analgesic at an appropriate dose. Do not administer Exalgo more frequently than every 24 hours.

Discontinuing Exalgo: Taper by gradually decreasing the dose by 25% to 50% every 2 to 3 days to a dose of 8 mg every 24 hours before discontinuing therapy.

Dosing adjustment in renal impairment:

Oral (immediate release), injectable: Initiate with 25% to 50% of the usual starting dose depending on the degree of impairment. Monitor closely for respiratory and CNS depression.

Oral (extended release; Exalgo):

Moderate impairment (CrCl 30 to 60 mL/minute): Initiate with 50% of the usual starting dose for patients with normal renal function; monitor closely for respiratory and CNS depression.

Severe impairment (CrCl <30 mL/minute): Initiate with 25% of the usual starting dose for patients with normal renal function; monitor closely for respiratory and CNS depression. Consider use of an alternate analgesic with better dosing flexibility.

Dosing adjustment in hepatic impairment:

Oral (immediate release), injectable:

Moderate impairment: Initiate with 25% to 50% of the usual starting dose for patients with normal hepatic function.

Severe impairment: Has not been studied; initial dose should be more conservative as compared to those with moderate impairment; use with caution.

Oral (extended release; Exalgo):

Moderate impairment: Initiate with 25% of the usual starting dose for patients with normal hepatic function; monitor closely for respiratory and CNS depression.

Severe impairment: Use alternate analgesic.

Administration

Parenteral: **Note: Vial stopper may contain latex.** May be given SubQ or IM; IM route is not recommended (APS, 2008).

IV: For IVP, must be given slowly over 2 to 3 minutes (rapid IVP has been associated with an increase in side effects, especially respiratory depression and hypotension)

Oral: Hydromorphone is available in an 8 mg immediate release tablet and an 8 mg extended release tablet. Extreme caution should be taken to avoid confusing dosage forms.

Exalgo: Tablets should be swallowed whole; do not crush, break, chew, dissolve or inject. May be taken with or without food.

Hydromorph Contin: Capsule should be swallowed whole; do not crush or chew; contents may be sprinkled on soft food and swallowed

Monitoring Parameters Pain relief, respiratory and mental status, blood pressure; signs or symptoms of hypogonadism or hypoadrenalism (Brennan, 2013)

Additional Information Equianalgesic doses: Morphine 10 mg IM = hydromorphone 1.5 mg IM

Exalgo is indicated for the management of moderate-to-severe pain in opioid-tolerant patients (requiring around-the-clock analgesia for an extended period of time). Patients are considered to be opioid tolerant if they have been taking oral morphine ≥60 mg/day, fentanyl transdermal ≥25 mcg/hour, oral oxycodone ≥30 mg/day, oral hydromorphone ≥8 mg/day, oral oxymorphone ≥25 mg/day, or an equianalgesic dose of another opioid for ≥1 week.

Dosage Forms

Liquid, Oral:

Dilaudid: 1 mg/mL (473 mL)

Generic: 1 mg/mL (473 mL)

Solution, Injection:

Dilaudid: 1 mg/mL (1 mL); 2 mg/mL (1 mL); 4 mg/mL (1 mL)

Dilaudid-HP: 10 mg/mL (1 mL, 5 mL, 50 mL)

Generic: 1 mg/mL (0.5 mL, 1 mL); 2 mg/mL (1 mL, 20 mL); 4 mg/mL (1 mL); 10 mg/mL (1 mL); 50 mg/5 mL (5 mL); 500 mg/50 mL (50 mL)

Solution, Injection [preservative free]:

Generic: 10 mg/mL (1 mL); 50 mg/5 mL (5 mL); 500 mg/50 mL (50 mL)

Solution Reconstituted, Injection:

Dilaudid-HP: 250 mg (1 ea)

Suppository, Rectal:

Generic: 3 mg (6 ea)

Tablet, Oral:

Dilaudid: 2 mg, 4 mg, 8 mg

Generic: 2 mg, 4 mg, 8 mg

Tablet ER 24 Hour Abuse-Deterrent, Oral:

Exalgo: 8 mg, 12 mg, 16 mg, 32 mg

Generic: 8 mg, 12 mg, 16 mg, 32 mg

Dosage Forms: Canada

Capsule, controlled release:

Hydromorph Contin: 3 mg, 6 mg, 12 mg, 18 mg, 24 mg, 30 mg [not available in U.S.]

◆ **Hydromorphone HP (Can)** *see* HYDROmorphone *on page 1016*

◆ **Hydromorphone HP 10 (Can)** *see* HYDROmorphone *on page 1016*

◆ **Hydromorphone HP 20 (Can)** *see* HYDROmorphone *on page 1016*

◆ **Hydromorphone HP 50 (Can)** *see* HYDROmorphone *on page 1016*

◆ **Hydromorphone HP Forte (Can)** *see* HYDROmorphone *on page 1016*

◆ **Hydromorphone Hydrochloride** *see* HYDROmorphone *on page 1016*

◆ **Hydromorphone Hydrochloride Injection, USP (Can)** *see* HYDROmorphone *on page 1016*

◆ **Hydroquinol** *see* Hydroquinone *on page 1020*

Hydroquinone (HYE droe kwin one)

Brand Names: U.S. Aclaro; Aclaro PD; Alphaquin HP; Eldopaque Forte [DSC]; Eldopaque [OTC] [DSC]; Eldoquin Forte [DSC]; Eldoquin [OTC] [DSC]; EpiQuin Micro; Esoterica Daytime [OTC]; Esoterica Facial [OTC]; Esoterica Fade Nighttime [OTC]; Esoterica Sensitive Skin [OTC]; Exuviance Lightening Complex [OTC]; Hydroquinone Time Release; Lustra; Lustra-AF; Lustra-Ultra; Melpaque HP; Melquin 3; Melquin HP; NAVA-SC; NeoCeuticals Post-Acne Fade [OTC]; NeoStrata HQ Skin Lightening [OTC]; Nuquin HP; Remergent HQ; Skin Bleaching; Skin Bleaching-Sunscreen; TL Hydroquinone

Brand Names: Canada Eldopaque®; Eldoquin®; Glyquin® XM; Lustra®; NeoStrata® HQ; Solaquin Forte®; Solaquin®; Ultraquin™

Index Terms Hydroquinol; Quinol

Pharmacologic Category Depigmenting Agent

Use Gradual bleaching of hyperpigmented skin conditions

Pregnancy Risk Factor C

Dosage Children >12 years and Adults: Topical: Apply thin layer and rub in twice daily

Additional Information Complete prescribing information should be consulted for additional detail.

Dosage Forms

Cream, External:

Alphaquin HP: 4% (28.4 g, 56.7 g)

EpiQuin Micro: 4% (30 g)

Esoterica Daytime [OTC]: 2% (70 g)

Esoterica Facial [OTC]: 2% (85 g)

Esoterica Fade Nighttime [OTC]: 2% (70 g)

Esoterica Sensitive Skin [OTC]: 1.5% (85 g)

Hydroquinone Time Release: 4% (30 g)

Lustra: 4% (56.8 g)

Lustra-AF: 4% (56.8 g)

Lustra-Ultra: 4% (28.4 g, 56.8 g)

Melpaque HP: 4% (28.4 g)

Melquin HP: 4% (28.4 g)

NAVA-SC: 4% (28.4 g)

Nuquin HP: 4% (28.4 g, 56.7 g)

Remergent HQ: 4% (30 mL)

Skin Bleaching: 4% (28.35 g)

Skin Bleaching-Sunscreen: 4% (28.35 g)

TL Hydroquinone: 4% (30 g)

Generic: 4% (28.35 g)

Emulsion, External:

Aclaro: 4% (48.2 g)

Aclaro PD: 4% (42.5 g)

Gel, External:

Exuviance Lightening Complex [OTC]: 2% (30 g)

NeoCeuticals Post-Acne Fade [OTC]: 2% (30 g)

NeoStrata HQ Skin Lightening [OTC]: 2% (30 g)

Nuquin HP: 4% (28.4 g)

Solution, External:

Melquin 3: 3% (29.57 mL)

◆ **Hydroquinone, Fluocinolone Acetonide, and Tretinoin** *see* Fluocinolone, Hydroquinone, and Tretinoin *on page 894*

◆ **Hydroquinone Time Release** *see* Hydroquinone *on page 1020*

◆ **HydroSKIN [OTC]** *see* Hydrocortisone (Topical) *on page 1014*

◆ **Hydro Skin Maximum Strength [OTC]** *see* Hydrocortisone (Topical) *on page 1014*

◆ **HydroVal® (Can)** *see* Hydrocortisone (Topical) *on page 1014*

Hydroxocobalamin (hye droks oh koe BAL a min)

Brand Names: U.S. Cyanokit

Brand Names: Canada Cyanokit

Index Terms Vitamin B_{12a}

Pharmacologic Category Antidote; Vitamin, Water Soluble

Use

IM injection: Treatment of pernicious anemia; treatment of vitamin B_{12} deficiency due to dietary deficiencies or malabsorption diseases, inadequate secretion of intrinsic factor, competition for vitamin B_{12} by intestinal parasites/bacteria, or inadequate utilization of B_{12} (eg, during neoplastic treatment)

IV infusion (Cyanokit®): Treatment of cyanide poisoning (known or suspected)

Pregnancy Risk Factor C

Dosage

Cyanide poisoning: IV: **Note:** If cyanide poisoning is suspected, antidotal therapy must be given immediately.

Children (off-label use): Initial: 70 mg/kg (maximum: 5 **g**) as a single infusion; may repeat a second dose of 35 mg/kg depending on the severity of poisoning and clinical response (Shepherd, 2008).

Adults: Initial: 5 **g** as a single infusion; may repeat a second 5 **g** dose depending on the severity of poisoning and clinical response. Maximum cumulative dose: 10 **g**.

Vitamin B_{12} deficiency: IM:

Children: Initial: 100 mcg once daily for ≥2 weeks (total dose: 1-5 **mg**); maintenance: 30-50 mcg once per month

Adults: Initial: 30 mcg once daily for 5-10 days; maintenance: 100-200 mcg once per month

Note: Larger doses may be required in critically-ill patients or if patient has neurologic disease, an infectious disease, or hyperthyroidism.

Dosage adjustment in renal impairment: No dosage adjustments provided in manufacturer's labeling (has not been studied).

Dosage adjustment in hepatic impairment: No dosage adjustments provided in manufacturer's labeling (has not been studied).

Additional Information Complete prescribing information should be consulted for additional detail.

Dosage Forms

Solution, Intramuscular:
Generic: 1000 mcg/mL (30 mL)

Solution Reconstituted, Intravenous:
Cyanokit: 5 g (1 ea)

◆ **4-Hydroxybutyrate** *see* Sodium Oxybate *on page 1908*

◆ **Hydroxycarbamide** *see* Hydroxyurea *on page 1021*

Hydroxychloroquine (hye droks ee KLOR oh kwin)

Brand Names: U.S. Plaquenil

Brand Names: Canada Apo-Hydroxyquine; Gen-Hydroxychloroquine; Mylan-Hydroxychloroquine; Plaquenil; PRO-Hydroxyquine

Index Terms Hydroxychloroquine Sulfate

Pharmacologic Category Aminoquinoline (Antimalarial)

Use Suppression and treatment of acute attacks of malaria; treatment of systemic lupus erythematosus (SLE) and rheumatoid arthritis

Dosage Note: Hydroxychloroquine sulfate 200 mg is equivalent to 155 mg hydroxychloroquine base and 250 mg chloroquine phosphate. All doses below expressed as hydroxychloroquine sulfate. Second-line alternative treatment for malaria (chloroquine is preferred).

Oral:

Children:

Malaria, chemoprophylaxis: 6.5 mg/kg once weekly (not to exceed 400 mg/dose); begin 2 weeks before exposure; continue for 4 weeks (per CDC guidelines) after leaving endemic area; if suppressive therapy is not begun prior to the exposure, double the initial dose and give in 2 doses, 6 hours apart and continue treatment for 8 weeks

Malaria, acute attack: 13 mg/kg initially (not to exceed 800 mg/dose), followed by 6.5 mg/kg (not to exceed 400 mg/dose) at 6, 24, and 48 hours

Adults:

Malaria, chemoprophylaxis: 400 mg weekly on same day each week; begin 2 weeks before exposure; continue for 4 weeks (per CDC guidelines) after leaving endemic area; if suppressive therapy is not begun prior to the exposure, double the initial dose and give in 2 doses, 6 hours apart and continue treatment for 8 weeks

Malaria, acute attack: 800 mg initially, followed by 400 mg at 6, 24, and 48 hours

Rheumatoid arthritis: Initial: 400-600 mg/day taken with food or milk; increase dose gradually until optimum response level is reached; usually after 4-12 weeks dose should be reduced by 1/2 to a maintenance dose of 200-400 mg/day

Lupus erythematosus: 400 mg every day or twice daily for several weeks-months depending on response; 200-400 mg/day for prolonged maintenance therapy

Q fever, chronic (off-label use; CDC, 2013): Oral:

Endocarditis or vascular infection: 200 mg every 8 hours in combination with doxycycline for ≥18 months

Noncardiac organ disease: 200 mg every 8 hours in combination with doxycycline (duration based on serologic response; ID consult recommended)

Postpartum with serologic evidence present >12 months after delivery: 200 mg every 8 hours in combination with doxycycline for 12 months

Dosage adjustment in renal impairment: Use with caution; dosage adjustment may be necessary in severe dysfunction (Bernstein, 1992); specific guidelines not available.

Additional Information Complete prescribing information should be consulted for additional detail.

Dosage Forms

Tablet, Oral:
Plaquenil: 200 mg
Generic: 200 mg

◆ **Hydroxychloroquine Sulfate** *see* Hydroxychloroquine *on page 1021*

◆ **Hydroxydaunomycin Hydrochloride** *see* DOXOrubicin (Conventional) *on page 679*

◆ **Hydroxyethyl Starch** *see* Hetastarch *on page 1004*

◆ **Hydroxyethyl Starch** *see* Tetrastarch *on page 2019*

◆ **Hydroxyldaunorubicin Hydrochloride** *see* DOXOrubicin (Conventional) *on page 679*

Hydroxyprogesterone Caproate
(hye droks ee proe JES te rone CAP ro ate)

Brand Names: U.S. Makena

Index Terms 17OHPC

Pharmacologic Category Progestin

Use To reduce the risk of preterm birth in women with singleton pregnancies who have a history of spontaneous preterm birth (delivery <37 weeks gestation) with previous singleton pregnancies

Pregnancy Risk Factor B

Dosage IM: Pregnant females ≥16 years: To reduce the risk of preterm birth: 250 mg once weekly (every 7 days). Treatment may begin between 16 weeks 0 days and 20 weeks 6 days of gestation. Continue weekly administration until 37 weeks gestation or until delivery, whichever comes first.

Dosage adjustment in renal impairment: No dosage adjustment provided in manufacturer's labeling (has not been studied).

Dosage adjustment in hepatic impairment: No dosage adjustment provided in manufacturer's labeling (has not been studied). However, hydroxyprogesterone caproate is extensively metabolized and hepatic impairment may reduce its elimination.

Additional Information Complete prescribing information should be consulted for additional detail.

Dosage Forms

Oil, Intramuscular:
Makena: 250 mg/mL (5 mL)

◆ **9-hydroxy-risperidone** *see* Paliperidone *on page 1556*

Hydroxyurea (hye droks ee yoor EE a)

Brand Names: U.S. Droxia; Hydrea

Brand Names: Canada Apo-Hydroxyurea; Gen-Hydroxyurea; Hydrea®; Mylan-Hydroxyurea

Index Terms HU; Hydroxycarbamide; Hydurea

Pharmacologic Category Antineoplastic Agent, Miscellaneous

Use Treatment of melanoma, refractory chronic myelocytic leukemia (CML); recurrent, metastatic, or inoperable ovarian cancer; management (with concomitant radiation therapy) of squamous cell head and neck cancer (excluding lip cancer); management of sickle cell patients who have had at least three painful crises in the previous 12 months (to reduce frequency of these crises and the need for blood transfusions)

Pregnancy Risk Factor D

Pregnancy Considerations Animal reproduction studies have demonstrated teratogenicity and embryotoxicity at doses lower than the usual human dose (based on BSA). Hydroxyurea may cause fetal harm if administered during pregnancy. Women of childbearing potential should be advised to avoid becoming pregnant during treatment and should use effective contraception.

Breast-Feeding Considerations Hydroxyurea is excreted in breast milk. Due to the potential for serious adverse reactions in the nursing infant, the decision to discontinue hydroxyurea or to discontinue breast-feeding should take into account the importance of treatment to the mother.

Contraindications Hypersensitivity to hydroxyurea or any component of the formulation

Hydrea: Marked bone marrow suppression (WBC <2500/mm^3 or platelet count <100,000/mm^3) or severe anemia

Warnings/Precautions Hazardous agent - use appropriate precautions for handling and disposal (NIOSH 2014 [group 1]); to decrease risk of exposure, wear gloves when handling and wash hands before and after contact. Leukopenia and neutropenia commonly occur (thrombocytopenia and anemia are less common); leukopenia/neutropenia occur first. Hematologic toxicity reversible (rapid) with treatment interruption. Correct severe anemia prior to initiating treatment. Hydrea® use is contraindicated in marked bone marrow suppression; should not be used in sickle cell anemia with severe bone marrow suppression (neutrophils <2000/mm^3, platelets <80,000/mm^3, hemoglobin <4.5 g/dL, or reticulocytes <80,000/mm^3 when hemoglobin <9 g/dL). Use with caution in patients with a history of prior chemotherapy or radiation therapy; myelosuppression is more common. Patients with a history of radiation therapy are also at risk for exacerbation of post irradiation erythema. Self-limiting megaloblastic erythropoiesis may be seen early in treatment (may resemble pernicious anemia, but is unrelated to vitamin B_{12} or folic acid deficiency). Plasma iron clearance may be delayed and iron utilization rate (by erythrocytes) may be reduced. Potentially significant drug-drug interactions may exist, requiring dose or frequency adjustment, additional monitoring, and/or selection of alternative therapy. When treated concurrently with hydroxyurea and antiretroviral agents (including didanosine and stavudine), HIV-infected patients are at higher risk for potentially fatal pancreatitis, hepatotoxicity, hepatic failure, and severe peripheral neuropathy; discontinue immediately if signs of these toxicities develop. Hyperuricemia may occur with antineoplastic treatment; adequate hydration and initiation or dosage adjustment of uricosuric agents (eg, allopurinol) may be necessary.

In patients with sickle cell anemia, use is not recommended if neutrophils <2000/mm^3, platelets <80,000/mm^3, hemoglobin <4.5 g/dL, or reticulocytes <80,000/mm^3 when hemoglobin <9 g/dL. May cause macrocytosis, which can mask folic acid deficiency; prophylactic folic acid supplementation is recommended. **[U.S. Boxed Warning]: Hydroxyurea is mutagenic and clastogenic; causes cellular transformation resulting in tumorigenicity; also considered genotoxic and may be carcinogenic. Treatment of myeloproliferative disorders (eg, polycythemia vera, thrombocythemia) with long-term hydroxyurea is associated with secondary leukemia;** it is unknown if this is drug-related or disease-related. Skin cancer has been reported with long-term hydroxyurea use. Cutaneous vasculitic toxicities (vasculitic ulceration and gangrene) have been reported with hydroxyurea treatment, most often in patients with a history of or receiving concurrent interferon therapy; discontinue hydroxyurea and consider alternate cytoreductive therapy if cutaneous vasculitic toxicity develops. Use caution with renal dysfunction; may require dose reductions. Elderly patients may be more sensitive to the effects of hydroxyurea; may require lower doses. **[U.S. Boxed Warning]: Should be administered under the supervision of a physician experienced in the treatment of sickle cell anemia** or in cancer chemotherapy.

Adverse Reactions

Cardiovascular: Edema

Central nervous system: Chills, disorientation, dizziness, drowsiness (dose-related), fever, hallucinations, headache, malaise, seizure

Dermatologic: Alopecia, cutaneous vasculitic toxicities, dermatomyositis-like skin changes, facial erythema, gangrene, hyperpigmentation, maculopapular rash, nail atrophy, nail discoloration, peripheral erythema, scaling, skin atrophy, skin cancer, skin ulcer, vasculitis ulcerations, violet papules

Endocrine & metabolic: Hyperuricemia

Gastrointestinal: Anorexia, constipation, diarrhea, gastrointestinal irritation and mucositis, (potentiated with radiation therapy), nausea, pancreatitis, stomatitis, vomiting

Genitourinary: Dysuria

Hematologic: Myelosuppression (anemia, leukopenia/neutropenia [common], thrombocytopenia; hematologic recovery: within 2 weeks); macrocytosis, megaloblastic erythropoiesis, secondary leukemias (long-term use)

Hepatic: Hepatic enzymes increased, hepatotoxicity

Neuromuscular & skeletal: Peripheral neuropathy, weakness

Renal: BUN increased, creatinine increased, renal tubular dysfunction

Respiratory: Acute diffuse pulmonary infiltrates (rare), dyspnea, pulmonary fibrosis (rare)

Drug Interactions

Metabolism/Transport Effects None known.

Avoid Concomitant Use

Avoid concomitant use of Hydroxyurea with any of the following: BCG; CloZAPine; Didanosine; Dipyrone; Natalizumab; Pimecrolimus; Stavudine; Tacrolimus (Topical); Tofacitinib; Vaccines (Live)

Increased Effect/Toxicity

Hydroxyurea may increase the levels/effects of: CloZAPine; Didanosine; Leflunomide; Natalizumab; Stavudine; Tofacitinib; Vaccines (Live)

The levels/effects of Hydroxyurea may be increased by: Denosumab; Didanosine; Dipyrone; Pimecrolimus; Roflumilast; Stavudine; Tacrolimus (Topical); Trastuzumab

Decreased Effect

Hydroxyurea may decrease the levels/effects of: BCG; Coccidioides immitis Skin Test; Sipuleucel-T; Vaccines (Inactivated); Vaccines (Live)

The levels/effects of Hydroxyurea may be decreased by: Echinacea

Storage/Stability Store at room temperature of 25°C (77°F); excursions permitted between 15°C and 30°C (59°F and 86°F).

Mechanism of Action Antimetabolite which selectively inhibits ribonucleoside diphosphate reductase, preventing the conversion of ribonucleotides to deoxyribonucleotides, halting the cell cycle at the G1/S phase and therefore has radiation sensitizing activity by maintaining cells in the G_1 phase and interfering with DNA repair. In sickle cell anemia, hydroxyurea increases red blood cell (RBC) hemoglobin F levels, RBC water content, deformability of sickled cells, and alters adhesion of RBCs to endothelium.

Pharmacodynamics/Kinetics

Onset: Sickle cell anemia: Fetal hemoglobin increase: 4-12 weeks

Absorption: Readily absorbed (≥80%)

Distribution: Distributes widely into tissues (including into the brain); estimated volume of distribution approximates total body water (Gwilt, 1998)

Metabolism: 60% via hepatic and GI tract

Protein binding: 75% to 80% bound to serum proteins (Gwilt, 1998)

Half-life elimination: 1.9-3.9 hours (Gwilt, 1998); Children: Sickle cell anemia: 1.7 hours (range: 0.7-3 hours) (Ware, 2011)

Time to peak: 1-4 hours

Excretion: Urine (sickle cell anemia: 40% of administered dose)

Dosage Oral: Doses should be based on ideal or actual body weight, whichever is less (per manufacturer):

Children ≥6 months: Sickle cell anemia (off-label use): Initial: 15-20 mg/kg once daily; may increase by 5 mg/kg/day every 2-6 months to a maximum dose of 30-35 mg/kg/day (Ferster, 2001; Hankins, 2005; Kinney, 1999; Thornburg, 2009; Wang, 2001; Wang, 2011; Zimmerman, 2004)

Adults:

Antineoplastic uses: Titrate dose to patient response; if WBC count falls to <2500/mm^3, or the platelet count to <100,000/mm^3, therapy should be stopped for at least 3 days and resumed when values rise toward normal

Chronic myeloid leukemia (resistant): Continuous therapy: 20-30 mg/kg once daily

Solid tumors (head and neck cancer, melanoma, ovarian cancer):

Intermittent therapy: 80 mg/kg as a single dose every third day

Continuous therapy: 20-30 mg/kg once daily

Concomitant therapy with irradiation (head and neck cancer): 80 mg/kg as a single dose every third day starting at least 7 days before initiation of irradiation

Sickle cell anemia: Initial: 15 mg/kg/day; if blood counts are in an acceptable range, may increase by 5 mg/kg every 12 weeks until the maximum tolerated dose of 35 mg/kg/day is achieved or the dose that does not produce toxic effects (do not increase dose if blood counts are between acceptable and toxic ranges). Monitor for toxicity every 2 weeks; if toxicity occurs, withhold treatment until the bone marrow recovers, then restart with a dose reduction of 2.5 mg/kg/day; if no toxicity occurs over the next 12 weeks, then the subsequent dose may be increased by 2.5 mg/kg/day every 12 weeks to a maximum tolerated dose (dose which does not produce hematologic toxicity for 24 consecutive weeks). If hematologic toxicity recurs a second time at a specific dose, do not retry that dose.

Acceptable hematologic ranges: Neutrophils ≥2500/mm^3; platelets ≥95,000/mm^3; hemoglobin >5.3 g/dL, and reticulocytes ≥95,000/mm^3 if the hemoglobin concentration is <9 g/dL

Toxic hematologic ranges: Neutrophils <2000/mm^3; platelets <80,000/mm^3; hemoglobin <4.5 g/dL; and reticulocytes <80,000/mm^3 if the hemoglobin concentration is <9 g/dL

Acute myeloid leukemia (AML), cytoreduction (off-label use): 50-100 mg/kg/day until WBC <100,000/mm^3 (Grund, 1977) **or** 50-60 mg/kg/day until WBC <10,000-20,000/mm^3 (Dohner, 2010)

Essential thrombocythemia, high-risk (off-label use): 500-1000 mg daily; adjust dose to maintain platelets <400,000/mm^3 (Harrison, 2005)

Head and neck cancer (off-label dosing; with concurrent radiation therapy and fluorouracil): 1000 mg every 12 hours for 11 doses per cycle (Garden, 2004)

Hypereosinophilic syndrome (off-label use): 1000-3000 mg/day (Klion, 2006)

Meningioma (off-label use): 20 mg/kg once daily (Newton, 2000; Rosenthal, 2002)

Polycythemia vera, high-risk (off-label use): 15-20 mg/kg/day (Finazzi, 2007)

Elderly: May require lower doses.

Dosage adjustment for toxicity:

Cutaneous vasculitic ulcerations: Discontinue

Gastrointestinal toxicity (severe nausea, vomiting, anorexia): Temporarily interrupt treatment

Mucositis (severe): Temporarily interrupt treatment

Pancreatitis: Discontinue permanently

Hematologic toxicity:

Antineoplastic uses (CML, head and neck cancer, melanoma, ovarian cancer): WBC <2500/mm^3 or platelets <100,000/mm^3: Interrupt treatment (for at least 3 days), may resume when values rise toward normal

Sickle cell anemia: Neutrophils <2000/mm^3, platelets <80,000/mm^3, hemoglobin <4.5 g/dL, or reticulocytes <80,000/mm^3 with hemoglobin <9 g/dL: Interrupt treatment; following recovery, may resume with a dose reduction of 2.5 mg/kg/day. If no toxicity occurs over the next 12 weeks, subsequent dose may be increased by 2.5 mg/kg/day every 12 weeks to a dose which does not produce hematologic toxicity for 24 consecutive weeks. If hematologic toxicity recurs a second time at a specific dose, do not retry that dose.

Dosage adjustment in renal impairment:

The manufacturer's labeling recommends the following adjustments:

Sickle cell anemia:

CrCl ≥60 mL/minute: No dosage adjustment (of initial dose) necessary.

CrCl <60 mL/minute: Reduce initial dose to 7.5 mg/kg/day (Yan, 2005); titrate to response/avoidance of toxicity (refer to usual dosing)

ESRD: Reduce initial dose to 7.5 mg/kg/dose (administer after dialysis on dialysis days); titrate to response/avoidance of toxicity

Other approved indications: Reduction in initial dose is recommended; however, no specific adjustments are available.

The following adjustments have also been reported:

Aronoff, 2007: Adults:

CrCl >50 mL/minute: No dosage adjustment necessary

CrCl 10-50 mL/minute: Administer 50% of dose

CrCl <10 mL/minute: Administer 20% of dose

Hemodialysis: Administer dose after dialysis on dialysis days

Continuous renal replacement therapy (CRRT): Administer 50% of dose

Kintzel, 1995:

CrCl 46-60 mL/minute: Administer 85% of dose

CrCl 31-45 mL/minute: Administer 80% of dose

CrCl <30 mL/minute: Administer 75% of dose

Dosing adjustment in hepatic impairment: No dosage adjustment provided in the manufacturer's labeling; closely monitor for bone marrow toxicity.

Dosing in obesity: *ASCO Guidelines for appropriate chemotherapy dosing in obese adults with cancer:* Utilize patient's actual body weight (full weight) for calculation of body surface area- or weight-based dosing, particularly when the intent of therapy is curative; manage regimen-related toxicities in the same manner as for nonobese patients; if a dose reduction is utilized due to toxicity, consider resumption of full weight-based dosing with subsequent cycles, especially if cause of toxicity (eg, hepatic or renal impairment) is resolved (Griggs, 2012). **Note:** The manufacturer recommends dosing based on ideal or actual body weight, whichever is less.

Dietary Considerations In sickle cell patients, supplemental administration of folic acid is recommended; hydroxyurea may mask development of folic acid deficiency.

Administration The manufacturer does not recommend opening the capsules.

Hazardous agent; use appropriate precautions for handling and disposal (NIOSH 2014 [group 1]). Impervious gloves should be worn when handling; avoid exposure to crushed or open capsules.

Monitoring Parameters CBC with differential and platelets, renal function and liver function tests, serum uric acid; hemoglobin F levels (sickle cell disease); monitor for cutaneous toxicities

Sickle cell disease: Monitor for toxicity every 2 weeks. If toxicity occurs, stop treatment until the bone marrow recovers; restart at 2.5 mg/kg/day less than the dose at which toxicity occurs. If no toxicity occurs over the next 12 weeks, then the subsequent dose should be increased by 2.5 mg/kg/day. Reduced dosage of hydroxyurea alternating with erythropoietin may decrease myelotoxicity and increase levels of fetal hemoglobin in patients who have not been helped by hydroxyurea alone.

Acceptable range: Neutrophils ≥2500 cells/mm^3, platelets ≥95,000/mm^3, hemoglobin >5.3 g/dL, and reticulocytes ≥95,000/mm^3 if the hemoglobin concentration is <9 g/dL

Toxic range: Neutrophils <2000 cells/mm^3, platelets <80,000/mm^3, hemoglobin <4.5 g/dL, and reticulocytes <80,000/mm^3 if the hemoglobin concentration is <9 g/dL

Dosage Forms

Capsule, Oral:

Droxia: 200 mg, 300 mg, 400 mg

Hydrea: 500 mg

Generic: 500 mg

Extemporaneous Preparations Hazardous agent: Use appropriate precautions for handling and disposal (NIOSH 2014 [group 1]).

A 40 mg/mL oral suspension may be prepared with capsules and either a 1:1 mixture of Ora-Sweet® and Ora-Plus® or a 1:1 mixture of methylcellulose 1% and simple syrup NF. Empty the contents of eight 500 mg capsules into a mortar. Add small portions of chosen vehicle and mix to a uniform paste; mix while incrementally adding the vehicle to **almost** 100 mL; transfer to a calibrated bottle, rinse mortar with vehicle, and add sufficient quantity of vehicle to make 100 mL. Label "shake well" and "refrigerate". Store in plastic prescription bottles. Stable for 14 days at room temperature or refrigerated (preferred) (Nahata, 2003).

A 100 mg/mL oral solution may be prepared with capsules. Mix the contents of twenty 500 mg capsules with enough room temperature sterile water (~50 mL) to initially result in a 200 mg/mL concentration. Stir vigorously using a magnetic stirrer for several hours, then filter to remove insoluble contents. Add 50 mL Syrpalta® (flavored syrup, HUMCO) to filtered solution, resulting in 100 mL of a 100 mg/mL hydroxyurea solution. Stable for 1 month at room temperature in amber plastic bottle (Heeney, 2004).

Heeney MM, Whorton MR, Howard TA, et al, "Chemical and Functional Analysis of Hydroxyurea Oral Solutions," *J Pediatr Hematol Oncol*, 2004, 26(3):179-84.

Nahata MC, Morosco RS, Boster EA, et al, "Stability of Hydroxyurea in Two Extemporaneously Prepared Oral Suspensions Stored at Two Temperatures," 2003, 38:P-161(E) [abstract from 2003 ASHP Midyear Clinical Meeting].

◆ **1-α-hydroxyvitamin D$_3$** *see* Alfacalcidol [CAN/INT] *on page 82*

HydrOXYzine (hye DROKS i zeen)

Brand Names: U.S. Vistaril

Brand Names: Canada Apo-Hydroxyzine; Atarax; Hydroxyzine Hydrochloride Injection, USP; Novo-Hydroxyzin; Nu-Hydroxyzine; PMS-Hydroxyzine; Riva-Hydroxyzine

Index Terms Hydroxyzine Hydrochloride; Hydroxyzine Pamoate

Pharmacologic Category Antiemetic; Histamine H$_1$ Antagonist; Histamine H$_1$ Antagonist, First Generation; Piperazine Derivative

Additional Appendix Information

Beers Criteria – Potentially Inappropriate Medications for Geriatrics *on page 2271*

Use Treatment of anxiety/agitation (including adjunctive therapy in alcoholism); adjunct to pre- and postoperative analgesia and anesthesia; antipruritic; antiemetic

Pregnancy Considerations Adverse events were observed in animal reproduction studies. Hydroxyzine crosses the placenta. Maternal hydroxyzine use has generally not resulted in an increased risk of birth defects. Use of hydroxyzine early in pregnancy is contraindicated but hydroxyzine is approved for pre- and postpartum adjunctive therapy to reduce opioid dosage, treat anxiety, and control emesis. Antihistamines are recommended for the treatment pruritus with rash in pregnant women (although second generation antihistamines may be preferred). Antihistamines are not recommended for treatment of pruritus associated with intrahepatic cholestasis in pregnancy. Possible withdrawal symptoms have been observed in neonates following chronic maternal use of hydroxyzine during pregnancy.

Breast-Feeding Considerations It is not known if hydroxyzine is excreted in breast milk. Breast-feeding is not recommended by the manufacturer. Antihistamines may decrease maternal serum prolactin concentrations when administered prior to the establishment of nursing.

Contraindications Hypersensitivity to hydroxyzine or any component of the formulation; early pregnancy; SubQ, intra-arterial, or IV injection

Warnings/Precautions Causes sedation, caution must be used in performing tasks which require alertness (eg, operating machinery or driving). Sedative effects of CNS depressants or ethanol are potentiated. Use with caution with narrow-angle glaucoma, prostatic hyperplasia, bladder neck obstruction, asthma, or COPD. In the elderly, avoid use of this potent anticholinergic agent due to increased risk of confusion, dry mouth, constipation, and other anticholinergic effects; clearance decreases in patients of advanced age (Beers Criteria).

For IM use only. Subcutaneous, IV, and intra-arterial routes of administration are contraindicated. Intravascular hemolysis, thrombosis, and digital gangrene have been reported with IV or intra-arterial administration (Baumgartner, 1979); SubQ administration may result in significant tissue damage. If inadvertent IV administration results in extravasation, stop infusion immediately and disconnect (leave cannula/needle in place); gently aspirate extravasated solution (do **NOT** flush the line); remove needle/cannula; elevate extremity.

Benzyl alcohol and derivatives: Some dosage forms may contain benzyl alcohol and/or sodium benzoate/benzoic acid; benzoic acid (benzoate) is a metabolite of benzyl alcohol; large amounts of benzyl alcohol (≥99 mg/kg/day) have been associated with a potentially fatal toxicity ("gasping syndrome") in neonates; the "gasping syndrome" consists of metabolic acidosis, respiratory distress, gasping respirations, CNS dysfunction (including convulsions, intracranial hemorrhage), hypotension and cardiovascular collapse (AAP, 1997; CDC, 1982); some data suggests that benzoate displaces bilirubin from protein binding sites (Ahlfors, 2001); avoid or use dosage forms containing benzyl alcohol and/or benzyl alcohol derivative with caution in neonates. See manufacturer's labeling.

Adverse Reactions

Central nervous system: Dizziness, drowsiness (transient), fatigue, involuntary movements

Gastrointestinal: Xerostomia

Hypersensitivity: Hypersensitivity reaction

Ophthalmic: Blurred vision

Respiratory: Respiratory depression (at higher than recommended doses)

Rare but important or life-threatening: Fixed drug eruption, hallucination, seizure (at considerably higher than recommended doses), skin rash, tremor (at considerably higher than recommended doses)

Drug Interactions

Metabolism/Transport Effects **Inhibits** CYP2D6 (weak)

Avoid Concomitant Use

Avoid concomitant use of HydrOXYzine with any of the following: Aclidinium; Azelastine (Nasal); Glucagon; Ipratropium (Oral Inhalation); Orphenadrine; Paraldehyde; Potassium Chloride; Thalidomide; Tiotropium; Umeclidinium

Increased Effect/Toxicity

HydrOXYzine may increase the levels/effects of: AbobotulinumtoxinA; Alcohol (Ethyl); Anticholinergic Agents; ARIPiprazole; Azelastine (Nasal); Barbiturates; Buprenorphine; CNS Depressants; Glucagon; Highest Risk QTc-Prolonging Agents; Hydrocodone; Meperidine; Methotrimeprazine; Metyrosine; Mirabegron; Mirtazapine; Moderate Risk QTc-Prolonging Agents; OnabotulinumtoxinA; Orphenadrine; Paraldehyde; Potassium Chloride; Pramipexole; RimabotulinumtoxinB; ROPINIRole; Rotigotine; Selective Serotonin Reuptake Inhibitors; Suvorexant; Thalidomide; Thiazide Diuretics; Tiotropium; Topiramate; Zolpidem

The levels/effects of HydrOXYzine may be increased by: Aclidinium; Brimonidine (Topical); Cannabis; Doxylamine; Dronabinol; Droperidol; Ipratropium (Oral Inhalation); Kava Kava; Magnesium Sulfate; Methotrimeprazine; Mianserin; Mifepristone; Nabilone; Perampanel; Pramlintide; Rufinamide; Sodium Oxybate; Tapentadol; Tetrahydrocannabinol; Umeclidinium

Decreased Effect

HydrOXYzine may decrease the levels/effects of: Acetylcholinesterase Inhibitors; Benzylpenicilloyl Polylysine; Betahistine; Hyaluronidase; Itopride; Secretin

The levels/effects of HydrOXYzine may be decreased by: Acetylcholinesterase Inhibitors; Amphetamines

Storage/Stability

Injection: Store at 20°C to 25°C (68°F to 77°F); excursions permitted to 15°C to 30°C (59°F to 86°F). Protect from light.

Capsules: Store below 30°C (86°F); protect from light.

Solution (hydrochloride salt): Store at 15°C to 30°C (59°F to 86°F); protect from light.

Tablets: Store at 20°C to 25°C (68°F to 77°F).

Mechanism of Action Competes with histamine for H_1-receptor sites on effector cells in the gastrointestinal tract, blood vessels, and respiratory tract. Possesses skeletal muscle relaxing, bronchodilator, antihistamine, antiemetic, and analgesic properties.

Pharmacodynamics/Kinetics

Onset of action: Oral: 15-30 minutes; Injection: Rapid

Duration: Decreased histamine-induced wheal and flare areas: 2 to ≥36 hours; Suppression of pruritus: 1-12 hours (Simons, 1984)

Absorption: Oral: Rapid

Distribution: Adults: V_d: ~16 L/kg (Simons, 1984); Elderly: ~23 L/kg (Simons K, 1989); Hepatic dysfunction: ~23 L/kg (Simons F, 1989)

Metabolism: Hepatic to multiple metabolites, including cetirizine (active) (Simons F, 1989)

Half-life elimination: Adults: ~20 hours (Simons, 1984); Elderly: ~29 hours (Simons K, 1989); Hepatic dysfunction: ~37 hours (Simons F, 1989)

Time to peak: Oral administration: Serum: ~2 hours; Peak suppression of antihistamine-induced wheal and flare: 4-12 hours (Simons, 1984)

Excretion: Urine

Dosage Note: Adjust dose based on patient response.

Children:

- Preoperative sedation:
  - Oral: 0.6 mg/kg/dose
  - IM: 1.1 mg/kg/dose
- Pruritus, anxiety: Oral:
  - <6 years: 50 mg daily in divided doses
  - ≥6 years: 50 to 100 mg daily in divided doses
- Antiemetic: IM: 1.1 mg/kg/dose

Adults:

- Antiemetic: IM: 25 to 100 mg/dose
- Anxiety:
  - Oral:
    - *Manufacturer's labeling:* 50 to 100 mg 4 times daily
    - *Alternative recommendations (off-label dosing):* 37.5 to 75 mg daily in divided doses (WFSBP [Bandelow, 2008]; WFSBP [Bandelow, 2012])
  - IM: Initial: 50 to 100 mg, then every 4 to 6 hours as needed
- Preoperative sedation:
  - Oral: 50 to 100 mg
  - IM: 25 to 100 mg
- Pruritus: Oral: 25 mg 3 to 4 times daily

Elderly: Initiate dosing using the lower end of the recommended dosage range due to an increased potential for anticholinergic side effects. Refer to adult dosing.

Dosing adjustment in renal impairment: No dosage adjustment provided in the manufacturer's labeling; however, the following guidelines have been used by some clinicians (Aronoff, 2007): Adults:

GFR >50 mL/minute: No adjustment recommended.

GFR ≤50 mL/minute: Administer 50% of normal dose.

Continuous renal replacement therapy (CRRT), hemodialysis, peritoneal dialysis: Administer 50% of the normal dose.

Dosing interval in hepatic impairment: Change dosing interval to every 24 hours in patients with primary biliary cirrhosis (Simons F, 1989).

Administration

Injection: For IM use only. Do **NOT** administer IV, SubQ, or intra-arterially. Administer IM deep in large muscle. In adults, the preferred site is the upper outer quadrant of the buttock or midlateral thigh. In children, the preferred site is the midlateral thigh. The upper outer quadrant of the gluteal region should be used only when necessary to minimize potential damage to the sciatic nerve.

Oral: Shake suspension vigorously prior to use.

Monitoring Parameters Relief of symptoms, mental status, blood pressure

Dosage Forms

Capsule, Oral:

Vistaril: 25 mg, 50 mg

Generic: 25 mg, 50 mg, 100 mg

Solution, Intramuscular:

Generic: 25 mg/mL (1 mL); 50 mg/mL (1 mL, 2 mL, 10 mL)

Solution, Oral:

Generic: 10 mg/5 mL (473 mL)

Syrup, Oral:

Generic: 10 mg/5 mL (118 mL, 473 mL)

Tablet, Oral:

Generic: 10 mg, 25 mg, 50 mg

- ◆ **Hydroxyzine Hydrochloride** *see* HydrOXYzine *on page 1024*
- ◆ **Hydroxyzine Hydrochloride Injection, USP (Can)** *see* HydrOXYzine *on page 1024*
- ◆ **Hydroxyzine Pamoate** *see* HydrOXYzine *on page 1024*
- ◆ **Hydurea** *see* Hydroxyurea *on page 1021*
- ◆ **Hygroton** *see* Chlorthalidone *on page 430*
- ◆ **Hylan G-F 20** *see* Hyaluronate and Derivatives *on page 1006*
- ◆ **Hylan Polymers** *see* Hyaluronate and Derivatives *on page 1006*
- ◆ **Hylase Wound** *see* Hyaluronate and Derivatives *on page 1006*
- ◆ **HyoMax-SL** *see* Hyoscyamine *on page 1026*
- ◆ **Hyonatol** *see* Hyoscyamine, Atropine, Scopolamine, and Phenobarbital *on page 1027*
- ◆ **Hyophen™** *see* Methenamine, Phenyl Salicylate, Methylene Blue, Benzoic Acid, and Hyoscyamine *on page 1318*
- ◆ **Hyoscine Butylbromide** *see* Scopolamine (Systemic) *on page 1870*

Hyoscyamine (hye oh SYE a meen)

Brand Names: U.S. Anaspaz; Ed-Spaz; HyoMax-SL; Hyosyne; Levbid; Levsin; Levsin/SL; NuLev; Oscimin; Oscimin SR; Symax Duotab; Symax FasTabs; Symax-SL; Symax-SR

Brand Names: Canada Levsin

Index Terms *l*-Hyoscyamine Sulfate; Hyoscyamine Sulfate

Pharmacologic Category Anticholinergic Agent

Additional Appendix Information

Beers Criteria – Potentially Inappropriate Medications for Geriatrics *on page 2271*

Use

Anesthesia:

Preoperative antimuscarinic: Preoperative antimuscarinic to reduce salivary, tracheobronchial, and pharyngeal secretions; to reduce volume and acidity of gastric secretions; to block cardiac vagal inhibitory reflexes during induction of anesthesia and intubation

Reversal of neuromuscular blockade and associated muscarinic effects: Protects against peripheral muscarinic effects (such as bradycardia and excessive secretions produced by halogenated hydrocarbons and cholinergic agents [such as physostigmine, neostigmine, and pyridostigmine]) given to reverse actions of curariform agents

Antidote for anticholinesterase agent poisoning: Antidote for poisoning by anticholinesterase agents

Biliary and renal colic: Adjunctive therapy with morphine or other opioids for the symptomatic relief of biliary and renal colic

Diagnostic procedures: Reduces GI motility to facilitate diagnostic procedures such as endoscopy or hypotonic duodenography; may also improve radiologic visibility of the kidneys

GI disorders:

Aid in the control of acute episodes of gastric secretion, visceral spasm, hypermotility in spastic colitis, pylorospasm, and associated abdominal cramps; relieve symptoms in functional intestinal disorders (eg, mild dysenteries, diverticulitis) and infant colic (elixir and oral solution)

Adjunctive therapy for treatment in peptic ulcer; irritable bowel syndrome (irritable colon, spastic colon, acute enterocolitis, mucous colitis) and other functional GI disorders; neurogenic bowel disturbances (including splenic flexure syndrome and neurogenic colon)

Pancreatitis: Reduce pain and hypersecretion in pancreatitis

Parkinsonism: In parkinsonism, to reduce rigidity and tremors and to control associated sialorrhea and hyperhidrosis

Partial heart block: For use in certain cases of partial heart block associated with vagal activity

Rhinitis: "Drying agent" in the relief of symptoms of acute rhinitis

Urinary system disorder: To control hypermotility in spastic bladder and cystitis; adjunctive therapy in the treatment of neurogenic bladder

Pregnancy Risk Factor C

Dosage

Gastrointestinal disorders: Oral:

Children <2 years: Drops (Hyosyne [0.125 mg/**mL**]): Dose as listed, based on age and weight (kg); repeat dose every 4 hours or as needed:

3.4 kg: 4 **drops**; maximum: 24 **drops** daily
5 kg: 5 **drops**; maximum: 30 **drops** daily
7 kg: 6 **drops**; maximum: 36 **drops** daily
10 kg: 8 **drops**; maximum: 48 **drops** daily

Children 2 to <12 years:

Tablets (regular release [Levsin], dispersible [Anaspaz, ED-SPAZ, NuLev, Symax FasTab]): 0.0625 to 0.125 mg every 4 hours or as needed; maximum: 0.75 mg daily

Drops (Hyosyne [0.125 mg/**mL**]): 0.03125 mg (0.25 mL) to 0.125 mg (1 mL) every 4 hours or as needed; maximum: 0.75 mg (6 mL) daily

Elixir (Hyosyne [0.125 mg/**5 mL**]): Dose as listed, based on age and weight (kg); repeat dose every 4 hours or as needed:

10 kg: 0.03125 mg (1.25 mL); maximum: 0.75 mg (30 mL) daily
20 kg: 0.0625 mg (2.5 mL); maximum: 0.75 mg (30 mL) daily
40 kg: 0.09375 mg (3.75 mL); maximum: 0.75 mg (30 mL) daily
50 kg: 0.125 mg (5 mL); maximum: 0.75 mg (30 mL) daily

Children ≥12 years, Adolescents, and Adults:

Tablet, dispersible:

Anaspaz, ED-SPAZ, NuLev, Symax FasTab: 0.125 to 0.25 mg every 4 hours or as needed; maximum: 1.5 mg daily

Oscimin: 0.125 to 0.25 mg 3 to 4 times daily; may increase to every 4 hours as needed; maximum: 1.5 mg daily

Tablet, extended release:

Levbid: 0.375 to 0.75 mg every 12 hours; maximum: 1.5 mg daily

Oscimin SR, Symax Duotab, Symax SR: 0.375 to 0.75 mg every 12 hours or 0.375 mg every 8 hours; maximum: 1.5 mg daily

Tablet, regular release:

Levsin: 0.125 to 0.25 mg every 4 hours or as needed; maximum: 1.5 mg daily

Oscimin: 0.125 to 0.25 mg 3 to 4 times daily; may increase to every 4 hours as needed; maximum: 1.5 mg daily

Tablet, sublingual (Oscimin, Symax SL): 0.125 to 0.25 mg 3 to 4 times daily; may increase to every 4 hours as needed; maximum: 1.5 mg daily

Drops (Hyosyne [0.125 mg/**mL**]): 0.125 mg (1 mL) to 0.25 mg (2 mL) every 4 hours or as needed; maximum: 1.5 mg (12 mL) daily

Elixir (Hyosyne [0.125 mg/**5 mL**]): 0.125 mg (5 mL) to 0.25 mg (10 mL) every 4 hours or as needed; maximum: 1.5 mg (60 mL) daily

IM, IV, SubQ: 0.25 to 0.5 mg; may repeat as needed up to 4 times daily, at 4-hour intervals

Diagnostic procedures: Adults: IV: 0.25 to 0.5 mg given 5 to 10 minutes prior to procedure

Preanesthesia: Children >2 years, Adolescents, and Adults: IM, IV, SubQ: 5 **mcg**/kg given 30 to 60 minutes prior to induction of anesthesia or at the time preoperative opioids or sedatives are administered

Reduce drug-induced bradycardia during surgery: Adults: IV: 0.125 mg; repeat as needed

Reverse neuromuscular blockade: Adults: IM, IV, SubQ: 0.2 mg for every 1 mg neostigmine (or the physostigmine/pyridostigmine equivalent)

Dosage adjustment in renal impairment: No dosage adjustment provided in manufacturer's labeling, use with caution.

Dosage adjustment in hepatic impairment: No dosage adjustment provided in manufacturer's labeling.

Additional Information Complete prescribing information should be consulted for additional detail.

Dosage Forms

Elixir, Oral:
- Hyosyne: 0.125 mg/5 mL (473 mL)
- Generic: 0.125 mg/5 mL (473 mL)

Solution, Injection:
- Levsin: 0.5 mg/mL (1 mL)

Solution, Oral:
- Hyosyne: 0.125 mg/mL (15 mL)
- Generic: 0.125 mg/mL (15 mL)

Tablet, Oral:
- Levsin: 0.125 mg
- Oscimin: 0.125 mg
- Generic: 0.125 mg

Tablet Dispersible, Oral:
- Anaspaz: 0.125 mg
- Ed-Spaz: 0.125 mg
- NuLev: 0.125 mg
- Oscimin: 0.125 mg
- Symax FasTabs: 0.125 mg
- Generic: 0.125 mg

Tablet Extended Release, Oral:
- Symax Duotab: 0.375 mg

Tablet Extended Release 12 Hour, Oral:
- Levbid: 0.375 mg
- Oscimin SR: 0.375 mg
- Symax-SR: 0.375 mg
- Generic: 0.375 mg

Tablet Sublingual, Sublingual:
- HyoMax-SL: 0.125 mg
- Levsin/SL: 0.125 mg
- Oscimin: 0.125 mg
- Symax-SL: 0.125 mg
- Generic: 0.125 mg

Hyoscyamine, Atropine, Scopolamine, and Phenobarbital

(hye oh SYE a meen, A troe peen, skoe POL a meen, & fee noe BAR bi tal)

Brand Names: U.S. Donnatal Extentabs®; Donnatal®; Hyonatol

Index Terms Atropine, Hyoscyamine, Phenobarbital, and Scopolamine; Belladonna Alkaloids With Phenobarbital; Phenobarbital, Hyoscyamine, Atropine, and Scopolamine; Scopolamine, Hyoscyamine, Atropine, and Phenobarbital

Pharmacologic Category Anticholinergic Agent; Antispasmodic Agent, Gastrointestinal

Use Adjunct in treatment of irritable bowel syndrome, acute enterocolitis, duodenal ulcer

Pregnancy Risk Factor C

Dosage Oral:

Children ≥2 years: Elixir: To be given every 4-6 hours; initial dose based on weight:
- 9.1 kg: 1 mL every 4 hours **or** 1.5 mL every 6 hours
- 13.6 kg: 1.5 mL every 4 hours **or** 2 mL every 6 hours
- 22.7 kg: 2.5 mL every 4 hours **or** 3.75 mL every 6 hours
- 34 kg: 3.75 mL every 4 hours **or** 5 mL every 6 hours
- 45.4 kg: 5 mL every 4 hours **or** 7.5 mL every 6 hours

Adults:
- Immediate release: 1-2 tablets or 5-10 mL of elixir 3-4 times/day
- Extended release: One tablet every 12 hours; may increase to 1 tablet every 8 hours if needed

Additional Information Complete prescribing information should be consulted for additional detail.

Dosage Forms Considerations Elixir contains ethanol (up to 23.8%).

Dosage Forms

Elixir:
- Donnatal®: Hyoscyamine 0.1037 mg, atropine 0.0194 mg, scopolamine 0.0065 mg, and phenobarbital 16.2 mg per 5 mL

Tablet:
- Donnatal®: Hyoscyamine 0.1037 mg, atropine 0.0194 mg, scopolamine 0.0065 mg, and phenobarbital 16.2 mg
- Hyonatol: Hyoscyamine 0.1037 mg, atropine 0.0194 mg, scopolamine 0.0065 mg, and phenobarbital 16.2 mg

Tablet, extended release:
- Donnatal Extentabs®: Hyoscyamine 0.3111 mg, atropine 0.0582 mg, scopolamine 0.0195 mg, and phenobarbital 48.6 mg

- ◆ **Hyoscyamine, Methenamine, Benzoic Acid, Phenyl Salicylate, and Methylene Blue** *see* Methenamine, Phenyl Salicylate, Methylene Blue, Benzoic Acid, and Hyoscyamine *on page 1318*
- ◆ **Hyoscyamine, Methenamine, Methylene Blue, Phenyl Salicylate, and Sodium Phosphate Monobasic** *see* Methenamine, Sodium Phosphate Monobasic, Phenyl Salicylate, Methylene Blue, and Hyoscyamine *on page 1318*
- ◆ **Hyoscyamine, Methenamine, Sodium Phosphate Monobasic, Phenyl Salicylate, and Methylene Blue** *see* Methenamine, Sodium Phosphate Monobasic, Phenyl Salicylate, Methylene Blue, and Hyoscyamine *on page 1318*
- ◆ **Hyoscyamine Sulfate** *see* Hyoscyamine *on page 1026*
- ◆ **Hyosyne** *see* Hyoscyamine *on page 1026*
- ◆ **Hyperal** *see* Total Parenteral Nutrition *on page 2073*
- ◆ **Hyperalimentation** *see* Total Parenteral Nutrition *on page 2073*
- ◆ **HyperHEP B S/D** *see* Hepatitis B Immune Globulin (Human) *on page 1002*
- ◆ **HyperRAB S/D** *see* Rabies Immune Globulin (Human) *on page 1764*
- ◆ **HyperRHO S/D** *see* Rh_o(D) Immune Globulin *on page 1794*
- ◆ **HyperSal** *see* Sodium Chloride *on page 1902*
- ◆ **HyperTET S/D** *see* Tetanus Immune Globulin (Human) *on page 2015*
- ◆ **Hypertonic Saline** *see* Sodium Chloride *on page 1902*
- ◆ **HyQvia** *see* Immune Globulin *on page 1056*
- ◆ **Hyqvia** *see* Immune Globulin *on page 1056*
- ◆ **HySept [OTC]** *see* Sodium Hypochlorite Solution *on page 1906*
- ◆ **Hytrin** *see* Terazosin *on page 2001*

◆ **Hyzaar** *see* Losartan and Hydrochlorothiazide *on page 1250*

◆ **Hyzaar DS (Can)** *see* Losartan and Hydrochlorothiazide *on page 1250*

◆ **HZV** *see* Zoster Vaccine *on page 2218*

Ibandronate (eye BAN droh nate)

Brand Names: U.S. Boniva

Index Terms Ibandronate Sodium; Ibandronic Acid

Pharmacologic Category Bisphosphonate Derivative

Use Treatment and prevention of osteoporosis in postmenopausal females

Pregnancy Risk Factor C

Pregnancy Considerations Adverse effects were observed in animal reproduction studies. It is not known if bisphosphonates cross the placenta, but fetal exposure is expected (Djokanovic, 2008; Stathopoulos, 2011). Bisphosphonates are incorporated into the bone matrix and gradually released over time. The amount available in the systemic circulation varies by dose and duration of therapy. Theoretically, there may be a risk of fetal harm when pregnancy follows the completion of therapy; however, available data have not shown that exposure to bisphosphonates during pregnancy significantly increases the risk of adverse fetal events (Djokanovic, 2008; Levy, 2009; Stathopoulos, 2011). Until additional data is available, most sources recommend discontinuing bisphosphonate therapy in women of reproductive potential as early as possible prior to a planned pregnancy; use in premenopausal women should be reserved for special circumstances when rapid bone loss is occurring (Bhalla, 2010; Pereira, 2012; Stathopoulos, 2011). Because hypocalcemia has been described following *in utero* bisphosphonate exposure, exposed infants should be monitored for hypocalcemia after birth (Djokanovic, 2008; Stathopoulos, 2011).

Breast-Feeding Considerations It is not known if ibandronate is excreted into breast milk. The manufacturer recommends caution be exercised when administering ibandronate to nursing women.

Contraindications Hypersensitivity to ibandronate or any component of the formulation; hypocalcemia; oral tablets are also contraindicated in patients unable to stand or sit upright for at least 60 minutes and in patients with abnormalities of the esophagus which delay esophageal emptying, such as stricture or achalasia

Warnings/Precautions Hypocalcemia must be corrected before therapy initiation. Ensure adequate calcium and vitamin D intake. Osteonecrosis of the jaw (ONJ) has been reported in patients receiving bisphosphonates. Risk factors include invasive dental procedures (eg, tooth extraction, dental implants, boney surgery); a diagnosis of cancer, with concomitant chemotherapy or corticosteroids; poor oral hygiene, ill-fitting dentures; and comorbid disorders (anemia, coagulopathy, infection, preexisting dental disease); risk may increase with duration of bisphosphonate use. Most reported cases occurred after IV bisphosphonate therapy; however, cases have been reported following oral therapy. A dental exam and preventive dentistry should be performed prior to placing patients with risk factors on chronic bisphosphonate therapy. The manufacturer's labeling states that discontinuing bisphosphonates in patients requiring invasive dental procedures may reduce the risk of ONJ. However, other experts suggest that there is no evidence that discontinuing therapy reduces the risk of developing ONJ (Assael, 2009). The benefit/risk must be assessed by the treating physician and/or dentist/surgeon prior to any invasive dental procedure. Patients developing ONJ while on bisphosphonates should receive care by an oral surgeon.

Atypical femur fractures have been reported in patients receiving bisphosphonates for treatment/prevention of osteoporosis. The fractures include subtrochanteric femur (bone just below the hip joint) and diaphyseal femur (long segment of the thigh bone). Some patients experience prodromal pain weeks or months before the fracture occurs. It is unclear if bisphosphonate therapy is the cause for these fractures, although the majority of cases have been reported in patients taking bisphosphonates. Patients receiving long-term (>3-5 years) therapy may be at an increased risk. Discontinue bisphosphonate therapy in patients who develop a femoral shaft fracture.

Infrequently, severe (and occasionally debilitating) bone, joint, and/or muscle pain have been reported during bisphosphonate treatment. The onset of pain ranged from a single day to several months. Discontinue intravenous ibandronate therapy in patients who experience severe symptoms; symptoms usually resolve upon discontinuation. Some patients experienced recurrence when rechallenged with same drug or another bisphosphonate; avoid use in patients with a history of these symptoms in association with bisphosphonate therapy.

Oral bisphosphonates may cause dysphagia, esophagitis, esophageal or gastric ulcer; risk may increase in patients unable to comply with dosing instructions; discontinue use if new or worsening symptoms develop. Intravenous bisphosphonates may cause transient decreases in serum calcium and have also been associated with renal toxicity.

Use not recommended with severe renal impairment (CrCl <30 mL/minute). In the management of osteoporosis, re-evaluate the need for continued therapy periodically; the optimal duration of treatment has not yet been determined. Consider discontinuing after 3-5 years of use in patients at low-risk for fracture; following discontinuation, re-evaluate fracture risk periodically. Potentially significant drug-drug interactions may exist, requiring dose or frequency adjustment, additional monitoring, and/or selection of alternative therapy.

Adverse Reactions

Cardiovascular: Hypertension

Central nervous system: Diarrhea, dizziness, headache, insomnia

Dermatologic: Skin rash

Endocrine & metabolic: Hypercholesterolemia

Gastrointestinal: Abdominal pain, constipation, diarrhea, dyspepsia, dysphagia, nausea, vomiting

Genitourinary: Urinary tract infection

Hepatic: Decreased serum alkaline phosphatase

Hypersensitivity: Hypersensitivity reaction

Infection: Infection

Local: Injection site reaction

Neuromuscular & skeletal: Arthralgia, arthropathy, back pain, limb pain, localized osteoarthritis, muscle cramps, myalgia, osteonecrosis of the jaw, weakness

Respiratory: Bronchitis, flu-like symptoms, nasopharyngitis, pneumonia, upper respiratory tract infection

Miscellaneous: Acute phase reaction-like symptoms

Rare but important or life-threatening: Acute renal failure, anaphylactic shock, anaphylaxis, angioedema, exacerbation of asthma, femur fracture (diaphyseal or subtrochanteric), hypocalcemia, iritis, malignant neoplasm of esophagus, musculoskeletal pain (bone, joint, or muscle; incapacitating), ophthalmic inflammation, prolonged Q-T interval on ECG (Bonilla, 2014), scleritis, uveitis

Drug Interactions

Metabolism/Transport Effects None known.

Avoid Concomitant Use There are no known interactions where it is recommended to avoid concomitant use.

Increased Effect/Toxicity

Ibandronate may increase the levels/effects of: Deferasirox; Highest Risk QTc-Prolonging Agents; Moderate Risk QTc-Prolonging Agents; Phosphate Supplements

The levels/effects of Ibandronate may be increased by: Aminoglycosides; Mifepristone; Nonsteroidal Anti-Inflammatory Agents; Systemic Angiogenesis Inhibitors

Decreased Effect

The levels/effects of Ibandronate may be decreased by: Antacids; Calcium Salts; Iron Salts; Magnesium Salts; Multivitamins/Minerals (with ADEK, Folate, Iron); Multivitamins/Minerals (with AE, No Iron); Proton Pump Inhibitors

Food Interactions Food may reduce absorption; mean oral bioavailability is decreased up to 90% when given with food. Management: Take with a full glass (6-8 oz) of plain water, at least 60 minutes prior to any food, beverages, or medications. Mineral water with a high calcium content should be avoided. Wait at least 60 minutes after taking ibandronate before taking anything else.

Storage/Stability Store at controlled room temperature of 25°C (77°F); excursions permitted to 15°C to 30°C (59°F to 86°F).

Mechanism of Action A bisphosphonate which inhibits bone resorption via actions on osteoclasts or on osteoclast precursors; decreases the rate of bone resorption, leading to an indirect increase in bone mineral density.

Pharmacodynamics/Kinetics

Distribution: Terminal V_d: 90 L; 40% to 50% of circulating ibandronate binds to bone

Protein binding: 85.7% to 99.5%

Metabolism: Not metabolized

Bioavailability: Oral: Minimal; reduced ~90% following standard breakfast

Half-life elimination:

Oral: 150 mg dose: Terminal: 37-157 hours

IV: Terminal: ~5-25 hours

Time to peak, plasma: Oral: 0.5-2 hours

Excretion: Urine (50% to 60% of absorbed dose, excreted as unchanged drug); feces (unabsorbed drug)

Dosage

Postmenopausal osteoporosis (treatment): Adults: **Note:** Consider discontinuing after 3-5 years of use for osteoporosis in patients at low-risk for fracture. Patients should receive supplemental calcium and vitamin D if dietary intake is inadequate.

Oral: 150 mg once monthly

IV: 3 mg every 3 months

Postmenopausal osteoporosis (prevention): Adults: Oral: 150 mg once monthly. **Note:** Patients should receive supplemental calcium and vitamin D if dietary intake is inadequate.

Hypercalcemia of malignancy (off-label use): Adults: IV: 2-6 mg over 1-2 hours (Pecherstorfer, 2003; Ralston, 1997)

Metastatic bone disease due to breast cancer (off-label use): Adults: IV: 6 mg every 3-4 weeks (Diel, 2004)

Missed doses:

Oral: If once-monthly oral dose is missed, it should be given the next morning after remembered if the next month's scheduled dose is >7 days away. If the next month's scheduled dose is within 7 days, wait until the next month's scheduled dose. May then return to the original monthly schedule (original scheduled day of the month). Do not give >150 mg within 7 days.

IV: If an IV dose is missed, it should be administered as soon as it can be rescheduled. Thereafter, it should be given every 3 months from the date of the last injection.

Dosage adjustment in renal impairment:

Osteoporosis: Oral, IV:

CrCl ≥30 mL/minute: No dosage adjustment necessary.

CrCl <30 mL/minute: Use not recommended.

Oncologic uses (off-label): IV: CrCl <30 mL/minute: 2 mg every 3-4 weeks (von Moos, 2005)

Dosage adjustment in hepatic impairment: No dosage adjustment necessary (has not been studied); however, ibandronate does not undergo hepatic metabolism.

Dietary Considerations

Ensure adequate calcium and vitamin D intake; if dietary intake is inadequate, dietary supplementation is recommended. Women and men should consume:

Calcium: 1000 mg/day (men: 50-70 years) **or** 1200 mg/day (women ≥51 years and men ≥71 years) (IOM, 2011; NOF, 2013)

Vitamin D: 800-1000 IU/day (men and women ≥50 years) (NOF, 2013). Recommended Dietary Allowance (RDA): 600 IU/day (men and women ≤70 years) **or** 800 IU/day (men and women ≥71 years) (IOM, 2011).

Ibandronate tablet should be taken with a full glass (6-8 oz) of plain water, at least 60 minutes prior to any food, beverages, or medications. Mineral water with a high calcium content should be avoided.

Administration

Oral: Administer 60 minutes before the first food or drink of the day (other than water) and prior to taking any oral medications or supplements (eg, calcium, antacids, vitamins). Ibandronate should be taken in an upright position with a full glass (6-8 oz) of plain water and the patient should avoid lying down for 60 minutes to minimize the possibility of GI side effects. Mineral water with a high calcium content should be avoided. The tablet should be swallowed whole; do not chew or suck. Do not eat or drink anything (except water) for 60 minutes following administration of ibandronate.

IV: Administer as a 15-30 second bolus intravenously; avoid paravenous or intraarterial administration (may cause tissue damage). Do not mix with calcium-containing solutions or other drugs. For osteoporosis, do not administer more frequently than every 3 months. Infuse over 1 hour for metastatic bone disease due to breast cancer (Diel, 2004) and over 1-2 hours for hypercalcemia of malignancy (Pecherstorfer, 2003; Ralston, 1997).

Monitoring Parameters

Osteoporosis: Bone mineral density (BMD) should be reevaluated every 2 years (or more frequently) after initiating therapy (NOF, 2013); annual measurements of height and weight, assessment of chronic back pain; serum calcium and 25(OH)D; may consider measuring biochemical markers of bone turnover

Serum creatinine prior to each IV dose

Reference Range

Calcium (total): Adults: 9.0-11.0 mg/dL (2.05-2.54 mmol/L), may slightly decrease with aging

Phosphorus: 2.5-4.5 mg/dL (0.81-1.45 mmol/L)

Vitamin D: There is no clear consensus on a reference range for total serum 25(OH)D concentrations or the validity of this level as it relates clinically to bone health. In addition, there is significant variability in the reporting of serum 25(OH)D levels as a result of different assay types in use; however, the following ranges have been suggested:

Adults (IOM, 2011): Sufficient levels in practically all persons: ≥20 ng/mL (50 nmol/L); concern for risk of toxicity: >50 ng/mL (125 nmol/L)

Osteoporosis patients (NOF, 2013): Recommended level to reach and maintain: ~30 ng/mL (75 nmol/L)

Dosage Forms

Solution, Intravenous:

Boniva: 3 mg/3 mL (3 mL)

Generic: 3 mg/3 mL (3 mL)

Solution, Intravenous [preservative free]:
Generic: 3 mg/3 mL (3 mL)

Tablet, Oral:
Boniva: 150 mg
Generic: 150 mg

◆ **Ibandronate Sodium** *see* Ibandronate *on page 1028*

Ibandronic Acid [INT] (i ban DRON ik AS id)

International Brand Names Bondronat (AT, CH, DE, DK, ES, FR, SE); Bonviva (AT, SE)

Pharmacologic Category Bisphosphonate Derivative

Reported Use Treatment of hypercalcemia of malignancy

Dosage Range IV: 2-4 mg infused over 2 hours

Product Availability Product available in various countries; not currently available in the U.S.

Dosage Forms
Injection, solution: 1 mg/mL (1 mL, 2 mL, 4 mL)

◆ **Ibandronic Acid** *see* Ibandronate *on page 1028*

◆ **Ibenzmethyzin** *see* Procarbazine *on page 1717*

◆ **Ibidomide Hydrochloride** *see* Labetalol *on page 1151*

Ibrutinib (eye BROO ti nib)

Brand Names: U.S. Imbruvica

Brand Names: Canada Imbruvica

Index Terms BTK inhibitor PCI-32765; CRA-032765; PCI-32765

Pharmacologic Category Antineoplastic Agent; Antineoplastic Agent, Bruton Tyrosine Kinase Inhibitor; Antineoplastic Agent, Tyrosine Kinase Inhibitor

Use

Chronic lymphocytic leukemia: Treatment of patients with chronic lymphocytic leukemia (CLL) who have received at least 1 prior therapy; treatment of CLL patients with 17p deletion.

Mantle cell lymphoma: Treatment of mantle cell lymphoma (MCL) in patients who have received at least 1 prior therapy

Pregnancy Risk Factor D

Pregnancy Considerations Adverse events were observed in animal reproduction studies. The U.S. labeling recommends women of reproductive potential avoid pregnancy during therapy. The Canadian labeling recommends women of reproductive potential use highly effective contraception during and for 3 months after completion of treatment; if using a hormonal method of contraception, add a barrier method; male patients should use a condom (during and for 3 months after completion of treatment) when engaging in sexual activity with a pregnant woman.

Breast-Feeding Considerations It is not known if ibrutinib is excreted in breast milk. Due to the potential for serious adverse reactions in the nursing infant, the manufacturer recommends a decision be made whether to discontinue nursing or to discontinue the drug, taking into account the importance of treatment to the mother.

Contraindications

U.S. labeling: There are no contraindications listed in the manufacturer's labeling.

Canadian labeling: Known hypersensitivity to ibrutinib or any component of the formulation.

Warnings/Precautions Hazardous agent – use appropriate precautions for handling and disposal (meets NIOSH 2014 criteria). Grade 3 and 4 neutropenia, thrombocytopenia, and anemia occurred commonly during clinical studies. Monitor blood counts monthly or as clinically necessary. Lymphocytosis (≥50% increase from baseline) may occur upon therapy initiation, generally within the first few weeks of therapy. The increase in lymphocytes is temporary, and resolves by a median of 8 weeks (mantle cell lymphoma) or 23 weeks (chronic lymphocytic leukemia). Some patients who developed lymphocytosis (lymphocytes >400,000/mcL) have developed intracranial hemorrhage, lethargy, headache, and gait instability (some cases may have been associated with disease progression). Monitor for leukostasis, particularly in patients experiencing a rapid increase in lymphocytes to >400,000/mcL. Grade 3 or higher bleeding events (subdural hematoma, gastrointestinal bleeding, hematuria, and post-procedural bleeding) have occurred. Bleeding events of any grade, including bruising and petechiae have occurred in approximately half of patients receiving ibrutinib. Patients receiving concurrent antiplatelet or anticoagulant treatment may have an increased risk for bleeding. Evaluate the risk-benefit of withholding ibrutinib for 3 to 7 days prior to and after surgery, depending on the procedure type and risk of bleeding. Serious infections (some fatal) have been observed; monitor closely for fever and other signs/symptoms of infection. Evaluate promptly. Patients treated with ibrutinib have developed second primary malignancies, including skin cancers and other carcinomas. Evaluate for sign/symptoms of malignancy during treatment.

Atrial fibrillation and atrial flutter have occurred, particularly in patients with cardiac risk factors, infections (acute), or with a history of atrial fibrillation. Monitor periodically for clinical symptoms of atrial fibrillation (eg, palpitations, lightheadedness); an ECG should be performed if symptoms or new onset dyspnea develop. For persistent atrial fibrillation, evaluate the risk-benefit of ibrutinib treatment and dose modification. Atrial fibrillation, hypertension, infections (eg, pneumonia, cellulitis), and gastrointestinal toxicity (eg, diarrhea and dehydration) were observed more frequently in elderly patients; maintain adequate hydration. Use with caution in patients with preexisting renal impairment; has not been studied in those with severe impairment or in patients on dialysis. Renal failure has been reported with use; some cases were fatal. Clinical trials report serum creatinine increases of up to 3 times ULN; monitor renal function periodically and maintain hydration. Increased uric acid levels have been observed, including grade 4 elevations; monitor for tumor lysis syndrome in patients at risk (eg, high tumor burden). Use with caution in patients with any degree of hepatic impairment. Patients with AST or ALT levels ≥3 times ULN were excluded from clinical trials; ibrutinib is hepatically metabolized, and exposure is expected to increase in patients with hepatic dysfunction. Monitor closely for toxicity. May cause dizziness, fatigue, and/or weakness which may impair physical or mental abilities; patients must be cautioned about performing tasks that require mental alertness (eg, operating machinery or driving). Potentially significant drug-drug/drug-food interactions may exist, requiring dose or frequency adjustment, additional monitoring, and/or selection of alternative therapy.

Adverse Reactions

Cardiovascular: Atrial fibrillation, atrial flutter, hypertension (more common in CLL patients), peripheral edema (more common in MCL patients)

Central nervous system: Anxiety (CLL), chills (CLL), dizziness, fatigue (more common in MCL patients), headache, insomnia (CLL), peripheral neuropathy (CLL)

Dermatologic: Skin infection, skin rash

Endocrine & metabolic: Dehydration (MCL), hyperuricemia (MCL), increased uric acid (MCL)

Gastrointestinal: abdominal pain (more common in MCL patients), constipation, decreased appetite, diarrhea (more common in CLL patients), dyspepsia, nausea (more common in MCL patients), stomatitis, vomiting

Genitourinary: Urinary tract infection

Hematologic & oncologic: Anemia, bruise (more common in CLL patients), decreased hemoglobin, decreased platelet count (more common in CLL patients), hemorrhage (bleeding events including gastrointestinal bleeding, hematuria, postprocedural bleeding, subdural hematoma, and other carcinomas), malignant neoplasm (secondary; includes one death due to histiocytic sarcoma), malignant neoplasm of skin, neutropenia, petechia

Infection: Infection

Neuromuscular & skeletal: Arthralgia (more common in CLL patients), musculoskeletal pain (more common in MCL patients), muscle spasm, weakness

Renal: Increased serum creatinine

Respiratory: Cough, dyspnea (more common in MCL patients), epistaxis (MCL), oropharyngeal pain (CLL), pneumonia, sinusitis, upper respiratory tract infection (more common in CLL patients)

Miscellaneous: Fever, laceration (CLL)

Rare but important or life-threatening: Renal failure

Drug Interactions

Metabolism/Transport Effects **Substrate** of CYP2D6 (minor), CYP3A4 (major); **Note:** Assignment of Major/Minor substrate status based on clinically relevant drug interaction potential; **Inhibits** BCRP, P-glycoprotein

Avoid Concomitant Use

Avoid concomitant use of Ibrutinib with any of the following: BCG; Bosutinib; CloZAPine; Conivaptan; CYP3A4 Inducers (Strong); CYP3A4 Inhibitors (Moderate); CYP3A4 Inhibitors (Strong); Dipyrone; Fusidic Acid (Systemic); Idelalisib; Natalizumab; PAZOPanib; Pimecrolimus; Silodosin; St Johns Wort; Tacrolimus (Topical); Tofacitinib; Topotecan; Vaccines (Live); VinCRIStine (Liposomal)

Increased Effect/Toxicity

Ibrutinib may increase the levels/effects of: Afatinib; Agents with Antiplatelet Properties; Anticoagulants; Bosutinib; Brentuximab Vedotin; CloZAPine; Colchicine; Dabigatran Etexilate; DOXOrubicin (Conventional); Edoxaban; Everolimus; Ledipasvir; Leflunomide; Naloxegol; Natalizumab; PAZOPanib; P-glycoprotein/ABCB1 Substrates; Prucalopride; Rifaximin; Rivaroxaban; Silodosin; Tofacitinib; Topotecan; Vaccines (Live); VinCRIStine (Liposomal)

The levels/effects of Ibrutinib may be increased by: Conivaptan; CYP3A4 Inhibitors (Moderate); CYP3A4 Inhibitors (Strong); Dasatinib; Denosumab; Dipyrone; Flaxseed Oil; Fusidic Acid (Systemic); Idelalisib; Ivacaftor; Luliconazole; Mifepristone; Omega-3 Fatty Acids; Pimecrolimus; Roflumilast; Simeprevir; Tacrolimus (Topical); Trastuzumab; Vitamin E

Decreased Effect

Ibrutinib may decrease the levels/effects of: BCG; Coccidioides immitis Skin Test; Sipuleucel-T; Vaccines (Inactivated); Vaccines (Live)

The levels/effects of Ibrutinib may be decreased by: CYP3A4 Inducers (Moderate); CYP3A4 Inducers (Strong); Dabrafenib; Deferasirox; Echinacea; Siltuximab; St Johns Wort; Tocilizumab

Food Interactions Grapefruit and Seville oranges moderately inhibit CYP3A and may increase ibrutinib exposure. Management: Avoid grapefruit and Seville oranges during therapy.

Storage/Stability Store at 20°C to 25°C (68°F to 77°F); excursions are permitted between 15°C and 30°C (59°F and 86°F). Keep in original container.

Mechanism of Action Ibrutinib is a potent and irreversible inhibitor of Bruton's tyrosine kinase (BTK), an integral component of the B-cell receptor (BCR) and cytokine receptor pathways. Constitutive activation of B-cell receptor signaling is important for survival of malignant B-cells; BTK inhibition results in decreased malignant B-cell proliferation and survival.

Pharmacodynamics/Kinetics

Distribution: ~10,000 L

Bioavailability: Administration with food increased the C_{max} by ~2- to 4-fold and the AUC 2-fold (compared with overnight fasting).

Protein binding: ~97%

Metabolism: Hepatic via CYP3A (major) and CYP2D6 (minor) to active metabolite PCI-45227

Half-life elimination: 4 to 6 hours

Time to peak: 1 to 2 hours

Excretion: Feces (80%; ~1% as unchanged drug); urine (<10%, as metabolites)

Dosage

Chronic lymphocytic leukemia (CLL), previously treated: Adults: Oral: 420 mg once daily (Byrd, 2014)

CLL with 17p deletion: Adults: Oral: 420 mg once daily (Byrd, 2014)

Mantle cell lymphoma (MCL), previously treated: Adults: Oral: 560 mg once daily (Wang, 2013)

Missed doses: Administer as soon as the missed dose is remembered on the same day; return to normal scheduling the following day. Do not take extra capsules to make up for the missed dose.

Dosage adjustment for concomitant therapy:

Moderate or strong CYP3A inhibitors:

U.S. labeling: Avoid concurrent use with moderate or strong CYP3A inhibitors which are taken chronically; consider an alternative agent with less CYP3A inhibition. If short term use (≤7 days) of a strong inhibitor is necessary, consider withholding ibrutinib therapy until the strong CYP3A inhibitor is discontinued. If concomitant use of a moderate inhibitor is necessary, reduce ibrutinib dose to 140 mg once daily. Monitor closely for toxicity during concomitant use.

Canadian labeling: Avoid concurrent use with moderate or strong CYP3A inhibitors; consider an alternative agent with less CYP3A inhibition. If use of a strong inhibitor is necessary, withhold ibrutinib temporarily until the strong CYP3A inhibitor is discontinued. If concomitant use of a moderate inhibitor is necessary, reduce ibrutinib dose to 140 mg once daily until the inhibitor is discontinued. Monitor closely for toxicity during concomitant use.

Strong CYP3A inducers: Avoid concurrent use with strong CYP3A inducers; consider alternative agents with less CYP3A induction.

Dosage adjustment for toxicity:

Hematologic toxicity: ≥ grade 3 neutropenia with infection or fever, or grade 4 toxicity: Interrupt therapy; upon improvement to grade 1 toxicity or baseline, resume dosing at the starting dose. If toxicity recurs, reduce daily dose by 140 mg. If toxicity recurs after first dose reduction, reduce daily dose by an additional 140 mg. If toxicity persists following 2 dose reductions, discontinue therapy.

Nonhematologic toxicity: ≥ grade 3 toxicity: Interrupt therapy; upon improvement to grade 1 toxicity or baseline, resume dosing at the starting dose. If toxicity recurs, reduce daily dose by 140 mg. If toxicity recurs after first dose reduction, reduce daily dose by an additional 140 mg. If toxicity persists following 2 dose reductions, discontinue therapy.

Recommend dose reductions for toxicity (following recovery):

Chronic lymphocytic leukemia:

First occurrence: Restart at 420 mg once daily

Second occurrence: Restart at 280 mg once daily

Third occurrence: Restart at 140 mg once daily

Fourth occurrence: Discontinue

Mantle cell lymphoma:
First occurrence: Restart at 560 mg once daily
Second occurrence: Restart at 420 mg once daily
Third occurrence: Restart at 280 mg once daily
Fourth occurrence: Discontinue

Dosage adjustment for renal impairment:

Mild to moderate impairment (CrCl ≥25 mL/minute [U.S. labeling] or CrCl >30 mL/minute [Canadian labeling]): There are no dosage adjustments provided in the manufacturer's labeling; however, renal excretion is minimal and drug exposure is not altered in patients with mild to moderate impairment.

Severe impairment (CrCl <25 mL/minute [U.S. labeling] or CrCl ≤30 mL/minute [Canadian labeling]): There are no dosage adjustments provided in the manufacturer's labeling (has not been studied).

End-stage renal disease (ESRD) requiring dialysis: There are no dosage adjustments provided in the manufacturer's labeling (has not been studied).

Dosage adjustment for hepatic impairment:

U.S. labeling: Mild, moderate, or severe impairment (Child-Pugh class A, B, or C): There are no dosage adjustments provided in the manufacturer's labeling. Ibrutinib is metabolized hepatically; significant increases in drug exposure are expected in patients with hepatic impairment. Patients with AST or ALT levels ≥3 times ULN were excluded from clinical trials.

Canadian labeling:

Mild impairment (Child-Pugh class A): May consider dose reduction to 140 mg once daily (based on preliminary data) only if clinically indicated; monitor closely.

Moderate and severe impairment (Child-Pugh class B and C): Avoid use.

Dietary Considerations Avoid grapefruit, grapefruit juice, and Seville oranges during therapy.

Administration Administer orally with water at approximately the same time every day. Swallow capsules whole; do not open, break, or chew the capsules. Maintain adequate hydration during treatment. Hazardous agent; use appropriate precautions for handling and disposal (meets NIOSH 2014 criteria).

Monitoring Parameters Monitor blood counts monthly or as clinically necessary; renal and hepatic function; uric acid levels as clinically necessary; sign/symptoms of bleeding, infections, and second primary malignancies; signs/symptoms of atrial fibrillation; ECG prior to initiation (patients with cardiac risk factors or history of atrial fibrillation) and during therapy if clinically indicated.

Dosage Forms

Capsule, Oral:

Imbruvica: 140 mg

◆ **IBU-200 [OTC]** *see* Ibuprofen *on page 1032*

◆ **Ibudone** *see* Hydrocodone and Ibuprofen *on page 1013*

Ibuprofen (eye byoo PROE fen)

Brand Names: U.S. Addaprin [OTC]; Advil Junior Strength [OTC]; Advil Migraine [OTC]; Advil [OTC]; Caldolor; Childrens Advil [OTC]; Childrens Ibuprofen [OTC]; Childrens Motrin Jr Strength [OTC]; Childrens Motrin [OTC]; Dyspel [OTC]; EnovaRX-Ibuprofen; Genpril [OTC]; I-Prin [OTC]; IBU-200 [OTC]; Ibuprofen Childrens [OTC]; Ibuprofen Comfort Pac; Ibuprofen Junior Strength [OTC]; Infants Advil [OTC]; Infants Ibuprofen [OTC]; KS Ibuprofen [OTC]; Motrin IB [OTC]; Motrin Infants Drops [OTC]; Motrin Junior Strength [OTC]; Motrin [OTC]; NeoProfen; Provil [OTC]

Brand Names: Canada Advil; Advil Pediatric Drops; Apo-Ibuprofen; Caldolor; Children's Advil; Children's Europrofen; Ibuprofen Muscle and Joint; Jamp-Ibuprofen; Motrin; Motrin (Children's); Motrin IB; Novo-Profen; Pamprin Ibuprofen Formula; PMS-Ibuprofen; Super Strength Motrin IB Liquid Gel Capsules

Index Terms *p*-Isobutylhydratropic Acid; Ibuprofen Lysine

Pharmacologic Category Nonsteroidal Anti-inflammatory Drug (NSAID), Oral; Nonsteroidal Anti-inflammatory Drug (NSAID), Parenteral

Additional Appendix Information

Beers Criteria – Potentially Inappropriate Medications for Geriatrics *on page 2271*

Use

Oral: Inflammatory diseases and rheumatoid disorders, mild to moderate pain, fever, dysmenorrhea, osteoarthritis

Ibuprofen injection (Caldolor): Management of mild-to-moderate pain; management moderate-to-severe pain when used concurrently with an opioid analgesic; reduction of fever

Ibuprofen lysine injection (NeoProfen): Patent ductus arteriosus (PDA): To close a clinically significant PDA in premature infants weighing between 500-1500 g who are no more than 32 weeks of gestational age when usual medical management (eg, diuretics, fluid restriction, respiratory support) is ineffective.

OTC labeling: Reduction of fever; management of pain due to headache, sore throat, arthritis, physical or athletic overexertion (eg, sprains/strains), menstrual pain, dental pain, minor muscle/bone/joint pain, backache, pain due to the common cold and flu

Pregnancy Risk Factor C/D ≥30 weeks gestation

Pregnancy Considerations Adverse events were not observed in the initial animal reproduction studies; therefore, the manufacturer classifies ibuprofen as pregnancy category C (category D: ≥30 weeks' gestation). NSAID exposure during the first trimester is not strongly associated with congenital malformations; however, cardiovascular anomalies and cleft palate have been observed following NSAID exposure in some studies. The use of a NSAID close to conception may be associated with an increased risk of miscarriage. Nonteratogenic effects have been observed following NSAID administration during the third trimester including: Myocardial degenerative changes, prenatal constriction of the ductus arteriosus, fetal tricuspid regurgitation, failure of the ductus arteriosus to close postnatally; renal dysfunction or failure, oligohydramnios; gastrointestinal bleeding or perforation, increased risk of necrotizing enterocolitis; intracranial bleeding (including intraventricular hemorrhage), platelet dysfunction with resultant bleeding; pulmonary hypertension. Because they may cause premature closure of the ductus arteriosus, use of NSAIDs late in pregnancy should be avoided (use after 31 or 32 weeks' gestation is not recommended by some clinicians). US labeling for Caldolor specifically notes that use at ≥30 weeks' gestation should be avoided and therefore classifies ibuprofen as pregnancy category D at this time. Canadian labeling contraindicates use of ibuprofen (IV and oral) during the third trimester. The chronic use of NSAIDs in women of reproductive age may be associated with infertility that is reversible upon discontinuation of the medication. A registry is available for pregnant women exposed to autoimmune medications including ibuprofen. For additional information contact the Organization of Teratology Information Specialists, OTIS Autoimmune Diseases Study, at 877-311-8972.

Breast-Feeding Considerations Based on limited data, only very small amounts of ibuprofen are excreted into breast milk. Adverse events have not been reported in nursing infants. Because there is a potential for adverse events to occur in nursing infants, the manufacturer does not recommend the use of ibuprofen while breast-feeding. Use with caution in nursing women with hypertensive disorders of pregnancy or preexisting renal disease.

Contraindications

Hypersensitivity to ibuprofen; history of asthma, urticaria, or allergic-type reaction to aspirin or other NSAIDs; aspirin triad (eg, bronchial asthma, aspirin intolerance, rhinitis); perioperative pain in the setting of coronary artery bypass graft (CABG) surgery

Ibuprofen lysine (NeoProfen): Preterm neonates: With proven or suspected infection that is untreated; congenital heart disease in whom patency of the PDA is necessary for satisfactory pulmonary or systemic blood flow (eg, pulmonary atresia, severe coarctation of the aorta, severe tetralogy of Fallot); bleeding (especially those with active intracranial hemorrhage or GI bleeding); thrombocytopenia; coagulation defects; proven or suspected necrotizing enterocolitis; or significant renal function impairment.

Canadian labeling: Additional contraindications (not in US labeling): Cerebrovascular bleeding or other bleeding disorders; active gastric/duodenal/peptic ulcer, active GI bleeding; inflammatory bowel disease; uncontrolled heart failure; moderate [IV formulation only] to severe renal impairment (creatinine clearance [CrCl] <30 mL/minute); deteriorating renal disease; moderate [IV formulation only] to severe hepatic impairment; active hepatic disease; hyperkalemia; third trimester of pregnancy; breastfeeding; patients <18 years of age [IV formulation only]; patients <12 years of age [oral formulation only]; systemic lupus erythematosus [oral formulation only]

OTC labeling: When used for self-medication, do not use if previous allergic reaction to any other pain reliever/fever reducer; prior to or following cardiac surgery.

Warnings/Precautions [U.S. Boxed Warning]: NSAIDs are associated with an increased risk of adverse cardiovascular thrombotic events, including fatal MI and stroke. Risk may be increased with duration of use or preexisting cardiovascular risk factors or disease. Carefully evaluate individual cardiovascular risk profiles prior to prescribing. May cause new-onset hypertension or worsening of existing hypertension. Response to ACE inhibitors, thiazides, or loop diuretics may be impaired with concurrent use of NSAIDs. Use caution with fluid retention. Avoid use in heart failure (ACCF/AHA [Yancy, 2013]). Concurrent administration of ibuprofen, and potentially other nonselective NSAIDs, may interfere with aspirin's cardioprotective effect. **[U.S. Boxed Warning]: Use is contraindicated for treatment of perioperative pain in the setting of coronary artery bypass graft (CABG) surgery.** Risk of MI and stroke may be increased with use following CABG surgery.

May increase the risk of aseptic meningitis, especially in patients with systemic lupus erythematosus (SLE) and mixed connective tissue disorders. Platelet adhesion and aggregation may be decreased; may prolong bleeding time; patients with coagulation disorders or who are receiving anticoagulants should be monitored closely. Anemia may occur; patients on long-term NSAID therapy should be monitored for anemia. Rarely, NSAID use may cause severe blood dyscrasias (eg, agranulocytosis, aplastic anemia, thrombocytopenia).

NSAID use may compromise existing renal function; dose-dependent decreases in prostaglandin synthesis may result from NSAID use, reducing renal blood flow which may cause renal decompensation. NSAID use may increase the risk for hyperkalemia. Patients with impaired renal function, dehydration, heart failure, liver dysfunction, those taking diuretics, and ACE inhibitors, and the elderly are at greater risk of renal toxicity and hyperkalemia. Rehydrate patient before starting therapy; monitor renal function closely. The Canadian labeling contraindicates use in moderate (IV only) to severe renal impairment, with deteriorating renal disease and in patients with hyperkalemia. Use of ibuprofen lysine (NeoProfen) is contraindicated in preterm infants with significant renal impairment. Long-term NSAID use may result in renal papillary necrosis.

NSAIDs may increase risk of gastrointestinal irritation, inflammation, ulceration, bleeding, and perforation. These events can be fatal and may occur at any time during therapy and without warning. Elderly patients are at increased risk for serious adverse events. Use caution with a history of GI disease (bleeding or ulcers), concurrent therapy with aspirin, anticoagulants and/or corticosteroids, smoking, use of ethanol, the elderly or debilitated patients. When used concomitantly with aspirin, a substantial increase in the risk of gastrointestinal complications (eg, ulcer) occurs; concomitant gastroprotective therapy (eg, proton pump inhibitors) is recommended (Bhatt, 2008). The Canadian labeling contraindicates use in patients with active GI disease (eg, peptic ulcer) or GI bleeding and inflammatory bowel disease.

Use the lowest effective dose for the shortest duration of time, consistent with individual patient goals, to reduce risk of cardiovascular or GI adverse events. Alternate therapies should be considered for patients at high risk.

NSAIDs may cause serious skin adverse events including exfoliative dermatitis, Stevens-Johnson Syndrome (SJS) and toxic epidermal necrolysis (TEN); discontinue use at first sign of skin rash or hypersensitivity. Anaphylactoid reactions may occur, even without prior exposure; patients with "aspirin triad" (bronchial asthma, aspirin intolerance, rhinitis) may be at increased risk. Do not use in patients who experience bronchospasm, asthma, rhinitis, or urticaria with NSAID or aspirin therapy. Use caution in other forms of asthma.

NSAIDS may cause drowsiness, dizziness, blurred vision and other neurologic effects which may impair physical or mental abilities; patients must be cautioned about performing tasks which require mental alertness (eg, operating machinery or driving). Monitor vision with long-term therapy. Blurred/diminished vision, scotomata, and changes in color vision have been reported. Discontinue use with altered vision and perform ophthalmologic exam.

Use with caution in patients with decreased hepatic function. Closely monitor patients with any abnormal LFT. Severe hepatic reactions (eg, fulminant hepatitis, jaundice, liver necrosis, liver failure) have occurred with NSAID use, rarely; discontinue if signs or symptoms of liver disease develop, or if systemic manifestations occur. The Canadian labeling contraindicates use in moderate (IV only) to severe impairment and with active hepatic disease.

In the elderly, avoid chronic use (unless alternative agents ineffective and patient can receive concomitant gastroprotective agent); nonselective oral NSAID use is associated with an increased risk of GI bleeding and peptic ulcer disease in older adults in high risk category (eg, >75 years or age or receiving concomitant oral/parenteral corticosteroids, anticoagulants, or antiplatelet agents) (Beers Criteria). Potentially significant drug interactions may exist, requiring dose or frequency adjustment, additional monitoring, and/or selection of alternative therapy.

Withhold for at least 4-6 half-lives prior to surgical or dental procedures.

Ibuprofen injection (Caldolor) must be diluted prior to administration; hemolysis can occur if not diluted.

Ibuprofen lysine injection (NeoProfen): Hold second or third doses if urinary output is <0.6 mL/kg/hour. May alter signs of infection. May inhibit platelet aggregation; monitor for signs of bleeding. May displace bilirubin; use caution when total bilirubin is elevated. Long-term evaluations of neurodevelopment, growth, or diseases associated with prematurity following treatment have not been conducted. A second course of treatment, alternative pharmacologic therapy or surgery may be needed if the ductus arteriosus fails to close or reopens following the initial course of therapy.

Benzyl alcohol and derivatives: Some dosage forms may contain sodium benzoate/benzoic acid; benzoic acid (benzoate) is a metabolite of benzyl alcohol; large amounts of benzyl alcohol (≥99 mg/kg/day) have been associated with a potentially fatal toxicity ("gasping syndrome") in neonates; the "gasping syndrome" consists of metabolic acidosis, respiratory distress, gasping respirations, CNS dysfunction (including convulsions, intracranial hemorrhage), hypotension, and cardiovascular collapse (AAP, 1997; CDC, 1982); some data suggests that benzoate displaces bilirubin from protein binding sites (Ahlfors, 2001); avoid or use dosage forms containing benzyl alcohol derivative with caution in neonates. See manufacturer's labeling.

Phenylalanine: Some products may contain phenylalanine.

Self medication (OTC use): Prior to self-medication, patients should contact healthcare provider if they have had recurring stomach pain or upset, ulcers, bleeding problems, high blood pressure, heart or kidney disease, other serious medical problems, are currently taking a diuretic, aspirin, anticoagulant, or are ≥60 years of age. If patients are using for migraines, they should also contact healthcare provider if they have not had a migraine diagnosis by healthcare provider, a headache that is different from usual migraine, worst headache of life, fever and neck stiffness, headache from head injury or coughing, first headache at ≥50 years of age, daily headache, or migraine requiring bed rest. Recommended dosages should not be exceeded, due to an increased risk of GI bleeding. Stop use and consult a healthcare provider if symptoms get worse, newly appear, fever lasts for >3 days or pain lasts >3 days (children) and >10 days (adults). Do not give for >10 days unless instructed by healthcare provider. Consuming ≥3 alcoholic beverages/day or taking longer than recommended may increase the risk of GI bleeding.

Adverse Reactions

Oral:

Cardiovascular: Edema

Central nervous system: Dizziness, headache, nervousness

Dermatologic: Itching, rash

Endocrine & metabolic: Fluid retention

Gastrointestinal: Abdominal pain/cramps/distress, appetite decreased, constipation, diarrhea, dyspepsia, epigastric pain, flatulence, heartburn, nausea, vomiting

Otic: Tinnitus

Rare but important or life-threatening: Acute renal failure, agranulocytosis, anaphylaxis, aplastic anemia, azotemia, blurred vision, bone marrow suppression, confusion, creatinine clearance decreased, duodenal ulcer, edema, eosinophilia, epistaxis, erythema multiforme, gastric ulcer, GI bleed, GI hemorrhage, GI ulceration, hallucinations, hearing decreased, hematuria, hematocrit decreased, hemoglobin decreased, hemolytic anemia, hepatitis, hypertension, inhibition of platelet aggregation, jaundice, liver function tests abnormal, leukopenia, melena, neutropenia, pancreatitis, photosensitivity, Stevens-Johnson syndrome, thrombocytopenia, toxic amblyopia, toxic epidermal necrolysis, urticaria, vesiculobullous eruptions, vision changes

Injection: Ibuprofen (Caldolor®):

Cardiovascular: Edema, hypertension

Central nervous system: Dizziness, headache

Dermatologic: Pruritus

Endocrine & metabolic: Hypernatremia, hypokalemia

Gastrointestinal: Abdominal pain, dyspepsia, flatulence, nausea, vomiting

Genitourinary: Urinary retention

Hematologic: Anemia, hemorrhage, neutropenia

Renal: BUN increased

Respiratory: Cough

Injection: Ibuprofen lysine (NeoProfen®):

Cardiovascular: Edema, heart failure, intraventricular hemorrhage, hypotension, tachycardia

Central nervous system: Seizure

Dermatologic: Skin irritation

Endocrine & metabolic: Adrenal insufficiency, hypernatremia, hypocalcemia, hyper-/hypoglycemia

Gastrointestinal: Abdominal distension, feeding problems, gastritis, GI disorders, GI reflux, ileus, non NEC

Genitourinary: Urinary tract infection

Hematologic: Anemia, neutropenia, thrombocytopenia

Hepatic: Cholestasis, jaundice

Local: Injection-site reaction

Respiratory: Apnea, respiratory infection

Renal: Urea increased, renal impairment, creatinine increased, renal failure, urine output decreased (small decrease reported on days 2-6 with compensatory increase in output on day 9)

Respiratory: Respiratory failure, atelectasis

Miscellaneous: Infection, inguinal hernia, sepsis

Rare but important or life-threatening: GI perforation, necrotizing enterocolitis

Drug Interactions

Metabolism/Transport Effects Substrate of CYP2C19 (minor), CYP2C9 (minor); **Note:** Assignment of Major/Minor substrate status based on clinically relevant drug interaction potential; **Inhibits** CYP2C9 (weak)

Avoid Concomitant Use

Avoid concomitant use of Ibuprofen with any of the following: Dexketoprofen; Floctafenine; Ketorolac (Nasal); Ketorolac (Systemic); NSAID (COX-2 Inhibitor); Omacetaxine; Urokinase

Increased Effect/Toxicity

Ibuprofen may increase the levels/effects of: 5-ASA Derivatives; Agents with Antiplatelet Properties; Aliskiren; Aminoglycosides; Anticoagulants; Apixaban; Bisphosphonate Derivatives; Collagenase (Systemic); CycloSPORINE (Systemic); Dabigatran Etexilate; Deferasirox; Desmopressin; Digoxin; Eplerenone; Haloperidol; Ibritumomab; Lithium; Methotrexate; Nonsteroidal Anti-Inflammatory Agents; NSAID (COX-2 Inhibitor); Obinutuzumab; Omacetaxine; PEMEtrexed; Porfimer; Potassium-Sparing Diuretics; PRALAtrexate; Quinolone Antibiotics; Rivaroxaban; Salicylates; Tacrolimus (Systemic); Tenofovir; Thrombolytic Agents; Tositumomab and Iodine I 131 Tositumomab; Urokinase; Vancomycin; Verteporfin; Vitamin K Antagonists

The levels/effects of Ibuprofen may be increased by: ACE Inhibitors; Angiotensin II Receptor Blockers; Antidepressants (Tricyclic, Tertiary Amine); Corticosteroids (Systemic); CycloSPORINE (Systemic); Dasatinib; Dexketoprofen; Diclofenac (Systemic); Floctafenine; Glucosamine; Herbs (Anticoagulant/Antiplatelet Properties); Ibrutinib; Ketorolac (Nasal); Ketorolac (Systemic); Limaprost; Multivitamins/Fluoride (with ADE); Multivitamins/Minerals (with ADEK, Folate, Iron); Multivitamins/Minerals (with AE, No Iron); Omega-3 Fatty Acids; Pentosan Polysulfate Sodium; Pentoxifylline; Probenecid; Prostacyclin Analogues; Selective Serotonin Reuptake Inhibitors; Serotonin/Norepinephrine Reuptake Inhibitors; Sodium Phosphates; Tipranavir; Treprostinil; Vitamin E; Voriconazole

Decreased Effect

Ibuprofen may decrease the levels/effects of: ACE Inhibitors; Aliskiren; Angiotensin II Receptor Blockers; Beta-Blockers; Eplerenone; HydrALAZINE; Imatinib; Loop

Diuretics; Potassium-Sparing Diuretics; Prostaglandins (Ophthalmic); Salicylates; Selective Serotonin Reuptake Inhibitors; Thiazide Diuretics

The levels/effects of Ibuprofen may be decreased by: Bile Acid Sequestrants; Salicylates

Food Interactions Ibuprofen peak serum levels may be decreased if taken with food. Management: Administer with food.

Preparation for Administration

Ibuprofen injection (Caldolor): Must be diluted prior to use. Dilute with D_5W, NS or LR to a final concentration ≤4 mg/mL.

Ibuprofen lysine injection (NeoProfen): Dilute with dextrose or saline to an appropriate volume.

Storage/Stability

Ibuprofen injection (Caldolor): Store intact vials at room temperature of 20°C to 25°C (68°F to 77°F). Must be diluted prior to use. Diluted solutions stable for 24 hours at room temperature.

Ibuprofen lysine injection (NeoProfen): Store at 20°C to 25°C (68°F to 77°F); excursions are permitted between 15°C and 30°C (59°F and 86°F). Protect from light. Store vials in carton until use. After first withdrawal from vial, discard remaining solution (preservative free). Following dilution, use within 30 minutes.

Suspension: Store at controlled room temperature of 15°C to 30°C (59°F to 86°F).

Tablet: Store at controlled room temperature of 20°C to 25°C (68°F to 77°F).

Mechanism of Action Reversibly inhibits cyclooxygenase-1 and 2 (COX-1 and 2) enzymes, which results in decreased formation of prostaglandin precursors; has antipyretic, analgesic, and anti-inflammatory properties

Other proposed mechanisms not fully elucidated (and possibly contributing to the anti-inflammatory effect to varying degrees), include inhibiting chemotaxis, altering lymphocyte activity, inhibiting neutrophil aggregation/activation, and decreasing proinflammatory cytokine levels.

Pharmacodynamics/Kinetics

Onset of action: Oral: Analgesic: Within 30 to 60 minutes (Davies, 1998; Mehlisch, 2013); Antipyretic: <1 hour (Sullivan, 2011)

Duration: Oral: Antipyretic: 6 to 8 hours (Sullivan, 2011)

Absorption: Oral: Rapid

Distribution: V_d: 6.35 L; Premature infants (highly variable between studies; Van Overmeire, 2001):

Day 3: 160 to 328 mL/kg; Subset with ductal closure: 145 to 349 mL/kg

Day 5: 94 to 248 mL/kg; Subset with ductal closure: 72 to 222 mL/kg

Protein binding: >99%; Premature infants: ~95% (Aranda, 1997)

Bioavailability: 80%

Metabolism: Hepatic via oxidation

Half-life elimination:

Premature infants (highly variable between studies): 23 to 75 hours (Aranda, 2006; Capparelli, 2007)

Children 3 months to 10 years: 1.6 ± 0.7 hours

Adults: ~2 hours; End-stage renal disease: Unchanged (Aronoff, 2007)

Time to peak: Oral: ~1 to 2 hours

Excretion: Urine (primarily as metabolites; 1% as unchanged drug); some feces

Dosage

IV:

Neonates: Ibuprofen lysine (NeoProfen): Infants weighing between 500 to 1,500 g and ≤32 weeks GA: Patent ductus arteriosus: Initial dose: Ibuprofen 10 mg/kg, followed by two doses of 5 mg/kg at 24 and 48 hours. Dose should be based on birth weight.

Adults (Caldolor): **Note**: Patients should be well hydrated prior to administration

Analgesic: 400 to 800 mg every 6 hours as needed (maximum: 3.2 g daily)

Antipyretic:

US labeling: Initial: 400 mg, then every 4 to 6 hours or 100 to 200 mg every 4 hours as needed (maximum: 3.2 g daily)

Canadian labeling: Initial: 200 to 400 mg, then every 4 to 6 hours as needed up to 24 hours (maximum: 2.4 g daily)

Oral:

Children:

Analgesic: Infants and Children <50 kg: Limited data available in infants <6 months: 4 to 10 mg/kg/dose every 6 to 8 hours; maximum single dose: 400 mg; maximum daily dose: 40 mg/kg/day (American Pain Society, 2008; Berde, 1990; Berde, 2002; Kliegman, 2011)

Antipyretic: Infants ≥6 months, Children, and Adolescents: 5 to 10 mg/kg/dose every 6 to 8 hours; maximum single dose: 400 mg; maximum daily dose: 40 mg/kg/day up to 1,200 mg daily, unless directed by physician (under physician supervision, not to exceed maximum of 2,400 mg daily) (Litalien, 2001; Sullivan, 2011)

Juvenile idiopathic arthritis (JIA) (off-label use): Children and Adolescents: 30 to 40 mg/kg/**day** divided in 3 to 4 divided doses; start at lower end of dosing range and titrate; patients with milder disease may be treated with 20 mg/kg/day; patients with more severe disease may require up to 50 mg/kg/day; maximum single dose: 800 mg; maximum daily dose: 2,400 mg (Giannini, 1990; Kliegman, 2011; Litalien, 2001)

OTC labeling (analgesic, antipyretic): **Note:** Discontinue use and consult health care provider if no improvement within 24 hours after initiating therapy or if symptoms persist >3 days or worsen.

Children 6 months to 11 years: See table; use of weight to select dose is preferred; doses may be repeated every 6 to 8 hours (maximum: 4 doses/day)

Children ≥12 years: Refer to adult dosing.

Ibuprofen Dosing

Weight (lb)	Age	Dosage (mg)
12-17	6-11 mo	50
18-23	12-23 mo	75
24-35	2-3 y	100
36-47	4-5 y	150
48-59	6-8 y	200
60-71	9-10 y	250
72-95	11 y	300

Adults:

Analgesia/pain/dysmenorrhea: 400 mg every 4 to 6 hours as needed

Osteoarthritis, rheumatoid arthritis:

US labeling: 400 to 800 mg/dose 3 to 4 times daily (maximum dose: 3.2 g daily)

Canadian labeling: Initial: 1,200 mg in divided doses (maximum: 2.4 g daily); Maintenance: 600 to 1,200 mg daily in divided doses

OTC labeling:

Analgesic, antipyretic: 200 mg every 4 to 6 hours as needed; if no relief may increase to 400 mg every 4 to 6 hours as needed (maximum: 1.2 g daily); Duration: treatment for >10 days as an analgesic or >3 days as an antipyretic is not recommended unless directed by health care provider.

Migraine: 400 mg at onset of symptoms (maximum: 400 mg/24 hours unless directed by health care provider)

Pericarditis (off-label use): 400 to 800 mg 3 to 4 times daily (maximum dose: 3.2 g daily) (Imazio, 2009); with pericarditis postmyocardial infarction, the ACCF/AHA prefers the use of aspirin (O'Gara, 2013).

Dosage adjustment in renal impairment:

US labeling: There are no dosage adjustments provided in the manufacturer's labeling; use with caution (has not been studied in advanced disease).

Canadian labeling:

Mild impairment: There are no dosage adjustments provided in the manufacturer's labeling (has not been studied).

Moderate impairment:

Oral: There are no dosage adjustments provided in the manufacturer's labeling; use with caution.

IV: Use is contraindicated.

Severe impairment (CrCl <30 mL/minute) or deteriorating renal disease: Use is contraindicated.

KDIGO 2012 guidelines provide the following recommendations for NSAIDs:

eGFR 30 to <60 mL/minute/1.73 m^2: Avoid use in patients with intercurrent disease that increases risk of acute kidney injury.

eGFR <30 mL/minute/1.73 m^2: Avoid use.

Neoprofen: If anuria or marked oliguria (urinary output <0.6 mL/kg/hour) evident at the scheduled time of the second or third dose, hold dose until renal function returns to normal. Use is contraindicated in preterm infants with significant renal impairment.

Dosage adjustment in severe hepatic impairment:

US labeling: There are no dosage adjustment provided in manufacturer's labeling; use caution and discontinue if hepatic function worsens.

Canadian labeling:

Mild impairment: There are no dosage adjustments provided in the manufacturer's labeling.

Moderate impairment:

Oral: There are no dosage adjustments provided in the manufacturer's labeling.

IV: Use is contraindicated.

Severe impairment or active hepatic disease: Use is contraindicated.

Dietary Considerations Should be taken with food. Some products may contain phenylalanine and/or potassium.

Administration

Oral: Administer with food

IV:

Caldolor: For IV administration only; infuse over at least 30 minutes

NeoProfen (ibuprofen lysine): For IV administration only; administration via umbilical arterial line has not been evaluated. Infuse over 15 minutes through port closest to insertion site. Avoid extravasation. Do not administer simultaneously via same line with TPN. If needed, interrupt TPN for 15 minutes prior to and after ibuprofen administration, keeping line open with dextrose or saline.

Monitoring Parameters CBC, chemistry profile, occult blood loss and periodic liver function tests; monitor response (pain, range of motion, grip strength, mobility, ADL function), inflammation; observe for weight gain, edema; monitor renal function (urine output, serum BUN and creatinine); observe for bleeding, bruising; evaluate gastrointestinal effects (abdominal pain, bleeding, dyspepsia); mental confusion, disorientation; blood pressure; periodic ophthalmic exams with long-term therapy; signs of infection (ibuprofen lysine)

Reference Range Plasma concentrations >200 mcg/mL may be associated with severe toxicity

Dosage Forms Considerations EnovaRX-Ibuprofen is a compounding kit. Refer to manufacturer's labeling for compounding instructions.

Dosage Forms

Capsule, Oral:

Advil [OTC]: 200 mg

Advil Migraine [OTC]: 200 mg

KS Ibuprofen [OTC]: 200 mg

Generic: 200 mg

Cream, External:

EnovaRX-Ibuprofen: 10% (60 g, 120 g)

Kit, Combination:

Ibuprofen Comfort Pac: 800 mg

Solution, Intravenous:

Caldolor: 400 mg/4 mL (4 mL); 800 mg/8 mL (8 mL)

Solution, Intravenous [preservative free]:

NeoProfen: 10 mg/mL (2 mL)

Suspension, Oral:

Childrens Advil [OTC]: 100 mg/5 mL (30 mL, 120 mL)

Childrens Ibuprofen [OTC]: 100 mg/5 mL (118 mL, 120 mL, 237 mL, 240 mL); 40 mg/mL (15 mL)

Childrens Motrin [OTC]: 100 mg/5 mL (60 mL, 120 mL); 40 mg/mL (15 mL)

Ibuprofen Childrens [OTC]: 100 mg/5 mL (118 mL, 120 mL, 240 mL)

Infants Advil [OTC]: 50 mg/1.25 mL (15 mL)

Infants Ibuprofen [OTC]: 50 mg/1.25 mL (15 mL, 30 mL)

Motrin [OTC]: 40 mg/mL (15 mL)

Motrin Infants Drops [OTC]: 50 mg/1.25 mL (15 mL, 30 mL)

Generic: 100 mg/5 mL (5 mL, 118 mL, 120 mL, 473 mL)

Tablet, Oral:

Addaprin [OTC]: 200 mg

Advil [OTC]: 200 mg

Advil Junior Strength [OTC]: 100 mg

Dyspel [OTC]: 200 mg

Genpril [OTC]: 200 mg

I-Prin [OTC]: 200 mg

IBU-200 [OTC]: 200 mg

Motrin IB [OTC]: 200 mg

Motrin Junior Strength [OTC]: 100 mg

Provil [OTC]: 200 mg

Generic: 200 mg, 400 mg, 600 mg, 800 mg

Tablet Chewable, Oral:

Advil Junior Strength [OTC]: 100 mg

Childrens Motrin [OTC]: 50 mg

Childrens Motrin Jr Strength [OTC]: 100 mg

Ibuprofen Junior Strength [OTC]: 100 mg

Motrin Junior Strength [OTC]: 100 mg

- **Ibuprofen and Hydrocodone** *see* Hydrocodone and Ibuprofen *on page 1013*
- **Ibuprofen and Oxycodone** *see* Oxycodone and Ibuprofen *on page 1542*
- **Ibuprofen and Pseudoephedrine** *see* Pseudoephedrine and Ibuprofen *on page 1743*
- **Ibuprofen Childrens [OTC]** *see* Ibuprofen *on page 1032*
- **Ibuprofen Comfort Pac** *see* Ibuprofen *on page 1032*
- **Ibuprofen Junior Strength [OTC]** *see* Ibuprofen *on page 1032*
- **Ibuprofen Lysine** *see* Ibuprofen *on page 1032*
- **Ibuprofen Muscle and Joint (Can)** *see* Ibuprofen *on page 1032*

Ibutilide (i BYOO ti lide)

Brand Names: U.S. Corvert

Index Terms Ibutilide Fumarate

Pharmacologic Category Antiarrhythmic Agent, Class III

Additional Appendix Information

Beers Criteria - Potentially Inappropriate Medications for Geriatrics *on page 2271*

Use Acute termination of atrial fibrillation or flutter of recent onset; the effectiveness of ibutilide has not been determined in patients with arrhythmias >90 days in duration

Note: According to the American Heart Association/American College of Cardiology/Heart Rhythm Society guidelines for the management of atrial fibrillation, in patients with pre-excited atrial fibrillation and rapid ventricular response who are not hemodynamically compromised, the use of ibutilide to restore sinus rhythm or slow the ventricular rate is recommended (AHA/ACC/HRS [January, 2014]).

Pregnancy Risk Factor C

Dosage IV: Initial:

Adults:

<60 kg: 0.01 mg/kg over 10 minutes

≥60 kg: 1 mg over 10 minutes

Note: Discontinue infusion if arrhythmia terminates, if sustained or nonsustained ventricular tachycardia occurs, or if marked prolongation of QT/QTc occurs. If the arrhythmia does not terminate within 10 minutes after the end of the initial infusion, a second infusion of equal strength may be infused over a 10-minute period.

Elderly: Refer to adult dosing. Dose selection should be cautious, usually starting at the lower end of the dosing range.

Dosage adjustment in renal impairment: No dosage adjustment necessary.

Dosage adjustment in hepatic impairment: No dosage adjustment necessary.

Additional Information Complete prescribing information should be consulted for additional detail.

Dosage Forms

Solution, Intravenous:

Corvert: 1 mg/10 mL (10 mL)

Generic: 1 mg/10 mL (10 mL)

- ◆ **Ibutilide Fumarate** *see* Ibutilide *on page 1036*
- ◆ **IC51** *see* Japanese Encephalitis Virus Vaccine (Inactivated) *on page 1141*

Icatibant (eye KAT i bant)

Brand Names: U.S. Firazyr

Brand Names: Canada Firazyr

Index Terms HOE 140; Icatibant Acetate

Pharmacologic Category Selective Bradykinin B2 Receptor Antagonist

Use Hereditary angioedema: Treatment of acute attacks of hereditary angioedema (HAE)

Pregnancy Risk Factor C

Dosage SubQ: Adults: Hereditary angioedema (HAE): 30 mg/dose; may repeat one dose every 6 hours if response is inadequate or symptoms recur (maximum: 3 doses/24 hours). **Note:** The safety of >8 injections/month has not been evaluated in clinical trials (Firazyr Canadian product monograph, 2014).

Dosing adjustment in renal impairment: No dosage adjustments are recommended.

Dosing adjustment in hepatic impairment: No dosage adjustments are recommended.

Additional Information Complete prescribing information should be consulted for additional detail.

Dosage Forms

Solution, Subcutaneous [preservative free]:

Firazyr: 30 mg/3 mL (3 mL)

- ◆ **Icatibant Acetate** *see* Icatibant *on page 1037*
- ◆ **ICI-182,780** *see* Fulvestrant *on page 939*
- ◆ **ICI-204,219** *see* Zafirlukast *on page 2192*
- ◆ **ICI-46474** *see* Tamoxifen *on page 1971*
- ◆ **ICI-118630** *see* Goserelin *on page 981*
- ◆ **ICI-176334** *see* Bicalutamide *on page 262*
- ◆ **ICI-D1033** *see* Anastrozole *on page 148*
- ◆ **ICI-D1694** *see* Raltitrexed [CAN/INT] *on page 1769*
- ◆ **ICL670** *see* Deferasirox *on page 582*
- ◆ **Iclusig** *see* PONATinib *on page 1680*

Icodextrin (eye KOE dex trin)

Brand Names: U.S. Adept; Extraneal

Pharmacologic Category Adhesiolytic; Peritoneal Dialysate, Osmotic

Use

Adept®: Reduction of postsurgical adhesions in gynecologic laparoscopic procedures

Extraneal®: Daily exchange for the long dwell (8- to 16-hour) during continuous ambulatory peritoneal dialysis (CAPD) or automated peritoneal dialysis (APD) for the management of end-stage renal disease (ESRD); improvement of long-dwell ultrafiltration and clearance of creatinine and urea nitrogen (compared to 4.25% dextrose) in patients with high/average or greater transport characteristics as measured by peritoneal equilibration test (PET)

Pregnancy Risk Factor C

Dosage Intraperitoneal: Adults:

CAPD or APD (Extraneal®): Given as a single daily exchange in CAPD or APD; dwell time of 8-16 hours is suggested

Laparoscopic gynecologic surgery (Adept®): Irrigate with at least 100 mL every 30 minutes during surgery; aspirate remaining fluid after surgery is completed, then instill 1 L into the cavity

Additional Information Complete prescribing information should be consulted for additional detail.

Dosage Forms

Solution, Intraperitoneal:

Adept: 4% (1000 mL, 1500 mL)

Extraneal: 7.5% (2000 mL, 2500 mL)

- ◆ **Icosapent Ethyl** *see* Omega-3 Fatty Acids *on page 1507*
- ◆ **ICRF-187** *see* Dexrazoxane *on page 606*
- ◆ **Icy Hot [OTC]** *see* Methyl Salicylate and Menthol *on page 1344*
- ◆ **Idamycin PFS** *see* IDArubicin *on page 1037*

IDArubicin (eye da ROO bi sin)

Brand Names: U.S. Idamycin PFS

Brand Names: Canada Idamycin PFS; Idarubicin Hydrochloride Injection

Index Terms 4-Demethoxydaunorubicin; 4-DMDR; Idarubicin Hydrochloride; IDR; IMI 30; SC 33428

Pharmacologic Category Antineoplastic Agent, Anthracycline; Antineoplastic Agent, Topoisomerase II Inhibitor

Use Treatment of acute myeloid leukemia (AML)

Pregnancy Risk Factor D

Dosage Note: Idarubicin is associated with a moderate emetic potential; antiemetics are recommended to prevent nausea and vomiting (Basch, 2011; Dupuis, 2011; Roila, 2010).

Children: AML (off-label use): IV: 10 to 12 mg/m^2/day for 3 days every 3 weeks

Adults: IV:

AML induction: 12 mg/m²/day for 3 days

AML consolidation: 10 to 12 mg/m²/day for 2 days

Dosage adjustment in renal impairment: There are no dosage adjustments provided in the manufacturer's labeling; however, it does recommend that dosage reductions be made. Patients with S_{cr}: ≥2 mg/dL did not receive treatment in many clinical trials. The following adjustments have also been recommended (Aronoff, 2007):

Children:

CrCl <50 mL/minute: Administer 75% of dose

Hemodialysis: Administer 75% of dose

Continuous ambulatory peritoneal dialysis (CAPD): Administer 75% of dose

Continuous renal replacement therapy (CRRT): Administer 75% of dose

Adults:

CrCl 10 to 50 mL/minute: Administer 75% of dose

CrCl <10 mL/minute: Administer 50% of dose

Hemodialysis/CAPD: Supplemental dose not needed

Dosage adjustment/comments in hepatic impairment:

Bilirubin 2.6 to 5 mg/dL: Administer 50% of dose

Bilirubin >5 mg/dL: Avoid use

Dosing in obesity: *ASCO Guidelines for appropriate chemotherapy dosing in obese adults with cancer:* Utilize patient's actual body weight (full weight) for calculation of body surface area- or weight-based dosing, particularly when the intent of therapy is curative; manage regimen-related toxicities in the same manner as for nonobese patients; if a dose reduction is utilized due to toxicity, consider resumption of full weight-based dosing with subsequent cycles, especially if cause of toxicity (eg, hepatic or renal impairment) is resolved (Griggs, 2012).

Additional Information Complete prescribing information should be consulted for additional detail.

Dosage Forms

Solution, Intravenous [preservative free]:

Idamycin PFS: 5 mg/5 mL (5 mL); 10 mg/10 mL (10 mL); 20 mg/20 mL (20 mL)

Generic: 5 mg/5 mL (5 mL); 10 mg/10 mL (10 mL); 20 mg/20 mL (20 mL)

◆ **Idarubicin Hydrochloride** *see* IDArubicin *on page 1037*

◆ **Idarubicin Hydrochloride Injection (Can)** *see* IDArubicin *on page 1037*

◆ **IDEC-C2B8** *see* RiTUXimab *on page 1825*

Idelalisib (eye del a LIS ib)

Brand Names: U.S. Zydelig

Index Terms CAL-101; GS-1101; PI_3K Delta Inhibitor CAL-101

Pharmacologic Category Antineoplastic Agent, Phosphatidylinositol 3-Kinase Inhibitor

Use

Chronic lymphocytic leukemia: Treatment of relapsed chronic lymphocytic leukemia (CLL) (in combination with rituximab) when rituximab alone is appropriate therapy due to other comorbidities

Follicular B-cell non-Hodgkin lymphoma: Treatment of relapsed follicular B-cell non-Hodgkin lymphoma after at least 2 prior systemic therapies

Small lymphocytic lymphoma: Treatment of relapsed small lymphocytic lymphoma (SLL) after at least 2 prior systemic therapies

Pregnancy Risk Factor D

Pregnancy Considerations Adverse events were observed in animal reproduction studies. Women of reproductive potential should use effective contraception during therapy and for at least 1 month after treatment discontinuation.

Breast-Feeding Considerations It is not known if idelalisib is excreted in breast milk. Due to the potential for serious adverse reactions in the nursing infant, the manufacturer recommends a decision be made whether to discontinue nursing or to discontinue the drug, taking into account the importance of treatment to the mother.

Contraindications Serious hypersensitivity reactions, including anaphylaxis and toxic epidermal necrolysis, to idelalisib or any component of the formulation

Warnings/Precautions Hazardous agent - use appropriate precautions for handling and disposal (meets NIOSH 2014 criteria). **[U.S. Boxed Warning]: Serious hepatotoxicity (some fatal) has been observed. Monitor hepatic function at baseline and during therapy. May require treatment interruption and/or dosage reduction.** ALT/AST elevations >5 times ULN have occurred, and were generally observed during the first 12 weeks of therapy; transaminase elevations were reversible upon therapy interruption. Hepatotoxicity may recur upon rechallenge, even if it a reduced dose; discontinue for recurrent hepatotoxicity. Avoid concomitant use with other hepatotoxic agents. Monitor ALT/AST every 2 weeks for the first 3 months, every 4 weeks for the next 3 months, then every 1 to 3 months thereafter, or as clinically necessary. Increase monitoring to weekly if ALT or AST >3 times ULN until resolved. Interrupt therapy if ALT/AST >5 times ULN; monitor LFTs weekly until resolved. **[U.S. Boxed Warning]: Serious and/or fatal diarrhea and colitis have been reported. Monitor closely; may require treatment interruption, dosage reduction, and/or discontinuation.** Grade 3 or higher diarrhea or colitis have been reported in clinical trials. Diarrhea may occur at any time during therapy and responds poorly to antidiarrheal (antimotility) medications. The median time to resolution of diarrhea was 1 week to 1 month (following therapy interruption); corticosteroids were used in some cases to manage toxicity. Avoid concomitant use with other promotility agents. **[U.S. Boxed Warning]: Serious and fatal intestinal perforation may occur; discontinue permanently if perforation develops.** In some patients, perforation was preceded by moderate to severe diarrhea. Monitor closely for new or worsening abdominal pain, chills, fever, nausea, or vomiting.

[U.S. Boxed Warning]: Serious and fatal pneumonitis may occur. Monitor for pulmonary symptoms and bilateral interstitial infiltrates. May require therapy interruption or discontinuation. Symptoms such as cough, dyspnea, hypoxia, interstitial infiltrates, or an oxygen saturation decrease of more than 5% should be promptly evaluated. Interrupt therapy for suspected pneumonitis; if diagnosis is confirmed, discontinue idelalisib and administer corticosteroids as appropriate. Serious allergic/hypersensitivity reactions, including anaphylaxis, have been reported. Discontinue permanently for serious reactions and manage appropriately.

Severe and/or life-threatening cutaneous reactions (grade 3 or higher), such as exfoliative dermatitis, rash (generalized, erythematous, macular-papular, pruritic, exfoliative), and skin disorder, have been observed. One case of toxic epidermal necrolysis (TEN) was reported when idelalisib was administered in combination with rituximab and bendamustine. Monitor closely for dermatologic toxicity and discontinue for severe reactions. Grade 3 or 4 neutropenia occurred in close to one-third of patients in clinical trials; thrombocytopenia and anemia (any grade) have also been reported. Monitor blood counts at least every 2 weeks for the first 3 months, and at least weekly in patients with neutropenia. May require treatment interruption and dosage reduction. Potentially significant interactions may exist, requiring dose or frequency adjustment, additional monitoring, and/or selection of alternative therapy. Consult drug interactions database for more detailed information.

Adverse Reactions As reported with monotherapy.

Cardiovascular: Peripheral edema

Central nervous system: Fatigue, headache, insomnia

Dermatologic: Night sweats, skin rash

Gastrointestinal: Abdominal pain, decreased appetite, diarrhea, nausea, vomiting

Hematologic & oncologic: Decreased hemoglobin, decreased neutrophils, decreased platelet count

Hepatic: Increased serum ALT, increased serum AST, severe hepatotoxicity

Neuromuscular & skeletal: Weakness

Respiratory: Cough, dyspnea, pneumonia, upper respiratory tract infection

Miscellaneous: Fever

Rare but important or life-threatening (reported with mono- or combination therapy): Anaphylaxis, hypersensitivity reaction, intestinal perforation, toxic epidermal necrolysis

Drug Interactions

Metabolism/Transport Effects Substrate of CYP3A4 (major), P-glycoprotein, UGT1A4; **Note:** Assignment of Major/Minor substrate status based on clinically relevant drug interaction potential; **Inhibits** CYP2C19 (weak), CYP2C8 (weak), CYP3A4 (strong), UGT1A1

Avoid Concomitant Use

Avoid concomitant use of Idelalisib with any of the following: Ado-Trastuzumab Emtansine; Alfuzosin; Apixaban; Astemizole; Avanafil; Axitinib; BCG; Bosutinib; Cabozantinib; Ceritinib; Conivaptan; Crizotinib; CYP3A4 Inducers (Strong); CYP3A4 Substrates; Dapoxetine; Dronedarone; Eplerenone; Everolimus; Halofantrine; Ibrutinib; Irinotecan; Ivabradine; Lapatinib; Lercanidipine; Lomitapide; Lovastatin; Lurasidone; Macitentan; Naloxegol; Natalizumab; Nilotinib; Nisoldipine; Olaparib; Pimecrolimus; Pimozide; Ranolazine; Red Yeast Rice; Regorafenib; Rivaroxaban; Salmeterol; Silodosin; Simeprevir; Simvastatin; St Johns Wort; Suvorexant; Tacrolimus (Topical); Tamsulosin; Terfenadine; Ticagrelor; Tofacitinib; Tolvaptan; Toremifene; Trabectedin; Ulipristal; Vaccines (Live); Vemurafenib; VinCRIStine (Liposomal); Vorapaxar

Increased Effect/Toxicity

Idelalisib may increase the levels/effects of: Ado-Trastuzumab Emtansine; Alfuzosin; Almotriptan; Alosetron; Apixaban; Astemizole; Avanafil; Axitinib; Bedaquiline; Bortezomib; Bosentan; Bosutinib; Brentuximab Vedotin; Brinzolamide; Budesonide (Nasal); Cabozantinib; Cannabis; Ceritinib; Conivaptan; Corticosteroids (Orally Inhaled); Corticosteroids (Systemic); Crizotinib; CYP3A4 Substrates; Dapoxetine; Dienogest; Dofetilide; Dronabinol; Dronedarone; Dutasteride; Eplerenone; Everolimus; Fluticasone (Nasal); Halofantrine; Ibrutinib; Iloperidone; Imatinib; Imidafenacin; Irinotecan; Ivabradine; Lacosamide; Lapatinib; Leflunomide; Lercanidipine; Levobupivacaine; Lomitapide; Lovastatin; Lumefantrine; Lurasidone; Macitentan; MethylPREDNISolone; Naloxegol; Natalizumab; Nilotinib; Nisoldipine; Olaparib; Ospemifene; Paricalcitol; Pimozide; PONATinib; Pranlukast; PrednisoLONE (Systemic); PredniSONE; Propafenone; Ranolazine; Red Yeast Rice; Regorafenib; Repaglinide; Retapamulin; Rilpivirine; Rivaroxaban; RomiDEPsin; Salmeterol; Silodosin; Simeprevir; Simvastatin; SORAfenib; Suvorexant; Tamsulosin; Terfenadine; Tetrahydrocannabinol; Ticagrelor; Tofacitinib; Tolvaptan; Toremifene; Trabectedin; Ulipristal; Vaccines (Live); Vemurafenib; Vilazodone; VinCRIStine (Liposomal); Vorapaxar; Zuclopenthixol

The levels/effects of Idelalisib may be increased by: CYP3A4 Inhibitors (Strong); Denosumab; Pimecrolimus; Roflumilast; Tacrolimus (Topical); Trastuzumab

Decreased Effect

Idelalisib may decrease the levels/effects of: BCG; Coccidioides immitis Skin Test; Ifosfamide; Prasugrel; Sipuleucel-T; Ticagrelor; Vaccines (Inactivated); Vaccines (Live)

The levels/effects of Idelalisib may be decreased by: Bosentan; CYP3A4 Inducers (Moderate); CYP3A4 Inducers (Strong); Deferasirox; Echinacea; Siltuximab; St Johns Wort; Tocilizumab

Storage/Stability Store at 20°C to 30°C (68°F to 86°F); excursions are permitted between 15°C and 30°C (59°F and 86°F). Dispense in the original container.

Mechanism of Action Potent small molecule inhibitor of the delta isoform of phosphatidylinositol 3-kinase (PI3Kδ), which is highly expressed in malignant lymphoid B-cells. PI3Kδ inhibition results in apoptosis of malignant tumor cells. In addition, idelalisib inhibits several signaling pathways, including B-cell receptor, CXCR4 and CXCR5 signaling which may play important roles in CLL pathophysiology (Furman, 2014).

Pharmacodynamics/Kinetics

Distribution: 23 L

Protein binding: >84%

Metabolism: Hepatic; primarily via aldehyde oxidase and CYP3A (to major metabolite GS-563117); minor metabolism via UGT1A4

Half-life elimination: ~8 hours

Time to peak: Median: 1.5 hours

Excretion: Feces (78%; 44% as GS-563117); urine (14%; 49% as GS-563117)

Dosage Note: Optimal duration and safety of therapy beyond several months is currently unknown.

Chronic lymphocytic leukemia, relapsed: Adults: Oral: 150 mg twice daily (in combination with rituximab); continue until disease progression or unacceptable toxicity (Furman, 2014)

Follicular B-cell non-Hodgkin lymphoma, relapsed: Adults: Oral: 150 mg twice daily; continue until disease progression or unacceptable toxicity (Gopal, 2014)

Small lymphocytic lymphoma, relapsed: Adults: Oral: 150 mg twice daily; continue until disease progression or unacceptable toxicity (Gopal, 2014)

Dosage adjustment for toxicity:

Anaphylaxis: Permanently discontinue.

Dermatologic toxicity: Severe cutaneous reactions: Discontinue.

Hematologic toxicity:

Neutropenia:

ANC 1000 to <1500 cells/mm^3: Continue current dose.

ANC 500 to <1000 cells/mm^3: Continue current dose; monitor blood counts at least weekly.

ANC <500 cells/mm^3: Temporarily interrupt therapy; monitor blood counts at least weekly until ANC ≥500 cells/mm^3, then may reinitiate therapy at 100 mg twice daily.

Thrombocytopenia:

Platelets 50,000 to <75,000 cells/mm^3: Continue current dose.

Platelets 25,000 to <50,000 cells/mm^3: Continue current dose; monitor platelet counts at least weekly.

Platelets <25,000 cells/mm^3: Temporarily interrupt therapy; monitor platelet counts at least weekly, may reinitiate therapy at 100 mg twice daily when platelets recover to ≥25,000 cells/mm^3.

Gastrointestinal toxicity:

Moderate diarrhea (increase of 4 to 6 stools/day over baseline): Continue current dose; monitor at least weekly until resolved.

Severe diarrhea (increase of ≥7 stools/day over baseline) or hospitalization: Temporarily interrupt therapy; monitor at least weekly until resolved, then may reinitiate therapy at 100 mg twice daily.

Life-threatening diarrhea: Discontinue permanently.

Pulmonary toxicity: Discontinue for symptomatic pneumonitis of any severity.

Other toxicity (not listed above): If severe or life-threatening toxicities occur, interrupt therapy until toxicity is resolved. If the decision is made to resume therapy, reduce the dose to 100 mg twice daily. Discontinue permanently if severe or life-threatening toxicities recur upon rechallenge.

Dosage adjustment for renal impairment:

CrCl ≥15 mL/minute: No dosage adjustment is necessary.

CrCl <15 mL/minute: There are no dosage adjustments provided in the manufacturer's labeling (has not been studied).

Dosage adjustment for hepatic impairment:

Preexisting hepatic impairment: Exposure is increased in patients with ALT/AST or bilirubin >ULN as compared to patients with normal hepatic function; patients with ALT/AST >2.5 times ULN or bilirubin >1.5 times ULN were excluded from some studies. Based on a pharmacokinetic study in patients with moderate and severe hepatic impairment, single oral doses of 150 mg were well tolerated; idelalisib and GS-563117 exposure differences were not considered clinically relevant (Jin, 2014). Monitor closely for toxicity.

Hepatotoxicity during treatment:

ALT/AST >3 to 5 times ULN or bilirubin >1.5 to 3 times ULN: Continue current dose; monitor LFTs at least weekly until ALT/AST and/or bilirubin ≤1 times ULN.

ALT/AST >5 to 20 times ULN or bilirubin >3 to 10 times ULN: Temporarily interrupt therapy. Monitor LFTs at least weekly until ALT/AST and/or bilirubin ≤1 times ULN, then may reinitiate therapy at 100 mg twice daily.

ALT/AST >20 times ULN or bilirubin >10 times ULN: Discontinue permanently.

Recurrent hepatotoxicity: Discontinue.

Administration Administer orally twice daily with or without food. Swallow tablets whole.

Missed doses: May administer a missed dose if within 6 hours of usual dosing time. If >6 hours, skip the missed dose and resume therapy with the next scheduled dose.

Hazardous agent; use appropriate precautions for handling and disposal (meets NIOSH 2014 criteria).

Monitoring Parameters Liver function tests every 2 weeks for the first 3 months, every 4 weeks for the next 3 months, then every 1 to 3 months thereafter, or as clinically necessary; complete blood counts at least every 2 weeks for the first 3 months, and at least weekly in patients with neutropenia, or as clinically necessary; signs/symptoms of diarrhea/colitis, intestinal perforation, pneumonitis, dermatologic toxicity, and hypersensitivity reactions

Dosage Forms

Tablet, Oral:

Zydelig: 100 mg, 150 mg

◆ **IDR** *see* IDArubicin *on page 1037*

Idrocilamide [INT] (i droe SIL a mide)

International Brand Names Srilane (BE, FR, LU); Talval (CH)

Pharmacologic Category Skeletal Muscle Relaxant

Reported Use Treatment of painful muscle spasms associated with musculoskeletal conditions

Dosage Range Adults: Topical: Apply to affected area 1-3 times/day

Product Availability Product available in various countries; not currently available in the U.S.

Dosage Forms

Cream: 5% (50 g, 100 g)

Idursulfase (eye dur SUL fase)

Brand Names: U.S. Elaprase

Brand Names: Canada Elaprase

Pharmacologic Category Enzyme

Use Hunter syndrome: Replacement therapy in Hunter syndrome (mucopolysaccharidosis II; MPS II) for improvement of walking capacity

Pregnancy Risk Factor C

Dosage Hunter syndrome (mucopolysaccharidosis II): Children ≥5 years, Adolescents, and Adults: IV: 0.5 mg/kg once weekly

Dosage adjustment in renal impairment: No dosage adjustment provided in manufacturer's labeling.

Dosage adjustment in hepatic impairment: No dosage adjustment provided in manufacturer's labeling.

Additional Information Complete prescribing information should be consulted for additional detail.

Dosage Forms

Solution, Intravenous [preservative free]:

Elaprase: 6 mg/3 mL (3 mL)

◆ **IDV** *see* Indinavir *on page 1066*

◆ **iFerex 150 [OTC]** *see* Polysaccharide-Iron Complex *on page 1677*

◆ **Ifex** *see* Ifosfamide *on page 1040*

Ifosfamide (eye FOSS fa mide)

Brand Names: U.S. Ifex

Brand Names: Canada Ifex

Index Terms Isophosphamide; Z4942

Pharmacologic Category Antineoplastic Agent, Alkylating Agent; Antineoplastic Agent, Alkylating Agent (Nitrogen Mustard)

Use

U.S. labeling: Treatment (third-line) of germ cell testicular cancer (in combination with other chemotherapy drugs and with concurrent mesna)

Canadian labeling (not approved indications in the U.S.): Treatment of soft tissue sarcoma, pancreatic cancer (relapsed or refractory), cervical cancer (advanced or recurrent; as monotherapy or in combination with cisplatin and bleomycin)

Pregnancy Risk Factor D

Pregnancy Considerations Embryotoxic and teratogenic effects have been observed in animal reproduction studies. Fetal growth retardation and neonatal anemia have been reported with exposure to ifosfamide-containing regimens during human pregnancy. Male and female fertility may be affected (dose and duration dependent). Ifosfamide interferes with oogenesis and spermatogenesis; amenorrhea, azoospermia, and sterility have been reported and may be irreversible. Avoid pregnancy during treatment; male patients should not father a child for at least 6 months after completion of therapy.

Breast-Feeding Considerations Breast-feeding should be avoided during ifosfamide treatment. According to the manufacturer, the decision to discontinue ifosfamide or discontinue breast-feeding should take into account the risk of exposure to the infant and the benefits of treatment to the mother.

Contraindications Hypersensitivity to ifosfamide or any component of the formulation; urinary outflow obstruction

Canadian labeling: Additional contraindications (not in U.S. labeling): Severe myelosuppression; severe renal or hepatic impairment; active infection (bacterial, fungal, viral); severe immunosuppression; urinary tract disease (eg, cystitis); advanced cerebral arteriosclerosis

Warnings/Precautions Hazardous agent: Use appropriate precautions for handling and disposal (NIOSH 2014 [group 1]). **[U.S. Boxed Warning]: Hemorrhagic cystitis may occur; concomitant mesna reduces the risk of hemorrhagic cystitis.** Hydration (at least 2 L/day in adults), dose fractionation, and/or mesna administration will reduce the incidence of hematuria and protect against hemorrhagic cystitis. Obtain urinalysis prior to each dose; if microscopic hematuria is detected, withhold until complete resolution. Exclude or correct urinary tract obstructions prior to treatment. Use with caution (if at all) in patients with active urinary tract infection. Hemorrhagic cystitis is dose-dependent and is increased with high single doses (compared with fractionated doses); past or concomitant bladder radiation or busulfan treatment may increase the risk for hemorrhagic cystitis. **[U.S. Boxed Warning]: May cause severe nephrotoxicity, resulting in renal failure.** Acute and chronic renal failure as well as renal parenchymal and tubular necrosis (including acute) have been reported; tubular damage may be delayed and may persist. Renal manifestations include decreased glomerular rate, increased creatinine, proteinuria, enzymuria, cylindruria, aminoaciduria, phosphaturia, and glycosuria. Syndrome of inappropriate antidiuretic hormone (SIADH), renal rickets, and Fanconi syndrome have been reported. Evaluate renal function prior to and during treatment; monitor urine for erythrocytes and signs of urotoxicity.

[U.S. Boxed Warning]: May cause CNS toxicity which may be severe, resulting in encephalopathy and death; monitor for CNS toxicity; discontinue for encephalopathy. Symptoms of CNS toxicity (somnolence, confusion, dizziness, disorientation, hallucinations, cranial nerve dysfunction, psychotic behavior, extrapyramidal symptoms, seizures, coma blurred vision, and/or incontinence) have been observed within a few hours to a few days after initial dose and generally resolve within 2-3 days of treatment discontinuation (although may persist longer); maintain supportive care until complete resolution. Risk factors may include hypoalbuminemia, renal dysfunction, and prior history of ifosfamide-induced encephalopathy. Concomitant centrally-acting medications may result in additive CNS effects. Peripheral neuropathy has been reported.

[U.S. Boxed Warning]: Severe bone marrow suppression may occur (dose-limiting toxicity); monitor blood counts before and after each cycle. Leukopenia, neutropenia, thrombocytopenia and anemia are associated with ifosfamide. Myelosuppression is dose dependent, increased with single high doses (compared to fractionated doses) and increased with decreased renal function. Severe myelosuppression may occur when administered in combination with other chemotherapy agents or radiation therapy. Use with caution in patients with compromised bone marrow reserve. Unless clinically necessary, avoid administering to patients with WBC <2000/mm^3 and platelets <50,000/mm^3. Antimicrobial prophylaxis may be necessary in some neutropenic patients; Administer antibiotics and/or antifungal agents for neutropenic fever. May cause significant suppression of the immune responses; may lead to serious infection, sepsis or septic shock; reported infections have included bacterial, viral, fungal, and parasitic; latent infections may be reactivated; use with caution with other immunosuppressants or in patients with infection.

Arrhythmias, ST-segment or T-wave changes, cardiomyopathy, pericardial effusion, pericarditis, and epicardial fibrosis have been observed; the risk for cardiotoxicity is dose-dependent; concomitant cardiotoxic agents (eg, anthracyclines), irradiation of the cardiac region, and renal impairment may also increase the risk; use with caution in patients with cardiac risk factors or preexisting cardiac disease. Interstitial pneumonitis, pulmonary fibrosis, and pulmonary toxicity leading to respiratory failure have been reported; monitor for signs and symptoms of pulmonary toxicity.

Anaphylactic/anaphylactoid reactions have been associated with ifosfamide; cross sensitivity with similar agents may occur. Hepatic sinusoidal obstruction syndrome (SOS), formerly called veno-occlusive disease (VOD), has been reported with ifosfamide-containing regimens. Secondary malignancies may occur; the risk for myelodysplastic syndrome (which may progress to acute leukemia) is increased with treatment. May interfere with wound healing. Use with caution in patients with prior radiation therapy. Ifosfamide is associated with a moderate emetic potential; antiemetics are recommended to prevent nausea and vomiting (Basch, 2011; Dupuis, 2011; Roila, 2010).

Adverse Reactions

Central nervous system: CNS toxicity or encephalopathy, fever

Dermatologic: Alopecia

Endocrine & metabolic: Metabolic acidosis

Gastrointestinal: Anorexia, nausea/vomiting

Hematologic: Anemia, leukopenia, neutropenic fever, thrombocytopenia

Hepatic: Bilirubin increased, liver dysfunction, transaminases increased

Local: Phlebitis

Renal: Hematuria (reduced with mesna), renal impairment

Miscellaneous: Infection

Rare but important or life-threatening: Acute respiratory distress syndrome, acute tubular necrosis, agranulocytosis, alkaline phosphatase increased, allergic reaction, alveolitis (allergic), amenorrhea, aminoaciduria, amnesia, anaphylactic reaction, angina, angioedema, anuria, arrhythmia, arthralgia, asterixis, atrial ectopy, atrial fibrillation/flutter, azoospermia, bladder irritation, bleeding, blurred vision, bone marrow failure, bradycardia, bradyphrenia, bronchospasm, bundle branch block, BUN increased, capillary leak syndrome, cardiac arrest, cardiogenic shock, cardiomyopathy, cardiotoxicity, catatonia, cecitis, chest pain, cholestasis, coagulopathy, colitis, conjunctivitis, creatinine clearance decreased/increased, creatinine increased, cylindruria, cytolytic hepatitis, delirium, delusion, dermatitis, diarrhea, DIC, DVT, dysesthesia, dyspnea, dysuria, echolalia, edema, ejection fraction decreased, enterocolitis, enuresis, enzymuria, erythema, extrapyramidal disorder, facial swelling, Fanconi syndrome, fatigue, gait disturbance, GGT increased, GI hemorrhage, glycosuria, gonadotropin increased, granulocytopenia, growth retardation (children), hemolytic anemia, hemolytic uremic syndrome, hemorrhagic cystitis, hepatic failure, hepatic sinusoidal obstruction syndrome (SOS; formerly veno-occlusive disease [VOD]), hepatitis fulminant, hepatitis (viral), hepatorenal syndrome, herpes zoster, hyperglycemia, hyper-/hypotension, hypersensitivity reactions, hypocalcemia, hypokalemia, hyponatremia, hypophosphatemia, hypoxia, ileus, immunosuppression, infertility, infusion site reactions (erythema, inflammation, pain, pruritus, swelling, tenderness), interstitial lung disease, jaundice, LDH increased, leukoencephalopathy, lymphopenia, malaise, mania, mental status change, methemoglobinemia, MI, mucosal inflammation/ulceration, multiorgan failure, mutism, myocardial hemorrhage, myocarditis, nephrogenic diabetes insipidus, neuralgia, neutropenia, oligospermia, oliguria, osteomalacia (adults), ovarian failure, ovulation disorder, palmar-plantar erythrodysesthesia syndrome, pancreatitis, pancytopenia, panic attack, paranoia, paresthesia, pericardial effusion, pericarditis, peripheral neuropathy, petechiae, phosphaturia, pleural effusion, *Pneumocystis jiroveci* pneumonia, pneumonia, pneumonitis, pollakiuria, polydipsia, polyneuropathy, polyuria, portal vein thrombosis, premature atrial contractions, premature menopause, progressive multifocal leukoencephalopathy, proteinuria, pruritus, pulmonary edema, pulmonary embolism, pulmonary fibrosis, pulmonary hypertension, QRS complex abnormal, radiation recall dermatitis, rash (including macular and papular), renal failure, renal parenchymal damage, renal tubular acidosis, respiratory failure, reversible posterior leukoencephalopathy syndrome (RPLS), rhabdomyolysis, rickets, salivation, secondary malignancy, seizure, sepsis, septic shock, SIADH, skin necrosis, spermatogenesis impaired, status epilepticus, sterility, Stevens-Johnson syndrome, stomatitis, ST segment abnormal, supraventricular extrasystoles, tachycardia, tinnitus, toxic epidermal necrolysis, tubulointerstitial nephritis, tumor lysis syndrome, T-wave inversion, uremia, urticaria, vasculitis, ventricular extrasystoles/fibrillation/tachycardia, ventricular failure, vertigo, visual impairment, wound healing impairment

Drug Interactions

Metabolism/Transport Effects **Substrate** of CYP2B6 (major), CYP2C19 (minor), CYP2C8 (minor), CYP2C9 (minor), CYP3A4 (minor); **Note:** Assignment of Major/Minor substrate status based on clinically relevant drug interaction potential; **Inhibits** CYP3A4 (weak); **Induces** CYP2C9 (moderate)

Avoid Concomitant Use

Avoid concomitant use of Ifosfamide with any of the following: BCG; CloZAPine; Dipyrone; Natalizumab; Pimecrolimus; Pimozide; Tacrolimus (Topical); Tofacitinib; Vaccines (Live)

Increased Effect/Toxicity

Ifosfamide may increase the levels/effects of: ARIPiprazole; CloZAPine; Dofetilide; Hydrocodone; Leflunomide; Lomitapide; Natalizumab; Pimozide; Tofacitinib; Vaccines (Live); Vitamin K Antagonists

The levels/effects of Ifosfamide may be increased by: Aprepitant; Busulfan; CYP2B6 Inhibitors (Moderate); CYP3A4 Inducers (Moderate); CYP3A4 Inducers (Strong); Denosumab; Dipyrone; Fosaprepitant; Pimecrolimus; Quazepam; Roflumilast; Tacrolimus (Topical); Trastuzumab

Decreased Effect

Ifosfamide may decrease the levels/effects of: BCG; Coccidioides immitis Skin Test; Sipuleucel-T; Vaccines (Inactivated); Vaccines (Live)

The levels/effects of Ifosfamide may be decreased by: CYP2B6 Inducers (Strong); CYP3A4 Inducers (Moderate); CYP3A4 Inducers (Strong); CYP3A4 Inhibitors (Moderate); CYP3A4 Inhibitors (Strong); Dabrafenib; Echinacea

Preparation for Administration Hazardous agent; use appropriate precautions for handling and disposal (NIOSH 2014 [group 1]). Reconstitute powder with SWFI or bacteriostatic SWFI (1 g in 20 mL or 3 g in 60 mL) to a concentration of 50 mg/mL. Further dilution in 50-1000 mL D_5W, NS, or lactated Ringer's (to a final concentration of 0.6-20 mg/mL) is recommended for IV infusion (may also dilute in $D_{2.5}W$, ½NS, or D_5NS).

Storage/Stability Store intact vials of powder for injection at room temperature of 20°C to 25°C (68°F to 77°F); avoid temperatures >30°C (86°F). Store intact vials of solution under refrigeration at 2°C to 8°C (36°F to 46°F). Reconstituted solutions and solutions diluted for administration are stable for 24 hours refrigerated.

Mechanism of Action Causes cross-linking of strands of DNA by binding with nucleic acids and other intracellular structures; inhibits protein synthesis and DNA synthesis

Pharmacodynamics/Kinetics Pharmacokinetics are dose dependent

Distribution: V_d: Approximates total body water; penetrates CNS, but not in therapeutic levels

Protein binding: Negligible

Metabolism: Hepatic to active metabolites isofosforamide mustard, 4-hydroxy-ifosfamide, acrolein, and inactive dichloroethylated and carboxy metabolites; acrolein is the agent implicated in development of hemorrhagic cystitis

Half-life elimination (increased in the elderly):

High dose (3800-5000 mg/m²): ~15 hours

Lower dose (1600-2400 mg/m²): ~7 hours

Excretion:

High dose (5000 mg/m²): Urine (70% to 86%; 61% as unchanged drug)

Lower dose (1600-2400 mg/m²): Urine (12% to 18% as unchanged drug)

Dosage Note: To prevent bladder toxicity, ifosfamide should be given with the urinary protector mesna and hydration of at least 2 L of oral or IV fluid per day. Ifosfamide is associated with a moderate emetic potential; antiemetics are recommended to prevent nausea and vomiting (Basch, 2011; Dupuis, 2011; Roila, 2010).

Children: IV:

Ewing sarcoma (off-label use):

VAC/IE regimen: IE: 1800 mg/m²/day for 5 days (in combination with mesna and etoposide) alternate with VAC (vincristine, doxorubicin, and cyclophosphamide) every 3 weeks for a total of 17 courses (Grier, 2003)

ICE-CAV regimen: ICE: 1800 mg/m²/day for 5 days every 3-4 weeks for 2 courses (in combination with carboplatin and etoposide [and mesna]), followed by CAV (cyclophosphamide, doxorubicin, and vincristine) (Milano, 2006)

VAIA regimen: 3000 mg/m²/day on days 1, 2, 22, 23, 43, and 44 for 4 courses (in combination with vincristine, doxorubicin, dactinomycin, and mesna) (Paulussen, 2001) **or** 2000 mg/m²/day for 3 days every 3 weeks for 14 courses (in combination with vincristine, doxorubicin, dactinomycin, and mesna) (Paulussen, 2008)

VIDE regimen: 3000 mg/m²/day over 1-3 hours for 3 days every 3 weeks for 6 courses (in combination with vincristine, doxorubicin, etoposide, and mesna) (Juergens, 2006)

IE regimen: 1800 mg/m²/day over 1 hour for 5 days every 3 weeks for 12 cycles (in combination with etoposide and mesna) (Miser, 1987)

ICE regimen: 1800 mg/m²/day for 5 days every 3 weeks for up to 12 cycles (in combination with carboplatin and etoposide [and mesna]) (van Winkle, 2005)

Osteosarcoma (off-label use):

Ifosfamide/cisplatin/doxorubicin/HDMT regimen: 3000 mg/m²/day continuous infusion for 5 days during weeks 4 and 10 (preop) and during weeks 16, 25, and 34 (postop) (in combination with cisplatin, doxorubicin, methotrexate [high-dose], and mesna) (Bacci, 2003)

Ifosfamide/cisplatin/epirubicin regimen: Children ≥15 years: 2000 mg/m²/day over 4 hours for 3 days (days 2, 3, and 4) every 3 weeks for 3 cycles (preop) and every 4 weeks for 3 cycles (postop) (in combination with cisplatin, epirubicin, and mesna) (Basaran, 2007)

IE regimen: 3000 mg/m²/day over 3 hours for 4 days every 3-4 weeks (in combination with etoposide and mesna) (Gentet, 1997)

ICE regimen: Children ≥1 year: 1800 mg/m²/day for 5 days every 3 weeks for up to 12 cycles (in combination with carboplatin and etoposide [and mesna]) (van Winkle, 2005)

Ifosfamide/HDMT/etoposide regimen: 3000 mg/m²/day over 3 hours for 4 days during weeks 4 and 9 (3 additional postop courses were administered in good responders) (in combination with methotrexate [high-dose], etoposide, and mesna) (Le Deley, 2007)

Adults: IV:

Testicular cancer:

U.S. manufacturer's labeling; as part of combination chemotherapy and with mesna: 1200 mg/m²/day for 5 days every 3 weeks or after hematologic recovery

VIP regimen: 1200 mg/m²/day for 5 days every 3 weeks for 4 cycles (in combination with etoposide, mesna, and cisplatin) (Nichols, 1998)

VeIP regimen: 1200 mg/m²/day for 5 days every 3 weeks for 4 cycles (in combination with vinblastine, mesna, and cisplatin) (Loehrer, 1998)

Canadian labeling: IV: Soft tissue sarcoma, cervical cancer (advanced or recurrent), pancreatic cancer (relapsed or refractory): 2000-2400 mg/m²/day for 5 consecutive days (with mesna), may repeat after 3-4 weeks (or longer depending on patient status) or if lower daily dosage or total dosage over a longer time period is indicated, administer every other day (eg, days 1, 3, 5, 7, 9) or over 10 consecutive days at reduced doses.

High **single-dose** infusions of up to 5000-8000 mg/m²/24 hour with continuous mesna may also be feasible; may repeat after 3-4 weeks (or longer depending on patient's condition).

Adult off-label uses and/or dosing: IV:

Testicular cancer:

TIP regimen (off-label dosing): 1500 mg/m²/day for 4 days (days 2-5) every 3 weeks for 4 cycles (in combination with paclitaxel, mesna, and cisplatin) (Kondagunta, 2005)

TICE regimen (off-label dosing): 2000 mg/m²/day for 3 days (days 2-4) over 4 hours every 2 weeks for 2 cycles (in combination with paclitaxel and mesna; followed by carboplatin and etoposide) (Kondagunta, 2007)

Cervical cancer, recurrent or metastatic: 1500 mg/m²/day for 5 days every 3 weeks (with mesna) (Coleman, 1986; Sutton, 1993)

Hodgkin lymphoma, relapsed or refractory:

ICE regimen: 5000 mg/m² (over 24 hours) beginning on day 2 every 2 weeks for 2 cycles (in combination with mesna, carboplatin, and etoposide) (Moskowitz, 2001)

IGEV regimen: 2000 mg/m²/day for 4 days every 3 weeks for 4 cycles (in combination with mesna, gemcitabine, vinorelbine, and prednisolone) (Santoro, 2007)

MINE-ESHAP regimen: 1500 mg/m²/day for 3 days every 4 weeks for up to 2 cycles (MINE is combination with mesna, mitoxantrone, and etoposide; MINE alternates with ESHAP for up to 2 cycles of each) (Fernandez, 2010)

Non-Hodgkin lymphomas:

CODOX-M/IVAC regimen:

Adults ≤65 years: Cycles 2 and 4 (IVAC): 1500 mg/m²/day for 5 days (IVAC is combination with cytarabine, mesna, and etoposide; IVAC alternates with CODOX-M) (Mead, 2008)

Adults >65 years: Cycles 2 and 4 (IVAC): 1000 mg/m²/day for 5 days (IVAC is combination with cytarabine, mesna, and etoposide; IVAC alternates with CODOX-M) (Mead, 2008)

MINE-ESHAP regimen: 1330 mg/m²/day for 3 days every 3 weeks for 6 cycles (MINE is combination with mesna, mitoxantrone, and etoposide; followed by ESHAP) (Rodriguez, 1995)

RICE regimen: 5000 mg/m² (over 24 hours) beginning on day 4 every 2 weeks for 3 cycles (in combination with mesna, carboplatin, etoposide, and rituximab) (Kewalramani, 2004)

Ewing sarcoma:

VAC/IE regimen: Adults ≤30 years: IE: 1800 mg/m²/day for 5 days (in combination with mesna and etoposide) alternate with VAC (vincristine, doxorubicin, and cyclophosphamide) every 3 weeks for a total of 17 courses (Grier, 2003)

VAIA regimen: 3000 mg/m²day on days 1, 2, 22, 23, 43, and 44 for 4 courses (in combination with vincristine, doxorubicin, dactinomycin, and mesna) (Paulussen, 2001) **or** Adults ≤35 years: 2000 mg/m²/day for 3 days every 3 weeks for 14 courses (in combination with vincristine, doxorubicin, dactinomycin, and mesna) (Paulussen, 2008)

VIDE regimen: Adults ≤50 years: 3000 mg/m²/day over 1-3 hours for 3 days every 3 weeks for 6 courses (in combination with vincristine, doxorubicin, etoposide, and mesna) (Juergens, 2006)

IE regimen: 1800 mg/m²/day over 1 hour for 5 days every 3 weeks for 12 cycles (in combination with etoposide and mesna) (Miser, 1987)

ICE regimen: Adults ≤22 years: 1800 mg/m²/day for 5 days every 3 weeks for up to 12 cycles (in combination with carboplatin and etoposide [and mesna]) (van Winkle, 2005)

Osteosarcoma:

Ifosfamide/cisplatin/doxorubicin/HDMT regimen: Adults <40 years: 3000 mg/m²/day continuous infusion for 5 days during weeks 4 and 10 (preop) and during weeks 16, 25, and 34 (postop) (in combination with cisplatin, doxorubicin, methotrexate [high-dose], and mesna) (Bacci, 2003)

Ifosfamide/cisplatin/epirubicin regimen: 2000 mg/m²/day over 4 hours for 3 days (days 2, 3, and 4) every 3 weeks for 3 cycles (preop) and every 4 weeks for 3 cycles (postop) (in combination with cisplatin, epirubicin, and mesna) (Basaran, 2007)

ICE regimen (adults ≤22 years): 1800 mg/m²/day for 5 days every 3 weeks for up to 12 cycles (in combination with carboplatin and etoposide [and mesna]) (van Winkle, 2005)

Soft tissue sarcoma:

Single-agent ifosfamide: 3000 mg/m²/day over 4 hours for 3 days every 3 weeks for at least 2 cycles or until disease progression (van Oosterom, 2002)

ICE regimen: 1500 mg/m²/day for 4 days every 4 weeks for 4-6 cycles (in combination with carboplatin, etoposide, and regional hyperthermia) (Nickenig, 2009)

MAID regimen: 2000 mg/m²/day continuous infusion for 3 days every 3 weeks (in combination with mesna, doxorubicin and dacarbazine) (Antman, 1993) **or** 2500 mg/m²/day continuous infusion for 3 days every 3 weeks (in combination with mesna, doxorubicin, and dacarbazine); reduce ifosfamide to 1500mg/m²/day if prior pelvic irradiation (Elias, 1989)

Ifosfamide/epirubicin: 1800 mg/m²/day over 1 hour for 5 days every 3 weeks for 5 cycles (in combination with mesna and epirubicin) (Frustaci, 2001)

AIM regimens: 1500 mg/m²/day over 2 hours for 4 days every 3 weeks for 4-6 cycles (in combination with mesna and doxorubicin) (Worden, 2005) **or** 2000-3000 mg/m²/day over 3 hours for 3 days (in combination with mesna and doxorubicin) (Grobmyer, 2004)

Dosing adjustment in renal impairment:
U.S. labeling: Consider dosage reduction in patients with renal impairment; however, no dosage adjustment is provided in the manufacturer's labeling; ifosfamide (and metabolites) are excreted renally and may accumulate in patients with renal dysfunction. Ifosfamide and metabolites are dialyzable.
Canadian labeling:
Mild-moderate impairment: No dosage adjustment provided in the manufacturer's labeling.
Severe impairment: Use is contraindicated.
The following adjustments have also been recommended:
Aronoff, 2007:
CrCl ≥10 mL/minute: Children and Adults: No dosage adjustment necessary.
CrCl <10 mL/minute: Children and Adults: Administer 75% of dose.
Hemodialysis (supplement for dialysis):
Children: 1 g/m^2 followed by hemodialysis 6-8 hours later
Adults: No supplemental dose needed.
Kintzel, 1995:
CrCl 46-60 mL/minute: Administer 80% of dose.
CrCl 31-45 mL/minute: Administer 75% of dose.
CrCl <30 mL/minute: Administer 70% of dose.

Dosing adjustment in hepatic impairment: No dosage adjustment provided in the manufacturer's labeling; however, ifosfamide is extensively hepatically metabolized to both active and inactive metabolites; use with caution. The following adjustments have been recommended:
Floyd, 2006: Bilirubin >3 mg/dL: Administer 25% of dose.
Canadian labeling:
Mild-to-moderate impairment: No dosage adjustment provided in manufacturer labeling; use with caution.
Severe impairment: Use is contraindicated.

Dosing in obesity: *ASCO Guidelines for appropriate chemotherapy dosing in obese adults with cancer:* Utilize patient's actual body weight (full weight) for calculation of body surface area- or weight-based dosing, particularly when the intent of therapy is curative; manage regimen-related toxicities in the same manner as for nonobese patients; if a dose reduction is utilized due to toxicity, consider resumption of full weight-based dosing with subsequent cycles, especially if cause of toxicity (eg, hepatic or renal impairment) is resolved (Griggs, 2012).

Administration Ifosfamide is associated with a moderate emetic potential; antiemetics are recommended to prevent nausea and vomiting (Basch, 2011; Dupuis, 2011; Roila, 2010).

Administer IV over at least 30 minutes (infusion times may vary by protocol; refer to specific protocol for infusion duration)

Hazardous agent; use appropriate precautions for handling and disposal (NIOSH 2014 [group 1]).

Monitoring Parameters CBC with differential (prior to each dose), urine output, urinalysis (prior to each dose), liver function, and renal function tests; signs and symptoms of neurotoxicity, pulmonary toxicity, and/or hemorrhagic cystitis

Dosage Forms
Solution, Intravenous:
Generic: 1 g/20 mL (20 mL); 3 g/60 mL (60 mL)
Solution, Intravenous [preservative free]:
Generic: 1 g/20 mL (20 mL); 3 g/60 mL (60 mL)
Solution Reconstituted, Intravenous:
Ifex: 1 g (1 ea); 3 g (1 ea)
Generic: 1 g (1 ea); 3 g (1 ea)

◆ **IG** *see* Immune Globulin *on page 1056*

◆ **IgG4-Kappa Monoclonal Antibody** *see* Natalizumab *on page 1432*

◆ **IGIM** *see* Immune Globulin *on page 1056*

◆ **IGIV** *see* Immune Globulin *on page 1056*

◆ **IGIVnex (Can)** *see* Immune Globulin *on page 1056*

◆ **IGSC** *see* Immune Globulin *on page 1056*

◆ **IIV** *see* Influenza Virus Vaccine (Inactivated) *on page 1075*

◆ **IIV3** *see* Influenza Virus Vaccine (Inactivated) *on page 1075*

◆ **IIV4** *see* Influenza Virus Vaccine (Inactivated) *on page 1075*

◆ **IL-1Ra** *see* Anakinra *on page 148*

◆ **IL-2** *see* Aldesleukin *on page 72*

◆ **IL-11** *see* Oprelvekin *on page 1519*

◆ **Ilaris** *see* Canakinumab *on page 335*

◆ **Ilevro** *see* Nepafenac *on page 1439*

Iloperidone (eye loe PER i done)

Brand Names: U.S. Fanapt; Fanapt Titration Pack

Pharmacologic Category Second Generation (Atypical) Antipsychotic

Additional Appendix Information
Beers Criteria – Potentially Inappropriate Medications for Geriatrics *on page 2271*

Use Schizophrenia: Treatment of adults with schizophrenia

Pregnancy Risk Factor C

Pregnancy Considerations Adverse events were observed in animal reproduction studies. Antipsychotic use during the third trimester of pregnancy has a risk for abnormal muscle movements (extrapyramidal symptoms [EPS]) and/or withdrawal symptoms in newborns following delivery. Symptoms in the newborn may include agitation, feeding disorder, hypertonia, hypotonia, respiratory distress, somnolence, and tremor; these effects may be self-limiting or require hospitalization. Iloperidone may cause hyperprolactinemia, which may decrease reproductive function in both males and females.

The ACOG recommends that therapy during pregnancy be individualized; treatment with psychiatric medications during pregnancy should incorporate the clinical expertise of the mental health clinician, obstetrician, primary healthcare provider, and pediatrician. Safety data related to atypical antipsychotics during pregnancy is limited and routine use is not recommended. However, if a woman is inadvertently exposed to an atypical antipsychotic while pregnant, continuing therapy may be preferable to switching to a typical antipsychotic that the fetus has not yet been exposed to; consider risk:benefit (ACOG, 2008).

Healthcare providers are encouraged to enroll women 18 to 45 years of age exposed to iloperidone during pregnancy in the Atypical Antipsychotics Pregnancy Registry (1-866-961-2388 or http://www.womensmentalhealth.org/pregnancyregistry).

Breast-Feeding Considerations It is not known if iloperidone is excreted into breast milk. Breast-feeding is not recommended by the manufacturer.

Contraindications Hypersensitivity to iloperidone or any component of the formulation

Warnings/Precautions [U.S. Boxed Warning]: Elderly patients with dementia-related psychosis treated with antipsychotics are at an increased risk of death compared to placebo. Most deaths appeared to be either cardiovascular (eg, heart failure, sudden death) or infectious (eg, pneumonia) in nature. In addition, an increased incidence of cerebrovascular effects (eg, transient ischemic attack, cerebrovascular accidents) has been reported in studies of placebo-controlled trials of antipsychotics in elderly patients with dementia-related psychosis. Iloperidone is not approved for the treatment of dementia-related psychosis.

May cause CNS depression, which may impair physical or mental abilities; patients must be cautioned about performing tasks that require mental alertness (eg, operating machinery or driving). Caution in patients with predisposition to seizures. Use is not recommended in patients with hepatic impairment. Esophageal dysmotility and aspiration have been associated with antipsychotic use; use with caution in patients at risk of aspiration pneumonia (ie, Alzheimer's disease). Use is associated with increased prolactin levels; clinical significance of hyperprolactinemia in patients with breast cancer or other prolactin-dependent tumors is unknown. May alter temperature regulation. Leukopenia, neutropenia, and agranulocytosis (sometimes fatal) have been reported in clinical trials and postmarketing reports; presence of risk factors (eg, preexisting low WBC or history of drug-induced leuko-/neutropenia) should prompt periodic blood count assessment and discontinuation at first signs of blood dyscrasias.

May alter cardiac conduction and prolong the QTc interval; life-threatening arrhythmias have occurred with therapeutic doses of antipsychotics. Risks may be increased by conditions or concomitant medications which cause bradycardia, hypokalemia, and/or hypomagnesemia. Avoid use in combination with QTc-prolonging drugs and in patients with congenital long QT syndrome, history of cardiac arrhythmia, recent MI, or uncompensated heart failure. Discontinue treatment in patients found to have persistent QTc intervals >500 msec. Further cardiac evaluation is warranted in patients with symptoms of dizziness, palpitations, or syncope. May cause orthostatic hypotension; use with caution in patients at risk of this effect (eg, concurrent medication use which may predispose to hypotension/bradycardia or presence of hypovolemia) or in those who would not tolerate transient hypotensive episodes. Use with caution in patients with cardiovascular diseases (eg, heart failure, history of myocardial infarction or ischemia, cerebrovascular disease, conduction abnormalities).

May cause anticholinergic effects (confusion, agitation, constipation, xerostomia, blurred vision, urinary retention); therefore, use with caution in patients with decreased gastrointestinal motility, urinary retention, BPH, xerostomia, or visual problems (including narrow-angle glaucoma). May cause extrapyramidal symptoms (EPS), including pseudoparkinsonism, acute dystonic reactions, akathisia, and tardive dyskinesia. Risk of dystonia (and probably other EPS) may be greater with increased doses, use of conventional antipsychotics, males, and younger patients. Risk of neuroleptic malignant syndrome (NMS) may be increased in patients with Parkinson's disease or Lewy body dementia. May cause hyperglycemia; in some cases may be extreme and associated with ketoacidosis, hyperosmolar coma, or death. Use with caution in patients with diabetes or other disorders of glucose regulation; monitor for worsening of glucose control. Dyslipidemia has been reported with atypical antipsychotics; risk profile may differ between agents. In clinical trials, changes in triglyceride and total cholesterol levels observed with iloperidone were similar to those observed with placebo or were clinically insignificant. Small reductions in cholesterol and triglycerides have been observed in longer term iloperidone trials.

Significant weight gain has been observed with antipsychotic therapy; incidence varies with product. Monitor waist circumference and BMI. Rare cases of priapism have been reported.

Use in elderly patients with dementia is associated with an increased risk of mortality and cerebrovascular accidents; avoid antipsychotic use for behavioral problems associated with dementia unless alternative nonpharmacologic therapies have failed and patient may harm self or others. In addition, use may cause or exacerbate syndrome of inappropriate antidiuretic hormone secretion or hyponatremia; monitor sodium closely with initiation or dosage adjustments in older adults (Beers Criteria).

Potentially significant interactions may exist, requiring dose or frequency adjustment, additional monitoring, and/or selection of alternative therapy. The possibility of a suicide attempt is inherent in psychotic illness; use caution in high-risk patients during initiation of therapy. Prescriptions should be written for the smallest quantity consistent with good patient care. Continued use for >6 weeks has not been evaluated.

Adverse Reactions

Cardiovascular: Hypotension, orthostatic hypotension, palpitations, tachycardia

Central nervous system: Aggression, akathisia, delusion, extrapyramidal symptoms, fatigue, lethargy, restlessness, somnolence, tremor

Dermatologic: Rash

Gastrointestinal: Abdominal discomfort, diarrhea, nausea, weight gain/loss, xerostomia

Genitourinary: Ejaculation failure, erectile dysfunction, urinary incontinence

Neuromuscular & skeletal: Arthralgia, dyskinesia, muscle spasm, myalgia, stiffness

Ocular: Blurred vision, conjunctivitis

Respiratory: Dyspnea, nasal congestion, nasopharyngitis, upper respiratory tract infection

Rare but important or life-threatening: Acute renal failure, amenorrhea, amnesia, anemia, anorgasmia, aphthous stomatitis, appetite increased, arrhythmia, asthma, AV block (first degree), blepharitis, bradykinesia, breast pain, bulimia nervosa, cataract, catatonia, cholelithiasis, confusion, dehydration, delirium, difficulty walking, dry eye, duodenal ulcer, dystonia, dysuria, edema, enuresis, epistaxis, esophageal reflux, eyelid edema, eye swelling, fecal incontinence, fluid retention, gastric acid secretion increased, gastritis, gynecomastia, heart failure, hematocrit/hemoglobin decreased, hiatal hernia, hostility, hyperemia, hyperthermia, hypokalemia, hypothyroidism, impulse control disorder, lenticular opacities, leukopenia, libido decreased, major depression, mania, menorrhagia, menstrual irregularities, metrorrhagia, mood swings, mouth ulceration, nasal dryness, nephrolithiasis, neutrophils increased, nystagmus, obsessive compulsive disorder, panic attack, paraesthesia, paranoia, parkinsonism, pollakiuria, polydipsia psychogenic, postmenopausal hemorrhage, prostatitis, pruritus, psychomotor hyperactivity, QTc interval prolongation, restless leg syndrome, retrograde ejaculation, rhinorrhea, salivation, sinus congestion, sleep apnea syndrome, stomatitis, testicular pain, thirst, tinnitus, torticollis, urinary retention, urticaria, vertigo

Drug Interactions

Metabolism/Transport Effects **Substrate** of CYP2D6 (major), CYP3A4 (minor); **Note:** Assignment of Major/Minor substrate status based on clinically relevant drug interaction potential; **Inhibits** CYP3A4 (weak)

Avoid Concomitant Use

Avoid concomitant use of Iloperidone with any of the following: Amisulpride; Azelastine (Nasal); Highest Risk QTc-Prolonging Agents; Ivabradine; Metoclopramide; Mifepristone; Moderate Risk QTc-Prolonging Agents; Orphenadrine; Paraldehyde; Pimozide; Sulpiride; Thalidomide

Increased Effect/Toxicity

Iloperidone may increase the levels/effects of: Alcohol (Ethyl); Amisulpride; Azelastine (Nasal); Buprenorphine; CNS Depressants; Highest Risk QTc-Prolonging Agents; Hydrocodone; Lomitapide; Methotrimeprazine; Methylphenidate; Metyrosine; Orphenadrine; Paraldehyde; Pimozide; Selective Serotonin Reuptake Inhibitors; Serotonin Modulators; Sulpiride; Suvorexant; Thalidomide; Zolpidem

The levels/effects of Iloperidone may be increased by: Abiraterone Acetate; Acetylcholinesterase Inhibitors (Central); Brimonidine (Topical); Cannabis; CYP2D6 Inhibitors (Moderate); CYP2D6 Inhibitors (Strong); CYP3A4 Inhibitors (Strong); Doxylamine; Dronabinol; Ivabradine; Kava Kava; Magnesium Sulfate; MAO Inhibitors; Methotrimeprazine; Methylphenidate; Metoclopramide; Metyrosine; Mifepristone; Moderate Risk QTc-Prolonging Agents; Nabilone; Peginterferon Alfa-2b; Perampanel; QTc-Prolonging Agents (Indeterminate Risk and Risk Modifying); Rufinamide; Serotonin Modulators; Sodium Oxybate; Tapentadol; Tetrahydrocannabinol

Decreased Effect

Iloperidone may decrease the levels/effects of: Amphetamines; Anti-Parkinson's Agents (Dopamine Agonist); Quinagolide

The levels/effects of Iloperidone may be decreased by: CYP2D6 Inhibitors (Strong); Peginterferon Alfa-2b

Storage/Stability Store at 25°C (77°F); excursions permitted to 15°C to 30°C (59°F to 86°F). Protect from light and moisture.

Mechanism of Action Iloperidone is a piperidinyl-benzisoxazole atypical antipsychotic with mixed D_2/5-HT_2 antagonist activity. It exhibits high affinity for 5-HT_{2A}, D_2, and D_3 receptors, low to moderate affinity for D_1, D_4, H_1, 5-HT_{1A}, 5-HT_6, 5-HT_7, and $NE_{\alpha 1}$ receptors, and no affinity for muscarinic receptors. The addition of serotonin antagonism to dopamine antagonism (classic neuroleptic mechanism) is thought to improve negative symptoms of psychoses and reduce the incidence of extrapyramidal side effects. Iloperidone's low affinity for histamine H_1 receptors may decrease the risk for weight gain and somnolence while its affinity for $NE_{\alpha 1/\alpha 2C}$ may provide antidepressant and anxiolytic activity and improved cognitive function.

Pharmacodynamics/Kinetics

Absorption: Well absorbed

Distribution: V_d: 1340 to 2800 L

Protein binding: ~97% iloperidone; ~92% active metabolites (P88 and P95)

Metabolism: Hepatic via carbonyl reduction, hydroxylation (CYP2D6) and O-demethylation (CYP3A4); forms active metabolites (P88 and P95)

Bioavailability: Oral: Tablet (relative to solution): 96%

Half-life elimination:

Extensive metabolizers: Iloperidone: 18 hours; P88: 26 hours; P95: 23 hours

Poor metabolizers: Iloperidone: 33 hours; P88: 37 hours; P95: 31 hours

Time to peak, plasma: 2 to 4 hours

Excretion: Urine (58% extensive metabolizers, 45% poor metabolizers); feces (20% extensive metabolizers, 22% poor metabolizers)

Dosage Oral: Adults: Schizophrenia: Initial: 1 mg twice daily; titrate to the recommended dosage range with dosage adjustments not to exceed 2 mg twice daily (4 mg daily) every 24 hours; recommended dosage range: 6 to 12 mg twice daily (maximum: 24 mg daily)

Note: Titrate dose to effect (to avoid orthostatic hypotensive effects); treatment >6 weeks has not been evaluated; when reinitiating treatment after discontinuation (>3 days), the initial titration schedule should be followed.

Dosage adjustment in patients receiving strong CYP2D6 inhibitors (eg, paroxetine, fluoxetine, quinidine): Decrease iloperidone dose by 50%; when the CYP2D6 inhibitor is discontinued, return to previous dose.

Dosage adjustment in patients receiving strong CYP3A4 inhibitors (eg, ketoconazole, clarithromycin): Decrease iloperidone dose by 50%; when the CYP3A4 inhibitor is discontinued, return to previous dose.

Dosage adjustment in poor metabolizers of CYP2D6: Decrease iloperidone dose by 50%.

Dosage adjustment in renal impairment: There are no dosage adjustments provided in manufacturer's labeling; however, pharmacokinetics of iloperidone do not appear to be altered by renal impairment due to extensive hepatic metabolism.

Dosage adjustment in hepatic impairment:

Mild impairment: No dosage adjustment necessary.

Moderate impairment: There are no dosage adjustments provided in the manufacturer's labeling; use with caution.

Severe hepatic impairment: Use is not recommended.

Administration Administer with or without food.

Monitoring Parameters Mental status; vital signs (as clinically indicated); blood pressure (baseline; repeat 3 months after antipsychotic initiation, then yearly); ECG (as clinically indicated); weight, height, BMI, waist circumference (baseline; repeat at 4, 8, and 12 weeks after initiating or changing therapy, then quarterly; consider switching to a different antipsychotic for a weight gain ≥5% of initial weight); CBC (as clinically indicated; monitor frequently during the first few months of therapy in patients with preexisting low WBC or history of drug-induced leukopenia/neutropenia); electrolytes (annually and as clinically indicated; perform baseline serum potassium and magnesium with periodic monitoring in patients at risk for significant electrolyte disturbances); liver function (annually and as clinically indicated); personal and family history of obesity, diabetes, dyslipidemia, hypertension, or cardiovascular disease (baseline; repeat annually); fasting plasma glucose level/HbA_{1c} (baseline; repeat 3 months after starting antipsychotic, then yearly); fasting lipid panel (baseline; repeat 3 months after initiation of antipsychotic; if LDL level is normal, repeat at 2- to 5-year intervals or more frequently if clinical indicated); changes in menstruation, libido, development of galactorrhea, erectile and ejaculatory function (at each visit for the first 12 weeks after the antipsychotic is initiated or until the dose is stable, then yearly); abnormal involuntary movements or parkinsonian signs (baseline; repeat weekly until dose stabilized for at least 2 weeks after introduction and for 2 weeks after any significant dose increase); tardive dyskinesia (every 12 months; high-risk patients every 6 months); ocular examination (yearly in patients >40 years; every 2 years in younger patients) (ADA, 2004; Lehman, 2004; Marder, 2004).

Dosage Forms

Tablet, Oral:

Fanapt: 1 mg, 2 mg, 4 mg, 6 mg, 8 mg, 10 mg, 12 mg

Fanapt Titration Pack: 1 mg (2s), 2 mg (2s), 4 mg (2s), and 6 mg (2s)

Iloprost (EYE loe prost)

Brand Names: U.S. Ventavis

Index Terms Iloprost Tromethamine; Prostacyclin PGI_2

Pharmacologic Category Prostacyclin; Prostaglandin; Vasodilator

Use Pulmonary arterial hypertension: Treatment of pulmonary arterial hypertension (World Health Organization [WHO] group I) in patients with New York Heart Association (NYHA) class III or IV symptoms to improve exercise tolerance, symptoms, and diminish clinical deterioration.

Pregnancy Risk Factor C

Dosage Inhalation: Adults: Pulmonary arterial hypertension (PAH): Initial: 2.5 mcg/dose; if tolerated, increase to 5 mcg/dose; administer 6-9 times daily (dosing at intervals ≥2 hours while awake according to individual need and tolerability); maintenance dose: 2.5-5 mcg/dose; maximum daily dose: 45 mcg (ie, 5 mcg/dose 9 times daily)

Dosage adjustment in renal impairment: Inhaled iloprost has not been studied in renal impairment; however, according to the manufacturer, no adjustment is required in patients with renal impairment who are not on dialysis (the effect of dialysis on iloprost is unknown).

Dosage adjustment in hepatic impairment: Child-Pugh class B or C: Consider increasing dosing interval (eg, every 3-4 hours) based on response at the end of the dose interval

Additional Information Complete prescribing information should be consulted for additional detail.

Dosage Forms

Solution, Inhalation [preservative free]:

Ventavis: 10 mcg/mL (1 mL); 20 mcg/mL (1 mL)

◆ **Iloprost Tromethamine** *see* Iloprost *on page 1046*

◆ **Ilotycin** *see* Erythromycin (Ophthalmic) *on page 764*

Imatinib (eye MAT eh nib)

Brand Names: U.S. Gleevec

Brand Names: Canada ACT-Imatinib; Apo-Imatinib; Gleevec; Teva-Imatinib

Index Terms CGP-57148B; Glivec; Imatinib Mesylate; STI-571

Pharmacologic Category Antineoplastic Agent, BCR-ABL Tyrosine Kinase Inhibitor; Antineoplastic Agent, Tyrosine Kinase Inhibitor

Use Treatment of:

Gastrointestinal stromal tumors (GIST) kit-positive (CD117), including unresectable and/or metastatic malignant and adjuvant treatment following complete resection

Philadelphia chromosome-positive (Ph+) chronic myeloid leukemia (CML) in chronic phase (newly-diagnosed) in children and adults

Ph+ CML in blast crisis, accelerated phase, or chronic phase after failure of interferon therapy

Ph+ acute lymphoblastic leukemia (ALL) (relapsed or refractory)

Ph+ ALL (newly diagnosed; in combination with chemotherapy) in children

Aggressive systemic mastocytosis (ASM) without D816V c-Kit mutation (or c-Kit mutation status unknown)

Dermatofibrosarcoma protuberans (DFSP) (unresectable, recurrent and/or metastatic)

Hypereosinophilic syndrome (HES) and/or chronic eosinophilic leukemia (CEL)

Myelodysplastic/myeloproliferative disease (MDS/MPD) associated with platelet-derived growth factor receptor (PDGFR) gene rearrangements

Canadian labeling (not an approved indication in the U.S.): Ph+ ALL induction therapy (newly diagnosed; as a single agent)

Pregnancy Risk Factor D

Pregnancy Considerations Animal reproduction studies have demonstrated teratogenic effects and fetal loss. Women of childbearing potential are advised not to become pregnant (female patients and female partners of male patients); highly effective contraception is recommended. Case reports of pregnancies while on therapy (both males and females) include reports of spontaneous abortion, minor abnormalities (hypospadias, pyloric stenosis, and small intestine rotation) at or shortly after birth, and other congenital abnormalities including skeletal malformations, hypoplastic lungs, exomphalos, kidney abnormalities, hydrocephalus, cerebellar hypoplasia, and cardiac defects.

Retrospective case reports of women with CML in complete hematologic response (CHR) with cytogenic response (partial or complete) who interrupted imatinib therapy due to pregnancy, demonstrated a loss of response in some patients while off treatment. At 18 months after treatment reinitiation following delivery, CHR was again achieved in all patients and cytogenic response was achieved in some patients. Cytogenetic response rates may not be at as high as compared to patients with 18 months of uninterrupted therapy (Ault, 2006; Pye, 2008).

Breast-Feeding Considerations Imatinib and its active metabolite are found in human breast milk; the milk/plasma ratio is 0.5 for imatinib and 0.9 for the active metabolite. Based on body weight, up to 10% of a therapeutic maternal dose could potentially be received by a breastfed infant, the decision to discontinue breast-feeding during therapy or to discontinue imatinib should take into account the benefits of treatment to the mother.

Contraindications There are no contraindications listed in the manufacturer's U.S. labeling.

Canadian labeling: Hypersensitivity to imatinib or any component of the formulation

Warnings/Precautions Hazardous agent - use appropriate precautions for handling and disposal (NIOSH 2014 [group 1]). Often associated with fluid retention, weight gain, and edema (risk increases with higher doses and age >65 years); occasionally serious and may lead to significant complications, including pleural effusion, pericardial effusion, pulmonary edema, and ascites. Monitor regularly for rapid weight gain or other signs/symptoms of fluid retention. Use with caution in patients where fluid accumulation may be poorly tolerated, such as in cardiovascular disease (heart failure [HF] or hypertension) and pulmonary disease. Severe HF and left ventricular dysfunction (LVD) have been reported occasionally, usually in patients with comorbidities and/or risk factors; carefully monitor patients with preexisting cardiac disease or risk factors for HF or history of renal failure. With initiation of imatinib treatment, cardiogenic shock and/or LVD have been reported in patients with hypereosinophilic syndrome and cardiac involvement (reversible with systemic steroids, circulatory support and temporary cessation of imatinib). Patients with high eosinophil levels and an abnormal echocardiogram or abnormal serum troponin level may benefit from prophylactic systemic steroids (for 1 to 2 weeks) with the initiation of imatinib.

Severe bullous dermatologic reactions (including erythema multiforme and Stevens-Johnson syndrome) have been reported; recurrence has been described with rechallenge. Case reports of successful resumption at a lower dose (with corticosteroids and/or antihistamine) have been described; however, some patients may experience recurrent reactions.

Hepatotoxicity may occur (may be severe); fatal hepatic failure and severe hepatic injury requiring liver transplantation have been reported with both short- and long-term use; monitor liver function prior to initiation and monthly or as needed thereafter; therapy interruption or dose reduction may be necessary. Transaminase and bilirubin elevations, and acute liver failure have been observed with imatinib in combination with chemotherapy. Use with caution in patients with preexisting hepatic impairment; dosage adjustment recommended in patients with severe impairment. Use with caution in renal impairment; dosage adjustment recommended for moderate and severe impairment. Tumor lysis syndrome (TLS), including fatalities, has been reported in patients with ALL, CML eosinophilic leukemias, and GIST; risk for TLS is higher in patients with a high tumor burden or high proliferation rate; monitor closely; correct clinically significant dehydration and treat high uric acid levels prior to initiation of imatinib.

Imatinib is associated with a moderate emetic potential; antiemetics may be recommended to prevent nausea and vomiting (Dupuis, 2011; Roila, 2010). May cause GI irritation, severe hemorrhage (grades 3 and 4; including gastrointestinal hemorrhage and/or tumor hemorrhage; hemorrhage incidence is higher in patients with GIST [gastrointestinal tumors may have been hemorrhage source]), or hematologic toxicity (anemia, neutropenia, and thrombocytopenia; usually occurring within the first several months of treatment); monitor blood counts weekly for the first month, biweekly for the second month, and as clinically necessary thereafter; median duration of neutropenia is 2 to 3 weeks; median duration of thrombocytopenia is 3 to 4 weeks; in CML, cytopenias are more common in accelerated or blast phase than in chronic phase. Hypothyroidism has been reported in patients who were receiving thyroid hormone replacement therapy prior to the initiation of imatinib; monitor thyroid function; the average onset for imatinib-induced hypothyroidism is 2 weeks; consider doubling levothyroxine doses upon initiation of imatinib (Hamnvik, 2011). Potentially significant drug-drug interactions may exist, requiring dose or frequency adjustment, additional monitoring, and/or selection of alternative therapy. Imatinib exposure may be reduced in patients who have had gastric surgery (eg, bypass, major gastrectomy, or resection); monitor imatinib trough concentrations (Liu, 2011; Pavlovsky, 2009; Yoo, 2010). Growth retardation has been reported in children receiving imatinib for the treatment of CML; generally where treatment was initiated in prepubertal children; growth velocity was usually restored as pubertal age was reached (Shima, 2011); monitor growth closely. Reports of accidents have been received but it is unclear if imatinib has been the direct cause in any case; advise patients regarding side effects such as dizziness, blurred vision, or somnolence; use caution when driving/operating motor vehicles and heavy machinery.

Adverse Reactions

Cardiovascular: Chest pain, edema (includes aggravated edema, anasarca, ascites, palpitation, pericardial effusion, peripheral edema, pulmonary edema, and superficial edema); facial edema, flushing, hypotension (children and adolescents), pleural effusion (children and adolescents)

Central nervous system: Anxiety, cerebral hemorrhage, chills, depression, dizziness, fatigue, headache, hypoesthesia, insomnia, pain, paresthesia, peripheral neuropathy, rigors, taste disorder

Dermatologic: Alopecia (GIST), dermatitis (GIST), diaphoresis (GIST), erythema, night sweats (CML), pruritus, skin photosensitivity, skin rash, xeroderma

Endocrine & metabolic: Decreased serum albumin, hyperglycemia, hypocalcemia (GIST), hypokalemia (more common in children and adolescents), increased lactate dehydrogenase (GIST), weight gain

Gastrointestinal: Abdominal distension, abdominal pain, anorexia, constipation, decreased appetite, diarrhea, dyspepsia, flatulence, gastritis, gastroesophageal reflux, gastrointestinal hemorrhage, nausea, stomatitis, vomiting, xerostomia

Hematologic & oncologic: Anemia, febrile neutropenia, hemorrhage, hypoproteinemia, leukopenia (GIST), lymphocytopenia (GIST), neutropenia, pancytopenia, thrombocytopenia

Hepatic: Increased alkaline phosphatase, increased serum ALT, increased serum AST, increased serum bilirubin, increased serum transaminases (children and adolescents)

Infection: Infection (more common in children and adolescents)

Neuromuscular & skeletal: Arthralgia, back pain (GIST), joint swelling, limb pain (GIST), muscle cramps, musculoskeletal pain (more common in adults), myalgia, ostealgia, weakness

Ophthalmic: Blurred vision, conjunctival hemorrhage, conjunctivitis, dry eyes, increased lacrimation (more common in DFSP), periorbital edema

Renal: Increased serum creatinine

Respiratory: Cough, dyspnea, epistaxis, flu-like symptoms, hypoxia, nasopharyngitis, pharyngitis (CML), pharyngolaryngeal pain, pneumonia (CML), pneumonitis (children and adolescents), rhinitis (DFSP), upper respiratory tract infection

Miscellaneous: Fever

Rare but important or life-threatening: Actinic keratosis, acute generalized exanthematous pustulosis, anaphylactic shock, angina pectoris, angioedema, aplastic anemia, arthritis, ascites, atrial fibrillation, avascular necrosis of bones, bullous rash, cardiac arrest, cardiac arrhythmia, cardiac failure (severe), cardiac tamponade, cardiogenic shock, cataract, cellulitis, cerebral edema, decreased linear skeletal growth rate (children), diverticulitis, DRESS syndrome, dyschromia, embolism, eosinophilia, erythema multiforme, exfoliative dermatitis, fungal infection, gastric ulcer, gastrointestinal obstruction, gastrointestinal perforation, glaucoma, gout, hearing loss, hematemesis, hematoma, hematuria, hemolytic anemia, hepatic failure, hepatic necrosis, hepatitis, hepatotoxicity, herpes simplex infection, herpes zoster, hypercalcemia, hyperkalemia, hypersensitivity angiitis, hypertension, hyperuricemia, hypomagnesemia, hyponatremia, hypophosphatemia, hypothyroidism, IgA vasculitis, increased intracranial pressure, inflammatory bowel disease, interstitial pneumonitis, interstitial pulmonary disease, intestinal obstruction, left ventricular dysfunction, lichen planus, lower respiratory tract infection, lymphadenopathy, macular edema, melena, memory impairment, migraine, myocardial infarction, myopathy, optic neuritis, osteonecrosis (hip), ovarian cyst (hemorrhagic), palmar-plantar erythrodysesthesia, pancreatitis, papilledema, pericarditis, psoriasis, pulmonary fibrosis, pulmonary hemorrhage, pulmonary hypertension, Raynaud's phenomenon, renal failure, respiratory failure, restless leg syndrome, retinal hemorrhage, rhabdomyolysis, ruptured corpus luteal cyst, sciatica, seizure, sepsis, Stevens-Johnson syndrome, subconjunctival hemorrhage, subdural hematoma, Sweet's syndrome, syncope, tachycardia, thrombocythemia, thrombosis, toxic epidermal necrolysis, tumor hemorrhage (GIST), tumor lysis syndrome, urinary tract infection, vitreous hemorrhage

Drug Interactions

Metabolism/Transport Effects Substrate of CYP1A2 (minor), CYP2C19 (minor), CYP2C8 (minor), CYP2C9 (minor), CYP2D6 (minor), CYP3A4 (major), P-glycoprotein; **Note:** Assignment of Major/Minor substrate status based on clinically relevant drug interaction potential; **Inhibits** BCRP, CYP2C9 (weak), CYP2D6 (weak), CYP3A4 (moderate), P-glycoprotein

Avoid Concomitant Use

Avoid concomitant use of Imatinib with any of the following: BCG; Bosutinib; CloZAPine; Dipyrone; Ibrutinib; Ivabradine; Lomitapide; Naloxegol; Natalizumab; Olaparib; PAZOPanib; Pimecrolimus; Pimozide; Simeprevir; Tacrolimus (Topical); Tofacitinib; Tolvaptan; Trabectedin; Ulipristal; Vaccines (Live)

Increased Effect/Toxicity

Imatinib may increase the levels/effects of: ARIPiprazole; Avanafil; Bosentan; Bosutinib; Budesonide (Systemic, Oral Inhalation); Cannabis; CloZAPine; Colchicine; CycloSPORINE (Systemic); CYP3A4 Substrates; Dapoxetine; Dofetilide; DOXOrubicin (Conventional);

Dronabinol; Eliglustat; Eplerenone; Everolimus; FentaNYL; Halofantrine; Hydrocodone; Ibrutinib; Ivabradine; Ivacaftor; Leflunomide; Lomitapide; Lurasidone; Naloxegol; Natalizumab; Olaparib; OxyCODONE; PAZOPanib; Pimozide; Propafenone; Ranolazine; Rivaroxaban; Salmeterol; Saxagliptin; Simeprevir; Simvastatin; Suvorexant; Tetrahydrocannabinol; Tofacitinib; Tolvaptan; Topotecan; Trabectedin; Ulipristal; Vaccines (Live); Vilazodone; Warfarin; Zopiclone; Zuclopenthixol

The levels/effects of Imatinib may be increased by: Acetaminophen; CYP3A4 Inhibitors (Moderate); CYP3A4 Inhibitors (Strong); Denosumab; Dipyrone; Lansoprazole; P-glycoprotein/ABCB1 Inhibitors; Pimecrolimus; Roflumilast; Tacrolimus (Topical); Trastuzumab

Decreased Effect

Imatinib may decrease the levels/effects of: BCG; Coccidioides immitis Skin Test; Fludarabine; Ifosfamide; Sipuleucel-T; Vaccines (Inactivated); Vaccines (Live)

The levels/effects of Imatinib may be decreased by: Bosentan; CYP3A4 Inducers (Moderate); CYP3A4 Inducers (Strong); Dabrafenib; Deferasirox; Dexamethasone (Systemic); Echinacea; Gemfibrozil; Ibuprofen; Mitotane; P-glycoprotein/ABCB1 Inducers; Rifamycin Derivatives; Siltuximab; St Johns Wort; Tocilizumab

Food Interactions Food may reduce GI irritation. Grapefruit juice may increase imatinib plasma concentration. Management: Take with a meal and a large glass of water. Avoid grapefruit juice. Maintain adequate hydration, unless instructed to restrict fluid intake.

Storage/Stability Store at 25°C (77°F); excursions permitted between 15°C to 30°C (59°F to 86°F). Protect from moisture.

Mechanism of Action Inhibits Bcr-Abl tyrosine kinase, the constitutive abnormal gene product of the Philadelphia chromosome in chronic myeloid leukemia (CML). Inhibition of this enzyme blocks proliferation and induces apoptosis in Bcr-Abl positive cell lines as well as in fresh leukemic cells in Philadelphia chromosome positive CML. Also inhibits tyrosine kinase for platelet-derived growth factor (PDGF), stem cell factor (SCF), c-Kit, and cellular events mediated by PDGF and SCF.

Pharmacodynamics/Kinetics

Absorption: Rapid

Protein binding: Parent drug and metabolite: ~95% to albumin and alpha$_1$-acid glycoprotein

Metabolism: Hepatic via CYP3A4 (minor metabolism via CYP1A2, CYP2D6, CYP2C9, CYP2C19); primary metabolite (active): N-demethylated piperazine derivative (CGP74588); severe hepatic impairment (bilirubin >3-10 times ULN) increases AUC by 45% to 55% for imatinib and its active metabolite, respectively

Bioavailability: 98%; may be decreased in patients who have had gastric surgery (eg, bypass, total or partial resection)

Half-life elimination: Adults: Parent drug: ~18 hours; N-desmethyl metabolite: ~40 hours; Children: Parent drug: ~15 hours

Time to peak: 2-4 hours

Excretion: Feces (68% primarily as metabolites, 20% as unchanged drug); urine (13% primarily as metabolites, 5% as unchanged drug)

Dosage Note: Treatment may be continued until disease progression or unacceptable toxicity. The optimal duration of therapy for chronic myeloid leukemia (CML) in complete remission is not yet determined. Discontinuing CML treatment is not recommended unless part of a clinical trial (Baccarani, 2009). Imatinib is associated with a moderate emetic potential; antiemetics may be recommended to prevent nausea and vomiting (Dupuis, 2011; Roila, 2010).

Children ≥1 year and Adolescents: Oral:

Ph+ ALL (newly diagnosed): 340 mg/m^2/day (in combination with chemotherapy); maximum: 600 mg daily

Ph+ CML (chronic phase, newly diagnosed): 340 mg/m^2/day; maximum: 600 mg daily

Adults: Oral:

Ph+ CML:

Chronic phase: 400 mg once daily; may be increased to 600 mg daily, if tolerated, for disease progression, lack of hematologic response after 3 months, lack of cytogenetic response after 6-12 months, or loss of previous hematologic or cytogenetic response. An increase to 800 mg daily has been used (Cortes, 2010; Hehlmann, 2014).

Canadian labeling: 400 mg once daily; may be increased to 600-800 mg daily

Accelerated phase or blast crisis: 600 mg once daily; may be increased to 800 mg daily (400 mg twice daily), if tolerated, for disease progression, lack of hematologic response after 3 months, lack of cytogenetic response after 6-12 months, or loss of previous hematologic or cytogenetic response

Ph+ ALL (relapsed or refractory): 600 mg once daily

GIST (adjuvant treatment following complete resection): 400 mg once daily; recommended treatment duration: 3 years

GIST (unresectable and/or metastatic malignant): 400 mg once daily; may be increased up to 800 mg daily (400 mg twice daily), if tolerated, for disease progression. **Note:** Significant improvement (progression-free survival, objective response rate) was demonstrated in patients with KIT exon 9 mutation with 800 mg (versus 400 mg), although overall survival (OS) was not impacted. The higher dose did not demonstrate a difference in time to progression or OS patients with Kit exon 11 mutation or wild-type status (Debiec-Rychter, 2006; Heinrich, 2009).

Canadian labeling: 400-600 mg daily (depending on disease stage/progression); may be increased to 600-800 mg daily

ASM with eosinophilia: Initiate at 100 mg once daily; titrate up to a maximum of 400 mg once daily (if tolerated) for insufficient response to lower dose

ASM without D816V c-Kit mutation or c-Kit mutation status unknown: 400 mg once daily

DFSP: 400 mg twice daily

HES/CEL: 400 mg once daily

HES/CEL with FIP1L1-PDGFRα fusion kinase: Initiate at 100 mg once daily; titrate up to a maximum of 400 mg once daily (if tolerated) if insufficient response to lower dose

MDS/MPD: 400 mg once daily

Ph+ ALL (induction, newly diagnosed): *Canadian labeling (not an approved use in the U.S.):* 600 mg once daily

Chordoma, progressive, advanced, or metastatic expressing PDGFRB and/or PDGFB (off-label use): 400 mg twice daily (Stacchiotti, 2012)

Desmoid tumors, unresectable and/or progressive (off-label use): 300 mg twice daily (BSA ≥1.5 m^2), 200 mg twice daily (BSA 1-1.49 m^2), 100 mg twice daily (BSA <1 m^2) (Chugh, 2010) **or** 400 mg once daily; may increase to 400 mg twice daily if progressive disease on 400 mg daily (Penel, 2011)

Melanoma, advanced or metastatic with C-KIT mutation (off-label use): 400 mg twice daily (Carvajal, 2011)

Stem cell transplant (SCT, off-label use) for CML (in patients who have not failed imatinib therapy prior to transplant):

Prophylactic use to prevent relapse post SCT: 400 mg daily starting after engraftment for 1 year post transplant (Carpenter, 2007) **or** 300 mg daily starting on day +35 post SCT (increased to 400 mg within 4 weeks) and continued until 12 months post transplant (Olavarria, 2007)

Relapse post SCT: Initial: 400 mg daily; if inferior response after 3 months, dose may be increased to 600-800 mg daily (Hess, 2005) **or** 400-600 mg daily (chronic phase) **or** 600 mg daily (blast or accelerated phase) (DeAngelo, 2004)

Dosage adjustment with concomitant strong CYP3A4 inducers: Avoid concomitant use of strong CYP3A4 inducers (eg, dexamethasone, carbamazepine, phenobarbital, phenytoin, rifabutin, rifampin); if concomitant use cannot be avoided, increase imatinib dose by at least 50% with careful monitoring.

Dosage adjustment for renal impairment:

U.S. labeling:

Mild impairment (CrCl 40-59 mL/minute): Maximum recommended dose: 600 mg

Moderate impairment (CrCl 20-39 mL/minute): Decrease recommended starting dose by 50%; dose may be increased as tolerated; maximum recommended dose: 400 mg

Severe impairment (CrCl <20 mL/minute): Use caution; a dose of 100 mg daily has been tolerated in a limited number of patients with severe impairment (Gibbons, 2008)

Canadian labeling:

Mild impairment (CrCl 40-59 mL/minute): Initial dose: 400 mg once daily (minimum effective dose); titrate to efficacy and tolerability

Moderate impairment (CrCl 20-39 mL/minute): Initial dose: 400 mg once daily (minimum effective dose); titrate to efficacy and tolerability; the use of 800 mg dose is not recommended

Severe impairment (CrCl <20 mL/minute): Use is not recommended

Dosage adjustment for hepatic impairment:

U.S. labeling:

Mild-to-moderate impairment: No dosage adjustment necessary

Severe impairment: Reduce dose by 25%

Canadian labeling:

Mild-to-moderate impairment: Initial dose: 400 mg once daily (minimum effective dose)

Severe impairment: Initial dose: 200 mg once daily; may increase up to 300 mg once daily in the absence of severe toxicity; decrease dose with unacceptable toxicity

Dosage adjustment for hepatotoxicity (during therapy): If elevations of bilirubin >3 times ULN or transaminases >5 times ULN occur, withhold treatment until bilirubin <1.5 times ULN and transaminases <2.5 times ULN. Resume treatment at a reduced dose as follows (**Note:** The decision to resume treatment should take into consideration the initial severity of hepatotoxicity):

Children ≥1 year and Adolescents: If current dose 340 mg/m²/day, reduce dose to 260 mg/m²/day

Adults:

If current dose 400 mg daily, reduce dose to 300 mg daily

If current dose 600 mg daily, reduce dose to 400 mg daily

If current dose 800 mg daily, reduce dose to 600 mg daily

Dosage adjustment for hematologic adverse reactions:

Chronic phase CML (initial dose 400 mg daily in adults or 340 mg/m²/day in children); ASM, MDS/MPD, and HES/CEL (initial dose 400 mg daily); or GIST (initial dose 400 mg daily [U.S. labeling] or 400-600 mg daily [Canadian labeling]): If ANC <1 x 10^9/L and/or platelets <50 x 10^9/L: Withhold until ANC ≥1.5 x 10^9/L and platelets ≥75 x 10^9/L; resume treatment at original starting dose. For recurrent neutropenia and/or thrombocytopenia, withhold until recovery, and reinstitute treatment at a reduced dose as follows:

Children ≥1 year and Adolescents: If initial dose 340 mg/m²/day, reduce dose to 260 mg/m²/day

Adults:

If initial dose 400 mg daily, reduce dose to 300 mg daily

If initial dose 600 mg daily (Canadian labeling; not in U.S. labeling), reduce dose to 400 mg daily

CML (accelerated phase or blast crisis): Adults (initial dose 600 mg daily): If ANC <0.5 x 10^9/L and/or platelets <10 x 10^9/L, establish whether cytopenia is related to leukemia (bone marrow aspirate or biopsy). If unrelated to leukemia, reduce dose to 400 mg daily. If cytopenia persists for an additional 2 weeks, further reduce dose to 300 mg daily. If cytopenia persists for 4 weeks and is still unrelated to leukemia, withhold treatment until ANC ≥1 x 10^9/L and platelets ≥20 x 10^9/L, then resume treatment at 300 mg daily.

ASM associated with eosinophilia and HES/CEL with FIP1L1-PDGFRα fusion kinase: Adults (starting dose 100 mg daily): If ANC <1 x 10^9/L and/or platelets <50 x 10^9/L: Withhold until ANC ≥1.5 x 10^9/L and platelets ≥75 x 10^9/L; resume treatment at previous dose.

DFSP: Adults (initial dose 800 mg daily): If ANC <1 x 10^9/L and/or platelets <50 x 10^9/L, withhold until ANC ≥1.5 x 10^9/L and platelets ≥75 x 10^9/L; resume treatment at reduced dose of 600 mg daily. For recurrent neutropenia and/or thrombocytopenia, withhold until recovery, and reinstitute treatment with a further dose reduction to 400 mg daily.

Ph+ ALL:

Pediatrics (Schultz, 2009): Hematologic toxicity requiring dosage adjustments was not observed in the study. No major toxicities were observed with imatinib at 340 mg/m²/day in combination with intensive chemotherapy.

Adults (initial dose 600 mg daily): If ANC <0.5 x 10^9/L and/or platelets <10 x 10^9/L, establish whether cytopenia is related to leukemia (bone marrow aspirate or biopsy). If unrelated to leukemia, reduce dose to 400 mg daily. If cytopenia persists for an additional 2 weeks, further reduce dose to 300 mg daily. If cytopenia persists for 4 weeks and is still unrelated to leukemia, withhold treatment until ANC ≥1 x 10^9/L and platelets ≥20 x 10^9/L, then resume treatment at 300 mg daily.

Dosage adjustment for nonhematologic adverse reactions (eg, severe edema): Withhold treatment until toxicity resolves; may resume if appropriate (depending on initial severity of adverse event).

Dietary Considerations Avoid grapefruit juice.

Administration Imatinib is associated with a moderate emetic potential; antiemetics may be recommended to prevent nausea and vomiting (Dupuis, 2011; Roila, 2010).

Should be administered with a meal and a large glass of water. It is not recommended to crush or chew tablets due to bitter taste. Tablets may be dispersed in water or apple juice (using ~50 mL for 100 mg tablet, ~200 mL for 400 mg tablet); stir until dissolved and administer immediately. In adults, doses ≤600 mg may be given once daily; 800 mg dose should be administered as 400 mg twice daily.

Dosing in children may be once or twice daily for CML and once daily for Ph+ ALL. For daily dosing ≥800 mg, the 400 mg tablets should be used in order to reduce iron exposure.

Hazardous agent; use appropriate precautions for handling and disposal (NIOSH 2014 [group 1]).

Monitoring Parameters CBC (weekly for first month, biweekly for second month, then periodically thereafter), liver function tests (at baseline and monthly or as clinically indicated; more frequently [at least weekly] in patients with moderate-to-severe hepatic impairment [Ramanathan, 2008]), renal function, serum electrolytes (including calcium, phosphorus, potassium and sodium levels); bone marrow cytogenetics (in CML; at 6-, 12-, and 18 months); fatigue, weight, and edema/fluid status; consider echocardiogram and serum troponin levels in patients with HES/CEL, and in patients with MDS/MPD or ASM with high eosinophil levels; in pediatric patients, also monitor serum glucose, albumin, and growth

Gastric surgery (eg, bypass, major gastrectomy, or resection) patients: Monitor imatinib trough concentrations (Liu, 2011; Pavlovsky, 2009; Yoo, 2010)

Thyroid function testing (Hamnvik, 2011):

Preexisting levothyroxine therapy: Obtain baseline TSH levels, then monitor every 4 weeks until levels and levothyroxine dose are stable, then monitor every 2 months

Without preexisting thyroid hormone replacement: TSH at baseline, then every 4 weeks for 4 months, then every 2-3 months

Monitor for signs/symptoms of CHF in patients with at risk for cardiac failure or patients with preexisting cardiac disease. In Canada, a baseline evaluation of left ventricular ejection fraction is recommended prior to initiation of imatinib therapy in all patients with known underlying heart disease or in elderly patients. Monitor for signs/symptoms of gastrointestinal irritation or perforation and dermatologic toxicities.

Dosage Forms

Tablet, Oral:

Gleevec: 100 mg, 400 mg

Extemporaneous Preparations Hazardous agent: Use appropriate precautions for handling and disposal (NIOSH 2014 [group 1]).

An oral suspension may be prepared by placing tablets (whole, do not crush) in a glass of water or apple juice. Use ~50 mL for 100 mg tablet, or ~200 mL for 400 mg tablet. Stir until tablets are disintegrated, then administer immediately. To ensure the full dose is administered, rinse the glass and administer residue.

Gleevec (imatinib) [prescribing information]. East Hanover, NJ: Novartis Pharmaceuticals; October 2013.

- ◆ **Imatinib Mesylate** *see* Imatinib *on page 1047*
- ◆ **Imbruvica** *see* Ibrutinib *on page 1030*
- ◆ **IMC-1121B** *see* Ramucirumab *on page 1775*
- ◆ **IMC-C225** *see* Cetuximab *on page 413*
- ◆ **Imdur [DSC]** *see* Isosorbide Mononitrate *on page 1126*
- ◆ **Imdur (Can)** *see* Isosorbide Mononitrate *on page 1126*
- ◆ **Imferon** *see* Iron Dextran Complex *on page 1117*
- ◆ **IMI 30** *see* IDArubicin *on page 1037*
- ◆ **IMid-1** *see* Lenalidomide *on page 1177*

Imidapril [INT] (i MID a pril)

International Brand Names Cardipril (PT, TR); Indopril (VN); Norten (PH); Novarok (JP); Tanapress (ID); Tanatril (AE, AR, AT, CN, CZ, DE, FR, GB, GR, HK, IN, IT, JP, KR, LB, MY, PK, PL, SG, VN); Tanattril (SA, SK, TH); Vascor (PH)

Index Terms Imidapril Hydrochloride

Pharmacologic Category Angiotensin-Converting Enzyme (ACE) Inhibitor

Reported Use Treatment of hypertension including renal parenchymal hypertension; treatment of diabetic nephropathy

Dosage Range Oral:

Hypertension:

Adults: 2.5 to 20 mg once daily

Elderly: 2.5 to 10 mg once daily

Diabetic nephropathy: Adults: 5 mg once daily

Product Availability Product available in various countries; not currently available in the U.S.

Dosage Forms

Tablet, oral, as hydrochloride: 2.5 mg, 5 mg, 10 mg, 20 mg

- ◆ **Imidapril Hydrochloride** *see* Imidapril [INT] *on page 1051*
- ◆ **Imidazole Carboxamide** *see* Dacarbazine *on page 549*
- ◆ **Imidazole Carboxamide Dimethyltriazene** *see* Dacarbazine *on page 549*
- ◆ **IMIG** *see* Immune Globulin *on page 1056*

Imiglucerase (i mi GLOO ser ace)

Brand Names: U.S. Cerezyme

Brand Names: Canada Cerezyme

Pharmacologic Category Enzyme

Use Gaucher disease:

U.S. labeling: Long-term enzyme replacement therapy for patients with type 1 Gaucher disease that results in at least one of the following: anemia, bone disease, hepatomegaly or splenomegaly, and thrombocytopenia

Canadian labeling: Long-term enzyme replacement therapy for patients with type 1 Gaucher disease or patients with type 3 Gaucher disease who display non-neurological manifestations (anemia, bone disease, hepatomegaly or splenomegaly, and thrombocytopenia) of the disease.

Pregnancy Risk Factor C

Dosage

Gaucher disease, type 1: Children ≥2 years, Adolescents, and Adults: IV (dose is individualized): Initial range: 2.5 units/kg 3 times weekly, up to 60 units/kg every 2 weeks. **Note:** Dosage adjustments are made based on assessment and therapeutic goals. Most benefits observed with doses of 30-60 units/kg every 2 weeks (Charrow, 2004).

Gaucher disease, type 3 (Canadian labeling; not in U.S. labeling): Children ≥2 years, Adolescents, and Adults: IV (dose is individualized): Initial range: 2.5 units/kg 3 times weekly, up to 60 units/kg every 2 weeks. Doses up to 120 units/kg every 2 weeks have been safely administered.

Dosage adjustment in renal impairment: No dosage adjustment provided in the manufacturer's labeling.

Dosage adjustment in hepatic impairment: No dosage adjustment provided in the manufacturer's labeling.

Additional Information Complete prescribing information should be consulted for additional detail.

Dosage Forms

Solution Reconstituted, Intravenous:

Cerezyme: 200 units (1 ea); 400 units (1 ea)

- ◆ **Imipemide** *see* Imipenem and Cilastatin *on page 1051*

Imipenem and Cilastatin
(i mi PEN em & sye la STAT in)

Brand Names: U.S. Primaxin® I.V.

Brand Names: Canada Imipenem and Cilastatin for Injection; Primaxin I.V. Infusion; RAN-Imipenem-Cilastatin

Index Terms Cilastatin and Imipenem; Imipemide; Primaxin I.M. [DSC]

Pharmacologic Category Antibiotic, Carbapenem

Use Treatment of lower respiratory tract, urinary tract, intra-abdominal, gynecologic, bone and joint, skin and skin structure, endocarditis (caused by *Staphylococcus aureus*) and polymicrobic infections as well as bacterial septicemia. Antibacterial activity includes gram-positive bacteria (methicillin-sensitive *S. aureus* and *Streptococcus* spp), resistant gram-negative bacilli (including extended spectrum beta-lactamase-producing *Escherichia coli* and *Klebsiella* spp, *Enterobacter* spp, and *Pseudomonas aeruginosa*), and anaerobes.

Pregnancy Risk Factor C

Pregnancy Considerations Teratogenic events have not been observed in animal reproduction studies. Due to pregnancy induced physiologic changes, some pharmacokinetic parameters of imipenem/cilastatin may be altered. Pregnant women have a larger volume of distribution resulting in lower serum peak levels than for the same dose in nonpregnant women. Clearance is also increased.

Breast-Feeding Considerations Imipenem is excreted in human milk. The low concentrations and low oral bioavailability suggest minimal exposure risk to the infant. The manufacturer recommends that caution be exercised when administering imipenem/cilastatin to nursing women. Nondose-related effects could include modification of bowel flora.

Contraindications Hypersensitivity to imipenem/cilastatin or any component of the formulation

Warnings/Precautions Dosage adjustment required in patients with impaired renal function; elderly patients often require lower doses (adjust to renal function). Prolonged use may result in fungal or bacterial superinfection, including *C. difficile*-associated diarrhea (CDAD) and pseudomembranous colitis; CDAD has been observed >2 months postantibiotic treatment. Carbapenems have been associated with CNS adverse effects, including confusional states and seizures (myoclonic); use caution with CNS disorders (eg, brain lesions and history of seizures) and adjust dose in renal impairment to avoid drug accumulation, which may increase seizure risk. Use with caution in patients with hypersensitivity to beta-lactams (including penicillins or cephalosporins); patients with impaired renal function are at increased risk of seizures if not properly dose adjusted. May decrease divalproex sodium/valproic acid concentrations leading to breakthrough seizures; concomitant use is not recommended. Not recommended in pediatric CNS infections due to seizure risk. Serious hypersensitivity reactions, including anaphylaxis, have been reported (some without a history of previous allergic reactions to beta-lactams).

Adverse Reactions

Cardiovascular: Phlebitis, tachycardia

Central nervous system: Seizure

Dermatologic: Skin rash

Gastrointestinal: Diarrhea, gastroenteritis, nausea, oral candidiasis, vomiting

Genitourinary: Oliguria, proteinuria, urine discoloration

Hematologic & oncologic: Decreased hematocrit (more common in infants and children 3 months to 12 years), decreased hemoglobin, decreased platelet count, eosinophilia, increased hematocrit, neutropenia, thrombocythemia,

Hepatic: Decreased serum bilirubin, increased serum alkaline phosphatase, increased serum ALT, increased serum AST (more common in infants and children 3 months to 12 years), increased serum bilirubin

Local: Irritation at injection site

Renal: Increased serum creatinine

Rare but important or life-threatening: Acute renal failure, agranulocytosis, back pain (thoracic spinal), basophilia, bilirubinuria, bone marrow depression, brain disease, candidiasis, casts in urine, change in prothrombin time, *Clostridium difficile* associated diarrhea, confusion, cyanosis, decreased serum sodium, dental discoloration, drug fever, dyskinesia, erythema multiforme, hallucination, hearing loss, heartburn, hematuria, hemolytic anemia, hemorrhagic colitis, hepatic failure, hepatitis (including fulminant onset), hyperchloremia, hypersensitivity, hyperventilation, hypotension, increased blood urea nitrogen, increased lactate dehydrogenase, increased serum potassium, increased urinary urobilinogen, injection site infection, jaundice, leukocytosis, leukocyturia, leukopenia, lymphocytosis, myoclonus, neutropenia, pancytopenia, positive direct Coombs' test, pseudomembranous colitis, pseudomonas infection (resistant *P. aeruginosa*), psychiatric disturbances, Stevens-Johnson syndrome, thrombocytopenia, toxic epidermal necrolysis

Drug Interactions

Metabolism/Transport Effects None known.

Avoid Concomitant Use

Avoid concomitant use of Imipenem and Cilastatin with any of the following: BCG; Ganciclovir-Valganciclovir

Increased Effect/Toxicity

Imipenem and Cilastatin may increase the levels/effects of: CycloSPORINE (Systemic)

The levels/effects of Imipenem and Cilastatin may be increased by: CycloSPORINE (Systemic); Ganciclovir-Valganciclovir; Probenecid

Decreased Effect

Imipenem and Cilastatin may decrease the levels/effects of: BCG; CycloSPORINE (Systemic); Sodium Picosulfate; Typhoid Vaccine; Valproic Acid and Derivatives

Preparation for Administration IV: Prior to use, dilute dose into 100-250 mL of an appropriate solution. Imipenem is inactivated at acidic or alkaline pH. Final concentration should not exceed 5 mg/mL.

Storage/Stability Imipenem/cilastatin powder for injection should be stored at <25°C (77°F).

IV: Reconstituted IV solutions are stable for 4 hours at room temperature and 24 hours when refrigerated. Do not freeze.

Mechanism of Action Inhibits bacterial cell wall synthesis by binding to one or more of the penicillin-binding proteins (PBPs); which in turn inhibits the final transpeptidation step of peptidoglycan synthesis in bacterial cell walls, thus inhibiting cell wall biosynthesis. Bacteria eventually lyse due to ongoing activity of cell wall autolytic enzymes (autolysins and murein hydrolases) while cell wall assembly is arrested. Cilastatin prevents renal metabolism of imipenem by competitive inhibition of dehydropeptidase along the brush border of the renal tubules.

Pharmacodynamics/Kinetics

Distribution: Rapidly and widely to most tissues and fluids including sputum, pleural fluid, peritoneal fluid, interstitial fluid, bile, aqueous humor, and bone; highest concentrations in pleural fluid, interstitial fluid, and peritoneal fluid; low concentrations in CSF

Protein binding: Imipenem: 20%; cilastatin: 40%

Metabolism: Imipenem is metabolized in the kidney by dehydropeptidase I; cilastatin prevents imipenem metabolism by this enzyme; cilastatin is partially metabolized renally

Half-life elimination: IV: Both drugs: 60 minutes; prolonged with renal impairment

Excretion: Both drugs: Urine (~70% as unchanged drug)

Dosage

Usual dosage ranges: Note: Dosage based on **imipenem** content:

Children >3 months: Non-CNS infections: IV: 15-25 mg/kg every 6 hours; maximum dosage: Susceptible infections: 2 g/day; moderately-susceptible organisms: 4 g/day

Adults: IV: Weight ≥70 kg: 250-1000 mg every 6-8 hours; maximum: 4 g/day. **Note:** For adults weighing <70 kg, refer to Dosing adjustment in renal impairment

Indication-specific dosing: Note: Doses based on imipenem content.

Infants, Children, and Adolescents: IV:

Cystic fibrosis: Up to 100 mg/kg/day divided every 6 hours; maximum dose: 4 g daily has been used. **Note:** Efficacy in exacerbations may be limited due to rapid development of resistance (Zobell, 2013).

Children: IV:

Burkholderia pseudomallei (melioidosis) (off-label use): IV: Initial: 20 mg/kg every 8 hours for at least 10 days (White, 2003) **or** 25 mg/kg (up to 1 g) every 6 hours for at least 10 days (Currie, 2003); continue parenteral therapy until clinical improvement, then switch to oral therapy if tolerated and/or appropriate

Adults:

Burkholderia pseudomallei (melioidosis) (off-label use): Initial: 20 mg/kg every 8 hours for at least 10 days (White, 2003) **or** 25 mg/kg (up to 1 g) every 6 hours for at least 10 days (Currie, 2003); continue parenteral therapy until clinical improvement, then switch to oral therapy if tolerated and/or appropriate

Intra-abdominal infections: IV:

Mild infection: 250-500 mg every 6 hours

Severe infection: 500 mg every 6 hours **or** 1 g every 8 hours for 4-7 days (provided source controlled). **Note:** Not recommended for mild-to-moderate, community-acquired intra-abdominal infections due to risk of toxicity and the development of resistant organisms (Solomkin, 2010)

Liver abscess (off-label use): IV: 500 mg every 6 hours for 4-6 weeks (Ulug, 2010)

Mild infection: Note: Rarely a suitable option in mild infections; normally reserved for moderate-severe cases: IV:

Fully-susceptible organisms: 250 mg every 6 hours

Moderately-susceptible organisms: 500 mg every 6 hours

Moderate infection: IV:

Fully-susceptible organisms: 500 mg every 6-8 hours

Moderately-susceptible organisms: 500 mg every 6 hours or 1 g every 8 hours

Neutropenic fever (off-label use): IV: 500 mg every 6 hours (Paul, 2006)

***Pseudomonas* infections:** IV: 500 mg every 6 hours; **Note:** Higher doses may be required based on organism sensitivity.

Severe infection: IV:

Fully-susceptible organisms: 500 mg every 6 hours

Moderately-susceptible organisms: 1 g every 6-8 hours

Maximum daily dose should not exceed 50 mg/kg or 4 g/day, whichever is lower

Urinary tract infection: IV:

Uncomplicated: 250 mg every 6 hours

Complicated: 500 mg every 6 hours

Dosage adjustment in hepatic impairment: Hepatic dysfunction may further impair cilastatin clearance in patients receiving chronic renal replacement therapy; consider decreasing the dosing frequency.

Dosage adjustment in renal impairment: IV: **Note:**

Patients with a CrCl ≤5 mL/minute/1.73 m^2 should not receive imipenem/cilastatin unless hemodialysis is instituted within 48 hours.

Patients weighing <30 kg with impaired renal function should not receive imipenem/cilastatin.

Reduced IV dosage regimen based on creatinine clearance and/or body weight: See table.

Intermittent hemodialysis (IHD) (administer after hemodialysis on dialysis days): Use the dosing recommendation for patients with a CrCl 6-20 mL/minute; administer dose after dialysis session and every 12 hours thereafter **or** 250-500 mg every 12 hours (Heintz, 2009). **Note:** Dosing dependent on the assumption of 3 times/week, complete IHD sessions.

Peritoneal dialysis (off-label dosing): Dose as for CrCl 6-20 mL/minute (Somani, 1988)

Continuous renal replacement therapy (CRRT) (Heintz, 2009; Trotman, 2005): Drug clearance is highly dependent on the method of renal replacement, filter type, and flow rate. Appropriate dosing requires close monitoring of pharmacologic response, signs of adverse reactions due to drug accumulation, as well as drug concentrations in relation to target trough (if appropriate). The following are general recommendations only (based on dialysate flow/ultrafiltration rates of 1-2 L/hour and minimal residual renal function) and should not supersede clinical judgment:

CVVH: Loading dose of 1 g followed by either 250 mg every 6 hours **or** 500 mg every 8 hours

CVVHD: Loading dose of 1 g followed by either 250 mg every 6 hours **or** 500 mg every 6-8 hours

CVVHDF: Loading dose of 1 g followed by either 250 mg every 6 hours **or** 500 mg every 6 hours

Note: Data suggest that 500 mg every 8-12 hours may provide sufficient time above MIC to cover organisms with MIC values ≤2 mg/L; however, a higher dose of 500 mg every 6 hours is recommended for resistant organisms (particularly *Pseudomonas* spp) with MIC ≥4 mg/L or deep-seated infections (Fish, 2005).

Reduced IV dosage regimen based on creatinine clearance and/or body weight:

U.S. labeling: See table.

Imipenem and Cilastatin Dosage in Renal Impairment

Reduced IV Dosage Regimen Based on Creatinine Clearance (mL/minute/1.73 m^2) and/or Body Weight <70 kg					
	Body Weight (kg)				
	≥70	60	50	40	30
Total daily dose for normal renal function: 1 g/day					
CrCl ≥71	250 mg q6h	250 mg q8h	125 mg q6h	125 mg q6h	125 mg q8h
CrCl 41-70	250 mg q8h	125 mg q6h	125 mg q6h	125 mg q8h	125 mg q8h
CrCl 21-40	250 mg q12h	250 mg q12h	125 mg q8h	125 mg q12h	125 mg q12h
CrCl 6-20	250 mg q12h	125 mg q12h	125 mg q12h	125 mg q12h	125 mg q12h
Total daily dose for normal renal function: 1.5 g/day					
CrCl ≥71	500 mg q8h	250 mg q6h	250 mg q6h	250 mg q8h	125 mg q6h
CrCl 41-70	250 mg q6h	250 mg q8h	250 mg q8h	125 mg q6h	125 mg q8h
CrCl 21-40	250 mg q8h	250 mg q8h	250 mg q12h	125 mg q8h	125 mg q8h
CrCl 6-20	250 mg q12h	250 mg q12h	250 mg q12h	125 mg q12h	125 mg q12h

(continued)

Imipenem and Cilastatin Dosage in Renal Impairment *(continued)*

Reduced IV Dosage Regimen Based on Creatinine Clearance (mL/minute/1.73 m²) and/or Body Weight <70 kg					
	Body Weight (kg)				
	≥70	60	50	40	30
Total daily dose for normal renal function: 2 g/day					
CrCl ≥71	500 mg q6h	500 mg q8h	250 mg q6h	250 mg q6h	250 mg q8h
CrCl 41-70	500 mg q8h	250 mg q6h	250 mg q6h	250 mg q8h	125 mg q6h
CrCl 21-40	250 mg q6h	250 mg q8h	250 mg q8h	250 mg q12h	125 mg q8h
CrCl 6-20	250 mg q12h	250 mg q12h	250 mg q12h	250 mg q12h	125 mg q12h
Total daily dose for normal renal function: 3 g/day					
CrCl ≥71	1000 mg q8h	750 mg q8h	500 mg q6h	500 mg q8h	250 mg q6h
CrCl 41-70	500 mg q6h	500 mg q8h	500 mg q8h	250 mg q6h	250 mg q8h
CrCl 21-40	500 mg q8h	500 mg q8h	250 mg q6h	250 mg q8h	250 mg q8h
CrCl 6-20	500 mg q12h	500 mg q12h	250 mg q12h	250 mg q12h	250 mg q12h
Total daily dose for normal renal function: 4 g/day					
CrCl ≥71	1000 mg q6h	1000 mg q8h	750 mg q8h	500 mg q6h	500 mg q8h
CrCl 41-70	750 mg q8h	750 mg q8h	500 mg q6h	500 mg q8h	250 mg q6h
CrCl 21-40	500 mg q6h	500 mg q8h	500 mg q8h	250 mg q6h	250 mg q8h
CrCl 6-20	500 mg q12h	500 mg q12h	500 mg q12h	250 mg q12h	250 mg q12h

Canadian labeling: Reduced IV dosage regimen based on creatinine clearance (mL/minute/1.73 m^2) and body weight ≥70 kg (**Note:** The manufacturer labeling recommends further proportionate dose reductions for patients <70 kg, but does not provide specific dosing recommendations):

Mild renal impairment (CrCl 31-70 mL/minute/1.73 m^2):

Fully-susceptible organisms: Maximum dosage: 500 mg every 8 hours

Less susceptible organisms (primarily some *Pseudomonas* strains): Maximum dosage: 500 mg every 6 hours

Moderate renal impairment (CrCl 21-30 mL/minute/1.73 m^2):

Fully-susceptible organisms: Maximum dosage: 500 mg every 12 hours

Less susceptible organisms (primarily some *Pseudomonas* strains): Maximum dosage: 500 mg every 8 hours

Severe renal impairment (CrCl 0-20 mL/minute/1.73 m^2):

Fully-susceptible organisms: Maximum dosage: 250 mg every 12 hours

Less susceptible organisms (primarily some *Pseudomonas* strains): Maximum dosage: 500 mg every 12 hours

Note: Patients with CrCl 6-20 mL/minute/1.73 m^2 should receive 250 mg every 12 hours or 3.5 mg/kg (whichever is lower) every 12 hours for most pathogens; seizure risk may increase with higher dosing.

Dietary Considerations Some products may contain sodium.

Administration IV: Do not administer IV push. Infuse doses ≤500 mg over 20-30 minutes; infuse doses ≥750 mg over 40-60 minutes.

Monitoring Parameters Periodic renal, hepatic, and hematologic function tests; monitor for signs of anaphylaxis during first dose

Dosage Forms

Injection, powder for reconstitution: Imipenem 250 mg and cilastatin 250 mg; imipenem 500 mg and cilastatin 500 mg

Primaxin® I.V.: Imipenem 250 mg and cilastatin 250 mg; imipenem 500 mg and cilastatin 500 mg

◆ **Imipenem and Cilastatin for Injection (Can)** *see* Imipenem and Cilastatin *on page 1051*

Imipramine (im IP ra meen)

Brand Names: U.S. Tofranil; Tofranil-PM

Brand Names: Canada Impril; Novo-Pramine; PMS Imipramine

Index Terms Imipramine Hydrochloride; Imipramine Pamoate

Pharmacologic Category Antidepressant, Tricyclic (Tertiary Amine)

Additional Appendix Information

Beers Criteria - Potentially Inappropriate Medications for Geriatrics *on page 2271*

Use

Childhood enuresis: As temporary adjunctive therapy in reducing enuresis in children ≥6 years of age, after possible organic causes have been excluded by appropriate tests

Depression: Treatment of depression

Dosage

Children and Adolescents: Oral: **Note:** Manufacturer labeling warns against use of doses >2.5 mg/kg/**day** in pediatric patients; ECG changes (of unknown significance) have been reported in pediatric patients who received twice this amount.

Depression: Adolescents: Initial: 25-50 mg daily; increase gradually; maximum: 100 mg daily in single or divided doses. **Note:** Controlled clinical trials have not shown tricyclic antidepressants to be superior to placebo for the treatment of depression in children and adolescents; not recommended as first line medication; may be beneficial for patient with comorbid conditions (ADHD, enuresis) (Birmaher, 2007; Dopheide, 2006; Wagner, 2005).

Enuresis: Children ≥6 years and Adolescents: Imipramine **hydrochloride**: Initial: 25 mg 1 hour before bedtime, if inadequate response still seen after 1 week of therapy, increase by 25 mg daily; dose should not exceed 2.5 mg/kg/**day** or 50 mg at bedtime if 6-12 years of age or 75 mg at bedtime if ≥12 years

Attention-deficit/hyperactivity disorder (off-label use): Children ≥6 years and Adolescents: Initial: 1 mg/kg/day in 1-3 divided doses; titrate as needed; maximum daily dose: 4 mg/kg/**day** or 200 mg **daily**; for doses >2 mg/kg/day, monitor serum concentrations (target: ≤200 ng/mL) (Himpel, 2005; Pliszka, 2007).

Neuropathic pain (off-label use): Children: Initial: 0.2-0.4 mg/kg at bedtime; dose may be increased by 50% every 2-3 days up to 1-3 mg/kg/dose at bedtime (Berde, 1990)

Adults: Oral:

Depression:

Outpatients: Initial: 75 mg daily; may increase gradually to 150 mg daily. May be given in divided doses or as a single bedtime dose; Maintenance: 50-150 mg daily; maximum: 200 mg daily.

Inpatients: Initial: 100-150 mg daily; may increase gradually to 200 mg daily; if no response after 2 weeks, may further increase to 250-300 mg daily. May be given in divided doses or as a single bedtime dose; maximum: 300 mg daily.

Neuropathic pain (off-label use): **Note:** Not the preferred TCA (Bril, 2011; Dworkin, 2007). Initial: 50 mg once daily or in divided doses twice daily; increase gradually up to 150 mg daily (Kvinesdal, 1984; Sindrup, 2003) or to a dosage sufficient to achieve an imipramine plus desipramine plasma concentration of 113-170 ng/mL (SI: 400-600 nmol/L) (Sindrup, 1989; Sindrup, 1990)

Panic disorder (off-label use): Initial: 10 mg once daily; increase gradually to a usual dose of 75-300 mg daily (APA, 2009; Bandelow, 2008)

Post-traumatic stress disorder (PTSD) (off-label use): Initial: 50 mg once daily; increase gradually to 200-300 mg once daily to achieve blood levels in the therapeutic range (>150 ng/mL) (Frank, 1988; Kosten, 1991)

Elderly: Depression: Initial: 25-50 mg at bedtime; may increase every 3 days for inpatients and weekly for outpatients if tolerated to a recommended maximum of 100 mg daily.

MAO inhibitor recommendations:

Switching to or from an MAO inhibitor intended to treat psychiatric disorders:

Allow 14 days to elapse between discontinuing an MAO inhibitor intended to treat psychiatric disorders and initiation of imipramine.

Allow 14 days to elapse between discontinuing imipramine and initiation of an MAO inhibitor intended to treat psychiatric disorders.

Use with other MAO inhibitors (linezolid or IV methylene blue):

Do not initiate imipramine in patients receiving linezolid or IV methylene blue; consider other interventions for psychiatric condition.

If urgent treatment with linezolid or IV methylene blue is required in a patient already receiving imipramine and potential benefits outweigh potential risks, discontinue imipramine promptly and administer linezolid or IV methylene blue. Monitor for serotonin syndrome for 2 weeks or until 24 hours after the last dose of linezolid or IV methylene blue, whichever comes first. May resume imipramine 24 hours after the last dose of linezolid or IV methylene blue.

Dosage adjustment in renal impairment: No dosage adjustment provided in manufacturer's labeling; use with caution.

Dosage adjustment in hepatic impairment: No dosage adjustment provided in manufacturer's labeling; use with caution.

Additional Information Complete prescribing information should be consulted for additional detail.

Dosage Forms

Capsule, Oral:

Tofranil-PM: 75 mg, 100 mg, 125 mg, 150 mg

Generic: 75 mg, 100 mg, 125 mg, 150 mg

Tablet, Oral:

Tofranil: 10 mg, 25 mg, 50 mg

Generic: 10 mg, 25 mg, 50 mg

Dosage Forms: Canada Note: Refer also to Dosage Forms.

Tablet, Oral: 75 mg

◆ **Imipramine Hydrochloride** *see* Imipramine *on page 1054*

◆ **Imipramine Pamoate** *see* Imipramine *on page 1054*

Imiquimod (i mi KWI mod)

Brand Names: U.S. Aldara; Zyclara; Zyclara Pump

Brand Names: Canada Aldara P; Apo-Imiquimod; Vyloma; Zyclara

Pharmacologic Category Skin and Mucous Membrane Agent; Topical Skin Product

Use

Aldara®: Treatment of external genital and perianal warts/condyloma acuminata; nonhyperkeratotic, nonhypertrophic actinic keratosis on face or scalp; superficial basal cell carcinoma (sBCC) with a maximum tumor diameter of 2 cm located on the trunk (excluding anogenital skin), neck, or extremities (excluding hands or feet)

Vyloma™ (Canadian availability; not available in the U.S.): Treatment of external genital and perianal warts/condyloma acuminata

Zyclara®:

U.S. labeling: Treatment of external genital and perianal warts/condyloma acuminata (3.75% formulation); treatment of clinically typical visible or palpable, actinic keratoses on face or scalp (2.5% or 3.75% formulation)

Canadian labeling: Treatment of clinically typical visible or palpable, actinic keratoses on face or scalp

Pregnancy Risk Factor C

Dosage Topical: **Note:** Imiquimod treatment should not be prolonged beyond recommended period due to missed doses or rest periods.

U.S. labeling:

Actinic keratosis: Adults: **Note:** Prescribed course of therapy should be completed even if all lesions appear to be gone. Safety and efficacy of repeated use in a previously treated area has not been established.

Aldara®: Treatment should be limited to areas ≤25 cm^2; apply 2 times/week for 16 weeks to a treatment area on face or scalp (but not both concurrently); no more than 1 packet should be applied at each application and no more than 36 packets applied per 16 weeks; apply prior to bedtime and leave on skin for ~8 hours. Remove with mild soap and water.

Zyclara® 2.5%, 3.75%: Treatment consists of 2 cycles (14 days each) separated by 1 rest period (14 days) with no treatment. Apply up to 2 packets or 2 full actuations of pump once daily at bedtime to affected area on either face or balding scalp (but not both concurrently); leave on skin for ~8 hours. Remove with mild soap and water. Patient should not receive more than 56 packets or 2 x 7.5 g pumps or 1 x 15 g pump per 2 cycles of treatment.

External genital and/or perianal warts/condyloma acuminata: Children ≥12 years and Adults:

Aldara®: Apply a thin layer 3 times/week prior to bedtime and leave on skin for 6-10 hours. Remove with mild soap and water. Examples of 3 times/week application schedules are: Monday, Wednesday, Friday; or Tuesday, Thursday, Saturday. Continue treatment until there is total clearance of the warts or a maximum duration of therapy of 16 weeks.

Zyclara® 3.75%: Apply a thin layer using up to 1 packet or 1 full actuation of pump once daily prior to bedtime and leave on skin for ~8 hours. Remove with mild soap and water. Continue treatment until there is total clearance of the warts or a maximum duration of therapy of 8 weeks. Patient should not receive more than 56 packets or 2 x 7.5 g pumps or 1 x 15 g pump per course of treatment.

Superficial basal cell carcinoma: Adults: Aldara®: Apply once daily prior to bedtime, 5 days/week for 6 weeks. No more than 36 packets should be used during the 6-week treatment period. Tumor treatment area should not exceed 3 cm (maximum of 2 cm tumor diameter plus a 1 cm margin of skin around the tumor). The diameter of cream droplet applied should range from 4 mm to 7 mm for tumor areas of 0.5 cm to 2 cm, respectively. Leave on skin for ~8 hours. Remove with mild soap and water. Safety and efficacy of repeated use in a previously treated area have not been established.

Canadian labeling:

Actinic keratosis: Adults: **Note:** Prescribed course of therapy should be completed even if all lesions appear to be gone; safety and efficacy of repeated use in a previously treated area have not been established.

Aldara®: Treatment should be limited to areas ≤25 cm^2; apply 2 times/week for 16 weeks to a treatment area on face or scalp (but not both concurrently); no more than 1 packet should be applied at each application; apply prior to bedtime and leave on skin for ~8 hours. Remove with mild soap and water.

Zyclara®: Treatment should be limited to an area <200 cm^2 on the face or scalp and consists of 2 cycles (14 days each) separated by 1 rest period (14 days) with no treatment. Apply up to 2 packets or 2 full actuations of pump once daily at bedtime to affected area on either face or balding scalp (but not both concurrently). Leave on skin for ~8 hours. Remove with mild soap and water. Patient should not receive more than 56 packets or 2 x 7.5 g pumps or 1 x 15 g pump per 2 cycles of treatment.

External genital and/or perianal warts/condyloma acuminata: Adults:

Aldara®: Apply a thin layer 3 times/week prior to bedtime and leave on skin for 6-10 hours. Remove with mild soap and water. Examples of 3 times/week application schedules are: Monday, Wednesday, Friday; or Tuesday, Thursday, Saturday. Continue treatment until there is total clearance of the warts or a maximum duration of therapy of 16 weeks.

Vyloma™: Apply a thin layer once daily prior to bedtime and leave on skin for ~8 hours. Remove with mild soap and water. Continue treatment until there is total clearance of the warts or maximum duration of therapy of 8 weeks.

Superficial basal cell carcinoma: Adults: Aldara®: Apply once daily prior to bedtime, 5 days/week for 6 weeks. Tumor treatment area should not exceed 3 cm (maximum of 2 cm tumor diameter plus a 1 cm margin of skin around the tumor). The diameter of cream droplet applied should range from 4 mm to 7 mm for tumor areas of 0.5 cm to 2 cm, respectively. Leave on skin for ~8 hours. Remove with mild soap and water. Safety and efficacy of repeated use in a previously treated area have not been established.

Off-label uses: Common warts (5% cream): Apply once daily prior to bedtime for 5 days/week for up to 16 weeks (Hengge, 2000) or apply twice daily for up to 24 weeks (Grussendorf-Conen, 2002)

Dosing adjustment for toxicity:

Local skin reactions (eg, erythema, edema, scabbing, etc): Temporarily interrupt treatment for up to several days for severe or intolerable reactions; may consider resuming therapy once reaction subsides.

Systemic/flu-like reactions (eg, malaise, fever, rigors, etc): Consider temporary interruption of therapy.

Vulvar swelling: Interrupt or discontinue therapy for severe vulvar swelling.

Dosing adjustment in renal impairment: No dosage adjustment provided in manufacturer's labeling.

Dosing adjustment in hepatic impairment: No dosage adjustment provided in manufacturer's labeling.

Additional Information Complete prescribing information should be consulted for additional detail.

Dosage Forms

Cream, External:

Aldara: 5% (12 ea)
Zyclara: 3.75% (28 ea)
Zyclara Pump: 2.5% (7.5 g); 3.75% (7.5 g)
Generic: 5% (1 ea, 12 ea, 24 ea)

Dosage Forms: Canada

Cream, topical:

Vyloma™: 3.75% (28s)

- **Imitrex** *see* SUMAtriptan *on page 1953*
- **Imitrex DF (Can)** *see* SUMAtriptan *on page 1953*
- **Imitrex Injection (Can)** *see* SUMAtriptan *on page 1953*
- **Imitrex Nasal Spray (Can)** *see* SUMAtriptan *on page 1953*
- **Imitrex STATdose Refill** *see* SUMAtriptan *on page 1953*
- **Imitrex STATdose System** *see* SUMAtriptan *on page 1953*
- **ImmuCyst (Can)** *see* BCG *on page 229*

Immune Globulin (i MYUN GLOB yoo lin)

Brand Names: U.S. Bivigam; Carimune NF; Flebogamma; Flebogamma DIF; GamaSTAN S/D; Gammagard; Gammagard S/D; Gammagard S/D Less IgA; Gammaked; Gammaplex; Gamunex-C; Hizentra; Hizentra 20%; Hyqvia; Octagam; Privigen

Brand Names: Canada Gamastan S/D; Gammagard Liquid; Gammagard S/D; Gamunex; Hizentra; IGIVnex; Octagam 10%; Privigen

Index Terms Gamma Globulin; Human Normal Immunoglobulin; HyQvia; IG; IGIM; IGIV; IGSC; IMIG; Immune Globulin Subcutaneous (Human); Immune Serum Globulin; ISG; IV Immune Globulin; IVIG; Normal Immunoglobulin; Octagam 10%; Panglobulin; SCIG

Pharmacologic Category Blood Product Derivative; Immune Globulin

Additional Appendix Information

Immunization Recommendations *on page 2255*

Use

Treatment of primary humoral immunodeficiency syndromes (congenital agammaglobulinemia, severe combined immunodeficiency syndromes [SCIDS], common variable immunodeficiency, X-linked immunodeficiency, Wiskott-Aldrich syndrome) (Bivigam, Carimune NF, Flebogamma DIF, HyQvia, Gammagard Liquid, Gammagard S/D, Gammaked, Gammaplex, Gamunex-C, Hizentra, Octagam 5%, Privigen)

Treatment of acute and chronic immune thrombocytopenia (ITP) (Carimune NF, Gammagard S/D, Gammaked, Gammaplex [chronic only], Gamunex-C, Octagam 10% [chronic only], Privigen [chronic only])

Treatment of chronic inflammatory demyelinating polyneuropathy (CIDP) (Gammaked, Gamunex-C)

Treatment of multifocal motor neuropathy (MMN) (Gammagard Liquid)

Prevention of coronary artery aneurysms associated with Kawasaki syndrome (in combination with aspirin) (Gammagard S/D)

Prevention of bacterial infection in patients with hypogammaglobulinemia and/or recurrent bacterial infections with B-cell chronic lymphocytic leukemia (CLL) (Gammagard S/D)

Prevention of serious infection in immunoglobulin deficiency (select agammaglobulinemias) (GamaSTAN S/D)

Provision of passive immunity in the following susceptible individuals (GamaSTAN S/D):

Hepatitis A: Pre-exposure prophylaxis; postexposure: within 14 days and/or prior to manifestation of disease

Measles: For use within 6 days of exposure in an unvaccinated person, who has not previously had measles

Rubella: Postexposure prophylaxis to reduce the risk of infection and fetal damage in exposed pregnant women who will not consider therapeutic abortion

Varicella: For immunosuppressed patients when varicella zoster immune globulin is not available

Pregnancy Risk Factor C

Pregnancy Considerations Animal reproduction studies have not been conducted. Immune globulins cross the placenta in increased amounts after 30 weeks gestation. Intravenous immune globulin has been recommended for use in fetal-neonatal alloimmune thrombocytopenia and pregnancy-associated ITP (Anderson, 2007). Intravenous immune globulin is recommended to prevent measles in nonimmune women exposed during pregnancy (CDC, 2013). May also be used in postexposure prophylaxis for rubella to reduce the risk of infection and fetal damage in exposed pregnant women who will not consider therapeutic abortion (per GamaSTAN S/D product labeling; use for postexposure rubella prophylaxis is not currently recommended [CDC, 2013]).

HyQvia: Women who become pregnant during treatment are encouraged to enroll in the HyQvia Pregnancy Registry (1-866-424-6724).

Breast-Feeding Considerations It is not known if immune globulin from these preparations is excreted in breast milk. The manufacturer recommends that caution be exercised when administering immune globulin to nursing women. The manufacturer of HyQvia recommends administration to nursing women only if clearly indicated.

Contraindications Hypersensitivity to immune globulin or any component of the formulation; IgA deficiency (with anti-IgA antibodies and history of hypersensitivity); hyperprolinemia (Hizentra, Privigen); isolated IgA deficiency (GamaSTAN S/D); severe thrombocytopenia or coagulation disorders where IM injections are contraindicated (GamaSTAN S/D); hypersensitivity to corn (Octagam); hereditary intolerance to fructose; infants/neonates for whom sucrose or fructose tolerance has not been established (Gammaplex); hypersensitivity to hyaluronidase or recombinant human hyaluronidase (HyQvia)

Warnings/Precautions [U.S. Boxed Warning]: IV administration only: Acute renal dysfunction (increased serum creatinine, oliguria, acute renal failure, osmotic nephrosis) can rarely occur and has been associated with fatalities; usually within 7 days of use (more likely with products stabilized with sucrose). Use with caution in the elderly, patients with renal disease, diabetes mellitus, volume depletion, sepsis, paraproteinemia, and nephrotoxic medications due to risk of renal dysfunction. In patients at risk of renal dysfunction, ensure adequate hydration prior to administration; the rate of infusion and concentration of solution should be minimized. Discontinue if renal function deteriorates.

[U.S. Boxed Warning]: Thrombosis may occur with immune globulin products even in the absence of risk factors for thrombosis. For patients at risk of thrombosis (eg, advanced age, history of atherosclerosis, impaired cardiac output, prolonged immobilization, hypercoagulable conditions, history of venous or arterial thrombosis, use of estrogens, indwelling central vascular catheters, hyperviscosity, and cardiovascular risk factors), administer at the minimum dose and infusion rate practicable. Ensure adequate hydration before administration. Monitor for signs and symptoms of thrombosis and assess blood viscosity in patients at risk for hyperviscosity such as those with cryoglobulins, fasting chylomicronemia/severe hypertriglyceridemia, or monoclonal gammopathies.

High-dose regimens (1 g/kg for 1 to 2 days) are not recommended for individuals with fluid overload or where fluid volume may be of concern. Hypersensitivity and anaphylactic reactions can occur (some severe); patients with anti-IgA antibodies are at greater risk; a severe fall in blood pressure may rarely occur with anaphylactic reaction; immediate treatment (including epinephrine 1:1000) should be available. Product of human plasma; may potentially contain infectious agents which could transmit disease, including unknown or emerging viruses and other pathogens. Screening of donors, as well as testing and/or inactivation or removal of certain viruses, reduces the risk. Infections thought to be transmitted by this product should be reported to the manufacturer. Aseptic meningitis may occur with high doses (≥1 g/kg) and/or rapid infusion; syndrome usually appears within several hours to 2 days following treatment; usually resolves within several days after product is discontinued; patients with a migraine history may be at higher risk for AMS. Increased risk of hypersensitivity, especially in patients with anti-IgA antibodies; use is contraindicated in patients with IgA deficiency (with antibodies against IgA and history of hypersensitivity) or isolated IgA deficiency (GamaSTAN S/D). Increased risk of hematoma formation when administered subcutaneously for the treatment of ITP.

Intravenous immune globulin has been associated with antiglobulin hemolysis (acute or delayed); monitor for signs of hemolytic anemia. Cases of hemolysis-related renal dysfunction/failure or disseminated intravascular coagulation (DIC) have been reported. Risk factors include high doses (≥2 g/kg) and non-O blood type (FDA, 2012). In chronic ITP, assess risk versus benefit of high-dose regimen in patients with increased risk of thrombosis, hemolysis, acute kidney injury, or volume overload.

Patients should be adequately hydrated prior to initiation of therapy. Hyperproteinemia, increased serum viscosity and hyponatremia may occur; distinguish hyponatremia from pseudohyponatremia to prevent volume depletion, a further increase in serum viscosity, and a higher risk of thrombotic events. Patients should be monitored for adverse events during and after the infusion. Stop administration with signs of infusion reaction (fever, chills, nausea, vomiting, and rarely shock). Risk may be increased with initial treatment, when switching brands of immune globulin, and with treatment interruptions of >8 weeks. Monitor for transfusion-related acute lung injury (TRALI); noncardiogenic pulmonary edema has been reported with immune globulin use. TRALI is characterized by severe respiratory distress, pulmonary edema, hypoxemia, and fever (in the presence of normal left ventricular function) and usually occurs within 1-6 hours after infusion. Response to live vaccinations may be impaired. Some clinicians may administer intravenous immune globulin products as a subcutaneous infusion based on patient tolerability and clinical judgment. SubQ infusion should begin 1 week after the last IV dose; dose should be individualized based on clinical response and serum IgG trough concentrations; consider premedicating with acetaminophen and diphenhydramine.

Some products may contain maltose, which may result in falsely elevated blood glucose readings; maltose-containing products may be contraindicated in patients with an allergy to corn. Some products may contain polysorbate 80, sodium, and/or sucrose. Some products may contain sorbitol; do not use in patients with fructose intolerance. Hizentra and Privigen contain the stabilizer L-proline and are contraindicated in patients with hyperprolinemia. Packaging of some products may contain natural latex/natural rubber; skin testing should not be performed with GamaSTAN S/D as local irritation can occur and be misinterpreted as a positive reaction.

Adverse Reactions Adverse effects are reported as class effects rather than for specific products.

Cardiovascular: Chest tightness, edema, facial flushing, hypertension, hypotension, palpitations, tachycardia

Central nervous system: Anxiety, aseptic meningitis, chills, dizziness, drowsiness, fatigue, headache, lethargy, malaise, migraine, pain, rigors

Dermatologic: Dermatitis, diaphoresis, eczema, erythema, hyperhidrosis, pruritus, skin rash, urticaria

Endocrine & metabolic: Dehydration, increased lactate dehydrogenase

Gastrointestinal: Abdominal cramps, abdominal pain, diarrhea, dyspepsia, gastroenteritis, gastrointestinal distress, nausea, sore throat, toothache, vomiting

Genitourinary: Anuria, oliguria, osmotic nephrosis, proximal tubular nephropathy

Hematologic & oncologic: Anemia, bruise, decreased hematocrit, hematoma, hemolysis (mild), hemolytic anemia, hemorrhage, petechia, purpura, thrombocytopenia

Hepatic: Increased serum bilirubin

Hypersensitivity: Anaphylaxis, angioedema, hypersensitivity reaction

Local: Infusion site reaction (including erythema at injection site, irritation at injection site, itching at injection site, pain at injection site, swelling at injection site, warm sensation at injection site)

Neuromuscular & skeletal: Arthralgia, back pain, leg cramps, limb pain, muscle cramps, muscle spasm, myalgia, neck pain, weakness

Ophthalmic: Conjunctivitis

Otic: Otalgia

Renal: Acute renal failure, increased blood urea nitrogen, increased serum creatinine, renal tubular necrosis

Respiratory: Bronchitis, cough, dyspnea, epistaxis, exacerbation of asthma, flu-like symptoms, nasal congestion, oropharyngeal pain, pharyngitis, rhinitis, rhinorrhea, sinusitis, upper respiratory tract infection, wheezing

Miscellaneous: Fever, infusion related reaction

Rare but important or life-threatening): Antibody development (nonneutralizing antibodies to recombinant human hyaluronidase), blurred vision, bronchospasm, burning sensation, cardiac failure, cerebrovascular accident, chest pain, circulatory shock, coma, cyanosis, decreased serum alkaline phosphatase, disseminated intravascular coagulation, epidermolysis, erythema multiforme, exacerbation of autoimmune pure red cell aplasia, hepatic insufficiency, insomnia, pancytopenia, positive direct Coombs test, pulmonary edema, pulmonary embolism, renal insufficiency, respiratory distress, seizure, Stevens-Johnson syndrome, syncope, thromboembolism, transfusion-related acute lung injury, transient ischemic attack, tremor

Drug Interactions

Metabolism/Transport Effects None known.

Avoid Concomitant Use There are no known interactions where it is recommended to avoid concomitant use.

Increased Effect/Toxicity

The levels/effects of Immune Globulin may be increased by: Estrogen Derivatives

Decreased Effect

Immune Globulin may decrease the levels/effects of: Vaccines (Live)

Preparation for Administration Dilution is dependent upon the manufacturer and brand. Gently swirl; do not shake; avoid foaming. Do not heat. Do not mix products from different manufacturers together. Discard unused portion of vials.

Bivigam: Dilution is not recommended.

Carimune NF: In a sterile laminar air flow environment, reconstitute with NS, D_5W, or SWFI. Complete dissolution may take up to 20 minutes. Begin infusion within 24 hours.

Flebogamma DIF: Dilution is not recommended.

Gammagard Liquid: May dilute in D_5W only.

Gammagard S/D: Reconstitute with SWFI.

Gammaked: May dilute in D_5W only.

Gamunex-C: May dilute in D_5W only.

HyQvia: Bring refrigerated product to room temperature before use. Do **not** mix hyaluronidase and immune globulin prior to administration.

Octagam 10%: Do not dilute. Bottles may be pooled into sterile infusion bags and infused within 8 hours after pooling.

Privigen: If necessary to further dilute, D_5W may be used.

Storage/Stability Stability is dependent upon the manufacturer and brand. Do not freeze (do not use if previously frozen). Do not shake. Do not heat (do not use if previously heated).

Bivigam: Store under refrigeration at 2°C to 8°C (36°F to 46°F). Dilution is not recommended.

Carimune NF: Prior to reconstitution, store at or below 30°C (86°F). Reconstitute with NS, D_5W, or SWFI. Following reconstitution in a sterile laminar air flow environment, store under refrigeration. Begin infusion within 24 hours.

Flebogamma DIF: Store at 2°C to 25°C (36°F to 77°F).

GamaSTAN S/D: Store under refrigeration at 2°C to 8°C (36°F to 46°F). The following stability information has also been reported for GamaSTAN S/D: May be exposed to room temperature for a cumulative 7 days (Cohen, 2007).

Gammagard Liquid: Prior to use, store at 2°C to 8°C (36°F to 46°F). May store at room temperature of 25°C (77°F) within the first 24 months of manufacturing. Storage time at room temperature varies with length of time previously refrigerated; refer to product labeling for details.

Gammagard S/D: Store at ≤25°C (≤77°F). May store diluted solution under refrigeration at 2°C to 8°C (36°F to 46°F) for up to 24 hours if originally prepared in a sterile laminar air flow environment.

Gammaked: Store at 2°C to 8°C (36°F to 46°F); may be stored at ≤25°C (≤77°F) for up to 6 months.

Gammaplex: Store at 2°C to 25°C (36°F to 77°F). Protect from light.

Gamunex-C: Store at 2°C to 8°C (36°F to 46°F); may be stored at ≤25°C (≤77°F) for up to 6 months.

Hizentra: Store at ≤25°C (≤77°F). Keep in original carton to protect from light.

HyQvia: Store at 2°C to 8°C (36°F to 46°F) for up to 36 months; may store at ≤25°C (≤77°F) for up to 3 months during the first 24 months from the date of manufacture (after 3 months at room temperature, discard); do not return vial to refrigerator after it has been stored at room temperature.

Octagam 5%: Store at 2°C to 25°C (36°F to 77°F).

Octagam 10%: Store at 2°C to 8°C (36°F to 46°F) for 24 months from the date of manufacture; within these first 12 months, may store up to 6 months at ≤25°C (77°F); after storage at ≤25°C (77°F), the product must be used or discarded.

Privigen: Store at ≤25°C (≤77°F). Protect from light.

Mechanism of Action Replacement therapy for primary and secondary immunodeficiencies, and IgG antibodies against bacteria, viral, parasitic and mycoplasma antigens; interference with F_c receptors on the cells of the reticuloendothelial system for autoimmune cytopenias and ITP; provides passive immunity by increasing the antibody titer and antigen-antibody reaction potential

Pharmacodynamics/Kinetics

Onset of action: IV: Provides immediate antibody levels

Duration: IM, IV: Immune effect: 3 to 4 weeks (variable)

Distribution: V_d: 0.05 to 0.13 L/kg

Intravascular portion (primarily): Healthy subjects: 41% to 57%; Patients with congenital humoral immunodeficiencies: ~70%

Half-life elimination: IM: ~23 days; SubQ: ~59 days (HyQvia); IV: IgG (variable among patients): Healthy subjects: 14 to 24 days; Patients with congenital humoral immunodeficiencies: 26 to 40 days; hypermetabolism associated with fever and infection have coincided with a shortened half-life

Time to peak:

Plasma: SubQ: Gammagard Liquid: 2.9 days; Hizentra: 2.9 days; HyQvia: ~5 days.

Serum: IM: ~48 hours

Dosage Note: Some clinicians may administer IVIG formulations FDA approved only for intravenous administration as a subcutaneous infusion based on clinical judgment and patient tolerability.

Children and Adolescents:

Kawasaki syndrome: IV:

Gammagard S/D: 1,000 mg/kg as a single dose **or** 400 mg/kg/day for 4 consecutive days. Begin within 7 days of onset of fever.

AHA guidelines (2004): 2,000 mg/kg as a single dose within 10 days of disease onset

Note: Must be used in combination with aspirin: 80 to 100 mg/kg/day orally, divided every 6 hours for up to 14 days (until fever resolves for at least 48 hours); then decrease dose to 3 to 5 mg/kg/day once daily. In patients without coronary artery abnormalities, give lower dose for 6 to 8 weeks. In patients with coronary artery abnormalities, low-dose aspirin should be continued indefinitely.

Children, Adolescents, and Adults:

B-cell chronic lymphocytic leukemia (CLL) (Gammagard S/D): IV: 400 mg/kg every 3 to 4 weeks

Chronic inflammatory demyelinating polyneuropathy (CIDP) (Gammaked, Gamunex-C): IV: Loading dose: 2,000 mg/kg (given in divided doses over 2 to 4 consecutive days); Maintenance: 1,000 mg/kg every 3 weeks. Alternatively, administer 500 mg/kg/day for 2 consecutive days every 3 weeks.

Hepatitis A (GamaSTAN S/D): IM:

Preexposure prophylaxis upon travel into endemic areas (hepatitis A vaccine preferred):

0.02 **mL**/kg for anticipated risk of exposure <3 months

0.06 **mL**/kg for anticipated risk of exposure ≥3 months; repeat every 4 to 6 months.

Postexposure prophylaxis: 0.02 **mL**/kg given within 14 days of exposure and/or prior to manifestation of disease; not needed if at least 1 dose of hepatitis A vaccine was given at ≥1 month before exposure

Immunoglobulin deficiency (GamaSTAN S/D): IM: 0.66 **mL**/kg (minimum dose should be 100 mg/kg) every 3 to 4 weeks. Administer a double dose at onset of therapy; some patients may require more frequent injections.

Immune thrombocytopenia (ITP):

Carimune NF: IV: Initial: 400 mg/kg/day for 2 to 5 days; Maintenance: 400 mg/kg as needed to maintain platelet count ≥30,000/mm^3 and/or to control significant bleeding; may increase dose if needed (range: 800 to 1,000 mg/kg)

Gammagard S/D: IV: 1,000 mg/kg; up to 3 additional doses may be given based on patient response and/or platelet count. **Note:** Additional doses should be given on alternate days.

Gammaked, Gamunex-C: IV: 1,000 mg/kg/day for 2 consecutive days (second dose may be withheld if adequate platelet response in 24 hours) **or** 400 mg/kg once daily for 5 consecutive days

Privigen: IV: 1,000 mg/kg/day for 2 consecutive days

Measles:

GamaSTAN S/D: IM:

Immunocompetent: 0.25 **mL**/kg given within 6 days of exposure

Immunocompromised children: 0.5 **mL**/kg (maximum dose: 15 **mL**) immediately following exposure

Postexposure prophylaxis, any nonimmune person (off-label): 0.5 **mL**/kg (maximum dose: 15 **mL**) within 6 days of exposure (CDC, 2013)

Gammaked, Gamunex-C, Octagam 5%: IV:

Prophylaxis in patients with primary humoral immunodeficiency (**ONLY** if routine dose is <400 mg/kg): ≥400 mg/kg immediately before expected exposure

Treatment in patients with primary immunodeficiency: 400 mg/kg administered as soon as possible after exposure

Postexposure prophylaxis, any nonimmune person (off-label population): 400 mg/kg within 6 days of exposure (CDC, 2013)

Hizentra: SubQ infusion: Measles exposure in patients with primary humoral immunodeficiency: Weekly dose: ≥200 mg/kg for 2 consecutive weeks for patients at risk of measles exposure (eg, during an outbreak; travel to endemic area). Biweekly dose: ≥400 mg/kg single infusion. In patients who have been exposed to measles, administer the minimum dose as soon as possible following exposure.

ACIP recommendations: The Advisory Committee on Immunization Practices (ACIP) recommends postexposure prophylaxis with immune globulin (IG) to any nonimmune person exposed to measles. The following patient groups are at risk for severe measles complications and should receive IG therapy: Infants <12 months of age, pregnant women without evidence of immunity; severely compromised persons (eg, persons with severe primary immunodeficiency; some bone marrow transplant patients; some ALL patients; and some patients with AIDS or HIV infection [refer to guidelines for additional details]). IGIM is recommended for infants <12 months of age. IGIV is recommended for pregnant women and immunocompromised persons. Although prophylaxis may be given to any nonimmune person, priority should be given to those at greatest risk for measles complications and also to persons exposed in settings with intense, prolonged, close contact (eg, households, daycare centers, classrooms). Following IG administration, any nonimmune person should then receive the measles mumps and rubella (MMR) vaccine if the person is ≥12 months of age at the time of vaccine administration and the vaccine is not otherwise contraindicated. MMR should not be given until 6 months following IGIM or 8 months following IGIV administration. If a person is already receiving IGIV therapy, a dose of 400 mg/kg IV within 3 weeks prior to exposure (or 200 mg/kg SubQ for 2 consecutive weeks prior to exposure if previously on SubQ therapy) should be sufficient to prevent measles infection. IG therapy is not indicated for any person who already received one dose of a measles-containing vaccine at ≥12 months of age unless they are severely immunocompromised (CDC, 2013).

Primary humoral immunodeficiency disorders:

IV infusion dosing:

Bivigam: IV: 300 to 800 mg/kg every 3 to 4 weeks; dose adjusted based on monitored trough serum IgG concentrations and clinical response

Carimune NF: IV: 400 to 800 mg/kg every 3 to 4 weeks

Flebogamma DIF, Gammagard Liquid, Gammagard S/D, Gammaked, Gamunex-C, Octagam 5%: IV: 300 to 600 mg/kg every 3 to 4 weeks; dose adjusted based on monitored trough serum IgG concentrations and clinical response

Privigen: IV: 200 to 800 mg/kg every 3 to 4 weeks; dose adjusted based on monitored trough serum IgG concentrations and clinical response

Switching to weekly subcutaneous infusion dosing:

Gammagard Liquid, Gammaked, Gamunex-C: SubQ infusion: Begin 1 week after last IV dose. Use the following equation to calculate initial dose:

Initial weekly dose (g) = [1.37 x IGIV dose (g)] divided by [IV dose interval (weeks)]

Note: For subsequent dose adjustments, refer to product labeling.

Hizentra: SubQ infusion: For weekly dosing, begin 1 week after last IV infusion. For biweekly dosing, begin 1 or 2 weeks after last IV infusion or 1 week after the last Hizentra weekly infusion. **Note:** Patient should have received an IV immune globulin routinely for at least 3 months before switching to SubQ. Use the following equation to calculate initial weekly dose:

Initial weekly dose (g) = [Previous IGIV dose (g)] divided by [IV dose interval (eg, 3 or 4 weeks)] then multiply by 1.53. To convert the dose (in g) to mL, multiply the calculated dose (in g) by 5.

Initial biweekly dose (g) = multiply the calculated weekly dose by 2.

Note: For subsequent dose adjustments, refer to product labeling.

Rubella (GamaSTAN S/D): IM: Prophylaxis during pregnancy: 0.55 **mL**/kg

Varicella (GamaSTAN S/D): IM: Prophylaxis: 0.6 to 1.2 **mL**/kg (varicella zoster immune globulin preferred) within 72 hours of exposure

Adults:

Immune thrombocytopenia (ITP) (Gammaplex, Octagam 10%): IV: 1,000 mg/kg/day for 2 consecutive days

Multifocal motor neuropathy (MMN) (Gammagard liquid): IV: 500 to 2,400 mg/kg/month based upon response

Primary humoral immunodeficiency disorders:

IV infusion dosing (Gammaplex): IV: 300 to 800 mg/kg every 3 to 4 weeks; dose adjusted based on monitored trough serum IgG concentrations and clinical response

SubQ infusion dosing (HyQvia): SubQ: See manufacturer's labeling for initial ramp-up schedule (initiating treatment with a full monthly dose has not been evaluated); dose adjusted based on monitored trough serum IgG concentrations and clinical response after initial ramp-up. **Note:** For patients previously on another IgG treatment, administer the first dose ~1 week after the last infusion of previous treatment.

Patients naive to IgG therapy or switching from IG SubQ therapy: SubQ: 300 to 600 mg/kg every 3 to 4 weeks, after the initial dose ramp-up

Patients switching from IGIV therapy: SubQ: Administer the same dose and frequency as the previous IGIV therapy every 3 to 4 weeks, after the initial dose ramp-up.

Off-label uses: IV:

Acquired hypogammaglobulinemia secondary to malignancy (off-label use): Adults: 400 mg/kg/dose every 3 weeks; reevaluate every 4 to 6 months (Anderson, 2007)

Guillain-Barré syndrome (off-label use): Children and Adults: Various regimens have been used, including:

400 mg/kg/day for 5 days (Hughes, 2003)

or

400 mg/kg/day for 6 days (Patwa, 2012)

or

2,000 mg/kg in divided doses administered over 2 to 5 days (Feasby, 2007)

Hematopoietic stem cell transplantation with hypogammaglobulinemia (CDC guidelines, 2000; off-label use):

Children: 400 mg/kg per month; increase dose or frequency to maintain IgG levels >400 mg/dL

Adolescents and Adults: 500 mg/kg/week

HIV-associated thrombocytopenia (off-label use): Adults: 1,000 mg/kg/day for 2 days (Anderson, 2007)

Lambert-Eaton myasthenic syndrome (LEMS) (off-label use): Adults: 1,000 mg/kg/day for 2 days (Bain, 1996; Patwa, 2012)

Multiple sclerosis (relapsing-remitting, when other therapies cannot be used) (off-label use): Children and Adults: 1,000 mg/kg per month, with or without an induction of 400 mg/kg/day for 5 days (Feasby, 2007)

Myasthenia gravis (severe exacerbation) (off-label use): Children and Adults: 2,000 mg/kg per treatment course administered in divided doses over 2 to 5 consecutive days (eg, 400 mg/kg/day for 5 days) (Feasby, 2007; Patwa, 2012). Although, in one study in adults, a single dose of 1,000 mg/kg had similar efficacy to 1,000 mg/kg given on 2 consecutive days (Gajdos, 2005).

Refractory dermatomyositis/polymyositis (off-label uses): Children and Adults: 2,000 mg/kg per treatment course administered in divided doses over 2 to 5 consecutive days (eg, 400 mg/kg/day for 5 days) (Feasby, 2007)

Dosage adjustment in renal impairment:

IV: Use with caution due to risk of immune globulin-induced renal dysfunction; the rate of infusion and concentration of solution should be minimized.

IM, SubQ infusion: There are no dosage adjustments provided in the manufacturer's labeling; risk of immune globulin-induced renal dysfunction has not been identified with IM and SubQ infusion administration.

Dosage adjustment in hepatic impairment: IM, IV, SubQ infusion: There are no dosage adjustments provided in the manufacturer's labeling.

Dosing in obesity: Some clinicians dose IVIG on ideal body weight or an adjusted ideal body weight in morbidly-obese patients (Siegel, 2010).

Dietary Considerations Some products may contain sodium.

Administration Note: If plasmapheresis employed for treatment of condition, administer immune globulin **after** completion of plasmapheresis session.

IM: Administer IM in the anterolateral aspects of the upper thigh or deltoid muscle of the upper arm. Avoid gluteal region due to risk of injury to sciatic nerve. Divide doses >10 mL and inject in multiple sites.

GamaSTAN S/D is for IM administration only.

IV infusion: Infuse over 2 to 24 hours; administer in separate infusion line from other medications; if using primary line, flush with NS or D_5W (product specific; consult product prescribing information) prior to administration. Decrease dose, rate and/or concentration of infusion in patients who may be at risk of renal failure. Decreasing the rate or stopping the infusion may help relieve some adverse effects (flushing, changes in pulse rate, changes in blood pressure). Epinephrine should be available during administration. For initial treatment or in the elderly, a lower concentration and/or a slower rate of infusion should be used. Initial rate of administration and titration is specific to each IVIG product. Refrigerated product should be warmed to room temperature prior to infusion. Some products require filtration; refer to individual product labeling. Antecubital veins should be used, especially with concentrations ≥10% to prevent injection site discomfort.

Bivigam 10%: Primary humoral immunodeficiency: Initial (first 10 minutes): 0.5 mg/kg/minute (0.3 **mL**/kg/**hour**); Maintenance: Increase every 20 minutes (if tolerated) by 0.8 mg/kg/minute (0.48 **mL**/kg/**hour)** up to 6 mg/kg/minute (3.6 **mL**/kg/**hour**)

Carimune NF: Refer to product labeling.

Flebogamma DIF 10%: Primary humoral immunodeficiency: Initial: 1 mg/kg/minute (0.6 **mL**/kg/**hour**); Maintenance: Increase slowly (if tolerated) up to 8 mg/kg/minute (4.8 **mL**/kg/**hour**)

Gammagard Liquid 10%:

Multifocal motor neuropathy (MMN): Initial: 0.8 mg/kg/minute (0.5 **mL**/kg/**hour**); Maintenance: Increase gradually (if tolerated) up to 9 mg/kg/minute (5.4 **mL**/kg/**hour**)

Primary humoral immunodeficiency: Initial (first 30 minutes): 0.8 mg/kg/minute (0.5 **mL/kg/hour**); Maintenance: Increase every 30 minutes (if tolerated) up to: 8 mg/kg/minute (5 **mL/kg/hour**)

Gammagard S/D: 5% solution: Initial: 0.5 **mL/kg/hour**; may increase (if tolerated) to a maximum rate of 4 **mL/kg/hour**. If 5% solution is tolerated at maximum rate, may administer 10% solution with an initial rate of 0.5 **mL/kg/hour**; may increase (if tolerated) to a maximum rate of 8 **mL/kg/hour**

Gammaked 10%:

CIDP: Initial (first 30 minutes): 2 mg/kg/minute (1.2 **mL/kg/hour**); Maintenance: Increase gradually (if tolerated) up to 8 mg/kg/minute (4.8 **mL/kg/hour**)

Primary humoral immunodeficiency or ITP: Initial (first 30 minutes): 1 mg/kg/minute (0.6 **mL/kg/hour**); Maintenance: Increase gradually (if tolerated) up to 8 mg/kg/minute (4.8 **mL/kg/hour**)

Gammaplex 5%: Primary humoral immunodeficiency or ITP: Initial (first 15 minutes): 0.5 mg/kg/minute (0.6 **mL/kg/hour**); Maintenance: Increase every 15 minutes (if tolerated) up to 4 mg/kg/minute (4.8 **mL/kg/hour**)

Gamunex-C 10%:

CIDP: Initial (first 30 minutes): 2 mg/kg/minute (1.2 **mL/kg/hour**); Maintenance: Increase gradually (if tolerated) up to 8 mg/kg/minute (4.8 **mL/kg/hour**)

Primary humoral immunodeficiency or ITP: Initial (first 30 minutes): 1 mg/kg/minute (0.6 **mL/kg/hour**); Maintenance: Increase gradually (if tolerated) up to 8 mg/kg/minute (4.8 **mL/kg/hour**)

Octagam 5%: Primary humoral immunodeficiency: Initial (first 30 minutes): 0.5 mg/kg/minute (0.6 **mL/kg/hour**); Maintenance: Double infusion rate (if tolerated) every 30 minutes up to a maximum rate of <3.33 mg/kg/minute (4.2 **mL/kg/hour**)

Octagam 10%: ITP: Initial (first 30 minutes):1 mg/kg/minute (0.6 **mL/kg/hour**); Maintenance: Increase every 30 minutes (if tolerated) up to a maximum rate of 12 mg/kg/minute (7.2 **mL/kg/hour**)

Privigen 10%

ITP: Initial: 0.5 mg/kg/minute (0.3 **mL/kg/hour**); Maintenance: Increase gradually (if tolerated) up to 4 mg/kg/minute (2.4 **mL/kg/hour**)

Primary humoral immunodeficiency: Initial: 0.5 mg/kg/minute (0.3 **mL/kg/hour**); Maintenance: Increase gradually (if tolerated) up to 8 mg/kg/minute (4.8 **mL/kg/hour**)

SubQ infusion: Initial dose should be administered in a healthcare setting capable of providing monitoring and treatment in the event of hypersensitivity. Using aseptic technique, follow the infusion device manufacturer's instructions for filling the reservoir and preparing the pump. Remove air from administration set and needle by priming. For products excluding HyQvia, appropriate injection sites include the abdomen, thigh, upper arm, lower back, and/or lateral hip; dose may be infused into multiple sites (spaced ≥2 inches apart) simultaneously. HyQvia may be injected into the middle to upper abdomen or thigh (avoid bony prominences, or areas that are scarred, inflamed, or infected). If two sites are used simultaneously for HyQvia, the two infusion sites should be on opposite sides of the body. After the sites are clean and dry, insert subcutaneous needle and prime administration set. Attach sterile needle to administration set, gently pull back on the syringe to assure a blood vessel has not been inadvertently accessed (do not use needle and tubing if blood present). Repeat for each injection site; deliver the dose following instructions for the infusion device. Rotate the site(s) between successive infusions. Treatment may be transitioned to the home/home care setting in the absence of adverse reactions.

Gammagard Liquid:

Injection sites: ≤8 simultaneous injection sites

Initial infusion rate:

<40 kg: 15 mL/hour per injection site (maximum volume: 20 mL per injection site)

≥40 kg: 20 mL/hour per injection site (maximum volume: 30 mL per injection site)

Maintenance infusion rate:

<40 kg: 15 to 20 mL/hour per injection site (maximum volume: 20 mL per injection site)

≥40 kg: 20 to 30 mL/hour per injection site (maximum volume: 30 mL per injection site)

Gammaked, Gamunex-C:

Injection sites: ≤8 simultaneous injection sites

Recommended infusion rate: 20 mL/hour per injection site

Hizentra:

Injection sites:

Weekly dosing: ≤4 simultaneous injection sites or ≤12 sites consecutively per infusion

Biweekly dosing: Increase the number of injection sites as needed.

Maximum infusion rate: First infusion: 15 mL/hour per injection site; subsequent infusions: 25 mL/hour per injection site

Maximum infusion volume: First 4 infusions: 15 mL per injection site; subsequent infusions: 20 mL per injection site (maximum: 25 mL per site as tolerated)

HyQvia: Administer components of HyQvia (immune globulin and hyaluronidase) sequentially; do not use either component alone. Infusion pump capable of infusing rates up to 300 mL/hour/site required; must also have the ability to titrate the flow rate. Use a 24 gauge subcutaneous needle set labeled for high flow rates. Infuse the two components of HyQvia sequentially, beginning with the hyaluronidase. Initiate the infusion of the full dose of the immune globulin through the same subcutaneous needle set within ~10 minutes of hyaluronidase infusion. For each full or partial vial of immune globulin used, administer the entire contents of the hyaluronidase vial. A second site can be used based on tolerability and total volume; if a second site is used, administer half of total volume of the hyaluronidase in each site. Flush the infusion line with NS or D_5W if required.

Injection sites:

Volume per site:

<40 kg: ≤300 mL per injection site

≥40 kg: ≤600 mL per injection site

Infusion rate:

Recombinant human hyaluronidase: ~1 to 2 mL/minute, or as tolerated.

Immune globulin:

First 2 infusions:

<40 kg: 5 mL/hour for 5 to 15 minutes; 10 mL/hour for 5 to 15 minutes; 20 mL/hour for 5 to 15 minutes; 40 mL/hour for 5 to 15 minutes; then 80 mL/hour for remainder of infusion

≥40 kg: 10 mL/hour for 5 to 15 minutes; 30 mL/hour for 5 to 15 minutes; 60 mL/hour for 5 to 15 minutes; 120 mL/hour for 5 to 15 minutes; then 240 mL/hour for remainder of infusion

Next 2 or 3 infusions:

<40 kg: 10 mL/hour for 5 to 15 minutes; 20 mL/hour for 5 to 15 minutes; 40 mL/hour for 5 to 15 minutes; 80 mL/hour for 5 to 15 minutes; then 160 mL/hour for remainder of infusion

≥40 kg: 10 mL/hour for 5 to 15 minutes; 30 mL/hour for 5 to 15 minutes; 120 mL/hour for 5 to 15 minutes; 240 mL/hour for 5 to 15 minutes; then 300 mL/hour for remainder of infusion

Monitoring Parameters Renal function, urine output, IgG concentrations, hemoglobin and hematocrit, platelets (in patients with ITP); infusion- or injection-related adverse reactions, anaphylaxis, signs and symptoms of hemolysis; blood viscosity (in patients at risk for hyperviscosity); presence of antineutrophil antibodies (if TRALI is suspected); volume status; neurologic symptoms (if AMS suspected); pulmonary adverse reactions; clinical response

For patients at high risk of hemolysis (dose ≥2 g/kg, given as a single dose or divided over several days, and non-O blood type): Hemoglobin or hematocrit prior to and 36 to 96 hours postinfusion.

SubQ infusion: Monitor IgG trough levels every 2-3 months before/after conversion from IV; subcutaneous infusions provide more constant IgG levels than usual IV immune globulin treatments.

Additional Information IM: When administering immune globulin for hepatitis A prophylaxis, use should be considered for the following close contacts of persons with confirmed hepatitis A: unvaccinated household and sexual contacts, persons who have shared illicit drugs, regular babysitters, staff and attendees of child care centers, food handlers within the same establishment (CDC, 2006).

For travelers, immune globulin is not an alternative to careful selection of foods and water; immune globulin can interfere with the antibody response to parenterally administered live virus vaccines. Frequent travelers should be tested for hepatitis A antibody, immune hemolytic anemia, and neutropenia (with ITP, IV route is usually used).

IgA content:

Bivigam: ≤200 mcg/mL
Carimune NF: 1000-2000 mcg/mL
Flebogamma 5% DIF: <50 mcg/mL
Flebogamma 10% DIF: <100 mcg/mL
Gammagard Liquid: 37 mcg/mL
Gammagard S/D 5% solution: <1 mcg/mL or <2.2 mcg/mL (product dependent) (see **Note**)
Gammaked: 46 mcg/mL
Gammaplex: <10 mcg/mL
Gamunex-C: 46 mcg/mL
Hizentra: ≤50 mcg/mL
Octagam 5%: ≤200 mcg/mL
Octagam 10%: 106 mcg/mL
Privigen: ≤25 mcg/mL

Note: Manufacturer has discontinued Gammagard S/D 5% solution; however, the lower IgA product will remain available by special request for patients with known reaction to IgA or IgA deficiency with antibodies.

Dosage Forms Considerations

Carimune NF may contain a significant amount of sodium and also contains sucrose.

Gammagard S/D may contain a significant amount of sodium and also contains glucose.

Hyqvia Kit is supplied with a Hyaluronidase (Human Recombinant) component intended for injection prior to Immune Globulin administration to improve dispersion and absorption of the Immune Globulin.

Dosage Forms

Injectable, Intramuscular [preservative free]:
GamaSTAN S/D: 15% to 18% [150 to 180 mg/mL] (2 mL, 10 mL)

Kit, Subcutaneous:
Hyqvia: 2.5 g/25 mL, 5 g/50 mL, 20 g/200 mL, 30 g/300 mL

Solution, Injection:
Gamunex-C: 1 g/10 mL (10 mL); 2.5 g/25 mL (25 mL); 5 g/50 mL (50 mL); 10 g/100 mL (100 mL); 20 g/200 mL (200 mL); 40 g/400 mL (400 mL)

Solution, Injection [preservative free]:
Gammagard: 1 g/10 mL (10 mL); 2.5 g/25 mL (25 mL); 5 g/50 mL (50 mL); 10 g/100 mL (100 mL); 20 g/200 mL (200 mL); 30 g/300 mL (300 mL)
Gammaked: 1 g/10 mL (10 mL); 2.5 g/25 mL (25 mL); 5 g/50 mL (50 mL); 10 g/100 mL (100 mL); 20 g/200 mL (200 mL)

Solution, Intravenous:
Flebogamma: 0.5 g/10 mL (10 mL)
Octagam: 1 g/20 mL (20 mL); 2.5 g/50 mL (50 mL); 5 g/100 mL (100 mL); 10 g/200 mL (200 mL); 25 g/500 mL (500 mL)

Solution, Intravenous [preservative free]:
Bivigam: 5 g/50 mL (50 mL); 10 g/100 mL (100 mL)
Flebogamma DIF: 0.5 g/10 mL (10 mL); 2.5 g/50 mL (50 mL); 5 g/50 mL (50 mL); 5 g/100 mL (100 mL); 10 g/100 mL (100 mL); 10 g/200 mL (200 mL); 20 g/200 mL (200 mL); 20 g/400 mL (400 mL)
Gammaplex: 2.5 g/50 mL (50 mL); 5 g/100 mL (100 mL); 10 g/200 mL (200 mL); 20 g/400 mL (400 mL)
Octagam: 2 g/20 mL (20 mL); 5 g/50 mL (50 mL); 10 g/100 mL (100 mL); 20 g/200 mL (200 mL)
Privigen: 5 g/50 mL (50 mL); 10 g/100 mL (100 mL); 20 g/200 mL (200 mL); 40 g/400 mL (400 mL)

Solution, Subcutaneous [preservative free]:
Hizentra: 10 g/50 mL (50 mL)
Hizentra 20%: 1 g/5 mL (5 mL); 2 g/10 mL (10 mL); 4 g/20 mL (20 mL)

Solution Reconstituted, Intravenous:
Carimune NF: 6 g (1 ea); 12 g (1 ea)
Gammagard S/D: 2.5 g (1 ea); 5 g (1 ea); 10 g (1 ea)

Solution Reconstituted, Intravenous [preservative free]:
Gammagard S/D Less IgA: 5 g (1 ea); 10 g (1 ea)

- ◆ **Immune Globulin Subcutaneous (Human)** *see* Immune Globulin *on page 1056*
- ◆ **Immune Serum Globulin** *see* Immune Globulin *on page 1056*
- ◆ **Immunine VH (Can)** *see* Factor IX (Human) *on page 840*
- ◆ **Imodium® (Can)** *see* Loperamide *on page 1236*
- ◆ **Imodium A-D [OTC]** *see* Loperamide *on page 1236*
- ◆ **Imodium® Advanced Multi-Symptom (Can)** *see* Loperamide and Simethicone *on page 1237*
- ◆ **Imodium® Multi-Symptom Relief [OTC]** *see* Loperamide and Simethicone *on page 1237*
- ◆ **Imogam Rabies-HT** *see* Rabies Immune Globulin (Human) *on page 1764*
- ◆ **Imogam Rabies Pasteurized (Can)** *see* Rabies Immune Globulin (Human) *on page 1764*
- ◆ **Imovane (Can)** *see* Zopiclone [CAN/INT] *on page 2217*
- ◆ **Imovax Polio (Can)** *see* Poliovirus Vaccine (Inactivated) *on page 1673*
- ◆ **Imovax Rabies** *see* Rabies Vaccine *on page 1764*
- ◆ **Impril (Can)** *see* Imipramine *on page 1054*
- ◆ **Imuran** *see* AzaTHIOprine *on page 210*
- ◆ **Inactivated Influenza Vaccine, Quadrivalent** *see* Influenza Virus Vaccine (Inactivated) *on page 1075*
- ◆ **Inactivated Influenza Vaccine, Trivalent** *see* Influenza Virus Vaccine (Inactivated) *on page 1075*
- ◆ **INCB424** *see* Ruxolitinib *on page 1856*
- ◆ **INCB 18424** *see* Ruxolitinib *on page 1856*
- ◆ **Incivek [DSC]** *see* Telaprevir *on page 1983*
- ◆ **Incivek™ (Can)** *see* Telaprevir *on page 1983*

IncobotulinumtoxinA

(in kuh BOT yoo lin num TOKS in aye)

Brand Names: U.S. Xeomin

Brand Names: Canada Xeomin Cosmetic™; Xeomin®
Index Terms Botulinum Toxin Type A
Pharmacologic Category Neuromuscular Blocker Agent, Toxin; Ophthalmic Agent, Toxin
Use
U.S. labeling: Treatment of blepharospasm in patients previously treated with onabotulinumtoxinA (Botox®); treatment of cervical dystonia in botulinum toxin-naïve and previously treated patients; temporary improvement in the appearance of moderate-to-severe glabellar lines associated with corrugator and/or procerus muscle activity

Canadian labeling:
Xeomin®: Treatment of hypertonicity disorders of the seventh nerve (eg, blepharospasm, hemifacial spasm); treatment of poststroke spasticity of upper limb(s); treatment of cervical dystonia (spasmodic torticollis)
Xeomin Cosmetic™: Temporary improvement in the appearance of moderate-to-severe glabellar lines
Pregnancy Risk Factor C
Dosage IM: Adults:
Blepharospasm:
U.S. labeling: Initial: Total dose should be the same as previously administered onabotulinumtoxinA dose. If prior onabotulinumtoxinA dose is not known: 1.25-2.5 units/injection site (maximum initial dose: 35 units/eye or 70 units/both eyes). Number and location of injection sites based on disease severity and previous dose/response to onabotulinumtoxinA (in clinical trials, a mean number of 6 injections per eye were administered). Cumulative dose should not exceed 35 units/eye or 70 units/both eyes administered no more frequently than every 3 months.
Canadian labeling: Initial: 1.25-2.5 units/injection site (maximum initial dose: 25 units/eye). Dose may be increased up to twice the previous dose if the response from the initial dose lasted ≤2 months; maximum dose per site: 5 units. Cumulative dose should not exceed 35 units/eye or 70 units/both eyes administered no more frequently than every 3 months.
Cervical dystonia:
U.S. labeling: Initial total dose: 120 units (in clinical trials, similar efficacy was noted with initial total doses of 120 and 240 units and between treatment experienced and treatment naïve patients). Dose and number of injection sites should be individualized based on prior treatment, response, duration of effect, adverse events, number/location of muscle(s) to be treated and disease severity. In clinical trials most patients received a total of 2-10 injections into treated muscles. Administer no more frequently than every 3 months
Canadian labeling: Usual total dose: 200 units (maximum: 300 units; maximum dose per injection site: 50 units); administer no more frequently than every 3 months
Reduction of glabellar lines: Inject 4 units into each of the 5 sites (2 injections in each corrugator muscle and 1 injection in the procerus muscle) for a total dose of 20 units per treatment session. Administer no more frequently than every 3 months.
Spasticity of upper limb (poststroke): Canadian labeling (not in U.S. labeling): Individualize dose based on patient size, extent, and location of muscle involvement, degree of spasticity, local muscle weakness, and response to prior treatment. In clinical trials, total doses up to 400 units were administered as separate injections typically divided among selected muscles; may repeat therapy at ≥3 months with appropriate dosage based upon the clinical condition of patient at time of retreatment.
Suggested guidelines for the treatment of stroke-related upper limb spasticity: Note: The lowest recommended starting dose should be used. Dosage and number of injection sites should be individualized. Multiple injections may minimize adverse effects. Dose listed is total dose administered to site:
Biceps: 80 units
Brachialis: 50 units
Brachioradialis: 60 units
Flexor carpi radialis: 50 units
Flexor carpi ulnaris: 40 units
Flexor digitorum profundus: 40 units
Flexor digitorum superficialis: 40 units
Adductor pollicis: 10 units
Flexor pollicis brevis: 10 units
Flexor pollicis longus: 20 units
Pronator quadratus 25 units
Pronator teres: 40 units

Elderly: Initiate therapy at lowest recommended dose and titrate upward cautiously.

Dosage adjustment in renal impairment: There are no dosage adjustments provided in manufacturer's labeling.
Dosage adjustment in hepatic impairment: There are no dosage adjustments provided in manufacturer's labeling.
Additional Information Complete prescribing information should be consulted for additional detail.
Dosage Forms
Solution Reconstituted, Intramuscular [preservative free]:
Xeomin: 50 units (1 ea); 100 units (1 ea)
Dosage Forms: Canada
Injection, powder for reconstitution:
Xeomin Cosmetic™: 100 units

◆ **Incruse Ellipta** *see* Umeclidinium *on page 2113*

Indacaterol (in da KA ter ol)

Brand Names: U.S. Arcapta Neohaler
Brand Names: Canada Onbrez® Breezhaler®
Index Terms Indacaterol Maleate; QAB149
Pharmacologic Category $Beta_2$ Agonist; $Beta_2$-Adrenergic Agonist, Long-Acting
Use Long-term maintenance treatment of airflow obstruction in chronic obstructive pulmonary disease (COPD) including chronic bronchitis and/or emphysema
Pregnancy Risk Factor C
Dosage Inhalation: Adults: COPD (maintenance): 75 mcg once daily (maximum: 75 mcg once daily). **Note:** A dose of 75 to 300 mcg once daily is recommended by the 2013 Updated GOLD Guidelines.

Dosage adjustment in renal impairment: No dosage adjustment necessary.
Dosage adjustment in hepatic impairment:
Mild-to-moderate impairment: No dosage adjustment necessary.
Severe impairment: There are no dosage adjustments provided in manufacturer's labeling.
Additional Information Complete prescribing information should be consulted for additional detail.
Dosage Forms
Capsule, Inhalation:
Arcapta Neohaler: 75 mcg

Indacaterol and Glycopyrronium [CAN/INT] (in da KA ter ol & glye koe PYE roe nee um)

Brand Names: Canada Ultibro Breezhaler

Index Terms Glycopyrronium and Indacaterol; Glycopyrronium Bromide and Indacaterol Maleate; Indacaterol Maleate and Glycopyrronium Bromide; QVA149

Pharmacologic Category Anticholinergic Agent; $Beta_2$ Agonist; $Beta_2$-Adrenergic Agonist, Long-Acting

Use Note: Not approved in U.S.

Chronic obstructive pulmonary disease: Long-term maintenance treatment of airflow obstruction in chronic obstructive pulmonary disease (COPD) including chronic bronchitis and/or emphysema

Pregnancy Considerations Refer to individual monographs.

Breast-Feeding Considerations It is not known if indacaterol or glycopyrronium are excreted into breast milk. The manufacturer recommends use only if the potential benefits to the mother are expected to be greater than the possible risks to the fetus. Also refer to individual monographs.

Contraindications Hypersensitivity to indacaterol maleate, or glycopyrronium bromide, or any component of the formulation; severe hypersensitivity to milk proteins; monotherapy in patients with asthma (ie, without concurrent use of a long-term asthma control medication such as an inhaled corticosteroid). **Note:** Combination product is not approved for treatment of asthma.

Warnings/Precautions [Canadian Boxed Warning]: COPD/Asthma: Ultibro Breezhaler is only indicated for COPD. It is not indicated for treatment of asthma. Do not use for acute bronchospastic episodes of COPD; always prescribe with an inhaled short-acting $beta_2$-agonist and educate patient on appropriate use. Upon initiation of the combination inhaler, use of short-acting $beta_2$-agonists should be limited to treat acute symptoms. Do not initiate in patients with significantly worsening or acutely deteriorating COPD. Do not increase the dose or frequency beyond what is recommended.

[Canadian Boxed Warning]: Long-acting $beta_2$-agonists (LABAs) increase the risk of asthma-related deaths. In a large, randomized, placebo-controlled U.S. clinical trial (SMART, 2006), salmeterol was associated with an increase in asthma-related deaths (when added to usual asthma therapy); risk is considered a class effect among all LABAs. It is unknown if indacaterol increases asthma-related deaths. No data exist associating LABA use with an increased risk of death in patients with COPD.

Rarely, paradoxical, life-threatening bronchospasm may occur with use of inhaled beta2-agonists; distinguish from inadequate response, discontinue medication immediately, institute alternative therapy. Use with caution in patients with cardiovascular disease (arrhythmia, coronary insufficiency, hypertension, or HF); beta-agonists may cause elevation in blood pressure and heart rate. $Beta_2$-agonists may also produce changes in the ECG (eg, T-wave flattening, QTc prolongation, ST segment depression).

Use with caution in patients with diabetes mellitus, severe hepatic impairment, or severe renal impairment (GFR <30 mL/minute/1.73 m^2) including ESRD on dialysis. Use with caution in seizure disorders, hyperthyroidism, hypokalemia, narrow angle glaucoma, prostatic hyperplasia or bladder neck obstruction.

Hypersensitivity reactions may occur; discontinue therapy if patient develops an allergic reaction; do not rechallenge. Product contains lactose; allergic reactions possible in patients with severe milk protein allergy. Use is contraindicated in patients with severe milk protein allergy. May cause drowsiness, dizziness, and/or blurred vision; patients must be cautioned about performing tasks which require mental alertness (eg, operating machinery or driving). Potentially significant drug-drug interactions may exist, requiring dose or frequency adjustment, additional monitoring, and/or selection of alternative therapy.

Adverse Reactions Also see indacaterol monograph.

Cardiovascular: Chest pain

Central nervous system: Dizziness, headache

Gastrointestinal: Dyspepsia, gastroenteritis, xerostomia

Genitourinary: Dysuria, urinary tract infection

Neuromuscular & skeletal: Musculoskeletal pain

Respiratory: Cough, nasopharyngitis, pneumonia, rhinitis, sinusitis, upper respiratory tract infection

Miscellaneous: Fever

Rare but important or life-threatening: Atrial fibrillation, bladder outflow obstruction, cardiac arrhythmia, cystitis, dental caries, diabetes mellitus, glaucoma, hypersensitivity reaction, ischemic heart disease, paradoxical bronchospasm, tachycardia

Drug Interactions

Metabolism/Transport Effects Refer to individual components.

Avoid Concomitant Use

Avoid concomitant use of Indacaterol and Glycopyrronium with any of the following: Aclidinium; Beta-Blockers (Nonselective); Glucagon; Highest Risk QTc-Prolonging Agents; Iobenguane I 123; Ipratropium (Oral Inhalation); Ivabradine; Long-Acting Beta2-Agonists; Mifepristone; Potassium Chloride; Tiotropium; Umeclidinium

Increased Effect/Toxicity

Indacaterol and Glycopyrronium may increase the levels/effects of: AbobotulinumtoxinA; Analgesics (Opioid); Anticholinergic Agents; Atosiban; Cannabinoid-Containing Products; Corticosteroids (Systemic); Glucagon; Highest Risk QTc-Prolonging Agents; Long-Acting Beta2-Agonists; Loop Diuretics; Mirabegron; Moderate Risk QTc-Prolonging Agents; OnabotulinumtoxinA; Potassium Chloride; RimabotulinumtoxinB; Sympathomimetics; Thiazide Diuretics; Tiotropium; Topiramate

The levels/effects of Indacaterol and Glycopyrronium may be increased by: Aclidinium; AtoMOXetine; Caffeine and Caffeine Containing Products; Cannabinoid-Containing Products; Ipratropium (Oral Inhalation); Ivabradine; Linezolid; MAO Inhibitors; Mifepristone; Pramlintide; QTc-Prolonging Agents (Indeterminate Risk and Risk Modifying); Tedizolid; Theophylline Derivatives; Tricyclic Antidepressants; Umeclidinium

Decreased Effect

Indacaterol and Glycopyrronium may decrease the levels/effects of: Acetylcholinesterase Inhibitors; Iobenguane I 123; Itopride; Secretin

The levels/effects of Indacaterol and Glycopyrronium may be decreased by: Acetylcholinesterase Inhibitors; Beta-Blockers (Beta1 Selective); Beta-Blockers (Nonselective); Betahistine

Storage/Stability Store at 15°C to 25°C (59°F to 77°F). Protect from moisture. Store capsules in blisters and remove immediately before use.

Mechanism of Action

Indacaterol: Relaxes bronchial smooth muscle by selective action on beta2-receptors with little effect on heart rate; acts locally in the lung.

Glycopyrronium: In COPD, competitively and reversibly inhibits the action of acetylcholine at muscarinic receptor subtypes 1-3 (greater affinity for subtypes 1 and 3) in bronchial smooth muscle thereby causing bronchodilation.

Pharmacodynamics/Kinetics Refer to individual agents

Dosage

COPD (maintenance): Adults: Oral Inhalation: Contents of 1 capsule (indacaterol 110 mcg/glycopyrronium 50 mcg) inhaled once daily using Ultibro Breezhaler device. **Note:** Dose delivered per capsule is equivalent to indacaterol 85 mcg/glycopyrronium 43 mcg.

Elderly: Refer to adult dosing.

Dosage adjustment in renal impairment:

Mild-to-moderate impairment: No dosage adjustment necessary.

Severe impairment (GFR <30 mL/minute/1.73 m^2): There are no dosage adjustments provided in manufacturer's labeling; use with caution.

Dosage adjustment in hepatic impairment:

Mild-to-moderate impairment: No dosage adjustment necessary.

Severe impairment: There are no dosage adjustments provided in manufacturer's labeling (has not been studied); use with caution.

Administration For inhalation using the Ultibro Breezhaler only. Not to be used for the relief of acute attacks. Administer once daily at the same time each day. Remove capsule from foil blister immediately before use. Avoid getting drug powder into eyes. Capsule should not be swallowed. Refer to manufacturer labeling for detailed administration information.

Monitoring Parameters Serum potassium (patients predisposed to hypokalemia); serum glucose (diabetic patients); relief of COPD symptoms

Product Availability Not available in the U.S.

Dosage Forms: Canada

Capsule, Inhalation:

Ultibro Breezhaler: Indacaterol 110 mcg and glycopyrronium 50 mcg [contains lactose monohydrate, milk protein, tartrazine]

◆ **Indacaterol Maleate** *see* Indacaterol *on page 1063*

◆ **Indacaterol Maleate and Glycopyrronium Bromide** *see* Indacaterol and Glycopyrronium [CAN/INT] *on page 1063*

Indapamide (in DAP a mide)

Brand Names: Canada Apo-Indapamide; Dom-Indapamide; JAMP-Indapamide; Lozide; Mylan-Indapamide; Novo-Indapamide; PHL-Indapamide; PMS-Indapamide; PRO-Indapamide; Riva-Indapamide

Pharmacologic Category Antihypertensive; Diuretic, Thiazide-Related

Use

Heart failure: Treatment of edema in heart failure

Hypertension: Management of mild-to-moderate hypertension

The 2014 guideline for the management of high blood pressure in adults (Eighth Joint National Committee [JNC 8]) recommends initiation of pharmacologic treatment to lower blood pressure for the following patients:

- Patients ≥60 years of age with systolic blood pressure (SBP) ≥150 mm Hg or diastolic blood pressure (DBP) ≥90 mm Hg. Goal of therapy is SBP <150 mm Hg and DBP <90 mm Hg.
- Patients <60 years of age with SBP ≥140 mm Hg or DBP is ≥90 mm Hg. Goal of therapy is SBP <140 mm Hg and DBP <90 mm Hg.
- Patients ≥18 years of age with diabetes and SBP ≥140 mm Hg or DBP ≥90 mm Hg. Goal of therapy is SBP <140 mm Hg and DBP <90 mm Hg.
- Patients ≥18 years of age with chronic kidney disease (CKD) and SBP ≥140 mm Hg or DBP ≥90 mm Hg. Goal of therapy is SBP <140 mm Hg and DBP <90 mm Hg.

In patients with CKD, regardless of race or diabetes status, the use of an ACE inhibitor (ACEI) or angiotensin receptor blocker (ARB) as initial therapy is recommended to improve kidney outcomes. In the general non-black population (without CKD) including those with diabetes, initial antihypertensive treatment should consist of a thiazide-type diuretic, calcium channel blocker, ACEI, or ARB. In the general black population (without CKD), including those with diabetes, initial antihypertensive treatment should consist of a thiazide-type diuretic or a calcium channel blocker **instead of** an ACEI or ARB.

Pregnancy Risk Factor B

Pregnancy Considerations Adverse events were not observed in animal reproduction studies. Diuretics cross the placenta and are found in cord blood. Maternal use may cause may cause fetal or neonatal jaundice, thrombocytopenia, or other adverse events observed in adults. Use of diuretics during normal pregnancies is not appropriate; use may be considered when edema is due to pathologic causes (as in the nonpregnant patient); monitor. Canadian labeling contraindicates use in pregnant women.

Breast-Feeding Considerations It is not known if indapamide is excreted in breast milk. If therapy is needed, the manufacturer recommends that nursing be discontinued.

Contraindications Hypersensitivity to indapamide or any component of the formulation or sulfonamide-derived drugs; anuria

Canadian labeling: Additional contraindications (not in U.S. labeling): Severe renal failure (CrCl <30 mL/minute); hepatic encephalopathy; severe hepatic impairment; hypokalemia; concomitant use with antiarrhythmic agents causing torsade de pointes; pregnancy; breast-feeding; hereditary problems of galactose intolerance, glucose-galactose malabsorption, or Lapp lactase deficiency

Warnings/Precautions Use with caution in severe renal disease; Canadian labeling contraindicates use in severe renal failure (CrCl <30 mL/minute). Electrolyte disturbances including severe hyponatremia (with hypokalemia, hypochloremic alkalosis, hypomagnesemia, or hypercalcemia) can occur; risk may be dose dependent. Correct hypokalemia before initiating therapy (Canadian labeling contraindicates use in hypokalemia). Use with caution in severe hepatic dysfunction; hepatic encephalopathy can be caused by electrolyte disturbances (Canadian labeling contraindicates use in severe hepatic impairment or hepatic encephalopathy). Gout may be precipitated in certain patients with a history of gout, a familial predisposition to gout, or chronic renal failure. Use caution in patients with prediabetes or diabetes; may alter glucose control. May cause SLE exacerbation or activation. Use with caution in patients with moderate or high cholesterol concentrations. Photosensitization may occur.

Chemical similarities are present among sulfonamides, sulfonylureas, carbonic anhydrase inhibitors, thiazides, and loop diuretics (except ethacrynic acid). Use in patients with sulfonamide allergy is specifically contraindicated in product labeling, however, a risk of cross-reaction exists in patients with allergy to any of these compounds; avoid use when previous reaction has been severe. Discontinue if signs of hypersensitivity are noted. Formulation may contain lactose; Canadian labeling recommends avoiding use in patients with hereditary conditions of galactose intolerance, glucose-galactose malabsorption, or lactase deficiency.

Adverse Reactions

Cardiovascular: Arrhythmia, chest pain, flushing, orthostatic hypotension, palpitation, peripheral edema, PVC, vasculitis

Central nervous system: Agitation, anxiety, depression, dizziness, drowsiness, fatigue, headache, insomnia, irritability, lethargy, lightheadedness, malaise, nervousness, (dose dependent), pain, tension, tiredness, vertigo

Dermatologic: Hives, pruritus, rash

Endocrine & metabolic: Hyperglycemia, hyperuricemia, hypochloremia, hypokalemia (dose dependent), hyponatremia, libido decreased

Gastrointestinal: Abdominal pain, anorexia, constipation, cramping, diarrhea, dyspepsia, gastric irritation, nausea, vomiting, weight loss, xerostomia

Neuromuscular & skeletal: Back pain, hypertonia, muscle cramps/spasm, paresthesia, weakness
Ocular: Blurred vision,conjunctivitis
Renal: BUN increased, creatinine increased, glycosuria
Respiratory: Cough, pharyngitis, rhinitis, rhinorrhea, sinusitis
Miscellaneous: Flu-like syndrome, infection
Rare but important or life-threatening: Agranulocytosis, anaphylactic reaction, aplastic anemia, bullous eruptions, erythema multiforme, fever, hepatitis, hypercalcemia, jaundice (cholestatic jaundice), leukopenia, liver function test abnormality, pancreatitis, photosensitivity, pneumonitis, purpura, Stevens-Johnson syndrome, thrombocytopenia, torsade de pointes

Drug Interactions

Metabolism/Transport Effects None known.

Avoid Concomitant Use

Avoid concomitant use of Indapamide with any of the following: Dofetilide

Increased Effect/Toxicity

Indapamide may increase the levels/effects of: ACE Inhibitors; Allopurinol; Amifostine; Antihypertensives; Calcium Salts; CarBAMazepine; Cardiac Glycosides; Cyclophosphamide; Diazoxide; Dofetilide; DULoxetine; Highest Risk QTc-Prolonging Agents; Hypotensive Agents; Levodopa; Lithium; Moderate Risk QTc-Prolonging Agents; Multivitamins/Minerals (with ADEK, Folate, Iron); Multivitamins/Minerals (with AE, No Iron); Obinutuzumab; OXcarbazepine; Porfimer; RisperiDONE; RiTUXimab; Sodium Phosphates; Topiramate; Verteporfin; Vitamin D Analogs

The levels/effects of Indapamide may be increased by: Alcohol (Ethyl); Alfuzosin; Analgesics (Opioid); Anticholinergic Agents; Barbiturates; Beta2-Agonists; Brimonidine (Topical); Corticosteroids (Orally Inhaled); Corticosteroids (Systemic); Dexketoprofen; Diazoxide; Herbs (Hypotensive Properties); Licorice; MAO Inhibitors; Mifepristone; Multivitamins/Fluoride (with ADE); Nicorandil; Pentoxifylline; Phosphodiesterase 5 Inhibitors; Prostacyclin Analogues; Selective Serotonin Reuptake Inhibitors

Decreased Effect

Indapamide may decrease the levels/effects of: Antidiabetic Agents

The levels/effects of Indapamide may be decreased by: Bile Acid Sequestrants; Herbs (Hypertensive Properties); Methylphenidate; Nonsteroidal Anti-Inflammatory Agents; Yohimbine

Storage/Stability Store at 20°C to 25°C (68°F to 77°F).

Mechanism of Action Diuretic effect is localized at the proximal segment of the distal tubule of the nephron; it does not appear to have significant effect on glomerular filtration rate nor renal blood flow; like other diuretics, it enhances sodium, chloride, and water excretion by interfering with the transport of sodium ions across the renal tubular epithelium

Pharmacodynamics/Kinetics

Absorption: Rapid and complete
Distribution: V_d: 25 L (Grebow, 1982)
Protein binding, plasma: 71% to 79%
Metabolism: Extensively hepatic
Bioavailability: 93% (Ernst, 2009)
Half-life elimination: Biphasic: 14 and 25 hours
Time to peak: 2 hours
Excretion: Urine (~70%; 7% as unchanged drug within 48 hours); feces (23%)

Dosage Adults: Oral:

Edema: Initial: 2.5 mg daily; if inadequate response after 1 week, may increase dose to 5 mg daily. **Note:** There is little therapeutic benefit to increasing the dose >5 mg daily; there is, however, an increased risk of electrolyte disturbances

Hypertension: Initial: 1.25 mg daily; if inadequate response, may increase dose once every 4 weeks to 2.5 mg daily and then to 5 mg daily if needed. Consider adding another antihypertensive and decreasing the dose if response is not adequate. Usual dosage range (ASH/ISH [Weber, 2014]): 1.25 to 2.5 mg daily. **Note:** Canadian labeling recommends a maximum dose of 2.5 mg daily.

Calcium nephrolithiasis (off-label use): 2.5 mg once daily (AUA [Pearle, 2014])

Dosage adjustment in renal impairment: There are no dosage adjustments provided in manufacturer's labeling; use with caution. Canadian labeling contraindicates use in severe impairment (CrCl <30 mL/min).

Dosage adjustment in hepatic impairment: There are no dosage adjustments provided in manufacturer's labeling; use with caution. Canadian labeling contraindicates use in severe hepatic impairment or hepatic encephalopathy.

Dietary Considerations May be taken without regard to meals (Caruso, 1983); however, administration with food or milk may to decrease GI adverse effects.

Administration May be administered without regard to meals (Caruso, 1983); however, administration with food or milk may decrease GI adverse effects. Administer early in day to avoid nocturia.

Monitoring Parameters Blood pressure (both standing and sitting/supine); serum electrolytes, hepatic function, renal function, uric acid; assess weight, I & O reports daily to determine fluid loss

Dosage Forms

Tablet, Oral:

Generic: 1.25 mg, 2.5 mg

◆ **Indapamide and Perindopril** *see* Perindopril and Indapamide [CAN/INT] *on page 1626*

◆ **Inderal (Can)** *see* Propranolol *on page 1731*

◆ **Inderal XL** *see* Propranolol *on page 1731*

◆ **Inderal LA** *see* Propranolol *on page 1731*

Indinavir (in DIN a veer)

Brand Names: U.S. Crixivan

Brand Names: Canada Crixivan

Index Terms IDV; Indinavir Sulfate

Pharmacologic Category Antiretroviral, Protease Inhibitor (Anti-HIV)

Use Treatment of HIV infection; should always be used as part of a multidrug regimen (at least three antiretroviral agents)

Pregnancy Risk Factor C

Dosage

Children and Adolescents 4 to 15 years (off-label use): 400 mg/m^2 every 12 hours is currently under study (HHS [pediatric], 2014)

Adults: Oral:

Unboosted regimen: 800 mg every 8 hours

Ritonavir-boosted regimen: Ritonavir 100-200 mg twice daily plus indinavir 800 mg twice daily

Dosage adjustments for indinavir when administered in combination therapy:

Delavirdine, itraconazole, or ketoconazole: Reduce indinavir dose to 600 mg every 8 hours

Efavirenz: Increase indinavir dose to 1000 mg every 8 hours

Lopinavir and ritonavir (Kaletra™): Indinavir 600 mg twice daily

Nelfinavir: Increase indinavir dose to 1200 mg twice daily

Nevirapine: Increase indinavir dose to 1000 mg every 8 hours

Rifabutin: Reduce rifabutin to 1/2 the standard dose plus increase indinavir to 1000 mg every 8 hours

Dosage adjustment in renal impairment: There are no dosage adjustments provided in the manufacturer's labeling (has not been studied).

Dosage adjustment in hepatic impairment:

Mild-moderate impairment due to cirrhosis, monotherapy: 600 mg every 8 hours

Severe impairment: There are no dosage adjustments provided in the manufacturer's labeling (has not been studied).

Additional Information Complete prescribing information should be consulted for additional detail.

Dosage Forms

Capsule, Oral:

Crixivan: 200 mg, 400 mg

◆ **Indinavir Sulfate** *see* Indinavir *on page 1066*

Indobufen [INT] (in doe BYOO fen)

International Brand Names Ibustrin (AT, CZ, HR, IT, MX, PT)

Pharmacologic Category Antiplatelet Agent

Reported Use Prevention of platelet aggregation which leads to thrombus formation

Dosage Range Adults: Oral: 200-400 mg/day given in divided doses every 12 hours

Product Availability Product available in various countries; not currently available in the U.S.

Dosage Forms

Tablet: 100 mg, 200 mg

◆ **Indocin** *see* Indomethacin *on page 1067*

◆ **Indometacin** *see* Indomethacin *on page 1067*

Indomethacin (in doe METH a sin)

Brand Names: U.S. Indocin

Brand Names: Canada Apo-Indomethacin; Novo-Methacin; Pro-Indo; ratio-Indomethacin; Sandoz-Indomethacin

Index Terms Indometacin; Indomethacin Sodium Trihydrate

Pharmacologic Category Nonsteroidal Anti-inflammatory Drug (NSAID), Oral; Nonsteroidal Anti-inflammatory Drug (NSAID), Parenteral

Additional Appendix Information

Beers Criteria - Potentially Inappropriate Medications for Geriatrics *on page 2271*

Use

Acute pain, mild to moderate (Tivorbex only): Treatment of mild to moderate acute pain in adults

Arthritis (excluding Tivorbex): Treatment of moderate to severe rheumatoid arthritis (RA), including acute flares of chronic disease; moderate to severe osteoarthritis (OA); acute gouty arthritis (except extended-release [ER] capsules)

Inflammatory conditions (excluding Tivorbex): Treatment of moderate to severe ankylosing spondylitis; acute painful shoulder (bursitis and/or tendinitis)

Patent ductus arteriosus (IV only): An alternative to surgery for closure of patent ductus arteriosus in neonates

Pregnancy Risk Factor C (<30 weeks gestation); C/D (≥30 weeks gestation [manufacturer specific])

Pregnancy Considerations Adverse events have been observed in animal reproduction studies; studies in pregnant women have demonstrated risk to the fetus if administered at ≥30 weeks gestation. Indomethacin crosses the placenta and can be detected in fetal plasma and amniotic fluid. Indomethacin exposure during the first trimester is not strongly associated with congenital malformations; however, cardiovascular anomalies and cleft palate have been observed following NSAID exposure in some studies. The use of an NSAID close to conception may be associated with an increased risk of miscarriage. Nonteratogenic effects have been observed following NSAID administration during the third trimester, including myocardial degenerative changes, prenatal constriction of the ductus arteriosus, failure of the ductus arteriosus to close postnatally, and fetal tricuspid regurgitation; renal dysfunction or failure, oligohydramnios; gastrointestinal bleeding or perforation, increased risk of necrotizing enterocolitis; intracranial bleeding (including intraventricular hemorrhage), platelet dysfunction with resultant bleeding; and pulmonary hypertension. The risk of fetal ductal constriction following maternal use of indomethacin is increased with gestational age and duration of therapy. Because they may cause premature closure of the ductus arteriosus, use of NSAIDs late in pregnancy should be avoided (use after 31 or 32 weeks gestation is not recommended by some clinicians). Indomethacin has been used for a short duration (eg, ≤48 hours) in the management of preterm labor. Indomethacin should be used with caution in pregnant women with hypertension. The chronic use of NSAIDs in women of reproductive age may be associated with infertility that is reversible upon discontinuation of the medication.

Breast-Feeding Considerations Indomethacin is excreted into breast milk and low amounts have been measured in the plasma of nursing infants. Seizures in a nursing infant were observed in one case report, although adverse events have not been noted in other cases. Breast-feeding is not recommended by most manufacturers; Tivorbex may be used with caution during breast-feeding. (The therapeutic use of indomethacin is contraindicated in neonates with significant renal failure.) Hypertensive crisis and psychiatric side effects have been noted in case reports following use of indomethacin for analgesia in postpartum women. Use with caution in nursing women with hypertensive disorders of pregnancy or preexisting renal disease.

Contraindications

Hypersensitivity (eg, anaphylactic reactions and serious skin reactions) to indomethacin, aspirin, other NSAIDs, or any component of the formulation; perioperative pain in the setting of coronary artery bypass graft (CABG) surgery;history of asthma, urticaria, or allergic-type reactions after taking aspirin or other NSAID agents (severe, even fatal, anaphylactic-like reactions have been reported); patients with a history of proctitis or recent rectal bleeding (suppositories)

Neonates: Necrotizing enterocolitis; impaired renal function; active bleeding (including intracranial hemorrhage and gastrointestinal bleeding), thrombocytopenia, coagulation defects; untreated infection; congenital heart disease where patent ductus arteriosus is necessary

Warnings/Precautions [U.S. Boxed Warning]: NSAIDs are associated with an increased risk of adverse cardiovascular thrombotic events, including MI and stroke. Risk may be increased with duration of use or preexisting cardiovascular risk factors or disease. May cause new-onset hypertension or worsening of existing hypertension. Monitor blood pressure closely during initiation of treatment and throughout the course of therapy. Use caution in patients with fluid retention. Avoid use in heart failure (ACCF/AHA [Yancy, 2013]). Concurrent administration of ibuprofen, and potentially other nonselective NSAIDs, may interfere with aspirin's cardioprotective effect. **[U.S. Boxed Warning]: Use is contraindicated for treatment of perioperative pain in the setting of coronary artery bypass graft (CABG) surgery.** Risk of MI and stroke may be increased with use following CABG surgery.

Platelet adhesion and aggregation may be decreased; may prolong bleeding time; patients with coagulation disorders or who are receiving anticoagulants should be monitored closely. Anemia may occur; patients on long-term NSAID therapy should be monitored for anemia. Rarely, NSAID use may cause severe blood dyscrasias (eg, agranulocytosis, aplastic anemia, thrombocytopenia).

NSAID use may compromise existing renal function; dose-dependent decreases in prostaglandin synthesis may result from NSAID use, reducing renal blood flow which may cause renal decompensation. NSAID use may increase the risk for hyperkalemia. Patients with impaired renal function, dehydration, heart failure, liver dysfunction, those taking diuretics, and ACE inhibitors are at greater risk of renal toxicity and hyperkalemia. Rehydrate patient before starting therapy; monitor renal function closely. Not recommended for use in patients with advanced renal disease. Long-term NSAID use may result in renal papillary necrosis.

[U.S. Boxed Warning]: NSAIDs may increase risk of gastrointestinal irritation, inflammation, ulceration, bleeding, and perforation. Use caution with a history of GI disease (bleeding or ulcers), concurrent therapy with aspirin, anticoagulants and/or corticosteroids, smoking, use of alcohol, the elderly or debilitated patients. When used concomitantly with aspirin, a substantial increase in the risk of gastrointestinal complications (eg, ulcer) occurs; concomitant gastroprotective therapy (eg, proton pump inhibitors) is recommended (Bhatt, 2008).

Use the lowest effective dose for the shortest duration of time, consistent with individual patient goals, to reduce risk of cardiovascular or GI adverse events. Alternate therapies should be considered for patients at high risk.

NSAIDS may cause drowsiness, dizziness, blurred vision and other neurologic effects which may impair physical or mental abilities; patients must be cautioned about performing tasks which require mental alertness (eg, operating machinery or driving). Discontinue use with blurred or diminished vision and perform ophthalmologic exam. Monitor vision with long-term therapy. Headache may occur; cessation of therapy required if headache persists after dosage reduction.

NSAIDs may cause potentially fatal serious skin adverse events including exfoliative dermatitis, Stevens-Johnson syndrome (SJS) and toxic epidermal necrolysis (TEN); discontinue use at first sign of skin rash or hypersensitivity. Anaphylactoid reactions may occur, even without prior exposure; patients with "aspirin triad" (bronchial asthma, aspirin intolerance, rhinitis) may be at increased risk. Use is contraindicated in patients who experience bronchospasm, asthma, rhinitis, or urticaria with NSAID or aspirin therapy. Use caution in other forms of asthma.

Use with caution in patients with decreased hepatic function. Closely monitor patients with any abnormal LFT. Severe hepatic reactions (eg, jaundice, fulminant hepatitis, liver necrosis, liver failure) have occurred with NSAID use, rarely; discontinue if signs or symptoms of liver disease develop, or if systemic manifestations occur. The elderly are at increased risk for adverse effects (especially peptic ulceration, CNS effects, renal toxicity) from NSAIDs even at low doses. Prolonged use may cause corneal deposits and retinal disturbances; discontinue if visual changes are observed. Use caution with depression, epilepsy, or Parkinson's disease.

Withhold for at least 4-6 half-lives prior to surgical or dental procedures. Potentially significant drug-drug interactions may exist, requiring dose or frequency adjustment, additional monitoring, and/or selection of alternative therapy. Consult drug interactions database for more detailed information.

Elderly: Nonselective oral NSAID use is associated with an increased risk of GI bleeding and peptic ulcer disease in older adults in high risk category (eg, >75 years or age or receiving concomitant oral/parenteral corticosteroids, anticoagulants, or antiplatelet agents). Risk of adverse events may be higher with indomethacin compared to other NSAIDs; avoid use in this age group (Beers Criteria). Indomethacin may cause confusion or, rarely, psychosis; remain alert to the possibility of such adverse reactions in elderly patients.

Oral: Hepatotoxicity has been reported in younger children treated for juvenile idiopathic arthritis (JIA). Closely monitor if use is needed in children ≥2 years of age.

Adverse Reactions

Cardiovascular: Presyncope, syncope

Central nervous system: Depression, dizziness, drowsiness, fatigue, headache, malaise, vertigo

Dermatologic: Hyperhidrosis, pruritus, skin rash

Endocrine & metabolic: Hot flash

Gastrointestinal: Abdominal pain, constipation, decreased appetite, diarrhea, dyspepsia, epigastric pain, heartburn, nausea, rectal irritation (suppository), tenesmus (suppository), vomiting

Hematologic & oncologic: Postoperative hemorrhage

Otic: Tinnitus

Miscellaneous: Swelling (postprocedural)

Rare but important or life-threatening: Acute respiratory distress, agranulocytosis, anaphylaxis, anemia, angioedema, aphthous stomatitis, aplastic anemia, aseptic meningitis, asthma, bone marrow depression, cardiac arrhythmia, cardiac failure, cerebrovascular accident, chest pain, cholestatic jaundice, coma, confusion, convulsions, corneal deposits, depersonalization, depression, diplopia, disseminated intravascular coagulation, dysarthria, edema, erythema multiforme, erythema nodosum, exacerbation of epilepsy, exacerbation of Parkinson's disease, exfoliative dermatitis, fluid retention, gastritis, gastroenteritis, gastrointestinal hemorrhage, gastrointestinal perforation (rare), gastrointestinal ulcer, glycosuria, gynecomastia, hearing loss, hematuria, hemodynamic deterioration (patients with severe heart failure and hyponatremia), hemolytic anemia, hepatic failure, hepatic necrosis, hepatitis (including fatal cases), hyperglycemia, hyperkalemia, hypersensitivity reaction, hypertension, hypotension, immune thrombocytopenia, interstitial nephritis, intestinal obstruction, intestinal stenosis, involuntary muscle movements, jaundice, leukopenia, maculopathy, myocardial infarction, necrotizing fasciitis, nephrotic syndrome, oliguria, peripheral neuropathy, proctitis, psychosis, pulmonary edema, purpura, rectal hemorrhage, regional ileitis, renal failure, renal insufficiency, retinal disturbance, shock, significant cardiovascular event, Stevens-Johnson syndrome, stomatitis, syncope, thrombocytopenia, thrombophlebitis, toxic amblyopia, toxic epidermal necrolysis, ulcerative colitis, vaginal hemorrhage

Drug Interactions

Metabolism/Transport Effects Substrate of CYP2C19 (minor), CYP2C9 (minor); **Note:** Assignment of Major/Minor substrate status based on clinically relevant drug interaction potential; **Inhibits** CYP2C19 (weak), CYP2C9 (weak)

Avoid Concomitant Use

Avoid concomitant use of Indomethacin with any of the following: Dexketoprofen; Floctafenine; Ketorolac (Nasal); Ketorolac (Systemic); NSAID (COX-2 Inhibitor); Omacetaxine; Urokinase

Increased Effect/Toxicity

Indomethacin may increase the levels/effects of: 5-ASA Derivatives; Agents with Antiplatelet Properties; Aliskiren; Aminoglycosides; Anticoagulants; Apixaban; Bisphosphonate Derivatives; Collagenase (Systemic); CycloSPORINE (Systemic); Dabigatran Etexilate; Deferasirox; Desmopressin; Digoxin; Eplerenone; Haloperidol; Ibritumomab; Lithium; Methotrexate; Nonsteroidal Anti-Inflammatory Agents; NSAID (COX-2 Inhibitor); Obinutuzumab; Omacetaxine; PEMEtrexed; Porfimer; Potassium-Sparing Diuretics; PRALAtrexate; Quinolone Antibiotics; Rivaroxaban; Salicylates; Tacrolimus (Systemic); Tenofovir; Thrombolytic Agents; Tiludronate; Tositumomab and Iodine I 131 Tositumomab; Triamterene; Urokinase; Vancomycin; Verteporfin; Vitamin K Antagonists

The levels/effects of Indomethacin may be increased by: ACE Inhibitors; Angiotensin II Receptor Blockers; Antidepressants (Tricyclic, Tertiary Amine); Corticosteroids (Systemic); CycloSPORINE (Systemic); Dasatinib; Dexketoprofen; Diclofenac (Systemic); Floctafenine; Glucosamine; Herbs (Anticoagulant/Antiplatelet Properties); Ibrutinib; Ketorolac (Nasal); Ketorolac (Systemic); Limaprost; Multivitamins/Fluoride (with ADE); Multivitamins/Minerals (with ADEK, Folate, Iron); Multivitamins/Minerals (with AE, No Iron); Omega-3 Fatty Acids; Pentosan Polysulfate Sodium; Pentoxifylline; Probenecid; Prostacyclin Analogues; Selective Serotonin Reuptake Inhibitors; Serotonin/Norepinephrine Reuptake Inhibitors; Sodium Phosphates; Tipranavir; Treprostinil; Vitamin E

Decreased Effect

Indomethacin may decrease the levels/effects of: ACE Inhibitors; Aliskiren; Angiotensin II Receptor Blockers; Beta-Blockers; Eplerenone; Glucagon; HydrALAZINE; Loop Diuretics; Potassium-Sparing Diuretics; Prostaglandins (Ophthalmic); Salicylates; Selective Serotonin Reuptake Inhibitors; Thiazide Diuretics

The levels/effects of Indomethacin may be decreased by: Bile Acid Sequestrants; Salicylates

Food Interactions Food may decrease the rate but not the extent of absorption. Indomethacin peak serum levels may be delayed if taken with food. Management: Administer with food or milk to minimize GI upset.

Preparation for Administration IV: Reconstitute with 1-2 mL preservative free NS or SWFI just prior to administration. Discard any unused portion. Do not use preservative-containing diluents for reconstitution.

Storage/Stability

Capsules: Store at 15°C to 30°C (59°F to 86°F). Protect from light. Protect ER capsules from moisture.

Tivorbex: Store Tivorbex capsules at 25°C (77°F); excursions permitted to 15°C to 30°C (59°F to 86°F). Store in the original container; protect from moisture and light.

IV: Store below 30°C (86°F). Protect from light.

Suppositories: Store refrigerated at 2°C to 8°C (36°F to 46°F).

Suspension: Store below 30°C (86°F). Avoid temperatures above 50°C (122°F). Protect from freezing.

Mechanism of Action Reversibly inhibits cyclooxygenase-1 and 2 (COX-1 and 2) enzymes, which results in decreased formation of prostaglandin precursors; has antipyretic, analgesic, and anti-inflammatory properties

Other proposed mechanisms not fully elucidated (and possibly contributing to the anti-inflammatory effect to varying degrees), include inhibiting chemotaxis, altering lymphocyte activity, inhibiting neutrophil aggregation/activation, and decreasing proinflammatory cytokine levels.

Pharmacodynamics/Kinetics

Onset of action: ~30 minutes

Duration: 4-6 hours

Absorption: Oral: Immediate release: Prompt and extensive; Extended release: 90% over 12 hours

Distribution: Crosses blood-brain barrier

Protein binding: 99%

Metabolism: Hepatic; significant enterohepatic recirculation; metabolites include desmethyl, desbenzoyl and desmethyl-desbenzoyl (all in unconjugated form)

Bioavailability: 100%

Half-life elimination: 4.5 hours; prolonged in neonates

Time to peak: Oral: Immediate release: 2 hours; Tivorbex capsules: 1.67 hours

Excretion: Urine (60%, primarily as glucuronide conjugates); feces (33%, primarily as metabolites)

Dosage

Patent ductus arteriosus:

Neonates: IV: Initial: 0.2 mg/kg, followed by 2 doses depending on postnatal age (PNA):

PNA **at time of first dose** <48 hours: 0.1 mg/kg at 12- to 24-hour intervals

PNA **at time of first dose** 2 to 7 days: 0.2 mg/kg at 12- to 24-hour intervals

PNA **at time of first dose** >7 days: 0.25 mg/kg at 12- to 24-hour intervals

In general, may use 12-hour dosing interval if urine output >1 mL/kg/hour after prior dose; use 24-hour dosing interval if urine output is <1 mL/kg/hour but >0.6 mL/kg/hour; doses should be withheld if patient has oliguria (urine output <0.6 mL/kg/hour) or anuria

Inflammatory/rheumatoid disorders: **Note:** Use lowest effective dose.

Children ≥2 years: Oral (excluding Tivorbex): 1 to 2 mg/kg/day in 2 to 4 divided doses; maximum dose: 4 mg/kg/day; not to exceed 150 to 200 mg daily

Adolescents >14 years and Adults: Oral (excluding Tivorbex), rectal: 25 to 50 mg/dose 2 to 3 times daily; maximum dose: 200 mg daily; extended release capsule should be given on a 1 to 2 times daily schedule (maximum dose for extended release: 150 mg daily). In patients with arthritis and persistent night pain and/or morning stiffness may give the larger portion (up to 100 mg) of the total daily dose at bedtime.

Bursitis/tendonitis: Oral (excluding Tivorbex), rectal: Adults: Initial dose: 75 to 150 mg daily in 3 to 4 divided doses **or** 1 to 2 divided doses for extended release; usual treatment is 7 to 14 days

Acute gouty arthritis: Oral (excluding Tivorbex), rectal: Adults: 50 mg 3 times daily until pain is tolerable then reduce dose; usual treatment <3 to 5 days

Acute pain (mild to moderate): Adults: Oral (Tivorbex only): 20 mg 3 times daily or 40 mg 2 or 3 times daily

Prevention of pancreatitis post-endoscopic retrograde cholangiopancreatography (ERCP) (off-label use): Rectal: Adults: 100 mg immediately after ERCP (Elmunzer, 2012)

Elderly: Refer to adult dosing. Use lowest recommended dose and frequency in elderly to initiate therapy for indications listed in adult dosing.

Dosage adjustment in renal impairment: There are no dosage adjustments provided in the manufacturer's labeling; not recommended in patients with advanced renal disease.

Dosage adjustment in hepatic impairment: There are no dosage adjustments provided in the manufacturer's labeling; use with caution.

Dietary Considerations May cause GI upset; take with food or milk to minimize

Administration

Oral: Administer with food, milk, or antacids to decrease GI adverse effects. Extended release capsules must be swallowed whole; do not crush.

IV: Administer over 20 to 30 minutes. Reconstitute IV formulation just prior to administration; discard any unused portion; avoid IV bolus administration or infusion via an umbilical catheter into vessels near the superior mesenteric artery as these may cause vasoconstriction and can compromise blood flow to the intestines. Do not administer intra-arterially.

Monitoring Parameters Monitor response (pain, range of motion, grip strength, mobility, ADL function), inflammation; observe for weight gain, edema; monitor renal function (serum creatinine, BUN); observe for bleeding, bruising; evaluate gastrointestinal effects (abdominal pain, bleeding, dyspepsia); mental confusion, disorientation, CBC, blood pressure, liver function tests (particularly with pediatric use); ophthalmologic exams with prolonged therapy

Product Availability Tivorbex: FDA approved February 2014; anticipated availability currently unknown. Refer to the prescribing information for additional information.

Dosage Forms

Capsule, Oral:

Generic: 25 mg, 50 mg

Capsule Extended Release, Oral:

Generic: 75 mg

Solution Reconstituted, Intravenous:

Indocin: 1 mg (1 ea)

Generic: 1 mg (1 ea)

Solution Reconstituted, Intravenous [preservative free]:

Generic: 1 mg (1 ea)

Suppository, Rectal:

Indocin: 50 mg (30 ea)

Suspension, Oral:

Indocin: 25 mg/5 mL (237 mL)

Dosage Forms: Canada Note: Refer also to Dosage Forms. Extended release capsule, intravenous solution, and oral suspension are not available in Canada.

Suppository, Rectal: 100 mg

◆ **Indomethacin Sodium Trihydrate** *see* Indomethacin *on page 1067*

Indoramin [INT] (in DOR a min)

International Brand Names Baratol (GB, IE, ZA); Doralese (GB, IE); Indorene (IT); Orfidora (ES); Vidora (FR); Wydora (DE); Wypresin (AT)

Index Terms Indoramin Hydrochloride

Pharmacologic Category Alpha-Adrenergic Blocking Agent, Oral

Reported Use Treatment of hypertension; benign prostatic hyperplasia

Dosage Range Adults: Oral:

Hypertension: 25 mg twice daily; increased if necessary by 25 mg every 2 weeks to maximum of 200 mg daily in divided doses

Benign prostatic hyperplasia: 20 mg twice daily; may increase dose by 20 mg every 2 weeks to a maximum of 100 mg/day

Product Availability Product available in various countries; not currently available in the U.S.

Dosage Forms

Tablet: 20 mg, 25 mg, 50 mg

◆ **Indoramin Hydrochloride** *see* Indoramin [INT] *on page 1070*

◆ **INF-alpha 2** *see* Interferon Alfa-2b *on page 1096*

◆ **Infanrix** *see* Diphtheria and Tetanus Toxoids, and Acellular Pertussis Vaccine *on page 649*

◆ **Infanrix Hexa™ (Can)** *see* Diphtheria and Tetanus Toxoids, Acellular Pertussis, Hepatitis B (Recombinant), Poliovirus (Inactivated), and *Haemophilus influenzae* B Conjugate (Adsorbed) Vaccine [CAN/INT] *on page 647*

◆ **Infants Advil [OTC]** *see* Ibuprofen *on page 1032*

◆ **Infants Ibuprofen [OTC]** *see* Ibuprofen *on page 1032*

◆ **Infasurf** *see* Calfactant *on page 334*

◆ **Infed** *see* Iron Dextran Complex *on page 1117*

◆ **Infergen [DSC]** *see* Interferon Alfacon-1 *on page 1100*

InFLIXimab (in FLIKS e mab)

Brand Names: U.S. Remicade

Brand Names: Canada Remicade

Index Terms Avakine; Infliximab, Recombinant

Pharmacologic Category Antirheumatic, Disease Modifying; Gastrointestinal Agent, Miscellaneous; Immunosuppressant Agent; Monoclonal Antibody; Tumor Necrosis Factor (TNF) Blocking Agent

Use

Treatment of moderately- to severely-active rheumatoid arthritis (with methotrexate) (to reduce signs/symptoms of active arthritis and inhibit progression of structural damage and improve physical function)

Treatment of moderately- to severely-active Crohn disease with inadequate response to conventional therapy (to reduce signs/symptoms and induce and maintain clinical remission) or to reduce the number of draining enterocutaneous and rectovaginal fistulas and maintain fistula closure

Treatment of psoriatic arthritis (to reduce signs/symptoms of active arthritis and inhibit progression of structural damage and improve physical function)

Treatment of chronic severe (extensive and/or disabling) plaque psoriasis as an alternative to other systemic therapy

Treatment of active ankylosing spondylitis (to reduce signs/symptoms)

Treatment of moderately- to severely-active ulcerative colitis with inadequate response to conventional therapy (to reduce signs/symptoms and induce and maintain clinical remission, mucosal healing and eliminate corticosteroid use)

Pregnancy Risk Factor B

Pregnancy Considerations Animal reproduction studies have not been conducted. Infliximab crosses the placenta and can be detected in the serum of infants for up to 6 months following *in utero* exposure. The safety of administering live or live-attenuated vaccines to exposed infants is not known. If a biologic agent such as infliximab is needed to treat inflammatory bowel disease during pregnancy, it is recommended to hold therapy after 30 weeks gestation (Habal, 2012).

Healthcare providers are also encouraged to enroll women exposed to infliximab during pregnancy in the Mother-ToBaby Autoimmune Diseases Study by contacting the Organization of Teratology Information Specialists (OTIS) (877-311-8972).

Breast-Feeding Considerations Small amounts of infliximab have been detected in breast milk. Information is available from three postpartum women who were administered infliximab 5 mg/kg 1-24 weeks after delivery. Infliximab was detected within 12 hours and the highest milk concentrations (0.09-0.105 mcg/mL) were seen 2-3 days after the dose. Corresponding maternal serum concentrations were 18-64 mcg/mL (Ben-Horin, 2011). Due to the potential for serious adverse reactions in the nursing infant, the manufacturer recommends a decision be made whether to discontinue nursing or to discontinue the drug, taking into account the importance of treatment to the mother.

Contraindications Hypersensitivity to infliximab, murine proteins or any component of the formulation; doses >5 mg/kg in patients with moderate or severe heart failure (NYHA Class III/IV)

Canadian labeling: Additional contraindications (not in U.S. labeling): Severe infections (eg, sepsis, abscesses, tuberculosis, and opportunistic infections)

Warnings/Precautions [U.S. Boxed Warning]: Patients receiving infliximab are at increased risk for serious infections which may result in hospitalization and/or fatality; infections usually developed in patients receiving concomitant immunosuppressive agents (eg, methotrexate or corticosteroids) and may present as disseminated (rather than local) disease. Active tuberculosis (or reactivation of latent tuberculosis), invasive fungal (including aspergillosis, blastomycosis, candidiasis, coccidioidomycosis, histoplasmosis, and pneumocystosis) and bacterial, viral or other opportunistic infections (including legionellosis and listeriosis) have been reported. Monitor closely for signs/symptoms of infection. Discontinue for serious infection or sepsis. Consider risks versus benefits prior to use in patients with a history of chronic or recurrent infection. Consider empiric antifungal therapy in patients who are at risk for invasive fungal infection and develop severe systemic illness. Caution should be exercised when considering use the elderly or in patients with conditions that predispose them to infections (eg, diabetes) or residence/travel from areas of endemic mycoses (blastomycosis, coccidioidomycosis, histoplasmosis), or with latent or localized infections. Do not initiate infliximab therapy in patients with an active infection, including clinically important localized infection. Patients who develop a new infection while undergoing treatment should be monitored closely. Potentially significant drug interactions may exist, requiring dose or frequency adjustment, additional monitoring, and/or selection of alternative therapy.

[U.S. Boxed Warning]: Infliximab treatment has been associated with active tuberculosis (may be disseminated or extrapulmonary) or reactivation of latent infections; evaluate patients for tuberculosis risk factors and latent tuberculosis infection (with a tuberculin skin test) prior to and during therapy; treatment of latent tuberculosis should be initiated before use. Patients with initial negative tuberculin skin tests should receive continued monitoring for tuberculosis throughout treatment. Most cases of reactivation have been reported within the first couple months of treatment. Caution should be exercised when considering the use of infliximab in patients who have been exposed to tuberculosis.

Patients should be brought up to date with all immunizations before initiating therapy. Live vaccines should not be given concurrently; there is no data available concerning secondary transmission of live vaccines in patients receiving therapy. Use caution when administering live vaccines to infants born to female patients who received infliximab therapy while pregnant; infliximab crosses the placenta and has been detected in infants' serum for up to 6 months. Reactivation of hepatitis B virus (HBV) has occurred in chronic virus carriers (may be fatal); use with caution; evaluate prior to initiation and during treatment.

[U.S. Boxed Warning]: Lymphoma and other malignancies (may be fatal) have been reported in children and adolescent patients receiving TNF-blocking agents including infliximab. Half the cases are lymphomas (Hodgkin's and non-Hodgkin's). **[U.S. Boxed Warning]: Postmarketing cases of hepatosplenic T-cell lymphoma have been reported in patients treated with infliximab. Almost all patients had received and concurrent or prior treatment with azathioprine or mercaptopurine at or prior to diagnosis and the majority of reported cases occurred in adolescent and young adult males with Crohn disease or ulcerative colitis.** Malignancies occurred after a median of 30 months (range 1 to 84 months) after the first dose of TNF blocker therapy; most patients were receiving concomitant immunosuppressants. The impact of infliximab on the development and course of malignancies is not fully defined. As compared to the general population, an increased risk of lymphoma has been noted in clinical trials; however, rheumatoid arthritis alone has been previously associated with an increased rate of lymphoma. Use caution in patients with a history of COPD, higher rates of malignancy were reported in COPD patients treated with infliximab. Psoriasis patients with a history of phototherapy had a higher incidence of nonmelanoma skin cancers. Melanoma and Merkel cell carcinoma have been reported in patients receiving TNF-blocking agents including infliximab. Perform periodic skin examinations in all patients during therapy, particularly those at increased risk for skin cancer.

Severe hepatic reactions (including hepatitis, jaundice, acute hepatic failure, and cholestasis) have been reported during treatment; reactions occurred between 2 weeks to >1 year after initiation of therapy and some cases were fatal or necessitated liver transplantation; discontinue with jaundice and/or marked increase in liver enzymes (≥5 times ULN). Use caution with heart failure; if a decision is made to use with heart failure, monitor closely and discontinue if exacerbated or new symptoms occur. Doses >5 mg/kg should not be administered in patients with moderate-to-severe heart failure (NYHA Class III/IV). Use caution with history of hematologic abnormalities; hematologic toxicities (eg, leukopenia, neutropenia, thrombocytopenia, pancytopenia) have been reported (may be fatal); discontinue if significant abnormalities occur. Positive antinuclear antibody titers have been detected in patients (with negative baselines). Rare cases of autoimmune disorder, including lupus-like syndrome, have been reported; monitor and discontinue if symptoms develop. Rare cases of optic neuritis and demyelinating disease (including multiple sclerosis, systemic vasculitis, and Guillain-Barré syndrome) have been reported; use with caution in patients with preexisting or recent onset CNS demyelinating disorders, or seizures; discontinue if significant CNS adverse reactions develop.

Acute infusion reactions may occur. Hypersensitivity reaction may occur within 2 hours of infusion. Medication and equipment for management of hypersensitivity reaction should be available for immediate use. Interruptions and/or reinstitution at a slower rate may be required (consult protocols). Pretreatment may be considered, and may be warranted in all patients with prior infusion reactions. Serum sickness-like reactions have occurred; may be associated with a decreased response to treatment. The development of antibodies to infliximab may increase the risk of hypersensitivity and/or infusion reactions; concomitant use of immunosuppressants may lessen the development of anti-infliximab antibodies. The risk of infusion reactions may be increased with retreatment after an interruption or discontinuation of prior maintenance therapy. Retreatment in psoriasis patients should be resumed as a scheduled maintenance regimen without any induction doses; use of an induction regimen should be used cautiously for retreatment of all other patients.

Efficacy was not established in a study to evaluate infliximab use in juvenile idiopathic arthritis (JIA).

Adverse Reactions

Reported in adults with rheumatoid arthritis:

Cardiovascular: Bradycardia, cardiac arrest, cardiac arrhythmia, cardiac failure, cerebral infarction, circulatory shock, edema, hypertension, hypotension, myocardial infarction, pulmonary embolism, syncope, tachycardia, thrombophlebitis (deep)

Central nervous system: Confusion, dizziness, fatigue, headache, meningitis, neuritis, pain, peripheral neuropathy, seizure, suicidal tendencies

Dermatologic: Cellulitis, diaphoresis, pruritus, skin rash

Endocrine & metabolic: Dehydration, menstrual disease

Gastrointestinal: Abdominal pain (more common in Crohn's patients), biliary colic, cholecystitis, cholelithiasis, constipation, diarrhea, dyspepsia, gastrointestinal hemorrhage, intestinal obstruction, intestinal perforation, intestinal stenosis, nausea, pancreatitis, peritonitis, rectal pain

Genitourinary: Urinary tract infection

Hematologic & oncologic: Anemia, basal cell carcinoma, hemolytic anemia, leukopenia, lymphadenopathy, malignant lymphoma, malignant neoplasm, malignant neoplasm of breast, pancytopenia, sarcoidosis, thrombocytopenia

Hepatic: Hepatitis, increased serum ALT (risk increased with concomitant methotrexate)

Hypersensitivity: Delayed hypersensitivity (plaque psoriasis), hypersensitivity reaction, serum sickness

Immunologic: Antibody development (anti-infliximab; Mayer, 2006), antibody development (double-stranded DNA), increased ANA titer

Infection: Abscess (including Crohn's patients with fistulizing disease), candidiasis, infection, sepsis

Neuromuscular & skeletal: Arthralgia, back pain, herniated disk, lupus-like syndrome, myalgia, tendon disease

Renal: Nephrolithiasis, renal failure

Respiratory: Adult respiratory distress syndrome, bronchitis, cough, dyspnea, pharyngitis, pleural effusion, pleurisy, pulmonary edema, respiratory insufficiency, rhinitis, sinusitis, upper respiratory tract infection

Miscellaneous: Fever, ulcer

The following adverse events were reported in children with Crohn's disease and were more common in children than adults:

Cardiovascular: Flushing

Gastrointestinal: Bloody stools

Hepatic: Increased liver enzymes

Hematologic & oncologic: Anemia, leukopenia, neutropenia

Hypersensitivity: Hypersensitivity reaction (respiratory)

Immunologic: Antibody development (anti-infliximab)

Infection: Bacterial infection, infection (more common with every 8-week vs every 12-week infusions), viral infection

Neuromuscular & skeletal: Bone fracture

Rare but important or life-threatening (adults or children): Agranulocytosis, anaphylactic shock, anaphylaxis, angina pectoris, angioedema, autoimmune hepatitis, cardiac failure (worsening), cholestasis, demyelinating disease of the central nervous system (eg, multiple sclerosis, optic neuritis), demyelinating disease (peripheral; eg, Guillain-Barré syndrome, chronic inflammatory demyelinating polyneuropathy, multifocal motor neuropathy), dysgeusia, erythema multiforme, hepatic carcinoma, hepatic failure, hepatic injury, hepatitis B (reactivation), Hodgkin lymphoma, immune thrombocytopenia, interstitial fibrosis, interstitial pneumonitis, jaundice, leukemia, liver function tests increased, lupus-like syndrome (drug-induced), malignant lymphoma (hepatosplenic T-cell [HSTCL]), malignant melanoma, malignant neoplasm (leiomyosarcoma), Merkel cell carcinoma, neuropathy, opportunistic infection, pericardial effusion, pneumonia, psoriasis (including new onset, palmoplantar, pustular, or exacerbation), reactivated tuberculosis, renal cell carcinoma, seizure, Stevens-Johnson syndrome, thrombotic thrombocytopenia purpura, toxic epidermal necrolysis, transverse myelitis, tuberculosis, vasculitis (systemic and cutaneous)

Drug Interactions

Metabolism/Transport Effects None known.

Avoid Concomitant Use

Avoid concomitant use of InFLIXimab with any of the following: Abatacept; Adalimumab; Anakinra; BCG; Belimumab; Canakinumab; Certolizumab Pegol; Etanercept; Golimumab; Natalizumab; Pimecrolimus; Rilonacept; Tacrolimus (Topical); Tocilizumab; Tofacitinib; Ustekinumab; Vaccines (Live); Vedolizumab

Increased Effect/Toxicity

InFLIXimab may increase the levels/effects of: Abatacept; Anakinra; Belimumab; Canakinumab; Certolizumab Pegol; Leflunomide; Natalizumab; Rilonacept; Tofacitinib; Vaccines (Live); Vedolizumab

The levels/effects of InFLIXimab may be increased by: Adalimumab; Denosumab; Etanercept; Golimumab; Pimecrolimus; Roflumilast; Tacrolimus (Topical); Tocilizumab; Trastuzumab; Ustekinumab

Decreased Effect

InFLIXimab may decrease the levels/effects of: BCG; Coccidioides immitis Skin Test; Sipuleucel-T; Vaccines (Inactivated); Vaccines (Live)

The levels/effects of InFLIXimab may be decreased by: Echinacea

Preparation for Administration Reconstitute vials with 10 mL sterile water for injection. Swirl vial gently to dissolve powder; do not shake. Allow solution to stand for 5 minutes. Total dose of reconstituted product should be further diluted to 250 mL of 0.9% sodium chloride injection to a final concentration of 0.4-4 mg/mL. Infusion of dose should begin within 3 hours of preparation.

Storage/Stability Store vials at 2°C to 8°C (36°F to 46°F).

Mechanism of Action Infliximab is a chimeric monoclonal antibody that binds to human tumor necrosis factor alpha (TNFα), thereby interfering with endogenous TNFα activity. Elevated TNFα levels have been found in involved tissues/fluids of patients with rheumatoid arthritis, ankylosing spondylitis, psoriatic arthritis, plaque psoriasis, Crohn disease and ulcerative colitis. Biological activities of TNFα include the induction of proinflammatory cytokines (interleukins), enhancement of leukocyte migration, activation of neutrophils and eosinophils, and the induction of acute phase reactants and tissue degrading enzymes. Animal models have shown TNFα expression causes polyarthritis, and infliximab can prevent disease as well as allow diseased joints to heal.

Pharmacodynamics/Kinetics

Onset of action: Crohn disease: ~2 weeks

Distribution: V_d: 3-6 L

Half-life elimination: 7-12 days

Dosage IV: **Note:** Premedication with antihistamines (H_1-antagonist +/- H_2-antagonist), acetaminophen, and/or corticosteroids may be considered to prevent and/or manage infusion-related reactions:

Children and Adolescents: U.S. labeling ≥6 years, Canadian labeling ≥9 years: Crohn disease: 5 mg/kg at 0, 2, and 6 weeks, followed by 5 mg/kg every 8 weeks thereafter; if no response by week 14, consider discontinuing therapy

Children ≥6 years and Adolescents: Ulcerative colitis: 5 mg/kg at 0, 2, and 6 weeks, followed by 5 mg/kg every 8 weeks thereafter

Children ≥4 years and Adolescents: Juvenile idiopathic arthritis (off-label use): Initial: 3 mg/kg at 0, 2, and 6 weeks; then 3 to 6 mg/kg/dose every 8 weeks thereafter, in combination with methotrexate during induction and maintenance (Ruperto, 2010). Alternatively, some studies used 6 mg/kg starting at week 14 of a methotrexate induction regimen (weeks 0 to 13); repeat dose (6 mg/kg) at week 16 and 20, then every 8 weeks thereafter (Ruperto, 2007; Visvanathan, 2012).

Adults:

Crohn disease: 5 mg/kg at 0, 2, and 6 weeks, followed by 5 mg/kg every 8 weeks thereafter; dose may be increased to 10 mg/kg in patients who respond but then lose their response. If no response by week 14, consider discontinuing therapy.

Psoriatic arthritis (with or without methotrexate): 5 mg/kg at 0, 2, and 6 weeks, followed by 5 mg/kg every 8 weeks thereafter

Rheumatoid arthritis (in combination with methotrexate therapy): 3 mg/kg at 0, 2, and 6 weeks, followed by 3 mg/kg every 8 weeks thereafter; doses have ranged from 3-10 mg/kg repeated at 4- to 8-week intervals

Ankylosing spondylitis: 5 mg/kg at 0, 2, and 6 weeks, followed by 5 mg/kg every 6 weeks thereafter (Canadian labeling recommends every 6-8 weeks thereafter)

Plaque psoriasis: 5 mg/kg at 0, 2, and 6 weeks, followed by 5 mg/kg every 8 weeks thereafter

Ulcerative colitis: 5 mg/kg at 0, 2, and 6 weeks, followed by 5 mg/kg every 8 weeks thereafter

Dosage adjustment with heart failure (HF): Weigh risk versus benefits for individual patient:

Moderate-to-severe HF (NYHA Class III or IV): ≤5 mg/kg

Dosage adjustment in renal impairment: There are no dosage adjustments provided in the manufacturer's labeling.

Dosage adjustment in hepatic impairment: There are no dosage adjustments provided in the manufacturer's labeling.

Administration The infusion should begin within 3 hours of reconstitution and dilution. Infuse over at least 2 hours; do not infuse with other agents; use in-line low protein binding filter (≤1.2 micron). Temporarily discontinue or decrease infusion rate with infusion-related reactions. Antihistamines (H_1-antagonist +/- H_2-antagonist), acetaminophen and/or corticosteroids may be used to manage reactions. Infusion may be reinitiated at a lower rate upon resolution of mild-to-moderate symptoms.

Canadian labeling (not approved in U.S. labeling): Infusion of doses ≤6 mg/kg over not less than 1 hour may be considered in patients treated for rheumatoid arthritis who have initially tolerated 3 infusions each over 2 hours. Safety of shortened infusion has not been studied with doses >6 mg/kg.

Guidelines for the treatment and prophylaxis of infusion reactions: (**Note:** Limited to adult patients and dosages used in Crohn disease; prospective data for other populations [pediatrics, other indications/dosing] are not available).

A protocol for the treatment of infusion reactions, as well as prophylactic therapy for repeat infusions, has been published (Mayer, 2006).

Treatment of infusion reactions: Medications for the treatment of hypersensitivity reactions should be available for immediate use. For mild reactions, the rate of infusion should be decreased to 10 mL/hour. Initiate a normal saline infusion (500-1000 mL/hour) and appropriate symptomatic treatment (eg, acetaminophen and diphenhydramine); monitor vital signs every 10 minutes until normal. After 20 minutes, the infusion may be increased at 15-minute intervals, as tolerated, to completion (initial increase to 20 mL/hour, then 40 mL/hour, then 80 mL/hour, etc [maximum of 125 mL/hour]). For moderate reactions, the infusion should be stopped or slowed. Initiate a normal saline infusion (500-1000 mL/hour) and appropriate symptomatic treatment. Monitor vital signs every 5 minutes until normal. After 20 minutes, the infusion may be reinstituted at 10 mL/hour; then increased at 15-minute intervals, as tolerated, to completion (initial increase 20 mL/hour, then 40 mL/hour, then 80 mL/hour, etc [maximum of 125 mL/hour]). For severe reactions, the infusion should be stopped with administration of appropriate symptomatic treatment (eg, hydrocortisone/methylprednisolone, diphenhydramine and epinephrine) and frequent monitoring of vitals (consult institutional policies, if available). Retreatment after a severe reaction should only be done if the benefits outweigh the risks and with appropriate prophylaxis. Delayed infusion reactions typically occur 1-7 days after an infusion. Treatment should consist of appropriate symptomatic treatment (eg, acetaminophen, antihistamine, methylprednisolone).

Prophylaxis of infusion reactions: Premedication with acetaminophen and diphenhydramine 90 minutes prior to infusion may be considered in all patients with prior infusion reactions, and in patients with severe reactions corticosteroid administration is recommended. Steroid dosing may be oral (prednisone 50 mg orally every 12 hours for 3 doses prior to infusion) or intravenous (a single dose of hydrocortisone 100 mg or methylprednisolone 20-40 mg administered 20 minutes prior to the infusion). On initiation of the infusion, begin with a test dose at 10 mL/hour for 15 minutes. Thereafter, the infusion may be increased at 15-minute intervals, as tolerated, to completion (initial increase 20 mL/hour, then 40 mL/hour, then 80 mL/hour, etc). A maximum rate of 125 mL/hour is recommended in patients who experienced prior mild-moderate reactions and 100 mL/hour is recommended in patients who experienced prior severe reactions. In patients with cutaneous flushing, aspirin may be considered (Becker, 2004). For delayed infusion reactions, premedicate with acetaminophen and diphenhydramine 90 minutes prior to infusion. On initiation of the infusion, begin with a test dose at 10 mL/hour for 15 minutes. Thereafter, the infusion may be increased to infuse over 3 hours. Postinfusion therapy with acetaminophen for 3 days and an antihistamine for 7 days is recommended.

Monitoring Parameters Monitor improvement of symptoms and physical function assessments. During infusion, if reaction is noted, monitor vital signs every 2-10 minutes, depending on reaction severity, until normal. Latent TB screening prior to initiating and during therapy; signs/symptoms of infection (prior to, during, and following therapy); CBC with differential; signs/symptoms/worsening of heart failure; HBV screening prior to initiating (all patients), HBV carriers (during and for several months following therapy); signs and symptoms of hypersensitivity reaction; symptoms of lupus-like syndrome; LFTs (discontinue if >5 times ULN); signs and symptoms of malignancy (eg, splenomegaly, hepatomegaly, abdominal pain, persistent fever, night sweats, weight loss).

Psoriasis patients with history of phototherapy should be monitored for nonmelanoma skin cancer.

Dosage Forms

Solution Reconstituted, Intravenous [preservative free]:

Remicade: 100 mg (1 ea)

◆ **Infliximab, Recombinant** *see* InFLIXimab *on page 1070*

Influenza A Virus Vaccine (H5N1)

(in floo EN za aye VYE rus vak SEEN H5N1)

Index Terms Avian Influenza Virus Vaccine; Bird Flu Vaccine; H5N1 Influenza Vaccine; Highly Pathogenic Avian Influenza (HPAI) A (H5N1) Virus Vaccine; Influenza Virus Vaccine (H5N1); Influenza Virus Vaccine (Monovalent); Q-Pan H5N1 Influenza Vaccine

Pharmacologic Category Vaccine, Inactivated (Viral)

Additional Appendix Information

Immunization Administration Recommendations *on page 2250*

Immunization Recommendations *on page 2255*

Use Influenza A (H5N1) immunization:

GlaxoSmithKline product (adjuvanted): For active immunization of persons ≥18 years of age at increased risk of exposure to the influenza A (H5N1) virus subtype contained in the vaccine

Sanofi Pasteur product: For active immunization of persons 18-64 years of age at increased risk of exposure to the influenza A (H5N1) virus subtype contained in the vaccine

Pregnancy Risk Factor B/C (product specific)

Pregnancy Considerations Adverse events were not observed in animal reproduction studies using the H5N1 vaccine GlaxoSmithKline adjuvanted product; animal reproduction studies have not been conducted with the Sanofi Pasteur product. Inactivated viral vaccines have not been shown to cause increased risks to the fetus (CDC, 2011).

Breast-Feeding Considerations It is not known if this vaccine is excreted into breast milk. Inactivated virus vaccines do not affect the safety of breast-feeding for the mother or the infant (CDC, 2011).

Contraindications

GlaxoSmithKline product (adjuvanted): Known severe allergic reactions (eg, anaphylaxis) to any component of the vaccine, including egg protein, or after a previous dose of an influenza vaccine.

Sanofi Pasteur product: There are no contraindications listed in the manufacturer's labeling.

Warnings/Precautions Immediate treatment (including epinephrine 1:1000) for anaphylactoid and/or hypersensitivity reactions should be available during vaccine use. Use with caution in patients with a history of Guillain-Barré syndrome (GBS); these patients may have a greater likelihood of developing GBS. If recent occurrence of GBS (≤6 weeks), decision to administer vaccine should entail careful consideration of risk:benefit. Recent studies of patients who received the trivalent inactivated influenza vaccine or the monovalent H1N1 influenza vaccine have shown the risk of GBS is lower with vaccination than with influenza infection (Baxter, 2013; Greene, 2013; Kwong, 2013). Vaccination may not result in effective immunity in all patients. Response depends upon multiple factors (eg, type of vaccine, age of patient) and may be improved by administering the vaccine at the recommended dose, route, and interval. Vaccines may not be effective if administered during periods of altered immune competence (CDC, 2011). Use with caution in severely immunocompromised patients (eg, patients receiving chemo/radiation therapy or other immunosuppressive therapy [including high-dose corticosteroids]); may have a reduced response to vaccination (CDC, 2011). In general, household and close contacts of persons with altered immunocompetence may receive all age appropriate vaccines (CDC, 2011); inactivated vaccines should be administered ≥2 weeks prior to planned immunosuppression when feasible (Rubin, 2014). Syncope has been reported with use of injectable vaccines and may be accompanied by transient visual disturbances, weakness, or tonic-clonic movements. Procedures should be in place to avoid injuries from falling and to restore cerebral perfusion if syncope occurs. Sanofi Pasteur product has not been evaluated in patients ≥65 years of age. Some products may be manufactured with chicken egg protein. Some products may contain thimerosal; hypersensitivity reactions may occur

Adverse Reactions All serious adverse reactions must be reported to the U.S. Department of Health and Human Services (DHHS) Vaccine Adverse Event Reporting System (VAERS) 1-800-822-7967 or online at https://vaers.hhs.gov/esub/index.

Central nervous system: Fatigue, headache, shivering

Dermatologic: Diaphoresis

Gastrointestinal: Diarrhea, nausea

Local: Burning sensation at injection site, erythema at injection site, itching at injection site, pain at injection site, swelling at injection site, tenderness at injection site

Neuromuscular & skeletal: Arthralgia, myalgia

Respiratory: Nasal congestion

Miscellaneous: Fever

<1% (Limited to important or life-threatening): Celiac disease, cerebrovascular accident, convulsions, cranial nerve palsy (IV), Crohn's disease, erythema nodosum, facial paralysis, giant-cell arteritis, hepatitis, malignant neoplasm of thyroid, organ transplant rejection (corneal), polymyalgia rheumatica, psoriasis, pulmonary embolism, radiculopathy, rheumatoid arthritis, rheumatoid lung

Drug Interactions

Metabolism/Transport Effects None known.

Avoid Concomitant Use There are no known interactions where it is recommended to avoid concomitant use.

Increased Effect/Toxicity There are no known significant interactions involving an increase in effect.

Decreased Effect

The levels/effects of Influenza A Virus Vaccine (H5N1) may be decreased by: Belimumab; Immunosuppressants

Preparation for Administration GlaxoSmithKline product (adjuvanted): Prior to mixing, bring one vial of H5N1 antigen and one vial of AS03 adjuvant to room temperature (minimum of 15 minutes). Invert each vial to mix; do not use if particulate matter or discoloration are present. Withdraw contents of adjuvant vial and add to the H5N1 antigen vial. Mix thoroughly by inversion and label with the time and date of mixing on vial. After mixing, the final volume provides 10 doses (0.5 mL each). Use within 24 hours of mixing.

Storage/Stability

Sanofi Pasteur product: Store in a refrigerator at 2°C to 8°C (35°F to 46°F). Do not freeze. Discard if frozen. Protect from light.

GlaxoSmithKline product (adjuvanted): Prior to mixing, the H5N1 antigen and AS03 adjuvant vials should be stored in a refrigerator between 2°C and 8°C (36°F and 46°F). Do not freeze. Discard if frozen. Protect from light. After mixing, the vaccine may be stored under refrigeration between 2°C and 8°C (36°F and 46°F) or at room temperature up to 30°C (86°F) for up to 24 hours. Do not freeze. Discard if frozen. Protect from light.

Mechanism of Action

The GlaxoSmithKline product is an adjuvanted monovalent split virus (inactivated) preparation of the type A, subtype H5N1 avian strain of influenza virus (A/Indonesia/05/2005)

The Sanofi Pasteur product is a monovalent, split virus (inactivated) preparation of the type A, subtype H5N1 avian strain of influenza virus (A/Vietnam/1203/2004)

Both promote active immunity to influenza A H5N1 (avian).

Pharmacodynamics/Kinetics Onset of action:

GlaxoSmithKline product (adjuvanted): Fourfold increase in antibody titers (measured by hemagglutination inhibition [HI]) occurred in up to 90% of patients 18-64 years of age and 74% of patients ≥65 years of age 21 days after the second dose

Sanofi Pasteur product: Fourfold increase in antibody titers (measured by HI) occurred in up to 58% of patients 28 days after the second dose (Treanor, 2006).

Dosage IM: Immunization:

GlaxoSmithKline product (adjuvanted): Adults ≥18 years: 0.5 mL, followed by a second 0.5 mL dose given 21 days later

Sanofi Pasteur product: Adults 18-64 years: 1 mL, followed by second 1 mL dose given 28 days later (acceptable range: 21-35 days)

Dosage adjustment in renal impairment: No dosage adjustment provided in manufacturer's labeling.

Dosage adjustment in hepatic impairment: No dosage adjustment provided in manufacturer's labeling.

Administration For IM administration only. Inspect for particulate matter and discoloration prior to administration. Vaccinate in the deltoid muscle using a ≥1 inch needle length. Suspension should be shaken well prior to use.

GlaxoSmithKline product (adjuvanted): If vaccine is stored under refrigeration after mixing, bring to room temperature prior to administration (minimum 15 minutes).

Note: For patients at risk of hemorrhage following intramuscular injection, the ACIP recommends "it should be administered intramuscularly if, in the opinion of the physician familiar with the patient's bleeding risk, the vaccine can be administered by this route with reasonable safety. If the patient receives antihemophilia or other similar therapy, intramuscular vaccination can be scheduled shortly after such therapy is administered. A fine needle (23 gauge or smaller) can be used for the vaccination and firm pressure applied to the site (without rubbing) for at least 2 minutes. The patient should be instructed concerning the risk of hematoma from the injection." Patients on anticoagulant therapy should be considered to have the same bleeding risks and treated as those with clotting factor disorders (CDC, 2011).

Simultaneous administration of vaccines helps ensure the patients will be fully vaccinated by the appropriate age. Simultaneous administration of vaccines is defined as administering >1 vaccine on the same day at different anatomic sites. Separate vaccines should not be combined in the same syringe unless indicated by product specific labeling. Separate needles and syringes should be used for each injection. The ACIP prefers each dose of a specific vaccine in a series come from the same manufacturer when possible. Adolescents and adults should be vaccinated while seated or lying down. In general, preterm infants should be vaccinated at the same chronological age as full-term infants (CDC, 2011).

Antipyretics have not been shown to prevent febrile seizures. Antipyretics may be used to treat fever or discomfort following vaccination (CDC, 2011). One study reported that routine prophylactic administration of acetaminophen to prevent fever prior to vaccination decreased the immune response of some vaccines; the clinical significance of this reduction in immune response has not been established (Prymula, 2009).

Monitoring Parameters Monitor for syncope for 15 minutes following administration. If seizure-like activity associated with syncope occurs, maintain patient in supine or Trendelenburg position to reestablish adequate cerebral perfusion (CDC, 2011).

Additional Information U.S. federal law requires that the name of medication, date of administration, the vaccine manufacturer, lot number of vaccine, and the administering person's name, title, and address be entered into the patient's permanent medical record.

Because there are many strains of the H5N1 virus, multiple vaccines are under development. The antibody level needed for protection is not well established (Abdel-Ghafar, 2008) and a fourfold increase in hemagglutination inhibition antibody titers is generally used to measure immune response in clinical trials. The 2-dose regimen studied using H5N1 vaccine (Sanofi Pasteur product) prompted antibody response consistent with a protective titer in up to 58% of patients (Treanor, 2006). A second study has shown that a third dose of the vaccine further increases the antibody response (Zangwill, 2008). The GlaxoSmithKline product (adjuvanted) was shown to increase the immune response while sparing the amount of antigen needed per dose. This would allow for more vaccine to be produced using available antigen; however, the risk of adverse events was also increased (Langley, 2011).

Health care workers involved in the care of patients with known or suspected H5N1 viral subtype influenza infection should be vaccinated with the most recent seasonal human influenza vaccine in order to reduce the risk of coinfection of human influenza A viruses (OSHA, 2006).

Product Availability Products will not be commercially available; distribution will be limited as part of the U.S. Strategic National Stockpile.

GlaxoSmithKline product (adjuvanted) product, (also referred to as Q-Pan H5N1 influenza vaccine): FDA approved November 2013.

Dosage Forms

Injection, emulsion [monovalent]: GlaxoSmithKline product: Adjuvanted Hemagglutinin [A/Indonesia/05/2005 (H5N1)] 3.75 mcg/0.5 mL (5 mL)

Injection, suspension [monovalent]: Sanofi Pasteur product: Hemagglutinin [A/Vietnam/1203/2004 (H5N1)] 90 mcg/mL (5 mL)

◆ **Influenza Vaccine** *see* Influenza Virus Vaccine (Inactivated) *on page 1075*

◆ **Influenza Vaccine** *see* Influenza Virus Vaccine (Live/Attenuated) *on page 1080*

◆ **Influenza Virus Vaccine (H5N1)** *see* Influenza A Virus Vaccine (H5N1) *on page 1074*

Influenza Virus Vaccine (Inactivated)

(in floo EN za VYE rus vak SEEN, in ak ti VAY ted)

Brand Names: U.S. Afluria; Afluria Preservative Free; Fluarix; Fluarix Quadrivalent; Flucelvax; Flulaval; Flulaval Quadrivalent; Fluvirin; Fluvirin Preservative Free; Fluzone; Fluzone High-Dose; Fluzone Pediatric PF [DSC]; Fluzone Preservative Free; Fluzone Quadrivalent; Medical Provider EZ Flu; Medical Provider EZ Flu PF; Physicians EZ Use Flu

Brand Names: Canada Agriflu; Fluad; Fluviral; Fluzone; Fluzone Quadrivalent; Influvac; Intanza; Vaxigrip

Index Terms ccIIV3 [Flucelvax]; Cell Culture Inactivated Influenza Vaccine, Trivalent [Flucelvax]; H1N1 Influenza Vaccine; IIV; IIV3; IIV4; Inactivated Influenza Vaccine, Quadrivalent; Inactivated Influenza Vaccine, Trivalent; Influenza Vaccine; Influenza Virus Vaccine (Purified Surface Antigen); Influenza Virus Vaccine (Split-Virus); TIV (Trivalent Inactivated Influenza Vaccine)

Pharmacologic Category Vaccine, Inactivated (Viral)

Additional Appendix Information

Immunization Administration Recommendations *on page 2250*

Immunization Recommendations *on page 2255*

Use Influenza disease prevention: Active immunization against influenza disease caused by influenza virus subtypes A and type B contained in the vaccine

The Advisory Committee on Immunization Practices (ACIP) recommends routine annual vaccination with the seasonal influenza vaccine for all persons ≥6 months of age who do not otherwise have contraindications to the vaccine (CDC/ACIP [Grohskopf, 2014]).

The ACIP recommends use of any age and risk factor appropriate product and does not have a preferential recommendation for use of the trivalent inactivated influenza vaccine (IIV_3) or the quadrivalent inactivated influenza vaccine (IIV_4). In addition to the IIV products, other alternative products are available for certain patient populations: Healthy nonpregnant persons aged 2 to 49 years may receive vaccination with the live attenuated influenza vaccine (LAIV). When readily available, LAIV is the preferred vaccine for healthy children aged 2 to 8 years who do not have contraindications or precautions; immunization should not be delayed to allow for acquisition of LAIV. Persons 18 years and older may receive vaccination with the recombinant influenza vaccine (RIV) (CDC 62[07], 2013; CDC/ACIP [Grohskopf, 2014]).

When vaccine supply is limited, target groups for vaccination (those at higher risk of complications from influenza infection and their close contacts) include the following (CDC 62[07], 2013):

- Children 6 to 59 months of age
- Persons ≥50 years of age
- Residents of nursing homes and other long-term care facilities
- Adults and children with chronic pulmonary disorders (including asthma) or cardiovascular systems disorders (except hypertension), renal, hepatic, neurologic, or metabolic disorders (including diabetes mellitus)
- Persons who have immunosuppression (including immunosuppression caused by medications or HIV)
- Children and adolescents (6 months to 18 years of age) who are receiving long-term aspirin therapy, and therefore, may be at risk for developing Reye's syndrome after influenza
- Women who are or will be pregnant during the influenza season
- Healthcare personnel
- Household contacts (including children) and caregivers of children <5 years (particularly children <6 months) and adults ≥50 years
- Household contacts (including children) and caregivers of persons with medical conditions which put them at high risk of complications from influenza infection
- American Indians/Alaska Natives
- Morbidly obese (BMI ≥40)

Pregnancy Risk Factor B/C (manufacturer specific)

Pregnancy Considerations Adverse events were not observed in animal reproduction studies. Inactivated influenza vaccine has not been shown to cause fetal harm when given to pregnant women, although information related to use in the first trimester is limited (CDC 62[07], 2013). Following maternal immunization with the inactivated influenza virus vaccine, vaccine specific antibodies are observed in the newborn (Englund, 1993; Steinhoff, 2010; Zaman, 2008; Zuccotti, 2010). Vaccination of pregnant women protects infants from influenza infection, including infants <6 months of age who are not able to be vaccinated (CDC 62[07], 2013).

Pregnant women are at an increased risk of complications from influenza infection (Rasmussen, 2008). Influenza vaccination with the inactivated influenza vaccine (IIV) is recommended for all women who are or will become pregnant during the influenza season and who do not otherwise have contraindications to the vaccine (CDC 62 [07], 2013). Pregnant women should observe the same precautions as nonpregnant women to reduce the risk of exposure to influenza and other respiratory infections (CDC, 2010). When vaccine supply is limited, focus on delivering the vaccine should be given to women who are pregnant or will be pregnant during the flu season, as well as mothers of newborns and contacts or caregivers of children <5 years of age (CDC 62[07], 2013)

Healthcare providers are encouraged to refer women exposed to the influenza vaccine during pregnancy to the Vaccines and Medications in Pregnancy Surveillance System (VAMPSS) by contacting The Organization of Teratology Information Specialists (OTIS) at (877) 311-8972.

Women exposed to Flulaval, Flulaval Quadrivalent, Fluarix, or Fluarix Quadrivalent vaccine during pregnancy or their healthcare provider may also contact the GlaxoSmithKline registry at 888-452-9622.

Healthcare providers may enroll women exposed to Fluzone Intradermal or Fluzone Quadrivalent during pregnancy in the Sanofi Pasteur vaccination registry at 800-822-2463.

Breast-Feeding Considerations It is not known if inactivated influenza vaccine is excreted into breast milk. The manufacturers recommend that caution be used if administered to nursing women. Anti-influenza IgA antibodies can be detected in breast milk following maternal vaccination with the trivalent IIV vaccine (Schlaudecker, 2013). Inactivated vaccines do not affect the safety of breastfeeding for the mother or the infant (NCIRD/ACIP, 2011). Postpartum women may be vaccinated with either IIV or LAIV (CDC 62[07], 2013). When vaccine supply is limited, focus on delivering the vaccine should be given to women who are pregnant or will be pregnant during the flu season, as well as mothers of newborns and contacts or caregivers of children <5 years of age (CDC 62[07], 2013). Breastfeeding infants should be vaccinated according to the recommended schedules (NCIRD/ACIP, 2011).

Contraindications Severe allergic reaction (eg, anaphylaxis) to a previous influenza vaccination; hypersensitivity to any component of the formulation

Additional manufacturer contraindications for Afluria, Fluarix, Fluarix Quadrivalent, FluLaval, FluLaval Quadrivalent, Fluvirin, Fluzone, Fluzone High-Dose, Fluzone Intradermal, Fluzone Intradermal Quadrivalent, Fluzone Quadrivalent: History of severe allergic reaction (eg, anaphylaxis) to egg protein

Fluviral (not available in U.S.): Canadian labeling: Additional contraindications: Presence of acute respiratory infection, other active infections, or serious febrile illness

Warnings/Precautions Immediate treatment (including epinephrine 1:1000) for anaphylactoid and/or hypersensitivity reactions should be available during vaccine use. Oculorespiratory syndrome (ORS) is an acute, self-limiting reaction to IIV with one or more of the following symptoms appearing within 2 to 24 hours after the dose: Chest tightness, cough, difficulty breathing, facial swelling, red eyes, sore throat, or wheezing. Symptoms resolve within 48 hours of onset. The cause of ORS has not been established, but studies have suggested that it is not IgE-mediated. However, because ORS symptoms may be similar to those of an IgE-mediated hypersensitivity reaction, health care providers unsure of etiology of symptoms should seek advice from an allergist/immunologist when determining whether a patient may be revaccinated in subsequent seasons (CDC 62[07], 2013).

Most products are manufactured with chicken egg protein (expressed as ovalbumin content when content is disclosed on prescribing information). The ovalbumin content may vary from season to season and lot to lot of vaccine. Allergy to eggs must be distinguished from allergy to the vaccine. Recommendations are available from the ACIP and NACI regarding influenza vaccination to persons who report egg allergies; however, ACIP states a prior severe allergic reaction to influenza vaccine, regardless of the component suspected, is a contraindication to vaccination. Patients with a history of egg allergy who have experienced only hives following egg exposure should receive influenza vaccine using IIV (egg- or cell-culture based) or RIV, if otherwise appropriate; however, the vaccine should only be administered by a health care provider familiar with the manifestations of egg allergy and patients be monitored for at least 30 minutes after vaccination (CDC/ACIP [Grohskopf, 2014]). NACI does not consider an egg allergy as a contraindication to vaccination (NACI July 2014). Flucelvax ($ccIIV_3$) is an inactivated influenza vaccine manufactured using cell culture technology and provides an alternative to vaccines cultured with chicken egg protein but should not be considered egg free. It may be used in persons with a mild egg allergy if age appropriate and there are no other contraindications; appropriate precautions should be observed (CDC/ACIP [Grohskopf, 2014]). Some products are manufactured with gentamicin, kanamycin, neomycin, polymyxin or thimerosal; some packaging may contain natural latex rubber.

Some dosage forms may contain polysorbate 80 (also known as Tweens). Hypersensitivity reactions, usually a delayed reaction, have been reported following exposure to pharmaceutical products containing polysorbate 80 in certain individuals (Isaksson, 2002; Lucente 2000; Shelley, 1995). Thrombocytopenia, ascites, pulmonary deterioration, and renal and hepatic failure have been reported in premature neonates after receiving parenteral products containing polysorbate 80 (Alade, 1986; CDC, 1984). See manufacturer's labeling.

May consider deferring administration in patients with moderate or severe acute illness (with or without fever); may administer to patients with mild acute illness (with or without fever) (NCIRD/ACIP, 2011). Postmarketing reports of increased incidence of fever and febrile seizures in children <5 years of age has been observed with the use of the 2010 Southern Hemisphere formulation of the Afluria vaccine. Febrile events have also been reported in children 5 to <9 years of age. Based on information from the CDC, an increased rate of febrile seizures has been reported in young children 6 months to 4 years who received vaccination with inactivated influenza vaccine (IIV) and the 13-valent pneumococcal conjugate vaccine (PCV13) simultaneously. However, due to the risks associated with delaying either vaccine, administering them at separate visits or deviating from the recommended vaccine schedule is not currently recommended. The ACIP does not recommend use of Afluria in children <9 years of age (CDC 62[07], 2013, CDC/ACIP [Grohskopf, 2014]). Syncope has been reported with use of injectable vaccines and may be accompanied by transient visual disturbances, weakness, or tonic-clonic movements. Procedures should be in place to avoid injuries from falling and to restore cerebral perfusion if syncope occurs (CDC 57[17], 2008).

Use with caution in patients with history of Guillain-Barré syndrome (GBS); patients with history of GBS have a greater likelihood of developing GBS than those without. As a precaution, the ACIP recommends that patients with a history of GBS and who are at low risk for severe influenza complications, and patients known to have experienced GBS within 6 weeks following previous vaccination should generally not be vaccinated (consider influenza antiviral chemoprophylaxis in these patients). The benefits of vaccination may outweigh the potential risks in persons with a history of GBS who are also at high risk for complications of influenza (CDC 62[07], 2013). Recent studies of patients who received the trivalent inactivated influenza vaccine or the monovalent H1N1 influenza vaccine have shown the risk of GBS is lower with vaccination than with influenza infection (Baxter, 2013; Greene, 2013; Kwong, 2013). Some Canadian product labeling recommends delaying therapy in patients with active neurologic disorders.

Use with caution in severely immunocompromised patients (eg, patients receiving chemo/radiation therapy or other immunosuppressive therapy [including high-dose corticosteroid]); may have a reduced response to vaccination. Inactivated vaccine (IIV or RIV) is preferred over live virus vaccine for household members, healthcare workers and others coming in close contact with severely-immunosuppressed persons requiring care in a protected environment (CDC/ACIP [Grohskopf, 2014]; NCIRD/ACIP, 2011). In general, inactivated vaccines should be administered ≥2 weeks prior to planned immunosuppression when feasible (IDSA [Rubin, 2014]). Antigenic response may not be as great as expected in HIV-infected persons with CD4 cells <100/mm^3 and viral copies of HIV type 1 >30,000/mL, and a second dose does not improve immune response in these persons (CDC 62[07], 2013). Antibody responses may be lower and decline faster in older adults ≥65 years compared to younger adults, especially by 6 months postvaccination; however, deferral to later in the season may result in missed vaccination opportunities or early season infection (CDC/ACIP [Grohskopf, 2014]). Use of this vaccine for specific medical and/or other indications (eg, immunocompromising conditions, hepatic or kidney disease, diabetes) is also addressed in the ACIP Recommended Immunization Schedule (CDC/ACIP [Akinsanya-Beysolow, 2014]; CDC/ACIP [Bridges, 2014];). Specific recommendations for use of this vaccine in immunocompromised patients with asplenia, cancer, HIV infection, cerebrospinal fluid leaks, cochlear implants, hematopoietic stem cell transplant (prior to or after), sickle cell disease, solid organ transplant (prior to or after), or those receiving immunosuppressive therapy for chronic conditions are available from the IDSA (Rubin, 2013).

Use with caution in patients with a history of bleeding disorders (including thrombocytopenia) and/or patients on anticoagulant therapy; bleeding/hematoma may occur from IM administration (NCIRD/ACIP, 2011). In order to maximize vaccination rates, the ACIP, as well as the Canadian National Advisory Committee on Immunization (NACI), recommends simultaneous administration of all age-appropriate vaccines (live or inactivated) for which a person is eligible at a single clinic visit, unless contraindications exist (NACI July 2014; NCIRD/ACIP, 2011). Vaccination may not result in effective immunity in all patients. Response depends upon multiple factors (eg, type of vaccine, age of patient) and may be improved by administering the vaccine at the recommended dose, route, and interval. Vaccines may not be effective if administered during periods of altered immune competence (NCIRD/ACIP, 2011). Influenza vaccines from previous seasons must not be used (CDC 62[07], 2013).

Adverse Reactions All serious adverse reactions must be reported to the U.S. Department of Health and Human Services (DHHS) Vaccine Adverse Event Reporting System (VAERS) 1-800-822-7967 or online at https://vaers.hhs.gov/esub/index. In Canada, adverse reactions may be reported to local provincial/territorial health agencies or to the Vaccine Safety Section at Public Health Agency of Canada (1-866-844-0018).

Adverse reactions in adults ≥65 years of age may be greater using the high-dose vaccine, but are typically mild and transient.

Cardiovascular: Chest tightness, facial edema

Central nervous system: Chills, drowsiness, fatigue, fever, headache, irritability, malaise, migraine, shivering

Endocrine & metabolic: Dysmenorrhea

Gastrointestinal: Appetite decreased, diarrhea, nausea, sore throat, upper abdominal pain, vomiting

Local: Injection site reactions (including bruising, erythema, induration, inflammation, pain, soreness [≤64%; may last up to 2 days], pruritus, swelling, tenderness)
Neuromuscular & skeletal: Arthralgia, back pain, myalgia (may start within 6-12 hours and last 1-2 days; incidence generally equal to placebo in adults; occurs more frequently than placebo in children)
Ocular: Red eyes
Otic: Earache
Respiratory: Cough, nasal congestion, nasopharyngitis, pharyngolaryngeal pain, rhinitis, upper respiratory tract infection, wheezing
Miscellaneous: Diaphoresis

Rare but important or life-threatening: Allergic reactions, anaphylaxis, angioedema, convulsions, erythema multiforme, facial palsy (Bell's palsy), Guillain-Barré syndrome (GBS), Henoch-Schönlein purpura (IgA vasculitis), hypersensitivity reaction, limb paralysis, lymphadenopathy, myelitis (including encephalomyelitis and transverse myelitis), neuralgia, oculorespiratory syndrome (ORS; acute, self-limited reaction with ocular and respiratory symptoms), optic neuritis/neuropathy, paralysis, photophobia, serum sickness, Stevens-Johnson syndrome, syncope, tachycardia, thrombocytopenia, urticaria, vasculitis, vertigo

Drug Interactions

Metabolism/Transport Effects None known.

Avoid Concomitant Use There are no known interactions where it is recommended to avoid concomitant use.

Increased Effect/Toxicity There are no known significant interactions involving an increase in effect.

Decreased Effect

Influenza Virus Vaccine (Inactivated) may decrease the levels/effects of: Pneumococcal Conjugate Vaccine (13-Valent)

The levels/effects of Influenza Virus Vaccine (Inactivated) may be decreased by: Belimumab; Immunosuppressants; Pneumococcal Conjugate Vaccine (13-Valent)

Storage/Stability Store all products between 2°C to 8°C (36°F to 46°F). Potency is destroyed by freezing; do not use if product has been frozen.

Afluria: Discard multiple dose vials 28 days after initial entry. Between uses, the multiple dose vial should be stored at 2°C to 8°C (36°F to 46°F).

Fluarix, Fluarix Quadrivalent, Flucelvax: Protect from light.

Agriflu, Fluad: Protect from light. May be used if exposed to temperatures between 8°C to 25°C for less than 2 hours.

FluLaval, Fluviral: Discard multiple dose vials 28 days after initial entry. Protect from light.

Flulaval Quadrivalent: Between uses, the multiple dose vial should be stored at 2°C to 8°C (36°F to 46°F). Protect from light. Discard multiple dose vials 28 days after initial entry.

Fluvirin: Between uses, the multiple dose vial should be stored at 2°C to 8°C (36°F to 46°F). Protect from light.

Fluzone: Between uses, the multiple dose vial should be stored at 2°C to 8°C (36°F to 46°F).

Vaxigrip: Between uses, the multiple dose vial should be stored at 2°C to 8°C (36°F to 46°F). Discard 7 days after initial entry. Protect from light.

Mechanism of Action Promotes immunity to seasonal influenza virus by inducing specific antibody production. Each year the formulation is standardized according to the U.S. Public Health Service. Preparations from previous seasons must not be used.

Pharmacodynamics/Kinetics

Onset of action: Most adults have antibody protection within 2 weeks of vaccination (CDC 62[07], 2013)

Duration: ≥6 to 8 months when vaccine is antigenically similar to circulating virus (CDC 62[07], 2013); response may be diminished in persons ≥65 years and limited evidence suggests titers may decline significantly 6 months following vaccination in this population (CDC/ACIP [Grohskopf, 2014]).

Dosage It is important to note that influenza seasons vary in their timing and duration from year to year. In general, vaccination should begin soon after the vaccine becomes available (and, if possible, by October) and prior to onset of influenza activity in the community. However, vaccination should continue throughout the influenza season as long as vaccine is available. Unless noted, the ACIP does not have a preference for any given inactivated influenza vaccine (IIV) formulation when used within their specified age indications.

Fluarix, Fluarix Quadrivalent, FluLaval, FluLaval Quadrivalent: IM:
Children 3 to 8 years: 0.5 mL/dose (1 or 2 doses per season; see **"Note"**)
Children ≥9 years years, Adolescents, and Adults: 0.5 mL/dose (1 dose per season)

Fluzone, Fluzone Quadrivalent: IM:
Children 6 to 35 months: 0.25 mL/dose (1 or 2 doses per season; see **"Note"**)
Children 3 to 8 years: 0.5 mL/dose (1 or 2 doses per season; see **"Note"**)
Children ≥9 years years, Adolescents, and Adults: 0.5 mL/dose (1 dose per season)

Fluzone High-Dose: IM: Adults ≥65 years: 0.5 mL/dose (1 dose per season)

Fluvirin: IM:
Children 4 to 8 years: 0.5 mL/dose (1 or 2 doses per season; see **"Note"**)
Children ≥9 years years, Adolescents, and Adults: 0.5 mL/dose (1 dose per season)

Afluria: Although FDA-approved for use in children ≥5 years of age, the ACIP does not recommend use of Afluria in children <9 years due to an increased incidence of fever and febrile seizures noted during the 2010 to 2011 influenza season. However, if other age-appropriate vaccines are not available, children 5 to 8 years of age who are also considered at risk for influenza complications may be given Afluria. The benefits and risks of this vaccine should be discussed with parents or caregivers prior to administration (CDC/ACIP [Grohskopf, 2014]).
Children 5 to 8 years: IM: 0.5 mL/dose (1 or 2 doses per season; see **"Note"**)
Children ≥9 years and Adolescents <18 years: IM: 0.5 mL/dose (1 dose per season)
Adolescents and Adults 18 to 64 years: IM or via PharmaJet Stratis Needle-Free Injection System: 0.5 mL per dose as a single dose (1 dose per season)
Adults >64 years: IM: 0.5 mL per dose as a single dose (1 dose per season)

Flucelvax: IM: Adults: 0.5 mL/dose (1 dose per season)

Fluzone Intradermal, Fluzone Intradermal Quadrivalent: Adults 18 to 64 years of age: Intradermal: 0.1 mL/dose (1 dose per season)

Canadian labeling (products not available in U.S.):

Agriflu, Fluviral, Vaxigrip: IM:
Children 6 to 35 months: Manufacturer labeling: 0.25 mL/dose; NACI recommendation: 0.5 mL/dose (NACI, 2014) (1 or 2 doses per season; see **"Note"**)
Children 3 to 8 years: 0.5 mL/dose (1 or 2 doses per season; see **"Note"**)
Children ≥9 years, Adolescents, and Adults: 0.5 mL/dose (1 dose per season)

Fluad: IM: Adults ≥65 years: 0.5 mL/dose (1 dose per season)

Influvac: IM, SubQ: Adults: 0.5 mL/dose (1 per season).

Intanza 9 mcg/strain: Intradermal: Adults 18 to 59 years: 0.1 mL/dose (1 per season)

Intanza 15 mcg/strain: Intradermal: Adults ≥60 years: 0.1 mL/dose (1 per season)

Note: Infants and children 6 months to <9 years who received at least one dose of the 2013-2014 seasonal influenza vaccine or a total of ≥2 doses of seasonal influenza vaccine since July 1, 2010, need only 1 dose of the 2014 to 2015 seasonal influenza vaccine. All other children <9 years (including those whose vaccination status cannot be determined) should receive 2 doses separated by ≥4 weeks, in order to achieve satisfactory antibody response. Additional dosing considerations are provided when vaccination history is available prior to the 2010 to 2011 season; see current guidelines for additional information (CDC/ACIP [Grohskopf, 2014]).

Dosage adjustment in renal impairment: There are no dosage adjustments provided in the manufacturer's labeling.

Dosage adjustment in hepatic impairment: There are no dosage adjustments provided in the manufacturer's labeling.

Administration *Fluzone Intradermal, Fluzone Intradermal Quadrivalent, Intanza (Canadian availability):* For intradermal administration, preferably into the skin over the deltoid muscle only. Fluzone Intradermal and Fluzone Intradermal Quadrivalent should be shaken gently prior to use. Intanza should not be shaken prior to use. Hold system using the thumb and middle finger (do not place fingers on windows). Insert needle perpendicular to the skin; inject using index finger to push on plunger. Do not aspirate.

Afluria, Fluarix, Fluarix Quadrivalent, Flucelvax, FluLaval, FluLaval Quadrivalent, Fluvirin, Fluzone, Fluzone High-Dose, Fluzone Quadrivalent, Agriflu (Canadian availability), Fluad (Canadian availability), Fluviral (Canadian availability), Vaxigrip (Canadian availability): For IM administration only. Suspensions should be shaken well prior to use. Some manufacturers recommend avoiding use if visible particles are present in the suspension after shaking. See manufacturer labeling for specific recommendations. Inspect for particulate matter and discoloration prior to administration. Adults and older children should be vaccinated in the deltoid muscle using a ≥1 inch needle length. Young children (≥6 months to <12 months of age) should be vaccinated in the anterolateral aspect of the thigh using a 1 inch needle length. Children ≥1 years with adequate deltoid muscle mass should be vaccinated using a 1 inch needle. A ⅝-inch needle may be adequate in younger children (refer to guidelines) (CDC 62[07], 2013; NCIRD/ACIP, 2011). Do not inject into the gluteal region or areas where there may be a major nerve trunk.

Afluria via PharmaJet Stratis Needle-free Injection System: For IM administration in adults 18 to 64 years of age only. For detailed instructions on preparation and administration of a dose, refer to the "Instructions For Use" available online at www.pharmajet.com.

Influvac (Canadian availability): May be administered by IM or deep subcutaneous injection. Shake well prior to use.

Unless otherwise indicated in product labeling, jet injectors should **not** be used to administer inactivated influenza vaccines. Currently, *Afluria* is the only influenza vaccine licensed in the United States that can be given IM by a jet-injector device.

If a pediatric vaccine (0.25 mL) is inadvertently administered to an adult, an additional 0.25 mL should be administered to provide the full adult dose (0.5 mL). If the error is discovered after the patient has left, an adult dose should be given as soon as the patient can return. If an adult vaccine (0.5 mL) is inadvertently given to a child, no action needs to be taken (CDC 62[07], 2013). *Agriflu (Canadian availability):* If 0.25 mL dose is to be given, discard half the contained syringe volume prior to administration.

Note: For patients at risk of hemorrhage following intramuscular injection, the ACIP recommends "it should be administered intramuscularly if, in the opinion of the physician familiar with the patient's bleeding risk, the vaccine can be administered by this route with reasonable safety. If the patient receives antihemophilia or other similar therapy, intramuscular vaccination can be scheduled shortly after such therapy is administered. A fine needle (23 gauge or smaller) can be used for the vaccination and firm pressure applied to the site (without rubbing) for at least 2 minutes. The patient should be instructed concerning the risk of hematoma from the injection." Patients on anticoagulant therapy should be considered to have the same bleeding risks and treated as those with clotting factor disorders (NCIRD/ACIP, 2011).

Simultaneous administration of vaccines helps ensure the patients will be fully vaccinated by the appropriate age. Simultaneous administration of vaccines is defined as administering >1 vaccine on the same day at different anatomic sites. Separate vaccines should not be combined in the same syringe unless indicated by product specific labeling. Separate needles and syringes should be used for each injection. However, in general, vaccination should not be deferred if the brand name or route of the previous dose is not available or not known (NCIRD/ACIP, 2011). Adolescents and adults should be vaccinated while seated or lying down. In general, preterm infants should be vaccinated at the same chronological age as full-term infants (NCIRD/ACIP, 2011).

Antipyretics have not been shown to prevent febrile seizures. Antipyretics may be used to treat fever or discomfort following vaccination (NCIRD/ACIP, 2011). One study reported that routine prophylactic administration of acetaminophen to prevent fever prior to vaccination decreased the immune response of some vaccines; the clinical significance of this reduction in immune response has not been established (Prymula, 2009).

Monitoring Parameters Monitor for syncope for 15 minutes following administration. If seizure-like activity associated with syncope occurs, maintain patient in supine or Trendelenburg position to reestablish adequate cerebral perfusion (NCIRD/ACIP, 2011). For those individuals who report a history of egg allergy but it is determined that the inactivated vaccine can be used, observe vaccine recipient for at least 30 minutes after receipt of vaccine (CDC/ACIP [Grohskopf, 2014]).

Additional Information Pharmacies will stock the formulations(s) standardized according to the USPHS requirements for the season. Influenza vaccines from previous seasons must not be used. U.S. federal law requires that the name of medication, date of administration, the vaccine manufacturer, lot number of vaccine, and the administering person's name, title, and address, and documentation of the vaccine information statement (VIS; date on VIS and date given to patient) be entered into the patient's permanent medical record.

It is important to note that influenza seasons vary in their timing and duration from year to year. In general, vaccination should begin soon after the vaccine becomes available and prior to onset of influenza activity in the community. However, vaccination should continue throughout the influenza season as long as vaccine is available.

Seasonal quadrivalent influenza vaccines contain two subtype A strains and two subtype B strains; trivalent influenza vaccines contain two subtype A strains and one subtype B strain.

When vaccine supply is not limited, either IIV or LAIV can be used in healthy, nonpregnant persons aged 2-49 years of age. RIV can be used in persons 18 years of age and older.

When vaccine supply is limited, administration should focus on the ACIP target groups. When IIV vaccine is in short supply, administering LAIV to eligible persons is encouraged to increase available IIV to those patients in whom LAIV cannot be used. During periods of inactivated influenza vaccine (IIV) shortage, the CDC and ACIP have recommended vaccination be prioritized based on the following three tiers. The grouping is based on influenza associated mortality and hospitalization rates. Those listed in group 1 should be vaccinated first, followed by persons in group 2, and then group 3. If the vaccine supply is extremely limited, group 1 has also been subdivided in three tiers, where those in group 1A should be vaccinated first, followed by 1B, then 1C.

Priority groups for vaccination with inactivated seasonal influenza vaccine during periods of vaccine shortage (CDC, 2005):

Tier 1A:
- Persons ≥65 years with comorbid conditions
- Residents of long-term-care facilities

Tier 1B:
- Persons 2-64 years with comorbid conditions
- Persons ≥65 years without comorbid conditions
- Children 6-23 months
- Pregnant women

Tier 1C:
- Healthcare personnel
- Household contacts and out-of-home caregivers of children <6 months

Tier 2:
- Household contacts of children and adults at increased risk of influenza-associated complications
- Healthy persons 50-64 years

Tier 3:
- Persons 2-49 years without high-risk conditions

Further information available at http://www.cdc.gov/mmwr/preview/mmwrhtml/mm5430a4.htm

Dosage Forms

Device, Intradermal [preservative free]:
Fluzone: 9 mcg/strain (0.1 mL)

Injectable, Intramuscular:
Flulaval: (5 mL)
Fluvirin: (5 mL)
Fluzone: (5 mL)

Kit, Intramuscular:
Medical Provider EZ Flu:
Physicians EZ Use Flu:

Kit, Intramuscular [preservative free]:
Medical Provider EZ Flu PF:

Suspension, Intramuscular:
Afluria: (5 mL)
Fluarix Quadrivalent: 0.5 mL (0.5 mL)
Flulaval Quadrivalent: (5 mL)
Fluzone Quadrivalent: (5 mL)

Suspension, Intramuscular [preservative free]:
Afluria Preservative Free: (0.5 mL)
Fluarix: (0.5 mL)
Flucelvax: (0.5 mL)
Flulaval Quadrivalent: 0.5 mL (0.5 mL)
Fluvirin Preservative Free: (0.5 mL)
Fluzone High-Dose: (0.5 mL)
Fluzone Preservative Free: (0.5 mL)
Fluzone Quadrivalent: 0.25 mL (0.25 mL); 0.5 mL (0.5 mL)

Suspension Pen-injector, Intradermal [preservative free]:
Fluzone Quadrivalent: 9 mcg/strain (0.1 mL)

Dosage Forms: Canada

Injection, suspension:
Fluviral: Hemagglutinin 45 mcg/0.5 mL (5 mL)
Vaxigrip: Hemagglutinin 45 mcg/0.5 mL (5 mL)

Injection, suspension [preservative free]:
Agriflu: Hemagglutinin 45 mcg/0.5 mL (0.5 mL)
Fluad: Hemagglutinin 45 mcg/0.5 mL (0.5 mL)
Influvac: Hemagglutinin 45 mcg/0.5 mL (0.5 mL)
Intanza: Hemagglutinin 27 mcg/0.1 mL (0.1 mL); Hemagglutinin 45 mcg/0.1 mL (0.1 mL)
Vaxigrip: Hemagglutinin 45 mcg/0.5 mL (0.25 mL, 0.5 mL)

Influenza Virus Vaccine (Live/Attenuated)

(in floo EN za VYE rus vak SEEN live ah TEN yoo aye ted)

Brand Names: U.S. FluMist; FluMist Quadrivalent

Brand Names: Canada FluMist

Index Terms H1N1 Influenza Vaccine; Influenza Vaccine; Influenza Virus Vaccine (Trivalent, Live); LAIV; $LAIV_4$; Live Attenuated Influenza Vaccine; Live Attenuated Influenza Vaccine (Quadrivalent)

Pharmacologic Category Vaccine, Live (Viral)

Additional Appendix Information

Immunization Administration Recommendations *on page 2250*

Immunization Recommendations *on page 2255*

Use Influenza disease prevention: Active immunization of individuals 2 to 49 years of age against influenza disease caused by influenza virus subtypes A and type B contained in the vaccine.

The Advisory Committee on Immunization Practices (ACIP) recommends routine annual vaccination with seasonal influenza vaccine for all persons ≥6 months who do not otherwise have contraindications to the vaccine. ACIP recommends use of any age and risk factor appropriate product. Healthy, nonpregnant persons aged 2 to 49 years may receive vaccination with the seasonal live, attenuated influenza vaccine (LAIV) (nasal spray). When readily available, LAIV is the preferred vaccine for healthy children aged 2 to 8 years who do not have contraindications or precautions to the vaccine; immunization should not be delayed to allow for acquisition of LAIV. In addition, other alternative products are available for certain patient populations: Persons ≥6 months of age may receive the trivalent inactivated influenza vaccine (IIV_3) or the quadrivalent inactivated influenza vaccine (IIV_4). Persons 18 years and older may receive vaccination with the recombinant influenza vaccine (RIV) (CDC/ACIP [Grohskopf 2014]).

Pregnancy Risk Factor B

Pregnancy Considerations Adverse events were not observed in animal reproduction studies. LAIV is not recommended for use during pregnancy. Influenza vaccination with the inactivated influenza vaccine (IIV) is recommended for all women who are or will become pregnant during the influenza season and who do not otherwise have contraindications to the vaccine (CDC 62[07], 2013).

Healthy pregnant women do not need to avoid contact with persons vaccinated with LAIV (CDC 62[07], 2013). The nasal vaccine contains the same strains of influenza A and B found in the injection. Information specific to the use of LAIV in pregnancy is limited.

Health care providers are encouraged to refer women exposed to the influenza vaccine during pregnancy to the Vaccines and Medications in Pregnancy Surveillance System (VAMPSS) by contacting The Organization of Teratology Information Specialists (OTIS) at (877) 311-8972.

Breast-Feeding Considerations It is not known if the vaccine is excreted into breast milk. LAIV should be used with caution in breast-feeding women (per manufacturer) due to the possibility of virus excretion into breast milk; however, LAIV may be administered to breast-feeding women unless contraindicated due to other reasons (per CDC). Postpartum women may be vaccinated with either IIV or LAIV. When vaccine supply is limited, focus on delivering the vaccine should be given to mothers of newborns and contacts or caregivers of children <5 years of age (CDC 62[07], 2013).

Contraindications Severe allergic reaction (eg, anaphylaxis) to previous influenza vaccination; hypersensitivity to any component of the formulation, including egg protein; children and adolescents through 17 years of age receiving aspirin therapy

Warnings/Precautions Immediate treatment (including epinephrine 1:1000) for anaphylactoid and/or hypersensitivity reactions should be available during vaccine use. Manufactured with chicken egg protein. Allergy to eggs must be distinguished from allergy to the vaccine. Recommendations are available from the CDC regarding influenza vaccination to persons who report egg allergies; however, a prior severe allergic reaction to influenza vaccine, regardless of the component suspected, is a contraindication to vaccination. ACIP recommends use of IIV or RIV (if RIV is age appropriate) over LAIV when considering vaccination in persons reporting an egg allergy (due to lack of data of LAIV use in this setting) (CDC/ACIP [Grohskopf 2014]). Also manufactured with arginine, gelatin, and gentamicin.

Use with caution in patients with history of Guillain-Barré syndrome (GBS); patients with history of GBS have a greater likelihood of developing GBS than those without. As a precaution, the ACIP recommends that patients with a history of GBS and who are at low risk for severe influenza complications, and patients known to have experienced GBS within 6 weeks following previous vaccination should generally not be vaccinated (consider influenza antiviral chemoprophylaxis in these patients). Based on limited data, the benefits of vaccinating persons with a history of GBS who are also at high risk for complications of influenza may outweigh the risks (CDC 62[07], 2013). Recent studies of patients who received the trivalent inactivated influenza vaccine or the monovalent H1N1 influenza vaccine have shown the risk of GBS is lower with vaccination than with influenza infection (Baxter, 2013; Greene, 2013; Kwong, 2013).

Data on the use of the nasal spray in immunocompromised patients is limited. **Avoid contact with severely immunocompromised individuals for at least 7 days following vaccination (at least 14 days per Canadian labeling).** ACIP does not recommend the use of LAIV in immunosuppressed patients (CDC/ACIP [Grohskopf 2014]). ACIP does not recommend the use of LAIV for persons who care for severely immunocompromised individuals who require a protective environment due to the theoretical risk of transmitting the live virus from the vaccine. Persons who care for the severely immunocompromised should receive either IIV or RIV. Persons who have received LAIV should avoid contact with severely immunocompromised individuals for at least 7 days following vaccination (at least 14 days per Canadian labeling) (CDC 62[07], 2013). In general, live vaccines should be administered ≥4 weeks prior to planned immunosuppression and avoided within 2 weeks of immunosuppression when feasible (IDSA [Rubin, 2014]).

Per the U.S. prescribing information, the nasal spray should not be used in patients with asthma or children <5 years of age with recurrent wheezing; risk of wheezing following vaccination is increased. Patients with severe asthma or active wheezing were not included in clinical trials. Children <24 months of age had increased wheezing and hospitalizations following administration in clinical trials; use of the nasal spray is not approved in this age group. ACIP does not recommend the use of LAIV in patients with chronic pulmonary disorders including asthma and children 2-4 years of age who have had asthma or wheezing episodes within the past year (CDC/ACIP [Grohskopf 2014]). The safety of LAIV has not been established in individuals with underlying medical conditions that may predispose them to complications following wild-type influenza infection.

May consider deferring administration in patients with moderate or severe acute illness (with or without fever); may administer to patients with mild acute illness (with or without fever) (NCIRD/ACIP, 2011). ACIP does not recommend the use of LAIV in patients with chronic disorders of the cardiovascular system (except isolated hypertension), chronic metabolic diseases, hematologic disorders and hemoglobinopathies, hepatic disease, persons with HIV, neurologic or neuromuscular disorders, renal disease, or pregnant women (CDC/ACIP [Grohskopf 2014]). Use of this vaccine for specific medical and/or other indications (eg, immunocompromising conditions, hepatic or kidney disease, diabetes) is also addressed in the ACIP Recommended Immunization Schedule (CDC/ACIP [Akinsanya-Beysolow, 2014]; CDC/ACIP [Bridges, 2014]). Specific recommendations for use of this vaccine in immunocompromised patients with asplenia, cancer, HIV infection, cerebrospinal fluid leaks, cochlear implants, hematopoietic stem cell transplant (prior to or after), sickle cell disease, solid organ transplant (prior to or after), or those receiving immunosuppressive therapy for chronic conditions as well as contacts of immunocompromised patients are available from the IDSA (Rubin, 2014).

Defer immunization if nasal congestion is present which may impede delivery of vaccine (CDC 62[07], 2013). In order to maximize vaccination rates, the ACIP recommends simultaneous administration of all age-appropriate vaccines (live or inactivated) for which a person is eligible at a single clinic visit, unless contraindications exist (NCIRD/ACIP, 2011).

Studies conducted in children using trivalent IIV and LAIV have shown significantly greater efficacy of LAIV in younger children. Information is not yet available for the quadrivalent LAIV vaccine (CDC 62[07], 2013). The safety and efficacy of the nasal spray have not been established in adults ≥50 years of age (U.S. labeling) or ≥60 years of age (Canadian labeling). Vaccination may not result in effective immunity in all patients. Response depends upon multiple factors (eg, type of vaccine, age of patient) and may be improved by administering the vaccine at the recommended dose, route, and interval. Vaccines may not be effective if administered during periods of altered immune competence (NCIRD/ACIP, 2011). Influenza vaccines from previous seasons must not be used (CDC 62 [07], 2013).

Adverse Reactions All serious adverse reactions must be reported to the U.S. Department of Health and Human Services (DHHS) Vaccine Adverse Event Reporting System (VAERS) 1-800-822-7967 or online at https://vaers.hhs.gov/esub/index. In Canada, adverse reactions may be reported to local provincial/territorial health agencies or to the Vaccine Safety Section at Public Health Agency of Canada (1-866-844-0018).

Central nervous system: Chills, fever, headache, irritability, lethargy

Gastrointestinal: Abdominal pain, appetite decreased

Neuromuscular & skeletal: Muscle aches, tiredness/weakness

Otic: Otitis media

Respiratory: Sinusitis, sneezing
Respiratory: Cough, nasal congestion/ runny nose, wheezing
Rare but important or life-threatening: Anaphylactic reactions, asthma exacerbations, Bell's palsy, encephalitis (vaccine associated), epistaxis, Guillain-Barré syndrome, hypersensitivity reaction, meningitis (including eosinophilic meningitis), mitochondrial encephalomyopathy (Leigh syndrome) exacerbation, pericarditis

Drug Interactions

Metabolism/Transport Effects None known.

Avoid Concomitant Use

Avoid concomitant use of Influenza Virus Vaccine (Live/Attenuated) with any of the following: Belimumab; Fingolimod; Immunosuppressants; Salicylates

Increased Effect/Toxicity

Influenza Virus Vaccine (Live/Attenuated) may increase the levels/effects of: Salicylates

The levels/effects of Influenza Virus Vaccine (Live/Attenuated) may be increased by: Belimumab; Corticosteroids (Systemic); Dimethyl Fumarate; Fingolimod; Hydroxychloroquine; Immunosuppressants; Leflunomide; Mercaptopurine; Methotrexate

Decreased Effect

Influenza Virus Vaccine (Live/Attenuated) may decrease the levels/effects of: Tuberculin Tests

The levels/effects of Influenza Virus Vaccine (Live/Attenuated) may be decreased by: Antiviral Agents (Influenza A and B); Dimethyl Fumarate; Fingolimod; Immune Globulins; Immunosuppressants

Storage/Stability Store in refrigerator at 2°C to 8°C (35°F to 46°F). **Do not freeze.** The vaccine may be exposed to temperatures of up to 25°C for up to 12 hours without adverse impact; return to refrigerator as soon as possible; only a single excursion outside of the recommended storage conditions is permitted.

Mechanism of Action The vaccine contains live attenuated viruses which infect and replicate within the cells lining the nasopharynx. Promotes immunity to seasonal influenza virus by inducing specific antibody production. Each year the formulation is standardized according to the U.S. Public Health Service. Preparations from previous seasons must not be used.

Pharmacodynamics/Kinetics

Onset of action: Most adults have antibody protection within 2 weeks of vaccination (CDC 62[07], 2013)
Duration: ≥6 to 8 months when vaccine is antigenically similar to circulating virus (CDC 62[07], 2013); response may be diminished in persons ≥65 years and limited evidence suggests titers may decline significantly 6 months following vaccination in this population (CDC/ACIP [Grohskopf 2014])
Distribution: Following nasal administration, vaccine is distributed in the nasal cavity (~90%), stomach (~3%), brain (~2%), and lung (0.4%)

Dosage It is important to note that influenza seasons vary in their timing and duration from year to year. In general, vaccination should begin soon after the vaccine becomes available (and, if possible, by October) and prior to onset of influenza activity in the community. However, vaccination should continue throughout the influenza season as long as vaccine is available (CDC/ACIP [Grohskopf 2014]).

Intranasal (FluMist):

U.S. labeling:

Children 2-8 years: 0.2 mL/dose (1 or 2 doses per season; see **"Note"**)
Children ≥9 years, Adolescents, and Adults ≤49 years: 0.2 mL/dose (1 dose per season)
Elderly: Not indicated for use in patients ≥50 years

Canadian labeling:

Children 2-8 years: 0.2 mL/dose (1 or 2 doses per season; see **"Note"**)
Children ≥9 years, Adolescents, and Adults ≤59 years: 0.2 mL/dose (1 dose per season)
Elderly: Not indicated for use in patients ≥60 years

Note: Infants and children 6 months to <9 years who received at least one dose of the 2013-2014 seasonal influenza vaccine or a total of ≥2 doses of seasonal influenza vaccine since July 1, 2010, need only 1 dose of the 2014 to 2015 seasonal influenza vaccine. All other children <9 years (including those whose vaccination status cannot be determined) should receive 2 doses separated by ≥4 weeks, in order to achieve satisfactory antibody response. Additional dosing considerations are provided when vaccination history is available prior to the 2010 to 2011 season; see current guidelines for additional information (CDC/ACIP [Grohskopf 2014]).

Dosage adjustment in renal impairment: There are no dosage adjustments provided in the manufacturer's labeling.

Dosage adjustment in hepatic impairment: There are no dosage adjustments provided in the manufacturer's labeling.

Administration LAIV: Intranasal: For intranasal administration only; do not inject. Half the dose (0.1 mL) is administered to each nostril; patient should be in upright position. A dose divider clip is provided to allow administration of 0.1 mL into each nostril. Place the tip of the sprayer inside the nostril and depress plunger as rapidly as possible to deliver the dose. Remove dose divider clip and repeat into opposite nostril. The patient does not need to inhale during administration (may breath normally). Severely immunocompromised persons should not administer the live vaccine. If recipient sneezes following administration, the dose should not be repeated. Defer immunization if nasal congestion is present which may impede delivery of vaccine (CDC 62[07], 2013).

Simultaneous administration of vaccines helps ensure the patients will be fully vaccinated by the appropriate age. Simultaneous administration of vaccines is defined as administering >1 vaccine on the same day at different anatomic sites. The ACIP prefers each dose of a specific vaccine in a series come from the same manufacturer when possible. However, in general, vaccination should not be deferred if the brand name or route of the previous dose is not available or not known (CDC, 2011).

Antipyretics have not been shown to prevent febrile seizures. Antipyretics may be used to treat fever or discomfort following vaccination (CDC, 2011). One study reported that routine prophylactic administration of acetaminophen to prevent fever prior to vaccination decreased the immune response of some vaccines; the clinical significance of this reduction in immune response has not been established (Prymula, 2009). Aspirin-containing products should be avoided for 4 weeks following vaccination in children and adolescents ≤17 years of age.

Vaccine administration with oral influenza antiviral medications: Live influenza virus vaccine (LAIV) should not be given until 48 hours after the completion of influenza antiviral therapy (influenza A and B). Influenza antiviral therapy (influenza A and B) should not be administered for 2 weeks after receiving LAIV. If influenza antiviral therapy (influenza A and B) and LAIV are administered concomitantly, revaccination should be considered.

Additional Information Pharmacies will stock the formulations(s) standardized according to the USPHS requirements for the season. Influenza vaccines from previous seasons must not be used. U.S. federal law requires that the name of medication, date of administration, the vaccine manufacturer, lot number of vaccine, and the administering person's name, title, and address, and documentation of the vaccine information statement (VIS; date on VIS and date given to patient) be entered into the patient's permanent medical record.

It is important to note that influenza seasons vary in their timing and duration from year to year. In general, vaccination should begin soon after the vaccine becomes available and prior to onset of influenza activity in the community. However, vaccination should continue throughout the influenza season as long as vaccine is available.

Seasonal quadrivalent influenza vaccines contain two subtype A strains and two subtype B strains; trivalent influenza vaccines contain two subtype A strains and one subtype B strain.

When vaccine supply is not limited, either IIV or LAIV can be used in healthy, nonpregnant persons aged 2-49 years of age. RIV can be used in persons 18 years of age or older.

When vaccine supply is limited, administration should focus on the ACIP target groups. When IIV vaccine is in short supply, administering LAIV to eligible persons is encouraged to increase available IIV to those patients in whom LAIV cannot be used. During periods of inactivated influenza vaccine (IIV) shortage, the CDC and ACIP have recommended vaccination be prioritized based on the following three tiers. The grouping is based on influenza-associated mortality and hospitalization rates. Those listed in group 1 should be vaccinated first, followed by persons in group 2, and then group 3. If the vaccine supply is extremely limited, group 1 has also been subdivided in three tiers, where those in group 1A should be vaccinated first, followed by 1B, then 1C.

Priority groups for vaccination with inactivated seasonal influenza vaccine during periods of vaccine shortage (CDC, 2005):

Tier 1A:
- Persons ≥65 years with comorbid conditions
- Residents of long-term-care facilities

Tier 1B:
- Persons 2-64 years with comorbid conditions
- Persons ≥65 years without comorbid conditions
- Children 6-23 months
- Pregnant women

Tier 1C:
- Healthcare personnel
- Household contacts and out-of-home caregivers of children <6 months

Tier 2:
- Household contacts of children and adults at increased risk of influenza-associated complications
- Healthy persons 50-64 years

Tier 3:
- Persons 2-49 years without high-risk conditions

Further information available at http://www.cdc.gov/mmwr/preview/mmwrhtml/mm5430a4.htm

Dosage Forms

Liquid, Nasal [preservative free]:
FluMist: (1 ea)

Suspension, Nasal [preservative free]:
FluMist Quadrivalent: (1 ea)

◆ **Influenza Virus Vaccine (Monovalent)** *see* Influenza A Virus Vaccine (H5N1) *on page 1074*

◆ **Influenza Virus Vaccine (Purified Surface Antigen)** *see* Influenza Virus Vaccine (Inactivated) *on page 1075*

◆ **Influenza Virus Vaccine (Split-Virus)** *see* Influenza Virus Vaccine (Inactivated) *on page 1075*

◆ **Influenza Virus Vaccine (Trivalent, Live)** *see* Influenza Virus Vaccine (Live/Attenuated) *on page 1080*

◆ **Influvac (Can)** *see* Influenza Virus Vaccine (Inactivated) *on page 1075*

◆ **Infufer (Can)** *see* Iron Dextran Complex *on page 1117*

◆ **Infumorph 200** *see* Morphine (Systemic) *on page 1394*

◆ **Infumorph 500** *see* Morphine (Systemic) *on page 1394*

Ingenol Mebutate (IN je nol MEB u tate)

Brand Names: U.S. Picato

Index Terms *Euphorbia peplus* Derivative; PEP005

Pharmacologic Category Topical Skin Product

Use Topical treatment of actinic keratosis

Pregnancy Risk Factor C

Dosage Topical: Adults: Actinic keratoses:
- Face and scalp: Apply 0.015% gel once daily to affected area for 3 consecutive days
- Trunk/extremities: Apply 0.05% gel once daily to affected area for 2 consecutive days

Additional Information Complete prescribing information should be consulted for additional detail.

Dosage Forms

Gel, External:
Picato: 0.015% (3 ea); 0.05% (2 ea)

◆ **INH** *see* Isoniazid *on page 1120*

◆ **Inhibace (Can)** *see* Cilazapril [CAN/INT] *on page 434*

◆ **Inhibace Plus (Can)** *see* Cilazapril and Hydrochlorothiazide [CAN/INT] *on page 436*

◆ **Injectafer** *see* Ferric Carboxymaltose *on page 868*

◆ **Inlyta** *see* Axitinib *on page 207*

◆ **Innohep® (Can)** *see* Tinzaparin *on page 2043*

◆ **InnoPran XL** *see* Propranolol *on page 1731*

◆ **Insoluble Prussian Blue** *see* Ferric Hexacyanoferrate *on page 870*

◆ **Inspra** *see* Eplerenone *on page 740*

◆ **Instacort 5 [OTC]** *see* Hydrocortisone (Topical) *on page 1014*

◆ **Instacort 10 [OTC]** *see* Hydrocortisone (Topical) *on page 1014*

Insulin Aspart (IN soo lin AS part)

Brand Names: U.S. NovoLOG; NovoLOG FlexPen; NovoLOG PenFill

Brand Names: Canada NovoRapid®

Index Terms Aspart Insulin

Pharmacologic Category Insulin, Rapid-Acting

Use Treatment of type 1 diabetes mellitus (insulin dependent, IDDM) and type 2 diabetes mellitus (noninsulin dependent, NIDDM) to improve glycemic control

Pregnancy Risk Factor B

Dosage Note: Insulin aspart is a rapid-acting insulin analog which is normally administered SubQ as a premeal component of the insulin regimen or as a continuous SubQ infusion and should be used with intermediate- or long-acting insulin. When compared to insulin regular, insulin aspart has a more rapid onset and shorter duration of activity. In carefully controlled clinical settings with close medical supervision and monitoring of blood glucose and potassium, insulin aspart may also be administered IV Insulin requirements vary dramatically between patients and dictate frequent monitoring and close medical supervision.

Diabetes mellitus: SubQ:

General insulin dosing:

Type 1: Children ≥2 years, Adolescents, and Adults: **Note:** Multiple daily doses or continuous subcutaneous infusions guided by blood glucose monitoring are the standard of diabetes care. Combinations of insulin formulations are commonly used. The daily doses presented below are expressed as the **total units/kg/day of all insulin formulations combined.**

Initial total insulin dose: 0.2-0.6 units/kg/day in divided doses. Conservative initial doses of 0.2-0.4 units/kg/day are often recommended to avoid the potential for hypoglycemia. A rapid-acting insulin may be the only insulin formulation used initially.

Usual maintenance range: 0.5-1 units/kg/day in divided doses. An estimate of anticipated needs may be based on body weight and/or activity factors as follows:

Nonobese: 0.4-0.6 units/kg/day

Obese: 0.8-1.2 units/kg/day

Pubescent Children and Adolescents: During puberty, requirements may substantially increase to >1 unit/kg/day and in some cases up to 2 units/kg/day (IDF-ISPAD, 2011).

Division of daily insulin requirement ("conventional therapy"): Generally, 50% to 75% of the total daily dose (TDD) is given as an intermediate- or long-acting form of insulin (in 1-2 daily injections). The remaining portion of the TDD is then divided and administered before or at mealtimes (depending on the formulation) as a rapid-acting (eg, insulin aspart) or short-acting form of insulin. Some patients may benefit from the use of CSII which delivers rapid-acting insulin (insulin aspart) as a continuous infusion throughout the day and as boluses at mealtimes via an external pump device.

Division of daily insulin requirement ("intensive therapy"): Basal insulin delivery with 1 or 2 doses of intermediate- or long-acting insulin formulations superimposed with doses of short- or rapid-acting insulin (eg, insulin aspart) formulations 3 or more times daily.

Adjustment of dose: Dosage must be titrated to achieve glucose control and avoid hypoglycemia. Adjust dose to maintain premeal and bedtime glucose in target range. Since combinations of agents are frequently used, dosage adjustment must address the individual component of the insulin regimen which most directly influences the blood glucose value in question, based on the known onset and duration of the insulin component. Treatment and monitoring regimens must be individualized.

Continuous SubQ insulin infusion (insulin pump): A combination of a "basal" continuous insulin infusion rate with preprogrammed, premeal bolus doses which are patient controlled. When converting from multiple daily SubQ doses of maintenance insulin, it is advisable to reduce the basal rate to less than the equivalent of the total daily units of the longer acting insulin (eg, NPH); divide the total number of units by 24 to get the basal rate in units/hour. Do not include the total units of regular insulin or other rapid-acting insulin formulations in this calculation. The same premeal regular insulin dosage may be used.

Type 2: Adults: Augmentation therapy (patients for which diet, exercise, weight reduction, and oral hypoglycemic agents have not been adequate): Initial dosage of 0.2 units/kg/day or 10 units/day of an intermediate-acting (eg, NPH) or long-acting insulin administered at bedtime has been recommended. As an alternative, regular insulin or rapid-acting insulin formulations administered before meals have also been used. Dosage must be carefully adjusted.

Diabetic ketoacidosis (DKA), mild-to-moderate (off-label use): Treatment should continue until reversal of acid-base derangement/ketonemia. Serum glucose is not a direct indicator of these abnormalities, and may decrease more rapidly than correction of the metabolic abnormalities. Also refer to institution-specific protocols where appropriate.

Children and Adolescents: SubQ (**Note:** Use of IV regular insulin is preferred; only use the SubQ route if IV infusion access is unavailable): 0.3 units/kg followed in 1 hour by 0.1 units/kg given every hour or 0.15-0.2 units/kg every 2 hours; continue until acidosis clears, then decrease to 0.05 units/kg given every hour until maintenance SubQ replacement dosing can be initiated (Kitabchi, 2004; Wolfsdorf, 2007).

Hyperglycemia, critically ill (off-label use): Adults: IV continuous infusion: Insulin therapy should be implemented when blood glucose ≥150 mg/dL with a goal to maintain blood glucose <150 mg/dL (with values absolutely <180 mg/dL) using a protocol that achieves a low rate of hypoglycemia (ie, ≤70 mg/dL). Before discontinuation, stable ICU patients should be transitioned to a protocol-driven basal/bolus insulin regimen, based on insulin infusion history and carbohydrate intake, to avoid loss of glycemic control. Subcutaneous insulin therapy may be considered for selected clinically stable ICU patients (Jacobi, 2012). **Note:** The Surviving Sepsis Campaign guidelines recommend initiating insulin dosing in patients with severe sepsis when 2 consecutive blood glucose concentrations are >180 mg/dL and to target an upper blood glucose ≤180 mg/dL (Dellinger, 2013).

Dosing adjustment in renal impairment: No dosage adjustment provided in manufacturer's labeling; insulin requirements may be reduced due to changes in insulin clearance or metabolism; monitor blood glucose closely.

Dosing adjustment in hepatic impairment: No dosage adjustment provided in manufacturer's labeling; insulin requirements may be reduced due to changes in insulin clearance or metabolism; monitor blood glucose closely.

Additional Information Complete prescribing information should be consulted for additional detail.

Dosage Forms

Solution, Subcutaneous:

NovoLOG: 100 units/mL (10 mL)

Solution Cartridge, Subcutaneous:

NovoLOG PenFill: 100 units/mL (3 mL)

Solution Pen-injector, Subcutaneous:

NovoLOG FlexPen: 100 units/mL (3 mL)

◆ **Insulin Aspart and Insulin Aspart Protamine** *see* Insulin Aspart Protamine and Insulin Aspart *on page 1084*

Insulin Aspart Protamine and Insulin Aspart (IN soo lin AS part PROE ta meen & IN soo lin AS part)

Brand Names: U.S. NovoLOG® Mix 70/30; NovoLOG® Mix 70/30 FlexPen®

Brand Names: Canada NovoMix® 30

Index Terms Insulin Aspart and Insulin Aspart Protamine; NovoLog 70/30

Pharmacologic Category Insulin, Combination

Use Treatment of type 1 diabetes mellitus (insulin dependent, IDDM) and type 2 diabetes mellitus (noninsulin dependent, NIDDM) to improve glycemic control

Pregnancy Risk Factor B

Dosage Note: Insulin aspart protamine is an intermediate-acting insulin and insulin aspart is a rapid-acting insulin administered by SubQ injection. Insulin aspart protamine and insulin aspart combination products are approximately equipotent to insulin NPH and insulin regular combination products with a similar duration of activity, but with a more rapid onset. With combination insulin products, the proportion of rapid-acting to long-acting insulin is fixed; basal vs prandial dose adjustments cannot be made. Fixed-ratio insulins (such as insulin aspart protamine and insulin aspart combination) are typically administered as 2 daily doses with each dose intended to cover two meals and a snack. Because of variability in the peak effect and individual patient variability in activities, meals, etc, it may be more difficult to achieve complete glycemic control using fixed combinations of insulins; frequent monitoring and close medical supervision may be necessary.

Diabetes mellitus: SubQ:

General insulin dosing:

Type 1: Children, Adolescents, and Adults: **Note:** Multiple daily doses are utilized and guided by blood glucose monitoring. Combinations of different insulin formulations are commonly used. The daily doses presented below are expressed as the **total units/kg/day of all insulin formulations combined.** Insulin aspart protamine and insulin aspart combination product is **not** intended for initial therapy; basal insulin requirements should be established **first** to direct dosing of combination insulin products.

Usual maintenance range: 0.5-1 units/kg/day in divided doses. An estimate of anticipated needs may be based on body weight and/or activity factors as follows:

Nonobese: 0.4-0.6 units/kg/day

Obese: 0.8-1.2 units/kg/day

Pubescent Children and Adolescents: During puberty, requirements may substantially increase to >1 unit/kg/day and in some cases up to 2 units/kg/day (IDF-ISPAD, 2011).

Division of daily insulin requirement ("conventional therapy"): Generally, 50% to 75% of the daily insulin dose is given as an intermediate- or long-acting form of insulin (in 1-2 daily injections). The remaining portion of the 24-hour insulin requirement is divided and administered as either regular insulin or a rapid-acting form of insulin at the same time before breakfast and dinner.

Adjustment of dose: Dosage must be titrated to achieve glucose control and avoid hypoglycemia. Adjust dose to maintain premeal and bedtime glucose in target range. Since combinations of agents are frequently used, dosage adjustment must address the individual component of the insulin regimen which most directly influences the blood glucose value in question, based on the known onset and duration of the insulin component. Treatment and monitoring regimens must be individualized.

Type 2: Adults: Augmentation therapy (patients for which diet, exercise, weight reduction, and oral hypoglycemic agents have not been adequate): **Note:** Insulin aspart protamine and insulin aspart combination product is **not** intended for initial therapy; basal insulin requirements should be established **first** to direct dosing of combination insulin products. Dosage must be carefully adjusted.

Dosing adjustment in renal impairment: No dosage adjustment provided in manufacturer's labeling; insulin requirements may be reduced due to changes in insulin clearance or metabolism; monitor blood glucose closely.

Dosing adjustment in hepatic impairment: No dosage adjustment provided in manufacturer's labeling; insulin requirements may be reduced due to changes in insulin clearance or metabolism; monitor blood glucose closely.

Additional Information Complete prescribing information should be consulted for additional detail.

Dosage Forms

Injection, suspension:

NovoLOG® Mix 70/30: Insulin aspart protamine suspension 70% [intermediate acting] and insulin aspart solution 30% [rapid acting]: 100 units/mL (10 mL)

NovoLOG® Mix 70/30 FlexPen®: Insulin aspart protamine suspension 70% [intermediate acting] and insulin aspart solution 30% [rapid acting]: 100 units/mL (3 mL)

Insulin Detemir (IN soo lin DE te mir)

Brand Names: U.S. Levemir; Levemir FlexPen [DSC]; Levemir FlexTouch

Brand Names: Canada Levemir®

Index Terms Detemir Insulin

Pharmacologic Category Insulin, Intermediate- to Long-Acting

Use Treatment of type 1 diabetes mellitus (insulin dependent, IDDM) and type 2 diabetes mellitus (noninsulin dependent, NIDDM) to improve glycemic control

Pregnancy Risk Factor B

Dosage Note: Insulin detemir is an intermediate-acting insulin administered by SubQ injection. When compared to insulin NPH, insulin detemir has slower, more prolonged absorption; duration of activity is dose-dependent. Insulin detemir may be given once or twice daily when used as the basal insulin component of therapy. Changing the basal insulin component from another insulin to insulin detemir can be done on a unit-to-unit basis. Insulin requirements vary dramatically between patients and dictate frequent monitoring and close medical supervision.

Diabetes mellitus: SubQ:

General insulin dosing:

Type 1: Children, Adolescents, and Adults: **Note:** Multiple daily doses are utilized and guided by blood glucose monitoring. Combinations of insulin formulations are commonly used. The daily doses presented below are expressed as the **total units/kg/day of all insulin formulations combined.**

Usual maintenance range: 0.5-1 units/kg/day in divided doses. An estimate of anticipated needs may be based on body weight and/or activity factors as follows:

Nonobese: 0.4-0.6 units/kg/day

Obese: 0.8-1.2 units/kg/day

Pubescent Children and Adolescents: During puberty, requirements may substantially increase to >1 unit/kg/day and in some cases up to 2 units/kg/day (IDF-ISPAD, 2011).

Division of daily insulin requirement ("conventional therapy"): Generally, 50% to 75% of the total daily dose (TDD) is given as an intermediate-acting (eg, insulin detemir) or a long-acting form of insulin (in 1-2 daily injections). The remaining portion of the TDD is then divided and administered before or at mealtimes (depending on the formulation) as a rapid-acting or short-acting form of insulin.

Division of daily insulin requirement ("intensive therapy"): Basal insulin delivery with 1 or 2 doses of intermediate-acting (eg, insulin detemir) or long-acting insulin formulations superimposed with doses of short- or rapid-acting insulin formulations 3 or more times daily.

Adjustment of dose: Dosage must be titrated to achieve glucose control and avoid hypoglycemia. Adjust dose to maintain premeal and bedtime glucose in target range. Since combinations of agents are frequently used, dosage adjustment must address the individual component of the insulin regimen which most directly influences the blood glucose value in question, based on the known onset and duration of the insulin component. Treatment and monitoring regimens must be individualized.

Insulin detemir-specific dosing: Manufacturer recommendations:

Type 1: Children ≥2 years, Adolescents, and Adults: Initial dose: Approximately one-third of the total daily insulin requirement administered in 1-2 divided doses. A rapid- or short-acting insulin should be used to complete the balance (~2/3) of the total daily insulin requirement.

Conversion from insulin glargine or NPH insulin: May be substituted on an equivalent unit-per-unit basis; in one Type 2 diabetes clinical trial, higher doses of insulin detemir were required than insulin NPH.

Type 2: Adults: Initial:

Inadequately controlled on oral antidiabetic agents: 10 units (or 0.1-0.2 units/kg) once daily in the evening; may also administer total daily dose in 2 divided doses.

Inadequately controlled on GLP-1 receptor agonist: 10 units once daily in the evening.

Conversion from insulin glargine or NPH insulin: May be substituted on an equivalent unit-per-unit basis; in one Type 2 diabetes clinical trial, higher doses of insulin detemir were required than insulin NPH.

Dosing adjustment in renal impairment: No dosage adjustment provided in manufacturer's labeling; insulin requirements may be reduced due to changes in insulin clearance or metabolism; monitor blood glucose closely.

Dosing adjustment in hepatic impairment: No dosage adjustment provided in manufacturer's labeling; insulin requirements may be reduced due to changes in insulin clearance or metabolism; monitor blood glucose closely.

Additional Information Complete prescribing information should be consulted for additional detail.

Dosage Forms

Solution, Subcutaneous:

Levemir: 100 units/mL (10 mL)

Solution Pen-injector, Subcutaneous:

Levemir FlexTouch: 100 units/mL (3 mL)

Insulin Glargine (IN soo lin GLAR jeen)

Brand Names: U.S. Lantus; Lantus SoloStar

Brand Names: Canada Lantus®; Lantus® OptiSet®

Index Terms Glargine Insulin

Pharmacologic Category Insulin, Long-Acting

Use Treatment of type 1 diabetes mellitus (insulin dependent, IDDM) and type 2 diabetes mellitus (noninsulin dependent, NIDDM) to improve glycemic control

Pregnancy Risk Factor C

Dosage Note: Insulin glargine is a long-acting insulin administered by SubQ injection. Insulin glargine is approximately equipotent to human insulin, but has a slower onset, no pronounced peak, and a longer duration of activity. Changing the basal insulin component from another insulin to insulin glargine can be done on a unit-to-unit basis. Insulin requirements vary dramatically between patients and dictates frequent monitoring and close medical supervision.

Diabetes mellitus: SubQ:

General insulin dosing:

Type 1: Children, Adolescents, and Adults: **Note:** Multiple daily doses are utilized and guided by blood glucose monitoring. Combinations of insulin formulations are commonly used. The daily doses presented below are expressed as the total units/kg/day of all insulin formulations used. Insulin glargine must be used in combination with a rapid- or short-acting insulin.

Usual maintenance range: 0.5-1 units/kg/day in divided doses. An estimate of anticipated needs may be based on body weight and/or activity factors as follows:

Nonobese: 0.4-0.6 units/kg/day

Obese: 0.8-1.2 units/kg/day

Pubescent Children and Adolescents: During puberty, requirements may substantially increase to >1 unit/kg/day and in some cases up to 2 units/kg/day (IDF-ISPAD, 2011).

Division of daily insulin requirement ("conventional therapy"): Generally, 50% to 75% of the total daily dose (TDD) is given as an intermediate-acting or a long-acting form of insulin (eg, insulin glargine) (in 1-2 daily injections). The remaining portion of the TDD is then divided and administered before or at mealtimes (depending on the formulation) as a rapid-acting or short-acting form of insulin.

Division of daily insulin requirement ("intensive therapy"): Basal insulin delivery with 1 or 2 doses of intermediate-acting or long-acting insulin formulations superimposed with doses of short- or rapid-acting insulin formulations 3 or more times daily.

Adjustment of dose: Dosage must be titrated to achieve glucose control and avoid hypoglycemia. Adjust dose to maintain premeal and bedtime glucose in target range. Since combinations of agents are frequently used, dosage adjustment must address the individual component of the insulin regimen which most directly influences the blood glucose value in question, based on the known onset and duration of the insulin component.

Insulin glargine-specific dosing: Manufacturer recommendations:

Type 1: Children ≥6 years, Adolescents, and Adults: Initial dose: Approximately one-third of the total daily insulin requirement administered once daily. A rapid-acting or short-acting insulin should also be used to complete the balance (~2/3) of the total daily insulin requirement.

Type 2: Adults: Initial basal insulin dose: 10 units (or 0.2 units/kg) once daily

Conversion to insulin glargine from other insulin therapies:

Converting from once-daily NPH insulin: May be substituted on an equivalent unit-per-unit basis

Converting from twice-daily NPH insulin: Initial dose: Use 80% of the total daily dose of NPH (eg, 20% reduction); administer once daily; adjust dosage according to patient response

Dosing adjustment in renal impairment: No dosage adjustment provided in manufacturer's labeling; insulin requirements may be reduced due to changes in insulin clearance or metabolism; monitor blood glucose closely.

Dosing adjustment in hepatic impairment: No dosage adjustment provided in manufacturer's labeling; insulin requirements may be reduced due to changes in insulin clearance or metabolism; monitor blood glucose closely.

Additional Information Complete prescribing information should be consulted for additional detail.

Dosage Forms

Solution, Subcutaneous:

Lantus: 100 units/mL (10 mL)

Solution Pen-injector, Subcutaneous:

Lantus SoloStar: 100 units/mL (3 mL)

Insulin Glulisine (IN soo lin gloo LIS een)

Brand Names: U.S. Apidra; Apidra SoloStar

Brand Names: Canada Apidra®

Index Terms Glulisine Insulin

Pharmacologic Category Insulin, Rapid-Acting

Use Treatment of type 1 diabetes mellitus (insulin dependent, IDDM) and type 2 diabetes mellitus (noninsulin dependent, NIDDM) to improve glycemic control

Pregnancy Risk Factor C

Dosage Note: Insulin glulisine is a rapid-acting insulin analog which is normally administered SubQ as a premeal component of the insulin regimen or as a continuous SubQ infusion and should be used with an intermediate- or long-acting insulin. When compared to insulin regular, insulin glulisine has a more rapid onset and shorter duration of activity. In carefully controlled clinical settings with close medical supervision and monitoring of blood glucose and potassium, insulin glulisine may be administered IV Insulin requirements vary dramatically between patients and dictate frequent monitoring and close medical supervision.

Diabetes mellitus: SubQ:

General insulin dosing:

Type 1: Children ≥4 years, Adolescents, and Adults: **Note:** Multiple daily doses or continuous subcutaneous infusions guided by blood glucose monitoring are the standard of diabetes care. Combinations of insulin formulations are commonly used. The daily doses presented below are expressed as the **total units/kg/day of all insulin formulations combined.**

Initial total insulin dose: 0.2-0.6 units/kg/day in divided doses. Conservative initial doses of 0.2-0.4 units/kg/day are often recommended to avoid the potential for hypoglycemia. A rapid-acting insulin may be the only insulin formulation used initially.

Usual maintenance range: 0.5-1 units/kg/day in divided doses. An estimate of anticipated needs may be based on body weight and/or activity factors as follows:

Nonobese: 0.4-0.6 units/kg/day

Obese: 0.8-1.2 units/kg/day

Pubescent Children and Adolescents: During puberty, requirements may substantially increase to >1 unit/kg/day and in some cases up to 2 units/kg/day (IDF-ISPAD, 2011).

Division of daily insulin requirement ("conventional therapy"): Generally, 50% to 75% of the total daily dose (TDD) is given as an intermediate- or long-acting form of insulin (in 1-2 daily injections). The remaining portion of the TDD is then divided and administered before or at mealtimes (depending on the formulation) as a rapid-acting insulin (eg, insulin glulisine) or short-acting form of insulin. Some patients may benefit from the use of CSII which delivers rapid-acting insulin (insulin aspart) as a continuous infusion throughout the day and as boluses at mealtimes via an external pump device.

Division of daily insulin requirement ("intensive therapy"): Basal insulin delivery with 1 or 2 doses of intermediate- or long-acting insulin formulations superimposed with doses of short- or rapid-acting insulin (eg, insulin glulisine) formulations 3 or more times daily.

Adjustment of dose: Dosage must be titrated to achieve glucose control and avoid hypoglycemia. Adjust dose to maintain premeal and bedtime glucose in target range. Since combinations of agents are frequently used, dosage adjustment must address the individual component of the insulin regimen which most directly influences the blood glucose value in question, based on the known onset and duration of the insulin component. Treatment and monitoring regimens must be individualized.

Continuous SubQ insulin infusion (insulin pump): A combination of a "basal" continuous insulin infusion rate with preprogrammed, premeal bolus doses which are patient controlled. When converting from multiple daily SubQ doses of maintenance insulin, it is advisable to reduce the basal rate to less than the equivalent of the total daily units of the longer-acting insulin (eg, NPH); divide the total number of units by 24 to get the basal rate in units/hour. Do not include the total units of regular insulin or other rapid-acting insulin formulations in this calculation. The same premeal regular insulin dosage may be used.

Type 2: Adults: Augmentation therapy (patients for which diet, exercise, weight reduction, and oral hypoglycemic agents have not been adequate): Initial dosage of 0.2 units/kg/day or 10 units/day of an intermediate-acting (eg, NPH) or long-acting insulin administered at bedtime has been recommended. As an alternative, regular insulin or rapid-acting insulin (eg, insulin glulisine) formulations administered before meals have also been used. Dosage must be carefully adjusted.

Hyperglycemia, critically ill (off-label use): Adults: IV continuous infusion: Insulin therapy should be implemented when blood glucose ≥150 mg/dL with a goal to maintain blood glucose <150 mg/dL (with values absolutely <180 mg/dL) using a protocol that achieves a low rate of hypoglycemia (ie, ≤70 mg/dL). Before discontinuation, stable ICU patients should be transitioned to a protocol-driven basal/bolus insulin regimen, based on insulin infusion history and carbohydrate intake, to avoid loss of glycemic control. Subcutaneous insulin therapy may be considered for selected clinically stable ICU patients (Jacobi, 2012). **Note:** The Surviving Sepsis Campaign guidelines recommend initiating insulin dosing in patients with severe sepsis when 2 consecutive blood glucose concentrations are >180 mg/dL and to target an upper blood glucose ≤180 mg/dL (Dellinger, 2013).

Dosing adjustment in renal impairment: No dosage adjustment provided in manufacturer's labeling; insulin requirements may be reduced due to changes in insulin clearance or metabolism; monitor blood glucose closely.

Dosing adjustment in hepatic impairment: No dosage adjustment provided in manufacturer's labeling; insulin requirements may be reduced due to changes in insulin clearance or metabolism; monitor blood glucose closely.

Additional Information Complete prescribing information should be consulted for additional detail.

Dosage Forms

Solution, Injection:

Apidra: 100 units/mL (10 mL)

Solution Pen-injector, Subcutaneous:

Apidra SoloStar: 100 units/mL (3 mL)

Insulin Lispro (IN soo lin LYE sproe)

Brand Names: U.S. HumaLOG; HumaLOG KwikPen

Brand Names: Canada Humalog®

Index Terms Lispro Insulin

Pharmacologic Category Insulin, Rapid-Acting

Use Treatment of type 1 diabetes mellitus (insulin dependent, IDDM) and type 2 diabetes mellitus (noninsulin dependent, NIDDM) to improve glycemic control

Pregnancy Risk Factor B

Dosage Note: Insulin lispro is a rapid-acting insulin analog which is normally administered SubQ as a premeal component of the insulin regimen or as a continuous SubQ infusion and should be used with intermediate- or long-acting insulin. When compared to insulin regular, insulin lispro has a more rapid onset and shorter duration of activity. In carefully controlled clinical settings with close medical supervision and monitoring of blood glucose and potassium, insulin lispro may also be administered IV Insulin requirements vary dramatically between patients and dictate frequent monitoring and close medical supervision.

Diabetes mellitus: SubQ:

General insulin dosing:

Type 1: Children ≥3 years, Adolescents, and Adults: **Note:** Multiple daily doses or continuous subcutaneous infusions guided by blood glucose monitoring are the standard of diabetes care. Combinations of insulin formulations are commonly used. The daily doses presented below are expressed as the **total units/kg/day of all insulin formulations combined.**

Initial total insulin dose: 0.2-0.6 units/kg/day in divided doses. Conservative initial doses of 0.2-0.4 units/kg/day are often recommended to avoid the potential for hypoglycemia. A rapid-acting insulin may be the only insulin formulation used initially.

Usual maintenance range: 0.5-1 units/kg/day in divided doses. An estimate of anticipated needs may be based on body weight and/or activity factors as follows:

Nonobese: 0.4-0.6 units/kg/day

Obese: 0.8-1.2 units/kg/day

Pubescent Children and Adolescents: During puberty, requirements may substantially increase to >1 unit/kg/day and in some cases up to 2 units/kg/day (IDF-ISPAD, 2011).

Division of daily insulin requirement ("conventional therapy"): Generally, 50% to 75% of the total daily dose (TDD) is given as an intermediate- or long-acting form of insulin (in 1-2 daily injections). The remaining portion of the TDD is then divided and administered as either before or at mealtimes (depending on the formulation) as a rapid-acting insulin (eg, insulin lispro) or short-acting form of insulin. Some patients may benefit from the use of CSII which delivers rapid-acting insulin (insulin lispro) as a continuous infusion throughout the day and as boluses at mealtimes via an external pump device.

Division of daily insulin requirement ("intensive therapy"): Basal insulin delivery with 1 or 2 doses of intermediate- or long-acting insulin formulations superimposed with doses of short- or rapid-acting insulin (eg, insulin lispro) formulations 3 or more times daily.

Adjustment of dose: Dosage must be titrated to achieve glucose control and avoid hypoglycemia. Adjust dose to maintain premeal and bedtime glucose in target range. Since combinations of agents are frequently used, dosage adjustment must address the individual component of the insulin regimen which most directly influences the blood glucose value in question, based on the known onset and duration of the insulin component. Treatment and monitoring regimens must be individualized.

Continuous SubQ insulin infusion (insulin pump): A combination of a "basal" continuous insulin infusion rate with preprogrammed, premeal bolus doses which are patient controlled. When converting from multiple daily SubQ doses of maintenance insulin, it is advisable to reduce the basal rate to less than the equivalent of the total daily units of the longer-acting insulin (eg, NPH); divide the total number of units by 24 to get the basal rate in units/hour. Do not include the total units of regular insulin or other rapid-acting insulin formulations in this calculation. The same premeal regular insulin dosage may be used.

Type 2: Adults: Augmentation therapy (patients for which diet, exercise, weight reduction, and oral hypoglycemic agents have not been adequate): Initial dosage of 0.2 units/kg/day or 10 units/day of an intermediate- acting (eg, NPH) or long-acting insulin administered at bedtime has been recommended. As an alternative, regular insulin or rapid-acting insulin (eg, insulin lispro) formulations administered before meals have also been used. Dosage must be carefully adjusted.

Diabetic ketoacidosis (DKA), mild-to-moderate (off-label use): Treatment should continue until reversal of acid-base derangement/ketonemia. Serum glucose is not a direct indicator of these abnormalities, and may decrease more rapidly than correction of the metabolic abnormalities. Also refer to institution-specific protocols where appropriate.

Children and Adolescents: SubQ (**Note:** Use of IV regular insulin is preferred; only use the SubQ route if IV infusion access is unavailable): 0.3 units/kg followed in one hour by 0.1 units/kg given every hour or 0.15-0.2 units/kg every 2 hours; continue until acidosis clears, then decrease to 0.05 units/kg given every hour until maintenance SubQ replacement dosing can be initiated (Kitabchi, 2004; Wolfsdorf, 2007).

Dosing adjustment in renal impairment: Adults: Insulin requirements are reduced due to changes in insulin clearance or metabolism. No dosage adjustment provided in manufacturer's labeling; however, the following adjustments have been recommended (Aronoff, 2007):

CrCl >50 mL/minute: No adjustment necessary

CrCl 10-50 mL/minute: Administer at 75% of recommended dose

CrCl <10 mL/minute: Administer at 50% of recommended dose and monitor glucose closely

Hemodialysis: Because of a large molecular weight (6000 daltons), insulin is not significantly removed by either peritoneal or hemodialysis; supplemental dose is not necessary

Peritoneal dialysis: Supplemental dose is not necessary

Continuous renal replacement therapy: Administer at 75% of recommended dose

Dosing adjustment in hepatic impairment: No dosage adjustment provided in manufacturer's labeling; insulin requirements may be reduced due to changes in insulin clearance or metabolism; monitor blood glucose closely.

Additional Information Complete prescribing information should be consulted for additional detail.

Dosage Forms

Solution, Subcutaneous:

HumaLOG: 100 units/mL (3 mL, 10 mL)

HumaLOG KwikPen: 100 units/mL (3 mL)

Solution Pen-injector, Subcutaneous:

HumaLOG KwikPen: 100 units/mL (3 mL)

◆ **Insulin Lispro and Insulin Lispro Protamine** *see* Insulin Lispro Protamine and Insulin Lispro *on page 1088*

Insulin Lispro Protamine and Insulin Lispro

(IN soo lin LYE sproe PROE ta meen & IN soo lin LYE sproe)

Brand Names: U.S. HumaLOG® Mix 50/50™; HumaLOG® Mix 50/50™ KwikPen™; HumaLOG® Mix 75/25™; HumaLOG® Mix 75/25™ KwikPen™

Brand Names: Canada Humalog® Mix 25

Index Terms Insulin Lispro and Insulin Lispro Protamine

Pharmacologic Category Insulin, Combination

Use Treatment of type 1 diabetes mellitus (insulin dependent, IDDM) and type 2 diabetes mellitus (noninsulin dependent, NIDDM) to improve glycemic control

Pregnancy Risk Factor B

Dosage Note: Lispro protamine is an intermediate-acting insulin and lispro is a rapid-acting insulin administered by SubQ injection. Insulin lispro protamine and insulin lispro combination products are approximately equipotent to insulin NPH and insulin regular combination products with a similar duration of activity but a more rapid onset. With combination insulin products, the proportion of rapid-acting to long-acting insulin is fixed; basal vs prandial dose adjustments cannot be made. Fixed-ratio insulins (such as insulin lispro protamine and insulin lispro combination) are typically administered as 2 daily doses with each dose intended to cover two meals and a snack. Because of variability in the peak effect and individual patient variability in activities, meals, etc, it may be more difficult to achieve complete glycemic control using fixed combinations of insulins; frequent monitoring and close medical supervision may be necessary.

Diabetes mellitus: SubQ:

General insulin dosing:

Type 1: Adults: **Note:** Multiple daily doses are utilized and guided by blood glucose monitoring. Combinations of insulin formulations are commonly used. The daily doses presented below are expressed as the **total units/kg/day of all insulin formulations combined.** Insulin lispro protamine and insulin lispro combination product is **not** intended for initial therapy; basal insulin requirements should be established **first** to direct dosing of combination insulin products.

Usual maintenance range: 0.5-1 units/kg/day in divided doses. An estimate of anticipated needs may be based on body weight and/or activity factors as follows:

Nonobese: 0.4-0.6 units/kg/day

Obese: 0.8-1.2 units/kg/day

Pubescent Children and Adolescents: During puberty, requirements may substantially increase to >1 unit/kg/day and in some cases up to 2 units/kg/day (IDF-ISPAD, 2011).

Division of daily insulin requirement ("conventional therapy"): Generally, 50% to 75% of the daily insulin dose is given as an intermediate- or long-acting form of insulin (in 1-2 daily injections). The remaining portion of the 24-hour insulin requirement is divided and administered as either regular insulin or a rapid-acting form of insulin at the same time before breakfast and dinner.

Adjustment of dose: Dosage must be titrated to achieve glucose control and avoid hypoglycemia. Adjust dose to maintain premeal and bedtime glucose in target range. Since combinations of agents are frequently used, dosage adjustment must address the individual component of the insulin regimen which most directly influences the blood glucose value in question, based on the known onset and duration of the insulin component. Treatment and monitoring regimens must be individualized.

Type 2: Adults: Augmentation therapy (patients for which diet, exercise, weight reduction, and oral hypoglycemic agents have not been adequate): **Note:** Insulin lispro protamine and insulin lispro combination product is **not** intended for initial therapy; basal insulin requirements should be established **first** to direct dosing of combination insulin products. Dosage must be carefully adjusted.

Dosing adjustment in renal impairment: No dosage adjustment provided in manufacturer's labeling; insulin requirements may be reduced due to changes in insulin clearance or metabolism; monitor blood glucose closely.

Dosing adjustment in hepatic impairment: No dosage adjustment provided in manufacturer's labeling; insulin requirements may be reduced due to changes in insulin clearance or metabolism; monitor blood glucose closely.

Additional Information Complete prescribing information should be consulted for additional detail.

Dosage Forms

Injection, suspension:

HumaLOG® Mix 50/50™: Insulin lispro protamine suspension 50% [intermediate acting] and insulin lispro solution 50% [rapid acting]: 100 units/mL (10 mL)

HumaLOG® Mix 50/50™ KwikPen™: Insulin lispro protamine suspension 50% [intermediate acting] and insulin lispro solution 50% [rapid acting]: 100 units/mL (3 mL)

HumaLOG® Mix 75/25™: Insulin lispro protamine suspension 75% [intermediate acting] and insulin lispro solution 25% [rapid acting]: 100 units/mL (10 mL)

HumaLOG® Mix 75/25™ KwikPen™: Insulin lispro protamine suspension 75% [intermediate acting] and insulin lispro solution 25% [rapid acting]: 100 units/mL (3 mL)

Insulin NPH (IN soo lin N P H)

Brand Names: U.S. HumuLIN N KwikPen [OTC]; HumuLIN N Pen [OTC] [DSC]; HumuLIN N [OTC]; NovoLIN N ReliOn [OTC]; NovoLIN N [OTC]

Brand Names: Canada Humulin® N; Novolin® ge NPH

Index Terms Isophane Insulin; NPH Insulin

Pharmacologic Category Insulin, Intermediate-Acting

Use Treatment of type 1 diabetes mellitus (insulin dependent, IDDM) and type 2 diabetes mellitus (noninsulin dependent, NIDDM) to improve glycemic control

Pregnancy Risk Factor B

Dosage Note: Insulin NPH is an intermediate-acting insulin formulation which is usually administered subcutaneously once or twice daily. When compared to insulin regular, insulin NPH has a slower onset and longer duration of activity. Insulin requirements vary dramatically between patients and dictate frequent monitoring and close medical supervision.

Diabetes mellitus: SubQ:

General insulin dosing:

Type 1: Children, Adolescents, and Adults: **Note:** Multiple daily doses are utilized and guided by blood glucose monitoring. Combinations of insulin formulations are commonly used. The daily doses presented below are expressed as the **total units/kg/day of all insulin formulations combined.** Insulin NPH is **not** intended for initial therapy; basal insulin requirements should be established **first** to direct dosing.

Usual maintenance range: 0.5-1 units/kg/day in divided doses. An estimate of anticipated needs may be based on body weight and/or activity factors as follows:

Nonobese: 0.4-0.6 units/kg/day

Obese: 0.8-1.2 units/kg/day

Pubescent Children and Adolescents: During puberty, requirements may substantially increase to >1 unit/kg/day and in some cases up to 2 units/kg/day (IDF-ISPAD, 2011).

Division of daily insulin requirement ("conventional therapy"): Generally, 50% to 75% of the total daily dose (TDD) is given as an intermediate-acting (eg, NPH) or a long-acting form of insulin (in 1-2 daily injections). The remaining portion of the TDD is then divided and administered before or at mealtimes (depending on the formulation) as a rapid-acting or short-acting form of insulin.

Division of daily insulin requirement ("intensive therapy"): Basal insulin delivery with 1 or 2 doses of intermediate-acting (eg, NPH) or long-acting insulin formulations superimposed with doses of short- or rapid-acting insulin formulations 3 or more times daily.

Adjustment of dose: Dosage must be titrated to achieve glucose control and avoid hypoglycemia. Adjust dose to maintain premeal and bedtime glucose in target range. Since combinations of agents are frequently used, dosage adjustment must address the individual component of the insulin regimen which most directly influences the blood glucose value in question, based on the known onset and duration of the insulin component.

Type 2: Augmentation therapy (patients for which diet, exercise, weight reduction, and oral hypoglycemic agents have not been adequate): Adults: Initial dosage of 0.2 units/kg/day or 10 units/day of an intermediate-acting (eg, NPH) or long-acting insulin administered at bedtime has been recommended. As an alternative, regular insulin or rapid-acting insulin formulations administered before meals have also been used. Dosage must be carefully adjusted.

Dosing adjustment in renal impairment: No dosage adjustment provided in manufacturer's labeling; insulin requirements may be reduced due to changes in insulin clearance or metabolism; monitor blood glucose closely.

Dosing adjustment in hepatic impairment: No dosage adjustment provided in manufacturer's labeling; insulin requirements may be reduced due to changes in insulin clearance or metabolism; monitor blood glucose closely.

Additional Information Complete prescribing information should be consulted for additional detail.

Dosage Forms

Suspension, Subcutaneous:

HumuLIN N [OTC]: 100 units/mL (3 mL, 10 mL)

NovoLIN N [OTC]: 100 units/mL (10 mL)

NovoLIN N ReliOn [OTC]: 100 units/mL (10 mL)

Suspension Pen-injector, Subcutaneous:

HumuLIN N KwikPen [OTC]: 100 units/mL (3 mL)

Dosage Forms: Canada

Injection, suspension:

Novolin® ge NPH: 100 units/mL (3 mL, 10 mL)

Insulin NPH and Insulin Regular

(IN soo lin N P H & IN soo lin REG yoo ler)

Brand Names: U.S. HumuLIN® 70/30; HumuLIN® 70/30 KwikPen; NovoLIN® 70/30

Brand Names: Canada Humulin® 20/80; Humulin® 70/30; Novolin® ge 30/70; Novolin® ge 40/60; Novolin® ge 50/50

Index Terms Insulin Regular and Insulin NPH; Isophane Insulin and Regular Insulin; NPH Insulin and Regular Insulin

Pharmacologic Category Insulin, Combination

Use Treatment of type 1 diabetes mellitus (insulin dependent, IDDM) and type 2 diabetes mellitus (noninsulin dependent, NIDDM) to improve glycemic control

Pregnancy Risk Factor B

Dosage Note: Insulin NPH is an intermediate-acting insulin and regular insulin is a short-acting insulin administered by SubQ injection. When compared to insulin NPH, the combination product (insulin NPH and insulin regular) has a shorter onset of action and a similar duration of action. With combination insulin products, the proportion of short-acting to long-acting insulin is fixed; basal vs prandial dose adjustments cannot be made. Fixed-ratio insulins (such as insulin NPH and insulin regular combination) are typically administered as 2 daily doses with each dose intended to cover two meals and a snack. Because of variability in the peak effect and individual patient variability in activities, meals, etc, it may be more difficult to achieve complete glycemic control using fixed combinations of insulins; frequent monitoring and close medical supervision may be necessary.

Diabetes mellitus: SubQ:

General insulin dosing:

Type 1: Children, Adolescents, and Adults: **Note:** Multiple daily doses are utilized and guided by blood glucose monitoring. Combinations of different insulin formulations are commonly used. The daily doses presented below are expressed as the **total units/kg/day of all insulin formulations combined.** Insulin NPH and insulin regular combination product is **not** intended for initial therapy; basal insulin requirements should be established **first** to direct dosing of combination insulin products.

Usual maintenance range: 0.5-1 units/kg/day in divided doses. An estimate of anticipated needs may be based on body weight and/or activity factors as follows:

Nonobese: 0.4-0.6 units/kg/day

Obese: 0.8-1.2 units/kg/day

Pubescent Children and Adolescents: During puberty, requirements may substantially increase to >1 unit/kg/day and in some cases up to 2 units/kg/day (IDF-ISPAD, 2011).

Division of daily insulin requirement ("conventional therapy"): Generally, 50% to 75% of the total daily dose (TDD) is given as an intermediate-acting (eg, NPH) or a long-acting form of insulin (in 1-2 daily injections). The remaining portion of the TDD is then divided and administered before or at mealtimes (depending on the formulation) as a rapid-acting or short-acting form of insulin.

Adjustment of dose: Dosage must be titrated to achieve glucose control and avoid hypoglycemia. Adjust dose to maintain premeal and bedtime glucose in target range. Since combinations of agents are frequently used, dosage adjustment must address the individual component of the insulin regimen which most directly influences the blood glucose value in question, based on the known onset and duration of the insulin component.

Type 2: Augmentation therapy (patients for which diet, exercise, weight reduction, and oral hypoglycemic agents have not been adequate): Adults: **Note:** Insulin NPH and insulin regular combination product is **not** intended for initial therapy; basal insulin requirements should be established **first** to direct dosing of combination insulin products. Dosage must be carefully adjusted.

Dosing adjustment in renal impairment: No dosage adjustment provided in manufacturer's labeling; insulin requirements may be reduced due to changes in insulin clearance or metabolism; monitor blood glucose closely.

Dosing adjustment in hepatic impairment: No dosage adjustment provided in manufacturer's labeling; insulin requirements may be reduced due to changes in insulin clearance or metabolism; monitor blood glucose closely.

Additional Information Complete prescribing information should be consulted for additional detail.

Dosage Forms

Injection, suspension:

HumuLIN® 70/30: Insulin NPH suspension 70% [intermediate acting] and insulin regular solution 30% [short acting]: 100 units/mL (3 mL, 10 mL)

HumuLIN® 70/30 KwikPen: Insulin NPH suspension 70% [intermediate acting] and insulin regular solution 30% [short acting]: 100 units/mL (3 mL)

NovoLIN® 70/30: Insulin NPH suspension 70% [intermediate acting] and insulin regular solution 30% [short acting]: 100 units/mL (10 mL)

Dosage Forms: Canada

Injection, suspension:

Humulin® 20/80: Insulin regular solution 20% [short acting] and insulin NPH suspension 80% [intermediate acting]: 100 units/mL (3 mL)

Novolin® ge 30/70: Insulin regular solution 30% [short acting] and insulin NPH suspension 70% [intermediate acting]: 100 units/mL (3 mL)

Novolin® ge 40/60: Insulin regular solution 40% [short acting] and insulin NPH suspension 60% [intermediate acting]: 100 units/mL (3 mL)

Novolin® ge 50/50: Insulin regular solution 50% [short acting] and insulin NPH suspension 50% [intermediate acting]: 100 units/mL (3 mL)

Insulin Regular (IN soo lin REG yoo ler)

Brand Names: U.S. HumuLIN R U-500 (CONCENTRATED); HumuLIN R [OTC]; NovoLIN R ReliOn [OTC]; NovoLIN R [OTC]

Brand Names: Canada Humulin R; Novolin ge Toronto

Index Terms Regular Insulin

Pharmacologic Category Insulin, Short-Acting

Additional Appendix Information

Beers Criteria - Potentially Inappropriate Medications for Geriatrics *on page 2271*

Use Diabetes mellitus, type 1 or type 2: Treatment of diabetes mellitus (type 1 or type 2) to improve glycemic control

Pregnancy Risk Factor B

Pregnancy Considerations Recombinant human insulin for injection is identical to endogenous insulin; therefore, animal reproduction studies have not been conducted. Minimal amounts of endogenous insulin cross the placenta. Exogenous insulin bound to anti-insulin antibodies can be detected in cord blood (Menon 1990)

In women with diabetes, maternal hyperglycemia can be associated with congenital malformations as well as adverse effects in the fetus, neonate, and the mother (ACOG 2005; ADA 2014; Kitzmiller 2008; Metzger 2007). To prevent adverse outcomes, prior to conception and throughout pregnancy maternal blood glucose and HbA_{1c} should be kept as close to normal as possible but without causing significant hypoglycemia (ACOG 2013; ADA 2014; Blumer 2013; Kitzmiller 2008; Lambert 2013). Prior to pregnancy, effective contraception should be used until glycemic control is achieved (ADA 2014; Kitzmiller 2008).

Insulin requirements tend to fall during the first trimester of pregnancy and increase in the later trimesters, peaking at 28 to 32 weeks of gestation. Following delivery, insulin requirements decrease rapidly (ACOG 2005).

Rapid acting insulins, such as insulin aspart or insulin lispro may be preferred over regular human insulin in women trying to conceive (Blumer 2013); however, there is no need to switch a pregnant woman who is well controlled on injectable human insulin to a short acting analogue (Lambert 2013).

Breast-Feeding Considerations Both exogenous and endogenous insulin are excreted into breast milk (study not conducted with this preparation) (Whitmore 2012). Breast-feeding is encouraged for all women, including those with type 1, type 2, or GDM (ACOG 2005; Blumer 2013; Metzger 2007). Small snacks before feeds may help decrease the risk of hypoglycemia in women with pregestational diabetes (ACOG 2005; Reader 2004).

Adverse events have not been reported in nursing infants following use of regular insulin for injection; adjustments of the mothers insulin dose may be needed.

Contraindications

Hypersensitivity to regular insulin or any component of the formulation; during episodes of hypoglycemia.

Documentation of allergenic cross-reactivity for insulin is limited. However, because of similarities in chemical structure and/or pharmacologic actions, the possibility of cross-sensitivity cannot be ruled out with certainty.

Warnings/Precautions Hypoglycemia is the most common adverse effect of insulin. The timing of hypoglycemia differs among various insulin formulations. Hypoglycemia may result from increased work or exercise without eating; use of long-acting insulin preparations (eg, insulin detemir, insulin glargine) may delay recovery from hypoglycemia. Profound and prolonged episodes of hypoglycemia may result in convulsions, unconsciousness, temporary or permanent brain damage or even death. Insulin requirements may be altered during illness, emotional disturbances or other stressors. Instruct patients to use caution with ethanol; may increase risk of hypoglycemia. Insulin may produce hypokalemia which, if left untreated, may result in respiratory paralysis, ventricular arrhythmia and even death. Use with caution in patients at risk for hypokalemia (eg, IV insulin use). Severe, life-threatening, generalized allergic reactions, including anaphylaxis, may occur. If hypersensitivity reactions occur, discontinue therapy, treat the patient with supportive care and monitor until signs and symptoms resolve. Use with caution in renal or hepatic impairment. In the elderly, avoid use of sliding scale injectable insulin in this population due to increased risk of hypoglycemia without benefits in management of hyperglycemia regardless of care setting (Beers Criteria).

Human insulin differs from animal-source insulin. Any change of insulin should be made cautiously; changing manufacturers, type, and/or method of manufacture may result in the need for a change of dosage. U-500 regular insulin is a concentrated insulin formulation which contains 500 units of insulin per mL; for SubQ administration only using a U-100 insulin syringe or tuberculin syringe; **not for IV administration**. To avoid dosing errors when using a U-100 insulin syringe, the prescribed dose should be written in actual insulin units and as unit markings on the U-100 insulin syringe (eg, 50 units [10 units on a U-100 insulin syringe]). To avoid dosing errors when using a tuberculin syringe, the prescribed dose should be written in actual insulin units and as a volume (eg, 50 units [0.1 mL]). Mixing U-500 regular insulin with other insulin formulations is not recommended.

Regular insulin may be administered IV or IM in selected clinical situations; close monitoring of blood glucose and serum potassium, as well as medical supervision, is required.

The general objective of exogenous insulin therapy is to approximate the physiologic pattern of insulin secretion which is characterized by two distinct phases. Phase 1 insulin secretion suppresses hepatic glucose production and phase 2 insulin secretion occurs in response to carbohydrate ingestion; therefore, exogenous insulin therapy may consist of basal insulin (eg, intermediate- or long-acting insulin or via continuous subcutaneous insulin infusion [CSII]) and/or preprandial insulin (eg, short- or rapid-acting insulin). Patients with type 1 diabetes do not produce endogenous insulin; therefore, these patients require both basal and preprandial insulin administration. Patients with type 2 diabetes retain some beta-cell function in the early stages of their disease; however, as the disease progresses, phase 1 insulin secretion may become completely impaired and phase 2 insulin secretion becomes delayed and/or inadequate in response to meals. Therefore, patients with type 2 diabetes may be treated with oral antidiabetic agents, basal insulin, and/or preprandial insulin depending on the stage of disease and current glycemic control. Since treatment regimens often consist of multiple agents, dosage adjustments must address the specific phase of insulin release that is primarily contributing to the patient's impaired glycemic control. Diabetes self-management education (DSME) is essential to maximize the effectiveness of therapy. Treatment and monitoring regimens must be individualized.

Potentially significant drug-drug interactions may exist, requiring dose or frequency adjustment, additional monitoring, and/or selection of alternative therapy. In particular, concurrent use with peroxisome proliferator-activated receptor (PPAR)-gamma agonists, including thiazolidinediones (TZDs) may cause dose-related fluid retention and lead to or exacerbate heart failure.

Adverse Reactions Primarily symptoms of hypoglycemia. Frequency not defined.

Cardiovascular: Palpitations, tachycardia

Central nervous system: Confusion, fatigue, headache, hypothermia, loss of consciousness, myasthenia, paresthesia

Dermatologic: Diaphoresis, erythema, pallor, urticaria

Endocrine & metabolic: Hypoglycemia, hypokalemia

Gastrointestinal: Hunger, nausea, oral hypoesthesia

Hypersensitivity: Anaphylaxis, hypersensitivity reaction (local and/or systemic)

Local: Lipoatrophy at injection site, lipotrophy at injection site, localized edema, local pruritus, pain at injection site, warm sensation at injection site

Neuromuscular & skeletal: Tremor

Ophthalmic: Blurred vision (transient), presbyopia (transient)

Drug Interactions

Metabolism/Transport Effects None known.

Avoid Concomitant Use There are no known interactions where it is recommended to avoid concomitant use.

Increased Effect/Toxicity

Insulin Regular may increase the levels/effects of: Hypoglycemic Agents; Quinolone Antibiotics

The levels/effects of Insulin Regular may be increased by: Androgens; Beta-Blockers; Edetate CALCIUM Disodium; Edetate Disodium; GLP-1 Agonists; Herbs (Hypoglycemic Properties); Liraglutide; MAO Inhibitors; Metreleptin; Pegvisomant; Pramlintide; Salicylates; Selective Serotonin Reuptake Inhibitors; SGLT2 Inhibitors

Decreased Effect

The levels/effects of Insulin Regular may be decreased by: Corticosteroids (Orally Inhaled); Corticosteroids (Systemic); Danazol; Loop Diuretics; Luteinizing Hormone-Releasing Hormone Analogs; Somatropin; Thiazide Diuretics

Preparation for Administration

For SubQ administration:

Humulin R: May be diluted with the universal diluent, Sterile Diluent for Humalog, Humulin N, Humulin R, Humulin 70/30, and Humulin R U-500, to a concentration of 10 units/mL (U-10) or 50 units/mL (U-50).

Novolin R: Insulin Diluting Medium for NovoLog is **not** intended for use with Novolin R or any insulin product other than insulin aspart.

For IV infusion:

Humulin R: May be diluted in NS or D_5W to concentrations of 0.1-1 unit/mL.

Novolin R: May be diluted in NS, D_5W, or $D_{10}W$ with 40 mEq/L potassium chloride at concentrations of 0.05 to 1 unit/mL.

Storage/Stability

Humulin R, Humulin R U-500: Store unopened vials in refrigerator between 2°C and 8°C (36°F to 46°F); do not freeze; keep away from heat and sunlight. Once punctured (in use), vials may be stored for up to 31 days in the refrigerator between 2°C and 8°C (36°F to 46°F) or at room temperature of ≤30°C (≤86°F).

Novolin R: Store unopened vials in refrigerator between 2°C and 8°C (36°F to 46°F) until product expiration date or at room temperature ≤25°C (≤77°F) for up to 42 days; do not freeze; keep away from heat and sunlight. Once punctured (in use), store vials at room temperature ≤25°C (≤77°F) for up to 42 days (this includes any days stored at room temperature prior to opening vial); refrigeration of in-use vials is not recommended.

Canadian labeling (not in U.S. labeling): All products: Unopened vials, cartridges, and pens should be stored under refrigeration between 2°C and 8°C (36°F to 46°F) until the expiration date; do not freeze; keep away from heat and sunlight. Once punctured (in use), Humulin vials, cartridges, and pens should be stored at room temperature <25°C (<77°F) for up to 4 weeks. Once punctured (in use), Novolin ge vials, cartridges, and pens may be stored for up to 1 month at room temperature <25°C (<77°F) for vials or <30°C (<86°F) for pens/cartridges; do not refrigerate.

For SubQ administration:

Humulin R: According to the manufacturer, diluted insulin should be stored at 30°C (86°F) and used within 14 days **or** at 5°C (41°F) and used within 28 days.

For IV infusion:

Humulin R: Stable for 48 hours at room temperature or for 48 hours under refrigeration followed by 48 hours at room temperature.

Novolin R: Stable for 24 hours at room temperature

Mechanism of Action Insulin acts via specific membrane-bound receptors on target tissues to regulate metabolism of carbohydrate, protein, and fats. Target organs for insulin include the liver, skeletal muscle, and adipose tissue.

Within the liver, insulin stimulates hepatic glycogen synthesis. Insulin promotes hepatic synthesis of fatty acids, which are released into the circulation as lipoproteins. Skeletal muscle effects of insulin include increased protein synthesis and increased glycogen synthesis. Within adipose tissue, insulin stimulates the processing of circulating lipoproteins to provide free fatty acids, facilitating triglyceride synthesis and storage by adipocytes; also directly inhibits the hydrolysis of triglycerides. In addition, insulin stimulates the cellular uptake of amino acids and increases cellular permeability to several ions, including potassium, magnesium, and phosphate. By activating sodium-potassium ATPases, insulin promotes the intracellular movement of potassium.

Normally secreted by the pancreas, insulin products are manufactured for pharmacologic use through recombinant DNA technology using either *E. coli* or *Saccharomyces cerevisiae*. Insulins are categorized based on the onset, peak, and duration of effect (eg, rapid-, short-, intermediate-, and long-acting insulin).

Pharmacodynamics/Kinetics Note: Rate of absorption, onset, and duration of activity may be affected by site of injection, exercise, presence of lipodystrophy, local blood supply, and/or temperature.

Onset of action: SubQ: 0.5 hours

Peak effect: SubQ: 2.5 to 5 hours

Duration: SubQ:

U-100: 4 to 12 hours (may increase with dose)

U-500: Up to 24 hours

Distribution: IV, SubQ: V_d: 0.26 to 0.36 L/kg

Bioavailability: SubQ: 55% to 77%

Half-life elimination: IV: ~0.5 to 1 hour (dose-dependent); SubQ: 1.5 hours

Time to peak, plasma: SubQ: 0.8 to 2 hours

Excretion: Urine

Dosage

Diabetes mellitus: Note: Insulin requirements vary dramatically between patients and therapy requires dosage adjustments with careful medical supervision. Specific formulations may require distinct administration procedures; please see individual agents.

SubQ: Children and Adults:

Diabetes mellitus, type 1: **Note:** Multiple daily injections (MDI) guided by blood glucose monitoring or the use of continuous subcutaneous insulin infusions (CSII) is the standard of care for patients with type 1 diabetes. Combinations of insulin formulations are commonly used.

Initial dose: 0.5 to 1 units/kg/day in divided doses. Conservative initial doses of 0.2 to 0.4 units/kg/day may be recommended to avoid the potential for hypoglycemia.

Division of daily insulin requirement: Generally, 50% to 75% of the total daily dose (TDD) is given as an intermediate- or long-acting form of insulin (in 1 to 2 daily injections). The remaining portion of the TDD is then divided and administered before or at mealtimes (depending on the formulation) as a rapid-acting or short-acting form of insulin.

Adjustment of dose: Dosage must be titrated to achieve glucose control and avoid hypoglycemia. Adjust dose to maintain preprandial plasma glucose between 70 to 130 mg/dL for most patients. Since treatment regimens often consist of multiple formulations, dosage adjustments must address the specific phase of insulin release that is primarily contributing to the patient's impaired glycemic control. Treatment and monitoring regimens must be individualized. Also see Additional Information.

Usual maintenance range: 0.5 to 1.2 units/kg/day in divided doses. Insulin requirements are patient-specific and may vary based on age, body weight, and/or activity factors:

Adolescents: May require as much as 1.5 units/kg/day during puberty (Silverstein, 2005)

Prepuberty: 0.7 to 1 unit/kg/day

Diabetes mellitus, type 2: The goal of therapy is to achieve an HbA_{1c} <7% as quickly as possible using the safe titration of medications. According to a consensus statement by the ADA and European Association for the Study of Diabetes (EASD), basal insulin therapy (eg, intermediate- or long-acting insulin) should be considered in patients with type 2 diabetes who fail to achieve glycemic goals with lifestyle interventions and metformin ± a sulfonylurea. Pioglitazone or a GLP-1 agonist may also be considered prior to initiation of basal insulin therapy. In patients who continue to fail to achieve glycemic goals despite the addition of basal insulin, intensification of insulin therapy should be considered; this generally consists of multiple daily injections with a combination of insulin formulations (Nathan, 2009).

Intensification of therapy: Add a second injection of a short-, rapid-, or intermediate-acting insulin as needed based on blood glucose monitoring; the timing of administration and type of insulin added for intensification of therapy depends on the blood glucose level that is consistently out of the target range (eg, preprandial glucose levels before lunch or dinner, postprandial glucose levels, and/or bedtime glucose levels). Additional injections and subsequent dosage adjustments must address the specific phase of insulin release that is primarily contributing to the patient's impaired glycemic control. Intensification of therapy can usually begin with a second injection of ~4 units/day followed by adjustments of ~2 units/day every 3 days until the targeted blood glucose is within range (Nathan, 2009).

In the setting of glucose toxicity (loss of beta-cell sensitivity to glucose concentrations), insulin therapy may be used for short-term management to restore sensitivity of beta-cells; in these cases, the dose may need to be rapidly reduced/withdrawn when sensitivity is re-established.

Diabetic ketoacidosis (DKA) (off-label use): Only IV regular insulin should be used for severe DKA (Kitabchi, 2009). Treatment should continue until reversal of acid-base derangement/ketonemia. Serum glucose is not a direct indicator of these abnormalities, and may decrease more rapidly than correction of the metabolic abnormalities. Also, refer to institution-specific protocols where appropriate.

Children and Adults <20 years (Kitabchi, 2004):

IV:

Infusion: 0.1 units/kg/hour

Adjustment: If serum glucose does not fall by 50 mg/dL in the first hour, check hydration status; if acceptable, double insulin dose hourly until glucose levels fall at rate of 50 to 75 mg/dL per hour. Once serum glucose reaches 250 mg/dL, decrease dose to 0.05 to 0.1 units/kg/hour; dextrose-containing IV fluids should be administered to maintain serum glucose between 150 to 250 mg/dL until the acidosis clears. After resolution of DKA, supplement IV insulin with SubQ insulin as needed until the patient is able to eat and transition fully to a SubQ insulin regimen. An overlap of ~1 to 2 hours between discontinuation of IV insulin and administration of SubQ insulin is recommended to ensure adequate plasma insulin levels.

SubQ, IM (**Note:** Only use the SubQ and IM route if IV infusion access is unavailable): 0.1 to 0.3 units/kg SubQ bolus, followed by 0.1 units/kg given every hour SubQ or IM or 0.15 to 0.2 units/kg every 2 hours SubQ; continue until acidosis clears, then decrease to 0.05 units/kg given every hour until SubQ replacement dosing can be initiated (Kitabchi, 2004; Wolfsdorf, 2007)

Adults ≥20 years (Kitabchi, 2009):

IV:

Bolus: 0.1 units/kg (optional)

Infusion: 0.1 to 0.14 units/kg/hour. **Note:** If no IV bolus was administered, patients should receive a continuous infusion of 0.14 units/kg/hour; lower doses may not achieve adequate insulin concentrations to suppress hepatic ketone body production.

Adjustment: If serum glucose does not fall by at least 10% in the first hour, give an IV bolus of 0.14 units/kg and continue previous regimen. In addition, if serum glucose does not fall by 50 to 70 mg/dL in the first hour, the insulin infusion dose should be increased hourly until a steady glucose decline is achieved Once serum glucose reaches 200 mg/dL, decrease infusion dose to 0.02 to 0.05 units/kg/hour or switch to SubQ rapid-acting insulin (eg, aspart, lispro) at 0.1 units/kg every 2 hours; dextrose-containing IV fluids should be administered to maintain serum glucose between 150 to 250 mg/dL until the acidosis clears. After resolution of DKA, supplement IV insulin with SubQ insulin as needed until the patient is able to eat and transition fully to a SubQ insulin regimen. An overlap of ~1 to 2 hours between discontinuation of IV insulin and administration of SubQ insulin is recommended to ensure adequate plasma insulin levels.

SubQ, IM: The following dosing regimen from the 2004 ADA position statement recommends regular insulin (Kitabchi, 2004):

Bolus: 0.4 units/kg; **Note:** Give half of the dose (0.2 units/kg) as an IV bolus and half of the dose (0.2 units/kg) as SubQ or IM

Intermittent: 0.1 units/kg given every hour SubQ or IM

Adjustment: If serum glucose does not fall by 50 to 70 mg/dL in the first hour, administer 10 units hourly by IV bolus until glucose levels fall at a rate of 50 to 70 mg/dL per hour. Once serum glucose reaches 250 mg/dL, decrease dose to 5 to 10 units SubQ every 2 hours; dextrose-containing IV fluids should be administered to maintain serum glucose between 150 to 250 mg/dL until the acidosis clears.

Gestational diabetes mellitus (off-label use): SubQ: Insulin therapy should be considered when medical nutrition therapy has not achieved GDM glycemic goals (fasting plasma glucose: <95 mg/dL; 1-hour postprandial levels: <130 to 140 mg/dL; 2-hour postprandial levels: <120 mg/dL); dose and timing of administration should be based on frequent monitoring of plasma glucose levels (ACOG, 2001; ADA, 2004). Human insulin may be preferred (ADA, 2004); however, rapid-acting insulin analogues may also be considered (ACOG, 2001).

Hyperglycemia, critically ill (off-label use): Adults: IV continuous infusion: Insulin therapy should be implemented when blood glucose ≥150 mg/dL with a goal to maintain blood glucose <150 mg/dL (with values absolutely <180 mg/dL) using a protocol that achieves a low rate of hypoglycemia (ie, ≤70 mg/dL). Alternatively, other rapid acting insulin analogues (eg, insulin aspart or insulin glulisine) may also be used as a continuous infusion to maintain glycemic control (in place of regular insulin). Before discontinuation, stable ICU patients should be transitioned to a protocol-driven basal/bolus insulin regimen, based on insulin infusion history and carbohydrate intake, to avoid loss of glycemic control. Subcutaneous insulin therapy may be considered for selected clinically stable ICU patients (Jacobi, 2012). **Note:** The Surviving Sepsis Campaign guidelines recommend initiating insulin dosing in patients with severe sepsis when 2 consecutive blood glucose concentrations are >180 mg/dL and to target an upper blood glucose ≤180 mg/dL (Dellinger, 2013).

Hyperkalemia, moderate-to-severe (off-label use): IV:

Children: 0.1 units/kg regular insulin with dextrose 400 mg/kg infused over 15 to 30 minutes; ratio of ~1 unit of insulin to every 4 g of dextrose (Hegenbarth, 2008). **Note:** Dextrose monotherapy may be sufficient to correct hyperkalemia.

Adults: 10 units regular insulin mixed with 25 g dextrose (50 mL $D_{50}W$) given over 15 to 30 minutes (ACLS, 2010); alternatively, 50 mL $D_{50}W$ over 5 minutes followed by 10 units regular insulin IV push over seconds may be administered in the setting of imminent cardiac arrest. In patients with ongoing cardiac arrest (eg, PEA with presumed hyperkalemia), administration of $D_{50}W$ over <5 minutes is routine. Effects on potassium are temporary. As appropriate, consider methods of enhancing potassium removal/excretion.

Hyperosmolar hyperglycemic state (HHS) (off-label use): Only regular injectable insulin should be used. Infusion should continue until reversal of mental status changes and hyperosmolality. Serum glucose is not a direct indicator of these abnormalities, and may decrease more rapidly than correction of the metabolic abnormalities. Also, refer to institution-specific protocols where appropriate.

Children and Adults <20 years (Kitabchi, 2004):

IV:

Infusion: 0.1 units/kg/hour

Adjustment: If serum glucose does not fall by 50 mg/dL in the first hour, check hydration status; if acceptable, double insulin dose hourly until glucose levels fall at rate of 50 to 75 mg/dL per hour. Once serum glucose reaches 300 mg/dL, decrease dose to 0.05 to 0.1 units/kg/hour; dextrose-containing IV fluids should be administered to maintain serum glucose between 250 to 300 mg/dL until hyperosmolality clears and mental status returns to normal. After resolution of HHS, supplement IV insulin with SubQ insulin as needed until the patient is able to eat and transition fully to a SubQ insulin regimen. An overlap of ~1 to 2 hours between discontinuation of IV insulin and administration of SubQ insulin is recommended to ensure adequate plasma insulin levels.

SubQ, IM (**Note:** Only use the SubQ and IM route if IV infusion access is unavailable): 0.1 to 0.3 units/kg SubQ bolus, followed by 0.1 units/kg given every hour SubQ or IM or 0.15 to 0.2 units/kg every 2 hours SubQ; continue until resolution of hyperosmolality, then decrease to 0.05 units/kg given every hour until SubQ replacement dosing can be initiated (Kitabchi, 2004; Wolfsdorf, 2007)

Adults ≥20 years (Kitabchi, 2009):

IV:

Bolus: 0.1 units/kg bolus (optional)

Infusion: 0.1 to 0.14 units/kg/hour. **Note:** If no IV bolus was administered, patients should receive a continuous infusion of 0.14 units/kg/hour.

Adjustment: If serum glucose does not fall by at least 10% in the first hour, give an IV bolus of 0.14 units/kg and continue previous regimen. In addition, if serum glucose does not fall by 50 to 70 mg/dL in the first hour, the insulin infusion dose should be increased hourly until a steady glucose decline is achieved. Once serum glucose reaches 300 mg/dL, decrease dose to 0.02 to 0.05 units/kg/hour; dextrose-containing IV fluids should be administered to maintain serum glucose between 200 to 300 mg/dL until the patient is mentally alert. After resolution of HHS, supplement IV insulin with SubQ insulin as needed until the patient is able to eat and transition fully to a SubQ insulin regimen. An overlap of ~1 to 2 hours between discontinuation of IV insulin and administration of SubQ insulin is recommended to ensure adequate plasma insulin levels.

Dosage adjustment in renal impairment: Note: Insulin requirements are reduced due to changes in insulin clearance or metabolism. Close monitoring of blood glucose and adjustment of therapy may be required in renal impairment.

SubQ, IV:

CrCl 10 to 50 mL/minute: Administer at 75% of normal dose and monitor glucose closely

CrCl <10 mL/minute: Administer at 25% to 50% of normal dose and monitor glucose closely

Hemodialysis: Because of a large molecular weight (6000 daltons), insulin is not significantly removed by hemodialysis; supplemental dose is not necessary

Peritoneal dialysis: Because of a large molecular weight (6000 daltons), insulin is not significantly removed by peritoneal dialysis; supplemental dose is not necessary

Continuous renal replacement therapy: Administer 75% of normal dose and monitor glucose closely; supplemental dose is not necessary

Dosage adjustment in hepatic impairment: Insulin requirements may be reduced. Close monitoring of blood glucose and adjustment of therapy may be required in hepatic impairment.

Dietary Considerations Individualized medical nutrition therapy (MNT) based on ADA recommendations is an integral part of therapy.

Usual Infusion Concentrations: Pediatric IV infusion: 0.1 unit/mL, 0.5 unit/mL, **or** 1 unit/mL

Usual Infusion Concentrations: Adult IV infusion: 100 units in 100 mL (concentration: 1 unit/mL) of NS

Administration

SubQ administration: Do not use if solution is viscous or cloudy; use only if clear and colorless. Regular insulin should be administered within 30 to 60 minutes before a meal. Cold injections should be avoided. SubQ administration is usually made into the thighs, arms, buttocks, or abdomen; rotate injection sites. When mixing regular insulin with other preparations of insulin, regular insulin should be drawn into syringe first. Regular insulin is not recommended for use in external SubQ insulin infusion pump.

IM administration: Do not use if solution is viscous or cloudy; use only if clear and colorless. May be administered IM in selected clinical situations; close monitoring of blood glucose and serum potassium as well as medical supervision is required.

IV administration: Do not use if solution is viscous or cloudy; use only if clear and colorless. May be administered IV with close monitoring of blood glucose and serum potassium; appropriate medical supervision is required. If possible, avoid IV bolus administration in pediatric patients with DKA; may increase risk of cerebral edema. **Do not administer mixtures of insulin formulations intravenously.** IV administration of U-500 regular insulin is not recommended.

IV infusions: To minimize insulin adsorption to IV tubing: Flush the IV tubing with a priming infusion of 20 mL from the insulin infusion, whenever a new IV tubing set is added to the insulin infusion container (Jacobi, 2012; Thompson, 2012).

Note: Also refer to institution-specific protocols where appropriate.

If insulin is required prior to the availability of the insulin drip, regular insulin should be administered by IV push injection.

Because of insulin adsorption to IV tubing or infusion bags, the actual amount of insulin being administered via IV infusion could be substantially less than the apparent amount. Therefore, adjustment of the IV infusion rate should be based on effect and not solely on the apparent insulin dose. The apparent dose may be used as a starting point for determining the subsequent SubQ dosing regimen (Moghissi, 2009); however, the transition to SubQ administration requires continuous medical supervision, frequent monitoring of blood glucose, and careful adjustment of therapy. In addition, SubQ insulin should be given 1 to 4 hours prior to the discontinuation of IV insulin to prevent hyperglycemia (Moghissi, 2009).

Monitoring Parameters

Critically-ill patients receiving insulin infusion: Blood glucose every 1 to 2 hours. **Note:** Every 4 hour blood glucose monitoring is not recommended unless a low hypoglycemia rate is demonstrated with the insulin protocol used. Arterial or venous whole blood sampling is recommended for patients in shock, on vasopressor therapy, or with severe edema, and when on a prolonged insulin infusion (Jacobi, 2012).

Diabetes mellitus: Plasma glucose, electrolytes, HbA_{1c}

DKA/HHS: Serum electrolytes, glucose, BUN, creatinine, osmolality, venous pH (repeat arterial blood gases are generally unnecessary), anion gap, urine output, urinalysis, mental status

Hyperkalemia: Serum potassium and glucose must be closely monitored to avoid hypokalemia, rebound hyperkalemia, and hypoglycemia.

Reference Range

Therapeutic, serum insulin (fasting): 5-20 µIU/mL (SI: 35-145 pmol/L)

Glucose, fasting:

Newborns: 60-110 mg/dL

Adults: 60-110 mg/dL

Elderly: 100-180 mg/dL

Recommendations for glycemic control in nonpregnant adults with diabetes mellitus (ADA, 2013):

HbA_{1c}: <7% (a more aggressive [<6.5%] or less aggressive [<8%] HbA_{1c} goal may be targeted based on patient-specific characteristics)

Preprandial capillary plasma glucose: 70-130 mg/dL

Peak postprandial capillary plasma glucose: <180 mg/dL

Additional Information

Split-mixed or basal-bolus regimens: Combination regimens which optimize differences in the onset and duration of different insulin products are commonly used to approximate physiologic secretion. In split-mixed regimens, an intermediate-acting insulin (eg, NPH insulin) is administered once or twice daily and supplemented by short-acting (regular) or rapid-acting (lispro, aspart, or glulisine) insulin. Blood glucose measurements are completed several times daily. Dosages are adjusted emphasizing the individual component of the regimen which most directly influences the blood sugar in question (either the intermediate-acting component or the shorter-acting component). Fixed-ratio formulations (eg, 70/30 mix) may be used as twice daily injections in this scenario; however, the ability to titrate the dosage of an individual component is limited. An example of a "split-mixed" regimen would be 21 units of NPH plus 9 units of regular insulin in the morning and an evening meal dose consisting of 14 units of NPH plus 6 units of regular insulin.

Basal-bolus regimens are designed to more closely mimic physiologic secretion. These regimens employ a long-acting insulin (eg, glargine) to simulate basal insulin secretion. The basal component is frequently administered at bedtime or in the early morning. This is supplemented by multiple daily injections of rapid-acting products (lispro, aspart, or glulisine) immediately prior to a meal, which provides insulin at the time when nutrients are absorbed. An example of a basal-bolus regimen would be 30 units of glargine at bedtime and 12 units of lispro insulin prior to each meal.

Estimation of the effect per unit: A "Rule of 1500" has been frequently used as a means to estimate the change in blood sugar relative to each unit of insulin administered. In fact, the recommended values used in these calculations may vary from 1500-2200 (a value of 1500 is generally recommended for regular insulin while 1800 is recommended for "rapid-acting insulins"). The higher values lead to more conservative estimates of the effect per unit of insulin, and therefore lead to more cautious adjustments. The effect per unit of insulin is approximated by dividing the selected numerical value (eg, 1500-2200) by the number of units/day received by the patient. This may be used as a crude approximation of the patient's insulin sensitivity as adjustments to individual components of the regimen are made. Each additional unit of insulin added to the corresponding insulin dose may be expected to lower the blood glucose by this amount.

To illustrate, in the "basal-bolus" regimen example presented above, the rule of 1800 would indicate an expected change of 27 mg/dL per unit of lispro insulin (the total daily insulin dose is 66 units; using the formula: 1800/66 = 27). A patient may be instructed to add additional insulin if the preprandial glucose is >125 mg/dL. For a prelunch glucose of 195 mg/dL, this would mean the patient would administer the scheduled 12 units of lispro along with an additional "correctional" 3 units for a total of 15 units prior to the meal. If correctional doses are required on a consistent basis, an adjustment of the patients diet and/or scheduled insulin dose may be necessary.

Dosage Forms

Solution, Injection:

HumuLIN R [OTC]: 100 units/mL (3 mL, 10 mL)

NovoLIN R [OTC]: 100 units/mL (10 mL)

NovoLIN R ReliOn [OTC]: 100 units/mL (10 mL)

Solution, Subcutaneous:

HumuLIN R U-500 (CONCENTRATED): 500 units/mL (20 mL)

◆ **Insulin Regular and Insulin NPH** *see* Insulin NPH and Insulin Regular *on page 1090*

◆ **Intanza (Can)** *see* Influenza Virus Vaccine (Inactivated) *on page 1075*

◆ **Integrilin** *see* Eptifibatide *on page 751*

◆ **Intelence** *see* Etravirine *on page 821*

◆ **Intelence® (Can)** *see* Etravirine *on page 821*

◆ **α-2-interferon** *see* Interferon Alfa-2b *on page 1096*

◆ **Interferon Alfa-2a (PEG Conjugate)** *see* Peginterferon Alfa-2a *on page 1590*

◆ **Interferon Alfa-2b (PEG Conjugate)** *see* Peginterferon Alfa-2b *on page 1596*

Interferon Alfa-2b (in ter FEER on AL fa too bee)

Brand Names: U.S. Intron A; Intron-A

Brand Names: Canada Intron A

Index Terms INF-alpha 2; Interferon Alpha-2b; rLFN-α2; α-2-interferon

Pharmacologic Category Antineoplastic Agent, Biological Response Modulator; Biological Response Modulator; Immunomodulator, Systemic; Interferon

Use

AIDS-related Kaposi sarcoma: Treatment of patients 18 years and older with AIDS-related Kaposi sarcoma

Chronic hepatitis B: Treatment of chronic hepatitis B in patients 1 year and older with compensated liver disease

Chronic hepatitis C: Treatment of chronic hepatitis C in patients 18 years and older with compensated liver disease who have a history of blood or blood-product exposure and/or are hepatitis C virus (HCV) antibody-positive; in combination with ribavirin for treatment of chronic hepatitis C in patients 3 years and older with compensated liver disease previously untreated with alpha interferon therapy and in patients 18 years and older who have relapsed following alpha interferon therapy

Condylomata acuminata: Treatment of patients 18 years and older with condylomata acuminata involving external surfaces of the genital and perianal areas

Follicular lymphoma: Initial treatment of clinically aggressive follicular non-Hodgkin lymphoma in conjunction with anthracycline-containing combination chemotherapy in patients 18 years and older

Hairy cell leukemia: Treatment of patients 18 years and older with hairy cell leukemia

Malignant melanoma: Adjuvant to surgical treatment in patients 18 years and older with malignant melanoma who are free of disease but at high risk for systemic recurrence, within 56 days of surgery

Pregnancy Risk Factor C / X in combination with ribavirin

Pregnancy Considerations Animal reproduction studies have demonstrated abortifacient effects. Disruption of the normal menstrual cycle was also observed in animal studies; therefore, the manufacturer recommends that reliable contraception is used in women of childbearing potential. Alfa interferon is endogenous to normal amniotic fluid. *In vitro* administration studies have reported that when administered to the mother, it does not cross the placenta. Case reports of use in pregnant women are limited. The Perinatal HIV Guidelines Working Group does not recommend that interferon-alfa be used during pregnancy. Interferon alfa-2b monotherapy should only be used in pregnancy when the potential benefit to the mother justifies the possible risk to the fetus. Combination therapy with ribavirin is contraindicated in pregnancy (refer to Ribavirin monograph); two forms of contraception should be used during combination therapy and patients should have monthly pregnancy tests. A pregnancy registry has been established for women inadvertently exposed to ribavirin while pregnant (800-593-2214).

Breast-Feeding Considerations Breast milk samples obtained from a lactating mother prior to and after administration of interferon alfa-2b showed that interferon alfa is present in breast milk and administration of the medication did not significantly affect endogenous levels. Breast-feeding is not linked to the spread of hepatitis C virus; however, if nipples are cracked or bleeding, breast-feeding is not recommended. Mothers coinfected with HIV are discouraged from breast-feeding to decrease potential transmission of HIV.

Contraindications

Hypersensitivity to interferon alfa or any component of the formulation; decompensated liver disease; autoimmune hepatitis

Combination therapy with interferon alfa-2b and ribavirin is also contraindicated in women who are pregnant, in males with pregnant partners; in patients with hemoglobinopathies (eg, thalassemia major, sickle-cell anemia); or creatinine clearance <50 mL/minute

Documentation of allergenic cross-reactivity for interferons is limited. However, because of similarities in chemical structure and/or pharmacologic actions, the possibility of cross-sensitivity cannot be ruled out with certainty.

Warnings/Precautions [U.S. Boxed Warning]: May cause or aggravate fatal or life-threatening autoimmune disorders, neuropsychiatric symptoms (including depression and/or suicidal thoughts/behaviors), ischemic, and/or infectious disorders; monitor closely with clinical and lab evaluations (periodic); discontinue treatment for severe persistent or worsening symptoms; some cases may resolve with discontinuation.

Neuropsychiatric disorders: May cause neuropsychiatric events, including depression, psychosis, mania, suicidal behavior/ideation, homicidal ideation; may occur in patients with or without previous psychiatric symptoms. Careful neuropsychiatric monitoring is recommended during and for 6 months after treatment in patients who develop psychiatric disorders (including clinical depression). New or exacerbated neuropsychiatric or substance abuse disorders are best managed with early intervention. Use with caution in patients with a history of psychiatric disorders. Drug screening and periodic health evaluation (including monitoring of psychiatric symptoms) is recommended if initiating treatment in patients with coexisting psychiatric condition or substance abuse disorders. Suicidal ideation or attempts may occur more frequently in pediatric patients when compared to adults. Higher doses in elderly patients, or diseases other than hairy cell leukemia, may result in increased CNS toxicity.

Hepatic disease: May cause hepatotoxicity; monitor closely if abnormal liver function tests develop. A transient increase in ALT (≥2 times baseline) may occur in patients treated with interferon alfa-2b for chronic hepatitis B. Therapy generally may continue; monitor. Worsening and potentially fatal liver disease, including jaundice, hepatic encephalopathy, and hepatic failure have been reported in patients receiving interferon alfa for chronic hepatitis B and C with decompensated liver disease, autoimmune hepatitis, history of autoimmune disease, and immunosuppressed transplant recipients; avoid use in these patients. Chronic hepatitis B or C patients with a history of autoimmune disease or who are immunosuppressed transplant recipients should not receive interferon alfa-2b. Discontinue treatment (if appropriate) in any patient developing signs or symptoms of liver failure.

Bone marrow suppression: Causes bone marrow suppression, including potentially severe cytopenias, and very rarely, aplastic anemia. Discontinue treatment for severe neutropenia (ANC <500/mm^3) or thrombocytopenia (platelets <25,000/mm^3). Hemolytic anemia (hemoglobin <10 g/dL) was observed when combined with ribavirin; anemia occurred within 1-2 weeks of initiation of therapy. Use caution in patients with preexisting myelosuppression and in patients with concomitant medications which cause myelosuppression.

Autoimmune disorders: Avoid use in patients with history of autoimmune disorders; development of autoimmune disorders (thrombocytopenia, vasculitis, Raynaud's disease, rheumatoid arthritis, lupus erythematosus and rhabdomyolysis) has been associated with use. Monitor closely; consider discontinuing. Worsening of psoriasis and sarcoidosis (and the development of new sarcoidosis) have been reported; use caution.

Cardiovascular disease/coagulation disorders: Use caution and monitor closely in patients with cardiovascular disease (ischemic or thromboembolic), arrhythmias, hypertension, and in patients with a history of MI or prior therapy with cardiotoxic drugs. Patients with preexisting cardiac disease and/or advanced cancer should have baseline and periodic ECGs. May cause hypotension (during administration or delayed), arrhythmia, tachycardia, cardiomyopathy (~2% in AIDS-related Kaposi Sarcoma patients) and/or MI. Hemorrhagic cerebrovascular events have been observed with therapy. Use caution in patients with coagulation disorders.

Endocrine disorders: Thyroid disorders (possibly reversible) have been reported; use caution in patients with preexisting thyroid disease. TSH levels should be within normal limits prior to initiating interferon. Discontinue interferon use in patients who cannot maintain normal ranges with thyroid medication. Diabetes mellitus has been reported; discontinue if cannot effectively manage with medication. Use with caution in patients with a history of diabetes mellitus, particularly if prone to DKA. Hypertriglyceridemia has been reported; discontinue if persistent and severe, and/or combined with symptoms of pancreatitis.

Pulmonary disease: Dyspnea, pulmonary infiltrates, pulmonary hypertension, interstitial pneumonitis, pneumonia, bronchiolitis obliterans, and sarcoidosis may be induced or aggravated by treatment, sometimes resulting in respiratory failure or fatality. Has been reported more in patients being treated for chronic hepatitis C, although has also occurred with use for oncology indications. Patients with fever, cough, dyspnea or other respiratory symptoms should be evaluated with a chest x-ray; monitor closely and consider discontinuing treatment with evidence of impaired pulmonary function. Use with caution in patients with a history of pulmonary disease.

Ophthalmic disorders: Decreased or loss of vision, macular edema, optic neuritis, retinal hemorrhages, cotton wool spots, papilledema, retinal detachment (serous), and retinal artery or vein thrombosis have occurred (or been aggravated) in patients receiving alpha interferons. Use caution in patients with preexisting eye disorders; monitor closely; a complete eye exam should be done promptly in patients who develop ocular symptoms; discontinue with new or worsening ophthalmic disorders.

Commonly associated with fever and flu-like symptoms; rule out other causes/infection with persistent fever; use with caution in patients with debilitating conditions. Acute hypersensitivity reactions have been reported. Do not treat patients with visceral AIDS-related Kaposi sarcoma associated with rapidly-progressing or life-threatening disease. Some formulations contain albumin, which may carry a remote risk of viral transmission. Due to differences in dosage, patients should not change brands of interferons without the concurrence of their healthcare provider. Combination therapy with ribavirin is associated with birth defects and/or fetal mortality and hemolytic anemia. Do not use combination therapy with ribavirin in patients with CrCl <50 mL/minute. Interferon alfa-2b at doses ≥10 million units/m^2 is associated with a moderate emetic potential; antiemetics may be recommended to prevent nausea and vomiting. Potentially significant drug-drug interactions may exist, requiring dose or frequency adjustment, additional monitoring, and/or selection of alternative therapy.

Benzyl alcohol and derivatives: Diluent for injection may contain benzyl alcohol; large amounts of benzyl alcohol (≥99 mg/kg/day) have been associated with a potentially fatal toxicity ("gasping syndrome") in neonates; the "gasping syndrome" consists of metabolic acidosis, respiratory distress, gasping respirations, CNS dysfunction (including convulsions, intracranial hemorrhage), hypotension, and cardiovascular collapse (AAP, 1997; CDC, 1982); some data suggests that benzoate displaces bilirubin from protein binding sites (Ahlfors, 2001); avoid or use dosage forms containing benzyl alcohol with caution in neonates.

Some dosage forms may contain polysorbate 80 (also known as Tweens). Hypersensitivity reactions, usually a delayed reaction, have been reported following exposure to pharmaceutical products containing polysorbate 80 in certain individuals (Isaksson, 2002; Lucente 2000; Shelley, 1995). Thrombocytopenia, ascites, pulmonary deterioration, and renal and hepatic failure have been reported in premature neonates after receiving parenteral products containing polysorbate 80 (Alade, 1986; CDC, 1984). See manufacturer's labeling.

Adverse Reactions Note: In a majority of patients, a flu-like symptom (fever, chills, tachycardia, malaise, myalgia, headache), occurs within 1-2 hours of administration; may last up to 24 hours and may be dose limiting.

Cardiovascular: Chest pain, edema, hypertension

Central nervous system: Agitation, amnesia, anxiety, chills, confusion, depression, dizziness, drowsiness, fatigue, headache, hypoesthesia, insomnia, irritability, lack of concentration, malaise, pain, paresthesia, right upper quadrant pain, rigors, vertigo

Dermatologic: Alopecia, dermatitis, diaphoresis, pruritus, skin rash, xeroderma

Endocrine & metabolic: Amenorrhea, decreased libido, weight loss

Gastrointestinal: Abdominal pain, anorexia, constipation, diarrhea, dysgeusia, dyspepsia, gingivitis, loose stools, nausea, vomiting (more common in children), xerostomia

Genitourinary: Urinary tract infection

Hematologic & oncologic: Anemia, leukopenia, neutropenia, purpura, thrombocytopenia

Hepatic: Increased serum alkaline phosphatase, increased serum ALT, increased serum AST

Infection: Candidiasis, infection, herpes virus infection

Local: Injection site reaction

Neuromuscular & skeletal: Arthralgia, back pain, myalgia, skeletal pain, weakness

Renal: Increased blood urea nitrogen, increased serum creatinine, polyuria

Respiratory: Bronchitis, cough, dyspnea, epistaxis, flu-like symptoms, nasal congestion, pharyngitis, sinusitis

Miscellaneous: Fever (more common in children)

Rare but important or life-threatening: Abnormal hepatic function tests, aggressive behavior, albuminuria, alcohol intolerance, amyotrophy, anaphylaxis, angina pectoris, angioedema, aphasia, aplastic anemia (rarely), ascites, asthma, atrial fibrillation, Bell's palsy, bradycardia, bronchiolitis obliterans, bronchoconstriction, bronchospasm, cardiac arrhythmia, cardiac failure, cardiomegaly, cardiomyopathy, cellulitis, cerebrovascular accident, colitis, coma, conjunctivitis, coronary artery disease, cyanosis, cystitis, dehydration, diabetes mellitus, dysphasia, dysuria, eczema, epidermal cyst, erythema, erythema multiforme, erythematous rash, exacerbation of psoriasis, exacerbation of sarcoidosis, extrapyramidal reaction, extrasystoles, gastrointestinal hemorrhage, granulocytopenia, hallucination, hearing loss, heart valve disease, hematuria, hemolytic anemia, hemoptysis, hepatic encephalopathy, hepatic failure, hepatitis, hepatotoxicity, hot flash, homicidal ideation, hyperbilirubinemia, hypercalcemia, hyperglycemia, hypermenorrhea, hypersensitivity reaction (acute), hypertriglyceridemia, hyperthyroidism, hypochromic anemia, hypotension, hypothermia, hypothyroidism, hypoventilation, immune thrombocytopenia, impotence, increased lactate dehydrogenase, interstitial pneumonitis, jaundice, leukorrhea, lupus erythematosus, lymphadenitis, lymphadenopathy, lymphocytopenia, lymphocytosis, macular edema, maculopapular rash, migraine, myocardial infarction, myositis, nephrotic syndrome, neuralgia, neuropathy, nystagmus, optic neuritis, palpitations, pancreatitis, pancytopenia, papilledema, paranoia, peripheral ischemia, peripheral neuropathy, photophobia, pituitary insufficiency, pleural effusion, pneumonia, psychoneurosis, pneumothorax, proteinuria, psychosis, pulmonary embolism, pulmonary fibrosis, pulmonary hypertension, pulmonary infiltrates, pure red cell aplasia, Raynaud's phenomenon, reduced ejection fraction, renal failure, renal insufficiency, respiratory insufficiency, retinal detachment (serous), retinal thrombosis, retinal cotton-wool spot, retinal vein occlusion, rhabdomyolysis, seizure, sepsis, sexual disorder, skin photosensitivity, Stevens-Johnson syndrome, stomatitis, suicidal ideation, syncope, systemic lupus erythematosus, tachycardia, tendonitis, tissue necrosis at injection site, thrombotic thrombocytopenic purpura, thrombosis, toxic epidermal necrolysis, upper respiratory tract infection, urinary incontinence, urticaria, uterine hemorrhage, vasculitis, Vogt-Koyanagi-Harada syndrome, wheezing

Drug Interactions

Metabolism/Transport Effects Inhibits CYP1A2 (weak)

Avoid Concomitant Use

Avoid concomitant use of Interferon Alfa-2b with any of the following: CloZAPine; Dipyrone; Telbivudine

Increased Effect/Toxicity

Interferon Alfa-2b may increase the levels/effects of: Aldesleukin; CloZAPine; Methadone; Ribavirin; Telbivudine; Theophylline Derivatives; Zidovudine

The levels/effects of Interferon Alfa-2b may be increased by: Dipyrone

Decreased Effect There are no known significant interactions involving a decrease in effect.

Preparation for Administration Powder for injection: The manufacturer recommends reconstituting vial with the diluent provided (SWFI). When reconstituted with SWFI 1 mL, the 10 million unit vial concentration is 10 million units/mL, the 18 million unit vial concentration is 18 million units/mL, and the 50 million unit vial concentration is 50 million units/mL. Swirl gently. To prepare solution for infusion, further dilute appropriate dose in NS 100 mL. Final concentration should be ≥10 million units/100 mL.

Storage/Stability Store intact vials under refrigeration at 2°C to 8°C (36°F to 46°F); do not freeze. After reconstitution of powder for injection, product should be used immediately, but may be stored under refrigeration for ≤24 hours.

Mechanism of Action Binds to a specific receptor on the cell wall to initiate intracellular activity; multiple effects can be detected including induction of gene transcription. Inhibits cellular growth, alters the state of cellular differentiation, interferes with oncogene expression, alters cell surface antigen expression, increases phagocytic activity of macrophages, and augments cytotoxicity of lymphocytes for target cells

Pharmacodynamics/Kinetics

Distribution: V_d: 31 L; but has been noted to be much greater (370-720 L) in leukemia patients receiving continuous infusion IFN; IFN does not penetrate the CSF

Metabolism: Primarily renal

Bioavailability: IM: 83%; SubQ: 90%

Half-life elimination: IV: ~2 hours; IM, SubQ: ~2-3 hours

Time to peak, serum: IM, SubQ: ~3-12 hours; IV: By the end of a 30-minute infusion

Dosage Consider premedication with acetaminophen prior to administration to reduce the incidence of some adverse reactions. Not all dosage forms and strengths are appropriate for all indications; refer to product labeling for details. Interferon alfa-2b at doses ≥10 million units/m^2 is associated with a moderate emetic potential; antiemetics may be recommended to prevent nausea and vomiting.

Children 1-17 years: **Note:** The following dosing may also be used in **infants** in the setting of HIV-exposure/-infection (CDC, 2009).

Chronic hepatitis B (including HIV coinfection): SubQ: 3 million units/m^2 3 times weekly for 1 week, followed by 6 million units/m^2 3 times weekly (maximum: 10 million units per dose); total duration of therapy 16-24 weeks (treat for 24 weeks in HIV-exposure/-infection)

Chronic hepatitis C with HIV coinfection: IM, SubQ: 3-5 million units/m^2 3 times weekly (maximum: 3 million units per dose) with ribavirin for 48 weeks, regardless of HCV genotype (CDC, 2009)

Adults:

Hairy cell leukemia: IM, SubQ: 2 million units/m^2 3 times weekly for up to 6 months (may continue treatment with sustained treatment response); discontinue for disease progression or failure to respond after 6 months

Lymphoma (follicular): SubQ: 5 million units 3 times weekly for up to 18 months

Malignant melanoma: Induction: 20 million units/m^2 IV for 5 consecutive days per week for 4 weeks, followed by maintenance dosing of 10 million units/m^2 SubQ 3 times weekly for 48 weeks

AIDS-related Kaposi sarcoma: IM, SubQ: 30 million units/m^2 3 times weekly; continue until disease progression or until maximal response has been achieved after 16 weeks

Chronic hepatitis B: IM, SubQ: 5 million units daily or 10 million units 3 times weekly for 16 weeks

Chronic hepatitis C: IM, SubQ: 3 million units 3 times weekly. In patients with normalization of ALT at 16 weeks, continue treatment (if tolerated) for 18-24 months; consider discontinuation if normalization does not occur at 16 weeks. **Note:** May be used in combination therapy with ribavirin in previously untreated patients or in patients who relapse following alpha interferon therapy.

Condyloma acuminata: Intralesionally: 1 million units/lesion (maximum: 5 lesions per treatment) 3 times weekly (on alternate days) for 3 weeks; may administer a second course at 12-16 weeks

Dosage adjustment for toxicity:

Neuropsychiatric disorders (during treatment):

Clinical depression or other psychiatric problem: Monitor closely during and for 6 months after treatment.

Severe depression or other psychiatric disorder: Discontinue treatment.

Persistent or worsening psychiatric symptoms, suicidal ideation, aggression towards others: Discontinue treatment and follow with appropriate psychiatric intervention.

Hypersensitivity reaction (acute, serious), ophthalmic disorders (new or worsening), thyroid abnormality development (which cannot be normalized with medication), signs or symptoms of liver failure: Discontinue treatment.

Hematologic toxicity (also refer to indication specified adjustments below): ANC <500/mm^3 or platelets <25,000/mm^3: Discontinue treatment.

Liver function abnormality, pulmonary infiltrate development, evidence of pulmonary function impairment, or autoimmune disorder development, triglycerides >1000 mg/dL: Monitor closely and discontinue if appropriate.

Manufacturer-recommended adjustments, listed according to indication:

Lymphoma (follicular):

Neutrophils >1000/mm^3 to <1500/mm^3: Reduce dose by 50%; may re-escalate to starting dose when neutrophils return to >1500/mm^3

Severe toxicity (neutrophils <1000/mm^3 or platelets <50,000/mm^3): Temporarily withhold.

AST >5 times ULN or serum creatinine >2 mg/dL: Permanently discontinue.

Hairy cell leukemia:

Platelet count <50,000/mm^3: Do not administer intramuscularly (administer SubQ instead).

Severe toxicity: Reduce dose by 50% or temporarily withhold and resume with 50% dose reduction; permanently discontinue if persistent or recurrent severe toxicity is noted.

Chronic hepatitis B:

WBC <1500/mm^3, granulocytes <750/mm^3, or platelet count <50,000/mm^3, or other laboratory abnormality or severe adverse reaction: Reduce dose by 50%; may re-escalate to starting dose upon resolution of hematologic toxicity. Discontinue for persistent intolerance.

WBC <1000/mm^3, granulocytes <500/mm^3, or platelet count <25,000/mm^3: Permanently discontinue.

Chronic hepatitis C: Severe toxicity: Reduce dose by 50% or temporarily withhold until subsides; permanently discontinue for persistent toxicities after dosage reduction.

AIDS-related Kaposi sarcoma: Severe toxicity: Reduce dose by 50% or temporarily withhold; may resume at reduced dose with toxicity resolution; permanently discontinue for persistent/recurrent toxicities.

Malignant melanoma (induction and maintenance):

Severe toxicity, including neutrophils >250/mm^3 to <500/mm^3 or ALT/AST >5-10 times ULN: Temporarily withhold; resume with a 50% dose reduction when adverse reaction abates.

Neutrophils <250/mm^3, ALT/AST >10 times ULN, or severe/persistent adverse reactions: Permanently discontinue.

Dosage adjustment in renal impairment:

Renal impairment at treatment initiation: Combination therapy with ribavirin (hepatitis C) is contraindicated in patients with CrCl <50 mL/minute; use combination therapy with ribavirin (hepatitis C) with caution in patients with impaired renal function and CrCl ≥50 mL/minute.

Renal toxicity during treatment: Indication-specific adjustments: Lymphoma (follicular): Serum creatinine >2 mg/dL: Permanently discontinue.

Dosage adjustment in hepatic impairment:

Hepatic impairment at treatment initiation: There are no dosage adjustments provided in the manufacturer's labeling. Contraindicated in patients with decompensated liver disease or autoimmune hepatitis.

Hepatotoxicity during treatment: Indication-specific adjustments:

Lymphoma (follicular): AST >5 times ULN: Permanently discontinue.

Malignant melanoma (induction and maintenance):

ALT/AST >5 to 10 times ULN: Temporarily withhold; resume with a 50% dose reduction when adverse reaction abates

ALT/AST >10 times ULN: Permanently discontinue.

Administration Administer dose in the evening (if possible) to enhance tolerability. Not all dosage forms are recommended for all administration routes; refer to manufacturer's labeling. Interferon alfa-2b at doses ≥10 million units/m^2 is associated with a moderate emetic potential; antiemetics may be recommended to prevent nausea and vomiting.

IM: Rotate injection sites; preferred sites for injection are anterior thigh, deltoid, and superolateral buttock. Some patients may be appropriate for self-administration with appropriate training. Allow to reach room temperature prior to injection. In hairy cell leukemia treatment, if platelets are <50,000/mm^3, do not administer intramuscularly (administer SubQ instead).

IV: Infuse over ~20 minutes

SubQ: Suggested for those who are at risk for bleeding or are thrombocytopenic. Rotate SubQ injection site; preferred sites for injection are abdomen (except around the navel), anterior thigh, and outer upper arm. Patient should be well hydrated. Some patients may be appropriate for self-administration with appropriate training. Allow to reach room temperature prior to injection.

Intralesional: Inject at an angle nearly parallel to the plane of the skin, directing the needle to center of the base of the wart to infiltrate the lesion core and cause a small wheal. Only infiltrate the keratinized layer; avoid administration which is too deep or shallow. Allow to reach room temperature prior to injection.

Monitoring Parameters

CBC with differential (baseline and periodic during treatment), liver function tests (baseline and periodic), electrolytes (baseline and periodic), serum creatinine (baseline), albumin, prothrombin time, triglycerides, thyroid-stimulating hormone (TSH) baseline and periodically during treatment (in patients with preexisting thyroid disorders, repeat TSH at 3 months and 6 months); chest x-ray (baseline), weight; ophthalmic exam (baseline and periodic, or with new ocular symptoms); ECG (baseline and during treatment; in patients with preexisting cardiac abnormalities or in advanced stages of cancer); neuropsychiatric changes during and for 6 months after therapy

Chronic hepatitis B: CBC with differential and platelets and liver function tests: Baseline, weeks 1, 2, 4, 8, 12, and 16, at the end of treatment, and then 3 and 6 months post treatment

Chronic hepatitis C:

CBC with differential and platelets: Baseline, weeks 1 and 2, then monthly

Liver function: Every 3 months

TSH: Baseline and periodically during treatment; in patients with preexisting thyroid disorders also repeat at 3 months and 6 months

Malignant melanoma: CBC with differential and platelets and liver function tests: Weekly during induction phase, then monthly during maintenance

Oncology patients: Thyroid function monitoring (Hamnvik, 2011): TSH and anti-TPO antibodies at baseline; if TPO antibody positive, monitor TSH every 2 months; if TPO antibody negative, monitor TSH every 6 months

Dosage Forms

Solution, Injection:

Intron-A: 6,000,000 units/mL (3.8 mL); 10,000,000 units/mL (3.2 mL)

Solution Reconstituted, Injection:

Intron-A: 10,000,000 units (1 ea); 18,000,000 units (1 ea); 50,000,000 units (1 ea)

Solution Reconstituted, Injection [preservative free]:

Intron A: 10,000,000 units (1 ea); 18,000,000 units (1 ea); 50,000,000 units (1 ea)

Interferon Alfacon-1 (in ter FEER on AL fa con one)

Brand Names: U.S. Infergen [DSC]

Pharmacologic Category Interferon

Use Treatment of chronic hepatitis C virus (HCV) infection in patients ≥18 years of age with compensated liver disease and anti-HCV serum antibodies or HCV RNA; concurrent use with ribavirin in HCV-infected patients who have failed treatment with pegylated interferon/ribavirin (Bacon, 2009)

Pregnancy Risk Factor C

Dosage Adults ≥18 years: SubQ:

Chronic HCV infection: 9 mcg 3 times/week for 24 weeks; allow 48 hours between doses

Combination therapy with ribavirin: 15 mcg/day with ribavirin for up to 48 weeks

Patients who have previously tolerated interferon therapy but did not respond or relapsed: 15 mcg 3 times/week for up to 48 weeks

Dose reduction for toxicity: Dose should be held in patients who experience a severe adverse reaction, and treatment should be stopped or decreased if the reaction does not become tolerable.

Doses were reduced from 9 mcg to 7.5 mcg in the pivotal study.

For patients receiving 15 mcg/dose, doses were reduced in 3 mcg decrements. Efficacy is decreased with doses <7.5 mcg

Elderly: No information available.

Dosage adjustment in renal impairment: CrCl <50 mL/minute: Hepatitis C: Avoid combination therapy with ribavirin

Dosage adjustment in hepatic impairment: Use in decompensated hepatic disease (Child-Pugh class B or C) is contraindicated

Additional Information Complete prescribing information should be consulted for additional detail.

Interferon Alfa-n3 (in ter FEER on AL fa en three)

Brand Names: U.S. Alferon N

Brand Names: Canada Alferon N

Pharmacologic Category Interferon

Use Condylomata acuminata: Intralesional treatment of refractory or recurring external condylomata acuminata (venereal or genital warts) in patients 18 years of age or older.

Pregnancy Risk Factor C

Dosage Adults: Condylomata acuminata: Intralesional: 250,000 units (0.05 mL) per wart twice weekly for a maximum of 8 weeks; maximum dose per treatment session: 2.5 million units (0.5 mL). Therapy should not be repeated for at least 3 months after the initial 8-week course of therapy (unless existing warts grow or new warts appear).

Dosage adjustment in renal impairment: There are no dosage adjustments provided in the manufacturer's labeling.

Dosage adjustment in hepatic impairment: There are no dosage adjustments provided in the manufacturer's labeling.

Additional Information Complete prescribing information should be consulted for additional detail.

Dosage Forms

Solution, Injection:

Alferon N: 5,000,000 units/mL (1 mL)

◆ **Interferon Alpha-2b** *see* Interferon Alfa-2b *on page 1096*

Interferon Alpha, Multi-Subtype [INT]
(in ter FEER on AL fa, MUL tee-sub tipe)

International Brand Names Multiferon (BG, IN, MX, SE, ZA)

Index Terms Alpha-Interferon Multi-Subtype; HuIFN-alpha-Le; Multi-Subtype Alpha-Interferon; Natural Human Alpha-Interferon; Natural IFN-alpha; nIFN-alpha

Pharmacologic Category Interferon

Reported Use First and/or second-line treatment (rescue therapy) of viral and malignant diseases include: Chronic myelogenous leukemia (CML), hairy cell leukemia, hepatitis B, hepatitis C, malignant melanoma, and renal cell carcinoma

Dosage Range Adults: SubQ: High-risk malignant melanoma (after resection and 2 doses of dacarbazine): 3 million international units 3 times per week for 6 months

Product Availability Product available in various countries; not currently available in the U.S.

Dosage Forms

Injection, solution: 6 int. units/mL (1 mL) [contains albumin]

Interferon Beta-1a (in ter FEER on BAY ta won aye)

Brand Names: U.S. Avonex; Avonex Pen; Rebif; Rebif Rebidose; Rebif Rebidose Titration Pack; Rebif Titration Pack

Brand Names: Canada Avonex; Rebif

Index Terms rIFN beta-1a

Pharmacologic Category Interferon

Use

Multiple sclerosis: Treatment of relapsing forms of multiple sclerosis (MS) to decrease the frequency of clinical exacerbations and delay the accumulation of physical disability

Canadian labeling: Additional uses (not in U.S. labeling): Avonex: To decrease the number and volume of active brain lesions, decrease overall disease burden, and delay onset of clinically definite MS in patients who have experienced a single demyelinating event.

Pregnancy Risk Factor C

Pregnancy Considerations Adverse events have not been observed in animal reproduction studies; however, the possibility of adverse effects cannot be ruled out. Preliminary data from the Avonex pregnancy registry (published in abstract) do not show an increased risk of adverse fetal events when exposure occurs during pregnancy (Richman, 2012; Tomczyk, 2013); however, other studies have reported conflicting results. Until additional information is available, consideration should be given to discontinuing treatment if a woman becomes pregnant, or 1 month prior to becoming pregnant in women with mild disease (Coyle, 2012; Houtchens, 2013; Lu, 2013).

Breast-Feeding Considerations Small amounts of interferon beta-1a are excreted in breast milk. Milk samples were obtained from six lactating women (6-23 months postpartum) receiving Avonex 30 mcg IM once weekly; sampling occurred at intervals for 72 hours after the dose. The highest reported concentration was 179 pg/mL and the relative infant dose was calculated to be <1% of the maternal dose. Adverse events were not observed in the nursing infants (Hale, 2012). The manufacturer recommends that caution be exercised when administering interferon beta-1a to nursing women.

Contraindications

Hypersensitivity to natural or recombinant interferon beta, human albumin (albumin-containing formulations only), or any other component of the formulation

Documentation of allergenic cross-reactivity for interferons is limited. However, because of similarities in chemical structure and/or pharmacologic actions, the possibility of cross-sensitivity cannot be ruled out with certainty.

Canadian labeling: Additional contraindications (not in U.S. labeling): Rebif: Pregnancy; decompensated liver disease

Warnings/Precautions Interferons have been associated with psychiatric adverse events (psychosis, depression, suicidal behavior/ideation) in patients with and without previous psychiatric symptoms; use with caution in patients with depression. Patients exhibiting depressive symptoms or other severe psychiatric symptoms should be closely monitored and discontinuation of therapy should be considered.

Autoimmune disorders including idiopathic thrombocytopenia, hyper- and hypothyroidism and rarely autoimmune hepatitis have been reported. Consider discontinuation of treatment if patient develops a new autoimmune disorder. Allergic reactions, including anaphylaxis, have been reported; some reactions may occur after prolonged use. Discontinue therapy if anaphylaxis or other allergic reactions occur. Rare cases of severe hepatic injury, including cases of hepatic failure requiring transplantation, have been reported in patients receiving interferon beta-1a; risk may be increased by ethanol use or concurrent therapy with hepatotoxic drugs. Some reports indicate symptoms began after 1-6 months of treatment. Transaminase elevations may be asymptomatic. Use with caution in patients with active or a history of liver disease, alcohol abuse, or increased serum ALT (>2.5 times ULN) at baseline. Obtain liver function tests at 1-, 3-, and 6 months post therapy initiation and periodically thereafter. Treatment should be suspended immediately if jaundice or symptoms of hepatic dysfunction occur. Consider dose reductions or temporary discontinuation if ALT >5 times ULN. Hematologic effects, including pancytopenia (rare), leukopenia, and thrombocytopenia, have been reported. Monitor blood counts at 1-, 3-, and 6 months post therapy initiation and periodically thereafter. Events may recur with rechallenge.

Associated with a high incidence of flu-like adverse effects; use of analgesics and/or antipyretics on treatment days may be helpful. Use caution in patients with preexisting cardiovascular disease. Rare cases of new-onset cardiomyopathy and/or HF have been reported. Use caution in patients with seizure disorders. Thyroid abnormalities may develop with use; may worsen preexisting thyroid conditions. Monitor thyroid function tests every 6 months or as clinically necessary. Safety and efficacy in patients with chronic progressive MS have not been established. Severe injection site reactions have occurred, including pain, erythema, edema, cellulitis, abscess, and necrosis. Necrosis may occur at single and multiple sites. Some reactions have occurred ≥2 years after initiation; reactions typically resolve with conservative treatment (antibiotics or surgical intervention may be required). Patient and/or caregiver competency in injection technique should be confirmed and periodically re-evaluated. Albumin is a component of some formulations (contraindicated in albumin-sensitive patients); rare risk of CJD or viral transmission. The packaging (prefilled syringe tip cap) may contain latex.

Adverse Reactions

Cardiovascular: Chest pain, vasodilation

Central nervous system: Ataxia, chills, depression, dizziness, drowsiness, fatigue, headache, hypertonia, malaise, migraine, pain, seizure, suicidal tendencies

Dermatologic: Alopecia, erythematous rash, maculopapular rash, urticaria

Endocrine & metabolic: Thyroid disease

Gastrointestinal: Abdominal pain, nausea, toothache, xerostomia

Genitourinary: Urine abnormality, urinary frequency, urinary incontinence, urinary tract infection

Hematologic & oncologic: Anemia, leukopenia, lymphadenopathy, thrombocytopenia

Hepatic: Hyperbilirubinemia, increased serum ALT, increased serum AST

Immunologic: Antibody development (neutralizing; significance not known)

Infection: Infection

Local: Bruising at injection site, inflammation at injection site, injection site reaction, pain at injection site, tissue necrosis at injection site

Neuromuscular & skeletal: Arthralgia, back pain, myalgia, rigors, skeletal pain, weakness

Ophthalmic: Eye disease, visual disturbance, xerophthalmia

Respiratory: Bronchitis, flu-like symptoms, sinusitis, upper respiratory tract infection

Miscellaneous: Fever

Rare but important or life-threatening: Abnormal healing, abscess, abscess at injection site, amnesia, anaphylaxis, arteritis, arthritis, bloody stools, breast fibroadenosis, cardiac arrest, cardiac failure, cellulitis at injection site, conjunctivitis, depersonalization, dermal ulcer, diverticulitis, drug dependence, emphysema, epididymitis, erythema multiforme, facial paralysis, fibrosis at injection site, furunculosis, gallbladder disease, gastritis, gastrointestinal hemorrhage, gingivitis, gynecomastia, hemolytic uremic syndrome, hemorrhage, hepatic failure, hepatic neoplasm, hepatitis, hepatomegaly, hernia, hypersensitivity reaction at injection site, hyperthyroidism, hypoglycemia, hypokalemia, hypomagnesemia, hypotension, hypothyroidism, immune thrombocytopenia, intestinal obstruction, intestinal perforation, lipoma, lupus erythematosus, menopause, neoplasm, nephrolithiasis, neurological signs and symptoms (transient; may mimic multiple sclerosis exacerbations), nevus, orthostatic hypotension, osteonecrosis, pancytopenia, pelvic inflammatory disease, pericarditis, periodontitis, peripheral vascular disease, Peyronie's disease, pneumonia, postmenopausal bleeding, proctitis, psychiatric disorders (new or worsening; including suicidal ideation), psychoneurosis, pulmonary embolism, pyelonephritis, retinal vascular disease, sepsis, severe weakness (transient), skin photosensitivity, Stevens-Johnson syndrome, synovitis, tachycardia, telangiectasia, testicular disease, thromboembolism, thrombotic thrombocytopenic purpura, uterine fibroids, vaginal hemorrhage, vascular disease, vesicular eruption

Drug Interactions

Metabolism/Transport Effects None known.

Avoid Concomitant Use There are no known interactions where it is recommended to avoid concomitant use.

Increased Effect/Toxicity

Interferon Beta-1a may increase the levels/effects of: Theophylline Derivatives; Zidovudine

Decreased Effect There are no known significant interactions involving a decrease in effect.

Preparation for Administration Avonex: Reconstitute with 1.1 mL of diluent (SWFI) and swirl gently to dissolve. Do not shake. The reconstituted product contains no preservative and is for single-use only; discard unused portion.

Storage/Stability

Avonex:

Prefilled syringe or pen: Store at 2°C to 8°C (36°F to 46°F); do not freeze. Protect from light. Allow to warm to room temperature prior to use (do not use external heat source). If refrigeration is not available, product may be stored at ≤25°C (77°F) for up to 7 days.

Vial: Store unreconstituted vial at 2°C to 8°C (36°F to 46°F). If refrigeration is not available, may be stored at 25°C (77°F) for up to 30 days; do not freeze. Protect from light. Following reconstitution, use immediately, but may be stored up to 6 hours at 2°C to 8°C (36°F to 46°F); do not freeze.

Rebif: Store at 2°C to 8°C (36°F to 46°F); do not freeze. Protect from heat and light. Allow to warm to room temperature prior to use (do not use external heat source). Refrigeration is preferred; however, if needed, may be stored at 2°C to 25°C (36°F to 77°F) for up to 30 days.

Mechanism of Action Interferon beta differs from naturally occurring human protein by a single amino acid substitution and the lack of carbohydrate side chains; alters the expression and response to surface antigens and can enhance immune cell activities. Properties of interferon beta that modify biologic responses are mediated by cell surface receptor interactions; mechanism in the treatment of MS is unknown.

Pharmacodynamics/Kinetics

Onset of action: Avonex: 12 hours (based on biological response markers)

Duration: Avonex: 4 days (based on biological response markers)

Half-life elimination: Avonex: ~19 hours (range: 8-54 hours); Rebif: 69 hours

Time to peak, serum: Avonex (IM): ~15 hours (range: 6-36 hours); Rebif (SubQ): 16 hours

Dosage

Multiple sclerosis (MS): Adults: **Note:** Analgesics and/or antipyretics may help decrease flu-like symptoms on treatment days:

IM (Avonex):

U.S. labeling: 30 mcg once weekly; to decrease flu-like symptoms, may initiate once-weekly dosing with 7.5 mcg (week 1) then increase dose in increments of 7.5 mcg once weekly (weeks 2 to 4) up to recommended dose (30 mcg once weekly)

Canadian labeling: 30 mcg once weekly; may consider increasing to 60 mcg once weekly in progressive relapsing MS or secondary progressive MS with recurrent neurologic dysfunction

SubQ (Rebif): Target dose is either 22 or 44 mcg 3 times weekly; doses should be separated by at least 48 hours:

Target dose 44 mcg 3 times weekly:

Initial: 8.8 mcg (20% of target dose) 3 times weekly for 2 weeks

Titration: 22 mcg (50% of target dose) 3 times weekly for 2 weeks

Target dose: 44 mcg 3 times weekly

Target dose 22 mcg 3 times weekly:

Initial: 4.4 mcg (20% of target dose) 3 times weekly for 2 weeks

Titration: 11 mcg (50% of target dose) 3 times weekly for 2 weeks

Target dose: 22 mcg 3 times weekly

Single demyelinating event (Canadian labeling [Rebif]; not in U.S. labeling): Adults: SubQ:

Target dose 44 mcg 3 times weekly: Note: Analgesics and/or antipyretics prior to and for 24 hours after dosing may help decrease flu-like symptoms:

Initial: 8.8 mcg (20% of target dose) 3 times weekly for 2 weeks

Titration: 22 mcg (50% of target dose) 3 times weekly for 2 weeks

Target dose: 44 mcg 3 times weekly

Dosage adjustment for toxicity:

Autoimmune disorder development: Consider discontinuing treatment.

Depression or other severe psychiatric symptoms: Consider discontinuing treatment.

Hepatotoxicity:

ALT >5 x ULN: Temporarily discontinue therapy or consider dose reduction until ALT normalizes, then may consider retitration of dose.

Symptomatic (eg, jaundice): Discontinue immediately.

Leukopenia: May require temporary discontinuation or dose reduction until resolution.

Dosage adjustment in renal impairment: There are no dosage adjustments provided in the manufacturer's labeling (has not been studied).

Dosage adjustment in hepatic impairment: There are no dosage adjustments provided in the manufacturer's labeling; use with caution in patients active liver disease, alcohol abuse, ALT >2.5 x ULN, or a history of significant liver disease.

Administration The first injection should be administered under the supervision of a health care professional.

Avonex: Administer IM; rotate injection site; do not inject into area where skin is irritated, red, bruised, scarred, or infected. Two hours after injection, examine site for redness, swelling, or tenderness. Discard any unused portion.

Rebif: Administer SubQ at the same time of day on the same 3 days each week (eg, Mon, Wed, Fri), preferably in the late afternoon or evening; doses should be at least 48 hours apart; rotate injection site; do not inject into area where skin is irritated, red, bruised, or scarred. Discard any unused portion.

Monitoring Parameters Thyroid function tests, CBC with differential, transaminase levels, blood chemistries, symptoms of autoimmune disorders, signs/symptoms of psychiatric disorder (including depression and/or suicidal ideation), signs/symptoms of new onset/worsening cardiovascular disease

Avonex: Frequency of monitoring for patients receiving Avonex® has not been specifically defined; in clinical trials, monitoring was at 6-month intervals. Canadian labeling recommends liver function testing monthly for first 6 months, then every 6 months thereafter or as clinically indicated.

Rebif: CBC and liver function testing at 1-, 3-, and 6 months, then periodically thereafter. Thyroid function every 6 months (in patients with preexisting abnormalities and/or clinical indications). Canadian labeling recommends liver function testing monthly for first 6 months, then every 6 months thereafter or as clinically indicated.

Dosage Forms

Injection, powder for reconstitution [preservative free]:

Avonex: 33 mcg [contains albumin (human); provides 30 mcg/mL following reconstitution; supplied with diluent]

Injection, solution:

Avonex, Avonex Pen: 30 mcg/0.5 mL (0.5 mL)

Injection, solution [preservative free]:

Rebif: 22 mcg/0.5 mL (0.5 mL), 44 mcg/0.5 mL (0.5 mL)

Rebif Rebidose: 22 mcg/0.5 mL (0.5 mL), 44 mcg/0.5 mL (0.5 mL)

Injection, solution [preservative free, combination package]:

Rebif Titration Pack: 8.8 mcg/0.2 mL (6s) and 22 mcg/0.5 mL (6s)

Rebif Rebidose Titration Pack: 8.8 mcg/0.2 mL (6s) and 22 mcg/0.5 mL (6s)

Interferon Beta-1b (in ter FEER on BAY ta won bee)

Brand Names: U.S. Betaseron; Extavia

Brand Names: Canada Betaseron; Extavia

Index Terms rIFN beta-1b

Pharmacologic Category Interferon

Use Treatment of relapsing forms of multiple sclerosis (MS); treatment of first clinical episode with MRI features consistent with MS

Canadian labeling: Additional use (not in U.S. labeling): Treatment of secondary-progressive MS

Pregnancy Risk Factor C

Pregnancy Considerations Adverse events have been observed in animal reproduction studies. Spontaneous abortions were reported in 4 women during a clinical trial. Women with multiple sclerosis are generally recommended to discontinue therapy prior to conception (Lu, 2012). The Canadian labeling contraindicates use in pregnant women.

Breast-Feeding Considerations It is not known if interferon beta-1b is excreted in breast milk. Due to the potential for serious adverse reactions in the nursing infant, the decision to continue or discontinue breastfeeding during therapy should take into account the risk of exposure to the infant and the benefits of treatment to the mother.

Contraindications

Hypersensitivity to natural or recombinant interferon beta, albumin human or any other component of the formulation

Canadian labeling: Additional contraindication (not in U.S. labeling): Pregnancy, decompensated liver disease (Betaseron, Extavia); current severe depression and/or suicidal ideation (Extavia)

Warnings/Precautions Allergic reactions (eg, bronchospasm, dyspnea, skin rash, tongue edema, urticaria), including anaphylaxis (rare), have been reported with use; discontinue use if anaphylaxis occurs. Associated with a high incidence of flu-like adverse effects; use of analgesics and/or antipyretics on treatment days may be helpful. Improvement in symptoms occurs over time. Hepatotoxicity has been reported with beta interferons, including rare reports of hepatitis (autoimmune) and hepatic failure requiring transplant; use with caution in patients with concurrent exposure to other hepatotoxic drugs. Monitor liver function tests as clinically necessary. Consider discontinuation if serum transaminase levels increase significantly or are associated with clinical symptoms (eg, jaundice). Interferons have been associated with severe psychiatric adverse events (psychosis, mania, depression, suicidal behavior/ideation) in patients with and without previous psychiatric symptoms; avoid use in severe psychiatric disorders and use caution in patients with a history of depression; patients exhibiting symptoms of depression should be closely monitored and discontinuation of therapy should be considered. Use with caution in patients with a history of seizure disorder.

Use with caution in patients with preexisting cardiovascular disease. Rare cases of new-onset cardiomyopathy and/or HF have been reported. If HF worsens in the absence of another etiology, consider discontinuation of therapy. Use with caution in patients with hepatic impairment or in combination with alcohol. The Canadian labeling contraindicates use in patients with decompensated hepatic disease. Use with caution in patients with bone marrow suppression; may require increased monitoring. Leukopenia has also been observed; routine monitoring of complete blood counts with differentials is recommended. Dose reduction may be required. Thyroid abnormalities may develop with use; may worsen preexisting thyroid conditions. Monitor thyroid function tests every 6 months or as clinically necessary.

Severe injection site reactions (necrosis) may occur, which may or may not heal with continued therapy. Reactions generally arise within the first 4 months of therapy, but have occurred ≥1 year after initiation. Incidence of reactions tend to improve over time. Patient and/or caregiver competency in injection technique should be confirmed and periodically re-evaluated. Do not inject into affected area until completely healed; if multiple lesions occur, discontinue use until they are fully healed. Contains albumin, which may carry a remote risk of transmitting viral diseases.

Adverse Reactions Note: Flu-like syndrome (including at least two of the following - chills, diaphoresis, fever, headache, malaise, and myalgia) are reported in the majority of patients (60%) and decrease over time (average duration ~1 week).

Cardiovascular: Chest pain, hypertension, palpitations, peripheral edema, peripheral vascular disease, tachycardia, vasodilatation

Central nervous system: Anxiety, ataxia, chills, dizziness, headache, hypertonia, insomnia, malaise, myasthenia, nervousness, pain

Dermatologic: Alopecia, dermatological disease, diaphoresis, skin rash

Endocrine & metabolic: Dysmenorrhea, hypermenorrhea, weight gain

Gastrointestinal: Abdominal pain, constipation, diarrhea, dyspepsia, nausea

Genitourinary: Cystitis, impotence, pelvic pain, prostatic disease, urinary frequency, urinary urgency, uterine hemorrhage

Hematologic & oncologic: Leukopenia, lymphadenopathy, lymphocytopenia, neutropenia

Hepatic: Increased serum ALT (>5x baseline), increased serum AST (>5x baseline)

Hypersensitivity: Hypersensitivity

Immunologic: Antibody development (neutralizing; significance not known)

Local: Injection site reaction (including inflammation, pain, tissue necrosis, hypersensitivity reaction, swelling, residual mass)

Neuromuscular & skeletal: Arthralgia, leg cramps, myalgia, weakness

Respiratory: Dyspnea, flu-like symptoms (decreases over treatment course)

Miscellaneous: Fever

Rare but important or life-threatening: Anaphylaxis, anorexia, apnea, ataxia, autoimmune hepatitis, capillary leak syndrome (in patients with preexisting monoclonal gammopathy), cardiac arrest, cardiac arrhythmia, cardiac failure, cardiomegaly, cardiomyopathy, cerebral hemorrhage, coma, confusion, convulsion, deep vein thrombosis, delirium, depersonalization, depression, emotional lability, erythema nodosum, ethanol sensitization, exfoliative dermatitis, gastrointestinal hemorrhage, hallucinations, hematemesis, hepatic failure, hepatitis, hyperthyroidism, hyperuricemia, hypocalcemia, increased gamma-glutamyl transferase, increased serum triglycerides maculopapular rash, manic behavior, myocardial infarction, pancreatitis, pericardial effusion, pneumonia, pruritus, psychosis, pulmonary embolism, rash, sepsis, shock, skin discoloration, skin photosensitivity, suicidal ideation, syncope, SIADH, thrombocytopenia, thyroid dysfunction, urinary tract infection, urosepsis, vasculitis, vaginal hemorrhage, vesiculobullous dermatitis, weight loss

Drug Interactions

Metabolism/Transport Effects None known.

Avoid Concomitant Use There are no known interactions where it is recommended to avoid concomitant use.

Increased Effect/Toxicity
Interferon Beta-1b may increase the levels/effects of: Theophylline Derivatives; Zidovudine

Decreased Effect There are no known significant interactions involving a decrease in effect.

Preparation for Administration To reconstitute solution, inject 1.2 mL of diluent (provided); gently swirl to dissolve, do not shake. Reconstituted solution provides 0.25 mg/mL. Use product within 3 hours of reconstitution. Discard unused portion of vial. Foaming may occur if swirled or shaken too vigorously; allow vial to sit until foam settles.

Storage/Stability Store intact vials at 20°C to 25°C (68°F to 77°F); excursions permitted to 15°C to 30°C (59°F to 86°F) for ≤3 months. If not used immediately following reconstitution, refrigerate solution at 2°C to 8°C (35°F to 46°F) and use within 3 hours; do not freeze or shake solution. Discard unused portion of vial.

Mechanism of Action Interferon beta-1b differs from naturally occurring human protein by a single amino acid substitution and the lack of carbohydrate side chains; mechanism in the treatment of MS is unknown; however, immunomodulatory effects attributed to interferon beta-1b include enhancement of suppressor T cell activity, reduction of proinflammatory cytokines, down-regulation of antigen presentation, and reduced trafficking of lymphocytes into the central nervous system. Improves MRI lesions, decreases relapse rate, and disease severity in patients with secondary progressive MS.

Pharmacodynamics/Kinetics Limited data due to small doses used

Half-life elimination: 8 minutes to 4.3 hours

Time to peak, serum: 1-8 hours

Dosage Note: Analgesics and/or antipyretics may help decrease flu-like symptoms on treatment days:

Multiple sclerosis (relapsing) or treatment of first clinical episode with MRI features consistent with MS: Adults: SubQ: Initial: 0.0625 mg (0.25 mL) every other day; gradually increase dose by 0.0625 mg every 2 weeks

Target dose: 0.25 mg (1 mL) every other day

Note: In clinical trials involving patients with a single clinical event suggestive of MS, dose was initiated at 0.0625 mg (2 million units [0.25 mL]) every other day and titrated weekly up to a target dose of 8 million units (1 mL) every other day (Kappos, 2006).

Multiple sclerosis (secondary-progressive) [Canadian labeling; not in U.S. labeling]: Adults: SubQ: Initial: 0.125 mg (4 million units [0.5 mL]) every other day for 2 weeks

Target dose: 0.25 mg (1 mL) every other day

Dosage adjustment in renal impairment: No dosage adjustment provided in manufacturer's labeling.

Dosage adjustment in hepatic impairment: No dosage adjustment provided in manufacturer's labeling. The Canadian labeling contraindicates use in decompensated liver disease.

Administration Withdraw dose of reconstituted solution from the vial into a sterile syringe fitted with a 27-gauge (Extavia) or 30-gauge (Betaseron) needle and inject the solution subcutaneously; sites for self-injection include outer surface of the arms, abdomen (**except** 2-inch area around the navel), hips, and thighs. Rotate SubQ injection site. Do not inject into area where skin is bruised, infected, or broken. Patient should be well hydrated. If a dose is missed, administer as soon as remembered; do not administer on 2 consecutive days. Time subsequent doses every 48 hours.

Monitoring Parameters Complete blood chemistries (including platelet count) and liver function tests are recommended at 1, 3, and 6 months following initiation of therapy and periodically thereafter. Thyroid function should be assessed every 6 months in patients with history of thyroid dysfunction or as clinically necessary. Monitor for flu-like symptoms, allergic or anaphylactic reactions, injection site reactions, and for sign/symptoms of depression.

Canadian labeling: Additional monitoring recommendations (not in U.S. labeling): Baseline pregnancy test, chest X-ray, and ECG

Additional Information American Academy of Neurology and MS Council guidelines suggest that, based upon published data, 6 million units of Avonex® (interferon beta-1a) (30 mcg) is equivalent to approximately 7-9 million units of Betaseron® (220-280 mcg).

Dosage Forms

Kit, Subcutaneous:
Betaseron: 0.3 mg

Kit, Subcutaneous [preservative free]:
Extavia: 0.3 mg

Interferon Gamma-1b

(in ter FEER on GAM ah won bee)

Brand Names: U.S. Actimmune

Brand Names: Canada Actimmune®

Pharmacologic Category Interferon

Use Reduce frequency and severity of serious infections associated with chronic granulomatous disease; delay time to disease progression in patients with severe, malignant osteopetrosis

Pregnancy Risk Factor C

Pregnancy Considerations Teratogenic effects were not observed in animal studies. A dose-related abortifacient activity was reported in Rhesus monkeys. Safety and efficacy in pregnant women has not been established.

Breast-Feeding Considerations Potential for serious adverse reactions. Because its use has not been evaluated during lactation, breast-feeding is not recommended

Contraindications Hypersensitivity to interferon gamma, *E. coli* derived proteins, or any component of the formulation

Warnings/Precautions Hypersensitivity reactions have been reported (rarely). Transient cutaneous rashes may occur. Dose-related bone marrow toxicity has been reported; use caution in patients with myelosuppression. May cause hepatotoxicity and the incidence may be increased in children <1 year of age. Doses >10 times the weekly recommended dose (used in studies for off-label indications) have been associated with a different pattern/frequency of adverse effects. Flu-like symptoms which may exacerbate preexisting cardiovascular disorders (including ischemia, HF, or arrhythmias) and the development of neurologic disorders have been noted at the higher doses. Caution should also be used in patients with seizure disorders or compromised CNS function.

Adverse Reactions Based on 50 mcg/m^2 dose administered 3 times weekly for chronic granulomatous disease

Central nervous system: Chills, depression, fatigue, fever, headache

Dermatologic: Rash

Gastrointestinal: Abdominal pain, diarrhea, nausea, vomiting

Local: Injection site erythema or tenderness

Neuromuscular & skeletal: Arthralgia, back pain, myalgia

Postmarketing and/or case reports: Alkaline phosphatase elevated, atopic dermatitis, granulomatous colitis, hepatomegaly, hypersensitivity reactions, hypokalemia, neutropenia, Stevens-Johnson syndrome

Additional adverse reactions noted at doses >100 mcg/m^2 administered 3 times weekly: ALT increased, AST increased, autoantibodies increased, bronchospasm, chest discomfort, confusion, dermatomyositis exacerbation, disorientation, DVT, gait disturbance, GI bleeding, hallucinations, heart block, heart failure, hepatic insufficiency, hyperglycemia, hypertriglyceridemia, hyponatremia, hypotension, interstitial pneumonitis, lupus-like syndrome, MI, neutropenia, pancreatitis (may be fatal), Parkinsonian symptoms, PE, proteinuria, renal insufficiency (reversible), seizure, syncope, tachyarrhythmia, tachypnea, thrombocytopenia, TIA

Drug Interactions

Metabolism/Transport Effects Inhibits CYP1A2 (weak), CYP2E1 (weak)

Avoid Concomitant Use There are no known interactions where it is recommended to avoid concomitant use.

Increased Effect/Toxicity

Interferon Gamma-1b may increase the levels/effects of: Theophylline Derivatives; Zidovudine

Decreased Effect There are no known significant interactions involving a decrease in effect.

Storage/Stability Store in refrigerator at 2°C to 8°C (36°F to 46°F); do not freeze. Do not shake. Discard if left unrefrigerated for >12 hours.

Mechanism of Action Interferon gamma participates in immunoregulation by enhancing the oxidative metabolism of macrophages; it also enhances antibody dependent cellular cytotoxicity, activates natural killer cells and has a role in the expression of Fc receptors and histocompatibility antigens. The exact mechanism of action for the treatment of chronic granulomatous disease or osteopetrosis has not been defined.

Pharmacodynamics/Kinetics

Absorption: IM, SubQ: >89%

Half-life elimination: IV: 38 minutes; IM: ~3 hours, SubQ: ~6 hours

Time to peak, plasma: IM: 4 hours (1.5 ng/mL); SubQ: 7 hours (0.6 ng/mL)

Dosage If severe reactions occur, reduce dose by 50% or therapy should be interrupted until adverse reaction abates.

Children: Severe, malignant osteopetrosis: SubQ:

BSA ≤0.5 m^2: 1.5 mcg/kg/dose 3 times/week

BSA >0.5 m^2: 50 mcg/m^2 (1 million units/m^2) 3 times/week

Children and Adults: Chronic granulomatous disease: SubQ:

BSA ≤0.5 m^2: 1.5 mcg/kg/dose 3 times/week

BSA >0.5 m^2: 50 mcg/m^2 (1 million units/m^2) 3 times/week

Note: Previously expressed as 1.5 million units/m^2; 50 mcg is equivalent to 1 million units/m^2.

Dosage adjustment in renal impairment: No dosage adjustment provided in manufacturer's labeling.

Dosage adjustment in hepatic impairment: No dosage adjustment provided in manufacturer's labeling.

Administration Administer by SubQ injection into the right and left deltoid or anterior thigh.

Monitoring Parameters CBC with differential, platelets, LFTs (monthly in children <1 year), electrolytes, BUN, creatinine, and urinalysis prior to therapy and at 3-month intervals

Dosage Forms

Solution, Subcutaneous:

Actimmune: 2,000,000 units/0.5 mL (0.5 mL)

- ◆ **Interleukin-1 Receptor Antagonist** *see* Anakinra *on page 148*
- ◆ **Interleukin 2** *see* Aldesleukin *on page 72*
- ◆ **Interleukin-11** *see* Oprelvekin *on page 1519*
- ◆ **Intermezzo** *see* Zolpidem *on page 2212*
- ◆ **Intralipid** *see* Fat Emulsion (Plant Based) *on page 848*
- ◆ **Intrapleural Talc** *see* Talc (Sterile) *on page 1971*
- ◆ **Intravenous Fat Emulsion** *see* Fat Emulsion (Plant Based) *on page 848*
- ◆ **Intravenous Fat Emulsion (Fish-Oil Based)** *see* Fat Emulsion (Fish Oil Based) [CAN/INT] *on page 847*
- ◆ **Intrifiban** *see* Eptifibatide *on page 751*
- ◆ **Intron A** *see* Interferon Alfa-2b *on page 1096*
- ◆ **Intropin** *see* DOPamine *on page 669*
- ◆ **Introvale** *see* Ethinyl Estradiol and Levonorgestrel *on page 803*
- ◆ **Intuniv** *see* GuanFACINE *on page 990*
- ◆ **Intuniv XR (Can)** *see* GuanFACINE *on page 990*
- ◆ **INVanz** *see* Ertapenem *on page 760*
- ◆ **Invanz (Can)** *see* Ertapenem *on page 760*
- ◆ **Invega** *see* Paliperidone *on page 1556*
- ◆ **Invega Sustenna** *see* Paliperidone *on page 1556*
- ◆ **Invirase** *see* Saquinavir *on page 1865*
- ◆ **Iodine and Potassium Iodide** *see* Potassium Iodide and Iodine *on page 1690*
- ◆ **Iodochlorhydroxyquin and Flumethasone** *see* Clioquinol and Flumethasone [CAN/INT] *on page 465*

Iodoquinol (eye oh doe KWIN ole)

Brand Names: U.S. Yodoxin

Brand Names: Canada Diodoquin®

Index Terms Diiodohydroxyquin

Pharmacologic Category Amebicide

Use Treatment of intestinal amebiasis due to trophozoite and cyst forms of *Entamoeba histolytica*

Dosage Oral:

Children: 30-40 mg/kg daily (maximum: 650 mg per dose) in 3 divided doses for 20 days; not to exceed 1.95 g daily

Adults: 650 mg 3 times daily after meals for 20 days; not to exceed 1.95 g daily

Additional Information Complete prescribing information should be consulted for additional detail.

Dosage Forms

Tablet, Oral:

Yodoxin: 210 mg, 650 mg

Iodoquinol and Hydrocortisone

(eye oh doe KWIN ole & hye droe KOR ti sone)

Brand Names: U.S. Alcortin A; Dermazene; Vytone

Index Terms Hydrocortisone and Iodoquinol

Pharmacologic Category Antifungal Agent, Topical; Corticosteroid, Topical

Use Treatment of eczema (including impetiginized, nuchal, and nummular); acne urticata; anogenital pruritus, atopic and contact dermatitis, endogenous chronic infectious dermatitis; chronic eczematoid otitis externa; folliculitis, intertrigo; lichen simplex chronicus; moniliasis; dermatoses (mycotic or bacterial); neurodermatitis (localized or systemic); pyoderma, stasis dermatitis

Pregnancy Risk Factor C

Dosage Dermatoses: Children ≥12 years, Adolescents, and Adults: Topical: Apply 3-4 times daily to affected area(s)

Additional Information Complete prescribing information should be consulted for additional detail.

Dosage Forms

Cream, topical: Iodoquinol 1% and hydrocortisone 1% (30 g)

Dermazene: Iodoquinol 1% and hydrocortisone 1% (30 g)

Vytone: Iodoquinol 1% and hydrocortisone 1.9% per 2 g packet (30s)

Gel, topical:

Alcortin A: Iodoquinol 1% and hydrocortisone 2% (2 g)

◆ **Iophen C-NR** *see* Guaifenesin and Codeine *on page 987*

◆ **Iophen DM-NR [OTC]** *see* Guaifenesin and Dextromethorphan *on page 987*

◆ **Iophen-NR [OTC]** *see* GuaiFENesin *on page 986*

◆ **Iopidine** *see* Apraclonidine *on page 165*

Ipilimumab (ip i LIM u mab)

Brand Names: U.S. Yervoy

Brand Names: Canada Yervoy®

Index Terms MDX-010; MDX-CTLA-4; MOAB-CTLA-4

Pharmacologic Category Antineoplastic Agent, Monoclonal Antibody

Use Treatment of unresectable or metastatic melanoma

Pregnancy Risk Factor C

Pregnancy Considerations Adverse effects were observed in animal reproduction studies. Ipilimumab is an IgG1 immunoglobulin and human IgG1 is known to cross the placenta, therefore, ipilimumab may be expected to reach the fetus.

Breast-Feeding Considerations Due to the potential for serious adverse reactions in the nursing infant, the decision to discontinue ipilimumab or to discontinue breast-feeding should take into account the importance of treatment to the mother.

Contraindications There are no contraindications listed within the manufacturer's labeling.

Canadian labeling: Hypersensitivity to ipilimumab or any component of the formulation; active life-threatening autoimmune disease, or with organ transplantation graft where further immune activation is potentially imminently life-threatening

Warnings/Precautions [U.S. Boxed Warning]: Severe and fatal immune-mediated adverse effects due to T-cell activation and proliferation may occur. While any organ system may be involved, common severe effects include dermatitis (including toxic epidermal necrolysis), endocrine disorder, enterocolitis, hepatitis, and neuropathy. Reactions generally occur during treatment, although some reactions have occurred weeks to months after treatment discontinuation. Discontinue treatment (permanently) and initiate high-dose corticosteroid treatment for severe immune mediated reactions. Evaluate liver function and thyroid function tests at baseline and prior to each dose. Assess for signs and symptoms of enterocolitis, dermatitis, neuropathy, and endocrine disorder at baseline and prior to each dose. Initiate prednisone 1-2 mg/kg/day (or equivalent) for severe reactions. Uncommon immune-mediated adverse effects reported include hemolytic anemia, iritis, meningitis, nephritis, pericarditis, pneumonitis, and uveitis. Administer corticosteroid ophthalmic drops in patients who develop episcleritis, iritis, or uveitis; permanently discontinue ipilimumab if unresponsive to topical ophthalmic immunosuppressive treatments. For severe immune-mediated episcleritis or uveitis, initiate prednisone 1-2 mg/kg/day (or equivalent); taper over at least 1 month (Weber, 2012).

Immune-mediated enterocolitis was reported to occur at a median onset of 6-7 weeks. Monitor for signs and symptoms of enterocolitis (abdominal pain, blood in stool, diarrhea, or mucous in stool; with or without fever) and intestinal perforation (peritoneal signs, ileus). If enterocolitis develops, infectious causes should be ruled out; consider endoscopy for persistent or severe symptoms. Withhold ipilimumab treatment and administer antidiarrheals for moderate enterocolitis (diarrhea with ≤6 stools over baseline abdominal pain, mucous or blood in stool); if persists for >1 week, initiate prednisone at 0.5 mg/kg/day (or equivalent). If severe enterocolitis (diarrhea ≥7 stools above baseline, fever, ileus, peritoneal signs) develops, permanently discontinue ipilimumab and initiate prednisone 1-2 mg/kg/day (or equivalent); when resolved to ≤ grade 1, taper corticosteroids slowly over ≥1 month (rapid tapering may worsen symptoms).

Severe, life-threatening or fatal hepatotoxicity and immune-mediated hepatitis have been observed. Monitor liver function tests (LFTs) and evaluate for signs of hepatotoxicity prior to each dose; if hepatotoxicity develops, infectious or malignant causes should be ruled out and liver function should be monitored more frequently until resolves. Withhold treatment for grade 2 hepatotoxicity (ALT or AST 2.5-5 times ULN or total bilirubin 1.5-3 times ULN). If severe hepatotoxicity develops (ALT or AST >5 times ULN or total bilirubin >3 times ULN), permanently discontinue ipilimumab and initiate prednisone 1-2 mg/kg/day (or equivalent). If transaminases do not decrease within 48 hours of steroid initiation, consider adding mycophenolate mofetil (Weber, 2012). May begin tapering corticosteroid (over 1 month) when LFTs show sustained improvement or return to baseline.

Severe, life-threatening, or fatal dermatitis has been reported. The median time to onset for dermatologic toxicity is 3 weeks (range: ≤17 weeks). Monitor for rash and pruritus; dermatitis should be considered immune-mediated unless identified otherwise. Mild-to-moderate dermatitis (localized rash and pruritus) should be treated symptomatically; topical or systemic corticosteroids should be administered if not resolved within 1 week. Withhold treatment for moderate to severe dermatologic symptoms. Permanently discontinue and initiate prednisone 1-2 mg/kg/day (or equivalent) for Stevens-Johnson syndrome, toxic epidermal necrolysis, or rash complicated by dermal ulceration (full thickness) or necrotic, bullous, or hemorrhagic manifestations; when dermatitis is controlled, taper corticosteroid over at least 1 month.

Severe or life-threatening endocrine disorders (hypopituitarism, adrenal insufficiency, hypogonadism and hypothyroidism) have been reported; may require hospitalization. Endocrine disorders of moderate severity (including hypothyroidism, adrenal insufficiency, hypopituitarism, and less commonly hyperthyroidism and Cushing's syndrome) which have required hormone replacement therapy or medical intervention have also been reported. The median onset for moderate-to-severe endocrine disorders was 11 weeks (range: ≤19 weeks); long-term hormone replacement therapy has been required in many cases. Monitor thyroid function tests and serum chemistries prior to each dose; also monitor for signs of hypophysitis, adrenal insufficiency and thyroid disorders (eg, abdominal pain, fatigue, headache, hypotension, mental status changes, unusual bowel habits); rule out other potential causes such as brain metastases. Endocrine disorders should be considered immune-mediated unless identified otherwise; consider endocrinology referral for further evaluation. If symptomatic, withhold ipilimumab treatment and initiate prednisone 1-2 mg/kg/day (or equivalent) and appropriate hormone replacement therapy.

Severe peripheral motor neuropathy and fatal Guillain-Barré syndrome have been reported (rare). Monitor for signs of motor or sensory neuropathy (unilateral or bilateral weakness, sensory changes or paresthesia). Withhold treatment in patients with neuropathy that does not interfere with daily activities (moderate neuropathy). Permanently discontinue for severe neuropathy (interferes with daily activities, including symptoms similar to Guillain-Barré syndrome). Consider initiating prednisone 1-2 mg/kg/day (or equivalent) for severe neuropathies.

Adverse Reactions

Central nervous system: Fatigue, fever, headache

Dermatologic: Dermatitis (includes Stevens-Johnson syndrome, toxic epidermal necrolysis, dermal ulceration, necrotic, bullous or hemorrhagic dermatitis), pruritus, rash, urticaria, vitiligo

Endocrine & metabolic: Adrenal insufficiency, hypophysitis, hypopituitarism, hypothyroidism

Gastrointestinal: Abdominal pain, appetite decreased, colitis, constipation, diarrhea, enterocolitis, intestinal perforation, nausea, vomiting

Hematologic: Anemia, eosinophilia

Hepatic: ALT increased, hepatotoxicity

Renal: Nephritis

Respiratory: Cough, dyspnea

Miscellaneous: Antibody formation

Rare but important or life-threatening: Acute respiratory distress syndrome, angiopathy, arthritis, blepharitis, bronchiolitis obliterans organizing pneumonia (Barjaktarevic 2013), conjunctivitis, Cushing's syndrome, decreased corticotrophin, encephalitis, episcleritis, erythema multiforme, esophagitis, gastrointestinal ulcer, Guillain-Barré syndrome, hemolytic anemia, hepatic failure, hepatitis (immune-mediated), hyperthyroidism, hypogonadism, increased serum AST, increased serum bilirubin, increased thyrotropin, infusion reaction, iritis, leukocytoclastic vasculitis, meningitis, myasthenia gravis, myelofibrosis, myocarditis, myositis, neuropathy (sensory and motor), neurosensory hypoacusis, ocular myositis, pancreatitis, pericarditis, peritonitis, pneumonitis, polymyalgia rheumatica, polymyositis, psoriasis, renal failure, sarcoidosis, scleritis, sepsis, temporal arteritis, thyroiditis (autoimmune), uveitis, vascular leak syndrome, vasculitis

Drug Interactions

Metabolism/Transport Effects None known.

Avoid Concomitant Use There are no known interactions where it is recommended to avoid concomitant use.

Increased Effect/Toxicity

Ipilimumab may increase the levels/effects of: Vemurafenib

Decreased Effect There are no known significant interactions involving a decrease in effect.

Preparation for Administration Prior to preparation, allow vials to sit at room temperature for ~5 minutes. Inspect vial prior to use; solution may have a pale yellow color or may contain translucent or white amorphous ipilimumab particles; discard if cloudy or discolored. Withdraw appropriate ipilimumab volume and transfer to IV bag, dilute with NS or D_5W to a final concentration between 1-2 mg/mL. Mix by gently inverting, do not shake.

Storage/Stability Store intact vials refrigerated at 2°C to 8°C (36°F to 46°C); do not freeze. Protect from light. Prior to preparation, allow vials to sit at room temperature for ~5 minutes. Solutions diluted for infusion are stable for up to 24 hours refrigerated or at room temperature.

Mechanism of Action Ipilimumab is a recombinant human IgG1 immunoglobulin monoclonal antibody which binds to the cytotoxic T-lymphocyte associated antigen 4 (CTLA-4). CTLA-4 is a down-regulator of T-cell activation pathways. Blocking CTLA-4 allows for enhanced T-cell activation and proliferation. In melanoma, ipilimumab may indirectly mediate T-cell immune responses against tumors.

Pharmacodynamics/Kinetics

Distribution: V_{ss}: 7.21 L

Half-life elimination: Terminal: 15.4 days

Dosage IV: Adults: Melanoma, unresectable or metastatic: 3 mg/kg every 3 weeks for 4 doses

Dosage adjustment for toxicity:

Temporarily withhold scheduled dose for the following:

Moderate immune-mediated reactions

Symptomatic endocrine disorder

Grade 2 hepatotoxicity (AST or ALT >2.5 to ≤5 x ULN or bilirubin >1.5 to ≤3 x ULN)

Note: If receiving prednisone <7.5 mg daily (or equivalent), may resume with complete or partial resolution (to ≤ grade 1) of symptoms. Resume ipilimumab treatment at 3 mg/kg every 3 weeks until all 4 planned doses have been administered or until 16 weeks from initial dose, whichever occurs first.

Permanently discontinue for the following:

Failure to complete treatment course within 16 weeks of initial dose

Persistent moderate adverse reactions or unable to reduce corticosteroid dose to prednisone 7.5 mg daily (or equivalent)

Severe or life-threatening adverse reactions including:

Central nervous system or neuromuscular toxicity: Severe motor or sensory neuropathy, Guillain-Barré syndrome, or myasthenia gravis

Dermatologic toxicities: Stevens-Johnson syndrome, toxic epidermal necrolysis, or rash complicated by full thickness dermal ulceration, or necrotic, bullous, or hemorrhagic manifestations

Gastrointestinal toxicities: Colitis with abdominal pain, fever, ileus, or peritoneal symptoms, increase in stool frequency (≥7 over baseline), stool incontinence, require IV hydration for >24 hours, or GI hemorrhage or perforation; grades 3/4 amylase or lipase increases (Weber, 2012)

Hepatotoxicities: ALT or AST >5 times ULN, or total bilirubin >3 times ULN

Ophthalmic toxicities: Immune-mediated ocular disease unresponsive to topical immunosuppressive treatment

Severe immune-mediated reactions involving any organ system (eg, myocarditis [noninfectious], nephritis, pancreatitis, pneumonitis)

Dosage adjustment in renal impairment: No dosage adjustment necessary.

Dosage adjustment in hepatic impairment:

Impairment at baseline:

Mild impairment (total bilirubin >1 to 1.5 x ULN **or** AST >ULN): No dosage adjustment necessary.

Moderate or severe impairment (total bilirubin >1.5 x ULN and any AST): No dosage adjustment provided in manufacturer's labeling (has not been studied).

Impairment during treatment:

AST or ALT >2.5 to ≤5 x ULN or bilirubin >1.5 to ≤3 x ULN: Temporarily withhold treatment.

ALT or AST >5 times ULN, or total bilirubin >3 times ULN: Permanently discontinue.

Administration IV: Infuse over 90 minutes through a low protein-binding in-line filter. Flush with NS or D_5W at the end of infusion

Monitoring Parameters Monitor liver function and evaluate for signs of hepatotoxicity prior to each dose; if hepatotoxicity develops, liver function should be monitored more frequently until resolves. If liver functions tests are >8 times ULN, monitor every other day until begin to fall, then weekly until normal (Weber, 2012). Monitor serum chemistries prior to each dose. Monitor for signs of hypophysitis, adrenal insufficiency and thyroid disorders (eg, abdominal pain, fatigue, headache, hypotension, mental status changes, unusual bowel habits). Monitor TSH, free T_4 and cortisol levels (morning) at baseline, prior to dose, and as clinically indicated. Monitor for signs and symptoms of enterocolitis (abdominal pain, blood or mucus in stool or diarrhea, and intestinal perforation (peritoneal signs, ileus). Monitor for rash and pruritus. Monitor for signs of motor or sensory neuropathy (unilateral or bilateral weakness, sensory changes or paresthesia). Monitor for ocular toxicity at baseline, then at 4-8 weeks with further evaluations as clinically indicated (Renouf, 2012).

Dosage Forms

Solution, Intravenous [preservative free]:

Yervoy: 50 mg/10 mL (10 mL); 200 mg/40 mL (40 mL)

◆ **IPOL** *see* Poliovirus Vaccine (Inactivated) *on page 1673*

Ipratropium (Systemic) (i pra TROE pee um)

Brand Names: U.S. Atrovent HFA

Brand Names: Canada Atrovent HFA; Gen-Ipratropium; Mylan-Ipratropium Sterinebs; Novo-Ipramide; Nu-Ipratropium; PMS-Ipratropium; ratio-Ipratropium UDV; Teva-Ipratropium Sterinebs

Index Terms Ipratropium Bromide

Pharmacologic Category Anticholinergic Agent

Use Anticholinergic bronchodilator used in bronchospasm associated with COPD, bronchitis, and emphysema

Pregnancy Risk Factor B

Pregnancy Considerations Teratogenic effects were not observed in animal studies. Inhaled ipratropium is recommended for use as additional therapy for pregnant women with severe asthma exacerbations.

Breast-Feeding Considerations It is not known if ipratropium (oral inhalation) is excreted in breast milk. The manufacturer recommends that caution be exercised when administering ipratropium (oral inhalation) to nursing women.

Contraindications Hypersensitivity to ipratropium, atropine (and its derivatives), or any component of the formulation

Warnings/Precautions Immediate hypersensitivity reactions (urticaria, angioedema, rash, bronchospasm) have been reported. Rarely, paradoxical bronchospasm may occur with use of inhaled bronchodilating agents; this should be distinguished from inadequate response. Not indicated for the initial treatment of acute episodes of bronchospasm where rescue therapy is required for rapid response. Should only be used in acute exacerbations of asthma in conjunction with short-acting beta-adrenergic agonists for acute episodes (NAEPP 2007). Use with caution in patients with myasthenia gravis, narrow-angle glaucoma, benign prostatic hyperplasia (BPH), or bladder neck obstruction

Adverse Reactions

Central nervous system: Dizziness, headache

Gastrointestinal: Dyspepsia, nausea, taste perversion, xerostomia

Genitourinary: Urinary tract infection

Neuromuscular & skeletal: Back pain

Respiratory: Bronchitis, COPD exacerbation, cough, dyspnea, rhinitis, sinusitis, upper respiratory infection

Miscellaneous: Flu-like syndrome

Rare but important or life-threatening: Accommodation disorder, anaphylactic reaction, angioedema, bronchospasm, corneal edema, eye pain (acute), glaucoma, hypersensitivity reactions, hypotension, intraocular pressure increased, laryngospasm, palpitations, stomatitis, tachycardia, urinary retention

Drug Interactions

Metabolism/Transport Effects None known.

Avoid Concomitant Use

Avoid concomitant use of Ipratropium (Oral Inhalation) with any of the following: Aclidinium; Anticholinergic Agents; Glucagon; Potassium Chloride; Tiotropium; Umeclidinium

Increased Effect/Toxicity

Ipratropium (Oral Inhalation) may increase the levels/effects of: AbobotulinumtoxinA; Analgesics (Opioid); Anticholinergic Agents; Cannabinoid-Containing Products; Glucagon; Mirabegron; OnabotulinumtoxinA; Potassium Chloride; RimabotulinumtoxinB; Thiazide Diuretics; Tiotropium; Topiramate

The levels/effects of Ipratropium (Oral Inhalation) may be increased by: Aclidinium; Mianserin; Pramlintide; Umeclidinium

Decreased Effect

Ipratropium (Oral Inhalation) may decrease the levels/effects of: Acetylcholinesterase Inhibitors; Itopride; Secretin

The levels/effects of Ipratropium (Oral Inhalation) may be decreased by: Acetylcholinesterase Inhibitors

Storage/Stability

Aerosol: Store at controlled room temperature of 25°C (77°F). Do not store near heat or open flame.

Solution: Store at 15°C to 30°C (59°F to 86°F). Protect from light.

Mechanism of Action Blocks the action of acetylcholine at parasympathetic sites in bronchial smooth muscle causing bronchodilation; local application to nasal mucosa inhibits serous and seromucous gland secretions.

Pharmacodynamics/Kinetics

Onset of action: Bronchodilation: Within 15 minutes

Peak effect: 1-2 hours

Duration: 2-5 hours

Absorption: Negligible

Distribution: 15% of dose reaches lower airways

Protein Binding: ≤9%

Half-life elimination: 2 hours

Excretion: Urine

Dosage

Nebulization:

Children ≤12 years: Asthma exacerbation, acute (NAEPP 2007): 250-500 mcg every 20 minutes for 3 doses, then as needed. **Note:** Should be given in combination with a short-acting beta-adrenergic agonist.

Children >12 years and Adults:

Bronchodilator for COPD: 500 mcg (one unit-dose vial) 3-4 times/day with doses 6-8 hours apart

Asthma exacerbation, acute (NAEPP 2007): 500 mcg every 20 minutes for 3 doses, then as needed. **Note:** Should be given in combination with a short-acting beta-adrenergic agonist.

Oral inhalation: MDI:

Children ≤12 years: Asthma exacerbation, acute (NAEPP 2007): 4-8 inhalations every 20 minutes as needed for up to 3 hours. **Note:** Should be given in combination with a short-acting beta-adrenergic agonist.

Children >12 years and Adults:

Bronchodilator for COPD: 2 inhalations 4 times/day, up to 12 inhalations/24 hours

Asthma exacerbation, acute (NAEPP 2007): 8 inhalations every 20 minutes as needed for up to 3 hours. **Note:** Should be given in combination with a short-acting beta-adrenergic agonist.

Dosage adjustment in renal impairment: No dosage adjustment provided in manufacturer's labeling (has not been studied).

Dosage adjustment in hepatic impairment: No dosage adjustment provided in manufacturer's labeling (has not been studied).

Administration Avoid spraying into the eyes.

Atrovent® HFA: Prior to initial use, prime inhaler by releasing 2 test sprays into the air. If the inhaler has not been used for >3 days, reprime.

Dosage Forms Considerations Atrovent HFA 12.9 g canister contains 200 inhalations.

Dosage Forms

Aerosol Solution, Inhalation:

Atrovent HFA: 17 mcg/actuation (12.9 g)

Solution, Inhalation:

Generic: 0.02% (2.5 mL)

Solution, Inhalation [preservative free]:

Generic: 0.02% (2.5 mL)

Ipratropium (Nasal) (i pra TROE pee um)

Brand Names: U.S. Atrovent

Brand Names: Canada Alti-Ipratropium; Apo-Ipravent®; Atrovent®; Mylan-Ipratropium Solution

Index Terms Ipratropium Bromide

Pharmacologic Category Anticholinergic Agent

Use Symptomatic relief of rhinorrhea associated with the common cold and allergic and nonallergic rhinitis

Pregnancy Risk Factor B

Dosage Intranasal: Nasal spray:

Symptomatic relief of rhinorrhea associated with the common cold (safety and efficacy of use beyond 4 days in patients with the common cold have not been established):

Children 5-11 years: 0.06%: 2 sprays in each nostril 3 times/day

Children ≥12 years and Adults: 0.06%: 2 sprays in each nostril 3-4 times/day

Symptomatic relief of rhinorrhea associated with allergic/nonallergic rhinitis: Children ≥6 years and Adults: 0.03%: 2 sprays in each nostril 2-3 times/day

Symptomatic relief of rhinorrhea associated with seasonal allergic rhinitis (safety and efficacy of use beyond 3 weeks in patients with seasonal allergic rhinitis has not been established): Children ≥5 years and Adults: 0.06%: 2 sprays in each nostril 4 times/day

Dosage adjustment in renal impairment: No dosage adjustment provided in manufacturer's labeling (has not been studied); use with caution.

Dosage adjustment in hepatic impairment: No dosage adjustment provided in manufacturer's labeling (has not been studied); use with caution.

Additional Information Complete prescribing information should be consulted for additional detail.

Dosage Forms Considerations

Atrovent 0.03% (21 mcg/spray) nasal solution 30 mL bottles contain 345 sprays, and the 0.06% (42 mcg/spray) 15 mL bottles contain 165 sprays.

Dosage Forms

Solution, Nasal:

Atrovent: 0.03% (30 mL); 0.06% (15 mL)

Generic: 0.03% (30 mL); 0.06% (15 mL)

Ipratropium and Albuterol
(i pra TROE pee um & al BYOO ter ole)

Brand Names: U.S. Combivent® Respimat®; Combivent® [DSC]; DuoNeb®

Brand Names: Canada Apo-Salvent-Ipravent Sterules; Combivent Respimat; Combivent UDV; ratio-Ipra Sal UDV; Teva-Combo Sterinebs

Index Terms Albuterol and Ipratropium; Salbutamol and Ipratropium

Pharmacologic Category Anticholinergic Agent; Beta$_2$-Adrenergic Agonist

Use Treatment of COPD in those patients who are currently on a regular bronchodilator who continue to have bronchospasms and require a second bronchodilator

Pregnancy Risk Factor C

Dosage COPD: Inhalation: Adults:

Aerosol for inhalation:

Combivent®: Two inhalations 4 times daily (maximum: 12 inhalations/24 hours)

Combivent® Respimat®: One inhalation 4 times daily (maximum: 6 inhalations/24 hours)

Solution for nebulization: Initial: 3 mL every 6 hours (maximum: 3 mL every 4 hours)

Dosage adjustment in renal impairment: No dosage adjustment provided in manufacturer's labeling (has not been studied); use with caution.

Dosage adjustment in hepatic impairment: No dosage adjustment provided in manufacturer's labeling (has not been studied); use with caution.

Additional Information Complete prescribing information should be consulted for additional detail.

Dosage Forms

Solution, for nebulization: Ipratropium 0.5 mg and albuterol (base) 2.5 mg per 3 mL (30s, 60s)

DuoNeb®: Ipratropium 0.5 mg and albuterol (base) 2.5 mg per 3 mL (30s, 60s)

Solution, for oral inhalation [spray]:

Combivent® Respimat®: Ipratropium bromide 20 mcg and albuterol (base) 100 mcg per inhalation (4 g) [120 metered actuations]

Ipratropium and Fenoterol [CAN/INT]
(i pra TROE pee um & fen oh TER ole)

Brand Names: Canada Duovent® UDV

Index Terms Fenoterol and Ipratropium; Fenoterol Hydrobromide and Ipratropium Bromide; Ipratropium Bromide and Fenoterol Hydrobromide

Pharmacologic Category Anticholinergic Agent; Beta$_2$-Adrenergic Agonist

Use Note: Not approved in U.S.

Treatment of bronchospasm associated with acute severe exacerbation of COPD or bronchial asthma

Pregnancy Considerations Adverse events were not observed in animal reproduction studies using this combination via inhalation.

Breast-Feeding Considerations It is not known if ipratropium or fenoterol are excreted into breast milk. The manufacturer recommends caution be used if administered to nursing women.

Contraindications Hypersensitivity to ipratropium, fenoterol, sympathomimetic amines, atropine (and its derivatives), or any component of the formulation; tachyarrhythmias; hypertrophic obstructive cardiomyopathy

Warnings/Precautions Use with caution in patients with cardiovascular disease (arrhythmia, hypertension, HF); beta-agonists may cause elevation in blood pressure and heart rate and may result in CNS stimulation/excitation. Beta$_2$-agonists may also increase risk of arrhythmias and myocardial ischemia. Use with caution in cystic fibrosis, diabetes mellitus, narrow-angle glaucoma, hyperthyroidism, pheochromocytoma, prostatic hyperplasia/bladder neck obstruction, and seizure disorders. Rarely, paradoxical bronchospasm may occur with the use of inhaled bronchodilating agents. Ipratropium is not indicated for the initial treatment of acute episodes of bronchospasm. Fenoterol may cause hypokalemia; use caution, particularly in severe asthmatic patients receiving concomitant therapy (eg, steroids, xanthine derivatives) capable of potentiating hypokalemia. Immediate hypersensitivity reactions (urticaria, angioedema, rash, bronchospasm) have been reported with use.

Symptom relief of <3 hours following an administered dose or failure of previous dosage regimen to provide relief indicates worsening of asthma and requires therapy adjustment; patients should be instructed to notify healthcare provider immediately and to not exceed recommended dose. Serious adverse events, including fatalities, have been associated with excessive use of inhaled sympathomimetics. Concomitant use with other sympathomimetic amines is not recommended; closely monitor patients receiving concomitant therapy with other sympathomimetics. Anti-inflammatory therapy should be administered to patients receiving beta$_2$-agonist inhalation therapy on a routine basis. Use in conjunction with IPPV may be ineffective in severe airway obstruction; fatal episodes of hypoxia and pneumothorax have been associated with the use of ipratropium/fenoterol in conjunction with IPPV in acute asthma attacks.

Adverse Reactions

Cardiovascular: Arrhythmias, atrial fibrillation, cardiac arrest, hyper-/hypotension, myocardial ischemia, palpitation, QTc prolongation, SVT, tachycardia

Central nervous system: Dizziness, headache, nervousness, psychological alterations

Gastrointestinal: Constipation, diarrhea, nausea, vomiting, xerostomia

Genitourinary: Urinary retention

Endocrine & metabolic: Hyperglycemia, hypokalemia

Neuromuscular & skeletal: Muscle cramps, myalgia, tremor, weakness

Ophthalmic: Accommodation disturbance, acute angle closure glaucoma, eye pain, intraocular pressure increased, mydriasis

Respiratory: Bronchospasm (inhalation induced), cough, pharyngitis, throat irritation

Miscellaneous: Allergic reactions (anaphylaxis, angioedema, bronchospasm, laryngospasm, oropharyngeal edema, skin rash, urticaria); diaphoresis

Drug Interactions

Metabolism/Transport Effects None known.

Avoid Concomitant Use

Avoid concomitant use of Ipratropium and Fenoterol with any of the following: Aclidinium; Anticholinergic Agents; Beta-Blockers (Nonselective); Glucagon; Iobenguane I 123; Potassium Chloride; Tiotropium; Umeclidinium

Increased Effect/Toxicity

Ipratropium and Fenoterol may increase the levels/effects of: AbobotulinumtoxinA; Analgesics (Opioid); Anticholinergic Agents; Atosiban; Cannabinoid-Containing Products; Glucagon; Loop Diuretics; Mirabegron; OnabotulinumtoxinA; Potassium Chloride; RimabotulinumtoxinB; Sympathomimetics; Thiazide Diuretics; Tiotropium; Topiramate

The levels/effects of Ipratropium and Fenoterol may be increased by: Aclidinium; AtoMOXetine; Cannabinoid-Containing Products; Linezolid; MAO Inhibitors; Mianserin; Pramlintide; Tedizolid; Umeclidinium

Decreased Effect

Ipratropium and Fenoterol may decrease the levels/effects of: Acetylcholinesterase Inhibitors; Iobenguane I 123; Itopride; Secretin

The levels/effects of Ipratropium and Fenoterol may be decreased by: Acetylcholinesterase Inhibitors; Beta-Blockers (Beta1 Selective); Beta-Blockers (Nonselective); Betahistine

Storage/Stability Store unopened vials at 15°C to 25°C (59°F to 77°F). Protect from light. May dilute with preservative-free NS. Use immediately following dilution. Discard unused portion of vial.

Mechanism of Action

Ipratropium: Blocks the action of acetylcholine at parasympathetic sites in bronchial smooth muscle causing bronchodilation

Fenoterol: Relaxes bronchial smooth muscle by action on $beta_2$-receptors

Pharmacodynamics/Kinetics

Onset of action:

Ipratropium: Bronchodilation: Within 15 minutes

Peak effect: 1-2 hours

Fenoterol: Bronchodilation: 5 minutes

Peak effect: 30-60 minutes

Duration:

Ipratropium: 6-8 hours

Fenoterol: 4-6 hours; In combination with ipratropium: 6-8 hours

Absorption: Ipratropium: Negligible

Distribution: Ipratropium: Inhalation: ~3% of dose reaches lower airways

Dosage Nebulization: Children ≥12 years and Adults: Usual dose: 4 mL; may repeat every 6 hours as needed

Administration Inhalation: Nebulization: Wash hands before and after treatment. Wash and dry nebulizer after each treatment. Twist open the top of one unit dose vial and squeeze the contents into the nebulizer reservoir. Connect the nebulizer reservoir to the face mask. Connect nebulizer to compressor. Sit in a comfortable, upright position. Put on the face mask and turn on the compressor. If a face mask is used, avoid leakage around the mask (temporary blurring of vision, worsening of narrow-angle glaucoma, or eye pain may occur if mist gets into eyes). Breathe calmly and deeply until no more mist is formed in the nebulizer (about 5 minutes). At this point, treatment is finished.

Monitoring Parameters Spirometry (FEV, FVC); potassium

Product Availability Not available in U.S.

Dosage Forms: Canada

Solution for nebulization:

Duovent® UDV: Ipratropium bromide 0.5 mg and fenoterol 1.25 mg per 4 mL (20s)

◆ **Ipratropium Bromide** *see* Ipratropium (Nasal) *on page 1109*

◆ **Ipratropium Bromide** *see* Ipratropium (Systemic) *on page 1108*

◆ **Ipratropium Bromide and Fenoterol Hydrobromide** *see* Ipratropium and Fenoterol [CAN/INT] *on page 1109*

◆ **I-Prin [OTC]** *see* Ibuprofen *on page 1032*

◆ **Iprivask** *see* Desirudin *on page 593*

◆ **Iproveratril Hydrochloride** *see* Verapamil *on page 2154*

◆ **IPV** *see* Poliovirus Vaccine (Inactivated) *on page 1673*

Irbesartan (ir be SAR tan)

Brand Names: U.S. Avapro

Brand Names: Canada ACT-Irbesartan; Apo-Irbesartan; Auro-Irbesartan; Ava-Irbesartan; Avapro; Dom-Irbesartan; JAMP-Irbesartan; Mylan-Irbesartan; PMS-Irbesartan; RAN-Irbesartan; ratio-Irbesartan; Sandoz-Irbesartan; Teva-Irbesartan

Pharmacologic Category Angiotensin II Receptor Blocker; Antihypertensive

Use

Hypertension: Treatment of hypertension alone or in combination with other antihypertensives

The 2014 guideline for the management of high blood pressure in adults (Eighth Joint National Committee [JNC 8; James, 2013]) recommends initiation of pharmacologic treatment to lower blood pressure for the following patients:

- Patients ≥60 years of age with systolic blood pressure (SBP) ≥150 mm Hg or diastolic blood pressure (DBP) ≥90 mm Hg. Goal of therapy is SBP <150 mm Hg and DBP <90 mm Hg.
- Patients <60 years of age with SBP ≥140 mm Hg or DBP ≥90 mm Hg. Goal of therapy is SBP <140 mm Hg and DBP <90 mm Hg.
- Patients ≥18 years of age with diabetes and SBP ≥140 mm Hg or DBP ≥90 mm Hg. Goal of therapy is SBP <140 mm Hg and DBP <90 mm Hg.
- Patients ≥18 years of age with chronic kidney disease (CKD) and SBP ≥140 mm Hg or DBP ≥90 mm Hg. Goal of therapy is SBP <140 mm Hg and DBP <90 mm Hg.

In patients with CKD, regardless of race or diabetes status, the use of an ACE inhibitor (ACEI) or angiotensin receptor blocker (ARB) as initial therapy is recommended to improve kidney outcomes. In the general nonblack population (without CKD), including those with diabetes, initial antihypertensive treatment should consist of a thiazide-type diuretic, calcium channel blocker, ACEI, or ARB. In the general black population (without CKD), including those with diabetes, initial antihypertensive treatment should consist of a thiazide-type diuretic or a calcium channel blocker instead of an ACEI or ARB.

Diabetic nephropathy: Treatment of diabetic nephropathy with an elevated serum creatinine and proteinuria (>300 mg/day) in patients with type 2 diabetes and hypertension.

Pregnancy Risk Factor D

Pregnancy Considerations **[U.S. Boxed Warning]: Drugs that act on the renin-angiotensin system can cause injury and death to the developing fetus. Discontinue as soon as possible once pregnancy is detected.** The use of drugs which act on the renin-angiotensin system are associated with oligohydramnios. Oligohydramnios, due to decreased fetal renal function, may lead to fetal lung hypoplasia and skeletal malformations. Use is also associated with anuria, hypotension, renal failure, skull hypoplasia, and death in the fetus/neonate. The exposed fetus should be monitored for fetal growth, amniotic fluid volume, and organ formation. Infants exposed *in utero* should be monitored for hyperkalemia, hypotension, and oliguria (exchange transfusions or dialysis may be needed). These adverse events are generally associated with maternal use in the second and third trimesters.

Untreated chronic maternal hypertension is also associated with adverse events in the fetus, infant, and mother. The use of angiotensin II receptor blockers is not recommended to treat chronic uncomplicated hypertension in pregnant women and should generally be avoided in women of reproductive potential (ACOG, 2013).

Breast-Feeding Considerations It is not known if irbesartan is excreted into breast milk. Due to the potential for serious adverse reactions in the nursing infant, the manufacturer recommends a decision be made whether to discontinue nursing or to discontinue the drug, taking into account the importance of treatment to the mother.

Contraindications

Hypersensitivity to irbesartan or any component of the formulation; concomitant use with aliskiren in patients with diabetes mellitus

Documentation of allergenic cross-reactivity for drugs in this class is limited. However, because of similarities in chemical structure and/or pharmacologic actions, the possibility of cross-sensitivity cannot be ruled out with certainty.

Canadian labeling: Additional contraindications (not in U.S. labeling): Concomitant use with aliskiren in patients with moderate to severe renal impairment (GFR <60 mL/minute/1.73 m^2)

Warnings/Precautions **[U.S. Boxed Warning]: Drugs that act on the renin-angiotensin system can cause injury and death to the developing fetus. Discontinue as soon as possible once pregnancy is detected.** May cause hyperkalemia; avoid potassium supplementation unless specifically required by health care provider. May be associated with deterioration of renal function and/or increases in serum creatinine, particularly in patients with low renal blood flow (eg, renal artery stenosis, heart failure) whose glomerular filtration rate (GFR) is dependent on efferent arteriolar vasoconstriction by angiotensin II. Avoid use or use a much smaller dose in patients who are intravascularly volume-depleted; use caution in patients with unstented unilateral or bilateral renal artery stenosis. When unstented bilateral renal artery stenosis is present, use is generally avoided due to the elevated risk of deterioration in renal function unless possible benefits outweigh risks. AUCs of irbesartan (not the active metabolite) are about 50% greater in patients with CrCl <30 mL/minute and are doubled in hemodialysis patients. In surgical patients on chronic angiotensin receptor blocker (ARB) therapy, intraoperative hypotension may occur with induction and maintenance of general anesthesia.

Potentially significant drug interactions may exist, requiring dose or frequency adjustment, additional monitoring, and/or selection of alternative therapy.

Angioedema has been reported rarely with some angiotensin II receptor antagonists (ARBs) and may occur at any time during treatment (especially following first dose). It may involve the head and neck (potentially compromising airway) or the intestine (presenting with abdominal pain). Patients with idiopathic or hereditary angioedema or previous angioedema associated with ACE-inhibitor therapy may be at an increased risk. Prolonged frequent monitoring may be required, especially if tongue, glottis, or larynx are involved, as they are associated with airway obstruction. Patients with a history of airway surgery may have a higher risk of airway obstruction. Discontinue therapy immediately if angioedema occurs. Aggressive early management is critical. Intramuscular (IM) administration of epinephrine may be necessary. Do not readminister to patients who have had angioedema with ARBs.

Adverse Reactions

Cardiovascular: Orthostatic hypotension

Central nervous system: Dizziness, fatigue

Endocrine & metabolic: Hyperkalemia

Gastrointestinal: Diarrhea, dyspepsia

Respiratory: Cough, upper respiratory infection

Rare but important or life-threatening: Anemia (case report; Simonetti, 2007), angina, angioedema, arrhythmia, cardiopulmonary arrest, conjunctivitis, depression, dyspnea, ecchymosis, epistaxis, gout, heart failure, hepatitis, hypotension, jaundice, libido decreased, MI, orthostatic hypotension, paresthesia, renal failure, renal function impaired, sexual dysfunction, stroke, thrombocytopenia, transaminases increased, urticaria

Drug Interactions

Metabolism/Transport Effects **Substrate** of CYP2C9 (minor); **Note:** Assignment of Major/Minor substrate status based on clinically relevant drug interaction potential; **Inhibits** CYP2C8 (moderate), CYP2C9 (moderate), CYP2D6 (weak), CYP3A4 (weak)

Avoid Concomitant Use

Avoid concomitant use of Irbesartan with any of the following: Pimozide

Increased Effect/Toxicity

Irbesartan may increase the levels/effects of: ACE Inhibitors; Amifostine; Antihypertensives; ARIPiprazole; Bosentan; Cannabis; Carvedilol; CycloSPORINE (Systemic); CYP2C8 Substrates; CYP2C9 Substrates; Dofetilide; Dronabinol; DULoxetine; Hydrocodone; Hypotensive Agents; Levodopa; Lithium; Lomitapide; Nonsteroidal Anti-Inflammatory Agents; Obinutuzumab; Pimozide; Potassium-Sparing Diuretics; RisperiDONE; RiTUXimab; Sodium Phosphates; Tetrahydrocannabinol

The levels/effects of Irbesartan may be increased by: Alfuzosin; Aliskiren; Barbiturates; Brimonidine (Topical); Canagliflozin; Dapoxetine; Diazoxide; Eplerenone; Heparin; Heparin (Low Molecular Weight); Herbs (Hypotensive Properties); MAO Inhibitors; Nicorandil; Pentoxifylline; Phosphodiesterase 5 Inhibitors; Potassium Salts; Prostacyclin Analogues; Tolvaptan; Trimethoprim

Decreased Effect
The levels/effects of Irbesartan may be decreased by: Herbs (Hypertensive Properties); Methylphenidate; Nonsteroidal Anti-Inflammatory Agents; Yohimbine

Storage/Stability Store at 25°C (77°F); excursions are permitted between 15°C and 30°C (59°F and 86°F).

Mechanism of Action Irbesartan is an angiotensin receptor antagonist. Angiotensin II acts as a vasoconstrictor. In addition to causing direct vasoconstriction, angiotensin II also stimulates the release of aldosterone. Once aldosterone is released, sodium as well as water are reabsorbed. The end result is an elevation in blood pressure. Irbesartan binds to the AT1 angiotensin II receptor. This binding prevents angiotensin II from binding to the receptor thereby blocking the vasoconstriction and the aldosterone secreting effects of angiotensin II.

Pharmacodynamics/Kinetics
Onset of action: Peak effect: 1 to 2 hours
Duration: >24 hours
Distribution: V_d: 53 to 93 L
Protein binding, plasma: 90%
Metabolism: Hepatic, primarily CYP2C9
Bioavailability: 60% to 80%
Half-life elimination: Terminal: 11 to 15 hours
Time to peak, serum: 1.5 to 2 hours
Excretion: Feces (80%); urine (20%)

Dosage
Hypertension: Oral:
Children ≥6 to 12 years (off-label use): Initial: 75 mg once daily; may be titrated to a maximum of 150 mg once daily (NHBPEP, 2004).
Adolescents (off-label use): Initial: 150 mg once daily; may be titrated to a maximum dose of 300 mg once daily (NHBPEP, 2004).
Adults: 150 mg once daily; patients may be titrated to 300 mg once daily; usual dosage range (ASH/ISH [Weber, 2014]): 150 to 300 mg daily; target dose (JNC 8 [James, 2013]): 300 mg once daily.
Note: Starting dose in volume-depleted patients should be 75 mg
Nephropathy in patients with type 2 diabetes and hypertension: Adults: Oral: Target dose: 300 mg once daily

Dosage adjustment in renal impairment: Mild to severe renal impairment: No dosage adjustment necessary unless the patient is also volume depleted.

Dosage adjustment in hepatic impairment: No dosage adjustment necessary.

Administration May be administered with or without food.

Monitoring Parameters Electrolytes, serum creatinine, BUN, urinalysis

Dosage Forms
Tablet, Oral:
Avapro: 75 mg, 150 mg, 300 mg
Generic: 75 mg, 150 mg, 300 mg

Irbesartan and Hydrochlorothiazide
(ir be SAR tan & hye droe klor oh THYE a zide)

Brand Names: U.S. Avalide

Brand Names: Canada ACT Irbesartan/HCT; Apo-Irbesartan/HCTZ; Avalide; Irbesartan-HCT; Irbesartan-HCTZ; JAMP-Irbesartan and Hydrochlorothiazide; Mint-Irbesartan/HCTZ; PMS-Irbesartan HCTZ; Ran-Irbesartan HCTZ; ratio-Irbesartan HCTZ; Sandoz-Irbesartan HCT; Teva-Irbesartan HCTZ

Index Terms Avapro HCT; Hydrochlorothiazide and Irbesartan

Pharmacologic Category Angiotensin II Receptor Blocker; Antihypertensive; Diuretic, Thiazide

Use Hypertension: Treatment of hypertension

Pregnancy Risk Factor D

Dosage Hypertension: Adults: Oral: **Note:** Maximum antihypertensive effects are attained within 2 to 4 weeks after initiation or a change in dose; however, if necessary, may carefully titrate dose as soon as after 1 week of treatment.
Add-on therapy: Dose must be individualized. A patient who is not controlled with either agent alone may be switched to the combination product. The lowest dosage available is irbesartan 150 mg/hydrochlorothiazide 12.5 mg.
Initial therapy: Irbesartan 150 mg/hydrochlorothiazide 12.5 mg once daily. If initial response is inadequate, may titrate dose after 1 to 2 weeks (maximum daily dose: irbesartan 300 mg/hydrochlorothiazide 25 mg).

Dosing adjustment in renal impairment:
Mild-to-moderate impairment (CrCl >30 mL/minute): No dosage adjustment necessary; use with caution.
Severe impairment (CrCl ≤30 mL/minute): Use not recommended.

Dosage adjustment in hepatic impairment: No dosage adjustment necessary; use with caution.

Additional Information Complete prescribing information should be consulted for additional detail.

Dosage Forms
Tablet, oral: 150/12.5: Irbesartan 150 mg and hydrochlorothiazide 12.5 mg; 300/12.5: Irbesartan 300 mg and hydrochlorothiazide 12.5 mg
Avalide: Irbesartan 150 mg and hydrochlorothiazide 12.5 mg; irbesartan 300 mg and hydrochlorothiazide 12.5 mg

- **Irbesartan-HCT (Can)** *see* Irbesartan and Hydrochlorothiazide *on page 1112*
- **Irbesartan-HCTZ (Can)** *see* Irbesartan and Hydrochlorothiazide *on page 1112*
- **IRESSA (Can)** *see* Gefitinib [CAN/INT] *on page 950*

Irinotecan (eye rye no TEE kan)

Brand Names: U.S. Camptosar

Brand Names: Canada Camptosar; Irinotecan For Injection; Irinotecan Hydrochloride Trihydrate Injection

Index Terms Camptothecin-11; CPT-11; Irinotecan HCl; Irinotecan Hydrochloride

Pharmacologic Category Antineoplastic Agent, Camptothecin; Antineoplastic Agent, Topoisomerase I Inhibitor

Use Colorectal cancer, metastatic: Treatment of metastatic carcinoma of the colon or rectum

Pregnancy Risk Factor D

Pregnancy Considerations Adverse events were observed in animal reproduction studies. May cause fetal harm if administered during pregnancy. Women of childbearing potential should avoid becoming pregnant while receiving treatment.

Breast-Feeding Considerations It is not known if irinotecan is excreted in breast milk. Due to the potential for serious adverse reactions in the nursing infant, the manufacturer recommends a decision be made whether to discontinue nursing or to discontinue the drug, taking into account the importance of treatment to the mother.

Contraindications Hypersensitivity to irinotecan or any component of the formulation

Warnings/Precautions Hazardous agent - use appropriate precautions for handling and disposal (NIOSH 2014 [group 1]). Severe hypersensitivity reactions (including anaphylaxis) have occurred. Monitor closely; discontinue therapy if hypersensitivity occurs. Irinotecan is an irritant; avoid extravasation. If extravasation occurs, the manufacturer recommends flushing the external site with sterile water and applying ice.

[U.S. Boxed Warning]: Severe diarrhea may be dose-limiting and potentially fatal; early-onset and late-onset diarrhea may occur. Early diarrhea occurs during or within 24 hours of receiving irinotecan and is characterized by cholinergic symptoms; may be prevented or treated with atropine. Late diarrhea may be life-threatening and should be promptly treated with loperamide. Antibiotics may be necessary if patient develops ileus, fever, or severe neutropenia. Interrupt treatment and reduce subsequent doses for severe diarrhea. Early diarrhea is generally transient and rarely severe; cholinergic symptoms may include increased salivation, rhinitis, miosis, diaphoresis, flushing, abdominal cramping, and lacrimation; bradycardia may also occur. Cholinergic symptoms may occur more frequently with higher irinotecan doses. Late diarrhea occurs more than 24 hours after treatment, which may lead to dehydration, electrolyte imbalance, or sepsis. Late diarrhea may be complicated by colitis, ulceration, bleeding, ileus, obstruction, or infection; cases of megacolon and intestinal perforation have been reported. The median time to onset for late diarrhea is 5 days with every-3-week irinotecan dosing and 11 days with weekly dosing. Advise patients to have loperamide readily available for the treatment of late diarrhea. Patients with diarrhea should be carefully monitored and treated promptly; may require fluid and electrolyte therapy. Bowel function should be returned to baseline for at least 24 hours prior to resumption of weekly irinotecan dosing. Avoid diuretics and laxatives in patients experiencing diarrhea. Patients >65 years of age are at greater risk for early and late diarrhea. A dose reduction is recommended for patients ≥70 years of age receiving the every-3-week regimen. Irinotecan is associated with a moderate emetic potential; antiemetics are recommended to prevent nausea and vomiting (Basch, 2011; Dupuis, 2011; Roila, 2010).

[U.S. Boxed Warning]: May cause severe myelosuppression. Deaths due to sepsis following severe neutropenia have been reported. Complications due to neutropenia should be promptly managed with antibiotics. Therapy should be temporarily withheld if neutropenic fever occurs or if the absolute neutrophil count is <1000/mm^3; reduce the dose upon recovery to an absolute neutrophil count ≥1000/mm^3. Patients who have previously received pelvic/abdominal radiation therapy have an increased risk of severe bone marrow suppression; the incidence of grade 3 or 4 neutropenia was higher in patients receiving weekly irinotecan who have previously received pelvic/abdominal radiation therapy. Concurrent radiation therapy is not recommended with irinotecan (based on limited data). Fatal cases of interstitial pulmonary disease (IPD)-like events have been reported with single-agent and combination therapy. Risk factors for pulmonary toxicity include preexisting lung disease, use of pulmonary toxic medications, radiation therapy, and colony-stimulating factors. Patients with risk factors should be monitored for respiratory symptoms before and during irinotecan treatment. Promptly evaluate progressive changes in baseline pulmonary symptoms or any new-onset pulmonary symptoms (eg, dyspnea, cough, fever). Discontinue all chemotherapy if IPD is diagnosed.

Patients with even modest elevations in total serum bilirubin levels (1-2 mg/dL) have a significantly greater likelihood of experiencing first-course grade 3 or 4 neutropenia than those with bilirubin levels that were <1 mg/dL. Patients with abnormal glucuronidation of bilirubin, such as those with Gilbert's syndrome, may also be at greater risk of myelosuppression when receiving therapy with irinotecan. Use caution when treating patients with known hepatic dysfunction or hyperbilirubinemia exposure to the active metabolite (SN-38) is increased; toxicities may be increased. Dosage adjustments should be considered.

Patients homozygous for the UGT1A1*28 allele are at increased risk of neutropenia; initial one-level dose reduction should be considered for both single-agent and combination regimens. Heterozygous carriers of the UGT1A1*28 allele may also be at increased risk; however, most patients have tolerated normal starting doses.

Renal impairment and acute renal failure have been reported, possibly due to dehydration secondary to diarrhea. Use with caution in patients with renal impairment; not recommended in patients on dialysis. Patients with bowel obstruction should not be treated with irinotecan until resolution of obstruction. Contains sorbitol; do not use in patients with hereditary fructose intolerance. Thromboembolic events have been reported. Higher rates of hospitalization, neutropenic fever, thromboembolism, first-cycle discontinuation, and early mortality were observed in patients with a performance status of 2 than in patients with a performance status of 0 or 1. Except as part of a clinical trial, use in combination with fluorouracil and leucovorin administered for 4 or 5 consecutive days ("Mayo Clinic" regimen) is not recommended due to increased toxicity. Potentially significant interactions may exist, requiring dose or frequency adjustment, additional monitoring, and/or selection of alternative therapy. CYP3A4 enzyme inducers may decrease exposure to irinotecan and SN-38 (active metabolite); enzyme inhibitors may increase exposure; for use in patients with CNS tumors (off-label use), selection of antiseizure medications that are not enzyme inducers is preferred.

Adverse Reactions

Cardiovascular: Edema, hypotension, thromboembolic events, vasodilation

Central nervous system: Chills, cholinergic toxicity (includes rhinitis, increased salivation, miosis, lacrimation, diaphoresis, flushing and intestinal hyperperistalsis); confusion, dizziness, fever, headache, insomnia, pain, somnolence

Dermatologic: Alopecia, rash

Endocrine & metabolic: Dehydration

Gastrointestinal: Abdominal fullness/pain, anorexia, constipation, cramps, diarrhea (early/late), dyspepsia, flatulence, mucositis, nausea, stomatitis, vomiting, weight loss

Hematologic: Anemia, hemorrhage, leukopenia, neutropenia, neutropenic fever/infection, thrombocytopenia

Hepatic: Alkaline phosphatase increased, ascites and/or jaundice, AST increased, bilirubin increased

Neuromuscular & skeletal: Back pain, weakness

Respiratory: Cough, dyspnea, pneumonia, rhinitis

Miscellaneous: Diaphoresis

Rare but important or life-threatening: ALT increased, amylase increased, anaphylactoid reaction, anaphylaxis, angina, arterial thrombosis, bleeding, bradycardia, cardiac arrest, cerebral infarct, cerebrovascular accident, circulatory failure, colitis, dysrhythmia, embolus, gastrointestinal bleeding, gastrointestinal obstruction, hepatomegaly, hyperglycemia, hypersensitivity, hyponatremia, ileus, interstitial pulmonary disease (IPD), intestinal perforation, ischemic colitis, lipase increased, lymphocytopenia, megacolon, MI, myocardial ischemia, neutropenic typhlitis, pancreatitis, paresthesia, peripheral vascular disorder, pulmonary embolus; pulmonary toxicity (dyspnea, fever, reticulonodular infiltrates on chest x-ray); renal failure (acute), renal impairment, thrombocytopenia (immune mediated), thrombophlebitis, thrombosis, typhlitis, ulcerative colitis

Note: In limited pediatric experience, dehydration (often associated with severe hypokalemia and hyponatremia) was among the most significant grade 3/4 adverse events.

Drug Interactions

Metabolism/Transport Effects Substrate of CYP2B6 (major), CYP3A4 (major), P-glycoprotein, SLCO1B1, UGT1A1; **Note:** Assignment of Major/Minor substrate status based on clinically relevant drug interaction potential

Avoid Concomitant Use

Avoid concomitant use of Irinotecan with any of the following: BCG; CloZAPine; Conivaptan; CYP3A4 Inducers (Strong); CYP3A4 Inhibitors (Strong); Dipyrone; Fusidic Acid (Systemic); Gemfibrozil; Grapefruit Juice; Idelalisib; Natalizumab; Pimecrolimus; St Johns Wort; Tacrolimus (Topical); Tofacitinib; Vaccines (Live)

Increased Effect/Toxicity

Irinotecan may increase the levels/effects of: CloZAPine; Leflunomide; Natalizumab; Tofacitinib; Vaccines (Live)

The levels/effects of Irinotecan may be increased by: Aprepitant; Bevacizumab; Ceritinib; Conivaptan; CYP2B6 Inhibitors (Moderate); CYP3A4 Inhibitors (Moderate); CYP3A4 Inhibitors (Strong); Dasatinib; Denosumab; Dipyrone; Eltrombopag; Fosaprepitant; Fusidic Acid (Systemic); Gemfibrozil; Grapefruit Juice; Idelalisib; Ivacaftor; Luliconazole; Mifepristone; Netupitant; P-glycoprotein/ABCB1 Inhibitors; Pimecrolimus; Quazepam; Regorafenib; Roflumilast; Simeprevir; SORAfenib; Tacrolimus (Topical); Teriflunomide; Trastuzumab

Decreased Effect

Irinotecan may decrease the levels/effects of: BCG; Coccidioides immitis Skin Test; Sipuleucel-T; Vaccines (Inactivated); Vaccines (Live)

The levels/effects of Irinotecan may be decreased by: Bosentan; CYP2B6 Inducers (Strong); CYP3A4 Inducers (Moderate); CYP3A4 Inducers (Strong); Dabrafenib; Deferasirox; Echinacea; P-glycoprotein/ABCB1 Inducers; Siltuximab; St Johns Wort; Tocilizumab

Preparation for Administration Hazardous agent; use appropriate precautions for handling and disposal (NIOSH 2014 [group 1]). Dilute in D_5W (preferred) or NS to a final concentration of 0.12-2.8 mg/mL.

Storage/Stability Store intact vials at 15°C to 30°C (59°F to 86°F). Protect from light; retain vials in original carton until use. Solutions diluted in NS may precipitate if refrigerated. Solutions diluted in D_5W are stable for 24 hours at room temperature or 48 hours under refrigeration at 2°C to 8°C (36°F to 46°F), although the manufacturer recommends use within 24 hours if refrigerated, or within 4 to 12 hours (manufacturer dependent; refer to specific prescribing information) at room temperature (including infusion time) only if prepared under strict aseptic conditions (eg, laminar flow hood). Do not freeze. Undiluted commercially available injectable solution prepared in oral syringes is stable for 21 days under refrigeration (Wagner, 2010).

Mechanism of Action Irinotecan and its active metabolite (SN-38) bind reversibly to topoisomerase I-DNA complex preventing religation of the cleaved DNA strand. This results in the accumulation of cleavable complexes and double-strand DNA breaks. As mammalian cells cannot efficiently repair these breaks, cell death consistent with S-phase cell cycle specificity occurs, leading to termination of cellular replication.

Pharmacodynamics/Kinetics

Protein binding, plasma: Predominantly albumin; Irinotecan: 30% to 68%, SN-38 (active metabolite): ~95%

Metabolism: Primarily hepatic to SN-38 (active metabolite) by carboxylesterase enzymes; SN-38 undergoes conjugation by UDP-glucuronosyl transferase 1A1 (UGT1A1) to form a glucuronide metabolite. SN-38 is increased by UGT1A1*28 polymorphism (10% of North Americans are homozygous for UGT1A1*28 allele).

Half-life elimination: Irinotecan: 6-12 hours; SN-38: ~10-20 hours

Time to peak: SN-38: Following 90-minute infusion: ~1 hour

Excretion: Urine: Irinotecan (11% to 20%), metabolites (SN-38 <1%, SN-38 glucuronide, 3%)

Dosage Note: A reduction in the starting dose by one dose level should be considered for prior pelvic/abdominal radiotherapy, performance status of 2, or known homozygosity for UGT1A1*28 allele (subsequent dosing/adjustments should be based on individual tolerance). Consider premedication of atropine 0.25-1 mg IV or SubQ in patients with cholinergic symptoms (eg, increased salivation, rhinitis, miosis, diaphoresis, abdominal cramping) or early-onset diarrhea. Irinotecan is associated with a moderate emetic potential; antiemetics are recommended to prevent nausea and vomiting (Basch, 2011; Dupuis, 2011; Roila, 2010).

Ewing's sarcoma, recurrent or progressive (off-label use): Children and Adults: IV: 20 mg/m² days 1-5 and days 8-12 every 3 weeks (in combination with temozolomide) (Casey, 2009)

Rhabdomyosarcoma, relapsed/refractory (off-label use; Vassal, 2007):

Children <10 kg: 20 mg/kg once every 3 weeks

Children ≥10 kg and Adolescents: 600 mg/m² once every 3 weeks

Colorectal cancer, metastatic (single-agent therapy):

Adults: IV:

Weekly regimen: 125 mg/m² over 90 minutes on days 1, 8, 15, and 22 of a 6-week treatment cycle (may adjust upward to 150 mg/m² if tolerated)

- Adjusted dose level -1: 100 mg/m²
- Adjusted dose level -2: 75 mg/m²
- Further adjust to 50 mg/m² (in decrements of 25-50 mg/m²) if needed

Once-every-3-week regimen: 350 mg/m² over 90 minutes, once every 3 weeks

- Adjusted dose level -1: 300 mg/m²
- Adjusted dose level -2: 250 mg/m²
- Further adjust to 200 mg/m² (in decrements of 25-50 mg/m²) if needed

Colorectal cancer, metastatic (in combination with fluorouracil and leucovorin): Adults: IV: Six-week (42-day) cycle:

Regimen 1: 125 mg/m² over 90 minutes on days 1, 8, 15, and 22; to be given in combination with bolus leucovorin and fluorouracil (leucovorin administered immediately following irinotecan; fluorouracil immediately following leucovorin)

- Adjusted dose level -1: 100 mg/m²
- Adjusted dose level -2: 75 mg/m²
- Further adjust if needed in decrements of ~20%

Regimen 2: 180 mg/m² over 90 minutes on days 1, 15, and 29; to be given in combination with infusional leucovorin and bolus/infusion fluorouracil (leucovorin administered immediately following irinotecan; fluorouracil immediately following leucovorin)

- Adjusted dose level -1: 150 mg/m²
- Adjusted dose level -2: 120 mg/m²
- Further adjust if needed in decrements of ~20%

Colorectal cancer, metastatic (off-label dosing): Adults: IV: FOLFOXIRI regimen: 165 mg/m² over 1 hour once every 2 weeks (in combination with oxaliplatin, leucovorin, and fluorouracil) (Falcone, 2007)

Cervical cancer, recurrent or metastatic (off-label use): Adults: IV: 125 mg/m² over 90 minutes once weekly for 4 consecutive weeks followed by a 2-week rest during each 6 week treatment cycle (Verschraegen, 1997)

CNS tumor, recurrent glioblastoma (off-label use): Adults: IV: 125 mg/m² over 90 minutes once every 2 weeks (in combination with bevacizumab). **NOTE:** In patients taking concurrent antiepileptic enzyme-inducing medications irinotecan dose was increased to 340 mg/m² (Friedman, 2009; Vredenburgh, 2007).

Esophageal cancer, metastatic or locally advanced (off-label use): Adults: IV: 65 mg/m² over 90 minutes days 1, 8, 15, and 22 of a 6-week treatment cycle (in combination with cisplatin) (Ajani, 2002; Ilson, 1999) **or** 80 mg/m² weekly for 6 weeks of a 7-week treatment cycle (in combination with leucovorin and fluorouracil) (Dank, 2008) **or** 250 mg/m² every 3 weeks (in combination with capecitabine) (Leary, 2009; Moehler, 2010)

Gastric cancer, metastatic or locally advanced (off-label use): Adults: IV: 65 mg/m² over 90 minutes days 1, 8, 15, and 22 of a 6-week treatment cycle (in combination with cisplatin) (Ajani, 2002) **or** 70 mg/m² over 90 minutes on days 1 and 15 of a 4-week treatment cycle (in combination with cisplatin) for up to 6 cycles (Park, 2005) **or** 180 mg/m² over 90 minutes every 2 weeks (in combination with leucovorin and fluorouracil) (Bouche, 2004) **or** 80 mg/m² weekly for 6 weeks of a 7-week treatment cycle (in combination with leucovorin and fluorouracil) (Dank, 2008) **or** 250 mg/m² every 3 weeks (in combination with capecitabine) (Moehler, 2010)

Non-small cell lung cancer, advanced (off-label use): Adults: IV: 60 mg/m² days 1, 8, and 15 every 4 weeks (in combination with cisplatin) (Ohe, 2007)

Pancreatic cancer, advanced (off-label use): Adults: IV: FOLFIRINOX regimen: 180 mg/m² over 90 minutes every 2 weeks (in combination with oxaliplatin, leucovorin, and fluorouracil) (Conroy, 2005; Conroy, 2011)

Small cell lung cancer, extensive stage (off-label use): Adults: IV: 60 mg/m² days 1, 8, and 15 every 4 weeks (in combination with cisplatin) (Noda, 2002) **or** 65 mg/m² days 1 and 8 every 3 weeks (in combination with cisplatin) (Hanna, 2006) **or** 175 mg/m² day 1 every 3 weeks (in combination with carboplatin) (Hermes, 2008) **or** 50 mg/m² days 1, 8 and 15 every 4 weeks (in combination with carboplatin) (Schmittel, 2006)

Elderly:
- Weekly dosing schedule: No dosing adjustment is recommended
- Every 3-week dosing colorectal cancer schedule: Recommended initial dose is 300 mg/m²/dose for patients ≥70 years

Dosing adjustment in renal impairment:
- Renal impairment: There is no dosage adjustment provided in manufacturer's labeling (has not been studied); use with caution.
- Dialysis: Use in patients with dialysis is not recommended by the manufacturer; however, literature suggests reducing weekly dose from 125 mg/m² to 50 mg/m² and administer after hemodialysis or on non-dialysis days (Janus, 2010).

Dosing adjustment in hepatic impairment:
Manufacturer's recommendations:
- Liver metastases with normal hepatic function: No dosage adjustment necessary.
- Bilirubin >ULN to ≤2 mg/dL: Consider reducing initial dose by one dose level
- Bilirubin >2 mg/dL: Use is not recommended

Alternate recommendations: The following adjustments have also been recommended:
- Bilirubin 1.5-3 mg/dL: Administer 75% of dose (Floyd, 2006)
- Bilirubin 1.51 to 3 times ULN: Reduce dose from 350 mg/m² every 3 weeks to 200 mg/m² every 3 weeks (Raymond, 2002)

Dosing in obesity: *ASCO Guidelines for appropriate chemotherapy dosing in obese adults with cancer:* Utilize patient's actual body weight (full weight) for calculation of body surface area- or weight-based dosing, particularly when the intent of therapy is curative; manage regimen-related toxicities in the same manner as for nonobese patients; if a dose reduction is utilized due to toxicity, consider resumption of full weight-based dosing with subsequent cycles, especially if cause of toxicity (eg, hepatic or renal impairment) is resolved (Griggs, 2012).

Dosage adjustment for toxicities: It is recommended that new courses begin only after the granulocyte count recovers to ≥1500/mm³, the platelet counts recovers to ≥100,000/mm³, and treatment-related diarrhea has fully resolved. Depending on the patient's ability to tolerate therapy, doses should be adjusted in increments of 25-50 mg/m². Treatment should be delayed 1-2 weeks to allow for recovery from treatment-related toxicities. If the patient has not recovered after a 2-week delay, consider discontinuing irinotecan. See tables below and on next page.

Colorectal Cancer: Single-Agent Schedule: Recommended Dosage Modifications[1]

Toxicity NCI Grade[2] (Value)	During a Cycle of Therapy	At Start of Subsequent Cycles of Therapy (After Adequate Recovery), Compared to Starting Dose in Previous Cycle[1]	
	Weekly	Weekly	Once Every 3 Weeks
No toxicity	Maintain dose level	↑ 25 mg/m² up to a maximum dose of 150 mg/m²	Maintain dose level
Neutropenia			
Grade 1 (1500-1999/mm³)	Maintain dose level	Maintain dose level	Maintain dose level
Grade 2 (1000-1499/mm³)	↓ 25 mg/m²	Maintain dose level	Maintain dose level
Grade 3 (500-999/mm³)	Omit dose until resolved to ≤ grade 2, then ↓ 25 mg/m²	↓ 25 mg/m²	↓ 50 mg/m²
Grade 4 (<500/mm³)	Omit dose until resolved to ≤ grade 2, then ↓ 50 mg/m²	↓ 50 mg/m²	↓ 50 mg/m²
Neutropenic Fever (grade 4 neutropenia and ≥ grade 2 fever)	Omit dose until resolved, then ↓ 50 mg/m²	↓ 50 mg/m²	↓ 50 mg/m²
Other Hematologic Toxicities	Dose modifications for leukopenia, thrombocytopenia, and anemia during a course of therapy and at the start of subsequent courses of therapy are also based on NCI toxicity criteria and are the same as recommended for neutropenia above.		
Diarrhea			
Grade 1 (2-3 stools/day > pretreatment)	Maintain dose level	Maintain dose level	Maintain dose level
Grade 2 (4-6 stools/day > pretreatment)	↓ 25 mg/m²	Maintain dose level	Maintain dose level
Grade 3 (7-9 stools/day > pretreatment)	Omit dose until resolved to ≤ grade 2, then ↓ 25 mg/m²	↓ 25 mg/m²	↓ 50 mg/m²
Grade 4 (≥10 stools/day > pretreatment)	Omit dose until resolved to ≤ grade 2, then ↓ 50 mg/m²	↓ 50 mg/m²	↓ 50 mg/m²

(continued)

Colorectal Cancer: Single-Agent Schedule: Recommended Dosage Modifications[1] *(continued)*

Toxicity NCI Grade[2] (Value)	During a Cycle of Therapy	At Start of Subsequent Cycles of Therapy (After Adequate Recovery), Compared to Starting Dose in Previous Cycle[1]	
	Weekly	Weekly	Once Every 3 Weeks
Other Nonhematologic Toxicities[3]			
Grade 1	Maintain dose level	Maintain dose level	Maintain dose level
Grade 2	↓ 25 mg/m^2	↓ 25 mg/m^2	↓ 50 mg/m^2
Grade 3	Omit dose until resolved to ≤ grade 2, then ↓ 25 mg/m^2	↓ 25 mg/m^2	↓ 50 mg/m^2
Grade 4	Omit dose until resolved to ≤ grade 2, then ↓ 50 mg/m^2	↓ 50 mg/m^2	↓ 50 mg/m^2

[1]All dose modifications should be based on the worst preceding toxicity.

[2]National Cancer Institute Common Toxicity Criteria (version 1.0).

[3]Excludes alopecia, anorexia, asthenia.

Colorectal Cancer: Combination Schedules: Recommended Dosage Modifications[1]

Toxicity NCI[2] Grade (Value)	During a Cycle of Therapy	At the Start of Subsequent Cycles of Therapy (After Adequate Recovery), Compared to the Starting Dose in the Previous Cycle[1]
No toxicity	Maintain dose level	Maintain dose level
Neutropenia		
Grade 1 (1500-1999/mm^3)	Maintain dose level	Maintain dose level
Grade 2 (1000-1499/mm^3)	↓ 1 dose level	Maintain dose level
Grade 3 (500-999/mm^3)	Omit dose until resolved to ≤ grade 2, then ↓ 1 dose level	↓ 1 dose level
Grade 4 (<500/mm^3)	Omit dose until resolved to ≤ grade 2, then ↓ 2 dose levels	↓ 2 dose levels
Neutropenic Fever (grade 4 neutropenia and ≥ grade 2 fever)	Omit dose until resolved, then ↓ 2 dose levels	
Other Hematologic Toxicities	Dose modifications for leukopenia or thrombocytopenia during a course of therapy and at the start of subsequent courses of therapy are also based on NCI toxicity criteria and are the same as recommended for neutropenia above.	
Diarrhea		
Grade 1 (2-3 stools/day > pretreatment)	Delay dose until resolved to baseline, then give same dose	Maintain dose level
Grade 2 (4-6 stools/day > pretreatment)	Omit dose until resolved to baseline, then ↓ 1 dose level	Maintain dose level
Grade 3 (7-9 stools/day > pretreatment)	Omit dose until resolved to baseline, then ↓ by 1 dose level	↓ 1 dose level
Grade 4 (≥10 stools/day > pretreatment)	Omit dose until resolved to baseline, then ↓ 2 dose levels	↓ 2 dose levels
Other Nonhematologic Toxicities[3]		
Grade 1	Maintain dose level	Maintain dose level
Grade 2	Omit dose until resolved to ≤ grade 1, then ↓ 1 dose level	Maintain dose level
Grade 3	Omit dose until resolved to ≤ grade 2, then ↓ 1 dose level	↓ 1 dose level
Grade 4	Omit dose until resolved to ≤ grade 2, then ↓ 2 dose levels	↓ 2 dose levels
Mucositis and/or stomatitis	Decrease only 5-FU, not irinotecan	Decrease only 5-FU, not irinotecan

[1]All dose modifications should be based on the worst preceding toxicity.

[2]National Cancer Institute Common Toxicity Criteria (version 1.0).

[3]Excludes alopecia, anorexia, asthenia.

Dietary Considerations Contains sorbitol; do not use in patients with hereditary fructose intolerance.

Administration Administer by IV infusion, usually over 90 minutes. Irinotecan is associated with a moderate emetic potential (Basch, 2011; Dupuis, 2011; Roila, 2010); premedication with dexamethasone and a 5-HT$_3$ blocker is recommended 30 minutes prior to administration; prochlorperazine may be considered for subsequent use (if needed). Consider atropine 0.25-1 mg IV or SubQ as premedication for or treatment of cholinergic symptoms (eg, increased salivation, rhinitis, miosis, diaphoresis, abdominal cramping) or early onset diarrhea.

The recommended regimen to manage late diarrhea is loperamide 4 mg orally at onset of late diarrhea, followed by 2 mg every 2 hours (or 4 mg every 4 hours at night) until 12 hours have passed without a bowel movement. If diarrhea recurs, then repeat administration. Loperamide should not be used for more than 48 consecutive hours.

Hazardous agent; use appropriate precautions for handling and disposal (NIOSH 2014 [group 1]).

Monitoring Parameters CBC with differential, platelet count, and hemoglobin with each dose; bilirubin, electrolytes (with severe diarrhea); bowel movements and hydration status; signs/symptoms of pulmonary toxicity or hypersensitivity reactions; monitor infusion site for signs of inflammation and avoid extravasation

A test is available for genotyping of UGT1A1; however, guidelines for use are not established and not recommended in patients who have experienced toxicity as a dose reduction is already recommended (NCCN Colon Cancer Guidelines v.3.2014)

Additional Information Patients who are homozygous for the UGT1A1*28 allele are at increased risk for neutropenia; a decreased dose is recommended. Clinical research of patients who are heterozygous for UGT1A1*28 have been variable for increased neutropenic risk and such patients have tolerated normal starting doses. An FDA-approved test (Invader Molecular Assay) is available for clinical determination of UGT phenotype.

Dosage Forms

Solution, Intravenous:

Camptosar: 40 mg/2 mL (2 mL); 100 mg/5 mL (5 mL); 300 mg/15 mL (15 mL)

Generic: 40 mg/2 mL (2 mL); 100 mg/5 mL (5 mL); 500 mg/25 mL (25 mL)

Solution, Intravenous [preservative free]:

Generic: 40 mg/2 mL (2 mL); 100 mg/5 mL (5 mL)

◆ **Irinotecan For Injection (Can)** *see* Irinotecan *on page 1112*

◆ **Irinotecan HCl** *see* Irinotecan *on page 1112*

◆ **Irinotecan Hydrochloride** *see* Irinotecan *on page 1112*

◆ **Irinotecan Hydrochloride Trihydrate Injection (Can)** *see* Irinotecan *on page 1112*

◆ **Iron Carboxymaltose** *see* Ferric Carboxymaltose *on page 868*

◆ **Iron Dextran** *see* Iron Dextran Complex *on page 1117*

Iron Dextran Complex

(EYE ern DEKS tran KOM pleks)

Brand Names: U.S. Dexferrum; Infed

Brand Names: Canada Dexiron; Infufer

Index Terms High-Molecular-Weight Iron Dextran (DexFerrum); Imferon; Iron Dextran; Low-Molecular-Weight Iron Dextran (INFeD)

Pharmacologic Category Iron Salt

Use Iron deficiency: Treatment of iron deficiency in patients in whom oral administration is unsatisfactory or infeasible

Pregnancy Risk Factor C

Pregnancy Considerations Adverse events have been observed in animal reproduction studies. It is not known if iron dextran (as iron dextran) crosses the placenta. It is recommended that pregnant women meet the dietary requirements of iron with diet and/or supplements in order to prevent adverse events associated with iron deficiency anemia in pregnancy. Treatment of iron deficiency anemia in pregnant women is the same as in nonpregnant women and in most cases, oral iron preparations may be used. Except in severe cases of maternal anemia, the fetus achieves normal iron stores regardless of maternal concentrations.

Breast-Feeding Considerations Trace amounts of iron dextran (as iron dextran) are found in human milk. Iron is normally found in breast milk. Breast milk or iron fortified formulas generally provide enough iron to meet the recommended dietary requirements of infants. The amount of iron in breast milk is generally not influenced by maternal iron status.

Contraindications Hypersensitivity to iron dextran or any component of the formulation; any anemia not associated with iron deficiency

Warnings/Precautions [U.S. Boxed Warning]: Deaths associated with parenteral administration following anaphylactic-type reactions have been reported (use only where resuscitation equipment and personnel are available). A test dose should be administered to all patients prior to the first therapeutic dose. Fatal reactions have occurred even in patients who tolerated the test dose. Monitor patients for signs/symptoms of anaphylactic reactions during any iron dextran administration; fatalities have occurred with the test dose. A history of drug allergy (including multiple drug allergies) and/or the concomitant use of an ACE inhibitor may increase the risk of anaphylactic-type reactions. Adverse events (including life-threatening) associated with iron dextran usually occur with the high-molecular-weight formulation (Dexferrum), compared to low-molecular-weight (INFeD) (Chertow, 2006). Delayed (1-2 days) infusion reaction (including arthralgia, back pain, chills, dizziness, and fever) may occur with large doses (eg, total dose infusion) of IV iron dextran; usually subsides within 3-4 days. Delayed reaction may also occur (less commonly) with IM administration; subsiding within 3-7 days. Use with caution in patients with a history of significant allergies, asthma, serious hepatic impairment, preexisting cardiac disease (may exacerbate cardiovascular complications), and rheumatoid arthritis (may exacerbate joint pain and swelling). Avoid use during acute kidney infection.

In patients with chronic kidney disease (CKD) requiring iron supplementation, the IV route is preferred for hemodialysis patients; either oral iron or IV iron may be used for nondialysis and peritoneal dialysis CKD patients. In patients with cancer-related anemia (either due to cancer or chemotherapy-induced) requiring iron supplementation, the IV route is superior to oral therapy; IM administration is not recommended for parenteral iron supplementation.

[U.S. Boxed Warning]: Use only in patients where the iron deficient state is not amenable to oral iron therapy. Discontinue oral iron prior to initiating parenteral iron therapy. Exogenous hemosiderosis may result from excess iron stores; patients with refractory anemias and/or hemoglobinopathies may be prone to iron overload with unwarranted iron supplementation. Anemia in the elderly is often caused by "anemia of chronic disease" or associated with inflammation rather than blood loss. Iron stores are usually normal or increased, with a serum ferritin >50 ng/mL and a decreased total iron binding capacity. IV administration of iron dextran is often preferred over IM in the elderly secondary to a decreased muscle mass and the need for daily injections. Intramuscular injections of iron-carbohydrate complexes may have a risk of delayed injection site tumor development. Iron dextran products differ in chemical characteristics. The high-molecular-weight formulation (Dexferrum) and the low-molecular-weight formulation (INFeD) are not clinically interchangeable. Intramuscular iron dextran use in neonates may be associated with an increased incidence of gram-negative sepsis.

Adverse Reactions Adverse event risk is reported to be higher with the high-molecular-weight iron dextran formulation.

Cardiovascular: Arrhythmia, bradycardia, cardiac arrest, chest pain, chest tightness, cyanosis, flushing, hyper-/hypotension, shock, syncope, tachycardia

Central nervous system: Chills, disorientation, dizziness, fever, headache, malaise, seizure, unconsciousness, unresponsiveness

Dermatologic: Pruritus, purpura, rash, urticaria

Gastrointestinal: Abdominal pain, diarrhea, nausea, taste alteration, vomiting

Genitourinary: Discoloration of urine

Hematologic: Leukocytosis, lymphadenopathy

Local: Injection site reactions (cellulitis, inflammation, pain, phlebitis, soreness, swelling), muscle atrophy/fibrosis (with IM injection), skin/tissue staining (at the site of IM injection), sterile abscess

Neuromuscular & skeletal: Arthralgia, arthritis/arthritis exacerbation, back pain, myalgia, paresthesia, weakness

Respiratory: Bronchospasm, dyspnea, respiratory arrest, wheezing

Renal: Hematuria

Miscellaneous: Anaphylactic reactions (sudden respiratory difficulty, cardiovascular collapse), diaphoresis

Postmarketing and/or case reports: Angioedema, tumor formation (at former injection site)

Drug Interactions

Metabolism/Transport Effects None known.

Avoid Concomitant Use

Avoid concomitant use of Iron Dextran Complex with any of the following: Dimercaprol

Increased Effect/Toxicity

The levels/effects of Iron Dextran Complex may be increased by: ACE Inhibitors; Dimercaprol

Decreased Effect There are no known significant interactions involving a decrease in effect.

Preparation for Administration Solutions for infusion should be diluted in 250-1000 mL NS.

Storage/Stability Store at 20°C to 25°C (68°F to 77°F); excursions permitted to 15°C to 30°C (59°F to 86°F).

Mechanism of Action The released iron, from the plasma, eventually replenishes the depleted iron stores in the bone marrow where it is incorporated into hemoglobin

Pharmacodynamics/Kinetics

Onset of action: IV: Serum ferritin peak: 7-9 days after dose

Absorption:

IM: 50% to 90% is promptly absorbed, balance is slowly absorbed over month

IV: Uptake of iron by the reticuloendothelial system appears to be constant at about 10-20 mg/hour

Excretion: Urine and feces via reticuloendothelial system

Dosage IM (INFeD; Z-track method should be used for IM injection), IV (Dexferrum, INFeD):

A 0.5 mL test dose (0.25 mL in infants) should be given prior to starting iron dextran therapy; total dose should be divided into a daily schedule for IM, total dose may be given as a single continuous infusion. Individual doses of ≤2 mL may be administered daily until calculated total dose is received.

Iron-deficiency anemia:

Children 5-15 kg: Should not normally be given in the first 4 months of life:

Dose (mL) = 0.0442 (desired hemoglobin - observed hemoglobin) x W + (0.26 x W)

Desired hemoglobin: Usually 12 g/dL

W = Total body weight in kg

Children >15 kg and Adults:

Dose (mL) = 0.0442 (desired hemoglobin - observed hemoglobin) x LBW + (0.26 x LBW)

Desired hemoglobin: Usually 14.8 g/dL

LBW = Lean body weight in kg

Iron replacement therapy for blood loss: Replacement iron (mg) = blood loss (mL) x hematocrit

Maximum daily dosage: Manufacturer's labeling: **Note:** Replacement of larger estimated iron deficits may be achieved by serial administration of smaller incremental dosages. Daily dosages should be limited to:

Children:

<5 kg: 25 mg iron (0.5 mL)

5-10 kg: 50 mg iron (1 mL)

Children ≥10 kg and Adults: 100 mg iron (2 mL)

Cancer-/chemotherapy-associated anemia: Adults: IV: **Note:** Use the iron-deficiency anemia equation for determining a calculated dose, when applicable.

Weekly administration (off-label dosing; INFed):

Weeks 1-3: Test dose of 25 mg (over 1-2 minutes), followed by 75 mg (bolus) once weekly

Weeks 4 and after: 100 mg over 5 minutes once weekly until the calculated dose is reached (Auerbach, 2004)

or

Week 1: Test dose of 25 mg (slow IV push), followed 1 hour later by 75 mg over 5 minutes

Weeks 2-10: 100 mg over 5 minutes once weekly for a total cumulative dose of 1000 mg (NCCN anemia guidelines v.2.2014)

Total dose infusion (off-label dosing; INFeD):

Test dose of 25 mg (over 1-2 minutes), followed 1 hour later by the balance of the calculated total dose mixed in 500 mL NS and infused at 175 mL/hour (Auerbach, 2004)

or

Test dose of 25 mg (slow IV push) followed 1 hour later by the balance of the total dose as a single infusion over several hours; if calculated dose exceeds 1000 mg, administer remaining dose in excess of 1000 mg after 4 weeks if inadequate hemoglobin response (NCCN anemia guidelines v.2.2014)

Dosage adjustment in renal impairment: No dosage adjustment provided in manufacturer's labeling.

Dosage adjustment in hepatic impairment: No dosage adjustment provided in manufacturer's labeling.

Administration Note: A test dose should be given on the first day of therapy; patient should be observed for 1 hour for hypersensitivity reaction, then the remainder of the day's dose (dose minus test dose) should be given. Resuscitation equipment, medication, and trained personnel should be available. An uneventful test dose does not ensure an anaphylactic-type reaction will not occur during administration of the therapeutic dose.

IM (INFeD): Use Z-track technique (displacement of the skin laterally prior to injection); injection should be deep into the upper outer quadrant of buttock; alternate buttocks with subsequent injections. Administer test dose at same recommended site using the same technique.

IV: Test dose should be given gradually over at least 30 seconds (INFeD) or 5 minutes (Dexferrum), or over 1-2 minutes (INFeD) for cancer-/chemotherapy-associated anemia (Auerbach, 2004). Subsequent dose(s) may be administered by IV bolus undiluted at a rate not to exceed 50 mg/minute (maximum 100 mg). For total dose infusion in patients with cancer-/chemotherapy-associated anemia (off-label dose): 1 hour after the test dose, administer the balance of the dose diluted in 500 mL NS and infuse at 175 mL/hour (Auerbach, 2004) or administer over several hours (NCCN Anemia guidelines v.2.2104). Avoid dilutions with dextrose (increased incidence of local pain and phlebitis).

Monitoring Parameters Hemoglobin, hematocrit, reticulocyte count, serum ferritin, serum iron, TIBC; monitor for anaphylaxis/hypersensitivity reaction (during test dose and therapeutic dose)

Reference Range

Hemoglobin: Adults:

Males: 13.5-16.5 g/dL

Females: 12.0-15.0 g/dL

Serum iron: 40-160 mcg/dL

Total iron binding capacity: 230-430 mcg/dL

Transferrin: 204-360 mg/dL

Percent transferrin saturation: 20% to 50%

Dosage Forms Considerations

Strength of iron dextran complex is expressed as elemental iron.

Dosage Forms

Solution, Injection:

Dexferrum: 50 mg/mL (1 mL, 2 mL)

Infed: 50 mg/mL (2 mL)

- ◆ **Iron Dextri-Maltose** *see* Ferric Carboxymaltose *on page 868*
- ◆ **Iron Fumarate** *see* Ferrous Fumarate *on page 870*
- ◆ **Iron Gluconate** *see* Ferrous Gluconate *on page 870*
- ◆ **Iron-Polysaccharide Complex** *see* Polysaccharide-Iron Complex *on page 1677*

Iron Sucrose (EYE ern SOO krose)

Brand Names: U.S. Venofer

Brand Names: Canada Venofer

Pharmacologic Category Iron Salt

Use Iron deficiency anemia: Treatment of iron-deficiency anemia in chronic kidney disease (CKD)

Pregnancy Risk Factor B

Pregnancy Considerations Teratogenic effects were not observed in animal studies. There are no adequate and well-controlled studies in pregnant women. Based on limited data, iron sucrose may be effective for the treatment of iron-deficiency anemia in pregnancy. It is recommended that pregnant women meet the dietary requirements of iron with diet and/or supplements in order to prevent adverse events associated with iron deficiency anemia in pregnancy. Treatment of iron deficiency anemia in pregnant women is the same as in nonpregnant women and in most cases, oral iron preparations may be used. Except in severe cases of maternal anemia, the fetus achieves normal iron stores regardless of maternal concentrations.

Breast-Feeding Considerations Iron is normally found in breast milk. Breast milk or iron fortified formulas generally provide enough iron to meet the recommended dietary requirements of infants. The amount of iron in breast milk is generally not influenced by maternal iron status.

Contraindications Known hypersensitivity to iron sucrose or any component of the formulation

Warnings/Precautions Hypersensitivity reactions, including rare postmarketing anaphylactic and anaphylactoid reactions (some fatal), have been reported; monitor patients during and for ≥30 minutes postadministration; discontinue immediately for signs/symptoms of a hypersensitivity reaction (shock, hypotension, loss of consciousness). Equipment for resuscitation and trained personnel experienced in handling medical emergencies should always be immediately available. Significant hypotension has been reported frequently in hemodialysis-dependent patients. Hypotension has also been reported in peritoneal dialysis and nondialysis patients. Hypotension may be related to total dose or rate of administration (avoid rapid IV injection), follow recommended guidelines. Withhold iron in the presence of tissue iron overload; periodic monitoring of hemoglobin, hematocrit, serum ferritin, and transferrin saturation is recommended.

Adverse Reactions Events are associated with use in adults unless otherwise specified.

Cardiovascular: Arteriovenous fistula thrombosis (children), chest pain, hyper-/hypotension, peripheral edema

Central nervous system: Dizziness, fever, headache

Dermatologic: Pruritus

Endocrine & metabolic: Fluid overload, gout, hyper-/hypoglycemia

Gastrointestinal: Abdominal pain, diarrhea, nausea, peritonitis (children), vomiting, taste perversion

Local: Injection site reaction

Neuromuscular & skeletal: Arthralgia, back pain, extremity pain, muscle cramps, myalgia, weakness

Ocular: Conjunctivitis

Otic: Ear pain

Respiratory: Cough, dyspnea, nasal congestion, nasopharyngitis, pharyngitis, sinusitis, upper respiratory infection

Miscellaneous: Graft complication, sepsis

Rare but important or life-threatening: Anaphylactic shock, anaphylactoid reactions, angioedema, bradycardia, cardiovascular collapse, hypersensitivity (including wheezing), loss of consciousness, necrotizing enterocolitis (reported in premature infants, no causal relationship established), seizure, shock, urine discoloration

Drug Interactions

Metabolism/Transport Effects None known.

Avoid Concomitant Use

Avoid concomitant use of Iron Sucrose with any of the following: Dimercaprol

Increased Effect/Toxicity

The levels/effects of Iron Sucrose may be increased by: Dimercaprol

Decreased Effect There are no known significant interactions involving a decrease in effect.

Preparation for Administration

Children: May administer undiluted or diluted in 25 mL of NS. Do not dilute to concentrations <1 mg/mL.

Adults: Doses ≤200 mg may be administered undiluted or diluted in a maximum of 100 mL NS. Doses >200 mg should be diluted in a maximum of 250 mL NS. Do not dilute to concentrations <1 mg/mL.

Storage/Stability Store intact vials at controlled room temperature of 20°C to 25°C (68°F to 77°F); excursions permitted to 15°C to 30°C (59°F to 86°F); do not freeze. Iron sucrose is stable for 7 days at room temperature (23°C to 27°C [73°F to 81°F]) or under refrigeration (2°C to 6°C [36°F to 43°F]) when undiluted in a plastic syringe or following dilution in normal saline in a plastic syringe (concentration 2-10 mg/mL) or for 7 days at room temperature (23°C to 27°C [73°F to 81°F]) following dilution in normal saline in an IV bag (concentration 1-2 mg/mL).

Mechanism of Action Iron sucrose is dissociated by the reticuloendothelial system into iron and sucrose. The released iron increases serum iron concentrations and is incorporated into hemoglobin.

Pharmacodynamics/Kinetics

Distribution: V_{dss}: Healthy adults: 7.9 L

Metabolism: Dissociated into iron and sucrose by the reticuloendothelial system

Half-life elimination: Healthy adults: 6 hours; Nondialysis-dependent adolescents: 8 hours

Excretion: Healthy adults: Urine (5%) within 24 hours

Dosage Doses expressed in mg of **elemental** iron. **Note:** Test dose: Product labeling does not indicate need for a test dose in product-naive patients.

Children ≥2 years and Adolescents: Iron-deficiency anemia in chronic kidney disease (CKD): IV: **Note:** Not indicated for iron replacement treatment in children and adolescents.

Hemodialysis-dependent patient: Maintenance therapy: 0.5 mg/kg/dose (maximum: 100 mg) every 2 weeks for 6 doses; may repeat if clinically indicated.

Nondialysis-dependent patient: Maintenance therapy: 0.5 mg/kg/dose (maximum: 100 mg) every 4 weeks for 3 doses; may repeat if clinically indicated

Peritoneal dialysis-dependent patient: Maintenance therapy: 0.5 mg/kg/dose (maximum: 100 mg) every 4 weeks for 3 doses; may repeat if clinically indicated

Adults:

Iron-deficiency anemia in CKD: IV:

Hemodialysis-dependent patient: 100 mg administered during consecutive dialysis sessions to a cumulative total dose of 1000 mg (10 doses); may repeat treatment if clinically indicated.

Peritoneal dialysis-dependent patient: Two infusions of 300 mg administered 14 days apart, followed by a single 400 mg infusion 14 days later (total cumulative dose of 1000 mg in 3 divided doses); may repeat treatment if clinically indicated.

Nondialysis-dependent patient: 200 mg administered on 5 different occasions within a 14-day period (total cumulative dose: 1000 mg in 14-day period); may repeat treatment if clinically indicated. **Note:** Dosage has also been administered as 2 infusions of 500 mg on day 1 and day 14 (limited experience).

Chemotherapy-associated anemia (off-label use): IV: 200 mg once every 3 weeks for 5 doses (Bastit, 2008) **or** 100 mg once weekly during weeks 0 to 6, followed by 100 mg every other week from weeks 8 to 14 (Hedenus, 2007)

Elderly: Refer to adult dosing.

Dosage adjustment in renal impairment: No dosage adjustment provided in manufacturer's labeling.

Dosage adjustment in hepatic impairment: No dosage adjustment provided in manufacturer's labeling.

Administration Administer intravenously as a slow IV injection (**not** for rapid IV injection) or as an IV infusion. Can be administered through dialysis line.

Children and Adolescents:

Slow IV injection: Administer undiluted over 5 minutes

Infusion: Infuse diluted solution over 5-60 minutes

Adults:

Slow IV injection: May administer doses ≤200 mg undiluted by slow IV injection over 2-5 minutes. When administering to hemodialysis-dependent patients, give iron sucrose early during the dialysis session.

Infusion: Infuse diluted doses ≤200 mg over at least 15 minutes; infuse diluted 300 mg dose over 1.5 hours; infuse diluted 400 mg dose over 2.5 hours; infuse diluted 500 mg dose over 3.5-4 hours (limited experience). When administering to hemodialysis-dependent patients, give iron sucrose early during the dialysis session.

Monitoring Parameters

CKD patients: Hematocrit, hemoglobin, serum ferritin, serum iron, transferrin, percent transferrin saturation, TIBC (takes ~4 weeks of treatment to see increased serum iron and ferritin, and decreased TIBC); iron status should be assessed ≥48 hours after last dose (due to rapid increase in values following administration); signs/ symptoms of hypersensitivity reactions (during and ≥30 minutes following infusion); hypotension (following infusion)

Chemotherapy-associated anemia (off-label use): Iron, total iron-binding capacity, transferrin saturation, or ferritin levels at baseline and periodically (Rizzo, 2011)

Reference Range

Hemoglobin: Adults:

Males: 13.5-16.5 g/dL

Females: 12.0-15.0 g/dL

Serum iron: 40-160 mcg/dL

Total iron binding capacity: 230-430 mcg/dL

Transferrin: 204-360 mg/dL

Percent transferrin saturation: 20% to 50%

Dosage Forms Considerations Strength of iron sucrose is expressed as elemental iron.

Dosage Forms

Solution, Intravenous [preservative free]:

Venofer: 20 mg/mL (2.5 mL, 5 mL, 10 mL)

◆ **Iron Sulfate** *see* Ferrous Sulfate *on page 871*

◆ **Iron Supplement Childrens [OTC]** *see* Ferrous Sulfate *on page 871*

◆ **ISD** *see* Isosorbide Dinitrate *on page 1124*

◆ **ISDN** *see* Isosorbide Dinitrate *on page 1124*

◆ **Isentress** *see* Raltegravir *on page 1767*

◆ **Isepacine Sulfate** *see* Isepamicin [INT] *on page 1120*

Isepamicin [INT] (eye SEP a mye sin)

International Brand Names Exacin (JP); Isepacin (AT, IT, JP, MX, PT); Isepacine (BE); Isepalline (FR)

Index Terms Isepacine Sulfate

Pharmacologic Category Antibiotic, Aminoglycoside

Reported Use Treatment of susceptible bacterial infections

Dosage Range Adults: IM, IV: 8-15 mg/kg daily in 2 divided doses; maximum: 1.5 g/day

Product Availability Product available in various countries; not currently available in the U.S.

Dosage Forms

Injection, solution: 250 mg/mL (1 mL, 2 mL)

◆ **ISG** *see* Immune Globulin *on page 1056*

◆ **ISIS 301012** *see* Mipomersen *on page 1375*

◆ **ISMN** *see* Isosorbide Mononitrate *on page 1126*

◆ **Isoamyl Nitrite** *see* Amyl Nitrite *on page 147*

◆ **Isobamate** *see* Carisoprodol *on page 363*

Isoconazole [INT] (eye soe KOE na zole)

International Brand Names Azonit (JO, LB); Epelon (TW); Fazol (FR); Gino-Travogen (PT); Gyno-Travogen (AE, AT, BH, CH); Icaden (BR, CO, CR, DO, EC, GT, HN, NI, PA, PE, PY, SV, UY, VE); Imefu (TW); Isocon (PK); Isogen (IL); Isonazol (KR); Micoderm (PE); Mupaten (AR); Travogen (AE, AT, BE, BH, CH, CY, EE, EG, GR, HK, JO, KW, LB, LT, MY, PH, PL, QA, RO, RU, SA, SG, SI, TH, TR); Ufarin (CL); Wazole (TW)

Index Terms Isoconazole Nitrate

Pharmacologic Category Antifungal Agent, Topical

Reported Use Treatment of topical and vaginal fungal infections

Dosage Range Adults:

Topical: Apply once daily

Vaginal tablet: 600 mg, insert once at bedtime

Product Availability Product available in various countries; not currently available in the U.S.

Dosage Forms

Cream: 10 mg/g (20 g)

Solution, topical: 10 mg/g (20 mL)

Tablet, vaginal: 300 mg, 600 mg

◆ **Isoconazole Nitrate** *see* Isoconazole [INT] *on page 1120*

◆ **IsoDitrate ER** *see* Isosorbide Dinitrate *on page 1124*

Isoniazid (eye soe NYE a zid)

Brand Names: Canada Dom-Isoniazid; Isotamine; PDP-Isoniazid

Index Terms INH; Isonicotinic Acid Hydrazide

Pharmacologic Category Antitubercular Agent

Use

Active tuberculosis infections: Treatment of susceptible active tuberculosis (eg, *Mycobacterium tuberculosis*) infections.

Latent tuberculosis infection (LTBI): Treatment of LTBI caused by *Mycobacterium tuberculosis* (also referred to as prophylaxis or preventive therapy). **Note:** To identify candidates for LTBI treatment, refer to CDC guidelines (http://www.cdc.gov/tb/publications/ltbi/pdf/Targeted-LTBI.pdf) for current recommendations.

Pregnancy Risk Factor C

Pregnancy Considerations Adverse events were observed in some animal reproduction studies. Isoniazid crosses the human placenta. Due to the risk of tuberculosis to the fetus, treatment is recommended when the probability of maternal disease is moderate to high. The CDC recommends isoniazid as part of the initial treatment regimen. Pyridoxine supplementation is recommended (25 mg/day) (CDC, 2003). Due to biologic changes during pregnancy and early postpartum, pregnant women may have increased susceptibility to tuberculosis infection or reactivation of latent disease (Mathad, 2012).

Breast-Feeding Considerations Small amounts of isoniazid are excreted in breast milk; concentrations are considered nontoxic and not therapeutic to the nursing infant. Women with tuberculosis taking isoniazid should not be discouraged from breast-feeding. Pyridoxine supplementation is recommended for the mother and infant (CDC, 2003). Women with tuberculosis mastitis should breast-feed using the unaffected breast (Mathad, 2012). In the United States, breast-feeding is not recommended for women with tuberculosis who are also coinfected with HIV (DHHS [adult], 2014).

Contraindications Hypersensitivity to isoniazid or any component of the formulation, including drug-induced hepatitis; acute liver disease; previous history of hepatic injury during isoniazid therapy; previous severe adverse reaction (drug fever, chills, arthritis) to isoniazid

Warnings/Precautions Use with caution in patients with severe renal impairment and liver disease. **[U.S. Boxed Warning]: Severe and sometimes fatal hepatitis may occur; usually occurs within the first 3 months of treatment, although may develop even after many months of treatment.** The risk of developing hepatitis is age-related, although isoniazid-induced hepatotoxicity has been reported in children; daily ethanol consumption, chronic liver disease, or injection drug use may also increase the risk. Contraindicated in patients with acute liver disease or previous isoniazid-associated hepatic injury. Fatal hepatitis associated with isoniazid may be increased in women (particularly black and Hispanic and in any woman in the postpartum period). Closer monitoring may be considered in these groups. Patients given isoniazid must be monitored carefully and interviewed at monthly intervals. Patients must report any prodromal symptoms of hepatitis, such as fatigue, paresthesias of hands and feet, weakness, dark urine, rash, anorexia, nausea, fever >3 days' duration, and/or abdominal pain (especially right upper quadrant discomfort), icterus, or vomiting. Patients should be instructed to immediately hold therapy if any of these symptoms occur, and contact their prescriber. If abnormalities of liver function exceed 3 to 5 times the upper limit of normal (ULN), strongly consider discontinuation of isoniazid. If isoniazid must be reinstituted, wait for symptoms and laboratory abnormalities to resolve and use very small and gradual increasing doses, withdrawing therapy immediately if an indication of recurrent hepatic involvement. Treatment with isoniazid for latent tuberculosis infection should be deferred in patients with acute hepatic diseases. Periodic ophthalmic examinations are recommended even when usual symptoms do not occur. Potentially significant drug interactions may exist, requiring dose or frequency adjustment, additional monitoring, and/or selection of alternative therapy. Use should be carefully monitored in the following groups: Daily users of alcohol, active chronic liver disease, severe renal dysfunction, age >35 years, concurrent use of any chronically administered drug, history of previous isoniazid discontinuation, existence of or conditions predisposing to peripheral neuropathy, pregnancy, injection drug use, women in minority groups (particularly postpartum), HIV seropositive patients. AST and ALT should be obtained at baseline and at least monthly during LTBI use. Discontinue temporarily or permanently if liver function tests >3 to 5 times ULN. Pyridoxine (10 to 50 mg/day) is recommended in individuals at risk for development of peripheral neuropathies (eg, HIV infection, nutritional deficiency, diabetes, pregnancy). Children with low milk and low meat intake should receive concomitant pyridoxine therapy. Multidrug regimens should be utilized for the treatment of active tuberculosis to prevent the emergence of drug resistance.

Adverse Reactions

Cardiovascular: Hypertension, palpitation, tachycardia, vasculitis

Central nervous system: Depression, dizziness, encephalopathy, fever, lethargy, memory impairment, psychosis, seizure, slurred speech, toxic encephalopathy

Dermatologic: Flushing, rash (morbilliform, maculopapular, pruritic, or exfoliative)

Endocrine & metabolic: Gynecomastia, hyperglycemia, metabolic acidosis, pellagra, pyridoxine deficiency

Gastrointestinal: Anorexia, epigastric distress, nausea, stomach pain, vomiting

Hematologic: Agranulocytosis, anemia (sideroblastic, hemolytic, or aplastic), eosinophilia, thrombocytopenia

Hepatic: Bilirubinuria, hepatic dysfunction, hepatitis (may involve progressive liver damage; risk increases with age), hyperbilirubinemia, jaundice, LFTs mildly increased

Neuromuscular & skeletal: Arthralgia, hyper-reflexia, paresthesia, peripheral neuropathy (dose-related incidence), weakness

Ocular: Blurred vision, loss of vision, optic neuritis/atrophy

Miscellaneous: Lupus-like syndrome, lymphadenopathy, rheumatic syndrome

Drug Interactions

Metabolism/Transport Effects **Substrate** of CYP2E1 (major); **Note:** Assignment of Major/Minor substrate status based on clinically relevant drug interaction potential; **Inhibits** CYP1A2 (weak), CYP2A6 (moderate), CYP2C19 (moderate), CYP2C9 (weak), CYP2D6 (moderate), CYP2E1 (moderate), CYP3A4 (weak); **Induces** CYP2E1 (moderate)

Avoid Concomitant Use

Avoid concomitant use of Isoniazid with any of the following: Pimozide; Tegafur; Thioridazine

Increased Effect/Toxicity

Isoniazid may increase the levels/effects of: Acetaminophen; ARIPiprazole; CarBAMazepine; Chlorzoxazone; Citalopram; CycloSERINE; CYP2A6 Substrates; CYP2C19 Substrates; CYP2D6 Substrates; CYP2E1 Substrates; Dofetilide; DOXOrubicin (Conventional); Eliglustat; Fesoterodine; Fosphenytoin; Hydrocodone; Lomitapide; Metoprolol; Nebivolol; Phenytoin; Pimozide; Theophylline Derivatives; Thioridazine

The levels/effects of Isoniazid may be increased by: Disulfiram; Ethionamide; Propafenone; Rifamycin Derivatives

Decreased Effect

Isoniazid may decrease the levels/effects of: Clopidogrel; Codeine; Itraconazole; Ketoconazole (Systemic); Levodopa; Tamoxifen; Tegafur; TraMADol

The levels/effects of Isoniazid may be decreased by: Antacids; Corticosteroids (Systemic); Cyproterone

Food Interactions

Isoniazid may decrease folic acid absorption and alters pyridoxine metabolism. Management: Increase dietary intake of folate, niacin, and magnesium.

Tyramine-containing food: Isoniazid has weak monoamine oxidase inhibiting activity and may potentially inhibit tyramine metabolism. Several case reports of mild reactions (flushing, palpitations, headache, mild increase in blood pressure, diaphoresis) after ingestion of certain types of cheese or red wine, have been reported (Self, 1999; Toutoungi, 1985). Management: Manufacturer's labeling recommends avoiding tyramine-containing foods (eg, aged or matured cheese, air-dried or cured meats including sausages and salamis; fava or broad bean pods, tap/draft beers, Marmite concentrate, sauerkraut, soy sauce, and other soybean condiments). However, the clinical relevance of the tyramine reaction for the vast majority of patients receiving isoniazid has been questioned due to isoniazid's weak MAO inhibition and the relatively few published case reports of the interaction. Although not fully investigated, it has been proposed that the reaction has a genetic component and may only be significant in poor or intermediate acetylators since isoniazid is primarily inactivated by acetylation (DiMartini, 1995; Toutoungi, 1985).

Histamine-containing food: Isoniazid may also inhibit diamine oxidase resulting in headache, sweating, palpitations, flushing, diarrhea, itching, wheezing, dyspnea or hypotension to histamine-containing foods (eg, skipjack, tuna, saury, other tropical fish). Management: Manufacturer's labeling recommends avoiding histamine-containing foods; corticosteroids and antihistamines may be administered if histamine intoxication occurs (Miki, 2005).

Storage/Stability

Tablet: Store at 20°C to 25°C (68°F to 77°F). Protect from light.

Oral solution: Store at 15°C to 30°C (59°F to 86°F). Protect from light.

Injection: Store at 20°C to 25°C (68°F to 77°F). Protect from light. Isoniazid injection may crystallize at low temperatures. If this occurs, warm the vial to room temperature before use to redissolve the crystals.

Mechanism of Action Isoniazid inhibits the synthesis of mycoloic acids, an essential component of the bacterial cell wall. At therapeutic levels isoniazid is bacteriocidal against actively growing intracellular and extracellular *Mycobacterium tuberculosis* organisms.

Pharmacodynamics/Kinetics

Distribution: All body tissues and fluids including CSF

Metabolism: Hepatic with rate determined genetically by acetylation phenotype

Time to peak, serum: 1 to 2 hours

Excretion: Urine (50% to 70%)

Pharmacokinetic note: Isoniazid is primarily metabolized by acetylation and dehydrazination. Rate of acetylation is genetically determined. Approximately 50% of blacks and whites are "slow inactivators" and the rest are "rapid inactivators". The large majority of Eskimo and Asian patients are "rapid inactivators". Acetylation rate does not significantly alter the effectiveness, but slow acetylation may lead to higher blood levels and possibly an increase in adverse effects.

Dosage

Usual dosage ranges: Oral, IM:

Infants, Children, and Adolescents: 10 to 15 mg/kg/day once daily (maximum: 300 mg daily) or 15 to 40 mg/kg given 1 to 3 times per week (maximum: 900 mg per dose)

Adults: 5 mg/kg/day (usual: 300 mg daily) as a single daily dose or 15 mg/kg (maximum: 900 mg per dose) given 1 to 3 times per week

Indication-specific dosing: Recommendations often change due to resistant strains and newly-developed information; consult CDC for current recommendations. Intramuscular injection is available for patients who are unable to either take or absorb oral therapy. Treatment may be defined by the number of doses administered (eg, CDC preferred regimen for active tuberculosis involves 182 doses of INH and rifampin, and 56 doses of pyrazinamide and ethambutol [CDC, 2011]).

Tuberculosis, active (drug susceptible; excludes meningitis): Always given in combination with other antitubercular drugs. In the initial dosing phase, ethambutol may be discontinued if drug susceptibility studies demonstrate susceptibility to isoniazid, rifampin and pyrazinamide (CDC, 2011).

Infants, Children, and Adolescents: Oral, IM:

CDC recommendations (MMWR, 2003): Initial: 10 to 15 mg/kg/day once daily (maximum dose: 300 mg daily) with concomitant rifampin and pyrazinamide, with or without ethambutol for 8 weeks.

Continuation phase: 10 to 15 mg/kg/day once daily (maximum dose: 300 mg daily) with concomitant rifampin for 18 weeks.

Note: The above is the CDC preferred regimen (CDC, 2011)

or

Initial phase 1: 10 to 15 mg/kg/day once daily (maximum dose: 300 mg daily) with concomitant rifampin, pyrazinamide and with or without ethambutol for 2 weeks, followed by:

Initial phase 2: 20 to 30 mg/kg/dose 2 times weekly (maximum: 900 mg per dose) with concomitant rifampin, pyrazinamide and with or without ethambutol for 6 weeks.

Continuation phase: 20 to 30 mg/kg/dose 2 times weekly (maximum: 900 mg per dose) with concomitant rifampin for 18 weeks.

Alternate recommendations: (Red Book [AAP], 2012): Initial: 10 to 15 mg/kg once daily (maximum dose: 300 mg) or 20 to 30 mg/kg 2 times weekly (maximum dose: 900 mg) with concomitant rifampin, pyrazinamide and ethambutol for 2 months.

Continuation phase: 10 to 15 mg/kg once daily (maximum dose: 300 mg) or 20 to 30 mg/kg 2 times weekly (maximum dose: 900 mg) with concomitant rifampin for 4 months.

Adults: Oral, IM: **Note:** Concomitant administration of pyridoxine is recommended in malnourished patients or those prone to neuropathy (eg, patients with HIV-infection, diabetes, renal failure,or chronic alcohol abusers).

CDC recommendations (MMWR, 2003): Initial: 5 mg/kg/day once daily (usual dose: 300 mg daily) with concomitant rifampin and pyrazinamide, with or without ethambutol for 8 weeks.

Continuation phase: 5 mg/kg/day once daily (usual dose: 300 mg daily) with concomitant rifampin for 18 weeks

Note: The above is the CDC preferred regimen; patients who are non-HIV exposed/infected, have no cavities on chest radiograph, and who also have negative acid fast bacilli sputum smears at the end of the initial phase can be treated with 15 mg/kg weekly (maximum dose: 900 mg) and rifapentine for 18 weeks in the continuation phase (CDC, 2011).

or

Initial phase: 5 mg/kg/day once daily (usual dose: 300 mg daily) with concomitant rifampin, pyrazinamide and with or without ethambutol for 2 weeks, followed by 15 mg/kg/dose 2 times weekly (maximum: 900 mg per dose) with concomitant rifampin, pyrazinamide and with or without ethambutol for 6 weeks.

Continuation phase: 15 mg/kg/dose 2 times weekly (maximum: 900 mg per dose) with concomitant rifampin for 18 weeks.

Note: In patients who are non-HIV exposed/infected, have no cavities on chest radiograph, and who also have negative acid fast bacilli sputum smears at the end of the initial phase can be treated with 15 mg/kg weekly (maximum dose: 900 mg) and rifapentine for 18 weeks in the continuation phase (CDC, 2011).

or

Initial: 15 mg/kg/dose 3 times weekly (maximum: 900 mg per dose) with concomitant rifampin, pyrazinamide and with or without ethambutol for 8 weeks.

Continuation phase: 15 mg/kg/dose 3 times weekly (maximum: 900 mg per dose) with concomitant rifampin for 18 weeks.

Note: In patients who are non-HIV exposed/infected, have no cavities on chest radiograph, and who also have negative acid fast bacilli sputum smears at the end of the initial phase can be treated with 15 mg/kg weekly (maximum dose: 900 mg) and rifapentine for 18 weeks in the continuation phase (CDC, 2011).

Tuberculosis, active, meningitis (drug susceptible): Always given in combination with other antitubercular drugs. **Note:** Concomitant administration of pyridoxine is recommended in malnourished patients or those prone to neuropathy (eg, patients with HIV-infection, diabetes, renal failure or chronic alcohol abusers).

Infants, Children, and Adolescents: Oral, IM:

CDC recommendations (MMWR, 2003): Initial: 10 to 15 mg/kg once daily (maximum dose: 300 mg) with concomitant rifampin, pyrazinamide and ethambutol for 8 weeks; dexamethasone is given concomitantly in the first 6 weeks.

Continuation phase: 10 to 15 mg/kg/day once daily (maximum: 300 mg daily) with concomitant rifampin for 7 to 10 months.

Note: The above is the CDC preferred regimen (MMWR, 2003).

Alternate recommendations (Red Book [AAP], 2012): Initial: 10 to 15 mg/kg once daily (maximum dose: 300 mg) with concomitant rifampin, pyrazinamide and an aminoglycoside, ethambutol or ethionamide for 8 weeks.

Continuation phase: 10 to 15 mg/kg once daily (maximum dose: 300 mg) or 20 to 30 mg/kg 2 times weekly (maximum dose: 900 mg) with concomitant rifampin for 7 to 10 months.

Adults:

CDC recommendations (MMWR, 2003): Initial: 5 mg/kg once daily (usual dose: 300 mg) with concomitant rifampin, pyrazinamide and ethambutol for 8 weeks; dexamethasone is given concomitantly in the first 6 weeks.

Continuation phase: 5 mg/kg/day once daily (maximum: 300 mg daily) with concomitant rifampin for 7 to 10 months.

Note: The above is the CDC preferred regimen (MMWR, 2003).

Tuberculosis, latent infection (LTBI):

Infants and Children <12 years: Oral, IM:

CDC recommendations (CDC, 2013): 10 to 20 mg/kg/day once daily (maximum: 300 mg per dose) (preferred regimen) or 20 to 40 mg/kg (maximum: 900 mg per dose) twice weekly for 9 months.

Note: Once weekly regimen of isoniazid and rifapentine may also be considered in children ≥2 or <12 years if completion of 9-month regimen (preferred) is unlikely and the hazard of tuberculosis is great (CDC, 2013). Refer to Children ≥12 years and Adolescents dosing.

Alternate recommendations (Red Book [AAP], 2012): 10 to 15 mg/kg/day once daily (maximum: 300 mg per dose) for 9 months.

Children ≥12 years and Adolescents: Oral, IM:

CDC recommendations (CDC, 2013): 10 to 20 mg/kg/day once daily (maximum: 300 mg per dose) (preferred regimen) or 20 to 40 mg/kg (maximum: 900 mg per dose) twice weekly for 9 months (CDC, 2013), or 15 mg/kg/dose (maximum: 900 mg per dose) once weekly in combination with rifapentine for 12 weeks (CDC, 2013). **Note:** Rifapentine-containing regimen is also recommended for HIV-infected patients not receiving antiretroviral therapy (ART), however, ART is recommended for **all** HIV-infected individuals to reduce the risk of disease progression and prevent HIV transmission (DHHS [adult], 2014).

Alternate recommendation (Red Book [AAP], 2012): 10 to 15 mg/kg/day once daily (maximum: 300 mg per dose) for 9 months.

Adults: **Note:** Concomitant administration of pyridoxine is recommended in malnourished patients or those prone to neuropathy (eg, patients with HIV-infection, diabetes, renal failure or chronic alcohol abusers).

CDC recommendations (CDC, 2013):

Non-HIV exposed/infected: 5 mg/kg (maximum: 300 mg per dose) once daily for 6 to 9 months or 15 mg/kg (maximum: 900 mg per dose) twice weekly for 9 months. **Note:** 6 months may be considered to reduce costs of therapy and improve adherence.

Alternate regimen: Not pregnant and/or not expecting to become pregnant: 15 mg/kg/dose (maximum 900 mg) once weekly in combination with rifapentine for 12 weeks. **Note:** Also recommended for HIV-infected patients not receiving antiretroviral therapy (ART), however, ART is recommended for **all** HIV-infected individuals to reduce the risk of disease progression and prevent HIV transmission (DHHS [adult], 2014).

HIV exposed/infected receiving antiretroviral therapy: 5 mg/kg (maximum: 300 mg per dose) once daily for 9 months or 15 mg/kg (maximum: 900 mg per dose) twice weekly for 9 months. **Note:** LTBI treatment is **not** recommended in HIV-infected persons who are anergic and have not had recent contact with anyone with infectious tuberculosis. (DHHS [adult], 2013).

Nontuberculous mycobacterium *(M. kansasii)* (off-label use): Adults: 5 mg/kg/day (maximum: 300 mg daily) for duration to include 12 months of culture-negative sputum; typically used in combination with ethambutol and rifampin (Griffith, 2007).

Dosage adjustment in renal impairment: No dosage adjustment necessary.

ESRD receiving intermittent hemodialysis (IHD): Administer dose post dialysis (Aronoff, 2007).

Dosage adjustment in hepatic impairment: There are no dosage adjustments provided in the manufacturer's labeling; however, use with caution; may accumulate and additional liver damage may occur in patients with preexisting liver disease. Contraindicated in patients with acute liver disease or previous isoniazid-associated hepatic injury. For ALT or AST >3 times the ULN: discontinue or temporarily withhold treatment. Treatment with isoniazid for latent tuberculosis infection should be deferred in patients with acute hepatic diseases.

Dietary Considerations Increase dietary intake of folate, niacin, magnesium.

Administration

Oral: May be administered with or without food.

Intramuscular: IM injection may be used for patients who are unable to either take or absorb oral therapy. Inject deep IM into a large muscle mass.

Monitoring Parameters Baseline and periodic (more frequently in patients with higher risk for hepatitis) liver function tests (ALT and AST); sputum cultures monthly (until 2 consecutive negative cultures reported); monitoring for prodromal signs of hepatitis

LTBI therapy: American Thoracic Society/Centers for Disease Control (ATS/CDC) recommendations: Monthly clinical evaluation, including brief physical exam for adverse events. Use should be carefully monitored in the following groups: daily users of alcohol, active chronic liver disease, severe renal dysfunction, age >35 years, concurrent use of any chronically administered drug, history of previous isoniazid discontinuation, existence of or conditions predisposing to peripheral neuropathy, pregnancy, injection drug use, women in minority groups (particularly postpartum), HIV seropositive patients. AST and ALT should be obtained at baseline and at least monthly during LTBI use. Discontinue temporarily or permanently if liver function tests >3 to 5 times ULN. Routine, periodic monitoring is recommended for any patient with an abnormal baseline or at increased risk for hepatotoxicity.

Additional Information The AAP recommends that pyridoxine supplementation (1 to 2 mg/kg/day) should be administered to malnourished children or adolescents on meat or milk-deficient diets, breast-feeding infants, and those predisposed to neuritis to prevent peripheral neuropathy; administration of isoniazid syrup has been associated with diarrhea.

Dosage Forms

Solution, Injection:

Generic: 100 mg/mL (10 mL)

Syrup, Oral:

Generic: 50 mg/5 mL (473 mL)

Tablet, Oral:

Generic: 100 mg, 300 mg

Extemporaneous Preparations Note: Commercial oral solution is available (50 mg/mL)

A 10 mg/mL oral suspension may be made with tablets, purified water, and sorbitol. Crush ten 100 mg tablets in a mortar and reduce to a fine powder. Add 10 mL of purified water and mix to a uniform paste. Mix while adding sorbitol in incremental proportions to **almost** 100 mL; transfer to a graduated cylinder, rinse mortar with sorbitol, and add quantity of sorbitol sufficient to make 100 mL (do not use sugar-based solutions). Label "shake well" and "refrigerate". Stable for 21 days refrigerated.

Nahata MC, Pai VB, and Hipple TF, *Pediatric Drug Formulations*, 5th ed, Cincinnati, OH: Harvey Whitney Books Co, 2004.

Isoniazid and Thiacetazone [INT]

(eye soe NYE a zid & thye ah SEE ta zone)

Index Terms Thiacetazone and Isoniazid

Pharmacologic Category Antitubercular Agent

Reported Use Treatment of pulmonary and extrapulmonary tuberculosis

Dosage Range Adults: Oral: 1 capsule (containing isoniazid 300 mg and thiacetazone 150 mg) daily

Product Availability Product available in various countries; not currently available in the U.S.

Dosage Forms

Capsule: Isoniazid 300 mg and thiacetazone 150 mg

◆ **Isonicotinic Acid Hydrazide** *see* Isoniazid *on page 1120*

◆ **Isonipecaine Hydrochloride** *see* Meperidine *on page 1293*

◆ **Isophane Insulin** *see* Insulin NPH *on page 1089*

◆ **Isophane Insulin and Regular Insulin** *see* Insulin NPH and Insulin Regular *on page 1090*

◆ **Isophosphamide** *see* Ifosfamide *on page 1040*

Isoproterenol (eye soe proe TER e nole)

Brand Names: U.S. Isuprel

Index Terms Isoproterenol Hydrochloride

Pharmacologic Category $Beta_1$- & $Beta_2$-Adrenergic Agonist Agent

Use Manufacturer's labeled indications (see **"Note"**): Mild or transient episodes of heart block that do not require electric shock or pacemaker therapy; serious episodes of heart block and Adams-Stokes attacks (except when caused by ventricular tachycardia or fibrillation); cardiac arrest until electric shock or pacemaker therapy is available; bronchospasm during anesthesia; adjunct to fluid and electrolyte replacement therapy and other drugs and procedures in the treatment of hypovolemic or septic shock and low cardiac output states (eg, decompensated heart failure, cardiogenic shock)

Note: The use of isoproterenol in advanced cardiac life support (ACLS) has largely been supplanted by the use of other adrenergic agents (eg, epinephrine and dopamine). The use of isoproterenol for bronchospasm during anesthesia and cardiogenic, hypovolemic, or septic shock is no longer recommended.

Pregnancy Risk Factor C

Dosage IV: **Note:** Patients may exhibit dose-dependent vasodilation due to unopposed $beta_2$-agonism elicited by isoproterenol.

Bradyarrhythmias, AV nodal block, or refractory torsade de pointes:

Children: Continuous infusion: Usual range: 0.05-2 mcg/**kg**/minute; titrate to patient response

Adults: Continuous infusion: Usual range: 2-10 mcg/minute; titrate to patient response

Brugada syndrome with electrical storm (off-label use): Adults: IV bolus: Initial: 1-2 mcg, followed by a continuous infusion of 0.15-0.3 mcg/minute for 1 day; may repeat sequence if ventricular tachycardia/fibrillation recurs (Watanabe, 2006; Zipes, 2006).

Tilt table testing for syncope (Benditt, 1996; Brignole, 2004): Adults: Continuous infusion: Initial: 1 mcg/minute; increase as necessary based on response; maximum dose: 5 mcg/minute. **Note:** Timing of initiation and dose adjustment during test may be institution-specific.

Dosage adjustment in renal impairment: No dosage adjustment provided in manufacturer's labeling.

Dosage adjustment in hepatic impairment: No dosage adjustment provided in manufacturer's labeling.

Additional Information Complete prescribing information should be consulted for additional detail.

Dosage Forms

Solution, Injection:

Isuprel: 0.2 mg/mL (1 mL, 5 mL)

◆ **Isoproterenol Hydrochloride** *see* Isoproterenol *on page 1124*

◆ **Isoptin SR** *see* Verapamil *on page 2154*

◆ **Isopto Atropine** *see* Atropine *on page 200*

◆ **Isopto® Atropine (Can)** *see* Atropine *on page 200*

◆ **Isopto Carbachol** *see* Carbachol *on page 346*

◆ **Isopto® Carbachol (Can)** *see* Carbachol *on page 346*

◆ **Isopto Carpine** *see* Pilocarpine (Ophthalmic) *on page 1649*

◆ **Isopto® Carpine (Can)** *see* Pilocarpine (Ophthalmic) *on page 1649*

◆ **Isopto Homatropine** *see* Homatropine *on page 1005*

◆ **Isordil Titradose** *see* Isosorbide Dinitrate *on page 1124*

◆ **Isosorbide (Can)** *see* Isosorbide Dinitrate *on page 1124*

Isosorbide Dinitrate (eye soe SOR bide dye NYE trate)

Brand Names: U.S. Dilatrate-SR; IsoDitrate ER; Isordil Titradose

Brand Names: Canada ISDN; Isosorbide; Novo-Sorbide; PMS-Isosorbide

Index Terms ISD; ISDN

Pharmacologic Category Antianginal Agent; Vasodilator

Use Angina pectoris: Prevention of angina pectoris

Note: Due to slower onset of action, not the drug of choice to abort an acute anginal episode.

Pregnancy Risk Factor C

Pregnancy Considerations Adverse events were observed in some animal reproduction studies. Nitric oxide donors, such as isosorbide, have been evaluated for preeclampsia and cervical ripening; isosorbide dinitrate use in these conditions is not currently recommended (Kalidindi, 2012; Ramirez, 2011).

Breast-Feeding Considerations It is not known if isosorbide dinitrate is excreted in breast milk. The manufacturer recommends that caution be exercised when administering isosorbide dinitrate to nursing women.

Contraindications

Hypersensitivity to isosorbide dinitrate or any component of the formulation; hypersensitivity to organic nitrates; concurrent use with phosphodiesterase inhibitors (sildenafil, tadalafil, vardenafil, or avanafil); concurrent use with riociguat

Canadian labeling: Additional contraindications (not in U.S. labeling): Cardiogenic shock or risk of cardiogenic shock developing

Warnings/Precautions Severe hypotension can occur; paradoxical bradycardia and increased angina pectoris can accompany hypotension. Postural hypotension can also occur; ethanol may potentiate this effect. Use with caution in volume depletion and moderate hypotension, and use with extreme caution with inferior wall MI and suspected right ventricular infarctions. Instruct patients to use caution with ethanol; may increase risk of hypotension. Avoid use in patients with hypertrophic cardiomyopathy (HCM) with outflow tract obstruction; nitrates may reduce preload, exacerbating obstruction and cause hypotension or syncope and/or worsening of heart failure (ACCF/AHA [Gersh, 2011]).

Avoid use of extended release formulations in acute MI or acute HF; cannot easily reverse effects if adverse events develop. Nitrates may precipitate or aggravate increased intracranial pressure and subsequently may worsen clinical outcomes in patients with neurologic injury (eg, intracranial hemorrhage, traumatic brain injury). Appropriate dosing intervals are needed to minimize tolerance development. Tolerance can only be overcome by short periods of nitrate absence from the body. Dose escalation does not overcome this effect. When used for HF in combination with hydralazine, tolerance is less of a concern (Gogia, 1995).

Potentially significant drug-drug interactions may exist, requiring dose or frequency adjustment, additional monitoring, and/or selection of alternative therapy.

Adverse Reactions

Cardiovascular: Crescendo angina (uncommon), hypotension, orthostatic hypotension, rebound hypertension (uncommon), syncope (uncommon)

Central nervous system: Headache (most common), lightheadedness (related to blood pressure changes)

Hematologic: Methemoglobinemia (rare, overdose)

Drug Interactions

Metabolism/Transport Effects **Substrate** of CYP3A4 (major); **Note:** Assignment of Major/Minor substrate status based on clinically relevant drug interaction potential

Avoid Concomitant Use

Avoid concomitant use of Isosorbide Dinitrate with any of the following: Conivaptan; Fusidic Acid (Systemic); Idelalisib; Phosphodiesterase 5 Inhibitors; Riociguat

Increased Effect/Toxicity

Isosorbide Dinitrate may increase the levels/effects of: DULoxetine; Hypotensive Agents; Levodopa; Prilocaine; Riociguat; RisperiDONE; Rosiglitazone; Sodium Nitrite

The levels/effects of Isosorbide Dinitrate may be increased by: Alcohol (Ethyl); Aprepitant; Barbiturates; Ceritinib; Conivaptan; CYP3A4 Inhibitors (Moderate); CYP3A4 Inhibitors (Strong); Dapoxetine; Dasatinib; Fosaprepitant; Fusidic Acid (Systemic); Idelalisib; Ivacaftor; Luliconazole; Mifepristone; Netupitant; Nicorandil; Nitric Oxide; Phosphodiesterase 5 Inhibitors; Simeprevir; Stiripentol

Decreased Effect

The levels/effects of Isosorbide Dinitrate may be decreased by: Bosentan; CYP3A4 Inducers (Moderate); CYP3A4 Inducers (Strong); Dabrafenib; Deferasirox; Mitotane; Siltuximab; St Johns Wort; Tocilizumab

Storage/Stability Store at room temperature. Protect from light and moisture.

Mechanism of Action Stimulation of intracellular cyclic-GMP results in vascular smooth muscle relaxation of both arterial and venous vasculature with more prominent effects on the veins. Primarily reduces cardiac oxygen demand by decreasing preload (left ventricular end-diastolic pressure); may modestly reduce afterload. Additionally, coronary artery dilation improves collateral flow to ischemic regions.

Pharmacodynamics/Kinetics

Onset of action: Sublingual tablet: ~2 to 5 minutes; Oral tablet and capsule (includes extended-release formulations): ~1 hour

Duration: Sublingual tablet: 1 to 2 hours; Oral tablet and capsule (includes extended-release formulations): Up to 8 hours

Distribution: V_d: 2 to 4 L/kg

Metabolism: Extensively hepatic to conjugated metabolites, including isosorbide 5-mononitrate (active) and 2-mononitrate (active)

Bioavailability: Oral immediate release formulations: Highly variable (10% to 90%); increases with chronic therapy

Half-life elimination: Parent drug: ~1 hour; Metabolites (5-mononitrate: 5 hours; 2-mononitrate: 2 hours)

Excretion: Urine and feces

Dosage Note: Due to slower onset of action, not the drug of choice to abort an acute anginal episode. Tolerance to nitrate effects develops with chronic exposure: Dose escalation does not overcome this effect. Tolerance can only be overcome by short periods of nitrate absence from the body. Nitrate-free intervals of ≥14 hours (immediate release products) or >18 hours (sustained release products) may help minimize tolerance.

Adults (elderly should be given lowest recommended daily doses initially and titrate upward):

Angina pectoris:

Oral:

Immediate release: Initial: 5 to 20 mg 2 to 3 times daily; Maintenance: 10 to 40 mg 2 to 3 times daily **or** 5 to 80 mg 2 to 3 times daily (Anderson, 2011)

Sustained release: 40 to 160 mg daily has been used in clinical trials (a nitrate free interval of >18 hours is recommended; however, a clinically efficacious dosage interval has not been clearly established) **or** 40 mg 1 to 2 times daily (Anderson, 2011). Maximum dose: 160 mg/day (Dilatrate-SR only).

Sublingual [Canadian product]: 5 to 10 mg every 2 to 4 hours for prophylaxis of acute angina; may supplement with 5 to 10 mg prior to activities which may provoke an anginal episode.

Heart failure (off-label use; ACCF/AHA [Yancy, 2013]):

Oral: Immediate release (**Note:** Use in combination with hydralazine):

Initial dose: 20 to 30 mg 3 to 4 times daily

Maximum dose: 120 mg daily in divided doses

Esophageal spastic disorders (off-label use; Goyal, 1998):

Oral (immediate release), sublingual: 10 to 30 mg before meals

Dosage adjustment in renal impairment: There are no dosage adjustments provided in manufacturer's labeling.

Hemodialysis: Supplemental dose is not necessary

Peritoneal dialysis: Supplemental dose is not necessary

Dosage adjustment in hepatic impairment: There are no dosage adjustments provided in manufacturer's labeling.

Administration May consider administration of first dose in physician office; observe for maximal cardiovascular dynamic effects and adverse effects (orthostatic hypotension, headache). Do not administer around the clock; allow nitrate-free interval ≥14 hours (immediate release products) and >18 hours (sustained release products). Do not crush sublingual tablets or extended release formulations.

Immediate release products: When prescribed twice daily, consider administering at 8 AM and 1 PM. For 3 times/day dosing, consider 8 AM, 1 PM, and 6 PM.

Sustained release products: Consider once daily in morning or twice-daily dosing at 8 AM and between 1-2 PM.

Monitoring Parameters Blood pressure, heart rate

Product Availability Sublingual tablets have been discontinued in the U.S. for more than 1 year.

Dosage Forms

Capsule Extended Release, Oral:

Dilatrate-SR: 40 mg

Tablet, Oral:

Isordil Titradose: 5 mg, 40 mg

Generic: 5 mg, 10 mg, 20 mg, 30 mg

Tablet Extended Release, Oral:

IsoDitrate ER: 40 mg

Generic: 40 mg

Dosage Forms: Canada

Tablet, Oral: 10 mg, 30 mg

Tablet, Sublingual: 5 mg

Isosorbide Dinitrate and Hydralazine

(eye soe SOR bide dye NYE trate & hye DRAL a zeen)

Brand Names: U.S. BiDil

Index Terms Hydralazine and Isosorbide Dinitrate

Pharmacologic Category Antihypertensive; Vasodilator

Use Treatment of heart failure (HF), adjunct to standard therapy, in self-identified African-Americans

American College of Cardiology/American Heart Association heart failure guidelines recommendations (ACCF/AHA [Yancy, 2013]). Patients who are African-American (self-identified) with heart failure with reduced ejection fraction (HFrEF) NYHA class III-IV remaining symptomatic despite optimal guideline-directed medical therapy; Patients with HFrEF who do not tolerate an ACE inhibitor or an angiotensin receptor blocker (ARB)

Pregnancy Risk Factor C

Dosage Heart failure: Oral: Adults: Initial: 1 tablet 3 times daily; may titrate to a maximum dose of 2 tablets 3 times daily

Dosage adjustment for toxicity: If patient experiences intolerable side effects, dose may be reduced to as little as one-half tablet 3 times/day; dose should be titrated upward as soon as tolerated.

Dosage adjustment in renal impairment: No dosage adjustment provided in manufacturer's labeling (has not been studied).

Dosage adjustment in hepatic impairment: No dosage adjustment provided in manufacturer's labeling (has not been studied).

Additional Information Complete prescribing information should be consulted for additional detail.

Dosage Forms

Tablet:

BiDil®: Isosorbide dinitrate 20 mg and hydralazine 37.5 mg

Isosorbide Mononitrate

(eye soe SOR bide mon oh NYE trate)

Brand Names: U.S. Imdur [DSC]

Brand Names: Canada Apo-ISMN; Imdur; PMS-ISMN; PRO-ISMN

Index Terms ISMN

Pharmacologic Category Antianginal Agent; Vasodilator

Use Prevention of angina pectoris

Pregnancy Risk Factor B/C (manufacturer dependent)

Pregnancy Considerations Adverse events were observed in some animal reproduction studies. Nitric oxide donors, such as isosorbide, have been evaluated for pre-eclampsia and cervical ripening; isosorbide mononitrate use in these conditions is not currently recommended (Kalidindi, 2012; Ramirez, 2011).

Breast-Feeding Considerations It is not known if isosorbide mononitrate is excreted in breast milk. The manufacturer recommends that caution be exercised when administering isosorbide mononitrate to nursing women.

Contraindications Hypersensitivity to isosorbide mononitrate or any component of the formulation; hypersensitivity to organic nitrates; concurrent use with phosphodiesterase-5 (PDE-5) inhibitors (sildenafil, tadalafil, or vardenafil)

Warnings/Precautions Avoid use in hypertrophic cardiomyopathy with outflow tract obstruction; nitrates may reduce preload, exacerbating obstruction and cause hypotension or syncope and/or worsening of heart failure (Gersh, 2011). Use with caution in volume depletion, moderate hypotension, and extreme caution with inferior wall MI and suspected right ventricular infarctions. Instruct patients to use caution with ethanol; may increase risk of hypotension. Nitrates may precipitate or aggravate increased intracranial pressure and subsequently may worsen clinical outcomes in patients with neurologic injury (eg, intracranial hemorrhage, traumatic brain injury). Postural hypotension, transient episodes of weakness, dizziness, or syncope may occur even with small doses; ethanol accentuates these effects; tolerance and cross-tolerance to nitrate antianginal and hemodynamic effects may occur during prolonged isosorbide mononitrate therapy; (minimized by using the smallest effective dose, by alternating coronary vasodilators or offering drug-free intervals of as little as 12 hours). Excessive doses may result in severe headache, blurred vision, or xerostomia; increased anginal symptoms may be a result of dosage increases. Avoid concurrent use with PDE-5 inhibitors (eg, sildenafil, tadalafil, vardenafil). When nitrate administration becomes medically necessary, may administer nitrates only if 24 hours have elapsed after use of sildenafil or vardenafil (48 hours after tadalafil use) (O'Connor, 2010).

Adverse Reactions

Cardiovascular: Angina, flushing

Central nervous system: Dizziness, emotional lability, fatigue, headache, pain

Dermatologic: Pruritus, rash

Gastrointestinal: Abdominal pain, diarrhea, nausea

Respiratory: Cough increased, upper respiratory infection

Miscellaneous: Allergic reaction

Rare but important or life-threatening: Apoplexy, arrhythmia, bradycardia, dyspnea, edema, hyper-/hypotension, methemoglobinemia (rare, overdose), MI, orthostatic hypotension, pallor, palpitation, paresthesia, tachycardia

Drug Interactions

Metabolism/Transport Effects Substrate of CYP3A4 (major); **Note:** Assignment of Major/Minor substrate status based on clinically relevant drug interaction potential

Avoid Concomitant Use

Avoid concomitant use of Isosorbide Mononitrate with any of the following: Conivaptan; Fusidic Acid (Systemic); Idelalisib; Phosphodiesterase 5 Inhibitors; Riociguat

Increased Effect/Toxicity

Isosorbide Mononitrate may increase the levels/effects of: DULoxetine; Hypotensive Agents; Levodopa; Prilocaine; Riociguat; RisperiDONE; Rosiglitazone; Sodium Nitrite

The levels/effects of Isosorbide Mononitrate may be increased by: Alcohol (Ethyl); Aprepitant; Barbiturates; Ceritinib; Conivaptan; CYP3A4 Inhibitors (Moderate); CYP3A4 Inhibitors (Strong); Dapoxetine; Dasatinib; Fosaprepitant; Fusidic Acid (Systemic); Idelalisib; Ivacaftor; Luliconazole; Mifepristone; Netupitant; Nicorandil; Nitric Oxide; Phosphodiesterase 5 Inhibitors; Simeprevir; Stiripentol

Decreased Effect

The levels/effects of Isosorbide Mononitrate may be decreased by: Bosentan; CYP3A4 Inducers (Moderate); CYP3A4 Inducers (Strong); Dabrafenib; Deferasirox; Mitotane; Siltuximab; St Johns Wort; Tocilizumab

Storage/Stability Tablets should be stored in a tight container at room temperature of 15°C to 30°C (59°F to 86°F).

Mechanism of Action Nitroglycerin and other nitrates form free radical nitric oxide. In smooth muscle, nitric oxide activates guanylate cyclase which increases guanosine 3'5' monophosphate (cGMP) leading to dephosphorylation of myosin light chains and smooth muscle relaxation. Produces a vasodilator effect on the peripheral veins and arteries with more prominent effects on the veins. Primarily reduces cardiac oxygen demand by decreasing preload (left ventricular end-diastolic pressure); may modestly reduce afterload; dilates coronary arteries and improves collateral flow to ischemic regions.

Pharmacodynamics/Kinetics

Onset of action: 30 to 60 minutes

Duration: Immediate release: ≥6 hours (Thadani, 1987); Extended release: ≥12 to 24 hours (Anderson, 2007)

Absorption: Nearly complete and low intersubject variability in its pharmacokinetic parameters and plasma concentrations

Distribution: V_d: ~0.6 L/kg

Protein binding: <5%

Metabolism: Hepatic

Bioavailability: ~100%

Half-life elimination: Mononitrate: ~5 to 6 hours

Excretion: Predominantly urine (2% as unchanged drug); feces (1% of dose)

Dosage Oral:

Adults:

Regular release tablet: Initial: 5 to 20 mg twice daily with the 2 doses given 7 hours apart (eg, 8 AM and 3 PM) to decrease tolerance development; patients initiating therapy with 5 mg twice daily (eg, small stature) should be titrated up to 10 mg twice daily in first 2 to 3 days.

Extended release tablet: Initial: 30 to 60 mg given once daily in the morning; titrate upward as needed, giving at least 3 days between increases; maximum daily single dose: 240 mg

Elderly: Start with lowest recommended adult dose.

Dosage adjustment in renal impairment: Dose adjustment not necessary

Hemodialysis: Dose supplementation is not necessary.

Peritoneal dialysis: Dose supplementation is not necessary.

Dosage adjustment in hepatic impairment: Dose adjustment not necessary

Note: Tolerance to nitrate effects develops with chronic exposure. Dose escalation does not overcome this effect. Tolerance can only be overcome by short periods of nitrate absence from the body. Short periods of nitrate withdrawal may help minimize tolerance. Recommended twice daily dosage regimens incorporate this interval. Administer sustained release tablet once daily in the morning.

Administration Do not administer around-the-clock. Immediate release tablet should be scheduled twice daily with doses 7 hours apart (8 AM and 3 PM); extended release tablet may be administered once daily in the morning upon rising with a half-glassful of fluid. Do not chew or crush extended release tablets. Due to insoluble matrix embedding, extended release tablets that are scored may be split (Gunasekara, 1999).

Monitoring Parameters Monitor for orthostasis, increased hypotension

Dosage Forms

Tablet, Oral:

Generic: 10 mg, 20 mg

Tablet Extended Release 24 Hour, Oral:

Generic: 30 mg, 60 mg, 120 mg

◆ **Isotamine (Can)** *see* Isoniazid *on page 1120*

ISOtretinoin (eye soe TRET i noyn)

Brand Names: U.S. Absorica; Amnesteem; Claravis; Myorisan; Zenatane

Brand Names: Canada Accutane; Clarus; Epuris

Index Terms 13-*cis*-Retinoic Acid; 13-*cis*-Vitamin A Acid; 13-CRA; *Cis*-Retinoic Acid; Accutane; Isotretinoinum

Pharmacologic Category Acne Products; Antineoplastic Agent, Retinoic Acid Derivative; Retinoic Acid Derivative

Use Treatment of severe recalcitrant nodular acne unresponsive to conventional therapy

Pregnancy Risk Factor X

Pregnancy Considerations Isotretinoin and its metabolites can be detected in fetal tissue following maternal use during pregnancy (Benifla, 1995; Kraft, 1989). **[U.S. Boxed Warnings]: Use of isotretinoin is contraindicated in females who are or may become pregnant. Birth defects (facial, eye, ear, skull, central nervous system, cardiovascular, thymus and parathyroid gland abnormalities) have been noted following isotretinoin exposure during pregnancy and the risk for severe birth defects is high, with any dose or even with short treatment duration. Low IQ scores have also been reported. The risk for spontaneous abortion and premature births is increased. Because of the high likelihood of teratogenic effects, all patients (male and female), prescribers, wholesalers, and dispensing pharmacists must register and be active in the iPLEDGE™ risk evaluation and mitigation strategy (REMS) program; do not prescribe isotretinoin for women who are or who are likely to become pregnant while using the drug. If pregnancy occurs during therapy, isotretinoin should be discontinued immediately and the patient referred to an obstetrician-gynecologist specializing in reproductive toxicity.** This medication is contraindicated in females of childbearing potential unless they are able to comply with the guidelines of the iPLEDGE™ pregnancy prevention program. Females of childbearing potential must have two negative pregnancy tests with a sensitivity of at least 25 mIU/mL prior to beginning therapy and testing should continue monthly during therapy. Females of childbearing potential should not become pregnant during therapy or for 1 month following discontinuation of isotretinoin. Upon discontinuation of treatment, females of childbearing potential should have a pregnancy test after their last dose and again one month after their last dose. Two forms of contraception should be continued during this time. Any pregnancies should be reported to the iPLEDGE™ program (www.ipledgeprogram.com or 866-495-0654) and the FDA through MedWatch (800-FDA-1088).

Breast-Feeding Considerations It is not known if isotretinoin is excreted in breast milk. A case report describes a green discharge from the breast of a nonlactating woman which was determined to be iatrogenic galactorrhea due to isotretinoin (Larsen, 1985). Due to the potential for serious adverse reactions in the nursing infant, the manufacturer recommends a decision be made whether to discontinue nursing or to discontinue the drug, taking into account the importance of treatment to the mother.

Contraindications Hypersensitivity to isotretinoin or any component of the formulation; sensitivity to parabens, vitamin A, or other retinoids; pregnant women or those who may become pregnant

Warnings/Precautions Hazardous agent - use appropriate precautions for handling and disposal (meets NIOSH 2014 criteria). This medication should only be prescribed by prescribers competent in treating severe recalcitrant nodular acne and experienced with the use of systemic retinoids. Anaphylaxis and other types of allergic reactions, including cutaneous reactions and allergic vasculitis, have been reported. **[U.S. Boxed Warnings]: Birth defects**

(facial, eye, ear, skull, central nervous system, cardiovascular, thymus and parathyroid gland abnormalities) have been noted following isotretinoin exposure during pregnancy and the risk for severe birth defects is high, with any dose or even with short treatment duration. Low IQ scores have also been reported. The risk for spontaneous abortion and premature births is increased. Because of the high likelihood of teratogenic effects, all patients (male and female), prescribers, wholesalers, and dispensing pharmacists must register and be active in the iPLEDGE™ risk evaluation and mitigation strategy (REMS) program; do not prescribe isotretinoin for women who are or who are likely to become pregnant while using the drug. If pregnancy occurs during therapy, isotretinoin should be discontinued immediately and the patient referred to an obstetrician-gynecologist specializing in reproductive toxicity (see Additional Information for details). Women of childbearing potential must be capable of complying with effective contraceptive measures. Patients must select and commit to two forms of contraception. Therapy is begun after two negative pregnancy tests; effective contraception must be used for at least 1 month before beginning therapy, during therapy, and for 1 month after discontinuation of therapy. Prescriptions should be written for no more than a 30-day supply, and pregnancy testing and counseling should be repeated monthly.

May cause depression, psychosis, aggressive or violent behavior, and changes in mood; use with extreme caution in patients with psychiatric disorders. Rarely, suicidal thoughts and actions have been reported during isotretinoin usage. All patients should be observed closely for symptoms of depression or suicidal thoughts. Discontinuation of treatment alone may not be sufficient, further evaluation may be necessary. Cases of pseudotumor cerebri (benign intracranial hypertension) have been reported, some with concomitant use of tetracycline (avoid using together). Patients with papilledema, headache, nausea, vomiting, and visual disturbances should be referred to a neurologist and treatment with isotretinoin discontinued. Hearing impairment, which can continue after therapy is discontinued, may occur. Clinical hepatitis, elevated liver enzymes, inflammatory bowel disease, skeletal hyperostosis, premature epiphyseal closure, vision impairment, corneal opacities, decreased tolerance to contact lenses (due to dry eyes), and decreased night vision have also been reported with the use of isotretinoin. Rare postmarketing cases of severe skin reactions (eg, Stevens-Johnson syndrome, erythema multiforme) have been reported with use.

Use with caution in patients with diabetes mellitus; impaired glucose control has been reported. Use caution in patients with hypertriglyceridemia; acute pancreatitis and fatal hemorrhagic pancreatitis (rare) have been reported. Instruct patients to avoid or limit ethanol; may increase triglyceride levels if taken in excess. Bone mineral density may decrease; use caution in patients with a genetic predisposition to bone disorders (ie, osteoporosis, osteomalacia) and with disease states or concomitant medications that can induce bone disorders. Patients may be at risk when participating in activities with repetitive impact (such as sports). Patients should be instructed not to donate blood during therapy and for 1 month following discontinuation of therapy due to risk of donated blood being given to a pregnant female. Safety of long-term use is not established and is not recommended.

Absorica™: Absorption is ~83% greater than Accutane® when administered under fasting conditions; they are bioequivalent when taken with a high-fat meal. Absorica™ is **not** interchangeable with other generic isotretinoin products. Isotretinoin and tretinoin (which is also known as all-*trans* retinoic acid, or ATRA) may be confused, while both products may be used in cancer treatment, they are **not** interchangeable; verify product prior to dispensing and administration to prevent medication errors.

Adverse Reactions

Cardiovascular: Chest pain, edema, flushing, palpitation, stroke, syncope, tachycardia, vascular thrombotic disease

Central nervous system: Aggressive behavior, depression, dizziness, drowsiness, emotional instability, fatigue, headache, insomnia, lethargy, malaise, nervousness, paresthesia, pseudotumor cerebri, psychosis, seizure, stroke, suicidal ideation, suicide attempts, suicide, violent behavior

Dermatologic: Abnormal wound healing acne fulminans, alopecia, bruising, cheilitis, cutaneous allergic reactions, dry nose, dry skin, eczema, eruptive xanthomas, facial erythema, fragility of skin, hair abnormalities, hirsutism, hyperpigmentation, hypopigmentation, increased sunburn susceptibility, nail dystrophy, paronychia, peeling of palms, peeling of soles, photoallergic reactions, photosensitizing reactions, pruritus, purpura, rash

Endocrine & metabolic: Abnormal menses, blood glucose increased, cholesterol increased, HDL decreased, hyperuricemia, triglycerides increased

Gastrointestinal: Bleeding and inflammation of the gums, colitis, esophagitis, esophageal ulceration, inflammatory bowel disease, nausea, nonspecific gastrointestinal symptoms, pancreatitis, weight loss, xerostomia

Genitourinary: Nonspecific urogenital findings

Hematologic: Agranulocytosis (rare), anemia, neutropenia, pyogenic granuloma, thrombocytopenia

Hepatic: Alkaline phosphatase increased, ALT increased, AST increased, GGTP increased, hepatitis, LDH increased

Neuromuscular & skeletal: Arthralgia, arthritis, back pain, bone abnormalities, bone mineral density decreased, calcification of tendons and ligaments, CPK increased, myalgia, premature epiphyseal closure, skeletal hyperostosis, tendonitis, weakness

Ocular: Blepharitis, cataracts, chalazion, color vision disorder, conjunctivitis, corneal opacities, eyelid inflammation, hordeolum, keratitis, night vision decreased, optic neuritis, photophobia, visual disturbances

Otic: Hearing impairment, tinnitus

Renal: Glomerulonephritis, hematuria, proteinuria, pyuria, vasculitis

Respiratory: Bronchospasms, epistaxis, respiratory infection, voice alteration, Wegener's granulomatosis

Miscellaneous: Allergic reactions, anaphylactic reactions, disseminated herpes simplex, diaphoresis, infection, lymphadenopathy

Rare but important or life-threatening: Abnormal meibomian gland secretion, erythema multiforme, meibomian gland atrophy, myopia, pseudotumor cerebri, rhabdomyolysis, Stevens-Johnson syndrome, toxic epidermal necrolysis, visual acuity decreased

Drug Interactions

Metabolism/Transport Effects None known.

Avoid Concomitant Use

Avoid concomitant use of ISOtretinoin with any of the following: Multivitamins/Fluoride (with ADE); Multivitamins/Minerals (with ADEK, Folate, Iron); Multivitamins/Minerals (with AE, No Iron); Tetracycline Derivatives; Vitamin A

Increased Effect/Toxicity

ISOtretinoin may increase the levels/effects of: Mipomersen; Porfimer; Verteporfin; Vitamin A

The levels/effects of ISOtretinoin may be increased by: Alcohol (Ethyl); Multivitamins/Fluoride (with ADE); Multivitamins/Minerals (with ADEK, Folate, Iron); Multivitamins/Minerals (with AE, No Iron); Tetracycline Derivatives

Decreased Effect

ISOtretinoin may decrease the levels/effects of: Contraceptives (Estrogens); Contraceptives (Progestins)

Food Interactions Isotretinoin bioavailability increased if taken with food or milk. Management: Administer orally with a meal (except Absorica™ which may be taken without regard to meals).

Storage/Stability Store at 20°C to 25°C (68°F to 77°F); excursions permitted between 15°C to 30°C (59°F to 86°F). Protect from light.

Mechanism of Action Reduces sebaceous gland size and reduces sebum production in acne treatment; in neuroblastoma, decreases cell proliferation and induces differentiation

Pharmacodynamics/Kinetics

Absorption: Enhanced with a high-fat meal; Absorica™ absorption is ~83% greater than Accutane® when administered under fasting conditions; they are bioequivalent when taken with a high-fat meal.

Protein binding: 99% to 100%; primarily albumin

Metabolism: Hepatic via CYP2B6, 2C8, 2C9, 2D6, 3A4; forms metabolites; major metabolite: 4-oxo-isotretinoin (active)

Half-life elimination: Terminal: Parent drug: 21 hours; Metabolite: 21-24 hours

Time to peak, serum: 3-5 hours

Excretion: Urine and feces (equal amounts)

Dosage Oral:

Children 1-17 years: Neuroblastoma, high-risk (off-label use): 160 mg/m^2/day (in 2 divided doses) days 1 through 14 every 28 days for 6 cycles, beginning after continuation chemotherapy or transplantation (Matthay, 1999)

Children 12-17 years and Adults:

Acne, severe recalcitrant nodular: 0.5-1 mg/kg/day in 2 divided doses for 15-20 weeks; may discontinue earlier if the total cyst count decreases by 70%. Adults with very severe disease/scarring or primarily involves the trunk may require dosage adjustment up to 2 mg/kg/day. A second course of therapy may be initiated after a period of ≥2 months off therapy. A dose of ≤0.5 mg/kg/day may be used to minimize initial flaring (Strauss, 2007).

Acne, moderate (off-label use): 20 mg/day (~0.3-0.4 mg/kg/day) for 6 months (Amichai, 2006)

Dosing adjustment in renal impairment: No dosage adjustment provided in the manufacturer's labeling.

Dosing adjustment in hepatic impairment:

Hepatic impairment prior to treatment: No dosage adjustment provided in the manufacturer's labeling.

Hepatotoxicity during treatment: Liver enzymes may normalize with dosage reduction or with continued treatment; discontinue if normalization does not readily occur or if hepatitis is suspected.

Dietary Considerations Should be taken with food, except Absorbica™ which may be taken without regard to meals. Limit intake of vitamin A; avoid use of other vitamin A products. Some formulations may contain soybean oil.

Administration Administer orally with a meal (except Absorica™ which may be taken without regard to meals). According to the manufacturers' labeling, capsules should be swallowed whole with a full glass of liquid. For patients unable to swallow capsule whole, an oral liquid may be prepared; may irritate esophagus if contents are removed from the capsule.

Hazardous agent; use appropriate precautions for handling and disposal (meets NIOSH 2014 criteria).

Monitoring Parameters CBC with differential and platelet count, baseline sedimentation rate, glucose, CPK; signs of depression, mood alteration, psychosis, aggression, severe skin reactions

Pregnancy test (for all female patients of childbearing potential): Two negative tests with a sensitivity of at least 25 mIU/mL prior to beginning therapy (the second performed at least 19 days after the first test and performed during the first 5 days of the menstrual period immediately preceding the start of therapy); monthly tests to rule out pregnancy prior to refilling prescription.

Lipids: Prior to treatment and at weekly or biweekly intervals until response to treatment is established. Test should not be performed <36 hours after consumption of ethanol.

Liver function tests: Prior to treatment and at weekly or biweekly intervals until response to treatment is established.

Additional Information All patients (male and female), must be registered in the iPLEDGE™ risk management program. Females of childbearing potential must receive oral and written information reviewing the hazards of therapy and the effects that isotretinoin can have on a fetus. Therapy should not begin without two negative pregnancy tests at least 19 days apart. Two forms of contraception (a primary and secondary form as described in the iPLEDGE™ program materials) must be used simultaneously beginning 1 month prior to treatment, during treatment, and for 1 month after therapy is discontinued; limitations to their use must be explained. Microdosed progesterone products that do not contain an estrogen ("mini-pills") are not an acceptable form of contraception during isotretinoin treatment. Prescriptions should be written for no more than a 30-day supply, and pregnancy testing and counseling should be repeated monthly. During therapy, pregnancy tests must be conducted by a CLIA-certified laboratory. Prescriptions must be filled and picked up from the pharmacy within 7 days of specimen collection for pregnancy test for women of childbearing potential. Prescriptions for males and females of nonchildbearing potential must be filled and picked up within 30 days of prescribing.

Any cases of accidental pregnancy should be reported to the iPLEDGE™ program or FDA MedWatch. All patients (male and female) must read and sign the informed consent material provided in the pregnancy prevention program.

Dosage Forms

Capsule, Oral:

Absorica: 10 mg, 20 mg, 25 mg, 30 mg, 35 mg, 40 mg

Amnesteem: 10 mg, 20 mg, 40 mg

Claravis: 10 mg, 20 mg, 30 mg, 40 mg

Myorisan: 10 mg, 20 mg, 40 mg

Zenatane: 10 mg, 20 mg, 40 mg

Extemporaneous Preparations Hazardous agent: Use appropriate precautions for handling and disposal of teratogenic capsule contents (meets NIOSH 2014 criteria).

For patients unable to swallow the capsules whole, an oral liquid may be prepared with softgel capsules (not recommended by the manufacturers) by one of the following methods:

Place capsules (softgel formulations only) in small container and add warm (~37°C [97°F]) water or milk to cover capsule(s); wait 2-3 minutes until capsule is softened and then drink the milk or water with the softened capsule, or swallow softened capsule.

Puncture capsule (softgel formulations only) with needle or cut with scissors; squeeze capsule contents into 5-10 mL of milk or tube feed formula; draw mixture up into oral syringe and administer via feeding tube; flush feeding tube with ≥30 mL additional milk or tube feeding formula.

Puncture capsule (softgel formulations only) with needle or cut with scissors and draw contents into oral syringe; add 1-5 mL of medium chain triglyceride, soybean, or safflower oil to the oral syringe; mix gently and administer via feeding tube; flush feeding tube with ≥30 mL milk or tube feeding formula.

Lam MS, "Extemporaneous Compounding of Oral Liquid Dosage Formulations and Alternative Drug Delivery Methods for Anticancer Drugs," *Pharmacotherapy*, 2011, 31(2):164-92.

◆ **Isotretinoinum** *see* ISOtretinoin *on page* *1127*

Isradipine (iz RA di peen)

Pharmacologic Category Antihypertensive; Calcium Channel Blocker; Calcium Channel Blocker, Dihydropyridine

Use Hypertension: Management of hypertension (may be used alone or concurrently with thiazide-type diuretics).

The 2014 guideline for the management of high blood pressure in adults (JNC 8) recommends initiation of pharmacologic treatment to lower blood pressure for the following patients (JNC8 [James, 2013]):

- Patients ≥60 years of age, with systolic blood pressure (SBP) ≥150 mm Hg or diastolic blood pressure (DBP) ≥90 mm Hg. Goal of therapy is SBP <150 mm Hg and DBP <90 mm Hg.
- Patients <60 years of age, with SBP ≥140 mm Hg or DBP ≥90 mm Hg. Goal of therapy is SBP <140 mm Hg and DBP <90 mm Hg.
- Patients ≥18 years of age with diabetes, with SBP ≥140 mm Hg or DBP ≥90 mm Hg. Goal of therapy is SBP <140 mm Hg and DBP <90 mm Hg.
- Patients ≥18 years of age with chronic kidney disease (CKD), with SBP ≥140 mm Hg or DBP ≥90 mm Hg. Goal of therapy is SBP <140 mm Hg and DBP <90 mm Hg.

In patients with chronic kidney disease (CKD), regardless of race or diabetes status, the use of an ACE inhibitor (ACEI) or angiotensin receptor blocker (ARB) as initial therapy is recommended to improve kidney outcomes. In the general nonblack population (without CKD) including those with diabetes, initial antihypertensive treatment should consist of a thiazide-type diuretic, calcium channel blocker, ACEI, or ARB. In the general black population (without CKD) including those with diabetes, initial antihypertensive treatment should consist of a thiazide-type diuretic or a calcium channel blocker **instead of** an ACEI or ARB.

Pregnancy Risk Factor C

Dosage Hypertension: Oral:

Children (off-label use): Initial: 0.15-0.2 mg/kg/day in 3-4 divided doses; maximum 0.8 mg/kg/day, up to 20 mg daily (NHBPEP, 2004).

Adults: 2.5 mg twice daily; antihypertensive response occurs in 2-3 hours; maximal response in 2-4 weeks; increase dose at 2- to 4-week intervals at 2.5-5 mg increments; usual dose range (ASH/ISH [Weber, 2014]): 5-10 mg twice daily. **Note:** Most patients show no improvement with doses >10 mg daily except adverse reaction rate increases; therefore, maximal dose in older adults should be 10 mg daily.

Elderly: Refer to adult dosing.

Dosage adjustment in renal impairment: There are no dosage adjustments provided in manufacturer's labeling; however, bioavailability is increased with mild renal impairment and decreased with severe renal impairment. Other sources recommend that no initial dosage adjustment is required (Aronoff, 2007). Isradipine is not removed by hemodialysis; therefore, supplemental doses after hemodialysis are not necessary (Schonholzer, 1992).

Dosage adjustment in hepatic impairment: There are no dosage adjustments provided in manufacturer's labeling; however, peak serum concentrations are increased by 32% and bioavailability is increased by 52%.

Additional Information Complete prescribing information should be consulted for additional detail.

Dosage Forms

Capsule, Oral:

Generic: 2.5 mg, 5 mg

◆ **Istalol** *see* Timolol (Ophthalmic) *on page* *2043*

◆ **Istodax** *see* RomiDEPsin *on page* *1841*

◆ **Isuprel** *see* Isoproterenol *on page* *1124*

Itopride [INT] (EYE to pride)

International Brand Names Aflusan (AR); Ampty (IN); Ao Wei Xian (CN); Dagla (DO, GT, MX); Elthon (CN, VN); Ganaton (IN, JP, KW, LB, PH, PK, RU, TH); Gapraton (KR); Gapride (KR); Gatof (KR); Itoprid (AR, IN); Itzodial (KR); Nogerd (PK); Tespral (PK); Wei Tai (CN); Zirid (EE)

Index Terms Itopride Hydrochloride

Pharmacologic Category Gastrointestinal Agent, Prokinetic

Reported Use Treatment of gastrointestinal symptoms caused by reduced gastrointestinal motility.

Dosage Range Adults: Oral: 50 mg 3 times/day before meals

Product Availability Product available in various countries; not currently available in the U.S.

Dosage Forms

Tablet: 50 mg

◆ **Itopride Hydrochloride** *see* Itopride [INT] *on page* *1130*

Itraconazole (i tra KOE na zole)

Brand Names: U.S. Onmel; Sporanox; Sporanox Pulsepak

Brand Names: Canada Sporanox

Pharmacologic Category Antifungal Agent, Oral

Use

Aspergillosis (capsules): Treatment of pulmonary and extrapulmonary aspergillosis in immunocompromised and nonimmunocompromised patients who are intolerant of or refractory to amphotericin B therapy.

Blastomycosis (capsules): Treatment of pulmonary and extrapulmonary blastomycosis in immunocompromised and nonimmunocompromised patients.

Histoplasmosis (capsules): Treatment of histoplasmosis, including chronic cavitary pulmonary disease and disseminated, nonmeningeal histoplasmosis in immunocompromised and nonimmunocompromised patients.

Onychomycosis:

Capsules: Treatment of onychomycosis of the toenail, with or without fingernail involvement, and onychomycosis of the fingernail caused by dermatophytes (tinea unguium) in nonimmunocompromised patients

Tablets: Treatment of onychomycosis of the toenail caused by *Trichophyton rubrum* or *Trichophyton mentagrophytes* in nonimmunocompromised patients

Oropharyngeal/Esophageal candidiasis (oral solution): Treatment of oropharyngeal and esophageal candidiasis

Canadian labeling: Oral capsules: Additional indications (not in U.S. labeling):

Candidiasis, oral and/or esophageal: Treatment of oral and/or esophageal candidiasis in immunocompromised and immunocompetent patients

Chromomycosis: Treatment of chromomycosis in immunocompromised and immunocompetent patients

Dermatomycoses: Treatment of dermatomycoses due to tinea pedis, tinea cruris, tinea corporis, and of pityriasis versicolor in patients for whom oral therapy is appropriate

Onychomycosis: Treatment of onychomycosis in immunocompromised and immunocompetent patients

Paracoccidioidomycosis: Treatment of paracoccidioidomycosis in immunocompromised and immunocompetent patients

Sporotrichosis: Treatment of cutaneous and lymphatic sporotrichosis in immunocompromised and immunocompetent patients

Pregnancy Risk Factor C

Pregnancy Considerations Dose related adverse events were observed in animal reproduction studies. Use is contraindicated for the treatment of onychomycosis during pregnancy. If used for the treatment of onychomycosis in women of reproductive potential, effective contraception should be used during treatment and for 2 months following treatment. Therapy should begin on the second or third day following menses. Congenital abnormalities have been reported during postmarketing surveillance, but a causal relationship has not been established. The Canadian labeling contraindicates use in the treatment of onychomycosis or dermatomycoses (tinea corporis, tinea cruris, tinea pedis, pityriasis versicolor) in women who are pregnant or intend to become pregnant.

Breast-Feeding Considerations Itraconazole is excreted in breast milk. According to the manufacturer, the decision to continue or discontinue breast-feeding during therapy should take into account the risk of exposure to the infant and the benefits of treatment to the mother.

Contraindications

Hypersensitivity to itraconazole or any component of the formulation; concurrent administration with cisapride, disopyramide, dofetilide, dronedarone, eplerenone, ergot derivatives, felodipine, irinotecan, lovastatin, lurasidone, methadone, midazolam (oral), nisoldipine, pimozide, quinidine, ranolazine, simvastatin, or triazolam; concurrent administration with colchicine in patients with renal or hepatic impairment; treatment of onychomycosis (or other non-life-threatening indications) in patients with evidence of ventricular dysfunction, heart failure (HF) or a history of HF; treatment of onychomycosis in women who are pregnant or intend to become pregnant

Canadian labeling: Additional contraindications (not in U.S. labeling): Concurrent administration with levacetylmethadol (not available in Canada) or eletriptan (capsule, oral solution); treatment of dermatomycosis (tinea pedis, tinea cruris, tinea corporis, pityriasis versicolor) in women who are pregnant or intend to become pregnant (capsule)

Warnings/Precautions [U.S. Boxed Warning]: Negative inotropic effects have been observed following intravenous administration. Discontinue or reassess use if signs or symptoms of HF (heart failure) occur during treatment. [U.S. Boxed Warning]: Use is contraindicated for treatment of onychomycosis in patients with ventricular dysfunction or a history of HF. Cases of HF, peripheral edema, and pulmonary edema have occurred in patients treated for onychomycosis. HF has been reported, particularly in patients receiving a total daily oral dose of 400 mg. Use with caution in patients with risk factors for HF (COPD, renal failure, edematous disorders, ischemic or valvular disease). Discontinue if signs or symptoms of HF or neuropathy occur during treatment. Due to potential toxicity, the manufacturer recommends confirmation of diagnosis testing of nail specimens prior to treatment of onychomycosis. The Canadian labeling contraindicates use in the treatment of dermatomycoses (tinea corporis, tinea cruris, tinea pedis, pityriasis versicolor) in patients with evidence of ventricular dysfunction or a history of HF.

[U.S. Boxed Warning]: Coadministration with itraconazole can cause elevated plasma concentrations of certain drugs and can lead to QT prolongation and ventricular tachyarrhythmias, including torsades de pointes. Coadministration with methadone, disopyramide, dofetilide, dronedarone, quinidine, ergot alkaloids, irinotecan, lurasidone, oral midazolam, pimozide, triazolam, felodipine, nisoldipine, ranolazine, eplerenone, cisapride, lovastatin, simvastatin and, in subjects with renal or hepatic impairment, colchicine, is contraindicated. The Canadian labeling additionally contraindicates coadministration with eletriptan. Additional potentially significant interactions may exist, requiring dose or frequency adjustment, additional monitoring, and/or selection of alternative therapy.

May cause CNS depression, which may impair physical or mental abilities; patients must be cautioned about performing tasks that require mental alertness (eg, operating machinery, driving). Use with caution in patients with renal impairment; dosage adjustment may be needed. Use caution in patients with a history of hypersensitivity to other azoles. Rare cases of serious hepatotoxicity (including liver failure and death) have been reported (including some cases occurring within the first week of therapy); hepatotoxicity was reported in some patients without preexisting liver disease or risk factors. Use with caution in patients with preexisting hepatic impairment; monitor liver function closely. Not recommended for use in patients with active liver disease, elevated liver enzymes, or prior hepatotoxic reactions to other drugs unless the expected benefit exceeds the risk of hepatotoxicity. Discontinue treatment if signs or symptoms of hepatotoxicity develop. Transient or permanent hearing loss has been reported. Quinidine (a contraindicated drug) was used concurrently in several of these cases. Hearing loss usually resolves after discontinuation, but may persist in some patients.

Large differences in itraconazole pharmacokinetic parameters have been observed in cystic fibrosis patients receiving the solution; if a patient with cystic fibrosis does not respond to therapy, alternate therapies should be considered. Due to differences in bioavailability, oral capsules and oral solution cannot be used interchangeably. Only the oral solution has proven efficacy for oral and esophageal candidiasis. Initiation of treatment with oral solution is not recommended in patients at immediate risk for systemic candidiasis (eg, patients with severe neutropenia). Absorption of itraconazole capsules is reduced when gastric acidity is reduced; administer capsules or tablets with an acidic beverage (eg, cola) in patients with reduced gastric acidity and separate administration from acid suppressive therapy. The Canadian labeling contraindicates use in the treatment of dermatomycoses (tinea corporis, tinea cruris, tinea pedis, pityriasis versicolor) in women who are pregnant or intend to become pregnant.

Adverse Reactions

Cardiovascular: Chest pain, edema, hypertension

Central nervous system: Abnormal dreams, anxiety, depression, dizziness, fatigue, headache, malaise, pain

Dermatologic: Diaphoresis, pruritus, skin rash

Endocrine & metabolic: Hypertriglyceridemia, hypokalemia

Gastrointestinal: Abdominal pain, aphthous stomatitis, constipation, diarrhea, dyspepsia, flatulence, gastritis, gastroenteritis, gastrointestinal disease, gingivitis, increased appetite, nausea, vomiting

Genitourinary: Cystitis, urinary tract infection

Hepatic: Abnormal hepatic function tests, increased liver enzymes
Infection: Herpes zoster
Neuromuscular & skeletal: Bursitis, myalgia, tremor, weakness
Respiratory: Cough, dyspnea, increased bronchial secretions, pharyngitis, pneumonia, rhinitis, sinusitis, upper respiratory tract infection
Miscellaneous: Fever
Rare but important or life-threatening: Abnormal urinalysis, acute generalized exanthematous pustulosis, adrenal insufficiency, albuminuria, anaphylactoid reaction, anaphylaxis, angioedema, cardiac arrhythmia, cardiac failure, confusion, congestive heart failure, dehydration, dysphagia, erythema multiforme, erythematous rash, exfoliative dermatitis, gastrointestinal disease, gynecomastia, hearing loss, hematuria, hepatic failure, hepatitis, hepatotoxicity, hyperbilirubinemia, hyperglycemia, hyperhidrosis, hyperkalemia, hypersensitivity angiitis, hypersensitivity reaction, hypomagnesemia, increased blood urea nitrogen, increased creatine phosphokinase, increased gamma-glutamyl transferase, increased lactate dehydrogenase, increased serum alkaline phosphatase, increased serum ALT, increased serum AST, left heart failure, leukopenia, menstrual disease, mucosal inflammation, neutropenia, orthostatic hypotension, pancreatitis, paresthesia, peripheral edema, pollakiuria, pulmonary edema, renal insufficiency, rigors, serum sickness, sinus bradycardia, Stevens-Johnson syndrome, tachycardia, thrombocytopenia, toxic epidermal necrolysis, vasculitis, voice disorder

Drug Interactions

Metabolism/Transport Effects Substrate of CYP3A4 (major); **Note:** Assignment of Major/Minor substrate status based on clinically relevant drug interaction potential; **Inhibits** CYP3A4 (strong), P-glycoprotein

Avoid Concomitant Use

Avoid concomitant use of Itraconazole with any of the following: Ado-Trastuzumab Emtansine; Alfuzosin; Aliskiren; ALPRAZolam; Apixaban; Astemizole; Avanafil; Axitinib; Bosutinib; Cabozantinib; Ceritinib; Cisapride; Conivaptan; Crizotinib; CYP3A4 Inducers (Strong); Dapoxetine; Dihydroergotamine; Disopyramide; Dofetilide; Dronedarone; Efavirenz; Eletriptan; Eplerenone; Ergoloid Mesylates; Ergonovine; Ergotamine; Estazolam; Everolimus; Felodipine; Fusidic Acid (Systemic); Halofantrine; Ibrutinib; Idelalisib; Irinotecan; Ivabradine; Lapatinib; Lercanidipine; Lomitapide; Lovastatin; Lurasidone; Macitentan; Methadone; Methylergonovine; Midazolam; Naloxegol; Nevirapine; Nilotinib; Nisoldipine; Olaparib; PAZOPanib; Pimozide; QuiNIDine; Ranolazine; Red Yeast Rice; Regorafenib; Rivaroxaban; Saccharomyces boulardii; Salmeterol; Silodosin; Simeprevir; Simvastatin; Suvorexant; Tamsulosin; Terfenadine; Ticagrelor; Tolvaptan; Topotecan; Toremifene; Trabectedin; Triazolam; Ulipristal; Vemurafenib; VinCRIStine (Liposomal); Vorapaxar

Increased Effect/Toxicity

Itraconazole may increase the levels/effects of: Ado-Trastuzumab Emtansine; Afatinib; Alfuzosin; Aliskiren; Almotriptan; Alosetron; ALPRAZolam; Apixaban; ARIPiprazole; Astemizole; AtorvaSTATin; Avanafil; Axitinib; Bedaquiline; Boceprevir; Bortezomib; Bosentan; Bosutinib; Brentuximab Vedotin; Brinzolamide; Budesonide (Nasal); Budesonide (Systemic, Oral Inhalation); BusPIRone; Busulfan; Cabazitaxel; Cabozantinib; Calcium Channel Blockers; Cannabis; Cardiac Glycosides; Ceritinib; Cilostazol; Cisapride; Cobicistat; Colchicine; Conivaptan; Corticosteroids (Orally Inhaled); Corticosteroids (Systemic); Crizotinib; CycloSPORINE (Systemic); CYP3A4 Substrates; Dabigatran Etexilate; Dapoxetine; Darunavir; Dasatinib; Dienogest; Dihydroergotamine; Disopyramide; DOCEtaxel; Dofetilide; DOXOrubicin (Conventional); Dronabinol; Dronedarone; Dutasteride; Edoxaban; Eletriptan; Eliglustat; Elvitegravir; Eplerenone; Ergoloid Mesylates; Ergonovine; Ergotamine; Erlotinib; Estazolam; Etizolam; Etravirine; Everolimus; Felodipine; FentaNYL; Fesoterodine; Fexofenadine; Fluticasone (Nasal); Fluticasone (Oral Inhalation); Fosamprenavir; GuanFACINE; Halofantrine; Highest Risk QTc-Prolonging Agents; Hydrocodone; Ibrutinib; Iloperidone; Imatinib; Imidafenacin; Indinavir; Irinotecan; Ivabradine; Ivacaftor; Ixabepilone; Lacosamide; Lapatinib; Ledipasvir; Lercanidipine; Levobupivacaine; Levomilnacipran; Lomitapide; Losartan; Lovastatin; Lurasidone; Macitentan; Macrolide Antibiotics; Maraviroc; Methadone; Methylergonovine; MethylPREDNISolone; Midazolam; Mifepristone; Moderate Risk QTc-Prolonging Agents; Naloxegol; Nilotinib; Nintedanib; Nisoldipine; Olaparib; Ospemifene; OxyCODONE; Paliperidone; Paricalcitol; PAZOPanib; P-glycoprotein/ABCB1 Substrates; Pimecrolimus; Pimozide; PONATinib; Pranlukast; Pravastatin; PrednisoLONE (Systemic); PredniSONE; Propafenone; Prucalopride; QUEtiapine; QuiNIDine; Ranolazine; Red Yeast Rice; Regorafenib; Repaglinide; Retapamulin; Rifaximin; Rilpivirine; Riociguat; Rivaroxaban; RomiDEPsin; Rosuvastatin; Ruxolitinib; Salmeterol; Saquinavir; Saxagliptin; Sildenafil; Silodosin; Simeprevir; Simvastatin; Sirolimus; Solifenacin; SORAfenib; SUNItinib; Suvorexant; Tacrolimus (Systemic); Tacrolimus (Topical); Tadalafil; Tamsulosin; Telaprevir; Temsirolimus; Terfenadine; Tetrahydrocannabinol; Ticagrelor; Tofacitinib; Tolterodine; Tolvaptan; Topotecan; Toremifene; Trabectedin; Triazolam; Ulipristal; Vardenafil; Vemurafenib; Vilazodone; VinBLAStine; VinCRIStine; VinCRIStine (Liposomal); Vinorelbine; Vitamin K Antagonists; Vorapaxar; Zolpidem; Zopiclone; Zuclopenthixol

The levels/effects of Itraconazole may be increased by: Boceprevir; Cobicistat; Conivaptan; CYP3A4 Inhibitors (Moderate); CYP3A4 Inhibitors (Strong); Darunavir; Etravirine; Fosamprenavir; Fusidic Acid (Systemic); Grapefruit Juice; Idelalisib; Indinavir; Lopinavir; Luliconazole; Macrolide Antibiotics; Mifepristone; Netupitant; Ritonavir; Saquinavir; Stiripentol; Telaprevir; Tipranavir

Decreased Effect

Itraconazole may decrease the levels/effects of: Amphotericin B; Ifosfamide; Meloxicam; Prasugrel; Saccharomyces boulardii; Ticagrelor

The levels/effects of Itraconazole may be decreased by: Antacids; Bosentan; CYP3A4 Inducers (Moderate); CYP3A4 Inducers (Strong); Dabrafenib; Deferasirox; Didanosine; Efavirenz; Etravirine; Grapefruit Juice; H2-Antagonists; Isoniazid; Nevirapine; Proton Pump Inhibitors; Siltuximab; St Johns Wort; Sucralfate; Tocilizumab

Food Interactions

Capsules: Absorption enhanced by food and possibly by gastric acidity. Cola drinks have been shown to increase the absorption of the capsules in patients with achlorhydria or those taking H_2-receptor antagonists or other gastric acid suppressors. Grapefruit/grapefruit juice may increase serum levels. Management: Take capsules immediately after meals. Avoid grapefruit juice.
Solution: Food decreases the bioavailability and increases the time to peak concentration. Management: Take solution on an empty stomach 1 hour before or 2 hours after meals.

Storage/Stability

Capsule: Store at room temperature of 15°C to 25°C (59°F to 77°F). Protect from light and moisture.
Oral solution: Store at ≤25°C (77°F); do not freeze.
Tablet: Store at room temperature 15°C to 25°C (59°F to 77°F); excursions are permitted between 15°C and 30°C (59°F and 86°F). Protect from light and moisture.

Mechanism of Action Interferes with cytochrome P450 activity, decreasing ergosterol synthesis (principal sterol in fungal cell membrane) and inhibiting cell membrane formation

Pharmacodynamics/Kinetics

Absorption: Requires gastric acidity; capsule or tablet better absorbed with food, solution better absorbed on empty stomach

Distribution: V_d (average): >700 L; highly lipophilic and tissue concentrations are higher than plasma concentrations. The highest concentrations: adipose, omentum, endometrium, cervical and vaginal mucus, and skin/nails. Aqueous fluids (eg, CSF and urine) contain negligible amounts.

Protein binding, plasma: 99.8%; metabolite hydroxy-itraconazole: 99.6%

Metabolism: Extensively hepatic via CYP3A4 into >30 metabolites including hydroxy-itraconazole (major metabolite); appears to have *in vitro* antifungal activity. Main metabolic pathway is oxidation; may undergo saturation metabolism with multiple dosing.

Bioavailability: Variable, ~55% increases by 30% under fasted conditions (oral solution); **Note:** Oral solution has a higher degree of bioavailability (149% ± 68%) relative to oral capsules; should not be interchanged

Half-life elimination: Oral: Single dose: 16 to 28 hours, Multiple doses: 34 to 42 hours; Cirrhosis (single dose): 37 hours (range: 20 to 54 hours)

Time to peak, plasma: Capsules/tablets: 2 to 5 hours; Oral solution: 2.5 hours

Excretion: Urine (<0.03% active drug, 35% as inactive metabolites); feces (54%; ~3% to 18% as unchanged drug)

Dosage

Children: Oral:

Indication-specific dosing:

Infants and Children (HIV-exposed/-positive; off-label use): **Note:** Doses >200 mg daily should be administered in 2 divided doses.

Candidiasis:

Oropharyngeal: Oral solution: 2.5 mg/kg/dose twice daily (maximum: 200 mg daily [400 mg daily if fluconazole-refractory]) for 7 to 14 days (CDC, 2009a)

Esophageal: Oral solution: 5 mg/kg/day once daily or divided twice daily for 4 to 21 days (CDC, 2009a)

Coccidioidomycosis:

Treatment: Oral: 5 to 10 mg/kg/dose twice daily for 3 days, followed by 2 to 5 mg/kg/dose orally twice daily (maximum: 400 mg daily) (CDC, 2009a)

Relapse prevention: Oral: 2 to 5 mg/kg/dose twice daily (maximum: 400 mg daily) (CDC, 2009a)

Cryptococcus:

Treatment, consolidation therapy: Oral solution (preferred): Initial: 2.5 to 5 mg/kg/dose 3 times daily (maximum daily dose: 600 mg daily) for 3 days (9 doses) followed by 5 to 10 mg/kg/day divided once or twice daily (maximum daily dose: 400 mg daily) for a minimum of 8 weeks (CDC, 2009a)

Relapse prevention: Oral solution: 5 mg/kg/dose once daily (maximum: 200 mg daily) (CDC, 2009a)

Histoplasmosis:

Treatment of mild disseminated disease: Oral solution: 2 to 5 mg/kg/dose 3 times daily for 3 days (9 doses), followed by twice daily for 12 months (maximum: 200 mg per dose) (CDC, 2009a)

Consolidation treatment for moderate-severe to severe disseminated disease, including CNS infection (following appropriate induction therapy): Oral solution: 2 to 5 mg/kg/dose 3 times daily for 3 days, followed by 2 to 5 mg/kg/dose (maximum: 200 mg per dose) twice daily for 12 months for non-CNS-disseminated disease or for ≥12 months for CNS infection as determined by clinical response (CDC, 2009a)

Relapse prevention: Oral solution: 5 mg/kg/dose twice daily (maximum: 400 mg daily) (CDC, 2009a)

Adults: **Note:** Doses >200 mg daily should be administered in 2 divided doses.

Aspergillosis: Oral capsule: 200 to 400 mg daily. **Note:** For life-threatening infections, the U.S. labeling recommends administering a loading dose of 200 mg 3 times daily (total: 600 mg daily) for the first 3 days of therapy. Continue treatment for at least 3 months and until clinical and laboratory evidence suggest that infection has resolved.

Aspergillosis, invasive (salvage therapy; voriconazole-susceptible): Duration of therapy should be a minimum of 6 to 12 weeks or throughout period of immunosuppression: Oral capsule: 200 to 400 mg daily; **Note:** 2008 IDSA guidelines recommend 600 mg daily for 3 days, followed by 400 mg daily (Walsh, 2008)

Aspergillosis, allergic (ABPA, sinusitis): Oral: 200 mg daily; may be used in conjunction with corticosteroids (Andes, 2000; Walsh, 2008)

Blastomycosis: Manufacturer labeling: Oral capsule: Initial: 200 mg once daily; if no clinical improvement or evidence of progressive infection, may increase dose in increments of 100 mg up to maximum of 400 mg daily. **Note:** For life-threatening infections, the U.S. labeling recommends administering a loading dose of 200 mg 3 times daily (total 600 mg daily) for the first 3 days of therapy. Continue treatment for at least 3 months and until clinical and laboratory evidence suggest that infection has resolved.

Alternative dosing: 200 mg 3 times daily for 3 days, then 200 mg twice daily for 6 to 12 months; in moderately-severe to severe infection, therapy should be initiated with ~2 weeks of amphotericin B (Chapman, 2008).

Candidiasis:

Esophageal:

U.S. labeling: Oral solution: 100 to 200 mg once daily for a minimum of 3 weeks; continue dosing for 2 weeks after resolution of symptoms

Canadian labeling:

Oral solution: 100 to 200 mg once daily for a minimum of 3 weeks; continue dosing for 2 weeks after resolution of symptoms

Oral capsule: 100 mg once daily for 4 weeks; increase dose to 200 mg once daily in patients with AIDS and neutropenic patients

Oropharyngeal:

U.S. labeling: Oral solution: 200 mg once daily for 1 to 2 weeks; in patients unresponsive or refractory to fluconazole: 100 mg twice daily (clinical response expected in 2 to 4 weeks)

Canadian labeling:

Oral solution: 200 mg once daily or in divided doses daily for 1 to 2 weeks

Oral capsule: 100 mg once daily for 2 weeks; increase dose to 200 mg once daily in patients with AIDS and neutropenic patients

Chromomycosis: Canadian labeling (not in U.S. labeling): Oral capsule: 200 mg once daily for 6 months (when due to *Fonsecaea pedrosoi*) or 100 mg once daily for 3 months (when due to *Cladosporium carrioni*)

Coccidioidomycosis (nonprogressive, nondisseminated disease): Oral: 200 mg twice daily or 3 times daily (Galgiani, 2005)

Histoplasmosis: Manufacturer labeling: Oral capsule: Initial: 200 mg once daily; if no clinical improvement or evidence of progressive infection, may increase dose in increments of 100 mg up to maximum of 400 mg daily. **Note:** For life-threatening infections, the U.S.

labeling recommends administering a loading dose of 200 mg 3 times daily (total: 600 mg daily) for the first 3 days of therapy. Continue treatment for at least 3 months and until clinical and laboratory evidence suggest that infection has resolved.

Alternative dosing: 200 mg 3 times daily for 3 days, then 200 mg twice daily (or once daily in mild-moderate disease) for 6 to 12 weeks in mild-moderate disease or ≥12 months in progressive disseminated or chronic cavitary pulmonary histoplasmosis; in moderately severe to severe infection, therapy should be initiated with ~2 weeks of a lipid formation of amphotericin B (Wheat, 2007).

Long-term suppression therapy: 200 mg daily (CDC, 2009b)

Meningitis: Oral:

Coccidioides: 400 to 600 mg daily (Galgiani, 2005)

Coccidioides, HIV-positive (off-label use): 200 mg 3 times daily for 3 days, then 200 mg twice daily; maintenance: 200 mg twice daily life-long (CDC, 2009b)

Appropriate use: Fluconazole is preferred for meningeal infections (CDC, 2009b; Galgiani, 2005)

Onychomycosis (fingernail involvement only): Oral capsule: 200 mg twice daily for 1 week; repeat 1-week course after 3-week off-time

Onychomycosis (toenails due to *Trichophyton rubrum* or *T. mentagrophytes*): Oral tablet: 200 mg once daily for 12 consecutive weeks.

Onychomycosis (toenails with or without fingernail involvement): Oral capsule: 200 mg once daily for 12 consecutive weeks

Canadian labeling (not in U.S. labeling): "Pulse-dosing": 200 mg twice daily for 1 week; repeat 1-week course twice with 3-week off-time between each course

Paracoccidioidomycosis: Canadian labeling (not in U.S. labeling): Oral capsule: 100 mg once daily for 6 months

Penicilliosis, HIV-positive (off-label use): Oral capsule: 400 mg daily for 8 weeks (mild disease) or 10 weeks (severe infections). In severely ill patients, initiate therapy with 2 weeks of amphotericin B. Maintenance: 200 mg daily (CDC, 2009b)

Pityriasis versicolor: Canadian labeling (not in U.S. labeling): Oral capsule: 200 mg once daily for 7 days

Pneumonia: Oral:

Coccidioides: Mild to moderate: 200 mg twice daily (Galgiani, 2005)

Coccidioides, HIV-positive (focal pneumonia): 200 mg 3 times daily for 3 days, then 200 mg twice daily (CDC, 2009b)

Sporotrichosis: Oral:

Lymphocutaneous: 200 mg daily for 3 to 6 months (Kauffman, 2007)

Canadian labeling (not in U.S. labeling): 100 mg once daily for 3 months

Osteoarticular and pulmonary: 200 mg twice daily for ≥1 years (may use amphotericin B initially for stabilization) (Kauffman, 2007)

Tinea corporis or tinea cruris: Canadian labeling (not in U.S. labeling): Oral capsule: 100 mg once daily for 14 consecutive days or 200 mg once daily for 7 consecutive days. **Note:** Equivalency between regimens not established.

Tinea pedis: Canadian labeling (not in U.S. labeling): Oral capsule: 100 mg once daily for 28 consecutive days or 200 mg twice daily for 7 consecutive days. **Note:** Equivalency between regimens not established. Patients with chronic resistant infection may benefit from lower dose and extended treatment time (100 mg once daily for 28 days).

Dosage adjustment in renal impairment: The manufacturer's labeling states to use with caution in patients with renal impairment; dosage adjustment may be needed. Limited data suggest that no dosage adjustments are required in renal impairment; wide variations observed in plasma concentrations versus time profiles in patients with uremia, or receiving hemodialysis or continuous ambulatory peritoneal dialysis (Boelaert, 1988).

Dosage adjustment in hepatic impairment: There are no dosage adjustments provided in the manufacturer's labeling; however, use caution and monitor closely for signs/symptoms of toxicity.

Dietary Considerations

Capsule, tablet: Take with food.

Solution: Take without food, if possible.

Administration Doses >200 mg/day are given in 2 divided doses; do not administer with antacids. Capsule and oral solution formulations are not bioequivalent and thus are not interchangeable. Capsule and tablet absorption is best if taken with food, therefore, it is best to administer itraconazole after meals at the same time each day; solution should be taken on an empty stomach. When treating oropharyngeal and esophageal candidiasis, solution should be swished vigorously in mouth (10 mL at a time), then swallowed.

Monitoring Parameters Liver function in patients with preexisting hepatic dysfunction, and in all patients being treated for longer than 1 month; serum concentrations particularly for oral therapy (due to erratic bioavailability with capsule formulation); renal function; signs/symptoms of CHF

Reference Range Serum concentrations may be performed to assure therapeutic levels. Itraconazole plus the metabolite hydroxyitraconazole concentrations should be >1 mcg/mL (not to exceed 10 mcg/mL).

Timing of serum samples: Obtain level after ~2 weeks of therapy, level may be drawn anytime during the dosing interval.

Dosage Forms

Capsule, Oral:

Sporanox: 100 mg

Sporanox Pulsepak: 100 mg

Generic: 100 mg

Solution, Oral:

Sporanox: 10 mg/mL (150 mL)

Tablet, Oral:

Onmel: 200 mg

Extemporaneous Preparations Note: Commercial oral solution is available (10 mg/mL)

A 20 mg/mL oral suspension may be made with capsules. Empty the contents of forty 100 mg capsules and add 15 mL of Alcohol, USP. Let stand for 5 minutes. Crush the beads in a mortar and reduce to a fine powder. Mix while adding a 1:1 mixture of Ora-Sweet and Ora-Plus in incremental proportions to **almost** 200 mL; transfer to a calibrated bottle, rinse mortar with vehicle, and add quantity of vehicle sufficient to make 200 mL. Label "shake well" and "refrigerate". Stable for 56 days refrigerated.

Nahata MC, Pai VB, and Hipple TF, *Pediatric Drug Formulations*, 5th ed, Cincinnati, OH: Harvey Whitney Books Co, 2004.

Ivabradine [INT] (eye VAB ra deen)

International Brand Names Coralan (AU, HK, ID, IL, IN, MY, PH, SG, TH); Coraxan (RU); Corlentor (EE, HR, NL, RO); Prociralan (RO); Procoralan (AE, AR, AT, BE, BH, BR, CH, CL, CO, CY, CZ, DE, DK, EC, EE, FR, GR, HN, HR, IE, IS, IT, KR, KW, LB, LT, NL, PL, PT, QA, SA, SE, SI, SK, TR, VN)

Index Terms Ivabradine Hydrochloride

Pharmacologic Category Cardiovascular Agent, Other

Reported Use Symptomatic treatment of chronic stable angina pectoris in patients with normal sinus rhythm, who have a contraindication or intolerance for beta-blockers; treatment of chronic heart failure (NYHA class II-IV) with systolic dysfunction in patients with normal sinus rhythm and heart rate ≥75 bpm, in combination with standard multidrug therapy, including beta-blockers (if tolerated) or excluding beta-blockers (if contraindicated or not tolerated)

Dosage Range Adults: Oral:

Angina: Initial dose: 5 mg twice daily; may increase dose after 3-4 weeks to 7.5 mg twice daily depending on response

Heart failure: Initial: 5 mg twice daily; after 2 weeks, adjust dose based on heart rate

Note: May decrease dose to 2.5 mg twice daily if heart rate decreases below 50 bpm at rest or if patient experiences symptoms of bradycardia; discontinue if decreased heart rate and/or bradycardia persist

Product Availability Product available in various countries; not currently available in the U.S.

Dosage Forms

Tablet, as hydrochloride: 5 mg, 7.5 mg

◆ **Ivabradine Hydrochloride** *see* Ivabradine [INT] *on page 1134*

Ivacaftor (eye va KAF tor)

Brand Names: U.S. Kalydeco

Brand Names: Canada Kalydeco

Index Terms VX-770

Pharmacologic Category Cystic Fibrosis Transmembrane Conductance Regulator Potentiator

Use Cystic fibrosis: For the treatment of cystic fibrosis (CF) in patients ≥6 years of age who have one of the following mutations in the cystic fibrosis transmembrane conductance regulator (CFTR) gene: G551D, G1244E, G1349D, G178R, G551S, R117H, S1251N, S1255P, S549N, or S549R. **Note:** Canadian labeling (not in U.S. labeling) also approves for use in patients with G970R mutation.

If the patient's genotype is unknown, a U.S. Food and Drug Administration-cleared cystic fibrosis mutation test should be used to detect the presence of a CFTR mutation followed by verification with bidirectional sequencing when recommended by the mutation test instructions for use.

Limitations of use: According to the manufacturer labeling, ivacaftor is not effective in patients with CF who are homozygous for the F508del mutation in the CTFR gene.

Pregnancy Risk Factor B

Pregnancy Considerations Adverse events have not been observed in animal reproduction studies.

Breast-Feeding Considerations Although unknown, the manufacturer suggests that excretion of ivacaftor in breast milk is probable; caution is recommended when administering ivacaftor to nursing women.

Contraindications There are no contraindications listed in the manufacturer's U.S. labeling.

Canadian labeling: Hypersensitivity to ivacaftor or any component of the formulation

Warnings/Precautions May increase hepatic transaminases; temporarily discontinue treatment if ALT or AST >5 times ULN. Use with caution in patients with moderate or severe hepatic impairment. Noncongenital lens opacities and cataracts have been reported in patients ≤12 years of age treated with ivacaftor; other risk factors were present in some cases (eg, corticosteroid use, exposure to radiation), but a possible risk related to ivacaftor cannot be excluded. Baseline and follow-up ophthalmological examinations are recommended in pediatric patients. Potentially significant drug-drug interactions may exist, requiring dose or frequency adjustment, additional monitoring, and/or selection of alternative therapy.

Adverse Reactions

Central nervous system: Dizziness, headache

Dermatologic: Acne, rash

Gastrointestinal: Abdominal pain, diarrhea, nausea

Endocrine & metabolic: Hyperglycemia

Hepatic: Transaminases increased

Neuromuscular & skeletal: Arthralgia, musculoskeletal chest pain, myalgia

Respiratory: Nasal congestion, nasopharyngitis, oropharyngeal pain, pharyngeal erythema, pleuritic chest pain, rhinitis, sinus congestion, upper respiratory tract infection, wheezing

Miscellaneous: Bacteria in sputum

Rare but important or life-threatening: Hypoglycemia

Drug Interactions

Metabolism/Transport Effects Substrate of CYP3A4 (major); **Note:** Assignment of Major/Minor substrate status based on clinically relevant drug interaction potential; **Inhibits** CYP2C8 (weak), CYP2C9 (weak), CYP3A4 (weak), P-glycoprotein

Avoid Concomitant Use

Avoid concomitant use of Ivacaftor with any of the following: Bosutinib; Conivaptan; CYP3A4 Inducers (Strong); Fusidic Acid (Systemic); Grapefruit Juice; Idelalisib; PAZOPanib; Pimozide; Silodosin; St Johns Wort; Topotecan; VinCRIStine (Liposomal)

Increased Effect/Toxicity

Ivacaftor may increase the levels/effects of: Afatinib; ARIPiprazole; Bosutinib; Brentuximab Vedotin; Colchicine; CYP3A4 Substrates; Dabigatran Etexilate; Dofetilide; DOXOrubicin (Conventional); Edoxaban; Everolimus; Hydrocodone; Ledipasvir; Lomitapide; Naloxegol; PAZOPanib; P-glycoprotein/ABCB1 Substrates; Pimozide; Prucalopride; Rifaximin; Rivaroxaban; Silodosin; Topotecan; VinCRIStine (Liposomal)

The levels/effects of Ivacaftor may be increased by: Conivaptan; CYP3A4 Inhibitors (Moderate); CYP3A4 Inhibitors (Strong); Dasatinib; Fusidic Acid (Systemic); Grapefruit Juice; Idelalisib; Luliconazole; Mifepristone; Simeprevir; Stiripentol

Decreased Effect

The levels/effects of Ivacaftor may be decreased by: Bosentan; CYP3A4 Inducers (Moderate); CYP3A4 Inducers (Strong); Dabrafenib; Deferasirox; Siltuximab; St Johns Wort; Tocilizumab

Food Interactions Ivacaftor serum concentrations may be increased when taken with grapefruit or Seville oranges. Management: Avoid concurrent use.

Storage/Stability Store at 20°C to 25°C (68°F to 77°F); excursions permitted to 15°C to 30°C (59°F to 86°F).

Mechanism of Action Potentiates epithelial cell chloride ion transport of defective (G551D mutant) cell-surface CFTR protein thereby improving the regulation of salt and water absorption and secretion in various tissues (eg, lung, gastrointestinal tract).

Pharmacodynamics/Kinetics

Onset of action: FEV_1 increased, sweat chloride decreased within ~2 weeks

Absorption: Variable; increased (by two- to fourfold) with fatty foods

Distribution: V_d: 353 L

Protein binding: ~99%; primarily to $alpha_1$ acid glycoprotein, albumin

Metabolism: Hepatic; extensive via CYP3A; forms 2 major metabolites (M1 [active; 1/6 potency] and M6 [inactive])

Half-life elimination: ~12 hours

Time to peak: ~4 hours

Excretion: Feces (88%, 65% of administered dose as metabolites); urine (minimal, as unchanged drug)

Dosage Oral: Children ≥6 years, Adolescents, and Adults: 150 mg every 12 hours

Dosage adjustment for ivacaftor with concomitant medications:

CYP3A strong inhibitors (eg, ketoconazole, itraconazole, posaconazole, voriconazole, clarithromycin, telithromycin): 150 mg twice **weekly**

CYP3A moderate inhibitors (eg, erythromycin, fluconazole): 150 mg once daily

CYP3A strong inducers (eg, carbamazepine, phenobarbital, phenytoin, rifabutin, rifampin, St John's wort): Use is not recommended

Dosage adjustment for toxicity: ALT or AST >5 times ULN: Hold ivacaftor; may resume if elevated transaminases resolved and after assessing benefits vs risks of continued treatment

Dosage adjustment in renal impairment:

CrCl >30 mL/minute: No dosage adjustment necessary (not studied).

CrCl ≤30 mL/minute: There are no dosage adjustments provided in manufacturer's labeling (not studied); use with caution.

End-stage renal disease (ESRD): There are no dosage adjustments provided in manufacturer's labeling (not studied); use with caution.

Dosage adjustment in hepatic impairment:

Mild impairment (Child-Pugh class A): No dosage adjustment necessary.

Moderate impairment (Child-Pugh class B): 150 mg once daily.

Severe impairment (Child-Pugh class C): Has not been studied; use with caution.

U.S. labeling: Initial: 150 mg once daily or less frequently.

Canadian labeling: Initial: 150 mg once every other day; adjust for tolerance and/or response.

Dietary Considerations Take with high-fat-containing foods (eg, butter, cheese pizza, eggs, peanut butter). Avoid grapefruit or Seville oranges.

Administration Oral: Administer with high-fat-containing foods (eg, butter, cheese pizza, eggs, peanut butter).

Monitoring Parameters CF mutation test (prior to therapy initiation if G551D mutation status unknown); ALT/AST at baseline, every 3 months for 1 year, then annually thereafter or as clinically indicated; FEV_1; baseline and follow-up ophthalmological exams in pediatric patients

Additional Information G551D mutation is present in approximately 4% to 5% of patients with CF. When used in addition to standard therapy (eg, dornase alfa, inhaled tobramycin), ivacaftor may provide further improvements in FEV_1, a reduction in pulmonary exacerbations, and a beneficial weight gain in CF patients. Long-term benefits on disease progression have not been established.

Dosage Forms

Tablet, Oral:

Kalydeco: 150 mg

Ivermectin (Systemic) (eye ver MEK tin)

Brand Names: U.S. Stromectol

Pharmacologic Category Anthelmintic

Use Treatment of the following infections: Strongyloidiasis of the intestinal tract due to the nematode parasite *Strongyloides stercoralis*. Onchocerciasis due to the immature form of the nematode parasite *Onchocerca volvulus*

Pregnancy Risk Factor C

Pregnancy Considerations Teratogenic effects have been observed in animal reproduction studies; therefore, the manufacturer classifies ivermectin as pregnancy category C. Ivermectin is not recommended for use in pregnancy. Although studies during pregnancy are limited, several mass treatment programs have not identified an increased risk of adverse fetal, neonatal, or maternal outcomes following ivermectin use in the first and second trimesters.

Breast-Feeding Considerations Ivermectin is measurable in low concentrations in breast milk and is less than maternal plasma concentrations. Peak concentrations of ivermectin in breast milk may occur 4-12 hours after the oral dose. In one study, the calculated infant daily dose was 2.75 mcg/kg in a 1-month-old infant and would not be expected to cause adverse effects in the infant. The manufacturer and the CDC do not have safety data in children <15 kg and the CDC does not recommend the use of ivermectin in lactating women.

Contraindications Hypersensitivity to ivermectin or any component of the formulation

Warnings/Precautions Data have shown that antihelmintic drugs like ivermectin may cause cutaneous and/or systemic reactions (Mazzoti reaction) of varying severity including ophthalmological reactions in patients with onchocerciasis. These reactions are probably due to allergic and inflammatory responses to the death of microfilariae. Patients with hyper-reactive onchodermatitis may be more likely than others to experience severe adverse reactions, especially edema and aggravation of the onchodermatitis. Repeated treatment may be required in immunocompromised patients (eg, HIV); control of extraintestinal strongyloidiasis may necessitate suppressive (once monthly) therapy. Pretreatment assessment for *Loa loa* infection is recommended in any patient with significant exposure to endemic areas (West and Central Africa); serious and/or fatal encephalopathy has been reported (rarely) during treatment in patients with loiasis. Ivermectin has no activity against adult *Onchocerca volvulus* parasites.

Adverse Reactions

Cardiovascular: Facial edema, orthostatic hypotension, peripheral edema, tachycardia

Central nervous system: Dizziness

Dermatologic: Pruritus

Gastrointestinal: Diarrhea, nausea

Hematologic: Eosinophilia, hemoglobin increased, leukocytes decreased

Hepatic: ALT increased, AST increased

Miscellaneous: Mazzotti-type reaction (with onchocerciasis): Arthralgia/synovitis, fever, lymph node enlargement/tenderness, pruritus, skin involvement (edema/urticarial rash)

Rare but important or life-threatening: Abdominal distention, abdominal pain, anemia, anorexia, anterior uveitis, asthma exacerbation, back pain, bilirubin increased, chest discomfort, chorioretinitis, choroiditis, coma, confusion, conjunctival hemorrhage (associated with onchocerciasis), conjunctivitis, constipation, dyspnea, encephalopathy (rare; associated with loiasis), eyelid edema, eye sensation abnormal, fatigue, fecal incontinence, headache, hepatitis, hypotension, INR increased (with concomitant warfarin), keratitis, lethargy, leukopenia, mental status changes, myalgia, neck pain, rash, red eye, seizure, somnolence, standing/walking difficulty, Stevens-Johnson syndrome, stupor, toxic epidermal necrolysis, tremor, urinary incontinence, urticaria, vertigo, vision loss (transient), vomiting, weakness

Drug Interactions

Metabolism/Transport Effects Substrate of CYP3A4 (minor), P-glycoprotein; **Note:** Assignment of Major/Minor substrate status based on clinically relevant drug interaction potential

Avoid Concomitant Use

Avoid concomitant use of Ivermectin (Systemic) with any of the following: BCG

Increased Effect/Toxicity

Ivermectin (Systemic) may increase the levels/effects of: Vitamin K Antagonists

The levels/effects of Ivermectin (Systemic) may be increased by: Azithromycin (Systemic); P-glycoprotein/ABCB1 Inhibitors

Decreased Effect

Ivermectin (Systemic) may decrease the levels/effects of: BCG; Sodium Picosulfate; Typhoid Vaccine

The levels/effects of Ivermectin (Systemic) may be decreased by: P-glycoprotein/ABCB1 Inducers

Food Interactions Bioavailability is increased 2.5-fold when administered following a high-fat meal. Management: Administer on an empty stomach.

Storage/Stability Store at <30°C (86°F).

Mechanism of Action Ivermectin is a semisynthetic anthelminthic agent; it binds selectively and with strong affinity to glutamate-gated chloride ion channels which occur in invertebrate nerve and muscle cells. This leads to increased permeability of cell membranes to chloride ions then hyperpolarization of the nerve or muscle cell, and death of the parasite.

Pharmacodynamics/Kinetics

Onset of action:

Peak effect in treatment of onchocerciasis: 3-6 months

Peak effect in treatment of strongyloides: 3 months

Absorption: Well absorbed

Distribution: V_d: 3-3.5 L/kg (healthy males); does not cross blood-brain barrier

Protein binding: ~93%

Metabolism: Hepatic via CYP3A4 (major), CYP2D6 (minor), and CYP2E1 (minor)

Bioavailability: Increased with high-fat meal

Half-life elimination: ~18 hours

Time to peak, serum: ~4 hours

Excretion: Feces; urine (<1%)

Dosage

Onchocerciasis: Children ≥15 kg and Adults: Oral: 150 mcg/kg as a single dose; retreatment may be required every 3-12 months until asymptomatic

Strongyloidiasis: Children ≥15 kg and Adults: Oral:

Manufacturer recommendations: 200 mcg/kg as a single dose; perform follow-up stool examinations.

Alternative dosing: 200 mcg/kg/day for 2 days (CDC, 2012)

Ascariasis due to *Ascaris lumbricoides* (off-label use): Children ≥15 kg and Adults: Oral: 200 mcg/kg as a single dose (Marti, 1996; Naquira, 1989)

Cutaneous larva migrans (CLM) due to *Ancylostoma braziliense* (off-label use): Children ≥15 kg and Adults: Oral: 200 mcg/kg as a single dose (Vanhaecke, 2013)

Demodicosis due to *Demodex folliculorum* and *Demodex brevis* (off-label use): Children ≥15 kg and Adults: Oral: 200 mcg/kg as a single dose, followed by topical permethrin (Eismann, 2010)

Filariasis due to *Mansonella ozzardi* (off-label use): Adults: Oral: 6 mg as a single dose (Gonzales, 1999)

Filariasis due to *Mansonella streptocerca* (off-label use): Children ≥15 kg and Adults: Oral: 150 mcg/kg as a single dose (Fischer, 1997)

Filariasis due to *Wucheria bancrofti* (off-label use): Children ≥15 kg and Adults: Oral: 200-400 mcg/kg as a single dose in combination with albendazole (Addiss, 1997; Ismail, 2001)

Gnathostomiasis due to *Gnathostoma spinigerum* (off-label use): Children ≥15 kg and Adults: Oral: 200 mcg/kg as a single dose (Nontasut, 2000; Kraivichian, 2004)

Lice due to *Pediculus humanus capitis, Pediculus humanus corporis, Phthirus pubis* (off-label use): Children ≥15 kg and Adults: Oral: 200 mcg/kg/dose; generally requires >1 dose; number of doses and dosage intervals have not been established

Pediculus humanus capitis: Children ≥15 kg and Adults: Oral: 400 mcg/kg/dose every 7 days for 2 doses (Chosidow, 2010)

Pediculus humanus corporis: Children ≥15 kg and Adults: Oral: 200 mcg/kg/dose every 7 days for 3 doses (Foucault, 2006)

Phthirus pubis: Children ≥15 kg and Adults: Oral: 250 mcg/kg/dose every 7 days for 2 doses (Burkhart, 2004)

Scabies due to *Sarcoptes scabiei* in immunocompromised patients (off-label use): Children ≥15 kg and Adults: Oral: 200 mcg/kg as a single dose; may repeat dose in 14 days (Meinking, 1995). **Note:** Preferred drug for immunocompromised patients with crusted scabies.

Trichuriasis due to *Trichuris trichiura* (off-label use): Children ≥15 kg and Adults: Oral: 200 mcg/kg as a single dose on day 1; may repeat dose on day 4 (Naquira, 1989)

Dosage adjustment in renal impairment: No dosage adjustment provided in manufacturer's labeling.

Dosage adjustment in hepatic impairment: No dosage adjustment provided in manufacturer's labeling.

Dietary Considerations Take on an empty stomach with water.

Administration Administer on an empty stomach with water.

Monitoring Parameters Skin and eye microfilarial counts, periodic ophthalmologic exams; follow up stool examinations

Dosage Forms

Tablet, Oral:

Stromectol: 3 mg

Generic: 3 mg

Ivermectin (Topical) (eye ver MEK tin)

Brand Names: U.S. Sklice; Soolantra

Index Terms Ivermectin Cream; Ivermectin Lotion; Soolantra

Pharmacologic Category Antiparasitic Agent, Topical; Pediculocide

Use

Head lice (*Pediculus capitis*) (Sklice lotion): Treatment of head lice infestations in patients 6 months and older.

Rosacea (Soolantra cream): Treatment of inflammatory lesions of rosacea in adult patients.

Pregnancy Risk Factor C

Dosage

Head lice: Topical: Lotion: Children ≥6 months, Adolescents, and Adults: Apply sufficient amount (up to 1 tube) to completely cover dry scalp and hair; for single-dose use only.

Rosacea: Topical: Cream: Adults: Apply to each affected area (eg, forehead, chin, nose, each cheek) once daily.

Dosage adjustment in renal impairment: There are no dosage adjustments provided in the manufacturer's labeling.

Dosage adjustment in hepatic impairment: There are no dosage adjustments provided in the manufacturer's labeling.

Additional Information Complete prescribing information should be consulted for additional detail.

Product Availability

Soolantra cream: FDA approved December 2014; Soolantra is indicated for the treatment of inflammatory lesions of rosacea.

Dosage Forms

Cream, External:

Soolantra: 1% (30 g)

Lotion, External:

Sklice: 0.5% (117 g)

- **Ivermectin Cream** *see* Ivermectin (Topical) *on page 1137*
- **Ivermectin Lotion** *see* Ivermectin (Topical) *on page 1137*
- **IVIG** *see* Immune Globulin *on page 1056*
- **IV Immune Globulin** *see* Immune Globulin *on page 1056*
- **IV-VIG** *see* Vaccinia Immune Globulin (Intravenous) *on page 2118*
- **Ivy Block [OTC]** *see* Bentoquatam *on page 246*
- **Ivy-Rid [OTC]** *see* Benzocaine *on page 246*

Ixabepilone (ix ab EP i lone)

Brand Names: U.S. Ixempra Kit

Index Terms Azaepothilone B; BMS-247550; Epothilone B Lactam

Pharmacologic Category Antineoplastic Agent, Antimicrotubular; Antineoplastic Agent, Epothilone B Analog

Use Breast cancer: Treatment of metastatic or locally-advanced breast cancer resistant to treatment with an anthracycline and a taxane, or if taxane-resistant and further anthracycline therapy is contraindicated (in combination with capecitabine) or as monotherapy in tumors are resistant or refractory to anthracyclines, taxanes, and capecitabine.

Anthracycline resistance is defined as progression during treatment or within 3 months in the metastatic setting (within 6 months in the adjuvant setting). Taxane resistance is defined as progression during treatment within 4 months in the metastatic setting (within 12 months in the adjuvant setting).

Pregnancy Risk Factor D

Pregnancy Considerations Adverse events were observed in animal reproduction studies. Women of childbearing potential should be advised to use effective contraception during treatment.

Breast-Feeding Considerations It is not known if ixabepilone is excreted in breast milk. Due to the potential for serious adverse reactions in the nursing infant, a decision should be made to discontinue breast-feeding or to discontinue the drug, taking into account the importance of treatment to the mother.

Contraindications History of severe (grade 3 or 4) hypersensitivity to polyoxyethylated castor oil (eg, Cremophor EL) or its derivatives; neutrophil count <1,500/mm^3 or platelet count <100,000/mm^3; combination therapy with ixabepilone and capecitabine in patients with AST or ALT >2.5 times ULN or bilirubin >1 times ULN

Warnings/Precautions Hazardous agent - use appropriate precautions for handling and disposal (NIOSH 2014 [group 1]). **[U.S. Boxed Warning]: Due to increased risk of toxicity and neutropenia-related mortality, combination therapy with capecitabine is contraindicated in patients with AST or ALT >2.5 times ULN or bilirubin >1 times ULN.** Use (as monotherapy) is not recommended if AST or ALT >10 times ULN or bilirubin >3 times ULN; use caution in patients with AST or ALT >5 times ULN. Toxicities and serious adverse reactions are increased (in mono- and combination therapy) with hepatic dysfunction; dosage reductions are necessary. Diluent contains Cremophor EL, which is associated with hypersensitivity reactions; use is contraindicated in patients with a history of severe hypersensitivity to Cremophor EL or its derivatives. Medications for the treatment of reaction should be available for immediate use; reactions may also be managed with a reduction of infusion rate. Premedicate with an H_1- and H_2-antagonist 1 hour prior to infusion; patients who experience hypersensitivity (eg, bronchospasm, dyspnea, flushing, rash) should also be premedicated with a corticosteroid for all subsequent cycles if treatment is continued.

Dose-dependent myelosuppression, particularly neutropenia, may occur with mono- or combination therapy. Neutropenic fever and infection have been reported with use. The risk for neutropenia is increased with hepatic dysfunction, especially when used in combination with capecitabine. Severe neutropenia and/or thrombocytopenia may require dosage adjustment and/or treatment delay. Peripheral (sensory and motor) neuropathy occurs commonly; may require dose reductions, treatment delays or discontinuation. Usually occurs during the first 3 cycles. Use with caution in patients with preexisting neuropathy. Patients with diabetes may have an increased risk for severe peripheral neuropathy. Use with caution in patients with a history of cardiovascular disease; the incidence of MI, ventricular dysfunction, and supraventricular arrhythmias is higher when ixabepilone is used in combination with capecitabine (as compared to capecitabine alone). Consider discontinuing ixabepilone in patients who develop cardiac ischemia or impaired cardiac function.

Potentially significant drug-drug interactions may exist, requiring dose or frequency adjustment, additional monitoring, and/or selection of alternative therapy. Due to the ethanol content in the diluent, may cause cognitive impairment; patients must be cautioned about performing tasks which require mental alertness (eg, operating machinery or driving). Toxicities or serious adverse events with combination therapy may be increased in the elderly.

Adverse Reactions

Monotherapy:

Cardiovascular: Chest pain, edema

Central nervous system: Dizziness, fever, headache, insomnia, pain

Dermatologic: Alopecia, hyperpigmentation, nail disorder, palmar-plantar erythrodysesthesia/hand-and-foot syndrome, pruritus, rash, skin exfoliation

Endocrine & metabolic: Dehydration, hot flush

Gastrointestinal: Abdominal pain, anorexia, constipation, diarrhea, gastroesophageal reflux disease, mucositis/stomatitis, nausea, taste perversion, vomiting, weight loss

Hematologic: Anemia, leukopenia, neutropenia, neutropenic fever, thrombocytopenia

Neuromuscular & skeletal: Motor neuropathy, musculoskeletal pain, myalgia/arthralgia, peripheral neuropathy (median onset cycle 4), sensory neuropathy, weakness

Ocular: Lacrimation increased

Respiratory: Cough, dyspnea, upper respiratory tract infection

Miscellaneous: Hypersensitivity, infection

Mono- and combination therapy: Rare but important or life-threatening: Alkaline phosphatase increased, angina, atrial flutter, autonomic neuropathy, cardiomyopathy, cerebral hemorrhage, coagulopathy, colitis, dysphagia, dysphonia, embolism, enterocolitis, erythema multiforme, gastrointestinal hemorrhage, gastroparesis, GGT increased, hemorrhage, hepatic failure (acute), hypokalemia, hyponatremia, hypotension, hypovolemia, hypovolemic shock, hypoxia, ileus, interstitial pneumonia, jaundice, left ventricular dysfunction, metabolic acidosis, MI, nephrolithiasis, neutropenic infection, orthostatic hypotension, pneumonia, pneumonitis, pulmonary edema (acute), radiation recall, renal failure, respiratory failure, sepsis, septic shock, supraventricular arrhythmia, syncope, thrombosis, transaminases increased, trismus, urinary tract infection, vasculitis

Drug Interactions

Metabolism/Transport Effects Substrate of CYP3A4 (major); **Note:** Assignment of Major/Minor substrate status based on clinically relevant drug interaction potential

Avoid Concomitant Use

Avoid concomitant use of Ixabepilone with any of the following: CloZAPine; Conivaptan; Dipyrone; Fusidic Acid (Systemic); Idelalisib; St Johns Wort

Increased Effect/Toxicity

Ixabepilone may increase the levels/effects of: CloZAPine

The levels/effects of Ixabepilone may be increased by: Aprepitant; Ceritinib; Conivaptan; CYP3A4 Inhibitors (Moderate); CYP3A4 Inhibitors (Strong); Dasatinib; Dipyrone; Fosaprepitant; Fusidic Acid (Systemic); Idelalisib; Ivacaftor; Luliconazole; Mifepristone; Netupitant; Simeprevir; Stiripentol

Decreased Effect

The levels/effects of Ixabepilone may be decreased by: Bosentan; CYP3A4 Inducers (Moderate); CYP3A4 Inducers (Strong); Dabrafenib; Deferasirox; Dexamethasone (Systemic); Mitotane; Siltuximab; St Johns Wort; Tocilizumab

Food Interactions Grapefruit juice may increase plasma concentrations of ixabepilone. Management: Avoid grapefruit juice.

Preparation for Administration Hazardous agent; use appropriate precautions for handling and disposal (NIOSH 2014 [group 1]). Allow to reach room temperature for ~30 minutes prior to reconstitution. Diluent vial may contain a white precipitate which should dissolve upon reaching room temperature. **Reconstitute only with the provided diluent.** Dilute the 15 mg vial with 8 mL and the 45 mg vial with 23.5 mL (using provided diluent) to a concentration of 2 mg/mL (contains overfill). Gently swirl and invert vial until dissolved completely. Prior to administration, further dilute using a non-DEHP container (eg, glass, polypropylene or polyolefin), to a final concentration of 0.2 to 0.6 mg/mL in ~250 mL lactated Ringer's, adjusted sodium chloride 0.9% (pH adjusted prior to ixabepilone addition with 2 mEq sodium bicarbonate per 250 to 500 mL sodium chloride) or PLASMA-LYTE A Injection pH 7.4. Mix thoroughly.

Storage/Stability Store intact vials under refrigeration at 2°C to 8°C (36°F to 46°F); protect from light. Reconstituted solution (in the vial) is stable for up to 1 hour at room temperature; infusion solution diluted in appropriate solution for infusion is stable for 6 hours at room temperature if a pH range of 6 to 9 is maintained (infusion must be completed within 6 hours).

Mechanism of Action Epothilone B analog; binds to the beta-tubulin subunit of the microtubule, stabilizing microtubular promoting tubulin polymerization and stabilizing microtubular function, thus arresting the cell cycle (at the G2/M phase) and inducing apoptosis. Activity in taxane-resistant cells has been demonstrated.

Pharmacodynamics/Kinetics

Distribution: >1,000 L

Protein binding: 67% to 77%

Metabolism: Extensively hepatic, via CYP3A4; >30 metabolites (inactive) formed

Half-life elimination: ~52 hours

Time to peak, plasma: At the end of infusion (3 hours)

Excretion: Feces (65%; 2% of the total dose as unchanged drug); urine (21%; 6% of the total dose as unchanged drug)

Dosage Note: Premedicate with an H_1-antagonist (eg, oral diphenhydramine 50 mg) and H_2-antagonist (eg, oral ranitidine 150 to 300 mg) ~1 hour prior to infusion. Patients with a history of hypersensitivity should also be premedicated with corticosteroids (dexamethasone 20 mg orally 1 hour before or IV 30 minutes before infusion). For dose calculation, body surface area (BSA) is capped at a maximum of 2.2 m^2.

Breast cancer (metastatic or locally advanced): Adults: IV: 40 mg/m^2/dose over 3 hours every 3 weeks (maximum dose: 88 mg) either as monotherapy or in combination with capecitabine

Dosage adjustment with concomitant strong CYP3A4 inhibitors/inducers:

CYP3A4 inhibitors: Avoid concomitant administration with strong CYP3A4 inhibitors (eg, itraconazole, ketoconazole, voriconazole, clarithromycin, telithromycin, nefazodone, atazanavir, delavirdine, indinavir, nelfinavir, ritonavir, saquinavir); if concomitant administration with a strong CYP3A4 inhibitor cannot be avoided, consider a dose reduction to 20 mg/m^2. When a strong CYP3A4 inhibitor is discontinued, allow ~1 week to elapse prior to adjusting ixabepilone dose upward to the indicated dose.

CYP3A4 inducers: Avoid concomitant administration with strong CYP3A4 inducers (eg, dexamethasone, phenytoin, carbamazepine, rifampin, phenobarbital); if concomitant administration with a strong CYP3A4 inducer cannot be avoided and after maintenance on the strong CYP3A4 inducer is established, consider adjusting the ixabepilone dose gradually up to 60 mg/m^2 (as a 4-hour infusion), with careful monitoring. If the strong CYP3A4 enzyme inducer is discontinued, reduce ixabepilone dose to the dose used prior to initiation of the CYP3A4 inducer.

Ixabepilone dosage adjustments for toxicity for monotherapy or combination therapy:

Hematologic:

Neutrophils <500/mm^3 for ≥7 days: Reduce ixabepilone dose by 20%

Neutropenic fever: Reduce ixabepilone dose by 20%

Platelets <25,000/mm^3 (or <50,000/mm^3 with bleeding): Reduce ixabepilone dose by 20%

Nonhematologic:

Neuropathy:

Grade 2 (moderate) for ≥7 days: Reduce ixabepilone dose by 20%

Grade 3 (severe) for <7 days: Reduce ixabepilone dose by 20%

Grade 3 (severe or disabling) for ≥7 days: Discontinue ixabepilone treatment

Grade 3 toxicity (severe; other than neuropathy): Reduce ixabepilone dose by 20%

Grade 3 arthralgia/myalgia or fatigue (transient): Continue ixabepilone at current dose

Grade 3 hand-foot syndrome: Continue ixabepilone at current dose

Grade 4 toxicity (disabling): Discontinue ixabepilone treatment

Note: Adjust dosage at the start of a cycle are based on toxicities (hematologic and nonhematologic) from the previous cycle; delay new cycles until neutrophils have recovered to ≥1,500/mm^3, platelets have recovered to ≥100,000/mm^3 and nonhematologic toxicities have resolved or improved to at least grade 1. If toxicities persist despite initial dose reduction, reduce dose an additional 20%.

Capecitabine dosage adjustments for toxicity in combination therapy with ixabepilone: Refer to Capecitabine monograph.

Dosage adjustment in renal impairment: There are no dosage adjustments provided in the manufacturer's labeling, however, renal excretion is minimal. Pharmacokinetics (monotherapy) are not affected in patients with mild-to-moderate renal insufficiency (CrCl >30 mL/minute); monotherapy has not been studied in patients with serum creatinine >1.5 times ULN. Combination therapy with capecitabine has not been studied in patients with CrCl <50 mL/minute.

Dosage adjustment in hepatic impairment:

Ixabepilone monotherapy (initial cycle; adjust doses for subsequent cycles based on toxicity):

AST and ALT ≤2.5 times ULN and bilirubin ≤1 times ULN: No dosage adjustment necessary

AST and ALT >2.5 to ≤10 times ULN and bilirubin >1 to ≤1.5 times ULN: Reduce dose to 32 mg/m^2

AST and ALT ≤10 times ULN and bilirubin >1.5 to ≤3 times ULN: Reduce dose to 20 to 30 mg/m^2 (initiate treatment at 20 mg/m^2, may escalate up to a maximum of 30 mg/m^2 in subsequent cycles if tolerated)

AST or ALT >10 times ULN or bilirubin >3 times ULN: Use is not recommended

Combination therapy of ixabepilone with capecitabine:

AST and ALT ≤2.5 times ULN and bilirubin ≤1 times ULN: No dosage adjustment necessary

AST or ALT >2.5 times ULN or bilirubin >1 times ULN: Use is contraindicated

Dosing in obesity: *ASCO Guidelines for appropriate chemotherapy dosing in obese adults with cancer:* In general, utilize patient's actual body weight (full weight) for calculation of body surface area- or weight-based dosing, particularly when the intent of therapy is curative; manage regimen-related toxicities in the same manner as for nonobese patients; if a dose reduction is utilized due to toxicity, consider resumption of full weight-based dosing with subsequent cycles, especially if cause of toxicity (eg, hepatic or renal impairment) is resolved (Griggs, 2012). **Note:** According to the manufacturer, patients with a body surface area (BSA) >2.2 m^2 should be dosed based upon a maximum BSA of 2.2 m^2

Dietary Considerations Avoid grapefruit juice (may increase plasma concentrations of ixabepilone).

Administration IV: Infuse over 3 hours. Use non-DEHP administration set (eg, polyethylene); filter with a 0.2 to 1.2 micron inline filter. Administration should be completed within 6 hours of preparation. If the dose is increased (above 40 mg/m^2) due to concomitant CYP3A4 inducer use, infuse over 4 hours.

Hazardous agent; use appropriate precautions for handling and disposal (NIOSH 2014 [group 1]).

Monitoring Parameters CBC with differential; hepatic function (ALT, AST, bilirubin); monitor for hypersensitivity, signs/symptoms of neuropathy

Dosage Forms

Solution Reconstituted, Intravenous:

Ixempra Kit: 15 mg (1 ea); 45 mg (1 ea)

- ◆ **Ixempra Kit** *see* Ixabepilone *on page 1138*
- ◆ **Ixiaro** *see* Japanese Encephalitis Virus Vaccine (Inactivated) *on page 1141*
- ◆ **Izba** *see* Travoprost *on page 2089*
- ◆ **Jakafi** *see* Ruxolitinib *on page 1856*
- ◆ **Jakavi (Can)** *see* Ruxolitinib *on page 1856*
- ◆ **Jalyn** *see* Dutasteride and Tamsulosin *on page 702*
- ◆ **JAMP-ACET-Tramadol (Can)** *see* Acetaminophen and Tramadol *on page 37*
- ◆ **JAMP-Alendronate (Can)** *see* Alendronate *on page 79*
- ◆ **JAMP-Allopurinol (Can)** *see* Allopurinol *on page 90*
- ◆ **JAMP-Amlodipine (Can)** *see* AmLODIPine *on page 123*
- ◆ **JAMP-Anastrozole (Can)** *see* Anastrozole *on page 148*
- ◆ **JAMP-Atenolol (Can)** *see* Atenolol *on page 189*
- ◆ **JAMP-Atorvastatin (Can)** *see* AtorvaSTATin *on page 194*
- ◆ **JAMP-Bicalutamide (Can)** *see* Bicalutamide *on page 262*
- ◆ **JAMP-Candesartan (Can)** *see* Candesartan *on page 335*
- ◆ **JAMP-Carvedilol (Can)** *see* Carvedilol *on page 367*
- ◆ **JAMP-Ciprofloxacin (Can)** *see* Ciprofloxacin (Systemic) *on page 441*
- ◆ **JAMP-Citalopram (Can)** *see* Citalopram *on page 451*
- ◆ **JAMP-Clopidogrel (Can)** *see* Clopidogrel *on page 484*
- ◆ **Jamp-Colchicine (Can)** *see* Colchicine *on page 500*
- ◆ **JAMP-Cyclobenzaprine (Can)** *see* Cyclobenzaprine *on page 516*
- ◆ **Jamp-Dicyclomine (Can)** *see* Dicyclomine *on page 622*
- ◆ **Jamp-Dimenhydrinate [OTC] (Can)** *see* DimenhyDRINATE *on page 637*
- ◆ **Jamp-Docusate [OTC] (Can)** *see* Docusate *on page 661*
- ◆ **Jamp-Domperidone (Can)** *see* Domperidone [CAN/INT] *on page 666*
- ◆ **JAMP-Donepezil (Can)** *see* Donepezil *on page 668*
- ◆ **JAMP-Escitalopram (Can)** *see* Escitalopram *on page 765*
- ◆ **JAMP-Ezetimibe (Can)** *see* Ezetimibe *on page 832*
- ◆ **JAMP-Finasteride (Can)** *see* Finasteride *on page 878*
- ◆ **JAMP-Fluoxetine (Can)** *see* FLUoxetine *on page 899*
- ◆ **Jamp-Fosinopril (Can)** *see* Fosinopril *on page 932*
- ◆ **JAMP-Gabapentin (Can)** *see* Gabapentin *on page 943*
- ◆ **Jamp-Ibuprofen (Can)** *see* Ibuprofen *on page 1032*
- ◆ **JAMP-Indapamide (Can)** *see* Indapamide *on page 1065*
- ◆ **JAMP-Irbesartan (Can)** *see* Irbesartan *on page 1110*
- ◆ **JAMP-Irbesartan and Hydrochlorothiazide (Can)** *see* Irbesartan and Hydrochlorothiazide *on page 1112*
- ◆ **Jamp-Lactulose (Can)** *see* Lactulose *on page 1156*
- ◆ **JAMP-Letrozole (Can)** *see* Letrozole *on page 1181*
- ◆ **JAMP-Levetiracetam (Can)** *see* LevETIRAcetam *on page 1191*
- ◆ **JAMP-Lisinopril (Can)** *see* Lisinopril *on page 1226*
- ◆ **JAMP-Losartan (Can)** *see* Losartan *on page 1248*
- ◆ **JAMP-Losartan HCTZ (Can)** *see* Losartan and Hydrochlorothiazide *on page 1250*
- ◆ **JAMP-Metformin (Can)** *see* MetFORMIN *on page 1307*
- ◆ **JAMP-Metformin Blackberry (Can)** *see* MetFORMIN *on page 1307*
- ◆ **JAMP-Methotrexate (Can)** *see* Methotrexate *on page 1322*
- ◆ **JAMP-Metoprolol-L (Can)** *see* Metoprolol *on page 1350*
- ◆ **Jamp-Mirtazapine (Can)** *see* Mirtazapine *on page 1376*
- ◆ **Jamp-Montelukast (Can)** *see* Montelukast *on page 1392*
- ◆ **JAMP-Mycophenolate (Can)** *see* Mycophenolate *on page 1405*
- ◆ **JAMP-Olanzapine ODT (Can)** *see* OLANZapine *on page 1491*
- ◆ **JAMP-Omeprazole DR (Can)** *see* Omeprazole *on page 1508*
- ◆ **JAMP-Ondansetron (Can)** *see* Ondansetron *on page 1513*
- ◆ **JAMP-Pantoprazole (Can)** *see* Pantoprazole *on page 1570*
- ◆ **JAMP-Paroxetine (Can)** *see* PARoxetine *on page 1579*
- ◆ **JAMP-Pioglitazone (Can)** *see* Pioglitazone *on page 1654*
- ◆ **JAMP-Pravastatin (Can)** *see* Pravastatin *on page 1700*

◆ **JAMP-Quetiapine (Can)** *see* QUEtiapine *on page 1751*
◆ **JAMP-Ramipril (Can)** *see* Ramipril *on page 1771*
◆ **JAMP-Risperidone (Can)** *see* RisperiDONE *on page 1818*
◆ **JAMP-Rizatriptan (Can)** *see* Rizatriptan *on page 1836*
◆ **JAMP-Rizatriptan IR (Can)** *see* Rizatriptan *on page 1836*
◆ **JAMP-Ropinirole (Can)** *see* ROPINIRole *on page 1844*
◆ **Jamp-Rosuvastatin (Can)** *see* Rosuvastatin *on page 1848*
◆ **JAMP-Sertraline (Can)** *see* Sertraline *on page 1878*
◆ **JAMP-Simvastatin (Can)** *see* Simvastatin *on page 1890*
◆ **JAMP-Terbinafine (Can)** *see* Terbinafine (Systemic) *on page 2002*
◆ **JAMP-Tobramycin (Can)** *see* Tobramycin (Systemic, Oral Inhalation) *on page 2052*
◆ **JAMP-Vancomycin (Can)** *see* Vancomycin *on page 2130*
◆ **JAMP-Zolmitriptan (Can)** *see* ZOLMitriptan *on page 2210*
◆ **JAMP-Zopiclone (Can)** *see* Zopiclone [CAN/INT] *on page 2217*
◆ **Jantoven** *see* Warfarin *on page 2186*
◆ **Janumet** *see* Sitagliptin and Metformin *on page 1898*
◆ **Janumet XR** *see* Sitagliptin and Metformin *on page 1898*
◆ **Januvia** *see* SitaGLIPtin *on page 1897*
◆ **Januvia® (Can)** *see* SitaGLIPtin *on page 1897*

Japanese Encephalitis Virus Vaccine (Inactivated)

(jap a NEESE en sef a LYE tis VYE rus vak SEEN, in ak ti VAY ted)

Brand Names: U.S. Ixiaro
Brand Names: Canada Ixiaro
Index Terms IC51; JE-VC (Ixiaro)
Pharmacologic Category Vaccine, Inactivated (Viral)
Additional Appendix Information

Immunization Administration Recommendations *on page 2250*
Immunization Recommendations *on page 2255*

Use Japanese encephalitis vaccination: For active immunization against Japanese encephalitis (JE) for persons 2 months of age and older

The Advisory Committee on Immunization Practices (ACIP) recommends vaccination for (CDC, 2010; CDC, 2013):

- Persons spending ≥1 month in endemic areas during transmission season
- Research laboratory workers who may be exposed to the Japanese encephalitis virus

Vaccination should also be considered for the following:

• Travelers to areas with an ongoing outbreak
• Travelers spending <30 days in endemic areas during the transmission season and planning to go outside of urban areas and have an increased risk of exposure. For example, high-risk activities include extensive outdoor activity in rural areas especially at night; extensive outdoor activities such as camping, hiking, etc; staying in accommodations without air conditioning, screens or bed nets.
• Travelers to endemic areas who are unsure of specific destination, activities, or duration of travel

Japanese encephalitis vaccine is not recommended for short-term travelers whose visit will be restricted to urban areas or periods outside of the well-defined JE virus transmission season.

Pregnancy Risk Factor B
Dosage U.S. recommended primary immunization schedule:

Children 2 months to <3 years: IM: 0.25 mL/dose; a total of 2 doses given on days 0 and 28. Series should be completed at least 1 week prior to potential exposure.

Children ≥3 years, Adolescents, and Adults: IM: 0.5 mL/dose; a total of 2 doses given on days 0 and 28. Series should be completed at least 1 week prior to potential exposure.

Booster dose: Adults ≥17 years: Booster dose may be given prior to potential re-exposure if the primary series was completed >1 year previously. The safety of booster doses in children and adolescents <17 years has not been established.

Note: If the second dose is missed, limited data from one clinical trial in adults demonstrate a 99% seroconversion rate when the second dose was administered 11 months after the initial dose.

Elderly: Refer to adult dosing.

Dosage adjustment in renal impairment: No dosage adjustment provided in manufacturer's labeling.

Dosage adjustment in hepatic impairment: No dosage adjustment provided in manufacturer's labeling.

Additional Information Complete prescribing information should be consulted for additional detail.

Dosage Forms

Suspension, Intramuscular:
Ixiaro: (0.5 mL)

◆ **Jardiance** *see* Empagliflozin *on page 718*
◆ **Jaydess (Can)** *see* Levonorgestrel *on page 1201*
◆ **Jencycla** *see* Norethindrone *on page 1473*
◆ **Jentadueto** *see* Linagliptin and Metformin *on page 1217*
◆ **Jetrea** *see* Ocriplasmin *on page 1484*
◆ **JE-VC (Ixiaro)** *see* Japanese Encephalitis Virus Vaccine (Inactivated) *on page 1141*
◆ **Jevtana** *see* Cabazitaxel *on page 316*
◆ **Jinteli** *see* Ethinyl Estradiol and Norethindrone *on page 808*
◆ **J-Max [OTC]** *see* Guaifenesin and Phenylephrine *on page 988*
◆ **Jock Itch Spray [OTC]** *see* Tolnaftate *on page 2063*
◆ **Jolessa** *see* Ethinyl Estradiol and Levonorgestrel *on page 803*
◆ **Jolivette** *see* Norethindrone *on page 1473*

Josamycin [INT] (joe sa MYE sin)

International Brand Names Alplucine[vet.] (FR); Beibeisha (CN); Iosalide (IT); Jomybel (BE); Josacin (DE); Josacine (FR); Josalid (AT); Josamina (ES); Josaxin (ES, IT, JP); Wilprafen (CZ, DE, HU, LU, RU)
Index Terms Josamycin Proprionate
Pharmacologic Category Antibiotic, Macrolide
Reported Use Treatment of infections caused by susceptible organisms including infections of the upper and lower respiratory system
Dosage Range Adults: Oral: 1-2 g every 24 hours in 2-3 divided doses
Product Availability Product available in various countries; not currently available in the U.S.
Dosage Forms

Suspension, oral: 125 mg/5 mL, 250 mg/5 mL, 375 mg/5 mL
Tablet: 500 mg, 750 mg, 1000 mg

◆ **Josamycin Proprionate** *see* Josamycin [INT] *on page 1141*

- ◆ **J-Tan PD [OTC]** *see* Brompheniramine *on page 292*
- ◆ **Jublia** *see* Efinaconazole *on page 710*
- ◆ **Junel 1.5/30** *see* Ethinyl Estradiol and Norethindrone *on page 808*
- ◆ **Junel 1/20** *see* Ethinyl Estradiol and Norethindrone *on page 808*
- ◆ **Junel Fe 1.5/30** *see* Ethinyl Estradiol and Norethindrone *on page 808*
- ◆ **Junel Fe 1/20** *see* Ethinyl Estradiol and Norethindrone *on page 808*
- ◆ **Jurnista (Can)** *see* HYDROmorphone *on page 1016*
- ◆ **Just For Kids [OTC]** *see* Fluoride *on page 895*
- ◆ **Juvederm Ultra** *see* Hyaluronate and Derivatives *on page 1006*
- ◆ **Juvederm Ultra XC** *see* Hyaluronate and Derivatives *on page 1006*
- ◆ **Juvederm Ultra Plus** *see* Hyaluronate and Derivatives *on page 1006*
- ◆ **Juvederm Ultra Plus XC** *see* Hyaluronate and Derivatives *on page 1006*
- ◆ **Juvederm Voluma XC** *see* Hyaluronate and Derivatives *on page 1006*
- ◆ **Juvisync™ [DSC]** *see* Sitagliptin and Simvastatin *on page 1899*
- ◆ **Juxtapid** *see* Lomitapide *on page 1233*
- ◆ **K-10 (Can)** *see* Potassium Chloride *on page 1687*
- ◆ **K-99 [OTC]** *see* Potassium Gluconate *on page 1690*
- ◆ **Kabiven** *see* Total Parenteral Nutrition *on page 2073*
- ◆ **Kadcyla** *see* Ado-Trastuzumab Emtansine *on page 58*
- ◆ **Kadian** *see* Morphine (Systemic) *on page 1394*
- ◆ **Kalbitor** *see* Ecallantide *on page 703*
- ◆ **Kaletra** *see* Lopinavir and Ritonavir *on page 1237*
- ◆ **Kalexate** *see* Sodium Polystyrene Sulfonate *on page 1912*
- ◆ **Kalydeco** *see* Ivacaftor *on page 1135*

Kanamycin (kan a MYE sin)

Index Terms Kanamycin Sulfate

Pharmacologic Category Antibiotic, Aminoglycoside

Use Treatment of serious infections caused by susceptible strains of *E. coli*, *Proteus* species, *Enterobacter aerogenes*, *Klebsiella pneumoniae*, *Serratia marcescens*, and *Acinetobacter* species; second-line treatment of *Mycobacterium tuberculosis*

Pregnancy Risk Factor D

Dosage Note: Dosing should be based on ideal body weight

Children: Infections: IM, IV: 15 mg/kg/day in divided doses every 8-12 hours

Adults:

Infections: IM, IV: 5-7.5 mg/kg/dose in divided doses every 8-12 hours (<15 mg/kg/day)

Intraperitoneal: After contamination in surgery: 500 mg

Irrigating solution: 0.25%; maximum 1.5 g/day (via all administration routes)

Aerosol: 250 mg 2-4 times/day

Dosage adjustment in renal impairment: Adults: IV: The following adjustments have been recommended (Aronoff, 2007). **Note:** Renally adjusted dose recommendations are based on a dose of 7.5 mg/kg every 12 hours.

CrCl >50 mL/minute: Administer every 12-24 hours

CrCl 10-50 mL/minute: Administer every 24-72 hours; monitor levels.

CrCl <10 mL/minute: Administer every 48-72 hours; monitor levels.

Intermittent hemodialysis (IHD): One-half the dose administered after hemodialysis on dialysis days.

Peritoneal dialysis (PD): Administration via PD fluid: 15-20 mg/L/day of PD fluid

Continuous renal replacement therapy (CRRT): Administer every 24-72 hours; monitor levels. **Note:** Drug clearance is highly dependent on the method of renal replacement, filter type, and flow rate. Appropriate dosing requires close monitoring of pharmacologic response, signs of adverse reactions due to drug accumulation, as well as drug concentrations in relation to target trough (if appropriate).

Dosage adjustment in hepatic impairment: No dosage adjustment provided in manufacturer's labeling.

Additional Information Complete prescribing information should be consulted for additional detail.

- ◆ **Kanamycin Sulfate** *see* Kanamycin *on page 1142*
- ◆ **Kank-A® (Can)** *see* Cetylpyridinium and Benzocaine [CAN/INT] *on page 415*
- ◆ **Kank-A Mouth Pain [OTC]** *see* Benzocaine *on page 246*
- ◆ **Kaopectate [OTC] (Can)** *see* Attapulgite [CAN/INT] *on page 204*
- ◆ **Kaopectate Children's [OTC] (Can)** *see* Attapulgite [CAN/INT] *on page 204*
- ◆ **Kaopectate Extra Strength [OTC] (Can)** *see* Attapulgite [CAN/INT] *on page 204*
- ◆ **Kaote DVI** *see* Antihemophilic Factor (Human) *on page 152*
- ◆ **Kao-Tin [OTC]** *see* Bismuth *on page 265*
- ◆ **Kao-Tin [OTC]** *see* Docusate *on page 661*
- ◆ **Kapidex** *see* Dexlansoprazole *on page 603*
- ◆ **Kapvay** *see* CloNIDine *on page 480*
- ◆ **Karbinal™ ER** *see* Carbinoxamine *on page 356*
- ◆ **Karbinal ER** *see* Carbinoxamine *on page 356*
- ◆ **Kariva** *see* Ethinyl Estradiol and Desogestrel *on page 799*
- ◆ **Kayexalate** *see* Sodium Polystyrene Sulfonate *on page 1912*
- ◆ **Kayexalate® (Can)** *see* Sodium Polystyrene Sulfonate *on page 1912*
- ◆ **Kcentra** *see* Prothrombin Complex Concentrate (Human) [(Factors II, VII, IX, X), Protein C, and Protein S] *on page 1738*
- ◆ **KCl** *see* Potassium Chloride *on page 1687*
- ◆ **Kdur** *see* Potassium Chloride *on page 1687*
- ◆ **K-Dur (Can)** *see* Potassium Chloride *on page 1687*
- ◆ **Kedbumin** *see* Albumin *on page 67*
- ◆ **K-Effervescent** *see* Potassium Bicarbonate and Potassium Citrate *on page 1687*
- ◆ **Keflex** *see* Cephalexin *on page 405*
- ◆ **Kefzol** *see* CeFAZolin *on page 373*
- ◆ **Kelnor™** *see* Ethinyl Estradiol and Ethynodiol Diacetate *on page 801*
- ◆ **Kenalog** *see* Triamcinolone (Systemic) *on page 2099*
- ◆ **Kenalog** *see* Triamcinolone (Topical) *on page 2100*
- ◆ **Kenalog® (Can)** *see* Triamcinolone (Topical) *on page 2100*
- ◆ **Keoxifene Hydrochloride** *see* Raloxifene *on page 1765*
- ◆ **Kepivance** *see* Palifermin *on page 1555*
- ◆ **Kepivance® (Can)** *see* Palifermin *on page 1555*
- ◆ **Keppra** *see* LevETIRAcetam *on page 1191*

- ◆ **Keppra XR** *see* LevETIRAcetam *on page 1191*
- ◆ **Kerafoam** *see* Urea *on page 2114*
- ◆ **Kerafoam 42** *see* Urea *on page 2114*
- ◆ **Keralac** *see* Urea *on page 2114*
- ◆ **Keratinocyte Growth Factor, Recombinant Human** *see* Palifermin *on page 1555*
- ◆ **Kerlone** *see* Betaxolol (Systemic) *on page 256*
- ◆ **Kerr Insta-Char [OTC]** *see* Charcoal, Activated *on page 416*
- ◆ **Kerr Insta-Char in Sorbitol [OTC]** *see* Charcoal, Activated *on page 416*
- ◆ **Kerydin** *see* Tavaborole *on page 1980*
- ◆ **Ketalar** *see* Ketamine *on page 1143*

Ketamine (KEET a meen)

Brand Names: U.S. Ketalar

Brand Names: Canada Ketalar; Ketamine Hydrochloride Injection, USP

Index Terms Ketamine Hydrochloride

Pharmacologic Category General Anesthetic

Use Induction and maintenance of general anesthesia

Pregnancy Considerations Adverse events have not been observed in animal reproduction studies. Ketamine crosses the placenta and can be detected in fetal tissue. Ketamine produces dose dependent increases in uterine contractions; effects may vary by trimester. The plasma clearance of ketamine is reduced during pregnancy. Dose related neonatal depression and decreased APGAR scores have been reported with large doses administered at delivery (Ghoneim, 1977; Little, 1972; White, 1982).

Breast-Feeding Considerations It is not known if ketamine is excreted in breast milk.

Contraindications Hypersensitivity to ketamine or any component of the formulation; conditions in which an increase in blood pressure would be hazardous

Warnings/Precautions Use with caution in patients with coronary artery disease, catecholamine depletion, hypertension, and tachycardia. Cardiac function should be continuously monitored in patients with increased blood pressure or cardiac decompensation. Postanesthetic emergence reactions which can manifest as vivid dreams, hallucinations, and/or frank delirium occur; these reactions are less common in patients <15 years of age and >65 years and when given intramuscularly. Emergence reactions, confusion, or irrational behavior may occur up to 24 hours postoperatively and may be reduced by pretreatment with a benzodiazepine and the use of ketamine at the lower end of the dosing range. Rapid IV administration or overdose may cause respiratory depression, apnea, and enhanced pressor response. Resuscitative equipment should be available during use. Use with caution in patients with CSF pressure elevation, the chronic alcoholic or acutely alcohol-intoxicated. May cause dependence (withdrawal symptoms on discontinuation) and tolerance with prolonged use. May cause CNS depression, which may impair physical or mental abilities; patients must be cautioned about performing tasks which require mental alertness (eg, operating machinery or driving). When used for outpatient surgery, the patient be accompanied by a responsible adult. Should be administered under the supervision of a physician experienced in administering general anesthetics.

Adverse Reactions

Cardiovascular: Arrhythmia, bradycardia/tachycardia, hyper-/hypotension

Central nervous system: Intracranial pressure increased

Dermatologic: Erythema (transient), morbilliform rash (transient)

Gastrointestinal: Anorexia, nausea, salivation increased, vomiting

Local: Pain at the injection site, exanthema at the injection site

Neuromuscular & skeletal: Skeletal muscle tone enhanced (tonic-clonic movements)

Ocular: Diplopia, intraocular pressure increased, nystagmus

Respiratory: Airway obstruction, apnea, bronchial secretions increased, respiratory depression, laryngospasm

Miscellaneous: Anaphylaxis, dependence with prolonged use, emergence reactions (includes confusion, delirium, dreamlike state, excitement, hallucinations, irrational behavior, vivid imagery)

Drug Interactions

Metabolism/Transport Effects Substrate of CYP2B6 (major), CYP2C9 (major), CYP3A4 (major); **Note:** Assignment of Major/Minor substrate status based on clinically relevant drug interaction potential

Avoid Concomitant Use

Avoid concomitant use of Ketamine with any of the following: Azelastine (Nasal); Conivaptan; Fusidic Acid (Systemic); Idelalisib; Orphenadrine; Paraldehyde; Thalidomide

Increased Effect/Toxicity

Ketamine may increase the levels/effects of: Alcohol (Ethyl); Azelastine (Nasal); Buprenorphine; CNS Depressants; Hydrocodone; Memantine; Methotrimeprazine; Metyrosine; Mirtazapine; Orphenadrine; Paraldehyde; Pramipexole; ROPINIRole; Rotigotine; Selective Serotonin Reuptake Inhibitors; Suvorexant; Thalidomide; Thiopental; Zolpidem

The levels/effects of Ketamine may be increased by: Brimonidine (Topical); Cannabis; Ceritinib; Conivaptan; CYP2B6 Inhibitors (Moderate); CYP2C9 Inhibitors (Moderate); CYP2C9 Inhibitors (Strong); CYP3A4 Inhibitors (Moderate); CYP3A4 Inhibitors (Strong); Dasatinib; Doxylamine; Dronabinol; Droperidol; Fosaprepitant; Fusidic Acid (Systemic); HydrOXYzine; Idelalisib; Ivacaftor; Kava Kava; Luliconazole; Magnesium Sulfate; Methotrimeprazine; Mifepristone; Nabilone; Netupitant; Perampanel; Quazepam; Rufinamide; Simeprevir; Sodium Oxybate; Stiripentol; Tapentadol; Tetrahydrocannabinol

Decreased Effect

The levels/effects of Ketamine may be decreased by: CYP2C9 Inducers (Strong); Dabrafenib

Preparation for Administration The 50 mg/mL and 100 mg/mL vials may be further diluted in D_5W or NS to prepare a maintenance infusion with a final concentration of 1 mg/mL (or 2 mg/mL in patients with fluid restrictions). The 10 mg/mL vials are not recommended to be further diluted. Do not mix with barbiturates or diazepam (precipitation may occur). **Note:** The 100 mg/mL concentration should not be administered IV unless properly diluted with an equal volume of SWFI, NS, or D_5W.

Storage/Stability Store at 20°C to 25°C (68°F to 77°F). Protect from light.

Mechanism of Action Produces a cataleptic-like state in which the patient is dissociated from the surrounding environment by direct action on the cortex and limbic system. Ketamine is a noncompetitive NMDA receptor antagonist that blocks glutamate. Low (subanesthetic) doses produce analgesia, and modulate central sensitization, hyperalgesia and opioid tolerance. Reduces polysynaptic spinal reflexes.

Pharmacodynamics/Kinetics

Onset of action:

IV: Anesthetic effect: 30 seconds

IM: Anesthetic effect: 3-4 minutes

Duration: Anesthetic effect: IV: 5-10 minutes; IM: 12-25 minutes

Distribution: V_d: 3 L/kg

Metabolism: Hepatic via hydroxylation and N-demethylation; the metabolite norketamine is 33% as potent as parent compound; greater conversion to norketamine occurs after oral administration as compared to parenteral administration

Bioavailability: Oral: 16%; Intranasal: 50%

Half-life elimination: Alpha: 10-15 minutes; Beta: 2.5 hours

Excretion: Primarily urine

Dosage May be used in combination with anticholinergic agents to decrease hypersalivation.

Adolescents ≥16 years and Adults: **Note:** Titrate dose for desired effect.

Sedation/analgesia (off-label use):

Procedural (operative or nonoperative):

IM: 2 to 4 mg/kg (Miller, 2010; White, 1982); may follow with a continuous infusion if necessary

IV: 0.2 to 0.8 mg/kg (Miller, 2010; Remérand, 2009; Zakine, 2008; White, 1982); a maximum bolus dose of 50 mg was used in one study (Remérand, 2009). May follow bolus dose with a continuous infusion if necessary.

Continuous IV infusion: 2 to 7 mcg/kg/minute (Hocking, 2003; Remérand, 2009; Zakine, 2008)

Critically ill patients (as an adjunct to an opioid analgesic for non-neuropathic pain): IV: Initial: 0.1 to 0.5 mg/kg bolus; followed by 0.83 to 6.7 mcg/kg/minute (equivalent to 0.05 to 0.4 **mg/kg/hour**) (SCCM [Barr, 2013])

Anesthesia:

Induction of anesthesia:

Manufacturer's labeling:

IM: 6.5 to 13 mg/kg

IV: 1 to 4.5 mg/kg

Alternate recommendations (off-label dosing): **Note:** lower doses may be used if adjuvant drugs (eg, midazolam) are administered (Miller, 2010).

IM: 4 to 10 mg/kg (Green, 1990; Miller, 2010; White, 1982)

IV: 0.5 to 2 mg/kg (Miller, 2010; White, 1982)

Maintenance of anesthesia: May administer supplemental doses of one-half to the full induction dose or a continuous infusion of 0.1 to 0.5 mg/minute (per manufacturer). **Note:** To maintain an adequate concentration of ketamine for maintenance of anesthesia, 1 to 2 mg/minute has been recommended (White, 1982); doses in the range of 15-90 mcg/kg/minute (~1 to 6 mg/minute in a 70-kg patient) have also been suggested (Miller, 2010). Concurrent use of nitrous oxide reduces ketamine requirements.

Dosage adjustment in renal impairment: There are no dosage adjustments provided in the manufacturer's labeling.

Dosage adjustment in hepatic impairment: There are no dosage adjustments provided in the manufacturer's labeling.

Administration

Oral: Mix the appropriate dose (using the 100 mg/mL injectable solution) in cola or other beverage; administer immediately after preparation.

IV: According to the manufacturer, may administer bolus/induction doses over 1 minute or at a rate of 0.5 mg/kg/minute; more rapid administration may result in respiratory depression and enhanced pressor response. Some experts suggest administration over 2 to 3 minutes (Miller, 2010).

Monitoring Parameters Heart rate, blood pressure, respiratory rate, transcutaneous O_2 saturation, emergence reactions; cardiac function should be continuously monitored in patients with increased blood pressure or cardiac decompensation

Additional Information May produce emergence psychosis including auditory and visual hallucinations, restlessness, disorientation, vivid dreams, and irrational behavior in ~12% of patients; pretreatment with a benzodiazepine reduces incidence of psychosis by >50%. Spontaneous involuntary movements, nystagmus, hypertonus, and vocalizations are also common.

The analgesia outlasts the general anesthetic component. Bronchodilation is beneficial in asthmatic or COPD patients. Laryngeal reflexes may remain intact or may be obtunded. The direct myocardial depressant action of ketamine can be seen in stressed, catecholamine-deficient patients. Ketamine increases cerebral metabolism and cerebral blood flow while producing a noncompetitive block of the glutaminergic postsynaptic NMDA receptor. It lowers seizure threshold and stimulates salivary secretions (atropine/scopolamine treatment is recommended).

Dosage Forms

Solution, Injection:

Ketalar: 10 mg/mL (20 mL); 50 mg/mL (10 mL); 100 mg/mL (5 mL)

Generic: 10 mg/mL (20 mL); 50 mg/mL (10 mL); 100 mg/mL (5 mL, 10 mL)

◆ **Ketamine Hydrochloride** *see* Ketamine *on page 1143*

◆ **Ketamine Hydrochloride Injection, USP (Can)** *see* Ketamine *on page 1143*

Ketanserin [INT] (keet AN ser in)

International Brand Names Aseranox (GR); Ketensin (NL); Perketan (IT); Serefrex (AR); Serepress (IT); Sufrexal (BE, CZ, IT, LU, MX, NL, NO, PT); Vulketan [vet.] (AT, CH)

Index Terms Ketanserin Tartrate

Pharmacologic Category Serotonin Antagonist

Reported Use Management of hypertension

Dosage Range Adults: Oral: 20 mg twice daily

Product Availability Product available in various countries; not currently available in the U.S.

Dosage Forms

Tablet: 20 mg, 40 mg

◆ **Ketanserin Tartrate** *see* Ketanserin [INT] *on page 1144*

Ketazolam [INT] (kee TAZ o lam)

International Brand Names Anseren (IT); Ansieten (AR); Ansietil (CL); Atenual (PE); Marcen (ES); Sedatival (CL, PE); Sedotime (ES, PE); Solatran (BE, CH, ZA); Unakalm (ES, NL, PT)

Pharmacologic Category Benzodiazepine

Reported Use Treatment of anxiety, tension, irritability, and similar stress related symptoms

Dosage Range Oral:

Adults: 15-60 mg/day in a single dose or divided doses taken prior to bedtime; usual dosage: 30 mg/day prior to bedtime

Dosage adjustment in the elderly and debilitated patients: Lower dose should be considered.

Product Availability Product available in various countries; not currently available in the U.S.

Dosage Forms

Capsule: 15 mg, 30 mg, 45 mg

◆ **Ketek** *see* Telithromycin *on page 1987*

Ketoconazole (Systemic) (kee toe KOE na zole)

Brand Names: Canada Apo-Ketoconazole; Teva-Ketoconazole

Index Terms Nizoral

Pharmacologic Category Antifungal Agent, Imidazole Derivative; Antifungal Agent, Oral

Use Fungal infections:

U.S. labeling: Systemic fungal infections: Treatment of susceptible fungal infections, including blastomycosis, histoplasmosis, paracoccidioidomycosis, coccidioidomycosis, and chromomycosis in patients who have failed or who are intolerant to other antifungal therapies

Canadian labeling: Treatment of serious or life-threatening systemic fungal infections (eg, systemic candidiasis, chronic mucocutaneous candidiasis, coccidioidomycosis, paracoccidioidomycosis, histoplasmosis, and chromomycosis) where alternate therapy is inappropriate or ineffective; may be considered for severe dermatophytoses unresponsive to other therapy

Pregnancy Risk Factor C

Dosage

Fungal infections: Oral:

Children ≥2 years: 3.3-6.6 mg/kg once daily

Adults: 200-400 mg once daily

Therapy duration: Continue therapy until active fungal infection has resolved (based on clinical and laboratory parameters); some infections may require at least 6 months of therapy.

Prostate cancer, advanced (off-label use): Adults: Oral: 400 mg 3 times daily (in combination with oral hydrocortisone) until disease progression (Ryan, 2007; Small, 2004)

Dosage adjustment in renal impairment: No dosage adjustment provided in manufacturer's labeling. Some clinicians suggest that no dosage adjustment is necessary in mild-to-severe impairment (Aronoff, 2007).

Hemodialysis: Not dialyzable

Dosage adjustment in hepatic impairment: No dosage adjustment provided in manufacturer's labeling; use with caution due to risks of hepatotoxicity.

Hepatotoxicity during treatment:

U.S. labeling: If ALT >ULN or 30% above baseline (or if patient is symptomatic), interrupt therapy and obtain full hepatic function panel. Upon normalization of liver function, may consider resuming therapy if benefit outweighs risk (hepatotoxicity has been reported on rechallenge).

Canadian labeling: Discontinue therapy for liver function tests >3 times ULN or if abnormalities persist, worsen, or are associated with hepatotoxicity symptoms.

Additional Information Complete prescribing information should be consulted for additional detail.

Dosage Forms

Tablet, Oral:

Generic: 200 mg

Ketoconazole (Topical) (kee toe KOE na zole)

Brand Names: U.S. Extina; Ketodan; Nizoral; Nizoral A-D [OTC]; Xolegel

Brand Names: Canada Ketoderm; Nizoral

Pharmacologic Category Antifungal Agent, Imidazole Derivative; Antifungal Agent, Topical

Use

Cream: Treatment of tinea corporis, tinea cruris, tinea versicolor, cutaneous candidiasis, seborrheic dermatitis

Foam, gel: Treatment of seborrheic dermatitis

Shampoo: Treatment of dandruff, seborrheic dermatitis, tinea versicolor

Pregnancy Risk Factor C

Dosage

Shampoo:

Seborrheic dermatitis (ketoconazole 1%): Children ≥12 years and Adults: Apply twice weekly for up to 8 weeks with at least 3 days between each shampoo

Tinea versicolor (ketoconazole 2%): Adults: Apply to damp skin, lather, leave on 5 minutes, and rinse (one application should be sufficient)

Topical:

Tinea infections: Adults: Cream: Rub gently into the affected area once daily. Duration of treatment: Tinea corporis, cruris: 2 weeks; tinea pedis: 6 weeks

Seborrheic dermatitis: Children ≥12 years and Adults:

Cream: Rub gently into the affected area twice daily for 4 weeks or until clinical response is noted

Foam: Apply to affected area twice daily for 4 weeks

Gel: Rub gently into the affected area once daily for 2 weeks

Susceptible fungal infections in the oral cavity (candidiasis, oral thrush, and chronic mucocutaneous candidiasis) (off-label use): Adults: Cream: Apply locally as directed with a thin coat to inner surface of denture and affected areas after meals

Additional Information Complete prescribing information should be consulted for additional detail.

Dosage Forms

Cream, External:

Generic: 2% (15 g, 30 g, 60 g)

Foam, External:

Extina: 2% (50 g, 100 g)

Ketodan: 2% (100 g)

Gel, External:

Xolegel: 2% (45 g)

Kit, External:

Ketodan: 2%

Shampoo, External:

Nizoral: 2% (120 mL)

Nizoral A-D [OTC]: 1% (125 mL, 200 mL)

Generic: 2% (120 mL)

◆ **Ketodan** *see* Ketoconazole (Topical) *on page 1145*

◆ **Ketoderm (Can)** *see* Ketoconazole (Topical) *on page 1145*

Ketoprofen (kee toe PROE fen)

Brand Names: U.S. Active-Ketoprofen

Brand Names: Canada Ketoprofen SR; Ketoprofen-E; PMS-Ketoprofen; PMS-Ketoprofen-E

Pharmacologic Category Nonsteroidal Anti-inflammatory Drug (NSAID), Oral

Additional Appendix Information

Beers Criteria – Potentially Inappropriate Medications for Geriatrics *on page 2271*

Use

Osteoarthritis: Treatment of osteoarthritis

Pain: Treatment of mild to moderate pain (regular release only)

Primary dysmenorrhea: Treatment of primary dysmenorrhea (regular release only)

Rheumatoid arthritis: Treatment of rheumatoid arthritis

Canadian labeling: Additional use (not in U.S. labeling): Treatment of ankylosing spondylitis

Pregnancy Risk Factor C

Dosage Note: The enteric coated tablet [Canadian product] and extended release formulations are not recommended for the treatment of acute pain. Lower doses should be considered in small, elderly, or debilitated patients.

Oral:
Adults:
Rheumatoid arthritis, osteoarthritis:
Regular release: *U.S. labeling:* 50 mg 4 times daily **or** 75 mg 3 times daily; up to a maximum of 300 mg daily
Regular release or enteric coated: *Canadian labeling:* 50 mg 3 or 4 times daily; up to 200 mg daily; twice daily regimen (eg, 100 mg twice daily) may be considered after maintenance dose is established although some patients respond more favorably to more frequent dosing. For severe rheumatic activity or an inadequate response to lower dosages, may consider dose increase up to a maximum 300 mg daily.
Extended release: 200 mg once daily
Dysmenorrhea, mild to moderate pain: Regular release: 25-50 mg every 6-8 hours up to a maximum of 300 mg daily
Elderly:
U.S. labeling: Manufacturer labeling recommends that initial dose should be decreased in patients >75 years but does not provide specific dosing recommendations; use caution when dosage changes are made
Canadian labeling: Reduce initial dose by 33% to 50%
Rectal suppository [Canadian product]:
Adults: Ankylosing spondylitis, osteoarthritis, or rheumatoid arthritis: Insert one suppository rectally in the morning and evening (twice daily) or at bedtime (once daily). May supplement with divided oral dosing up to a combined rectal/oral maximum of 200 mg daily; for severe rheumatic activity or an inadequate response to lower dosages, a combined rectal/oral dose up to 300 mg daily may be considered. Patients should be maintained at the lowest effective dose.
Elderly: Manufacturer labeling recommends that the initial dose should be decreased but does not provide specific dosing recommendation.

Dosage adjustment in renal impairment: In general, NSAIDs are not recommended for use in patients with advanced renal disease, but the manufacturer of ketoprofen does provide some guidelines for adjustment in renal dysfunction:
U.S. labeling:
Mild impairment: Maximum dose: 150 mg daily
Severe impairment: GFR <25 mL/minute/1.73 m^2: Maximum dose: 100 mg daily
Canadian labeling: Reduce initial dose by 33% to 50%.
Dosage adjustment in hepatic impairment: Hepatic impairment and serum albumin <3.5 g/dL: Maximum initial dose: 100 mg daily

Additional Information Complete prescribing information should be consulted for additional detail.

Dosage Forms Considerations Active-Ketoprofen is a compounding kit. Refer to manufacturer's labeling for compounding instructions.

Dosage Forms
Capsule, Oral:
Generic: 50 mg, 75 mg
Capsule Extended Release 24 Hour, Oral:
Generic: 200 mg
Cream, External:
Active-Ketoprofen: 5% (120 g)

Dosage Forms: Canada Note: Refer also to Dosage Forms. Extended release capsule and external cream are not available in Canada.
Enteric coated tablet, Oral: 50 mg, 100 mg
Extended release tablet, Oral: 200 mg
Suppository, Rectal: 50 mg, 100 mg

◆ **Ketoprofen-E (Can)** *see* Ketoprofen *on page 1145*
◆ **Ketoprofen SR (Can)** *see* Ketoprofen *on page 1145*

Ketorolac (Systemic) (KEE toe role ak)

Brand Names: Canada Apo-Ketorolac Injectable®; Apo-Ketorolac®; Ketorolac Tromethamine Injection, USP; Novo-Ketorolac; Toradol®; Toradol® IM

Index Terms Ketorolac Tromethamine; Toradol

Pharmacologic Category Nonsteroidal Anti-inflammatory Drug (NSAID), Oral; Nonsteroidal Anti-inflammatory Drug (NSAID), Parenteral

Additional Appendix Information
Beers Criteria – Potentially Inappropriate Medications for Geriatrics *on page 2271*

Use Short-term (≤5 days) management of moderate-to-severe acute pain requiring analgesia at the opioid level

Pregnancy Risk Factor C

Pregnancy Considerations Adverse events were observed in some animal reproduction studies. Ketorolac crosses the placenta (Walker, 1988). NSAID exposure during the first trimester is not strongly associated with congenital malformations; however, cardiovascular anomalies and cleft palate have been observed following NSAID exposure in some studies (Ericson, 2001). The use of an NSAID close to conception may be associated with an increased risk of miscarriage (Li, 2003; Nielsen, 2001). Nonteratogenic effects have been observed following NSAID administration during the third trimester, including myocardial degenerative changes, prenatal constriction of the ductus arteriosus, fetal tricuspid regurgitation, failure of the ductus arteriosus to close postnatally; renal dysfunction or failure, oligohydramnios; gastrointestinal bleeding or perforation, increased risk of necrotizing enterocolitis; intracranial bleeding (including intraventricular hemorrhage), platelet dysfunction with resultant bleeding; pulmonary hypertension (Van den Veyver, 1993). Because they may cause premature closure of the ductus arteriosus, use of NSAIDs late in pregnancy should be avoided (use after 31 or 32 weeks gestation is not recommended by some clinicians) (Moise, 1993). **[U.S. Boxed Warning]: Ketorolac is contraindicated during labor and delivery (may inhibit uterine contractions and adversely affect fetal circulation).** The chronic use of NSAIDs in women of reproductive age may be associated with infertility that is reversible upon discontinuation of the medication.

Breast-Feeding Considerations Low concentrations of ketorolac are found in breast milk (milk concentrations were <1% of the weight-adjusted maternal dose in one study [Wischnik, 1989]). The manufacturer recommends that caution be used if administered to nursing women.

Contraindications Hypersensitivity to ketorolac, aspirin, other NSAIDs, or any component of the formulation; active or history of peptic ulcer disease; recent or history of GI bleeding or perforation; patients with advanced renal disease or risk of renal failure (due to volume depletion); prophylaxis before major surgery; suspected or confirmed cerebrovascular bleeding; hemorrhagic diathesis, incomplete hemostasis, or high risk of bleeding; concurrent use with ASA, other NSAIDs, probenecid or pentoxifylline; epidural or intrathecal administration; perioperative pain in the setting of coronary artery bypass graft (CABG) surgery; labor and delivery

Warnings/Precautions [U.S. Boxed Warning]: Inhibits platelet function; contraindicated in patients with cerebrovascular bleeding (suspected or confirmed), hemorrhagic diathesis, incomplete hemostasis and patients at high risk for bleeding. Effects on platelet adhesion and aggregation may prolong bleeding time. Anemia may occur; patients on long-term NSAID therapy should be monitored for anemia. Rarely, NSAID use has been associated with potentially severe blood dyscrasias (eg, agranulocytosis, thrombocytopenia, aplastic anemia).

[U.S. Boxed Warning]: NSAIDs are associated with an increased risk of adverse cardiovascular thrombotic events, including MI and stroke. Risk may be increased with duration of use or preexisting cardiovascular risk factors or disease. Carefully evaluate individual cardiovascular risk profiles prior to prescribing. May cause new-onset hypertension or worsening of existing hypertension. Use caution with fluid retention. Avoid use in heart failure (ACCF/AHA [Yancy, 2013]). Concurrent use of aspirin has not been shown to consistently reduce thromboembolic events. **[U.S. Boxed Warning]: Use is contraindicated as prophylactic analgesic before any major surgery and is contraindicated for treatment of perioperative pain in the setting of coronary artery bypass graft (CABG) surgery.** Risk of MI and stroke may be increased with use following CABG surgery. Wound bleeding and postoperative hematomas have been associated with ketorolac use in the perioperative setting.

[U.S. Boxed Warning]: Ketorolac is contraindicated in patients with advanced renal impairment and in patients at risk for renal failure due to volume depletion. NSAID use may compromise existing renal function; dose-dependent decreases in prostaglandin synthesis may result from NSAID use, reducing renal blood flow which may cause renal decompensation. NSAID use may increase the risk for hyperkalemia. Patients with impaired renal function, dehydration, heart failure, liver dysfunction, those taking diuretics and ACE inhibitors, and the elderly are at greater risk of renal toxicity. Use with caution in patients with impaired renal function or history of kidney disease; dosage adjustment is required in patients with moderate elevation in serum creatinine. Monitor renal function closely. Acute renal failure, interstitial nephritis, and nephrotic syndrome have been reported with ketorolac use; papillary necrosis and renal injury have been reported with the use of NSAIDs. Use of NSAIDs can compromise existing renal function. Rehydrate patient before starting therapy.

[U.S. Boxed Warning]: NSAIDs may increase risk of gastrointestinal irritation, inflammation, ulceration, bleeding, and perforation. These events may occur at any time during therapy and without warning. Use is contraindicated in patients with active/history of peptic ulcer disease and recent/history of GI bleeding or perforation. Use caution with a history of inflammatory bowel disease, concurrent therapy with anticoagulants, and/or corticosteroids, smoking, use of alcohol, the elderly, or debilitated patients.

[U.S. Boxed Warning]: Ketorolac injection is contraindicated in patients with prior hypersensitivity reaction to aspirin or NSAIDs. NSAIDs may cause serious skin adverse events including exfoliative dermatitis, Stevens-Johnson syndrome (SJS), and toxic epidermal necrolysis (TEN); discontinue use at first sign of skin rash or hypersensitivity. Hypersensitivity or anaphylactoid reactions may occur, even without prior exposure; patients with "aspirin triad" (bronchial asthma, aspirin intolerance, rhinitis) may be at increased risk. Do not use in patients who experience bronchospasm, asthma, rhinitis, or urticaria with NSAID or aspirin therapy. Use caution in other forms of asthma.

Use with caution in patients with hepatic impairment or a history of liver disease. Closely monitor patients with any abnormal LFT. Rarely, severe hepatic reactions (eg, fulminant hepatitis, hepatic necrosis, liver failure) have occurred with NSAID use; discontinue if signs or symptoms of liver disease develop, or if systemic manifestations occur.

[U.S. Boxed Warning]: Dosage adjustment is required for patients ≥65 years of age. Avoid use in older adults; use is associated with an increased risk of GI bleeding and peptic ulcer disease in older adults in high risk category (eg, >75 years or age or receiving concomitant oral/parenteral corticosteroids, anticoagulants, or antiplatelet agents) (Beers Criteria). **[U.S. Boxed Warning]: Dosage adjustment is required for patients weighing <50 kg (<110 pounds). [U.S. Boxed Warning]: Ketorolac is contraindicated during labor and delivery (may inhibit uterine contractions and adversely affect fetal circulation). [U.S. Boxed Warning]: Concurrent use of ketorolac with aspirin or other NSAIDs is contraindicated due to the increased risk of adverse reactions.**

[U.S. Boxed Warning]: Contraindicated for epidural or intrathecal administration (formulation contains alcohol). [U.S. Boxed Warning]: Systemic ketorolac is indicated for short term (≤5 days) use in adults for treatment of moderately severe acute pain requiring opioid-level analgesia. Low doses of opioids may be needed for breakthrough pain. **[U.S. Boxed Warning]: Oral therapy is only indicated for use as continuation treatment, following parenteral ketorolac and is not indicated for minor or chronic painful conditions. Do not exceed maximum daily recommended doses; does not improve efficacy but may increase the risk of serious adverse effects.** The combined therapy duration (oral and parenteral) should not exceed 5 days. Use the lowest effective dose for the shortest duration of time, consistent with individual patient goals, to reduce risk of cardiovascular or GI adverse events. Alternate therapies should be considered for patients at high risk. **[U.S. Boxed Warning]: Ketorolac is not indicated for use in children.**

Potentially significant drug-drug interactions may exist, requiring dose or frequency adjustment, additional monitoring, and/or selection of alternative therapy.

NSAIDS may cause drowsiness, dizziness, blurred vision and other neurologic effects which may impair physical or mental abilities; patients must be cautioned about performing tasks which require mental alertness (eg, operating machinery or driving). Discontinue use with blurred or diminished vision and perform ophthalmologic exam.

Adverse Reactions

Cardiovascular: Edema, hypertension

Central nervous system: Dizziness, drowsiness, headache

Dermatologic: Diaphoresis, pruritus, skin rash

Gastrointestinal: Constipation, diarrhea, dyspepsia, flatulence, gastrointestinal fullness, gastrointestinal hemorrhage, gastrointestinal pain, gastrointestinal perforation, gastrointestinal ulcer, heartburn, nausea, stomatitis, vomiting

Hematologic & oncologic: Anemia, prolonged bleeding time, purpura

Hepatic: Increased liver enzymes

Local: Pain at injection site

Otic: Tinnitus

Renal: Renal function abnormality

Rare but important or life-threatening: Abnormality in thinking, acute pancreatitis, acute renal failure, agranulocytosis, alopecia, anaphylactoid reaction, anaphylaxis, angioedema, aplastic anemia, aseptic meningitis, asthma, azotemia, bradycardia, bronchospasm, bruise, cardiac arrhythmia, cholestatic jaundice, coma, confusion, congestive heart failure, conjunctivitis, cough, cystitis, depression, dysuria, eosinophilia, epistaxis, eructation, erythema multiforme, euphoria, exacerbation of urinary frequency, exfoliative dermatitis, extrapyramidal reaction, flank pain, gastritis, glossitis, hallucination, hearing loss, hematemesis, hematuria, hemolytic anemia, hemolytic-uremic syndrome, hepatic failure, hepatitis, hyperglycemia, hyperkalemia, hyperkinesis, hypersensitivity reaction, hyponatremia, hypotension, increased susceptibility to infection, increased thirst, infertility, inflammatory bowel disease, insomnia, interstitial nephritis, jaundice, lack of concentration, laryngeal edema, leukopenia, lymphadenopathy, maculopapular rash, melena, myocardial infarction, nephritis, oliguria, palpitations, pancytopenia, paresthesia, pneumonia, polyuria, proteinuria, psychosis, pulmonary edema, rectal hemorrhage, renal failure, respiratory depression, rhinitis, seizure, sepsis, skin photosensitivity, Stevens-Johnson syndrome, stomatitis (ulcerative), stupor, syncope, tachycardia, thrombocytopenia, tongue edema, toxic epidermal necrolysis, urinary retention, urticaria, vasculitis, weight gain, wound hemorrhage (postoperative)

Drug Interactions

Metabolism/Transport Effects None known.

Avoid Concomitant Use

Avoid concomitant use of Ketorolac (Systemic) with any of the following: Aspirin; Dexketoprofen; Floctafenine; Ketorolac (Nasal); Nonsteroidal Anti-Inflammatory Agents; Omacetaxine; Pentoxifylline; Probenecid; Urokinase

Increased Effect/Toxicity

Ketorolac (Systemic) may increase the levels/effects of: 5-ASA Derivatives; Agents with Antiplatelet Properties; Aliskiren; Aminoglycosides; Anticoagulants; Apixaban; Aspirin; Bisphosphonate Derivatives; Collagenase (Systemic); CycloSPORINE (Systemic); Dabigatran Etexilate; Deferasirox; Desmopressin; Digoxin; Eplerenone; Haloperidol; Ibritumomab; Lithium; Methotrexate; Neuromuscular-Blocking Agents (Nondepolarizing); Nonsteroidal Anti-Inflammatory Agents; Obinutuzumab; Omacetaxine; PEMEtrexed; Pentoxifylline; Porfimer; Potassium-Sparing Diuretics; PRALAtrexate; Quinolone Antibiotics; Rivaroxaban; Salicylates; Tacrolimus (Systemic); Tenofovir; Thrombolytic Agents; Tositumomab and Iodine I 131 Tositumomab; Urokinase; Vancomycin; Verteporfin; Vitamin K Antagonists

The levels/effects of Ketorolac (Systemic) may be increased by: ACE Inhibitors; Angiotensin II Receptor Blockers; Antidepressants (Tricyclic, Tertiary Amine); Corticosteroids (Systemic); CycloSPORINE (Systemic); Dasatinib; Dexketoprofen; Floctafenine; Glucosamine; Herbs (Anticoagulant/Antiplatelet Properties); Ibrutinib; Ketorolac (Nasal); Limaprost; Multivitamins/Fluoride (with ADE); Multivitamins/Minerals (with ADEK, Folate, Iron); Multivitamins/Minerals (with AE, No Iron); Omega-3 Fatty Acids; Pentosan Polysulfate Sodium; Probenecid; Prostacyclin Analogues; Selective Serotonin Reuptake Inhibitors; Serotonin/Norepinephrine Reuptake Inhibitors; Sodium Phosphates; Tipranavir; Treprostinil; Vitamin E

Decreased Effect

Ketorolac (Systemic) may decrease the levels/effects of: ACE Inhibitors; Aliskiren; Angiotensin II Receptor Blockers; Aspirin; Beta-Blockers; Eplerenone; HydrALAZINE; Loop Diuretics; Potassium-Sparing Diuretics; Prostaglandins (Ophthalmic); Salicylates; Selective Serotonin Reuptake Inhibitors; Thiazide Diuretics

The levels/effects of Ketorolac (Systemic) may be decreased by: Bile Acid Sequestrants; Salicylates

Food Interactions High-fat meals may delay time to peak (by ~1 hour) and decrease peak concentrations. Management: Administer tablet with food or milk to decrease gastrointestinal distress.

Storage/Stability

Injection: Store at room temperature of 15°C to 30°C (59°F to 86°F). Protect from light. Injection is clear and has a slight yellow color. Precipitation may occur at relatively low pH values.

Tablet: Store at room temperature of 15°C to 30°C (59°F to 86°F).

Mechanism of Action Reversibly inhibits cyclooxygenase-1 and 2 (COX-1 and 2) enzymes, which results in decreased formation of prostaglandin precursors; has antipyretic, analgesic, and anti-inflammatory properties

Other proposed mechanisms not fully elucidated (and possibly contributing to the anti-inflammatory effect to varying degrees), include inhibiting chemotaxis, altering lymphocyte activity, inhibiting neutrophil aggregation/activation, and decreasing proinflammatory cytokine levels.

Pharmacodynamics/Kinetics

Onset of action: Analgesic: IM, IV: ~30 minutes

Peak effect: Analgesic: ≤2-3 hours

Duration: Analgesic: 4-6 hours

Absorption: Oral: Well absorbed (100%)

Distribution: ~13 L; poor penetration into CSF

Protein binding: 99%

Metabolism: Hepatic

Half-life elimination: 2-6 hours; prolonged 30% to 50% in elderly; up to 19 hours in renal impairment

Time to peak, serum: IM: 30-60 minutes

Excretion: Urine (92%, ~60% as unchanged drug); feces ~6%

Dosage Pain management (acute; moderately severe): **Note:** The maximum combined duration of treatment (for parenteral and oral) is 5 days; do not increase dose or frequency; supplement with low-dose opioids if needed for breakthrough pain.

Adolescents ≥17 years and Adults ≥50 kg:

IM: 60 mg as a single dose or 30 mg every 6 hours (maximum daily dose: 120 mg)

IV: 30 mg as a single dose or 30 mg every 6 hours (maximum daily dose: 120 mg)

Oral: 20 mg, followed by 10 mg every 4-6 hours as needed; do not exceed 40 mg daily; oral dosing is intended to be a continuation of IM or IV therapy only

Adults, critically-ill (off-label dose): IM, IV: 30 mg once, followed by 15-30 mg every 6 hours for up to 5 days (maximum daily dose: 120 mg) (Barr, 2013)

Elderly ≥65 years: **Note:** May have an increased incidence of GI bleeding, ulceration, and perforation. The maximum combined duration of treatment (for parenteral and oral) is 5 days.

IM: 30 mg as a single dose or 15 mg every 6 hours (maximum daily dose: 60 mg)

IV: 15 mg as a single dose or 15 mg every 6 hours (maximum daily dose: 60 mg)

Oral: 10 mg, followed by 10 mg every 4-6 hours as needed; do not exceed 40 mg daily; oral dosing is intended to be a continuation of IM or IV therapy only

Dosage adjustments for low body weight (<50 kg): Refer to elderly dosing.

Dosage adjustment in renal impairment: Use is contraindicated in patients with advanced renal impairment or patients at risk for renal failure due to volume depletion.

Mild-to-moderate impairment:

IM: 30 mg as a single dose or 15 mg every 6 hours (maximum daily dose: 60 mg)

IV: 15 mg as a single dose or 15 mg every 6 hours (maximum daily dose: 60 mg)

Oral: 10 mg, followed by 10 mg every 4-6 hours as needed; do not exceed 40 mg daily; oral dosing is intended to be a continuation of IM or IV therapy only

Note: The maximum combined duration of treatment (for parenteral and oral) is 5 days.

Advanced impairment or patients at risk for renal failure due to volume depletion: Use is contraindicated.

Dosage adjustment in hepatic impairment: No dosage adjustment provided in manufacturer's labeling. Use with caution, may cause elevation of liver enzymes; discontinue if clinical signs and symptoms of liver disease develop.

Dietary Considerations Administer tablet with food or milk to decrease gastrointestinal distress.

Administration

Oral: May take with food to reduce GI upset.

IM: Administer slowly and deeply into the muscle.

IV: Administer IV bolus over a minimum of 15 seconds.

Monitoring Parameters Monitor response (pain, range of motion, grip strength, mobility, ADL function), inflammation; observe for weight gain, edema; monitor renal function (serum creatinine, BUN, urine output); CBC and platelets, liver function tests; chemistry profile; blood pressure; observe for bleeding, bruising; evaluate gastrointestinal effects (abdominal pain, bleeding, dyspepsia); mental confusion, disorientation

Reference Range Serum concentration: Therapeutic: 0.3-5 mcg/mL; Toxic: >5 mcg/mL

Additional Information Ketorolac 30 mg IM provides analgesia comparable to morphine ≤12 mg or meperidine ≤100 mg (Buckley, 1990).

Dosage Forms

Solution, Injection:

Generic: 15 mg/mL (1 mL); 30 mg/mL (1 mL); 60 mg/2 mL (2 mL); 300 mg/10 mL (10 mL)

Solution, Injection [preservative free]:

Generic: 15 mg/mL (1 mL); 30 mg/mL (1 mL); 60 mg/2 mL (2 mL)

Solution, Intramuscular:

Generic: 30 mg/mL (1 mL); 60 mg/2 mL (2 mL)

Tablet, Oral:

Generic: 10 mg

Ketorolac (Nasal) (KEE toe role ak)

Brand Names: U.S. Sprix

Index Terms Ketorolac Tromethamine

Pharmacologic Category Nonsteroidal Anti-inflammatory Drug (NSAID), Nasal

Use Moderate to moderately severe pain: Short-term (up to 5 days) management of moderate to moderately severe pain in adults that requires analgesia at the opioid level.

Pregnancy Risk Factor C/D ≥30 weeks gestation

Dosage Intranasal: **Note:** The maximum combined duration of treatment (for nasal spray or other ketorolac formulations) is 5 days.

Adults<65 years and ≥50 kg: One spray (15.75 mg) in each nostril (total dose: 31.5 mg) every 6-8 hours; maximum dose: 4 doses (126 mg)/day

Dosage adjustments in adults with low body weight (<50 kg): One spray (15.75 mg) in 1 nostril (total dose: 15.75 mg) every 6-8 hours; maximum dose: 4 doses (63 mg)/day

Elderly (≥65 years): Intranasal: One spray (15.75 mg) in 1 nostril (total dose: 15.75 mg) every 6-8 hours; maximum dose: 4 doses (63 mg)/day

Dosage adjustment in renal impairment:

Renal insufficiency: Intranasal: One spray (15.75 mg) in 1 nostril (total dose: 15.75 mg) every 6-8 hours; maximum dose: 4 doses (63 mg)/day

Advanced renal impairment (or at risk for renal failure due to volume depletion): Use is contraindicated

Dosage adjustment in hepatic impairment: Use with caution with hepatic impairment or history of hepatic disease; use may cause elevation of liver enzymes; discontinue if clinical signs and symptoms of liver disease develop.

Additional Information Complete prescribing information should be consulted for additional detail.

Dosage Forms

Solution, Nasal [preservative free]:

Sprix: 15.75 mg/spray (1 ea)

Ketorolac (Ophthalmic) (KEE toe role ak)

Brand Names: U.S. Acular; Acular LS; Acuvail

Brand Names: Canada Acular LS®; Acular®; Apo-Ketorolac® Ophthalmic; ratio-Ketorolac

Index Terms Ketorolac Tromethamine

Pharmacologic Category Nonsteroidal Anti-inflammatory Drug (NSAID), Ophthalmic

Use Temporary relief of ocular itching due to seasonal allergic conjunctivitis; postoperative pain and/or inflammation following cataract extraction; reduction of ocular pain, burning, and stinging following corneal refractive surgery

Pregnancy Risk Factor C

Dosage Ophthalmic:

Children ≥2 years, Adolescents, and Adults: Acular®:

Allergic conjunctivitis (relief of ocular itching): Instill 1 drop to affected eye(s) 4 times daily

Inflammation following cataract extraction: Instill 1 drop to affected eye(s) 4 times daily beginning 24 hours after surgery; continue for 2 weeks

Children ≥3 years, Adolescents, and Adults: Acular LS®:

Pain, burning/stinging following corneal refractive surgery: Instill 1 drop to affected eye(s) 4 times daily as needed for up to 4 days after surgery

Adults: Acuvail®: Pain and inflammation associated with cataract surgery: Instill 1 drop to affected eye(s) 2 times daily 24 hours before surgery and on the day of surgery; continue for 2 weeks

Dosage adjustment in renal impairment: No dosage adjustment provided in manufacturer's labeling.

Dosage adjustment in hepatic impairment: No dosage adjustment provided in manufacturer's labeling.

Additional Information Complete prescribing information should be consulted for additional detail.

Dosage Forms

Solution, Ophthalmic:

Acular: 0.5% (5 mL)

Acular LS: 0.4% (5 mL)

Generic: 0.4% (5 mL); 0.5% (3 mL, 5 mL, 10 mL)

Solution, Ophthalmic [preservative free]:

Acuvail: 0.45% (30 ea)

◆ **Ketorolac Tromethamine** *see* Ketorolac (Nasal) *on page 1149*

◆ **Ketorolac Tromethamine** *see* Ketorolac (Ophthalmic) *on page 1149*

◆ **Ketorolac Tromethamine** *see* Ketorolac (Systemic) *on page 1146*

◆ **Ketorolac Tromethamine Injection, USP (Can)** *see* Ketorolac (Systemic) *on page 1146*

Ketotifen (Systemic) [CAN/INT]

(kee toe TYE fen)

Brand Names: Canada APO-Ketotifen®; Novo-Ketotifen; Nu-Ketotifen®; PMS-Ketotifen; Zaditen®

Index Terms Ketotifen Fumarate

Pharmacologic Category Histamine H_1 Antagonist; Histamine H_1 Antagonist, Second Generation; Mast Cell Stabilizer; Piperidine Derivative

Use Note: Not approved in U.S.

Adjunctive therapy in the chronic treatment of pediatric patients ≥6 months of age with mild, atopic asthma

Pregnancy Considerations Adverse fetal effects were found in some but not all animal studies. Safety in human pregnancy has not been established.

Contraindications Hypersensitivity to ketotifen or any component of the formulation; use of ketotifen syrup in patients sensitive to benzoate compounds

Warnings/Precautions Indicated for prophylactic treatment; not effective for the prevention or treatment of acute asthma attacks. Therapy for acute symptoms of asthma (eg, corticosteroids, beta$_2$-agonists, xanthine derivatives) should be maintained and gradually reduced. Several weeks of oral ketotifen therapy may be needed to observe clinical response while maximum therapeutic response usually requires duration of therapy ≥10 weeks. Therapy should be maintained for at least 2-3 months to determine effectiveness. If therapy requires discontinuation, gradually reduce over 2-4 weeks. Oral dosage forms may cause sedation early in therapy. Sedative effects may be reduced by initiating therapy at one-half the recommended daily dose with gradual increase over 5 days to maintenance dose.

Caution patients about performing tasks which require mental alertness (eg, driving or operating machinery). Thrombocytopenia has occurred rarely when used concomitantly with oral antidiabetic agents. Use with caution in epileptic patients; may lower seizure threshold. Use caution in diabetics and individuals with benzoate allergies as the syrup preparation contains carbohydrates and benzoate compounds.

Adverse Reactions

Central nervous system: Headache, sedation, sleep disturbance

Dermatologic: Rash, urticaria

Gastrointestinal: Abdominal pain, appetite increased, weight gain

Respiratory: Respiratory infection (4%), epistaxis (1%)

Miscellaneous: Flu (3%), puffy eyelid (1%)

Rare but important or life-threatening: Cystitis, dizziness, erythema multiforme, excitation, hepatitis, insomnia, irritability, nervousness, Stevens-Johnson syndrome, thrombocytopenia, transaminases increased, xerostomia

Storage/Stability

Syrup: Store at up to 25°C (up to 77°F).

Tablet: Store at up to 25°C (up to 77°F). Protect from moisture.

Mechanism of Action Exhibits noncompetitive H$_1$-receptor antagonist and mast cell stabilizer properties. Efficacy in asthma likely results from a combination of anti-inflammatory and antihistaminergic actions including interference with chemokine-induced migration of eosinophils into inflamed airways, inhibition of airway hyper-reactivity due to platelet activating factor (PAF), antagonism of leukotriene-induced bronchoconstriction.

Pharmacodynamics/Kinetics

Absorption: Rapid, ≥60%

Protein binding: 75%

Metabolism: Hepatic via N-glucuronidation to inactive metabolite ketotifen-N-glucoronide; N-demethylation to active metabolite nor-ketotifen; and keto-reduction to hydroxyl derivative

Clearance: Increased in children >3 years; decreased in children ≤3 years

Bioavailability: ~50%

Half-life elimination: ~9-9.5 hours

Time to peak, plasma: 2-4 hours

Excretion: Urine (>60% as metabolites, 1% as unchanged drug)

Dosage Oral: Atopic asthma (prophylactic treatment):

Children 6 months to 3 years: Initial: 0.05 mg/kg once daily or in 2 divided doses for 5 days; Maintenance: 0.05 mg/kg twice daily (maximum dose: 1 mg twice daily)

Children >3 years: Initial: 1 mg once daily or in 2 divided doses for 5 days; Maintenance: 1 mg twice daily

Dosage adjustment in renal impairment: There are no dosage adjustments provided in manufacturer's labeling.

Dosage adjustment in hepatic impairment: There are no dosage adjustments provided in manufacturer's labeling.

Dietary Considerations May be taken without regard to meals. Syrup contains carbohydrate 4 g/5 mL.

Administration Administer without regards to meals.

Product Availability Not available in the U.S.

Dosage Forms: Canada

Syrup, oral:

Zaditen®: 1 mg/5 mL (250 mL)

Tablet, oral:

Zaditen®: 1 mg

Ketotifen (Ophthalmic) (kee toe TYE fen)

Brand Names: U.S. Alaway Childrens Allergy [OTC]; Alaway [OTC]; Claritin Eye [OTC]; Zaditor [OTC]; ZyrTEC Itchy Eye [OTC]

Brand Names: Canada Zaditor®

Index Terms Ketotifen Fumarate

Pharmacologic Category Histamine H$_1$ Antagonist; Histamine H$_1$ Antagonist, Second Generation; Mast Cell Stabilizer; Piperidine Derivative

Use Temporary relief of eye itching due to allergic conjunctivitis

Pregnancy Risk Factor C

Dosage Ophthalmic: Allergic conjunctivitis: Children ≥3 years and Adults: Instill 1 drop into the affected eye(s) twice daily, every 8-12 hours

Additional Information Complete prescribing information should be consulted for additional detail.

Dosage Forms

Solution, Ophthalmic:

Alaway [OTC]: 0.025% (10 mL)

Alaway Childrens Allergy [OTC]: 0.025% (5 mL)

Claritin Eye [OTC]: 0.025% (5 mL)

Zaditor [OTC]: 0.025% (5 mL)

ZyrTEC Itchy Eye [OTC]: 0.025% (5 mL)

Generic: 0.025% (5 mL)

Dosage Forms: Canada

Solution, ophthalmic [drops]:

Zaditor®: 0.025% (5 mL)

Solution, ophthalmic [drops], preservative free:

Zaditor®: 0.025% (0.4 mL) (30s)

- **Ketotifen Fumarate** *see* Ketotifen (Ophthalmic) *on page* *1150*
- **Ketotifen Fumarate** *see* Ketotifen (Systemic) [CAN/INT] *on page* *1149*
- **Keytruda** *see* Pembrolizumab *on page* *1604*
- **Khedezla** *see* Desvenlafaxine *on page* *598*
- **Khloditan** *see* Mitotane *on page* *1382*
- **KI** *see* Potassium Iodide *on page* *1690*
- **Kidkare Children's Cough/Cold [OTC]** *see* Chlorpheniramine, Pseudoephedrine, and Dextromethorphan *on page* *428*
- **Kidrolase (Can)** *see* Asparaginase (*E. coli*) *on page* *179*
- **Kineret** *see* Anakinra *on page* *148*
- **Kinrix®** *see* Diphtheria and Tetanus Toxoids, Acellular Pertussis, and Poliovirus Vaccine *on page* *646*
- **Kionex** *see* Sodium Polystyrene Sulfonate *on page* *1912*
- **Kitabis Pak** *see* Tobramycin (Systemic, Oral Inhalation) *on page* *2052*
- **Kitabis Pak** *see* Tobramycin (Systemic, Oral Inhalation) *on page* *2052*
- **Kivexa (Can)** *see* Abacavir and Lamivudine *on page* *22*
- **Klaron** *see* Sulfacetamide (Topical) *on page* *1943*
- **Klean-Prep (Can)** *see* Polyethylene Glycol-Electrolyte Solution *on page* *1674*
- **Klofatsimiini** *see* Clofazimine [INT] *on page* *473*
- **Klofatzimin** *see* Clofazimine [INT] *on page* *473*

- ◆ **Klofaziminos** *see* Clofazimine [INT] *on page 473*
- ◆ **KlonoPIN** *see* ClonazePAM *on page 478*
- ◆ **Klor-Con** *see* Potassium Chloride *on page 1687*
- ◆ **Klor-Con 10** *see* Potassium Chloride *on page 1687*
- ◆ **Klor-Con/EF** *see* Potassium Bicarbonate and Potassium Citrate *on page 1687*
- ◆ **Klor-Con M10** *see* Potassium Chloride *on page 1687*
- ◆ **Klor-Con M15** *see* Potassium Chloride *on page 1687*
- ◆ **Klor-Con M20** *see* Potassium Chloride *on page 1687*
- ◆ **K-Lyte/Cl** *see* Potassium Bicarbonate and Potassium Chloride *on page 1687*
- ◆ **KMD 3213** *see* Silodosin *on page 1885*
- ◆ **Koate-DVI** *see* Antihemophilic Factor (Human) *on page 152*
- ◆ **Koffex DM-D (Can)** *see* Pseudoephedrine and Dextromethorphan *on page 1743*
- ◆ **Koffex Expectorant (Can)** *see* GuaiFENesin *on page 986*
- ◆ **Kogenate FS** *see* Antihemophilic Factor (Recombinant) *on page 152*
- ◆ **Kogenate FS Bio-Set** *see* Antihemophilic Factor (Recombinant) *on page 152*
- ◆ **Kolephrin GG/DM [OTC]** *see* Guaifenesin and Dextromethorphan *on page 987*
- ◆ **Kombiglyze™ XR** *see* Saxagliptin and Metformin *on page 1869*
- ◆ **Komboglyze™ (Can)** *see* Saxagliptin and Metformin *on page 1869*
- ◆ **Konakion (Can)** *see* Phytonadione *on page 1647*
- ◆ **Konsyl [OTC]** *see* Psyllium *on page 1744*
- ◆ **Konsyl-D [OTC]** *see* Psyllium *on page 1744*
- ◆ **Korlym** *see* Mifepristone *on page 1366*
- ◆ **K-Phos** *see* Potassium Acid Phosphate *on page 1687*
- ◆ **K-Phos Neutral** *see* Potassium Phosphate and Sodium Phosphate *on page 1692*
- ◆ **K-Phos No. 2** *see* Potassium Phosphate and Sodium Phosphate *on page 1692*
- ◆ **K-Prime** *see* Potassium Bicarbonate and Potassium Citrate *on page 1687*
- ◆ **Kristalose** *see* Lactulose *on page 1156*
- ◆ **Krystexxa** *see* Pegloticase *on page 1602*
- ◆ **KS Ibuprofen [OTC]** *see* Ibuprofen *on page 1032*
- ◆ **K-Sol** *see* Potassium Chloride *on page 1687*
- ◆ **KS Stool Softener [OTC]** *see* Docusate *on page 661*
- ◆ **K-Tab** *see* Potassium Chloride *on page 1687*
- ◆ **Kurvelo** *see* Ethinyl Estradiol and Levonorgestrel *on page 803*
- ◆ **Kuvan** *see* Sapropterin *on page 1864*
- ◆ **K-Vescent** *see* Potassium Bicarbonate and Potassium Citrate *on page 1687*
- ◆ **K-Vescent** *see* Potassium Chloride *on page 1687*
- ◆ **Kwell** *see* Lindane *on page 1217*
- ◆ **Kwellada-P [OTC] (Can)** *see* Permethrin *on page 1627*
- ◆ **Kynamro** *see* Mipomersen *on page 1375*
- ◆ **Kynesia (Can)** *see* Benztropine *on page 248*
- ◆ **Kyprolis** *see* Carfilzomib *on page 361*
- ◆ **Kytril** *see* Granisetron *on page 983*
- ◆ **L-749,345** *see* Ertapenem *on page 760*
- ◆ **L-758,298** *see* Fosaprepitant *on page 929*
- ◆ **L 754030** *see* Aprepitant *on page 166*
- ◆ **LA 20304a** *see* Gemifloxacin *on page 957*

Labetalol (la BET a lole)

Brand Names: U.S. Trandate

Brand Names: Canada Apo-Labetalol; Labetalol Hydrochloride Injection, USP; Normodyne; Trandate

Index Terms Ibidomide Hydrochloride; Labetalol Hydrochloride

Pharmacologic Category Antihypertensive; Beta-Blocker With Alpha-Blocking Activity

Use Hypertenstion: Treatment of mild-to-severe hypertension; IV for severe hypertension (eg, hypertensive emergencies)

The 2014 guideline for the management of high blood pressure in adults (Eighth Joint National Committee [JNC 8]) recommends initiation of pharmacologic treatment to lower blood pressure for the following patients (JNC8 [James, 2013]):

- Patients ≥60 years of age, with systolic blood pressure (SBP) ≥150 mm Hg or diastolic blood pressure (DBP) ≥90 mm Hg. Goal of therapy is SBP <150 mm Hg and DBP <90 mm Hg.
- Patients <60 years of age, with SBP ≥140 mm Hg or DBP ≥90 mm Hg. Goal of therapy is SBP <140 mm Hg and DBP <90 mm Hg.
- Patients ≥18 years of age with diabetes, with SBP ≥140 mm Hg or DBP ≥90 mm Hg. Goal of therapy is SBP <140 mm Hg and DBP <90 mm Hg.
- Patients ≥18 years of age with chronic kidney disease (CKD), with SBP ≥140 mm Hg or DBP ≥90 mm Hg. Goal of therapy is SBP <140 mm Hg and DBP <90 mm Hg.

In patients with CKD, regardless of race or diabetes status, the use of an ACE inhibitor (ACEI) or angiotensin receptor blocker (ARB) as initial therapy is recommended to improve kidney outcomes. In the general nonblack population (without CKD) including those with diabetes, initial antihypertensive treatment should consist of a thiazide-type diuretic, calcium channel blocker, ACEI, or ARB. In the general black population (without CKD) including those with diabetes, initial antihypertensive treatment should consist of a thiazide-type diuretic or a calcium channel blocker **instead of** an ACEI or ARB.

Pregnancy Risk Factor C

Pregnancy Considerations Adverse events have been observed in some animal reproduction studies. Labetalol crosses the placenta and can be detected in cord blood and infant serum after delivery (Haraldsson, 1989; Rogers, 1990). Fetal/neonatal bradycardia, hypoglycemia, hypotension, and/or respiratory depression have been observed following in utero exposure to labetalol. Adequate facilities for monitoring infants at birth should be available.

Untreated chronic maternal hypertension and pre-eclampsia are also associated with adverse events in the fetus, infant, and mother. Oral labetalol is considered an appropriate agent for the treatment of chronic hypertension in pregnancy; intravenous labetalol is recommended for use in the management of acute onset severe hypertension in pregnancy and hypertension associated with pre-eclampsia (ACOG, 2011; ACOG 2013).

Breast-Feeding Considerations Low amounts of labetalol are found in breast milk and can be detected in the serum of nursing infants. The manufacturer recommends that caution be exercised when administering labetalol to nursing women.

Contraindications Hypersensitivity to labetalol or any component of the formulation; severe bradycardia; heart block greater than first degree (except in patients with a functioning artificial pacemaker); cardiogenic shock;

bronchial asthma; uncompensated cardiac failure; conditions associated with severe and prolonged hypotension

Warnings/Precautions Consider preexisting conditions such as sick sinus syndrome before initiating. Symptomatic hypotension with or without syncope may occur with labetalol; close monitoring of patient is required especially with initial dosing and dosing increases; blood pressure must be lowered at a rate appropriate for the patient's clinical condition. Initiation with a low dose and gradual up-titration may help to decrease the occurrence of hypotension or syncope. Patients should be advised to avoid driving or other hazardous tasks during initiation of therapy due to the risk of syncope. Orthostatic hypotension may occur with IV administration; patient should remain supine during and for up to 3 hours after IV administration. Use with caution in impaired hepatic function; bioavailability is increased due to decreased first-pass metabolism. Severe hepatic injury including some fatalities have also been rarely reported with use: periodically monitor LFTs with prolonged use. Use with caution in patients with diabetes mellitus; may potentiate hypoglycemia and/or mask signs and symptoms. Bradycardia may be observed more frequently in elderly patients (>65 years of age); dosage reductions may be necessary. May also reduce release of insulin in response to hyperglycemia; dosage of antidiabetic agents may need to be adjusted. May mask signs of hyperthyroidism (eg, tachycardia); if hyperthyroidism is suspected, carefully manage and monitor; abrupt withdrawal may exacerbate symptoms of hyperthyroidism or precipitate thyroid storm. Elimination of labetalol is reduced in elderly patients; lower maintenance doses may be required.

Use only with extreme caution in compensated heart failure and monitor for a worsening of the condition. Beta-blocker therapy should not be withdrawn abruptly (particularly in patients with CAD), but gradually tapered to avoid acute tachycardia, hypertension, and/or ischemia. Chronic beta-blocker therapy should not be routinely withdrawn prior to major surgery. Use caution with concurrent use of digoxin, verapamil, or diltiazem; bradycardia or heart block can occur. Use with caution in patients receiving inhaled anesthetic agents known to depress myocardial contractility. Patients with bronchospastic disease should not receive beta-blockers; if used at all, should be used cautiously with close monitoring. Use with caution in patients with myasthenia gravis or psychiatric disease (may cause or exacerbate CNS depression). Can precipitate or aggravate symptoms of arterial insufficiency in patients with PVD and Raynaud's disease; use with caution and monitor for progression of arterial obstruction. If possible, obtain diagnostic tests for pheochromocytoma prior to use. May induce or exacerbate psoriasis. Labetalol has been shown to be effective in lowering blood pressure and relieving symptoms in patients with pheochromocytoma. However, some patients have experienced paradoxical hypertensive responses; use with caution in patients with pheochromocytoma. Additional alpha-blockade may be required during use of labetalol. Use caution with history of severe anaphylaxis to allergens; patients taking beta-blockers may become more sensitive to repeated challenges. Treatment of anaphylaxis (eg, epinephrine) in patients taking beta-blockers may be ineffective or promote undesirable effects.

Intraoperative floppy iris syndrome has been observed in cataract surgery patients who were on or were previously treated with alpha$_1$-blockers; causality has not been established and there appears to be no benefit in discontinuing alpha-blocker therapy prior to surgery. Instruct patients to inform ophthalmologist of labetalol use when considering eye surgery.

Benzyl alcohol and derivatives: Some dosage forms may contain sodium benzoate/benzoic acid; benzoic acid (benzoate) is a metabolite of benzyl alcohol; large amounts of benzyl alcohol (≥99 mg/kg/day) have been associated with a potentially fatal toxicity ("gasping syndrome") in neonates; the "gasping syndrome" consists of metabolic acidosis, respiratory distress, gasping respirations, CNS dysfunction (including convulsions, intracranial hemorrhage), hypotension, and cardiovascular collapse (AAP, 1997; CDC, 1982); some data suggests that benzoate displaces bilirubin from protein binding sites (Ahlfors, 2001); avoid or use dosage forms containing benzyl alcohol derivative with caution in neonates. See manufacturer's labeling.

Adverse Reactions

Cardiovascular: Edema, flushing, hypotension, orthostatic hypotension (IV use), ventricular arrhythmia (IV use)

Central nervous system: Dizziness, fatigue, headache, somnolence, vertigo

Dermatologic: Pruritus, rash, scalp tingling

Gastrointestinal: Dyspepsia, nausea, taste disturbance, vomiting

Genitourinary: Ejaculatory failure, impotence

Hepatic: Transaminases increased

Neuromuscular & skeletal: Paresthesia, weakness

Ocular: Vision abnormal

Renal: BUN increased

Respiratory: Dyspnea, nasal congestion

Miscellaneous: Diaphoresis

Rare but important or life-threatening: Alopecia (reversible), anaphylactoid reaction, ANA positive, angioedema, bradycardia, bronchospasm, cholestatic jaundice, CHF, diabetes insipidus, heart block, hepatic necrosis, hepatitis, hypersensitivity, Peyronie's disease, psoriaform rash, Raynaud's syndrome, syncope, systemic lupus erythematosus, toxic myopathy, urinary retention, urticaria

Other adverse reactions noted with beta-adrenergic blocking agents include agranulocytosis, catatonia, emotional lability, intensification of preexisting AV block, ischemic colitis. laryngospasm, mental depression, mesenteric artery thrombosis, nonthrombocytopenic purpura, respiratory distress, short-term memory loss, and thrombocytopenic purpura.

Drug Interactions

Metabolism/Transport Effects None known.

Avoid Concomitant Use

Avoid concomitant use of Labetalol with any of the following: Beta2-Agonists; Ceritinib; Floctafenine; Methacholine

Increased Effect/Toxicity

Labetalol may increase the levels/effects of: Alpha-/Beta-Agonists (Direct-Acting); Alpha1-Blockers; Alpha2-Agonists; Amifostine; Antihypertensives; Antipsychotic Agents (Phenothiazines); Bradycardia-Causing Agents; Bupivacaine; Cardiac Glycosides; Ceritinib; Cholinergic Agonists; Disopyramide; DULoxetine; Ergot Derivatives; Fingolimod; Grass Pollen Allergen Extract (5 Grass Extract); Hypotensive Agents; Insulin; Lacosamide; Levodopa; Lidocaine (Systemic); Lidocaine (Topical); Mepivacaine; Methacholine; Midodrine; Obinutuzumab; RisperiDONE; RiTUXimab; Sulfonylureas

The levels/effects of Labetalol may be increased by: Acetylcholinesterase Inhibitors; Alpha2-Agonists; Aminoquinolines (Antimalarial); Amiodarone; Anilidopiperidine Opioids; Antipsychotic Agents (Phenothiazines); Barbiturates; Bretylium; Brimonidine (Topical); Calcium Channel Blockers (Dihydropyridine); Calcium Channel Blockers (Nondihydropyridine); Diazoxide; Dipyridamole; Disopyramide; Dronedarone; Floctafenine; Herbs (Hypotensive Properties); MAO Inhibitors; Nicorandil; Pentoxifylline; Phosphodiesterase 5 Inhibitors; Propafenone; Prostacyclin Analogues; Regorafenib; Reserpine; Tofacitinib

Decreased Effect

Labetalol may decrease the levels/effects of: Beta2-Agonists; Theophylline Derivatives

The levels/effects of Labetalol may be decreased by: Barbiturates; Herbs (Hypertensive Properties); Methylphenidate; Nonsteroidal Anti-Inflammatory Agents; Rifamycin Derivatives; Yohimbine

Food Interactions Labetalol serum concentrations may be increased if taken with food. Management: Administer with food.

Storage/Stability

Tablets: Store at room temperature (refer to manufacturer's labeling for detailed storage requirements). Protect from light and excessive moisture.

Injectable: Store at room temperature (refer to manufacturer's labeling for detailed storage requirements); do not freeze. Protect from light. The solution is clear to slightly yellow.

Parenteral admixture: Stability of parenteral admixture at room temperature (25°C) and refrigeration temperature (4°C): 3 days.

Mechanism of Action Blocks alpha-, $beta_1$-, and $beta_2$-adrenergic receptor sites; elevated renins are reduced. The ratios of alpha- to beta-blockade differ depending on the route of administration: 1:3 (oral) and 1:7 (IV).

Pharmacodynamics/Kinetics

Onset of action: Oral: 20 minutes to 2 hours; IV: 2 to 5 minutes

Peak effect: Oral: 1-4 hours; IV: 5 to 15 minutes

Duration: Blood pressure response:

Oral: 8 to 12 hours (dose dependent)

IV: 2 to 18 hours (dose dependent; based on single and multiple sequential doses of 0.25 to 0.5 mg/kg with cumulative dosing up to 3.25 mg/kg)

Absorption: Complete

Distribution: V_d: Adults: 3 to 16 L/kg; mean: <9.4 L/kg; moderately lipid soluble, therefore, can enter CNS

Protein binding: 50%

Metabolism: Hepatic, primarily via glucuronide conjugation; extensive first-pass effect

Bioavailability: Oral: 25%; increased with liver disease, elderly, and concurrent cimetidine

Half-life elimination: Oral: 6 to 8 hours; IV: ~5.5 hours

Time to peak, plasma: Oral: 1 to 2 hours

Excretion: Urine (55% to 60% as glucuronide conjugates, <5% as unchanged drug)

Clearance: Possibly decreased in neonates/infants

Dosage

Children: Due to limited documentation of its use, labetalol should be initiated cautiously in pediatric patients with careful dosage adjustment and blood pressure monitoring.

Oral: Hypertension (off-label use): Initial: 1 to 3 mg/kg/day, in 2 divided doses; maximum: 10 to 12 mg/kg/day, up to 1200 mg/day

IV, intermittent bolus doses of 0.3 to 1 mg/kg/dose have been reported.

For treatment of pediatric hypertensive emergencies, initial continuous infusions of 0.4 to 1 mg/kg/hour with a maximum of 3 mg/kg/hour have been used. Administration requires the use of an infusion pump.

Adults:

Hypertension: Oral: Initial: 100 mg twice daily, may increase as needed every 2 to 3 days by 100 mg twice daily (titration increments not to exceed 200 mg twice daily) until desired response is obtained; usual dosage range (ASH/ISH [Weber, 2014]): 100 to 300 mg twice daily; may require up to 2400 mg daily.

Acute hypertension (hypertensive emergency/urgency):

IV bolus: Per the manufacturer: Initial: 20 mg IV push over 2 minutes; may administer 40 to 80 mg at 10-minute intervals, up to 300 mg total cumulative dose; as appropriate, follow with oral antihypertensive regimen

IV infusion (acute loading): Per the manufacturer: Initial: 2 mg/minute; titrate to response up to 300 mg total cumulative dose (eg, discontinue after 2.5 hours of 2 mg/minute); usual total dose required: 50 to 200 mg; as appropriate, follow with oral antihypertensive regimen

Note: Although loading infusions are well described in the product labeling, the labeling is silent in specific clinical situations, such as in the patient who has an initial response to labetalol infusions but cannot be converted to an oral route for subsequent dosing. There is limited documentation of prolonged continuous infusions (ie, >300 mg/day). In rare clinical situations, higher continuous infusion doses up to 6 mg/minute have been used in the critical care setting (eg, aortic dissection) and up to 8 mg/minute (eg, hypertension with ongoing acute ischemic stroke). At these doses, it may be best to consider an alternative agent if the labetalol infusion is not meeting the goals of therapy. At the other extreme, continuous infusions at relatively low doses (0.03 to 0.1 mg/minute) have been used in some settings (following loading infusion in patients who are unable to be converted to oral regimens or in some cases as a continuation of outpatient oral regimens). These prolonged infusions should not be confused with loading infusions. Because of wide variation in the use of infusions, an awareness of institutional policies and practices is extremely important. Careful clarification of orders and specific infusion rates/units is required to avoid confusion. Due to the prolonged duration of action, careful monitoring should be extended for the duration of the infusion and for several hours after the infusion. Excessive administration may result in prolonged hypotension and/or bradycardia.

Arterial hypertension in acute ischemic stroke (off-label use [Jauch, 2013]): IV:

Patient otherwise eligible for reperfusion treatment (eg, alteplase) except blood pressure (BP) >185/110 mm Hg: 10 to 20 mg over 1 to 2 minutes; may repeat once. If BP does not decline and remains >185/110 mm Hg, alteplase should not be administered.

Management of BP during and after reperfusion treatment (eg, alteplase) to maintain BP ≤180/105 mm Hg: If systolic BP >180 to 230 mm Hg or diastolic >105 to 120 mm Hg, then administer 10 mg over 1 to 2 minutes followed by an infusion of 2 to 8 mg/minute. If hypertension is refractory or diastolic BP >140 mm Hg, consider other IV antihypertensives (eg, nitroprusside).

IV to oral conversion: Upon discontinuation of IV infusion, may initiate oral dose of 200 mg followed in 6 to 12 hours with an additional dose of 200 to 400 mg. Thereafter, dose patients with 400 to 2400 mg/day in divided doses depending on blood pressure response.

Elderly: Refer to adult dosing.

Hypertension: Oral:

Manufacturer's recommendations: Initial: 100 mg twice daily; may titrate in increments of 100 mg twice daily; usual maintenance: 100 to 200 mg twice daily

ACCF/AHA Expert Consensus recommendations: Consider lower initial doses and titrating to response (Aronow, 2011)

Dosage adjustment in renal impairment: There are no dosage adjustments provided in manufacturer's labeling. Not removed by hemo- or peritoneal dialysis; supplemental dose is not necessary.

Dosage adjustment in hepatic impairment: There are no dosage adjustments provided in manufacturer's labeling. However, dosage reduction may be necessary in hepatic impairment due to decreased metabolism and increased oral bioavailability, use with caution.

Usual Infusion Concentrations: Pediatric IV infusion: 1 mg/mL

Usual Infusion Concentrations: Adult IV infusion: 500 mg in 250 mL (concentration: 2 mg/mL) of D_5W

Administration Bolus dose may be administered IV push at a rate of 10 mg/minute; may follow with continuous IV infusion

Monitoring Parameters Blood pressure, standing and sitting/supine, pulse, cardiac monitor and blood pressure monitor required for IV administration; consult individual institutional policies and procedures

Dosage Forms

Solution, Intravenous:

Generic: 5 mg/mL (4 mL, 20 mL, 40 mL)

Tablet, Oral:

Trandate: 100 mg, 200 mg, 300 mg

Generic: 100 mg, 200 mg, 300 mg

Extemporaneous Preparations A 40 mg/mL labetalol hydrochloride oral suspension may be made with tablets and one of three different vehicles (cherry syrup, a 1:1 mixture of Ora-Sweet® and Ora-Plus®, or a 1:1 mixture of Ora-Sweet® SF and Ora-Plus®). Crush sixteen 300 mg tablets in a mortar and reduce to a fine powder. Add 20 mL of the chosen vehicle and mix to a uniform paste; mix while adding the vehicle in incremental proportions to **almost** 120 mL; transfer to a calibrated bottle, rinse mortar with vehicle, and add quantity of vehicle sufficient to make 120 mL. Label "shake well" and "protect from light". Stable for 60 days when stored in amber plastic prescription bottles in the dark at room temperature or refrigerated (Allen, 1996).

Extemporaneously prepared solutions of labetalol hydrochloride (approximate concentrations 7-10 mg/mL) prepared in distilled water, simple syrup, apple juice, grape juice, and orange juice were stable for 4 weeks when stored in amber glass or plastic prescription bottles at room temperature or refrigerated (Nahata, 1991).

Allen LV Jr and Erickson MA 3rd, "Stability of Labetalol Hydrochloride, Metoprolol Tartrate, Verapamil Hydrochloride, and Spironolactone with Hydrochlorothiazide in Extemporaneously Compounded Oral Liquids," *Am J Health Syst Pharm*, 1996, 53(19):2304-9.

Nahata MC, "Stability of Labetalol Hydrochloride in Distilled Water, Simple Syrup, and Three Fruit Juices," *DICP*, 1991, 25(5):465-9.

◆ **Labetalol Hydrochloride** *see* Labetalol *on page 1151*

◆ **Labetalol Hydrochloride Injection, USP (Can)** *see* Labetalol *on page 1151*

Lacidipin [INT] (la SI di peen)

International Brand Names Caldine (FR); Fecipil (TW); Lacibloc (PH); Lacipil (BG, BR, CL, CO, CZ, EE, EG, HN, HR, IT, LT, MY, NZ, PH, PL, PT, RO, RU, SG, SI, SK, TR, TW, VE, VN); Lacivas FC (IN); Lanidem (KR); Lasyn (TW); Midotens (BR); Motens (BE, CH, DK, GB, GR, NL); Tens (CO); Vaxar (KR)

Pharmacologic Category Calcium Channel Blocker

Reported Use Treatment of hypertension

Dosage Range Adults: Oral: Initial: 2 mg as a single daily dose, preferably in the morning; may increase after 3-4 weeks to 4 mg/day; maximum dose: 6 mg/day

Product Availability Product available in various countries; not currently available in the U.S.

Dosage Forms

Tablet: 2 mg, 4 mg

Lacosamide (la KOE sa mide)

Brand Names: U.S. Vimpat

Brand Names: Canada Vimpat

Index Terms ADD 234037; Harkoseride; LCM; SPM 927

Pharmacologic Category Anticonvulsant, Miscellaneous

Use Partial-onset seizures: Monotherapy or adjunctive therapy in the treatment of partial-onset seizures

Pregnancy Risk Factor C

Pregnancy Considerations Adverse events were observed in animal reproduction studies. Available information related to use in pregnancy is limited; if inadvertent exposure occurs during pregnancy, close monitoring of the mother and fetus/newborn is recommended (Hoeltzenbein, 2011). A registry is available for women exposed to lacosamide during pregnancy: Pregnant women may contact the North American Antiepileptic Drug (AED) Pregnancy Registry (888-233-2334 or http://www.aedpregnancyregistry.org).

Breast-Feeding Considerations It is unknown if lacosamide is excreted in human milk. The manufacturer recommends a decision be made whether to discontinue nursing or to discontinue the drug, taking into account the importance of treatment to the mother.

Contraindications

U.S. labeling: There are no contraindications listed in manufacturer's labeling.

Canadian labeling: Hypersensitivity to lacosamide or any component of the formulation; second- or third-degree atrioventricular (AV) block (current or history of).

Warnings/Precautions Antiepileptics are associated with an increased risk of suicidal behavior/thoughts with use (regardless of indication); patients should be monitored for signs/symptoms of depression, suicidal tendencies, and other unusual behavior changes during therapy and instructed to inform their healthcare provider immediately if symptoms occur. CNS effects may occur; patients should be cautioned about performing tasks which require alertness (eg, operating machinery or driving). Lacosamide may prolong PR interval; second degree and complete AV block has also been reported. Use caution in patients with conduction problems (eg, first/second degree atrioventricular block and sick sinus syndrome without pacemaker), sodium channelopathies (eg, Brugada Syndrome), myocardial ischemia, heart failure, structural heart disease, or if concurrent use with other drugs that prolong the PR interval; ECG is recommended prior to initiating therapy and when at the steady state maintenance dose. Monitor closely with IV lacosamide administration; bradycardia and AV block have occurred during infusions. Instruct patients to contact their healthcare provider if signs or symptoms of conduction problems occur (eg, low or irregular pulse, feeling of lightheadedness and fainting). During short-term trials, atrial fibrillation/flutter, or syncope occurred slightly more often in patients with diabetic neuropathy and/or cardiovascular disease. In addition, in open-label studies, syncope has been associated with a history of cardiac disease risk factors and use of drugs that slow AV conduction. Use caution with renal or hepatic impairment and if these patients are taking strong inhibitors of CYP3A4 and CYP2C9; dosage adjustment may be necessary. Multiorgan hypersensitivity reactions can occur (rare); monitor patient and discontinue therapy if necessary. Withdraw therapy gradually (≥1 week) to minimize the potential of increased seizure frequency. Blurred vision and diplopia may occur during therapy. If visual disturbances persist, further assessment, including dose reduction and discontinuation should be considered. Monitor patients with known vision-related issues or ocular conditions. Effects with ethanol may be potentiated. Some products may contain phenylalanine.

Adverse Reactions

Cardiovascular: Syncope (adults; dose-related: >400 mg/day)

Central nervous system: Abnormal gait, ataxia, depression, dizziness, drowsiness, equilibrium disturbance, fatigue, headache, memory impairment, vertigo

Dermatologic: Pruritus

Gastrointestinal: Diarrhea, nausea, vomiting

Hematologic & oncologic: Bruise

Hepatic: Increased serum ALT

Local: Local irritation, pain at injection site

Neuromuscular & skeletal: Tremor, weakness

Ophthalmic: Blurred vision, diplopia, nystagmus

Miscellaneous: Laceration

Rare but important or life-threatening: Abnormal hepatic function tests, acute psychosis, aggressive behavior, agitation, agranulocytosis, anemia, angioedema, atrial fibrillation, atrial flutter, atrioventricular block, bradycardia, cerebellar syndrome, cognitive dysfunction, disturbance in attention, DRESS syndrome, euphoria, falling, hallucination, hepatitis, insomnia, nephritis, neutropenia, Stevens-Johnson syndrome, toxic epidermal necrolysis, urticaria

Drug Interactions

Metabolism/Transport Effects Substrate of CYP2C19 (minor); **Note:** Assignment of Major/Minor substrate status based on clinically relevant drug interaction potential; **Inhibits** CYP2C19 (weak)

Avoid Concomitant Use There are no known interactions where it is recommended to avoid concomitant use.

Increased Effect/Toxicity

The levels/effects of Lacosamide may be increased by: Bradycardia-Causing Agents; CarBAMazepine; CYP2C9 Inhibitors (Strong); CYP3A4 Inhibitors (Strong); Delavirdine; NiCARdipine

Decreased Effect

The levels/effects of Lacosamide may be decreased by: CarBAMazepine; Fosphenytoin; Mefloquine; Mianserin; Orlistat; PHENobarbital; Phenytoin

Preparation for Administration Injection: May be mixed with compatible diluents (NS, LR, D_5W) in glass or PVC.

Storage/Stability

Injection: Store at 20°C to 25°C (68°F to 77°F); excursions are permitted between 15°C and 30°C (59°F and 86°F). Do not freeze. Stable when mixed with compatible diluents (NS, LR, D_5W) for up to 4 hours at room temperature. Discard any unused portion.

Oral solution, tablets: Store at 20°C to 25°C (68°F to 77°F); excursions are permitted between 15°C and 30°C (59°F and 86°F). Do not freeze oral solution. Discard any unused portion of oral solution after 7 weeks.

Mechanism of Action *In vitro* studies have shown that lacosamide stabilizes hyperexcitable neuronal membranes and inhibits repetitive neuronal firing by enhancing the slow inactivation of sodium channels (with no effects on fast inactivation of sodium channels).

Pharmacodynamics/Kinetics

Absorption: Oral: Completely

Distribution: V_d: ~0.6 L/kg

Protein binding: <15%

Metabolism: Hepatic via CYP3A4, CYP2C9, and CYP2C19; forms metabolite, O-desmethyl-lacosamide (inactive)

Bioavailability: ~100%

Half-life elimination: ~13 hours

Time to peak, plasma: Oral: 1-4 hours

Excretion: Urine (95%; 40% as unchanged drug, 30% as inactive metabolite, 20% as uncharacterized metabolite); feces (<0.5%)

Dosage

Partial onset seizure:

Monotherapy: Adolescents ≥17 years and Adults: Oral, IV:

Initial: 100 mg twice daily; may be increased at weekly intervals by 50 mg twice daily based on response and tolerability.

Alternative initial dosage: Loading dose: 200 mg followed approximately 12 hours later by 100 mg twice daily for 1 week; may be increased at weekly intervals by 50 mg twice daily based on response and tolerability. **Note:** Administer loading doses under medical supervision because of the increased incidence of CNS adverse reactions.

Maintenance: 150 to 200 mg twice daily. **Note:** For patients already on a single antiepileptic and converting to lacosamide monotherapy, maintain the maintenance dose for 3 days before beginning withdrawal of the concomitant antiepileptic drug. Gradually taper the concomitant antiepileptic drug over ≥6 weeks.

Adjunctive therapy: Adolescents ≥17 years and Adults: Oral, IV:

Initial: 50 mg twice daily; may be increased at weekly intervals by 50 mg twice daily based on response and tolerability.

Alternative initial dosage: Loading dose of 200 mg followed approximately 12 hours later by 100 mg twice daily for 1 week; may be increased at weekly intervals by 50 mg twice daily based on response and tolerability. **Note:** Administer loading doses under medical supervision because of the increased incidence of CNS adverse reactions.

Maintenance dose: 100 to 200 mg twice daily

Switching from oral to IV dosing: When switching from oral to IV formulations, the total daily dose and frequency should be the same; IV therapy should only be used temporarily. Clinical study experience of IV lacosamide is limited to 5 days of consecutive treatment.

Dosage adjustment in renal impairment: Use caution when titrating dose.

Mild-to-moderate renal impairment: No dosage adjustment necessary. However, in patients with renal impairment taking concomitant strong CYP3A4 and/or CYP2C9 inhibitors, dosage reduction may be necessary.

Severe renal impairment (CrCl ≤30 mL/minute): Maximum dose: 300 mg daily. Further dosage reduction/limitation may be necessary with concomitant use of strong CYP3A4 and/or CYP2C9 inhibitors.

End-stage renal disease (ESRD) requiring hemodialysis: Maximum dose: 300 mg daily. Further dosage reduction/limitation may be necessary with concomitant use of strong CYP3A4 and/or CYP2C9 inhibitors. Removed by hemodialysis; after 4-hour hemodialysis treatment, a supplemental dose of up to 50% should be considered.

Dosage adjustment in hepatic impairment: Use caution when titrating dose.

Mild-to-moderate hepatic impairment: Maximum dose: 300 mg daily. Further dosage reduction/limitation may be necessary in patients taking concomitant strong CYP3A4 and/or CYP2C9 inhibitors.

Severe hepatic impairment: Use is not recommended.

Dietary Considerations Some products may contain phenylalanine.

Administration

Injection: Administer over 15 to 60 minutes; infusions over 30 to 60 minutes are preferred to minimize adverse effects. IV administration has been used for up to 5 days. Can be administered without further dilution or may be mixed with compatible diluents (NS, LR, D_5W).

Oral solution, tablets: May be administered with or without food. Oral solution should be administered with a calibrated measuring device (not a household teaspoon or tablespoon).

Monitoring Parameters Patients with conduction problems, sodium channelopathies, concomitant medications that prolong PR interval or severe cardiac disease should have ECG tracing prior to start of therapy and when at steady-state. Monitor these patients closely during IV infusions (cases of bradycardia and AV block have occurred during infusions). Monitor for suicidality (eg, suicidal thoughts, depression, behavioral changes).

Dosage Forms

Solution, Intravenous:

Vimpat: 200 mg/20 mL (20 mL)

Solution, Oral:

Vimpat: 10 mg/mL (200 mL, 465 mL)

Tablet, Oral:

Vimpat: 50 mg, 100 mg, 150 mg, 200 mg

◆ **LaCrosse Complete [OTC]** *see* Sodium Phosphates *on page 1909*

◆ **Lactoflavin** *see* Riboflavin *on page 1803*

Lactulose (LAK tyoo lose)

Brand Names: U.S. Constulose; Enulose; Generlac; Kristalose

Brand Names: Canada Apo-Lactulose; Euro-Lac; Jamp-Lactulose; PMS-Lactulose; Ratio-Lactulose; Teva-Lactulose

Pharmacologic Category Ammonium Detoxicant; Laxative, Osmotic

Use Prevention and treatment of portal-systemic encephalopathy (including hepatic precoma and coma); treatment of constipation

Pregnancy Risk Factor B

Pregnancy Considerations Adverse events have not been observed in animal reproduction studies. Lactulose is poorly absorbed following oral administration. Use of dietary fiber or bulk-forming laxatives along with increased fluid intake is generally considered first line therapy for treating constipation in pregnant women. Short-term use of lactulose is also considered to be safe/low risk when therapy is needed; however, side effects may limit its use (Cullen, 2007; Mahadevan, 2006; Prather, 2004; Wald, 2003).

Breast-Feeding Considerations It is not known if lactulose is excreted into breast milk; however, lactulose is poorly absorbed following oral administration. The manufacturer recommends that caution be used if administered to a nursing woman.

Contraindications Use in patients requiring a low galactose diet

Warnings/Precautions Use with caution in patients with diabetes mellitus; solution contains galactose and lactose. Monitor periodically for electrolyte imbalance when lactulose is used >6 months or in patients predisposed to electrolyte abnormalities (eg, elderly). Hepatic disease may predispose patients to electrolyte imbalance. Infants receiving lactulose may develop hyponatremia and dehydration. Patients receiving lactulose and an oral anti-infective agent should be monitored for possible inadequate response to lactulose. During proctoscopy or colonoscopy procedures involving electrocautery, a theoretical risk of reaction between H_2 gas accumulation and electrical spark may exist; thorough bowel cleansing with a nonfermentable solution is recommended.

Adverse Reactions

Endocrine & metabolic: Dehydration, hypernatremia, hypokalemia

Gastrointestinal: Abdominal discomfort, abdominal distention, belching, cramping, diarrhea (excessive dose), flatulence, nausea, vomiting

Drug Interactions

Metabolism/Transport Effects None known.

Avoid Concomitant Use There are no known interactions where it is recommended to avoid concomitant use.

Increased Effect/Toxicity There are no known significant interactions involving an increase in effect.

Decreased Effect There are no known significant interactions involving a decrease in effect.

Storage/Stability Store at room temperature; do not freeze. Protect from light. Discard solution if cloudy or very dark. Prolonged exposure to cold temperatures will cause thickening which will return to normal upon warming to room temperature.

Mechanism of Action The bacterial degradation of lactulose resulting in an acidic pH inhibits the diffusion of NH_3 into the blood by causing the conversion of NH_3 to NH_4+; also enhances the diffusion of NH_3 from the blood into the gut where conversion to NH_4+ occurs; produces an osmotic effect in the colon with resultant distention promoting peristalsis; reduces blood ammonia concentration to reduce the degree of portal systemic encephalopathy

Pharmacodynamics/Kinetics

Onset:

Constipation: Up to 24 to 48 hours to produce a normal bowel movement

Encephalopathy: At least 24 to 48 hours

Absorption: Not appreciable

Metabolism: Via colonic flora to lactic acid and acetic acid; requires colonic flora for drug activation

Excretion: Primarily feces; urine (≤3%)

Dosage

Constipation: Oral:

Children (off-label use): 0.7 to 2 g/kg/day (1 to 3 mL/kg/day) in divided doses, maximum: 40 g/day (60 mL/day) (NASPGHAN, 2006)

Adults: 10 to 20 g (15 to 30 mL) daily; may increase to 40 g (60 mL) daily if necessary

Prevention of portal systemic encephalopathy (PSE): Oral:

Infants: 1.7 to 6.7 g/day (2.5 to 10 mL/day) in divided doses; adjust dosage to produce 2 to 3 stools/day

Children: 26.7 to 60 g/day (40 to 90 mL/day) in divided doses; adjust dosage to produce 2 to 3 stools/day

Adults: 20 to 30 g (30 to 45 mL) 3 to 4 times/day; adjust dose every 1 to 2 days to produce 2 to 3 soft stools/day

Treatment of acute PSE: Adults:

Oral: 20 to 30 g (30 to 45 mL) every 1 hour to induce rapid laxation; reduce to 20 to 30 g (30 to 45 mL) 3 to 4 times/day after laxation is achieved titrate to produce 2 to 3 soft stools/day

Rectal administration (retention enema): 200 g (300 mL) diluted with 700 mL of water or NS via rectal balloon catheter; retain for 30 to 60 minutes; may repeat every 4 to 6 hours; transition to oral treatment prior to discontinuing rectal administration

Treatment of overt hepatic encephalopathy (OHE) episodes: Adults (route not specified): 16.7 g (25 mL) every 1 to 2 hours until at least 2 soft or loose bowel movements are produced daily; titrate to maintain 2 to 3 bowel movements daily (AASLD [Vilstrup 2014]).

Dosage adjustment in renal impairment: There are no dosage adjustments provided in the manufacturer's labeling.

Dosage adjustment in hepatic impairment: There are no dosage adjustments provided in the manufacturer's labeling.

Dietary Considerations Contraindicated in patients on galactose-restricted diet.

Administration

Oral solution: May mix with fruit juice, water or milk.

Crystals for oral solution: Dissolve contents of packet in 120 mL water.

Rectal: Mix with water or normal saline; administer as retention enema using a rectal balloon catheter; retain for 30 to 60 minutes. Transition to oral lactulose when appropriate (able to take oral medication and no longer a risk for aspiration) prior to discontinuing rectal administration

Monitoring Parameters Blood pressure, standing/supine; serum electrolytes, serum ammonia; bowel movement patterns, fluid status

Dosage Forms

Packet, Oral:

Kristalose: 10 g (30 ea); 20 g (30 ea)

Solution, Oral:

Constulose: 10 g/15 mL (237 mL, 946 mL)

Enulose: 10 g/15 mL (473 mL)

Generlac: 10 g/15 mL (473 mL, 1892 mL)

Generic: 10 g/15 mL (15 mL, 30 mL, 236 mL, 237 mL, 473 mL, 500 mL, 946 mL, 1892 mL); 20 g/30 mL (30 mL)

- **Ladakamycin** *see* AzaCITIDine *on page 209*

Lafutidine [INT] (la FU ti deen)

International Brand Names He Ke DiSi (CN); Lafaxid (IN); Lafuca (KR); Lafumac (IN); Nuo Fei (CN); Stodine (KR); Stogar (JP, KR); Storan (KR); Stotidin (KR); Weisida (CN)

Pharmacologic Category Histamine H_2 Antagonist

Reported Use Treatment of gastric, duodenal, and stomal ulcers; acute gastritis and acute exacerbation of chronic gastritis; preanesthetic

Dosage Range Adults: Oral:

Gastritis (acute) and acute exacerbation of chronic gastritis: 10 mg/day after evening meal or before bedtime

Preanesthetic: 10 mg prior to bedtime the day before operation and 2 hours before introduction of anesthetic on day of operation

Ulcers, gastric, duodenal, and stomal: 10 mg twice daily, once after breakfast and once after evening meal or before bedtime

Dosage adjustment in the elderly: Decrease dose and/or interval according to physiologic function

Dosage adjustment in the renal/hepatic impairment: Decreased dose and/or interval may be required

Product Availability Product available in various countries; not currently available in the U.S.

Dosage Forms Tablet: 5 mg, 10 mg

- **LAIV** *see* Influenza Virus Vaccine (Live/Attenuated) *on page 1080*
- **LAIV$_4$** *see* Influenza Virus Vaccine (Live/Attenuated) *on page 1080*
- **L-AmB** *see* Amphotericin B (Liposomal) *on page 139*
- **Lambrolizumab** *see* Pembrolizumab *on page 1604*
- **LaMICtal** *see* LamoTRIgine *on page 1160*
- **Lamictal (Can)** *see* LamoTRIgine *on page 1160*
- **LaMICtal ODT** *see* LamoTRIgine *on page 1160*
- **LaMICtal Starter** *see* LamoTRIgine *on page 1160*
- **LaMICtal XR** *see* LamoTRIgine *on page 1160*
- **LamISIL** *see* Terbinafine (Systemic) *on page 2002*
- **Lamisil (Can)** *see* Terbinafine (Systemic) *on page 2002*
- **Lamisil (Can)** *see* Terbinafine (Topical) *on page 2004*
- **LamISIL Advanced [OTC]** *see* Terbinafine (Topical) *on page 2004*
- **LamISIL AF Defense [OTC]** *see* Tolnaftate *on page 2063*
- **LamISIL AT [OTC]** *see* Terbinafine (Topical) *on page 2004*
- **LamISIL AT Jock Itch [OTC]** *see* Terbinafine (Topical) *on page 2004*
- **LamISIL AT Spray [OTC]** *see* Terbinafine (Topical) *on page 2004*
- **LamISIL Spray** *see* Terbinafine (Topical) *on page 2004*

LamiVUDine (la MI vyoo deen)

Brand Names: U.S. Epivir; Epivir HBV

Brand Names: Canada 3TC; Apo-Lamivudine; Apo-Lamivudine HBV; Heptovir

Index Terms 3TC

Pharmacologic Category Antihepadnaviral, Reverse Transcriptase Inhibitor, Nucleoside (Anti-HBV); Antiretroviral, Reverse Transcriptase Inhibitor, Nucleoside (Anti-HIV)

Use

Chronic hepatitis B (Epivir HBV): For the treatment of chronic hepatitis B associated with evidence of hepatitis B viral replication and active liver inflammation.

Limitations of use: Use only when an alternative antiviral agent with a higher genetic barrier to resistance is not available or appropriate; has not been evaluated in patients with HBV-HIV-1 coinfection, hepatitis C virus or hepatitis delta virus; has also not been evaluated in patients with chronic HBV infection with decompensated liver disease or in liver transplant recipients.

HIV infection (Epivir): In combination with other antiretroviral agents for the treatment of HIV

Pregnancy Risk Factor C

Pregnancy Considerations Adverse events were observed in some animal reproduction studies. Lamivudine has a high level of transfer acrosses the human placenta. No increased risk of overall birth defects has been observed following first trimester exposure according to data collected by the antiretroviral pregnancy registry. The pharmacokinetics of lamivudine during pregnancy are not significantly altered and dosage adjustment is not required. Cases of lactic acidosis/hepatic steatosis syndrome related to mitochondrial toxicity have been reported in pregnant women with prolonged use of nucleoside analogues. It is not known if pregnancy itself potentiates this known side effect; however, women may be at increased risk of lactic acidosis and liver damage. In addition, these adverse events are similar to other rare but life-threatening syndromes which occur during pregnancy (eg, HELLP syndrome). Hepatic enzymes and electrolytes should be monitored in women receiving nucleoside analogues and clinicians should watch for early signs of the syndrome. In addition, mitochondrial dysfunction may develop in infants following in utero exposure. The DHHS Perinatal HIV Guidelines consider lamivudine in combination with either abacavir, tenofovir, or zidovudine to be a preferred NRTI backbone for antiretroviral-naïve pregnant women. The DHHS Perinatal HIV Guidelines also consider lamivudine plus tenofovir a recommended dual NRTI/NtRTI backbone for HIV/HBV coinfected pregnant women. Use caution with hepatitis B coinfection; hepatitis B flare may occur if lamivudine is discontinued postpartum.

Regardless of CD4 count or HIV RNA copy number, all HIV-infected pregnant women should receive a combination antiretroviral (ARV) drug regimen. A combination of antepartum, intrapartum, and infant ARV prophylaxis is recommended. ARV therapy should be started as soon as possible in women with symptomatic infection. Although earlier initiation may be more effective in reducing the perinatal transmission of HIV, initiation may be delayed until after 12 weeks gestation in women who do not require immediate treatment after careful consideration of maternal conditions (eg, nausea and vomiting) and the potential risks of first trimester fetal exposure for specific agents. A scheduled cesarean delivery at 38 weeks gestation is recommended for all women with HIV RNA >1000 copies/mL or unknown concentrations near delivery in order to decrease transmission. If ARV therapy must be interrupted for <24 hours during the peripartum period, stop then restart all medications simultaneously in order to decrease the chance of developing resistance. Long-term follow-up is recommended for all infants exposed to ARV medications. In couples who want to conceive, the HIV-infected partner should attain maximum viral suppression prior to conception.

Health care providers are encouraged to enroll pregnant women exposed to antiretroviral medications in the Antiretroviral Pregnancy Registry (1-800-258-4263 or www.APRegistry.com). Health care providers caring for HIV-infected women and their infants may contact the National Perinatal HIV Hotline (888-448-8765) for clinical consultation (HHS [perinatal], 2014).

Breast-Feeding Considerations Lamivudine is excreted into breast milk and can be detected in the serum of nursing infants.

Maternal or infant antiretroviral therapy does not completely eliminate the risk of postnatal HIV transmission. In addition, multiclass-resistant virus has been detected in breast-feeding infants despite maternal therapy. Therefore, in the United States, where formula is accessible, affordable, safe, and sustainable, and the risk of infant mortality due to diarrhea and respiratory infections is low, complete avoidance of breast-feeding by HIV-infected women is recommended to decrease potential transmission of HIV (HHS [perinatal], 2014).

Contraindications Clinically significant hypersensitivity (eg, anaphylaxis) to lamivudine or any component of the formulation

Warnings/Precautions Use caution with renal impairment; dosage reduction recommended. Use with extreme caution in children with history of pancreatitis or risk factors for development of pancreatitis. Pancreatitis has been reported, particularly in HIV-infected children with a history of nucleoside use. Do not use as monotherapy in treatment of HIV. Lamivudine combined with emtricitabine is not recommended as a dual-NRTI combination due to similar resistance patterns and negligible additive antiviral activity; lamivudine and abacavir or tenofovir combination is recommended as the NRTIs in a fully suppressive antiretroviral regimen (HHS [adult], 2014). Treatment of HBV in patients with unrecognized/untreated HIV may lead to rapid HIV resistance. In addition, treatment of HIV in patients with unrecognized/untreated HBV may lead to rapid HBV resistance. Use with caution in combination with interferon alfa with or without ribavirin in HIV/HBV coinfected patients; monitor closely for hepatic decompensation, anemia, or neutropenia; dose reduction or discontinuation of interferon and/or ribavirin may be required if toxicity evident. In HIV/HBV coinfection, lamivudine and tenofovir are a recommended NRTI backbone in a fully suppressive antiretroviral regimen to provide activity against both HIV and HBV (HHS [adult], 2014). **[U.S. Boxed Warning]: Do not use Epivir HBV tablets or Epivir HBV oral solution for the treatment of HIV.**

[U.S. Boxed Warning]: Lactic acidosis and severe hepatomegaly with steatosis have been reported, including fatal cases. Use caution in hepatic impairment. Pregnancy, obesity, and/or prolonged therapy may increase the risk of lactic acidosis and liver damage.

Immune reconstitution syndrome may develop resulting in the occurrence of an inflammatory response to an indolent or residual opportunistic infection during initial HIV treatment or activation of autoimmune disorders (eg, Graves' disease, polymyositis, Guillain-Barré syndrome) later in therapy. May be associated with fat redistribution. Concomitant use of other lamivudine-containing products should be avoided.

[U.S. Boxed Warning]: Monitor patients closely for several months following discontinuation of therapy for chronic hepatitis B; clinical exacerbations may occur, including fatal cases. **Monitor hepatic function with clinical and laboratory follow up for at least several months after hepatitis B treatment discontinuation. Initiate antihepatitis B (HBV) medications if clinically appropriate. [U.S. Boxed Warning]: HIV-1 resistance may emerge in chronic hepatitis B-infection patients with unrecognized or untreated HIV-1 infection. Counseling and (HIV) testing should be offered to all patients before beginning treatment with lamivudine for hepatitis B and then periodically during treatment. Lamivudine dosing for hepatitis B is subtherapeutic if used for HIV-1 infection treatment. Lamivudine monotherapy is not appropriate for HIV-1 infection treatment.** Lamivudine resistant HIV-1 can develop rapidly and limit treatment options if used in unrecognized or untreated HIV-1 infection or if a patient becomes coinfected during HBV treatment. Lamivudine dosing for hepatitis B is also subtherapeutic if used for HIV-1/HBV coinfection treatment. If lamivudine is chosen as part of a HIV-1 treatment regimen in coinfected patients, the higher lamivudine dosage indicated for HIV-1 therapy should be used, with other drugs, in an appropriate combination regimen.

Not recommended as first-line therapy of chronic HBV due to high rate of resistance. Consider use only if other anti-HBV antiviral regimens with more favorable resistance patterns cannot be used. May be appropriate for short-term treatment of acute HBV (Lok, 2009). Potential compliance problems, frequency of administration, and adverse effects should be discussed with patients before initiating therapy to help prevent the emergence of resistance.

Adverse Reactions

Central nervous system: Chills, depression, dizziness, fatigue, fever, headache, insomnia

Dermatologic: Rash

Gastrointestinal: Abdominal pain, amylase increased, anorexia, diarrhea, dyspepsia, heartburn, lipase increased, nausea, pancreatitis, vomiting

Hematologic: Hemoglobinemia, neutropenia, thrombocytopenia

Hepatic: Transaminases increased

Neuromuscular & skeletal: Arthralgia, creatine phosphokinase increased, musculoskeletal pain, myalgia, neuropathy

Miscellaneous: Infections (includes ear, nose, and throat)

Rare but important or life-threatening: Alopecia, anaphylaxis, anemia, body fat redistribution, hepatitis B exacerbation, hepatomegaly, hyperbilirubinemia, hyperglycemia, immune reconstitution syndrome, lactic acidosis, lymphadenopathy, muscle weakness, paresthesia, peripheral neuropathy, pruritus, red cell aplasia, rhabdomyolysis, splenomegaly, steatosis, stomatitis, urticaria, weakness, wheezing

Drug Interactions

Metabolism/Transport Effects None known.

Avoid Concomitant Use

Avoid concomitant use of LamiVUDine with any of the following: Emtricitabine

Increased Effect/Toxicity

LamiVUDine may increase the levels/effects of: Emtricitabine

The levels/effects of LamiVUDine may be increased by: Ganciclovir-Valganciclovir; Ribavirin; Trimethoprim

Decreased Effect There are no known significant interactions involving a decrease in effect.

Food Interactions Food decreases the rate of absorption and C_{max}; however, there is no change in the systemic AUC. Management: Administer with or without food.

Storage/Stability

Oral solution:

Epivir: Store at 25°C (77°F) tightly closed.

Epivir HBV: Store at 20°C to 25°C (68°F to 77°F) tightly closed.

Tablet: Store at 25°C (77°F); excursions are permitted between 15°C and 30°C (59°F and 86°F).

Mechanism of Action Lamivudine is a cytosine analog. *In vitro*, lamivudine is triphosphorylated, the principle mode of action is inhibition of HIV reverse transcription via viral DNA chain termination; inhibits RNA- and DNA-dependent DNA polymerase activities of reverse transcriptase. In hepatitis B, the monophosphate form of lamivudine is incorporated into the viral DNA by hepatitis B virus polymerase, resulting in DNA chain termination.

Pharmacodynamics/Kinetics

Absorption: Rapid

Distribution: V_d: 1.3 L/kg

Protein binding, plasma: <36%

Metabolism: Minor; only known metabolite is trans-sulfoxide metabolite

Bioavailability: Absolute; Cp_{max} decreased with food although AUC not significantly affected

Children: 66%

Adults: 86% to 87%

Half-life elimination: Children: 2 hours; Adults: 5-7 hours

Time to peak, plasma: Fed: 3.2 hours; Fasted: 0.9 hours

Excretion: Primarily urine (majority as unchanged drug)

Dosage Oral:

HIV: Note: Use with at least two other antiretroviral agents when treating HIV.

Infants 1-3 months (HHS [pediatric], 2014): 4 mg/kg/dose twice daily

Infants and Children 3 months to 16 years: 4 mg/kg/dose twice daily (maximum: 150 mg twice daily)

Alternate weight-based dosing using scored 150 mg tablets (HHS [pediatric], 2014):

14-21 kg: 75 mg twice daily (150 mg/day)

22-29 kg: 75 mg in the morning, 150 mg in the evening (225 mg/day)

≥30 kg: 150 mg twice daily (300 mg/day)

Adults: **Note:** For patients who are HLA-B*5701 negative, lamivudine plus abacavir is a component of a recommended regimen (with dolutegravir) for all treatment-naïve patients and a component of a recommended regimen (with efavirenz or ritonavir boosted atazanavir) for patients with pre-ART plasma HIV RNA <100,000 copies/mL (HHS [adult], 2014)

<50 kg (HHS [pediatric], 2014): 4 mg/kg/dose twice daily (maximum: 150 mg twice daily)

≥50 kg: 150 mg twice daily or 300 mg once daily

Treatment of hepatitis B (Epivir HBV): Note: Not a preferred agent in chronic HBV treatment due to high rates of resistance; consider alternative agents. Tablets and oral solution may be used interchangeably; for doses <100 mg, oral solution is recommended.

Children 2-17 years: 3 mg/kg/dose once daily (maximum: 100 mg/day)

Adults: 100 mg/day

Treatment duration (AASLD practice guidelines):

Hepatitis Be antigen (HBeAg) positive chronic hepatitis: Treat ≥1 year until HBeAg seroconversion and undetectable serum HBV DNA; continue therapy for ≥6 months after HBeAg seroconversion

HBeAg negative chronic hepatitis: Treat >1 year until hepatitis B surface antigen (HBsAg) clearance

Note: Patients not achieving <2 log decrease in serum HBV DNA after at least 6 months of therapy should either receive additional treatment or be switched to an alternative therapy (Lok, 2009).

Treatment of hepatitis B/HIV coinfection (in patients with both infections requiring treatment): Note: The formulation and dosage of Epivir HBV are not appropriate for patients infected with both HBV and HIV. Tenofovir and lamivudine are a preferred NRTI backbone in a fully suppressive antiretroviral regimen for the treatment of HIV/HBV coinfection (HHS [adult], 2014).

Infants and Children: 4 mg/kg/dose (maximum: 150 mg) twice daily, in combination with other antiretrovirals in an antiretroviral (ARV) regimen (DHHS [pediatric], 2013).

Adolescents and Adults: 150 mg twice daily or 300 mg once daily, in combination with other antiretrovirals in an ARV regimen (HHS [adult], 2014)

Postexposure prophylaxis for HIV exposure (off-label use [CDC, 2005]): Adolescents ≥16 years and Adults: 150 mg twice daily or 300 mg once daily, in combination with zidovudine, tenofovir, stavudine, or didanosine, with or without a protease inhibitor depending on risk

Dosage adjustment in renal impairment: HIV:

Patients ≤16 years: Insufficient data; however, dose reduction should be considered.

Patients >16 years:

CrCl ≥50 mL/minute: No dosage adjustment necessary.

CrCl 30-49 mL/minute: Administer 150 mg once daily

CrCl 15-29 mL/minute: Administer 150 mg first dose, then 100 mg once daily

CrCl 5-14 mL/minute: Administer 150 mg first dose, then 50 mg once daily

CrCl <5 mL/minute: Administer 50 mg first dose, then 25 mg once daily

Dosage adjustment in renal impairment: Hepatitis B:

Adults:

CrCl ≥50 mL/minute: No dosage adjustment necessary.

CrCl 30-49 mL/minute: Administer 100 mg first dose then 50 mg once daily

CrCl 15-29 mL/minute: Administer 100 mg first dose then 25 mg once daily

CrCl 5-14 mL/minute: Administer 35 mg first dose then 15 mg once daily

CrCl <5 mL/minute: Administer 35 mg first dose then 10 mg once daily

Dialysis: Negligible amounts are removed by 4-hour hemodialysis or peritoneal dialysis. Supplemental dosing not needed; however, dosing after dialysis is recommended (HHS [adult], 2014).

Dosage adjustment in hepatic impairment: No dosage adjustment necessary. However, has not been studied in the setting of decompensated liver disease.

Dietary Considerations May be taken without regard to meals. Some products may contain sucrose.

Administration May be administered without regard to meals. Adjust dosage in renal failure.

Monitoring Parameters Amylase, bilirubin, liver enzymes (every 3 months during therapy), hematologic parameters, HIV viral load, and CD4 count; signs/symptoms of pancreatitis or hepatonecroinflammation (Epivir HBV), HBV DNA (regularly during therapy), HBeAg and anti-HBe (after 1 year of therapy and every 3-6 months thereafter); signs/symptoms of HBV relapse/exacerbation (for at least several months after stopping treatment)

Dosage Forms

Solution, Oral:

Epivir: 10 mg/mL (240 mL)

Epivir HBV: 5 mg/mL (240 mL)

Generic: 10 mg/mL (240 mL)

Tablet, Oral:

Epivir: 150 mg, 300 mg

Epivir HBV: 100 mg

Generic: 100 mg, 150 mg, 300 mg

◆ **Lamivudine, Abacavir, and Dolutegravir** *see* Abacavir, Dolutegravir, and Lamivudine *on page* 22

◆ **Lamivudine, Abacavir, and Zidovudine** *see* Abacavir, Lamivudine, and Zidovudine *on page* 22

◆ **Lamivudine and Abacavir** *see* Abacavir and Lamivudine *on page* 22

Lamivudine and Zidovudine

(la MI vyoo deen & zye DOE vyoo deen)

Brand Names: U.S. Combivir

Brand Names: Canada Combivir; Teva-Lamivudine/Zidovudine

Index Terms AZT + 3TC (error-prone abbreviation); Zidovudine and Lamivudine

Pharmacologic Category Antiretroviral, Reverse Transcriptase Inhibitor, Nucleoside (Anti-HIV)

Use Treatment of HIV infection when therapy is warranted based on clinical and/or immunological evidence of disease progression

Pregnancy Risk Factor C

Dosage Adolescents ≥30 kg and Adults: Oral: One tablet twice daily

Note: Because this is a fixed-dose combination product, avoid use in patients requiring dosage reduction including children <30 kg, renally-impaired patients with a creatinine clearance <50 mL/minute, hepatic impairment, or those patients experiencing dose-limiting adverse effects.

Dosage adjustment in renal impairment: CrCl <50 mL/minute: Fixed-dose combination lamivudine/zidovudine is not recommended; use individual components for patients requiring dose adjustments.

Dosage adjustment in hepatic impairment: Fixed-dose combination lamivudine/zidovudine is not recommended; use individual components for patients requiring dose adjustments.

Additional Information Complete prescribing information should be consulted for additional detail.

Dosage Forms

Tablet, oral: Lamivudine 150 mg and zidovudine 300 mg

Combivir: Lamivudine 150 mg and zidovudine 300 mg [scored]

LamoTRIgine

(la MOE tri jeen)

Brand Names: U.S. LaMICtal; LaMICtal ODT; LaMICtal Starter; LaMICtal XR

Brand Names: Canada Apo-Lamotrigine; Auro-Lamotrigine; Lamictal; Mylan-Lamotrigine; PMS-Lamotrigine; ratio-Lamotrigine; Teva-Lamotrigine

Index Terms BW-430C; LTG

Pharmacologic Category Anticonvulsant, Miscellaneous

Use

U.S. labeling:

Bipolar disorder (immediate release only): Maintenance treatment of bipolar I disorder to delay the time to occurrence of mood episodes (depression, mania, hypomania, mixed episodes) in adults treated for acute mood episodes with standard therapy.

Epilepsy:

Adjunctive therapy:

Immediate release: Adjunctive therapy for partial-onset seizures, generalized seizures of Lennox-Gastaut syndrome, and primary generalized tonic-clonic seizures in adults and children 2 years and older.

Extended release: Adjunctive therapy for primary generalized tonic-clonic seizures and partial-onset seizures with or without secondary generalization in patients 13 years and older.

Monotherapy:

Immediate release: Conversion to monotherapy in adults (16 years and older) with partial-onset seizures who are receiving treatment with carbamazepine, phenytoin, phenobarbital, primidone, or valproate as the single antiepileptic drug (AED).

Extended release: Conversion to monotherapy in patients 13 years and older with partial-onset seizures who are receiving treatment with a single AED.

Canadian labeling: **Epilepsy:** Immediate release:

Adjunctive therapy: Adjunctive therapy for epilepsy uncontrolled by conventional therapy in adults; seizures associated with Lennox-Gastaut syndrome in children ≥9 kg and adults.

Monotherapy: Monotherapy in adults with epilepsy following withdrawal of concurrent AEDs

Pregnancy Risk Factor C

Pregnancy Considerations Adverse events have been observed in animal reproduction studies. Lamotrigine crosses the human placenta and can be measured in the plasma of exposed newborns (Harden and Pennell, 2009; Ohman, 2000). An overall increase in major congenital malformations has not been observed in available studies; however, an increased risk for cleft lip or cleft palate has not been ruled out (Cunnington, 2011; Hernández-Díaz, 2012; Holmes, 2012). An increased risk of malformations following maternal lamotrigine use may be associated with larger doses (Cunnington, 2007; Tomson, 2011). Polytherapy may increase the risk of congenital malformations; monotherapy with the lowest effective dose is recommended (Harden and Meader, 2009).

Due to pregnancy-induced physiologic changes, women who are pregnant may require dose adjustments of lamotrigine in order to maintain clinical response; monitoring during pregnancy should be considered (Harden and Pennell, 2009). For women with epilepsy who are planning a pregnancy in advance, baseline serum concentrations should be measured once or twice prior to pregnancy during a period when seizure control is optimal. Monitoring can then be continued up to once a month during pregnancy and every second day during the first week post partum (Patsalos, 2008). In women taking lamotrigine who are trying to avoid pregnancy, potentially significant interactions may exist with hormone-containing contraceptives; consult drug interactions database for more detailed information.

Pregnancy registries are available for women who have been exposed to lamotrigine. Patients may enroll themselves in the North American Antiepileptic Drug (NAAED) Pregnancy Registry by calling (888) 233-2334. Additional information is available at www.aedpregnancyregistry.org.

Breast-Feeding Considerations Lamotrigine is excreted in breast milk and may be as high as 50% of the maternal serum concentration. Adverse events observed in breast-feeding infants include apnea, drowsiness, and poor sucking. The manufacturer recommends that caution be exercised when administering lamotrigine to nursing women and to monitor the nursing infant.

Contraindications Hypersensitivity (eg, rash, angioedema, acute urticaria, extensive pruritus, mucosal ulceration) to lamotrigine or any component of the formulation

Warnings/Precautions [U.S. Boxed Warning]: Severe and potentially life-threatening skin rashes requiring hospitalization have been reported; incidence of serious rash is higher in pediatric patients than adults; risk may be increased by coadministration with valproic acid, higher than recommended starting doses, and exceeding recommended dose titration. The majority of cases occur in the first 8 weeks; however, isolated cases may occur after prolonged treatment or in patients without these risk factors. Discontinue at first sign of rash and do not reinitiate therapy unless rash is clearly not drug related. Rare cases of Stevens-Johnson syndrome, toxic epidermal necrolysis, and angioedema have been reported.

Antiepileptics are associated with an increased risk of suicidal behavior/thoughts with use (regardless of indication); patients should be monitored for signs/symptoms of depression, suicidal tendencies, and other unusual behavior changes during therapy and instructed to inform their healthcare provider immediately if symptoms occur.

A spectrum of hematologic effects have been reported with use (eg, neutropenia, leukopenia, thrombocytopenia, pancytopenia, anemias, and rarely, aplastic anemia and pure red cell aplasia); patients with a previous history of adverse hematologic reaction to any drug may be at increased risk. Early detection of hematologic change is important; advise patients of early signs and symptoms including fever, sore throat, mouth ulcers, infections, easy bruising, petechial or purpuric hemorrhage. May be associated with hypersensitivity syndrome (eg, anticonvulsant hypersensitivity syndrome). Multiorgan hypersensitivity reactions (drug reaction with eosinophilia and systemic symptoms [DRESS]) have been reported. Symptoms may include fever, rash, and/or lymphadenopathy; monitor for signs and symptoms of possible disparate manifestations associated with lymphatic, hepatic, renal, and/or hematologic organ systems. Evaluate patient with fever and lymphadenopathy, even if rash is not present; discontinuation and conversion to alternate therapy may be required. Increased risk of developing aseptic meningitis has been reported; symptoms (eg, headache, nuchal rigidity, fever, nausea/vomiting, rash, photophobia) have generally occurred within 1 to 45 days following therapy initiation. Use caution in patients with renal or hepatic impairment. Avoid abrupt cessation, taper over at least 2 weeks if possible.

May cause CNS depression, which may impair physical or mental abilities. Patients must be cautioned about performing tasks which require mental alertness (eg, operating machinery or driving). Effects with other sedative drugs or ethanol may be potentiated. Binds to melanin and may accumulate in the eye and other melanin-rich tissues; the clinical significance of this is not known. Safety and efficacy have not been established for use as initial monotherapy, conversion to monotherapy from antiepileptic drugs (AED) other than carbamazepine, phenytoin, phenobarbital, primidone or valproic acid or conversion to monotherapy from two or more AEDs. Patients treated for bipolar disorder should be monitored closely for clinical worsening or suicidality; prescriptions should be written for the smallest quantity consistent with good patient care. Efficacy in the acute treatment of mood episodes has not been established. Potentially significant drug-drug interactions may exist, requiring dose or frequency adjustment, additional monitoring, and/or selection of alternative therapy. There is a potential for medication errors with similar-sounding medications and among different lamotrigine formulations; medication errors have occurred.

Some dosage forms may contain polysorbate 80 (also known as Tweens). Hypersensitivity reactions, usually a delayed reaction, have been reported following exposure to pharmaceutical products containing polysorbate 80 in certain individuals (Isaksson, 2002; Lucente 2000; Shelley, 1995). Thrombocytopenia, ascites, pulmonary deterioration, and renal and hepatic failure have been reported in premature neonates after receiving parenteral products containing polysorbate 80 (Alade, 1986; CDC, 1984). See manufacturer's labeling.

Adverse Reactions

Cardiovascular: Chest pain, edema, peripheral edema

Central nervous system: Abnormal dreams, abnormality in thinking, agitation, amnesia, anxiety, ataxia, confusion, depression, dizziness, drowsiness, dyspraxia, emotional lability, fatigue, hyperreflexia, hypoesthesia, hyporeflexia, insomnia, irritability, migraine, pain, paresthesia, suicidal ideation

Dermatologic: Skin rash (nonserious is more common), dermatitis, diaphoresis, xeroderma

Endocrine & metabolic: Dysmenorrhea, weight gain, weight loss

Gastrointestinal: Abdominal pain, anorexia, constipation, dyspepsia, flatulence, peptic ulcer, vomiting, xerostomia

Gastrointestinal: Nausea

Genitourinary: Increased libido, urinary frequency

Hematologic & oncologic: Rectal hemorrhage

Infection: Infection

Neuromuscular & skeletal: Arthralgia, back pain, myalgia, neck pain, weakness

Ophthalmic: Amblyopia, nystagmus, visual disturbance

Respiratory: Bronchitis, cough, dyspnea, epistaxis, nasopharyngitis, pharyngitis, rhinitis, sinusitis, upper respiratory tract infection

Miscellaneous: Fever

Rare but important or life-threatening: Abnormal hepatic function tests, abnormal lacrimation, accommodation disturbance, acne vulgaris, acute renal failure, ageusia, agranulocytosis, akathisia, alcohol intolerance, alopecia, altered sense of smell, amyotrophy, anemia, anorgasmia, apathy, aphasia, apnea, arthritis, aseptic meningitis, blepharoptosis, breast abscess, breast neoplasm, bursitis, central nervous system depression, cerebellar syndrome, conjunctivitis, cystitis, deafness, decreased fibrin, decreased libido, decreased serum fibrinogen, deep vein thrombophlebitis, delirium, delusions, depersonalization, depression, dermatitis (exfoliative, fungal), disseminated intravascular coagulation, DRESS syndrome, dry eye syndrome, dysphagia, dysphoria, dysuria, ecchymosis, ejaculatory disorder, eosinophilia, epididymitis, eructation, erythema multiforme, esophagitis, exacerbation of Parkinson disease, extrapyramidal reaction, gastritis, gastrointestinal hemorrhage, gingival hemorrhage, gingival hyperplasia, gingivitis, glossitis, hallucination, hemiplegia, hemorrhage, hepatitis, herpes zoster, hirsutism, hostility, hot flash, hyperalgesia, hyperbilirubinemia, hyperesthesia, hyperglycemia, hypermenorrhagia, hypersensitivity reaction, hypertension, hyperventilation, hypokinesia, hypothyroidism, hypotonia, immunosuppression (progressive), impotence, increased appetite, increased gamma glutamyl transpeptidase, increased serum alkaline phosphatase, increased serum ALT, increased serum AST, lactation, leg cramps, leukocytosis, leukoderma, leukopenia, lupus-like syndrome, lymphadenopathy, lymphocytosis, maculopapular rash, malaise, manic depressive reaction, memory impairment, multiorgan failure, muscle spasm, myasthenia, myoclonus, neuralgia, neutropenia, nightmares, oral mucosa ulcer, orthostatic hypotension, oscillopsia, otalgia, palpitations, pancreatitis, pancytopenia, panic attack, paralysis, paranoid reaction, pathological fracture, peripheral neuritis, personality disorder, petechia, photophobia, polyuria, psychosis, pure red cell aplasia, pustular rash, racing mind, renal pain, rhabdomyolysis, sialorrhea, skin discoloration, sleep disorder, status epilepticus, Stevens-Johnson syndrome, strabismus, suicidal tendencies, syncope, tachycardia, tendinous contracture, thrombocytopenia, tics, tinnitus, tonic-clonic seizures (exacerbation), urinary incontinence, urinary retention, urinary urgency, uveitis, vasculitis, vasodilation, vesiculobullous dermatitis, visual field defect, withdrawal seizures

Drug Interactions

Metabolism/Transport Effects None known.

Avoid Concomitant Use

Avoid concomitant use of LamoTRIgine with any of the following: Azelastine (Nasal); Orphenadrine; Paraldehyde; Thalidomide

Increased Effect/Toxicity

LamoTRIgine may increase the levels/effects of: Alcohol (Ethyl); Azelastine (Nasal); Buprenorphine; CarBAMazepine; CNS Depressants; Desmopressin; Hydrocodone; MetFORMIN; Methotrimeprazine; Metyrosine; Mirtazapine; OLANZapine; Orphenadrine; Paraldehyde; Pramipexole; Procainamide; ROPINIRole; Rotigotine; Selective Serotonin Reuptake Inhibitors; Suvorexant; Thalidomide; Zolpidem

The levels/effects of LamoTRIgine may be increased by: Brimonidine (Topical); Cannabis; Doxylamine; Dronabinol; Droperidol; HydrOXYzine; Kava Kava; Magnesium Sulfate; Methotrimeprazine; Nabilone; Perampanel; Rufinamide; Sodium Oxybate; Tapentadol; Tetrahydrocannabinol; Valproic Acid and Derivatives

Decreased Effect

LamoTRIgine may decrease the levels/effects of: Contraceptives (Progestins)

The levels/effects of LamoTRIgine may be decreased by: Atazanavir; Barbiturates; CarBAMazepine; Contraceptives (Estrogens); Ezogabine; Fosphenytoin; Mefloquine; Mianserin; Orlistat; Phenytoin; Primidone; Rifampin; Ritonavir

Food Interactions Food has no effect on absorption.

Storage/Stability Store at 15°C to 30°C (59°F to 86°F). Protect from light.

Mechanism of Action A triazine derivative which inhibits release of glutamate (an excitatory amino acid) and inhibits voltage-sensitive sodium channels, which stabilizes neuronal membranes. Lamotrigine has weak inhibitory effect on the 5-HT_3 receptor; *in vitro* inhibits dihydrofolate reductase.

Pharmacodynamics/Kinetics

Absorption: Immediate release: Rapid and complete

Distribution: V_d: 0.9 to 1.3 L/kg

Protein binding: ~55%

Metabolism: Hepatic and renal; metabolized primarily by glucuronic acid conjugation to inactive metabolites

Bioavailability: Immediate release: 98%; **Note:** AUCs were similar for immediate release and extended release preparations in patients receiving nonenzyme-inducing AEDs. In subjects receiving concomitant enzyme-inducing AEDs, bioavailability of extended release product was ~21% lower than immediate release product; in some of these subjects, a decrease in AUC of up to 70% was observed when switching from immediate release to extended release tablets.

Half-life elimination: Immediate release: Adults: 25 to 33 hours, Elderly: 25 to 43 hours; Extended release: Similar to immediate release

- Concomitant valproic acid therapy: Adults: 48 to 70 hours; Children 5 to 11 years: 66 hours; Children 10 months to 5 years: 45 hours
- Concomitant phenytoin, phenobarbital, primidone, or carbamazepine therapy: Adults: 13 to 14 hours; Children 10 months to 11 years: 7 to 8 hours
- Concomitant phenytoin, phenobarbital, primidone, or carbamazepine plus valproate therapy: Adults: 27 hours; Children 5 to 11 years: 19 hours
- Chronic renal failure: 43 hours
- Hemodialysis: 13 hours during dialysis; 57 hours between dialysis (~20% of a dose is eliminated in a 4-hour dialysis session)
- Hepatic impairment:
  - Mild: 26 to 66 hours
  - Moderate: 28 to 116 hours
  - Severe without ascites: 56 to 78 hours
  - Severe with ascites: 52 to 148 hours

Time to peak, plasma: Immediate release: ~1 to 5 hours (dependent on adjunct therapy); Extended release: 4 to 11 hours (dependent on adjunct therapy)

Excretion: Urine (94%, ~90% as glucuronide conjugates and ~10% unchanged); feces (2%)

Dosage Oral: **Note:** Drugs that induce lamotrigine glucuronidation include carbamazepine, phenytoin, phenobarbital, primidone, rifampin, lopinavir/ritonavir, and atazanavir/ritonavir. Valproic acid inhibits lamotrigine glucuronidation. Extended release formulation not FDA approved for children ≤12 years of age.

U.S. labeling:

Children 2-12 years: Lennox-Gastaut syndrome (adjunctive), partial seizures (adjunctive), or primary generalized tonic-clonic seizures (adjunctive): **Note:** Whole tablets should be used for dosing, round calculated dose down to the nearest whole tablet. Alternatively, a suspension may be prepared using immediate release tablets (see also Extemporaneous Preparations). Children <30 kg will likely require maintenance doses to be increased by as much as 50% based on clinical response regardless of regimen below:

Immediate release formulation:

- Regimens **not containing** carbamazepine, phenytoin, phenobarbital, primidone, rifampin, lopinavir/ritonavir, or valproic acid: Initial: Weeks 1 and 2: 0.3 mg/kg/day in 1-2 divided doses; Weeks 3 and 4: 0.6 mg/kg/day in 2 divided doses; Week 5 and beyond: Increase by 0.6 mg/kg/day every 1-2 weeks; Usual maintenance: 4.5-7.5 mg/kg/day (maximum: 300 mg daily) in 2 divided doses
- Regimens **containing** valproic acid: Initial: Weeks 1 and 2: 0.15 mg/kg/day in 1-2 divided doses (if calculated dose is equal to or rounds down to 1 mg daily, give 2 mg every other day instead); Weeks 3 and 4: 0.3 mg/kg/day in 1-2 divided doses; Week 5 and beyond: Increase by 0.3 mg/kg/day every 1-2 weeks; Usual maintenance: 1-5 mg/kg/day (maximum: 200 mg daily) in 1 or 2 divided doses or 1 to 3 mg/kg/day with valproic acid alone (maximum: 200 mg daily)
- Regimens **containing** carbamazepine, phenytoin, phenobarbital, primidone, rifampin, or lopinavir/ritonavir, and without valproic acid: Initial: Weeks 1 and 2: 0.6 mg/kg/day in 2 divided doses; Weeks 3 and 4: 1.2 mg/kg/day in 2 divided doses; Week 5 and beyond: Increase by 1.2 mg/kg/day every 1-2 weeks; Usual maintenance: 5-15 mg/kg/day (maximum: 400 mg daily) in 2 divided doses

Adolescents >12 years:

- Lennox-Gastaut syndrome (adjunctive): *Immediate release formulation:* Refer to adult dosing.
- Partial seizures (adjunctive) or primary generalized tonic-clonic seizures (adjunctive): *Immediate release or extended release formulation*: Refer to adult dosing.
- Conversion from adjunctive therapy with drugs that inhibit or induce lamotrigine glucuronidation to monotherapy with lamotrigine:
  - *Immediate release formulation:* Adolescents ≥16 years: Refer to adult dosing.
  - *Extended release formulation:* Adolescents ≥13 years: Refer to adult dosing.

Adults:

Lennox-Gastaut syndrome (adjunctive): *Immediate release formulation:*

Regimens **not containing** carbamazepine, phenytoin, phenobarbital, primidone, rifampin, lopinavir/ritonavir, or valproic acid: Initial: Weeks 1 and 2: 25 mg once daily; Weeks 3 and 4: 50 mg once daily; Week 5 and beyond: Increase by 50 mg daily every 1-2 weeks; Usual maintenance: 225 to 375 mg daily in 2 divided doses

Regimens **containing** valproic acid: Initial: Weeks 1 and 2: 25 mg every other day; Weeks 3 and 4: 25 mg once daily; Week 5 and beyond: Increase by 25 to 50 mg daily every 1 to 2 weeks; Usual maintenance: 100 to 200 mg daily (valproic acid alone) or 100 to 400 mg daily (valproic acid and other drugs that induce glucuronidation) in 1 or 2 divided doses

Regimens **containing** carbamazepine, phenytoin, phenobarbital, primidone, rifampin, or lopinavir/ritonavir, and without valproic acid: Initial: Weeks 1 and 2: 50 mg once daily; Weeks 3 and 4: 100 mg daily in 2 divided doses; Week 5 and beyond: Increase by 100 mg daily every 1-2 weeks; Usual maintenance: 300 to 500 mg daily in 2 divided doses (doses as high as 700 mg/day have been used)

Partial seizures (adjunctive) and primary generalized tonic-clonic seizures (adjunctive):

Immediate release formulation:

Regimens **not containing** carbamazepine, phenytoin, phenobarbital, primidone, rifampin, lopinavir/ritonavir, or valproic acid: Initial: Weeks 1 and 2: 25 mg once daily; Weeks 3 and 4: 50 mg once daily; Week 5 and beyond: Increase by 50 mg daily every 1 to 2 weeks; Usual maintenance: 225 to 375 mg daily in 2 divided doses

Regimens **containing** valproic acid: Initial: Weeks 1 and 2: 25 mg every other day; Weeks 3 and 4: 25 mg once daily; Week 5 and beyond: Increase by 25-50 mg daily every 1 to 2 weeks; Usual maintenance: 100-200 mg daily (valproic acid alone) or 100 to 400 mg daily (valproic acid and other drugs that induce glucuronidation) in 1 or 2 divided doses

Regimens **containing** carbamazepine, phenytoin, phenobarbital, primidone, rifampin, or lopinavir/ritonavir, and without valproic acid: Initial: Weeks 1 and 2: 50 mg once daily; Weeks 3 and 4: 100 mg daily in 2 divided doses; Week 5 and beyond: Increase by 100 mg daily every 1 to 2 weeks; Usual maintenance: 300 to 500 mg daily in 2 divided doses (doses as high as 700 mg/day have been used)

Extended release formulation:

Regimens **not containing** carbamazepine, phenytoin, phenobarbital, primidone, rifampin, lopinavir/ritonavir, or valproic acid: Initial: Weeks 1 and 2: 25 mg once daily; Weeks 3 and 4: 50 mg once daily; Week 5: 100 mg once daily; Week 6: 150 mg once daily; Week 7: 200 mg once daily; Week 8 and beyond: Dose increases should not exceed 100 mg daily at weekly intervals; Usual maintenance: 300 to 400 mg once daily

Regimens **containing** valproic acid: Initial: Weeks 1 and 2: 25 mg every other day; Weeks 3 and 4: 25 mg once daily; Week 5: 50 mg once daily; Week 6: 100 mg once daily; Week 7: 150 mg once daily; Week 8 and beyond: Dose increases should not exceed 100 mg daily at weekly intervals; Usual maintenance: 200 to 250 mg once daily

Regimens **containing** carbamazepine, phenytoin, phenobarbital, primidone, rifampin, or lopinavir/ritonavir, and without valproic acid: Initial: Weeks 1 and 2: 50 mg once daily; Weeks 3 and 4: 100 mg once daily; Week 5: 200 mg once daily; Week 6: 300 mg once daily; Week 7: 400 mg once daily; Week 8 and beyond: Dose increases should not exceed 100 mg daily at weekly intervals; Usual maintenance: 400 to 600 mg once daily

<u>Conversion strategy from adjunctive therapy with valproic acid to monotherapy with lamotrigine:</u>

Immediate release formulation:

- Initiate and titrate as per escalation recommendations for adjunctive therapy to a lamotrigine dose of 200 mg daily.
- Then taper valproic acid dose in decrements of not >500 mg/day/week to a valproic acid dosage of 500 mg daily; this dosage should be maintained for 1 week. The lamotrigine dosage should then be increased to 300 mg daily while valproic acid is simultaneously decreased to 250 mg daily; this dosage should be maintained for 1 week.
- Valproic acid may then be discontinued, while the lamotrigine dose is increased by 100 mg daily at weekly intervals to achieve a lamotrigine maintenance dose of 500 mg daily in 2 divided doses.

Extended release formulation:

- Initiate and titrate as per escalation recommendations for adjunctive therapy to a lamotrigine dose of 150 mg daily.
- Then taper valproic acid dose in decrements of not >500 mg/day/week to a valproic acid dose of 500 mg daily; this dosage should be maintained for 1 week. The lamotrigine dosage should then be increased to 200 mg daily while valproic acid is simultaneously decreased to 250 mg daily; this dosage should be maintained for 1 week.
- Valproic acid may then be discontinued, while the lamotrigine dose is increased to achieve a maintenance dosage range of 250-300 mg once daily.

<u>Conversion strategy from adjunctive therapy with drugs that induce lamotrigine glucuronidation (carbamazepine, phenytoin, phenobarbital, primidone) to monotherapy with lamotrigine:</u> *Immediate release formulation and extended release formulation:*

- Initiate and titrate as per escalation recommendations for adjunctive therapy to a lamotrigine dose of 500 mg daily
- Concomitant enzyme-inducing drug should then be withdrawn by 20% decrements each week over a 4-week period.
- Two weeks after withdrawal of the enzyme-inducing drug, the dosage of lamotrigine extended release may be tapered in decrements of not >100 mg/day at intervals of 1 week to achieve a maintenance dosage range of 250-300 mg once daily; no further dosage reduction is required for lamotrigine immediate release.

<u>Conversion strategy from adjunctive therapy with drugs that do **not** inhibit or induce lamotrigine glucuronidation to monotherapy with lamotrigine:</u>

Immediate release formulation: No specific guidelines available

Extended release formulation: Initiate and titrate as per escalation recommendations for adjunctive therapy to a lamotrigine dose of 250-300 mg daily. Concomitant drug should then be withdrawn by 20% decrements each week over a 4-week period.

<u>Conversion from immediate release to extended release (Lamictal XR):</u> Initial dose of the extended release tablet should match the total daily dose of the immediate-release formulation. Adjust dose as needed within the recommended dosing guidelines.

Bipolar disorder: *Immediate release formulation:*

Regimens **not containing** carbamazepine, phenytoin, phenobarbital, primidone, rifampin, lopinavir/ritonavir, or valproic acid: Initial: Weeks 1 and 2: 25 mg once daily; Weeks 3 and 4: 50 mg once daily; Week 5: 100 mg once daily; Week 6 and maintenance: 200 mg once daily

Regimens **containing** valproic acid: Initial: Weeks 1 and 2: 25 mg every other day; Weeks 3 and 4: 25 mg once daily; Week 5: 50 mg once daily; Week 6 and maintenance: 100 mg once daily

Regimens **containing** carbamazepine, phenytoin, phenobarbital, primidone, rifampin, or lopinavir/ritonavir, and without valproic acid: Initial: Weeks 1 and 2: 50 mg once daily; Weeks 3 and 4: 100 mg daily in divided doses; Week 5: 200 mg daily in divided doses; Week 6: 300 mg daily in divided doses; Maintenance: Up to 400 mg daily in divided doses

Adjustment following discontinuation of drugs that inhibit or induce lamotrigine glucuronidation:

Discontinuing valproic acid with current dose of lamotrigine 100 mg daily: 150 mg daily for week 1, then increase to 200 mg daily beginning week 2

Discontinuing carbamazepine, phenytoin, phenobarbital, primidone, rifampin, or lopinavir/ritonavir with current dose of lamotrigine 400 mg daily: 400 mg daily for week 1, then decrease to 300 mg daily for week 2, then decrease to 200 mg daily beginning week 3

Canadian labeling:

Children ≤12 years (and ≥9 kg): Lennox-Gastaut syndrome (adjunctive therapy): **Note:** Whole tablets should be used for dosing, round calculated dose down to the nearest whole tablet. Alternatively, a suspension may be prepared using immediate release tablets (see also Extemporaneous Preparations). Several weeks to months may be required to achieve individualized maintenance dose. Use is not recommended in children <9 kg.

Regimens **containing** valproic acid regardless of any other concomitant medication: Initial: Weeks 1 and 2: 0.15 mg/kg once daily (if calculated dose is equal to or rounds down to 1 mg daily give 2 mg every other day instead); Weeks 3 and 4: 0.3 mg/kg once daily; Week 5 and beyond: Increase dose by 0.3 mg/kg every 1-2 weeks (usual maintenance dose: 1-5 mg/kg daily in 1 or 2 divided doses) up to a maximum dose of 200 mg daily. **Note:** Alternatively, refer to manufacturer's labeling for recommended weight-based rounding regimen.

Regimens **containing** carbamazepine, phenytoin, phenobarbital, primidone, or other drugs that induce glucuronidation and without valproic acid: Initial: Weeks 1 and 2: 0.3 mg/kg twice daily; Weeks 3 and 4: 0.6 mg/kg twice daily; Week 5 and beyond: Increase dose by 1.2 mg/kg every 1-2 weeks (usual maintenance dose: 2.5-7.5 mg/kg twice daily) up to a maximum dose of 400 mg daily. **Note:** When necessary, round doses down to closest 5 mg interval (eg, calculated dose >5 mg and <10 mg would be rounded to 5 mg; calculated dose >10 mg and <15 mg would be rounded to 10 mg). For week 5 and beyond, dose increases made every 1-2 weeks should not exceed previous daily dose administered in week 4 (eg, if week 4 dose was 20 mg daily than dose increase in week 5 or beyond should not exceed 20 mg daily). Manufacturer labeling suggests that insufficient data exists to support weight based dosing in patients >59 kg.

Adolescents >12 years: Lennox-Gastaut syndrome (adjunctive therapy): Refer to adult dosing.

Adolescents ≥16 years: Uncontrolled epilepsy (adjunctive therapy); conversion from adjunctive therapy with concomitant drugs that inhibit or induce lamotrigine glucuronidation to monotherapy with lamotrigine: Refer to adult dosing

Adults: Uncontrolled epilepsy (adjunctive) or Lennox-Gastaut syndrome (adjunctive):

Regimens **containing** inducers of lamotrigine glucuronidation and valproic acid or regimens not containing agents that induce or inhibit lamotrigine glucuronidation: Initial: Weeks 1 and 2: 25 mg once daily; Weeks 3 and 4: 25 mg twice daily; Week 5 and beyond: Increase dose by 25-50 mg every 1-2 weeks until maintenance dose established (usual maintenance dose: 100-200 mg daily in 2 divided doses)

Regimens **containing** inducers of lamotrigine glucuronidation and without valproic acid: Initial: Weeks 1 and 2: 50 mg once daily; Weeks 3 and 4: 50 mg twice daily; Week 5 and beyond: Increase dose by 100 mg every 1-2 weeks until maintenance dose established (usual maintenance dose: 300-500 mg daily in 2 divided doses)

Conversion from adjunctive therapy with concomitant drugs that inhibit or induce lamotrigine glucuronidation to lamotrigine monotherapy: Decrease dose of concomitant antiepileptic agent by ~20% of original dose every week for 5 weeks (slower taper may be considered if clinically indicated). Lamotrigine dosage adjustments during this period should be determined by changes in lamotrigine pharmacokinetics due to withdrawal of the concomitant drugs that inhibit or induce lamotrigine glucuronidation, and by the clinical response of patient.

Additional considerations:

Discontinuing therapy: Decrease dose by ~50% per week, over at least 2 weeks unless safety concerns require a more rapid withdrawal. Discontinuing carbamazepine, phenytoin, phenobarbital, primidone, rifampin, lopinavir/ritonavir, or atazanavir/ritonavir should prolong the half-life of lamotrigine; discontinuing valproic acid should shorten the half-life of lamotrigine

Restarting therapy after discontinuation: If lamotrigine has been withheld for >5 half-lives, consider restarting according to initial dosing recommendations. **Note:** Concomitant medications may affect the half-life of lamotrigine; consider pharmacokinetic interactions when restarting therapy.

Concomitant therapy:

Dosage adjustment with atazanavir/ritonavir: Follow initial lamotrigine dosing guidelines, maintenance dose should be adjusted as follows:

Patients **not** taking concomitant carbamazepine, phenytoin, phenobarbital, primidone, rifampin, estrogen-containing contraceptives, or lopinavir/ritonavir: Lamotrigine maintenance dose may need to be increased if atazanavir/ritonavir is added or decreased if atazanavir/ritonavir is discontinued.

Dosage adjustment with estrogen-containing hormonal contraceptives: Follow initial lamotrigine dosing guidelines, maintenance dose should be adjusted as follows, based on concomitant medications:

Patients taking concomitant carbamazepine, phenytoin, phenobarbital, primidone, rifampin, lopinavir/ritonavir, or atazanavir/ritonavir: No dosing adjustment required

Patients **not** taking concomitant carbamazepine, phenytoin, phenobarbital, primidone, rifampin, lopinavir/ritonavir, or atazanavir/ritonavir: Lamotrigine maintenance dose may need increased by twofold over target dose. If already taking a stable dose of lamotrigine and starting contraceptive, maintenance dose may need increased by twofold. Dose increases should start when contraceptive is started and titrated to clinical response increasing no more rapidly than

50-100 mg daily every week. Gradual increases of lamotrigine plasma levels may occur during the inactive "pill-free" week and will be greater when dose increases are made the week before. If increased adverse events consistently occur during "pill-free" week, overall maintenance dose adjustments may be required. When discontinuing estrogen-containing hormonal contraceptive, dose of lamotrigine may need decreased by as much as 50%; do not decrease by more than 25% of total daily dose over a 2-week period unless clinical response or plasma levels indicate otherwise. Dose adjustments during "pill-free" week are not recommended.

Dosage adjustment in renal impairment: There are no dosage adjustments provided in the manufacturer's labeling. Decreased maintenance dosage may be effective in patients with significant renal impairment; has not been adequately studied; use with caution

Dosage adjustment in hepatic impairment:

U.S. labeling:

Mild impairment: No dosage adjustment necessary.

Moderate-to-severe impairment without ascites: Decrease initial, escalation, and maintenance doses by ~25%; adjust according to clinical response and tolerance.

Moderate-to-severe impairment with ascites: Decrease initial, escalation, and maintenance doses by ~50%; adjust according to clinical response and tolerance.

Canadian labeling:

Mild and moderate impairment (Child-Pugh classes A and B): Reduce initial, escalation, and maintenance dosing by ~50%; adjust according to clinical response and tolerance.

Severe impairment (Child-Pugh class C): Reduce initial, escalation, and maintenance dosing by ~75%; adjust according to clinical response and tolerance.

Administration Doses should be rounded down to the nearest whole tablet.

Lamictal chewable/dispersible tablets: May be chewed, dispersed in water or diluted fruit juice, or swallowed whole. To disperse tablets, add to a small amount of liquid (just enough to cover tablet); let sit ~1 minute until dispersed; swirl solution and consume immediately. Do not administer partial amounts of liquid. If tablets are chewed, a small amount of water or diluted fruit juice should be used to aid in swallowing.

Lamictal ODT: Place tablets on tongue and move around in the mouth. Tablets will dissolve rapidly and can be swallowed with or without food or water.

Lamictal XR: Administer without regard to meals. Swallow whole; do not chew, crush, or cut.

Monitoring Parameters Serum levels of concurrent anticonvulsants, LFTs, renal function, hypersensitivity reactions (especially rash); seizure, frequency and duration; suicidality (eg, suicidal thoughts, depression, behavioral changes); signs/symptoms of aseptic meningitis

Reference Range A therapeutic serum concentration range has not been established for lamotrigine. Dosing should be based on therapeutic response. Lamotrigine plasma concentrations of 0.25-29.1 mcg/mL have been reported in the literature.

Dosage Forms Considerations

LaMICtal Kits are available as follows:

Blue - for patients already taking valproate

LaMICtal Starter: 25 mg (35s)

LaMICtal ODT (Titration): 25 mg (21s) and 50 mg (7s)

LaMICtal XR (Titration): 25 mg (21s) and 50 mg (7s)

Green- for patients already taking carbamazepine, phenytoin, phenobarbital, or primidone, and **not** taking valproate

LaMICtal Starter: 25 mg (84s) and 100 mg (14s)

LaMICtal ODT (Titration): 50 mg (42s) and 100 mg (14s)

LaMICtal XR (Titration): 50 mg (14s) and 100 mg (14s) and 200 mg (7s)

Orange - for patients not taking carbamazepine, phenytoin, phenobarbital, primidone, or valproate

LaMICtal Starter: 25 mg (42s) and 100 mg (7s)

LaMICtal ODT (Titration): 25 mg (14s) and 50 mg (14s) and 100 mg (7s)

LaMICtal XR (Titration): 25 mg (14s) and 50 mg (14s) and 100 mg (7s)

Dosage Forms

Kit, Oral:

LaMICtal ODT: Blue Kit: 25 mg (21s) & 50 mg (7s), Orange Kit: 25 mg (14s) & 50 mg (14s) & 100 mg (7s), Green Kit: 50 mg (42s) & 100 mg (14s)

LaMICtal Starter: Blue Kit: 25 mg (35s), Orange Kit: 25 mg (42s) & 100 mg (7s), Green Kit: 25 mg (84s) & 100 mg (14s)

LaMICtal XR: Blue Kit: 25 mg (21s) & 50 mg (7s), Green Kit: 50 mg (14s) & 100 mg (14s) & 200 mg (7s), Orange Kit: 25 mg (14s) & 50 mg (14s) & 100 mg (7s)

Tablet, Oral:

LaMICtal: 25 mg, 100 mg, 150 mg, 200 mg

Generic: 25 mg, 100 mg, 150 mg, 200 mg

Tablet Chewable, Oral:

LaMICtal: 5 mg, 25 mg

Generic: 5 mg, 25 mg

Tablet Dispersible, Oral:

LaMICtal ODT: 25 mg, 50 mg, 100 mg, 200 mg

Generic: 25 mg, 50 mg, 100 mg, 200 mg

Tablet Extended Release 24 Hour, Oral:

LaMICtal XR: 25 mg, 50 mg, 100 mg, 200 mg, 250 mg, 300 mg

Generic: 25 mg, 50 mg, 100 mg, 200 mg, 250 mg, 300 mg

Extemporaneous Preparations A 1 mg/mL oral suspension may be made with tablets and one of two different vehicles (a 1:1 mixture of Ora-Sweet and Ora-Plus or a 1:1 mixture of Ora-Sweet SF and Ora-Plus). Crush one 100 mg tablet in a mortar and reduce to a fine powder. Add small portions of the chosen vehicle and mix to a uniform paste; mix while adding the vehicle in incremental proportions to **almost** 100 mL; transfer to a graduated cylinder, rinse mortar with vehicle, and add quantity of vehicle sufficient to make 100 mL. Label "shake well" and "protect from light". Stable for 91 days when stored in amber plastic prescription bottles in the dark at room temperature or refrigerated.

Nahata M, Morosco R, Hipple T. "Stability of Lamotrigine in Two Extemporaneously Prepared Oral Suspensions at 4 and 25 Degrees C," *Am J Health Syst Pharm*, 1999, 56(3):240-2.

◆ **Lanaphilic/Urea [OTC]** *see* Urea *on page 2114*

◆ **Lanoxin** *see* Digoxin *on page 627*

◆ **Lanoxin Pediatric** *see* Digoxin *on page 627*

Lanreotide (lan REE oh tide)

Brand Names: U.S. Somatuline Depot

Brand Names: Canada Somatuline Autogel

Index Terms Lanreotide Acetate

Pharmacologic Category Somatostatin Analog

Use

Acromegaly: Long-term treatment of acromegalic patients who have had an inadequate response to surgery and/or radiotherapy, or for whom surgery and/or radiotherapy is not an option.

Gastroenteropancreatic neuroendocrine tumors: Treatment of patients with unresectable, well- or moderately-differentiated, locally advanced or metastatic gastroenteropancreatic neuroendocrine tumors (GEP-NETs).

Pregnancy Risk Factor C

Dosage

Acromegaly: Adults *(U.S. labeling)* **or** Adolescents ≥16 years and Adults *(Canadian labeling)*: SubQ: Initial dose: 90 mg once every 4 weeks for 3 months; after initial 90 days of therapy, adjust dose based on clinical response of patient, growth hormone (GH) levels, and/or insulin-like growth factor 1 (IGF-1) levels as follows:

GH ≤1 ng/mL, IGF-1 normal, symptoms stable: 60 mg once every 4 weeks; once stabilized on 60 mg once every 4 weeks, may consider regimen of 120 mg once every 6 or 8 weeks (extended-interval dosing)

GH >1 to 2.5 ng/mL, IGF-1 normal, symptoms stable: 90 mg once every 4 weeks; once stabilized on 90 mg once every 4 weeks, may consider regimen of 120 mg once every 6 or 8 weeks (extended-interval dosing)

GH >2.5 ng/mL, IGF-1 elevated and/or uncontrolled symptoms: 120 mg once every 4 weeks

Gastroenteropancreatic neuroendocrine tumors (GEP-NETs): Adults: SubQ: 120 mg once every 4 weeks

Dosage adjustment in renal impairment:

Acromegaly:

Mild impairment (CrCl 60 to 89 mL/minute): No dosage adjustment necessary.

Moderate to severe impairment (CrCl ≤59 mL/minute): Initial dose: 60 mg once every 4 weeks for 3 months; adjust dose based on clinical response of patient, GH levels, and/or IGF-1 levels; use of an extended-interval dose of 120 mg once every 6 or 8 weeks should be done with caution.

Gastroenteropancreatic neuroendocrine tumors:

Mild to moderate impairment (CrCl ≥30 mL/minute): No dosage adjustment necessary.

Severe impairment (CrCl <30 mL/minute): There are no dosage adjustments provided in the manufacturer's labeling (has not been studied).

Dosage adjustment in hepatic impairment:

Acromegaly:

Mild impairment: No dosage adjustment necessary.

Moderate to severe impairment: Initial dose: 60 mg once every 4 weeks for 3 months; adjust dose based on clinical response of patient, GH levels, and/or IGF-1 levels; use of an extended-interval dose of 120 mg once every 6 or 8 weeks should be done with caution.

Gastroenteropancreatic neuroendocrine tumors: There are no dosage adjustments provided in the manufacturer's labeling (has not been studied).

Additional Information Complete prescribing information should be consulted for additional detail.

Dosage Forms

Solution, Subcutaneous:

Somatuline Depot: 120 mg/0.5 mL (0.5 mL); 60 mg/0.2 mL (0.2 mL); 90 mg/0.3 mL (0.3 mL)

Dosage Forms: Canada

Injection, solution:

Somatuline® Autogel®: 60 mg/~0.3 mL (~0.3 mL); 90 mg/~0.4 mL (~0.4 mL); 120 mg/~0.5 mL (~0.5 mL)

◆ **Lanreotide Acetate** *see* Lanreotide *on page 1165*

Lansoprazole (lan SOE pra zole)

Brand Names: U.S. First-Lansoprazole; Heartburn Relief 24 Hour [OTC] [DSC]; Heartburn Treatment 24 Hour [OTC]; Prevacid; Prevacid 24HR [OTC]; Prevacid SoluTab

Brand Names: Canada Apo-Lansoprazole; Mylan-Lansoprazole; PMS-Lansoprazole; Prevacid; Prevacid FasTab; Q-Lansoprazole; RAN-Lansoprazole; Riva-Lansoprazole; Sandoz-Lansoprazole; Teva-Lansoprazole

Pharmacologic Category Proton Pump Inhibitor; Substituted Benzimidazole

Use Short-term (4 weeks) treatment of active duodenal ulcers; maintenance treatment of healed duodenal ulcers; as part of a multidrug regimen for *H. pylori* eradication to reduce the risk of duodenal ulcer recurrence; short-term (up to 8 weeks) treatment of active benign gastric ulcer; treatment of NSAID-associated gastric ulcer; to reduce the risk of NSAID-associated gastric ulcer in patients with a history of gastric ulcer who require an NSAID; short-term treatment of symptomatic GERD; short-term (up to 8 weeks) treatment for all grades of erosive esophagitis; to maintain healing of erosive esophagitis; long-term treatment of pathological hypersecretory conditions, including Zollinger-Ellison syndrome

OTC labeling: Relief of frequent heartburn (≥2 days/week)

Pregnancy Risk Factor B

Pregnancy Considerations Adverse events were not observed in animal reproduction studies. An increased risk of hypospadias was reported following maternal use of proton pump inhibitors (PPIs) during pregnancy (Anderka, 2012), but this was based on a small number of exposures and the same association was not found in another study (Erichsen, 2012). Most available studies have not shown an increased risk of major birth defects following maternal use of PPIs during pregnancy (Diav-Citrin, 2005; Matok, 2012; Pasternak, 2010). When treating GERD in pregnancy, PPIs may be used when clinically indicated (Katz, 2013).

Breast-Feeding Considerations It is not known if lansoprazole is excreted into breast milk. Due to the potential for serious adverse reactions in the nursing infant, the manufacturer recommends a decision be made whether to discontinue nursing or to discontinue the drug, taking into account the importance of treatment to the mother.

Contraindications Hypersensitivity to lansoprazole or any component of the formulation

Warnings/Precautions Use of proton pump inhibitors (PPIs) may increase the risk of gastrointestinal infections (eg, *Salmonella, Campylobacter*). Relief of symptoms does not preclude the presence of a gastric malignancy. Atrophic gastritis (by biopsy) has been noted with long-term omeprazole therapy; this may also occur with lansoprazole. No reports of enterochromaffin-like (ECL) cell carcinoids, dysplasia, or neoplasia have occurred. Use of proton pump inhibitors (PPIs) may increase risk of CDAD, especially in hospitalized patients; consider CDAD diagnosis in patients with persistent diarrhea that does not improve. Use the lowest dose and shortest duration of PPI therapy appropriate for the condition being treated. Severe liver dysfunction may require dosage reductions. Decreased *H. pylori* eradication rates have been observed with short-term (≤7 days) combination therapy. The American College of Gastroenterology recommends 10-14 days of therapy (triple or quadruple) for eradication of *H. pylori* (Chey, 2007).

PPIs may diminish the therapeutic effect of clopidogrel thought to be due to reduced formation of the active metabolite of clopidogrel. The manufacturer of clopidogrel recommends either avoidance of both omeprazole (even when scheduled 12 hours apart) and esomeprazole or use of a PPI with comparatively less effect on the active metabolite of clopidogrel (eg, pantoprazole). Although lansoprazole exhibits the most potent CYP2C19 inhibition *in vitro* (Li, 2004; Ogilvie, 2011), an *in vivo* study of extensive CYP2C19 metabolizers showed less reduction of the active metabolite of clopidogrel by lansoprazole/dexlansoprazole compared to esomeprazole/omeprazole (Frelinger, 2012). The manufacturer of lansoprazole states that no dosage adjustment is necessary for clopidogrel when used concurrently. In contrast to these warnings, others have recommended the continued use of PPIs, regardless of the degree of inhibition, in patients with a history of GI bleeding or multiple risk factors for GI bleeding who are also receiving clopidogrel since no evidence has established clinically meaningful differences in outcome; however, a clinically-significant interaction cannot be excluded in those who are poor metabolizers of clopidogrel (Abraham, 2010; Levine, 2011). Additionally, concomitant use of lansoprazole with some drugs may require cautious use, may not be recommended, or may require dosage adjustments.

Increased incidence of osteoporosis-related bone fractures of the hip, spine, or wrist may occur with PPI therapy. Patients on high-dose or long-term therapy should be monitored. Use the lowest effective dose for the shortest duration of time, use vitamin D and calcium supplementation, and follow appropriate guidelines to reduce risk of fractures in patients at risk.

Hypomagnesemia, reported rarely, usually with prolonged PPI use of >3 months (most cases >1 year of therapy); may be symptomatic or asymptomatic; severe cases may cause tetany, seizures, and cardiac arrhythmias. Consider obtaining serum magnesium concentrations prior to beginning long-term therapy, especially if taking concomitant digoxin, diuretics, or other drugs known to cause hypomagnesemia; and periodically thereafter. Hypomagnesemia may be corrected by magnesium supplementation, although discontinuation of lansoprazole may be necessary; magnesium levels typically return to normal within 1 week of stopping.

Prolonged treatment (≥2 years) may lead to vitamin B_{12} malabsorption and subsequent vitamin B_{12} deficiency. The magnitude of the deficiency is dose-related and the association is stronger in females and those younger in age (<30 years); prevalence is decreased after discontinuation of therapy (Lam, 2013).

Benzyl alcohol and derivatives: Some dosage forms may contain benzyl alcohol; large amounts of benzyl alcohol (≥99 mg/kg/day) have been associated with a potentially fatal toxicity ("gasping syndrome") in neonates; the "gasping syndrome" consists of metabolic acidosis, respiratory distress, gasping respirations, CNS dysfunction (including convulsions, intracranial hemorrhage), hypotension, and cardiovascular collapse (AAP, 1997; CDC, 1982); some data suggests that benzoate displaces bilirubin from protein binding sites (Ahlfors, 2001); avoid or use dosage forms containing benzyl alcohol with caution in neonates. See manufacturer's labeling.

When used for self-medication, patients should be instructed not to use if they have difficulty swallowing, are vomiting blood, or have bloody or black stools. Prior to use, patients should contact healthcare provider if they have liver disease, heartburn for >3 months, heartburn with dizziness, lightheadedness, or sweating, MI symptoms, frequent chest pain, frequent wheezing (especially with heartburn), unexplained weight loss, nausea/vomiting, stomach pain, or are taking antifungals, atazanavir, digoxin, tacrolimus, theophylline, or warfarin. Patients should stop use and consult a healthcare provider if heartburn continues or worsens, or if they need to take for >14 days or more often than every 4 months. Patients should be informed that it may take 1-4 days for full effect to be seen; should not be used for immediate relief.

Adverse Reactions

Central nervous system: Dizziness, headache

Gastrointestinal: Abdominal pain, constipation, diarrhea, nausea

Rare but important or life-threatening: Abdomen enlarged, abnormal dreams, abnormal menses, abnormal stools, abnormal vision, agitation, agranulocytosis, albuminuria, allergic reaction, alkaline phosphatase increased, ALT increased, alopecia, amblyopia, amnesia, anaphylactoid reaction, anemia, angina, anorexia, anxiety, aplastic anemia, appetite increased, arrhythmia, AST increased, arthralgia, arthritis, asthma, avitaminosis, bezoar, bilirubinemia, blepharitis, blurred vision, bradycardia, breast enlargement, breast pain, breast tenderness, bronchitis, candidiasis, carcinoma, cardiospasm, cataract, cerebrovascular accident, cerebral infarction, chest pain, chills, cholelithiasis, cholesterol increased/decreased, *Clostridium difficile*-associated diarrhea (CDAD), colitis, confusion, conjunctivitis, cough increased, creatinine increased, deafness, dehydration, dementia, depersonalization, depression, diabetes mellitus, diaphoresis, diplopia, dry eyes, dry skin, dyspepsia, dysphagia, dyspnea, dysmenorrhea, dysuria, edema, electrolyte imbalance, emotional lability, enteritis, eosinophilia, epistaxis, eructation, erythema multiforme, esophageal stenosis, esophageal ulcer, esophagitis, fecal discoloration, fever, fixed eruption, flatulence, flu-like syndrome, fracture, fundic gland polyps, gastric nodules, gastrin levels increased, gastritis, gastroenteritis, gastrointestinal anomaly, gastrointestinal hemorrhage, GGTP increased/decreased, glaucoma, glucocorticoid levels increased, glossitis, glycosuria, goiter, gout, gum hemorrhage, gynecomastia, halitosis, hallucinations, hematemesis, hematuria, hemiplegia, hemolysis, hemolytic anemia, hemoptysis, hepatotoxicity, hostility aggravated, hyper-/hypoglycemia, hyperkinesia, hyperlipemia, hypertonia, hypoesthesia, hyper-/hypotension, hypomagnesemia, hypothyroidism, impotence, infection, insomnia, interstitial nephritis, kidney calculus, laryngeal neoplasia, LDH increased, leg cramps, leukopenia, leukorrhea, libido decreased/increased, liver function test abnormal, lung fibrosis, lymphadenopathy, maculopapular rash, malaise, melena, menorrhagia, migraine, moniliasis (oral), mouth ulceration, musculoskeletal pain, myalgia, myasthenia, myositis, MI, nervousness, neurosis, neutropenia, pain, palpitation, pancreatitis, pancytopenia, paresthesia, parosmia, pelvic pain, peripheral edema, pharyngitis, photophobia, platelet abnormalities, pneumonia, polyuria, pruritus, ptosis, rash, rectal hemorrhage, retinal degeneration, rhinitis, salivation increased, seizure, shock, sinusitis, skin carcinoma, sleep disorder, somnolence, speech disorder, Stevens-Johnson syndrome, stomatitis, stridor, syncope, synovitis, tachycardia, taste loss, taste perversion, tenesmus, thirst, thrombocytopenia, thrombotic thrombocytopenic purpura, tinnitus, tremor, tongue disorder, toxic epidermal necrolysis, ulcerative colitis, ulcerative stomatitis, upper respiratory inflammation, upper respiratory infection, urethral pain, urinary frequency/urgency, urination impaired, urinary retention, urinary tract infection, urticaria, vaginitis, vasodilation, vertigo, visual field defect, vomiting, weakness, WBC abnormal, weight gain/loss, xerostomia

Drug Interactions

Metabolism/Transport Effects Substrate of CYP2C19 (major), CYP2C9 (minor), CYP3A4 (major); **Note:** Assignment of Major/Minor substrate status based on clinically relevant drug interaction potential; **Inhibits** CYP2C19 (weak), CYP2C9 (weak), CYP2D6 (weak), CYP3A4 (weak); **Induces** CYP1A2 (moderate)

Avoid Concomitant Use

Avoid concomitant use of Lansoprazole with any of the following: Dasatinib; Delavirdine; Erlotinib; Nelfinavir; PAZOPanib; Pimozide; Rilpivirine; Risedronate

Increased Effect/Toxicity

Lansoprazole may increase the levels/effects of: Amphetamine; ARIPiprazole; Dexmethylphenidate; Dextroamphetamine; Dofetilide; Hydrocodone; Imatinib; Lomitapide; Methotrexate; Methylphenidate; Pimozide; Raltegravir; Risedronate; Saquinavir; Tacrolimus (Systemic); Vitamin K Antagonists; Voriconazole

The levels/effects of Lansoprazole may be increased by: Fluconazole; Ketoconazole (Systemic); Voriconazole

Decreased Effect

Lansoprazole may decrease the levels/effects of: Atazanavir; Bisphosphonate Derivatives; Bosutinib; Cefditoren; Clopidogrel; Dabigatran Etexilate; Dabrafenib; Dasatinib; Delavirdine; Erlotinib; Gefitinib; Indinavir; Iron Salts; Itraconazole; Ketoconazole (Systemic); Ledipasvir; Mesalamine; Multivitamins/Minerals (with ADEK, Folate, Iron); Mycophenolate; Nelfinavir; Nilotinib; PAZOPanib; Posaconazole; Rilpivirine; Riociguat; Risedronate; Vismodegib

The levels/effects of Lansoprazole may be decreased by: Bosentan; CYP2C19 Inducers (Strong); CYP3A4 Inducers (Moderate); CYP3A4 Inducers (Strong); Dabrafenib; Deferasirox; Mitotane; Siltuximab; St Johns Wort; Tipranavir; Tocilizumab

Food Interactions Prolonged treatment (≥2 years) may lead to malabsorption of dietary vitamin B_{12} and subsequent vitamin B_{12} deficiency (Lam, 2013).

Storage/Stability

Capsules, orally disintegrating tablets: Store at 25°C (77°F); excursions permitted to 15°C to 30°C (59°F to 86°F). Protect from light and moisture.

Powder for suspension (First® compounding kit): Prior to compounding, store at 15°C to 30°C (59°F to 86°F). Once compounded, the product is stable for 30 days at room temperature and under refrigeration; manufacturer recommendation is for the compounded product to be stored under refrigeration; protect from freezing. Protect from light.

Mechanism of Action Decreases acid secretion in gastric parietal cells through inhibition of (H+, K+)-ATPase enzyme system, blocking the final step in gastric acid production.

Pharmacodynamics/Kinetics

Onset of action: Gastric acid suppression: Oral: 1-3 hours

Duration: Gastric acid suppression: Oral: >1 day

Absorption: Rapid

Distribution: V_d: 14-18 L

Protein binding: 97%

Metabolism: Hepatic via CYP2C19 and 3A4, and in parietal cells to two active metabolites that are not present in systemic circulation

Bioavailability: ≥80%; decreased 50% to 70% if given 30 minutes after food

Half-life elimination: 1.5 ± 1 hours; Elderly: 2-3 hours; Hepatic impairment: 3-7 hours

Time to peak, plasma: 1.7 hours

Excretion: Feces (67%); urine (33%)

Dosage

Children 1-11 years: GERD, erosive esophagitis: Oral:

≤30 kg: 15 mg once daily for up to 12 weeks

>30 kg: 30 mg once daily for up to 12 weeks

Note: Doses were increased in some pediatric patients if still symptomatic after 2 or more weeks of treatment (maximum dose: 30 mg twice daily)

Children 12-17 years: Oral:

Nonerosive GERD: 15 mg once daily for up to 8 weeks

Erosive esophagitis: 30 mg once daily for up to 8 weeks

Adults: Oral:

Duodenal ulcer: Short-term treatment: 15 mg once daily for 4 weeks; maintenance therapy: 15 mg once daily

Gastric ulcer: Short-term treatment: 30 mg once daily for up to 8 weeks

NSAID-associated gastric ulcer (healing): 30 mg once daily for 8 weeks; controlled studies did not extend past 8 weeks of therapy

NSAID-associated gastric ulcer (to reduce risk): 15 mg once daily for up to 12 weeks; controlled studies did not extend past 12 weeks of therapy

Symptomatic GERD: Short-term treatment: 15 mg once daily for up to 8 weeks

Erosive esophagitis: Short-term treatment: 30 mg once daily for up to 8 weeks; continued treatment for an additional 8 weeks may be considered for recurrence or for patients who do not heal after the first 8 weeks of therapy; maintenance therapy: 15 mg once daily

Hypersecretory conditions: Initial: 60 mg once daily; adjust dose based upon patient response and to reduce acid secretion to <10 mEq/hour (5 mEq/hour in patients with prior gastric surgery); doses of 90 mg twice daily have been used; administer doses >120 mg/day in divided doses

Helicobacter pylori eradication:

Manufacturer labeling: 30 mg 3 times daily administered with amoxicillin 1000 mg 3 times daily for 14 days **or** 30 mg twice daily administered with amoxicillin 1000 mg *and* clarithromycin 500 mg twice daily for 10-14 days

American College of Gastroenterology guidelines (Chey, 2007):

Nonpenicillin allergy: 30 mg twice daily administered with amoxicillin 1000 mg *and* clarithromycin 500 mg twice daily for 10-14 days

Penicillin allergy: 30 mg twice daily administered with clarithromycin 500 mg *and* metronidazole 500 mg twice daily for 10-14 days **or** 30 mg once or twice daily administered with bismuth subsalicylate 525 mg *and* metronidazole 250 mg *plus* tetracycline 500 mg 4 times daily for 10-14 days

Heartburn: OTC labeling: 15 mg once daily for 14 days; may repeat 14 days of therapy every 4 months. Do not take for >14 days or more often than every 4 months, unless instructed by healthcare provider.

Stress ulcer prophylaxis, ICU patients (off-label use): 30 mg once daily (Brophy, 2010; Olsen, 2008). **Note:** Intended for patients with associated risk factors (eg, coagulopathy, mechanical ventilation for ≥48 hours, severe sepsis); discontinue use once risk factors have resolved (Dellinger, 2013).

Dosage adjustment in renal impairment: No dosage adjustment necessary.

Dosage adjustment in hepatic impairment: Bioavailability increased in hepatic impairment. Consider dose reduction in severe impairment.

Dietary Considerations Should be taken before eating; best if taken before breakfast. Some products may contain phenylalanine.

Administration

Oral: Administer before food; best if taken before breakfast. The intact granules should not be chewed or crushed; however, several options are available for those patients unable to swallow capsules:

Capsules may be opened and the intact granules sprinkled on 1 tablespoon of applesauce, Ensure® pudding, cottage cheese, yogurt, or strained pears. The granules should then be swallowed immediately.

Capsules may be opened and emptied into ~60 mL orange juice, apple juice, or tomato juice; mix and swallow immediately. Rinse the glass with additional juice and swallow to assure complete delivery of the dose.

Orally-disintegrating tablets: Should not be swallowed whole, broken, cut, or chewed. Place tablet on tongue; allow to dissolve (with or without water) until particles can be swallowed. Orally-disintegrating tablets may also be administered via an oral syringe: Place the 15 mg tablet in an oral syringe and draw up ~4 mL water, or place the 30 mg tablet in an oral syringe and draw up ~10 mL water. After tablet has dispersed, administer within 15 minutes. Refill the syringe with water (2 mL for the 15 mg tablet; 5 mL for the 30 mg tablet), shake gently, then administer any remaining contents.

Nasogastric tube administration:

Capsule: Capsule can be opened, the granules mixed (not crushed) with 40 mL of apple juice and then administered through the NG tube into the stomach, then flush tube with additional apple juice. Do not mix with other liquids. Thirty milligrams has also been suspended in 10 mL of 8.4% sodium bicarbonate solution (or apple juice) and administered via NG tube (Brophy, 2010).

Orally-disintegrating tablet: Nasogastric tube ≥8 French: Place a 15 mg tablet in a syringe and draw up ~4 mL water, or place the 30 mg tablet in a syringe and draw up ~10 mL water. After tablet has dispersed, administer within 15 minutes. Refill the syringe with ~5 mL water, shake gently, and then flush the nasogastric tube.

Monitoring Parameters Patients with Zollinger-Ellison syndrome should be monitored for gastric acid output, which should be maintained at ≤10 mEq/hour during the last hour before the next lansoprazole dose; lab monitoring should include CBC, liver function, renal function, and serum gastrin levels

Dosage Forms

Capsule Delayed Release, Oral:
- Heartburn Treatment 24 Hour [OTC]: 15 mg
- Prevacid: 15 mg, 30 mg
- Prevacid 24HR [OTC]: 15 mg
- Generic: 15 mg, 30 mg

Suspension, Oral:
- First-Lansoprazole: 3 mg/mL (90 mL, 150 mL, 300 mL)

Tablet Dispersible, Oral:
- Prevacid SoluTab: 15 mg, 30 mg

Extemporaneous Preparations A 3 mg/mL oral solution (Simplified Lansoprazole Solution [SLS]) may be made with capsules and sodium bicarbonate. Empty the contents of ten lansoprazole 30 mg capsules into a beaker. Add 100 mL sodium bicarbonate 8.4% and gently stir until dissolved (about 15 minutes). Transfer solution to an amber-colored syringe or bottle. A prior study showed that SLS was stable for 8 hours at room temperature or for 14 days refrigerated (DiGiancinto, 2000). However, a more recent study, demonstrated SLS to be stable for 48 hours at room temperature in oral syringes and for only 7 days when refrigerated (Morrison, 2013).

Note: A more palatable lansoprazole (3 mg/mL) suspension is commercially available as a compounding kit (First-Lansoprazole).

DiGiancinto JL, Olsen KM, Bergman KL, et al, "Stability of Suspension Formulations of Lansoprazole and Omeprazole Stored in Amber-Colored Plastic Oral Syringes," *Ann Pharmacother*, 2000, 34(5):600-5

Morrison JT, Lugo RA, Thigpen JC, et al, "Stability of Extemporaneously Prepared Lansoprazole Suspension at Two Temperatures," *J Pediatr Pharmacol Ther*, 2013, 18(2):122-7.

Sharma V, "Comparison of 24-hour Intragastric pH Using Four Liquid Formulations of Lansoprazole and Omeprazole," *Am J Health Syst Pharm*, 1999, 56(Suppl 4):18-21.

Sharma VK, Vasudeva R, and Howden CW, "Simplified Lansoprazole Suspension - Liquid Formulations of Lansoprazole - Effectively Suppresses Intragastric Acidity When Administered Through a Gastrostomy," *Am J Gastroenterol*, 1999, 94(7):1813-7.

Lansoprazole, Amoxicillin, and Clarithromycin

(lan SOE pra zole, a moks i SIL in, & kla RITH roe mye sin)

Brand Names: U.S. Prevpac®

Brand Names: Canada Hp-PAC®

Index Terms Amoxicillin, Clarithromycin, and Lansoprazole; Clarithromycin, Lansoprazole, and Amoxicillin; Lansoprazole, Amoxicillin, and Clarithromycin

Pharmacologic Category Antibiotic, Macrolide Combination; Antibiotic, Penicillin; Gastrointestinal Agent, Miscellaneous; Proton Pump Inhibitor; Substituted Benzimidazole

Use Eradication of *H. pylori* to reduce the risk of recurrent duodenal ulcer

Pregnancy Risk Factor C

Dosage Oral: Adults: Lansoprazole 30 mg, amoxicillin 1 g, and clarithromycin 500 mg taken together twice daily for 10 or 14 days

Dosage adjustment in renal impairment: CrCl <30 mL/minute: Use is not recommended.

Dosage adjustment in hepatic impairment: Bioavailability of lansoprazole increased in hepatic impairment. Consider dose reduction in severe hepatic impairment

Additional Information Complete prescribing information should be consulted for additional detail.

Dosage Forms

Combination package [each administration card contains]:

Prevpac®:
- Capsule: Amoxicillin 500 mg (4 capsules/day)
- Capsule, delayed release (Prevacid®): Lansoprazole 30 mg (2 capsules/day)
- Tablet (Biaxin®): Clarithromycin 500 mg (2 tablets/day)

Generic:
- Capsule: Amoxicillin 500 mg (4 capsules/day)
- Capsule, delayed release: Lansoprazole 30 mg (2 capsules/day)
- Tablet: Clarithromycin 500 mg (2 tablets/day)

◆ **Lansoprazole, Amoxicillin, and Clarithromycin** *see* Lansoprazole, Amoxicillin, and Clarithromycin *on page 1169*

Lanthanum (LAN tha num)

Brand Names: U.S. Fosrenol

Brand Names: Canada Fosrenol

Index Terms Lanthanum Carbonate

Pharmacologic Category Phosphate Binder

Use Reduction of serum phosphate in patients with stage 5 chronic kidney disease (end-stage renal disease [ESRD]; kidney failure: GFR <15 mL/minute/1.73 m^2 or dialysis)

Pregnancy Risk Factor C

Dosage Oral: Adults: Reduction of serum phosphorous: Initial: 1500 mg daily (U.S. labeling) or 750 to 1500 mg daily (Canadian labeling) divided and taken with meals; typical increases of 750 mg daily every 2 to 3 weeks are suggested as needed to reduce the serum phosphate level <6 mg/dL; usual dosage range: 1500 to 3000 mg daily; doses of up to 4500 mg have been evaluated

Dosage adjustment in renal impairment: No dosage adjustment necessary.

Dosage adjustment in hepatic impairment: There is no dosage adjustment provided in manufacturer's labeling.

Additional Information Complete prescribing information should be consulted for additional detail.

Dosage Forms

Tablet Chewable, Oral:
- Fosrenol: 500 mg, 750 mg, 1000 mg

◆ **Lanthanum Carbonate** *see* Lanthanum *on page 1169*

◆ **Lantus** *see* Insulin Glargine *on page 1086*

◆ **Lantus® (Can)** *see* Insulin Glargine *on page 1086*

◆ **Lantus® OptiSet® (Can)** *see* Insulin Glargine *on page 1086*

◆ **Lantus SoloStar** *see* Insulin Glargine *on page 1086*

◆ **Lanvis® (Can)** *see* Thioguanine *on page 2029*

Lapatinib (la PA ti nib)

Brand Names: U.S. Tykerb

Brand Names: Canada Tykerb

Index Terms GW572016; Lapatinib Ditosylate

Pharmacologic Category Antineoplastic Agent, Anti-HER2; Antineoplastic Agent, Epidermal Growth Factor Receptor (EGFR) Inhibitor; Antineoplastic Agent, Tyrosine Kinase Inhibitor

Use

Breast cancer: Treatment of human epidermal growth receptor type 2 (HER2) overexpressing advanced or metastatic breast cancer (in combination with capecitabine) in patients who have received prior therapy (with an anthracycline, a taxane, and trastuzumab); HER2 over-expressing hormone receptor–positive metastatic breast cancer in postmenopausal women where hormone therapy is indicated (in combination with letrozole)

Limitations of use: Patients should have disease progression on trastuzumab prior to initiation of treatment with lapatinib in combination with capecitabine.

Pregnancy Risk Factor D

Pregnancy Considerations Adverse events were demonstrated in animal reproduction studies. Lapatinib may cause fetal harm if administered during pregnancy. Women of childbearing potential should be advised to avoid pregnancy during treatment.

Breast-Feeding Considerations It is not known if lapatinib is excreted in breast milk. Due to the potential for serious adverse reactions in the nursing infant, the decision to discontinue lapatinib or discontinue breast-feeding during treatment should take in account the benefits of treatment to the mother.

Contraindications Known severe hypersensitivity to lapatinib or any component of the formulation

Warnings/Precautions Hazardous agent - use appropriate precautions for handling and disposal (meets NIOSH 2014 criteria). Decreases in left ventricular ejection fraction (LVEF) have been reported (usually within the first 3 months of treatment); baseline and periodic LVEF evaluations are recommended; interrupt treatment with decreased LVEF ≥ grade 2 or LVEF <LLN; may reinitiate with a reduced dose after a minimum of 2 weeks if the LVEF recovers and the patient is asymptomatic. QTc prolongation has been observed; use caution in patients with a history of QTc prolongation or with medications known to prolong the QT interval; a baseline and periodic 12-lead ECG should be considered; correct electrolyte (potassium, calcium and magnesium) abnormalities prior to and during treatment. Use with caution in conditions which may impair left ventricular function and in patients with a history of or predisposed to (prior treatment with anthracyclines, chest wall irradiation) left ventricular dysfunction. Interstitial lung disease (ILD) and pneumonitis have been reported (with lapatinib monotherapy and with combination chemotherapy); monitor for pulmonary symptoms which may indicate ILD or pneumonitis; discontinue treatment for grade 3 (or higher) pulmonary symptoms indicative of ILD or pneumonitis (eg, dyspnea, dry cough).

[U.S. Boxed Warning]: Hepatotoxicity (ALT or AST >3 times ULN and total bilirubin >2 times ULN) has been reported with lapatinib; may be severe and/or fatal. Onset of hepatotoxicity may occur within days to several months after treatment initiation. Monitor (at baseline and every 4 to 6 weeks during treatment, and as clinically indicated); discontinue with severe changes in liver function; do not reinitiate. Use caution in patients with hepatic dysfunction; dose reductions should be considered in patients with preexisting severe (Child-Pugh class C) hepatic impairment. Potentially significant drug-drug interactions may exist, requiring dose or frequency adjustment, additional monitoring, and/or selection of alternative therapy. Patients who carry the HLA alleles DQA1*02:01 and DRB1*07:01 may experience a greater incidence of severe liver injury than patients who are noncarriers. These alleles are present in ~15% to 25% of Caucasian, Asian, African, and Hispanic patient populations and 1% in Japanese populations. May cause diarrhea (onset is generally within 6 days and duration is 4 to 5 days); may be severe and/or fatal; instruct patients to immediately report any bowel pattern changes. After first unformed stool, administer antidiarrheal agents; severe diarrhea may require hydration, electrolytes, antibiotics (if duration >24 hours, fever, or grade 3/4 neutropenia), and/or treatment interruption, dose reduction, or discontinuation. Severe cutaneous reactions have been reported with use. Discontinue therapy if life-threatening dermatologic reactions (eg, progressive skin rash with blisters or mucosal lesions) such as erythema multiforme, Stevens-Johnson syndrome, or toxic epidermal necrolysis occur.

Adverse Reactions

Cardiovascular: LVEF decreased

Central nervous system: Fatigue, headache, insomnia

Dermatologic: Alopecia, dry skin, nail disorder, palmar-plantar erythrodysesthesia (hand-and-foot syndrome), pruritus, rash

Gastrointestinal: Abdominal pain, anorexia, diarrhea, dyspepsia, mucosal inflammation, stomatitis, vomiting

Hematologic: Anemia, neutropenia, thrombocytopenia

Hepatic: ALT increased, AST increased, total bilirubin increased

Neuromuscular & skeletal: Back pain, limb pain, weakness

Respiratory: Dyspnea, epistaxis

Rare but important or life-threatening: Anaphylaxis, hepatotoxicity, hypersensitivity, interstitial lung disease, paronychia, pneumonitis, Prinzmetal's angina, QTc prolongation

Drug Interactions

Metabolism/Transport Effects **Substrate** of CYP3A4 (major), P-glycoprotein; **Note:** Assignment of Major/Minor substrate status based on clinically relevant drug interaction potential; **Inhibits** BCRP, CYP2C8 (moderate), CYP3A4 (weak), P-glycoprotein

Avoid Concomitant Use

Avoid concomitant use of Lapatinib with any of the following: Bosutinib; Conivaptan; CYP3A4 Inducers (Strong); CYP3A4 Inhibitors (Strong); Dexamethasone (Systemic); Fusidic Acid (Systemic); Grapefruit Juice; Highest Risk QTc-Prolonging Agents; Idelalisib; Ivabradine; Mifepristone; PAZOPanib; Pimozide; Silodosin; St Johns Wort; Topotecan; VinCRIStine (Liposomal)

Increased Effect/Toxicity

Lapatinib may increase the levels/effects of: Afatinib; ARIPiprazole; Bosutinib; Brentuximab Vedotin; Colchicine; CYP2C8 Substrates; Dabigatran Etexilate; DOXOrubicin (Conventional); Edoxaban; Everolimus; Highest Risk QTc-Prolonging Agents; Hydrocodone; Ledipasvir; Lomitapide; Moderate Risk QTc-Prolonging Agents; Naloxegol; PAZOPanib; P-glycoprotein/ABCB1 Substrates; Pimozide; Prucalopride; Rifaximin; Rivaroxaban; Silodosin; Topotecan; VinCRIStine (Liposomal)

The levels/effects of Lapatinib may be increased by: Aprepitant; Conivaptan; CYP3A4 Inhibitors (Moderate); CYP3A4 Inhibitors (Strong); Dasatinib; Fosaprepitant; Fusidic Acid (Systemic); Grapefruit Juice; Idelalisib; Ivabradine; Ivacaftor; Luliconazole; Mifepristone; Netupitant; P-glycoprotein/ABCB1 Inhibitors; QTc-Prolonging Agents (Indeterminate Risk and Risk Modifying); Simeprevir

Decreased Effect

The levels/effects of Lapatinib may be decreased by: Bosentan; CYP3A4 Inducers (Moderate); CYP3A4 Inducers (Strong); Dabrafenib; Deferasirox; Dexamethasone (Systemic); P-glycoprotein/ABCB1 Inducers; Siltuximab; St Johns Wort; Tocilizumab

Food Interactions Systemic exposure of lapatinib is increased when administered with food (AUC three- to fourfold higher). Grapefruit juice may increase the levels/effects of lapatinib. Management: Administer once daily on an empty stomach, 1 hour before or 1 hour after a meal at the same time each day. Avoid grapefruit juice. Maintain adequate hydration, unless instructed to restrict fluid intake.

Storage/Stability Store at room temperature of 25°C (77°F); excursions permitted between 15°C and 30°C (59°F and 86°F).

Mechanism of Action Tyrosine kinase (dual kinase) inhibitor; inhibits EGFR (ErbB1) and HER2 (ErbB2) by reversibly binding to tyrosine kinase, blocking phosphorylation and activation of downstream second messengers (Erk1/2 and Akt), regulating cellular proliferation and survival in ErbB- and ErbB2-expressing tumors. Combination therapy with lapatinib and endocrine therapy may overcome endocrine resistance occurring in HER2+ and hormone receptor positive disease.

Pharmacodynamics/Kinetics

Absorption: Incomplete and variable

Protein binding: >99% to albumin and alpha$_1$-acid glycoprotein

Metabolism: Hepatic; extensive via CYP3A4 and 3A5, and to a lesser extent via CYP2C19 and 2C8 to oxidized metabolites

Half-life elimination: ~24 hours

Time to peak, plasma: ~4 hours (Burris, 2009)

Excretion: Feces (27% as unchanged drug; range 3% to 67%); urine (<2%)

Dosage Note: Patients should have disease progression on trastuzumab prior to initiation of treatment with lapatinib in combination with capecitabine.

Breast cancer, metastatic, HER2+ (with prior anthracycline, taxane, and trastuzumab therapy): Adults: Oral: 1250 mg once daily (in combination with capecitabine) until disease progression or unacceptable toxicity (Geyer, 2006)

Breast cancer, metastatic, HER2+, hormonal therapy indicated: Adults: Oral: 1500 mg once daily (in combination with letrozole) until disease progression (Johnston, 2009)

Breast cancer, metastatic, HER2+ with brain metastases, first-line therapy (off-label use): Adults: Oral: 1250 mg once daily (in combination with capecitabine) until disease progression or unacceptable toxicity (Bachelot, 2013)

Breast cancer, metastatic, HER2+, with progression on prior trastuzumab therapy (off-label use): Adults: Oral: 1000 mg once daily (in combination with trastuzumab) (Blackwell, 2010; Blackwell, 2012)

Missed doses: If a dose is missed, resume with the next scheduled daily dose; do not double the dose the next day.

Dosage adjustment for concomitant CYP3A4 inhibitors/inducers:

CYP3A4 inhibitors: Avoid the use of concomitant strong CYP3A4 inhibitors. If concomitant use cannot be avoided, consider reducing lapatinib to 500 mg once daily with careful monitoring. When a strong CYP3A4 inhibitor is discontinued, allow ~1 week to elapse prior to adjusting the lapatinib dose upward.

CYP3A4 inducers: Avoid the use of concomitant strong CYP3A4 inducers.

U.S. labeling: If concomitant use cannot be avoided, consider gradually titrating lapatinib from 1250 mg once daily up to 4500 mg daily (in combination with capecitabine) **or** from 1500 mg once daily up to 5500 mg daily (in combination with letrozole), based on tolerability and with careful monitoring. If the strong CYP3A4 enzyme inducer is discontinued, reduce the lapatinib dose to the indicated dose.

Canadian labeling: If concomitant use cannot be avoided, titrate lapatinib dose gradually upward based on tolerability. If the strong CYP3A4 enzyme inducer is discontinued, reduce the lapatinib dose over 2 weeks.

Dosage adjustment for toxicity:

Cardiac toxicity: Discontinue treatment for at least 2 weeks for LVEF < LLN or decreased LVEF ≥ grade 2 (U.S. labeling) or decreased LVEF ≥ grade 3 (Canadian labeling); may be restarted at 1000 mg once daily (in combination with capecitabine) **or** 1250 mg once daily (in combination with letrozole) if LVEF recovers to normal and patient is asymptomatic.

Dermatologic toxicity: Discontinue treatment for suspected erythema multiforme, Stevens-Johnson syndrome, or toxic epidermal necrolysis.

Diarrhea:

Grade 3 diarrhea or grade 1 or 2 diarrhea with complicating features (moderate-to-severe abdominal cramping, grade 2 or higher nausea/vomiting, decreased performance status, fever, sepsis, neutropenia, frank bleeding, or dehydration):

U.S. labeling: Interrupt treatment; may restart at a reduced dose (from 1500 mg once daily to 1250 mg once daily or from 1250 mg once daily to 1000 mg once daily) when diarrhea resolves to ≤ grade 1.

Canadian labeling: Interrupt treatment; may restart at a reduced dose (from 1500 mg once daily to 1250 mg once daily or from 1250 mg once daily to 1000 mg once daily or from 1000 mg once daily to 750 mg once daily) when diarrhea resolves to ≤ grade 1.

Grade 4 diarrhea: Permanently discontinue.

Pulmonary toxicity: Discontinue treatment with pulmonary symptoms indicative of interstitial lung disease or pneumonitis which are ≥ grade 3

Other toxicities: Withhold for any toxicity (other than cardiac) ≥ grade 2 until toxicity resolves to ≤ grade 1 and reinitiate at the standard dose of 1250 mg or 1500 mg once daily; for persistent toxicity, reduce dosage to 1000 mg once daily (in combination with capecitabine) **or** 1250 mg once daily (in combination with letrozole)

Dosage adjustment in renal impairment: There are no dosage adjustments provided in the manufacturer's labeling (has not been studied); however, due to the minimal renal elimination (<2%), dosage adjustments may not be necessary.

Dosage adjustment in hepatic impairment:

Severe preexisting impairment (Child-Pugh class C):

In combination with capecitabine: Reduce dose from 1250 mg once daily to 750 mg once daily

In combination with letrozole: Reduce dose from 1500 mg once daily to 1000 mg once daily

Severe hepatotoxicity during treatment: Discontinue permanently (do not rechallenge).

Dietary Considerations Avoid grapefruit juice.

Administration Administer once daily, on an empty stomach, 1 hour before or 1 hour after a meal. Take full dose at the same time each day; dividing dose throughout the day is not recommended.

Note: For combination treatment with capecitabine, capecitabine should be administered in 2 doses (approximately 12 hours apart) and taken with food or within 30 minutes after a meal.

Hazardous agent; use appropriate precautions for handling and disposal (meets NIOSH 2014 criteria).

Monitoring Parameters LVEF (baseline and periodic), CBC with differential, liver function tests, including transaminases, bilirubin, and alkaline phosphatase (baseline and every 4-6 weeks during treatment); electrolytes including calcium, potassium, magnesium; monitor for fluid retention; ECG monitoring if at risk for QTc prolongation; symptoms of ILD or pneumonitis; monitor for diarrhea and dermatologic toxicity

Dosage Forms

Tablet, Oral:

Tykerb: 250 mg

- **Lapatinib Ditosylate** *see* Lapatinib *on page 1169*
- **L-Arginine** *see* Arginine *on page 171*
- **L-Arginine Hydrochloride** *see* Arginine *on page 171*
- **Larin 1.5/30** *see* Ethinyl Estradiol and Norethindrone *on page 808*
- **Larin 1/20** *see* Ethinyl Estradiol and Norethindrone *on page 808*
- **Larin Fe 1.5/30** *see* Ethinyl Estradiol and Norethindrone *on page 808*
- **Larin Fe 1/20** *see* Ethinyl Estradiol and Norethindrone *on page 808*

Laronidase (lair OH ni days)

Brand Names: U.S. Aldurazyme

Brand Names: Canada Aldurazyme®

Index Terms Recombinant α-L-Iduronidase (Glycosaminoglycan α-L-Iduronohydrolase)

Pharmacologic Category Enzyme

Use Treatment of Hurler and Hurler-Scheie forms of mucopolysaccharidosis I (MPS I); treatment of Scheie form of MPS I in patients with moderate-to-severe symptoms

Pregnancy Risk Factor B

Dosage Note: Premedicate with antipyretic and/or antihistamines 1 hour prior to start of infusion.

IV: Children ≥6 months and Adults: 0.58 mg/kg once weekly; dose should be rounded up to the nearest whole vial

Dosage adjustment in renal impairment: No dosage adjustment provided in manufacturer's labeling.

Dosage adjustment in hepatic impairment: No dosage adjustment provided in manufacturer's labeling.

Additional Information Complete prescribing information should be consulted for additional detail.

Dosage Forms

Solution, Intravenous:

Aldurazyme: 2.9 mg/5 mL (5 mL)

- **Lasix** *see* Furosemide *on page 940*
- **Lasix Special (Can)** *see* Furosemide *on page 940*
- **L-ASP** *see* Asparaginase (*E. coli*) *on page 179*
- **L-asparaginase (*E. coli*)** *see* Asparaginase (*E. coli*) *on page 179*
- **L-asparaginase (*Erwinia*)** *see* Asparaginase (*Erwinia*) *on page 180*
- **L-asparaginase with Polyethylene Glycol** *see* Pegaspargase *on page 1588*
- **Lassar's Zinc Paste** *see* Zinc Oxide *on page 2200*

Latanoprost (la TA noe prost)

Brand Names: U.S. Xalatan

Brand Names: Canada Apo-Latanoprost; CO Latanoprost; GD-Latanoprost; Xalatan

Pharmacologic Category Ophthalmic Agent, Antiglaucoma; Prostaglandin, Ophthalmic

Use Elevated intraocular pressure: Reduction of elevated intraocular pressure (IOP) in patients with open-angle glaucoma and ocular hypertension.

Pregnancy Risk Factor C

Dosage Elevated intraocular pressure: Adults: Ophthalmic: One drop in the affected eye(s) once daily in the evening; do not exceed the once daily dosage (may decrease the IOP-lowering effect)

Dosage adjustment in renal impairment: There is no dosage adjustment provided in manufacturer's labeling. However, dosage adjustment unlikely due to low systemic absorption.

Dosage adjustment in hepatic impairment: There is no dosage adjustment provided in manufacturer's labeling. However, dosage adjustment unlikely due to low systemic absorption.

Additional Information Complete prescribing information should be consulted for additional detail.

Dosage Forms

Solution, Ophthalmic:

Xalatan: 0.005% (2.5 mL)

Generic: 0.005% (2.5 mL)

Latanoprost and Timolol [CAN/INT]

(la TA noe prost & TIM oh lol)

Brand Names: Canada Xalacom

Index Terms Timolol Maleate and Latanoprost

Pharmacologic Category Beta-Blocker, Nonselective; Ophthalmic Agent, Antiglaucoma; Prostaglandin, Ophthalmic

Use Note: Not approved in U.S.

Reduction of intraocular pressure (IOP) in patients with open-angle glaucoma or ocular hypertension who are insufficiently responsive to topical beta-blockers, prostaglandin analogues, or other IOP-reducing agents and in whom combination therapy is appropriate

Pregnancy Considerations Reproductive studies have not been conducted with this combination. See individual agents.

Breast-Feeding Considerations Timolol has been detected in human breast milk following ophthalmic administration. Latanoprost may enter human breast milk. See individual agents.

Contraindications Hypersensitivity to latanoprost, timolol, benzalkonium chloride, or any component of the formulation; reactive airway disease including severe chronic obstructive pulmonary disease (COPD) and presence or history of bronchial asthma; sinus bradycardia, second-/third-degree atrioventricular block, overt cardiac failure, cardiogenic shock

Warnings/Precautions See individual agents.

Adverse Reactions Also see individual agents.

Cardiovascular: Chest pain, hypertension

Central nervous system: Depression, headache

Dermatologic: Rash, skin disorder

Endocrine & metabolic: Diabetes mellitus, hypercholesterolemia

Neuromuscular & skeletal: Arthritis, back pain

Ocular: Blepharitis, cataract, conjunctival disorder, conjunctivitis, corneal disorder, eye irritation, eyelash alterations (including darkening, lengthening, thickening), eye pain, hyperemia, iris pigmentation increased, keratitis, meibomianitis, photophobia, refraction errors, skin disorder, vision abnormal, visual field defect

Respiratory: Bronchitis, sinusitis, upper respiratory infection

Miscellaneous: Flu-like symptoms, infection

Rare but important or life-threatening: Bradycardia, cardiac failure, corneal ulceration, cough, cystitis, cystoid macular edema, dizziness, dyspepsia, dyspnea, epiphora, eyelid edema, glycosuria, hyperglycemia, insomnia, intraocular pressure increased, optic atrophy, pneumonia, retinal disorder, seborrhea, skin discoloration, tachycardia, urinary tract infection, uveitis

Drug Interactions

Metabolism/Transport Effects Refer to individual components.

Avoid Concomitant Use

Avoid concomitant use of Latanoprost and Timolol with any of the following: Beta2-Agonists; Ceritinib; Floctafenine; Methacholine

Increased Effect/Toxicity

Latanoprost and Timolol may increase the levels/effects of: Alpha-/Beta-Agonists (Direct-Acting); Alpha1-Blockers; Alpha2-Agonists; Antipsychotic Agents (Phenothiazines); ARIPiprazole; Bimatoprost; Bradycardia-Causing Agents; Bupivacaine; Cardiac Glycosides; Ceritinib; Cholinergic Agonists; Disopyramide; DULoxetine; Ergot Derivatives; Fingolimod; Grass Pollen Allergen Extract (5 Grass Extract); Hypotensive Agents; Insulin; Lacosamide; Levodopa; Lidocaine (Systemic); Lidocaine (Topical); Mepivacaine; Methacholine; Midodrine; RisperiDONE; Sulfonylureas

The levels/effects of Latanoprost and Timolol may be increased by: Abiraterone Acetate; Acetylcholinesterase Inhibitors; Alpha2-Agonists; Aminoquinolines (Antimalarial); Amiodarone; Anilidopiperidine Opioids; Antipsychotic Agents (Phenothiazines); Barbiturates; Bretylium; Calcium Channel Blockers (Dihydropyridine); Calcium Channel Blockers (Nondihydropyridine); Cobicistat; CYP2D6 Inhibitors (Moderate); CYP2D6 Inhibitors (Strong); Darunavir; Dipyridamole; Disopyramide; Dronedarone; Floctafenine; MAO Inhibitors; Nicorandil; Peginterferon Alfa-2b; Propafenone; Regorafenib; Reserpine; Selective Serotonin Reuptake Inhibitors; Tofacitinib

Decreased Effect

Latanoprost and Timolol may decrease the levels/effects of: Beta2-Agonists; Theophylline Derivatives

The levels/effects of Latanoprost and Timolol may be decreased by: Barbiturates; Nonsteroidal Anti-Inflammatory Agents; Peginterferon Alfa-2b; Rifamycin Derivatives

Storage/Stability Prior to opening, store under refrigeration at 2°C to 8°C (36°F to 46°F). After opening may store at room temperature up to 25°C (77°F) up to 10 weeks. Protect from light.

Mechanism of Action

Latanoprost: A prostaglandin F_2-alpha analog believed to reduce intraocular pressure by increasing the outflow of the aqueous humor

Timolol: Blocks both $beta_1$- and $beta_2$-adrenergic receptors, reduces intraocular pressure by reducing aqueous humor production or possibly outflow; reduces blood pressure by blocking adrenergic receptors and decreasing sympathetic outflow, produces a negative chronotropic and inotropic activity through an unknown mechanism

Pharmacodynamics/Kinetics See individual agents.

Dosage Ophthalmic: Adults: Instill 1 drop into affected eye(s) once daily

Administration Wash hands prior to use. Remove contact lenses prior to administration; wait 15 minutes before reinserting if using products containing benzalkonium chloride. Separate administration of other ophthalmic agents by 5 minutes.

Monitoring Parameters IOP, iris color changes, eyelash changes; systemic effects of beta blockade

Product Availability Not available in U.S.

Dosage Forms: Canada

Solution, ophthalmic:

Xalacom™: Latanoprost (0.005%) and timolol 0.5% (as base) (2.5 mL)

- **Latisse** *see* Bimatoprost *on page 264*
- **Latrix XM** *see* Urea *on page 2114*
- **Latuda** *see* Lurasidone *on page 1256*
- **Laxa Basic [OTC]** *see* Docusate *on page 661*
- **Laxative [OTC]** *see* Bisacodyl *on page 265*
- **Lazanda** *see* FentaNYL *on page 857*
- ***l*-Bunolol Hydrochloride** *see* Levobunolol *on page 1194*
- **L(-)-Bupivacaine** *see* Levobupivacaine [INT] *on page 1194*
- **LC-4 Lidocaine [OTC]** *see* Lidocaine (Topical) *on page 1211*
- **LC-5 Lidocaine [OTC]** *see* Lidocaine (Topical) *on page 1211*
- **LCM** *see* Lacosamide *on page 1154*
- **L-Deprenyl** *see* Selegiline *on page 1873*
- **LDK378** *see* Ceritinib *on page 407*
- **LDP-341** *see* Bortezomib *on page 276*
- **LEA29Y** *see* Belatacept *on page 233*
- **Lectopam® (Can)** *see* Bromazepam [CAN/INT] *on page 290*
- **Lederle Leucovorin (Can)** *see* Leucovorin Calcium *on page 1183*

Ledipasvir and Sofosbuvir

(le DIP as vir & soe FOS bue vir)

Brand Names: U.S. Harvoni

Brand Names: Canada Harvoni

Index Terms GS-5885; Sofosbuvir and Ledipasvir

Pharmacologic Category Antihepaciviral, NS5A Inhibitor; Antihepaciviral, Polymerase Inhibitor (Anti-HCV)

Use Chronic hepatitis C: Treatment of chronic hepatitis C (CHC) genotype 1 in adults.

Pregnancy Risk Factor B

Pregnancy Considerations Adverse events were not observed in animal reproduction studies using the components of this combination.

Breast-Feeding Considerations It is not known if ledipasvir or sofosbuvir are excreted into breast milk. According to the U.S. labeling, the decision to breastfeed during therapy should take into account the risk of exposure to the infant and the benefits of treatment to the mother. The Canadian labeling recommends discontinuing breast-feeding prior to initiating therapy.

Contraindications

There are no contraindications listed in the manufacturer's U.S. labeling.

Canadian labeling: Hypersensitivity to any component of the formulation.

Warnings/Precautions Potentially significant drug-drug interactions may exist, requiring dose or frequency adjustment, additional monitoring, and/or selection of alternative therapy, including use with potent P-gp inducers (eg, rifampin, St John's wort). Avoid concurrent use with other sofosbuvir-containing products. Therapy should be initiated by a physician experienced in the treatment of chronic hepatitis C. Tablets may contain lactose; consider lactose content prior to initiating therapy in patients with rare hereditary problems of galactose intolerance.

Adverse Reactions

Central nervous system: Fatigue, headache, insomnia

Gastrointestinal: Diarrhea, increased serum lipase, nausea

Hepatic: Hyperbilirubinemia

Drug Interactions

Metabolism/Transport Effects Refer to individual components.

Avoid Concomitant Use

Avoid concomitant use of Ledipasvir and Sofosbuvir with any of the following: Bosutinib; Modafinil; OXcarbazepine; PAZOPanib; P-glycoprotein/ABCB1 Inducers; Rifabutin; Rifapentine; Rosuvastatin; Silodosin; Simeprevir; Topotecan; VinCRIStine (Liposomal)

Increased Effect/Toxicity

Ledipasvir and Sofosbuvir may increase the levels/effects of: Afatinib; Bosutinib; Brentuximab Vedotin; Colchicine; Dabigatran Etexilate; Edoxaban; Everolimus; Naloxegol; PAZOPanib; P-glycoprotein/ABCB1 Substrates; Prucalopride; Rifaximin; Rivaroxaban; Rosuvastatin; Silodosin; Simeprevir; Tenofovir; Topotecan; VinCRIStine (Liposomal)

The levels/effects of Ledipasvir and Sofosbuvir may be increased by: P-glycoprotein/ABCB1 Inhibitors; Simeprevir

Decreased Effect

The levels/effects of Ledipasvir and Sofosbuvir may be decreased by: Antacids; H2-Antagonists; Modafinil; OXcarbazepine; P-glycoprotein/ABCB1 Inducers; Proton Pump Inhibitors; Rifabutin; Rifapentine

Storage/Stability Store below 30°C (86°F). Dispense in original container.

Mechanism of Action Ledipasvir inhibits the HCV NS5A protein necessary for viral replication; sofosbuvir is a prodrug converted to its pharmacologically active form (GS-461203), inhibits NS5B RNA-dependent RNA polymerase, also essential for viral replication, and acts as a chain terminator.

Pharmacodynamics/Kinetics

Absorption: Ledipasvir and sofosbuvir are well absorbed

Protein binding: Ledipasvir: >99.8%; Sofosbuvir: 61% to 65%

Metabolism: Ledipasvir: Slow oxidative metabolism via an unknown mechanism; Sofosbuvir: Hepatic; forms pharmacologically active nucleoside (uridine) analog triphosphate GS-461203; Dephosphorylation results in the formation of nucleoside inactive metabolite GS-331007

Half-life elimination: Ledipasvir: 47 hours; Sofosbuvir: ~0.5 hours

Time to peak: Ledipasvir: 4 to 4.5 hours; Sofosbuvir: ~0.8 to 1 hour

Excretion: Ledipasvir: Feces (~86%), urine (1%); Sofosbuvir: Urine (80%), feces (14%)

Dosage

Chronic hepatitis C (CHC) infection in monoinfected (HCV) genotype 1 patients: Adults: Oral: Treatment regimen and duration based on clinical scenario as noted below; fixed-dose tablet is ledipasvir 90 mg and sofosbuvir 400 mg:

Treatment-naive patients with or without cirrhosis or treatment-experienced patients without cirrhosis: One tablet once daily for 12 weeks.

Treatment-experienced patients with cirrhosis: One tablet once daily for 24 weeks.

Note: Treatment-naive patients without cirrhosis who have HCV RNA <6 million units/mL may be considered for therapy of 8 weeks duration. Treatment experienced patients are defined as those who have failed treatment with either a regimen of peginterferon alfa and ribavirin or a regimen of an HCV protease inhibitor and peginterferon alfa and ribavirin.

Missed dose: Canadian labeling: If missed dose is within 18 hours of regularly scheduled time, administer as soon as possible; if >18 hours from regularly scheduled time, resume at next regularly scheduled dose (do not double dose). If patient vomits <5 hours after administration dose should be repeated; if >5 hours, resume administer at next regularly scheduled dose.

Dosage adjustment in renal impairment

CrCl >30 mL/minute/1.73 m^2: No dosage adjustment necessary.

CrCl ≤30 mL/minute/1.73 m^2: There are no dosage adjustments provided in the manufacturer's labeling. However, sofosbuvir and metabolite accumulate in patients with severely impaired renal function.

End stage renal disease (ESRD), including those requiring intermittent hemodialysis (IHD): There are no dosage adjustments provided in the manufacturer's labeling However, sofosbuvir and metabolite accumulate in patients with severely impaired renal function.

Dosage adjustment in hepatic impairment

Child-Pugh class A, B, or C: No dosage adjustment necessary.

Decompensated cirrhosis: There are no dosage adjustments provided in the manufacturer's labeling (has not been studied).

Administration Oral: Administer with or without food.

Monitoring Parameters Bilirubin, liver enzymes, and serum creatinine at baseline and periodically when clinically indicated. Serum HCV-RNA at baseline, during treatment, at the end of treatment, during treatment follow-up, and when clinically indicated.

Dosage Forms

Tablet, Oral:

Harvoni: Ledipasvir 90 mg and sofosbuvir 400 mg

◆ **Leena** *see* Ethinyl Estradiol and Norethindrone *on page 808*

Leflunomide (le FLOO noh mide)

Brand Names: U.S. Arava

Brand Names: Canada Apo-Leflunomide; Arava; Mylan-Leflunomide; PHL-Leflunomide; PMS-Leflunomide; Sandoz-Leflunomide; Teva-Leflunomide

Pharmacologic Category Antirheumatic, Disease Modifying

Use Rheumatoid arthritis: Treatment of active rheumatoid arthritis (RA) in adults to reduce signs and symptoms, to inhibit structural damage as evidenced by x-ray erosions and joint-space narrowing, and to improve physical function.

Pregnancy Risk Factor X

Pregnancy Considerations Has been associated with teratogenic and embryolethal effects in animal models at low doses. Leflunomide is contraindicated in pregnant women or women of childbearing potential who are not using reliable contraception. Pregnancy must be excluded prior to initiating treatment. **[U.S. Boxed Warning]: Women of childbearing potential should not receive therapy until pregnancy has been excluded,** they have been counseled concerning fetal risk, and reliable contraceptive measures have been confirmed. Following treatment, pregnancy should be avoided until undetectable serum concentrations (<0.02 mg/L) are verified. This may be accomplished by the use of an enhanced drug elimination procedure using cholestyramine. Serum concentrations <0.02 mg/L should be verified by two separate tests performed at least 14 days apart. If serum concentrations are >0.02 mg/L, additional cholestyramine treatment should be considered. As an alternative to cholestyramine, the Canadian labeling recommends that activated charcoal may be used to enhance drug elimination. Pregnant women exposed to leflunomide should be registered with the pregnancy registry (877-311-8972). It is not known if males taking leflunomide may contribute to fetal toxicity. Males taking leflunomide who wish to father a child should consider discontinuing therapy and using the cholestyramine procedure to eliminate the medication. The Canadian labeling recommends avoiding use in males capable of fathering a child and who are not using reliable contraception during and for a total of 2 years after treatment unless an elimination procedure is used; for men receiving treatment and desiring to father a child, serum concentrations of the active metabolite should be verified by two separate tests performed at least 14 days apart. If levels <0.02 mg/L are confirmed with the second test, an additional waiting period of 3 months is recommended.

Breast-Feeding Considerations It is not known whether leflunomide is secreted in human milk. Because the potential for serious adverse reactions exists in the nursing infant, a decision should be made whether to discontinue nursing or discontinue the drug, taking into account the importance of the drug to the mother.

Contraindications

Hypersensitivity to leflunomide, teriflunomide, or any component of the formulation; pregnancy

Canadian labeling: Additional contraindications (not in U.S. labeling): Moderate to severe renal impairment; immunodeficiency states; impaired bone marrow function or significant anemia, leukopenia, neutropenia, or thrombocytopenia due to causes other than rheumatoid arthritis; serious infections; impaired liver function; severe hypoproteinemia; women of childbearing potential who are not using reliable contraception before, during, and for a period of 2 years after treatment with leflunomide (or as long as plasma levels of the active metabolite are above 0.02 mg/L); breast-feeding; patients younger than 18 years of age

Warnings/Precautions Hazardous agent - use appropriate precautions for handling and disposal (NIOSH 2014 [group 2]).

[U.S. Boxed Warning]: Use has been associated with rare reports of hepatotoxicity, hepatic failure, and death. Treatment should not be initiated in patients with preexisting acute or chronic liver disease or ALT >2 x ULN. Use caution in patients with concurrent exposure to potentially hepatotoxic drugs. Monitor ALT levels during therapy; discontinue if ALT >3 x ULN occurs and, if hepatotoxicity is likely leflunomide-induced, start drug elimination procedures (eg, cholestyramine, activated charcoal). **If leflunomide-induced liver injury is unlikely because another probable cause has been found, resumption of therapy may be considered.**

Use has been associated (rarely) with interstitial lung disease; discontinue in patients who develop new onset or worsening of pulmonary symptoms. Drug elimination procedures should be considered (eg, cholestyramine, activated charcoal) if interstitial lung disease occurs (with some fatalities reported). May increase susceptibility to infection, including opportunistic pathogens (especially *Pneumocystis jiroveci* pneumonia, tuberculosis [including extrapulmonary tuberculosis], and aspergillosis). Severe infections, sepsis, and fatalities have been reported. Not recommended in patients with severe immunodeficiency, bone marrow dysplasia, or severe, uncontrolled infections. Caution should be exercised when considering the use in patients with a history of new/recurrent infections, with conditions that predispose them to infections, or with chronic, latent, or localized infections. Patients who develop a new infection while undergoing treatment should be monitored closely; consider discontinuation of therapy and drug elimination procedures if infection is serious.

Use of some immunosuppressive medications may affect defenses against malignancies; impact on the development and course of malignancies is not fully defined. Use with caution in patients with a prior history of significant hematologic abnormalities; avoid use with bone marrow dysplasia. The Canadian labeling contraindicates use with impaired bone marrow function or significant anemia, leukopenia, neutropenia, or thrombocytopenia due to causes other than rheumatoid arthritis. Use has been associated with rare pancytopenia, agranulocytosis, and thrombocytopenia, generally when given concurrently or recently with methotrexate or other immunosuppressive agents. Monitoring of hematologic function is required; discontinue if evidence of bone marrow suppression and begin drug elimination procedures (eg, cholestyramine or activated charcoal). Rare cases of dermatologic reactions (including Stevens-Johnson syndrome, toxic epidermal necrolysis, and drug reaction with eosinophilia and systemic symptoms [DRESS]) have been reported; discontinue if evidence of severe dermatologic reaction occurs, and begin drug elimination procedures (eg, cholestyramine or activated charcoal). Cases of peripheral neuropathy have been reported; use with caution in patients >60 years of age, receiving concomitant neurotoxic medications, or patients with diabetes; discontinue if evidence of peripheral neuropathy occurs and begin drug elimination procedures (eg, cholestyramine, activated charcoal).

Safety has not been established in patients with latent tuberculosis infection. Patients should be screened for tuberculosis and if necessary, treated prior to initiating therapy. Use with caution in patients with renal impairment. The Canadian labeling contraindicates use in moderate to severe impairment. Use in patients with hepatic impairment is not recommended due to risk of increased hepatotoxicity. **[U.S. Boxed Warning]: Women of childbearing potential should not receive therapy until pregnancy has been excluded,** they have been counseled concerning fetal risk and reliable contraceptive measures have been confirmed. Women of childbearing potential should also undergo drug elimination procedures (eg, cholestyramine, activated charcoal) following discontinuation of therapy. The Canadian labeling contraindicates use in women of childbearing potential who are not using reliable contraception before, during, and for a period of 2 years after treatment with leflunomide (or as long as plasma levels of the active metabolite are above 0.02 mg/L). Patients should be brought up to date with all immunizations before initiating therapy. Live vaccines should not be given concurrently; there is no data available concerning secondary transmission of live vaccines in patients receiving therapy. Due to variations in clearance, it may take up to 2 years to reach low levels of leflunomide metabolite serum concentrations. A drug elimination procedure using cholestyramine or activated charcoal is recommended when a more rapid elimination is needed. Potentially significant drug-drug interactions may exist, requiring dose or frequency adjustment, additional monitoring, and/or selection of alternative therapy.

Adverse Reactions

Cardiovascular: Angina pectoris, chest pain, hypertension, palpitations, peripheral edema, tachycardia, varicose veins, vasculitis, vasodilatation

Central nervous system: Anxiety, depression, dizziness, headache, insomnia, malaise, migraine, neuralgia, neuritis, pain, paresthesia, sleep disorder, vertigo

Dermatologic: Acne vulgaris, alopecia, contact dermatitis, cutaneous nodule, dermal ulcer, dermatological disease, diaphoresis, dry skin, eczema, fungal dermatitis, hair discoloration, maculopapular rash, nail disease, pruritus, skin discoloration, skin rash, subcutaneous nodule

Endocrine & metabolic: Albuminuria, diabetes mellitus, hyperglycemia, hyperlipidemia, hyperthyroidism, hypokalemia, menstrual disease, weight loss

Gastrointestinal: Abdominal pain, anorexia, cholelithiasis, colitis, constipation, diarrhea, dysgeusia, dyspepsia, enlargement of salivary glands, esophagitis, flatulence, gastritis, gastroenteritis, gastrointestinal pain, gingivitis, hernia, melena, nausea, oral candidiasis, oral mucosa ulcer, stomatitis, vomiting, xerostomia

Genitourinary: Cystitis, dysuria, hematuria, pelvic pain, prostatic disease, urinary frequency, urinary tract infection, vulvo candidiasis

Hematologic & oncologic: Anemia, ecchymoses, hematoma
Hepatic: Abnormal hepatic function tests, increased serum ALT (>3 x ULN; reversible)
Hypersensitivity: Hypersensitivity reaction
Infection: Abscess, herpes simplex infection, herpes zoster
Neuromuscular & skeletal: Arthralgia, arthropathy, back pain, bursitis, increased creatine phosphokinase, leg cramps, muscle cramps, myalgia, neck pain, ostealgia, osteoarthritis, osteonecrosis, rupture of tendon, synovitis, tenosynovitis, weakness,
Ophthalmic: Blurred vision, cataract, conjunctivitis, eye disease
Respiratory: Asthma, bronchitis, cough, dyspnea, epistaxis, flu-like symptoms, pharyngitis, pneumonia, pulmonary disease, respiratory tract infection, rhinitis, sinusitis, upper respiratory tract infection
Miscellaneous: Accidental injury, cyst, fever
Rare but important or life-threatening: Agranulocytosis, cholestasis, cutaneous lupus erythematosus, DRESS syndrome, eosinophilia, erythema multiforme, exacerbation of psoriasis, hepatitis, hepatotoxicity (rare, including hepatic necrosis and hepatic failure), hypophosphaturia, interstitial pulmonary disease, necrotizing angiitis (cutaneous), opportunistic infection, pancreatitis, pancytopenia, peripheral neuropathy, pustular psoriasis, sepsis, Stevens-Johnson syndrome, thrombocytopenia, toxic epidermal necrolysis, uricosuria

Drug Interactions

Metabolism/Transport Effects Inhibits CYP2C9 (moderate)

Avoid Concomitant Use

Avoid concomitant use of Leflunomide with any of the following: BCG; Natalizumab; Pimecrolimus; Tacrolimus (Topical); Teriflunomide; Tofacitinib

Increased Effect/Toxicity

Leflunomide may increase the levels/effects of: Bosentan; Cannabis; Carvedilol; CYP2C9 Substrates; Dronabinol; Natalizumab; Teriflunomide; Tetrahydrocannabinol; Tofacitinib; TOLBUTamide; Vaccines (Live); Vitamin K Antagonists

The levels/effects of Leflunomide may be increased by: Denosumab; Immunosuppressants; Methotrexate; Pimecrolimus; Rifampin; Roflumilast; Tacrolimus (Topical); TOLBUTamide; Trastuzumab

Decreased Effect

Leflunomide may decrease the levels/effects of: BCG; Coccidioides immitis Skin Test; Sipuleucel-T; Vaccines (Inactivated)

The levels/effects of Leflunomide may be decreased by: Bile Acid Sequestrants; Charcoal, Activated; Echinacea

Food Interactions No interactions with food have been noted. Management: Maintain adequate hydration, unless instructed to restrict fluid intake.

Storage/Stability Store at 25°C (77°F); excursions permitted to 15°C to 30°C (59°F to 86°F). Protect from light.

Mechanism of Action Leflunomide is an immunomodulatory agent that inhibits pyrimidine synthesis, resulting in antiproliferative and anti-inflammatory effects. Leflunomide is a prodrug; the active metabolite is responsible for activity. For CMV, may interfere with virion assembly.

Pharmacodynamics/Kinetics

Distribution: V_d: M1: 0.13 L/kg
Protein binding: M1: >99% to albumin
Metabolism: Hepatic to an active metabolite M1 (also known as A77 1726 or teriflunomide), which accounts for nearly all pharmacologic activity; further metabolism to multiple inactive metabolites; undergoes enterohepatic recirculation
Bioavailability: 80% (relative to oral solution)
Half-life elimination: M1: Mean: 14 to 15 days; enterohepatic recycling appears to contribute to the long half-life of this agent, since activated charcoal and cholestyramine substantially reduce plasma half-life
Time to peak: M1: 6 to 12 hours
Excretion: Feces (48%); urine (43%)

Dosage

Adults:

Rheumatoid arthritis: Oral: Loading dose: 100 mg once daily for 3 days; maintenance dose: 20 mg once daily, may reduce dose to 10 mg once daily if higher dose is not tolerated (maximum dose: 20 mg once daily). **Note:** The loading dose may be omitted in patients at increased risk of hepatic or hematologic toxicity (eg, recent concomitant methotrexate or other immunosuppressive agents). Due to the long half-life of the active metabolite, serum concentrations may require a prolonged period to decline after dosage reduction.

CMV disease, resistant to standard antivirals (off-label use): Some authors recommend 100 to 200 mg/day for 5 to 7 days, followed by 40 to 60 mg/day (Avery, 2004; Avery, 2010). Others have utilized the standard rheumatoid arthritis dosing (John, 2004). Adjust dose based on serum concentrations of metabolite and adverse events (Avery, 2008; Avery, 2010; Williams, 2002).

Children ≥3 years and Adolescents: Juvenile idiopathic arthritis (off-label use) (Silverman, 2005):

<20 kg: 100 mg as a single dose followed by 10 mg every other day
20 kg to 40 kg: 100 mg once daily for 2 days followed by 10 mg once daily
>40 kg: 100 mg once daily for 3 days followed by 20 mg once daily

Dosage adjustment in renal impairment:

U.S. labeling: There are no dosage adjustments provided in the manufacturer's labeling; use with caution.

Canadian labeling:

Mild impairment: There are no dosage adjustments provided in the manufacturer's labeling; use with caution.
Moderate to severe impairment: Use is contraindicated.

Dosage adjustment in hepatic impairment:

U.S. labeling: Not recommended for use in patients with preexisting liver disease or those with ALT >2 time ULN; monitor liver function closely.

Canadian labeling: Use is contraindicated.

Dosage adjustment in hepatic toxicity:

U.S. labeling: ALT elevations >3 x ULN: Discontinue drug therapy and investigate probable cause; if leflunomide induced, initiate cholestyramine drug elimination process.

Canadian labeling:

ALT elevations 2 to 3 x ULN: May reduce maintenance dose to 10 mg once daily; monitor ALT weekly.
Persistent ALT elevations >2 x ULN or ALT elevations >3 x ULN: Discontinue treatment and initiate drug elimination procedures.

Drug elimination procedure: To achieve nondetectable serum concentrations (<0.02 mg/L) of the active metabolite (M1) of leflunomide administer the following:

Cholestyramine: 8 g 3 times daily for 11 days. The 11 days do not need to be consecutive unless plasma concentrations need to be lowered rapidly. Verify serum concentrations by 2 separate tests ≥14 days apart. If plasma concentrations are still high, additional cholestyramine treatment may be considered. In healthy volunteers, cholestyramine 8 g 3 times daily for 24 hours decreased M1 concentrations by 40% in 24 hours and 49% to 65% in 48 hours.

Activated charcoal: 50 g (orally or via nasogastric tube) every 6 hours for 24 hours was shown to decrease plasma concentrations of M1 by 37% in 24 hours and 48% in 48 hours. **Note:** As an alternative to cholestyramine, the Canadian labeling recommends activated charcoal 50 g 4 times daily for 11 days (may modify duration based on clinical response or laboratory results).

Administration Administer without regard to meals.

Hazardous agent; use appropriate precautions for handling and disposal (NIOSH 2014 [group 2]).

Monitoring Parameters A complete blood count (WBC, platelet count, hemoglobin or hematocrit), serum phosphate, as well as serum transaminase determinations should be monitored at baseline and monthly during the initial 6 months of treatment; if stable, monitoring frequency may be decreased to every 6 to 8 weeks thereafter (continue monthly when used in combination with other immunosuppressive agents). ALT should be monitored at least monthly for the first 6 months of treatment, then every 6 to 8 weeks thereafter (discontinue if ALT >3 x ULN, treat with cholestyramine, and monitor liver function at least weekly until normal). In addition, monitor for signs/symptoms of severe infection, pulmonary symptoms (eg, cough, dyspnea), abnormalities in hepatic function tests, symptoms of hepatotoxicity, and blood pressure. If coadministered with methotrexate, monthly transaminases (ALT, AST) and serum albumin levels are recommended. Screen for tuberculosis and pregnancy prior to therapy.

When used for CMV disease, monitor serum trough concentrations of active metabolite (also see Reference Range).

Reference Range CMV disease:

Timing of serum samples: Initial: Obtain 24 hours after last dose of loading regimen and periodically thereafter

Therapeutic concentration: Active metabolite (A77 1726, M1, or teriflunomide): Trough: 50-80 mcg/mL (Avery, 2010) or up to 100 mcg/mL (Williams, 2002)

Dosage Forms

Tablet, Oral:

Arava: 10 mg, 20 mg

Generic: 10 mg, 20 mg

◆ **Legatrin PM® [OTC]** *see* Acetaminophen and Diphenhydramine *on page 36*

◆ **Lemtrada** *see* Alemtuzumab *on page 75*

Lenalidomide (le na LID oh mide)

Brand Names: U.S. Revlimid

Brand Names: Canada Revlimid

Index Terms CC-5013; IMid-1

Pharmacologic Category Angiogenesis Inhibitor; Antineoplastic Agent; Immunomodulator, Systemic

Use

Mantle cell lymphoma: Treatment of patients with mantle cell lymphoma that has relapsed or progressed after 2 prior therapies (one of which included bortezomib).

Multiple myeloma: Treatment of multiple myeloma (in combination with dexamethasone) in patients who have received at least one prior therapy

Myelodysplastic syndromes: Treatment of patients with transfusion-dependent anemia due to low- or intermediate-1-risk myelodysplastic syndromes (MDS) associated with a deletion 5q (del 5q) cytogenetic abnormality with or without additional cytogenetic abnormalities

Limitations of use: Lenalidomide is not indicated and is not recommended for the treatment of chronic lymphocytic leukemia (CLL) outside of controlled clinical trials.

Pregnancy Risk Factor X

Pregnancy Considerations [U.S. Boxed Warning]: Lenalidomide is an analogue of thalidomide (a human teratogen) and could potentially cause severe birth defects or embryo-fetal death; do not use during pregnancy (contraindication); avoid pregnancy while taking lenalidomide. Obtain 2 negative pregnancy tests prior to initiation of treatment; 2 forms of contraception (or abstain from heterosexual intercourse) must be used at least 4 weeks prior to, during, and for 4 weeks after lenalidomide treatment (and during treatment interruptions). In order to decrease the risk of embryo-fetal exposure, lenalidomide is available only through a restricted distribution program (Revlimid REMS). Animal reproduction studies with lenalidomide in nonhuman primates have demonstrated malformations similar to those observed in humans with thalidomide.

Women of childbearing potential should be treated only if they are able to comply with the conditions of the Revlimid REMS program. Women of reproductive potential must avoid pregnancy 4 weeks prior to therapy, during therapy, during therapy interruptions, and for ≥4 weeks after therapy is discontinued. Two forms of effective contraception (eg, tubal ligation, IUD, hormonal birth control methods, male latex or synthetic condom, diaphragm, or cervical cap) or total abstinence from heterosexual intercourse must be used by females who are not infertile or who have not had a hysterectomy. A negative pregnancy test (sensitivity of at least 50 mIU/mL) 10-14 days prior to therapy, within 24 hours prior to beginning therapy, weekly during the first 4 weeks, and every 4 weeks (every 2 weeks for women with irregular menstrual cycles) thereafter is required for women of childbearing potential. Lenalidomide must be immediately discontinued for a missed period, abnormal pregnancy test or abnormal menstrual bleeding; refer patient to a reproductive toxicity specialist if pregnancy occurs during treatment.

Lenalidomide is also present in the semen of males. Males (including those vasectomized) should use a latex or synthetic condom during any sexual contact with women of childbearing age during treatment, during treatment interruptions, and for 4 weeks after discontinuation. Male patients should not donate sperm during, and for 4 weeks after treatment, and during therapy interruptions.

The parent or legal guardian for patients between 12 and 18 years of age must agree to ensure compliance with the required guidelines. Any suspected fetal exposure should be reported to the FDA via the MedWatch program (1-800-FDA-1088) and to Celgene Corporation (1-888-423-5436).

Breast-Feeding Considerations It is not known if lenalidomide is excreted in breast milk. Due to the potential for serious adverse reactions in the infant, a decision should be made to discontinue nursing or discontinue treatment. Use in breast-feeding women is contraindicated in the Canadian labeling.

Contraindications Hypersensitivity (eg, angioedema, Stevens-Johnson syndrome, toxic epidermal necrolysis) to lenalidomide or any component of the formulation; pregnancy

Canadian labeling: Additional contraindications (not in U.S. labeling): Platelet count <50,000/mm^3 (in MDS patients); hypersensitivity to thalidomide; women capable of becoming pregnant; breast-feeding women

Warnings/Precautions Hazardous agent - use appropriate precautions for handling and disposal (NIOSH 2014 [group 2]).

[U.S. Boxed Warning]: Hematologic toxicity (neutropenia and thrombocytopenia) occurs in a majority of patients (grade 3/4: 80% in patients with del 5q myelodysplastic syndrome) and may require dose

reductions and/or delays; the use of blood product support and/or growth factors may be needed. CBC should be monitored weekly for the first 8 weeks and at least monthly thereafter in patients being treated for del 5q myelodysplastic syndromes. In patients being treated for multiple myeloma, monitor CBC every 2 weeks for 12 weeks and monthly thereafter. In patients receiving lenalidomide for mantle cell lymphoma (MCL), monitor CBC weekly for the first cycle, every 2 weeks during cycles 2 to 4, and monthly thereafter. **[U.S. Boxed Warning]: Lenalidomide has been associated with a significant increase in risk for arterial and venous thromboembolic events in multiple myeloma patients treated with lenalidomide and dexamethasone combination therapy. Deep vein thrombosis (DVT), pulmonary embolism (PE), myocardial infarction, and stroke have occurred; monitor for signs and symptoms of thromboembolism (shortness of breath, chest pain, or arm or leg swelling) and seek prompt medical attention with development of these symptoms. Thromboprophylaxis is recommended; the choice of regimen should be based on assessment of the patient's underlying risk factors.** Erythropoietin-stimulating agents (ESAs) and estrogens may contribute to thromboembolic risk; use with caution. Patients with a prior history of arterial thromboembolic events may be at greater risk; minimize modifiable factors such as hyperlipidemia, hypertension, and smoking. Anticoagulant prophylaxis should be individualized and selected based on the thromboembolism risk of the combination treatment regimen, using the safest and easiest to administer (Palumbo, 2008).

In a clinical trial comparing lenalidomide versus chlorambucil single agent therapy in patients >65 years of age with chronic lymphocytic leukemia patients (not an FDA-approved indication), increased mortality was observed in the lenalidomide treatment arm. Atrial fibrillation, cardiac failure, and MI were observed more frequently in lenalidomide-treated patients; lenalidomide (alone or in combination) is not currently recommended for first-line treatment of CLL. Second primary malignancies (SPMs), including hematologic (AML and lymphoma) and solid tumor malignancies, and skin cancers, have been reported with lenalidomide when used for the treatment of MDS and multiple myeloma; the incidence may be higher when lenalidomide is used in combination with an alkylating agent.

Angioedema, Stevens-Johnson syndrome (SJS), and toxic epidermal necrolysis (TEN) have been reported; may be fatal. Consider interrupting or discontinuing treatment with grade 2 or 3 skin rash; discontinue and do not reinitiate treatment with grade 4 rash, exfoliative or bullous rash, or for suspected SJS or TEN. Patients with a history of grade 4 rash with thalidomide should not receive lenalidomide. Discontinue treatment with angioedema. Use caution in renal impairment; may experience an increased rate of toxicities (due to reduced clearance and increased half-life); initial dosage adjustments are recommended for moderate-to-severe and dialysis-dependent renal impairment. Tumor lysis syndrome (with fatalities) has been reported with lenalidomide; patients with a high tumor burden may be at risk for tumor lysis syndrome; monitor closely; institute appropriate management for hyperuricemia. Tumor flare reaction has been observed in studies of lenalidomide for the treatment of chronic lymphocytic leukemia (CLL) and lymphoma; clinical presentation includes low grade fever, pain, rash, and tender lymph node swelling. In patients with MCL, tumor flare may mimic disease progression; monitor closely. In clinical trials, the majority of tumor flare events occurred in the first cycle of therapy. Treatment with corticosteroids, nonsteroidal anti-inflammatory drugs (NSAIDs), and/or analgesics may be considered; therapy interruption may be necessary as well. Hepatic failure, including fatalities, has occurred in patients treated with combination lenalidomide and dexamethasone therapy; may have hepatocellular, cholestatic, or mixed characteristics. Risk factors may include preexisting viral liver disease, elevated liver enzymes at baseline, and concomitant medications. Monitor closely; interrupt therapy in patients with abnormal hepatic function tests. May consider resuming treatment at a lower dose upon return to baseline. Certain adverse reactions (DVT, pulmonary embolism, atrial fibrillation, renal failure) are more likely in elderly patients. Monitor renal function closely, and select dose accordingly.

[U.S. Boxed Warning]: Lenalidomide is an analogue of thalidomide (a human teratogen) and could potentially cause severe birth defects or embryo-fetal death; do not use during pregnancy (contraindication); avoid pregnancy while taking lenalidomide. Obtain 2 negative pregnancy testes prior to initiation of treatment; 2 forms of contraception (or abstain from heterosexual intercourse) must be used at least 4 weeks prior to, during and for 4 weeks after lenalidomide treatment (and during treatment interruptions). Distribution is restricted; physicians, pharmacies, and patients must be registered with the Revlimid REMS program. In order to decrease the risk of embryo-fetal exposure, lenalidomide is available only through a restricted distribution program (Revlimid REMS). Prescribers and pharmacies must be certified with the program to prescribe or dispense lenalidomide. Males taking lenalidomide (even those vasectomized) must use a latex or synthetic condom during any sexual contact with women of childbearing potential and for up to 28 days following discontinuation of therapy. Males taking lenalidomide must not donate sperm. Patients should be advised not to donate blood during therapy and for 1 month following completion of therapy. May cause dizziness or fatigue; caution patients about performing tasks which require mental alertness (eg, operating machinery or driving). Potentially significant drug-drug interactions may exist, requiring dose or frequency adjustment, additional monitoring, and/or selection of alternative therapy. Formulation contains lactose; avoid use in patients with Lapp lactase deficiency, glucose-galactose malabsorption, or glucose intolerance. Lenalidomide should only be prescribed to patients (male and female) who can understand and comply with the conditions of the Revlimid REMS program. If used in patients between 12 to 18 years of age, the parent or legal guardian must agree to ensure compliance with the Revlimid REMS program.

Adverse Reactions

Cardiovascular: Angina pectoris, atrial fibrillation, bradycardia, cardiac failure, cerebral ischemia, cerebrovascular accident, chest pain, deep vein thrombosis, edema, hypertension, hypotension, myocardial infarction, palpitations, peripheral edema, pulmonary embolism, syncope, tachycardia

Central nervous system: Depression, dizziness, emotional lability, fatigue, glossalgia, hallucination, headache, hypoesthesia, insomnia, lethargy, local pain, malaise, peripheral neuropathy, rigors

Dermatologic: Cellulitis, diaphoresis, ecchymoses, erythema, hyperpigmentation, night sweats, pruritus, skin rash, xeroderma

Endocrine & metabolic: Dehydration, hirsutism, hypokalemia, hypomagnesemia, hyponatremia, hypophosphatemia, hypothyroidism, loss of libido, weight loss

Gastrointestinal: Abdominal pain, anorexia, constipation, decreased appetite, diarrhea, dysgeusia, gastrointestinal hemorrhage, hypocalcemia, loose stools, nausea, vomiting, xerostomia

Genitourinary: Dysuria, erectile dysfunction, urinary tract infection

Hematologic & oncologic: Anemia, autoimmune hemolytic anemia, febrile neutropenia, granulocytopenia, leukopenia, lymphocytopenia, neutropenia (MDS: Onset: 42 days [range: 14-411 days]; recovery: 17 days [range: 2-170 days]), pancytopenia, squamous cell carcinoma of skin, thrombocytopenia (MDS: Onset: 28 days [range: 8-290 days]; recovery: 22 days [range: 5-224 days]), tumor flare

Hepatic: Abnormal hepatic function tests, increased serum ALT

Infection: Bacteremia, sepsis

Neuromuscular & skeletal: Arthralgia, back pain, limb pain, muscle cramps, muscle spasm, myalgia, ostealgia, tremor, weakness

Ophthalmic: Blindness, blurred vision, cataract, ocular hypertension

Renal: Renal failure

Respiratory: Bronchitis, cough, dyspnea, epistaxis, hoarseness, hypoxia, nasopharyngitis, pharyngitis, pleural effusion, pneumonia, pneumonitis, pulmonary hypertension, respiratory distress, rhinitis, sinusitis, upper respiratory tract infection

Miscellaneous: Fever, multi-organ failure, physical health deterioration

Rare but important or life-threatening: Abnormal gait, acute leukemia, adrenocortical insufficiency, angioedema, aphasia, arthritis, atrial flutter, azotemia, bacterial infection, biliary obstruction, bone fracture, bone marrow depression, calcium pyrophosphate deposition disease, cardiogenic shock, cardiorespiratory arrest, cerebral edema, cholecystitis, chronic obstructive pulmonary disease, circulatory shock, clostridial infection, colonic polyps, decreased hemoglobin, delirium, desquamation, diabetes mellitus, diabetic ketoacidosis, diverticulitis, drug overdose, dysphagia, encephalitis, erythema multiforme, falling, Fanconi's syndrome, fungal infection, gastritis, gastroenteritis, gastroesophageal reflux disease, gout, Graves' disease, hematuria, hemolysis, hemolytic anemia, hemorrhage, hemorrhagic diathesis, hepatic failure, hepatitis, hyperbilirubinemia, hypernatremia, hypersensitivity reaction, hypoglycemia, impaired consciousness, increased cardiac enzymes (troponin I), increased serum creatinine, influenza, inguinal hernia, interstitial pulmonary disease, intestinal obstruction, intestinal perforation, intracranial hemorrhage, irritable bowel syndrome, ischemia, ischemic colitis, Klebsiella infection, leukoencephalopathy, localized infection, lung carcinoma, malignant lymphoma, melena, migraine, myelocytic leukemia, myopathy, neck pain, nephrolithiasis, neutropenic infection, nodule, orthostatic hypotension, otic infection, pancreatitis, pelvic pain, peripheral ischemia, perirectal abscess, prostate carcinoma, pseudomembranous colitis, pseudomonas infection, pulmonary edema, pulmonary infiltrates, rectal hemorrhage, renal cyst, renal tubular necrosis, respiratory failure, second primary malignant neoplasms (AML, lymphomas, solid tumors), septic shock, spinal cord compression, splenic infarction, staphylococcal infection, Stevens-Johnson syndrome, stomatitis, subarachnoid hemorrhage, supraventricular cardiac, Sweet's Syndrome, tachyarrhythmia, thrombophlebitis, toxic epidermal necrolysis, transfusion reaction, transient ischemic attacks, tumor lysis syndrome, urinary retention, urosepsis, urticaria, ventricular dysfunction, viral infection

Drug Interactions

Metabolism/Transport Effects **Substrate** of P-glycoprotein

Avoid Concomitant Use

Avoid concomitant use of Lenalidomide with any of the following: Abatacept; Anakinra; BCG; Canakinumab; Certolizumab Pegol; CloZAPine; Dipyrone; Natalizumab; Pimecrolimus; Rilonacept; Tacrolimus (Topical); Tocilizumab; Tofacitinib; Vaccines (Live); Vedolizumab

Increased Effect/Toxicity

Lenalidomide may increase the levels/effects of: Abatacept; Anakinra; Bisphosphonate Derivatives; Canakinumab; Certolizumab Pegol; CloZAPine; Digoxin; Leflunomide; Natalizumab; Rilonacept; Tofacitinib; Vaccines (Live); Vedolizumab

The levels/effects of Lenalidomide may be increased by: Denosumab; Dexamethasone (Systemic); Dipyrone; Erythropoiesis-Stimulating Agents; Estrogen Derivatives; Pimecrolimus; Roflumilast; Tacrolimus (Topical); Tocilizumab; Trastuzumab

Decreased Effect

Lenalidomide may decrease the levels/effects of: BCG; Coccidioides immitis Skin Test; Sipuleucel-T; Vaccines (Inactivated); Vaccines (Live)

The levels/effects of Lenalidomide may be decreased by: Echinacea

Storage/Stability Store at 20°C to 25°C (68°F to 77°F); excursions permitted to 15°C and 30°C (59°F and 86°F).

Mechanism of Action Immunomodulatory, antiangiogenic, and antineoplastic characteristics via multiple mechanisms. Selectively inhibits secretion of proinflammatory cytokines (potent inhibitor of tumor necrosis factor-alpha secretion); enhances cell-mediated immunity by stimulating proliferation of anti-CD3 stimulated T cells (resulting in increased IL-2 and interferon gamma secretion); inhibits trophic signals to angiogenic factors in cells. Inhibits the growth of myeloma cells by inducing cell cycle arrest and cell death.

Pharmacodynamics/Kinetics

Absorption: Rapid

Protein binding: ~30%

Half-life elimination: 3 to 5 hours; Moderate to severe renal impairment: Increased threefold; Hemodialysis patients: Increased ~4.5-fold

Time, to peak, plasma: MDS or myeloma patients: 0.5 to 6 hours

Excretion: Urine (~82%; as unchanged drug)

Hemodialysis effect: ~40% of a dose is removed in a single dialysis session

Dosage

Mantle cell lymphoma (MCL): Adults: Oral: 25 mg once daily for 21 days of a 28-day treatment cycle; continue until disease progression or unacceptable toxicity

Multiple myeloma: Adults: Oral: 25 mg once daily for 21 days of a 28-day treatment cycle (in combination with dexamethasone)

Myelodysplastic syndrome (MDS) with deletion 5q: Adults: Oral: 10 mg once daily

Chronic lymphocytic leukemia (CLL), relapsed/refractory (off-label use): Adults: Oral: 10 mg once daily beginning on day 9 of cycle 1; administer continuously in combination with cyclic rituximab (Badoux, 2013)

Diffuse large B-cell lymphoma, relapsed/refractory (off-label use): Adults: Oral: 25 mg once daily for 21 days of a 28-day treatment cycle for up to 1 year (Wiernik, 2008)

Multiple myeloma, newly diagnosed (off-label use): Adults: Oral: 25 mg once daily for 14 days of a 21-day cycle (in combination with bortezomib and dexamethasone) for 8 cycles (Kumar, 2012; Richardson, 2010)

Multiple myeloma, maintenance (following autologous stem cell transplant; off-label use): Adults: Oral: 10 mg once daily for 3 months, then increased to 15 mg daily if tolerated; continue until relapse (Attal, 2012; McCarthy, 2012) **or** 10 mg once daily for 21 days of a 28-day treatment cycle until relapse (Palumbo, 2010)

Myelodysplastic syndrome (MDS), lower risk, without deletion 5q (off-label use): Adults: Oral: 10 mg once daily (Raza, 2008)

Systemic light chain amyloidosis (off-label use): Adults: Oral: 15 mg once daily for 21 days of a 28-day cycle (in combination with dexamethasone) (Nair, 2012; Sanchorawala, 2007)

Elderly: Refer to adult dosing; due to the potential for decreased renal function in the elderly, select dose carefully and closely monitor renal function

Dosage adjustment in renal impairment:

Recommended initial dose adjustment in the FDA-approved labeling; further individualize based on tolerance:

MCL:

CrCl >60 mL/minute: No adjustment required

CrCl 30 to 60 mL/minute: 10 mg once daily

CrCl <30 mL/minute (nondialysis dependent): 15 mg every 48 hours

ESRD: CrCl <30 mL/minute and dialysis dependent: 5 mg once daily (administer after dialysis on dialysis days)

MDS:

CrCl >60 mL/minute: No adjustment required

CrCl 30 to 60 mL/minute: 5 mg once daily

CrCl <30 mL/minute (nondialysis dependent): 2.5 mg once daily

ESRD: CrCl <30 mL/minute and dialysis dependent: 2.5 mg once daily (administer after dialysis on dialysis days)

Multiple myeloma:

CrCl >60 mL/minute: No adjustment required

CrCl 30 to 60 mL/minute: 10 mg once daily (may increase to 15 mg once daily after 2 cycles if nonresponsive but tolerating treatment; Chen, 2007)

CrCl <30 mL/minute (nondialysis dependent): 15 mg every 48 hours

ESRD: CrCl <30 mL/minute and dialysis dependent: 5 mg once daily (administer after dialysis on dialysis days)

Recommended adjustment in Canadian labeling:

MDS:

CrCl ≥60 mL/minute: No adjustment required

CrCl 30 to 59 mL/minute: 5 mg once daily

CrCl <30 mL/minute (nondialysis dependent): 5 mg every 48 hours

ESRD: CrCl <30 mL/minute and dialysis dependent: 5 mg 3 times weekly (administer after each dialysis)

Multiple myeloma:

CrCl ≥60 mL/minute: No adjustment required

CrCl 30 to 59 mL/minute: 10 mg once daily (may increase to 15 mg once daily after 2 cycles if nonresponsive but tolerating treatment; Chen, 2007)

CrCl <30 mL/minute (nondialysis dependent): 15 mg every 48 hours

ESRD: CrCl <30 mL/minute and dialysis dependent: 5 mg once daily (administer after dialysis on dialysis days)

Dosage adjustment in hepatic impairment: There are no dosage adjustments provided in the manufacturer's labeling (has not been studied). However, lenalidomide undergoes minimal hepatic metabolism.

Dosage adjustment for NONHEMATOLOGIC toxicities:

Dermatologic toxicities:

Skin rash, grade 2 or 3: Consider interrupting or discontinuing treatment

Angioedema, grade 4 rash, exfoliative or bullous rash, or suspected Stevens-Johnson syndrome or toxic epidermal necrolysis: Discontinue treatment; do not rechallenge

Tumor flare reaction:

Grade 1 or 2: Continue therapy at physician's discretion; may consider symptom management with corticosteroids, nonsteroidal anti-inflammatory drugs (NSAIDs) and/or analgesic therapy.

Grade 3 or 4: Interrupt therapy until resolved to ≤ grade 1; consider symptom management with corticosteroids, nonsteroidal anti-inflammatory drugs (NSAIDs) and/or analgesic therapy.

Other toxicities: For additional treatment-related grade 3/4 toxicities, hold treatment and restart at next lower dose level when toxicity has resolved to ≤ grade 2.

Dosage adjustment for HEMATOLOGIC toxicities:

Adjustment for thrombocytopenia in MCL:

Platelets <50,000/mm^3: Hold treatment, check CBC weekly

When platelets return to ≥50,000/mm^3: Resume treatment at 5 mg below previous dose; do not dose below 5 mg daily

Adjustment for neutropenia in MCL:

ANC <1,000/mm^3 for at least 7 days or associated with fever (≥38.5°C [101°F]): Hold treatment, check CBC weekly

ANC <500/mm^3: Hold treatment, check CBC weekly

When ANC returns to ≥1,000/mm^3: Resume treatment at 5 mg below previous dose; do not dose below 5 mg daily

Adjustment for thrombocytopenia in MDS:

Thrombocytopenia developing within 4 weeks of beginning treatment at 10 mg daily:

Baseline platelets ≥100,000/mm^3:

If platelets <50,000/mm^3: Hold treatment

When platelets return to ≥50,000/mm^3: Resume treatment at 5 mg daily

Baseline platelets <100,000/mm^3:

If platelets fall to 50% of baseline: Hold treatment

If baseline ≥60,000/mm^3 and platelet level returns to ≥50,000/mm^3: Resume at 5 mg daily

If baseline <60,000/mm^3 and platelet level returns to ≥30,000/mm^3: Resume at 5 mg daily

Thrombocytopenia developing after 4 weeks of beginning treatment at 10 mg daily:

Platelets <30,000/mm^3 **or** <50,000/mm^3 with platelet transfusions: Hold treatment

When platelets return to ≥30,000/mm^3 (without hemostatic failure): Resume at 5 mg daily

Thrombocytopenia developing with treatment at 5 mg daily:

Platelets <30,000/mm^3 **or** <50,000/mm^3 with platelet transfusions: Hold treatment

When platelets return to ≥30,000/mm^3 (without hemostatic failure):

U.S. labeling: Resume at 2.5 mg once daily

Canadian labeling: Resume at 5 mg every other day

Adjustment for neutropenia in MDS:

Neutropenia developing within 4 weeks of beginning treatment at 10 mg daily:

For baseline absolute neutrophil count (ANC) ≥1,000/mm^3:

ANC <750/mm^3: Hold treatment

When ANC returns to ≥1,000/mm^3: Resume at 5 mg daily

For baseline absolute neutrophil count (ANC) <1,000/mm^3:

ANC <500/mm^3: Hold treatment

When ANC returns to ≥500/mm^3: Resume at 5 mg daily

Neutropenia developing after 4 weeks of beginning treatment at 10 mg daily:

ANC <500/mm^3 for ≥7 days or associated with fever (≥38.5°C [101°F]): Hold treatment

When ANC returns to ≥500/mm^3: Resume at 5 mg daily

Neutropenia developing with treatment at 5 mg daily:
ANC <500/mm³ for ≥7 days or associated with fever (≥38.5°C [101°F]): Hold treatment
When ANC returns to ≥500/mm³:
U.S. labeling: Resume at 2.5 mg once daily
Canadian labeling: Resume at 5 mg every other day

Adjustment for thrombocytopenia in multiple myeloma:
Platelets <30,000/mm³: Hold treatment, check CBC weekly
When platelets return to ≥30,000/mm³: Resume at 15 mg daily
Additional occurrence of platelets <30,000/mm³: Hold treatment
When platelets return to ≥30,000/mm³: Resume treatment at 5 mg below previous dose; do not dose below 5 mg daily

Adjustment for neutropenia in multiple myeloma:
ANC <1,000/mm³: Hold treatment, add G-CSF, check CBC weekly
When ANC returns to ≥1,000/mm³ (with neutropenia as only toxicity): Resume at 25 mg daily
When ANC returns to ≥1,000/mm³ (with additional toxicities): Resume at 15 mg daily
Additional occurrence of ANC <1,000/mm³: Hold treatment
When ANC returns to ≥1,000/mm³: Resume treatment at 5 mg below previous dose; do not dose below 5 mg daily.

Administration Administer at about the same time each day with water; administer with or without food. Swallow capsule whole; do not break, open, or chew.

Missed doses: May administer a missed dose if within 12 hours of usual dosing time. If greater than 12 hours, patient should skip dose for that day and resume usual dosing the following day. Patient should **not** take 2 doses to make up for a missed dose.

Hazardous agent; use appropriate precautions for handling and disposal (NIOSH 2014 [group 2]).

Monitoring Parameters CBC with differential (MCL - weekly for the first cycle, every 2 weeks during cycles 2-4; MDS - weekly for first 8 weeks; multiple myeloma - every 2 weeks for the first 3 months), then monthly thereafter; serum creatinine, liver function tests, thyroid function tests (TSH at baseline then every 2-3 months during lenalidomide treatment [Hamnvik, 2011]); ECG when clinically indicated; monitor for signs and symptoms of thromboembolism, tumor lysis syndrome, or tumor flare reaction

Women of childbearing potential: Pregnancy test 10-14 days **and** 24 hours prior to initiating therapy, weekly during the first 4 weeks of treatment, then every 2-4 weeks through 4 weeks after therapy discontinued

Dosage Forms
Capsule, Oral:
Revlimid: 2.5 mg, 5 mg, 10 mg, 15 mg, 20 mg, 25 mg

Lenograstim [INT] (len oh GRA stim)

International Brand Names Granocyte (AR, AT, BE, BG, BR, CH, CL, CN, CY, DE, DK, EE, FI, FR, GB, GR, HN, HR, ID, IE, IL, IN, IT, KW, LT, MY, NL, NO, PH, PK, PL, QA, RU, SE, SG, SI, TH, TR, TW, VE); Neutrogin (JP, KR)

Pharmacologic Category Colony Stimulating Factor

Reported Use To reduce the duration of neutropenia and associated complications in patients with nonmyeloid malignancy following bone marrow transplant or following treatment with cytotoxic chemotherapy; mobilisation of peripheral blood progenitor cells for harvesting and subsequent infusion; treatment of severe chronic neutropenia

Dosage Range Adults:
Severe chronic neutropenia or following chemotherapy: SubQ: 150 mcg/m²/day
Bone marrow transplant: IV, SubQ: 150 mcg/m²/day

Product Availability Product available in various countries; not currently available in the U.S.

Dosage Forms
Injection, powder for reconstitution: 13.4 million units [105 mcg]; 33.6 million units [263 mcg]

◆ **Lepargylic Acid** *see* Azelaic Acid *on page 213*

Lercanidipine [INT] (ler ca NID i peen)

International Brand Names Anadip (KR); Areta (BG); Cardiovasc (IT); Carmen (DE); Corifeo (DE); Kapidin (BG, CZ); Landip (IN); Lecadin (KR); Lercadip (AE, BH, ES, GR, IT, KW, LB, QA, SA, SE, TH); Lercal (SK); Lercamen (RU); Lercan (AU, FR); Lercapin (EE, KR, LT); Lercaton (HU); Lerdip (NL); Lervasc (IN); Lerzam (ES); Nircadel (DK); Oridip (FI); Pegfel (RO); Pinox (HR); Renovia (BG); Vasodip (IL); Zanedip (IT, KR, VN); Zanicor (PT); Zanidip (AT, AU, BE, CH, CN, DK, ES, FI, FR, GB, GR, HU, NL, NO, NZ, PT, SE, TH); Zircol (AU)

Index Terms Lercanidipine Hydrochloride

Pharmacologic Category Calcium Channel Blocker

Reported Use Treatment of mild to moderate hypertension

Dosage Range Adults: Oral: Initial: 10 mg once daily; may increase, if necessary, after at least 2 weeks to 20 mg/day

Product Availability Product available in various countries; not currently available in the U.S.

Dosage Forms
Tablet: 10 mg

◆ **Lercanidipine Hydrochloride** *see* Lercanidipine [INT] *on page 1181*

◆ **Lescol** *see* Fluvastatin *on page 915*

◆ **Lescol XL** *see* Fluvastatin *on page 915*

◆ **Lessina** *see* Ethinyl Estradiol and Levonorgestrel *on page 803*

◆ **Letairis** *see* Ambrisentan *on page 107*

Letrozole (LET roe zole)

Brand Names: U.S. Femara

Brand Names: Canada ACH-Letrozole; Apo-Letrozole; Auro-Letrozole; Bio-Letrozole; Femara; JAMP-Letrozole; Mar-Letrozole; MED-Letrozole; Myl-Letrozole; PMS-Letrozole; RAN-Letrozole; Riva-Letrozole; Sandoz-Letrozole; Teva-Letrozole; Zinda-Letrozole

Index Terms CGS-20267

Pharmacologic Category Antineoplastic Agent, Aromatase Inhibitor

Use Breast cancer in postmenopausal women: Adjuvant treatment of hormone receptor positive early breast cancer, extended adjuvant treatment of early breast cancer after 5 years of tamoxifen; treatment of advanced breast cancer with disease progression following antiestrogen therapy; first-line treatment of hormone receptor positive or hormone receptor unknown, locally-advanced, or metastatic breast cancer

Pregnancy Risk Factor X

Pregnancy Considerations Adverse events were observed in animal reproduction studies. Letrozole is FDA approved for postmenopausal women only (no clinical benefit for breast cancer has been demonstrated in premenopausal women). Use in women who are or who may become pregnant is contraindicated. Women who are perimenopausal or recently postmenopausal should use adequate contraception until postmenopausal status is fully established.

Breast-Feeding Considerations It is not known if letrozole is excreted in breast milk. Due to the potential for serious adverse reactions in the nursing infant, a decision should be made whether to discontinue nursing or to discontinue the drug, taking into account the importance of treatment to the mother. Use in nursing women is contraindicated in the Canadian labeling.

Contraindications Use in women who are or may become pregnant

Canadian labeling: Additional contraindications (not in U.S. labeling): Hypersensitivity to letrozole, other aromatase inhibitors, or any component of the formulation; use in patients <18 years of age; breast-feeding

Warnings/Precautions Hazardous agent - use appropriate precautions for handling and disposal (NIOSH 2014 [group 1]). Not generally indicated for known hormone-receptor negative disease. Use caution with hepatic impairment; dose adjustment recommended in patients with cirrhosis or severe hepatic dysfunction. May cause dizziness, fatigue, and somnolence; patients should be cautioned before performing tasks which require mental alertness (eg, operating machinery or driving). May increase total serum cholesterol; in patients treated with adjuvant therapy and cholesterol levels within normal limits, an increase of ≥1.5 x ULN in total cholesterol has been demonstrated in 8.2% of letrozole-treated patients (25% requiring lipid-lowering medications) vs 3.2% of tamoxifen-treated patients (16% requiring medications); monitor cholesterol panel; may require antihyperlipidemics. May cause decreases in bone mineral density (BMD); a decrease in hip BMD by 3.8% from baseline in letrozole-treated patients vs 2% in placebo at 2 years has been demonstrated; however, there was no statistical difference in changes to the lumbar spine BMD scores; monitor BMD. Potentially significant drug-drug interactions may exist, requiring dose or frequency adjustment, additional monitoring, and/or selection of alternative therapy.

Adverse Reactions

Cardiovascular: Angina; cerebrovascular accident including hemorrhagic stroke, thrombotic stroke; chest pain, hypertension, MI, peripheral edema; thromboembolic event including venous thrombosis, thrombophlebitis, portal vein thrombosis, pulmonary embolism; transient ischemic attack

Central nervous system: Anxiety, depression, dizziness, fatigue, headache, insomnia, pain, somnolence, vertigo

Dermatologic: Alopecia, pruritus, rash

Endocrine & metabolic: Breast pain, hot flashes, hypercholesterolemia, hypercalcemia

Gastrointestinal: Abdominal pain, anorexia, constipation, diarrhea, dyspepsia, nausea, vomiting, weight gain, weight loss

Genitourinary: Urinary tract infection, vaginal bleeding, vaginal dryness, vaginal hemorrhage, vaginal irritation

Neuromuscular & skeletal: Arthralgia, arthritis, back pain, bone fracture, bone mineral density decreased, bone pain, limb pain, musculoskeletal pain, myalgia, osteoporosis, weakness

Ocular: Cataract

Renal: Renal disorder

Respiratory: Cough, dyspnea, pleural effusion

Miscellaneous: Diaphoresis, infection, influenza, night sweats, secondary malignancy, viral infection

Rare but important or life-threatening: Anaphylactic reaction, angioedema, arterial thrombosis, cardiac failure, carpal tunnel syndrome, endometrial cancer, endometrial hyperplasia, endometrial proliferation, erythema multiforme, hepatitis, leukopenia, memory impairment, stomatitis, tachycardia, thrombocytopenia, toxic epidermal necrolysis, trigger finger

Drug Interactions

Metabolism/Transport Effects **Substrate** of CYP2A6 (minor), CYP3A4 (minor); **Note:** Assignment of Major/Minor substrate status based on clinically relevant drug interaction potential; **Inhibits** CYP2A6 (strong), CYP2C19 (weak)

Avoid Concomitant Use

Avoid concomitant use of Letrozole with any of the following: Tegafur

Increased Effect/Toxicity

Letrozole may increase the levels/effects of: CYP2A6 Substrates; Methadone

Decreased Effect

Letrozole may decrease the levels/effects of: Tegafur

The levels/effects of Letrozole may be decreased by: Tamoxifen

Storage/Stability Store at room temperature of 25°C (77°F); excursions permitted to 15°C to 30°C (59°F to 86°F).

Mechanism of Action Nonsteroidal competitive inhibitor of the aromatase enzyme system which binds to the heme group of aromatase, a cytochrome P450 enzyme which catalyzes conversion of androgens to estrogens (specifically, androstenedione to estrone and testosterone to estradiol). This leads to inhibition of the enzyme and a significant reduction in plasma estrogen (estrone, estradiol and estrone sulfate) levels. Does not affect synthesis of adrenal or thyroid hormones, aldosterone, or androgens.

Pharmacodynamics/Kinetics

Absorption: Rapid and well absorbed; not affected by food

Distribution: V_d: ~1.9 L/kg

Protein binding, plasma: Weak

Metabolism: Hepatic via CYP3A4 and 2A6 to an inactive carbinol metabolite

Half-life elimination: Terminal: ~2 days

Time to steady state, plasma: 2 to 6 weeks

Excretion: Urine (90%; 6% as unchanged drug, 75% as glucuronide carbinol metabolite, 9% as unidentified metabolites)

Dosage

Breast cancer, advanced (first- or second-line treatment): Adults: Females: Postmenopausal: Oral: 2.5 mg once daily; continue until tumor progression

Breast cancer, early (adjuvant treatment): Adults: Females: Postmenopausal: Oral: 2.5 mg once daily; optimal duration unknown, duration in clinical trial is 5 years; discontinue at relapse

Breast cancer, early (extended adjuvant treatment): Adults: Females: Postmenopausal: Oral: 2.5 mg once daily; optimal duration unknown, duration in clinical trials is 5 years (after 5 years of tamoxifen); discontinue at relapse. In clinical trials letrozole was initiated within 3 months of discontinuing tamoxifen (Goss, 2003; Jin, 2012).

Infertility/ovulation stimulation in anovulatory women with polycystic ovarian syndrome (PCOS; off-label use): Oral: 2.5 to 7.5 mg daily on cycle days 3 to 7 (Franik, 2014; Legro, 2013; Legro, 2014; Misso, 2012). Up to 5 treatment cycles may be administered with the dose increased in subsequent cycles for nonresponse or poor ovulatory response as determined by progesterone levels; maximum dose 7.5 mg daily (Legro, 2014). Additional trials may be necessary to further define the routine use of letrozole in infertile women with PCOS.

Ovarian (epithelial) cancer (off-label use): 2.5 mg once daily; continue until disease progression (Ramirez, 2008)

Elderly: No dosage adjustments required

Dosage adjustment in renal impairment:

CrCl ≥10 mL/minute: No dosage adjustment necessary.

CrCl <10 mL/minute: There are no dosage adjustments provided in the manufacturer's labeling.

Dosage adjustment in hepatic impairment:

U.S. labeling:

Mild to moderate impairment (Child-Pugh class A or B): No dosage adjustment necessary.

Severe impairment (Child-Pugh class C) and cirrhosis: 2.5 mg every other day

Noncirrhotic patients with elevated bilirubin: There are no dosage adjustments provided in the manufacturer's labeling (effect has not been determined).

Canadian labeling:

Mild to moderate impairment (Child-Pugh class A or B): No dosage adjustment necessary.

Severe impairment (Child-Pugh class C): There are no dosage adjustments provided in the manufacturer's labeling (insufficient data). Monitor closely.

Dietary Considerations Calcium and vitamin D supplementation are recommended.

Administration Administer orally with or without food. Hazardous agent; use appropriate precautions for handling and disposal (NIOSH 2014 [group 1]).

Monitoring Parameters Monitor periodically during therapy: Complete blood counts, thyroid function tests; serum electrolytes, cholesterol, transaminases, and creatinine; blood pressure; bone density

Canadian labeling recommends monitoring LH, FSH, and/or estradiol prior to initiating therapy and regularly for the first 6 months in women whose menopausal status is unclear or who become amenorrheic following chemotherapy. For infertility/ovarian stimulation (off-label use), a pregnancy test is recommended prior to initiation. Midluteal progestin concentrations (in a clinical study, nonresponse to treatment was defined as a progesterone concentration <3 ng/mL during the midluteal phase; poor ovulatory response was defined as progesterone concentrations indicating ovulation but just above the cutoff point) (Legro, 2014).

Dosage Forms

Tablet, Oral:

Femara: 2.5 mg

Generic: 2.5 mg

◆ **Leucovorin** *see* Leucovorin Calcium *on page 1183*

Leucovorin Calcium (loo koe VOR in KAL see um)

Brand Names: Canada Lederle Leucovorin; Leucovorin Calcium Injection; Leucovorin Calcium Injection USP

Index Terms 5-Formyl Tetrahydrofolate; Calcium Folinate; Calcium Leucovorin; Citrovorum Factor; Folinate Calcium; Folinic Acid (error prone synonym); Leucovorin

Pharmacologic Category Antidote; Chemotherapy Modulating Agent; Rescue Agent (Chemotherapy); Vitamin, Water Soluble

Use

Methotrexate toxicity:

Injection: Rescue agent after high-dose methotrexate treatment in osteosarcoma and to diminish the toxicity and counteract the effects of impaired methotrexate elimination and of inadvertent overdosage of folic acid antagonists.

Oral: Rescue agent to diminish toxicity and counteract effects of impaired methotrexate elimination and inadvertent overdoses of folic acid antagonists.

Megaloblastic anemia: Injection: Treatment of megaloblastic anemias due to folic acid deficiency (when oral therapy is not feasible).

Advanced colorectal cancer: Injection: Palliative treatment of advanced colorectal cancer to prolong survival (in combination with 5-fluorouracil).

Pregnancy Risk Factor C

Pregnancy Considerations Animal reproduction studies have not been conducted. Leucovorin is a biologically active form of folic acid. Adequate amounts of folic acid are recommended during pregnancy. Refer to Folic Acid monograph.

Breast-Feeding Considerations Leucovorin is a biologically active form of folic acid. Adequate amounts of folic acid are recommended in breast-feeding women. Refer to Folic Acid monograph.

Contraindications Pernicious anemia and other megaloblastic anemias secondary to vitamin B_{12}-deficiency

Warnings/Precautions When used for the treatment of accidental folic acid antagonist overdose, administer as soon as possible. When used for the treatment of a methotrexate overdose, administer IV leucovorin as soon as possible. Monitoring of the serum methotrexate concentration is essential to determine the optimal dose/duration of leucovorin; however, do not wait for the results of a methotrexate level before initiating therapy. It is important to adjust the leucovorin dose once a methotrexate level is known. When used for methotrexate rescue therapy, methotrexate serum concentrations should be monitored to determine dose and duration of leucovorin therapy. The dose may need to be increased or administration prolonged in situations where methotrexate excretion may be delayed (eg, ascites, pleural effusion, renal insufficiency, inadequate hydration); **never administer leucovorin intrathecally**. Parenteral administration may be preferred to oral if vomiting or malabsorption is likely. Potentially significant drug-drug interactions may exist, requiring dose or frequency adjustment, additional monitoring, and/or selection of alternative therapy. Combination of leucovorin and sulfamethoxazole-trimethoprim for the acute treatment of PCP in patients with HIV infection has been reported to cause increased rates of treatment failure. Leucovorin may increase the toxicity of 5-fluorouracil; deaths from severe enterocolitis, diarrhea, and dehydration have been reported (in elderly patients); granulocytopenia and fever have also been reported. Hypersensitivity, including allergic reactions, anaphylactoid reactions, and urticaria have been reported with leucovorin.

Leucovorin is inappropriate treatment for pernicious anemia and other megaloblastic anemias secondary to a lack of vitamin B_{12}; a hematologic remission may occur while neurologic manifestations progress. Leucovorin is excreted renally; the risk for toxicities may be increased in patients with renal impairment.

Benzyl alcohol and derivatives: When doses >10 mg/m^2 are required using the powder for injection, reconstitute using sterile water for injection, not a solution containing benzyl alcohol; large amounts of benzyl alcohol (≥99 mg/kg/day) have been associated with a potentially fatal toxicity ("gasping syndrome") in neonates; the "gasping syndrome" consists of metabolic acidosis, respiratory distress, gasping respirations, CNS dysfunction (including convulsions, intracranial hemorrhage), hypotension, and cardiovascular collapse (AAP, 1997; CDC, 1982); some data suggests that benzoate displaces bilirubin from protein binding sites (Ahlfors, 2001); avoid or use dosage forms containing benzyl alcohol with caution in neonates. See manufacturer's labeling.

Injection: Due to calcium content, do not administer IV solutions at a rate >160 mg/minute. Not intended for intrathecal use.

Adverse Reactions

Dermatologic: Rash, pruritus, erythema, urticaria

Hematologic: Thrombocytosis

Respiratory: Wheezing

Miscellaneous: Allergic reactions, anaphylactoid reactions

Drug Interactions

Metabolism/Transport Effects None known.

Avoid Concomitant Use

Avoid concomitant use of Leucovorin Calcium with any of the following: Raltitrexed; Trimethoprim

Increased Effect/Toxicity

Leucovorin Calcium may increase the levels/effects of: Capecitabine; Fluorouracil (Systemic); Fluorouracil (Topical); Tegafur

Decreased Effect

Leucovorin Calcium may decrease the levels/effects of: Fosphenytoin; PHENobarbital; Phenytoin; Primidone; Raltitrexed; Trimethoprim

The levels/effects of Leucovorin Calcium may be decreased by: Glucarpidase

Preparation for Administration

Powder for injection: Reconstitute with SWFI or BWFI; dilute in D_5W or NS for infusion. When doses >10 mg/m^2 are required, reconstitute using sterile water for injection, not a solution containing benzyl alcohol.

For methanol toxicity, dilute in D_5W (Barceloux, 2002).

Storage/Stability

Powder for injection: Store at room temperature of 25°C (77°F). Protect from light. Solutions reconstituted with bacteriostatic water for injection U.S.P., must be used within 7 days. Solutions reconstituted with SWFI must be used immediately. Parenteral admixture is stable for 24 hours stored at room temperature (25°C) and for 4 days when stored under refrigeration (4°C).

Solution for injection: Prior to dilution, store vials under refrigeration at 2°C to 8°C (36°F to 46°F). Protect from light.

Tablet: Store at room temperature of 15°C to 30°C (59°F to 86°F).

Mechanism of Action A reduced form of folic acid, leucovorin supplies the necessary cofactor blocked by methotrexate. Leucovorin actively competes with methotrexate for transport sites, displaces methotrexate from intracellular binding sites, and restores active folate stores required for DNA/RNA synthesis. Stabilizes the binding of 5-dUMP and thymidylate synthetase, enhancing the activity of fluorouracil. When administered with pyrimethamine for the treatment of opportunistic infections, leucovorin reduces the risk for hematologic toxicity (DHHS, 2013).

Methanol toxicity treatment: Formic acid (methanol's toxic metabolite) is normally metabolized to carbon dioxide and water by 10-formyltetrahydrofolate dehydrogenase after being bound to tetrahydrofolate. Administering a source of tetrahydrofolate may aid the body in eliminating formic acid (Barceloux, 2002).

Pharmacodynamics/Kinetics

Absorption: Oral, IM: Well absorbed

Metabolism: Intestinal mucosa and hepatically to 5-methyltetrahydrofolate (5MTHF; active)

Bioavailability: Saturable at oral doses >25 mg; 25 mg (97%), 50 mg (75%), 100 mg (37%)

Half-life elimination: ~4-8 hours

Time to peak: Oral: ~2 hours; IV: Total folates: 10 minutes; 5MTHF: ~1 hour

Excretion: Urine (primarily); feces

Dosage

Colorectal cancer (also refer to Combination Regimens): Adults: IV: 200 mg/m^2/day over at least 3 minutes for 5 days every 4 weeks for 2 cycles, then every 4 to 5 weeks (in combination with fluorouracil) **or** 20 mg/m^2/day for 5 days every 4 weeks for 2 cycles, then every 4 to 5 weeks (in combination with fluorouracil)

Folic acid antagonist (eg, trimethoprim, pyrimethamine) overdose: Children and Adults: Oral: 5 to 15 mg once daily

Folate-deficient megaloblastic anemia: Children and Adults: IM, IV: ≤1 mg once daily

High-dose methotrexate-rescue: Children and Adults: Initial: Oral, IM, IV: 15 mg (~10 mg/m^2); start 24 hours after beginning methotrexate infusion; continue every 6 hours for 10 doses, until methotrexate level is <0.05 micromolar. Adjust dose as follows:

Normal methotrexate elimination (serum methotrexate level ~10 micromolar at 24 hours after administration, 1 micromolar at 48 hours, and <0.2 micromolar at 72 hours): Oral, IM, IV: 15 mg every 6 hours for 60 hours (10 doses) beginning 24 hours after the start of methotrexate infusion Delayed late methotrexate elimination (serum methotrexate level remaining >0.2 micromolar at 72 hours and >0.05 micromolar at 96 hours after administration): Continue leucovorin calcium 15 mg (oral, IM, or IV) every 6 hours until methotrexate level is <0.05 micromolar

Delayed early methotrexate elimination and/or acute renal injury (serum methotrexate level ≥50 micromolar at 24 hours, or ≥5 micromolar at 48 hours, or a doubling of serum creatinine level at 24 hours after methotrexate administration): IV: 150 mg every 3 hours until methotrexate level is <1 micromolar, then 15 mg every 3 hours until methotrexate level is <0.05 micromolar

High-dose methotrexate overexposure: Children and Adults: Leucovorin nomogram dosing for high-dose methotrexate overexposure (off-label dosing; generalized dosing derived from reference nomogram figures, refer to each reference [Bleyer, 1978; Bleyer, 1981; Widemann, 2006] or institution-specific nomogram for details):

At 24 hours:

For methotrexate levels of ≥100 micromolar at ~24 hours, leucovorin is initially dosed at 1000 mg/m^2 every 6 hours

For methotrexate levels of ≥10 to <100 micromolar at 24 hours, leucovorin is initially dosed at 100 mg/m^2 every 3 or 6 hours

For methotrexate levels of ~1 to 10 micromolar at 24 hours, leucovorin is initially dosed at 10 mg/m^2 every 3 or 6 hours

At 48 hours:

For methotrexate levels of ≥100 micromolar at 48 hours, leucovorin is dosed at 1000 mg/m^2 every 6 hours

For methotrexate levels of ≥10 to <100 micromolar at 48 hours, leucovorin is dosed at 100 mg/m^2 every 3 hours

For methotrexate levels of ~1 to 10 micromolar at 48 hours, leucovorin is dosed at 100 mg/m^2 every 6 hours **or** 10 to 100 mg/m^2 every 3 hours

At 72 hours:

For methotrexate levels of ≥10 micromolar at 72 hours, leucovorin is dosed at 100 to 1000 mg/m^2 every 3 to 6 hours

For methotrexate levels of ~1 to 10 micromolar at 72 hours, leucovorin is dosed at 10 to 100 mg/m^2 every 3 hours

For methotrexate levels of ~0.1 to 1 micromolar at 72 hours, leucovorin is dosed at 10 mg/m^2 every 3 to 6 hours

If serum creatinine is increased more than 50% above baseline, increase the standard leucovorin dose to 100 mg/m^2 every 3 hours, then adjust according to methotrexate levels above.

Follow methotrexate levels daily, leucovorin may be discontinued when methotrexate level is <0.1 micromolar

Methotrexate overdose (inadvertent): Children and Adults (begin as soon as possible after overdose): Oral, IM, IV: 10 mg/m^2 every 6 hours until the methotrexate level is <0.01 micromolar. If serum creatinine is increased more than 50% above baseline 24 hours after methotrexate administration, if 24 hour methotrexate level is >5 micromolar, or if 48 hour methotrexate level is >0.9 micromolar, increase leucovorin dose to 100 mg/m^2 IV every 3 hours until the methotrexate level is <0.01 micromolar.

Do not administer leucovorin intrathecally; the use of intrathecal leucovorin is not advised (Jardine, 1996; Smith, 2008).

Cofactor therapy in methanol toxicity (off-label use): Children, Adolescents, and Adults: IV: 1 mg/kg (maximum dose: 50 mg) over 30 to 60 minutes every 4 to 6 hours. Therapy should continue until methanol and formic acid have been completely eliminated (Barceloux, 2002)

Pemetrexed toxicity (off-label dose): Adults: IV: 100 mg/m^2 once, followed by 50 mg/m^2 every 6 hours for 8 days (used in clinical trial for CTC grade 4 leukopenia ≥3 days; CTC grade 4 neutropenia ≥3 days; immediately for CTC grade 4 thrombocytopenia, bleeding associated with grade 3 thrombocytopenia, or grade 3 or 4 mucositis) (Alimta [prescribing information], 2013)

Prevention of pyrimethamine hematologic toxicity in HIV-positive patients (off-label uses; CDC, 2009):

Infants and Children >1 month of age: **Note:** Leucovorin should continue for 1 week after pyrimethamine is discontinued.

Toxoplasmosis (*Toxoplasma gondii*):

Primary prophylaxis: Oral: 5 mg once every 3 days (in combination with pyrimethamine [with either dapsone or atovaquone])

Secondary prophylaxis: Oral: 5 mg once every 3 days (in combination with pyrimethamine [with either sulfadiazine, atovaquone, or clindamycin])

Treatment (congenital): Oral or IM: 10 mg with every pyrimethamine dose (in combination with either sulfadiazine or clindamycin); treatment duration: 12 months

Treatment (acquired): Acute induction: Oral: 10 to 25 mg once daily (in combination with pyrimethamine [with either sulfadiazine, clindamycin, or atovaquone]) for ≥6 weeks

Adults: Oral:

Isosporiasis (*Isospora belli*):

Treatment: 10 to 25 mg once daily (in combination with pyrimethamine)

Chronic maintenance (secondary prophylaxis): 5 to 10 mg once daily (in combination with pyrimethamine)

Pneumocystis jirovecii pneumonia (PCP): Prophylaxis (primary and secondary): 25 mg once weekly (in combination with pyrimethamine [with dapsone]) **or** 10 mg once daily (in combination with pyrimethamine [with atovaquone])

Toxoplasmosis (*Toxoplasma gondii*):

Primary prophylaxis: 25 mg once weekly (in combination with pyrimethamine [with dapsone]) **or** 10 mg once daily (in combination with pyrimethamine [with atovaquone])

Treatment: 10 to 25 mg once daily (in combination with pyrimethamine [with either sulfadiazine, clindamycin, atovaquone, or azithromycin]). **Note:** May increase leucovorin to 50 to 100 mg/day in divided doses in cases of pyrimethamine toxicity (rash, nausea, bone marrow suppression).

Chronic maintenance (secondary prophylaxis): 10 to 25 mg once daily (in combination with pyrimethamine [with either sulfadiazine or clindamycin]) **or** 10 mg once daily (in combination with pyrimethamine [with atovaquone])

Dosage adjustment in renal impairment: There are no dosage adjustments provided in manufacturer's labeling.

Dosage adjustment in hepatic impairment: There are no dosage adjustments provided in manufacturer's labeling.

Dietary Considerations Solutions for injection contain calcium 0.004 mEq per leucovorin 1 mg

Administration Due to calcium content, do not administer IV solutions at a rate >160 mg/minute; not intended for intrathecal use.

Refer to individual protocols. Should be administered IM, IV push, or IV infusion (15 minutes to 2 hours). Leucovorin should not be administered concurrently with methotrexate. It is commonly initiated 24 hours after the start of methotrexate. Toxicity to normal tissues may be irreversible if leucovorin is not initiated by ~40 hours after the start of methotrexate.

As a rescue after folate antagonists: Administer by IV bolus, IM, or orally.

Do not administer orally in the presence of nausea or vomiting. Doses >25 mg should be administered parenterally.

Combination therapy with fluorouracil: Fluorouracil is usually given after, or at the midpoint, of the leucovorin infusion. Leucovorin is usually administered by IV bolus injection or short (10-120 minutes) IV infusion. Other administration schedules have been used; refer to individual protocols.

For the treatment of methanol toxicity, infuse over 30 to 60 minutes (Barceloux, 2002)

Monitoring Parameters

High-dose methotrexate therapy: Plasma methotrexate concentration; leucovorin is continued until the plasma methotrexate level <0.05 micromolar. With 4- to 6-hour high-dose methotrexate infusions, plasma drug values in excess of 50 and 1 micromolar at 24 and 48 hours after starting the infusion, respectively, are often predictive of delayed methotrexate clearance.

Fluorouracil therapy: CBC with differential and platelets, liver function tests, electrolytes

Dosage Forms

Solution, Injection:

Generic: 300 mg/30 mL (30 mL)

Solution Reconstituted, Injection:

Generic: 100 mg (1 ea); 200 mg (1 ea); 350 mg (1 ea); 500 mg (1 ea)

Solution Reconstituted, Injection [preservative free]:

Generic: 50 mg (1 ea); 100 mg (1 ea); 200 mg (1 ea); 350 mg (1 ea)

Tablet, Oral:

Generic: 5 mg, 10 mg, 15 mg, 25 mg

Extemporaneous Preparations A 5 mg/mL oral suspension may be prepared with tablets, Cologel, and a 2:1 mixture of simple syrup and wild cherry syrup. Crush twenty-four 25 mg tablets in a glass mortar and reduce to a fine powder; transfer powder to amber bottle. Add 30 mL Cologel and shake mixture thoroughly. Add a quantity of syrup mixture sufficient to make 120 mL. Label "shake well" and "refrigerate". Stable for 28 days refrigerated.

Lam MS. Extemporaneous Compounding of Oral Liquid Dosage Formulations and Alternative Drug Delivery Methods for Anticancer Drugs. *Pharmacotherapy*. 2011;31(2):164-192.

◆ **Leucovorin Calcium Injection (Can)** *see* Leucovorin Calcium *on page 1183*

◆ **Leucovorin Calcium Injection USP (Can)** *see* Leucovorin Calcium *on page 1183*

◆ **Leukeran** *see* Chlorambucil *on page 419*

◆ **Leukeran® (Can)** *see* Chlorambucil *on page 419*

◆ **Leukine** *see* Sargramostim *on page 1865*

Leuprolide (loo PROE lide)

Brand Names: U.S. Eligard; Lupron Depot; Lupron Depot-Ped

Brand Names: Canada Eligard; Lupron; Lupron Depot

Index Terms Abbott-43818; Leuprolide Acetate; Leuprorelin Acetate; TAP-144

Pharmacologic Category Antineoplastic Agent, Gonadotropin-Releasing Hormone Agonist; Gonadotropin Releasing Hormone Agonist

Use

Central precocious puberty: Treatment of children with central precocious puberty

Endometriosis: Management of endometriosis, including pain relief and reduction of endometriotic lesions

Prostate cancer: Palliative treatment of advanced prostate cancer

Uterine leiomyomata (fibroids): Treatment of anemia caused by uterine leiomyomata (fibroids)

Pregnancy Risk Factor X

Pregnancy Considerations Adverse events were observed in animal reproduction studies. Pregnancy must be excluded prior to the start of treatment. Although leuprolide usually inhibits ovulation and stops menstruation, contraception is not ensured and a nonhormonal contraceptive should be used. Use is contraindicated in pregnant women.

Breast-Feeding Considerations It is not known if leuprolide is excreted into breast milk; use is contraindicated in nursing women.

Contraindications

Hypersensitivity to leuprolide, GnRH, GnRH-agonist analogs, or any component of the formulation; undiagnosed abnormal vaginal bleeding (Lupron Depot 3.75 mg [monthly] and Lupron Depot 11.25 mg [3-month]); pregnancy; breast-feeding (Lupron Depot 3.75 mg [monthly] and Lupron Depot 11.25 mg [3-month])

Lupron Depot 22.5 mg, 30 mg, and 45 mg are also not indicated for use in women

Warnings/Precautions Hazardous agent - use appropriate precautions for handling and disposal (NIOSH 2014 [group 1]). Transient increases in testosterone serum levels (~50% above baseline) occur at the start of treatment. Androgen-deprivation therapy (ADT) may increase the risk for cardiovascular disease (Levine, 2010); sudden cardiac death and stroke have been reported in men receiving GnRH agonists; ADT may prolong the QT/QTc interval; consider the benefits of ADT versus the risk for QT prolongation in patients with a history of QTc prolongation, congenital long QT syndrome, heart failure, frequent electrolyte abnormalities, and in patients with medications known to prolong the QT interval, or with preexisting cardiac disease. Consider periodic monitoring of electrocardiograms and electrolytes in at-risk patients. Tumor flare, bone pain, neuropathy, urinary tract obstruction, and spinal cord compression have been reported when used for prostate cancer; closely observe patients for weakness, paresthesias, hematuria, and urinary tract obstruction in first few weeks of therapy. Observe patients with metastatic vertebral lesions or urinary obstruction closely. Exacerbation of endometriosis or uterine leiomyomata may occur initially. Decreased bone density has been reported when used for ≥6 months; use caution in patients with additional risk factors for bone loss (eg, chronic alcohol use, corticosteroid therapy). In patients with prostate cancer, androgen deprivation therapy may increase the risk for cardiovascular disease, diabetes, insulin resistance, obesity, alterations in lipids, and fractures; monitor as clinically necessary. Use caution in patients with a history of psychiatric illness; alteration in mood, memory impairment, and depression have been associated with use. Rare cases of pituitary apoplexy (frequently secondary to pituitary adenoma) have been observed with GnRH agonist administration (onset from 1 hour to usually <2 weeks); may present as sudden headache, vomiting, visual or mental status changes, and infrequently cardiovascular collapse; immediate medical attention required. Convulsions have been observed in postmarketing reports; patients affected included both those with and without a history of cerebrovascular disorders, central nervous system anomalies or tumors, epilepsy, seizures, and those on concomitant medications which may lower the seizure threshold. If seizures occur, manage accordingly. Females treated for precocious puberty may experience menses or spotting during the first 2 months of treatment; notify healthcare provider if bleeding continues after the second month.

Benzyl alcohol and derivatives: Some dosage forms may contain benzyl alcohol; large amounts of benzyl alcohol (≥99 mg/kg/day) have been associated with a potentially fatal toxicity ("gasping syndrome") in neonates; the "gasping syndrome" consists of metabolic acidosis, respiratory distress, gasping respirations, CNS dysfunction (including convulsions, intracranial hemorrhage), hypotension, and cardiovascular collapse (AAP, 1997; CDC, 1982); some data suggests that benzoate displaces bilirubin from protein binding sites (Ahlfors, 2001); avoid or use dosage forms containing benzyl alcohol with caution in neonates.

Some dosage forms may contain polysorbate 80 (also known as Tweens). Hypersensitivity reactions, usually a delayed reaction, have been reported following exposure to pharmaceutical products containing polysorbate 80 in certain individuals (Isaksson, 2002; Lucente 2000; Shelley, 1995). Thrombocytopenia, ascites, pulmonary deterioration, and renal and hepatic failure have been reported in premature neonates after receiving parenteral products containing polysorbate 80 (Alade, 1986; CDC, 1984). See manufacturer's labeling.

Vehicle used in depot injectable formulations (polylactide-co-glycolide microspheres) has rarely been associated with retinal artery occlusion in patients with abnormal arteriovenous anastomosis. Due to different release properties, combinations of dosage forms or fractions of dosage forms should not be interchanged.

Adverse Reactions

Children (based on 1-month and 3-month pediatric formulations combined)

Cardiovascular: Vasodilation

Central nervous system: Emotional lability, headache, mood changes, pain

Dermatologic: Acne vulgaris, seborrhea, skin rash (including erythema multiforme)

Endocrine & metabolic: Weight gain

Genitourinary: Vaginal discharge, vaginal hemorrhage, vaginitis

Local: Injection site reaction, pain at injection site

Rare but important or life-threatening: Abnormal gait, alopecia, arthralgia, asthma, body odor, bradycardia, cervix disease, decreased visual acuity, depression, dysmenorrhea, dysphagia, epistaxis, excessive crying, feminization, gingivitis, goiter, growth suppression, gynecomastia, hirsutism, hyperhidrosis, hyperkinesia, hypersensitivity reaction, hypertension, infection, leukoderma, myopathy, obesity, peripheral edema, personality disorder, precocious puberty, purpura, skin striae, syncope, urinary incontinence

Adults: Note: For prostate cancer treatment, an initial rise in serum testosterone concentrations may cause "tumor flare" or worsening of symptoms, including bone pain, neuropathy, hematuria, or ureteral or bladder outlet obstruction during the first 2 weeks. Similarly, an initial increase in estradiol levels, with a temporary worsening of symptoms, may occur in women treated with leuprolide.

Delayed release formulations:

Cardiovascular: Angina pectoris, atrial fibrillation, bradycardia, cardiac arrhythmia, cardiac failure, edema, hypertension, hypotension, palpitations, syncope, tachycardia, thrombophlebitis (deep)

Central nervous system: Agitation, anxiety, confusion, delusions, dementia, depression, dizziness, fatigue, fever, headache, insomnia, nervousness, neuropathy, ostealgia, pain, paralysis, paresthesia, seizure

Dermatologic: Acne vulgaris, allergic skin reaction, alopecia, cellulitis, diaphoresis, hair disease, pruritus, skin rash

Endocrine & metabolic: Decreased libido, decreased serum bicarbonate, dehydration, gynecomastia, hirsutism, hot flash, hypercholesterolemia, hyperglycemia, hyperlipidemia, hyperuricemia, hypoalbuminemia, hypocholesterolemia, hypoproteinemia, increased lactate dehydrogenase, increased prostatic acid phosphatase, menstrual disorder, weight changes

Gastrointestinal: Anorexia, change in bowel habits, constipation, diarrhea, dysphagia, eruction, gastric ulcer, gastroenteritis, gastrointestinal disease, gastrointestinal hemorrhage, intestinal obstruction, nausea and vomiting, peptic ulcer

Genitourinary: Balanitis, bladder spasm, dysuria, erectile dysfunction, genitourinary complaint, hematuria, impotence, lactation, mastalgia, nocturia, penile disease, testicular atrophy, testicular disease, testicular pain, urinary incontinence, urinary retention, urinary tract infection, urinary urgency, vaginitis

Hematologic & oncologic: Anemia, bruise, change in platelet count (increased), decreased hemocrit, decreased hemoglobin, decreased prostatic acid phosphatase, ecchymoses, eosinophilia, leukopenia, lymphadenopathy, neoplasm

Hepatic: Abnormal hepatic function tests, hepatomegaly, increased serum AST, prolonged partial thromboplastin time, prolonged prothrombin time

Hypersensitivity: Hypersensitivity reaction

Infection: Infection

Local: Burning sensation at injection site (transient), erythema at injection site, injection site reaction, pain at injection site

Neuromuscular & skeletal: Arthralgia, arthropathy, myalgia, neuromuscular disease, pathological fracture, weakness

Renal: Decreased urine specific gravity, increased blood urea nitrogen, increased serum creatinine, increased urine specific gravity, polyuria

Respiratory: Cough, dyspnea, emphysema, epistaxis, flu-like symptoms, hemoptysis, increased bronchial secretions, pleural effusion, pulmonary edema, respiratory tract disease

Miscellaneous: Fever

Immediate release formulation:

Cardiovascular: Angina pectoris, cardiac arrhythmia, cardiac failure, ECG changes, heart murmur, hypertension, myocardial infarction, peripheral edema, pulmonary embolism, syncope, thrombophlebitis

Central nervous system: Anxiety, depression, dizziness, headache, insomnia, fatigue, fever, nervousness, ostealgia, pain, peripheral neuropathy

Endocrine & metabolic: decreased libido, diabetes mellitus, goiter, gynecomastia, hot flash, hypercalcemia, hypoglycemia

Dermatologic: Alopecia, dermatitis, hyperpigmentation, pruritus, skin lesion

Gastrointestinal: Anorexia, constipation, diarrhea, dysphagia, diarrhea, dysphagia, gastrointestinal hemorrhage, nausea and vomiting, peptic ulcer, rectal polyps

Genitourinary: Bladder spasm, decreased testicular size, dysuria, hematuria, impotence, incontinence, mastalgia, testicular pain, urinary frequency, urinary tract infection, urinary tract obstruction

Hematologic & oncologic: Anemia, bruise

Infection: Infection

Local: Injection site reaction

Neuromuscular & skeletal: Weakness

Ophthalmic: Blurred vision

Renal: Hematuria, increased blood urea nitrogen, increased serum creatinine

Respiratory: Cough, dyspnea, pneumonia, pulmonary fibrosis

Miscellaneous: Fever, inflammation

Children and Adults: *Any formulations:* Rare but important or life-threatening: Abscess at injection site, anaphylaxis, anaphylactoid reaction, asthma, bone fracture (spine), cerebrovascular accident, convulsions, coronary artery disease, decreased white blood cell count, diabetes mellitus, fibromyalgia syndrome (arthralgia/myalgia, headaches, GI distress), hemoptysis, hepatic injury, hepatic insufficiency, hepatotoxicity, hyperuricemia, hypokalemia, hypoproteinemia, induration at injection site, interstitial pulmonary disease, leukocytosis, myocardial infarction, osteopenia, paralysis, penile swelling, peripheral neuropathy, pituitary apoplexy (cardiovascular collapse, mental status altered, ophthalmoplegia, sudden headache, visual changes, vomiting), prolonged QT interval on ECG, prostate pain, pulmonary embolism, pulmonary infiltrates, retroperitoneal fibrosis (pelvic), seizure, skin photosensitivity, suicidal ideation (rare), tenosynovitis (symptoms), thrombocytopenia, transient ischemic attacks

Drug Interactions

Metabolism/Transport Effects None known.

Avoid Concomitant Use

Avoid concomitant use of Leuprolide with any of the following: Corifollitropin Alfa; Highest Risk QTc-Prolonging Agents; Indium 111 Capromab Pendetide; Ivabradine; Mifepristone

Increased Effect/Toxicity

Leuprolide may increase the levels/effects of: Corifollitropin Alfa; Highest Risk QTc-Prolonging Agents; Moderate Risk QTc-Prolonging Agents

The levels/effects of Leuprolide may be increased by: Ivabradine; Mifepristone; QTc-Prolonging Agents (Indeterminate Risk and Risk Modifying)

Decreased Effect

Leuprolide may decrease the levels/effects of: Antidiabetic Agents; Indium 111 Capromab Pendetide

Preparation for Administration Hazardous agent; use appropriate precautions for handling and disposal (NIOSH 2014 [group 1]).

Eligard: Packaged in two syringes; one contains the Atrigel polymer system and the second contains leuprolide acetate powder; follow package instructions for mixing

Lupron Depot, Lupron Depot-Ped: Reconstitute only with diluent provided

Storage/Stability

Eligard: Store at 2°C to 8°C (36°F to 46°C). Allow to reach room temperature prior to using; once mixed, must be administered within 30 minutes.

Lupron Depot, Lupron Depot-Ped: Store at room temperature of 25°C (77°F); excursions permitted to 15°C to 30°C (59°F to 86°F). Upon reconstitution, the suspension does not contain a preservative and should be used immediately; discard if not used within 2 hours.

Leuprolide acetate 5 mg/mL solution: Store at 20°C to 25°C (68°F to 77°F); excursions permitted to 15°C to 30°C (59°F to 86°F). Protect from light and store vial in carton until use. Do not freeze.

Mechanism of Action Leuprolide, is an agonist of gonadotropin releasing hormone (GnRH). Acting as a potent inhibitor of gonadotropin secretion; continuous administration results in suppression of ovarian and testicular steroidogenesis due to decreased levels of LH and FSH with subsequent decrease in testosterone (male) and estrogen (female) levels. In males, testosterone levels are reduced to below castrate levels. Leuprolide may also have a direct inhibitory effect on the testes, and act by a different mechanism not directly related to reduction in serum testosterone.

Pharmacodynamics/Kinetics

Onset of action: Following transient increase, testosterone suppression occurs in ~2-4 weeks of continued therapy

Distribution: Males: V_d: 27 L

Protein binding: 43% to 49%

Metabolism: Major metabolite, pentapeptide (M-1)

Bioavailability: SubQ: 94%

Excretion: Urine (<5% as parent and major metabolite)

Dosage

Children: Precocious puberty (consider discontinuing by age 11 for females and by age 12 for males):

IM:

Lupron Depot-Ped (monthly):

≤25 kg: 7.5 mg every month

>25-37.5 kg: 11.25 mg every month

>37.5 kg: 15 mg every month

Titrate dose upward in increments of 3.75 mg every 4 weeks if down-regulation is not achieved.

Lupron Depot-Ped (3 month): 11.25 mg or 30 mg every 12 weeks

SubQ (leuprolide acetate 5 mg/mL solution): Initial: 50 mcg/kg/day; titrate dose upward by 10 mcg/kg/day if down-regulation is not achieved. **Note:** Higher mg/kg doses may be required in younger children.

Adults:

Prostate cancer, advanced:

IM:

Lupron Depot 7.5 mg (monthly): 7.5 mg every month **or**

Lupron Depot 22.5 mg (3 month): 22.5 mg every 12 weeks **or**

Lupron Depot 30 mg (4 month): 30 mg every 16 weeks **or**

Lupron Depot 45 mg (6 month): 45 mg every 24 weeks

SubQ:

Eligard: 7.5 mg monthly **or** 22.5 mg every 3 months **or** 30 mg every 4 months **or** 45 mg every 6 months

Leuprolide acetate 5 mg/mL solution: 1 mg daily

Endometriosis: IM: Initial therapy may be with leuprolide alone or in combination with norethindrone; if retreatment for an additional 6 months is necessary, concomitant norethindrone should be used. Retreatment is not recommended for longer than one additional 6-month course.

Lupron Depot: 3.75 mg every month for up to 6 months **or**

Lupron Depot-3 month: 11.25 mg every 3 months for up to 2 doses (6 months total duration of treatment)

Uterine leiomyomata (fibroids): IM (in combination with iron):

Lupron Depot: 3.75 mg every month for up to 3 months **or**

Lupron Depot-3 month: 11.25 mg as a single injection

Breast cancer, premenopausal ovarian ablation (off-label use): IM:

Lupron Depot: 3.75 mg every 28 days for up to 24 months (Boccardo, 1999) **or**

Lupron Depot-3 month: 11.25 mg every 3 months for up to 24 months (Boccardo, 1999; Schmid, 2007)

Adults: Males: Treatment of paraphilia/hypersexuality (off-label use; Guay, 2009; Reilly, 2000):

Note: May cause an initial increase in androgen concentrations which may be treated with an antiandrogen (eg, flutamide, cyproterone) for 1-2 months (Guay, 2009). Avoid use in patients with osteoporosis or active pituitary pathology.

SubQ: Test dose: 1 mg (observe for hypersensitivity)

Depot IM: 3.75-7.5 mg monthly

Dosage adjustment in renal impairment: There are no dosage adjustments provided in the manufacturer's labeling (has not been studied).

Dosage adjustment in hepatic impairment: There are no dosage adjustments provided in the manufacturer's labeling (has not been studied).

Administration

Do not use concurrently a fractional dose of the 3-, 4-, or 6-month depot formulation, or a combination of doses of the monthly depot formulation or any depot formulation due to different release characteristics. Do not use a combination of syringes to achieve a particular dose.

IM: Lupron Depot, Lupron Depot-Ped: Administer as a single injection into the gluteal area, anterior thigh, or deltoid. Vary injection site periodically

SubQ:

Eligard: Vary injection site; choose site with adequate subcutaneous tissue (eg, upper or mid-abdomen, upper buttocks); avoid areas that may be compressed or rubbed (eg, belt or waistband)

Leuprolide acetate 5 mg/mL solution: Vary injection site; if an alternate syringe from the syringe provided is required, insulin syringes should be used

Hazardous agent; use appropriate precautions for handling and disposal (NIOSH 2014 [group 1]).

Monitoring Parameters Bone mineral density

Precocious puberty: GnRH testing (blood LH and FSH levels), measurement of height and bone age every 6-12 months, testosterone in males and estradiol in females (IM [monthly] and SubQ formulations: 1-2 months after initiation of therapy or with dosage change; IM [3 month] formulation: 2-3 months after initiation of therapy, month 6, and as clinically indicated thereafter); Tanner staging

Prostatic cancer: LH and FSH levels, serum testosterone (~4 weeks after initiation of therapy), PSA; weakness, paresthesias, and urinary tract obstruction in first few weeks of therapy. Screen for diabetes (blood glucose and HbA_{1c}) and cardiovascular risk prior to initiating and periodically during treatment. Consider periodic monitoring of electrocardiograms and electrolytes.

Treatment of paraphilia/hypersexuality (off-label use; Reilly, 2000): CBC (baseline, monthly for 4 months then every 6 months); serum testosterone (baseline, monthly for 4 months then every 6 months); serum LH (baseline and every 6 months), FSH (baseline), serum BUN and creatinine (baseline and every 6 months); bone density (baseline and yearly); ECG (baseline)

Additional Information

Eligard Atrigel: A nongelatin-based, biodegradable, polymer matrix

Oncology Comment: Guidelines from the American Society of Clinical Oncology (ASCO) for hormonal management of advanced prostate cancer which is androgen-sensitive (Loblaw, 2007) recommend either orchiectomy or luteinizing hormone-releasing hormone (LHRH) agonists as initial treatment for androgen deprivation.

Dosage Forms

Kit, Injection:

Generic: 1 mg/0.2 mL

Kit, Intramuscular:

Lupron Depot: 7.5 mg, 45 mg

Kit, Intramuscular [preservative free]:
Lupron Depot: 3.75 mg, 11.25 mg, 22.5 mg, 30 mg
Lupron Depot-Ped: 7.5 mg, 11.25 mg, 15 mg, 30 mg (Ped), 11.25 mg (Ped)
Kit, Subcutaneous:
Eligard: 7.5 mg, 22.5 mg, 30 mg, 45 mg

◆ **Leuprolide Acetate** *see* Leuprolide *on page 1186*

◆ **Leuprolide Acetate and Norethindrone Acetate** *see* Leuprolide and Norethindrone *on page 1189*

Leuprolide and Norethindrone
(loo PROE lide & nor eth IN drone)

Brand Names: U.S. Lupaneta Pack
Index Terms Leuprolide Acetate and Norethindrone Acetate; Norethindrone and Leuprolide
Pharmacologic Category Gonadotropin Releasing Hormone Agonist; Progestin
Use Endometriosis: Management of initial and recurrent painful symptoms of endometriosis
Pregnancy Risk Factor X
Dosage Endometriosis: Adults: Females: **Note:** Treatment consists of an oral norethindrone tablet used in conjunction with an IM leuprolide injection. The initial therapy should be limited to 6 months duration; a single retreatment of not more than 6 additional months may be administered if symptoms recur. Maximum total duration of therapy is 12 months.
1 month:
Injection: IM: Leuprolide 3.75 mg as a single dose administered by healthcare provider once every month for up to 6 doses (maximum initial therapy: 6 months; maximum cumulative therapy: 12 months)
Tablet: Oral: Norethindrone 5 mg once daily for up to 6 months (maximum initial therapy: 6 months; maximum cumulative therapy: 12 months)
3 month:
Injection: IM: Leuprolide 11.25 mg as a single dose administered by healthcare provider once every 3 months for up to 2 doses (maximum initial therapy: 6 months; maximum cumulative therapy: 12 months)
Tablet: Oral: Norethindrone 5 mg once daily for up to 6 months (maximum initial therapy: 6 months; maximum cumulative therapy: 12 months)

Dosage adjustment in renal Impairment: No dosage adjustment provided in manufacturer's labeling (has not been studied).
Dosage adjustment in hepatic Impairment: No dosage adjustment provided in manufacturer's labeling (has not been studied). Use is contraindicated with hepatic tumors or disease.
Additional Information Complete prescribing information should be consulted for additional detail.
Dosage Forms
Kit, Combination:
Lupaneta Pack: 1-month kit: leuprolide acetate 3.75 mg depot suspension for injection (1) and norethindrone acetate 5 mg oral tablets (30), 3-month kit: leuprolide acetate 11.25 mg depot suspension for injection (1) and norethindrone acetate 5 mg oral tablets (90)

◆ **Leuprorelin Acetate** *see* Leuprolide *on page 1186*

◆ **Leurocristine Sulfate** *see* VinCRIStine *on page 2163*

◆ **Leustatin** *see* Cladribine *on page 455*

Levalbuterol (leve al BYOO ter ole)

Brand Names: U.S. Xopenex; Xopenex Concentrate; Xopenex HFA
Index Terms Levalbuterol Hydrochloride; Levalbuterol Tartrate; Levosalbutamol; R-albuterol
Pharmacologic Category $Beta_2$ Agonist
Use Bronchospasm: Treatment or prevention of bronchospasm in patients with reversible obstructive airway disease
Pregnancy Risk Factor C
Pregnancy Considerations Teratogenic effects were not observed in animal reproduction studies; however, racemic albuterol was teratogenic in some species. Beta-agonists may interfere with uterine contractility if administered during labor.

Uncontrolled asthma is associated with adverse events on pregnancy (increased risk of perinatal mortality, pre-eclampsia, preterm birth, low birth weight infants). Other $beta_2$-receptor agonists are currently preferred for the treatment of asthma during pregnancy (NAEPP, 2005).
Breast-Feeding Considerations It is not known whether levalbuterol is excreted in human milk. Although breast-feeding is not recommended by the manufacturer, the use of $beta_2$-receptor agonists are not considered a contraindication to breast-feeding (NAEPP, 2005).
Contraindications Hypersensitivity to levalbuterol, albuterol, or any component of the formulation
Warnings/Precautions Optimize anti-inflammatory treatment before initiating maintenance treatment with levalbuterol. Do not use as a component of chronic therapy without an anti-inflammatory agent. Only the mildest form of asthma (Step 1 and/or exercise-induced) would not require concurrent use based upon asthma guidelines (NAEPP, 2007). Patient must be instructed to seek medical attention in cases where acute symptoms are not relieved or a previous level of response is diminished. The need to increase frequency of use may indicate deterioration of asthma, and treatment must not be delayed.

Use caution in patients with cardiovascular disease (arrhythmia or hypertension or HF), convulsive disorders, diabetes, glaucoma, hyperthyroidism, or hypokalemia. Beta-agonists may cause elevation in blood pressure, heart rate, and result in CNS stimulation/excitation. $Beta_2$-agonists may increase risk of arrhythmia, increase serum glucose, or decrease serum potassium.

Immediate hypersensitivity reactions (urticaria, angioedema, rash, bronchospasm, anaphylaxis, oropharyngeal edema) have been reported. Do not exceed recommended dose; serious adverse events including fatalities, have been associated with excessive use of inhaled sympathomimetics. Rarely, paradoxical bronchospasm may occur with use of inhaled bronchodilating agents; this should be distinguished from inadequate response. Potentially significant interactions may exist, requiring dose or frequency adjustment, additional monitoring, and/or selection of alternative therapy.
Adverse Reactions
Cardiovascular: Tachycardia
Central nervous system: Anxiety, dizziness, headache, migraine, nervousness, weakness
Dermatologic: Rash
Endocrine & metabolic: Serum glucose increased, serum potassium decreased
Gastrointestinal: Diarrhea, dyspepsia
Neuromuscular & skeletal: Leg cramps, tremor
Respiratory: Asthma, cough, nasal edema, pharyngitis, rhinitis, sinusitis, viral infection
Miscellaneous: Accidental injury, flu-like syndrome, viral infection,
Rare but important or life-threatening: Abnormal ECG, acne, anaphylaxis, angina, angioedema, arrhythmia, atrial fibrillation, chest pain, dysmenorrhea, epistaxis, extrasystole, gastroenteritis, gastroesophageal reflux disease, hematuria, hypertension, hypoesthesia (hand),

hypokalemia, lymphadenopathy, metabolic acidosis, myalgia, nausea, oropharyngeal dryness, paresthesia, supraventricular arrhythmia, syncope, vaginal moniliasis

Note: Immediate hypersensitivity reactions have occurred (including angioedema, oropharyngeal edema, urticaria, and anaphylaxis).

Drug Interactions

Metabolism/Transport Effects None known.

Avoid Concomitant Use

Avoid concomitant use of Levalbuterol with any of the following: Beta-Blockers (Nonselective); Iobenguane I 123

Increased Effect/Toxicity

Levalbuterol may increase the levels/effects of: Atosiban; Loop Diuretics; Sympathomimetics; Thiazide Diuretics

The levels/effects of Levalbuterol may be increased by: AtoMOXetine; Cannabinoid-Containing Products; Linezolid; MAO Inhibitors; Tedizolid; Tricyclic Antidepressants

Decreased Effect

Levalbuterol may decrease the levels/effects of: Iobenguane I 123

The levels/effects of Levalbuterol may be decreased by: Beta-Blockers (Beta1 Selective); Beta-Blockers (Nonselective); Betahistine

Preparation for Administration Concentrated solution should be diluted with 2.5 mL NS prior to use.

Storage/Stability

Aerosol: Store at 20°C to 25°C (68°F to 77°F); protect from freezing and direct sunlight. Store with mouthpiece down. Discard after 200 actuations (15 g canister) or 80 actuations (8.4 g canister).

Solution for nebulization: Store in protective foil pouch at 20°C to 25°C (68°F to 77°F). Protect from light and excessive heat. Vials should be used within 2 weeks after opening protective pouch. Use within 1 week and protect from light if removed from pouch. Vials of concentrated solution should be used immediately after removing from protective pouch.

Mechanism of Action Relaxes bronchial smooth muscle by action on $beta_2$-receptors with little effect on heart rate

Pharmacodynamics/Kinetics

Onset of action (as measured by a 15% increase in FEV_1):

Aerosol: 5.5 to 10.2 minutes

Peak effect: ~77 minutes

Nebulization: 10 to 17 minutes

Peak effect: 1.5 hours

Duration (as measured by a 15% increase in FEV_1):

Aerosol: 3 to 4 hours (up to 6 hours in some patients)

Nebulization: 5 to 6 hours (up to 8 hours in some patients)

Absorption: A portion of inhaled dose is absorbed to systemic circulation

Half-life elimination: 3.3 to 4 hours

Time to peak, serum:

Aerosol: Children: 0.8 hours, Adults: 0.5 hours

Nebulization: Children: 0.3 to 0.6 hours, Adults: 0.2 hours

Dosage

Bronchospasm:

Metered-dose inhaler:

Children ≥4 years, Adolescents, and Adults: 2 puffs every 4 to 6 hours as needed; in some patients, 1 inhalation every 4 hours may be sufficient (maximum: 2 inhalations every 4 hours).

Elderly: Refer to adult dosing, starting with lowest dose; titrate cautiously

Solution for nebulization:

Asthma Guidelines (off-label; NAEPP, 2007):

Children ≤4 years: 0.31 to 1.25 mg every 4 to 6 hours as needed

Children 5 to 11 years: 0.31 to 0.63 mg every 8 hours as needed

Manufacturer's labeling:

Children 6 to 11 years: 0.31 mg 3 times daily (maximum: 0.63 mg 3 times daily)

Children ≥12 years, Adolescents, and Adults: Initial: 0.63 mg 3 times daily at intervals of 6 to 8 hours; dosage may be increased to 1.25 mg 3 times daily with close monitoring for adverse effects (maximum: 1.25 mg 3 times daily)

Elderly: Refer to adult dosing, starting with lowest dose; titrate cautiously.

Exacerbation of asthma (acute, severe) (off-label; NAEPP, 2007):

Metered-dose inhaler:

Children <12 years: 4 to 8 puffs every 20 minutes for 3 doses, then every 1 to 4 hours as needed

Children ≥12 years, Adolescents, and Adults: 4 to 8 puffs every 20 minutes for up to 4 hours, then every 1 to 4 hours as needed

Solution for nebulization:

Children <12 years: 0.075 mg/kg (minimum: 1.25 mg) every 20 minutes for 3 doses, then 0.075 to 0.15 mg/kg (maximum: 5 mg) every 1 to 4 hours as needed

Children ≥12 years, Adolescents, and Adults: 1.25 to 2.5 mg every 20 minutes for 3 doses, then 1.25 to 5 mg every 1 to 4 hours as needed

Dosage adjustment in renal impairment: There are no dosage adjustments provided in the manufacturer's labeling. Use with caution.

Dosage adjustment in hepatic impairment: There are no dosage adjustments provided in the manufacturer's labeling (has not been studied).

Administration Inhalation:

Metered-dose inhaler: Shake well before use; prime with 4 test sprays prior to first use or if inhaler has not been used for more than 3 days. Clean actuator (mouthpiece) weekly. A spacer device or valved holding chamber is recommended when using a metered-dose inhaler.

Solution for nebulization: Safety and efficacy were established when administered with the following nebulizers: PARI LC Jet, PARI LC Plus, as well as the following compressors: PARI Master, Dura-Neb 2000, and Dura-Neb 3000. Concentrated solution should be diluted prior to use. Blow-by administration is not recommended, use a mask device if patient unable to hold mouthpiece in mouth for administration.

Monitoring Parameters Asthma symptoms; FEV_1, peak flow, and/or other pulmonary function tests; heart rate, blood pressure, CNS stimulation; arterial blood gases (if condition warrants); serum potassium, serum glucose (in selected patients)

Dosage Forms Considerations Xopenex HFA 15 g canisters contain 200 inhalations and 8.4 g canisters contain 80 inhalations.

Dosage Forms

Aerosol, Inhalation:

Xopenex HFA: 45 mcg/actuation (15 g)

Nebulization Solution, Inhalation:

Xopenex: 0.63 mg/3 mL (3 mL); 1.25 mg/3 mL (3 mL)

Generic: 0.63 mg/3 mL (3 mL)

Nebulization Solution, Inhalation [preservative free]:

Xopenex: 0.31 mg/3 mL (3 mL)

Xopenex Concentrate: 1.25 mg/0.5 mL (30 ea)

Generic: 0.31 mg/3 mL (3 mL); 0.63 mg/3 mL (3 mL); 1.25 mg/3 mL (3 mL); 1.25 mg/0.5 mL (1 ea, 30 ea)

◆ **Levalbuterol Hydrochloride** *see* Levalbuterol *on page 1189*

◆ **Levalbuterol Tartrate** *see* Levalbuterol *on page 1189*

◆ **Levaquin** *see* Levofloxacin (Systemic) *on page 1197*

◆ **Levaquin in 5% Dextrose Injection (Can)** *see* Levofloxacin (Systemic) *on page 1197*

- ◆ **Levarterenol Bitartrate** *see* Norepinephrine *on page 1472*
- ◆ **Levate (Can)** *see* Amitriptyline *on page 119*
- ◆ **Levbid** *see* Hyoscyamine *on page 1026*
- ◆ **Levemir** *see* Insulin Detemir *on page 1085*
- ◆ **Levemir® (Can)** *see* Insulin Detemir *on page 1085*
- ◆ **Levemir FlexPen [DSC]** *see* Insulin Detemir *on page 1085*
- ◆ **Levemir FlexTouch** *see* Insulin Detemir *on page 1085*

LevETIRAcetam (lee va tye RA se tam)

Brand Names: U.S. Keppra; Keppra XR

Brand Names: Canada Abbott-Levetiracetam; ACT Levetiracetam; Apo-Levetiracetam; Auro-Levetiracetam; Dom-Levetiracetam; JAMP-Levetiracetam; Keppra; PHL-Levetiracetam; PMS-Levetiracetam; PRO-Levetiracetam; RAN-Levetiracetam

Pharmacologic Category Anticonvulsant, Miscellaneous

Use

Myoclonic seizures:

*Immediate-release tablets/oral solution:*Adjunctive therapy in the treatment of myoclonic seizures in adults and adolescents 12 years and older with juvenile myoclonic epilepsy.

IV: Adjunctive therapy in the treatment of myoclonic seizures in adults and adolescents 12 years and older with juvenile myoclonic epilepsy.

Partial-onset seizures:

Immediate-release tablets/oral solution: Adjunctive therapy in the treatment of partial-onset seizures in adults and children 1 month and older with epilepsy.

Extended-release tablets: Adjunctive therapy in the treatment of partial-onset seizures in adults and adolescents 12 years and older with epilepsy.

IV: Adjunctive therapy in the treatment of partial-onset seizures in adults and children 1 month and older with epilepsy.

Primary generalized tonic-clonic seizures:

Immediate-release tablets/oral solution: Adjunctive therapy in the treatment of primary generalized tonic-clonic seizures in adults and children 6 years and older with idiopathic generalized epilepsy.

IV: Adjunctive therapy in the treatment of primary generalized tonic-clonic seizures in adults and children 6 years and older with idiopathic generalized epilepsy.

Pregnancy Risk Factor C

Pregnancy Considerations Developmental toxicities were observed in animal reproduction studies. Levetiracetam crosses the placenta and can be detected in the neonate at birth. Concentrations in the umbilical cord at delivery are similar to those in the maternal plasma. Serum concentrations of levetiracetam may decrease as pregnancy progresses; monitor carefully throughout pregnancy and postpartum (Tomson, 2007).

A registry is available for women exposed to levetiracetam during pregnancy: Pregnant women may enroll themselves into the North American Antiepileptic Drug (AED) Pregnancy Registry (888-233-2334 or http://www.aedpregnancyregistry.org/).

The North American AED registry has published data collected from pregnant women taking levetiracetam monotherapy from 1997 to 2011 (n=450). Eleven major malformations were diagnosed within 12 weeks of birth. The relative risk of major malformations was not increased in comparison to women with epilepsy not taking AEDs (n=442; RR 2.2, 95% CI 0.8 to 6.4) or in comparison to women using lamotrigine monotherapy (n=1,562; RR 1.2, 95% CI 0.6 to 2.5) (Hernández-Díaz, 2012).

Breast-Feeding Considerations Levetiracetam can be detected in breast milk. Using data from 11 women collected 4-23 days after delivery, the estimated exposure of levetiracetam to the breast-feeding infant would be ~2 mg/kg/day (relative infant dose 7.9% of the weight-adjusted maternal dose). Adverse events were not reported in the nursing infants (Tomson, 2007). Due to the potential for serious adverse reactions in the nursing infant, the manufacturer recommends a decision be made whether to discontinue nursing or to discontinue the drug, taking into account the importance of treatment to the mother.

Contraindications There are no contraindications listed in the U.S. manufacturer's labeling.

Canadian labeling: Hypersensitivity to levetiracetam or any component of the formulation

Warnings/Precautions Antiepileptics are associated with an increased risk of suicidal behavior/thoughts with use (regardless of indication); patients should be monitored for signs/symptoms of depression, suicidal tendencies, and other unusual behavior changes during therapy and instructed to inform their health care provider immediately if symptoms occur.

Severe reactions, including toxic epidermal necrolysis (TEN) and Stevens-Johnson syndrome (SJS), have been reported in adults and children. Onset is usually within ~2 weeks of treatment initiation, but may be delayed (>4 months); recurrence following rechallenge has been reported. Drug should be discontinued if there are any signs of a hypersensitivity reaction or unspecified rash; if signs or symptoms suggest SJS or TEN, do not resume therapy and consider alternative treatment.

Psychosis, paranoia, hallucinations, and behavioral symptoms (including aggression, agitation, anger, anxiety, apathy, confusion, depersonalization, depression, emotional lability, hostility, hyperkinesias, irritability, nervousness, neurosis, and personality disorder) may occur; incidence may be increased in children. Dose reduction or discontinuation may be required. Levetiracetam should be withdrawn gradually, when possible, to minimize the potential of increased seizure frequency. Use caution with renal impairment; dosage adjustment may be necessary. May cause CNS depression (impaired coordination, weakness, dizziness, and somnolence), which may impair physical or mental abilities. Symptoms occur most commonly during the first month of therapy. Patients must be cautioned about performing tasks that require mental alertness (eg, operating machinery or driving). Although rare, decreases in red blood cell counts, hemoglobin, hematocrit, white blood cell counts and neutrophils have been observed. Cases of eosinophilia and lymphocytosis have also been reported. Isolated elevations in diastolic blood pressure measurements have been reported in children <4 years of age; however, no observable differences were noted in mean diastolic measurements of children receiving levetiracetam vs placebo. Similar effects have not been observed in older children and adults. Potentially significant interactions may exist, requiring dose or frequency adjustment, additional monitoring, and/or selection of alternative therapy.

Adverse Reactions Information given for all indications and populations (adults and children) unless otherwise specified.

Cardiovascular: Increased blood pressure (diastolic; infants and children <4 years)

Central nervous system: Aggressive behavior (children and adolescents 4 to 16 years), agitation (children and adolescents 4 to 16 years), amnesia, anxiety, ataxia (partial-onset seizures; includes abnormal gait, incoordination), behavioral problems (includes aggression, agitation, anger, anxiety, apathy, depersonalization, depression, dizziness, emotional lability, irritability, neurosis), confusion, depression, dizziness, drowsiness, emotional lability, falling (children and adolescents 4 to 16 years), fatigue, headache, hostility, insomnia (children and adolescents 4 to 16 years), irritability (infants, children and adolescents 1 month to 16 years), lethargy (children and adolescents 4 to 16 years), mood changes (children and adolescents 4 to 16 years), nervousness, pain, paranoia (children and adolescents 4 to 16 years), paresthesia, psychotic symptoms, sedation (children and adolescents 4 to 16 years), vertigo

Gastrointestinal: Anorexia, constipation (children and adolescents 4 to 16 years), decreased appetite (children and adolescents 4 to 16 years), diarrhea, gastroenteritis (children and adolescents 4 to 16 years), nausea, upper abdominal pain (children and adolescents 4 to 16 years), vomiting (children and adolescents 4 to 16 years)

Hematologic & oncologic: Bruise (children and adolescents 4 to 16 years), decreased neutrophils, decreased white blood cell count, eosinophilia (children and adolescents 4 to 16 years)

Infection: Infection, influenza

Neuromuscular & skeletal: Arthralgia (children and adolescents 4 to 16 years), joint sprain (children and adolescents 4 to 16 years), neck pain, weakness

Ophthalmic: Conjunctivitis (children and adolescents 4 to 16 years), diplopia

Otic: Otalgia (children and adolescents 4 to 16 years)

Respiratory: Cough, nasal congestion (children and adolescents 4 to 16 years), nasopharyngitis, pharyngolaryngeal pain (children and adolescents 4 to 16 years), pharyngitis, rhinitis, sinusitis

Miscellaneous: Head trauma (children and adolescents 4 to 16 years)

Rare but important or life-threatening: Alopecia, decreased red blood cells, dyskinesia, eczema, equilibrium disturbance, erythema multiforme, hepatic failure, hepatitis, hyperkinesia, hyponatremia, memory impairment, myalgia, myasthenia, pancreatitis, pancytopenia (with bone marrow suppression in some cases), panic attack, personality disorder, skin rash, Stevens-Johnson syndrome, suicidal tendencies, thrombocytopenia, toxic epidermal necrolysis, weight loss

Drug Interactions

Metabolism/Transport Effects None known.

Avoid Concomitant Use

Avoid concomitant use of LevETIRAcetam with any of the following: Azelastine (Nasal); Orphenadrine; Paraldehyde; Thalidomide

Increased Effect/Toxicity

LevETIRAcetam may increase the levels/effects of: Alcohol (Ethyl); Azelastine (Nasal); Buprenorphine; CNS Depressants; Hydrocodone; Methotrimeprazine; Metyrosine; Mirtazapine; Orphenadrine; Paraldehyde; Pramipexole; ROPINIRole; Rotigotine; Selective Serotonin Reuptake Inhibitors; Suvorexant; Thalidomide; Zolpidem

The levels/effects of LevETIRAcetam may be increased by: Brimonidine (Topical); Cannabis; Doxylamine; Dronabinol; Droperidol; HydrOXYzine; Kava Kava; Magnesium Sulfate; Methotrimeprazine; Nabilone; Perampanel; Rufinamide; Sodium Oxybate; Tapentadol; Tetrahydrocannabinol

Decreased Effect

The levels/effects of LevETIRAcetam may be decreased by: Mefloquine; Mianserin; Orlistat

Food Interactions Food may delay, but does not affect the extent of absorption. Management: Administer without regard to meals.

Preparation for Administration Vials for injection: Must dilute dose in 100 mL of NS, LR, or D_5W. If a smaller volume is required (eg, pediatric patients) the amount of diluent should be calculated to not exceed a maximum levetiracetam concentration of 15 mg/mL of diluted solution.

Storage/Stability

Oral solution, tablets: Store at 25°C (77°F); excursions permitted to 15°C to 30°C (59°F to 86°F).

Premixed solution for infusion: Store at 20°C to 25°C (68°F to 77°F).

Vials for injection: Store at 25°C (77°F); excursions permitted to 15°C to 30°C (59°F to 86°F). Admixed solution is stable for 24 hours in PVC bags kept at room temperature.

Mechanism of Action The precise mechanism by which levetiracetam exerts its antiepileptic effect is unknown. However, several studies have suggested the mechanism may involve one or more of the following central pharmacologic effects: inhibition of voltage-dependent N-type calcium channels; facilitation of GABA-ergic inhibitory transmission through displacement of negative modulators; reduction of delayed rectifier potassium current; and/or binding to synaptic proteins which modulate neurotransmitter release.

Pharmacodynamics/Kinetics

Absorption: Oral: Rapid and almost complete

Immediate release: Food decreases C_{max} by 20% and delays time to C_{max} (T_{max}) by 1.5 hours.

Extended release: Intake of a high-fat, high-calorie breakfast before the administration results in a higher C_{max} and longer median T_{max}; the median T_{max} is 2 hours longer in the fed state.

Distribution: V_d: Similar to total body water

Protein binding: <10%

Metabolism: Not extensive; primarily by enzymatic hydrolysis; forms metabolites (inactive)

Bioavailability: 100%

Half-life elimination: ~6 to 8 hours; extended release tablet: ~7 hours; half-life increased in renal dysfunction

Time to peak, plasma: Oral: Immediate release: ~1 hour; Extended release: ~4 hours

Excretion: Urine (66% as unchanged drug)

Dosage Note: Use oral solution in children ≤20 kg; oral solution or immediate release tablets may be used in children >20 kg. When switching from oral to IV formulations, the total daily dose should be the same.

Myoclonic seizures:

Oral: Immediate release: Children ≥12 years, Adolescents, and Adults: Initial: 500 mg twice daily; may increase every 2 weeks by 500 mg/dose to the recommended dose of 1,500 mg twice daily. Efficacy of doses other than 3000 mg/day has not been established.

IV: Children ≥ 12 years, Adolescents, and Adults: Initial: 500 mg twice daily; may increase every 2 weeks by 500 mg/dose to the recommended dose of 1,500 mg twice daily. Efficacy of doses other than 3,000 mg/day has not been established.

Partial onset seizures:

Oral:

Immediate release:

Children 1 month to <6 months: Initial: 7 mg/kg/dose twice daily; may increase every 2 weeks by 7 mg/kg/dose to a recommended dose of 21 mg/kg/dose twice daily

Children 6 months to <4 years: Initial: 10 mg/kg/dose twice daily; may increase every 2 weeks by 10 mg/kg/dose to a recommended dose of 25 mg/kg/dose twice daily

Children and Adolescents 4 to <16 years: Initial: 10 mg/kg/dose twice daily; may increase every 2 weeks by 10 mg/kg/dose to a recommended dose of 30 mg/kg/dose twice daily (maximum daily dose: 3000 mg/day)

Alternate immediate-release fixed tablet dosing for partial onset seizures:

20 to 40 kg: Initial: 250 mg twice daily, increase every 2 weeks by 250 mg twice daily to the maximum recommended dose of 750 mg twice daily

>40 kg: Initial: 500 mg twice daily, increase every 2 weeks by 500 mg twice daily to the maximum recommended dose of 1,500 mg twice daily

Adolescents ≥16 years and Adults: Initial: 500 mg twice daily; may increase every 2 weeks by 500 mg/dose to a maximum of 1,500 mg twice daily. Doses >3000 mg/day have been used in trials; however, there is no evidence of increased benefit.

Extended release: Children ≥12 years, Adolescents, and Adults: Initial: 1,000 mg once daily; may increase every 2 weeks by 1,000 mg/day to a maximum of 3000 mg once daily.

IV:

Children 1 month to <6 months: Initial: 7 mg/kg twice daily; increase every 2 weeks by 7 mg/kg/dose to a recommended dose of 21 mg/kg twice daily. In clinical trials the average daily dose was 35 mg/kg/day. Efficacy of lower doses has not been established.

Children 6 months to <4 years: Initial: 10 mg/kg twice daily; increase every 2 weeks by 10 mg/kg/dose to a recommended dose of 25 mg/kg twice daily. If the patient cannot tolerate 50 mg/kg/day, reduce the daily dose. In clinical trials the average daily dose was 47 mg/kg/day.

Children and Adolescents 4 to <16 years: Initial: 10 mg/kg twice daily; increase every 2 weeks by 10 mg/kg/dose to the recommended dose of 30 mg/kg twice daily. If the patient cannot tolerate 60 mg/kg/day, reduce the daily dose. In clinical trials the average daily dose was 44 mg/kg/day and the maximum daily dose was 3,000 mg/day.

Adolescents ≥16 years and Adults: Initial: 500 mg twice daily; may increase every 2 weeks by 500 mg/dose to a maximum of 1,500 mg twice daily. Doses >3,000 mg/day have been used in trials; however, there is no evidence of increased benefit.

Tonic-clonic seizures:

Oral: Immediate release:

Children and Adolescents 6 to <16 years: Initial: 10 mg/kg/dose twice daily; may increase every 2 weeks by 10 mg/kg/dose to the recommended dose of 30 mg/kg twice daily. Efficacy of doses other than 60 mg/kg/day has not been established.

Adolescents ≥16 years and Adults: Initial: 500 mg twice daily; may increase every 2 weeks by 500 mg/dose to the recommended dose of 1,500 mg twice daily. Efficacy of doses other than 3,000 mg/day has not been established.

IV:

Children and Adolescents 6 to <16 years: Initial: 10 mg/kg twice daily; increase every 2 weeks by 10 mg/kg/dose to the recommended dose of 30 mg/kg twice daily. Efficacy of doses lower than 60 mg/kg/day has not been established.

Adolescents ≥16 years and Adults: Initial: 500 mg twice daily; may increase every 2 weeks by 500 mg/dose to the recommended dose of 1,500 mg twice daily. Efficacy of doses other than 3,000 mg/day has not been established.

Loading dose (off-label): Adults: Immediate release: Initial doses of 1500 to 2000 mg have been well-tolerated (Betts, 2000; Koubeissi, 2008), although the necessity of a loading dose has not been established.

Refractory status epilepticus (off-label use): Adults: 1,000 to 3,000 mg administered over 15 minutes (Meierkord, 2010); 2,500 mg has been safely administered over 5 minutes in one report (Uges, 2009). **Note:** Levetiracetam has not been well studied in comparison to other agents routinely used in this setting.

Dosing adjustment in renal impairment: Adults:

Immediate-release and IV formulations:

CrCl >80 mL/minute/1.73 m^2: 500 to 1,500 mg every 12 hours

CrCl 50 to 80 mL/minute/1.73 m^2: 500 to 1,000 mg every 12 hours

CrCl 30 to 50 mL/minute/1.73 m^2: 250 to 750 mg every 12 hours

CrCl <30 mL/minute/1.73 m^2: 250 to 500 mg every 12 hours

End-stage renal disease (ESRD) requiring hemodialysis: 500 to 1,000 mg every 24 hours; supplemental dose of 250 to 500 mg is recommended posthemodialysis

Peritoneal dialysis (PD): 500 to 1000 mg every 24 hours (Aronoff, 2007)

Continuous renal replacement therapy (CRRT): 250 to 750 mg every 12 hours (Aronoff, 2007)

Extended-release tablets:

CrCl >80 mL/minute/1.73 m^2: 1,000 to 3,000 mg every 24 hours

CrCl 50 to 80 mL/minute/1.73 m^2: 1,000 to 2,000 mg every 24 hours

CrCl 30 to 50 mL/minute/1.73 m^2: 500 to 1,500 mg every 24 hours

CrCl <30 mL/minute/1.73 m^2: 500 to 1,000 mg every 24 hours

ESRD requiring hemodialysis: Use of immediate release formulation is recommended.

Dosing adjustment in hepatic impairment:

U.S. labeling: No dosage adjustment necessary

Canadian labeling:

Mild to moderate impairment: No dosage adjustment necessary

Severe impairment: Reduce maintenance dose by 50% in patients who **also** have CrCl <60 mL/minute/1.73 m^2

Dietary Considerations May be taken without regard to meals.

Administration

IV: Infuse over 15 minutes

Oral: Administer without regard to meals.

Oral solution: Administer with a calibrated measuring device (not a household teaspoon or tablespoon)

Tablet (immediate release and extended release): Only administer as whole tablet; do not crush, break or chew.

Monitoring Parameters CNS depression (impaired coordination, weakness, dizziness, and somnolence); psychiatric and behavioral symptoms (aggression, agitation, anger, anxiety, apathy, confusion, depersonalization, depression, emotional lability, hostility, hyperkinesias, irritability, nervousness, neurosis, suicidal thoughts and personality disorder); diastolic blood pressure in children 1 month to <4 years of age

Dosage Forms

Solution, Intravenous:

Keppra: 500 mg/5 mL (5 mL)

Generic: 500 mg/100 mL (100 mL); 1000 mg/100 mL (100 mL); 1500 mg/100 mL (100 mL); 500 mg/5 mL (5 mL)

Solution, Intravenous [preservative free]:
Generic: 500 mg/5 mL (5 mL)
Solution, Oral:
Keppra: 100 mg/mL (473 mL)
Generic: 100 mg/mL (5 mL, 473 mL, 500 mL)
Tablet, Oral:
Keppra: 250 mg, 500 mg, 750 mg, 1000 mg
Generic: 250 mg, 500 mg, 750 mg, 1000 mg
Tablet Extended Release 24 Hour, Oral:
Keppra XR: 500 mg, 750 mg
Generic: 500 mg, 750 mg

◆ **Levitra** *see* Vardenafil *on page 2138*

Levobunolol (lee voe BYOO noe lole)

Brand Names: U.S. Betagan
Brand Names: Canada Apo-Levobunolol®; Betagan®; Novo-Levobunolol; PMS-Levobunolol; Ratio-Levobunolol; Sandoz-Levobunolol
Index Terms *l*-Bunolol Hydrochloride; Levobunolol Hydrochloride
Pharmacologic Category Beta-Adrenergic Blocker, Nonselective; Ophthalmic Agent, Antiglaucoma
Use To lower intraocular pressure in chronic open-angle glaucoma or ocular hypertension
Pregnancy Risk Factor C
Dosage Glaucoma (open-angle, chronic), intraocular hypertension: Adults: Ophthalmic:
0.25% solution: Instill 1-2 drops into affected eye(s) twice daily
0.5% solution: Instill 1-2 drops into affected eye(s) once daily; may increase to 1 drop twice daily in patients with severe or uncontrolled glaucoma; Maximum dose: Doses >1 drop twice daily (0.5%) are generally not more effective.
Dosage adjustment in renal impairment: No dosage adjustment provided in manufacturer's labeling.
Dosage adjustment in hepatic impairment: No dosage adjustment provided in manufacturer's labeling.
Additional Information Complete prescribing information should be consulted for additional detail.
Dosage Forms
Solution, Ophthalmic:
Betagan: 0.5% (5 mL, 10 mL, 15 mL)
Generic: 0.25% (5 mL, 10 mL); 0.5% (5 mL, 10 mL, 15 mL)

◆ **Levobunolol Hydrochloride** *see* Levobunolol *on page 1194*

Levobupivacaine [INT] (LEE voe byoo PIV a kane)

International Brand Names Chirocaina (CL, VE); Chirocaine (AT, AU, BE, BH, CH, CN, CZ, FI, FR, GB, GR, HK, HN, HR, ID, IE, IT, JP, KR, KW, MY, NL, NO, PE, PH, PL, QA, SE, SG, SI, SK, TH, TR, TW, VN); Popscaine (JP)
Index Terms (-)-bupivacaine; (S)-bupivacaine; L(-)-Bupivacaine; Levobupivacaine Hydrochloride
Pharmacologic Category Local Anesthetic
Reported Use Pain management; surgical anesthesia (0.25%, 0.5%, and 0.75% solutions only)
Dosage Range Note: Dose ranges are not intended to guide prescribing; consult local prescribing information for additional dosage and administration information.
Children >6 months to <12 years: Surgical anesthesia: Local infiltration (Ilioinguinal/iliohypogastric block): 0.5 **mL**/kg/side of 0.25% solution (maximum: 1.25 **mg**/kg/side) or 0.25 **mL**/kg/side of 0.5% solution (maximum: 1.25 **mg**/kg/side)
Adults:
Surgical anesthesia:
Dental: 5 to 10 **mL** of 0.5% to 0.75% solution
Epidural:
Cesarean section: 15 to 30 **mL** of 0.5% solution; maximum single dose: 150 **mg**
Surgery, **not** cesarean section: 10 to 20 **mL** of 0.5% to 0.75% solution; maximum single dose: 150 **mg**; prolonged surgeries may require a maximum cumulative dose of 400 **mg**/24 hours
Intrathecal: 3 **mL** of 0.5% solution
Local infiltration: 1 to 60 **mL** of 0.25% solution; maximum: 150 **mg**
Ophthalmic: 5 to 15 **mL** of 0.75% solution
Peripheral nerve: 1 to 40 **mL** of 0.25% to 0.5% solution; maximum: 150 **mg**
Pain management:
Labor pain (epidural bolus): 6 to 20 **mL** of 0.25% solution
Labor pain (epidural infusion): 10 to 15 **mL**/hour of 0.0625% solution or 4 to 10 **mL**/hour of 0.125% solution (maximum: 12.5 **mg**/hour; a maximum cumulative dose of 400 **mg** per 24 hours is recommended)
Peri- and postoperative pain (epidural infusion): 10 to 30 **mL**/hour of 0.0625% solution, or 10 to 15 **mL**/hour of 0.125% solution, or 5 to 7.5 **mL**/hour of 0.25% solution (maximum: 18.75 **mg**/hour; a maximum cumulative dose of 400 **mg** per 24 hours is recommended; however, postoperative doses of to 570 **mg**/24 hours have been well tolerated)
Product Availability Product available in various countries; not currently available in the U.S.
Dosage Forms
Solution, Infusion/Injection: 2.5 mg/mL, 5 mg/mL, 7.5 mg/mL (10 mL)
Solution, Infusion [premixed]: 0.625 mg/mL, 1.25 mg/mL (100 mL, 200 mL)

◆ **Levobupivacaine Hydrochloride** *see* Levobupivacaine [INT] *on page 1194*

◆ **Levocabastine Hydrochloride** *see* Levocabastine (Nasal) [CAN/INT] *on page 1194*

◆ **Levocabastine Hydrochloride** *see* Levocabastine (Ophthalmic) [CAN/INT] *on page 1195*

Levocabastine (Nasal) [CAN/INT]
(LEE voe kab as teen)

Brand Names: Canada Livostin
Index Terms Levocabastine Hydrochloride
Pharmacologic Category Histamine H_1 Antagonist; Histamine H_1 Antagonist, Second Generation; Piperidine Derivative
Use Note: Not approved in U.S.
Allergic rhinitis: Symptomatic treatment of allergic rhinitis in patients 12 years and older.
Pregnancy Considerations Adverse events were observed in some animal reproduction studies when using oral doses much larger than the equivalent maximum human nasal dose.
Breast-Feeding Considerations Following intranasal application, minute amounts of levocabastine have been detected in human breast milk (Simons 1999). The manufacturer recommends that caution be exercised when administering levocabastine to nursing women.
Contraindications Hypersensitivity to levocabastine or any component of the formulation
Warnings/Precautions Use with caution in renal impairment; limited data available regarding use in this population. Not generally associated with significant sedation; patients experiencing drowsiness must be cautioned about performing dangerous tasks that require mental alertness

(eg, driving or operating machinery). Potentially significant drug-drug interactions may exist, requiring dose or frequency adjustment, additional monitoring, and/or selection of alternative therapy.

Adverse Reactions Note: Most adverse reactions are transient; incidence often similar to placebo.

Central nervous system: Fatigue, headache, somnolence

Gastrointestinal: Xerostomia

Respiratory: Epistaxis, nasal irritation

Rare but important or life-threatening: Abdominal pain, aggravated nasal obstruction, allergic reactions, appetite increased, application site reactions (nasal discomfort, nasal edema), bronchospasm, coughing, dizziness, dry nose, dyspnea, eyelid edema, external ear pruritus, facial edema, hearing decreased, hypersensitivity, malaise, nasal congestion, nasal pruritus, nausea, rash, respiratory disorder, rhinorrhea, tachycardia, taste abnormal, throat irritation, weight gain

Drug Interactions

Metabolism/Transport Effects None known.

Avoid Concomitant Use

Avoid concomitant use of Levocabastine (Nasal) with any of the following: Aclidinium; Azelastine (Nasal); Glucagon; Ipratropium (Oral Inhalation); Orphenadrine; Paraldehyde; Potassium Chloride; Thalidomide; Tiotropium; Umeclidinium

Increased Effect/Toxicity

Levocabastine (Nasal) may increase the levels/effects of: AbobotulinumtoxinA; Analgesics (Opioid); Azelastine (Nasal); Buprenorphine; Glucagon; Hydrocodone; Metyrosine; Mirabegron; Mirtazapine; OnabotulinumtoxinA; Orphenadrine; Paraldehyde; Potassium Chloride; Pramipexole; RimabotulinumtoxinB; ROPINIRole; Rotigotine; Selective Serotonin Reuptake Inhibitors; Suvorexant; Thalidomide; Thiazide Diuretics; Tiotropium; Topiramate; Zolpidem

The levels/effects of Levocabastine (Nasal) may be increased by: Aclidinium; Brimonidine (Topical); Cannabis; Doxylamine; Dronabinol; HydrOXYzine; Ipratropium (Oral Inhalation); Kava Kava; Magnesium Sulfate; Mianserin; Nabilone; Perampanel; Rufinamide; Sodium Oxybate; Tapentadol; Tetrahydrocannabinol; Umeclidinium

Decreased Effect

Levocabastine (Nasal) may decrease the levels/effects of: Acetylcholinesterase Inhibitors; Hyaluronidase; Itopride; Secretin

The levels/effects of Levocabastine (Nasal) may be decreased by: Acetylcholinesterase Inhibitors

Storage/Stability Store at 15°C to 30°C (59°F to 86°F).

Mechanism of Action Potent, selective histamine H_1-receptor antagonist

Pharmacodynamics/Kinetics

Onset of action: 10 minutes

Absorption: Incomplete

Distribution: V_{dss}: 1.13 L/kg

Protein binding: ~55%

Metabolism: Hepatic (minimal)

Bioavailability: 60% to 80%

Half-life elimination: 35 to 40 hours

Time to peak: 3 hours

Excretion: Urine (65% to 70% as unchanged drug); feces (10% to 20% as unchanged drug) (Simons, 1999)

Dosage Allergic rhinitis: Children ≥12 years, Adolescents, and Adults ≤65 years: Intranasal: Two sprays in each nostril twice daily; if necessary, may increase dose to 2 sprays 3 to 4 times daily; consider therapy discontinuation if no response within 3 days. Continuous treatment >10 weeks has not been evaluated.

Dosage adjustment in renal impairment: There are no dosage adjustments provided in the manufacturer's labeling; use with caution.

Dosage adjustment in hepatic impairment: There are no dosage adjustments provided in the manufacturer's labeling.

Administration Intranasal: Shake bottle well before each use. Prior to initial use, bottle should be primed until a fine spray is delivered. Instruct patients to blow nose and clear nasal passages before administering spray and to inhale nasally while spraying.

Product Availability Not available in U.S.

Dosage Forms: Canada

Microsuspension, intranasal, as hydrochloride [spray]:

Livostin: 0.05% [50 mcg/spray] (15 mL) [contains benzalkonium chloride]

Levocabastine (Ophthalmic) [CAN/INT]

(LEE voe kab as teen)

Brand Names: Canada Livostin Eye Drops

Index Terms Levocabastine Hydrochloride

Pharmacologic Category Histamine H_1 Antagonist; Histamine H_1 Antagonist, Second Generation; Piperidine Derivative

Use Note: Not approved in U.S.

Treatment of seasonal allergic conjunctivitis

Pregnancy Considerations Adverse events were observed in animal reproduction studies when using doses much larger than the equivalent maximum human ophthalmic dose.

Breast-Feeding Considerations Following ophthalmic application, minute amounts of levocabastine have been detected in human breast milk (Simons 1999).

Contraindications Hypersensitivity to levocabastine or any component of the formulation

Warnings/Precautions For topical ophthalmic use only. Solution contains benzalkonium chloride which may be absorbed by soft contact lenses. Not for use in patients wearing soft contact lenses during treatment.

Adverse Reactions

Central nervous system: Fatigue

Ocular: Irritation (similar to placebo)

Respiratory: Epistaxis

Rare but important or life-threatening: Dry eye, fever, insomnia, keratitis, nasal congestion, nausea, pruritus, rash

Drug Interactions

Metabolism/Transport Effects None known.

Avoid Concomitant Use There are no known interactions where it is recommended to avoid concomitant use.

Increased Effect/Toxicity There are no known significant interactions involving an increase in effect.

Decreased Effect There are no known significant interactions involving a decrease in effect.

Storage/Stability Store between 15°C and 30°C (59°F and 86°F). Discard 1 month after initially opening bottle.

Mechanism of Action Potent, selective histamine H_1-receptor antagonist for topical ophthalmic use

Pharmacodynamics/Kinetics

Onset of action: 10-15 minutes

Absorption: Incomplete, within 1-2 hours

Metabolism: Hepatic (minimal)

Bioavailability: ~30% in patients with allergic conjunctivitis

Half-life, elimination: 33 hours

Excretion: Urine (65% to 70% as unchanged drug); feces (10% to 20% as unchanged drug)

Dosage Children ≥12 years and Adults ≤65 years: Allergic conjunctivitis: Usual dosel: Instill 1 drop in affected eye(s) 2 times/day; may increase to 1 drop 3-4 times/day. If no improvement within 3 days, consider discontinuation of therapy. Continuous therapy >16 weeks has not been studied.

Dosage adjustment in renal impairment: No dosage adjustment provided in manufacturer's labeling. However, dosage adjustment unlikely due to low systemic absorption.

Dosage adjustment in hepatic impairment: No dosage adjustment provided in manufacturer's labeling. However, dosage adjustment unlikely due to low systemic absorption.

Administration For topical ophthalmic use only. Shake bottle well. Wash hands prior to use. Avoid touching the dropper tip to surfaces to avoid contamination.

Product Availability Not available in U.S.

Dosage Forms: Canada

Suspension, ophthalmic:

Livostin®: 0.05% (5 mL, 10 mL)

◆ **Levocarb CR (Can)** *see* Carbidopa and Levodopa *on page 351*

Levocetirizine (LEE vo se TI ra zeen)

Brand Names: U.S. Xyzal

Index Terms Levocetirizine Dihydrochloride

Pharmacologic Category Histamine H_1 Antagonist; Histamine H_1 Antagonist, Second Generation; Piperazine Derivative

Use Relief of symptoms of perennial and seasonal allergic rhinitis; treatment of skin manifestations (uncomplicated) of chronic idiopathic urticaria

Pregnancy Risk Factor B

Dosage Oral:

Perennial allergic rhinitis, chronic urticaria:

Children 6 months to 5 years: 1.25 mg once daily (in the evening); maximum: 1.25 mg

Children 6-11 years: 2.5 mg once daily (in the evening); maximum: 2.5 mg/day

Children ≥12 years and Adults: 5 mg once daily (in the evening); some patients may experience relief of symptoms with 2.5 mg once daily

Seasonal allergic rhinitis:

Children 2-5 years: 1.25 mg once daily (in the evening); maximum: 1.25 mg

Children 6-11 years: 2.5 mg once daily (in the evening); maximum: 2.5 mg/day

Children ≥12 years and Adults: 5 mg once daily (in the evening); some patients may experience relief of symptoms with 2.5 mg once daily

Elderly: Refer to adult dosing; dosing should begin at the lower end of the dosing range

Dosage adjustments in renal impairment:

Children 6 months to 11 years with renal impairment: Contraindicated

Children ≥12 and Adults:

CrCl 50-80 mL/minute: 2.5 mg once daily

CrCl 30-50 mL/minute: 2.5 mg once every other day

CrCl 10-30 mL/minute: 2.5 mg twice weekly (every 3 or 4 days)

CrCl <10 mL/minute, hemodialysis patients: Contraindicated

Dosage adjustments in hepatic impairment: No adjustment required.

Additional Information Complete prescribing information should be consulted for additional detail.

Dosage Forms

Solution, Oral:

Xyzal: 2.5 mg/5 mL (148 mL)

Generic: 2.5 mg/5 mL (148 mL)

Tablet, Oral:

Xyzal: 5 mg

Generic: 5 mg

◆ **Levocetirizine Dihydrochloride** *see* Levocetirizine *on page 1196*

◆ **Levodopa and Benserazide** *see* Benserazide and Levodopa [CAN/INT] *on page 244*

◆ **Levodopa and Carbidopa** *see* Carbidopa and Levodopa *on page 351*

Levodopa, Carbidopa, and Entacapone

(lee voe DOE pa, kar bi DOE pa, & en TA ka pone)

Brand Names: U.S. Stalevo

Brand Names: Canada Stalevo

Index Terms Carbidopa, Entacapone, and Levodopa; Carbidopa, Levodopa, and Entacapone; Entacapone, Carbidopa, and Levodopa

Pharmacologic Category Anti-Parkinson's Agent, COMT Inhibitor; Anti-Parkinson's Agent, Decarboxylase Inhibitor; Anti-Parkinson's Agent, Dopamine Precursor

Additional Appendix Information

Oral Dosages That Should Not Be Crushed *on page 2276*

Use Parkinson disease: Treatment of Parkinson disease.

Pregnancy Risk Factor C

Dosage Parkinson disease: Adults: Oral

Note: All strengths of Stalevo contain a carbidopa/levodopa ratio of 1:4 plus entacapone 200 mg.

Dose should be individualized based on therapeutic response; doses may be adjusted by changing strength or adjusting interval. Fractionated doses are not recommended and only 1 tablet should be given at each dosing interval; maximum daily dose: 8 tablets of Stalevo 50, 75, 100, 125, or 150, **or** 6 tablets of Stalevo 200. Patients receiving <70 to 100 mg of the carbidopa component may experience nausea and vomiting.

Patients previously treated with carbidopa/levodopa immediate release tablets (ratio of 1:4):

With current entacapone therapy: May switch directly to corresponding strength of combination tablet. No data available on transferring patients from controlled release preparations or products with a 1:10 ratio of carbidopa/levodopa.

Without entacapone therapy:

If current levodopa dose is >600 mg daily or history of moderate or severe dyskinesias: Levodopa dose reduction may be required when adding entacapone to therapy; therefore, titrate dose using individual products first (carbidopa/levodopa immediate release with a ratio of 1:4 plus entacapone 200 mg); then transfer to combination product once stabilized.

If current levodopa dose is <600 mg and without a history of dyskinesias: May transfer to corresponding dose of combination product; monitor, dose reduction of levodopa may be required.

Patients previously treated with benserazide/levodopa immediate release tablets [Canadian product]: With current entacapone therapy: Prior to switching to combination product (carbidopa/levodopa/entacapone), withhold treatment for 1 night, then initiate (carbidopa/levodopa/entacapone) therapy the following morning at a dose that provides either an equivalent amount or ~5% to 10% more levodopa.

Dosage adjustment in renal impairment:

U.S. labeling: There are no dosage adjustments provided in manufacturer's labeling. Use of levodopa and carbidopa has not been studied in patients with renal impairment. Use with caution.

Canadian labeling: There are no dosage adjustments provided in the manufacturer's labeling; titrate dose cautiously in severe impairment. Use is contraindicated in uncompensated renal disease.

Dosage adjustment in hepatic impairment:

U.S. labeling: There are no dosage adjustments provided in manufacturer's labeling (has not been studied); use with caution in biliary obstruction or hepatic disease.

Canadian labeling: Use is contraindicated. There are no dosage adjustments provided in the manufacturer's labeling; titrate dose cautiously in severe impairment. Use is contraindicated in uncompensated hepatic disease.

Additional Information Complete prescribing information should be consulted for additional detail.

Dosage Forms

Tablet:

Stalevo: 50: Levodopa 50 mg, carbidopa 12.5 mg, and entacapone 200 mg; 75: Levodopa 75 mg, carbidopa 18.75 mg, and entacapone 200 mg; 100: Levodopa 100 mg, carbidopa 25 mg, and entacapone 200 mg; 125: Levodopa 125 mg, carbidopa 31.25 mg, and entacapone 200 mg; 150: Levodopa 150 mg, carbidopa 37.5 mg, and entacapone 200 mg; 200: Levodopa 200 mg, carbidopa 50 mg, and entacapone 200 mg

Generic: Levodopa 50 mg, carbidopa 12.5 mg, and entacapone 200 mg; Levodopa 75 mg, carbidopa 18.75 mg, and entacapone 200 mg; Levodopa 100 mg, carbidopa 25 mg, and entacapone 200 mg; Levodopa 125 mg, carbidopa 31.25 mg, and entacapone 200 mg; Levodopa 150 mg, carbidopa 37.5 mg, and entacapone 200 mg; Levodopa 200 mg, carbidopa 50 mg, and entacapone 200 mg

◆ **Levo-Dromoran** *see* Levorphanol *on page 1204*

Levofloxacin (Systemic) (lee voe FLOKS a sin)

Brand Names: U.S. Levaquin

Brand Names: Canada ACT Levofloxacin; APO-Levofloxacin; Levaquin; Levaquin in 5% Dextrose Injection; Mylan-Levofloxacin; Novo-Levofloxacin; PMS-Levofloxacin; Sandoz-Levofloxacin

Pharmacologic Category Antibiotic, Fluoroquinolone; Antibiotic, Respiratory Fluoroquinolone

Use Treatment of community-acquired pneumonia, including multidrug resistant strains of *S. pneumoniae* (MDRSP); nosocomial pneumonia; chronic bronchitis (acute bacterial exacerbation); acute bacterial rhinosinusitis (ABRS); prostatitis (chronic bacterial), urinary tract infection (uncomplicated or complicated); acute pyelonephritis; skin or skin structure infections (uncomplicated or complicated); reduce incidence or disease progression of inhalational anthrax (postexposure); prophylaxis and treatment of plague (pneumonic and septicemic) due to *Y. pestis*

Pregnancy Risk Factor C

Pregnancy Considerations Adverse events have been observed in some animal reproduction studies. Levofloxacin crosses the placenta and can be detected in the amniotic fluid and cord blood (Ozyüncü and Beksac 2010; Ozyuncu and Nemutl, 2010). Information specific to levofloxacin use during pregnancy is limited (Padberg 2014).

Breast-Feeding Considerations Based on data from a case report, small amounts of levofloxacin are excreted in breast milk (Cahill 2005). Due to the potential for serious adverse reactions in the nursing infant, the manufacturer recommends a decision be made whether to discontinue nursing or to discontinue the drug, taking into account the importance of treatment to the mother.

Contraindications Hypersensitivity to levofloxacin, any component of the formulation, or other quinolones

Canadian labeling: Additional contraindications (not in U.S. labeling): History of tendonitis or tendon rupture associated with use of any quinolone antimicrobial agent

Warnings/Precautions **[U.S. Boxed Warning]: There have been reports of tendon inflammation and/or rupture with quinolone antibiotics; risk may be increased with concurrent corticosteroids, organ transplant recipients, and in patients >60 years of age.** Rupture of the Achilles tendon sometimes requiring surgical repair has been reported most frequently; but other tendon sites (eg, rotator cuff, biceps) have also been reported. Strenuous physical activity, rheumatoid arthritis, and renal impairment may be an independent risk factor for tendonitis. Discontinue at first sign of tendon inflammation or pain. May occur even after discontinuation of therapy. Use with caution in patients with rheumatoid arthritis; may increase risk of tendon rupture. Safety of use in pediatric patients for >14 days of therapy has not been studied; increased incidence of musculoskeletal disorders (eg, arthralgia, tendon rupture) has been observed in children. CNS effects may occur (toxic psychoses, tremor, restlessness, anxiety, lightheadedness, paranoia, depression, nightmares, confusion, and very rarely hallucinations increased intracranial pressure (including pseudotumor cerebri, seizures, or toxic psychosis). Potential for seizures, although very rare, may be increased with concomitant NSAID therapy. Use with caution in individuals at risk of seizures, with known or suspected CNS disorders or renal dysfunction. Avoid excessive sunlight and take precautions to limit exposure (eg, loose fitting clothing, sunscreen); may cause moderate-to-severe phototoxicity reactions. Discontinue use if photosensitivity occurs.

Rare cases of torsade de pointes have been reported in patients receiving levofloxacin. Use caution in patients with known prolongation of QT interval, bradycardia, hypokalemia, hypomagnesemia, or in those receiving concurrent therapy with Class Ia or Class III antiarrhythmics.

Severe hypersensitivity reactions, including anaphylaxis, have occurred with quinolone therapy. Reactions may present as typical allergic symptoms after a single dose, or may manifest as severe idiosyncratic dermatologic, vascular, pulmonary, renal, hepatic, and/or hematologic events, usually after multiple doses. Prompt discontinuation of drug should occur if skin rash or other symptoms arise. Prolonged use may result in fungal or bacterial superinfection, including *C. difficile*-associated diarrhea (CDAD) and pseudomembranous colitis; CDAD has been observed >2 months postantibiotic treatment. Peripheral neuropathy has been reported (rare); may occur soon after initiation of therapy and may be irreversible; discontinue if symptoms of sensory or sensorimotor neuropathy occur. **[U.S. Boxed Warning]: Quinolones may exacerbate myasthenia gravis; avoid use (rare, potentially life-threatening weakness of respiratory muscles may occur).** Unrelated to hypersensitivity, severe hepatotoxicity (including acute hepatitis and fatalities) has been reported. Elderly patients may be at greater risk. Discontinue therapy immediately if signs and symptoms of hepatitis occur. Hemolytic reactions may (rarely) occur with quinolone use in patients with latent or actual G6PD deficiency.

Fluoroquinolones have been associated with the development of serious, and sometimes fatal, hypoglycemia, most often in elderly diabetics, but also in patients without diabetes. This occurred most frequently with gatifloxacin (no longer available systemically) but may occur at a lower frequency with other quinolones.

Benzyl alcohol and derivatives: Some dosage forms may contain benzyl alcohol; large amounts of benzyl alcohol (≥99 mg/kg/day) have been associated with a potentially fatal toxicity ("gasping syndrome") in neonates; the "gasping syndrome" consists of metabolic acidosis, respiratory distress, gasping respirations, CNS dysfunction (including convulsions, intracranial hemorrhage), hypotension, and cardiovascular collapse (AAP, 1997; CDC, 1982); some data suggests that benzoate displaces bilirubin from protein binding sites (Ahlfors, 2001); avoid or use dosage forms containing benzyl alcohol with caution in neonates. See manufacturer's labeling.

Adverse Reactions

Cardiovascular: Chest pain, edema

Central nervous system: Dizziness, headache, insomnia

Dermatologic: Pruritus, skin rash

Gastrointestinal: Abdominal pain, constipation, diarrhea, dyspepsia, nausea, vomiting

Genitourinary: Vaginitis

Infection: Candidiasis

Local: Injection site reaction

Respiratory: Dyspnea

Rare but important or life-threatening: Abnormal electroencephalogram, abnormal gait, acute renal failure, ageusia, agranulocytosis, anaphylactoid reaction, anemia (including aplastic and hemolytic), anorexia, anosmia, brain disease (rare), cardiac arrest, cardiac arrhythmia (including ventricular tachycardia/fibrillation and torsade de pointes), *Clostridium difficile*-associated diarrhea, confusion, convulsions, crystalluria, cylindruria, depression, elevation in serum levels of skeletal-muscle enzymes, eosinophilia, epistaxis, erythema multiforme, esophagitis, exacerbation of myasthenia gravis, gastritis (including gastroenteritis), glossitis, granulocytopenia, hallucination, hepatic failure (some fatal), hepatic insufficiency, hepatitis, hyperglycemia, hyperkalemia, hyperkinesias, hypersensitivity reaction (including anaphylaxis, angioedema, rash, pneumonitis, and serum sickness), hypertension, hypertonia, hypoacusis, hypoglycemia, hypotension, increased INR, increased intracranial pressure, increased serum alkaline phosphatase, increased serum transaminases, interstitial nephritis, intestinal obstruction, jaundice, leukocytosis, leukopenia, leukorrhea, lymphadenopathy, multiorgan failure, muscle injury, muscle spasm, pancreatitis, pancytopenia, paralysis, paranoia, peripheral neuropathy (may be irreversible), phlebitis, phototoxicity, prolonged prothrombin time, prolonged Q-T interval on ECG, pseudotumor cerebri, psychosis, renal function abnormality, rhabdomyolysis, rupture of tendon, scotoma, seizure, skeletal pain, skin photosensitivity, sleep disorder (including abnormal dreams and nightmares), Stevens-Johnson syndrome, stomatitis, suicidal ideation, syncope, tachycardia, tendonitis, toxic epidermal necrolysis, toxic psychosis, thrombocytopenia (including thrombotic thrombocytopenic purpura), uveitis, vasculitis (leukocytoclastic), vasodilatation, visual disturbances(including diplopia), voice disorder

Drug Interactions

Metabolism/Transport Effects None known.

Avoid Concomitant Use

Avoid concomitant use of Levofloxacin (Systemic) with any of the following: BCG; Highest Risk QTc-Prolonging Agents; Ivabradine; Mifepristone; Strontium Ranelate

Increased Effect/Toxicity

Levofloxacin (Systemic) may increase the levels/effects of: Highest Risk QTc-Prolonging Agents; Moderate Risk QTc-Prolonging Agents; Porfimer; Sulfonylureas; Tacrolimus (Systemic); Varenicline; Verteporfin; Vitamin K Antagonists

The levels/effects of Levofloxacin (Systemic) may be increased by: Corticosteroids (Systemic); Insulin; Ivabradine; Mifepristone; Nonsteroidal Anti-Inflammatory Agents; Probenecid; QTc-Prolonging Agents (Indeterminate Risk and Risk Modifying)

Decreased Effect

Levofloxacin (Systemic) may decrease the levels/effects of: BCG; Didanosine; Mycophenolate; Sodium Picosulfate; Sulfonylureas; Typhoid Vaccine

The levels/effects of Levofloxacin (Systemic) may be decreased by: Antacids; Calcium Salts; Didanosine; Iron Salts; Lanthanum; Magnesium Salts; Multivitamins/Minerals (with ADEK, Folate, Iron); Multivitamins/Minerals (with AE, No Iron); Quinapril; Sevelamer; Strontium Ranelate; Sucralfate; Zinc Salts

Preparation for Administration Solution for injection: Single-use vials must be further diluted in compatible solution to a final concentration of 5 mg/mL prior to infusion.

Storage/Stability

Solution for injection:

Vial: Store at room temperature. Protect from light. Diluted solution (5 mg/mL) is stable for 72 hours when stored at room temperature; stable for 14 days when stored under refrigeration. When frozen, stable for 6 months; do not refreeze. Do not thaw in microwave or by bath immersion.

Premixed: Store at ≤25°C (77°F); do not freeze. Brief exposure to 40°C (104°F) does not affect product. Protect from light.

Tablet, oral solution: Store at 25°C (77°F); excursions permitted to 15°C to 30°C (59°F to 86°F).

Mechanism of Action As the S(-) enantiomer of the fluoroquinolone, ofloxacin, levofloxacin, inhibits DNA-gyrase in susceptible organisms thereby inhibits relaxation of supercoiled DNA and promotes breakage of DNA strands. DNA gyrase (topoisomerase II), is an essential bacterial enzyme that maintains the superhelical structure of DNA and is required for DNA replication and transcription, DNA repair, recombination, and transposition.

Pharmacodynamics/Kinetics

Absorption: Rapid and complete

Distribution: V_d: 74-112 L; CSF concentrations ~15% of serum levels; high concentrations are achieved in prostate, lung, and gynecological tissues, sinus, saliva

Protein binding: ~24% to 38%; primarily to albumin

Metabolism: Minimally hepatic

Bioavailability: ~99%

Half-life elimination: ~6-8 hours

Time to peak, serum: Oral: 1-2 hours

Excretion: Urine (~87% as unchanged drug, <5% as metabolites); feces (<4%)

Dosage Note: Sequential therapy (intravenous to oral) may be instituted based on prescriber's discretion.

Usual dosage range: Adults: Oral, IV: 250-500 mg every 24 hours; severe or complicated infections: 750 mg every 24 hours

Indication-specific dosing:

Infants ≥6 months and Children ≤4 years:

Community-acquired pneumonia (CAP) (IDSA/PIDS, 2011): Note: May consider addition of vancomycin or clindamycin to empiric therapy if community-acquired MRSA suspected; alternative to ceftriaxone or cefotaxime in patients not fully immunized for *H. influenzae* type b and *S. pneumoniae*, or significant local resistance to penicillin in invasive pneumococcal strains.

S. pneumoniae (MICs to penicillin ≤2.0 mcg/mL), mild infection or step-down therapy (alternative to amoxicillin): Oral: 8-10 mg/kg/dose every 12 hours (maximum: 750 mg daily)

S. pneumoniae (MICs to penicillin ≥4.0 mcg/mL):

Moderate-to-severe infection (alternative to ceftriaxone): IV: 8-10 mg/kg/dose every 12 hours (maximum: 750 mg daily)

Mild infection, step-down therapy (preferred): Oral: 8-10 mg/kg/dose every 12 hours (maximum: 750 mg daily)

H. influenzae, moderate-to-severe infection (alternative to ampicillin, ceftriaxone, or cefotaxime): IV: 8-10 mg/kg/dose every 12 hours (maximum: 750 mg daily)

Atypical pathogens, moderate-to-severe infection (alternative to azithromycin) or empiric treatment (alternative to azithromycin +/- beta-lactam; should be limited to macrolide allergic/intolerant patients): Oral, IV: 8-10 mg/kg/dose every 12 hours (maximum: 750 mg daily)

Infants ≥6 months, Children, and Adults: Oral, IV:

Anthrax (inhalational, postexposure):

≤50 kg: 8 mg/kg every 12 hours for 60 days (do not exceed 250 mg/dose), beginning as soon as possible after exposure

>50 kg and Adults: 500 mg every 24 hours for 60 days, beginning as soon as possible after exposure

Plague (prophylaxis and treatment):

≤50 kg: 8 mg/kg every 12 hours for 10-14 days (do not exceed 250 mg/dose), beginning as soon as possible after exposure

>50 kg and Adults: 500 mg every 24 hours for 10-14 days, beginning as soon as possible after exposure. **Note:** Dose of 750 mg once daily may be considered if clinically warranted.

Children ≥1 year:

Surgical (preoperative) prophylaxis (off-label use): IV: 10 mg/kg within 120 minutes prior to surgical incision (maximum: 500 mg) (Bratzler, 2013)

Children:

Acute bacterial rhinosinusitis (off-label use): Oral, IV: 10-20 mg/kg/day divided every 12-24 hours for 10-14 days (maximum: 500 mg daily). **Note:** Recommended in patients with a type I penicillin allergy, after failure of initial therapy or in patients at risk for antibiotic resistance (eg, daycare attendance, age <2 years, recent hospitalization, antibiotic use within the past month) (Chow, 2012).

Children 5-16 years:

Community-acquired pneumonia (CAP) (IDSA/PIDS, 2011): Note: May consider addition of vancomycin or clindamycin to empiric therapy if community-acquired MRSA suspected; alternative to ceftriaxone or cefotaxime in patients not fully immunized for *H. influenzae* type b and *S. pneumoniae*, or significant local resistance to penicillin in invasive pneumococcal strains.

S. pneumoniae (MICs to penicillin ≤2.0 mcg/mL), mild infection or step-down therapy (alternative to amoxicillin): Oral: 8-10 mg/kg/dose once daily (maximum: 750 mg daily)

S. pneumoniae (MICs to penicillin ≥4.0 mcg/mL):

Moderate-to-severe infection (alternative to ceftriaxone): IV: 8-10 mg/kg/dose once daily (maximum: 750 mg daily)

Mild infection, step-down therapy (preferred): Oral: 8-10 mg/kg/dose once daily (maximum: 750 mg daily)

H. influenzae, moderate-to-severe infection (alternative to ampicillin, ceftriaxone, or cefotaxime): IV: 8-10 mg/kg/dose once daily (maximum: 750 mg daily)

Atypical pathogens:

Moderate-to-severe infection (alternative to azithromycin): IV: 8-10 mg/kg/dose once daily (maximum: 750 mg daily)

Mild infection, step-down therapy (alternative to azithromycin in adolescents with skeletal maturity): Oral: 500 mg once daily

Adults: Oral, IV:

Acute bacterial rhinosinusitis:

Manufacturer's recommendations: 750 mg every 24 hours for 5 days or 500 mg every 24 hours for 10-14 days

Alternate recommendations: 500 mg every 24 hours for 5-7 days (Chow, 2012)

***Chlamydia trachomatis* sexually-transmitted infections (off-label use) (CDC, 2010):** Oral: 500 mg every 24 hours for 7 days

Chronic bronchitis (acute bacterial exacerbation): Oral: 500 mg every 24 hours for 7 days; Canadian labeling (not in U.S. labeling) also includes a dosage regimen of 750 mg every 24 hours for 5 days

Diverticulitis, peritonitis (off-label use) (Solomkin, [IDSA] 2010): 750 mg every 24 hours for 7-10 days; use adjunctive metronidazole therapy

Epididymitis, nongonococcal (off-label use) (CDC, 2010): Oral: 500 mg once daily for 10 days

Gonococcal infection (off-label use) (CDC, 2010): As of April 2007, the CDC no longer recommends the use of fluoroquinolones for the treatment of uncomplicated or more serious gonococcal disease, unless no other options exist and susceptibility can be confirmed via culture.

Intra-abdominal infection, complicated, community-acquired (in combination with metronidazole) (off-label use) (Solomkin, [IDSA] 2010): IV: 750 mg once daily for 4-7 days (provided source controlled). **Note:** Avoid using in settings where *E. coli* susceptibility to fluoroquinolones is <90%.

Pelvic inflammatory disease (off-label use) (CDC, 2010): Oral: 500 mg once daily for 14 days with or without concomitant metronidazole; **Note:** The CDC recommends use as an alternative therapy only if standard parenteral cephalosporin therapy is not feasible and community prevalence of quinolone-resistant gonococcal organisms is low. Culture sensitivity must be confirmed.

Pneumonia:

Community-acquired (CAP): 500 mg every 24 hours for 7-14 days or 750 mg every 24 hours for 5 days (efficacy of 5-day regimen for MDRSP not established)

Healthcare-associated (HAP): 750 mg every 24 hours for 7-14 days

Prostatitis (chronic bacterial): Oral: 500 mg every 24 hours for 28 days

Skin and skin structure infections:

Uncomplicated: 500 mg every 24 hours for 7-10 days

Complicated: 750 mg every 24 hours for 7-14 days

Surgical (preoperative) prophylaxis (off-label use): IV: 500 mg within 120 minutes prior to surgical incision (Bratzler, 2013)

Traveler's diarrhea (off-label use): Oral: 500 mg for one dose (Sanders, 2007)

Tuberculosis, drug-resistant tuberculosis, or intolerance to first-line agents (off-label use): Oral: 500-1000 mg every 24 hours (CDC, 2003)

Urethritis, nongonococcal (off-label use) (CDC, 2010): Oral: 500 mg every 24 hours for 7 days

Urinary tract infections:

Uncomplicated: 250 mg once daily for 3 days

Complicated, including pyelonephritis: 250 mg once daily for 10 days **or** 750 mg once daily for 5 days

Dosage adjustment in renal impairment: IV, Oral:

Normal renal function dosing of 250 mg daily:

CrCl 20-49 mL/minute: No dosage adjustment required

CrCl 10-19 mL/minute: Administer 250 mg every 48 hours (except in uncomplicated UTI, where no dosage adjustment is required)

Hemodialysis/chronic ambulatory peritoneal dialysis (CAPD): No information available

Normal renal function dosing of 500 mg daily:

CrCl 20-49 mL/minute: Administer 500 mg initial dose, followed by 250 mg every 24 hours

CrCl 10-19 mL/minute: Administer 500 mg initial dose, followed by 250 mg every 48 hours

Hemodialysis/chronic ambulatory peritoneal dialysis (CAPD): Administer 500 mg initial dose, followed by 250 mg every 48 hours; supplemental doses are not required following either hemodialysis or CAPD.

Normal renal function dosing of 750 mg daily:

CrCl 20-49 mL/minute: Administer 750 mg every 48 hours

CrCl 10-19 mL/minute: Administer 750 mg initial dose, followed by 500 mg every 48 hours

Hemodialysis/chronic ambulatory peritoneal dialysis (CAPD): Administer 750 mg initial dose, followed by 500 mg every 48 hours; supplemental doses are not required following either hemodialysis or CAPD.

Normal renal function dosing of 750 or 1000 mg daily (treatment of tuberculosis **only**) (CDC, 2003): CrCl <30 mL/minute: Administer 750 or 1000 mg 3 times per week (in hemodialysis patients administer after dialysis on dialysis days).

Continuous renal replacement therapy (CRRT) (Heintz, 2009; Trotman, 2005): Drug clearance is highly dependent on the method of renal replacement, filter type, and flow rate. Appropriate dosing requires close monitoring of pharmacologic response, signs of adverse reactions due to drug accumulation, as well as drug concentrations in relation to target trough (if appropriate). The following are general recommendations only (based on dialysate flow/ultrafiltration rates of 1-2 L/hour and minimal residual renal function) and should not supersede clinical judgment:

CVVH: Loading dose of 500-750 mg followed by 250 mg every 24 hours

CVVHD: Loading dose of 500-750 mg followed by 250-500 mg every 24 hours

CVVHDF: Loading dose of 500-750 mg followed by 250-750 mg every 24 hours

Dosage adjustment in hepatic impairment: IV, Oral: No dosage adjustment provided in manufacturer's labeling (has not been studied). However, dosage adjustment unlikely due to limited hepatic metabolism.

Dietary Considerations Tablets may be taken without regard to meals. Oral solution should be administered on an empty stomach (1 hour before or 2 hours after a meal). Take 2 hours before or 2 hours after multiple vitamins, antacids, or other products containing magnesium, aluminum, iron, or zinc.

Administration

Oral: Tablets may be administered without regard to meals. Oral solution should be administered 1 hour before or 2 hours after meals. Maintain adequate hydration of patient to prevent crystalluria.

IV: Infuse 250-500 mg IV solution over 60 minutes; infuse 750 mg IV solution over 90 minutes. Too rapid of infusion can lead to hypotension. Avoid administration through an intravenous line with a solution containing multivalent cations (eg, magnesium, calcium). Maintain adequate hydration of patient to prevent crystalluria or cylindruria.

Monitoring Parameters Evaluation of organ system functions (renal, hepatic, and hematopoietic) is recommended periodically during therapy; the possibility of crystalluria should be assessed; WBC and signs of infection

Dosage Forms

Solution, Intravenous [preservative free]:

Levaquin: 500 mg/100 mL (100 mL); 750 mg/150 mL (150 mL)

Generic: 250 mg/50 mL (50 mL); 500 mg/100 mL (100 mL); 750 mg/150 mL (150 mL); 25 mg/mL (20 mL, 30 mL)

Solution, Oral:

Levaquin: 25 mg/mL (480 mL)

Generic: 25 mg/mL (10 mL, 20 mL, 100 mL, 200 mL, 480 mL)

Tablet, Oral:

Levaquin: 250 mg, 500 mg, 750 mg

Generic: 250 mg, 500 mg, 750 mg

Extemporaneous Preparations Note: Commercial oral solution is available (25 mg/mL)

A 50 mg/mL oral suspension may be made with tablets and a 1:1 mixture of Ora-Plus® and strawberry syrup NF. Crush six 500 mg levofloxacin tablets in a mortar and reduce to a fine powder. Add small portions of the vehicle and mix to a uniform paste; mix while adding the vehicle in incremental proportions to **almost** 60 mL; transfer to a graduated cylinder, rinse mortar with vehicle, and add quantity of vehicle sufficient to make 60 mL. Label "shake well". Stable for 57 days when stored in amber plastic prescription bottles at room temperature or refrigerated.

VandenBussche HL, Johnson CE, and Fontana EM, et al, "Stability of Levofloxacin in an Extemporaneously Compounded Oral Liquid," *Am J Health Syst Pharm*, 1999, 56(22):2316-8.

Levofloxacin (Ophthalmic) (lee voe FLOKS a sin)

Pharmacologic Category Antibiotic, Fluoroquinolone; Antibiotic, Ophthalmic

Use Treatment of bacterial conjunctivitis caused by susceptible organisms (Quixin® 0.5% ophthalmic solution); treatment of corneal ulcer caused by susceptible organisms (Iquix® 1.5% ophthalmic solution)

Pregnancy Risk Factor C

Dosage Ophthalmic:

Usual dosage range:

Children ≥1 year: 1-2 drops every 2-6 hours

Adults: 1-2 drops every 2-6 hours

Indication-specific dosing:

Children ≥1 year and Adults:

Conjunctivitis (0.5% ophthalmic solution):

Treatment day 1 and day 2: Instill 1-2 drops into affected eye(s) every 2 hours while awake, up to 8 times/day

Treatment day 3 through day 7: Instill 1-2 drops into affected eye(s) every 4 hours while awake, up to 4 times/day

Children ≥6 years and Adults:

Corneal ulceration (1.5% ophthalmic solution):

Treatment day 1 through day 3: Instill 1-2 drops into affected eye(s) every 30 minutes to 2 hours while awake and 4-6 hours after retiring

Treatment day 4 through completion: Instill 1-2 drops into affected eye(s) every 1-4 hours while awake

Dosage adjustment in renal impairment: No dosage adjustment provided in manufacturer's labeling. However, dosage adjustment unlikely due to low systemic absorption.

Dosage adjustment in hepatic impairment: No dosage adjustment provided in manufacturer's labeling. However, dosage adjustment unlikely due to low systemic absorption.

Additional Information Complete prescribing information should be consulted for additional detail.

Dosage Forms

Solution, Ophthalmic:

Generic: 0.5% (5 mL)

◆ **Levo-folinic Acid** *see* LEVOleucovorin *on page 1200*

LEVOleucovorin (lee voe loo koe VOR in)

Brand Names: U.S. Fusilev

Index Terms 6S-leucovorin; Calcium Levoleucovorin; L-leucovorin; Levo-folinic Acid; Levo-leucovorin; Levoleucovorin Calcium Pentahydrate; S-leucovorin

Pharmacologic Category Antidote; Chemotherapy Modulating Agent; Rescue Agent (Chemotherapy)

Use Treatment of advanced, metastatic colorectal cancer (palliative) in combination with fluorouracil; rescue agent after high-dose methotrexate therapy in osteosarcoma; antidote for impaired methotrexate elimination and for inadvertent overdosage of folic acid antagonists

Pregnancy Risk Factor C

Dosage Note: Levoleucovorin, when substituted in place of leucovorin calcium (the racemic form), is dosed at **one-half** the usual dose of leucovorin calcium:

Colorectal cancer: Adults IV: The following regimens have been used (in combination with fluorouracil; fluorouracil doses may need to be adjusted for toxicity; no adjustment required for the levoleucovorin dose):

100 mg/m²/day over at least 3 minutes (followed by fluorouracil 370 mg/m²/day) for 5 days every 4 weeks for 2 cycles, then every 4-5 weeks depending on recovery from toxicities, **or**

10 mg/m²/day (followed by fluorouracil 425 mg/m²/day) for 5 days every 4 weeks for 2 cycles, then every 4-5 weeks depending on recovery from toxicities, **or**

Alternative dosing: Levoleucovorin, when substituted in place of leucovorin calcium within a chemotherapy regimen, is dosed at **one-half** the usual dose of leucovorin calcium (Goldberg, 1997; NCCN colon cancer guidelines v.2.2013)

High-dose methotrexate rescue: Children and Adults: IV: Usual dose: 7.5 mg (~5 mg/m²) every 6 hours for 10 doses, beginning 24 hours after the start of the methotrexate infusion (based on a methotrexate dose of 12 g/m² IV over 4 hours). Levoleucovorin (and hydration and urinary alkalinization) should be continued and/or adjusted until the methotrexate level is <0.05 micromolar (5 x 10^{-8} M) as follows:

Normal methotrexate elimination (serum methotrexate levels ~10 micromolar at 24 hours post administration, 1 micromolar at 48 hours and <0.2 micromolar at 72 hours post infusion): 7.5 mg IV every 6 hours for 10 doses

Delayed late methotrexate elimination (serum methotrexate levels >0.2 micromolar at 72 hours and >0.05 micromolar at 96 hours post methotrexate infusion): Continue 7.5 mg IV every 6 hours until methotrexate level is <0.05 micromolar

Delayed early methotrexate elimination and/or evidence of acute renal injury (serum methotrexate level ≥50 micromolar at 24 hours, ≥5 micromolar at 48 hours or a doubling or more of the serum creatinine level at 24 hours post methotrexate infusion): 75 mg IV every 3 hours until methotrexate level is <1 micromolar, followed by 7.5 mg IV every 3 hours until methotrexate level is <0.05 micromolar

Significant clinical toxicity in the presence of less severe abnormalities in methotrexate elimination or renal function (as described above): Extend levoleucovorin treatment for an additional 24 hours (total of 14 doses) in subsequent treatment cycles.

Delayed methotrexate elimination due to third space fluid accumulation, renal insufficiency, or inadequate hydration: May require higher levoleucovorin doses or prolonged administration.

Methotrexate overdose (inadvertent): Children and Adults: IV: 7.5 mg (~5 mg/m²) every 6 hours; continue until the methotrexate level is <0.01 micromolar (10^{-8} M). Initiate treatment as soon as possible after methotrexate overdose. Increase the levoleucovorin dose to 50 mg/m² IV every 3 hours if the 24 hour serum creatinine has increased 50% over baseline, or if the 24-hour methotrexate level is >5 micromolar (5 x 10^{-6} M), or if the 48-hour methotrexate level is >0.9 micromolar (9 x 10^{-7} M); continue levoleucovorin until the methotrexate level is <0.01 micromolar (10^{-8} M). Hydration (aggressive) and urinary alkalinization (with sodium bicarbonate) should also be maintained.

Dosage adjustment in renal impairment: No dosage adjustment provided in manufacturer's labeling.

Dosage adjustment in hepatic impairment: No dosage adjustment provided in manufacturer's labeling.

Additional Information Complete prescribing information should be consulted for additional detail.

Dosage Forms

Solution Reconstituted, Intravenous:

Fusilev: 50 mg (1 ea)

◆ **Levo-leucovorin** *see* LEVOleucovorin *on page 1200*

◆ **Levoleucovorin Calcium Pentahydrate** *see* LEVOleucovorin *on page 1200*

◆ **Levomefolate Calcium, Drospirenone, and Ethinyl Estradiol** *see* Ethinyl Estradiol, Drospirenone, and Levomefolate *on page 812*

◆ **Levomefolate, Drospirenone, and Ethinyl Estradiol** *see* Ethinyl Estradiol, Drospirenone, and Levomefolate *on page 812*

◆ **Levomepromazine** *see* Methotrimeprazine [CAN/INT] *on page 1329*

◆ **Levonest** *see* Ethinyl Estradiol and Levonorgestrel *on page 803*

Levonorgestrel (LEE voe nor jes trel)

Brand Names: U.S. Mirena; My Way [DSC]; Next Choice One Dose [DSC]; Opcicon One-Step [OTC]; Plan B; Plan B One-Step; Plan B One-Step [OTC]; Skyla; Take Action [OTC]

Brand Names: Canada Jaydess; Mirena; Next Choice; NorLevo; Option 2; Plan B

Index Terms LNg 20; Plan B

Pharmacologic Category Contraceptive; Progestin

Use

Intrauterine device (IUD): Prevention of pregnancy; treatment of heavy menstrual bleeding in women who also choose to use an IUD for contraception

Oral: Emergency contraception following unprotected intercourse or possible contraceptive failure

Pregnancy Considerations Use during pregnancy is contraindicated. When pregnancies have continued following levonorgestrel exposure, congenital anomalies have been infrequent. Significant adverse effects on infant growth and development have not been observed (limited data). In doses larger than those used for oral contraception, progestins have been reported to increase the risk of masculinization of female genitalia.

Intrauterine device: Pregnancy should be ruled out prior to insertion. Women who become pregnant with an IUD in place risk septic abortion (septic shock and death may occur). Removal of the device is recommended, however, removal or manipulation of IUD may result in pregnancy loss. In addition, miscarriage, premature labor, and premature delivery may occur if pregnancy is continued with IUD in place. Following pregnancy, insertion of the device should not take place until 6 weeks postpartum or until involution of the uterus is complete. The device may be inserted immediately following a first trimester abortion. Following removal of the device, ~80% of women who wished to conceive became pregnant within 12 months.

Oral tablet: A rapid return of fertility is expected following use for emergency contraception; routine contraceptive measures should be initiated or continued following use to ensure ongoing prevention of pregnancy. Barrier contraception is recommended immediately following emergency contraception. Short-term contraception (eg, oral hormonal contraceptive pills, patches, rings) may be started with barrier contraception or after the next menstrual period. Long term contraception (eg, IUD, depot medroxyprogesterone, progestin implant) should be started after the next menstrual period (ACOG, 2010).

Breast-Feeding Considerations Following maternal use of the oral tablets or intrauterine device, levonorgestrel is found in breast milk and can be detected in the serum of nursing infants (Shikary, 1987). In general, no adverse effects on the growth or development if the infant have been observed. Isolated cases of decreased milk production have been reported. Risk of perforation with IUD is increased in lactating women. Following pregnancy, insertion of the device should not take place until 6 weeks postpartum or until involution of the uterus is complete. Women who are breast-feeding may use levonorgestrel for emergency contraception (ACOG, 2010).

Contraindications Hypersensitivity to levonorgestrel or any component of the formulation; pregnancy

Additional product-specific contraindications:

Intrauterine device: Postcoital contraception, congenital or acquired uterine anomaly including fibroids that distort the uterine cavity, acute pelvic inflammatory disease, history of pelvic inflammatory disease (unless there has been a subsequent intrauterine pregnancy), postpartum endometritis or infected abortion within past 3 months, known or suspected uterine or cervical neoplasia, untreated acute cervicitis or vaginitis or other lower genital tract infections until infection is controlled, conditions which increase susceptibility to pelvic infections, unremoved IUD, undiagnosed uterine bleeding, active hepatic disease or hepatic tumors, current or history of known or suspected carcinoma of the breast or other progestin-sensitive cancer

Canadian labeling: Additional contraindications (not in U.S. labeling): Bacterial endocarditis, known immunodeficiency, hematologic malignancy, recent trophoblastic disease while human chorionic gonadotropin (hCG) hormone levels are elevated; cervical dysplasia

Oral: It is not known if the same contraindications associated with long-term progestin-only contraceptives apply to the levonorgestrel emergency contraception dose regimens. A history of ectopic pregnancy is not a contraindication to use in emergency contraception. Canadian labeling contraindicates use in patients with undiagnosed vaginal bleeding.

Warnings/Precautions Hazardous agent - use appropriate precautions for handling and disposal (NIOSH 2014 [group 2]).

These products do not protect against HIV infection or other sexually transmitted diseases (CDC, 2013). Menstrual bleeding patterns may be altered with use of the intrauterine device; the possibility of pregnancy should be considered if menstruation does not occur within 6 weeks of the previous menstrual period. If bleeding irregularities continue with prolonged use, appropriate diagnostic measures should be taken to rule out endometrial pathology. An increase in menstrual bleeding may indicate a partial or complete expulsion of the IUD. The risk of expulsion may be increased when the uterus is not completely involuted. If expulsion occurs, device may be replaced within 7 days of a menstrual period once pregnancy is ruled out. When using the oral tablet, spotting may occur following use; the possibility of pregnancy should be considered if menstruation is delayed for >7 days of the expected menstrual period.

Patients taking progestin-only contraceptives and presenting with lower abdominal pain should be evaluated for delayed follicular atresia (ovarian cysts) and ectopic pregnancy. Use caution in patients with previous ectopic pregnancy. Women with history of ectopic pregnancy were excluded from clinical trials; women with previous ectopic pregnancy, tubal surgery, or pelvic infection may be at increased risk for ectopic pregnancy. The possibility of ectopic pregnancy should be considered in patients with lower abdominal pain, especially in association with missed periods or vaginal bleeding in women with prior amenorrhea. Ectopic pregnancy may result in loss of fertility. May have adverse effects on glucose tolerance; use caution in women with diabetes. Use of the IUD is contraindicated with active hepatic disease or hepatic tumors. Use with caution in patients with depression; may be more susceptible to recurrence of depressive episodes; consider removal of IUD for serious recurrence. Depression is not a contraindication to use of the intrauterine device (CDC, 2010). Not indicated for use in postmenopausal women.

The use of combination hormonal contraceptives has been associated with a slight increase in the frequency of breast cancer, however, studies are not consistent. Data is insufficient to determine if progestin only contraceptives also increase this risk. Use of the intrauterine device is contraindicated in patients who have or who have had breast cancer or other progestin-sensitive cancers. The risk of cardiovascular side effects increases in women using estrogen containing combined hormonal contraceptives and who smoke cigarettes, especially those who are >35 years of age. This risk relative to progestin-only contraceptives has not been established. Women who take contraceptives should be advised not to smoke. Smoking is not a contraindication to use of the intrauterine device (CDC, 2010). The use of estrogens and/or progestins may change the results of some laboratory tests (eg, coagulation factors, lipids, glucose tolerance, binding proteins). The dose, route, and the specific estrogen/progestin influences these changes. In addition, personal risk factors (eg, cardiovascular disease, smoking, diabetes, age) also contribute to adverse events; use of specific products may be contraindicated in women with certain risk factors.

Additional formulation-specific warnings:

Intrauterine device: An increased incidence of group A streptococcal sepsis, pelvic inflammatory disease (may be asymptomatic), and actinomycosis have been reported with use. Using aseptic technique during insertion is essential to minimizing the risk of serious infections. Pelvic inflammatory disease occurs more frequently within the first year and most often within the first month after insertion; risk is increased with multiple sexual partners. May perforate uterus or cervix; risk of perforation is increased in lactating women and when the uterus is fixed retroverted or not completely involuted during the postpartum period. Pregnancy may result if perforation occurs; delayed detection of perforation may result in migration of IUD outside of uterine cavity, adhesions, peritonitis, intestinal perforations, intestinal obstruction, abscesses, and erosion of adjacent viscera. Insertion should be done by a trained health care provider. Insertion may be associated with pain, bleeding, or vasovagal reactions (eg, syncope, bradycardia), or seizure in an epileptic patients. Removal of the device may be necessary for the following reasons: pelvic infection, symptomatic genital actinomycosis, endometrial or cervical cancer, uterine or cervical perforation, and pregnancy. Use the intrauterine system with caution if any of the following conditions exist and consider removal if any of them arise during use: Coagulopathy or are receiving anticoagulants; marked increase of blood pressure; severe arterial disease, such as stroke or MI; exceptionally severe headache; and migraine, focal migraine with asymmetrical visual loss, or other symptoms indicating transient cerebral ischemia. In addition, consider removal if uterine or cervical malignancy or jaundice occurs during use. Embedded devices should also be removed. Not effective for emergency contraception.

Skyla, Jaydess [Canadian product]: Only under specific conditions may this device be scanned safely by MRI. Image quality may also be impaired if area of interest is relatively close to the device

Oral tablet: Not intended to be used for routine contraception and will not terminate an existing pregnancy. Barrier contraception is recommended immediately following emergency contraception and throughout the same menstrual cycle; efficacy of hormonal contraception may be decreased. When used for emergency contraception, reduced efficacy has been reported in women ≥75 kg to 80 kg and lack of efficacy has been reported in women >80 kg; the Canadian labeling recommends that alternative emergency contraceptive methods be considered (Plan B Canadian product monograph, 2014). The CDC recommends that obese women can generally use any type of contraceptive but suggests that levonorgestrel may be less efficacious in obese women compared to ulipristal acetate (CDC, 2013).

Adverse Reactions

Intrauterine device:

Cardiovascular: Edema

Central nervous system: Depression, headache, migraine, nervousness

Dermatologic: Acne, alopecia, eczema, hirsutism, pruritus, rash, urticaria

Endocrine & metabolic: Amenorrhea, breast pain/tenderness, dysmenorrhea, enlarged follicles, libido decreased, menorrhagia, ovarian cysts

Gastrointestinal: Abdominal distension, abdominal pain, nausea, weight gain

Genitourinary: Cervicitis, dyspareunia, intermenstrual bleeding/spotting, leukorrhea, pelvic infection, pelvic pain, uterine/vaginal bleeding alterations, vaginal discharge, vaginitis, vulvovaginitis

Hematologic: Anemia

Neuromuscular & skeletal: Back pain

Miscellaneous: Ectopic pregnancy, IUD expulsion

Rare but important or life-threatening: Angioedema, cervical wall perforation, device breakage, failed insertion, hypersensitivity reactions, jaundice, sepsis, uterine bleeding, uterine wall perforation

Oral tablets:

Central nervous system: Dizziness, fatigue, headache

Endocrine & metabolic: Breast tenderness, heavier menstrual bleeding, lighter menstrual bleeding, menses delayed

Gastrointestinal: Abdominal pain, diarrhea, nausea, vomiting

Rare but important or life-threatening: Dysmenorrhea, menstruation irregularities, oligomenorrhea, pelvic pain

Drug Interactions

Metabolism/Transport Effects Substrate of CYP3A4 (major); **Note:** Assignment of Major/Minor substrate status based on clinically relevant drug interaction potential

Avoid Concomitant Use

Avoid concomitant use of Levonorgestrel with any of the following: Griseofulvin; Tranexamic Acid; Ulipristal

Increased Effect/Toxicity

Levonorgestrel may increase the levels/effects of: C1 inhibitors; Selegiline; Thalidomide; Tranexamic Acid; Voriconazole

The levels/effects of Levonorgestrel may be increased by: Atazanavir; Boceprevir; Cobicistat; Herbs (Progestogenic Properties); Lopinavir; Metreleptin; Mifepristone; Tipranavir; Voriconazole

Decreased Effect

Levonorgestrel may decrease the levels/effects of: Anticoagulants; Fosamprenavir; Vitamin K Antagonists

The levels/effects of Levonorgestrel may be decreased by: Acitretin; Aminoglutethimide; Aprepitant; Artemether; Barbiturates; Bexarotene (Systemic); Bile Acid Sequestrants; Bosentan; CarBAMazepine; CloBAZam; CYP3A4 Inducers (Moderate); CYP3A4 Inducers (Strong); Dabrafenib; Darunavir; Deferasirox; Efavirenz; Eslicarbazepine; Exenatide; Felbamate; Fosamprenavir; Fosaprepitant; Fosphenytoin; Griseofulvin; LamoTRIgine; Lopinavir; Metreleptin; Mifepristone; Mitotane; Mycophenolate; Nelfinavir; Nevirapine; OXcarbazepine; Perampanel; Phenytoin; Primidone; Prucalopride; Retinoic Acid Derivatives; Rifamycin Derivatives; Saquinavir; Siltuximab; St Johns Wort; Sugammadex; Telaprevir; Tocilizumab; Topiramate; Ulipristal

Storage/Stability

Intrauterine device: Store at 25°C (77°F); excursions permitted between 15°C to 30°C (59°F to 86°F).

Oral tablet: Store at 20°C to 25°C (68°F to 77°F).

Mechanism of Action Pregnancy may be prevented through several mechanisms: Thickening of cervical mucus, which inhibits sperm passage through the uterus and sperm survival; inhibition of ovulation, from a negative feedback mechanism on the hypothalamus, leading to reduced secretion of follicle stimulating hormone (FSH) and luteinizing hormone (LH); altering the endometrium, which may affect implantation. Levonorgestrel is not effective once the implantation process has begun.

Pharmacodynamics/Kinetics

Duration: Intrauterine device: Mirena: Up to 5 years; Skyla, Jaydess [Canadian product]: Up to 3 years

Absorption: Oral: Rapid and complete

Distribution: V_d: ~1.8 L/kg

Protein binding: Highly bound to albumin (~50%) and sex hormone-binding globulin (~47%) (Fotherby, 1995)

Metabolism: Hepatic via CYP3A4; forms inactive metabolites

Half-life elimination: Oral: ~27 hours

Time to peak: Oral: ~2 hours

Excretion: Urine (45%); feces (32%)

Dosage Adults: Females:

Long-term prevention of pregnancy: Intrauterine device (Skyla, Jaydess [Canadian product]): To be inserted into uterine cavity; should be inserted within 7 days of onset of menstruation or immediately after first trimester abortion; releases levonorgestrel ~6 mcg per day over 3 years. May be removed and replaced with a new unit at any time during menstrual cycle; do not leave any one system in place for >3 years.

Long-term prevention of pregnancy, treatment of heavy menstrual bleeding: Intrauterine device (Mirena): To be inserted into uterine cavity; should be inserted within 7 days of onset of menstruation or immediately after first trimester abortion; initially releases levonorgestrel 20 mcg per day, then rate subsequently decreases; mean release rate over 5 years is levonorgestrel ~14 mcg per day. May be removed and replaced with a new unit at anytime during menstrual cycle; do not leave any one system in place for >5 years.

Back up contraception: If the intrauterine device is inserted within the first 7 days of the onset of menstruation, backup contraception is not needed. However, the device may be inserted at any time once it is determined that the woman is not pregnant. If insertion occurs >7 days after menstrual bleeding started, an additional form of contraception must be used for 7 days unless the woman abstains from sexual intercourse (CDC, 2013).

Continuation of therapy or switching to different contraceptive (Skyla, Mirena, Jaydess [Canadian product]): At the time of device removal, a new device may be inserted immediately if continuation of therapy is desired. If the patient wishes to change to a different method of birth control, remove the device during the first 7 days of menstrual cycle and begin the new therapy. If the device is not removed during menstruation (or if the patient has irregular menstrual cycles) and wants to start a different method of birth control, consider starting the new method 7 days prior to device removal.

Emergency contraception: Oral: May be used at any time during menstrual cycle:

Two-dose regimen: One 0.75 mg tablet as soon as possible within 72 hours of unprotected sexual intercourse; a second 0.75 mg tablet should be taken 12 hours after the first dose

Single-dose regimen: One 1.5 mg tablet as soon as possible within 72 hours of unprotected sexual intercourse

Elderly: Not indicated for use in postmenopausal women

Dosage adjustment in renal impairment: There are no dosage adjustments provided in the manufacturer's labeling (has not been studied).

Dosage adjustment in hepatic impairment: There are no dosage adjustments provided in the manufacturer's labeling (has not been studied); use of the intrauterine device is contraindicated with active hepatic disease or hepatic tumor.

Administration

Intrauterine device: Consider administering analgesics prior to insertion. Insert into the uterine cavity to the recommended depth with the provided insertion device; should not be forced into the uterus. If necessary, dilate the cervical canal and consider using a paracervical block. Transvaginal ultrasound may be used to check proper placement. Remove if not positioned properly and insert a new IUD; do not reinsert removed IUD. Exclude perforation if exceptional pain or bleeding occurs after insertion.

Oral: Consider repeating the dose if vomiting occurs within 2 hours. If severe vomiting occurs, may consider administering the oral tablets vaginally (ACOG, 2010).

Hazardous agent; use appropriate precautions for handling and disposal (NIOSH 2014 [group 2]).

Monitoring Parameters

IUD: Prior to insertion: Assessment of pregnancy status; cervical examination; weight (optional; BMI at baseline may be helpful to monitor changes during therapy); STD screen (unless already screened according to CDC STD Treatment guidelines) (CDC, 2013). Re-examine following insertion (4-6 weeks Mirena, Skyla; 4-12 weeks Jaydess [Canadian product]) and then yearly or more frequently if necessary. Threads should be visible; if length of thread has changed device may have become displaced, broken, perforated the uterus, or expelled. Transvaginal ultrasound may be used to check placement. Monitor for prolonged menstrual bleeding, amenorrhea, irregularity of menses, Pap smear, blood pressure, serum glucose in patients with diabetes, LDL levels in patients with hyperlipidemias; re-examine following first menses postinsertion of IUD. Patients presenting with lower abdominal pain should be evaluated for follicular atresia and ectopic pregnancy. Signs of infection following IUD insertion, especially in patients at increased risk (eg, patients on chronic corticosteroids, patients with type 1 diabetes mellitus). Monitor for signs/symptoms of thromboembolism in women who require surgery with prolonged immobilization.

Oral tablet: Evaluate for pregnancy, spontaneous abortion or ectopic pregnancy if menses is delayed for ≥1 week following emergency contraception, or if lower abdominal pain or persistent irregular bleeding develops.

Reference Range Intrauterine device:

Mirena: Plasma concentrations range from 150-200 pg/mL

Skyla, Jaydess [Canadian product]: Plasma concentrations range from a peak of 192 pg/mL (2 days following insertion) to 59-61 pg/mL (after 3 years)

Additional Information

Intrauterine device (IUD):

Mirena: The cumulative 5-year pregnancy rate is ~0.7 pregnancies/100 users. Over 70% of women in the trials had previously used IUDs. The reported pregnancy rate after 12 months was ≤0.2 pregnancies/100 users. Approximately 80% of women who wish to conceive have become pregnant within 12 months of device removal. The recommended patient profile for this product: A woman who has at least one child, is in a stable and mutually-monogamous relationship, no history of pelvic inflammatory disease, and no history of ectopic pregnancy or predisposition to ectopic pregnancy. Keep a copy of the consent form and record lot number of device.

Skyla: The cumulative 3-year pregnancy rate is ~0.9 pregnancies/100 users. Approximately 77% of women who wish to conceive have become pregnant within 12 months of device removal.

Oral tablet: Treatment for emergency contraception should begin as soon as possible; however, treatment is still moderately effective if used within 5 days and should be made available to women up to 5 days after unprotected or inadequately protected intercourse. May be used in women with contraindications to conventional oral contraceptive agents (eg, cardiovascular disease, migraines, liver disease). When used as directed for emergency contraception, the expected pregnancy rate is decreased from 8% to 1%. Approximately 87% of women have their next menstrual period at approximately the expected time. A rapid return to fertility following use is expected. When using the two-dose emergency contraceptive regimen, the second dose is equally effective if taken 12-24 hours after the first (ACOG, 2010).

Dosage Forms

Intrauterine Device, Intrauterine:

Mirena: 20 mcg/24 hr

Skyla: 13.5 mg

Tablet, Oral:

Opcicon One-Step [OTC]: 1.5 mg

Plan B: 0.75 mg

Plan B One-Step [OTC]: 1.5 mg, 1.5 mg

Take Action [OTC]: 1.5 mg

Generic: 0.75 mg, 1.5 mg

- ◆ **Levonorgestrel and Estradiol** *see* Estradiol and Levonorgestrel *on page* *781*
- ◆ **Levonorgestrel and Ethinyl Estradiol** *see* Ethinyl Estradiol and Levonorgestrel *on page* *803*
- ◆ **Levophed** *see* Norepinephrine *on page* *1472*
- ◆ **Levophed® (Can)** *see* Norepinephrine *on page* *1472*
- ◆ **Levora** *see* Ethinyl Estradiol and Levonorgestrel *on page* *803*

Levorphanol (lee VOR fa nole)

Index Terms Levo-Dromoran; Levorphan Tartrate; Levorphanol Tartrate

Pharmacologic Category Analgesic, Opioid

Additional Appendix Information

Opioid Conversion Table *on page* *2232*

Use Relief of moderate-to-severe pain; preoperative sedation/analgesia; management of chronic pain (eg, cancer) requiring opioid therapy

Pregnancy Risk Factor C

Dosage Adults: **Note:** These are guidelines and do not represent the maximum doses that may be required in all patients. Doses should be titrated to pain relief/prevention.

Acute pain (moderate-to-severe): Oral: Initial: Opioid-naive: 2 mg every 6-8 hours as needed; patients with prior opioid exposure may require higher initial doses; usual dosage range: 2-4 mg every 6-8 hours as needed

Note: The American Pain Society recommends an initial dose of 4 mg for severe pain in adults (APS, 6th ed)

Chronic pain: Patients taking opioids chronically may become tolerant and require doses higher than the usual dosage range to maintain the desired effect. Tolerance can be managed by appropriate dose titration. **There is no optimal or maximal dose for levorphanol in chronic pain. The appropriate dose is one that relieves pain throughout its dosing interval without causing unmanageable side effects.**

Dosing adjustment in renal impairment: Use with caution; initial dose should be reduced in severe renal impairment

Dosing adjustment in hepatic impairment: Use with caution; initial dose should be reduced in severe hepatic impairment

Additional Information Complete prescribing information should be consulted for additional detail.

Dosage Forms

Tablet, Oral:

Generic: 2 mg

◆ **Levorphanol Tartrate** *see* Levorphanol *on page 1204*

◆ **Levorphan Tartrate** *see* Levorphanol *on page 1204*

◆ **Levosalbutamol** *see* Levalbuterol *on page 1189*

Levosimendan [INT] (LEE voe si men dan)

International Brand Names Daxim (CL, VE); Simdak (IS, SI, SK); Simdax (AE, AR, AT, BG, BR, CY, CZ, ES, FI, GR, HR, HU, IL, IT, KW, MX, NO, NZ, PE, PT, QA, RO, RU, SE, SG, TR, UY); Simenda (IN)

Pharmacologic Category Vasodilator

Reported Use Management of congestive heart failure (CHF)

Dosage Range Adults: IV: Loading dose: 6-24 mcg/kg over 10 minutes followed by a continuous infusion of 0.05-0.2 mcg/kg/minute, adjusted according to response.

Product Availability Product available in various countries; not currently available in the U.S.

Dosage Forms

Injection: 2.5 mg/mL (5 mL, 10 mL)

◆ **Levothroid [DSC]** *see* Levothyroxine *on page 1205*

Levothyroxine (lee voe thye ROKS een)

Brand Names: U.S. Levothroid [DSC]; Levoxyl; Synthroid; Tirosint; Unithroid; Unithroid Direct

Brand Names: Canada Eltroxin; Levothyroxine Sodium; Levothyroxine Sodium for Injection; Synthroid

Index Terms *L*-Thyroxine Sodium; Levothyroxine Sodium; T_4

Pharmacologic Category Thyroid Product

Use

Oral:

Hypothyroidism: Replacement or supplemental therapy in congenital or acquired hypothyroidism of any etiology, except transient hypothyroidism during the recovery phase of subacute thyroiditis. Specific indications include primary (thyroidal), secondary (pituitary), and tertiary (hypothalamic) hypothyroidism and subclinical hypothyroidism. Primary hypothyroidism may result from functional deficiency, primary atrophy, partial or total congenital absence of the thyroid gland, or from the effects of surgery, radiation, or drugs, with or without the presence of goiter.

Pituitary thyrotropin-stimulating hormone suppression: Prevention or treatment of various types of euthyroid goiters, including thyroid nodules, subacute or chronic lymphocytic thyroiditis (Hashimoto thyroiditis), multinodular goiter and as an adjunct to surgery and radioiodine therapy in the management of thyrotropin-dependent well-differentiated thyroid cancer.

Injectable:

U.S. labeling: Treatment of myxedema coma

Canadian labeling: Refer to oral indications; IV may be substituted for oral when rapid repletion is required; IV or IM may be used when oral administration is not possible.

Pregnancy Risk Factor A

Pregnancy Considerations Endogenous thyroid hormones minimally cross the placenta; the fetal thyroid becomes active around the end of the first trimester. Levothyroxine has not been shown to increase the risk of congenital abnormalities.

Uncontrolled maternal hypothyroidism may result in adverse neonatal outcomes (eg, premature birth, low birth weight, and respiratory distress) and adverse maternal outcomes (eg, spontaneous abortion, pre-eclampsia, stillbirth, and premature delivery). To prevent adverse events, normal maternal thyroid function should be maintained prior to conception and throughout pregnancy. Levothyroxine is considered the treatment of choice for the control of hypothyroidism during pregnancy. Due to alterations of endogenous maternal thyroid hormones, the levothyroxine dose may need to be increased during pregnancy and the dose usually needs to be decreased after delivery.

Breast-Feeding Considerations Endogenous thyroid hormones are minimally found in breast milk. The amount of endogenous thyroxine found in breast milk does not influence infant plasma thyroid values. Levothyroxine was not found to cause adverse events to the infant or mother during breast-feeding. Adequate thyroid hormone concentrations are required to maintain normal lactation. Appropriate levothyroxine doses should be continued during breast-feeding.

Contraindications

Hypersensitivity to levothyroxine sodium or any component of the formulation; acute MI; thyrotoxicosis of any etiology; uncorrected adrenal insufficiency

Capsule: Additional contraindication: Inability to swallow capsules (eg, infants, small children)

Injection:

U.S. labeling: There are no contraindications listed in the manufacturer's labeling when used for labeled indication (treatment of myxedema coma); consider contraindications for oral therapy if using as a temporary substitute for oral treatment (off-label use) in patients with chronic hypothyroidism.

Canadian labeling: Hypersensitivity to levothyroxine sodium or any component of the formulation; acute MI; thyrotoxicosis of any etiology; uncorrected adrenal insufficiency.

Warnings/Precautions [U.S. Boxed Warning]: Thyroid supplements are ineffective and potentially toxic when used for the treatment of obesity or for weight reduction, especially in euthyroid patients. High doses may produce serious or even life-threatening toxic effects particularly when used with some anorectic drugs (eg, sympathomimetic amines). Levothyroxine, either alone or with other concomitant therapeutic agents, should not be used for the treatment of obesity or for weight loss. Routine use of T_4 for TSH suppression is not recommended in patients with benign thyroid nodules. In patients deemed appropriate candidates, treatment should never be fully suppressive (TSH <0.1 mIU/L). Use with caution and reduce dosage in patients with cardiovascular disease; patients with developing or worsening cardiac ▶

symptoms should have their dose reduced or therapy withheld for 7 days then resumed at a reduced dose. Use cautiously in the elderly since they may be more likely to have compromised cardiovascular functions. Patients with adrenal insufficiency, myxedema, diabetes mellitus and insipidus may have symptoms exaggerated or aggravated. Use is contraindicated in patients with uncorrected adrenal insufficiency. Chronic hypothyroidism predisposes patients to coronary artery disease. Long-term therapy can decrease bone mineral density. Levoxyl may rapidly swell and disintegrate causing choking or gagging (should be administered with a full glass of water); use caution in patients with dysphagia or other swallowing disorders.

Adverse Reactions

Cardiovascular: Angina pectoris, cardiac arrest, cardiac arrhythmia, congestive heart failure, flushing, hypertension, increased pulse, myocardial infarction, palpitations, tachycardia

Central nervous system: Anxiety, choking sensation (Levoxyl), emotional lability, fatigue, headache, heat intolerance, hyperactivity, insomnia, irritability, myasthenia, nervousness, pseudotumor cerebri (children), seizure (rare)

Dermatologic: Alopecia, diaphoresis

Endocrine & metabolic: Menstrual disease, weight loss

Gastrointestinal: Abdominal cramps, diarrhea, dysphagia (Levoxyl), gag reflex (Levoxyl), increased appetite, vomiting

Genitourinary: Infertility

Hepatic: Increased liver enzymes

Hypersensitivity: Hypersensitivity (to inactive ingredients; symptoms include urticaria, pruritus, rash, flushing, angioedema, GI symptoms, fever, arthralgia, serum sickness, wheezing)

Neuromuscular & skeletal: Decreased bone mineral density, slipped capital femoral epiphysis (children), tremor

Respiratory: Dyspnea

Miscellaneous: Fever

Drug Interactions

Metabolism/Transport Effects None known.

Avoid Concomitant Use

Avoid concomitant use of Levothyroxine with any of the following: Sodium Iodide I131; Sucroferric Oxyhydroxide

Increased Effect/Toxicity

Levothyroxine may increase the levels/effects of: Tricyclic Antidepressants; Vitamin K Antagonists

The levels/effects of Levothyroxine may be increased by: Piracetam

Decreased Effect

Levothyroxine may decrease the levels/effects of: Sodium Iodide I131; Theophylline Derivatives

The levels/effects of Levothyroxine may be decreased by: Aluminum Hydroxide; Bile Acid Sequestrants; Calcium Polystyrene Sulfonate; Calcium Salts; CarBAMazepine; Ciprofloxacin (Systemic); Estrogen Derivatives; Fosphenytoin; Iron Salts; Lanthanum; Magnesium Salts; Multivitamins/Minerals (with ADEK, Folate, Iron); Orlistat; Phenytoin; Raloxifene; Rifampin; Selective Serotonin Reuptake Inhibitors; Sevelamer; Sodium Polystyrene Sulfonate; Sucralfate; Sucroferric Oxyhydroxide

Food Interactions Taking levothyroxine with enteral nutrition may cause reduced bioavailability and may lower serum thyroxine levels leading to signs or symptoms of hypothyroidism. Soybean flour (infant formula), cottonseed meal, walnuts, and dietary fiber may decrease absorption of levothyroxine from the GI tract. Management: Take in the morning on an empty stomach at least 30 minutes before food. Consider an increase in dose if taken with enteral tube feed.

Preparation for Administration Dilute vial for injection with 5 mL normal saline. Reconstituted concentrations for the 100 mcg, 200 mcg and 500 mcg vials are 20 mcg/mL, 40 mcg/mL, and 100 mcg/mL, respectively. Shake well and use immediately after reconstitution (manufacturer labeling suggests reconstituted vial is stable for 4 hours); discard any unused portions.

Storage/Stability

Capsules and tablets: Store at 25°C (77°F); excursions are permitted between 15°C and 30°C (59°F and 86°F). Protect from light and moisture.

Injection: Store at 20°C to 25°C (68°F to 77°F). Protect from light.

Additional stability data:

Stability in polypropylene syringes (100 mcg/mL in NS) at 5°C ± 1°C is 7 days (Gupta, 2000).

Stability in latex-free, PVC minibags protected from light and stored at 15°C to 30°C (59°F to 86°F) was 12 hours for a 2 mcg/mL concentration or 18 hours for a 0.4 mcg/mL concentration in NS. May be exposed to light; however, stability time is significantly reduced, especially for the 2 mcg/mL concentration (Strong, 2010).

Mechanism of Action Levothyroxine (T_4) is a synthetic form of thyroxine, an endogenous hormone secreted by the thyroid gland. T_4 is converted to its active metabolite, L-triiodothyronine (T_3). Thyroid hormones (T_4 and T_3) then bind to thyroid receptor proteins in the cell nucleus and exert metabolic effects through control of DNA transcription and protein synthesis; involved in normal metabolism, growth, and development; promotes gluconeogenesis, increases utilization and mobilization of glycogen stores, and stimulates protein synthesis, increases basal metabolic rate

Pharmacodynamics/Kinetics

Absorption: Oral: Erratic (40% to 80% [per manufacturer]); may be decreased by age and specific foods and drugs

Protein binding: >99% bound to plasma proteins including thyroxine-binding globulin, thyroxine-binding prealbumin, and albumin

Metabolism: Hepatic to triiodothyronine (T_3; active); ~80% thyroxine (T_4) deiodinated in kidney and periphery; glucuronidation/conjugation also occurs; undergoes enterohepatic recirculation

Bioavailability: Oral tablets: 64% (nonfasting state) to 79% to 81% (fasting state)

Time to peak, serum: 2 hours

Half-life elimination: Euthyroid: 6 to 8 days; Hypothyroid: 9 to 10 days; Hyperthyroid: 3 to 4 days

Excretion: Urine (major route of elimination; decreases with age); feces (~20%)

Dosage Doses should be adjusted based on clinical response and laboratory parameters.

Oral:

Hypothyroidism:

Infants and Children: Daily dosage based on body weight and age as listed below:

1 to 3 months: 10 to 15 mcg/kg/day; if the infant is at risk for development of cardiac failure, use a lower starting dose of 25 mcg daily; if the initial serum T_4 is very low (<5 mcg/dL), begin treatment at a higher dosage of approximately 50 mcg daily. (12 to 17 mcg/kg/day) (AAP, 2006; Selva, 2002)

3 to 6 months: 8 to 10 mcg/kg/day

6 to 12 months: 6 to 8 mcg/kg/day

1 to 5 years: 5 to 6 mcg/kg/day

6 to 12 years: 4 to 5 mcg/kg/day

>12 years: 2 to 3 mcg/kg/day

Growth and puberty complete: 1.7 mcg/kg/day; refer to Adult dosing (U.S. labeling) or 1.6 to 1.7 mcg/kg/day (Canadian labeling)

Dosing modifications:

Hyperactivity in older children may be minimized by starting at 1/4 of the recommended dose and increasing each week by that amount until the full dose is achieved (4 weeks).

Children with severe or chronic hypothyroidism should be started at 25 mcg daily; adjust dose by 25 mcg every 2 to 4 weeks.

Adults (including children in whom growth and puberty are complete, healthy adults <50 years of age, and older adults who have been recently treated for hyperthyroidism or who have been hypothyroid for only a few months): ~1.7 mcg/kg/day; usual doses are ≤200 mcg daily (range: 100 to 125 mcg daily [70 kg adult]); doses ≥300 mcg daily are rare (consider poor compliance, malabsorption, and/or drug interactions). Titrate dose every 6 weeks.

Adults >50 years without cardiac disease **or** <50 years with cardiac disease: Initial: 25 to 50 mcg daily; adjust dose by 12.5 to 25 mcg increments at 6- to 8-week intervals as needed

Adults >50 years with cardiac disease: Initial: 12.5 to 25 mcg daily; adjust dose by 12.5 to 25 mcg increments at 4- to 6-week intervals (many clinicians prefer to adjust at 6- to 8-week intervals)

Note: Elderly patients may require <1 mcg/kg/day. Patients with combined hypothyroidism and cardiac disease should be monitored carefully for changes in stability.

Severe hypothyroidism: Adults: Initial: 12.5 to 25 mcg daily; adjust dose by 25 mcg daily every 2 to 4 weeks as appropriate

Myxedema: Adults: Oral agents are not recommended for myxedema: Refer to IV dosing.

Subclinical hypothyroidism: Adults: 1 mcg/kg/day

TSH suppression: Adults:

Well-differentiated thyroid cancer: Highly individualized; Doses >2 mcg/kg/day may be needed to suppress TSH to <0.1 mIU/L in intermediate- to high-risk tumors. Low-risk tumors may be maintained at or slightly below the lower limit of normal (0.1 to 0.5 mIU/L) (Cooper, 2009).

Benign nodules and nontoxic multinodular goiter: Routine use of T_4 for TSH suppression is not recommended in patients with benign thyroid nodules. In patients deemed appropriate candidates, treatment should never be fully suppressive (TSH <0.1 mIU/L) (Cooper, 2009; Gharib, 2010). Avoid use if TSH is already suppressed.

IM, IV: Children, Adolescents, Adults, and Elderly: Hypothyroidism (Canadian labeling; off-label route [IM] and off-label use in U.S.): 50% of the oral dose; alternatively, some clinicians administer up to 80% of the oral dose. **Note:** Bioavailability of the oral formulation is highly variable, but absorption has been measured to be ~80%, when the oral tablet formulation was administered in the recommended fasting state (Dickerson, 2010; Fish, 1987).

IV:

Adults: Myxedema coma or stupor: Initial: 300 to 500 mcg initially, followed by 50 to 100 mcg once daily until patient is able to tolerate oral administration; smaller doses should be considered in patients with cardiovascular disease

Elderly: Myxedema coma: Refer to adult dosing; lower doses may be needed

Dosage adjustment for toxicity: Cardiac symptoms (onset or worsening): Manufacturer labeling recommends reducing dosage or withholding therapy for 7 days and then resuming therapy at reduced dosage. Specific dosing recommendations are not provided.

Dosage adjustment in renal impairment: There are no dosage adjustments provided in manufacturer's labeling.

Dosage adjustment in hepatic impairment: There are no dosage adjustments provided in manufacturer's labeling.

Administration

Oral: Administer in the morning on an empty stomach, at least 30 minutes before food.

Capsule: Must be swallowed whole; do not cut, crush, or attempt to dissolve capsules in water to prepare a suspension.

Tablet: May be crushed and suspended in 5 to 10 mL of water; suspension should be used immediately. Levoxyl should be administered with a full glass of water to prevent gagging (due to tablet swelling). **Note:** The Canadian labeling suggests that crushed tablets may also be suspended in breast milk or non-soybean based formula or sprinkled over a small amount of food (eg, apple sauce); avoid the use of foods with high content of iron, fiber, or soybean.

Nasogastric tube: Bioavailability of levothyroxine is reduced if administered with enteral tube feeds. Since holding feedings for at least 1 hour before and after levothyroxine administration may not completely resolve the interaction, an increase in dose (eg, additional 25 mcg) may be necessary (Dickerson, 2010).

Parenteral: May be administered by IV injection; may also be administered IM when oral administration is not feasible (Canadian labeling; off-label route in U.S.).

Monitoring Parameters Thyroid function test (serum thyroxine, thyrotropin concentrations), resin triiodothyronine uptake (rT_3U), free thyroxine index (FTI), T_4, TSH, heart rate, blood pressure, clinical signs of hypo- and hyperthyroidism; TSH is the most reliable guide for evaluating adequacy of thyroid replacement dosage. TSH may be elevated during the first few months of thyroid replacement despite patients being clinically euthyroid. In cases where T_4 remains low and TSH is within normal limits, an evaluation of "free" (unbound) T_4 is needed to evaluate further increase in dosage

Infants: Monitor closely for cardiac overload, arrhythmias, and aspiration from avid suckling

Infants/children: Monitor closely for under/overtreatment. Undertreatment may decrease intellectual development and linear growth, and lead to poor school performance due to impaired concentration and slowed mentation. Overtreatment may adversely affect brain maturation, accelerate bone age (leading to premature closure of the epiphyses and reduced adult height); craniosynostosis has been reported in infants. Treated children may experience a period of catch-up growth. Monitor TSH and total or free T_4 at 2 and 4 weeks after starting treatment; every 1-2 months for first year of life; every 2-3 months during years 1-3; every 3-12 months until growth completed. Perform routine clinical examinations at regular intervals (to assess mental and physical growth and development).

Adults: Monitor TSH every 6-8 weeks until normalized; 8-12 weeks after dosage changes; every 6-12 months throughout therapy

Reference Range Pediatrics: Cord T_4 and values in the first few weeks are much higher, falling over the first months and years. ≥10 years: ~5.8-11 mcg/dL (SI: 75-142 nmol/L). Borderline low: ≤4.5-5.7 mcg/dL (SI: 58-73 nmol/L); low: ≤4.4 mcg/dL (SI: 57 nmol/L); results <2.5 mcg/dL (SI: <32 nmol/L) are strong evidence for hypothyroidism.

Approximate adult normal range: 4-12 mcg/dL (SI: 51-154 nmol/L). Borderline high: 11.1-13 mcg/dL (SI: 143-167 nmol/L); high: ≥13.1 mcg/dL (SI: 169 nmol/L). Normal range is increased in women on birth control pills (5.5-12 mcg/dL); normal range in pregnancy: ~5.5-16 mcg/dL (SI: ~71-206 nmol/L). TSH: 0.4-10 (for those ≥80 years) mIU/L; T_4: 4-12 mcg/dL (SI: 51-154 nmol/L); T_3 (RIA) (total T_3): 80-230 ng/dL (SI: 1.2-3.5 nmol/L); T_4 free (free T_4): 0.7-1.8 ng/dL (SI: 9-23 pmol/L).

Additional Information Equivalent doses: The following statement on relative potency of thyroid products is included in a joint statement by American Thyroid Association (ATA), American Association of Clinical Endocrinologists (AACE) and The Endocrine Society (TES): For purposes of conversion, levothyroxine sodium (T_4) 100 mcg is usually considered equivalent to desiccated thyroid 60 to 65 mg (1 grain), liothyronine sodium (T_3) 25 mcg, or liotrix 12.5 mcg T_3/50 mcg T_4. However, these are rough guidelines only and do not obviate the careful re-evaluation of a patient when switching thyroid hormone preparations, including a change from one brand of levothyroxine to another. Joint position statement is available at http://www.thyroid.org/thyroxine-products-joint-position-statement/.

Note: Several medications have effects on thyroid production or conversion. The impact in thyroid replacement has not been specifically evaluated, but patient response should be monitored:

Methimazole: Decreases thyroid hormone secretion, while propylthiouracil decrease thyroid hormone secretion and decreases conversion of T_4 to T_3.

Beta-adrenergic antagonists: Decrease conversion of T_4 to T_3 (dose related, propranolol ≥160 mg/day); patients may be clinically euthyroid.

Iodide, iodine-containing radiographic contrast agents may decrease thyroid hormone secretion; may also increase thyroid hormone secretion, especially in patients with Graves' disease.

Other agents reported to impact on thyroid production/conversion include aminoglutethimide, amiodarone, chloral hydrate, diazepam, ethionamide, interferon-alpha, interleukin-2, lithium, lovastatin (case report), glucocorticoids (dose-related), mercaptopurine, sulfonamides, thiazide diuretics, and tolbutamide.

In addition, a number of medications have been noted to cause transient depression in TSH secretion, which may complicate interpretation of monitoring tests for levothyroxine, including corticosteroids, octreotide, and dopamine. Metoclopramide may increase TSH secretion

Dosage Forms

Capsule, Oral:

Tirosint: 13 mcg, 25 mcg, 50 mcg, 75 mcg, 88 mcg, 100 mcg, 112 mcg, 125 mcg, 137 mcg, 150 mcg

Solution Reconstituted, Intravenous [preservative free]:

Generic: 100 mcg (1 ea); 200 mcg (1 ea); 500 mcg (1 ea)

Tablet, Oral:

Levoxyl: 25 mcg, 50 mcg, 75 mcg, 88 mcg, 100 mcg, 112 mcg, 125 mcg, 137 mcg, 150 mcg, 175 mcg, 200 mcg

Synthroid: 25 mcg, 50 mcg, 75 mcg, 88 mcg, 100 mcg, 112 mcg, 125 mcg, 137 mcg, 150 mcg, 175 mcg, 200 mcg, 300 mcg

Unithroid: 25 mcg, 50 mcg, 75 mcg, 88 mcg, 100 mcg, 112 mcg, 125 mcg, 137 mcg, 150 mcg, 175 mcg, 200 mcg, 300 mcg

Unithroid Direct: 25 mcg, 50 mcg, 75 mcg, 88 mcg, 100 mcg, 112 mcg, 125 mcg, 150 mcg, 175 mcg, 200 mcg, 300 mcg

Generic: 25 mcg, 50 mcg, 75 mcg, 88 mcg, 100 mcg, 112 mcg, 125 mcg, 137 mcg, 150 mcg, 175 mcg, 200 mcg, 300 mcg

Dosage Forms: Canada Refer also to Dosage Forms.

Note: Capsules are not available in Canada.

Tablet, Oral, as sodium:

Eltroxin: 50 mcg, 100 mcg, 150 mcg, 200 mcg, 300 mcg

Extemporaneous Preparations A 25 mcg/mL oral suspension may be made with tablets and 40 mL glycerol. Crush twenty-five 0.1 mg levothyroxine tablets in a mortar and reduce to a fine powder. Add small portions of glycerol and mix to a uniform suspension. Transfer to a calibrated 100 mL amber bottle; rinse the mortar with about 10 mL of glycerol and pour into the bottle; repeat until all 40 mL of glycerol is used. Add quantity of water sufficient to make 100 mL. Label "shake well" and "refrigerate". Stable for 8 days refrigerated.

Boulton DW, Fawcett JP, and Woods DJ, "Stability of an Extemporaneously Compounded Levothyroxine Sodium Oral Liquid," *Am J Health Syst Pharm*, 1996, 53(10):1157-61.

◆ **Levothyroxine and Liothyronine** *see* Liotrix *on page 1221*

◆ **Levothyroxine and Liothyronine** *see* Thyroid, Desiccated *on page 2031*

◆ **Levothyroxine Sodium** *see* Levothyroxine *on page 1205*

◆ **Levothyroxine Sodium for Injection (Can)** *see* Levothyroxine *on page 1205*

◆ **Levoxyl** *see* Levothyroxine *on page 1205*

◆ **Levsin** *see* Hyoscyamine *on page 1026*

◆ **Levsin/SL** *see* Hyoscyamine *on page 1026*

◆ **Lev-Tov [OTC]** *see* Folic Acid, Cyanocobalamin, and Pyridoxine *on page 921*

◆ **Levulan Kerastick** *see* Aminolevulinic Acid *on page 114*

◆ **Lexapro** *see* Escitalopram *on page 765*

◆ **Lexiva** *see* Fosamprenavir *on page 928*

◆ **L-Glutamine** *see* Glutamine *on page 971*

◆ **LHRH** *see* Gonadorelin [CAN/INT] *on page 980*

◆ **LH-RH Agonist** *see* Histrelin *on page 1005*

◆ ***l*-Hyoscyamine Sulfate** *see* Hyoscyamine *on page 1026*

◆ **Lialda** *see* Mesalamine *on page 1301*

◆ **Librax** *see* Clidinium and Chlordiazepoxide *on page 460*

◆ **Librium** *see* ChlordiazePOXIDE *on page 422*

◆ **LiceMD [OTC]** *see* Pyrethrins and Piperonyl Butoxide *on page 1746*

◆ **Licide [OTC]** *see* Pyrethrins and Piperonyl Butoxide *on page 1746*

◆ **Lidemol® (Can)** *see* Fluocinonide *on page 894*

◆ **Lidex** *see* Fluocinonide *on page 894*

◆ **Lidex® (Can)** *see* Fluocinonide *on page 894*

Lidocaine (Systemic) (LYE doe kane)

Brand Names: U.S. Xylocaine; Xylocaine (Cardiac); Xylocaine-MPF

Brand Names: Canada Xylocard

Index Terms Lidocaine Hydrochloride; Lignocaine Hydrochloride

Pharmacologic Category Antiarrhythmic Agent, Class Ib; Local Anesthetic

Use Local and regional anesthesia by infiltration, nerve block, epidural, or spinal techniques; acute treatment of ventricular arrhythmias from myocardial infarction or cardiac manipulation (eg, cardiac surgery)

Note: The routine prophylactic use of lidocaine to prevent arrhythmia associated with fibrinolytic administration or to suppress isolated ventricular premature beats, couplets, runs of accelerated idioventricular rhythm, and nonsustained ventricular tachycardia (VT) is not recommended (ACCF/AHA [O'Gara, 2013]).

Pregnancy Risk Factor B

Pregnancy Considerations Adverse events were not observed in animal reproduction studies. Lidocaine and its metabolites cross the placenta and can be detected in the fetal circulation following injection (Cavalli, 2004; Mitani, 1987). Adverse reactions in the fetus/neonate may affect the CNS, heart, or peripheral vascular tone. Fetal heart monitoring is recommended. Lidocaine injection is approved for obstetric analgesia. Lidocaine administered by local infiltration is used to provide analgesia prior to episiotomy and during repair of obstetric lacerations (ACOG, 2002). Administration by the perineal route may result in greater absorption than administration by the epidural route (Cavalli, 2004). Cumulative exposure from all routes of administration should be considered. When used as an antiarrhythmic, ACLS guidelines recommend using the same dose that would be used in a nonpregnant woman (Vanden Hoek, 2010).

Breast-Feeding Considerations Lidocaine is excreted into breast milk. The manufacturer recommends that caution be used when administered to a nursing woman. When administered by injection for dental or obstetric analgesia, small amounts are detected in breast milk; oral bioavailability to the nursing infant is expected to be low and the amount of lidocaine available to the nursing infant would not be expected to cause adverse events (Lebedevs, 1993; Ortega, 1999). Cumulative exposure from all routes of administration should be considered.

Contraindications Hypersensitivity to lidocaine or any component of the formulation; hypersensitivity to another local anesthetic of the amide type; Adam-Stokes syndrome; Wolff-Parkinson-White syndrome; severe degrees of SA, AV, or intraventricular heart block (except in patients with a functioning artificial pacemaker); premixed injection may contain corn-derived dextrose and its use is contraindicated in patients with allergy to corn or corn-related products

Warnings/Precautions Use caution in patients with severe hepatic dysfunction or pseudocholinesterase deficiency; may have increased risk of lidocaine toxicity.

Intravenous: Constant ECG monitoring is necessary during IV administration. Use cautiously in hepatic impairment, HF, marked hypoxia, severe respiratory depression, hypovolemia, history of malignant hyperthermia, or shock. Increased ventricular rate may be seen when administered to a patient with atrial fibrillation. Correct electrolyte disturbances, especially hypokalemia or hypomagnesemia, prior to use and throughout therapy. Use is contraindicated in patients with Wolff-Parkinson-White syndrome and severe degrees of SA, AV, or intraventricular heart block (except in patients with a functioning artificial pacemaker). Correct any underlying causes of ventricular arrhythmias. Monitor closely for signs and symptoms of CNS toxicity. The elderly may be prone to increased CNS and cardiovascular side effects. Reduce dose in hepatic dysfunction and CHF.

Benzyl alcohol and derivatives: Some dosage forms may contain benzyl alcohol; large amounts of benzyl alcohol (≥99 mg/kg/day) have been associated with a potentially fatal toxicity ("gasping syndrome") in neonates; the "gasping syndrome" consists of metabolic acidosis, respiratory distress, gasping respirations, CNS dysfunction (including convulsions, intracranial hemorrhage), hypotension, and cardiovascular collapse (AAP, 1997; CDC, 1982); some data suggests that benzoate displaces bilirubin from protein binding sites (Ahlfors, 2001); avoid or use dosage forms containing benzyl alcohol with caution in neonates. See manufacturer's labeling.

Injectable anesthetic: Follow appropriate administration techniques so as not to administer any intravascularly. Continuous intra-articular infusion of local anesthetics after arthroscopic or other surgical procedures is **not** an approved use; chondrolysis (primarily in the shoulder joint) has occurred following infusion, with some cases requiring arthroplasty or shoulder replacement. Solutions containing antimicrobial preservatives should not be used for epidural or spinal anesthesia. Some solutions contain a bisulfite; avoid in patients who are allergic to bisulfite. Resuscitative equipment, medicine and oxygen should be available in case of emergency. Use products containing epinephrine cautiously in patients with significant vascular disease, compromised blood flow, or during or following general anesthesia (increased risk of arrhythmias). Adjust the dose for the elderly, pediatric, acutely ill, and debilitated patients.

Adverse Reactions Effects vary with route of administration. Many effects are dose related.

Cardiovascular: Arrhythmia, bradycardia, arterial spasms, cardiovascular collapse, defibrillator threshold increased, edema, flushing, heart block, hypotension, sinus node supression, vascular insufficiency (periarticular injections)

Central nervous system: Agitation, anxiety, apprehension, coma, confusion, disorientation, dizziness, drowsiness, euphoria, hallucinations, headache, hyperesthesia, hypoesthesia, lethargy, lightheadedness, nervousness, psychosis, seizure, slurred speech, somnolence, unconsciousness

Gastrointestinal: Metallic taste, nausea, vomiting

Local: Thrombophlebitis

Intradermal system: Application site reactions: Bruising/burning/contusion/hemorrhage/pain, edema, erythema, petechiae, pruritus

Neuromuscular & skeletal: Paresthesia, transient radicular pain (subarachnoid administration), tremor, twitching, weakness

Otic: Tinnitus

Respiratory: Bronchospasm, dyspnea, respiratory depression or arrest

Miscellaneous: Allergic reactions, anaphylactic reaction, anaphylactoid reaction, sensitivity to temperature extremes

Following spinal anesthesia: Cauda equina syndrome, double vision, hypotension, nausea, peripheral nerve symptoms, positional headache, respiratory inadequacy, shivering

Rare but important or life-threatening: Asystole, confusion, disorientation, flushing, headache, hyper-/hypoesthesia, hypersensitivity, methemoglobinemia, nervousness, skin reaction, weakness

Drug Interactions

Metabolism/Transport Effects Substrate of CYP1A2 (major), CYP2A6 (minor), CYP2B6 (minor), CYP2C9 (minor), CYP3A4 (major); **Note:** Assignment of Major/Minor substrate status based on clinically relevant drug interaction potential; **Inhibits** CYP1A2 (weak)

Avoid Concomitant Use

Avoid concomitant use of Lidocaine (Systemic) with any of the following: Conivaptan; Fusidic Acid (Systemic); Idelalisib; Saquinavir

Increased Effect/Toxicity

Lidocaine (Systemic) may increase the levels/effects of: Prilocaine; Sodium Nitrite

The levels/effects of Lidocaine (Systemic) may be increased by: Abiraterone Acetate; Amiodarone; Aprepitant; Beta-Blockers; Ceritinib; Conivaptan; CYP1A2 Inhibitors (Moderate); CYP1A2 Inhibitors (Strong); CYP3A4 Inhibitors (Moderate); CYP3A4 Inhibitors (Strong); Dasatinib; Deferasirox; Disopyramide; Fosaprepitant; Fusidic Acid (Systemic); Hyaluronidase; Idelalisib; Ivacaftor; Luliconazole; Mifepristone; Netupitant; Nitric Oxide; Peginterferon Alfa-2b; Saquinavir; Simeprevir; Stiripentol; Telaprevir; Vemurafenib

Decreased Effect

Lidocaine (Systemic) may decrease the levels/effects of: Technetium Tc 99m Tilmanocept

The levels/effects of Lidocaine (Systemic) may be decreased by: Bosentan; Cannabis; CYP1A2 Inducers (Strong); CYP3A4 Inducers (Moderate); CYP3A4 Inducers (Strong); Cyproterone; Dabrafenib; Deferasirox; Etravirine; Mitotane; Siltuximab; St Johns Wort; Teriflunomide; Tocilizumab

Preparation for Administration Local infiltration: Buffered lidocaine for injectable local anesthetic may be prepared: Add 2 mL of sodium bicarbonate 8.4% to 18 mL of lidocaine 1% (Christoph, 1988).

Storage/Stability Injection: Stable at room temperature. Stability of parenteral admixture at room temperature (25°C) is the expiration date on premixed bag; out of overwrap stability is 30 days.

Mechanism of Action Class Ib antiarrhythmic; suppresses automaticity of conduction tissue, by increasing electrical stimulation threshold of ventricle, His-Purkinje system, and spontaneous depolarization of the ventricles during diastole by a direct action on the tissues; blocks both the initiation and conduction of nerve impulses by decreasing the neuronal membrane's permeability to sodium ions, which results in inhibition of depolarization with resultant blockade of conduction

Pharmacodynamics/Kinetics

Onset of action: Single bolus dose: 45 to 90 seconds

Duration: 10 to 20 minutes

Distribution: V_d: 1.1 to 2.1 L/kg; alterable by many patient factors; decreased in CHF and liver disease; crosses blood-brain barrier

Protein binding: 60% to 80% to alpha$_1$ acid glycoprotein

Metabolism: 90% hepatic; active metabolites monoethylglycinexylidide (MEGX) and glycinexylidide (GX) can accumulate and may cause CNS toxicity

Half-life elimination: Biphasic: Prolonged with congestive heart failure, liver disease, shock, severe renal disease; Initial: 7 to 30 minutes; Terminal: Infants, premature: 3.2 hours, Adults: 1.5 to 2 hours

Excretion: Urine (<10% as unchanged drug, ~90% as metabolites)

Dosage

Antiarrhythmic:

Children:

IV, intraosseous (I.O.): **Note:** For use in VF or pulseless VT if amiodarone is not available; give after defibrillation attempts, CPR, and epinephrine:

Loading dose: 1 mg/kg (maximum: 100 mg); follow with continuous infusion; may administer second bolus of 0.5 to 1 mg/kg if delay between bolus and start of infusion is >15 minutes (PALS, 2000; PALS, 2010)

Continuous infusion: 20 to 50 mcg/kg/minute (PALS, 2010). Per the manufacturer, do not exceed 20 mcg/kg/minute in patients with shock, hepatic disease, cardiac arrest, or CHF.

Endotracheal: 2 to 3 mg/kg; flush with 5 mL of NS and follow with 5 assisted manual ventilations (PALS, 2010)

Adults (ACLS, 2010):

VF or pulseless VT (after defibrillation attempts, CPR, and vasopressor administration) if amiodarone is not available: IV, intraosseous (I.O.): Initial: 1 to 1.5 mg/kg. If refractory VF or pulseless VT, repeat with 0.5 to 0.75 mg/kg bolus every 5 to 10 minutes (maximum cumulative dose: 3 mg/kg). Follow with continuous infusion (1 to 4 mg/minute) after return of perfusion. Reappearance of arrhythmia during constant infusion: 0.5 mg/kg bolus and reassessment of infusion (Zipes, 2000).

Endotracheal (loading dose only): 2 to 3.75 mg/kg (2 to 2.5 times the recommended IV dose); dilute in 5 to 10 mL NS or sterile water. **Note:** Absorption is greater with sterile water and results in less impairment of PaO_2.

Hemodynamically stable monomorphic VT: IV: 1 to 1.5 mg/kg; repeat with 0.5 to 0.75 mg/kg every 5 to 10 minutes as necessary (maximum cumulative dose: 3 mg/kg). Follow with continuous infusion of 1 to 4 mg/minute (or 14 to 57 mcg/kg/minute).

Note: Reduce maintenance infusion in patients with CHF, shock, or hepatic disease; initiate infusion at 10 mcg/kg/minute (maximum dose: 1.5 mg/minute or 20 mcg/kg/minute).

Anesthetic, local injectable: Children and Adults: Varies with procedure, degree of anesthesia needed, vascularity of tissue, duration of anesthesia required, and physical condition of patient; maximum: 4.5 mg/kg/dose not to exceed 300 mg; do not repeat within 2 hours.

Interstitial cystitis (bladder pain syndrome) (off-label use): Adults: Intravesical:

Various dosage regimens of alkalinized lidocaine alone or with heparin (20,000 to 50,000 units) have been used. There is a risk of precipitation if proper alkalinization does not occur. Lidocaine stability and pH should be determined after the components have been mixed, prior to administration (Parsons, 2012)

Single instillation: Single intravesical administration of lidocaine (200 mg)/heparin (50,000 units)/sodium bicarbonate (420 mg) in 15 mL of sterile water, instilled into the bladder via catheter and allowed to dwell for 30 minutes before drainage (Parsons, 2012).

Weekly instillation: Weekly bladder instillations for 12 consecutive weeks with lidocaine 4% (5 mL)/heparin (20,000 units)/sodium bicarbonate 7% (25 mL), instilled into an empty bladder via catheter and allowed to dwell for 30 minutes before drainage (Nomiya, 2013).

Daily instillation: Daily bladder instillations for 5 days with lidocaine (200 mg)/sodium bicarbonate 8.4% solution (final volume of 10 mL), instilled into an empty bladder and allowed to dwell for 1 hour before drainage (Nickel, 2009).

Dosage adjustment in renal impairment: No dosage adjustment provided in manufacturer's labeling. However, accumulation of metabolites may be increased in renal dysfunction. Not dialyzable (0% to 5%) by hemo- or peritoneal dialysis; supplemental dose is not necessary.

Dosage adjustment in hepatic impairment: Use with caution; reduce maintenance infusion. Initial: 0.75 mg/minute or 10 mcg/kg/minute; maximum dose: 1.5 mg/minute or 20 mcg/kg/minute. Monitor lidocaine concentrations closely and adjust infusion rate as necessary; consider alternative therapy.

Dietary Considerations Premixed injection may contain corn-derived dextrose and its use is contraindicated in patients with allergy to corn-related products.

Usual Infusion Concentrations: Pediatric Note: Premixed solutions available

IV infusion: 8000 **mcg**/mL

Usual Infusion Concentrations: Adult Note: Premixed solutions available

IV infusion: 1000 mg in 250 mL (concentration: 4 mg/mL) **or** 2000 mg in 250 mL (concentration: 8 mg/mL) of D_5W

Administration

IV:

Bolus: According to the manufacturer, may administer at 25 to 50 mg/minute. In the setting of cardiac arrest (eg, ventricular fibrillation or pulseless ventricular tachycardia), may be infused rapidly into a peripheral vein (Dorian, 2002).

Continuous infusion: After initial bolus dosing, may administer as a continuous infusion; refer to indication-specific infusion rates in dosing for detailed recommendations. In the setting of cardiac arrest, infusion may be initiated once patient has return of spontaneous circulation resulting from lidocaine administration; however, there is no evidence to support subsequent continuous infusion to prevent recurrence (ACLS [Peberdy, 2010]). Local thrombophlebitis may occur in patients receiving prolonged IV infusions.

Endotracheal (off-label administration route): Dilute in NS or sterile water. Absorption is greater with sterile water and results in less impairment of PaO_2 (Hahnel, 1990). Stop compressions, spray drug quickly down tube. Flush with 5 mL of NS and follow immediately with several quick insufflations and continue chest compressions.

Intraosseous (IO; off-label administration route): Intraosseous administration is a safe and effective alternative to venous access in children with cardiac arrest; the onset for most medications is similar to that of IV administration (PALS, 2010). In adults, I.O. administration is a reasonable alternative when quick IV access is not feasible (ACLS, 2010).

Intravesical (off-label use): Various regimens of alkalinized lidocaine (with or without heparin) have been instilled into the bladder

Monitoring Parameters Liver function tests, lidocaine concentrations, ECG; consult individual institutional policies and procedures

Reference Range

Therapeutic: 1.5 to 5.0 mcg/mL (SI: 6 to 21 micromole/L)
Potentially toxic: >6 mcg/mL (SI: >26 micromole/L)
Toxic: >9 mcg/mL (SI: >38 micromole/L)

Dosage Forms

Solution, Injection:

Xylocaine: 0.5% (50 mL); 1% (20 mL, 50 mL); 2% (10 mL, 20 mL, 50 mL)

Xylocaine-MPF: 0.5% (50 mL); 1% (2 mL, 5 mL, 10 mL, 30 mL); 1.5% (10 mL, 20 mL); 2% (2 mL, 5 mL, 10 mL); 4% (5 mL)

Generic: 0.5% (50 mL); 1% (2 mL, 5 mL, 10 mL, 20 mL, 30 mL, 50 mL); 1.5% (20 mL); 2% (2 mL, 5 mL, 20 mL, 50 mL)

Solution, Injection [preservative free]:

Generic: 0.5% (50 mL); 1% (2 mL, 5 mL, 30 mL); 1.5% (20 mL); 2% (2 mL, 5 mL, 10 mL); 4% (5 mL)

Solution, Intravenous:

Xylocaine (Cardiac): 20 mg/mL (5 mL)

Generic: 10 mg/mL (5 mL); 20 mg/mL (5 mL); 0.4% [4 mg/mL] (250 mL, 500 mL); 0.8% [8 mg/mL] (250 mL); 2% (5 mL); 5% [50 mg/mL] (2 mL)

Solution, Intravenous [preservative free]:

Generic: 10 mg/mL (5 mL); 20 mg/mL (5 mL)

Lidocaine (Topical) (LYE doe kane)

Brand Names: U.S. AneCream [OTC]; AneCream5 [OTC]; EnovaRX-Lidocaine HCl; Glydo; LC-4 Lidocaine [OTC]; LC-5 Lidocaine [OTC]; Lidoderm; Lidopin; LidoRx; Lidovex; LMX 4 Plus [OTC]; LMX 4 [OTC]; LMX 5 [OTC]; LTA 360 Kit; Predator [OTC]; RectiCare [OTC]; Tecnu First Aid [OTC]; Topicaine 5 [OTC]; Topicaine [OTC]; Xolido XP [OTC]; Xylocaine; Zingo

Brand Names: Canada Betacaine; Lidodan; Lidoderm; Maxilene; Xylocaine

Index Terms Lidocaine Hydrochloride; Lidocaine Patch; Lignocaine Hydrochloride; Viscous Lidocaine; Xylocaine Viscous

Pharmacologic Category Analgesic, Topical; Local Anesthetic

Use

Intradermal injection (Zingo): Topical local analgesia prior to venipuncture or peripheral intravenous (IV) cannulation in children ≥3 years; topical local analgesia prior to venipuncture in adults.

Jelly: Prevention and control of pain in procedures involving the male and female urethra; for topical treatment of painful urethritis

Oral topical solution (2% viscous): Topical anesthesia of irritated or inflamed oral mucous membranes and pharyngeal tissue; reducing gagging during the taking of x-ray. **Note:** Not approved for relief of teething pain and discomfort in infants and children; serious adverse (toxic) effects have been reported (AAP, 2011; AAPD, 2012; ISMP, 2014).

Oral topical solution (4%): Topical anesthesia of accessible mucous membranes of the oral and nasal cavities and proximal portions of the digestive tract. **Note:** Not approved for relief of teething pain and discomfort in infants and children; serious adverse (toxic) effects have been reported (AAP, 2011; AAPD, 2012; ISMP, 2014).

Patch (Lidoderm): Relief of pain associated with postherpetic neuralgia

Patch (LidoPatch): Temporary relief of localized pain

Rectal: Temporary relief of pain and itching due to anorectal disorders

Topical: Local anesthetic for oral mucous membrane; use in laser/cosmetic surgeries; pruritus, pruritic eczemas, insect bites, pain, soreness, minor burns, cuts, and abrasions of the skin; discomfort due to pruritus ani, pruritus vulvae, hemorrhoids, anal fissures, and similar conditions of the skin and mucous membranes.

Pregnancy Risk Factor B

Dosage Anesthesia, topical:

Cream:

LidaMantle, Lidovex: Skin irritation: Children, Adolescents, and Adults: Apply a thin film to affected area 2 to 3 times daily as needed

L-M-X 4: Skin irritation: Children ≥2 years, Adolescents, and Adults: Apply up to 3 to 4 times daily to intact skin

L-M-X 5: Relief of anorectal pain and itching: Children ≥12 years, Adolescents, and Adults: Apply to affected area up to 6 times daily

Gel, ointment: Adults: Apply to affected area ≤4 times daily as needed (maximum dose: 4.5 mg/kg, not to exceed 300 mg)

Intradermal injection:

Children ≥3 years and Adolescents: Apply one intradermal lidocaine (0.5 mg) device to the site planned for venipuncture or IV cannulation, 1 to 3 minutes prior to needle insertion.

Adults: Apply one intradermal lidocaine (0.5 mg) device to the site planned for venipuncture, 1 to 3 minutes prior to needle insertion.

Jelly:

Children and Adolescents: Dose varies with age and weight (maximum dose: 4.5 mg/kg)

Adults (maximum dose: 30 mL [600 mg] in any 12-hour period):

Anesthesia of male urethra: 5 to 30 mL (100 to 600 mg)
Anesthesia of female urethra: 3 to 5 mL (60 to 100 mg)

Oral topical solution (2% viscous): **Note:** Not approved for relief of teething pain and discomfort in infants and children; serious adverse (toxic) effects have been reported; AAP, AAPD, and ISMP strongly discourage use (AAP, 2011; AAPD, 2012; ISMP, 2014).

Infants and Children <3 years: ≤1.2 mL applied to area with a cotton-tipped applicator no more frequently than every 3 hours (maximum: 4 doses per 12-hour period; use only if the underlying condition requires treatment with product volume of ≤1.2 mL)

Children ≥3 years and Adolescents: Do not exceed 4.5 mg/kg/dose (or 300 mg per dose); swished in the mouth and spit out no more frequently than every 3 hours (maximum: 4 doses per 12-hour period)

Adults:

Anesthesia of the mouth: 15 mL swished in the mouth and spit out no more frequently than every 3 hours (maximum: 4.5 mg/kg [or 300 mg per dose]; 8 doses per 24-hour period)

Anesthesia of the pharynx: 15 mL gargled no more frequently than every 3 hours (maximum: 4.5 mg/kg [or 300 mg per dose]; 8 doses per 24-hour period); may be swallowed

Patch: Adults:

Lidoderm: Postherpetic neuralgia: Apply patch to most painful area. Up to 3 patches may be applied in a single application. Patch(es) may remain in place for up to 12 hours in any 24-hour period.

LidoPatch: Pain (localized): Apply patch to painful area. Patch may remain in place for up to 12 hours in any 24-hour period. No more than 1 patch should be used in a 24-hour period.

Topical solution (4%): **Note:** For use in mucous membranes of oral and nasal cavities and proximal GI tract.

Children and Adolescents: Dose varies with age and weight (maximum dose: 4.5 mg/kg)

Adults: Apply 1 to 5 mL (40 to 200 mg) to affected area (maximum dose: 4.5 mg/kg, not to exceed 300 mg per dose)

Dosage adjustment in renal impairment: There are no dosage adjustments provided in the manufacturer's labeling.

Dosage adjustment in hepatic impairment: There are no dosage adjustments provided in the manufacturer's labeling; use caution in patients with severe hepatic disease.

Additional Information Complete prescribing information should be consulted for additional detail.

Dosage Forms Considerations

EnovaRX-Lidocaine is a compounding kit. Refer to manufacturer's package insert for compounding instructions.

Dosage Forms

Cream, External:

AneCream [OTC]: 4% (5 g, 15 g, 30 g)
AneCream5 [OTC]: 5% (15 g, 30 g)
EnovaRX-Lidocaine HCl: 5% (60 g, 120 g); 10% (60 g, 120 g)
LC-4 Lidocaine [OTC]: 4% (45 g)
LC-5 Lidocaine [OTC]: 5% (45 g)
Lidopin: 3% (28 g, 85 g); 3.25% (28 g, 85 g)
Lidovex: 3.75% (60 g)
LMX 4 [OTC]: 4% (5 g, 15 g, 30 g)
LMX 5 [OTC]: 5% (15 g, 30 g)
Predator [OTC]: 4% (63 g)
RectiCare [OTC]: 5% (30 g)
Xolido XP [OTC]: 4% (118 mL)
Generic: 3% (28.3 g, 28.35 g, 85 g)

Device, Intradermal:

Zingo: 0.5 mg (1 ea)

Gel, External:

LidoRx: 3% (10 mL, 30 mL)
Tecnu First Aid [OTC]: 0.2-2.5% (56.7 g)
Topicaine [OTC]: 4% (10 g, 30 g, 113 g)
Topicaine 5 [OTC]: 5% (10 g, 30 g, 113 g)
Generic: 2% (5 mL, 20 mL, 30 mL)

Gel, External [preservative free]:

Glydo: 2% (6 mL, 11 mL)
Generic: 2% (5 mL, 10 mL)

Kit, External:

AneCream [OTC]: 4%
LMX 4 Plus [OTC]: 4%

Lotion, External:

Generic: 3% (177 mL)

Ointment, External:

Generic: 5% (30 g, 35.44 g, 50 g)

Patch, External:

Lidoderm: 5% (1 ea, 30 ea)
Generic: 5% (1 ea, 30 ea)

Solution, External:

Xylocaine: 4% (50 mL)
Generic: 4% (50 mL)

Solution, Mouth/Throat:

Generic: 2% (15 mL, 100 mL)

Solution, Mouth/Throat [preservative free]:

LTA 360 Kit: 4% (4 mL)
Generic: 4% (4 mL)

Lidocaine and Epinephrine

(LYE doe kane & ep i NEF rin)

Brand Names: U.S. Lignospan® Forte; Lignospan® Standard; Xylocaine® MPF With Epinephrine; Xylocaine® With Epinephrine

Brand Names: Canada Xylocaine® With Epinephrine

Index Terms Epinephrine and Lidocaine

Pharmacologic Category Local Anesthetic

Use Local infiltration anesthesia; AVS for nerve block

Pregnancy Risk Factor B

Dosage Dosage varies with the anesthetic procedure, degree of anesthesia needed, vascularity of tissue, duration of anesthesia required, and physical condition of patient.

Dental anesthesia, infiltration, or conduction block:

Children <12 years: 20-30 mg (1-1.5 mL) of lidocaine hydrochloride as a 2% solution with epinephrine 1:100,000; maximum: 4.5 mg of lidocaine hydrochloride/kg of body weight or 100-150 mg as a single dose

Children ≥12 years and Adults: Do not exceed 7 mg/kg body weight up to a maximum range of 300 mg (usual dental practice) to 500 mg (approved product labeling) of lidocaine hydrochloride and 3 mcg (0.003 mg) of epinephrine/kg of body weight or 0.2 mg epinephrine per dental appointment. The effective anesthetic dose varies with procedure, intensity of anesthesia needed, duration of anesthesia required, and physical condition of the patient. Always use the lowest effective dose along with careful aspiration.

Note: For most routine dental procedures, lidocaine hydrochloride 2% with epinephrine 1:100,000 is preferred. When a more pronounced hemostasis is required, a 1:50,000 epinephrine concentration should be used.

Dosage adjustment in renal impairment: No dosage adjustment provided in manufacturer's labeling. However, accumulation of metabolites may be increased in renal dysfunction.

Dosage adjustment in hepatic impairment: No dosage adjustment provided in manufacturer's labeling; use with caution.

Additional Information Complete prescribing information should be consulted for additional detail.

Dosage Forms

Injection, solution:

Generics:

0.5% / 1:200,000: Lidocaine hydrochloride 0.5% [5 mg/mL] and epinephrine 1:200,000 (50 mL)

1% / 1:100,000: Lidocaine hydrochloride 1% [10 mg/mL] and epinephrine 1:100,000 (20 mL, 30 mL, 50 mL)

2% / 1:100,000: Lidocaine hydrochloride 2% [20 mg/mL] and epinephrine 1:100,000 (30 mL, 50 mL)

Brands:

Xylocaine® with Epinephrine:

0.5% / 1:200,000: Lidocaine hydrochloride 0.5% [5 mg/mL] and epinephrine 1:200,000 (50 mL)

1% / 1:100,000: Lidocaine hydrochloride 1% [10 mg/mL] and epinephrine 1:100,000 (10 mL, 20 mL, 50 mL)

2% / 1:100,000: Lidocaine hydrochloride 2% [20 mg/mL] and epinephrine 1:100,000 (10 mL, 20 mL, 50 mL)

Injection, solution [preservative free]:

Generics:

1.5% / 1:200,000: Lidocaine hydrochloride 1.5% [15 mg/mL] and epinephrine 1:200,000 (5 mL, 30 mL)

2% / 1:200,000: Lidocaine hydrochloride 2% [20 mg/mL] and epinephrine 1:200,000 (20 mL)

Brands:

Xylocaine®-MPF with Epinephrine:

1% / 1:200,000: Lidocaine hydrochloride 1% [10 mg/mL] and epinephrine 1:200,000 (5 mL, 10 mL, 30 mL)

1.5% / 1:200,000: Lidocaine hydrochloride 1.5% [15 mg/mL] and epinephrine 1:200,000 (5 mL, 10 mL, 30 mL)

2% / 1:200,000: Lidocaine hydrochloride 2% [20 mg/mL] and epinephrine 1:200,000 (5 mL, 10 mL, 20 mL)

Injection, solution [for dental use]:

Generics:

2% / 1:50,000: Lidocaine hydrochloride 2% [20 mg/mL] and epinephrine 1:50,000 (1.7 mL, 1.8 mL)

2% / 1:100,000: Lidocaine hydrochloride 2% [20 mg/mL] and epinephrine 1:100,000 (1.7 mL, 1.8 mL)

Brands:

Lignospan® Forte: 2% / 1:50,000: Lidocaine hydrochloride 2% [20 mg/mL] and epinephrine 1:50,000 (1.7 mL)

Lignospan® Standard: 2% / 1:100,000: Lidocaine hydrochloride 2% [20 mg/mL] and epinephrine 1:100,000 (1.7 mL)

Lidocaine and Prilocaine

(LYE doe kane & PRIL oh kane)

Brand Names: U.S. EMLA®; Oraqix®

Brand Names: Canada EMLA®; Oraqix®

Index Terms Prilocaine and Lidocaine

Pharmacologic Category Local Anesthetic

Use

U.S. labeling:

Cream: Topical anesthetic for use on normal intact skin to provide local analgesia for minor procedures such as IV cannulation or venipuncture; has also been used for painful procedures such as lumbar puncture and skin graft harvesting; for superficial minor surgery of genital mucous membranes and as an adjunct for local infiltration anesthesia in genital mucous membranes.

Periodontal gel: Topical anesthetic for use in periodontal pockets during scaling or root planing procedures

Canadian labeling:

Cream: Topical anesthetic to provide local analgesia for the following: minor procedures on intact skin such as IV cannulation or venipuncture, superficial procedures such as skin grafting and electrolysis, laser treatment for superficial skin surgery (eg, warts, moles, skin nodules, scar tissue); superficial minor surgery of genital mucous membranes and as an adjunct for local infiltration anesthesia in genital mucous membranes; mechanical cleansing/debridement of leg ulcers; vaccination with measles-mumps-rubella (MMR), diphtheria-pertussis-tetanus-poliovirus (DPTP), *Haemophilus influenzae* b, and hepatitis B.

Patch: Topical anesthetic of intact skin for IV cannulation or venipuncture; vaccination with measles-mumps-rubella (MMR), diphtheria-pertussis-tetanus-poliovirus (DPTP), *Haemophilus influenzae* b, and hepatitis B.

Periodontal gel: Topical anesthetic for use in periodontal pockets during scaling or root planing procedures

Pregnancy Risk Factor B

Dosage Although the incidence of systemic adverse effects is very low, caution should be exercised, particularly when applying over large areas and leaving on for >2 hours

Infants and Children (intact skin): **Note:** If a patient >3 months of age does not meet the minimum weight requirement, the maximum total dose should be restricted to the corresponding maximum based on patient weight.

Cream: Should **not** be used in neonates with a gestation age <37 weeks nor in infants <12 months of age who are receiving treatment with methemoglobin-inducing agents

Dosing is based on child's age and weight:

Age 0-3 months or <5 kg: Apply a maximum of 1 g over no more than 10 cm^2 of skin; leave on for no longer than 1 hour

Age 3 months to 12 months and >5 kg: Apply no more than a maximum 2 g total over no more than 20 cm^2 of skin; leave on for no longer than 4 hours

Age 1-6 years and >10 kg: Apply no more than a maximum of 10 g total over no more than 100 cm^2 of skin; leave on for no longer than 4 hours. U.S. labeling recommends leaving on for no longer than 4 hours. Canadian labeling recommends leaving on for no longer than 5 hours.

Age 7-12 years and >20 kg: Apply no more than a maximum 20 g total over no more than 200 cm^2 of skin; leave on for no longer than 4 hours. U.S. labeling recommends leaving on for no longer than 4 hours. Canadian labeling recommends leaving on for no longer than 5 hours.

Transdermal patch [Canadian product]: **Note:** Should not be used in neonates with a gestation age <37 weeks nor in infants <12 months of age who are receiving treatment with methemoglobin-inducing agents

Dosing is based on child's age and weight: Apply patch(es) to skin area(s) <10 cm^2:

Age 0-3 months or <5 kg: Apply 1 patch and leave on for ~1 hour (do not exceed 1-hour application time); do not apply more than 1 patch at same time; safety of repeated dosing not established

Age 3 months to 12 months and >5 kg: Apply 1-2 patches for ~1 hour (maximum application time: 4 hours); do not apply more than 2 patches at the same time

Age 1-6 years and >10 kg: Apply 1 or more patches for minimum of 1 hour (maximum application time: 5 hours); maximum dose: 10 patches

Age 7-12 years and >20 kg: Apply 1 or more patches for a minimum of 1 hour (maximum application time: 5 hours); maximum dose: 20 patches

Adults (intact skin):

Cream: **Note:** Apply a thick layer to intact skin and cover with an occlusive dressing. Dermal analgesia can be expected to increase for up to 3 hours under occlusive dressing and persist for 1-2 hours after removal of the cream.

U.S. labeling:

Minor dermal procedures (eg, IV cannulation or venipuncture): Apply 2.5 g of cream (1/2 of the 5 g tube) over 20-25 cm^2 of skin surface area) for at least 1 hour

Major dermal procedures (eg, more painful dermatological procedures involving a larger skin area such as split thickness skin graft harvesting): Apply 2 g of cream per 10 cm^2 of skin and allow to remain in contact with the skin for at least 2 hours.

Adult male genital skin (eg, pretreatment prior to local anesthetic infiltration): Apply a thick layer of cream (1 g per 10 cm^2) to the skin surface for 15 minutes. Local anesthetic infiltration should be performed immediately after removal of cream.

Adult female genital mucous membranes: Minor procedures (eg, removal of condylomata acuminata, pretreatment for local anesthetic infiltration): Apply a thick layer of cream (5-10 g) for 5-10 minutes. The local anesthetic infiltration or procedure should be performed immediately after removal of cream.

Canadian labeling:

Minor dermal procedures (eg, IV cannulation, venipuncture, surgical or laser treatment): Apply 2 g (~1/2 of the 5 g tube) over ~13.5 cm^2 for at least 1 hour but no longer than 5 hours

Major dermal procedures (eg, split-skin grafting): 1.5-2 g per 10 cm^2 (maximum: 60 g per 400 cm^2) for at least 2 hours but no longer than 5 hours

Genital mucosa (eg, surgical procedures ≤10 minutes such as localized wart removal, and prior to local anesthetic infiltration): Apply 2 g (~1/2 of 5 g tube) per lesion (maximum: 10 g) for 5-10 minutes. Initiate procedure immediately after removing cream.

Leg ulcers (eg, mechanical cleansing/surgical debridement): Apply ~1-2 g per 10 cm^2 (maximum: 10 g) for at least 30 minutes and up to 60 minutes for necrotic tissue that is more difficult to penetrate. Initiate procedure immediately after removing cream.

Periodontal gel (Oraqix®): Apply on gingival margin around selected teeth using the blunt-tipped applicator included in package. Wait 30 seconds, then fill the periodontal pockets using the blunt-tipped applicator until gel becomes visible at the gingival margin. Wait another 30 seconds before starting treatment. May reapply; maximum recommended dose: One treatment session: 5 cartridges (8.5 g)

Transdermal patch [Canadian product]: Apply 1 or more patches to intact skin surface area <10 cm^2 for at least 1 hour (maximum application time: 5 hours)

Elderly: Smaller areas of treatment may be necessary depending on status of patient (eg, debilitated, impaired hepatic function). Refer to adult dosing.

Dosage adjustment in renal impairment: No dosage adjustment provided in manufacturer labeling. Lidocaine and prilocaine primarily undergo hepatic metabolism and their pharmacokinetics are not expected to be changed significantly in renal impairment.

Dosage adjustment in hepatic impairment: Smaller areas of treatment are recommended for patients with severe hepatic impairment.

Additional Information Complete prescribing information should be consulted for additional detail.

Dosage Forms

Cream, topical: Lidocaine 2.5% and prilocaine 2.5% (5 g, 30 g)

EMLA®: Lidocaine 2.5% and prilocaine 2.5% (5 g, 30 g)

Gel, periodontal:

Oraqix®: Lidocaine 2.5% and prilocaine 2.5% (1.7 g)

Dosage Forms: Canada

Patch, transdermal:

EMLA® Patch: Lidocaine 2.5% and prilocaine 2.5% per patch (2s, 20s)

Lidocaine and Tetracaine

(LYE doe kane & TET ra kane)

Brand Names: U.S. Pliaglis; Synera

Index Terms Eutectic Mixture of Lidocaine and Tetracaine; Tetracaine and Lidocaine

Pharmacologic Category Analgesic, Topical; Local Anesthetic

Use

Cream: For use on intact skin in adults to provide topical local analgesia for superficial dermatological procedures.

Patch: For use on intact skin in patients ≥3 years to provide local analgesia for superficial venous access and superficial dermatological procedures.

Pregnancy Risk Factor B

Dosage Anesthesia, topical:

Cream: Adults: Superficial dermatological procedures: Prior to procedure, apply to intact skin for 20 to 60 minutes. Amount of cream varies depending on size of the surface area to be treated; see manufacturer's labeling for detailed information.

Patch: Children ≥3 years, Adolescents, and Adults:

Venipuncture or intravenous cannulation: Prior to procedure, apply to intact skin for 20 to 30 minutes; **Note:** May use another patch at a new location to facilitate venous access after a failed attempt; remove previous patch.

Superficial dermatological procedures: Prior to procedure, apply to intact skin for 30 minutes

Dosage adjustment in renal impairment: There are no dosage adjustments provided in the manufacturer's labeling. Lidocaine primarily undergoes hepatic metabolism and its pharmacokinetics are not expected to be changed significantly following topical administration of recommended doses in renal impairment.

Dosage adjustment in hepatic impairment: There are no dosage adjustments provided in the manufacturer's labeling (has not been studied). Use caution in patients with severe hepatic dysfunction.

Additional Information Complete prescribing information should be consulted for additional detail.

Dosage Forms

Cream, external:

Pliaglis: Lidocaine 7% and tetracaine 7% (30 g, 100 g)

Patch, transdermal:

Synera: Lidocaine 70 mg and tetracaine 70 mg (10s)

◆ **Lidocaine Hydrochloride** *see* Lidocaine (Systemic) *on page 1208*

◆ **Lidocaine Hydrochloride** *see* Lidocaine (Topical) *on page 1211*

◆ **Lidocaine Patch** *see* Lidocaine (Topical) *on page 1211*

◆ **Lidodan (Can)** *see* Lidocaine (Topical) *on page 1211*

◆ **Lidoderm** *see* Lidocaine (Topical) *on page 1211*

◆ **Lidopin** *see* Lidocaine (Topical) *on page 1211*

◆ **LidoRx** *see* Lidocaine (Topical) *on page 1211*

◆ **Lidovex** *see* Lidocaine (Topical) *on page 1211*

◆ **LID-Pack® (Can)** *see* Bacitracin and Polymyxin B *on page 222*

- ◆ **Lignocaine Hydrochloride** *see* Lidocaine (Systemic) *on page 1208*
- ◆ **Lignocaine Hydrochloride** *see* Lidocaine (Topical) *on page 1211*
- ◆ **Lignospan® Forte** *see* Lidocaine and Epinephrine *on page 1212*
- ◆ **Lignospan® Standard** *see* Lidocaine and Epinephrine *on page 1212*
- ◆ **Limbitrol** *see* Amitriptyline and Chlordiazepoxide *on page 122*

Linaclotide (lin AK loe tide)

Brand Names: U.S. Linzess

Brand Names: Canada Constella

Index Terms Linaclotide Acetate

Pharmacologic Category Gastrointestinal Agent, Miscellaneous

Use

Chronic idiopathic constipation: Treatment of chronic idiopathic constipation (CIC) in adults

Irritable bowel syndrome with constipation: Treatment of irritable bowel syndrome with constipation (IBS-C) in adults

Pregnancy Risk Factor C

Pregnancy Considerations Adverse events were observed in some animal reproduction studies. Linaclotide and its metabolite are not measurable in plasma when used at recommended doses.

Breast-Feeding Considerations It is not known if linaclotide is excreted in breast milk; linaclotide and its metabolite are not measurable in plasma when used at recommended doses. The manufacturer recommends to use caution if administered to breast-feeding women.

Contraindications

Use in pediatric patients <6 years of age; known or suspected mechanical gastrointestinal obstruction

Canadian labeling: Additional contraindications (not in U.S. labeling): Hypersensitivity to linaclotide or any component of the formulation

Warnings/Precautions [U.S. Boxed Warning]: Use is contraindicated in pediatric patients <6 years of age. Use in pediatric patients 6-17 years of age should be avoided. Deaths due to dehydration were observed in young juvenile animals during nonclinical studies; deaths were not observed in older juvenile animals. There are not sufficient safety and efficacy data to support use in pediatric patients. May cause diarrhea. Patients should be instructed to discontinue use and contact their health care provider if severe diarrhea occurs. Administration with a high-fat meal may worsen diarrhea.

Adverse Reactions Adverse reactions reported with use in IBS-C and CIC.

Central nervous system: Fatigue, headache

Endocrine & metabolic: Dehydration

Gastrointestinal: Abdominal distension, abdominal pain, diarrhea (including severe), dyspepsia, fecal incontinence, flatulence, gastroesophageal reflux disease, viral gastroenteritis, vomiting

Respiratory: Sinusitis, upper respiratory tract infection

Rare but important or life-threatening: Hematochezia, hypersensitivity reaction, rectal hemorrhage

Drug Interactions

Metabolism/Transport Effects None known.

Avoid Concomitant Use There are no known interactions where it is recommended to avoid concomitant use.

Increased Effect/Toxicity There are no known significant interactions involving an increase in effect.

Decreased Effect There are no known significant interactions involving a decrease in effect.

Storage/Stability Store at 25°C (77°F) in tightly closed, original container with included desiccant packet; excursions permitted between 15°C and 30°C (59°F and 86°F). Do not repackage; protect from moisture.

Mechanism of Action Linaclotide and its active metabolite bind and agonize guanylate cyclase-C on the luminal surface of intestinal epithelium. Intracellular and extracellular cyclic guanosine monophosphate (cGMP) concentrations are subsequently increased resulting in chloride and bicarbonate secretion into the intestinal lumen. Intestinal fluid increases and GI transit time is decreased. Increased extracellular cGMP may decrease visceral pain by reducing pain-sensing nerve activity.

Pharmacodynamics/Kinetics

Absorption: Minimal systemic availability; plasma concentrations are not measurable when used at recommended doses.

Distribution: Minimal tissue distribution is expected given immeasurable plasma concentrations when used at recommended doses.

Metabolism: Metabolized within GI tract to active metabolite; parent drug and metabolite undergo proteolytic degradation within the intestinal lumen to smaller peptides and amino acids

Excretion: Primarily feces (3% to 5%; as the active metabolite)

Dosage

Adults: Oral:

Chronic idiopathic constipation (CIC): 145 mcg once daily

Irritable bowel syndrome with constipation (IBS-C): 290 mcg once daily

Elderly: Not adequately studied in the elderly. Refer to adult dosing.

Dosage adjustment in renal impairment: No dosage adjustment necessary.

Dosage adjustment in hepatic impairment: No dosage adjustment necessary.

Dietary Considerations Administer at least 30 minutes before the first meal of the day on an empty stomach. Loose stools and greater stool frequency may occur after administration with a high-fat breakfast.

Administration Oral: Administer at least 30 minutes before the first meal of the day on an empty stomach; loose stools and greater stool frequency may occur after administration with a high-fat breakfast. Swallow capsule whole; do not break or chew capsules.

Monitoring Parameters

IBS-C: Abdominal pain, spontaneous bowel movement quality and frequency

CIC: Frequency of straining during bowel movements; spontaneous bowel movement quality and frequency

Dosage Forms

Capsule, Oral:

Linzess: 145 mcg, 290 mcg

◆ **Linaclotide Acetate** *see* Linaclotide *on page 1215*

Linagliptin (lin a GLIP tin)

Brand Names: U.S. Tradjenta

Brand Names: Canada Trajenta

Index Terms BI-1356; Trajenta

Pharmacologic Category Antidiabetic Agent, Dipeptidyl Peptidase IV (DPP-IV) Inhibitor

Use Type 2 diabetes mellitus: As an adjunct to diet and exercise to improve glycemic control in adults with type 2 diabetes (noninsulin dependent, NIDDM) as monotherapy or in combination with other antidiabetic agents

Pregnancy Risk Factor B

Pregnancy Considerations Adverse events were not observed in animal reproduction studies, except with doses that were also maternally toxic.

In women with diabetes, maternal hyperglycemia can be associated with congenital malformations as well as adverse effects in the fetus, neonate, and the mother (ACOG, 2005; ADA, 2014; Kitzmiller, 2008; Metzger, 2007). To prevent adverse outcomes, prior to conception and throughout pregnancy maternal blood glucose and HbA_{1c} should be kept as close to normal as possible but without causing significant hypoglycemia (ACOG, 2013; ADA, 2014; Blumer, 2013; Kitzmiller, 2008). Prior to pregnancy, effective contraception should be used until glycemic control is achieved (ADA, 2014; Kitzmiller, 2008). Other agents are currently recommended to treat diabetes in pregnant women (ACOG, 2013; Blumer, 2013).

Breast-Feeding Considerations It is not known if linagliptin is excreted in breast milk. The manufacturer recommends that caution be used if administered to breast-feeding women.

Contraindications

Hypersensitivity (eg, anaphylaxis, angioedema, exfoliative skin conditions, urticaria, or bronchial hyperreactivity) to linagliptin or any component of the formulation

Canadian labeling: Additional contraindications: Use in type 1 diabetes mellitus or diabetic ketoacidosis

Warnings/Precautions Avoid use in type 1 diabetes mellitus (insulin dependent, IDDM) and diabetic ketoacidosis (DKA) due to lack of efficacy in these populations. Diabetes self-management education (DSME) is essential to maximize the effectiveness of therapy. Cases of acute pancreatitis, including fatalities, have been reported with use. Monitor for signs/symptoms of pancreatitis; discontinue use immediately if pancreatitis is suspected and initiate appropriate management. Use with caution in patients with a history of pancreatitis as it is not known if this population is at greater risk. Clinical trials included only a limited number of patients with heart failure (HF). No specific recommendations regarding this population are provided in the approved U.S. labeling (Canadian labeling recommends against use in this population). Potentially significant drug-drug interactions may exist, requiring dose or frequency adjustment, additional monitoring, and/or selection of alternative therapy. Rare hypersensitivity reactions including anaphylaxis, angioedema, and exfoliative skin conditions have been reported in patients treated with linagliptin; discontinue if signs/symptoms of hypersensitivity reactions occur. Events have generally been noted within the first 3 months of therapy, and may occur with the initial dose. Use with caution if patient has experienced angioedema with other DPP-IV inhibitor use.

Adverse Reactions

Reported for patients on monotherapy unless otherwise specified

Central nervous system: Headache (combination therapy)

Endocrine & metabolic: Hypertriglyceridemia (combination therapy), hypoglycemia (more common or severe in combination therapy), increased uric acid, severe hypoglycemia (combination therapy), weight gain (combination therapy)

Gastrointestinal: Constipation (combination therapy)

Genitourinary: Urinary tract infection (combination therapy)

Neuromuscular & skeletal: Arthralgia (combination therapy), back pain (combination therapy), limb pain (combination therapy)

Respiratory: Cough (monotherapy and combination therapy), nasopharyngitis

<1% (Rare, but important or life-threatening): Acute pancreatitis, anaphylaxis, angioedema, severe hypersensitivity

Drug Interactions

Metabolism/Transport Effects Substrate of CYP3A4 (major), P-glycoprotein; **Note:** Assignment of Major/Minor substrate status based on clinically relevant drug interaction potential

Avoid Concomitant Use There are no known interactions where it is recommended to avoid concomitant use.

Increased Effect/Toxicity

Linagliptin may increase the levels/effects of: ACE Inhibitors

The levels/effects of Linagliptin may be increased by: Androgens; Pegvisomant; P-glycoprotein/ABCB1 Inhibitors; Ritonavir

Decreased Effect

The levels/effects of Linagliptin may be decreased by: Bosentan; Corticosteroids (Orally Inhaled); Corticosteroids (Systemic); CYP3A4 Inducers (Moderate); CYP3A4 Inducers (Strong); Dabrafenib; Danazol; Deferasirox; Luteinizing Hormone-Releasing Hormone Analogs; Mitotane; P-glycoprotein/ABCB1 Inducers; Siltuximab; Somatropin; St Johns Wort; Thiazide Diuretics; Tocilizumab

Storage/Stability Store at 25°C (77°F); excursions permitted between 15°C to 30°C (59°F to 86°F).

Mechanism of Action Linagliptin inhibits dipeptidyl peptidase IV (DPP-IV) enzyme resulting in prolonged active incretin levels. Incretin hormones (eg, glucagon-like peptide-1 [GLP-1] and glucose-dependent insulinotropic polypeptide [GIP]) regulate glucose homeostasis by increasing insulin synthesis and release from pancreatic beta cells and decreasing glucagon secretion from pancreatic alpha cells. Decreased glucagon secretion results in decreased hepatic glucose production. Under normal physiologic circumstances, incretin hormones are released by the intestine throughout the day and levels are increased in response to a meal; incretin hormones are rapidly inactivated by the DPP-IV enzyme.

Pharmacodynamics/Kinetics

Absorption: Rapid

Distribution: Extensive

Protein binding: 70% to 80%; concentration dependent

Metabolism: Not extensively metabolized

Bioavailability: ~30%

Half-life elimination: Effective (therapeutic): ~12 hours; Terminal (DPP-IV saturable binding): >100 hours

Time to peak: 1.5 hours

Excretion: 80% feces unchanged; 5% urine unchanged

Dosage Oral: Adults: Type 2 diabetes: 5 mg once daily

Concomitant use with insulin and/or insulin secretagogues (eg, sulfonylureas): Reduced dose of insulin and/or insulin secretagogues may be needed.

Dosage adjustment in renal impairment: No dosage adjustment necessary.

Dosage adjustment in hepatic impairment: No dosage adjustment necessary. **Note:** Canadian labeling does not recommend use in severe hepatic impairment.

Dietary Considerations Individualized medical nutrition therapy (MNT) based on ADA recommendations is an integral part of therapy.

Administration May be administered with or without food.

Monitoring Parameters HbA_{1c}, serum glucose; signs/symptoms of pancreatitis

Reference Range

Recommendations for glycemic control in nonpregnant adults with diabetes (ADA, 2015):

HbA_{1c}: <7% (a more aggressive [<6.5%] or less aggressive [<8%] HbA_{1c} goal may be targeted based on patient-specific characteristics)

Preprandial capillary plasma glucose: 80 to 130 mg/dL

Peak postprandial capillary blood glucose: <180 mg/dL

Recommendations for glycemic control in pediatric (all age groups) patients with type 1 diabetes (ADA, 2015):

HbA_{1c}: <7.5% (individualization may be appropriate based on patient-specific characteristics; <7% is reasonable if it can be achieved without excessive hypoglycemia)

Preprandial capillary plasma glucose: 90 to 130 mg/dL

Bedtime and overnight capillary blood glucose: 90 to 150 mg/dL

Dosage Forms

Tablet, Oral:

Tradjenta: 5 mg

Linagliptin and Metformin
(lin a GLIP tin & met FOR min)

Brand Names: U.S. Jentadueto

Brand Names: Canada Jentadueto

Index Terms Linagliptin and Metformin Hydrochloride; Metformin and Linagliptin; Metformin Hydrochloride and Linagliptin

Pharmacologic Category Antidiabetic Agent, Biguanide; Antidiabetic Agent, Dipeptidyl Peptidase IV (DPP-IV) Inhibitor

Use Diabetes mellitus type 2: As an adjunct to diet and exercise to improve glycemic control in adults with type 2 diabetes mellitus (noninsulin dependent, NIDDM) when treatment with both linagliptin and metformin is appropriate.

Pregnancy Risk Factor B

Dosage

Type 2 diabetes mellitus: Adults: Oral: Initial doses should be based on current dose of linagliptin and metformin.

Patients currently on metformin: Initial dose: Linagliptin 5 mg daily plus current daily dose of metformin given in 2 equally divided doses; maximum: linagliptin 5 mg/metformin 2000 mg daily.

Patients not on metformin: Initial dose: Linagliptin 5 mg daily plus metformin 1000 mg daily given in 2 equally divided doses; maximum: linagliptin 5 mg/metformin 2000 mg daily.

Concomitant use with insulin and/or insulin secretagogues (eg, sulfonylureas): Reduced dose of insulin and/or insulin secretagogues may be needed.

Dosing adjustment: Metformin component may be gradually increased up to the maximum dose. Maximum dose: Linagliptin 5 mg/metformin 2000 mg daily

Elderly: Refer to adult dosing. The initial and maintenance dosing should be conservative, due to the potential for decreased renal function (monitor). Do not use in patients ≥80 years of age unless normal renal function has been established.

Dosage adjustment in renal impairment: Use is contraindicated in patients with renal disease or renal impairment (serum creatinine ≥1.5 mg/dL [≥136 micromole/L] in males or ≥1.4 mg/dL [≥124 micromole/L] in females or abnormal clearance [<60 mL/minute per Canadian labeling]).

Dosage adjustment in hepatic impairment: Avoid metformin; liver disease is a risk factor for the development of lactic acidosis during metformin therapy.

Additional Information Complete prescribing information should be consulted for additional detail.

Dosage Forms

Tablet, oral:

Jentadueto 2.5/500: Linagliptin 2.5 mg and metformin 500 mg

Jentadueto 2.5/850: Linagliptin 2.5 mg and metformin 850 mg

Jentadueto 2.5/1000: Linagliptin 2.5 mg and metformin 1000 mg

◆ **Linagliptin and Metformin Hydrochloride** *see* Linagliptin and Metformin *on page 1217*

Lindane (LIN dane)

Index Terms Benzene Hexachloride; Gamma Benzene Hexachloride; Hexachlorocyclohexane; Kwell

Pharmacologic Category Antiparasitic Agent, Topical; Pediculocide; Scabicidal Agent

Use

Lotion: Treatment of *Sarcoptes scabiei* (scabies)

Shampoo: Treatment of *Pediculus capitis* (head lice) and *Phthirus pubis* (crab lice)

Note: Not recommended for first line-treatment; use should be reserved for patients who are intolerant to or have failed first-line agents.

Pregnancy Risk Factor C

Dosage Infants, Children, Adolescents, and Adults: Topical:

Scabies: Apply a thin layer of lotion and massage it on skin from the neck to the toes; after 8-12 hours, bathe and remove the drug; most patients will require 30 mL; larger adults may require up to 60 mL. Do not retreat. Do not leave on for more than 12 hours.

Head lice, crab lice: Apply shampoo to dry hair and massage into hair for 4 minutes; add small quantities of water to hair until lather forms, then rinse hair thoroughly and comb with a fine tooth comb to remove nits. Amount of shampoo needed is based on length and density of hair; most patients will require 30 mL (maximum: 60 mL). Do not retreat.

Additional Information Complete prescribing information should be consulted for additional detail.

Dosage Forms

Lotion, External:

Generic: 1% (60 mL)

Shampoo, External:

Generic: 1% (60 mL)

◆ **Linessa (Can)** *see* Ethinyl Estradiol and Desogestrel *on page 799*

Linezolid (li NE zoh lid)

Brand Names: U.S. Zyvox

Brand Names: Canada Apo-Linezolid; Linezolid Injection; Sandoz-Linezolid; Zyvoxam

Pharmacologic Category Antibiotic, Oxazolidinone

Use Treatment of vancomycin-resistant *Enterococcus faecium* (VRE) infections, nosocomial pneumonia caused by *Staphylococcus aureus* (including MRSA) or *Streptococcus pneumoniae* (including multidrug-resistant strains [MDRSP]), complicated and uncomplicated skin and skin structure infections (including diabetic foot infections without concomitant osteomyelitis), and community-acquired pneumonia caused by susceptible gram-positive organisms

Pregnancy Risk Factor C

Pregnancy Considerations Adverse effects were observed in some animal reproduction studies at doses that were also maternally toxic. Information related to linezolid use during pregnancy is limited.

Breast-Feeding Considerations Linezolid is excreted into breast milk. The manufacturer advises caution if administering linezolid to a breast-feeding woman. Non-dose-related effects could include modification of bowel flora.

Contraindications Hypersensitivity to linezolid or any other component of the formulation; concurrent use or within 2 weeks of MAO inhibitors

Warnings/Precautions Myelosuppression has been reported and may be dependent on duration of therapy (generally >2 weeks of treatment); use with caution in patients with preexisting myelosuppression, in patients receiving other drugs which may cause bone marrow suppression, or in chronic infection (previous or concurrent antibiotic therapy). Weekly CBC monitoring is recommended. Consider discontinuation in patients developing myelosuppression (or in whom myelosuppression worsens during treatment).

Lactic acidosis has been reported with use. Linezolid exhibits mild MAO inhibitor properties and has the potential to have the same interactions as other MAO inhibitors; use with caution and monitor closely in patients with uncontrolled hypertension, pheochromocytoma, carcinoid syndrome, or untreated hyperthyroidism; do not use in the absence of close monitoring. Hypoglycemic episodes have been reported; use with caution and closely monitor glucose in diabetic patients. Dose reductions/discontinuation of concurrent hypoglycemic agents or discontinuation of linezolid may be required. Symptoms of agitation, confusion, hallucinations, hyper-reflexia, myoclonus, shivering, and tachycardia may occur with concomitant proserotonergic drugs (eg, SSRIs/SNRIs, tricyclic antidepressants, triptans, meperidine, bupropion) or agents which reduce linezolid's metabolism; these medications should not be used concurrently unless patient is closely monitored for signs/symptoms of serotonin syndrome or neuroleptic malignant syndrome-like reactions. Patients maintained on proserotonergic drugs requiring urgent treatment with linezolid may receive linezolid if the other proserotonergic drug is discontinued promptly and the benefits of linezolid outweigh risks; monitor for 2 weeks (5 weeks for fluoxetine) after discontinuation of maintenance drug or 24 hours after last linezolid dose, whichever comes first. Unnecessary use may lead to the development of resistance to linezolid; consider alternatives before initiating outpatient treatment.

Peripheral and optic neuropathy (with vision loss) has been reported in adults and children and may occur primarily with extended courses of therapy >28 days; any symptoms of visual change or impairment warrant immediate ophthalmic evaluation and possible discontinuation of therapy. Seizures have been reported; use with caution in patients with a history of seizures. Prolonged use may result in fungal or bacterial superinfection, including *C. difficile*-associated diarrhea (CDAD) and pseudomembranous colitis; CDAD has been observed >2 months post-antibiotic treatment.

Due to inconsistent concentrations in the CSF, empiric use in pediatric patients with CNS infections is not recommended by the manufacturer; however, there are multiple case reports describing successful treatment of documented VRE and *Staphylococcus aureus* CNS and shunt infections in the literature. Linezolid should not be used in the empiric treatment of catheter-related bloodstream infection (CRBSI), but may be appropriate for targeted therapy (Mermel, 2009).

Benzyl alcohol and derivatives: Some dosage forms may contain sodium benzoate/benzoic acid; benzoic acid (benzoate) is a metabolite of benzyl alcohol; large amounts of benzyl alcohol (≥99 mg/kg/day) have been associated with a potentially fatal toxicity ("gasping syndrome") in neonates; the "gasping syndrome" consists of metabolic acidosis, respiratory distress, gasping respirations, CNS dysfunction (including convulsions, intracranial hemorrhage), hypotension, and cardiovascular collapse (AAP, 1997; CDC, 1982); some data suggests that benzoate displaces bilirubin from protein binding sites (Ahlfors, 2001); avoid or use dosage forms containing benzyl alcohol derivative with caution in neonates. See manufacturer's labeling.

Oral suspension contains phenylalanine.

Adverse Reactions

Central nervous system: Dizziness, headache, insomnia, vertigo (children)

Dermatologic: Pruritus (children), skin rash

Endocrine & metabolic: Increased amylase, increased lactate dehydrogenase

Gastrointestinal: Abdominal pain, constipation, diarrhea, dysgeusia, increased serum lipase, loose stools (children), nausea, oral candidiasis, pancreatitis, tongue discoloration, vomiting

Genitourinary: Vulvovaginal candidiasis

Hematologic & oncologic: Anemia, decreased hemoglobin, eosinophilia (children), leukopenia (more common in children), neutropenia (more common in children), thrombocytopenia

Hepatic: Abnormal hepatic function tests, increased serum alkaline phosphatase, increased serum ALT, increased serum AST (adults), increased serum bilirubin (more common in children)

Infection: Fungal infection

Renal: Increased blood urea nitrogen, increased serum creatinine

Miscellaneous: Fever

Rare but important or life-threatening: Anaphylaxis, angioedema, bullous skin disease, *Clostridium difficile*-associated diarrhea, convulsions, hypertension, hypoglycemia, lactic acidosis, optic neuropathy, pancytopenia, peripheral neuropathy, rhabdomyolysis, seizures, serotonin syndrome (with concurrent use of other serotonergic agents), Stevens-Johnson syndrome, vision loss

Drug Interactions

Metabolism/Transport Effects Inhibits Monoamine Oxidase

Avoid Concomitant Use

Avoid concomitant use of Linezolid with any of the following: Alcohol (Ethyl); Anilidopiperidine Opioids; Apraclonidine; AtoMOXetine; BCG; Bezafibrate; Buprenorphine; BuPROPion; BusPIRone; CarBAMazepine; CloZAPine; Cyclobenzaprine; Cyproheptadine; Dapoxetine; Dexmethylphenidate; Dextromethorphan; Diethylpropion; Dipyrone; Hydrocodone; HYDROmorphone; Isometheptene; Levonordefrin; MAO Inhibitors; Maprotiline; Meperidine; Methyldopa; Methylene Blue; Methylphenidate; Mianserin; Mirtazapine; Morphine (Liposomal); Morphine (Systemic); Nefazodone; Oxymorphone; Pholcodine; Pizotifen; Selective Serotonin Reuptake Inhibitors; Serotonin 5-HT1D Receptor Agonists; Serotonin/Norepinephrine Reuptake Inhibitors; Tapentadol; Tetrabenazine; Tetrahydrozoline (Nasal); TraZODone; Tricyclic Antidepressants; Tryptophan

Increased Effect/Toxicity

Linezolid may increase the levels/effects of: Antipsychotic Agents; Apraclonidine; AtoMOXetine; Betahistine; Bezafibrate; Brimonidine (Ophthalmic); Brimonidine (Topical); BuPROPion; CloZAPine; Cyproheptadine; Dexmethylphenidate; Dextromethorphan; Diethylpropion; Domperidone; Doxylamine; Hydrocodone; HYDROmorphone; Hypoglycemic Agents; Isometheptene; Levonordefrin; Lithium; Meperidine; Methadone; Methyldopa; Methylene Blue; Methylphenidate; Metoclopramide; Mianserin; Mirtazapine; Morphine (Liposomal); Morphine (Systemic); Nefazodone; OxyCODONE; Pizotifen; Reserpine; Selective Serotonin Reuptake Inhibitors; Serotonin 5-HT1D Receptor Agonists; Serotonin Modulators; Serotonin/Norepinephrine Reuptake Inhibitors; Sympathomimetics; Tetrahydrozoline (Nasal); TraZODone; Tricyclic Antidepressants

The levels/effects of Linezolid may be increased by: Alcohol (Ethyl); Anilidopiperidine Opioids; Antiemetics (5HT3 Antagonists); Antipsychotic Agents; Buprenorphine; BusPIRone; CarBAMazepine; COMT Inhibitors; Cyclobenzaprine; Dapoxetine; Dipyrone; Levodopa; MAO Inhibitors; Maprotiline; Oxymorphone; Pholcodine; Tapentadol; Tetrabenazine; TraMADol; Tryptophan

Decreased Effect

Linezolid may decrease the levels/effects of: BCG; Domperidone; Sodium Picosulfate; Typhoid Vaccine

The levels/effects of Linezolid may be decreased by: Cyproheptadine; Domperidone

Food Interactions Concurrent ingestion of foods rich in tyramine, dopamine, tyrosine, phenylalanine, tryptophan, or caffeine may cause sudden and severe high blood pressure (hypertensive crisis or serotonin syndrome). Beverages containing tyramine (eg, hearty red wine and beer) may increase toxic effects. Management: Avoid tyramine-containing foods (aged or matured cheese, air-dried or cured meats including sausages and salamis; fava or broad bean pods, tap/draft beers, Marmite concentrate, sauerkraut, soy sauce, and other soybean condiments). Food's freshness is also an important concern; improperly stored or spoiled food can create an environment in which tyramine concentrations may increase. Avoid foods containing dopamine, tyrosine, phenylalanine, tryptophan, or caffeine. Avoid beverages containing tyramine.

Preparation for Administration Oral suspension: Reconstitute with 123 mL of distilled water (in 2 portions); shake vigorously. Concentration is 100 mg/5 mL. Prior to administration mix gently by inverting bottle; do not shake.

Storage/Stability

Infusion: Store at 25°C (77°F); excursions permitted to 15°C to 30°C (59°F to 86°F). Protect from light. Keep infusion bags in overwrap until ready for use. Protect infusion bags from freezing.

Oral suspension: Following reconstitution, store at 25°C (77°F); excursions permitted to 15°C to 30°C (59°F to 86°F). Use reconstituted suspension within 21 days. Protect from light.

Tablet: Store at 25°C (77°F); excursions permitted to 15°C to 30°C (59°F to 86°F). Protect from light; protect from moisture.

Mechanism of Action Inhibits bacterial protein synthesis by binding to bacterial 23S ribosomal RNA of the 50S subunit. This prevents the formation of a functional 70S initiation complex that is essential for the bacterial translation process. Linezolid is bacteriostatic against enterococci and staphylococci and bactericidal against most strains of streptococci.

Pharmacodynamics/Kinetics

Absorption: Rapid and extensive

Distribution: V_{dss}: Adults: 40-50 L

Protein binding: Adults: 31%

Metabolism: Hepatic via oxidation of the morpholine ring, resulting in two inactive metabolites (aminoethoxyacetic acid, hydroxyethyl glycine); minimally metabolized, may be mediated by cytochrome P450

Bioavailability: Oral: ~100%

Half-life elimination: Children ≥1 week (full-term) to 11 years: 1.5-3 hours; Adults: 4-5 hours

Time to peak: Adults: Oral: 1-2 hours

Excretion: Urine (~30% of total dose as parent drug, ~50% of total dose as metabolites); feces (~9% of total dose as metabolites)

Nonrenal clearance: Adults: ~65%

Dosage

Usual dosage: Oral, IV:

Children ≤11 years: 10 mg/kg (maximum: 600 mg/dose) every 8 hours

Children ≥12 years and Adults: 600 mg every 12 hours

Indication-specific dosing:

Pneumonia:

Community-acquired pneumonia (CAP):

Manufacturer's recommendation (includes concurrent bacteremia): Oral, IV:

Infants (excluding preterm neonates <1 week) and Children ≤11 years: 10 mg/kg/dose every 8 hours for 10-14 days

Children ≥12 years and Adults: 600 mg every 12 hours for 10-14 days. **Note**: May consider 7-day treatment course (versus manufacturer recommended 10-14 days) in patients with healthcare-, hospital-, and ventilator-associated pneumonia who have demonstrated good clinical response (ATS/IDSA, 2005).

Alternate recommendations:

Infants >3 months and Children ≤11 years (IDSA/PIDS, 2011):

S. pneumoniae (MICs to penicillin ≤2.0 mcg/mL), mild infection or step-down therapy (alternative to amoxicillin): Oral: 10 mg/kg/dose every 8 hours

S. pneumoniae (MICs to penicillin ≥4.0 mcg/mL):

Severe infection (alternative to ceftriaxone): IV: 10 mg/kg/dose every 8 hours

Mild infection, step-down therapy (preferred): Oral: 10 mg/kg/dose every 8 hours

S. aureus (methicillin-resistant/clindamycin-susceptible):

Severe infection (alternative to vancomycin or clindamycin): IV: 10 mg/kg/dose every 8 hours

Mild infection, step-down therapy (alternative to clindamycin): Oral: 10 mg/kg/dose every 8 hours

S. aureus (methicillin- and clindamycin-resistant):

Severe infection (alternative to vancomycin): IV: 10 mg/kg/dose every 8 hours

Mild infection, step-down therapy (preferred): Oral: 10 mg/kg/dose every 8 hours

Children ≤11 years (Liu, 2011): Oral, IV: *S. aureus* (methicillin-resistant): 10 mg/kg/dose every 8 hours for 7-21 days (maximum: 600 mg/dose)

Children ≥12 years (IDSA/PIDS, 2011):

S. pneumoniae (MICs to penicillin ≤2.0 mcg/mL), mild infection or step-down therapy (alternative to amoxicillin): Oral: 10 mg/kg/dose every 12 hours

S. pneumoniae (MICs to penicillin ≥4.0 mcg/mL)

Severe infection (alternative to ceftriaxone): IV: 10 mg/kg/dose every 12 hours

Mild infection, step-down therapy (preferred): Oral: 10 mg/kg/dose every 12 hours

S. aureus (methicillin-resistant/clindamycin-susceptible):

Severe infection (alternative to vancomycin/clindamycin): IV: 10 mg/kg/dose every 12 hours

Mild infection, step-down therapy (alternative to clindamycin): Oral: 10 mg/kg/dose every 12 hours

S. aureus (methicillin- and clindamycin-resistant):

Severe infection (alternative to vancomycin): IV: 10 mg/kg/dose every 12 hours

Mild infection, step-down therapy (preferred): Oral: 10 mg/kg/dose every 12 hours

Children ≥12 years and Adults: (Liu, 2011): Oral, IV: *S. aureus* (methicillin-resistant): 600 mg every 12 hours for 7-21 days

Healthcare-associated (HA) pneumonia: Oral, IV:

Manufacturer's recommendation:

Infants (excluding preterm neonates <1 week) and Children ≤11 years: 10 mg/kg every 8 hours for 10-14 days

Children ≥12 years and Adults: 600 mg every 12 hours for 10-14 days.

Note: May consider 7-day treatment course (versus manufacturer recommended 10-14 days) in patients with healthcare-, hospital-, and ventilator-associated pneumonia who have demonstrated good clinical response (ATS/IDSA, 2005).

Alternate recommendations (Liu, 2011): *S. aureus* (methicillin-resistant):

Children ≤11 years: 10 mg/kg/dose every 8 hours for 7-21 days (maximum: 600 mg/dose)

Children ≥12 years and Adults: 600 mg every 12 hours for 7-21 days

Skin and skin structure infections, complicated: Oral, IV:

Infants (excluding preterm neonates <1 week) and Children ≤11 years: 10 mg/kg every 8 hours for 10-14 days

Children ≥12 years and Adults: 600 mg every 12 hours for 10-14 days. **Note:** For diabetic foot infections, initial treatment duration is up to 4 weeks depending on severity of infection and response to therapy (Lipsky, 2012).

Skin and skin structure infections, uncomplicated: Oral:

Infants (excluding preterm neonates <1 week) and Children <5 years: 10 mg/kg every 8 hours for 10-14 days

Children 5-11 years: 10 mg/kg every 12 hours for 10-14 days

Children ≥12-18 years: 600 mg every 12 hours for 10-14 days

Adults: 400 mg every 12 hours for 10-14 days; **Note:** 400 mg dose is recommended in the product labeling; however, 600 mg dose is commonly employed clinically; consider 5- to 10-day treatment course as opposed to the manufacturer recommended 10-14 days (Liu, 2011; Stevens, 2005). For diabetic foot infections, may extend treatment duration up to 4 weeks if slow to resolve (Lipsky, 2012).

VRE infections including concurrent bacteremia: Oral, IV:

Infants (excluding preterm neonates <1 week) and Children ≤11 years: 10 mg/kg every 8 hours for 14-28 days

Children ≥12 years and Adults: 600 mg every 12 hours for 14-28 days

Brain abscess, subdural empyema, spinal epidural abscess (*S. aureus* [methicillin-resistant]) (off-label use; Liu, 2011): Oral, IV:

Children ≤11 years: 10 mg/kg every 8 hours for 4-6 weeks (maximum: 600 mg/dose)

Children ≥12 years and Adults: 600 mg every 12 hours for 4-6 weeks

Meningitis (*S. aureus* [methicillin-resistant]) (off-label use; Liu, 2011): Oral, IV: Children ≥12 years and Adults: 600 mg every 12 hours for 2 weeks

Osteomyelitis (*S. aureus* [methicillin-resistant]) (off-label use; Liu, 2011): Oral, IV:

Infants (excluding preterm neonates <1 week) and Children ≤11 years: 10 mg/kg every 8 hours for a minimum of 4-6 weeks (maximum: 600 mg/dose)

Children ≥12 years and Adults: 600 mg every 12 hours for a minimum of 8 weeks (some experts combine with rifampin)

Prosthetic joint infection (off-label use): Oral, IV:

Enterococcus spp (penicillin-susceptible or -resistant) (alternative treatment): 600 mg every 12 hours for 4-6 weeks (consider adding an aminoglycoside) followed by an oral antibiotic suppressive regimen (Osmon, 2013)

Staphylococci (oxacillin-sensitive or -resistant) (alternative treatment): 600 mg every 12 hours for 2-6 weeks used in combination with rifampin followed by oral antibiotic treatment and suppressive regimens (Osmon, 2013)

Septic arthritis (*S. aureus* [methicillin-resistant]) (off-label use; Liu, 2011): Oral, IV:

Infants (excluding preterm neonates <1 week) and Children ≤11 years: 10 mg/kg every 8 hours for 3-4 weeks (maximum: 600 mg/dose)

Children ≥12 years and Adults: 600 mg every 12 hours for 3-4 weeks

Septic thrombosis of cavernous or dural venous sinus (*S. aureus* [methicillin-resistant]) (off-label use; Liu, 2011): Oral, IV:

Children ≤11 years: 10 mg/kg every 8 hours for 4-6 weeks (maximum: 600 mg/dose)

Children ≥12 years and Adults: 600 mg every 12 hours for 4-6 weeks

Elderly: No dosage adjustment required

Dosage adjustment in renal impairment: No adjustment is recommended. The two primary metabolites may accumulate in patients with renal impairment but the clinical significance is unknown. Weigh the risk of accumulation of metabolites versus the benefit of therapy. Monitor for hematopoietic (eg, anemia, leukopenia, thrombocytopenia) and neuropathic (eg, peripheral neuropathy) adverse events when administering for extended periods.

Intermittent hemodialysis (administer after hemodialysis on dialysis days): Dialyzable (~30% removed during 3-hour dialysis session): If administration time is not immediately after dialysis session, may consider administration of a supplemental dose especially early in the treatment course to maintain levels above the MIC (Brier, 2003). Others have recommended no supplemental dose or dosage adjustment for patients on intermittent hemodialysis, peritoneal dialysis, or continuous renal replacement therapy (eg, CVVHD) (Heintz, 2009; Trotman, 2005)

Dosage adjustment in hepatic impairment:

Mild-to-moderate hepatic impairment (Child-Pugh class A or B): No dosage adjustment required

Severe hepatic impairment (Child-Pugh class C): Use has not been adequately evaluated

Dietary Considerations Take without regard to meals. Some products may contain sodium and/or phenylalanine. Avoid consuming large amounts of tyramine-containing foods/beverages. Some examples include aged or matured cheese, air-dried or cured meats (including sausages and salamis), fava or broad bean pods, tap/draft beers, Marmite concentrate, sauerkraut, soy sauce, and other soybean condiments.

Administration

IV: Administer intravenous infusion over 30-120 minutes. Do not mix or infuse with other medications. When the same intravenous line is used for sequential infusion of other medications, flush line with D_5W, NS, or LR before and after infusing linezolid. The yellow color of the injection may intensify over time without affecting potency.

Oral suspension: Invert gently to mix prior to administration, do not shake. Administer without regard to meals.

Monitoring Parameters Weekly CBC, particularly in patients at increased risk of bleeding, with preexisting myelosuppression, on concomitant medications that cause bone marrow suppression, in those who require >2 weeks of therapy, or in those with chronic infection who have received previous or concomitant antibiotic therapy; visual function with extended therapy (≥3 months) or in patients with new onset visual symptoms, regardless of therapy length

Dosage Forms

Solution, Intravenous:

Zyvox: 2 mg/mL (100 mL, 300 mL)

Generic: 2 mg/mL (300 mL)

Suspension Reconstituted, Oral:
Zyvox: 100 mg/5 mL (150 mL)
Tablet, Oral:
Zyvox: 600 mg

- ◆ **Linezolid Injection (Can)** *see* Linezolid *on page 1217*
- ◆ **Linzess** *see* Linaclotide *on page 1215*
- ◆ **Lioresal** *see* Baclofen *on page 223*
- ◆ **Lioresal D.S. (Can)** *see* Baclofen *on page 223*
- ◆ **Lioresal Intrathecal (Can)** *see* Baclofen *on page 223*

Liothyronine (lye oh THYE roe neen)

Brand Names: U.S. Cytomel; Triostat
Brand Names: Canada Cytomel®
Index Terms Liothyronine Sodium; Sodium *L*-Triiodothyronine; T_3 Sodium (error-prone abbreviation)
Pharmacologic Category Thyroid Product
Use
Oral: Replacement or supplemental therapy in hypothyroidism; management of nontoxic goiter; a diagnostic aid
IV: Treatment of myxedema coma/precoma
Pregnancy Risk Factor A
Dosage Doses should be adjusted based on clinical response and laboratory parameters.
Children: Congenital hypothyroidism: Oral: 5 mcg/day increase by 5 mcg every 3-4 days until the desired response is achieved. Usual maintenance dose: 20 mcg/day for infants, 50 mcg/day for children 1-3 years of age, and adult dose for children >3 years.
Adults:
Hypothyroidism: Oral: 25 mcg/day increase by increments of 12.5-25 mcg/day every 1-2 weeks to a maximum of 100 mcg/day; usual maintenance dose: 25-75 mcg/day.
Patients with cardiovascular disease: Refer to Elderly dosing.
T_3 suppression test: Oral: 75-100 mcg/day for 7 days; use lowest dose for elderly
Myxedema: Oral: Initial: 5 mcg/day; increase in increments of 5-10 mcg/day every 1-2 weeks. When 25 mcg/day is reached, dosage may be increased at intervals of 5-25 mcg/day every 1-2 weeks. Usual maintenance dose: 50-100 mcg/day.
Myxedema coma: IV: 25-50 mcg
Patients with known or suspected cardiovascular disease: 10-20 mcg
Note: Normally, at least 4 hours should be allowed between doses to adequately assess therapeutic response and no more than 12 hours should elapse between doses to avoid fluctuations in hormone levels. Oral therapy should be resumed as soon as the clinical situation has been stabilized and the patient is able to take oral medication. If levothyroxine rather than liothyronine sodium is used in initiating oral therapy, the physician should bear in mind that there is a delay of several days in the onset of levothyroxine activity and that IV therapy should be discontinued gradually.
Simple (nontoxic) goiter: Oral: Initial: 5 mcg/day; increase by 5-10 mcg every 1-2 weeks; after 25 mcg/day is reached, may increase dose by 12.5-25 mcg. Usual maintenance dose: 75 mcg/day
Elderly: Oral: 5 mcg/day; increase by 5 mcg/day every 2 weeks

Dosage adjustment in renal impairment: No dosage adjustment provided in manufacturer's labeling.
Dosage adjustment in hepatic impairment: No dosage adjustment provided in manufacturer's labeling.
Additional Information Complete prescribing information should be consulted for additional detail.
Dosage Forms
Solution, Intravenous:
Triostat: 10 mcg/mL (1 mL)
Generic: 10 mcg/mL (1 mL)
Tablet, Oral:
Cytomel: 5 mcg, 25 mcg, 50 mcg
Generic: 5 mcg, 25 mcg, 50 mcg

- ◆ **Liothyronine and Levothyroxine** *see* Liotrix *on page 1221*
- ◆ **Liothyronine Sodium** *see* Liothyronine *on page 1221*

Liotrix (LYE oh triks)

Brand Names: U.S. Thyrolar®
Brand Names: Canada Thyrolar®
Index Terms Levothyroxine and Liothyronine; Liothyronine and Levothyroxine; T_3/T_4 Liotrix
Pharmacologic Category Thyroid Product
Use
Replacement or supplemental therapy in hypothyroidism (uniform mixture of T_4:T_3 in 4:1 ratio by weight)
Thyroid-stimulating hormone (TSH) suppressant therapy used in the management of thyroid cancer (levothyroxine is generally recommended for this indication); prevention or treatment of euthyroid goiters (eg, thyroid nodules, subacute or chronic lymphocytic thyroiditis [Hashimoto's], multinodular goiters)
Diagnostic agent in suppression tests to diagnose suspected mild hyperthyroidism or to demonstrate thyroid gland autonomy
Pregnancy Risk Factor A
Dosage Oral:
Congenital hypothyroidism:
Children: **Note:** In newly diagnosed infants, begin therapy with full dose.
0-6 months: Levothyroxine 12.5-25 mcg/Liothyronine 3.1-6.25 mcg once daily
6-12 months: Levothyroxine 25-37.5 mcg/Liothyronine 6.25-9.35 mcg once daily
1-5 years: Levothyroxine 37.5-50 mcg/Liothyronine 9.35-12.5 mcg once daily
6-12 years: Levothyroxine 50-75 mcg/Liothyronine 12.5-18.75 mcg once daily
>12 years: Levothyroxine 75 mcg/Liothyronine 18.75 mcg once daily
Also see individual agents.
Hypothyroidism:
Adults: Initial: Levothyroxine 25 mcg/Liothyronine 6.25 mcg once daily; may increase by levothyroxine 12.5 mcg/Liothyronine 3.1 mcg every 2-3 weeks. A lower initial dose (levothyroxine 12.5 mcg/Liothyronine 3.1 mcg) is recommended in patients with long-standing myxedema, especially if cardiovascular impairment coexists. If angina occurs, reduce dose (usual maintenance dose: levothyroxine 50-100 mcg/Liothyronine 12.5-25 mcg)
Elderly: Initial: Levothyroxine 12.5-25 mcg/Liothyronine 3.1-6.25 mcg once daily; may increase by levothyroxine 12.5 mcg/Liothyronine 3.1 mcg every 2-3 weeks
Additional Information Complete prescribing information should be consulted for additional detail.
Dosage Forms
Tablet, oral:
Thyrolar®:
1/4 [levothyroxine 12.5 mcg and liothyronine 3.1 mcg]
1/2 [levothyroxine 25 mcg and liothyronine 6.25 mcg]
1 [levothyroxine 50 mcg and liothyronine 12.5 mcg]
2 [levothyroxine 100 mcg and liothyronine 25 mcg]
3 [levothyroxine 150 mcg and liothyronine 37.5 mcg]

- ◆ **Lipancreatin** *see* Pancrelipase *on page 1566*

- ◆ **Lipase, Protease, and Amylase** *see* Pancrelipase *on page 1566*
- ◆ **Lipiarrmycin** *see* Fidaxomicin *on page 875*
- ◆ **Lipidil EZ (Can)** *see* Fenofibrate and Derivatives *on page 852*
- ◆ **Lipidil Micro (Can)** *see* Fenofibrate and Derivatives *on page 852*
- ◆ **Lipidil Supra (Can)** *see* Fenofibrate and Derivatives *on page 852*
- ◆ **Lipitor** *see* AtorvaSTATin *on page 194*
- ◆ **Lipodox** *see* DOXOrubicin (Liposomal) *on page 684*
- ◆ **Lipodox 50** *see* DOXOrubicin (Liposomal) *on page 684*
- ◆ **Lipofen** *see* Fenofibrate and Derivatives *on page 852*
- ◆ **Liposomal Bupivacaine** *see* Bupivacaine (Liposomal) *on page 299*
- ◆ **Liposomal Cytarabine** *see* Cytarabine (Liposomal) *on page 540*
- ◆ **Liposomal DAUNOrubicin** *see* DAUNOrubicin (Liposomal) *on page 580*
- ◆ **Liposomal DOXOrubicin** *see* DOXOrubicin (Liposomal) *on page 684*
- ◆ **Liposomal Vincristine** *see* VinCRIStine (Liposomal) *on page 2166*
- ◆ **Liposome Vincristine** *see* VinCRIStine (Liposomal) *on page 2166*
- ◆ **Liposyn III** *see* Fat Emulsion (Plant Based) *on page 848*
- ◆ **Liptruzet** *see* Ezetimibe and Atorvastatin *on page 833*
- ◆ **Liqua-Cal [OTC]** *see* Calcium and Vitamin D *on page 326*
- ◆ **Liquibid [OTC]** *see* GuaiFENesin *on page 986*
- ◆ **Liquibid® D-R [OTC]** *see* Guaifenesin and Phenylephrine *on page 988*
- ◆ **Liquibid® PD-R [OTC]** *see* Guaifenesin and Phenylephrine *on page 988*
- ◆ **Liquid Antidote** *see* Charcoal, Activated *on page 416*
- ◆ **Liquituss GG [OTC]** *see* GuaiFENesin *on page 986*

Liraglutide (lir a GLOO tide)

Brand Names: U.S. Victoza

Brand Names: Canada Victoza

Index Terms NN2211; Saxenda

Pharmacologic Category Antidiabetic Agent, Glucagon-Like Peptide-1 (GLP-1) Receptor Agonist

Use

Chronic weight management (Saxenda): As an adjunct to a reduced-calorie diet and increased physical activity for chronic weight management in adult patients with an initial body mass index of 30 kg/m^2 or greater (obese) or 27 kg/m^2 or greater (overweight) in the presence of at least one weight-related comorbid condition (eg, hypertension, type 2 diabetes mellitus, dyslipidemia)

Diabetes mellitus, type 2 (Victoza): As an adjunct to diet and exercise to improve glycemic control in adults with type 2 diabetes mellitus.

Pregnancy Risk Factor X (Saxenda)/C (Victoza)

Pregnancy Considerations Adverse events were observed in animal reproduction studies.

Use for chronic weight management is contraindicated in pregnant women. Weight loss therapy is generally not recommended for pregnant women. Obese and overweight women should be encouraged to participate in weight reduction programs prior to attempting pregnancy; weight gain during pregnancy should be determined by prepregnancy BMI and current guidelines (ACOG 2005; IOM 2009; NHLBI 1998).

In women with diabetes, maternal hyperglycemia can be associated with congenital malformations as well as adverse effects in the fetus, neonate, and the mother (ACOG 2005; ADA 2014; Kitzmiller 2008; Metzger 2007). To prevent adverse outcomes, prior to conception and throughout pregnancy maternal blood glucose and HbA_{1c} should be kept as close to normal as possible but without causing significant hypoglycemia (ACOG 2013; ADA 2014; Blumer 2013; Kitzmiller 2008). Prior to pregnancy, effective contraception should be used until glycemic control is achieved (ADA 2014; Kitzmiller 2008). Other agents are currently recommended to treat diabetes in pregnant women (ACOG 2013; Blumer 2013).

Breast-Feeding Considerations It is not known if liraglutide is excreted into breast milk. Because tumors were observed in animal studies, the manufacturer recommends that a decision be made whether to discontinue nursing or to discontinue the drug, taking into account the importance of treatment to the mother.

Weight loss therapy is generally not recommended for lactating women (NHLBI 1998). Weight loss programs which include physical activity and nutrition components should be discussed at the 6-week postpartum visit (ADA 2009).

Contraindications Hypersensitivity to liraglutide or any component of the formulation; history of or family history of MTC; patients with multiple endocrine neoplasia syndrome type 2 (MEN2); pregnancy (Saxenda).

Canadian labeling: Additional contraindications (not in US labeling): Pregnancy; breast-feeding

Warnings/Precautions Hazardous agent - use appropriate precautions for handling and disposal (NIOSH 2014 [group 2]).

[U.S. Boxed Warning] Dose- and duration- dependent thyroid C-cell tumors have developed in animal studies with liraglutide therapy; relevance in humans unknown. Due to the finding in animal studies, patients were monitored with serum calcitonin or thyroid ultrasound during clinical trials; however, it is unknown if this is beneficial in decreasing the risk of thyroid tumors. Patients should be counseled on the risk and symptoms (eg, neck mass, dysphagia, dyspnea, persistent hoarseness) of thyroid tumors. Use is contraindicated in patients with or a family history of medullary thyroid cancer and in patients with multiple endocrine neoplasia syndrome type 2 (MEN2). During clinical studies, a few cases of thyroid C-cell hyperplasia were reported. Consultation with an endocrinologist is recommended in patients who develop elevated calcitonin concentrations or have thyroid nodules detected during imaging studies or physical exam; routine monitoring of serum calcitonin or using thyroid ultrasound for early detection of medullary thyroid carcinoma (MTC) is of unknown value (due to risk of unnecessary procedures and low specificity of serum calcitonin testing for MTC).

Serious hypersensitivity reactions, including anaphylactic reactions and angioedema, have been reported with use; discontinue therapy in the event of a hypersensitivity reaction. Use with caution in patients with a history of angioedema to other GLP-1 receptor agonists (angioedema has been reported with other GLP-1 receptor agonists); potential for cross-sensitivity is unknown. Cases of acute and chronic pancreatitis (including fatal and nonfatal, hemorrhagic or necrotizing pancreatitis) have been reported; monitor for signs and symptoms of pancreatitis (eg, persistent severe abdominal pain which may radiate to the back and which may or may not be accompanied by vomiting. If pancreatitis is suspected, discontinue use. Do not resume unless an alternative etiology of pancreatitis is confirmed. Use with caution in patients with a history of pancreatitis or consider antidiabetic therapies other than liraglutide. Use with caution in patients with cholelithiasis and/or alcohol abuse. Cholelithiasis and cholecystitis have been reported in patients treated with liraglutide for obesity. Most common reactions are gastrointestinal related; these symptoms may be dose-related and may decrease in frequency/severity with gradual titration and continued use. Slows gastric emptying; has not been studied in patients with preexisting gastroparesis. Use may be associated with weight loss (likely due to reduced intake) independent of the change in hemoglobin A_{1c}. Use with caution in patients with hepatic impairment. Use with caution in renal impairment, particularly during initiation of therapy and dose escalation; cases of acute renal failure and chronic renal failure exacerbation have been reported; some cases have been reported in patients with no known preexisting renal disease.

Suicidal behavior, with one case of attempted suicide, has been reported in patients treated for obesity; monitor for new or worsening depression, suicidal thoughts or behavior, or unusual changes in mood or behavior. Discontinue use if suicidal thoughts or behaviors occur. Avoid use in patients with history of suicidal attempts or active suicidal ideation. Increased resting heart rate has been reported in patients treated for obesity; monitoring is recommended. Discontinue use in patients who experience a sustained increase in resting heart rate.

Victoza is not recommended for first-line therapy; use as adjunct to diet and exercise. Do not use in patients with type 1 diabetes mellitus or for the treatment of diabetic ketoacidosis; not a substitute for insulin. Saxenda is not indicated for the treatment of type 2 diabetes and concomitant use with insulin is not recommended. Diabetes self-management education (DSME) is essential to maximize the effectiveness of therapy. According to the Centers for Disease Control and Prevention (CDC), pen-shaped injection devices should never be used for more than one person (even when the needle is changed) because of the risk of infection. The injection device should be clearly labeled with individual patient information to ensure that the correct pen is used (CDC, 2012). Potentially significant interactions may exist, requiring dose or frequency adjustment, additional monitoring, and/or selection of alternative therapy.

Adverse Reactions

Obesity:

>10%:

Cardiovascular: Increased heart rate (>10 bpm from baseline: 34%; >20 bpm from baseline: 5%)

Central nervous system: Headache (14%)

Endocrine & metabolic: Hypoglycemia (Type 2 diabetics: combination therapy with sulfonylurea: 44%; monotherapy: 16%; nondiabetic patients 2% to 3%)

Gastrointestinal: Nausea (39%), diarrhea (21%), constipation (19%), vomiting (16%)

1% to 10%:

Cardiovascular: Tachycardia (6%; one resting heart rate >100 bpm)

Central nervous system: Fatigue (8%), dizziness (7%)

Gastrointestinal: Decreased appetite (10%), dyspepsia (10%), abdominal distension (5%), abdominal pain (5%), eructation (5%), gastroenteritis (5%), gastroesophageal reflux disease (5%), increased serum lipase (5%; >3 x ULN: 2%), upper abdominal pain (5%), flatulence (4%), viral gastroenteritis (3%), cholelithiasis (2%), xerostomia (2%)

Genitourinary: Urinary tract infection (4%)

Immunologic: Antibody development (3%; neutralizing: 1%)

Local: Injection site reactions (3% to 14%; including erythema [1% to 3%], itching [1% to 3%], rash [1% to 3%])

Neuromuscular & skeletal: Weakness (2%)

Type 2 diabetes mellitus: Incidence reported in monotherapy trials unless otherwise specified.

>10%: Gastrointestinal: Nausea (28%), diarrhea (17%), vomiting (11%)

1% to 10%:

Central nervous system: Headache (9%)

Gastrointestinal: Constipation (10%), dyspepsia (combination trials: 9%)

Hepatic: Hyperbilirubinemia (monotherapy and combination trials: 4%)

Immunologic: Antibody development: Antiliraglutide antibodies (low titers [concentrations not requiring dilution of serum]; monotherapy and combination trials: 9%), cross-reacting antiliraglutide antibodies to native GLP-1 (monotherapy: 7%; combination trials: 5%)

Local: Injection site reactions (monotherapy and combination trials: 2% [includes rash, erythema])

<Rare but important or life-threatening: Acute renal failure, asthma, benign gastrointestinal neoplasm (colorectal), carcinoma (papillary thyroid), cholecystitis, cholestasis, chronic renal failure (exacerbation), first degree atrioventricular block, hepatitis, hypersensitivity reaction, increased susceptibility to infection, left bundle branch block, malignant neoplasm (including colorectal carcinoma), malignant neoplasm of breast, medullary thyroid carcinoma, pancreatitis (including acute, chronic, hemorrhagic, and necrotizing), papillary thyroid carcinoma, right bundle branch block, suicidal ideation, systolic hypotension, thyroid disease (C-cell hyperplasia), upper respiratory tract infection

Drug Interactions

Metabolism/Transport Effects None known.

Avoid Concomitant Use There are no known interactions where it is recommended to avoid concomitant use.

Increased Effect/Toxicity

Liraglutide may increase the levels/effects of: Insulin; Sulfonylureas

The levels/effects of Liraglutide may be increased by: Androgens; Pegvisomant

Decreased Effect

The levels/effects of Liraglutide may be decreased by: Corticosteroids (Orally Inhaled); Corticosteroids (Systemic); Danazol; Luteinizing Hormone-Releasing Hormone Analogs; Somatropin; Thiazide Diuretics

Storage/Stability Prior to initial use, store under refrigeration at 2°C to 8°C (36°F to 46°F); after initial use, may be stored in refrigerator or at room temperature of 15°C to 30°C (59°F to 86°F). Do not freeze (discard if freezing occurs). Protect from heat and light. Pen should be discarded 30 days after initial use.

Mechanism of Action Liraglutide is a long acting analog of human glucagon-like peptide-1 (GLP-1) (an incretin hormone) which increases glucose-dependent insulin secretion, decreases inappropriate glucagon secretion, increases B-cell growth/replication, slows gastric emptying, and decreases food intake. Liraglutide administration results in decreases in hemoglobin A_{1c} by approximately 1%.

Pharmacodynamics/Kinetics

Distribution: V_d: SubQ: ~13 to 25 L; IV: 0.07 L/kg

Protein binding: >98%

Metabolism: Endogenously metabolized by dipeptidyl peptidase IV (DPP-IV) and endogenous endopeptidases (Croom, 2009); metabolism occurs slower than that seen with native GLP-1

Bioavailability: SubQ: ~55%

Half-life, elimination: ~13 hours

Time to peak, plasma: 8 to 12 hours

Excretion: Urine (6%, as metabolites); feces (5%, as metabolites)

Dosage Chronic weight management: Adults: SubQ: Initial: 0.6 mg once daily for one week; increase by 0.6 mg daily at weekly intervals to a target dose of 3 mg once daily. If the patient cannot tolerate an increased dose during dose escalation, consider delaying dose escalation for one week. If the 3 mg daily dose is not tolerated, discontinue use as efficacy has not been established at lower doses.

Note: Evaluate change in body weight 16 weeks after initiation of therapy; discontinue if at least 4% of baseline body weight loss has not been achieved.

Diabetes mellitus, type 2: Adults: SubQ: Initial: 0.6 mg once daily for 1 week; then increase to 1.2 mg once daily; may increase further to 1.8 mg once daily if optimal glycemic response not achieved with 1.2 mg daily.

Note: Initial dose is intended to reduce GI symptoms; does not provide effective glycemic control.

Missed doses: In the event of a missed dose, the once daily regimen can be resumed with the next scheduled dose (an extra dose or an increase in the next dose should **not** be attempted); if >3 days have passed since the last liraglutide dose, reinitiate therapy at 0.6 mg/day to avoid GI symptoms and titrate according to prescriber discretion.

Dosage adjustment in renal impairment:

U.S. labeling: Mild-to-severe impairment: There are no dosage adjustments provided in the manufacturer's labeling; however, use with caution, due to limited experience and reports of acute renal failure and exacerbation of chronic renal failure.

Canadian labeling:

Mild impairment: No dosage adjustment necessary.

Moderate-to-severe impairment: Use is not recommended.

Dosage adjustment in hepatic impairment:

U.S. labeling: Mild-to-severe impairment: There are no dosage adjustments provided in the manufacturer's labeling; use with caution, due to limited experience.

Canadian labeling: Mild-to-severe impairment: Use is not recommended.

Dietary Considerations Individualized medical nutrition therapy (MNT) based on ADA recommendations is an integral part of therapy.

Administration Do not inject intravenously or intramuscularly. Inject subcutaneously in the upper arm, thigh, or abdomen. Administer without regard to meals or time of day. Change needle with each administration. Use only if clear, colorless, and free of particulate matter. Do not share pens between patients even if needle is changed. If using concomitantly with insulin, administer as separate injections (do **not** mix); may inject in the same body region as insulin, but not adjacent to one another.

Hazardous agent; use appropriate precautions for handling and disposal (NIOSH 2014 [group 2]).

Monitoring Parameters Plasma glucose, HbA_{1c}; renal function; signs/symptoms of pancreatitis; emergence of worsening depression, suicidal thoughts/behavior, changes in behavior; heart rate

Reference Range Recommendations for glycemic control in nonpregnant adults with diabetes (ADA, 2013):

HbA_{1c}: <7% (a more aggressive [<6.5%] or less aggressive [<8%] HbA_{1c} goal may be targeted based on patient-specific characteristics)

Preprandial capillary plasma glucose: 70-130 mg/dL

Peak postprandial capillary blood glucose: <180 mg/dL

Product Availability

Saxenda: FDA approved December 2014; anticipated availability is unknown.

Saxenda (liraglutide injection) is approved as a treatment option for chronic weight management (in conjunction with a reduced-calorie diet and physical activity).

Dosage Forms

Solution Pen-injector, Subcutaneous:

Victoza: 18 mg/3 mL (3 mL)

Lisdexamfetamine (lis dex am FET a meen)

Brand Names: U.S. Vyvanse

Brand Names: Canada Vyvanse

Index Terms Lisdexamfetamine Dimesylate; Lisdexamphetamine; NRP104

Pharmacologic Category Central Nervous System Stimulant

Use Attention deficit hyperactivity disorder: Treatment of attention-deficit/hyperactivity disorder (ADHD)

Pregnancy Risk Factor C

Pregnancy Considerations Adverse effects have not been observed in animal reproduction studies. Lisdexamfetamine is converted to dextroamphetamine. The majority of human data is based on illicit amphetamine/methamphetamine exposure and not from therapeutic maternal use (Golub, 2005). Use of amphetamines during pregnancy may lead to an increased risk of premature birth and low birth weight; newborns may experience symptoms of withdrawal. Behavioral problems may also occur later in childhood (LaGasse, 2012).

Breast-Feeding Considerations The majority of human data is based on illicit amphetamine/methamphetamine exposure and not from therapeutic maternal use (Golub, 2005). Amphetamines are excreted into breast milk and use may decrease milk production. Increased irritability, agitation, and crying have been reported in nursing infants (ACOG, 2011). According to the manufacturer, the decision to continue or discontinue breast-feeding during therapy should take into account the risk of exposure to the infant and the benefits of treatment to the mother.

Contraindications

Hypersensitivity to amphetamine products or any component of the formulation; concurrent use of MAO inhibitor, or within 14 days of the last MAO inhibitor dose.

Canadian labeling: Additional contraindications (not in U.S. labeling): Known hypersensitivity or idiosyncrasy to sympathomimetic amines; advanced arteriosclerosis; symptomatic cardiovascular disease; moderate-to-severe hypertension; hyperthyroidism; glaucoma; agitated states; history of drug abuse

Warnings/Precautions Sudden death, stroke, and myocardial infarction have been reported in adults receiving the recommended doses of CNS stimulants. In children and adolescents with preexisting structural cardiac abnormalities or other serious heart problems, sudden death has been reported while receiving the recommended doses of CNS stimulants for ADHD. These products should be avoided in the patients with known serious structural cardiac abnormalities, cardiomyopathy, serious heart rhythm abnormalities, coronary artery disease (adults), or other serious cardiac problems that could increase the risk of sudden death. Patients should be carefully evaluated for these cardiac disorders prior to initiation of therapy. Patients who develop exertional chest pain, unexplained syncope, or arrhythmias during therapy should be evaluated promptly. CNS stimulants may increase heart rate (mean increase: 3 to 6 bpm) and blood pressure (mean increase: 2 to 4 mm Hg); monitor for adverse events related to tachycardia or hypertension. Stimulants are associated with peripheral vasculopathy, including Raynaud phenomenon; signs/symptoms are usually mild and intermittent, and generally improve with dose reduction or discontinuation. Digital ulceration and/or soft tissue breakdown have been observed rarely; monitor for digital changes during therapy and seek further evaluation (eg, rheumatology) if necessary.

Use with caution in patients with preexisting psychosis or bipolar disorder (may induce mixed/manic episode). May exacerbate symptoms of behavior and thought disorder in psychotic patients; new onset psychosis or mania may occur in children or adolescents with stimulant use. Patients should be screened for bipolar disorder prior to treatment; consider discontinuation if such symptoms (eg, delusional thinking, hallucinations, or mania) occur. May be associated with aggressive behavior or hostility (causal relationship not established); monitor for development or worsening of these behaviors. Use with caution in patients with Tourette syndrome; stimulants may exacerbate tics (motor and phonic) and Tourette syndrome. Evaluate for tics and Tourette syndrome prior to therapy initiation. **[U.S. Boxed Warning]: CNS stimulants (including lisdexamfetamine) have a high potential for abuse and dependence; assess for abuse potential prior to use and monitor for signs of abuse and dependence while on therapy.** Use with caution in patients with history of ethanol or drug abuse (Canadian labeling contraindicates use if history of drug abuse). Prescriptions should be written for the smallest quantity consistent with good patient care to minimize possibility of overdose. Abrupt discontinuation following high doses or for prolonged periods may result in symptoms for withdrawal (eg, depression, extreme fatigue). Canadian labeling recommends discontinuing therapy if improvement is not observed after 1 month of dosage titration.

Elderly patients may have decreased renal, hepatic or cardiac function or other concomitant disease or drug therapy; initiate dose at the low end of the dosing range. Appetite suppression may occur; particularly in children. Use of stimulants has been associated with weight loss and slowing of growth rate; monitor growth rate and weight during treatment. Treatment interruption may be necessary in patients who are not increasing in height or gaining weight as expected. Hypersensitivity, including anaphylaxis, Stevens-Johnson syndrome, angioedema, and urticaria have been observed. Potentially significant drug-drug interactions may exist, requiring dose or frequency adjustment, additional monitoring, and/or selection of alternative therapy.

Adverse Reactions

Cardiovascular: Increased blood pressure (adults), increased heart rate (adults)

Central nervous system: Agitation (adults), anxiety (adults), dizziness (children), drowsiness (children), emotional lability (children), insomnia, irritability (children), jitteriness (adults), restlessness (adults), tics (children)

Dermatologic: Hyperhidrosis (adults), skin rash (children)

Endocrine & metabolic: Decreased libido (adults), weight loss (more common in children and adolescents)

Gastrointestinal: Abdominal pain (children), anorexia (adults), appetite decreased (more common in children and adolescents), diarrhea (adults), nausea, vomiting (children), xerostomia (more common in adults)

Genitourinary: Erectile dysfunction (adults)

Neuromuscular & skeletal: Tremor (adults)

Respiratory: Dyspnea (adults)

Miscellaneous: Fever (children)

Rare but important or life-threatening: Accommodation disturbance, bruxism, cardiomyopathy, cerebrovascular accident, decreased linear skeletal growth rate, depression, dermatillomania, diplopia, exacerbation of tics, excoriation, frequent erections, hallucination, headache, hepatitis (eosinophilic), hypersensitivity, hypertension, incoherent speech, mania, mydriasis, myocardial infarction, overstimulation, peripheral vascular insufficiency, prolonged erection, psychotic reaction, Raynaud's phenomenon, seizure, Stevens-Johnson syndrome, suicidal tendencies, tachycardia

Drug Interactions

Metabolism/Transport Effects None known.

Avoid Concomitant Use

Avoid concomitant use of Lisdexamfetamine with any of the following: Iobenguane I 123; MAO Inhibitors

Increased Effect/Toxicity

Lisdexamfetamine may increase the levels/effects of: Analgesics (Opioid); Sympathomimetics

The levels/effects of Lisdexamfetamine may be increased by: Alkalinizing Agents; Antacids; AtoMOXetine; Cannabinoid-Containing Products; Carbonic Anhydrase Inhibitors; Linezolid; MAO Inhibitors; Tedizolid; Tricyclic Antidepressants

Decreased Effect

Lisdexamfetamine may decrease the levels/effects of: Antihistamines; Ethosuximide; Iobenguane I 123; Ioflupane I 123; PHENobarbital; Phenytoin

The levels/effects of Lisdexamfetamine may be decreased by: Ammonium Chloride; Antipsychotic Agents; Ascorbic Acid; Gastrointestinal Acidifying Agents; Lithium; Methenamine; Multivitamins/Fluoride (with ADE); Multivitamins/Minerals (with ADEK, Folate, Iron); Multivitamins/Minerals (with AE, No Iron); Urinary Acidifying Agents

Food Interactions High-fat meal prolongs T_{max} by ~1 hour. Management: Administer without regard to meals.

Storage/Stability Store at 25°C (77°F) excursions are permitted between 15°C and 30°C (59°F and 86°F). Protect from light.

Mechanism of Action Lisdexamfetamine dimesylate is a prodrug that is converted to the active component dextroamphetamine (a noncatecholamine, sympathomimetic amine). Amphetamines are noncatecholamine, sympathomimetic amines that cause release of catecholamines (primarily dopamine and norepinephrine) from their storage sites in the presynaptic nerve terminals. A less significant mechanism may include their ability to block the reuptake of catecholamines by competitive inhibition.

Pharmacodynamics/Kinetics

Absorption: Rapid

Distribution: Dextroamphetamine: V_d: Adults: 3.5 to 4.6 L/kg; distributes into CNS; mean CSF concentrations are 80% of plasma

Metabolism: Metabolized in the blood by hydrolytic activity of red blood cells to dextroamphetamine and l-lysine; does not undergo CYP mediated metabolism

Half-life elimination: Lisdexamfetamine: <1 hour; Dextroamphetamine: 10 to 13 hours

Time to peak, serum: T_{max}: Lisdexamfetamine: ~1 hour; Dextroamphetamine: ~3.5 hours

Excretion: Urine (96%, 42% as amphetamine-related compounds, 2% as lisdexamfetamine, 25% hippuric acid); feces (minimal)

Dosage Note: Individualize dosage based on patient need and response to therapy. Administer at the lowest effective dose.

Attention-deficit/hyperactivity disorder (ADHD): Children ≥6 years, Adolescents, and Adults: Oral:

U.S. labeling: Initial: 30 mg once daily in the morning; may increase in increments of 10 mg or 20 mg daily at weekly intervals until optimal response is obtained; maximum: 70 mg daily

Canadian labeling: Initial: 20 to 30 mg once daily in the morning; per clinical discretion, dose may be increased at weekly intervals up to a maximum dose of 60 mg daily. Discontinue therapy if improvement is not observed after 1 month of dosage titration. **Note:** For patients requiring dose titration, the Canadian ADHD Resource Alliance (CADDRA) 2011 practice guidelines recommend weekly increases of 10 mg daily up to a maximum of 60 mg daily for children or 70 mg daily for adolescent and adult patients.

Dosage adjustment in renal impairment:

U.S. labeling:

GFR ≥30 mL/minute/1.73 m^2: There are no dosage adjustments provided in the manufacturer's labeling.

GFR 15 to <30 mL/minute/1.73 m^2: Maximum dose: 50 mg daily.

GFR <15 mL/minute/1.73 m^2: Maximum dose: 30 mg daily.

ESRD requiring hemodialysis: Maximum dose: 30 mg daily; lisdexamfetamine and dextroamphetamine are not dialyzable.

Canadian labeling:

Mild to moderate impairment (GFR ≥30 mL/minute/1.73 m^2): There are no dosage adjustments provided in the manufacturer's labeling.

Severe impairment (GFR <30 mL/minute/1.73 m^2): Maximum dose: 50 mg daily.

Dialysis: There is no specific dosage recommendation provided in the manufacturer's labeling; however, the manufacturer recommends considering further maximum dosage reductions (compared to that recommended for severe impairment).

Dosage adjustment in hepatic impairment: There are no dosage adjustments provided in the manufacturer's labeling.

Administration Administer in the morning without regard to meals; swallow capsule whole, do not chew. Capsule may be opened and the entire contents dissolved in glass of water, yogurt, or orange juice; stir until dispersed completely and consume the entire mixture immediately; do not store mixture. The active ingredient dissolves completely once dispersed; however, a film containing the inactive ingredients may remain in the glass or container once the mixture is consumed. Do not take less than one capsule daily; a single capsule should not be divided.

Monitoring Parameters Cardiac evaluation should be completed on any patient who develops exertional chest pain, unexplained syncope, and any symptom of cardiac disease during treatment with stimulants; growth (height and weight) in children; CNS activity in all patients; signs of peripheral vasculopathy (eg, digital changes); behavioral changes; signs of misuse, abuse, or addiction

When used for the treatment of ADHD, thoroughly evaluate for cardiovascular risk. Monitor heart rate, blood pressure, and consider obtaining ECG prior to initiation (Vetter, 2008).

Dosage Forms

Capsule, Oral:

Vyvanse: 10 mg, 20 mg, 30 mg, 40 mg, 50 mg, 60 mg, 70 mg

Dosage Forms: Canada Refer to Dosage Forms. **Note:** Vyvanse 70 mg capsule is not available in Canada.

◆ **Lisdexamfetamine Dimesylate** *see* Lisdexamfetamine *on page 1224*

◆ **Lisdexamphetamine** *see* Lisdexamfetamine *on page 1224*

Lisinopril (lyse IN oh pril)

Brand Names: U.S. Prinivil; Zestril

Brand Names: Canada Apo-Lisinopril; Auro-Lisinopril; CO Lisinopril; Dom-Lisinopril; JAMP-Lisinopril; Mylan-Lisinopril; PMS-Lisinopril; Prinivil; PRO-Lisinopril; RAN-Lisinopril; Riva-Lisinopril; Sandoz-Lisinopril; Teva-Lisinopril (Type P); Teva-Lisinopril (Type Z); Zestril

Pharmacologic Category Angiotensin-Converting Enzyme (ACE) Inhibitor; Antihypertensive

Use

Acute myocardial infarction: Treatment of acute myocardial infarction (MI) within 24 hours in hemodynamically-stable patients to improve survival

Note: The 2013 American College of Cardiology Foundation/American Heart Association (ACCF/AHA) guidelines for the management of patients with ST-elevation myocardial infarction (STEMI) states that an ACE inhibitor should be initiated within the first 24 hours after STEMI in patients with anterior MI, heart failure, or left ventricular ejection fraction (LVEF) of 0.4 or less. It is also reasonable to initiate an ACE inhibitor in all patients with STEMI (O'Gara, 2013).

Heart failure: Adjunctive therapy in treatment systolic of heart failure (HF)

Note: The ACCF/AHA 2013 heart failure guidelines recommend the use of ACE inhibitors, along with other guideline directed medical therapies, to prevent HF in patients with a reduced ejection fraction who have a history of MI (stage B HF), to prevent HF in any patient with a reduced ejection fraction (stage B HF), or to treat those with HF and reduced ejection fraction (stage C HFrEF) (Yancy, 2013).

Hypertension: Treatment of hypertension, either alone or in combination with other antihypertensive agents in adult and pediatric patients 6 years and older

The 2014 guideline for the management of high blood pressure in adults (Eighth Joint National Committee [JNC 8]) recommends initiation of pharmacologic treatment to lower blood pressure for the following patients:

- Patients ≥60 years of age with systolic blood pressure (SBP) ≥150 mm Hg or diastolic blood pressure (DBP) ≥90 mm Hg. Goal of therapy is SBP <150 mm Hg and DBP <90 mm Hg.
- Patients <60 years of age with SBP ≥140 mm Hg or DBP is ≥90 mm Hg. Goal of therapy is SBP <140 mm Hg and DBP <90 mm Hg.
- Patients ≥18 years of age with diabetes and SBP ≥140 mm Hg or DBP ≥90 mm Hg. Goal of therapy is SBP <140 mm Hg and DBP <90 mm Hg.
- Patients ≥18 years of age with chronic kidney disease (CKD) and SBP ≥140 mm Hg or DBP ≥90 mm Hg. Goal of therapy is SBP <140 mm Hg and DBP <90 mm Hg.

In patients with CKD, regardless of race or diabetes status, the use of an ACE inhibitor (ACEI) or angiotensin receptor blocker (ARB) as initial therapy is recommended to improve kidney outcomes. In the general nonblack population (without CKD) including those with diabetes, initial antihypertensive treatment should consist of a thiazide-type diuretic, calcium channel blocker, ACEI, or ARB. In the general black population (without CKD) including those with diabetes, initial antihypertensive treatment should consist of a thiazide-type diuretic or a calcium channel blocker **instead of** an ACEI or ARB.

Pregnancy Risk Factor D

Pregnancy Considerations [U.S. Boxed Warning]: Drugs that act on the renin-angiotensin system can cause injury and death to the developing fetus. Discontinue as soon as possible once pregnancy is detected. Lisinopril crosses the placenta; teratogenic effects may occur following maternal use during pregnancy. Drugs that act on the renin-angiotensin system are associated with oligohydramnios. Oligohydramnios, due to decreased fetal renal function, may lead to fetal lung hypoplasia and skeletal malformations. Their use in pregnancy is also associated with anuria, hypotension, renal failure, skull hypoplasia, and death in the fetus/neonate. Chronic maternal hypertension itself is also associated with adverse events in the fetus/infant. ACE inhibitors are not recommended during pregnancy to treat maternal hypertension or heart failure. Use of an ACE inhibitor should also be avoided in any woman of reproductive age. Women who are planning a pregnancy should be considered for other medication options if an ACE inhibitor is currently prescribed or the ACE inhibitor should be discontinued as soon as possible once pregnancy is detected. The exposed fetus should be monitored for fetal growth, amniotic fluid volume, and organ formation. Infants exposed to an ACE inhibitor *in utero* should be monitored for hyperkalemia, hypotension, and oliguria (exchange transfusions or dialysis may be needed). These adverse events are generally associated with maternal use in the second and third trimesters.

Untreated chronic maternal hypertension is also associated with adverse events in the fetus, infant, and mother. The use of ACE inhibitors is not recommended to treat chronic uncomplicated hypertension in pregnant women and should generally be avoided in women of reproductive potential (ACOG, 2013).

Breast-Feeding Considerations It is not known if lisinopril is excreted in breast milk. The manufacturer recommends discontinuing use of lisinopril or discontinuing breast-feeding taking into account the importance of therapy to the mother.

Contraindications

Hypersensitivity to lisinopril or any component of the formulation; angioedema related to previous treatment with an ACE inhibitor; patients with idiopathic or hereditary angioedema; concomitant use with aliskiren in patients with diabetes mellitus

Documentation of allergenic cross-reactivity for ACE inhibitors is limited. However, because of similarities in chemical structure and/or pharmacologic actions, the possibility of cross-sensitivity cannot be ruled out with certainty.

Canadian labeling: Additional contraindications (not in U.S. labeling): Concomitant use with aliskiren-containing drugs in patients with moderate-to-severe renal impairment (GFR <60 mL/minute/1.73 m^2)

Warnings/Precautions Anaphylactic reactions may occur rarely with ACE inhibitors. At any time during treatment (especially following first dose), angioedema may occur rarely with ACE inhibitors; it may involve the head and neck (potentially compromising airway) or the intestine (presenting with abdominal pain). African-Americans may be at an increased risk. Prolonged frequent monitoring may be required especially if tongue, glottis, or larynx are involved as they are associated with airway obstruction. Patients with a history of airway surgery may have a higher risk of airway obstruction. Aggressive early and appropriate management is critical. Use in patients with idiopathic or hereditary angioedema or previous angioedema associated with ACE inhibitor therapy is contraindicated. Severe anaphylactoid reactions may be seen during hemodialysis (eg, CVVHD) with high-flux dialysis membranes (eg, AN69), and rarely, during low density lipoprotein apheresis with dextran sulfate cellulose. Rare cases of anaphylactoid reactions have been reported in patients undergoing sensitization treatment with hymenoptera (bee, wasp) venom while receiving ACE inhibitors.

Symptomatic hypotension with or without syncope can occur with ACE inhibitors (usually with the first several doses). Effects are most often observed in volume depleted patients; correct volume depletion prior to initiation. Other patients at risk include those with heart failure and systolic blood pressure <100 mm Hg, ischemic heart disease, cerebrovascular disease, renal dialysis, hyponatremia, high-dose diuretic therapy, severe aortic stenosis, or hypertrophic cardiomyopathy. Close monitoring of patient is required especially within the first few weeks of initial dosing and with dosing increases; blood pressure must be lowered at a rate appropriate for the patient's clinical condition. Initiation of therapy in patients with ischemic heart disease or cerebrovascular disease warrants close observation due to the potential consequences posed by falling blood pressure (eg, MI, stroke). Avoid use in hemodynamically unstable patients after acute MI. Use with caution in hypertrophic cardiomyopathy with outflow tract obstruction, severe aortic stenosis, or before, during, or immediately after major surgery. **[U.S. Boxed Warning]: Drugs that act on the renin-angiotensin system can cause injury and death to the developing fetus. Discontinue as soon as possible once pregnancy is detected.**

Hyperkalemia may occur with ACE inhibitors; risk factors include renal dysfunction, diabetes mellitus, concomitant use of potassium-sparing diuretics, potassium supplements, and/or potassium-containing salts. Use cautiously, if at all, with these agents and monitor potassium closely. Cough may occur with ACE inhibitors. Other causes of cough should be considered (eg, pulmonary congestion in patients with heart failure) and excluded prior to discontinuation.

May be associated with deterioration of renal function and/or increases in serum creatinine, particularly in patients with low renal blood flow (eg, renal artery stenosis, heart failure) whose glomerular filtration rate (GFR) is dependent on efferent arteriolar vasoconstriction by angiotensin II; deterioration may result in oliguria, acute renal failure, and progressive azotemia. Small increases in serum creatinine may occur following initiation; consider discontinuation only in patients with progressive and/or significant deterioration in renal function. Use with caution in patients with unstented unilateral/bilateral renal artery stenosis. When unstented bilateral renal artery stenosis is present, use is generally avoided due to the elevated risk of deterioration in renal function unless possible benefits outweigh risks. Potentially significant drug-drug interactions may exist, requiring dose or frequency adjustment, additional monitoring, and/or selection of alternative therapy.

Rare toxicities associated with ACE inhibitors include cholestatic jaundice or hepatitis (which may progress to fulminant hepatic necrosis), agranulocytosis, neutropenia, or leukopenia with myeloid hypoplasia. Patients with collagen vascular diseases (especially with concomitant renal impairment) or renal impairment alone may be at increased risk for hematologic toxicity; periodically monitor CBC with differential in these patients.

Adverse Reactions Note: Higher rates of adverse reactions have generally been noted in patients with heart failure. However, the frequency of adverse effects associated with placebo is also increased in this population.

Cardiovascular: Chest pain, flushing, hypotension, orthostatic effect, syncope

Central nervous system: Altered sense of smell, dizziness, fatigue, headache

Dermatologic: Alopecia, diaphoresis, erythema, pruritus, skin photosensitivity, Stevens-Johnson syndrome, toxic epidermal necrolysis, urticaria

Endocrine & metabolic: Diabetes mellitus, gout, hyperkalemia, increased nonprotein nitrogen, SIADH

Gastrointestinal: Constipation, diarrhea, dysgeusia, flatulence, pancreatitis, xerostomia

Genitourinary: Impotence

Hematologic & oncologic: Bone marrow suppression, decreased hematocrit (small), decreased hemoglobin (small), hemolytic anemia, leukopenia, neutropenia, thrombocytopenia

Infection: Common cold

Neuromuscular & skeletal: Weakness

Ophthalmic: Blurred vision, diplopia, photophobia, vision loss

Otic: Tinnitus

Renal: Increased blood urea nitrogen, increased serum creatinine (often transient), renal insufficiency (in patients with acute myocardial infarction)

Respiratory: Cough

Rare but important or life-threatening: Acute renal failure, anaphylactoid reactions, angioedema, anuria, arthralgia, arthritis, asthma, ataxia, azotemia, bronchitis, bronchospasm, cardiac arrest, cardiac arrhythmia, chills, confusion, cutaneous pseudolymphoma, dehydration, drowsiness, dyspepsia, dyspnea, dysuria, eosinophilia, eosinophilic pneumonitis, epistaxis, facial edema, fever, gastritis, hallucination, heartburn, hemoptysis, hepatic necrosis, hepatitis (hepatocellular jaundice or cholestatic jaundice), herpes zoster, hypersomnia, hypervolemia, hypoglycemia (diabetic patients on oral antidiabetic agents or insulin), hyponatremia, increased erythrocyte sedimentation rate, insomnia, intestinal angioedema, irritability, laryngitis, leukocytosis, malaise, malignant neoplasm of lung, mastalgia, memory impairment, mood changes (including depressive symptoms), muscle spasm, musculoskeletal pain, myalgia, myocardial infarction, oliguria, orthopnea, orthostatic hypotension, palpitations, paresthesia, paroxysmal nocturnal dyspnea, pemphigus, peripheral edema, peripheral neuropathy, pharyngitis, pleural effusion, pneumonia, positive ANA titer, psoriasis, pulmonary embolism, pulmonary infarct, pulmonary infiltrates, pyelonephritis, rhinitis, rhinorrhea, sinusitis, skin infection, skin lesion, skin rash, sore throat, systemic lupus erythematosus, transient ischemic attacks, tremor, uremia, urinary tract infection, vasculitis, vertigo, viral infection, visual hallucination (Doane, 2013), weight gain, weight loss, wheezing

Drug Interactions

Metabolism/Transport Effects None known.

Avoid Concomitant Use There are no known interactions where it is recommended to avoid concomitant use.

Increased Effect/Toxicity

Lisinopril may increase the levels/effects of: Allopurinol; Amifostine; Antihypertensives; AzaTHIOprine; DULoxetine; Ferric Gluconate; Gold Sodium Thiomalate; Grass Pollen Allergen Extract (5 Grass Extract); Hypotensive Agents; Iron Dextran Complex; Levodopa; Lithium; Nonsteroidal Anti-Inflammatory Agents; Obinutuzumab; RisperiDONE; RiTUXimab; Sodium Phosphates

The levels/effects of Lisinopril may be increased by: Alfuzosin; Aliskiren; Angiotensin II Receptor Blockers; Barbiturates; Brimonidine (Topical); Canagliflozin; Dapoxetine; Diazoxide; DPP-IV Inhibitors; Eplerenone; Everolimus; Heparin; Heparin (Low Molecular Weight); Herbs (Hypotensive Properties); Loop Diuretics; MAO Inhibitors; Nicorandil; Pentoxifylline; Phosphodiesterase 5 Inhibitors; Potassium Salts; Potassium-Sparing Diuretics; Prostacyclin Analogues; Sirolimus; Temsirolimus; Thiazide Diuretics; TiZANidine; Tolvaptan; Trimethoprim

Decreased Effect

The levels/effects of Lisinopril may be decreased by: Aprotinin; Herbs (Hypertensive Properties); Icatibant; Lanthanum; Methylphenidate; Nonsteroidal Anti-Inflammatory Agents; Salicylates; Yohimbine

Storage/Stability Store at controlled room temperature. Protect from moisture, freezing, and excessive heat.

Mechanism of Action Competitive inhibitor of angiotensin-converting enzyme (ACE); prevents conversion of angiotensin I to angiotensin II, a potent vasoconstrictor; results in lower levels of angiotensin II which causes an increase in plasma renin activity and a reduction in aldosterone secretion; a CNS mechanism may also be involved in hypotensive effect as angiotensin II increases adrenergic outflow from CNS; vasoactive kallikreins may be decreased in conversion to active hormones by ACE inhibitors, thus reducing blood pressure

Pharmacodynamics/Kinetics

Onset of action: 1 hour

Peak effect: Hypotensive: Oral: ~6 hours

Duration: 24 hours

Absorption: Unaffected by food

Metabolism: Not metabolized

Bioavailability: Adults: ~25% (range: 6% to 60%); decreased to 16% with NYHA Class II-IV heart failure; Children: ~28%

Half-life elimination: 12 hours

Time to peak: ~7 hours

Excretion: Primarily urine (as unchanged drug)

Dosage

Acute myocardial infarction (within 24 hours in hemodynamically stable patients): Adults: Oral: 5 mg immediately, then 5 mg at 24 hours, 10 mg at 48 hours, and 10 mg every day thereafter for 6 weeks. Patients should continue to receive standard treatments such as thrombolytics, aspirin, and beta-blockers.

According to the 2013 ACCF/AHA guidelines for STEMI: Initial: 2.5 to 5 mg once daily; titrate to 10 mg daily or higher as tolerated (O'Gara, 2013).

Note: For patients with SBP 100 to 120 mm Hg following infarct, initiate therapy with 2.5 mg once daily for 3 days; if SBP falls to <100 mm Hg give maintenance dose of 5 mg once daily (may temporarily reduce to 2.5 mg once daily if necessary). Discontinue if SBP <90 mm Hg for >1 hour.

Heart failure: Adults: Oral: Initial: 2.5 to 5 mg once daily; then increase by no more than 10 mg increments at intervals no less than 2 weeks to a maximum daily dose of 40 mg. Usual maintenance: 5 to 40 mg daily as a single dose. Target dose: 20 to 40 mg once daily (ACCF/AHA [Yancy, 2013])

Note: If patient has hyponatremia (serum sodium <130 mEq/L) or renal impairment (CrCl <30 mL/minute or creatinine >3 mg/dL), then initial dose should be 2.5 mg daily

Hypertension:

Children ≥6 years: Oral: Initial: 0.07 mg/kg once daily (up to 5 mg); increase dose at 1- to 2-week intervals up to a maximum dose of 0.61 mg/kg or 40 mg once daily; doses >0.61 mg/kg or >40 mg have not been evaluated.

Adults: Oral: Initial: 10 mg once daily (not maintained on a diuretic) or 5 mg once daily (maintained on a diuretic). Target dose (JNC 8 [James, 2013]): 40 mg once daily; usual dosage range (ASH/ISH [Weber, 2014]): 10 to 40 mg daily

Note: Antihypertensive effect may diminish toward the end of the dosing interval especially with doses of 10 mg/day. An increased dose may aid in extending the duration of antihypertensive effect. Doses up to 80 mg/day have been used, but do not appear to give greater effect.

Patients taking diuretics should have them discontinued 2 to 3 days prior to initiating lisinopril if possible. Restart diuretic after blood pressure is stable if needed.

Elderly: Consider lower initial doses (eg, 2.5 to 5 mg daily) and titrate to response (Aronow, 2011)

Dosage adjustment in renal impairment:

Acute myocardial infarction (within 24 hours in hemodynamically stable patients): Adults:

CrCl >30 mL/minute: No dosage adjustment necessary.

CrCl 10 to 30 mL/minute: Initial: 2.5 mg daily

CrCl <10 mL/minute: Initial: 2.5 mg daily

Hemodialysis: Initial: 2.5 mg daily (dialyzable)

Heart failure: Adults: Initial doses should be modified and upward titration should be cautious, based on response (maximum: 40 mg/day)

CrCl >30 mL/minute: No dosage adjustment necessary.

CrCl 10 to 30 mL/minute or creatinine >3 mg/dL: Initial: 2.5 mg daily
CrCl <10 mL/minute: Initial: 2.5 mg daily
Hemodialysis: Initial: 2.5 mg daily (dialyzable)

Hypertension:

Children:

GFR >30 mL/minute/1.73 m^2: No dosage adjustment necessary.

GFR <30 mL/minute/1.73 m^2: Use is not recommended.

Adults: Initial doses should be modified and upward titration should be cautious, based on response (maximum: 40 mg/day)

CrCl >30 mL/minute: No dosage adjustment necessary.

CrCl 10 to 30 mL/minute: Initial: 5 mg daily

CrCl <10 mL/minute: Initial: 2.5 mg once daily

Hemodialysis: Initial: 2.5 mg daily (dialyzable)

Dosage adjustment in hepatic impairment: There are no dosage adjustments provided in the manufacturer's labeling.

Dietary Considerations Use potassium-containing salt substitutes cautiously in patients with diabetes, patients with renal dysfunction, or those maintained on potassium supplements or potassium-sparing diuretics.

Administration Administer as a single daily dose and without regard to meals.

Monitoring Parameters BUN, serum creatinine, renal function, WBC, and potassium; if patient has collagen vascular disease and/or renal impairment, periodically monitor CBC with differential; hypotensive effects within 1 to 3 hours of initial dose or with increased dosages.

2013 ACCF/AHA Heart Failure guideline recommendations: Within 1-2 weeks after initiation and periodically thereafter, reassess renal function and serum potassium especially in patients with preexisting hypotension, hyponatremia, diabetes mellitus, azotemia, or those taking potassium supplements (ACCF/AHA [Yancy, 2013]).

Dosage Forms

Tablet, Oral:

Prinivil: 5 mg, 10 mg, 20 mg

Zestril: 2.5 mg, 5 mg, 10 mg, 20 mg, 30 mg, 40 mg

Generic: 2.5 mg, 5 mg, 10 mg, 20 mg, 30 mg, 40 mg

Extemporaneous Preparations A 1 mg/mL lisinopril oral suspension may be made with tablets and a mixture of Bicitra and Ora-Sweet SF. Place ten 20 mg tablets into an 8 ounce amber polyethylene terephthalate (PET) bottle and then add 10 mL purified water and shake for at least 1 minute. Gradually add 30 mL of Bicitra and 160 mL of Ora-Sweet SF to the bottle and gently shake after each addition to disperse the contents. Store resulting suspension at ≤25°C (77°F) for up to 4 weeks. Label bottle "shake well" (Prinivil prescribing information, 2013; Thompson, 2003).

A 1 mg/mL lisinopril oral suspension may be made with tablets and a 1:1 mixture of Ora-Plus® and Ora-Sweet®. Crush ten 10 mg tablets in a mortar and reduce to a fine powder. Add small portions of the vehicle and mix to a uniform paste; mix while adding the vehicle in incremental proportions to **almost** 100 mL; transfer to a graduated cylinder; rinse mortar with vehicle, and add quantity of vehicle sufficient to make 100 mL. Store in amber plastic prescription bottles; label "shake well". Stable for 13 weeks at room temperature or refrigerated (Nahata, 2004).

A 1 mg/mL lisinopril oral suspension also be made with tablets, methylcellulose 1% with parabens, and simple syrup NF. Crush ten 10 mg tablets in a mortar and reduce to a fine powder. Add 7.7 mL of methylcellulose gel and mix to a uniform paste; mix while adding the simple syrup in incremental proportions to **almost** 100 mL; transfer to a graduated cylinder; rinse mortar with vehicle, and add quantity of vehicle sufficient to make 100 mL. Store in amber plastic prescription bottles; label "shake well". Stable for 13 weeks refrigerated or 8 weeks at room temperature (Nahata, 2004).

A 2 mg/mL lisinopril syrup may be made with powder (Sigma Chemical Company, St. Louis, MO) and simple syrup. Dissolve 1 g of lisinopril powder in 30 mL of distilled water. Mix while adding simple syrup in incremental proportions in a quantity sufficient to make 500 mL. Label "shake well" and "refrigerate". Stable for 30 days when stored in amber plastic prescription bottles at room temperature or refrigerated. **Note:** Although no visual evidence of microbial growth was observed, the authors recommend refrigeration to inhibit microbial growth (Webster, 1997).

Nahata MC and Morosco RS, "Stability of Lisinopril in Two Liquid Dosage Forms," *Ann Pharmacother*, 2004, 38(3):396-9.

Prinivil (lisinopril) [prescribing information]. Whitehouse Station, NJ: Merck & Co., Inc; February 2013.

Thompson KC, Zhao Z, Mazakas JM, et al, "Characterization of an Extemporaneous Liquid Formulation of Lisinopril," *Am J Health Syst Pharm*, 2003, 60(1):69-74.

Webster AA, English BA, and Rose DJ, "The Stability of Lisinopril as an Extemporaneous Syrup," *Intr J Pharmaceut Compound*, 1997, 1:352-3.

Lisinopril and Hydrochlorothiazide

(lyse IN oh pril & hye droe klor oh THYE a zide)

Brand Names: U.S. Prinzide; Zestoretic

Brand Names: Canada Apo-Lisinopril/Hctz; Ava-Lisinopril/Hctz; Mylan-Lisinopril/Hctz; Prinzide; Sandoz-Lisinopril/Hctz; Teva-Lisinopril/Hctz (Type P); Teva-Lisinopril/Hctz (Type Z); Zestoretic

Index Terms Hydrochlorothiazide and Lisinopril

Pharmacologic Category Angiotensin-Converting Enzyme (ACE) Inhibitor; Antihypertensive; Diuretic, Thiazide

Use Treatment of hypertension

Pregnancy Risk Factor D

Dosage Adults: Oral: Dosage is individualized; see each component for appropriate dosing suggestions; doses >80 mg/day lisinopril or >50 mg/day hydrochlorothiazide are not recommended.

Dosage adjustment in renal impairment: Dosage adjustments should be made with caution. Usual regimens of therapy need not be adjusted as long as patient's CrCl >30 mL/minute. In patients with more severe renal impairment, loop diuretics are preferred.

Dosage adjustment in hepatic impairment: No dosage adjustment provided in manufacturer's labeling; use with caution.

Additional Information Complete prescribing information should be consulted for additional detail.

Dosage Forms

Tablet, oral: 10/12.5: Lisinopril 10 mg and hydrochlorothiazide 12.5 mg; 20/12.5: Lisinopril 20 mg and hydrochlorothiazide 12.5 mg; 20/25: Lisinopril 20 mg and hydrochlorothiazide 25 mg

Prinzide®:

10/12.5: Lisinopril 10 mg and hydrochlorothiazide 12.5 mg

Zestoretic®:

10/12.5: Lisinopril 10 mg and hydrochlorothiazide 12.5 mg

20/12.5: Lisinopril 20 mg and hydrochlorothiazide 12.5 mg

20/25: Lisinopril 20 mg and hydrochlorothiazide 25 mg

◆ **Lispro Insulin** *see* Insulin Lispro *on page 1087*

◆ **Lithane (Can)** *see* Lithium *on page 1230*

Lithium (LITH ee um)

Brand Names: U.S. Lithobid

Brand Names: Canada Apo-Lithium Carbonate; Carbolith; Lithane; Lithmax; PMS-Lithium Carbonate; PMS-Lithium Citrate

Index Terms Eskalith; Lithium Carbonate; Lithium Citrate

Pharmacologic Category Antimanic Agent

Use Bipolar disorder: Acute treatment of manic episodes and maintenance therapy for patients with a diagnosis of bipolar disorder.

Pregnancy Risk Factor D

Pregnancy Considerations Adverse events have been observed in animal reproduction studies. Lithium crosses the placenta in concentrations similar to those in the maternal plasma (Newport, 2005). Cardiac malformations in the infant, including Ebstein's anomaly, are associated with use of lithium during the first trimester of pregnancy. Other adverse events including polyhydramnios, fetal/neonatal cardiac arrhythmias, hypoglycemia, diabetes insipidus, changes in thyroid function, premature delivery, floppy infant syndrome, or neonatal lithium toxicity are associated with lithium exposure when used later in pregnancy (ACOG, 2008). The incidence of adverse events may be associated with higher maternal doses (Newport, 2005).

Due to pregnancy-induced physiologic changes, women who are pregnant may require dose adjustments of lithium to achieve euthymia and avoid toxicity (ACOG, 2008; Grandjean, 2009; Yonkers, 2011).

For planned pregnancies, use of lithium during the first trimester should be avoided if possible (Grandjean, 2009). If lithium is needed during pregnancy, the minimum effective dose should be used, maternal serum concentrations should be monitored, and consideration should be given to start therapy after the period of organogenesis; lithium should be suspended 24 to 48 hours prior to delivery or at the onset of labor when delivery is spontaneous, then restarted when the patient is medically stable after delivery (ACOG, 2008; Grandjean, 2009; Newport, 2005). Fetal echocardiography should be considered if first trimester exposure occurs (ACOG, 2008).

Breast-Feeding Considerations Lithium is excreted into breast milk and serum concentrations of nursing infants may be 10% to 50% of the maternal serum concentration (Grandjean, 2009). Hypotonia, hypothermia, cyanosis, electrocardiogram changes, and lethargy have been reported in nursing infants (ACOG, 2008). It is generally recommended that breast-feeding be avoided during maternal use of lithium; however, treatment may be continued in appropriately selected patients (Grandjean, 2009; Sharma, 2009; Viguera, 2007). The hydration status of the nursing infant and maternal serum concentrations of lithium should be monitored (ACOG, 2008). In addition, monitor the infant for lethargy, growth, and feeding problems; obtain infant serum concentrations only if clinical concerns arise (Bogen, 2012; Yonkers, 2011). Long-term effects on development and behavior have not been studied (ACOG, 2008; Grandjean, 2009).

Contraindications Hypersensitivity to lithium or any component of the formulation; avoid use in patients with severe cardiovascular or renal disease, or with severe debilitation, dehydration, or sodium depletion

Warnings/Precautions [U.S. Boxed Warning]: Lithium toxicity is closely related to serum levels and can occur at therapeutic doses; serum lithium determinations are required to monitor therapy. Use with caution in patients with mild-moderate renal impairment mild-moderate cardiovascular disease, debilitated patients, and elderly patients due to an increased risk of lithium toxicity. Likewise, use caution in patients in patients with significant fluid loss (protracted sweating, diarrhea, or prolonged fever); temporary reduction or cessation of therapy may be warranted. Lithium may unmask Brugada syndrome; avoid use in patients with or suspected of having Brugada Syndrome. Consult with a cardiologist if a patient is suspected of having Brugada Syndrome or has risk factors for Brugada syndrome (eg, unexplained syncope, a family history of Brugada Syndrome, a family history of sudden death before the age of 45 years), or if unexplained syncope or palpitations develop after starting therapy. Use with caution in patients with thyroid disease; hypothyroidism may occur with treatment. Chronic therapy results in diminished renal concentrating ability (nephrogenic diabetes insipidus); this is usually reversible when lithium is discontinued. Changes in renal function should be monitored, and re-evaluation of treatment may be necessary. Use caution in patients at risk of suicide (suicidal thoughts or behavior) by drug overdose; lithium has a narrow therapeutic index. Lithium may impair the patient's alertness, affecting the ability to operate machinery or driving a vehicle. Neuromuscular-blocking agents should be administered with caution; the response may be prolonged. Higher serum concentrations may be required and tolerated during an acute manic phase; however, the tolerance decreases when symptoms subside. Normal fluid and salt intake must be maintained during therapy.

Benzyl alcohol and derivatives: Some dosage forms may contain benzyl alcohol; large amounts of benzyl alcohol (≥99 mg/kg/day) have been associated with a potentially fatal toxicity ("gasping syndrome") in neonates; the "gasping syndrome" consists of metabolic acidosis, respiratory distress, gasping respirations, CNS dysfunction (including convulsions, intracranial hemorrhage), hypotension, and cardiovascular collapse (AAP, 1997; CDC, 1982); some data suggests that benzoate displaces bilirubin from protein binding sites (Ahlfors, 2001); avoid or use dosage forms containing benzyl alcohol with caution in neonates. See manufacturer's labeling.

Adverse Reactions

Cardiovascular: Abnormal T waves on ECG, bradycardia, cardiac arrhythmia, chest tightness, circulatory shock, cold extremities, edema, hypotension, myxedema, sinus node dysfunction, startled response, syncope

Central nervous system: Ataxia, blackout spells, cogwheel rigidity, coma, confusion, dizziness, drowsiness, dystonia, EEG pattern changes, extrapyramidal reaction, fatigue, hallucination, headache, hyperactive deep tendon reflex, hypertonia, involuntary choreoathetoid movements, lethargy, local anesthesia, memory impairment, loss of consciousness, metallic taste, myasthenia gravis (rare), pseudotumor cerebri, psychomotor retardation, reduced intellectual ability, restlessness, salty taste, sedation, seizure, slowed intellectual functioning, slurred speech, stupor, tics, vertigo, worsening of organic brain syndromes

Dermatologic: Acne vulgaris, alopecia, blue-gray skin pigmentation, dermal ulcer, dry or thinning of hair, exacerbation of psoriasis, folliculitis, pruritus, psoriasis, skin rash, xerosis

Endocrine & metabolic: Albuminuria, dehydration, diabetes insipidus, euthyroid goiter, glycosuria, hypercalcemia, hyperglycemia, hyperparathyroidism, hyperthyroidism, hypothyroidism, increased radioactive iodine uptake, increased thirst, polydipsia, weight gain, weight loss

Gastrointestinal: Abdominal pain, anorexia, dental caries, diarrhea, dysgeusia, dyspepsia, excessive salivation, flatulence, gastritis, nausea, sialadenitis, sialorrhea, swelling of lips, vomiting, xerostomia

Genitourinary: Impotence, incontinence, oliguria

Hematologic & oncologic: Leukocytosis

Hypersensitivity: Angioedema

Neuromuscular & skeletal: Joint swelling, muscle hyperirritability, neuromuscular excitability, polyarthralgia, tremor
Ophthalmic: Blurred vision, exophthalmos, nystagmus, transient scotoma
Otic: Tinnitus
Renal: Decreased creatinine clearance, polyuria
Miscellaneous: Fever
Rare but important or life-threatening: Brugada syndrome

Drug Interactions

Metabolism/Transport Effects None known.

Avoid Concomitant Use

Avoid concomitant use of Lithium with any of the following: Dapoxetine

Increased Effect/Toxicity

Lithium may increase the levels/effects of: Antipsychotic Agents; Highest Risk QTc-Prolonging Agents; Metoclopramide; Moderate Risk QTc-Prolonging Agents; Neuromuscular-Blocking Agents; Selective Serotonin Reuptake Inhibitors; Serotonin Modulators; Tricyclic Antidepressants

The levels/effects of Lithium may be increased by: ACE Inhibitors; Angiotensin II Receptor Blockers; Antiemetics (5HT3 Antagonists); Calcium Channel Blockers (Nondihydropyridine); CarBAMazepine; Dapoxetine; Desmopressin; Eplerenone; Fosphenytoin; Loop Diuretics; MAO Inhibitors; Methyldopa; Mifepristone; Nonsteroidal Anti-Inflammatory Agents; Phenytoin; Potassium Iodide; Thiazide Diuretics; Topiramate

Decreased Effect

Lithium may decrease the levels/effects of: Amphetamines; Antipsychotic Agents; Desmopressin

The levels/effects of Lithium may be decreased by: Caffeine and Caffeine Containing Products; Calcitonin; Calcium Polystyrene Sulfonate; Carbonic Anhydrase Inhibitors; Loop Diuretics; Sodium Bicarbonate; Sodium Chloride; Sodium Polystyrene Sulfonate; Theophylline Derivatives

Storage/Stability Store between 15°C and 30°C (59°F to 86°F). Protect tablets and capsules from moisture.

Mechanism of Action The precise mechanism of action in mood disorders is unknown. Traditionally thought to alter cation transport across cell membranes in nerve and muscle cells, influence the reuptake of serotonin and/or norepinephrine, and inhibit second messenger systems involving the phosphatidylinositol cycle (Ward, 1994). May also provide neuroprotective effects by increasing glutamate clearance, inhibiting apoptoctic glycogen synthase kinase activity, increasing the levels of antiapoptotic protein Bcl-2 and, enhancing the expression of neurotropic factors, including brain-derived neurotrophic factor (Sanacora, 2008).

Pharmacodynamics/Kinetics

Absorption: Rapid and complete
Distribution: V_d: Initial: 0.307 L/kg; V_{dss}: 0.7 to 1 L/kg
Protein binding: Not protein bound
Metabolism: Not metabolized
Bioavailability: 80% to 100%
Half-life elimination: 18 to 36 hours
Time to peak, serum: Immediate release: ~0.5 to 3 hours; Extended release: 2 to 6 hours; Solution: 15 to 60 minutes
Excretion: Urine (primarily; unchanged drug); sweat, saliva, and feces (negligible amounts)
Clearance: 80% of filtered lithium is reabsorbed in the proximal convoluted tubules (Ward, 1994)

Dosage Oral: **Note:** Monitor serum concentrations and clinical response (efficacy and toxicity) to determine proper dose. Each 5 mL of lithium citrate oral solution contains 8 mEq of lithium ion, equivalent to the amount of lithium in 300 mg of lithium carbonate immediate release capsules/tablets.

Bipolar disorder (acute mania, acute depression [off-label use], and maintenance):

Children 6 to 12 years (off-label use): Oral: 15 to 60 mg/kg/day in 3 to 4 divided doses; dose not to exceed usual adult dosage. Monitor serum concentrations and clinical response (efficacy and toxicity) to determine proper dose (Nelson, 1996)

Children >12 years, Adolescents, and Adults: Oral:

Immediate release: Initial: Initiate at low dose (eg, 300 mg 3 times daily or less); increase gradually based on response and tolerability (APA, 2002); usual dosage: 900 to 1,800 mg daily in 3 to 4 divided doses

Extended release: Initiate at low dose (eg, 450 mg 2 times daily or less); increase gradually based on response and tolerability (APA, 2002); usual dosage: 900 to 1,800 mg daily in 2 divided doses

Elderly: Initiate therapy with lower doses; refer to adult dosing.

Depression, augmentation of antidepressant (off-label use): Adults: Oral: Initial: Initiate at a low dose (eg, 300 mg once daily or 300 mg twice daily); increase gradually based on response and tolerability; usual dosage: 600 to 1200 mg daily in divided doses (Bauer, 2003a; Bauer 2003b; Nelson, 2014)

Dosage adjustment in renal impairment:

CrCl 10 to 50 mL/minute: Administer 50% to 75% of normal dose
CrCl <10 mL/minute: Administer 25% to 50% of normal dose
End stage renal disease (ESRD) with hemodialysis: Dose after dialysis (Aronoff, 2007).

Dosage adjustment in hepatic impairment: There are no dosage adjustments provided in the manufacturer's labeling.

Dietary Considerations May be taken with meals to avoid GI upset; maintain adequate fluid intake.

Administration Administer with meals to decrease GI upset. Extended release tablets must be swallowed whole; do not crush or chew.

Monitoring Parameters Renal function including BUN and SrCr (baseline, every 2 to 3 months during the first 6 months of treatment, then once a year in stable patients or as clinically indicated); serum electrolytes (baseline, then periodically), thyroid (baseline, 1 to 2 times with in the first 6 months of treatment, then once a year in stable patients or as clinically indicated); beta-hCG pregnancy test for all females not known to be sterile (baseline); ECG with rhythm strip (baseline for all patients over 40 years, repeat as clinical indicated), CBC with differential (baseline, repeat as clinically indicated); serum lithium levels (twice weekly until both patient's clinical status and levels are stable, then repeat levels every 1 to 3 months or as clinically indicated); weight (baseline, then periodically) (APA, 2002).

Canadian labeling (additional monitoring recommendations): Serum calcium prior to initiation of therapy, at 6 months, and annually thereafter during prolonged therapy.

Reference Range Levels should be obtained twice weekly until both patient's clinical status and levels are stable then levels may be obtained no less than every 6 months (APA, 2002).

Timing of serum samples: Draw trough just before next dose (8-12 hours after previous dose)

Therapeutic levels:

Acute mania: 0.5 to 1.2 mEq/L (SI: 0.5 to 1.2 mmol/L)

Maintenance: 0.6 to 1 mEq/L (SI: 0.6 to 1.0 mmol/L); a higher rate of relapse is described in subjects who are maintained at <0.4 mEq/L (SI: 0.4 mmol/L) (APA, 2002)

Toxic concentrations

>1.5 mEq/L (SI: >1.5 mmol/L): Early signs and symptoms of intoxication may include marked tremor, nausea, diarrhea, blurred vision, vertigo, confusion, and decreased deep tendon reflexes.

>2.5 mEq/L (SI: >2.5 mmol/L): Intoxication symptoms may progress to include severe neurological complications, seizures, coma, cardiac dysrhythmia, and permanent neurological impairment.

>3.5 mEq/L (SI: >3.5 mmol/L): Potentially lethal toxicity (APA, 2002; Mitchell, 2001).

Note: A 10% to 26% increase in levels can be expected if there is a change to once daily (usually night-time) dosing (Mitchell, 2001).

Dosage Forms

Capsule, Oral:

Generic: 150 mg, 300 mg, 600 mg

Solution, Oral:

Generic: 8 mEq/5 mL (5 mL, 500 mL)

Tablet, Oral:

Generic: 300 mg

Tablet Extended Release, Oral:

Lithobid: 300 mg

Generic: 300 mg, 450 mg

- ◆ **Lithium Carbonate** *see* Lithium *on page* 1230
- ◆ **Lithium Citrate** *see* Lithium *on page* 1230
- ◆ **Lithmax (Can)** *see* Lithium *on page* 1230
- ◆ **Lithobid** *see* Lithium *on page* 1230
- ◆ **Little Colds Decongestant [OTC]** *see* Phenylephrine (Systemic) *on page* 1638
- ◆ **Little Fevers [OTC]** *see* Acetaminophen *on page* 32
- ◆ **Livalo** *see* Pitavastatin *on page* 1663
- ◆ **Live Attenuated Influenza Vaccine** *see* Influenza Virus Vaccine (Live/Attenuated) *on page* 1080
- ◆ **Live Attenuated Influenza Vaccine (Quadrivalent)** *see* Influenza Virus Vaccine (Live/Attenuated) *on page* 1080
- ◆ **Live Smallpox Vaccine** *see* Smallpox Vaccine *on page* 1900
- ◆ **Livostin (Can)** *see* Levocabastine (Nasal) [CAN/INT] *on page* 1194
- ◆ **Livostin Eye Drops (Can)** *see* Levocabastine (Ophthalmic) [CAN/INT] *on page* 1195
- ◆ **L-leucovorin** *see* LEVOleucovorin *on page* 1200
- ◆ **LM3100** *see* Plerixafor *on page* 1665
- ◆ **10% LMD** *see* Dextran *on page* 607
- ◆ **LMD in D5W** *see* Dextran *on page* 607
- ◆ **LMD in NaCl** *see* Dextran *on page* 607
- ◆ **L-methylfolate, Methylcobalamin, and N-acetylcysteine** *see* Methylfolate, Methylcobalamin, and Acetylcysteine *on page* 1334
- ◆ **LMX 4 [OTC]** *see* Lidocaine (Topical) *on page* 1211
- ◆ **LMX 4 Plus [OTC]** *see* Lidocaine (Topical) *on page* 1211
- ◆ **LMX 5 [OTC]** *see* Lidocaine (Topical) *on page* 1211
- ◆ **LNg 20** *see* Levonorgestrel *on page* 1201
- ◆ **Locacorten® Vioform® (Can)** *see* Clioquinol and Flumethasone [CAN/INT] *on page* 465
- ◆ **Locoid** *see* Hydrocortisone (Topical) *on page* 1014
- ◆ **Locoid® (Can)** *see* Hydrocortisone (Topical) *on page* 1014
- ◆ **Locoid Lipocream** *see* Hydrocortisone (Topical) *on page* 1014
- ◆ **Lodalis (Can)** *see* Colesevelam *on page* 503
- ◆ **Lodine** *see* Etodolac *on page* 815
- ◆ **Lodosyn** *see* Carbidopa *on page* 351

Lodoxamide (loe DOKS a mide)

Brand Names: U.S. Alomide

Brand Names: Canada Alomide®

Index Terms Lodoxamide Tromethamine

Pharmacologic Category Mast Cell Stabilizer

Use Treatment of vernal keratoconjunctivitis, vernal conjunctivitis, and vernal keratitis

Pregnancy Risk Factor B

Dosage Ophthalmic: Children >2 years and Adults: Instill 1-2 drops in eye(s) 4 times/day for up to 3 months

Dosage adjustment in renal impairment: No dosage adjustment provided in manufacturer's labeling. However, dosage adjustment unlikely due to low systemic absorption.

Dosage adjustment in hepatic impairment: No dosage adjustment provided in manufacturer's labeling. However, dosage adjustment unlikely due to low systemic absorption.

Additional Information Complete prescribing information should be consulted for additional detail.

Dosage Forms

Solution, Ophthalmic:

Alomide: 0.1% (10 mL)

- ◆ **Lodoxamide Tromethamine** *see* Lodoxamide *on page* 1232
- ◆ **Loestrin 1.5/30 (Can)** *see* Ethinyl Estradiol and Norethindrone *on page* 808
- ◆ **Loestrin 21 1.5/30** *see* Ethinyl Estradiol and Norethindrone *on page* 808
- ◆ **Loestrin 21 1/20** *see* Ethinyl Estradiol and Norethindrone *on page* 808
- ◆ **Loestrin 24 Fe** *see* Ethinyl Estradiol and Norethindrone *on page* 808
- ◆ **Loestrin Fe 1.5/30** *see* Ethinyl Estradiol and Norethindrone *on page* 808
- ◆ **Loestrin Fe 1/20** *see* Ethinyl Estradiol and Norethindrone *on page* 808
- ◆ **Lo-Femenal 21 (Can)** *see* Ethinyl Estradiol and Norgestrel *on page* 812

Lofepramine [INT] (loe FE pra meen)

International Brand Names Deftan (ES); Deprimil (PT); Emdalen (ZA); Feprapax (GB); Gamanil (GB, IE); Gamonil (CH, DE); Lomont (GB); Tymelyt (AT, BE, CZ, DK, LU, SE)

Pharmacologic Category Antidepressant, Tricyclic (Tertiary Amine)

Reported Use Treatment of depression

Dosage Range Adults: Oral: 140-210 mg/day in divided doses

Product Availability Product available in various countries; not currently available in the U.S.

Dosage Forms

Suspension, oral: 70 mg/5 mL (150 mL)

Tablet: 70 mg

Lofexidine [INT] (loe FEX i deen)

International Brand Names BritLofex (GB); Kai Er Ding (CN)

Index Terms Lofexidine Hydrochloride

Pharmacologic Category $Alpha_2$-Adrenergic Agonist

Reported Use Relief of symptoms associated with opiate (eg, methadone, heroin, hydrocodone) withdrawal such as chills, sweating, stomach cramps, muscle pain, and runny nose. Does not relieve symptoms of craving.

Dosage Range Adults: Oral: Initial: 0.8 mg/day in divided doses; titrate by 0.4-0.8 mg/day; maximum: 2.4 mg/day, should not exceed 0.8 mg/dose. Duration of treatment without concurrent opioid use: 7-10 days (longer durations may be considered).

Product Availability Product available in various countries; not currently available in the U.S.

Dosage Forms

Tablet: 0.2 mg

- ◆ **Lofexidine Hydrochloride** *see* Lofexidine [INT] *on page 1232*
- ◆ **Lofibra** *see* Fenofibrate and Derivatives *on page 852*
- ◆ **LoHist-D [OTC]** *see* Chlorpheniramine and Pseudoephedrine *on page 427*
- ◆ **L-OHP** *see* Oxaliplatin *on page 1528*
- ◆ **LoKara** *see* Desonide *on page 597*
- ◆ **Lo Loestrin Fe** *see* Ethinyl Estradiol and Norethindrone *on page 808*
- ◆ **Lomedia 24 Fe** *see* Ethinyl Estradiol and Norethindrone *on page 808*

Lomefloxacin [INT] (loe me FLOKS a sin)

International Brand Names Decalogiflox (FR); Ge Tai (CN); Keqi (CL); Logiflox (FR); Lomaday (MY); Lomax (AE, BH, KW, SA); Lomaxacin (KR); Lomebact (TW); Lomeflon (JP); Lomeflox (DO, HK); Lomflox (IN, SG); Maxaquin (AU, CZ, EC, HK, IT, KR, MX, PK, PT, VE, ZA); Okacin (BE, BH, DK, JO, KW, LU, PH, PY, QA, SG, UY, VE); Okacyn (ZA); Uniquin (AT)

Index Terms Lomefloxacin Hydrochloride

Pharmacologic Category Antibiotic, Quinolone

Reported Use Acute bacterial exacerbation of chronic bronchitis caused by susceptible gram-negative organisms; urinary tract infections (uncomplicated and complicated) caused by susceptible organisms; surgical prophylaxis (transrectal prostate biopsy or transurethral procedures)

Dosage Range Adults: Oral: 400 mg once daily

Product Availability Product available in various countries; not currently available in the U.S.

Dosage Forms

Tablet: 400 mg

- ◆ **Lomefloxacin Hydrochloride** *see* Lomefloxacin [INT] *on page 1233*
- ◆ **Lo Minastrin Fe [DSC]** *see* Ethinyl Estradiol and Norethindrone *on page 808*

Lomitapide (loe MI ta pide)

Brand Names: U.S. Juxtapid

Brand Names: Canada Juxtapid

Index Terms AEGR-733; BMS 201038; Lomitapide Mesylate

Pharmacologic Category Antilipemic Agent, Microsomal Triglyceride Transfer Protein (MTP) Inhibitor

Use Homozygous familial hypercholesterolemia: Adjunct to a low-fat diet and other lipid-lowering treatments, including low-density lipoprotein (LDL) apheresis where available, to reduce LDL cholesterol, total cholesterol, apolipoprotein B (apo B), and non-high-density lipoprotein cholesterol (non-HDL-C) in patients with homozygous familial hypercholesterolemia.

Pregnancy Risk Factor X

Pregnancy Considerations Teratogenic effects have been observed in animal reproduction studies using doses lower than equivalent human doses. Use is contraindicated in pregnant women. Discontinue immediately if pregnancy occurs during treatment. Women of reproductive potential should have a negative pregnancy test prior to therapy and effective contraception must be used during treatment. Dose adjustment may be required for women using oral contraceptives.

Health care providers are encouraged to enroll women exposed to lomitapide during pregnancy in the Global Lomitapide Pregnancy Exposure Registry by calling 1-877-902-4099.

Breast-Feeding Considerations It is not known if lomitapide is excreted into breast milk. Due to the potential for serious adverse reactions in the nursing infant, a decision should be made whether to discontinue nursing or to discontinue the drug, taking into account the importance of treatment to the mother.

Contraindications

Pregnancy; coadministration with moderate or strong CYP3A4 inhibitors; moderate or severe hepatic impairment (Child-Pugh class B or C) and patients with active liver disease, including unexplained persistent elevations of serum transaminases.

Canadian labeling: Additional contraindications (not in U.S. labeling): Hypersensitivity to lomitapide or any component of the formulation; known significant, chronic bowel disease (eg, inflammatory bowel disease, malabsorption); concomitant administration of simvastatin >20 mg daily (concomitant use with simvastatin 40 mg daily is permitted in patients previously tolerant of simvastatin 80 mg daily for ≥1 year without evidence of myotoxicity); galactose intolerance, Lapp-lactase deficiency, or glucose-galactose malabsorption

Warnings/Precautions [U.S. Boxed Warning]: May cause transaminase elevations; elevations in ALT or AST ≥3 times upper limit of normal occurred during clinical trials (no clinically meaningful concomitant bilirubin, INR, or alkaline phosphatase elevation was observed). Lomitapide also increases hepatic fat, with or without concomitant transaminase elevations. Hepatic steatosis associated with lomitapide (reversible upon discontinuation) may be a risk factor for progressive liver disease including steatohepatitis and cirrhosis. Monitor hepatic function (ALT, AST, alkaline phosphatase and total bilirubin) prior to treatment; monitor ALT and AST regularly as recommended during treatment; dosage adjustment or discontinuation may be necessary; transaminases typically reduce within 1-4 weeks after discontinuation. Alcohol ingestion may increase the risk of hepatic steatosis; alcohol consumption should be limited to ≤1 drink/day. Use caution when administered concomitantly with other hepatotoxic medications (eg, acetaminophen (>4 g/day for ≥3 days/ week), amiodarone, isotretinoin, methotrexate, tetracyclines, and tamoxifen); may require more frequent monitoring of liver function tests. Concomitant administration with other LDL-lowering agents that also have the potential to increase hepatic fat is not recommended (has not been studied). Use with caution in patients with mild (Child-Pugh class A) hepatic impairment due to increased drug exposure; a reduced maximum dose is recommended. Use is contraindicated in patients with moderate to severe (Child-Pugh class B or C) impairment or active liver disease including unexplained persistent elevations of serum transaminases. Monitor liver function as recommended. Use with caution in patients with mild-to-severe renal impairment including end-stage renal disease (ESRD) not receiving dialysis (has not been evaluated); drug exposure may significantly increase. Use with caution in patients with ESRD receiving dialysis; a reduced maximum dose of 40 mg daily is recommended.

Safety and effectiveness have not been established in patients with hypercholesterolemia who do not have homozygous familial hypercholesterolemia. The effect of lomitapide on cardiovascular morbidity and mortality has not been determined.

Significant gastrointestinal events (eg, diarrhea, nausea, dyspepsia, vomiting) occurred during treatment with lomitapide; absorption of other oral medications may be affected; adherence to a low-fat diet (<20% of energy from fat) and gradual titration of dosage will reduce the risk of gastrointestinal adverse events. Lomitapide may reduce the absorption of fat-soluble nutrients (eg, vitamin E, linoleic acid, alpha-linolenic acid, eicosapentaenoic acid, and docosahexaenoic acid); supplementation is recommended; patients with chronic bowel or pancreatic diseases predisposed to malabsorption are at increased risk for deficiency. Canadian labeling contraindicates use in patients with known significant, chronic bowel disease (eg, inflammatory bowel disease, malabsorption).

Potentially significant drug-drug interactions may exist, requiring dose or frequency adjustment, additional monitoring, and/or selection of alternative therapy. Contains lactose; avoid use in patients with hereditary galactose intolerance, Lapp lactase deficiency, or glucose-galactose malabsorption; may result in diarrhea and malabsorption. **[U.S. Boxed Warning]: Due to the risk for hepatotoxicity, access is restricted through a REMS program (Juxtapid REMS program).** Only certified health care providers and pharmacies may prescribe and dispense lomitapide.

Adverse Reactions

Cardiovascular: Angina pectoris, chest pain, palpitation

Central nervous system: Dizziness, fatigue, fever, headache

Gastrointestinal: Abdominal discomfort, abdominal distension, abdominal pain, constipation, diarrhea, dyspepsia, flatulence, frequent bowel movement, gastroenteritis, gastroesophageal reflux disease, nausea, rectal tenesmus, vomiting, weight loss

Hepatic: Hepatotoxicity, increased serum transaminases, increased serum transaminases ≥3 times upper limit of normal, liver steatosis

Neuromuscular & skeletal: Back pain

Respiratory: Nasal congestion, nasopharyngitis, pharyngolaryngeal pain

Miscellaneous: Influenza

Rare but important or life-threatening: Abnormal pulmonary function test, anemia, cough, decreased appetite, dehydration, early satiety, eructation, eye swelling, gait disturbance, gastroenteritis, hematemesis, hematuria, hepatomegaly, hyperhidrosis, hypersensitivity, increase neutrophil, increased appetite, increased gamma-glutamyl transferase, increased serum bilirubin, increased white blood cell count, joint swelling, lower gastrointestinal hemorrhage, myalgia, myocardial infarction, pain in extremity, paresthesia, pharyngeal lesion, prolonged prothrombin time, proteinuria, pyrexia, rsinusitis, skin rash, somnolence, transiet ischemic attack, xeroderma

Drug Interactions

Metabolism/Transport Effects Substrate of CYP1A2 (minor), CYP2B6 (minor), CYP2C19 (minor), CYP2C8 (minor), CYP3A4 (major); **Note:** Assignment of Major/Minor substrate status based on clinically relevant drug interaction potential; **Inhibits** CYP3A4 (moderate), P-glycoprotein

Avoid Concomitant Use

Avoid concomitant use of Lomitapide with any of the following: Bosutinib; Conivaptan; CYP3A4 Inhibitors (Moderate); CYP3A4 Inhibitors (Strong); Fusidic Acid (Systemic); Ibrutinib; Idelalisib; Ivabradine; Lovastatin; Mipomersen; Naloxegol; Olaparib; PAZOPanib; Pimozide; Silodosin; Simeprevir; Tipranavir; Tolvaptan; Topotecan; Trabectedin; Ulipristal; VinCRIStine (Liposomal)

Increased Effect/Toxicity

Lomitapide may increase the levels/effects of: Afatinib; ARIPiprazole; Avanafil; Bosentan; Bosutinib; Brentuximab Vedotin; Budesonide (Systemic, Oral Inhalation); Cannabis; Colchicine; CYP3A4 Substrates; Dabigatran Etexilate; Dapoxetine; Dofetilide; DOXOrubicin (Conventional); Dronabinol; Edoxaban; Eliglustat; Eplerenone; Everolimus; FentaNYL; Halofantrine; Hydrocodone; Ibrutinib; Ivabradine; Ivacaftor; Ledipasvir; Lovastatin; Lurasidone; Mipomersen; Naloxegol; Nintedanib; Olaparib; OxyCODONE; PAZOPanib; P-glycoprotein/ABCB1 Substrates; Pimecrolimus; Pimozide; Propafenone; Prucalopride; Ranolazine; Rifaximin; Rivaroxaban; Salmeterol; Saxagliptin; Silodosin; Simeprevir; Simvastatin; Suvorexant; Tetrahydrocannabinol; Tolvaptan; Topotecan; Trabectedin; Ulipristal; Vilazodone; VinCRIStine (Liposomal); Warfarin; Zopiclone; Zuclopenthixol

The levels/effects of Lomitapide may be increased by: Alcohol (Ethyl); Conivaptan; CYP3A4 Inhibitors (Moderate); CYP3A4 Inhibitors (Strong); CYP3A4 Inhibitors (Weak); Fusidic Acid (Systemic); Idelalisib; Luliconazole; Mifepristone; Tipranavir

Decreased Effect

The levels/effects of Lomitapide may be decreased by: Bile Acid Sequestrants; Bosentan; CYP3A4 Inducers (Moderate); CYP3A4 Inducers (Strong); Dabrafenib; Deferasirox; Mitotane; Siltuximab; St Johns Wort; Tocilizumab

Food Interactions High-fat diets containing ≥20% of total calories from fat may increase the risk of gastrointestinal adverse reactions (eg, abdominal pain/discomfort, constipation, diarrhea, flatulence, and nausea/vomiting). Grapefruit juice may increase lomitapide plasma concentration. Absorption of fat-soluble nutrients may be reduced. Management: Avoid administering with high fat diets. Avoid grapefruit juice. Take recommended daily supplements of vitamin E, alpha-linolenic acid (ALA), linoleic acid, eicosapentaenoic acid (EPA), and docosahexaenoic acid (DHA).

Storage/Stability Store at 20°C to 25°C (68°F to 77°F); excursions permitted between 15°C to 30°C (59°F to 86°F). Brief exposure up to 40°C (104°F) may be tolerated provided the mean temperature does not exceed 25°C (77°F); minimize this type of exposure. Protect from moisture.

Mechanism of Action Lomitapide directly binds to and inhibits microsomal triglyceride transfer protein (MTP) which is located in the lumen of the endoplasmic reticulum. MTP inhibition prevents the assembly of apo-B containing lipoproteins in enterocytes and hepatocytes resulting in reduced production of chylomicrons and VLDL and subsequently reduces plasma LDL-C concentrations.

Pharmacodynamics/Kinetics

Distribution: Mean V_d: 985-1292 L

Protein binding: 99.8% to plasma proteins

Metabolism: Primarily hepatic (extensive) through CYP3A4 to M1 and M3 (major [inactive *in vitro*] metabolites); CYP1A2, CYP2B6, CYP2C8, and CYP2C19 are also involved in metabolism to a minor degree.

Bioavailability: ~7%

Half-life elimination: 39.7 hours

Time to peak: ~6 hours

Excretion: Urine (53% to 60%; major component: M1 metabolite); feces (33% to 35%; major component: parent drug)

Dosage Homozygous familial hypercholesterolemia (HoFH):

Note: Transaminases should be measured prior to initiation and any dose increase; obtain a negative pregnancy test in female patients of reproductive potential prior to beginning treatment. Maintenance dose should be individualized, taking into account patient characteristics such as goal of therapy and response to treatment. To reduce development of fat-soluble nutrient deficiency, administer daily supplements containing vitamin E 400 units, linoleic acid ≥200 mg, alpha-linolenic acid (ALA) ≥210 mg, eicosapentaenoic acid (EPA) ≥110 mg, and docosahexaenoic acid (DHA) ≥80 mg. Initiate and maintain a low-fat diet supplying <20% of energy from fat.

Adults: Oral: Initial: 5 mg once daily; after 2 weeks of therapy, may increase dose to 10 mg once daily, as tolerated; *then at 4-week intervals,* the dose may be increased to 20 mg once daily, *then* to 40 mg once daily, *and finally* to a maximum dose of 60 mg once daily.

*Dosage adjustment for lomitapide with **weak** CYP3A inhibitors (eg, amiodarone, amlodipine, atorvastatin, cyclosporine, fluoxetine, oral contraceptives):* Maximum dose: 30 mg once daily

Dosage adjustment for toxicity: *Hepatotoxicity:* **Note:** If patient experiences clinical symptoms of liver injury (eg, nausea, vomiting, abdominal pain, fever, jaundice, lethargy, flu-like symptoms) with transaminase elevation, increases in bilirubin ≥2 times ULN, or active liver disease, discontinue use and investigate for probable cause.

AST or ALT ≥ 3 to <5 times ULN: Confirm measurement (within 1 week); once confirmed, reduce dose and obtain additional liver function tests (LFTs) (eg, alkaline phosphatase, total bilirubin, and INR); repeat tests weekly and withhold subsequent doses if signs of abnormal liver function (eg, increased bilirubin or INR), if transaminases rise to >5 times ULN, or if they do not fall to <3 times ULN within ~4 weeks; investigate for probable cause. If resuming after transaminase resolution to <3 times ULN, consider reducing dose and monitor LFTs more frequently.

AST or ALT ≥ 5 times ULN: Withhold doses, obtain additional LFTs (eg, alkaline phosphatase, total bilirubin, and INR); investigate for probable cause. If resuming after transaminase resolution to <3 times ULN, reduce dose and monitor LFTs more frequently.

Dosage adjustment for renal impairment:

Mild-to-severe impairment (not receiving dialysis): There are no dosage adjustments provided in the manufacturer's labeling (has not been studied); however, it is possible that patients with renal impairment not receiving dialysis may experience increases in lomitapide exposure exceeding 50%.

End stage renal disease (ESRD; receiving dialysis): Maximum dose: 40 mg once daily

Dosage adjustment for hepatic impairment:

Mild impairment (Child-Pugh class A): Maximum dose: 40 mg once daily

Moderate-to-severe impairment (Child-Pugh class B or C), active liver disease (including unexplained persistent transaminase elevations): Use is contraindicated.

Administration Oral: Administer with a glass of water and without food; administer at least 2 hours after the evening meal since administration with food may increase risk of gastrointestinal adverse effects. Swallow capsules whole (do not open, crush, dissolve, or chew).

Monitoring Parameters Baseline: ALT, AST, alkaline phosphatase, total bilirubin; pregnancy test in females of reproductive potential; measure transaminases prior to any increase in dose or monthly (whichever occurs first) during the first year, and then at least every 3 months and prior to dosage increases (also see Dosage adjustment for toxicity)

Dosage Forms

Capsule, Oral:

Juxtapid: 5 mg, 10 mg, 20 mg

◆ **Lomitapide Mesylate** *see* Lomitapide *on page 1233*

◆ **Lomotil** *see* Diphenoxylate and Atropine *on page 644*

Lomustine (loe MUS teen)

Brand Names: U.S. Gleostine

Brand Names: Canada CeeNU

Index Terms CCNU; CeeNU; Lomustinum

Pharmacologic Category Antineoplastic Agent, Alkylating Agent; Antineoplastic Agent, Alkylating Agent (Nitrosourea)

Use

Brain tumors: Treatment of primary and metastatic brain tumors (after appropriate surgical and/or radiotherapeutic procedures).

Hodgkin lymphoma: Treatment of relapsed or refractory Hodgkin lymphoma (secondary therapy) in combination with other chemotherapy agents; however, its use is limited in the management of Hodgkin lymphoma due to efficacy of other chemotherapy agents/regimens.

Pregnancy Risk Factor D

Dosage Note: Dispense only enough capsules for a single dose; do not dispense more than one dose at a time (ISMP, 2014). Repeat courses should only be administered after adequate recovery of leukocytes to >4000/mm^3 and platelets to >100,000/mm^3. Doses should be rounded to the nearest 10 mg. Lomustine is associated with a moderate emetic potential; antiemetics are recommended to prevent nausea and vomiting (Dupuis, 2011).

Brain tumors: Pediatrics and Adults: *Manufacturer's labeling:* Oral: 130 mg/m^2 as a single dose once every 6 weeks; reduce dose to 100 mg/m^2 as a single dose once every 6 weeks in patients with compromised bone marrow function (dosage reductions may be recommended for combination chemotherapy regimens).

Anaplastic oligodendroglioma: PCV regimen (off-label combination): Adults: Oral: 130 mg/m^2 on day 1 every 6 weeks for up to 4 cycles prior to radiation therapy (in combination with procarbazine and vincristine) (Cairncross, 2006; Cairncross, 2013).

Astrocytoma, high grade: POC regimen (off-label dosing): Children ≥18 months, Adolescents, and Adults ≤21 years: Oral: 100 mg/m^2 on day 1 every 6 weeks for 8 cycles (in combination with vincristine and prednisone) (Finlay, 1995).

Glioblastoma, recurrent: Adults:

PCV regimen (off-label dosing): Oral: 110 mg/m^2 on day 1 every 6 weeks for 7 cycles (in combination with procarbazine and vincristine) (Levin, 2000)

Single-agent therapy: Oral: 100 to 130 mg/m^2 every 6 weeks until disease progression or unacceptable toxicity (Wick, 2010).

Medulloblastoma (off-label dosing): Children ≥3 years, Adolescents, and Adults ≤21 years: Oral: 75 mg/m^2 on day 1 every 6 weeks for 8 cycles (in combination with cisplatin and vincristine) (Packer, 2006; Packer, 1999).

Hodgkin lymphoma: Pediatrics and Adults: *Manufacturer's labeling:* Oral: 130 mg/m^2 as a single dose once every 6 weeks; reduce dose to 100 mg/m^2 as a single dose once every 6 weeks in patients with compromised bone marrow function (dosage reductions may be recommended for combination chemotherapy regimens)

Dosing adjustment (based on nadir) for subsequent cycles:
Leukocytes >3000/mm^3, platelets >75,000/mm^3: No dosage adjustment required
Leukocytes 2000 to 2999/mm^3, platelets 25,000 to 74,999/mm^3: Administer 70% of prior dose
Leukocytes <2000/mm^3, platelets <25,000/mm^3: Administer 50% of prior dose

Dosage adjustment in renal impairment: There is no dosage adjustment provided in the manufacturer's labeling. The following adjustments have been recommended:
Aronoff, 2007: Adults:
CrCl 10 to 50 mL/minute: Administer 75% of dose
CrCl <10 mL/minute: Administer 25% to 50% of dose
Hemodialysis: Supplemental dose is not necessary
Continuous ambulatory peritoneal dialysis (CAPD): Administer 25% to 50% of dose
Kintzel, 1995:
CrCl 46 to 60 mL/minute: Administer 75% of normal dose
CrCl 31 to 45 mL/minute: Administer 70% of normal dose
CrCl ≤30 mL/minute: Avoid use

Dosage adjustment in hepatic impairment: There are no dosage adjustments provided in the manufacturer's labeling. However, lomustine is hepatically metabolized and caution should be used in patients with hepatic dysfunction.

Dosing in obesity: *ASCO Guidelines for appropriate chemotherapy dosing in obese adults with cancer:* Utilize patient's actual body weight (full weight) for calculation of body surface area- or weight-based dosing, particularly when the intent of therapy is curative; manage regimen-related toxicities in the same manner as for nonobese patients; if a dose reduction is utilized due to toxicity, consider resumption of full weight-based dosing with subsequent cycles, especially if cause of toxicity (eg, hepatic or renal impairment) is resolved (Griggs, 2012).

Additional Information Complete prescribing information should be consulted for additional detail.

Dosage Forms
Capsule, Oral:
Gleostine: 10 mg, 40 mg, 100 mg
Generic: 10 mg, 40 mg, 100 mg

◆ **Lomustinum** *see* Lomustine *on page 1235*
◆ **Longastatin** *see* Octreotide *on page 1485*
◆ **Loniten (Can)** *see* Minoxidil (Systemic) *on page 1374*
◆ **Lo Ovral** *see* Ethinyl Estradiol and Norgestrel *on page 812*
◆ **Loperacap (Can)** *see* Loperamide *on page 1236*

Loperamide (loe PER a mide)

Brand Names: U.S. Anti-Diarrheal [OTC]; Diamode [OTC]; Imodium A-D [OTC]; Loperamide A-D [OTC]

Brand Names: Canada Apo-Loperamide®; Diarr-Eze; Dom-Loperamide; Imodium®; Loperacap; Novo-Loperamide; PMS-Loperamine; Rhoxal-loperamide; Rho®-Loperamine; Riva-Loperamide; Sandoz-Loperamide

Index Terms Loperamide Hydrochloride

Pharmacologic Category Antidiarrheal

Use Control and symptomatic relief of chronic diarrhea associated with inflammatory bowel disease and of acute nonspecific diarrhea; to reduce volume of ileostomy discharge
OTC labeling: Control of symptoms of diarrhea, including Traveler's diarrhea

Pregnancy Risk Factor C

Pregnancy Considerations Teratogenic effects were not observed in animal reproduction studies. Information related to loperamide use in pregnancy is limited and data is conflicting (Einarson, 2000; Källén, 2008). For acute diarrhea in pregnant women, some clinicians recommend oral rehydration and dietary changes; loperamide in small amounts may be used only if symptoms are disabling (Wald, 2003).

Breast-Feeding Considerations Small amounts of loperamide are excreted in human breast milk (information is based on studies using loperamide oxide, the prodrug of loperamide [Nikodem, 1992]). The manufacturer does not recommend use in nursing women.

Contraindications Hypersensitivity to loperamide or any component of the formulation; abdominal pain without diarrhea; children <2 years of age
Avoid use as primary therapy in patients with acute dysentery (bloody stools and high fever), acute ulcerative colitis, bacterial enterocolitis (caused by *Salmonella, Shigella*, and *Campylobacter*), pseudomembranous colitis associated with broad-spectrum antibiotic use

Warnings/Precautions Loperamide is a symptom-directed treatment; if an underlying diagnosis is made, other disease-specific treatment may be indicated. Rare cases of anaphylaxis and anaphylactic shock have been reported. Use is contraindicated if diarrhea is accompanied by high fever or blood in stool. Use caution in young children as response may be variable because of dehydration; contraindicated in children <2 years of age. Concurrent fluid and electrolyte replacement is often necessary in all age groups depending upon severity of diarrhea. Should not be used when inhibition of peristalsis is undesirable or dangerous. Discontinue promptly if constipation, abdominal pain, abdominal distension, blood in stool, or ileus develop. Do not use when peristalsis inhibition should be avoided due to potential for ileus, megacolon, and/or toxic megacolon. Stop therapy in AIDS patients at the first sign of abdominal distention; cases of toxic megacolon have occurred in AIDS patients with infectious colitis (due to viral or bacterial pathogens). Use caution in patients with hepatic impairment due to reduced first-pass metabolism; monitor for signs of CNS toxicity. May cause drowsiness or dizziness, which may impair physical or mental abilities; patients must be cautioned about performing tasks which require mental alertness (eg, operating machinery or driving). Discontinue use and consult health care provider if diarrhea lasts longer than 2 days, symptoms worsen, or abdominal swelling or bulging develops.

Benzyl alcohol and derivatives: Some dosage forms may contain sodium benzoate/benzoic acid; benzoic acid (benzoate) is a metabolite of benzyl alcohol; large amounts of benzyl alcohol (≥99 mg/kg/day) have been associated with a potentially fatal toxicity ("gasping syndrome") in neonates; the "gasping syndrome" consists of metabolic acidosis, respiratory distress, gasping respirations, CNS dysfunction (including convulsions, intracranial hemorrhage), hypotension, and cardiovascular collapse (AAP, 1997; CDC, 1982); some data suggests that benzoate displaces bilirubin from protein binding sites (Ahlfors, 2001); avoid or use dosage forms containing benzyl alcohol derivative with caution in neonates. See manufacturer's labeling.

Adverse Reactions
Central nervous system: Dizziness
Gastrointestinal: Abdominal cramping, constipation, nausea
Postmarketing and/or case reports: Abdominal distention, abdominal pain, allergic reactions, anaphylactic shock, anaphylactoid reactions, angioedema, bullous eruption (rare), drowsiness, dyspepsia, erythema multiforme (rare), fatigue, flatulence, hypersensitivity, paralytic ileus,

megacolon, pruritus, rash, Stevens-Johnson syndrome (rare), toxic epidermal necrolysis (rare), toxic megacolon, urinary retention, urticaria, vomiting, xerostomia

Drug Interactions

Metabolism/Transport Effects **Substrate** of P-glycoprotein

Avoid Concomitant Use There are no known interactions where it is recommended to avoid concomitant use.

Increased Effect/Toxicity

The levels/effects of Loperamide may be increased by: P-glycoprotein/ABCB1 Inhibitors

Decreased Effect

The levels/effects of Loperamide may be decreased by: P-glycoprotein/ABCB1 Inducers

Storage/Stability Store at 20°C to 25°C (68°F to 77°F).

Mechanism of Action Acts directly on circular and longitudinal intestinal muscles, through the opioid receptor, to inhibit peristalsis and prolong transit time; reduces fecal volume, increases viscosity, and diminishes fluid and electrolyte loss; demonstrates antisecretory activity. Loperamide increases tone on the anal sphincter

Pharmacodynamics/Kinetics

Absorption: Poor
Distribution: Poor penetration into brain
Metabolism: Hepatic via oxidative N-demethylation
Half-life elimination: 9-14 hours
Time to peak, plasma: Liquid: 2.5 hours; Capsule: 5 hours

Dosage Oral:

Children:

- Acute diarrhea: Initial doses (in first 24 hours):
  - 2-5 years (13-20 kg): 1 mg 3 times/day
  - 6-8 years (20-30 kg): 2 mg twice daily
  - 8-12 years (>30 kg): 2 mg 3 times/day
  - Maintenance: After initial dosing, 0.1 mg/kg doses after each loose stool, daily dose should not exceed the recommended dose for the initial 24 hours
- Traveler's diarrhea:
  - 6-8 years: 2 mg after first loose stool, followed by 1 mg after each subsequent stool (maximum dose: 4 mg/day)
  - 9-11 years: 2 mg after first loose stool, followed by 1 mg after each subsequent stool (maximum dose: 6 mg/day)
  - ≥12 years: Refer to adult dosing.

Adults:

- Acute diarrhea: Initial: 4 mg, followed by 2 mg after each loose stool, up to 16 mg/day
- Chronic diarrhea: Initial: Follow acute diarrhea; maintenance dose should be slowly titrated downward to minimum required to control symptoms (typically, 4-8 mg/day as a single dose or in divided doses)
- Traveler's diarrhea: Initial: 4 mg after first loose stool, followed by 2 mg after each subsequent stool (maximum dose: 8 mg/day)
- Cancer treatment-induced diarrhea (off-label use): 4 mg followed by 2 mg every 4 hours or after each unformed stool; Maximum: 16 mg/day (Benson, 2004) **or** 4 mg followed by 2 mg every 2 hours (4 mg every 4 hours at night) until 12 hours have passed without a loose bowel movement (Sharma, 2005)
- Irinotecan-induced delayed diarrhea (off-label use): 4 mg after first loose or frequent bowel movement, then 2 mg every 2 hours (4 mg every 4 hours at night) until 12 hours have passed without a bowel movement (Rothenberg, 1996)

Dosage adjustment in renal impairment: No dosage adjustment necessary.

Dosage adjustment in hepatic impairment: No dosage adjustment provided in manufacturer's labeling; use with caution.

Dietary Considerations Some products may contain sodium.

Dosage Forms

Capsule, Oral:
Generic: 2 mg

Liquid, Oral:
Imodium A-D [OTC]: 1 mg/7.5 mL (30 mL, 120 mL, 240 mL, 360 mL)
Generic: 1 mg/5 mL (5 mL, 10 mL, 118 mL)

Suspension, Oral:
Generic: 1 mg/7.5 mL (120 mL)

Tablet, Oral:
Anti-Diarrheal [OTC]: 2 mg
Diamode [OTC]: 2 mg
Imodium A-D [OTC]: 2 mg
Loperamide A-D [OTC]: 2 mg

Tablet Chewable, Oral:
Imodium A-D [OTC]: 2 mg

◆ **Loperamide A-D [OTC]** *see* Loperamide *on page 1236*

Loperamide and Simethicone

(loe PER a mide & sye METH i kone)

Brand Names: U.S. Imodium® Multi-Symptom Relief [OTC]

Brand Names: Canada Imodium® Advanced Multi-Symptom

Index Terms Simethicone and Loperamide Hydrochloride

Pharmacologic Category Antidiarrheal; Antiflatulent

Use Control of symptoms of diarrhea and gas (bloating, pressure, and cramps)

Dosage Oral: Acute diarrhea (weight-based dosing is preferred):

Children:

- 6-8 years (48-59 lbs): 1 caplet or tablet after first loose stool, followed by 1/2 caplet/tablet with each subsequent loose stool (maximum: 2 caplets or tablets/24 hours)
- 9-11 years (60-95 lbs): 1 caplet or tablet after first loose stool, followed by 1/2 caplet or tablet with each subsequent loose stool (maximum: 3 caplets or tablets/24 hours)

Children >12 years and Adults: One caplet or tablet after first loose stool, followed by 1 caplet or tablet with each subsequent loose stool (maximum: 4 caplets or tablets/ 24 hours)

Additional Information Complete prescribing information should be consulted for additional detail.

Dosage Forms

Caplet:
Imodium® Multi-Symptom Relief: Loperamide hydrochloride 2 mg and simethicone 125 mg

Tablet, chewable:
Imodium® Muliti-Symptom Relief: Loperamide hydrochloride 2 mg and simethicone 125 mg

◆ **Loperamide Hydrochloride** *see* Loperamide *on page 1236*

◆ **Lopid** *see* Gemfibrozil *on page 956*

Lopinavir and Ritonavir

(loe PIN a veer & ri TOE na vir)

Brand Names: U.S. Kaletra

Brand Names: Canada Kaletra

Index Terms Ritonavir and Lopinavir

Pharmacologic Category Antiretroviral, Protease Inhibitor (Anti-HIV)

Use Treatment of HIV infection in combination with other antiretroviral agents

Pregnancy Risk Factor C

Pregnancy Considerations Adverse events were not seen in animal reproduction studies, except at doses which were also maternally toxic. Lopinavir/ritonavir has a low level of transfer across the human placenta. Based on information collected by the Antiretroviral Pregnancy Registry, an increased risk of teratogenic effects has not been observed in humans. The HHS Perinatal HIV Guidelines consider lopinavir/ritonavir to be a preferred protease inhibitor for use in antiretroviral-naive pregnant women. Due to a decrease in bioavailability, a dose increase is suggested during the second and third trimesters of pregnancy, especially in PI-experienced women. Monitor virologic response (and lopinavir serum concentrations if available) if the standard dose is used. Once-daily dosing is not recommended during pregnancy. A small increased risk of preterm birth has been associated with maternal use of protease inhibitor-based combination antiretroviral (ARV) therapy during pregnancy; however, the benefits of use generally outweigh this risk and protease inhibitors (PIs) should not be withheld if otherwise recommended. Hyperglycemia, new onset of diabetes mellitus, or diabetic ketoacidosis have been reported with PIs; it is not clear if pregnancy increases this risk.

Regardless of CD4 count or HIV RNA copy number, all HIV-infected pregnant women should receive a combination antiretroviral ARV drug regimen. A combination of antepartum, intrapartum, and infant ARV prophylaxis is recommended. ARV therapy should be started as soon as possible in women with symptomatic infection. Although earlier initiation may be more effective in reducing the perinatal transmission of HIV, initiation may be delayed until after 12 weeks gestation in women who do not require immediate treatment after careful consideration of maternal conditions (eg, nausea and vomiting) and the potential risks of first trimester fetal exposure for specific agents. A scheduled cesarean delivery at 38 weeks gestation is recommended for all women with HIV RNA >1000 copies/mL or unknown concentrations near delivery in order to decrease transmission. If ARV therapy must be interrupted for <24 hours during the peripartum period, stop then restart all medications simultaneously in order to decrease the chance of developing resistance. Long-term follow-up is recommended for all infants exposed to ARV medications. In couples who want to conceive, the HIV-infected partner should attain maximum viral suppression prior to conception.

Health care providers are encouraged to enroll pregnant women exposed to antiretroviral medications in the Antiretroviral Pregnancy Registry (1-800-258-4263 or www.APRegistry.com). Health care providers caring for HIV-infected women and their infants may contact the National Perinatal HIV Hotline (888-448-8765) for clinical consultation (HHS [perinatal], 2014).

Breast-Feeding Considerations Lopinavir/ritonavir concentrations are very low to undetectable in breast milk and undetectable in the serum of nursing infants. Maternal or infant antiretroviral therapy does not completely eliminate the risk of postnatal HIV transmission. In addition, multiclass-resistant virus has been detected in breast-feeding infants despite maternal therapy. Therefore, in the United States, where formula is accessible, affordable, safe, and sustainable, and the risk of infant mortality due to diarrhea and respiratory infections is low, complete avoidance of breast-feeding by HIV-infected women is recommended to decrease potential transmission of HIV (HHS [perinatal], 2014).

Contraindications Hypersensitivity (eg, toxic epidermal necrolysis, Stevens-Johnson syndrome, erythema multiforme, urticaria, angioedema) to any of the ingredients, including ritonavir; coadministration with drugs that are highly dependent on CYP3A for clearance and for which elevated plasma concentrations are associated with serious and/or life-threatening reactions; coadministration with the potent CYP3A inducers (where significantly decreased lopinavir levels may be associated with a potential for loss of virologic response and resistance and cross-resistance to develop): Alfuzosin, cisapride, ergot derivatives (eg, dihydroergotamine, ergotamine, methylergonovine), lovastatin, oral midazolam, pimozide, rifampin, sildenafil (when used to treat pulmonary arterial hypertension), simvastatin, St John's wort, and triazolam.

Warnings/Precautions Potentially significant interactions may exist, requiring dose or frequency adjustment, additional monitoring, and/or selection of alternative therapy. Cases of pancreatitis, some fatal, have been associated with lopinavir/ritonavir; use caution in patients with a history of pancreatitis or advanced HIV-1 disease (may be at increased risk). Patients with signs or symptoms of pancreatitis should be evaluated and therapy suspended as clinically appropriate. May alter cardiac conduction and prolong the QTc and/or PR interval; second and third degree AV block and torsade de pointes have been observed. Possible higher risk of myocardial infarction associated with the cumulative use of lopinavir/ritonavir. Use with caution in patients with underlying structural heart disease, preexisting conduction system abnormalities, ischemic heart disease or cardiomyopathies. Avoid use in combination with QTc- or PR-interval prolonging drugs or in patients with hypokalemia or congenital long QT syndrome.

Changes in glucose tolerance, hyperglycemia, exacerbation of diabetes, DKA, and new-onset diabetes mellitus have been reported in patients receiving protease inhibitors. May cause hepatitis or exacerbate preexisting hepatic dysfunction; use with caution in patients with hepatitis B or C and in hepatic disease; patients with hepatitis or elevations in transaminases prior to the start of therapy may be at increased risk for further increases in transaminases or hepatic dysfunction (rare fatalities reported postmarketing). Consider more frequent liver function test monitoring during therapy initiation in patients with preexisting hepatic dysfunction. Large increases in total cholesterol and triglycerides have been reported; screening should be done prior to therapy and periodically throughout treatment. Increased bleeding may be seen in patients with hemophilia A or B who are taking protease inhibitors. Redistribution or accumulation of body fat has been observed in patients using antiretroviral therapy. Patients may develop immune reconstitution syndrome resulting in the occurrence of an inflammatory response to an indolent or residual opportunistic infection during initial HIV treatment or activation of autoimmune disorders (eg, Graves' disease, polymyositis, Guillain-Barré syndrome) later in therapy; further evaluation and treatment may be required.

The oral solution is highly concentrated and contains large amounts of alcohol. Healthcare providers should pay special attention to accurate calculation, measurement, and administration of dose. Overdose in a child may lead to lethal ethanol or propylene glycol toxicity. Once-daily dosing is not recommended in patients with ≥3 lopinavir-resistance-associated substitutions; those receiving efavirenz, nevirapine, or nelfinavir, carbamazepine, phenobarbital, phenytoin, or in children <18 years of age. Safety, efficacy, and pharmacokinetic profiles of lopinavir and ritonavir have not been established for neonates <14 days of age. Neonates <14 days of age, particularly preterm neonates, are at risk for developing propylene glycol toxicity with use of the lopinavir/ritonavir oral solution. Oral solution contains ethanol and propylene glycol; ethanol competitively inhibits propylene glycol metabolism. Postmarketing reports in preterm neonates following use of the oral solution include cardiotoxicity (complete AV block, bradycardia, cardiomyopathy), lactic acidosis, CNS depression, respiratory complications, acute renal failure, and death. The oral solution should not be used in the immediate postnatal period, including full term neonates age <14 days or preterm neonates until 14 days after their due date, unless the infant is closely monitored and benefits clearly outweigh risk.

Adverse Reactions Data presented for short- and long-term combination antiretroviral therapy in both protease inhibitor experienced and naïve patients.

Cardiovascular: Vasodilation

Central nervous system: Anxiety, fatigue (including weakness), headache, insomnia

Dermatologic: Skin infection (including cellulitis, folliculitis, furuncle), skin rash (more common in children)

Endocrine & metabolic: Alteration in sodium (children), hypercholesterolemia, hyperglycemia, hypertriglyceridemia, hyperuricemia, increased gamma-glutamyl transferase, increased serum triglycerides, weight loss

Gastrointestinal: Abdominal pain, diarrhea, dysgeusia (more common in children), dyspepsia, flatulence, gastroenteritis, increased serum amylase, increased serum lipase, nausea, vomiting (more common in children)

Hematologic & oncologic: Neutropenia, thrombocytopenia (children)

Hepatic: Hepatitis (including increased AST, ALT, and gamma-glutamyl transferase), increased serum ALT, increased serum AST, increased serum bilirubin (more common in children)

Hypersensitivity: Hypersensitivity (including urticaria and angioedema)

Neuromuscular & skeletal: Musculoskeletal pain, weakness

Respiratory: Lower respiratory tract infection, upper respiratory tract infection

Rare but important or life-threatening: Acne vulgaris, alopecia, amenorrhea, amnesia, anemia, anorexia, asthma, atherosclerotic disease, atrial fibrillation, atrioventricular block (second and third degree), atrophic striae, bacterial infection, benign neoplasm, bradycardia, brain disease, breast hypertrophy, bronchitis, cerebral infarction, cerebrovascular accident, cholangitis, cholecystitis, confusion, Cushing's syndrome, cyst, decreased creatine clearance, decreased glucose tolerance, deep vein thrombosis, dehydration, depression, dermal ulcer, diabetes mellitus, duodenitis, dyskinesia, eczema, edema, enteritis, enterocolitis, erythema multiforme, exfoliative dermatitis, extrapyramidal reaction, facial paralysis, fecal incontinence, first degree atrioventricular block, gastritis, gastroesophageal reflux disease, gastrointestinal hemorrhage, gastrointestinal ulcer, gynecomastia, hematuria, hemorrhagic colitis, hemorrhoids, hepatic insufficiency, hepatomegaly, hyperacusis, hyperhidrosis, hypermenorrhea, hypersensitivity reaction, hypertension, hypertonia, hypogonadism (males), hypophosphatemia, hypothyroidism, immune reconstitution syndrome, impotence, jaundice, lactic acidosis, leukopenia, lipoma, liver steatosis, liver tenderness, lymphadenopathy, maculopapular rash, migraine, myocardial infarction, neoplasm, nephritis, neuropathy, obesity, oral mucosa ulcer, orthostatic hypotension, osteonecrosis, otitis media, pancreatitis, periodontitis, peripheral edema, peripheral neuropathy, prolonged Q-T interval on ECG, propylene glycol toxicity (preterm neonates [includes cardiomyopathy, lactic acidosis, acute renal failure, respiratory complications]), pulmonary edema, rectal hemorrhage, redistribution of body fat (including facial wasting), renal failure, rhabdomyolysis, seborrhea, seizure, sialadenitis, skin discoloration, splenomegaly, Stevens-Johnson syndrome, stomatitis, thrombophlebitis, torsades de pointes, tricuspid regurgitation, vasculitis, viral infection, vitamin deficiency, weight gain

Drug Interactions

Metabolism/Transport Effects Refer to individual components.

Avoid Concomitant Use

Avoid concomitant use of Lopinavir and Ritonavir with any of the following: Ado-Trastuzumab Emtansine; Alfuzosin; Amiodarone; Apixaban; Astemizole; Atovaquone; Avanafil; Axitinib; Bosutinib; Cabozantinib; Ceritinib; Cisapride; Conivaptan; Crizotinib; Dapoxetine; Darunavir; Dasabuvir; Disulfiram; Dronedarone; Enzalutamide; Eplerenone; Ergot Derivatives; Etravirine; Everolimus; Flecainide; Fluticasone (Nasal); Fusidic Acid (Systemic); Halofantrine; Highest Risk QTc-Prolonging Agents; Ibrutinib; Irinotecan; Ivabradine; Lapatinib; Lercanidipine; Lomitapide; Lovastatin; Lurasidone; Macitentan; Methadone; Midazolam; Mifepristone; Moderate Risk QTc-Prolonging Agents; Naloxegol; Nilotinib; Nisoldipine; Olaparib; PAZOPanib; Pimozide; Propafenone; QuiNIDine; QuiNINE; Ranolazine; Red Yeast Rice; Regorafenib; Rifampin; Rivaroxaban; Salmeterol; Silodosin; Simeprevir; Simvastatin; St Johns Wort; Suvorexant; Tamoxifen; Tamsulosin; Telaprevir; Terfenadine; Thioridazine; Ticagrelor; Tipranavir; Tolvaptan; Topotecan; Toremifene; Trabectedin; TraZODone; Triazolam; Ulipristal; Vemurafenib; VinCRIStine (Liposomal); Vorapaxar; Voriconazole

Increased Effect/Toxicity

Lopinavir and Ritonavir may increase the levels/effects of: Ado-Trastuzumab Emtansine; Afatinib; Alfuzosin; Almotriptan; Alosetron; ALPRAZolam; Amiodarone; Apixaban; ARIPiprazole; Astemizole; AtoMOXetine; AtorvaSTATin; Avanafil; Axitinib; Bosentan; Bosutinib; Brentuximab Vedotin; Brinzolamide; Budesonide (Nasal); Budesonide (Systemic, Oral Inhalation); Cabazitaxel; Cabozantinib; Calcium Channel Blockers (Dihydropyridine); Calcium Channel Blockers (Nondihydropyridine); Cannabis; Ceritinib; Cisapride; Colchicine; Conivaptan; Contraceptives (Progestins); Corticosteroids (Orally Inhaled); Corticosteroids (Systemic); Crizotinib; Cyclophosphamide; CycloSPORINE (Systemic); CYP2C8 Substrates; CYP2D6 Substrates; CYP3A4 Substrates; Dabigatran Etexilate; Dapoxetine; Dasabuvir; Dasatinib; Digoxin; DOXOrubicin (Conventional); Dronabinol; Dronedarone; Dutasteride; Edoxaban; Enfuvirtide; Enzalutamide; Eplerenone; Ergot Derivatives; Erlotinib; Estazolam; Etizolam; Everolimus; FentaNYL; Fesoterodine; Flecainide; Fluticasone (Nasal); Fluticasone (Oral Inhalation); Fusidic Acid (Systemic); GuanFACINE; Halofantrine; Highest Risk QTc-Prolonging Agents; Hydrocodone; Ibrutinib; Idelalisib; Imatinib; Imidafenacin; Irinotecan; Itraconazole; Ivabradine; Ivacaftor; Ixabepilone; Ketoconazole (Systemic); Lacosamide; Lapatinib; Ledipasvir; Lercanidipine; Levobupivacaine; Levomilnacipran; Linagliptin; Lomitapide; Lovastatin; Lurasidone; Macitentan; Maraviroc; Meperidine; MethylPREDNISolone; Metoprolol; Midazolam; Naloxegol; Nebivolol; Nefazodone; Nelfinavir; Nilotinib; Nintedanib; Nisoldipine; Olaparib; Ospemifene; OxyCODONE; Paricalcitol; PAZOPanib; P-glycoprotein/ABCB1 Substrates; Pimecrolimus; Pimozide; Pioglitazone; PONATinib; Pranlukast; PrednisoLONE (Systemic); PredniSONE; Propafenone; Protease Inhibitors; Prucalopride; QuiNIDine; QuiNINE; Ranolazine; Red Yeast Rice; Regorafenib; Retapamulin; Rifabutin; Rifaximin; Rilpivirine; Riociguat; Rivaroxaban; Rosuvastatin; Ruxolitinib; Salmeterol; Saxagliptin; Sildenafil; Silodosin; Simeprevir; Simvastatin; Suvorexant; Tacrolimus (Systemic); Tacrolimus (Topical); Tadalafil; Tamsulosin; Temsirolimus; Tenofovir; Terfenadine; Tetrahydrocannabinol; Thioridazine; Ticagrelor; Tofacitinib; Tolterodine; Tolvaptan; Topotecan; Toremifene; Trabectedin; TraZODone; Treprostinil; Triamcinolone (Systemic); Triazolam; Ulipristal; Vardenafil; Vemurafenib; Vilazodone; VinBLAStine; VinCRIStine;

VinCRIStine (Liposomal); Vorapaxar; Vortioxetine; Zopiclone

The levels/effects of Lopinavir and Ritonavir may be increased by: ARIPiprazole; Delavirdine; Disulfiram; Enfuvirtide; Fusidic Acid (Systemic); Ivabradine; Ketoconazole (Systemic); Methadone; MetroNIDAZOLE (Systemic); MetroNIDAZOLE (Topical); Mifepristone; Moderate Risk QTc-Prolonging Agents; P-glycoprotein/ABCB1 Inhibitors; QTc-Prolonging Agents (Indeterminate Risk and Risk Modifying); QuiNINE; Rifabutin; Rifampin; Simeprevir

Decreased Effect

Lopinavir and Ritonavir may decrease the levels/effects of: Abacavir; Atovaquone; Boceprevir; BuPROPion; Canagliflozin; Codeine; Contraceptives (Estrogens); Contraceptives (Progestins); CYP2C19 Substrates; Darunavir; Deferasirox; Delavirdine; Didanosine; Etravirine; Fosphenytoin; Hydrocodone; Ifosfamide; LamoTRIgine; Meperidine; Methadone; Phenytoin; Prasugrel; Proguanil; QuiNINE; Tamoxifen; Telaprevir; Ticagrelor; Valproic Acid and Derivatives; Voriconazole; Warfarin; Zidovudine

The levels/effects of Lopinavir and Ritonavir may be decreased by: Antacids; Boceprevir; Bosentan; CarBAMazepine; CYP3A4 Inducers (Moderate); CYP3A4 Inducers (Strong); Dabrafenib; Efavirenz; Fosamprenavir; Fosphenytoin; Garlic; Mitotane; Nelfinavir; Nevirapine; PHENobarbital; Phenytoin; Rifampin; Siltuximab; St Johns Wort; Tipranavir; Tocilizumab

Food Interactions Moderate- to high-fat meals increase the C_{max} and AUC of lopinavir/ritonavir oral solution; no significant changes observed with oral tablets. Management: Take oral solution with food; take tablet with or without food.

Storage/Stability

Oral solution: Store at 2°C to 8°C (36°F to 46°F). Avoid exposure to excessive heat. If stored at room temperature (25°C or 77°F), use within 2 months.

Tablet: Store at USP controlled room temperature of 20°C to 25°C (68°F to 77°F). Exposure to high humidity outside of the original container for >2 weeks is not recommended.

Mechanism of Action A coformulation of lopinavir and ritonavir. The lopinavir component binds to the site of HIV-1 protease activity and inhibits the cleavage of viral Gag-Pol polyprotein precursors into individual functional proteins required for infectious HIV. This results in the formation of immature, noninfectious viral particles. The ritonavir component inhibits the CYP3A metabolism of lopinavir, allowing increased plasma levels of lopinavir.

Pharmacodynamics/Kinetics

Ritonavir: See Ritonavir monograph.

Lopinavir:

Protein binding: 98% to 99%; decreased with mild-to-moderate hepatic dysfunction

Metabolism: Hepatic via CYP3A4; 13 metabolites identified

Half-life elimination: 5-6 hours

Time to peak, plasma: ~4 hours

Excretion: Feces (83%, 20% as unchanged drug); urine (10%; <3% as unchanged drug)

Dosage Oral:

Children: Dosage based on weight or body surface area (BSA), **presented based on lopinavir component** (maximum dose: Lopinavir 400 mg/ritonavir 100 mg).

14 days to 6 months: 16 mg/kg or 300 mg/m^2 twice daily; **Note:** Should not be administered to neonates age <14 days (defined as postmenstrual age of 42 weeks [first day of mother's last menstrual period to birth plus postnatal age]) and a postnatal age of at least 14 days

6 months to 18 years: **Note:** FDA-approved dose is approximately equivalent to lopinavir 230 mg/m^2 per dose.

<15 kg: 12 mg/kg twice daily

15-40 kg: 10 mg/kg twice daily

>40 kg: Lopinavir 400 mg/ritonavir 100 mg twice daily

Adults:

Twice-daily dosing:

Therapy-naive or therapy-experienced: Lopinavir 400 mg/ritonavir 100 mg twice daily.

Therapy-naive or therapy-experienced patients receiving efavirenz, fosamprenavir, nelfinavir, nevirapine: Lopinavir 500 mg/ritonavir 125 mg tablets twice daily **or** lopinavir 533 mg/ritonavir 133 mg solution twice daily

Once-daily dosing: Therapy-naive or experienced patients with <3 lopinavir resistance-associated substitutions: Lopinavir 800 mg/ritonavir 200 mg once daily

Elderly: Initial studies did not include enough elderly patients to determine effects based on age. Use with caution due to possible decreased hepatic, renal, and cardiac function.

Dosage adjustment for combination therapy with efavirenz, fosamprenavir, nelfinavir, or nevirapine:

Twice-daily dosing:

Children 14 days to 6 months: Combination therapy with these agents is not recommended due to lack of data.

Children 6 months to 18 years: Solution or tablet (**based on mg of lopinavir component**): FDA-approved dose is approximately equivalent to lopinavir 300 mg/m^2 per dose:

<15 kg: 13 mg/kg twice daily (**Note:** Tablets are not recommended)

15-45 kg: 11 mg/kg twice daily

>45 kg: Refer to adult dosing

Children >45 kg and Adults: Therapy-naive and therapy-experienced patients:

Solution: Lopinavir 533 mg/ritonavir 133 mg (6.5 mL) twice daily

Tablet: Lopinavir 500 mg/ritonavir 125 mg twice daily

Once-daily dosing:

Children: Not recommended

Adults: Not recommended in those receiving efavirenz, fosamprenavir, nevirapine, nelfinavir, carbamazepine, phenobarbital, phenytoin.

Dosage adjustment in renal impairment: Has not been studied in patients with renal impairment; however, a decrease in clearance is not expected

Hemodialysis: Avoid once-daily dosing in hemodialysis patients (HHS [adult], 2014)

Dosage adjustment in hepatic impairment: Use caution in hepatic impairment (metabolized primarily by the liver)

Mild-to-moderate impairment: Lopinavir AUC may be increased ~30%

Severe impairment: No data available

Dietary Considerations Solution must be taken with food. Tablet may be taken with or without food

Administration

Solution: Must be administered with food; if using didanosine, take didanosine 1 hour before or 2 hours after lopinavir/ritonavir. Administer using calibrated dosing syringe.

Tablet: May be taken with or without food. Swallow whole, do not break, crush, or chew. May be taken with didanosine when taken without food. Tablets are not recommended in patients <15 kg.

Monitoring Parameters Triglycerides, cholesterol, LFTs, electrolytes, basic HIV monitoring, viral load and CD4 count, glucose

Dosage Forms

Solution, oral:

Kaletra: Lopinavir 80 mg and ritonavir 20 mg per mL

Tablet:

Kaletra:

Lopinavir 100 mg and ritonavir 25 mg

Lopinavir 200 mg and ritonavir 50 mg

Loprazolam [INT] (loe PRA zoe lam)

International Brand Names Abran (KR); Dormonoct (AR, BE, GB, IE, NL, PT, ZA); Havlane (FR); Somnovit (ES); Sonin (DE)

Index Terms Loprazolam Mesylate

Pharmacologic Category Benzodiazepine

Reported Use Treatment of insomnia

Dosage Range Oral: 1-2 mg at bedtime

Product Availability Product available in various countries; not currently available in the U.S.

Dosage Forms

Tablet, as mesylate: 2 mg

- ◆ **Loprazolam Mesylate** *see* Loprazolam [INT] *on page 1241*
- ◆ **Lopreeza** *see* Estradiol and Norethindrone *on page 781*
- ◆ **Lopresor (Can)** *see* Metoprolol *on page 1350*
- ◆ **Lopresor SR (Can)** *see* Metoprolol *on page 1350*
- ◆ **Lopressor** *see* Metoprolol *on page 1350*
- ◆ **Loprox** *see* Ciclopirox *on page 433*
- ◆ **Loradamed [OTC]** *see* Loratadine *on page 1241*

Loratadine (lor AT a deen)

Brand Names: U.S. Alavert [OTC]; Allergy Relief For Kids [OTC]; Allergy Relief [OTC]; Allergy [OTC]; Childrens Loratadine [OTC]; Claritin Reditabs [OTC]; Claritin [OTC]; Loradamed [OTC]; Loratadine Childrens [OTC]; Loratadine Hives Relief [OTC]; QlearQuil 24 Hour Relief [OTC]; Triaminic Allerchews [OTC]

Brand Names: Canada Apo-Loratadine; Claritin®; Claritin® Kids

Index Terms Tavist ND

Pharmacologic Category Histamine H_1 Antagonist; Histamine H_1 Antagonist, Second Generation; Piperidine Derivative

Additional Appendix Information

Beers Criteria – Potentially Inappropriate Medications for Geriatrics *on page 2271*

Use

Allergic rhinitis: Relief of nasal and non-nasal symptoms of seasonal allergic rhinitis

Urticaria: Treatment of itching due to hives (urticarial)

Pregnancy Considerations Maternal use of loratadine has not been associated with an increased risk of major malformations. The use of antihistamines for the treatment of rhinitis during pregnancy is generally considered to be safe at recommended doses. Although safety data is limited, loratadine may be the preferred second generation antihistamine for the treatment of rhinitis or urticaria during pregnancy.

Breast-Feeding Considerations Small amounts of loratadine and its active metabolite, desloratadine, are excreted into breast milk.

Contraindications Hypersensitivity to loratadine or any component of the formulation

Warnings/Precautions Use with caution in patients with liver or renal impairment. Hepatic impairment increases systemic exposure. Some products may contain phenylalanine. May be inappropriate in older adults depending on comorbidities (eg, dementia, delirium) due to its potent anticholinergic effects (Beers Criteria). Effects may be potentiated when used with other sedative drugs or ethanol.

Benzyl alcohol and derivatives: Some dosage forms may contain sodium benzoate/benzoic acid; benzoic acid (benzoate) is a metabolite of benzyl alcohol; large amounts of benzyl alcohol (≥99 mg/kg/day) have been associated with a potentially fatal toxicity ("gasping syndrome") in neonates; the "gasping syndrome" consists of metabolic acidosis, respiratory distress, gasping respirations, CNS dysfunction (including convulsions, intracranial hemorrhage), hypotension, and cardiovascular collapse (AAP, 1997; CDC, 1982); some data suggests that benzoate displaces bilirubin from protein binding sites (Ahlfors, 2001); avoid or use dosage forms containing benzyl alcohol derivative with caution in neonates. See manufacturer's labeling.

Adverse Reactions

Central nervous system: Fatigue, headache, malaise, nervousness, somnolence

Dermatologic: Rash

Gastrointestinal: Abdominal pain, stomatitis, xerostomia

Neuromuscular & skeletal: Hyperkinesia

Ocular: Conjunctivitis

Respiratory: Dysphonia, epistaxis, pharyngitis, upper respiratory infection, wheezing

Miscellaneous: Flu-like syndrome, viral infection

Rare but important or life-threatening: Abnormal hepatic function, agitation, alopecia, altered lacrimation, altered micturition, altered salivation, altered taste, amnesia, anaphylaxis, angioneurotic edema, anorexia, arthralgia, back pain, blepharospasm, blurred vision, breast enlargement, breast pain, bronchospasm, chest pain, confusion, depression, dizziness, dysmenorrhea, dyspnea, erythema multiforme, hemoptysis, hepatic necrosis, hepatitis, hypotension, impaired concentration, impotence, insomnia, irritability, jaundice, menorrhagia, migraine, nausea, palpitation, paresthesia, paroniria, peripheral edema, photosensitivity, pruritus, purpura, rigors, seizure, supraventricular tachyarrhythmia, syncope, tachycardia, tremor, urinary discoloration, urticaria, thrombocytopenia, vaginitis, vertigo, vomiting, weight gain

Drug Interactions

Metabolism/Transport Effects Substrate of CYP2D6 (minor), CYP3A4 (minor), P-glycoprotein; **Note:** Assignment of Major/Minor substrate status based on clinically relevant drug interaction potential; **Inhibits** CYP2C19 (weak), CYP2C8 (weak), CYP2D6 (weak)

Avoid Concomitant Use

Avoid concomitant use of Loratadine with any of the following: Aclidinium; Azelastine (Nasal); Glucagon; Ipratropium (Oral Inhalation); Orphenadrine; Paraldehyde; Potassium Chloride; Thalidomide; Tiotropium; Umeclidinium

Increased Effect/Toxicity

Loratadine may increase the levels/effects of: AbobotulinumtoxinA; Alcohol (Ethyl); Analgesics (Opioid); Anticholinergic Agents; ARIPiprazole; Azelastine (Nasal); Buprenorphine; CNS Depressants; Glucagon; Hydrocodone; Methotrimeprazine; Metyrosine; Mirabegron; Mirtazapine; OnabotulinumtoxinA; Orphenadrine; Paraldehyde; Potassium Chloride; Pramipexole; RimabotulinumtoxinB; ROPINIRole; Rotigotine; Selective Serotonin Reuptake Inhibitors; Suvorexant; Thalidomide; Thiazide Diuretics; Tiotropium; Topiramate; Zolpidem

The levels/effects of Loratadine may be increased by: Aclidinium; Amiodarone; Brimonidine (Topical); Cannabis; Doxylamine; Dronabinol; Droperidol; HydrOXYzine; Ipratropium (Oral Inhalation); Kava Kava; Magnesium Sulfate; Methotrimeprazine; Mianserin; Nabilone; Perampanel; P-glycoprotein/ABCB1 Inhibitors; Pramlintide; Rufinamide; Sodium Oxybate; Tapentadol; Tetrahydrocannabinol; Umeclidinium

Decreased Effect

Loratadine may decrease the levels/effects of: Acetylcholinesterase Inhibitors; Benzylpenicilloyl Polylysine; Betahistine; Hyaluronidase; Itopride; Secretin

The levels/effects of Loratadine may be decreased by: Acetylcholinesterase Inhibitors; Amphetamines; P-glycoprotein/ABCB1 Inducers

Food Interactions Food increases bioavailability and delays peak. Management: Administer without regard to meals.

Storage/Stability Store at 20°C to 25°C (68°F to 77°F).

Rapidly-disintegrating tablets: Use within 6 months of opening foil pouch, and immediately after opening individual tablet blister. Store in a dry place.

Mechanism of Action Long-acting tricyclic antihistamine with selective peripheral histamine H_1-receptor antagonistic properties

Pharmacodynamics/Kinetics

Onset of action: 1-3 hours

Peak effect: 8-12 hours

Duration: >24 hours

Absorption: Rapid

Metabolism: Extensively hepatic via CYP2D6 and 3A4 to active metabolite (descarboethoxyloratadine)

Half-life elimination: Mean: 8.4 hours (range: 3-20 hours)

Excretion: Urine (40%) and feces (40%) as metabolites

Dosage Oral: Seasonal allergic rhinitis, urticaria:

Children 2-5 years: 5 mg once daily

Children ≥6 years and Adults: 10 mg once daily or 5 mg twice daily (RediTabs)

Elderly: Peak plasma levels are increased; elimination half-life is slightly increased; specific dosing adjustments are not available

Dosage adjustment in renal impairment: No dosage adjustment provided in manufacturer's labeling; however, the following recommendations have been recommended (Aronoff, 2007):

Children ≥2 years: No dosage adjustment necessary for any degree of renal impairment.

Adults:

CrCl 10-50 mL/minute: Recommended dose every 24 to 48 hours.

CrCl <10 mL/minute: Recommended dose every 48 hours.

Dialysis: Recommended dose every 48 hours.

Continuous renal replacement therapy (CRRT): No dosage adjustment necessary if clearance is 2000 mL/minute.

Dosage adjustment in hepatic impairment: No dosage adjustment provided in manufacturer's labeling. However, hepatic impairment increases systemic exposure to loratadine.

Dietary Considerations May be taken without regard to meals. Some products may contain phenylalanine and/or sodium.

Administration May be administered without regard to meals.

Dispersible tablet: Place in mouth and allow to dissolve. Swallow with or without water.

Dosage Forms

Capsule, Oral:

Claritin [OTC]: 10 mg

Solution, Oral:

Childrens Loratadine [OTC]: 5 mg/5 mL (120 mL)

Loratadine Childrens [OTC]: 5 mg/5 mL (120 mL)

Loratadine Hives Relief [OTC]: 5 mg/5 mL (120 mL)

Syrup, Oral:

Allergy Relief [OTC]: 5 mg/5 mL (236 mL)

Allergy Relief For Kids [OTC]: 5 mg/5 mL (120 mL)

Childrens Loratadine [OTC]: 5 mg/5 mL (120 mL)

Claritin [OTC]: 5 mg/5 mL (60 mL, 120 mL, 150 mL)

Loratadine Childrens [OTC]: 5 mg/5 mL (120 mL)

Tablet, Oral:

Alavert [OTC]: 10 mg

Allergy [OTC]: 10 mg

Allergy Relief [OTC]: 10 mg

Claritin [OTC]: 10 mg

Loradamed [OTC]: 10 mg

QlearQuil 24 Hour Relief [OTC]: 10 mg

Generic: 10 mg

Tablet Chewable, Oral:

Claritin [OTC]: 5 mg

Tablet Dispersible, Oral:

Alavert [OTC]: 10 mg

Allergy [OTC]: 10 mg

Allergy Relief [OTC]: 10 mg

Claritin Reditabs [OTC]: 5 mg, 10 mg

Triaminic Allerchews [OTC]: 10 mg

◆ **Loratadine-D 12 Hour [OTC]** *see* Loratadine and Pseudoephedrine *on page 1242*

Loratadine and Pseudoephedrine

(lor AT a deen & soo doe e FED rin)

Brand Names: U.S. Alavert™ Allergy and Sinus [OTC]; Claritin-D® 12 Hour Allergy & Congestion [OTC]; Claritin-D® 24 Hour Allergy & Congestion [OTC]; Loratadine-D 12 Hour [OTC]

Brand Names: Canada Chlor-Tripolon ND®; Claritin® Extra; Claritin® Liberator

Index Terms Pseudoephedrine and Loratadine

Pharmacologic Category Alpha/Beta Agonist; Decongestant; Histamine H_1 Antagonist; Histamine H_1 Antagonist, Second Generation; Piperidine Derivative

Use Temporary relief of symptoms of seasonal allergic rhinitis, other upper respiratory allergies, or the common cold

Dosage Children ≥12 years and Adults: Oral:

Claritin-D® 12-Hour: 1 tablet every 12 hours

Alavert™ Allergy and Sinus, Claritin-D® 24-Hour: 1 tablet daily

Dosage adjustment in renal impairment: CrCl ≤30 mL/minute:

Claritin-D® 12-Hour: 1 tablet daily

Claritin-D® 24-Hour: 1 tablet every other day

Dosage adjustment in hepatic impairment: Should be avoided

Additional Information Complete prescribing information should be consulted for additional detail.

Dosage Forms

Tablet, extended release: Loratadine 10 mg and pseudoephedrine 240 mg

Alavert™ Allergy and Sinus [OTC]: Loratadine 5 mg and pseudoephedrine 120 mg

Claritin-D® 12 Hour Allergy & Congestion [OTC]: Loratadine 5 mg and pseudoephedrine 120 mg

Claritin-D® 24 Hour Allergy & Congestion [OTC]: Loratadine 10 mg and pseudoephedrine 240 mg

Loratadine-D 12 Hour [OTC]: Loratadine 5 mg and pseudoephedrine sulfate 120 mg

◆ **Loratadine Childrens [OTC]** *see* Loratadine *on page 1241*

◆ **Loratadine Hives Relief [OTC]** *see* Loratadine *on page 1241*

LORazepam (lor A ze pam)

Brand Names: U.S. Ativan; LORazepam Intensol

Brand Names: Canada Apo-Lorazepam; Ativan; Dom-Lorazepam; Lorazepam Injection, USP; PHL-Lorazepam; PMS-Lorazepam; PRO-Lorazepam; Teva-Lorazepam

Pharmacologic Category Benzodiazepine

Additional Appendix Information

Beers Criteria - Potentially Inappropriate Medications for Geriatrics *on page 2271*

Use

Anxiety (oral): Management of anxiety disorders, short-term (≤4 months) relief of anxiety symptoms, or anxiety associated with depressive symptoms, or anxiety/stress-associated insomnia

Anesthesia premedication (parenteral): Anesthesia premedication to relieve anxiety or to produce amnesia (diminish recall) or sedation

Anesthesia premedication (sublingual): *Canadian labeling:* Anesthesia premedication to relieve anxiety prior to surgical procedures

Status epilepticus (parenteral): Treatment of status epilepticus

Pregnancy Risk Factor D

Pregnancy Considerations Teratogenic effects have been observed in some animal reproduction studies. Lorazepam and its metabolite cross the human placenta. Teratogenic effects in humans have been observed with some benzodiazepines (including lorazepam); however, additional studies are needed. The incidence of premature birth and low birth weights may be increased following maternal use of benzodiazepines; hypoglycemia and respiratory problems in the neonate may occur following exposure late in pregnancy. Neonatal withdrawal symptoms may occur within days to weeks after birth and "floppy infant syndrome" (which also includes withdrawal symptoms) have been reported with some benzodiazepines (including lorazepam). Elimination of lorazepam in the newborn infant is slow; following *in utero* exposure, term infants may excrete lorazepam for up to 8 days (Bergman, 1992; Iqbal, 2002; Wikner, 2007).

Breast-Feeding Considerations Lorazepam can be detected in breast milk. Drowsiness, lethargy, or weight loss in nursing infants have been observed in case reports following maternal use of some benzodiazepines (Iqbal, 2002). Breast-feeding is not recommended by the manufacturer.

Contraindications

Hypersensitivity to lorazepam, any component of the formulation, or other benzodiazepines (cross-sensitivity with other benzodiazepines may exist); acute narrow-angle glaucoma; sleep apnea (parenteral); intra-arterial injection of parenteral formulation; severe respiratory insufficiency (except during mechanical ventilation)

Canadian labeling: Additional contraindications (not in U.S. labeling): Myasthenia gravis

Warnings/Precautions Use with caution in elderly or debilitated patients, patients with hepatic disease (including alcoholics) or renal impairment. In older adults, benzodiazepines increase the risk of impaired cognition, delirium, falls, fractures, and motor vehicle accidents. Due to increased sensitivity in this age group, avoid use for treatment of insomnia, agitation, or delirium. (Beers Criteria). Use with caution in patients with respiratory disease (COPD or sleep apnea) or limited pulmonary reserve, or impaired gag reflex. Initial doses in elderly or debilitated patients should be at the lower end of the dosing range. May worsen hepatic encephalopathy.

Causes CNS depression (dose-related) resulting in sedation, dizziness, confusion, or ataxia which may impair physical and mental capabilities. Patients must be cautioned about performing tasks which require mental alertness (eg, operating machinery or driving). Effects may be potentiated when used with other sedative drugs or ethanol. Potentially significant drug-drug interactions may exist, requiring dose or frequency adjustment, additional monitoring, and/or selection of alternative therapy. Benzodiazepines have been associated with falls and traumatic injury and should be used with extreme caution in patients who are at risk of these events.

Lorazepam may cause anterograde amnesia. Paradoxical reactions, including hyperactive or aggressive behavior have been reported with benzodiazepines, particularly in adolescent/pediatric or psychiatric patients. Does not have analgesic, antidepressant, or antipsychotic properties.

Preexisting depression may worsen or emerge during therapy. Not recommended for use in primary depressive or psychotic disorders. Should not be used in patients at risk for suicide without adequate antidepressant treatment. Risk of dependence increases in patients with a history of alcohol or drug abuse and those with significant personality disorders; use with caution in these patients. Tolerance, psychological and physical dependence may also occur with higher dosages and prolonged use. The risk of dependence is decreased with short-term treatment (2-4 weeks); evaluate the need for continued treatment prior to extending therapy duration. Benzodiazepines have been associated with dependence and acute withdrawal symptoms on discontinuation or reduction in dose. Acute withdrawal, including seizures, may be precipitated after administration of flumazenil to patients receiving long-term benzodiazepine therapy. Lorazepam is a short half-life benzodiazepine. Tolerance develops to the sedative, hypnotic, and anticonvulsant effects. It does not develop to the anxiolytic effects (Vinkers, 2012). Chronic use of this agent may increase the perioperative benzodiazepine dose needed to achieve desired effect.

As a hypnotic agent, should be used only after evaluation of potential causes of sleep disturbance. Failure of sleep disturbance to resolve after 7-10 days may indicate psychiatric or medical illness. A worsening of insomnia or the emergence of new abnormalities of thought or behavior may represent unrecognized psychiatric or medical illness and requires immediate and careful evaluation.

Status epilepticus should not be treated with injectable benzodiazepines alone; requires close observation and management and possibly ventilatory support. When used as a component of preanesthesia, monitor for heavy sedation and airway obstruction; equipment necessary to maintain airway and ventilatory support should be available. Parenteral formulation of lorazepam contains polyethylene glycol which has resulted in toxicity during high-dose and/or longer-term infusions. Parenteral formulation also contains propylene glycol (PG); may be associated with dose-related toxicity and can occur ≥48 hours after initiation of lorazepam. Limited data suggest increased risk of PG accumulation at doses of ≥6 mg/hour for 48 hours or more (Nelson, 2008). Monitor for signs of toxicity which may include acute renal failure, lactic acidosis, and/or osmol gap. May consider using enteral delivery of lorazepam tablets to decrease the risk of PG toxicity (Lugo, 1999).

Benzyl alcohol and derivatives: Some dosage forms may contain benzyl alcohol; large amounts of benzyl alcohol (≥99 mg/kg/day) have been associated with a potentially fatal toxicity ("gasping syndrome") in neonates; the "gasping syndrome" consists of metabolic acidosis, respiratory distress, gasping respirations, CNS dysfunction (including convulsions, intracranial hemorrhage), hypotension, and cardiovascular collapse (AAP, 1997; CDC, 1982); some data suggests that benzoate displaces bilirubin from protein binding sites (Ahlfors, 2001); avoid or use dosage forms containing benzyl alcohol with caution in neonates. See manufacturer's labeling.

Adverse Reactions

Cardiovascular: Hypotension

Central nervous system: Aggressive behavior, agitation, akathisia, amnesia, anxiety, central nervous system stimulation, coma, disinhibition, disorientation, dizziness, drowsiness, dysarthria, euphoria, excitement, extrapyramidal reaction, fatigue, headache, hostility, hypothermia, irritability, mania, memory impairment, outbursts of anger, psychosis, sedation, seizures, sleep apnea (exacerbation), sleep disturbances, slurred speech, stupor, suicidal behavior, suicidal ideation, unsteadiness, vertigo

Dermatologic: Alopecia, skin rash

Gastrointestinal: Changes in appetite, constipation

Endocrine & metabolic: Change in libido, hyponatremia, SIADH

Genitourinary: Impotence, orgasm disturbance

Hematologic & oncologic: Agranulocytosis, pancytopenia, thrombocytopenia

Hepatic: Increased serum alkaline phosphatase, increased serum bilirubin, increased serum transaminases, jaundice

Hypersensitivity: Anaphylaxis, anaphylactoid reaction, hypersensitivity reaction

Local: Erythema at injection site, pain at injection site

Neuromuscular & skeletal: Weakness

Ophthalmic: Visual disturbances (including diplopia and blurred vision)

Respiratory: Apnea, exacerbation of obstructive pulmonary disease, hypoventilation, nasal congestion, respiratory depression, respiratory failure, worsening of sleep apnea

Rare but important or life-threatening: Abnormal gait, abnormal hepatic function tests, abnormality in thinking, acidosis, cardiac arrhythmia, ataxia, blood coagulation disorder, bradycardia, cardiac arrest, cardiac failure, cerebral edema, confusion, convulsions, cystitis, decreased mental acuity, delirium, depression, drug dependence (with prolonged use), drug toxicity (polyethylene glycol or propylene glycol poisoning [prolonged IV infusion]), excessive crying, gastrointestinal hemorrhage, hallucinations, hearing loss, heart block, hematologic abnormality, hepatotoxicity, hypertension, hyperventilation, hyporeflexia, infection, injection site reaction, myoclonus, neuroleptic malignant syndrome, paralysis, pericardial effusion, pheochromocytoma (aggravation), pneumothorax, pulmonary edema, pulmonary hemorrhage, pulmonary hypertension, seizure, tachycardia, urinary incontinence, ventricular arrhythmia, withdrawal syndrome

Drug Interactions

Metabolism/Transport Effects None known.

Avoid Concomitant Use

Avoid concomitant use of LORazepam with any of the following: Azelastine (Nasal); Methadone; OLANZapine; Orphenadrine; Paraldehyde; Sodium Oxybate; Thalidomide

Increased Effect/Toxicity

LORazepam may increase the levels/effects of: Alcohol (Ethyl); Azelastine (Nasal); Buprenorphine; CloZAPine; CNS Depressants; Fosphenytoin; Hydrocodone; Methadone; Methotrimeprazine; Metyrosine; Mirtazapine; Orphenadrine; Paraldehyde; Phenytoin; Pramipexole; ROPINIRole; Rotigotine; Selective Serotonin Reuptake Inhibitors; Sodium Oxybate; Suvorexant; Thalidomide; Zolpidem

The levels/effects of LORazepam may be increased by: Brimonidine (Topical); Cannabis; Doxylamine; Dronabinol; Droperidol; HydrOXYzine; Kava Kava; Loxapine; Magnesium Sulfate; Methotrimeprazine; Nabilone; OLANZapine; Perampanel; Probenecid; Rufinamide; Tapentadol; Teduglutide; Tetrahydrocannabinol; Valproic Acid and Derivatives

Decreased Effect

The levels/effects of LORazepam may be decreased by: Theophylline Derivatives; Yohimbine

Preparation for Administration

IV injection: Dilute IV dose prior to use with an equal volume of compatible diluent (D_5W, NS, SWFI).

Infusion: Use 2 mg/mL injectable vial to prepare; there may be decreased stability when using 4 mg/mL vial. Dilute to ≤1 mg/mL and mix in glass bottle. Precipitation may occur. Can also be administered undiluted via infusion.

IM: Administer undiluted.

Storage/Stability

Parenteral: Intact vials should be refrigerated (room temperature storage information may be available; contact product manufacturer to obtain current recommendations). Protect from light. Do not use discolored or precipitate-containing solutions. Parenteral admixture is stable at room temperature (25°C) for 24 hours.

Oral concentrate: Store at colder room temperature or refrigerate at 2°C to 8°C (36°F to 46°F). Discard open bottle after 90 days.

Oral tablet: Store at 25°C (77°F); excursions are permitted between 15°C and 30°C (59°F and 86°F).

Sublingual tablet [Canadian product]: Store at 15°C to 25°C (59°F to 77°F). Protect from light.

Mechanism of Action Binds to stereospecific benzodiazepine receptors on the postsynaptic GABA neuron at several sites within the central nervous system, including the limbic system, reticular formation. Enhancement of the inhibitory effect of GABA on neuronal excitability results by increased neuronal membrane permeability to chloride ions. This shift in chloride ions results in hyperpolarization (a less excitable state) and stabilization. Benzodiazepine receptors and effects appear to be linked to the GABA-A receptors. Benzodiazepines do not bind to GABA-B receptors.

Pharmacodynamics/Kinetics

Onset of action:

- Hypnosis: IM: 20-30 minutes
- Sedation: IV: Within 2-3 minutes (Greenblatt, 1983)
- Anticonvulsant: IV: Within 10 minutes; Oral: 30-60 minutes

Duration: Up to 8 hours

Absorption: IM: Rapid and complete absorption; Oral: Readily absorbed

Distribution: V_d: Neonates: 0.78 L/kg; Children and Adolescents: 1.9 L/kg; Adults: 1.3 L/kg

Protein binding: ~85% to 93%; free fraction may be significantly higher in elderly

Metabolism: Hepatic; rapidly conjugated to inactive compounds

Bioavailability: Oral: 90%

Half-life elimination: Neonates: ~42 hours; Children 2-12 years: ~18 hours; Adolescents: ~28 hours; Adults: Oral: ~14 hours; End-stage renal disease (ESRD): ~18 hours

Time to peak: IM: ≤3 hours; Oral: ~2 hours; Sublingual tablet [Canadian product]: 1 hour

Excretion: Urine (~88%; predominantly as inactive metabolites); feces (~7%)

Dosage

Anxiety disorder:

- Adults: Oral: 1-10 mg daily in 2-3 divided doses; usual dose: 2-6 mg daily in divided doses
- Elderly or debilitated: Oral:
  - *U.S. labeling:* Initial: 1-2 mg daily in divided doses; Beers Criteria: Avoid maintenance doses >3 mg daily
  - *Canadian labeling:* Initial: 0.5 mg daily; titrate cautiously as tolerated

Insomnia due to anxiety or stress: Adults: Oral: 2-4 mg at bedtime

Premedication for anesthesia:

Adults:

IM: 0.05 mg/kg administered 2 hours before surgery (maximum dose: 4 mg)

IV: 0.044 mg/kg administered 15-20 minutes before surgery (usual dose: 2 mg; maximum dose: 4 mg); **Note:** Doses >2 mg should generally not be exceeded in patients >50 years.

Sublingual tablet [Canadian product]: 0.05 mg/kg 1-2 hours before surgery (maximum dose: 4 mg)

Elderly or debilitated: *Canadian labeling:* IM, IV: Reduce the initial dose by approximately 50% and adjust as needed and tolerated; IV dose should generally not exceed 2 mg in patients >50 years

Status epilepticus:

Infants, Children, and Adolescents (off-label use):

IV: 0.1 mg/kg (maximum dose: 4 mg) slow IV (maximum rate: 2 mg/minute); may repeat in 5-10 minutes (Brophy, 2012)

or

IV, IM: 0.05-0.1 mg/kg; repeat doses every 10-15 minutes for clinical effect (American Academy of Pediatrics, 1998)

Adults: IV: 4 mg slow IV (maximum rate: 2 mg/minute); may repeat in 5-10 minutes (Brophy, 2012). May be given IM, but IV preferred.

Elderly or debilitated: *Canadian labeling:* IV: Reduce the initial dose by approximately 50% and adjust as needed and tolerated

Agitation in the ICU patient (off-label use): Adults: IV: Loading dose: 0.02-0.04 mg/kg (maximum single dose: 2 mg); Maintenance: 0.02-0.06 mg/kg every 2-6 hours as needed **or** 0.01-0.1 mg/kg/hour; maximum dose: ≤10 mg/hour (Barr, 2013)

Alcohol withdrawal delirium (off-label use) (Mayo-Smith, 2004): Adults:

IV: 1-4 mg every 5-15 minutes until calm, then every hour as needed to maintain light somnolence

IM: 1-4 mg every 30-60 minutes until calm, then every hour as needed to maintain light somnolence

Alcohol withdrawal syndrome (off-label use) (Mayo-Smith, 1997): Adults:

Oral, IM, IV (fixed-dose regimen): 2 mg every 6 hours for 4 doses, then 1 mg every 6 hours for 8 additional doses

Oral, IM, IV (symptom-triggered regimen): 2-4 mg every 1 hour as needed; dose determined by a validated severity assessment scale

Chemotherapy-associated nausea and vomiting (off-label use):

Anticipatory nausea/vomiting (prevention and treatment): Infants ≥1 month, Children, and Adolescents: Oral: 0.04 to 0.08 mg/kg/dose (maximum dose: 2 mg) once at bedtime the evening prior to chemotherapy and once the next day before chemotherapy (Dupuis, 2014)

Breakthrough nausea/vomiting: Children ≥2 years and Adolescents: IV: 0.025-0.05 mg/kg/dose (maximum dose: 2 mg) every 6 hours as needed (Dupuis, 2003); however, additional data may be necessary to further define the role of lorazepam in children for chemotherapy-associated nausea and vomiting

Breakthrough nausea/vomiting or as adjunct to standard antiemetics: Adults: Oral, IV, Sublingual (off-label route): 0.5-2 mg every 4-6 hours as needed (NCCN Antiemesis guidelines v.1.2013)

Partial complex seizures, refractory (off-label use): Adults: Oral: 1 mg twice daily; increase biweekly in increments of 1 mg twice daily until seizures stop or side effects occur (Walker, 1984); however, additional data may be necessary to further define the role of lorazepam in this condition

Psychogenic catatonia (off-label use): Adults:

IM, Sublingual (off-label route): 1-2 mg; repeat dose in 3 hours then again in another 3 hours if initial and subsequent doses, respectively, are ineffective (Rosebush, 1990; Rosebush, 2010); however, additional data may be necessary to further define the role of lorazepam in this condition

or

Oral, IM, IV: Initial: 1 mg; may repeat in 5 minutes if necessary. If initial challenge is unsuccessful, may increase dose up to 4-8 mg per day; may continue treatment for up to 5 days (Bush, 1996); however, additional data may be necessary to further define the role of lorazepam in this condition

Rapid tranquilization of the agitated patient (off-label use): Adults: Oral, IM: 1-3 mg administered every 30-60 minutes; may be administered with an antipsychotic (eg, haloperidol) (Allen, 2005; Battaglia, 2005; De Fruyt, 2004). **Note:** When administering IM, may consider a lower initial dose (eg, 0.5 mg) (Allen, 2005).

Dosage adjustment for lorazepam with concomitant medications: *Probenecid or valproic acid:* Reduce lorazepam dose by 50%

Dosage adjustment in renal impairment:

Oral: No dosage adjustment necessary (Aronoff, 2007).

IM, IV: Risk of propylene glycol toxicity. Monitor closely if using for prolonged periods of time or at high doses.

Mild-to-moderate disease: Use with caution.

Severe disease or failure: Use is not recommended.

Dosage adjustment in hepatic impairment:

Oral:

Mild-to-moderate disease: No dose adjustment necessary.

Severe insufficiency and/or encephalopathy: Use with caution; may require lower doses.

IM, IV:

Mild-to-moderate disease: Use with caution.

Severe disease or failure: Use is not recommended.

Administration

IM: Should be administered (undiluted) deep into the muscle mass.

IV injection: Dilute prior to use. Do not exceed 2 mg/minute or 0.05 mg/kg over 2-5 minutes. Monitor IV site during administration. Avoid intra-arterial administration. Avoid extravasation.

Continuous IV infusion (off-label administration mode; Barr, 2013) solutions should have an in-line filter and the solution should be checked frequently for possible precipitation (Grillo, 1996).

Oral: Lorazepam oral concentrate: Use only the provided calibrated dropper to withdraw the prescribed dose. Mix the dose with liquid (eg, water, juice, soda, soda-like beverage) or semisolid food (eg, applesauce, pudding), and stir for a few seconds to blend completely. The prepared mixture should be administered immediately.

Sublingual tablet [Canadian product]: Place under tongue; patient should not swallow for at least 2 minutes.

Monitoring Parameters Respiratory and cardiovascular status, blood pressure, heart rate, symptoms of anxiety

CBC, liver function tests; clinical signs of propylene glycol toxicity (for continuous high-dose and/or long duration intravenous use) including serum creatinine, BUN, serum lactate, osmol gap

Critically-ill patients: Monitor depth of sedation with either the Richmond Agitation-Sedation Scale (RASS) or Sedation-Agitation Scale (SAS) (Barr, 2013)

Reference Range Therapeutic: 50-240 ng/mL (SI: 156-746 nmol/L)

Dosage Forms

Concentrate, Oral:

LORazepam Intensol: 2 mg/mL (30 mL)

Generic: 2 mg/mL (30 mL)

Solution, Injection:
Ativan: 2 mg/mL (1 mL, 10 mL); 4 mg/mL (1 mL, 10 mL)
Generic: 2 mg/mL (1 mL, 10 mL); 4 mg/mL (1 mL, 10 mL)
Tablet, Oral:
Ativan: 0.5 mg, 1 mg, 2 mg
Generic: 0.5 mg, 1 mg, 2 mg

Dosage Forms: Canada
Tablet, Sublingual: 0.5 mg, 1 mg, 2 mg

Extemporaneous Preparations Note: Commercial oral solution is available (2 mg/mL)

Two different 1 mg/mL oral suspensions may be made from different generic lorazepam tablets (Mylan Pharmaceuticals or Watson Laboratories), sterile water, Ora-Sweet, and Ora-Plus.

Mylan tablets: Place one-hundred-eighty 2 mg tablets in a 12-ounce amber glass bottle; add 144 mL of sterile water to disperse the tablets; shake until slurry is formed. Add 108 mL Ora-Plus in incremental proportions; then add a quantity of Ora-Sweet sufficient to make 360 mL. Label "shake well" and "refrigerate". Stable for 91 days when stored in amber glass prescription bottles at room temperature or refrigerated (preferred).

Watson tablets: Place one-hundred-eighty 2 mg tablets in a 12-ounce amber glass bottle; add 48 mL sterile water to disperse the tablets; shake until slurry is formed. Add 156 mL of Ora-Plus in incremental proportions; then add a quantity of Ora-Sweet sufficient to make 360 mL. Label "shake well" and "refrigerate". Store in amber glass prescription bottles. Stable for 63 days at room temperature or 91 days refrigerated.

Lee ME, Lugo RA, Rusho WJ, et al, "Chemical Stability of Extemporaneously Prepared Lorazepam Suspension at Two Temperatures," *J Pediatr Pharmacol Ther*, 2004, 9(4):254-58.

◆ **Lorazepam Injection, USP (Can)** *see* LORazepam *on page 1243*

◆ **LORazepam Intensol** *see* LORazepam *on page 1243*

Lorcaserin (lor KA ser in)

Brand Names: U.S. Belviq
Index Terms Lorcaserin Hydrochloride
Pharmacologic Category Anorexiant; Serotonin 5-HT_{2C} Receptor Agonist
Use Chronic weight management, as an adjunct to a reduced-calorie diet and increased physical activity, in patients with either an initial body mass index (BMI) of ≥30 kg/m^2 **or** an initial BMI of ≥27 kg/m^2 and at least one weight-related comorbid condition (eg, hypertension, dyslipidemia, type 2 diabetes)
Pregnancy Risk Factor X
Pregnancy Considerations Adverse fetal effects were observed in some animal reproduction studies. Due to the fact that weight loss during pregnancy offers no clinical benefit, lorcaserin is contraindicated in pregnancy. Obese and overweight women should be encouraged to participate in weight reduction programs prior to attempting pregnancy; weight gain during pregnancy should be determined by their prepregnancy BMI and current guidelines (ADA, 2009; IOM, 2009).
Breast-Feeding Considerations Lorcaserin may alter maternal serum prolactin concentrations. It is not known if lorcaserin is excreted into breast milk. According to the manufacturer, the decision to continue or discontinue breast-feeding during therapy should take into account the risk of exposure to the infant and the benefits of treatment to the mother. Weight-loss therapy is generally not recommended for lactating women. Weight-loss programs which include physical activity and nutrition components should be discussed at the 6-week postpartum visit (ADA, 2009; IOM, 2009).
Contraindications Pregnancy
Warnings/Precautions Use may cause confusion, somnolence, fatigue, and cognitive impairment (difficulty with concentration/attention/memory); patients must be cautioned about performing tasks which require mental alertness (eg, operating machinery or driving). Agents affecting the CNS have been associated with depression and suicidal ideation; monitor patients closely during use; discontinue for suicidal thoughts or behaviors. Priapism may occur with use; men with erections >4 hours should immediately discontinue lorcaserin and seek emergency medical attention to avoid irreversible damage to erectile tissue. Use with caution in men with conditions that increase the risk for priapism (eg, sickle cell anemia, multiple myeloma, leukemia) or men with anatomical penis deformities (eg, angulation, cavernosal fibrosis, Peyronie's disease). Rare WBC and RBC count decreases (including leukopenia, lymphopenia, neutropenia, anemia, decreases in hematocrit and hemoglobin) have been observed; consider monitoring CBC periodically during use. Increased prolactin levels may occur; obtain prolactin levels if signs or symptoms of hyperprolactinemia occur (eg, galactorrhea, gynecomastia).

Primary pulmonary hypertension (PPH) is a rare and frequently fatal pulmonary disease, which has been reported in patients receiving other centrally acting, serotonergic weight loss agents. Available data from clinical trials are inadequate to determine if lorcaserin increases the risk for pulmonary hypertension (due to the low incidence of PPH occurring in the general population); however, a theoretical risk cannot be excluded. Cardiac valvular disease has been associated with the use of agents exhibiting potent 5-HT_{2B} agonist activity (eg, cabergoline, fenfluramine [not currently on the U.S. market], dexfenfluramine [not currently on the U.S. market]). Cardiac valvular disease is believed to result from activation of 5-HT_{2B} receptors in interstitial cardiac cells. Lorcaserin has greater affinity for 5-HT_{2C} receptors compared to 5-HT_{2B} receptors (at therapeutic doses). However, a slight increase in incidence of regurgitant cardiac valve disease (mitral and/or aortic) has been observed with lorcaserin compared to placebo in some clinical trials (pooled RR: 1.16; 95% CI: 0.81-1.67). The incidence observed in both groups was low, making it difficult to ascertain the risk of valvular disease with lorcaserin therapy based on available data. Evaluate patients if signs/symptoms of valvular heart disease (eg, dyspnea, dependent edema, heart failure, new onset cardiac murmur) arise during therapy; consider discontinuing therapy if present. Use has not been studied in patients with hemodynamically-significant valvular heart disease. Do not use lorcaserin in combination with potent serotonergic and dopaminergic agents that are potent 5-HT_{2B} receptor agonists (eg, cabergoline) due to the risk for cardiac valvulopathy.

Serotonin syndrome (SS)/neuroleptic malignant syndrome (NMS)-like reactions have occurred with serotonergic agents such as lorcaserin, particularly when used in combination with other serotonergic agents (eg, triptans, SNRIs, SSRIs, TCAs, bupropion, St John's wort, tryptophan), agents that impair metabolism of serotonin (eg, MAO inhibitors, dextromethorphan, tramadol, lithium), or antidopaminergic agents (eg, antipsychotics). Concurrent use with these agents should be avoided. If concomitant use cannot be avoided, coadminister with extreme caution, and closely monitor patients, particularly during treatment initiation. Discontinue treatment (and any concomitant serotonergic and/or antidopaminergic agents) immediately if signs/symptoms of SS or NMS-like reactions arise.

Use with caution in patients with bradycardia or heart block (second or third degree); bradycardia has been observed rarely with use. Use with caution in patients with heart failure (has not been studied). Effect of lorcaserin on cardiovascular morbidity and mortality has not been established. Use with caution in patients with type 2 diabetes mellitus; weight loss from therapy may result in decreased requirements of antidiabetic agents and an increased risk of hypoglycemia; monitor blood glucose. Use with caution in patients with severe hepatic impairment (not studied); lorcaserin undergoes extensive hepatic metabolism. Use is not recommended in patients with severe renal impairment or end stage renal disease. Use with caution in patients with moderate renal impairment. Serum concentrations and principal metabolite (M1 and M5) half-lives are increased in renal impairment.

In short-term studies, euphoria, hallucinations, and dissociation have been observed with lorcaserin at supratherapeutic doses. Data suggest lorcaserin may produce psychic dependence. Physical dependence or a withdrawal syndrome has not been observed. Pharmacotherapy for weight loss should be used in conjunction with a comprehensive weight management program including diet and exercise. Discontinue if significant weight loss has not occurred (ie, <5% within the first 12 weeks of treatment). Concomitant use of lorcaserin with other agents intended for weight loss (eg, phentermine, orlistat, OTC, or herbal preparations) has not been evaluated; safety and efficacy of coadministration with other weight loss agents are unknown.

Adverse Reactions

Cardiovascular: Hypertension, peripheral edema, valvulopathy

Central nervous system: Anxiety, cognitive impairment, depression, dizziness, fatigue, headache, insomnia, psychiatric disorders

Dermatologic: Rash

Endocrine & metabolic: Diabetes mellitus exacerbation, hyper-/hypoglycemia, prolactin increased

Gastrointestinal: Appetite decreased, constipation, diarrhea, gastroenteritis, nausea, toothache, vomiting, xerostomia

Genitourinary: Urinary tract infection

Hematologic: Hemoglobin decreased, lymphocytes decreased, neutrophils decreased

Neuromuscular & skeletal: Back pain, muscle spasms, musculoskeletal pain

Ocular: Eye disorders

Respiratory: Cough, nasopharyngitis, oropharyngeal pain, sinus congestion, upper respiratory tract infection,

Miscellaneous: Seasonal allergy, stress

Rare but important or life-threatening: Bradycardia, dissociation, euphoria, serotonin syndrome, suicidal ideation

Drug Interactions

Metabolism/Transport Effects Inhibits CYP2D6 (moderate)

Avoid Concomitant Use

Avoid concomitant use of Lorcaserin with any of the following: Dapoxetine; Ergot Derivatives; Thioridazine

Increased Effect/Toxicity

Lorcaserin may increase the levels/effects of: Antipsychotic Agents; ARIPiprazole; CYP2D6 Substrates; DOXOrubicin (Conventional); Eliglustat; Ergot Derivatives; Fesoterodine; Metoclopramide; Metoprolol; Nebivolol; Phosphodiesterase 5 Inhibitors; Serotonin Modulators; Thioridazine

The levels/effects of Lorcaserin may be increased by: Antiemetics (5HT3 Antagonists); Antipsychotic Agents; BuPROPion; Dapoxetine; Propafenone; Tedizolid

Decreased Effect

Lorcaserin may decrease the levels/effects of: Codeine; Tamoxifen

Storage/Stability Store at 25°C (77°F); excursions permitted to 15°C to 30°C (59°F to 86°F).

Mechanism of Action Lorcaserin is believed to activate serotonin 5-HT_{2C} receptors, which stimulate pro-opiomelanocortin (POMC) neurons in the arcuate nucleus of the hypothalamus, leading to increased alpha-melanocortin stimulating hormone release at melanocortin-4 receptors and resulting in satiety and decreased food intake. At recommended doses, lorcaserin has greater affinity for 5-HT_{2C} receptors compared to other 5-HT receptor subtypes (including 5-HT_{2A} and 5-HT_{2B}), the 5-HT receptor transporter, and 5-HT reuptake sites (Hurren, 2011).

Pharmacodynamics/Kinetics

Distribution: Distributes to the CNS and cerebrospinal fluid

Protein binding: ~70% to plasma proteins

Metabolism: Extensive hepatic metabolism, via multiple enzymatic pathways, producing two major metabolites (inactive), lorcaserin sulfamate (M1) and N-carbamoyl glucuronide lorcaserin (M5), as well as minor metabolites (glucuronide and sulfate conjugates)

Half-life elimination: ~11 hours

Time to peak: 1.5-2 hours

Excretion: Urine (92%, as metabolites); feces (2%, as metabolites)

Dosage Weight management: Adults: Oral: 10 mg twice daily (maximum: 10 mg twice daily); evaluate response by week 12; if patient has not lost ≥5% of baseline body weight, discontinue therapy

Dosage adjustment in renal impairment: Note: Renal function was estimated in studies using ideal body weight (IBW) with the Cockcroft-Gault formula.

Mild impairment (CrCl >50 mL/minute): No dosage adjustment necessary.

Moderate impairment (CrCl 30-50 mL/minute): Use with caution; serum concentrations and half-life of major metabolites are increased.

Severe impairment (CrCl <30 mL/minute): Use is not recommended.

ESRD: Use is not recommended; hemodialysis does not remove lorcaserin or M1 metabolite

Dosage adjustment in hepatic impairment:

Mild-to-moderate impairment (Child-Pugh score 5-9): No dosage adjustment necessary.

Severe impairment: Use with caution (has not been studied); undergoes extensive hepatic metabolism.

Administration Administer orally with or without food.

Monitoring Parameters Weight, waist circumference; CBC (periodically during use); blood glucose (in diabetics); prolactin levels (if galactorrhea, gynecomastia or other signs/symptoms of hyperprolactinemia arise); monitor for depression or suicidal thoughts/behavior; signs/symptoms of SS/NMS-like reaction; signs/symptoms of valvular heart disease (dyspnea, dependent edema)

Additional Information *In vitro*, lorcaserin has an 18-fold and 104-fold greater affinity for $5HT_{2C}$ receptors compared to 5-HT_{2A} and $5HT_{2B}$ receptors, respectively (Hurren, 2011).

Dosage Forms

Tablet, Oral:

Belviq: 10 mg

◆ **Lorcaserin Hydrochloride** *see* Lorcaserin *on page 1246*

◆ **Lorcet® 10/650 [DSC]** *see* Hydrocodone and Acetaminophen *on page 1012*

◆ **Lorcet® Plus [DSC]** *see* Hydrocodone and Acetaminophen *on page 1012*

Lormetazepam [INT] (lor met A ze pam)

International Brand Names Aldosomnil (ES); Axilium (IT); Dilamet (AR); Ergocalm (DE); Loramet (BE, CH, ES, GR, HK, NL, SG, TH, ZA); Loranka (BE); Loretam (DE); Luzul (IT); Minias (IT); Noctamid (AT, BE, CH, CY, DE, EG, ES, GR, IE, NL, NZ, PT, TR, ZA); Noctamide (FR);

Noctofer (PL); Nocton (CL); Octonox (BE); Pronoctan (DK); Sedaben (BE); Stilaze (BE)

Pharmacologic Category Benzodiazepine

Reported Use Short-term treatment of insomnia

Dosage Range Usual dose:

Adults: 0.5-1.5 mg once daily prior to bedtime

Elderly: 0.5 mg once daily prior to bedtime; maximum dose: 1 mg

Product Availability Product available in various countries; not currently available in the U.S.

Dosage Forms

Capsule: 0.5 mg, 1 mg, 2 mg

Tablet: 0.5 mg, 1 mg, 2 mg

Lornoxicam [INT] (lor NOKS i kam)

International Brand Names Acabel (AR, ES, PT, VE); Artok (AT); Bosporon (ES, PT); Camri (IN); Da Lu (CN); Flexilor (VN); Hypodol (AR); Lenor (IN); Lonocam (KR); Lorcam (JP); Lornica (IN); Lornicam (CO); Lornox (AT); Mediloxan (MX); Noxi (IN); Noxon (IT); Qinda (CN); Taigalor (IT); Telos (DE); Xafon (CN); Xefo (AE, AR, AT, BG, BR, CH, DK, EG, GR, HU, IE, IL, KR, LB, LT, PL, RO, SA, SE, SI, SK, TH, TR, ZA); Xefo Rapid (AR, BG, CZ, LT, RO, SI, SK); Xefocam (RU)

Pharmacologic Category Nonsteroidal Anti-inflammatory Drug (NSAID), Oral; Nonsteroidal Anti-inflammatory Drug (NSAID), Parenteral

Reported Use Treatment of osteoarthritis, rheumatoid arthritis, and painful conditions including postoperative pain

Dosage Range Adults:

IM, IV: Acute pain, osteoarthritis, rheumatoid arthritis: 8-16 mg/day; in rare cases maximum initial daily dose may be increased to 24 mg; treatment should be limited to 2 days

Oral:

Rheumatoid arthritis and osteoarthritis: Initial dose: 12 mg/day in 2-3 divided doses; total dose should not exceed 16 mg/day

Acute pain: 8-16 mg/day; doses >8 mg/day should be given in 2-3 divided doses

Product Availability Product available in various countries; not currently available in the U.S.

Dosage Forms

Injection, solution: 8 mg

Tablet: 4 mg, 8 mg

◆ **Lortab®** *see* Hydrocodone and Acetaminophen *on page 1012*

◆ **Lortuss EX** *see* Guaifenesin, Pseudoephedrine, and Codeine *on page 989*

◆ **Loryna** *see* Ethinyl Estradiol and Drospirenone *on page 801*

◆ **Lorzone** *see* Chlorzoxazone *on page 430*

Losartan (loe SAR tan)

Brand Names: U.S. Cozaar

Brand Names: Canada ACT Losartan; Apo-Losartan; Auro-Losartan; Cozaar; JAMP-Losartan; Mint-Losartan; Mylan-Losartan; PMS-Losartan; RAN-Losartan; Sandoz Losartan; Septa Losartan; Teva-Losartan

Index Terms DuP 753; Losartan Potassium; MK594

Pharmacologic Category Angiotensin II Receptor Blocker; Antihypertensive

Use

Diabetic nephropathy: Treatment of diabetic nephropathy with an elevated serum creatinine and proteinuria (urinary albumin to creatinine ratio ≥300 mg/g) in patients with type 2 diabetes and a history of hypertension.

Hypertension:

Treatment of hypertension, alone or in combination with other antihypertensive agents.

The 2014 guideline for the management of high blood pressure in adults (Eighth Joint National Committee [JNC 8]) recommends initiation of pharmacologic treatment to lower blood pressure for the following patients:

- Patients ≥60 years of age with systolic blood pressure (SBP) ≥150 mm Hg or diastolic blood pressure (DBP) ≥90 mm Hg. Goal of therapy is SBP <150 mm Hg and DBP <90 mm Hg.
- Patients <60 years of age with SBP ≥140 mm Hg or DBP is ≥90 mm Hg. Goal of therapy is SBP <140 mm Hg and DBP <90 mm Hg.
- Patients ≥18 years of age with diabetes and SBP ≥140 mm Hg or DBP ≥90 mm Hg. Goal of therapy is SBP <140 mm Hg and DBP <90 mm Hg.
- Patients ≥18 years of age with chronic kidney disease (CKD) and SBP ≥140 mm Hg or DBP ≥90 mm Hg. Goal of therapy is SBP <140 mm Hg and DBP <90 mm Hg.

In patients with CKD, regardless of race or diabetes status, the use of an ACE inhibitor (ACEI) or angiotensin receptor blocker (ARB) as initial therapy is recommended to improve kidney outcomes. In the general nonblack population (without CKD) including those with diabetes, initial antihypertensive treatment should consist of a thiazide-type diuretic, calcium channel blocker, ACEI, or ARB. In the general black population (without CKD) including those with diabetes, initial antihypertensive treatment should consist of a thiazide-type diuretic or a calcium channel blocker instead of an ACEI or ARB.

Hypertension with left ventricular hypertrophy: To reduce the risk of stroke in patients with hypertension and left ventricular hypertrophy (LVH). Evidence suggests that this benefit does not apply to black patients.

Pregnancy Risk Factor D

Pregnancy Considerations [U.S. Boxed Warning]: Drugs that act on the renin-angiotensin system can cause injury and death to the developing fetus. Discontinue as soon as possible once pregnancy is detected. The use of drugs which act on the renin-angiotensin system are associated with oligohydramnios. Oligohydramnios, due to decreased fetal renal function, may lead to fetal lung hypoplasia and skeletal malformations. Use is also associated with anuria, hypotension, renal failure, skull hypoplasia, and death in the fetus/neonate. The exposed fetus should be monitored for fetal growth, amniotic fluid volume, and organ formation. Infants exposed *in utero* should be monitored for hyperkalemia, hypotension, and oliguria (exchange transfusions or dialysis may be needed). These adverse events are generally associated with maternal use in the second and third trimesters.

Untreated chronic maternal hypertension is also associated with adverse events in the fetus, infant, and mother. The use of angiotensin II receptor blockers is not recommended to treat chronic uncomplicated hypertension in pregnant women and should generally be avoided in women of reproductive potential (ACOG, 2013).

Breast-Feeding Considerations It is not known if losartan is found in breast milk. Due to the potential for serious adverse reactions in the nursing infant, the manufacturer recommends a decision be made whether to discontinue nursing or to discontinue the drug, taking into account the importance of treatment to the mother.

Contraindications

Hypersensitivity to losartan or any component of the formulation; concomitant use with aliskiren in patients with diabetes mellitus

Documentation of allergenic cross-reactivity for angiotensin receptor blockers is limited. However, because of similarities in chemical structure and/or pharmacologic actions, the possibility of cross-sensitivity cannot be ruled out with certainty.

Canadian labeling: Additional contraindications (not in U.S. labeling): Concomitant use with aliskiren in patients with moderate-to-severe renal impairment (GFR <60 mL/minute/1.73 m^2)

Warnings/Precautions [U.S. Boxed Warning]: Drugs that act on the renin-angiotensin system can cause injury and death to the developing fetus. Discontinue as soon as possible once pregnancy is detected. Avoid use or use a much smaller dose in patients who are volume-depleted; correct depletion first. Use with caution in patients with significant aortic/mitral stenosis. May cause hyperkalemia; avoid potassium supplementation unless specifically required by healthcare provider. May be associated with deterioration of renal function and/or increases in serum creatinine, particularly in patients with low renal blood flow (eg, renal artery stenosis, heart failure) whose glomerular filtration rate (GFR) is dependent on efferent arteriolar vasoconstriction by angiotensin II. Use caution in patients with unstented unilateral/bilateral renal artery stenosis. When unstented bilateral renal artery stenosis is present, use is generally avoided due to the elevated risk of deterioration in renal function unless possible benefits outweigh risks. Use with caution with preexisting renal insufficiency. AUCs of losartan (not the active metabolite) are about 50% greater in patients with CrCl <30 mL/minute and are doubled in hemodialysis patients. Potentially significant drug interactions may exist, requiring dose or frequency adjustment, additional monitoring, and/or selection of alternative therapy. In surgical patients on chronic angiotensin receptor blocker (ARB) therapy, intraoperative hypotension may occur with induction and maintenance of general anesthesia.

Angioedema has been reported rarely with some angiotensin II receptor antagonists (ARBs) and may occur at any time during treatment (especially following first dose). It may involve the head and neck (potentially compromising airway) or the intestine (presenting with abdominal pain). Patients with idiopathic or hereditary angioedema or previous angioedema associated with ACE-inhibitor therapy may be at an increased risk. Prolonged frequent monitoring may be required, especially if tongue, glottis, or larynx are involved, as they are associated with airway obstruction. Patients with a history of airway surgery may have a higher risk of airway obstruction. Discontinue therapy immediately if angioedema occurs. Aggressive early management is critical. Intramuscular (IM) administration of epinephrine may be necessary. Do not readminister to patients who have had angioedema with ARBs.

When used to reduce the risk of stroke in patients with HTN and LVH, may not be effective in the black population. Use caution with hepatic dysfunction, dose adjustment may be needed.

Adverse Reactions

Cardiovascular: Chest pain, hypotension, orthostatic hypotension, first-dose hypotension (dose related)

Central nervous system: Dizziness, fatigue, fever, hypoesthesia, insomnia

Dermatology: Cellulitis

Endocrine: Hyperkalemia, hypoglycemia

Gastrointestinal: Abdominal pain, diarrhea, dyspepsia, gastritis, nausea, weight gain

Genitourinary: Urinary tract infection

Hematologic: Anemia

Neuromuscular & skeletal: Back pain, knee pain, leg pain, muscle cramps, muscular weakness, myalgia, weakness

Respiratory: Bronchitis, cough, nasal congestion, sinusitis upper respiratory infection

Miscellaneous: Flu-like syndrome, infection

Frequency ≤ placebo: Abdominal pain, edema, headache, nausea, pharyngitis

Rare but important or life-threatening: Acute psychosis with paranoid delusions, ageusia, allergic reaction, alopecia, anaphylactic reactions, anemia, angina, angioedema, anorexia, anxiety, arrhythmia, arthralgia, arthritis, ataxia, AV block (second degree), bilirubin increased, blurred vision, bradycardia, bronchitis, BUN increased, confusion, conjunctivitis, constipation, CVA, depression, dermatitis, dysgeusia, dyspnea, ecchymosis, epistaxis, erythroderma, erythema, facial edema, fever, flatulence, flushing, gastritis, gout, hematocrit decreased, hemoglobin decreased, Henoch-Schönlein purpura (IgA vasculitis), hepatitis, hyponatremia, hypotension, impotence, joint swelling, maculopapular rash, malaise, memory impairment, MI, migraine, muscle weakness, myositis, neoplasm, nervousness, orthostatic effects, pancreatitis, paresthesia, peripheral neuropathy, pharyngitis, photosensitivity, pruritus, rash, rhabdomyolysis, rhinitis, serum creatinine increased, sleep disorder, somnolence, syncope, tachycardia, taste perversion, thrombocytopenia, tinnitus, transaminases increased, tremor, urinary frequency, urticaria, vasculitis, ventricular arrhythmia, vertigo, visual acuity decreased, vomiting, xerostomia

Drug Interactions

Metabolism/Transport Effects Substrate of CYP2C9 (major), CYP3A4 (major); **Note:** Assignment of Major/Minor substrate status based on clinically relevant drug interaction potential; **Inhibits** CYP1A2 (weak), CYP2C19 (weak), CYP2C8 (moderate), CYP2C9 (moderate), CYP3A4 (weak)

Avoid Concomitant Use

Avoid concomitant use of Losartan with any of the following: Pimozide

Increased Effect/Toxicity

Losartan may increase the levels/effects of: ACE Inhibitors; Amifostine; Antihypertensives; ARIPiprazole; Bosentan; Cannabis; Carvedilol; CycloSPORINE (Systemic); CYP2C8 Substrates; CYP2C9 Substrates; Dofetilide; Dronabinol; DULoxetine; Hydrocodone; Hypotensive Agents; Levodopa; Lithium; Lomitapide; Nonsteroidal Anti-Inflammatory Agents; Obinutuzumab; Pimozide; Potassium-Sparing Diuretics; RisperiDONE; RiTUXimab; Sodium Phosphates; Tetrahydrocannabinol

The levels/effects of Losartan may be increased by: Alfuzosin; Aliskiren; Antifungal Agents (Azole Derivatives, Systemic); Barbiturates; Brimonidine (Topical); Canagliflozin; Ceritinib; CYP2C9 Inhibitors (Moderate); CYP2C9 Inhibitors (Strong); Dapoxetine; Diazoxide; Eplerenone; Heparin; Heparin (Low Molecular Weight); Herbs (Hypotensive Properties); MAO Inhibitors; Mifepristone; Nicorandil; Pentoxifylline; Phosphodiesterase 5 Inhibitors; Potassium Salts; Prostacyclin Analogues; Tolvaptan; Trimethoprim

Decreased Effect

The levels/effects of Losartan may be decreased by: Bosentan; CYP2C9 Inducers (Strong); CYP3A4 Inducers (Moderate); CYP3A4 Inducers (Strong); Dabrafenib; Deferasirox; Fluconazole; Herbs (Hypertensive Properties); Methylphenidate; Mitotane; Nonsteroidal Anti-Inflammatory Agents; Rifampin; Siltuximab; St Johns Wort; Tocilizumab; Yohimbine

Storage/Stability Store at 25°C (77°F); excursions are permitted to 15°C to 30°C (59°F to 86°F). Protect from light.

Mechanism of Action As a selective and competitive, nonpeptide angiotensin II receptor antagonist, losartan blocks the vasoconstrictor and aldosterone-secreting effects of angiotensin II; losartan interacts reversibly at the AT1 and AT2 receptors of many tissues and has slow dissociation kinetics; its affinity for the AT1 receptor is 1000 times greater than the AT2 receptor. Angiotensin II receptor antagonists may induce a more complete inhibition of the renin-angiotensin system than ACE inhibitors, they do not affect the response to bradykinin, and are less likely to be associated with nonrenin-angiotensin effects (eg, cough and angioedema). Losartan increases urinary flow rate and in addition to being natriuretic and kaliuretic, increases excretion of chloride, magnesium, uric acid, calcium, and phosphate.

Pharmacodynamics/Kinetics

Onset of action: 6 hours

Distribution: V_d: Losartan: 34 L; E-3174: 12 L; animal studies suggest that losartan does not cross the blood-brain barrier

Protein binding, plasma: High

Metabolism: Hepatic (14%) via CYP2C9 and 3A4 to active metabolite, E-3174 (10 to 40 times more potent than losartan); extensive first-pass effect

Bioavailability: ~33%; AUC of E-3174 is four times greater than that of losartan

Half-life elimination: Losartan: 2 hours; E-3174: 6 to 9 hours

Time to peak, serum: Losartan: 1 to 2 hours; E-3174: 3.5 to 4 hours

Excretion: Urine (4% as unchanged drug, 6% as active metabolite); feces

Dosage Oral:

Hypertension:

Children and Adolescents 6 to 16 years:

U.S. labeling: Initial: 0.7 mg/kg once daily (maximum: 50 mg daily); doses >1.4 mg/kg (>100 mg daily) have not been studied

Canadian labeling:

≥20 kg to <50 kg: 25 mg once daily (maximum: 50 mg once daily)

≥50 kg: 50 mg once daily (maximum: 100 mg once daily)

Adults: Initial: 50 mg once daily; can be administered once or twice daily with total daily doses ranging from 25 to 100 mg; usual dosage range (ASH/ISH [Weber, 2014]): 50 to 100 mg daily; target dose (JNC 8 [James, 2013]): 100 mg daily in 1 or 2 divided doses

Patients receiving diuretics or with intravascular volume depletion: Initial: 25 mg once daily

Diabetic nephropathy: Adults: Initial: 50 mg once daily; can be increased to 100 mg once daily based on blood pressure response

Hypertension with left ventricular hypertrophy: Adults: Initial: 50 mg once daily, can be increased to 100 mg once daily based on blood pressure response. May be used in combination with a thiazide diuretic

Aortic-root dilation with Marfan's syndrome (off-label use): Children 14 months to 16 years: Initial: 0.6 mg/kg/day; can be increased to a maximum of 1.4 mg/kg/day (not to exceed adult maximum of 100 mg daily) (Brooke, 2008)

Heart failure (off-label use): Adults: Initial: 12.5 to 25 mg once daily; target dose: 150 mg once daily (HFSA, 2010; Konstam, 2009). The ACCF/AHA 2013 heart failure guidelines recommend an initial dose of 25 to 50 mg once daily; target dose: 150 mg once daily (Yancy, 2013).

Dosing adjustment in renal impairment:

Children: Use is not recommended if GFR <30 mL/minute/1.73 m^2

Adults: Initial: No dosage adjustment necessary.

Dosing adjustment in hepatic impairment:

Children 6 to 16 years:

U.S. labeling: No specific dosing recommendations are provided in the manufacturer's labeling, however it may be advisable to initiate therapy at a reduced dosage.

Canadian labeling: Use is not recommended.

Adults: Reduce the initial dose to 25 mg daily

Dietary Considerations May be taken without regard to meals. Some products may contain potassium.

Administration May be administered without regard to meals.

Monitoring Parameters

Supine blood pressure, electrolytes, serum creatinine, BUN, urinalysis, symptomatic hypotension and tachycardia, CBC

Neonates exposed *in utero* should be monitored for oliguria and hypotension.

2013 ACCF/AHA Heart Failure guideline recommendations:

Within 1 to 2 weeks after initiation, reassess blood pressure (including postural blood pressure changes), renal function, and serum potassium; follow closely after dose changes. Patients with systolic blood pressure <80 mm Hg, low serum sodium, diabetes mellitus, and impaired renal function should be closely monitored (ACCF/AHA [Yancy, 2013]).

Dosage Forms

Tablet, Oral:

Cozaar: 25 mg, 50 mg, 100 mg

Generic: 25 mg, 50 mg, 100 mg

Extemporaneous Preparations A 2.5 mg/mL losartan oral suspension may be made with tablets and a 1:1 mixture of Ora-Plus® and Ora-Sweet® SF. Combine 10 mL of purified water and ten losartan 50 mg tablets in an 8-ounce amber polyethylene terephthalate bottle. Shake well for at least 2 minutes. Allow concentrate to stand for 1 hour, then shake for 1 minute. Separately, prepare 190 mL of a 1:1 mixture of Ora-Plus® and Ora-Sweet® SF; add to tablet and water mixture in the bottle and shake for 1 minute. Label "shake well" and "refrigerate". Return promptly to refrigerator after each use. Stable for 4 weeks when stored in amber polyethylene terephthalate prescription bottles and refrigerated (Cozaar prescribing information, 2014).

Cozaar prescribing information, Merck & Co, Inc, Whitehouse Station, NJ, 2014.

Losartan and Hydrochlorothiazide

(loe SAR tan & hye droe klor oh THYE a zide)

Brand Names: U.S. Hyzaar

Brand Names: Canada ACT Losartan/HCT; Apo-Losartan/HCTZ; Auro-Losartan HCT; Hyzaar; Hyzaar DS; JAMP-Losartan HCTZ; Losartan-HCT; Losartan-HCTZ; Mint-Losartan/HCTZ; Mint-Losartan/HCTZ DS; Mylan-Losartan/HCTZ; PMS-Losartan/HCTZ; Sandoz-Losartan HCT; Sandoz-Losartan HCT DS; Teva-Losartan/HCTZ

Index Terms Hydrochlorothiazide and Losartan

Pharmacologic Category Angiotensin II Receptor Blocker; Antihypertensive; Diuretic, Thiazide

Use

Hypertension: Treatment of hypertension.

Hypertension with left ventricular hypertrophy: To reduce the risk of stroke in patients with hypertension and left ventricular hypertrophy (LVH). Evidence suggests that this benefit does not apply to black patients.

Pregnancy Risk Factor D

Dosage

Hypertension: Adults: Oral: **Note:** Dose must be individualized; combination product may be substituted for individual components in patients currently maintained on both agents separately or in patients not adequately controlled with monotherapy.

Replacement therapy: Losartan 50 to 100 mg/hydrochlorothiazide 12.5 to 25 mg once daily; as appropriate, dose may be titrated after ~3 weeks of therapy as necessary until maximum daily dose is reached. Maximum daily dose: Losartan 100 mg/hydrochlorothiazide 25 mg once daily.

Severe hypertension: Initial: Losartan 50 mg/hydrochlorothiazide 12.5 mg once daily; dose may be titrated after 2 to 4 weeks of therapy as necessary until maximum daily dose is reached. Maximum daily dose: Losartan 100 mg/hydrochlorothiazide 25 mg once daily.

Hypertension with left ventricular hypertrophy: Adults: Oral: **Note:** Initiate treatment with losartan monotherapy. If blood pressure reduction inadequate, then may initiate losartan/hydrochlorothiazide combination.

Losartan 50 mg/hydrochlorothiazide 12.5 mg once daily; may increase to losartan 100 mg/hydrochlorothiazide 12.5 mg once daily, followed by losartan 100 mg/hydrochlorothiazide 25 mg once daily if needed to control blood pressure.

Dosage adjustment in renal impairment:

Mild to moderate impairment (CrCl >30 mL/minute): No dosage adjustment necessary.

Severe impairment (CrCl ≤30 mL/minute): Use is not recommended.

Dosage adjustment in hepatic impairment: Use is not recommended as initial therapy.

Additional Information Complete prescribing information should be consulted for additional detail.

Dosage Forms

Tablet, oral: 50/12.5: Losartan 50 mg and hydrochlorothiazide 12.5 mg; 100/12.5: Losartan 100 mg and hydrochlorothiazide 12.5 mg; 100/25: Losartan 100 mg and hydrochlorothiazide 25 mg

Hyzaar: 50/12.5: Losartan 50 mg and hydrochlorothiazide 12.5 mg; 100/12.5: Losartan 100 mg and hydrochlorothiazide 12.5 mg; 100/25: Losartan 100 mg and hydrochlorothiazide 25 mg

- ◆ **Losartan-HCT (Can)** *see* Losartan and Hydrochlorothiazide *on page 1250*
- ◆ **Losartan-HCTZ (Can)** *see* Losartan and Hydrochlorothiazide *on page 1250*
- ◆ **Losartan Potassium** *see* Losartan *on page 1248*
- ◆ **LoSeasonique** *see* Ethinyl Estradiol and Levonorgestrel *on page 803*
- ◆ **Losec (Can)** *see* Omeprazole *on page 1508*
- ◆ **Lotemax** *see* Loteprednol *on page 1251*
- ◆ **Lotemax® (Can)** *see* Loteprednol *on page 1251*
- ◆ **Lotensin** *see* Benazepril *on page 238*
- ◆ **Lotensin HCT®** *see* Benazepril and Hydrochlorothiazide *on page 240*

Loteprednol (loe te PRED nol)

Brand Names: U.S. Alrex; Lotemax

Brand Names: Canada Alrex®; Lotemax®

Index Terms Loteprednol Etabonate

Pharmacologic Category Corticosteroid, Ophthalmic

Use

Alrex®: Temporary relief of signs and symptoms of seasonal allergic conjunctivitis

Lotemax®: Treatment of postoperative inflammation and pain following ocular surgery; treatment of inflammatory conditions (eg, steroid-responsive inflammatory conditions of the palpebral and bulbar conjunctiva, cornea, and anterior segment of the globe such as allergic conjunctivitis, acne rosacea, superficial punctate keratitis, herpes zoster keratitis, iritis, cyclitis, selected infective conjunctivitis, when the inherent hazard of steroid use is accepted to obtain an advisable diminution in edema and inflammation)

Pregnancy Risk Factor C

Dosage

Seasonal allergic conjunctivitis: Ophthalmic: Alrex® 0.2% suspension: Instill 1 drop into affected eye(s) 4 times daily.

Inflammatory conditions: Ophthalmic: Lotemax® 0.5% suspension: Instill 1-2 drops into the conjunctival sac of the affected eye(s) 4 times daily. During the initial treatment within the first week, the dosing may be increased up to 1 drop every hour. Advise patients not to discontinue therapy prematurely. If signs and symptoms fail to improve after 2 days, re-evaluate the patient.

Postoperative inflammation: Ophthalmic:

Lotemax® 0.5% ointment: Apply ~1/2 inch ribbon into the conjunctival sac of the affected eye(s) 4 times daily beginning 24 hours after surgery and continuing throughout the first 2 weeks of the postoperative period.

Lotemax® 0.5% gel, 0.5% suspension: Instill 1-2 drops into the conjunctival sac of the affected eye(s) 4 times daily beginning 24 hours after surgery and continuing throughout the first 2 weeks of the postoperative period.

Dosage adjustment in renal impairment: No dosage adjustment provided in manufacturer's labeling. However, dosage adjustment unlikely due to low systemic absorption.

Dosage adjustment in hepatic impairment: No dosage adjustment provided in manufacturer's labeling. However, dosage adjustment unlikely due to low systemic absorption.

Additional Information Complete prescribing information should be consulted for additional detail.

Dosage Forms

Gel, Ophthalmic:

Lotemax: 0.5% (5 g)

Ointment, Ophthalmic:

Lotemax: 0.5% (3.5 g)

Suspension, Ophthalmic:

Alrex: 0.2% (5 mL, 10 mL)

Lotemax: 0.5% (5 mL, 10 mL, 15 mL)

Loteprednol and Tobramycin
(loe te PRED nol & toe bra MYE sin)

Brand Names: U.S. Zylet®

Index Terms Loteprednol Etabonate and Tobramycin; Tobramycin and Loteprednol Etabonate

Pharmacologic Category Antibiotic/Corticosteroid, Ophthalmic

Use Treatment of steroid-responsive ocular inflammatory conditions where either a superficial bacterial ocular infection or the risk of a superficial bacterial ocular infection exists

Pregnancy Risk Factor C

Dosage Ophthalmic: Children and Adults: Instill 1-2 drops into the affected eye(s) every 4-6 hours; may increase frequency during the first 24-48 hours to every 1-2 hours. Interval should increase as signs and symptoms improve. Further evaluation should occur for use of greater than 20 mL.

Dosage adjustment in renal impairment: No dosage adjustment provided in manufacturer's labeling. However, dosage adjustment unlikely due to low systemic absorption.

Dosage adjustment in hepatic impairment: No dosage adjustment provided in manufacturer's labeling. However, dosage adjustment unlikely due to low systemic absorption.

Additional Information Complete prescribing information should be consulted for additional detail.

Dosage Forms

Suspension, ophthalmic [drops]:

Zylet®: Loteprednol 0.5% and tobramycin 0.3% (2.5 mL, 5 mL, 10 mL)

- **Loteprednol Etabonate** *see* Loteprednol *on page 1251*
- **Loteprednol Etabonate and Tobramycin** *see* Loteprednol and Tobramycin *on page 1251*
- **Lotrel®** *see* Amlodipine and Benazepril *on page 125*
- **Lotriderm (Can)** *see* Betamethasone and Clotrimazole *on page 256*
- **Lotrimin AF [OTC]** *see* Clotrimazole (Topical) *on page 488*
- **Lotrimin AF [OTC]** *see* Miconazole (Topical) *on page 1360*
- **Lotrimin AF Deodorant Powder [OTC]** *see* Miconazole (Topical) *on page 1360*
- **Lotrimin AF For Her [OTC]** *see* Clotrimazole (Topical) *on page 488*
- **Lotrimin AF Jock Itch Powder [OTC]** *see* Miconazole (Topical) *on page 1360*
- **Lotrimin AF Powder [OTC]** *see* Miconazole (Topical) *on page 1360*
- **Lotrimin Ultra [OTC]** *see* Butenafine *on page 314*
- **Lotrisone** *see* Betamethasone and Clotrimazole *on page 256*

Lovastatin (LOE va sta tin)

Brand Names: U.S. Altoprev; Mevacor

Brand Names: Canada Apo-Lovastatin; Ava-Lovastatin; CO Lovastatin; Dom-Lovastatin; Mevacor; Mylan-Lovastatin; PHL-Lovastatin; PMS-Lovastatin; PRO-Lovastatin; Riva-Lovastatin; Sandoz-Lovastatin; Teva-Lovastatin

Index Terms Mevinolin; Monacolin K

Pharmacologic Category Antilipemic Agent, HMG-CoA Reductase Inhibitor

Use

Adjunct to dietary therapy to decrease elevated serum total and LDL-cholesterol concentrations in primary hypercholesterolemia

Primary prevention of coronary artery disease (patients without symptomatic disease with average to moderately elevated total and LDL-cholesterol and below average HDL-cholesterol); slow progression of coronary atherosclerosis in patients with coronary heart disease and reduce the risk of myocardial infarction, unstable angina, and coronary revascularization procedures.

Adjunct to dietary therapy in adolescent patients (10-17 years of age, females >1 year postmenarche) with heterozygous familial hypercholesterolemia having LDL >189 mg/dL, **or** LDL >160 mg/dL with positive family history of premature cardiovascular disease (CVD), **or** LDL >160 mg/dL with the presence of at least two other CVD risk factors

Primary and secondary prevention of atherosclerotic cardiovascular disease (ASCVD) according to the American College of Cardiology/American Heart Association: To reduce the risk of ASCVD in patients with clinical ASCVD (eg, coronary heart disease, stroke/TIA, or peripheral arterial disease presumed to be of atherosclerotic origin) who are greater than 75 years of age or not a candidate for high-intensity statin therapy; in patients without clinical ASCVD if LDL-C is 190 mg/dL or greater and not a candidate for high-intensity statin therapy; in patients without clinical ASCVD who have type 1 or type 2 diabetes and are between 40 and 75 years of age; in patients with an estimated 10-year ASCVD risk 7.5% or greater and who are between 40 and 75 years of age (Stone, 2013). Specific recommendations from the Kidney Disease: Improving Global Outcomes (KDIGO) organization have also been released for patients with chronic kidney disease (KDIGO [Tonelli, 2013]).

Pregnancy Risk Factor X

Pregnancy Considerations Adverse events were observed in animal reproduction studies. There are reports of congenital anomalies following maternal use of HMG-CoA reductase inhibitors in pregnancy; however, maternal disease, differences in specific agents used, and the low rates of exposure limit the interpretation of the available data (Godfrey, 2012; Lecarpentier, 2012). Cholesterol biosynthesis may be important in fetal development; serum cholesterol and triglycerides increase normally during pregnancy. The discontinuation of lipid lowering medications temporarily during pregnancy is not expected to have significant impact on the long term outcomes of primary hypercholesterolemia treatment.

Use of lovastatin is contraindicated in pregnancy. HMG-CoA reductase inhibitors should be discontinued prior to pregnancy (ADA, 2013). If treatment of dyslipidemias is needed in pregnant women or in women of reproductive age, other agents are preferred (Berglund, 2012; Stone, 2013). The manufacturer recommends administration to women of childbearing potential only when conception is highly unlikely and patients have been informed of potential hazards.

Breast-Feeding Considerations It is not known if lovastatin is excreted into breast milk. Due to the potential for serious adverse reactions in a nursing infant, use while breast-feeding is contraindicated by the manufacturer.

Contraindications

Hypersensitivity to lovastatin or any component of the formulation; active liver disease; unexplained persistent elevations of serum transaminases; concomitant use of strong CYP3A4 inhibitors (eg, clarithromycin, erythromycin, itraconazole, ketoconazole, nefazodone, posaconazole, voriconazole, protease inhibitors [including boceprevir and telaprevir], telithromycin, cobicistat-containing products); pregnancy; breast-feeding

Canadian labeling: Additional contraindications (not in U.S. labeling): Concomitant use of cyclosporine

Warnings/Precautions Secondary causes of hyperlipidemia should be ruled out prior to therapy. Liver enzyme tests should be obtained at baseline and as clinically indicated; routine periodic monitoring of liver enzymes is not necessary. Use with caution in patients who consume large amounts of ethanol or have a history of liver disease; use is contraindicated with active liver disease and with unexplained transaminase elevations. Rhabdomyolysis with or without acute renal failure has occurred. Risk of rhabdomyolysis is dose-related and increased with concurrent use of lipid-lowering agents which may also cause rhabdomyolysis (fibric acid derivatives or niacin at doses ≥1 g/day) or during concurrent use with potent CYP3A4 inhibitors. Use is contraindicated in patients taking strong CYP3A4 inhibitors. Concomitant use of lovastatin with some drugs may require cautious use, may not be recommended, may require dosage adjustments, or may be contraindicated. Increases in HbA_{1c} and fasting blood glucose have been reported with HMG-CoA reductase inhibitors; however, the benefits of statin therapy far outweigh the risk of dysglycemia. Monitor closely if used with other drugs associated with myopathy (eg, colchicine). Patients should be instructed to report unexplained muscle pain or weakness; lovastatin should be discontinued if myopathy is suspected/confirmed. Immune-mediated necrotizing myopathy (IMNM), an autoimmune-mediated myopathy, has been reported (rarely) with HMG-CoA reductase inhibitor therapy. IMNM presents as proximal muscle weakness with elevated CPK levels, which persists despite discontinuation of HMG-CoA reductase inhibitor therapy; additionally, muscle biopsy may show necrotizing myopathy with limited inflammation; immunosuppressive therapy (eg, corticosteroids, azathioprine) may be used for treatment. The manufacturer recommends temporary discontinuation for elective major surgery, acute medical or surgical conditions, or in any patient experiencing an acute or serious condition predisposing to renal failure (eg, sepsis, hypotension, trauma, uncontrolled seizures). Based on current research and clinical guidelines (Fleisher, 2009), HMG-CoA reductase inhibitors should be continued in the perioperative period. Use with caution in patients with advanced age; these patients are predisposed to myopathy.

Adverse Reactions

Central nervous system: Dizziness, headache

Dermatologic: Rash

Gastrointestinal: Abdominal pain, constipation, diarrhea, dyspepsia, flatulence, nausea

Neuromuscular & skeletal: Increased CPK (>2x normal), muscle cramps, myalgia, weakness

Ocular: Blurred vision

Rare but important or life-threatening: Acid regurgitation, alopecia, amnesia (reversible), arthralgia, blood glucose increased, chest pain, cognitive impairment (reversible), confusion (reversible), dermatomyositis, diabetes mellitus (new onset), eye irritation, glycosylated hemoglobin (Hb A_{1c}) increased, insomnia, leg pain, memory disturbance (reversible), memory impairment (reversible), paresthesia, pruritus, vomiting, xerostomia

Additional class-related events or case reports (not necessarily reported with lovastatin therapy): Alkaline phosphatase increased, alteration in taste, anaphylaxis, angioedema, anorexia, anxiety, arthritis, cataracts, chills, cholestatic jaundice, cirrhosis, depression, dryness of skin/mucous membranes, dyspnea, eosinophilia, erectile dysfunction, erythema multiforme, ESR increased, facial paresis, fatty liver, fever, flushing, fulminant hepatic necrosis, GGT increased, gynecomastia, hemolytic anemia, hepatic failure (fatal and nonfatal), hepatitis, hepatoma, hyperbilirubinemia, hypersensitivity reaction, immune-mediated necrotizing myopathy (IMNM), impaired extraocular muscle movement, impotence, interstitial lung disease, leukopenia, libido decreased, malaise, myopathy, nail changes, nodules, ophthalmoplegia, pancreatitis, peripheral nerve palsy, peripheral neuropathy, photosensitivity, polymyalgia rheumatica, positive ANA, psychic disturbance, purpura, renal failure (secondary to rhabdomyolysis), rhabdomyolysis, skin discoloration, Stevens-Johnson syndrome, systemic lupus erythematosus-like syndrome, thrombocytopenia, thyroid dysfunction, toxic epidermal necrolysis, transaminases increased, tremor, urticaria, vasculitis, vertigo

Drug Interactions

Metabolism/Transport Effects **Substrate** of CYP3A4 (major), P-glycoprotein; **Note:** Assignment of Major/Minor substrate status based on clinically relevant drug interaction potential; **Inhibits** CYP2C9 (weak), CYP3A4 (weak)

Avoid Concomitant Use

Avoid concomitant use of Lovastatin with any of the following: Boceprevir; Clarithromycin; Conivaptan; CycloSPORINE (Systemic); CYP3A4 Inhibitors (Strong); Erythromycin (Systemic); Fusidic Acid (Systemic); Gemfibrozil; Idelalisib; Lomitapide; Mifepristone; Pimozide; Protease Inhibitors; Red Yeast Rice; Telaprevir; Telithromycin

Increased Effect/Toxicity

Lovastatin may increase the levels/effects of: ARIPiprazole; DAPTOmycin; Diltiazem; Dofetilide; Hydrocodone; PAZOPanib; Pimozide; Trabectedin; Vitamin K Antagonists

The levels/effects of Lovastatin may be increased by: Acipimox; Amiodarone; Aprepitant; Azithromycin (Systemic); Bezafibrate; Boceprevir; Ceritinib; Ciprofibrate; Clarithromycin; Colchicine; Conivaptan; CycloSPORINE (Systemic); CYP3A4 Inhibitors (Moderate); CYP3A4 Inhibitors (Strong); Cyproterone; Danazol; Dasatinib; Diltiazem; Dronedarone; Erythromycin (Systemic); Fenofibrate and Derivatives; Fluconazole; Fosaprepitant; Fusidic Acid (Systemic); Gemfibrozil; Grapefruit Juice; Idelalisib; Ivacaftor; Lomitapide; Luliconazole; Mifepristone; Netupitant; Niacin; Niacinamide; P-glycoprotein/ABCB1 Inhibitors; Protease Inhibitors; QuiNINE; Raltegravir; Ranolazine; Red Yeast Rice; Sildenafil; Simeprevir; Telaprevir; Telithromycin; Ticagrelor; Verapamil

Decreased Effect

Lovastatin may decrease the levels/effects of: Lanthanum

The levels/effects of Lovastatin may be decreased by: Antacids; Bosentan; CYP3A4 Inducers (Moderate); CYP3A4 Inducers (Strong); Dabrafenib; Deferasirox; Efavirenz; Etravirine; Fosphenytoin; Mitotane; P-glycoprotein/ABCB1 Inducers; Phenytoin; Rifamycin Derivatives; Siltuximab; St Johns Wort; Tocilizumab

Food Interactions Food decreases the bioavailability of lovastatin extended release tablets and increases the bioavailability of lovastatin immediate release tablets. Lovastatin serum concentrations may be increased if taken with grapefruit juice. Management: Avoid concurrent intake of large quantities (>1 quart/day) of grapefruit juice.

Storage/Stability

Tablet, immediate release: Store at 20°C to 25°C (68°F to 77°F). Protect from light

Tablet, extended release: Store at 20°C to 25°C (68°F to 77°F); excursions permitted between 15°C to 30°C (59°F to 86°F). Avoid excessive heat and humidity.

Mechanism of Action Lovastatin acts by competitively inhibiting 3-hydroxyl-3-methylglutaryl-coenzyme A (HMG-CoA) reductase, the enzyme that catalyzes the rate-limiting step in cholesterol biosynthesis

Pharmacodynamics/Kinetics

Onset of action: LDL-cholesterol reductions: 3 days

Absorption: 30%; increased with extended release tablets when taken in the fasting state

Protein binding: >95%

Metabolism: Hepatic; extensive first-pass effect; hydrolyzed to β-hydroxyacid (active)

Bioavailability: Increased with extended release tablets

Half-life elimination: 1.1-1.7 hours

Time to peak, serum: Immediate release: 2-4 hours; extended release: 12-14 hours

Excretion: Feces (~80% to 85%); urine (10%)

Dosage

Adolescents 10-17 years: Oral: Immediate release tablet:

- LDL reduction <20%: Initial: 10 mg daily with evening meal
- LDL reduction ≥20%: Initial: 20 mg daily with evening meal
- Usual range: 10-40 mg once daily with evening meal, then adjust dose at 4-week intervals; maximum dose per manufacturer: 40 mg daily

Adults: Oral:

- Immediate release: Initial: 20 mg once daily with evening meal, then adjust at 4-week intervals; maximum dose: 80 mg daily

Extended release: Initial: 20, 40, or 60 mg once daily at bedtime, then adjust at 4-week intervals; maximum dose: 60 mg daily

Note: Doses should be individualized according to the baseline LDL-cholesterol levels, the recommended goal of therapy, and patient response. For patients requiring smaller reductions in cholesterol, the use of the extended release tablet is not recommended; consider use of immediate release formulation.

ACC/AHA Blood Cholesterol Guideline recommendations to reduce the risk of atherosclerotic cardiovascular disease (ASCVD) (Stone, 2013): Adults ≥21 years: Oral:

Primary prevention:

LDL-C ≥190 mg/dL: High intensity therapy necessary; use alternate statin therapy (eg, atorvastatin or rosuvastatin)

Type 1 or 2 diabetes and age 40-75 years: Moderate intensity therapy: Immediate release: 40 mg once daily

Type 1 or 2 diabetes, age 40-75 years, and an estimated 10-year ASCVD risk ≥7.5%: High intensity therapy necessary; use alternate statin therapy (eg, atorvastatin or rosuvastatin)

Age 40-75 years and an estimated 10-year ASCVD risk ≥7.5%: Moderate to high intensity therapy: Immediate release: 40 mg once daily or consider using high intensity statin therapy (eg, atorvastatin or rosuvastatin)

Secondary prevention:

Patient has clinical ASCVD (eg, coronary heart disease, stroke/TIA, or peripheral arterial disease presumed to be of atherosclerotic origin) **and:**

Age ≤75 years: High intensity therapy necessary; use alternate statin therapy (eg, atorvastatin or rosuvastatin)

Age >75 years or not a candidate for high intensity therapy: Moderate intensity therapy: Immediate release: 40 mg once daily

Elderly: Immediate release: Refer to adult dosing; Extended release: Initial: 20 mg once daily at bedtime

Dosage adjustment for lovastatin with concomitant medications:

Amiodarone: Maximum recommended lovastatin dose (extended release and immediate release): 40 mg daily

Danazol, diltiazem, dronedarone, or verapamil: Initial lovastatin (immediate release) dose: 10 mg daily; Maximum recommended lovastatin (extended release and immediate release) dose: 20 mg daily

Lomitapide: Consider lovastatin dose reduction (per lomitapide manufacturer).

Dosage adjustment for toxicity:

Severe muscle symptoms or fatigue: Promptly discontinue use; evaluate CPK, creatinine, and urinalysis for myoglobinuria (Stone, 2013).

Mild to moderate muscle symptoms: Discontinue use until symptoms can be evaluated; evaluate patient for conditions that may increase the risk for muscle symptoms (eg, hypothyroidism, reduced renal or hepatic function, rheumatologic disorders such as polymyalgia rheumatica, steroid myopathy, vitamin D deficiency, or primary muscle diseases). Upon resolution, resume the original or lower dose of lovastatin. If muscle symptoms recur, discontinue lovastatin use. After muscle symptom resolution, may then use a low dose of a different statin; gradually increase if tolerated. In the absence of continued statin use, if muscle symptoms or elevated CPK continues after 2 months, consider other causes of muscle symptoms. If determined to be due to another condition aside from statin use, may resume statin therapy at the original dose (Stone, 2013).

Dosage adjustment in renal impairment: CrCl <30 mL/minute: Use with caution and carefully consider doses >20 mg/day.

Dosage adjustment in hepatic impairment: No dosage adjustment provided in manufacturer's labeling (has not been studied).

Dietary Considerations Before initiation of therapy, patients should be placed on a standard cholesterol-lowering diet for 6 weeks and the diet should be continued during drug therapy. Avoid intake of large quantities of grapefruit juice (≥1 quart/day); may increase toxicity. Immediate release tablet should be taken with the evening meal.

Red yeast rice contains variable amounts of several compounds that are structurally similar to HMG-CoA reductase inhibitors, primarily monacolin K (or mevinolin) which is structurally identical to lovastatin; concurrent use of red yeast rice with HMG-CoA reductase inhibitors may increase the incidence of adverse and toxic effects (Lapi, 2008; Smith, 2003).

Administration Administer immediate release tablet with the evening meal. Administer extended release tablet at bedtime; do not crush or chew.

Monitoring Parameters

2013 ACC/AHA Blood Cholesterol Guideline recommendations (Stone, 2013):

Lipid panel (total cholesterol, HDL, LDL, triglycerides): Baseline lipid panel; fasting lipid profile within 4-12 weeks after initiation or dose adjustment and every 3-12 months (as clinically indicated) thereafter. If 2 consecutive LDL levels are <40 mg/dL, consider decreasing the dose.

Hepatic transaminase levels: Baseline measurement of hepatic transaminase levels (ie, ALT); measure hepatic function if symptoms suggest hepatotoxicity (eg, unusual fatigue or weakness, loss of appetite, abdominal pain, dark-colored urine or yellowing of skin or sclera) during therapy.

CPK: CPK should not be routinely measured. Baseline CPK measurement is reasonable for some individuals (eg, family history of statin intolerance or muscle disease, clinical presentation, concomitant drug therapy that may increase risk of myopathy). May measure CPK in any patient with symptoms suggestive of myopathy (pain, tenderness, stiffness, cramping, weakness, or generalized fatigue).

Evaluate for new-onset diabetes mellitus during therapy; if diabetes develops, continue statin therapy and encourage adherence to a heart-healthy diet, physical activity, a healthy body weight, and tobacco cessation.

If patient develops a confusional state or memory impairment, may evaluate patient for nonstatin causes (eg, exposure to other drugs), systemic and neuropsychiatric causes, and the possibility of adverse effects associated with statin therapy.

Manufacturer recommendations: Liver enzyme tests at baseline and repeated when clinically indicated. Measure CPK when myopathy is being considered or may measure CPK periodically in patients starting therapy or when dosage increase is necessary. Analyze lipid panel at intervals of 4 weeks or more.

Dosage Forms

Tablet, Oral:

Mevacor: 20 mg, 40 mg

Generic: 10 mg, 20 mg, 40 mg

Tablet Extended Release 24 Hour, Oral:

Altoprev: 20 mg, 40 mg, 60 mg

Dosage Forms: Canada Refer to Dosage Forms. **Note:** Extended release tablet is not available in Canada.

◆ **Lovastatin and Niacin** *see* Niacin and Lovastatin *on page 1446*

◆ **Lovaza** *see* Omega-3 Fatty Acids *on page 1507*
◆ **Lovenox** *see* Enoxaparin *on page 726*
◆ **Lovenox HP (Can)** *see* Enoxaparin *on page 726*
◆ **Lovenox With Preservative (Can)** *see* Enoxaparin *on page 726*
◆ **Low-Molecular-Weight Iron Dextran (INFeD)** *see* Iron Dextran Complex *on page 1117*
◆ **Low-Ogestrel** *see* Ethinyl Estradiol and Norgestrel *on page 812*
◆ **Loxapac (Can)** *see* Loxapine *on page 1255*

Loxapine (LOKS a peen)

Brand Names: U.S. Adasuve; Loxitane [DSC]
Brand Names: Canada Apo-Loxapine; Dom-Loxapine; Loxapac; PHL-Loxapine; Xylac
Index Terms Loxapine Succinate; Oxilapine Succinate
Pharmacologic Category First Generation (Typical) Antipsychotic
Additional Appendix Information
Beers Criteria - Potentially Inappropriate Medications for Geriatrics *on page 2271*
Use
Schizophrenia: IM, Oral: Treatment of schizophrenia.
Agitation associated with schizophrenia or bipolar I disorder: Inhalation: Acute treatment of agitation associated with schizophrenia or bipolar I disorder in adults.
Pregnancy Risk Factor C
Dosage
Schizophrenia:
Oral:
Adults: Initial: 10 mg twice daily (up to 50 mg daily may be considered in severely disturbed patients), increase dose until psychotic symptoms are controlled; usual maintenance: 60-100 mg daily in divided doses 2-4 times daily; satisfactory response often observed with doses of 20-60 mg daily (maximum: 250 mg daily). Therapy should be maintained at lowest effective dose.
Elderly: Reduced dosing may be indicated due to risks of adverse events associated with high-dose therapy.
IM (Canadian availability; not available in the U.S.): Adults: 12.5-50 mg every 4-6 hours or longer; individualize dose early in therapy; some patients respond satisfactorily to twice-daily dosing
Acute treatment of agitation associated with schizophrenia or bipolar I disorder: Inhalation: 10 mg once daily; maximum dose 10 mg per 24-hour period

Dosage adjustment in renal impairment: No dosage adjustment provided in manufacturer's labeling.
Dosage adjustment in hepatic impairment: No dosage adjustment provided in manufacturer's labeling. Canadian labeling does not recommend use in severe hepatic disease.
Additional Information Complete prescribing information should be consulted for additional detail.
Dosage Forms
Aerosol Powder Breath Activated, Inhalation [preservative free]:
Adasuve: 10 mg (1 ea)
Capsule, Oral:
Generic: 5 mg, 10 mg, 25 mg, 50 mg
Dosage Forms: Canada
Injection, solution:
Loxapac: 50 mg/mL (1 mL)
Solution, oral [concentrate]:
Xylac: 25 mg/mL (100 mL)
Tablet, oral:
Xylac: 2.5 mg, 5 mg, 10 mg, 25 mg, 50 mg

◆ **Loxapine Succinate** *see* Loxapine *on page 1255*
◆ **Loxitane [DSC]** *see* Loxapine *on page 1255*

Loxoprofen [INT] (loks oh PRO fen)

International Brand Names Ajuloxon (KR); An Pu Luo (CN); Bei Luo (CN); Japrolox (VN); Lopen (KR); Lopentac (KR); Loxfen (VN); Loxfin (KR); Loxonin (BR, CN, JP, MX, PE, TH, VE); Oxeno (AR); Reloc (KR); Roxonin (AE, BH, KW, LB, QA, SA); Ruo Mai (CN)
Index Terms Loxoprofen Sodium
Pharmacologic Category Nonsteroidal Anti-inflammatory Drug (NSAID), Oral
Reported Use Management of pain and inflammation associated with musculoskeletal and joint disorders or operative procedures
Dosage Range Adults: Oral: Immediate release: 60 mg 3 times/day
Product Availability Product available in various countries; not currently available in the U.S.
Dosage Forms
Tablet, immediate release: 60 mg

◆ **Loxoprofen Sodium** *see* Loxoprofen [INT] *on page 1255*
◆ **Lozide (Can)** *see* Indapamide *on page 1065*
◆ **Lozi-Flur** *see* Fluoride *on page 895*
◆ **L-PAM** *see* Melphalan *on page 1283*
◆ **L-Phenylalanine Mustard** *see* Melphalan *on page 1283*
◆ **LRH** *see* Gonadorelin [CAN/INT] *on page 980*
◆ **L-Sarcolysin** *see* Melphalan *on page 1283*
◆ **LTA 360 Kit** *see* Lidocaine (Topical) *on page 1211*
◆ **LTG** *see* LamoTRIgine *on page 1160*
◆ ***L*-Thyroxine Sodium** *see* Levothyroxine *on page 1205*
◆ **Lu-26-054** *see* Escitalopram *on page 765*
◆ **Lu AA21004** *see* Vortioxetine *on page 2183*

Lubiprostone (loo bi PROS tone)

Brand Names: U.S. Amitiza
Index Terms RU 0211; SPI 0211
Pharmacologic Category Chloride Channel Activator; Gastrointestinal Agent, Miscellaneous
Use Treatment of chronic idiopathic constipation; treatment of opioid-induced constipation with chronic non-cancer pain; treatment of irritable bowel syndrome with constipation in adult women
Pregnancy Risk Factor C
Dosage
Chronic idiopathic constipation: Adults: Oral: 24 mcg twice daily
Irritable bowel syndrome with constipation: Females ≥18 years: Oral: 8 mcg twice daily
Opioid-induced constipation: Adults: Oral: 24 mcg twice daily

Dosage adjustment for renal impairment: No dosage adjustment necessary.
Dosage adjustment for hepatic impairment:
Mild hepatic impairment (Child-Pugh class A): No dosage adjustment necessary.
Moderate hepatic impairment (Child-Pugh class B):
Chronic idiopathic constipation: Initial: 16 mcg twice daily; may increase to 24 mcg twice daily if tolerated and an adequate response has not been obtained with lower dosage.
Irritable bowel syndrome with constipation: No dosage adjustment necessary.

Opioid-induced constipation: Initial: 16 mcg twice daily; may increase to 24 mcg twice daily if tolerated and an adequate response has not been obtained with lower dosage.

Severe hepatic impairment (Child-Pugh class C):

Chronic idiopathic constipation: Initial: 8 mcg twice daily; may increase to 16-24 mcg twice daily if tolerated and an adequate response has not been obtained with lower dosage.

Irritable bowel syndrome with constipation: Initial: 8 mcg once daily; may increase to 8 mcg twice daily if tolerated and an adequate response has not been obtained at lower dosage.

Opioid-induced constipation: Initial: 8 mcg twice daily; may increase to 16-24 mcg twice daily if tolerated and an adequate response has not been obtained with lower dosage.

Additional Information Complete prescribing information should be consulted for additional detail.

Dosage Forms

Capsule, Oral:

Amitiza: 8 mcg, 24 mcg

◆ **Lucentis** *see* Ranibizumab *on page 1776*

Lucinactant (loo sin AK tant)

Brand Names: U.S. Surfaxin

Pharmacologic Category Lung Surfactant

Use Prevention of respiratory distress syndrome (RDS) in premature infants at high risk for RDS

Dosage Endotracheal: Respiratory distress prophylaxis: Premature infants: 5.8 mL/kg birth weight; up to 3 subsequent doses (total of 4 doses) may be administered at ≥6-hour intervals within the first 48 hours of life

Dosage adjustment in renal impairment: No dosage adjustment provided in manufacturer's labeling.

Dosage adjustment in hepatic impairment: No dosage adjustment provided in manufacturer's labeling.

Additional Information Complete prescribing information should be consulted for additional detail.

Dosage Forms

Suspension, Inhalation:

Surfaxin: 30 mg/mL (8.5 mL)

◆ **Ludiomil** *see* Maprotiline *on page 1271*

◆ **Lugol's Solution** *see* Potassium Iodide and Iodine *on page 1690*

Luliconazole (loo li KON a zole)

Brand Names: U.S. Luzu

Pharmacologic Category Antifungal Agent, Topical

Use Fungal infections: Topical treatment of tinea pedis, tinea cruris, and tinea corporis caused by the organisms *Trichophyton rubrum* and *Epidermophyton floccosum*

Pregnancy Risk Factor C

Dosage Fungal Infection: Adults: Topical:

Tinea pedis: Apply to affected area and ~1 inch of immediate surrounding area(s) once daily for 2 weeks

Tinea cruris or tinea corporis: Apply to affected area and ~1 inch of immediate surrounding area(s) once daily for 1 week

Dosage adjustment in renal impairment: No dosage adjustment provided in the manufacturer's labeling.

Dosage adjustment in hepatic impairment: No dosage adjustment provided in the manufacturer's labeling.

Additional Information Complete prescribing information should be consulted for additional detail.

Dosage Forms

Cream, External:

Luzu: 1% (60 g)

◆ **Lumefantrine and Artemether** *see* Artemether and Lumefantrine *on page 177*

◆ **Lumigan** *see* Bimatoprost *on page 264*

◆ **Lumigan RC (Can)** *see* Bimatoprost *on page 264*

◆ **Luminal Sodium** *see* PHENobarbital *on page 1632*

◆ **Lumizyme** *see* Alglucosidase Alfa *on page 85*

◆ **Lunesta** *see* Eszopiclone *on page 793*

◆ **Lupaneta Pack** *see* Leuprolide and Norethindrone *on page 1189*

◆ **Lupron (Can)** *see* Leuprolide *on page 1186*

◆ **Lupron Depot** *see* Leuprolide *on page 1186*

◆ **Lupron Depot-Ped** *see* Leuprolide *on page 1186*

Lurasidone (loo RAS i done)

Brand Names: U.S. Latuda

Brand Names: Canada Latuda

Index Terms Lurasidone Hydrochloride; SM-13496

Pharmacologic Category Second Generation (Atypical) Antipsychotic

Additional Appendix Information

Beers Criteria – Potentially Inappropriate Medications for Geriatrics *on page 2271*

Use Psychiatric issues: Treatment of schizophrenia; monotherapy or adjunctive therapy of depressive episodes associated with bipolar I disorder

Pregnancy Risk Factor B

Pregnancy Considerations Adverse events were not observed in animal reproduction studies. Antipsychotic use during the third trimester of pregnancy has a risk for abnormal muscle movements (extrapyramidal symptoms [EPS]) and/or withdrawal symptoms in newborns following delivery. Symptoms in the newborn may include agitation, feeding disorder, hypertonia, hypotonia, respiratory distress, somnolence, and tremor; these effects may be self-limiting or require hospitalization. Lurasidone may cause hyperprolactinemia, which may decrease reproductive function in both males and females.

The ACOG recommends that therapy during pregnancy be individualized; treatment with psychiatric medications during pregnancy should incorporate the clinical expertise of the mental health clinician, obstetrician, primary healthcare provider, and pediatrician. Safety data related to atypical antipsychotics during pregnancy is limited and routine use is not recommended. However, if a woman is inadvertently exposed to an atypical antipsychotic while pregnant, continuing therapy may be preferable to switching to a typical antipsychotic that the fetus has not yet been exposed to; consider risk:benefit (ACOG, 2008).

Healthcare providers are encouraged to enroll women 18-45 years of age exposed to lurasidone during pregnancy in the Atypical Antipsychotics Pregnancy Registry (866-961-2388 or http://www.womensmentalhealth.org/pregnancyregistry).

Breast-Feeding Considerations It is not known if lurasidone is excreted in breast milk. Due to the potential for serious adverse reactions in the nursing infant, the manufacturer recommends a decision be made whether to discontinue nursing or to discontinue the drug, taking into account the importance of the treatment to the mother.

Contraindications Hypersensitivity to lurasidone or any component of the formulation; concomitant use with strong CYP3A4 inhibitors (eg, ketoconazole) and inducers (eg, rifampin)

Warnings/Precautions [U.S. Boxed Warning]: Antidepressants increase the risk of suicidal thinking and behavior in children, adolescents, and young adults (18-24 years of age) with major depressive disorder and other psychiatric disorders; consider risk prior to prescribing. Lurasidone is not approved in the U.S. for use in children. Short-term studies did not show an increased risk in patients >24 years of age and showed a decreased risk in patients ≥65 years. **[U.S. Boxed Warning]: Closely monitor all patients for clinical worsening, suicidality, or unusual changes in behavior,** particularly during the initial 1-2 months of therapy or during periods of dosage adjustments (increases or decreases); the patient's family or caregiver should be instructed to closely observe the patient and communicate condition with healthcare provider. A medication guide concerning the use of antidepressants should be dispensed with each prescription.

The possibility of a suicide attempt is inherent in major depression and may persist until remission occurs. Patients treated with antidepressants (for any indication) should be observed for clinical worsening and suicidality, especially during the initial few months of a course of drug therapy, or at times of dose changes (increases or decreases). Worsening depression and severe abrupt suicidality that are not part of the presenting symptoms may require discontinuation or modification of drug therapy. Use caution in high-risk patients during initiation of therapy.

Prescriptions should be written for the smallest quantity consistent with good patient care. The patient's family or caregiver should be alerted to monitor patients for the emergence of suicidality and associated behaviors such as anxiety, agitation, panic attacks, insomnia, irritability, hostility, impulsivity, akathisia, hypomania, and mania; patients should be instructed to notify their healthcare provider if any of these symptoms or worsening depression or psychosis occur.

[U.S. Boxed Warning]: Elderly patients with dementia-related psychosis treated with antipsychotics are at an increased risk of death compared to placebo. Most deaths appeared to be either cardiovascular (eg, heart failure, sudden death) or infectious (eg, pneumonia) in nature. **Lurasidone is not approved for the treatment of dementia-related psychosis.** An increased incidence of cerebrovascular effects (eg, transient ischemic attack, stroke), including fatalities, has been reported in placebo-controlled trials of antipsychotics for the unapproved use in elderly patients with dementia-related psychosis.

Leukopenia, neutropenia, and agranulocytosis (sometimes fatal) have been reported in clinical trials and postmarketing reports with antipsychotic use; presence of risk factors (eg, preexisting low WBC or history of drug-induced leuko-/neutropenia) should prompt periodic blood count assessment. Discontinue therapy at first signs of blood dyscrasias or if absolute neutrophil count <1000/mm^3.

Low to moderately sedating, use with caution in disorders where CNS depression is a feature; patients must be cautioned about performing tasks which require mental alertness (eg, operating machinery or driving). Effects may be potentiated when used with other sedative drugs or ethanol. Use with caution in Parkinson's disease. Caution in patients with predisposition to seizures, including those with a history of seizures, head trauma, brain damage, alcoholism, or concurrent therapy with medications which may lower seizure threshold. Elderly patients may be at increased risk of seizures due to an increased prevalence of predisposing factors. Use with caution in renal or hepatic dysfunction; dose reduction recommended in moderate-to-severe impairment. Esophageal dysmotility and aspiration have been associated with antipsychotic use; use with caution in patients at risk of aspiration pneumonia (ie, Alzheimer's disease). Use is associated with increased prolactin levels; clinical significance of hyperprolactinemia in patients with breast cancer or other prolactin-dependent tumors is unknown. May alter temperature regulation.

Use with caution in patients with severe cardiac disease, hemodynamic instability, prior myocardial infarction or ischemic heart disease. May cause orthostatic hypotension; use with caution in patients at risk of this effect (eg, concurrent medication use which may predispose to hypotension/bradycardia or presence of hypovolemia) or in those who would not tolerate transient hypotensive episodes. Antipsychotics may alter cardiac conduction; life-threatening arrhythmias have occurred with therapeutic doses of antipsychotics. Relative to other antipsychotics, lurasidone has minimal effects on the QTc interval and therefore, risk for arrhythmias is low. However, Canadian labeling recommends avoiding use of lurasidone in patients with a history of cardiac arrhythmias, situations that may increase the risk of torsade de pointes and/or sudden death due to QT prolongation including bradycardia, congenital QT prolongation, electrolyte disturbances (ie, hypokalemia or hypomagnesemia), or in combination with other QTc-prolonging agents. Increases in total cholesterol and triglyceride concentrations have been observed with atypical antipsychotic use; during clinical trials of lurasidone, there were no significant changes in total cholesterol or triglycerides observed. Potentially significant drug-drug interactions may exist, requiring dose or frequency adjustment, additional monitoring, and/or selection of alternative therapy. Consult drug interactions database for more detailed information.

May cause extrapyramidal symptoms (EPS), including pseudoparkinsonism, acute dystonic reactions, akathisia, and tardive dyskinesia (potentially irreversible). Risk of tardive dyskinesia may be increased in elderly patients, particularly elderly women. Risk of dystonia (and probably other EPS) may be greater with increased doses, use of conventional antipsychotics, males, and younger patients. Use may be associated with neuroleptic malignant syndrome (NMS); monitor for mental status changes, fever, muscle rigidity and/or autonomic instability (risk may be increased in patients with Parkinson's disease or Lewy body dementia). May cause hyperglycemia; in some cases may be extreme and associated with ketoacidosis, hyperosmolar coma, or death. Use with caution in patients with diabetes or other disorders of glucose regulation; monitor for worsening of glucose control. Significant weight gain has been observed with antipsychotic therapy; incidence varies with product. Monitor waist circumference and BMI.

Use in elderly patients with dementia is associated with an increased risk of mortality and cerebrovascular accidents; avoid antipsychotic use for behavioral problems associated with dementia unless alternative nonpharmacologic therapies have failed and patient may harm self or others. In addition, use may cause or exacerbate syndrome of inappropriate antidiuretic hormone secretion or hyponatremia; monitor sodium closely with initiation or dosage adjustments in older adults (Beers Criteria).

Adverse Reactions

Cardiovascular: Orthostatic hypotension, tachycardia

Central nervous system: Agitation, akathisia (dose-related), anxiety, dizziness, drowsiness (dose-related), dystonia, extrapyramidal reaction, insomnia, parkinsonian-like syndrome, restlessness

Dermatologic: Pruritus, skin rash

Endocrine & metabolic: Increased serum cholesterol, increased serum glucose (fasting), increased serum prolactin (≥5 x ULN), increased serum triglycerides, weight gain (≥7% increase in baseline body weight)

Gastrointestinal: Abdominal pain, decreased appetite, diarrhea, dyspepsia, nausea, sialorrhea, vomiting, xerostomia
Genitourinary: Urinary tract infection
Infection: Influenza
Neuromuscular & skeletal: Back pain, increased creatine phosphokinase
Ophthalmic: Blurred vision
Renal: Increased serum creatinine
Respiratory: Nasopharyngitis
Rare but important or life-threatening: Amenorrhea, anemia, angina pectoris, angioedema, atrioventricular block, breast hypertrophy, cerebrovascular accident, gastritis, dysmenorrhea, erectile dysfunction, galactorrhea, hypomania, leukopenia, mania, neuroleptic malignant syndrome, panic attack, renal failure, rhabdomyolysis, seizure, suicidal ideation, tardive dyskinesia, venous thromboembolism

Drug Interactions

Metabolism/Transport Effects Substrate of CYP3A4 (major); **Note:** Assignment of Major/Minor substrate status based on clinically relevant drug interaction potential; **Inhibits** CYP3A4 (weak)

Avoid Concomitant Use

Avoid concomitant use of Lurasidone with any of the following: Amisulpride; Azelastine (Nasal); Conivaptan; CYP3A4 Inducers (Strong); CYP3A4 Inhibitors (Strong); DOPamine; EPINEPHrine (Systemic, Oral Inhalation); Fusidic Acid (Systemic); Grapefruit Juice; Idelalisib; Metoclopramide; Orphenadrine; Paraldehyde; Pimozide; St Johns Wort; Sulpiride; Thalidomide

Increased Effect/Toxicity

Lurasidone may increase the levels/effects of: Alcohol (Ethyl); Amisulpride; ARIPiprazole; Azelastine (Nasal); Buprenorphine; CNS Depressants; Disopyramide; Dofetilide; Hydrocodone; Lomitapide; Methotrimeprazine; Methylphenidate; Metyrosine; Mirtazapine; Orphenadrine; Paraldehyde; Pimozide; Procainamide; QuiNIDine; Selective Serotonin Reuptake Inhibitors; Serotonin Modulators; Sulpiride; Suvorexant; Thalidomide; Zolpidem

The levels/effects of Lurasidone may be increased by: Acetylcholinesterase Inhibitors (Central); Brimonidine (Topical); Cannabis; Conivaptan; CYP3A4 Inhibitors (Moderate); CYP3A4 Inhibitors (Strong); Dasatinib; DOPamine; Doxylamine; Dronabinol; Droperidol; EPINEPHrine (Systemic, Oral Inhalation); Fusidic Acid (Systemic); Grapefruit Juice; HydrOXYzine; Idelalisib; Ivacaftor; Kava Kava; Lithium; Luliconazole; Magnesium Sulfate; MAO Inhibitors; Methotrimeprazine; Methylphenidate; Metoclopramide; Metyrosine; Mifepristone; Nabilone; Perampanel; Rufinamide; Serotonin Modulators; Simeprevir; Sodium Oxybate; Tapentadol; Tetrabenazine; Tetrahydrocannabinol

Decreased Effect

Lurasidone may decrease the levels/effects of: Amphetamines; Anti-Parkinson's Agents (Dopamine Agonist); Quinagolide

The levels/effects of Lurasidone may be decreased by: Bosentan; CYP3A4 Inducers (Moderate); CYP3A4 Inducers (Strong); Dabrafenib; Deferasirox; Lithium; Siltuximab; St Johns Wort; Tocilizumab

Food Interactions Administration with food (≥350 calories) increased C_{max} and AUC of lurasidone ~3 times and 2 times, respectively, compared to administration under fasting conditions. Lurasidone exposure was not affected by the fat content of the meal. Management: Administer with food (≥350 calories).

Storage/Stability Store at controlled room temperature of 25°C (77°F); excursions permitted to 15°C to 30°C (59°F to 86°F).

Mechanism of Action Lurasidone is a benzoisothiazol-derivative atypical antipsychotic with mixed serotonin-dopamine antagonist activity. It exhibits high affinity for D_2, 5-HT_{2A}, and 5-HT_7 receptors; moderate affinity for alpha$_{2C}$-adrenergic receptors; and is a partial agonist for 5-HT_{1A} receptors. Lurasidone has no significant affinity for muscarinic M_1 and histamine H_1 receptors. The addition of serotonin antagonism to dopamine antagonism (classic neuroleptic mechanism) is thought to improve negative symptoms of psychoses and reduce the incidence of extrapyramidal side effects as compared to typical antipsychotics.

Pharmacodynamics/Kinetics

Distribution: V_d: 6173 L
Protein binding: ~99%
Metabolism: Primarily via CYP3A4; two active metabolites (ID-14283 and ID-14326) and two major nonactive metabolites (ID-20219 and ID-20220) produced
Bioavailability: 9% to 19%
Half-life elimination: 18 hours; Main active metabolite, ID-14283 (exo-hydroxy metabolite), exhibits a half-life of 7.5-10 hours
Time to peak: 1-3 hours; steady state concentrations achieved within 7 days
Excretion: Urine (~9%); feces (~80%)

Dosage

Depressive episodes associated with bipolar I disorder (monotherapy or as an adjunct to lithium or valproic acid): Adults: Oral: Initial: 20 mg once daily; titration is not required; maximum recommended dose: 120 mg daily. **Note:** Doses ≥80 mg daily during monotherapy studies did not provide additional efficacy compared to lower doses (eg, 20-60 mg daily).

Schizophrenia: Adults: Oral: Initial: 40 mg once daily; titration is not required; maximum recommended dose: 160 mg daily

Concomitant CYP3A4 inhibitors/inducers:

CYP3A4 inhibitors:

Concomitant administration with a **strong** CYP3A4 inhibitor (eg, ketoconazole) is contraindicated.

Concomitant administration with a **moderate** CYP3A4 inhibitor (eg, diltiazem):

U.S. labeling: Initial dose: 20 mg once daily; do not exceed 80 mg daily of lurasidone

Canadian labeling: Do not exceed 40 mg daily of lurasidone

CYP3A4 inducers:

Concomitant administration with a **strong** CYP3A4 inducer (eg, rifampin) is contraindicated.

Concomitant administration with a **moderate** CYP3A4 inducer: Lurasidone dose may need to be increased when combined with a moderate CYP3A4 inducer for ≥7 days.

Dosing adjustment in renal impairment:

U.S. labeling:
CrCl ≥50 mL/minute: No dosage adjustment necessary.
CrCl <50 mL/minute: Initial: 20 mg daily; maximum: 80 mg daily

Canadian labeling:
CrCl ≥50 mL/minute: No dosage adjustment necessary.
CrCl <50 mL/minute: Maximum: 40 mg daily

Dosing adjustment in hepatic impairment:

U.S. labeling:
Mild impairment (Child-Pugh class A): No dosage adjustment necessary.
Moderate impairment (Child-Pugh class B): Initial: 20 mg daily; maximum: 80 mg daily
Severe impairment (Child-Pugh class C): Initial: 20 mg daily; maximum: 40 mg daily

Canadian labeling:

Mild impairment (Child-Pugh class A): No dosage adjustment necessary.

Moderate and severe impairment (Child-Pugh class B and C): Maximum: 40 mg daily

Dietary Considerations Should be taken with food (≥350 calories).

Administration Administer with food (≥350 calories).

Monitoring Parameters Mental status; vital signs (as clinically indicated); blood pressure (baseline; repeat 3 months after antipsychotic initiation, then yearly); weight, height, BMI, waist circumference (baseline; repeat at 4, 8, and 12 weeks after initiating or changing therapy, then quarterly; consider switching to a different antipsychotic for a weight gain ≥5% of initial weight); CBC (as clinically indicated; monitor frequently during the first few months of therapy in patients with preexisting low WBC or history of drug-induced leukopenia/neutropenia); electrolytes, renal and liver function (annually and as clinically indicated); personal and family history of obesity, diabetes, dyslipidemia, hypertension, or cardiovascular disease (baseline; repeat annually); fasting plasma glucose level/HbA_{1c} (baseline; repeat 3 months after starting antipsychotic, then yearly); fasting lipid panel (baseline; repeat 3 months after initiation of antipsychotic; if LDL level is normal repeat at 2- to 5-year intervals or more frequently if clinically indicated); changes in menstruation, libido, development of galactorrhea, erectile and ejaculatory function (at each visit for the first 12 weeks after the antipsychotic is initiated or until the dose is stable, then yearly); abnormal involuntary movements or parkinsonian signs (baseline; repeat weekly until dose stabilized for at least 2 weeks after introduction and for 2 weeks after any significant dose increase); tardive dyskinesia (every 12 months; high-risk patients every 6 months); ocular examination (yearly in patients >40 years; every 2 years in younger patients) (ADA, 2004; Lehman, 2004; Marder, 2004).

Dosage Forms

Tablet, Oral:

Latuda: 20 mg, 40 mg, 60 mg, 80 mg, 120 mg

◆ **Lurasidone Hydrochloride** *see* Lurasidone *on page 1256*

◆ **Lustra** *see* Hydroquinone *on page 1020*

◆ **Lustra® (Can)** *see* Hydroquinone *on page 1020*

◆ **Lustra-AF** *see* Hydroquinone *on page 1020*

◆ **Lustra-Ultra** *see* Hydroquinone *on page 1020*

◆ **Luteinizing Hormone Releasing Hormone** *see* Gonadorelin [CAN/INT] *on page 980*

◆ **Lutera** *see* Ethinyl Estradiol and Levonorgestrel *on page 803*

◆ **Lutrepulse (Can)** *see* Gonadorelin [CAN/INT] *on page 980*

Lutropin Alfa [CAN/INT] (LOO troe pin AL fa)

Brand Names: Canada Luveris

Index Terms r-hLH; Recombinant Human Luteinizing Hormone

Pharmacologic Category Gonadotropin; Ovulation Stimulator

Use Note: Not approved in U.S.

Infertility: Stimulation of follicular development in infertile hypogonadotropic hypogonadal (HH) women with profound luteinizing hormone (LH) deficiency (<1.2 units/L); to be used in combination with follitropin alfa

Pregnancy Considerations Adverse events have been observed in animal reproduction studies. Ectopic pregnancy, miscarriage, spontaneous abortion, and multiple births have been reported. The incidence of congenital abnormality may be slightly higher after assisted reproductive techniques than with spontaneous conception; higher incidence may be related to parenteral characteristics (maternal age, sperm characteristics). Lutropin alfa is used to stimulate follicular development; use is contraindicated in women who are already pregnant.

Breast-Feeding Considerations It is not known if lutropin alfa is excreted into breast milk. Use in breast-feeding women is contraindicated per the manufacturer labeling.

Contraindications Hypersensitivity to lutropin alfa or any component of the formulation; primary ovarian failure; uncontrolled thyroid or adrenal dysfunction; active, untreated tumors of the hypothalamus and pituitary gland; ovarian, uterine, or breast cancer; abnormal uterine bleeding of undetermined origin; ovarian cyst or enlargement unrelated to polycystic ovarian disease and of undetermined origin; malformations of sexual organs incompatible with pregnancy; fibroid tumors of the uterus incompatible with pregnancy; pregnancy; breast-feeding

Warnings/Precautions These medications should only be used by physicians who are thoroughly familiar with infertility problems and their management. To minimize risks, use only at the lowest effective dose. Monitor ovarian response with serum estradiol and vaginal ultrasound on a regular basis.

Ovarian enlargement, which may be accompanied by abdominal distention or abdominal pain, generally regresses without treatment within 2 to 3 weeks; more common in women with polycystic ovarian syndrome. If ovaries are abnormally enlarged on the last day of treatment, withhold hCG to reduce the risk of ovarian hyperstimulation syndrome (OHSS). OHSS, an exaggerated response to ovulation induction therapy, is characterized by an increase in vascular permeability, which causes a fluid shift from intravascular space to third space compartments (eg, peritoneal cavity, thoracic cavity) (ASRM, 2008; SOGC-CFAS, 2011). This syndrome may begin within 24 hours of treatment, but may become most severe 7 to 10 days after therapy (SOGC-CFAS, 2011). OHSS is typically self-limiting with spontaneous resolution, although it may be more severe and protracted if pregnancy occurs (ASRM, 2008). Symptoms of mild/moderate OHSS may include abdominal distention/discomfort, diarrhea, nausea, and/or vomiting. Severe OHSS symptoms may include abdominal pain that is severe, acute respiratory distress syndrome, anuria/oliguria, ascites, dyspnea, hypotension, nausea/vomiting (intractable), pericardial effusions, tachycardia, or thromboembolism. Decreased creatinine clearance, hemoconcentration, hypoproteinemia, elevated liver enzymes, elevated WBC, and electrolyte imbalances may also be present (ASRM, 2008; Fiedler, 2012; SOGC-CFAS, 2011). If severe OHSS occurs, stop treatment and consider hospitalizing the patient. (ASRM, 2008; SOGC-CFAS, 2011). Treatment is primarily symptomatic and includes fluid and electrolyte management, analgesics, and prevention of thromboembolic complications (ASRM, 2008; SOGC-CFAS, 2011). The ascitic, pleural, and pericardial fluids may be removed if needed to relieve symptoms (eg, pulmonary distress, cardiac tamponade) (ASRM, 2008; SOGC-CFAS, 2011). Women with OHSS should avoid pelvic examination and/or intercourse (ASRM, 2008; SOGC-CFAS, 2011).

Thromboembolic events, both in association with and separate from OHSS, have been reported. Multiple births may result from the use of these medications; advise patient of the potential risk of multiple births before starting the treatment. Discontinuation of therapy is recommended if there is a high risk for multiple pregnancies. Use with caution in patients with renal or hepatic dysfunction. Gonadotropins may increase the risk of an acute porphyric attack in patients with porphyria or a family history of porphyria; discontinuation of therapy may be necessary with onset or worsening of condition. Benign and malignant neoplasms have been reported with multiple drug infertility treatment; causative association between gonadotropin therapy and increased risk of malignancy has not yet been established. Not indicated for use in females <16 years of age or >60 years of age.

Adverse Reactions

Central nervous system: Fatigue, headache, pain

Endocrine & metabolic: Increased serum cholesterol, ovarian cyst, ovarian disease, ovarian hyperstimulation

Gastrointestinal: Abdominal pain, constipation, diarrhea, flatulence, nausea

Genitourinary: Dysmenorrhea, mastalgia

Hepatic: Increased serum ALT, increased serum AST

Local: Injection site reaction

Respiratory: Upper respiratory tract infection

Rare but important or life-threatening: Anaphylaxis, breast hypertrophy, conjunctivitis, dental caries, depression, ectopic pregnancy, edema, hemorrhage (in pregnancy), herpes simplex infection, hypersensitivity reaction, infection, Klebsiella species, ovarian hyperstimulation syndrome, ovary enlargement, pelvic congestion syndrome, porphyria, shock, spontaneous abortion, thromboembolism, uterine spasm, vaginal hemorrhage, vaginitis, vasodilatation, vulvovaginal candidiasis

Drug Interactions

Metabolism/Transport Effects None known.

Avoid Concomitant Use There are no known interactions where it is recommended to avoid concomitant use.

Increased Effect/Toxicity There are no known significant interactions involving an increase in effect.

Decreased Effect There are no known significant interactions involving a decrease in effect.

Preparation for Administration Reconstitute lutropin alfa powder with 1 mL SWFI. Mix gently; do not shake. If bubbles appear, allow to settle prior to use. May add follitropin alfa to lutropin alfa vial and administer in the same syringe.

Storage/Stability

Powder for reconstitution: Store at 2°C to 25°C (36°F to 77°F). Protect from light. Use immediately after reconstitution.

Solution for injection: Store at 2°C to 8°C (36°F to 46°F). Do not freeze. Protect from light. After opening, store at 2°C to 8°C (36°F to 46°F) for up to 28 days.

Mechanism of Action Lutropin alfa is a recombinant luteinizing hormone prepared using Chinese hamster cell ovaries. Administration leads to increased follicular estradiol secretion needed for follicle stimulating hormone induced follicular development.

Pharmacodynamics/Kinetics

Distribution: V_{dss}: 10 to 14 L

Bioavailability: 56%

Half-life elimination: Terminal: 21 hours

Time to peak, serum: 9 hours

Excretion: Urine (<5% unchanged)

Dosage Infertility: Adults: Females (≥16 years to ≤60 years): SubQ: 75 units daily until adequate follicular development is noted (maximum dose: 75 units daily); maximum duration of treatment: 14 days, unless signs of imminent follicular development are present. Duration of stimulation may be extended in any one cycle up to 5 weeks (treatment should be individualized based on response to prior cycle). Administer concomitantly with follitropin alfa. Administer hCG one day after the last dose of lutropin alfa and follitropin alfa. Encourage patients to have daily intercourse beginning the day prior to hCG administration and until ovulation is apparent. If the ovaries are abnormally enlarged or if abdominal pain occurs, withhold hCG, discontinue lutropin alfa and follitropin alfa, and advise patient to avoid intercourse.

Dosage adjustment in renal impairment: There are no dosage adjustments provided in the manufacturer's labeling (has not been studied).

Dosage adjustment in hepatic impairment: There are no dosage adjustments provided in the manufacturer's labeling (has not been studied).

Administration SubQ: Administer in the stomach or thigh; rotate injection sites. Do not shake solution; allow any bubbles to settle prior to administration. Contents of lutropin alfa vial may be mixed in the same syringe with follitropin alfa. Refer to manufacturer labeling for instructions on how to use lutropin alfa prefilled syringe.

Monitoring Parameters

Prior to therapy: Baseline LH <1.2 units/L, FSH <5 units/L

Monitor sufficient follicular maturation. This may be directly estimated by sonographic visualization of the ovaries and endometrial lining or measuring serum estradiol levels. The combination of both ultrasonography and measurement of estradiol levels is useful for monitoring for the growth and development of follicles and timing hCG administration.

The clinical evaluation of estrogenic activity (changes in vaginal cytology and changes in appearance and volume of cervical mucus) provides an indirect estimate of the estrogenic effect upon the target organs and, therefore, it should only be used adjunctively with more direct estimates of follicular development (ultrasonography and serum estradiol determinations).

The clinical confirmation of ovulation is obtained by direct and indirect indices of progesterone production. The indices most generally used are: rise in basal body temperature, increase in serum progesterone, and menstruation following the shift in basal body temperature. Sonographic evidence of ovulation includes collapsed follicle, fluid in the cul-de-sac, ovarian stigmata, and secretory endometrium.

Monitor for signs and symptoms of OHSS for at least 2 weeks following hCG administration.

OHSS: Monitoring of hospitalized patients should include abdominal circumference, albumin, cardiorespiratory status, electrolytes, fluid balance, hematocrit, hemoglobin, serum creatinine, urine output, urine specific gravity, vital signs, weight (all daily or as necessary) and liver enzymes (weekly) (ASRM, 2008; SOGC-CFAS, 2011).

Product Availability Not available in the U.S.

Dosage Forms: Canada Excipient information presented when available (limited, particularly for generics); consult specific product labeling.

Solution Reconstituted, Subcutaneous:

Luveris: 75 units

Solution, Subcutaneous:

Luveris: 450 units/0.72 mL

- ◆ **Luveris (Can)** *see* Lutropin Alfa [CAN/INT] *on page 1259*
- ◆ **Luvox** *see* FluvoxaMINE *on page 916*
- ◆ **Luvox CR [DSC]** *see* FluvoxaMINE *on page 916*
- ◆ **Luxiq** *see* Betamethasone (Topical) *on page 255*
- ◆ **Luzu** *see* Luliconazole *on page 1256*
- ◆ **LY139603** *see* AtoMOXetine *on page 191*
- ◆ **LY146032** *see* DAPTOmycin *on page 563*
- ◆ **LY170053** *see* OLANZapine *on page 1491*
- ◆ **LY-188011** *see* Gemcitabine *on page 952*
- ◆ **LY231514** *see* PEMEtrexed *on page 1606*
- ◆ **LY246736** *see* Alvimopan *on page 104*
- ◆ **LY248686** *see* DULoxetine *on page 698*
- ◆ **LY303366** *see* Anidulafungin *on page 150*
- ◆ **LY333328** *see* Oritavancin *on page 1519*
- ◆ **LY570310** *see* Telaprevir *on page 1983*

◆ **LY-640315** *see* Prasugrel *on page 1699*

◆ **LY2148568** *see* Exenatide *on page 830*

◆ **LY2189265** *see* Dulaglutide *on page 697*

◆ **Lybrel** *see* Ethinyl Estradiol and Levonorgestrel *on page 803*

◆ **Lyderm® (Can)** *see* Fluocinonide *on page 894*

◆ **Lymphocyte Immune Globulin** *see* Antithymocyte Globulin (Equine) *on page 157*

◆ **Lymphocyte Mitogenic Factor** *see* Aldesleukin *on page 72*

Lynestrenol [INT] (lin ES tre nole)

International Brand Names Exlutena (SE); Exluton (AR, BE, CZ, FI, FR, LU, MX, NL, PT, ZA); Exlutona (CH, DE, NO); Orgametril (AT, BE, CH, CZ, DE, DK, ES, FI, FR, HU, IN, LU, NL, PT, SE)

Index Terms Lynoestrenol

Pharmacologic Category Progestin

Reported Use Treatment of endometriosis; prevention of pregnancy

Dosage Range Adults: Oral: One tablet daily

Product Availability Product available in various countries; not currently available in the U.S.

Dosage Forms

Tablet: 0.5 mg, 5 mg

◆ **Lynoestrenol** *see* Lynestrenol [INT] *on page 1261*

◆ **Lyrica** *see* Pregabalin *on page 1710*

◆ **Lysodren** *see* Mitotane *on page 1382*

◆ **Lysteda** *see* Tranexamic Acid *on page 2081*

◆ **Lyza** *see* Norethindrone *on page 1473*

◆ **Maalox [OTC]** *see* Calcium Carbonate *on page 327*

◆ **Maalox Advanced Maximum Strength [OTC]** *see* Aluminum Hydroxide, Magnesium Hydroxide, and Simethicone *on page 104*

◆ **Maalox Advanced Regular Strength [OTC]** *see* Aluminum Hydroxide, Magnesium Hydroxide, and Simethicone *on page 104*

◆ **Maalox Childrens [OTC]** *see* Calcium Carbonate *on page 327*

◆ **MabCampath (Can)** *see* Alemtuzumab *on page 75*

◆ **Macrobid** *see* Nitrofurantoin *on page 1463*

◆ **Macrodantin** *see* Nitrofurantoin *on page 1463*

◆ **Macrogol** *see* Polyethylene Glycol 3350 *on page 1674*

◆ **Macugen** *see* Pegaptanib *on page 1588*

Mafenide (MA fe nide)

Brand Names: U.S. Sulfamylon

Index Terms Mafenide Acetate

Pharmacologic Category Antibiotic, Topical

Use

Cream: Adjunctive antibacterial agent in the treatment of second- and third-degree burns

Solution: Adjunctive antibacterial agent for use under moist dressings over meshed autografts on excised burn wounds

Pregnancy Risk Factor C

Dosage Children and Adults: Topical:

Cream: Apply once or twice daily with a sterile-gloved hand; apply to a thickness of approximately 1/16 inch; the burned area should be covered with cream at all times

Solution: Cover graft area with 1 layer of fine mesh gauze. Wet an 8-ply burn dressing with mafenide solution and cover graft area. Keep dressing wet using syringe or irrigation tubing every 4 hours (or as necessary), or by moistening dressing every 6-8 hours (or as necessary). Irrigation dressing should be secured with bolster dressing and wrapped as appropriate. May leave dressings in place for up to 5 days.

Dosage adjustment for acidosis: Discontinuing treatment for 24-48 hours may aid in restoring acid-base balance

Additional Information Complete prescribing information should be consulted for additional detail.

Dosage Forms

Cream, External:

Sulfamylon: 85 mg/g (56.7 g, 113.4 g, 453.6 g)

Packet, External:

Sulfamylon: 50 g (1 ea, 5 ea)

Generic: 50 g (1 ea, 5 ea)

◆ **Mafenide Acetate** *see* Mafenide *on page 1261*

◆ **Mag-200 [OTC]** *see* Magnesium Oxide *on page 1265*

◆ **Mag-Al [OTC]** *see* Aluminum Hydroxide and Magnesium Hydroxide *on page 103*

Magaldrate and Simethicone

(MAG al drate & sye METH i kone)

Index Terms Riopan Plus; Simethicone and Magaldrate

Pharmacologic Category Antacid; Antiflatulent

Use Relief of hyperacidity associated with peptic ulcer, gastritis, peptic esophagitis, and hiatal hernia which are accompanied by symptoms of gas

Dosage Adults: Oral: 5-10 mL (540-1080 mg magaldrate) between meals and at bedtime

Additional Information Complete prescribing information should be consulted for additional detail.

Dosage Forms

Suspension, oral: Magaldrate 540 mg and simethicone 20 mg per 5 mL

◆ **Mag-Al Ultimate [OTC]** *see* Aluminum Hydroxide and Magnesium Hydroxide *on page 103*

◆ **Mag Citrate** *see* Magnesium Citrate *on page 1262*

◆ **Mag-Delay [OTC]** *see* Magnesium Chloride *on page 1261*

◆ **Mag-G [OTC]** *see* Magnesium Gluconate *on page 1263*

◆ **Maginex™ [OTC]** *see* Magnesium L-aspartate Hydrochloride *on page 1264*

◆ **Maginex™ DS [OTC]** *see* Magnesium L-aspartate Hydrochloride *on page 1264*

◆ **Magnesia Magma** *see* Magnesium Hydroxide *on page 1263*

◆ **Magnesium L-lactate Dihydrate** *see* Magnesium L-lactate *on page 1264*

◆ **Magnesium Carbonate and Aluminum Hydroxide** *see* Aluminum Hydroxide and Magnesium Carbonate *on page 103*

Magnesium Chloride (mag NEE zhum KLOR ide)

Brand Names: U.S. Chloromag; Mag-Delay [OTC]; Mag-SR Plus Calcium [OTC]; Mag-SR [OTC]; Slow Magnesium/Calcium [OTC]; Slow-Mag [OTC]

Pharmacologic Category Electrolyte Supplement, Oral; Electrolyte Supplement, Parenteral; Magnesium Salt

Use Correction or prevention of hypomagnesemia; dietary supplement

Pregnancy Risk Factor C

Dosage Note: Serum magnesium is poor reflection of repletional status as the majority of magnesium is intracellular; serum levels may be transiently normal for a few hours after a dose is given; therefore, aim for consistently high normal serum levels in patients with normal renal function for most efficient repletion.

Dietary supplement: Adults: Oral (Mag 64®, Mag Delay™, Slow-Mag®): 2 tablets once daily

Parenteral nutrition supplementation: IV (elemental magnesium):

Children:

<50 kg: 0.3-0.5 mEq/kg/day

>50 kg: 10-30 mEq/day

Adults: 8-24 mEq/day

RDA (elemental magnesium) (IOM, 1997):

Children:

1-3 years: 80 mg/day

4-8 years: 130 mg/day

9-13 years: 240 mg/day

14-18 years:

Females: 360 mg/day

Pregnancy: 400 mg/day

Lactation: 360 mg/day

Males: 410 mg/day

Adults:

19-30 years:

Females: 310 mg/day

Pregnancy: 350 mg/day

Lactation: 310 mg/day

Males: 400 mg/day

≥31 years:

Females: 320 mg/day

Pregnancy: 360 mg/day

Lactation: 320 mg/day

Males: 420 mg/day

Dosage adjustment in renal impairment: CrCl <30 mL/minute: Use with caution; monitor for hypermagnesemia

Dosage adjustment in hepatic impairment: No dosage adjustment provided in manufacturer's labeling.

Additional Information Complete prescribing information should be consulted for additional detail.

Dosage Forms Considerations

1 g magnesium chloride = elemental magnesium 120 mg = magnesium 9.85 mEq = magnesium 4.93 mmol

Elemental magnesium 64 mg = magnesium 5.26 mEq = magnesium 2.62 mmol

Dosage Forms

Solution, Injection:

Chloromag: 200 mg/mL (50 mL)

Generic: 200 mg/mL (50 mL)

Tablet Delayed Release, Oral:

Mag-SR Plus Calcium [OTC]: 64-106 mg

Slow Magnesium/Calcium [OTC]: 64-106 mg

Slow-Mag [OTC]: 71.5-119 mg

Tablet Extended Release, Oral:

Mag-Delay [OTC]: 535 (64 mg) mg

Mag-SR [OTC]: 535 (64 mg) mg

Magnesium Citrate (mag NEE zhum SIT rate)

Brand Names: U.S. Citroma [OTC]

Brand Names: Canada Citro-Mag

Index Terms Citrate of Magnesia; Mag Citrate

Pharmacologic Category Laxative, Saline; Magnesium Salt

Use Relieves occasional constipation

Dosage Laxative: Oral: Solution:

Children:

2-6 years: 60-90 mL given once or in divided doses (maximum: 90 mL/24 hours)

6-12 years: 90-210 mL given once or in divided doses

Children ≥12 years, Adolescents, and Adults: 195-300 mL given once or in divided doses

Dosage adjustment in renal impairment: No dosage adjustment provided in manufacturer's labeling; however, magnesium is renally excreted. Use caution; accumulation of magnesium in renal impairment may lead to magnesium toxicity.

Additional Information Complete prescribing information should be consulted for additional detail.

Dosage Forms Considerations 1 g magnesium citrate ≈ elemental magnesium 160 mg = magnesium 13 mEq = magnesium 6.5 mmol

Dosage Forms

Solution, Oral:

Citroma [OTC]: 1.745 g/30 mL (296 mL)

Generic: 1.745 g/30 mL (296 mL)

Tablet, Oral:

Generic: 100 mg

◆ **Magnesium Gluceptate** *see* Magnesium Glucoheptonate [CAN/INT] *on page 1262*

Magnesium Glucoheptonate [CAN/INT]

(mag NEE zhum gloo koh HEP toh nate)

Brand Names: Canada Magnesium Glucoheptonate

Index Terms Magnesium Gluceptate

Pharmacologic Category Magnesium Salt

Use Note: Not approved in U.S.

Dietary supplement

Pregnancy Considerations Magnesium crosses the placenta; serum concentrations in the fetus are similar to those in the mother (Idama, 1998; Osada, 2002).

Breast-Feeding Considerations Magnesium is found in breast milk; concentrations remain constant during the first year of lactation and are not influenced by dietary intake under normal conditions. Magnesium requirements are the same in lactating and nonlactating females (IOM, 1997).

Contraindications Severe renal impairment and/or lesions

Warnings/Precautions Use magnesium with caution in patients with impaired renal function; accumulation of magnesium may lead to magnesium intoxication. Use is contraindicated in patients with severe renal impairment and/or lesions. Concurrent hypokalemia or hypocalcemia can accompany a magnesium deficit. Hypomagnesemia is frequently associated with hypokalemia and requires correction in order to normalize potassium.

Use with extreme caution in patients with myasthenia gravis or other neuromuscular disease. Hypermagnesemia may result in heart block; use with caution in patients with preexisting heart block.

Adverse Reactions Gastrointestinal: Diarrhea, nausea, vomiting

Drug Interactions

Metabolism/Transport Effects None known.

Avoid Concomitant Use

Avoid concomitant use of Magnesium Glucoheptonate with any of the following: Raltegravir

Increased Effect/Toxicity

Magnesium Glucoheptonate may increase the levels/effects of: Calcium Channel Blockers; Gabapentin; Neuromuscular-Blocking Agents

The levels/effects of Magnesium Glucoheptonate may be increased by: Alfacalcidol; Calcitriol; Calcium Channel Blockers

Decreased Effect

Magnesium Glucoheptonate may decrease the levels/effects of: Bisphosphonate Derivatives; Deferiprone; Dolutegravir; Eltrombopag; Gabapentin; Levothyroxine; Multivitamins/Fluoride (with ADE); Mycophenolate; Phosphate Supplements; Quinolone Antibiotics; Raltegravir; Tetracycline Derivatives; Trientine

The levels/effects of Magnesium Glucoheptonate may be decreased by: Trientine

Mechanism of Action Magnesium is important as a cofactor in many enzymatic reactions in the body involving protein synthesis and carbohydrate metabolism (at least 300 enzymatic reactions require magnesium). Actions on lipoprotein lipase have been found to be important in reducing serum cholesterol and on sodium/potassium ATPase in promoting polarization (eg, neuromuscular functioning).

Pharmacodynamics/Kinetics Excretion: Urine (as magnesium)

Dosage Note: Serum magnesium is poor reflection of repletional status as the majority of magnesium is intracellular; serum levels may be transiently normal for a few hours after a dose is given, therefore, aim for consistently high normal serum levels in patients with normal renal function for most efficient repletion.

RDA (elemental magnesium):

1-3 years: 80 mg/day
4-8 years: 130 mg/day
9-13 years: 240 mg/day
14-18 years:
Females: 360 mg/day
Pregnant females: 400 mg/day
Males: 410 mg/day
19-30 years:
Females: 310 mg/day
Pregnant females: 350 mg/day
Males: 400 mg/day
≥31 years:
Females: 320 mg/day
Pregnant females: 360 mg/day
Males: 420 mg/day

Hypomagnesemia: Adults: Oral: 1500-3000 mg (75-150 mg elemental magnesium) 1-3 times/day

Dosing adjustment in renal impairment:

Mild-to-moderate renal impairment: Use with caution; monitor serum magnesium levels carefully
Severe renal impairment: Use is contraindicated

Dietary Considerations Take with meals.

Administration Administer with meals.

Monitoring Parameters Serum magnesium levels should be monitored to avoid overdose; monitor for diarrhea

Reference Range Serum total magnesium: 1.5-2.3 mg/dL (SI: 0.62-0.95 mmol/L or 1.2-1.9 mEq/L); slightly different ranges are reported by different laboratories

Product Availability Not available in U.S.

Dosage Forms Considerations 1 g magnesium glucoheptonate = elemental magnesium 50 mg = magnesium 4.2 mEq = magnesium 2.1 mmol

Dosage Forms: Canada

Solution, oral: 100 mg/mL

◆ **Magnesium Glucoheptonate (Can)** *see* Magnesium Glucoheptonate [CAN/INT] *on page* 1262

Magnesium Gluconate

(mag NEE zhum GLOO koe nate)

Brand Names: U.S. Mag-G [OTC]; Magonate [OTC]

Pharmacologic Category Electrolyte Supplement, Oral; Magnesium Salt

Use Dietary supplement

Dosage RDA (elemental magnesium):

Children:
1-3 years: 80 mg/day
4-8 years: 130 mg/day
9-13 years: 240 mg/day
14-18 years:
Females: 360 mg/day
Pregnant females: 400 mg/day
Males: 410 mg/day
Adults:
19-30 years:
Females: 310 mg/day
Pregnant females: 350 mg/day
Males: 400 mg/day
≥31 years:
Females: 320 mg/day
Pregnant females: 360 mg/day
Males: 420 mg/day

Dosing in renal impairment: CrCl <30 mL/minute: Use with caution; monitor for hypermagnesemia

Additional Information Complete prescribing information should be consulted for additional detail.

Dosage Forms Considerations 1 g magnesium gluconate = elemental magnesium 54 mg = magnesium 4.5 mEq = magnesium 2.25 mmol

Dosage Forms

Liquid, Oral:

Magonate [OTC]: Magnesium carbonate equivalent to magnesium gluconate 1000 mg (54 mg elemental magnesium) per 5 mL (355 mL)

Tablet, Oral:

Mag-G [OTC]: 500 mg (27 mg elemental magnesium)
Magonate [OTC]: 500 mg (27 mg elemental magnesium)
Generic: Elemental magnesium 27.5 mg

Tablet, Oral [preservative free]:

Generic: 500 mg (27 mg elemental magnesium)

Magnesium Hydroxide

(mag NEE zhum hye DROKS ide)

Brand Names: U.S. Dulcolax Milk of Magnesia [OTC]; Milk of Magnesia Concentrate [OTC]; Milk of Magnesia [OTC]; Pedia-Lax [OTC]

Index Terms Magnesia Magma; Milk of Magnesia; MOM

Pharmacologic Category Antacid; Laxative; Magnesium Salt

Use Short-term treatment of occasional constipation and symptoms of hyperacidity, laxative

Dosage Oral:

Laxative:
Liquid:
Children: Magnesium hydroxide 400 mg/5 mL: 1-3 mL/kg/day; adjust dose to induce daily bowel movement
OTC labeling:
<2 years: Use not recommended
2-5 years: Magnesium hydroxide 400 mg/5 mL: 5-15 mL/day once daily at bedtime or in divided doses
6-11 years:
Magnesium hydroxide 400 mg/5 mL: 15-30 mL/day once daily at bedtime or in divided doses
Magnesium hydroxide 800 mg/5 mL: 7.5-15 mL/day once daily at bedtime or in divided doses
Children ≥12 years and Adults:
Magnesium hydroxide 400 mg/5 mL: 30-60 mL/day once daily at bedtime or in divided doses
Magnesium hydroxide 800 mg/5 mL: 15-30 mL/day once daily at bedtime or in divided doses

Tablet: OTC labeling:
Children:
<3 years: Use not recommended
3-5 years: Magnesium hydroxide 311 mg/tablet: 2 tablets/day once daily at bedtime or in divided doses
6-11 years: Magnesium hydroxide 311 mg/tablet: 4 tablets/day once daily at bedtime or in divided doses
Children ≥12 years and Adults: Magnesium hydroxide 311 mg/tablet: 8 tablets/day once daily at bedtime or in divided doses
Antacid: OTC labeling:
Liquid: Children ≥12 years and Adults: Magnesium hydroxide 400 mg/5 mL: 5-15 mL as needed up to 4 times/day
Tablet:
Children <12 years: Use not recommended
Children ≥12 years and Adults: Magnesium hydroxide 311 mg/tablet: 2-4 tablets every 4 hours up to 4 times/day

Dosing in renal impairment: Patients in severe renal failure should not receive magnesium due to toxicity from accumulation. Patients with a CrCl <30 mL/minute receiving magnesium should be monitored by serum magnesium levels.

Additional Information Complete prescribing information should be consulted for additional detail.

Dosage Forms
Suspension, Oral:
Dulcolax Milk of Magnesia [OTC]: 400 mg/5 mL (355 mL)
Milk of Magnesia [OTC]: 400 mg/5 mL (355 mL, 473 mL, 480 mL, 769 mL); 1200 mg/15 mL (355 mL); 7.75% (30 mL, 355 mL, 360 mL, 473 mL, 480 mL)
Milk of Magnesia Concentrate [OTC]: 2400 mg/10 mL (10 mL, 100 mL, 400 mL)
Tablet Chewable, Oral:
Pedia-Lax [OTC]: 400 mg

- **Magnesium Hydroxide, Aluminum Hydroxide, and Simethicone** *see* Aluminum Hydroxide, Magnesium Hydroxide, and Simethicone *on page 104*
- **Magnesium Hydroxide and Aluminum Hydroxide** *see* Aluminum Hydroxide and Magnesium Hydroxide *on page 103*
- **Magnesium Hydroxide and Calcium Carbonate** *see* Calcium Carbonate and Magnesium Hydroxide *on page 328*

Magnesium Hydroxide and Mineral Oil
(mag NEE zhum hye DROKS ide & MIN er al oyl)

Brand Names: U.S. Phillips'® M-O [OTC]
Index Terms Haley's M-O; MOM/Mineral Oil Emulsion
Pharmacologic Category Laxative
Use Short-term treatment of occasional constipation
Dosage Oral: Laxative: OTC labeling:
Children <6 years: Use not recommended
Children 6-11 years: 20-30 mL at bedtime
Children ≥12 years and Adults: 45-60 mL at bedtime

Dosage adjustment in renal impairment: Patients in severe renal failure should not receive magnesium due to toxicity from accumulation. Patients with a CrCl <30 mL/minute should be monitored by serum magnesium levels.

Additional Information Complete prescribing information should be consulted for additional detail.

Dosage Forms
Suspension, oral:
Phillips'® M-O [OTC]: Magnesium hydroxide 300 mg and mineral oil 1.25 mL per 5 mL

Magnesium L-aspartate Hydrochloride
(mag NEE zhum el as PAR tate hye droe KLOR ide)

Brand Names: U.S. Maginex™ DS [OTC]; Maginex™ [OTC]
Index Terms MAH
Pharmacologic Category Electrolyte Supplement, Oral; Magnesium Salt
Use Dietary supplement
Dosage
Dietary Reference Intake for Magnesium: Dosage is in terms of elemental magnesium (IOM, 1997): Oral:
Children:
1-6 months: Adequate intake: 30 mg daily
7-12 months: Adequate intake: 75 mg daily
1-3 years: RDA: 80 mg daily
4-8 years: RDA: 130 mg daily
9-13 years: RDA: 240 mg daily
14-18 years: RDA:
Females: 360 mg daily
Pregnant females: 400 mg daily
Lactation: 360 mg daily
Males: 410 mg daily
Adults: RDA:
19-30 years:
Females: 310 mg daily
Pregnant females: 350 mg daily
Lactation: 310 mg daily
Males: 400 mg daily
≥31 years:
Females: 320 mg daily
Pregnant females: 360 mg daily
Lactation: 320 mg daily
Males: 420 mg daily

OTC labeling:
Dietary supplement (dosage in terms of magnesium-L-aspartate hydrochloride salt): Adults: Oral: One packet or 2 tablets (1230 mg) up to 3 times daily

Dosage adjustment in renal impairment: No dosage adjustment provided in manufacturer's labeling; however, magnesium is renally excreted. Use caution; accumulation of magnesium in renal impairment may lead to magnesium toxicity.

Additional Information Complete prescribing information should be consulted for additional detail.

Dosage Forms Considerations 1 g magnesium L-aspartate Hydrochloride ≈ elemental magnesium 100 mg = magnesium 8.1 mEq = magnesium 4.05 mmol

Dosage Forms
Granules for solution, oral [preservative free]:
Maginex™ DS [OTC]: 1230 mg/packet (30s)
Tablet, enteric coated, oral [preservative free]:
Maginex™ [OTC]: 615 mg

Magnesium L-lactate (mag NEE zhum el LAK tate)

Brand Names: U.S. Mag-Tab SR [OTC]
Index Terms Magnesium L-lactate Dihydrate
Pharmacologic Category Electrolyte Supplement; Magnesium Salt
Use Dietary supplement
Dosage
Dietary supplement: Oral: Adults: 1-2 caplets every 12 hours
RDA (elemental magnesium):
Children:
1-3 years: 80 mg/day
4-8 years: 130 mg/day
9-13 years: 240 mg/day

14-18 years:
Females: 360 mg/day
Pregnant females: 400 mg/day
Males: 410 mg/day
Adults:
19-30 years:
Females: 310 mg/day
Pregnant females: 350 mg/day
Males: 400 mg/day
≥31 years:
Females: 320 mg/day
Pregnant females: 360 mg/day
Males: 420 mg/day

Dosage adjustment in renal impairment: CrCl <30 mL/minute: Use with caution; monitor for hypermagnesemia

Additional Information Complete prescribing information should be consulted for additional detail.

Dosage Forms Considerations 1 g Magnesium L-lactate ≈ elemental magnesium 120 mg = magnesium 9.8 mEq = magnesium 4.9 mmol

Dosage Forms

Tablet Extended Release, Oral:
Mag-Tab SR [OTC]: Elemental magnesium 84 mg [7 mEq]

Magnesium Oxide (mag NEE zhum OKS ide)

Brand Names: U.S. Mag-200 [OTC]; Maox [OTC]; Uro-Mag [OTC]

Index Terms Mag Oxide

Pharmacologic Category Electrolyte Supplement, Oral; Magnesium Salt

Use Dietary supplement; relief of acid indigestion and upset stomach; short-term treatment of occasional constipation

Dosage

Dietary Reference Intake for Magnesium: Dosage is in terms of elemental magnesium (IOM, 1997): Oral:
Children:
1-6 months: Adequate intake: 30 mg daily
7-12 months: Adequate intake: 75 mg daily
1-3 years: RDA: 80 mg daily
4-8 years: RDA: 130 mg daily
9-13 years: RDA: 240 mg daily
14-18 years: RDA:
Females: 360 mg daily
Pregnant females: 400 mg daily
Lactation: 360 mg daily
Males: 410 mg daily
Adults: RDA:
19-30 years:
Females: 310 mg daily
Pregnant females: 350 mg daily
Lactation: 310 mg daily
Males: 400 mg daily
≥31 years:
Females: 320 mg daily
Pregnant females: 360 mg daily
Lactation: 320 mg daily
Males: 420 mg daily

OTC labeling:

Antacid (dosage in terms of magnesium oxide salt): Adults: Oral: Tablet: 1-2 tablets (400-800 mg) daily or in divided doses; maximum: 2 tablets daily

Dietary supplement (dosage in terms of magnesium oxide salt): Adults: Oral:
Mag-Ox 400®: Two tablets (800 mg) daily with food (maximum: 2 tablets/24 hours)
Uro-Mag®: 3-4 capsules (420-560 mg) daily with food

Laxative (dosage in terms of elemental magnesium): Children ≥12 years, Adolescents, and Adults: Oral: Caplet: 2-4 caplets (1000-2000 mg) at bedtime or in divided doses

Dosing in renal impairment: No dosage adjustment provided in manufacturer's labeling; however, magnesium is renally excreted. Use with caution; accumulation in renal impairment may lead to magnesium toxicity.

Additional Information Complete prescribing information should be consulted for additional detail.

Dosage Forms Considerations 400 mg magnesium oxide = elemental magnesium 240 mg = magnesium 19.9 mEq = magnesium 9.85 mmol

Dosage Forms

Capsule, Oral:
Uro-Mag [OTC]: 140 mg

Tablet, Oral:
Mag-200 [OTC]: 200 mg
Maox [OTC]: 420 mg
Generic: 250 mg, 400 mg, 420 mg

Tablet, Oral [preservative free]:
Generic: 400 mg, 500 mg

◆ **Magnesium Oxide, Sodium Picosulfate, and Citric Acid** *see* Sodium Picosulfate, Magnesium Oxide, and Citric Acid *on page 1911*

Magnesium Salicylate (mag NEE zhum sa LIS i late)

Brand Names: U.S. Doans Extra Strength [OTC]; Doans Pills [OTC]; MST 600

Pharmacologic Category Salicylate

Use Mild-to-moderate pain, fever, various inflammatory conditions; relief of pain and inflammation of rheumatoid arthritis and osteoarthritis

Dosage Oral:
Children ≥12 years and Adults: Relief of mild-to-moderate pain:
Doan's® Extra Strength, Momentum®: Two caplets every 6 hours as needed (maximum: 8 caplets/24 hours)
Keygesic: One tablet every 4 hours as needed (maximum: 4 tablets/24 hours)

Additional Information Complete prescribing information should be consulted for additional detail.

Dosage Forms

Tablet, Oral:
Doans Extra Strength [OTC]: 580 mg
Doans Pills [OTC]: 325 mg
MST 600: 600 mg

Magnesium Sulfate (mag NEE zhum SUL fate)

Brand Names: U.S. Epsom Salt [OTC]

Index Terms Epsom Salts; $MgSO_4$ (error-prone abbreviation)

Pharmacologic Category Anticonvulsant, Miscellaneous; Electrolyte Supplement, Parenteral; Magnesium Salt

Use

Treatment and prevention of hypomagnesemia; prevention and treatment of seizures in severe pre-eclampsia or eclampsia, pediatric acute nephritis; treatment of cardiac arrhythmias (VT/VF) caused by hypomagnesemia

OTC labeling: Soaking aid for minor cuts and bruises; laxative for the relief of occasional constipation

Pregnancy Risk Factor D

Pregnancy Considerations Magnesium crosses the placenta; serum concentrations in the fetus are similar to those in the mother (Idama, 1998; Osada, 2002). Continuous maternal use for >5-7 days (in doses such as those used for preterm labor, an off-label use) may cause fetal hypocalcemia and bone abnormalities, as well as fractures in the neonate. Magnesium sulfate injection is used for the prevention and treatment of seizures in pregnant or postpartum women with severe pre-eclampsia or eclampsia (ACOG, 2013). Magnesium sulfate may also be used prior to early preterm delivery to reduce the risk of cerebral palsy (ACOG, 2010; Reeves, 2011). Tocolytics may be used for the short-term (48 hour) prolongation of pregnancy to allow for the administration of antenatal steroids and should not be used prior to fetal viability or when the risks of use to the fetus or mother are greater than the risk of preterm birth; maintenance therapy with tocolytics is ineffective and not recommended. Magnesium sulfate injection may be used in conjunction with tocolytics for neuroprotection (it is not preferred for use as a tocolytic); however, an increased risk of maternal complications may be observed when used in combination with some tocolytic agents (ACOG, 2012).

Breast-Feeding Considerations Magnesium is found in breast milk; concentrations remain constant during the first year of lactation and are not influenced by dietary intake under normal conditions. Magnesium requirements are the same in lactating and nonlactating females (IOM, 1997). When magnesium sulfate is used in the intrapartum management of eclampsia, breast milk concentrations are generally increased for only ~24 hours after the end of treatment (Idama, 1998). The manufacturer recommends that caution be used if administered to nursing women.

Contraindications Hypersensitivity to any component of the formulation; heart block; myocardial damage; IV use for pre-eclampsia/eclampsia during the 2 hours prior to delivery

Warnings/Precautions Use magnesium with caution in patients with impaired renal function (accumulation of magnesium may lead to magnesium intoxication). Use with extreme caution in patients with myasthenia gravis or other neuromuscular disease. Magnesium toxicity can lead to fatal cardiovascular arrest and/or respiratory paralysis. The parenteral product may contain aluminum; toxic aluminum concentrations may be seen with high doses, prolonged use, or renal dysfunction. Premature neonates are at higher risk due to immature renal function and aluminum intake from other parenteral sources. Parenteral aluminum exposure of >4 to 5 mcg/kg/day is associated with CNS and bone toxicity; tissue loading may occur at lower doses (Federal Register, 2002). See manufacturer's labeling. Concurrent hypokalemia or hypocalcemia can accompany a magnesium deficit. Unlikely to effectively terminate irregular/polymorphic VT (with normal baseline QT interval) (Neumar, 2010).

Obstetric use: Vigilant monitoring and safe administration techniques (ISMP, 2005) recommended to avoid potential for errors resulting in toxicity. Monitor mother and fetus closely. Use longer than 5-7 days may cause adverse fetal events.

Self-medication (OTC Use): When used as a soaking aid, patients should not use if there is evidence of infection or prompt relief is not obtained. When used as a laxative, patients should consult a healthcare provider prior to use if they have: kidney disease; are on a magnesium-restricted diet; have abdominal pain, nausea, or vomiting; change in bowel habits lasting >2 weeks; have already used a laxative for >1 week

Adverse Reactions Adverse effects on neuromuscular function may occur at lower concentrations in patients with neuromuscular disease (eg, myasthenia gravis).

Cardiovascular: Flushing (IV; dose related), hypotension (IV; rate related), vasodilation (IV; rate related)

Endocrine & metabolic: Hypermagnesemia

Drug Interactions

Metabolism/Transport Effects None known.

Avoid Concomitant Use

Avoid concomitant use of Magnesium Sulfate with any of the following: Calcium Polystyrene Sulfonate; Raltegravir; Sodium Polystyrene Sulfonate

Increased Effect/Toxicity

Magnesium Sulfate may increase the levels/effects of: Calcium Channel Blockers; Calcium Polystyrene Sulfonate; CNS Depressants; Gabapentin; Neuromuscular-Blocking Agents; Sodium Polystyrene Sulfonate

The levels/effects of Magnesium Sulfate may be increased by: Alfacalcidol; Calcitriol; Calcium Channel Blockers

Decreased Effect

Magnesium Sulfate may decrease the levels/effects of: Bisphosphonate Derivatives; Deferiprone; Dolutegravir; Eltrombopag; Gabapentin; Levothyroxine; Multivitamins/Fluoride (with ADE); Mycophenolate; Phosphate Supplements; Quinolone Antibiotics; Raltegravir; Tetracycline Derivatives; Trientine

The levels/effects of Magnesium Sulfate may be decreased by: Trientine

Food Interactions Increased alcohol intake can deplete magnesium stores (IOM, 1997).

Preparation for Administration

IV: Dilute to a ≤20% solution for IV infusion.

IM: A 25% or 50% concentration may be used for adults and dilution to a ≤20% solution is recommended for children.

Oral: Dissolve granules in 8 ounces of water prior to administration.

Topical: Dissolve 2 cups of granules per gallon of warm water to use as a soaking aid.

Storage/Stability Prior to use, store at room temperature of 20°C to 25°C (68°F to 77°F). Do not freeze. Refrigeration of solution may result in precipitation or crystallization.

Mechanism of Action When taken orally, magnesium promotes bowel evacuation by causing osmotic retention of fluid which distends the colon with increased peristaltic activity; parenterally, magnesium decreases acetylcholine in motor nerve terminals and acts on myocardium by slowing rate of S-A node impulse formation and prolonging conduction time. Magnesium is necessary for the movement of calcium, sodium, and potassium in and out of cells, as well as stabilizing excitable membranes.

Intravenous magnesium may improve pulmonary function in patients with asthma; causes relaxation of bronchial smooth muscle independent of serum magnesium concentration.

Pharmacodynamics/Kinetics

Onset of action: Anticonvulsant: IM: 1 hour; IV: Immediate

Duration of anticonvulsant activity: IM: 3-4 hours; IV: 30 minutes

Distribution: Bone (50% to 60%); extracellular fluid (1% to 2%) (IOM, 1997)

Protein binding: 30%, to albumin

Excretion: Urine (as magnesium)

Dosage Dose represented as magnesium sulfate unless stated otherwise. **Note:** Serum magnesium is poor reflection of repletional status as the majority of magnesium is intracellular; serum concentrations may be transiently normal for a few hours after a dose is given, therefore, aim for consistently high normal serum concentrations in patients with normal renal function for most efficient repletion.

Note: 1 g of magnesium sulfate = 98.6 mg elemental magnesium = 8.12 mEq elemental magnesium = magnesium 4.06 mmol

Hypomagnesemia: Note: Treatment depends on severity and clinical status. In asymptomatic patients (when oral route is available), oral replacement therapy is a better replacement method than IV administration.

Children: IV, I.O.: 25-50 mg/kg/dose over 10-20 minutes (over several minutes for torsade de pointes); maximum single dose: 2000 mg (PALS, 2010)

Adults:

Mild deficiency: IM: Manufacturer's labeling: 1 g every 6 hours for 4 doses, or as indicated by serum magnesium concentrations

Mild-to-moderate (serum concentration 1-1.5 mg/dL): IV: 1-4 g (up to 0.125 g/kg), administer at ≤1 g/hour if asymptomatic; do not exceed 12 g over 12 hours (Kraft, 2005). **Note:** Additional supplementation may be required after the initial dose with replenishment occurring over several days.

Severe deficiency:

IM: Manufacturer's labeling: Up to 250 mg/kg within a 4-hour period

IV:

Severe (<1 mg/dL): 4-8 g (up to 0.1875 g/kg), administer at ≤1 g/hour if asymptomatic; in symptomatic patients, may administer ≤4 g over 4-5 minutes (Kraft, 2005)

With polymorphic VT (including torsade de pointes): IV push: 1-2 g (ACLS, 2010)

Obesity: Weight >130% of ideal body weight (IBW) or body mass index (BMI) ≥30 kg/m^2: When determining maximum per kg dose for replacement, some clinicians suggest using adjusted body weight (AdjBW) (Kraft, 2005).

AdjBW (men) = ([wt (kg) -IBW (kg)] x 0.3) + IBW

AdjBW (women) = ([wt (kg) -IBW (kg)] x 0.25) + IBW

Asthma (off-label use): IV (NAEPP, 2007):

Children: 25-75 mg/kg (maximum: 2 g)

Adults: 2 g

Eclampsia/pre-eclampsia (severe): Adults:

Manufacturer's labeling: IV: An initial total dose of 10-14 g administered as follows: 4 g infusion with simultaneous IM injections of 4-5 g in each buttock. After the initial IV/IM doses, may administer a 1-2 g/hour continuous infusion or may follow with IM doses of 4-5 g into alternate buttocks every 4 hours as necessary. Maximum: 40 g/24 hours. IV use for pre-eclampsia/eclampsia is contraindicated during the 2 hours prior to delivery.

Alternate dosing (off-label): IV: 4-6 g loading dose followed by 1-2 g/hour continuous infusion for at least 24 hours (ACOG, 2013)

Torsade de pointes or VF/pulseless VT associated with torsade de pointes (off-label use): Adults: IV, I.O.: 1-2 g over 15 minutes (ACLS, 2010)

Parenteral nutrition supplementation: IV:

Children:

<50 kg: 0.3-0.5 mEq elemental magnesium/kg/day (Mirtallo, 2004)

>50 kg: 10-30 mEq elemental magnesium daily (Mirtallo, 2004)

Adults: 8-24 mEq elemental magnesium daily

Laxative: Oral:

Children 6-12 years: 1-2 teaspoons of granules dissolved in water once daily

Children >12 years, Adolescents, and Adults: 2-6 teaspoons of granules dissolved in water once daily

Soaking aid: Topical: Adults: Dissolve 2 cupfuls of granules per gallon of warm water

RDA (IOM, 1997):

Children:

1-3 years: 80 mg elemental magnesium daily

4-8 years: 130 mg elemental magnesium daily

9-13 years: 240 mg elemental magnesium daily

14-18 years:

Females: 360 mg elemental magnesium daily

Pregnant females: 400 mg elemental magnesium daily

Breast-feeding females: 360 mg elemental magnesium daily

Males: 410 mg elemental magnesium daily

Adults:

19-30 years:

Females: 310 mg elemental magnesium daily

Pregnant females: 350 mg elemental magnesium daily

Breast-feeding females: 310 mg elemental magnesium daily

Males: 400 mg elemental magnesium daily

≥31 years:

Females: 320 mg elemental magnesium daily

Pregnant females: 360 mg elemental magnesium daily

Breast-feeding females: 320 mg elemental magnesium daily

Males: 420 mg elemental magnesium daily

Dosage adjustment in renal impairment:

Hypomagnesemia: Renal dysfunction: Reduce dose by 50% (Kraft, 2005). Use with caution; monitor for hypermagnesemia; Close monitoring is required.

Pre-eclampsia/eclampsia: Severe renal impairment: Per the manufacturer, do not exceed 20 grams during a 48 hour period.

Dosage adjustment in hepatic impairment: No dosage adjustment necessary.

Dietary Considerations Whole grains, legumes and dark-green leafy vegetables are dietary sources of magnesium (IOM, 1997).

Administration

Injection: May be administered IM or IV

IM: Must be diluted prior to administration for children (Adults: 25% or 50% concentration; Children: ≤20% diluted solution)

IV: Must be diluted to a ≤20% solution for IV infusion and may be administered IV push, IVPB, or continuous IV infusion. When giving IV push, must dilute first and should generally not be given any faster than 150 mg/minute; may administer over 1 to 2 minutes in patients with persistent pulseless VT or VF with known hypomagnesemia (Dager, 2006). ACLS guidelines recommend administration over 15 minutes in patients with torsade de pointes (ACLS, 2010). In patients not in cardiac arrest, hypotension and asystole may occur with rapid administration.

Maximal rate of infusion: Up to 50% of an IV dose may be eliminated in the urine, therefore, slower administration may improve retention (maximum rate: 1 g/hour in asymptomatic patients). For doses <6 g, infuse over 8 to 12 hours and for larger doses infuse over 24 hours if patient is asymptomatic. If patient is severely symptomatic (or has conditions such as preeclampsia or eclampsia) more aggressive therapy (≤4 g over 4 to 5 minutes) may be required; patients should be closely monitored (Kraft, 2005).

Oral: When used as a laxative, the patient should drink a full 8 ounces of liquid following each dose. Lemon juice may be added to the initial solution to improve the taste.

Topical: May dissolve granules to prepare a solution for use as a soaking aid or as a compress. To make a compress, use a towel to apply as a wet dressing.

Monitoring Parameters
IV: Rapid administration: ECG monitoring, vital signs, deep tendon reflexes; magnesium concentrations if frequent or prolonged dosing required particularly in patients with renal dysfunction, calcium, and potassium concentrations; renal function
Obstetrics: Patient status including vital signs, oxygen saturation, deep tendon reflexes, level of consciousness, fetal heart rate, maternal uterine activity.

Reference Range Serum magnesium: 1.5-2.5 mg/dL; slightly different ranges are reported by different laboratories

Dosage Forms Considerations
1 g of magnesium sulfate = elemental magnesium 98.6 mg = magnesium 8.12 mEq = magnesium 4.06 mmol

Magnesium sulfate 1% [10 mg/mL] in Dextrose 5% injection is equivalent to elemental magnesium 0.081 mEq/mL.
Magnesium sulfate 2% [20 mg/mL] in Dextrose 5% injection is equivalent to elemental magnesium 0.162 mEq/mL.
Magnesium sulfate 4% [40 mg/mL] in Water injection is equivalent to elemental magnesium 0.325 mEq/mL.
Magnesium sulfate 8% [80 mg/mL] in Water injection is equivalent to elemental magnesium 0.65 mEq/mL.
Magnesium sulfate 50% injection is equivalent to elemental magnesium 4 mEq/mL.

Dosage Forms
Capsule, Oral:
Generic: 70 mg
Granules, Oral:
Epsom Salt [OTC]: (454 g, 1810 g, 1816 g)
Solution, Injection:
Generic: 40 mg/mL (50 mL, 100 mL, 500 mL, 1000 mL); 80 mg/mL (50 mL); 50% (2 mL, 10 mL, 20 mL, 50 mL)
Solution, Intravenous:
Generic: 10 mg/mL (100 mL); 20 mg/mL (500 mL)

◆ **Magnesium Sulfate, Potassium Sulfate, and Sodium Sulfate** *see* Sodium Sulfate, Potassium Sulfate, and Magnesium Sulfate *on page 1914*

◆ **Magnesium Sulfate, Sodium Sulfate, and Potassium Sulfate** *see* Sodium Sulfate, Potassium Sulfate, and Magnesium Sulfate *on page 1914*

◆ **Magnesium Trisilicate and Aluminum Hydroxide** *see* Aluminum Hydroxide and Magnesium Trisilicate *on page 103*

◆ **Magonate [OTC]** *see* Magnesium Gluconate *on page 1263*

◆ **Mag Oxide** *see* Magnesium Oxide *on page 1265*

◆ **Mag-SR [OTC]** *see* Magnesium Chloride *on page 1261*

◆ **Mag-SR Plus Calcium [OTC]** *see* Magnesium Chloride *on page 1261*

◆ **Mag-Tab SR [OTC]** *see* Magnesium L-lactate *on page 1264*

◆ **MAH** *see* Magnesium L-aspartate Hydrochloride *on page 1264*

◆ **Makena** *see* Hydroxyprogesterone Caproate *on page 1021*

◆ **Malarone®** *see* Atovaquone and Proguanil *on page 198*

◆ **Malarone® Pediatric (Can)** *see* Atovaquone and Proguanil *on page 198*

Malathion (mal a THYE on)

Brand Names: U.S. Ovide
Pharmacologic Category Antiparasitic Agent, Topical; Pediculocide; Scabicidal Agent
Use Head lice infection: Topical treatment of *Pediculus humanus capitis* (head lice and their ova) of the scalp hair
Pregnancy Risk Factor B
Dosage Head lice (*Pediculus humanus capitis*): Children ≥6 years, Adolescents, and Adults: Topical: Apply sufficient amount to cover and thoroughly moisten dry hair and scalp; allow hair to dry naturally and shampoo after 8 to 12 hours. If required, repeat with second application in 7 to 9 days. Further treatment is generally not necessary.

Dosage adjustment in renal function impairment: There are no dosage adjustments provided in the manufacturer's labeling.
Dosage adjustment in hepatic function impairment: There are no dosage adjustments provided in the manufacturer's labeling.

Additional Information Complete prescribing information should be consulted for additional detail.
Dosage Forms
Lotion, External:
Ovide: 0.5% (59 mL)
Generic: 0.5% (59 mL)

◆ **Mandelamine® (Can)** *see* Methenamine *on page 1317*

◆ **Mandrake** *see* Podophyllum Resin *on page 1672*

◆ **Manerix (Can)** *see* Moclobemide [CAN/INT] *on page 1384*

Manganese (MAN ga nees)

Brand Names: U.S. Mangimin [OTC]; MN-50 [OTC]
Index Terms Manganese Chloride; Manganese Sulfate
Pharmacologic Category Dietary Supplement; Trace Element, Parenteral
Use Trace element added to total parenteral nutrition (TPN) solution to prevent manganese deficiency; orally as a dietary supplement
Pregnancy Risk Factor C
Dosage
Oral: **Adequate intake:**
0-6 months: 0.003 mg/day
7-12 months: 0.6 mg/day
1-3 years: 1.2 mg/day
4-8 years: 1.5 mg/day
9-13 years: Males: 1.9 mg/day; Females: 1.6 mg/day
14-18 years: Males: 2.2 mg/day; Females: 1.6 mg/day
Adults: Males: 2.3 mg/day; Females: 1.8 mg/day
Pregnancy: 2 mg/day
Lactation: 2.6 mg/day
IV:
Children: 2-10 **mcg**/kg/day usually administered in TPN solutions
Note: Use caution in premature neonates; manganese chloride solution for injection contains aluminum
Adults: 150-800 **mcg**/day usually administered in TPN solutions

Dosage adjustment in renal impairment: Use caution; manganese chloride solution for injection contains aluminum
Dosage adjustment in hepatic impairment: Use caution; dose may need to be decreased or withheld

Additional Information Complete prescribing information should be consulted for additional detail.
Dosage Forms
Capsule, Oral:
MN-50 [OTC]: Elemental manganese 16.67 mg
Solution, Intravenous:
Generic: Elemental manganese 0.1 mg/mL (10 mL)
Tablet, Oral:
Mangimin [OTC]: Elemental manganese 10 mg

Generic: Elemental manganese 15 mg, 50 mg [elemental manganese 5.7 mg], Elemental manganese 50 mg, 93 mg [elemental manganese 25 mg]

- ◆ **Manganese Chloride** *see* Manganese *on page 1268*
- ◆ **Manganese Sulfate** *see* Manganese *on page 1268*
- ◆ **Mangimin [OTC]** *see* Manganese *on page 1268*

Manidipine [INT] (ma NID i peen)

International Brand Names Artedil (ES); Caldine (PH); Calslot (JP); Iperten (FR, HU, IT); Kerdica (TH); Madipine (KR); Madiplot (TH); Manivasc (BR); Manyper (DE, GR); Vascoman (IT)

Index Terms Manidipine Dihydrochloride

Pharmacologic Category Calcium Channel Blocker

Reported Use Management of hypertension

Dosage Range Adults: Oral: Initial: 10 mg once daily; may increase to 20 mg once daily after 1-2 weeks if needed

Product Availability Product available in various countries; not currently available in the U.S.

Dosage Forms

Tablet, as dihydrochloride: 10 mg, 20 mg

- ◆ **Manidipine Dihydrochloride** *see* Manidipine [INT] *on page 1269*

Mannitol (MAN i tole)

Brand Names: U.S. Aridol; Osmitrol; Resectisol

Brand Names: Canada Osmitrol®

Index Terms *D*-Mannitol

Pharmacologic Category Diagnostic Agent; Diuretic, Osmotic; Genitourinary Irrigant

Use

Injection: Reduction of increased intracranial pressure associated with cerebral edema; reduction of increased intraocular pressure; promoting urinary excretion of toxic substances; genitourinary irrigant in transurethral prostatic resection or other transurethral surgical procedures

Note: Although FDA-labeled indications, the use of mannitol for the prevention of acute renal failure and/or promotion of diuresis is not routinely recommended (Kellum, 2008).

Genitourinary irrigation solution: Irrigation in transurethral prostatic resection or other transurethral surgical procedures

Powder for inhalation: Assessment of bronchial hyperresponsiveness

Pregnancy Risk Factor C

Pregnancy Considerations Reproduction studies have not been conducted.

Breast-Feeding Considerations It is not known if mannitol is excreted in breast milk. The manufacturer recommends that caution be exercised when administering mannitol to nursing women.

Contraindications

Injection: Hypersensitivity to mannitol or any component of the formulation; severe renal disease (anuria); severe dehydration; active intracranial bleeding except during craniotomy; progressive heart failure, pulmonary congestion, or renal dysfunction after mannitol administration; severe pulmonary edema or congestion

Genitourinary irrigation solution: Anuria

Powder for inhalation: Hypersensitivity to mannitol, gelatin, or any component of the formulation; conditions that may be compromised by induced bronchospasm or repeated spirometry (eg, aortic or cerebral aneurysm, uncontrolled hypertension, recent MI or cerebral vascular accident)

Warnings/Precautions Should not be administered until adequacy of renal function and urine flow is established; use 1-2 test doses to assess renal response. Excess amounts can lead to profound diuresis with fluid and electrolyte loss; close medical supervision and dose evaluation are required. Watch for and correct electrolyte disturbances; adjust dose to avoid dehydration. May cause renal dysfunction especially with high doses; use caution in patients taking other nephrotoxic agents, with sepsis or preexisting renal disease. To minimize adverse renal effects, adjust to keep serum osmolality less than 320 mOsm/L. Discontinue if evidence of acute tubular necrosis.

In patients being treated for cerebral edema, mannitol may accumulate in the brain (causing rebound increases in intracranial pressure) if circulating for long periods of time as with continuous infusion; intermittent boluses preferred. Cardiovascular status should also be evaluated; do not administer electrolyte-free mannitol solutions with blood. If hypotension occurs monitor cerebral perfusion pressure to ensure adequate. Vesicant (at concentrations >5%); ensure proper catheter or needle position prior to and during IV infusion; avoid extravasation of IV infusions.

Powder for inhalation (Aridol): **[U.S. Boxed Warning] Use may result in severe bronchospasm; use only for bronchial challenge testing. Testing should only be done by trained professionals. Not for use in patients with asthma or very low baseline pulmonary function. Medications (eg, short-acting inhaled beta-agonist) and equipment for the treatment of severe bronchospasm should be readily available.** Use with caution in patients with conditions that may increase sensitivity to bronchoconstriction (eg, severe cough, ventilatory impairment, spirometry-induced bronchoconstriction, hemoptysis of unknown origin, pneumothorax, recent abdominal, thoracic, or intraocular surgery, unstable angina, active upper or lower respiratory tract infection). Patients who have ≥10% reduction in FEV_1 on administration of the 0 mg capsule, patients with a positive response to bronchial challenge testing, or patients who develop significant respiratory symptoms should receive short acting inhaled beta-agonist; monitor until full recovery to baseline. Bronchial challenge testing should not be performed in children <6 years of age as these patients are unable to provide reliable spirometric results.

Adverse Reactions

Inhalation:

Cardiovascular: Chest discomfort

Central nervous system: Dizziness, headache

Gastrointestinal: Nausea, retching, throat irritation

Respiratory: Cough, dyspnea, pharyngolaryngeal pain, rhinorrhea, wheezing

Rare but important or life-threatening: FEV_1 decreased, gagging

Injection:

Cardiovascular: Chest pain, CHF, circulatory overload, hyper-/hypotension, peripheral edema, tachycardia

Central nervous system: Chills, convulsions, dizziness, fever, headache

Dermatologic: Bullous eruption, urticaria

Endocrine & metabolic: Fluid and electrolyte imbalance, dehydration and hypovolemia secondary to rapid diuresis, hyperglycemia, hypernatremia, hyponatremia (dilutional), hyperosmolality-induced hyperkalemia, metabolic acidosis (dilutional), osmolar gap increased, water intoxication

Gastrointestinal: Nausea, vomiting, xerostomia

Genitourinary: Dysuria, polyuria

Local: Pain, thrombophlebitis, tissue necrosis

Ocular: Blurred vision

Renal: Acute renal failure, acute tubular necrosis (adult dose >200 g/day; serum osmolality >320 mOsm/L)

Respiratory: Pulmonary edema, rhinitis

Miscellaneous: Allergic reactions

Drug Interactions

Metabolism/Transport Effects None known.

Avoid Concomitant Use

Avoid concomitant use of Mannitol with any of the following: Aminoglycosides

Increased Effect/Toxicity

Mannitol may increase the levels/effects of: Amifostine; Aminoglycosides; Antihypertensives; DULoxetine; Hypotensive Agents; Levodopa; Obinutuzumab; RisperiDONE; RiTUXimab; Sodium Phosphates

The levels/effects of Mannitol may be increased by: Alfuzosin; Analgesics (Opioid); Barbiturates; Brimonidine (Topical); Diazoxide; Herbs (Hypotensive Properties); MAO Inhibitors; Nicorandil; Pentoxifylline; Phosphodiesterase 5 Inhibitors; Prostacyclin Analogues

Decreased Effect

The levels/effects of Mannitol may be decreased by: Herbs (Hypertensive Properties); Methylphenidate; Yohimbine

Storage/Stability

Injection: Should be stored at room temperature of 15°C to 30°C (59°F to 86°F); do not freeze. In concentrations ≥15%, crystallization may occur at low temperatures; do not use solutions that contain crystals. Heating in a hot water bath and vigorous shaking may be utilized for resolubilization. Cool solutions to body temperature before using.

Irrigation: Store at room temperature of 25°C (77°F); excursions permitted up to 40°C. Avoid excessive heat; do not warm above 150°F (66°C). Do not freeze.

Powder for inhalation: Store at <25°C (<77°F); excursions permitted between 15°C to 30°C (59°F to 86°F). Do not freeze.

Mechanism of Action Produces an osmotic diuresis by increasing the osmotic pressure of glomerular filtrate, which inhibits tubular reabsorption of water and electrolytes and increases urinary output. Mechanism of action in reduction of intracranial pressure (ICP) is controversial. However, it is thought that mannitol reduces ICP by reducing blood viscosity which transiently increases cerebral blood flow and oxygen transport. This in turn reduces cerebral blood volume and ICP. Furthermore, mannitol reduces ICP by withdrawing water from the brain parenchyma and excretes water in the urine (Allen, 2009; Bratton, 2007; Miller, 2010).

Pharmacodynamics/Kinetics

Onset of action: Diuresis: Injection: 1-3 hours; Reduction in intracranial pressure: ~15-30 minutes

Duration: Reduction in intracranial pressure: 1.5-6 hours

Distribution: 34.3 L; remains confined to extracellular space (except in extreme concentrations); does not penetrate the blood-brain barrier (generally, penetration is low)

Metabolism: Minimally hepatic to glycogen

Bioavailability: Inhaled: 59% (relative to oral administration: 96%)

Half-life elimination: Terminal: 4.7 hours

Time to peak, plasma: Inhaled: 1.5 hours

Excretion: Urine (~55% to 87% as unchanged drug)

Dosage

Children: IV:

Increased intracranial pressure (off-label dosing): 0.25-1 g/kg/dose; repeat as needed to maintain serum osmolality <300-320 mOsm/kg (Adelson, 2003; Broderick, 2007; Hegenbarth, 2008)

Reduction of intraocular pressure: 1-2 g/kg or 30-60 g/m^2 administered over 30-60 minutes 1-1.5 hours prior to surgery

Reduction of intraocular pressure (traumatic hyphema): 1.5 g/kg administered over 45 minutes twice daily for IOP >35 mm Hg; may administer every 8 hours in patients with extremely high pressure (Crouch, 1999)

Children ≥6 years and Adults: Inhalation: Assessment of bronchial hyper-responsiveness: Administer in a stepwise fashion (measuring FEV_1 in duplicate after each administration) until the patient has a positive response or 635 mg of mannitol has been administered (whichever comes first).

Positive test: 15% reduction in FEV_1 from baseline or 10% incremental reduction in FEV_1 between consecutive doses

Negative test: Administration of full dose (635 mg) without reduction in FEV_1 sufficient to meet criteria for a positive test

Administration should be as follows:

Stepwise Administration Schedule

Dose #	Dose (mg)	Cumulative Dose (mg)	Capsules/Dose
1	0	0	1
2	5	5	1
3	10	15	1
4	20	35	1
5	40	75	1
6	80	155	2 x 40 mg caps
7	160	315	4 x 40 mg caps
8	160	475	4 x 40 mg caps
9	160	635	4 x 40 mg caps

Children ≥12 years and Adults:

IV:

Increased intracranial pressure, cerebral edema (off-label dosing): 0.25-1 g/kg/dose; may repeat every 6-8 hours as needed (Adelson, 2003; Bratton, 2007); maintain serum osmolality <300-320 mOsm/kg (Adelson, 2003; Rabinstein, 2006)

Reduction of intraocular pressure: 0.25-2 g/kg administered over 30-60 minutes 1-1.5 hours prior to surgery

Reduction of intraocular pressure (traumatic hyphema): 1.5 g/kg administered over 45 minutes twice daily for IOP >35 mm Hg; may administer every 8 hours in patients with extremely high pressure (Crouch, 1999)

Severe traumatic brain injury (off-label use): ~1.4 g/kg as initial management prior to neurosurgery with concurrent fluid replacement (Cruz, 2001; Cruz, 2002; Cruz, 2004)

Kidney transplant:

Donor: 12.5 g (with adequate hydration) prior to nephrectomy; may repeat (Morris, 2008)

Recipient: 50 g before kidney revascularization (Sprung, 2000; Tiggeler, 1984; van Valenberg, 1987; Weimar, 1983)

Topical: Transurethral irrigation: Use 5% urogenital solution as required for irrigation

Elderly: Refer to adult dosing. Consider initiation at lower end of dosing range.

Dosage adjustment in renal impairment: Contraindicated in severe renal impairment. Use caution in patients with underlying renal disease. May be used to reduce the incidence of acute tubular necrosis when administered prior to revascularization during kidney transplantation.

Dosage adjustment in hepatic impairment: No adjustment required.

Administration

IV: Concentration and rate of administration depends on indication/severity, or may be adjusted to urine flow. For cerebral edema or elevated ICP, administer over 30-60 minutes. Inspect for crystals prior to administration. If crystals are present, redissolve by warming solution. Use filter-type administration set for infusion solutions containing mannitol ≥20%. Do not administer with blood.

Crenation and agglutination of red blood cells may occur if administered with whole blood.

Vesicant (at concentrations >5%); ensure proper catheter or needle position prior to and during IV infusion. Avoid extravasation of IV infusions.

Extravasation management: If extravasation occurs, stop infusion immediately and disconnect (leave needle/cannula in place); gently aspirate extravasated solution (do **NOT** flush the line); initiate hyaluronidase antidote; remove needle/cannula; apply dry cold compresses (Hurst, 2004); elevate extremity.

Hyaluronidase: SubQ: Administer multiple 0.5-1 mL injections of a 15 units/mL solution around the periphery of the extravasation (Kumar, 2003).

Inhalation (Aridol): Administer using supplied single patient use inhaler; do not puncture capsule more than once; do not swallow capsules. A nose clip may be used if preferred. The patient should exhale completely, followed by a controlled rapid deep inspiration from the device; hold breath for 5 seconds and exhale through the mouth. Measure FEV_1 in duplicate 60 seconds after inhalation; repeat process until positive response or full dose (635 mg) has been administered.

Irrigation: Administer using only the appropriate transurethral urologic instrumentation.

Monitoring Parameters Renal function, daily fluid I & O, serum electrolytes, serum and urine osmolality; for treatment of elevated intracranial pressure, maintain serum osmolality in the range of 300-320 mOsm/kg (serum osmolality >320 mOsm/kg may increase the risk of acute renal tubular damage).

Bronchial challenge test: Standard spirometry prior to bronchial challenge test; FEV_1 in duplicate 60 seconds after administration of each step of test

Additional Information May autoclave or heat to redissolve crystals; mannitol 20% has an approximate osmolarity of 1100 mOsm/L and mannitol 25% has an approximate osmolarity of 1375 mOsm/L

Bronchial challenge testing: The dose of inhaled mannitol which causes a 15% reduction in FEV_1 is expressed as PD_{15}

Dosage Forms

Kit, Inhalation:

Aridol:

Solution, Intravenous:

Osmitrol: 5% (1000 mL); 10% (500 mL); 15% (500 mL); 20% (250 mL, 500 mL)

Generic: 5% (1000 mL); 10% (1000 mL); 15% (500 mL); 20% (250 mL, 500 mL); 25% (50 mL)

Solution, Intravenous [preservative free]:

Generic: 25% (50 mL)

Solution, Irrigation:

Resectisol: 5% (2000 mL)

- ◆ **Mantoux** *see* Tuberculin Tests *on page 2110*
- ◆ **Maox [OTC]** *see* Magnesium Oxide *on page 1265*
- ◆ **Mapap [OTC]** *see* Acetaminophen *on page 32*
- ◆ **Mapap Arthritis Pain [OTC]** *see* Acetaminophen *on page 32*
- ◆ **Mapap Children's [OTC]** *see* Acetaminophen *on page 32*
- ◆ **Mapap Extra Strength [OTC]** *see* Acetaminophen *on page 32*
- ◆ **Mapap Infant's [OTC]** *see* Acetaminophen *on page 32*
- ◆ **Mapap Junior Rapid Tabs [OTC]** *see* Acetaminophen *on page 32*
- ◆ **Mapap PM [OTC]** *see* Acetaminophen and Diphenhydramine *on page 36*
- ◆ **Mapezine (Can)** *see* CarBAMazepine *on page 346*

Maprotiline (ma PROE ti leen)

Brand Names: Canada Teva-Maprotiline

Index Terms Ludiomil; Maprotiline Hydrochloride

Pharmacologic Category Antidepressant, Tetracyclic

Use

Anxiety: Relief of anxiety associated with depression

Depression: Treatment of major depressive disorder (MDD)

Pregnancy Risk Factor B

Dosage

Depression or anxiety: Oral:

Adults: Initial: 25 to 75 mg once daily or in divided doses; increase gradually in 25 mg increments after 2 weeks based on response and tolerability. Usual dosage: 100 to 225 mg once daily or in divided doses; maximum dose: 225 mg daily. **Note:** Initial doses of 100 to 150 mg daily may be considered in severely depressed, hospitalized patients (APA, 2010; Bauer, 2013).

Elderly: Initial: 25 mg once daily; increase gradually in 25 mg increments after 2 weeks based on response and tolerability. Usual dose: 50 to75 mg once daily or in divided doses

Discontinuation of therapy: Upon discontinuation of antidepressant therapy, gradually taper the dose to minimize the incidence of withdrawal symptoms and allow for the detection of re-emerging symptoms. Evidence supporting ideal taper rates is limited. APA and NICE guidelines suggest tapering therapy over at least several weeks with consideration to the half-life of the antidepressant; antidepressants with a shorter half-life may need to be tapered more conservatively. In addition for long-term treated patients, WFSBP guidelines recommend tapering over 4-6 months. If intolerable withdrawal symptoms occur following a dose reduction, consider resuming the previously prescribed dose and/or decrease dose at a more gradual rate (APA, 2010; Bauer, 2002; Haddad, 2001; NCCMH, 2010; Schatzberg, 2006; Shelton, 2001; Warner, 2006).

MAO inhibitor recommendations:

Switching to or from an MAO inhibitor intended to treat psychiatric disorders:

Allow 14 days to elapse between discontinuing an MAO inhibitor intended to treat psychiatric disorders and initiation of maprotiline.

Allow 14 days to elapse between discontinuing maprotiline and initiation of an MAO inhibitor intended to treat psychiatric disorders.

Use with other MAO inhibitors (such as linezolid or IV methylene blue):

Do not initiate maprotiline in patients receiving linezolid or IV methylene blue; consider other interventions for psychiatric condition.

If urgent treatment with linezolid or IV methylene blue is required in a patient already receiving maprotiline and potential benefits outweigh potential risks, discontinue maprotiline promptly and administer linezolid or IV methylene blue. Monitor for serotonin syndrome for 2 weeks or until 24 hours after the last dose of linezolid or IV methylene blue, whichever comes first. May resume maprotiline 24 hours after the last dose of linezolid or IV methylene blue.

Dosage adjustment in renal impairment: There are no dosage adjustments provided in the manufacturer's labeling.

Dosage adjustment in hepatic impairment: There are no dosage adjustments provided in the manufacturer's labeling.

Additional Information Complete prescribing information should be consulted for additional detail.

Dosage Forms

Tablet, Oral:

Generic: 25 mg, 50 mg, 75 mg

- ◆ **Maprotiline Hydrochloride** *see* Maprotiline *on page 1271*
- ◆ **Mar-Allopurinol (Can)** *see* Allopurinol *on page 90*
- ◆ **Mar-Amlodipine (Can)** *see* AmLODIPine *on page 123*
- ◆ **Mar-Anastrozole (Can)** *see* Anastrozole *on page 148*

Maraviroc (mah RAV er rock)

Brand Names: U.S. Selzentry

Brand Names: Canada Celsentri

Index Terms UK-427,857

Pharmacologic Category Antiretroviral, CCR5 Antagonist (Anti-HIV)

Use HIV infection: Treatment of CCR5-tropic HIV-1 infection, in combination with other antiretroviral agents

Pregnancy Risk Factor B

Dosage Oral:

Adolescents ≥16 years (HHS [pediatric], 2014) and Adults: 300 mg twice daily (when administered concomitantly with tipranavir/ritonavir, nevirapine, raltegravir, all NRTIs and enfuvirtide)

Dosage adjustment for concomitant CYP3A inhibitors/inducers:

CYP3A inhibitors (with or without a CYP3A inducer): 150 mg twice daily; dose recommended when maraviroc administered concomitantly with strong CYP3A inhibitors including (but not limited to) protease inhibitors (excluding tipranavir/ritonavir), delavirdine, ketoconazole, itraconazole, clarithromycin, nefazodone, telithromycin, boceprevir, or telaprevir.

CYP3A inducers (without a strong CYP3A inhibitor): 600 mg twice daily; dose recommended when maraviroc administered concomitantly with CYP3A inducers including (but not limited to) efavirenz, etravirine, rifampin, carbamazepine, phenobarbital, and phenytoin

Dosage adjustment in renal impairment:

CrCl ≥30 mL/minute:

CrCl ≥30 mL/minute and concomitant potent CYP3A inhibitors (with or without a CYP3A inducer): 150 mg twice daily

CrCl ≥30 mL/minute and concomitant potent CYP3A inducer (without a CYP3A inhibitor): 600 mg twice daily

CrCl ≥30 mL/minute and other concomitant medications (eg, tipranavir/ritonavir, nevirapine, raltegravir, all NRTIs, and enfuvirtide): 300 mg twice daily

CrCl <30 mL/minute:

CrCl <30 mL/minute and concomitant potent CYP3A inhibitors (with or without a CYP3A inducer) **or** concomitant potent CYP3A inducer (without a CYP3A inhibitor): Not recommended

CrCl <30 mL/minute and other concomitant medications (eg, tipranavir/ritonavir, nevirapine, raltegravir, all NRTIs, and enfuvirtide): 300 mg twice daily. If postural hypotension occurs, reduce dose to 150 mg twice daily

CrCl <30 mL/minute and experiencing postural hypotension: Reduce dose to 150 mg twice daily

ESRD requiring intermittent hemodialysis (IHD):

With concomitant potent CYP3A inhibitors (with or without a CYP3A inducer) or concomitant potent CYP3A inducer (without a CYP3A inhibitor): Not recommended. **Note:** Hemodialysis has minimal effect on clearance.

With other concomitant medications (eg, tipranavir/ritonavir, nevirapine, raltegravir, all NRTIs, and enfuvirtide): 300 mg twice daily. If postural hypotension occurs, reduce dose to 150 mg twice daily. **Note:** Hemodialysis has minimal effect on clearance.

Dosage adjustment in hepatic impairment:

Mild-to-moderate impairment: Use caution; maraviroc concentrations are increased although dosage adjustment is not recommended.

Moderate impairment (with concomitant strong CYP3A inhibitor): Use caution; maraviroc concentrations may be increased; monitor closely for adverse events.

Severe impairment: No dosage adjustment provided in manufacturer's labeling (has not been studied).

Additional Information Complete prescribing information should be consulted for additional detail.

Dosage Forms

Tablet, Oral:

Selzentry: 150 mg, 300 mg

- ◆ **Marcaine** *see* Bupivacaine *on page 299*
- ◆ **Marcaine® (Can)** *see* Bupivacaine *on page 299*
- ◆ **Marcaine Preservative Free** *see* Bupivacaine *on page 299*
- ◆ **Marcaine Spinal** *see* Bupivacaine *on page 299*
- ◆ **Mar-Ciprofloxacin (Can)** *see* Ciprofloxacin (Systemic) *on page 441*
- ◆ **Mar-Citalopram (Can)** *see* Citalopram *on page 451*
- ◆ **Mar-Cof CG** *see* Guaifenesin and Codeine *on page 987*
- ◆ **Mar-Donepezil (Can)** *see* Donepezil *on page 668*
- ◆ **Mar-Escitalopram (Can)** *see* Escitalopram *on page 765*
- ◆ **Mar-Ezetimibe (Can)** *see* Ezetimibe *on page 832*
- ◆ **Margesic** *see* Butalbital, Acetaminophen, and Caffeine *on page 313*
- ◆ **Marine Lipid Concentrate [OTC]** *see* Omega-3 Fatty Acids *on page 1507*
- ◆ **Marinol** *see* Dronabinol *on page 694*
- ◆ **Marinol® (Can)** *see* Dronabinol *on page 694*
- ◆ **Mark 1** *see* Atropine and Pralidoxime *on page 203*
- ◆ **Mar-Letrozole (Can)** *see* Letrozole *on page 1181*
- ◆ **Marlissa** *see* Ethinyl Estradiol and Levonorgestrel *on page 803*
- ◆ **Mar-Metformin (Can)** *see* MetFORMIN *on page 1307*
- ◆ **Mar-Montelukast (Can)** *see* Montelukast *on page 1392*
- ◆ **Mar-Olanzapine (Can)** *see* OLANZapine *on page 1491*
- ◆ **Mar-Olanzapine ODT (Can)** *see* OLANZapine *on page 1491*
- ◆ **Mar-Ondansetron (Can)** *see* Ondansetron *on page 1513*
- ◆ **Marqibo** *see* VinCRIStine (Liposomal) *on page 2166*
- ◆ **Mar-Quetiapine (Can)** *see* QUEtiapine *on page 1751*
- ◆ **Mar-Ramipril (Can)** *see* Ramipril *on page 1771*
- ◆ **Mar-Risperidone (Can)** *see* RisperiDONE *on page 1818*
- ◆ **Mar-Rizatriptan (Can)** *see* Rizatriptan *on page 1836*
- ◆ **Mar-Sertraline (Can)** *see* Sertraline *on page 1878*
- ◆ **Mar-Simvastatin (Can)** *see* Simvastatin *on page 1890*
- ◆ **Mar-Tramadol/Acet (Can)** *see* Acetaminophen and Tramadol *on page 37*
- ◆ **Marvelon (Can)** *see* Ethinyl Estradiol and Desogestrel *on page 799*
- ◆ **Mar-Zopiclone (Can)** *see* Zopiclone [CAN/INT] *on page 2217*
- ◆ **Matulane** *see* Procarbazine *on page 1717*
- ◆ **Matzim LA** *see* Diltiazem *on page 634*

- **3M Avagard [OTC]** *see* Chlorhexidine Gluconate *on page 422*
- **Mavik** *see* Trandolapril *on page 2080*
- **Maxair Autohaler [DSC]** *see* Pirbuterol *on page 1662*
- **Maxalt** *see* Rizatriptan *on page 1836*
- **Maxalt-MLT** *see* Rizatriptan *on page 1836*
- **Maxalt RPD (Can)** *see* Rizatriptan *on page 1836*
- **MaxEPA [OTC]** *see* Omega-3 Fatty Acids *on page 1507*
- **Maxichlor PEH [OTC] [DSC]** *see* Chlorpheniramine and Phenylephrine *on page 426*
- **Maxichlor PEH DM [OTC] [DSC]** *see* Chlorpheniramine, Phenylephrine, and Dextromethorphan *on page 428*
- **Maxichlor PSE [OTC]** *see* Chlorpheniramine and Pseudoephedrine *on page 427*
- **Maxichlor PSE DM [OTC] [DSC]** *see* Chlorpheniramine, Pseudoephedrine, and Dextromethorphan *on page 428*
- **Maxidex** *see* Dexamethasone (Ophthalmic) *on page 602*
- **Maxidol (Can)** *see* Naproxen *on page 1427*
- **Maxidone [DSC]** *see* Hydrocodone and Acetaminophen *on page 1012*
- **Maxifed [OTC]** *see* Guaifenesin and Pseudoephedrine *on page 989*
- **Maxifed-G [OTC] [DSC]** *see* Guaifenesin and Pseudoephedrine *on page 989*
- **Maxilene (Can)** *see* Lidocaine (Topical) *on page 1211*
- **Maximum Strength Pepcid AC (Can)** *see* Famotidine *on page 845*
- **Maxipime** *see* Cefepime *on page 378*
- **Maxitrol®** *see* Neomycin, Polymyxin B, and Dexamethasone *on page 1437*
- **Maxzide** *see* Hydrochlorothiazide and Triamterene *on page 1012*
- **Maxzide-25** *see* Hydrochlorothiazide and Triamterene *on page 1012*
- **May Apple** *see* Podophyllum Resin *on page 1672*
- **M-Clear** *see* Guaifenesin and Codeine *on page 987*
- **M-Clear WC** *see* Guaifenesin and Codeine *on page 987*
- **MCV** *see* Meningococcal (Groups A / C / Y and W-135) Diphtheria Conjugate Vaccine *on page 1289*
- **MCV4** *see* Meningococcal (Groups A / C / Y and W-135) Diphtheria Conjugate Vaccine *on page 1289*
- **MDL 73,147EF** *see* Dolasetron *on page 663*
- **MDV3100** *see* Enzalutamide *on page 733*
- **MDX-010** *see* Ipilimumab *on page 1106*
- **MDX-1106** *see* Nivolumab *on page 1469*
- **MDX-CTLA-4** *see* Ipilimumab *on page 1106*

Measles, Mumps, and Rubella Virus Vaccine (MEE zels, mumpz & roo BEL a VYE rus vak SEEN)

Brand Names: U.S. M-M-R II

Brand Names: Canada M-M-R II; Priorix

Index Terms MMR; Mumps, Measles and Rubella Vaccines; Rubella, Measles and Mumps Vaccines

Pharmacologic Category Vaccine, Live (Viral)

Additional Appendix Information

Immunization Administration Recommendations *on page 2250*

Immunization Recommendations *on page 2255*

Use Measles, mumps, and rubella prophylaxis

The Advisory Committee on Immunization Practices (ACIP) recommends routine vaccination for the following (CDC/ACIP [McLean, 2013]):

- All children (first dose given at 12 to 15 months of age)
- Adults born 1957 or later (without evidence of immunity or documentation of vaccination). Vaccine may be given to adults born prior to 1957 if they do not have contraindications to the MMR vaccine.
- Adults at higher risk for exposure to and transmission of measles mumps and rubella should receive special consideration for vaccination, unless an acceptable evidence of immunity exists. This includes international travelers, persons attending colleges and other post high school education, persons working in healthcare facilities.

Pregnancy Risk Factor C

Dosage SubQ: **Note:** The minimum interval between 2 doses of MMR vaccine is 28 days (CDC/ACIP [McLean, 2013]).

Infants 6 to 11 months: 0.5 mL per dose

International travel: Children without evidence of immunity traveling internationally should receive 1 dose of MMR before departure from the United States; these children should be revaccinated with 2 doses of MMR with the first dose between 12 to 15 months of age (and at least 28 days after the previous dose) and the second dose at least 28 days later (CDC/ACIP [Akinsanya-Beysolow, 2014]; CDC/ACIP [McLean, 2013]).

Measles outbreak: If there is risk of exposure to measles involving infants, one dose of MMR vaccine may be administered (CDC/ACIP [McLean, 2013]).

Children ≥12 months and Adolescents: 0.5 mL per dose

Primary immunization is recommended at 12 to 15 months of age and repeated at 4 to 6 years of age; the second dose is recommended prior to entering kindergarten or first grade. The second dose may be administered at any time provided at least 28 days have elapsed since the first dose (CDC/ACIP [McLean, 2013]).

HIV infection without evidence of MMR immunity: Children and adolescents with HIV infection and without evidence of severe immunosuppression should have 2 doses of MMR. Those with perinatal HIV infection who were vaccinated prior to effective ART should have 2 additional doses of MMR once ART is established (CDC/ACIP [McLean, 2013]).

Household/close contacts of immunocompromised persons: Two doses of MMR administered at least 28 days apart unless they have acceptable evidence of immunity (CDC/ACIP [McLean, 2013]).

International travel: Children without evidence of immunity traveling internationally should receive 2 doses of MMR before departure from the United States. The second dose 28 days later (CDC/ACIP [McLean, 2013]).

Measles or mumps outbreak: Children ages 1 to 4 years who received 1 dose of MMR should be considered for a second dose if the outbreak involves preschool-aged children (CDC/ACIP [McLean, 2013]).

Adults: 0.5 mL per dose; 1 or 2 doses administered at least 28 days apart based upon the following criteria (CDC/ACIP [McLean, 2013]):

Adults born in or after 1957 should be vaccinated unless they have acceptable evidence of immunity.

Adults born prior to 1957 are considered immune to measles, mumps, and rubella but may be vaccinated if they do not have contraindications to the vaccine. Pregnant adults born prior to 1957 are not considered immune to rubella.

Healthcare personnel: Persons born in or after 1957 should have 2 doses of vaccine unless they have acceptable evidence of immunity. Unvaccinated persons born prior to 1957 should also consider vaccination with 2 doses unless they have laboratory evidence or laboratory confirmation of disease.

HIV infection (without severe immunosuppression): Two doses of MMR unless there is acceptable evidence of immunity.

Household/close contacts of immunocompromised persons: Two doses of MMR unless there is acceptable evidence of immunity.

International travelers: Two doses of MMR prior to travel unless there is acceptable evidence of immunity.

Measles, mumps, or rubella outbreak (community): Adults who received 1 dose of MMR should be considered for a second dose if the outbreak involves measles or mumps in adults. Vaccination should also be considered for persons born prior to 1957 without evidence of immunity who may be exposed to mumps. A single dose of a rubella-containing vaccine is considered adequate vaccination during a rubella outbreak.

Measles, mumps, or rubella outbreak (healthcare facility): Unvaccinated health care personnel without evidence of immunity regardless of birth year should receive 2 doses during a measles or mumps outbreak and one dose during a rubella outbreak.

Students: Persons entering post-high school educational facilities should receive 2 doses of MMR unless they have acceptable evidence of immunity prior to enrollment.

Women of childbearing potential: One dose of MMR unless they have acceptable evidence of immunity. Vaccination should not be given during pregnancy and pregnancy should be avoided for 28 days after vaccine administration.

Dosage adjustment in renal impairment: There are no dosage adjustments provided in manufacturer's labeling.

Dosage adjustment in hepatic impairment: There are no dosage adjustments provided in manufacturer's labeling.

Additional Information Complete prescribing information should be consulted for additional detail.

Dosage Forms

Injection, powder for reconstitution [preservative free]:
M-M-R II: Measles virus ≥1000 $TCID_{50}$, mumps virus ≥20,000 $TCID_{50}$, and rubella virus ≥1000 $TCID_{50}$

Measles, Mumps, Rubella, and Varicella Virus Vaccine

(MEE zels, mumpz, roo BEL a, & var i SEL a VYE rus vak SEEN)

Brand Names: U.S. ProQuad

Brand Names: Canada Priorix-Tetra

Index Terms MMRV; Mumps, Rubella, Varicella, and Measles Vaccine; Rubella, Varicella, Measles, and Mumps Vaccine; Varicella, Measles, Mumps, and Rubella Vaccine

Pharmacologic Category Vaccine, Live (Viral)

Additional Appendix Information

Immunization Administration Recommendations *on page 2250*

Immunization Recommendations *on page 2255*

Use

Measles, mumps, rubella, and varicella vaccination: To provide active immunization for the prevention of measles, mumps, rubella, and varicella in children 12 months to 12 years of age.

The Advisory Committee on Immunization Practices (ACIP) recommends routine vaccination against measles, mumps, rubella, and varicella in healthy children; the first dose should be given at 12-15 months of age and the second dose at 4-6 years of age. For children receiving their first dose at 12-47 months of age, either the MMRV combination vaccine or separate MMR and varicella vaccines can be used. (The ACIP prefers administration of separate MMR and varicella vaccines as the first dose in this age group unless the parent or caregiver expresses preference for the MMRV combination.) For children receiving the first dose at ≥48 months or their second dose at any age, use of MMRV is preferred. For children with a personal or family history of seizures, the ACIP recommends vaccination with separate MMR and varicella vaccines, as opposed to the MMRV combination vaccine (CDC, 2010).

Canadian labeling (not in U.S. labeling): MMRV combination vaccine is approved for use in healthy children 9 months to 6 years; may consider use in healthy children ≤12 years of age based upon prior experience with the separate component (live-attenuated MMR or live-attenuated varicella [OKA-strain]) vaccines.

Dosage *U.S. labeling:* SubQ: Children 12 months to 12 years: One dose (0.5 mL). The first dose is usually administered at 12-15 months of age. If a second dose of measles, mumps, rubella, and varicella vaccine is needed, ProQuad can be used with the second dose usually administered at 4-6 years of age. At least 1 month should elapse between a previous dose of a measles-containing vaccine (eg, MMR) and at least 3 months should elapse between a dose of varicella-containing vaccine.

ACIP recommendations: For children receiving their first dose at 12-47 months of age, either the MMRV combination vaccine or separate MMR and varicella vaccines can be used. (The ACIP prefers administration of separate MMR and varicella vaccines as the first dose in this age group unless the parent or caregiver expresses preference for the MMRV combination.) For children receiving the first dose at ≥48 months or their second dose at any age, use of MMRV is preferred. The ACIP recommends that children with a personal or family history of seizures be vaccinated with separate MMR and varicella vaccines, as opposed to the MMRV combination vaccine (CDC, 2010)

Canadian labeling: IM, SubQ: Children 9 months to 6 years: Two doses (0.5 mL each dose) administered at least 4-6 weeks apart (minimum interval between doses: 4 weeks)

Dosage adjustment in renal impairment: No dosage adjustment provided in manufacturer's labeling.

Dosage adjustment in hepatic impairment: No dosage adjustment provided in manufacturer's labeling.

Additional Information Complete prescribing information should be consulted for additional detail.

Dosage Forms

Injection, powder for reconstitution [preservative free]:
ProQuad: Measles virus ≥3.00 log_{10} $TCID_{50}$, mumps virus ≥4.30 log_{10} $TCID_{50}$, rubella virus ≥3.00 log_{10} $TCID_{50}$, and varicella virus ≥3.99 log_{10} PFU

Dosage Forms: Canada

Injection, powder for reconstitution [preservative free]:
Priorix-Tetra (CAN): Measles virus ≥3.00 log_{10} $CCID_{50}$, mumps virus ≥4.4 log_{10} $CCID_{50}$, rubella virus ≥3.00 log_{10} $CCID_{50}$, and varicella virus ≥3.3 log_{10} PFU

Mebendazole [CAN/INT] (me BEN da zole)

Brand Names: Canada Vermox

Index Terms Vermox

Pharmacologic Category Anthelmintic

Use Note: Not approved in U.S.

Treatment of *Ancylostoma duodenale* or *Necator americanus* (hookworms), *Ascaris lumbricoides* (roundworms), *Enterobius vermicularis* (pinworms), *Strongyloides stercoralis* (roundworm), *Taenia solium* (tapeworms), *Trichuris trichiura* (whipworms)

Pregnancy Risk Factor C

Pregnancy Considerations Adverse events have been observed in animal reproduction studies; adverse pregnancy outcomes have not been observed following use in pregnancy (Diav-Citrin, 2003; Gyorkos, 2006). Treatment of pinworm in pregnancy may be considered; however, the CDC suggests postponing therapy until the third trimester when possible (CDC, 2010).

Breast-Feeding Considerations Since only 2% to 10% of mebendazole is absorbed, it is unlikely that it is excreted in breast milk in significant quantities (CDC, 2010)

Contraindications Hypersensitivity to mebendazole or any component of the formulation

Warnings/Precautions Use with caution in hepatic impairment; systemic exposure may be increased. Not effective for hydatid disease. Neutropenia and agranulocytosis have been reported with high doses and prolonged use. Concomitant use with metronidazole should be avoided; may increase the risk of adverse events including Stevens-Johnson syndrome and toxic epidermal necrolysis. Experience with use in children <2 years of age is limited; convulsions in infants <1 year have been reported (rare) postmarketing.

Adverse Reactions

Central nervous system: Dizziness, drowsiness, headache, seizure

Dermatologic: Alopecia, angioedema, exanthema, itching, rash, Stevens-Johnson syndrome, toxic epidermal necrolysis, urticaria

Gastrointestinal: Abdominal pain, diarrhea, vomiting

Hematologic: Agranulocytosis, eosinophilia, hemoglobin decreased, leukopenia, neutropenia

Hepatic: Alkaline phosphatase increased, ALT increased, AST increased, GGT increased, hepatitis

Renal: BUN increased, cylindruria, glomerulonephritis, hematuria

Miscellaneous: Hypersensitivity reactions (anaphylactic, anaphylactoid)

Drug Interactions

Metabolism/Transport Effects None known.

Avoid Concomitant Use

Avoid concomitant use of Mebendazole with any of the following: MetroNIDAZOLE (Systemic)

Increased Effect/Toxicity

Mebendazole may increase the levels/effects of: MetroNIDAZOLE (Systemic)

The levels/effects of Mebendazole may be increased by: Cimetidine

Decreased Effect

The levels/effects of Mebendazole may be decreased by: Aminoquinolines (Antimalarial); CarBAMazepine; Fosphenytoin; Phenytoin

Food Interactions Mebendazole serum levels may be increased if taken with food. Management: Administer without regard to meals.

Storage/Stability Store at 15°C to 30°C (59°F to 86°F). Protect from light.

Mechanism of Action Inhibits the formation of helminth microtubules; selectively and irreversibly blocks glucose uptake and other nutrients in susceptible adult intestine-dwelling helminths

Pharmacodynamics/Kinetics

Distribution: V_d: 1-2 L/kg; to liver, fat, muscle, plasma, and hepatic cysts

Protein binding: 90% to 95%

Metabolism: Extensively hepatic

Bioavailability: ~20%

Half-life elimination: 3-6 hours

Time to peak, serum: 2-4 hours

Excretion: Primarily feces; urine (~2%)

Dosage Oral: Children ≥2 years; Adolescents, and Adults:

Canadian labeling:

Ancylostoma duodenale (hookworm), *Necator americanus* (hookworm), *Ascaris lumbricoides* (roundworm), *Strongyloides stercoralis* (roundworm), *Taenia solium* (tapeworms), *Trichuris trichiura* (whipworm), mixed infection: 100 mg twice daily for 3 days; repeat in 3 weeks if not cured with initial treatment

Enterobius vermicularis (pinworm): 100 mg as a single dose; repeat in 2 and 4 weeks (manufacturer's labeling); treatment should include family members in close contact with patient (*Med Lett*, 2007)

Off-label dosing:

Ancylostoma duodenale (hookworm), *Ascaris lumbricoides* (roundworm), *Necator americanus* (hookworm), *Trichuris trichiura* (whipworm): 500 mg as a single dose (*Med Lett*, 2007)

Off-label uses:

Ancylostoma caninum (eosinophilic enterocolitis): 100 mg twice daily for 3 days (*Med Lett*, 2007)

Capillaria philippinensis (capillariasis): 200 mg twice daily for 20 days (*Med Lett*, 2007)

Giardia duodenalis (giardiasis): 200 mg 3 times daily for 5 days (Canete, 2006; Chandy, 2009)

Mansonella perstans (filariasis): 100 mg twice daily for 30 days (*Med Lett*, 2007)

Visceral larva migrans (toxocariasis): 100-200 mg twice daily for 5 days (*Med Lett*, 2007)

Dosage adjustment in renal impairment: No dosage adjustment provided in manufacturer's labeling.

Dosage adjustment in hepatic impairment: No dosage adjustment provided in manufacturer's labeling; however, undergoes extensive hepatic metabolism; use with caution as systemic exposure may be increased.

Administration Tablets may be chewed, swallowed whole, or crushed and mixed with food. Tablets may be administered with or without food.

Monitoring Parameters Periodic hematologic, hepatic, and renal function; check for helminth ova in feces within 3-4 weeks following the initial therapy

Product Availability Not available in U.S.

Dosage Forms: Canada

Tablet, oral:

Vermox® 100 mg

Mebeverine [INT] (me BEV er een)

International Brand Names Arluy (MX); Bevacol (JO, LB, SA); Bevispas (ZA); Colese (AU); Colofac (AT, AU, GB, IE, PK, TH, ZA); Colopriv (FR); Colospa (ID, IN); Colospa Retard (HR); Colospasmin (AE, BH, EG, KW, QA, RO); Colotal (IL); Cuspa (IN); Doloverina (PY); Duspamen (SA); Duspatal (CL, DE, IT, NL, PT); Duspatalin (AE, AR, BE, BH, BR, CH, CN, CY, CZ, DK, ES, FR, HK, HN, HU, ID, JO, KR, KW, LT, LU, MX, MY, PE, PH, PY, QA, RO, SA, SK, TW, UY, VN); Duspatalin Retard (CO, EC, LB); Duspatin (TH); Irbosyd (ID); MBC (IN); Mebagen (SA); Mebemerck (DE); Mebemint (CO); Mebetin (HK, MY, SG); Mebeverine EG (BE); Mebeverine Hydrochloride (GB); Mebrin (IN); Menosor (TH); Merverin (UY); Meva (SA); Meverina (PY); Rudakol (HR); Spasmonal (BE, LU); Spasmopriv (FR); Spasmotalin (SA); Verimed (VN); Verine (AE, SA); Verine SR (QA)

Index Terms Mebeverine Hydrochloride

Pharmacologic Category Antispasmodic Agent, Gastrointestinal

Reported Use Treatment of irritable bowel syndrome

Dosage Range Adults: Oral: 100-135 mg 3 times/day before meals or 200 mg 2 times/day (modified release capsule)

Product Availability Product available in various countries; not currently available in the U.S.

Dosage Forms

Capsule: 200 mg

Granules: 135 mg/packet

Suspension: 10 mg/mL

Tablet: 100 mg, 135 mg

◆ **Mebeverine Hydrochloride** *see* Mebeverine [INT] *on page 1275*

Mebhydrolin [INT] (meb HYE dro lin)

International Brand Names Fabahistin (GB, ZA); Incidal (NL)

Index Terms Mebhydrolin Napadisylate

Pharmacologic Category Antihistamine

Reported Use Symptomatic relief of allergic symptoms caused by histamine release, including nasal allergies and allergic dermatosis

Dosage Range Oral:

Children 2-5 years: 50-150 mg/day

Children 5-10 years: 100-200 mg/day

Children >10 years and Adults: 100-300 mg/day

Product Availability Product available in various countries; not currently available in the U.S.

Dosage Forms

Tablet: 50 mg

◆ **Mebhydrolin Napadisylate** *see* Mebhydrolin [INT] *on page 1276*

Mechlorethamine (Systemic)

(me klor ETH a meen)

Brand Names: U.S. Mustargen

Index Terms Chlorethazine; Chlorethazine Mustard; HN_2; Mechlorethamine Hydrochloride; Mustine; Nitrogen Mustard

Pharmacologic Category Antineoplastic Agent, Alkylating Agent; Antineoplastic Agent, Alkylating Agent (Nitrogen Mustard)

Use

Hodgkin lymphoma: Palliative treatment of Hodgkin lymphoma

Malignant effusion: Palliative treatment of effusions from metastatic carcinomas

Additional approved uses (manufacturer labeling): Treatment of lymphosarcoma, chronic myelocytic or chronic lymphocytic leukemia, polycythemia vera, mycosis fungoides, and bronchogenic carcinoma

Pregnancy Risk Factor D

Dosage Dosage should be based on ideal dry weight (evaluate the presence of edema or ascites so that dosage is based on actual weight unaugmented by edema/ascites). Mechlorethamine is associated with a high emetic potential (Basch, 2011; Dupuis, 2011; Roila, 2010); antiemetics are recommended to prevent nausea and vomiting.

Hodgkin lymphoma (off-label dosing): Adults: IV:

MOPP regimen: 6 mg/m^2 on days 1 and 8 of a 28-day cycle for 6 to 8 cycles (Canelos, 1992; DeVita, 1970)

Stanford V regimen: 6 mg/m^2 as a single dose on day 1 in weeks 1, 5, and 9 (Horning, 2000; Horning, 2002)

Malignant effusion: Intracavitary: 0.4 mg/kg as a single dose, although 0.2 mg/kg (10-20 mg) as a single dose has been used by the *intrapericardial* route

Dosage adjustment in renal impairment: No dosage adjustment provided in manufacturer's labeling.

Dosage adjustment in hepatic impairment: No dosage adjustment provided in manufacturer's labeling. The following have also been reported:

Mild-to-moderate impairment: No dosage adjustment necessary (Ecklund, 2005).

Severe liver impairment: No dosage adjustment necessary; concomitant chemotherapy may require alteration until improvement in hepatic function (Ecklund, 2005).

Dosing in obesity: *ASCO Guidelines for appropriate chemotherapy dosing in obese adults with cancer:* In general, utilize patient's actual body weight (full weight) for calculation of body surface area- or weight-based dosing, particularly when the intent of therapy is curative; manage regimen-related toxicities in the same manner as for nonobese patients; if a dose reduction is utilized due to toxicity, consider resumption of full weight-based dosing with subsequent cycles, especially if cause of toxicity (eg, hepatic or renal impairment) is resolved (Griggs, 2012). **Note:** The manufacturer recommends dosing be based on ideal dry body weight and the presence of edema or ascites should be considered so the dose will be based on unaugmented weight.

Additional Information Complete prescribing information should be consulted for additional detail.

Product Availability Mustargen: Mustargen was acquired by Recordati Rare Diseases in 2013; availability information is currently unknown.

Dosage Forms

Solution Reconstituted, Injection:

Mustargen: 10 mg (1 ea)

Mechlorethamine (Topical) (me klor ETH a meen)

Brand Names: U.S. Valchlor

Index Terms Mechlorethamine HCl (Topical); Mechlorethamine Topical Gel

Pharmacologic Category Antineoplastic Agent, Alkylating Agent; Antineoplastic Agent, Alkylating Agent (Nitrogen Mustard)

Use Cutaneous T-cell lymphoma: Topical treatment of stage IA and IB mycosis fungoides-type cutaneous T-cell lymphoma in patients who have received prior skin-directed therapy

Pregnancy Risk Factor D

Dosage

Cutaneous T-cell lymphoma (mycosis fungoides-type): Adults: Topical: Apply a thin film once daily to affected areas of skin

Note: Concurrent use of topical or systemic corticosteroids was not allowed in the clinical study (Lessin, 2013).

Dosage adjustment for toxicity: Skin ulceration (any grade), blistering, or dermatitis (moderately severe-to-severe): Withhold treatment; upon improvement, may reinitiate treatment with a reduced frequency of once every 3 days; if every 3-day application is tolerated for at least 1 week, may increase to every other day for at least 1 week, then (if tolerated) may increase to once daily.

Dosage adjustment in renal impairment: No dosage adjustment provided in the manufacturer's labeling; however, dosage adjustment is unlikely based on the lack of systemic exposure.

Dosage adjustment in hepatic impairment: No dosage adjustment provided in the manufacturer's labeling; however, dosage adjustment is unlikely based on the lack of systemic exposure.

Additional Information Complete prescribing information should be consulted for additional detail.

Dosage Forms Considerations Valchlor 0.016% is equivalent to 0.02% mechlorethamine hydrochloride

Dosage Forms

Gel, External:

Valchlor: 0.016% (60 g)

- **Mechlorethamine HCl (Topical)** *see* Mechlorethamine (Topical) *on page 1276*
- **Mechlorethamine Hydrochloride** *see* Mechlorethamine (Systemic) *on page 1276*
- **Mechlorethamine Topical Gel** *see* Mechlorethamine (Topical) *on page 1276*

Meclizine (MEK li zeen)

Brand Names: U.S. Dramamine Less Drowsy [OTC]; Medi-Meclizine [OTC]; Motion-Time [OTC]; Travel Sickness [OTC]; UniVert; Vertin-32 [OTC]

Index Terms Antivert; Meclizine Hydrochloride; Meclozine Hydrochloride

Pharmacologic Category Antiemetic; Histamine H_1 Antagonist; Histamine H_1 Antagonist, First Generation; Piperazine Derivative

Additional Appendix Information

Beers Criteria – Potentially Inappropriate Medications for Geriatrics *on page 2271*

Use Prevention and treatment of symptoms of motion sickness; management of vertigo with diseases affecting the vestibular system

Pregnancy Risk Factor B

Dosage Children ≥12 years and Adults: Oral:

Motion sickness: 25-50 mg 1 hour before travel, repeat dose every 24 hours if needed

Vertigo: 25-100 mg daily in divided doses

Dosage adjustment in renal impairment: No dosage adjustment provided in manufacturer's labeling.

Dosage adjustment in hepatic impairment: No dosage adjustment provided in manufacturer's labeling.

Additional Information Complete prescribing information should be consulted for additional detail.

Dosage Forms

Tablet, Oral:

Dramamine Less Drowsy [OTC]: 25 mg
Medi-Meclizine [OTC]: 25 mg
UniVert: 32 mg
Vertin-32 [OTC]: 32 mg
Generic: 12.5 mg, 25 mg

Tablet Chewable, Oral:

Motion-Time [OTC]: 25 mg
Travel Sickness [OTC]: 25 mg
Generic: 25 mg

- **Meclizine Hydrochloride** *see* Meclizine *on page 1277*
- **Meclozine Hydrochloride** *see* Meclizine *on page 1277*

Mecysteine [INT] (me SIS te een)

International Brand Names Acthiol (BR); Actiol (IT); Chistait (JP); Epecoal (JP); Moltanine (JP); Pectite (JP); Pelmain (JP); Visclair (GB, IE)

Index Terms Mecysteine Hydrochloride; Methyl Cysteine

Pharmacologic Category Mucolytic Agent

Reported Use To reduce sputum viscosity

Dosage Range Oral:

Children >5 years: 100 mg 3 times/day

Adults: 100-200 mg 3-4 times/day before meals; reduce to 200 mg twice daily after 6 weeks

Prophylaxis: 100-200 mg 2-3 times every other day during winter months

Product Availability Product available in various countries; not currently available in the U.S.

Dosage Forms

Tablet, as hydrochloride: 100 mg

- **Mecysteine Hydrochloride** *see* Mecysteine [INT] *on page 1277*
- **Med-Anastrozole (Can)** *see* Anastrozole *on page 148*

Medazepam [INT] (me DA ze pam)

International Brand Names Ansilan (CZ); Celium (TH); Medazine (TH); Narsis (PK); Nobrium (AE); Rudotel (DE, HU, LT, PL, RU, SK); Rusedal (DE)

Index Terms Medazepam Hydrochloride

Pharmacologic Category Benzodiazepine

Reported Use Short-term treatment of anxiety disorders

Dosage Range Adults: Oral: 10-30 mg/day in divided doses; doses up to 60 mg/day have been given

Product Availability Product available in various countries; not currently available in the U.S.

Dosage Forms

Tablet: 10 mg

- **Medazepam Hydrochloride** *see* Medazepam [INT] *on page 1277*
- **Med-Derm Hydrocortisone [OTC]** *see* Hydrocortisone (Topical) *on page 1014*
- **Med-Dutasteride (Can)** *see* Dutasteride *on page 702*
- **Medent®-PEI [OTC]** *see* Guaifenesin and Phenylephrine *on page 988*
- **Medical Provider EZ Flu** *see* Influenza Virus Vaccine (Inactivated) *on page 1075*
- **Medical Provider EZ Flu PF** *see* Influenza Virus Vaccine (Inactivated) *on page 1075*
- **Medicinal Carbon** *see* Charcoal, Activated *on page 416*
- **Medicinal Charcoal** *see* Charcoal, Activated *on page 416*
- **Medi-First Anti-Fungal [OTC]** *see* Tolnaftate *on page 2063*
- **Medi-First Hydrocortisone [OTC]** *see* Hydrocortisone (Topical) *on page 1014*
- **Medi-Meclizine [OTC]** *see* Meclizine *on page 1277*
- **Medi-Phenyl [OTC]** *see* Phenylephrine (Systemic) *on page 1638*
- **Mediproxen [OTC]** *see* Naproxen *on page 1427*
- **MED-Letrozole (Can)** *see* Letrozole *on page 1181*
- **Medrol** *see* MethylPREDNISolone *on page 1340*
- **Medrol Dose Pack** *see* MethylPREDNISolone *on page 1340*
- **Medrol (Pak)** *see* MethylPREDNISolone *on page 1340*
- **Med-Rosuvastatin (Can)** *see* Rosuvastatin *on page 1848*
- **Medroxy (Can)** *see* MedroxyPROGESTERone *on page 1277*

MedroxyPROGESTERone

(me DROKS ee proe JES te rone)

Brand Names: U.S. Depo-Provera; Depo-SubQ Provera 104; Provera

Brand Names: Canada Alti-MPA; Apo-Medroxy; Depo-Prevera; Depo-Provera; Dom-Medroxyprogesterone; Gen-Medroxy; Medroxy; Medroxyprogesterone Acetate Injectable Suspension USP; Novo-Medrone; PMS-Medroxyprogesterone; Provera; Provera-Pak; Teva-Medroxyprogesterone

Index Terms Acetoxymethylprogesterone; Medroxyprogesterone Acetate; Methylacetoxyprogesterone; MPA

Pharmacologic Category Contraceptive; Progestin

Use Secondary amenorrhea or abnormal uterine bleeding due to hormonal imbalance; reduction of endometrial hyperplasia in nonhysterectomized postmenopausal women receiving conjugated estrogens; prevention of pregnancy; management of endometriosis-associated pain; adjunctive therapy and palliative treatment of recurrent and metastatic endometrial carcinoma

Pregnancy Risk Factor X

Pregnancy Considerations Use is contraindicated in women who are pregnant, as a diagnostic test for pregnancy, or for missed abortion. In general, there is not an increased risk of birth defects following inadvertent use of the injectable medroxyprogesterone (MPA) contraceptives early in pregnancy. Hypospadias has been reported in male babies and clitoral enlargement and labial fusion have been reported in female babies exposed to MPA during the first trimester of pregnancy. High doses impair fertility. Ectopic pregnancies have been reported with use of the MPA contraceptive injection. Median time to conception/return to ovulation following discontinuation of MPA contraceptive injection is 10 months following the last injection.

Breast-Feeding Considerations Medroxyprogesterone (MPA) is excreted into breast milk. Composition, quality, and quantity of breast milk are not affected; adverse developmental and behavioral effects have not been noted following exposure of infant to MPA while breast-feeding. The manufacturer does not recommend the use of MPA tablets in breast-feeding mothers; however, guidelines note that the injectable MPA contraceptives can be initiated immediately postpartum in women who are nursing (CDC, 2010; CDC, 2011; CDC, 2013).

Contraindications Hypersensitivity to medroxyprogesterone or any component of the formulation; history of or current thrombophlebitis or venous thromboembolic disorders (including DVT, PE); cerebral vascular disease; severe hepatic dysfunction or disease; carcinoma of the breast or other estrogen- or progesterone-dependent neoplasia; undiagnosed vaginal bleeding; missed abortion, diagnostic test for pregnancy, pregnancy

Warnings/Precautions Hazardous agent - use appropriate precautions for handling and disposal (NIOSH 2014 [group 2]).

[U.S. Boxed Warning]: Prolonged use of medroxyprogesterone contraceptive injection may result in a loss of bone mineral density (BMD). It is not known if use during adolescence or early adulthood will decrease peak bone mass accretion or increase the risk for osteoporotic fractures later in life. Loss is related to the duration of use, may not be completely reversible on discontinuation of the drug, and incidence is not significantly different between the SubQ and IM dosage forms. The impact on peak bone mass in adolescents should be weighed against the potential for unintended pregnancies in treatment decision. Consider alternative contraceptive methods in patients at risk for osteoporosis (eg, metabolic bone disease, family history of osteoporosis, chronic use of medications associated with osteoporosis such as corticosteroids). **[U.S. Boxed Warning]: Long-term use (ie, >2 years) should be limited to situations where other birth control methods are inadequate.** Consider other methods of birth control in women with (or at risk for) osteoporosis. **[U.S. Boxed Warning]: Inform patients that injectable contraceptives do not protect against HIV infection or other sexually-transmitted diseases.** When used for contraception, the possibility of ectopic pregnancy should be considered in patients with abdominal pain. Anaphylaxis or anaphylactoid reactions have been reported with use of the injection; medication for the treatment of hypersensitivity reactions should be available for immediate use.

[U.S. Boxed Warning]: Estrogens with or without progestin should not be used to prevent cardiovascular disease. Using data from the Women's Health Initiative (WHI) studies, an increased risk of deep vein thrombosis (DVT) and stroke has been reported with CE and an increased risk of DVT, stroke, pulmonary emboli (PE) and myocardial infarction (MI) has been reported with CE with MPA in postmenopausal women. Additional risk factors include diabetes mellitus, hypercholesterolemia, hypertension, SLE, obesity, tobacco use, and/or history of venous thromboembolism (VTE). Risk factors should be managed appropriately; discontinue use if adverse cardiovascular events occur or are suspected. If thrombosis develops with contraceptive treatment, discontinue treatment (unless no other acceptable contraceptive alternative). Whenever possible, progestins in combination with estrogens should be discontinued at least 4-6 weeks prior to and for 2 weeks following elective surgery associated with an increased risk of thromboembolism or during periods of prolonged immobilization.

[U.S. Boxed Warning]: Estrogens with or without progestin should not be used to prevent dementia. In the Women's Health Initiative Memory Study (WHIMS), an increased incidence of dementia was observed in women ≥65 years of age taking CE alone or in combination with MPA.

[U.S. Boxed Warning]: Based on data from the Women's Health Initiative (WHI) studies, an increased risk of invasive breast cancer was observed in postmenopausal women using conjugated estrogens (CE) in combination with medroxyprogesterone acetate (MPA). This risk may be associated with duration of use and declines once combined therapy is discontinued (Chlebowski, 2009). The risk of invasive breast cancer was decreased in postmenopausal women with a hysterectomy using CE only, regardless of weight. However, the risk was not significantly decreased in women at high risk for breast cancer (family history of breast cancer, personal history of benign breast disease) (Anderson, 2012). An increase in abnormal mammogram findings has also been reported with estrogen alone or in combination with progestin therapy. Use is contraindicated in patients with known or suspected breast cancer.

MPA is used to reduce the risk of endometrial hyperplasia in nonhysterectomized postmenopausal women receiving conjugated estrogens. The use of unopposed estrogen in women with an intact uterus is associated with an increased risk of endometrial cancer. The addition of a progestin to estrogen therapy may decrease the risk of endometrial hyperplasia, a precursor to endometrial cancer. Adequate diagnostic measures, including endometrial sampling if indicated, should be performed to rule out malignancy in postmenopausal women with undiagnosed abnormal vaginal bleeding. Estrogens may exacerbate endometriosis. Malignant transformation of residual endometrial implants has been reported posthysterectomy with unopposed estrogen therapy. Consider adding a progestin in women with residual endometriosis posthysterectomy. Postmenopausal estrogen therapy and combined estrogen/progesterone therapy may increase the risk of ovarian cancer; however, the absolute risk to an individual woman is small. Although results from various studies are not consistent, risk does not appear to be significantly associated with the duration, route, or dose of therapy. In one study, the risk decreased after 2 years following discontinuation of therapy (Mørch, 2009). Although the risk of ovarian cancer is rare, women who are at an increased risk (eg, family history) should be counseled about the association (NAMS, 2012).

[U.S. Boxed Warning]: Estrogens with or without progestin should be used for the shortest duration possible at the lowest effective dose consistent with treatment goals. Before prescribing estrogen therapy to postmenopausal women, the risks and benefits must be weighed for each patient. Women should be informed of these risks and benefits, as well as possible effects of progestin when added to estrogen therapy. Patients should be reevaluated as clinically appropriate to determine if treatment is still necessary. Available data related to treatment risks are from Women's Health Initiative (WHI) studies, which evaluated oral CE 0.625 mg with or without MPA 2.5 mg relative to placebo in postmenopausal women. Other combinations and dosage forms of estrogens and progestins were not studied. **Outcomes reported from clinical trials using CE with or without MPA should be assumed to be similar for other doses and other dosage forms of estrogens and progestins until comparable data becomes available.**

Discontinue pending examination in cases of sudden partial or complete vision loss, sudden onset of proptosis, diplopia, or migraine; discontinue permanently if papilledema or retinal vascular lesions are observed on examination. Use with caution in patients with diseases that may be exacerbated by fluid retention (including asthma, epilepsy, migraine, cardiac, or renal dysfunction). Contraceptive therapy with medroxyprogesterone commonly results in an average weight gain of ~2.5 kg after 1 year and ~3.7 kg after 2 years of treatment. Use caution with history of depression.

May have adverse effects on glucose tolerance; use caution in women with diabetes. MPA is extensively metabolized in the liver. Discontinue if jaundice develops or if acute or chronic hepatic disturbances occur. Use is contraindicated with severe hepatic disease. Unscheduled bleeding/spotting may occur. Presentation of irregular, unresolving vaginal bleeding following previously regular cycles warrants further evaluation including endometrial sampling, if indicated, to rule out malignancy. Not for use prior to menarche. The use of estrogens and/or progestins may change the results of some laboratory tests (eg, coagulation factors, lipids, glucose tolerance, binding proteins). The dose, route, and the specific estrogen/progestin influences these changes. In addition, personal risk factors (eg, cardiovascular disease, smoking, diabetes, age) also contribute to adverse events; use of specific products may be contraindicated in women with certain risk factors.

Some dosage forms may contain polysorbate 80 (also known as Tweens). Hypersensitivity reactions, usually a delayed reaction, have been reported following exposure to pharmaceutical products containing polysorbate 80 in certain individuals (Isaksson, 2002; Lucente 2000; Shelley, 1995). Thrombocytopenia, ascites, pulmonary deterioration, and renal and hepatic failure have been reported in premature neonates after receiving parenteral products containing polysorbate 80 (Alade, 1986; CDC, 1984). See manufacturer's labeling.

Adverse Reactions Adverse effects as reported with any dosage form

Cardiovascular: Edema

Central nervous system: Depression, dizziness, fatigue, headache, insomnia, nervousness

Dermatologic: Acne, alopecia, rash

Endocrine & metabolic: Breast pain, hot flashes, libido decreased, menstrual irregularities (includes bleeding, amenorrhea, or both)

Gastrointestinal: Abdominal pain/discomfort, bloating, nausea, weight gain (>10 lbs at 24 months)

Genitourinary: Cervical smear abnormal, leukorrhea, menometrorrhagia, menorrhagia, pelvic pain, urinary tract infection, vaginitis

Genitourinary: Dysmenorrhea, leukorrhea, vaginitis

Local: Injection site reaction (SubQ administration): Atrophy, induration, pain

Rare but important or life-threatening: Allergic reaction, anaphylaxis, anaphylactoid reactions, angioedema, asthma, blood dyscrasia, bone mineral density decreased, breast cancer, breast changes, cervical cancer, chest pain, chloasma, cholestatic jaundice, deep vein thrombosis, diaphoresis, dyspnea, facial palsy, galactorrhea, glucose tolerance decreased, hirsutism, hoarseness, injection site reactions, jaundice, lack of return to fertility, lactation decreased, melasma, nipple bleeding, optic neuritis, osteoporosis, osteoporotic fractures, paralysis, paresthesia, pulmonary embolus, rectal bleeding, retinal thrombosis, scleroderma, seizure, syncope, tachycardia, thrombophlebitis, urticaria

Drug Interactions

Metabolism/Transport Effects **Substrate** of CYP3A4 (major); **Note:** Assignment of Major/Minor substrate status based on clinically relevant drug interaction potential; **Induces** CYP3A4 (weak)

Avoid Concomitant Use

Avoid concomitant use of MedroxyPROGESTERone with any of the following: Griseofulvin; Indium 111 Capromab Pendetide; Tranexamic Acid; Ulipristal

Increased Effect/Toxicity

MedroxyPROGESTERone may increase the levels/effects of: C1 inhibitors; Selegiline; Thalidomide; Tranexamic Acid; Voriconazole

The levels/effects of MedroxyPROGESTERone may be increased by: Atazanavir; Boceprevir; Cobicistat; Herbs (Progestogenic Properties); Lopinavir; Metreleptin; Mifepristone; Tipranavir; Voriconazole

Decreased Effect

MedroxyPROGESTERone may decrease the levels/effects of: Anticoagulants; ARIPiprazole; Fosamprenavir; Hydrocodone; Indium 111 Capromab Pendetide; Saxagliptin; Vitamin K Antagonists

The levels/effects of MedroxyPROGESTERone may be decreased by: Acitretin; Aminoglutethimide; Aprepitant; Artemether; Barbiturates; Bexarotene (Systemic); Bile Acid Sequestrants; Bosentan; CarBAMazepine; CloBAZam; CYP3A4 Inducers (Moderate); CYP3A4 Inducers (Strong); Dabrafenib; Darunavir; Deferasirox; Efavirenz; Eslicarbazepine; Felbamate; Fosamprenavir; Fosaprepitant; Fosphenytoin; Griseofulvin; LamoTRIgine; Lopinavir; Metreleptin; Mifepristone; Mitotane; Mycophenolate; Nelfinavir; Nevirapine; OXcarbazepine; Perampanel; Phenytoin; Primidone; Prucalopride; Retinoic Acid Derivatives; Rifamycin Derivatives; Saquinavir; Siltuximab; St Johns Wort; Sugammadex; Telaprevir; Tocilizumab; Topiramate; Ulipristal

Food Interactions Bioavailability of the oral tablet is increased when taken with food; half-life is unchanged. Management: Administer without regard to food.

Storage/Stability Store at room temperature.

Mechanism of Action Inhibits secretion of pituitary gonadotropins, which prevents follicular maturation and ovulation; causes endometrial thinning

Pharmacodynamics/Kinetics

Absorption: Oral: Well absorbed; IM: Slow

Protein binding: 86% to 90% primarily to albumin; does not bind to sex hormone–binding globulin

Metabolism: Extensively hepatic via hydroxylation and conjugation; forms metabolites

Half-life elimination: Oral: 12 to 17 hours; IM (Depo-Provera Contraceptive): ~50 days; SubQ: ~40 days

Time to peak: Oral: 2 to 4 hours; IM (Depo-Provera Contraceptive): ~3 weeks; SubQ: ~1 week

Excretion: Urine

Dosage

Adolescents and Adults:

Amenorrhea: Oral: 5 to 10 mg/day for 5 to 10 days

Abnormal uterine bleeding: Oral: 5 to 10 mg for 5 to 10 days starting on day 16 or 21 of cycle

Contraception:

Depo-Provera Contraceptive: IM: 150 mg every 3 months (every 13 weeks)

depo-subQ provera 104: SubQ: 104 mg every 3 months (every 12 to 14 weeks)

Endometriosis (depo-subQ provera 104): SubQ: 104 mg every 3 months (every 12 to 14 weeks)

Adults:

Endometrial carcinoma, recurrent or metastatic (adjunctive/palliative treatment) (Depo-Provera): IM: 400 to 1,000 mg/week

Accompanying cyclic estrogen therapy, postmenopausal: Oral: 5 to 10 mg for 12 to 14 consecutive days each month, starting on day 1 or day 16 of the cycle; lower doses may be used if given with estrogen continuously throughout the cycle

Treatment of paraphilia/hypersexuality (off-label use; Reilly, 2000): Males (**Note:** Avoid use if active pituitary pathology, hepatic failure, or thromboembolic disease): IM (Depo-Provera): 100 to 600 mg weekly

Oral: 100 to 500 mg daily

Dosage adjustment in renal impairment: There are no dosage adjustments provided in the manufacturer's labeling (has not been studied).

Dosage adjustment in hepatic impairment: Use is contraindicated with severe impairment. Discontinue with jaundice or if liver function disturbances occur. Consider lower dose or less frequent administration with mild to moderate impairment. Use of the contraceptive injection has not been studied in patients with hepatic impairment; consideration should be given to not readminister if jaundice develops

Dietary Considerations Ensure adequate calcium and vitamin D intake

Administration

IM: Depo-Provera Contraceptive: Administer first dose during the first 5 days of menstrual period, or within the first 5 days postpartum if not breast-feeding, or at the sixth week postpartum if breast-feeding exclusively. Shake vigorously prior to administration. Administer by deep IM injection in the gluteal or deltoid muscle.

When switching from combined hormonal contraceptives (estrogen plus progestin), the first injection should be on the day after the last active tablet or (at the latest) the day after the final inactive tablet. When switching from other contraceptive methods, ensure continuous contraceptive coverage.

SubQ: depo-subQ provera 104: Administer first dose during the first 5 days of menstrual period, or at the sixth week postpartum if breast-feeding. Shake vigorously for at least 1 minute prior to administration. Administer by SubQ injection in the anterior thigh or abdomen; avoid boney areas and the umbilicus. Administer slowly over 5 to 7 seconds. Do not rub the injection area.

When switching from combined hormonal contraceptives (estrogen plus progestin), the first injection should be within 7 days after the last active pill, or removal of patch or ring. If switching from the IM to SubQ formulation, the next dose should be given within the prescribed dosing period for the IM injection to ensure continuous coverage.

Hazardous agent; use appropriate precautions for handling and disposal (NIOSH 2014 [group 2]).

Monitoring Parameters Before starting therapy, a physical exam with reference to the breasts and pelvis are recommended, including a Papanicolaou smear. Exam may be deferred if appropriate prior to administration of MPA contraceptive injection; pregnancy should be ruled out prior to use. Monitor patient closely for loss of vision; sudden onset of proptosis, diplopia, or migraine; signs and symptoms of thromboembolic disorders; signs or symptoms of depression; glucose in patients with diabetes; or blood pressure. BMD with long-term use (per manufacturer).

Adequate diagnostic measures, including endometrial sampling, if indicated, should be performed to rule out malignancy in all cases of undiagnosed abnormal vaginal bleeding.

Treatment of paraphilia/hypersexuality (Guay, 2009; Reilly, 2000): Hepatic function test (baseline and during treatment if suspected hepatotoxicity); CBC (baseline); serum testosterone (baseline then monthly for 4 months then every 6 months); serum LH and prolactin (baseline and every 6 months); FSH (baseline); glucose; bone scan (baseline then annually) if serum testosterone significantly suppressed; gallbladder function; blood pressure; weight gain

Dosage Forms

Suspension, Intramuscular:

Depo-Provera: 150 mg/mL (1 mL); 400 mg/mL (2.5 mL)

Generic: 150 mg/mL (1 mL)

Suspension, Subcutaneous:

Depo-SubQ Provera 104: 104 mg/0.65 mL (0.65 mL)

Tablet, Oral:

Provera: 2.5 mg, 5 mg, 10 mg

Generic: 2.5 mg, 5 mg, 10 mg

◆ **Medroxyprogesterone Acetate** *see* MedroxyPROGESTERone *on page* 1277

◆ **Medroxyprogesterone Acetate Injectable Suspension USP (Can)** *see* MedroxyPROGESTERone *on page* 1277

◆ **Med-Sotalol (Can)** *see* Sotalol *on page* 1927

◆ **Mefenamic (Can)** *see* Mefenamic Acid *on page* 1280

Mefenamic Acid (me fe NAM ik AS id)

Brand Names: U.S. Ponstel

Brand Names: Canada Dom-Mefenamic Acid; Mefenamic; PMS-Mefenamic Acid; Ponstan

Pharmacologic Category Nonsteroidal Anti-inflammatory Drug (NSAID), Oral

Additional Appendix Information

Beers Criteria − Potentially Inappropriate Medications for Geriatrics *on page* 2271

Use Short-term relief of mild-to-moderate pain including primary dysmenorrhea

Pregnancy Risk Factor C

Dosage Children >14 years and Adults: Oral: 500 mg to start then 250 mg every 6 hours as needed; maximum therapy: 1 week

Dosage adjustment in renal impairment: Use is not recommended.

Dosage adjustment in hepatic impairment: No dosage adjustment provided in manufacturer's labeling (has not been studied). However, adjustment may be necessary due to extensive hepatic metabolism.

Additional Information Complete prescribing information should be consulted for additional detail.

Dosage Forms

Capsule, Oral:

Ponstel: 250 mg

Generic: 250 mg

Mefloquine (ME floe kwin)

Index Terms Mefloquine Hydrochloride

Pharmacologic Category Antimalarial Agent

Use Treatment of mild-to-moderate acute malarial infections and prevention of malaria caused by *Plasmodium falciparum* (including chloroquine-resistant strains) or *P. vivax*

Note: Due to geographical resistance and cross-resistance, consult current CDC guidelines.

Pregnancy Risk Factor B

Dosage Oral (dose expressed as mg of mefloquine hydrochloride):

Malaria:

Mild-to-moderate, treatment: **Note:** If clinical improvement is not seen within 48-72 hours, an alternative therapy should be used for retreatment.

Children ≥6 months: 20-25 mg/kg/day in 2 divided doses, taken 6-8 hours apart (maximum total dose: 1250 mg)

Adults: 1250 mg (5 tablets) as a single dose

Uncomplicated, treatment (off-label dose):

Children ≥6 months: 15 mg/kg, followed 6-12 hours later by 10 mg/kg/dose (maximum total dose: 1250 mg) (CDC, 2013b)

Adults: 750 mg (3 tablets) as initial dose, followed 6-12 hours later by 500 mg (2 tablets) (CDC, 2013b)

Uncomplicated, chloroquine-resistant *P. vivax* malaria treatment (off-label use):

Children ≥6 months: 15 mg/kg, followed 6-12 hours later by 10 mg/kg/dose (maximum total dose: 1250 mg) with concomitant primaquine (CDC, 2013b)

Adults: 750 mg (3 tablets) as initial dose, followed 6-12 hours later by 500 mg (2 tablets) with concomitant primaquine (CDC, 2013b)

Chemoprophylaxis:

Children ≥6 months: 5 mg/kg/dose once weekly (maximum dose: 250 mg) starting 1 week (CDC, 2014: ≥2 weeks) before arrival in endemic area, continuing weekly during travel and for 4 weeks after leaving endemic area. **Note:** Prophylaxis may begin 2-3 weeks prior to travel to ensure tolerance.

Manufacturer's labeling:

20-30 kg: 1/2 of 250 mg tablet (125 mg) once weekly

30-45 kg: 3/4 of 250 mg tablet (187.5 mg) once weekly

>45 kg: One tablet (250 mg) once weekly

Off-label dosing (CDC, 2014):

≤9 kg: 5 mg/kg/dose once weekly

>9-19 kg: 1/4 of 250 mg tablet (62.5 mg) once weekly

>19-30 kg: 1/2 of 250 mg tablet (125 mg) once weekly

>30-45 kg: 3/4 of 250 mg tablet (187.5 mg) once weekly

>45 kg: One tablet (250 mg) once weekly

Adults: 250 mg weekly starting 1 week (CDC, 2014: ≥2 weeks) before arrival in endemic area, continuing weekly during travel and for 4 weeks after leaving endemic area. **Note:** Prophylaxis may begin 2-3 weeks prior to travel to ensure tolerance.

Dosage adjustment in renal impairment: No dosage adjustment necessary; only a small amount of mefloquine is renally eliminated.

Dosage adjustment in hepatic impairment: No dosage adjustment provided in manufacturer's labeling; however; half-life may be prolonged and plasma levels may be higher in patients with hepatic impairment

Additional Information Complete prescribing information should be consulted for additional detail.

Dosage Forms

Tablet, Oral:

Generic: 250 mg

◆ **Mefloquine Hydrochloride** *see* Mefloquine *on page 1280*

◆ **Mefoxin** *see* CefOXitin *on page 386*

Mefruside [INT] (MEF ru side)

International Brand Names Baycaron (DE, GB, IE, NL, NO); duranifin (DE); Gomsid (KR)

Pharmacologic Category Diuretic, Miscellaneous

Reported Use Treatment of edema and hypertension

Dosage Range Adults: Oral: 25-50 mg/day

Product Availability Product available in various countries; not currently available in the U.S.

Dosage Forms

Tablet: 25 mg

◆ **Mega-C/A Plus** *see* Ascorbic Acid *on page 178*

◆ **Megace ES** *see* Megestrol *on page 1281*

◆ **Megace Oral** *see* Megestrol *on page 1281*

◆ **Megace OS (Can)** *see* Megestrol *on page 1281*

Megestrol (me JES trole)

Brand Names: U.S. Megace ES; Megace Oral

Brand Names: Canada Megace OS; Megestrol

Index Terms 5071-1DL(6); Megestrol Acetate

Pharmacologic Category Antineoplastic Agent, Hormone; Appetite Stimulant; Progestin

Additional Appendix Information

Beers Criteria – Potentially Inappropriate Medications for Geriatrics *on page 2271*

Use

Anorexia or cachexia: *Suspension:* Treatment of anorexia, cachexia, or unexplained significant weight loss in patients with AIDS

Limitations of use: Treatment of AIDS-related weight loss should only be initiated after addressing the treatable causes (eg, malignancy, infection, malabsorption, endocrine disease, renal disease, psychiatric disorder) for weight loss. Megestrol is not intended to prevent weight loss.

Breast cancer: *Tablet:* Treatment (palliative) of advanced breast cancer

Endometrial cancer: *Tablet:* Treatment (palliative) of advanced endometrial carcinoma

Additional Canadian use (not an approved use in the U.S.): *Tablet:* Treatment of anorexia, cachexia, or weight loss secondary to metastatic cancer

Pregnancy Risk Factor D (tablet) / X (suspension)

Pregnancy Considerations Adverse events were demonstrated in animal reproduction studies. May cause fetal harm if administered to a pregnant woman. Use during pregnancy is contraindicated (suspension) and appropriate contraception is recommended in women who may become pregnant. In clinical studies, megestrol was shown to cause breakthrough vaginal bleeding in women.

Breast-Feeding Considerations Megestrol is excreted into breast milk. Information is available from five nursing women, ~8 weeks postpartum, who were administered megestrol 4 mg in combination with ethinyl estradiol 50 mcg daily for contraception. Maternal serum and milk samples were obtained over 5 days, beginning 10 days after therapy began. The highest concentrations of megestrol were found at the samples taken 3 hours after the maternal dose. Mean concentrations of megestrol were 6.5 ng/mL (maternal serum; range: 3.7 to 10.8 ng/mL), 4.6 ng/mL (foremilk; range: 1.1 to 12.7 ng/mL), and 5.6 ng/mL (hindmilk; range: 1.2 to 18.5 ng/mL) (Nilsson, 1977). Due to the potential for adverse reaction in the newborn, the manufacturer recommends discontinuing breast-feeding while receiving megestrol. In addition, in the United States, where formula is accessible, affordable, safe, and sustainable, and the risk of infant mortality due to diarrhea and respiratory infections is low, complete avoidance of breast-feeding by HIV-infected women is recommended to decrease potential transmission of HIV (DHHS [perinatal], 2012).

Contraindications Hypersensitivity to megestrol or any component of the formulation; known or suspected pregnancy (suspension)

Warnings/Precautions Hazardous agent - use appropriate precautions for handling and disposal (NIOSH 2014 [group 1]). May suppress hypothalamic-pituitary-adrenal (HPA) axis during chronic administration; consider the possibility of adrenal suppression in any patient receiving or being withdrawn from chronic therapy when signs/symptoms suggestive of hypoadrenalism are noted (during stress or in unstressed state). Laboratory evaluation and replacement/stress doses of rapid-acting glucocorticoid should be considered. Cushing syndrome has been reported with long-term use. New-onset diabetes and exacerbation of preexisting diabetes have been reported with long-term use. Use with caution in patients with a history of thromboembolic disease. Avoid use in older adults due to minimal effect on weight, and an increased risk of thrombosis and possibly death (Beers Criteria). Vaginal bleeding or discharge may occur in females. The effects on HIV viral replications are unknown in patients with AIDS-related cachexia. Potentially significant drug-drug interactions may exist, requiring dose or frequency adjustment, additional monitoring, and/or selection of alternative therapy.

Megace ES suspension is not equivalent to other formulations on a mg per mg basis; Megace ES suspension 625 mg/5 mL is equivalent to megestrol acetate suspension 800 mg/20 mL.

Benzyl alcohol and derivatives: Some dosage forms may contain sodium benzoate/benzoic acid; benzoic acid (benzoate) is a metabolite of benzyl alcohol; large amounts of benzyl alcohol (≥99 mg/kg/day) have been associated with a potentially fatal toxicity ("gasping syndrome") in neonates; the "gasping syndrome" consists of metabolic acidosis, respiratory distress, gasping respirations, CNS dysfunction (including convulsions, intracranial hemorrhage), hypotension, and cardiovascular collapse (AAP, 1997; CDC, 1982); some data suggests that benzoate displaces bilirubin from protein binding sites (Ahlfors, 2001); avoid or use dosage forms containing benzyl alcohol derivative with caution in neonates. See manufacturer's labeling.

Adverse Reactions

Cardiovascular: Cardiac failure, cardiomyopathy, chest pain, edema, hypertension, palpitations, peripheral edema

Central nervous system: Abnormality in thinking, carpal tunnel syndrome, confusion, convulsions, depression, headache, hypoesthesia, insomnia, lethargy, malaise, mood change, neuropathy, pain (similar to placebo), paresthesia

Dermatologic: Alopecia, dermatological disease, diaphoresis, pruritus, skin rash, vesicobullous dermatitis

Endocrine & metabolic: Adrenocortical insufficiency, albuminuria, amenorrhea, Cushing's syndrome, decreased libido, diabetes mellitus, gynecomastia, hot flash, HPA-axis suppression, hypercalcemia, hyperglycemia, increased lactate dehydrogenase, weight gain (not attributed to edema or fluid retention)

Gastrointestinal: Abdominal pain, constipation, diarrhea (similar to placebo), dyspepsia, flatulence, nausea, oral moniliasis, sialorrhea, vomiting, xerostomia

Genitourinary: Breakthrough bleeding, impotence, urinary frequency, urinary incontinence, urinary tract infection

Hematologic & oncologic: Leukopenia, sarcoma, tumor flare

Hepatic: Hepatomegaly

Infection: Candidiasis, herpes virus infection, infection

Neuromuscular & skeletal: Weakness

Ophthalmic: Amblyopia

Respiratory: Cough, dyspnea, hyperventilation, pharyngitis, pneumonia, pulmonary disorder

Miscellaneous: Fever

Rare but important or life-threatening: Decreased glucose tolerance, thromboembolic phenomena (including deep vein thrombosis, pulmonary embolism, thrombophlebitis)

Drug Interactions

Metabolism/Transport Effects None known.

Avoid Concomitant Use

Avoid concomitant use of Megestrol with any of the following: Dofetilide; Indium 111 Capromab Pendetide; Ulipristal

Increased Effect/Toxicity

Megestrol may increase the levels/effects of: C1 inhibitors; Dofetilide

The levels/effects of Megestrol may be increased by: Herbs (Progestogenic Properties)

Decreased Effect

Megestrol may decrease the levels/effects of: Anticoagulants; Indium 111 Capromab Pendetide

The levels/effects of Megestrol may be decreased by: Aminoglutethimide; Ulipristal

Storage/Stability

Suspension: Store at 15°C to 25°C (59°F to 77°F); protect from heat. Store/dispense in a tight container.

Tablet: Store at 20°C to 25°C (68°F to 77°F); protect from light.

Mechanism of Action A synthetic progestin with antiestrogenic properties which disrupt the estrogen receptor cycle. Megestrol interferes with the normal estrogen cycle and results in a lower LH titer. May also have a direct effect on the endometrium. Megestrol is an antineoplastic progestin thought to act through an antileutenizing effect mediated via the pituitary. May stimulate appetite by antagonizing the metabolic effects of catabolic cytokines.

Pharmacodynamics/Kinetics

Metabolism: Hepatic (to free steroids and glucuronide conjugates)

Half-life elimination: Suspension: 20 to 50 hours; Tablet: 13 to 105 hours

Time to peak, serum: 1 to 3 hours

Excretion: Urine (57% to 78%; 5% to 8% as metabolites); feces (8% to 30%)

Dosage Note: Megace ES suspension is not equivalent to other formulations on a mg-per-mg basis:

Anorexia or cachexia associated with AIDS: Adults: Oral: Suspension:

U.S. labeling: Initial: 625 mg daily (of the 125 mg/mL suspension) or 800 mg daily (of the 40 mg/mL suspension); daily doses of 400 mg to 800 mg have been found to be effective

Canadian labeling: Usual dose: 400 to 800 mg once daily for at least 2 months

Breast cancer, advanced: Adults: Oral: Tablet:

U.S. labeling: 160 mg per day in divided doses of 40 mg 4 times daily for at least 2 months

Canadian labeling: 160 mg or 125 mg/m^2 daily (40 mg 4 times daily or 160 mg once daily) for at least 2 months

Endometrial cancer, advanced: Adults: Oral: Tablet:

U.S. labeling: 40 to 320 mg daily in divided doses for at least 2 months; maximum doses used (off-label) have been up to 800 mg/day in advanced or recurrent carcinomas (Lentz, 1996)

Canadian labeling: 80 to 320 mg or 62.5 to 250 mg/m^2 daily in divided doses (40 to 80 mg 1 to 4 times daily or 160 to 320 mg daily) for at least 2 months

Cancer-related cachexia: *Canadian labeling:* Adults: Oral: Tablet: 400 to 800 mg once daily for at least 2 months

Cancer-related cachexia (off-label use/dosing in U.S.): Adults: Oral: Doses ranging from 160 to 800 mg per day were effective in achieving weight gain, higher doses (>160 mg) were associated with more weight gain (Beller, 1997; Loprinzi, 1990; Loprinzi, 1993; Vadell, 1998); based on a meta-analysis, an optimal dose has not been determined (Ruiz Garcia, 2013)

Elderly: Use with caution; refer to adult dosing.

Dosage adjustment in renal impairment: There are no dosage adjustments provided in the manufacturer's labeling; urinary excretion of megestrol acetate is substantial, use caution.

Dosage adjustment in hepatic impairment: There are no dosage adjustments provided in the manufacturer's labeling.

Administration Oral: Shake suspension well before use. Hazardous agent; use appropriate precautions for handling and disposal (NIOSH 2014 [group 1]).

Monitoring Parameters Observe for signs of thromboembolic events; blood pressure, weight; serum glucose

Dosage Forms

Suspension, Oral:
Megace ES: 625 mg/5 mL (150 mL)
Megace Oral: 40 mg/mL (240 mL)
Generic: 40 mg/mL (10 mL, 240 mL, 480 mL); 400 mg/10 mL (10 mL)

Tablet, Oral:
Generic: 20 mg, 40 mg

Dosage Forms: Canada Refer also to Dosage Forms. **Note:** Megace ES not available in Canada.
Tablet, Oral, as acetate: 160 mg

◆ **Megestrol Acetate** *see* Megestrol *on page 1281*

Meglumine Antimoniate [INT]

(ME gloo meen an tee MO nee ate)

International Brand Names Glucantim (IT); Glucantime (BR, ES, FR)

Pharmacologic Category Antiprotozoal

Reported Use Treatment of leishmaniasis (except *L. aethiopica*)

Dosage Range Adults: IM, IV: 20 mg/kg/day

Product Availability Product available in various countries; not currently available in the U.S.

Dosage Forms
Injection, solution: Equivalent to 85 mg of pentavalent antimony/mL

◆ **Mekinist** *see* Trametinib *on page 2077*

Melitracen [INT] (mel i TRAY sen)

International Brand Names Dixeran (AT, BE, CH); Thymeol (JP)

Index Terms Melitracen Hydrochloride

Pharmacologic Category Antidepressant, Tricyclic

Reported Use Treatment of depression

Dosage Range Adults: Oral: 25 mg 2-3 times/day

Product Availability Product available in various countries; not currently available in the U.S.

Dosage Forms
Tablet, as hydrochloride: 25 mg

◆ **Melitracen Hydrochloride** *see* Melitracen [INT] *on page 1283*

◆ **Mellaril** *see* Thioridazine *on page 2030*

Meloxicam (mel OKS i kam)

Brand Names: U.S. Meloxicam Comfort Pac; Mobic

Brand Names: Canada Apo-Meloxicam; Auro-Meloxicam; Ava-Meloxicam; CO Meloxicam; Dom-Meloxicam; Mobicox; Mylan-Meloxicam; PHL-Meloxicam; PMS-Meloxicam; ratio-Meloxicam; Teva-Meloxicam

Pharmacologic Category Nonsteroidal Anti-inflammatory Drug (NSAID), Oral

Additional Appendix Information
Beers Criteria – Potentially Inappropriate Medications for Geriatrics *on page 2271*

Use Relief of signs and symptoms of osteoarthritis, rheumatoid arthritis, and juvenile idiopathic arthritis (JIA)

Pregnancy Risk Factor C / D ≥30 weeks gestation

Dosage Oral:

Children ≥2 years: Juvenile idiopathic arthritis (JIA): 0.125 mg/kg/day; maximum dose: 7.5 mg/day

Adults: Osteoarthritis, rheumatoid arthritis: Initial: 7.5 mg once daily; some patients may receive additional benefit from increasing dose to 15 mg once daily; maximum dose: 15 mg/day

Elderly: Increased concentrations may occur in elderly patients (particularly in females); however, no specific dosage adjustment is recommended

Dosage adjustment in renal impairment:
Mild-to-moderate impairment: No specific dosage recommendations
Significant impairment (CrCl ≤20 mL/minute): Patients with severe renal impairment have not been adequately studied; use not recommended.
Hemodialysis: Maximum dose: 7.5 mg/day

Dosage adjustment in hepatic impairment:
Mild-to-moderate hepatic impairment (Child-Pugh class A or B): No dosage adjustment is necessary
Severe hepatic impairment: Patients with severe hepatic impairment have not been adequately studied

Additional Information Complete prescribing information should be consulted for additional detail.

Dosage Forms Considerations
Meloxicam Comfort Pac is a kit containing meloxicam oral tablets 15 mg, and Duraflex topical gel.

Dosage Forms

Kit, Combination:
Meloxicam Comfort Pac: 15 mg

Suspension, Oral:
Mobic: 7.5 mg/5 mL (100 mL)
Generic: 7.5 mg/5 mL (100 mL)

Tablet, Oral:
Mobic: 7.5 mg, 15 mg
Generic: 7.5 mg, 15 mg

Dosage Forms: Canada Note: Refer also to Dosage Forms. Combination kit and oral suspension are not available in Canada.
Tablet, Oral:
Mobicox: 7.5 mg, 15 mg

◆ **Meloxicam Comfort Pac** *see* Meloxicam *on page 1283*

◆ **Melpaque HP** *see* Hydroquinone *on page 1020*

Melphalan (MEL fa lan)

Brand Names: U.S. Alkeran

Brand Names: Canada Alkeran

Index Terms L-PAM; L-Phenylalanine Mustard; L-Sarcolysin; Phenylalanine Mustard

Pharmacologic Category Antineoplastic Agent, Alkylating Agent; Antineoplastic Agent, Alkylating Agent (Nitrogen Mustard)

Use

Multiple myeloma: Palliative treatment of multiple myeloma (injection and tablets).

Ovarian carcinoma: Palliative treatment of nonresectable epithelial ovarian carcinoma (tablets)

Pregnancy Risk Factor D

Pregnancy Considerations Animal studies have demonstrated embryotoxicity and teratogenicity. Therapy may suppress ovarian function leading to amenorrhea. There are no adequate and well-controlled studies in pregnant women. May cause fetal harm if administered during pregnancy. Women of childbearing potential should be advised to avoid pregnancy while on melphalan therapy.

Breast-Feeding Considerations According to the manufacturer, melphalan should not be administered if breast-feeding.

Contraindications Hypersensitivity to melphalan or any component of the formulation; patients whose disease was resistant to prior melphalan therapy

Warnings/Precautions Hazardous agent; use appropriate precautions for handling and disposal (NIOSH 2014 [group 1]).

[U.S. Boxed Warning]: Bone marrow suppression is common; may be severe and result in infection or bleeding; has been demonstrated more with the IV formulation (compared to oral); myelosuppression is dose-related. Monitor blood counts; may require treatment delay or dose modification for thrombocytopenia or neutropenia. Use with caution in patients with prior bone marrow suppression, impaired renal function (consider dose reduction), or who have received prior (or concurrent) chemotherapy or irradiation. Myelotoxicity is generally reversible, although irreversible bone marrow failure has been reported. In patients who are candidates for autologous transplantation, avoid melphalan-containing regimens prior to transplant (due to the effects on stem cell reserve). Signs of infection, such as fever and WBC rise, may not occur; lethargy and confusion may be more prominent signs of infection.

[U.S. Boxed Warning]: Hypersensitivity reactions (including anaphylaxis) have occurred in ~2% of patients receiving IV melphalan, usually after multiple treatment cycles. Discontinue infusion and treat symptomatically. Hypersensitivity may also occur (rarely) with oral melphalan. Do not readminister (oral or IV) in patients who experience hypersensitivity to melphalan.

Gastrointestinal toxicities, including nausea, vomiting, diarrhea and mucositis, are common. When administering high-dose melphalan in autologous transplantation, cryotherapy is recommended to prevent oral mucositis (Lalla, 2014). Melphalan is associated with a moderate emetic potential (depending on dose and/or administration route); antiemetics may be recommended to prevent nausea and vomiting (Dupuis, 2011). Abnormal liver function tests may occur; hepatitis and jaundice have also been reported; hepatic sinusoidal obstruction syndrome (SOS; formerly called veno-occlusive disease) has been reported with IV melphalan. Pulmonary fibrosis (some fatal) and interstitial pneumonitis have been observed with treatment. Dosage reduction is recommended with IV melphalan in patients with renal impairment; reduced initial doses may also be recommended with oral melphalan. Closely monitor patients with azotemia.

[U.S. Boxed Warning]: Produces chromosomal changes and is leukemogenic and potentially mutagenic; secondary malignancies (including acute myeloid leukemia, myeloproliferative disease, and carcinoma) have been reported reported (some patients were receiving combination chemotherapy or radiation therapy); the risk is increased with increased treatment duration and cumulative doses. Suppresses ovarian function and produces amenorrhea; may also cause testicular suppression.

Extravasation may cause local tissue damage; administration by slow injection into a fast running IV solution into an injection port or via a central line is recommended; do not administer directly into a peripheral vein. **[U.S. Boxed Warning]: Should be administered under the supervision of an experienced cancer chemotherapy physician.** Avoid vaccination with live vaccines during treatment if immunocompromised. Toxicity may be increased in elderly; start with lowest recommended adult doses. Potentially significant drug-drug interactions may exist, requiring dose or frequency adjustment, additional monitoring, and/or selection of alternative therapy.

Adverse Reactions

Gastrointestinal: Nausea, diarrhea, oral ulceration, vomiting

Hematologic: Anemia, leukopenia (nadir: 14-21 days; recovery: 28-35 days), myelosuppression, thrombocytopenia (nadir: 14-21 days; recovery: 28-35 days)

Miscellaneous: Hypersensitivity (includes bronchospasm, dyspnea, edema, hypotension, pruritus, rash, tachycardia, urticaria); secondary malignancy (cumulative dose and duration dependent, includes acute myeloid leukemia, myeloproliferative syndrome, carcinoma)

Rare by important or life-threatening: Agranulocytosis, allergic reactions, alopecia, amenorrhea, anaphylaxis (rare), bleeding (with high-dose therapy),, bone marrow failure (irreversible), BUN increased, cardiac arrest, cardiotoxicity (angina, arrhythmia, hypertension, MI; with high-dose therapy), encephalopathy, hemolytic anemia, hemorrhagic cystitis, hepatic sinusoidal obstruction syndrome (SOS; veno-occlusive disease; high-dose IV melphalan), hepatitis, infection, injection site reactions (ulceration, necrosis), interstitial pneumonitis, jaundice, mucositis (with high-dose therapy), ovarian suppression, paralytic ileus (with high-dose therapy), pruritus, pulmonary fibrosis, radiation myelopathy, rash (maculopapular), renal toxicity (with high-dose therapy), seizure (with high-dose therapy), sepsis, SIADH, skin hypersensitivity, sterility, stomatitis, testicular suppression, tingling sensation, transaminases increased, vasculitis, warmth sensation

Drug Interactions

Metabolism/Transport Effects None known.

Avoid Concomitant Use

Avoid concomitant use of Melphalan with any of the following: BCG; CloZAPine; Dipyrone; Nalidixic Acid; Natalizumab; Pimecrolimus; Tacrolimus (Topical); Tofacitinib; Vaccines (Live)

Increased Effect/Toxicity

Melphalan may increase the levels/effects of: Carmustine; CloZAPine; CycloSPORINE (Systemic); Leflunomide; Natalizumab; Tofacitinib; Vaccines (Live)

The levels/effects of Melphalan may be increased by: Denosumab; Dipyrone; Nalidixic Acid; Pimecrolimus; Roflumilast; Tacrolimus (Topical); Trastuzumab

Decreased Effect

Melphalan may decrease the levels/effects of: BCG; Coccidioides immitis Skin Test; Sipuleucel-T; Vaccines (Inactivated); Vaccines (Live)

The levels/effects of Melphalan may be decreased by: Echinacea

Food Interactions Food interferes with oral absorption. Management: Administer on an empty stomach.

Preparation for Administration Hazardous agent; use appropriate precautions for handling and disposal (NIOSH 2014 [group 1]).

Injection: Stability is limited; must be prepared fresh. **The time between reconstitution/dilution and administration of parenteral melphalan must be kept to a minimum (manufacturer recommends <60 minutes) because reconstituted and diluted solutions are unstable.** Dissolve powder initially with 10 mL of supplied diluent to a concentration of 5 mg/mL; shake immediately and vigorously to dissolve. **Immediately** dilute dose in NS to a concentration of ≤0.45 mg/mL (manufacturer recommended concentration). Do not refrigerate solution; precipitation occurs if stored at 5°C. The manufacturer recommends administration within 60 minutes of reconstitution.

Storage/Stability

Tablet: Store in refrigerator at 2°C to 8°C (36°F to 46°F). Protect from light.

Injection: Store intact vials at 20°C to 25°C (68°F to 77°F). Protect from light. The manufacturer recommends administration be completed within 60 minutes of reconstitution; **immediately** dilute dose in NS. Do not refrigerate solution; precipitation occurs.

Mechanism of Action Alkylating agent which is a derivative of mechlorethamine that inhibits DNA and RNA synthesis via formation of carbonium ions; cross-links strands of DNA; acts on both resting and rapidly dividing tumor cells.

Pharmacodynamics/Kinetics Note: Pharmacokinetics listed are for FDA-approved doses.

Absorption: Oral: Variable and incomplete

Distribution: V_d: 0.5 L/kg; low penetration into CSF

Protein binding: 53% to 92%; primarily to albumin (40% to 60%), ~20% to alpha$_1$-acid glycoprotein

Metabolism: Hepatic; chemical hydrolysis to monohydroxymelphalan and dihydroxymelphalan

Bioavailability: Oral: Variable; 56% to 93%; exposure is reduced with a high-fat meal

Half-life elimination: Terminal: IV: 75 minutes; Oral: 1 to 2 hours

Time to peak, serum: Oral: ~1 to 2 hours

Excretion: Oral: Feces (20% to 50%); urine (~10% as unchanged drug)

Dosage Note: Melphalan is associated with a moderate emetic potential (depending on dose and/or administration route); antiemetics may be recommended to prevent nausea and vomiting (Dupuis, 2011).

Oral: Adults (adjust dose based on patient response and weekly blood counts):

Multiple myeloma (palliative treatment): **Note:** Response is gradual; may require repeated courses to realize benefit:

Usual dose (as described in the manufacturer's labeling):

6 mg once daily for 2 to 3 weeks initially, followed by up to 4 weeks rest, then a maintenance dose of 2 mg daily as hematologic recovery begins **or**

10 mg daily for 7 to 10 days; institute 2 mg daily maintenance dose after WBC >4,000 cells/mm^3 and platelets >100,000 cells/mm^3 (~4 to 8 weeks); titrate maintenance dose to hematologic response **or**

0.15 mg/kg/day for 7 days, with a 2 to 6 week rest, followed by a maintenance dose of ≤0.05 mg/kg/day as hematologic recovery begins **or**

0.25 mg/kg/day for 4 days (or 0.2 mg/kg/day for 5 days); repeat at 4- to 6-week intervals as ANC and platelet counts return to normal

Other dosing regimens in **combination therapy** (off-label doses):

4 mg/m^2/day for 7 days every 4 weeks (in combination with prednisone **or** with prednisone and thalidomide) (Palumbo, 2006; Palumbo, 2008) **or**

6 mg/m^2/day for 7 days every 4 weeks (in combination with prednisone) (Palumbo, 2004) **or**

0.25 mg/kg/day for 4 days every 6 weeks (in combination with prednisone [Facon, 2006; Facon, 2007] **or** with prednisone and thalidomide [Facon, 2007]) **or**

9 mg/m^2/day for 4 days every 6 weeks (in combination with prednisone **or** with prednisone and bortezomib) (Dimopoulos, 2009; San Miguel, 2008)

Ovarian carcinoma: 0.2 mg/kg/day for 5 days, repeat every 4 to 5 weeks **or**

Off-label dosing: 7 mg/m^2/day in 2 divided doses for 5 days, repeat every 28 days (Wadler, 1996)

Amyloidosis, light chain (off-label use): 0.22 mg/kg/day for 4 days every 28 days (in combination with oral dexamethasone) (Palladini, 2004) **or** 10 mg/m^2/day for 4 days every month (in combination with oral dexamethasone) for 12 to 18 treatment cycles (Jaccard, 2007)

IV:

Children (off-label use): Conditioning regimen for autologous hematopoietic stem cell transplantation:

140 mg/m^2 2 days prior to transplantation (combined with busulfan) (Canete, 2009; Oberlin, 2006) **or**

180 mg/m^2 (with pre- and posthydration) 12 to 30 hours prior to transplantation (Pritchard, 2005) **or**

45 mg/m^2/day for 4 days starting 8 days prior to transplantation (combined with busulfan or etoposide and carboplatin) (Berthold, 2005)

Adults:

Multiple myeloma (palliative treatment): 16 mg/m^2 administered at 2-week intervals for 4 doses, then administer at 4-week intervals after adequate hematologic recovery.

Conditioning regimen for autologous hematopoietic stem cell transplantation (off-label use):

200 mg/m^2 alone 2 days prior to transplantation (Fermand, 2005; Moreau, 2002) **or**

140 mg/m^2 2 days prior to transplantation (combined with busulfan) (Fermand, 2005) **or**

140 mg/m^2 2 days prior to transplantation (combined with total body irradiation [TBI]) (Moreau, 2002) **or**

140 mg/m^2 5 days prior to transplantation (combined with TBI) (Barlogie, 2006)

Hodgkin lymphoma, relapsed/refractory (off-label use): 30 mg/m^2 on day 6 of combination chemotherapy (mini-BEAM) regimen (Colwill, 1995; Martin, 2001)

Elderly: Refer to adult dosing; use caution and begin at the lower end of dosing range

Dosage adjustment for toxicity:

Oral:

WBC <3,000/mm^3: Withhold treatment until recovery

Platelets <100,000/mm^3: Withhold treatment until recovery

IV: Adjust dose based on blood cell count at the nadir and day of treatment

Dosing adjustment in renal impairment:

The manufacturer's labeling contains the following adjustment recommendations (for approved dosing levels) based on route of administration:

Oral: Moderate-to-severe renal impairment: Consider a reduced dose initially

IV: BUN ≥30 mg/dL: Reduce dose by up to 50%

The following adjustments have also been recommended:

Aronoff, 2007: Adults: Oral (based on a 6 mg once-daily dose):

CrCl 10 to 50 mL/minute: Administer 75% of dose

CrCl <10 mL/minute: Administer 50% of dose

Hemodialysis: Administer dose after hemodialysis

Continuous ambulatory peritoneal dialysis (CAPD): Administer 50% of dose

Continuous renal replacement therapy (CRRT): Administer 75% of dose

Carlson, 2005: Oral (for melphalan-prednisone combination therapy; based on a study evaluating toxicity with melphalan dosed at 0.25 mg/kg/day for 4 days/cycle):

CrCl >10 to <30 mL/minute: Administer 75% of dose

CrCl ≤10 mL/minute: Data is insufficient for a recommendation

Kintzel, 1995:

Oral: Adjust dose in the presence of hematologic toxicity

IV:

CrCl 46 to 60 mL/minute: Administer 85% of normal dose

CrCl 31 to 45 mL/minute: Administer 75% of normal dose

CrCl <30 mL/minute: Administer 70% of normal dose

Badros, 2001: IV: Autologous stem cell transplant (single-agent conditioning regimen; no busulfan or irradiation): Serum creatinine >2 mg/dL: Reduce dose from 200 mg/m^2 over 2 days (as 100 mg/m^2/day for 2 days) to 140 mg/m^2 given as a single-dose infusion

Dosing adjustment in hepatic impairment: Melphalan is hepatically metabolized; however, dosage adjustment does not appear to be necessary (King, 2001).

Dosing in obesity:

*American Society of Clinical Oncology (ASCO) Guidelines for appropriate chemotherapy dosing in obese adults with cancer (**Note:** Excludes HSCT dosing):* Utilize patient's actual body weight (full weight) for calculation of body surface area- or weight-based dosing, particularly when the intent of therapy is curative; manage regimen-related toxicities in the same manner as for nonobese patients; if a dose reduction is utilized due to toxicity, consider resumption of full weight-based dosing with subsequent cycles, especially if cause of toxicity (eg, hepatic or renal impairment) is resolved (Griggs, 2012).

American Society for Blood and Marrow Transplantation (ASBMT) practice guideline committee position statement on chemotherapy dosing in obesity: Utilize actual body weight (full weight) for calculation of body surface area in melphalan dosing for hematopoietic stem cell transplant conditioning regimens in adults (Bubalo, 2014).

Administration Melphalan is associated with a moderate emetic potential (depending on dose and/or administration route); antiemetics may be recommended to prevent nausea and vomiting (Dupuis, 2011).

Oral: Administer on an empty stomach (Schmidt, 2002)

Parenteral: Due to limited stability, complete administration of IV dose should occur within 60 minutes of reconstitution

IV: Infuse over 15 to 20 minutes. Extravasation may cause local tissue damage; administration by slow injection into a fast running IV solution into an injection port or via a central line is recommended; do not administer by direct injection into a peripheral vein.

Hazardous agent; use appropriate precautions for handling and disposal (NIOSH 2014 [group 1]).

Monitoring Parameters CBC with differential and platelet count, serum electrolytes, serum uric acid

Dosage Forms

Solution Reconstituted, Intravenous:

Alkeran: 50 mg (1 ea)

Generic: 50 mg (1 ea)

Tablet, Oral:

Alkeran: 2 mg

◆ **Melquin 3** *see* Hydroquinone *on page 1020*

◆ **Melquin HP** *see* Hydroquinone *on page 1020*

Memantine (me MAN teen)

Brand Names: U.S. Namenda; Namenda Titration Pak; Namenda XR; Namenda XR Titration Pack

Brand Names: Canada ACT Memantine; Apo-Memantine; Ebixa; PMS-Memantine; RAN-Memantine; ratio-Memantine; Riva-Memantine; Sandoz-Memantine

Index Terms Memantine Hydrochloride

Pharmacologic Category N-Methyl-D-Aspartate Receptor Antagonist

Use Alzheimer disease: Treatment of moderate to severe dementia of the Alzheimer type.

Pregnancy Risk Factor B

Pregnancy Considerations Adverse events have been observed in animal reproduction studies.

Breast-Feeding Considerations It is not known if memantine is excreted in breast milk. The manufacturer recommends that caution be exercised when administering memantine to nursing women.

Contraindications Hypersensitivity to memantine or any component of the formulation

Warnings/Precautions Use with caution in patients with cardiovascular disease; an increased incidence of cardiac failure, angina, bradycardia, and hypertension (compared with placebo) was observed in clinical trials. Use caution with seizure disorders or severe hepatic impairment. Use with caution in severe renal impairment; dose adjustments may be required. Worsening of corneal condition has been observed in a clinical trial; periodic ophthalmic exams during use have been recommended (Canadian labeling). Clearance is significantly reduced by alkaline urine; use caution with medications, dietary changes, or patient conditions which may alter urine pH.

Adverse Reactions Adverse reactions similar in immediate and extended release formulations except as noted.

Cardiovascular: Hypertension, hypotension (extended release)

Central nervous system: Aggressive behavior, anxiety (extended release), confusion, depression (extended release), dizziness, drowsiness, fatigue, hallucination, headache, pain

Endocrine & metabolic: Weight gain (extended release)

Gastrointestinal: Abdominal pain, constipation, diarrhea, vomiting

Genitourinary: Urinary incontinence

Infection: Influenza

Neuromuscular & skeletal: Back pain

Respiratory: Cough, dyspnea

Rare but important or life-threatening: Anorexia, aspiration pneumonia, atrioventricular block, bone fracture, bradycardia, brain disease, bronchitis, cardiac failure, carpal tunnel syndrome, cerebral infarction, cerebrovascular accident, cholelithiasis, colitis, complete atrioventricular block, deep vein thrombosis, drug-induced Parkinson disease, fecal incontinence, gastritis, gastroesophageal reflux disease, hepatic failure, hepatitis (including cytolytic and cholestatic), hyperglycemia, hypoglycemia, increased INR, increased serum alkaline phosphatase, neuroleptic malignant syndrome, otitis media, pancreatitis, pancytopenia, peripheral edema, prolonged Q-T interval on ECG, psychotic reaction, renal failure, second-degree atrioventricular block, sepsis, SIADH, Stevens-Johnson syndrome, suicidal tendencies, supraventricular tachycardia, thrombotic thrombocytopenic purpura, tonic-clonic seizures, torsades de pointes, upper respiratory tract infection, urinary tract infection

Drug Interactions

Metabolism/Transport Effects Substrate of OCT2

Avoid Concomitant Use There are no known interactions where it is recommended to avoid concomitant use.

Increased Effect/Toxicity

Memantine may increase the levels/effects of: Trimethoprim

The levels/effects of Memantine may be increased by: Alkalinizing Agents; BuPROPion; Carbonic Anhydrase Inhibitors; NMDA Receptor Antagonists; Trimethoprim

Decreased Effect There are no known significant interactions involving a decrease in effect.

Storage/Stability

Capsule (extended release): Store between 20°C to 25°C (68°F to 77°F).

Tablet, oral solution: Store at 25°C (77°C); excursions are permitted between 15°C and 30°C (59°F and 86°F).

Mechanism of Action Glutamate, the primary excitatory amino acid in the CNS, may contribute to the pathogenesis of Alzheimer's disease (AD) by overstimulating various glutamate receptors leading to excitotoxicity and neuronal cell death. Memantine is an uncompetitive antagonist of the N-methyl-D-aspartate (NMDA) type of glutamate receptors, located ubiquitously throughout the brain. Under normal physiologic conditions, the (unstimulated) NMDA receptor ion channel is blocked by magnesium ions, which are displaced after agonist-induced depolarization. Pathologic or excessive receptor activation, as postulated to occur during AD, prevents magnesium from reentering and blocking the channel pore resulting in a chronically open state and excessive calcium influx. Memantine binds to the intra-pore magnesium site, but with longer dwell time, and thus functions as an effective receptor blocker only under conditions of excessive stimulation; memantine does not affect normal neurotransmission.

Pharmacodynamics/Kinetics

Absorption: Well absorbed

Distribution: 9 to 11 L/kg

Protein binding: 45%

Metabolism: Partially hepatic, primarily independent of the CYP enzyme system; forms 3 metabolites (minimal activity)

Half-life elimination: Terminal: ~60 to 80 hours

Time to peak, serum: Immediate release: 3 to 7 hours; Extended release: 9 to 12 hours

Excretion: Urine (74%; ~48% of the total dose as unchanged drug; undergoes active tubular secretion moderated by pH-dependent tubular reabsorption; excretion reduced by alkaline urine pH)

Dosage

Alzheimer disease (moderate-to-severe): Adults: Oral:

Immediate release: Initial: 5 mg daily; increase dose by 5 mg daily to a target dose of 20 mg daily; wait ≥1 week between dosage changes. Doses >5 mg daily should be given in 2 divided doses. **Note:** If treatment is interrupted for longer than several days, the treatment may need to be restarted at a lower dose and retitrated.

Suggested titration: 5 mg daily for ≥1 week; 5 mg twice daily for ≥1 week; 15 mg daily given in 5 mg and 10 mg separate doses for ≥1 week; then 10 mg twice daily

Extended release: Initial: 7 mg once daily, increase dose by 7 mg daily to a target maximum dose of 28 mg once daily; wait ≥1 week between dosage changes (if previous dose well tolerated)

Note: When switching from immediate release product to the extended release product, begin the extended release product the day after the last dose of the immediate release product. Patients on immediate release 10 mg twice daily should be switched to extended release 28 mg once daily.

Missed dose: If a single dose is missed, do not double up on the next dose; take the next dose as scheduled. If several days of dosing are missed, dosing may need to be resumed at lower doses and retitrated.

Mild-to-moderate vascular dementia (off-label use): Adults: Oral: Immediate release: Initial: 5 mg daily, titrated by 5 mg daily weekly to a target dose of 10 mg twice daily (Orgogozo, 2002)

Dosage adjustment in renal impairment: Note: Renal function may be estimated using the Cockcroft-Gault formula for dosage adjustment purposes.

Mild impairment: No dosage adjustment necessary.

Moderate impairment:

U.S. labeling: No dosage adjustment necessary.

Canadian labeling: (CrCl 30-49 mL/minute): Initial: 5 mg once daily; after at least 1 week of therapy and if tolerated, titrate up to 5 mg twice daily; based on clinical response (and if well tolerated), may further titrate dosage upward in weekly increments to 20 mg daily according to suggested titration schedule

Severe impairment:

U.S. labeling: CrCl 5-29 mL/minute: Immediate release: Initial: 5 mg once daily; after at least 1 week of therapy and if tolerated, may titrate up to a target dose of 5 mg twice daily; Extended release: Target dose of 14 mg once daily.

Note: When switching from immediate release product to the extended release product, begin the extended release product the day after the last dose of the immediate release product. Patients on immediate release 5 mg twice daily should be switched to extended release 14 mg once daily.

Canadian labeling: CrCl 15-29 mL/minute: Initial: 5 mg once daily; after at least 1 week of therapy and if tolerated, may titrate up to a target dose of 5 mg twice daily

Dosage adjustment in hepatic impairment:

Mild-to-moderate impairment: No dosage adjustment necessary.

Severe impairment:

U.S. labeling: There are no dosage adjustments provided in the manufacturer's labeling (has not been studied); use with caution.

Canadian labeling: There are no dosage adjustments provided in the manufacturer's labeling (has not been studied); avoid use.

Administration Administer without regard to meals. Extended release capsules may be swallowed whole or entire contents of capsule may be sprinkled on applesauce and swallowed immediately; do not chew, crush, or divide. Withdraw and administer oral solution with provided dosing device; dose should be slowly squirted into the corner of the patient's mouth. Do not mix oral solution with any other liquid.

Monitoring Parameters Cognitive function; periodic ophthalmic exam (Canadian labeling)

Dosage Forms

Capsule Extended Release 24 Hour, Oral:

Namenda XR: 7 mg, 14 mg, 21 mg, 28 mg

Namenda XR Titration Pack: 7 mg (7s) and 14 mg (7s) and 21 mg (7s) and 28 mg (7s)

Solution, Oral:

Namenda: 10 mg/5 mL (360 mL)

Tablet, Oral:

Namenda: 5 mg, 10 mg

Namenda Titration Pak: 5 mg (28s) and 10 mg (21s)

- ◆ **Memantine Hydrochloride** *see* Memantine *on page 1286*
- ◆ **Menactra** *see* Meningococcal (Groups A / C / Y and W-135) Diphtheria Conjugate Vaccine *on page 1289*
- ◆ **MenACWY** *see* Meningococcal (Groups A / C / Y and W-135) Diphtheria Conjugate Vaccine *on page 1289*
- ◆ **MenACWY-D (Menactra)** *see* Meningococcal (Groups A / C / Y and W-135) Diphtheria Conjugate Vaccine *on page 1289*
- ◆ **MenACWY-CRM (Menveo)** *see* Meningococcal (Groups A / C / Y and W-135) Diphtheria Conjugate Vaccine *on page 1289*
- ◆ **MenACWY-TT** *see* Meningococcal Polysaccharide (Groups A / C / Y and W-135) Tetanus Toxoid Conjugate Vaccine [CAN/INT] *on page 1290*
- ◆ **MenCC** *see* Meningococcal Group C-CRM197 Conjugate Vaccine [CAN/INT] *on page 1288*
- ◆ **MenC-CRM197** *see* Meningococcal Group C-CRM197 Conjugate Vaccine [CAN/INT] *on page 1288*

- **M-END DM [OTC] [DSC]** *see* Chlorpheniramine, Pseudoephedrine, and Dextromethorphan *on page 428*
- **Menest** *see* Estrogens (Esterified) *on page 790*
- **Menest® (Can)** *see* Estrogens (Esterified) *on page 790*
- **Menhibrix** *see* Meningococcal Polysaccharide (Groups C and Y) and *Haemophilus* b Tetanus Toxoid Conjugate Vaccine *on page 1291*
- **Meningitec (Can)** *see* Meningococcal Group C-CRM197 Conjugate Vaccine [CAN/INT] *on page 1288*
- **Meningococcal Conjugate Vaccine** *see* Meningococcal (Groups A / C / Y and W-135) Diphtheria Conjugate Vaccine *on page 1289*

Meningococcal Group C-CRM197 Conjugate Vaccine [CAN/INT]

(me NIN joe kok al groop see see ahr em wuhn nahyn tee sev uhn KON joo gate vak SEEN)

Brand Names: Canada Meningitec; Menjugate

Index Terms MenC-CRM197; MenCC

Pharmacologic Category Vaccine

Additional Appendix Information

Immunization Administration Recommendations *on page 2250*

Immunization Recommendations *on page 2255*

Use Note: Not approved in U.S.

To provide active immunization against invasive meningococcal disease caused by *N. meningitidis* serogroup C, in children ≥2 months and adults

The National Advisory Committee on Immunization (NACI) recommendations for persons considered at an increased risk for meningococcal disease:

Chemoprophylaxis and immunoprophylaxis: Selection of meningococcal vaccination to be based upon serogroup(s):

Individuals living in the same household or with close contact (eg, kissing, shared cigarettes, shared eating or drinking utensils) of infected patient

Employees and children of nursery schools or day care

Immunoprophylaxis: Selection of meningococcal vaccination to be based upon serogroup(s):

Adolescents and young adults

Laboratory workers routinely exposed to isolates of *N. meningitidis*

Military recruits

Persons traveling to or who reside in countries where *N. meningitidis* is hyperendemic or epidemic, particularly if contact with local population will be prolonged

Persons with terminal complement component deficiencies

Persons with anatomic or functional asplenia

Note: Use is also recommended during meningococcal outbreaks caused by serogroup C.

Chemoprophylaxis:

Healthcare workers with intensive unprotected contact with infected patients

Airline passengers sitting directly next to an infected patient for duration of at least 8 hours

See NACI guidelines for specific drug treatment at http://www.phac-aspc.gc.ca/naci-ccni

Pregnancy Considerations Animal reproduction studies have not demonstrated risks to the fetus.

Breast-Feeding Considerations It is not known if this vaccine is found in breast milk. The manufacturer recommends evaluating the risk to benefit ratio prior to administering to a nursing woman.

Contraindications Hypersensitivity to meningococcal group C-CRM197 conjugate vaccine or any component of the formulation

Warnings/Precautions Anaphylactoid and/or hypersensitivity reactions may occur with use. Immediate treatment including epinephrine 1:1000 should be available for immediate use. Defer treatment in patients with moderate-to-severe acute illness (with/without fever). Patients with mild acute illness without fever may receive vaccination as scheduled. Use caution in patients on anticoagulants and/or with bleeding disorders (eg, thrombocytopenia, hemophilia). Deep IM administration of vaccine may lead to bleeding or hematoma. Vaccination may not result in effective immunity in all patients. Response depends upon multiple factors (eg, type of vaccine, age of patient) and may be improved by administering the vaccine at the recommended dose, route, and interval. Vaccines may not be effective if administered during periods of altered immune competence (CDC, 2011). Use caution in immunocompromised patients. Response to vaccine may be reduced. Syncope has been reported with use of injectable vaccines and may be accompanied by transient visual disturbances, weakness, or tonic-clonic movements. Procedures should be in place to avoid injuries from falling and to restore cerebral perfusion if syncope occurs. Vaccination does not protect against other serogroups of *Neisseria meningitidis* or diphtheria. Regularly scheduled vaccinations for diphtheria should be administered. Allow at least a 2-week interval between administration of Menjugate® and vaccinations against other serogroups of *Neisseria meningitidis*.

Adverse Reactions

Central nervous system: Chills, crying (unusual/persistent), fever, headache, irritability, malaise, sleepiness

Dermatologic: Rash

Gastrointestinal: Appetite changes, diarrhea, nausea, vomiting

Local: Injection site: Erythema, induration, pain

Neuromuscular & skeletal: Arthralgia, myalgia

Rare but important or life-threatening: Agitation, anaphylaxis, angioedema, bronchospasm, dizziness, facial edema, hypersensitivity reactions, hypoesthesia, hypotonia, lymphadenopathy, maculopapular rash, paresthesia, pruritus, seizure, syncope, urticaria

Drug Interactions

Metabolism/Transport Effects None known.

Avoid Concomitant Use There are no known interactions where it is recommended to avoid concomitant use.

Increased Effect/Toxicity There are no known significant interactions involving an increase in effect.

Decreased Effect

The levels/effects of Meningococcal Group C-CRM197 Conjugate Vaccine may be decreased by: Belimumab; Immunosuppressants

Preparation for Administration

Menjugate® vial: Gently agitate diluent vial, then withdraw 0.6 mL of diluent and inject into Menjugate® vial. Gently shake vial until content dissolves.

Menjugate® syringe: Gently agitate diluent syringe, then inject entire content of syringe into Menjugate® vial. Gently shake vial until contents dissolves and then withdraw contents of vial back into syringe. Change needle prior to administration.

Storage/Stability Store at 2°C to 8°C (36°F to 46°F); do not freeze. Protect from light. Upon reconstitution, use immediately.

Alternative storage: Prior to reconstitution; store up to 25°C (77°F); do not freeze. Protect from light. Use or discard within 6 months of date removed from refrigerator or upon reaching expiration date on outside packaging (whichever comes first).

Mechanism of Action Induces immunity against meningococcal disease via the formation of bactericidal antibodies directed toward the polysaccharide capsular components of *Neisseria meningitidis* serogroup C.

Dosage IM:

Infants:

≥2-12 months: 0.5 mL as a single dose for a total of 3 doses administered at least 4 weeks apart

≥4-11 months without prior vaccination: 0.5 mL as a single dose for a total of 2 doses administered at least 4 weeks apart

Note: The NACI recommends at least 1 of the 3 sequential doses for infants ≥2-12 months be administered beyond 5 months of age.

Children ≥1 year and Adults: 0.5 mL as a single dose

Administration Administer by deep intramuscular injection only; do not administer via IV, SubQ, or I.D. routes. Administer into the anterolateral thigh in infants and the deltoid area in older children, adolescents, and adults. Use separate injection sites if administering multiple vaccinations on the same day.

Acetaminophen may be used when needed to provide comfort; however, routine prophylactic administration of acetaminophen to prevent fever due to vaccine use is not recommended. There is evidence of a decreased immune response to some vaccines associated with acetaminophen administration; the clinical significance of this reduction in immune response has not been established.

Monitoring Parameters Monitor for syncope for 15 minutes following administration. If seizure-like activity associated with syncope occurs, maintain patient in supine or Trendelenburg position to reestablish adequate cerebral perfusion.

Product Availability Not available in U.S.

Dosage Forms: Canada

Injection, powder for reconstitution:

Menjugate®: 10 mcg of oligosaccharide antigen group C

Meningococcal (Groups A / C / Y and W-135) Diphtheria Conjugate Vaccine

(me NIN joe kok al groops aye, see, why & dubl yoo won thur tee fyve dif THEER ee a KON joo gate vak SEEN)

Brand Names: U.S. Menactra; Menveo

Brand Names: Canada Menactra; Menveo

Index Terms MCV; MCV4; MenACWY; MenACWY-CRM (Menveo); MenACWY-D (Menactra); Meningococcal Conjugate Vaccine

Pharmacologic Category Vaccine, Inactivated (Bacterial)

Additional Appendix Information

Immunization Administration Recommendations *on page 2250*

Immunization Recommendations *on page 2255*

Use

Meningococcal disease prevention: Provide active immunization of children and adults against invasive meningococcal disease caused by *N. meningitidis* serogroups A, C, Y, and W-135.

The Advisory Committee on Immunization Practices (ACIP) (CDC/ACIP [Cohn, 2013]):

ACIP recommends routine vaccination of the following:
- Children and adolescents 11-18 years of age
- Persons ≥2 months of age who are at increased risk of meningococcal disease
- Persons (in all recommended age groups) at increased risk who are part of outbreaks caused by vaccine preventable serogroups

Those at increased risk of meningococcal disease include the following:
- Persons ≥2 months of age with medical conditions such as anatomical or functional asplenia or persistent compliment component deficiencies (eg, C_5-C_9, properdin, factor H, or factor D)
- Persons ≥9 months of age that travel to or reside in countries where meningococcal disease is hyperendemic or epidemic, especially if contact with the local population will be prolonged
- Unvaccinated or incompletely vaccinated first year college students living in residence halls
- Military recruits
- Microbiologists with occupational exposure

The Canadian National Advisory Committee on Immunization (NACI): NACI recommends a routine vaccination at ~12 years of age but no booster unless at a continued high risk of exposure. Either quadrivalent vaccine may be used; NACI does not have a preference. NACI recommends use of Menveo (off-label use) for high risk persons 2 months to 2 years of age if vaccination with a quadrivalent vaccine is needed; may also be considered for use in persons ≥56 years of age (NACI, 39[1], 2013). Additional recommendations may be found at www.phac-aspc.gc.ca/publicat/ccdr-rmtc/13vol39/acs-dcc-1/index-eng.php

Pregnancy Risk Factor B/C (manufacturer dependent)

Dosage IM:

Menactra:

Infants ≥9 months and Children <2 years: 0.5 mL/dose given as a 2-dose series, 3 months apart

Children ≥2 years, Adolescents, and Adults ≤55 years: 0.5 mL/dose given as a single dose

Menveo: Age at initial vaccination:

Infants ≥2 months to <7 months: 0.5 mL/dose given as a 4-dose series at 2, 4, 6, and 12 months of age

Infants ≥7 months and Children <2 years: 0.5 mL/dose given as a 2-dose series, with the second dose given during the second year of life and at least 3 months after the first dose

Children ≥2 to <6 years: 0.5 mL/dose given as a single dose; for children at continued high risk of meningococcal disease, may consider an additional dose given 2 months after the first dose

Children ≥6 years, Adolescents, and Adults ≤55 years: 0.5 mL/dose given as a single dose

ACIP recommendations (CDC/ACIP [Akinsanya-Beysolow, 2014]; CDC/ACIP [Bridges, 2014]): **Note:** Use of the abbreviation, MenACWY, refers to either meningococcal quadrivalent polysaccharide vaccine. MenACWY-CRM refers specifically to Menveo; MenACWY-D refers specifically to Menactra.

Primary vaccination:

Infants, Children, and Adolescents: **Note:** Patients who are HIV positive should receive two doses two months apart.

<11 years: Not routinely recommended; see dosing for persons at increased risk

11 to 12 years: One 0.5 mL dose. Children not at increased risk for meningococcal disease who may have been previously vaccinated with Hib-MenCY-TT (MenHibrix) or MenACWY (Menactra or Menveo) prior to their tenth birthday, should receive the routinely recommended doses of MenACWY (Menactra or Menveo) at 11 to 12 years

13 to 18 years: One 0.5 mL dose if not previously vaccinated

Adults:

19 to 21 years: Not routinely recommended; may receive one 0.5 mL dose as a catch-up vaccination if no dose was received after the sixteenth birthday

≥22 years: Not routinely recommended; see dosing for persons at increased risk

Primary vaccination: Persons at increased risk for meningococcal disease:

Infants and Children <2 years with anatomic or functional asplenia, including sickle-cell disease:

Infants and Children <19 months: MenACWY-CRM (Menveo): IM: 0.5 mL per dose for a total of 4 doses given as follows: 2, 4, 6, and 12 to 15 months

Children 19 to 23 months (incomplete vaccination): MenACWY-CRM (Menveo): IM: 0.5 mL per dose for a total of 2 doses given at least three months apart.

Infants and Children <2 years with persistent complement component deficiency:

Infants and Children <19 months: MenACWY-CRM (Menveo): IM: 0.5 mL per dose for a total of 4 doses given as follows: 2, 4, 6, and 12 to 15 months

Infants and Children 7 to 23 months (unvaccinated):

MenACWY-CRM (Menveo): IM: 0.5 mL per dose for a total of 2 doses; the second dose should be given at age ≥12 months and at least three months after the first dose.

MenACWY-D (Menactra): IM: 0.5 mL per dose for a total of 2 doses; the first dose should be given at age ≥9 months and the second dose should be given at least three months after the first dose. May be given as early as 8 weeks apart if needed prior to travel.

Infants and Children <2 years for community outbreak (due to vaccine serogroup): Infants ≥2 months to Children 23 months: Initiate or complete an age appropriate series of MenACWY-CRM (Menveo) or MenACWY-D (Menactra); see Primary vaccination above for dosing.

Infants and Children <2 years with travel to or residence in countries with hyperendemic or epidemic meningococcal disease: Infants ≥9 months to Children 23 months: Initiate or complete an age appropriate series of MenACWY-CRM (Menveo) or MenACWY-D (Menactra); see Primary vaccination above for dosing.

Children ≥2 years, Adolescents, and Adults ≤55 years not previously vaccinated and who have persistent complement deficiencies, functional or anatomic asplenia, or who have HIV infection and another indication for vaccination: Two 0.5 mL doses, given ≥2 months apart. If using MenACWY-D (Menactra), administer ≥4 weeks after completion of all PCV doses

Children ≥2 years, Adolescents, and Adults ≤55 years not previously vaccinated and who are either: First year college students ≤21 years of age living in residential housing, traveling to or residents of areas where meningococcal disease is endemic/hyperendemic, at risk during a community outbreak, military recruits, or microbiologists routinely exposed to *Neisseria meningitidis*: One 0.5 mL dose. If using MenACWY-D (Menactra), administer ≥4 weeks after completion of all PCV doses. College students ≤21 years should have documentation of a vaccination not more than 5 years before enrollment (preferably a dose on their sixteenth birthday)

Adults ≥56 years: Meningococcal polysaccharide vaccine (MPSV4, Menomune) is preferred for meningococcal vaccine-naive persons in this age group who require a single dose. If multiple doses are anticipated, see booster dosing for persons at increased risk.

Booster dose: Children ≥11 years, Adolescents, and Adults ≤21 years: One 0.5 mL dose if the first dose was given prior to the sixteenth birthday. If primary vaccination was at 11 to 12 years, the booster dose should be given at age 16. If the primary vaccination was given at 13 to 15 years, the booster dose should be given at age 16 to 18. Minimum interval between MenACWY (Menveo or Menactra) doses is 8 weeks. A booster dose is not needed if the primary dose was given after the sixteenth birthday unless the person becomes at increased risk for meningococcal disease.

Booster vaccination: Persons at increased risk for meningococcal disease:

Manufacturer labeling: Menactra: Adolescents ≥15 years and Adults ≤55 years: Repeat a single dose ≥4 years after prior dose.

ACIP recommendations (CDC/ACIP [Bridges, 2014]; CDC/ACIP [Cohn, 2013]):

If first dose received at 2 months to 6 years of age: Repeat dose 3 years after primary vaccination, and every 5 years thereafter if the person remains at increased risk.

If first dose received at ≥7 years of age: Repeat dose 5 years after primary vaccination, and every 5 years thereafter if the person remains at increased risk.

Adults ≥56 years: Persons previously vaccinated with MenACWY and who require revaccination or for whom multiple doses are anticipated, MenACWY-D (Menactra) is preferred. Otherwise, meningococcal polysaccharide vaccine (MPSV4, Menomune) is preferred for meningococcal vaccine naïve persons in this age group who require a single dose.

Dosage adjustment in renal impairment: There are no dosage adjustments provided in the manufacturer's labeling.

Dosage adjustment in hepatic impairment: There are no dosage adjustments provided in the manufacturer's labeling.

Additional Information Complete prescribing information should be consulted for additional detail.

Dosage Forms

Injection, solution [preservative free]:

Menactra: 4 mcg each of polysaccharide antigen groups A, C, Y, and W-135 [bound to diphtheria toxoid 48 mcg] per 0.5 mL

Menveo: MenA oligosaccharide 10 mcg, MenC oligosaccharide 5 mcg, MenY oligosaccharide 5 mcg, and MenW-135 oligosaccharide 5 mcg [bound to CRM_{197} protein 32.7-64.1 mcg] per 0.5 mL

Meningococcal Polysaccharide (Groups A / C / Y and W-135) Tetanus Toxoid Conjugate Vaccine [CAN/INT]

(me NIN joe kok al pol i SAK a ride groops aye, see, why & dubl yoo won thur tee fyve TET a nus TOKS oyd KON joo gate vak SEEN)

Brand Names: Canada Nimenrix

Index Terms MenACWY-TT

Pharmacologic Category Vaccine, Inactivated (Bacterial)

Additional Appendix Information

Immunization Administration Recommendations *on page 2250*

Immunization Recommendations *on page 2255*

Use Note: Not approved in U.S.

Meningococcal disease prevention: Provides active immunization against invasive meningococcal disease caused by *Neisseria meningitidis* serogroups A, C, Y, and W-135

Pregnancy Considerations Adverse effects were not observed in animal reproduction studies.

Breast-Feeding Considerations It is not known if this vaccine is found in breast milk. According to the manufacturer, the decision to continue or discontinue breastfeeding during therapy should take into account the risk of exposure to the infant and the benefits of treatment to the mother.

Contraindications Hypersensitivity to any component of the vaccine.

Warnings/Precautions Immediate treatment (including epinephrine 1:1000) for anaphylactoid and/or hypersensitivity reactions should be available during vaccine use.

Syncope may occur before or following vaccination. Procedures should be in place to avoid injuries from falling. Defer administration in patients with severe acute febrile illness; may administer to patients with mild acute illness.

Use with caution in patients with a history of bleeding disorders (including thrombocytopenia) and/or patients on anticoagulant therapy; bleeding/hematoma may occur from IM administration. Use with caution in terminal complement deficiencies, functional or anatomic asplenia, and severely immunocompromised patients (eg, patients receiving chemo/radiation therapy or other immunosuppressive therapy [including high-dose corticosteroids]); may have a reduced response to vaccination. In general, household and close contacts of persons with altered immunocompetence may receive all age appropriate vaccines (CDC 60[2], 2011); inactivated vaccines should be administered ≥2 weeks prior to planned immunosuppression when feasible (Rubin, 2014).

For intramuscular injection only. Not intended for intravascular, intradermal, or subcutaneous administration. Confers protection only against *Neisseria meningitidis* serogroups contained in the vaccine. May be administered to patients previously vaccinated with a plain polysaccharide meningococcal vaccine; administration in patients previously vaccinated with a conjugated meningococcal C vaccine has not been studied. Vaccine contains tetanus toxoid but is not a substitute for tetanus immunization.

Vaccination may not result in effective immunity in all patients. Response depends upon multiple factors (eg, type of vaccine, age of patient) and may be improved by administering the vaccine at the recommended dose, route, and interval. Compared with other meningococcal serogroups, a more rapid decline of antibodies to meningococcal serogroup A has been observed in some clinical trials. Vaccines may not be effective if administered during periods of altered immune competence (CDC 60[2], 2011).

Adverse Reactions In Canada, adverse reactions may be reported to local provincial/territorial health agencies or to the Vaccine Safety Section at Public Health Agency of Canada (1-866-844-0018).

Central nervous system: Drowsiness (more common in children 12 to 23 months), fatigue (more common in children, adolescents, and adults 6 to 25 years), irritability (more common in children 12 to 23 months), headache (more common in children, adolescents, and adults 6 to 25 years)

Gastrointestinal: Decreased appetite (more common in children 12 to 23 months), gastrointestinal symptoms (more common in children, adolescents, and adults 6 to 25 years)

Local: Erythema at injection site (more common in children 12 months to 10 years), hematoma at injection site, pain at injection site (more common in children, adolescents, and adults 6 to 25 years), swelling at injection site (more common in children, adolescents, and adults 12 months to 25 years)

Miscellaneous: Fever

Rare but important or life-threatening: Local anesthesia (injection site), syncope

Drug Interactions

Metabolism/Transport Effects None known.

Avoid Concomitant Use There are no known interactions where it is recommended to avoid concomitant use.

Increased Effect/Toxicity There are no known significant interactions involving an increase in effect.

Decreased Effect

Meningococcal Polysaccharide (Groups A / C / Y and W-135) Tetanus Toxoid Conjugate Vaccine may decrease the levels/effects of: Tetanus Toxoids Vaccines

The levels/effects of Meningococcal Polysaccharide (Groups A / C / Y and W-135) Tetanus Toxoid Conjugate Vaccine may be decreased by: Belimumab; Immunosuppressants

Preparation for Administration Add entire contents of prefilled syringe containing diluent to the vial containing powder. Shake the vial until the powder completely dissolves. Resulting solution should be clear and colorless. Withdraw solution from vial using new needle. Use immediately after reconstitution.

Storage/Stability Prior to reconstitution, store between 2°C to 8°C (36°F to 46°F). Prefilled syringe containing diluent may also be stored at 25°C (77°F). Do not freeze. Protect from light. After reconstitution, administer vaccine immediately. Do not mix with other vaccines in the same syringe.

Mechanism of Action Induces immunity against meningococcal disease via the formation of bactericidal antibodies directed toward the polysaccharide capsular components of *Neisseria meningitidis* serogroups A, C, Y and W-135.

Dosage Meningococcal disease prevention: Children ≥1 year, Adolescents, and Adults ≤55 years: IM: 0.5 mL as single dose. **Note:** The need for a booster dose has not been established. Manufacturer labeling suggests that a second dose may be considered for patients at increased risk of exposure to meningococcal serogroup A and who received the first Nimenrix dose >1 year prior.

Dosage adjustment in renal impairment: There are no dosage adjustments provided in the manufacturer's labeling.

Dosage adjustment in hepatic impairment: There are no dosage adjustments provided in the manufacturer's labeling.

Administration For IM injection. Do not administer intravascularly, intradermally, or subcutaneously. Administer into the deltoid muscle. May consider administering into the anterolateral aspect of the thigh for children 1 year to 23 months of age.

Monitoring Parameters Monitor for syncope for at least 15 minutes following administration (Canadian Immunization Guide, 2013).

Product Availability Not available in the U.S.

Dosage Forms: Canada

Injection, powder for reconstitution [preservative free]:

Nimenrix: 5 mcg each of polysaccharide antigen groups A, C, Y, and W-135 [bound to tetanus toxoid 44 mcg] per 0.5 mL dose

Meningococcal Polysaccharide (Groups C and Y) and *Haemophilus* b Tetanus Toxoid Conjugate Vaccine

(me NIN joe kok al pol i SAK a ride groops see & why & he MOF i lus bee TET a nus TOKS oyd KON joo gate vak SEEN)

Brand Names: U.S. Menhibrix

Index Terms Hib-MenCY-TT

Pharmacologic Category Vaccine, Inactivated (Bacterial)

Additional Appendix Information

Immunization Administration Recommendations *on page 2250*

Immunization Recommendations *on page 2255*

Use To provide active immunity to prevent invasive disease caused by meningococcal serogroups C and Y and *Haemophilus influenzae* type b

The Advisory Committee on Immunization Practices (ACIP) recommends vaccination only for infants 2-18 months of age who are at increased risk for meningococcal disease, including:

- Infants with persistent complement pathway deficiencies
- Infants with anatomic or functional asplenia, including sickle cell disease
- Infants in communities with serogroups C and Y meningococcal disease outbreaks

The ACIP does not recommend routine vaccination for infants not at increased risk for meningococcal disease. In addition, infants traveling to certain areas (eg, meningitis belt of sub-Saharan Africa) will require a meningococcal vaccine with serogroups A and W_{135}; vaccination with Hib-MenCY-TT will not be adequate (CDC, 2013).

Pregnancy Risk Factor C

Dosage Primary immunization: Infants ≥6 weeks and Children ≤18 months: IM: 0.5 mL/dose given as a four-dose series at 2, 4, 6, and 12-15 months of age. The first dose may be given as early as 6 weeks of age and the fourth dose may be given as late as 18 months of age.

Note: The ACIP recommends vaccination only for infants ≥2 months and children ≤18 months of age who are at an increased risk for meningococcal disease. The first dose may be given as early as 6 weeks of age and the fourth dose may be given as late as 18 months of age. If an infant at increased risk is behind on Hib vaccine doses, Hib-MenCY-TT may be used to catch up using the current Hib schedule. If the first dose of Hib-MenCY-TT is given ≥12 months of age, two doses should be given 8 weeks apart. If infants have/will receive a different Hib vaccine, a two-dose series of a quadrivalent meningococcal vaccine is recommended (Menactra® for ages 9-23 months; Menactra® or Menveo® for ages >23 months) (CDC, 2013).

Dosage adjustment in renal impairment: No dosage adjustment provided in manufacturer's labeling.

Dosage adjustment in hepatic impairment: No dosage adjustment provided in manufacturer's labeling.

Additional Information Complete prescribing information should be consulted for additional detail.

Dosage Forms

Solution Reconstituted, Intramuscular [preservative free]:

Menhibrix: 5 mcg each of polysaccharide antigen groups C and Y, and 2.5 mcg Haemophilus b capsular polysaccharide per 0.5 mL dose (1 ea)

◆ **Meningococcal Polysaccharide Vaccine** *see* Meningococcal Polysaccharide Vaccine (Groups A / C / Y and W-135) *on page* 1292

Meningococcal Polysaccharide Vaccine (Groups A / C / Y and W-135)

(me NIN joe kok al pol i SAK a ride vak SEEN groops aye, see, why & dubl yoo won thur tee fyve)

Brand Names: U.S. Menomune-A/C/Y/W-135

Brand Names: Canada Menomune-A/C/Y/W-135

Index Terms Meningococcal Polysaccharide Vaccine; MPSV; MPSV4

Pharmacologic Category Vaccine, Inactivated (Bacterial)

Additional Appendix Information

Immunization Administration Recommendations *on page* 2250

Immunization Recommendations *on page* 2255

Use Provide active immunity to meningococcal serogroups contained in the vaccine

The Advisory Committee on Immunization Practices (ACIP) recommends routine vaccination for persons at increased risk for meningococcal disease. Meningococcal quadrivalent conjugate vaccine (MenACWY) is preferred; meningococcal polysaccharide vaccine (MPSV4) is preferred in meningococcal vaccine-naive adults ≥56 years of age requiring only a single vaccination (CDC/ACIP [Cohn, 2013]).

Those at increased risk of meningococcal disease include the following:

- Persons ≥2 months of age with medical conditions such as anatomical or functional asplenia or persistent compliment component deficiencies (eg, C_5-C_9, properdin, factor H, or factor D)
- Persons ≥9 months of age that travel to or reside in countries where meningococcal disease is hyperendemic or epidemic, especially if contact with the local population will be prolonged
- Unvaccinated or incompletely vaccinated first year college students living in residence halls
- Military recruits
- Microbiologists with occupational exposure
- Persons (in all recommended age groups) at risk who are part of outbreaks caused by vaccine preventable serogroups

Pregnancy Risk Factor C

Dosage

Immunization: Children ≥2 years, Adolescents, and Adults: SubQ: 0.5 mL/dose

ACIP recommendations (CDC/ACIP [Cohn, 2013]):

Children, Adolescents, and Adults <56 years: Not routinely recommended

Adults ≥56 years: Meningococcal polysaccharide vaccine (MPSV4, Menomune) is preferred for meningococcal vaccine-naive persons in this age group who are at increased risk of meningococcal infection and require a single dose (eg, travelers or during a community outbreak). Persons previously vaccinated with a quadrivalent meningococcal conjugate vaccine (MenACWY, Menveo, or Menactra) and who require revaccination or for whom multiple doses are anticipated, MenACWY-D (Menactra) is preferred (eg, persons with asplenia or microbiologists).

Dosage adjustment in renal impairment: There are no dosage adjustments provided in manufacturer's labeling.

Dosage adjustment in hepatic impairment: There are no dosage adjustments provided in manufacturer's labeling.

Additional Information Complete prescribing information should be consulted for additional detail.

Dosage Forms

Injection, powder for reconstitution [MPSV4]:

Menomune-A/C/Y/W-135: 50 mcg each of polysaccharide antigen groups A, C, Y, and W-135 per 0.5 mL dose

◆ **Menjugate (Can)** *see* Meningococcal Group C-CRM197 Conjugate Vaccine [CAN/INT] *on page* 1288

◆ **Menomune-A/C/Y/W-135** *see* Meningococcal Polysaccharide Vaccine (Groups A / C / Y and W-135) *on page* 1292

◆ **Menopur** *see* Menotropins *on page* 1292

◆ **Menostar** *see* Estradiol (Systemic) *on page* 775

Menotropins (men oh TROE pins)

Brand Names: U.S. Menopur; Repronex

Brand Names: Canada Menopur; Repronex

Index Terms hMG; Human Menopausal Gonadotropin

Pharmacologic Category Gonadotropin; Ovulation Stimulator

Use

Menopur: For multiple follicle development and pregnancy in ovulatory women as part of an assisted reproductive technology (ART) cycle

Repronex: In conjunction with hCG to for multiple follicular development (controlled ovarian stimulation) and ovulation induction in women who have previously received GnRH agonist or antagonist for pituitary suppression

Limitations of use: Prior to therapy, preform a complete gynecologic exam and endocrinologic evaluation to diagnose the cause of infertility; exclude the possibility of pregnancy; evaluate the fertility status of the male partner; exclude a diagnosis of primary ovarian failure.

Pregnancy Risk Factor X

Dosage Adults:

Ovulation induction (females): *Repronex:* IM, SubQ: Initial: 150 units once daily for the first 5 days of treatment. Adjustments should not be made more frequently than once every 2 days and should not exceed 75-150 units per adjustment based on ultrasound monitoring of ovarian response and/or measurement of serum estradiol levels. Maximum daily dose: 450 units; treatment >12 days is not recommended. If patient's response is appropriate, administer hCG one day following the last dose of Repronex. Hold dose if serum estradiol is >2000 pg/mL, if the ovaries are abnormally enlarged, or if abdominal pain occurs; the patient should also be advised to refrain from intercourse. May repeat process if follicular development is inadequate or if pregnancy does not occur.

Assisted reproductive technologies (ART) (females):

Menopur: SubQ: Initial: 225 units once daily beginning on cycle day 2 or 3; Menotropins may be administered together with urofollitropin and the total initial dose of both products combined should not exceed 225 units (menotropins 150 units and urofollitropin 75 units; or menotropins 75 units and urofollitropin 150 units). Dose should be adjusted after 5 days based on ultrasound monitoring of ovarian response and/or measurement of serum estradiol levels. Do not make additional adjustments more frequently than once every 2 days or by >150 units. Maximum daily dose: 450 units (of menotropins, or menotropins plus urofollitropin); treatment >20 days is not recommended. Once adequate follicular development is evident, hCG should be administered. Withhold the hCG dose if ovarian monitoring suggests an increased risk of ovarian hyperstimulation syndrome (OHSS).

Repronex: IM, SubQ: Initial: 225 units once daily; adjustments in dose based on ultrasound monitoring of ovarian response and/or measurement of serum estradiol levels should not be made more frequently than once every 2 days and should not exceed more than 75-150 units per adjustment. Maximum daily dose: 450 units; treatment >12 days is not recommended. Once adequate follicular development is evident, hCG should be administered to induce final follicular maturation in preparation for oocyte retrieval. Withhold the hCG dose if ovarian monitoring suggests an increased risk of OHSS.

Spermatogenesis (males) (off-label use): IM: Following pretreatment with hCG: 75 units 3 times per week with hCG twice weekly until sperm is detected in the ejaculate (4-6 months); if response is inadequate after 6 months, may increase menotropins dosage to 150 units 3 times per week for another 6 months (AACE, 2002)

Dosage adjustment in renal impairment: There are no dosage adjustments provided in manufacturer's labeling (has not been studied).

Dosage adjustment in hepatic impairment: There are no dosage adjustments provided in manufacturer's labeling (has not been studied).

Additional Information Complete prescribing information should be consulted for additional detail.

Dosage Forms Considerations 75 units of menotropins represents 75 units each of FSH activity and LH activity

Dosage Forms

Injection, powder for reconstitution:

Menopur, Repronex: 75 units

◆ **Mentax** *see* Butenafine *on page 314*

◆ **Menthol and Methyl Salicylate** *see* Methyl Salicylate and Menthol *on page 1344*

◆ **Menveo** *see* Meningococcal (Groups A / C / Y and W-135) Diphtheria Conjugate Vaccine *on page 1289*

Meperidine (me PER i deen)

Brand Names: U.S. Demerol; Meperitab

Brand Names: Canada Demerol

Index Terms Isonipecaine Hydrochloride; Meperidine Hydrochloride; Pethidine Hydrochloride

Pharmacologic Category Analgesic, Opioid

Additional Appendix Information

Beers Criteria - Potentially Inappropriate Medications for Geriatrics *on page 2271*

Opioid Conversion Table *on page 2232*

Use Management of moderate-to-severe pain; adjunct to anesthesia and preoperative sedation

Pregnancy Risk Factor C

Pregnancy Considerations Animal reproduction studies have not been conducted by the manufacturer. Meperidine crosses the placenta; meperidine and its active metabolite accumulate in the fetus. Respiratory or CNS depression should be expected to occur in the newborn if maternal IM administration occurs within a few hours of delivery (Mattingly, 2003). When used for pain relief during labor, opioids may temporarily affect the heart rate of the fetus. Due to the prolonged half-life of the active metabolite, dose-dependant sedation in the neonate may be observed for 2-3 days following delivery. Meperidine has been used for the management of pain during labor; however, due to adverse maternal and fetal effects, other opioids may be preferred. Meperidine should also be avoided following delivery when postoperative analgesia is needed (ACOG, 2002).

If chronic opioid exposure occurs in pregnancy, adverse events in the newborn (including withdrawal) may occur; monitoring of the neonate is recommended. The minimum effective dose should be used if opioids are needed (Chou, 2009). Neonatal abstinence syndrome following opioid exposure may present with autonomic (eg, fever, temperature instability), gastrointestinal (eg, diarrhea, vomiting, poor feeding/weight gain), or neurologic (eg, high-pitched crying, increased muscle tone, irritability, seizure, tremor) symptoms (Dow, 2012; Hudak, 2012).

Breast-Feeding Considerations Meperidine is excreted in breast milk and may cause CNS and/or respiratory depression in the nursing infant. Due to the potential for serious adverse reactions in the nursing infant, the manufacturer recommends a decision be made whether to discontinue nursing or to discontinue the drug, taking into account the importance of treatment to the mother.

Small concentrations of meperidine are excreted into breast milk following single doses. With multiple doses, concentrations of meperidine and the active metabolite may increase and both are slowly eliminated by a nursing infant (Spigset, 2000). Parenteral opioids used during labor have the potential to interfere with a newborns natural reflex to nurse within the first few hours after birth. Nursing infants exposed to large doses of opioids should be monitored for apnea and sedation. If treatment for pain in nursing women is needed, other agents are preferred (Montgomery, 2012)

Contraindications Hypersensitivity to meperidine or any component of the formulation; use with or within 14 days of MAO inhibitors; severe respiratory insufficiency

Warnings/Precautions Oral meperidine is not recommended for acute/chronic pain management. Meperidine should not be used for acute/cancer pain because of the risk of neurotoxicity. Normeperidine (an active metabolite and CNS stimulant) may accumulate and precipitate anxiety, tremors, or seizures; risk increases with CNS or renal dysfunction, prolonged use (>48 hours), and cumulative dose (>600 mg/24 hours in adults). The Institute for Safe Medication Practice recommends avoiding the use of meperidine for pain control, especially in the elderly and renally impaired (ISMP, 2007). In the elderly; meperidine is not an effective oral analgesic at commonly used doses; may cause neurotoxicity; other agents are preferred in the elderly (Beers Criteria).

May cause CNS depression, which may impair physical or mental abilities; patients must be cautioned about performing tasks which require mental alertness (eg, operating machinery or driving). Potentially significant drug interactions may exist, requiring dose or frequency adjustment, additional monitoring, and/or selection of alternative therapy. Effects (eg, sedation, respiratory depression, hypotension) may be potentiated when used with other sedative/hypnotic drugs, general anesthetics, phenothiazines, or ethanol; consider reduced dose of meperidine if using concomitantly. Use only with extreme caution (if at all) in patients with head injury or increased intracranial pressure (ICP). Avoid use in patients with CNS depression or coma as these patients are susceptible to intracranial effects of CO_2 retention. Use caution with pulmonary, hepatic, or renal disorders, supraventricular tachycardias (including atrial flutter), acute abdominal conditions, biliary tract dysfunction, pancreatitis, delirium tremens, hypothyroidism, myxedema, toxic psychosis, kyphoscoliosis, morbid obesity, adrenal insufficiency, Addison's disease, seizure disorders, pheochromocytoma, BPH, or urethral stricture. May cause hypotension (including orthostatic hypotension); use with caution in patients with depleted blood volume or drugs which may exaggerate hypotensive effects (including phenothiazines or general anesthetics).

In patients with sickle cell anemia, use with caution and decrease initial dose; normeperidine (active metabolite) may accumulate and induce seizures in these patients; Note: Meperidine is not considered a first-line agent for treatment of acute sickle cell pain (NHLBI, 2002); it is not recommended for use in sickle cell patients by the American Pain Society (APS, 2008); use of meperidine should be reserved for brief episodes of treatment in sickle cell patients who have previously benefited from meperidine therapy, or in those who have allergies or are intolerant to other opioids (NHLBI, 2002).

An opioid-containing analgesic regimen should be tailored to each patient's needs and based upon the type of pain being treated (acute versus chronic), the route of administration, degree of tolerance for opioids (naive versus chronic user), age, weight, and medical condition. The optimal analgesic dose varies widely among patients. Some preparations contain sulfites which may cause allergic reaction. Tolerance or drug dependence may result from extended use. Healthcare provider should be alert to problems of abuse, misuse, and diversion. Concurrent use of agonist/antagonist analgesics may precipitate withdrawal symptoms and/or reduced analgesic efficacy in patients following prolonged therapy with mu opioid agonists. Abrupt discontinuation following prolonged use may also lead to withdrawal symptoms. Avoid use in the elderly. After chronic maternal exposure to opioids, neonatal withdrawal syndrome may occur in the newborn; monitor neonate closely. Signs and symptoms include irritability, hyperactivity and abnormal sleep pattern, high-pitched cry, tremor, vomiting, diarrhea, and failure to gain weight. Onset, duration and severity depend on the drug used, duration of use, maternal dose, and rate of drug elimination by the newborn. Opioid withdrawal syndrome in the neonate, unlike in adults, may be life-threatening and should be treated according to protocols developed by neonatology experts.

Benzyl alcohol and derivatives: Some dosage forms may contain sodium benzoate/benzoic acid; benzoic acid (benzoate) is a metabolite of benzyl alcohol; large amounts of benzyl alcohol (≥99 mg/kg/day) have been associated with a potentially fatal toxicity ("gasping syndrome") in neonates; the "gasping syndrome" consists of metabolic acidosis, respiratory distress, gasping respirations, CNS dysfunction (including convulsions, intracranial hemorrhage), hypotension, and cardiovascular collapse (AAP, 1997; CDC, 1982); some data suggests that benzoate displaces bilirubin from protein binding sites (Ahlfors, 2001); avoid or use dosage forms containing benzyl alcohol derivative with caution in neonates. See manufacturer's labeling.

Adverse Reactions

Cardiovascular: Bradycardia, cardiac arrest, circulatory depression, flushing, hypotension, palpitations, shock, syncope, tachycardia

Central nervous system: Agitation, confusion, delirium, depression, disorientation, dizziness, drowsiness, drug dependence (physical dependence), dysphoria, euphoria, fatigue, habituation, hallucination, headache, increased intracranial pressure, malaise, myoclonus, nervousness, paradoxical central nervous system stimulation, restlessness, sedation, seizure (associated with metabolite accumulation), serotonin syndrome

Dermatologic: Diaphoresis, pruritus, skin rash, urticaria

Gastrointestinal: Abdominal cramps, anorexia, biliary colic, constipation, nausea, paralytic ileus, spasm of sphincter of Oddi, vomiting, xerostomia

Genitourinary: Ureteral spasm, urinary retention

Hypersensitivity: Anaphylaxis, histamine release, hypersensitivity reaction

Local: Injection site reaction (including pain, wheal, and flare)

Neuromuscular & skeletal: Muscle twitching, tremor, weakness

Ophthalmic: Visual disturbance

Respiratory: Dyspnea, respiratory arrest, respiratory depression

Rare but important or life-threatening: Hypogonadism (Brennan, 2013; Debono, 2011)

Drug Interactions

Metabolism/Transport Effects None known.

Avoid Concomitant Use

Avoid concomitant use of Meperidine with any of the following: Azelastine (Nasal); Dapoxetine; MAO Inhibitors; Orphenadrine; Paraldehyde; Thalidomide

Increased Effect/Toxicity

Meperidine may increase the levels/effects of: Alcohol (Ethyl); Alvimopan; Antipsychotic Agents; Azelastine (Nasal); Buprenorphine; CNS Depressants; Desmopressin; Diuretics; Hydrocodone; Methotrimeprazine; Metoclopramide; Metyrosine; Orphenadrine; Paraldehyde; Pramipexole; ROPINIRole; Rotigotine; Serotonin Modulators; Suvorexant; Thalidomide; Zolpidem

The levels/effects of Meperidine may be increased by: Amphetamines; Anticholinergic Agents; Antiemetics (5HT3 Antagonists); Antipsychotic Agents; Antipsychotic Agents (Phenothiazines); Barbiturates; Brimonidine (Topical); Cannabis; Dapoxetine; Doxylamine; Dronabinol;

Droperidol; HydrOXYzine; Kava Kava; Magnesium Sulfate; MAO Inhibitors; Methotrimeprazine; Nabilone; Perampanel; Protease Inhibitors; Rufinamide; Sodium Oxybate; Succinylcholine; Tapentadol; Tetrahydrocannabinol

Decreased Effect

Meperidine may decrease the levels/effects of: Pegvisomant

The levels/effects of Meperidine may be decreased by: Ammonium Chloride; Fosphenytoin; Mixed Agonist / Antagonist Opioids; Naltrexone; Phenytoin; Protease Inhibitors

Storage/Stability

Injection solution: Store at 20°C to 25°C (68°F to 77°F); excursions permitted to 15°C to 30°C (59°F to 86°F).

Tablets: Store at 25°C (77°F); excursions permitted to 15°C to 30°C (59°F to 86°F).

Mechanism of Action Binds to opioid receptors in the CNS, causing inhibition of ascending pain pathways, altering the perception of and response to pain; produces generalized CNS depression

Pharmacodynamics/Kinetics

Onset of action: Analgesic: Oral, SubQ: 10-15 minutes; IV: ~5 minutes

Peak effect: SubQ.: ~1 hour; Oral: 2 hours

Duration: Oral, SubQ.: 2-4 hours

Absorption: IM: Erratic and highly variable

Protein binding: 65% to 75%

Metabolism: Hepatic; hydrolyzed to meperidinic acid (inactive) or undergoes N-demethylation to normeperidine (active; has 1/2 the analgesic effect and 2-3 times the CNS effects of meperidine)

Bioavailability: ~50% to 60%; increased with liver disease

Half-life elimination:

Parent drug: Terminal phase: Adults: 2.5-4 hours, Liver disease: 7-11 hours

Normeperidine (active metabolite): 15-30 hours; can accumulate with high doses (>600 mg/day) or with decreased renal function

Excretion: Urine (as metabolites)

Dosage Note: The American Pain Society (2008) and ISMP (2007) do not recommend meperidine's use as an analgesic. If use in acute pain (in patients without renal or CNS disease) cannot be avoided, treatment should be limited to ≤48 hours and doses should not exceed 600 mg/24 hours. Oral route is not recommended for treatment of acute or chronic pain. If IV route is required, consider a reduced dose. Patients with prior opioid exposure may require higher initial doses.

Children: Pain: Oral, IM, SubQ: 1.1-1.8 mg/kg/dose every 3-4 hours as needed (maximum: 50-150 mg/dose)

Preoperatively: IM, SubQ: 1.1-2.2 mg/kg given 30-90 minutes before the beginning of anesthesia (maximum: 50-150 mg/dose)

Adults:

Pain: Oral, IM, SubQ: 50-150 mg every 3-4 hours as needed

Preoperatively: IM, SubQ: 50-150 mg given 30-90 minutes before the beginning of anesthesia

Obstetrical analgesia: IM, SubQ: 50-100 mg when pain becomes regular; may repeat at every 1-3 hours

Postoperative shivering (off-label use): IV: 25-50 mg once (Crowley, 2008; Kranke, 2002; Mercandante, 1994; Wang, 1999)

Elderly: Avoid use (American Pain Society, 2008; ISMP, 2007)

Dosing adjustment in renal impairment: Avoid use in renal impairment (American Pain Society, 2008; ISMP, 2007)

Dosing adjustment in hepatic impairment: Use with caution in severe hepatic impairment; consider a lower initial dose when initiating therapy. An increased opioid effect may be seen in patients with cirrhosis; dose reduction is more important for the oral than IV route.

Administration

Solution for injection: Meperidine may be administered IM, SubQ, or IV; IV push should be administered slowly using a diluted solution, use of a 10 mg/mL concentration has been recommended.

Oral solution: Administer solution in 1/2 glass of water; undiluted solution may exert topical anesthetic effect on mucous membranes

Monitoring Parameters Pain relief, respiratory and mental status, blood pressure; observe patient for excessive sedation, CNS depression, seizures, respiratory depression; signs or symptoms of hypogonadism or hypoadrenalism (Brennan, 2013)

Dosage Forms

Solution, Injection:

Demerol: 25 mg/mL (1 mL); 25 mg/0.5 mL (0.5 mL); 50 mg/mL (1 mL, 30 mL); 75 mg/1.5 mL (1.5 mL); 100 mg/2 mL (2 mL); 75 mg/mL (1 mL); 100 mg/mL (1 mL, 20 mL)

Generic: 10 mg/mL (30 mL); 25 mg/mL (1 mL); 50 mg/mL (1 mL); 100 mg/mL (1 mL)

Solution, Oral:

Generic: 50 mg/5 mL (500 mL)

Tablet, Oral:

Demerol: 50 mg, 100 mg

Meperitab: 50 mg, 100 mg

Generic: 50 mg, 100 mg

- **Meperidine Hydrochloride** *see* Meperidine *on page 1293*
- **Meperitab** *see* Meperidine *on page 1293*
- **Mephyton®** *see* Phytonadione *on page 1647*

Mepivacaine (me PIV a kane)

Brand Names: U.S. Carbocaine; Carbocaine Preservative-Free; Polocaine; Polocaine-MPF

Brand Names: Canada Carbocaine®; Polocaine®

Index Terms Mepivacaine Hydrochloride

Pharmacologic Category Local Anesthetic

Use Local or regional analgesia; anesthesia by local infiltration, peripheral and central neural techniques (epidural and caudal); **not** for use in spinal anesthesia

Pregnancy Risk Factor C

Dosage

Injectable local anesthetic: Dose varies with procedure, degree of anesthesia needed, vascularity of tissue, duration of anesthesia required, and physical condition of patient. The smallest dose and concentration required to produce the desired effect should be used.

Children: Injection: According to the manufacturer, a mepivacaine dose up to 6.6 mg/kg or 400 mg (whichever is less) may be administered during any single dental sitting. For most procedures, doses >180 mg are unnecessary. The American Academy of Pediatric Dentistry (AAPD) recommends a maximum mepivacaine dose of 4.4 mg/kg or a maximum total dose of 300 mg in any single dental sitting (AAPD, 2009).

Adults: Maximum single or total dose given for one procedure: 400 mg; 500 mg if epinephrine has been added (Barash, 2009)

Cervical, brachial, intercostal, pudendal nerve block: 5-40 mL of a 1% solution (maximum: 400 mg) **or** 5-20 mL of a 2% solution (maximum: 400 mg). For pudendal block, inject one-half the total dose each side.

Transvaginal block (paracervical plus pudendal): Up to 30 mL (total for both sides) of a 1% solution (maximum: 300 mg). Inject one-half the total dose each side.

Paracervical block: Up to 20 mL (total for both sides) of a 1% solution (maximum: 200 mg). Inject one-half the total dose to each side. This is the maximum recommended dose per 90-minute procedure; inject slowly with 5 minutes between sides.

Caudal and epidural block (preservative free solutions only): 15-30 mL of a 1% solution (maximum: 300 mg) **or** 10-25 mL of a 1.5% solution (maximum: 375 mg) **or** 10-20 mL of a 2% solution (maximum: 400 mg)

Infiltration: Up to 40 mL of a 1% solution (maximum: 400 mg); up to 50 mL if epinephrine has been added (maximum: 500 mg) (Barash, 2009); an equivalent amount of a 0.5% solution (prepared by diluting the 1% solution with NS) may be used for large areas

Peripheral nerve block to provide a surgical level of anesthesia (Miller, 2010):

Major nerve block (blockade of two or more distinct nerves, a nerve plexus, or very large nerves at more proximal sites: 30-50 mL of a 1% or 1.5% solution (maximum: 500 mg)

Minor nerve block (blockade of a single nerve [eg, ulnar or radial]): 5-20 mL of a 1% solution (maximum: 200 mg)

Therapeutic block: 1-5 mL of 1% solution (maximum: 50 mg) **or** 1-5 mL of 2% solution (maximum: 100 mg)

Elderly: Decreased doses suggested by manufacturer's labeling; however, no dosing adjustments provided. Refer to adult dosing.

Dosage adjustment in renal impairment: No dosage adjustment provided in manufacturer's labeling; use with caution.

Dosage adjustment in hepatic impairment: No dosage adjustment provided in manufacturer's labeling; use with caution.

Additional Information Complete prescribing information should be consulted for additional detail.

Dosage Forms

Solution, Injection:

Carbocaine: 1% (50 mL); 2% (50 mL)

Polocaine: 1% (50 mL); 2% (50 mL)

Generic: 3% (1.8 mL)

Solution, Injection [preservative free]:

Carbocaine Preservative-Free: 1% (30 mL); 1.5% (30 mL); 2% (20 mL)

Polocaine-MPF: 1% (30 mL); 1.5% (30 mL); 2% (20 mL)

◆ **Mepivacaine Hydrochloride** *see* Mepivacaine *on page 1295*

Meprobamate (me proe BA mate)

Index Terms Equanil

Pharmacologic Category Antianxiety Agent, Miscellaneous

Additional Appendix Information

Beers Criteria – Potentially Inappropriate Medications for Geriatrics *on page 2271*

Use Management of anxiety disorders

Dosage Oral:

Anxiety:

Children 6-12 years: 200-600 mg/day in 2-3 divided doses

Adults: 1200-1600 mg/day in 3-4 divided doses, up to 2400 mg/day

Muscle spasm (TMJ) pain (off-label use): Adults: 1200-1600 mg/day in 3-4 divided doses, up to 2400 mg/day

Dosing interval in renal impairment: No dosage adjustment provided in manufacturer's labeling; however, the following adjustments have been recommended (Aronoff, 2007): Adults:

CrCl 10-50 mL/minute: Administer every 9-12 hours.

CrCl <10 mL/minute: Administer every 12-18 hours.

Hemodialysis: No dosage adjustment necessary.

Peritoneal dialysis: Administer every 12-18 hours.

Continuous renal replacement therapy (CRRT): Administer every 9-12 hours.

Dosing adjustment in hepatic impairment: No dosage adjustment provided in manufacturer's labeling; use with caution.

Additional Information Complete prescribing information should be consulted for additional detail.

Dosage Forms

Tablet, Oral:

Generic: 200 mg, 400 mg

◆ **Mepron** *see* Atovaquone *on page 197*

◆ **Mepron® (Can)** *see* Atovaquone *on page 197*

◆ **Mercaptoethane Sulfonate** *see* Mesna *on page 1305*

Mercaptopurine (mer kap toe PURE een)

Brand Names: U.S. Purinethol; Purixan

Brand Names: Canada Purinethol

Index Terms 6-Mercaptopurine (error-prone abbreviation); 6-MP (error-prone abbreviation)

Pharmacologic Category Antineoplastic Agent, Antimetabolite; Antineoplastic Agent, Antimetabolite (Purine Analog); Immunosuppressant Agent

Use Acute lymphoblastic leukemia: Treatment maintenance treatment of acute lymphoblastic leukemia (ALL), as part of a combination chemotherapy regimen

Pregnancy Risk Factor D

Pregnancy Considerations May cause fetal harm if administered during pregnancy. Case reports of fetal loss have been noted with mercaptopurine administration during the first trimester; adverse effects have also been noted with second and third trimester use. Women of child bearing potential should avoid becoming pregnant during treatment.

Breast-Feeding Considerations Mercaptopurine is the active metabolite of azathioprine. Following administration of azathioprine, mercaptopurine can be detected in breast milk (Gardiner, 2006). It is not known if/how much mercaptopurine is found in breast milk following oral administration. According to the manufacturer, the decision to discontinue mercaptopurine or discontinue breast-feeding during therapy should take into account the benefits of treatment to the mother.

Contraindications Hypersensitivity to mercaptopurine or any component of the formulation; patients whose disease showed prior resistance to mercaptopurine

Warnings/Precautions Hazardous agent - use appropriate precautions for handling and disposal (NIOSH 2014 [group 1]).

Hepatotoxicity has been reported, including jaundice, ascites, hepatic necrosis (may be fatal), intrahepatic cholestasis, parenchymal cell necrosis, and/or hepatic encephalopathy; may be due to direct hepatic cell damage or hypersensitivity. While hepatotoxicity or hepatic injury may occur at any dose, dosages >2.5 mg/kg/day are associated with a higher incidence. Signs of jaundice generally appear early in treatment, after ~1-2 months (range: 1 week to 8 years) and may resolve following discontinuation; recurrence with rechallenge has been noted. Monitor liver function tests, including transaminases, alkaline phosphatase, and bilirubin weekly with treatment initiation, then monthly thereafter (monitor more frequently if used in combination with other hepatotoxic drugs or in patients with preexisting hepatic impairment). Consider a reduced dose in patients with baseline hepatic impairment; monitor closely for toxicity. Withhold treatment for clinical signs of jaundice (hepatomegaly, anorexia, tenderness), deterioration in liver function tests, toxic hepatitis, or biliary stasis until hepatotoxicity is ruled out.

Dose-related leukopenia, thrombocytopenia, and anemia are common; however, may be indicative of disease progression. Hematologic toxicity may be delayed. Bone marrow may appear hypoplastic (could also appear normal). Monitor blood counts; dose may require adjusting for severe neutropenia or thrombocytopenia. Monitor for bleeding (due to thrombocytopenia) or infection (due to neutropenia). Profound severe or repeated hematologic toxicity may be indicative of TPMT deficiency. Patients with homozygous genetic defect of thiopurine methyltransferase (TPMT) are more sensitive to myelosuppressive effects; generally associated with rapid myelosuppression. Significant mercaptopurine dose reductions will be necessary (possibly with continued concomitant chemotherapy at normal doses). Patients who are heterozygous for TPMT defects will have intermediate activity; may have increased toxicity (primarily myelosuppression) although will generally tolerate normal mercaptopurine doses. Consider TPMT testing for severe toxicities/excessive myelosuppression. Potentially significant drug-drug interactions may exist, requiring dose or frequency adjustment, additional monitoring, and/or selection of alternative therapy. Because azathioprine is metabolized to mercaptopurine, concomitant use with azathioprine may result in profound myelosuppression and should be avoided. Concurrent use of allopurinol and mercaptopurine may result in a significant increase in hematologic toxicity; avoid concurrent use. Hematologic toxicity may be exacerbated by other medications which inhibit TPMT (eg, mesalamine, olsalazine, sulfasalazine) or by other myelosuppressive drugs.

Immunosuppressive agents, including mercaptopurine, are associated with the development of lymphoma and other malignancies including hepatosplenic T-cell lymphoma (HSTCL). Mercaptopurine is immunosuppressive; immune responses to infections may be impaired and the risk for infection is increased; common signs of infection, such as fever and leukocytosis may not occur; lethargy and confusion may be more prominent signs of infection. Immune response to vaccines may be diminished; live virus vaccines impose a risk for infection. Consider adjusting dosage in patients with renal impairment. Some renal adverse effects may be minimized with hydration and prophylactic antihyperuricemic therapy. To avoid potentially serious dosage errors, the terms "6-mercaptopurine" or "6-MP" should be avoided; use of these terms has been associated with sixfold overdosages.

Adverse Reactions

Central nervous system: Drug fever, malaise

Dermatologic: Alopecia, hyperpigmentation, skin rash, urticaria

Endocrine & metabolic: Hyperuricemia

Gastrointestinal: Anorexia, cholestasis, diarrhea, mucositis, oral lesion, nausea (minimal), pancreatitis, sprue-like symptoms, stomach pain, ulcerative bowel lesion, vomiting (minimal)

Genitourinary: Oligospermia, renal toxicity, uricosuria

Hematologic: Anemia, bone marrow depression (onset 7-10 days; nadir 14 days; recovery: 21 days), granulocytopenia, hemorrhage, hepatosplenic T-cell lymphomas, leukopenia, lymphocytopenia, metastases, neutropenia, thrombocytopenia

Hepatic: Ascites, hepatic encephalopathy, hepatic fibrosis, hepatic injury, hepatic necrosis, hepatomegaly, hepatotoxicity, hyperbilirubinemia, increased serum transaminases, intrahepatic cholestasis, jaundice, toxic hepatitis

Immunologic: Immunosuppression

Infection: Infection

Respiratory: Pulmonary fibrosis

Drug Interactions

Metabolism/Transport Effects None known.

Avoid Concomitant Use

Avoid concomitant use of Mercaptopurine with any of the following: AzaTHIOprine; BCG; CloZAPine; Dipyrone; Febuxostat; Natalizumab; Pimecrolimus; Tacrolimus (Topical); Tofacitinib

Increased Effect/Toxicity

Mercaptopurine may increase the levels/effects of: CloZAPine; Leflunomide; Natalizumab; Tofacitinib; Vaccines (Live)

The levels/effects of Mercaptopurine may be increased by: 5-ASA Derivatives; Allopurinol; AzaTHIOprine; Denosumab; Dipyrone; DOXOrubicin (Conventional); Febuxostat; Pimecrolimus; Roflumilast; Sulfamethoxazole; Tacrolimus (Topical); Trastuzumab; Trimethoprim

Decreased Effect

Mercaptopurine may decrease the levels/effects of: BCG; Coccidioides immitis Skin Test; Sipuleucel-T; Vaccines (Inactivated); Vitamin K Antagonists

The levels/effects of Mercaptopurine may be decreased by: Echinacea

Food Interactions Absorption is variable with food. Management: Take on an empty stomach at the same time each day 1 hour before or 2 hours after a meal. Maintain adequate hydration, unless instructed to restrict fluid intake.

Preparation for Administration

Hazardous agent; use appropriate precautions for handling and disposal (NIOSH 2014 [group 1]).

Measure dose with an oral dosing syringe to assure proper dose is administered. If oral syringe is intended to be reused, wash with warm soapy water and rinse well (hold syringe under water and move plunger several times to ensure inside of syringe is clean); allow to dry completely.

Storage/Stability

Tablets: Store at 15°C to 25°C (59°F to 77°F). Store in a dry place.

Suspension: Store at 15°C to 25°C (59°F to 77°F). Store in a dry place. Use within 6 weeks after opening.

Mechanism of Action Mercaptopurine is a purine antagonist which inhibits DNA and RNA synthesis; acts as false metabolite and is incorporated into DNA and RNA, eventually inhibiting their synthesis; specific for the S phase of the cell cycle

Pharmacodynamics/Kinetics

Absorption: Variable and incomplete (~50% of a dose is absorbed); C_{max} of suspension is 34% higher than the tablet

Distribution: V_d: > total body water; CNS penetration is poor

Protein binding: ~19%

Metabolism: Hepatic and in GI mucosa; hepatically via xanthine oxidase and methylation via TPMT to sulfate conjugates, 6-thiouric acid, and other inactive compounds; first-pass effect

Half-life elimination (age dependent): ~2 hours

Excretion: Urine (46% as mercaptopurine and metabolites)

Dosage Note: Patients with minimal or no thiopurine S-methyltransferase (TPMT) activity are at increased risk for severe toxicity at conventional mercaptopurine doses and generally require dose reduction; consider TPMT gene polymorphism testing in patients who experience severe bone marrow suppression (homozygous deficient patients may require up to a 90% dosage reduction; heterozygous patients usually tolerate recommended doses, although some may require dosage reduction).

Children and Adolescents: Oral:

Acute lymphocytic leukemia (ALL): Maintenance: 1.5 to 2.5 mg/kg once daily (50 to 75 mg/m^2 once daily); continue based on blood counts **or**

Off-label ALL dosing (combination chemotherapy; refer to specific reference for combinations): Adolescents ≥15 years:

Consolidation phase: 60 mg/m^2/day days 0 to 27 days (5-week course) (Stock, 2008) **or** 60 mg/m^2/day days 0 to 13 and days 28 to 41 (9-week course) (Stock, 2008)

Early intensification (two 4-week courses): 60 mg/m^2/day days 1 to 14 (Larson, 1995; Larson, 1998; Stock, 2008)

Interim maintenance: 60 mg/m^2/day days 0 to 41 (8-week course) (Stock, 2008) **or** 60 mg/m^2/day days 1 to 70 (12-week course) (Larson, 1995; Larson, 1998; Stock, 2008)

Maintenance (prolonged): 50 mg 3 times/day for 2 years (Kantarjian, 2000; Thomas, 2004) **or** 60 mg/m^2/day for 2 years from diagnosis (Larson, 1995; Larson, 1998; Stock, 2008) **or** 75 mg/m^2/day for 2 years (girls) or 3 years (boys) from first interim maintenance (Stock, 2008)

Acute promyelocytic leukemia (APL): Maintenance (off-label use): Adolescents ≥15 years: 60 mg/m^2/day for 1 year (in combination with tretinoin and methotrexate) (Powell, 2010)

Autoimmune hepatitis (off-label use): 1.5 mg/kg/day (in combination with prednisone) (Manns, 2010)

Crohn disease, remission maintenance (off-label use): Doses range from 1 to 1.5 mg/kg/day (Grossman, 2008; Markowitz, 2000); children <6 years may require higher doses to achieve clinical improvement (Grossman, 2008)

Ulcerative colitis, remission maintenance (off-label use): Doses range from 1 to 1.5 mg/kg/day (Grossman, 2008; Sandhu, 2010); children <6 years may require higher doses to achieve clinical improvement (Grossman, 2008); additional trials may be necessary to further define the role of mercaptopurine in pediatric patients with this condition.

Dosage adjustment with concurrent allopurinol: Reduce mercaptopurine dosage to 25% to 33% of the usual dose.

Dosage adjustment in TPMT-deficiency: Not always established; substantial reductions are generally required only in homozygous deficiency.

Adults: Oral:

ALL: Maintenance: 1.5 to 2.5 mg/kg once daily (50 to 75 mg/m^2 once daily); continue based on blood counts **or**

Off-label ALL dosing (combination chemotherapy; refer to specific reference for combinations):

Early intensification (two 4-week courses): 60 mg/m^2/day days 1 to 14 (Larson, 1995; Larson, 1998)

Interim maintenance (12-week course): 60 mg/m^2/day days 1 to 70 (Larson, 1995; Larson, 1998)

Maintenance (prolonged): 50 mg 3 times daily for 2 years (Kantarjian, 2000; Thomas, 2004) **or** 60 mg/m^2/day for 2 years from diagnosis (Larson, 1995; Larson, 1998)

APL maintenance (off-label use): 60 mg/m^2/day for 1 year (in combination with tretinoin and methotrexate) (Powell, 2010)

Crohn disease, remission maintenance or reduction of steroid use (off-label use): 1 to 1.5 mg/kg/day (Lichtenstein, 2009)

Ulcerative colitis (off-label use):

Initial: 50 mg once daily; titrate dose up if clinical remission not achieved or down if leukopenia occurs (Lobel, 2004) **or**

Initial: 50 mg (25 mg if heterozygous for TPMT activity) once daily; titrate up to goal of 1.5 mg/kg (0.75 mg/kg if heterozygous for TPMT activity) if WBC >4,000/mm^3 (and at least 50% of baseline) and LFTs and amylase are stable (Siegel, 2005) **or**

Maintenance: 1 to 1.5 mg/kg/day (Carter, 2004) **or**

Remission maintenance: 1.5 mg/kg/day (Danese, 2011)

Dosage adjustment with concurrent allopurinol: Reduce mercaptopurine dosage to 25% to 33% of the usual dose.

Elderly: Due to renal decline with age, initiate treatment at the low end of recommended dose range

Dosing adjustment in renal impairment: The manufacturer's labeling recommends starting with reduced doses (starting at the low end of the dosing range) or increasing the dosing interval to every 36 to 48 hours in patients with renal impairment to avoid accumulation; however, no specific dosage adjustment is provided.

The following adjustments have also been recommended (Aronoff, 2007): Children:

CrCl <50 mL/minute/1.73 m^2: Administer every 48 hours

Hemodialysis: Administer every 48 hours

Continuous ambulatory peritoneal dialysis (CAPD): Administer every 48 hours

Continuous renal replacement therapy (CRRT): Administer every 48 hours

Dosing adjustment in hepatic impairment: The manufacturer's labeling recommends considering a reduced dose (starting at the low end of the dosing range) with close monitoring for toxicity in patients with hepatic baseline impairment; however, no specific dosage adjustment is provided.

Dosing in obesity: *ASCO Guidelines for appropriate chemotherapy dosing in obese adults with cancer:* Utilize patient's actual body weight (full weight) for calculation of body surface area- or weight-based dosing, particularly when the intent of therapy is curative; manage regimen-related toxicities in the same manner as for nonobese patients; if a dose reduction is utilized due to toxicity, consider resumption of full weight-based dosing with subsequent cycles, especially if cause of toxicity (eg, hepatic or renal impairment) is resolved (Griggs, 2012).

Administration Administer preferably on an empty stomach (1 hour before or 2 hours after meals)

ALL treatment in children (Schmiegelow, 1997): Administration in the evening has demonstration superior outcome; administration with food did not significantly affect outcome.

Suspension: Shake well for at least 30 seconds to ensure suspension is mixed thoroughly (suspension is viscous). Measure dose with an oral dosing syringe to assure proper dose is administered. Use within 6 weeks after opening.

Hazardous agent; use appropriate precautions for handling and disposal (NIOSH 2014 [group 1]).

Monitoring Parameters CBC with differential (weekly initially, although clinical status may require increased frequency), bone marrow exam (to evaluate marrow status), liver function tests (transaminases, alkaline phosphatase, and bilirubin; weekly initially, then monthly; monitor more frequently if on concomitant hepatotoxic agents or in patients with preexisting hepatic impairment), renal function, urinalysis; consider TPMT genotyping to identify TPMT defect (if severe hematologic toxicity occurs)

For use as immunomodulatory therapy in CD or UC, monitor CBC with differential weekly for 1 month, then biweekly for 1 month, followed by monitoring every 1 to 2 months throughout the course of therapy. LFTs should be assessed every 3 months. Monitor for signs/symptoms of malignancy (eg, splenomegaly, hepatomegaly, abdominal pain, persistent fever, night sweats, weight loss).

Dosage Forms

Suspension, Oral:

Purixan: 2000 mg/100 mL (100 mL)

Tablet, Oral:

Purinethol: 50 mg

Generic: 50 mg

Extemporaneous Preparations Hazardous agent: Use appropriate precautions for handling and disposal (NIOSH 2014 [group 1]).

A 50 mg/mL oral suspension may be prepared in a vertical flow hood with tablets and a mixture of sterile water for injection (SWFI), simple syrup, and cherry syrup. Crush thirty 50 mg tablets in a mortar and reduce to a fine powder. Add ~5 mL SWFI and mix to a uniform paste; then add ~10 mL simple syrup; mix while continuing to add cherry syrup to make a final volume of 30 mL; transfer to a calibrated bottle. Label "shake well" and "caution chemotherapy". Stable for 35 days at room temperature.

Aliabadi HM, Romanick M, Desai, S, et al, "Effect of Buffer and Antioxidant on Stability of a Mercaptopurine Suspension," *Am J Health Syst Pharm*, 2008, 65(5):441-7.

◆ **6-Mercaptopurine (error-prone abbreviation)** *see* Mercaptopurine *on page 1296*

◆ **Mercapturic Acid** *see* Acetylcysteine *on page 40*

Meropenem (mer oh PEN em)

Brand Names: U.S. Merrem

Brand Names: Canada Meropenem For Injection; Merrem

Pharmacologic Category Antibiotic, Carbapenem

Use

Bacterial meningitis: Treatment of bacterial meningitis in pediatric patients 3 months and older caused by *Streptococcus pneumoniae*, *Haemophilus influenzae*, and *Neisseria meningitidis*

Complicated skin and skin structure infections: Treatment of complicated skin and skin structure infections in adults and pediatric patients 3 months and older caused by *Staphylococcus aureus* (methicillin-susceptible isolates only), *Streptococcus pyogenes*, *S. agalactiae*, viridans group streptococci, *Enterococcus faecalis* (vancomycin-susceptible isolates only), *Pseudomonas aeruginosa*, *Escherichia coli*, *Proteus mirabilis*, *Bacteroides fragilis*, and *Peptostreptococcus* species

Intra-abdominal infections: Treatment of complicated appendicitis and peritonitis in adult and pediatric patients caused by viridans group streptococci, *E. coli*, *Klebsiella pneumoniae*, *P. aeruginosa*, *B. fragilis*, *B. thetaiotaomicron*, and *Peptostreptococcus* species

Canadian labeling: Additional indications (not in U.S. labeling): Treatment of lower respiratory tract infections (community-acquired and nosocomial pneumonias), uncomplicated skin and skin structure infections, complicated urinary tract infections, gynecologic infections (excluding chlamydia), and septicemia; treatment of bacterial meningitis in adults caused by *S. pneumoniae*, *H. influenzae*, and *N. meningitidis* (use in adult meningitis based on pediatric data)

Pregnancy Risk Factor B

Pregnancy Considerations Adverse events were not observed in animal reproduction studies. Incomplete transplacental transfer of meropenem was found using an *ex vivo* human perfusion model.

Breast-Feeding Considerations Small amounts of meropenem are excreted into breast milk (case report). The manufacturer recommends that caution be exercised when administering meropenem to breast-feeding women. Nondose-related effects could include modification of bowel flora.

Contraindications Hypersensitivity to meropenem, other drugs in the same class, or any component of the formulation; patients who have experienced anaphylactic reactions to beta-lactams

Warnings/Precautions Serious hypersensitivity reactions, including anaphylaxis, have been reported (some without a history of previous allergic reactions to beta-lactams). Carbapenems have been associated with CNS adverse effects, including confusional states and seizures (myoclonic); use caution with CNS disorders (eg, brain lesions and history of seizures) and adjust dose in renal impairment to avoid drug accumulation, which may increase seizure risk. Outpatient use may result in paresthesias, seizures, or headaches that can impair neuromotor function and alertness; patients should not operate machinery or drive until it is established that meropenem is well tolerated. Prolonged use may result in fungal or bacterial superinfection, including *C. difficile*-associated diarrhea (CDAD) and pseudomembranous colitis; CDAD has been observed >2 months postantibiotic treatment. Use with caution in patients with renal impairment; dosage adjustment required in patients with moderate-to-severe renal dysfunction. Thrombocytopenia has been reported in patients with renal dysfunction. Lower doses (based upon renal function) are often required in the elderly. Potentially significant drug-drug interactions may exist, requiring dose or frequency adjustment, additional monitoring, and/or selection of alternative therapy.

Adverse Reactions

Central nervous system: Headache, pain

Dermatologic: Pruritus, rash (includes diaper-area moniliasis in infants)

Endocrine & metabolic: Hypoglycemia

Gastrointestinal: Constipation, diarrhea, glossitis, nausea, oral moniliasis, vomiting

Hematologic: Anemia

Local: Inflammation at the injection site, injection site reaction, phlebitis/thrombophlebitis

Respiratory: Apnea, pharyngitis, pneumonia

Miscellaneous: Sepsis, shock

Rare but important or life-threatening: Abdominal enlargement, abdominal pain, agitation/delirium, agranulocytosis, alkaline phosphatase increased, ALT increased, AST increased, anemia (hypochromic), angioedema, anorexia, anxiety, aPTT decreased, asthma, back pain, bilirubin increased, bradycardia, BUN increased, cardiac arrest, chest pain, chills, cholestatic jaundice/jaundice, confusion, cough, creatinine increased, depression, diaphoresis, dizziness, dyspepsia, dyspnea, dysuria, eosinophilia, epistaxis, erythema multiforme, fever, flatulence, gastrointestinal hemorrhage, hallucinations, heart failure, hematuria, hemoglobin/hematocrit decreased, hemolytic anemia, hemoperitoneum, hepatic failure, hyper-/hypotension, hypervolemia, hypokalemia, hypoxia, ileus, injection site edema, injection site pain, insomnia, intestinal obstruction, LDH increased, leukocytosis, leukopenia, melena, MI, nervousness, neutropenia, paresthesia, pelvic pain, peripheral edema, platelets decreased/increased, pleural effusion, PT decreased, pulmonary edema, positive Coombs test, pulmonary embolism, renal failure, respiratory disorder, seizure, skin ulcer, somnolence, Stevens-Johnson syndrome, syncope, tachycardia, toxic epidermal necrolysis, urinary incontinence, urticaria, vaginal moniliasis, weakness, WBC decreased, whole body pain

Drug Interactions

Metabolism/Transport Effects None known.

Avoid Concomitant Use
Avoid concomitant use of Meropenem with any of the following: BCG; Probenecid

Increased Effect/Toxicity
The levels/effects of Meropenem may be increased by: Probenecid

Decreased Effect
Meropenem may decrease the levels/effects of: BCG; Sodium Picosulfate; Typhoid Vaccine; Valproic Acid and Derivatives

Preparation for Administration Meropenem infusion vials may be reconstituted with SWFI. The 500 mg vials should be reconstituted with 10 mL, and 1 g vials with 20 mL. May be further diluted with compatible solutions for infusion. Consult detailed reference/product labeling for compatibility.

Storage/Stability Freshly prepared solutions should be used. However, constituted solutions maintain satisfactory potency under the conditions described below. Solutions should not be frozen.

Dry powder should be stored at controlled room temperature 20°C to 25°C (68°F to 77°F).

Injection reconstitution: Stability in vial when constituted (up to 50 mg/mL) with:

SWFI:

U.S. labeling: Stable for up to 3 hours at up to 25°C (77°F) or for up to 13 hours at up to 5°C (41°F).

Canadian labeling: Stable for up to 3 hours at 15°C to 25°C (59°F to 77°F) or for up to 16 hours at 2°C to 8°C (36°F to 46°F).

Infusion admixture (1 to 20 mg/mL): Solution is stable when diluted in NS for 1 hour at up to 25°C (77°F) or 15 hours at up to 5°C (41°F). Solutions constituted with dextrose injection 5% should be used immediately. **Note:** Meropenem stability (admixed with NS at a concentration of 20 mg/mL) at room temperature for >1 hour or under refrigeration for >15 hours is not supported by the manufacturer. Data exist supporting stability (admixed with NS at a concentration of 20 mg/mL) at room temperature for ≤4 hours and under refrigeration ≤24 hours (Patel, 1997).

Mechanism of Action Inhibits bacterial cell wall synthesis by binding to several of the penicillin-binding proteins, which in turn inhibit the final transpeptidation step of peptidoglycan synthesis in bacterial cell walls, thus inhibiting cell wall biosynthesis; bacteria eventually lyse due to ongoing activity of cell wall autolytic enzymes (autolysins and murein hydrolases) while cell wall assembly is arrested

Pharmacodynamics/Kinetics Note: In the elderly, reduction in plasma clearance correlates with age-associated reduction in creatinine clearance (Craig, 1997). Clearance correlates with creatinine clearance in patients with renal impairment.

Distribution: V_d: Adults: 15 to 20 L, Children: 0.37 to 0.49 L/kg; penetrates well into most body fluids and tissues (Craig, 1997)

Protein binding: ~2%

Metabolism: Hepatic; hydrolysis of beta-lactam bond to open beta-lactam form (inactive) (Craig, 1997)

Half-life elimination: Infants <3 months: ~2.5 hours (mean); Infants ≥3 months, Children, Adolescents, and Adults: Normal renal function: 1 to 1.5 hours

Time to peak: Tissue: ~1 hour following infusion; CSF: 2 to 3 hours with inflamed meninges

Excretion: Urine (~70% as unchanged drug; ~28% inactive metabolite); feces (2%)

Dosage

Usual dosage ranges:

Infants <3 months: IV:

Gestational age <32 weeks:

Postnatal age <14 days: 20 mg/kg/dose every 12 hours

Postnatal age ≥14 days: 20 mg/kg/dose every 8 hours

Gestational age ≥32 weeks:

Postnatal age <14 days: 20 mg/kg/dose every 8 hours

Postnatal age ≥14 days: 30 mg/kg/dose every 8 hours

Infants ≥3 months, Children, and Adolescents (≤50 kg): IV: 30 to 120 mg/kg/day divided every 8 hours (maximum dose: 6 **g** daily)

Children and Adolescents (>50 kg): IV: 1.5 to 6 g daily divided every 8 hours

Adults: IV: 1.5 to 6 **g** daily divided every 8 hours

Extended infusion method (off-label dosing): IV: 0.5 to 2 **g** over 3 hours every 8 hours (Crandon, 2011; Dandekar, 2003). **Note:** Dosing used at some centers and is based on pharmacokinetic/pharmacodynamic modeling and not clinical efficacy data. Meropenem stability (admixed with NS at a concentration of 20 mg/mL) at room temperature for >1 hour or under refrigeration for >15 hours is not supported by the manufacturer. Data exist supporting stability (admixed with NS at a concentration of 20 mg/mL) at room temperature for ≤4 hours and under refrigeration ≤24 hours (Patel, 1997).

Indication-specific dosing:

Infants <3 months: IV: **Note:** Administer as an IV infusion over 30 minutes; do not administer as an IV bolus

Intra-abdominal infections (complicated):

Gestational age <32 weeks:

Postnatal age <14 days: 20 mg/kg/dose every 12 hours

Postnatal age ≥14 days: 20 mg/kg/dose every 8 hours

Gestational age ≥32 weeks:

Postnatal age <14 days: 20 mg/kg/dose every 8 hours

Postnatal age ≥14 days: 30 mg/kg/dose every 8 hours

Infants ≥3 months, Children, and Adolescents (≤50 kg): IV:

Catheter-related blood stream infections (off-label use): 20 mg/kg every 8 hours; maximum single dose: 1,000 mg (Mermel, 2009)

Cystic fibrosis, pulmonary exacerbation (off-label use): 40 mg/kg every 8 hours; maximum single dose: 2,000 mg (Zobell, 2012)

Febrile neutropenia (off-label use): 20 mg/kg every 8 hours (maximum dose: 1,000 mg every 8 hours) (Lehrnbecher, 2012; Yildirim, 2008)

Intra-abdominal infections (complicated): 20 mg/kg every 8 hours (maximum dose: 1,000 mg every 8 hours) (Solomkin, 2010)

Meningitis: 40 mg/kg every 8 hours (maximum dose: 2,000 mg every 8 hours)

Pneumonia (community-acquired): Canadian labeling (not in U.S. labeling): 10 to 20 mg/kg every 8 hours (maximum dose: 1,000 mg every 8 hours)

Skin and skin structure infections:

Complicated: U.S. labeling:

Pseudomonas aeruginosa-suspected or confirmed: 20 mg/kg every 8 hours

Pseudomonas aeruginosa not suspected: 10 mg/kg every 8 hours (maximum dose: 500 mg every 8 hours)

Uncomplicated: Canadian labeling (not in U.S. labeling): 10 to 20 mg/kg every 8 hours (maximum dose: 1,000 mg every 8 hours)

Urinary tract infection (complicated): Canadian labeling (not in U.S. labeling): 10 mg/kg every 8 hours (maximum dose: 500 mg every 8 hours)

Children and Adolescents (>50 kg): IV: **Meningitis:** 2 g every 8 hours

Children and Adolescents (>50 kg) and Adults: IV:

***Burkholderia pseudomallei* (melioidosis) (off-label use):** 1 g every 8 hours (Cheng, 2004; Inglis, 2006)

Catheter-related bloodstream infections (off-label use): 1 g every 8 hours (Mermel, 2009)

Cholangitis, intra-abdominal infections, complicated: 1 g every 8 hours. **Note:** 2010 IDSA guidelines recommend treatment duration of 4 to 7 days (provided source controlled). Not recommended for mild to moderate, community-acquired intra-abdominal infections due to risk of toxicity and the development of resistant organisms (Solomkin, 2010).

Cystic fibrosis, pulmonary exacerbation (off-label use): 40 mg/kg every 8 hours; maximum single dose: 2 g (Zobell, 2012)

Febrile neutropenia (off-label use): 1 g every 8 hours (Ohata, 2011; Paul, 2010)

Pneumonia (community-acquired): Canadian labeling (not in U.S. labeling): 500 mg every 8 hours

Pneumonia (hospital-acquired, health care-associated, or ventilator-associated) (off-label use): 1 g every 8 hours (ATS/IDSA, 2005)

Prosthetic joint infection, *Pseudomonas aeruginosa* (off-label use): 1 g every 8 hours for 4 to 6 weeks (consider addition of aminoglycoside) (Osmon, 2013)

Skin and skin structure infections:

Complicated: U.S. labeling:

Pseudomonas aeruginosa-suspected or confirmed: 1 g every 8 hours

Pseudomonas aeruginosa not suspected: 500 mg every 8 hours

Uncomplicated: Canadian labeling (not in U.S. labeling): 500 mg every 8 hours

Urinary tract infections (complicated): Canadian labeling (not in U.S. labeling): 500 mg every 8 hours. **Note:** Up to 1 g every 8 hours may be administered (Pallett, 2010).

Adults:

Meningitis: IV:

Off-label use in U.S.: 2 g every 8 hours; duration of therapy dependent upon pathogen: *N. meningitides*, *H. influenza*: 7 days; *S. pneumoniae*: 10 to 14 days; aerobic gram-negative bacilli: 21 days (Tunkel, 2004)

Canadian labeling (not in U.S. labeling): 2 g every 8 hours

Gynecologic and pelvic inflammatory disease: Canadian labeling (not in U.S. labeling): IV: 500 mg every 8 hours

Pneumonia (nosocomial): Canadian labeling (not in U.S. labeling): IV: 1 g every 8 hours

Septicemia: Canadian labeling (not in U.S. labeling): IV: 1 g every 8 hours

Dosage adjustment in renal impairment:

Children:

Manufacturer's labeling: There are no dosage adjustments provided in the manufacturer's labeling (has not been studied)

Alternate recommendations: (off-label dosing; Aronoff, 2007):

GFR 30 to 50 mL/minute: Administer 20 to 40 mg/kg every 12 hours

GFR 10 to 29 mL/minute: Administer 10 to 20 mg/kg every 12 hours

GFR <10 mL/minute: Administer 10 to 20 mg/kg every 24 hours

Intermittent hemodialysis (IHD): 10 to 20 mg/kg every 24 hours (administer after hemodialysis on dialysis days)

Peritoneal dialysis (PD): 10 to 20 mg/kg every 24 hours

Continuous renal replacement therapy (CRRT): 20 to 40 mg/kg every 12 hours

Adults:

Manufacturer's labeling:

CrCl >50 mL/minute: No dosage adjustment necessary.

CrCl 26 to 50 mL/minute: Administer recommended dose based on indication every 12 hours

CrCl 10 to 25 mL/minute: Administer one-half recommended dose based on indication every 12 hours

CrCl <10 mL/minute: Administer one-half recommended dose based on indication every 24 hours

Alternative dosing recommendations: (off-label dosing; Aronoff, 2007):

GFR 10 to 50 mL/minute: Administer recommended dose (based on indication) every 12 hours

GFR <10 mL/minute: Administer recommended dose (based on indication) every 24 hours

Intermittent hemodialysis (IHD) (administer after hemodialysis on dialysis days): Meropenem and its metabolite are readily dialyzable: 500 mg every 24 hours. **Note:** Dosing dependent on the assumption of 3 times weekly, complete IHD sessions.

Peritoneal dialysis (off-label dose): Administer recommended dose (based on indication) every 24 hours (Aronoff, 2007).

Continuous renal replacement therapy (CRRT) (Heintz, 2009; Trotman, 2005): Drug clearance is highly dependent on the method of renal replacement, filter type, and flow rate. Appropriate dosing requires close monitoring of pharmacologic response, signs of adverse reactions due to drug accumulation, as well as drug concentrations in relation to target trough (if appropriate). The following are general recommendations only (based on dialysate flow/ultrafiltration rates of 1 to 2 L/hour and minimal residual renal function) and should not supersede clinical judgment:

CVVH: Loading dose of 1 **g** followed by either 500 mg every 8 hours **or** 1 **g** every 12 hours

CVVHD/CVVHDF: Loading dose of 1 **g** followed by either 500 mg every 6 to 8 hours **or** 1 **g** every 8 to 12 hours

Note: Consider giving patients receiving CVVHDF dosages of 750 mg every 8 hours **or** 1.5 **g** every 12 hours (Heintz, 2009). Substantial variability exists in various published recommendations, ranging from 1 to 3 **g** daily in 2 to 3 divided doses. One gram every 12 hours achieves a target trough of ~4 mg/L.

Dosage adjustment in hepatic impairment: No dosage adjustment necessary.

Dietary Considerations Some products may contain sodium.

Administration IV:

Infants <3 months: Administer as an IV infusion over 30 minutes

Infants ≥3 months, Children, Adolescents, and Adults: Administer IV infusion over 15 to 30 minutes; IV bolus injection (5 to 20 mL) over 3 to 5 minutes

Extended infusion administration (off-label dosing): Adults: Administer over 3 hours (Crandon 2011; Dandekar, 2003). **Note:** Must consider meropenem's limited room temperature stability if using extended infusions

Monitoring Parameters Perform culture and sensitivity testing prior to initiating therapy. Monitor for signs of anaphylaxis during first dose. During prolonged therapy, monitor renal function, liver function, CBC.

Dosage Forms

Solution Reconstituted, Intravenous:

Merrem: 500 mg (1 ea); 1 g (1 ea)

Generic: 500 mg (1 ea); 1 g (1 ea)

◆ **Meropenem For Injection (Can)** *see* Meropenem *on page 1299*

◆ **Merrem** *see* Meropenem *on page 1299*

◆ **Mersyndol® With Codeine (Can)** *see* Acetaminophen, Codeine, and Doxylamine [CAN/INT] *on page 37*

Mesalamine (me SAL a meen)

Brand Names: U.S. Apriso; Asacol HD; Canasa; Delzicol; Lialda; Pentasa; Rowasa; SfRowasa

Brand Names: Canada Asacol; Asacol 800; Mesasal; Mezavant; Novo-5 ASA; Pentasa; Salofalk

Index Terms 5-Aminosalicylic Acid; 5-ASA; Fisalamine; Mesalazine

Pharmacologic Category 5-Aminosalicylic Acid Derivative

Use

U.S. labeling:

Oral:

Apriso: Maintenance of remission of ulcerative colitis in patients ≥18 years

Asacol HD: Treatment of moderately active ulcerative colitis in adults

Lialda, Pentasa: Treatment and maintenance of remission of mildly to moderately active ulcerative colitis

Delzicol: Treatment of mildly to moderately active ulcerative colitis in patients ≥12 years; maintenance of remission of ulcerative colitis in adults

Rectal: Treatment of active mild to moderate distal ulcerative colitis (suspension only), proctosigmoiditis (suspension only), or proctitis (suspension and suppository)

Canadian labeling:

Oral:

Asacol, Mezavant: Treatment and maintenance of remission of mildly- to moderately-active ulcerative colitis

Asacol 800: Treatment of moderately active ulcerative colitis

Mesasal: Treatment and maintenance of remission of ulcerative colitis

Pentasa: Treatment and maintenance of remission of mildly to moderately active ulcerative colitis; treatment and maintenance of remission of mild to moderate Crohn disease

Rectal: Treatment and maintenance of remission of distal ulcerative colitis (extending to splenic flexure) and as adjunctive therapy in more extensive disease (suspension only); treatment and maintenance of ulcerative proctitis (suppository only)

Pregnancy Risk Factor B/C (product specific)

Pregnancy Considerations Adverse events were not observed in animal reproduction studies. Dibutyl phthalate (DBP) is an inactive ingredient in the enteric coating of Asacol and Asacol HD; adverse effects in male rats were noted at doses greater than the recommended human dose. Mesalamine is known to cross the placenta. An increased rate of congenital malformations has not been observed in human studies. Preterm birth, still birth and decreased birth weight have been observed; however, these events may also be due to maternal disease. When treatment for inflammatory bowel disease is needed during pregnancy, mesalamine may be used, although products with DBP should be avoided (Habal, 2012; Mottet, 2009).

Breast-Feeding Considerations Low concentrations of the parent drug (undetectable to 0.11 mg/L) and higher concentrations of the N-acetyl metabolite of the parent drug (5-18 mg/L) have been detected in human breast milk following oral or rectal maternal doses of 500 mg to 3 g daily. Adverse effects (diarrhea) in a nursing infant have been reported while the mother received rectal administration of mesalamine within 12 hours after the first dose (Nelis, 1989). The manufacturer recommends that caution be used if administered to a nursing woman. Other sources consider use of mesalamine to be safe while breast-feeding (Habal, 2012; Mottet, 2009).

Contraindications

U.S. labeling: Hypersensitivity to mesalamine, aminosalicylates, salicylates, or any component of the formulation (including suppository vehicle of vegetable fatty acid esters)

Canadian labeling: Hypersensitivity to mesalamine, salicylates, or any component of the formulation; severe renal impairment (GFR <30 mL/minute/1.73 m^2); severe hepatic impairment

Additional contraindications per specific Canadian product labeling: Existing gastric or duodenal ulcer, urinary tract obstruction, use in children <2 years of age (Asacol, Asacol 800, Mesasal, Pentasa, Salofalk); hemorrhagic diathesis (Mesasal); patients unable to swallow intact tablet (Asacol, Asacol 800); renal parenchymal disease (Pentasa)

Warnings/Precautions May cause an acute intolerance syndrome (cramping, acute abdominal pain, bloody diarrhea; sometimes fever, headache, rash); discontinue if this occurs. Use caution in patients with active peptic ulcers. Patients with pyloric stenosis or other gastrointestinal obstructive disorders may have prolonged gastric retention of tablets, delaying the release of mesalamine in the colon. Pericarditis or myocarditis (mesalamine-induced cardiac hypersensitivity reactions) should be considered in patients with chest pain; use with caution in patients predisposed to these conditions. Pancreatitis should be considered in patients with new abdominal discomfort. Symptomatic worsening of colitis/IBD may occur following initiation of therapy. Oligospermia (rare, reversible) has been reported in males. Use caution in patients with sulfasalazine hypersensitivity. Use caution in patients with impaired hepatic function; hepatic failure has been reported. Canadian labeling contraindicates use in severe hepatic impairment. Renal disease (including minimal change nephropathy, acute/chronic interstitial nephritis, nephrotic syndrome, and rarely renal failure) has been reported; use caution with other medications converted to mesalamine. An evaluation of renal function is recommended prior to initiation of mesalamine products and periodically during treatment. Use caution in patients with renal impairment. Canadian labeling contraindicates use in severe renal impairment GFR <30 mL/minute/1.73 m^2; urinary tract obstruction and renal parenchymal disease are also included as contraindications in specific Canadian labels (refer to Contraindications). Use caution with other medications converted to mesalamine. Postmarketing reports suggest an increased incidence of blood dyscrasias in patients >65 years of age. In addition, elderly may have difficulty administering and retaining rectal suppositories or may have decreased renal function; use with caution and monitor.

Apriso contains phenylalanine. The Asacol HD 800 mg tablet has not been shown to be bioequivalent to two Asacol 400 mg tablets [Canadian product] or two Delzicol 400 mg capsules. Canasa suppositories contain saturated vegetable fatty acid esters (contraindicated in patients with allergy to these components). Rowasa, Salofalk [Canadian product] and Pentasa [Canadian product] enema contain metabisulfite salts that may cause severe hypersensitivity reactions (ie, anaphylaxis) in patients with sulfite allergies.

Adverse Reactions Adverse effects vary depending upon dosage form.

Cardiovascular: Chest pain, hypertension, peripheral edema, vasodilation

Central nervous system: Anxiety, chills, dizziness, fatigue, headache (more common in adults), insomnia, malaise, migraine, nervousness, pain, paresthesia, vertigo

Dermatologic: Acne vulgaris, alopecia, diaphoresis, pruritus, skin rash

Endocrine & metabolic: Increased serum triglycerides, weight loss (children and adolescents)

Gastrointestinal: Abdominal distention, abdominal pain, abnormal stools, anorectal pain (on insertion of enema tip), bloody diarrhea (children and adolescents), constipation, diarrhea, dyspepsia, eructation, exacerbation of ulcerative colitis (more common in children and adolescents), flatulence, gastroenteritis, gastrointestinal hemorrhage, hemorrhoids, intolerance syndrome, nausea, pancreatitis (children and adolescents), rectal hemorrhage, rectal pain, sclerosing cholangitis (children and adolescents), tenesmus, vomiting

Genitourinary: Polyuria

Hematologic & oncologic: Hematocrit/hemoglobin decreased

Hepatic: Abnormal hepatic function tests, cholestatic hepatitis, increased serum ALT increased, increased serum transaminases

Hypersensitivity: Anaphylaxis

Infection: Infection, viral infection (adenovirus; children and adolescents)

Neuromuscular & skeletal: Arthralgia, arthritis, back pain, hypertonia, musculoskeletal pain (leg/joint), myalgia, weakness

Ophthalmic: Conjunctivitis, visual disturbance

Otic: Otalgia, tinnitus

Renal: Decreased creatinine clearance, hematuria

Respiratory: Bronchitis, cough, dyspnea, flu-like symptoms, nasopharyngitis (more common in children and adolescents), pharyngitis, rhinitis, sinusitis (more common in children and adolescents)

Miscellaneous: Fever

Rare but important or life-threatening: Abdominal distention, abnormal T waves on ECG, agranulocytosis, albuminuria, alopecia, anemia, angioedema, aplastic anemia, cholecystitis, cholestatic jaundice, DRESS syndrome, drug fever, dysuria, edema, eosinophilia, eosinophilic pneumonitis, erythema nodosum, exacerbation of asthma, fecal discoloration, frequent bowel movements, granulocytopenia, Guillain-Barré syndrome, hepatic failure, hepatic injury, hepatic necrosis, hepatitis, hepatotoxicity, hypersensitivity pneumonitis, hypersensitivity reactions, idiopathic nephrotic syndrome, increased blood urea nitrogen, increased serum bilirubin, increased serum creatinine, interstitial nephritis, interstitial pneumonitis, jaundice, Kawasaki-like syndrome, leukopenia, lupus-like syndrome, lymphadenopathy, mucus stools, myocarditis, nephrotoxicity, neutropenia, oligospermia, painful defecation, palpitations, pancytopenia, paresthesia, perforated peptic ulcer, perianal skin irritation, pericardial effusion, pericarditis, peripheral neuropathy, pharyngolaryngeal pain, pleurisy, pneumonitis, pruritus, pulmonary interstitial fibrosis, pyoderma gangrenosum, rectal discharge, rectal polyp, renal disease, renal failure, skin photosensitivity, Stevens-Johnson syndrome, systemic lupus erythematosus, tachycardia, tenesmus, thrombocythemia, thrombocytopenia, transverse myelitis, vasodilation

Drug Interactions

Metabolism/Transport Effects None known.

Avoid Concomitant Use There are no known interactions where it is recommended to avoid concomitant use.

Increased Effect/Toxicity

Mesalamine may increase the levels/effects of: Heparin; Heparin (Low Molecular Weight); Thiopurine Analogs; Varicella Virus-Containing Vaccines

The levels/effects of Mesalamine may be increased by: Nonsteroidal Anti-Inflammatory Agents

Decreased Effect

Mesalamine may decrease the levels/effects of: Cardiac Glycosides

The levels/effects of Mesalamine may be decreased by: Antacids; H2-Antagonists; Proton Pump Inhibitors

Storage/Stability

Capsule:

Apriso: Store between 20°C to 25°C (68°F to 77°F)

Delzicol: Store between 20°C to 25°C (68°F to 77°F); excursions permitted between 15°C and 30°C (59°F and 86°F).

Pentasa: Store between 15°C to 30°C (59°F to 86°F). Protect from light.

Enema: Store at room temperature. Use promptly once foil wrap is removed. Contents may darken with time (do not use if dark brown).

Suppository: Store below 25°C (below 77°F). May store under refrigeration; do not freeze. Protect from direct heat, light, and humidity.

Tablet: Store at room temperature:

Asacol HD: 20°C to 25°C (68°F to 77°F); excursions permitted between 15°C and 30°C (59°F and 86°F).

Asacol, Asacol 800 [Canadian products]: 15°C to 30°C (59°F to 86°F)

Lialda: 15°C to 30°C (59°F to 86°F)

Mezavant [Canadian product]: 15°C to 25°C (59°F to 77°F)

Mechanism of Action Mesalamine (5-aminosalicylic acid) is the active component of sulfasalazine; the specific mechanism of action of mesalamine is unknown; however, it is thought that it modulates local chemical mediators of the inflammatory response, especially leukotrienes, and is also postulated to be a free radical scavenger or an inhibitor of tumor necrosis factor (TNF); action appears topical rather than systemic

Pharmacodynamics/Kinetics

Absorption: Rectal: Variable and dependent upon retention time, underlying GI disease, and colonic pH; Oral: Tablet: ~20% to 28%, Capsule: ~20% to 40%

Distribution: ~18 L

Protein binding: Mesalamine (5-ASA): ~43%; N-acetyl-5-ASA: ~78%

Metabolism: Hepatic and via GI tract to N-acetyl-5-aminosalicylic acid

Half-life elimination: 5-ASA: 0.5 to 10 hours; N-acetyl-5-ASA: 2 to 15 hours

Time to peak, serum:

Capsule: Apriso: ~4 hours; Delzicol: 4 to 16 hours; Pentasa: 3 hours

Rectal: 4 to 7 hours; Pentasa, Salofalk [Canadian products]: 2 to 6 hours

Tablet: Asacol HD: 10 to 16 hours; Lialda: 9 to 12 hours

Canadian products: Asacol: 7 hours; Asacol 800: 10 hours; Mesasal: ~7 hours; Mezavant: 8 hours (range: 4 to 34 hours)

Excretion: Urine (primarily as metabolites, <8% as unchanged drug); feces (<2%)

Dosage

Oral:

Children and Adolescents ≥12 years: Treatment of ulcerative colitis: Delzicol:

17 to <33 kg: 36 to 71 mg/kg/day in divided doses twice daily for 6 weeks; maximum dose: 1200 mg daily

33 to <54 kg: 37 to 61 mg/kg/day in divided doses twice daily for 6 weeks; maximum dose: 2000 mg daily

54 to 90 kg: 27 to 44 mg/kg/day in divided doses twice daily for 6 weeks; maximum dose: 2400 mg daily

Adults:

Treatment of ulcerative colitis (usual course of therapy is 3 to 8 weeks):

U.S. labeling:

Asacol HD: 1.6 g 3 times daily for 6 weeks (**Note:** Approved for treatment only)

Delzicol: 800 mg 3 times daily for 6 weeks

Lialda: 2.4 to 4.8 g once daily for up to 8 weeks

Pentasa: 1 g 4 times daily

Canadian labeling:

Asacol: 800 mg to 3.2 g in divided doses daily; for severe active disease may increase to 4.8 g daily

Asacol 800: 1.6 g 3 times daily for 6 weeks (**Note:** Approved for treatment only)

Mesasal: 1.5 to 3 g daily in 3 divided doses

Mezavant: 2.4 to 4.8 g once daily for up to 8 weeks

Pentasa: 500 mg 4 times daily; may increase to 1 g 4 times daily if needed

Maintenance of remission of ulcerative colitis:

U.S. labeling:

Apriso: 1.5 g once daily in the morning

Delzicol: 1.6 g in 4 divided doses

Lialda: 2.4 g once daily

Pentasa: 1 g 4 times daily

Canadian labeling:

Asacol: 1.6 g daily in divided doses

Mesasal: 1.5 g daily in 3 divided doses

Mezavant: 2.4 g once daily

Pentasa: 500 mg 4 times daily; may increase to 1 g 4 times daily if needed

Treatment of mild to moderate Crohn disease: Pentasa (Canadian labeling; not in U.S. labeling): Initial: 1 g 4 times daily

Maintenance of remission of mild to moderate Crohn disease: Pentasa (Canadian labeling; not in U.S. labeling): 1 g 3 times daily

Rectal: Adults: **Note:** Duration of rectal therapy is 3 to 6 weeks; some patients may require rectal and oral therapy concurrently.

Treatment of active mild to moderate distal ulcerative colitis or proctosigmoiditis:

U.S. labeling: Retention enema: 4 g at bedtime, retained overnight, approximately 8 hours

Canadian labeling: Retention enema: Salofalk 4 g or Pentasa 1 to 4 g at bedtime; retained overnight, approximately 8 hours

Maintenance of remission of distal ulcerative colitis:

Canadian labeling: Retention enema: 2 g at bedtime daily or 4 g at bedtime every 2 to 3 days

Active ulcerative proctitis:

U.S. labeling:

Retention enema: 4 g at bedtime, retained overnight, approximately 8 hours

Suppository: Insert one 1000 mg suppository in rectum daily at bedtime; retained for at least 1 to 3 hours to achieve maximum benefit

Canadian labeling: Suppository:

Pentasa: Insert one 1000 mg suppository in rectum daily at bedtime; retained for at least 1 to 3 hours to achieve maximum benefit

Salofalk: Insert 500 mg suppository in rectum 2 to 3 times daily or 1000 mg suppository in rectum once daily at bedtime; retained for at least 1 to 3 hours to achieve maximum benefit. Usual dose: 1 to 1.5 g daily until significant clinical response or remission. Taper off gradually; avoid abrupt discontinuation.

Elderly: See adult dosing; use with caution

Dosage adjustment in renal impairment: There are no dosage adjustments provided in manufacturer's labeling; however, dosage adjustment may be necessary since mesalamine is renally eliminated. Use with caution. Canadian labeling contraindicates use in severe impairment (GFR <30 mL/minute/1.73 m^2); urinary tract obstruction and renal parenchymal disease are also contraindicated in specific Canadian labels (refer to Contraindications).

Dosage adjustment in hepatic impairment: There are no dosage adjustments provided in manufacturer's labeling; use with caution. Canadian labeling contraindicates use in severe impairment.

Dietary Considerations Some products may contain phenylalanine.

Apriso: Do not administer with antacids.

Canasa rectal suppository contains saturated vegetable fatty acid esters.

Administration Oral:

Capsules:

Apriso: Administer with or without food; do not administer with antacids. The capsule should be swallowed whole per the manufacturer's labeling; however, opening the capsule and placing the contents (delayed release granules) on food with a pH <6 is not expected to affect the release of mesalamine once ingested (data on file, Salix Pharmaceuticals Medical Information). There is no safety/efficacy information regarding this practice. The contents of the capsules should not be chewed or crushed.

Delzicol: Administer with or without food. The capsule should be swallowed whole with water per the manufacturer's labeling; do not break, chew, crush, or open.

Pentasa: Administer with or without food. Although the manufacturer recommends swallowing the capsule whole, if a patient is unable to swallow the capsule, some clinicians support opening the capsules and placing the contents (controlled-release beads) on yogurt or peanut butter (Crohn's & Colitis Foundation of America). There are currently no published data evaluating the safety/efficacy of this practice. The contents of the capsules should not be chewed or crushed.

Tablets: Swallow whole; do not break, chew, or crush.

Asacol [Canadian product]: Do not break outer coating; administer with or without food.

Asacol HD, Asacol 800 [Canadian product]: Do not break outer coating; administer with or without food.

Lialda: Do not break outer coating; should be administered once daily with a meal.

Mesasal [Canadian product]: Administer before meals.

Mezavant [Canadian product]: Do not break outer coating; should be administered once daily with a meal.

Pentasa [Canadian product]: Administer with meals.

Rectal enema: Shake bottle well. Retain enemas for 8 hours or as long as practical.

Suppository: Remove foil wrapper; avoid excessive handling. Should be retained for at least 1 to 3 hours to achieve maximum benefit.

Monitoring Parameters Renal function (prior to and periodically during therapy); CBC (particularly in elderly patients); hepatic function

Dosage Forms

Capsule Delayed Release, Oral:

Delzicol: 400 mg

Capsule Extended Release, Oral:

Pentasa: 250 mg, 500 mg

Capsule Extended Release 24 Hour, Oral:

Apriso: 0.375 g

Enema, Rectal:

SfRowasa: 4 g/60 mL (60 mL)

Generic: 4 g (60 mL)

Kit, Rectal:

Rowasa: 4 g

Generic: 4 g

Suppository, Rectal:

Canasa: 1000 mg (30 ea, 42 ea)

Tablet Delayed Release, Oral:

Asacol HD: 800 mg

Lialda: 1.2 g

Dosage Forms: Canada

Enema, Rectal:

Pentasa: 1 g/100 mL, 4 g/100 mL

Salofalk: 2 g/60 mL, 4 g/60 mL

Suppository, Rectal:

Pentasa: 1000 mg

Salofalk: 500 mg, 1000 mg

Tablet Delayed Release, Oral:
Asacol: 400 mg
Asacol 800: 800 mg
Mesasal: 500 mg
Pentasa: 500 mg, 1 g
Tablet, delayed and extended release: Mezavant: 1.2 g

◆ **Mesalazine** *see* Mesalamine *on page 1301*

◆ **Mesasal (Can)** *see* Mesalamine *on page 1301*

◆ **M-Eslon (Can)** *see* Morphine (Systemic) *on page 1394*

Mesna (MES na)

Brand Names: U.S. Mesnex

Brand Names: Canada Mesna for injection; Uromitexan

Index Terms Mercaptoethane Sulfonate; Sodium 2-Mercaptoethane Sulfonate

Pharmacologic Category Antidote; Chemoprotective Agent

Use

Prevention of ifosfamide-induced hemorrhagic cystitis: Preventive agent to reduce the incidence of ifosfamide-induced hemorrhagic cystitis

Limitations of use: Mesna is not indicted to reduce the risk of hematuria due to other conditions such as thrombocytopenia

Pregnancy Risk Factor B

Pregnancy Considerations Adverse effects were not observed in animal reproduction studies. Use during pregnancy only if clearly needed.

Breast-Feeding Considerations It is not known if mesna is excreted in breast milk. Benzyl alcohol, a component in some formulations, does enter breast milk and may be absorbed by a nursing infant. Due to the potential for adverse reactions in the nursing infant, a decision should be made to discontinue breast-feeding or to discontinue mesna, taking into account the importance of treatment to the mother.

Contraindications Hypersensitivity to mesna or any component of the formulation

Warnings/Precautions Monitor urine for hematuria. Severe hematuria despite utilization of mesna may require ifosfamide dose reduction or discontinuation. Examine morning urine specimen for hematuria prior to ifosfamide or cyclophosphamide treatment; if hematuria (>50 RBC/HPF) develops, reduce the ifosfamide/cyclophosphamide dose or discontinue the drug; will not prevent hemorrhagic cystitis in all patients. Mesna will not reduce the risk of hematuria related to thrombocytopenia. Patients should receive adequate hydration during treatment. Mesna is intended for the prevention of hemorrhagic cystitis and will not prevent or alleviate other toxicities associated with ifosfamide or cyclophosphamide.

Hypersensitivity reactions have been reported; symptoms ranged from mild hypersensitivity to systemic anaphylactic reactions and may include fever, hypotension, tachycardia, acute renal impairment, hypoxia, respiratory distress, urticaria, angioedema, signs of disseminated intravascular coagulation, hematologic abnormalities, increased liver enzymes, nausea, vomiting, arthralgia, and myalgia. Reactions may occur with the first exposure, or after several months of treatment. Monitor for signs/symptoms of reactions. May require discontinuation. Patients with autoimmune disorders receiving cyclophosphamide and mesna may be at increased risk. Mesna is a thiol compound; it is unknown if the risk for reaction is increased in patients who have had a reaction to other thiol compounds (eg, amifostine). Drug rash with eosinophilia and systemic symptoms and bullous/ulcerative skin and mucosal reactions consistent with Stevens-Johnson syndrome (SJS) or toxic epidermal necrolysis (TEN) have been reported. The skin and mucosal reactions may be characterized by rash, pruritus, urticaria, erythema, burning sensation, angioedema, periorbital edema, flushing, and stomatitis. Reactions may occur with the first exposure, or after several months of treatment. May require discontinuation.

Benzyl alcohol and derivatives: Some dosage forms may contain benzyl alcohol; large amounts of benzyl alcohol (≥99 mg/kg/day) have been associated with a potentially fatal toxicity ("gasping syndrome") in neonates; the "gasping syndrome" consists of metabolic acidosis, respiratory distress, gasping respirations, CNS dysfunction (including convulsions, intracranial hemorrhage), hypotension, and cardiovascular collapse (AAP, 1997; CDC, 1982); some data suggests that benzoate displaces bilirubin from protein binding sites (Ahlfors, 2001); avoid or use dosage forms containing benzyl alcohol with caution in neonates. See manufacturer's labeling.

Adverse Reactions

Mesna alone (frequency not defined):

Cardiovascular: Flushing

Central nervous system: Dizziness, fever, headache, hyperesthesia, somnolence

Dermatologic: Rash

Gastrointestinal: Anorexia, constipation, diarrhea, flatulence, nausea, taste alteration/bad taste (with oral administration), vomiting

Local: Injection site reactions

Neuromuscular: Arthralgia, back pain, rigors

Ocular: Conjunctivitis

Respiratory: Cough, pharyngitis, rhinitis

Miscellaneous: Flu-like syndrome

Mesna alone or in combination: Rare but important or life-threatening: Allergic reaction, anaphylactic reaction, hypersensitivity, hyper-/hypotension, injection site erythema, injection site pain, limb pain, malaise, myalgia, platelets decreased, ST-segment increased, tachycardia, tachypnea, transaminases increased

Drug Interactions

Metabolism/Transport Effects None known.

Avoid Concomitant Use There are no known interactions where it is recommended to avoid concomitant use.

Increased Effect/Toxicity There are no known significant interactions involving an increase in effect.

Decreased Effect There are no known significant interactions involving a decrease in effect.

Preparation for Administration IV: Dilute in D_5W, NS, $D_5{}^1/_4NS$, $D_5{}^1/_3NS$, $D_5{}^1/_2NS$, or lactated Ringer's to a final concentration of 20 mg/mL.

Storage/Stability Store intact vials and tablets at room temperature of 20°C to 25°C (68°F to 77°F); excursions are permitted between 15°C and 30°C (59°F and 86°F). Opened multidose vials may be stored and used for use up to 8 days after initial puncture. Solutions diluted for infusion stored at room temperature should be used within 24 hours. According to the manufacturer, mesna and ifosfamide may be mixed in the same bag if the final ifosfamide concentration is ≤50 mg/mL. Solutions of mesna and ifosfamide (1:1) in NS at a concentration of up to 20 mg/mL are stable for 14 days in PVC bags (Zhang, 2014). Solutions of mesna (0.5 to 3.2 mg/mL) and cyclophosphamide (1.8 to 10.8 mg/mL) in D_5W are stable for 48 hours refrigerated or 6 hours at room temperature (Menard, 2003). Mesna injection prepared for oral administration is stable for at least 9 days undiluted in polypropylene syringes and stored at 5°C, 24°C, 35°C; for 7 days when diluted 1:2 or 1:5 with syrups and stored at 24°C in capped tubes; or for 24 hours at 5°C when diluted to 1:2, 1:10, and 1:100 in orange or apple juice, milk, or carbonated beverages (Goren, 1991).

Mechanism of Action In blood, mesna is oxidized to dimesna which in turn is reduced in the kidney back to mesna, supplying a free thiol group which binds to and inactivates acrolein, the urotoxic metabolite of ifosfamide and cyclophosphamide

Pharmacodynamics/Kinetics

Distribution: 0.65 ± 0.24 L/kg; distributed to total body water

Metabolism: Rapidly oxidized to mesna disulfide (dimesna)

Bioavailability: Oral: Free mesna: 58% (range: 45% to 71%); not affected by food

Half-life elimination: Mesna: ~22 minutes; Dimesna: ~70 minutes

Time to peak, plasma: Oral: Free mesna: 1.5 to 4 hours

Excretion: Urine (32% as mesna; 33% as dimesna)

Dosage Note: Mesna dosing schedule should be repeated each day ifosfamide is received. If ifosfamide dose is adjusted (decreased or increased), the mesna dose should also be modified to maintain the mesna-to-ifosfamide ratio.

Prevention of ifosfamide-induced hemorrhagic cystitis:

Standard-dose ifosfamide (manufacturer's labeling): Adults: IV: Mesna dose is equal to 20% of the ifosfamide dose given for 3 doses: With the ifosfamide dose, at hour 4, and at hour 8 after the ifosfamide dose (total daily mesna dose is 60% of the ifosfamide dose)

Oral mesna (following IV mesna; for ifosfamide doses ≤2 g/m²/day): Adults: Mesna dose (IV) is equal to 20% of the ifosfamide dose at hour 0, followed by mesna dose (orally) equal to 40% of the ifosfamide dose given 2 and 6 hours after the ifosfamide dose (total daily mesna dose is 100% of the ifosfamide dose). **Note:** If the oral mesna dose is vomited within 2 hours of administration, repeat the dose or administer IV mesna.

Short infusion standard-dose ifosfamide (<2.5 g/m²/day): ASCO guidelines: Children (off-label) and Adults: IV: Total mesna dose is equal to 60% of the ifosfamide dose, in 3 divided doses (each mesna dose as 20% of ifosfamide dose), given 15 minutes before the ifosfamide dose, and 4 and 8 hours after each dose of ifosfamide (Hensley, 2009).

Continuous infusion standard-dose ifosfamide (<2.5 g/m²/day): ASCO guidelines: Children (off-label) and Adults: IV: Mesna dose (as a bolus) is equal to 20% of the ifosfamide dose, followed by a continuous infusion of mesna at 40% of the ifosfamide dose; continue mesna infusion for 12-24 hours after completion of ifosfamide infusion (Hensley, 2009)

High-dose ifosfamide (>2.5 g/m²/day): ASCO guidelines: Children (off-label) and Adults: Evidence for use is inadequate; more frequent and prolonged mesna administration regimens may be required (Hensley, 2009)

Other dosing strategies used in combination with ifosfamide (off-label dosing):

Mesna continuous infusion: Children and Adults: IV: 1.8 g/m²/day to 5 g/m²/day as a continuous infusion (100% of the ifosfamide dose), repeated each day ifosfamide is received; see protocols for specific details (Bacci, 2003; Kolb, 2003; Moskowitz, 2011)

Mesna bolus followed by continuous infusion: Children and Adults: IV: 1000 mg/m² 1 hour prior to ifosfamide on day 1, followed by 3000 mg/m²/day continuous infusion (continuous infusion is 100% of the ifosfamide dose) on days 1, 2, and 3 (with sufficient hydration) every 3 weeks for 6 courses (Juergens, 2006)

Mesna (20% higher than ifosfamide) continuous infusion: Children: IV: 3600 mg/m²/day continuous infusion for 4 days (mesna dose is 20% higher than ifosfamide), with hydration, during weeks 4 and 9 (3 additional postop courses were administered in good responders) (Le Deley, 2007)

Prevention of cyclophosphamide-induced hemorrhagic cystitis (off-label use):

HDCAV/IE regimen for Ewing sarcoma: Children ≥4 years and Adults <40 years: IV: 2100 mg/m²/day continuous infusion (mesna dose is equivalent to the cyclophosphamide dose) for 2 days with cyclophosphamide infusion during cycles 1, 2, 3, and 6 (Kolb, 2003)

Hyper-CVAD regimen for ALL: Adults: IV: 600 mg/m²/day continuous infusion (mesna continuous infusion is same total dose as cyclophosphamide) on days 1, 2, and 3, beginning with cyclophosphamide and ending 6 hours after the last cyclophosphamide dose during odd-numbered cycles (cycles 1, 3, 5, 7) of an 8-cycle phase (Kantarjian, 2000)

Dosage adjustment in renal impairment: There are no dosage adjustments provided in the manufacturer's labeling (has not been studied).

Dosage adjustment in hepatic impairment: There are no dosage adjustments provided in the manufacturer's labeling (has not been studied).

Administration Maintain adequate hydration and urinary output during ifosfamide treatment

IV: Administer as an IV bolus (per manufacturer); may also be administered by short infusion or continuous infusion (maintain continuous infusion for 12-24 hours after completion of ifosfamide infusion) (Hensley, 2009); refer to specific protocol for administration rate/details

Oral: Administer orally in tablet formulation; patients who vomit within 2 hours after taking oral mesna should repeat the dose or receive IV mesna. A solution may be prepared from solution for injection by dilution in syrup, juice, carbonate beverages, or milk (Goren, 1991); see Extemporaneous Preparations section.

Monitoring Parameters Monitor urine for hematuria; urine output and hydration status; monitor for signs/symptoms of hypersensitivity or dermatologic toxicity

Additional Information Oncology Comment: Guidelines from the American Society of Clinical Oncology (ASCO) for the use of chemotherapy and radiotherapy protectants (Hensley, 2009 [update]; Schuchter, 2002) recommend mesna to decrease the incidence of ifosfamide-induced urotoxicity associated with short infusion and continuous infusion standard-dose ifosfamide (<2.5 g/m²/day). Although evidence is inadequate regarding mesna's uroprotective effects in high-dose ifosfamide (>2.5 g/m²/day), the guidelines suggest more frequent and prolonged mesna administration times may be required. For prevention of high-dose cyclophosphamide-induced urotoxicity (associated with stem cell transplantation), the guidelines recommend mesna in conjunction with saline diuresis (or forced saline diuresis alone).

Dosage Forms

Solution, Intravenous:

Mesnex: 100 mg/mL (10 mL)

Generic: 100 mg/mL (10 mL)

Tablet, Oral:

Mesnex: 400 mg

Dosage Forms: Canada

Note: Tablets are not available in Canada.

Solution, Intravenous:

Mesna for injection: 100 mg/mL (10 mL)

Uromitexan: 100 mg/mL (4 mL, 10 mL, 50 mL)

Extemporaneous Preparations An oral solution may be prepared from mesna solution for injection. Dilute solution for injection to 20 mg/mL or 50 mg/mL with orange or grape syrup. Prior to administration, syrup-diluted solutions may be diluted to a final concentration of 1, 10, or 50 mg/mL with any of the following: carbonated beverages, apple juice, orange juice, or milk. Mesna injection prepared for oral administration is stable for at least 9 days undiluted in polypropylene syringes and stored at 5°C, 24°C, 35°C; for 7 days when diluted 1:2 or 1:5 with syrups and stored at 24°C in capped tubes; or for 24 hours at 5°C when diluted to 1:2, 1:10, and 1:100 in orange or apple juice, milk, or carbonated beverages. Dilution of mesna with diet or sugar-free preparations has not been evaluated.

Goren MP, Lyman BA, Li JT. The stability of mesna in beverages and syrup for oral administration. *Cancer Chemother Pharmacol.* 1991;28 (4):298-301.

◆ **Mesna for injection (Can)** *see* Mesna *on page 1305*

◆ **Mesnex** *see* Mesna *on page 1305*

Mesterolone [INT] (mes TER oh lone)

International Brand Names Mestoranum (DE, DK, NO); Proviron (AT, AU, BE, BR, CH, CL, CZ, DE, ES, FI, FR, GB, HR, HU, IT, LU, MX, NL, PT); Provironum (IN); Vistimon (DE)

Pharmacologic Category Androgen

Reported Use Male: Androgen replacement, hypogonadism, infertility

Dosage Range Adults: Male: Oral: 50-100 mg/day in divided doses

Product Availability Product available in various countries; not currently available in the U.S.

Dosage Forms

Tablet: 25 mg, 50 mg

◆ **Mestinon** *see* Pyridostigmine *on page 1746*

◆ **Mestinon® (Can)** *see* Pyridostigmine *on page 1746*

◆ **Mestinon®-SR (Can)** *see* Pyridostigmine *on page 1746*

◆ **Mestranol and Norethindrone** *see* Norethindrone and Mestranol *on page 1475*

◆ **Metadate CD** *see* Methylphenidate *on page 1336*

◆ **Metadate ER** *see* Methylphenidate *on page 1336*

◆ **Metadol (Can)** *see* Methadone *on page 1311*

◆ **Metadol-D (Can)** *see* Methadone *on page 1311*

◆ **Metafolbic Plus** *see* Methylfolate, Methylcobalamin, and Acetylcysteine *on page 1334*

◆ **Metafolbic Plus RF** *see* Methylfolate, Methylcobalamin, and Acetylcysteine *on page 1334*

◆ **Metamizole** *see* Dipyrone [INT] *on page 653*

◆ **Metamizole Sodium** *see* Dipyrone [INT] *on page 653*

◆ **Metamizol Sodico** *see* Dipyrone [INT] *on page 653*

◆ **Metamucil® (Can)** *see* Psyllium *on page 1744*

◆ **Metamucil MultiHealth Fiber [OTC]** *see* Psyllium *on page 1744*

Metaproterenol (met a proe TER e nol)

Brand Names: Canada Apo-Orciprenaline®; ratio-Orciprenaline®; Tanta-Orciprenaline®

Index Terms Alupent; Metaproterenol Sulfate; Orciprenaline Sulfate

Pharmacologic Category $Beta_2$ Agonist

Use Bronchodilator in reversible airway obstruction due to asthma or COPD

Pregnancy Risk Factor C

Dosage Oral:

Children:

<6 years (limited experience): 1.3-2.6 mg/kg/day divided every 6-8 hours

6-9 years (or <27 kg): 10 mg/dose 3-4 times/day

Children >9 years (or ≥27 kg) and Adults: 20 mg 3-4 times/day

Elderly: Refer to adult dosing.

Dosage adjustment in renal impairment: No dosage adjustment provided in manufacturer's labeling.

Dosage adjustment in hepatic impairment: No dosage adjustment provided in manufacturer's labeling.

Additional Information Complete prescribing information should be consulted for additional detail.

Dosage Forms

Syrup, Oral:

Generic: 10 mg/5 mL (473 mL)

Tablet, Oral:

Generic: 10 mg, 20 mg

◆ **Metaproterenol Sulfate** *see* Metaproterenol *on page 1307*

Metaxalone (me TAKS a lone)

Brand Names: U.S. Skelaxin

Brand Names: Canada Skelaxin®

Pharmacologic Category Skeletal Muscle Relaxant

Additional Appendix Information

Beers Criteria - Potentially Inappropriate Medications for Geriatrics *on page 2271*

Use Relief of discomfort associated with acute, painful musculoskeletal conditions

Dosage Oral: Children >12 years and Adults: Muscle discomfort: 800 mg 3-4 times/day

Dosage adjustment in renal impairment: Use caution in patients with mild-to-moderate renal impairment; contraindicated with significant impairment. No specific recommendation are provided in approved labeling.

Dosage adjustment in hepatic impairment: Use caution in patients with mild-to-moderate hepatic impairment; contraindicated with significant impairment. No specific recommendation are provided in approved labeling.

Additional Information Complete prescribing information should be consulted for additional detail.

Dosage Forms

Tablet, Oral:

Skelaxin: 800 mg

Generic: 800 mg

MetFORMIN (met FOR min)

Brand Names: U.S. Fortamet; Glucophage; Glucophage XR; Glumetza; Riomet

Brand Names: Canada Apo-Metformin; Ava-Metformin; CO Metformin; Dom-Metformin; Glucophage; Glumetza; Glycon; JAMP-Metformin; JAMP-Metformin Blackberry; Mar-Metformin; Metformin FC; Mint-Metformin; Mylan-Metformin; Novo-Metformin; PHL-Metformin; PMS-Metformin; PRO-Metformin; Q-Metformin; RAN™-Metformin; ratio-Metformin; Riva-Metformin; Sandoz-Metformin FC; Septa-Metformin; Teva-Metformin

Index Terms Metformin Hydrochloride

Pharmacologic Category Antidiabetic Agent, Biguanide

Use Management of type 2 diabetes mellitus (noninsulin dependent, NIDDM) when hyperglycemia cannot be managed with diet and exercise alone.

Note: If not contraindicated and if tolerated, metformin is the preferred initial pharmacologic agent for type 2 diabetes management (ADA, 2013).

Pregnancy Risk Factor B

Pregnancy Considerations Adverse events have not been observed in animal reproduction studies. Metformin has been found to cross the placenta in concentrations which may be comparable to those found in the maternal plasma. Pharmacokinetic studies suggest that clearance of metformin may increase during pregnancy and dosing may need adjusted in some women when used during the third trimester (Charles, 2006; de Oliveira Baraldi, 2011; Eyal, 2010; Gardiner, 2003; Hughes, 2006; Vanky, 2005).

An increased risk of birth defects or adverse fetal/neonatal outcomes has not been observed following maternal use of metformin for GDM or type 2 diabetes when glycemic control is maintained (Balani, 2009; Coetzee, 1979; Coetzee, 1984; Ekpebegh, 2007; Niromanesh, 2012; Rowan, 2008; Rowan, 2010; Tertti, 2008). In women with diabetes, maternal hyperglycemia can be associated with congenital malformations as well as adverse effects in the fetus, neonate, and the mother (ACOG, 2005; ADA, 2014; Kitzmiller, 2008; Metzger, 2007). To prevent adverse outcomes, prior to conception and throughout pregnancy maternal blood glucose and HbA_{1c} should be kept as close to normal as possible but without causing significant hypoglycemia (ACOG, 2013; ADA, 2014; Blumer, 2013; Kitzmiller, 2008). Prior to pregnancy, effective contraception should be used until glycemic control is achieved (ADA, 2014; Kitzmiller, 2008).

Metformin may be used to treat GDM when non-pharmacologic therapy is not effective in maintaining glucose control (ACOG, 2013). Metformin or lifestyle intervention may also be used in women with a history of GDM who later develop prediabetes in order to prevent or delay type 2 diabetes (ADA, 2014).

Metformin is recommended to treat insulin resistance associated with PCOS; however, its use may also restore spontaneous ovulation. Women with PCOS who do not desire to become pregnant should use effective contraception. Although studied for use in women with anovulatory PCOS, there is no evidence that it improves live birth rates or decreases pregnancy complications. Routine use to treat infertility related to PCOS is not currently recommended (ACOG, 2009; Fauser, 2012).

Breast-Feeding Considerations Low amounts of metformin (generally ≤1% of the weight-adjusted maternal dose) are excreted into breast milk. Small amounts of metformin have been detected in the serum of nursing infants. Because breast milk concentrations of metformin stay relatively constant, avoiding nursing around peak plasma concentrations in the mother would not be helpful in reducing metformin exposure to the infant (Briggs, 2005; Eyal, 2010; Gardiner, 2003; Hale, 2002).

According to the manufacturer, due to the potential for hypoglycemia in the nursing infant, a decision should be made whether to discontinue nursing or to discontinue the drug, taking into account the importance of treatment to the mother. Breast-feeding is encouraged for all women, including those with diabetes (ACOG, 2005; Blumer, 2013; Metzger, 2007). Small snacks before feeds may help decrease the risk of hypoglycemia in women with pregestational diabetes (ACOG, 2005; Reader, 2004); metformin may be used in breast-feeding women (Blumer, 2013).

Contraindications

U.S. labeling: Hypersensitivity to metformin or any component of the formulation; renal disease or renal dysfunction (serum creatinine ≥1.5 mg/dL in males or ≥1.4 mg/dL in females) or abnormal creatinine clearance from any cause, including shock, acute myocardial infarction, or septicemia; acute or chronic metabolic acidosis with or without coma (including diabetic ketoacidosis)

Canadian labeling: Hypersensitivity to metformin or any component of the formulation; renal function unknown, renal impairment, and serum creatinine levels above the upper limit of normal range; renal disease or renal dysfunction (serum creatinine ≥136 micromol/L in males or ≥124 micromol/L in females or abnormal creatinine clearance <60 mL/minute) which may result from conditions such as cardiovascular collapse (shock), acute myocardial infarction, and septicemia; unstable and/or insulin-dependent (Type I) diabetes mellitus; history of ketoacidosis with or without coma; history of lactic acidosis (regardless of precipitating factors); excessive alcohol intake (acute or chronic); severe hepatic dysfunction or clinical or laboratory evidence of hepatic disease; cardiovascular collapse and disease states associated with hypoxemia including cardiorespiratory insufficiency, which are often associated with hyperlactacidemia; stress conditions (eg, severe infection, trauma, surgery and postoperative recovery phase); severe dehydration; pregnancy; breast-feeding

Note: The manufacturer recommends to temporarily discontinue metformin in patients undergoing radiologic studies in which intravascular iodinated contrast media are utilized.

Warnings/Precautions [U.S. Boxed Warning]: Lactic acidosis is a rare, but potentially severe consequence of therapy with metformin that requires urgent care and hospitalization. The risk is increased in patients with acute congestive heart failure, dehydration, excessive alcohol intake, hepatic or renal impairment, or sepsis. Symptoms may be nonspecific (eg, abdominal distress, malaise, myalgia, respiratory distress, somnolence); low pH, increased anion gap and elevated blood lactate may be observed. Discontinue immediately if acidosis is suspected. Lactic acidosis should be suspected in any patient with diabetes receiving metformin with evidence of acidosis but without evidence of ketoacidosis. Discontinue metformin in patients with conditions associated with dehydration, sepsis, or hypoxemia. The risk of accumulation and lactic acidosis increases with the degree of impairment of renal function. Use caution in patients with congestive heart failure requiring pharmacologic management, particularly in patients with unstable or acute CHF; risk of lactic acidosis may be increased secondary to hypoperfusion.

Metformin is substantially excreted by the kidney. The risk of accumulation and lactic acidosis increases with the degree of impairment of renal function. Patients with renal function below the limit of normal for their age should not receive metformin. Metformin should be withheld in patients with prerenal azotemia. In elderly patients, renal function should be monitored regularly; should not be initiated in patients ≥80 years of age unless normal renal function is confirmed. Use of concomitant medications that may affect renal function (ie, affect tubular secretion) may also affect metformin disposition. Therapy should be suspended for any surgical procedures (Canadian labeling recommends discontinuing use 48 hours prior to surgical procedures excluding minor procedures not associated with restricted food and fluid intake). Restart only after normal oral intake resumed and normal renal function is verified. Due to the risk of acute alteration in renal function, the manufacturer's labeling states to temporarily discontinue metformin prior to or at the time of intravascular administration of iodinated contrast media, withhold for 48 hours after the radiologic study, and restart only after renal function has been confirmed as normal. The American College of Radiology (ACR) guidelines also recommend to temporarily discontinue metformin at the time of contrast injection but only for certain patients: Patients with known renal dysfunction (and withhold until renal function monitoring assures safe reinstitution) and patients with normal renal function, but with multiple comorbidities (liver dysfunction, alcohol abuse, cardiac failure, myocardial/peripheral muscle ischemia, sepsis, severe infection) (and withhold for 48 hours). In patients with normal renal function and no known comorbidities, ACR states that discontinuation of metformin is not necessary (ACR, 2013). It may be necessary to discontinue metformin and administer insulin if the patient is exposed to stress (fever, trauma, infection, surgery).

Avoid use in patients with impaired liver function. Patient must be instructed to avoid excessive acute or chronic ethanol use; ethanol may potentiate metformin's effect on lactate metabolism. Administration of oral antidiabetic drugs has been reported to be associated with increased cardiovascular mortality; metformin does not appear to share this risk. Insoluble tablet shell of Glumetza 1000 mg extended release tablet may remain intact and be visible in the stool. Other extended released tablets (Fortamet, Glucophage XR, Glumetza 500 mg) may appear in the stool as a soft mass resembling the tablet.

Adverse Reactions

Cardiovascular: Chest discomfort, flushing, palpitation

Central nervous system: Chills, dizziness, headache, lightheadedness

Dermatologic: Rash

Endocrine & metabolic: Hypoglycemia

Gastrointestinal: Abdominal discomfort, abdominal distention, abnormal stools, constipation, diarrhea, dyspepsia, flatulence, heartburn, indigestion, nausea, taste disorder, vomiting

Neuromuscular & skeletal: Myalgia, weakness

Respiratory: Dyspnea, upper respiratory tract infection

Miscellaneous: Decreased vitamin B_{12} levels, flu-like syndrome, increased diaphoresis, nail disorder

Rare but important or life-threatening: Lactic acidosis, leukocytoclastic vasculitis, megaloblastic anemia, pneumonitis

Drug Interactions

Metabolism/Transport Effects Substrate of OCT2

Avoid Concomitant Use

Avoid concomitant use of MetFORMIN with any of the following: Alcohol (Ethyl)

Increased Effect/Toxicity

MetFORMIN may increase the levels/effects of: Dalfampridine; Dofetilide

The levels/effects of MetFORMIN may be increased by: Alcohol (Ethyl); Androgens; BuPROPion; Carbonic Anhydrase Inhibitors; Cephalexin; Cimetidine; Dalfampridine; Dolutegravir; Glycopyrrolate; Iodinated Contrast Agents; LamoTRIgine; Pegvisomant; Ranolazine; Topiramate; Trimethoprim; Vandetanib

Decreased Effect

MetFORMIN may decrease the levels/effects of: Trospium

The levels/effects of MetFORMIN may be decreased by: Corticosteroids (Orally Inhaled); Corticosteroids (Systemic); Danazol; Luteinizing Hormone-Releasing Hormone Analogs; Somatropin; Thiazide Diuretics; Verapamil

Food Interactions Food decreases the extent and slightly delays the absorption. Management: Administer with a meal.

Storage/Stability

Oral solution: Store at 15°C to 30°C (59°F to 86°F).

Tablets: Store at 20°C to 25°C (68°F to 77°F); excursion permitted to 15°C to 30°C (59°F to 86°F). Protect from light and moisture.

Mechanism of Action Decreases hepatic glucose production, decreasing intestinal absorption of glucose and improves insulin sensitivity (increases peripheral glucose uptake and utilization)

Pharmacodynamics/Kinetics

Onset of action: Within days; maximum effects up to 2 weeks

Distribution: V_d: 654 ± 358 L; partitions into erythrocytes

Protein binding: Negligible

Metabolism: Not metabolized by the liver

Bioavailability: Absolute: Fasting: 50% to 60%

Half-life elimination: Plasma: 4-9 hours

Time to peak, serum: Immediate release: 2-3 hours; Extended release: 7 hours (range: 4-8 hours)

Excretion: Urine (90% as unchanged drug; active secretion)

Dosage

Type 2 diabetes management: **Note:** Allow 1 to 2 weeks between dose titrations: Generally, clinically significant responses are not seen at doses <1,500 mg daily; however, a lower recommended starting dose and gradual increased dosage is recommended to minimize gastrointestinal symptoms.

Immediate-release tablet or solution: Oral:

Children 10 to 16 years: Initial: 500 mg twice daily; increases in daily dosage should be made in increments of 500 mg at weekly intervals, given in divided doses, up to a maximum of 2,000 mg daily

Children ≥17 years and Adults: Initial: 500 mg twice daily **or** 850 mg once daily; titrate in increments of 500 mg weekly or 850 mg every other week; may also titrate from 500 mg twice a day to 850 mg twice a day after 2 weeks

If a dose >2,000 mg daily is required, it may be better tolerated in 3 divided doses. Maximum recommended dose 2,550 mg daily.

Extended-release tablet: Oral: **Note:** If glycemic control is not achieved at maximum dose, may divide dose and administer twice daily.

Children ≥17 years and Adults:

Fortamet: Initial: 500 to 1,000 mg once daily; dosage may be increased by 500 mg weekly; maximum dose: 2,500 mg once daily

Glucophage XR: Initial: 500 mg once daily; dosage may be increased by 500 mg weekly; maximum dose: 2,000 mg once daily

Adults: Glumetza: Initial: 1,000 mg once daily; dosage may be increased by 500 mg weekly; maximum dose: 2,000 mg once daily

Elderly: The initial and maintenance dosing should be conservative, due to the potential for decreased renal function. Generally, elderly patients should not be titrated to the maximum dose of metformin. Do not use in patients ≥80 years of age unless normal renal function has been established.

Transfer from other antidiabetic agents: No transition period is generally necessary except when transferring from chlorpropamide. When transferring from chlorpropamide, care should be exercised during the first 2 weeks because of the prolonged retention of chlorpropamide in the body, leading to overlapping drug effects and possible hypoglycemia.

Concomitant metformin and oral sulfonylurea therapy: If patients have not responded to 4 weeks of the maximum dose of metformin monotherapy, consider a gradual addition of an oral sulfonylurea, even if prior primary or secondary failure to a sulfonylurea has occurred. Continue metformin at the maximum dose. If adequate response has not occurred following 3 months of metformin and sulfonylurea combination therapy, consider switching to insulin with or without metformin.

Failed sulfonylurea therapy: Patients with prior failure on glyburide may be treated by gradual addition of metformin. Initiate with glyburide 20 mg and metformin 500 mg daily. Metformin dosage may be increased by 500 mg/day at weekly intervals, up to a maximum metformin dose (dosage of glyburide maintained at 20 mg daily).

Concomitant metformin and insulin therapy: Initial: 500 mg metformin once daily, continue current insulin dose; increase by 500 mg metformin weekly until adequate glycemic control is achieved

Maximum daily dose: Immediate release and solution: 2,550 mg metformin; Extended release: 2,000 to 2,500 mg (varies by product)

Decrease insulin dose 10% to 25% when FPG <120 mg/dL; monitor and make further adjustments as needed

Type 2 diabetes prevention (off-label use): **Immediate release tablet or solution:** Oral: Adults: Initial: 850 mg once daily; Target: 850 mg twice daily (Knowler, 2002)

Dosing adjustment in renal impairment:

Manufacturer's recommendations:

Serum creatinine (SCr) ≥1.5 mg/dL (males) or ≥1.4 mg/dL (females): Use is contraindicated.

Abnormal CrCl (U.S. labeling: Not defined; Canadian labeling: <60 mL/minute): Use is contraindicated.

Alternate recommendations:

Note: The United Kingdom National Institute for Health and Clinical Excellence (NICE) Guidelines recommends prescribing metformin with caution in those patients who are at risk of sudden deterioration in renal function and at risk of an estimated glomerular filtration rate (eGFR) <45 mL/minute/1.73 m^2 (NICE, 2008]). Some evidence suggests that use of metformin is unsafe when eGFR <30 ml/minute/1.73 m^2 (calculated using MDRD) (Shaw, 2007). A review of the available data by members of the American Diabetes Association proposed the following recommendations based on eGFR (Lipska, 2011):

eGFR ≥60 mL/minute/1.73 m^2: No contraindications, monitor renal function annually

eGFR ≥45 to <60 mL/minute/1.73 m^2: Continue use; monitor renal function every 3 to 6 months

eGFR ≥30 to <45 mL/minute/1.73 m^2: In patients currently receiving metformin, use with caution, consider dosage reduction (eg, 50% reduction or 50% of maximal dose), monitor renal function every 3 months. Do not initiate therapy in patients with eGFR <45 mL/minute/1.73 m^2

eGFR <30 mL/minute/1.73 m^2: Discontinue use.

Dosing adjustment in hepatic impairment: Avoid metformin; liver disease is a risk factor for the development of lactic acidosis during metformin therapy.

Dietary Considerations Drug may cause GI upset; take with food (to decrease GI upset). Take at the same time(s) each day. Dietary modification based on ADA recommendations is a part of therapy. Monitor for signs and symptoms of vitamin B_{12} and/or folic acid deficiency; supplementation may be required.

Administration Administer with a meal (to decrease GI upset).

Extended release: Swallow whole; do not crush, break, or chew. Administer once daily doses with the evening meal. Fortamet should also be administered with a full glass of water.

Monitoring Parameters Urine for glucose and ketones, fasting blood glucose, hemoglobin A_{1c}, and fructosamine. Initial and periodic monitoring of hematologic parameters (eg, hemoglobin/hematocrit and red blood cell indices) and renal function should be performed, at least annually (Canadian labeling recommends monitoring renal function every 6 months or more frequently if necessary). While megaloblastic anemia has been rarely seen with metformin, if suspected, vitamin B_{12} deficiency should be excluded.

Reference Range Recommendations for glycemic control in nonpregnant adults with diabetes (ADA, 2013):

HbA_{1c}: <7% (a more aggressive [<6.5%] or less aggressive [<8%] HbA_{1c} goal may be targeted based on patient-specific characteristics)

Preprandial capillary plasma glucose: 70-130 mg/dL

Peak postprandial capillary blood glucose: <180 mg/dL

Dosage Forms Considerations Extended release tablets utilize differing release mechanisms: Glucophage XR uses dual hydrophilic polymer matrix systems, Fortamet uses single-composition osmotic technology, and Glumetza uses gastric retention technology.

Dosage Forms

Solution, Oral:

Riomet: 500 mg/5 mL (118 mL, 473 mL)

Tablet, Oral:

Glucophage: 500 mg, 850 mg, 1000 mg

Generic: 500 mg, 850 mg, 1000 mg

Tablet Extended Release 24 Hour, Oral:

Fortamet: 500 mg, 1000 mg

Glucophage XR: 500 mg, 750 mg

Glumetza: 500 mg, 1000 mg

Generic: 500 mg, 750 mg, 1000 mg

Dosage Forms: Canada

Tablet, oral:

Glycon: 500 mg, 850 mg

- ◆ **Metformin and Dapagliflozin** *see* Dapagliflozin and Metformin *on page 561*
- ◆ **Metformin and Glipizide** *see* Glipizide and Metformin *on page 969*
- ◆ **Metformin and Glyburide** *see* Glyburide and Metformin *on page 974*
- ◆ **Metformin and Linagliptin** *see* Linagliptin and Metformin *on page 1217*
- ◆ **Metformin and Repaglinide** *see* Repaglinide and Metformin *on page 1792*
- ◆ **Metformin and Rosiglitazone** *see* Rosiglitazone and Metformin *on page 1847*
- ◆ **Metformin and Saxagliptin** *see* Saxagliptin and Metformin *on page 1869*
- ◆ **Metformin and Sitagliptin** *see* Sitagliptin and Metformin *on page 1898*
- ◆ **Metformin FC (Can)** *see* MetFORMIN *on page 1307*
- ◆ **Metformin Hydrochloride** *see* MetFORMIN *on page 1307*
- ◆ **Metformin Hydrochloride and Dapagliflozin** *see* Dapagliflozin and Metformin *on page 561*
- ◆ **Metformin Hydrochloride and Linagliptin** *see* Linagliptin and Metformin *on page 1217*
- ◆ **Metformin Hydrochloride and Pioglitazone Hydrochloride** *see* Pioglitazone and Metformin *on page 1655*
- ◆ **Metformin Hydrochloride and Rosiglitazone Maleate** *see* Rosiglitazone and Metformin *on page 1847*
- ◆ **Metformin Hydrochloride and Saxagliptin** *see* Saxagliptin and Metformin *on page 1869*

Methacholine (meth a KOLE leen)

Brand Names: U.S. Provocholine

Brand Names: Canada Methacholine Omega; Provocholine®

Index Terms Methacholine Chloride

Pharmacologic Category Diagnostic Agent

Use Diagnosis of bronchial airway hyperactivity

Pregnancy Risk Factor C

Dosage Note: For inhalation only: Children ≥5 years and Adults:

Before inhalation challenge, perform baseline pulmonary function tests; the patient must have an FEV_1 of at least 70% of the predicted value. The following is a suggested schedule for administration of methacholine challenge. Calculate cumulative units by multiplying number of breaths by concentration given. Total cumulative units is the sum of cumulative units for each concentration given. See table.

Methacholine

Vial	Serial Concentration (mg/mL)	No. of Breaths	Cumulative Units per Concentration	Total Cumulative Units
E	0.025	5	0.125	0.125
D	0.25	5	1.25	1.375
C	2.5	5	12.5	13.88
B	10	5	50	63.88
A	25	5	125	188.88

Determine FEV_1 within 5 minutes of challenge, a positive challenge is a 20% reduction in FEV_1

Dosage adjustment in renal impairment: No dosage adjustment provided in manufacturer's labeling.

Dosage adjustment in hepatic impairment: No dosage adjustment provided in manufacturer's labeling.

Additional Information Complete prescribing information should be consulted for additional detail.

Dosage Forms

Solution Reconstituted, Inhalation:

Provocholine: 100 mg (1 ea)

◆ **Methacholine Chloride** *see* Methacholine *on page 1310*

◆ **Methacholine Omega (Can)** *see* Methacholine *on page 1310*

Methadone (METH a done)

Brand Names: U.S. Dolophine; Methadone HCl Intensol; Methadose; Methadose Sugar-Free

Brand Names: Canada Metadol; Metadol-D; Methadose

Index Terms Methadone Hydrochloride

Pharmacologic Category Analgesic, Opioid

Additional Appendix Information

Opioid Conversion Table *on page 2232*

Use

Chronic pain (except for oral soluble tablets for suspension): Management of pain severe enough to require daily, around-the-clock, long-term opioid treatment and for which alternative treatment options are inadequate.

Limitations of use: Because of the risks of addiction, abuse, and misuse with opioids, even at recommended doses, and because of the greater risks of overdose and death with long-acting opioids, reserve methadone for use in patients for whom alternative analgesic treatment options (eg, nonopioid analgesics, immediate-release opioid analgesics) are ineffective, not tolerated, or would be otherwise inadequate to provide sufficient management of pain. Methadone is not for use as an as-needed analgesic.

Detoxification: Detoxification and maintenance treatment of opioid addiction (heroin or other morphine-like drugs), in conjunction with appropriate social and medical services.

Pregnancy Risk Factor C

Pregnancy Considerations Adverse events were observed in animal reproduction studies. Methadone crosses the placenta and can be detected in cord blood, amniotic fluid, and newborn urine.

Methadone is considered the standard of care when treating opioid addiction in pregnant women. Women receiving methadone for the treatment of addiction should be maintained on their daily dose of methadone in addition to receiving the same pain management options during labor and delivery as opioid-naïve women; maintenance doses of methadone will not provide adequate pain relief. Narcotic agonist-antagonists should be avoided for the treatment of labor pain in women maintained on methadone due to the risk of precipitating acute withdrawal (ACOG, 2012; Dow, 2012).

Data is available related to fetal/neonatal outcomes following maternal use of methadone during pregnancy. Information collected by the Teratogen Information System is complicated by maternal use of illicit drugs, nutrition, infection, and psychosocial circumstances. However, pregnant women in methadone treatment programs are reported to have improved fetal outcomes compared to pregnant women using illicit drugs. Fetal growth, birth weight, length, and/or head circumference may be decreased in infants born to opioid-addicted mothers treated with methadone during pregnancy. Growth deficits do not appear to persist; however, decreased performance on psychometric and behavioral tests has been found to continue into childhood. Abnormal fetal nonstress tests have also been reported.

[U.S. Boxed Warning]: Prolonged maternal use of opioids during pregnancy can cause neonatal withdrawal syndrome in the newborn, which may be life-threatening if not recognized and treated according to protocols developed by neonatology experts. If prolonged opioid therapy is required in a pregnant woman, ensure treatment is available and warn patient of risk to the neonate. Withdrawal symptoms in the neonate may be observed up to 2 to 4 weeks after delivery and should be expected (ACOG, 2012). Neonatal abstinence syndrome following opioid exposure may present with autonomic (eg, fever, temperature instability), gastrointestinal (eg, diarrhea, vomiting, poor feeding/weight gain), or neurologic (eg, high-pitched crying, increased muscle tone, irritability, seizure, tremor) symptoms (Dow, 2012; Hudak, 2012). Monitoring is recommended for neonates born to mothers receiving methadone for neonatal abstinence syndrome (Chou, 2014).

Methadone clearance in pregnant women is increased and half-life is decreased during the 2nd and 3rd trimesters of pregnancy; the dosage of methadone may need increased or dosing interval decreased during pregnancy to avoid withdrawal symptoms in the mother. Dosage may need decreased following delivery (ACOG, 2012).

Long-term opioid use may cause secondary hypogonadism, which may lead to sexual dysfunction or infertility (Brennan, 2013). Amenorrhea may also develop secondary to substance abuse; pregnancy may occur following the initiation of buprenorphine or methadone maintenance treatment. Contraception counseling is recommended to prevent unplanned pregnancies (Dow, 2012).

Breast-Feeding Considerations Methadone is excreted into breast milk; the dose to a nursing infant has been calculated to be 2% to 3% of the maternal dose (following oral doses of 10 to 80 mg/day). Peak methadone levels appear in breast milk 4 to 5 hours after an oral dose. Methadone has been detected in the plasma of some breast-fed infants whose mothers are taking methadone. Sedation and respiratory depression have been reported in nursing infants. The manufacturer recommends that women monitor their nursing infants for sedation and that they should be instructed as to when to contact their healthcare provider for emergency care. In addition, the manufacturer recommends slowly weaning to prevent withdrawal symptoms in the nursing infant.

When methadone is used to treat opioid addiction in nursing women, guidelines do not contraindicate breast-feeding as long as the infant is tolerant to the dose and other contraindications do not exist (ACOG, 2012). If additional illicit substances are being abused, women treated with methadone should pump and discard breast milk until sobriety is established (ACOG, 2012; Dow, 2012).

Contraindications

Hypersensitivity to methadone or any component of the formulation; significant respiratory depression (in the absence of resuscitative equipment or in an unmonitored setting); acute or severe bronchial asthma (in the absence of resuscitative equipment or in an unmonitored setting) or hypercarbia; known or suspected paralytic ileus; concurrent use of selegiline (Emsam product labeling)

Methadone is not to be used on an as-needed basis; it is not for pain that is mild or not expected to persist; it is not for acute pain or postoperative pain.

Canadian labeling: Additional contraindications (not in U.S. labeling): Diarrhea associated with pseudomembranous colitis or caused by poisoning until toxic material has been eliminated from the gastrointestinal tract

Warnings/Precautions The optimal analgesic dose varies widely among patients. Doses should be titrated to pain relief/prevention. Patients maintained on stable doses of methadone may need rescue doses of a immediate release analgesic in case of acute pain (eg, postoperative pain, physical trauma). Methadone is ineffective for the relief of anxiety. May cause CNS depression, which may impair physical or mental abilities. Patients must be cautioned about performing tasks which require mental alertness (eg, operating machinery or driving). Effects may be potentiated when used with other CNS depressants (eg, sedatives, anxiolytics, hypnotics, neuroleptics, other opioids). Contraindicated in patients with respiratory depression and in those with conditions that increase the risk of life-threatening respiratory depression. Use with caution and monitor for respiratory depression in patients with significant chronic obstructive pulmonary disease or cor pulmonale, and patients having a substantially decreased respiratory reserve, hypoxia, hypercarbia, or preexisting respiratory depression, particularly when initiating therapy and titrating with methadone; even therapeutic doses may decrease respiratory drive to the point of apnea. Consider the use of alternative nonopioid analgesics in these patients. Use with caution in patients with depression or suicidal tendencies, or in patients with a history of drug or ethanol abuse. Avoid use of methadone in patients with CNS depression or coma as these patients are susceptible to intracranial effects of CO_2 retention. Use with caution in patients with head injury or increased intracranial pressure; reduced respiratory drive and resultant CO_2 retention may increase intracranial pressure. Elderly may be more susceptible to adverse effects (eg, CNS, respiratory, gastrointestinal). Decrease initial dose and use caution in the elderly, debilitated or cachectic; with hyper/hypothyroidism, morbid obesity, adrenal insufficiency, prostatic hyperplasia, or urethral stricture; or with severe renal or hepatic failure. Should only be prescribed by healthcare professionals who are knowledgeable in the use of potent opioids for chronic pain management.

[U.S. Boxed Warning]: QTc interval prolongation and serious arrhythmias (eg, torsades de pointes) have occurred during treatment. Closely monitor patients during initiation and titration for changes in cardiac rhythm. Patients should be informed of the potential arrhythmia risk, evaluated for any history of structural heart disease, arrhythmia, syncope, and for existence of potential drug interactions including drugs that possess QTc interval-prolonging properties, promote hypokalemia, hypomagnesemia, or hypocalcemia, or reduce elimination of methadone (eg, CYP3A4 inhibitors). Obtain baseline ECG for all patients and risk stratify according to QTc interval; QTc interval prolongation and torsades de pointes may be associated with doses >200 mg/day, but have also been observed with lower doses. Other agents should be used in patients with a baseline QTc interval ≥500 msecs (Chou, 2014).

Potentially significant drug-drug interactions may exist, requiring dose or frequency adjustment, additional monitoring, and/or selection of alternative therapy. May cause severe hypotension; use caution with severe volume depletion or other conditions which may compromise maintenance of normal blood pressure. Use caution with cardiovascular disease or patients predisposed to dysrhythmias. Concurrent use of mixed agonist/antagonist analgesics (eg, pentazocine, nalbuphine, butorphanol) or partial agonist (eg, buprenorphine) analgesics may precipitate withdrawal symptoms and/or reduced analgesic efficacy in patients following prolonged therapy with mu opioid agonists. Abrupt discontinuation following prolonged use may also lead to withdrawal symptoms. Abrupt cessation may precipitate withdrawal symptoms. Gradually taper dose. **[U.S. Boxed Warning]: When used for treatment of opioid addiction:** May only be dispensed by certified opioid treatment programs. Exceptions include inpatient treatment of other conditions and emergency period (not >3 days) while definitive substance abuse treatment is being sought.

Benzyl alcohol and derivatives: Some dosage forms may contain sodium benzoate/benzoic acid; benzoic acid (benzoate) is a metabolite of benzyl alcohol; large amounts of benzyl alcohol (≥99 mg/kg/day) have been associated with a potentially fatal toxicity ("gasping syndrome") in neonates; the "gasping syndrome" consists of metabolic acidosis, respiratory distress, gasping respirations, CNS dysfunction (including convulsions, intracranial hemorrhage), hypotension, and cardiovascular collapse (AAP, 1997; CDC, 1982); some data suggests that benzoate displaces bilirubin from protein binding sites (Ahlfors, 2001); avoid or use dosage forms containing benzyl alcohol derivative with caution in neonates. See manufacturer's labeling.

Oral formulations:

[U.S. Boxed Warning]: May cause serious, life-threatening, or fatal respiratory depression. Monitor closely for respiratory depression, especially during initiation or dose escalation. Carbon dioxide retention from opioid-induced respiratory depression can exacerbate the sedating effects of opioids. Peak respiratory depressant effect of methadone occurs later and persists longer than the peak analgesic effect, particularly during the initial dosing phase. Misuse or abuse (chewing, swallowing, snorting, or injecting the dissolved product) causes uncontrolled medication delivery resulting in a significant risk of overdose and death. Incomplete cross tolerance may occur; patients tolerant to other mu opioid agonists may not be tolerant to methadone.

[U.S. Boxed Warning]: Prolonged maternal use of opioids during pregnancy can cause neonatal withdrawal syndrome in the newborn which may be life-threatening if not recognized and treated according to protocols developed by neonatology experts. If prolonged opioid therapy is required in a pregnant woman, ensure treatment is available and warn patient of risk to the neonate. Signs and symptoms include irritability, hyperactivity and abnormal sleep pattern, high pitched cry, tremor, vomiting, diarrhea, and failure to gain weight. Onset, duration, and severity depend on the drug used, duration of use, maternal dose, and rate of drug elimination by the newborn. **[U.S. Boxed Warning]: Users**

are exposed to the risks of addiction, abuse, and misuse, potentially leading to overdose and death. Assess each patient's risk prior to prescribing; monitor all patients regularly for development of these behaviors or conditions. Risk of opioid abuse is increased in patients with a history or family history of alcohol or drug abuse or mental illness. **[U.S. Boxed Warning]: Accidental ingestion of even one dose, especially in children, can result in a fatal overdose of methadone.** Use with caution in patients with biliary tract dysfunction including acute pancreatitis; may cause constriction of sphincter of Oddi. May obscure diagnosis or clinical course of patients with acute abdominal conditions. Avoid use in gastrointestinal obstruction.

Soluble tablets (diskets): **[U.S. Boxed Warning]: For oral administration only;** excipients to deter use by injection are contained in tablets.

Adverse Reactions During prolonged administration, adverse effects may decrease over several weeks; however, constipation and sweating may persist.

Cardiovascular: Bigeminy, bradycardia, cardiac arrest, cardiac arrhythmia, cardiac failure, cardiomyopathy, ECG changes, edema, extrasystoles, flushing, hypotension, inversion T wave on ECG, orthostatic hypotension, palpitations, peripheral vasodilation, phlebitis, prolonged Q-T interval on ECG, shock, syncope, tachycardia, torsades de pointes, ventricular fibrillation, ventricular tachycardia

Central nervous system: Agitation, confusion, disorientation, dizziness, drowsiness, drug dependence (physical dependence), dysphoria, euphoria, habituation, hallucination, headache, insomnia, sedation, seizure

Dermatologic: Diaphoresis, hemorrhagic urticaria (can occur locally with intravenous administration [rare]), localized erythema (intravenous/subcutaneous), pruritus, rash at injection site (intravenous), skin rash, urticaria, urticaria at injection site (intravenous)

Endocrine & metabolic: Amenorrhea, antidiuretic effect, decreased libido, hypokalemia, hypomagnesemia, weight gain

Gastrointestinal: Abdominal pain, anorexia, biliary tract spasm, constipation, glossitis, nausea, stomach cramps, vomiting, xerostomia

Genitourinary: Impotence, urinary hesitancy, urinary retention

Hematologic: Thrombocytopenia (reversible, reported in patients with chronic hepatitis)

Local: Local pruritus (intravenous), local pain (intravenous/subcutaneous), local swelling (intravenous/subcutaneous)

Neuromuscular & skeletal: Weakness

Ophthalmic: Miosis, visual disturbance

Respiratory: Pulmonary edema, respiratory arrest, respiratory depression

Rare but important or life-threatening): Hypogonadism (Brennan, 2013; Debono, 2011)

Drug Interactions

Metabolism/Transport Effects Substrate of CYP2B6 (major), CYP2C19 (minor), CYP2C9 (minor), CYP2D6 (minor), CYP3A4 (major); **Note:** Assignment of Major/Minor substrate status based on clinically relevant drug interaction potential; **Inhibits** CYP2D6 (moderate), CYP3A4 (weak)

Avoid Concomitant Use

Avoid concomitant use of Methadone with any of the following: Alcohol (Ethyl); Azelastine (Nasal); Benzodiazepines; Conivaptan; Dapoxetine; Fusidic Acid (Systemic); Highest Risk QTc-Prolonging Agents; Idelalisib; Itraconazole; Ivabradine; Ketoconazole (Systemic); Lopinavir; Mifepristone; Orphenadrine; Paraldehyde; Pimozide; Posaconazole; Thalidomide; Thioridazine

Increased Effect/Toxicity

Methadone may increase the levels/effects of: Alvimopan; Antipsychotic Agents; ARIPiprazole; Azelastine (Nasal); Buprenorphine; CNS Depressants; CYP2D6 Substrates; Desmopressin; Diuretics; DOXOrubicin (Conventional); Fesoterodine; Highest Risk QTc-Prolonging Agents; Hydrocodone; Lomitapide; Lopinavir; Methotrimeprazine; Metoclopramide; Metoprolol; Metyrosine; Moderate Risk QTc-Prolonging Agents; Nebivolol; Orphenadrine; Paraldehyde; Pimozide; Pramipexole; ROPINIRole; Rotigotine; Saquinavir; Serotonin Modulators; Suvorexant; Thalidomide; Thioridazine; Zidovudine; Zolpidem

The levels/effects of Methadone may be increased by: Alcohol (Ethyl); Amphetamines; Anticholinergic Agents; Antiemetics (5HT3 Antagonists); Antipsychotic Agents; Antipsychotic Agents (Phenothiazines); Aprepitant; ARIPiprazole; Aromatase Inhibitors; Benzodiazepines; Boceprevir; Brimonidine (Topical); Cannabis; Cobicistat; Conivaptan; CYP2B6 Inhibitors (Moderate); CYP3A4 Inhibitors (Moderate); CYP3A4 Inhibitors (Strong); Dapoxetine; Dasatinib; Doxylamine; Dronabinol; Droperidol; Fluconazole; Fosaprepitant; Fusidic Acid (Systemic); HydrOXYzine; Idelalisib; Interferons (Alfa); Itraconazole; Ivabradine; Ivacaftor; Kava Kava; Ketoconazole (Systemic); Luliconazole; Magnesium Sulfate; MAO Inhibitors; Methotrimeprazine; Mifepristone; Nabilone; Netupitant; Perampanel; Posaconazole; QTc-Prolonging Agents (Indeterminate Risk and Risk Modifying); Rufinamide; Selective Serotonin Reuptake Inhibitors; Simeprevir; Sodium Oxybate; Stiripentol; Succinylcholine; Tapentadol; Tetrahydrocannabinol; Voriconazole

Decreased Effect

Methadone may decrease the levels/effects of: Codeine; Didanosine; Fosamprenavir; Lubiprostone; Pegvisomant; Tamoxifen

The levels/effects of Methadone may be decreased by: Ammonium Chloride; Boceprevir; Bosentan; CarBAMazepine; CYP3A4 Inducers (Moderate); CYP3A4 Inducers (Strong); Dabrafenib; Darunavir; Deferasirox; Etravirine; Fosamprenavir; Fosphenytoin; Lopinavir; Mitotane; Mixed Agonist / Antagonist Opioids; Naltrexone; Nelfinavir; PHENobarbital; Phenytoin; Primidone; Reverse Transcriptase Inhibitors (Non-Nucleoside); Rifamycin Derivatives; Ritonavir; Saquinavir; Siltuximab; St Johns Wort; Telaprevir; Tipranavir; Tocilizumab

Food Interactions Grapefruit/grapefruit juice may increase levels of methadone. Management: Avoid concurrent use of grapefruit juice.

Storage/Stability

Injection: Store at controlled room temperature of 15°C to 30°C (59°F to 86°F). Protect from light.

Oral concentrate, oral solution, tablet: Store at 25°C (77°F); excursions are permitted between 15°C and 30°C (59°F and 86°F).

Mechanism of Action Binds to opiate receptors in the CNS, causing inhibition of ascending pain pathways, altering the perception of and response to pain; produces generalized CNS depression. Methadone has also been shown to have weak N-methyl-D-aspartate (NMDA) receptor antagonism (Callahan, 2004).

Pharmacodynamics/Kinetics

Onset of action: Oral: Analgesic: 0.5 to 1 hour; Parenteral: 10 to 20 minutes

Peak effect: Parenteral: 1 to 2 hours; Oral: Continuous dosing: 3 to 5 days

Duration of analgesia: Oral: 4 to 8 hours (single-dose studies), increases to 22 to 48 hours with repeated doses; slow release from the liver and other tissues may prolong duration of action

Distribution: Lipophilic; V_{dss}: 1 to 8 L/kg

Protein binding: 85% to 90% primarily to alpha-1 acid glycoprotein
Metabolism: Hepatic; N-demethylation primarily via CYP3A4, CYP2B6, and CYP2C19 to inactive metabolites
Bioavailability: Oral: 36% to 100%
Half-life elimination: Terminal: 8 to 59 hours; may be prolonged with alkaline pH
Time to peak, plasma: 1 to 7.5 hours
Excretion: Urine (<10% as unchanged drug); increased with urine pH <6

Dosage Regulations regarding methadone use may vary by state and/or country. Obtain advice from appropriate regulatory agencies and/or consult with pain management/ palliative care specialists. **Note:** These are guidelines and do not represent the maximum doses that may be required. Consider total daily dose, potency, prior opioid use, degree of opioid experience and tolerance, conversion from previous opioid, patient's general condition, concurrent medications, and type and severity of pain during prescribing process. Other factors to consider:

- Interpatient variability in absorption, metabolism, and relative analgesic potency.
- Population-based equianalgesic conversion ratios between methadone and other opioids are not accurate when applied to individuals.
- Duration of analgesic action is much shorter than plasma elimination half-life.
- Steady-state plasma concentrations and full analgesic effects are not attained until 3 to 5 days after initiation.
- Methadone has a narrow therapeutic index, particularly when used concomitantly with other medications.

Chronic pain: Adults:

Manufacturer's labeling: Opioid-naive: Use as the first opioid analgesic:

Oral: Initial: 2.5 mg every 8 to 12 hours

IV: Initial: 2.5 to 10 mg every 8 to 12 hours; titrate slowly to effect; may also be administered by SubQ or IM injection (manufacturer's labeling)

Alternative recommendations: Opioid-naive: Oral:

Gradual titration (for chronic noncancer pain and situations where frequent monitoring is unnecessary): Initial: 2.5 mg every 8 hours; may increase dose by 2.5 mg per dose (Va/DoD, 2010) or 5 mg per day (Chou, 2014) every 5 to 7 days. Once a stable dose is reached, the dosing interval may be extended to every 8 to 12 hours, or longer (Va/DOD, 2010).

Faster titration (for cancer pain and situations where frequent monitoring is possible): Initial: 2.5 mg every 6 to 8 hours; may increase dose by 2.5 mg per dose as often as every day over about 4 days. Once a stable dose is reached, the dosing interval may be extended to every 8 to 12 hours, or longer (Va/DoD, 2010).

Conversion recommendations:

Manufacturer's labeling:

Conversion from oral opioids to oral methadone: Discontinue all other around-the-clock opioids when methadone therapy is initiated; fatalities have occurred in opioid-tolerant patients during conversion to methadone. Substantial interpatient variability exists in relative potency. Therefore, it is safer to underestimate a patient's daily oral methadone requirement and provide breakthrough pain relief with rescue medication (eg, immediate release opioid) than to overestimate requirements. Patient response to methadone needs to be monitored closely throughout the process of the conversion. Sum the current total daily dose of oral opioid, convert it to a morphine equivalent dose according to conversion factor for that specific opioid, then multiply the morphine equivalent dose by the corresponding percentage in the table to calculate the approximate oral methadone daily dose. Divide total daily methadone dose by intended dosing schedule (ie, divide by 3 for administration every 8 hours). Round down, if necessary, to the nearest strength available. For patients on a regimen of more than one opioid, calculate the approximate oral methadone dose for each opioid and sum the totals to obtain the approximate total methadone daily dose, and divide the total daily methadone dose by the intended dosing schedule (ie, divide by 3 for administration every 8 hours). For patients on a regimen of fixed-ratio opioid/nonopioid analgesic medications, only the opioid component of these medications should be used in the conversion. **Note:** Conversion factors in table are only for the conversion from another oral opioid analgesic to methadone. Table cannot be used to convert from methadone to another opioid (doing so may lead to fatal overdose due to overestimation of the new opioid). This is not a table of equianalgesic doses.

Daily oral morphine dose <100 mg: Estimated daily oral methadone dose: 20% to 30% of total daily morphine dose

Daily oral morphine dose 100 to 300 mg: Estimated daily oral methadone dose: 10% to 20% of total daily morphine dose

Daily oral morphine dose 300 to 600 mg: Estimated daily oral methadone dose: 8% to 12% of total daily morphine dose

Daily oral morphine dose 600 to 1000 mg: Estimated daily oral methadone dose: 5% to 10% of total daily morphine dose.

Daily oral morphine dose >1000 mg: Estimated daily oral methadone dose: <5% of total daily morphine dose.

Conversion from parenteral methadone to oral methadone: Initial dose: Parenteral: Oral ratio: 1:2 (eg, 5 mg parenteral methadone equals 10 mg oral methadone)

Alternative recommendations: Opioid-tolerant:

Conversion from oral morphine to oral methadone: 1) There is not a linear relationship when converting to methadone from oral morphine. The higher the daily morphine equivalent dose the more potent methadone is, and 2) conversion to methadone is more of a process than a calculation. In general, the starting methadone dose should not exceed 30 to 40 mg/day, even in patients on high doses of other opioids. Patient response to methadone needs to be monitored closely throughout the process of the conversion. There are several proposed ratios for converting from oral morphine to oral methadone (Ayonrinde, 2000; Mercadente, 2001; Ripamonti, 1998). The estimated total daily methadone dose should then be divided to reflect the intended dosing schedule (eg, divide by 3 and administer every 8 hours). Patients who have not taken an opioid for 1 to 2 weeks should be considered opioid naïve (Chou, 2014).

Titration and maintenance: Manufacturer's labeling: May adjust dosage every 1 to 2 days to a dose providing adequate analgesia and minimal adverse reactions. Breakthrough pain may require a dose increase or rescue medication with an immediate-release analgesic. Some guidelines note that dose increases should not be more than 10 mg per day every 5 to 7 days (Chou, 2014).

Discontinuation: Manufacturer's labeling: When pain management is no longer required, do not abruptly discontinue. Reduce dose every 2 to 4 days to prevent signs or symptoms of withdrawal.

Critically-ill patients (off-label use; Barr, 2013): Note: May be used to slow development of tolerance when escalation with other opioids is required. Enteral methadone has also been used to wean prolonged continuous opioid infusions (Al Qadheeb, 2012)

Oral: 10 to 40 mg every 6 to 12 hours

IV: 2.5 to 10 mg every 8 to 12 hours

Detoxification: Adults: Oral:

Initial: A single dose of 20 to 30 mg is usually sufficient to suppress symptoms. Should not exceed 30 mg; lower doses should be considered in patients with low tolerance at initiation (eg, absence of opioids ≥5 days); an additional 5 to 10 mg of methadone may be provided if withdrawal symptoms have not been suppressed or if symptoms reappear after 2 to 4 hours; total daily dose on the first day should not exceed 40 mg. Do not increase dose without waiting for steady-state to be achieved. Levels will accumulate over the first few days; deaths have occurred in early treatment due to cumulative effects. Reassure the patient that duration of effect will increase as methadone accumulates.

Maintenance: Titrate to a dosage which prevents opioid withdrawal symptoms for 24 hours, prevents craving, attenuates euphoric effect of self-administered opioids, and tolerance to sedative effects of methadone. Usual range: 80 to 120 mg/day (titration should occur cautiously)

Withdrawal: Dose reductions should be <10% of the maintenance dose, every 10 to 14 days

Detoxification (short-term): Adults: Oral:

Initial: Titrate to ~40 mg/day in divided doses to achieve stabilization.

Maintenance: May continue 40 mg dose for 2 to 3 days.

Withdrawal: After 2 to 3 days of stabilization at 40 mg, gradually decrease the dose on a daily basis or at 2-day intervals. Keep dose at a level sufficient to keep withdrawal symptoms at a tolerable level. Hospitalized patients may tolerate a total daily dose decrease of 20%; ambulatory patients may require a slower reduction.

Dosage adjustment during pregnancy: Methadone dose may need to be increased or the dosing interval decreased when chronic doses are used during the second or third trimesters. Use is not appropriate for short term analgesia during labor and delivery.

Dosage adjustment for toxicity:

Excessive opioid-related adverse events: Reduce next dose. Assess and reduce both the maintenance dose and dosing interval if necessary. Some guidelines recommend holding the dose if there is evidence of sedation (Chou, 2014).

QTc prolongation (Chou, 2014):

QTc >450 to 499 msecs: Discuss potential risks and benefits. Evaluate and correct potential causes of QTc interval prolongation prior to initiating therapy. Consider alternative therapies or reduced methadone dose if QTc interval becomes ≥450 to 499 msecs during treatment.

QTc ≥500 msecs: Alternative therapies for opioid addiction or chronic pain are recommended. If QTc ≥500 msecs occurs during therapy, switch to an alternative therapy or immediately decrease the dose of methadone; correct any reversible causes of QTc interval prolongation and repeat ECG.

Dosage adjustment in renal impairment: Off-label dosing (Aronoff, 2007): Adults:

CrCl ≥10 mL/minute: No dosage adjustment necessary

CrCl <10 mL/minute: Administer 50% to 75% of normal dose

Dosage adjustment in hepatic impairment: There are no dosage adjustments provided in the manufacturer's labeling; however, undergoes hepatic metabolism and systemic exposure may be increased after repeated dosing. Avoid in severe liver disease.

Administration Oral dose for detoxification and maintenance may be administered in fruit juice or water. Dispersible tablet should not be chewed or swallowed; add to liquid and allow to dissolve before administering. May rinse if residual remains. Injectable solution can be administered IM, SubQ, or IV; rate of IV administration not defined.

Monitoring Parameters

Assess efficacy of pain control; vital signs and mental status; signs of drug abuse, addiction, or diversion; signs or symptoms of hypogonadism or hypoadrenalism (Brennan, 2013). Also evaluate constipation, nausea, pruritus, respiratory depression, and sedation (Chou, 2014).

Obtain baseline ECG (evaluate QTc interval) prior to therapy in patients with risk factors for QTc interval prolongation, a prior ECG with a QTc >450 msecs, or a history suggesting prior ventricular arrhythmia. If an ECG was obtained within the previous 3 months and it showed a QTc interval <450 msecs, it can be used as a baseline for patients without new risk factors. Repeat ECG 2 to 4 weeks after initiating therapy and after significant dose increases; follow-up ECG should also be done if new risk factors present or signs/symptoms of arrhythmia occur. Repeat ECG when the methadone dose reaches 30 to 40 mg per day (when started at lower doses) and again at 100 mg per day (Chou, 2014).

Reference Range Prevention of opioid withdrawal: Therapeutic: 100 to 400 ng/mL (SI: 0.32 to 1.29 micromole/L); Toxic: >2 mcg/mL (SI: >6.46 micromole/L)

Dosage Forms

Concentrate, Oral:

Methadone HCl Intensol: 10 mg/mL (30 mL)

Methadose: 10 mg/mL (1000 mL)

Methadose Sugar-Free: 10 mg/mL (1000 mL)

Generic: 10 mg/mL (30 mL, 1000 mL)

Solution, Injection:

Generic: 10 mg/mL (20 mL)

Solution, Oral:

Generic: 5 mg/5 mL (500 mL); 10 mg/5 mL (500 mL)

Tablet, Oral:

Dolophine: 5 mg, 10 mg

Methadose: 10 mg

Generic: 5 mg, 10 mg

Tablet Soluble, Oral:

Methadose: 40 mg

Generic: 40 mg

Dosage Forms: Canada

Concentrate, Oral:

Metadol: 10 mg/mL

Methadose: 10 mg/mL

Methadose Sugar-Free: 10 mg/mL

Solution, Oral:

Metadol: 1 mg/mL [unflavored]

Tablet, Oral:

Metadol: 1 mg, 5 mg, 10 mg, 25 mg

- ◆ **Methadone HCl Intensol** *see* Methadone *on page 1311*
- ◆ **Methadone Hydrochloride** *see* Methadone *on page 1311*
- ◆ **Methadose** *see* Methadone *on page 1311*
- ◆ **Methadose Sugar-Free** *see* Methadone *on page 1311*
- ◆ **Methaminodiazepoxide Hydrochloride** *see* ChlordiazePOXIDE *on page 422*

Methamphetamine (meth am FET a meen)

Brand Names: U.S. Desoxyn

Brand Names: Canada Desoxyn

Index Terms Desoxyephedrine Hydrochloride; Methamphetamine Hydrochloride

Pharmacologic Category Anorexiant; Central Nervous System Stimulant; Sympathomimetic

Use

Attention-deficit/hyperactivity disorder (ADHD): For a stabilizing effect in children >6 years with a behavioral syndrome characterized by the following group of developmentally inappropriate symptoms: Moderate to severe distractibility, short attention span, hyperactivity, emotional lability, and impulsivity

Exogenous obesity: Short-term (ie, a few weeks) adjunct in a regimen of weight reduction based on caloric restriction, for patients in whom obesity is refractory to alternative therapy (eg, repeated diets, group programs, other drugs)

Pregnancy Risk Factor C

Pregnancy Considerations Adverse effects have been observed in animal reproduction studies. Methamphetamine and amphetamine were detected in newborn tissues following intermittent maternal use of Desoxyn during pregnancy (Garriott, 1973). The majority of human data is based on illicit amphetamine/methamphetamine exposure and not from therapeutic maternal use (Golub, 2005). Use of amphetamines during pregnancy may lead to an increased risk of premature birth and low birth weight; newborns may experience symptoms of withdrawal. Behavioral problems may also occur later in childhood (LaGasse, 2012).

Breast-Feeding Considerations Methamphetamine is excreted in breast milk. The majority of human data is based on illicit amphetamine/methamphetamine exposure and not from therapeutic maternal use (Golub, 2005). Amphetamines may decrease milk production. Increased irritability, agitation, and crying have been reported in nursing infants (ACOG, 2011). Due to the potential for serious adverse reactions in the nursing infant, breast-feeding is not recommended by the manufacturer.

Contraindications

During or within 14 days following MAO inhibitors; glaucoma; advanced arteriosclerosis; symptomatic cardiovascular disease; moderate to severe hypertension; hyperthyroidism; hypersensitivity or idiosyncrasy to sympathomimetic amines; agitated state; patients with a history of drug abuse

Documentation of allergenic cross-reactivity for amphetamines is limited. However, because of similarities in chemical structure and/or pharmacologic actions, the possibility of cross-sensitivity cannot be ruled out with certainty.

Warnings/Precautions CNS stimulant use has been associated with serious cardiovascular events including sudden death in patients with preexisting structural cardiac abnormalities or other serious heart problems (sudden death in children and adolescents; sudden death, stroke and MI in adults). These products should be avoided in the patients with known serious structural cardiac abnormalities, cardiomyopathy, serious heart rhythm abnormalities, or other serious cardiac problems that could increase the risk of sudden death that these conditions alone carry. Patients should be carefully evaluated for cardiac disease prior to initiation of therapy. Patients who develop angina, unexplained syncope, or other symptoms of cardiac disease during therapy should be evaluated immediately. Use with caution in patients with hypertension and other cardiovascular conditions (heart failure, recent MI, ventricular arrhythmia) that might be exacerbated by increases in blood pressure or heart rate. Use is contraindicated in patients with moderate-to-severe hypertension. Amphetamines may impair the ability to engage in potentially hazardous activities; patients must be cautioned about performing tasks which require mental alertness (eg, operating machinery or driving). Stimulants are associated with peripheral vasculopathy, including Raynaud's phenomenon; signs/symptoms are usually mild and intermittent, and generally improve with dose reduction or discontinuation. Digital ulceration and/or soft tissue breakdown have been observed rarely; monitor for digital changes during therapy and seek further evaluation (eg, rheumatology) if necessary. Difficulty in accommodation and blurred vision has been reported with the use of stimulants.

Use with caution in patients with psychiatric disorders, diabetes, or seizure disorders. May exacerbate symptoms of behavior and thought disorder in psychotic patients; new onset psychosis or mania may occur with stimulant use. Patients should be screened for bipolar disorder prior to treatment; consider discontinuation if such symptoms (eg, delusional thinking, hallucinations, or mania) occur. May be associated with aggressive behavior or hostility (causal relationship not established); monitor for development or worsening of these behaviors. May exacerbate motor and phonic tics and Tourette's syndrome. **[U.S. Boxed Warning]: Potential for drug dependency and abuse exists.** Use is contraindicated in patients with history of drug abuse. Prescriptions should be written for the smallest quantity consistent with good patient care to minimize possibility of overdose. Recommended to be used as part of a comprehensive treatment program for attention deficit disorders. Aggression and hostility has been reported with use of medications for ADHD treatment; no evidence suggests that stimulants cause aggressive behavior, but patient should be monitored for the onset or exacerbation of these behaviors. **[U.S. Boxed Warning]: Use in weight reduction programs only when alternative therapy has been ineffective.** Avoid prolonged treatment durations due to potential for drug dependence. Abrupt discontinuation following high doses or for prolonged periods may result in symptoms for withdrawal. Discontinue if satisfactory weight loss has not occurred within the first 4 weeks of treatment, or if tolerance develops.

Therapy is not appropriate for the treatment of fatigue in normal patients. Use caution in the elderly due to the risk for causing dependence, hypertension, angina, and myocardial infarction. Use of stimulants in pediatric patients has been associated with suppression of growth; monitor growth rate during treatment.

Adverse Reactions

Cardiovascular: Cardiorespiratory arrest, hypertension, palpitations, tachycardia

Central nervous system: Dizziness, drug dependence (prolonged use), drug withdrawal, dysphoria, euphoria, exacerbation of tics (motor, phonic, and Tourette's syndrome), headache, insomnia, overstimulation, psychosis, restlessness

Dermatologic: Skin rash, urticaria

Endocrine & metabolic: Change in libido, growth suppression (children), weight loss

Gastrointestinal: Anorexia, constipation, diarrhea, unpleasant taste, xerostomia

Genitourinary: Frequent erections, impotence, prolonged erection

Neuromuscular & skeletal: Tremor

Miscellaneous: Drug tolerance (prolonged use)

Drug Interactions

Metabolism/Transport Effects Substrate of CYP2D6 (major); **Note:** Assignment of Major/Minor substrate status based on clinically relevant drug interaction potential

Avoid Concomitant Use

Avoid concomitant use of Methamphetamine with any of the following: Iobenguane I 123; MAO Inhibitors

Increased Effect/Toxicity

Methamphetamine may increase the levels/effects of: Analgesics (Opioid); Sympathomimetics

The levels/effects of Methamphetamine may be increased by: Abiraterone Acetate; Alkalinizing Agents; Antacids; AtoMOXetine; Cannabinoid-Containing Products; Carbonic Anhydrase Inhibitors; Cobicistat; CYP2D6 Inhibitors (Moderate); CYP2D6 Inhibitors (Strong); Darunavir; Linezolid; MAO Inhibitors; Peginterferon Alfa-2b; Tedizolid; Tricyclic Antidepressants

Decreased Effect

Methamphetamine may decrease the levels/effects of: Antihistamines; Ethosuximide; Iobenguane I 123; Ioflupane I 123; PHENobarbital; Phenytoin

The levels/effects of Methamphetamine may be decreased by: Ammonium Chloride; Antipsychotic Agents; Ascorbic Acid; Gastrointestinal Acidifying Agents; Lithium; Methenamine; Multivitamins/Fluoride (with ADE); Multivitamins/Minerals (with ADEK, Folate, Iron); Multivitamins/Minerals (with AE, No Iron); Peginterferon Alfa-2b; Urinary Acidifying Agents

Food Interactions Amphetamine serum levels may be altered if taken with acidic food, juices, or vitamin C. Management: Administer 30 minutes before a meal.

Storage/Stability Store below 30°C (86°F).

Mechanism of Action A sympathomimetic amine related to ephedrine and amphetamine with CNS stimulant activity; causes release of catecholamines (primarily dopamine and other catecholamines) from their storage sites in the presynaptic nerve terminals. Inhibits reuptake and metabolism of catecholamines through inhibition of monoamine transporters and oxidase.

Pharmacodynamics/Kinetics

Absorption: Rapid from GI tract

Metabolism: Predominately hepatic via aromatic hydroxylation, N-dealkylation and deamination; forms ≥7 metabolites

Half-life elimination: 4-5 hours

Excretion: Urine primarily (dependent on urine pH; alkaline urine increases the half-life); 62% of dose eliminated within first 24 hours as ~33% unchanged drug with remainder as metabolites

Dosage Oral:

ADHD: Children ≥6 years: Oral: Initial: 5 mg 1-2 times daily; may increase by 5 mg increments at weekly intervals until optimum response is achieved; usual effective dose range: 20-25 mg daily in 1 or 2 divided doses

Exogenous obesity: Children ≥12 years and Adults: Oral: 5 mg given 30 minutes before each meal; treatment duration should not exceed a few weeks

Dosage adjustment in renal impairment: No dosage adjustment provided in manufacturer's labeling.

Dosage adjustment in hepatic impairment: No dosage adjustment provided in manufacturer's labeling.

Dietary Considerations Most effective when combined with a low calorie diet and behavior modification counseling.

Administration For obesity, administer 30 minutes before each meal. Late evening doses should be avoided due to potential for insomnia.

Monitoring Parameters Heart rate, respiratory rate, blood pressure, CNS activity, body weight (BMI), signs of peripheral vasculopathy (eg, digital changes); growth rate in children

When used for the treatment of ADHD, thoroughly evaluate for cardiovascular risk. Monitor heart rate, blood pressure, and consider obtaining ECG prior to initiation (Vetter, 2008). Monitor for aggression and hostility.

Reference Range

Adult classification of weight by BMI (kg/m^2):

- Underweight: <18.5
- Normal: 18.5-24.9
- Overweight: 25-29.9
- Obese, class I: 30-34.9
- Obese, class II: 35-39.9
- Extreme obesity (class III): ≥40

Waist circumference: In adults with a BMI of 25-34.9 kg/m^2, high-risk waist circumference is defined as:

- Men >102 cm (>40 in)
- Women >88 cm (>35 in)

Additional Information Illicit methamphetamine may contain lead; alkalinizing urine can result in longer methamphetamine half-life and elevated blood level; ephedrine is a precursor in the illicit manufacture of methamphetamine; ephedrine is extracted by dissolving ephedrine tablets in water or alcohol (50,000 tablets can result in 1 kg of ephedrine); conversion to methamphetamine occurs at a rate of 50% to 70% of the weight of ephedrine. 3,4-methylene dioxymethamphetamine (slang: XTC, Ecstasy, Adam) affects the serotonergic, dopaminergic, and noradrenergic pathways. As such, it can cause the serotonin syndrome associated with malignant hyperthermia and rhabdomyolysis.

Dosage Forms

Tablet, Oral:

Desoxyn: 5 mg

Generic: 5 mg

◆ **Methamphetamine Hydrochloride** *see* Methamphetamine *on page 1315*

◆ **Methampyrone** *see* Dipyrone [INT] *on page 653*

Methazolamide (meth a ZOE la mide)

Brand Names: U.S. Neptazane

Brand Names: Canada Apo-Methazolamide®

Pharmacologic Category Carbonic Anhydrase Inhibitor; Diuretic, Carbonic Anhydrase Inhibitor; Ophthalmic Agent, Antiglaucoma

Use Treatment of chronic open-angle or secondary glaucoma; short-term therapy of acute angle-closure glaucoma prior to surgery

Pregnancy Risk Factor C

Dosage Adults: Oral: 50-100 mg 2-3 times/day

Dosage adjustment in renal impairment: Contraindicated in marked renal dysfunction.

Dosage adjustment in hepatic impairment: Contraindicated in marked hepatic dysfunction.

Additional Information Complete prescribing information should be consulted for additional detail.

Dosage Forms

Tablet, Oral:

Neptazane: 25 mg, 50 mg

Generic: 25 mg, 50 mg

Methenamine (meth EN a meen)

Brand Names: U.S. Hiprex; Urex

Brand Names: Canada Dehydral®; Hiprex®; Mandelamine®; Urasal®

Index Terms Hexamethylenetetramine; Methenamine Hippurate; Methenamine Mandelate; Urex

Pharmacologic Category Antibiotic, Miscellaneous

Use Prophylaxis or suppression of recurrent urinary tract infections; urinary tract discomfort secondary to hypermotility

Pregnancy Risk Factor C (methenamine mandelate)

Dosage Oral:

Children:

>2-6 years: *Mandelate:* 50-75 mg/kg/day in 3-4 doses or 0.25 g/30 lb 4 times/day

6-12 years:

Hippurate: 0.5-1 g twice daily

Mandelate: 50-75 mg/kg/day in 3-4 doses or 0.5 g 4 times/day

>12 years and Adults:
Hippurate: 1 g twice daily
Mandelate: 1 g 4 times/day after meals and at bedtime

Dosage adjustment in renal impairment: Contraindicated in renal insufficiency.

Dosage adjustment in hepatic impairment: Contraindicated in severe hepatic impairment.

Additional Information Complete prescribing information should be consulted for additional detail.

Dosage Forms

Tablet, Oral:
Hiprex: 1 g
Urex: 1 g
Generic: 0.5 g, 1 g

Methenamine and Sodium Acid Phosphate

(meth EN a meen & SOW dee um AS id FOS fate)

Brand Names: U.S. Uroqid-Acid® No. 2

Index Terms Methenamine Mandelate and Sodium Acid Phosphate; Sodium Acid Phosphate and Methenamine

Pharmacologic Category Antibiotic, Miscellaneous

Use Prophylaxis or suppression of bacteriuria associated with recurrent urinary tract infections

Pregnancy Risk Factor C

Dosage Oral: Adults: Initial: 2 tablets 4 times daily; maintenance: 2-4 tablets daily in divided doses

Additional Information Complete prescribing information should be consulted for additional detail.

Dosage Forms

Tablet:
Uroqid-Acid® No. 2: Methenamine 500 mg and sodium acid phosphate 500 mg

◆ **Methenamine Hippurate** *see* Methenamine *on page 1317*

◆ **Methenamine Mandelate** *see* Methenamine *on page 1317*

◆ **Methenamine Mandelate and Sodium Acid Phosphate** *see* Methenamine and Sodium Acid Phosphate *on page 1318*

Methenamine, Phenyl Salicylate, Methylene Blue, Benzoic Acid, and Hyoscyamine

(meth EN a meen, fen nil sa LIS i late, METH i leen bloo, ben ZOE ik AS id & hye oh SYE a meen)

Brand Names: U.S. Hyophen™; Prosed®/DS

Index Terms Benzoic Acid, Hyoscyamine, Methenamine, Methylene Blue, and Phenyl Salicylate; Benzoic Acid, Methenamine, Methylene Blue, Phenyl Salicylate, and Hyoscyamine; Hyoscyamine, Methenamine, Benzoic Acid, Phenyl Salicylate, and Methylene Blue; Methylene Blue, Methenamine, Benzoic Acid, Phenyl Salicylate, and Hyoscyamine; Phenyl Salicylate, Methenamine, Methylene Blue, Benzoic Acid, and Hyoscyamine

Pharmacologic Category Antibiotic, Miscellaneous

Use Urinary tract discomfort secondary to hypermotility resulting from infection or diagnostic procedures

Pregnancy Risk Factor C

Dosage Oral:
Children >6 years: Dosage must be individualized
Adults: One tablet 4 times/day

Dosage adjustment in renal impairment: No dosage adjustment provided in manufacturer's labeling.

Dosage adjustment in hepatic impairment: No dosage adjustment provided in manufacturer's labeling.

Additional Information Complete prescribing information should be consulted for additional detail.

Dosage Forms

Tablet, oral:
Hyophen™, Prosed®/DS: Methenamine 81.6 mg, phenyl salicylate 36.2 mg, methylene blue 10.8 mg, benzoic acid 9 mg, hyoscyamine sulfate 0.12 mg

Methenamine, Sodium Phosphate Monobasic, Phenyl Salicylate, Methylene Blue, and Hyoscyamine

(meth EN a meen, SOW dee um FOS fate mon oh BAY sik, fen nil sa LIS i late, METH i leen bloo, & hye oh SYE a meen)

Brand Names: U.S. Phosphasal; Urelle; Uribel; Urimar-T; Uro-L; Uro-MP; Ustell; Utira-C

Index Terms Hyoscyamine, Methenamine, Methylene Blue, Phenyl Salicylate, and Sodium Phosphate Monobasic; Hyoscyamine, Methenamine, Sodium Phosphate Monobasic, Phenyl Salicylate, and Methylene Blue; Methylene Blue, Methenamine, Sodium Phosphate Monobasic, Phenyl Salicylate, and Hyoscyamine; Phenyl Salicylate, Methenamine, Methylene Blue, Sodium Biphosphate, and Hyoscyamine; Sodium Phosphate Monobasic, Methenamine, Methylene Blue, Phenyl Salicylate, and Hyoscyamine

Pharmacologic Category Antibiotic, Miscellaneous

Use Treatment of symptoms of irritative voiding; relief of local symptoms associated with urinary tract infections; relief of urinary tract symptoms caused by diagnostic procedures

Pregnancy Risk Factor C

Dosage Oral:
Children >6 years: Dosage must be individualized
Adults: One tablet 4 times daily (followed by liberal fluid intake)

Dosage adjustment in renal impairment: No dosage adjustment provided in manufacturer's labeling.

Dosage adjustment in hepatic impairment: No dosage adjustment provided in manufacturer's labeling.

Additional Information Complete prescribing information should be consulted for additional detail.

Dosage Forms

Capsule, oral:
Uribel: Methenamine 118 mg, sodium phosphate monobasic 40.8 mg, phenyl salicylate 36 mg, methylene blue 10 mg, hyoscyamine sulfate 0.12 mg
Uro-MP: Methenamine 118 mg, sodium phosphate monobasic 40.8 mg, phenyl salicylate 36 mg, methylene blue 10 mg, hyoscyamine sulfate 0.12 mg
Ustell: Methenamine 120 mg, sodium phosphate monobasic 40.8 mg, phenyl salicylate 36 mg, methylene blue 10 mg, hyoscyamine sulfate 0.12 mg

Tablet, oral:
Phosphasal: Methenamine 81.6 mg, sodium phosphate monobasic 40.8 mg, phenyl salicylate 36.2 mg, methylene blue 10.8 mg, hyoscyamine sulfate 0.12 mg
Urelle: Methenamine 81 mg, sodium phosphate monobasic 40.8 mg, phenyl salicylate 32.4 mg, methylene blue 10.8 mg, hyoscyamine sulfate 0.12 mg
Urimar-T: Methenamine 120 mg, sodium phosphate monobasic 40.8 mg, phenyl salicylate 36.2 mg, methylene blue 10.8 mg, hyoscyamine sulfate 0.12 mg
Uro-L: Methenamine 81 mg, sodium phosphate monobasic 40.8 mg, phenyl salicylate 32.4 mg, methylene blue 10.8 mg, hyoscyamine sulfate 0.12 mg
Utira-C: Methenamine 81.6 mg, sodium phosphate monobasic 40.8 mg, phenyl salicylate 36.2 mg, methylene blue 10.8 mg, hyoscyamine sulfate 0.12 mg

◆ **Methergine® (Can)** *see* Methylergonovine *on page 1333*

Methimazole (meth IM a zole)

Brand Names: U.S. Tapazole

Brand Names: Canada Dom-Methimazole; PHL-Methimazole; Tapazole

Index Terms MMI; Thiamazole

Pharmacologic Category Antithyroid Agent; Thioamide

Use Hyperthyroidism: Treatment of hyperthyroidism in patients with Graves' disease or toxic multinodular goiter (surgery or radioactive iodine therapy is not appropriate); amelioration of hyperthyroid symptoms in preparation for thyroidectomy or radioactive iodine therapy.

Pregnancy Risk Factor D

Pregnancy Considerations Methimazole has been found to readily cross the placenta. Congenital anomalies, including esophageal atresia, choanal atresia, aplasia cutis, and dysmorphic facies, have been observed in neonates born to mothers taking methimazole during pregnancy (Stangaro-Green, 2011). Nonteratogenic adverse events, including fetal and neonatal hypothyroidism, have been observed following maternal methimazole use. The transfer of thyroid-stimulating immunoglobulins can stimulate the fetal thyroid *in utero* and transiently after delivery and may increase the risk of fetal or neonatal hyperthyroidism (De Groot, 2012; Stangaro-Green, 2011).

Uncontrolled maternal hyperthyroidism may result in adverse neonatal outcomes (eg, prematurity, low birth weight, infants born small for gestational age) and adverse maternal outcomes (eg, pre-eclampsia, congestive heart failure) (ACOG, 2002; Stangaro-Green, 2011). To prevent adverse fetal and maternal events, normal maternal thyroid function should be maintained prior to conception and throughout pregnancy. Antithyroid treatment is recommended for the control of hyperthyroidism during pregnancy. Due to an increased risk of congenital anomalies with methimazole, propylthiouracil is preferred during the first trimester of pregnancy and methimazole is preferred during the second and third trimesters of pregnancy (ACOG, 2002; De Groot, 2012; Stangaro-Green, 2011). If drug therapy is changed, maternal thyroid function should be monitored after 2 weeks and then every 2 to 4 weeks (De Groot, 2012).

The severity of hyperthyroidism may fluctuate throughout pregnancy and may result in decreased dose requirements or discontinuation of methimazole 2 to 3 weeks prior to delivery.

Breast-Feeding Considerations Methimazole is excreted into human breast milk. The thyroid function and intellectual development of breast-fed infants are not affected by exposure to maternal methimazole during breast-feeding. The American Thyroid Association considers doses of methimazole <30 mg/day to be safe during breast-feeding. Methimazole should be administered after nursing and in divided doses (Stagnaro-Green, 2011).

Contraindications Hypersensitivity to methimazole or any component of the formulation

Warnings/Precautions May cause significant bone marrow depression; the most severe manifestation is agranulocytosis. Aplastic anemia, thrombocytopenia, and leukopenia may also occur. and with concomitant use of other drugs known to cause myelosuppression (particularly agranulocytosis). Monitor patients closely; discontinue if significant bone marrow suppression occurs, particularly agranulocytosis or aplastic anemia.

May cause hypoprothrombinemia and bleeding. Monitoring is recommended, especially before surgical procedures. Antithyroid agents have been associated with rare but severe dermatologic reactions. Discontinue in the presence of exfoliative dermatitis. Hepatotoxicity (including acute liver failure) may occur. Symptoms suggestive of hepatic dysfunction (eg, anorexia, pruritus, right upper quadrant pain) should prompt evaluation. Discontinue in the presence of hepatitis and clinically significant hepatic abnormality, including transaminase >3 times upper limit of normal. May cause hypothyroidism; routinely monitor TSH and free T_4 levels, adjust dose to maintain euthyroid state. ANCA-positive vasculitis may develop during therapy discontinue use in the presence of vasculitis use. Discontinue in the presence of unexplained fever. A lupus-like syndrome may occur. Potentially significant drug-drug interactions may exist, requiring dose or frequency adjustment, additional monitoring, and/or selection of alternative therapy.

Adverse Reactions

Cardiovascular: ANCA-positive vasculitis, edema, leukocytoclastic vasculitis, periarteritis

Central nervous system: Drowsiness, fever, headache, neuritis, vertigo

Dermatologic: Alopecia, exfoliative dermatitis, pruritus, skin pigmentation, skin rash, urticaria

Endocrine & metabolic: Goiter, hypoglycemic coma

Gastrointestinal: Constipation, epigastric distress, loss of taste perception, nausea, salivary gland swelling, vomiting, weight gain

Hematologic: Agranulocytosis, aplastic anemia, granulocytopenia, hypoprothrombinemia, leukopenia, thrombocytopenia

Hepatic: Hepatic necrosis, hepatitis, jaundice

Neuromuscular & skeletal: Arthralgia, myalgia, paresthesia

Renal: Nephritis

Miscellaneous: Insulin autoimmune syndrome, lymphadenopathy, SLE-like syndrome

Drug Interactions

Metabolism/Transport Effects Inhibits CYP1A2 (weak), CYP2A6 (weak), CYP2B6 (weak), CYP2C19 (weak), CYP2C9 (weak), CYP2D6 (weak), CYP2E1 (weak), CYP3A4 (weak)

Avoid Concomitant Use

Avoid concomitant use of Methimazole with any of the following: CloZAPine; Dipyrone; Pimozide; Sodium Iodide I131

Increased Effect/Toxicity

Methimazole may increase the levels/effects of: ARIPiprazole; Cardiac Glycosides; CloZAPine; Dofetilide; Hydrocodone; Lomitapide; Pimozide; Theophylline Derivatives

The levels/effects of Methimazole may be increased by: Dipyrone

Decreased Effect

Methimazole may decrease the levels/effects of: PredniSoLONE (Systemic); Sodium Iodide I131; Vitamin K Antagonists

Storage/Stability Store at 15°C to 30°C (59°F to 86°F).

Mechanism of Action Inhibits the synthesis of thyroid hormones by blocking the oxidation of iodine in the thyroid gland; blocks synthesis of thyroxine and triiodothyronine (T_3); does not inactivate circulating T_4 and T_3

Pharmacodynamics/Kinetics

Onset of action: Antithyroid: Oral: 12 to 18 hours (Clark, 2006)

Duration: 36 to 72 hours (Clark, 2006)

Distribution: Concentrated in thyroid gland

Protein binding, plasma: None (Cooper, 2005)

Metabolism: Hepatic

Excretion: Urine

Dosage Oral: Administer in equally divided doses every 8 hours

Children and Adolescents:

Hyperthyroidism: Initial: 0.4 mg/kg/day in 3 divided doses; maintenance: 0.2 mg/kg/day in 3 divided doses

Hyperthyroidism associated with Graves' disease

Manufacturer's labeling: Initial: 0.4 mg/kg/day in 3 divided doses; maintenance: 0.2 mg/kg/day in 3 divided doses

Alternate dosing: Initial: 0.2 to 0.5 mg/kg once daily (range: 0.1 to 1 mg/kg/day) to restore euthyroidism, then reduce dose by 50% or more and continue for a total of 1 to 2 years; may then discontinue or reduce dose to assess if patient is in remission. **Note:** In severe cases, initial doses that are 50% to 100% higher may be used (Bahn, 2011).

The following dosing approach may also be used (Bahn, 2011):

Infants: 1.25 mg daily

Children 1 to 5 years: 2.5 to 5 mg daily

Children 5 to 10 years: 5 to 10 mg daily

Children and Adolescents 10 to 18 years: 10 to 20 mg daily

Adults:

Hyperthyroidism: Initial: 15 mg daily in 3 divided doses for mild hyperthyroidism; 30 to 40 mg daily in 3 divided doses for moderately severe hyperthyroidism; 60 mg daily in 3 divided doses for severe hyperthyroidism; maintenance: 5 to 15 mg daily (may be given as a single daily dose in many cases) (Mandana, 2004)

Adjust dosage as required to achieve and maintain serum T_3, T_4, and TSH levels in the normal range. An elevated T_3 may be the sole indicator of inadequate treatment. An elevated TSH indicates excessive antithyroid treatment.

Hyperthyroidism associated with Graves' disease:

Manufacturer's labeling: Initial: 15 mg daily in 3 divided doses for mild hyperthyroidism; 30 to 40 mg daily in 3 divided doses for moderately severe hyperthyroidism; 60 mg daily in 3 divided doses for severe hyperthyroidism; maintenance: 5 to 15 mg daily (may be given as a single daily dose in many cases) (Mandana, 2004)

Alternate dosing: Initial: 10 to 20 mg once daily to restore euthyroidism; maintenance: 5 to 10 mg once daily for a total of 12 to 18 months, then taper or discontinue if TSH is normal at that time (Bahn, 2011)

Iodine-induced thyrotoxicosis (off-label use): 20 to 40 mg daily given either once or twice daily (Bahn, 2011)

Thyrotoxic crisis (off-label use): **Note:** Recommendations vary; use in combination with other specific agents. Dosages of 20 to 25 mg every 6 hours have been used; once stable, dosing frequency may be reduced to once or twice daily (Nayak, 2006). The American Thyroid Association and the American Association of Clinical Endocrinologists recommend 60 to 80 mg daily (Bahn, 2011). Rectal administration has also been described (Nabil, 1982).

Thyrotoxicosis (type I amiodarone-induced; off-label use): 40 mg once daily to restore euthyroidism (generally 3 to 6 months). **Note:** If high doses continue to be required, dividing the dose may be more effective (Bahn, 2011).

Dosage adjustment in renal impairment: There are no dosage adjustments provided in the manufacturer's labeling.

Dosage adjustment in hepatic impairment: There are no dosage adjustments provided in the manufacturer's labeling.

Administration In thyrotoxic crisis, rectal administration has been described (Nabil, 1982).

Monitoring Parameters Monitor for signs of hypothyroidism, hyperthyroidism, free T_4, T_3; CBC with differential, liver function (baseline and as needed), serum thyroxine, free thyroxine index; prothrombin time (especially before surgical procedures)

Additional Information A potency ratio of methimazole to propylthiouracil of at least 20-30:1 is recommended when changing from one drug to another (eg, 300 mg of propylthiouracil would be roughly equivalent to 10-15 mg of methimazole) (Bahn, 2011).

Dosage Forms

Tablet, Oral:

Tapazole: 5 mg, 10 mg

Generic: 5 mg, 10 mg

Extemporaneous Preparations Suppositories can be made from methimazole tablets; dissolve 1200 mg methimazole in 12 mL of water and add to 52 mL cocoa butter containing 2 drops of Span 80. Stir the resulting mixture to form a water-oil emulsion and pour into 2.6 mL suppository molds to cool.

Nabil N, Miner DJ, and Amatruda JM, "Methimazole: An Alternative Route of Administration," *J Clin Endo Metab*, 1982, 54(1):180-1.

◆ **Methitest** *see* MethylTESTOSTERone *on page 1345*

Methocarbamol (meth oh KAR ba mole)

Brand Names: U.S. Robaxin; Robaxin-750

Brand Names: Canada Robaxin®

Pharmacologic Category Skeletal Muscle Relaxant

Additional Appendix Information

Beers Criteria – Potentially Inappropriate Medications for Geriatrics *on page 2271*

Use Adjunctive treatment of muscle spasm associated with acute painful musculoskeletal conditions (eg, tetanus)

Pregnancy Risk Factor C

Pregnancy Considerations Animal reproduction studies have not been conducted. The manufacturer notes that fetal and congenital abnormalities have been rarely reported following *in utero* exposure. Use during pregnancy only if clearly needed.

Breast-Feeding Considerations It is not known if methocarbamol is excreted in breast milk. The manufacturer recommends that caution be exercised when administering methocarbamol to nursing women.

Contraindications Hypersensitivity to methocarbamol or any component of the formulation; renal impairment (injection formulation)

Warnings/Precautions May cause CNS depression, which may impair physical or mental abilities; patients must be cautioned about performing tasks which require mental alertness (eg, operating machinery or driving). Effects may be potentiated when used with other sedative drugs or ethanol. Plasma protein binding and clearance are decreased and the half-life is increased in patients with hepatic impairment. Muscle relaxants are poorly tolerated by the elderly due to potent anticholinergic effects, sedation, and risk of fracture. Efficacy is questionable at dosages tolerated by elderly patients; avoid use (Beers Criteria).

Injection: Contraindicated in renal impairment. Contains polyethylene glycol. Rate of injection should not exceed 3 mL/minute; solution is hypertonic; avoid extravasation. Use with caution in patients with a history of seizures. Use caution with hepatic impairment. Vial stopper contains latex. Recommended only for the treatment of tetanus in pediatric patients.

Adverse Reactions

Cardiovascular: Bradycardia, flushing, hypotension, syncope

Central nervous system: Amnesia, confusion, coordination impaired (mild), dizziness, drowsiness, fever, headache, insomnia, lightheadedness, sedation, seizures, vertigo

Dermatologic: Angioneurotic edema, pruritus, rash, urticaria

Gastrointestinal: Dyspepsia, metallic taste, nausea, vomiting

Hematologic: Leukopenia
Hepatic: Jaundice
Local: Pain at injection site, thrombophlebitis
Ocular: Blurred vision, conjunctivitis, diplopia, nystagmus
Respiratory: Nasal congestion
Miscellaneous: Hypersensitivity reactions including anaphylaxis

Drug Interactions

Metabolism/Transport Effects None known.

Avoid Concomitant Use

Avoid concomitant use of Methocarbamol with any of the following: Azelastine (Nasal); Orphenadrine; Paraldehyde; Thalidomide

Increased Effect/Toxicity

Methocarbamol may increase the levels/effects of: Alcohol (Ethyl); Azelastine (Nasal); Buprenorphine; CNS Depressants; Hydrocodone; Methotrimeprazine; Metyrosine; Mirtazapine; Orphenadrine; Paraldehyde; Pramipexole; ROPINIRole; Rotigotine; Selective Serotonin Reuptake Inhibitors; Suvorexant; Thalidomide; Zolpidem

The levels/effects of Methocarbamol may be increased by: Brimonidine (Topical); Cannabis; Doxylamine; Dronabinol; Droperidol; Eperisone; HydrOXYzine; Kava Kava; Magnesium Sulfate; Methotrimeprazine; Nabilone; Perampanel; Rufinamide; Sodium Oxybate; Tapentadol; Tetrahydrocannabinol

Decreased Effect

Methocarbamol may decrease the levels/effects of: Pyridostigmine

Preparation for Administration Solution for injection: May administer undiluted or diluted in D_5W or NS (1 vial/ ≤250 mL diluent).

Storage/Stability

Solution for injection: Prior to dilution, store at controlled room temperature of 20°C to 25°C (68°F to 77°F); excursions permitted to 15°C to 30°C (59°F to 86°F).
Tablet: Store at controlled room temperature of 20°C to 25°C (68°F to 77°F).

Mechanism of Action Causes skeletal muscle relaxation by general CNS depression

Pharmacodynamics/Kinetics

Onset of action: Muscle relaxation: Oral: ~30 minutes
Protein binding: 46% to 50%
Metabolism: Hepatic via dealkylation and hydroxylation
Half-life elimination: 1-2 hours
Time to peak, serum: Oral: 1-2 hours
Excretion: Urine (primarily as metabolites)

Dosage

Tetanus: IV:
Children: Recommended **only** for use in tetanus: 15 mg/kg/dose or 500 mg/m^2/dose, may repeat every 6 hours if needed; maximum dose: 1.8 g/m^2/day for 3 days only
Adults: Initial dose: 1-2 g by direct IV injection, which may be followed by an additional 1-2 g by infusion (maximum initial dose: 3 g total); followed by 1-2 g every 6 hours until oral administration by mouth or via NG tube is possible; total oral daily doses of up to 24 g may be needed; injection should not be used for more than 3 consecutive days
Muscle spasm:
Oral: Children ≥16 years and Adults: 1.5 g 4 times/day for 2-3 days (up to 8 g/day may be given in severe conditions), then decrease to 4-4.5 g/day in 3-6 divided doses
IM, IV: Adults: Initial: 1 g; may repeat every 8 hours if oral administration not possible; maximum dose: 3 g/day for no more than 3 consecutive days. If condition persists, may repeat course of therapy after a drug-free interval of 48 hours.

Dosage adjustment in renal impairment: No dosage adjustment provided in manufacturer's labeling. However, administration of the parenteral formulation is contraindicated in patients with renal dysfunction due to the presence of polyethylene glycol.

Dosage adjustment in hepatic impairment: No dosage adjustment provided in manufacturer's labeling. However, elimination may be reduced in patients with cirrhosis.

Administration

Solution for injection:
IM: A maximum of 5 mL can be administered into each gluteal region.
IV: Maximum rate: 3 mL/minute; may be administered undiluted or diluted. Monitor closely for extravasation. Administer IV while in recumbent position. Maintain position for at least 10-15 minutes following infusion.
Tablet: May be crushed and mixed with food or liquid if needed.

Monitoring Parameters Monitor closely for extravasation (IV administration).

Dosage Forms

Solution, Injection:
Robaxin: 100 mg/mL (10 mL)
Solution, Injection [preservative free]:
Generic: 100 mg/mL (10 mL)
Tablet, Oral:
Robaxin: 500 mg
Robaxin-750: 750 mg
Generic: 500 mg, 750 mg

Methohexital (meth oh HEKS i tal)

Brand Names: U.S. Brevital Sodium

Brand Names: Canada Brevital

Index Terms Methohexital Sodium

Pharmacologic Category Barbiturate; General Anesthetic

Use Induction of anesthesia; procedural sedation

Pregnancy Risk Factor B

Dosage Doses must be titrated to effect.

Infants <1 month: Safety and efficacy not established.
Infants ≥1 month and Children:
Anesthesia induction:
IM: 6.6-10 mg/kg of a 5% solution
Rectal: Usual: 25 mg/kg of a 1% solution
IV (off-label dose): 1-2 mg/kg/dose of a 1% solution
Procedural sedation (off-label dose):
IV: Initial: 0.5 mg/kg; may repeat 0.5 mg/kg to a maximum total dose of 2 mg/kg
Rectal: 25 mg/kg of a 10% (100 mg/mL) solution given 5-15 minutes prior to procedure; maximum dose 500 mg
Adults: IV:
Induction: 1-1.5 mg/kg
Procedural sedation (off-label dose): 0.75-1 mg/kg; can redose 0.5 mg/kg every 2-5 minutes as needed (Bahn, 2005)
Wada test (off-label use): 3-4 mg over 3 seconds; following signs of recovery, administer a second dose of 2 mg over 2 seconds (Buchtel, 2002)
Elderly: IV: Refer to adult dosing. Reduce dose or administer at the low end of the dosage range.

Dosage adjustment in renal impairment: No dosage adjustment provided in manufacturer's labeling; use with caution.

Dosage adjustment in hepatic impairment: No dosage adjustment provided in manufacturer's labeling. However, adjustment may be necessary due to hepatic metabolism. Use with caution.

Additional Information Complete prescribing information should be consulted for additional detail.

Dosage Forms

Solution Reconstituted, Injection:

Brevital Sodium: 500 mg (1 ea); 2.5 g (1 ea)

- **Methohexital Sodium** *see* Methohexital *on page 1321*

Methotrexate (meth oh TREKS ate)

Brand Names: U.S. Otrexup; Rasuvo; Rheumatrex; Trexall

Brand Names: Canada Apo-Methotrexate; JAMP-Methotrexate; Methotrexate Injection USP; Methotrexate Injection, BP; Methotrexate Sodium Injection; Metoject; ratio-Methotrexate Sodium

Index Terms Amethopterin; Methotrexate Sodium; Methotrexatum; MTX (error-prone abbreviation)

Pharmacologic Category Antineoplastic Agent, Antimetabolite (Antifolate); Antirheumatic, Disease Modifying; Immunosuppressant Agent

Use

Oncology-related uses: Acute lymphoblastic leukemia (ALL) maintenance treatment, ALL meningeal leukemia (prophylaxis and treatment); treatment of trophoblastic neoplasms (gestational choriocarcinoma, chorioadenoma destruens and hydatidiform mole), breast cancer, head and neck cancer (epidermoid), cutaneous T-Cell lymphoma (advanced mycosis fungoides), lung cancer (squamous cell and small cell), advanced non-Hodgkin lymphomas (NHL), osteosarcoma

Nononcology uses: Treatment of psoriasis (severe, recalcitrant, disabling); severe, active rheumatoid arthritis (RA); active polyarticular-course juvenile idiopathic arthritis (pJIA)

Limitations of use: Otrexup and Rasuvo are not indicated for the treatment of neoplastic diseases.

Pregnancy Risk Factor X (psoriasis, rheumatoid arthritis)

Pregnancy Considerations [U.S. Boxed Warning]: Methotrexate may cause fetal death and/or congenital abnormalities. Studies in animals and pregnant women have shown evidence of fetal abnormalities; therefore, the manufacturer classifies methotrexate as pregnancy category X (for psoriasis or RA). A pattern of congenital malformations associated with maternal methotrexate use is referred to as the aminopterin/methotrexate syndrome. Features of the syndrome include CNS, skeletal, and cardiac abnormalities. Low birth weight and developmental delay have also been reported. The use of methotrexate may impair fertility and cause menstrual irregularities or oligospermia during treatment and following therapy. Methotrexate is approved for the treatment of trophoblastic neoplasms (gestational choriocarcinoma, chorioadenoma destruens, and hydatidiform mole) and has been used for the medical management of ectopic pregnancy and the medical management of abortion. **[U.S. Boxed Warning]: Use is contraindicated for the treatment of psoriasis or RA in pregnant women.** Pregnancy should be excluded prior to therapy in women of childbearing potential. Use for the treatment of neoplastic diseases only when the potential benefit to the mother outweighs the possible risk to the fetus. Pregnancy should be avoided for ≥3 months following treatment in male patients and ≥1 ovulatory cycle in female patients. A registry is available for pregnant women exposed to autoimmune medications including methotrexate. For additional information contact the Organization of Teratology Information Specialists, OTIS Autoimmune Diseases Study, at 877-311-8972.

Breast-Feeding Considerations Low amounts of methotrexate are excreted into breast milk. Due to the potential for serious adverse reactions in a breast-feeding infant, use is contraindicated in nursing mothers.

Contraindications Known hypersensitivity to methotrexate or any component of the formulation; breast-feeding

Additional contraindications for patients with psoriasis or rheumatoid arthritis: Pregnancy, alcoholism, alcoholic liver disease or other chronic liver disease, immunodeficiency syndrome (overt or laboratory evidence); preexisting blood dyscrasias (eg, bone marrow hypoplasia, leukopenia, thrombocytopenia, significant anemia)

Warnings/Precautions Hazardous agent - use appropriate precautions for handling and disposal (NIOSH 2014 [group 1]).

[U.S. Boxed Warning]: Methotrexate has been associated with acute (elevated transaminases) and potentially fatal chronic (fibrosis, cirrhosis) hepatotoxicity. Risk is related to cumulative dose (≥1.5 g) and prolonged exposure. Monitor closely (with liver function tests, including serum albumin) for liver toxicities. Liver enzyme elevations may be noted, but may not be predictive of hepatic disease in long term treatment for psoriasis (but generally is predictive in rheumatoid arthritis [RA] treatment). With long-term use, liver biopsy may show histologic changes, fibrosis, or cirrhosis; periodic liver biopsy is recommended with long-term use for psoriasis patients with risk factors for hepatotoxicity and for persistent abnormal liver function tests in psoriasis patients without risk factors for hepatotoxicity and in RA patients; discontinue methotrexate with moderate-to-severe change in liver biopsy. Risk factors for hepatotoxicity include history of above moderate ethanol consumption, persistent abnormal liver chemistries, history of chronic liver disease (including hepatitis B or C), family history of inheritable liver disease, diabetes, obesity, hyperlipidemia, lack of folate supplementation during methotrexate therapy, cumulative methotrexate dose exceeding 1.5 g, continuous daily methotrexate dosing and history of significant exposure to hepatotoxic drugs. Use caution with preexisting liver impairment; may require dosage reduction. Use caution when used with other hepatotoxic agents (azathioprine, retinoids, sulfasalazine). **[U.S. Boxed Warning]: Methotrexate elimination is reduced in patients with ascites and pleural effusions;** resulting in prolonged half-life and toxicity; may require dose reduction or discontinuation. Monitor closely for toxicity.

[U.S. Boxed Warning]: May cause renal damage leading to acute renal failure, especially with high-dose methotrexate; monitor renal function and methotrexate levels closely, maintain adequate hydration and urinary alkalinization. Use caution in osteosarcoma patients treated with high-dose methotrexate in combination with nephrotoxic chemotherapy (eg, cisplatin). **[U.S. Boxed Warning]: Methotrexate elimination is reduced in patients with renal impairment;** may require dose reduction or discontinuation; monitor closely for toxicity. **[U.S. Boxed Warning]: Tumor lysis syndrome may occur in patients with high tumor burden;** use appropriate prevention and treatment.

[U.S. Boxed Warning]: May cause potentially life-threatening pneumonitis (acute or chronic); may require treatment interruption; may be irreversible. Pulmonary symptoms may occur at any time during therapy and at any dosage; monitor closely for pulmonary symptoms, particularly dry, nonproductive cough. Other potential symptoms include fever, dyspnea, hypoxemia, or pulmonary infiltrate. **[U.S. Boxed Warning]: Methotrexate elimination is reduced in patients with pleural effusions;** may require dose reduction or discontinuation. Monitor closely for toxicity.

[U.S. Boxed Warning]: Bone marrow suppression may occur (sometimes fatal); aplastic anemia has been reported; anemia, pancytopenia, leukopenia, neutropenia, and/or thrombocytopenia may occur. Use caution in patients with preexisting bone marrow suppression. Discontinue treatment (immediately) in RA or psoriasis if a significant decrease in hematologic components is noted. **[U.S. Boxed Warning]: Use of low-dose methotrexate has been associated with the development of malignant lymphomas;** may regress upon treatment discontinuation; treat lymphoma appropriately if regression is not induced by cessation of methotrexate. Discontinue methotrexate if lymphoma does not regress. Other secondary tumors have been reported.

[U.S. Boxed Warning]: Gastrointestinal toxicity may occur; diarrhea and ulcerative stomatitis may require treatment interruption; hemorrhagic enteritis or intestinal perforation (with fatality) may occur. Use with caution in patients with peptic ulcer disease, ulcerative colitis. In children, doses ≥12 g/m^2 (IV) are associated with a high emetic potential; doses ≥250 mg/m^2 (IV) in adults and children are associated with moderate emetic potential (Dupuis, 2011). Antiemetics may be recommended to prevent nausea and vomiting.

May cause neurotoxicity including seizures (usually in pediatric ALL patients receiving intermediate-dose (1 g/m^2 methotrexate), leukoencephalopathy (usually in patients who have received cranial irradiation) and stroke-like encephalopathy (usually with high-dose regimens). Chemical arachnoiditis (headache, back pain, nuchal rigidity, fever) and myelopathy may result from intrathecal administration. Chronic leukoencephalopathy has been reported with high-dose and with intrathecal methotrexate; may be progressive and fatal. May cause dizziness and fatigue; may affect the ability to drive or operate heavy machinery.

[U.S. Boxed Warning]: Any dose level, route of administration, or duration of therapy may cause severe and potentially fatal dermatologic reactions, including toxic epidermal necrolysis, Stevens-Johnson syndrome, exfoliative dermatitis, skin necrosis, and erythema multiforme. Recovery has been reported with treatment discontinuation. Radiation dermatitis and sunburn may be precipitated by methotrexate administration. Psoriatic lesions may be worsened by concomitant exposure to ultraviolet radiation.

Potentially significant drug-drug interactions may exist, requiring dose or frequency adjustment, additional monitoring, and/or selection of alternative therapy. **[U.S. Boxed Warning]: Concomitant administration with NSAIDs may cause severe bone marrow suppression, aplastic anemia, and GI toxicity.** Do not administer NSAIDs prior to or during high-dose methotrexate therapy; may increase and prolong serum methotrexate levels. Doses used for psoriasis may still lead to unexpected toxicities; use caution when administering NSAIDs or salicylates with lower doses of methotrexate for RA. Methotrexate may increase the levels and effects of mercaptopurine; may require dosage adjustments. Vitamins containing folate may decrease response to systemic methotrexate; folate deficiency may increase methotrexate toxicity. Concomitant use of proton pump inhibitors with methotrexate (primarily high-dose methotrexate) may elevate and prolong serum methotrexate and metabolite (hydroxymethotrexate) levels; may lead to toxicities; use with caution. Immunization may be ineffective during methotrexate treatment. Immunization with live vaccines is not recommended; cases of disseminated vaccinia infections due to live vaccines have been reported. **[U.S. Boxed Warning]: Concomitant methotrexate administration with radiotherapy may increase the risk of soft tissue necrosis and osteonecrosis.**

[U.S. Boxed Warnings]: Should be administered under the supervision of a physician experienced in the use of antimetabolite therapy; serious and fatal toxicities have occurred at all dose levels. Immune suppression may lead to potentially fatal opportunistic infections, including *Pneumocystis jirovecii* pneumonia (PCP). Use methotrexate with extreme caution in patients with an active infection (contraindicated in patients with immunodeficiency syndrome). **[U.S. Boxed Warnings]: For rheumatoid arthritis and psoriasis, immunosuppressive therapy should only be used when disease is active, severe, recalcitrant, and disabling; and where less toxic, traditional therapy is ineffective. Methotrexate formulations and/or diluents containing preservatives should not be used for intrathecal or high-dose methotrexate therapy. May cause fetal death or congenital abnormalities; do not use for psoriasis or RA treatment in pregnant women.** May cause impairment of fertility, oligospermia, and menstrual dysfunction. Toxicity from methotrexate or any immunosuppressive is increased in the elderly. Methotrexate injection may contain benzyl alcohol and should not be used in neonates. Errors have occurred (some resulting in death) when methotrexate was administered as a "daily" dose instead of a "weekly" dose intended for some indications. The ISMP Targeted Medication Safety Best Practices for Hospitals recommends hospitals use a weekly dosage regimen default for oral methotrexate orders, with a hard stop override requiring verification of appropriate oncology indication; manual systems should require verification of an oncology indication prior to dispensing oral methotrexate for daily administration. Pharmacists should provide patient education for patients discharged on weekly oral methotrexate; education should include written leaflets that contain clear instructions about the weekly dosing schedule and explain the danger of taking extra doses (ISMP, 2014).

When used for intrathecal administration, should not be prepared during the preparation of any other agents; after preparation, store intrathecal medications in an isolated location or container clearly marked with a label identifying as "intrathecal" use only; delivery of intrathecal medications to the patient should only be with other medications intended for administration into the central nervous system (Jacobson, 2009).

Benzyl alcohol and derivatives: Some dosage forms may contain benzyl alcohol; large amounts of benzyl alcohol (≥99 mg/kg/day) have been associated with a potentially fatal toxicity ("gasping syndrome") in neonates; the "gasping syndrome" consists of metabolic acidosis, respiratory distress, gasping respirations, CNS dysfunction (including convulsions, intracranial hemorrhage), hypotension, and cardiovascular collapse (AAP, 1997; CDC, 1982); some data suggests that benzoate displaces bilirubin from protein binding sites (Ahlfors, 2001); avoid or use dosage forms containing benzyl alcohol with caution in neonates. See manufacturer's labeling.

Adverse Reactions Note: Adverse reactions vary by route and dosage.

Cardiovascular: Arterial thrombosis, cerebral thrombosis, chest pain, deep vein thrombosis, hypotension, pericardial effusion, pericarditis, plaque erosion (psoriasis), pulmonary embolism, retinal thrombosis, thrombophlebitis, vasculitis

Central nervous system: Abnormal cranial sensation, brain disease, chemical arachnoiditis (intrathecal; acute), chills, cognitive dysfunction (has been reported at low dosage), dizziness, drowsiness, fatigue, headache (pJIA), leukoencephalopathy (intravenous administration after craniospinal irradiation or repeated high-dose therapy; may be chronic), malaise, mood changes (has been reported at low dosage), neurological signs and symptoms (at high dosages; including confusion, hemiparesis, transient blindness, seizures, and coma), severe neurotoxicity (reported with unexpectedly increased frequency among pediatric patients with acute lymphoblastic leukemia who were treated with intermediate-dose intravenous methotrexate), speech disturbance

Dermatologic: Acne vulgaris, alopecia, burning sensation of skin (psoriasis), dermal ulcer, dermatitis (rheumatoid arthritis), diaphoresis, ecchymoses, erythema multiforme, erythematous rash, exfoliative dermatitis, furunculosis, hyperpigmentation, hypopigmentation, pruritus (rheumatoid arthritis), skin abnormalities related to radiation recall, skin necrosis, skin photosensitivity, skin rash, Stevens-Johnson syndrome, telangiectasia, toxic epidermal necrolysis, urticaria

Endocrine & metabolic: Decreased libido, decreased serum albumin, diabetes mellitus, gynecomastia, menstrual disease

Gastrointestinal: Abdominal distress, anorexia, aphthous stomatitis, diarrhea, enteritis, gastrointestinal hemorrhage, gingivitis, hematemesis, intestinal perforation, melena, nausea and vomiting, stomatitis

Genitourinary: Azotemia, cystitis, defective oogenesis, defective spermatogenesis, dysuria, hematuria, impotence, infertility, oligospermia, pancreatitis, proteinuria, severe renal disease, vaginal discharge

Hematologic & oncologic: Agranulocytosis, anemia, aplastic anemia, bone marrow depression (nadir: 7-10 days), decreased hematocrit, eosinophilia, gastric ulcer, hypogammaglobulinemia, leukopenia (WBC <3000/mm^3), lymphadenopathy, lymphoma, lymphoproliferative disorder, neutropenia, non-Hodgkin's lymphoma (in patients receiving low-dose oral methotrexate), pancytopenia (rheumatoid arthritis), thrombocytopenia (rheumatoid arthritis; platelet count <100,000/mm^3), tumor lysis syndrome

Hepatic: Cirrhosis (chronic therapy), hepatic failure, hepatic fibrosis (chronic therapy), hepatitis (acute), hepatotoxicity, increased liver enzymes

Hypersensitivity: Anaphylactoid reaction

Infection: Cryptococcosis, cytomegalovirus disease (including cytomegaloviral pneumonia, sepsis, nocardiosis), herpes simplex infection, herpes zoster, histoplasmosis, infection, pneumonia due to *pneumocystis jiroveci*, vaccinia (disseminated; following smallpox immunization)

Neuromuscular & skeletal: Arthralgia, myalgia, myelopathy (subacute), osteonecrosis (with radiotherapy), osteoporosis, stress fracture

Ophthalmic: Blurred vision, conjunctivitis, eye pain, visual disturbance

Otic: Tinnitus

Renal: Renal failure

Respiratory: Chronic obstructive pulmonary disease, cough, epistaxis, interstitial pneumonitis (rheumatoid arthritis), pharyngitis, pneumonia, pulmonary alveolitis, pulmonary disease, pulmonary fibrosis, respiratory failure, upper respiratory tract infection

Miscellaneous: Fever, nodule, tissue necrosis

Drug Interactions

Metabolism/Transport Effects Substrate of OAT3, P-glycoprotein, SLCO1B1

Avoid Concomitant Use

Avoid concomitant use of Methotrexate with any of the following: Acitretin; BCG; CloZAPine; Dipyrone; Foscarnet; Natalizumab; Pimecrolimus; Tacrolimus (Topical)

Increased Effect/Toxicity

Methotrexate may increase the levels/effects of: CloZAPine; CycloSPORINE (Systemic); Dipyrone; Leflunomide; Loop Diuretics; Natalizumab; Tegafur; Theophylline Derivatives; Tofacitinib; Vaccines (Live)

The levels/effects of Methotrexate may be increased by: Acitretin; Alitretinoin (Systemic); Ciprofloxacin (Systemic); CycloSPORINE (Systemic); Denosumab; Dexketoprofen; Dipyrone; Eltrombopag; Foscarnet; Fosphenytoin-Phenytoin; Loop Diuretics; Mipomersen; Nonsteroidal Anti-Inflammatory Agents; Penicillins; P-glycoprotein/ABCB1 Inhibitors; Pimecrolimus; Probenecid; Proton Pump Inhibitors; Roflumilast; Salicylates; SulfaSALAzine; Sulfonamide Derivatives; Tacrolimus (Topical); Teriflunomide; Trastuzumab; Trimethoprim

Decreased Effect

Methotrexate may decrease the levels/effects of: BCG; Coccidioides immitis Skin Test; Fosphenytoin-Phenytoin; Loop Diuretics; Sapropterin; Sipuleucel-T; Vaccines (Inactivated)

The levels/effects of Methotrexate may be decreased by: Bile Acid Sequestrants; Echinacea; P-glycoprotein/ABCB1 Inducers

Food Interactions Methotrexate peak serum levels may be decreased if taken with food. Milk-rich foods may decrease methotrexate absorption. Management: Administer without regard to food.

Preparation for Administration Hazardous agent; use appropriate precautions for handling and disposal (NIOSH 2014 [group 1]). **Use preservative-free preparations for intrathecal or high-dose methotrexate administration.**

IV: Dilute powder with D_5W or NS to a concentration of ≤25 mg/mL (20 mg and 50 mg vials) and 50 mg/mL (1 g vial). May further dilute in D_5W or NS.

Intrathecal: Prepare intrathecal solutions with preservative-free NS, lactated Ringer's, or Elliot's B solution to a final volume of up to 12 mL (volume generally based on institution or practitioner preference). Intrathecal methotrexate concentrations may be institution specific or based on practitioner preference, generally ranging from a final concentration of 1 mg/mL (per prescribing information; Grossman, 1993; Lin, 2008) up to ~2 to 4 mg/mL (de Lemos, 2009; Glantz, 1999). For triple intrathecal therapy (methotrexate 12 mg/hydrocortisone 24 mg/cytarabine 36 mg), preparation to final volume of 12 mL is reported (Lin, 2008). Intrathecal medications should **NOT** be prepared during the preparation of any other agents.

Storage/Stability

Tablets: Store between 20°C and 25°C (68°F and 77°F); excursions are permitted between 15°C and 30°C (59°F and 86°F). Protect from light.

Injection: Store intact vials and autoinjectors between 20°C and 25°C (68°F and 77°F); excursions may be permitted between 15°C and 30°C (59°F and 86°F). Protect from light.

IV: Solution diluted in D_5W or NS is stable for 24 hours at room temperature (21°C to 25°C).

Intrathecal: Intrathecal dilutions are preservative free and should be used as soon as possible after preparation. After preparation, store intrathecal medications (until use) in an isolated location or container clearly marked with a label identifying as "intrathecal" use only.

Mechanism of Action Methotrexate is a folate antimetabolite that inhibits DNA synthesis, repair, and cellular replication. Methotrexate irreversibly binds to and inhibits dihydrofolate reductase, inhibiting the formation of reduced folates, and thymidylate synthetase, resulting in inhibition of purine and thymidylic acid synthesis, thus interfering with DNA synthesis, repair, and cellular replication. Methotrexate is cell cycle specific for the S phase of the cycle. Actively proliferative tissues are more susceptible to the effects of methotrexate.

The MOA in the treatment of rheumatoid arthritis is unknown, but may affect immune function. In psoriasis, methotrexate is thought to target rapidly proliferating epithelial cells in the skin.

In Crohn disease, it may have immune modulator and anti-inflammatory activity.

Pharmacodynamics/Kinetics

Onset of action: Antirheumatic: 3 to 6 weeks; additional improvement may continue longer than 12 weeks

Absorption:
  Oral: Highly variable; dose dependent
  IM injection: Complete
Distribution: Penetrates slowly into 3rd space fluids (eg, pleural effusions, ascites), exits slowly from these compartments (slower than from plasma); sustained concentrations retained in kidney and liver
V_d: IV: 0.18 L/kg (initial); 0.4 to 0.8 L/kg (steady state)
Protein binding: ~50%
Metabolism: Partially metabolized by intestinal flora (after oral administration) to DAMPA by carboxypeptidase; hepatic aldehyde oxidase converts methotrexate to 7-hydroxy methotrexate; polyglutamates are produced intracellularly and are just as potent as methotrexate; their production is dose- and duration-dependent and they are slowly eliminated by the cell once formed. Polyglutamated forms can be converted back to methotrexate.
Bioavailability: Oral: ~20% to 95%; in general, bioavailability is dose dependent and decreases as the dose increases (especially at doses >80 mg/m^2)
Half-life elimination: Low dose: 3 to 10 hours; High dose: 8 to 15 hours; Children: 1 to 6 hours
Time to peak, serum: Oral: 1 to 2 hours; IM: 30 to 60 minutes
Excretion: Dose and route dependent; IV: Urine (80% to 90% as unchanged drug; 5% to 7% as 7-hydroxy methotrexate); feces (<10%)

Dosage Note: Methotrexate doses between 100 and 500 mg/m^2 **may require** leucovorin calcium rescue. Doses >500 mg/m^2 **require** leucovorin calcium rescue (refer to Dosage adjustment for toxicity leucovorin calcium dosing). In children, doses ≥12 g/m^2 (IV) are associated with a high emetic potential; doses ≥250 mg/m^2 (IV) in adults and children are associated with moderate emetic potential (Dupuis, 2011). Antiemetics may be recommended to prevent nausea and vomiting.

Children:
Polyarticular juvenile idiopathic arthritis (pJIA): Oral, IM, SubQ: Initial: 10 mg/m^2 once weekly; adjust dose gradually to optimal response; doses up to 20 to 30 mg/m^2 once weekly have been used (doses above 20 mg/m^2 once weekly may be associated with an increased risk of toxicity).
Acute lymphoblastic leukemia (ALL; intrathecal therapy is also administered [refer to specific reference]):
  Consolidation/intensification phases (as part of a combination regimen): 1,000 mg/m^2 IV over 24 hours in week 1 of intensification and 20 mg/m^2 IM (use 50% dose reduction if on same day as intrathecal methotrexate) on day 1 of week 2 of intensification phase; Intensification repeats every 2 weeks for a total of 12 courses (Mahoney, 2000) **or** 5,000 mg/m^2 IV over 24 hours days 8, 22, 36, and 50 of consolidation phase (Schrappe, 2000) with leucovorin rescue
  Interim maintenance (as part of a combination regimen): 15 mg/m^2 orally days 0, 7, 14, 21, 28, and 35 of interim maintenance phase (Seibel, 2008) **or** 100 mg/m^2 (escalate dose by 50 mg/m^2 each dose) IV days 0, 10, 20, 30, and 40 of increased intensity interim maintenance phase (Seibel, 2008)
  Maintenance (as part of a combination regimen): 20 mg/m^2 IM weekly on day 1 of weeks 25 to 130 (Mahoney, 2000) **or** 20 mg/m^2 orally days 7, 14, 21, 28, 35, 42, 49, 56, 63, 70, and 77 (Seibel, 2008)
  T-cell acute lymphoblastic leukemia (Asselin, 2011; triple intrathecal therapy is also administered [refer to specific reference]):
  Induction (weeks 1 to 6; as part of a combination regimen): IV:
    Low dose: 40 mg/m^2 day 2
    High dose: 500 mg/m^2 over 30 minutes followed by 4500 mg/m^2 over 23.5 hours (with leucovorin rescue) day 22
  Consolidation (weeks 7 to 33; combination chemotherapy): IV: High dose: 500 mg/m^2 over 30 minutes followed by 4,500 mg/m^2 over 23.5 hours (with leucovorin rescue) in weeks 7, 10, and 13 with leucovorin rescue
  Continuation (weeks 34 to 108; combination chemotherapy): IV, IM: 30 mg/m^2 weekly until 2 years after documented complete remission
  ALL, CNS prophylaxis triple intrathecal therapy (off-label dosing): Intrathecal: Age-based dosing (in combination with cytarabine and hydrocortisone): Days of administration vary based on risk status and protocol; refer to institutional protocols or reference for details (Matloub, 2006):
    <2 years: 8 mg
    2 to <3 years: 10 mg
    3 to ≤8 years: 12 mg
    >8 years: 15 mg
Meningeal leukemia, prophylaxis or treatment: Intrathecal: 6 to 12 mg/dose (based on age) every 2 to 7 days; continue for 1 dose beyond CSF cell count normalization. **Note:** Optimal intrathecal chemotherapy dosing should be based on age rather than on body surface area (BSA); CSF volume correlates with age and not to BSA (Bleyer, 1983; Kerr, 2001):
  <1 year: 6 mg/dose
  1 year: 8 mg/dose
  2 years: 10 mg/dose
  ≥3 years: 12 mg/dose
Osteosarcoma: IV: MAP regimen: 12 g/m^2 (maximum dose: 20 g) over 4 hours (followed by leucovorin rescue) for 4 doses during induction (before surgery) at weeks 3, 4, 8, and 9, and for 8 doses during maintenance (after surgery) at weeks 15, 16, 20, 21, 25, 26, 30, and 31 (in combination with doxorubicin and cisplatin) (Meyers, 2005); other combinations, intervals, and doses (8 to 14 g/m^2/dose) have been described (with leucovorin rescue), refer to specific reference for details (Bacci, 2000; Bacci, 2003; Goorin, 2003; Le Deley, 2007; Meyers, 1992; Weiner, 1986; Winkler, 1988)
Crohn disease, induction and maintenance (off-label use): SubQ: 15 mg/m^2 once weekly; maximum dose: 25 mg (Rufo, 2012)
Dermatomyositis (off-label use): Oral, SubQ (preferred): The lesser of 15 mg/m^2 or 1 mg/kg once weekly (maximum dose: 40 mg/week) in combination with corticosteroids (Huber, 2010) **or** 15 mg/m^2 once weekly (range: 10 to 20 mg/m^2 once weekly; maximum dose: 25 mg/week) in combination with prednisone (Ramanan, 2005)
Graft-versus-host disease, acute (aGVHD) prophylaxis (off-label use): IV: Refer to adult dosing.

Adults:
Acute lymphoblastic leukemia (ALL):
  Meningeal leukemia prophylaxis or treatment: Intrathecal: Manufacturer's labeling: 12 mg (maximum:15 mg/dose) every 2 to 7 days; continue for 1 dose beyond CSF cell count normalization. **Note:** Optimal intrathecal chemotherapy dosing should be based on age rather than on body surface area (BSA); CSF volume correlates with age and not to BSA (Bleyer, 1983; Kerr, 2001).
  CALGB 8811 regimen (Larson, 1995; combination therapy):
  Early intensification: Intrathecal: 15 mg day 1 of early intensification phase, repeat in 4 weeks
  CNS prophylaxis/interim maintenance phase:
    Intrathecal: 15 mg days 1, 8, 15, 22, and 29
    Oral: 20 mg/m^2 days 36, 43, 50, 57, and 64

Prolonged maintenance: Oral: 20 mg/m^2 days 1, 8, 15, and 22 every 4 weeks for 24 months from diagnosis

Dose-intensive regimen (Kantarjian, 2000; combination therapy):

IV: 200 mg/m^2 over 2 hours, followed by 800 mg/m^2 over 24 hours beginning day 1, (followed by leucovorin rescue) of even numbered cycles (in combination with cytarabine; alternates with Hyper-CVAD)

CNS prophylaxis: Intrathecal: 12 mg on day 2 of each cycle; duration depends on risk

Maintenance: IV: 10 mg/m^2/day for 5 days every month for 2 years (in combination with prednisone, vincristine, and mercaptopurine)

Breast cancer: IV: CMF regimen: 40 mg/m^2 days 1 and 8 every 4 weeks (in combination with cyclophosphamide and fluorouracil) for 6 to 12 cycles (Bonadonna, 1995; Levine, 1998)

Choriocarcinoma, chorioadenoma, gestational trophoblastic diseases: 15 to 30 mg oral or IM daily for a 5-day course; may repeat for 3 to 5 courses (manufacturer's labeling) **or** 100 mg/m^2 IV over 30 minutes followed by 200 mg/m^2 IV over 12 hours (with leucovorin 24 hours after the start of methotrexate), administer a second course if hCG levels plateau for 3 consecutive weeks (Garrett, 2002)

Head and neck cancer, advanced: IV: 40 mg/m^2 once weekly until disease progression or unacceptable toxicity (Forastiere, 1992; Guardiola, 2004; Stewart, 2009)

Lymphoma, non-Hodgkin: IV:

CODOX-M/IVAC regimen (Mead, 2008): Cycles 1 and 3 of CODOX-M (CODOX-M alternates with IVAC)

Adults ≤65 years: IV: 300 mg/m^2 over 1 hour (on day 10) followed by 2700 mg/m^2 over 23 hours (with leucovorin rescue)

Adults >65 years: IV: 100 mg/m^2 over 1 hour (on day 10) followed by 900 mg/m^2 over 23 hours (with leucovorin rescue)

Hyper-CVAD alternating with high dose methotrexate/cytarabine regimen: IV: 1000 mg/m^2 over 24 hours on day 1 during even courses (2, 4, 6, and 8) of 21-day treatment cycles (Thomas, 2006) **or** 200 mg/m^2 bolus day 1 followed by 800 mg/m^2 over 24 hours during even courses (2, 4, 6, and 8) of 21-day treatment cycles (Khouri, 1998) with leucovorin rescue

Mycosis fungoides (cutaneous T-cell lymphoma): 5 to 50 mg once weekly or 15 to 37.5 mg twice weekly orally or IM for early stages (manufacturer's labeling) **or** 25 mg orally once weekly, may increase to 50 mg once weekly (Zackheim, 2003)

Osteosarcoma: Adults ≤30 years: IV: MAP regimen: 12 g/m^2 (maximum dose: 20 g) over 4 hours (followed by leucovorin rescue) for 4 doses during induction (before surgery) at weeks 3, 4, 8, and 9, and for 8 doses during maintenance (after surgery) at weeks 15, 16, 20, 21, 25, 26, 30, and 31 (in combination with doxorubicin and cisplatin) (Meyers, 2005); other combinations, intervals, age ranges, and doses (8 to 14 g/m^2/dose) have been described (with leucovorin rescue), refer to specific reference for details (Bacci, 2000; Bacci, 2003; Goorin, 2003; Le Deley, 2007; Meyers, 1992; Weiner, 1986; Winkler, 1988)

Psoriasis: **Note:** Some experts recommend concomitant folic acid 1 to 5 mg daily (except the day of methotrexate) to reduce hematologic, gastrointestinal, and hepatic adverse events related to methotrexate.

Oral: Initial: 2.5 to 5 mg/dose every 12 hours for 3 doses per week **or**

Oral, IM, IV, SubQ: Initial: 10 to 25 mg once weekly; adjust dose gradually to optimal response (doses above 20 mg once weekly are associated with an increased incidence of toxicity); doses >30 mg per week should not be exceeded.

Note: An initial test dose of 2.5 to 5 mg is recommended in patients with risk factors for hematologic toxicity or renal impairment (Kalb, 2009).

Rheumatoid arthritis: **Note:** Some experts recommend concomitant folic acid at a dose of least 5 mg per week (except the day of methotrexate) to reduce hematologic, gastrointestinal, and hepatic adverse events related to methotrexate.

Oral (manufacturer labeling): Initial: 7.5 mg once weekly or 2.5 mg every 12 hours for 3 doses per week; adjust dose gradually to optimal response (dosage above 20 mg once weekly are associated with an increased incidence of toxicity); *alternatively*, 10 to 15 mg once weekly, increased by 5 mg every 2 to 4 weeks to a maximum of 20 to 30 mg once weekly has been recommended by some experts (Visser, 2009)

SubQ: Initial: 7.5 mg once weekly; adjust dose gradually to optimal response (doses above 20 mg once weekly are associated with an increased incidence of toxicity) **or** Initial: 15 mg once weekly; if insufficient response, after 16 weeks, may increase to 20 mg once weekly (Braun, 2008)

IM: Initial: 7.5 mg once weekly; adjust dose gradually to optimal response (doses above 20 mg once weekly are associated with an increased incidence of toxicity)

Off-label uses:

Bladder cancer (off-label use): IV:

Dose-dense MVAC regimen: 30 mg/m^2 day 1 every 2 weeks (in combination with vinblastine, doxorubicin, and cisplatin) (Sternberg, 2001)

CMV regimen: 30 mg/m^2 days 1 and 8 every 3 weeks for 3 cycles (in combination with cisplatin, vinblastine and leucovorin rescue) (Griffiths, 2011)

CNS Lymphoma (off-label use): IV: 8000 mg/m^2 over 4 hours (followed by leucovorin rescue) every 14 days until complete response or a maximum of 8 cycles; if complete response, follow with 2 consolidation cycles at the same dose every 14 days (with leucovorin rescue), followed by 11 maintenance cycles of 8000 mg/m^2 every 28 days with leucovorin rescue (Batchelor, 2003) **or** 2500 mg/m^2 over 2 to 3 hours every 14 days for 5 doses (in combination with vincristine, procarbazine, intrathecal methotrexate, leucovorin, dexamethasone, and cytarabine) (De Angelis, 2002) **or** 3500 mg/m^2 over 2 hours on day 2 every 2 weeks (in combination with rituximab, vincristine, procarbazine, and leucovorin [with intra-omaya methotrexate 12 mg between days 5 and 12 of each cycle if positive CSF cytology]) for 5 to 7 induction cycles (Shah, 2007)

Crohn disease, moderate/severe, corticosteroid-dependent or refractory (off-label use):

Remission induction or reduction of steroid use: IM, SubQ: 25 mg once weekly (Lichtenstein, 2009)

Remission maintenance: IM: 15 mg once weekly (Feagan, 2000; Lichtenstein, 2009)

Dermatomyositis/polymyositis (off-label uses):

Oral: Initial: 7.5 to 15 mg per week, often adjunctively with high-dose corticosteroid therapy; may increase in weekly 2.5 mg increments to target dose of 10 to 25 mg per week (**Note:** Administration of folate 5 to 7 mg per week has been used to reduce side effects) (Briemberg, 2003; Newman, 1995; Wiendl, 2008).

IV, IM: Doses of 20 to 60 mg per week have been employed if failure with oral therapy (doses >50 mg per week may require leucovorin calcium rescue) (Briemberg, 2003)

Ectopic pregnancy (off-label use): IM:

Single-dose regimen: Methotrexate 50 mg/m^2 on day 1; Measure serum hCG levels on days 4 and 7; if needed, repeat dose on day 7 (Barnhart, 2009)

Two-dose regimen: Methotrexate 50 mg/m^2 on day 1; Measure serum hCG levels on day 4 and administer a second dose of methotrexate 50 mg/m^2; Measure serum hCG levels on day 7 and if needed, administer a third dose of 50 mg/m^2 (Barnhart, 2009)

Multidose regimen: Methotrexate 1 mg/kg on day 1; leucovorin calcium 0.1 mg/kg IM on day 2; measure serum hCG on day 2; methotrexate 1 mg/kg on day 3; leucovorin calcium 0.1 mg/kg on day 4; measure serum hCG on day 4; continue up to a total of 4 courses based on hCG concentrations (Barnhart, 2009)

Graft-versus-host disease, acute (aGVHD), prophylaxis (off-label use): IV: 15 mg/m^2/dose on day 1 and 10 mg/m^2/dose on days 3 and 6 after allogeneic transplant (in combination with cyclosporine and prednisone) (Chao, 1993; Chao, 2000; Ross, 1999) **or** 15 mg/m^2/dose on day 1 and 10 mg/m^2/dose on days 3, 6, and 11 after allogeneic transplant (in combination with cyclosporine) (Chao, 2000) **or** 15 mg/m^2/dose on day 1 and 10 mg/m^2/dose on days 3, 6, and 11 after allogeneic transplant (in combination with cyclosporine, followed by leucovorin); may omit day 11 methotrexate for grade 2 or higher toxicity (Ruutu, 2013)

Nonleukemic meningeal cancer (off-label use): Intrathecal: 12 mg/dose twice weekly for 4 weeks, then weekly for 4 doses, then monthly for 4 doses (Glantz, 1998) **or** 10 mg twice weekly for 4 weeks, then weekly for 1 month, then every 2 weeks for 2 months (Glantz, 1999) **or** 10 to 15 mg twice weekly for 4 weeks, then once weekly for 4 weeks, then a maintenance regimen of once a month (Chamberlain, 2010)

Soft tissue sarcoma (desmoid tumors, aggressive fibromatosis), advanced (off-label use): IV: 30 mg/m^2 every 7 to 10 days (dose usually rounded to 50 mg) in combination with vinblastine for 1 year (Azzarelli, 2001)

Systemic lupus erythematosus, moderate-to-severe (off-label use): Oral: Initial: 7.5 mg once weekly; may increase by 2.5 mg increments weekly (maximum: 20 mg once weekly), in combination with prednisone (Fortin, 2008)

Takayasu arteritis, refractory or relapsing disease (off-label use): Oral: Initial dose: 0.3 mg/kg/week (maximum: 15 mg per week), titrated by 2.5 mg increments every 1 to 2 weeks until reaching a maximum tolerated weekly dose of 25 mg (use in combination with a corticosteroid; Hoffman, 1994)

Elderly:

Breast cancer: Patients >60 years: IV: CMF regimen: 30 mg/m^2 days 1 and 8 every 4 weeks (in combination with cyclophosphamide and fluorouracil) for up to 12 cycles (Bonadonna, 1995)

Meningeal leukemia: Intrathecal: Consider a dose reduction (CSF volume and turnover may decrease with age)

Non-Hodgkin lymphoma: CODOX-M/IVAC regimen (Mead, 2008): Cycles 1 and 3 of CODOX-M (CODOX-M alternates with IVAC): IV: 100 mg/m^2 over 1 hour (on day 10) followed by 900 mg/m^2 over 23 hours (with leucovorin rescue)

Rheumatoid arthritis/psoriasis: Oral: Initial: 5 to 7.5 mg per week, not to exceed 20 mg per week

Dosage adjustment for toxicity:

Methotrexate toxicities:

Nonhematologic toxicity: Diarrhea, stomatitis, or vomiting which may lead to dehydration: Discontinue until recovery

Hematologic toxicity:

Psoriasis, rheumatoid arthritis: Significant blood count decrease: Discontinue immediately.

Oncologic uses: Profound granulocytopenia and fever: Evaluate immediately; consider broad-spectrum parenteral antimicrobial coverage

Leucovorin calcium dosing (from methotrexate injection prescribing information; other leucovorin dosing/schedules may be specific to chemotherapy protocols):

Normal methotrexate elimination (serum methotrexate level ~10 micromolar at 24 hours after administration, 1 micromolar at 48 hours, and <0.2 micromolar at 72 hours): Leucovorin calcium 15 mg (oral, IM, or IV) every 6 hours for 60 hours (10 doses) beginning 24 hours after the start of methotrexate infusion

Delayed late methotrexate elimination (serum methotrexate level remaining >0.2 micromolar at 72 hours and >0.05 micromolar at 96 hours after administration): Continue leucovorin calcium 15 mg (oral, IM or IV) every 6 hours until methotrexate level is <0.05 micromolar

Delayed early methotrexate elimination and/or acute renal injury (serum methotrexate level ≥50 micromolar at 24 hours, or ≥5 micromolar at 48 hours, or a doubling of serum creatinine level at 24 hours after methotrexate administration): Leucovorin calcium 150 mg IV every 3 hours until methotrexate level is <1 micromolar, then 15 mg IV every 3 hours until methotrexate level <0.05 micromolar

Leucovorin nomogram dosing for high-dose methotrexate overexposure (**generalized dosing** derived from reference nomogram figures, refer to each reference [Bleyer, 1978; Bleyer, 1981; Widemann, 2006] or institution-specific nomogram for details):

At 24 hours:

For methotrexate levels of ≥100 micromolar at ~24 hours, leucovorin is initially dosed at 1000 mg/m^2 every 6 hours

For methotrexate levels of ≥10 to <100 micromolar at 24 hours, leucovorin is initially dosed at 100 mg/m^2 every 3 or 6 hours

For methotrexate levels of ~1 to 10 micromolar at 24 hours, leucovorin is initially dosed at 10 mg/m^2 every 3 or 6 hours

At 48 hours:

For methotrexate levels of ≥100 micromolar at 48 hours, leucovorin is dosed at 1000 mg/m^2 every 6 hours

For methotrexate levels of ≥10 to <100 micromolar at 48 hours, leucovorin is dosed at 100 mg/m^2 every 3 hours

For methotrexate levels of ~1 to 10 micromolar at 48 hours, leucovorin is dosed at 100 mg/m^2 every 6 hours **or** 10 to 100 mg/m^2 every 3 hours

At 72 hours:

For methotrexate levels of ≥10 micromolar at 72 hours, leucovorin is dosed at 100 to 1000 mg/m^2 every 3 to 6 hours

For methotrexate levels of ~1 to 10 micromolar at 72 hours, leucovorin is dosed at 10 to 100 mg/m^2 every 3 hours

For methotrexate levels of ~0.1 to 1 micromolar at 72 hours, leucovorin is dosed at 10 mg/m^2 every 3 to 6 hours

If serum creatinine is increased more than 50% above baseline, increase the standard leucovorin dose to 100 mg/m^2 every 3 hours, then adjust according to methotrexate levels above.

Follow methotrexate levels daily, leucovorin may be discontinued when methotrexate level is <0.1 micromolar

Dosage adjustment in renal impairment: There are no dosage adjustments provided in the manufacturer's labeling. The following adjustments have been recommended:

Aronoff, 2007:

Children:

CrCl 10 to 50 mL/minute/1.73 m^2: Administer 50% of dose

CrCl <10 mL/minute/1.73 m^2: Administer 30% of dose
Intermittent hemodialysis: Administer 30% of dose (post dialysis)
Continuous ambulatory peritoneal dialysis (CAPD): Administer 30% of dose
Continuous renal replacement therapy (CRRT): Administer 50% of dose

Adults:
CrCl 10 to 50 mL/minute: Administer 50% of dose
CrCl <10 mL/minute: Avoid use
Intermittent hemodialysis: Administer 50% of dose (post dialysis)
Continuous renal replacement therapy (CRRT): Administer 50% of dose

Kintzel, 1995:
CrCl 46 to 60 mL/minute: Administer 65% of normal dose
CrCl 31 to 45 mL/minute: Administer 50% of normal dose
CrCl <30 mL/minute: Avoid use

Hemodialysis patients with cancer (Janus, 2010): Administer 25% of dose after hemodialysis; monitor closely for toxicity

High-dose methotrexate, dose intensive regimen for ALL (200 mg/m^2 over 2 hours, followed by 800 mg/m^2 over 24 hours with leucovorin rescue [Kantarjian, 2000]):
Serum creatinine <1.5 mg/dL: No dosage adjustment necessary
Serum creatinine 1.5 to 2 mg/dL: Administer 75% of dose
Serum creatinine >2 mg/dL: Administer 50% of dose

Dosage adjustment in hepatic impairment: There are no dosage adjustments provided in the manufacturer's labeling; use with caution in patients with impaired hepatic function or preexisting hepatic damage. The following adjustments have been recommended (Floyd, 2006):
Bilirubin 3.1 to 5 mg/dL **or** transaminases >3 times ULN: Administer 75% of dose
Bilirubin >5 mg/dL: Avoid use

Dosing in obesity: *ASCO Guidelines for appropriate chemotherapy dosing in obese adults with cancer:* Utilize patient's actual body weight (full weight) for calculation of body surface area- or weight-based dosing, particularly when the intent of therapy is curative; manage regimen-related toxicities in the same manner as for nonobese patients; if a dose reduction is utilized due to toxicity, consider resumption of full weight-based dosing with subsequent cycles, especially if cause of toxicity (eg, hepatic or renal impairment) is resolved (Griggs, 2012).

Dietary Considerations Some products may contain sodium.

Administration In children, doses ≥12 g/m^2 are associated with a high emetic potential; doses ≥250 mg/m^2 (IV) in adults and children are associated with moderate emetic potential (Dupuis, 2011). Antiemetics may be recommended to prevent nausea and vomiting.

Methotrexate may be administered orally, IM, IV, intrathecally, or SubQ; IV administration may be as slow push (10 mg/minute), bolus infusion, or 24-hour continuous infusion (route and rate of administration depend on indication and/or protocol; refer to specific references). Must use preservative-free formulation for intrathecal or high-dose methotrexate administration.

Specific dosing schemes vary, but high doses should be followed by leucovorin calcium rescue to prevent toxicity; refer to Additional Information.

Otrexup and Rasuvo are autoinjectors for once weekly subcutaneous use in the abdomen or thigh; patient may self-administer after appropriate training. All schedules should be continually tailored to the individual patient. An initial test dose may be given prior to the regular dosing schedule to detect any extreme sensitivity to adverse effects.

Hazardous agent; use appropriate precautions for handling and disposal (NIOSH 2014 [group 1]).

Monitoring Parameters

Oncologic uses: Baseline and frequently during treatment: CBC with differential and platelets, serum creatinine, BUN, liver function tests (LFTs); methotrexate levels and urine pH (with high-dose methotrexate); closely monitor fluid and electrolyte status in patients with impaired methotrexate elimination; chest x-ray (baseline); pulmonary function test (if methotrexate-induced lung disease suspected); monitor carefully for toxicities (due to impaired elimination) in patients with ascites, pleural effusion, decreased folate stores, renal impairment, and/or hepatic impairment

Psoriasis (Kalb, 2009; Menter, 2009):
CBC with differential and platelets (baseline, 7 to 14 days after initiating therapy or dosage increase, every 2 to 4 weeks for first few months, then every 1 to 3 months depending on leukocyte count and stability of patient) monitor more closely in patients with risk factors for hematologic toxicity (eg, renal insufficiency, advanced age, hypoalbuminemia); BUN and serum creatinine (baseline and every 2 to 3 months) calculate glomerular filtration rate if at risk for renal dysfunction; consider PPD for latent TB screening (baseline); LFTs (baseline, monthly for first 6 months, then every 1 to 2 months; more frequently if at risk for hepatotoxicity or if clinically indicated; liver function tests should be performed at least 5 days after the last dose); pregnancy test (if female of reproductive potential); chest x-ray (baseline if underlying lung disease); pulmonary function test (if methotrexate-induced lung disease suspected)
Liver biopsy for patients **with** risk factors for hepatotoxicity: Baseline or after 2 to 6 months of therapy and with each 1 to 1.5 g cumulative dose interval
Liver biopsy for patients **without** risk factors for hepatotoxicity: If persistent elevations in 5 of 9 AST levels during a 12-month period, or decline of serum albumin below the normal range with normal nutritional status. Consider biopsy after cumulative dose of 3.5 to 4 g and after each additional 1.5 g.

Rheumatoid arthritis (American College of Rheumatology Subcommittee, 2002; Kremer, 1994; Saag, 2008; Singh, 2012):
CBC with differential and platelets serum creatinine, and LFTs at baseline and every 2 to 4 weeks for 3 months after initiation or following dose increases, then every 8 to 12 weeks for 3 to 6 months, then every 12 weeks for 6 months; monitor more frequently if clinically indicated.
Chest x-ray (within 1 year prior to initiation), Hepatitis B and C serology (if at high risk); tuberculosis testing annually for patients who live, travel or work in areas with likely TB exposure
Liver biopsy: Baseline (if persistent abnormal baseline LFTs, history of alcoholism, or chronic hepatitis B or C) or during treatment if persistent LFT elevations (6 of 12 tests abnormal over 1 year or 5 of 9 results when LFTs performed at 6-week intervals)

Crohn disease (off-label use; Lichtenstein, 2009): CBC with differential and platelets (baseline and periodic) and liver function tests (baseline and every 1 to 2 months); baseline liver biopsy (in patients with abnormal baseline LFTs or with chronic liver disease); liver biopsy at 1 year if (over a 1-year span) AST consistently elevated or serum albumin consistently decreased; chest x-ray (baseline)

Ectopic pregnancy (off-label use; Barnhart, 2009): Prior to therapy, measure serum hCG, CBC with differential and platelets, liver function tests, serum creatinine. Serum hCG concentrations should decrease between treatment days 4 and 7. If hCG decreases by >15%, additional courses are not needed however, continue to measure hCG weekly until no longer detectable. If <15% decrease is observed, repeat dose per regimen.

Reference Range Therapeutic levels: Variable; Toxic concentration: Variable; therapeutic range is dependent upon therapeutic approach.

High-dose regimens produce drug levels that are between 0.1 to 1 micromole/L 24 to 72 hours after drug infusion

Toxic: Low-dose therapy: >0.2 micromole/L; high-dose therapy: >1 micromole/L

Additional Information Oncology Comment:

Glucarpidase: Methotrexate overexposure: The rescue agent, glucarpidase, is an enzyme which rapidly hydrolyzes extracellular methotrexate into inactive metabolites, resulting in a rapid reduction of methotrexate concentrations. Glucarpidase is approved for the treatment of toxic plasma methotrexate concentrations (>1 micromole/L) in patients with delayed clearance due to renal impairment. Glucarpidase has also been administered intrathecally (off-label use/route) for inadvertent intrathecal methotrexate overexposure. Refer to Glucarpidase monograph.

Dosage Forms

Solution, Injection:

Generic: 25 mg/mL (2 mL, 10 mL)

Solution, Injection [preservative free]:

Generic: 25 mg/mL (2 mL, 4 mL, 8 mL, 10 mL, 40 mL); 50 mg/2 mL (2 mL); 100 mg/4 mL (4 mL); 250 mg/10 mL (10 mL); 1 g/40 mL (40 mL)

Solution Auto-injector, Subcutaneous [preservative free]:

Otrexup: 10 mg/0.4 mL (0.4 mL); 15 mg/0.4 mL (0.4 mL); 20 mg/0.4 mL (0.4 mL); 25 mg/0.4 mL (0.4 mL)

Rasuvo: 7.5 mg/0.15 mL (0.15 mL); 10 mg/0.2 mL (0.2 mL); 12.5 mg/0.25 mL (0.25 mL); 15 mg/0.3 mL (0.3 mL); 17.5 mg/0.35 mL (0.35 mL); 20 mg/0.4 mL (0.4 mL); 22.5 mg/0.45 mL (0.45 mL); 25 mg/0.5 mL (0.5 mL); 27.5 mg/0.55 mL (0.55 mL); 30 mg/0.6 mL (0.6 mL)

Solution Reconstituted, Injection [preservative free]:

Generic: 1 g (1 ea)

Tablet, Oral:

Rheumatrex: 2.5 mg

Trexall: 5 mg, 7.5 mg, 10 mg, 15 mg

Generic: 2.5 mg

◆ **Methotrexate Injection, BP (Can)** *see* Methotrexate *on page 1322*

◆ **Methotrexate Injection USP (Can)** *see* Methotrexate *on page 1322*

◆ **Methotrexate Sodium** *see* Methotrexate *on page 1322*

◆ **Methotrexate Sodium Injection (Can)** *see* Methotrexate *on page 1322*

◆ **Methotrexatum** *see* Methotrexate *on page 1322*

Methotrimeprazine [CAN/INT]

(meth oh trye MEP ra zeen)

Brand Names: Canada Apo-Methoprazine; Novo-Meprazine; Nozinan; PMS-Methotrimeprazine

Index Terms Levomepromazine; Methotrimeprazine Hydrochloride

Pharmacologic Category Analgesic, Nonopioid; Antimanic Agent; First Generation (Typical) Antipsychotic

Use Note: Not approved in U.S.

Treatment of schizophrenia; psychosis; manic-depressive syndromes; anxiety or tension disorders; management of pain, including pain caused by neuralgia or cancer; adjunct to general anesthesia; management of nausea and vomiting; sedation

Pregnancy Considerations Antipsychotic use during the third trimester of pregnancy has a risk for abnormal muscle movements (extrapyramidal symptoms [EPS]) and withdrawal symptoms in newborns following delivery. Symptoms in the newborn may include agitation, feeding disorder, hypertonia, hypotonia, respiratory distress, somnolence, and tremor; these effects may be self-limiting or require hospitalization.

Contraindications Hypersensitivity to methotrimeprazine, phenothiazines, or any component of the formulation; hepatic disease; hematologic disorders (blood dyscrasia); coma or CNS depression due to ethanol, hypnotics, analgesics, or opioids

Warnings/Precautions Not approved for the treatment of dementia or dementia-related psychosis in elderly patients. May be sedating; use with caution in disorders where CNS depression is a feature. May impair physical or mental abilities; patients must cautioned about performing tasks which require mental alertness (eg, operating machinery or driving). Effects with other sedative drugs or ethanol may be potentiated. Use in hepatic disease is contraindicated. Use with caution in Parkinson's disease; hemodynamic instability; bone marrow suppression; predisposition to seizures; and in cardiac, renal, or respiratory disease. Caution in breast cancer or other prolactin-dependent tumors (may elevate prolactin levels). May alter temperature regulation or mask toxicity of other drugs due to antiemetic effects. May alter cardiac conduction; life-threatening arrhythmias have occurred with therapeutic doses of phenothiazines. May cause orthostatic hypotension; use with caution in patients at risk of hypotension or where transient hypotensive episodes would be poorly tolerated (cardiovascular disease or cerebrovascular disease). Hypotension may occur following administration, particularly when parenteral form is used or in high dosages.

Phenothiazines may cause anticholinergic effects (constipation, xerostomia, blurred vision, urinary retention); therefore, they should be used with caution in patients with decreased gastrointestinal motility, urinary retention, BPH, xerostomia, or visual problems. Conditions which also may be exacerbated by cholinergic blockade include narrow-angle glaucoma (screening is recommended) and worsening of myasthenia gravis. May cause extrapyramidal symptoms and/or tardive dyskinesia. May be associated with neuroleptic malignant syndrome (NMS). Priapism has been reported rarely with use.

Adverse Reactions Note: Some reactions listed are based on reports for other agents in this same pharmacologic class, and may not be specifically reported for methotrimeprazine.

Cardiovascular: Orthostatic hypotension, QTc prolongation (rare), tachycardia, venous thromboembolism

Central nervous system: Dizziness, drowsiness; extrapyramidal symptoms (akathisia, dystonias, pseudoparkinsonism, tardive dyskinesia); headache, impairment of temperature regulation, neuroleptic malignant syndrome (NMS), seizure

Dermatologic: Photosensitivity (rare), rash

Endocrine & metabolic: Gynecomastia, hyperglycemia or glucose intolerance, libido changes, menstrual irregularity

Gastrointestinal: Constipation, ileus, nausea, necrotizing enterocolitis, vomiting, weight gain, xerostomia

Genitourinary: Ejaculatory disturbances or dysfunction, incontinence, polyuria, priapism, urinary retention

Hematologic: Agranulocytosis (rare), eosinophilia, hemolytic anemia, leukopenia, pancytopenia, thrombocytopenic purpura
Hepatic: Cholestatic jaundice, hepatotoxicity
Respiratory: Pulmonary embolus
Miscellaneous: Diaphoresis

Drug Interactions

Metabolism/Transport Effects Inhibits CYP2D6 (strong)

Avoid Concomitant Use

Avoid concomitant use of Methotrimeprazine with any of the following: Aclidinium; Amisulpride; Azelastine (Nasal); Glucagon; Ipratropium (Oral Inhalation); Metoclopramide; Orphenadrine; Paraldehyde; Pimozide; Potassium Chloride; Sulpiride; Tamoxifen; Thalidomide; Thioridazine; Tiotropium; Umeclidinium

Increased Effect/Toxicity

Methotrimeprazine may increase the levels/effects of: AbobotulinumtoxinA; Alcohol (Ethyl); Amisulpride; Anticholinergic Agents; Antidepressants (Serotonin Reuptake Inhibitor/Antagonist); ARIPiprazole; AtoMOXetine; Azelastine (Nasal); Beta-Blockers; Buprenorphine; CNS Depressants; CYP2D6 Substrates; DOXOrubicin (Conventional); Eliglustat; Fesoterodine; Glucagon; Highest Risk QTc-Prolonging Agents; Hydrocodone; Iloperidone; Methylphenidate; Metoprolol; Metyrosine; Mirabegron; Moderate Risk QTc-Prolonging Agents; Nebivolol; OnabotulinumtoxinA; Orphenadrine; Paraldehyde; Pimozide; Porfimer; Potassium Chloride; Propafenone; RimabotulinumtoxinB; Selective Serotonin Reuptake Inhibitors; Serotonin Modulators; Sulpiride; Suvorexant; Tetrabenazine; Thalidomide; Thiazide Diuretics; Thioridazine; Tiotropium; Verteporfin; Vortioxetine; Zolpidem

The levels/effects of Methotrimeprazine may be increased by: Acetylcholinesterase Inhibitors (Central); Aclidinium; Antidepressants (Serotonin Reuptake Inhibitor/Antagonist); Antimalarial Agents; Beta-Blockers; Brimonidine (Topical); Cannabis; CNS Depressants; Dronabinol; Droperidol; Ipratropium (Oral Inhalation); Kava Kava; Lithium; Magnesium Sulfate; MAO Inhibitors; Methylphenidate; Metoclopramide; Metyrosine; Mifepristone; Nabilone; Perampanel; Pramlintide; Rufinamide; Serotonin Modulators; Sodium Oxybate; Tapentadol; Tetrahydrocannabinol; Umeclidinium

Decreased Effect

Methotrimeprazine may decrease the levels/effects of: Acetylcholinesterase Inhibitors; Amphetamines; Anti-Parkinson's Agents (Dopamine Agonist); Codeine; Iloperidone; Itopride; Quinagolide; Secretin; Tamoxifen

The levels/effects of Methotrimeprazine may be decreased by: Acetylcholinesterase Inhibitors; Antacids; Anti-Parkinson's Agents (Dopamine Agonist); Lithium

Storage/Stability

Injection solution: Store at 15°C to 30°C (59°F to 86°F). Protect from light. Methotrimeprazine diluted to 0.13-6.25 mg/mL with 0.9% sodium chloride in a polypropylene syringe has been shown to be stable for ≤14 days at room temperature (Hardy, 2011).

Tablet: Store at 15°C to 30°C (59°F to 86°F). Protect from light.

Mechanism of Action Aliphatic phenothiazine that antagonizes D1 and D2 dopamine receptor subtypes; also binds alpha-1, alpha-2, serotonin (5-HT_1 and 5-HT_2), and muscarinic (M_1 and M_2) receptors

Pharmacodynamics/Kinetics

Onset of action: Injection: 1 hour
Duration: 2-4 hours
Distribution: V_d: 23-42 L/kg
Bioavailability: 50%
Time to peak, serum: IM: 0.5-1.5 hours; Oral: 1-3 hours
Half-life elimination: 15-30 hours
Excretion: Urine; feces

Dosage Note: Patients receiving parenteral therapy should be switched to oral therapy as soon as possible. If pronounced sedation occurs, administer smaller doses during the day and higher doses at night.

Children:

Oral: 0.25 mg/kg/day in 2-3 divided doses; may increase gradually based on response

Children <12 years: Maximum dose: 40 mg/day

IM: 0.063-0.125 mg/kg/day in 1-3 divided doses

IV: Intraoperative: 0.063 mg/kg in 250 mL D_5W infused slowly at a rate of 20-40 drops/minute

Adults:

Oral:

Anxiety, mild-moderate pain: Initial: 6-25 mg/day in 3 divided doses; titrate to effect

Psychoses, severe pain: Initial: 50-75 mg/day in 2-3 divided doses; titrate to effect (doses up to 1000 mg/day or greater have been used in treatment of some patients with psychoses). If higher dosages are used to initiate therapy (100-200 mg/day), patients should be restricted to bed for the first few days of therapy.

Sedative: 10-25 mg at bedtime

IM:

Psychoses, severe pain: 75-100 mg (administered in 3-4 deep IM injections)

Analgesia:

Preoperative: 10-25 mg every 8 hours (final preoperative dose may be 25-50 mg administered ~1 hour prior to surgery)

Postoperative: 10-25 mg every 8 hours

IV: Intraoperative/labor: 10-25 mg in 500 mL D_5W infused slowly at a rate of 20-40 drops/minute

SubQ (off-label route): Palliative care:

Continuous infusion: 6.25-250 mg/day (via syringe driver) (Adam, 1997)

Bolus administration: Median dose: 6.25 mg/day (range: 3.12-25 mg/day) administered as 1-2 divided doses (Eisenchlas, 2005)

Dosage adjustment in renal impairment: No dosage adjustment provided in manufacturer's labeling; use with caution.

Dosage adjustment in hepatic impairment: Contraindicated in patients with hepatic disease.

Administration Administer tablet orally with meals. Injection may be administered parenterally by slow IV infusion or deep IM injection; or subcutaneously (off-label route) as bolus injection (Eisenchlas, 2005) or as continuous infusion over 24 hours (Adam, 1997). For intermittent dosing, may administer smaller doses during day and higher doses at night if pronounced sedation occurs.

Monitoring Parameters Liver function tests (baseline and periodically thereafter); CBC (baseline, during the first 2-3 months of therapy, and regularly thereafter); blood pressure; plasma glucose (patients with or at risk of diabetes); abnormal involuntary movement scale (AIMS); extrapyramidal symptoms (EPS)

Product Availability Not available in U.S.

Dosage Forms: Canada

Injection, solution:

Nozinan®: 25 mg/mL (1 mL)

Tablet, oral: 2 mg, 5 mg, 25 mg, 50 mg

◆ **Methotrimeprazine Hydrochloride** *see* Methotrimeprazine [CAN/INT] *on page 1329*

Methoxsalen (Systemic) (meth OKS a len)

Brand Names: U.S. 8-Mop; Oxsoralen Ultra; Uvadex

Brand Names: Canada Uvadex

Index Terms 8-Methoxypsoralen; 8-MOP; Methoxypsoralen

Pharmacologic Category Psoralen

Use

Oral: Symptomatic control of severe, recalcitrant disabling psoriasis; repigmentation of idiopathic vitiligo; palliative treatment of skin manifestations of cutaneous T-cell lymphoma (CTCL)

Extracorporeal: Palliative treatment of skin manifestations of CTCL that is unresponsive to other forms of treatment

Pregnancy Risk Factor C/D (Uvadex)

Dosage Adults: **Note:** Refer to treatment protocols for UVA exposure guidelines.

Psoriasis: Oral:

Initial: 10 to 70 mg 1.5 to 2 hours (Oxsoralen Ultra) or 2 hours (8-MOP) before exposure to UVA light; dose may be repeated 2 to 3 times per week, based on UVA exposure; doses must be given at least 48 hours apart. Dosage is based upon patient's body weight and skin type:

<30 kg: 10 mg
30 to 50 kg: 20 mg
51 to 65 kg: 30 mg
66 to 80 kg: 40 mg
81 to 90 kg: 50 mg
91 to 115 kg: 60 mg
>115 kg: 70 mg

Note: Dosage may be increased (one time) by 10 mg after 15th treatment if minimal or no response.

Maintenance: When 95% psoriasis clearing achieved, may begin 1 treatment every week for at least 2 treatments; followed by 1 treatment every 2 weeks for at least 2 treatments; then every 3 weeks for at least 2 treatments then as needed to maintain response while minimizing UVA exposure.

Vitiligo: Oral (8-MOP): 20 mg 2 to 4 hours before exposure to UVA light; dose may be repeated based on erythema and tenderness of skin; do not give on 2 consecutive days

Cutaneous T-cell lymphoma (CTCL): Extracorporeal (Uvadex): Dose is determined by treatment volume; amount of Uvadex needed for each treatment may be calculated using the following equation: Treatment volume x 0.017 = mL of Uvadex needed. Inject this amount into the recirculation bag prior to the photoactivation phase using the UVAR XTS or CELLEX photopheresis system (consult user's guide).

Treatment schedule: Two consecutive days every 4 weeks for a minimum of 7 treatment cycles, may accelerate to 2 consecutive days every 2 weeks if skin score worsens (eg, increases from baseline) after assessment during the fourth treatment cycle. If skin score improves by 25% after 4 consecutive weeks of accelerated therapy, may resume regular treatment schedule. Patients maintained on accelerated therapy may receive a maximum of 20 accelerated therapy cycles. There is no clinical evidence to show that treatment with methoxsalen for more than 6 months or using a different schedule provides additional benefit.

Dosage adjustment in renal impairment: There are no dosage adjustments provided in manufacturer's labeling.

Dosage adjustment in hepatic impairment: There are no dosage adjustments provided in manufacturer's labeling; use with caution.

Additional Information Complete prescribing information should be consulted for additional detail.

Dosage Forms

Capsule, Oral:

8-Mop: 10 mg
Oxsoralen Ultra: 10 mg
Generic: 10 mg

Solution, Injection:

Uvadex: 20 mcg/mL (10 mL)

Methoxsalen (Topical) (meth OKS a len)

Brand Names: U.S. Oxsoralen

Index Terms Methoxypsoralen

Pharmacologic Category Psoralen

Use Repigmentation of idiopathic vitiligo

Pregnancy Risk Factor C

Dosage Topical: **Note:** Refer to treatment protocols for UVA exposure guidelines.

Children ≥12 years and Adults: Vitiligo: Lotion is applied by healthcare provider prior to UVA light exposure, usually no more than once weekly; frequency is determined by erythema response

Additional Information Complete prescribing information should be consulted for additional detail.

Dosage Forms

Lotion, External:

Oxsoralen: 1% (29.57 mL)

◆ **Methoxypsoralen** *see* Methoxsalen (Systemic) *on page 1330*

◆ **Methoxypsoralen** *see* Methoxsalen (Topical) *on page 1331*

◆ **8-Methoxypsoralen** *see* Methoxsalen (Systemic) *on page 1330*

Methsuximide (meth SUKS i mide)

Brand Names: U.S. Celontin

Brand Names: Canada Celontin®

Pharmacologic Category Anticonvulsant, Succinimide

Use Control of absence (petit mal) seizures that are refractory to other drugs

Dosage Oral: Adults: Anticonvulsant: 300 mg/day for the first week; may increase by 300 mg/day at weekly intervals up to 1.2 g/day in 2-4 divided doses/day

Dosage adjustment in renal impairment: No dosage adjustment provided in manufacturer's labeling; use with caution.

Dosage adjustment in hepatic impairment: No dosage adjustment provided in manufacturer's labeling; use with caution.

Additional Information Complete prescribing information should be consulted for additional detail.

Dosage Forms

Capsule, Oral:

Celontin: 300 mg

Methyclothiazide (meth i kloe THYE a zide)

Index Terms Enduron

Pharmacologic Category Antihypertensive; Diuretic, Thiazide

Use Management of hypertension; adjunctive therapy of edema

The 2014 guideline for the management of high blood pressure in adults (Eighth Joint National Committee [JNC 8]) recommends initiation of pharmacologic treatment to lower blood pressure for the following patients:

- Patients ≥60 years of age with systolic blood pressure (SBP) ≥150 mm Hg or diastolic blood pressure (DBP) ≥90 mm Hg. Goal of therapy is SBP <150 mm Hg and DBP <90 mm Hg.
- Patients <60 years of age with SBP ≥140 mm Hg or DBP is ≥90 mm Hg. Goal of therapy is SBP <140 mm Hg and DBP <90 mm Hg.
- Patients ≥18 years of age with diabetes and SBP ≥140 mm Hg or DBP ≥90 mm Hg. Goal of therapy is SBP <140 mm Hg and DBP <90 mm Hg.

- Patients ≥18 years of age with chronic kidney disease (CKD) and SBP ≥140 mm Hg or DBP ≥90 mm Hg. Goal of therapy is SBP <140 mm Hg and DBP <90 mm Hg.

In patients with CKD, regardless of race or diabetes status, the use of an ACE inhibitor (ACEI) or angiotensin receptor blocker (ARB) as initial therapy is recommended to improve kidney outcomes. In the general nonblack population (without CKD) including those with diabetes, initial antihypertensive treatment should consist of a thiazide-type diuretic, calcium channel blocker, ACEI, or ARB. In the general black population (without CKD), including those with diabetes, initial antihypertensive treatment should consist of a thiazide-type diuretic or a calcium channel blocker **instead of** an ACEI or ARB.

Pregnancy Risk Factor B

Dosage Adults: Oral:

Edema: 2.5 to 10 mg daily

Hypertension: 2.5 to 5 mg daily; may add another antihypertensive if 5 mg is not adequate after a trial of 8 to 12 weeks of therapy

Dosage adjustment in renal impairment: There are no dosage adjustments provided in manufacturer's labeling. However, thiazides are usually ineffective with CrCl <30 mL/minute; use with caution.

Dosage adjustment in hepatic impairment: There are no dosage adjustments provided in manufacturer's labeling; use with caution.

Additional Information Complete prescribing information should be consulted for additional detail.

Dosage Forms

Tablet, Oral:

Generic: 5 mg

◆ **Methylacetoxyprogesterone** *see* MedroxyPROGESTERone *on page 1277*

Methyl Aminolevulinate

(METH il a mee noe LEV ue lin ate)

Brand Names: U.S. Metvixia

Brand Names: Canada Metvix

Index Terms Methyl Aminolevulinate Hydrochloride; P-1202

Pharmacologic Category Photosensitizing Agent, Topical; Topical Skin Product

Use

Actinic keratosis: Treatment of thin and moderately thick, nonhyperkeratotic, nonpigmented actinic keratoses of the face and scalp in immunocompetent patients (photodynamic therapy [PDT] to be used in conjunction with red light illumination).

Limitations of use: Safety and efficacy have not been established for treatment of cutaneous malignancies or for skin lesions other than nonhyperkeratotic face and scalp actinic keratoses using PDT with methyl aminolevulinate cream; safety and efficacy of methyl aminolevulinate cream have not been established in patients with immunosuppression, porphyria, or pigmented actinic keratosis; has not been tested on patients with inherited or acquired coagulation defects; use without subsequent red light illumination is not recommended.

Pregnancy Risk Factor C

Dosage Actinic keratoses: Adults: Topical: Apply up to 1 g to prepared actinic keratoses, occlude for 3 hours, followed by red light illumination; repeat in 1 week. **Note:** If multiple lesions being treated, 1 g should not be exceeded for all lesions combined per treatment session.

Additional Information Complete prescribing information should be consulted for additional detail.

Dosage Forms

Cream, External:

Metvixia: 16.8% (2 g)

◆ **Methyl Aminolevulinate Hydrochloride** *see* Methyl Aminolevulinate *on page 1332*

◆ **Methylcobalamin, Acetylcysteine, and Methylfolate** *see* Methylfolate, Methylcobalamin, and Acetylcysteine *on page 1334*

◆ **Methyl Cysteine** *see* Mecysteine [INT] *on page 1277*

Methyldopa (meth il DOE pa)

Brand Names: Canada Methyldopa; Novo-Medopa

Index Terms Aldomet; Methyldopate Hydrochloride

Pharmacologic Category $Alpha_2$-Adrenergic Agonist; Antihypertensive

Additional Appendix Information

Beers Criteria – Potentially Inappropriate Medications for Geriatrics *on page 2271*

Use

Hypertension: Management of moderate to severe hypertension

Note: According to the Eighth Joint National Committee (JNC 8) guidelines, methyldopa is **not** recommended for the initial treatment of hypertension (James, 2013).

Pregnancy Risk Factor B/C (injectable)

Dosage

Hypertension:

Children:

Oral: Initial: 10 mg/kg/day in 2 to 4 divided doses; increase every 2 days as needed to maximum dose of 65 mg/kg/day; do not exceed 3 g daily.

IV: 5-10 mg/kg/dose every 6 to 8 hours up to a total maximum daily dose of 65 mg/kg/day or 3 g daily

Adults:

Oral: Initial: 250 mg 2 to 3 times daily; increase every 2 days as needed (maximum dose: 3 g daily); usual dose range (ASH/ISH [Weber, 2014]): 250 to 500 mg twice daily. **Note:** When administered with other antihypertensives other than thiazide diuretics, limit initial daily dose of methyldopa to 500 mg daily.

IV: 250 to 500 mg every 6 to 8 hours; maximum dose: 1 g every 6 hours

Elderly: Initiate at the lower end of the dosage range.

Dosage adjustment in renal impairment:

There are no dosage adjustments provided in manufacturer's labeling; however, the following adjustments have been recommended (Aronoff, 2007):

CrCl >50 mL/minute: Administer every 8 hours.

CrCl 10 to 50 mL/minute: Administer every 8 to 12 hours.

CrCl <10 mL/minute: Administer every 12 to 24 hours.

Intermittent hemodialysis (administer after hemodialysis on dialysis days): Moderately dialyzable (up to 60% with a 6-hour session) (Yeh, 1970).

Peritoneal dialysis (PD): Administer every 12 to 24 hours.

Continuous renal replacement therapy (CRRT): Administer every 8 to 12 hours. **Note:** Use of antihypertensives in patients requiring CRRT is generally not recommended since CRRT is typically employed when patient cannot tolerate intermittent hemodialysis due to hypotension.

Dosage adjustment in hepatic impairment: Use is contraindicated in patients with active hepatic disease.

Additional Information Complete prescribing information should be consulted for additional detail.

Dosage Forms

Solution, Intravenous:

Generic: 250 mg/5 mL (5 mL)

Tablet, Oral:

Generic: 250 mg, 500 mg

Dosage Forms: Canada Note: Also refer to Dosage Forms. Intravenous solution is not available in Canada.

Tablet, Oral: 125 mg

◆ **Methyldopate Hydrochloride** *see* Methyldopa *on page 1332*

Methylene Blue (METH i leen bloo)

Index Terms Methylthionine Chloride; Methylthioninium Chloride

Pharmacologic Category Antidote

Use Methemoglobinemia: Treatment of drug-induced methemoglobinemia

Pregnancy Risk Factor X

Dosage

Children, Adolescents, and Adults: Methemoglobinemia: IV: 1 to 2 mg/kg or 25 to 50 mg/m^2 over 5 to 10 minutes; may be repeated in 1 hour if necessary

Adults:

Chromoendoscopy (off-label use): Topical: 0.1% to 1% solution sprayed via catheter or directly applied onto gastrointestinal mucosa during procedure (Areia 2008; Ichimasa 2014; Kaminski 2014; Ngamruengphong 2009)

Ifosfamide-induced encephalopathy (off-label use): **Note:** Treatment may not be necessary; encephalopathy may improve spontaneously (Patel 2006): Oral, IV:

Prevention: 50 mg every 6 to 8 hours (Turner 2003)

Treatment: 50 mg as a single dose or every 4 to 8 hours until symptoms resolve (Patel 2006; Turner 2003)

Onychomycosis (toenail; off-label use): Topical: 2% solution applied to lesions at 15 day intervals for 6 months; used in conjunction with photodynamic therapy (Figueiredo Souza 2014)

Sentinel node mapping in breast cancer surgery (off-label use): Intraparenchymal: 5 mg in 3 to 5 mL NS administered once during procedure (Simmons 2001; Simmons 2003; Thevarajah 2005)

Vasoplegia syndrome associated with cardiac surgery (off-label use): IV: 1.5 to 2 mg/kg over 20 to 60 minutes administered once (Levin 2004; Leyh 2003). **Note:** Improvement of vasoplegia (eg, increased systemic vascular resistance, reduced vasopressor dosage) has been observed within 1 to 2 hours following methylene blue administration. Some have employed the use of continuous infusion (0.5 to 1 mg/kg/hour) after administration of the bolus dose; however, prospective clinical trials are necessary to validate this dosing schema (Grayling 2003; Omar 2014; Weiner 2013).

Dosage adjustment in renal impairment: There are no dosage adjustments provided in the manufacturer's labeling. However, use with caution in severe renal impairment.

Dosage adjustment in hepatic impairment: There are no dosage adjustments provided in the manufacturer's labeling.

Additional Information Complete prescribing information should be consulted for additional detail.

Dosage Forms

Solution, Injection:

Generic: 1% (1 mL, 10 mL)

◆ **Methylene Blue, Methenamine, Benzoic Acid, Phenyl Salicylate, and Hyoscyamine** *see* Methenamine, Phenyl Salicylate, Methylene Blue, Benzoic Acid, and Hyoscyamine *on page 1318*

◆ **Methylene Blue, Methenamine, Sodium Phosphate Monobasic, Phenyl Salicylate, and Hyoscyamine** *see* Methenamine, Sodium Phosphate Monobasic, Phenyl Salicylate, Methylene Blue, and Hyoscyamine *on page 1318*

◆ **Methylergometrine Maleate** *see* Methylergonovine *on page 1333*

Methylergonovine (meth il er goe NOE veen)

Brand Names: Canada Methergine®

Index Terms Methylergometrine Maleate; Methylergonovine Maleate

Pharmacologic Category Ergot Derivative

Use Management of uterine atony, hemorrhage and subinvolution of the uterus following delivery of the placenta; control of uterine hemorrhage following delivery of the anterior shoulder in the second stage of labor

Pregnancy Risk Factor C

Pregnancy Considerations Animal reproduction studies have not been conducted. Methylergonovine is intended for use after delivery of the infant; use is contraindicated during pregnancy.

Breast-Feeding Considerations At normal doses used to control postpartum uterine bleeding, small amounts are excreted in breast milk. In one study, ten women were given a single dose of methylergonovine 0.5 mg once lactation was established. Simultaneous maternal milk and plasma samples were taken 1 and 2 hours later. Maximum milk concentrations were 410-830 pg/mL, 2-3 hours after the dose and declined to 0.2 pg/mL (median) at 5 hours. The mean M/P ratios were 0.18 (at 1 hour) and 0.17 (at 2 hours) (Vogel, 2004). Methylergonovine may decrease breast milk production. Some manufacturers do not recommend breast-feeding during therapy or for 12 hours after the last dose due to adverse reactions reported in breast-feeding infants.

Contraindications Hypersensitivity to methylergonovine or any component of the formulation; hypertension; toxemia; pregnancy

Warnings/Precautions Hazardous agent - use appropriate precautions for handling and disposal (NIOSH 2014 [group 3]).

Use caution in patients with sepsis, obliterative vascular disease, cardiovascular disease, hepatic or renal involvement, or second stage of labor; administer with extreme caution if using intravenously. Patients with coronary artery disease (CAD) or risk factors for CAD may be more likely to develop myocardial ischemia and infarction following methylergonovine-induced vasospasm. Pleural and peritoneal fibrosis have been reported with prolonged daily use of other ergot alkaloids. Ergot alkaloid use may result in ergotism (intense vasoconstriction) resulting in peripheral vascular ischemia and possible gangrene. Concomitant use with potent inhibitors of CYP3A4 (includes protease inhibitors, azole antifungals, and some macrolide antibiotics) and ergot alkaloids has been associated with acute ergot toxicity (ergotism); concurrent use of certain ergot alkaloids (eg, ergotamine and dihydroergotamine) are not recommended by the manufacturer. Not for routine IV administration due to risk of inducing sudden hypertensive and cerebrovascular accidents. IV administration should only be considered during life-threatening situations. Inadvertent administration to newborns has been reported.

Adverse Reactions

Cardiovascular: Acute MI, angina pectoris, arterial spasm, atrioventricular block, bradycardia, cerebrovascular accident, chest pain, hyper-/hypotension, palpitation, tachycardia, vasospasm, ventricular fibrillation

Central nervous system: Dizziness, hallucinations, headache, seizure

Dermatologic: Rash

Endocrine & metabolic: Water intoxication

Gastrointestinal: Abdominal pain, diarrhea, foul taste, nausea, vomiting

Local: Thrombophlebitis

Neuromuscular & skeletal: Leg cramps, paresthesia

Otic: Tinnitus

Renal: Hematuria

Respiratory: Dyspnea, nasal congestion
Miscellaneous: Anaphylaxis, diaphoresis

Drug Interactions

Metabolism/Transport Effects Substrate of CYP3A4 (major); **Note:** Assignment of Major/Minor substrate status based on clinically relevant drug interaction potential

Avoid Concomitant Use

Avoid concomitant use of Methylergonovine with any of the following: Alpha-/Beta-Agonists; Alpha1-Agonists; Boceprevir; Cobicistat; Conivaptan; Dapoxetine; Fusidic Acid (Systemic); Idelalisib; Itraconazole; Ketoconazole (Systemic); Lorcaserin; Nitroglycerin; Posaconazole; Protease Inhibitors; Serotonin 5-HT1D Receptor Agonists; Telaprevir; Voriconazole

Increased Effect/Toxicity

Methylergonovine may increase the levels/effects of: Alpha-/Beta-Agonists; Alpha1-Agonists; Antipsychotic Agents; Metoclopramide; Serotonin 5-HT1D Receptor Agonists; Serotonin Modulators

The levels/effects of Methylergonovine may be increased by: Antiemetics (5HT3 Antagonists); Antipsychotic Agents; Aprepitant; Beta-Blockers; Boceprevir; Ceritinib; Cobicistat; Conivaptan; CYP3A4 Inhibitors (Moderate); CYP3A4 Inhibitors (Strong); Dapoxetine; Dasatinib; Fosaprepitant; Fusidic Acid (Systemic); Idelalisib; Itraconazole; Ivacaftor; Ketoconazole (Systemic); Lorcaserin; Luliconazole; Macrolide Antibiotics; Mifepristone; Netupitant; Nitroglycerin; Posaconazole; Protease Inhibitors; Serotonin 5-HT1D Receptor Agonists; Simeprevir; Stiripentol; Tedizolid; Telaprevir; Voriconazole

Decreased Effect

Methylergonovine may decrease the levels/effects of: Nitroglycerin

Storage/Stability

Injection: Store under refrigeration at 2°C to 8°C (36°F to 46°F). Protect from light. The following stability information has also been reported: May be stored at room temperature for up to 14 days (Cohen, 2007).

Tablet: Store below 25°C (77°F).

Mechanism of Action Increases the tone, rate and amplitude of contractions on the smooth muscles of the uterus, producing sustained contractions which shortens the third stage of labor and reduces blood loss.

Pharmacodynamics/Kinetics

Onset of action: Oxytocic: Oral: 5-10 minutes; IM: 2-5 minutes; IV: Immediately
Duration: Oral: ~3 hours; IM: ~3 hours; IV: 45 minutes
Absorption: Rapid
Distribution: V_d: 39-73 L
Metabolism: Hepatic
Bioavailability: Oral: 60%; IM: 78%
Half-life elimination: ~3 hours (range: 1.5-12.7 hours)
Time to peak, serum: Oral: 0.3-2 hours; IM: 0.2-0.6 hours
Excretion: Urine and feces

Dosage Adults:

Oral: 0.2 mg 3-4 times daily in the puerperium for up to 7 days (maximum duration: 1 week)

IM, IV: 0.2 mg after delivery of anterior shoulder, after delivery of placenta, or during puerperium; may be repeated every 2-4 hours as needed. **Note:** IV administration should only be considered during life-threatening situations.

Dosage adjustment in renal impairment: No dosage adjustment provided in manufacturer's labeling; use with caution.

Dosage adjustment in hepatic impairment: No dosage adjustment provided in manufacturer's labeling; use with caution.

Administration

IV: Administer over ≥60 seconds. Should not be routinely administered IV because of possibility of inducing sudden hypertension and cerebrovascular accident. IV administration should only be considered during life-threatening situations.

IM: May be administered intramuscularly.

Oral: Available in tablets for oral administration.

Hazardous agent; use appropriate precautions for handling and disposal (NIOSH 2014 [group 3]).

Monitoring Parameters Blood pressure

Dosage Forms

Solution, Injection:
Generic: 0.2 mg/mL (1 mL)

Solution, Injection [preservative free]:
Generic: 0.2 mg/mL (1 mL)

Tablet, Oral:
Generic: 0.2 mg

◆ **Methylergonovine Maleate** *see* Methylergonovine *on page 1333*

Methylfolate, Methylcobalamin, and Acetylcysteine

(meth il FO late meth il koe BAL a min & a se teel SIS teen)

Brand Names: U.S. Cerefolin® NAC; Metafolbic Plus; Metafolbic Plus RF

Index Terms Acetylcysteine, Methylcobalamin, and Methylfolate; Acetylcysteine, Methylfolate, and Methylcobalamin; L-methylfolate, Methylcobalamin, and N-acetylcysteine; Methylcobalamin, Acetylcysteine, and Methylfolate

Pharmacologic Category Dietary Supplement

Use Medicinal food for use in patients with neurovascular oxidative stress and/or hyperhomocysteinemia

Dosage Oral: Children ≥12 years and Adults: One tablet daily

Additional Information Complete prescribing information should be consulted for additional detail.

Dosage Forms

Tablet, oral:

Cerefolin® NAC: L-methylfolate 6 mg, methylcobalamin 2 mg, N-acetylcysteine 600 mg, and Schizochytrium algae [contains soy; gluten free, lactose free, yeast free]

Metafolbic Plus: L-methylfolate 6 mg, methylcobalamin 2 mg, and N-acetylcysteine 600 mg [gluten free, lactose free, sugar free, yeast free]

Metafolbic Plus RF: L-methylfolate 6 mg, methylcobalamin 2 mg, N-acetylcysteine 600 mg, and Schizochytrium algae [contains soy; gluten free, yeast free]

◆ **Methylin** *see* Methylphenidate *on page 1336*
◆ **Methylmorphine** *see* Codeine *on page 497*

Methylnaltrexone (meth il nal TREKS one)

Brand Names: U.S. Relistor

Brand Names: Canada Relistor

Index Terms Methylnaltrexone Bromide; N-methylnaltrexone Bromide

Pharmacologic Category Gastrointestinal Agent, Miscellaneous; Opioid Antagonist, Peripherally-Acting

Use

Opioid-induced constipation with advanced illness: Treatment of opioid-induced constipation in adult patients with advanced illness (receiving palliative care) who have an inadequate response to conventional laxative regimens.

Opioid-induced constipation with chronic non-cancer pain: Treatment of opioid-induced constipation in adult patients with chronic non-cancer pain.

Pregnancy Risk Factor C

Pregnancy Considerations Adverse effects were not observed in animal reproduction studies. Maternal use of methylnaltrexone during pregnancy may precipitate opioid withdrawal effects in newborn.

Breast-Feeding Considerations It is not known if methylnaltrexone is excreted in breast milk. Due to the potential for serious adverse reactions in the nursing infant, the manufacturer recommends a decision be made whether to discontinue nursing or to discontinue the drug, taking into account the importance of treatment to the mother.

Contraindications

Known or suspected gastrointestinal obstruction; patients at increased risk of recurrent obstruction due to the potential for gastrointestinal perforation.

Canadian labeling: Additional contraindications (not in U.S. labeling): Hypersensitivity to methylnaltrexone or any component of the formulation

Warnings/Precautions Discontinue treatment for severe or persistent diarrhea. Gastrointestinal perforations have been reported in patients with advanced illnesses associated with impaired structural integrity of the GI wall (eg, Ogilvie's syndrome, peptic ulcer disease, diverticular disease, infiltrative GI tract malignancies, or peritoneal metastases). Use with caution in these patients or in patients with other conditions that may result in impaired integrity of the GI wall (eg, Crohn disease); Monitor for development of severe, persistent or worsening abdominal pain; discontinue therapy if this occurs. Use is contraindicated in patients with known or suspected GI obstruction or at increased risk of recurrent obstruction. Use with caution in patients with renal impairment; dosage adjustment recommended for severe renal impairment (CrCl <30 mL/minute). Has not been studied in patients with end-stage renal impairment requiring dialysis. May precipitate symptoms of opioid withdrawal (eg, abdominal pain, anxiety, chills, diarrhea, hyperhidrosis, and yawning). Use with caution in patients with disruptions to the blood-brain barrier; may increase the risk for withdrawal and/or reduced analgesia. Monitor for symptoms of opioid withdrawal in such patients. Discontinue methylnaltrexone if opioids are discontinued. Use beyond 4 months has not been studied.

Appropriate use for patients with opioid-induced constipation with chronic non-cancer pain: Efficacy has been established in patients who have taken opioids for ≥4 weeks; sustained exposure to opioids prior to initiation of methylnaltrexone may increase sensitivity to effects. All laxative maintenance therapy should be discontinued prior to initiation of therapy; laxative therapy may be added if a suboptimal response to therapy is noted after 3 days. When the opioid regimen has been changed, the patient should be re-evaluated for the need to continue methylnaltrexone therapy.

Adverse Reactions

Central nervous system: Chills, dizziness

Dermatologic: Hyperhidrosis

Endocrine & metabolic: Hot flash

Gastrointestinal: Abdominal pain, diarrhea, flatulence, nausea

Neuromuscular & skeletal: Tremor

Rare but important or life-threatening: Abdominal cramps, gastrointestinal perforation, increased body temperature, muscle spasm, opioid withdrawal syndrome, piloerection, syncope

Drug Interactions

Metabolism/Transport Effects Substrate of CYP2D6 (minor); **Note:** Assignment of Major/Minor substrate status based on clinically relevant drug interaction potential

Avoid Concomitant Use

Avoid concomitant use of Methylnaltrexone with any of the following: Naloxegol; Opioid Antagonists

Increased Effect/Toxicity

Methylnaltrexone may increase the levels/effects of: Naloxegol; Opioid Antagonists

Decreased Effect There are no known significant interactions involving a decrease in effect.

Storage/Stability Store intact vials and prefilled syringes between 20°C and 25°C (68°F and 77°F); excursions are permitted between 15°C and 30°C (59°F and 86°F). Do not freeze. Protect from light. Solution withdrawn from the single use vial is stable in a syringe for 24 hours at room temperature. Do not remove the prefilled syringe from the tray until ready to administer.

Mechanism of Action An opioid receptor antagonist which blocks opioid binding at the mu receptor, methylnaltrexone is a quaternary derivative of naltrexone with restricted ability to cross the blood-brain barrier. It therefore functions as a peripheral acting opioid antagonist, including actions on the gastrointestinal tract to inhibit opioid-induced decreased gastrointestinal motility and delay in gastrointestinal transit time, thereby decreasing opioid-induced constipation. Does not affect opioid analgesic effects.

Pharmacodynamics/Kinetics

Onset of action: Usually within 30-60 minutes (in responding patients)

Absorption: SubQ: Rapid

Distribution: V_{dss}: ~1.1 L/kg

Protein binding: 11% to 15%

Metabolism: Metabolized to methyl-6-naltrexol isomers, methylnaltrexone sulfate, and other minor metabolites

Half-life elimination: Terminal: ~8 hours

Time to peak, plasma: SubQ: 30 minutes

Excretion: Urine (~54%, primarily as unchanged drug); feces (~17%, primarily as unchanged drug)

Dosage Adults: SubQ:

Opioid-induced constipation with chronic non-cancer pain: 12 mg once daily. **Note:** Discontinue all laxatives prior to use; if response is not optimal after 3 days, laxative therapy may be reinitiated.

Opioid-induced constipation with advanced illness: Dosing is according to body weight: Administer 1 dose every other day as needed; maximum: 1 dose/24 hours.

<38 kg: 0.15 mg/kg (round dose up to nearest 0.1 mL of volume)

38 to <62 kg: 8 mg

62 to 114 kg: 12 mg

>114 kg: 0.15 mg/kg (round dose up to nearest 0.1 mL of volume)

Dosage adjustment in renal impairment:

Mild-to-moderate impairment: No dosage adjustment necessary

Severe impairment (CrCl <30 mL/minute): Administer 50% of normal dose

End-stage renal impairment (dialysis-dependent): There are no dosage adjustments provided in the manufacturer's labeling (has not been studied)

Dosage adjustment in hepatic impairment:

Mild-to-moderate impairment (Child-Pugh class A or B): No dosage adjustment necessary

Severe impairment: There are no dosage adjustments provided in the manufacturer's labeling (has not been studied)

Administration Administer by subcutaneous injection into the upper arm, abdomen, or thigh. Rotate injection sites at each dose. Toilet facilities should be nearby immediately following administration. Discard any unused medication that remains in the vial.

Monitoring Parameters Severe, persistent, or worsening abdominal pain; symptoms of opioid withdrawal; adequate analgesia; signs or symptoms of orthostatic hypotension.

Additional Information In some clinical trials, patients who received methylnaltrexone were on a palliative opioid therapy equivalent to a mean daily oral morphine dose of 172 mg, at a stable dose for ≥3 days. Constipation was defined as <3 bowel movements/week or no bowel movement for >2 days. Patients maintained their regular laxative regimen for at least 3 days prior to treatment and throughout the study.

Dosage Forms

Kit, Subcutaneous:

Relistor: 12 mg/0.6 mL

Solution, Subcutaneous:

Relistor: 8 mg/0.4 mL (0.4 mL); 12 mg/0.6 mL (0.6 mL)

◆ **Methylnaltrexone Bromide** *see* Methylnaltrexone *on page 1334*

Methylphenidate (meth il FEN i date)

Brand Names: U.S. Concerta; Daytrana; Metadate CD; Metadate ER; Methylin; Quillivant XR; Ritalin; Ritalin LA; Ritalin SR [DSC]

Brand Names: Canada Apo-Methylphenidate; Apo-Methylphenidate SR; Biphentin; Concerta; PHL-Methylphenidate; PMS-Methylphenidate; ratio-Methylphenidate; Ritalin; Ritalin SR; Sandoz-Methylphenidate SR; Teva-Methylphenidate ER-C

Index Terms Methylphenidate Hydrochloride

Pharmacologic Category Central Nervous System Stimulant

Use

U.S. labeling: Treatment of attention-deficit/hyperactivity disorder (ADHD); symptomatic management of narcolepsy (except Concerta, Daytrana, Metadate CD, Ritalin LA, and Quillivant XR)

Canadian labeling: Treatment of attention-deficit/hyperactivity disorder (ADHD); symptomatic management of narcolepsy (except Biphentin, Concerta)

Pregnancy Risk Factor C

Pregnancy Considerations Adverse events were observed in animal reproduction studies. Information related to the use of methylphenidate in pregnant women with attention-deficit/hyperactivity disorder (Bolea-Akmanac, 2013; Dideriksen, 2013) or narcolepsy (Maurovich-Horvat, 2013; Thorpy, 2013) is limited.

Breast-Feeding Considerations Methylphenidate excretion into breast milk has been noted in case reports. In both cases, the authors calculated the relative infant dose to be ≤0.2% of the weight adjusted maternal dose. Adverse events were not noted in either infant, however, both were older (6 months of age and 11 months of age) and exposure was limited (Hackett, 2006; Spigset, 2007). The manufacturer recommends that caution be used if administered to a nursing woman.

Contraindications

U.S. labeling: Hypersensitivity to methylphenidate or any component of the formulation; marked anxiety, tension, and agitation; glaucoma; use during or within 14 days following MAO inhibitor therapy; family history or diagnosis of Tourette's syndrome or tics

Additional contraindications: Metadate CD and Metadate ER: Severe hypertension, heart failure, arrhythmia, hyperthyroidism, recent MI or angina; concomitant use of halogenated anesthetics

Canadian labeling: Hypersensitivity to methylphenidate or any component of the formulation; marked anxiety, tension, and agitation; glaucoma; use during or within 14 days following MAO inhibitor therapy; family history or diagnosis of Tourette's syndrome or tics, thyrotoxicosis, advanced arteriosclerosis, symptomatic cardiovascular disease, or moderate-to-severe hypertension

Additional contraindications: Ritalin and Ritalin SR: Pheochromocytoma

Warnings/Precautions CNS stimulant use has been associated with serious cardiovascular events (eg, sudden death in children and adolescents; sudden death, stroke, and MI in adults) in patients with preexisting structural cardiac abnormalities or other serious heart problems. These products should be avoided in patients with known serious structural cardiac abnormalities, cardiomyopathy, serious heart rhythm abnormalities, or other serious cardiac problems that could further increase their risk of sudden death. Patients should be carefully evaluated for cardiac disease prior to initiation of therapy. Use of stimulants can cause an increase in blood pressure (average 2 to 4 mm Hg) and increases in heart rate (average 3 to 6 bpm), although some patients may have larger than average increases. Use caution with hypertension, hyperthyroidism, or other cardiovascular conditions that might be exacerbated by increases in blood pressure or heart rate. Some products are contraindicated in patients with heart failure, arrhythmias, severe hypertension, hyperthyroidism, angina, or recent MI. Stimulants are associated with peripheral vasculopathy, including Raynaud's phenomenon; signs/symptoms are usually mild and intermittent, and generally improve with dose reduction or discontinuation. Digital ulceration and/or soft tissue breakdown have been observed rarely; monitor for digital changes during therapy and seek further evaluation (eg, rheumatology) if necessary. Prolonged and painful erections (priapism), sometimes requiring surgical intervention, have been reported (rarely) with methylphenidate and atomoxetine use in pediatric and adult patients. Priapism has been reported to develop after some time on the drug, often subsequent to an increase in dose but also during a period of drug withdrawal (drug holidays or discontinuation). Patients with certain hematological dyscrasias (eg, sickle cell disease), malignancies, perineal trauma, or concomitant use of alcohol, illicit drugs, or other medications associated with priapism may be at increased risk. Patients who develop abnormally sustained or frequent and painful erections should discontinue therapy and seek immediate medical attention. An emergent urological consultation should be obtained in severe cases. Priapism has been associated with different dosage forms and products; it is not known if rechallenge with a different formulation will risk recurrence. Avoidance of stimulants and atomoxetine may be preferred in patients with severe cases that were slow to resolve and/or required detumescence (Eiland, 2014).

Has demonstrated value as part of a comprehensive treatment program for ADHD. Use with caution in patients with bipolar disorder (may induce mixed/manic episode). May exacerbate symptoms of behavior and thought disorder in psychotic patients; new-onset psychosis or mania may occur with stimulant use. Patients should be screened for bipolar disorder prior to treatment; consider discontinuation if such symptoms (eg, delusional thinking, hallucinations, mania) occur. May be associated with aggressive behavior or hostility (causal relationship not established); monitor for development or worsening of these behaviors. Use caution with seizure disorders (may reduce seizure threshold). Use caution in patients with history of ethanol or drug abuse. May exacerbate symptoms of behavior and thought disorder in psychotic patients. **[U.S. Boxed Warning]: Potential for drug dependency exists - avoid abrupt discontinuation in patients who have received for prolonged periods.** Visual disturbances have been reported (rare). Not labeled for use in children <6 years of age. Use of stimulants has been associated with suppression of growth in children; monitor growth rate during treatment.

Concerta should not be used in patients with esophageal motility disorders or preexisting severe gastrointestinal narrowing (small bowel disease, short gut syndrome, history of peritonitis, cystic fibrosis, chronic intestinal pseudo-obstruction, Meckel's diverticulum). Concomitant use of Metadate CD and Metadate ER with halogenated anesthetics is contraindicated; may cause sudden elevations in blood pressure; if surgery is planned, do not administer Metadate CD or Metadate ER on the day of surgery. Transdermal system may cause allergic contact sensitization, characterized by intense local reactions (edema, papules) that may spread beyond the patch site; sensitization may subsequently manifest systemically with other routes of methylphenidate administration; monitor closely. Avoid exposure of application site to any direct external heat sources (eg, hair dryers, heating pads, electric blankets); may increase the rate and extent of absorption and risk of overdose. Efficacy of transdermal methylphenidate therapy for >7 weeks has not been established. Potentially significant drug-drug interactions may exist, requiring dose or frequency adjustment, additional monitoring, and/or selection of alternative therapy. Biphentin [Canadian product] controlled release capsules are not interchangeable with other controlled release formulations. Some dosage forms may contain lactose or sucrose; use with caution in patients intolerant to either component (some manufacturer labels recommend avoiding use in such patients).

Benzyl alcohol and derivatives: Some dosage forms may contain sodium benzoate/benzoic acid; benzoic acid (benzoate) is a metabolite of benzyl alcohol; large amounts of benzyl alcohol (≥99 mg/kg/day) have been associated with a potentially fatal toxicity ("gasping syndrome") in neonates; the "gasping syndrome" consists of metabolic acidosis, respiratory distress, gasping respirations, CNS dysfunction (including convulsions, intracranial hemorrhage), hypotension, and cardiovascular collapse (AAP, 1997; CDC, 1982); some data suggests that benzoate displaces bilirubin from protein binding sites (Ahlfors, 2001); avoid or use dosage forms containing benzyl alcohol derivative with caution in neonates. See manufacturer's labeling.

Adverse Reactions

All dosage forms:

Cardiovascular: Angina pectoris, cardiac arrhythmia, cerebrovascular accident, cerebrovascular occlusion, decreased pulse, heart murmur, hypertension, hypotension, increased pulse, myocardial infarction, necrotizing angiitis, palpitations, Raynaud's phenomenon, tachycardia, vasculitis

Central nervous system: Aggressive behavior, agitation, anxiety, cerebral arteritis, cerebral hemorrhage, confusion, depression, dizziness (more common in adults), drowsiness, emotional lability (more common in children), fatigue, Gilles de la Tourette's syndrome (rare), headache (more common in adults), hypertonia, hypervigilance, irritability, insomnia, lethargy, nervousness, neuroleptic malignant syndrome (NMS) (rare), outbursts of anger, paresthesia, restlessness, tension, toxic psychosis, vertigo, vocal tics (children)

Dermatologic: Alopecia, erythema multiforme, excoriation (children), exfoliative dermatitis, hyperhidrosis, skin rash (children), urticaria

Endocrine & metabolic: Decreased libido, growth suppression, weight loss

Gastrointestinal: Abdominal pain (children & adolescents), anorexia (more common in children & adolescents), bruxism, constipation, decreased appetite (more common in adults), diarrhea, dyspepsia, motion sickness (children), nausea, vomiting, xerostomia

Genitourinary: Dysmenorrhea, erectile dysfunction

Hematologic & oncologic: Anemia, immune thrombocytopenia, leukopenia, pancytopenia, thrombocytopenia

Hepatic: Abnormal hepatic function tests, hepatic coma, increased serum bilirubin, increased serum transaminases

Hypersensitivity: Hypersensitivity reaction

Neuromuscular & skeletal: Arthralgia, dyskinesia, tremor

Ophthalmic: Accommodation disturbance, blurred vision, dry eye syndrome, eye pain (children), mydriasis

Respiratory: Dyspnea, increased cough, pharyngitis, pharyngolaryngeal pain, rhinitis, sinusitis, upper respiratory tract infection

Miscellaneous: Accidental injury, fever (children & adolescents)

Rare but important or life-threatening: Bradycardia, disorientation, extrasystoles, hallucination, increased serum alkaline phosphatase, mania, migraine, obsessive-compulsive disorder, peripheral vascular insufficiency, priapism, seizure, supraventricular tachycardia, ventricular premature contractions

Transdermal system:

Central nervous system: Headache, insomnia, irritability

Gastrointestinal: Decreased appetite, nausea

Infection: Viral infection

Cardiovascular: Tachycardia

Central nervous system: Dizziness (adolescents), emotional lability, vocal tic

Endocrine & metabolic: Weight loss

Gastrointestinal: Abdominal pain, anorexia, vomiting

Local: Application site reaction

Respiratory: Nasal congestion, nasopharyngitis

Rare but important or life-threatening: Allergic contact dermatitis, allergic contact sensitivity, anaphylaxis, angioedema, hallucination, seizure

Drug Interactions

Metabolism/Transport Effects Inhibits CYP2D6 (weak)

Avoid Concomitant Use

Avoid concomitant use of Methylphenidate with any of the following: Alcohol (Ethyl); Inhalational Anesthetics; Iobenguane I 123; MAO Inhibitors

Increased Effect/Toxicity

Methylphenidate may increase the levels/effects of: Anti-Parkinson's Agents (Dopamine Agonist); Antipsychotic Agents; ARIPiprazole; CloNIDine; Fosphenytoin; Inhalational Anesthetics; PHENobarbital; Phenytoin; Primidone; Sympathomimetics; Tricyclic Antidepressants; Vitamin K Antagonists

The levels/effects of Methylphenidate may be increased by: Alcohol (Ethyl); Antacids; Antipsychotic Agents; AtoMOXetine; Cannabinoid-Containing Products; H2-Antagonists; MAO Inhibitors; Proton Pump Inhibitors

Decreased Effect

Methylphenidate may decrease the levels/effects of: Antihypertensives; Iobenguane I 123; Ioflupane I 123

Food Interactions

Ethanol: Alcohol consumption increases the rate of methylphenidate release from Metadate CD and Ritalin LA (extended-release capsules), but not from Concerta (extended-release tablet); an *in vitro* study involving Metadate CD and Ritalin LA showed that an alcohol concentration of 40% resulted in 84% and 98% of the methylphenidate being released in the first hour, respectively. Management: Avoid consuming alcohol during therapy.

Food: Food may increase oral absorption of immediate release tablet/solution and chewable tablet. Management: Administer 30-45 minutes before meals.

Preparation for Administration

Suspension: *Extended release (Quillivant XR):* Prior to dispensing, reconstitute with an appropriate amount of water (refer to bottle).

Storage/Stability

Capsule:

Extended release (Metadate CD, Ritalin LA): Store at 25°C (77°F); excursions permitted to 15°C to 30°C (59°F to 86°F). Protect from light.

Controlled release (Biphentin [Canadian product]): Store at 15°C to 30°C (59°F to 86°F).

Solution: *Immediate release (Methylin):* Store at 20°C to 25°C (68°F to 77°F).

Suspension: *Extended release (Quillivant XR):* Store at 25°C (77°F); excursions permitted to 15°C to 30°C (59°F to 86°F), before and after reconstitution. Reconstituted bottle must be used within 4 months.

Tablet:

Chewable (Methylin): Store at 20°C to 25°C (68°F to 77°F). Protect from light and moisture.

Extended release:

Metadate ER: Store at 20°C to 25°C (68°F to 77°F); excursions permitted to 15°C to 30°C (59°F to 86°F). Protect from light and moisture.

Concerta: Store at 25°C (77°F); excursions permitted to 15°C to 30°C (59°F to 86°F). Protect from humidity.

Immediate release (Ritalin): Store at 25°C (77°F); excursions permitted to 15°C to 30°C (59°F to 86°F). Protect from light and moisture.

Sustained release (Ritalin-SR): Store at 25°C (77°F); excursions permitted to 15°C to 30°C (59°F to 86°F). Protect from light and moisture.

Transdermal system: *Daytrana:* Store at 25°C (77°F); excursions permitted to 15°C to 30°C (59°F to 86°F). Keep patches stored in protective pouch. Once tray is opened, use patches within 2 months; once an individual patch has been removed from the pouch and the protective liner removed, use immediately. Do not refrigerate or freeze.

Mechanism of Action Mild CNS stimulant; blocks the reuptake of norepinephrine and dopamine into presynaptic neurons; appears to stimulate the cerebral cortex and subcortical structures similar to amphetamines

Pharmacodynamics/Kinetics

Onset of action: Peak effect:

Immediate release tablet: Cerebral stimulation: ~2 hours

Controlled release capsule: Biphentin [Canadian product]: Initial: within 1 hour

Extended release capsule: Metadate CD, Ritalin LA: Biphasic; initial peak similar to immediate release product, followed by second rising portion (corresponding to extended release portion)

Extended release tablet: Concerta: Initial: 1-2 hours

Sustained release tablet: Ritalin-SR: 4-7 hours

Transdermal: ~2 hours; may be expedited by the application of external heat

Duration: Immediate release tablet: 3-6 hours; Sustained release tablet: Ritalin-SR: 8 hours; Extended release tablet: Metadate ER: 8 hours, Concerta: 12 hours; Controlled release capsule: Biphentin [Canadian product]: ~10-12 hours

Absorption:

Oral: Readily absorbed

Chewable tablet: Methylin: A high-fat meal delayed peak time (~1 hour) and increased AUC (~20%).

Controlled release capsule: Biphentin [Canadian product]: Food delayed initial peak slightly (~18 minutes); relative to immediate release tablets, AUC is similar in fed or fasted state (~100%)

Extended release capsule:

Metadate CD: A high-fat meal delayed the early peak (~1 hour), and increased C_{max} (~30%) and AUC (~17%).

Ritalin LA: A high-fat meal delayed absorption and peak times, but not the amount absorbed nor initial peak concentration (second peak lowered by ~25%).

Extended release suspension: Quillivant XR: A high-fat meal led to an earlier peak (~1 hour), and increased C_{max} (~28%) and AUC (~19%).

Extended release tablet: Metadate ER: Food resulted in greater C_{max} and AUC compared to fasting.

Immediate release solution: Methylin: A high-fat meal delayed peak time (~1 hour), and increased C_{max} (~13%) and AUC (~25%).

Transdermal: Absorption increased when applied to inflamed skin or exposed to heat. Absorption is continuous for 9 hours after application.

Distribution: V_d: *d*-methylphenidate: 2.65 ± 1.11 L/kg, *l*-methylphenidate: 1.80 ± 0.91 L/kg

Protein binding: 10% to 33%

Metabolism: Extensive metabolism, predominately via de-esterification by carboxylesterase CES1A1 to alpha-phenyl-piperidine acetic acid (PPAA; ritalinic acid) which has little to no pharmacologic activity.

Bioavailability: Extended release suspension: Quillivant XR: 95% (relative to immediate release oral solution)

Half-life elimination: *d*-methylphenidate: 3-6 hours; *l*-methylphenidate: 1-3 hours

Time to peak: Biphentin [Canadian product]: ~2-3 hours; Concerta: C_{max}: 6-8 hours; Daytrana: 7.5-10.5 hours; Quillivant XR: ~4 hours

Excretion: Urine (90% as metabolites and unchanged drug)

Dosage

ADHD:

Oral, immediate release (IR) products (tablets, chewable tablets, and solution): Children ≥6 years, Adolescents, and Adults: Initial: 5 mg twice daily, before breakfast and lunch; increase by 5-10 mg daily at weekly intervals; maximum dose: 60 mg daily (in 2-3 divided doses).

Oral, extended release (ER), sustained release (SR) products (capsules, tablets, and oral suspension): Children ≥6 years and Adolescents <18 years: *Concerta:*

Patients not currently taking methylphenidate: Initial: 18 mg once daily in the morning

Patients currently taking immediate release (IR) methylphenidate: Initial: **Note:** Dosing based on current regimen and clinical judgment; suggested dosing listed below:

- Patients taking IR methylphenidate 5 mg 2-3 times daily **or** (Canadian labeling; not in U.S. labeling) methylphenidate SR 20 mg daily: 18 mg once every morning
- Patients taking IR methylphenidate 10 mg 2-3 times daily **or** (Canadian labeling; not in U.S. labeling) methylphenidate SR 40 mg daily: 36 mg once every morning
- Patients taking IR methylphenidate 15 mg 2-3 times daily **or** (Canadian labeling; not in U.S. labeling) methylphenidate SR 60 mg daily: 54 mg once every morning
- Patients taking IR methylphenidate 20 mg 2-3 times daily: 72 mg once every morning

Dose adjustment: May increase dose in increments of 18 mg at weekly intervals. A dosage strength of 27 mg is available for situations in which a dosage between 18-36 mg is desired.

Maximum dose:

U.S. labeling: 54 mg daily in children 6-12 years **or** 2 mg/kg/day (up to 72 mg daily) in adolescents <18 years

Canadian labeling: 54 mg daily in children and adolescents 6-18 years

Children ≥6 years, Adolescents, and Adults:

Biphentin [Canadian product]: Patients not currently taking methylphenidate: Initial: 10-20 mg once daily; may be adjusted in 10 mg increments at weekly intervals. Maximum: 60 mg daily (children ≥6 years, adolescents) or 80 mg daily (adults). **Note:** In some children >60 kg, a maximum dose of 1 mg/kg/daily (not to exceed 80 mg daily) may be necessary; however, close monitoring for adverse events is required. Reduce dose or discontinue if adverse events arise.

Conversion from immediate release methylphenidate formulations to Biphentin: Use equivalent total daily dose administered once daily.

Metadate ER, Ritalin-SR: May be given in place of immediate release products (duration of action ~8 hours), once the immediate release formulation daily dose is titrated and the titrated 8-hour dosage corresponds to sustained or extended release tablet size; maximum: 60 mg daily

Metadate CD, Quillivant XR: Initial: 20 mg once daily; may be adjusted in 10-20 mg increments at weekly intervals; maximum: 60 mg daily

Ritalin LA: Initial: 20 mg once daily (10 mg once daily may be considered for some patients); may be adjusted in 10 mg increments at weekly intervals; maximum: 60 mg daily

Conversion from immediate release or sustained release methylphenidate formulation to Ritalin LA: Use equivalent total daily dose administered once daily.

Adolescent ≥18 years and Adults (<65 years): *Concerta:*

Patients not currently taking methylphenidate: Initial:
U.S. labeling: 18-36 mg once every morning
Canadian labeling: 18 mg once every morning

Patients currently taking immediate release (IR) methylphenidate: Initial: **Note:** Dosing based on current regimen and clinical judgment; suggested dosing listed below:

- Patients taking IR methylphenidate 5 mg 2-3 times daily **or** (Canadian labeling; not in U.S. labeling) methylphenidate SR 20 mg daily: 18 mg once every morning
- Patients taking IR methylphenidate 10 mg 2-3 times daily **or** (Canadian labeling; not in U.S. labeling) methylphenidate SR 40 mg daily: 36 mg once every morning
- Patients taking IR methylphenidate 15 mg 2-3 times daily **or** (Canadian labeling; not in U.S. labeling) methylphenidate SR 60 mg daily: 54 mg once every morning
- Patients taking IR methylphenidate 20 mg 2-3 times daily: 72 mg once every morning

Dose adjustment: May increase dose in increments of 18 mg at weekly intervals. A dosage strength of 27 mg is available for situations in which a dosage between 18-36 mg is desired. Maximum dose: 72 mg daily.

Transdermal: (Daytrana): Children ≥6 years and Adolescents <18 years: Initial: 10 mg patch once daily; remove up to 9 hours after application. Titrate based on response and tolerability; may increase to next transdermal dose no more frequently than every week. **Note:** Application should occur 2 hours prior to desired effect. Drug absorption may continue for a period of time after patch removal. The prescribing information recommends patients converting from another formulation of methylphenidate should be initiated at 10 mg regardless of their previous dose and titrated as needed due to the differences in bioavailability of the transdermal formulation. However, some clinicians have supported higher starting patch doses for patients converting from oral methylphenidate doses of >20 mg daily; for example, the 15 mg (18.75 cm^2) patch has been investigated to have the same effect as 22.5 mg daily of the immediate release preparation, 27 mg/day of the osmotic release preparation, or 20 mg daily of the encapsulated bead preparation (Arnold, 2007).

Narcolepsy: Oral: Children ≥6 years, Adolescents, Adults:

Immediate release tablets and solution *(Methylin, Ritalin):* Initial: 5 mg twice daily before breakfast and lunch; increase by 5-10 mg daily at weekly intervals; maximum dose: 60 mg daily (in 2-3 divided doses).

Extended and sustained release tablets *(Metadate ER, Ritalin-SR):* May be given in place of immediate release products (duration of action ~8 hours), once the immediate release formulation daily dose is titrated and the titrated 8-hour dosage corresponds to sustained or extended release tablet size; maximum: 60 mg daily.

Depression in medically-ill older adults or adult patients with terminal illness and/or receiving palliative care (off-label use): Adults: Oral: Initial: ***Immediate release:*** 2.5-5 mg once daily before breakfast or twice daily before breakfast and lunch; increase by 2.5-5 mg daily every 1-3 days in divided doses before breakfast and lunch as tolerated; maximum dose: 20-40 mg daily (Hardy, 2009; Kerr 2012). *Do **not** use sustained release product.*

Dosage adjustment in renal impairment:

Oral: No dosage adjustment provided in manufacturer's labeling (has not been studied); undergoes extensive metabolism to a renally eliminated metabolite with little or no pharmacologic activity.

Transdermal: No dosage adjustment provided in manufacturer's labeling (has not been studied).

Dosage adjustment in hepatic impairment:

Oral: No dosage adjustment provided in manufacturer's labeling (has not been studied).

Transdermal: No dosage adjustment provided in manufacturer's labeling (has not been studied).

Dietary Considerations Administer immediate release (IR) tablet (Ritalin), IR solution (Methylin), chewable tablet (Methylin), and sustained released tablet (Ritalin-SR) 30-45 minutes before meals. Some products may contain phenylalanine.

Administration

Oral:

Controlled release capsule (Biphentin; Canadian product): Administer in the morning with breakfast. Swallow whole; do not crush or chew capsule. Alternatively, capsules may be opened and the contents sprinkled onto applesauce, ice cream, or yogurt, but the beads must not be crushed or chewed.

Immediate release (IR) tablet (Ritalin), IR solution (Methylin), chewable tablet (Methylin): Administer each dose 30-45 minutes before a meal. Ensure last daily dose is administered before 6 pm if difficulty sleeping occurs. Administer chewable tablet with at least 8 ounces of water or other fluid.

Extended release capsule (Metadate CD, Ritalin LA): Administer in the morning. May be taken with or without food. Alternatively, capsules may be opened and the contents sprinkled onto a small amount (equal to 1 tablespoon) of cold applesauce. Swallow applesauce without chewing. Do not crush or chew capsule contents.

Extended release suspension (Quillivant XR): Administer in the morning with or without food. Shake bottle ≥10 seconds prior to administration. Use the oral dosing dispenser provided; wash after each use.

Extended release tablet:

Metadate ER: May be taken with or without food. Swallow whole with water or other fluid; do not crush or chew tablet.

Concerta: Administer in the morning. May be taken with or without food, but must be taken with water or other fluid. Do not crush, chew, or divide tablet.

Sustained release tablet (Ritalin-SR): Administer 30-45 minutes before a meal. Swallow whole; do not crush or chew tablet.

Topical: Transdermal (Daytrana): Apply to clean, dry, non-oily, intact skin to the hip area, avoiding the waistline; do not premedicate the patch site with hydrocortisone or other solutions, creams, ointments, or emollients. Apply at the same time each day to alternating hips. Press firmly for 30 seconds to ensure proper adherence. Avoid exposure of application site to external heat source, which may increase the amount of drug absorbed. If difficulty is experienced when separating the patch from the liner or if any medication (sticky substance) remains on the liner after separation; discard that patch and apply a new patch. Do not use a patch that has been damaged or torn; do not cut patch. If patch should dislodge, may replace with new patch (to different site) but total wear time should not exceed 9 hours; do not reapply with dressings, tape, or common adhesives. Patch may be removed early if a shorter duration of effect is desired or if late day side effects occur. Wash hands with soap and water after handling. Avoid touching the sticky side of the patch. If patch removal is difficult, an oil-based product (eg, petroleum jelly, olive oil) may be applied to the patch edges to aid removal; never apply acetone-based products (eg, nail polish remover) to patch. Dispose of used patch by folding adhesive side onto itself, and discard in toilet or appropriate lidded container.

Monitoring Parameters Periodic CBC, differential, and platelet counts with prolonged use; blood pressure, heart rate; signs and symptoms of depression, aggression, or hostility; growth rate in children; signs of central nervous system stimulation; signs of peripheral vasculopathy (eg, digital changes)

Transdermal: Signs of worsening erythema, blistering or edema which does not improve within 48 hours of patch removal, or spreads beyond patch site.

When used for the treatment of ADHD, thoroughly evaluate for cardiovascular risk. Monitor heart rate, blood pressure, and consider obtaining ECG prior to initiation (Vetter, 2008).

Additional Information Treatment with methylphenidate may include "drug holidays" or periodic discontinuation in order to assess the patient's requirements and to decrease tolerance and limit suppression of linear growth and weight. Specific patients may require 3 doses/day for treatment of ADHD (ie, additional dose at 4 PM).

Concerta is an osmotic controlled release formulation (OROS) of methylphenidate. The tablet has an immediate-release overcoat that provides an initial dose of methylphenidate within 1 hour. The overcoat covers a trilayer core. The trilayer core is composed of two layers containing the drug and excipients, and one layer of osmotic components. As water from the gastrointestinal tract enters the core, the osmotic components expand and methylphenidate is released.

Metadate CD capsules contain a mixture of immediate release and extended release beads, designed to release 30% of the dose immediately and 70% over an extended period.

Ritalin LA uses a combination of immediate release and enteric coated, delayed release beads.

Dosage Forms

Capsule Extended Release, Oral:

Metadate CD: 10 mg, 20 mg, 30 mg, 40 mg, 50 mg, 60 mg

Generic: 10 mg, 20 mg, 30 mg, 40 mg, 50 mg, 60 mg

Capsule Extended Release 24 Hour, Oral:

Ritalin LA: 10 mg, 20 mg, 30 mg, 40 mg

Generic: 20 mg, 30 mg, 40 mg

Patch, Transdermal:

Daytrana: 10 mg/9 hr (30 ea); 15 mg/9 hr (30 ea); 20 mg/9 hr (30 ea); 30 mg/9 hr (30 ea)

Solution, Oral:

Methylin: 5 mg/5 mL (500 mL); 10 mg/5 mL (500 mL)

Generic: 5 mg/5 mL (500 mL); 10 mg/5 mL (500 mL)

Suspension Reconstituted, Oral:

Quillivant XR: 25 mg/5 mL (60 mL, 120 mL, 150 mL, 180 mL)

Tablet, Oral:

Ritalin: 5 mg, 10 mg, 20 mg

Generic: 5 mg, 10 mg, 20 mg

Tablet Chewable, Oral:

Methylin: 2.5 mg, 5 mg, 10 mg

Tablet Extended Release, Oral:

Concerta: 18 mg, 27 mg, 36 mg, 54 mg

Metadate ER: 20 mg

Generic: 10 mg, 18 mg, 20 mg, 27 mg, 36 mg, 54 mg

Dosage Forms: Canada

Capsule, controlled release, oral:

Biphentin®: 10 mg, 15 mg, 20 mg, 30 mg, 40 mg, 50 mg, 60 mg, 80 mg

◆ **Methylphenidate Hydrochloride** *see* Methylphenidate *on page 1336*

◆ **Methylphenoxy-Benzene Propanamine** *see* AtoMOXetine *on page 191*

◆ **Methylphenyl Isoxazolyl Penicillin** *see* Oxacillin *on page 1528*

◆ **Methylphytyl Napthoquinone** *see* Phytonadione *on page 1647*

MethylPREDNISolone (meth il pred NIS oh lone)

Brand Names: U.S. A-Methapred; Depo-Medrol; Medrol; Medrol (Pak); Solu-MEDROL

Brand Names: Canada Depo-Medrol; Medrol; Methylprednisolone Acetate; Methylprednisolone Sodium Succinate For Injection; Methylprednisolone Sodium Succinate For Injection USP; Solu-Medrol

Index Terms 6-α-Methylprednisolone; A-Methapred; Medrol Dose Pack; Methylprednisolone Acetate; Methylprednisolone Sodium Succinate; Solumedrol

Pharmacologic Category Corticosteroid, Systemic

Additional Appendix Information

Corticosteroids Systemic Equivalencies *on page 2228*

Use Primarily as an anti-inflammatory or immunosuppressant agent in the treatment of a variety of diseases including those of dermatologic, endocrine, GI, hematologic, allergic, inflammatory, neoplastic, neurologic, ophthalmic, renal, respiratory, and autoimmune origin. Prevention and treatment of graft-versus-host disease following allogeneic bone marrow transplantation.

Pregnancy Risk Factor C

Pregnancy Considerations Adverse events have been observed with corticosteroids in animal reproduction studies. Methylprednisolone crosses the placenta (Anderson, 1981). Some studies have shown an association between first trimester systemic corticosteroid use and oral clefts (Park-Wyllie, 2000; Pradat, 2003). Systemic corticosteroids may also influence fetal growth (decreased birth weight); however, information is conflicting (Lunghi, 2010). Hypoadrenalism may occur in newborns following maternal use of corticosteroids in pregnancy; monitor.

When systemic corticosteroids are needed in pregnancy, it is generally recommended to use the lowest effective dose for the shortest duration of time, avoiding high doses during the first trimester (Leachman, 2006; Lunghi, 2010; Makol, 2011; Østensen, 2009). Inhaled corticosteroids are preferred for the treatment of asthma during pregnancy. Systemic corticosteroids such as methylprednisolone may be used for the treatment of severe persistent asthma if needed; the lowest dose administered on alternate days (if possible) should be used (NAEPP, 2005).

Pregnant women exposed to methylprednisolone for antirejection therapy following a transplant may contact the National Transplantation Pregnancy Registry (NTPR) at 215-955-4820. Women exposed to methylprednisolone during pregnancy for the treatment of an autoimmune disease may contact the OTIS Autoimmune Diseases Study at 877-311-8972.

Breast-Feeding Considerations Corticosteroids are excreted in human milk. The manufacturer notes that when used systemically, maternal use of corticosteroids have the potential to cause adverse events in a nursing infant (eg, growth suppression, interfere with endogenous corticosteroid production) and therefore recommends a decision be made whether to discontinue nursing or to discontinue the drug, taking into account the importance of treatment to the mother. If there is concern about exposure to the infant, some guidelines recommend waiting 4 hours after the maternal dose of an oral systemic corticosteroid before breast-feeding in order to decrease potential exposure to the nursing infant (based on a study using prednisolone) (Bae, 2011; Leachman, 2006; Makol, 2011; Ost, 1985). Other guidelines note that maternal use of systemic corticosteroids is not a contraindication to breast-feeding (NAEPP, 2005).

Contraindications Hypersensitivity to methylprednisolone or any component of the formulation; systemic fungal infection; administration of live virus vaccines; methylprednisolone formulations containing benzyl alcohol preservative are contraindicated in premature infants; IM administration in idiopathic thrombocytopenic purpura; intrathecal administration

Warnings/Precautions Corticosteroids are not approved for epidural injection. Serious neurologic events (eg, spinal cord infarction, paraplegia, quadriplegia, cortical blindness, stroke), some resulting in death, have been reported with epidural injection of corticosteroids, with and without use of fluoroscopy.

Use with caution in patients with thyroid disease, hepatic impairment, renal impairment, cardiovascular disease, diabetes, glaucoma, cataracts, myasthenia gravis, multiple sclerosis, osteoporosis, seizures, or GI diseases (diverticulitis, intestinal anastomoses, peptic ulcer, ulcerative colitis) due to perforation risk. Avoid ethanol may enhance gastric mucosal irritation. Not recommended for the treatment of optic neuritis; may increase frequency of new episodes. Use with caution in patients with a history of ocular herpes simplex; corneal perforation has occurred; do not use in active ocular herpes simplex, Use caution following acute MI (corticosteroids have been associated with myocardial rupture). Cardiomegaly and congestive heart failure have been reported following concurrent use of amphotericin B and hydrocortisone for the management of fungal infections.

Because of the risk of adverse effects, systemic corticosteroids should be used cautiously in the elderly in the smallest possible effective dose for the shortest duration. May affect growth velocity; growth should be routinely monitored in pediatric patients. Withdraw therapy with gradual tapering of dose. Patients may require higher doses when subject to stress (ie, trauma, surgery, severe infection).

May cause hypercorticism or suppression of hypothalamic-pituitary-adrenal (HPA) axis, particularly in younger children or in patients receiving high doses for prolonged periods. HPA axis suppression may lead to adrenal crisis. Withdrawal and discontinuation of a corticosteroid should be done slowly and carefully. Particular care is required when patients are transferred from systemic corticosteroids to inhaled products due to possible adrenal insufficiency or withdrawal from steroids, including an increase in allergic symptoms. Adult patients receiving >20 mg per day of prednisone (or equivalent) may be most susceptible. Fatalities have occurred due to adrenal insufficiency in asthmatic patients during and after transfer from systemic corticosteroids to aerosol steroids; aerosol steroids do not provide the systemic steroid needed to treat patients having trauma, surgery, or infections. Use in septic shock or sepsis syndrome may increase mortality in some populations (eg, patients with elevated serum creatinine, patients who develop secondary infections after use).

Acute myopathy has been reported with high dose corticosteroids, usually in patients with neuromuscular transmission disorders; may involve ocular and/or respiratory muscles; monitor creatine kinase; recovery may be delayed. Corticosteroid use may cause psychiatric disturbances, including depression, euphoria, insomnia, mood swings, and personality changes. Preexisting psychiatric conditions may be exacerbated by corticosteroid use. Prolonged use of corticosteroids may increase the incidence of secondary infection, cause activation of latent infections, mask acute infection (including fungal infections), prolong or exacerbate viral or parasitic infections, or limit response to vaccines. Exposure to chickenpox or measles should be avoided; corticosteroids should not be used to treat ocular herpes simplex. Corticosteroids should not be used for cerebral malaria, fungal infections, or viral hepatitis. Close observation is required in patients with latent tuberculosis and/or TB reactivity; restrict use in active TB (only fulminating or disseminated TB in conjunction with antituberculosis treatment). Amebiasis should be ruled out in any patient with recent travel to tropic climates or unexplained diarrhea prior to initiation of corticosteroids. Use with extreme caution in patients with *Strongyloides* infections; hyperinfection, dissemination and fatalities have occurred. Prolonged treatment with corticosteroids has been associated with the development of Kaposi's sarcoma (case reports); discontinuation may result in clinical improvement.

High-dose corticosteroids should not be used to manage acute head injury. Rare cases of anaphylactoid reactions have been observed in patients receiving corticosteroids. Avoid injection or leakage into the dermis; dermal and/or subdermal skin depression may occur at the site of injection. Avoid deltoid muscle injection; subcutaneous atrophy may occur. Potentially significant drug-drug interactions may exist, requiring dose or frequency adjustment, additional monitoring, and/or selection of alternative therapy.

Benzyl alcohol and derivatives: Methylprednisolone **acetate** I.M. injection (multiple-dose vial) and the diluent for methylprednisolone **sodium succinate** injection may contain benzyl alcohol; large amounts of benzyl alcohol (≥99 mg/kg/day) have been associated with a potentially fatal toxicity ("gasping syndrome") in neonates; the "gasping syndrome" consists of metabolic acidosis, respiratory distress, gasping respirations, CNS dysfunction (including convulsions, intracranial hemorrhage), hypotension, and cardiovascular collapse (AAP, 1997; CDC, 1982); some data suggests that benzoate displaces bilirubin from protein binding sites (Ahlfors, 2001); avoid or use dosage forms containing benzyl alcohol with caution in neonates.

Some dosage forms may contain polysorbate 80 (also known as Tweens). Hypersensitivity reactions, usually a delayed reaction, have been reported following exposure to pharmaceutical products containing polysorbate 80 in certain individuals (Isaksson, 2002; Lucente 2000; Shelley, 1995). Thrombocytopenia, ascites, pulmonary deterioration, and renal and hepatic failure have been reported in premature neonates after receiving parenteral products containing polysorbate 80 (Alade, 1986; CDC, 1984). See manufacturer's labeling.

Adverse Reactions

Cardiovascular: Arrhythmias, bradycardia, cardiac arrest, cardiomegaly, circulatory collapse, congestive heart failure, edema, fat embolism, hypertension, hypertrophic cardiomyopathy in premature infants, myocardial rupture (post MI), syncope, tachycardia, thromboembolism, vasculitis

Central nervous system: Delirium, depression, emotional instability, euphoria, hallucinations, headache, intracranial pressure increased, insomnia, malaise, mood swings, nervousness, neuritis, personality changes, psychic disorders, pseudotumor cerebri (usually following discontinuation), seizure, vertigo

Dermatologic: Acne, allergic dermatitis, alopecia, dry scaly skin, ecchymoses, edema, erythema, hirsutism, hyper-/hypopigmentation, hypertrichosis, impaired wound healing, petechiae, rash, skin atrophy, sterile abscess, skin test reaction impaired, striae, urticaria

Endocrine & metabolic: Adrenal suppression, amenorrhea, carbohydrate intolerance increased, Cushing's syndrome, diabetes mellitus, fluid retention, glucose intolerance, growth suppression (children), hyperglycemia, hyperlipidemia, hypokalemia, hypokalemic alkalosis, menstrual irregularities, negative nitrogen balance, pituitary-adrenal axis suppression, protein catabolism, sodium and water retention

Gastrointestinal: Abdominal distention, appetite increased, bowel/bladder dysfunction (after intrathecal administration), gastrointestinal hemorrhage, gastrointestinal perforation, nausea, pancreatitis, peptic ulcer, perforation of the small and large intestine, ulcerative esophagitis, vomiting, weight gain

Hematologic: Leukocytosis (transient)

Hepatic: Hepatomegaly, transaminases increased

Local: Postinjection flare (intra-articular use), thrombophlebitis

Neuromuscular & skeletal: Arthralgia, arthropathy, aseptic necrosis (femoral and humoral heads), fractures, muscle mass loss, muscle weakness, myopathy (particularly in conjunction with neuromuscular disease or neuromuscular-blocking agents), neuropathy, osteoporosis, parasthesia, tendon rupture, vertebral compression fractures, weakness

Ocular: Cataracts, exophthalmoses, glaucoma, intraocular pressure increased

Renal: Glycosuria

Respiratory: Pulmonary edema

Miscellaneous: Abnormal fat disposition, anaphylactoid reaction, anaphylaxis, angioedema, avascular necrosis, diaphoresis, hiccups, hypersensitivity reactions, infections, secondary malignancy

Rare but important or life-threatening: Venous thrombosis (Johannesdottir, 2013)

Drug Interactions

Metabolism/Transport Effects Substrate of CYP3A4 (minor); **Note:** Assignment of Major/Minor substrate status based on clinically relevant drug interaction potential; **Inhibits** CYP2C8 (weak), CYP3A4 (weak)

Avoid Concomitant Use

Avoid concomitant use of MethylPREDNISolone with any of the following: Aldesleukin; BCG; Indium 111 Capromab Pendetide; Mifepristone; Natalizumab; Pimecrolimus; Pimozide; Tacrolimus (Topical); Tofacitinib

Increased Effect/Toxicity

MethylPREDNISolone may increase the levels/effects of: Acetylcholinesterase Inhibitors; Amphotericin B; Androgens; ARIPiprazole; Ceritinib; CycloSPORINE (Systemic); Deferasirox; Dofetilide; Hydrocodone; Leflunomide; Lomitapide; Loop Diuretics; Natalizumab; Nicorandil; NSAID (COX-2 Inhibitor); NSAID (Nonselective); Pimozide; Quinolone Antibiotics; Thiazide Diuretics; Tofacitinib; Vaccines (Live); Warfarin

The levels/effects of MethylPREDNISolone may be increased by: Aprepitant; CycloSPORINE (Systemic); CYP3A4 Inhibitors (Strong); Denosumab; Estrogen Derivatives; Fosaprepitant; Indacaterol; Mifepristone; Neuromuscular-Blocking Agents (Nondepolarizing); Pimecrolimus; Roflumilast; Salicylates; Tacrolimus (Topical); Telaprevir; Trastuzumab

Decreased Effect

MethylPREDNISolone may decrease the levels/effects of: Aldesleukin; Antidiabetic Agents; BCG; Calcitriol; Coccidioides immitis Skin Test; Corticorelin; CycloSPORINE (Systemic); Hyaluronidase; Indium 111 Capromab Pendetide; Isoniazid; Salicylates; Sipuleucel-T; Telaprevir; Urea Cycle Disorder Agents; Vaccines (Inactivated)

The levels/effects of MethylPREDNISolone may be decreased by: Aminoglutethimide; Antacids; Barbiturates; Bile Acid Sequestrants; CarBAMazepine; Echinacea; Fosphenytoin; Mifepristone; Mitotane; Phenytoin; Primidone; Rifamycin Derivatives

Preparation for Administration

Standard diluent (Solu-Medrol): 40 mg/50 mL D_5W; 125 mg/50 mL D_5W.

Minimum volume (Solu-Medrol): 50 mL D_5W.

Storage/Stability

Methylprednisolone acetate; tablets: Store at 20°C to 25°C (68°F to 77°F).

Methylprednisolone sodium succinate: Store intact vials at controlled room temperature of 20°C to 25°C (68°F to 77°F). Protect from light. Reconstituted solutions of methylprednisolone sodium succinate should be stored at room temperature of 20°C to 25°C (68°F to 77°F) and used within 48 hours. Stability of parenteral admixture at room temperature (25°C) and at refrigeration temperature (4°C) is 48 hours.

Mechanism of Action In a tissue-specific manner, corticosteroids regulate gene expression subsequent to binding specific intracellular receptors and translocation into the nucleus. Corticosteroids exert a wide array of physiologic effects including modulation of carbohydrate, protein, and lipid metabolism and maintenance of fluid and electrolyte homeostasis. Moreover cardiovascular, immunologic, musculoskeletal, endocrine, and neurologic physiology are influenced by corticosteroids. Decreases inflammation by suppression of migration of polymorphonuclear leukocytes and reversal of increased capillary permeability.

Pharmacodynamics/Kinetics

Onset of action: Peak effect (route dependent): Oral: 1 to 2 hours; IM: 4 to 8 days; Intra-articular: 1 week; methylprednisolone sodium succinate is highly soluble and has a rapid effect by IM and IV routes

Duration (route dependent): Oral: 30 to 36 hours; IM: 1 to 4 weeks; Intra-articular: 1 to 5 weeks; methylprednisolone acetate has a low solubility and has a sustained IM effect

Distribution: V_d: 0.7 to 1.5 L/kg

Half-life elimination: 3 to 3.5 hours; reduced in obese

Excretion: Clearance: Reduced in obese

Dosage Dosing should be based on the lesser of ideal body weight or actual body weight

Children: **Only sodium succinate may be given IV;** methylprednisolone sodium succinate is highly soluble and has a rapid effect by IM and IV routes. Methylprednisolone acetate has a low solubility and has a sustained IM effect.

Acute spinal cord injury (off-label use): IV (sodium succinate): 30 mg/kg over 15 minutes, followed in 45 minutes by a continuous infusion of 5.4 mg/kg/hour for 23 hours. **Note:** Due to insufficient evidence of clinical efficacy (ie, preserving or improving spinal cord function), the routine use of methylprednisolone in the treatment of acute spinal cord injury is no longer recommended. If used in this setting, methylprednisolone should not be initiated >8 hours after the injury; not effective in penetrating trauma (eg, gunshot) (Consortium for Spinal Cord Medicine, 2008).

Anti-inflammatory or immunosuppressive: Oral, IM, IV (sodium succinate): 0.5-1.7 mg/kg/day **or** 5-25 mg/m^2/day in divided doses every 6-12 hours; "Pulse" therapy: 15-30 mg/kg/dose over ≥30 minutes given once daily for 3 days

Asthma exacerbations, including status asthmaticus (emergency medical care or hospital doses) (NAEPP, 2007): Children ≤12 years: Oral, IV: 1-2 mg/kg/day in 2 divided doses (maximum: 60 mg/day) until peak expiratory flow is 70% of predicted or personal best

Lupus nephritis: IV (sodium succinate): 30 mg/kg over ≥30 minutes every other day for 6 doses

Adults: **Only sodium succinate may be given IV;** methylprednisolone sodium succinate is highly soluble and has a rapid effect by IM and IV routes. Methylprednisolone acetate has a low solubility and has a sustained IM effect.

Acute spinal cord injury (off-label use): IV (sodium succinate): 30 mg/kg over 15 minutes, followed in 45 minutes by a continuous infusion of 5.4 mg/kg/hour for 23 hours. **Note:** Due to insufficient evidence of clinical efficacy (ie, preserving or improving spinal cord function), the routine use of methylprednisolone in the treatment of acute spinal cord injury is no longer recommended. If used in this setting, methylprednisolone should not be initiated >8 hours after the injury; not effective in penetrating trauma (eg, gunshot) (Consortium for Spinal Cord Medicine, 2008).

Allergic conditions: Oral: Tapered-dosage schedule (eg, dose-pack containing 21 x 4 mg tablets):

Day 1: 24 mg on day 1 administered as 8 mg (2 tablets) before breakfast, 4 mg (1 tablet) after lunch, 4 mg (1 tablet) after supper, and 8 mg (2 tablets) at bedtime **OR** 24 mg (6 tablets) as a single dose or divided into 2 or 3 doses upon initiation (regardless of time of day)

Day 2: 20 mg on day 2 administered as 4 mg (1 tablet) before breakfast, 4 mg (1 tablet) after lunch, 4 mg (1 tablet) after supper, and 8 mg (2 tablets) at bedtime

Day 3: 16 mg on day 3 administered as 4 mg (1 tablet) before breakfast, 4 mg (1 tablet) after lunch, 4 mg (1 tablet) after supper, and 4 mg (1 tablet) at bedtime

Day 4: 12 mg on day 4 administered as 4 mg (1 tablet) before breakfast, 4 mg (1 tablet) after lunch, and 4 mg (1 tablet) at bedtime

Day 5: 8 mg on day 5 administered as 4 mg (1 tablet) before breakfast and 4 mg (1 tablet) at bedtime

Day 6: 4 mg on day 6 administered as 4 mg (1 tablet) before breakfast

Anti-inflammatory or immunosuppressive:

Oral: 2-60 mg/day in 1-4 divided doses to start, followed by gradual reduction in dosage to the lowest possible level consistent with maintaining an adequate clinical response.

IM (sodium succinate): 10-80 mg/day once daily

IM (acetate): 10-80 mg every 1-2 weeks

IV (sodium succinate): 10-40 mg over a period of several minutes and repeated IV or IM at intervals depending on clinical response; when high dosages are needed, give 30 mg/kg over a period ≥30 minutes and may be repeated every 4-6 hours for 48 hours.

Arthritis: Intra-articular (acetate): Administer every 1-5 weeks.

Large joints (eg, knee, ankle): 20-80 mg

Medium joints (eg, elbow, wrist): 10-40 mg

Small joints: 4-10 mg

Asthma exacerbations, including status asthmaticus (emergency medical care or hospital doses): Oral, IV: 40-80 mg/day in 1-2 divided doses until peak expiratory flow is 70% of predicted or personal best (NAEPP, 2007)

Asthma, severe persistent, long-term control: Oral: 7.5-60 mg/day (or on alternate days) (NAEPP, 2007)

COPD exacerbation (off-label use): **Note:** Dose, frequency, and duration of therapy not established. GOLD guidelines recommend the use of oral prednisone; however, methylprednisolone may be used as an alternative (GOLD [Decramer, 2014]). No comparative studies exist to examine safety and efficacy between low-, medium-, or high-dose regimens. The following regimens have been evaluated:

Oral:

Low dose: 32 mg once daily for 1 week followed by 24 mg daily for 4 additional days then 4 mg once weekly (Willaert, 2002). Although tapering was employed, tapering is not necessary at this dosage range (Vrondracek, 2006).

Medium dose: 40 mg every 6 hours until wheeze-free, followed by 40 mg once daily (Shortall, 2002).

IV:

Low dose: 40 mg once daily for 10 days followed by 20 mg once daily (duration not specified) followed by 4 mg orally once daily for 4 additional days (Willaert, 2002). Although tapering was employed, tapering is not necessary at this dosage range (Vrondracek, 2006).

Medium dose: 0.5 mg/kg every 6 hours for 72 hours (Albert, 1980) **or** 0.5 mg/kg every 6 hours for 3 days followed by 0.5 mg/kg every 12 hours for 3 days then 0.5 mg/kg daily for 4 additional days (Sayiner, 2001) **or** 0.5 mg/kg every 6 hours for 72 hours followed by 0.5 mg/kg every 12 hours for 3 days (days 4 through 6) followed by 0.5 mg/kg once daily for 4 days (days 7 through 10) for patients on ventilatory support (Alía, 2011) **or** 40 mg every 6 hours until wheeze-free, followed by *oral* 40 mg once daily (Shortall, 2002).

High dose: 125 mg every 6 hours for 3 days followed by an oral prednisone taper (treatment duration of combined IV and oral therapy was 2 or 8 weeks) (Niewoehner, 1999)

Note: Dosing is empiric and has not been established by clinical trials. Based on expert opinion, commonly used regimens ranging from 60 to 125 mg IV administered 1 to 4 times daily followed by oral therapy (eg, prednisone 40 mg once daily) for a total of 5 to 14 days of therapy may be employed. IV administration with a higher dose (eg, ≥60 mg) may be preferred for those patients with impending or actual acute respiratory failure; outcome trials not available for this approach.

Dermatitis, acute severe: IM (acetate): 80 to 120 mg as a single dose

Dermatitis, chronic: IM (acetate): 40 to 120 mg every 5 to 10 days

Dermatologic conditions (eg, keloids, lichen planus): Intralesional (acetate): 20 to 60 mg

Dermatomyositis/polymyositis: IV (sodium succinate): 1 g/day for 3 to 5 days for severe muscle weakness, followed by conversion to oral prednisone (Drake, 1996)

Gout, acute: IM, IV: Initial: 0.5 to 2 mg/kg; may be repeated as clinically indicated (ACR guidelines [Khanna, 2012])

Lupus nephritis: High-dose "pulse" therapy: IV (sodium succinate): 0.5 to 1 g/day for 3 days (Ponticelli, 2010)

Pneumocystis pneumonia in AIDS patients: IV: 30 mg twice daily for 5 days, then 30 mg once daily for 5 days, then 15 mg once daily for 11 days

Dosage adjustment in renal impairment: There are no dosage adjustments provided in the manufacturer's labeling; use with caution.

Dosage adjustment in hepatic impairment: There are no dosage adjustments provided in the manufacturer's labeling.

Dietary Considerations Take with meals to decrease GI upset; need diet rich in pyridoxine, vitamin C, vitamin D, folate, calcium, phosphorus, and protein.

Administration

Administer with meals to decrease GI upset.

Parenteral: Methylprednisolone sodium succinate may be administered IM or IV; IV administration may be IVP over one to several minutes or IVPB or continuous IV infusion. **Acetate salt should not be given IV.** Avoid injection into the deltoid muscle due to a high incidence of subcutaneous atrophy. Avoid injection or leakage into the dermis; dermal and/or subdermal skin depression may occur at the site of injection.

IV: Succinate:

Low dose: ≤1.8 mg/kg or ≤125 mg/dose: IV push over 3 to 15 minutes

Moderate dose: ≥2 mg/kg or 250 mg/dose: IV over 15 to 30 minutes

High dose: 15 mg/kg or ≥500 mg/dose: IV over ≥30 minutes

Doses >15 mg/kg or ≥1 g: Administer over 1 hour

Do **not** administer high-dose IV push; hypotension, cardiac arrhythmia, and sudden death have been reported in patients given high-dose methylprednisolone IV push (>0.5 g over <10 minutes); intermittent infusion over 15 to 60 minutes; maximum concentration: IV push 125 mg/mL

IM: Avoid injection into the deltoid muscle due to a high incidence of subcutaneous atrophy. Avoid injection or leakage into the dermis; dermal and/or subdermal skin depression may occur at the site of injection. Do not inject into areas that have evidence of acute local infection.

Monitoring Parameters Blood pressure, blood glucose, electrolytes, growth in children

Additional Information Sodium content of 1 g sodium succinate injection: 2.01 mEq; 53 mg of sodium succinate salt is equivalent to 40 mg of methylprednisolone base

Methylprednisolone acetate: Depo-Medrol

Methylprednisolone sodium succinate: Solu-Medrol

Dosage Forms

Solution Reconstituted, Injection:

A-Methapred: 40 mg (1 ea); 125 mg (1 ea)

Solu-MEDROL: 500 mg (1 ea); 1000 mg (1 ea); 2 g (1 ea)

Generic: 40 mg (1 ea); 125 mg (1 ea); 1000 mg (1 ea)

Solution Reconstituted, Injection [preservative free]:

Solu-MEDROL: 40 mg (1 ea); 125 mg (1 ea); 500 mg (1 ea); 1000 mg (1 ea)

Suspension, Injection:

Depo-Medrol: 20 mg/mL (5 mL); 40 mg/mL (1 mL, 5 mL, 10 mL); 80 mg/mL (1 mL, 5 mL)

Generic: 40 mg/mL (1 mL, 5 mL, 10 mL); 80 mg/mL (1 mL, 5 mL)

Tablet, Oral:

Medrol: 2 mg, 4 mg, 8 mg, 16 mg, 32 mg

Medrol (Pak): 4 mg

Generic: 4 mg, 8 mg, 16 mg, 32 mg

- **6-α-Methylprednisolone** *see* MethylPREDNISolone *on page 1340*
- **Methylprednisolone Acetate** *see* MethylPREDNISolone *on page 1340*
- **Methylprednisolone Sodium Succinate** *see* MethylPREDNISolone *on page 1340*
- **Methylprednisolone Sodium Succinate For Injection (Can)** *see* MethylPREDNISolone *on page 1340*
- **Methylprednisolone Sodium Succinate For Injection USP (Can)** *see* MethylPREDNISolone *on page 1340*
- **4-Methylpyrazole** *see* Fomepizole *on page 922*
- **Methylrosaniline Chloride** *see* Gentian Violet *on page 962*

Methyl Salicylate and Menthol

(METH il sa LIS i late & MEN thol)

Brand Names: U.S. BenGay [OTC]; Icy Hot [OTC]; Precise [OTC]; Salonpas Arthritis Pain [OTC]; Salonpas Jet Spray [OTC]; Salonpas Massage Foam [OTC]; Salonpas Pain Relief Patch [OTC]; Thera-Gesic Plus [OTC]; Thera-Gesic [OTC]

Index Terms Menthol and Methyl Salicylate

Pharmacologic Category Analgesic, Topical; Salicylate; Topical Skin Product

Use Temporary relief of minor aches and pains of muscle and joints associated with arthritis, bruises, simple backache, sprains, and strains

Dosage Topical: Pain relief:

Balm, cream, foam, spray, stick: Children ≥12 years and Adults: Apply to affected area; may repeat up to 3-4 times/day

Patch:

Methyl salicylate 10% and menthol 1.5%: Children ≥12 years and Adults: Apply 1 patch to affected area not more than 3-4 times daily; leave in place for no more than 8 hours

Methyl salicylate 10% and menthol 3%: Adults: Apply 1 patch to affected area and leave in place for up to 8-12 hours; do not exceed 1 patch/application. If pain still present, a second patch may be applied for up to 8-12 hours (maximum: 2 patches/24 hours; 3 days of consecutive use)

Additional Information Complete prescribing information should be consulted for additional detail.

Dosage Forms

Aerosol, foam, topical:

Salonpas Massage Foam [OTC]: Methyl salicylate 10% and menthol 3% (118 mL)

Aerosol, spray, topical:

Salonpas Jet Spray [OTC]: Methyl salicylate 10% and menthol 3% (118 mL)

Balm, topical:

Icy Hot Balm [OTC]: Methyl salicylate 29% and menthol 7.6% (99.2 g)

Cream, topical:

BenGay Arthritis Formula [OTC]: Methyl salicylate 30% and menthol 8% (57 g, 113 g)

BenGay Greaseless [OTC]: Methyl salicylate 15% and menthol 10% (57 g, 113 g)

Icy Hot [OTC]: Methyl salicylate 30% and menthol 10% (35.4 g, 85 g)

Precise [OTC]: Methyl salicylate 30% and menthol 10% (75 g)

Thera-Gesic [OTC]: Methyl salicylate 15% and menthol 1% (85 g, 142 g)

Thera-Gesic Plus [OTC]: Methyl salicylate 15% and menthol 4% (85 g) [contains aloe]

Patch, topical:

Salonpas Arthritis Pain [OTC]: Methyl salicylate 10% and menthol 3% (5s)

Salonpas Pain Relief Patch: Methyl salicylate 10% and menthol 1.5% (3s)

Salonpas Pain Relief Patch: Methyl salicylate 10% and menthol 3% (5s)

Stick, topical:

Icy Hot [OTC]: Methyl salicylate 30% and menthol 10% (49 g)

MethylTESTOSTERone (meth il tes TOS te rone)

Brand Names: U.S. Android; Methitest; Testred

Pharmacologic Category Androgen

Additional Appendix Information

Beers Criteria – Potentially Inappropriate Medications for Geriatrics *on page 2271*

Use

Males:

Delayed puberty: To stimulate puberty in carefully selected males with clearly delayed puberty.

Hypogonadotropic hypogonadism (congenital or acquired): Treatment of idiopathic gonadotropin or luteinizing hormone-releasing hormone (LHRH) deficiency, or pituitary hypothalamic injury from tumors, trauma, or radiation.

Primary hypogonadism (congenital or acquired): Treatment of testicular failure caused by cryptorchidism, bilateral torsion, orchitis, vanishing testis syndrome; or orchidectomy.

Females:

Breast cancer, metastatic: Secondarily in women with advancing inoperable metastatic (skeletal) mammary cancer who are 1 to 5 years postmenopausal; has also been used in premenopausal women with breast cancer who have benefited from oophorectomy and are considered to have a hormone responsive tumor.

Pregnancy Risk Factor X

Dosage

Breast cancer, metastatic (females): Adults: Oral: 50 to 200 mg daily

Hypogonadism; delayed puberty (males): **Note:** Individualize dose based on response and tolerability: Adolescents and Adults: Oral: 10 to 50 mg daily

Dosage adjustment in renal impairment: There are no dosage adjustments provided in the manufacturer's labeling. However, patients with renal disease may be at an increased risk of fluid retention.

Dosage adjustment in hepatic impairment: There are no dosage adjustments provided in the manufacturer's labeling. However, patients with hepatic disease may be at an increased risk of fluid retention.

Additional Information Complete prescribing information should be consulted for additional detail.

Dosage Forms

Capsule, Oral:

Android: 10 mg

Testred: 10 mg

Tablet, Oral:

Methitest: 10 mg

◆ **Methylthionine Chloride** *see* Methylene Blue *on page 1333*

◆ **Methylthioninium Chloride** *see* Methylene Blue *on page 1333*

Metipranolol (met i PRAN oh lol)

Index Terms Metipranolol Hydrochloride

Pharmacologic Category Beta-Blocker, Nonselective; Ophthalmic Agent, Antiglaucoma

Use Treatment of chronic open-angle glaucoma or ocular hypertension

Pregnancy Risk Factor C

Dosage Ophthalmic: Adults: Instill 1 drop in the affected eye(s) twice daily

Dosage adjustment in renal impairment: No dosage adjustment provided in manufacturer's labeling. However, dosage adjustment unlikely due to low systemic absorption.

Dosage adjustment in hepatic impairment: No dosage adjustment provided in manufacturer's labeling. However, dosage adjustment unlikely due to low systemic absorption.

Additional Information Complete prescribing information should be consulted for additional detail.

Dosage Forms

Solution, Ophthalmic:

Generic: 0.3% (5 mL, 10 mL)

◆ **Metipranolol Hydrochloride** *see* Metipranolol *on page 1345*

Metoclopramide (met oh KLOE pra mide)

Brand Names: U.S. Metozolv ODT; Reglan

Brand Names: Canada Apo-Metoclop; Metoclopramide Hydrochloride Injection; Metoclopramide Omega; Metonia; Nu-Metoclopramide; PMS-Metoclopramide

Pharmacologic Category Antiemetic; Gastrointestinal Agent, Prokinetic

Additional Appendix Information

Beers Criteria – Potentially Inappropriate Medications for Geriatrics *on page 2271*

Use

Injection:

Diabetic gastroparesis (diabetic gastric stasis): Relief of symptoms associated with acute and recurrent diabetic gastric stasis.

Prevention of nausea and vomiting associated with emetogenic cancer chemotherapy: Prophylaxis of vomiting associated with emetogenic cancer chemotherapy.

Prevention of postoperative nausea and vomiting: Prophylaxis of postoperative nausea and vomiting in circumstances where nasogastric suction is undesirable.

Radiological examination: To stimulate gastric emptying and intestinal transit of barium when delayed emptying interferes with radiological examination of the stomach and/or small intestine.

Small bowel intubation: To facilitate small bowel intubation in adults and pediatrics in whom the tube does not pass the pylorus with conventional maneuvers.

Oral:

Diabetic gastroparesis (diabetic gastric stasis): Relief of symptoms associated with acute and recurrent diabetic gastroparesis (gastric stasis) in adults.

Gastroesophageal reflux: Short-term (4 to 12 weeks) therapy for adults with documented symptomatic gastroesophageal reflux disease (GERD) who fail to respond to conventional therapy.

Limitations of use: Oral metoclopramide is indicated for adults only. Treatment should not exceed 12-week duration.

Pregnancy Risk Factor B

Pregnancy Considerations Adverse events were not observed in animal reproduction studies. Metoclopramide crosses the placenta and can be detected in cord blood and amniotic fluid (Arvela, 1983; Bylsma-Howell, 1983). Available evidence suggests safe use during pregnancy (Berkovitch, 2002; Matok, 2009; Sørensen, 2000). Metoclopramide may be used for the treatment of nausea and vomiting of pregnancy (ACOG, 2004; Levichek, 2002) and prophylaxis for nausea and vomiting associated with cesarean delivery (ASA, 2007; Mahadevan, 2006; Smith, 2011). Other agents are preferred for gastroesophageal reflux (Mahadevan, 2006).

Breast-Feeding Considerations Metoclopramide is excreted in breast milk. Information is available from studies conducted in mothers nursing preterm infants (n=14; delivered at 23-34 weeks gestation) or term infants (n=18) and taking metoclopramide 10 mg 3 times daily. The median concentration of metoclopramide in breast milk was ~45 ng/mL in the preterm infants and the mean concentration was ~48 ng/mL in the full term infants. The authors of both studies calculated the relative infant dose to be 3% to 5%, based on a therapeutic infant dose of 0.5 mg/kg/day. Metoclopramide was also detected in the serum of one nursing full term infant (Hansen, 2005; Kauppila, 1983). Metoclopramide may increase prolactin concentrations and cause galactorrhea and gynecomastia, but studies which evaluated its use to increase milk production for women who want to nurse have had mixed results. In addition, due to the potential for adverse events, nonpharmacologic measure should be considered prior to the use of medications as galactagogues (ABM, 2011). The manufacturer recommends that caution be used if administered to a nursing woman.

Contraindications Known sensitivity or intolerance to metoclopramide or any component of the formulation; situations where gastrointestinal (GI) motility may be dangerous, including mechanical GI obstruction, perforation or hemorrhage; pheochromocytoma; history of seizure disorder (eg, epilepsy), concomitant use with other agents likely to increase extrapyramidal reactions

Warnings/Precautions **[U.S. Boxed Warning]: May cause tardive dyskinesia, a serious movement disorder which is often irreversible; the risk of developing tardive dyskinesia increases with duration of treatment and total cumulative dose. Discontinue metoclopramide in patients who develop signs/symptoms of tardive dyskinesia. There is no known treatment for tardive dyskinesia. In some patients, symptoms lessen or resolve after metoclopramide treatment is stopped. Avoid metoclopramide treatment longer than 12 weeks in all but rare cases in which therapeutic benefit is thought to outweigh the risk of developing tardive dyskinesia.** Tardive dyskinesia is characterized by involuntary movements of the face, tongue, or extremities and may be disfiguring. An analysis of utilization patterns showed that ~20% of patients who used metoclopramide took it for longer than 12 weeks. Metoclopramide may mask underlying tardive disease by suppressing or partially suppressing tardive dyskinesia signs (metoclopramide should not be used to control tardive dyskinesia symptoms as the long-term course is unknown). The risk for tardive dyskinesia appears to be increased in the elderly, women, and diabetics, although it is not possible to predict which patients will develop tardive dyskinesia. There is no known effective treatment for established cases of tardive dyskinesia, although in some patients, tardive dyskinesia may remit (partially or completely) within several weeks to months after metoclopramide is withdrawn.

May cause extrapyramidal symptoms (EPS), generally manifested as acute dystonic reactions within the initial 24 to 48 hours of use at the usual adult dose (30 to 40 mg/day). Risk of these reactions is increased at higher doses, and in pediatric patients and adults <30 years of age. Symptoms may include involuntary limb movements, facial grimacing, torticollis, oculogyric crisis, rhythmic tongue protrusion, bulbar type speech, trismus, or dystonic reactions resembling tetanus. May also rarely present as stridor and dyspnea (may be due to laryngospasm). Dystonic symptoms may be managed with IM diphenhydramine or benztropine. Pseudoparkinsonism (eg, bradykinesia, tremor, rigidity, mask-like facies) may also occur (usually within first 6 months of therapy) and is generally reversible within 2 to 3 months following discontinuation. Symptoms of Parkinson disease may be exacerbated by metoclopramide; use with extreme caution (or avoid use) in patients with Parkinson disease.

Metoclopramide use may be associated (rarely) with neuroleptic malignant syndrome (NMS); may be fatal. Monitor for manifestations of NMS, which include hyperthermia, muscle rigidity, altered consciousness, and autonomic instability (irregular pulse or blood pressure, tachycardia, diaphoresis, and cardiac arrhythmias). Discontinue immediately if signs/symptoms of NMS appear and begin intensive symptomatic management and monitoring. Bromocriptine and dantrolene have been used to manage NMS, although effectiveness have not been established.

Mental depression has occurred (in patients with and without a history of depression), symptoms range from mild to severe (suicidal ideation and suicide); use in patients with a history of depression only if anticipated benefits outweigh potential risks.

In a study in hypertensive patients, IV metoclopramide was associated with catecholamine release. Use with caution in patients with hypertension. There are reports of hypertensive crises in some patients with undiagnosed pheochromocytoma. Immediately discontinue with any rapid rise in blood pressure that is associated with metoclopramide. Hypertensive crises may be managed with phentolamine. Use with caution in patients who are at risk of fluid overload (HF, cirrhosis); metoclopramide causes a transient increase in serum aldosterone and increases the risk for fluid retention/overload; discontinue if adverse events or signs/symptoms appear.

Patients with NADH-cytochrome b5 reductase deficiency are at increased risk of methemoglobinemia and/or sulfhemoglobinemia. Use with caution in patients with renal impairment; dosage adjustment may be needed. Use with caution following surgical anastomosis/closure; promotility agents may theoretically increase pressure in suture lines.

For patients with diabetic gastroparesis, the usual manifestations of delayed gastric emptying (eg, nausea, vomiting, heartburn, persistent fullness after meals, anorexia) appear to respond to metoclopramide within different time intervals. Significant relief of nausea occurs early and continues to improve over a 3-week period; relief of vomiting and anorexia may precede the relief of abdominal fullness by a week or more. If gastroesophageal reflux symptoms are confined to particular situations, such as following the evening meal, consider use of metoclopramide as a single dose prior to the provocative situation, rather than using the drug throughout the day. Symptoms of postprandial and daytime heartburn respond better to metoclopramide, with less observed effect on nocturnal symptoms. Because there is no documented correlation between symptoms and healing of esophageal lesions, patients with documented lesions should be monitored endoscopically. Healing of esophageal ulcers and erosions has been endoscopically demonstrated at the end of a 12-week trial using a dosage of 15 mg 4 times daily.

Avoid use in older adults (except for diabetic gastroparesis) due to risk of extrapyramidal effects, including tardive dyskinesia; risk potentially even greater in frail older adults (Beers Criteria). In addition, risk of tardive dyskinesia may be increased in older women. EPS are increased in pediatric patients. In neonates, prolonged clearance of metoclopramide may lead to increased serum concentrations. Neonates may also have decreased levels of NADH-cytochrome b5 reductase which increases the risk of methemoglobinemia. Potentially significant drug-drug interactions may exist, requiring dose or frequency adjustment, additional monitoring, and/or selection of alternative therapy. CNS effects may be potentiated when used with other sedative drugs or ethanol. Abrupt discontinuation may (rarely) result in withdrawal symptoms (dizziness, headache, nervousness).

Benzyl alcohol and derivatives: Some dosage forms may contain sodium benzoate/benzoic acid; benzoic acid (benzoate) is a metabolite of benzyl alcohol; large amounts of benzyl alcohol (≥99 mg/kg/day) have been associated with a potentially fatal toxicity ("gasping syndrome") in neonates; the "gasping syndrome" consists of metabolic acidosis, respiratory distress, gasping respirations, CNS dysfunction (including convulsions, intracranial hemorrhage), hypotension, and cardiovascular collapse (AAP, 1997; CDC, 1982); some data suggests that benzoate displaces bilirubin from protein binding sites (Ahlfors, 2001); avoid or use dosage forms containing benzyl alcohol derivative with caution in neonates. See manufacturer's labeling.

Adverse Reactions

Cardiovascular: Atrioventricular block, bradycardia, congestive heart failure, flushing (following high IV doses), hypertension, hypotension, supraventricular tachycardia

Central nervous system: Akathisia, confusion, depression, dizziness, drowsiness (dose related), drug-induced Parkinson's disease, dystonic reaction (dose and age related), fatigue, hallucination (rare), headache, insomnia, lassitude, neuroleptic malignant syndrome (rare), restlessness, seizure, somnolence, suicidal ideation, tardive dyskinesia

Dermatologic: Skin rash, urticaria

Endocrine & metabolic: Amenorrhea, fluid retention, galactorrhea, gynecomastia, hyperprolactinemia, porphyria

Gastrointestinal: Diarrhea, nausea, vomiting

Genitourinary: Impotence, urinary frequency, urinary incontinence

Hematologic & oncologic: Agranulocytosis, leukopenia, methemoglobinemia, neutropenia, sulfhemoglobinemia

Hepatic: Hepatotoxicity (rare)

Hypersensitivity: Angioedema (rare), hypersensitivity reaction

Neuromuscular & skeletal: Laryngospasm (rare)

Ophthalmic: Visual disturbance

Respiratory: Bronchospasm, laryngeal edema (rare)

Drug Interactions

Metabolism/Transport Effects **Substrate** of CYP1A2 (minor), CYP2D6 (minor); **Note:** Assignment of Major/Minor substrate status based on clinically relevant drug interaction potential; **Inhibits** CYP2D6 (weak)

Avoid Concomitant Use

Avoid concomitant use of Metoclopramide with any of the following: Antipsychotic Agents; Droperidol; Promethazine; Tetrabenazine; Trimetazidine

Increased Effect/Toxicity

Metoclopramide may increase the levels/effects of: Antipsychotic Agents; CycloSPORINE (Systemic); Highest Risk QTc-Prolonging Agents; Moderate Risk QTc-Prolonging Agents; Prilocaine; Promethazine; Selective Serotonin Reuptake Inhibitors; Sodium Nitrite; Tetrabenazine; Tricyclic Antidepressants; Trimetazidine; Venlafaxine

The levels/effects of Metoclopramide may be increased by: Droperidol; Metyrosine; Mifepristone; Nitric Oxide; Serotonin Modulators

Decreased Effect

Metoclopramide may decrease the levels/effects of: Anti-Parkinson's Agents (Dopamine Agonist); Atovaquone; Posaconazole; Quinagolide

Preparation for Administration Injection: Lower doses (≤10 mg): No dilution required; Higher doses (>10 mg): Dilute in 50 mL of compatible solution (preferably NS).

Storage/Stability

Injection: Store intact vials at room temperature of 20°C to 25°C (68°F to 77°F); injection is photosensitive and should be protected from light during storage; parenteral admixtures in D_5W, $D_5{}^{1/2}NS$, NS, LR, or Ringer's injection are stable for up to 24 hours after preparation at normal light conditions or up to 48 hours if protected from light. When mixed with NS, can be stored frozen for up to 4 weeks; metoclopramide is degraded when admixed and frozen with D_5W.

Tablet: Store at room temperature of 20°C to 25°C (68°F to 77°F). Dispense in tight, light-resistant container.

Tablet, orally disintegrating: Store at room temperature of 20°C to 25°C (68°F to 77°F). Keep in original packaging until just prior to use.

Mechanism of Action Blocks dopamine receptors and (when given in higher doses) also blocks serotonin receptors in chemoreceptor trigger zone of the CNS; enhances the response to acetylcholine of tissue in upper GI tract causing enhanced motility and accelerated gastric emptying without stimulating gastric, biliary, or pancreatic secretions; increases lower esophageal sphincter tone

Pharmacodynamics/Kinetics

Onset of action: Oral: 30 to 60 minutes; IV: 1 to 3 minutes; IM: 10 to 15 minutes

Duration: Therapeutic: 1 to 2 hours, regardless of route

Absorption: Oral: Rapid, well absorbed

Distribution: V_d: ~3.5 L/kg

Protein binding: ~30%

Bioavailability: Oral: Range: 65% to 95%

Half-life elimination: Normal renal function: Pediatric: ~4 hours; Adults: 5 to 6 hours (may be dose dependent)

Time to peak, serum: Oral: 1 to 2 hours

Excretion: Urine (~85%)

Dosage

Children:

Small bowel intubation (postpyloric feeding tube placement): IV:

<6 years: 0.1 mg/kg as a single dose

6-14 years: 2.5 to 5 mg as a single dose

>14 years: Refer to adult dosing.

Prevention of chemotherapy-associated nausea and vomiting (off-label use): Moderately emetogenic chemotherapy (patients who cannot receive corticosteroids): IV: 1 mg/kg prior to chemotherapy, followed by Oral: 0.0375 mg/kg every 6 hours; regimen also includes ondansetron or granisetron; concurrent administration of diphenhydramine or benztropine is recommended to prevent metoclopramide-induced adverse effects (Dupuis, 2013)

Adults:

Diabetic gastroparesis:

Oral: 10 mg up to 4 times daily 30 minutes before meals and at bedtime for 2 to 8 weeks. Treatment >12 weeks is not recommended.

IM, IV (for severe symptoms): 10 mg over 1 to 2 minutes IV; up to 10 days of therapy may be necessary before symptoms are controlled to allow transition to oral administration.

Gastroparesis management, regardless of etiology (off-label use): American College of Gastroenterology Guidelines: Oral: Initial: 5 mg 3 times daily before meals. Dosage range: 5 to 10 mg 2 to 3 times daily before meals (maximum: 40 mg daily). Liquid formulation is preferred (to increase absorption) and the use of drug holidays or dose reductions (eg, 5 mg before the two main meals of the day) is also recommended when clinically possible (Camilleri, 2013).

Gastroesophageal reflux: Oral: 10 to 15 mg up to 4 times daily 30 minutes before meals and at bedtime; alternatively, single doses of up to 20 mg (rather than continuous treatment) may be administered prior to provoking situation if symptoms are intermittent. More sensitive patients may require only 5 mg/dose. Treatment >12 weeks is not recommended.

Prevention of nausea and vomiting associated with emetogenic chemotherapy: IV: **Note:** pretreatment with diphenhydramine will decrease risk of extrapyramidal reactions

Highly emetogenic: Initial dose: 2 mg/kg over 15 minutes 30 minutes before chemotherapy; repeat every 2 hours for 2 doses, then every 3 hours for 3 doses

Less emetogenic: Initial dose: 1 mg/kg over 15 minutes 30 minutes before chemotherapy; repeat every 2 hours for 2 doses, then every 3 hours for 3 doses

Delayed-emesis prophylaxis (off-label): Oral: 20 to 40 mg (or 0.5 mg/kg/dose) 2 to 4 times daily for 3 to 4 days in combination with dexamethasone (ASCO guidelines [Kris, 2006])

Refractory or intolerant to antiemetics with a higher therapeutic index (off-label; Hesketh, 2008):

IV: 1 to 2 mg/kg/dose before chemotherapy and repeat 2 hours after chemotherapy

Oral: 0.5 mg/kg every 6 hours on days 2 to 4

Prevention of postoperative nausea and vomiting: IM, IV (off-label route): Usual dose: 10 mg near end of surgery; some patients may require 20 mg. **Note:** Guidelines discourage use of 10 mg metoclopramide due to lack of effectiveness (Gan, 2007); comparative study indicates higher dose (20 mg) may be efficacious (Quaynor, 2002)

Radiological exam: IV: 10 mg as a single dose

Small bowel intubation (postpyloric feeding tube placement): IV: 10 mg as a single dose

Prevention of radiation therapy-induced nausea and vomiting (minimal emetic risk) (off-label use): Oral: 20 mg as rescue therapy; if rescue therapy is used, then administer prior to each fraction until the end of radiation therapy (Basch, 2011)

Elderly: Initial: Dose at the lower end of the recommended range (may require only 5 mg/dose). Use the lowest effective dose. Refer to adult dosing.

Dosage adjustment in renal impairment: CrCl <40 mL/minute: Administer at 50% of normal dose

Hemodialysis: Not dialyzable (0% to 5%); supplemental dose is not necessary

Dosage adjustment in hepatic impairment: There are no dosage adjustments provided in the manufacturer's labeling. However, metoclopramide has been used safely in patients with advanced liver disease with normal renal function.

Administration

Injection: May be given IM, direct IV push, short infusion (at least 15 minutes), or continuous infusion; lower doses (≤10 mg) of metoclopramide can be given IV push undiluted over 1 to 2 minutes; higher doses (>10 mg) to be diluted in 50 mL of compatible solution (preferably NS) and given IVPB over at least 15 minutes. **Note:** Rapid IV administration may be associated with a transient (but intense) feeling of anxiety and restlessness, followed by drowsiness.

Tablets: When used for gastroparesis/reflux, administer 30 minutes prior to meals and at bedtime.

Orally disintegrating tablets: When used for gastroparesis/reflux, administer on an empty stomach at least 30 minutes prior to food and at bedtime (do not repeat if inadvertently taken with food). Do not remove from packaging until time of administration. If tablet breaks or crumbles while handling, discard and remove new tablet. Using dry hands, place tablet on tongue and allow to dissolve (disintegrates within ~1 minute [range: 10 seconds to 14 minutes]). Swallow with saliva.

Monitoring Parameters Signs of tardive dyskinesias, extrapyramidal symptoms; signs/symptoms of neuroleptic malignant syndrome

Dosage Forms

Solution, Injection:

Generic: 5 mg/mL (2 mL)

Solution, Injection [preservative free]:

Generic: 5 mg/mL (2 mL)

Solution, Oral:

Generic: 5 mg/5 mL (10 mL, 473 mL); 10 mg/10 mL (10 mL)

Tablet, Oral:

Reglan: 5 mg, 10 mg

Generic: 5 mg, 10 mg

Tablet Dispersible, Oral:

Metozolv ODT: 5 mg

◆ **Metoclopramide Hydrochloride Injection (Can)** *see* Metoclopramide *on page 1345*

◆ **Metoclopramide Omega (Can)** *see* Metoclopramide *on page 1345*

◆ **Metoject (Can)** *see* Methotrexate *on page 1322*

Metolazone (me TOLE a zone)

Brand Names: U.S. Zaroxolyn [DSC]

Brand Names: Canada Zaroxolyn

Pharmacologic Category Diuretic, Thiazide-Related

Use

Edema: Treatment of edema in congestive heart failure and edema accompanying renal diseases, including the nephrotic syndrome and states of diminished renal function.

Hypertension: Treatment of hypertension.

Pregnancy Risk Factor B

Pregnancy Considerations Adverse events have not been observed in animal reproduction studies. Metolazone crosses the placenta and appears in cord blood. Hypoglycemia, hypokalemia, hyponatremia, jaundice, and thrombocytopenia are reported as complications to the fetus or newborn following maternal use of thiazide diuretics.

Breast-Feeding Considerations Metolazone is excreted in breast milk. Due to the potential for serious adverse reactions in the nursing infant, the manufacturer recommends a decision be made whether to discontinue nursing or to discontinue the drug, taking into account the importance of treatment to the mother.

Contraindications

Hypersensitivity to metolazone or any component of the formulation; anuria; hepatic coma or precoma.

Documentation of allergenic cross-reactivity for diuretics is limited. However, because of similarities in chemical structure and/or pharmacologic actions, the possibility of cross-sensitivity cannot be ruled out with certainty.

Warnings/Precautions Severe hypokalemia and/or hyponatremia can occur rapidly following initial doses. Hypercalcemia, hypochloremic alkalosis, and/or hypomagnesemia can also occur. Correct hypokalemia before initiating therapy. Sensitivity reactions, including angioedema and bronchospasm, may occur. Orthostatic hypotension may also occur. Ethanol may potentiate orthostatic hypotensive effect of metolazone. Instruct patients to avoid ethanol during therapy. If taken concurrently, monitor for hypotensive effects. Use with caution in severe hepatic dysfunction. Hyperuricemia can occur and gout can be precipitated. Cautious use in patients with prediabetes or diabetes; may see a change in glucose control. Can cause SLE exacerbation or activation. Azotemia and oliguria may occur. Use caution in severe renal impairment. If azotemia and oliguria worsen during treatment in these patients, discontinue therapy. Photosensitization may occur.

Chemical similarities are present among sulfonamides, sulfonylureas, carbonic anhydrase inhibitors, thiazides, and loop diuretics (except ethacrynic acid). Use with caution in patients with thiazide or sulfonamide allergy; avoid use when previous reaction has been severe. Discontinue if signs of hypersensitivity are noted. Potentially significant drug-drug interactions may exist, requiring dose or frequency adjustment, additional monitoring, and/or selection of alternative therapy. Do not interchange Zaroxolyn with other formulations of metolazone that are not therapeutically equivalent at the same doses (eg, Mykrox, no longer available in the US).

Adverse Reactions

Cardiovascular: Chest pain/discomfort, necrotizing angiitis, orthostatic hypotension, palpitation, syncope, venous thrombosis, vertigo, volume depletion

Central nervous system: Chills, depression, dizziness, drowsiness, fatigue, headache, lightheadedness, restlessness

Dermatologic: Petechiae, photosensitivity, pruritus, purpura, rash, skin necrosis, Stevens-Johnson syndrome, toxic epidermal necrolysis, urticaria

Endocrine & metabolic: Gout attacks, hypercalcemia, hyperglycemia, hyperuricemia, hypochloremia, hypochloremic alkalosis, hypokalemia, hypomagnesemia, hyponatremia, hypophosphatemia

Gastrointestinal: Abdominal bloating, abdominal pain, anorexia, constipation, diarrhea, epigastric distress, nausea, pancreatitis, vomiting, xerostomia

Genitourinary: Impotence

Hematologic: Agranulocytosis, aplastic/hypoplastic anemia, hemoconcentration, leukopenia, thrombocytopenia

Hepatic: Cholestatic jaundice, hepatitis

Neuromuscular & skeletal: Joint pain, muscle cramps/spasm, neuropathy, paresthesia, weakness

Ocular: Blurred vision (transient)

Renal: BUN increased, glucosuria

Drug Interactions

Metabolism/Transport Effects None known.

Avoid Concomitant Use

Avoid concomitant use of Metolazone with any of the following: Dofetilide

Increased Effect/Toxicity

Metolazone may increase the levels/effects of: ACE Inhibitors; Allopurinol; Amifostine; Antihypertensives; Calcium Salts; CarBAMazepine; Cardiac Glycosides; Cyclophosphamide; Diazoxide; Dofetilide; DULoxetine; Hypotensive Agents; Ivabradine; Levodopa; Lithium; Multivitamins/Minerals (with ADEK, Folate, Iron); Multivitamins/Minerals (with AE, No Iron); Obinutuzumab; OXcarbazepine; Porfimer; RisperiDONE; RiTUXimab; Sodium Phosphates; Topiramate; Toremifene; Verteporfin; Vitamin D Analogs

The levels/effects of Metolazone may be increased by: Alcohol (Ethyl); Alfuzosin; Analgesics (Opioid); Anticholinergic Agents; Barbiturates; Beta2-Agonists; Brimonidine (Topical); Corticosteroids (Orally Inhaled); Corticosteroids (Systemic); Dexketoprofen; Diazoxide; Herbs (Hypotensive Properties); Licorice; MAO Inhibitors; Multivitamins/Fluoride (with ADE); Nicorandil; Pentoxifylline; Phosphodiesterase 5 Inhibitors; Prostacyclin Analogues; Selective Serotonin Reuptake Inhibitors

Decreased Effect

Metolazone may decrease the levels/effects of: Antidiabetic Agents

The levels/effects of Metolazone may be decreased by: Bile Acid Sequestrants; Herbs (Hypertensive Properties); Methylphenidate; Nonsteroidal Anti-Inflammatory Agents; Yohimbine

Storage/Stability Store at 25°C (77°F); excursions are permitted between 15°C and 30°C (59°Fand 86°F). Protect from light.

Mechanism of Action Inhibits sodium reabsorption in the distal tubules causing increased excretion of sodium and water, as well as, potassium and hydrogen ions

Pharmacodynamics/Kinetics

Onset of action: Diuresis: ~60 minutes

Duration: ≥24 hours

Absorption: Incomplete

Distribution: Crosses placenta; enters breast milk

Protein binding: 90% to 95%

Time to peak, serum: ~8 hours

Excretion: Urine (unchanged)

Dosage Oral:

Adults:

Edema associated with renal disease: Initial: 5-20 mg once daily.

Edema associated with heart failure (off-label dose): Initial: 2.5 mg once daily; maximum daily dose: 20 mg. (ACCF/AHA [Yancy, 2013]); **Note:** Dosing frequency may be adjusted based on patient-specific diuretic needs (eg, administration every other day or weekly) (HFSA [Lindenfeld, 2010]).

Hypertension: Initial: 2.5-5 mg once daily; adjust dose as necessary to achieve maximum therapeutic effect.

Elderly: Refer to adult dosing.

Dosage adjustment in renal impairment: There are no dosage adjustments provided in the manufacturer's labeling; use caution in patients with severe renal impairment, as most of the drug is excreted by the renal route and accumulation may occur.

Dosage adjustment in hepatic impairment: There are no dosage adjustments provided in manufacturer's labeling; contraindicated in hepatic coma or precoma.

Dietary Considerations May require potassium supplementation

Administration Administer orally as a single daily dose with or without food. Take early in day to avoid nocturia.

Monitoring Parameters Serum electrolytes, uric acid, fluid balance, renal function, blood pressure (standing, sitting/supine)

Additional Information Metolazone 5 mg is approximately equivalent to hydrochlorothiazide 50 mg.

Dosage Forms

Tablet, Oral:

Generic: 2.5 mg, 5 mg, 10 mg

Extemporaneous Preparations A 1 mg/mL oral suspension may be made by with tablets and one of three different vehicles (cherry syrup diluted 1:4 with simple syrup; a 1:1 mixture of Ora-Sweet and Ora-Plus; or a 1:1 mixture of Ora-Sweet SF and Ora-Plus). Crush twelve 10 mg tablets in a mortar and reduce to a fine powder. Add small portions of the chosen vehicle and mix to a uniform paste; mix while adding the vehicle in incremental proportions to **almost**

120 mL; transfer to a calibrated bottle, rinse mortar with vehicle, and add quantity of vehicle sufficient to make 120 mL. Label "shake well" and "refrigerate". Stable for 60 days.

A 0.25 mg/mL oral suspension may be made with tablets and a 1:1 mixture of methylcellulose 1% and simple syrup. Crush one 2.5 mg tablet in a mortar and reduce to a fine powder. Add small portions of the vehicle and mix to a uniform paste; mix while adding the vehicle in incremental proportions to **almost** 10 mL; transfer to a calibrated bottle, rinse mortar with vehicle, and add quantity of vehicle sufficient to make 10 mL. Label "shake well" and "refrigerate". Stable for 91 days refrigerated (preferred), 28 days at room temperature in plastic, and 14 days at room temperature in glass.

Nahata, MC, Pai VB, and Hipple TF, *Pediatric Drug Formulations*, 5th ed, Cincinnati, OH: Harvey Whitney Books Co, 2004.

◆ **Metonia (Can)** *see* Metoclopramide *on page 1345*

Metoprolol (me toe PROE lole)

Brand Names: U.S. Lopressor; Toprol XL

Brand Names: Canada Apo-Metoprolol; Apo-Metoprolol (Type L); Apo-Metoprolol SR; Ava-Metoprolol; Ava-Metoprolol (Type L); Betaloc; Dom-Metoprolol-B; Dom-Metoprolol-L; JAMP-Metoprolol-L; Lopresor; Lopresor SR; Metoprolol Tartrate Injection, USP; Metoprolol-25; Metoprolol-L; Mylan-Metoprolol (Type L); Nu-Metop; PMS-Metoprolol-B; PMS-Metoprolol-L; Riva-Metoprolol-L; Sandoz-Metoprolol (Type L); Sandoz-Metoprolol SR; Teva-Metoprolol

Index Terms Metoprolol Succinate; Metoprolol Tartrate

Pharmacologic Category Antianginal Agent; Antihypertensive; Beta-Blocker, Beta-1 Selective

Use Treatment of angina pectoris, hypertension, or hemodynamically-stable acute myocardial infarction

According to the ACCF/AHA 2013 guidelines for the management of ST-elevation myocardial infarction (STEMI) and the guidelines for the management of unstable angina/non-STEMI, oral beta-blockers should be initiated within the first 24 hours unless the patient has signs of heart failure, evidence of a low-output state, an increased risk for cardiogenic shock, or other contraindications. Intravenous use should be reserved for those patients who have refractory hypertension or ongoing ischemia (ACCF/AHA [Anderson, 2013]; ACCF/AHA [O'Gara, 2013]).

Extended release: Treatment of angina pectoris or hypertension; to reduce mortality/hospitalization in patients with heart failure (HF) (stable NYHA Class II or III) already receiving ACE inhibitors, diuretics, and/or digoxin

The ACCF/AHA 2013 heart failure guidelines recommend the use of 1 of 3 beta blockers (ie, bisoprolol, carvedilol, or extended-release metoprolol succinate) for all patients with recent or remote history of MI or ACS and reduced ejection fraction (rEF) to reduce mortality, for all patients with rEF to prevent symptomatic HF (even if no history of MI), and for all patients with current or prior symptoms of HF with reduced ejection fraction (HFrEF), unless contraindicated, to reduce morbidity and mortality (ACCF/AHA [Yancy, 2013]).

The 2014 guideline for the management of high blood pressure in adults (Eighth Joint National Committee [JNC 8]) recommends initiation of pharmacologic treatment to lower blood pressure for the following patients (JNC8 [James, 2013]):

- Patients ≥60 years of age, with systolic blood pressure (SBP) ≥150 mm Hg or diastolic blood pressure (DBP) ≥90 mm Hg. Goal of therapy is SBP <150 mm Hg and DBP <90 mm Hg.
- Patients <60 years of age, with SBP ≥140 mm Hg or DBP ≥90 mm Hg. Goal of therapy is SBP <140 mm Hg and DBP <90 mm Hg.
- Patients ≥18 years of age with diabetes, with SBP ≥140 mm Hg or DBP ≥90 mm Hg. Goal of therapy is SBP <140 mm Hg and DBP <90 mm Hg.
- Patients ≥18 years of age with chronic kidney disease (CKD), with SBP ≥140 mm Hg or DBP ≥90 mm Hg. Goal of therapy is SBP <140 mm Hg and DBP <90 mm Hg.

In patients with CKD, regardless of race or diabetes status, the use of an ACE inhibitor (ACEI) or angiotensin receptor blocker (ARB) as initial therapy is recommended to improve kidney outcomes. In the general nonblack population (without CKD) including those with diabetes, initial antihypertensive treatment should consist of a thiazide-type diuretic, calcium channel blocker, ACEI, or ARB. In the general black population (without CKD) including those with diabetes, initial antihypertensive treatment should consist of a thiazide-type diuretic or a calcium channel blocker **instead of** an ACEI or ARB.

Pregnancy Risk Factor C

Pregnancy Considerations Adverse events were observed in animal studies; therefore, the manufacturer classifies metoprolol as pregnancy category C. Metoprolol crosses the placenta and can be detected in cord blood, amniotic fluid, and the serum of newborn infants. In a cohort study, an increased risk of cardiovascular defects was observed following maternal use of beta-blockers during pregnancy. Intrauterine growth restriction (IUGR), small placentas, as well as fetal/neonatal bradycardia, hypoglycemia, and/or respiratory depression have been observed following *in utero* exposure to beta-blockers as a class. Adequate facilities for monitoring infants at birth should be available. Untreated chronic maternal hypertension and pre-eclampsia are also associated with adverse events in the fetus, infant, and mother. The clearance of metoprolol is increased and serum concentrations and AUC of metoprolol are decreased during pregnancy. Metoprolol has been evaluated for the treatment of hypertension in pregnancy, but other agents may be more appropriate for use.

Breast-Feeding Considerations Small amounts of metoprolol can be detected in breast milk. The manufacturer recommends that caution be exercised when administering metoprolol to nursing women.

Contraindications

Hypersensitivity to metoprolol, any component of the formulation, or other beta-blockers

Note: Additional contraindications are formulation and/or indication specific.

Immediate release tablets/injectable formulation:

Hypertension and angina: Sinus bradycardia; second- and third-degree heart block; cardiogenic shock; overt heart failure; sick sinus syndrome (except in patients with a functioning artificial pacemaker); severe peripheral arterial disease; pheochromocytoma (without alpha blockade)

Myocardial infarction: Severe sinus bradycardia (heart rate <45 beats/minute); significant first-degree heart block (P-R interval ≥0.24 seconds); second- and third-degree heart block; systolic blood pressure <100 mm Hg; moderate-to-severe cardiac failure

Extended release tablet: Severe bradycardia, second- and third degree heart block; cardiogenic shock; decompensated heart failure; sick sinus syndrome (except in patients with a functioning artificial pacemaker)

Warnings/Precautions [U.S. Boxed Warning]: Beta-blocker therapy should not be withdrawn abruptly (particularly in patients with CAD), but gradually tapered over 1-2 weeks to avoid acute tachycardia, hypertension, and/or ischemia. Consider preexisting conditions such as sick sinus syndrome before initiating. Metoprolol commonly produces mild first-degree heart block (P-R interval >0.2-0.24 sec). May also produce severe first- (P-R interval ≥0.26 sec), second-, or third-degree heart block. Patients with acute MI (especially right ventricular MI) have a high risk of developing heart block of varying degrees. If severe heart block occurs, metoprolol should be discontinued and measures to increase heart rate should be employed. Symptomatic hypotension may occur with use. May precipitate or aggravate symptoms of arterial insufficiency in patients with PVD and Raynaud's disease; use with caution and monitor for progression of arterial obstruction. Potentially significant interactions may exist, requiring dose or frequency adjustment, additional monitoring, and/or selection of alternative therapy. Consult drug interactions database for more detailed information.

In general, beta-blockers should be avoided in patients with bronchospastic disease. Metoprolol, with B_1 selectivity, should be used cautiously in bronchospastic disease with close monitoring. Use cautiously in patients with diabetes because it can mask prominent hypoglycemic symptoms. May mask signs of hyperthyroidism (eg, tachycardia); if hyperthyroidism is suspected, carefully manage and monitor; abrupt withdrawal may exacerbate symptoms of hyperthyroidism or precipitate thyroid storm. Alterations in thyroid function tests may be observed. Use caution with hepatic dysfunction. Use with caution in patients with myasthenia gravis or psychiatric disease (may cause CNS depression). Although perioperative beta-blocker therapy is recommended prior to elective surgery in selected patients, use of high-dose extended release metoprolol in patients naïve to beta-blocker therapy undergoing noncardiac surgery has been associated with bradycardia, hypotension, stroke, and death. Chronic beta-blocker therapy should not be routinely withdrawn prior to major surgery. Use of beta-blockers may unmask cardiac failure in patients without a history of dysfunction. Adequate alpha-blockade is required prior to use of any beta-blocker for patients with untreated pheochromocytoma. May induce or exacerbate psoriasis. Use caution with history of severe anaphylaxis to allergens; patients taking beta-blockers may become more sensitive to repeated allergen challenges. Treatment of anaphylaxis (eg, epinephrine) in patients taking beta-blockers may be ineffective or promote undesirable effects. Bradycardia may be observed more frequently in elderly patients (>65 years of age); dosage reductions may be necessary.

Extended release: Use with caution in patients with compensated heart failure; monitor for a worsening of heart failure.

Adverse Reactions

Cardiovascular: Arterial insufficiency (usually Raynaud type), bradycardia, chest pain, CHF, edema (peripheral), first-degree heart block (P-R interval ≥0.26 sec), hypotension, palpitation, syncope

Central nervous system: Confusion, depression, dizziness, fatigue, hallucination, headache, insomnia, memory loss (short-term), nightmares, sleep disturbances, somnolence, vertigo

Dermatology: Photosensitivity, pruritus, psoriasis exacerbated, rash

Endocrine & metabolic: Diabetes exacerbated, libido decreased, Peyronie's disease

Gastrointestinal: Constipation, diarrhea, flatulence, gastrointestinal pain, heartburn, nausea, vomiting, xerostomia

Hematologic: Claudication

Neuromuscular & skeletal: Musculoskeletal pain

Ocular: Blurred vision, visual disturbances

Otic: Tinnitus

Respiratory: Dyspnea, rhinitis, shortness of breath, wheezing

Miscellaneous: Cold extremities

Rare but important or life-threatening: Agranulocytosis, alkaline phosphatase increased, alopecia (reversible), anxiety, arthralgia, arthritis, cardiogenic shock, diaphoresis increased, dry eyes, gangrene, hepatitis, HDL decreased, impotence, jaundice, lactate dehydrogenase increased, nervousness, paresthesia, retroperitoneal fibrosis, second-degree heart block, taste disturbance, third-degree heart block, thrombocytopenia, transaminases increased, triglycerides increased, urticaria, vomiting, weight gain

Other events reported with beta-blockers: Catatonia, emotional lability, fever, hypersensitivity reactions, laryngospasm, nonthrombocytopenic purpura, respiratory distress, thrombocytopenic purpura

Drug Interactions

Metabolism/Transport Effects **Substrate** of CYP2C19 (minor), CYP2D6 (major); **Note:** Assignment of Major/Minor substrate status based on clinically relevant drug interaction potential; **Inhibits** CYP2D6 (weak)

Avoid Concomitant Use

Avoid concomitant use of Metoprolol with any of the following: Ceritinib; Floctafenine; Methacholine

Increased Effect/Toxicity

Metoprolol may increase the levels/effects of: Alpha-/Beta-Agonists (Direct-Acting); Alpha1-Blockers; Alpha2-Agonists; Amifostine; Antihypertensives; Antipsychotic Agents (Phenothiazines); ARIPiprazole; Bradycardia-Causing Agents; Bupivacaine; Cardiac Glycosides; Ceritinib; Cholinergic Agonists; Disopyramide; Ergot Derivatives; Fingolimod; Grass Pollen Allergen Extract (5 Grass Extract); Hypotensive Agents; Insulin; Lacosamide; Levodopa; Lidocaine (Systemic); Lidocaine (Topical); Mepivacaine; Methacholine; Midodrine; Obinutuzumab; RisperiDONE; RiTUXimab; Sulfonylureas

The levels/effects of Metoprolol may be increased by: Abiraterone Acetate; Acetylcholinesterase Inhibitors; Alpha2-Agonists; Aminoquinolines (Antimalarial); Anilidopiperidine Opioids; Antipsychotic Agents (Phenothiazines); Barbiturates; Bretylium; Brimonidine (Topical); Calcium Channel Blockers (Dihydropyridine); Calcium Channel Blockers (Nondihydropyridine); Cobicistat; CYP2D6 Inhibitors; Darunavir; Diazoxide; Dipyridamole; Disopyramide; Dronedarone; Floctafenine; Herbs (Hypotensive Properties); Lercanidipine; MAO Inhibitors; Mirabegron; Nicorandil; Peginterferon Alfa-2b; Pentoxifylline; Phosphodiesterase 5 Inhibitors; Propafenone; Prostacyclin Analogues; Regorafenib; Reserpine; Selective Serotonin Reuptake Inhibitors; Tofacitinib

Decreased Effect

Metoprolol may decrease the levels/effects of: Beta2-Agonists; Lercanidipine; Theophylline Derivatives

The levels/effects of Metoprolol may be decreased by: Barbiturates; Herbs (Hypertensive Properties); Methylphenidate; Mirabegron; Nonsteroidal Anti-Inflammatory Agents; Peginterferon Alfa-2b; Rifamycin Derivatives; Yohimbine

Food Interactions Food increases absorption. Metoprolol serum levels may be increased if taken with food. Management: Take immediate release tartrate tablets with food; succinate can be taken with or without food.

Storage/Stability

Injection: Store at 25°C (77°F); excursions permitted to 15°C to 30°C (59°F to 86°F). Protect from light and heat.

Tablet: Store at 25°C (77°F); excursions permitted to 15°C to 30°C (59°F to 86°F). Protect from moisture and heat.

Mechanism of Action Selective inhibitor of $beta_1$-adrenergic receptors; competitively blocks $beta_1$-receptors, with little or no effect on $beta_2$-receptors at doses <100 mg; does not exhibit any membrane stabilizing or intrinsic sympathomimetic activity

Pharmacodynamics/Kinetics

Onset of action: Peak effect: Oral: 1 to 2 hours (Regårdh, 1980); IV: 20 minutes (when infused over 10 minutes)

Duration: Oral: Immediate release: Variable (dose-related; 50% reduction in maximum heart rate after single doses of 20, 50, and 100 mg occurred at 3.3, 5, and 6.4 hours, respectively), Extended release: ~24 hours; IV: 5 to 8 hours

Absorption: Rapid and complete

Distribution: V_d: 3.2 to 5.6 L/kg

Protein binding: ~10% to albumin

Metabolism: Extensively hepatic via CYP2D6; significant first-pass effect (~50%)

Bioavailability: Oral: Immediate release: ~40% to 50% (Johnsson, 1975); Extended release: 77% relative to immediate release

Half-life elimination: 3 to 4 hours (7 to 9 hours in poor CYP2D6 metabolizers)

Excretion: Urine (<10% as unchanged drug; increased to 30% to 40% in poor CYP2D6 metabolizers)

Dosage

Children: Hypertension: Oral:

1 to 17 years: Immediate release tablet: (National High Blood Pressure Education Program Working Group on High Blood Pressure in Children and Adolescents, 2004): Initial: 1 to 2 mg/kg/day; maximum 6 mg/kg/day (≤200 mg daily); administer in 2 divided doses

≥6 years: Extended release tablet: Initial: 1 mg/kg once daily (maximum initial dose: 50 mg daily). Adjust dose based on patient response (maximum: 2 mg/kg/day or 200 mg daily)

Adults:

Angina: Oral:

Immediate release: Initial: 50 mg twice daily; usual dosage range: 50 to 200 mg twice daily; maximum: 400 mg daily; increase dose at weekly intervals to desired effect

Extended release: Initial: 100 mg daily (maximum: 400 mg daily)

Atrial fibrillation/flutter (ventricular rate control), supraventricular tachycardia (SVT) (acute treatment; off-label use; AHA/ACC/HRS [January 2014]; AHA [Neumar, 2010]): IV: 2.5 to 5 mg every 2 to 5 minutes (maximum total dose: 15 mg over a 10- to 15-minute period). **Note:** Initiate cautiously in patients with concomitant heart failure; avoid in patients with decompensated heart failure; electrical cardioversion preferred.

Maintenance: Oral (immediate release): 25 to 100 mg twice daily; Oral (extended release): 50 to 400 mg once daily

Heart failure: **Note:** Initiate only in stable patients or hospitalized patients after volume status has been optimized and IV diuretics, vasodilators, and inotropic agents have all been successfully discontinued. Caution should be used when initiating in patients who required inotropes during their hospital course. Increase dose gradually and monitor for congestive signs and symptoms of HF making every effort to achieve target dose shown to be effective (ACCF/AHA [Yancy, 2013]; HFSA [Lindenfeld, 2010]; MERIT-HF Study Group, 1999).

Oral (extended release): Initial: 25 mg once daily (reduce to 12.5 mg once daily in NYHA class higher than class II); may double dosage every 2 weeks as tolerated (target dose: 200 mg daily)

ACCF/AHA 2013 Heart Failure Guidelines: Oral (extended release): Initial: 12.5 to 25 mg once daily; maximum daily dose: 200 mg (Yancy, 2013)

Hypertension: Oral:

Immediate release: Initial: 50 mg twice daily; effective dosage range: 100 to 450 mg daily in 2 to 3 divided doses; increase dose at weekly intervals to desired effect; maximum total daily dose: 450 mg; usual dosage range (ASH/ISH [Weber, 2014]): 50 to 100 mg twice daily; target dose (JNC 8 [James, 2013]): 100 to 200 mg daily

Extended release: Initial: 25 to 100 mg once daily; increase doses at weekly (or longer) intervals to desired effect; maximum: 400 mg daily

Hypertension/ventricular rate control: IV (in patients having nonfunctioning GI tract): Initial: 1.25 to 5 mg every 6 to 12 hours; titrate initial dose to response. Initially, low doses may be appropriate to establish response; however, although not routine, up to 15 mg administered as frequently as every 3 hours has been employed in patients with refractory tachycardia.

Myocardial infarction:

Early treatment:

IV: 5 mg every 5 minutes as tolerated for up to 3 doses in the early treatment of ST elevation myocardial infarction; titrate to heart rate and blood pressure; then begin oral therapy. Note: The ACCF/AHA guidelines for the management of STEMI recommend the use of IV metoprolol at the time of presentation in patients with STEMI who are hypertensive or have ongoing ischemia without contraindications. Do not initiate this regimen in those with signs of heart failure, a low output state, increased risk of cardiogenic shock, or other contraindications (eg, second- or third-degree heart block) (ACCF/AHA [O'Gara, 2013]).

Oral: 25 to 50 mg orally every 6 to 12 hours; transition over the next 2 to 3 days to twice daily dosing of metoprolol tartrate (immediate release) or to daily metoprolol succinate (extended release) and increase as tolerated to a maximum daily dose of 200 mg. **Note:** The ACCF/AHA guidelines for the management of STEMI recommend initiation within the first 24 hours. Do not initiate this regimen in those with signs of heart failure, a low output state, increased risk of cardiogenic shock, or other contraindications (eg, second- or third-degree heart block) (ACCF/AHA [O'Gara, 2013]).

Secondary prevention (off-label use): Oral: Immediate release: 25 to 100 mg twice daily; optimize dose based on heart rate and blood pressure; continue indefinitely (Olsson, 1992).

Thyrotoxicosis (off-label use): Oral: Immediate release: 25 to 50 mg every 6 hours; may also consider administering extended release formulation (Bahn, 2011)

Elderly: Hypertension: Initiate at the lower end of the dosage range and titrate to response

Note: Switching dosage forms:

When switching from immediate release metoprolol to extended release, the same total daily dose of metoprolol should be used.

When switching between oral and intravenous dosage forms, in most cases, equivalent beta-blocking effect is achieved when doses in a 2.5:1 (Oral:IV) ratio is used. However, in one bioavailability study including healthy volunteers, a range of Oral:IV conversion ratios was found to be approximately 2:1 to 5:1 (Regardh, 1974). Therefore, patient variability may exist and a specific ratio may not apply to all patients, especially if comorbid conditions are present. For example, based on a range of 2.5:1 to 5:1 ratios, if the patient is receiving a chronic oral dose of 25 mg twice daily (50 mg daily), this would translate to 2.5 to 5 mg IV every 6 hours. Recognizing that patients receiving larger chronic oral doses should not automatically be converted to a large IV dose, consideration should be given to further reducing the initial IV dose and basing subsequent doses on the clinical response (Huckleberry, 2003).

Dosage adjustment in renal impairment: No dosage adjustment necessary.

Dosage adjustment in hepatic impairment: There are no dosage adjustments provided in manufacturer's labeling. However, reduced dose may be necessary due to extensive hepatic metabolism.

Dietary Considerations Immediate release tablets should be taken with food. Extended release tablets may be taken without regard to meals.

Administration

Oral: Extended release tablets may be divided in half; do not crush or chew. Administer immediate release tablets with or immediately following food.

IV: IV dose is much smaller than oral dose. When administered acutely for cardiac treatment, monitor ECG and blood pressure; may administer by rapid infusion (IV push) over 1 minute. May also be administered by slow infusion (ie, 5 to 10 mg of metoprolol in 50 mL of fluid) over ~30 to 60 minutes during less urgent situations (eg, substitution for oral metoprolol).

Monitoring Parameters Acute cardiac treatment: Monitor ECG and blood pressure with IV administration; heart rate and blood pressure with oral administration. IV use in a nonemergency situation: Necessary monitoring for surgical patients who are unable to take oral beta-blockers (because of prolonged ileus) has not been defined. Some institutions require monitoring of baseline and postinfusion heart rate and blood pressure when a patient's response to beta-blockade has not been characterized (ie, the patient's initial dose or following a change in dose). Consult individual institutional policies and procedures.

Dosage Forms

Solution, Intravenous:

Lopressor: 1 mg/mL (5 mL)

Generic: 1 mg/mL (5 mL); 5 mg/5 mL (5 mL)

Tablet, Oral:

Lopressor: 50 mg, 100 mg

Generic: 25 mg, 50 mg, 100 mg

Tablet Extended Release 24 Hour, Oral:

Toprol XL: 25 mg, 50 mg, 100 mg, 200 mg

Generic: 25 mg, 50 mg, 100 mg, 200 mg

Extemporaneous Preparations A 10 mg/mL oral suspension may be made with metoprolol tartrate tablets and one of three different vehicles (cherry syrup; a 1:1 mixture of Ora-Sweet® and Ora-Plus®; or a 1:1 mixture of Ora-Sweet® SF and Ora-Plus®). Crush twelve 100 mg tablets in a mortar and reduce to a fine powder. Add 20 mL of the chosen vehicle and mix to a uniform paste; mix while adding the vehicle in incremental proportions to **almost** 120 mL; transfer to a calibrated bottle, rinse mortar with vehicle, and add quantity of vehicle sufficient to make 120 mL. Label "shake well" and "protect from light". Stable for 60 days.

Allen LV Jr and Erickson MA 3rd, "Stability of Labetalol Hydrochloride, Metoprolol Tartrate, Verapamil Hydrochloride, and Spironolactone With Hydrochlorothiazide in Extemporaneously Compounded Oral Liquids," *Am J Health Syst Pharm*, 1996, 53(19):2304-9.

- ◆ **Metoprolol-25 (Can)** *see* Metoprolol *on page 1350*
- ◆ **Metoprolol-L (Can)** *see* Metoprolol *on page 1350*
- ◆ **Metoprolol Succinate** *see* Metoprolol *on page 1350*
- ◆ **Metoprolol Tartrate** *see* Metoprolol *on page 1350*
- ◆ **Metoprolol Tartrate Injection, USP (Can)** *see* Metoprolol *on page 1350*
- ◆ **Metozolv ODT** *see* Metoclopramide *on page 1345*

Metreleptin (met re LEP tin)

Brand Names: U.S. Myalept

Index Terms Recombinant Methionyl-Human Leptin

Pharmacologic Category Leptin Analog

Use Lipodystrophy: Replacement therapy to treat the complications of leptin deficiency, in addition to diet, in patients with congenital or acquired generalized lipodystrophy. **Note:** Not indicated for use in patients with HIV-related lipodystrophy or for use in patients with metabolic disease (eg, diabetes mellitus, hypertriglyceridemia) without concurrent evidence of congenital or acquired generalized lipodystrophy.

Pregnancy Risk Factor C

Dosage Lipodystrophy: Infants, Children, Adolescents, and Adults: SubQ:

Note: Increase or decrease dose based on clinical response (eg, inadequate metabolic control) or other considerations (eg, tolerability issues, excessive weight loss [especially in pediatric patients]).

Baseline weight ≤40 kg: Initial dose: 0.06 mg/kg once daily; increase or decrease by 0.02 mg/kg daily based on response or adverse effects. Maximum dose: 0.13 mg/kg once daily.

Baseline weight >40 kg: Initial dose: 2.5 mg (males) or 5 mg (females) once daily; increase or decrease by 1.25-2.5 mg daily based on response or adverse effects. Maximum dose: 10 mg once daily.

Discontinuation: When discontinuing therapy in patients with risk factors for pancreatitis (eg, history of pancreatitis, severe hypertriglyceridemia), taper the dose over a 1-week period and monitor triglyceride levels; consider initiating or adjusting the dose of lipid-lowering medications as needed.

Dosage adjustment in renal impairment: There are no dosage adjustments provided in the manufacturer's labeling (has not been studied).

Dosage adjustment in hepatic impairment: There are no dosage adjustments provided in the manufacturer's labeling (has not been studied).

Additional Information Complete prescribing information should be consulted for additional detail.

Dosage Forms

Solution Reconstituted, Subcutaneous:

Myalept: 11.3 mg (1 ea)

- ◆ **Metro** *see* MetroNIDAZOLE (Systemic) *on page 1353*
- ◆ **MetroCream** *see* MetroNIDAZOLE (Topical) *on page 1357*
- ◆ **Metrogel** *see* MetroNIDAZOLE (Topical) *on page 1357*
- ◆ **MetroGel-Vaginal** *see* MetroNIDAZOLE (Topical) *on page 1357*
- ◆ **MetroLotion** *see* MetroNIDAZOLE (Topical) *on page 1357*

MetroNIDAZOLE (Systemic)

(met roe NYE da zole)

Brand Names: U.S. Flagyl; Flagyl ER; Metro

Brand Names: Canada Flagyl; Metronidazole Injection USP; Novo-Nidazol; PMS-Metronidazole

Index Terms Metronidazole Hydrochloride

Pharmacologic Category Amebicide; Antibiotic, Miscellaneous; Antiprotozoal, Nitroimidazole

Use

Amebiasis: Oral immediate release tablet and capsule: Treatment of acute intestinal amebiasis (amebic dysentery) and amebic liver abscess

Limitations of use (oral immediate-release tablet, capsule and injection): When used for amebic liver abscess, may be used concurrently with percutaneous needle aspiration when it is clinically indicated

Anaerobic bacterial infections (caused by *Bacteroides spp*, including the *B. fragilis* group): Oral immediate-release tablet, capsule, and injection:

Bacterial septicemia: Treatment of bacterial septicemia (also caused by *Clostridium spp*)

Bone and joint infections: Treatment (adjunctive therapy) of bone and joint infections

CNS Infections: Treatment of CNS infections, including meningitis and brain abscess

Endocarditis: Treatment of endocarditis

Gynecologic infections: Treatment of gynecologic infections including endometritis, endomyometritis, tubo-ovarian abscess, or postsurgical vaginal cuff infection (also caused by *Clostridium spp*, *Peptococcus spp*, *Peptostreptococcus spp*, and *Fusobacterium spp*)

Intra-abdominal infections: Treatment of intra-abdominal infections, including peritonitis, intra-abdominal abscess and liver abscess (also caused by *Clostridium spp*, *Eubacterium spp*, *Peptococcus spp*, and *Peptostreptococcus spp*)

Lower respiratory tract infections: Treatment of lower respiratory tract infections, including pneumonia, empyema and lung abscess

Skin and skin structure infections: Treatment of skin and skin structure infections (also caused by *Clostridium spp*, *Peptococcus spp*, *Peptostreptococcus spp*, and *Fusobacterium spp*)

Bacterial vaginosis: Oral extended-release tablet: Treatment of bacterial vaginosis in nonpregnant women

Surgical prophylaxis (colorectal surgery): Injection: Preoperative, intraoperative, and postoperative prophylaxis to reduce the incidence of postoperative infection in patients undergoing elective colorectal surgery classified as contaminated or potentially contaminated.

Trichomoniasis: Oral immediate-release tablet, capsule, and injection: Treatment of infections caused by *Trichomonas vaginalis*, including treatment of asymptomatic sexual partners

Pregnancy Risk Factor B

Pregnancy Considerations Adverse events were not observed in animal reproduction studies. Metronidazole crosses the placenta. Cleft lip with or without cleft palate has been reported following first trimester exposure to metronidazole; however, most studies have not shown an increased risk of congenital anomalies or other adverse events to the fetus following maternal use during pregnancy. Because metronidazole was carcinogenic in some animal species, concern has been raised whether metronidazole should be used during pregnancy. Available studies have not shown an increased risk of infant cancer following metronidazole exposure during pregnancy; however, the ability to detect a signal for this may have been limited. Use of metronidazole during the first trimester of pregnancy is contraindicated by the manufacturer.

Metronidazole pharmacokinetics are similar between pregnant and nonpregnant patients (Amon, 1981; Visser, 1984; Wang, 2011). Bacterial vaginosis has been associated with adverse pregnancy outcomes (including preterm labor); metronidazole is recommended for the treatment of symptomatic bacterial vaginosis in pregnant patients (CDC, 2010). Vaginal trichomoniasis has been also associated with adverse pregnancy outcomes (including preterm labor). Treatment may relieve symptoms and prevent sexual transmission; however, metronidazole use has not resulted in reduced perinatal morbidity and should not be used solely to prevent preterm delivery. Some clinicians consider deferring therapy in asymptomatic women until >37 weeks gestation (CDC, 2010). Metronidazole may also be used for the treatment of giardiasis in pregnant women (some sources recommend second and third trimester administration only) (DHHS, 2013; Gardner, 2001) and symptomatic amebiasis during pregnancy (DHHS, 2013; Li, 1996). The use of other agents is preferred when treatment is needed during pregnancy for *Clostridium difficile* (Surawicz, 2013), *Helicobacter pylori* (Mahadevan, 2006), or Crohn disease (Mottet, 2009). Consult current guidelines for appropriate use in pregnant women.

Breast-Feeding Considerations Metronidazole can be detected in breast milk in concentrations similar to the maternal serum. Infant serum concentrations may be near maternal therapeutic concentrations. Due to the potential for tumorigenicity observed in animal studies, the manufacturer recommends a decision be made whether to discontinue nursing or to discontinue the drug, taking into account the importance of treatment to the mother. Alternately, the mother may pump and discard breast milk for 24 hours after the last dose. Some guidelines note if metronidazole is given, breast-feeding should be withheld for 12 to 24 hours after the dose (CDC, 2010). Use of other agents is preferred in some cases, such as when treating breast-feeding women for Crohn disease (Mottet, 2009) or *Clostridium difficile* infection (Surawicz, 2013).

Contraindications Hypersensitivity to metronidazole, nitroimidazole derivatives, or any component of the formulation; pregnant patients (first trimester) with trichomoniasis; use of disulfiram within the past 2 weeks; use of alcohol or propylene glycol-containing products during therapy or within 3 days of therapy discontinuation

Warnings/Precautions [U.S. Boxed Warning]: Possibly carcinogenic based on animal data. Reserve use for conditions described in Use; unnecessary use should be avoided. Use with caution in patients with severe liver impairment and ESRD due to potential accumulation; reduce dosage in patients with severe liver impairment and consider dosage reduction in patients with severe renal impairment (CrCl <10 mL/minute) who are receiving prolonged therapy. Dose should not specifically be reduced in anuric patients (accumulated metabolites may be rapidly removed by dialysis). Hemodialysis patients may need supplemental dosing. Use with caution in patients with blood dyscrasias (monitor CBC with differential at baseline, during and after treatment) or history of seizures.

Aseptic meningitis (symptoms may occur within hours of a dose); encephalopathy (cerebellar toxicity with ataxia, dizziness, dysarthria and/or CNS lesions); seizures; and peripheral and optic neuropathies have been reported especially with increased doses and chronic treatment; monitor and consider discontinuation of therapy if symptoms occur. Prolonged use may result in fungal or bacterial superinfection, including *C. difficile*-associated diarrhea (CDAD) and pseudomembranous colitis; CDAD has been observed >2 months postantibiotic treatment. Guidelines recommend the use of oral metronidazole for initial treatment of mild to moderate *C. difficile* infection and the use of oral vancomycin for initial treatment of severe *C. difficile* infection (with or without IV metronidazole depending on the presence of complications). May treat recurrent mild to moderate infection once with oral metronidazole; avoid use beyond first reoccurrence (Cohen, 2010, Surawicz, 2013). Candidiasis infection (known or unknown) maybe more prominent during metronidazole treatment, antifungal treatment required. If *H. pylori* is not eradicated in patients being treated with metronidazole in a regimen, it should be assumed that metronidazole resistance has occurred and it should not again be used.

Abdominal cramps, nausea, vomiting, headaches, and flushing have been reported with oral and injectable metronidazole and concomitant alcohol consumption; avoid alcoholic beverages or products containing propylene glycol during oral and injectable therapy and for at least 3 days after oral therapy. Use with caution in the elderly; dosage adjustment may be required based on renal and/or hepatic function. Do not use extended-release tablets in patients with severe hepatic impairment (Child-Pugh class C) unless benefit outweighs risk. Use injection with caution in patients with heart failure, edema or other sodium retaining states, including corticosteroid treatment. In patients receiving continuous nasogastric secretion aspiration, sufficient metronidazole may be removed in the aspirate to cause a reduction in serum levels. Potentially significant drug-drug interactions may exist, requiring dose or frequency adjustment, additional monitoring, and/or selection of alternative therapy.

Adverse Reactions

Cardiovascular: Flattened T-wave on ECG, flushing, local thrombophlebitis (IV), syncope

Central nervous system: Aseptic meningitis, ataxia, brain disease, confusion, depression, disulfiram-like reaction (with alcohol), dizziness, dysarthria, dyspareunia, headache, insomnia, irritability, metallic taste, peripheral neuropathy, seizure, vertigo

Dermatologic: Erythematous rash, pruritus, Stevens-Johnson syndrome, toxic epidermal necrolysis, urticaria

Gastrointestinal: Abdominal cramps, abdominal pain, anorexia, constipation, diarrhea, epigastric distress, glossitis, hairy tongue, nausea, pancreatitis (rare), proctitis, stomatitis, vomiting, xerostomia

Genitourinary: Cystitis, dark urine (rare), decreased libido, dysmenorrhea, dysuria, genital pruritus, sensation of pelvic pressure, urinary incontinence, urinary tract infection, urine abnormality, vaginal dryness, vaginitis, vulvovaginal candidiasis

Hematologic & oncologic: Leukopenia (reversible), thrombocytopenia (reversible, rare)

Immunologic: Serum sickness-like reaction (joint pains)

Infection: Bacterial infection, candidiasis

Neuromuscular & skeletal: Weakness

Ophthalmic: Optic neuropathy

Renal: Polyuria

Respiratory: Flu-like symptoms, nasal congestion, pharyngitis, rhinitis, sinusitis, upper respiratory tract infection

Miscellaneous: Fever, lesion (central nervous system, reversible)

Drug Interactions

Metabolism/Transport Effects Substrate of CYP2A6 (minor); **Note:** Assignment of Major/Minor substrate status based on clinically relevant drug interaction potential; **Inhibits** CYP2C9 (weak), CYP3A4 (weak)

Avoid Concomitant Use

Avoid concomitant use of MetroNIDAZOLE (Systemic) with any of the following: Alcohol (Ethyl); BCG; Carbocisteine; Disulfiram; Mebendazole; Pimozide

Increased Effect/Toxicity

MetroNIDAZOLE (Systemic) may increase the levels/effects of: Alcohol (Ethyl); ARIPiprazole; Busulfan; Carbocisteine; Fluorouracil (Systemic); Fosphenytoin; Highest Risk QTc-Prolonging Agents; Hydrocodone; Lomitapide; Lopinavir; Moderate Risk QTc-Prolonging Agents; Phenytoin; Pimozide; Tegafur; Tipranavir; Vitamin K Antagonists

The levels/effects of MetroNIDAZOLE (Systemic) may be increased by: Disulfiram; Mebendazole; Mifepristone

Decreased Effect

MetroNIDAZOLE (Systemic) may decrease the levels/effects of: BCG; Mycophenolate; Sodium Picosulfate; Typhoid Vaccine

The levels/effects of MetroNIDAZOLE (Systemic) may be decreased by: Fosphenytoin; PHENobarbital; Phenytoin; Primidone

Food Interactions Peak antibiotic serum concentration lowered and delayed, but total drug absorbed not affected.

Storage/Stability

Oral:

Extended release: Store at 25°C (77°F); excursions are permitted between 15°C and 30°C (59°F and 86°F).

Immediate release: Store at 15°C to 25°C (59°F to 77°F). Protect the tablets from light.

Injection: Store at 20°C to 25°C (68°F to 77°F). Protect from light. Avoid excessive heat. Do not refrigerate. Do not remove unit from overwrap until ready for use. Discard unused solution.

Mechanism of Action After diffusing into the organism, interacts with DNA to cause a loss of helical DNA structure and strand breakage resulting in inhibition of protein synthesis and cell death in susceptible organisms

Pharmacodynamics/Kinetics

Absorption: Oral: Well absorbed

Distribution: To bile, seminal fluid, bone, liver, and liver abscesses, lung and vaginal secretions; crosses blood-brain barrier; saliva and CSF concentrations similar to those in plasma

Protein binding: <20%

Metabolism: Hepatic (30% to 60%) to several metabolites including an active hydroxyl metabolite

Half-life elimination: ~8 hours

Time to peak, serum: Oral: Immediate release: 1 to 2 hours; Extended release: ~5 hours

Excretion: Urine (unchanged drug and metabolites: 60% to 80%; ~20% of total as unchanged drug); feces (6% to 15%)

Dosage

Indication-specific dosing

Note: Appropriate aerobic organism treatment should be added to regimens, as clinically indicated

Infants, Children, and Adolescents:

Amebiasis: Oral: 35 to 50 mg/kg/day in divided doses every 8 hours for 7 to 10 days (*Red Book* [AAP, 2012])

Trichomoniasis: Oral: 15 mg/kg/day in divided doses every 8 hours for 7 days (*Red Book* [AAP, 2012])

Anaerobic infections (off-label dosing):

Oral: 30 to 50 mg/kg/day in divided doses every 8 hours (maximum: 2250 mg/day) (*Red Book* [AAP, 2012])

IV: 22.5 to 40 mg/kg/day in divided doses every 8 hours (maximum: 1500 mg/day) (*Red Book* [AAP, 2012])

Balantidiasis (off-label use): Oral: 35 to 50 mg/kg/day in 3 divided doses for 5 days (*Red Book* [AAP, 2012]; Schuster, 2008)

Clostridium difficile-associated diarrhea (CDAD; off-label use): Oral: 30 mg/kg/day divided every 6 hours for ≥10 days (maximum: 2 g/day) (*Red Book* [AAP, 2012]; Schutze, 2013). **Note:** Recommended agent for the initial treatment of mild to moderate disease and for first relapse (*Red Book* [AAP, 2012]; Schutze, 2013).

Giardiasis (off-label use): Oral: 15 mg/kg/day in divided doses every 8 hours for 5 to 10 days (Granados, 2012; *Red Book* [AAP, 2012])

Helicobacter pylori eradication (off-label use): Oral: 20 mg/kg/day in 2 divided doses for 10 to 14 days in combination therapy with amoxicillin and either a proton pump inhibitor or bismuth subsalicylate **or** 20 mg/kg/day in 2 divided doses on days 6 through 10 in combination therapy with a proton pump inhibitor and clarithromycin (after treatment with amoxicillin and a proton pump inhibitor for days 1 through 5) (maximum: 1 g/day) (Koletzko, 2011)

Surgical (preoperative) prophylaxis (off-label use):

Infants <1200 g: IV: 7.5 mg/kg within 60 minutes prior to surgical incision in combination with other antibiotics (Bratzler, 2013).

Infants ≥1200 g and Children ≥1 year:

IV: 15 mg/kg within 60 minutes prior to surgical incision in combination with other antibiotics (maximum: 500 mg per dose) (Bratzler, 2013).

Oral (for colorectal surgical prophylaxis only): 15 mg/kg (maximum: 1000 mg) every 3 to 4 hours for 3 doses, starting after mechanical bowel preparation the afternoon and evening before the procedure, with or without additional oral antibiotics and with an appropriate IV antibiotic prophylaxis regimen (Bratzler, 2013).

Tetanus (*Clostridium tetani* infection; off-label use): Oral, IV: 30 mg/kg per day (maximum: 4 g/day) in divided doses every 6 hours for 10 to 14 days in combination with tetanus immune globulin and supportive therapy (*Red Book* [AAP, 2012])

Adolescents: Oral:

Pelvic inflammatory disease (off-label dosing): Refer to adult dosing

Sexual assault (prophylaxis; off-label use): Refer to adult dosing

Vaginal infections:

Vaginitis: (*Trichomonas vaginalis*; off-label use): 2 g as a single dose (*Red Book* [AAP, 2012])

Vaginosis (bacterial; off-label use): 500 mg twice daily for 7 days (*Red Book* [AAP, 2012])

Adults:

Amebiasis (acute dysentery): Oral: Immediate-release tablets and capsules: 750 mg every 8 hours for 5 to 10 days

Amebic liver abscess: Oral:

Immediate-release tablets: 500 to 750 mg every 8 hours for 5 to 10 days

Capsules: 750 mg every 8 hours for 5 to 10 days

Anaerobic infections (diverticulitis, peritonitis, cholangitis, or abscess): Oral (immediate release), IV: 500 mg every 6 to 8 hours (maximum: 4 g/day); **Note:** Initial: 1 g IV loading dose may be administered

Bacterial vaginosis or vaginitis due to *Gardnerella*, *Mobiluncus*: Oral:

Immediate-release tablet: 500 mg twice daily for 7 days (off-label use; CDC, 2010)

Extended-release tablet: 750 mg once daily for 7 days

Intra-abdominal infection:

Manufacturer's labeling: Oral (immediate release), IV: 500 mg every 6 hours (maximum: 4 g/day); **Note:** Initial: 1 g IV loading dose may be administered

Alternate dosing: Complicated, community-acquired, mild to moderate (in combination with cephalosporin or fluoroquinolone; off-label dosing): IV: 500 mg every 8 to 12 hours **or** 1.5 g every 24 hours for 4 to 7 days (provided source controlled) (Solomkin, 2010)

Pelvic inflammatory disease (off-label dosing): Oral (immediate release): 500 mg twice daily for 14 days (in combination with a third generation parenteral cephalosporin and doxycycline) (CDC, 2010)

Trichomoniasis (index case and sex partner): Oral:

Immediate-release tablets:

Manufacturer's labeling: 250 mg every 8 hours for 7 days **or** 1 g twice daily for 2 doses (on same day) **or** 2 g as a single dose

Alternate dosing: 500 mg twice daily for 7 days (CDC, 2010)

Capsules: 375 mg twice daily for 7 days

Trichomoniasis (failure of nitroimidazole [eg metronidazole] therapy in index case; treatment of sex partner; off-label dosing): Oral (immediate release): 500 mg twice daily for 7 days (CDC, 2010)

Balantidiasis (off-label use): IV, Oral (immediate release): 750 mg 3 times daily for ≥5 days (Anagyrou, 2003; Schuster, 2008)

Clostridium difficile-associated diarrhea (CDAD) (off-label use):

Mild to moderate infection: Oral (immediate release): 500 mg 3 times daily for 10 to 14 days (Cohen, 2010; Surawicz, 2013)

Severe complicated infection (no abdominal distention): IV: 500 mg 3 times daily with oral vancomycin for 10 to 14 days (Surawicz, 2013)

Severe complicated infection (with ileus, toxic colitis, and/or abdominal distention): IV: 500 mg 3 times daily with oral and rectal vancomycin for 10 to 14 days (Surawicz, 2013)

Note: Recent guideline recommends converting to oral vancomycin therapy if the patient does not show a clear clinical response after 5 to 7 days of metronidazole therapy (Surawicz, 2013)

Crohn disease (off-label use): Oral. (immediate release): 10 to 20 mg/kg/day; long-term (eg, several months) safety has not been established (Lichtenstein, 2009). **Note:** Reserved for mild to moderate disease in patients not responsive to sulfasalazine and/or who have colonic involvement (eg, ileocolitis and colitis) (Lichtenstein, 2009; Sutherland, 1991).

Dientamoeba fragilis infections (off-label use): Oral (immediate release): 500 to 750 mg 3 times daily for 10 days (CDC, 2012)

Giardiasis (off-label use): Oral (immediate release): 250 to 500 mg 3 times daily for 5 to 10 days (Granados, 2012)

Helicobacter pylori eradication (off-label use): Oral (immediate release):

Triple therapy: Metronidazole 500 mg twice daily for 10 to 14 days, in combination with clarithromycin and a proton pump inhibitor (Chey, 2007)

Quadruple therapy: Metronidazole 250 mg 4 times daily for 10 to 14 days, in combination with bismuth subsalicylate, a tetracycline, and either ranitidine or a proton pump inhibitor (Chey, 2007)

Periodontitis (associated with aggressive disease; off-label use): Oral (immediate release): 250 mg every 8 hours in combination with amoxicillin for 10 days; used in addition to scaling, root planing and pocket irrigation (Silva-Senem, 2013)

Pouchitits (post ileal pouch-anal anastomosis, acute treatment; off-label use): Oral (immediate release): 400 to 500 mg 3 times daily for 7 days (Holubar, 2010; Wall, 2011)

Sexual assault (prophylaxis; off-label use): Oral (immediate release): 2 g as a single dose in combination with ceftriaxone and azithromycin or doxycycline (CDC, 2010; CDC, 2012)

Surgical prophylaxis:

Manufacturer's labeling: IV: 15 mg/kg 1 hour prior to surgical incision; followed by 7.5 mg/kg 6 and 12 hours after initial dose

Alternate dosing:

IV: 500 mg within 60 minutes prior to surgical incision in combination with other antibiotics **Note:** Considered a recommended agent for select procedures other than colorectal surgery (off-label use; Bratzler, 2013).

Oral (for colorectal surgical prophylaxis only; immediate release) (off-label use): 1 g every 3 to 4 hours for 3 doses, starting after mechanical bowel preparation the afternoon and evening before the procedure with or without additional oral antibiotics and with an appropriate IV antibiotic prophylaxis regimen (Bratzler, 2013).

Tetanus (*Clostridium tetani* infection; off-label use): Oral (immediate release): 500 mg every 6 hours for 7 to 10 days in combination with supportive therapy (Ahmadsyah, 1985)

Urethritis (for recurrent or persistent urethritis; off-label use): Oral (immediate release): 2 g as a single dose with azithromycin. **Note:** Compliance with initial regimen and lack of re-exposure to an untreated sex partner should be excluded prior to use (CDC, 2010)

Elderly: Refer to adult dosing.

Dosage adjustment in renal impairment:

Manufacturer's labeling:

Mild, moderate, or severe impairment: There are no dosage adjustments provided in the manufacturer's labeling; however, decreased renal function does not alter the single-dose pharmacokinetics

End-stage renal disease (ESRD) requiring dialysis: Metronidazole metabolites may accumulate; monitor for adverse events. Accumulated metabolites may be rapidly removed by dialysis:

Intermittent hemodialysis (IHD): If administration cannot be separated from hemodialysis, consider supplemental dose following hemodialysis.

Peritoneal dialysis (PD): No dosage adjustment necessary.

Alternate dosing:

Intermittent hemodialysis (IHD) (administer after hemodialysis on dialysis days): Dialyzable (50% to 100%): 500 mg every 8 to 12 hours. **Note:** Dosing regimen highly dependent on clinical indication (trichomoniasis vs *C. difficile* colitis) (Heintz, 2009). **Note:** Dosing dependent on the assumption of thrice weekly, complete IHD sessions.

Continuous renal replacement therapy (CRRT) (Heintz, 2009; Trotman, 2005): Drug clearance is highly dependent on the method of renal replacement, filter type, and flow rate. Appropriate dosing requires close monitoring of pharmacologic response, signs of adverse reactions due to drug accumulation, as well as drug concentrations in relation to target trough (if appropriate). The following are general recommendations only (based on dialysate flow/ultrafiltration rates of 1 to 2 L/hour and minimal residual renal function) and should not supersede clinical judgment:

CVVH/CVVHD/CVVHDF: 500 mg every 6 to 12 hours (or per clinical indication; dosage reduction generally not necessary)

Dosage adjustment in hepatic impairment:

Manufacturer's labeling:

Mild or moderate impairment (Child-Pugh class A or B): No dosage adjustment necessary; use with caution and monitor for adverse events

Severe impairment (Child-Pugh class C):

Extended-release tablets: Use is not recommended.

Immediate-release capsules:

Amebiasis: 375 mg 3 times daily

Trichomoniasis: 375 mg once daily

Immediate-release tablets, injection: Reduce dose by 50%

Alternate dosing: The pharmacokinetics of a single oral 500 mg dose were not altered in patients with cirrhosis; initial dose reduction is therefore not necessary (Daneshmend, 1982). In one study of IV metronidazole, patients with alcoholic liver disease (with or without cirrhosis), demonstrated a prolonged elimination half-life (eg, ~18 hours). The authors recommended the dose be reduced accordingly (clearance was reduced by ~62%) and the frequency may be prolonged (eg, every 12 hours instead of every 6 hours) (Lau, 1987). In another single IV dose study using metronidazole metabolism to predict hepatic function, patients classified as Child-Pugh class C demonstrated a half-life of ~21.5 hours (Muscara, 1995).

Dietary Considerations

Immediate-release tablets and capsules may be administered with food to minimize stomach upset. Extended-release tablets should be taken on an empty stomach (1 hour before or 2 hours after meals).

Sodium: Injectable dosage form may contain sodium.

Ethanol: Use of ethanol is contraindicated during therapy and for 3 days after therapy discontinuation.

Administration

IV: Infuse intravenously over 30 to 60 minutes. Avoid contact of drug solution with equipment containing aluminum.

Oral: Immediate-release tablets and capsules may be administered with food to minimize stomach upset. Extended-release tablets should be administered on an empty stomach (1 hour before or 2 hours after meals); do not split, crush, or chew.

Monitoring Parameters Monitor CBC with differential at baseline and after prolonged or repeated courses of therapy. Closely monitor elderly patients and patients with severe hepatic impairment or ESRD for adverse reactions. Observe patients carefully if neurologic symptoms occur and consider discontinuation of therapy.

Dosage Forms Considerations Parenteral solution contains 28 mEq of sodium/gram of metronidazole.

Dosage Forms

Capsule, Oral:

Flagyl: 375 mg

Generic: 375 mg

Solution, Intravenous:

Metro: 500 mg (100 mL)

Generic: 500 mg (100 mL)

Solution, Intravenous [preservative free]:

Generic: 500 mg (100 mL)

Tablet, Oral:

Flagyl: 250 mg, 500 mg

Generic: 250 mg, 500 mg

Tablet Extended Release 24 Hour, Oral:

Flagyl ER: 750 mg

Extemporaneous Preparations A 50 mg/mL oral suspension may be made with tablets and a 1:1 mixture of Ora-Sweet and Ora-Plus. Crush twenty-four 250 mg tablets in a mortar and reduce to a fine powder. Add small portions of the vehicle and mix to a uniform paste; mix while adding the vehicle in incremental portions to **almost** 120 mL; transfer to a calibrated bottle, rinse mortar with vehicle, and add quantity of vehicle sufficient to make 120 mL. Label "shake well". Stable for 60 days at room temperature or refrigerated (Allen, 1996).

MetroNIDAZOLE (Topical) (met roe NYE da zole)

Brand Names: U.S. MetroCream; Metrogel; MetroGel-Vaginal; MetroLotion; Noritate; Rosadan; Vandazole

Brand Names: Canada MetroCream; Metrogel; MetroLotion; Nidagel; Noritate; Rosasol

Index Terms Metronidazole Hydrochloride

Pharmacologic Category Antibiotic, Topical

Use

Bacterial vaginosis: Vaginal gel: Treatment of bacterial vaginosis

Rosacea: Topical: Treatment of inflammatory lesions and erythema of rosacea

Pregnancy Risk Factor B

Dosage Adults:

Bacterial vaginosis: Vaginal:

0.75% (Vandazole): One applicatorful (~37.5 mg metronidazole) intravaginally once daily for 5 days

0.75% (MetroGel-vaginal, other products): One applicatorful (~37.5 mg metronidazole) intravaginally once or twice daily for 5 days

1.3%: One applicatorful (~65 mg metronidazole) intravaginally as a single dose

Rosacea: Topical:

0.75%: Apply and rub a thin film twice daily, morning and evening, to entire affected areas after washing.

1%: Apply thin film to affected area once daily

Dosage adjustment in renal impairment: There are no dosage adjustments provided in the manufacturer's labeling.

Dosage adjustment in hepatic impairment: There are no dosage adjustments provided in the manufacturer's labeling; use with caution in severe hepatic impairment.

Additional Information Complete prescribing information should be consulted for additional detail.

Dosage Forms

Cream, External:
MetroCream: 0.75% (45 g)
Noritate: 1% (60 g)
Rosadan: 0.75% (45 g)
Generic: 0.75% (45 g)

Gel, External:
Metrogel: 1% (55 g, 60 g)
Rosadan: 0.75% (45 g)
Generic: 0.75% (45 g); 1% (55 g, 60 g)

Gel, Vaginal:
MetroGel-Vaginal: 0.75% (70 g)
Vandazole: 0.75% (70 g)
Generic: 0.75% (70 g)

Kit, External:
Rosadan: 0.75%

Lotion, External:
MetroLotion: 0.75% (59 mL)
Generic: 0.75% (59 mL)

Metronidazole and Nystatin [CAN/INT]

(met roe NYE da zole & nye STAT in)

Brand Names: Canada Flagystatin

Index Terms Nystatin and Metronidazole

Pharmacologic Category Antifungal Agent, Vaginal; Antiprotozoal, Nitroimidazole

Use Note: Not approved in U.S.

Treatment of mixed vaginal infection due to *T. vaginalis* and *C. albicans*

Pregnancy Considerations Metronidazole crosses the placenta; information for nystatin is not available although systemic absorption is unlikely. The manufacturer does not recommend use of metronidazole during the first trimester of pregnancy or use of this combination product with the applicator after the seventh month of pregnancy. This combination product may decrease the effectiveness of condoms or diaphragms; other forms of contraception should be used during therapy. Also refer to individual agents.

Breast-Feeding Considerations Metronidazole is excreted in breast milk; information for nystatin is not available although systemic absorption is unlikely. The manufacturer of this combination product recommends that use in breast-feeding women be avoided. Also refer to individual agents.

Contraindications Hypersensitivity to metronidazole, nystatin, imidazoles, or any component of the formulation. Combined treatment with oral metronidazole should be avoided in active neurological disorders or in patients with a history of blood dyscrasia, hypothyroidism, or hypoadrenalism (unless the benefits outweigh the possible risk to the patient).

Also refer to Metronidazole (Systemic) monograph.

Warnings/Precautions Metronidazole is possibly carcinogenic based on animal studies. Flagystatin® may not be effective in bacterial vaginal infections and should not be prescribed unless there is direct evidence of trichomonal infestation or candidiasis. Nystatin possesses little or no antibacterial activity while metronidazole is selective against certain anaerobic bacteria. Candidiasis confirmation should be followed up with identification of promoting factors so they can be offset or eliminated. It is recommended that treatment of *Candida* involve all associated sites concurrently (intestinal, vaginal, or other infections).

Sexual partners should receive concurrent treatment (oral metronidazole) when there is evidence of trichomonal infestation. Systemic absorption of metronidazole from vaginal administration may occur. Adverse effects normally associated with systemic administration of metronidazole may occur following the vaginal administration. Prolonged use may result in fungal or bacterial superinfection, including *C. difficile*-associated diarrhea (CDAD) and pseudomembranous colitis; CDAD has been observed >2 months postantibiotic treatment.

Consult additional warnings in Metronidazole (Systemic) monograph when used concurrently with systemic metronidazole. Disulfiram-like reactions to ethanol have been reported with systemic metronidazole and may occur with topical metronidazole; consider avoidance of alcoholic beverages during therapy with topical products and for at least 1 day after. Central or peripheral neuropathy may occur with metronidazole treatment. Monitor and consider discontinuation of therapy if ataxia or other CNS signs/symptoms occur; use with caution in patients with CNS disease. Use caution in patients with hepatic encephalopathy. Total and differential leukocyte counts should be conducted before and after treatment. Patients should be informed that urine may become a darker color.

Use of soaps with an acid pH, vaginal injections, and tampons may promote fungal replication and should be avoided during treatment. Use may limit the effectiveness of diaphragms and condoms; concurrent use with treatment is not recommended.

Adverse Reactions See individual agents.

Drug Interactions

Metabolism/Transport Effects None known.

Avoid Concomitant Use

Avoid concomitant use of Metronidazole and Nystatin with any of the following: BCG

Increased Effect/Toxicity

Metronidazole and Nystatin may increase the levels/effects of: Alcohol (Ethyl); Disulfiram; Lopinavir; Tipranavir

Decreased Effect

Metronidazole and Nystatin may decrease the levels/effects of: BCG; Sodium Picosulfate

Storage/Stability

Vaginal ovules: Store at room temperature of 15°C to 25°C (59°F to 77°F). Protect from light.

Vaginal cream: Store at room temperature of 15°C to 30°C (59°F to 86°F).

Mechanism of Action See individual agents.

Pharmacodynamics/Kinetics See individual agents.

Dosage Intravaginal: Adults:

Vaginal tablet (ovule): Insert 1 tablet daily at bedtime for 10 consecutive days. May repeat for an additional 10 days if cure is not achieved.

Vaginal cream: Insert 1 applicatorful daily at bedtime for 10 consecutive days. May repeat for an additional 10 days if cure is not achieved.

Note: Applicator should not be used after the seventh month of pregnancy. If *Trichomonas vaginalis* is not completely eliminated, oral (systemic) metronidazole (250 mg twice daily for 10 days) should be administered.

Product Availability Not available in U.S.

Dosage Forms: Canada

Cream, vaginal:
Flagystatin®: Metronidazole 500 mg and nystatin 100,000 units per applicatorful (55 g)

Tablet, vaginal:
Flagystatin® Ovule: Metronidazole 500 mg and nystatin 100,000 units (10s)

◆ **Metronidazole Hydrochloride** *see* MetroNIDAZOLE (Systemic) *on page 1353*

◆ **Metronidazole Hydrochloride** *see* MetroNIDAZOLE (Topical) *on page 1357*

◆ **Metronidazole Injection USP (Can)** *see* MetroNIDAZOLE (Systemic) *on page 1353*

◆ **MET Tyrosine Kinase Inhibitor PF-02341066** *see* Crizotinib *on page 511*

◆ **Metvix (Can)** *see* Methyl Aminolevulinate *on page 1332*

◆ **Metvixia** *see* Methyl Aminolevulinate *on page 1332*

Metyrosine (me TYE roe seen)

Brand Names: U.S. Demser
Index Terms AMPT; OGMT
Pharmacologic Category Tyrosine Hydroxylase Inhibitor
Use Short-term management of pheochromocytoma before surgery, long-term management when surgery is contraindicated or when chronic malignant pheochromocytoma exists
Pregnancy Risk Factor C
Dosage Oral: Children ≥12 years and Adults: Initial: 250 mg 4 times/day, increased by 250-500 mg/day up to 4 g/day in 4 divided doses; titrate hypertensive patients to achieve normal blood pressure and symptom control and titrate normotensive patients to reduce catecholamines by ≥50%. Usual maintenance: 2-3 g/day in 4 divided doses; for preoperative preparation, administer optimum effective dosage for 5-7 days.

Dosing adjustment in renal impairment: No dosage adjustment provided in manufacturer's labeling.
Dosing adjustment in hepatic impairment: No dosage adjustment provided in manufacturer's labeling.

Additional Information Complete prescribing information should be consulted for additional detail.
Dosage Forms
Capsule, Oral:
Demser: 250 mg

◆ **Mevacor** *see* Lovastatin *on page 1252*

◆ **Mevinolin** *see* Lovastatin *on page 1252*

Mexiletine (meks IL e teen)

Brand Names: Canada Novo-Mexiletine
Pharmacologic Category Antiarrhythmic Agent, Class Ib
Use Management of serious ventricular arrhythmias; suppression of PVCs
Pregnancy Risk Factor C
Dosage Adults: Oral: Initial: 200 mg every 8 hours (may load with 400 mg if necessary); adjust dose every 2-3 days; usual dose: 200-300 mg every 8 hours; maximum dose: 1.2 g/day (some patients respond to every 12-hour dosing). When switching from another antiarrhythmic, initiate a 200 mg dose 6-12 hours after stopping former agents, 3-6 hours after stopping procainamide.

Dosage adjustment in renal impairment: No dosage adjustment necessary.
Dosage adjustment in hepatic impairment: Patients with hepatic impairment or hepatic congestion secondary to heart failure may require dose reduction; half-life is approximately doubled in patients with hepatic impairment.

Additional Information Complete prescribing information should be consulted for additional detail.
Dosage Forms
Capsule, Oral:
Generic: 150 mg, 200 mg, 250 mg

◆ **Mezavant (Can)** *see* Mesalamine *on page 1301*

◆ **$MgSO_4$ (error-prone abbreviation)** *see* Magnesium Sulfate *on page 1265*

◆ **Miacalcin** *see* Calcitonin *on page 322*

◆ **Mi-Acid [OTC]** *see* Aluminum Hydroxide, Magnesium Hydroxide, and Simethicone *on page 104*

◆ **Mi-Acid Double Strength [OTC]** *see* Calcium Carbonate and Magnesium Hydroxide *on page 328*

◆ **Mi-Acid Maximum Strength [OTC] [DSC]** *see* Aluminum Hydroxide, Magnesium Hydroxide, and Simethicone *on page 104*

◆ **Micaderm [OTC]** *see* Miconazole (Topical) *on page 1360*

Micafungin (mi ka FUN gin)

Brand Names: U.S. Mycamine
Brand Names: Canada Mycamine
Index Terms Micafungin Sodium
Pharmacologic Category Antifungal Agent, Parenteral; Echinocandin
Use
Candidemia, acute disseminated candidiasis, *Candida* peritonitis and abscesses: Treatment of candidemia, acute disseminated candidiasis, *Candida* peritonitis and abscesses
Esophageal candidiasis: Treatment of esophageal candidiasis
Prophylaxis of *Candida* infections: Prophylaxis of *Candida* infections in patients undergoing hematopoietic stem cell transplantation (HSCT)

Pregnancy Risk Factor C
Pregnancy Considerations Adverse events have been observed in animal reproduction studies. There are no adequate and well-controlled studies in pregnant women. Use only if benefit outweighs risk.
Breast-Feeding Considerations It is not known if micafungin is excreted in breast milk. The manufacturer recommends that caution be exercised when administering micafungin to nursing women.
Contraindications Hypersensitivity to micafungin, other echinocandins, or any component of the formulation
Warnings/Precautions Severe anaphylactic reactions, including shock, have been reported. New-onset or worsening hepatic impairment, including hepatitis and hepatic failure, has been reported. Monitor closely and evaluate appropriateness of continued use in patients who develop abnormal liver function tests during treatment. Hemolytic anemia and hemoglobinuria have been reported. Increased BUN, serum creatinine, renal dysfunction, and/or acute renal failure has been reported; use with caution in patients that develop worsening renal function during treatment; monitor closely.
Adverse Reactions
Cardiovascular: Atrial fibrillation, bradycardia, cardiac arrest, edema, hypertension, hypotension, localized phlebitis, myocardial infarction, pericardial effusion, peripheral edema, tachycardia
Central nervous system: Anxiety, brain disease, convulsions, delirium, dizziness, fatigue, headache, insomnia, intracranial hemorrhage, rigors
Dermatologic: Pruritus (more common in pediatric patients ages 3 days through 16 years), skin rash, urticaria (more common in pediatric patients ages 3 days through 16 years)
Endocrine & metabolic: Hyperglycemia, hyperkalemia, hypernatremia, hypervolemia, hypocalcemia, hypoglycemia, hypokalemia, hypomagnesemia
Gastrointestinal: Abdominal distension, abdominal pain, anorexia, constipation, diarrhea, dyspepsia, mucositis, nausea, vomiting

Genitourinary: Decreased urine output, hematuria
Hematologic & oncologic: Anemia (more common in pediatric patients ages 3 days through 16 years), blood coagulation disorder, febrile neutropenia, neutropenia, pancytopenia, thrombocytopenia, thrombotic thrombocytopenic purpura
Hepatic: Abnormal hepatic function tests (more common in pediatric patients ages 3 days through 16 years), hepatic failure, hepatic injury, hepatomegaly, hyperbilirubinemia (more common in pediatric patients ages 3 days through 16 years), increased serum alkaline phosphatase, increased serum ALT (more common in pediatric patients ages 3 days through 16 years), increased serum AST, jaundice
Hypersensitivity: Anaphylaxis, hypersensivity reaction
Infection: Bacteremia, sepsis
Local: Venous thrombosis at injection site
Neuromuscular & skeletal: Back pain
Renal: Renal failure
Respiratory: Cough, dyspnea, epistaxis
Miscellaneous: Fever (more common in pediatric patients ages 3 days through 16 years), infusion related reaction (more common in pediatric patients ages 3 days through 16 years)
Rare but important or life-threatening: Acidosis, acute renal failure, anaphylactoid reaction, anuria, apnea, cardiac arrhythmia, cyanosis, decreased white blood cell count, deep vein thrombosis, disseminated intravascular coagulation, erythema multiforme, hemoglobinuria, hemolysis, hemolytic anemia, hepatic insufficiency, hepatitis, hiccups, hyponatremia, hypoxia, increased blood urea nitrogen, increased serum creatinine, infection, injection site reaction, oliguria, pneumonia, pulmonary embolism, renal insufficiency, renal tubular necrosis, seizure, shock, skin necrosis, Stevens-Johnson syndrome, thrombophlebitis, tissue necrosis at injection site, toxic epidermal necrolysis, vasodilatation

Drug Interactions

Metabolism/Transport Effects Substrate of CYP3A4 (minor); **Note:** Assignment of Major/Minor substrate status based on clinically relevant drug interaction potential; **Inhibits** CYP3A4 (weak)

Avoid Concomitant Use

Avoid concomitant use of Micafungin with any of the following: Pimozide; Saccharomyces boulardii

Increased Effect/Toxicity

Micafungin may increase the levels/effects of: ARIPiprazole; Dofetilide; Hydrocodone; Lomitapide; Pimozide

Decreased Effect

Micafungin may decrease the levels/effects of: Saccharomyces boulardii

Preparation for Administration Aseptically add 5 mL of NS (preservative free) or D_5W to each 50 or 100 mg vial. To minimize foaming, gently swirl to dissolve; do not shake. Further dilute 50-150 mg in 100 mL NS or D_5W (when used in children the final concentration should be between 0.5-4 mg/mL; concentrations >1.5 mg/mL should be administered via central catheter). Protect infusion solution from light (it is not necessary to protect the drip chamber or tubing from light).

Storage/Stability Store at 25°C (77°F); excursions permitted to 15°C to 30°C (59°F to 86°F). Reconstituted and diluted solutions are stable for 24 hours at room temperature. Protect infusion solution from light (it is not necessary to protect the drip chamber or tubing from light).

Mechanism of Action Concentration-dependent inhibition of 1,3-beta-D-glucan synthase resulting in reduced formation of 1,3-beta-D-glucan, an essential polysaccharide comprising 30% to 60% of *Candida* cell walls (absent in mammalian cells); decreased glucan content leads to osmotic instability and cellular lysis

Pharmacodynamics/Kinetics

Distribution: 0.28-0.5 L/kg
Protein binding: >99%; primarily to albumin
Metabolism: Hepatic; forms M-1 (catechol), M-2 (methoxy), and M-5 metabolites (activity unknown)
Half-life elimination: Children: 5-22 hours; Adults: 11-21 hours
Excretion: Primarily feces (71%); urine (<15%)

Dosage

Candidemia, acute disseminated candidiasis, and *Candida* peritonitis and abscesses: IV:
Infants ≥4 months, Children, and Adolescents: 2 mg/kg once daily; maximum: 100 mg once daily
Adults: 100 mg once daily; mean duration of therapy (from clinical trials) was 15 days (range: 10 to 47 days)
Esophageal candidiasis: IV:
Infants ≥4 months, Children, and Adolescents:
≤30 kg: 3 mg/kg once daily
>30 kg: 2.5 mg/kg once daily; maximum: 150 mg once daily
Adults: 150 mg once daily; mean duration of therapy (from clinical trials) was 15 days (range: 10 to 30 days)
Prophylaxis of *Candida* infection in hematopoietic stem cell transplantation: IV:
Infants ≥4 months, Children, and Adolescents: 1 mg/kg once daily; maximum: 50 mg once daily
Adults: 50 mg once daily; mean duration of therapy (from clinical trials) was 19 days (range: 6 to 51 days)
Primary antifungal prophylaxis in allogeneic HSCT (when fluconazole is contraindicated; off-label dosing/population; pediatric guideline recommendation): Infants ≥1 month, Children, and Adolescents <19 years: IV: 1 mg/kg once daily; maximum: 50 mg once daily (Science, 2014)

Dosage adjustment in renal impairment: No dosage adjustment necessary.
Poorly dialyzed; no supplemental dose or dosage adjustment necessary, including patients on intermittent hemodialysis.

Dosage adjustment in hepatic impairment: No dosage adjustment necessary.

Administration For intravenous use only; infuse over 1 hour. When used in children, administer infusions >1.5 mg/mL via central catheter to minimize risk of infusion reactions. Flush line with NS prior to administration.

Monitoring Parameters Liver function tests

Dosage Forms

Solution Reconstituted, Intravenous:
Mycamine: 50 mg (1 ea); 100 mg (1 ea)

Solution Reconstituted, Intravenous [preservative free]:
Mycamine: 50 mg (1 ea); 100 mg (1 ea)

- ◆ **Micafungin Sodium** *see* Micafungin *on page 1359*
- ◆ **Micanol® (Can)** *see* Anthralin *on page 150*
- ◆ **Micardis** *see* Telmisartan *on page 1988*
- ◆ **Micardis HCT** *see* Telmisartan and Hydrochlorothiazide *on page 1990*
- ◆ **Micardis Plus (Can)** *see* Telmisartan and Hydrochlorothiazide *on page 1990*
- ◆ **Micatin [OTC]** *see* Miconazole (Topical) *on page 1360*
- ◆ **Micatin® (Can)** *see* Miconazole (Topical) *on page 1360*
- ◆ **Miconazole 3** *see* Miconazole (Topical) *on page 1360*
- ◆ **Miconazole 3 Combo Pack [OTC]** *see* Miconazole (Topical) *on page 1360*
- ◆ **Miconazole 7 [OTC]** *see* Miconazole (Topical) *on page 1360*

Miconazole (Topical) (mi KON a zole)

Brand Names: U.S. Aloe Vesta Antifungal [OTC]; Antifungal [OTC]; Azolen Tincture [OTC]; Baza Antifungal [OTC]; Carrington Antifungal [OTC]; Critic-Aid Clear AF [OTC]; Cruex Prescription Strength [OTC]; DermaFungal

[OTC]; Desenex Jock Itch [OTC]; Desenex Spray [OTC]; Desenex [OTC]; Fungoid Tincture [OTC]; Lotrimin AF Deodorant Powder [OTC]; Lotrimin AF Jock Itch Powder [OTC]; Lotrimin AF Powder [OTC]; Lotrimin AF [OTC]; Micaderm [OTC]; Micatin [OTC]; Miconazole 3; Miconazole 3 Combo Pack [OTC]; Miconazole 7 [OTC]; Micro Guard [OTC]; Miranel AF [OTC]; Mitrazol [OTC]; Podactin [OTC]; Remedy Antifungal [OTC]; Secura Antifungal Extra Thick [OTC]; Secura Antifungal [OTC]; Soothe & Cool INZO Antifungal [OTC]; Triple Paste AF [OTC]; Vagistat-3 [OTC]; Zeasorb-AF [OTC]

Brand Names: Canada Dermazole; Micatin®; Micozole; Monistat®; Monistat® 3

Index Terms Miconazole Nitrate

Pharmacologic Category Antifungal Agent, Imidazole Derivative; Antifungal Agent, Topical; Antifungal Agent, Vaginal

Use Treatment of vulvovaginal candidiasis and a variety of skin and mucous membrane fungal infections

Dosage

Topical: Children and Adults: **Note:** Not for OTC use in children <2 years:

- Tinea corporis: Apply twice daily for 4 weeks
- Tinea pedis: Apply twice daily for 4 weeks
  - Effervescent tablet: Dissolve 1 tablet in ~1 gallon of water; soak feet for 15-30 minutes; pat dry
- Tinea cruris: Apply twice daily for 2 weeks

Vaginal: Children ≥12 years and Adults: Vulvovaginal candidiasis:

- Cream, 2%: Insert 1 applicatorful at bedtime for 7 days
- Cream, 4%: Insert 1 applicatorful at bedtime for 3 days
- Suppository, 100 mg: Insert 1 suppository at bedtime for 7 days
- Suppository, 200 mg: Insert 1 suppository at bedtime for 3 days
- Suppository, 1200 mg: Insert 1 suppository (a one-time dose); may be used at bedtime or during the day

Note: Many products are available as a combination pack, with a suppository for vaginal instillation and cream to relieve external symptoms. External cream may be used twice daily, as needed, for up to 7 days.

Additional Information Complete prescribing information should be consulted for additional detail.

Dosage Forms

Aerosol, External:
- Desenex Spray [OTC]: 2% (133 g)
- Lotrimin AF [OTC]: 2% (150 g)

Aerosol Powder, External:
- Cruex Prescription Strength [OTC]: 2% (85 g)
- Desenex Jock Itch [OTC]: 2% (113 g)
- Desenex Spray [OTC]: 2% (113 g)
- Lotrimin AF Deodorant Powder [OTC]: 2% (133 g)
- Lotrimin AF Jock Itch Powder [OTC]: 2% (133 g)
- Lotrimin AF Powder [OTC]: 2% (133 g)

Cream, External:
- Antifungal [OTC]: 2% (14 g, 28 g, 42.5 g, 113 g, 198 g)
- Baza Antifungal [OTC]: 2% (4 g, 57 g, 142 g)
- Carrington Antifungal [OTC]: 2% (141 g)
- Micaderm [OTC]: 2% (30 g)
- Micatin [OTC]: 2% (14 g)
- Micro Guard [OTC]: 2% (57 g)
- Podactin [OTC]: 2% (28.35 g)
- Remedy Antifungal [OTC]: 2% (118 mL)
- Secura Antifungal [OTC]: 2% (57 g)
- Secura Antifungal Extra Thick [OTC]: 2% (92 g)
- Soothe & Cool INZO Antifungal [OTC]: 2% (56.7 g, 141.7 g)
- Generic: 2% (15 g, 28.4 g, 30 g)

Cream, Vaginal:
- Miconazole 7 [OTC]: 2% (45 g)
- Generic: 2% (45 g)

Kit, External:
- Fungoid Tincture [OTC]: 2%

Kit, Vaginal:
- Miconazole 3 Combo Pack [OTC]: Cream, topical: 2% (9 g) and Suppository, vaginal: 200 mg (3s)
- Vagistat-3 [OTC]: Cream, topical: 2% (9 g) and Suppository, vaginal: 200 mg (3s)

Lotion, External:
- Zeasorb-AF [OTC]: 2% (56 g)

Ointment, External:
- Aloe Vesta Antifungal [OTC]: 2% (56 g, 141 g)
- Critic-Aid Clear AF [OTC]: 2% (4 g, 57 g, 142 g)
- DermaFungal [OTC]: 2% (113 g)
- Triple Paste AF [OTC]: 2% (56.7 g)

Powder, External:
- Desenex [OTC]: 2% (43 g, 85 g)
- Lotrimin AF [OTC]: 2% (90 g)
- Micro Guard [OTC]: 2% (85 g)
- Mitrazol [OTC]: 2% (30 g)
- Remedy Antifungal [OTC]: 2% (85 g)
- Zeasorb-AF [OTC]: 2% (71 g)

Solution, External:
- Azolen Tincture [OTC]: 2% (29.57 mL)
- Fungoid Tincture [OTC]: 2% (29.57 mL)
- Miranel AF [OTC]: 2% (28 g)

Suppository, Vaginal:
- Miconazole 7 [OTC]: 100 mg (7 ea)
- Miconazole 3: 200 mg (3 ea)
- Generic: 100 mg (7 ea)

- ◆ **Miconazole Nitrate** *see* Miconazole (Topical) *on page 1360*
- ◆ **Micozole (Can)** *see* Miconazole (Topical) *on page 1360*
- ◆ **MICRhoGAM Ultra-Filtered Plus** *see* Rh_o(D) Immune Globulin *on page 1794*
- ◆ **Microgestin 1.5/30** *see* Ethinyl Estradiol and Norethindrone *on page 808*
- ◆ **Microgestin 1/20** *see* Ethinyl Estradiol and Norethindrone *on page 808*
- ◆ **Microgestin Fe 1.5/30** *see* Ethinyl Estradiol and Norethindrone *on page 808*
- ◆ **Microgestin Fe 1/20** *see* Ethinyl Estradiol and Norethindrone *on page 808*
- ◆ **Micro Guard [OTC]** *see* Miconazole (Topical) *on page 1360*
- ◆ **Micro-K** *see* Potassium Chloride *on page 1687*
- ◆ **Micro-K Extencaps (Can)** *see* Potassium Chloride *on page 1687*
- ◆ **Micronase** *see* GlyBURIDE *on page 972*
- ◆ **Micronefrin [OTC] [DSC]** *see* EPINEPHrine (Systemic, Oral Inhalation) *on page 735*
- ◆ **Micronized Colestipol HCl** *see* Colestipol *on page 504*
- ◆ **Micronor® (Can)** *see* Norethindrone *on page 1473*
- ◆ **Microzide** *see* Hydrochlorothiazide *on page 1009*
- ◆ **Midamor (Can)** *see* AMILoride *on page 113*

Midazolam (MID aye zoe lam)

Brand Names: Canada Midazolam Injection

Index Terms Midazolam Hydrochloride; Versed

Pharmacologic Category Benzodiazepine

Use Preoperative sedation; moderate sedation prior to diagnostic or radiographic procedures; ICU sedation (continuous infusion); induction and maintenance of general anesthesia

Pregnancy Risk Factor D

Pregnancy Considerations Adverse events were not observed in animal reproduction studies. Midazolam has been found to cross the human placenta and can be detected in the serum of the umbilical vein and artery, as well as the amniotic fluid. Teratogenic effects have been observed with some benzodiazepines; however, additional studies are needed. The incidence of premature birth and low birth weights may be increased following maternal use of benzodiazepines; hypoglycemia and respiratory problems in the neonate may occur following exposure late in pregnancy. Neonatal withdrawal symptoms may occur within days to weeks after birth and "floppy infant syndrome" (which also includes withdrawal symptoms) have been reported with some benzodiazepines (Bergman, 1992; Iqbal, 2002; Wikner, 2007).

Breast-Feeding Considerations Midazolam and hydroxymidazolam can be detected in breast milk. Based on information from two women, 2-3 months postpartum, the half-life of midazolam in breast milk is ~1 hour. Milk concentrations were below the limit of detection (<5 nmol/L) 4 hours after a single maternal dose of midazolam 15 mg. Drowsiness, lethargy, or weight loss in nursing infants have been observed in case reports following maternal use of some benzodiazepines (Iqbal, 2002; Matheson, 1990). The manufacturer recommends that caution be exercised when administering midazolam to nursing women.

Contraindications Hypersensitivity to midazolam or any component of the formulation; intrathecal or epidural injection of parenteral forms containing preservatives (ie, benzyl alcohol); acute narrow-angle glaucoma; concurrent use of potent inhibitors of CYP3A4 (amprenavir, atazanavir, or ritonavir)

Per respective protease inhibitor manufacturer's labeling: Concurrent use of oral midazolam with amprenavir, atazanavir, darunavir, indinavir, lopinavir-ritonavir, nelfinavir, ritonavir, saquinavir, tipranavir and concurrent use of oral or injectable midazolam with fosamprenavir

Warnings/Precautions **[U.S. Boxed Warning]: May cause severe respiratory depression, respiratory arrest, or apnea. Use with extreme caution, particularly in noncritical care settings.** Appropriate resuscitative equipment and qualified personnel must be available for administration and monitoring. Initial dosing must be cautiously titrated and individualized, particularly in elderly or debilitated patients, patients with hepatic impairment (including alcoholics), or in renal impairment, particularly if other CNS depressants (including opioids) are used concurrently. **[U.S. Boxed Warning]: Initial doses in elderly or debilitated patients should be conservative; as little as 1 mg, but not to exceed 2.5 mg.** Use with caution in patients with respiratory disease or impaired gag reflex. Use during upper airway procedures may increase risk of hypoventilation. Prolonged responses have been noted following extended administration by continuous infusion (possibly due to metabolite accumulation) or in the presence of drugs which inhibit midazolam metabolism.

Causes CNS depression (dose-related) resulting in sedation, dizziness, confusion, or ataxia which may impair physical and mental capabilities. Patients must be cautioned about performing tasks which require mental alertness (eg, operating machinery or driving). A minimum of 1 day should elapse after midazolam administration before attempting these tasks. Use with caution in patients receiving other CNS depressants or psychoactive agents. Effects with other sedative drugs or ethanol may be potentiated. Benzodiazepines have been associated with falls and traumatic injury and should be used with extreme caution in patients who are at risk of these events (especially the elderly).

Use with caution in patients receiving CYP3A4 inhibitors; may result in more intense and prolonged sedation; consider reducing midazolam dose and anticipate potential for prolongation and intensity of effect. The concurrent use of all protease inhibitors is contraindicated with oral midazolam per their respective manufacturer's labeling. The concurrent use of fosamprenavir is contraindicated with both oral and parenteral forms of midazolam.

May cause hypotension - hemodynamic events are more common in pediatric patients or patients with hemodynamic instability. Hypotension and/or respiratory depression may occur more frequently in patients who have received opioid analgesics. Use with caution in obese patients, chronic renal failure, and HF. Does not protect against increases in heart rate or blood pressure during intubation. Should not be used in shock, coma, or acute alcohol intoxication. **[U.S. Boxed Warning]: Do not administer by rapid IV injection in neonates; severe hypotension and seizures have been reported; risk may be increased with concomitant fentanyl use.**

Avoid intra-arterial administration or extravasation of parenteral formulation. Some formulations may contain cherry flavoring.

Midazolam causes anterograde amnesia. Paradoxical reactions, including hyperactive or aggressive behavior have been reported with benzodiazepines, particularly in adolescent/pediatric or psychiatric patients; may consider treatment with flumazenil (Massanari, 1997). Does not have analgesic, antidepressant, or antipsychotic properties.

Benzodiazepines have been associated with dependence and acute withdrawal symptoms on discontinuation or reduction in dose. Acute withdrawal, including seizures, may be precipitated after administration of flumazenil to patients receiving long-term benzodiazepine therapy. Midazolam is a short half-life benzodiazepine and may be of benefit in patients where a rapidly and short-acting agent is desired (acute agitation). Tolerance develops to the sedative and anticonvulsant effects. It does not develop to the anxiolytic effects (Vinkers, 2012).

Benzyl alcohol and derivatives: Some dosage forms may contain benzyl alcohol; large amounts of benzyl alcohol (≥99 mg/kg/day) have been associated with a potentially fatal toxicity ("gasping syndrome") in neonates; the "gasping syndrome" consists of metabolic acidosis, respiratory distress, gasping respirations, CNS dysfunction (including convulsions, intracranial hemorrhage), hypotension, and cardiovascular collapse (AAP, 1997; CDC, 1982); some data suggests that benzoate displaces bilirubin from protein binding sites (Ahlfors, 2001); avoid or use dosage forms containing benzyl alcohol with caution in neonates. See manufacturer's labeling.

Adverse Reactions

Cardiovascular: Hypotension

Central nervous system: Drowsiness, headache, oversedation, seizure-like activity

Gastrointestinal: Nausea, vomiting

Local: Pain and local reactions at injection site

Neuromuscular & skeletal: Myoclonic jerks (preterm infants)

Ocular: Nystagmus

Respiratory: Apnea, cough, decreased tidal volume and/or respiratory rate

Miscellaneous: Hiccups, paradoxical reaction, physical and psychological dependence with prolonged use

Rare but important or life-threatening: Agitation, amnesia, bigeminy, bronchospasm, emergence delirium, euphoria, hallucinations, laryngospasm, rash

Drug Interactions

Metabolism/Transport Effects Substrate of CYP2B6 (minor), CYP3A4 (major); **Note:** Assignment of Major/Minor substrate status based on clinically relevant drug interaction potential; **Inhibits** CYP2C8 (weak), CYP2C9 (weak), CYP3A4 (weak)

Avoid Concomitant Use

Avoid concomitant use of Midazolam with any of the following: Azelastine (Nasal); Boceprevir; Cobicistat; Conivaptan; Fusidic Acid (Systemic); Idelalisib; Itraconazole; Ketoconazole (Systemic); Methadone; OLANZapine; Orphenadrine; Paraldehyde; Pimozide; Protease Inhibitors; Sodium Oxybate; Telaprevir; Thalidomide

Increased Effect/Toxicity

Midazolam may increase the levels/effects of: Alcohol (Ethyl); ARIPiprazole; Azelastine (Nasal); Buprenorphine; CloZAPine; CNS Depressants; Dofetilide; Hydrocodone; Lomitapide; Methadone; Methotrimeprazine; Metyrosine; Mirtazapine; Orphenadrine; Paraldehyde; Pimozide; Pramipexole; Propofol; ROPINIRole; Rotigotine; Selective Serotonin Reuptake Inhibitors; Sodium Oxybate; Suvorexant; Thalidomide; Zolpidem

The levels/effects of Midazolam may be increased by: Aprepitant; AtorvaSTATin; Boceprevir; Brimonidine (Topical); Cannabis; Ceritinib; Cobicistat; Conivaptan; CYP3A4 Inhibitors (Moderate); CYP3A4 Inhibitors (Strong); Dasatinib; Doxylamine; Dronabinol; Droperidol; Fosaprepitant; Fusidic Acid (Systemic); HydrOXYzine; Idelalisib; Itraconazole; Ivacaftor; Kava Kava; Ketoconazole (Systemic); Luliconazole; Macrolide Antibiotics; Magnesium Sulfate; Methotrimeprazine; Mifepristone; Nabilone; Netupitant; OLANZapine; Perampanel; Propofol; Protease Inhibitors; Rufinamide; Simeprevir; Stiripentol; Tapentadol; Teduglutide; Telaprevir; Tetrahydrocannabinol

Decreased Effect

The levels/effects of Midazolam may be decreased by: Bosentan; CYP3A4 Inducers (Moderate); CYP3A4 Inducers (Strong); Dabrafenib; Deferasirox; Ginkgo Biloba; Mitotane; Siltuximab; St Johns Wort; Theophylline Derivatives; Tocilizumab; Yohimbine

Food Interactions Grapefruit juice may increase serum concentrations of midazolam. Management: Avoid concurrent use of grapefruit juice with oral midazolam.

Storage/Stability

Oral: Store at 25°C (77°F); excursions permitted to 15°C to 30°C (59°F to 86°F).

Injection: Store at 20°C to 25°C (68°F to 77°F), excursions permitted to 15°C to 30°C (59°F to 86°F). The manufacturer states that midazolam, at a final concentration of 0.5 mg/mL, is stable for up to 24 hours when diluted with D_5W or NS. A final concentration of 1 mg/mL in NS has been documented to be stable for up to 10 days (McMullin, 1995). Admixtures do not require protection from light for short-term storage.

Mechanism of Action Binds to stereospecific benzodiazepine receptors on the postsynaptic GABA neuron at several sites within the central nervous system, including the limbic system, reticular formation. Enhancement of the inhibitory effect of GABA on neuronal excitability results by increased neuronal membrane permeability to chloride ions. This shift in chloride ions results in hyperpolarization (a less excitable state) and stabilization. Benzodiazepine receptors and effects appear to be linked to the GABA-A receptors. Benzodiazepines do not bind to GABA-B receptors.

Pharmacodynamics/Kinetics

Onset of action: IM: Sedation: ~15 minutes; IV: 3-5 minutes; Oral: 10-20 minutes; Intranasal: Children: 4-8 minutes (Lee-Kim, 2004)

Peak effect: IM: 0.5-1 hour

Duration: IM: Up to 6 hours; Mean: 2 hours; Intranasal: Children: 18-41 minutes (Lee-Kim, 2004); IV: Single dose: <2 hours (dose-dependent) (Fragen, 1997); Cirrhosis: Up to 6 hours (MacGilcrhist, 1986)

Absorption: IM: Rapid, complete; Oral: Rapid

Distribution: V_d: 1-3.1 L/kg; increased in females, elderly, and obesity

Protein binding: ~97%; in patients with cirrhosis, protein binding is reduced with a free fraction of ~5% (Trouvin, 1988)

Metabolism: Extensively hepatic CYP3A4; 60% to 70% of biotransformed midazolam is the active metabolite 1-hydroxy-midazolam (or alpha-hydroxymidazolam)

Bioavailability: Oral: 40% to 50% (Kanto, 1985), ~36% (children); IM: >90%

Half-life elimination: 2-6 hours; prolonged in cirrhosis, congestive heart failure, obesity, renal failure, and elderly. **Note:** In patients with renal failure, reduced elimination of active hydroxylated metabolites leads to drug accumulation and prolonged sedation.

Excretion: IV: Urine (primarily as glucuronide conjugates of the hydroxylated metabolites); Oral: Urine (~90% within 24 hours; primarily [60% to 70%] as glucuronide conjugates of the hydroxylated metabolites; <0.03% as unchanged drug); feces (~2% to 10% over 5 days) (Kanto, 1985; Smith, 1981)

Dosage Note: The dose of midazolam needs to be individualized based on the patient's age, underlying diseases, and concurrent medications. Decrease dose (by ~30%) if opioids or other CNS depressants are administered concomitantly. Children <6 years may require higher doses and closer monitoring than older children; in children with obesity, calculate dose based on ideal body weight.

Conscious sedation for procedures or preoperative sedation: Infants ≥6 months, Children, and Adolescents ≤16 years:

Oral: 0.25 to 0.5 mg/kg (maximum: 20 mg) as a single dose 20 to 30 minutes prior to procedure. Children <6 years or less cooperative patients may require as much as 1 mg/kg as a single dose; 0.25 mg/kg may suffice for children 6 to 16 years of age or for cooperative patients. Doses of 0.5 to 0.75 mg/kg administered 20 to 30 minutes prior to procedure have also been suggested; however, doses above 0.5 mg/kg typically do not improve the sedative and anxiolytic effects but increase side effects during recovery (Bozkurt, 2007).

Rectal (off-label route): 0.5 to 0.75 mg/kg (maximum: 20 mg) as a single dose 20 to 30 minutes prior to procedure (Bozkurt, 2007).

Intranasal (off-label route): 0.2 to 0.5 mg/kg (maximum total dose: 10 mg or 5 mg per nare); may be administered 10 to 20 minutes prior to procedure (Bozkurt, 2007; Chiaretti, 2011). **Note:** Use 5 mg/mL injectable concentrated solution to deliver dose. Due to the low pH of the solution, burning upon administration is likely to occur.

IM: 0.1 to 0.15 mg/kg 30 to 60 minutes before surgery or procedure; range: 0.05 to 0.15 mg/kg; doses up to 0.5 mg/kg have been used in more anxious patients; maximum total dose: 10 mg

IV:

Infants <6 months: Limited information is available in nonintubated infants; dosing recommendations not clear; infants <6 months are at higher risk for airway obstruction and hypoventilation; titrate dose in small increments to desired effect

Infants 6 months to Children 5 years: Initial: 0.05 to 0.1 mg/kg; total dose of 0.6 mg/kg may be required; maximum total dose: 6 mg

Children 6 to 12 years: Initial: 0.025 to 0.05 mg/kg; total doses of 0.4 mg/kg may be required; maximum total dose: 10 mg

Children 12 to 16 years: Dose as adults; maximum total dose: 10 mg

Conscious sedation during mechanical ventilation: Infants, Children, and Adolescents: IV: Loading dose: 0.05 to 0.2 mg/kg, followed by initial continuous infusion: 0.06 to 0.12 mg/kg/**hour** (1 to 2 **mcg**/kg/minute); range in clinical trials: 0.024 to 0.564 mg/kg/**hour** (0.4 to 9.4 **mcg**/kg/minute) (Hartman, 2009)

Status epilepticus refractory to standard therapy (off-label use): Infants, Children, and Adolescents: IV: **Note:** Intubation required; adjust dose based on hemodynamics, seizure activity, and EEG. Loading dose: 0.15 mg/kg followed by a continuous infusion of 0.06 mg/kg/**hour** (1 **mcg**/kg/minute); titrate dose upward every 5 minutes until clinical seizure activity is controlled; mean infusion rate required in 24 children was 0.14 mg/kg/**hour** (2.3 **mcg**/kg/minute) with a range of 0.06 to 1.1 mg/kg/**hour** (1 to 18.3 **mcg**/kg/minute) (Rivera, 1993).

A more aggressive approach has been demonstrated to provide control of status epilepticus within 30 minutes of initiation: Loading dose: 0.5 mg/kg followed by 0.12 mg/kg/**hour** (2 **mcg**/kg/minute). If seizures persist or recur, administer 0.5 mg/kg bolus with an increase in the infusion rate to 0.24 mg/kg/**hour** (4 **mcg**/kg/minute); if seizures continue to persist/recur, administer 0.1 mg/kg bolus and increase infusion to 0.48 mg/kg/**hour** (8 **mcg**/kg/minute); continue to repeat this last incremental increase until seizure control or a maximum dose of 1.44 mg/kg/**hour** (24 **mcg**/kg/minute) is reached; do not allow >5 minutes to elapse between each dose increment while seizures persist (dose range within clinical trial: 0.12 to 1.92 mg/kg/**hour** or 2 to 32 **mcg**/kg/minute) (Morrison, 2006).

Status epilepticus, prehospital treatment (off-label use; Silbergleit, 2012): Children and Adolescents: IM: **Note:** Administered by paramedics when convulsions last >5 minutes **or** if convulsions are occurring after having intermittent seizures without regaining consciousness for >5 minutes.

13 to 40 kg: 5 mg once

>40 kg: Refer to adult dosing

Adults: The dose of midazolam needs to be individualized based on the patient's age, underlying diseases, and concurrent medications. Consider reducing dose by 20% to 50% in elderly, chronically ill, or debilitated patients and those receiving opioids or other CNS depressants.

Preoperative/preprocedural sedation: Healthy adults <60 years:

IM: 0.07 to 0.08 mg/kg 30 to 60 minutes prior to surgery/procedure; usual dose: 5 mg

IV: 0.02 to 0.04 mg/kg; repeat every 5 minutes as needed to desired effect or up to 0.1 to 0.2 mg/kg

Intranasal (off-label route): 0.1 mg/kg; administer 10 to 20 minutes prior to surgery/procedure (Uygur-Bayramiçli, 2002). **Note:** Use 5 mg/mL injectable solution to deliver dose. Due to the low pH of the solution, burning upon administration is likely to occur.

Conscious sedation: IV:

Manufacturer's labeling:

Healthy adults <60 years:

Initial: Some patients respond to doses as low as 1 mg; no more than 2.5 mg should be administered over a period of 2 minutes. Additional doses of midazolam may be administered after a 2-minute waiting period and evaluation of sedation after each dose increment. A total dose >5 mg is generally not needed.

Maintenance: 25% of dose used to reach sedative effect

Adults ≥60 years, debilitated, or chronically ill: Refer to elderly dosing.

Alternate recommendations: American Society for Gastrointestinal Endoscopy: Initial: 0.5 to 2 mg slow IV over at least 2 minutes; slowly titrate to effect by repeating doses every 2 to 3 minutes if needed; usual total dose: 2.5 to 5 mg (Waring, 2003)

Anesthesia: IV:

Induction: Adults <55 years:

Unpremedicated patients: 0.3 to 0.35 mg/kg over 20 to 30 seconds; after 2 minutes, may repeat if necessary at 25% of initial dose every 2 minutes, up to a total dose of 0.6 mg/kg in resistant cases

Premedicated patients: Usual dosage range: 0.05 to 0.2 mg/kg (Barash, 2009; Miller, 2010). Use of 0.2 mg/kg administered over 5 to 10 seconds has been shown to safely produce anesthesia within 30 seconds (Samuelson, 1981) and is recommended for ASA physical status P1 and P2 patients. When used with other anesthetic drugs (ie, coinduction), the dose is <0.1 mg/kg (Miller, 2010).

ASA physical status >P3 or debilitation: Reduce dose by at least 20% (Miller, 2010)

Maintenance: 0.05 mg/kg as needed (Miller, 2010), or continuous infusion 0.015 to 0.06 mg/kg/**hour** (0.25 to 1 **mcg**/kg/minute) (Barash, 2009; Miller, 2010)

Sedation in mechanically-ventilated patients: IV: Initial dose: 0.01 to 0.05 mg/kg (~0.5 to 4 mg); may repeat at 5- to 15-minute intervals until adequate sedation achieved; maintenance infusion: 0.02 to 0.1 mg/kg/**hour** (0.3 to 1.7 **mcg**/kg/minute). Titrate to reach desired level of sedation. Titration to maintain a light rather than a deep level of sedation is recommended unless clinically contraindicated (Barr, 2013). May consider a trial of daily awakening; if agitated after discontinuation of drip, then restart at 50% of the previous dose (Kress, 2000).

Status epilepticus refractory to standard therapy (off-label use): **Note:** Intubation required; adjust dose based on hemodynamics, seizure activity, and EEG. IV: 0.15 to 0.3 mg/kg (usual dose: 5 to 15 mg); may repeat every 10 to 15 minutes as needed **or** 0.2 mg/kg bolus followed by a continuous infusion of 0.05 to 0.6 mg/kg/**hour** (0.83 to 10 **mcg**/kg/minute) (Lowenstein, 2005; Meierkord, 2010)

Status epilepticus, prehospital treatment (off-label use): **Note:** Administered by paramedics when convulsions last >5 minutes **or** if convulsions are occurring after having intermittent seizures without regaining consciousness for >5 minutes. IM: 10 mg once (Silbergleit, 2012)

Elderly:

Anesthesia: IV: Induction: Adults >55 years:

Unpremedicated patients: Initial dose: 0.3 mg/kg

Premedicated patients: Reduce dose by at least 20% (Miller, 2010).

Conscious sedation: IV: Initial: 0.5 mg slow IV; give no more than 1.5 mg in a 2-minute period; if additional titration is needed, give no more than 1 mg over 2 minutes, waiting another 2 or more minutes to evaluate sedative effect; a total dose of >3.5 mg is rarely necessary

Preoperative/preprocedural sedation: Adults >60 years (without concomitant opioid administration): IM: 2 to 3 mg (or 0.02 to 0.05 mg/kg) 30 to 60 minutes prior to surgery/procedure; some may only require 1 mg (or 0.01 mg/kg) if anticipated intensity and duration of sedation is less critical.

Dosage adjustment in renal impairment: There are no dosage adjustments provided in manufacturer's labeling; however, patients with renal failure receiving a continuous infusion cannot adequately eliminate the active hydroxylated metabolites (eg, 1-hydroxymidazolam) contributing to prolonged sedation sometimes for days after discontinuation (Spina, 2007).

Intermittent hemodialysis: Supplemental dose is not necessary.

Continuous venovenous hemofiltration (CVVH): Unconjugated 1-hydroxymidazolam not effectively removed; 1-hydroxymidazolamglucuronide effectively removed; sieving coefficient = 0.45 (Swart, 2005).

Peritoneal dialysis: Significant drug removal is unlikely based on physiochemical characteristics.

Dosage adjustment in hepatic impairment:

Severe hepatic impairment (eg, cirrhosis): **Note:** Use with caution in patients with any degree of hepatic impairment; patients with hepatic encephalopathy likely to be more sensitive to midazolam.

Single dose (eg, induction): No dosage adjustment recommended; patients with hepatic impairment may be more sensitive compared to patients without hepatic impairment; anticipate longer duration of action (MacGilchrist, 1986; Trouvin, 1988).

Multiple dosing or continuous infusion: Expect longer duration of action and accumulation; based on patient response, dosage reduction likely to be necessary (Trouvin, 1988).

Dietary Considerations Avoid grapefruit juice with oral syrup.

Usual Infusion Concentrations: Pediatric IV infusion: 0.5 mg/mL **or** 1 mg/mL

Usual Infusion Concentrations: Adult IV infusion: 100 mg in 100 mL (concentration: 1 mg/mL) of D_5W or NS

Administration

Intranasal: **Note:** Due to the low pH of the solution, burning upon administration is likely to occur. Use of an atomizer, such as the MAD 300 Mucosal Atomizer which attaches to a tuberculin syringe, can reduce irritation. If possible, based upon dose to be administered, use higher concentration injectable solution to minimize volume administered intranasal. Smaller volume will reduce irritation and swallowing of administered dose. The maximum recommended dose volume per nare is 1 mL.

Using the 5 mg/mL injectable solution, draw up desired dose with a 1-3 mL needleless syringe; may attach a nasal mucosal atomization device prior to delivering dose. Deliver half of the total dose volume (of the 5 mg/mL concentration) into the first nare using the atomizer device or by dripping slowly into nostril, then deliver the other half of the dose into the second nare.

Oral: Do not mix with any liquid (such as grapefruit juice) prior to administration

Parenteral:

IM: Administer deep IM into large muscle.

IV: Administer by slow IV injection over at least 2-5 minutes at a concentration of 1-5 mg/mL or by IV infusion. For induction of anesthesia, administer IV bolus over 5-30 seconds. Continuous infusions should be administered via an infusion pump.

Monitoring Parameters Respiratory and cardiovascular status, blood pressure, blood pressure monitor required during IV administration

Critically-ill patients: Monitor depth of sedation with either the Richmond Agitation-Sedation Scale (RASS) or Sedation-Agitation Scale (SAS) (Barr, 2013)

Additional Information Abrupt discontinuation after sustained use (generally >10 days) may cause withdrawal symptoms. For neonates, since both concentrations of the injection contain 1% benzyl alcohol, use the 5 mg/mL injection and dilute to 0.5 mg/mL with SWI without preservatives to decrease the amount of benzyl alcohol delivered to the neonate; with continuous infusion, midazolam may accumulate in peripheral tissues; use lowest effective infusion rate to reduce accumulation effects; midazolam is 3-4 times as potent as diazepam; paradoxical reactions associated with midazolam use in children (eg, agitation, restlessness, combativeness) have been successfully treated with flumazenil (Massanari, 1997).

Dosage Forms

Solution, Injection:

Generic: 2 mg/2 mL (2 mL); 5 mg/5 mL (5 mL); 10 mg/10 mL (10 mL); 5 mg/mL (1 mL, 2 mL, 5 mL, 10 mL); 10 mg/2 mL (2 mL); 25 mg/5 mL (5 mL); 50 mg/10 mL (10 mL)

Solution, Injection [preservative free]:

Generic: 2 mg/2 mL (2 mL); 5 mg/5 mL (5 mL); 5 mg/mL (1 mL); 10 mg/2 mL (2 mL)

Syrup, Oral:

Generic: 2 mg/mL (118 mL)

◆ **Midazolam Hydrochloride** *see* Midazolam *on page 1361*

◆ **Midazolam Injection (Can)** *see* Midazolam *on page 1361*

Midecamycin [INT] (mi DEK a mye sin)

International Brand Names Aboren (AR); Macropen (BG, HR, JP, RU); Macroral (IT); Medemycin (HK, JP); Mei Jia Xin (CN); Mei Ou Ka (CN); Meilital (CN); Midecin (IT); Miocacin (GR, PT); Miocamen (CY, EG, GR, IT, LU); Miocamycin (JP); Miomax (PK); Miotin (TH, VN); Momicine (ES); Mosil (FR); Myoxam (ES)

Index Terms Midecamycin Acetate

Pharmacologic Category Antibiotic, Macrolide

Reported Use Treatment of infections caused by susceptible strains of *Staphylococcus*, *Streptococcus*, *Streptococcus pneumoniae*, and *Mycoplasma*

Dosage Range Adults: Oral: 900-1800 mg/day in 2-3 divided doses

Product Availability Product available in various countries; not currently available in the U.S.

Dosage Forms

Tablet: 600 mg, 900 mg

◆ **Midecamycin Acetate** *see* Midecamycin [INT] *on page 1365*

Midodrine (MI doe dreen)

Brand Names: Canada Amatine; Apo-Midodrine

Index Terms Midodrine Hydrochloride; ProAmatine

Pharmacologic Category $Alpha_1$ Agonist

Use Orthostatic hypotension: Treatment of symptomatic orthostatic hypotension

Pregnancy Risk Factor C

Pregnancy Considerations Adverse events were observed in animal reproduction studies. Information related to the use of midodrine in pregnancy is limited (Glatter, 2005).

Breast-Feeding Considerations It is not known if midodrine is excreted in breast milk. The manufacturer recommends that caution be exercised when administering midodrine to nursing women.

Contraindications Severe organic heart disease, acute renal disease, urinary retention, pheochromocytoma, thyrotoxicosis, persistent and excessive supine hypertension

Warnings/Precautions [U.S. Boxed Warning]: Indicated for patients for whom orthostatic hypotension significantly impairs their daily life despite standard clinical care. May cause hypertension. Use is not recommended with supine hypertension. Continue therapy only in patients who appear to attain symptomatic improvement during initial treatment. May cause supine hypertension; discontinue use immediately if supine hypertension persists. Use with caution when administered concurrently with vasoconstrictors (eg, phenylephrine, ephedrine, dihydroergotamine, phenylpropanolamine, pseudoephedrine). Use is not recommended in patients with initial supine systolic pressure >180 mm Hg. Due to marked elevation of supine blood pressure (BP greater than 200 mm Hg systolic), use in patients whose lives are considerably impaired despite standard clinical care, including nonpharmacologic treatment (such as support stockings), fluid expansion, and lifestyle alterations. Supine and sitting blood pressure should be monitored. May slow heart rate primarily due to vagal reflex. Use caution when administered concurrently with negative chronotropes (eg, digoxin, beta blockers). Discontinue use if signs or symptoms of bradycardia occur. Desglymidodrine, the active metabolite, is primarily renally excreted; assess renal function prior to initial dose; use with caution in patients with renal impairment (has not been studied) and initiate with a reduced dose; contraindicated in patients with acute renal failure. Caution should be exercised in patients with diabetes, visual problems (especially if receiving fludrocortisone), or hepatic dysfunction.

Adverse Reactions

Cardiovascular: Supine hypertension
Central nervous system: Chills, pain
Dermatologic: Dry skin, piloerection, pruritus, rash
Gastrointestinal: Abdominal pain
Genitourinary: Dysuria, polyuria, urinary urgency or retention
Neuromuscular & skeletal: Paresthesia
Rare but important or life-threatening: Anxiety, backache, canker sore, confusion, dizziness, dry skin, erythema multiforme, facial flushing, flatulence, flushing, GI distress, headache, heartburn, hyperesthesia, insomnia, ICP increased, leg cramps, nausea, somnolence, visual field defect, weakness, xerostomia

Drug Interactions

Metabolism/Transport Effects None known.

Avoid Concomitant Use

Avoid concomitant use of Midodrine with any of the following: Ergot Derivatives; Iobenguane I 123; MAO Inhibitors

Increased Effect/Toxicity

Midodrine may increase the levels/effects of: Droxidopa; Sympathomimetics

The levels/effects of Midodrine may be increased by: AtoMOXetine; Beta-Blockers; Calcium Channel Blockers (Nondihydropyridine); Cannabinoid-Containing Products; Cardiac Glycosides; Ergot Derivatives; Linezolid; MAO Inhibitors; Tedizolid; Tricyclic Antidepressants

Decreased Effect

Midodrine may decrease the levels/effects of: Benzylpenicilloyl Polylysine; Iobenguane I 123

The levels/effects of Midodrine may be decreased by: Alpha1-Blockers; Tricyclic Antidepressants

Storage/Stability Store at 20°C to 25°C (68°F to 77°F). Protect light and moisture.

Mechanism of Action Midodrine forms an active metabolite, desglymidodrine, which is an alpha$_1$-agonist. This agent increases arteriolar and venous tone resulting in a rise in standing, sitting, and supine systolic and diastolic blood pressure in patients with orthostatic hypotension.

Pharmacodynamics/Kinetics

Onset of action: ~1 hour
Duration: 2 to 3 hours
Absorption: Rapid
Distribution: Poorly crosses blood-brain barrier
Protein binding: Minimal
Metabolism: Hepatic and many other tissues; midodrine is a prodrug which undergoes rapid deglycination to desglymidodrine (active metabolite)
Bioavailability: Desglymidodrine: 93%
Half-life elimination: Desglymidodrine: ~3 to 4 hours; Midodrine: 25 minutes
Time to peak, serum: Desglymidodrine: 1 to 2 hours; Midodrine: 30 minutes
Excretion: Urine (Midodrine: Insignificant; Desglymidodrine: 80% by active renal secretion)

Dosage Adults: Oral:

Orthostatic hypotension: 10 mg 3 times daily during daytime hours (every 3 to 4 hours) when patient is upright
Prevention of hemodialysis-induced hypotension (off-label use): 2.5 to 10 mg given 15 to 30 minutes prior to dialysis session (Cruz, 1998; KDOQI, 2005; Prakash, 2004)
Vasovagal syncope (off-label use): Initial: 5 mg 3 times/day during daytime hours (every 6 hours) increased up to 15 mg/dose if necessary (Perez-Lugones, 2001; Ward, 1998)

Dosage adjustment in renal impairment: 2.5 mg 3 times daily, gradually increasing as tolerated
Hemodialysis: Dialyzable

Dosage adjustment in hepatic impairment: No dosage adjustment provided in manufacturer's labeling (has not been studied); use with caution.

Administration Doses may be given in approximately 3- to 4-hour intervals (eg, shortly before or upon rising in the morning, at midday, in the late afternoon not later than 6 PM). Avoid dosing after the evening meal or within 4 hours of bedtime. Continue therapy only in patients who appear to attain symptomatic improvement during initial treatment. Standing systolic blood pressure may be elevated 15-30 mm Hg at 1 hour after a 10 mg dose. Some effect may persist for 2-3 hours.

Monitoring Parameters Blood pressure; renal and hepatic function

Additional Information Single doses as high as 20 mg have been given to patients, but severe and persistent systolic supine hypertension occurs at a high rate (approximately 45%) at this dose. Total daily doses greater than 30 mg have been tolerated by some patients, but their safety and usefulness have not been studied systematically or established.

Dosage Forms

Tablet, Oral:

Generic: 2.5 mg, 5 mg, 10 mg

◆ **Midodrine Hydrochloride** *see* Midodrine *on page 1365*

◆ **Mifeprex** *see* Mifepristone *on page 1366*

Mifepristone (mi FE pris tone)

Brand Names: U.S. Korlym; Mifeprex

Index Terms RU-38486; RU-486

Pharmacologic Category Abortifacient; Antineoplastic Agent, Hormone Antagonist; Antiprogestin; Cortisol Receptor Blocker

Use

Korlym: To control hyperglycemia occurring secondary to hypercortisolism in patients with endogenous Cushing's syndrome who have type 2 diabetes mellitus or glucose intolerance and who failed surgery or who are not surgical candidates
Mifeprex: Medical termination of intrauterine pregnancy, through day 49 of pregnancy. Patients may need treatment with misoprostol and possibly surgery to complete therapy.

Pregnancy Risk Factor X

Dosage Oral:

Adults:

Hyperglycemia in patients with Cushing syndrome (Korlym): Initial dose: 300 mg once daily. Dose may be increased in 300 mg increments at intervals of ≥2-4 weeks based on tolerability and symptom control. Maximum dose: 1200 mg once daily, not to exceed

20 mg/kg/day. If treatment is interrupted, reinitiate at 300 mg daily or a dose lower than the dose that caused the treatment to be stopped if interruption due to adverse reactions

Dosage adjustment with concurrent use of strong CYP450 inhibitor therapy (eg, ketoconazole): Maximum dose 300 mg/day

Termination of pregnancy (Mifeprex): Treatment consists of 3 office visits by the patient; the patient must read medication guide and sign patient agreement prior to treatment:

Day 1 (mifepristone administration): 600 mg (three 200 mg tablets) taken as a single dose under physician supervision

Day 3 (misoprostol administration): Patient must return to the health care provider 2 days following administration of mifepristone; unless abortion has occurred (confirmed using ultrasound or clinical examination): Misoprostol 400 mcg (two 200 mcg tablets); **Note:** Patient may need treatment for cramps or gastrointestinal symptoms at this time

Day 14 (post-treatment exam): Patient must return to the health care provider ~14 days after administration of mifepristone; confirm complete termination of pregnancy by ultrasound or clinical exam. Surgical termination is recommended to manage treatment failures.

Termination of pregnancy (off-label dosing): Mifepristone 200 mg orally, followed by misoprostol 800 mcg vaginally 24 to 48 hours later (ACOG, 2014; FIGO, 2011)

Elderly: Hyperglycemia in patients with Cushing syndrome: Refer to adult dosing.

Dosage adjustment in renal impairment:

Hyperglycemia in patients with Cushing syndrome: Maximum dose 600 mg daily; **Note:** Following doses of 1200 mg daily for 7 days in patients with severe renal impairment (CrCl <30 mL/minute), exposure to mifepristone and its metabolites was increased and a large variability in exposure was observed.

Termination of pregnancy: There are no dosage adjustments provided in the manufacturer's labeling (has not been studied)

Dosage adjustment in hepatic impairment:

Hyperglycemia in patients with Cushing syndrome:

Mild-to-moderate impairment: Maximum dose 600 mg daily

Severe impairment: Use is not recommended

Note: Following single and multiple doses of 600 mg daily in patients with moderate hepatic impairment (Child-Pugh class B), a large variability in exposure to mifepristone and its metabolites was observed.

Termination of pregnancy: There are no dosage adjustments provided in the manufacturer's labeling (has not been studied); use with caution due to CYP3A4 metabolism.

Additional Information Complete prescribing information should be consulted for additional detail.

Dosage Forms

Tablet, Oral:

Korlym: 300 mg

Mifeprex: 200 mg

Miglitol (MIG li tol)

Brand Names: U.S. Glyset

Pharmacologic Category Antidiabetic Agent, Alpha-Glucosidase Inhibitor

Use Type 2 diabetes mellitus (noninsulin-dependent, NIDDM):

Monotherapy as an adjunct to diet to improve glycemic control in patients with type 2 diabetes mellitus (noninsulin-dependent, NIDDM) whose hyperglycemia cannot be managed with diet alone

Combination therapy with a sulfonylurea when diet plus either miglitol or a sulfonylurea alone do not result in adequate glycemic control. The effect of miglitol to enhance glycemic control is additive to that of sulfonylureas when used in combination.

Pregnancy Risk Factor B

Dosage Adults: Oral: Initial: 25 mg 3 times daily at the start of each meal; the dose may be increased to 50 mg 3 times daily after 4-8 weeks and continued for ~3 months; if glycosylated hemoglobin is not satisfactory, may further increase to maximum recommended dose: 100 mg 3 times daily

Dosing adjustment in renal impairment:

CrCl ≥25 mL/minute: No dosage adjustment necessary. Although miglitol is primarily excreted unchanged, the increased plasma levels in renal impairment are not expected to affect efficacy (clinical response is localized to the GI tract); however, the effects on adverse effects are unknown.

CrCl <25 mL/minute or S_{cr} >2 mg/dL: Use not recommended (not adequately studied).

Dosing adjustment in hepatic impairment: No dosage adjustment necessary.

Additional Information Complete prescribing information should be consulted for additional detail.

Dosage Forms

Tablet, Oral:

Glyset: 25 mg, 50 mg, 100 mg

Miglustat (MIG loo stat)

Brand Names: U.S. Zavesca

Brand Names: Canada Zavesca

Index Terms OGT-918

Pharmacologic Category Enzyme Inhibitor; Glucosylceramide Synthase Inhibitor

Use

Gaucher disease: Treatment of adult patients with mild-to-moderate type 1 Gaucher disease for whom enzyme replacement therapy is not a therapeutic option (eg, due to allergy, hypersensitivity, or poor venous access)

Canadian labeling: Additional use (not in U.S. labeling): Treatment to delay the progression of neurological manifestations in Niemann-Pick type C disease

Pregnancy Risk Factor C

Dosage Oral:

Type 1 Gaucher disease: Adults: 100 mg 3 times daily; dose may be reduced to 100 mg 1-2 times daily in patients with adverse effects (ie, tremor, GI distress)

Niemann-Pick Type C disease (Canadian labeling; not in U.S. labeling):

Children <12 years: **Note:** Children <4 years of age were not included in clinical trials; dose based on body surface area (BSA):

BSA >1.25 m^2: Miglustat 200 mg 3 times daily

BSA >0.88-1.25 m^2: Miglustat 200 mg 2 times daily

BSA >0.73-0.88 m^2: Miglustat 100 mg 3 times daily

BSA >0.47-0.73 m^2: Miglustat 100 mg 2 times daily

BSA ≤0.47 m^2: Miglustat 100 mg once daily

Children ≥12 and Adults: 200 mg 3 times daily

Dosage adjustment in renal impairment:

Gaucher disease: Adults:

CrCl 50-70 mL/minute/1.73 m^2: 100 mg twice daily

CrCl 30-50 mL/minute/1.73 m^2: 100 mg once daily

CrCl <30 mL/minute/1.73 m^2: Not recommended

Niemann-Pick Type C disease Canadian labeling (not in U.S. labeling):

Children <12 years:

CrCl 50-70 mL/minute/1.73 m^2: Administer two-thirds of regular dose in 2 equal doses (adjusted for BSA)

CrCl 30-50 mL/minute/1.73 m^2: Administer one-third of regular dose in 2 equal doses (adjusted for BSA)

CrCl <30 mL/minute/1.73 m^2: Not recommended

Children ≥12 years and Adults:

CrCl 50-70 mL/minute/1.73 m^2: 200 mg twice daily

CrCl 30-50 mL/minute/1.73 m^2: 100 mg twice daily

CrCl <30 mL/minute/1.73 m^2: Not recommended

Dosage adjustment in hepatic impairment: No dosage adjustment provided in manufacturer's labeling (has not been studied). However, dosage adjustment unlikely because miglustat is not metabolized by the liver.

Additional Information Complete prescribing information should be consulted for additional detail.

Dosage Forms

Capsule, Oral:

Zavesca: 100 mg

◆ **Migranal** *see* Dihydroergotamine *on page 633*

◆ **Migranal® (Can)** *see* Dihydroergotamine *on page 633*

◆ **Milk of Magnesia** *see* Magnesium Hydroxide *on page 1263*

◆ **Milk of Magnesia [OTC]** *see* Magnesium Hydroxide *on page 1263*

◆ **Milk of Magnesia Concentrate [OTC]** *see* Magnesium Hydroxide *on page 1263*

◆ **Millipred** *see* PrednisoLONE (Systemic) *on page 1703*

◆ **Millipred DP** *see* PrednisoLONE (Systemic) *on page 1703*

◆ **Millipred DP 12-Day** *see* PrednisoLONE (Systemic) *on page 1703*

Milnacipran (mil NAY ci pran)

Brand Names: U.S. Savella; Savella Titration Pack

Pharmacologic Category Antidepressant, Serotonin/Norepinephrine Reuptake Inhibitor

Use Management of fibromyalgia

Pregnancy Risk Factor C

Pregnancy Considerations Adverse events were observed in some animal reproduction studies. Nonteratogenic effects in the newborn following SSRI/SNRI exposure late in the third trimester include respiratory distress, cyanosis, apnea, seizures, temperature instability, feeding difficulty, vomiting, hypoglycemia, hyper- or hypotonia, hyper-reflexia, jitteriness, irritability, constant crying, and tremor. Symptoms may be due to the toxicity of the SNRIs/SSRIs or a discontinuation syndrome and may be consistent with serotonin syndrome associated with SSRI treatment. The long-term effects of *in utero* SNRI/SSRI exposure on infant development and behavior are not known.

Women inadvertently exposed to milnacipran during pregnancy may be enrolled in the Savella Pregnancy Registry (877-643-3010 or http://www.savellapregnancyregistry.com).

Breast-Feeding Considerations Milnacipran is excreted into breast milk. The manufacturer recommends that caution be exercised when administering milnacipran to nursing women.

Contraindications Use of MAOIs intended to treat psychiatric disorders (concurrently or within 5 days of discontinuing milnacipran, or within 2 weeks of discontinuing the MAOI); initiation of milnacipran in a patient receiving linezolid or methylene blue IV

Warnings/Precautions [U.S. Boxed Warning]: Milnacipran is a serotonin/norepinephrine reuptake inhibitor (SNRI) similar to SNRIs used to treat depression and other psychiatric disorders. Antidepressants increase the risk of suicidal thinking and behavior in children, adolescents, and young adults (18-24 years of age) with major depressive disorder (MDD) and other psychiatric disorders; consider risk prior to prescribing. Short-term studies did not show an increased risk in patients >24 years of age and showed a decreased risk in patients ≥65 years. Closely monitor for clinical worsening, suicidality, or unusual changes in behavior; the patient's family or caregiver should be instructed to closely observe the patient and communicate condition with healthcare provider. A medication guide concerning the use of antidepressants in children and teenagers should be dispensed with each prescription. **Milnacipran is not FDA approved for the treatment of major depressive disorder or for use in children.**

Suicide risks should be monitored in patients treated with SNRIs regardless of the indication. The possibility of a suicide attempt is inherent in major depression and may persist until remission occurs. Patients treated with antidepressants should be observed for clinical worsening and suicidality, especially during initial few months of a course of drug therapy, or at times of dose changes, either increases or decreases. Use caution in high-risk patients. Worsening depression and severe abrupt suicidality that are not part of the presenting symptoms may require discontinuation or modification of drug therapy. Prescriptions should be written for the smallest quantity consistent with good patient care. The patient's family or caregiver should be alerted to monitor patients for the emergence of suicidality and associated behaviors (such as anxiety, agitation, panic attacks, insomnia, irritability, hostility, impulsivity, akathisia, mania, and hypomania); patients should be instructed to notify their health care provider if any of these symptoms or worsening depression or psychosis occur.

Patients with major depressive disorder were excluded from clinical trials evaluating milnacipran for fibromyalgia; however, mania has been reported in patients with mood disorders taking similar medications. May worsen psychosis in some patients or precipitate a shift to mania or hypomania in patients with bipolar disorder. Patients presenting with depressive symptoms should be screened for bipolar disorder. Monotherapy in patients with bipolar disorder should be avoided. **Milnacipran is not FDA approved for the treatment of bipolar depression.**

Potentially life-threatening serotonin syndrome (SS) has occurred with serotonergic agents (eg, SSRIs, SNRIs), particularly when used in combination with other serotonergic agents (eg, triptans, TCAs, fentanyl, lithium, tramadol, buspirone, St John's wort, tryptophan) or agents that impair metabolism of serotonin (eg, MAO inhibitors intended to treat psychiatric disorders, other MAO inhibitors [ie, linezolid and intravenous methylene blue]). Monitor patients closely for signs of SS such as mental status changes (eg, agitation, hallucinations, delirium, coma); autonomic instability (eg, tachycardia, labile blood pressure, dizziness, diaphoresis, flushing, hyperthermia, incoordination); neuromuscular changes (eg, tremor, rigidity, myoclonus, hyperreflexia, incoordination); GI symptoms (eg, nausea, vomiting, diarrhea); and/or seizures. Discontinue treatment (and any concomitant serotonergic agent) immediately if signs/symptoms arise. Potential for severe reaction when used with MAO inhibitors; autonomic instability, coma, death, delirium, diaphoresis, hyperthermia, mental status changes/agitation, muscular rigidity, myoclonus, neuroleptic malignant syndrome features, and seizures may occur; concurrent use with MAO inhibitors is contraindicated. Do not use milnacipran in combination with an MAO inhibitor or within 14 days of discontinuing an MAO inhibitor; do not start an MAO inhibitor until ≥5 days after discontinuing milnacipran. Symptoms of serotonin syndrome may occur with concomitant proserotonergic drugs (ie, SSRIs/SNRIs or triptans), agents which reduce milnacipran's metabolism, or antidopaminergic agents (including antipsychotics). Concurrent use of serotonin precursors (eg, tryptophan) is not recommended. Effects may be potentiated when used with other sedative drugs or ethanol.

May increase blood pressure and heart rate. Preexisting cardiovascular disease (including hypertension and tachyarrhythmias) should be treated prior to initiating therapy. Blood pressure and heart rate should be evaluated prior to initiating therapy and periodically thereafter; consider dose reduction or gradual discontinuation of therapy in individuals with sustained hypertension or tachycardia during therapy. Use with caution in patients with preexisting hypertension, tachyarrhythmias (eg, atrial fibrillation), or other cardiovascular disease; and with concomitant medications known to increase blood pressure or heart rate. May impair platelet aggregation resulting in increased risk of bleeding events, particularly if used concomitantly with aspirin or NSAIDs due to ulcerogenic potential. Data are inconclusive regarding extent of bleeding risk of SNRIs in combination with warfarin or other anticoagulants. Bleeding related to SNRI use has been reported to range from relatively minor bruising and epistaxis to life-threatening hemorrhage. Avoid use in patients with substantial ethanol intake, evidence of chronic liver disease or hepatic impairment. Cases of increased liver enzymes and severe liver injury (including fulminant hepatitis) have been reported. Discontinue therapy with the presentation of jaundice or other signs of hepatic dysfunction and do not reinitiate therapy unless another source or cause is identified. Use caution in patients with a history of seizures. Use caution in patients with a history of dysuria, especially males with prostatic hypertrophy, prostatitis, or other lower urinary tract disorders. May cause mild pupillary dilation which in susceptible individuals can lead to an episode of narrow-angle glaucoma. Consider evaluating patients who have not had an iridectomy for narrow-angle glaucoma risk factors. SSRIs and SNRIs have been associated with the development of SIADH; hyponatremia has been reported rarely (including severe cases with serum sodium <110 mmol/L), predominately in the elderly. Volume depletion and/or concurrent use of diuretics likely increases risk. Bone fractures have been associated with antidepressant treatment. Use caution in elderly patients; may cause or exacerbate syndrome of inappropriate antidiuretic hormone secretion or hyponatremia. Consider the possibility of a fragility fracture if an antidepressant-treated patient presents with unexplained bone pain, point tenderness, swelling, or bruising (Rabenda, 2013; Rizzoli, 2012).

Abrupt discontinuation or interruption of antidepressant therapy has been associated with a discontinuation syndrome. Symptoms arising may vary with antidepressant however commonly include nausea, vomiting, diarrhea, headaches, light-headedness, dizziness, diminished appetite, sweating, chills, tremors, paresthesias, fatigue, somnolence, and sleep disturbances (eg, vivid dreams, insomnia). Greater risks for developing a discontinuation syndrome have been associated with antidepressants with shorter half-lives, longer durations of treatment, and abrupt discontinuation. For antidepressants of short or intermediate half-lives, symptoms may emerge within 2-5 days after treatment discontinuation and last 7-14 days (APA, 2010; Fava, 2006; Haddad, 2001; Shelton, 2001; Warner, 2006).

Adverse Reactions

Cardiovascular: Flushing, hypertension, increased blood pressure, increased heart rate, palpitations, peripheral edema, tachycardia

Central nervous system: Chills, depression, dizziness, drowsiness, falling, fatigue, headache, insomnia, irritability, migraine

Dermatologic: Hyperhidrosis, night sweats, skin rash

Endocrine & metabolic: Decreased libido, hot flash, hypercholesterolemia, weight changes

Gastrointestinal: Abdominal distension, abdominal pain, decreased appetite, constipation, diarrhea, dysgeusia, dyspepsia, flatulence, gastroesophageal reflux disease, nausea, vomiting, xerostomia

Genitourinary: Cystitis, decreased urine output, dysuria, ejaculatory disorder, ejaculation failure, erectile dysfunction, prostatitis, scrotal pain, testicular pain, testicular swelling, urethral pain, urinary hesitancy, urinary retention, urinary tract infection

Neuromuscular & skeletal: Tremor

Ophthalmic: Blurred vision

Respiratory: Dyspnea

Miscellaneous: Fever

Rare but important or life-threatening: Accommodation disturbance, acute renal failure, aggressive behavior, angle-closure glaucoma, anorexia, delirium, erythema multiforme, galactorrhea, hallucination, hepatitis, homicidal ideation, hyperprolactinemia, hypertensive crisis, hyponatremia, leukopenia, loss of consciousness, neuroleptic malignant syndrome (Stevens, 2008), neutropenia, outbursts of anger, parkinsonian-like syndrome, rhabdomyolysis, seizure, serotonin syndrome, Stevens-Johnson syndrome, supraventricular tachycardia, thrombocytopenia

Drug Interactions

Metabolism/Transport Effects None known.

Avoid Concomitant Use

Avoid concomitant use of Milnacipran with any of the following: Dapoxetine; Iobenguane I 123; Linezolid; MAO Inhibitors; Methylene Blue; Urokinase

Increased Effect/Toxicity

Milnacipran may increase the levels/effects of: Agents with Antiplatelet Properties; Alpha-/Beta-Agonists; Anticoagulants; Antipsychotic Agents; Apixaban; Aspirin; Collagenase (Systemic); Dabigatran Etexilate; Digoxin; Ibritumomab; Methylene Blue; Metoclopramide; NSAID (Nonselective); Obinutuzumab; Rivaroxaban; Salicylates; Serotonin Modulators; Thrombolytic Agents; Tositumomab and Iodine I 131 Tositumomab; Urokinase; Vitamin K Antagonists

The levels/effects of Milnacipran may be increased by: Alcohol (Ethyl); Antiemetics (5HT3 Antagonists); Antipsychotic Agents; ClomiPRAMINE; Dapoxetine; Dasatinib; Glucosamine; Herbs (Anticoagulant/Antiplatelet Properties); Ibrutinib; Limaprost; Linezolid; MAO Inhibitors; Multivitamins/Fluoride (with ADE); Multivitamins/Minerals (with ADEK, Folate, Iron); Multivitamins/Minerals (with AE, No Iron); Omega-3 Fatty Acids; Pentosan Polysulfate Sodium; Pentoxifylline; Prostacyclin Analogues; Tedizolid; Tipranavir; Vitamin E

Decreased Effect

Milnacipran may decrease the levels/effects of: Alpha2-Agonists; Iobenguane I 123; Ioflupane I 123

Storage/Stability Store at 25°C (77°F); excursions permitted between 15°C to 30°C (59°F to 86°F).

Mechanism of Action Potent inhibitor of norepinephrine and serotonin reuptake (3:1). Milnacipran has no significant activity for serotonergic, alpha- and beta-adrenergic, muscarinic, histaminergic, dopaminergic, opiate, benzodiazepine, and GABA receptors. It does not possess MAO-inhibitory activity.

Pharmacodynamics/Kinetics

Absorption: Well absorbed

Distribution: IV: V_d: ~400 L

Protein binding: 13%

Metabolism: Hepatic to inactive metabolites

Bioavailability: 85% to 90%

Half-life elimination: 6-8 hours

Time to peak, plasma: Oral: 2-4 hours

Excretion: Urine (55% as unchanged drug)

Dosage

Oral: Adults: 50 mg twice daily

Titration schedule: 12.5 mg once on day 1, then 12.5 mg twice daily on days 2-3, 25 mg twice daily on days 4-7, then 50 mg twice daily thereafter. Dose may be increased to 100 mg twice daily, based on individual response. Doses >200 mg daily have not been studied.

Discontinuation of therapy: Upon discontinuation of antidepressant therapy, gradually taper the dose to minimize the incidence of withdrawal symptoms and allow for the detection of re-emerging symptoms. Evidence supporting ideal taper rates is limited. APA and NICE guidelines suggest tapering therapy over at least several weeks with consideration to the half-life of the antidepressant; antidepressants with a shorter half-life may need to be tapered more conservatively. In addition for long-term treated patients, WFSBP guidelines recommend tapering over 4-6 months. If intolerable withdrawal symptoms occur following a dose reduction, consider resuming the previously prescribed dose and/or decrease dose at a more gradual rate (APA, 2010; Bauer, 2002; Haddad, 2001; NCCMH, 2010; Schatzberg, 2006; Shelton, 2001; Warner, 2006).

MAO inhibitor recommendations:

Switching to or from an MAO inhibitor intended to treat psychiatric disorders:

Allow ≥14 days to elapse between discontinuing an MAO inhibitor intended to treat psychiatric disorders and initiation of milnacipran.

Allow ≥5 days to elapse between discontinuing milnacipran and initiation of MAO inhibitor intended to treat psychiatric disorders.

Use with other MAO inhibitors (linezolid or IV methylene blue):

Do not initiate milnacipran in patients receiving linezolid or IV methylene blue; consider other interventions for psychiatric condition.

If urgent treatment with linezolid or IV methylene blue is required in a patient already receiving milnacipran and potential benefits outweigh potential risks, discontinue milnacipran promptly and administer linezolid or IV methylene blue. Monitor for serotonin syndrome for 5 days or until 24 hours after the last dose of linezolid or IV methylene blue, whichever comes first. May resume milnacipran 24 hours after the last dose of linezolid or IV methylene blue.

Dosage adjustment in renal impairment:

Mild renal impairment: No dosage adjustment necessary.

Moderate renal impairment: Use with caution

Severe renal impairment (CrCl ≤29 mL/minute): Reduce maintenance dose to 25 mg twice daily; dose may be increased to 50 mg twice daily, based on individual tolerance

End-stage renal disease (ESRD): Use not recommended

Dosage adjustment in hepatic impairment:

Mild-to-moderate hepatic impairment: No dosage adjustment necessary.

Severe hepatic impairment: No dosage adjustment necessary; use with caution.

Administration Oral: Administer with or without food; food may improve tolerability.

Monitoring Parameters Blood pressure and heart rate should be regularly monitored; renal function should be monitored for dosing purposes; mental status for suicidal ideation (especially at the beginning of therapy or when doses are increased or decreased); intraocular pressure should be monitored in those with baseline elevations or a history of glaucoma

Dosage Forms

Miscellaneous, Oral:

Savella Titration Pack: 12.5 & 25 & 50 mg (55 ea)

Tablet, Oral:

Savella: 12.5 mg, 25 mg, 50 mg, 100 mg

Milrinone (MIL ri none)

Brand Names: Canada Milrinone Injection; Milrinone Lactate Injection

Index Terms Milrinone Lactate

Pharmacologic Category Inotrope; Phosphodiesterase-3 Enzyme Inhibitor

Use Short-term IV therapy of acutely-decompensated heart failure

American College of Cardiology/American Heart Association heart failure (HF) guideline recommendations (ACCF/AHA [Yancy, 2013]): To maintain systemic perfusion and preserve end-organ performance in patients with cardiogenic shock; bridge therapy in stage D HF unresponsive to guideline-directed medical therapy and device therapy in patients awaiting heart transplant or mechanical circulatory support; short-term management of hospitalized patients with severe systolic dysfunction presenting with low blood pressure and significantly depressed cardiac output; long-term management (palliative therapy) in select patients with stage D HF unresponsive to guideline-directed medical therapy and device therapy who are not candidates for heart transplant or mechanical circulatory support.

Pregnancy Risk Factor C

Pregnancy Considerations Teratogenic effects have not been observed in animal reproduction studies; however, increased resorption was reported in some studies.

Breast-Feeding Considerations It is not known if milrinone is excreted in breast milk. The manufacturer recommends that caution be exercised when administering milrinone to nursing women.

Contraindications Hypersensitivity to milrinone, inamrinone, or any component of the formulation; concurrent use of inamrinone

Warnings/Precautions Monitor closely for hypotension. Avoid in severe obstructive aortic or pulmonic valvular disease. Milrinone may aggravate outflow tract obstruction in hypertrophic subaortic stenosis. Supraventricular and ventricular arrhythmias have developed in high-risk patients. Ensure that ventricular rate controlled in atrial fibrillation/flutter prior to initiating milrinone. Not recommended for use in acute MI patients. Monitor and correct fluid and electrolyte problems. Adjust dose in renal dysfunction. Discontinue therapy if dose-related elevations in LFTs and clinical symptoms of hepatotoxicity occur. According to the ACCF/AHA 2013 heart failure guidelines, long-term use of intravenous inotropic therapy without a specific indication or for reasons other than palliation is potentially harmful.

Adverse Reactions

Cardiovascular: Angina, hypotension, supraventricular arrhythmia, ventricular arrhythmia

Central nervous system: Headache

Rare but important or life-threatening: Anaphylaxis, atrial fibrillation, bronchospasm, hypokalemia, injection site reaction, liver function abnormalities, MI, rash, thrombocytopenia, torsade de pointes, tremor, ventricular fibrillation

Drug Interactions

Metabolism/Transport Effects None known.

Avoid Concomitant Use There are no known interactions where it is recommended to avoid concomitant use.

Increased Effect/Toxicity

Milrinone may increase the levels/effects of: Riociguat

Decreased Effect There are no known significant interactions involving a decrease in effect.

Preparation for Administration Standard dilution: For a final concentration of 0.2 mg/mL: Dilute Primacor® 1 mg/mL (20 mL) with 80 mL diluent (final volume: 100 mL) of ½NS, NS or D_5W. May also dilute 1 mg/mL (10 mL) with 40 mL diluent (final volume: 50 mL).

Storage/Stability

Injection: Store at 15°C to 30°C (59°F to 86°F); avoid freezing. Stable at 0.2 mg/mL in ½NS, NS, or D_5W for 72 hours at room temperature in normal light.

Premixed infusion: Store at room temperature at 25°C (77°F); brief exposure up to 40°C (104°F) will not adversely affect drug; minimize exposure to heat; avoid excessive heat; protect from freezing.

Mechanism of Action A selective phosphodiesterase inhibitor in cardiac and vascular tissue, resulting in vasodilation and inotropic effects with little chronotropic activity.

Pharmacodynamics/Kinetics

Onset of action: IV: 5-15 minutes

Distribution: V_{dss}: 0.32-0.45 L/kg

Protein binding, plasma: ~70%

Metabolism: Hepatic (12%)

Half-life elimination: Normal renal function: ~2.5 hours; CVVH: 20.1 hours (Taniguchi, 2000)

Excretion: Urine (85% as unchanged drug) within 24 hours; active tubular secretion is a major elimination pathway for milrinone

Dosage Inotropic support in heart failure: Adults: IV: Loading dose (optional, not recommended by ACCF/AHA 2013 heart failure guidelines; also see **"Note"**): 50 mcg/kg administered over 10 minutes followed by a maintenance dose titrated according to hemodynamic and clinical response; Maintenance dose: IV infusion: 0.375-0.75 mcg/kg/minute; lower initial doses of 0.1 mcg/kg/minute (with final maintenance doses of 0.2-0.3 mcg/kg/minute) have also been recommended (HFSA [Lindenfeld, 2010]). The ACCF/AHA 2013 heart failure guidelines recommend a maintenance dose of 0.125-0.75 mcg/kg/minute (ACCF/AHA [Yancy, 2013]).

Note: When initiating an infusion of 0.5 mcg/kg/minute without a loading dose, significant hemodynamic changes seen at 30 minutes with similar effects on pulmonary capillary wedge pressure and cardiac index seen at 2 and 3 hours, respectively, compared to loading dose regimen (Baruch, 2011).

Dosage adjustment in renal impairment:

Manufacturer recommended adjustment:

CrCl 50 mL/minute/1.73 m^2: Administer 0.43 mcg/kg/minute

CrCl 40 mL/minute/1.73 m^2: Administer 0.38 mcg/kg/minute

CrCl 30 mL/minute/1.73 m^2: Administer 0.33 mcg/kg/minute

CrCl 20 mL/minute/ 1.73 m^2: Administer 0.28 mcg/kg/minute

CrCl 10 mL/minute/1.73 m^2: Administer 0.23 mcg/kg/minute

CrCl 5 mL/minute/1.73 m^2: Administer 0.2 mcg/kg/minute

Alternative Dosing Adjustments in Patients with Renal Impairment[1]

CrCl (mL/min)	Starting dose (mcg/kg/min)		
	0.375	**0.5**	**0.75**
50	0.25	0.375	0.5
40	0.125	0.25	0.375
30	0.0625	0.125	0.25
20	Consider alternative therapy	0.0625	0.125
10	Consider alternative therapy		0.0625
5	Consider alternative therapy		

[1]Based on expert opinion

Usual Infusion Concentrations: Pediatric Note: Premixed solutions available

IV infusion: 200 **mcg**/mL

Usual Infusion Concentrations: Adult Note: Premixed solutions available

IV infusion: 20 mg in 100 mL (total volume) (concentration: 200 **mcg**/mL) of D_5W

Administration Infuse via infusion pump

Monitoring Parameters Platelet count, CBC, electrolytes (especially potassium and magnesium), liver function and renal function tests; ECG, CVP, SBP, DBP, heart rate; infusion site

If pulmonary artery catheter is in place, monitor cardiac index, stroke volume, systemic vascular resistance, pulmonary capillary wedge pressure and pulmonary vascular resistance.

Consult individual institutional policies and procedures.

Dosage Forms

Solution, Intravenous:

Generic: 200 mcg/mL (100 mL, 200 mL); 10 mg/10 mL (10 mL); 20 mg/20 mL (20 mL); 50 mg/50 mL (50 mL)

Solution, Intravenous [preservative free]:

Generic: 200 mcg/mL (100 mL, 200 mL)

- ◆ **Milrinone Injection (Can)** *see* Milrinone *on page 1370*
- ◆ **Milrinone Lactate** *see* Milrinone *on page 1370*
- ◆ **Milrinone Lactate Injection (Can)** *see* Milrinone *on page 1370*
- ◆ **Mimvey** *see* Estradiol and Norethindrone *on page 781*
- ◆ **Mimvey Lo** *see* Estradiol and Norethindrone *on page 781*
- ◆ **Minastrin 24 Fe** *see* Ethinyl Estradiol and Norethindrone *on page 808*
- ◆ **Minestrin 1/20 (Can)** *see* Ethinyl Estradiol and Norethindrone *on page 808*
- ◆ **MiniCaps Omega-3 [OTC]** *see* Omega-3 Fatty Acids *on page 1507*
- ◆ **Minims Cyclopentolate (Can)** *see* Cyclopentolate *on page 517*
- ◆ **Minims Prednisolone Sodium Phosphate (Can)** *see* PrednisoLONE (Ophthalmic) *on page 1706*
- ◆ **Minipress** *see* Prazosin *on page 1703*
- ◆ **Minirin (Can)** *see* Desmopressin *on page 594*
- ◆ **Minitran** *see* Nitroglycerin *on page 1465*
- ◆ **Minivelle** *see* Estradiol (Systemic) *on page 775*
- ◆ **Minocin** *see* Minocycline *on page 1371*

Minocycline (mi noe SYE kleen)

Brand Names: U.S. Minocin; Solodyn

Brand Names: Canada Apo-Minocycline; Arestin Microspheres; Dom-Minocycline; Minocin; Mylan-Minocycline; Novo-Minocycline; PHL-Minocycline; PMS-Minocycline; ratio-Minocycline; Riva-Minocycline; Sandoz-Minocycline

Index Terms Minocycline Hydrochloride; Ximino™

Pharmacologic Category Antibiotic, Tetracycline Derivative

Use

Treatment of susceptible bacterial infections of both gram-negative and gram-positive organisms; treatment of anthrax (inhalational, cutaneous, and gastrointestinal); moderate-to-severe acne; meningococcal (asymptomatic) carrier state; Rickettsial diseases (including Rocky Mountain spotted fever, Q fever); nongonococcal urethritis, gonorrhea; acute intestinal amebiasis; respiratory tract infection; skin/soft tissue infections; chlamydial infections

Extended release (Solodyn): Only indicated for treatment of inflammatory lesions of non-nodular moderate-to-severe acne

Pregnancy Risk Factor D

Pregnancy Considerations Tetracyclines cross the placenta and accumulate in developing teeth and long tubular bones. Rare spontaneous reports of congenital anomalies, including limb reduction, have been reported following maternal minocycline use. Due to limited information, a causal association cannot be established. Tetracyclines may discolor fetal teeth following maternal use during pregnancy; the specific teeth involved and the portion of the tooth affected depends on the timing and duration of exposure relative to tooth calcification. As a class, tetracyclines are generally considered second-line antibiotics in pregnant women and their use should be avoided (Mylonas, 2011). Minocycline should not be used for the treatment of acne in pregnant women, or in males or females attempting to conceive a child.

Breast-Feeding Considerations Minocycline is excreted in breast milk (Brogden, 1975). According to the manufacturer, the decision to continue or discontinue breast-feeding during therapy should take into account the risk of exposure to the infant and the benefits of treatment to the mother. Oral absorption is not affected by dairy products; therefore, oral absorption of minocycline by the breast-feeding infant would not be expected to be diminished by the calcium in the maternal milk. Nondose-related effects could include modification of bowel flora. There have been case reports of black discoloration of breast milk in women taking minocycline (Basler, 1985; Hunt, 1996).

Contraindications Hypersensitivity to minocycline, other tetracyclines, or any component of the formulation

Warnings/Precautions May be associated with increases in BUN secondary to antianabolic effects; use caution in patients with renal impairment (CrCl <80 mL/minute). Hepatotoxicity has been reported; use caution in patients with hepatic insufficiency. Autoimmune syndromes (eg, lupus-like, hepatitis, and vasculitis) have been reported; discontinue if symptoms occur. CNS effects (lightheadedness, vertigo) may occur; patients must be cautioned about performing tasks which require mental alertness (eg, operating machinery or driving). Intracranial hypertension (headache, blurred vision, diplopia, vision loss, and/or papilledema) has been associated with use. Women of childbearing age who are overweight or have a history of intracranial hypertension are at greater risk. Concomitant use of isotretinoin (known to cause pseudotumor cerebri) and minocycline should be avoided. Intracranial hypertension typically resolves after discontinuation of treatment; however, permanent visual loss is possible. If visual symptoms develop during treatment, prompt ophthalmologic evaluation is warranted. Intracranial pressure can remain elevated for weeks after drug discontinuation; monitor patients until they stabilize. May cause photosensitivity; discontinue if skin erythema occurs. Prolonged use may result in fungal or bacterial superinfection, including *C. difficile*-associated diarrhea (CDAD) and pseudomembranous colitis; CDAD has been observed >2 months postantibiotic treatment. May cause tissue hyperpigmentation, tooth enamel hypoplasia, or permanent tooth discoloration; more common with long-term use, but observed with repeated, short courses; use of tetracyclines should be avoided during tooth development (infancy and children <8 years of age) unless other drugs are not likely to be effective or are contraindicated. Do not use during pregnancy. In addition to affecting tooth development, tetracycline use has been associated with retardation of skeletal development and reduced bone growth. Rash, along with eosinophilia, fever, and organ failure (Drug Rash with Eosinophilia and Systemic Symptoms [DRESS] syndrome) has been reported; discontinue treatment immediately if DRESS syndrome is suspected. Potentially significant drug-drug interactions may exist, requiring dose or frequency adjustment, additional monitoring, and/or selection of alternative therapy.

Adverse Reactions

Cardiovascular: Myocarditis, pericarditis, vasculitis

Central nervous system: Bulging fontanels, dizziness, fatigue, fever, headache, hypoesthesia, malaise, mood changes, paresthesia, pseudotumor cerebri, sedation, seizure, somnolence, vertigo

Dermatologic: Alopecia, angioedema, drug rash with eosinophilia and systemic symptoms (DRESS), erythema multiforme, erythema nodosum, erythematous rash, exfoliative dermatitis, hyperpigmentation of nails, maculopapular rash, photosensitivity, pigmentation of the skin and mucous membranes, pruritus, Stevens-Johnson syndrome, toxic epidermal necrolysis, urticaria

Endocrine & metabolic: Thyroid cancer, thyroid discoloration, thyroid dysfunction

Gastrointestinal: Anorexia, diarrhea, dyspepsia, dysphagia, enamel hypoplasia, enterocolitis, esophageal ulcerations, esophagitis, glossitis, inflammatory lesions (oral/anogenital), moniliasis, nausea, oral cavity discoloration, pancreatitis, pseudomembranous colitis, stomatitis, tooth discoloration, vomiting, xerostomia

Genitourinary: Balanitis, vulvovaginitis

Hematologic: Agranulocytosis, eosinophilia, hemolytic anemia, leukopenia, neutropenia, pancytopenia, thrombocytopenia

Hepatic: Autoimmune hepatitis, hepatic cholestasis, hepatic failure, hepatitis, hyperbilirubinemia, jaundice, liver enzyme increases

Local: Injection site reaction (IV administration)

Neuromuscular & skeletal: Arthralgia, arthritis, bone discoloration, joint stiffness, joint swelling, myalgia

Otic: Hearing loss, tinnitus

Renal: Acute renal failure, BUN increased, interstitial nephritis

Respiratory: Asthma, bronchospasm, cough, dyspnea, pneumonitis, pulmonary infiltrate (with eosinophilia)

Miscellaneous: Anaphylaxis, hypersensitivity, lupus erythematosus, lupus-like syndrome, serum sickness

Drug Interactions

Metabolism/Transport Effects None known.

Avoid Concomitant Use

Avoid concomitant use of Minocycline with any of the following: BCG; Retinoic Acid Derivatives; Strontium Ranelate

Increased Effect/Toxicity

Minocycline may increase the levels/effects of: Mipomersen; Neuromuscular-Blocking Agents; Porfimer; Retinoic Acid Derivatives; Verteporfin; Vitamin K Antagonists

Decreased Effect

Minocycline may decrease the levels/effects of: Atazanavir; BCG; Iron Salts; Penicillins; Sodium Picosulfate; Typhoid Vaccine

The levels/effects of Minocycline may be decreased by: Antacids; Bile Acid Sequestrants; Bismuth; Bismuth Subsalicylate; Calcium Salts; Iron Salts; Lanthanum; Magnesium Salts; Multivitamins/Minerals (with ADEK, Folate, Iron); Multivitamins/Minerals (with AE, No Iron); Quinapril; Strontium Ranelate; Sucralfate; Sucroferric Oxyhydroxide; Zinc Salts

Food Interactions Minocycline serum concentrations are not significantly altered if taken with food or dairy products. Management: Administer without regard to food.

Preparation for Administration Injection: Reconstitute with 5 mL of sterile water for injection, and further dilute in 500-1000 mL of NS, D_5W, D_5NS, Ringer's injection, or LR.

Storage/Stability

Capsule (including pellet-filled), tablet: Store at 20°C to 25°C (68°F to 77°F); protect from heat. Protect from light and moisture.

Extended release tablet: Store at 15°C to 30°C (59°F to 86°F); protect from heat. Protect from light and moisture.

Injection: Store vials at 20°C to 25°C (68°F to 77°F) prior to reconstitution. Reconstituted solution is stable at room temperature for 24 hours. Final dilutions should be administered immediately.

Mechanism of Action Inhibits bacterial protein synthesis by binding with the 30S and possibly the 50S ribosomal subunit(s) of susceptible bacteria; cell wall synthesis is not affected

Rheumatoid arthritis: The mechanism of action of minocycline in rheumatoid arthritis is not completely understood. It is thought to have antimicrobial, anti-inflammatory, immunomodulatory, and chondroprotective effects. More specifically, it is thought to be a potent inhibitor of metalloproteinases, which are active in rheumatoid arthritis joint destruction.

Pharmacodynamics/Kinetics

Absorption: Oral: Well absorbed

Protein binding: 70% to 75%

Metabolism: Hepatic to inactive metabolites

Half-life elimination: IV: 15 to 23 hours; Oral: 16 hours (range: 11 to 22 hours)

Time to peak: Capsule, pellet filled: 1 to 4 hours; Extended release tablet: 3.5 to 4 hours

Excretion: Urine, feces

Dosage

Usual dosage range:

IV:

Children >8 years: Initial: 4 mg/kg, followed by 2 mg/kg/dose every 12 hours (maximum: 400 mg daily)

Adults: Initial: 200 mg, followed by 100 mg every 12 hours (maximum: 400 mg daily)

Oral:

Capsule or immediate release tablet:

Children >8 years: Oral: Initial: 4 mg/kg, followed by 2 mg/kg/dose every 12 hours (maximum: 400 mg daily)

Adults: Oral: Initial: 200 mg, followed by 100 mg every 12 hours; more frequent dosing intervals may be used (100 to 200 mg initially, followed by 50 mg 4 times daily)

Extended release tablet (Solodyn®): Children ≥12 years and Adults (≥45 kg): Oral: 45 to 135 mg once daily (weight based)

Indication-specific dosing:

Children ≥12 years and Adults:

Acne, inflammatory, non-nodular, moderate-to-severe (Solodyn®): Oral:

45 to 49 kg: 45 mg once daily
50 to 59 kg: 55 mg once daily
60 to 71 kg: 65 mg once daily
72 to 84 kg: 80 mg once daily
85 to 96 kg: 90 mg once daily
97 to 110 kg: 105 mg once daily
111 to 125 kg: 115 mg once daily
126 to 136 kg: 135 mg once daily

Note: Therapy should be continued for 12 weeks. Higher doses do not confer greater efficacy and may be associated with more acute vestibular side effects. Safety of use beyond 12 weeks has not been established.

Cellulitis (purulent) infection due to community-acquired MRSA (off-label use): Oral: Children >8 years: Initial: 4 mg/kg (maximum: 200 mg); Maintenance: 2 mg/kg/dose (maximum: 100 mg) every 12 hours for 5 to 10 days (Liu, 2011)

Adults:

Acne: Oral: Capsule or immediate-release tablet: 50 to 100 mg twice daily

Cellulitis (purulent) due to community-acquired MRSA (off-label use): Oral: Initial: 200 mg; Maintenance: 100 mg twice daily for 5 to 10 days (Liu, 2011)

Chlamydial or *Ureaplasma urealyticum* infection, uncomplicated: Oral, IV: Urethral, endocervical, or rectal: 100 mg every 12 hours for at least 7 days

Gonococcal infection, uncomplicated (males): Oral, IV:

Without urethritis or anorectal infection: Initial: 200 mg, followed by 100 mg every 12 hours for at least 4 days (cultures 2 to 3 days post-therapy)

Urethritis: 100 mg every 12 hours for 5 days

Meningococcal carrier state (manufacturer's labeling): Oral: 100 mg every 12 hours for 5 days. **Note:** CDC recommendations do not mention use of minocycline for eradicating nasopharyngeal carriage of meningococcal

Mycobacterium marinum: Oral: 100 mg every 12 hours for 6 to 8 weeks

Nocardiosis, cutaneous (non-CNS) (off-label use): Oral: 100 to 200 mg every 12 hours

Prosthetic joint infection:

Staphylococci (oxacillin-sensitive or -resistant) oral phase treatment (after completion of pathogen-specific IV therapy) following 1-stage exchange:

Total ankle, elbow, hip, or shoulder arthroplasty: 100 mg twice daily for 3 months; **Note:** Must be used in combination with rifampin (Osmon, 2013)

Total knee arthroplasty: 100 mg twice daily for 6 months; **Note:** Must be used in combination with rifampin (Osmon, 2013)

Chronic oral antimicrobial suppression (off-label use): Oral:

Propionibacterium spp (alternative to penicillin or amoxicillin): 100 mg twice daily (Osmon, 2013)

Staphylococci (oxacillin-resistant): 100 mg twice daily (Osmon, 2013)

Rheumatoid arthritis (off-label use): Oral: 100 mg twice daily (O'Dell, 2001)

Syphilis: Oral, IV: Initial: 200 mg, followed by 100 mg every 12 hours for 10 to 15 days

Elderly: Refer to adult dosing.

Dosage adjustment in renal impairment: Use with caution; monitor BUN and creatinine clearance. Consider decreasing dose or increasing dosing interval (extended release).

CrCl <80 mL/minute: Do not exceed 200 mg daily

Dosage adjustment in hepatic impairment: No dosage adjustment provided in manufacturer's labeling; however, hepatotoxicity has been reported. Use with caution in patients with hepatic impairment.

Dietary Considerations May be taken with or without food.

Administration

IV: Infuse slowly; avoid rapid administration. The manufacturer's labeling does not provide a recommended administration rate. The injectable route should be used only if the oral route is not feasible or adequate. Prolonged intravenous therapy may be associated with thrombophlebitis.

Oral: May be administered with or without food. Administer with adequate fluid to decrease the risk of esophageal irritation and ulceration. Swallow pellet-filled capsule and extended release tablet whole; do not chew, crush, or split.

Monitoring Parameters LFTs, BUN, renal function with long-term treatment; if symptomatic for autoimmune disorder, include ANA, CBC; ophthalmologic evaluation if visual disturbances occur

Product Availability Ximino™ extended-release capsules: FDA approved July 2012; anticipated availability currently unknown. Consult prescribing information for additional information.

Dosage Forms

Capsule, Oral:
Minocin: 50 mg, 75 mg, 100 mg
Generic: 50 mg, 75 mg, 100 mg

Kit, Combination:
Minocin: 50 mg, 100 mg

Solution Reconstituted, Intravenous:
Minocin: 100 mg (1 ea)

Tablet, Oral:
Generic: 50 mg, 75 mg, 100 mg

Tablet Extended Release 24 Hour, Oral:
Solodyn: 55 mg, 65 mg, 80 mg, 105 mg, 115 mg
Generic: 45 mg, 90 mg, 135 mg

◆ **Minocycline Hydrochloride** *see* Minocycline *on page 1371*

◆ **Min-Ovral (Can)** *see* Ethinyl Estradiol and Levonorgestrel *on page 803*

Minoxidil (Systemic) (mi NOKS i dil)

Brand Names: Canada Loniten

Pharmacologic Category Antihypertensive; Vasodilator, Direct-Acting

Use

Hypertension: Management of severe hypertension (usually in combination with a diuretic and beta-blocker)

Note: According to the Eighth Joint National Committee (JNC 8) guidelines, minoxidil is **not** recommended for the initial treatment of hypertension (James, 2013).

Pregnancy Risk Factor C

Dosage Oral:

Children <12 years: Hypertension: Initial: 0.1-0.2 mg/kg once daily; maximum: 5 mg/day; increase gradually every 3 days; usual dosage range: 0.25-1 mg/kg/day in 1-2 divided doses; maximum: 50 mg daily

Children ≥12 years and Adults: Hypertension: Initial: 5 mg once daily, increase gradually every 3 days (maximum: 100 mg daily); usual dosage range (ASH/ISH [Weber, 2014]): 5-10 mg daily

Note: Dosage adjustment is needed when added to concomitant therapy.

Elderly: Hypertension: Initial: 2.5 mg once daily; increase gradually.

Dosage adjustment in renal impairment: Patient with renal failure and/or receiving dialysis may require dosage reduction.

Supplemental dose is not necessary after hemo- or peritoneal dialysis.

Dosage adjustment in hepatic impairment: No dosage adjustment provided in manufacturer's labeling.

Additional Information Complete prescribing information should be consulted for additional detail.

Dosage Forms

Tablet, Oral:
Generic: 2.5 mg, 10 mg

Dosage Forms: Canada

Tablet, Oral:
Loniten: 2.5 mg, 10 mg

Minoxidil (Topical) (mi NOKS i dil)

Brand Names: U.S. Hair Regrowth Treatment Men [OTC]; Minoxidil for Men [OTC]; Rogaine Mens Extra Strength [OTC]

Brand Names: Canada Apo-Gain®; Rogaine®

Pharmacologic Category Topical Skin Product

Use Treatment of alopecia androgenetica in males and females

Dosage Topical: Adults: Alopecia: Apply twice daily; 4 months of therapy may be necessary for hair growth.

Additional Information Complete prescribing information should be consulted for additional detail.

Dosage Forms

Foam, External:
Rogaine Mens Extra Strength [OTC]: 5% (60 g)

Solution, External:
Hair Regrowth Treatment Men [OTC]: 5% (60 mL)
Minoxidil for Men [OTC]: 2% (60 mL); 5% (60 mL, 120 mL)
Generic: 5% (60 mL)

◆ **Minoxidil for Men [OTC]** *see* Minoxidil (Topical) *on page 1374*

◆ **Mint-Alendronate (Can)** *see* Alendronate *on page 79*

◆ **Mint-Amlodipine (Can)** *see* AmLODIPine *on page 123*

◆ **Mint-Anastrozole (Can)** *see* Anastrozole *on page 148*

◆ **Mint-Atenolol (Can)** *see* Atenolol *on page 189*

◆ **Mint-Ciproflox (Can)** *see* Ciprofloxacin (Systemic) *on page 441*

◆ **Mint-Ciprofloxacin (Can)** *see* Ciprofloxacin (Systemic) *on page 441*

◆ **Mint-Citalopram (Can)** *see* Citalopram *on page 451*

◆ **Mint-Dutasteride (Can)** *see* Dutasteride *on page 702*

◆ **Mint-Ezetimibe (Can)** *see* Ezetimibe *on page 832*

◆ **Mint-Finasteride (Can)** *see* Finasteride *on page 878*

◆ **Mint-Fluoxetine (Can)** *see* FLUoxetine *on page 899*

◆ **Mint-Gliclazide MR (Can)** *see* Gliclazide [CAN/INT] *on page 964*

◆ **Mint-Irbesartan/HCTZ (Can)** *see* Irbesartan and Hydrochlorothiazide *on page 1112*

◆ **Mint-Losartan (Can)** *see* Losartan *on page 1248*

◆ **Mint-Losartan/HCTZ (Can)** *see* Losartan and Hydrochlorothiazide *on page 1250*

◆ **Mint-Losartan/HCTZ DS (Can)** *see* Losartan and Hydrochlorothiazide *on page 1250*

◆ **Mint-Metformin (Can)** *see* MetFORMIN *on page 1307*

◆ **Mint-Montelukast (Can)** *see* Montelukast *on page 1392*

◆ **Mint-Ondansetron (Can)** *see* Ondansetron *on page 1513*

◆ **Mintox Plus [OTC]** *see* Aluminum Hydroxide, Magnesium Hydroxide, and Simethicone *on page 104*

◆ **Mint-Pantoprazole (Can)** *see* Pantoprazole *on page 1570*

◆ **Mint-Pioglitazone (Can)** *see* Pioglitazone *on page 1654*

◆ **Mint-Pravastatin (Can)** *see* Pravastatin *on page 1700*

◆ **Mint-Pregabalin (Can)** *see* Pregabalin *on page 1710*

- **Mint-Ramipril (Can)** *see* Ramipril *on page 1771*
- **Mint-Risperidon (Can)** *see* RisperiDONE *on page 1818*
- **Mint-Rosuvastatin (Can)** *see* Rosuvastatin *on page 1848*
- **MINT-Sertraline (Can)** *see* Sertraline *on page 1878*
- **Mint-Sildenafil (Can)** *see* Sildenafil *on page 1882*
- **Mint-Simvastatin (Can)** *see* Simvastatin *on page 1890*
- **Mint-Topiramate (Can)** *see* Topiramate *on page 2065*
- **Mint-Tramadol/Acet (Can)** *see* Acetaminophen and Tramadol *on page 37*
- **Mint-Zopiclone (Can)** *see* Zopiclone [CAN/INT] *on page 2217*
- **Miochol-E** *see* Acetylcholine *on page 40*
- **Miochol®-E (Can)** *see* Acetylcholine *on page 40*
- **Miostat** *see* Carbachol *on page 346*
- **Miostat® (Can)** *see* Carbachol *on page 346*

Mipomersen (mi poe MER sen)

Brand Names: U.S. Kynamro

Index Terms ISIS 301012; Mipomersen Sodium

Pharmacologic Category Antihyperlipidemic Agent, Apolipoprotein B Antisense Oligonucleotide

Use Adjunct to dietary therapy and other lipid-lowering treatments to reduce low-density lipoprotein cholesterol (LDL-C), total cholesterol, apolipoprotein B, and non-high-density lipoprotein cholesterol (non-HDL-C) in patients with homozygous familial hypercholesterolemia (HoFH)

Pregnancy Risk Factor B

Dosage Homozygous familial hypercholesterolemia (HoFH): Adults: SubQ: 200 mg once weekly. **Note:** Maximal LDL-C reduction seen after ~6 months.

Dosage adjustment for toxicity:

ALT or AST ≥3 x and <5 x ULN: First, repeat measurement within 1 week to confirm elevation. Once confirmed, withhold mipomersen and obtain additional liver function tests (eg, total bilirubin, alkaline phosphatase, and INR); investigate for probable cause. If resumed when AST or ALT <3 x ULN, monitor liver function tests more frequently.

ALT or AST ≥5 x ULN: Withhold mipomersen and obtain additional liver function tests (eg, total bilirubin, alkaline phosphatase, and INR); investigate for probable cause. If resumed when AST or ALT <3 x ULN, monitor liver function tests more frequently.

Clinical symptoms of liver injury (eg, nausea, vomiting, abdominal pain, fever, jaundice, lethargy, flu-like symptoms), bilirubin increase ≥2 x ULN, or active liver disease: Discontinue mipomersen; investigate for probable cause.

Dosage adjustment in renal impairment: No dosage adjustment provided in manufacturer's labeling (has not been studied); use is not recommended in patients with severe renal impairment, clinically significant proteinuria, or receiving hemodialysis.

Dosage adjustment in hepatic impairment: No dosage adjustment provided in manufacturer's labeling (has not been studied); use is contraindicated in patients with moderate or severe hepatic impairment (Child-Pugh class B or C), active liver disease, or unexplained persistent elevations of hepatic transaminases.

Additional Information Complete prescribing information should be consulted for additional detail.

Dosage Forms

Solution Prefilled Syringe, Subcutaneous [preservative free]:

Kynamro: 200 mg/mL (1 mL)

- **Mipomersen Sodium** *see* Mipomersen *on page 1375*

Mirabegron (mir a BEG ron)

Brand Names: U.S. Myrbetriq

Brand Names: Canada Myrbetriq

Index Terms YM-178

Pharmacologic Category $Beta_3$ Agonist

Use Treatment of overactive bladder (OAB) with symptoms of urinary frequency, urgency, or urge incontinence

Pregnancy Risk Factor C

Pregnancy Considerations Adverse effects were observed in some animal reproduction studies. The Canadian labeling contraindicates use in pregnancy.

Breast-Feeding Considerations Excretion of mirabegron into breast milk is expected. According to the manufacturer, the decision to continue or discontinue breast-feeding during therapy should take into account the risk of exposure to the infant and the benefits of treatment to the mother.

Contraindications There are no contraindications listed in the manufacturer's U.S. product labeling.

Canadian labeling: Hypersensitivity to mirabegron or any component of the formulation; severe uncontrolled hypertension (systolic blood pressure ≥180 mm Hg and/or diastolic blood pressure ≥110 mm Hg); pregnancy

Warnings/Precautions Dose-related increases in blood pressure were observed in clinical trials (mean increase of ~0.5-1 mm Hg compared to placebo in overactive bladder patients treated with 50 mg); monitor blood pressure periodically during therapy. Not recommended for use in patients with severe uncontrolled hypertension (SBP ≥180 and/or DBP ≥110 mm Hg); if used in patients with controlled and less severe hypertension, use with caution and monitor blood pressure closely; exacerbation of pre-existing hypertension has been reported. Use with caution in patients with bladder outlet obstruction (BOO) or in patients taking concomitant antimuscarinic medications; the risk of urinary retention may be increased. Use with caution in patients with a history of QT interval prolongation or those receiving medications known to prolong the QT interval. In one thorough QT study, supratherapeutic doses prolonged the QTc interval based on the individual subject-specific correction method (QTcI) in females but not in males (Malik, 2012). In general, mirabegron at the recommended dose has a low risk of QT interval prolongation (Sanford, 2013).

Mirabegron is a moderate CYP2D6 inhibitor; potentially significant drug-drug interactions may exist, requiring dose or frequency adjustment, additional monitoring, and/or selection of alternative therapy. Use with caution in patients with mild-to-moderate hepatic impairment; dosage adjustment is required in patients with moderate hepatic impairment. Use is not recommended in severe hepatic impairment. Use with caution in patients with renal impairment; dosage adjustment is required in patients with severe renal impairment. Use is not recommended in ESRD. Systemic exposure is increased in females compared to males; however, dosage adjustments are not necessary or recommended.

Adverse Reactions

Cardiovascular: Hypertension, tachycardia
Central nervous system: Dizziness, headache
Gastrointestinal: Constipation, diarrhea, xerostomia
Genitourinary: Cystitis, urinary tract infection
Neuromuscular & skeletal: Arthralgia, back pain
Respiratory: Nasopharyngitis, sinusitis
Miscellaneous: Flu-like syndrome

Rare but important or life-threatening: ALT/AST increased, atrial fibrillation, breast cancer, cerebrovascular accident, GGT increased, glaucoma, LDH increased, leukocytoclastic vasculitis, lung cancer, nephrolithiasis, osteoarthritis, palpitations, prostate cancer, Stevens-Johnson syndrome, urinary retention, vaginal infection, vulvovaginal pruritus

Drug Interactions

Metabolism/Transport Effects Substrate of CYP2D6 (minor), CYP3A4 (minor), P-glycoprotein; **Note:** Assignment of Major/Minor substrate status based on clinically relevant drug interaction potential; **Inhibits** CYP2D6 (moderate), CYP3A4 (weak)

Avoid Concomitant Use

Avoid concomitant use of Mirabegron with any of the following: Pimozide; Thioridazine

Increased Effect/Toxicity

Mirabegron may increase the levels/effects of: ARIPiprazole; CYP2D6 Substrates; Desipramine; Digoxin; DOXOrubicin (Conventional); Eliglustat; Fesoterodine; Flecainide; Highest Risk QTc-Prolonging Agents; Hydrocodone; Lomitapide; Metoprolol; Moderate Risk QTc-Prolonging Agents; Nebivolol; Pimozide; Propafenone; Solifenacin; Thioridazine

The levels/effects of Mirabegron may be increased by: Anticholinergic Agents; Ketoconazole (Systemic); Mifepristone

Decreased Effect

Mirabegron may decrease the levels/effects of: Codeine; Metoprolol; Tamoxifen; TraMADol

The levels/effects of Mirabegron may be decreased by: Rifampin

Food Interactions Coadministration with a high-fat meal decreased C_{max} and AUC by 45% and 17%, respectively. Coadministration with a low-fat meal decreased C_{max} and AUC by 75% and 51%, respectively. However, safety and efficacy were unaffected by food intake. Management: Mirabegron may be administered without regard to food.

Storage/Stability Store at 25°C (77°F); excursions permitted to 15°C to 30°C (59°F to 86°F).

Mechanism of Action Mirabegron, a beta-3 adrenergic receptor agonist, activates beta-3 adrenergic receptors in the bladder resulting in relaxation of the detrusor smooth muscle during the urine storage phase, thus increasing bladder capacity. At usual doses, mirabegron is believed to display selectivity for the beta-3 adrenergic receptor subtype compared to its affinity for the beta-1 and -2 adrenoceptor subtypes. Data have shown that beta-adrenoceptors, predominately the beta-3 subtype, mediate detrusor smooth muscle tone and promote the storage function of the human bladder.

Pharmacodynamics/Kinetics

Onset of action: Efficacy is seen within 8 weeks; steady state achieved within 7 days

Distribution: V_{ss}: ~1670 L (following IV administration)

Protein binding: ~71%; binds mainly to albumin and $alpha_1$-acid glycoprotein

Metabolism: Extensive metabolism via multiple pathways (eg, dealkylation, oxidation, glucuronidation, amide hydrolysis) via multiple enzymes (eg, UGT, esterase, CYP3A4, CYP2D6); two major pharmacologically inactive metabolites produced

Bioavailability: 29% to 35% (following 25 mg and 50 mg oral dosing, respectively); bioavailability is dose-dependent; C_{max} and AUC are higher in females compared to males

Half-life elimination: ~50 hours

Time to peak: ~3.5 hours

Excretion: Urine (radiolabeled drug: 55%; unchanged drug: ~25%); feces (radiolabeled drug: 34%; unchanged drug: 0%)

Dosage Overactive bladder (OAB): Adults: Oral: Initial: 25 mg once daily; efficacy is observed within 8 weeks for 25 mg dose. May increase to 50 mg once daily based on individual patient efficacy and tolerability.

Dosing with concomitant therapy: CYP2D6 substrates: Appropriate monitoring and possible dose adjustment of the CYP2D6 substrate (especially those with a narrow therapeutic index) may be necessary. The Canadian labeling specifically recommends limiting mirabegron to 25 mg once daily in patients receiving concomitant CYP2D6 substrates with a narrow therapeutic index (eg, flecainide, propafenone, thioridazine).

Dosing adjustment in renal impairment:

Mild-to-moderate impairment (CrCl 30-89 mL/minute or eGFR 30-89 mL/minute/1.73 m^2): No dosage adjustment necessary

Severe impairment (CrCl 15-29 mL/minute or eGFR 15-29 mL/minute/1.73 m^2): Do not exceed 25 mg once daily

ESRD (CrCl <15 mL/minute or eGFR <15 mL/minute/1.73 m^2) or patients requiring hemodialysis: Not recommended (has not been studied)

Dosing adjustment in hepatic impairment:

Mild impairment (Child-Pugh Class A): No dosage adjustment necessary

Moderate impairment (Child-Pugh Class B): Do not exceed 25 mg once daily

Severe impairment (Child-Pugh Class C): Not recommended (has not been studied)

Administration Administer orally without regard to food. Swallow the tablet whole with water; do not chew, divide, or crush.

Monitoring Parameters Monitor blood pressure at baseline and then periodically during therapy

Dosage Forms

Tablet Extended Release 24 Hour, Oral:

Myrbetriq: 25 mg, 50 mg

◆ **MiraLax [OTC]** *see* Polyethylene Glycol 3350 *on page 1674*

◆ **Miranel AF [OTC]** *see* Miconazole (Topical) *on page 1360*

◆ **Mirapex** *see* Pramipexole *on page 1695*

◆ **Mirapex ER** *see* Pramipexole *on page 1695*

◆ **Mircette** *see* Ethinyl Estradiol and Desogestrel *on page 799*

◆ **Mirena** *see* Levonorgestrel *on page 1201*

Mirtazapine (mir TAZ a peen)

Brand Names: U.S. Remeron; Remeron SolTab

Brand Names: Canada Apo-Mirtazapine; Auro-Mirtazapine; Auro-Mirtazapine OD; Ava-Mirtazapine; Dom-Mirtazapine; GD-Mirtazapine OD; Jamp-Mirtazapine; Mylan-Mirtazapine; PMS-Mirtazapine; PRO-Mirtazapine; ratio-Mirtazapine; Remeron; Remeron RD; Riva-Mirtazapine; Sandoz-Mirtazapine; Teva-Mirtazapine; Teva-Mirtazapine OD; ZYM-Mirtazapine

Pharmacologic Category Antidepressant, Alpha-2 Antagonist

Additional Appendix Information

Beers Criteria – Potentially Inappropriate Medications for Geriatrics *on page 2271*

Use Major depressive disorder: Treatment of major depressive disorder (MDD)

Pregnancy Risk Factor C

Pregnancy Considerations Adverse events were observed in some animal reproduction studies. A significant increase in major teratogenic effects has not been observed in humans following exposure to mirtazapine during pregnancy; however, some nonteratogenic adverse events (similar to those observed with SSRI agents) have been reported (Djulus, 2006; Einarson, 2009; Lennestål, 2007). Mirtazapine was found to cross the placenta following a maternal overdose (Hatzidaki, 2008).

The ACOG recommends that therapy with antidepressants during pregnancy be individualized; treatment of depression during pregnancy should incorporate the clinical expertise of the mental health clinician, obstetrician, primary healthcare provider, and pediatrician. According to the American Psychiatric Association (APA), the risks of medication treatment should be weighed against other treatment options and untreated depression. Consideration should be given to using agents with safety data in pregnancy. For women who discontinue antidepressant medications during pregnancy and who may be at high risk for postpartum depression, the medications can be restarted following delivery. Treatment algorithms have been developed by the ACOG and the APA for the management of depression in women prior to conception and during pregnancy (ACOG, 2008; APA, 2010; Yonkers, 2009).

Breast-Feeding Considerations Mirtazapine and its active metabolite are found in breast milk, with higher levels in the hindmilk than foremilk. Mirtazapine can also be detected in the serum of nursing infants; adverse events have generally not been observed, although possible sedation and weight gain was noted in one case report (Kristensen, 2007; Tonn, 2009). The manufacturer recommends that caution be used if administered to a breast-feeding woman.

Contraindications Hypersensitivity to mirtazapine or any component of the formulation; use of MAO inhibitors intended to treat psychiatric disorders (concurrently or within 14 days of discontinuing either mirtazapine or the MAO inhibitor); initiation of mirtazapine in a patient receiving linezolid or intravenous methylene blue

Warnings/Precautions [U.S. Boxed Warning]: Antidepressants increase the risk of suicidal thinking and behavior in children, adolescents, and young adults (18-24 years of age) with major depressive disorder (MDD) and other psychiatric disorders; consider risk prior to prescribing. Short-term studies did not show an increased risk in patients >24 years of age and showed a decreased risk in patients ≥65 years. Closely monitor for clinical worsening, suicidality, or unusual changes in behavior, particularly during the initial 1 to 2 months of therapy or during periods of dosage adjustments (increases or decreases); the patient's family or caregiver should be instructed to closely observe the patient and communicate condition with healthcare provider. A medication guide should be dispensed with each prescription. **Mirtazapine is not FDA approved for use in children.**

The possibility of a suicide attempt is inherent in major depression and may persist until remission occurs. Worsening depression and severe abrupt suicidality that are not part of the presenting symptoms may require discontinuation or modification of drug therapy. The patient's family or caregiver should be alerted to monitor patients for the emergence of suicidality and associated behaviors (such as agitation, irritability, hostility, impulsivity, and hypomania) and call health care provider.

May precipitate a shift to mania or hypomania in patients with bipolar disorder. Patients presenting with depressive symptoms should be screened for bipolar disorder. Monotherapy in patients with bipolar disorder should be avoided. **Mirtazapine is not FDA approved for the treatment of bipolar depression.**

Potentially life-threatening serotonin syndrome (SS) has occurred with serotonergic agents (eg, SSRIs, SNRIs), particularly when used in combination with other serotonergic agents (eg, triptans, TCAs, fentanyl, lithium, tramadol, buspirone, St John's wort, tryptophan) or agents that impair metabolism of serotonin (eg, MAO inhibitors intended to treat psychiatric disorders, other MAO inhibitors such as linezolid and intravenous methylene blue). Discontinue treatment (and any concomitant serotonergic agent) immediately if signs/symptoms arise. Discontinue immediately if signs and symptoms of neutropenia/agranulocytosis occur. May cause CNS depression, which may impair physical or mental abilities; patients must be cautioned about performing tasks that require mental alertness (eg, operating machinery or driving). The degree of sedation is moderate-high relative to other antidepressants. Conversely, may increase psychomotor restlessness within first few weeks of therapy. Dizziness may occur; it is unclear whether or not tolerance may develop to dizziness. The risks of orthostatic hypotension or anticholinergic effects are low relative to other antidepressants. The incidence of sexual dysfunction with mirtazapine is generally lower than with selective serotonin reuptake inhibitors (SSRIs) (Bauer, 2013). May increase appetite and stimulate weight gain. May increase serum cholesterol and triglyceride levels. Potentially significant interactions may exist, requiring dose or frequency adjustment, additional monitoring, and/or selection of alternative therapy.

QT prolongation, torsade de pointes, and ventricular fibrillation have been reported (rarely) (Remeron Canadian product monograph, 2014); case reports are mostly associated with mirtazapine overdose (although one case series of single-agent mirtazapine overdose in 84 patients did not identify any cases of QT prolongation [Berling, 2014]) or patients with risk factors for QT prolongation or receiving concomitant QT-prolonging agents. Use caution in patients with cardiovascular disease, history of QT prolongation, or receiving concomitant QT-prolonging agents.

Use caution in patients with a previous seizure disorder or condition predisposing to seizures such as brain damage, alcoholism, or concurrent therapy with other drugs which lower the seizure threshold. May cause mild pupillary dilation which in susceptible individuals can lead to an episode of narrow-angle glaucoma. Consider evaluating patients who have not had an iridectomy for narrow-angle glaucoma risk factors. Bone fractures have been associated with antidepressant treatment. Consider the possibility of a fragility fracture if an antidepressant-treated patient presents with unexplained bone pain, point tenderness, swelling, or bruising (Rabenda, 2013; Rizzoli, 2012). Use with caution in patients with hepatic or renal dysfunction. Use caution in elderly patients; may cause or exacerbate syndrome of inappropriate antidiuretic hormone secretion or hyponatremia; monitor sodium closely with initiation or dosage adjustments in older adults (Beers Criteria). Clinically significant transaminase elevations have been observed. SolTab formulation contains phenylalanine.

Abrupt discontinuation or interruption of antidepressant therapy has been associated with a discontinuation syndrome. Symptoms arising may vary with antidepressant however commonly include nausea, vomiting, diarrhea, headaches, lightheadedness, dizziness, diminished appetite, sweating, chills, tremors, paresthesias, fatigue, somnolence, and sleep disturbances (eg, vivid dreams, insomnia). Greater risks for developing a discontinuation syndrome have been associated with antidepressants with shorter half-lives, longer durations of treatment, and abrupt discontinuation. For antidepressants of short or intermediate half-lives, symptoms may emerge within 2 to 5 days after treatment discontinuation and last 7 to 14 days (APA, 2010; Fava, 2006; Haddad, 2001; Shelton, 2001; Warner, 2006).

Adverse Reactions

Cardiovascular: Edema, hypertension, peripheral edema, vasodilatation

Central nervous system: Abnormal dreams, abnormality in thinking, agitation, amnesia, anxiety, apathy, confusion, depression, dizziness, drowsiness, hypoesthesia, malaise, myasthenia, paresthesia, twitching, vertigo

Dermatologic: Pruritus, skin rash

Endocrine & metabolic: Increased serum cholesterol, increased serum triglycerides, increased thirst, weight gain (more common in pediatric patients)

Gastrointestinal: Abdominal pain, anorexia, constipation, increased appetite, vomiting, xerostomia

Genitourinary: Urinary frequency, urinary tract infection

Hepatic: Increased serum ALT (≥3 times ULN)

Neuromuscular & skeletal: Arthralgia, back pain, hyperkinesia, hypokinesia, myalgia, tremor, weakness

Respiratory: Dyspnea, flu-like symptoms, increased cough, sinusitis

Rare but important or life-threatening: Abnormal accommodation, abnormal healing, abnormal hepatic function tests, abnormal lacrimation, alopecia, altered sense of smell, amenorrhea, aphasia, arthritis, asphyxia, asthma, atrial arrhythmia, bigeminy, blepharitis, bradycardia, breast engorgement, breast hypertrophy, bursitis, cellulitis, cerebral ischemia, cholecystitis, colitis, conjunctivitis, cystitis, deafness, dehydration, delirium, dementia, depersonalization, diabetes mellitus, diarrhea, diplopia, drug dependence, dysmenorrhea, ejaculatory disorder, emotional lability, enlargement of abdomen, eosinophilia, erythema multiforme, exfoliative dermatitis, extrapyramidal reaction, facial edema, gastroenteritis, gingival hemorrhage, glaucoma, glossitis, gout, hepatic cirrhosis, herpes simplex infection, herpes zoster, hyperacusis, hyper-reflexia, hypotension, hypothyroidism, hypotonia, impotence, increased acid phosphatase, increased libido, insomnia, intestinal obstruction, laryngitis, left heart failure, leukorrhea, lymphadenopathy, lymphocytosis, migraine, myocardial infarction, myoclonus, myositis, neck pain, nephrolithiasis, nystagmus, oral candidiasis, ostealgia, osteoporosis, otalgia, pancreatitis, pancytopenia, paralysis, phlebitis, pneumonia, pneumothorax, prolonged Q-T interval on ECG, psychomotor agitation, psychoneurosis, psychotic depression, pulmonary embolism, restless leg syndrome, seborrhea, sedation, seizure, serotonin syndrome, skin hypertrophy, skin photosensitivity, stomatitis, suicidal behavior, syncope, tenosynovitis, torsade de pointes (rare), urethritis, urinary incontinence, urinary retention, urinary urgency, uterine hemorrhage, vaginitis, vascular headache, ventricular fibrillation, ventricular premature contractions, ventricular tachycardia

Drug Interactions

Metabolism/Transport Effects Substrate of CYP1A2 (major), CYP2C9 (minor), CYP2D6 (major), CYP3A4 (major); **Note:** Assignment of Major/Minor substrate status based on clinically relevant drug interaction potential; **Inhibits** CYP1A2 (weak), CYP3A4 (weak)

Avoid Concomitant Use

Avoid concomitant use of Mirtazapine with any of the following: Alcohol (Ethyl); Azelastine (Nasal); Conivaptan; Dapoxetine; Fusidic Acid (Systemic); Idelalisib; Linezolid; MAO Inhibitors; Methylene Blue; Orphenadrine; Paraldehyde; Pimozide; Thalidomide; Tryptophan

Increased Effect/Toxicity

Mirtazapine may increase the levels/effects of: ARIPiprazole; Azelastine (Nasal); Buprenorphine; Highest Risk QTc-Prolonging Agents; Hydrocodone; Lomitapide; Methotrimeprazine; Methylene Blue; Metoclopramide; Metyrosine; Moderate Risk QTc-Prolonging Agents; Orphenadrine; Paraldehyde; Pimozide; Pramipexole; ROPINIRole; Rotigotine; Serotonin Modulators; Suvorexant; Thalidomide; Warfarin; Zolpidem

The levels/effects of Mirtazapine may be increased by: Abiraterone Acetate; Alcohol (Ethyl); Antiemetics (5HT3 Antagonists); Aprepitant; Brimonidine (Topical); Cannabis; Ceritinib; CNS Depressants; Conivaptan; CYP1A2 Inhibitors (Moderate); CYP1A2 Inhibitors (Strong); CYP2D6 Inhibitors (Moderate); CYP2D6 Inhibitors (Strong); CYP3A4 Inhibitors (Moderate); CYP3A4 Inhibitors (Strong); Dapoxetine; Dasatinib; Deferasirox; Doxylamine; Dronabinol; Droperidol; Fosaprepitant; Fusidic Acid (Systemic); HydrOXYzine; Idelalisib; Ivacaftor; Kava Kava; Linezolid; Luliconazole; Magnesium Sulfate; MAO Inhibitors; Methotrimeprazine; Mifepristone; Nabilone; Netupitant; Peginterferon Alfa-2b; Perampanel; Rufinamide; Simeprevir; Sodium Oxybate; Stiripentol; Tapentadol; Tedizolid; Tetrahydrocannabinol; Tryptophan; Vemurafenib

Decreased Effect

Mirtazapine may decrease the levels/effects of: Alpha2-Agonists

The levels/effects of Mirtazapine may be decreased by: Bosentan; Cannabis; CYP1A2 Inducers (Strong); CYP3A4 Inducers (Moderate); CYP3A4 Inducers (Strong); Cyproterone; Dabrafenib; Deferasirox; Mitotane; Peginterferon Alfa-2b; Siltuximab; St Johns Wort; Teriflunomide; Tocilizumab

Storage/Stability Store at 25°C (77°F); excursions are permitted between 15°C and 30°C (59°F and 86°F). Protect from light and moisture. Use orally disintegrating tablets immediately upon opening individual tablet blister; once removed it cannot be stored.

Mechanism of Action Mirtazapine is a tetracyclic antidepressant that works by its central presynaptic $alpha_2$-adrenergic antagonist effects, which results in increased release of norepinephrine and serotonin. It is also a potent antagonist of 5-HT_2 and 5-HT_3 serotonin receptors and H_1 histamine receptors and a moderate peripheral $alpha_1$-adrenergic and muscarinic antagonist; it does not inhibit the reuptake of norepinephrine or serotonin.

Pharmacodynamics/Kinetics

Absorption: Rapid and complete

Protein binding: ~85%

Metabolism: Extensively hepatic via CYP1A2, 2D6, 3A4 and via demethylation and hydroxylation

Bioavailability: ~50%

Half-life elimination: 20 to 40 hours; increased with renal or hepatic impairment

Time to peak, serum: ~2 hours

Excretion: Urine (75%) and feces (15%) as metabolites

Dosage Oral:

Adults: Major depressive disorder (MDD): Initial: 15 mg nightly, may titrate dose up no more frequently than every 1 to 2 weeks to a maximum of 45 mg daily; dosage range: 15 to 45 mg daily

Elderly: There are no dosage adjustments provided in the manufacturer's labeling; however, clearance may be decreased in the elderly. Use with caution.

Discontinuation of therapy: Upon discontinuation of antidepressant therapy, gradually taper the dose to minimize the incidence of withdrawal symptoms and allow for the detection of re-emerging symptoms. Evidence supporting ideal taper rates is limited. APA and NICE guidelines suggest tapering therapy over at least several weeks with consideration to the half-life of the antidepressant; antidepressants with a shorter half-life may need to be tapered more conservatively. In addition for long-term treated patients, WFSBP guidelines recommend tapering over 4-6 months. If intolerable withdrawal symptoms occur following a dose reduction, consider resuming the previously prescribed dose and/or decrease dose at a more gradual rate (APA, 2010; Bauer, 2002; Haddad, 2001; NCCMH, 2010; Schatzberg, 2006; Shelton, 2001; Warner, 2006).

MAO inhibitor recommendations:

Switching to or from an MAO inhibitor intended to treat psychiatric disorders:

Allow 14 days to elapse between discontinuing an MAO inhibitor intended to treat psychiatric disorders and initiation of mirtazapine.

Allow 14 days to elapse between discontinuing mirtazapine and initiation of an MAO inhibitor intended to treat psychiatric disorders.

Use with other MAO inhibitors (linezolid or IV methylene blue):

Do not initiate mirtazapine in patients receiving linezolid or IV methylene blue; consider other interventions for psychiatric condition.

If urgent treatment with linezolid or IV methylene blue is required in a patient already receiving mirtazapine and potential benefits outweigh potential risks, discontinue mirtazapine promptly and administer linezolid or IV methylene blue. Monitor for serotonin syndrome for 2 weeks or until 24 hours after the last dose of linezolid or IV methylene blue, whichever comes first. May resume mirtazapine 24 hours after the last dose of linezolid or IV methylene blue.

Dosage adjustment in renal impairment: There are no dosage adjustments provided in the manufacturer's labeling; however, clearance is decreased with moderate and severe renal impairment. Use with caution.

Dosage adjustment in hepatic impairment: There are no dosage adjustments provided in the manufacturer's labeling; however, clearance may be decreased with hepatic impairment. Use with caution.

Dietary Considerations Some products may contain phenylalanine.

Administration

Orally disintegrating tablet: Administer without regard to meals. Open blister pack and place tablet on the tongue; tablet is formulated to dissolve on the tongue without water; do not split tablet.

Tablet: Administer without regard to meals. Canadian labeling does not recommend chewing tablet.

Monitoring Parameters Patients should be monitored for signs of agranulocytosis or severe neutropenia such as sore throat, stomatitis or other signs of infection or a low WBC; renal and hepatic function; mental status for depression, suicide ideation (especially at the beginning of therapy or when doses are increased or decreased), anxiety, social functioning, mania, panic attacks; signs/symptoms of serotonin syndrome; lipid profile; weight gain

Dosage Forms

Tablet, Oral:

Remeron: 15 mg, 30 mg, 45 mg

Generic: 7.5 mg, 15 mg, 30 mg, 45 mg

Tablet Dispersible, Oral:

Remeron SolTab: 15 mg, 30 mg, 45 mg

Generic: 15 mg, 30 mg, 45 mg

◆ **Mirvaso** *see* Brimonidine (Topical) *on page* 288

Misoprostol (mye soe PROST ole)

Brand Names: U.S. Cytotec

Brand Names: Canada Novo-Misoprostol; PMS-Misoprostol

Pharmacologic Category Prostaglandin

Use

Prevention of NSAID-induced gastric ulcers

Medical termination of pregnancy of ≤49 days in conjunction with mifepristone (refer to Mifepristone monograph for details)

Pregnancy Risk Factor X

Pregnancy Considerations Teratogenic effects were not observed in animal reproduction studies. Congenital anomalies following first trimester exposure have been reported, including skull defects, cranial nerve palsies, falcial malformations, and limb defects. Misoprostol may produce uterine contractions; fetal death, uterine perforation, and abortion may occur. **[U.S. Boxed Warning]: Use of misoprostol during pregnancy may cause abortion, birth defects, or premature birth. It is not to be used to reduce NSAID-induced ulcers in a woman of childbearing potential unless she is capable of complying with effective contraceptive measures and is at high risk of developing gastric ulcers and/or their complications.** If needed, the patient must have a negative pregnancy test within 2 weeks of starting therapy, she must use effective contraception during treatment, and therapy should begin on the second or third day of next normal menstrual period. Written and verbal warnings concerning the hazards of misoprostol should be provided.

Misoprostol is FDA approved for the medical termination of pregnancy of ≤49 days in conjunction with mifepristone.

Because misoprostol may induce or augment uterine contractions, it has been used off-label as a cervical-ripening agent for induction of labor in women who have not had a prior cesarean delivery or major uterine surgery. Hyperstimulation of the uterus, uterine rupture, or adverse events in the fetus or mother may occur with this use.

Breast-Feeding Considerations Misoprostol acid (the active metabolite of misoprostol) has been detected in breast milk. Concentrations following a single oral dose were 7.6-20.9 pg/mL after 1 hour and decreased to <1 pg/mL by 5 hours. Adverse events have not been reported in nursing infants (FIGO, 2012).

Contraindications Hypersensitivity to prostaglandins; pregnancy (when used to reduce NSAID-induced ulcers)

Warnings/Precautions Hazardous agent; use appropriate precautions for handling and disposal (NIOSH 2014 [group 3]).

[U.S. Boxed Warning]: Due to the abortifacient property of this medication, patients must be warned not to give this drug to others. [U.S. Boxed Warning]: Use of misoprostol during pregnancy may cause abortion, birth defects, or premature birth. It is not to be used to reduce NSAID-induced ulcers in a woman of childbearing potential unless she is capable of complying with effective contraceptive measures and is at high risk of developing gastric ulcers and/or their complications. If needed, the patient must have a negative pregnancy test within two weeks of starting therapy, she must use effective contraception during treatment and therapy should begin on the second or third day of next normal menstrual period. Women of childbearing potential taking this for reducing the risk of NSAID-induced gastric ulcers should be given oral and written warnings of the potential adverse events if pregnancy occurs during treatment. Adverse events have been reported when used outside of current product labeling (cervical ripening, induction of labor, postpartum hemorrhage). Uterine tachysystole may occur and progress to uterine tetany; uteroplacental blood flow may be impaired and uterine rupture or amniotic fluid embolism may occur. The risk of uterine rupture may be increased with advanced gestational age, grand multiparity, or prior uterine surgery. Uterine activity and fetal status should be monitored in a hospital setting. Misoprostol should not be used in situations where uterotonic drugs are otherwise contraindicated or inappropriate. ▶

When used for ulcers, use only in patients at high risk of complications from gastric ulcers (eg, the elderly or patients with concomitant diseases) or patients at high risk for developing gastric ulcers (eg, those with a history of ulcers) taking NSAIDs. Misoprostol must be taken during the duration of NSAID therapy. It is not effective in preventing duodenal ulcers in patients taking NSAIDs.

Use with caution in patients with cardiovascular disease, renal impairment, and the elderly.

Adverse Reactions

Central nervous system: Headache

Gastrointestinal: Abdominal pain, constipation, diarrhea, dyspepsia, flatulence, nausea, vomiting

Rare but important or life-threatening: Abnormal taste, abnormal vision, alkaline phosphatase increased, alopecia, anaphylaxis, anemia, amylase increase, anxiety, arrhythmia, arterial thrombosis, arthralgia, cardiac enzymes increased, chest pain, chills, confusion, CVA, deafness, depression, diaphoresis, dizziness, drowsiness, dysphagia, dyspnea, dysuria, edema, epistaxis, ESR increased, fatigue, fever, GI bleeding, GI inflammation, gingivitis, glycosuria, gout; gynecological disorders, hematuria, hepatobiliary function abnormal, hyper-/hypotension, impotence, loss of libido, MI, muscle cramps, myalgia, neuropathy, neurosis, nitrogen increased, pallor, phlebitis, polyuria, pulmonary embolism, purpura, rash, reflux, rigors, stiffness, syncope, thirst, thrombocytopenia, tinnitus, uterine rupture, weakness, weight changes

Drug Interactions

Metabolism/Transport Effects None known.

Avoid Concomitant Use

Avoid concomitant use of Misoprostol with any of the following: Carbetocin

Increased Effect/Toxicity

Misoprostol may increase the levels/effects of: Carbetocin; Oxytocin

The levels/effects of Misoprostol may be increased by: Antacids

Decreased Effect There are no known significant interactions involving a decrease in effect.

Food Interactions Misoprostol peak serum concentrations may be decreased if taken with food (not clinically significant).

Storage/Stability Store at or below 25°C (77°F).

Mechanism of Action Misoprostol is a synthetic prostaglandin E_1 analog that replaces the protective prostaglandins consumed with prostaglandin-inhibiting therapies (eg, NSAIDs); has been shown to induce uterine contractions

Pharmacodynamics/Kinetics

Absorption: Rapid and extensive

Metabolism: Hepatic; rapidly de-esterified to misoprostol acid (active)

Protein binding: Misoprostol acid: <90%

Half-life elimination: Misoprostol acid: 20-40 minutes

Time to peak, serum: Misoprostol acid: Fasting: 6-22 minutes

Excretion: Urine (80%)

Dosage

Oral: Adults:

Prevention of NSAID-induced gastric ulcers: 200 mcg 4 times daily with food; if not tolerated, may decrease dose to 100 mcg 4 times daily with food; last dose of the day should be taken at bedtime

Medical termination of pregnancy: Refer to Mifepristone monograph.

Prevention of postpartum hemorrhage (off-label use): 600 mcg as a single dose administered immediately after delivery; to be used in settings where oxytocin is not available (FIGO, 2012).

Treatment of incomplete abortion (off-label use): 600 mcg as a single dose (ACOG, 2009a).

Sublingual: Adults:

Treatment of missed abortion (off-label use): 600 mcg; may repeat every 3 hours for 2 additional doses if needed (ACOG, 2009a).

Treatment of postpartum hemorrhage (off-label use): 800 mcg as a single dose; to be used in settings where oxytocin is not available. Use caution if a prophylactic dose was already given, especially if adverse events were observed (FIGO, 2012).

Intravaginal: Adults:

Labor induction or cervical ripening (off-label uses): 25 mcg (1/4 of 100 mcg tablet); may repeat at intervals no more frequent than every 3-6 hours. Do not use in patients with previous cesarean delivery or prior major uterine surgery (ACOG, 2009b).

Treatment of missed abortion (off-label use): 800 mcg; may repeat every 3 hours for 2 additional doses if needed (ACOG, 2009a).

Dosage adjustment in renal impairment: Dose adjustment is not routinely needed; however, the dose may be reduced if the recommended dose is not tolerated. It is not known if misoprostol is removed by dialysis.

Dosage adjustment in hepatic impairment: No dosage adjustment provided in manufacturer's labeling.

Dietary Considerations Should be taken with food.

Administration Incidence of diarrhea may be lessened by having patient take dose right after meals and avoiding magnesium-containing antacids. When used for the prevention of NSAID-induced ulcers, therapy is usually begun on the second or third day of the next normal menstrual period in women of childbearing potential.

Hazardous agent; use appropriate precautions for handling and disposal (NIOSH 2014 [group 3]).

Monitoring Parameters

Prevention of NSAID-induced gastric ulcers: Pregnancy test in women of reproductive potential prior to therapy; adequate diagnostic measures in all cases of undiagnosed abnormal vaginal bleeding

Off-label pregnancy-related uses: Uterine activity and fetal status. When used for incomplete or missed abortion, reevaluate 1-2 weeks after dosing

Dosage Forms

Tablet, Oral:

Cytotec: 100 mcg, 200 mcg

Generic: 100 mcg, 200 mcg

◆ **Misoprostol and Diclofenac** *see* Diclofenac and Misoprostol *on page 621*

◆ **MITC** *see* MitoMYcin (Systemic) *on page 1380*

◆ **Mitigare** *see* Colchicine *on page 500*

◆ **MITO** *see* MitoMYcin (Systemic) *on page 1380*

◆ **MITO-C** *see* MitoMYcin (Systemic) *on page 1380*

◆ **Mitomycin-X** *see* MitoMYcin (Systemic) *on page 1380*

◆ **Mitomycin-C** *see* MitoMYcin (Ophthalmic) *on page 1382*

◆ **Mitomycin-C** *see* MitoMYcin (Systemic) *on page 1380*

MitoMYcin (Systemic) (mye toe MYE sin)

Brand Names: Canada Mitomycin For Injection; Mitomycin For Injection USP; Mutamycin®

Index Terms MITC; MITO; MITO-C; Mitomycin-C; Mitomycin-X; MMC; MTC; Mutamycin

Pharmacologic Category Antineoplastic Agent, Antibiotic

Use Treatment of adenocarcinoma of stomach or pancreas

Pregnancy Considerations Teratogenic effects have been observed in animal reproduction studies.

Breast-Feeding Considerations It is not known if mitomycin is excreted in human milk; the manufacturer recommends against breast-feeding during treatment.

Contraindications Hypersensitivity to mitomycin or any component of the formulation; thrombocytopenia; coagulation disorders, or other increased bleeding tendency

Warnings/Precautions Hazardous agent - use appropriate precautions for handling and disposal (NIOSH 2014 [group 1]). **[U.S. Boxed Warning]: Bone marrow suppression (thrombocytopenia and leukopenia) is common and may be severe and/or contribute to infections.** Fatalities due to sepsis have been reported; monitor for infections. Myelosuppression is dose-limiting, delayed in onset, and cumulative; therefore, monitor blood counts closely during and for ≥8 weeks following treatment; treatment delay or dosage adjustment may be required for significant thrombocytopenia (platelets <100,000/mm^3) or leukopenia (WBC<4000/mm^3) or a progressive decline in either value. Use with caution in patients who have received radiation therapy or in the presence of hepatobiliary dysfunction; reduce dosage in patients who are receiving radiation therapy simultaneously. Monitor for renal toxicity; do not administer if serum creatinine is >1.7 mg/dL. **[U.S. Boxed Warning]: Hemolytic-uremic syndrome (HUS) has been reported (incidence not defined); condition usually involves microangiopathic hemolytic anemia (hematocrit ≤5%), thrombocytopenia (≤100,000/mm^3), and irreversible renal failure (serum creatinine ≥1.6 mg/dL). HUS may occur at any time, is generally associated with single doses ≥60 mg, and HUS symptoms may be exacerbated by blood transfusion.** Other less common effects may include pulmonary edema, neurologic abnormalities, and hypertension. High mortality from HUS development has been reported, and is largely the result of renal failure. HUS may also be associated with cumulative doses ≥50 mg/m^2. Bladder fibrosis/contraction has been reported with intravesical administration (unapproved administration route). Mitomycin is a potent vesicant; ensure proper needle or catheter placement prior to and during infusion. Avoid extravasation. May cause necrosis and tissue sloughing; delayed erythema and/or ulceration have been reported.

Cases of acute respiratory distress syndrome (ARDS) have been reported in patients receiving mitomycin in combination with other chemotherapy who were maintained at FIO_2 concentrations >50% perioperatively; use caution to provide only enough oxygen to maintain adequate arterial saturation and avoid overhydration. Pulmonary toxicity has also been reported as dyspnea with nonproductive cough and appearance of pulmonary infiltrates on radiograph; discontinue therapy if pulmonary toxicity occurs and other potential etiologies have been ruled out. Shortness of breath and bronchospasm have been reported in patients receiving vinca alkaloids in combination with mitomycin or who received mitomycin previously; this acute respiratory distress has occurred within minutes to hours following the vinca alkaloid; may be managed with bronchodilators, steroids and/or oxygen. **[U.S. Boxed Warning]: Should be administered under the supervision of an experienced cancer chemotherapy physician.**

Adverse Reactions

Central nervous system: Fever

Dermatologic: Alopecia, mucous membrane toxicity

Gastrointestinal: Anorexia, nausea, stomatitis, vomiting

Hematologic: Myelosuppression (onset: 4 weeks; recovery: 8-10 weeks)

Renal: Serum creatinine increased

Miscellaneous: Thrombotic thrombocytopenic purpura (TTP)/hemolytic uremic syndrome (HUS)

Rare but important or life-threatening: Adult respiratory distress syndrome (ARDS), bladder fibrosis/contraction (intravesical administration), dyspnea, extravasation reactions, heart failure, hepatic sinusoidal obstruction syndrome (SOS, veno-occlusive liver disease), interstitial fibrosis, nonproductive cough, pulmonary infiltrates, rash, renal failure (irreversible)

Drug Interactions

Metabolism/Transport Effects **Substrate** of P-glycoprotein

Avoid Concomitant Use

Avoid concomitant use of MitoMYcin (Systemic) with any of the following: BCG; CloZAPine; Dipyrone; Natalizumab; Pimecrolimus; Tacrolimus (Topical); Tofacitinib; Vaccines (Live)

Increased Effect/Toxicity

MitoMYcin (Systemic) may increase the levels/effects of: CloZAPine; Leflunomide; Natalizumab; Tofacitinib; Vaccines (Live)

The levels/effects of MitoMYcin (Systemic) may be increased by: Antineoplastic Agents (Vinca Alkaloids); Denosumab; Dipyrone; P-glycoprotein/ABCB1 Inhibitors; Pimecrolimus; Roflumilast; Tacrolimus (Topical); Trastuzumab

Decreased Effect

MitoMYcin (Systemic) may decrease the levels/effects of: BCG; Coccidioides immitis Skin Test; Sipuleucel-T; Vaccines (Inactivated); Vaccines (Live)

The levels/effects of MitoMYcin (Systemic) may be decreased by: Echinacea; P-glycoprotein/ABCB1 Inducers

Preparation for Administration Hazardous agent; use appropriate precautions for handling and disposal (NIOSH 2014 [group 1]). Dilute powder with SWFI to a concentration of 0.5 mg/mL. May further dilute in NS or sodium lactate to 20-40 mcg/mL.

Storage/Stability Store intact vials at controlled room temperature; avoid exposure to temperatures >40°C (104°F). Reconstituted solution is stable for 7 days at room temperature and 14 days when refrigerated. Protect reconstituted solution from light. Solution of 0.5 mg/mL in a syringe is stable for 7 days at room temperature and 28 days when refrigerated and protected from light.

Further dilution to 20-40 mcg/mL:

In normal saline: Stable for 12 hours at room temperature.

In sodium lactate: Stable for 24 hours at room temperature.

Mechanism of Action Acts like an alkylating agent and produces DNA cross-linking (primarily with guanine and cytosine pairs); cell-cycle nonspecific; inhibits DNA and RNA synthesis; degrades preformed DNA, causes nuclear lysis and formation of giant cells. While not phase-specific *per se*, mitomycin has its maximum effect against cells in late G and early S phases.

Pharmacodynamics/Kinetics

Metabolism: Hepatic

Half-life elimination: 17-78 minutes; Terminal: 50 minutes

Excretion: Urine (~10% as unchanged drug)

Dosage Details concerning dosing in combination regimens should also be consulted. Adults:

Stomach or pancreas adenocarcinoma (manufacturer's labeling): IV: 20 mg/m^2 every 6-8 weeks

Anal carcinoma (off-label use): IV: 10 mg/m^2 as an IV bolus on days 1 and 29 (maximum: 20 mg/dose) in combination with fluorouracil and radiation therapy (Ajani, 2008)

Bladder cancer, nonmuscle invasive (off-label use/route): Intravesicular instillation:

Low risk of recurrence (uncomplicated): 40 mg as a single dose postoperatively; retain in bladder for 2 hours (Hall, 2007)

Increased risk of recurrence: 20 mg weekly for 6 weeks, followed by 20 mg monthly for 3 years; retain in bladder for 1-2 hours (Friedrich, 2007)

Dosage adjustment based on toxicity:

Leukocytes 2000 to <3000/mm^3: Hold therapy until leukocyte count ≥4000/mm^3; reduce to 70% of dose in subsequent cycles

Leukocytes <2000/mm^3: Hold therapy until leukocyte count ≥4000/mm^3; reduce to 50% of dose in subsequent cycles

Platelets 25,000 to <75,000/mm^3: Hold therapy until platelets ≥100,000/mm^3; reduce to 70% of dose in subsequent cycles

Platelets <25,000/mm^3: Hold therapy until platelets ≥100,000 mm^3; reduce to 50% of dose in subsequent cycles

Dosage adjustment in renal impairment: The manufacturer's labeling states to avoid use in patients with serum creatine >1.7 mg/dL, but no dosage adjustments are provided. The following adjustments have been used by some clinicians (Aronoff, 2007): Adults:

CrCl <10 mL/minute: Administer 75% of dose

Continuous ambulatory peritoneal dialysis (CAPD): Administer 75% of dose

Dosage adjustment in hepatic impairment: No dosage adjustment provided in manufacturer's labeling (has not been studied).

Dosing in obesity: *ASCO Guidelines for appropriate chemotherapy dosing in obese adults with cancer:* Utilize patient's actual body weight (full weight) for calculation of body surface area- or weight-based dosing, particularly when the intent of therapy is curative; manage regimen-related toxicities in the same manner as for nonobese patients; if a dose reduction is utilized due to toxicity, consider resumption of full weight-based dosing with subsequent cycles, especially if cause of toxicity (eg, hepatic or renal impairment) is resolved (Griggs, 2012).

Administration

IV: Administer slow IV push or by slow (15-30 minute) infusion via a freely-running saline infusion. Consider using a central venous catheter.

Vesicant; ensure proper needle or catheter placement prior to and during infusion; avoid extravasation.

Extravasation management: If extravasation occurs, stop infusion immediately and disconnect (leave cannula/needle in place); gently aspirate extravasated solution (do **NOT** flush the line); remove needle/cannula; elevate extremity. Initiate dimethyl sulfate (DMSO) antidote. Apply dry cold compress for 20 minutes 4 times/day for 1-2 days (Pérez Fidalgo, 2012).

DMSO: Apply topically to a region covering twice the affected area every 8 hours for 7 days; begin within 10 minutes of extravasation; do not cover with a dressing (Perez Fidalgo, 2012).

Intravesicular (off-label route): Instill into bladder and retain for up to 2 hours (Friedrich, 2007; Hall, 2007); rotate patient every 15-30 minutes

Hazardous agent; use appropriate precautions for handling and disposal (NIOSH 2014 [group 1]).

Monitoring Parameters Monitor CBC with differential (repeatedly during therapy and for ≥8 weeks following therapy); serum creatinine; pulmonary function tests; monitor for signs/symptoms of HUS

Dosage Forms

Solution Reconstituted, Intravenous:

Generic: 5 mg (1 ea); 20 mg (1 ea); 40 mg (1 ea)

MitoMYcin (Ophthalmic) (mye toe MYE sin)

Brand Names: U.S. Mitosol

Index Terms Mitomycin-C; MMC

Pharmacologic Category Antineoplastic Agent, Antibiotic; Ophthalmic Agent, Miscellaneous

Use Adjunct to *ab externo* glaucoma surgery

Pregnancy Risk Factor X

Dosage Topical ophthalmic: Adults: Glaucoma surgery, adjunctive therapy: 0.2 mg solution is aseptically applied via saturated sponges to surgical site of glaucoma filtration surgery for 2 minutes

Additional Information Complete prescribing information should be consulted for additional detail.

Dosage Forms

Kit, Ophthalmic:

Mitosol: 0.2 mg

◆ **Mitomycin For Injection (Can)** *see* MitoMYcin (Systemic) *on page* 1380

◆ **Mitomycin For Injection USP (Can)** *see* MitoMYcin (Systemic) *on page* 1380

◆ **Mitosol** *see* MitoMYcin (Ophthalmic) *on page* 1382

Mitotane (MYE toe tane)

Brand Names: U.S. Lysodren

Brand Names: Canada Lysodren

Index Terms Chloditan; Chlodithane; Khloditan; Mytotan; o,p'-DDD; Ortho,para-DDD

Pharmacologic Category Antineoplastic Agent, Miscellaneous

Use Adrenocortical carcinoma: Treatment of inoperable adrenocortical carcinoma (both functional and non-functional types)

Pregnancy Risk Factor D

Dosage Note: Mitotane is associated with a moderate emetic potential; antiemetics may be needed to prevent nausea and vomiting.

Adrenocortical carcinoma: Adults: Oral: Initial: 2 to 6 g daily in 3 to 4 divided doses, then increase incrementally to 9 to 10 g daily in 3 to 4 divided doses (maximum tolerated range: 2 to 16 g daily, usually 9 to 10 g daily; maximum dose studied: 18 to 19 g daily); continue as long as clinical benefit is demonstrated

Off-label dosing: Initial 1 to 2 g daily; increase by 1 to 2 g daily at 1 to 2 week intervals as tolerated to a maximum of 6 to 10 g daily; usual dose 4 to 5 g daily (Veytsman, 2009)

Cushing syndrome (off-label use): Adults: Oral: Initial dose: 500 mg 3 times daily; maximum dose: 3 g 3 times daily (Biller, 2008)

Dosage adjustment for toxicity:

Severe side effects: Reduce dose until a maximum tolerated dose is achieved

Significant neuropsychiatric adverse effects: Withhold treatment for at least 1 week and restart at a lower dose (Allolio, 2006)

Dosage adjustment in renal impairment: No dosage adjustment provided in manufacturer's labeling.

Dosage adjustment in hepatic impairment: No dosage adjustment provided in manufacturer's labeling. However, drug accumulation may occur in patients with liver disease; use with caution.

Additional Information Complete prescribing information should be consulted for additional detail.

Dosage Forms

Tablet, Oral:

Lysodren: 500 mg

MitoXANtrone (mye toe ZAN trone)

Brand Names: Canada Mitoxantrone Injection; Mitoxantrone Injection USP

Index Terms CL-232315; DHAD; DHAQ; Dihydroxyanthracenedione; Dihydroxyanthracenedione Dihydrochloride;

Mitoxantrone Dihydrochloride; Mitoxantrone HCl; Mitoxantrone Hydrochloride; Mitozantrone; Novantrone

Pharmacologic Category Antineoplastic Agent, Anthracenedione; Antineoplastic Agent, Topoisomerase II Inhibitor

Use Initial treatment of acute nonlymphocytic leukemias (ANLL [includes myelogenous, promyelocytic, monocytic and erythroid leukemias]); treatment of advanced hormone-refractory prostate cancer; secondary progressive or relapsing-remitting multiple sclerosis (MS)

Canadian labeling: Additional uses (not in U.S. labeling): Treatment of metastatic breast cancer, relapsed leukemia (adults), lymphoma, and hepatocellular carcinoma

Pregnancy Risk Factor D

Dosage Details concerning dosing in combination regimens should also be consulted. IV:

Children: Acute nonlymphocytic leukemias:

Acute myeloid leukemia (AML) consolidation phase (second course; off-label use): 10 mg/m^2 once daily for 5 days (in combination with cytarabine) (Stevens, 1998)

Acute promyelocytic leukemia (APL) consolidation phase (second course; off-label use): 10 mg/m^2 once daily for 5 days (Ortega, 2005; Sanz, 2004)

Adults:

U.S. labeling:

Acute nonlymphocytic leukemias (ANLL):

AML induction: 12 mg/m^2 once daily for 3 days (in combination with cytarabine); for incomplete response, may repeat (7-10 days later) at 12 mg/m^2 once daily for 2 days (in combination with cytarabine) (Arlin, 1990)

AML consolidation (beginning ~6 weeks after initiation of the final induction course): 12 mg/m^2 once daily for 2 days (in combination with cytarabine), repeat in 4 weeks (Arlin, 1990)

Multiple sclerosis: 12 mg/m^2 every 3 months (maximum lifetime cumulative dose: 140 mg/m^2; discontinue use with LVEF <50% or clinically significant reduction in LVEF)

Prostate cancer (advanced, hormone-refractory): 12-14 mg/m^2 every 3 weeks (in combination with corticosteroids)

Canadian labeling:

Acute nonlymphocytic leukemias (ANLL):

AML induction: 10-12 mg/m^2 once daily for 3 days (in combination with cytarabine); for incomplete response, may repeat at 10-12 mg/m^2 once daily for 2 days (in combination with cytarabine)

AML consolidation (beginning ~6 weeks after initiation of the final induction course): 12 mg/m^2 once daily for 2 days (in combination with cytarabine), repeat in 4 weeks

Acute leukemias (relapsed): Induction: 12 mg/m^2 once daily for 5 consecutive days; may repeat once if needed (at the same dose and duration)

Breast cancer (metastatic), lymphoma: Initial: Single agent: 14 mg/m^2 every 21 days; reduce initial dose to ≤12 mg/m^2 for myelosuppression due to previous treatment or for poor general health. When used in combination with other agents, reduce initial dose to 10-12 mg/m^2.

Hepatocellular cancer: Initial: Single agent: 14 mg/m^2 every 21 days; reduce initial dose to ≤12 mg/m^2 for myelosuppression due to previous treatment or for poor general health

Adult off-label uses and/or dosing:

AML, refractory:

CLAG-M regimen: 10 mg/m^2 once daily for 3 days (in combination with cladribine, cytarabine, and filgrastim), may repeat once if needed (Wierzbowska, 2008)

MEC or EMA regimen: 6 mg/m^2 once daily for 6 days (in combination with cytarabine and etoposide) (Amadori, 1991)

Mitoxantrone/Etoposide: 10 mg/m^2 once daily for 5 days (in combination with etoposide) (Ho, 1988)

APL consolidation phase (second course): 10 mg/m^2 once daily for 5 days (Sanz, 2004)

Hodgkin lymphoma, refractory:

MINE-ESHAP regimen: 10 mg/m^2 on day 1 every 28 days for up to 2 cycles (MINE is combination with mesna, ifosfamide, mitoxantrone, and etoposide; MINE alternates with ESHAP for up to 2 cycles of each) (Fernandez, 2010)

VIM-D regimen: 10 mg/m^2 on day 1 every 28 days (in combination with etoposide, ifosfamide, mesna, and dexamethasone) (Phillips, 1990)

Non-Hodgkin lymphoma (as part of combination chemotherapy regimens):

CNOP regimen: 10 mg/m^2 every 21 days (Bessell, 2003)

FCMR regimen: 8 mg/m^2 every 28 days (Forstpointner, 2004)

FMR regimen: 10 mg/m^2 every 21 days (Zinzani, 2004)

FND regimen: 10 mg/m^2 every 28 days (Tsimberidou, 2002)

MINE-ESHAP regimen: 8 mg/m^2 every 21 days for 6 cycles (MINE is combination with mesna, ifosfamide, mitoxantrone, and etoposide; followed by ESHAP) (Rodriguez, 1995)

Stem cell transplantation, autologous: 60 mg/m^2 administered 4-5 days prior to autografting (as 3 divided doses over 1 hour each at 1-2 hour intervals on the same day; in combination with other chemotherapeutic agent[s]) (Oyan, 2006; Tarella, 2001)

Dosage adjustment for toxicity:

ANLL patients: Severe or life-threatening nonhematologic toxicity: Withhold treatment until toxicity resolves

MS patients:

Neutrophils <1500/mm^3: Use is not recommended

Signs/symptoms of HF: Evaluate for cardiac signs/symptoms and LVEF

LVEF <50% or baseline LVEF below the lower limit of normal (LLN): Use is not recommended

Canadian labeling (not in U.S. labeling): Hepatocellular cancer, lymphoma, or breast cancer (metastatic):

WBC nadir >1500/mm^3 **and** platelet nadir >50,000/mm^3 and recovery ≤21 days: Repeat previous dose or increase dose by 2 mg/m^2 if myelosuppression is inadequate.

WBC nadir >1500/mm^3 **and** platelet nadir >50,000/mm^3 and recovery >21 days: Withhold treatment until recovery then resume at previous dose.

WBC nadir <1500/mm^3 **or** platelet nadir <50,000/mm^3 (regardless of recovery time): Withhold treatment until recovery then decrease previous dose by 2 mg/m^2.

WBC nadir <1000/mm^3 **or** platelet nadir <25,000/mm^3 (regardless of recovery time): Withhold treatment until recovery then decrease previous dose by 4 mg/m^2.

Dosage adjustment in renal impairment: No dosage adjustment provided in manufacturer's labeling (has not been studied).

Hemodialysis: Supplemental dose is not necessary

Peritoneal dialysis: Supplemental dose is not necessary

Elderly: Clearance is decreased in elderly patients; use with caution

Dosage adjustment in hepatic impairment:

U.S. labeling: No dosage adjustment provided in the manufacturer's labeling; however, clearance is reduced in hepatic dysfunction. Patients with severe hepatic dysfunction (bilirubin >3.4 mg/dL) have an AUC of 3 times greater than patients with normal hepatic function; consider dose adjustments. **Note:** MS patients with hepatic impairment should not receive mitoxantrone.

Canadian labeling:

Mild-to-moderate impairment: No specific dosage adjustment provided; consider dose adjustments and monitor closely.

Severe impairment: Use is contraindicated.

Dosing in obesity: *ASCO Guidelines for appropriate chemotherapy dosing in obese adults with cancer:* Utilize patient's actual body weight (full weight) for calculation of body surface area- or weight-based dosing, particularly when the intent of therapy is curative; manage regimen-related toxicities in the same manner as for nonobese patients; if a dose reduction is utilized due to toxicity, consider resumption of full weight-based dosing with subsequent cycles, especially if cause of toxicity (eg, hepatic or renal impairment) is resolved (Griggs, 2012).

Additional Information Complete prescribing information should be consulted for additional detail.

Dosage Forms

Concentrate, Intravenous:

Generic: 20 mg/10 mL (10 mL); 25 mg/12.5 mL (12.5 mL); 30 mg/15 mL (15 mL)

- ◆ **Mitoxantrone Dihydrochloride** *see* MitoXANtrone *on page* 1382
- ◆ **Mitoxantrone HCl** *see* MitoXANtrone *on page* 1382
- ◆ **Mitoxantrone Hydrochloride** *see* MitoXANtrone *on page* 1382
- ◆ **Mitoxantrone Injection (Can)** *see* MitoXANtrone *on page* 1382
- ◆ **Mitoxantrone Injection USP (Can)** *see* MitoXANtrone *on page* 1382
- ◆ **Mitozantrone** *see* MitoXANtrone *on page* 1382
- ◆ **Mitrazol [OTC]** *see* Miconazole (Topical) *on page* 1360

Mizolastine [INT] (mi zoe LAS teen)

International Brand Names Mistaline (FR); Mistamine (BE, CH, GB); Mizollen (BE, CH, DE, DK, FR, GB, IT, NL, SE); Zolim (DE); Zolistam (IT)

Pharmacologic Category Antihistamine, Low-Sedating

Reported Use Symptomatic relief of allergy such as hay fever, urticaria

Dosage Range Adults: Oral: 10 mg tablet daily

Product Availability Product available in various countries; not currently available in the U.S.

Dosage Forms

Tablet: 10 mg

- ◆ **MK-217** *see* Alendronate *on page* 79
- ◆ **MK383** *see* Tirofiban *on page* 2049
- ◆ **MK-0431** *see* SitaGLIPtin *on page* 1897
- ◆ **MK462** *see* Rizatriptan *on page* 1836
- ◆ **MK 0517** *see* Fosaprepitant *on page* 929
- ◆ **MK-0518** *see* Raltegravir *on page* 1767
- ◆ **MK594** *see* Losartan *on page* 1248
- ◆ **MK0826** *see* Ertapenem *on page* 760
- ◆ **MK 869** *see* Aprepitant *on page* 166
- ◆ **MK-3475** *see* Pembrolizumab *on page* 1604
- ◆ **MK4305** *see* Suvorexant *on page* 1961
- ◆ **MLN341** *see* Bortezomib *on page* 276
- ◆ **MMC** *see* MitoMYcin (Ophthalmic) *on page* 1382
- ◆ **MMC** *see* MitoMYcin (Systemic) *on page* 1380
- ◆ **MMF** *see* Mycophenolate *on page* 1405
- ◆ **MMI** *see* Methimazole *on page* 1319
- ◆ **MMR** *see* Measles, Mumps, and Rubella Virus Vaccine *on page* 1273
- ◆ **M-M-R II** *see* Measles, Mumps, and Rubella Virus Vaccine *on page* 1273
- ◆ **MMRV** *see* Measles, Mumps, Rubella, and Varicella Virus Vaccine *on page* 1274
- ◆ **MN-50 [OTC]** *see* Manganese *on page* 1268
- ◆ **MOAB 2C4** *see* Pertuzumab *on page* 1627
- ◆ **MOAB ABX-EGF** *see* Panitumumab *on page* 1568
- ◆ **MOAB C225** *see* Cetuximab *on page* 413
- ◆ **MoAb CD52** *see* Alemtuzumab *on page* 75
- ◆ **MOAB-CTLA-4** *see* Ipilimumab *on page* 1106
- ◆ **MOAB HER2** *see* Trastuzumab *on page* 2085
- ◆ **Mobic** *see* Meloxicam *on page* 1283
- ◆ **Mobicox (Can)** *see* Meloxicam *on page* 1283

Moclobemide [CAN/INT] (moe KLOE be mide)

Brand Names: Canada Apo-Moclobemide; Dom-Moclobemide; Manerix; Novo-Moclobemide; Nu-Moclobemide; PMS-Moclobemide; Teva-Moclobemide

Pharmacologic Category Antidepressant, Monoamine Oxidase Inhibitor, Reversible

Use Note: Not approved in U.S.

Symptomatic relief of depressive illness

Pregnancy Considerations Safety has not been established, use only if benefits outweigh the risks.

Breast-Feeding Considerations Less than 1% of maternal dose is excreted in breast milk; benefits should outweigh risks.

Contraindications Hypersensitivity to moclobemide or any component of the formulation; acute confusional states; concurrent use of sympathomimetics (and related compounds), MAO inhibitors, meperidine, tricyclic antidepressants, thioridazine, serotonergic drugs (including SSRIs)

Warnings/Precautions The possibility of a suicide attempt is inherent in major depression and may persist until remission occurs. Use caution in high-risk patients during initiation of therapy. Prescriptions should be written for the smallest quantity consistent with good patient care. Use caution in patients with thyrotoxicosis, pheochromocytoma, and renal dysfunction. Use caution in patients receiving concurrent CNS depressants, ethanol, or buspirone. Severe reactions may occur when used concurrently with MAO inhibitors and serotonergic agents, including SSRIs; do not use within 5 weeks of fluoxetine discontinuation. Do not initiate tricyclic antidepressant therapy until moclobemide has been discontinued for ≥2 days. Discontinue at least 2 days prior to local or general anesthesia. Use caution in hepatic impairment (dose adjustment required with severe impairment). Serum concentrations may be increased in patients who are slow CYP2D6 and/or CYP2C19 metabolizers. Dietary restriction of tyramine does not appear to be necessary for patients receiving moclobemide (patients must be informed of signs/symptoms of reaction).

Abrupt discontinuation or interruption of antidepressant therapy has been associated with a discontinuation syndrome. Symptoms arising may vary with antidepressant however commonly include nausea, vomiting, diarrhea, headaches, lightheadedness, dizziness, diminished appetite, sweating, chills, tremors, paresthesias, fatigue, somnolence, and sleep disturbances (eg, vivid dreams, insomnia). Greater risks for developing a discontinuation syndrome have been associated with antidepressants with shorter half-lives, longer durations of treatment, and abrupt discontinuation. More severe symptoms have also been associated with MAO inhibitors. For antidepressants of short or intermediate half-lives, symptoms may emerge within 2-5 days after treatment discontinuation and last 7-14 days (APA, 2010; Fava, 2006; Haddad, 2001; Shelton, 2001; Warner, 2006).

Adverse Reactions

Cardiovascular: Hypotension, tachycardia

Central nervous system: Agitation, anxiety, nervousness, sleep disturbance

Gastrointestinal: Constipation, diarrhea, vomiting

Neuromuscular & skeletal: Tremor

Ocular: Blurred vision

Rare but important or life-threatening: Aggression, allergic reaction, angina, apathy, bradycardia, cold sensation, confusion, conjunctivitis, delusions, disorientation, dry skin, dysarthria, dyspnea, dysuria, excitation, extrapyramidal effects, extrasystoles, flushing, gastritis, gingivitis, hallucinations, heartburn, hypertension, indigestion, insomnia, irritability, malaise, mania, memory disturbances, meteorism, metrorrhagia, migraine, muscular pain, nightmares, paresthesia, phlebitic symptoms, photopsia, polyuria, prolonged menstruation, pruritus, rash, skeletal pain, stomatitis, taste alteration, tenesmus, tension, tinnitus, transaminases increased, urticaria, visual disturbances

Drug Interactions

Metabolism/Transport Effects Substrate of CYP2C19 (major), CYP2D6 (minor); **Note:** Assignment of Major/Minor substrate status based on clinically relevant drug interaction potential; **Inhibits** CYP1A2 (weak), CYP2C19 (moderate), CYP2D6 (weak), Monoamine Oxidase

Avoid Concomitant Use

Avoid concomitant use of Moclobemide with any of the following: Aclidinium; Alcohol (Ethyl); Alpha-/Beta-Agonists (Indirect-Acting); Alpha1-Agonists; Amphetamines; Anilidopiperidine Opioids; Antidepressants (Serotonin Reuptake Inhibitor/Antagonist); Apraclonidine; AtoMOXetine; Bezafibrate; Buprenorphine; BuPROPion; BusPIRone; CarBAMazepine; Cyclobenzaprine; Cyproheptadine; Dapoxetine; Dexmethylphenidate; Dextromethorphan; Diethylpropion; Glucagon; Hydrocodone; HYDROmorphone; Ipratropium (Oral Inhalation); Isometheptene; Levonordefrin; Linezolid; Maprotiline; Meperidine; Methyldopa; Methylene Blue; Methylphenidate; Mianserin; Mirtazapine; Morphine (Liposomal); Morphine (Systemic); Oxymorphone; Pholcodine; Pizotifen; Potassium Chloride; Selective Serotonin Reuptake Inhibitors; Serotonin 5-HT1D Receptor Agonists; Serotonin/Norepinephrine Reuptake Inhibitors; Tapentadol; Tetrabenazine; Tetrahydrozoline (Nasal); Thioridazine; Tiotropium; Tricyclic Antidepressants; Tryptophan; Umeclidinium

Increased Effect/Toxicity

Moclobemide may increase the levels/effects of: AbobotulinumtoxinA; Alpha-/Beta-Agonists (Indirect-Acting); Alpha1-Agonists; Amphetamines; Analgesics (Opioid); Anticholinergic Agents; Antidepressants (Serotonin Reuptake Inhibitor/Antagonist); Antihypertensives; Antipsychotic Agents; Apraclonidine; ARIPiprazole; AtoMOXetine; Beta2-Agonists; Betahistine; Bezafibrate; Brimonidine (Ophthalmic); Brimonidine (Topical); BuPROPion; Cannabinoid-Containing Products; CYP2C19 Substrates; Cyproheptadine; Dexmethylphenidate; Dextromethorphan; Diethylpropion; Domperidone; Doxapram; Doxylamine; EPINEPHrine (Nasal); Epinephrine (Racemic); EPINEPHrine (Systemic, Oral Inhalation); Glucagon; Hydrocodone; HYDROmorphone; Hypoglycemic Agents; Isometheptene; Levonordefrin; Linezolid; Meperidine; Methadone; Methyldopa; Methylene Blue; Methylphenidate; Metoclopramide; Mianserin; Mirabegron; Mirtazapine; Morphine (Liposomal); Morphine (Systemic); Norepinephrine; OnabotulinumtoxinA; Orthostatic Hypotension Producing Agents; OxyCODONE; Pizotifen; Potassium Chloride; Reserpine; RimabotulinumtoxinB; Selective Serotonin Reuptake Inhibitors; Serotonin 5-HT1D Receptor Agonists; Serotonin Modulators; Serotonin/Norepinephrine Reuptake Inhibitors; Tetrahydrozoline (Nasal); Thiazide Diuretics; Thioridazine; Tiotropium; Topiramate; Tricyclic Antidepressants

The levels/effects of Moclobemide may be increased by: Aclidinium; Alcohol (Ethyl); Altretamine; Anilidopiperidine Opioids; Antiemetics (5HT3 Antagonists); Antipsychotic Agents; Buprenorphine; BusPIRone; CarBAMazepine; Cimetidine; COMT Inhibitors; Cyclobenzaprine; CYP2C19 Inhibitors (Moderate); CYP2C19 Inhibitors (Strong); Dapoxetine; Ipratropium (Oral Inhalation); Levodopa; Luliconazole; MAO Inhibitors; Maprotiline; Oxymorphone; Pholcodine; Pramlintide; Tapentadol; Tedizolid; Tetrabenazine; TraMADol; Tryptophan; Umeclidinium

Decreased Effect

Moclobemide may decrease the levels/effects of: Acetylcholinesterase Inhibitors; Clopidogrel; Domperidone; Itopride; Secretin

The levels/effects of Moclobemide may be decreased by: Acetylcholinesterase Inhibitors; CYP2C19 Inducers (Strong); Cyproheptadine; Dabrafenib; Domperidone

Food Interactions Dietary restriction of tyramine does not appear to be necessary.

Storage/Stability Store at 15°C to 30°C (59°F to 86°F).

Mechanism of Action Moclobemide is a benzamide derivative which acts as a short-acting reversible inhibitor of monoamine oxidase (MAO), which inhibits the metabolism (deamination) of serotonin, norepinephrine, and dopamine. It has a relative specificity for the A subtype of monoamine oxidase (MAO type A). Its action leads to increased concentrations of these neurotransmitters, which may account for the antidepressant activity of moclobemide.

Pharmacodynamics/Kinetics

Absorption: 98% from GI tract

Distribution: 1.2 L/kg

Protein binding: ~50% (primarily to albumin)

Metabolism: Extensively metabolized via hepatic oxidative reactions; partial metabolism via CYP2C19 and 2D6

Bioavailability: ~55% (single dose); 90% (repeated dosing)

Half-life elimination: Terminal: 1-2 hours

Excretion: Urine (95%, as metabolites; <1% as unchanged drug)

Dosage Oral: Adults: Initial: 300 mg/day in 2 divided doses; may increase dose gradually beginning 1 week after therapy initiation. Maximum dose: 600 mg/day. **Note:** Individual patient response may allow a reduction in daily dose in long-term therapy.

Coadministration with cimetidine: A 50% reduction in the dose of moclobemide may be necessary

Discontinuation of therapy: Upon discontinuation of antidepressant therapy, gradually taper the dose to minimize the incidence of withdrawal symptoms and allow for the detection of re-emerging symptoms. Evidence supporting ideal taper rates is limited. APA and NICE guidelines suggest tapering therapy over at least several weeks with consideration to the half-life of the antidepressant; antidepressants with a shorter half-life and MOA inhibitors may need to be tapered more conservatively. In addition for long-term treated patients, WFSBP guidelines recommend tapering over 4-6 months. If intolerable withdrawal symptoms occur following a dose reduction, consider resuming the previously prescribed dose and/or decrease dose at a more gradual rate (APA, 2010; Bauer,

2002; Haddad, 2001; NCCMH, 2010; Schatzberg, 2006; Shelton, 2001; Warner, 2006).

MAO inhibitor recommendations:

Switching to or from an MAO inhibitor intended to treat psychiatric disorders:

Allow 14 days to elapse between discontinuing an alternative antidepressant without long half-life metabolites (eg, TCAs, paroxetine, fluvoxamine, venlafaxine) or MAO inhibitor intended to treat psychiatric disorders and initiation of moclobemide.

Allow 5 weeks to elapse between discontinuing fluoxetine (with long half-life metabolites) intended to treat psychiatric disorders and initiation of moclobemide.

Allow at least 2-14 days to elapse between discontinuing moclobemide and initiation of an alternative antidepressant or MAO inhibitor intended to treat psychiatric disorders.

Use with other MAO inhibitors (such as linezolid or IV methylene blue):

Do not initiate moclobemide in patients receiving linezolid or IV methylene blue; consider other interventions for psychiatric condition.

If urgent treatment with linezolid or IV methylene blue is required in a patient already receiving moclobemide and potential benefits outweigh potential risks, discontinue moclobemide promptly and administer linezolid or IV methylene blue. Monitor for serotonin syndrome for 2 weeks or until 24 hours after the last dose of linezolid or IV methylene blue, whichever comes first. May resume moclobemide 24 hours after the last dose of linezolid or IV methylene blue.

Dosage adjustment in renal impairment: No dosage adjustment provided in manufacturer's labeling. Use with caution; however, single-dose pharmacokinetic data suggests that dosage adjustments are not necessary (multiple-dose studies have not been performed).

Dosage adjustment in hepatic impairment: Severe hepatic impairment: Decrease daily dose by 33% to 50%.

Dietary Considerations Should be taken immediately after meals. Manufacturer states no special dietary restrictions are required; tyramine-containing foods may be ingested during therapy. However, as a precaution, patients should be instructed to recognize occipital headache, palpitations, neck stiffness, or other potential signs of a severe reaction.

Administration Administer immediately after meals.

Monitoring Parameters Blood pressure, warning signs of suicide

Product Availability Not available in U.S.

Dosage Forms: Canada

Tablet, oral:

Apo-Moclobemide®, Dom-Moclobemide, Manerix®, Novo-Moclobemide, Nu-Moclobemide, PMS-Moclobemide: 100 mg, 150 mg, 300 mg

Modafinil (moe DAF i nil)

Brand Names: U.S. Provigil

Brand Names: Canada Alertec; Apo-Modafinil; Teva-Modafinil

Pharmacologic Category Central Nervous System Stimulant

Use Improve wakefulness in patients with excessive daytime sleepiness associated with narcolepsy and shift work sleep disorder (SWSD); adjunctive therapy for obstructive sleep apnea/hypopnea syndrome (OSAHS)

Pregnancy Risk Factor C

Pregnancy Considerations Adverse events were observed in some animal reproduction studies. Healthcare providers are encouraged to register pregnant patients exposed to modafinil by calling (866-404-4106). Efficacy of steroidal contraceptives (including depot and implantable contraceptives) may be decreased; alternate means of contraception should be considered during therapy and for 1 month after modafinil is discontinued.

Breast-Feeding Considerations It is not known if modafinil is excreted into breast milk. The manufacturer recommends caution be used if administered to nursing women.

Contraindications Hypersensitivity to modafinil, armodafinil, or any component of the formulation

Canadian labeling: Additional contraindications (not in U.S. labeling): Patients in agitated states or with severe anxiety

Warnings/Precautions For use following complete evaluation of sleepiness and in conjunction with other standard treatments (eg, CPAP). The degree of sleepiness should be reassessed frequently; some patients may not return to a normal level of wakefulness. Use is not recommended with a history of angina, cardiac ischemia, recent history of myocardial infarction, left ventricular hypertrophy, or patients with mitral valve prolapse who have developed mitral valve prolapse syndrome with previous CNS stimulant use.

Serious and life-threatening rashes (including Stevens-Johnson syndrome and toxic epidermal necrolysis) have been reported with modafinil. Most cases have occurred within the first 5 weeks of therapy; however, rare cases have occurred after long-term use. No risk factors have been identified to predict occurrence or severity. Patients should be advised to discontinue at first sign of rash. The serious nature of these dermatologic adverse effects, as well reports of psychiatric events, resulted in the FDA's Pediatric Advisory Committee unanimously recommending that a specific warning against the use of modafinil in children be added to the manufacturer's labeling. Modafinil is not FDA-approved for use in pediatrics for any indication.

In addition, rare cases of multiorgan hypersensitivity reactions in association with modafinil use, and lone cases of angioedema and anaphylactoid reactions with armodafinil, have been reported. Signs and symptoms are diverse, reflecting the involvement of specific organs. Patients typically present with fever and rash associated with organ-system dysfunction. Patients should be advised to report any signs and symptoms related to these effects; discontinuation of therapy is recommended.

Caution should be exercised when modafinil is given to patients with a history of psychosis; may impair the ability to engage in potentially hazardous activities. Stimulants may unmask tics in individuals with coexisting Tourette's syndrome. Use caution with renal or hepatic impairment (dosage adjustment in severe hepatic dysfunction is recommended). Instruct patients to avoid concomitant ethanol consumption.

Adverse Reactions

Cardiovascular: Chest pain, edema, hypertension, palpitation, tachycardia, vasodilation

Central nervous system: Agitation, anxiety (dose related), chills, confusion, depression, dizziness, emotional lability, headache (occurs more frequently in adults; dose related), insomnia, nervousness, somnolence, vertigo

Dermatologic: Rash (includes some severe cases requiring hospitalization)

Gastrointestinal: Abdominal pain (occurs more frequently in children), anorexia, appetite decreased (occurs more frequently in children), constipation, diarrhea, dyspepsia, flatulence, mouth ulceration, nausea, taste perversion, weight loss (occurs more frequently in children), xerostomia

Genitourinary: Abnormal urine, hematuria, pyuria

Hematologic: Eosinophilia

Hepatic: LFTs abnormal

Neuromuscular & skeletal: Back pain, dyskinesia, hyperkinesia, hypertonia, neck rigidity, paresthesia, tremor
Ocular: Abnormal vision, amblyopia, eye pain
Respiratory: Asthma, epistaxis, lung disorder, pharyngitis, rhinitis
Miscellaneous: Diaphoresis, flu-like syndrome, herpes simplex infection, thirst
Postmarketing and/or case reports: Agranulocytosis, anaphylactic reaction, angioedema, DRESS syndrome, erythema multiforme, hypersensitivity syndrome (multiorgan), mania, psychosis, Stevens-Johnson syndrome, toxic epidermal necrolysis

Drug Interactions

Metabolism/Transport Effects Substrate of CYP3A4 (major); **Note:** Assignment of Major/Minor substrate status based on clinically relevant drug interaction potential; **Inhibits** CYP2A6 (weak), CYP2C19 (moderate), CYP2C9 (weak), CYP2E1 (weak), CYP3A4 (weak); **Induces** CYP1A2 (moderate), CYP2B6 (moderate), CYP3A4 (moderate)

Avoid Concomitant Use

Avoid concomitant use of Modafinil with any of the following: Axitinib; Bosutinib; Conivaptan; Enzalutamide; Fusidic Acid (Systemic); Idelalisib; Iobenguane I 123; Nisoldipine; Olaparib; Pimozide; Simeprevir; Sofosbuvir

Increased Effect/Toxicity

Modafinil may increase the levels/effects of: Citalopram; Clarithromycin; CYP2C19 Substrates; Dofetilide; Hydrocodone; Ifosfamide; Lomitapide; Pimozide; Sympathomimetics

The levels/effects of Modafinil may be increased by: Aprepitant; AtoMOXetine; Cannabinoid-Containing Products; Ceritinib; Conivaptan; CYP3A4 Inhibitors (Moderate); CYP3A4 Inhibitors (Strong); Dasatinib; Fosaprepitant; Fusidic Acid (Systemic); Idelalisib; Ivacaftor; Linezolid; Luliconazole; Mifepristone; Netupitant; Stiripentol; Tedizolid

Decreased Effect

Modafinil may decrease the levels/effects of: ARIPiprazole; Axitinib; Bosutinib; Clarithromycin; Clopidogrel; Contraceptives (Estrogens); CycloSPORINE (Systemic); CYP3A4 Substrates; Dasabuvir; Enzalutamide; FentaNYL; Hydrocodone; Ibrutinib; Ifosfamide; Iobenguane I 123; Nisoldipine; Olaparib; Ombitasvir; Paritaprevir; Saxagliptin; Simeprevir; Sofosbuvir

The levels/effects of Modafinil may be decreased by: Bosentan; CYP3A4 Inducers (Moderate); CYP3A4 Inducers (Strong); Dabrafenib; Deferasirox; Mitotane; Siltuximab; St Johns Wort; Tocilizumab

Food Interactions Food delays absorption, but does not affect bioavailability. Management: Administer without regard to meals.

Storage/Stability

Provigil®: Store at 20°C to 25°C (68°F to 77°F).
Alertec® (Canadian availability; not available in U.S.): Store at 15°C to 30°C (59°F to 86°F).

Mechanism of Action The exact mechanism of action is unclear, it does not appear to alter the release of dopamine or norepinephrine, it may exert its stimulant effects by decreasing GABA-mediated neurotransmission, although this theory has not yet been fully evaluated; several studies also suggest that an intact central alpha-adrenergic system is required for modafinil's activity; the drug increases high-frequency alpha waves while decreasing both delta and theta wave activity, and these effects are consistent with generalized increases in mental alertness

Pharmacodynamics/Kinetics Modafinil is a racemic compound (10% *d*-isomer and 90% *l*-isomer at steady state) whose enantiomers have different pharmacokinetics

Distribution: V_d: 0.9 L/kg
Protein binding: ~60%, primarily to albumin
Metabolism: Hepatic; multiple pathways including CYP3A4
Half-life elimination: Effective half-life: 15 hours
Time to peak, serum: 2-4 hours
Excretion: Urine (as metabolites, <10% as unchanged drug)

Dosage

U.S. labeling:

Narcolepsy, obstructive sleep apnea/hypopnea syndrome (OSAHS): Adults: Oral: Initial: 200 mg as a single daily dose in the morning
Shift work sleep disorder (SWSD): Adults: Oral: Initial: 200 mg as a single dose taken ~1 hour prior to start of work shift

Note: Doses up to 400 mg daily, given as a single dose, have been well tolerated, but there is no consistent evidence that this dose confers additional benefit.

Canadian labeling:

Narcolepsy: Adults: Oral: Initial: 200 mg daily in 2 divided doses (first dose in the morning and second dose at noon [or no later than early afternoon]); may titrate dose upward in 100 mg increments as needed and tolerated (maximum single dose: <300 mg; maximum daily dose: 400 mg). Single doses ≥300 mg and daily doses >400 mg are associated with increased side effects and are not recommended.
Obstructive sleep apnea: Adults: Oral: 200 mg once daily in the morning.
Shift work sleep disorder: Adults: Oral: 200 mg as a single dose taken ~1 hour prior to start of work shift

Off-label use: ADHD: 100-400 mg daily (Taylor, 2000)

Elderly: Elimination of modafinil and its metabolites may be reduced as a consequence of aging and as a result, consider initiating at lower doses in this patient population.

Dosage adjustment in renal impairment: Severe impairment: There are no dosage adjustments provided in the manufacturer's labeling (insufficient data).

Dosage adjustment in hepatic impairment: Severe hepatic impairment: Dose should be reduced to one-half of that recommended for patients with normal liver function.

Administration

U.S. labeling: For the treatment of narcolepsy and obstructive sleep apnea/hypopnea syndrome, administer dose in the morning. For the treatment of shift work sleep disorder, administer dose ~1 hour prior to start of work shift.
Canadian labeling: For the treatment of narcolepsy, administer in 2 divided doses with first dose given in the morning and the second dose given at noon (or no later than early afternoon) to avoid potential for insomnia. For treatment of obstructive sleep apnea, administer as a single dose in the morning. For the treatment of shift work sleep disorder, administer dose ~1 hour prior to start of work shift.

Monitoring Parameters Levels of sleepiness; blood pressure in patients with hypertension; body mass index and weight loss; development of severe skin reactions; development or exacerbation of psychiatric symptoms (eg, agitation, anxiety, depression)

When used for the treatment of ADHD, thoroughly evaluate for cardiovascular risk. Monitor heart rate, blood pressure, and consider obtaining ECG prior to initiation (Vetter, 2008).

Dosage Forms

Tablet, Oral:

Provigil: 100 mg, 200 mg
Generic: 100 mg, 200 mg

Dosage Forms: Canada

Tablet, oral: 100 mg

Alertec®: 100 mg

◆ **Modecate® (Can)** *see* FluPHENAZine *on page* 905

◆ **Modecate® Concentrate (Can)** *see* FluPHENAZine *on page 905*

◆ **Moderiba** *see* Ribavirin *on page 1797*

◆ **Modicon** *see* Ethinyl Estradiol and Norethindrone *on page 808*

◆ **Modified Dakin's Solution** *see* Sodium Hypochlorite Solution *on page 1906*

◆ **Modified Shohl's Solution** *see* Sodium Citrate and Citric Acid *on page 1905*

◆ **Modulon (Can)** *see* Trimebutine [CAN/INT] *on page 2103*

Moexipril (mo EKS i pril)

Brand Names: U.S. Univasc [DSC]

Index Terms Moexipril Hydrochloride

Pharmacologic Category Angiotensin-Converting Enzyme (ACE) Inhibitor; Antihypertensive

Use Hypertension: Treatment of hypertension, alone or in combination with thiazide diuretics

The 2014 guideline for the management of high blood pressure in adults (Eighth Joint National Committee [JNC 8]) recommends initiation of pharmacologic treatment to lower blood pressure for the following patients:

- Patients ≥60 years of age with systolic blood pressure (SBP) ≥150 mm Hg or diastolic blood pressure (DBP) ≥90 mm Hg. Goal of therapy is SBP <150 mm Hg and DBP <90 mm Hg.
- Patients <60 years of age with SBP ≥140 mm Hg or DBP is ≥90 mm Hg. Goal of therapy is SBP <140 mm Hg and DBP <90 mm Hg.
- Patients ≥18 years of age with diabetes and SBP ≥140 mm Hg or DBP ≥90 mm Hg. Goal of therapy is SBP <140 mm Hg and DBP <90 mm Hg.
- Patients ≥18 years of age with chronic kidney disease (CKD) and SBP ≥140 mm Hg or DBP ≥90 mm Hg. Goal of therapy is SBP <140 mm Hg and DBP <90 mm Hg.

In patients with CKD, regardless of race or diabetes status, the use of an ACE inhibitor (ACEI) or angiotensin receptor blocker (ARB) as initial therapy is recommended to improve kidney outcomes. In the general nonblack population (without CKD) including those with diabetes, initial antihypertensive treatment should consist of a thiazide-type diuretic, calcium channel blocker, ACEI, or ARB. In the general black population (without CKD) including those with diabetes, initial antihypertensive treatment should consist of a thiazide-type diuretic or a calcium channel blocker **instead of** an ACEI or ARB.

Pregnancy Risk Factor D

Dosage Adults: Oral: Initial: 7.5 mg once daily (in patients **not** receiving diuretics), 1 hour prior to a meal **or** 3.75 mg once daily (when combined with thiazide diuretics); maintenance dose: 7.5-30 mg/day in 1 or 2 divided doses 1 hour before meals

Dosage adjustment in renal impairment: CrCl ≤40 mL/minute: Patients may be cautiously placed on 3.75 mg once daily, then upwardly titrated to a maximum of 15 mg/day.

Dosage adjustment in hepatic impairment: No dosage adjustment provided in manufacturer's labeling. However, hepatic impairment increases systemic exposure.

Additional Information Complete prescribing information should be consulted for additional detail.

Dosage Forms

Tablet, Oral:

Generic: 7.5 mg, 15 mg

Moexipril and Hydrochlorothiazide

(mo EKS i pril & hye droe klor oh THYE a zide)

Brand Names: U.S. Uniretic®

Brand Names: Canada Uniretic®

Index Terms Hydrochlorothiazide and Moexipril

Pharmacologic Category Angiotensin-Converting Enzyme (ACE) Inhibitor; Antihypertensive; Diuretic, Thiazide

Use Treatment of hypertension; not indicated for initial treatment of hypertension

Pregnancy Risk Factor D

Dosage Adults: Oral: 7.5-30 mg of moexipril, taken either in a single or divided dose 1 hour before meals; hydrochlorothiazide dose should be ≤50 mg/day

Dosage adjustment in renal impairment:

CrCl >40 mL/minute: No dosage adjustment necessary.

CrCl ≤40 mL/minute: Use not recommended.

Dosage adjustment in hepatic impairment: No dosage adjustment provided in manufacturer's labeling (has not been studied). However, hepatic impairment increases systemic exposure. Use with caution.

Additional Information Complete prescribing information should be consulted for additional detail.

Dosage Forms

Tablet, oral: 7.5/12.5: Moexipril 7.5 mg and hydrochlorothiazide 12.5; 15/12.5: Moexipril 15 mg and hydrochlorothiazide 12.5; 15/25: Moexipril 15 mg and hydrochlorothiazide 25

Uniretic®: 7.5/12.5: Moexipril 7.5 mg and hydrochlorothiazide 12.5 mg [scored]; 15/12.5: Moexipril 15 mg and hydrochlorothiazide 12.5 mg [scored]; 15/25: Moexipril 15 mg and hydrochlorothiazide 25 mg [scored]

◆ **Moexipril Hydrochloride** *see* Moexipril *on page 1388*

◆ **Mogadon (Can)** *see* Nitrazepam [CAN/INT] *on page 1461*

Molgramostim [INT] (mol GRA moe stim)

International Brand Names Gramal (MX); Growgen-GM (AR); Leucomax (AR, AT, BE, BR, CH, CZ, DE, DK, ES, FI, FR, GB, HR, HU, IE, IT, LU, MX, NL, NO, PT, SE); Mielogen (IT)

Index Terms rHu-GM-CSF

Pharmacologic Category Colony Stimulating Factor

Reported Use Treatment or prevention of neutropenia in patients receiving myelosuppressive therapy; acceleration of myeloid recovery following bone marrow transplantation

Dosage Range Note: Dose varies by indication, maximum dose: 10 mcg/kg

Cancer chemotherapy: SubQ: 5-10 mcg/kg/day; starting 24 hours after last dose of chemotherapy, continued for 7-10 days

Bone marrow transplantation: IV: 10 mcg/kg/day infused over 4-6 hours, starting day after transplantation, continued until absolute neutrophil count is in desirable range; maximum duration of treatment: 30 days

Product Availability Product available in various countries; not currently available in the U.S.

Dosage Forms

Injection, powder for reconstitution: 150 mcg (1.67 million units); 300 mcg (3.33 million units); 400 mcg (4.4 million units)

◆ **MOM** *see* Magnesium Hydroxide *on page 1263*

Mometasone (Oral Inhalation)

(moe MET a sone)

Brand Names: U.S. Asmanex 120 Metered Doses; Asmanex 14 Metered Doses; Asmanex 30 Metered Doses; Asmanex 60 Metered Doses; Asmanex 7 Metered Doses; Asmanex HFA

Brand Names: Canada Asmanex Twisthaler

Index Terms Mometasone Furoate

Pharmacologic Category Corticosteroid, Inhalant (Oral)

Additional Appendix Information

Inhaled Corticosteroids *on page 2229*

Use

Maintenance treatment of asthma as prophylactic therapy in patients 4 years and older (Asmanex Twisthaler) and 12 years and older (Asmanex HFA)

Limitations of use: Not indicated for the relief of acute bronchospasm.

Pregnancy Risk Factor C

Pregnancy Considerations Adverse events were observed in some animal reproduction studies. Hypoadrenalism may occur in infants born to mothers receiving corticosteroids during pregnancy. Based on available data, an overall increased risk of congenital malformations or a decrease in fetal growth has not been associated with maternal use of inhaled corticosteroids during pregnancy (Bakhireva, 2005; NAEPP, 2005; Namazy, 2004). Uncontrolled asthma is associated with adverse events in pregnancy (increased risk of perinatal mortality, pre-eclampsia, preterm birth, low birth weight infants). Inhaled corticosteroids are recommended for the treatment of asthma during pregnancy (most information available using budesonide) (ACOG, 2008; NAEPP, 2005).

Breast-Feeding Considerations Systemic corticosteroids are excreted in human milk. It is not known if sufficient quantities of mometasone are absorbed following oral inhalation to produce detectable amounts in breast milk; however, oral absorption is limited (<1%). The manufacturer recommends that caution be exercised when administering mometasone to nursing women. The use of inhaled corticosteroids is not considered a contraindication to breast-feeding (NAEPP, 2005).

Contraindications

Hypersensitivity to mometasone or any component of the formulation; hypersensitivity to milk proteins (Asmanex Twisthaler only); primary treatment of status asthmaticus or other acute episodes of asthma where intensive measures are required

Documentation of allergenic cross-reactivity for corticosteroids is limited. However, because of similarities in chemical structure and/or pharmacologic actions, the possibility of cross-sensitivity can not be ruled out with certainty.

Canadian labeling: Additional contraindications (not in U.S. labeling): Untreated systemic fungal, bacterial, viral, or parasitic infections; active or quiet tuberculosis infection of the respiratory tract; ocular herpes simplex

Warnings/Precautions May cause hypercorticism or suppression of hypothalamic-pituitary-adrenal (HPA) axis, particularly in younger children or in patients receiving high doses for prolonged periods. HPA axis suppression may lead to adrenal crisis. Withdrawal and discontinuation of a corticosteroid should be done slowly and carefully. Particular care is required when patients are transferred from systemic corticosteroids to inhaled products due to possible adrenal insufficiency or withdrawal from steroids, including an increase in allergic symptoms. Adult patients receiving >20 mg per day of prednisone (or equivalent) may be most susceptible. Fatalities have occurred due to adrenal insufficiency in asthmatic patients during and after transfer from systemic corticosteroids to aerosol steroids; aerosol steroids do not provide the systemic steroid needed to treat patients having trauma, surgery, or infections. When transferring to oral inhaler, previously-suppressed allergic conditions (rhinitis, conjunctivitis, eczema) may be unmasked.

Paradoxical bronchospasm may occur with wheezing after inhalation; if this occurs, stop steroid and treat with a fast-acting bronchodilator. Supplemental steroids (oral or parenteral) may be needed during stress or severe asthma attacks. Not to be used in status asthmaticus or for the relief of acute bronchospasm. Corticosteroid use may cause psychiatric disturbances, including depression, euphoria, insomnia, mood swings, and personality changes. Preexisting psychiatric conditions may be exacerbated by corticosteroid use. Prolonged use of corticosteroids may also increase the incidence of secondary infection, mask acute infection (including fungal infections), prolong or exacerbate viral infections, or limit response to vaccines. Exposure to chickenpox and measles should be avoided; corticosteroids should not be used to treat ocular herpes simplex. Corticosteroids should not be used for cerebral malaria or viral hepatitis. Close observation is required in patients with latent tuberculosis and/or TB reactivity; restrict use in active TB (only in conjunction with antituberculosis treatment). Use with extreme caution in untreated systemic fungal, bacterial, viral, or parasitic infections. Canadian labeling contraindicates use in patients with untreated systemic fungal, bacterial, viral, or parasitic infections, active or quiet tuberculosis infection of the respiratory tract and ocular herpes simplex.

Prolonged treatment with corticosteroids has been associated with the development of Kaposi sarcoma (case reports); if noted, discontinuation of therapy should be considered (Goedert, 2002). Local oropharyngeal *Candida* infections have been reported; if occurs treat appropriately while continuing mometasone therapy. Patients should be instructed to rinse mouth after each use.

Hypersensitivity reactions including, allergic dermatitis, anaphylaxis, angioedema, bronchospasm, flushing, pruritus, and rash, and urticaria have been reported; if these symptoms occur discontinue use. Use with caution in patients with thyroid disease, hepatic impairment, renal impairment, cardiovascular disease, diabetes, glaucoma, cataracts, myasthenia gravis, patients with or who are at risk for osteoporosis, patients at risk for seizures, or GI diseases (diverticulitis, peptic ulcer, ulcerative colitis) due to perforation risk. Use caution following acute MI (corticosteroids have been associated with myocardial rupture). Because of the risk of adverse effects, systemic corticosteroids should be used cautiously in the elderly in the smallest possible effective dose for the shortest duration.

Orally-inhaled corticosteroids may cause a reduction in growth velocity in pediatric patients (~1 centimeter per year [range: 0.3 to 1.8 cm per year] and related to dose and duration of exposure). To minimize the systemic effects of orally-inhaled corticosteroids, each patient should be titrated to the lowest effective dose. Growth should be routinely monitored in pediatric patients. Prior to use, the dose and duration of treatment should be based on the risk versus benefit for each individual patient. In general, use the smallest effective dose for the shortest duration of time to minimize adverse events. A gradual tapering of dose may be required prior to discontinuing therapy. There have been reports of systemic corticosteroid withdrawal symptoms (eg, joint/muscle pain, lassitude, depression) when withdrawing inhalation therapy. Asmanex Twisthaler may contain lactose; very rare anaphylactic reactions have been reported in patients with severe milk protein allergy. Potentially significant interactions may exist, requiring dose or frequency adjustment, additional monitoring, and/or selection of alternative therapy.

Adverse Reactions

Central nervous system: Depression, fatigue, headache, pain

Gastrointestinal: Abdominal pain, anorexia, dyspepsia, gastroenteritis, nausea, oral candidiasis, vomiting

Genitourinary: Dysmenorrhea, urinary tract infection

Hematologic & oncologic: Bruise

Infection: Infection, influenza

Neuromuscular & skeletal: Arthralgia, back pain, musculoskeletal pain, myalgia

Ophthalmic: Increased intraocular pressure

Otic: Otalgia

Respiratory: Allergic rhinitis (more common in adolescents & adults), bronchitis, dry throat, epistaxis, flu-like symptoms, nasal discomfort, nasopharyngitis, pharyngitis, sinus congestion, sinusitis, upper respiratory tract infection, voice disorder

Miscellaneous: Fever

Rare but important or life-threatening: Cataract, exacerbation of asthma, glaucoma, growth suppression, hypersensitivity

Drug Interactions

Metabolism/Transport Effects Substrate of CYP3A4 (minor); **Note:** Assignment of Major/Minor substrate status based on clinically relevant drug interaction potential

Avoid Concomitant Use

Avoid concomitant use of Mometasone (Oral Inhalation) with any of the following: Aldesleukin

Increased Effect/Toxicity

Mometasone (Oral Inhalation) may increase the levels/effects of: Amphotericin B; Ceritinib; Deferasirox; Loop Diuretics; Thiazide Diuretics

The levels/effects of Mometasone (Oral Inhalation) may be increased by: CYP3A4 Inhibitors (Strong); Telaprevir

Decreased Effect

Mometasone (Oral Inhalation) may decrease the levels/effects of: Aldesleukin; Antidiabetic Agents; Corticorelin; Hyaluronidase; Telaprevir

Storage/Stability

Asmanex HFA: Store at 20°C to 25°C (68°F to 77°F); excursions permitted to 15°C to 30°C (59°F to 86°F). Do not puncture. Do not use or store near heat or open flame. Exposure to temperatures above 120°F may cause bursting. Discard when the dose counter reads "0".

Asmanex Twisthaler: Store at 25°C (77°F); excursions permitted to 15°C to 30°C (59°F to 86°F). Discard when oral dose counter reads "00" (or 45 days [U.S. labeling] or 60 days [Canadian labeling] after opening the foil pouch).

Mechanism of Action May depress the formation, release, and activity of endogenous chemical mediators of inflammation (kinins, histamine, liposomal enzymes, prostaglandins). Leukocytes and macrophages may have to be present for the initiation of responses mediated by the above substances. Inhibits the margination and subsequent cell migration to the area of injury, and also reverses the dilatation and increased vessel permeability in the area resulting in decreased access of cells to the sites of injury.

Pharmacodynamics/Kinetics

Onset of action: Maximum effects may not be evident for ≥1 to 2 weeks

Absorption: <1%

Distribution: V_d: 152 L

Protein binding: 98% to 99%

Metabolism: Hepatic via CYP3A4; forms metabolite

Half-life elimination: ~5 hours

Time to peak, plasma: 0.5 to 2.5 hours

Excretion: Feces (~74%), urine (~8%)

Dosage Oral inhalation: **Note:** Dosage forms of Asmanex Twisthaler available in the U.S. (110 mcg and 220 mcg Twisthaler) deliver 100 mcg and 200 mcg mometasone furoate per actuation respectively. Maximum effects may not be evident for 1 to 2 weeks or longer; dose should be titrated to effect, using the lowest possible dose.

U.S. labeling:

Children 4 to 11 years: Asmanex Twisthaler: 110 mcg once daily in the evening (maximum: 110 mcg daily)

Children ≥12 years, Adolescents, and Adults: Previous therapy:

Bronchodilators: Asmanex Twisthaler: Initial: 220 mcg daily (maximum: 440 mcg daily); may be given in the evening or in divided doses twice daily

Inhaled corticosteroids:

Asmanex HFA: Maximum: 400 mcg twice daily (800 mcg daily)

Inhaled medium-dose corticosteroids: Asmanex HFA 100 mcg inhaler: 200 mcg twice daily

Inhaled high-dose corticosteroids: Asmanex HFA 200 mcg inhaler: 400 mcg twice daily

Asmanex Twisthaler: Initial: 220 mcg daily (maximum: 440 mcg daily); may be given in the evening or in divided doses twice daily

Oral corticosteroids: **Note:** Prednisone should be reduced slowly (ie, no faster than 2.5 mg daily on a weekly basis), beginning after at least 1 week of mometasone use

Asmanex HFA: Initial: 400 mcg twice daily (maximum: 800 mcg daily)

Asmanex Twisthaler: Initial: 440 mcg twice daily (maximum: 880 mcg daily)

Canadian labeling: Children ≥12 years, Adolescents, and Adults:

Usual dose: 200 to 400 mcg once daily in the evening or 200 mcg twice daily administered in the morning and evening. **Note:** Manufacturer suggests that there is a greater chance of achieving asthma control if once daily dosing is administered in the evening. Some patients (eg, previously receiving high-dose inhaled corticosteroids) may respond more favorably to 400 mcg daily administered in 2 divided doses. Titrate to the lowest effective dose.

Severe asthma and requiring oral corticosteroids: Initial: 400 mcg twice daily administered in the morning and evening; (maximum: 800 mcg daily). Taper off oral corticosteroid gradually by decreasing daily prednisone dose by 1 mg daily (or equivalent of other corticosteroid) no sooner than on a weekly basis, beginning after at least 1 week of mometasone use; upon successful taper off of oral steroids, titrate mometasone to lowest effective dose.

Asthma Guidelines (NAEPP, 2007): Children ≥12 years, Adolescents, and Adults:

"Low" dose: 200 mcg daily

"Medium" dose: 400 mcg daily

"High" dose: >400 mcg daily

Dosage adjustment in renal impairment: There are no dosage adjustments provided in the manufacturer's labeling (has not been studied).

Dosage adjustment in hepatic impairment: There are no dosage adjustments provided in the manufacturer's labeling (has not been studied). However, mometasone exposure is increased with hepatic impairment.

Dietary Considerations Asmanex Twisthaler contains lactose.

Administration

Asmanex HFA: Shake well prior to each inhalation. Administer as 2 inhalations twice daily (morning and evening). Prime before first use by releasing 4 test sprays into the air, away from the face, shaking well before each spray. If the inhaler has not been used for more than 5 days, prime the inhaler again with 4 test sprays. Rinse mouth with water without swallowing.

Asmanex Twisthaler: Exhale fully prior to bringing the Twisthaler up to the mouth. Place between lips and inhale quickly and deeply. Do not breathe out through the inhaler. Remove inhaler and hold breath for 10 seconds if possible. Rinse mouth after use.

Monitoring Parameters

HPA axis suppression; signs/symptoms of oral candidiasis; ocular effects (eg, cataracts, increased intraocular pressure, glaucoma)

Asthma: FEV_1, peak flow, and/or other pulmonary function tests

Product Availability Asmanex HFA: FDA approved April 2014; anticipated availability is currently unknown.

Dosage Forms

Aerosol, Inhalation:

Asmanex HFA: 100 mcg/actuation (13 g); 200 mcg/actuation (13 g)

Aerosol Powder Breath Activated, Inhalation:

Asmanex 120 Metered Doses: 220 mcg/INH (1 ea)

Asmanex 14 Metered Doses: 220 mcg/INH (1 ea)

Asmanex 30 Metered Doses: 110 mcg/INH (1 ea); 220 mcg/INH (1 ea)

Asmanex 60 Metered Doses: 220 mcg/INH (1 ea)

Asmanex 7 Metered Doses: 110 mcg/INH (1 ea)

Dosage Forms: Canada

Powder, for oral inhalation:

Asmanex Twisthaler: 200 mcg (30 doses, 60 doses); 400 mcg (30 doses, 60 doses)

Mometasone (Nasal) (moe MET a sone)

Brand Names: U.S. Nasonex

Brand Names: Canada Apo-Mometasone®; Nasonex®

Index Terms Mometasone Furoate

Pharmacologic Category Corticosteroid, Nasal

Additional Appendix Information

Inhaled Corticosteroids *on page 2229*

Use Treatment of nasal symptoms of seasonal and perennial allergic rhinitis; prevention of nasal symptoms associated with seasonal allergic rhinitis; treatment of nasal polyps in adults

Canadian labeling: Additional use (not in U.S. labeling): Treatment of mild-to-moderate uncomplicated rhinosinusitis or as adjunctive treatment (with antimicrobials) in acute rhinosinusitis

Pregnancy Risk Factor C

Dosage Intranasal:

Allergic rhinitis (seasonal and perennial):

U.S. labeling:

Children 2-11 years: 1 spray (50 mcg) in each nostril once daily

Children ≥12 years and Adults: 2 sprays (100 mcg) in each nostril once daily; when used for the prevention of allergic rhinitis, treatment should begin 2-4 weeks prior to pollen season

Canadian labeling:

Children 3-11 years: 1 spray (50 mcg) in each nostril once daily

Children ≥12 years and Adults: Initial: 2 sprays (100 mcg) in each nostril once daily; upon symptom control, may consider dose reduction to 1 spray (50 mcg) in each nostril once daily as maintenance therapy. **Note:** If adequate symptom control is not achieved with initial dosing, may increase dose to 4 sprays (200 mcg) in each nostril once daily (total daily dose: 400 mcg). Dose reduction is recommended upon symptom control.

Nasal polyps treatment: Adults: 2 sprays (100 mcg) in each nostril twice daily; 2 sprays (100 mcg) once daily may be effective in some patients

Rhinosinusitis, adjunctive treatment (acute): Canadian labeling (not in U.S. labeling): Children ≥12 years and Adults: 2 sprays (100 mcg) in each nostril twice daily; if inadequate symptom control, may increase to 4 sprays (200 mcg) in each nostril twice daily (total daily dose: 800 mcg)

Rhinosinusitis treatment (acute, mild-to-moderate, uncomplicated): Canadian labeling (not in U.S. labeling): Children ≥12 years and Adults: 2 sprays (100 mcg) in each nostril twice daily; use beyond 15 days has not been studied.

Elderly: Refer to adult dosing.

Additional Information Complete prescribing information should be consulted for additional detail.

Dosage Forms Considerations Nasonex 17 g bottles contain 120 sprays.

Dosage Forms

Suspension, Nasal:

Nasonex: 50 mcg/actuation (17 g)

Dosage Forms: Canada Excipient information presented when available (limited, particularly for generics); consult specific product labeling.

Suspension, intranasal:

Nasonex®: 50 mcg/spray [delivers 140 sprays]

Mometasone (Topical) (moe MET a sone)

Brand Names: U.S. Elocon

Brand Names: Canada Elocom; PMS-Mometasone; ratio-Mometasone; Taro-Mometasone

Index Terms Mometasone Furoate

Pharmacologic Category Corticosteroid, Topical

Additional Appendix Information

Topical Corticosteroids *on page 2230*

Use Corticosteroid-responsive dermatoses: Relief of the inflammatory and pruritic manifestations of corticosteroid-responsive dermatoses (medium potency topical corticosteroid)

Pregnancy Risk Factor C

Dosage Corticosteroid-responsive dermatoses: Topical: Apply sparingly, do not use occlusive dressings. Therapy should be discontinued when control is achieved; consider reassessment of diagnosis if no improvement is seen within 2 weeks.

U.S. labeling:

Cream, ointment: Children ≥2 years, Adolescents, and Adults: Apply a thin film to affected area once daily; do not use in pediatric patients for longer than 3 weeks

Lotion: Children ≥12 years, Adolescents, and Adults: Apply a few drops to affected area once daily

Canadian labeling:

Cream, ointment: Adults: Apply a thin film to affected area once daily; do not use on face, axillae or scrotum for more than 5 days and on the body for more than 3 weeks

Lotion: Adults: Apply a few drops to the affected area once daily; do not use on the face, scalp, axillae or scrotum for more than 5 days and on the body for more than 3 weeks

Dosage adjustment in renal impairment:

U.S. labeling: There are no dosage adjustments provided in the manufacturer's labeling.

Canadian labeling: There are no specific dosage adjustments provided in the manufacturer's labeling; however, the manufacturer recommends applying a minimum quantity for the shortest duration

Dosage adjustment in hepatic impairment:

U.S. labeling: There are no dosage adjustments provided in the manufacturer's labeling.

Canadian labeling: There are no specific dosage adjustments provided in the manufacturer's labeling; however, the manufacturer recommends applying a minimum quantity for the shortest duration

Additional Information Complete prescribing information should be consulted for additional detail.

Dosage Forms

Cream, External:

Elocon: 0.1% (15 g, 45 g, 50 g)

Generic: 0.1% (15 g, 45 g)

Lotion, External:

Elocon: 0.1% (30 mL, 60 mL)

Ointment, External:

Elocon: 0.1% (15 g, 45 g)

Generic: 0.1% (15 g, 45 g)

Solution, External:

Generic: 0.1% (30 mL, 60 mL)

◆ **Mometasone and Eformoterol** *see* Mometasone and Formoterol *on page 1392*

Mometasone and Formoterol

(moe MET a sone & for MOH te rol)

Brand Names: U.S. Dulera

Brand Names: Canada Zenhale

Index Terms Eformoterol and Mometasone; Formoterol and Mometasone; Formoterol and Mometasone Furoate; Formoterol Fumarate Dihydrate and Mometasone; Mometasone and Eformoterol

Pharmacologic Category $Beta_2$ Agonist, Long-Acting; $Beta_2$-Adrenergic Agonist, Long-Acting; Corticosteroid, Inhalant (Oral)

Use Asthma: Treatment of asthma in patients 12 years and older.

Limitations of use: Mometasone/formoterol is not indicated for the relief of acute bronchospasm.

Pregnancy Risk Factor C

Dosage

Asthma: Oral inhalation: Children ≥12 years, Adolescents, and Adults:

Previous therapy included inhaled low-dose corticosteroids: Canadian labeling (not in US labeling): Mometasone 50 mcg/formoterol 5 mcg: Two inhalations twice daily. Maximum daily dose: Mometasone 200 mcg/formoterol 20 mcg (4 inhalations).

Previous therapy included inhaled medium-dose corticosteroids: Mometasone 100 mcg/formoterol 5 mcg: Two inhalations twice daily. Consider the higher dose combination for patients not adequately controlled on the lower combination following 2 weeks of therapy. Maximum daily dose: Mometasone 400 mcg/formoterol 20 mcg (4 inhalations).

Previous therapy included inhaled high-dose corticosteroids: Mometasone 200 mcg/formoterol 5 mcg: following 2 weeks of therapy. Maximum daily dose: Mometasone 800 mcg/formoterol 20 mcg (4 inhalations).

Chronic obstructive pulmonary disease (stable) (off-label use): Adults: Oral inhalation: Mometasone 200 mcg/formoterol 10 mcg to mometasone 400 mcg/formoterol 10 mcg twice daily (Doherty, 2012; GOLD, 2014).

Dosage adjustment in renal impairment: There are no dosage adjustments provided in the manufacturer's labeling (has not been studied).

Dosage adjustment in hepatic impairment: There are no dosage adjustments provided in the manufacturer's labeling (has not been studied). However, mometasone exposure is increased with hepatic impairment.

Additional Information Complete prescribing information should be consulted for additional detail.

Dosage Forms

Aerosol, for oral inhalation:

Dulera: Mometasone 100 mcg and formoterol 5 mcg per inhalation (8.8 g) [60 metered actuations]

Dulera: Mometasone 100 mcg and formoterol 5 mcg per inhalation (13 g) [120 metered actuations]

Dulera: Mometasone 200 mcg and formoterol 5 mcg per inhalation (8.8 g) [60 metered actuations]

Dulera: Mometasone 200 mcg and formoterol 5 mcg per inhalation (13 g) [120 metered actuations]

Dosage Forms: Canada

Aerosol, for oral inhalation:

Zenhale: Mometasone furoate 50 mcg and formoterol fumarate dihydrate 5 mcg per inhalation [120 metered actuations]

◆ **Mometasone Furoate** *see* Mometasone (Nasal) *on page 1391*

◆ **Mometasone Furoate** *see* Mometasone (Oral Inhalation) *on page 1389*

◆ **Mometasone Furoate** *see* Mometasone (Topical) *on page 1391*

◆ **MOM/Mineral Oil Emulsion** *see* Magnesium Hydroxide and Mineral Oil *on page 1264*

◆ **Monacolin K** *see* Lovastatin *on page 1252*

◆ **Monicure (Can)** *see* Fluconazole *on page 885*

◆ **Monistat® (Can)** *see* Miconazole (Topical) *on page 1360*

◆ **Monistat® 3 (Can)** *see* Miconazole (Topical) *on page 1360*

◆ **Monoclate-P** *see* Antihemophilic Factor (Human) *on page 152*

◆ **Monoclonal Antibody 2C4** *see* Pertuzumab *on page 1627*

◆ **Monoclonal Antibody 5G1.1** *see* Eculizumab *on page 703*

◆ **Monoclonal Antibody ABX-EGF** *see* Panitumumab *on page 1568*

◆ **Monoclonal Antibody Anti-C5** *see* Eculizumab *on page 703*

◆ **Monoclonal Antibody Campath-1H** *see* Alemtuzumab *on page 75*

◆ **Monoclonal Antibody CD52** *see* Alemtuzumab *on page 75*

◆ **Monodox** *see* Doxycycline *on page 689*

◆ **Monoethanolamine** *see* Ethanolamine Oleate *on page 799*

◆ **MonoNessa** *see* Ethinyl Estradiol and Norgestimate *on page 810*

◆ **Mononine** *see* Factor IX (Human) *on page 840*

◆ **Monopril** *see* Fosinopril *on page 932*

◆ **Monovisc** *see* Hyaluronate and Derivatives *on page 1006*

Montelukast

(mon te LOO kast)

Brand Names: U.S. Singulair

Brand Names: Canada ACH-Montelukast; Apo-Montelukast; Auro-Montelukast; Auro-Montelukast Chewable Tablets; Dom-Montelukast; Dom-Montelukast FC; Jamp-Montelukast; Mar-Montelukast; Mint-Montelukast; Montelukast Sodium Tablets; Mylan-Montelukast; PMS-Montelukast; PMS-Montelukast FC; RAN-Montelukast; Riva-Montelukast FC; Sandoz-Montelukast; Sandoz-Montelukast Granules; Singulair; Teva-Montelukast

Index Terms Montelukast Sodium

Pharmacologic Category Leukotriene-Receptor Antagonist

Use Prophylaxis and chronic treatment of asthma; relief of symptoms of seasonal allergic rhinitis and perennial allergic rhinitis; prevention of exercise-induced bronchoconstriction

Pregnancy Risk Factor B

Pregnancy Considerations Adverse events have not been observed in animal reproduction studies. Structural defects have been reported in neonates exposed to montelukast *in utero*; however, a specific pattern and relationship to montelukast has not been established. Based on available data, an increased risk of teratogenic effects has not been observed with montelukast use in pregnancy (Bakhireva, 2007; Nelsen, 2012; Sarkar, 2009). Uncontrolled asthma is associated with adverse events on pregnancy (increased risk of perinatal mortality, pre-eclampsia, preterm birth, low birth weight infants). Montelukast may be considered for use in women who had a favorable response prior to becoming pregnant; however, initiating a leukotriene receptor antagonist during pregnancy is an alternative (but not preferred) treatment option for mild persistent asthma (NAEPP, 2005).

Breast-Feeding Considerations It is not known if montelukast is excreted into breast milk. The manufacturer recommends that caution be exercised when administering montelukast to nursing women.

Contraindications Hypersensitivity to montelukast or any component of the formulation

Warnings/Precautions Montelukast is not FDA approved for use in the reversal of bronchospasm in acute asthma attacks, including status asthmaticus; some studies, however, support its use as adjunctive therapy (Cylly, 2003; Ferreira, 2001; Harmancik, 2006). Appropriate rescue medication should be available. Montelukast treatment should continue during acute asthma exacerbation. When inhaled or systemic corticosteroid reduction is considered in patients initiating or receiving montelukast, appropriate clinical monitoring and a gradual dose reduction of the steroid are recommended.

Postmarketing reports of behavioral changes (eg, agitation, aggression, anxiety, attention deficit, depression, hallucinations, hostility, insomnia, irritability, restlessness, sleep disturbance, suicide ideation/behavior) have been noted in pediatric, adolescent, and adult patients. In a retrospective analysis performed by Merck, serious behavior-related events were rare (Philip, 2009a); assess patients for behavioral changes. Patients should be instructed to notify the prescriber if behavioral changes occur.

Potentially significant drug-drug interactions may exist, requiring dose or frequency adjustment, additional monitoring, and/or selection of alternative therapy. In rare cases, patients on therapy with montelukast may present with systemic eosinophilia, sometimes presenting with clinical features of vasculitis consistent with Churg-Strauss syndrome, a condition which is often treated with systemic corticosteroid therapy. Healthcare providers should be alert to eosinophilia, vasculitic rash, worsening pulmonary symptoms, cardiac complications, and/or neuropathy presenting in their patients. A causal association between montelukast and these underlying conditions has not been established. Montelukast will not interrupt bronchoconstrictor response to aspirin or other NSAIDs; aspirin sensitive asthmatics should continue to avoid these agents. The chewable tablet contains phenylalanine.

Adverse Reactions

Children ≥15 years and Adults:

Central nervous system: Dizziness, fatigue, fever, headache

Dermatologic: Skin rash

Gastrointestinal: Dyspepsia, gastroenteritis, toothache

Hepatic: Increased serum ALT, increased serum AST

Neuromuscular & skeletal: Weakness

Respiratory: Cough, epistaxis, nasal congestion, sinusitis, upper respiratory tract infection

Children 2 to ≤14 years:

Central nervous system: Fever, headache

Dermatologic: Dermatitis, eczema, skin rash, urticaria

Gastrointestinal: Abdominal pain, dyspepsia, gastroenteritis, nausea

Infection: Influenza, varicella, viral infection

Ophthalmic: Conjunctivitis

Otic: Otalgia, otitis

Respiratory: Laryngitis, pharyngitis, pneumonia, rhinorrhea, sinusitis, upper respiratory tract infection

Children 6 to 23 months:

Respiratory: Cough, otitis media, pharyngitis, rhinitis, tonsillitis, upper respiratory tract infection, wheezing

Rare but important or life-threatening: Anaphylaxis, angioedema, Churg-Strauss syndrome, depression, disorientation, eosinophilia (systemic), eosinophilic pneumonitis, erythema multiforme, erythema nodosum, hallucination, hepatic eosinophilic infiltration, hepatitis (mixed pattern, hepatocellular, and cholestatic), hypersensitivity, insomnia, memory impairment, pancreatitis, paresthesia, seizure, somnambulism, Stevens-Johnson syndrome, suicidal ideation, suicidal tendencies, thrombocytopenia, toxic epidermal necrolysis, vasculitis

Drug Interactions

Metabolism/Transport Effects Substrate of CYP2C9 (major), CYP3A4 (major); **Note:** Assignment of Major/Minor substrate status based on clinically relevant drug interaction potential; **Inhibits** CYP2C8 (weak), CYP2C9 (weak)

Avoid Concomitant Use There are no known interactions where it is recommended to avoid concomitant use.

Increased Effect/Toxicity

The levels/effects of Montelukast may be increased by: Ceritinib; CYP2C9 Inhibitors (Moderate); CYP2C9 Inhibitors (Strong); Mifepristone

Decreased Effect

The levels/effects of Montelukast may be decreased by: Bosentan; CYP2C9 Inducers (Strong); CYP3A4 Inducers (Moderate); CYP3A4 Inducers (Strong); Dabrafenib; Deferasirox; Mitotane; Siltuximab; St Johns Wort; Tocilizumab

Storage/Stability Store at room temperature of 25°C (77°F); excursions permitted to 15°C to 30°C (59°F to 86°F). Store in original package. Protect from moisture and light. Granules must be used within 15 minutes of opening packet.

Mechanism of Action Selective leukotriene receptor antagonist that inhibits the cysteinyl leukotriene receptor. Cysteinyl leukotrienes and leukotriene receptor occupation have been correlated with the pathophysiology of asthma, including airway edema, smooth muscle contraction, and altered cellular activity associated with the inflammatory process, which contribute to the signs and symptoms of asthma. Cysteinyl leukotrienes are also released from the nasal mucosa following allergen exposure leading to symptoms associated with allergic rhinitis (Jarvis, 2000).

Pharmacodynamics/Kinetics

Duration: >24 hours

Absorption: Rapid

Distribution: V_d: 8-11 L

Protein binding, plasma: >99%

Metabolism: Extensively hepatic via CYP3A4, 2C8, and 2C9

Bioavailability: Tablet: 10 mg, Mean: 64%; Chewable tablet: 5 mg: 73% (63% when administered with a standard meal)

Half-life elimination: 2.7-5.5 hours; Mild-to-moderate hepatic impairment: 7.4 hours

Time to peak: Tablet: 10 mg: 3-4 hours; Chewable tablet: 2-2.5 hours; granules: 1-3 hours (fasting) and 3.5 to ~9 hours (with high-fat meal)

Excretion: Feces (86%); urine (<0.2%)

Dosage Note: Patients with **both** asthma and allergic rhinitis should take only one dose in the evening.

Asthma: Oral:

Children ≥1 to <2 years: 4 mg (oral granules) once daily (in the evening)

Children ≥2 to <6 years: 4 mg (chewable tablet or oral granules) once daily (in the evening)

Children ≥6 years and Adolescents <15 years: 5 mg (chewable tablet) once daily (in the evening)

Adolescents ≥15 years and Adults: 10 mg once daily (in the evening)

Bronchoconstriction, exercise-induced (prevention): Note: Additional doses should not be administered within 24 hours. Daily administration to prevent exercise-induced bronchoconstriction has not been evaluated. Patients receiving montelukast for another indication should not take an additional dose to prevent exercise-induced bronchoconstriction. Oral:

Children ≥6 years and Adolescents <15 years: 5 mg (chewable tablet) at least 2 hours prior to exercise

Adolescents ≥15 years and Adults: 10 mg once daily at least 2 hours prior to exercise

Perennial allergic rhinitis: Oral:

Children 6 months to <2 years: 4 mg (oral granules) once daily

Children ≥2 to <6 years: 4 mg (chewable tablet or oral granules) once daily

Children ≥6 years and Adolescents <15 years: 5 mg (chewable tablet) once daily

Adolescents ≥15 years and Adults: 10 mg once daily

Seasonal allergic rhinitis: Oral:

Children ≥2 to <6 years: 4 mg (chewable tablet or oral granules) once daily

Children ≥6 years and Adolescents <15 years: 5 mg (chewable tablet) once daily

Adolescents ≥15 years and Adults: 10 mg once daily

Urticaria (nonsteroidal anti-inflammatory drug–induced) (off-label use): Oral: Adolescents ≥15 years and Adults: 10 mg once daily (Pacor, 2001)

Dosage adjustment in renal impairment: No dosage adjustment necessary

Dosage adjustment in hepatic impairment:

Mild-to-moderate impairment: No dosage adjustment necessary.

Severe impairment: No dosage adjustment provided in manufacturer's labeling; has not been studied.

Dietary Considerations Some products may contain phenylalanine.

Administration When treating asthma, administer dose in the evening. Patients with allergic rhinitis may individualize administration time (morning or evening). Patients with **both** asthma and allergic rhinitis should take a single dose in the evening. May administer without regard to food or meals.

Granules: May be administered directly in the mouth, dissolved in 5 mL of baby formula or breast milk, or mixed with a spoonful of applesauce, carrots, rice, or ice cream; do not add to any other liquids or foods. Administer within 15 minutes of opening packet.

Monitoring Parameters Mood or behavior changes, including suicidal thinking/behavior

Dosage Forms

Packet, Oral:

Singulair: 4 mg (30 ea)

Generic: 4 mg (1 ea, 30 ea)

Tablet, Oral:

Singulair: 10 mg

Generic: 10 mg

Tablet Chewable, Oral:

Singulair: 4 mg, 5 mg

Generic: 4 mg, 5 mg

- ◆ **Montelukast Sodium** *see* Montelukast *on page 1392*
- ◆ **Montelukast Sodium Tablets (Can)** *see* Montelukast *on page 1392*
- ◆ **Monurol** *see* Fosfomycin *on page 932*
- ◆ **Monurol® (Can)** *see* Fosfomycin *on page 932*
- ◆ **8-MOP** *see* Methoxsalen (Systemic) *on page 1330*
- ◆ **8-Mop** *see* Methoxsalen (Systemic) *on page 1330*
- ◆ **Morgidox** *see* Doxycycline *on page 689*
- ◆ **Morning After Pill** *see* Ethinyl Estradiol and Norgestrel *on page 812*
- ◆ **Moroctocog Alfa** *see* Antihemophilic Factor (Recombinant) *on page 152*

Morphine (Systemic) (MOR feen)

Brand Names: U.S. Astramorph; AVINza; Duramorph; Infumorph 200; Infumorph 500; Kadian; MS Contin

Brand Names: Canada Doloral; Kadian; M-Eslon; M.O.S. 10; M.O.S. 20; M.O.S. 30; M.O.S.-SR; M.O.S.-Sulfate; Morphine Extra Forte Injection; Morphine Forte Injection; Morphine HP; Morphine LP Epidural; Morphine SR; Morphine-EPD; MS Contin; MS Contin SRT; MS-IR; Novo-Morphine SR; PMS-Morphine Sulfate SR; ratio-Morphine; ratio-Morphine SR; Sandoz-Morphine SR; Statex; Teva-Morphine SR

Index Terms MS (error-prone abbreviation and should not be used); MSO_4 (error-prone abbreviation and should not be used); Roxanol

Pharmacologic Category Analgesic, Opioid

Additional Appendix Information

Opioid Conversion Table *on page 2232*

Use

Immediate-release oral products: Relief of moderate to severe acute and chronic pain for which use of an opioid analgesic is appropriate.

Injection: Relief of severe pain, such as myocardial infarction and severe injuries; relief of dyspnea of acute left ventricular failure and pulmonary edema; preanesthetic medication

Preservative-free injectable solution:

Infumorph: Used in continuous microinfusion devices for intrathecal or epidural administration in treatment of intractable chronic pain

Duramorph: For intravenous, epidural, or intrathecal administration in the management of pain for extended periods without attendant loss of motor, sensory, or sympathetic function. **Note: Not** for use in continuous microinfusion devices.

Extended-release oral products: Management of pain severe enough to require daily, around-the-clock, long-term opioid treatment and for which alternative treatment options are inadequate.

Limitations of use: Because of the risks of addiction, abuse, and misuse with opioids, even at recommended doses, and because of the greater risks of overdose and death with extended-release formulations, reserve extended-release formulations for use in patients for whom alternative treatment options (eg, nonopioid analgesics, immediate-release opioids) are ineffective, not tolerated, or would be otherwise inadequate to provide sufficient management of pain. MS Contin, Kadian, and Avinza are not indicated as as-needed analgesics.

Pregnancy Risk Factor C

Pregnancy Considerations Adverse events have been observed in some animal reproduction studies. Morphine crosses the human placenta. The frequency of congenital malformations has not been reported to be greater than expected in children from mothers treated with morphine during pregnancy. However, following *in utero* exposure, infants may exhibit withdrawal, decreased brain volume (reversible), small size, decreased ventilatory response to CO_2, and increased risk of sudden infant death syndrome.

Morphine sulfate injection may be used for the management of pain during labor (ACOG, 2002); however, some manufacturers specifically contraindicate use of the injection during labor when a premature birth is anticipated. When used for pain relief during labor, opioids may temporarily affect the heart rate of the fetus. Morphine injection may also be used to treat pain following delivery (ACOG, 2002).

[U.S. Boxed Warning]: Prolonged maternal use of opioids during pregnancy can cause neonatal withdrawal syndrome in the newborn, which may be life-threatening if not recognized and treated according to protocols developed by neonatology experts. If prolonged opioid therapy is required in a pregnant woman, ensure treatment is available and warn patient of risk to the neonate. If chronic opioid exposure occurs in pregnancy, adverse events in the newborn (including withdrawal) may occur; monitoring of the neonate is recommended. The minimum effective dose should be used if opioids are needed (Chou, 2009). Neonatal abstinence syndrome following opioid exposure may present with autonomic (eg, fever, temperature instability), gastrointestinal (eg, diarrhea, vomiting, poor feeding/weight gain), or neurologic (eg, high-pitched crying, increased muscle tone, irritability, seizure, tremor) symptoms (Dow, 2012; Hudak, 2012).

Long-term opioid use may cause secondary hypogonadism, which may lead to sexual dysfunction or infertility (Brennan, 2013).

Breast-Feeding Considerations Morphine concentrates in breast milk, with a milk to plasma AUC ratio of 2.5:1. Detectable serum levels of morphine can be found in infants following morphine administration to nursing mothers.

Parenteral opioids used during labor have the potential to interfere with a newborn's natural reflex to nurse within the first few hours after birth. Morphine is recommended as an analgesic in nursing women due to the limited amounts found in breast milk and poor oral bioavailability in nursing infants. Nursing infants exposed to large doses of opioids should be monitored for apnea and sedation (Montgomery, 2012).

Treatment of the mother with single doses of morphine is not expected to cause detrimental effects in nursing infants. Breast-feeding following chronic use or in neonates with hepatic or renal dysfunction may lead to higher levels of morphine in the infant and a risk of adverse effects (Spigset, 2000).

The manufacturers of extended release products note that due to the potential for serious adverse reactions in the nursing infant, a decision should be made whether to discontinue nursing or to discontinue the drug, taking into account the importance of treatment to the mother.

Contraindications Note: Some contraindications are product specific. For details, please see detailed product prescribing information.

Hypersensitivity to morphine sulfate or any component of the formulation; severe respiratory depression, acute or severe asthma (in an unmonitored setting or without resuscitative equipment); known or suspected paralytic ileus

Additional contraindication information (based on formulation):

- Epidural/intrathecal:
  - Astramorph/PF, Duramorph: Upper airway obstruction
  - Astramorph/PF, Duramorph, Infumorph: Usual contraindications related to neuraxial analgesia apply (eg, presence of infection at infusion site, concomitant anticoagulant therapy, uncontrolled bleeding diathesis)
- Extended release: GI obstruction
- Immediate release tablets/solution: Hypercarbia
- Injectable formulation: Heart failure due to chronic lung disease, cardiac arrhythmias; increased intracranial pressure, head injuries, brain tumors; acute alcoholism, deliriums tremens; seizure disorders; use during labor when a premature birth is anticipated
- Suppository: Severe CNS depression; cardiac arrhythmias, heart failure due to chronic lung disease; increased intracranial or cerebrospinal pressure, head injuries, brain tumor; acute alcoholism, delirium tremens; seizure disorder; use after biliary tract surgery, suspected surgical abdomen, surgical anastomosis; concurrent use or within 2 weeks of MAO inhibitors

Warnings/Precautions An opioid-containing analgesic regimen should be tailored to each patient's needs and based upon the type of pain being treated (acute versus chronic), the route of administration, degree of tolerance for opioids (naive versus chronic user), age, weight, and medical condition. The optimal analgesic dose varies widely among patients. Doses should be titrated to pain relief/prevention. When used as an epidural injection, monitor for delayed sedation.

All morphine sulfate formulations are capable of causing respiratory depression; risk increased in elderly patients, debilitated patients, and patients with conditions associated with hypoxia or hypercapnia. Monitor for respiratory depression, especially during initiation and titration. Extended-release formulations: **[U.S. Boxed Warning]: May cause serious, life-threatening, or fatal respiratory depression. Monitor closely for respiratory depression, especially during initiation or dose escalation. Instruct patients to swallow extended-release morphine formulations whole (or may sprinkle the contents of the Avinza capsule on applesauce and swallow without chewing); crushing, chewing, or dissolving the extended-release formulations can cause rapid release and absorption of a potentially fatal dose of morphine.** Carbon dioxide retention from opioid-induced respiratory depression can exacerbate the sedating effects of opioids. Use with caution and monitor for respiratory depression in patients with significant chronic obstructive pulmonary disease or cor pulmonale, and patients having a substantially decreased respiratory reserve, hypoxia, hypercarbia, or preexisting respiratory depression, particularly when initiating therapy and titrating with morphine; even therapeutic doses may decrease respiratory drive to the point of apnea. Consider the use of alternative nonopioid analgesics in these patients. Some dosage forms may be contraindicated in patients with severe respiratory disorders. Infants <3 months of age are more susceptible to respiratory depression, use with caution and generally in reduced doses in this age group.

Use caution in morbid obesity, adrenal insufficiency, prostatic hyperplasia, thyroid dysfunction, urinary stricture, renal impairment, or severe hepatic dysfunction and in patients with hypersensitivity reactions to other phenanthrene derivative opioid agonists (codeine, hydrocodone, hydromorphone, levorphanol, oxycodone, oxymorphone). Avoid use in patients with CNS depression or coma as these patients are susceptible to intracranial effects of CO_2 retention. Use with caution in patients with biliary tract dysfunction including acute pancreatitis as may cause constriction of sphincter of Oddi. May obscure diagnosis or clinical course of patients with acute abdominal conditions. May cause constipation which may be problematic in patients with unstable angina and patients post-myocardial infarction. Some preparations contain sulfites which may cause allergic reactions.

May cause CNS depression, which may impair physical or mental abilities; patients must be cautioned about performing tasks which require mental alertness (eg, operating machinery or driving). Potentially significant drug interactions may exist, requiring dose or frequency adjustment, additional monitoring, and/or selection of alternative therapy. Effects may be potentiated when used with other CNS depressants (eg, sedatives, anxiolytics, hypnotics, neuroleptics, other opioids). **[U.S. Boxed Warning]: Patients should not consume alcoholic beverages or medication containing ethanol while taking Avinza or Kadian; ethanol may increase morphine plasma levels resulting in a potentially fatal overdose.**

May cause hypotension; use with caution in patients with hypovolemia, cardiovascular disease (including acute MI), circulatory shock, or drugs which may exaggerate hypotensive effects (including phenothiazines or general anesthetics). May cause orthostatic hypotension and syncope in ambulatory patients. Use with extreme caution in patients with head injury, intracranial lesions, or elevated intracranial pressure; exaggerated elevation of ICP may occur if respiratory drive is depressed and CO_2 retention occurs. Use with caution in patients with seizure disorders, may exacerbate preexisting seizures. Tolerance or drug dependence may result from extended use. Concurrent use of mixed agonist/antagonist analgesics (eg, pentazocine, nalbuphine, butorphanol) or partial agonist (eg, buprenorphine) analgesics may precipitate withdrawal symptoms and/or reduced analgesic efficacy in patients following prolonged therapy with mu opioid agonists. Abrupt discontinuation following prolonged use may also lead to withdrawal symptoms; taper dose gradually when discontinuing.

Use epidural/intrathecal formulations with extreme caution in elderly patients.

Extended-release formulations: **[U.S. Boxed Warning]: Users are exposed to the risks of addiction, abuse, and misuse, potentially leading to overdose and death. Assess each patient's risk prior to prescribing; monitor all patients regularly for development of these behaviors or conditions.** Risk of opioid abuse is increased in patients with a history or family history of alcohol or drug abuse or mental illness. Avinza capsules contain fumaric acid; dangerous quantities of fumaric acid may be ingested when >1600 mg/day is used; serious renal toxicity may occur above the maximum dose. **Extended-release products are not interchangeable;** when determining a generic equivalent or switching from one extended-release product to another, review pharmacokinetic properties. **[U.S. Boxed Warning]: Prolonged maternal use of opioids during pregnancy can cause neonatal withdrawal syndrome in the newborn which may be life-threatening if not recognized and treated according to protocols developed by neonatology experts. If prolonged opioid therapy is required in a pregnant woman, ensure treatment is available and warn patient of risk to the neonate.** Signs and symptoms include irritability, hyperactivity, abnormal sleep pattern, high-pitched cry, tremor, vomiting, diarrhea, and failure to gain weight. Onset, duration, and severity depend on the drug used, duration of use, maternal dose, and rate of drug elimination by the newborn. **[U.S. Boxed Warning]: Accidental ingestion of even one dose, especially in children, can result in a fatal overdose of morphine.**

Highly concentrated oral solutions: **[U.S. Boxed Warning]: Check doses carefully when using highly concentrated oral solutions. The 100 mg/5 mL (20 mg/mL) concentration is indicated for use in opioid-tolerant patients only.**

Injections: Products are designed for administration by specific routes (ie, IV, intrathecal, epidural). Use caution when prescribing, dispensing, or administering to use formulations only by intended route(s).

Astramorph/PF, Duramorph, Infumorph: **[U.S. Boxed Warning]: Due to the risk of severe and/or sustained cardiopulmonary depressant effects, must be administered in a fully equipped room for resuscitation and staffed environment.** Naloxone injection should be immediately available. Patient should remain in this environment for at least 24 hours following the initial dose. **[U.S. Boxed Warning]: Accidental dermal exposure to Astramorph/PF, Duramorph, Infumorph should be rinsed with water. Contaminated clothing should be removed.** For patients receiving Infumorph via microinfusion device, patient may be observed, as appropriate, for the first several days after catheter implantation. Thoracic epidural administration has been shown to dramatically increase the risk of early and late respiratory depression.

[U.S. Boxed Warning]: Improper or erroneous substitution of Infumorph for regular Duramorph is likely to result in serious overdosage, leading to seizures, respiratory depression and possibly a fatal outcome. Infumorph should only be used in microinfusion devices; not for IV, IM, or SubQ administration or for single-dose administration. Monitor closely, especially in the first 24 hours. Inflammatory masses (eg, granulomas), some resulting in severe neurologic impairment have occurred when receiving Infumorph via indwelling intrathecal catheter; monitor carefully for new neurologic signs/symptoms. **[U.S. Boxed Warning]: Intrathecal dosage is usually 1/10 (one-tenth) that of epidural dosage.**

Benzyl alcohol and derivatives: Some dosage forms may contain sodium benzoate/benzoic acid; benzoic acid (benzoate) is a metabolite of benzyl alcohol; large amounts of benzyl alcohol (≥99 mg/kg/day) have been associated with a potentially fatal toxicity ("gasping syndrome") in neonates; the "gasping syndrome" consists of metabolic acidosis, respiratory distress, gasping respirations, CNS dysfunction (including convulsions, intracranial hemorrhage), hypotension, and cardiovascular collapse (AAP, 1997; CDC, 1982); some data suggests that benzoate displaces bilirubin from protein binding sites (Ahlfors, 2001); avoid or use dosage forms containing benzyl alcohol derivative with caution in neonates. See manufacturer's labeling.

Adverse Reactions Note: Individual patient differences are unpredictable. Reactions may be dose-, formulation-, and/or route-dependent.

Cardiovascular: Atrial fibrillation, bradycardia, chest pain, circulatory depression, edema, flushing, hyper-/hypotension, palpitation, peripheral edema, shock, syncope, tachycardia, vasodilation

Central nervous system: Amnesia, agitation, anxiety, apathy, apprehension, ataxia, chills, coma, confusion, delirium, depression, dizziness, dream abnormalities, drowsiness (tolerance usually develops to drowsiness with regular dosing for 1-2 weeks), dysphonia, euphoria, false sense of well being, fever, hallucination, headache (following epidural or intrathecal use), hypoesthesia, insomnia, lethargy, malaise, nervousness, physical and psychological dependence, restlessness, sedation, seizure, slurred speech, somnolence, vertigo

Dermatologic: Dry skin, pruritus (may be dose related), rash, urticaria

Endocrine & metabolic: Antidiuretic hormone release, gynecomastia, hypogonadism, hypokalemia, hyponatremia, libido decreased

Gastrointestinal: Abdominal distension, anorexia, abdominal pain, biliary colic, constipation (tolerance develops very slowly if at all), diarrhea, dyspepsia, dysphagia, flatulence, gastroenteritis, GERD, GI irritation, nausea (tolerance usually develops to nausea and vomiting with chronic use), paralytic ileus, rectal disorder, taste perversion, vomiting, weight loss, xerostomia

Genitourinary: Urinary retention (may be prolonged, up to 20 hours, following epidural or intrathecal use), bladder spasm, dysuria, ejaculation abnormal, impotence, urination decreased

Hematologic: Anemia (following intrathecal use), hematocrit decreased, leukopenia, thrombocytopenia

Hepatic: Liver function tests increased

Local: Pain at injection site

Neuromuscular & skeletal: Arthralgia, back pain, bone mineral density decreased, bone pain, foot drop, gait abnormalities, myoclonus, paresthesia, rigors, skeletal muscle rigidity, tremor, weakness

Ocular: Amblyopia, conjunctivitis, eye pain, vision problems/disturbance

Renal: Oliguria

Respiratory: Asthma, atelectasis, dyspnea, hiccups, hypercapnia, hypoxia, oxygen saturation decreased,pulmonary edema (noncardiogenic), respiratory depression, rhinitis

Miscellaneous: Diaphoresis, flu-like syndrome, histamine release, infection, thirst, voice alteration, withdrawal syndrome

Rare but important or life-threatening: Amenorrhea, anaphylaxis, apnea, biliary tract spasm, blurred vision, bronchospasm, cardiac arrest, cough reflex decreased, dehydration, diplopia, disorientation, hemorrhagic urticaria, intestinal obstruction, intracranial pressure increased, laryngospasm, menstrual irregularities, miosis, myoclonus, nystagmus, paradoxical CNS stimulation, respiratory arrest, sepsis, urinary tract spasm, thermal dysregulation, toxic psychoses

Drug Interactions

Metabolism/Transport Effects Substrate of CYP2D6 (minor), P-glycoprotein; **Note:** Assignment of Major/Minor substrate status based on clinically relevant drug interaction potential

Avoid Concomitant Use

Avoid concomitant use of Morphine (Systemic) with any of the following: Azelastine (Nasal); MAO Inhibitors; Orphenadrine; Paraldehyde; Thalidomide

Increased Effect/Toxicity

Morphine (Systemic) may increase the levels/effects of: Alcohol (Ethyl); Alvimopan; Azelastine (Nasal); Buprenorphine; CNS Depressants; Desmopressin; Diuretics; Hydrocodone; Methotrimeprazine; Metyrosine; Mirtazapine; Orphenadrine; Paraldehyde; Pramipexole; ROPINIRole; Rotigotine; Selective Serotonin Reuptake Inhibitors; Suvorexant; Thalidomide; Zolpidem

The levels/effects of Morphine (Systemic) may be increased by: Amphetamines; Anticholinergic Agents; Antipsychotic Agents (Phenothiazines); Brimonidine (Topical); Cannabis; Doxylamine; Dronabinol; Droperidol; HydrOXYzine; Kava Kava; Magnesium Sulfate; MAO Inhibitors; Methotrimeprazine; Nabilone; Perampanel; P-glycoprotein/ABCB1 Inhibitors; Rufinamide; Sodium Oxybate; Succinylcholine; Tapentadol; Tetrahydrocannabinol

Decreased Effect

Morphine (Systemic) may decrease the levels/effects of: Clopidogrel; Pegvisomant

The levels/effects of Morphine (Systemic) may be decreased by: Ammonium Chloride; Mixed Agonist / Antagonist Opioids; Naltrexone; P-glycoprotein/ABCB1 Inducers; Rifamycin Derivatives

Food Interactions

Ethanol: Alcoholic beverages or ethanol-containing products may disrupt extended release formulation resulting in rapid release of entire morphine dose. Management: Avoid alcohol. **Do not administer Avinza with alcoholic beverages or ethanol-containing prescription or nonprescription products.**

Food: Administration of oral morphine solution with food may increase bioavailability (ie, a report of 34% increase in morphine AUC when morphine oral solution followed a high-fat meal). The bioavailability of Avinza, MS Contin, or Kadian does not appear to be affected by food. Management: Take consistently with or without meals.

Storage/Stability

Capsule, extended release: Store at 25°C (77°F); excursions permitted to 15°C to 30°C (59°F to 86°F). Protect from light and moisture.

Injection: Store at controlled room temperature of 20°C to 25°C (68°F to 77°F); do not freeze. Protect from light. Degradation depends on pH and presence of oxygen; relatively stable in pH ≤4; darkening of solutions indicate degradation.

Astramorph/PF, Duramorph, Infumorph: Store in carton until use at controlled room temperature of 20°C to 25°C (68°F to 77°F); excursions permitted to 15°C to 30°C (59°F to 86°F); do not freeze; do not heat-sterilize. Contains no preservative or antioxidant. Protect from light.

Oral solution: Store at controlled room temperature of 15°C to 30°C (59°F to 86°F); do not freeze. Protect from moisture.

Suppositories: Store below controlled room temperature 25°C (77°F).

Tablet, extended release: Store at controlled room temperature of 25°C (77°F); excursions permitted to 15°C to 30°C (59°F to 86°F).

Tablet, immediate release: Store at controlled room temperature of 15°C to 30°C (59°F to 86°F). Protect from moisture.

Mechanism of Action Binds to opioid receptors in the CNS, causing inhibition of ascending pain pathways, altering the perception of and response to pain; produces generalized CNS depression

Pharmacodynamics/Kinetics

Onset of action (patient dependent; dosing must be individualized): Oral (immediate release): ~30 minutes; IV: 5 to 10 minutes

Duration (patient dependent; dosing must be individualized): Pain relief:

Immediate-release formulations: 4 hours

Extended-release capsule and tablet: 8 to 24 hours (formulation dependent)

Absorption: Variable

Distribution: V_d: 1 to 6 L/kg; binds to opioid receptors in the CNS and periphery (eg, GI tract)

Protein binding: 20% to 35%

Metabolism: Hepatic via conjugation with glucuronic acid primarily to morphine-6-glucuronide (active analgesic) morphine-3-glucuronide (inactive as analgesic); minor metabolites include morphine-3-6-diglucuronide; other minor metabolites include normorphine (active) and morphine 3-ethereal sulfate

Bioavailability: Oral: 17% to 33% (first-pass effect limits oral bioavailability; oral:parenteral effectiveness reportedly varies from 1:6 in opioid-naive patients to 1:3 with chronic use)

Half-life elimination: Adults: Immediate-release forms: 2 to 4 hours; Avinza: ~24 hours; Kadian: 11 to 13 hours

Time to peak, plasma: Avinza: 30 minutes (maintained for 24 hours); Kadian: ~10 hours

Excretion: Urine (primarily as morphine-3-glucuronide, ~2% to 12% excreted unchanged); feces (~7% to 10%). It has been suggested that accumulation of morphine-6-glucuronide might cause toxicity with renal insufficiency. All of the metabolites (ie, morphine-3-glucuronide, morphine-6-glucuronide, and normorphine) have been suggested as possible causes of neurotoxicity (eg, myoclonus).

Dosage These are guidelines and do not represent the doses that may be required in all patients. Doses and dosage intervals should be titrated to pain relief/prevention.

Children >6 months and <50 kg: *Acute pain (moderate to severe):*

Oral (immediate-release formulations): 0.15 to 0.3 mg/kg every 3 to 4 hours as needed. **Note:** The American Pain Society recommends an initial dose of 0.3 mg/kg for children with severe pain (American Pain Society [APS], 2008)

IM, SubQ: 0.1 to 0.2 mg/kg; **Note:** Repeated SubQ administration causes local tissue irritation, pain, and induration. The use of IM injections is no longer recommended especially for repeated administration due to painful administration, variable absorption and lag time to peak effect.

IV: 0.05 to 0.3 mg/kg every 3 to 4 hours as needed, not to exceed 10 mg per dose

Continuous infusion: Initial: 10 to 30 **mcg/kg/hour**; titrate as needed to control pain

Patient-controlled analgesia (PCA) (APS, 2008): **Note:**

Opioid naive: Consider lower end of dosing range:

Usual concentration: 1 mg/mL

Demand dose: Usual: 0.02 mg/kg/dose; range: 0.01 to 0.03 mg/kg/dose

Lockout interval: 8 to 10 minutes

Usual basal rate: 0 to 0.03 mg/kg/hour

Adults:

Acute pain (moderate to severe):

Oral (immediate-release formulations): Opioid naive: Initial: **Note:** Usual dosage range: 10 to 30 mg every 4 hours as needed. Patients with prior opioid exposure may require higher initial doses.

Solution: 10 to 20 mg every 4 hours as needed

Tablet: 15 to 30 mg every 4 hours as needed

IM, SubQ: **Note:** Repeated SubQ administration causes local tissue irritation, pain, and induration. The use of IM injections is no longer recommended especially for repeated administration due to painful administration, variable absorption and lag time to peak effect; other routes are more reliable and less painful (APS, 2008).

Initial: Opioid naive: 5 to 10 mg every 4 hours as needed; usual dosage range: 5 to 15 mg every 4 hours as needed. Patients with prior opioid exposure may require higher initial doses.

IV: Initial: Opioid naive: 2.5 to 5 mg every 3 to 4 hours; patients with prior opioid exposure may require higher initial doses. **Note:** Administration of 2 to 3 mg every 5 minutes until pain relief or if associated sedation, oxygen saturation <95%, or serious adverse event occurs may be appropriate in treating acute moderate to severe pain in settings such as the immediate postoperative period or the emergency department (Aubrun, 2012; Lvovschi, 2008); dose reduction in the immediate postoperative period (postanesthesia care unit) in elderly patients is usually not necessary (Aubrun, 2002). A maximum cumulative dose (eg, 10 mg) prompting reevaluation of continued morphine use and/or dose should be included as part of any medication order intended for short-term use (eg, PACU orders). Refer to institution-specific protocols as appropriate.

Acute myocardial infarction, analgesia (off-label use): Initial management: 4 to 8 mg (lower doses in elderly patients); subsequently may give 2 to 8 mg every 5 to 15 minutes as needed (ACCF/AHA [O'Gara, 2013]).

Critically ill patients, analgesia (off-label dose): 2 to 4 mg every 1 to 2 hours **or** 4 to 8 mg every 3 to 4 hours as needed (Barr, 2013)

IV, SubQ continuous infusion: 0.8 to 10 mg/hour; usual range: Up to 80 mg/hour. **Note:** May administer a loading dose (amount administered should depend on severity of pain) prior to initiating the infusion. A continuous (basal) infusion is not recommended in an opioid-naive patient (ISMP, 2009)

Continuous infusion for critically ill patients: Usual dosage range: 2 to 30 mg/hour (Barr, 2013)

Patient-controlled analgesia (PCA) (APS, 2008): **Note:** In opioid-naive patients, consider lower end of dosing range:

Usual concentration: 1 mg/mL

Demand dose: Usual: 1 mg; range: 0.5 to 2.5 mg

Lockout interval: 5 to 10 minutes

Epidural: Pain management: **Note: Must be preservative free.** Administer with extreme caution and in reduced dosage to geriatric or debilitated patients. Vigilant monitoring is particularly important in these patients.

Single-dose: **Lumbar region:** Astramorph/PF, Duramorph: 30 to 100 mcg/kg (optimal range: 2.5 to 3.75 mg; may depend upon patient comorbidities; Bujedo, 2012; Sultan, 2011)

Continuous infusion (may be combined with bupivacaine): 0.2 to 0.4 mg/hour (Bujedo, 2012)

Continuous microinfusion (Infumorph):

Opioid naive: Initial: 3.5 to 7.5 mg over 24 hours

Opioid tolerant: Initial: 4.5 to 10 mg over 24 hours, titrate to effect; usual maximum is ~30 mg per 24 hours

Intrathecal: **Note: Must be preservative free.** Administer with extreme caution and in reduced dosage to geriatric or debilitated patients. Intrathecal dose is usually 1/10 (one-tenth) that of epidural dosage.

Opioid naive: Single dose: Lumbar region: Astramorph/PF, Duramorph: 0.1 to 0.3 mg (may provide adequate relief for up to 24 hours; APS, 2008); repeat doses are **not** recommended. If pain recurs within 24 hours of administration, use of an alternate route of administration is recommended. **Note:** Although product labeling recommends doses up to 1 mg, an analgesic ceiling exists with doses >0.3 mg and the risk of respiratory depression is higher with doses >0.3 mg (Rathmell, 2005).

Continuous microinfusion (Infumorph): Lumbar region: After initial in-hospital evaluation of response to single-dose injections (Astramorph/PF, Duramorph) the initial dose of Infumorph is 0.2 to 1 mg over 24 hours

Opioid-tolerant: Continuous microinfusion (Infumorph): Lumbar region: Dosage range: 1 to 10 mg over 24 hours, titrate to effect; usual maximum is ~20 mg over 24 hours

Rectal: 10 to 20 mg every 3 to 4 hours

Chronic pain: **Note:** Patients taking opioids chronically may become tolerant and require doses higher than the usual dosage range to maintain the desired effect. Tolerance can be managed by appropriate dose titration. There is no optimal or maximal dose for morphine in chronic pain. The appropriate dose is one that relieves pain throughout its dosing interval without causing unmanageable side effects. Consider total daily dose, potency, prior opioid use, degree of opioid experience and tolerance, conversion from previous opioid (including opioid formulation), patient's general condition, concurrent medications, and type and severity of pain during prescribing process. Opioid tolerance is defined as: Patients already taking at least 60 mg of oral morphine daily, 25 mcg transdermal fentanyl per hour, 30 mg of oral oxycodone daily, 8 mg oral hydromorphone daily, 25 mg of oral oxymorphone daily, or an equivalent dose of another opioid for at least 1 week.

Oral (extended-release formulations): A patient's morphine requirement should be established using immediate-release formulations. Conversion to long-acting products may be considered when chronic, continuous treatment is required. Higher dosages should be reserved for use only in opioid-tolerant patients.

Capsules, extended release (Avinza): Daily dose administered once daily (for best results, administer at same time each day). **Note:** Avinza 90 mg and 120 mg are only indicated for use in opioid-tolerant patents.

Use as the first opioid analgesic or use in patients who are **not** opioid tolerant: Initial: 30 mg once daily

Conversion from other oral morphine formulations to Avinza: Total daily morphine dose given as once daily. The first dose of Avinza may be taken with the last dose of the immediate-release morphine. Maximum: 1600 mg daily due to fumaric acid content.

Conversion from other opioids to Avinza: Discontinue all other around-the-clock opioids when Avinza is initiated. Initial dose: 30 mg once daily; there are no established conversion ratios from other opioids to Avinza. Substantial interpatient variability exists in relative potency. Therefore, it is safer to underestimate a patient's daily oral morphine requirement and provide rescue medication (eg, immediate-release morphine) than to overestimate requirements. The first dose of Avinza may be taken with the last dose of the immediate-release opioids.

Titration and maintenance: Adjust in increments ≤30 mg daily every 3 to 4 days. Maximum: 1600 mg daily due to fumaric acid content.

Discontinuation of Avinza: Gradually titrate dose downward every 2 to 4 days. Do not discontinue abruptly.

Capsules, extended release (Kadian): **Note:** Kadian 100 mg, 130 mg, 150 mg, and 200 mg are only indicated for use in opioid-tolerant patients.

Use as the first opioid analgesic: Has not been evaluated. Use an immediate-release morphine formulation and then convert patients to Kadian in the same fashion as initiating therapy in a non–opioid-tolerant patient.

Use in patients who are **not** opioid tolerant: Initial: 30 mg once daily.

Conversion from other oral morphine formulations to Kadian: Total daily oral morphine dose may be either administered once daily or in 2 divided doses daily (every 12 hours).

Conversion from other opioids to Kadian: Discontinue all other around-the-clock opioids when Kadian is initiated. Initial dose: 30 mg once daily; there are no established conversion ratios from other opioids to Kadian. Substantial interpatient variability exists in relative potency. Therefore, it is safer to underestimate a patient's daily oral morphine requirement and provide rescue medication (eg, immediate-release morphine) than to overestimate requirements.

Titration and maintenance: Dose adjustments may be done every 1 to 2 days.

Discontinuation of Kadian: Gradually titrate dose downward every 2 to 4 days. Do not discontinue abruptly.

Tablets, extended release (MS Contin): Daily dose divided and administered every 8 or every 12 hours. **Note:** MS Contin 100 mg and 200 mg tablets are only indicated for use in opioid-tolerant patients.

Use as the first opioid analgesic: Initial: 15 mg every 8 to 12 hours.

Use in patients who are **not** opioid tolerant: Initial: 15 mg every 12 hours.

Conversion from other oral morphine formulations to MS Contin: Total daily oral morphine dose may be either administered in 2 divided doses daily (every 12 hours) **or** in 3 divided doses (every 8 hours).

Conversion from other opioids to MS Contin: Discontinue all other around-the-clock opioids when MS Contin is initiated. Initial: 15 mg every 8 to 12 hours; there are no established conversion ratios from other opioids to MS Contin. Substantial interpatient variability exists in relative potency. Therefore, it is safer to underestimate a patient's daily oral morphine requirement and provide rescue medication (eg, immediate-release morphine) than to overestimate requirements.

Titration and maintenance: Dose adjustments may be done every 1 to 2 days.

Discontinuation of MS Contin: Gradually titrate dose downward. Do not discontinue abruptly.

Conversion from parenteral morphine or other opioids to extended-release formulations: Substantial interpatient variability exists in relative potency. Therefore, it is safer to underestimate a patient's daily oral morphine requirement and provide breakthrough pain relief with immediate-release morphine than to overestimate requirements. Consider the parenteral to oral morphine ratio or other oral or parenteral opioids to oral morphine conversions.

Parenteral to oral morphine ratio: Between 2 to 6 mg of oral morphine may be required for analgesia equivalent to 1 mg of parenteral morphine. An oral dose 3 times the daily parenteral dose may be sufficient in chronic pain settings.

Other parenteral or oral nonmorphine opioids to oral morphine: Specific recommendations are not available; refer to published relative potency data realizing that such ratios are only approximations. In general, it is safest to administer half of the estimated daily morphine requirement as the initial dose, and to manage inadequate analgesia by supplementation with immediate-release morphine.

Conversion from methadone to extended-release formulations: Close monitoring is required when converting methadone to another opioid. Ratio between methadone and other opioid agonists varies widely according to previous dose exposure. Methadone has a long half-life and can accumulate in the plasma.

Elderly or debilitated patients: Use with caution; may require dose reduction.

Dosing adjustment in renal impairment:

CrCl 10 to 50 mL/minute: Children and Adults: Administer at 75% of normal dose.

CrCl <10 mL/minute: Children and Adults: Administer at 50% of normal dose.

Intermittent HD:

Children: Administer 50% of normal dose.

Adults: No dosage adjustment necessary.

Peritoneal dialysis: Children: Administer 50% of normal dose.

CRRT: Children and Adults: Administer 75% of normal dose, titrate.

Dosing adjustment/comments in hepatic disease: No dosage adjustment provided in manufacturer's labeling. Pharmacokinetics unchanged in mild liver disease; substantial extrahepatic metabolism may occur. In cirrhosis, increases in half-life and AUC suggest dosage adjustment required.

Dietary Considerations Morphine may cause GI upset; take with food if GI upset occurs. Be consistent when taking morphine with or without meals.

Usual Infusion Concentrations: Pediatric IV infusion: 0.1 mg/mL, 0.5 mg/mL, **or** 1 mg/mL

Usual Infusion Concentrations: Adult IV infusion: 1 mg/mL

Administration

Oral: Do not crush, chew, or dissolve extended release drug product; swallow whole. Kadian and Avinza can be opened and sprinkled on applesauce and eaten immediately without chewing; do not crush, dissolve, or chew the beads as it can result in a rapid release of a potentially fatal dose of morphine. Ensure all pellets have been swallowed by rinsing mouth. Contents of Kadian capsules may be opened and sprinkled over 10 mL water and flushed through prewetted 16F gastrostomy tube; do not administer Kadian through gastric/nasogastric tubes.

IV: When giving morphine IV push, it is best to first dilute with sterile water or NS for a final concentration of 1 to 2 mg/mL and then administer slowly over 4 to 5 minutes.

Epidural, intrathecal: Use preservative-free solutions for intrathecal or epidural use. Infumorph may **only** be used as a continuous microinfusion via catheter.

Monitoring Parameters Assess efficacy of pain control, vital signs, and mental status; signs of drug abuse, addiction, or diversion; signs or symptoms of hypogonadism or hypoadrenalism (Brennan, 2013)

Astramorph/PF, Duramorph, Infumorph: Patients should be observed in a fully-equipped and staffed environment for at least 24 hours following initiation, and as appropriate for the first several days after catheter implantation. Naloxone injection should be immediately available. Patient should remain in this environment for at least 24 hours following the initial dose. For patients receiving Infumorph via microinfusion device, patient may be observed, as appropriate, for the first several days after catheter implantation.

Note: Also refer to institution specific protocols as appropriate.

Dosage Forms

Capsule Extended Release 24 Hour, Oral:

AVINza: 30 mg, 45 mg, 60 mg, 75 mg, 90 mg, 120 mg

Kadian: 10 mg, 20 mg, 30 mg, 40 mg, 50 mg, 60 mg, 80 mg, 100 mg, 200 mg

Generic: 10 mg, 20 mg, 30 mg, 45 mg, 50 mg, 60 mg, 75 mg, 80 mg, 90 mg, 100 mg, 120 mg

Device, Intramuscular:

Generic: 10 mg/0.7 mL (0.7 mL)

Solution, Injection:

Generic: 2 mg/mL (1 mL); 4 mg/mL (1 mL); 5 mg/mL (1 mL); 8 mg/mL (1 mL); 10 mg/mL (1 mL, 10 mL); 15 mg/mL (1 mL, 20 mL)

Solution, Injection [preservative free]:

Astramorph: 0.5 mg/mL (2 mL); 1 mg/mL (2 mL)

Duramorph: 0.5 mg/mL (10 mL); 1 mg/mL (10 mL)

Infumorph 200: 200 mg/20 mL (10 mg/mL) (20 mL)

Infumorph 500: 500 mg/20 mL (25 mg/mL) (20 mL)

Generic: 0.5 mg/mL (10 mL); 1 mg/mL (10 mL)

Solution, Intravenous:

Generic: 1 mg/mL (10 mL, 30 mL); 25 mg/mL (4 mL, 10 mL); 50 mg/mL (20 mL, 50 mL)

Solution, Intravenous [preservative free]:

Generic: 1 mg/mL (30 mL); 2 mg/mL (1 mL); 4 mg/mL (1 mL); 150 mg/30 mL (30 mL); 8 mg/mL (1 mL); 10 mg/mL (1 mL); 15 mg/mL (1 mL); 25 mg/mL (10 mL)

Solution, Oral:

Generic: 10 mg/5 mL (5 mL, 15 mL, 100 mL, 500 mL); 20 mg/5 mL (5 mL, 100 mL, 500 mL); 20 mg/mL (15 mL, 30 mL, 120 mL, 240 mL); 100 mg/5 mL (30 mL, 120 mL)

Suppository, Rectal:

Generic: 5 mg (12 ea); 10 mg (12 ea); 20 mg (12 ea); 30 mg (12 ea)

Tablet, Oral:

Generic: 15 mg, 30 mg

Tablet Extended Release, Oral:

MS Contin: 15 mg, 30 mg, 60 mg, 100 mg, 200 mg

Generic: 15 mg, 30 mg, 60 mg, 100 mg, 200 mg

Dosage Forms: Canada

Solution, oral:

Doloral: 1 mg/mL; 5 mg/mL [not available in U.S.]

Morphine (Liposomal) (MOR feen)

Brand Names: U.S. DepoDur

Index Terms Extended Release Epidural Morphine; MS (error-prone abbreviation and should not be used); MSO_4 (error-prone abbreviation and should not be used)

Pharmacologic Category Analgesic, Opioid

Additional Appendix Information

Opioid Conversion Table *on page 2232*

Use Epidural (lumbar) single-dose management of surgical pain

Pregnancy Risk Factor C

Dosage Epidural:

Adults: Surgical anesthesia: Single-dose (extended release, DepoDur®): Lumbar epidural only; not recommended in patients <18 years of age:

Cesarean section: 10 mg (after clamping umbilical cord)

Lower abdominal/pelvic surgery: 10-15 mg

Major orthopedic surgery of lower extremity: 15 mg

To minimize the pharmacokinetic interaction resulting in higher peak serum concentrations of morphine, administer the test dose of the local anesthetic at least 15 minutes prior to administration. Use of DepoDur® with epidural local anesthetics has not been studied. Other medications should not be administered into the epidural space for at least 48 hours after administration.

Note: Some patients may benefit from a 20 mg dose; however, the incidence of adverse effects may be increased.

Elderly or debilitated patients: Use with caution; may require dose reduction

Dosage adjustment in renal impairment: No dosage adjustment necessary.

Dosage adjustment/comments in hepatic disease: No dosage adjustment necessary.

Additional Information Complete prescribing information should be consulted for additional detail.

Dosage Forms

Suspension, Epidural:

DepoDur: 10 mg/mL (1 mL); 15 mg/1.5 mL (1.5 mL)

- **Morphine-EPD (Can)** *see* Morphine (Systemic) *on page 1394*
- **Morphine Extra Forte Injection (Can)** *see* Morphine (Systemic) *on page 1394*
- **Morphine Forte Injection (Can)** *see* Morphine (Systemic) *on page 1394*
- **Morphine HP (Can)** *see* Morphine (Systemic) *on page 1394*

◆ **Morphine LP Epidural (Can)** *see* Morphine (Systemic) *on page 1394*

◆ **Morphine SR (Can)** *see* Morphine (Systemic) *on page 1394*

Morrhuate Sodium (MOR yoo ate SOW dee um)

Brand Names: U.S. Scleromate

Pharmacologic Category Sclerosing Agent

Use Treatment of small, uncomplicated varicose veins of the lower extremities

Pregnancy Risk Factor C

Dosage IV: Adults:

Note: A test dose of 0.25-1 mL of a 5% injection may be given (into a varicosity) 24 hours before full-dose treatment.

Full-dose treatment: 50-250 mg, depending on the size and degree of varicosity (50-100 mg for small or medium veins, 150-250 mg for large veins); may be given as multiple injections at one time or in single doses.

Dosage adjustment in renal impairment: No dosage adjustment provided in manufacturer's labeling.

Dosage adjustment in hepatic impairment: No dosage adjustment provided in manufacturer's labeling.

Additional Information Complete prescribing information should be consulted for additional detail.

Dosage Forms

Solution, Intravenous:

Scleromate: 5% (30 mL)

Generic: 5% (30 mL)

◆ **M.O.S. 10 (Can)** *see* Morphine (Systemic) *on page 1394*

◆ **M.O.S. 20 (Can)** *see* Morphine (Systemic) *on page 1394*

◆ **M.O.S. 30 (Can)** *see* Morphine (Systemic) *on page 1394*

Mosapride [INT] (MOE sa pride)

International Brand Names Alprida (AR); Biotonus (PE); Dosier (DO, EC, GT, HN, MX, NI, SV); Galopran (AR); Gamocid (KR); Gasmotin (CN, JP, PH, TH, VN); Gasprid (UY); Gastride (CO); Gastrokin (AR); Intesul (AR); Kinetix (IN); MIC (IN); Mopride (TW); Mosadil (KR); Mosamet (EC); Mosap (IN); Mosar (AR, KR, LB, UY); Mosaro (KR); Mosasone (KR); Motide (PE, PY); Moxar (CO); Wimotin (KR); Zurma (VN)

Index Terms Mosapride Citrate

Pharmacologic Category Gastrointestinal Agent, Prokinetic

Reported Use Treatment of gastrointestinal symptoms associated with gastritis including heartburn, nausea, and vomiting

Dosage Range Oral:

Adults: 5 mg 3 times/day before or after meals

Dosage adjustment for the elderly: 2.5 mg 3 times/day before or after meals

Product Availability Product available in various countries; not currently available in the U.S.

Dosage Forms

Tablet: 2.5 mg, 5 mg

◆ **Mosapride Citrate** *see* Mosapride [INT] *on page 1401*

◆ **M.O.S.-SR (Can)** *see* Morphine (Systemic) *on page 1394*

◆ **M.O.S.-Sulfate (Can)** *see* Morphine (Systemic) *on page 1394*

◆ **Motion Sickness [OTC]** *see* DimenhyDRINATE *on page 637*

◆ **Motion-Time [OTC]** *see* Meclizine *on page 1277*

◆ **Motrin [OTC]** *see* Ibuprofen *on page 1032*

◆ **Motrin (Can)** *see* Ibuprofen *on page 1032*

◆ **Motrin (Children's) (Can)** *see* Ibuprofen *on page 1032*

◆ **Motrin IB [OTC]** *see* Ibuprofen *on page 1032*

◆ **Motrin IB (Can)** *see* Ibuprofen *on page 1032*

◆ **Motrin Infants Drops [OTC]** *see* Ibuprofen *on page 1032*

◆ **Motrin Junior Strength [OTC]** *see* Ibuprofen *on page 1032*

◆ **Movantik** *see* Naloxegol *on page 1418*

◆ **MoviPrep** *see* Polyethylene Glycol-Electrolyte Solution *on page 1674*

◆ **Moxatag** *see* Amoxicillin *on page 130*

◆ **Moxeza** *see* Moxifloxacin (Ophthalmic) *on page 1403*

Moxifloxacin (Systemic) (moxs i FLOKS a sin)

Brand Names: U.S. Avelox; Avelox ABC Pack

Brand Names: Canada Avelox; Avelox I.V.

Index Terms Moxifloxacin Hydrochloride

Pharmacologic Category Antibiotic, Fluoroquinolone; Antibiotic, Respiratory Fluoroquinolone

Use Treatment of mild-to-moderate community-acquired pneumonia, including multidrug-resistant *Streptococcus pneumoniae* (MDRSP); acute bacterial exacerbation of chronic bronchitis; acute bacterial rhinosinusitis (ABRS); complicated and uncomplicated skin and skin structure infections; complicated intra-abdominal infections

Pregnancy Risk Factor C

Pregnancy Considerations Adverse events have been observed in some animal reproduction studies. Moxifloxacin crosses the placenta and can be detected in the amniotic fluid and cord blood (Ozyüncü and Beksac 2010; Ozyüncü and Nemutlu, 2010). Information specific to moxifloxacin use in pregnant women is limited (Padberg, 2014).

Breast-Feeding Considerations It is not known if moxifloxacin is excreted into breast milk. Due to the potential for serious adverse reactions in the nursing infant, the manufacturer recommends a decision be made whether to discontinue nursing or to discontinue the drug, taking into account the importance of treatment to the mother.

Contraindications Hypersensitivity to moxifloxacin, other quinolone antibiotics, or any component of the formulation

Warnings/Precautions [U.S. Boxed Warning]: There have been reports of tendon inflammation and/or rupture with quinolone antibiotics in all ages; risk may be increased with concurrent corticosteroids, solid organ transplant recipients, and in patients >60 years of age. Rupture of the Achilles tendon sometimes requiring surgical repair has been reported most frequently; but other tendon sites (eg, rotator cuff, biceps) have also been reported. Strenuous physical activity, rheumatoid arthritis, and renal impairment may be an independent risk factor for tendonitis. Inflammation and rupture may occur bilaterally. Cases have been reported within the first 48 hours, during, and up to several months after discontinuation of therapy. Discontinue at first sign of tendon inflammation or pain. Use with caution in patients with rheumatoid arthritis; may increase risk of tendon rupture. Use with caution in patients with a history of tendon disorders.

Use with caution in patients with significant bradycardia or acute myocardial ischemia. Moxifloxacin causes a concentration-dependent QT prolongation. Do not exceed recommended dose or infusion rate. Avoid use with uncorrected hypokalemia, with other drugs that prolong the QT interval or induce bradycardia, or with class Ia or III antiarrhythmic agents. CNS effects may occur (tremor, restlessness, confusion, and very rarely hallucinations, increased intracranial pressure [including pseudotumor cerebri] or seizures). Use with caution in patients with known or suspected CNS disorder. Potential for seizures, although very rare, may be increased with concomitant NSAID therapy. Use with caution in individuals at risk of seizures. Use with caution in patients with mild, moderate, or severe hepatic impairment or liver cirrhosis; may increase the risk of QT prolongation. Fulminant hepatitis potentially leading to liver failure (including fatalities) has been reported with use. Use with caution in diabetes; glucose regulation may be altered.

Fluoroquinolones have been associated with the development of serious, and sometimes fatal, hypoglycemia, most often in elderly diabetics, but also in patients without diabetes. This occurred most frequently with gatifloxacin (no longer available systemically) but may occur at a lower frequency with other quinolones.

Severe hypersensitivity reactions, including anaphylaxis, have occurred with quinolone therapy. Reactions may present as typical allergic symptoms after a single dose, or may manifest as severe idiosyncratic dermatologic, vascular, pulmonary, renal, hepatic, and/or hematologic events, usually after multiple doses. Prompt discontinuation of drug should occur if skin rash or other symptoms arise. Avoid excessive sunlight and take precautions to limit exposure (eg, loose fitting clothing, sunscreen); may cause moderate-to-severe phototoxicity reactions. Discontinue use if photosensitivity occurs. Prolonged use may result in fungal or bacterial superinfection, including *C. difficile*-associated diarrhea (CDAD) and pseudomembranous colitis; CDAD has been observed >2 months post-antibiotic treatment.

[U.S. Boxed Warning]: Quinolones may exacerbate myasthenia gravis; avoid use (rare, potentially life-threatening weakness of respiratory muscles may occur). Peripheral neuropathy has been reported (rare); may occur soon after initiation of therapy and may be irreversible; discontinue if symptoms of sensory or sensorimotor neuropathy occur. Hemolytic reactions may (rarely) occur with quinolone use in patients with latent or actual G6PD deficiency. Adverse effects (eg, tendon rupture, QT changes) may be increased in the elderly. Some quinolones may exacerbate myasthenia gravis, use with caution (rare, potentially life-threatening weakness of respiratory muscles may occur). Safety and efficacy of systemically administered moxifloxacin (oral, intravenous) in patients <18 years of age have not been established.

Adverse Reactions

Cardiovascular: Angina pectoris, atrial fibrillation, bradycardia, cardiac arrest, cardiac failure, chest discomfort, chest pain, edema, hypertension, hypotension, increased blood pressure, palpitations, peripheral edema, phlebitis, prolonged Q-T interval on ECG, syncope, tachycardia

Central nervous system: Agitation, anxiety, chills, confusion, depression, disorientation, dizziness, drowsiness, facial pain, fatigue, hallucination, headache, hypoesthesia, insomnia, lethargy, malaise, nervousness, noncardiac chest pain, pain, paresthesia, restlessness, vertigo

Dermatologic: Allergic dermatitis, erythema, hyperhidrosis, night sweats, pruritus, skin rash, urticaria

Endocrine & metabolic: Decreased serum glucose, dehydration, hyperchloremia, hyperglycemia, hyperlipidemia, hypokalemia, increased gamma-glutamyl transferase, increased lactate dehydrogenase, increased serum albumin, increased serum glucose, increased serum triglycerides, increased uric acid

Gastrointestinal: Abdominal discomfort, abdominal distension, abdominal pain, anorexia, constipation, decreased amylase, decreased appetite, diarrhea, dysgeusia, dyspepsia, flatulence, gastritis, gastroenteritis, gastroesophageal reflux disease, increased amylase, increased serum lipase, nausea, oral candidiasis, vomiting, xerostomia

Genitourinary: Dysuria, fungal vaginosis, vaginal infection, vulvovaginal candidiasis, vulvovaginal pruritus

Hematologic & oncologic: Anemia, decreased basophils, decreased hematocrit, decreased hemoglobin, decreased neutrophils, decreased prothrombin time, decreased red blood cells, eosinopenia, eosinophilia, increased MCH, increased neutrophils, leukocytosis, leukopenia, prolonged partial thromboplastin time, prolonged prothrombin time, thrombocythemia, thrombocytopenia

Hepatic: Abnormal hepatic function tests, decreased serum bilirubin, increased liver enzymes, increased serum alkaline phosphatase, increased serum ALT, increased serum AST, increased serum bilirubin, increased serum transaminases

Hypersensitivity: Hypersensitivity reaction

Immunologic: Increased serum globulins

Infection: Candidiasis, fungal infection (including oral)

Local: Extravasation

Neuromuscular & skeletal: Arthralgia, back pain, limb pain, muscle spasms, musculoskeletal pain, myalgia, tremor, weakness

Ophthalmic: Blurred vision

Otic: Tinnitus

Renal: Increased blood urea nitrogen, increased ionized serum calcium, increased serum creatinine, renal failure

Respiratory: Asthma, bronchospasm, dyspnea, hypoxia, wheezing

Miscellaneous: Fever

Rare but important or life-threatening: Agranulocytosis, anaphylactic shock, anaphylaxis, aplastic anemia, ataxia, auditory impairment, cholestatic jaundice, *Clostridium difficile* associated diarrhea, deafness (reversible), decreased INR, ECG abnormality, exacerbation of myasthenia gravis, hemolytic anemia, hepatic failure, hepatic necrosis, hepatitis (predominantly cholestatic), hepatotoxicity (idiosyncratic) (Chalasani 2014), hypoglycemia, increased intracranial pressure, interstitial nephritis, jaundice, pancytopenia, peripheral neuropathy (may be irreversible), phototoxicity, pneumonitis (allergic), polyneuropathy, pseudomembranous colitis, pseudotumor cerebri, psychotic reaction, renal insufficiency, rupture of tendon, seizure, skin photosensitivity, Stevens-Johnson syndrome, suicidal ideation, suicidal tendencies, tendonitis, thrombotic thrombocytopenic purpura, toxic epidermal necrolysis, ventricular tachyarrhythmias (including torsade de pointes and cardiac arrest [usually in patients with concurrent, severe proarrhythmic conditions]), vasculitis, vision loss (transient)

Drug Interactions

Metabolism/Transport Effects None known.

Avoid Concomitant Use

Avoid concomitant use of Moxifloxacin (Systemic) with any of the following: BCG; Highest Risk QTc-Prolonging Agents; Ivabradine; Mifepristone; Strontium Ranelate

Increased Effect/Toxicity

Moxifloxacin (Systemic) may increase the levels/effects of: Highest Risk QTc-Prolonging Agents; Moderate Risk QTc-Prolonging Agents; Porfimer; Sulfonylureas; Varenicline; Verteporfin; Vitamin K Antagonists

The levels/effects of Moxifloxacin (Systemic) may be increased by: Corticosteroids (Systemic); Insulin; Ivabradine; Mifepristone; Nonsteroidal Anti-Inflammatory Agents; Probenecid; QTc-Prolonging Agents (Indeterminate Risk and Risk Modifying)

Decreased Effect

Moxifloxacin (Systemic) may decrease the levels/effects of: BCG; Didanosine; Mycophenolate; Sodium Picosulfate; Sulfonylureas; Typhoid Vaccine

The levels/effects of Moxifloxacin (Systemic) may be decreased by: Antacids; Didanosine; Iron Salts; Lanthanum; Magnesium Salts; Multivitamins/Minerals (with ADEK, Folate, Iron); Multivitamins/Minerals (with AE, No Iron); Quinapril; Sevelamer; Strontium Ranelate; Sucralfate; Zinc Salts

Food Interactions Absorption is not affected by administration with a high-fat meal or yogurt.

Storage/Stability Store at controlled room temperature of 25°C (77°F). Do not refrigerate infusion solution.

Mechanism of Action Moxifloxacin is a DNA gyrase inhibitor, and also inhibits topoisomerase IV. DNA gyrase (topoisomerase II) is an essential bacterial enzyme that maintains the superhelical structure of DNA. DNA gyrase is required for DNA replication and transcription, DNA repair, recombination, and transposition; inhibition is bactericidal.

Pharmacodynamics/Kinetics

Absorption: Well absorbed; not affected by high-fat meal or yogurt

Distribution: V_d: 1.7 to 2.7 L/kg; tissue concentrations often exceed plasma concentrations in respiratory tissues, alveolar macrophages, abdominal tissues/fluids, uterine tissue (endometrium, myometrium), and sinus tissues

Protein binding: ~30% to 50%

Metabolism: Hepatic (~52% of dose) via glucuronide (~14%) and sulfate (~38%) conjugation

Bioavailability: ~90%

Half-life elimination: Single dose: Oral: 12-16 hours; IV: 8-15 hours

Excretion: Urine (as unchanged drug [20%] and glucuronide conjugates); feces (as unchanged drug [25%] and sulfate conjugates)

Dosage

Children ≥1 year (off-label use): **Surgical (perioperative) prophylaxis (off-label use):** IV: 10 mg/kg within 120 minutes prior to surgical incision (maximum dose: 400 mg) (Bratzler, 2013).

Adolescents (off-label use): **Community-acquired pneumonia (CAP) due to atypical pathogens (*M. pneumoniae, C. trachomatis, or C. pneumoniae*), mild infection or step-down therapy in adolescents with skeletal maturity, (alternative to azithromycin) (IDSA/PIDS, 2011):** Oral: 400 mg once daily

Adults: Oral, IV: Usual dosage range: 400 mg every 24 hours

Indication-specific dosing:

Acute bacterial rhinosinusitis: 400 mg every 24 hours for 10 days or 5-7 days (Chow, 2012). **Note:** Recommended in patients with beta-lactam allergy; may also be used if initial therapy fails, in areas with high endemic rates of penicillin nonsusceptible *S. pneumoniae*, those with severe infections, age >65 years, recent hospitalization, antibiotic use within the past month, or who are immunocompromised.

Chronic bronchitis, acute bacterial exacerbation: 400 mg every 24 hours for 5 days

Community-acquired pneumonia (CAP) (including MDRSP): 400 mg every 24 hours for 7-14 days

Intra-abdominal infections, complicated: 400 mg every 24 hours for 5-14 days (initiate with IV); **Note:** 2010 IDSA guidelines recommend a treatment duration of 4-7 days (provided source controlled) for community-acquired, mild-to-moderate IAI

***M. genitalium* infections** (including confirmed cases or clinically significant persistent cervicitis, pelvic inflammatory disease or urethritis in patients who previously received azithromycin or doxycycline; off-label use): Oral, IV: 400 mg every 24 hours for 7-10 days (Manhart, 2011)

Skin and skin structure infections:

Complicated: 400 mg every 24 hours for 7-21 days

Uncomplicated: 400 mg every 24 hours for 7 days

Surgical (perioperative) prophylaxis (off-label use): IV: 400 mg within 120 minutes prior to surgical incision (Bratzler, 2013).

Tuberculosis, drug-resistant tuberculosis, or intolerance to first-line agents (off-label use): Oral: 400 mg every 24 hours (*MMWR*, 2003)

Elderly: No dosage adjustments are required based on age

Dosage adjustment in renal impairment: No dosage adjustment required in renal impairment.

Poorly dialyzed; no supplemental dose or dosage adjustment necessary, including patients on intermittent hemodialysis, peritoneal dialysis, or continuous renal replacement therapy (eg, CVVHD).

Dosage adjustment in hepatic impairment: No dosage adjustment is required in mild, moderate, or severe hepatic insufficiency (Child-Pugh class A, B, or C); however, use with caution in this patient population secondary to the risk of QT prolongation.

Dietary Considerations May be taken without regard to meals. Take 4 hours before or 8 hours after multiple vitamins, antacids, or other products containing magnesium, aluminum, iron, or zinc.

Avelox IV infusion (premixed in sodium chloride 0.8%) contains sodium 34.2 mEq (~787 mg)/250 mL.

Administration Administer without regard to meals.

IV: Infuse over 60 minutes; do not infuse by rapid or bolus intravenous infusion

Monitoring Parameters WBC, signs of infection, signs/symptoms of disordered glucose regulation, blood glucose in diabetic patients

Dosage Forms

Solution, Intravenous [preservative free]:

Avelox: 400 mg/250 mL (250 mL)

Tablet, Oral:

Avelox: 400 mg

Avelox ABC Pack: 400 mg

Generic: 400 mg

Extemporaneous Preparations A 20 mg/mL oral suspension may be made using tablets. Crush three 400 mg tablets and reduce to a fine powder. Carefully sieve powder from enteric-coating remnants to improve pharmaceutical elegance. Add a small amount of a 1:1 mixture of Ora-Plus® and Ora-Sweet® or Ora-Sweet® SF and mix to a uniform paste; mix while adding the vehicle in geometric proportions to **almost** 60 mL; transfer to a calibrated bottle, rinse mortar with vehicle, and add quantity of vehicle sufficient to make 60 mL. Label "shake well". Stable 90 days at room temperature.

Hutchinson DJ, Johnson CE, and Klein KC, "Stability of Extemporaneously Prepared Moxifloxacin Oral Suspensions," *Am J Health Syst Pharm*, 2009, 66(7):665-7.

Moxifloxacin (Ophthalmic) (moxs i FLOKS a sin)

Brand Names: U.S. Moxeza; Vigamox

Brand Names: Canada Vigamox

Index Terms Moxifloxacin Hydrochloride

Pharmacologic Category Antibiotic, Fluoroquinolone; Antibiotic, Ophthalmic

Use Bacterial conjunctivitis: Treatment of bacterial conjunctivitis caused by susceptible organisms: *Acinetobacter lwoffii, Aerococcus viridams, Corynebacterium spp, Enterococcus faecalis, Micrococcus luteus, Staphylococcus arlettae, S. aureus, S. capitis, S. epidermidis, S. haemolyticus, S. hominis, S. saprophyticus, S. warneri, Streptococcus viridans spp., S. pneumoniae, Escherichia coli, Haemophilus influenzae, H. parainfluenzae, Klebsiella pneumoniae, Propionibacterium acnes, Chlamydia trachomatis*

Pregnancy Risk Factor C

Dosage Ophthalmic: Bacterial conjunctivitis:
Children ≥4 months, Adolescents, and Adults (Moxeza): Instill 1 drop into affected eye(s) 2 times daily for 7 days
Children ≥1 year, Adolescents, and Adults (Vigamox): Instill 1 drop into affected eye(s) 3 times daily for 7 days

Dosage adjustment in renal impairment: There are no dosage adjustments provided in the manufacturer's labeling. However, dosage adjustment unlikely due to low systemic absorption.

Dosage adjustment in hepatic impairment: There are no dosage adjustments provided in the manufacturer's labeling. However, dosage adjustment unlikely due to low systemic absorption.

Additional Information Complete prescribing information should be consulted for additional detail.

Dosage Forms

Solution, Ophthalmic:
Moxeza: 0.5% (3 mL)
Vigamox: 0.5% (3 mL)

- ◆ **Moxifloxacin Hydrochloride** *see* Moxifloxacin (Ophthalmic) *on page 1403*
- ◆ **Moxifloxacin Hydrochloride** *see* Moxifloxacin (Systemic) *on page 1401*
- ◆ **Mozobil** *see* Plerixafor *on page 1665*
- ◆ **4-MP** *see* Fomepizole *on page 922*
- ◆ **MP-424** *see* Telaprevir *on page 1983*
- ◆ **MPA** *see* MedroxyPROGESTERone *on page 1277*
- ◆ **MPA** *see* Mycophenolate *on page 1405*
- ◆ **6-MP (error-prone abbreviation)** *see* Mercaptopurine *on page 1296*
- ◆ **MPSV** *see* Meningococcal Polysaccharide Vaccine (Groups A / C / Y and W-135) *on page 1292*
- ◆ **MPSV4** *see* Meningococcal Polysaccharide Vaccine (Groups A / C / Y and W-135) *on page 1292*
- ◆ **MRA** *see* Tocilizumab *on page 2057*
- ◆ **MS Contin** *see* Morphine (Systemic) *on page 1394*
- ◆ **MS Contin SRT (Can)** *see* Morphine (Systemic) *on page 1394*
- ◆ **MS (error-prone abbreviation and should not be used)** *see* Morphine (Liposomal) *on page 1400*
- ◆ **MS (error-prone abbreviation and should not be used)** *see* Morphine (Systemic) *on page 1394*
- ◆ **MS-IR (Can)** *see* Morphine (Systemic) *on page 1394*
- ◆ **MSO_4 (error-prone abbreviation and should not be used)** *see* Morphine (Liposomal) *on page 1400*
- ◆ **MSO_4 (error-prone abbreviation and should not be used)** *see* Morphine (Systemic) *on page 1394*
- ◆ **MST 600** *see* Magnesium Salicylate *on page 1265*
- ◆ **MT103** *see* Blinatumomab *on page 271*
- ◆ **MTC** *see* MitoMYcin (Systemic) *on page 1380*
- ◆ **MTX (error-prone abbreviation)** *see* Methotrexate *on page 1322*
- ◆ **MucaphEd [OTC]** *see* Guaifenesin and Phenylephrine *on page 988*
- ◆ **Mucinex [OTC]** *see* GuaiFENesin *on page 986*
- ◆ **Mucinex® D [OTC]** *see* Guaifenesin and Pseudoephedrine *on page 989*
- ◆ **Mucinex® D Maximum Strength [OTC]** *see* Guaifenesin and Pseudoephedrine *on page 989*
- ◆ **Mucinex Allergy [OTC]** *see* Fexofenadine *on page 873*
- ◆ **Mucinex Chest Congestion Child [OTC]** *see* GuaiFENesin *on page 986*
- ◆ **Mucinex® Cold [OTC]** *see* Guaifenesin and Phenylephrine *on page 988*
- ◆ **Mucinex DM [OTC]** *see* Guaifenesin and Dextromethorphan *on page 987*
- ◆ **Mucinex DM Maximum Strength [OTC]** *see* Guaifenesin and Dextromethorphan *on page 987*
- ◆ **Mucinex Fast-Max DM Max [OTC]** *see* Guaifenesin and Dextromethorphan *on page 987*
- ◆ **Mucinex For Kids [OTC]** *see* GuaiFENesin *on page 986*
- ◆ **Mucinex Kid's Cough [OTC]** *see* Guaifenesin and Dextromethorphan *on page 987*
- ◆ **Mucinex Kid's Cough Mini-Melts [OTC]** *see* Guaifenesin and Dextromethorphan *on page 987*
- ◆ **Mucinex Maximum Strength [OTC]** *see* GuaiFENesin *on page 986*
- ◆ **Mucomyst** *see* Acetylcysteine *on page 40*
- ◆ **Mucomyst® (Can)** *see* Acetylcysteine *on page 40*
- ◆ **Mucosa [OTC]** *see* GuaiFENesin *on page 986*
- ◆ **Mucus-ER [OTC]** *see* GuaiFENesin *on page 986*
- ◆ **Mucus Relief [OTC]** *see* GuaiFENesin *on page 986*
- ◆ **Mucus Relief Childrens [OTC]** *see* GuaiFENesin *on page 986*
- ◆ **Mucus Relief Sinus [OTC]** *see* Guaifenesin and Phenylephrine *on page 988*
- ◆ **Multaq** *see* Dronedarone *on page 695*
- ◆ **Multi-Subtype Alpha-Interferon** *see* Interferon Alpha, Multi-Subtype [INT] *on page 1100*
- ◆ **Mumps, Measles and Rubella Vaccines** *see* Measles, Mumps, and Rubella Virus Vaccine *on page 1273*
- ◆ **Mumps, Rubella, Varicella, and Measles Vaccine** *see* Measles, Mumps, Rubella, and Varicella Virus Vaccine *on page 1274*

Mupirocin (myoo PEER oh sin)

Brand Names: U.S. Bactroban; Bactroban Nasal; Centany; Centany AT

Brand Names: Canada Bactroban

Index Terms Mupirocin Calcium; Pseudomonic Acid A

Pharmacologic Category Antibiotic, Topical

Use Topical infection:

Intranasal: Eradication of nasal colonization with methicillin-resistant *S. aureus* (MRSA) in adult patients and healthcare workers during institutional outbreaks of infections with this pathogen

Topical cream: Treatment of secondary infected traumatic skin lesions (up to 10 cm in length or 100 cm^2 in area) due to susceptible strains of *S. aureus* and *S. pyogenes*

Topical ointment: Treatment of impetigo due to *S. aureus* and *S. pyogenes*

Pregnancy Risk Factor B

Dosage

Intranasal: Children ≥12 years, Adolescents, and Adults: Eradication of nasal MRSA: Approximately one-half of the ointment from the single-use tube should be applied into one nostril and the other half into the other nostril twice daily for 5 days

Topical:
Infants ≥2 months, Children, Adolescents, and Adults: Impetigo: Ointment: Apply to affected area 3 times daily; re-evaluate after 3 to 5 days if no clinical response
Infants ≥3 months, Children, Adolescents, and Adults: Secondary skin infections: Cream: Apply to affected area 3 times daily for 10 days; re-evaluate after 3 to 5 days if no clinical response

Surgical prophylaxis in methicillin-resistant *S. aureus* (MRSA) carriers (off-label use): Intranasal: Approximately one-half of the ointment from the single-use tube should be applied into 1 nostril and the other half into the other nostril twice daily for 5 days (Bode, 2010; Lee, 2013)

Dosage adjustment in renal impairment: There are no dosage adjustments provided in the manufacturer's labeling (has not been studied).

Dosage adjustment in hepatic impairment: There are no dosage adjustments provided in the manufacturer's labeling.

Additional Information Complete prescribing information should be consulted for additional detail.

Dosage Forms

Cream, External:
Bactroban: 2% (15 g, 30 g)
Generic: 2% (15 g, 30 g)

Kit, External:
Centany AT: 2%

Ointment, External:
Bactroban: 2% (22 g)
Centany: 2% (30 g)
Generic: 2% (22 g)

Ointment, Nasal:
Bactroban Nasal: 2% (1 g)

- ◆ **Mupirocin Calcium** *see* Mupirocin *on page 1404*
- ◆ **Muro 128 [OTC]** *see* Sodium Chloride *on page 1902*
- ◆ **Muse** *see* Alprostadil *on page 96*
- ◆ **Muse Pellet (Can)** *see* Alprostadil *on page 96*
- ◆ **Mustargen** *see* Mechlorethamine (Systemic) *on page 1276*
- ◆ **Mustine** *see* Mechlorethamine (Systemic) *on page 1276*
- ◆ **Mutamycin** *see* MitoMYcin (Systemic) *on page 1380*
- ◆ **Mutamycin® (Can)** *see* MitoMYcin (Systemic) *on page 1380*
- ◆ **Mya (Can)** *see* Ethinyl Estradiol and Drospirenone *on page 801*
- ◆ **Myalept** *see* Metreleptin *on page 1353*
- ◆ **Myambutol** *see* Ethambutol *on page 798*
- ◆ **Mycamine** *see* Micafungin *on page 1359*
- ◆ **Mycelex** *see* Clotrimazole (Oral) *on page 488*
- ◆ **Mycobutin** *see* Rifabutin *on page 1803*
- ◆ **Mycocide CX Callus Exfoliator [OTC]** *see* Urea *on page 2114*
- ◆ **Mycocide Clinical NS [OTC]** *see* Tolnaftate *on page 2063*

Mycophenolate (mye koe FEN oh late)

Brand Names: U.S. CellCept; CellCept Intravenous; Myfortic

Brand Names: Canada Ach-Mycophenolate; Apo-Mycophenolate; CellCept; CellCept I.V.; CO Mycophenolate; JAMP-Mycophenolate; Myfortic; Mylan-Mycophenolate; Novo-Mycophenolate; Sandoz-Mycophenolate Mofetil

Index Terms MMF; MPA; Mycophenolate Mofetil; Mycophenolate Sodium; Mycophenolic Acid

Pharmacologic Category Immunosuppressant Agent

Use Prophylaxis of organ rejection concomitantly with cyclosporine and corticosteroids in patients receiving allogeneic renal (CellCept, Myfortic), cardiac (CellCept), or hepatic (CellCept) transplants

Pregnancy Risk Factor D

Pregnancy Considerations **[U.S. Boxed Warning]: Mycophenolate is associated with an increased risk of congenital malformations and first trimester pregnancy loss when used by pregnant women. Females of reproductive potential must be counseled about pregnancy prevention and planning.** Alternative agents should be considered for women planning a pregnancy. Adverse events have been reported in animal reproduction studies. In humans, the following congenital malformations have been reported: external ear abnormalities, cleft lip and palate, anomalies of the distal limbs, heart, esophagus and kidney. Spontaneous abortions have also been noted. Females of reproductive potential (girls who have entered puberty, women with a uterus who have not passed through clinically confirmed menopause) should have a negative pregnancy test with a sensitivity of ≥25 mIU/mL immediately before therapy and the test should be repeated 8-10 days later. Pregnancy tests should be repeated during routine follow-up visits. Acceptable forms of contraception should be used during treatment and for 6 weeks after therapy is discontinued. The effectiveness of hormonal contraceptive agents may be affected by mycophenolate. For women with lupus nephritis taking mycophenolate and who are planning a pregnancy, mycophenolate should be discontinued at least 6 weeks prior to trying to conceive (Hahn, 2012).

Healthcare providers should report female exposures to mycophenolate during pregnancy or within 6 weeks of discontinuing therapy to the Mycophenolate Pregnancy Registry (800-617-8191). The National Transplantation Pregnancy Registry (NTPR, Temple University) is a registry for pregnant women taking immunosuppressants following any solid organ transplant. The NTPR encourages reporting of all immunosuppressant exposures during pregnancy in transplant recipients at 877-955-6877.

Breast-Feeding Considerations It is unknown if mycophenolate is excreted in human milk. Due to potentially serious adverse reactions, the decision to discontinue the drug or discontinue breast-feeding should be considered. Breast-feeding is not recommended during therapy or for 6 weeks after treatment is complete.

Contraindications Hypersensitivity to mycophenolate mofetil, mycophenolic acid, mycophenolate sodium, or any component of the formulation
Cellcept: Intravenous formulation is also contraindicated in patients who are allergic to polysorbate 80

Warnings/Precautions Hazardous agent - use appropriate precautions for handling and disposal (NIOSH 2014 [group 2]).

[U.S. Boxed Warning]: Risk for bacterial, viral, fungal, and protozoal infections, including opportunistic infections, is increased with immunosuppressant therapy; infections may be serious and potentially fatal. Due to the risk of oversuppression of the immune system, which may increase susceptibility to infection, combination immunosuppressant therapy should be used with caution. Polyomavirus associated nephropathy (PVAN), JC virus-associated progressive multifocal leukoencephalopathy (PML), cytomegalovirus (CMV) infections, reactivation of hepatitis B (HBV) or hepatitis C (HCV), have been reported with use. A reduction in immunosuppression should be considered for patients with new or reactivated viral infections; however, in transplant recipients, the risk that reduced immunosuppression presents to the functioning graft should also be considered. PVAN, primarily from activation of BK virus, may lead to the deterioration of renal function and/or renal graft loss. PML, a potentially fatal condition, commonly presents with hemiparesis, apathy, ataxia, cognitive deficiencies, confusion, and hemiparesis. Risk factors for development of PML include treatment with immunosuppressants and immune function impairment; consultation with a neurologist should be considered in any patient with neurological symptoms receiving immunosuppressants. Risk of CMV viremia or disease is increased in transplant recipients CMV ▶

seronegative at the time of transplant who receive a graft from a CMV seropositive donor. In patients infected with HBV or HCV, viral reactivation may occur; these patients should be monitored for signs of active HBV or HCV. **[U.S. Boxed Warning]: Risk of development of lymphoma and skin malignancy is increased.** The risk for malignancies is related to intensity/duration of therapy. Patients should be monitored appropriately, instructed to limit exposure to sunlight/UV light to decrease the risk of skin cancer, and given supportive treatment should these conditions occur. Post-transplant lymphoproliferative disorder related to EBV infection has been reported in immunosuppressed organ transplant patients; risk is highest in EBV seronegative patients (including many young children). Neutropenia (including severe neutropenia) may occur, requiring dose reduction or interruption of treatment (risk greater from day 31-180 post-transplant). Use may rarely be associated with gastric or duodenal ulcers, GI bleeding and/or perforation. Use caution in patients with active serious digestive system disease; patients with active peptic ulcers were not included in clinical studies. Use caution in renal impairment as toxicity may be increased; may require dosage adjustment in severe impairment.

[U.S. Boxed Warning]: Mycophenolate is associated with an increased risk of congenital malformations and first trimester pregnancy loss when used by pregnant women. Females of reproductive potential must be counseled about pregnancy prevention and planning. Alternative agents should be considered for women planning a pregnancy. Females of reproductive potential should have a negative pregnancy test with a sensitivity of ≥25 mIU/mL immediately before therapy and the test should be repeated 8-10 days later. Pregnancy tests should be repeated during routine follow-up visits. Acceptable forms of contraception should be used during treatment and for 6 weeks after therapy is discontinued. Females of childbearing potential should have a negative pregnancy test within 1 week prior to beginning therapy. Two reliable forms of contraception should be used beginning 4 weeks prior to, during, and for 6 weeks after therapy. Because mycophenolate mofetil has demonstrated teratogenic effects in rats and rabbits, tablets should not be crushed, and capsules should not be opened or crushed. Avoid inhalation or direct contact with skin or mucous membranes of the powder contained in the capsules and the powder for oral suspension. Caution should be exercised in the handling and preparation of solutions of intravenous mycophenolate. Avoid skin contact with the intravenous solution and reconstituted suspension. If such contact occurs, wash thoroughly with soap and water, rinse eyes with plain water.

Theoretically, use should be avoided in patients with the rare hereditary deficiency of hypoxanthine-guanine phosphoribosyltransferase (such as Lesch-Nyhan or Kelley-Seegmiller syndrome). Intravenous solutions should be given over at least 2 hours; never administer intravenous solution by rapid or bolus injection. Live attenuated vaccines should be avoided during use; vaccinations may be less effective during therapy. **[U.S. Boxed Warning]: Should be administered under the supervision of a physician experienced in immunosuppressive therapy.**

Note: CellCept and Myfortic dosage forms should not be used interchangeably due to differences in absorption. Some dosage forms may contain phenylalanine. Some dosage forms may contain polysorbate 80 (also known as Tweens). Hypersensitivity reactions, usually a delayed reaction, have been reported following exposure to pharmaceutical products containing polysorbate 80 in certain individuals (Isaksson, 2002; Lucente 2000; Shelley, 1995). Thrombocytopenia, ascites, pulmonary deterioration, and renal and hepatic failure have been reported in premature neonates after receiving parenteral products containing polysorbate 80 (Alade, 1986; CDC, 1984). See manufacturer's labeling.

Adverse Reactions Note: In general, lower doses used in renal rejection patients had less adverse effects than higher doses. Rates of adverse effects were similar for each indication, except for those unique to the specific organ involved. The type of adverse effects observed in pediatric patients was similar to those seen in adults, with the exception of abdominal pain, anemia, diarrhea, fever, hypertension, infection, pharyngitis, respiratory tract infection, sepsis, and vomiting; lymphoproliferative disorder was the only type of malignancy observed.

As reported in adults following oral dosing of CellCept alone in renal, cardiac, and hepatic allograft rejection studies:

Cardiovascular: Chest pain, edema, hyper-/hypotension, peripheral edema, tachycardia

Central nervous system: Anxiety, dizziness, fever, headache, insomnia, pain

Dermatologic: Rash

Endocrine & metabolic: Hypercholesterolemia, hyperglycemia, hypocalcemia, hyper-/hypokalemia, hypomagnesemia

Gastrointestinal: Abdominal pain, anorexia, constipation, diarrhea, dyspepsia, nausea, vomiting

Genitourinary: Urinary tract infection

Hematologic: Anemia (including hypochromic), leukocytosis, leukopenia, thrombocytopenia

Hepatic: Ascites, liver function tests abnormal

Neuromuscular & skeletal: Back pain, paresthesia, tremor, weakness

Renal: BUN increased, creatinine increased, kidney function abnormal

Respiratory: Cough, dyspnea, lung disorder, pleural effusion, respiratory tract infection, sinusitis

Miscellaneous: *Candida*, herpes simplex, lactate dehydrogenase increased, sepsis

Use in combination with cyclosporine and corticosteroids:

Cardiovascular: Angina, arrhythmia, arterial thrombosis, atrial fibrillation, atrial flutter, bradycardia, cardiac arrest, cardiac failure, CHF, extrasystole, facial edema, hyper-/hypovolemia, orthostatic hypotension, pallor, palpitation, pericardial effusion, peripheral vascular disorder, supraventricular extrasystoles, supraventricular tachycardia, syncope, thrombosis, vasodilation, vasospasm, venous pressure increased, ventricular extrasystole, ventricular tachycardia

Central nervous system: Agitation, chills with fever, confusion, delirium, depression, emotional lability, hallucinations, hypoesthesia, malaise, nervousness, psychosis, seizure, somnolence, thinking abnormal, vertigo

Dermatologic: Acne, alopecia, bruising, cellulitis, fungal dermatitis, hirsutism, petechia, pruritus, skin carcinoma, skin hypertrophy, skin ulcer, vesiculobullous rash

Endocrine & metabolic: Acidosis, alkalosis, Cushing's syndrome, dehydration, diabetes mellitus, gout, hypercalcemia, hyper-hypophosphatemia, hyperlipemia, hyperuricemia, hypochloremia, hypoglycemia, hyponatremia, hypoproteinemia, hypothyroidism, parathyroid disorder

Gastrointestinal: Abdomen enlarged, dysphagia, esophagitis, flatulence, gastritis, gastroenteritis, gastrointestinal hemorrhage, gastrointestinal moniliasis, gingivitis, gum hyperplasia, ileus, melena, mouth ulceration, oral moniliasis, stomach disorder, stomach ulcer, stomatitis, xerostomia, weight gain/loss

Genitourinary: Impotence, nocturia, pelvic pain, prostatic disorder, scrotal edema, urinary frequency, urinary incontinence, urinary retention, urinary tract disorder

Hematologic: Coagulation disorder, hemorrhage, neutropenia, pancytopenia, polycythemia, prothrombin time increased, thromboplastin time increased

Hepatic: Alkaline phosphatase increased, bilirubinemia, cholangitis, cholestatic jaundice, GGT increased, hepatitis, jaundice, liver damage, transaminases increased

Local: Abscess

Neuromuscular & skeletal: Arthralgia, hypertonia, joint disorder, leg cramps, myalgia, myasthenia, neck pain, neuropathy, osteoporosis

Ocular: Amblyopia, cataract, conjunctivitis, eye hemorrhage, lacrimation disorder, vision abnormal

Otic: Deafness, ear disorder, ear pain, tinnitus

Renal: Albuminuria, creatinine increased, dysuria, hematuria, hydronephrosis, oliguria, pyelonephritis, renal failure, renal tubular necrosis

Respiratory: Apnea, asthma, atelectasis, bronchitis, epistaxis, hemoptysis, hiccup, hyperventilation, hypoxia, respiratory acidosis, pharyngitis, pneumonia, pneumothorax, pulmonary edema, pulmonary hypertension, respiratory moniliasis, rhinitis, sputum increased, voice alteration

Miscellaneous: *Candida* (mucocutaneous), CMV tissue invasive disease, CMV viremia/syndrome, herpes zoster cutaneous disease, cyst, diaphoresis, flu-like syndrome, healing abnormal, hernia, ileus infection, neoplasm, peritonitis, thirst

Rare but important or life-threatening: Atypical mycobacterial infection, BK virus-associated nephropathy, colitis, gastrointestinal perforation, infectious endocarditis, interstitial lung disorder, intestinal villous atrophy, lymphoma, lymphoproliferative disease, malignancy, meningitis, pancreatitis, progressive multifocal leukoencephalopathy (sometimes fatal), pulmonary fibrosis (fatal), pure red cell aplasia, tuberculosis

Drug Interactions

Metabolism/Transport Effects **Substrate** of OAT3, SLCO1B1, UGT1A10, UGT1A8, UGT1A9, UGT2B7

Avoid Concomitant Use

Avoid concomitant use of Mycophenolate with any of the following: BCG; Bile Acid Sequestrants; Cholestyramine Resin; Natalizumab; Pimecrolimus; Rifamycin Derivatives; Tacrolimus (Topical); Tofacitinib; Vaccines (Live)

Increased Effect/Toxicity

Mycophenolate may increase the levels/effects of: Acyclovir-Valacyclovir; Ganciclovir-Valganciclovir; Leflunomide; Natalizumab; Tofacitinib; Vaccines (Live)

The levels/effects of Mycophenolate may be increased by: Acyclovir-Valacyclovir; Denosumab; Ganciclovir-Valganciclovir; Pimecrolimus; Probenecid; Roflumilast; Tacrolimus (Topical); Teriflunomide; Trastuzumab

Decreased Effect

Mycophenolate may decrease the levels/effects of: BCG; Coccidioides immitis Skin Test; Contraceptives (Estrogens); Contraceptives (Progestins); Sipuleucel-T; Vaccines (Inactivated); Vaccines (Live)

The levels/effects of Mycophenolate may be decreased by: Antacids; Bile Acid Sequestrants; Cholestyramine Resin; CycloSPORINE (Systemic); Echinacea; Magnesium Salts; MetroNIDAZOLE (Systemic); Penicillins; Proton Pump Inhibitors; Quinolone Antibiotics; Rifamycin Derivatives; Sevelamer

Food Interactions Food decreases C_{max} of MPA by 40% following CellCept administration and 33% following Myfortic use; the extent of absorption is not changed. Management: Take CellCept or Myfortic on an empty stomach to decrease variability; however, Cellcept may be taken with food if necessary in stable renal transplant patients.

Preparation for Administration Hazardous agent; use appropriate precautions for handling and disposal (NIOSH 2014 [group 2]).

Oral suspension: Should be constituted prior to dispensing to the patient and **not** mixed with any other medication. Add 47 mL of water to the bottle and shake well for ~1 minute. Add another 47 mL of water to the bottle and shake well for an additional minute. Final concentration is 200 mg/mL of mycophenolate mofetil.

IV: Reconstitute the contents of each vial with 14 mL of 5% dextrose injection; dilute the contents of a vial with 5% dextrose in water to a final concentration of 6 mg mycophenolate mofetil per mL. **Note:** Vial is vacuum-sealed; if a lack of vacuum is noted during preparation, the vial should not be used.

Storage/Stability

Capsules: Store at 25°C (77°F); excursions permitted to 15°C to 30°C (59°F to 86°F).

Tablets: Store at 25°C (77°F); excursions permitted to 15°C to 30°C (59°F to 86°F). Protect from moisture and light.

Oral suspension: Store powder for oral suspension at 25°C (77°F); excursions permitted to 15°C to 30°C (59°F to 86°F). Once reconstituted, the oral solution may be stored at room temperature or under refrigeration. Do not freeze. The mixed suspension is stable for 60 days.

Injection: Store intact vials and diluted solutions at 25°C (77°F); excursions permitted to 15°C to 30°C (59°F to 86°F). Begin infusion within 4 hours of reconstitution.

Mechanism of Action MPA exhibits a cytostatic effect on T and B lymphocytes. It is an inhibitor of inosine monophosphate dehydrogenase (IMPDH) which inhibits *de novo* guanosine nucleotide synthesis. T and B lymphocytes are dependent on this pathway for proliferation.

Pharmacodynamics/Kinetics

Onset of action: Peak effect: Correlation of toxicity or efficacy is still being developed, however, one study indicated that 12-hour AUCs >40 mcg/mL/hour were correlated with efficacy and decreased episodes of rejection

Absorption: AUC values for MPA are lower in the early post-transplant period versus later (>3 months) post-transplant period. The extent of absorption in pediatrics is similar to that seen in adults, although there was wide variability reported.

Oral: Myfortic: 93%

Distribution:

CellCept: MPA: Oral: 4 L/kg; IV: 3.6 L/kg

Myfortic: MPA: Oral: 54 L (at steady state); 112 L (elimination phase)

Protein binding: MPA: >97%, MPAG 82%

Metabolism: Hepatic and via GI tract; CellCept is completely hydrolyzed in the liver to mycophenolic acid (MPA; active metabolite); enterohepatic recirculation of MPA may occur; MPA is glucuronidated to MPAG (inactive metabolite)

Bioavailability: Oral: CellCept: 94%; Myfortic: 72%

Half-life elimination:

CellCept: MPA: Oral: 18 hours; IV: 17 hours

Myfortic: MPA: Oral: 8-16 hours; MPAG: 13-17 hours

Time to peak, plasma: Oral: MPA:

CellCept: 1-1.5 hours

Myfortic: 1.5-2.75 hours

Excretion:

CellCept: MPA: Urine (<1%), feces (6%); MPAG: Urine (87%)

Myfortic: MPA: Urine (3%), feces; MPAG: Urine (>60%)

Dosage

Infants ≥3 months, Children, and Adolescents: Renal transplant: Oral:

CellCept suspension: 600 mg/m^2/dose twice daily; maximum dose: 1 g twice daily

Alternatively, may use Cellcept solid dosage forms according to BSA as follows:

BSA 1.25-1.5 m^2: 750 mg capsule twice daily

BSA >1.5 m^2: 1 g capsule or tablet twice daily

Children ≥5 years and Adolescents: Renal transplant: Oral:

Myfortic: Usual dosage: 400 mg/m^2/dose twice daily; maximum dose: 720 mg twice daily

BSA <1.19 m^2: Use of this formulation is not recommended

BSA 1.19-1.58 m^2: 540 mg twice daily (maximum: 1080 mg/day)

BSA >1.58 m^2: 720 mg twice daily (maximum: 1440 mg/day)

Adults: **Note:** May be used IV for up to 14 days; transition to oral therapy as soon as tolerated.

Renal transplant:

CellCept:

Oral: 1 g twice daily. Doses >2 g/day are not recommended.

IV: 1 g twice daily

Myfortic: Oral: 720 mg twice daily (total daily dose: 1440 mg)

Cardiac transplantation: CellCept:

Oral: 1.5 g twice daily

IV: 1.5 g twice daily

Hepatic transplantation: CellCept:

Oral: 1.5 g twice daily

IV: 1 g twice daily

Autoimmune hepatitis, refractory (off-label use): CellCept: Oral: 2 g/day (Manns, 2010)

Lupus nephritis (off-label use): CellCept: Oral:

Induction: 1 g twice daily for 6 months in combination with a glucocorticoid (Ong, 2005) **or** 2-3 g daily for 6 months in combination with glucocorticoids (Hahn, 2012)

Maintenance: 0.5-3 g daily (Contreras, 2004) **or** 1 g twice daily (Dooley, 2011) **or** 1-2 g daily (Hahn, 2012)

Myasthenia gravis (off-label use): CellCept: Oral: 1 g twice daily (range: 1-3 g daily) (Cahoon, 2006; Ciafaloni, 2001; Merriggioli, 2003)

Psoriasis, moderate-to-severe (off-label use): CellCept: Oral: 2-3 g daily (Menter, 2009)

Elderly: Dosage is the same as younger patients, however, dosing should be cautious due to possibility of increased hepatic, renal or cardiac dysfunction; elderly patients may be at an increased risk of certain infections, gastrointestinal hemorrhage, and pulmonary edema, as compared to younger patients

Dosing adjustment for toxicity (neutropenia): Neutropenia (ANC <1.3 x $10^3/\mu L$): Dosing should be interrupted or the dose reduced, appropriate diagnostic tests performed and patients managed appropriately

Dosing adjustment in renal impairment:

Renal transplant: GFR <25 mL/minute/1.73 m^2 in patients outside the immediate post-transplant period:

CellCept: Doses of >1 g administered twice daily should be avoided; patients should also be carefully observed; no dose adjustments are needed in renal transplant patients experiencing delayed graft function postoperatively

Myfortic: No dose adjustments are needed in renal transplant patients experiencing delayed graft function postoperatively; however, monitor carefully for potential concentration dependent adverse events

Cardiac or liver transplant: No data available; mycophenolate may be used in cardiac or hepatic transplant patients with severe chronic renal impairment if the potential benefit outweighs the potential risk

Autoimmune disease (off-label use): There have been no specific dosage adjustments identified, although use of lower doses may be required. MPA exposure appears to be inversely related to renal function (Abd Rahman, 2013); monitor closely for efficacy and adverse effects, especially in patients with end-stage renal disease (Haubitz, 2002; MacPhee, 2000).

Hemodialysis: Not removed; supplemental dose is not necessary

Peritoneal dialysis: Supplemental dose is not necessary

Dosage adjustment in hepatic impairment: No dosage adjustment is recommended for renal patients with severe hepatic parenchymal disease; however, it is not currently known whether dosage adjustments are necessary for hepatic disease with other etiologies

Dietary Considerations Oral dosage formulations should be taken on an empty stomach to avoid variability in MPA absorption. However, in stable renal transplant patients, Cellcept may be administered with food if necessary. Some products may contain phenylalanine.

Administration

Oral dosage formulations (tablet, capsule, suspension) should be administered on an empty stomach (1 hour before or 2 hours after meals) to avoid variability in MPA absorption. The oral solution may be administered via a nasogastric tube (minimum 8 French, 1.7 mm interior diameter); oral suspension should not be mixed with other medications. Delayed release tablets should not be crushed, cut, or chewed. Cellcept may be administered with food in stable renal transplant patients when necessary. If a dose is missed, administer as soon as it is remembered. If it is close to the next scheduled dose, skip the missed dose and resume at next regularly scheduled time; do not double a dose to make up for a missed dose.

Intravenous solutions should be administered over at least 2 hours (either peripheral or central vein); do **not** administer intravenous solution by rapid or bolus injection.

Hazardous agent; use appropriate precautions for handling and disposal (NIOSH 2014 [group 2]).

Monitoring Parameters Complete blood count (weekly for first month, twice monthly during months 2 and 3, then monthly thereafter through the first year); renal and liver function; signs and symptoms of organ rejection; signs and symptoms of bacterial, fungal, protozoal, new or reactivated viral, or opportunistic infections; neurological symptoms (eg, hemiparesis, confusion, cognitive deficiencies, ataxia) suggestive of PML, pregnancy test (immediately prior to initiation and 8-10 days later in females of childbearing potential, followed by repeat tests during therapy); monitor skin (for lesions suspicious of skin cancer); monitor for signs of lymphoma

Additional Information Females of reproductive potential are required to have contraceptive counseling and use acceptable birth control unless heterosexual intercourse is completely avoided. Use of an intrauterine device (IUD), tubal sterilization, or vasectomy of the female patient's partner are acceptable contraceptive methods that can be used alone. If a hormonal contraceptive is used (eg, combination oral contraceptive pills, transdermal patches, vaginal rings, or progestin only products), then one barrier method must also be used (eg, diaphragm or cervical cap with spermicide, contraceptive sponge, male or female condom). Alternatively, the use of two barrier methods is also acceptable (eg, diaphragm or cervical cap with spermicide, or contraceptive sponge **PLUS** male or female condom). Refer to manufacturer's labeling for full details.

Dosage Forms Considerations Single dose pharmacokinetic studies in adult renal transplant patients suggest that bioavailability is similar between oral mycophenolate mofetil (1000 mg) and delayed release mycophenolic acid (720 mg) (Arns, 2005). In clinical trials, comparative efficacy and safety profiles have been observed in adult renal transplant patients randomized to either oral mycophenolate mofetil (1000 mg twice daily) or delayed release mycophenolic acid (720 mg twice daily) (Budde, 2004; Salvadori, 2003).

Dosage Forms

Capsule, Oral:
CellCept: 250 mg
Generic: 250 mg

Solution Reconstituted, Intravenous:
CellCept Intravenous: 500 mg (1 ea)

Suspension Reconstituted, Oral:
CellCept: 200 mg/mL (160 mL)
Generic: 200 mg/mL (160 mL)

Tablet, Oral:
CellCept: 500 mg
Generic: 500 mg

Tablet Delayed Release, Oral:
Myfortic: 180 mg, 360 mg
Generic: 180 mg, 360 mg

Extemporaneous Preparations Hazardous agent; use appropriate precautions for handling and disposal (NIOSH 2014 [group 2]).

A 50 mg/mL oral suspension may be made with mycophenolate mofetil capsules, Ora-Plus, and cherry syrup. In a vertical flow hood, empty six 250 mg capsules into a mortar; add 7.5 mL Ora-Plus and mix to a uniform paste. Mix while adding 15 mL of cherry syrup in incremental proportions; transfer to a calibrated bottle, rinse mortar with cherry syrup, and add sufficient quantity of cherry syrup to make 30 mL. Label "shake well". Stable for 210 days at 5°C, for 28 days at 25°C to 37°C, and for 11 days at 45°C.

Venkataramanan R, McCombs JR, Zuckerman S, et al, "Stability of Mycophenolate Mofetil as an Extemporaneous Suspension," *Ann Pharmacother*, 1998, 32(7-8):755-7.

- ◆ **Mycophenolate Mofetil** *see* Mycophenolate *on page 1405*
- ◆ **Mycophenolate Sodium** *see* Mycophenolate *on page 1405*
- ◆ **Mycophenolic Acid** *see* Mycophenolate *on page 1405*
- ◆ **Mydral** *see* Tropicamide *on page 2108*
- ◆ **Mydriacyl** *see* Tropicamide *on page 2108*
- ◆ **Mydriacyl® (Can)** *see* Tropicamide *on page 2108*
- ◆ **Myferon 150 [OTC]** *see* Polysaccharide-Iron Complex *on page 1677*
- ◆ **Myfortic** *see* Mycophenolate *on page 1405*
- ◆ **Mylan-Acebutolol (Can)** *see* Acebutolol *on page 29*
- ◆ **Mylan-Acebutolol (Type S) (Can)** *see* Acebutolol *on page 29*
- ◆ **Mylan-Acyclovir (Can)** *see* Acyclovir (Systemic) *on page 47*
- ◆ **Mylan-Alendronate (Can)** *see* Alendronate *on page 79*
- ◆ **Mylan-Almotriptan (Can)** *see* Almotriptan *on page 92*
- ◆ **Mylan-Alprazolam (Can)** *see* ALPRAZolam *on page 94*
- ◆ **Mylan-Amantadine (Can)** *see* Amantadine *on page 105*
- ◆ **Mylan-Amiodarone (Can)** *see* Amiodarone *on page 114*
- ◆ **Mylan-Amlodipine (Can)** *see* AmLODIPine *on page 123*
- ◆ **Mylan-Amoxicillin (Can)** *see* Amoxicillin *on page 130*
- ◆ **Mylan-Anagrelide (Can)** *see* Anagrelide *on page 147*
- ◆ **Mylan-Anastrozole (Can)** *see* Anastrozole *on page 148*
- ◆ **Mylan-Atenolol (Can)** *see* Atenolol *on page 189*
- ◆ **Mylan-Atomoxetine (Can)** *see* AtoMOXetine *on page 191*
- ◆ **Mylan-Atorvastatin (Can)** *see* AtorvaSTATin *on page 194*
- ◆ **Mylan-Azathioprine (Can)** *see* AzaTHIOprine *on page 210*
- ◆ **Mylan-Azithromycin (Can)** *see* Azithromycin (Systemic) *on page 216*
- ◆ **Mylan-Baclofen (Can)** *see* Baclofen *on page 223*
- ◆ **Mylan-Beclo AQ (Can)** *see* Beclomethasone (Nasal) *on page 232*
- ◆ **Mylan-Bicalutamide (Can)** *see* Bicalutamide *on page 262*
- ◆ **Mylan-Bisoprolol (Can)** *see* Bisoprolol *on page 266*
- ◆ **Mylan-Bosentan (Can)** *see* Bosentan *on page 280*
- ◆ **Mylan-Bromazepam (Can)** *see* Bromazepam [CAN/INT] *on page 290*
- ◆ **Mylan-Budesonide AQ (Can)** *see* Budesonide (Nasal) *on page 296*
- ◆ **Mylan-Bupropion XL (Can)** *see* BuPROPion *on page 305*
- ◆ **Mylan-Candesartan (Can)** *see* Candesartan *on page 335*
- ◆ **Mylan-Candesartan HCTZ (Can)** *see* Candesartan and Hydrochlorothiazide *on page 338*
- ◆ **Mylan-Captopril (Can)** *see* Captopril *on page 342*
- ◆ **Mylan-Carbamazepine CR (Can)** *see* CarBAMazepine *on page 346*
- ◆ **Mylan-Carvedilol (Can)** *see* Carvedilol *on page 367*
- ◆ **Mylan-Cilazapril (Can)** *see* Cilazapril [CAN/INT] *on page 434*
- ◆ **Mylan-Cimetidine (Can)** *see* Cimetidine *on page 438*
- ◆ **Mylan-Ciprofloxacin (Can)** *see* Ciprofloxacin (Systemic) *on page 441*
- ◆ **Mylan-Citalopram (Can)** *see* Citalopram *on page 451*
- ◆ **Mylan-Clarithromycin (Can)** *see* Clarithromycin *on page 456*
- ◆ **Mylan-Clindamycin (Can)** *see* Clindamycin (Systemic) *on page 460*
- ◆ **Mylan-Clobetasol (Can)** *see* Clobetasol *on page 468*
- ◆ **Mylan-Clonazepam (Can)** *see* ClonazePAM *on page 478*
- ◆ **Mylan-Clopidogrel (Can)** *see* Clopidogrel *on page 484*
- ◆ **Mylan-Cyclobenzaprine (Can)** *see* Cyclobenzaprine *on page 516*
- ◆ **Mylan-Divalproex (Can)** *see* Valproic Acid and Derivatives *on page 2123*
- ◆ **Mylan-Domperidone (Can)** *see* Domperidone [CAN/INT] *on page 666*
- ◆ **Mylan-Donepezil (Can)** *see* Donepezil *on page 668*
- ◆ **Mylan-Doxazosin (Can)** *see* Doxazosin *on page 674*
- ◆ **Mylan-Efavirenz (Can)** *see* Efavirenz *on page 707*
- ◆ **Mylan-Enalapril (Can)** *see* Enalapril *on page 722*
- ◆ **Mylan-Entacapone (Can)** *see* Entacapone *on page 730*
- ◆ **Mylan-Escitalopram (Can)** *see* Escitalopram *on page 765*
- ◆ **Mylan-Esomeprazole (Can)** *see* Esomeprazole *on page 771*
- ◆ **Mylan-Eti-Cal Carepac (Can)** *see* Etidronate and Calcium Carbonate [CAN/INT] *on page 814*
- ◆ **Mylan-Etidronate (Can)** *see* Etidronate *on page 813*
- ◆ **Mylan-Ezetimibe (Can)** *see* Ezetimibe *on page 832*
- ◆ **Mylan-Famotidine (Can)** *see* Famotidine *on page 845*
- ◆ **Mylan-Fenofibrate Micro (Can)** *see* Fenofibrate and Derivatives *on page 852*

- **Mylan-Fentanyl Matrix Patch (Can)** *see* FentaNYL *on page* 857
- **Mylan-Finasteride (Can)** *see* Finasteride *on page* 878
- **Mylan-Fluconazole (Can)** *see* Fluconazole *on page* 885
- **Mylan-Fluoxetine (Can)** *see* FLUoxetine *on page* 899
- **Mylan-Fosinopril (Can)** *see* Fosinopril *on page* 932
- **Mylan-Gabapentin (Can)** *see* Gabapentin *on page* 943
- **Mylan-Galantamine ER (Can)** *see* Galantamine *on page* 946
- **Mylan-Gemfibrozil (Can)** *see* Gemfibrozil *on page* 956
- **Mylan-Gliclazide (Can)** *see* Gliclazide [CAN/INT] *on page* 964
- **Mylan-Glybe (Can)** *see* GlyBURIDE *on page* 972
- **Mylan-Hydroxychloroquine (Can)** *see* Hydroxychloroquine *on page* 1021
- **Mylan-Hydroxyurea (Can)** *see* Hydroxyurea *on page* 1021
- **Mylan-Indapamide (Can)** *see* Indapamide *on page* 1065
- **Mylan-Ipratropium Solution (Can)** *see* Ipratropium (Nasal) *on page* 1109
- **Mylan-Ipratropium Sterinebs (Can)** *see* Ipratropium (Systemic) *on page* 1108
- **Mylan-Irbesartan (Can)** *see* Irbesartan *on page* 1110
- **Mylan-Lamotrigine (Can)** *see* LamoTRIgine *on page* 1160
- **Mylan-Lansoprazole (Can)** *see* Lansoprazole *on page* 1166
- **Mylan-Leflunomide (Can)** *see* Leflunomide *on page* 1174
- **Mylan-Levofloxacin (Can)** *see* Levofloxacin (Systemic) *on page* 1197
- **Mylan-Lisinopril (Can)** *see* Lisinopril *on page* 1226
- **Mylan-Lisinopril/Hctz (Can)** *see* Lisinopril and Hydrochlorothiazide *on page* 1229
- **Mylan-Losartan (Can)** *see* Losartan *on page* 1248
- **Mylan-Losartan/HCTZ (Can)** *see* Losartan and Hydrochlorothiazide *on page* 1250
- **Mylan-Lovastatin (Can)** *see* Lovastatin *on page* 1252
- **Mylan-Meloxicam (Can)** *see* Meloxicam *on page* 1283
- **Mylan-Metformin (Can)** *see* MetFORMIN *on page* 1307
- **Mylan-Metoprolol (Type L) (Can)** *see* Metoprolol *on page* 1350
- **Mylan-Minocycline (Can)** *see* Minocycline *on page* 1371
- **Mylan-Mirtazapine (Can)** *see* Mirtazapine *on page* 1376
- **Mylan-Montelukast (Can)** *see* Montelukast *on page* 1392
- **Mylan-Mycophenolate (Can)** *see* Mycophenolate *on page* 1405
- **Mylan-Nabumetone (Can)** *see* Nabumetone *on page* 1411
- **Mylan-Naproxen EC (Can)** *see* Naproxen *on page* 1427
- **Mylan-Nevirapine (Can)** *see* Nevirapine *on page* 1440
- **Mylan-Nifedipine Extended Release (Can)** *see* NIFEdipine *on page* 1451
- **Mylan-Nitro Sublingual Spray (Can)** *see* Nitroglycerin *on page* 1465
- **Mylan-Olanzapine (Can)** *see* OLANZapine *on page* 1491
- **Mylan-Olanzapine ODT (Can)** *see* OLANZapine *on page* 1491
- **Mylan-Omeprazole (Can)** *see* Omeprazole *on page* 1508
- **Mylan-Ondansetron (Can)** *see* Ondansetron *on page* 1513
- **Mylan-Oxybutynin (Can)** *see* Oxybutynin *on page* 1536
- **Mylan-Pantoprazole (Can)** *see* Pantoprazole *on page* 1570
- **Mylan-Paroxetine (Can)** *see* PARoxetine *on page* 1579
- **Mylan-Pioglitazone (Can)** *see* Pioglitazone *on page* 1654
- **Mylan-Pramipexole (Can)** *see* Pramipexole *on page* 1695
- **Mylan-Pravastatin (Can)** *see* Pravastatin *on page* 1700
- **Mylan-Propafenone (Can)** *see* Propafenone *on page* 1725
- **Mylan-Quetiapine (Can)** *see* QUEtiapine *on page* 1751
- **Mylan-Ramipril (Can)** *see* Ramipril *on page* 1771
- **Mylan-Ranitidine (Can)** *see* Ranitidine *on page* 1777
- **Mylan-Riluzole (Can)** *see* Riluzole *on page* 1812
- **Mylan-Risperidone (Can)** *see* RisperiDONE *on page* 1818
- **Mylan-Risperidone ODT (Can)** *see* RisperiDONE *on page* 1818
- **Mylan-Rivastigmine (Can)** *see* Rivastigmine *on page* 1833
- **Mylan-Rizatriptan ODT (Can)** *see* Rizatriptan *on page* 1836
- **Mylan-Rosuvastatin (Can)** *see* Rosuvastatin *on page* 1848
- **Mylan-Selegiline (Can)** *see* Selegiline *on page* 1873
- **Mylan-Sertraline (Can)** *see* Sertraline *on page* 1878
- **Mylan-Simvastatin (Can)** *see* Simvastatin *on page* 1890
- **Mylan-Sotalol (Can)** *see* Sotalol *on page* 1927
- **Mylan-Sumatriptan (Can)** *see* SUMAtriptan *on page* 1953
- **Mylanta™ (Can)** *see* Aluminum Hydroxide and Magnesium Hydroxide *on page* 103
- **Mylanta Classic Maximum Strength Liquid [OTC]** *see* Aluminum Hydroxide, Magnesium Hydroxide, and Simethicone *on page* 104
- **Mylanta Classic Regular Strength Liquid [OTC]** *see* Aluminum Hydroxide, Magnesium Hydroxide, and Simethicone *on page* 104
- **Mylanta Double Strength (Can)** *see* Aluminum Hydroxide, Magnesium Hydroxide, and Simethicone *on page* 104
- **Mylanta Extra Strength (Can)** *see* Aluminum Hydroxide, Magnesium Hydroxide, and Simethicone *on page* 104
- **Mylan-Tamoxifen (Can)** *see* Tamoxifen *on page* 1971
- **Mylan-Tamsulosin (Can)** *see* Tamsulosin *on page* 1974
- **Mylanta Regular Strength (Can)** *see* Aluminum Hydroxide, Magnesium Hydroxide, and Simethicone *on page* 104
- **Mylanta Supreme [OTC]** *see* Calcium Carbonate and Magnesium Hydroxide *on page* 328
- **Mylanta Ultra [OTC]** *see* Calcium Carbonate and Magnesium Hydroxide *on page* 328
- **Mylan-Telmisartan (Can)** *see* Telmisartan *on page* 1988
- **Mylan-Telmisartan HCTZ (Can)** *see* Telmisartan and Hydrochlorothiazide *on page* 1990
- **Mylan-Terbinafine (Can)** *see* Terbinafine (Systemic) *on page* 2002
- **Mylan-Ticlopidine (Can)** *see* Ticlopidine *on page* 2040

- ◆ **Mylan-Timolol (Can)** *see* Timolol (Ophthalmic) *on page 2043*
- ◆ **Mylan-Tizanidine (Can)** *see* TiZANidine *on page 2051*
- ◆ **Mylan-Topiramate (Can)** *see* Topiramate *on page 2065*
- ◆ **Mylan-Trazodone (Can)** *see* TraZODone *on page 2091*
- ◆ **Mylan-Valacyclovir (Can)** *see* ValACYclovir *on page 2119*
- ◆ **Mylan-Valproic (Can)** *see* Valproic Acid and Derivatives *on page 2123*
- ◆ **Mylan-Valsartan (Can)** *see* Valsartan *on page 2127*
- ◆ **Mylan-Valsartan HCTZ (Can)** *see* Valsartan and Hydrochlorothiazide *on page 2129*
- ◆ **Mylan-Venlafaxine XR (Can)** *see* Venlafaxine *on page 2150*
- ◆ **Mylan-Verapamil (Can)** *see* Verapamil *on page 2154*
- ◆ **Mylan-Verapamil SR (Can)** *see* Verapamil *on page 2154*
- ◆ **Mylan-Warfarin (Can)** *see* Warfarin *on page 2186*
- ◆ **Mylan-Zolmitriptan (Can)** *see* ZOLMitriptan *on page 2210*
- ◆ **Mylan-Zolmitriptan ODT (Can)** *see* ZOLMitriptan *on page 2210*
- ◆ **Mylan-Zopiclone (Can)** *see* Zopiclone [CAN/INT] *on page 2217*
- ◆ **Myleran** *see* Busulfan *on page 312*
- ◆ **Myl-Letrozole (Can)** *see* Letrozole *on page 1181*
- ◆ **Mylotarg** *see* Gemtuzumab Ozogamicin *on page 957*
- ◆ **MYL Pregabalin (Can)** *see* Pregabalin *on page 1710*
- ◆ **Myl-Ranitidine (Can)** *see* Ranitidine *on page 1777*
- ◆ **MYL-Sildenafil (Can)** *see* Sildenafil *on page 1882*
- ◆ **Myobloc** *see* RimabotulinumtoxinB *on page 1813*
- ◆ **Myocet (Can)** *see* DOXOrubicin (Liposomal) *on page 684*
- ◆ **Myorisan** *see* ISOtretinoin *on page 1127*
- ◆ **Myozyme** *see* Alglucosidase Alfa *on page 85*
- ◆ **Myrbetriq** *see* Mirabegron *on page 1375*
- ◆ **Mysoline** *see* Primidone *on page 1714*
- ◆ **Mytotan** *see* Mitotane *on page 1382*
- ◆ **Mytussin® DAC** *see* Guaifenesin, Pseudoephedrine, and Codeine *on page 989*
- ◆ **My Way [DSC]** *see* Levonorgestrel *on page 1201*
- ◆ **Myzilra** *see* Ethinyl Estradiol and Levonorgestrel *on page 803*
- ◆ **N-9** *see* Nonoxynol 9 *on page 1471*
- ◆ **N-0923** *see* Rotigotine *on page 1851*
- ◆ **NAAK** *see* Atropine and Pralidoxime *on page 203*
- ◆ **Nabi-HB** *see* Hepatitis B Immune Globulin (Human) *on page 1002*
- ◆ **Nabiximols** *see* Tetrahydrocannabinol and Cannabidiol [CAN/INT] *on page 2018*
- ◆ **nab-Paclitaxel** *see* PACLitaxel (Protein Bound) *on page 1554*

Nabumetone (na BYOO me tone)

Brand Names: Canada Apo-Nabumetone; Gen-Nabumetone; Mylan-Nabumetone; Novo-Nabumetone; Relafen; Rhoxal-nabumetone; Sandoz-Nabumetone

Index Terms Relafen

Pharmacologic Category Nonsteroidal Anti-inflammatory Drug (NSAID), Oral

Additional Appendix Information

Beers Criteria – Potentially Inappropriate Medications for Geriatrics *on page 2271*

Use Management of osteoarthritis and rheumatoid arthritis

Pregnancy Risk Factor C

Dosage Adults: Oral: 1000 mg/day; an additional 500-1000 mg may be needed in some patients to obtain more symptomatic relief; may be administered once or twice daily (maximum dose: 2000 mg/day)

Note: Patients <50 kg are less likely to require doses >1000 mg/day.

Dosage adjustment in renal impairment: In general, NSAIDs are not recommended for use in patients with advanced renal disease, but the manufacturer of nabumetone does provide some guidelines for adjustment in renal dysfunction:

Moderate impairment (CrCl 30-49 mL/minute): Initial dose: 750 mg/day; maximum dose: 1500 mg/day

Severe impairment (CrCl <30 mL/minute): Initial dose: 500 mg/day; maximum dose: 1000 mg/day

Dosage adjustment in hepatic impairment: No dosage adjustment provided in manufacturer's labeling (has not been studied). Prodrug activation and metabolism are hepatic function dependent and may be reduced in severe hepatic impairment.

Additional Information Complete prescribing information should be consulted for additional detail.

Dosage Forms

Tablet, Oral:

Generic: 500 mg, 750 mg

- ◆ **NAC** *see* Acetylcysteine *on page 40*
- ◆ ***N*-Acetyl-L-cysteine** *see* Acetylcysteine *on page 40*
- ◆ ***N* Acetylcysteine** *see* Acetylcysteine *on page 40*
- ◆ **N-acetylgalactosamine-6-sulfatase** *see* Elosulfase Alfa *on page 714*
- ◆ **N-Acetyl-P-Aminophenol** *see* Acetaminophen *on page 32*
- ◆ **NaCl** *see* Sodium Chloride *on page 1902*

Nadifloxacin [INT] (na di FLOKS a sin)

International Brand Names Acuatim (ID, JP); Nadibact (IN); Nadixa (BG, CO, CR, DE, DO, EC, ES, GR, GT, HN, IT, KR, LB, MX, NI, PA, PE, PT, PY, SV, TR); Nadoxin (LB, PH); Pingfu (CN); Xin Ke Fei (CN); Yi You Ning (CN)

Pharmacologic Category Antibiotic, Quinolone

Reported Use Treatment of acne vulgaris and bacterial skin infections

Dosage Range Topical: Apply to lesions twice daily

Product Availability Product available in various countries; not currently available in the U.S.

Dosage Forms

Cream, topical: 1%

Nadolol (NAY doe lol)

Brand Names: U.S. Corgard

Brand Names: Canada Apo-Nadol; Teva-Nadolol

Pharmacologic Category Antianginal Agent; Antihypertensive; Beta-Blocker, Nonselective

Use Treatment of hypertension and angina pectoris

The 2014 guideline for the management of high blood pressure in adults (Eighth Joint National Committee [JNC 8]) recommends initiation of pharmacologic treatment to lower blood pressure for the following patients (JNC8 [James, 2013]):

- Patients ≥60 years of age, with systolic blood pressure (SBP) ≥150 mm Hg or diastolic blood pressure (DBP) ≥90 mm Hg. Goal of therapy is SBP <150 mm Hg and DBP <90 mm Hg.
- Patients <60 years of age, with SBP ≥140 mm Hg or DBP ≥90 mm Hg. Goal of therapy is SBP <140 mm Hg and DBP <90 mm Hg.
- Patients ≥18 years of age with diabetes, with SBP ≥140 mm Hg or DBP ≥90 mm Hg. Goal of therapy is SBP <140 mm Hg and DBP <90 mm Hg.
- Patients ≥18 years of age with chronic kidney disease (CKD), with SBP ≥140 mm Hg or DBP ≥90 mm Hg. Goal of therapy is SBP <140 mm Hg and DBP <90 mm Hg.

In patients with CKD, regardless of race or diabetes status, the use of an ACE inhibitor (ACEI) or angiotensin receptor blocker (ARB) as initial therapy is recommended to improve kidney outcomes. In the general nonblack population (without CKD) including those with diabetes, initial antihypertensive treatment should consist of a thiazide-type diuretic, calcium channel blocker, ACEI, or ARB. In the general black population (without CKD) including those with diabetes, initial antihypertensive treatment should consist of a thiazide-type diuretic or a calcium channel blocker **instead of** an ACEI or ARB.

Pregnancy Risk Factor C

Dosage

U.S. labeling: Adults: Oral:

Angina: Initial: 40 mg once daily, increase dosage gradually by 40 to 80 mg increments at 3- to 7-day intervals until optimum clinical response is obtained usual dose: 40 to 80 mg daily; maximum dose: 240 mg daily

Hypertension: 40 mg once daily, increase dosage gradually by 40 to 80 mg increments until optimum blood pressure reduction achieved. Usual dosage range (ASH/ISH [Weber, 2014]): 40 to 80 mg once daily. Doses up to 240 to 320 mg once daily in hypertension may be necessary

Canadian labeling: Adults: Oral:

Angina: Initial: 80 mg once daily, increase dosage gradually by 80 mg increments at 7-day intervals until optimum clinical response is obtained; may consider dose reduction to 40 mg once daily for patients stable on 80 mg daily; maximum dose: 240 mg daily

Hypertension: Initial: 80 mg once daily; increase dosage gradually by 80 mg increments at 7-day intervals until optimum blood pressure reduction achieved. Doses ≤ 240 mg daily are typically effective; maximum dose: 320 mg once daily

Off-label uses: Adults: Oral:

Atrial fibrillation (rate control): Usual maintenance dose: 10 to 240 mg once daily (AHA/ACC/HRS [January, 2014])

Variceal hemorrhage prophylaxis (Garcia-Tsao, 2007):

Primary prophylaxis: Initial: 40 mg once daily; adjust to maximal tolerated dose. **Note:** Risk factors for hemorrhage include Child-Pugh class B/C or variceal red wale markings on endoscopy.

Secondary prophylaxis: Initial: 40 mg once daily; adjust to maximal tolerated dose

Thyrotoxicosis: 40 to 160 mg once daily (Bahn, 2011)

Elderly: Hypertension: Consider lower initial doses (eg, 20 mg daily) and titrate to response (Aronow, 2011)

Dosing adjustment in renal impairment:

CrCl >50 mL/minute/1.73 m^2: Administer every 24 hours

CrCl 31 to 50 mL/minute/1.73 m^2: Administer every 24 to 36 hours

CrCl 10 to 30 mL/minute/1.73 m^2: Administer every 24 to 48 hours

CrCl <10 mL/minute/1.73 m^2: Administer every 40 to 60 hours

Dosage adjustments for dialysis are not provided in the manufacturer's labeling; however, the following guidelines have been used by some clinicians (Aronoff, 2007):

ESRD requiring hemodialysis: Administer dose postdialysis.

Peritoneal dialysis: Administer every 40 to 60 hours

Dosing adjustment in hepatic impairment: There are no dosage adjustments provided in the manufacturer's labeling.

Additional Information Complete prescribing information should be consulted for additional detail.

Dosage Forms

Tablet, Oral:

Corgard: 20 mg, 40 mg, 80 mg

Generic: 20 mg, 40 mg, 80 mg

Nadroparin [CAN/INT] (nad roe PA rin)

Brand Names: Canada Fraxiparine; Fraxiparine Forte

Index Terms Nadroparin Calcium

Pharmacologic Category Anticoagulant; Anticoagulant, Low Molecular Weight Heparin

Use Note: Not approved in U.S.

Prophylaxis of thromboembolic disorders (particularly deep venous thrombosis and pulmonary embolism) in general and orthopedic surgery; treatment of deep venous thrombosis; prevention of clotting during hemodialysis; treatment of unstable angina and non-Q-wave myocardial infarction

Pregnancy Considerations Adverse events were not observed in animal reproduction studies. Low molecular weight heparin (LMWH) does not cross the placenta; increased risks of fetal bleeding or teratogenic effects have not been reported. LMWH is recommended over unfractionated heparin for the treatment of acute venous thromboembolism (VTE) in pregnant women. LMWH is also recommended over unfractionated heparin for VTE prophylaxis in pregnant women with certain risk factors. LMWH should be discontinued prior to induction of labor or a planned cesarean delivery. When choosing therapy, fetal outcomes (ie, pregnancy loss, malformations), maternal outcomes (ie, VTE, hemorrhage), burden of therapy, and maternal preference should be considered (Guyatt, 2012).

Breast-Feeding Considerations Small amounts of LMWH have been detected in breast milk; however, because it has a low oral bioavailability, it is unlikely to cause adverse events in a nursing infant. Use of LMWH may be continued in breast-feeding women (Guyatt, 2012).

Contraindications Hypersensitivity to nadroparin, any component of the formulation, or to other low molecular weight heparins and/or heparin; acute infective endocarditis; active bleeding or increased risk of hemorrhage (hemostasis disorder); history of confirmed or suspected immunologically mediated heparin-induced thrombocytopenia (HIT) (delayed-onset severe thrombocytopenia) or positive *in vitro* test for antiplatelet antibodies in the presence of nadroparin; major blood clotting disorders; hemorrhagic tendency or other conditions involving increase risk of bleeding; organic lesions likely to bleed (active peptic ulceration); hemorrhagic cerebrovascular event (unless systemic emboli present); severe uncontrolled hypertension; diabetic or hemorrhagic retinopathy; injuries to or operations on the CNS, eyes, or ears; severe renal insufficiency (creatinine clearance <30 mL/minute when used for treatment); concomitant use of spinal/epidural anesthesia with repeated high-dose nadroparin

Note: Use of nadroparin in patients with current HIT or HIT with thrombosis is **not** recommended and considered contraindicated due to high cross-reactivity to heparin-platelet factor-4 antibody (Guyatt [ACCP], 2012; Warkentin, 1999).

Warnings/Precautions Spinal or epidural hematomas, including subsequent paralysis, may occur with recent or anticipated neuraxial anesthesia (epidural or spinal) or spinal puncture in patients anticoagulated with low molecular weight heparins (LMWHs) or heparinoids. Consider risk versus benefit prior to spinal procedures; risk is increased by concomitant agents which may alter hemostasis, the use of indwelling epidural catheters for analgesia, a history of spinal deformity or spinal surgery, as well as traumatic or repeated epidural or spinal punctures. Avoid lumbar puncture or spinal or epidural anesthesia for 12 hours following the last nadroparin prophylactic dose or 24 hours following the last nadroparin treatment dose. Nadroparin therapy should not be resumed for at least 2 hours after anesthesia procedures. Longer intervals should be considered for patients with renal impairment. Observe patient closely for bleeding if nadroparin is administered.

Not to be used interchangeably (unit for unit) with heparin or any other low molecular weight heparins (LMWHs). Cases of thrombocytopenia including thrombocytopenia with thrombosis have occurred. Use with caution in patients with history of thrombocytopenia (drug-induced or congenital) or platelet defects; monitor platelet count closely. Use is contraindicated in patients with a history of confirmed or suspected heparin-induced thrombocytopenia or positive *in vitro* test for antiplatelet antibodies in the presence of nadroparin. Discontinue therapy and consider alternative treatment if platelets are <100,000/mm^3 and/or thrombosis develops. Prosthetic valve thrombosis has been reported in patients receiving thromboprophylaxis therapy with LMWHs. Pregnant women may be at increased risk.

Monitor patient closely for signs or symptoms of bleeding. Certain patients are at increased risk of bleeding. Risk factors include bacterial endocarditis; congenital or acquired bleeding disorders; active ulcerative or angiodysplastic GI diseases; severe uncontrolled hypertension; hemorrhagic stroke; recent brain, spinal, or ophthalmology surgery; concomitant treatment with platelet inhibitors; recent GI bleeding; thrombocytopenia or platelet defects; severe liver disease; hypertensive or diabetic retinopathy; or in patients undergoing invasive procedures (particularly knee surgery). Use with caution in patients with hepatic or renal disease, or with a history of peptic ulcer disease; use is contraindicated in patients with active ulceration or in severe renal insufficiency (when used for treatment of thromboembolic disorders, unstable angina, or NSTEMI).

Can cause hyperkalemia possibly by affecting aldosterone production; monitor for hyperkalemia. Cutaneous necrosis preceded by purpura or infiltrated or painful erythematous blotches has been reported rarely; discontinue treatment immediately if suspected. Packaging may contain natural latex rubber. Do **not** administer intramuscularly.

Adverse Reactions Note: As with all anticoagulants, bleeding is the major adverse effect of nadroparin. Hemorrhage may occur at virtually any site. Risk is dependent on multiple variables.

Cardiovascular: Arterial/venous thrombosis, thromboembolism

Dermatologic: Angioedema (very rare), cutaneous necrosis (rare), rash

Endocrine & metabolic: Hypoaldosteronism (causing hyperkalemia and/or hyponatremia)

Genitourinary: Priapism (very rare)

Hematological: Bleeding, eosinophilia (very rare), thrombocytopenia, thrombocytosis

Hepatic: ALT increased, AST increased

Local: Calcinosis, injection site hematoma, pain at injection site

Neuromuscular & skeletal: Osteopenic effects

Miscellaneous: Allergic reactions, anaphylactoid reactions (very rare)

Rare but important or life-threatening: Erythema, pruritus, urticaria

Drug Interactions

Metabolism/Transport Effects None known.

Avoid Concomitant Use

Avoid concomitant use of Nadroparin with any of the following: Apixaban; Dabigatran Etexilate; Edoxaban; Omacetaxine; Rivaroxaban; Urokinase; Vorapaxar

Increased Effect/Toxicity

Nadroparin may increase the levels/effects of: ACE Inhibitors; Aliskiren; Angiotensin II Receptor Blockers; Anticoagulants; Canagliflozin; Collagenase (Systemic); Deferasirox; Eplerenone; Ibritumomab; Nintedanib; Obinutuzumab; Omacetaxine; Palifermin; Potassium Salts; Potassium-Sparing Diuretics; Rivaroxaban; Tositumomab and Iodine I 131 Tositumomab

The levels/effects of Nadroparin may be increased by: 5-ASA Derivatives; Agents with Antiplatelet Properties; Apixaban; Dabigatran Etexilate; Dasatinib; Edoxaban; Herbs (Anticoagulant/Antiplatelet Properties); Ibrutinib; Limaprost; Nonsteroidal Anti-Inflammatory Agents; Omega-3 Fatty Acids; Pentosan Polysulfate Sodium; Pentoxifylline; Prostacyclin Analogues; Salicylates; Sugammadex; Thrombolytic Agents; Tibolone; Tipranavir; Urokinase; Vitamin E; Vorapaxar

Decreased Effect

The levels/effects of Nadroparin may be decreased by: Estrogen Derivatives; Progestins

Storage/Stability Store between 15°C to 30°C (59°F to 86°F); do not freeze or refrigerate.

Mechanism of Action Nadroparin has high anti-Xa activity, but low anti-IIa activity. The greater ratio of anti-Xa activity has the potential to provide equivalent antithrombic efficacy with reduced hemorrhagic complications.

Pharmacodynamics/Kinetics

Duration: Anti-Xa activity: 18 hours

Distribution: V_d: ~3.6 L

Bioavailability: SubQ: ≥89%

Half-life elimination: 3.5 hours (prolonged in renal impairment)

Time to peak, serum: 3-6 hours

Excretion: Urine

Dosage Adults: **Note:** Dose expressed as anti-Xa international units

Prevention of clotting during hemodialysis: Single dose of 65 units/kg into arterial line at start of each dialysis session; may give additional dose if session lasts longer than 4 hours; adjust dose during subsequent dialysis sessions to plasma anti-Xa levels of 0.5-1 anti-Xa units/mL

Patients at risk of hemorrhage: Administer 32.5 units/kg; may give additional smaller dose if session lasts longer than 4 hours; adjust dose during subsequent dialysis sessions to plasma anti-Xa levels of 0.2-0.4 anti-Xa units/mL.

Thromboprophylaxis therapy: SubQ:

General surgery: Initial: 2850 units administered 2-4 hours preoperatively; Maintenance: SubQ: 2850 units once daily. Continue therapy for at least 7 days and until ambulant or no longer at DVT risk.

Hip replacement surgery: 38 units/kg (maximum dose: 3800 units) administered 12 hours preoperatively and repeated at 12 hours postoperatively then followed by 38 units/kg once daily (maximum dose: 3800 units) up to and including postoperative day 3; postoperative day 4 begin 57 units/kg once daily (maximum dose: 5700 units). Continue therapy for at least 10 days and until ambulant or no longer at DVT risk.

Treatment of DVT: SubQ: 171 units/kg once daily (maximum dose: 17,100 units/day); expected plasma anti-Xa levels are 1.2-1.8 anti-Xa units/mL 3-4 hours postinjection. **Note:** Patients at an increased risk of bleeding should receive a dose of 86 units/kg every 12 hours with expected plasma anti-Xa levels of 0.5-1.1 anti-Xa units/mL 3-4 hours postinjection.

Treatment of unstable angina and non-Q-wave myocardial infarction (in conjunction with aspirin): Initial: IV: 86 units/kg bolus. Maintenance: SubQ: 86 units/kg every 12 hours (usual treatment duration: 6 days); plasma anti-Xa levels should be <1.2 anti-Xa units/mL 3-4 hours postinjection

Conversion to oral anticoagulation therapy: Continue nadroparin until therapeutic INR has been achieved with vitamin K antagonist (usually at least 5 days).

Dosage adjustment in renal impairment:

CrCl ≥50 mL/minute: No dosage adjustment necessary.

CrCl ≥30-50 mL/minute: Reduce dose by 25% to 33%

CrCl <30 mL/minute:

Prophylaxis: Reduce dose by 25% to 33%

Treatment: Use is contraindicated

Dosage adjustment in hepatic impairment: No dosage adjustment provided in manufacturer's labeling (has not been studied).

Administration Administer by SubQ injection into anterolateral abdominal wall with subsequent doses to be administered alternately on right and left side of abdominal wall. The thigh may also be used. Do **not** administer intramuscularly.

May be administered IV only as initial bolus dose for unstable angina and non-Q-wave myocardial infarction.

Monitoring Parameters Platelet counts (at baseline and then twice weekly during therapy), bleeding complications including stool occult blood tests, hemoglobin, antifactor Xa levels (recommended to obtain levels 4 hours postdose in patients at increased risk for bleeding [eg, elderly, body weight <45 kg or >120 kg, renal impairment, pregnant women, and children]); renal function, hepatic function

Reference Range Anti-Xa level target (measured 4 hours after administration): Treatment of venous thromboembolism (Garcia, 2012):

Once-daily dosing: 1.3 Anti-Xa units/mL

Twice-daily dosing: 0.6-1 Anti-Xa units/mL

Additional Information Peak anti-Xa levels (~4 hours after dosing) should be maintained at ≤1.5 units/mL in patients at increased risk for bleeding (eg, elderly, renal impairment).

Product Availability Not available in U.S.

Dosage Forms: Canada

Injection, solution:

Fraxiparine: 9500 anti-Xa units/mL (0.2 mL, 0.3 mL, 0.4 mL, 0.6 mL, 0.8 mL, 1 mL)

Fraxiparine Forte: 19,000 anti-Xa units/mL (0.6 mL, 0.8 mL, 1 mL)

◆ **Nadroparin Calcium** *see* Nadroparin [CAN/INT] *on page 1412*

Nafarelin (naf a REL in)

Brand Names: U.S. Synarel

Brand Names: Canada Synarel®

Index Terms Nafarelin Acetate

Pharmacologic Category Gonadotropin Releasing Hormone Agonist

Use Treatment of endometriosis, including pain and reduction of lesions; treatment of central precocious puberty (CPP; gonadotropin-dependent precocious puberty) in children of both sexes

Pregnancy Risk Factor X

Dosage Intranasal:

Endometriosis: Adults: Females: 1 spray (200 mcg) in 1 nostril each morning and the other nostril each evening starting on days 2-4 of menstrual cycle (total: 2 sprays/day). Dose may be increased to 2 sprays (400 mcg; 1 spray in each nostril) in the morning and evening if amenorrhea is not achieved (total: 4 sprays [800 mcg]/day). Total duration of therapy should not exceed 6 months due to decreases in bone mineral density; retreatment is not recommended by the manufacturer.

Central precocious puberty: Children: Males/Females: 2 sprays (400 mcg) into each nostril in the morning and 2 sprays (400 mcg) into each nostril in the evening (total: 8 sprays [1600 mcg]/day). If inadequate suppression, may increase dose to 3 sprays (600 mcg) into alternating nostrils 3 times/day (total: 9 sprays [1800 mcg]/day).

Dosage adjustment in renal impairment: No dosage adjustment provided in manufacturer's labeling (has not been studied).

Dosage adjustment in hepatic impairment: No dosage adjustment provided in manufacturer's labeling (has not been studied).

Additional Information Complete prescribing information should be consulted for additional detail.

Dosage Forms

Solution, Nasal:

Synarel: 2 mg/mL (8 mL)

◆ **Nafarelin Acetate** *see* Nafarelin *on page 1414*

Nafcillin (naf SIL in)

Brand Names: U.S. Nallpen in Dextrose

Index Terms Ethoxynaphthamido Penicillin Sodium; Nafcillin Sodium; Nallpen; Sodium Nafcillin

Pharmacologic Category Antibiotic, Penicillin

Use Treatment of infections such as osteomyelitis, bacteremia, septicemia, endocarditis, and CNS infections caused by susceptible strains of *Staphylococcus* species

Pregnancy Risk Factor B

Pregnancy Considerations Adverse events have not been observed in animal reproduction studies. Information specific to nafcillin use in pregnancy is limited. Maternal use of penicillins has generally not resulted in an increased risk of birth defects.

Breast-Feeding Considerations Penicillins are excreted into breast milk. The manufacturer recommends that caution be exercised when administering nafcillin to nursing women. Nondose-related effects could include modification of bowel flora.

Contraindications Hypersensitivity to nafcillin, or any component of the formulation, or penicillins

Warnings/Precautions Serious and occasionally severe or fatal hypersensitivity (anaphylactoid) reactions have been reported in patients on penicillin therapy, especially with a history of beta-lactam hypersensitivity, history of sensitivity to multiple allergens, or previous IgE-mediated reactions (eg, anaphylaxis, angioedema, urticaria). Use with caution in asthmatic patients. Contains sodium; use with caution in patients with heart failure. Vesicant; ensure proper catheter or needle position prior to and during IV infusion; avoid extravasation of IV infusions. Large IV or intraventricular doses have been associated with neurotoxicity. Modification of dosage is necessary in patients with both severe renal and hepatic impairment. Elimination may be decreased in pediatric patients. Prolonged use may result in fungal or bacterial superinfection, including *C. difficile*-associated diarrhea (CDAD) and pseudomembranous colitis; CDAD has been observed >2 months postantibiotic treatment. Potentially significant drug-drug interactions may exist, requiring dose or frequency adjustment, additional monitoring, and/or selection of alternative therapy.

Adverse Reactions

Central nervous system: Neurotoxicity (high doses)

Gastrointestinal: *C. difficile*-associated diarrhea

Hematologic: Agranulocytosis, bone marrow depression, neutropenia

Local: Inflammation, pain, phlebitis, skin sloughing, swelling, and thrombophlebitis at the injection site; tissue necrosis with sloughing (SubQ extravasation)

Renal: Interstitial nephritis (rare), renal tubular damage (rare)

Miscellaneous: Anaphylaxis, hypersensitivity reactions (immediate and delayed; general incidence of 1% to 10% for penicillins), serum sickness

Rare but important or life-threatening: ALT increased, AST increased, bilirubin increased, cholestatic hepatitis, diarrhea, drug-induced lupus erythematosus, fever, hypokalemia, itching, nausea, rash (including bullous skin eruptions), vomiting

Drug Interactions

Metabolism/Transport Effects **Induces** CYP3A4 (moderate)

Avoid Concomitant Use

Avoid concomitant use of Nafcillin with any of the following: Axitinib; BCG; Bosutinib; Enzalutamide; Nisoldipine; Olaparib; Probenecid; Simeprevir

Increased Effect/Toxicity

Nafcillin may increase the levels/effects of: Clarithromycin; Ifosfamide; Methotrexate

The levels/effects of Nafcillin may be increased by: Probenecid

Decreased Effect

Nafcillin may decrease the levels/effects of: ARIPiprazole; Axitinib; BCG; Bosutinib; Calcium Channel Blockers; Clarithromycin; Contraceptives (Estrogens); CycloSPORINE (Systemic); CYP3A4 Substrates; Dasabuvir; Enzalutamide; FentaNYL; Hydrocodone; Ibrutinib; Ifosfamide; Mycophenolate; Nisoldipine; Olaparib; Ombitasvir; Paritaprevir; Saxagliptin; Simeprevir; Sodium Picosulfate; Typhoid Vaccine; Vitamin K Antagonists

The levels/effects of Nafcillin may be decreased by: Tetracycline Derivatives

Storage/Stability

Premixed infusions: Store in a freezer at -20°C (-4°F). Thaw at room temperature or under refrigeration only. Thawed bags are stable for 21 days under refrigeration or 72 hours at room temperature. Do not refreeze.

Vials: Reconstituted parenteral solution is stable for 3 days at room temperature and 7 days when refrigerated. For IV infusion in NS or D_5W, solution is stable for 24 hours at room temperature and 7 days when refrigerated.

Solutions for ambulatory IV infusion reservoirs (eg, >24-hour supply) may be subject to inadvertent exposure to temperatures higher than recommended due to heat radiation from patient's skin; lower concentrations of preparation may be needed to prevent precipitation of solution in some circumstances (Chan, 2005).

Mechanism of Action Interferes with bacterial cell wall synthesis during active multiplication, causing cell wall destruction and resultant bactericidal activity against susceptible bacteria; resistant to inactivation by staphylococcal penicillinase

Pharmacodynamics/Kinetics

Distribution: Widely distributed; CSF penetration is poor but enhanced by meningeal inflammation

Protein binding: ~90%; primarily to albumin

Metabolism: Primarily hepatic; undergoes enterohepatic recirculation

Half-life elimination:

Neonates: <3 weeks: 2.2-5.5 hours; 4-9 weeks: 1.2-2.3 hours

Children 1 month to 14 years: 0.75-1.9 hours

Adults: Normal renal/hepatic function: 30-60 minutes

Time to peak, serum: IM: 30-60 minutes

Excretion: Primarily feces; urine (~30% as unchanged drug)

Dosage

Indication-specific dosing:

Children:

Mild-to-moderate infections: IM, IV: 100-150 mg/kg/day in divided doses every 6 hours (maximum dose: 4000 mg daily)

Severe infections: IM, IV: 150-200 mg/kg/day in divided doses every 4-6 hours; for life-threatening infection (eg, meningitis) daily doses up to 200 mg/kg are used (maximum dose: 12 g daily)

Adults: IV:

Endocarditis: Methicillin-susceptible *Staphylococcus aureus* (MSSA):

Native valve: 12 g/24 hours in 4-6 divided doses (ie, 2 g every 4 hours or 3 g every 6 hours) for 6 weeks. **Note:** Dosing intended for ***complicated*** right-sided infective endocarditis (IE) or left-sided IE. For ***uncomplicated*** right-sided IE, 2 weeks of therapy may be adequate (Baddour, 2005). The British Society for Antimicrobial Chemotherapy (BSAC) recommends 4 weeks of therapy with a penicillinase-resistant penicillin for all patients with native valve IE due to MSSA unless patient has intracardiac prostheses, secondary lung abscesses, or osteomyelitis, then extend treatment to ≥6 weeks (Gould, 2012).

Prosthetic valve: 12 g/24 hours in 6 divided doses (ie, 2 g every 4 hours) for ≥6 weeks (use with rifampin for entire course and gentamicin for first 2 weeks) (Baddour, 2005)

Prosthetic joint infections: *Staphylococci (oxacillin-susceptible):* 1500-2000 mg every 4-6 hours for 4-6 weeks (2-6 weeks if in combination with rifampin), followed by oral antibiotic treatment and suppressive regimens (Osmon, 2013)

Skin and soft tissue infections: *Methicillin-susceptible Staphylococcus aureus (including necrotizing infection of fascia, muscle, skin):* 1000-2000 mg every 4 hours (Stevens, 2005)

Dosing adjustment in renal impairment: No dosage adjustment is necessary unless in the setting of concomitant hepatic impairment; however, manufacturer labeling does not provide specific dosage adjustments.

Poorly dialyzed. No supplemental dose or dosage adjustment necessary, including patients on intermittent hemodialysis, peritoneal dialysis, or continuous renal replacement therapy (eg, CVVHD) (Aronoff, 2007; Heintz, 2009).

Dosing adjustment in hepatic impairment: No specific dosage adjustments provided in manufacturer's labeling; however, dosage adjustment may be necessary particularly in the setting of concomitant renal impairment; nafcillin primarily undergoes hepatic metabolism. In patients with both hepatic and renal impairment, monitoring of serum drug levels and modification of dosage may be necessary.

Dietary Considerations Some products may contain sodium.

Administration

IM: Administer as a deep intragluteal injection; rotate injection sites.

IV: Infuse over 30-60 minutes. Vesicant; ensure proper needle or catheter placement prior to and during IV infusion. Avoid extravasation.

Extravasation management: If extravasation occurs, stop infusion immediately and disconnect (leave needle/cannula in place); gently aspirate extravasated solution (do **NOT** flush the line); initiate hyaluronidase antidote; remove needle/cannula (if not using IV hyaluronidase antidote), apply dry cold compresses (Hurst, 2004); elevate extremity.

Hyaluronidase: Intradermal or SubQ: Inject a total of 1 mL (15 units/mL) as five separate 0.2 mL injections (using a 25-gauge needle) into area of extravasation at the leading edge in a clockwise manner (MacCara, 1983; Zenk, 1981).

Monitoring Parameters Baseline and periodic CBC with differential; periodic urinalysis, BUN, serum creatinine, AST and ALT; observe for signs and symptoms of anaphylaxis during first dose

Dosage Forms

Solution, Intravenous:

Nallpen in Dextrose: 1 g/50 mL (50 mL); 2 g/100 mL (100 mL)

Solution Reconstituted, Injection:

Generic: 1 g (1 ea); 2 g (1 ea); 10 g (1 ea)

Solution Reconstituted, Injection [preservative free]:

Generic: 1 g (1 ea); 2 g (1 ea); 10 g (1 ea)

Solution Reconstituted, Intravenous:

Generic: 1 g (1 ea); 2 g (1 ea)

◆ **Nafcillin Sodium** *see* Nafcillin *on page 1414*

Naftidrofuryl [INT] (naf ti DROE fu ril)

International Brand Names Artocoron (DE); Azunaftil (DE); Di-Actane (FR); Dusodril (AT, CZ, DE, HR); Esdedril (IT); Gevatran (FR); Iridus (AR); Iridux (BR); Iridux F200 (BR); Luctor (DE); Nafrolen (CY); nafti von ct (DE); Nafti-Puren (DE); Nafti-ratiopharm (DE); Naftilong (DE, HU, LU); Naftilux (FR); Naftisol (AT); Naftodril (AT); Praxilene (BE, CH, ES, FR, GB, IE, IT, LU, PT); Sodipryl (CH)

Index Terms Naftidrofuryl Oxalate

Pharmacologic Category Vasodilator

Reported Use Treatment of peripheral and cerebral vascular disorders

Dosage Range Adults: Oral:

Cerebral vascular disorders: 100 mg 3 times/day

Peripheral vascular disorders: 100-200 mg 3 times/day

Product Availability Product available in various countries; not currently available in the U.S.

Dosage Forms

Capsule: 100 mg

Tablet: 200 mg

◆ **Naftidrofuryl Oxalate** *see* Naftidrofuryl [INT] *on page 1416*

Naftifine (NAF ti feen)

Brand Names: U.S. Naftin

Index Terms Naftifine Hydrochloride

Pharmacologic Category Antifungal Agent, Topical

Use

Tinea infections: Cream 1% and 2%, Gel 1%: Topical treatment of tinea cruris (jock itch), tinea corporis (ringworm), and tinea pedis (athlete's foot).

Tinea pedis: Gel 2%: Topical treatment of tinea pedis (athlete's foot).

Pregnancy Risk Factor B

Dosage

Tinea corporis, tinea cruris:

Children ≥12 years, Adolescents, and Adults: Topical: Cream 2%: Apply a thin layer once daily to affected area and healthy surrounding skin (1/2 inch margin) for 2 weeks

Adults: Topical: Cream 1% and gel 1%: Apply once daily (cream) or twice daily (gel; morning and evening) to affected area and surrounding skin for up to 4 weeks

Tinea pedis:

Children ≥12 years, Adolescents, and Adults: Topical: Cream 2% and gel 2%: Apply a thin layer once daily to affected area and healthy surrounding skin (1/2 inch margin) for 2 weeks

Adults: Topical: Cream 1% and gel 1%: Apply once daily (cream) or twice daily (gel; morning and evening) to affected area and surrounding skin for up to 4 weeks

Additional Information Complete prescribing information should be consulted for additional detail.

Dosage Forms

Cream, External:

Naftin: 1% (60 g, 90 g); 2% (45 g, 60 g)

Gel, External:

Naftin: 1% (40 g, 60 g, 90 g); 2% (45 g, 60 g)

◆ **Naftifine Hydrochloride** *see* Naftifine *on page 1416*

◆ **Naftin** *see* Naftifine *on page 1416*

◆ **$NaHCO_3$** *see* Sodium Bicarbonate *on page 1901*

Nalbuphine (NAL byoo feen)

Index Terms Nalbuphine Hydrochloride; Nubain

Pharmacologic Category Analgesic, Opioid; Analgesic, Opioid Partial Agonist

Additional Appendix Information

Opioid Conversion Table *on page 2232*

Use Relief of moderate-to-severe pain; preoperative analgesia, postoperative and surgical anesthesia, and obstetrical analgesia during labor and delivery

Pregnancy Risk Factor C

Pregnancy Considerations Adverse events were observed in some animal reproduction studies. Nalbuphine crosses the placenta. Nalbuphine is approved for use in obstetrical analgesia during labor and delivery. When used for pain relief during labor, opioids may temporarily affect the heart rate of the fetus (ACOG, 2002) and severe fetal bradycardia has been reported following use of nalbuphine in labor/delivery. Fetal bradycardia may occur when administered earlier in pregnancy (not documented). Use only if clearly needed, with monitoring to detect and manage possible adverse fetal effects. Naloxone has been reported to reverse bradycardia. Newborn should be monitored for respiratory depression or bradycardia following nalbuphine use in labor.

If chronic opioid exposure occurs in pregnancy, adverse events in the newborn (including withdrawal) may occur; monitoring of the neonate is recommended. The minimum effective dose should be used if opioids are needed (Chou, 2009). Neonatal abstinence syndrome following opioid exposure may present with autonomic (eg, fever, temperature instability), gastrointestinal (eg, diarrhea, vomiting, poor feeding/weight gain), or neurologic (eg, high-pitched crying, increased muscle tone, irritability, seizure, tremor) symptoms (Dow, 2012; Hudak, 2012).

Breast-Feeding Considerations Small amounts (<1% of maternal dose) of nalbuphine are excreted in breast milk. The manufacturer recommends that caution be exercised when administering nalbuphine to nursing women.

Parenteral opioids used during labor have the potential to interfere with a newborns natural reflex to nurse within the first few hours after birth. If nalbuphine is administered to a nursing woman, it is recommended to monitor both the mother and baby for psychotomimetic reactions. Nursing infants exposed to large doses of opioids should also be monitored for apnea and sedation (Montgomery, 2012).

Contraindications Hypersensitivity to nalbuphine or any component of the formulation

Warnings/Precautions Use caution in CNS depression. Sedation and psychomotor impairment are likely, and are additive with other CNS depressants or ethanol. May cause respiratory depression. Ambulatory patients must be cautioned about performing tasks which require mental alertness (eg, operating machinery or driving). Potentially significant drug interactions may exist, requiring dose or frequency adjustment, additional monitoring, and/or selection of alternative therapy. Effects may be potentiated when used with other sedative drugs or ethanol. Use with caution in patients with recent myocardial infarction, biliary tract impairment, pancreatitis, morbid obesity, thyroid dysfunction, head trauma, or increased intracranial pressure. Avoid use in patients with CNS depression or coma as these patients are susceptible to intracranial effects of CO_2 retention. Use caution in patients with prostatic hyperplasia and/or urinary stricture, adrenal insufficiency, decreased hepatic or renal function. Use with caution in patients with preexisting respiratory compromise (hypoxia and/or hypercapnia), COPD or other obstructive pulmonary disease; critical respiratory depression may occur, even at therapeutic dosages. May cause hypotension; use with caution in patients with hypovolemia, cardiovascular disease (including acute MI), or drugs which may exaggerate hypotensive effects (including phenothiazines or general anesthetics). May obscure diagnosis or clinical course of patients with acute abdominal conditions. May result in tolerance and/or drug dependence with chronic use; use with caution in patients with a history of drug dependence. Abrupt discontinuation following prolonged use may lead to withdrawal symptoms. May precipitate withdrawal symptoms in patients following prolonged therapy with mu opioid agonists.

Use with caution in pregnancy (close neonatal monitoring required when used in labor and delivery). After chronic maternal exposure to opioids, neonatal withdrawal syndrome may occur in the newborn; monitor neonate closely. Signs and symptoms include irritability, hyperactivity and abnormal sleep pattern, high pitched cry, tremor, vomiting, diarrhea and failure to gain weight. Onset, duration and severity depend on the drug used, duration of use, maternal dose, and rate of drug elimination by the newborn. Opioid withdrawal syndrome in the neonate, unlike in adults, may be life-threatening and should be treated according to protocols developed by neonatology experts. Use with caution in the elderly and debilitated patients; may be more sensitive to adverse effects.

Adverse Reactions

Central nervous system: Dizziness, headache, sedation

Dermatologic: Cold and clammy skin

Gastrointestinal: Nausea/vomiting, xerostomia

Rare but important or life-threatening: Abdominal pain, abnormal dreams, agitation, anaphylactoid reaction, anaphylaxis, anxiety, asthma, bitter taste, blurred vision, bradycardia, burning sensation, cardiac arrest, confusion, crying, delusions, depersonalization, depression, derealization, diaphoresis, drowsiness, dyspepsia, dysphoria, euphoria, fever, floating feeling, flushing, hallucination, hostility, hypersensitivity reaction, hypertension, hypogonadism (Brennan, 2013; Debono, 2011), hypotension, injection site reaction (pain, swelling, redness, burning), intestinal cramps, laryngeal edema, loss of consciousness, nervousness, numbness, pruritus, pulmonary edema, respiratory depression, respiratory distress, restlessness, seizure, skin rash, speech disturbance, stridor, tachycardia, tingling sensation, tremor, urinary urgency, urticaria

Drug Interactions

Metabolism/Transport Effects None known.

Avoid Concomitant Use

Avoid concomitant use of Nalbuphine with any of the following: Azelastine (Nasal); Orphenadrine; Paraldehyde; Thalidomide

Increased Effect/Toxicity

Nalbuphine may increase the levels/effects of: Alcohol (Ethyl); Alvimopan; Azelastine (Nasal); Buprenorphine; CNS Depressants; Desmopressin; Diuretics; Hydrocodone; Methotrimeprazine; Metyrosine; Mirtazapine; Orphenadrine; Paraldehyde; Pramipexole; ROPINIRole; Rotigotine; Selective Serotonin Reuptake Inhibitors; Suvorexant; Thalidomide; Zolpidem

The levels/effects of Nalbuphine may be increased by: Amphetamines; Anticholinergic Agents; Antipsychotic Agents (Phenothiazines); Brimonidine (Topical); Cannabis; Doxylamine; Dronabinol; Droperidol; HydrOXYzine; Kava Kava; Magnesium Sulfate; Methotrimeprazine; Nabilone; Perampanel; Rufinamide; Sodium Oxybate; Succinylcholine; Tapentadol; Tetrahydrocannabinol

Decreased Effect

Nalbuphine may decrease the levels/effects of: Analgesics (Opioid); Pegvisomant

The levels/effects of Nalbuphine may be decreased by: Ammonium Chloride; Mixed Agonist / Antagonist Opioids; Naltrexone

Storage/Stability Store at 20°C to 25°C (68°F to 77°F). Protect from light.

Mechanism of Action Agonist of kappa opiate receptors and partial antagonist of mu opiate receptors in the CNS, causing inhibition of ascending pain pathways, altering the perception of and response to pain; produces generalized CNS depression

Pharmacodynamics/Kinetics

Onset of action: Peak effect: SubQ, IM: <15 minutes; IV: 2-3 minutes

Metabolism: Hepatic

Half-life elimination: 5 hours

Excretion: Feces; urine (~7% as metabolites)

Dosage

Children ≥1 year (off-label use): Pain management: IM, IV, SubQ: 0.1-0.2 mg/kg every 3-4 hours as needed; maximum: 20 mg/dose and/or 160 mg/day

Adults:

Pain management: IM, IV, SubQ: 10 mg/70 kg every 3-6 hours; maximum single dose in nonopioid-tolerant patients: 20 mg; maximum daily dose: 160 mg

Surgical anesthesia supplement: IV: Induction: 0.3-3 mg/kg over 10-15 minutes; maintenance doses of 0.25-0.5 mg/kg may be given as required

Opioid-induced pruritus (off-label use): IV 2.5-5 mg; may repeat dose

Dosing adjustment in renal impairment: Use with caution and reduce dose; monitor.

Dosing adjustment in hepatic impairment: Use with caution and reduce dose.

Administration Administer IM, SubQ, or IV

Monitoring Parameters Relief of pain, respiratory and mental status, blood pressure; signs or symptoms of hypogonadism or hypoadrenalism (Brennan, 2013)

Dosage Forms

Solution, Injection:

Generic: 10 mg/mL (1 mL, 10 mL); 20 mg/mL (1 mL, 10 mL)

◆ **Nalbuphine Hydrochloride** *see* Nalbuphine *on page 1416*

◆ **Nalfon** *see* Fenoprofen *on page 857*

Nalidixic Acid [INT] (nal i DIKS ik AS id)

International Brand Names Acido Nalidixico Prodes (ES); Entolon (JP); Gramazine (TW); Gramoneg (IN, TH); Innoxalon (JP); Jicsron (JP); Kusnarin (JP); Mictral (GB); Nal-Acid (GR); Naldix (AE, BH, CY, EG, IL, IQ, IR, JO, KW, LB, LY, OM, QA, SA, SY, YE); Nali 500 (UY); Nalidix (AE, BH, CY, EG, IL, IQ, IR, JO, KW, LB, LY, OM, QA, SA, SY, YE); Nalidixic (VN); Nalidixin (CZ); Nalidixol (ES); Nalitucsan (JP); Nalixan (FI); Nalixone (MX); Narigix (JP); NegGram (IT); Negadix (IN); Negram (AE, AU, BH, CY, DE, EG, FR, GB, IE, IL, IQ, IR, JO, KW, LB, LY, NL, NO, OM, PK, QA, RU, SA, SY, TR, YE); Neladix (BG); Nevigramon (HN, HU, PL); Nicelate (JP); Nogermin (ES); Nogram (DE); Perry (TW); Poleon (JP); Puromylon (ZA); Renogram (HR); Sicmylon (JP); Unaserus (JP); Uriben (GB); Urineg (ID); Urogram (HR); Windol (TW); Winlomylon (BF, BJ, CI, ET, GH, GM, GN, KE, LR, MA, ML, MR, MU, MW, NE, NG, SC, SD, SL, SN, TN, TZ, UG, ZA, ZM, ZW); Wintomilon (PT); Wintomylon (AR, BF, BJ, BR, CI, CO, EC, ET, GH, GM, GN, KE, LR, MA, ML, MR, MU, MW, MX, MY, NE, NG, PE, SC, SD, SL, SN, TH, TN, TZ, UG, ZM, ZW); Wintron (JP)

Index Terms Nalidixinic Acid

Pharmacologic Category Antibiotic, Quinolone

Reported Use Treatment of urinary tract infections

Dosage Range Oral:

Children 3 months to 12 years: 55 mg/kg/day divided every 6 hours; suppressive therapy is 30 mg/kg/day divided every 6 hours

Adults: 1 g 4 times/day for 2 weeks; then suppressive therapy of 500 mg 4 times/day

Dosing comments in renal impairment: CrCl <50 mL/minute: Avoid use

Product Availability Product available in various countries; not currently available in the U.S.

Dosage Forms

Suspension, oral: 250 mg/5 mL (473 mL) [raspberry flavor] [Not available in the U.S.]

Tablet: 500 mg [Not available in the U.S.]

◆ **Nalidixinic Acid** *see* Nalidixic Acid [INT] *on page 1418*

◆ **Nallpen** *see* Nafcillin *on page 1414*

◆ **Nallpen in Dextrose** *see* Nafcillin *on page 1414*

◆ ***N*-allylnoroxymorphine Hydrochloride** *see* Naloxone *on page 1419*

Naloxegol (nal OX ee gol)

Brand Names: U.S. Movantik

Index Terms Movantik; Naloxegol Oxalate; NKTR-118

Pharmacologic Category Gastrointestinal Agent, Miscellaneous; Opioid Antagonist, Peripherally-Acting

Use Opioid-induced constipation: Treatment of opioid-induced constipation (OIC) in adult patients with chronic noncancer pain.

Pregnancy Risk Factor C

Pregnancy Considerations Adverse events were not observed in animal reproduction studies. However, exposure during pregnancy may potentiate opioid withdrawal in the fetus.

Breast-Feeding Considerations It is not known if naloxegol is excreted into breast milk. Due to the potential for serious adverse reactions (which could include opioid withdrawal in the nursing infant), the manufacturer recommends a decision be made whether to discontinue nursing or to discontinue the drug, taking into account the importance of treatment to the mother.

Contraindications Serious or severe hypersensitivity reaction to naloxegol or any component of the formulation; known or suspected GI obstruction or at increased risk of recurrent obstruction; concomitant use with strong CYP3A4 inhibitors (eg, clarithromycin, ketoconazole)

Warnings/Precautions GI perforation has been reported with use of another peripherally acting opioid antagonist (ie, methylnaltrexone) in patients with reduced wall integrity of the GI tract (eg, peptic ulcer disease, Ogilvie syndrome, diverticular disease, infiltrative gastrointestinal tract malignancies, peritoneal metastases). Consider the overall risk-benefit profile when using naloxegol in patients with these conditions or other conditions which might result in impaired integrity of the GI tract wall (eg, Crohn disease). Monitor for development of severe, persistent or worsening abdominal pain; discontinue naloxegol if this occurs. Use is contraindicated in patients with known or suspected GI obstruction or at increased risk of recurrent obstruction.

Symptoms consistent with opioid withdrawal (eg, hyperhidrosis, chills, abdominal pain, anxiety, irritability) have occurred. In clinical trials, patients receiving methadone for pain management were observed to have a higher frequency of GI adverse reactions that may have been related to opioid withdrawal than patients receiving other opioids. Patients having disruptions to the blood-brain barrier may be at increased risk for opioid withdrawal or reduced analgesia. Consider the overall risk-benefit profile when using naloxegol in such patients. Monitor for symptoms of opioid withdrawal in such patients.

Avoid use of naloxegol in patients with severe hepatic impairment (dosage has not been determined). No dosage adjustment is necessary for patients with mild or moderate hepatic impairment. Dosage reduction recommended for patients with CrCl <60 mL/minute (ie, moderate, severe, or end-stage renal disease). No dosage adjustment is necessary for patients with mild renal impairment. Potentially significant interactions may exist, requiring dose or frequency adjustment, additional monitoring, and/or selection of alternative therapy. Discontinue naloxegol if opioids are discontinued.

Adverse Reactions

Central nervous system: Headache

Dermatologic: Hyperhidrosis

Gastrointestinal: Abdominal pain, diarrhea, flatulence, nausea, vomiting

Rare but important or life-threatening:Anxiety, arthritis, back pain, chills, gastrointestinal perforation, irritability, joint pain, yawning

Drug Interactions

Metabolism/Transport Effects Substrate of CYP3A4 (major), P-glycoprotein; **Note:** Assignment of Major/Minor substrate status based on clinically relevant drug interaction potential

Avoid Concomitant Use

Avoid concomitant use of Naloxegol with any of the following: Conivaptan; CYP3A4 Inducers (Strong); CYP3A4 Inhibitors (Moderate); CYP3A4 Inhibitors (Strong); Fusidic Acid (Systemic); Grapefruit Juice; Idelalisib; Methylnaltrexone; Opioid Antagonists; St Johns Wort

Increased Effect/Toxicity

The levels/effects of Naloxegol may be increased by: Conivaptan; CYP3A4 Inhibitors (Moderate); CYP3A4 Inhibitors (Strong); Dasatinib; Fusidic Acid (Systemic); Grapefruit Juice; Idelalisib; Ivacaftor; Luliconazole; Methylnaltrexone; Mifepristone; Opioid Antagonists; P-glycoprotein/ABCB1 Inhibitors; Simeprevir

Decreased Effect

The levels/effects of Naloxegol may be decreased by: Bosentan; CYP3A4 Inducers (Moderate); CYP3A4 Inducers (Strong); Dabrafenib; Deferasirox; P-glycoprotein/ABCB1 Inducers; Siltuximab; St Johns Wort; Tocilizumab

Storage/Stability Store at 20°C to 25°C (68°F to 77°F); excursions are permitted between 15°C and 30°C (59°F and 86°F).

Mechanism of Action Naloxegol is a mu-opioid receptor antagonist. It is composed of naloxone conjugated with a polyethylene glycol polymer, which limits its ability to cross the blood-brain barrier. When administered at the recommended dose, naloxegol functions peripherally in tissues such as the GI tract, thereby decreasing the constipation associated with opioids (Webster, 2013).

Pharmacodynamics/Kinetics

Absorption: Rapid. With a high-fat meal, C_{max} and AUC increased by 30% and 45%, respectively.

Distribution: V_d: 968 to 2,140 L

Protein binding: ~4.2%

Metabolism: Hepatic via CYP3A (primarily). Data suggests no major metabolites. Minor metabolites formed via N-dealkylation, O-demethylation, oxidation and partial loss of the PEG chain.

Half-life elimination: 6 to 11 hours

Time to peak: <2 hours; in majority of subjects, a secondary C_{max} occurs ~0.4 to 3 hours after the first C_{max}

Excretion: Feces (68%; ~16% as unchanged drug); Urine (16%; <6% as unchanged drug)

Dosage Note: Discontinue all maintenance laxative therapy prior to use; may reintroduce laxatives as needed if suboptimal response to naloxegol after 3 days. Alteration in analgesic dosing regimen prior to initiating naloxegol is not required.

Opioid-induced constipation: Adults: Oral: 25 mg once daily in the morning on an empty stomach. If not tolerated, reduce dose to 12.5 mg once daily. Discontinue treatment if opioid pain medication is discontinued.

Dosing adjustment with concomitant medications:

Moderate CYP3A4 Inhibitors (eg, diltiazem, erythromycin, verapamil): Avoid concomitant use. If concurrent use is unavoidable, reduce dose of naloxegol to 12.5 mg once daily and monitor for adverse reactions.

Strong CYP3A4 inhibitors (eg, clarithromycin, ketoconazole): Concomitant use is contraindicated.

Dosage adjustment in renal impairment:

CrCl ≥60 mL/minute: No dosage adjustment necessary.

CrCl <60 mL/minute: Initial dose 12.5 mg once daily; if well tolerated but opioid-induced constipation symptoms continue, may increase to 25 mg once daily, taking into consideration the potential for markedly increased exposures in some patients with renal impairment and the increased risk of adverse reactions with higher exposures.

Dosage adjustment in hepatic impairment:

Mild to moderate impairment: No dosage adjustment necessary.

Severe impairment: Avoid use (has not been studied).

Dietary Considerations Take on an empty stomach. Avoid grapefruit or grapefruit juice.

Administration Oral: Administer naloxegol on an empty stomach at least 1 hour prior to or 2 hours after the first meal of the day. Swallow tablets whole, do not crush or chew. Avoid consumption of grapefruit or grapefruit juice during treatment.

Monitoring Parameters Symptoms of GI obstruction (eg, severe, persistent, or worsening abdominal pain); symptoms of opioid withdrawal (eg, chills, diaphoresis, anxiety, irritability, changes in blood pressure or heart rate).

Product Availability Movantik: FDA approved September 2014; anticipated availability is first half of 2015.

Dosage Forms

Tablet, Oral:

Movantik: 12.5 mg, 25 mg

◆ **Naloxegol Oxalate** *see* Naloxegol *on page 1418*

Naloxone (nal OKS one)

Brand Names: U.S. Evzio

Brand Names: Canada Naloxone Hydrochloride Injection; Naloxone Hydrochloride Injection USP

Index Terms *N*-allylnoroxymorphine Hydrochloride; Naloxone Hydrochloride; Narcan

Pharmacologic Category Antidote; Opioid Antagonist

Use

Opioid overdose: For the complete or partial reversal of opioid depression (including respiratory depression) induced by natural and synthetic opioids (eg, propoxyphene, methadone, nalbuphine, butorphanol, pentazocine). Naloxone is also indicated for the diagnosis of suspected or known acute opioid overdosage.

Evzio: For the emergency treatment of known or suspected opioid overdose as manifested by respiratory and/or CNS depression. Intended for immediate administration as emergency therapy in settings where opioids may be present. Not a substitute for emergency medical care.

Septic shock: For use as an adjunctive agent to increase blood pressure in the management of septic shock. **Note:** Naloxone is no longer a recommended adjunctive agent for the treatment of septic shock (Dellinger, 2013).

Pregnancy Risk Factor B/C (product-specific)

Pregnancy Considerations Adverse events were not observed in animal reproduction studies. Naloxone crosses the placenta. Consider the benefit to the mother and the risk to the fetus before administering to a pregnant woman who is known or suspected to be opioid dependent; may precipitate withdrawal in both the mother and fetus. In general, medications used as antidotes should take into consideration the health and prognosis of the mother; antidotes should be administered to pregnant women if there is a clear indication for use and should not be withheld because of fears of teratogenicity (Bailey, 2003). Use caution in pregnant women with mild-to-moderate hypertension during labor; severe hypertension may occur.

Breast-Feeding Considerations It is not known if naloxone is excreted into breast milk, however, systemic absorption following oral administration is low (Smith, 2012) and any exposure of naloxone to a nursing infant would therefore be limited. Since naloxone is used for opioid reversal, the opioid concentrations in the milk of a breast-feeding mother and potential transfer of the opioid to the infant should be considered.

Contraindications Hypersensitivity to naloxone or any component of the formulation

Warnings/Precautions Use with caution in patients with cardiovascular disease or in patients receiving medications with potential adverse cardiovascular effects (eg, hypotension, pulmonary edema, or arrhythmias); pulmonary edema and cardiovascular instability, including ventricular fibrillation, have been reported in association with abrupt reversal when using opioid antagonists. Administration of naloxone causes the release of catecholamines, which may precipitate acute withdrawal or unmask pain in those who regularly take opioids. Symptoms of acute withdrawal in opioid-dependent patients may include pain, hypertension, sweating, agitation, and irritability. In neonates born to mothers with narcotic dependence, opioid withdrawal may be life-threatening and symptoms may include shrill cry, failure to feed, seizures, and hyperactive reflexes. Carefully titrate the dose to reverse hypoventilation; do not fully awaken patient or reverse analgesic effect (postoperative patient). Excessive dosages should be avoided after use of opioids in surgery. Abrupt postoperative reversal may result in nausea, vomiting, sweating, tachycardia, hypertension, seizures, and other cardiovascular events (including pulmonary edema and ▶

arrhythmias). Reversal of partial opioid agonists or mixed opioid agonist/antagonists (eg, buprenorphine, pentazocine) may be incomplete and large doses of naloxone may be required. Recurrence of respiratory depression is possible if the opioid involved is long-acting; observe patients until there is no reasonable risk of recurrent respiratory depression.

To prevent overdose deaths, there are initiatives to dispense naloxone for self- or buddy-administration to patients at risk of opioid overdose (eg, recipients of high-dose opioids, suspected or confirmed history of illicit opioid use) and individuals likely to be present in an overdose situation (eg, family members of illicit drug users) (Albert, 2011; Bennett, 2011); Evzio is indicated for emergency treatment. Needleless administration via nebulization and the intranasal route by first responders and bystanders has also been described (Doe-Simkins, 2009; Weber, 2012). Needleless administration provides an alternative route of administration in patients with venous scarring due to illicit drug use (eg, heroin). There is a low incidence of death following naloxone reversal of opioid toxicity in patients who refuse transport to a healthcare facility (Wampler, 2011). Nevertheless, patients who received naloxone in the out-of-hospital setting should seek immediate emergency medical assistance after the first dose due to the likelihood that respiratory and/or central nervous system depression will return.

When the auto-injector (Evzio) is administered to infants <1 year of age, monitor the injection site for residual needle parts and signs of infection.

Adverse Reactions Adverse reactions are related to reversing dependency and precipitating withdrawal. Withdrawal symptoms are the result of sympathetic excess. Adverse events occur secondarily to reversal (withdrawal) of opioid analgesia and sedation.

Cardiovascular: Cardiac arrest, fever, flushing, hypertension, hypotension, tachycardia, ventricular fibrillation ventricular tachycardia

Central nervous system: Agitation, coma, crying (excessive [neonates]), encephalopathy, hallucination, irritability, nervousness, restlessness, seizure (neonates), tremulousness

Gastrointestinal: Abdominal cramps, diarrhea, nausea, vomiting

Local: Injection site reaction

Neuromuscular & skeletal: Ache, hyperreflexia (neonates), paresthesia, piloerection, tremor, weakness

Respiratory: Dyspnea, hypoxia, pulmonary edema, respiratory depression, rhinorrhea, sneezing

Miscellaneous: Diaphoresis, hot flashes, shivering, yawning

Drug Interactions

Metabolism/Transport Effects None known.

Avoid Concomitant Use

Avoid concomitant use of Naloxone with any of the following: Methylnaltrexone; Naloxegol

Increased Effect/Toxicity

Naloxone may increase the levels/effects of: Naloxegol

The levels/effects of Naloxone may be increased by: Methylnaltrexone

Decreased Effect There are no known significant interactions involving a decrease in effect.

Preparation for Administration

IV push: Dilute naloxone 0.4 mg (1 mL ampul) with 9 mL of NS for a total volume of 10 mL to achieve a concentration of 0.04 mg/mL (APS, 2008)

IV infusion: Dilute naloxone 2 mg in 500 mL of NS or D_5W to make a final concentration of 4 **mcg**/mL

Inhalation via nebulization (off-label route): Dilute 2 mg of naloxone with 3 mL of normal saline (Mycyk, 2003; Weber, 2012)

Storage/Stability

Solution, injection: Store at 20°C to 25°C (68°F to 77°F). Protect from light. Use IV infusion within 24 hours of preparation.

Solution, auto-injector (Evzio): Store at 15°C to 25°C (59°F to 77°F); excursions are permitted between 4°C and 40°C (39°F and 104°F). Store in the outer case provided.

Mechanism of Action Pure opioid antagonist that competes and displaces opioids at opioid receptor sites

Pharmacodynamics/Kinetics

Onset of action: Endotracheal, IM, SubQ: 2 to 5 minutes; Inhalation via nebulization: ~5 minutes (Mycyk, 2003); Intranasal: ~8 to 13 minutes (Kelley, 2005; Robertson, 2009); IV: ~2 minutes

Duration: ~30 to 120 minutes depending on route of administration; IV has a shorter duration of action than IM administration; since naloxone's action is shorter than that of most opioids, repeated doses are usually needed

Metabolism: Primarily hepatic via glucuronidation

Time to peak: IM, SubQ (Evzio): 15 minutes

Half-life elimination: Neonates: 3 to 4 hours; Adults: 0.5 to 1.5 hours

Excretion: Urine (as metabolites)

Dosage Note: Available routes of administration include IV (preferred), IM, and SubQ; other available routes (off-label) include endotracheal, inhalation via nebulization (adults only), intranasal (adults only), and intraosseous (I.O.). Endotracheal administration is the least desirable and is supported by only anecdotal evidence (case report) (Neumar, 2010); nebulized naloxone has been shown to be an effective alternative to parenteral administration when needleless administration is desired (Weber, 2012):

Infants, Children, and Adolescents:

Opioid overdose (with standard PALS protocols): IV, IM, SubQ, intraosseous (I.O.) (off-label route), endotracheal (off-label route): **Note:** IV administration is preferred; I.O. and endotracheal routes are alternative routes recommended by the PALS guidelines (Kleinman, 2010):

<5 years or ≤20 kg (off-label dose): 0.1 mg/kg/dose (maximum dose: 2 mg); repeat every 2 to 3 minutes if needed (Hegenbarth, 2008; Kleinman, 2010)

≥5 years or >20 kg: 2 mg; if no response, repeat every 2 to 3 minutes. If no response is observed after 10 mg total, consider other causes of respiratory depression (Hegenbarth, 2008; Kleinman, 2010).

Manufacturer's labeling: IV (preferred), IM, SubQ: Initial: 0.01 mg/kg/dose; if no response, a subsequent dose of 0.1 mg/kg may be given; **Note:** if using IM or SubQ route, dose should be given in divided doses.

Continuous infusion (off-label dosing): IV: If continuous infusion is required, calculate dosage/hour based on effective intermittent dose used and duration of adequate response seen (Tenenbein, 1984) **or** use two-thirds (2/3) of the initial effective naloxone bolus on an hourly basis; titrate dose (typically 0.04 to 0.16 mg/kg/hour for 2 to 5 days in children); one-half (1/2) of the initial bolus dose should be readministered 15 minutes after initiation of the continuous infusion to prevent a drop in naloxone levels; increase infusion rate as needed to assure adequate ventilation and prevent withdrawal symptoms (Goldfrank, 1986). **Note:** The infusion should be discontinued by reducing the infusion in decrements of 25%; closely monitor the patient (eg, pulse oximetry) after each adjustment and after discontinuation of the infusion for recurrence of opioid-induced respiratory depression (Perry, 1996).

IM, SubQ (Evzio): 0.4 mg (contents of 1 auto-injector) as a single dose; may repeat every 2 to 3 minutes until emergency medical assistance becomes available.

Reversal of respiratory depression with therapeutic opioid dosing: IV: 0.001 to 0.015 mg/kg/dose; dose may be repeated as needed (Hegenbarth, 2008; Kleinman, 2010)

Postoperative reversal: IV: 0.005 to 0.01 mg/kg (Fischer, 1974); may repeat every 2 to 3 minutes as needed based on response (adequate ventilation without significant pain)

Adults:

Opioid overdose (with standard ACLS protocols):

IV, IM, SubQ: Initial: 0.4 to 2 mg; may need to repeat doses every 2 to 3 minutes; after reversal, may need to readminister dose(s) at a later interval (ie, 20 to 60 minutes) depending on type/duration of opioid. If no response is observed after 10 mg total, consider other causes of respiratory depression. **Note:** May be given endotracheally (off-label route) as 2 to 2.5 times the initial IV dose (ie, 0.8 to 5 mg) (Neumar, 2010).

Continuous infusion (off-label dosing): IV: **Note:** For use with exposures to long-acting opioids (eg, methadone), sustained release product, and symptomatic body packers after initial naloxone response. Calculate dosage/hour based on effective intermittent dose used and duration of adequate response seen (Tenenbein, 1984) **or** use two-thirds (2/3) of the initial effective naloxone bolus on an hourly basis (typically 0.25 to 6.25 mg/hour); one-half (1/2) of the initial bolus dose should be readministered 15 minutes after initiation of the continuous infusion to prevent a drop in naloxone levels; adjust infusion rate as needed to assure adequate ventilation and prevent withdrawal symptoms (Goldfrank, 1986).

IM, SubQ (Evzio): 0.4 mg (contents of 1 auto-injector) as a single dose; may repeat every 2 to 3 minutes until emergency medical assistance becomes available.

Inhalation via nebulization (off-label route): 2 mg; may repeat. Switch to IV or IM administration when possible (Weber, 2012).

Intranasal administration (off-label route): 2 mg (1 mg per nostril); may repeat in 5 minutes if respiratory depression persists. **Note:** Onset of action is slightly delayed compared to IM or IV routes (Kelly, 2005; Robertson, 2009; Vanden Hoek, 2010).

Reversal of respiratory depression with therapeutic opioid doses: IV, IM, SubQ.: Initial: 0.04 to 0.4 mg; may repeat until desired response achieved. If desired response is not observed after 0.8 mg total, consider other causes of respiratory depression. **Note:** May be given endotracheally (off-label route) as 2 to 2.5 times the initial IV dose (ie, 0.08 to 1 mg) (Neumar, 2010).

Continuous infusion (off-label dosing): IV: **Note:** For use with exposures to long-acting opioids (eg, methadone) or sustained release products. Calculate dosage/hour based on effective intermittent dose used and duration of adequate response seen (Tenenbein, 1984) **or** use two-thirds (2/3) of the initial effective naloxone bolus on an hourly basis (typically 0.2 to 0.6 mg/hour); one-half (1/2) of the initial bolus dose should be readministered 15 minutes after initiation of the continuous infusion to prevent a drop in naloxone levels; adjust infusion rate as needed to assure adequate ventilation and prevent withdrawal symptoms (Goldfrank, 1986).

Opioid-dependent patients being treated for cancer pain (NCCN guidelines, v.2.2011): IV: 0.04 to 0.08 mg (40 to 80 **mcg**) slow IV push; administer every 30 to 60 seconds until improvement in symptoms; if no response is observed after total naloxone dose 1 mg, consider other causes of respiratory depression. **Note:** May dilute 0.4 mg/mL (1 mL) ampul into 9 mL of normal saline for a total volume of 10 mL to achieve a 0.04 mg/mL (40 **mcg**/mL) concentration.

Postoperative reversal: IV: 0.1 to 0.2 mg every 2 to 3 minutes until desired response (adequate ventilation and alertness without significant pain). **Note:** Repeat doses may be needed within 1 to 2 hour intervals depending on type, dose, and timing of the last dose of opioid administered.

Opioid-induced pruritus (off-label use): IV infusion: 0.25 **mcg/kg/hour**; **Note:** Monitor pain control; verify that the naloxone is not reversing analgesia (Gan, 1997)

Dosage adjustment in renal impairment: There are no dosage adjustments provided in the manufacturer's labeling.

Dosage adjustment in hepatic impairment: There are no dosage adjustments provided in the manufacturer's labeling.

Administration

IV push: Administer over 30 seconds as undiluted preparation **or** administer as diluted preparation slow IV push by diluting 0.4 mg (1 mL) ampul with 9 mL of normal saline for a total volume of 10 mL to achieve a concentration of 0.04 mg/mL (APS, 2008)

IV continuous infusion: Dilute to 4 **mcg**/mL in D_5W or normal saline

IM, SubQ: May administer IM or SubQ if unable to obtain IV access

Auto-injector: Evzio: For IM or SubQ use only. Intended for buddy administration; the person administering the medication should follow the printed instructions on the device or the electronic voice instructions coming from the speaker on the device. If the voice instruction system does not operate properly, the device will still deliver the intended dose of naloxone when properly administered. Administer IM or SubQ into the anterolateral aspect of the thigh; may be injected through clothing. When being administered to infants <1 year of age, the thigh muscle should be pinched during administration. Following proper administration, a red indicator appears in the viewing window; the needle is not visible before, during, or after the injection. Patients who received naloxone in the out-of-hospital setting should seek immediate emergency medical assistance after the first dose due to the likelihood that respiratory and/or central nervous system depression will return. Repeat doses may be required until emergency medical assistance becomes available; a new device must be used as each device contains a single dose of naloxone.

Endotracheal (off-label route): There is only anecdotal support for this route of administration. May require a slightly higher dose than used in other routes. Dilute to 1 to 2 mL with normal saline; flush with 5 mL of saline and then administer 5 ventilations (Neumar, 2010).

Inhalation via nebulization (off-label route): Dilute 2 mg of naloxone with 3 mL of normal saline and administer via nebulizer face mask (Mycyk, 2003; Weber, 2012).

Intranasal (off-label route): Administer total dose equally divided into each nostril using a mucosal atomizer device (MAD) (Kelly, 2005; Robertson, 2009; Vanden Hoek, 2010).

Monitoring Parameters Respiratory rate, heart rate, blood pressure, temperature, level of consciousness, ABGs or pulse oximetry

Additional Information May contain methyl and propylparabens

Dosage Forms

Solution, Injection:

Generic: 0.4 mg/mL (1 mL, 10 mL)

Solution, Injection [preservative free]:

Generic: 1 mg/mL (2 mL)

Solution Auto-injector, Injection:

Evzio: 0.4 mg/0.4 mL (0.4 mL)

◆ **Naloxone and Buprenorphine** *see* Buprenorphine and Naloxone *on page 304*

◆ **Naloxone and Oxycodone** *see* Oxycodone and Naloxone *on page 1542*

◆ **Naloxone Hydrochloride** *see* Naloxone *on page 1419*

◆ **Naloxone Hydrochloride Dihydrate and Buprenorphine Hydrochloride** *see* Buprenorphine and Naloxone *on page 304*

◆ **Naloxone Hydrochloride Injection (Can)** *see* Naloxone *on page 1419*

◆ **Naloxone Hydrochloride Injection USP (Can)** *see* Naloxone *on page 1419*

Naltrexone (nal TREKS one)

Brand Names: U.S. ReVia; Vivitrol

Brand Names: Canada ReVia

Index Terms Naltrexone Hydrochloride

Pharmacologic Category Antidote; Opioid Antagonist

Use

Alcohol dependence: Treatment of alcohol dependence.

Opioid dependence: For the blockade of the effects of exogenously administered opioids.

Pregnancy Risk Factor C

Pregnancy Considerations Adverse events were observed in animal reproduction studies.

Breast-Feeding Considerations Naltrexone is excreted into breast milk. Due to the potential for serious adverse reactions in the nursing infant, the manufacturer recommends a decision be made whether to discontinue nursing or to discontinue the drug, taking into account the importance of treatment to the mother.

Contraindications Hypersensitivity to naltrexone or any component of the formulation; opioid dependence or current use of opioid analgesics (including partial opioid agonists); acute opioid withdrawal; failure to pass naloxone challenge or positive urine screen for opioids

Warnings/Precautions Dose-related hepatocellular injury is possible; the margin of separation between the apparent safe and hepatotoxic doses appears to be ≤5-fold. Discontinue therapy if signs/symptoms of acute hepatitis develop. Clinicians should note that elevated transaminases may be a result of preexisting alcoholic liver disease, hepatitis B and/or C infection, or concomitant use of other hepatotoxic drugs; abrupt opioid withdrawal may also lead to acute liver injury. Therapy may precipitate withdrawal symptoms in patients addicted to opioids; patients should be opioid-free (including tramadol) for a minimum of 7-10 days; a naloxone challenge test may help to confirm patient is opioid-free prior to therapy if there is any suspicion since urinary opioid screen may not be sufficient proof. Patients transitioning from buprenorphine or methadone may be vulnerable to precipitation of withdrawal symptoms for as long as 2 weeks. Use of naltrexone does not eliminate or diminish withdrawal symptoms. Patients who had been treated with naltrexone may respond to lower opioid doses than previously used. This could result in potentially life-threatening opioid intoxication. Patients should be aware that they may be more sensitive to lower doses of opioids after naltrexone treatment is discontinued, after a missed dose, or near the end of the dosing interval. Warn patients that any attempt to overcome opioid blockade during naltrexone therapy, could potentially lead to fatal opioid overdose; the opioid competitive receptor blockade produced by naltrexone is potentially surmountable in the presence of large amounts of opioids. In naltrexone-treated patients requiring emergency pain management, consider alternatives to opioid therapy (eg, regional analgesia, nonopioid analgesics, general anesthesia). If opioid therapy is required for pain therapy, patients should be under the direct care of a trained anesthesia provider.

Suicidal thoughts, attempted suicide, and depression have been reported postmarketing; monitor closely. Hypersensitivity, including anaphylaxis, has been reported. Cases of eosinophilic pneumonia have been reported and should be considered in patients presenting with progressive hypoxia and dyspnea. Use with caution in patients with severe hepatic impairment (has not been studied; if coagulopathy presents, IM injection may cause hematoma formation). Use with caution in patients with moderate-to-severe renal impairment (has not been studied). Use IM injection with caution in patients with thrombocytopenia or any bleeding disorder (hemophilia and severe hepatic failure), and patients on anticoagulant therapy; bleeding/hematoma may occur from IM administration. Serious injection site reactions (eg, cellulitis, induration, hematoma, abscess, necrosis) have been reported with use, including severe cases requiring surgical debridement. Females appear to be at a higher risk. Patients should report any injection site pain, swelling, bruising, pruritus, or redness that does not improve (or worsens). For IM use only in the gluteal muscle; do **not** administer IV, SubQ, or into fatty tissue; incorrect administration may increase the risk of injection site reactions. Vehicle used in the injectable naltrexone formulation (polylactide-co-glycolide microspheres) has rarely been associated with retinal artery occlusion in patients with abnormal arteriovenous anastomosis following injection of other drug products that also use the polylactide-co-glycolide microspheres vehicle.

Adverse Reactions Combined reporting of adverse events from oral and injectable formulations:

Cardiovascular: Hypertension, syncope

Central nervous system: Anxiety, chills, decreased energy, depression, dizziness, energy increased, fatigue, feeling down, headache, insomnia, irritability, nervousness, suicidal ideation

Dermatologic: Skin rash

Gastrointestinal: Abdominal cramping, abdominal pain, appetite decreased, constipation, diarrhea, dry mouth, nausea, toothache, vomiting

Genitourinary: Delayed ejaculation, impotency

Endocrine & metabolic: Increased thirst, polydipsia

Hepatic: ALT increased, AST increased, GGT increased

Local: Injection site reaction (includes bruising, induration, nodules, pain, pruritus, swelling, tenderness)

Neuromuscular & skeletal: Arthralgia, back pain, CPK increased, muscle cramps, myalgia

Respiratory: Pharyngitis

Miscellaneous: Influenza

Rare but important or life-threatening: Abnormality in thinking, acne vulgaris, alopecia, angina, anorexia, atrial fibrillation, blood pressure increased, cerebral aneurysm, chest tightness, cholecystitis, colitis, COPD, dehydration, delirium, depression, DVT, dysuria, ECG changes, edema, eosinophilia (transient), eosinophilic pneumonia, epistaxis, GI hemorrhage, hemorrhoids, hepatic insufficiency, hepatitis, HF, hypercholesterolemia, hyperkinesia, hypersensitivity reaction (includes anaphylaxis, angioedema, and urticaria), ischemic stroke, leukocytosis, lymphadenopathy, MI, opioid withdrawal, palpitation, pancreatitis, paralytic ileus, paranoia, PE, perirectal abscess, photophobia, pneumonia, rhinorrhea, rigors, seizure, shortness of breath, swelling of eye, tachycardia, thrombocytopenia, ulcer

Drug Interactions

Metabolism/Transport Effects None known.

Avoid Concomitant Use

Avoid concomitant use of Naltrexone with any of the following: Methylnaltrexone; Naloxegol

Increased Effect/Toxicity

Naltrexone may increase the levels/effects of: Naloxegol

The levels/effects of Naltrexone may be increased by: Methylnaltrexone

Decreased Effect

Naltrexone may decrease the levels/effects of: Analgesics (Opioid)

Preparation for Administration Injection: Prior to reconstitution, allow drug vial and provided diluent to reach room temperature (~45 minutes). Using the provided 1-inch *preparation* needle, reconstitute with 3.4 mL of the diluent and allow to dissolve by vigorously shaking the vial for ~1 minute. Mixed suspension will be milky white, free of clumps, and will move freely down the walls of the vial. Immediately after suspension, withdraw 4.2 mL of the suspension using the same preparation needle.

Prior to administration, replace the preparation needle with the appropriate size provided *administration* needle (use the 2-inch needle with the needle protection device for patients with a larger amount of subcutaneous tissue overlying the gluteal muscle; for very lean patients, the 1.5-inch needle may be appropriate; either needle may be used for patients with average body habitus). Prior to injection, remove any air bubbles and push on the plunger until 4 mL of the suspension remains in the syringe. Following reconstitution of the suspension, administer immediately.

Storage/Stability

Injection: Store unopened kit at 2°C to 8°C (36°F to 46°F). Kit may be kept at room temperature of ≤25°C (77°F) for ≤7 days prior to use; do not freeze. Following reconstitution of the suspension, administer immediately.

Tablet: Store at 20°C to 25°C (68°F to 77°F).

Mechanism of Action Naltrexone (a pure opioid antagonist) is a cyclopropyl derivative of oxymorphone similar in structure to naloxone and nalorphine (a morphine derivative); it acts as a competitive antagonist at opioid receptor sites, showing the highest affinity for mu receptors.

Pharmacodynamics/Kinetics

Duration: Oral: 50 mg: 24 hours; 100 mg: 48 hours; 150 mg: 72 hours; IM: 4 weeks

Absorption: Oral: Almost complete

Distribution: V_d: ~1350 L; widely throughout the body but considerable interindividual variation exists

Metabolism: Extensively metabolized via noncytochrome-mediated dehydrogenase conversion to 6-beta-naltrexol (primary metabolite) and related minor metabolites; glucuronide conjugates are also formed from naltrexone and its metabolites

Oral: Extensive first-pass effect

Protein binding: 21%

Bioavailability: Oral: Variable range (5% to 40%)

Half-life elimination: Oral: 4 hours; 6-beta-naltrexol: 13 hours; IM: naltrexone and 6-beta-naltrexol: 5-10 days (dependent upon erosion of polymer)

Time to peak, serum: Oral: ~60 minutes; IM: Biphasic: ~2 hours (first peak), ~2-3 days (second peak)

Excretion: Primarily urine (as metabolites and small amounts of unchanged drug)

Dosage Adults: **Note:** Do not initiate therapy until patient is opioid-free (including tramadol) for at least 7-10 days as determined by urinalysis; consider naloxone challenge test to confirm patient is opioid-free if there is any suspicion since urinary opioid screen may not be sufficient proof.

Alcohol dependence:

Oral: 50 mg daily; alternative maintenance regimens may be used and include: 50 mg on weekdays with a 100 mg dose on Saturday; 100 mg every other day; or 150 mg every 3 days (degree of blockade may be reduced with extended dosing interval regimens and doses >50 mg may increase risk of hepatocellular injury)

IM: 380 mg once every 4 weeks

Opioid dependence:

Oral: Initial: 25 mg; if no withdrawal signs occur, administer 50 mg daily thereafter; alternative maintenance regimens may be used and include: 50 mg on weekdays with a 100 mg dose on Saturday; 100 mg every other day; or 150 mg every 3 days (degree of blockade may be reduced with extended dosing interval regimens and doses >50 mg may increase risk of hepatocellular injury)

IM: 380 mg once every 4 weeks

Dosage adjustment in renal impairment:

Mild impairment: No dosage adjustment necessary.

Moderate-to-severe impairment: No dosage adjustment provided in manufacturer's labeling (has not been studied); use with caution since naltrexone and its primary metabolite are primarily excreted in urine.

Dosage adjustment in hepatic impairment:

Mild-to-moderate impairment: No dosage adjustment necessary.

Severe impairment: No dosage adjustment provided in manufacturer's labeling (has not been studied); naltrexone AUC increased ~5- and 10-fold in patients with compensated or decompensated hepatic cirrhosis respectively.

Administration

Oral: May be administered with or without food. Administration with food or after meals may minimize adverse gastrointestinal effects. Advise patient not to self-administer opioids while receiving naltrexone therapy.

IM: Vivitrol: Administer IM into the upper outer quadrant of the gluteal area; must inject dose using one of the provided needles for administration. Use either the 1.5-inch needle (for very lean patients) or the 2-inch needle (for patients with a larger amount of subcutaneous tissue overlying the gluteal muscle). Either needle may be used for patients with average body habitus. Avoid inadvertent injection into a blood vessel; do not administer IV, SubQ, or into fatty tissue (the risk of serious injection site reaction is increased if given incorrectly as a SubQ injection or into fatty tissue instead of the gluteal muscle). Injection should alternate between the 2 buttocks. Do not substitute any components of the dose-pack.

Monitoring Parameters Liver function tests (baseline and periodic); monitor for opioid withdrawal, injection site reactions with IM administration, and depression and/or suicidal thinking

Dosage Forms

Suspension Reconstituted, Intramuscular:

Vivitrol: 380 mg (1 ea)

Tablet, Oral:

ReVia: 50 mg

Generic: 50 mg

Naltrexone and Bupropion

(nal TREKS one & byoo PROE pee on)

Brand Names: U.S. Contrave

Index Terms Bupropion and Naltrexone; Bupropion Hydrochloride and Naltrexone Hydrochloride

Pharmacologic Category Anorexiant; Antidepressant, Dopamine/Norepinephrine-Reuptake Inhibitor; Opioid Antagonist

Use Weight management: Adjunct to a reduced-calorie diet and increased physical activity for chronic weight management in adults with an initial body mass index (BMI) of ≥30 kg/m^2 or ≥27 kg/m^2 in the presence of at least one weight-related comorbid condition (eg, hypertension, type 2 diabetes mellitus, and/or dyslipidemia)

Limitations of use: The effect of naltrexone/bupropion on cardiovascular morbidity and mortality has not been established. The safety and effectiveness of naltrexone/bupropion in combination with other products intended for weight loss, including prescription drugs, over-the-counter drugs, and herbal preparations, have not been established.

Pregnancy Risk Factor X

Pregnancy Considerations Animal reproduction studies have not been conducted with this combination. Adverse fetal events following maternal use of bupropion during pregnancy have been reported in some studies. Weight-loss therapy is not recommended for pregnant women. Obese and overweight women should be encouraged to participate in weight reduction programs prior to attempting pregnancy; weight gain during pregnancy should be determined by their prepregnancy BMI and current guidelines (ADA, 2009; IOM, 2009). Use of this product is contraindicated in pregnant women.

Breast-Feeding Considerations Bupropion and naltrexone are excreted into breast milk. Breast-feeding is not recommended by the manufacturer.

Contraindications Hypersensitivity to bupropion, naltrexone, or any other component of the formulation; concomitant use of other bupropion-containing products; chronic opioid, opiate agonist (eg, methadone) or partial agonist (eg, buprenorphine) use; acute opioid withdrawal; uncontrolled hypertension; seizure disorder or a history of seizures; bulimia or anorexia nervosa; abrupt discontinuation of alcohol, benzodiazepines, barbiturates, and antiepileptic drugs; concomitant use of MAO inhibitors (concurrently or within 14 days of discontinuing the MAO inhibitor or naltrexone/bupropion); initiation of naltrexone/bupropion in a patient receiving linezolid or intravenous (IV) methylene blue; pregnancy

Warnings/Precautions [U.S. Boxed Warning]: Naltrexone/bupropion is not approved for use in the treatment of major depressive or psychiatric disorders; it contains bupropion the same active ingredient in some other antidepressant medications. Antidepressants increase the risk of suicidal thinking and behavior in children, adolescents, and young adults (18 to 24 years of age) with major depressive disorder (MDD) and other psychiatric disorders; consider risk prior to prescribing. Short-term studies of antidepressants did not show an increased risk in patients >24 years of age and showed a decreased risk in patients ≥65 years. Closely monitor patients for clinical worsening, suicidality, or unusual changes in behavior, particularly during the initial 1 to 2 months of therapy or during periods of dosage adjustments (increases or decreases); the patient's family or caregiver should be instructed to closely observe the patient and communicate condition with health care provider. A medication guide concerning the use of antidepressants should be dispensed with each prescription. The possibility of a suicide attempt is inherent in major depression and may persist until remission occurs. Worsening depression and severe abrupt suicidality that are not part of the presenting symptoms may require discontinuation or modification of drug therapy. Use caution in high-risk patients during initiation of therapy. Prescriptions should be written for the smallest quantity consistent with good patient care. The patient's family or caregiver should be alerted to monitor patients for the emergence of suicidality and associated behaviors such as anxiety, agitation, panic attacks, insomnia, irritability, hostility, impulsivity, akathisia, hypomania, and mania; patients should be instructed to notify their health care provider if any of these symptoms or worsening depression or psychosis occur.

Bupropion may precipitate a manic, mixed, or hypomanic episode; risk is increased in patients with bipolar disorder or who have risk factors for bipolar disorder. Screen patients for a history of bipolar disorder and the presence of risk factors including a family history of bipolar disorder, suicide, or depression. Naltrexone/bupropion is not FDA approved for bipolar depression. **[U.S. Boxed Warning]: Although naltrexone/bupropion is not approved for smoking cessation treatment, but serious neuropsychiatric events have occurred in patients taking bupropion for smoking cessation,** including changes in mood (eg, depression, mania), psychosis, hallucinations, paranoia, delusions, homicidal ideation, hostility, agitation, aggression, anxiety, panic, suicidal ideation, suicide attempt and completed suicide. **The majority of these reactions occurred during bupropion treatment; however some occurred during treatment discontinuation. A causal relationship is uncertain as depressed mood may be a symptom of nicotine withdrawal. Some cases also occurred in patients taking bupropion who continued to smoke. Observe all patients taking bupropion for neuropsychiatric reactions. Instruct patients to contact a health care provider if neuropsychiatric reactions occur.** Depression, suicide, attempted suicide, and suicidal ideation have also been reported with naltrexone use for the treatment of opioid dependence; however, no causal relationship has been demonstrated.

May precipitate symptoms of acute withdrawal in opioid-dependent patients. An opioid-free interval of a at least 7 to 10 days (including tramadol) is recommended for patients previously dependent on short-acting opioids (including tramadol); consider an opioid-free interval of up to 2 weeks in patients transitioning from buprenorphine or methadone. Patients who had been treated with naltrexone may respond to lower opioid doses than previously used. This could result in potentially life-threatening opioid intoxication. Warn patients that any attempt to overcome opioid blockade during naltrexone therapy, is dangerous and could potentially lead to fatal opioid overdose; the opioid competitive receptor blockade produced by naltrexone is potentially surmountable in the presence of large amounts of opioids. If chronic opiate therapy is required, treatment naltrexone/bupropion should be stopped; if intermittent opiate therapy is required, temporarily discontinue treatment naltrexone/bupropion and lower doses of opioids may be needed.

Bupropion may cause a dose-related risk of seizures. Use is contraindicated in patients with a seizure disorder or a history of seizures, current or past diagnosis of bulimia or anorexia nervosa or undergoing abrupt discontinuation of alcohol, benzodiazepines, barbiturates, and antiepileptic drugs. Use caution with concurrent use of antipsychotics, antidepressants, theophylline, systemic corticosteroids, stimulants (including cocaine), or hypoglycemic agents, or with excessive use of ethanol, benzodiazepines, sedative/hypnotics, or opioids. Use with caution in seizure-potentiating metabolic disorders (hypoglycemia, hyponatremia, severe hepatic impairment, and hypoxia), and in patients with an addiction to cocaine or stimulants, in patients withdrawing from sedatives, and in patients with a history of head trauma, severe stroke, arteriovenous malformation, or central nervous system tumor or infection. To minimize the risk of seizures, increase the dose gradually, administer the dose twice daily with no more than 2 tablets taken at a time, avoid administration with high-fat meals, skip missed doses, and limit the daily dose of to bupropion hydrochloride to ≤360 mg. Use of multiple bupropion formulations is contraindicated. Permanently discontinue if seizure occurs during therapy.

May elevate heart rate, blood pressure and cause hypertension; use is contraindicated in patients with uncontrolled hypertension. Events have been observed in patients with or without evidence of preexisting hypertension. Risks may be greater during the initial 3 months of therapy. Assess heart rate and blood pressure before initiating treatment and monitor periodically. Use with caution in patients with cardiovascular disease. Anaphylactoid/anaphylactic reactions have occurred, with symptoms of including pruritus, urticaria, angioedema, and dyspnea. Serious reactions have been (rarely) reported with bupropion, including erythema multiforme, Stevens-Johnson syndrome (SJS), and anaphylactic shock. Arthralgia, myalgia, and fever with rash and other symptoms suggestive of delayed hypersensitivity resembling serum sickness have been reported with bupropion. Weight loss may increase the risk of hypoglycemia in patients with type 2 diabetes mellitus treated with insulin and/or insulin secretagogues. Monitor blood glucose levels at baseline and periodically during treatment. Consider decreases in doses for concurrent antidiabetic medications which are non-glucose-dependent; and make adjustments to antidiabetic drug regimens if hypoglycemia develops during treatment. Bupropion may cause mild pupillary dilation, which in susceptible individuals can lead to an episode of narrow-angle glaucoma. Consider evaluating patients who have not had an iridectomy for narrow-angle glaucoma risk factors. Cases of hepatitis, significant liver dysfunction, and transient, asymptomatic hepatic transaminase elevations have been observed with naltrexone use. Discontinue therapy if signs/symptoms of acute hepatitis develop. Clinicians should note that elevated transaminases may be a result of preexisting alcoholic liver disease, hepatitis B and/or C infection, or concomitant use of other hepatotoxic drugs; abrupt opioid withdrawal may also lead to acute liver injury. Use with caution in patients with hepatic impairment; reduced doses are recommended. Use with caution in patients with mild renal impairment. Dosage reductions are necessary with moderate to severe impairment; avoid use in patients with end-stage renal disease. Use with caution in the elderly; may be at greater risk of drug accumulation during chronic dosing. Potentially significant drug-drug interactions may exist, requiring dose or frequency adjustment, additional monitoring, and/or selection of alternative therapy.

Adverse Reactions

Cardiovascular: Hypertension, increased blood pressure, myocardial infarction, palpitations, presyncope, tachycardia

Central nervous system: abnormal dreams, agitation, altered mental status, amnesia, anxiety, disturbance in attention, dizziness, fatigue, insomnia (more common in partients ≥65 years of age), depression (more common in patients ≥65 years of age), irritability, derealization, emotional lability, equilibrium disturbance, feeling abnormal, feeling hot, intention tremor, jitteriness, lethargy, memory impairment, nervousness, tension, vertigo

Central nervous system: Headache (18%), sleep disorder (14%)

Dermatologic: Alopecia, hyperhidrosis

Endocrine: Dehydration, hot flash, increased thirst

Gastrointestinal: Abdominal pain, cholecystitis, diarrhea, dysgeusia, eructation, hematochezia, hernia, lower abdominal pain, motion sickness, swelling of lips, upper abdominal pain, viral gastroenteritis, xerostomia

Gastrointestinal: Constipation, nausea, vomiting

Genitourinary: Erectile dysfunction, irregular menses, urinary tract infection, urinary urgency, vaginal dryness, vaginal hemorrhage

Hematologic & oncologic: Decreased hematocrit

Hepatic: Increased liver enzymes

Infection: Kidney infection, staphylococcal infection

Neuromuscular & skeletal: Herniated disk, jaw pain, strain, tremor, weakness

Otic: Tinnitus

Renal: Increased serum creatinine

Respiratory: Pneumonia

Rare but important or life-threatening: Hypoglycemia (concomitant use of antidiabetic medications), increased heart rate (resting), syncope

Drug Interactions

Metabolism/Transport Effects Refer to individual components.

Avoid Concomitant Use

Avoid concomitant use of Naltrexone and Bupropion with any of the following: MAO Inhibitors; Methylnaltrexone; Naloxegol; Pimozide; Tamoxifen; Thioridazine

Increased Effect/Toxicity

Naltrexone and Bupropion may increase the levels/effects of: Alcohol (Ethyl); ARIPiprazole; AtoMOXetine; Citalopram; CYP2D6 Substrates; DOXOrubicin (Conventional); Eliglustat; Fesoterodine; FLUoxetine; FluvoxaMINE; Iloperidone; Lorcaserin; Metoprolol; Naloxegol; Nebivolol; OCT2 Substrates; PARoxetine; Pimozide; Propafenone; Tetrabenazine; Thioridazine; Tricyclic Antidepressants; Vortioxetine

The levels/effects of Naltrexone and Bupropion may be increased by: Alcohol (Ethyl); Anti-Parkinson's Agents (Dopamine Agonist); CYP2B6 Inhibitors (Moderate); MAO Inhibitors; Methylnaltrexone; Mifepristone; Quazepam

Decreased Effect

Naltrexone and Bupropion may decrease the levels/effects of: Analgesics (Opioid); Codeine; Iloperidone; Ioflupane I 123; Tamoxifen

The levels/effects of Naltrexone and Bupropion may be decreased by: CYP2B6 Inducers (Strong); Dabrafenib; Efavirenz; Lopinavir; Ritonavir

Storage/Stability Store at 25°C (77°F); excursions are permitted between 15°C and 30°C (59°F and 86°F).

Mechanism of Action Naltrexone is a pure opioid antagonist, and bupropion is a relatively weak inhibitor of the neuronal reuptake of dopamine and norepinephrine. The exact neurochemical effects of naltrexone/bupropion leading to weight loss are not fully understood. Effects may result from action on areas of the brain involved in the regulation of food intake: the hypothalamus (appetite regulatory center) and the mesolimbic dopamine circuit (reward system).

Pharmacodynamics/Kinetics See individual agents.

Dosage

Weight management: Adults: Oral:

Initial: One tablet (naltrexone 8 mg/bupropion 90 mg) once daily in the morning for 1 week; at week 2, increase to 1 tablet twice daily administered in the morning and evening and continue for 1 week; at week 3, increase to 2 tablets in the morning and 1 tablet in the evening and continue for 1 week; at week 4, increase to 2 tablets twice daily administered in the morning and evening and continue for the remainder of the treatment course.

Usual dosage: Two tablets (naltrexone 16 mg/bupropion 180 mg) twice daily (maximum dose: naltrexone 32 mg/bupropion 360 mg daily).

Concomitant use with CYP2B6 inhibitors (eg, ticlopidine, clopidogrel): Maximum dose: One tablet (naltrexone 8 mg/bupropion 90 mg) twice daily

Discontinuation of therapy: If the patient has not lost at least 5% of baseline body weight after 12 weeks at the maintenance dosage, discontinue therapy; clinically meaningful weight loss is unlikely with continued treatment.

MAO inhibitor recommendations:

Switching to or from an MAO inhibitor antidepressant:

Allow 14 days to elapse between discontinuing an MAO inhibitor intended to treat depression and initiation of naltrexone/bupropion.

Allow 14 days to elapse between discontinuing naltrexone/bupropion and initiation of an MAO inhibitor intended to treat depression.

Use with reversible MAO inhibitors (such as linezolid or IV methylene blue):

Do not initiate naltrexone/bupropion in patients receiving linezolid or IV methylene blue; consider other interventions for psychiatric condition.

If urgent treatment with linezolid or IV methylene blue is required in a patient already receiving naltrexone/bupropion and potential benefits outweigh potential risks, discontinue naltrexone/bupropion promptly and administer linezolid or IV methylene blue. Monitor for increased risk of hypertensive reactions for 2 weeks or until 24 hours after the last dose of linezolid or IV methylene blue, whichever comes first. May resume naltrexone/bupropion 24 hours after the last dose of linezolid or IV methylene blue (Wellbutrin prescribing information, 2013).

Dosage adjustment with renal impairment:

Mild impairment: There are no dosage adjustments provided in the manufacturer's labeling (has not been studied); use with caution.

Moderate or severe impairment: Maximum dose: One tablet (naltrexone 8 mg/bupropion 90 mg) twice daily

End-stage renal disease (ESRD): Use is not recommended.

Dosage adjustment with hepatic impairment: Maximum dose: One tablet (naltrexone 8 mg/bupropion 90 mg) daily

Dietary Considerations Do not administer with high-fat meals; may result in a significant increase in bupropion and naltrexone systemic exposure.

Administration Administer twice daily doses in the morning and in the evening; do not administer with high-fat meals. Do not cut, chew, or crush tablets.

Monitoring Parameters Blood pressure and heart rate (baseline and periodic); blood glucose (baseline and periodic); weight; BMI; renal and liver function (base and periodic); mental status for depression, suicidal ideation (especially at the beginning of therapy or when doses are increased or decreased), anxiety, social functioning, mania, and panic attacks.

Dosage Forms

Tablet Extended Release 12 Hour, Oral:

Contrave: Naltrexone hydrochloride 8 mg and bupropion hydrochloride 90 mg

◆ **Naltrexone Hydrochloride** *see* Naltrexone *on page 1422*

◆ **Namenda** *see* Memantine *on page 1286*

◆ **Namenda Titration Pak** *see* Memantine *on page 1286*

◆ **Namenda XR** *see* Memantine *on page 1286*

◆ **Namenda XR Titration Pack** *see* Memantine *on page 1286*

◆ **Nanoparticle Albumin-Bound Paclitaxel** *see* PACLitaxel (Protein Bound) *on page 1554*

◆ **NAPA and NABZ** *see* Sodium Phenylacetate and Sodium Benzoate *on page 1908*

Naphazoline (Nasal) (naf AZ oh leen)

Brand Names: U.S. Privine® [OTC]

Index Terms Naphazoline Hydrochloride

Pharmacologic Category Alpha$_1$ Agonist; Imidazoline Derivative

Use Temporary relief of nasal congestion associated with the common cold, upper respiratory allergies, or sinusitis

Dosage Intranasal: Children ≥12 years and Adults: 0.05% instill 1-2 drops or sprays every 6 hours if needed; therapy should not exceed 3 days

Additional Information Complete prescribing information should be consulted for additional detail.

Dosage Forms

Solution, intranasal:

Privine® [OTC]: 0.05% (20 mL, 25 mL)

Naphazoline (Ophthalmic) (naf AZ oh leen)

Brand Names: U.S. Clear Eyes Redness Relief [OTC]; VasoClear [OTC]; VasoClear-A [OTC]

Brand Names: Canada Naphcon Forte®; Vasocon®

Index Terms Naphazoline Hydrochloride

Pharmacologic Category Alpha$_1$ Agonist; Imidazoline Derivative; Ophthalmic Agent, Vasoconstrictor

Use Topical ocular vasoconstrictor; relief of redness of the eye due to minor irritation

Pregnancy Risk Factor C

Dosage Ophthalmic: Adults:

0.1% solution (prescription): 1-2 drops into conjunctival sac every 3-4 hours as needed

0.012% or 0.025% solution (OTC): 1-2 drops into affected eye(s) up to 4 times/day; therapy should not exceed 3 days

Dosage adjustment in renal impairment: No dosage adjustment provided in manufacturer's labeling.

Dosage adjustment in hepatic impairment: No dosage adjustment provided in manufacturer's labeling.

Additional Information Complete prescribing information should be consulted for additional detail.

Dosage Forms

Solution, Ophthalmic:

Clear Eyes Redness Relief [OTC]: 0.012% (6 mL)
VasoClear [OTC]: 0.02% (15 mL)
VasoClear-A [OTC]: 0.02% (15 mL)
Generic: 0.1% (15 mL)

Naphazoline and Pheniramine

(naf AZ oh leen & fen NIR a meen)

Brand Names: U.S. Naphcon-A [OTC]; Opcon-A [OTC]; Visine-A [OTC]

Brand Names: Canada Naphcon-A; Visine Advanced Allergy

Index Terms Pheniramine and Naphazoline

Pharmacologic Category Alkylamine Derivative; Alpha$_1$ Agonist; Histamine H_1 Antagonist; Histamine H_1 Antagonist, First Generation; Imidazoline Derivative; Ophthalmic Agent, Vasoconstrictor

Use Treatment of ocular congestion, irritation, and itching

Dosage Ophthalmic: Children ≥6 years and Adults: 1-2 drops into the affected eye(s) up to 4 times/day

Additional Information Complete prescribing information should be consulted for additional detail.

Dosage Forms

Solution, ophthalmic:

Naphcon-A [OTC]: Naphazoline 0.025% and pheniramine 0.3%

Opcon-A [OTC]: Naphazoline 0.027% and pheniramine 0.3%

Visine-A [OTC]: Naphazoline 0.025% and pheniramine 0.3%

Generic: Naphazoline hydrochloride 0.027% and pheniramine maleate 0.315%

◆ **Naphazoline Hydrochloride** *see* Naphazoline (Nasal) *on page 1426*

◆ **Naphazoline Hydrochloride** *see* Naphazoline (Ophthalmic) *on page 1426*

◆ **Naphcon-A [OTC]** *see* Naphazoline and Pheniramine *on page 1426*

◆ **Naphcon-A (Can)** *see* Naphazoline and Pheniramine *on page 1426*

◆ **Naphcon Forte® (Can)** *see* Naphazoline (Ophthalmic) *on page 1426*

◆ **Naprelan** *see* Naproxen *on page 1427*

◆ **Naprosyn** *see* Naproxen *on page 1427*

Naproxen (na PROKS en)

Brand Names: U.S. Aleve [OTC]; All Day Pain Relief [OTC]; All Day Relief [OTC]; Anaprox; Anaprox DS; EC-Naprosyn; EnovaRX-Naproxen; Flanax Pain Relief [OTC]; Mediproxen [OTC]; Naprelan; Naprosyn; Naproxen Comfort Pac; Naproxen DR

Brand Names: Canada Aleve; Anaprox; Anaprox DS; Apo-Napro-Na; Apo-Napro-Na DS; Apo-Naproxen; Apo-Naproxen EC; Apo-Naproxen SR; Ava-Naproxen EC; Maxidol; Mylan-Naproxen EC; Naprelan; Naprosyn; Naproxen EC; Naproxen Sodium DS; Naproxen-NA; Naproxen-NA DF; Pediapharm Naproxen Suspension; PMS-Naproxen; PMS-Naproxen EC; PRO-Naproxen EC; Teva-Naproxen; Teva-Naproxen EC; Teva-Naproxen Sodium; Teva-Naproxen Sodium DS; Teva-Naproxen SR

Index Terms Naproxen Sodium

Pharmacologic Category Nonsteroidal Anti-inflammatory Drug (NSAID), Oral

Additional Appendix Information

Beers Criteria - Potentially Inappropriate Medications for Geriatrics *on page 2271*

Use

Acute gout/Ankylosing spondylitis/Bursitis/Juvenile arthritis/Juvenile rheumatoid arthritis/Osteoarthritis/Rheumatoid arthritis/Tendonitis (Rx products only): For the relief of the signs and symptoms of acute gout, ankylosing spondylitis, bursitis, juvenile arthritis (excluding ER tablets), juvenile rheumatoid arthritis (oral suspension only), osteoarthritis, rheumatoid arthritis, and tendonitis. Delayed-release naproxen is not recommended for initial treatment of acute pain.

Pain/Primary dysmenorrhea (Rx and OTC products): For the relief of mild-to-moderate pain and the treatment of primary dysmenorrhea. Delayed-release naproxen is not recommended for initial treatment of acute pain.

Pregnancy Risk Factor C

Pregnancy Considerations Adverse events were not observed in the initial animal reproduction studies; therefore, the manufacturer classifies naproxen as pregnancy category C. Naproxen crosses the placenta and can be detected in fetal tissue and the serum of newborn infants following *in utero* exposure. NSAID exposure during the first trimester is not strongly associated with congenital malformations; however, cardiovascular anomalies and cleft palate have been observed following NSAID exposure in some studies. The use of a NSAID close to conception may be associated with an increased risk of miscarriage. Nonteratogenic effects have been observed following NSAID administration during the third trimester including: Myocardial degenerative changes, prenatal constriction of the ductus arteriosus, fetal tricuspid regurgitation, failure of the ductus arteriosus to close postnatally; renal dysfunction or failure, oligohydramnios; gastrointestinal bleeding or perforation, increased risk of necrotizing enterocolitis; intracranial bleeding (including intraventricular hemorrhage), platelet dysfunction with resultant bleeding; pulmonary hypertension. Because they may cause premature closure of the ductus arteriosus, use of NSAIDs late in pregnancy should be avoided (use after 31 or 32 weeks gestation is not recommended by some clinicians). The Canadian labeling contraindicates use during the third trimester of pregnancy. The chronic use of NSAIDs in women of reproductive age may be associated with infertility that is reversible upon discontinuation of the medication. A registry is available for pregnant women exposed to autoimmune medications including naproxen. For additional information contact the Organization of Teratology Information Specialists, OTIS Autoimmune Diseases Study, at (877) 311-8972.

Breast-Feeding Considerations Small amounts of naproxen are excreted into breast milk. Naproxen has been detected in the urine of a breast-feeding infant. Breast-feeding is not recommended per the U.S. manufacturer labeling and is contraindicated per the Canadian manufacturer labeling. In a study which included 20 mother-infant pairs, there were two cases of drowsiness and one case of vomiting in the breast-fed infants. Maternal naproxen dose, duration, and relationship to breast-feeding were not provided.

Contraindications

Hypersensitivity to naproxen, aspirin, other NSAIDs, or any component of the formulation; treatment of perioperative pain in the setting of coronary artery bypass graft (CABG) surgery

Canadian labeling: Additional contraindications (not in U.S. labeling): Active peptic ulcers; active GI bleeding; cerebrovascular bleeding or other bleeding disorders; active GI inflammatory disease; severe liver impairment or active liver disease; severe renal impairment (Clcr <30 mL/minute) or deteriorating renal disease; severe uncontrolled heart failure; known hyperkalemia; third trimester of pregnancy; breast-feeding; inflammatory lesions or recent bleeding of the rectum or anus (suppository only); use in patients <16 years of age (suppository only); use in patients <18 years of age (naproxen enteric coated and sustained release tablets and naproxen sodium tablets); use in children <2 years (naproxen tablets and suspension).

Warnings/Precautions [U.S. Boxed Warning]: NSAIDs are associated with an increased risk of adverse cardiovascular thrombotic events, including MI and stroke. Risk may be increased with duration of use or preexisting cardiovascular risk factors or disease. Carefully evaluate individual cardiovascular risk profiles prior to prescribing. May cause new-onset hypertension or worsening of existing hypertension. Monitor blood pressure closely with initiation and during therapy. Use caution with fluid retention. Avoid use in heart failure (ACCF/AHA [Yancy, 2013]). Use the lowest effective dose for the shortest duration of time, consistent with individual patient goals, to reduce risk of cardiovascular or GI adverse events. Alternate therapies should be considered for patients at high risk. Concurrent administration of ibuprofen, and potentially other nonselective NSAIDs, may interfere with aspirin's cardioprotective effect. **[U.S. Boxed Warning]: Use is contraindicated for treatment of perioperative pain in the setting of coronary artery bypass graft (CABG) surgery.** Risk of MI and stroke may be increased with use following CABG surgery.

[U.S. Boxed Warning]: NSAIDs may increase risk of gastrointestinal irritation, inflammation, ulceration, bleeding, and perforation. These events may occur at any time during therapy and without warning. Risk for serious events is greater in elderly patients. Use caution with a history of GI disease (bleeding or ulcers). Canadian labeling contraindicates use with active peptic ulcers, GI bleeding, or inflammatory bowel disease. Use caution with concurrent therapy with aspirin, anticoagulants and/or corticosteroids, smoking, use of alcohol, the elderly or debilitated patients. When used concomitantly with aspirin, a substantial increase in the risk of gastrointestinal complications (eg, ulcer) occurs; concomitant gastroprotective therapy (eg, proton pump inhibitors) is recommended (Bhatt, 2008).

May increase the risk of aseptic meningitis, especially in patients with systemic lupus erythematosus (SLE) and mixed connective tissue disorders. Platelet adhesion and aggregation may be decreased; may prolong bleeding time; patients with coagulation disorders or who are receiving anticoagulants should be monitored closely. Anemia may occur; patients on long-term NSAID therapy should be monitored for anemia. Rarely, NSAID use may cause severe blood dyscrasias (eg, agranulocytosis, aplastic anemia, thrombocytopenia).

NSAID use may compromise existing renal function; dose-dependent decreases in prostaglandin synthesis may result from NSAID use, reducing renal blood flow which may cause renal decompensation. NSAID use may increase the risk for hyperkalemia (Canadian labeling contraindicates use in patients with known hyperkalemia). Patients with impaired renal function, dehydration, heart failure, liver dysfunction, those taking diuretics, and ACE inhibitors, and the elderly are at greater risk of renal toxicity and hyperkalemia. Rehydrate patient before starting therapy; monitor renal function closely. Not recommended for use in patients with advanced renal disease. Canadian labeling contraindicates use in severe renal impairment (Clcr <30 mL/minute) or deteriorating renal disease. Long-term NSAID use may result in renal papillary necrosis.

NSAIDs may cause serious skin adverse events including exfoliative dermatitis, Stevens-Johnson Syndrome (SJS) and toxic epidermal necrolysis (TEN); discontinue use at first sign of skin rash or hypersensitivity. Anaphylactoid reactions may occur, even without prior exposure; patients with "aspirin triad" (bronchial asthma, aspirin intolerance, rhinitis) may be at increased risk. Do not use in patients who experience bronchospasm, asthma, rhinitis, or urticaria with NSAID or aspirin therapy. Use caution in other forms of asthma.

Use with caution in patients with decreased hepatic function. Closely monitor patients with any abnormal LFT. Severe hepatic reactions (eg, fulminant hepatitis, liver failure) have occurred with NSAID use, rarely; discontinue if signs or symptoms of liver disease develop, or if systemic manifestations occur. Canadian labeling contraindicates use in severe impairment or with active liver disease.

NSAIDS may cause drowsiness, dizziness, blurred vision and other neurologic effects which may impair physical or mental abilities; patients must be cautioned about performing tasks which require mental alertness (eg, operating machinery or driving). Discontinue use with blurred or diminished vision and perform ophthalmologic exam. Monitor vision with long-term therapy. Withhold for at least 4-6 half-lives prior to surgical or dental procedures.

Use with caution in the elderly, particularly at higher doses; unbound plasma fraction increased. Dose adjustments may be necessary; avoid chronic use (unless alternative agents ineffective and patient can receive concomitant gastroprotective agent); nonselective oral NSAID use is associated with an increased risk of GI bleeding and peptic ulcer disease in older adults in high risk category (eg, >75 years or age or receiving concomitant oral/parenteral corticosteroids, anticoagulants, or antiplatelet agents) (Beers Criteria).

OTC labeling: Prior to self-medication, patients should contact healthcare provider if they have had recurring stomach pain or upset, ulcers, bleeding problems, asthma, high blood pressure, heart or kidney disease, other serious medical problems, are currently taking a diuretic, anticoagulant, other NSAIDs, or are ≥60 years of age. Recommended dosages and duration should not be exceeded, due to an increased risk of GI bleeding, MI, and stroke. Patients should stop use and consult a healthcare provider if symptoms get worse, newly appear, or continue; if an allergic reaction occurs; if feeling faint, vomit blood or have bloody/black stools; if having difficulty swallowing or heartburn, or if fever lasts for >3 days or pain >10 days. Consuming ≥3 alcoholic beverages/day or taking longer than recommended may increase the risk of GI bleeding. Not for self-medication (OTC use) in children <12 years of age. Canadian labeling contraindicates use of certain dosage forms based on age (refer to Contraindications for specific recommendations).

Adverse Reactions

Cardiovascular: Edema, palpitations

Central nervous system: Dizziness, drowsiness, headache, lightheadedness, vertigo

Dermatologic: Ecchymosis, pruritus, purpura, rash, skin eruption

Endocrine & metabolic: Fluid retention

Gastrointestinal: Abdominal pain, constipation, diarrhea, dyspepsia, flatulence, gross bleeding/perforation, heartburn, indigestion, nausea, stomatitis, ulcers, vomiting

Genitourinary: Abnormal renal function

Hematologic: Anemia, bleeding time increased, ecchymosis, hemolysis

Hepatic: LFTs increased

Ocular: Visual disturbances

Otic: Hearing disturbances, tinnitus

Respiratory: Dyspnea

Miscellaneous: Diaphoresis, thirst

Rare but important or life-threatening: Agranulocytosis, alopecia, anaphylactic/anaphylactoid reaction, angioneurotic edema, arrhythmia, aseptic meningitis, asthma, blurred vision, cognitive dysfunction, colitis, coma, confusion, CHF, conjunctivitis, cystitis, depression, dream abnormalities, dysuria, eosinophilia, eosinophilic pneumonitis, erythema multiforme, exfoliative dermatitis, glossitis, granulocytopenia, hallucinations, hematemesis, hepatitis, hyper-/hypoglycemia, hyper-/hypotension, infection, interstitial nephritis, melena, jaundice, leukopenia, liver failure, lymphadenopathy, menstrual disorders, malaise, MI, muscle weakness, myalgia, oliguria, pancreatitis, pancytopenia, paresthesia, photosensitivity, pneumonia, polyuria, proteinuria, pyrexia, rectal bleeding, renal failure, renal papillary necrosis, respiratory depression, sepsis, Stevens-Johnson syndrome, tachycardia, seizure, syncope, thrombocytopenia, toxic epidermal necrolysis ulcerative stomatitis, vasculitis

Drug Interactions

Metabolism/Transport Effects Substrate of CYP1A2 (minor), CYP2C9 (minor); **Note:** Assignment of Major/Minor substrate status based on clinically relevant drug interaction potential

Avoid Concomitant Use

Avoid concomitant use of Naproxen with any of the following: Dexketoprofen; Floctafenine; Ketorolac (Nasal); Ketorolac (Systemic); NSAID (COX-2 Inhibitor); Omacetaxine; Urokinase

Increased Effect/Toxicity

Naproxen may increase the levels/effects of: 5-ASA Derivatives; Agents with Antiplatelet Properties; Aliskiren; Aminoglycosides; Anticoagulants; Apixaban; Bisphosphonate Derivatives; Collagenase (Systemic); CycloSPORINE (Systemic); Dabigatran Etexilate; Deferasirox; Desmopressin; Digoxin; Eplerenone; Haloperidol; Ibritumomab; Lithium; Methotrexate; Nonsteroidal Anti-Inflammatory Agents; NSAID (COX-2 Inhibitor); Obinutuzumab; Omacetaxine; PEMEtrexed; Porfimer; Potassium-Sparing Diuretics; PRALAtrexate; Quinolone Antibiotics; Rivaroxaban; Salicylates; Tacrolimus (Systemic); Tenofovir; Thrombolytic Agents; Tositumomab and Iodine I 131

Tositumomab; Urokinase; Vancomycin; Verteporfin; Vitamin K Antagonists

The levels/effects of Naproxen may be increased by: ACE Inhibitors; Angiotensin II Receptor Blockers; Antidepressants (Tricyclic, Tertiary Amine); Corticosteroids (Systemic); CycloSPORINE (Systemic); Dasatinib; Dexketoprofen; Diclofenac (Systemic); Floctafenine; Glucosamine; Herbs (Anticoagulant/Antiplatelet Properties); Ibrutinib; Ketorolac (Nasal); Ketorolac (Systemic); Limaprost; Multivitamins/Fluoride (with ADE); Multivitamins/Minerals (with ADEK, Folate, Iron); Multivitamins/Minerals (with AE, No Iron); Omega-3 Fatty Acids; Pentosan Polysulfate Sodium; Pentoxifylline; Probenecid; Prostacyclin Analogues; Selective Serotonin Reuptake Inhibitors; Serotonin/Norepinephrine Reuptake Inhibitors; Sodium Phosphates; Tipranavir; Treprostinil; Vitamin E

Decreased Effect

Naproxen may decrease the levels/effects of: ACE Inhibitors; Aliskiren; Angiotensin II Receptor Blockers; Beta-Blockers; Eplerenone; HydrALAZINE; Loop Diuretics; Potassium-Sparing Diuretics; Prostaglandins (Ophthalmic); Salicylates; Selective Serotonin Reuptake Inhibitors; Thiazide Diuretics

The levels/effects of Naproxen may be decreased by: Bile Acid Sequestrants; Salicylates

Food Interactions Naproxen absorption rate/levels may be decreased if taken with food. Management: Administer with food, milk, or antacids to decrease GI adverse effects.

Storage/Stability Store at 15°C to 30°C (59°F to 86°F); suspension should not be exposed to excessive heat (>40°C [104°F]).

Mechanism of Action Reversibly inhibits cyclooxygenase-1 and 2 (COX-1 and 2) enzymes, which results in decreased formation of prostaglandin precursors; has antipyretic, analgesic, and anti-inflammatory properties

Other proposed mechanisms not fully elucidated (and possibly contributing to the anti-inflammatory effect to varying degrees), include inhibiting chemotaxis, altering lymphocyte activity, inhibiting neutrophil aggregation/activation, and decreasing proinflammatory cytokine levels.

Pharmacodynamics/Kinetics

Onset of action: Analgesic: 30 to 60 minutes

Duration: Analgesic: <12 hours

Absorption: Oral: Almost 100%

Distribution: 0.16 L/kg

Protein binding: >99% to albumin; increased free fraction in elderly

Metabolism: Hepatic to metabolites

Bioavailability: 95%

Half-life elimination: Normal renal function: 12 to 17 hours; Moderate-to-severe renal impairment: ~15 to 21 hours (Anttila, 1980)

Time to peak, serum:

Tablets, naproxen: 2 to 4 hours

Tablets, naproxen sodium: 1 to 2 hours

Tablets, delayed-release (empty stomach): 4 to 6 hours; range: 2 to 12 hours

Tablets, delayed-release (with food): 12 hours; range: 4 to 24 hours

Suspension: 1 to 4 hours

Suppository [Canadian product]: 2 to 3 hours

Excretion: Urine (95%; primarily as metabolites); feces (≤3%)

Dosage

Oral: **Note:** Dosage expressed as naproxen base; 200 mg naproxen base is equivalent to 220 mg naproxen sodium.

Children >2 years: Juvenile idiopathic arthritis: **Note:** Oral suspension is recommended: 10 mg/kg/day in 2 divided doses (up to 15 mg/kg/day has been tolerated). Do not exceed 15 mg/kg/day.

Adults: **Note:** For relief of acute pain, naproxen sodium may be preferred due to more rapid absorption and onset; naproxen base may also be used, however, EC-Naprosyn is not recommended.

Ankylosing spondylitis, osteoarthritis, rheumatoid arthritis: 500 to 1000 mg daily in 2 divided doses; if tolerating well and clinically indicated, may increase to 1500 mg daily of naproxen base for limited time period (<6 months)

Naproxen extended-release tablets: Initial: 750 to 1000 mg once daily; may temporarily increase to 1500 mg daily of naproxen base if tolerating well and clinically indicated

Gout, acute: Initial: 750 mg, followed by 250 mg every 8 hours until attack subsides

Naproxen extended-release tablets: Initial: 1000 to 1500 mg once daily followed by 1000 mg once daily until attack subsides

Pain (mild-to-moderate), dysmenorrhea, acute tendonitis, bursitis: Initial: 500 mg, followed by 500 mg every 12 hours **or** 250 mg every 6 to 8 hours; maximum daily dose: Day 1: 1250 mg naproxen base; subsequent daily doses should not exceed 1000 mg naproxen base

Naproxen extended-release tablets: Initial: 1000 mg once daily; may temporarily increase to 1500 mg once daily if greater pain relief is needed. Dose should be subsequently reduced to a maximum of 1000 mg daily.

Migraine, acute (off-label use): Initial: 750 mg; an additional 250 to 500 mg may be given if needed (maximum: 1250 mg in 24 hours) (Andersson, 1989; Nestvold, 1985).

Rectal suppository [Canadian product]: Adolescents ≥16 years and Adults: Ankylosing spondylitis, osteoarthritis, rheumatoid arthritis: Insert one 500 mg suppository into the rectum once daily (**Note:** Suppository may be used to substitute for one oral dose in patients receiving 1000 mg naproxen daily).

Elderly: Use with caution; dosage adjustment may be required. Refer to adult dosing.

OTC labeling: Pain, fever: Children ≥12 years, Adolescents, and Adults: 200 mg naproxen base every 8 to 12 hours; if needed, may take 400 mg naproxen base for the initial dose; maximum: 400 mg naproxen base in any 8- to 12-hour period or 600 mg naproxen base/24 hours

Dosage adjustment in renal impairment: CrCl <30 mL/minute: Use is not recommended

U.S. labeling: Use is not recommended.

Canadian labeling: Use is contraindicated.

Dosage adjustment in hepatic impairment: Manufacturer's labeling suggests that a reduced dose should be considered; use with caution in chronic disease (eg, alcoholic liver disease), particularly at higher doses; dose adjustment may be required. Canadian labeling contraindicates use in severe impairment or active liver disease.

Dietary Considerations Drug may cause GI upset, bleeding, ulceration, perforation; take with food or milk to minimize GI upset.

Administration

Oral: Administer with food, milk, or antacids to decrease GI adverse effects

Suspension: Shake suspension well before administration.

Tablet, delayed or extended release: Swallow tablet whole; do not break, crush, or chew.

Rectal suppository [Canadian product]: Insert suppository into rectum.

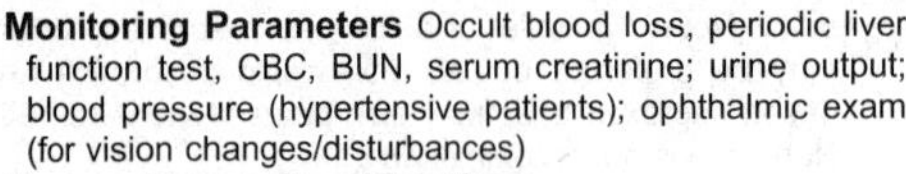

Monitoring Parameters Occult blood loss, periodic liver function test, CBC, BUN, serum creatinine; urine output; blood pressure (hypertensive patients); ophthalmic exam (for vision changes/disturbances)

Dosage Forms Considerations

EnovaRX-Naproxen is a compounding kit. Refer to manufacturer's package insert for compounding instructions.

Naproxen Comfort Pac is a combination kit containing naproxen tablets and Duraflex Comfort Gel

Dosage Forms

Capsule, Oral:
Aleve [OTC]: 220 mg

Cream, External:
EnovaRX-Naproxen: 10% (60 g, 120 g)

Kit, Combination:
Naproxen Comfort Pac: 500 mg

Suspension, Oral:
Naprosyn: 125 mg/5 mL (480 mL)
Generic: 125 mg/5 mL (500 mL)

Tablet, Oral:
Aleve [OTC]: 220 mg
All Day Pain Relief [OTC]: 220 mg
All Day Relief [OTC]: 220 mg
Anaprox: 275 mg
Anaprox DS: 550 mg
Flanax Pain Relief [OTC]: 220 mg
Mediproxen [OTC]: 220 mg
Naprosyn: 250 mg, 375 mg, 500 mg
Generic: 220 mg, 250 mg, 275 mg, 375 mg, 500 mg, 550 mg

Tablet Delayed Release, Oral:
EC-Naprosyn: 375 mg, 500 mg
Naproxen DR: 375 mg, 500 mg

Tablet Extended Release 24 Hour, Oral:
Naprelan: 375 mg, 500 mg, 750 mg

◆ **Naproxen and Sumatriptan** *see* Sumatriptan and Naproxen *on page 1957*

◆ **Naproxen Comfort Pac** *see* Naproxen *on page 1427*

◆ **Naproxen DR** *see* Naproxen *on page 1427*

◆ **Naproxen EC (Can)** *see* Naproxen *on page 1427*

◆ **Naproxen-NA (Can)** *see* Naproxen *on page 1427*

◆ **Naproxen-NA DF (Can)** *see* Naproxen *on page 1427*

◆ **Naproxen Sodium** *see* Naproxen *on page 1427*

◆ **Naproxen Sodium and Sumatriptan** *see* Sumatriptan and Naproxen *on page 1957*

◆ **Naproxen Sodium and Sumatriptan Succinate** *see* Sumatriptan and Naproxen *on page 1957*

◆ **Naproxen Sodium DS (Can)** *see* Naproxen *on page 1427*

◆ **Naramin [OTC]** *see* DiphenhydrAMINE (Systemic) *on page 641*

Naratriptan (NAR a trip tan)

Brand Names: U.S. Amerge

Brand Names: Canada Amerge; Sandoz-Naratriptan; Teva-Naratriptan

Index Terms Naratriptan Hydrochloride

Pharmacologic Category Antimigraine Agent; Serotonin 5-HT$_{1B, 1D}$ Receptor Agonist

Use Migraines: Acute treatment of migraine attacks with or without aura in adults.

Pregnancy Risk Factor C

Pregnancy Considerations Adverse events were observed in animal reproduction studies. Pregnancy outcome information for naratriptan is available from a pregnancy registry sponsored by GlaxoSmithKline. As of October 2008, data was available for 55 infants/fetuses exposed to naratriptan, and seven exposed to both naratriptan and sumatriptan. Following naratriptan exposure, there was one infant born with a birth defect; this infant was also exposed to sumatriptan during the first trimester of pregnancy (Cunnington, 2009). The pregnancy registry was closed in January, 2012 and additional information may be obtained from the manufacturer (800-336-2176). Additional information related to the use of naratriptan in pregnancy is limited (Källén, 2011; Nezvalová-Henriksen, 2010; Nezvalová-Henriksen, 2012). Until additional information is available, other agents are preferred for the initial treatment of migraine in pregnancy (Da Silva, 2012; MacGregor, 2012; Williams, 2012).

Breast-Feeding Considerations It is not known if naratriptan is excreted in breast milk. Due to the potential for serious adverse reactions in the nursing infant, the manufacturer recommends a decision be made whether to discontinue nursing or to discontinue the drug, taking into account the importance of treatment to the mother.

Contraindications

Ischemic coronary artery disease (CAD) (angina pectoris, history of myocardial infarction [MI], or documented silent ischemia); coronary artery vasospasm, including Prinzmetal's angina; Wolff-Parkinson-White syndrome or arrhythmias associated with other cardiac accessory conduction pathway disorders; history of stroke, transient ischemic attack (TIA), or history of hemiplegic or basilar migraine; peripheral vascular disease; ischemic bowel disease; uncontrolled hypertension; recent use (within 24 hours) of another 5-HT$_1$ agonist, ergotamine-containing medication, or ergot-type medication (eg, dihydroergotamine or methysergide); severe renal impairment (CrCl <15 mL/minute) or severe hepatic impairment; hypersensitivity to naratriptan or any component of the formulation

Canadian labeling: Additional contraindications (not in U.S. labeling): Severe hypertension, cardiac arrhythmias (especially tachycardias); valvular heart disease, congenital heart disease, atherosclerotic disease; management of ophthalmoplegic migraine

Documentation of allergenic cross-reactivity for triptans is limited. However, because of similarities in chemical structure and/or pharmacologic actions, the possibility of cross-sensitivity cannot be ruled out with certainty.

Warnings/Precautions Use only if there is a clear diagnosis of migraine. Use is contraindicated in patients with severe hepatic or renal impairment. Do not give to patients with risk factors for CAD until a cardiovascular evaluation has been performed; if evaluation is satisfactory, the health care provider should administer the first dose (consider ECG monitoring) and cardiovascular status should be periodically re-evaluated. Use is contraindicated in patients with ischemic or vasospastic CAD and Wolff-Parkinson-White syndrome or arrhythmias associated with other cardiac accessory conduction pathway disorders. Additionally, the Canadian labeling contraindicates use in patients with valvular heart disease, cardiac arrhythmias (especially tachycardias) and congenital heart disease. Cardiac events (coronary artery vasospasm, transient ischemia, myocardial infarction, ventricular tachycardia/fibrillation, cardiac arrest, and death), cerebral/subarachnoid hemorrhage, stroke (some fatal), peripheral vascular ischemia, gastrointestinal vascular ischemia/infarction, splenic infarction, and Raynaud's syndrome have been reported with 5-HT$_1$ agonist administration. Partial vision loss and blindness (transient and permanent) have been reported with use of 5-HT$_1$ agonists; a causal relationship between these events and 5-HT$_1$ agonist administration has not been clearly determined. Patients who experience sensations of chest pain/pressure/tightness or symptoms suggestive of angina following dosing should be evaluated for coronary artery disease or Prinzmetal's angina before receiving additional doses; if dosing is resumed and similar symptoms recur, monitor with ECG. Significant elevation in blood pressure, including hypertensive crisis with acute impairment of organ systems, has been reported on rare occasions in patients with and without a history of hypertension; monitor blood pressure. Blood pressure increases may be more pronounced in the elderly. Use in patients with uncontrolled hypertension is contraindicated; the Canadian labeling also contraindicates use in patients with severe hypertension.

May cause CNS depression, such as dizziness, weakness, or drowsiness, which may impair physical or mental abilities; patients must be cautioned about performing tasks which require mental alertness (eg, operating machinery or driving). Only indicated for the acute treatment of migraine; not indicated for migraine prophylaxis, or for the treatment of cluster headache, hemiplegic, basilar, or ophthalmoplegic (Canadian labeling) migraine. Acute migraine agents (eg, triptans, opioids, ergotamine, or a combination of the agents) used for 10 or more days per month may lead to worsening of headaches (medication overuse headache); withdrawal treatment may be necessary in the setting of overuse. If a patient does not respond to the first dose, the diagnosis of migraine should be reconsidered; rule out underlying neurologic disease in patients with atypical headache and in patients with no prior history of migraine.

Potentially significant drug-drug interactions may exist, requiring dose or frequency adjustment, additional monitoring, and/or selection of alternative therapy. Symptoms of agitation, confusion, hallucinations, hyper-reflexia, myoclonus, shivering, and tachycardia may occur with concomitant proserotonergic drugs (ie, SSRIs/SNRIs or triptans) or agents which reduce naratriptan's metabolism. Concurrent use of serotonin precursors (eg, tryptophan) is not recommended. If concomitant administration with SSRIs is warranted, monitor closely, especially at initiation and with dose increases. Discontinue naratriptan if serotonin syndrome is suspected. Anaphylaxis, anaphylactoid, and hypersensitivity reactions (including angioedema) have occurred; may be life-threatening or fatal.

Adverse Reactions

Central nervous system: Dizziness, drowsiness, fatigue, hot and cold flashes, pain, paresthesia, sensation of pressure (chest/neck/throat/jaw), vertigo

Gastrointestinal: Nausea, vomiting, xerostomia

Neuromuscular & skeletal: Neck pain

Ophthalmic: Photophobia

Respiratory: Constriction of the pharynx, ENT infection

Rare but important or life-threatening: Abnormal bilirubin levels, abnormal hepatic function tests, anaphylactoid reaction, anaphylaxis, anemia, angina pectoris, angioedema, bradycardia, cerebral infarction, colonic ischemia, coronary artery vasospasm, depression, ECG changes (atrial fibrillation, atrial flutter, premature ventricular contractions, PR prolongation, or QTc prolongation), glycosuria, hallucination, heart murmur, hypersensitivity reaction (some cases severe, including circulatory collapse), hypertension, hypothyroidism, ischemic heart disease, ketonuria, myocardial infarction, palpitations, seizure, serotonin syndrome, skin rash, subarachnoid hemorrhage, subconjunctival hemorrhage, syncope, thrombocytopenia, transient ischemic attacks, ventricular fibrillation, ventricular tachycardia

Drug Interactions

Metabolism/Transport Effects None known.

Avoid Concomitant Use

Avoid concomitant use of Naratriptan with any of the following: Dapoxetine; Ergot Derivatives

Increased Effect/Toxicity

Naratriptan may increase the levels/effects of: Antipsychotic Agents; Droxidopa; Ergot Derivatives; Metoclopramide; Serotonin Modulators

The levels/effects of Naratriptan may be increased by: Antiemetics (5HT3 Antagonists); Antipsychotic Agents; Dapoxetine; Ergot Derivatives; Tedizolid

Decreased Effect There are no known significant interactions involving a decrease in effect.

Storage/Stability Store at 20°C to 25°C (68°F to 77°F).

Mechanism of Action Selective agonist for serotonin ($5\text{-}HT_{1B}$ and $5\text{-}HT_{1D}$ receptors) in cranial arteries; causes vasoconstriction and reduces sterile inflammation associated with antidromic neuronal transmission correlating with relief of migraine

Pharmacodynamics/Kinetics

Onset of action: ~1-2 hours (Bomhof, 1999; Tfelt-Hansen, 2000)

Absorption: Well absorbed

Distribution: V_{dss}: 170 L

Protein binding, plasma: 28% to 31%

Metabolism: Hepatic via CYP

Bioavailability: ~70%

Half-life, elimination: 6 hours; increased in renal impairment (moderate impairment; mean: 11 hours; range: 7-20 hours); increased in hepatic impairment (moderate impairment: 8-16 hours)

Time to peak: 2-3 hours

Excretion: Urine (50% of total dose as unchanged drug; 30% of total dose as metabolites)

Dosage Note: If the first dose is ineffective, diagnosis needs to be re-evaluated. The safety of treating >4 migraines/month has not been established.

Acute migraine: Adults: Oral: Initial: 1-2.5 mg; if headache recurs or does not fully resolve, a second dose may be administered after 4 hours (maximum: 5 mg daily).

Elderly:

U.S. labeling: Refer to adult dosing. Dosing should generally start at the lower end of the dosing range due to possible increased incidence of hepatic, renal, and cardiac impairment.

Canadian labeling: Use is not recommended

Dosing in renal impairment:

Mild-to-moderate renal impairment:

U.S. labeling: Initial: 1 mg; do not exceed 2.5 mg in 24 hours

Canadian labeling: Initial: 1 mg; do not exceed 2 mg in 24 hours

Severe renal impairment (CrCl <15 mL/minute): Use is contraindicated

Dosing in hepatic impairment:

Mild-to-moderate hepatic impairment (Child-Pugh grade A or B):

U.S. labeling: Initial: 1 mg; do not exceed 2.5 mg in 24 hours

Canadian labeling: Initial: 1 mg; do not exceed 2 mg in 24 hours

Severe hepatic impairment (Child-Pugh grade C): Use is contraindicated

Administration Administer orally as soon as symptoms appear; may take with or without food. Do **not** crush or chew tablet; swallow whole with water.

Monitoring Parameters Headache severity, blood pressure, signs/symptoms suggestive of angina; perform a cardiovascular evaluation in triptan-naïve patients who have multiple cardiovascular risk factors (eg, increased age, diabetes, hypertension, smoking, obesity, strong family history of CAD), monitor ECG with first dose in patients with multiple cardiovascular risk factors who have a negative cardiovascular evaluation and consider periodic cardiovascular evaluation in such patients if they are intermittent long-term users; signs/symptoms of serotonin syndrome and hypersensitivity reactions.

Dosage Forms

Tablet, Oral:

Amerge: 1 mg, 2.5 mg

Generic: 1 mg, 2.5 mg

Extemporaneous Preparations A 0.5 mg/mL oral suspension may be made using tablets. Crush fifty 2.5 mg tablets and reduce to a fine powder. In small amounts, add 125 mL of Ora-Plus® and mix well after each addition. Transfer to a calibrated bottle, rinse mortar with vehicle, then add quantity of Ora-Sweet® or Ora-Sweet® SF sufficient to make 250 mL. Label "shake well" and "refrigerate". Stable 90 days refrigerated.

Nahata MC, Pai VB, and Hipple TF, *Pediatric Drug Formulations*, 5th ed, Cincinnati, OH: Harvey Whitney Books Co, 2004.

- **Naratriptan Hydrochloride** *see* Naratriptan *on page 1430*
- **Narcan** *see* Naloxone *on page 1419*
- **Nardil** *see* Phenelzine *on page 1630*
- **Nardil® (Can)** *see* Phenelzine *on page 1630*
- **Naropin** *see* Ropivacaine *on page 1846*
- **Naropin® (Can)** *see* Ropivacaine *on page 1846*
- **Nasacort Allergy 24HR [OTC]** *see* Triamcinolone (Nasal) *on page 2100*
- **Nasacort AQ** *see* Triamcinolone (Nasal) *on page 2100*
- **NasalCrom [OTC]** *see* Cromolyn (Nasal) *on page 514*
- **Nasal Decongestant [OTC]** *see* Phenylephrine (Systemic) *on page 1638*
- **Nasal Decongestant [OTC]** *see* Pseudoephedrine *on page 1742*
- **Nasal Decongestant PE Max St [OTC]** *see* Phenylephrine (Systemic) *on page 1638*
- **Nasalide® (Can)** *see* Flunisolide (Nasal) *on page 893*
- **Nasal Moist [OTC]** *see* Sodium Chloride *on page 1902*
- **Nascobal** *see* Cyanocobalamin *on page 515*
- **nasohist™ [OTC] [DSC]** *see* Chlorpheniramine and Phenylephrine *on page 426*
- **nasohist™ DM pediatric [OTC] [DSC]** *see* Chlorpheniramine, Phenylephrine, and Dextromethorphan *on page 428*
- **Nasonex** *see* Mometasone (Nasal) *on page 1391*
- **Nasonex® (Can)** *see* Mometasone (Nasal) *on page 1391*
- **Natacyn** *see* Natamycin *on page 1432*
- **Natacyn® (Can)** *see* Natamycin *on page 1432*

Natalizumab (na ta LIZ u mab)

Brand Names: U.S. Tysabri

Brand Names: Canada Tysabri

Index Terms AN100226; Anti-4 Alpha Integrin; IgG4-Kappa Monoclonal Antibody

Pharmacologic Category Gastrointestinal Agent, Miscellaneous; Monoclonal Antibody, Selective Adhesion-Molecule Inhibitor

Use

Crohn disease: For inducing and maintaining clinical response and remission in adult patients with moderately to severely active Crohn disease with evidence of inflammation who have had an inadequate response to, or are unable to tolerate, conventional Crohn disease therapies and inhibitors of tumor necrosis factor-alpha (TNF-alpha).

Multiple sclerosis: As monotherapy for the treatment of patients with relapsing forms of multiple sclerosis (MS). Natalizumab increases the risk of PML. When initiating and continuing treatment with natalizumab, consider whether the expected benefit of natalizumab is sufficient to offset this risk.

Canada labeling: Treatment of relapsing forms of multiple sclerosis

Pregnancy Risk Factor C

Dosage IV: Adults:

Multiple sclerosis: 300 mg infused over 1 hour every 4 weeks

Crohn disease: 300 mg infused over 1 hour every 4 weeks; discontinue if therapeutic benefit is not observed within initial 12 weeks of therapy

Concomitant use with corticosteroids: For patients who begin treatment while on chronic oral corticosteroids, begin tapering oral steroids when the onset of natalizumab therapeutic benefit is observed; discontinue use if patient cannot be tapered off of oral corticosteroids within 6 months of therapy initiation. If additional concomitant corticosteroids are required and exceed 3 months/year (in addition to initial corticosteroid taper), consider discontinuing therapy.

Dosage adjustment in renal impairment: No dosage adjustment provided in manufacturer's labeling (has not been studied).

Dosage adjustment in hepatic impairment: No dosage adjustment provided in manufacturer's labeling (has not been studied). Discontinue use with jaundice or signs/symptoms of hepatic injury.

Additional Information Complete prescribing information should be consulted for additional detail.

Dosage Forms

Concentrate, Intravenous [preservative free]:

Tysabri: 300 mg/15 mL (15 mL)

Natamycin (na ta MYE sin)

Brand Names: U.S. Natacyn

Brand Names: Canada Natacyn®

Index Terms Pimaricin

Pharmacologic Category Antifungal Agent, Ophthalmic

Use Treatment of blepharitis, conjunctivitis, and keratitis caused by susceptible fungi (*Aspergillus*, *Candida*, *Cephalosporium*, *Fusarium*, and *Penicillium*)

Pregnancy Risk Factor C

Dosage Adults: Ophthalmic:

Fungal keratitis: Instill 1 drop in conjunctival sac every 1-2 hours, after 3-4 days reduce to one drop 6-8 times/day; usual course of therapy is 2-3 weeks or until resolution of active fungal keratitis (may be useful to gradually reduce dosage at 4-7 day intervals to assure elimination of organism)

Fungal blepharitis or conjunctivitis: Instill 1 drop in conjunctival sac every 4-6 hours

Dosage adjustment in renal impairment: No dosage adjustment provided in manufacturer's labeling. However, dosage adjustment unlikely due to low systemic absorption.

Dosage adjustment in hepatic impairment: No dosage adjustment provided in manufacturer's labeling. However, dosage adjustment unlikely due to low systemic absorption.

Additional Information Complete prescribing information should be consulted for additional detail.

Dosage Forms

Suspension, Ophthalmic:

Natacyn: 5% (15 mL)

- **Natazia®** *see* Estradiol and Dienogest *on page 780*
- **Nat-Citalopram (Can)** *see* Citalopram *on page 451*

Nateglinide (na te GLYE nide)

Brand Names: U.S. Starlix

Brand Names: Canada Starlix

Pharmacologic Category Antidiabetic Agent, Meglitinide Analog

Use Type 2 diabetes mellitus: For the treatment of adults with type 2 diabetes mellitus as an adjunct to diet and exercise to improve glycemic control.

Pregnancy Risk Factor C

Pregnancy Considerations Adverse events have been observed in animal reproduction studies. Information describing the effects of nateglinide on pregnancy outcomes is limited (Twaites, 2007).

In women with diabetes, maternal hyperglycemia can be associated with congenital malformations as well as adverse effects in the fetus, neonate, and the mother (ACOG, 2005; ADA, 2014; Kitzmiller, 2008; Metzger, 2007). To prevent adverse outcomes, prior to conception and throughout pregnancy maternal blood glucose and HbA_{1c} should be kept as close to normal as possible but without causing significant hypoglycemia (ACOG, 2013; ADA, 2014; Blumer, 2013; Kitzmiller, 2008). Prior to pregnancy, effective contraception should be used until glycemic control is achieved (ADA, 2014; Kitzmiller, 2008). Other agents are currently recommended to treat diabetes in pregnant women (ACOG, 2013; Blumer, 2013).

Breast-Feeding Considerations It is not known if nateglinide is excreted in breast milk. Breast-feeding is not recommended by the manufacturer.

Contraindications Hypersensitivity to nateglinide or any component of the formulation; type 1 diabetes; diabetic ketoacidosis (this condition should be treated with insulin)

Warnings/Precautions Use with caution in patients with moderate-to-severe hepatic impairment. Use caution in severe renal dysfunction, elderly, malnourished, or patients with adrenal/pituitary dysfunction; may be more susceptible to glucose-lowering effects. All oral hypoglycemic agents are capable of producing hypoglycemia. Proper patient selection, dosage, and instructions to the patients are important to avoid hypoglycemic episodes. Ethanol may increase the risk of hypoglycemia; instruct patients to avoid ethanol. It may be necessary to discontinue nateglinide and administer insulin if the patient is exposed to stress (eg, fever, trauma, infection, surgery). Indicated for adjunctive therapy with metformin; not to be used as a substitute for metformin monotherapy. Combination treatment with sulfonylureas is not recommended (no additional benefit). Patients not adequately controlled on oral agents which stimulate insulin release (eg, glyburide) should not be switched to nateglinide or have nateglinide added to therapy.

Adverse Reactions As reported with nateglinide monotherapy:

Central nervous system: Dizziness

Endocrine & metabolic: Hypoglycemia, increased uric acid, weight gain

Neuromuscular & skeletal: Arthropathy

Respiratory: Flu-like symptoms, upper respiratory infection

Miscellaneous: Accidental injury

Rare but important or life-threatening: Cholestatic hepatitis, hypersensitivity reactions (including pruritus, rash, urticaria), increased liver enzymes, jaundice

Drug Interactions

Metabolism/Transport Effects Substrate of CYP2C9 (major), CYP3A4 (major), SLCO1B1; **Note:** Assignment of Major/Minor substrate status based on clinically relevant drug interaction potential; **Inhibits** CYP2C9 (weak)

Avoid Concomitant Use

Avoid concomitant use of Nateglinide with any of the following: Conivaptan; Fusidic Acid (Systemic); Idelalisib

Increased Effect/Toxicity

Nateglinide may increase the levels/effects of: Hypoglycemic Agents

The levels/effects of Nateglinide may be increased by: Androgens; Ceritinib; Conivaptan; CYP2C9 Inhibitors (Moderate); CYP2C9 Inhibitors (Strong); CYP3A4 Inhibitors (Moderate); CYP3A4 Inhibitors (Strong); Dasatinib; Eltrombopag; Fosaprepitant; Fusidic Acid (Systemic); Herbs (Hypoglycemic Properties); Idelalisib; Ivacaftor; Luliconazole; MAO Inhibitors; Mifepristone; Netupitant; Pegvisomant; Salicylates; Selective Serotonin Reuptake Inhibitors; SGLT2 Inhibitors; Simeprevir; Stiripentol; Teriflunomide

Decreased Effect

The levels/effects of Nateglinide may be decreased by: Bosentan; Corticosteroids (Orally Inhaled); Corticosteroids (Systemic); CYP2C9 Inducers (Strong); CYP3A4 Inducers (Moderate); CYP3A4 Inducers (Strong); Dabrafenib; Danazol; Deferasirox; Loop Diuretics; Luteinizing Hormone-Releasing Hormone Analogs; Mitotane; Siltuximab; Somatropin; St Johns Wort; Thiazide Diuretics; Tocilizumab

Food Interactions Rate of absorption is decreased and T_{max} is delayed when taken with food. Food does not affect AUC. Multiple peak plasma concentrations may be observed if fasting. Not affected by composition of meal. Management: Administer 1-30 minutes prior to meals.

Storage/Stability Store at 25°C (77°F); excursions are permitted between 15°C and 30°C (59°F and 86°F).

Mechanism of Action Nonsulfonylurea hypoglycemic agent which blocks ATP-dependent potassium channels, depolarizing the membrane and facilitating calcium entry through calcium channels. Increased intracellular calcium stimulates insulin release from the pancreatic beta cells. Nateglinide-induced insulin release is glucose-dependent.

Pharmacodynamics/Kinetics

Onset of action: Insulin secretion: ~20 minutes

Peak effect: 1 hour

Duration: 4 hours

Absorption: Rapid

Distribution: 10 L

Protein binding: 98%, primarily to albumin

Metabolism: Hepatic via hydroxylation followed by glucuronide conjugation via CYP2C9 (70%) and CYP3A4 (30%) to metabolites

Bioavailability: 73%

Half-life elimination: 1.5 hours

Time to peak: ≤1 hour

Excretion: Urine (83%, 16% as unchanged drug); feces (10%)

Dosage

Adults: Management of type 2 diabetes mellitus: Oral: Initial and maintenance dose: 120 mg 3 times daily; may be given alone or in combination with metformin or a thiazolidinedione. Patients close to HbA_{1c} goal at initiation of therapy may be started at 60 mg 3 times daily

Elderly: Refer to adult dosing

Dosage adjustment in renal impairment:

Mild to moderate impairment: No dosage adjustment necessary.

Severe impairment: No dosage adjustment necessary. Use with caution; may be more susceptible to glucose-lowering effects.

Dosage adjustment in hepatic impairment:

Mild impairment (Child-Pugh class A): No dosage adjustment necessary.

Moderate to severe impairment (Child-Pugh class B or C): No dosage adjustment provided in manufacturer's labeling. Use with caution; has not been studied.

Dietary Considerations Nateglinide should be taken 1-30 minutes prior to meals. Scheduled dose should not be taken if meal is missed to avoid hypoglycemia. Dietary modification based on ADA recommendations is a part of therapy. Decreases blood glucose concentration. Hypoglycemia may occur. Must be able to recognize symptoms of hypoglycemia (sweating, dizziness, palpitations, increased appetite, trembling).

Administration Administer 1-30 minutes prior to meals. Scheduled dose should not be administered if a meal is missed to avoid hypoglycemia.

Monitoring Parameters Monitor weight and lipid profile. Monitor fasting blood glucose (periodically) and glycosylated hemoglobin (HbA_{1c}) levels (every 3 months) with a goal of decreasing these levels towards the normal range. During dose adjustment, fasting glucose can be used to determine response.

Reference Range

Recommendations for glycemic control in nonpregnant adults with diabetes (ADA, 2015):

HbA_{1c}: <7% (a more aggressive [<6.5%] or less aggressive [<8%] HbA_{1c} goal may be targeted based on patient-specific characteristics)

Preprandial capillary plasma glucose: 80 to 130 mg/dL

Peak postprandial capillary blood glucose: <180 mg/dL

Recommendations for glycemic control in pediatric (all age groups) patients with type 1 diabetes (ADA, 2015):

HbA_{1c}: <7.5% (individualization may be appropriate based on patient-specific characteristics; <7% is reasonable if it can be achieved without excessive hypoglycemia)

Preprandial capillary plasma glucose: 90 to 130 mg/dL

Bedtime and overnight capillary blood glucose: 90 to 150 mg/dL

Additional Information An increase in weight was seen in nateglinide monotherapy, which was not seen when used in combination with metformin.

Dosage Forms

Tablet, Oral:

Starlix: 60 mg, 120 mg

Generic: 60 mg, 120 mg

◆ **Natesto** *see* Testosterone *on page* 2010

◆ **Natrecor** *see* Nesiritide *on page* 1439

◆ **Natriuretic Peptide** *see* Nesiritide *on page* 1439

◆ **Natroba** *see* Spinosad *on page* 1930

◆ **NatrOVA** *see* Spinosad *on page* 1930

◆ **Natulan (Can)** *see* Procarbazine *on page* 1717

◆ **Natural Fiber Therapy [OTC]** *see* Psyllium *on page* 1744

◆ **Natural Human Alpha-Interferon** *see* Interferon Alpha, Multi-Subtype [INT] *on page* 1100

◆ **Natural IFN-alpha** *see* Interferon Alpha, Multi-Subtype [INT] *on page* 1100

◆ **Natural Lung Surfactant** *see* Beractant *on page* 250

◆ **Natural Psyllium Seed [OTC]** *see* Psyllium *on page* 1744

◆ **Natural Vegetable Fiber [OTC]** *see* Psyllium *on page* 1744

◆ **Natural Vitamin E [OTC]** *see* Vitamin E *on page* 2174

◆ **Nature-Throid** *see* Thyroid, Desiccated *on page* 2031

◆ **Nauseatol [OTC] (Can)** *see* DimenhyDRINATE *on page* 637

◆ **Navane** *see* Thiothixene *on page* 2031

◆ **NAVA-SC** *see* Hydroquinone *on page* 1020

◆ **Navelbine** *see* Vinorelbine *on page* 2168

◆ **Na-Zone [OTC]** *see* Sodium Chloride *on page* 1902

◆ **N-Carbamoyl-L-Glutamic Acid** *see* Carglumic Acid *on page* 362

◆ **N-Carbamylglutamate** *see* Carglumic Acid *on page* 362

◆ ***n*-Docosanol** *see* Docosanol *on page* 661

Nebivolol (ne BIV oh lole)

Brand Names: U.S. Bystolic

Brand Names: Canada Bystolic

Index Terms Nebivolol Hydrochloride

Pharmacologic Category Antihypertensive; Beta-Blocker, Beta-1 Selective

Use Hypertension: Treatment of hypertension, alone or in combination with other agents

The 2014 guideline for the management of high blood pressure in adults (Eighth Joint National Committee [JNC 8]) recommends initiation of pharmacologic treatment to lower blood pressure for the following patients (JNC8 [James, 2013]):

- Patients ≥60 years of age, with systolic blood pressure (SBP) ≥150 mm Hg or diastolic blood pressure (DBP) ≥90 mm Hg. Goal of therapy is SBP <150 mm Hg and DBP <90 mm Hg.
- Patients <60 years of age, with SBP ≥140 mm Hg or DBP ≥90 mm Hg. Goal of therapy is SBP <140 mm Hg and DBP <90 mm Hg.
- Patients ≥18 years of age with diabetes, with SBP ≥140 mm Hg or DBP ≥90 mm Hg. Goal of therapy is SBP <140 mm Hg and DBP <90 mm Hg.
- Patients ≥18 years of age with chronic kidney disease (CKD), with SBP ≥140 mm Hg or DBP ≥90 mm Hg. Goal of therapy is SBP <140 mm Hg and DBP <90 mm Hg.

In patients with CKD, regardless of race or diabetes status, the use of an ACE inhibitor (ACEI) or angiotensin receptor blocker (ARB) as initial therapy is recommended to improve kidney outcomes. In the general nonblack population (without CKD) including those with diabetes, initial antihypertensive treatment should consist of a thiazide-type diuretic, calcium channel blocker, ACEI, or ARB. In the general black population (without CKD) including those with diabetes, initial antihypertensive treatment should consist of a thiazide-type diuretic or a calcium channel blocker **instead of** an ACEI or ARB.

Pregnancy Risk Factor C

Dosage

Adults: Oral:

U.S. labeling: Hypertension: Initial: 5 mg once daily; if initial response is inadequate, may be increased at 2-week intervals to a maximum dose of 40 mg once daily; usual dosage range (ASH/ISH [Weber, 2014]): 5 to 10 mg once daily

Canadian labeling: Hypertension: Initial: 5 mg once daily; if initial response is inadequate, may be increased at 2-week intervals to a maximum dose of 20 mg once daily; usual dosage range (ASH/ISH [Weber, 2014]): 5 to 10 mg once daily

Off-label use: Heart failure: Adults ≥70 years: Initial: 1.25 mg once daily; if tolerated, may increase by 2.5 mg at 1- to 2-week intervals to a maximum dose of 10 mg once daily (Flather, 2005). **Note:** Nebivolol has not been shown to reduce mortality in the general HF population.

Elderly: Refer to adult dosing.

Dosing adjustment in renal impairment: Severe impairment (CrCl <30 mL/minute): Initial: 2.5 mg daily; if initial response is inadequate, may increase cautiously.

Dosage adjustment in hepatic impairment:

Moderate impairment (Child-Pugh class B): Initial: 2.5 mg daily; if initial response is inadequate, may increase cautiously

Severe impairment (Child-Pugh class C): Use is contraindicated.

Additional Information Complete prescribing information should be consulted for additional detail.

Dosage Forms

Tablet, Oral:

Bystolic: 2.5 mg, 5 mg, 10 mg, 20 mg

- ◆ **Nebivolol Hydrochloride** *see* Nebivolol *on page 1434*
- ◆ **Nebupent** *see* Pentamidine *on page 1616*
- ◆ **Nebusal** *see* Sodium Chloride *on page 1902*
- ◆ **Necon 0.5/35** *see* Ethinyl Estradiol and Norethindrone *on page 808*
- ◆ **Necon 1/35** *see* Ethinyl Estradiol and Norethindrone *on page 808*
- ◆ **Necon® 1/50** *see* Norethindrone and Mestranol *on page 1475*
- ◆ **Necon 7/7/7** *see* Ethinyl Estradiol and Norethindrone *on page 808*
- ◆ **Necon 10/11** *see* Ethinyl Estradiol and Norethindrone *on page 808*

Nedocromil (ne doe KROE mil)

Brand Names: U.S. Alocril

Brand Names: Canada Alocril®

Index Terms Nedocromil Sodium

Pharmacologic Category Mast Cell Stabilizer

Use Treatment of itching associated with allergic conjunctivitis

Pregnancy Risk Factor B

Dosage Ophthalmic: Children ≥3 years and Adults: 1-2 drops in each eye twice daily daily throughout the period of exposure to allergen

Dosage adjustment in renal impairment: No dosage adjustment provided in manufacturer's labeling. However, dosage adjustment unlikely due to low systemic absorption.

Dosage adjustment in hepatic impairment: No dosage adjustment provided in manufacturer's labeling. However, dosage adjustment unlikely due to low systemic absorption.

Additional Information Complete prescribing information should be consulted for additional detail.

Dosage Forms

Solution, Ophthalmic:

Alocril: 2% (5 mL)

- ◆ **Nedocromil Sodium** *see* Nedocromil *on page 1435*

Nefazodone (nef AY zoe done)

Index Terms Nefazodone Hydrochloride; Serzone

Pharmacologic Category Antidepressant, Serotonin Reuptake Inhibitor/Antagonist

Use Depression: Treatment of depression

Pregnancy Risk Factor C

Dosage

Depression: Oral:

Adults: Initial: 100 mg twice daily; alternatively, depression treatment guidelines suggest starting doses of 50 to 100 mg daily (APA, 2010; Bauer 2013). Based on response and tolerability, gradually increase dose in increments of 100 to 200 mg daily (in 2 divided doses) and intervals of no less than 1 week to a usual dose of 150 to 600 mg daily in 2 divided doses

Elderly/Debilitated: Initial: 50 mg twice daily; gradually increase dose based on response and tolerability

Discontinuation of therapy: Upon discontinuation of antidepressant therapy, gradually taper the dose to minimize the incidence of withdrawal symptoms and allow for the detection of re-emerging symptoms. Evidence supporting ideal taper rates is limited. APA and NICE guidelines suggest tapering therapy over at least several weeks with consideration to the half-life of the antidepressant; antidepressants with a shorter half-life may need to be tapered more conservatively. In addition for long-term treated patients, WFSBP guidelines recommend tapering over 4 to 6 months. If intolerable withdrawal symptoms occur following a dose reduction, consider resuming the previously prescribed dose and/or decrease dose at a more gradual rate (APA, 2010; Bauer, 2002; Haddad, 2001; NCCMH, 2010; Schatzberg, 2006; Shelton, 2001; Warner, 2006).

MAO inhibitor recommendations:

Switching to or from an MAO inhibitor intended to treat psychiatric disorders:

Allow 14 days to elapse between discontinuing an MAO inhibitor intended to treat psychiatric disorders and initiation of nefazodone.

Allow 14 days to elapse between discontinuing nefazodone and initiation of an MAO inhibitor intended to treat psychiatric disorders.

Use with other MAO inhibitors (such as linezolid or IV methylene blue):

Do not initiate nefazodone in patients receiving linezolid or IV methylene blue; consider other interventions for psychiatric condition.

If urgent treatment with linezolid or IV methylene blue is required in a patient already receiving nefazodone and potential benefits outweigh potential risks, discontinue nefazodone promptly and administer linezolid or IV methylene blue. Monitor for serotonin syndrome for 2 weeks or until 24 hours after the last dose of linezolid or IV methylene blue, whichever comes first. May resume nefazodone 24 hours after the last dose of linezolid or IV methylene blue.

Dosage adjustment in renal impairment: There are no dosage adjustments provided in the manufacturer's labeling; however, adjustment unlikely since renal impairment does not alter steady state nefazodone plasma concentrations.

Dosage adjustment in hepatic impairment: There are no dosage adjustments provided in the manufacturer's labeling; however, use with caution since the AUC of nefazodone and its metabolites are ~25% greater in patients with cirrhosis

Additional Information Complete prescribing information should be consulted for additional detail.

Dosage Forms

Tablet, Oral:

Generic: 50 mg, 100 mg, 150 mg, 200 mg, 250 mg

- ◆ **Nefazodone Hydrochloride** *see* Nefazodone *on page 1435*

Nelarabine (nel AY re been)

Brand Names: U.S. Arranon

Brand Names: Canada Atriance™

Index Terms 2-Amino-6-Methoxypurine Arabinoside; 506U78; GW506U78

Pharmacologic Category Antineoplastic Agent, Antimetabolite; Antineoplastic Agent, Antimetabolite (Purine Analog)

Use Treatment of relapsed or refractory T-cell acute lymphoblastic leukemia (ALL) and T-cell lymphoblastic lymphoma

Pregnancy Risk Factor D

Dosage IV: T-cell ALL, T-cell lymphoblastic lymphoma:

Children: 650 mg/m^2/dose on days 1 through 5; repeat every 21 days until transplant, disease progression, or unacceptable toxicity

Adults: 1500 mg/m²/dose on days 1, 3, and 5; repeat every 21 days until transplant, disease progression, or unacceptable toxicity

Dosage adjustment for toxicity:

Neurologic toxicity ≥ grade 2: Discontinue treatment.

Hematologic or other (non-neurologic) toxicity: Consider treatment delay.

Dosage adjustment in renal impairment:

CrCl ≥50 mL/minute: No dosage adjustment necessary.

CrCl <50 mL/minute: No dosage adjustment provided in manufacturer's labeling, (although ARA-G clearance is decreased as renal function declines, data is insufficient for a dosing recommendation); monitor closely.

Dosage adjustment in hepatic impairment: No dosage adjustment provided in manufacturer's labeling (has not been studied); closely monitor with severe impairment (total bilirubin >3 times ULN)

Dosing in obesity: *ASCO Guidelines for appropriate chemotherapy dosing in obese adults with cancer:* Utilize patient's actual body weight (full weight) for calculation of body surface area- or weight-based dosing, particularly when the intent of therapy is curative; manage regimen-related toxicities in the same manner as for nonobese patients; if a dose reduction is utilized due to toxicity, consider resumption of full weight-based dosing with subsequent cycles, especially if cause of toxicity (eg, hepatic or renal impairment) is resolved (Griggs, 2012).

Additional Information Complete prescribing information should be consulted for additional detail.

Dosage Forms

Solution, Intravenous:

Arranon: 5 mg/mL (50 mL)

Dosage Forms: Canada

Injection, solution:

Atriance™: 5 mg/mL (50 mL)

Nelfinavir (nel FIN a veer)

Brand Names: U.S. Viracept

Brand Names: Canada Viracept

Index Terms NFV

Pharmacologic Category Antiretroviral, Protease Inhibitor (Anti-HIV)

Use In combination with other antiretroviral therapy in the treatment of HIV infection

Pregnancy Risk Factor B

Dosage

HIV infection: Oral:

Children 2 to <13 years:

U.S. labeling:

Weight-directed dosing: 45 to 55 mg/kg twice daily or 25 to 35 mg/kg 3 times daily (maximum: 2500 mg daily)

Fixed dosing:

10 to 12 kg: 500 mg (2 tablets) twice daily **or** 250 mg (1 tablet) 3 times daily

13 to 18 kg: 750 mg (3 tablets) twice daily **or** 500 mg (2 tablets) 3 times daily

19 to 20 kg: 1000 mg (4 tablets) twice daily **or** 500 mg (2 tablets) 3 times daily

>20 kg: 1000 to 1250 mg (4 to 5 tablets) twice daily **or** 750 mg (3 tablets) 3 times daily

Canadian labeling: 25 to 30 mg/kg 3 times daily (maximum: 2500 mg daily).

Adolescents and Adults: 750 mg 3 times daily or 1250 mg twice daily with meals in combination with other antiretroviral therapies. **Note:** The HHS Perinatal HIV Guidelines do not recommend the 3-times-daily dosing in pregnant women (HHS [perinatal], 2014).

Dosage adjustment in renal impairment: There are no dosage adjustments provided in the manufacturer's labeling (has not been studied). However, since <2% excreted in urine a dosage reduction would not be expected. Guidelines suggest that no dosage adjustment is necessary (HHS [adult], 2014).

Dosage adjustment in hepatic impairment:

U.S. labeling:

Mild impairment (Child-Pugh class A): No dosage adjustment necessary.

Moderate to severe impairment (Child-Pugh class B or C): Use not recommended.

Canadian labeling: There is no dosage adjustment provided in the manufacturer's labeling; use with caution.

Additional Information Complete prescribing information should be consulted for additional detail.

Dosage Forms

Tablet, Oral:

Viracept: 250 mg, 625 mg

- **Nembutal** *see* PENTobarbital *on page 1617*
- **Nembutal® Sodium (Can)** *see* PENTobarbital *on page 1617*
- **NeoCeuticals Post-Acne Fade [OTC]** *see* Hydroquinone *on page 1020*
- **Neo DM [OTC] [DSC]** *see* Chlorpheniramine, Phenylephrine, and Dextromethorphan *on page 428*
- **Neo-Fradin [DSC]** *see* Neomycin *on page 1436*

Neomycin (nee oh MYE sin)

Brand Names: U.S. Neo-Fradin [DSC]

Index Terms Neomycin Sulfate

Pharmacologic Category Ammonium Detoxicant; Antibiotic, Aminoglycoside; Antibiotic, Topical

Use Surgical (perioperative) prophylaxis for GI surgery; treatment of diarrhea caused by *E. coli*; adjunct in the treatment of hepatic encephalopathy

Pregnancy Risk Factor D

Dosage

Children: Oral:

Surgical (perioperative) prophylaxis: Oral: 15 mg/kg/dose for 3 doses administered over 10 hours (eg, at 1 PM, 2 PM, and 11 PM) on the day preceding surgery; maximum dose: 1000 mg; (Bratzler, 2013); used as an adjunct to mechanical cleansing of the intestine and in combination with erythromycin base and perioperative IV antibiotics

Hepatic encephalopathy: 50-100 mg/kg/day in divided doses every 6-8 hours or 2.5-7 g/m²/day divided every 4-6 hours for 5-6 days not to exceed 12 g daily

Adults: Oral:

Surgical (perioperative) prophylaxis:

Manufacturer's recommendations: 1 g at 1 PM, 2 PM, and 11 PM on the day preceding 8 AM surgery as an adjunct to mechanical cleansing of the bowel and oral erythromycin

Alternative recommendation: 1 g at 1 PM, 2 PM, and 11 PM on the day preceding 8 AM surgery combined with mechanical cleansing of the large intestine and oral erythromycin or metronidazole, and IV antibiotics on the day of surgery (Bratzler, 2013)

Hepatic encephalopathy: 500-2000 mg every 6-8 hours or 4-12 g daily divided every 4-6 hours for 5-6 days

Chronic hepatic insufficiency: 4 g daily for an indefinite period

Dosage adjustment in renal impairment: No specific dosage adjustment provided in manufacturer's labeling; however, dosage reduction or discontinuation of therapy should be considered if a patient develops renal insufficiency. The risk of nephro- and/or ototoxicity is increased in patients with renal impairment.

Dosage adjustment in hepatic impairment: No dosage adjustment provided in manufacturer's labeling.

Additional Information Complete prescribing information should be consulted for additional detail.

Dosage Forms

Tablet, Oral:

Generic: 500 mg

Neomycin and Polymyxin B

(nee oh MYE sin & pol i MIKS in bee)

Brand Names: U.S. Neosporin® G.U. Irrigant

Brand Names: Canada Neosporin® Irrigating Solution

Index Terms Polymyxin B and Neomycin

Pharmacologic Category Antibiotic, Topical; Genitourinary Irrigant

Use Short-term as a continuous irrigant or rinse in the urinary bladder to prevent bacteriuria and gram-negative rod septicemia associated with the use of indwelling catheters

Pregnancy Risk Factor D

Dosage Children and Adults: Bladder irrigation: **Not for injection**; add 1 mL irrigant to 1 L isotonic saline solution and connect container to the inflow of lumen of 3-way catheter. Continuous irrigant or rinse in the urinary bladder for up to a maximum of 10 days with administration rate adjusted to patient's urine output; usually no more than 1 L of irrigant is used per day.

Additional Information Complete prescribing information should be consulted for additional detail.

Dosage Forms

Solution, irrigation: Neomycin 40 mg and polymyxin B sulfate 200,000 units per 1 mL (1 mL, 20 mL)

Neosporin® G.U. Irrigant: Neomycin 40 mg and polymyxin sulfate B 200,000 units per 1 mL (1 mL, 20 mL)

◆ **Neomycin, Bacitracin, and Polymyxin B** *see* Bacitracin, Neomycin, and Polymyxin B *on page 223*

◆ **Neomycin, Bacitracin, Polymyxin B, and Hydrocortisone** *see* Bacitracin, Neomycin, Polymyxin B, and Hydrocortisone *on page 223*

Neomycin, Colistin, Hydrocortisone, and Thonzonium

(nee oh MYE sin, koe LIS tin, hye droe KOR ti sone, & thon ZOE nee um)

Brand Names: U.S. Coly-Mycin® S; Cortisporin®-TC

Index Terms Colistin, Hydrocortisone, Neomycin, and Thonzonium; Hydrocortisone, Neomycin, Colistin, and Thonzonium; Thonzonium, Neomycin, Colistin, and Hydrocortisone

Pharmacologic Category Antibiotic, Otic; Antibiotic/Corticosteroid, Otic; Corticosteroid, Otic

Use Treatment of superficial and susceptible bacterial infections of the external auditory canal; for treatment of susceptible bacterial infections of mastoidectomy and fenestration cavities

Pregnancy Risk Factor C

Dosage Otic:

Calibrated dropper:

Children: 4 drops in affected ear 3-4 times/day

Adults: 5 drops in affected ear 3-4 times/day

Dropper bottle:

Children: 3 drops in affected ear 3-4 times/day

Adults: 4 drops in affected ear 3-4 times/day

Note: Alternatively, a cotton wick may be inserted in the ear canal and saturated with suspension every 4 hours; wick should be replaced at least every 24 hours

Dosage adjustment in renal impairment: No dosage adjustment provided in manufacturer's labeling. However, dosage adjustment unlikely due to low systemic absorption.

Dosage adjustment in hepatic impairment: No dosage adjustment provided in manufacturer's labeling. However, dosage adjustment unlikely due to low systemic absorption.

Additional Information Complete prescribing information should be consulted for additional detail.

Dosage Forms

Suspension, otic [drops]:

Coly-Mycin® S: Neomycin 0.33%, colistin 0.3%, hydrocortisone 1%, and thonzonium 0.05% (5 mL)

Cortisporin®-TC: Neomycin 0.33%, colistin 0.3%, hydrocortisone 1%, and thonzonium 0.05% (10 mL)

Neomycin, Polymyxin B, and Dexamethasone

(nee oh MYE sin, pol i MIKS in bee, & deks a METH a sone)

Brand Names: U.S. Maxitrol®

Brand Names: Canada Dioptrol®; Maxitrol®

Index Terms Dexamethasone, Neomycin, and Polymyxin B; Polymyxin B, Neomycin, and Dexamethasone

Pharmacologic Category Antibiotic/Corticosteroid, Ophthalmic

Use Steroid-responsive inflammatory ocular conditions in which a corticosteroid is indicated and where bacterial infection or a risk of bacterial infection exists

Pregnancy Risk Factor C

Dosage Ophthalmic:

Children ≥2 years and Adults: Suspension: Instill 1-2 drops into the conjunctival sac of the affected eye(s) 4-6 times/day; in severe disease, drops may be used hourly and tapered to discontinuation

Adults: Ointment: Place ~1/2" ribbon in the conjunctival sac of the affected eye(s) 3-4 times/day or apply at bedtime as an adjunct with suspension

Note: If signs and symptoms do not improve after 2 days of treatment, the patient should be re-evaluated.

Dosage adjustment in renal impairment: No dosage adjustment provided in manufacturer's labeling. However, dosage adjustment unlikely due to insignificant systemic absorption.

Dosage adjustment in hepatic impairment: No dosage adjustment provided in manufacturer's labeling. However, dosage adjustment unlikely due to insignificant systemic absorption.

Additional Information Complete prescribing information should be consulted for additional detail.

Dosage Forms

Ointment, ophthalmic: Neomycin 3.5 mg, polymyxin B 10,000 units, and dexamethasone 0.1% per g (3.5 g)

Maxitrol®: Neomycin 3.5 mg, polymyxin B 10,000 units, and dexamethasone 0.1% per g (3.5 g)

Suspension, ophthalmic: Neomycin 3.5 mg, polymyxin B 10,000 units, and dexamethasone 0.1% per 1 mL (5 mL)

Maxitrol®: Neomycin 3.5 mg, polymyxin B10,000 units, and dexamethasone 0.1% per 1 mL (5 mL)

Neomycin, Polymyxin B, and Gramicidin

(nee oh MYE sin, pol i MIKS in bee, & gram i SYE din)

Brand Names: U.S. Neosporin® Ophthalmic Solution

Brand Names: Canada Neosporin®; Optimyxin Plus®

Index Terms Gramicidin, Neomycin, and Polymyxin B; Polymyxin B, Neomycin, and Gramicidin

Pharmacologic Category Antibiotic, Ophthalmic

Use Treatment of superficial ocular infection

Pregnancy Risk Factor C

Dosage Children and Adults: Ophthalmic: Instill 1-2 drops 4-6 times/day or more frequently as required for severe infections

Additional Information Complete prescribing information should be consulted for additional detail.

Dosage Forms

Solution, ophthalmic [drops]: Neomycin 1.75 mg, polymyxin B 10,000 units, and gramicidin 0.025 mg per 1 mL (10 mL)

Neosporin® Ophthalmic Solution: Neomycin 1.75 mg, polymyxin B 10,000 units, and gramicidin 0.025 mg per 1 mL (10 mL)

Neomycin, Polymyxin B, and Hydrocortisone

(nee oh MYE sin, pol i MIKS in bee, & hye droe KOR ti sone)

Brand Names: U.S. Cortisporin; Cortomycin

Brand Names: Canada Cortimyxin; Cortisporin Otic

Index Terms Hydrocortisone, Neomycin, and Polymyxin B; Polymyxin B, Neomycin, and Hydrocortisone

Pharmacologic Category Antibiotic, Ophthalmic; Antibiotic, Otic; Antibiotic, Topical; Antibiotic/Corticosteroid, Ophthalmic; Antibiotic/Corticosteroid, Otic; Antibiotic/Corticosteroid, Topical; Corticosteroid, Ophthalmic; Corticosteroid, Otic; Corticosteroid, Topical

Use Steroid-responsive inflammatory condition for which a corticosteroid is indicated and where bacterial infection or a risk of bacterial infection exists

Pregnancy Risk Factor C

Dosage Note: Duration of use of ophthalmic and otic preparations should be limited to 10 days unless otherwise directed by the healthcare provider.

Ophthalmic:

Children (off-label use): Instill 1-2 drops 2-4 times/day, or more frequently as required for severe infections

Adults: Instill 1-2 drops 2-4 times/day, or more frequently as required for severe infections

Otic: Otic solution is used **only** for bacterial infections of external auditory canal (eg, swimmer's ear).

Children 6 months to 2 years (off-label use): Instill 3 drops into affected ear 3-4 times/day

Children ≥2 years: Instill 3 drops into affected ear 3-4 times/day

Adults: Instill 4 drops into affected ear 3-4 times/day; otic suspension is the preferred otic preparation

Topical:

Children (off-label use): Apply a thin layer 1-4 times/day. Therapy should be discontinued when control is achieved; if no improvement is seen, reassessment of diagnosis may be necessary.

Adults: Apply a thin layer 1-4 times/day. Therapy should be discontinued when control is achieved; if no improvement is seen, reassessment of diagnosis may be necessary.

Dosage adjustment in renal impairment: No dosage adjustment provided in manufacturer's labeling. However, dosage adjustment unlikely due to low systemic absorption.

Dosage adjustment in hepatic impairment: No dosage adjustment provided in manufacturer's labeling. However, dosage adjustment unlikely due to low systemic absorption.

Additional Information Complete prescribing information should be consulted for additional detail.

Dosage Forms

Cream, topical:

Cortisporin®: Neomycin 3.5 mg, polymyxin B 10,000 units, and hydrocortisone 5 mg per g (7.5 g)

Solution, otic: Neomycin 3.5 mg, polymyxin B 10,000 units, and hydrocortisone 10 mg per mL (10 mL)

Cortisporin®, Cortomycin: Neomycin 3.5 mg, polymyxin B 10,000 units, and hydrocortisone 10 mg per mL (10 mL)

Suspension, ophthalmic [drops]: Neomycin 3.5 mg, polymyxin B 10,000 units, and hydrocortisone 10 mg per mL (7.5 mL)

Suspension, otic: Neomycin 3.5 mg, polymyxin B 10,000 units, and hydrocortisone 10 mg per mL (10 mL)

Cortomycin: Neomycin 3.5 mg, polymyxin B 10,000 units, and hydrocortisone 10 mg per mL (10 mL)

- ◆ **Neomycin Sulfate** *see* Neomycin *on page 1436*
- ◆ **Neo-Polycin™** *see* Bacitracin, Neomycin, and Polymyxin B *on page 223*
- ◆ **Neo-Polycin™ HC** *see* Bacitracin, Neomycin, Polymyxin B, and Hydrocortisone *on page 223*
- ◆ **NeoProfen** *see* Ibuprofen *on page 1032*
- ◆ **Neoral** *see* CycloSPORINE (Systemic) *on page 522*
- ◆ **Neosar** *see* Cyclophosphamide *on page 517*
- ◆ **Neosporin® (Can)** *see* Neomycin, Polymyxin B, and Gramicidin *on page 1437*
- ◆ **Neosporin® G.U. Irrigant** *see* Neomycin and Polymyxin B *on page 1437*
- ◆ **Neosporin® Irrigating Solution (Can)** *see* Neomycin and Polymyxin B *on page 1437*
- ◆ **Neosporin® Neo To Go® [OTC]** *see* Bacitracin, Neomycin, and Polymyxin B *on page 223*
- ◆ **Neosporin® Ophthalmic Solution** *see* Neomycin, Polymyxin B, and Gramicidin *on page 1437*
- ◆ **Neosporin® Topical [OTC]** *see* Bacitracin, Neomycin, and Polymyxin B *on page 223*

Neostigmine (nee oh STIG meen)

Brand Names: U.S. Bloxiverz; Prostigmin

Brand Names: Canada Prostigmin

Index Terms Neostigmine Bromide; Neostigmine Methylsulfate

Pharmacologic Category Acetylcholinesterase Inhibitor

Use

Myasthenia gravis (excluding Bloxiverz): Symptomatic control of myasthenia gravis

Postoperative bladder distention/Urinary retention (excluding Bloxiverz and Prostigmin tablets): Prevention and treatment of postoperative bladder distention and urinary retention after mechanical obstruction has been excluded.

Reversal of nondepolarizing muscle relaxants (excluding Prostigmin tablets): Reversal of effects of nondepolarizing neuromuscular blocking agents (eg, tubocurarine, or pancuronium) after surgery.

Pregnancy Risk Factor C

Dosage

Myasthenia gravis: Diagnosis (off-label use): IM:

Children: 0.025-0.04 mg/kg as a single dose

Adults: 0.02 mg/kg as a single dose

Myasthenia gravis: Treatment:

Children (off-label use):

Oral: 2 mg/kg/day, not to exceed 375 mg daily

IM, IV, SubQ: 0.01-0.04 mg/kg every 2-4 hours as needed

Adults:

Manufacturer's labeling:

Oral: Usual dose: 150 mg administered over a 24-hour period; interval between doses is of paramount importance and therapy is frequently required day and night. Dosage range: 15-375 mg daily in divided doses.

IM, SubQ: 0.5 mg; subsequent dosing based on individual patient response

Alternative recommendations (off-label dosing):

Oral: Initial: 15 mg every 8 hours; may increase every 1-2 days up to 375 mg daily maximum; interval between doses must be individualized to maximal response

IM, IV, SubQ: 0.5-2.5 mg every 1-3 hours as needed up to 10 mg/24 hours maximum

Reversal of nondepolarizing neuromuscular-blocking agents (NMBAs) after surgery:

Bloxiverz: IV: **Note:** An anticholinergic agent (atropine or glycopyrrolate) should be given prior to or in conjunction with neostigmine; in the presence of bradycardia, administer the anticholinergic prior to neostigmine. Peripheral nerve stimulation delivering train-of-four (TOF) stimulus must also be used to determine time of neostigmine initiation and need for additional doses.

Infants, Children, Adolescents, and Adults: Usual dose: 0.03-0.07 mg/kg generally achieves a TOF twitch ratio of 90% within 10-20 minutes of administration; maximum total dose: 0.07 mg/kg or 5 mg (whichever is less)

Dose selection guide:

The 0.03 mg/kg dose is recommended for reversal of NMBAs with shorter half-lives (eg, rocuronium); **or** when the first twitch response to the TOF stimulus is substantially >10% of baseline or when a second twitch is present.

The 0.07 mg/kg dose is recommended for NMBAs with longer half-lives (eg, vecuronium, pancuronium); **or** when the first twitch response is relatively weak (ie, not substantially >10% of baseline); or rapid recovery is needed.

Generic products: IV: **Note:** Administer with atropine 0.6-1.2 mg in a separate syringe several minutes before neostigmine.

Adults: 0.5-2 mg; repeat as required. Only in exceptional cases should the total dose exceed 5 mg.

Postoperative urinary retention: Adults: IM, SubQ:

Prevention: 0.25 mg as soon as possible after operation; repeat every 4-6 hours for 2-3 days

Treatment: 0.5 mg; if urination does not occur within an hour, patient should be catheterized. After the bladder has emptied or patient has voided, continue 0.5 mg every 3 hours for at least 5 doses.

Postoperative bladder distention: Adults: IM, SubQ:

Prevention: 0.25 mg as soon as possible after operation; repeat every 4-6 hours for 2-3 days

Treatment: 0.5 mg as needed

Dosage adjustment in renal impairment:

No dosage adjustment provided in manufacturer's labeling; however, the following adjustments have been recommended (Aronoff, 2007): Adults: Oral

CrCl >50 mL/minute: No dosage adjustment necessary

CrCl 10-50 mL/minute: Administer 50% of normal dose

CrCl <10 mL/minute: Administer 25% of normal dose

Hemodialysis: No dosage adjustment necessary

Peritoneal dialysis: No dosage adjustment necessary

Continuous renal replacement therapy (CRRT): Administer 50% of normal dose

Dosage adjustment in hepatic impairment: No dosage adjustment provided in manufacturer's labeling.

Additional Information Complete prescribing information should be consulted for additional detail.

Dosage Forms

Solution, Injection:

Prostigmin: 0.5 mg/mL (1 mL, 10 mL)

Generic: 0.5 mg/mL (10 mL); 1 mg/mL (10 mL)

Solution, Intravenous:

Bloxiverz: 5 mg/10 mL (10 mL); 10 mg/10 mL (10 mL)

- **Neostigmine Bromide** *see* Neostigmine *on page 1438*
- **Neostigmine Methylsulfate** *see* Neostigmine *on page 1438*
- **NeoStrata® HQ (Can)** *see* Hydroquinone *on page 1020*
- **NeoStrata HQ Skin Lightening [OTC]** *see* Hydroquinone *on page 1020*
- **NEPA** *see* Netupitant and Palonosetron *on page 1440*

Nepafenac (ne pa FEN ak)

Brand Names: U.S. Ilevro; Nevanac

Brand Names: Canada Nevanac®

Pharmacologic Category Nonsteroidal Anti-inflammatory Drug (NSAID), Ophthalmic

Use Treatment of pain and inflammation associated with cataract surgery

Pregnancy Risk Factor C

Dosage

Ophthalmic: Children ≥10 years, Adolescents, and Adults:

Ilevro™: Instill 1 drop into affected eye(s) once daily, beginning 1 day prior to surgery, the day of surgery, and through the first 2 weeks of the postoperative period. Instill 1 additional drop 30-120 minutes prior to surgery.

Nevanac®: Instill 1 drop into affected eye(s) 3 times/day, beginning 1 day prior to surgery, the day of surgery, and through the first 2 weeks of the postoperative period.

Dosage adjustment in renal impairment: No dosage adjustment provided in manufacturer's labeling.

Dosage adjustment in hepatic impairment: No dosage adjustment provided in manufacturer's labeling.

Additional Information Complete prescribing information should be consulted for additional detail.

Dosage Forms

Suspension, Ophthalmic:

Ilevro: 0.3% (1.7 mL, 3 mL)

Nevanac: 0.1% (3 mL)

- **Neptazane** *see* Methazolamide *on page 1317*
- **Nerisone Cream (Can)** *see* Diflucortolone [CAN/INT] *on page 625*
- **Nerisone Oily Cream (Can)** *see* Diflucortolone [CAN/INT] *on page 625*
- **Nerisone Ointment (Can)** *see* Diflucortolone [CAN/INT] *on page 625*
- **Nerve Agent Antidote Kit** *see* Atropine and Pralidoxime *on page 203*
- **Nesacaine** *see* Chloroprocaine *on page 423*
- **Nesacaine®-CE (Can)** *see* Chloroprocaine *on page 423*
- **Nesacaine-MPF** *see* Chloroprocaine *on page 423*

Nesiritide (ni SIR i tide)

Brand Names: U.S. Natrecor

Index Terms B-type Natriuretic Peptide (Human); hBNP; Natriuretic Peptide

Pharmacologic Category Natriuretic Peptide, B-Type, Human

Use Treatment of acutely decompensated heart failure (HF) with dyspnea at rest or with minimal activity

Pregnancy Risk Factor C

Dosage Adults: IV: Initial: 2 mcg/kg (bolus optional); followed by continuous infusion at 0.01 mcg/kg/minute. **Note:** Should not be initiated at a dosage higher than initial recommended dose. There is limited experience with increasing the dose >0.01 mcg/kg/minute; in one trial, a limited number of patients received higher doses that were increased no faster than every 3 hours by 0.005 mcg/kg/minute (preceded by a bolus of 1 mcg/kg), up to a maximum of 0.03 mcg/kg/minute. Increases beyond the initial infusion rate should be limited to selected patients and accompanied by close hemodynamic and renal function monitoring.

Patients experiencing hypotension during the infusion: Infusion dose should be reduced or discontinued. Other measures to support blood pressure should be initiated (eg, IV fluids, Trendelenburg position). Hypotension may be prolonged (up to hours); once patient is stabilized, may attempt to restart at a lower dose (reduce previous infusion dose by 30% and omit bolus).

Maximum dosing weight: According to the manufacturer, the PRECEDENT Trial capped dosing weight at 160 kg and the VMAC Trial capped dosing weight at 175 kg. There are no specific guidelines on maximum dosing weight and clinical judgment should be used.

Dosage adjustment in renal impairment: No dosage adjustment necessary. Use cautiously in patients with renal impairment or those patients who rely on the renin-angiotensin-aldosterone system for renal perfusion. Monitor renal function closely.

Dosage adjustment in hepatic impairment: No dosage adjustment provided in manufacturer's labeling.

Additional Information Complete prescribing information should be consulted for additional detail.

Dosage Forms

Solution Reconstituted, Intravenous:

Natrecor: 1.5 mg (1 ea)

◆ **NESP** *see* Darbepoetin Alfa *on page* 565

Netupitant and Palonosetron

(net UE pi tant & pal oh NOE se tron)

Brand Names: U.S. Akynzeo

Index Terms NEPA; Palonosetron and Netupitant

Pharmacologic Category Antiemetic; Selective 5-HT_3 Receptor Antagonist; Substance P/Neurokinin 1 Receptor Antagonist

Use Chemotherapy-induced nausea and vomiting: Prevention of acute and delayed nausea and vomiting associated with initial and repeat courses of cancer chemotherapy, including, but not limited to, highly emetogenic chemotherapy.

Dosage

Highly-emetogenic chemotherapy (including cisplatin-based): Adults: Oral: One capsule ~1 hour prior to initiation of chemotherapy on day 1 (Gralla, 2014). **Note:** Antiemetic regimen also includes dexamethasone 12 mg orally ~30 minutes prior to initiation of chemotherapy on day 1, and 8 mg orally once daily on days 2 to 4.

Anthracycline and cyclophosphamide-based chemotherapy and chemotherapy not considered highly emetogenic: Adults: Oral: One capsule ~1 hour prior to initiation of chemotherapy on day 1 (Gralla, 2014). **Note:** Antiemetic regimen also includes dexamethasone 12 mg orally ~30 minutes prior to chemotherapy on day 1.

Elderly: No dosage adjustment necessary. Refer to adult dosing.

Dosage adjustment in renal impairment:

Mild or moderate impairment: No dosage adjustment necessary.

Severe impairment or ESRD: Avoid use.

Dosage adjustment in hepatic impairment:

Mild or moderate impairment (Child-Pugh score 5 to 8): No dosage adjustment is necessary.

Severe impairment (Child-Pugh score >9): Avoid use.

Additional Information Complete prescribing information should be consulted for additional detail.

Dosage Forms

Capsule, Oral:

Akynzeo: Netupitant 300 mg and palonosetron 0.5 mg

◆ **Neulasta** *see* Pegfilgrastim *on page* 1589
◆ **Neulasta Delivery Kit** *see* Pegfilgrastim *on page* 1589
◆ **Neuleptil® (Can)** *see* Periciazine [CAN/INT] *on page* 1621
◆ **Neumega** *see* Oprelvekin *on page* 1519
◆ **Neupogen** *see* Filgrastim *on page* 875
◆ **Neupro** *see* Rotigotine *on page* 1851
◆ **Neuro-K-50 [OTC]** *see* Pyridoxine *on page* 1747
◆ **Neuro-K-250 T.D. [OTC]** *see* Pyridoxine *on page* 1747
◆ **Neuro-K-250 Vitamin B6 [OTC]** *see* Pyridoxine *on page* 1747
◆ **Neuro-K-500 [OTC]** *see* Pyridoxine *on page* 1747
◆ **Neurontin** *see* Gabapentin *on page* 943
◆ **Neut** *see* Sodium Bicarbonate *on page* 1901
◆ **NeutraCare** *see* Fluoride *on page* 895
◆ **NeutraGard Advanced** *see* Fluoride *on page* 895
◆ **Neutrahist PDX [OTC] [DSC]** *see* Chlorpheniramine, Pseudoephedrine, and Dextromethorphan *on page* 428
◆ **Neutrahist Pediatric [OTC]** *see* Chlorpheniramine and Pseudoephedrine *on page* 427
◆ **Neutra-Phos** *see* Potassium Phosphate and Sodium Phosphate *on page* 1692
◆ **Neutra-Phos®-K [OTC] [DSC]** *see* Potassium Phosphate *on page* 1691
◆ **Nevanac** *see* Nepafenac *on page* 1439
◆ **Nevanac® (Can)** *see* Nepafenac *on page* 1439

Nevirapine (ne VYE ra peen)

Brand Names: U.S. Viramune; Viramune XR

Brand Names: Canada Auro-Nevirapine; Mylan-Nevirapine; Teva-Nevirapine; Viramune; Viramune XR

Index Terms NVP

Pharmacologic Category Antiretroviral, Reverse Transcriptase Inhibitor, Non-nucleoside (Anti-HIV)

Use In combination therapy with other antiretroviral agents for the treatment of HIV-1

Pregnancy Risk Factor B

Pregnancy Considerations Teratogenic effects were not observed in animal reproduction studies. Nevirapine has a high level of transfer across the human placenta. No increased risk of overall birth defects has been observed following first trimester exposure according to data collected by the antiretroviral pregnancy registry. Pharmacokinetics are not altered during pregnancy and dose adjustment is not needed. The HHS Perinatal HIV Guidelines consider nevirapine to be an alternative NNRTI for use in antiretroviral-naïve pregnant patients. Nevirapine may be initiated in pregnant women with a $CD4^+$ lymphocyte count <250/mm^3 or continued in women who are virologically suppressed and tolerating therapy once pregnancy is detected (regardless of CD4+ lymphocyte count); however, **do not** initiate therapy in pregnant women with a $CD4^+$ lymphocyte count >250/mm^3 unless the benefit of therapy clearly outweighs the risk. Elevated transaminase concentrations at baseline may increase the risk of toxicity; the monitoring recommendation for transaminase levels is generally the same as in nonpregnant women. Hypersensitivity reactions (including hepatic toxicity and rash) are more common in women on NNRTI.

Regardless of CD4 count or HIV RNA copy number, all HIV-infected pregnant women should receive a combination antiretroviral (ARV) drug regimen. A combination of antepartum, intrapartum, and infant ARV prophylaxis is recommended. ARV therapy should be started as soon as possible in women with symptomatic infection. Although earlier initiation may be more effective in reducing the perinatal transmission of HIV, initiation may be delayed until after 12 weeks gestation in women who do not require immediate treatment after careful consideration of maternal conditions (eg, nausea and vomiting) and the potential risks of first trimester fetal exposure for specific agents. A scheduled cesarean delivery at 38 weeks gestation is recommended for all women with HIV RNA >1000 copies/mL or unknown concentrations near delivery in order to decrease transmission. If ARV therapy must be interrupted for <24 hours during the peripartum period, stop then restart all medications simultaneously in order to decrease the chance of developing resistance. Long-term follow-up is recommended for all infants exposed to ARV medications. In couples who want to conceive, the HIV-infected partner should attain maximum viral suppression prior to conception.

Health care providers are encouraged to enroll pregnant women exposed to antiretroviral medications in the Antiretroviral Pregnancy Registry (1-800-258-4263 or www.APRegistry.com). Health care providers caring for HIV-infected women and their infants may contact the National Perinatal HIV Hotline (888-448-8765) for clinical consultation (HHS [perinatal], 2014).

Breast-Feeding Considerations Nevirapine is excreted into breast milk and measurable in the serum of nursing infants. Maternal or infant antiretroviral therapy does not completely eliminate the risk of postnatal HIV transmission. In addition, multiclass resistant virus has been detected in breast-feeding infants despite maternal therapy. Therefore, in the United States, where formula is accessible, affordable, safe, and sustainable, and the risk of infant mortality due to diarrhea and respiratory infections is low, complete avoidance of breast-feeding by HIV-infected women is recommended to decrease potential transmission of HIV (HHS [perinatal], 2014).

Contraindications Moderate-to-severe hepatic impairment (Child-Pugh class B or C); use in occupational or nonoccupational postexposure prophylaxis (PEP) regimens

Canadian labeling: Additional contraindications (not in U.S. labeling): Clinically significant hypersensitivity to nevirapine or any component of the formulation; therapy rechallenge in patients with prior hypersensitivity reactions, severe rash, rash accompanied by constitutional symptoms, or clinical hepatitis due to nevirapine; severe hepatic dysfunction or AST or ALT >5 times ULN (pretreatment or during prior use of nevirapine); hereditary conditions of galactose intolerance (eg, galactosemia, Lapp lactase deficiency, glucose-galactose malabsorption); concomitant use of herbal products containing St John's wort

Warnings/Precautions Hazardous agent - use appropriate precautions for handling and disposal (NIOSH 2014 [group 2]).

[U.S. Boxed Warning]: Severe hepatotoxic reactions may occur (fulminant and cholestatic hepatitis, hepatic necrosis) and, in some cases, have resulted in hepatic failure and death. The greatest risk of these reactions is within the initial 6 weeks of treatment. Patients with a history of chronic hepatitis (B or C) or increased baseline transaminase levels may be at increased risk of hepatotoxic reactions. Female gender and patients with increased $CD4^+$-cell counts may be at substantially greater risk of hepatic events (often associated with rash). Therapy in antiretroviral naive patients should not be started with elevated $CD4^+$-cell counts unless the benefit of therapy outweighs the risk of serious hepatotoxicity (adult/postpubertal females: $CD4^+$-cell counts >250 cells/mm^3; adult males: $CD4^+$-cell counts >400 cells/mm^3). Use with caution in patients with preexisting dysfunction; monitor closely for drug-induced hepatotoxicity. U.S. labeling contraindicates use in patients with moderate-to-severe impairment (Child-Pugh class B or C). Canadian labeling contraindicates use in severe impairment.

[U.S. Boxed Warning]: Severe life-threatening skin reactions (eg, Stevens-Johnson syndrome, toxic epidermal necrolysis, hypersensitivity reactions with rash and organ dysfunction), including fatal cases, have occurred. The greatest risk of these reactions is within the initial 6 weeks of treatment; intensive monitoring is required during the initial 18 weeks of therapy to detect potentially life-threatening dermatologic and hypersensitivity reactions. If a rash occurs within the first 18 weeks of therapy, immediately check serum transaminases. Risk is greatest in African-Americans, Asian, or Hispanic race/ethnicity or in females (DHHS, 2011). If a severe dermatologic or hypersensitivity reaction occurs, nevirapine should be permanently discontinued; these events may include a severe rash, or a rash associated with fever, blisters, oral lesions, conjunctivitis, facial edema, muscle or joint aches, transaminase increases, general malaise, hepatitis, eosinophilia, granulocytopenia, lymphadenopathy, or renal dysfunction. Use of the 14-day lead-in dosing period is necessary to decrease the incidence of rash events. If nonsevere rash (in absence of transaminase elevations) occurs, do not increase dose until resolution of rash. If rash continues beyond 28 days, consider an alternative regimen. Coadministration of prednisone during the first 6 weeks of therapy increases incidence and severity of rash; concomitant prednisone is not recommended to prevent rash.

May cause redistribution of fat (eg, buffalo hump, peripheral wasting with increased abdominal girth, cushingoid appearance). Patients may develop immune reconstitution syndrome resulting in the occurrence of an inflammatory response to an indolent or residual opportunistic infection during initial HIV treatment or activation of autoimmune disorders (eg, Graves' disease, polymyositis, Guillain-Barré syndrome) later in therapy; further evaluation and treatment may be required. Rhabdomyolysis has been observed in conjunction with skin and/or hepatic adverse events during postmarketing surveillance. Termination of therapy is warranted with evidence of severe skin or liver toxicity.

Use with caution in patients taking strong CYP3A4 inhibitors, moderate or strong CYP3A4 inducers and major CYP3A4 substrates (see Drug Interactions); consider alternative agents that avoid or lessen the potential for CYP-mediated interactions. Concurrent use of St John's wort or efavirenz is not recommended; may decrease the therapeutic efficacy (St John's wort) or increase adverse effects (efavirenz). Canadian labeling contraindicates concurrent use with products containing St John's wort.

Nevirapine-based initial regimens should not be used in children <3 years of age if previously exposed to nevirapine during prevention of maternal-to-child transmission of HIV due to increased risk of resistance and treatment failure. Protease inhibitor-based initial regimens preferred in this population.

Due to rapid emergence of resistance, nevirapine should not be used as monotherapy or the only agent added to a failing regimen for the treatment of HIV. Consider alteration of antiretroviral therapies if disease progression occurs while patients are receiving nevirapine. Use care when timing discontinuation of regimens containing nevirapine; levels are sustained after levels of other medications decrease, leading to nevirapine resistance. Cross-resistance may be conferred to other non-nucleoside reverse transcriptase inhibitors (HHS [adult], 2014).

Some dosage forms may contain polysorbate 80 (also known as Tweens). Hypersensitivity reactions, usually a delayed reaction, have been reported following exposure to pharmaceutical products containing polysorbate 80 in certain individuals (Isaksson, 2002; Lucente 2000; Shelley, 1995). Thrombocytopenia, ascites, pulmonary deterioration, and renal and hepatic failure have been reported in premature neonates after receiving parenteral products containing polysorbate 80 (Alade, 1986; CDC, 1984). See manufacturer's labeling.

Adverse Reactions Note: Potentially life-threatening nevirapine-associated adverse effects may present with the following symptoms: Abrupt onset of flu-like symptoms, abdominal pain, jaundice, or fever with or without rash; may progress to hepatic failure with encephalopathy.

Central nervous system: Fatigue, fever, headache

Dermatologic: Rash

Endocrine & metabolic: Cholesterol increased, LDL increased

Gastrointestinal: Abdominal pain, amylase increased, diarrhea, nausea

Hematologic: Neutropenia

Hepatic: ALT increased, AST increased, symptomatic hepatic events (including hepatitis and hepatic failure)

Neuromuscular & skeletal: Arthralgia

Rare but important or life-threatening: Allergic reactions, anaphylaxis, anemia, angioedema, bullous eruptions, conjunctivitis, drug reaction with eosinophilia and systemic symptoms (DRESS), eosinophilia, hypersensitivity syndrome, hypophosphatemia, immune reconstitution syndrome, lymphadenopathy, oral lesions, redistribution/accumulation of body fat, renal dysfunction, rhabdomyolysis, Stevens-Johnson syndrome, toxic epidermal necrolysis, ulcerative stomatitis

Drug Interactions

Metabolism/Transport Effects Substrate of CYP2B6 (minor), CYP2D6 (minor), CYP3A4 (major); **Note:** Assignment of Major/Minor substrate status based on clinically relevant drug interaction potential; **Inhibits** CYP1A2 (weak), CYP2D6 (weak), CYP3A4 (weak); **Induces** CYP2B6 (strong), CYP3A4 (weak)

Avoid Concomitant Use

Avoid concomitant use of Nevirapine with any of the following: Atazanavir; CarBAMazepine; Dolutegravir; Efavirenz; Elvitegravir; Etravirine; Itraconazole; Ketoconazole (Systemic); Pimozide; Rilpivirine; St Johns Wort

Increased Effect/Toxicity

Nevirapine may increase the levels/effects of: Dofetilide; Efavirenz; Etravirine; Hydrocodone; Lomitapide; Pimozide; Rifabutin; Rilpivirine

The levels/effects of Nevirapine may be increased by: Atazanavir; Efavirenz; Fluconazole; Voriconazole

Decreased Effect

Nevirapine may decrease the levels/effects of: ARIPiprazole; Atazanavir; CarBAMazepine; Caspofungin; Contraceptives (Estrogens); Contraceptives (Progestins); CYP2B6 Substrates; Dolutegravir; Efavirenz; Elvitegravir; Etravirine; Fosamprenavir; Hydrocodone; Indinavir; Itraconazole; Ketoconazole (Systemic); Lopinavir; Methadone; Nelfinavir; Rifabutin; Rilpivirine; Saquinavir; Saxagliptin; Voriconazole

The levels/effects of Nevirapine may be decreased by: Bosentan; CarBAMazepine; CYP3A4 Inducers (Moderate); CYP3A4 Inducers (Strong); Dabrafenib; Deferasirox; Mitotane; Rifabutin; Rifampin; Siltuximab; St Johns Wort; Tocilizumab

Storage/Stability Store at 25°C (77°F); excursion permitted to 15°C to 30°C (59°F to 86°F).

Mechanism of Action As a non-nucleoside reverse transcriptase inhibitor, nevirapine has activity against HIV-1 by binding to reverse transcriptase. It consequently blocks the RNA-dependent and DNA-dependent DNA polymerase activities including HIV-1 replication. It does not require intracellular phosphorylation for antiviral activity.

Pharmacodynamics/Kinetics

Absorption: >90%

Distribution: Widely; V_d: 1.2 L/kg; CSF penetration approximates 40% to 50% of plasma

Protein binding, plasma: ~60%

Metabolism: Extensively hepatic via CYP3A4 and CYP2B6 (hydroxylation to inactive compounds); may undergo enterohepatic recycling

Bioavailability: 93% (immediate release tablet); ~75% (extended release tablet [relative to immediate release]); 91% (oral solution)

Half-life elimination: Decreases over 2- to 4-week time with chronic dosing due to autoinduction (ie, half-life = 45 hours initially and decreases to 25-30 hours)

Time to peak, serum: Immediate release: 4 hours; Extended release:~24 hours

Excretion: Urine (~81%, primarily as metabolites, <3% as unchanged drug); feces (~10%)

Dosage

HIV infection: Oral: **Note:** If patient experiences a rash during the 14-day lead-in period, dose should not be increased until the rash has resolved. A lead-in period must always be done with immediate release formulation and regimen should not exceed 28 days; alternative treatment should be considered at that point. If a rash occurs within the first 18 weeks of therapy, immediately check serum transaminases. Discontinue if severe rash, rash with constitutional symptoms, or rash with elevated hepatic transaminases is noted. Coadministration of prednisone during the first 6 weeks of therapy increases incidence and severity of rash; concomitant prednisone is not recommended to prevent rash. Permanently discontinue if symptomatic hepatic events occur. If therapy with any formulation is interrupted for >7 days, restart with initial dose of immediate release formulation for 14 days. Use of nevirapine in children <15 years of age is not approved in the Canadian labeling.

Manufacturer's labeling:

Infants and Children: *Immediate release:* 150 mg/m^2/dose once daily for first 14 days (maximum: 200 mg daily); increase dose to 150 mg/m^2/dose twice daily if no rash or untoward effects (maximum: 400 mg daily).

Children 6 to <18 years: *Extended release:* Dose based on body surface area (Mosteller formula); maintenance therapy using the extended release must follow a 14-day initial dosing period (lead-in) using the immediate release formulation unless patient is already maintained on a nevirapine immediate release regimen.

0.58 m^2 to 0.83 m^2: 200 mg once daily

0.84 m^2 to 1.16 m^2: 300 mg once daily

≥1.17 m^2: 400 mg once daily (do not exceed 400 mg daily)

Alternate recommendations (HHS [pediatric], 2014):

Note: Children <3 years of age: Nevirapine-based initial regimens should not be used in children previously exposed to nevirapine during prevention of maternal-to-child transmission of HIV

Children <8 years: *Immediate release:* 200 mg/m^2/dose once daily for first 14 days (maximum dose: 200 mg); increase dose to 200 mg/m^2/dose twice daily if no rash or untoward effects (maximum: 400 mg daily)

Children ≥8 years: *Immediate release:* 120-150 mg/m^2/dose once daily for 14 days (maximum dose: 200 mg); increase dose to 120-150 mg/m^2/dose twice daily if no rash or untoward effects (maximum: 400 mg daily)

Adolescents and Adults: **Note:** Therapy should not be initiated in patients with elevated CD4$^+$-cell counts unless the benefit of therapy outweighs the risk of serious hepatotoxicity (adult/post-pubertal females: CD4$^+$-cell counts >250 cells/mm^3; adult males: CD4$^+$-cell counts >400 cells/mm^3)

Immediate release:

Initial: 200 mg once daily for first 14 days

Maintenance: 200 mg twice daily (in combination with additional antiretroviral agents) if there is no rash or untoward effects during initial dosing period

Adults: *Extended release:* Maintenance: 400 mg once daily; maintenance therapy using the extended release must follow a 14-day initial dosing period (lead-in) using the immediate release formulation unless patient is already maintained on a nevirapine immediate release regimen.

Prevention of perinatal HIV transmission (HHS [perinatal], 2014): Oral: **Note:** Nevirapine is used in combination with zidovudine in select situations (eg, infants born to mothers with only intrapartum therapy or no therapy). Use is not recommended in women receiving standard recommended antenatal antiretroviral prophylaxis.

Dosage adjustment in renal impairment: Oral:

Immediate release:

CrCl ≥20 mL/minute: No dosage adjustment necessary.

CrCl <20 mL/minute: There are no dosage adjustments provided in the manufacturer's labeling (has not been studied).

Extended release: There are no dosage adjustments provided in the manufacturer's labeling (has not been studied).

Hemodialysis: An additional 200 mg *immediate release* dose is recommended following dialysis.

Dosage adjustment in hepatic impairment: Permanently discontinue if symptomatic hepatic events occur.

U.S. labeling:

Mild impairment (Child-Pugh class A):

Immediate release: There are no dosage adjustments provided in the manufacturer's labeling; use with caution.

Extended release: There are no dosage adjustments provided in the manufacturer's labeling (has not been studied).

Moderate-to-severe impairment (Child-Pugh class B or C): Use is contraindicated.

Canadian labeling:

Mild impairment (Child-Pugh class A): No dosage adjustment necessary.

Moderate impairment (Child-Pugh class B): There are no dosage adjustments provided in the manufacturer's labeling. Use with caution.

Severe impairment (Child-Pugh class C): Use is contraindicated.

Administration Oral: May be administered with or without food; may be administered with an antacid or didanosine. Shake suspension gently prior to administration; the use of an oral dosing syringe is recommended, especially if the dose is ≤5 mL; if using a dosing cup, after administration, rinse cup with water and also administer rinse. Extended release tablets must be swallowed whole and not crushed, chewed, or divided.

Hazardous agent; use appropriate precautions for handling and disposal (NIOSH 2014 [group 2]).

Monitoring Parameters Monitor CBC and viral load. Baseline liver function tests should be obtained prior to nevirapine's initiation. HHS adult guidelines recommend serum transaminase monitoring every 2 weeks for the first 4 weeks of therapy, monthly for the first 18 weeks, then frequently thereafter. Patients receiving maintenance immediate release nevirapine who change to the extended release formulation should adhere to their regular monitoring schedule. HHS adult guidelines recommend serum transaminase monitoring every 2 weeks for the first 4 weeks of therapy, then monthly for 3 months, followed by every 3-4 months. HHS pediatric guidelines recommend serum transaminase monitoring every 2 weeks for the first 4 weeks of therapy, followed by every 4 months. Assess/evaluate AST/ALT immediately in any patients with a rash. Permanently discontinue if patient experiences severe rash, constitutional symptoms associated with rash, rash with elevated AST/ALT, or clinical hepatitis. Mild-to-moderate rash without AST/ALT elevation may continue treatment per discretion of prescriber. If mild-to-moderate urticarial rash, do not restart if treatment is interrupted.

Additional Information Patients should never be taking more than one form (ie, immediate release or extended release) of nevirapine concomitantly. Potential compliance problems, frequency of administration, and adverse effects should be discussed with patients before initiating therapy to help prevent the emergence of resistance. Early virologic failure was observed with tenofovir and didanosine delayed release capsules, plus either efavirenz or nevirapine; use caution in treatment-naive patients with high baseline viral loads. Due to rapid emergence of resistance, nevirapine should not be used as monotherapy or as the only agent added to a failing regimen for the treatment of HIV. Use care when timing discontinuation of regimens containing nevirapine; levels of nevirapine are sustained after levels of other medications decrease, potentially leading to nevirapine resistance. Cross-resistance may be conferred to other non-nucleoside reverse transcriptase inhibitors.

Dosage Forms

Suspension, Oral:

Viramune: 50 mg/5 mL (240 mL)

Generic: 50 mg/5 mL (240 mL)

Tablet, Oral:

Viramune: 200 mg

Generic: 200 mg

Tablet Extended Release 24 Hour, Oral:

Viramune XR: 100 mg, 400 mg

Generic: 400 mg

- **New-Fill®** *see* Poly-L-Lactic Acid *on page 1676*
- **Nexafed [OTC]** *see* Pseudoephedrine *on page 1742*
- **NexAVAR** *see* SORAfenib *on page 1923*
- **Nexavar (Can)** *see* SORAfenib *on page 1923*
- **NexIUM** *see* Esomeprazole *on page 771*
- **Nexium (Can)** *see* Esomeprazole *on page 771*
- **Nexium 24HR** *see* Esomeprazole *on page 771*
- **NexIUM I.V.** *see* Esomeprazole *on page 771*
- **Next Choice (Can)** *see* Levonorgestrel *on page 1201*
- **Next Choice One Dose [DSC]** *see* Levonorgestrel *on page 1201*
- **Nexterone** *see* Amiodarone *on page 114*
- **NFV** *see* Nelfinavir *on page 1436*

Niacin (NYE a sin)

Brand Names: U.S. Niacin-50 [OTC]; Niacor; Niaspan; Slo-Niacin [OTC]

Brand Names: Canada Niaspan; Niaspan FCT; Niodan

Index Terms Nicotinic Acid; Vitamin B_3

Pharmacologic Category Antilipemic Agent, Miscellaneous; Vitamin, Water Soluble

Use Treatment of dyslipidemias (Fredrickson types IIa and IIb or primary hypercholesterolemia) as mono- or adjunctive therapy; to lower the risk of recurrent MI in patients with a history of MI and hyperlipidemia; to slow progression or promote regression of coronary artery disease; treatment of hypertriglyceridemia in patients at risk of pancreatitis; dietary supplement

Pregnancy Risk Factor C

Pregnancy Considerations Animal reproduction studies have not been conducted. Water soluble vitamins cross the placenta. When used as a dietary supplement, niacin requirements may be increased in pregnant women compared to nonpregnant women (IOM, 1998). It is not known if niacin at lipid-lowering doses is harmful to the developing fetus. If a woman becomes pregnant while receiving niacin for primary hypercholesterolemia, niacin should be discontinued. If a woman becomes pregnant while receiving niacin for hypertriglyceridemia, the benefits and risks of continuing niacin should be assessed on an individual basis.

Breast-Feeding Considerations Niacin is excreted in human breast milk. When used as a dietary supplement, niacin requirements may be increased in nursing women compared to non-nursing women (IOM, 1998). Because lipid-lowering doses of niacin may cause serious adverse reactions in nursing infants, a decision should be made whether to discontinue nursing or discontinue the drug, taking into account the importance of the drug to the mother.

Contraindications Hypersensitivity to niacin, niacinamide, or any component of the formulation; active hepatic disease or significant or unexplained persistent elevations in hepatic transaminases; active peptic ulcer; arterial hemorrhage

Warnings/Precautions Prior to initiation, secondary causes for hypercholesterolemia (eg, poorly controlled diabetes mellitus, hypothyroidism) should be excluded; management with diet and other nonpharmacologic measures (eg, exercise or weight reduction) should be attempted prior to initiation. Use has not been evaluated in Fredrickson type I or III dyslipidemias. Use with caution in patients with unstable angina or MI, renal disease, or with anticoagulants (may slightly increase prothrombin time). In patients with preexisting coronary artery disease, the incidence of atrial fibrillation was observed more frequently in those receiving immediate release (crystalline) niacin as compared to placebo (Coronary Drug Project Research Group, 1975). Niacin should not be used if patient experiences new-onset atrial fibrillation during therapy (Stone, 2013). Niacin may increase fasting blood glucose, although clinical data suggest increases are generally modest (<5%) (Guyton, 2007). Use niacin with caution in patients with diabetes. Monitor glucose; adjustment of diet and/or hypoglycemic therapy may be necessary. Niacin should not be used if patient experiences persistent hyperglycemia during therapy (Stone, 2013). Use with caution in patients with gout; niacin should not be used if patient experiences acute gout during therapy (Stone, 2013).

Use with caution in patients with a past history of hepatic impairment and/or who consume substantial amounts of ethanol; contraindicated with active liver disease or unexplained persistent transaminase elevation. Niacin should not be used if hepatic transaminase elevations >2 to 3 times upper limit of normal occur during therapy (Stone, 2013). Rare cases of rhabdomyolysis have occurred during concomitant use with HMG-CoA reductase inhibitors. With concurrent use or if symptoms suggestive of myopathy occur, monitor creatine phosphokinase (CPK) and potassium; use with caution in patients with renal impairment, inadequately treated hypothyroidism, patients with diabetes or the elderly; risk for myopathy and rhabdomyolysis may be increased. May cause gastrointestinal distress, vomiting, diarrhea, or aggravate peptic ulcer. Gastrointestinal distress may be attenuated with a gradual increase in dose and administration with food. Use is contraindicated in patients with active peptic ulcer disease; use with caution in patients with a past history of peptic ulcer. Niacin should not be used if patient experiences unexplained abdominal pain or gastrointestinal symptoms or unexplained weight loss during therapy (Stone, 2013). Dose-related reductions in platelet count and increases of prothrombin time may occur. Has been associated with small but statistically significant dose-related reductions in phosphorus levels. Monitor phosphorus levels periodically in patients at risk for hypophosphatemia.

Formulations of niacin (immediate release versus extended release) are not interchangeable (bioavailability varies); cases of severe hepatotoxicity, including fulminant hepatic necrosis, have occurred in patients who have substituted niacin products at equivalent doses. Patients should be initiated with low doses (eg, niacin extended release 500 mg at bedtime) with titration to achieve desired response. Flushing and pruritus, common adverse effects of niacin, may be attenuated with a gradual increase in dose, administering with food, avoidance of concurrent ingestion of ethanol or hot liquids, and/or by taking aspirin (adults: 325 mg) (Stone, 2013). May also use other NSAIDs according to the manufacturer. Flushing associated with extended release preparation is significantly reduced (Guyton, 2007). For immediate release preparations, may administer in 2 to 3 divided doses to reduce the frequency and severity. Niacin should not be used if patient experiences persistent severe cutaneous symptoms during therapy (Stone, 2013).

Adverse Reactions

Cardiovascular: Arrhythmias, atrial fibrillation, edema, flushing, hypotension, orthostasis, palpitation, syncope (rare), tachycardia

Central nervous system: Chills, dizziness, headache, insomnia, migraine, nervousness, pain

Dermatologic: Acanthosis nigricans, burning skin, dry skin, hyperpigmentation, maculopapular rash, pruritus, rash, skin discoloration, urticaria

Endocrine & metabolic: Glucose tolerance decreased, gout, phosphorous levels decreased, hyperuricemia

Gastrointestinal: Abdominal pain, amylase increased, diarrhea, dyspepsia, eructation, flatulence, nausea, peptic ulcers, vomiting

Hematologic: Platelet counts decreased

Hepatic: Hepatic necrosis (rare), hepatitis, jaundice, transaminases increased (dose-related), prothrombin time increased, total bilirubin increased

Neuromuscular & skeletal: CPK increased, leg cramps, myalgia, myasthenia, myopathy (with concurrent HMG-CoA reductase inhibitor), paresthesia, rhabdomyolysis (with concurrent HMG-CoA reductase inhibitor; rare), weakness

Ocular: Blurred vision, cystoid macular edema, toxic amblyopia

Respiratory: Cough, dyspnea

Miscellaneous: Diaphoresis, hypersensitivity reactions (rare; includes anaphylaxis, angioedema, laryngismus, vesiculobullous rash), LDH increased

Drug Interactions

Metabolism/Transport Effects None known.

Avoid Concomitant Use There are no known interactions where it is recommended to avoid concomitant use.

Increased Effect/Toxicity

Niacin may increase the levels/effects of: HMG-CoA Reductase Inhibitors

The levels/effects of Niacin may be increased by: Alcohol (Ethyl)

Decreased Effect

The levels/effects of Niacin may be decreased by: Bile Acid Sequestrants

Storage/Stability

Niaspan: Store at room temperature of 20°C to 25°C (68°F to 77°F).

Niacor: Store at controlled room temperature of 15°C to 30°C (59°F to 86°F).

Mechanism of Action Niacin (nicotinic acid) is bioconverted to nicotinamide which is further converted to nicotinamide adenine dinucleotide (NAD+) and the hydride equivalent (NADH) which are coenzymes necessary for tissue metabolism, lipid metabolism, and glycogenolysis (Belenky, 2006; Suave, 2008). The mechanism by which niacin (in lipid-lowering doses) affects plasma lipoproteins is not fully understood. It may involve several actions including partial inhibition of release of free fatty acids from adipose tissue, and increased lipoprotein lipase activity, which may increase the rate of chylomicron triglyceride removal from plasma. Ultimately, niacin reduces total cholesterol, apolipoprotein (apo) B, triglycerides, VLDL, LDL, lipoprotein (a), and increases HDL and other important components and subfractions (eg, LPA-I) (Kamanna, 2000)

Pharmacodynamics/Kinetics

Absorption: Immediate release formulation: Rapid and extensive. Extent of niacin ER absorption from niacin ER/lovastatin is increased (22% to 30%) with food.

Protein binding: <20% bound to serum proteins

Metabolism: Extensive first-pass metabolism; converted to nicotinamide adenine dinucleotide, nicotinuric acid (after conjugation with glycine), and other metabolites. At doses used to treat hyperlipidemia, metabolic pathways are saturable.

Half-life elimination: 20 to 48 minutes

Time to peak, serum: Immediate release formulation: 30 to 60 minutes; extended release formulation: 4 to 5 hours

Excretion: Urine 60% to 88% (unchanged drug [up to 12% recovered after multiple dosing] and metabolites)

Dosage Oral: **Note:** Formulations of niacin (regular release versus extended release) are not interchangeable.

Children:

Pellagra (off-label use): 50-100 mg/dose 3 times daily (some experts prefer niacinamide for treatment due to more favorable side effect profile)

Adequate intake (National Academy of Sciences, 1998):

0-5 months: 2 mg daily

6-11 months: 3 mg daily

Recommended daily allowances (National Academy of Sciences, 1998):

1-3 years: 6 mg daily

4-8 years: 8 mg daily

9-13 years: 12 mg daily

14-18 years: Females: 14 mg daily; Males: 16 mg daily

≥19 years: Refer to adult dosing

Adults:

Recommended daily allowances (National Academy of Sciences, 1998):

≥19 years: Females: 14 mg daily; Males: 16 mg daily

Pregnancy (all ages): 18 mg daily

Lactation (all ages): 17 mg daily

Dietary supplement (OTC labeling): 50 mg twice daily or 100 mg once daily. **Note:** Many over-the-counter formulations exist.

Hyperlipidemia:

Regular release formulation (Niacor): Initial: 250 mg once daily (with evening meal); increase frequency and/or dose every 4-7 days to desired response or first-level therapeutic dose (1.5-2 g daily in 2-3 divided doses); after 2 months, may increase at 2- to 4-week intervals to 3 g daily in 3 divided doses (maximum dose: 6 g daily in 3 divided doses). **Note:** Many over-the-counter formulations exist.

ACC/AHA Blood Cholesterol Guideline recommendations: Initial: 100 mg administered 3 times daily; increase dose gradually as tolerated to 3 g daily divided in 2-3 doses (Stone, 2013)

Sustained release (or controlled release) formulations: **Note:** Several over-the-counter formulations exist. Slo-Niacin: Usual dosage is 250-750 mg once daily, taken morning or evening, or as directed. Before using more than 500 mg daily, patient should consult health care provider.

Extended release formulation (Niaspan): Initial: 500 mg at bedtime for 4 weeks, then 1 g at bedtime for 4 weeks; adjust dose to response and tolerance; may increase dose every 4 weeks by 500 mg daily to a maximum of 2 g daily.

If additional LDL-lowering is necessary with lovastatin or simvastatin: Recommended initial lovastatin or simvastatin dose: 20 mg daily (maximum lovastatin or simvastatin dose: 40 mg daily); **Note:** Lovastatin prescribing information recommends a maximum dose of 20 mg daily with concurrent use of niacin (>1 g daily).

ACC/AHA Blood Cholesterol Guideline recommendations: Initial: 500 mg once daily; increase dose gradually (ie, no sooner than at weekly intervals) over 4-8 weeks as tolerated to a maximum dose of 2 g once daily (Stone, 2013)

Pellagra (off-label use): 50-100 mg 3-4 times daily; maximum: 500 mg daily (some experts prefer niacinamide for treatment due to more favorable side effect profile)

Dosage adjustment in renal impairment: No dosage adjustment provided in manufacturer's labeling (has not been studied); use with caution.

Dosage adjustment in hepatic impairment: No dosage adjustment provided in manufacturer's labeling (has not been studied). However, contraindicated in patients with significant or unexplained hepatic dysfunction, active liver disease or unexplained persistent transaminase elevations.

Dosage adjustment for hepatic toxicity: Transaminases rise ≥3 times ULN, either persistent or if symptoms of nausea, fever, and/or malaise occur: Discontinue therapy.

Dietary Considerations Should be taken with meal; low-fat meal if treating hyperlipidemia. Avoid hot drinks around the time of niacin dose.

Administration Administer with food. To attenuate flushing symptoms, may premedicate with aspirin 325 mg administered 30 minutes before dose; avoid ingestion of hot liquids or alcohol concurrently with niacin (Stone, 2013). May also use other NSAIDs to prevent flushing according to the manufacturer.

Niaspan: Administer at bedtime. Tablet strengths are not interchangeable. When switching from immediate release tablet, initiate Niaspan at lower dose and titrate. If therapy is interrupted for an extended period, dose should be retitrated.

Long-acting forms should not be crushed, broken, or chewed. Slo-Niacin may be broken along the score line. Do not substitute long-acting forms for immediate release ones.

Monitoring Parameters

2013 ACC/AHA Blood Cholesterol Guideline recommendations (Stone, 2013): Baseline hepatic transaminases, fasting blood glucose or hemoglobin A1c, and uric acid before initiation and repeat during uptitration to maintenance dose and every 6 months thereafter.

Manufacturer recommendations: Blood glucose (in diabetic patients); if on concurrent HMG-CoA reductase inhibitor, may periodically check CPK and serum potassium; liver function tests pretreatment, every 6-12 weeks for first year, then periodically (approximately every 6 months), monitor liver function more frequently if history of transaminase elevation with prior use; lipid profile; platelets (if on anticoagulants); PT (if on anticoagulants); uric acid (if predisposed to gout); phosphorus (if predisposed to hypophosphatemia)

Dosage Forms

Capsule Extended Release, Oral:
Generic: 250 mg, 500 mg

Capsule Extended Release, Oral [preservative free]:
Generic: 250 mg, 500 mg

Tablet, Oral:
Niacin-50 [OTC]: 50 mg
Niacor: 500 mg
Generic: 50 mg, 100 mg, 250 mg, 500 mg

Tablet, Oral [preservative free]:
Generic: 50 mg, 100 mg, 500 mg

Tablet Extended Release, Oral:
Niaspan: 500 mg, 750 mg, 1000 mg
Slo-Niacin [OTC]: 250 mg, 500 mg, 750 mg
Generic: 500 mg, 750 mg, 1000 mg

Tablet Extended Release, Oral [preservative free]:
Generic: 250 mg, 500 mg, 1000 mg

◆ **Niacin-50 [OTC]** *see* Niacin *on page 1443*

Niacinamide (nye a SIN a mide)

Index Terms Nicomide-T; Nicotinamide; Nicotinic Acid Amide; Vitamin B_3

Pharmacologic Category Vitamin, Water Soluble

Use Dietary supplement

Dosage Pellagra (off-label use): Oral:

Children: 10-50 mg every 6 hours until resolution of signs and symptoms (Hegyi, 2004)

Adults: 100 mg every 6 hours for several days (or until resolution of major signs and symptoms), followed by 50 mg every 8-12 hours until skin lesions heal (Hegyi, 2004)

Additional Information Complete prescribing information should be consulted for additional detail.

Dosage Forms

Tablet, Oral:
Generic: 100 mg, 500 mg

Tablet, Oral [preservative free]:
Generic: 100 mg, 500 mg

Niacin and Lovastatin (NYE a sin & LOE va sta tin)

Brand Names: U.S. Advicor

Index Terms Lovastatin and Niacin

Pharmacologic Category Antilipemic Agent, HMG-CoA Reductase Inhibitor; Antilipemic Agent, Miscellaneous

Use Primary hypercholesterolemia/mixed dyslipidemia: Treatment of primary hypercholesterolemia (heterozygous familial and nonfamilial) and mixed dyslipidemia (Fredrickson types IIa and IIb) in combination with a standard cholesterol-lowering diet.

Pregnancy Risk Factor X

Dosage Dosage forms are a fixed combination of niacin and lovastatin. Patients not currently on niacin extended release must start niacin extended release/lovastatin at the lowest dose.

Primary hypercholesterolemia/mixed dyslipidemia: Adults: Oral: Lowest dose: Niacin extended release 500 mg/lovastatin 20 mg once daily at bedtime with a low-fat snack; may increase by not more than 500 mg (niacin extended release) once daily at bedtime at 4-week intervals. Maximum dose: Niacin extended release 2000 mg/lovastatin 40 mg daily). **Note:** If therapy is interrupted for >7 days, reinstitution of therapy should begin with the lowest dose followed by retitration as needed.

Not for use as initial therapy of dyslipidemias. May be substituted for equivalent dose of Niaspan; however, manufacturer does not recommend direct substitution with other niacin products.

Dosage adjustment for lovastatin component with concomitant medications:

Amiodarone: Maximum recommended lovastatin dose: 40 mg daily

Danazol, diltiazem, dronedarone, or verapamil: Initial lovastatin dose: 10 mg daily (dosage unavailable with combination product; use separate components); Maximum recommended lovastatin dose: 20 mg daily

Dosage adjustment in renal impairment:

Mild to moderate impairment (CrCl ≥30 mL/minute): No dosage adjustment necessary

Severe impairment (CrCl <30 mL/minute): There are no dosage adjustments provided in the manufacturer's labeling; use doses of lovastatin >20 mg daily with caution

Dosage adjustment in hepatic impairment: There are no dosage adjustments provided in the manufacturer's labeling; contraindicated in active liver disease or unexplained persistent elevations of serum transaminases.

Additional Information Complete prescribing information should be consulted for additional detail.

Dosage Forms

Tablet, variable release, oral:
Advicor: 500/20: Niacin 500 mg [extended release] and lovastatin 20 mg [immediate release]; 750/20: Niacin 750 mg [extended release] and lovastatin 20 mg [immediate release]; 1000/20: Niacin 1000 mg [extended release] and lovastatin 20 mg [immediate release]; 1000/40: Niacin 1000 mg [extended release] and lovastatin 40 mg [immediate release]

◆ **Niacor** *see* Niacin *on page 1443*

◆ **Niaspan** *see* Niacin *on page 1443*

◆ **Niaspan FCT (Can)** *see* Niacin *on page 1443*

◆ **Niastase (Can)** *see* Factor VIIa (Recombinant) *on page 836*

◆ **Niastase RT (Can)** *see* Factor VIIa (Recombinant) *on page 836*

NiCARdipine (nye KAR de peen)

Brand Names: U.S. Cardene IV; Cardene SR [DSC]

Index Terms Nicardipine Hydrochloride

Pharmacologic Category Antianginal Agent; Antihypertensive; Calcium Channel Blocker; Calcium Channel Blocker, Dihydropyridine

Use Chronic stable angina (immediate-release product only); management of hypertension (immediate and sustained release products); parenteral only for short-term use when oral treatment is not feasible

The 2014 guideline for the management of high blood pressure in adults (JNC 8) recommends initiation of pharmacologic treatment to lower blood pressure for the following patients (JNC 8 [James, 2013]):

- Patients ≥60 years of age with systolic blood pressure (SBP) ≥150 mm Hg or diastolic blood pressure (DBP) ≥90 mm Hg. Goal of therapy is SBP <150 mm Hg and DBP <90 mm Hg.
- Patients <60 years of age with SBP ≥140 mm Hg or DBP ≥90 mm Hg. Goal of therapy is SBP <140 mm Hg and DBP <90 mm Hg.
- Patients ≥18 years of age with diabetes with SBP ≥140 mm Hg or DBP ≥90 mm Hg. Goal of therapy is SBP <140 mm Hg and DBP <90 mm Hg.
- Patients ≥18 years of age with chronic kidney disease (CKD) with SBP ≥140 mm Hg or DBP ≥90 mm Hg. Goal of therapy is SBP <140 mm Hg and DBP <90 mm Hg.

In patients with chronic kidney disease (CKD), regardless of race or diabetes status, the use of an ACE inhibitor (ACEI) or angiotensin receptor blocker (ARB) as initial therapy is recommended to improve kidney outcomes. In the general nonblack population (without CKD) including those with diabetes, initial antihypertensive treatment should consist of a thiazide-type diuretic, calcium channel blocker, ACEI, or ARB. In the general black population (without CKD) including those with diabetes, initial antihypertensive treatment should consist of a thiazide-type diuretic or a calcium channel blocker instead of an ACEI or ARB.

Pregnancy Risk Factor C

Pregnancy Considerations Adverse events were observed in some animal reproduction studies. Nicardipine has been used for the treatment of severe hypertension in pregnancy and preterm labor. Nicardipine crosses the placenta; changes in fetal heart rate, neonatal hypotension and neonatal acidosis have been observed following maternal use (rare; based on limited data). Adverse effects reported in pregnant women are generally similar to those reported in nonpregnant patients; however, pulmonary edema has been observed (Nij, 2010). Untreated chronic maternal hypertension is also associated with adverse events in the fetus, infant, and mother. If treatment for hypertension during pregnancy is needed, other agents are preferred (ACOG, 2013).

Breast-Feeding Considerations Nicardipine is minimally excreted into breast milk. Per the manufacturer, the possibility of infant exposure should be considered. In one study, peak milk concentrations ranged from 1.9-18.8 mcg/mL following oral maternal doses of 40-150 mg/day. The estimated exposure to the breast-feeding infant was calculated to be 0.073% of the weight-adjusted maternal oral dose or 0.14% of the weight-adjusted maternal IV dose. Adverse events were not noted in the infants.

Contraindications Hypersensitivity to nicardipine or any component of the formulation; advanced aortic stenosis

Warnings/Precautions Symptomatic hypotension with or without syncope can rarely occur; blood pressure must be lowered at a rate appropriate for the patient's clinical condition. Close monitoring of blood pressure and heart rate is required. Reflex tachycardia may occur resulting in angina and/or MI in patients with obstructive coronary disease especially in the absence of concurrent beta blockade. The most common side effect is peripheral edema (dose-dependent); occurs within 2-3 weeks of starting therapy. Use with caution in CAD (can cause increase in angina), aortic stenosis (may reduce coronary perfusion resulting in ischemia; use is contraindicated in patients with advanced aortic stenosis), and hypertrophic cardiomyopathy with outflow tract obstruction. The ACCF/AHA heart failure guidelines recommend to avoid use in patients with heart failure due to lack of benefit and/or worse outcomes with calcium channel blockers in general (Yancy, 2013). To minimize infusion site reactions, peripheral infusion sites (for IV therapy) should be changed every 12 hours; use of small peripheral veins should be avoided. Titrate IV dose cautiously in patients with renal or hepatic dysfunction. Use the IV form cautiously in patients with portal hypertension (can cause increase in hepatic pressure gradient). Initiate at the low end of the dosage range in the elderly.

Adverse Reactions

Cardiovascular: Chest pain (IV), edema, exacerbation of angina pectoris (dose related), extrasystoles (IV), flushing, hemopericardium (IV), hypertension (IV), hypotension (IV), palpitations, pedal edema (dose related), supraventricular tachycardia (IV), tachycardia

Central nervous system: Dizziness, headache, hypoesthesia, intracranial hemorrhage, pain, somnolence

Dermatologic: Diaphoresis, skin rash

Endocrine & metabolic: Hypokalemia (IV)

Gastrointestinal: Abdominal pain (IV), dyspepsia, nausea, nausea and vomiting (IV), xerostomia

Genitourinary: Hematuria

Local: Injection site reaction (IV), pain at injection site (IV)

Neuromuscular & skeletal: Myalgia, paresthesia, weakness

Rare but important or life-threatening: Abnormal dreams, abnormal hepatic function tests, abnormal vision, angina pectoris, arthralgia, atrial fibrillation (not distinguishable from natural history of atherosclerotic vascular disease), cerebral ischemia (not distinguishable from natural history of atherosclerotic vascular disease), conjunctivitis, deep vein thrombophlebitis, depression, ECG abnormal, gingival hyperplasia, heart block (not distinguishable from natural history of atherosclerotic vascular disease), hot flash, hyperkinesia, hypersensitivity reaction, hypertonia, hypophosphatemia, hypotension (exertional; not distinguishable from natural history of atherosclerotic vascular disease), myocardial infarction (chronic therapy; may be due to disease progression), neck pain, nervousness, oxygen saturation decreased (possible pulmonary shunting), parotitis, pericarditis (not distinguishable from natural history of atherosclerotic vascular disease), peripheral vascular disease, respiratory tract disease, sinus node dysfunction (chronic therapy; may be due to disease progression), sustained tachycardia, thrombocytopenia, tinnitus, tremor, urinary frequency, ventricular extrasystoles, ventricular tachycardia, vertigo

Drug Interactions

Metabolism/Transport Effects **Substrate** of CYP1A2 (minor), CYP2C9 (minor), CYP2D6 (minor), CYP2E1 (minor), CYP3A4 (major), P-glycoprotein; **Note:** Assignment of Major/Minor substrate status based on clinically relevant drug interaction potential; **Inhibits** CYP2C19 (moderate), CYP2C9 (strong), CYP2D6 (moderate), CYP3A4 (weak), P-glycoprotein

Avoid Concomitant Use

Avoid concomitant use of NiCARdipine with any of the following: Bosutinib; Conivaptan; Fusidic Acid (Systemic); Idelalisib; PAZOPanib; Pimozide; Silodosin; Thioridazine; Topotecan; VinCRIStine (Liposomal)

Increased Effect/Toxicity

NiCARdipine may increase the levels/effects of: Afatinib; Amifostine; Antihypertensives; ARIPiprazole; Atosiban; Beta-Blockers; Bosentan; Bosutinib; Brentuximab Vedotin; Calcium Channel Blockers (Nondihydropyridine); Carvedilol; Citalopram; Colchicine; CYP2C19 Substrates; CYP2C9 Substrates; CYP2D6 Substrates; Dabigatran Etexilate; Diclofenac (Systemic); DOXOrubicin (Conventional); Dronabinol; DULoxetine; Edoxaban; Eliglustat; Everolimus; Fesoterodine; Fosphenytoin; Highest Risk QTc-Prolonging Agents; Hydrocodone; Hypotensive Agents; Lacosamide; Ledipasvir; Levodopa; Lomitapide; Magnesium Salts; Metoprolol; Moderate Risk QTc-Prolonging Agents; Naloxegol; Nebivolol; Neuromuscular-Blocking Agents (Nondepolarizing);

Nitroprusside; Obinutuzumab; Ospemifene; PAZOPanib; P-glycoprotein/ABCB1 Substrates; Phenytoin; Pimozide; Propranolol; Prucalopride; Rifaximin; RisperiDONE; RiTUXimab; Rivaroxaban; Silodosin; Tacrolimus (Systemic); Tetrahydrocannabinol; Thioridazine; Topotecan; VinCRIStine (Liposomal)

The levels/effects of NiCARdipine may be increased by: Alfuzosin; Alpha1-Blockers; Antifungal Agents (Azole Derivatives, Systemic); Aprepitant; Barbiturates; Brimonidine (Topical); Calcium Channel Blockers (Nondihydropyridine); Cannabis; Ceritinib; Conivaptan; CycloSPORINE (Systemic); CYP3A4 Inhibitors (Moderate); CYP3A4 Inhibitors (Strong); Dapoxetine; Dasatinib; Diazoxide; Fluconazole; Fosaprepitant; Fusidic Acid (Systemic); Grapefruit Juice; Herbs (Hypotensive Properties); Idelalisib; Ivacaftor; Luliconazole; Macrolide Antibiotics; Magnesium Salts; MAO Inhibitors; Mifepristone; Netupitant; Nicorandil; Pentoxifylline; P-glycoprotein/ABCB1 Inhibitors; Phosphodiesterase 5 Inhibitors; Propafenone; Prostacyclin Analogues; Protease Inhibitors; Simeprevir; Stiripentol

Decreased Effect

NiCARdipine may decrease the levels/effects of: Clopidogrel; Codeine; Tamoxifen; TraMADol

The levels/effects of NiCARdipine may be decreased by: Barbiturates; Bosentan; Calcium Salts; CarBAMazepine; CYP3A4 Inducers (Moderate); CYP3A4 Inducers (Strong); Dabrafenib; Deferasirox; Efavirenz; Herbs (Hypertensive Properties); Melatonin; Methylphenidate; Mitotane; Nafcillin; P-glycoprotein/ABCB1 Inducers; Rifamycin Derivatives; Siltuximab; St Johns Wort; Tocilizumab; Yohimbine

Food Interactions Nicardipine average peak concentrations may be decreased if taken with food. Serum concentrations/toxicity of nicardipine may be increased by grapefruit juice. Management: Avoid grapefruit juice.

Preparation for Administration IV: Vial: Dilute 25 mg vial with 240 mL of compatible solution to provide a 250 mL total volume solution and a final concentration of 0.1 mg/mL.

Storage/Stability

IV:

Premixed bags: Store at controlled room temperature of 20°C to 25°C (68°F to 77°F). Protect from light and excessive heat. Do not freeze.

Vials: Store at controlled room temperature of 20°C to 25°C (68°F to 77°F). Protect from light. Diluted solution (0.1 mg/mL) is stable at room temperature for 24 hours in glass or PVC containers. Stability has also been demonstrated at room temperature at concentrations up to 0.5 mg/mL in PVC containers for 24 hours or in glass containers for up to 7 days (Baaske, 1996).

Oral (Cardene®, Cardene SR®): Store at 15°C to 30°C (59°F to 86°F). Protect from light. Freezing does not affect stability.

Mechanism of Action Inhibits calcium ion from entering the "slow channels" or select voltage-sensitive areas of vascular smooth muscle and myocardium during depolarization, producing a relaxation of coronary vascular smooth muscle and coronary vasodilation; increases myocardial oxygen delivery in patients with vasospastic angina

Pharmacodynamics/Kinetics

Onset of action: Oral: 0.5-2 hours; IV: 10 minutes; Hypotension: ~20 minutes

Duration:

IV: ≤8 hours

Oral: Immediate release capsules: ≤8 hours; Sustained release capsules: 8-12 hours

Absorption: Oral: ~100%

Protein binding: >95%

Metabolism: Hepatic; CYP3A4 substrate (major); extensive first-pass effect (saturable)

Bioavailability: 35%

Half-life elimination: 2-4 hours

Time to peak, serum: Oral: Immediate release: 30-120 minutes; Sustained release: 60-240 minutes

Excretion: Urine (49% to 60% as metabolites); feces (43% as metabolites)

Dosage

Adults:

Oral:

Immediate release: Initial: 20 mg 3 times/day; usual: 20-40 mg 3 times/day (allow 3 days between dose increases)

Sustained release: Initial: 30 mg twice daily, titrate up to 60 mg twice daily

Note: The total daily dose of immediate-release product may not automatically be equivalent to the daily sustained-release dose; use caution in converting.

IV:

Acute hypertension: Initial: 5 mg/hour increased by 2.5 mg/hour every 5 minutes (for rapid titration) to every 15 minutes (for gradual titration) up to a maximum of 15 mg/hour; in rapidly titrated patients, consider reduction to 3 mg/hour after response is achieved.

Arterial hypertension in acute ischemic stroke (off-label use [Jauch, 2013]):

Patient otherwise eligible for reperfusion treatment (eg, alteplase) except blood pressure (BP) >185/110 mm Hg: Initiate 5 mg/hour; titrate by 2.5 mg/hour at 5- to 15-minute intervals (maximum dose: 15 mg/hour). When goal BP obtained, adjust dose to maintain proper BP limits. If BP does not decline and remains >185/110 mm Hg, alteplase should not be administered.

Management of BP during and after reperfusion treatment (eg, alteplase) to maintain BP ≤180/105 mm Hg: If systolic BP >180-230 mm Hg or diastolic >105-120 mm Hg: Initiate 5 mg/hour; titrate by 2.5 mg/hour at 5- to 15-minute intervals (maximum dose: 15 mg/hour). If hypertension is refractory or diastolic BP >140 mm Hg, consider other IV antihypertensives (eg, nitroprusside).

Substitution for oral therapy (approximate equivalents):

20 mg every 8 hours oral, equivalent to 0.5 mg/hour IV infusion

30 mg every 8 hours oral, equivalent to 1.2 mg/hour IV infusion

40 mg every 8 hours oral, equivalent to 2.2 mg/hour IV infusion

Conversion to oral antihypertensive agent: Initiate oral antihypertensive at the same time that IV nicardipine is discontinued, if transitioning to oral nicardipine, start oral nicardipine 1 hour prior to IV discontinuation.

Elderly: Initiate at the low end of the dosage range. Specific guidelines for adjustment of nicardipine are not available, but careful monitoring is warranted and adjustment may be necessary.

Dosing adjustment in renal impairment:

Oral: Per the manufacturer: Titrate dose beginning with 20 mg 3 times/day (immediate release capsule) or 30 mg twice daily (sustained release capsule).

IV: Specific guidelines for adjustment of nicardipine are not available, but careful monitoring is warranted and adjustment may be necessary.

Dosing adjustment in hepatic impairment:

Oral: Per the manufacturer: Starting dose: 20 mg twice daily (immediate release) with titration. Refer to **"Note"** in adult dosing.

IV: Specific guidelines for adjustment of nicardipine are not available, but careful monitoring is warranted and adjustment may be necessary.

Dietary Considerations Avoid grapefruit juice.

Usual Infusion Concentrations: Pediatric Note: Premixed solutions available

IV infusion: 100 **mcg**/mL **or** 500 **mcg**/mL

Usual Infusion Concentrations: Adult Note: Premixed solutions available

IV infusion: 25 mg in 250 mL (total volume) (concentration: 0.1 mg/mL) **or** 25 mg in 50 mL (total volume) (concentration: 0.5 mg/mL) of D_5W or NS

Administration

Oral: The total daily dose of immediate-release product may not automatically be equivalent to the daily sustained-release dose; use caution in converting. Do not chew or crush the sustained release formulation, swallow whole. Do not open or cut capsules.

IV:

Vials must be diluted before use. Administer as a slow continuous infusion at a concentration of 0.1 mg/mL or 0.2 mg/mL. Peripheral venous irritation may be minimized by changing the site of infusion every 12 hours. Concentrations of 0.5 mg/mL may be administered via a central line only.

Premixed bags: No further dilution needed. For single use only, discard any unused portion. Use only if solution is clear; the manufacturer recommends not to admix or run in the same line as other medications.

Monitoring Parameters Blood pressure, heart rate; consult individual institutional policies and procedures

Dosage Forms

Capsule, Oral:

Generic: 20 mg, 30 mg

Solution, Intravenous:

Cardene IV: 20 mg (200 mL); 40 mg (200 mL); 40 mg (200 mL)

Generic: 2.5 mg/mL (10 mL)

- ◆ **Nicardipine Hydrochloride** *see* NiCARdipine *on page 1446*
- ◆ **NicAzelDoxy 30** *see* Doxycycline *on page 689*
- ◆ **NicAzelDoxy 60** *see* Doxycycline *on page 689*
- ◆ **Nicoderm (Can)** *see* Nicotine *on page 1449*
- ◆ **Nicoderm CQ [OTC]** *see* Nicotine *on page 1449*
- ◆ **Nicomide-T** *see* Niacinamide *on page 1446*

Nicorandil [INT] (ni KORE an dil)

International Brand Names Adancor (FR); Angicor (DK); Aprior (PH); Corflo (IN); Dancor (AT, CH, NL); Ikorel (AU, DK, FR, GR, IE, NL, NZ, TR); K-Cor (IN); Nicomen (VN); Nidil (TW); Nikoril (PT); Orandil (VN); Sigmart (CN, JP, KR, TW); Zynicor (IN)

Pharmacologic Category Vasodilator

Reported Use Prophylaxis and treatment of angina

Dosage Range Adults: Oral: Initial: 10 mg twice daily; dose may be titrated to 30 mg twice daily; may use 5 mg twice daily in patients prone to headache

Product Availability Product available in various countries; not currently available in the U.S.

Dosage Forms

Tablet: 10 mg, 20 mg

- ◆ **Nicorelief [OTC]** *see* Nicotine *on page 1449*
- ◆ **Nicorette [OTC]** *see* Nicotine *on page 1449*
- ◆ **Nicorette (Can)** *see* Nicotine *on page 1449*
- ◆ **Nicorette Mini [OTC]** *see* Nicotine *on page 1449*
- ◆ **Nicorette Plus (Can)** *see* Nicotine *on page 1449*
- ◆ **Nicorette Starter Kit [OTC]** *see* Nicotine *on page 1449*
- ◆ **Nicotinamide** *see* Niacinamide *on page 1446*

Nicotine (nik oh TEEN)

Brand Names: U.S. Nicoderm CQ [OTC]; Nicorelief [OTC]; Nicorette Mini [OTC]; Nicorette Starter Kit [OTC]; Nicorette [OTC]; Nicotrol; Nicotrol NS; Thrive [OTC]

Brand Names: Canada Habitrol; Nicoderm; Nicorette; Nicorette Plus; Nicotrol

Index Terms Habitrol; Nicotine Patch

Pharmacologic Category Smoking Cessation Aid

Use Smoking cessation: Treatment to aid smoking cessation for the relief of nicotine withdrawal symptoms (including nicotine craving)

Pregnancy Risk Factor D (nasal)

Pregnancy Considerations Nicotine is teratogenic in animal studies. Nicotine exposure via cigarette smoke may cause increased ectopic pregnancy, low birth weight, increased risk of spontaneous abortion, increased perinatal mortality; increased aortic blood flow, increased heart rate, decreased uterine blood flow, and decreased breathing have been reported in the fetus. Smoking during pregnancy is associated with sudden infant death syndrome (SIDS), an increased risk of asthma, infantile colic, and childhood obesity. Women who are pregnant should be encouraged not to smoke. The use of nicotine replacement products to aid in smoking cessation has not been adequately studied in pregnant women (amount of nicotine exposure is varied). Nonpharmacologic treatments are recommended. If the benefits of nicotine replacement therapy outweigh the unknown risks, products with intermittent dosing are suggested to be tried first. If a patch is used, it is suggested to remove it overnight while sleeping to decrease fetal exposure.

Breast-Feeding Considerations Nicotine from cigarette smoke is found in breast milk at 1.5-3 times the maternal plasma concentrations. The amount from nicotine replacement products is not known. Women who are breast-feeding are encouraged not to smoke.

Contraindications Hypersensitivity to nicotine or any component of the formulation; patients who are smoking during the postmyocardial infarction period; patients with life-threatening arrhythmias, or severe or worsening angina pectoris; active temporomandibular joint disease (gum); pregnancy; not for use in nonsmokers

Warnings/Precautions Hazardous agent - use appropriate precautions for handling and disposal (EPA, P-listed). Use with caution in oropharyngeal inflammation and in patients with history of esophagitis, peptic ulcer, coronary artery disease, recent MI, serious cardiac arrhythmias, vasospastic disease, angina, hypertension, hyperthyroidism, pheochromocytoma, diabetes, severe renal dysfunction, and hepatic dysfunction. Nicotine can increase heart rate and blood pressure; discontinue use if irregular heartbeat or palpitations occur. The oral inhaler and nasal spray should be used with caution in patients with bronchospastic disease (other forms of nicotine replacement may be preferred). Use of nasal product is not recommended with chronic nasal disorders (eg, allergy, rhinitis, nasal polyps, and sinusitis). Use with caution in patients who have an allergy to adhesive tape or who have skin problems. Discontinue use if skin redness caused by the patch does not resolve after 4 days or if inflammation or rash occurs. If vivid dreams or other sleep disturbances occur, remove the patch at bedtime and apply another patch in the morning. Cautious use of topical nicotine in patients with certain skin diseases. Hypersensitivity to the topical products can occur. Dental problems may be worsened by chewing the gum. Urge patients to stop smoking completely when initiating therapy.

Adverse Reactions

Nasal spray/inhaler:

Central nervous system: Headache

Gastrointestinal: Inhaler: Dyspepsia, mouth/throat irritation

Respiratory: Inhaler: Cough, rhinitis

Dermatologic: Acne

Endocrine & metabolic: Dysmenorrhea

Gastrointestinal: Diarrhea, flatulence, gum problems, hiccup, nausea, taste disturbance, tooth abrasions

Neuromuscular & skeletal: Arthralgia, back pain, jaw/neck pain

Respiratory: Nasal burning (nasal spray), sinusitis

Miscellaneous: Withdrawal symptoms

Rare but important or life-threatening: Allergy, amnesia, aphasia, bronchitis, bronchospasm, edema, migraine, numbness, pain, purpura, rash, sputum increased, vision abnormalities, xerostomia

Adverse events previously reported in prescription labeling for chewing gum, lozenge, and/or transdermal systems. May be product or dose specific:

Central nervous system: Concentration impaired, depression, dizziness, headache, insomnia, nervousness, pain

Gastrointestinal: Aphthous stomatitis, constipation, cough, diarrhea, dyspepsia, flatulence, gingival bleeding, glossitis, hiccups, jaw pain, nausea, salivation increased, stomatitis, taste perversion, tooth abrasions, ulcerative stomatitis, xerostomia

Dermatologic: Rash

Local: Application site reaction, local edema, local erythema

Neuromuscular & skeletal: Arthralgia, myalgia, paresthesia

Respiratory: Cough, sinusitis

Miscellaneous: Allergic reaction, diaphoresis

Drug Interactions

Metabolism/Transport Effects Substrate of CYP1A2 (minor), CYP2A6 (minor), CYP2B6 (minor), CYP2C19 (minor), CYP2C9 (minor), CYP2D6 (minor), CYP2E1 (minor), CYP3A4 (minor); **Note:** Assignment of Major/Minor substrate status based on clinically relevant drug interaction potential; **Inhibits** CYP2A6 (weak), CYP2E1 (weak)

Avoid Concomitant Use There are no known interactions where it is recommended to avoid concomitant use.

Increased Effect/Toxicity

Nicotine may increase the levels/effects of: Adenosine

The levels/effects of Nicotine may be increased by: Cimetidine

Decreased Effect There are no known significant interactions involving a decrease in effect.

Food Interactions Lozenge: Acidic foods/beverages decrease absorption of nicotine.

Storage/Stability Store at controlled room temperature.

NicoDerm CQ: Dispose of used patches by folding sticky ends together; place in pouch and discard.

Nicotrol: Protect cartridges from light.

Mechanism of Action Nicotine is one of two naturally-occurring alkaloids which exhibit their primary effects via autonomic ganglia stimulation. The other alkaloid is lobeline which has many actions similar to those of nicotine but is less potent. Nicotine is a potent ganglionic and central nervous system stimulant, the actions of which are mediated via nicotine-specific receptors. Biphasic actions are observed depending upon the dose administered. The main effect of nicotine in small doses is stimulation of all autonomic ganglia; with larger doses, initial stimulation is followed by blockade of transmission. Biphasic effects are also evident in the adrenal medulla; discharge of catecholamines occurs with small doses, whereas prevention of catecholamines release is seen with higher doses as a response to splanchnic nerve stimulation. Stimulation of the central nervous system (CNS) is characterized by tremors and respiratory excitation. However, convulsions may occur with higher doses, along with respiratory failure secondary to both central paralysis and peripheral blockade to respiratory muscles.

Pharmacodynamics/Kinetics

Onset of action: Intranasal: More closely approximate the time course of plasma nicotine levels observed after cigarette smoking than other dosage forms

Duration: Transdermal: 24 hours

Absorption: Transdermal: Slow

Metabolism: Hepatic, primarily to cotinine (1/5 as active)

Half-life elimination: Transdermal: ~4 hours (Bannon, 1989); Nasal spray: 1-2 hours; Inhaler: 1-2 hours

Time to peak, serum: Transdermal: ~2-8 hours (Bannon, 1989; DeVeaugh-Geiss, 2010); Nasal spray: 10-20 minutes

Excretion: Urine

Clearance: Renal: pH dependent

Dosage

Smoking deterrent: Patients should be advised to completely stop smoking upon initiation of therapy.

Oral:

Gum: Chew 1 piece of gum when urge to smoke, up to 24 pieces/day. Patients who smoke <25 cigarettes/day should start with 2-mg strength; patients smoking ≥25 cigarettes/day should start with the 4-mg strength. Use according to the following 12-week dosing schedule:

Weeks 1-6: Chew 1 piece of gum every 1-2 hours; to increase chances of quitting, chew at least 9 pieces/day during the first 6 weeks

Weeks 7-9: Chew 1 piece of gum every 2-4 hours

Weeks 10-12: Chew 1 piece of gum every 4-8 hours

Inhaler: Usually 6 to 16 cartridges per day; best effect was achieved by frequent continuous puffing (20 minutes); recommended duration of treatment is 3 months, after which patients may be weaned from the inhaler by gradual reduction of the daily dose over 6-12 weeks

Lozenge: Patients who smoke their first cigarette within 30 minutes of waking should use the 4 mg strength; otherwise the 2 mg strength is recommended. Use according to the following 12-week dosing schedule:

Weeks 1-6: One lozenge every 1-2 hours

Weeks 7-9: One lozenge every 2-4 hours

Weeks 10-12: One lozenge every 4-8 hours

Note: Use at least 9 lozenges/day during first 6 weeks to improve chances of quitting; do not use more than one lozenge at a time (maximum: 5 lozenges every 6 hours, 20 lozenges/day)

Topical: Transdermal patch: **Note:** Adjustment may be required during initial treatment (move to higher dose if experiencing withdrawal symptoms; lower dose if side effects are experienced).

NicoDerm CQ:

Patients smoking >10 cigarettes/day: Begin with **step 1** (21 mg/day) for 6 weeks, followed by **step 2** (14 mg/day) for 2 weeks; finish with **step 3** (7 mg/day) for 2 weeks

Patients smoking ≤10 cigarettes/day: Begin with **step 2** (14 mg/day) for 6 weeks, followed by **step 3** (7 mg/day) for 2 weeks

Nasal: Spray: 1-2 sprays/hour; do not exceed more than 5 doses (10 sprays) per hour [maximum: 40 doses/day (80 sprays); each dose (2 sprays) contains 1 mg of nicotine]

Dietary Considerations Some products may contain phenylalanine and/or sodium.

Administration

Gum: Should be chewed slowly to avoid jaw ache and to maximize benefit. Chew slowly until it tingles, then park gum between cheek and gum until tingle is gone; repeat process until most of tingle is gone (~30 minutes).

Lozenge: Should not be chewed or swallowed; allow to dissolve slowly (~20-30 minutes)

Nasal spray: Prime pump prior to first use (pump 6-8 times until fine spray appears) or if it has not been used for 24 hours (pump 1-2 times). Blow nose prior to use. Tilt head back slightly and insert tip of bottle into nostril. Breathe through mouth and spray once in each nostril. Do not sniff, swallow, or inhale through the nose during administration. After administration, wait 2-3 minutes before blowing nose.

Oral Inhalant: Insert cartridge into inhaler and push hard until it pops into place. Replace mouthpiece and twist the top and bottom so that markings do not line up. Inhale deeply into the back of the throat or puff in short breaths. Nicotine in cartridge is used up after about 20 minutes of active puffing.

Transdermal patch: Apply new patch to nonhairy, clean, dry skin on the upper body or upper outer arm; each patch should be applied to a different site. Apply immediately after removing backing from patch; press onto skin for ~10 seconds. Patch may be worn for 16 or 24 hours. If cigarette cravings occur upon awakening, wear for 24 hours; if vivid dreams or other sleep disturbances occur, remove the patch at bedtime and apply a new patch in the morning. Do not cut patch; causes rapid evaporation, rendering the patch useless. Do not wear more than 1 patch at a time; do not leave patch on for more than 24 hours. Wash hands after applying or removing patch.

Hazardous agent; use appropriate precautions for handling and disposal (EPA, P-listed).

Monitoring Parameters Heart rate and blood pressure periodically during therapy; discontinue therapy if signs of nicotine toxicity occur (eg, severe headache, dizziness, mental confusion, disturbed hearing and vision, abdominal pain; rapid, weak and irregular pulse; salivation, nausea, vomiting, diarrhea, cold sweat, weakness)

Additional Information A cigarette has 10-25 mg nicotine.

Dosage Forms

Gum, Mouth/Throat:

Nicorelief [OTC]: 2 mg (50 ea, 110 ea); 4 mg (50 ea, 110 ea)

Nicorette [OTC]: 2 mg (20 ea, 40 ea, 100 ea, 110 ea, 160 ea, 170 ea, 190 ea, 200 ea); 4 mg (20 ea, 40 ea, 100 ea, 110 ea, 160 ea, 170 ea, 190 ea, 200 ea)

Nicorette Starter Kit [OTC]: 2 mg (100 ea, 110 ea); 4 mg (110 ea)

Thrive [OTC]: 2 mg (100 ea, 110 ea); 4 mg (100 ea, 110 ea)

Generic: 2 mg (20 ea, 40 ea, 50 ea, 100 ea, 110 ea); 4 mg (20 ea, 40 ea, 50 ea, 100 ea, 110 ea)

Inhaler, Inhalation:

Nicotrol: 10 mg (168 ea)

Kit, Transdermal:

Generic: 21-14-7 mg/24 hr

Lozenge, Mouth/Throat:

Nicorette [OTC]: 2 mg (72 ea, 81 ea, 108 ea, 168 ea); 4 mg (72 ea, 81 ea, 108 ea, 168 ea)

Nicorette Mini [OTC]: 2 mg (81 ea, 135 ea); 4 mg (81 ea, 135 ea)

Generic: 2 mg (27 ea, 72 ea); 4 mg (27 ea, 72 ea)

Patch 24 Hour, Transdermal:

Nicoderm CQ [OTC]: 7 mg/24 hr (14 ea); 14 mg/24 hr (14 ea, 21 ea); 21 mg/24 hr (7 ea, 14 ea, 21 ea)

Generic: 7 mg/24 hr (7 ea, 14 ea); 14 mg/24 hr (7 ea, 14 ea); 21 mg/24 hr (1 ea, 7 ea, 14 ea, 28 ea)

Solution, Nasal:

Nicotrol NS: 10 mg/mL (10 mL)

◆ **Nicotine Patch** *see* Nicotine *on page 1449*

◆ **Nicotinic Acid** *see* Niacin *on page 1443*

◆ **Nicotinic Acid Amide** *see* Niacinamide *on page 1446*

◆ **Nicotrol** *see* Nicotine *on page 1449*

◆ **Nicotrol NS** *see* Nicotine *on page 1449*

◆ **Nicoumalone** *see* Acenocoumarol [CAN/INT] *on page 30*

◆ **Nidagel (Can)** *see* MetroNIDAZOLE (Topical) *on page 1357*

◆ **Nifediac CC** *see* NIFEdipine *on page 1451*

◆ **Nifedical XL** *see* NIFEdipine *on page 1451*

NIFEdipine (nye FED i peen)

Brand Names: U.S. Adalat CC; Afeditab CR; Nifediac CC; Nifedical XL; Procardia; Procardia XL

Brand Names: Canada Adalat XL; Apo-Nifed PA; Mylan-Nifedipine Extended Release; PMS-Nifedipine

Pharmacologic Category Antianginal Agent; Antihypertensive; Calcium Channel Blocker; Calcium Channel Blocker, Dihydropyridine

Additional Appendix Information

Beers Criteria – Potentially Inappropriate Medications for Geriatrics *on page 2271*

Use

Management of chronic stable or vasospastic angina; treatment of hypertension (sustained release products only)

The 2014 guideline for the management of high blood pressure in adults (JNC 8) recommends initiation of pharmacologic treatment to lower blood pressure for the following patients (JNC 8 [James, 2013]):

- Patients ≥60 years of age with systolic blood pressure (SBP) ≥150 mm Hg or diastolic blood pressure (DBP) ≥90 mm Hg. Goal of therapy is SBP <150 mm Hg and DBP <90 mm Hg.
- Patients <60 years of age with SBP ≥140 mm Hg or DBP ≥90 mm Hg. Goal of therapy is SBP <140 mm Hg and DBP <90 mm Hg.
- Patients ≥18 years of age with diabetes with SBP ≥140 mm Hg or DBP ≥90 mm Hg. Goal of therapy is SBP <140 mm Hg and DBP <90 mm Hg.
- Patients ≥18 years of age with chronic kidney disease (CKD) with SBP ≥140 mm Hg or DBP ≥90 mm Hg. Goal of therapy is SBP <140 mm Hg and DBP <90 mm Hg.

In patients with chronic kidney disease (CKD), regardless of race or diabetes status, the use of an ACE inhibitor (ACEI) or angiotensin receptor blocker (ARB) as initial therapy is recommended to improve kidney outcomes. In the general nonblack population (without CKD) including those with diabetes, initial antihypertensive treatment should consist of a thiazide-type diuretic, calcium channel blocker, ACEI, or ARB. In the general black population (without CKD) including those with diabetes, initial antihypertensive treatment should consist of a thiazide-type diuretic or a calcium channel blocker instead of an ACEI or ARB.

Pregnancy Risk Factor C

Pregnancy Considerations Adverse events were observed in animal reproduction studies. Nifedipine crosses the placenta and small amounts can be detected in the urine of newborn infants (Manninen, 1991; Silberschmidt, 2008). An increase in perinatal asphyxia, cesarean delivery, prematurity, and intrauterine growth retardation have been reported following maternal use. Untreated chronic maternal hypertension is also associated with adverse events in the fetus, infant, and mother. If treatment for hypertension during pregnancy is needed, nifedipine is one of the preferred agents (ACOG, 2013; SOGC [Magee, 2008]).

Nifedipine has also been evaluated for the treatment of preterm labor. Tocolytics may be used for the short-term (48 hour) prolongation of pregnancy to allow for the administration of antenatal steroids and should not be used prior to fetal viability or when the risks of use to the fetus or mother are greater than the risk of preterm birth (ACOG, 2012). Nifedipine is ineffective for maintenance tocolytic therapy (ACOG, 2012; Roos, 2013).

Breast-Feeding Considerations Nifedipine is excreted into breast milk. Reported concentrations are low and similar to those in the maternal serum (Ehrenkranz, 1989; Manninen, 1991; Penny, 1989). Breast-feeding is not recommended by the U.S. manufacturer (Canadian labeling contraindicates use). Nifedipine has been used for the treatment of Raynaud's phenomenon of the nipple in breast-feeding mothers (Barrett, 2013; Wu, 2012).

Contraindications

Hypersensitivity to nifedipine or any component of the formulation; concomitant use with strong CYP3A4 inducers (eg, rifampin); cardiogenic shock

Note: Considered contraindicated in patients with ST-elevation myocardial infarction (STEMI) (ACCF/AHA [O'Gara, 2013]).

Canadian labeling: Additional contraindications (not in U.S. labeling): Severe hypotension; patients with a Kock pouch (ileostomy after proctocolectomy; extended release tablets only); breast-feeding; pregnancy or women of childbearing potential. **Note:** SOGC and ACOG guidelines recommend nifedipine as a preferred agent for maternal hypertension (ACOG, 2013; SOGC [Magee, 2008]).

Warnings/Precautions Symptomatic hypotension with or without syncope can rarely occur; blood pressure must be lowered at a rate appropriate for the patient's clinical condition. **The use of immediate release nifedipine (sublingually or orally) in hypertensive emergencies and urgencies is neither safe nor effective.** Serious adverse events (eg, death, cerebrovascular ischemia, syncope, stroke, acute myocardial infarction, and fetal distress) have been reported. **Immediate release nifedipine should not be used for acute blood pressure reduction.**

Blood pressure lowering should be done at a rate appropriate for the patient's condition. Rapid drops in blood pressure can lead to arterial insufficiency. Increased angina and/or MI have occurred with initiation or dosage titration of dihydropyridine calcium channel blockers; use with caution in patients with obstructive coronary disease especially in the absence of concurrent beta-blockade. In patients with unstable angina/non-STEMI, the use of immediate-release nifedipine is not recommended except with concomitant beta-blockade (ACCF/AHA [Anderson, 2013]). Use with caution before major surgery. Cardiopulmonary bypass, intraoperative blood loss or vasodilating anesthesia may result in severe hypotension and/or increased fluid requirements. Consider withdrawing nifedipine (>36 hours) before surgery if possible.

The most common side effect is peripheral edema; occurs within 2-3 weeks of starting therapy. Reflex tachycardia may occur with use. Use with caution in severe aortic stenosis (especially with concomitant beta-adrenergic blocker), severe left ventricular dysfunction, renal impairment, hypertrophic cardiomyopathy (especially obstructive), concomitant therapy with beta-blockers or digoxin, and edema. The ACCF/AHA heart failure guidelines recommend to avoid use in patients with heart failure due to lack of benefit and/or worse outcomes with calcium channel blockers in general (Yancy, 2013). Use caution in patients with severe hepatic impairment. Clearance of nifedipine is reduced in cirrhotic patients leading to increased systemic exposure; monitor closely for adverse effects/toxicity and consider dose adjustments. Mild and transient elevations in liver function enzymes may be apparent within 8 weeks of therapy initiation. Abrupt withdrawal may cause rebound angina in patients with CAD. In the elderly, immediate release nifedipine should be avoided in due to potential to cause hypotension and risk of precipitating myocardial ischemia (Beers Criteria). Immediate release formulations should not be used to manage primary hypertension, adequate studies to evaluate outcomes have not been conducted. Avoid use of extended release tablets (Procardia XL) in patients with known stricture/narrowing of the GI tract. Adalat CC tablets contain lactose; do not use with galactose intolerance, Lapp lactase deficiency, or glucose-galactose malabsorption syndromes.

Potentially significant drug-drug interactions may exist, requiring dose or frequency adjustment, additional monitoring, and/or selection of alternative therapy.

Adverse Reactions

Cardiovascular: CHF, flushing, palpitation, peripheral edema (dose related), transient hypotension (dose related)

Central nervous system: Chills difficulties in balance, dizziness, fatigue, fever, giddiness, headache, jitteriness, lightheadedness, mood changes, nervousness, shakiness, sleep disturbances

Dermatologic: Dermatitis, pruritus, urticaria

Endocrine & metabolic: Sexual difficulties

Gastrointestinal: Constipation, cramps, diarrhea, flatulence, gingival hyperplasia, heartburn, nausea

Neuromuscular & skeletal: Inflammation, joint stiffness, muscle cramps, tremor, weakness

Ocular: Blurred vision

Respiratory: Chest congestion, cough, dyspnea, nasal congestion, sore throat, wheezing

Miscellaneous: Diaphoresis

Rare but important or life-threatening: Agranulocytosis, allergic hepatitis, alopecia, anemia, angina, angioedema, aplastic anemia, arrhythmia, arthritis with positive ANA, bezoars (Procardia XL®), cerebral ischemia, depression, dysosmia, epistaxis, EPS, erectile dysfunction, erythema multiforme, erythromelalgia, exanthematous pustulosis, exfoliative dermatitis, facial edema, gastroesophageal reflux, gastrointestinal obstruction (Procardia XL®), gastrointestinal ulceration (Procardia XL®), gynecomastia, hematuria, ischemia, leukopenia, lip cancer (Friedman, 2012), memory dysfunction, migraine, myalgia, myoclonus, nocturia, paranoid syndrome, parotitis, periorbital edema, photosensitivity, polyuria, purpura, Stevens-Johnson syndrome, syncope, tachycardia, taste perversion, thrombocytopenia, tinnitus, toxic epidermal necrolysis, transient blindness, ventricular arrhythmia

Reported with use of sublingual short-acting nifedipine: Acute MI, cerebrovascular ischemia, ECG changes, fetal distress, heart block, severe hypotension, sinus arrest, stroke, syncope

Drug Interactions

Metabolism/Transport Effects Substrate of CYP2D6 (minor), CYP3A4 (major); **Note:** Assignment of Major/Minor substrate status based on clinically relevant drug interaction potential; **Inhibits** CYP1A2 (weak), CYP2C9 (weak), CYP2D6 (weak), CYP3A4 (weak)

Avoid Concomitant Use

Avoid concomitant use of NIFEdipine with any of the following: Conivaptan; CYP3A4 Inducers (Strong); Fusidic Acid (Systemic); Grapefruit Juice; Idelalisib; Pimozide; St Johns Wort

Increased Effect/Toxicity

NIFEdipine may increase the levels/effects of: Amifostine; Antihypertensives; ARIPiprazole; Atosiban; Beta-Blockers; Calcium Channel Blockers (Nondihydropyridine); Digoxin; Dofetilide; DULoxetine; Hydrocodone; Hypotensive Agents; Levodopa; Lomitapide; Magnesium

Salts; Neuromuscular-Blocking Agents (Nondepolarizing); Nitroprusside; Obinutuzumab; Pimozide; QuiNIDine; RisperiDONE; RiTUXimab; Tacrolimus (Systemic); VinCRIStine; VinCRIStine (Liposomal)

The levels/effects of NIFEdipine may be increased by: Alcohol (Ethyl); Alfuzosin; Alpha1-Blockers; Antifungal Agents (Azole Derivatives, Systemic); Aprepitant; Barbiturates; Brimonidine (Topical); Calcium Channel Blockers (Nondihydropyridine); Ceritinib; Cimetidine; Cisapride; Conivaptan; CycloSPORINE (Systemic); CYP3A4 Inhibitors (Moderate); CYP3A4 Inhibitors (Strong); Dapoxetine; Dasatinib; Diazoxide; Fluconazole; FLUoxetine; Fosaprepitant; Fusidic Acid (Systemic); Grapefruit Juice; Herbs (Hypotensive Properties); Idelalisib; Ivacaftor; Luliconazole; Macrolide Antibiotics; Magnesium Salts; MAO Inhibitors; Mifepristone; Netupitant; Nicorandil; Pentoxifylline; Phosphodiesterase 5 Inhibitors; Prostacyclin Analogues; Protease Inhibitors; QuiNIDine; Simeprevir; Stiripentol

Decreased Effect

NIFEdipine may decrease the levels/effects of: Clopidogrel; QuiNIDine

The levels/effects of NIFEdipine may be decreased by: Barbiturates; Bosentan; Calcium Salts; CYP3A4 Inducers (Moderate); CYP3A4 Inducers (Strong); Dabrafenib; Deferasirox; Efavirenz; Herbs (Hypertensive Properties); Melatonin; Methylphenidate; Nafcillin; Siltuximab; St Johns Wort; Tocilizumab; Yohimbine

Food Interactions Nifedipine serum levels may be decreased if taken with food. Food may decrease the rate but not the extent of absorption of Procardia XL®. Increased nifedipine concentrations resulting in therapeutic and vasodilator side effects, including severe hypotension and myocardial ischemia, may occur if nifedipine is taken by patients ingesting grapefruit. Management: Avoid grapefruit/grapefruit juice.

Storage/Stability

Adalat CC, Afeditab CR, Procardia XL: Store below 30°C (86°F); protect from light and moisture.

Nifediac CC, Nifedical XL: Store at 25°C (77°F); excursions permitted to 15°C to 30°C (59°F to 86°F); protect from light and moisture.

Immediate release capsules (Procardia): Store at 15°C to 25°C (59°F to 77°F); prevent capsules from freezing; protect from light and moisture.

Mechanism of Action Inhibits calcium ion from entering the "slow channels" or select voltage-sensitive areas of vascular smooth muscle and myocardium during depolarization, producing a relaxation of coronary vascular smooth muscle and coronary vasodilation; increases myocardial oxygen delivery in patients with vasospastic angina; also reduces peripheral vascular resistance, producing a reduction in arterial blood pressure.

Pharmacodynamics/Kinetics

Onset of action: Immediate release: ~20 minutes

Protein binding (concentration dependent): 92% to 98%

Metabolism: Hepatic via CYP3A4 to inactive metabolites

Bioavailability: Capsule: 40% to 77%; Sustained release: 65% to 89% relative to immediate release capsules; bioavailability increased with significant hepatic disease

Half-life elimination: Adults: Healthy: 2-5 hours; Cirrhosis: 7 hours; Elderly: 7 hours (extended release tablet)

Excretion: Urine (60% to 80% as inactive metabolites); feces

Dosage Oral:

Children 1 to 17 years:

High altitude pulmonary edema (off-label use; Pollard, 2001): **Note:** Treatment with nifedipine is only necessary if response to oxygen and/or descent is unsatisfactory; extended release preparation is preferred at equivalent dose with proper frequency adjustment:

Immediate release: 0.5 mg/kg/dose (maximum: 20 mg per dose) every 8 hours

Hypertension (off-label use): Extended release tablet: Initial: 0.25 to 0.5 mg/kg/day once daily or in 2 divided doses; maximum: 3 mg/kg/day up to 120 mg daily

Adults: **Note:** Dosage adjustments should occur at 7- to 14-day intervals to allow for adequate assessment of new dose; however, if clinically indicated, titration may be done more rapidly with appropriate monitoring; when switching from immediate-release to sustained-release formulations, use same total daily dose.

Chronic stable or vasospastic angina:

Immediate release: Initial: 10 mg 3 times daily; usual dose: 10 to 20 mg 3 times daily; coronary artery spasm may require up to 20 to 30 mg 3 to 4 times daily; single doses >30 mg and total daily doses >120 mg are rarely needed; maximum: 180 mg daily (U.S. labeling) or 120 mg daily (Canadian labeling); **Note:** Do not use for acute anginal episodes; may precipitate myocardial infarction

Extended release:

U.S. labeling: Initial: 30 or 60 mg once daily; titrate as clinically indicated. Doses >90 mg daily should be used with caution and only if necessary (maximum: 120 mg daily)

Canadian labeling: Initial: 30 mg once daily; titrate as clinically indicated (maximum dose: 90 mg daily)

Hypertension: Extended release:

U.S. labeling: Initial: 30 or 60 mg once daily; usual dosage range (ASH/ISH [Weber, 2014]): 30 to 90 mg daily; maximum: 90 to 120 mg daily

Canadian labeling: Initial: 20 or 30 mg once daily; usual maintenance: 30 to 60 mg once daily (maximum: 90 mg daily)

Hypertension in pregnancy (ACOG, 2013):

Urgent blood pressure control: Oral: Immediate release: 10 to 20 mg; may repeat in 30 minutes if needed, then 10 to 20 mg every 2 to 6 hours

Chronic hypertension: Oral: Extended release tablet: 30 to 120 mg daily

High altitude pulmonary edema (off-label use; Luks, 2010):

Prevention: Extended release: 30 mg every 12 hours starting the day before ascent and may be discontinued after staying at the same elevation for 5 days or if descent initiated

Treatment: Extended release: 30 mg every 12 hours

Pulmonary hypertension (off-label use; Galie, 2004): Extended release: Initial: 30 mg twice daily; may increase cautiously to 120 to 240 mg daily

Raynaud's phenomenon (off-label use; Wigley, 2002): Extended release: Dosage range: 30 to 120 mg once daily

Elderly: Hypertension: Consider lower initial doses and titrate to response (Aronow, 2011)

Dosage adjustment in renal impairment: There are no dosage adjustments provided in manufacturer's labeling (has not been studied); the pharmacokinetics of nifedipine are not significantly influenced by the degree of renal impairment (only trace amounts of unchanged drug are found in urine).

Hemodialysis: Supplemental dose is not necessary

Peritoneal dialysis effects: Supplemental dose is not necessary

Dosage adjustment in hepatic impairment: There are no dosage adjustments provided in manufacturer's labeling (has not been studied); use with caution. Clearance of nifedipine is reduced in cirrhotic patients, which may lead to increased systemic exposure; monitor closely for adverse effects/toxicity and consider dose adjustments.

Dietary Considerations Avoid grapefruit juice with all products.

Immediate release: Capsule is rapidly absorbed orally if it is administered without food, but may result in vasodilator side effects; if flushing is problematic, administration with low-fat meals may decrease. In general, can take with or without food.

Extended release: Adalat CC, Afeditab CR, Nifediac CC: Take on an empty stomach (manufacturer recommendation). Other extended release products may not have this recommendation; consult product labeling.

Administration

Immediate release: In general, may be administered with or without food.

Extended release: Tablets should be swallowed whole; do not crush, split, or chew.

Adalat CC, Afeditab CR, Nifediac CC: Administer on an empty stomach (per manufacturer). Other extended release products may not have this recommendation; consult product labeling.

Monitoring Parameters Heart rate, blood pressure, signs and symptoms of CHF, peripheral edema

Additional Information When measuring smaller doses from the liquid-filled capsules, consider the following concentrations (for Procardia) 10 mg capsule = 10 mg/0.34 mL; 20 mg capsule = 20 mg/0.45 mL; may be used preoperative to treat hypertensive urgency.

Considerable attention has been directed to potential increases in mortality and morbidity when short-acting nifedipine is used in treating hypertension. The rapid reduction in blood pressure may precipitate adverse cardiovascular events.

Short-acting nifedipine should not be used for acute anginal episodes since this may precipitate myocardial infarction. Extended-release formulations are preferred for the management of chronic or vasospastic angina (Poole-Wilson, 2004).

Equivalency of extended release formulation (Adalat CC): The manufacturer states that it is acceptable to interchange two 30 mg tablets with one 60 mg tablet to effectively deliver a 60 mg dose. However, it is not recommended to substitute one 90 mg tablet with three 30 mg tablets, since the resulting C_{max} is 29% higher compared to giving the single 90 mg tablet.

Dosage Forms

Capsule, Oral:

Procardia: 10 mg

Generic: 10 mg, 20 mg

Tablet Extended Release 24 Hour, Oral:

Adalat CC: 30 mg, 60 mg, 90 mg

Afeditab CR: 30 mg, 60 mg

Nifediac CC: 30 mg, 60 mg, 90 mg

Nifedical XL: 30 mg, 60 mg

Procardia XL: 30 mg, 60 mg, 90 mg

Generic: 30 mg, 60 mg, 90 mg

Extemporaneous Preparations A 4 mg/mL oral suspension may be made with liquid capsules (**Note:** Concentration inside capsule may vary depending on manufacturer. Procardia: 10 mg capsule contains a concentration of 10 mg/0.34 mL [29.4 mg/mL]). Puncture the top of twelve 10 mg liquid capsules with one needle to create a vent. Insert a second needle attached to a syringe and extract the liquid; transfer to a calibrated bottle and add sufficient quantity of a 1:1 mixture of Ora-Sweet and Ora-Plus to make 30 mL. Label "shake well". Stable 90 days under refrigeration or at room temperature.

Nahata MC, Morosco RS, and Willhite EA, "Stability of Nifedipine in Two Oral Suspensions Stored at Two Temperatures," *J Am Pharm Assoc*, 2002, 42(6):865-7.

Niflumic Acid [INT] (nye FLU mik AS id)

International Brand Names Actol (AT, DE, ES); Donalgin (HU); Felalgyl (FR); Flogovital (AR); Flunir (FR); Niflactol (ES); Niflam (IT); Niflugel (BE, CH, CZ, FR); Nifluril (BE, CH, CZ, FR, LU, PT); Sabrinin (AT); Sepvadol (FR)

Index Terms Niflumic Acid Glycinamide

Pharmacologic Category Analgesic, Nonsteroidal Anti-inflammatory Drug; Nonsteroidal Anti-inflammatory Drug (NSAID), Oral

Reported Use Anti-inflammatory used in musculoskeletal and joint disorders

Dosage Range Adults:

Oral: 250 mg 3-4 times/day

Topical: Apply 3 times/day

Product Availability Product available in various countries; not currently available in the U.S.

Dosage Forms

Capsule: 250 mg

Cream: 3% (120 g)

Gel, topical: 2.5% (60 g)

◆ **Niflumic Acid Glycinamide** *see* Niflumic Acid [INT] *on page 1454*

◆ **nIFN-alpha** *see* Interferon Alpha, Multi-Subtype [INT] *on page 1100*

◆ **Niftolid** *see* Flutamide *on page 907*

Nifuroxazide [INT] (nye fyoor OKS a zide)

International Brand Names Akabar (MX); Antinal (BE, CH); Bacifurane (BE, LU); Bifix (FR); Diarret (IT); Ercefuryl (BE, ES, FR, IT, LU); Erceryl (FR); Eskapar (MX); Lumifurex (FR); Nifuroxazide EG (BE); Nifuroxazide-Eurogenerics (LU); Nifuroxazide-Ratiopharm (FR); Panfurex (FR, LU); Passifuril (BR); Pentofuryl (DE); Septidiaryl (FR); Topron (MX)

Pharmacologic Category Antidiarrheal

Reported Use Treatment of diarrhea

Dosage Range Adults: Oral: 200 mg 4 times/day

Product Availability Product available in various countries; not currently available in the U.S.

Dosage Forms

Capsule: 200 mg

Suspension, oral: 220 mg/5 mL

◆ **Nighttime Sleep Aid [OTC]** *see* DiphenhydrAMINE (Systemic) *on page 641*

◆ **Nikki** *see* Ethinyl Estradiol and Drospirenone *on page 801*

◆ **Nilandron** *see* Nilutamide *on page 1455*

Nilotinib (nye LOE ti nib)

Brand Names: U.S. Tasigna

Brand Names: Canada Tasigna

Index Terms AMN107; Nilotinib Hydrochloride Monohydrate

Pharmacologic Category Antineoplastic Agent, BCR-ABL Tyrosine Kinase Inhibitor; Antineoplastic Agent, Tyrosine Kinase Inhibitor

Use Chronic myelogenous leukemia:

Treatment of adults with newly diagnosed Philadelphia chromosome-positive chronic myelogenous leukemia (CML) in chronic phase.

Treatment of chronic- and accelerated-phase Philadelphia chromosome-positive CML in adults resistant or intolerant to prior therapy that included imatinib.

Pregnancy Risk Factor D

Dosage

Chronic myeloid leukemia (CML), Ph+, newly-diagnosed in chronic phase: Adults: Oral: 300 mg twice daily

CML, Ph+, resistant or intolerant in chronic or accelerated phase: Adults: Oral: 400 mg twice daily

Gastrointestinal stromal tumor (GIST), refractory (off-label use): Adults: Oral: 400 mg twice daily until disease progression or unacceptable toxicity (Reichardt, 2012)

Missed doses: If a dose is missed, do not make up, resume with next scheduled dose.

Dosage adjustment for concomitant CYP3A4 inhibitors/inducers:

CYP3A4 inhibitors: Avoid the concomitant use of a strong CYP3A4 inhibitor with nilotinib. If a strong CYP3A4 inhibitor is required, interruption of nilotinib treatment is recommended.

If therapy cannot be interrupted and concurrent use with a strong CYP3A4 inhibitor cannot be avoided:

U.S. labeling: Consider reducing the nilotinib dose to 300 mg once daily in patients with resistant or intolerant Ph+ CML (chronic or accelerated phase) or to 200 mg once daily in newly-diagnosed chronic phase Ph+ CML, with careful monitoring, especially of the QT interval. When a strong CYP3A4 inhibitor is discontinued, allow a washout period prior to adjusting nilotinib dose upward.

Canadian labeling: There are no dosage adjustments provided in the manufacturer's labeling; use caution and monitor QT interval closely

CYP3A4 inducers: Avoid the concomitant use of a strong CYP3A4 inducer with nilotinib (based on pharmacokinetic parameters, an increased nilotinib dose is not likely to compensate for decreased exposure).

Dosage adjustment in renal impairment: There are no dosage adjustments provided in the manufacturer's labeling (has not been studied in patients with serum creatinine >1.5 times ULN), however, nilotinib and its metabolites have minimal renal excretion; dosage adjustments for renal dysfunction may not be necessary.

Dosage adjustment in hepatic impairment:

For hepatic impairment at treatment initiation: **Note:** Consider alternative therapies first if possible; recommendations vary by indication

U.S. labeling:

Newly-diagnosed Ph+ CML in chronic phase: Mild-to-severe impairment (Child-Pugh class A, B, or C): Initial: 200 mg twice daily; may increase to 300 mg twice daily based on patient tolerability

Resistant or intolerant Ph+ CML in chronic or accelerated phase:

Mild-to-moderate impairment (Child-Pugh class A or B): Initial: 300 mg twice daily; may increase to 400 mg twice daily based on patient tolerability

Severe impairment (Child-Pugh class C): Initial: 200 mg twice daily; may increase to 300 mg twice daily and then further increased to 400 mg twice daily based on patient tolerability

Canadian labeling: No dosage adjustment necessary; use caution and monitor (including QT interval) closely.

For hepatotoxicity during treatment:

If bilirubin >3 times ULN (≥ grade 3): Withhold treatment, monitor bilirubin, resume treatment at 400 mg once daily when bilirubin returns to ≤1.5 times ULN (≤ grade 1)

If ALT or AST >5 times ULN (≥ grade 3): Withhold treatment, monitor transaminases, resume treatment at 400 mg once daily when ALT or AST returns to ≤2.5 times ULN (≤ grade 1)

Dosage adjustment for hematologic toxicity unrelated to underlying leukemia:

ANC <1000/mm^3 and/or platelets <50,000/mm^3: Withhold treatment, monitor blood counts

If ANC >1000/mm^3 and platelets >50,000/mm^3 within 2 weeks: Resume at prior dose

If ANC <1000/mm^3 and/or platelets <50,000/mm^3 for >2 weeks: Reduce dose to 400 mg once daily

Dosage adjustment for nonhematologic toxicity:

Amylase or lipase >2 times ULN (≥ grade 3): Withhold treatment, monitor serum amylase or lipase, resume treatment at 400 mg once daily when lipase or amylase returns to ≤1.5 times ULN (≤ grade 1)

Lipase increases in conjunction with abdominal symptoms: Withhold treatment and consider diagnostics to exclude pancreatitis

Clinically-significant moderate or severe nonhematologic toxicity: Withhold treatment, upon resolution of toxicity, resume at 400 mg once daily; may escalate back to initial dose (300 mg twice daily or 400 mg twice daily depending on indication) if clinically appropriate.

Dosage adjustment for QT prolongation: Note: Repeat ECG ~7 days after any dosage adjustment.

QTc >480 msec: Withhold treatment, monitor and correct potassium and magnesium levels; review concurrent medications.

If QT_cF returns to <450 msec and to within 20 msec of baseline within 2 weeks: Resume at prior dose

If QT_cF returns to 450 to 480 msec after 2 weeks: Reduce dose to 400 mg once daily

If QT_cF >480 msec after dosage reduction to 400 mg once daily: Discontinue treatment

Additional Information Complete prescribing information should be consulted for additional detail.

Dosage Forms

Capsule, Oral:

Tasigna: 150 mg, 200 mg

◆ **Nilotinib Hydrochloride Monohydrate** *see* Nilotinib *on page 1454*

Nilutamide (ni LOO ta mide)

Brand Names: U.S. Nilandron

Brand Names: Canada Anandron®

Index Terms RU-23908

Pharmacologic Category Antineoplastic Agent, Antiandrogen

Use Treatment of metastatic prostate cancer (in combination with surgical castration)

Pregnancy Risk Factor C

Dosage Oral: Adults: Prostate cancer, metastatic: 300 mg once daily (starting the same day or day after surgical castration) for 30 days, followed by 150 mg once daily

Dosage adjustment in renal impairment: No dosage adjustment provided in manufacturer's labeling.

Dosage adjustment in hepatic impairment:

No dosage adjustment provided in manufacturer's labeling. However, use is contraindicated in severe hepatic impairment.

During treatment: ALT >2 times ULN or jaundice: Discontinue treatment.

Additional Information Complete prescribing information should be consulted for additional detail.

Dosage Forms

Tablet, Oral:

Nilandron: 150 mg

Nilvadipine [INT] (nil VAD i peen)

International Brand Names Arcadipin (AT); Escor (AT, DE, DK, FI, LU); Nivadil (CH, DE, JP); Tensan (AT)

Index Terms Nivadipine

Pharmacologic Category Calcium Channel Blocker

Dosage Range

Hypertension: 4-16 mg/day; reduce dosage to a maximum dose of 8 mg in patients with cirrhosis or with concomitant use with cimetidine

Cerebrovascular disease: 2-4 mg twice daily

Angina pectoris: 8-16 mg/day

Product Availability Product available in various countries; not currently available in the U.S.

◆ **Nimbex** *see* Cisatracurium *on page 447*

◆ **Nimenrix (Can)** *see* Meningococcal Polysaccharide (Groups A / C / Y and W-135) Tetanus Toxoid Conjugate Vaccine [CAN/INT] *on page 1290*

Nimesulide [INT] (ni ME su lide)

International Brand Names Agudol (PY); Ainex (CO); Aldoron (AR); Algimesil (IT); Algolider (IT); AllDone (BG); Antalgo (IT); Antiflogil (BR); Antifloxil (ES); Apolide (MX); Aponil (TR); Arflex Retard (BR); Arslide (PK); Aulin (AR, BG, CH, CZ, GR, HR, IE, IT, PL, PT, RO, VE); Auronim (IN, RU); BangNi (CN); Biosal (IT); Blunid (PK); Coxtral (PL, RU); Defam (MX); Deflogen (BR); Delfos (IT); Doloc (CL); Doloctaprin (AR); Dolonime (CO); Domes (IT); Donulide (PT); Drexel (VE); Efridol (IT); Elinap (TR); Emdon (TH); Enetra (BG); Eskaflam (MX); Fansidol (IT); Fasulide (BR); Flamide (MX); Flogovital N.F. (AR); Flolid (IT); Gravx (PK); Guaxan (ES); Inflalid (BR); Isodol (IT); Jabasulide (PT); Laidor (IT); Ledoren (IT); Li Nuo Ke (CN); Manaslu (KR); Mesid (IT); Mesulid (BE, CZ, GR, HK, HU, IL, IN, IT, KR, LU, MX, PY); Metaflex (AR); MF/110 (IT); Molden (KR); Nerelid (IT); Nexen (FR); Nide (IT); Nidol (HK, HU, PK, TH); Nidolid (PH); Nimax (KR); Nimed (BG, CZ, ID, PT); Nimel (IN); Nimelid (VE); Nimepast (CL); Nimesil (IT, PL); Nimesol (PY); Nimesulene (IT); Nimesulide Dorom (IT); Nimesulide GNR (IT); Nimesulide UCB (IT); Nimind (IN); Nimm (HK, TR); Nimotop (PT); Nims (IT); Nimulid (IN); Nisal (IT); Nise (PE); Nisulid (BR, CH); Nisural (CL); Noalgos (IT); Nodo (UY); Noxalide (IT); Octaprin (AR); Pacisulide (HK); Penalgin (CO); Precoxi (MY); Prolid (RU); Pu Wei (CN); Quimoral Plus (PE); Redaflam (MX); Remov (IT); Resulin (IT); RuiLi (CN); Scaflam (BR, CO, VE); Scalid (BR); Severin (MX); Sharonim (HK); Sintalgin (BR); Solving (IT); Sulidamor (IT); Sulide (IT); Sulidene [vet.] (FR); Sulidin (PH); Sulidor (PT); Sulimed (ES); Tenesmin (UY); Teonim (IT); Veedol (TH); Ventor (GR); Virobron (AR); Xilox (HU); Ximede (ID)

Pharmacologic Category Analgesic, Nonsteroidal Anti-inflammatory Drug; Nonsteroidal Anti-inflammatory Drug (NSAID), Oral

Reported Use Treatment of dysmenorrhea, migraine, and other painful inflammatory conditions

Dosage Range Note: To reduce the risk of hepatotoxicity duration should be limited to 15 days.

Adults: Oral: 100 mg twice daily

Product Availability Product available in various countries; not currently available in the U.S.

Dosage Forms

Tablet: 100 mg

NiMODipine (nye MOE di peen)

Brand Names: U.S. Nymalize

Brand Names: Canada Nimotop

Pharmacologic Category Calcium Channel Blocker; Calcium Channel Blocker, Dihydropyridine

Use Subarachnoid hemorrhage: For the improvement of neurological outcome by reducing the incidence and severity of ischemic deficits in adult patients with subarachnoid hemorrhage (SAH) from ruptured intracranial berry aneurysms regardless of their postictus neurological condition (ie, Hunt and Hess grades I to V)

Pregnancy Risk Factor C

Pregnancy Considerations Adverse events have been observed in animal reproduction studies. Nimodipine crosses the placenta (Belfort, 1994). Nimodipine has been evaluated for the management of pre-eclampsia (Belfort, 1994; Belfort, 2003), but it is not one of the agents currently recommended for this condition (ACOG, 2011).

Breast-Feeding Considerations Nimodipine is excreted into breast milk; two case reports note concentrations to be <1% of the weight-adjusted maternal dose (Carcas, 1996; Tonks, 1995). Breast-feeding is not recommended by the manufacturer.

Contraindications There are no contraindications listed in the manufacturer's labeling.

Warnings/Precautions [U.S. Boxed Warning]: Nimodipine has inadvertently been administered IV when withdrawn from capsules into a syringe for subsequent nasogastric administration. Severe cardiovascular adverse events, including fatalities, have resulted; precautions (eg, adequate labeling, use of oral syringes) should be employed against such an event.

Increased angina and/or MI have occurred with initiation or dosage titration of calcium channel blockers. Reflex tachycardia may occur resulting in angina and/or MI in patients with obstructive coronary disease, especially in the absence of concurrent beta-blockade. Peripheral edema is a common adverse event; occurs within 2-3 weeks of starting therapy. Symptomatic hypotension with or without syncope can occur; blood pressure must be lowered at a rate appropriate for the patient's clinical condition. Monitor blood pressure closely during treatment. Use with caution in patients with cirrhosis due to the increased plasma concentrations of nimodipine and an increased risk of adverse reactions; a lower dose and close monitoring of blood pressure and heart rate is required. Intestinal pseudo-obstruction and ileus have been reported (rarely) during therapy.

Potentially significant drug-drug interactions may exist, requiring dose or frequency adjustment, additional monitoring, and/or selection of alternative therapy.

Adverse Reactions

Cardiovascular: Bradycardia, decreased blood pressure

Central nervous system: Headache

Gastrointestinal: Nausea

Rare but important or life-threatening: Anemia, decreased platelet count, disseminated intravascular coagulation, edema, gastrointestinal hemorrhage, gastrointestinal pseudo-obstruction, hematoma, hepatitis, hypertension, increased lactate dehydrogenase, increased serum alkaline phosphatase, increased serum ALT, increased serum glucose, intestinal obstruction, jaundice, rebound vasospasm, thrombocytopenia

Drug Interactions

Metabolism/Transport Effects Substrate of CYP3A4 (major); **Note:** Assignment of Major/Minor substrate status based on clinically relevant drug interaction potential

Avoid Concomitant Use

Avoid concomitant use of NiMODipine with any of the following: Conivaptan; Fusidic Acid (Systemic); Grapefruit Juice; Idelalisib

Increased Effect/Toxicity

NiMODipine may increase the levels/effects of: Amifostine; Antihypertensives; Atosiban; Beta-Blockers; Calcium Channel Blockers (Nondihydropyridine); DULoxetine; Fosphenytoin; Hypotensive Agents; Levodopa; Magnesium Salts; Neuromuscular-Blocking Agents (Nondepolarizing); Nitroprusside; Obinutuzumab; Phenytoin; QuiNIDine; RisperiDONE; RiTUXimab; Tacrolimus (Systemic)

The levels/effects of NiMODipine may be increased by: Alfuzosin; Alpha1-Blockers; Antifungal Agents (Azole Derivatives, Systemic); Aprepitant; Barbiturates; Brimonidine (Topical); Calcium Channel Blockers (Nondihydropyridine); Ceritinib; Cimetidine; Conivaptan; CycloSPORINE (Systemic); CYP3A4 Inhibitors (Moderate); CYP3A4 Inhibitors (Strong); Dapoxetine; Dasatinib; Diazoxide; Fluconazole; FLUoxetine; Fosaprepitant; Fusidic Acid (Systemic); Grapefruit Juice; Herbs (Hypotensive Properties); Idelalisib; Ivacaftor; Luliconazole; Macrolide Antibiotics; Magnesium Salts; MAO Inhibitors; Mifepristone; Netupitant; Nicorandil; Pentoxifylline; Phosphodiesterase 5 Inhibitors; Prostacyclin Analogues; Protease Inhibitors; QuiNIDine; Simeprevir; Stiripentol

Decreased Effect

NiMODipine may decrease the levels/effects of: Clopidogrel; QuiNIDine

The levels/effects of NiMODipine may be decreased by: Barbiturates; Bosentan; Calcium Salts; CarBAMazepine; CYP3A4 Inducers (Moderate); CYP3A4 Inducers (Strong); Dabrafenib; Deferasirox; Efavirenz; Herbs (Hypertensive Properties); Melatonin; Methylphenidate; Mitotane; Nafcillin; Rifamycin Derivatives; Siltuximab; St Johns Wort; Tocilizumab; Yohimbine

Food Interactions Administration with a standard breakfast results in a 68% lower maximum plasma concentration and 38% lower bioavailability as compared to administration under fasted conditions. In addition, AUC and maximum plasma concentration were increased by an average of 51% and 24%, respectively, following administration of nimodipine with grapefruit juice (Fuhr, 1998). Management: Administer on an empty stomach, at least 1 hour before or 2 hours after meals. Avoid concurrent use of grapefruit juice and nimodipine.

Storage/Stability Store at 25°C (77°F); excursions are permitted to 15°C to 30°C (59°F to 86°F). Protect capsules from light and freezing. Protect solution from light and do not refrigerate.

Mechanism of Action Nimodipine shares the pharmacology of other calcium channel blockers; animal studies indicate that nimodipine has a greater effect on cerebral arterials than other arterials; this increased specificity may be due to the drug's increased lipophilicity and cerebral distribution as compared to nifedipine; inhibits calcium ion from entering the "slow channels" or select voltage sensitive areas of vascular smooth muscle and myocardium during depolarization

Pharmacodynamics/Kinetics

Protein binding: >95%

Metabolism: Extensively hepatic via CYP3A4; undergoes first-pass metabolism

Bioavailability: 13%

Half-life elimination: 1-2 hours; prolonged with renal impairment

Time to peak, serum: ~1 hour

Excretion: Urine (<1% as unchanged drug); feces

Dosage Note: For oral administration **ONLY.**

Adults: Oral: 60 mg every 4 hours for 21 consecutive days. **Note:** Start therapy within 96 hours of the onset of subarachnoid hemorrhage.

Dosage adjustment in renal impairment: No dosage adjustment provided in manufacturer's labeling. However, nimodipine undergoes minimal renal elimination and dose adjustment may not be necessary. Not removed by hemo- or peritoneal dialysis; supplemental dose is not necessary.

Dosage adjustment in hepatic impairment: Reduce dosage to 30 mg every 4 hours in patients with cirrhosis.

Administration For enteral administration ONLY. Life-threatening adverse events have occurred when administered parenterally. Administer on an empty stomach at least 1 hour before or 2 hours after meals.

Nasogastric (NG) or gastric tube administration:

Oral solution (Nymalzine): Administer using the supplied oral syringe labeled **"ORAL USE ONLY"**. Following administration, refill the oral syringe with 20 mL of NS and flush any remaining contents from NG or gastric tube into the stomach.

Capsules: If the capsules cannot be swallowed, the liquid may be removed by making a hole in each end of the capsule with an 18-gauge needle and extracting the contents into a syringe; transfer these contents into an oral syringe (amber-colored oral syringe preferred). It is strongly recommended that preparation be done in the pharmacy. Label oral syringe with **"WARNING: For ORAL use only"** or **"Not for IV use."** Follow with a flush of 30 mL NS.

Dosage Forms

Capsule, Oral:

Generic: 30 mg

Solution, Oral:

Nymalize: 60 mg/20 mL (20 mL, 473 mL)

◆ **Nimotop (Can)** *see* NiMODipine *on page 1456*

Nimotuzumab [INT] (nye mo TOOSE zu mab)

International Brand Names Biomab EGFR (IN); CIMAher (AR, BR, CO); Taxinsheng (CN); Theracim (ID, PH, TH); TherCIM (AR, CO, CU, IN)

Index Terms TheraCIM hR3; Theraloc

Pharmacologic Category Antineoplastic Agent, Monoclonal Antibody; Epidermal Growth Factor Receptor (EGFR) Inhibitor

Reported Use Nasopharyngeal and head and neck cancer; relapsed high-grade glioma in children and adolescents

Dosage Range I.V.: Refer to individual protocols:

Children: Glioma: Induction phase: 150 mg/m^2/week as a weekly infusion for 6 weeks; consolidation phase: 150 mg/m^2 every 3 weeks until disease progression

Adults: 200 mg/week for 6-8 weeks with radiation or chemoradiotherapy

Product Availability Product available in various countries; not currently available in the U.S.

Nimustine [INT] (nye MYU steen)

International Brand Names Acnu (CH, DE, NL); Nidran (CN, JP, KR)

Index Terms ACNU; Nimustine Hydrochloride

Pharmacologic Category Antineoplastic Agent, Alkylating Agent (Nitrosourea)

Reported Use Treatment of cancer

Dosage Range Adults: I.V.: Refer to individual protocols: 2-3 mg/kg or 90-100 mg/m^2 as a single dose by slow I.V. administration; repeat in 6 weeks depending on hematological response

Product Availability Product available in various countries; not currently available in the U.S.

Dosage Forms Injection: 50 mg

◆ **Nimustine Hydrochloride** *see* Nimustine [INT] *on page 1457*

Nintedanib (nin TED a nib)

Brand Names: U.S. Ofev

Index Terms BIBF1120; Nintedanib Esylate

Pharmacologic Category Tyrosine Kinase Inhibitor

Use Idiopathic pulmonary fibrosis: Treatment of idiopathic pulmonary fibrosis (IPF).

Pregnancy Risk Factor D

Pregnancy Considerations Adverse events were observed in animal reproduction studies. Women of reproductive potential should use adequate contraception; pregnancy should be avoided during therapy and for at least 3 months after the last dose.

Breast-Feeding Considerations It is not known if nintedanib is excreted in breast milk; however it is probable. Due to the potential for serious adverse reactions in the nursing infant, the manufacturer recommends a decision be made whether to discontinue nursing or to discontinue the drug, taking into account the importance of treatment to the mother.

Contraindications There are no contraindications listed in the manufacturer's labeling.

Warnings/Precautions Hazardous agent – use appropriate precautions for handling and disposal (meets NIOSH 2014 criteria). Arterial thromboembolic events, including MI, have been reported. Use caution in patients at high cardiovascular risk, including in patients with known coronary artery disease. Consider treatment interruption in patients who develop signs or symptoms of acute myocardial ischemia. Diarrhea, nausea, and vomiting may occur. Diarrhea occurred in over 50% of nintedanib-treated patients, and was generally mild to moderate. Treat with appropriate supportive care (eg, adequate hydration, antidiarrheals, antiemetics); dose reduction and/or treatment interruption may be required. If gastrointestinal events do not resolve, discontinue treatment. May increase the risk of GI perforation; only use in patients with risk of GI perforation if the benefit outweighs the risk. Use caution in patients with recent abdominal surgery; discontinue in patients who develop GI perforation. Elevations of ALT, AST, GGT, alkaline phosphatase, and bilirubin have occurred; increases were reversible with dose modification/interruption. Obtain LFTs prior to treatment, monthly for 3 months, and every 3 months thereafter (or as clinically indicated).

May increase the risk of bleeding. Use in patients with known risk of bleeding only if the benefit outweighs the risk. Not recommended in patients with moderate or severe hepatic impairment (has not been studied). Patients should stop smoking prior to treatment and avoid smoking during therapy; smoking may decrease exposure to nintedanib.

Adverse Reactions

Cardiovascular: Arterial thrombosis, hypertension (includes hypertensive cardiomyopathy, hypertensive crisis), myocardial infarction

Central nervous system: Headache

Endocrine & metabolic: Hypothyroidism, weight loss

Gastrointestinal: Abdominal pain (includes abdominal tenderness, gastrointestinal pain, lower abdominal pain, upper abdominal pain), decreased appetite, diarrhea, nausea, vomiting

Hematologic and oncologic: Hemorrhage

Hepatic: Increased liver enzymes (includes abnormal alanine aminotransferase, abnormal aspartate aminotransferase, abnormal gamma-glutamyl transferase, abnormal hepatic function tests, hepatic insufficiency, increased serum ALT, increased serum AST, increased gamma-glutamyl transferase, increased serum alkaline phosphatase, increased serum transaminases)

Respiratory: Bronchitis

Rare but important or life-threatening: Gastrointestinal perforation

Drug Interactions

Metabolism/Transport Effects Substrate of CYP3A4 (minor), P-glycoprotein; **Note:** Assignment of Major/Minor substrate status based on clinically relevant drug interaction potential

Avoid Concomitant Use

Avoid concomitant use of Nintedanib with any of the following: Inducers of CYP3A4 and P-glycoprotein

Increased Effect/Toxicity

The levels/effects of Nintedanib may be increased by: Anticoagulants; Inhibitors of CYP3A4 and P-glycoprotein; P-glycoprotein/ABCB1 Inhibitors

Decreased Effect

The levels/effects of Nintedanib may be decreased by: Inducers of CYP3A4 and P-glycoprotein; P-glycoprotein/ABCB1 Inducers; Pirfenidone

Storage/Stability Store at 25°C (77°F); excursions are permitted between 15°C and 30°C (59°F and 86°F). Protect from humidity and avoid excessive heat.

Mechanism of Action Inhibits multiple receptor tyrosine kinases (RTKs) and nonreceptor tyrosine kinases (nRTKs), including platelet-derived growth factor (PDGFR alpha and PDGFR beta); fibroblast growth factor receptor (FGFR1, FGFR2, FGFR3); vascular endothelial growth factor (VEGFR1, VEGFR2, and VEGFR3); and Fms-like tyrosine kinase-3 (FLT3). Nintedanib binds competitively to the adenosine triphosphate (ATP) binding pocket of these receptors and blocks the intracellular signaling which is crucial for the proliferation, migration, and transformation of fibroblasts.

Pharmacodynamics/Kinetics

Absorption: Food increases exposure ~20% and delays absorption

Distribution: V_{ss}: 1050 L

Protein binding: ~98%

Metabolism: Hydrolytic cleavage by esterases to free acid moiety BIBF 1202; which is then glucuronidated by UGT 1A1, UGT 1A7, UGT 1A8, and UGT 1A10 to BIBF 1202 glucuronide; CYP 3A4 (minor).

Bioavailability: ~5%

Half-life elimination: 9.5 hours

Time to peak, plasma: 2 hours (4 hours with food)

Excretion: Feces (~93%); urine (<1%)

Dosage

Idiopathic pulmonary fibrosis (IPF): Adults: Oral: 150 mg every 12 hours (maximum: 300 mg daily)

Missed dose: If a dose is missed, the next dose should be taken at the next scheduled time. Do not make up a missed dose.

Dosage adjustment for toxicity:

Gastrointestinal toxicity (eg, diarrhea, nausea, vomiting) or other adverse reactions/toxicity: Dose reduction or temporary interruption may be needed. Treatment may be resumed at 150 mg every 12 hours or 100 mg every 12 hours, which may subsequently be increased to 150 mg every 12 hours. If a patient does not tolerate 100 mg twice daily, discontinue treatment.

Dosage adjustment in renal impairment:

Mild to moderate impairment (CrCl ≥30 mL/minute): No initial dosage adjustment necessary.

Severe impairment (CrCl <30 mL/minute): There are no dosage adjustments provided in the manufacturer's labeling (has not been studied)

Dosage adjustment in hepatic impairment:

Hepatic impairment at baseline:

Mild impairment: There are no dosage adjustments provided in the manufacturer's labeling (has not been studied); consider dose modification or discontinuation as needed.

Moderate to severe impairment: Use is not recommended (has not been studied).

Hepatotoxicity during treatment:

AST or ALT >3 times to <5 times ULN (without signs of severe liver damage): Interrupt treatment or reduce dosage to 100 mg every 12 hours. Once liver enzymes have returned to baseline values, reintroduce therapy at 100 mg every 12 hours, which may be subsequently increased to 150 mg every 12 hours. If a patient does not tolerate 100 mg twice daily, discontinue treatment.

AST or ALT >5 times ULN or >3 times ULN with signs or symptoms of severe liver damage: Discontinue therapy.

Dietary Considerations Take with food

Administration Oral: Administer with food. Swallow whole with liquid; do not chew or crush (bitter taste). Hazardous agent; use appropriate precautions for handling and disposal (meets NIOSH 2014 criteria).

Monitoring Parameters Obtain LFTs prior to treatment, monthly for 3 months, and every 3 months thereafter (or as clinically indicated). Monitor for gastrointestinal events (eg, diarrhea, nausea, vomiting), arterial thromboembolic events, bleeding, and gastrointestinal perforation.

Dosage Forms

Capsule, Oral:

Ofev: 100 mg, 150 mg

◆ **Nintedanib Esylate** *see* Nintedanib *on page 1458*

◆ **Niodan (Can)** *see* Niacin *on page 1443*

◆ **Nipent** *see* Pentostatin *on page 1618*

◆ **Nipride (Can)** *see* Nitroprusside *on page 1467*

◆ **Niravam** *see* ALPRAZolam *on page 94*

Nisoldipine (nye SOL di peen)

Brand Names: U.S. Sular

Pharmacologic Category Antihypertensive; Calcium Channel Blocker; Calcium Channel Blocker, Dihydropyridine

Use

Hypertension: Management of hypertension, alone or in combination with other antihypertensive agents

The 2014 guideline for the management of high blood pressure in adults (JNC 8) recommends initiation of pharmacologic treatment to lower blood pressure for the following patients (JNC 8 [James, 2013]):

- Patients ≥60 years of age with systolic blood pressure (SBP) ≥150 mm Hg or diastolic blood pressure (DBP) ≥90 mm Hg. Goal of therapy is SBP <150 mm Hg and DBP <90 mm Hg.
- Patients <60 years of age with SBP ≥140 mm Hg or DBP ≥90 mm Hg. Goal of therapy is SBP <140 mm Hg and DBP <90 mm Hg.
- Patients ≥18 years of age with diabetes with SBP ≥140 mm Hg or DBP ≥90 mm Hg. Goal of therapy is SBP <140 mm Hg and DBP <90 mm Hg.
- Patients ≥18 years of age with chronic kidney disease (CKD) with SBP ≥140 mm Hg or DBP ≥90 mm Hg. Goal of therapy is SBP <140 mm Hg and DBP <90 mm Hg.

In patients with chronic kidney disease (CKD), regardless of race or diabetes status, the use of an ACE inhibitor (ACEI) or angiotensin receptor blocker (ARB) as initial therapy is recommended to improve kidney outcomes. In the general nonblack population (without CKD) including those with diabetes, initial antihypertensive treatment should consist of a thiazide-type diuretic, calcium channel blocker, ACEI, or ARB. In the general black population (without CKD) including those with diabetes, initial antihypertensive treatment should consist of a thiazide-type diuretic or a calcium channel blocker instead of an ACEI or ARB.

Pregnancy Risk Factor C

Pregnancy Considerations Adverse events were not observed in animal reproduction studies when using doses that were not maternally toxic. Untreated chronic maternal hypertension is associated with adverse events in the fetus, infant, and mother. If treatment for hypertension during pregnancy is needed, other agents are preferred (ACOG, 2013).

Breast-Feeding Considerations It is not known if nisoldipine is excreted into breast milk. The manufacturer recommends a decision be made whether to discontinue nursing or to discontinue the drug, taking into account the importance of treatment to the mother.

Contraindications Hypersensitivity to nisoldipine, any component of the formulation, or other dihydropyridine calcium channel blockers

Warnings/Precautions With initiation or dosage titration of dihydropyridine calcium channel blockers, reflex tachycardia may occur resulting in angina and/or MI in patients with obstructive coronary disease especially in the absence of concurrent beta-blockade. Use with caution in patients with severe aortic stenosis, and hypertrophic cardiomyopathy with outflow tract obstruction. The ACCF/AHA heart failure guidelines recommend to avoid use in patients with heart failure due to lack of benefit and/or worse outcomes with calcium channel blockers in general (Yancy, 2013). Use with caution in hepatic impairment; lower starting dose required. The most common side effect is peripheral edema; occurs within 2-3 weeks of starting therapy. Symptomatic hypotension with or without syncope can rarely occur; blood pressure must be lowered at a rate appropriate for the patient's clinical condition. Some dosage forms contain tartrazine, which may cause allergic reactions in certain individuals (eg, aspirin hypersensitivity). Use with caution in patients >65 years of age; lower starting dose recommended.

Adverse Reactions

Cardiovascular: Angina exacerbation, chest pain, palpitation, peripheral edema (dose related), vasodilation

Central nervous system: Dizziness, headache

Dermatologic: Rash

Gastrointestinal: Nausea

Respiratory: Cough, dyspnea, pharyngitis, sinusitis,

Rare but important or life-threatening: Alopecia, amblyopia, amnesia, anemia, anorexia, anxiety, appetite increased, arthralgia, arthritis, asthma, ataxia, atrial fibrillation, blepharitis, BUN increased, bruising, cellulitis, cerebral ischemia, colitis, conjunctivitis, creatinine increased, creatine kinase increased, CVA, depression, diabetes mellitus, diaphoresis, diarrhea, dreams abnormal, dyspepsia, dysphagia, dyspnea, dysuria, end inspiratory wheeze, epistaxis, exfoliative dermatitis, facial edema, fever, first-degree AV block, flu-like syndrome, gastritis, gastrointestinal hemorrhage, gingival hyperplasia, glaucoma, glossitis, gout, gynecomastia, heart failure (decompensated), hematuria, hepatomegaly, herpes simplex, herpes zoster; hypersensitivity reaction (eg, angioedema, shortness of breath, tachycardia, chest tightness, hypotension, and rash); hyper-/hypotension, hypertonia, hypoesthesia, hypokalemia, insomnia, jugular venous distention, keratoconjunctivitis, leukopenia, libido decreased, liver function tests abnormal, maculopapular rash, malaise, melena, migraine, mouth ulceration, myalgia, myasthenia, MI, myositis, nocturia, nonprotein nitrogen increased, orthostatic hypotension, paresthesia, petechiae, photosensitivity, pleural effusion, pruritus, pustular rash, rales, retinal detachment, skin discoloration, skin ulcer, somnolence, supraventricular tachycardia, syncope, systolic ejection murmur, taste disturbance, temporary unilateral loss of vision, tenosynovitis, thyroiditis, tremor; T-wave abnormalities on ECG (flattening, inversion, nonspecific changes); urinary frequency, urticaria, vaginal hemorrhage, venous insufficiency, ventricular extrasystoles, vertigo, vitreous floater, weight gain/loss, xerostomia

Drug Interactions

Metabolism/Transport Effects Substrate of CYP3A4 (major); **Note:** Assignment of Major/Minor substrate status based on clinically relevant drug interaction potential; **Inhibits** CYP1A2 (weak), CYP3A4 (weak)

Avoid Concomitant Use

Avoid concomitant use of Nisoldipine with any of the following: Conivaptan; CYP3A4 Inducers (Moderate); CYP3A4 Inducers (Strong); CYP3A4 Inhibitors (Strong); Fusidic Acid (Systemic); Grapefruit Juice; Idelalisib; Pimozide

Increased Effect/Toxicity

Nisoldipine may increase the levels/effects of: Amifostine; Antihypertensives; ARIPiprazole; Atosiban; Beta-Blockers; Calcium Channel Blockers (Nondihydropyridine); Dofetilide; DULoxetine; Hydrocodone; Hypotensive Agents; Levodopa; Lomitapide; Magnesium Salts; Neuromuscular-Blocking Agents (Nondepolarizing); Nitroprusside; Obinutuzumab; Pimozide; RisperiDONE; RiTUXimab; Tacrolimus (Systemic)

The levels/effects of Nisoldipine may be increased by: Alfuzosin; Alpha1-Blockers; Aprepitant; Barbiturates; Brimonidine (Topical); Calcium Channel Blockers (Nondihydropyridine); Ceritinib; Cimetidine; Conivaptan; CycloSPORINE (Systemic); CYP3A4 Inhibitors (Moderate); CYP3A4 Inhibitors (Strong); Dapoxetine; Dasatinib; Diazoxide; Fluconazole; Fosaprepitant; Fusidic Acid (Systemic); Grapefruit Juice; Herbs (Hypotensive Properties); Idelalisib; Ivacaftor; Luliconazole; Macrolide Antibiotics; Magnesium Salts; MAO Inhibitors; Mifepristone; Netupitant; Nicorandil; Pentoxifylline; Phosphodiesterase 5 Inhibitors; Prostacyclin Analogues; Protease Inhibitors; Simeprevir

Decreased Effect

Nisoldipine may decrease the levels/effects of: Clopidogrel

The levels/effects of Nisoldipine may be decreased by: Barbiturates; Calcium Salts; CYP3A4 Inducers (Moderate); CYP3A4 Inducers (Strong); Deferasirox; Herbs (Hypertensive Properties); Melatonin; Methylphenidate; Siltuximab; Tocilizumab; Yohimbine

Food Interactions Peak concentrations of nisoldipine may be significantly increased if taken with high-lipid foods; however, total exposure (AUC) may be reduced. Grapefruit juice has been shown to significantly increase the bioavailability of nisoldipine. Management: Take on an empty stomach 1 hour before or 2 hours after a meal. Avoid a high-fat diet. Avoid grapefruit products before and after dosing.

Storage/Stability Store at controlled room temperature of 20°C to 25°C (68°F to 77°F). Protect from light; protect from moisture.

Mechanism of Action As a dihydropyridine calcium channel blocker, structurally similar to nifedipine, nisoldipine impedes the movement of calcium ions into vascular smooth muscle and cardiac muscle. Dihydropyridines are potent vasodilators and are not as likely to suppress cardiac contractility and slow cardiac conduction as other calcium antagonists such as verapamil and diltiazem; nisoldipine is 5-10 times as potent a vasodilator as nifedipine.

Pharmacodynamics/Kinetics

Duration: >24 hours

Absorption: Well absorbed. Peak concentrations significantly increased with high-lipid meals; however, AUC is reduced.

Protein binding: >99%

Metabolism: Extensively hepatic; 1 active metabolite (10% of activity of parent); first-pass effect

Bioavailability: ~5%

Half-life elimination: 9-18 hours

Time to peak: 4-14 hours

Excretion: Urine (60% to 80% as inactive metabolites); feces

Dosage Oral:

Sular (Geomatrix delivery system):

Adults: Initial: 17 mg once daily, then increase by 8.5 mg/week (or longer intervals) to attain adequate control of blood pressure

Usual dose range: 17-34 mg once daily; doses >34 mg once daily are not recommended

Elderly: Initial dose: 8.5 mg once daily, increase by 8.5 mg/week (or longer intervals) to attain adequate blood pressure control

Nisoldipine extended-release tablet (original formulation):

Adults: Oral: Initial: 20 mg once daily, then increase by 10 mg/week (or longer intervals) to attain adequate control of blood pressure

Usual dose range: 20-40 mg once daily; doses >60 mg once daily are not recommended

Elderly: Initial dose: 10 mg once daily, increase by 10 mg/week (or longer intervals) to attain adequate blood pressure control

Conversion from nisoldipine extended-release (original formulation) to Sular Geomatrix delivery system:

Nisoldipine Extended Release Dosing Equivalency

Original Extended Release Formulation	Sular Extended Release (Geomatrix delivery system)
10 mg	8.5 mg
20 mg	17 mg
30 mg	25.5 mg
40 mg	34 mg

Dosage adjustment in renal impairment:

Mild to moderate impairment: No dosage adjustment necessary.

Severe impairment: No dosage adjustment provided in manufacturer's labeling.

Dosage adjustment in hepatic impairment:

Sular (Geomatrix delivery system): An initial dose exceeding 8.5 mg once daily is not recommended for patients with hepatic impairment.

Nisoldipine extended-release (original formulation): An initial dose exceeding 10 mg once daily is not recommended for patients with hepatic impairment.

Dietary Considerations Take on an empty stomach (1 hour before or 2 hours after a meal). Avoid grapefruit juice before and after dosing. Avoid grapefuit juice; avoid high-fat diet.

Administration Administer at the same time each day to ensure minimal fluctuation of serum levels. Avoid high-fat diet. Administer on an empty stomach (1 hour before or 2 hours after a meal). Swallow whole; do not crush, break, split, or chew.

Monitoring Parameters Blood pressure, heart rate

Dosage Forms

Tablet Extended Release 24 Hour, Oral:

Sular: 8.5 mg, 17 mg, 34 mg

Generic: 8.5 mg, 17 mg, 20 mg, 25.5 mg, 30 mg, 34 mg, 40 mg

◆ **Nitalapram** *see* Citalopram *on page 451*

Nitazoxanide (nye ta ZOX a nide)

Brand Names: U.S. Alinia

Index Terms NTZ

Pharmacologic Category Antiprotozoal

Use Treatment of diarrhea caused by *Cryptosporidium parvum* or *Giardia lamblia*

Pregnancy Risk Factor B

Dosage Oral:

Children: Diarrhea caused by *Cryptosporidium parvum* or *Giardia lamblia*:

Children 1-3 years: Oral suspension: 100 mg every 12 hours for 3 days; may consider increasing duration up to 14 days in HIV-exposed/-infected pediatric patients with cryptosporidiosis (CDC, 2009)

Children 4-11 years: Oral suspension: 200 mg every 12 hours for 3 days; may consider increasing duration up to 14 days in HIV-exposed/-infected pediatric patients with cryptosporidiosis (CDC, 2009)

Children ≥12 years: Refer to adult dosing.

Adults:

Diarrhea caused by *Cryptosporidium parvum* or *Giardia lamblia*: Oral suspension or tablets: 500 mg every 12 hours for 3 days

Clostridium difficile-associated diarrhea (off-label use): Oral suspension or tablets: 500 mg every 12 hours for 7 to 10 days (Musher 2006; Musher 2009)

Dosage adjustment in renal impairment: No dosage adjustment provided in manufacturer's labeling (has not been studied); use with caution.

Dosage adjustment in hepatic impairment: No dosage adjustment provided in manufacturer's labeling (has not been studied); use with caution.

Additional Information Complete prescribing information should be consulted for additional detail.

Dosage Forms

Suspension Reconstituted, Oral:

Alinia: 100 mg/5 mL (60 mL)

Tablet, Oral:

Alinia: 500 mg

◆ **Nithiodote** *see* Sodium Nitrite and Sodium Thiosulfate *on page 1907*

Nitisinone (ni TIS i known)

Brand Names: U.S. Orfadin

Index Terms NTBC

Pharmacologic Category 4-Hydroxyphenylpyruvate Dioxygenase Inhibitor

Use Hereditary tyrosinemia type 1: Treatment of hereditary tyrosinemia type 1 (HT-1) as an adjunct to dietary restriction of tyrosine and phenylalanine

Pregnancy Risk Factor C

Dosage Hereditary tyrosinemia type 1 (HT-1): Oral: **Note:** Must be used in conjunction with a diet restricted in tyrosine and phenylalanine.

Children, Adolescents, and Adults: Initial: 1 mg/kg/day in 2 divided doses

Dosage adjustment for inadequate response: Note: Inadequate response is defined as continued abnormal biological parameters (erythrocyte PBG-synthase activity, urine 5-ALA, and urine and plasma succinylacetone) despite treatment. Plasma succinylacetone may take up to 3 months to normalize after start of therapy. If the aforementioned parameters are not available, may use urine succinylacetone, liver function tests, alpha-fetoprotein, serum tyrosine, and serum phenylalanine to evaluate response (exceptions may include during initiation of therapy and exacerbations).

Abnormal biological parameters (erythrocyte PBG-synthase activity, urine 5-ALA, and urine succinylacetone) at 1 month: Increase dose to 1.5 mg/kg/day

Abnormal biological parameters (erythrocyte PBG-synthase activity, urine 5-ALA, and urine and plasma succinylacetone) at 3 months: Further increase to maximum dose of 2 mg/kg/day

Dosage adjustment in renal impairment: There are no dosage adjustments provided in the manufacturer's labeling (has not been studied).

Dosage adjustment in hepatic impairment: There are no dosage adjustments provided in the manufacturer's labeling (has not been studied).

Additional Information Complete prescribing information should be consulted for additional detail.

Dosage Forms

Capsule, Oral:

Orfadin: 2 mg, 5 mg, 10 mg

◆ **Nitoman (Can)** *see* Tetrabenazine *on page 2016*

◆ **Nitrazadon (Can)** *see* Nitrazepam [CAN/INT] *on page 1461*

Nitrazepam [CAN/INT] (nye TRA ze pam)

Brand Names: Canada Apo-Nitrazepam; Mogadon; Nitrazadon; Sandoz-Nitrazepam

Index Terms Nitrozepamum

Pharmacologic Category Benzodiazepine

Use Note: Not approved in U.S.

Short-term management of insomnia; treatment of myoclonic seizures

Pregnancy Considerations Use during pregnancy is not recommended. Nitrazepam crosses the human placenta. Teratogenic effects have been observed with some benzodiazepines; however, additional studies are needed. The incidence of premature birth and low birth weights may be increased following maternal use of benzodiazepines; hypoglycemia and respiratory problems in the neonate may occur following exposure late in pregnancy. Neonatal withdrawal symptoms may occur within days to weeks after birth and "floppy infant syndrome" (which also includes withdrawal symptoms) have been reported with some benzodiazepines (Bergman, 1992; Iqbal, 2002; Wikner, 2007).

Breast-Feeding Considerations Nitrazepam is excreted into breast milk. Drowsiness, lethargy, or weight loss in nursing infants have been observed in case reports following maternal use of some benzodiazepines (Iqbal, 2002). Breast-feeding is not recommended by the manufacturer.

Contraindications Hypersensitivity to nitrazepam or any component of the formulation (cross sensitivity with other benzodiazepines may exist); myasthenia gravis; severe respiratory insufficiency (eg, significant sleep apnea syndrome); severe hepatic insufficiency; use as hypnotic in children

Warnings/Precautions Anaphylaxis/anaphylactoid reactions have been reported with use; patients who develop angioedema should not be rechallenged with nitrazepam. Nitrazepam has been implicated with sudden death in children <5 years of age being treated for seizure disorders. Use should be restricted to children unresponsive to other antiepileptic agents. Should be used only after evaluation of potential causes of sleep disturbance. Failure of sleep disturbance to resolve after 7-10 days may indicate psychiatric or medical illness. A worsening of insomnia or the emergence of new abnormalities of thought or behavior may represent unrecognized psychiatric or medical illness and requires immediate and careful evaluation. Not recommended for primary treatment of psychotic illness. Nitrazepam should not be used alone to treat depression (or anxiety associated with depression) since suicide may be precipitated in these patients.

Prescribed quantities should typically be for short term (7-10 days) and not exceed a 1-month supply. Use with caution in patients with history of drug dependence. Benzodiazepines have been associated with dependence and acute withdrawal symptoms upon discontinuation or reduction in dose. Acute withdrawal, including seizures, may be precipitated after administration of flumazenil to patients receiving long-term benzodiazepine therapy.

Use with caution in patients receiving other CNS depressant drugs; may potentiate effects of other sedative drugs or ethanol. Use with caution in patients with hepatic or renal disease and in patients with respiratory disease and limited pulmonary reserve. Use in severe hepatic impairment or severe respiratory insufficiency (eg, severe sleep apnea syndrome) is contraindicated. Caution patients about performing tasks which require mental alertness (eg, operating machinery or driving). Nitrazepam may rarely induce anterograde amnesia (particularly in the elderly); caution patients to ensure they have uninterrupted sleep of 7-8 hours after ingestion of dose. An increased risk for hazardous sleep-related activities such as sleep-driving; cooking and eating food, and making phone calls while asleep have also been noted. Paradoxical reactions, including hyperactive or aggressive behavior, have been reported with benzodiazepines, particularly in adolescent/pediatric or psychiatric patients. Nitrazepam is a long half-life benzodiazepine. Tolerance develops to the hypnotic and anticonvulsant effects (Vinkers, 2012). Chronic use of this agent may increase the perioperative benzodiazepine dose needed to achieve desired effect.

Use with caution in elderly or debilitated patients. Benzodiazepines have been associated with falls and traumatic injury and should be used with extreme caution in patients who are at risk of these events (especially the elderly). Bronchial hypersecretion and excessive salivation/drooling leading to aspiration pneumonia in young and elderly patients may occur rarely. Safety and efficacy for use as a hypnotic not established in children <18 years of age.

Adverse Reactions

Cardiovascular: Hypotension, palpitation

Central nervous system: Agitation, aggressiveness, amnesia, ataxia, confusion, delusions, depression, disorientation, dizziness, excitement, fatigue, hallucination, hangover, headache, hyperactivity, irritability, lethargy, lightheadedness, nervousness, nightmares, psychoses, rage, restlessness, sedation, staggering

Dermatologic: Cutaneous reactions

Endocrine & metabolic: Changes in libido

Gastrointestinal: Constipation, diarrhea, excessive salivation, heartburn, nausea, vomiting

Hematologic: Granulocytopenia, leukopenia

Hepatic: Hepatic function tests abnormal

Neuromuscular & skeletal: Delirium tremens, falling, muscle spasticity increased, muscle weakness

Ocular: Blurred vision

Respiratory: Aspiration, bronchial hypersecretion, dyspnea

Miscellaneous: Anaphylaxis/anaphylactoid reactions (angioedema, dyspnea, throat closing, nausea/vomiting)

Drug Interactions

Metabolism/Transport Effects None known.

Avoid Concomitant Use

Avoid concomitant use of Nitrazepam with any of the following: Azelastine (Nasal); Methadone; OLANZapine; Orphenadrine; Paraldehyde; Sodium Oxybate; Thalidomide

Increased Effect/Toxicity

Nitrazepam may increase the levels/effects of: Alcohol (Ethyl); Azelastine (Nasal); Buprenorphine; CloZAPine; CNS Depressants; Fosphenytoin; Hydrocodone; Methadone; Methotrimeprazine; Metyrosine; Mirtazapine; Orphenadrine; Paraldehyde; Phenytoin; Pramipexole; ROPINIRole; Rotigotine; Selective Serotonin Reuptake Inhibitors; Sodium Oxybate; Suvorexant; Thalidomide; Zolpidem

The levels/effects of Nitrazepam may be increased by: Brimonidine (Topical); Cannabis; Cosyntropin; Doxylamine; Dronabinol; Droperidol; HydrOXYzine; Kava Kava; Magnesium Sulfate; Methotrimeprazine; Nabilone; OLANZapine; Perampanel; Rufinamide; Tapentadol; Teduglutide; Tetrahydrocannabinol

Decreased Effect

The levels/effects of Nitrazepam may be decreased by: Rifampin; Theophylline Derivatives; Yohimbine

Storage/Stability Store 15°C to 30°C (59°F to 86°F). Protect from light.

Mechanism of Action Binds to stereospecific benzodiazepine receptors on the postsynaptic GABA neuron at several sites within the CNS, including the limbic system, reticular formation. Enhancement of the inhibitory effect of GABA on neuronal excitability results by increased neuronal membrane permeability to chloride ions. This shift in chloride ions results in hyperpolarization (a less excitable state) and stabilization. Benzodiazepine receptors and effects appear to be linked to the GABA-A receptors. Benzodiazepines do not bind to GABA-B receptors.

Pharmacodynamics/Kinetics

Onset of action: 20-50 minutes

Absorption: Rapid

Distribution: V_d: 2.4 L/kg, Elderly: 4.8 L/kg; also distributes into CSF, saliva

Protein binding: 87%

Metabolism: Hepatic: Nitroreduction, acetylation; no active metabolites

Bioavailability: ~80%

Half-life elimination: 30 hours, Elderly/ill patients: 40 hours

Time to peak, plasma: ~3 hours

Excretion: Urine (65% to 70%, ~1% as unchanged drug); feces (14% to 20%)

Dosage Oral:

Children ≤30 kg: Myoclonic seizures: Usual dosage: 0.3-1 mg/kg/day in 3 divided doses; **Note:** Therapy should be initiated below the usual dosage range and titrated carefully based on response. If inadequate response to usual dosage, may gradually increase dose further. Manufacturer labeling does not specify a maximum dosage.

Adults: Insomnia: 5-10 mg at bedtime; treatment should not exceed 7-10 consecutive days; use for more than 2-3 consecutive weeks requires complete re-evaluation of patient

Elderly or debilitated patients: 2.5 mg at bedtime; may increase dose to 5 mg if tolerated (maximum dose: 5 mg/day)

Administration Tablets may be swallowed whole, crushed, or dissolved in liquid. For insomnia, administer at bedtime. For myoclonic seizures, administer in 3 equally divided doses, or if doses are not divided equally, give larger dose at bedtime.

Monitoring Parameters Respiratory and cardiovascular status

Reference Range Steady state levels after 4 days: 40 ng/mL

Product Availability Not available in U.S.
Dosage Forms: Canada
Tablet, Oral: 5 mg, 10 mg

Nitrendipine [INT] (NYE tren di peen)

International Brand Names !Nitrendipin Basics (DE); Balminil (ES); Baylotensin (JP); Bayotensin (DE); Baypresol (ES); Baypress (AR, AT, BE, CH, CZ, DK, FR, HU, IT, LU, NL, PL); Deiten (IT); Farnitran (PT); Gericin (ES); Hiperdipina (PT); Jutapress (DE); Lusopress (IT); Monopress (ES); Nidrel (FR); Niprina (ES); Nirapel (AR); Nitre AbZ (DE); Nitre-Puren (DE); Nitregamma (DE); Nitren 1A Pharma (DE); Nitren acis (DE); Nitren Lich (DE); Nitrencord (BR); Nitrendepat (DE); Nitrendi-BASF (DE); Nitrendil (AR); Nitrendimerck (DE); Nitrendipin AL (DE); Nitrendipin Apogepha (DE); Nitrendipin Atid (DE); Nitrendipin Basics (DE); Nitrendipin beta (DE); nitrendipin corax (DE); Nitrendipin Heumann (DE); Nitrendipin Jenapharm (DE); Nitrendipin Lindo (DE); Nitrendipin Stada (DE); nitrendipin von ct (DE); Nitrendipin-ratiopharm (DE); Nitrendipino Bayvit (ES); Nitrendipino Ratiopharm (ES); Nitrendypina (PL); Nitrensal (DE); Nitrepress (DE); Sub Tensin (ES); Tensogradal (ES); Tocrat (AR); Tracil (AR); Trendinol (ES); Unipres (CZ, HR, HU, PL); Vastensium (ES); Veraxin (HR); Xasmun (ES)

Pharmacologic Category Calcium Channel Blocker

Dosage Range 20 mg/day (in patients with liver disease or in the elderly, an initial dose of 10 mg is recommended); maximum dose: 40 mg/day

Product Availability Product available in various countries; not currently available in the U.S.

◆ **Nitro-Bid** *see* Nitroglycerin *on page 1465*
◆ **Nitro-Dur** *see* Nitroglycerin *on page 1465*

Nitrofurantoin (nye troe fyoor AN toyn)

Brand Names: U.S. Furadantin; Macrobid; Macrodantin

Brand Names: Canada Apo-Nitrofurantoin; Macrobid; Macrodantin; Novo-Furantoin; Teva-Nitrofurantoin

Pharmacologic Category Antibiotic, Miscellaneous

Additional Appendix Information

Beers Criteria - Potentially Inappropriate Medications for Geriatrics *on page 2271*

Use

Urinary tract infections: For the treatment of urinary tract infections (UTIs) when caused by susceptible strains of *Escherichia coli*, enterococci, *Staphylococcus aureus*, and certain susceptible strains of *Klebsiella* and *Enterobacter* species.

Acute cystitis: Nitrofurantoin monohydrate/macrocrystals: Indicated only for the treatment of acute uncomplicated UTIs (acute cystitis) caused by susceptible strains of *E. coli* or *Staphylococcus saprophyticus* in patients ≥12 years of age.

Pregnancy Risk Factor B (contraindicated at term)

Pregnancy Considerations Adverse effects have not been observed in animal reproduction studies. Nitrofurantoin crosses the placenta (Perry, 1967) and maternal serum concentrations may be lower in pregnancy (Philipson, 1979). Current studies evaluating maternal use of nitrofurantoin during pregnancy and the development of birth defects have had mixed results (ACOG, 2011). An increased risk of neonatal jaundice was observed following maternal nitrofurantoin use during the last 30 days of pregnancy (Nordeng, 2013). Nitrofurantoin may be used to treat infections in pregnant women; use during the first trimester should be limited to situations where no alternative therapies are available. Prescriptions should be written when clinically appropriate and for the shortest effective duration for confirmed infections (ACOG, 2011).

Nitrofurantoin is contraindicated in pregnant patients at term (38-42 weeks gestation), during labor and delivery, or when the onset of labor is imminent due to the possibility of hemolytic anemia in the neonate. Alternative antibiotics should be considered in pregnant women with G-6-PD deficiency (Nordeng, 2013).

Breast-Feeding Considerations Trace amounts of nitrofurantoin can be detected in breast milk. Due to the potential for serious adverse reactions in the nursing infant, the manufacturer recommends a decision be made whether to discontinue nursing or to discontinue the drug, taking into account the importance of treatment to the mother. The therapeutic use of nitrofurantoin is contraindicated in neonates (<1 month of age) due to the possibility of hemolytic anemia caused by immature erythrocyte enzyme systems. In case reports, diarrhea was reported in two nursing infants and decreased milk volume was reported by one mother (dose, duration, relationship to breast-feeding not provided) (Ito, 1993).

Contraindications

Anuria, oliguria, or significant impairment of renal function (creatinine clearance [CrCl] <60 mL/minute or clinically significant elevated serum creatinine); previous history of cholestatic jaundice or hepatic dysfunction associated with prior nitrofurantoin use; hypersensitivity to drug or any component of the formulation.

Note: The manufacturer's contraindication in patients with CrCl <60 mL/minute has been challenged in the literature; limited data suggest that an alternative creatinine clearance threshold may be considered (Oplinger, 2013).

Because of the possibility of hemolytic anemia caused by immature erythrocyte enzyme systems (glutathione instability), the drug is contraindicated in pregnant patients at term (38 to 42 weeks gestation), during labor and delivery, or when the onset of labor is imminent; also contraindicated in neonates younger than 1 month of age.

Warnings/Precautions Use with caution in patients with G6PD deficiency (increased risk of hemolytic anemia). Urinary nitrofurantoin concentrations are variable in patients with impaired renal function. The manufacturer contraindicates use in CrCl <60 mL/minute; however, limited data suggest clinicians may consider using a lower threshold of CrCl ≥40 mL/minute when treatment is short term (≤1 week) for an uncomplicated UTI (Oplinger, 2013).

Use with caution if prolonged therapy is anticipated due to possible pulmonary toxicity. Acute, subacute, or chronic (usually after 6 months of therapy) pulmonary reactions (possibly fatal) have been observed in patients treated with nitrofurantoin; if these occur, discontinue therapy immediately; monitor closely for malaise, dyspnea, cough, fever, radiologic evidence of diffuse interstitial pneumonitis or fibrosis. Rare, but severe and sometimes fatal hepatic reactions (eg, cholestatic jaundice, hepatitis, hepatic necrosis) have been associated with nitrofurantoin (onset may be insidious); discontinue immediately if hepatitis occurs. Use is contraindicated in patients with a history of nitrofurantoin associated cholestatic jaundice or hepatic dysfunction. Monitor liver function test periodically. Has been associated with peripheral neuropathy (rare); risk may be increased in patients with anemia, renal impairment (CrCl <60 mL/minute), diabetes, vitamin B deficiency, debilitating disease, or electrolyte imbalance; use caution. Potentially significant drug-drug interactions may exist, requiring dose or frequency adjustment, additional monitoring, and/or selection of alternative therapy. Effects may be potentiated when used with other sedative drugs or ethanol. Use in the elderly, particularly females receiving long-term prophylaxis for recurrent UTIs, has been associated with an increased risk of hepatic and pulmonary toxicity, and peripheral neuropathy. In the elderly, avoid use for long-term suppression due to potential for pulmonary toxicity and availability of safer alternative agents (Beers Criteria). Use in the elderly, particularly females receiving long-term prophylaxis for recurrent UTIs, has also been associated with an increased risk of hepatic toxicity and peripheral neuropathy; monitor closely for toxicities during use. Prolonged use may result in fungal or bacterial superinfection, including *C. difficile*-associated diarrhea (CDAD) and pseudomembranous colitis; CDAD has been observed >2 months postantibiotic treatment. Use is contraindicated in children <1 month of age (at increased risk for hemolytic anemia). Not indicated for the treatment of pyelonephritis or perinephric abscesses. Postmarketing cases of optic neuritis have been reported.

Adverse Reactions

Cardiovascular: ECG changes (nonspecific ST/T wave changes, bundle branch block)

Central nervous system: Bulging fontanel (infants), chills, confusion, depression, dizziness, drowsiness, headache, malaise, numbness, paresthesia, peripheral neuropathy, pseudotumor cerebri, psychotic reaction, vertigo

Dermatologic: Alopecia, erythema multiforme, exfoliative dermatitis, pruritus, skin rash (eczematous, erythematous, maculopapular), Stevens-Johnson syndrome, urticaria

Endocrine & metabolic: Hyperphosphatemia

Gastrointestinal: Abdominal pain, anorexia, *Clostridium difficile* associated diarrhea, constipation, diarrhea, dyspepsia, flatulence, nausea, pancreatitis, pseudomembranous colitis, sialadenitis, vomiting

Genitourinary: Urine discoloration (brown)

Hematologic & oncologic: Agranulocytosis, aplastic anemia, eosinophilia, glucose-6-phosphate dehydrogenase deficiency anemia, granulocytopenia, hemoglobin decreased, hemolytic anemia, leukopenia, megaloblastic anemia, thrombocytopenia

Hepatic: Cholestatic jaundice, hepatitis, hepatic necrosis, increased serum transaminases

Hypersensitivity: Anaphylaxis, angioedema, hypersensitivity (including acute pulmonary hypersensitivity)

Infection: Superinfection (eg, *Pseudomonas* or *Candida*)

Neuromuscular & skeletal: Arthralgia, lupus-like syndrome, myalgia, weakness

Ophthalmic: Amblyopia, nystagmus, optic neuritis

Respiratory: Acute pulmonary reaction (symptoms include chills, chest pain, cough, dyspnea, fever, and eosinophilia), cough, cyanosis, dyspnea, pneumonitis, pulmonary fibrosis (with long-term use), pulmonary infiltration

Miscellaneous: Fever

Drug Interactions

Metabolism/Transport Effects None known.

Avoid Concomitant Use

Avoid concomitant use of Nitrofurantoin with any of the following: BCG; Magnesium Trisilicate; Norfloxacin

Increased Effect/Toxicity

Nitrofurantoin may increase the levels/effects of: Eplerenone; Prilocaine; Sodium Nitrite; Spironolactone

The levels/effects of Nitrofurantoin may be increased by: Nitric Oxide; Probenecid

Decreased Effect

Nitrofurantoin may decrease the levels/effects of: BCG; Norfloxacin; Sodium Picosulfate; Typhoid Vaccine

The levels/effects of Nitrofurantoin may be decreased by: Magnesium Trisilicate

Food Interactions Nitrofurantoin serum concentrations may be increased if taken with food. Management: Administer with meals.

Storage/Stability

Capsules: Store at controlled room temperature, 15°C to 30°C (59°F to 86°F). Dispense in a tight container using a child-resistant closure.

Oral suspension: Avoid exposure to strong light, which may darken the drug. It is stable when stored between 20°C and 25°C (68°F and 77°F). Protect from freezing. Dispense in glass amber bottles.

Mechanism of Action Nitrofurantoin is reduced by bacterial flavoproteins to reactive intermediates that inactivate or alter bacterial ribosomal proteins leading to inhibition of protein synthesis, aerobic energy metabolism, DNA, RNA, and cell wall synthesis. Nitrofurantoin is bactericidal in urine at therapeutic doses. The broad-based nature of this mode of action may explain the lack of acquired bacterial resistance to nitrofurantoin, as the necessary multiple and simultaneous mutations of the target macromolecules would likely be lethal to the bacteria.

Pharmacodynamics/Kinetics

Absorption: Well absorbed; macrocrystalline form absorbed more slowly due to slower dissolution (causes less GI distress)

Distribution: V_d: 0.8 L/kg

Protein binding: 60% to 90%

Metabolism: Body tissues (except plasma) metabolize 60% of drug to inactive metabolites

Bioavailability: Increased with food by ~40%

Half-life elimination: 20-60 minutes; prolonged with renal impairment

Excretion:

Suspension: Urine (~40%) and feces (small amounts) as metabolites and unchanged drug

Macrocrystals: Urine (20% to 25% as unchanged drug)

Dosage Oral:

Children >1 month:

UTI treatment (Furadantin, Macrodantin): 5-7 mg/kg/day in divided doses every 6 hours; maximum: 400 mg daily. Administer for 7 days or at least 3 days after obtaining sterile urine

UTI prophylaxis (Furadantin, Macrodantin): 1-2 mg/kg/day in divided doses every 12-24 hours; maximum: 100 mg daily (Redbook [AAP], 2012)

Children >12 years: UTI treatment (Macrobid): 100 mg twice daily for 7 days

Adults:

UTI treatment:

Furadantin, Macrodantin: 50-100 mg/dose every 6 hours; administer for 7 days or at least 3 days after obtaining sterile urine

Macrobid: 100 mg twice daily for 7 days

UTI prophylaxis (Furadantin, Macrodantin): 50-100 mg/dose at bedtime

Elderly: Avoid use; alternative agents preferred.

Dosage adjustment in renal impairment:

CrCl ≥60 mL/minute: No dosage adjustment provided in manufacturer's labeling.

CrCl <60 mL/minute: Use is contraindicated. **Note:** Although more evidence is needed, limited data suggest clinicians consider use in patients with CrCl ≥40 mL/minute when treatment is short term (≤1 week) for an uncomplicated UTI (Oplinger, 2013).

Dosage adjustment in hepatic impairment: No dosage adjustment provided in manufacturer's labeling. Contraindicated in patients with a previous history of cholestatic jaundice or hepatic dysfunction associated with nitrofurantoin.

Dietary Considerations Take with meals to improve absorption and decrease adverse effects.

Administration Administer with meals to improve absorption and decrease adverse effects; suspension may be mixed with water, milk, fruit juice, or infant formula. Shake suspension well before use.

Monitoring Parameters Signs of pulmonary reaction; signs of numbness or tingling of the extremities; CBC, periodic liver function tests, periodic renal function tests with long-term use

Dosage Forms

Capsule, Oral:

Macrobid: 100 mg

Macrodantin: 25 mg, 50 mg, 100 mg

Generic: 50 mg, 100 mg

Suspension, Oral:

Furadantin: 25 mg/5 mL (230 mL)

Generic: 25 mg/5 mL (230 mL, 240 mL)

◆ **Nitrogen Mustard** *see* Mechlorethamine (Systemic) *on page 1276*

Nitroglycerin (nye troe GLI ser in)

Brand Names: U.S. Minitran; Nitro-Bid; Nitro-Dur; Nitro-Time; Nitrolingual; NitroMist; Nitronal; Nitrostat; Rectiv

Brand Names: Canada Minitran; Mylan-Nitro Sublingual Spray; Nitro-Dur; Nitroglycerin Injection, USP; Nitrol; Nitrostat; Rho-Nitro Pump Spray; Transderm-Nitro; Trinipatch

Index Terms Glyceryl Trinitrate; GTN; Nitroglycerol; Nitronal; NTG; TNG; Tridil

Pharmacologic Category Antianginal Agent; Antidote, Extravasation; Vasodilator

Use Treatment or prevention of angina pectoris

Intravenous (IV) administration: Treatment or prevention of angina pectoris; acute decompensated heart failure (especially when associated with acute myocardial infarction); perioperative hypertension (especially during cardiovascular surgery); induction of intraoperative hypotension

Intra-anal administration (Rectiv ointment): Treatment of moderate-to-severe pain associated with chronic anal fissure

Pregnancy Risk Factor B/C (product specific)

Pregnancy Considerations Animal reproduction studies have not been conducted with all products; adverse events were not observed in animal reproduction studies conducted using the ointment. Nitroglycerin crosses the placenta (David, 2000). Concentrations following application of a transdermal patch 0.4 mg/hour were low but detectable in the fetal serum (fetal/maternal ratio: 0.23) (Bustard, 2003). Nitroglycerin may be used in pregnancy when immediate relaxation of the uterus is needed (ACOG, 2006; Axemo, 1998; Chandraharan, 2005). Intravenous nitroglycerin may be used to treat pre-eclampsia with pulmonary edema (ESG, 2011).

Breast-Feeding Considerations It is not known if nitroglycerin is excreted in breast milk. The manufacturer recommends that caution be exercised when administering nitroglycerin to nursing women. Information related to the use of nitroglycerin and breast-feeding is limited (Böttiger, 2010; O'Sullivan, 2011).

Contraindications

Hypersensitivity to organic nitrates or any component of the formulation (includes adhesives for transdermal product); concurrent use with phosphodiesterase-5 (PDE-5) inhibitors (sildenafil, tadalafil, or vardenafil); concurrent use with riociguat

Additional contraindications for IV product: Hypersensitivity to corn or corn products (solutions containing dextrose); constrictive pericarditis; pericardial tamponade; restrictive cardiomyopathy

Additional contraindications for sublingual product and rectal ointment: Early myocardial infarction (sublingual product only; see **Note**); increased intracranial pressure; severe anemia

Note: According to the 2013 American College of Cardiology Foundation/American Heart Association (ACCF/AHA) guidelines of the management of ST-elevation myocardial infarction (STEMI) and the 2013 ACCF/AHA guidelines for the management of unstable angina/non-ST-elevation myocardial infarction, avoid nitrates in the following conditions: Hypotension (SBP <90 mm Hg or ≥30 mm Hg below baseline), marked bradycardia or tachycardia, and right ventricular infarction. Sublingual nitroglycerin may be used as initial treatment of ongoing chest pain in patients who may have STEMI or UA/NSTEMI (Anderson, 2013; O'Gara, 2013).

Warnings/Precautions Severe hypotension can occur. Use with caution in volume depletion, moderate hypotension, and extreme caution with inferior wall MI and suspected right ventricular involvement. According to the ACCF/AHA, avoid use in patients with severe hypotension (SBP <90 mm Hg or ≥30 mm Hg below baseline), marked bradycardia or tachycardia, and right ventricular MI (ACCF/AHA [Anderson, 2013]; ACCF/AHA [O'Gara, 2013]). Avoid use in patients with hypertrophic cardiomyopathy (HCM) with outflow tract obstruction; nitrates may reduce preload, exacerbating obstruction and cause hypotension or syncope and/or worsening of heart failure (ACCF/AHA [Gersh, 2011]).

Paradoxical bradycardia and increased angina pectoris can accompany hypotension. Orthostatic hypotension can also occur. Ethanol can accentuate this. Tolerance does develop to nitrates and appropriate dosing is needed to minimize this (drug-free interval). Avoid use of long-acting agents in acute MI or acute HF; cannot easily reverse effects. Nitrates may aggravate angina caused by hypertrophic cardiomyopathy. Nitroglycerin may precipitate or aggravate increased intracranial pressure and subsequently may worsen clinical outcomes in patients with neurologic injury (eg, intracranial hemorrhage, traumatic brain injury). Nitroglycerin transdermal patches may contain conducting metal (eg, aluminum); remove patch prior to MRI. Potentially significant drug-drug interactions may exist, requiring dose or frequency adjustment, additional monitoring, and/or selection of alternative therapy.

Use caution when treating rectal anal fissures with nitroglycerin ointment formulation in patients with suspected or known significant cardiovascular disorders (eg, cardiomyopathies, heart failure, acute MI); intra-anal nitroglycerin administration may decrease systolic blood pressure and decrease arterial vascular resistance.

Adverse Reactions

Cardiovascular: Bradycardia, flushing, hypotension, orthostatic hypotension, peripheral edema, syncope, tachycardia

Central nervous system: Headache (common), dizziness, lightheadedness

Gastrointestinal: Nausea, vomiting, xerostomia

Neuromuscular & skeletal: Paresthesia, weakness

Respiratory: Dyspnea, pharyngitis, rhinitis

Miscellaneous: Diaphoresis

Rare but important or life-threatening): Allergic reactions, anaphylactoid reaction, application site irritation (patch), blurred vision, cardiovascular collapse, contact dermatitis (ointment, patch), crescendo angina, exfoliative dermatitis, fixed drug eruption (ointment, patch), methemoglobinemia (rare; overdose), pallor, palpitation, rash, rebound hypertension, restlessness, shock, vertigo

Drug Interactions

Metabolism/Transport Effects None known.

Avoid Concomitant Use

Avoid concomitant use of Nitroglycerin with any of the following: Ergot Derivatives; Phosphodiesterase 5 Inhibitors; Riociguat

Increased Effect/Toxicity

Nitroglycerin may increase the levels/effects of: DULoxetine; Ergot Derivatives; Hypotensive Agents; Levodopa; Prilocaine; Riociguat; RisperiDONE; Rosiglitazone; Sodium Nitrite

The levels/effects of Nitroglycerin may be increased by: Alcohol (Ethyl); Alfuzosin; Barbiturates; Dapoxetine; Nicorandil; Nitric Oxide; Phosphodiesterase 5 Inhibitors

Decreased Effect

Nitroglycerin may decrease the levels/effects of: Alteplase; Heparin

The levels/effects of Nitroglycerin may be decreased by: Ergot Derivatives

Preparation for Administration Nitronal (glyceryl trinitrate) 1 mg/mL (temporarily available in the U.S.):

To prepare a 100 **mcg**/mL solution: Withdraw 25 mL D_5W from a 250 mL bottle of D_5W and replace volume with 25 mg (25 mL) of Nitronal.

To prepare a 200 **mcg**/mL solution: Withdraw 50 mL D_5W from a 250 mL bottle of D_5W and replace volume with 50 mg (50 mL) of Nitronal.

Storage/Stability

IV solution: Doses should be made in glass bottles, EXCEL® or PAB® containers. Adsorption occurs to soft plastic (eg, PVC). Nitroglycerin diluted in D_5W or NS in glass containers is physically and chemically stable for 48 hours at room temperature and 7 days under refrigeration. In D_5W or NS in EXCEL®/PAB® containers it is physically and chemically stable for 24 hours at room temperature.

Store sublingual tablets, topical ointment, and rectal ointment in tightly closed containers at 20°C to 25°C (68°F to 77°F); slow release capsules at 20°C to 25°C (68°F to 77°F); translingual spray and transdermal patch at 15°C to 30°C (59°F to 86°F).

Mechanism of Action Nitroglycerin forms free radical nitric oxide. In smooth muscle, nitric oxide activates guanylate cyclase which increases guanosine 3'5' monophosphate (cGMP) leading to dephosphorylation of myosin light chains and smooth muscle relaxation. Produces a vasodilator effect on the peripheral veins and arteries with more prominent effects on the veins. Primarily reduces cardiac oxygen demand by decreasing preload (left ventricular end-diastolic pressure); may modestly reduce afterload; dilates coronary arteries and improves collateral flow to ischemic regions. For use in rectal fissures, intra-anal administration results in decreased sphincter tone and intra-anal pressure.

Pharmacodynamics/Kinetics

Onset of action: Sublingual tablet: 1 to 3 minutes; Translingual spray: Similar to sublingual tablet; Extended release: ~60 minutes; Topical: 15 to 30 minutes; Transdermal: ~30 minutes; IV: Immediate

Peak effect: Sublingual tablet: 5 minutes; Translingual spray: 4 to 10 minutes; Extended release: 2.5 to 4 hours; Topical: ~60 minutes; Transdermal: 120 minutes; IV: Immediate

Duration: Sublingual tablet: At least 25 minutes; Translingual spray: Similar to sublingual tablet; Extended release: 4 to 8 hours (Gibbons, 2002); Topical: 7 hours; Transdermal: 10 to 12 hours; IV: 3 to 5 minutes

Distribution: V_d: ~3 L/kg

Protein binding: 60%

Metabolism: Extensive first-pass effect; metabolized hepatically to glycerol di- and mononitrate metabolites via liver reductase enzyme; subsequent metabolism to glycerol and organic nitrate; nonhepatic metabolism via red blood cells and vascular walls also occurs

Half-life elimination: ~1 to 4 minutes

Excretion: Urine (as inactive metabolites)

Dosage Note: Hemodynamic and antianginal tolerance often develop within 24 to 48 hours of continuous nitrate administration. Nitrate-free interval (10 to 12 hours/day) is recommended to avoid tolerance development; gradually decrease dose in patients receiving NTG for prolonged period to avoid withdrawal reaction.

Extravasation (sympathomimetic vasopressors), treatment (alternative to phentolamine; off-label use): **Based on limited data in neonates; optimal dosing has not been established:** Pediatrics and Adults: Topical 2% ointment: 4 mm/kg applied as a thin ribbon to the affected area has been reported in a case series; after 8 hours, if no improvement, the dose may be reapplied to the affected site (Wong, 1992). Application of a 1-inch strip on the affected site has also been described to be successful (Denkler, 1989); may also be considered for adults as an alternative to phentolamine (Hurst, 2004).

Angina/coronary artery disease: Adults:

Oral: Initial: 2.5 to 6.5 mg 3 to 4 times/day; may titrate up to 26 mg 4 times/day

IV: 5 mcg/minute, increase by 5 mcg/minute every 3 to 5 minutes to 20 mcg/minute; if no response at 20 mcg/minute, may increase by 10 to 20 mcg/minute every 3 to 5 minutes (generally accepted maximum dose: 400 mcg/minute)

According to the 2013 ACCF/AHA guideline for the management of unstable angina/non-ST-elevation myocardial infarction (off-label dosing): Initial: 10 mcg/minute, increase by 10 mcg/minute every 3 to 5 minutes until relief of symptoms or blood pressure response noted; if no response at 20 mcg/minute, may increase by 10 mcg/minute and later by 20 mcg/minute may be used (Anderson, 2013). The 2013 ACCF/AHA guidelines for STEMI also recommend an initial dose of 10 mcg/minute with subsequent titration to desired blood pressure effect (O'Gara, 2013).

Sublingual: 0.3 to 0.6 mg every 5 minutes for maximum of 3 doses in 15 minutes; may also use prophylactically 5 to 10 minutes prior to activities which may provoke an attack

According to the 2013 ACCF/AHA guidelines for STEMI and the guidelines for the management of unstable angina/NSTEMI: If nitroglycerin is prescribed, advise the patient to take 1 dose promptly in response to chest pain. If pain is unrelieved or worsened 5 minutes after 1 dose, the patient or caregiver should call 9-1-1 immediately (Anderson, 2013; O'Gara, 2013).

Topical 2% ointment: 1/2" upon rising and 1/2" 6 hours later; if necessary, the dose may be doubled to 1" and subsequently doubled again to 2" if response is inadequate. Doses of 1/2" to 2" were used in clinical trials. Recommended maximum: 2 doses/day; include a nitrate free-interval ~10 to 12 hours/day.

Topical patch, transdermal: Initial: 0.2 to 0.4 mg/hour, titrate to 0.4 to 0.8 mg/hour; tolerance is minimized by using a patch-on period of 12 to 14 hours and patch-off period of 10 to 12 hours

Translingual: 1 to 2 sprays onto or under tongue every 3 to 5 minutes for maximum of 3 doses in 15 minutes, may also be used prophylactically 5 to 10 minutes prior to activities which may provoke an angina attack

According to the 2013 ACCF/AHA guidelines for STEMI and the guidelines for the management of unstable angina/NSTEMI: If nitroglycerin is prescribed, advise the patient to take 1 dose promptly in response to chest pain. If pain is unrelieved or worsened 5 minutes after 1 dose, the patient or caregiver should call 9-1-1 immediately (Anderson, 2013; O'Gara, 2013).

Anal fissure, chronic (0.4% ointment): Adults: Intra-anal: 1 inch (equals 1.5 mg of nitroglycerin) every 12 hours for up to 3 weeks

Esophageal spastic disorders (off-label use): Adults: Sublingual: 0.3 to 0.6 mg (Swamy, 1977)

Uterine relaxation (off-label use): Adults: IV bolus: 100 to 200 mcg; may repeat dose every 2 minutes as necessary (Axemo, 1998; Chandraharan, 2005)

Elderly: In general, dose selection should be cautious, usually starting at the low end of the dosing range

Dosage adjustment in renal impairment: There are no dosage adjustments provided in the manufacturer's labeling.

Dosage adjustment in hepatic impairment: There are no dosage adjustments provided in the manufacturer's labeling.

Usual Infusion Concentrations: Pediatric Note: Premixed solutions available

IV infusion: 100 **mcg**/mL, 200 **mcg**/mL, or 400 **mcg**/mL

Usual Infusion Concentrations: Adult Note: Premixed solutions available

IV infusion: 50 mg in 250 mL (concentration: 200 **mcg**/mL) **or** 100 mg in 250 mL (concentration: 400 **mcg**/mL) of D_5W

Administration

IV: Prepare in glass bottles, EXCEL or PAB containers. Adsorption occurs to soft plastic (eg, PVC); use administration sets intended for nitroglycerin. Administer via infusion pump.

Intra-anal ointment: Using a finger covering (eg, plastic wrap, surgical glove, finger cot), place finger beside 1 inch measuring guide on the box and squeeze ointment the length of the measuring line directly onto covered finger. Insert ointment into the anal canal using the covered finger up to first finger joint (do not insert further than the first finger joint) and apply ointment around the side of the anal canal. If intra-anal application is too painful, may apply the ointment to the outside of the anus. Wash hands following application.

Oral (extended release capsule): Swallow whole. Do not chew, break, or crush. Take with a full glass of water.

Sublingual: Do not chew, crush, or swallow sublingual tablet. Place under tongue and allow to dissolve. Alternately, may be placed in the buccal pouch.

Topical ointment: Wash hands prior to and after use. Application site should be clean, dry, and hair-free. Apply to chest or back with the applicator or dose-measuring paper. Spread in a thin layer over a 2.25 x 3.5 inch area. Do not rub into skin. Tape applicator into place.

Drug extravasation management, (treatment), sympathomimetic vasopressors (alternative to phentolamine) (off-label use): Stop vesicant infusion immediately and disconnect IV line (leave needle/cannula in place); gently aspirate extravasated solution from the IV line (do **NOT** flush the line); remove needle/cannula; elevate extremity. Apply nitroglycerin ointment as a thin ribbon to the affected area (Wong, 1992). May also apply dry warm compresses (Hurst, 2004).

Topical patch, transdermal: Application site should be clean, dry and hair-free. Remove patch after 12 to 14 hours. Rotate patch sites.

Translingual spray: Do not shake container. Prior to initial use, the pump must be primed by spraying 5 times (Nitrolingual) or 10 times (Nitromist) into the air. Priming sprays should be directed away from patient and others. Release spray onto or under tongue. Close mouth after administration. Do not rinse the mouth for at least 5 to 10 minutes. The end of the pump should be covered by the fluid in the bottle. If pump is unused for 6 weeks, a single priming spray (Nitrolingual) or 2 priming sprays (Nitromist) should be completed.

Monitoring Parameters Blood pressure, heart rate; consult individual institutional policies and procedures

Dosage Forms

Aerosol Solution, Translingual:
NitroMist: 400 mcg/spray (4.1 g, 8.5 g)
Generic: 400 mcg/spray (4.1 g, 8.5 g)

Capsule Extended Release, Oral:
Nitro-Time: 2.5 mg, 6.5 mg, 9 mg
Generic: 2.5 mg, 6.5 mg, 9 mg

Ointment, Rectal:
Rectiv: 0.4% (30 g)

Ointment, Transdermal:
Nitro-Bid: 2% (1 g, 30 g, 60 g)

Patch 24 Hour, Transdermal:
Minitran: 0.1 mg/hr (30 ea); 0.2 mg/hr (30 ea); 0.4 mg/hr (30 ea); 0.6 mg/hr (30 ea)
Nitro-Dur: 0.1 mg/hr (30 ea, 100 ea); 0.2 mg/hr (30 ea, 100 ea); 0.3 mg/hr (30 ea, 100 ea); 0.4 mg/hr (30 ea, 100 ea); 0.6 mg/hr (30 ea, 100 ea); 0.8 mg/hr (30 ea, 100 ea)
Generic: 0.1 mg/hr (30 ea, 4350 ea); 0.2 mg/hr (30 ea, 4350 ea); 0.4 mg/hr (30 ea, 4350 ea); 0.6 mg/hr (30 ea, 4350 ea)

Solution, Intravenous:
Nitronal: 1 mg/mL (25 mL, 50 mL)
Generic: 25 mg (250 mL); 50 mg (250 mL, 500 mL); 100 mg (250 mL); 200 mg (500 mL); 5 mg/mL (10 mL)

Solution, Translingual:
Nitrolingual: 0.4 mg/spray (4.9 g, 12 g)
Generic: 0.4 mg/spray (4.9 g, 12 g)

Tablet Sublingual, Sublingual:
Nitrostat: 0.3 mg, 0.4 mg, 0.6 mg

- **Nitroglycerin Injection, USP (Can)** *see* Nitroglycerin *on page 1465*
- **Nitroglycerol** *see* Nitroglycerin *on page 1465*
- **Nitrol (Can)** *see* Nitroglycerin *on page 1465*
- **Nitrolingual** *see* Nitroglycerin *on page 1465*
- **NitroMist** *see* Nitroglycerin *on page 1465*
- **Nitronal** *see* Nitroglycerin *on page 1465*
- **Nitropress** *see* Nitroprusside *on page 1467*

Nitroprusside (nye troe PRUS ide)

Brand Names: U.S. Nitropress

Brand Names: Canada Nipride

Index Terms Nitroprusside Sodium; Sodium Nitroferricyanide; Sodium Nitroprusside

Pharmacologic Category Antihypertensive; Vasodilator

Use Management of hypertensive crises; acute decompensated heart failure (HF); used for controlled hypotension to reduce bleeding during surgery

Pregnancy Risk Factor C

Pregnancy Considerations Animal studies have shown that nitroprusside may cross the placental barrier and result in fetal cyanide levels that are dose-related to maternal nitroprusside levels. However, information related to use in pregnancy is limited.

Breast-Feeding Considerations It is not known if nitroprusside is excreted in breast milk. Due to the potential for serious adverse reactions in the nursing infant, a decision should be made whether to discontinue nursing or to discontinue the drug, taking into account the importance of treatment to the mother.

Contraindications Treatment of compensatory hypertension (aortic coarctation, arteriovenous shunting); to produce controlled hypotension during surgery in patients with known inadequate cerebral circulation or in moribund patients requiring emergency surgery; high output heart failure associated with reduced systemic vascular resistance (eg, septic shock); congenital optic atrophy or tobacco amblyopia

Warnings/Precautions **[U.S. Boxed Warning] Excessive hypotension resulting in compromised perfusion of vital organs may occur; continuous blood pressure monitoring by experienced personnel is required. Except when used briefly or at low (<2 mcg/kg/minute) infusion rates, nitroprusside gives rise to large**

cyanide quantities. Do not use the maximum dose for more than 10 minutes; if blood pressure is not controlled by the maximum rate (ie, 10 mcg/kg/minute) after 10 minutes, discontinue infusion. Monitor for cyanide toxicity via acid-base balance and venous oxygen concentration; however, clinicians should note that these indicators may not always reliably indicate cyanide toxicity. Patients at risk of cyanide toxicity include those who are malnourished, have hepatic impairment, or those undergoing cardiopulmonary bypass, or therapeutic hypothermia (Rindone, 1992). Discontinue use of nitroprusside if signs and/or symptoms of cyanide toxicity (eg, metabolic acidosis, decreased oxygen saturation, bradycardia, confusion, convulsions) occur. Although not routinely done, sodium thiosulfate has been co-administered with nitroprusside using a 10:1 ratio of sodium thiosulfate to nitroprusside when higher doses of nitroprusside are used (eg, 4-10 mcg/kg/minute) for extended periods of time in order to prevent cyanide toxicity (Varon, 2008; Shulz, 2010); thiocyanate toxicity may still occur with this approach (Rindone, 1992). The use of other agents (eg, clevidipine, labetalol, nicardipine) should be considered if blood pressure is not controlled with nitroprusside. Use the lowest end of the dosage range with renal impairment. Cyanide toxicity may occur in patients with decreased liver function. Thiocyanate toxicity occurs in patients with renal impairment or those on prolonged infusions.

When nitroprusside is used for controlled hypotension during surgery, correct preexisting anemia and hypovolemia prior to use when possible. Use with extreme caution in patients with elevated intracranial pressure (head trauma, cerebral hemorrhage), severe renal impairment, hepatic failure, hypothyroidism. **[U.S. Boxed Warning]: Solution must be further diluted with 5% dextrose in water. Do not administer by direct injection.**

Adverse Reactions

Cardiovascular: Bradycardia, ECG changes, flushing, hypotension (excessive), palpitation, substernal distress, tachycardia

Central nervous system: Apprehension, dizziness, headache, intracranial pressure increased, restlessness

Dermatologic: Rash

Endocrine & metabolic: Metabolic acidosis (secondary to cyanide toxicity), hypothyroidism

Gastrointestinal: Abdominal pain, ileus, nausea, retching, vomiting

Hematologic: Methemoglobinemia, platelet aggregation decreased

Local: Injection site irritation

Neuromuscular & skeletal: Hyperreflexia (secondary to thiocyanate toxicity), muscle twitching

Ocular: Miosis (secondary to thiocyanate toxicity)

Otic: Tinnitus (secondary to thiocyanate toxicity)

Respiratory: Hyperoxemia (secondary to cyanide toxicity)

Miscellaneous: Cyanide toxicity, diaphoresis, thiocyanate toxicity

Drug Interactions

Metabolism/Transport Effects None known.

Avoid Concomitant Use There are no known interactions where it is recommended to avoid concomitant use.

Increased Effect/Toxicity

Nitroprusside may increase the levels/effects of: Amifostine; Antihypertensives; DULoxetine; Hypotensive Agents; Levodopa; Obinutuzumab; Prilocaine; RisperiDONE; RiTUXimab; Sodium Nitrite

The levels/effects of Nitroprusside may be increased by: Alfuzosin; Barbiturates; Brimonidine (Topical); Calcium Channel Blockers; Diazoxide; Herbs (Hypotensive Properties); MAO Inhibitors; Nicorandil; Nitric Oxide; Pentoxifylline; Phosphodiesterase 5 Inhibitors; Prostacyclin Analogues

Decreased Effect

The levels/effects of Nitroprusside may be decreased by: Herbs (Hypertensive Properties); Methylphenidate; Yohimbine

Preparation for Administration

Prior to administration, nitroprusside sodium should be further diluted by diluting 50 mg in 250-1000 mL of D_5W (preferred), LR, or NS.

Use only clear solutions; solutions of nitroprusside exhibit a color described as brownish, brown, brownish-pink, light orange, and straw. Solutions are highly sensitive to light. Exposure to light causes decomposition, resulting in a highly colored solution of orange, dark brown or blue. **A blue color indicates almost complete decomposition.** Do not use discolored solutions (eg, blue, green, red) or solutions in which particulate matter is visible.

Prepared solutions should be wrapped with aluminum foil or other opaque material to protect from light (do as soon as possible).

Storage/Stability Store the intact vial at 20°C to 25°C (68°F to 77°F). Protect from light.

Stability of parenteral admixture at room temperature (25°C) and at refrigeration temperature (4°C) is 24 hours.

Mechanism of Action Causes peripheral vasodilation by direct action on venous and arteriolar smooth muscle, thus reducing peripheral resistance; will increase cardiac output by decreasing afterload; reduces aortal and left ventricular impedance

Pharmacodynamics/Kinetics

Onset of action: Hypotensive effect: <2 minutes

Duration: Hypotensive effect: 1-10 minutes

Metabolism: Nitroprusside combines with hemoglobin to produce cyanide and cyanmethemoglobin. Cyanide detoxification occurs via rhodanase-mediated conversion of cyanide to thiocyanate; rhodanase couples cyanide molecules to sulfane sulfur groups from a sulfur donor (eg, thiosulfate, cystine, cysteine). This process has limited capacity and may become overwhelmed with large exposures once sulfur donor supplies are exhausted resulting in toxicity.

Half-life elimination: Nitroprusside, circulatory: ~2 minutes; Thiocyanate, elimination: ~3 days (may be doubled or tripled in renal failure)

Excretion: Urine (as thiocyanate)

Dosage IV:

Children: Acute hypertension: Initial: 0.3-0.5 mcg/kg/minute; may be titrated every few minutes to achieve desired hemodynamic effect; maximum dose: 10 mcg/kg/minute (Hegenbarth, 2008; NHBPEP, 2005). Doses ≥1.8 mcg/kg/minute are associated with increased cyanide concentration in pediatric patients (Moffett, 2008); monitor cyanide levels with prolonged use (eg, >72 hours) (NHBPEP, 2005).

Adults:

Acute hypertension: Initial: 0.3-0.5 mcg/kg/minute; may be titrated by 0.5 mcg/kg/minute every few minutes to achieve desired hemodynamic effect (Rhoney, 2009); maximum dose: 10 mcg/kg/minute. To avoid toxicity, some recommend a maximum dose of 2 mcg/kg/minute (Marik, 2007).

Acute decompensated heart failure: Initial: 5-10 **mcg/minute**; may be titrated rapidly (eg, up to every 5 minutes) to achieve desired hemodynamic effect; usual dosage range: 5-300 **mcg/minute**. Doses >400 **mcg/minute** are not recommended due to minimal added benefit and increased risk for thiocyanate toxicity (HFSA, 2010).

Dosage adjustment in renal impairment: No dosage adjustment provided in manufacturer's labeling. However, use in patients with renal impairment may lead to the accumulation of thiocyanate and subsequent toxicity; limit use.

Dosage adjustment in hepatic impairment: No dosage adjustment provided in manufacturer's labeling; due to the risk of cyanide toxicity, use with caution.

Usual Infusion Concentrations: Pediatric IV infusion: 100 **mcg**/mL **or** 200 **mcg**/mL

Usual Infusion Concentrations: Adult IV infusion: 50 mg in 250 mL (concentration: 200 **mcg**/mL) **or** 100 mg in 250 mL (concentration: 400 **mcg**/mL) of D_5W

Administration IV infusion only; infusion pump required; must be diluted prior to administration; not for direct injection. Due to potential for excessive hypotension, continuously monitor patient's blood pressure during therapy.

Monitoring Parameters Blood pressure, heart rate (cardiac monitor and blood pressure monitor required); monitor for cyanide and thiocyanate toxicity; monitor venous oxygen saturation; monitor acid-base status as acidosis can be the earliest sign of cyanide toxicity; monitor thiocyanate levels if requiring prolonged infusion (>3 days) or dose >3 mcg/kg/minute or patient has renal dysfunction; monitor cyanide blood levels (if available with appropriate turnaround time) in patients with decreased hepatic function

Consult individual institutional policies and procedures.

Reference Range Serum thiocyanate levels are not helpful in detecting toxicity. A level may be confirmatory if a patient is exhibiting signs and symptoms of thiocyanate toxicity. Initial signs of toxicity (eg, tinnitus) may be observed at levels >35 mcg/mL (manufacturer suggests 60 mcg/mL), but serious toxicity typically may not occur with levels <100 mcg/mL.

Dosage Forms

Solution, Intravenous:

Nitropress: 25 mg/mL (2 mL)

◆ **Nitroprusside Sodium** *see* Nitroprusside *on page 1467*

◆ **Nitrostat** *see* Nitroglycerin *on page 1465*

◆ **Nitro-Time** *see* Nitroglycerin *on page 1465*

Nitroxoline [INT] (ni TROKS o leen)

International Brand Names Cysto-Saar (DE); Nibiol (FR, VN); Nicene N (ZA); Nilox (DE); Nitroxolin-MIP Forte (BG)

Pharmacologic Category Antibiotic, Miscellaneous

Reported Use Acute and chronic uncomplicated lower urinary tract infection

Dosage Range Adults: Oral: 400-600 mg/day in divided doses after meals

Product Availability Product available in various countries; not currently available in the U.S.

Dosage Forms

Tablet: 100 mg

◆ **Nitrozepamum** *see* Nitrazepam [CAN/INT] *on page 1461*

◆ **Nivadipine** *see* Nilvadipine [INT] *on page 1456*

Nivolumab (nye VOL ue mab)

Brand Names: U.S. Opdivo

Index Terms Anti-PD-1 human monoclonal antibody MDX-1106; BMS-936558; MDX-1106; ONO-4538

Pharmacologic Category Antineoplastic Agent, Anti-PD-1 Monoclonal Antibody; Antineoplastic Agent, Monoclonal Antibody

Use Melanoma, unresectable or metastatic: Treatment of unresectable or metastatic melanoma and disease progression following ipilimumab and (if BRAF V600 mutation positive) a BRAF inhibitor

Pregnancy Considerations Adverse events were observed in animal reproduction studies. Nivolumab may be expected to cross the placenta; effects to the fetus may be greater in the second and third trimesters. Based on its mechanism of action, nivolumab is expected to cause fetal harm if used during pregnancy. Women of reproductive potential should use highly-effective contraception during therapy and for at least 5 months after treatment has been discontinued.

Breast-Feeding Considerations It is not known if nivolumab is excreted into breast milk. Due to the potential for serious adverse reactions in the nursing infant, the manufacturer recommends a decision be made to discontinue nursing or to discontinue the drug, taking into account the importance of treatment to the mother.

Contraindications There are no contraindications listed in the manufacturer's labeling.

Warnings/Precautions Immune-mediated pneumonitis (severe pneumonitis or interstitial lung disease) has been observed, including cases which were fatal. Immune-mediated pneumonitis is defined as no other clear etiology and requiring corticosteroid use. The median time to development was 2.2 months (range: 25 days to 3.5 months). Some cases developed after nivolumab was discontinued for other reasons. Patients with pneumonitis were managed with high-dose systemic corticosteroids (prednisone dose of ≥40 mg/day or equivalent) followed by a corticosteroid taper. Some patients with grade 2 pneumonitis had complete resolution and nivolumab was reinitiated without recurrence. Monitor for signs and symptoms of pneumonitis. May require treatment interruption, corticosteroid therapy, or permanent discontinuation. Grade 2 or higher pneumonitis should be managed with prednisone 1 to 2 mg/kg daily (or equivalent) followed by a corticosteroid taper. Withhold treatment until resolution for moderate (grade 2) immune-mediated pneumonitis; permanently discontinue for severe (grade 3) or life-threatening (grade 4) immune-mediated pneumonitis.

Diarrhea or colitis occurred in about one-fifth of patients receiving nivolumab. Immune-mediated colitis (defined as no other clear etiology and requiring corticosteroid use) including cases of grades 2 and 3 colitis occurred in some patients. The median time to onset of colitis was 2.5 months (range: 1 to 6 months) from nivolumab initiation; some cases developed after nivolumab was discontinued for other reasons. Grade 2 or 3 colitis was managed with high-dose systemic corticosteroids (prednisone ≥40 mg/day or equivalent) for a median duration of 1.4 months (range: 3 days to 2.4 months) followed by a corticosteroid taper. Most patients with grade 2 or 3 colitis had complete resolution (improvement to grade 0); after resolution, nivolumab was reinitiated in 1 patient without recurrence. Monitor for signs and symptoms of immune-mediated colitis. May require treatment interruption, corticosteroid therapy, or permanent discontinuation. Severe colitis (grade 3) or life-threatening colitis (grade 4) should be managed with prednisone 1 to 2 mg/kg daily (or equivalent) followed by a corticosteroid taper. Moderate colitis (grade 2) of >5 days duration should be managed with prednisone 0.5 to 1 mg/kg daily (or equivalent) followed by a corticosteroid taper; may increase to prednisone 1 to 2 mg/kg daily (or equivalent) if colitis worsens or does not improve despite corticosteroid therapy. Permanently discontinue nivolumab for grade 4 colitis or colitis that recurs upon reinitiation.

ALT, AST, alkaline phosphatase, and total bilirubin elevations occurred more frequently in nivolumab-treated patients (compared to chemotherapy-treated patients) in one clinical trial. Immune-mediated hepatitis (defined as no other clear etiology and requiring corticosteroid use) occurred in a small percentage of patients receiving nivolumab; cases included grade 2 and grade 3 hepatitis. The time to onset was ~3 to 4 months after nivolumab initiation (one case developed after nivolumab was discontinued for other reasons). Immune-mediated hepatitis was managed with high-dose systemic corticosteroids (prednisone ≥40 mg/day or equivalent); liver function tests improved to grade 1 within 15 days of corticosteroid initiation. Immune-mediated hepatitis resolved and did not recur with continued corticosteroid use in some patients, although one patient experienced grade 3 recurrence and permanently discontinued treatment. Monitor liver function at baseline and periodically for changes. Initiate prednisone 1 to 2 mg/kg daily (or equivalent) for grade 2 or higher transaminase elevations (with or without total bilirubin elevations). Withhold treatment for moderate (grade 2) immune-mediated hepatitis; permanently discontinue for severe (grade 3) or life-threatening (grade 4) immune-mediated hepatitis.

Creatinine elevations occurred more frequently in nivolumab-treated patients (compared to chemotherapy-treated patients) in one clinical trial. Two cases of grade 2 or 3 immune-mediated nephritis or renal dysfunction (defined as ≥ grade 2 creatinine elevations with no other clear etiology and requiring corticosteroid use) occurred at 3.5 and 6 months after nivolumab initiation (treatment was discontinued permanently in both cases and patients received high-dose systemic corticosteroids (prednisone ≥40 mg/day or equivalent). Immune-mediated nephritis resolved and did not recur with continued corticosteroid use in one patient, although the other patient experienced ongoing renal dysfunction. Monitor serum creatinine at baseline and periodically during treatment. Initiate prednisone 1 to 2 mg/kg daily (or equivalent) followed by a corticosteroid taper for life-threatening (grade 4) serum creatinine elevation and permanently discontinue nivolumab. Withhold treatment for moderate (grade 2) and severe (grade 3) creatinine elevations and administer prednisone 0.5 to 1 mg/kg daily (or equivalent) followed by a corticosteroid taper; if toxicity worsens or does not improve, permanently discontinue and increase to prednisone 1 to 2 mg/kg daily (or equivalent).

Immune-mediated hyperthyroidism and hypothyroidism have occurred, including grades 1 and 2 hyper-/hypothyroidism. The median onset for hyperthyroidism was 1.6 months (range: Up to 3.3 months); most cases resolved (may require medical management). Hypothyroidism occurred with a median onset of 2.5 months (range: 24 days to 11.7 months). Hypothyroidism was generally managed with thyroid hormone replacement therapy. Most patients received subsequent nivolumab treatment while continuing thyroid replacement therapy. Monitor thyroid function at baseline and for changes periodically during treatment. Isolated hypothyroidism may be managed with replacement therapy; initiate medical management to control hyperthyroidism.

Other clinically relevant other immune-mediated disorders may occur; may develop after discontinuation of nivolumab. Immune-mediated adverse reactions observed at the approved dose included adrenal insufficiency, autoimmune neuropathy, demyelination, facial/abducens nerve paresis, pancreatitis, and uveitis; at varying nivolumab doses diabetic ketoacidosis, Guillain-Barre syndrome, hypophysitis, hypopituitarism, and myasthenic syndrome were also observed. If an immune-mediated adverse event is suspected, evaluate to exclude other causes. Based on symptom severity, withhold nivolumab, administer high-dose corticosteroids, and if appropriate, initiate hormone-replacement therapy. Upon improvement to grade 0 or 1, begin corticosteroid taper (over at least 1 month). After corticosteroid taper is completed and based on the severity of the reaction, may consider reinitiating nivolumab.

Drug Interactions

Metabolism/Transport Effects None known.

Avoid Concomitant Use There are no known interactions where it is recommended to avoid concomitant use.

Increased Effect/Toxicity There are no known significant interactions involving an increase in effect.

Decreased Effect There are no known significant interactions involving a decrease in effect.

Preparation for Administration Withdraw the required volume and transfer into an IV container. Dilute with either NS or D_5W to a final concentration of 1 to 10 mg/mL. Mix by gentle inversion; do not shake.

Storage/Stability Store intact vials refrigerated at 2°C to 8°C (36°F to 46°F); do not freeze. Protect from light. Do not shake. After preparation, store the infusion solution at room temperature for no more than 4 hours (including infusion time) or refrigerated at 2°C to 8°C (36°F to 46°F) for up to 24 hours (including infusion time). Do not freeze solutions prepared for infusion.

Mechanism of Action Nivolumab is a fully human immunoglobulin G4 (IgG4) monoclonal antibody that selectively inhibits programmed cell death-1 (PD-1) activity by binding to the PD-1 receptor to block the ligands PD-L1 and PD-L2 from binding. The negative PD-1 receptor signaling that regulates T-cell activation and proliferation is therefore disrupted (Robert, 2014). This releases PD-1 pathway-mediated inhibition of the immune response, including the antitumor immune response.

Pharmacodynamics/Kinetics

Distribution: V_d: 8 L

Half-life elimination: ~27 days

Dosage Melanoma, unresectable or metastatic: Adults: IV: 3 mg/kg once every 2 weeks until disease progression or unacceptable toxicity

Dosage adjustment for toxicity:

Withhold treatment for any of the following (may resume upon recovery to grade 0 or 1 toxicity):

Colitis:

Grade 2 (duration >5 days): Also administer systemic corticosteroids (prednisone 0.5 to 1 mg/kg daily or equivalent) followed by a corticosteroid taper; may increase to prednisone 1 to 2 mg/kg daily (or equivalent) if colitis worsens or does not improve despite corticosteroid use

Grade 3: Also administer systemic corticosteroids (prednisone 1 to 2 mg/kg daily or equivalent) followed by a corticosteroid taper

Pneumonitis (grade 2); also administer high-dose systemic corticosteroids (prednisone 1 to 2 mg/kg daily or equivalent) followed by a corticosteroid taper

Other immune-mediated toxicities; also administer high-dose systemic corticosteroids followed by a corticosteroid taper (over 1 month)

Other treatment-related toxicity (severe or grade 3)

Permanently discontinue for:

Colitis (grade 4); also administer high-dose systemic corticosteroids (prednisone 1 to 2 mg/kg daily or equivalent) followed by a corticosteroid taper

Colitis (recurrent)

Pneumonitis (grade 3 or 4); also administer high-dose systemic corticosteroids (prednisone 1 to 2 mg/kg daily or equivalent) followed by a corticosteroid taper

Inability to reduce corticosteroid dose to prednisone ≤10 mg/day (or equivalent) within 12 weeks.

Other adverse reactions that are life-threatening or grade 4, severe or grade 3 adverse reactions that recur, or persistent grade 2 or 3 treatment-related toxicity that does not recover to grade 0 or 1 within 12 weeks after the last nivolumab dose.

Thyroid disorder (hyperthyroidism or hypothyroidism): There are no recommended dosage modifications.

Dosage adjustment for renal impairment:

Renal impairment prior to treatment initiation: No dosage adjustment necessary.

*Renal toxicity **during** treatment:*

Creatinine >1.5 to 6 times ULN or >1.5 times baseline: Withhold treatment; administer prednisone 0.5 to 1 mg/kg daily (or equivalent) followed by a corticosteroid taper; may resume therapy upon recovery to grade 0 or 1 toxicity. If toxicity worsens or does not improve, permanently discontinue and increase corticosteroid dose to prednisone 1 to 2 mg/kg daily (or equivalent).

Creatinine >6 times ULN: Permanently discontinue; initiate high-dose systemic corticosteroids (prednisone 1 to 2 mg/kg daily or equivalent) followed by a corticosteroid taper.

Dosage adjustment for hepatic impairment:

*Hepatic impairment **prior** to treatment initiation:*

Mild impairment (total bilirubin ≤ ULN and AST > ULN or total bilirubin <1 to 1.5 times ULN and any AST): No dosage adjustment necessary.

Moderate (total bilirubin >1.5 to 3 times ULN and any AST) to severe (total bilirubin >3 times ULN and any AST) impairment: There are no dosage adjustments provided in the manufacturer's labeling (has not been studied).

*Hepatotoxicity **during** treatment:*

AST or ALT >3 to 5 times ULN or total bilirubin >1.5 to 3 times ULN: Withhold treatment; may resume therapy upon recovery to grade 0 or 1 toxicity.

AST or ALT >5 times ULN or total bilirubin >3 times ULN or severe/life-threatening immune-mediated hepatitis: Permanently discontinue.

Immune-mediated hepatitis:

Grade 2 or higher transaminase elevations (with or without total bilirubin elevations): Withhold treatment and initiate high-dose systemic corticosteroids (prednisone 1 to 2 mg/kg daily or equivalent)

Severe (grade 3) or life-threatening (grade 4): Permanently discontinue treatment and initiate high-dose systemic corticosteroids (prednisone 1 to 2 mg/kg daily or equivalent)

Administration IV: Administer over 60 minutes through a line with a sterile, nonpyrogenic, low protein binding 0.2 to 1.2 micrometer in-line filter. Do not administer other medications through the same IV line. Flush IV line at the end of the infusion.

Monitoring Parameters Hepatic and renal function tests (baseline and periodic), thyroid function (baseline and periodic). Monitor for signs/symptoms of immune-mediated colitis and pneumonitis

Dosage Forms

Solution, Intravenous [preservative free]:

Opdivo: 40 mg/4 mL (4 mL); 100 mg/10 mL (10 mL)

◆ **Nix [OTC] (Can)** *see* Permethrin *on page 1627*

Nizatidine (ni ZA ti deen)

Brand Names: U.S. Axid; Axid AR [OTC]

Brand Names: Canada Apo-Nizatidine; Axid; Gen-Nizatidine; Novo-Nizatidine; Nu-Nizatidine; PMS-Nizatidine

Pharmacologic Category Histamine H_2 Antagonist

Use Treatment and maintenance of duodenal ulcer; treatment of benign gastric ulcer; treatment of gastroesophageal reflux disease (GERD)

Pregnancy Risk Factor B

Dosage Oral:

Children:

<12 years: GERD (off-label use): 10 mg/kg/day in divided doses given twice daily; may not be as effective in children <12 years

≥12 years:

GERD: Refer to adult dosing

Adults:

Duodenal ulcer:

Treatment of active ulcer: 300 mg at bedtime or 150 mg twice daily

Maintenance of healed ulcer: 150 mg/day at bedtime

Gastric ulcer: 150 mg twice daily or 300 mg at bedtime

GERD: 150 mg twice daily

Helicobacter pylori eradication (off-label use): 150 mg twice daily; requires combination therapy

Dosage adjustment in renal impairment:

Active treatment:

CrCl 20-50 mL/minute: 150 mg/day

CrCl <20 mL/minute: 150 mg every other day

Maintenance treatment:

CrCl 20-50 mL/minute: 150 mg every other day

CrCl <20 mL/minute: 150 mg every 3 days

Dosage adjustment in hepatic impairment: No dosage adjustment provided in manufacturer's labeling.

Additional Information Complete prescribing information should be consulted for additional detail.

Dosage Forms

Capsule, Oral:

Axid: 300 mg

Generic: 150 mg, 300 mg

Solution, Oral:

Axid: 15 mg/mL (480 mL)

Generic: 15 mg/mL (473 mL, 480 mL)

Tablet, Oral:

Axid AR [OTC]: 75 mg

◆ **Nizoral** *see* Ketoconazole (Systemic) *on page 1144*

◆ **Nizoral** *see* Ketoconazole (Topical) *on page 1145*

◆ **Nizoral A-D [OTC]** *see* Ketoconazole (Topical) *on page 1145*

◆ **NKTR-118** *see* Naloxegol *on page 1418*

◆ **N-Methylhydrazine** *see* Procarbazine *on page 1717*

◆ **N-methylnaltrexone Bromide** *see* Methylnaltrexone *on page 1334*

◆ **NN2211** *see* Liraglutide *on page 1222*

◆ **No Doz® Maximum Strength [OTC]** *see* Caffeine *on page 319*

◆ **NoHist DM [OTC]** *see* Chlorpheniramine, Phenylephrine, and Dextromethorphan *on page 428*

◆ **NoHist LQ [OTC]** *see* Chlorpheniramine and Phenylephrine *on page 426*

◆ **Nolvadex** *see* Tamoxifen *on page 1971*

◆ **Nolvadex-D (Can)** *see* Tamoxifen *on page 1971*

◆ **Non-Aspirin Pain Reliever [OTC]** *see* Acetaminophen *on page 32*

Nonoxynol 9 (non OKS i nole nine)

Brand Names: U.S. Shur-Seal Contraceptive [OTC]; Today Sponge [OTC]; VCF Vaginal Contraceptive [OTC]

Index Terms N-9

Pharmacologic Category Contraceptive; Spermicide

Use Prevention of pregnancy

Dosage Adolescents and Adults: **Note:** Prior to use, refer to specific product labeling for complete instructions.

Prevention of pregnancy: Vaginal:

Encare: Unwrap and insert 1 suppository vaginally at least 10 minutes prior to intercourse; effective for 1 hour

Today: Insert 1 sponge vaginally prior to intercourse; allow to remain in place for 6 hours after intercourse before removing; effective for use up to 24 continuous hours. Do not leave in place for >30 hours.

VCF:
Film: Insert 1 film vaginally at least 15 minutes, but no more than 3 hours, prior to intercourse. Insert new film for each act of intercourse or if more than 3 hours have elapsed.
Foam: Insert 1 applicatorful at least 15 minutes prior to intercourse; effective for up to 1 hour

Additional Information Complete prescribing information should be consulted for additional detail.

Dosage Forms

Film, Vaginal:
VCF Vaginal Contraceptive [OTC]: 28% (3 ea, 6 ea, 9 ea)

Foam, Vaginal:
VCF Vaginal Contraceptive [OTC]: 12.5% (17 g)

Gel, Vaginal:
Shur-Seal Contraceptive [OTC]: 2% (24 ea)

Miscellaneous, Vaginal:
Today Sponge [OTC]: 1000 mg (3 ea)

◆ **Non-Pseudo Sinus Decongestant [OTC]** *see* Phenylephrine (Systemic) *on page 1638*

◆ **Nora-BE** *see* Norethindrone *on page 1473*

◆ **Noradrenaline** *see* Norepinephrine *on page 1472*

◆ **Noradrenaline Acid Tartrate** *see* Norepinephrine *on page 1472*

◆ **Norco** *see* Hydrocodone and Acetaminophen *on page 1012*

◆ **Norcuron** *see* Vecuronium *on page 2144*

◆ **Norcuron® (Can)** *see* Vecuronium *on page 2144*

◆ **Nordeoxyguanosine** *see* Ganciclovir (Systemic) *on page 948*

◆ **Norditropin FlexPro** *see* Somatropin *on page 1918*

◆ **Norditropin Nordiflex (Can)** *see* Somatropin *on page 1918*

◆ **Norditropin NordiFlex Pen** *see* Somatropin *on page 1918*

◆ **Norditropin Simplexx (Can)** *see* Somatropin *on page 1918*

◆ **Norel CS [OTC]** *see* Chlorpheniramine, Phenylephrine, and Dextromethorphan *on page 428*

◆ **Norelgestromin and Ethinyl Estradiol** *see* Ethinyl Estradiol and Norelgestromin *on page 807*

Norepinephrine (nor ep i NEF rin)

Brand Names: U.S. Levophed

Brand Names: Canada Levophed®

Index Terms Levarterenol Bitartrate; Noradrenaline; Noradrenaline Acid Tartrate; Norepinephrine Bitartrate

Pharmacologic Category Alpha/Beta Agonist

Use Treatment of shock which persists after adequate fluid volume replacement; severe hypotension

Note: Recommended as the first-choice vasopressor for the treatment of sepsis and septic shock in adult patients (Dellinger, 2013)

Pregnancy Risk Factor C

Pregnancy Considerations Animal reproduction studies have not been conducted. Norepinephrine is an endogenous catecholamine and crosses the placenta (Minzter, 2010; Wang, 1999).

Breast-Feeding Considerations It is not known if norepinephrine is excreted in breast milk. The manufacturer recommends that caution be exercised when administering norepinephrine to nursing women.

Contraindications Hypersensitivity to norepinephrine, bisulfites (contains metabisulfite), or any component of the formulation; hypotension from hypovolemia except as an emergency measure to maintain coronary and cerebral perfusion until volume could be replaced; mesenteric or peripheral vascular thrombosis unless it is a lifesaving procedure; during anesthesia with cyclopropane (not available in U.S.) or halothane (not available in U.S.) anesthesia (risk of ventricular arrhythmias)

Warnings/Precautions Assure adequate circulatory volume to minimize need for vasoconstrictors. Avoid hypertension; monitor blood pressure closely and adjust infusion rate. Use with extreme caution in patients taking MAO-Inhibitors. Vesicant; ensure proper needle or catheter placement prior to and during infusion. Avoid extravasation; infuse into a large vein if possible. Avoid infusion into leg veins. Montior IV site closely. **[U.S. Boxed Warning]: If extravasation occurs, infiltrate the area with diluted phentolamine (5-10 mg in 10-15 mL of saline) with a fine hypodermic needle. Phentolamine should be administered as soon as possible after extravasation is noted to prevent sloughing/necrosis**. Product may contain sodium metabisulfite.

Adverse Reactions

Cardiovascular: Arrhythmias, bradycardia, peripheral (digital) ischemia
Central nervous system: Anxiety, headache (transient)
Local: Skin necrosis (with extravasation)
Respiratory: Dyspnea, respiratory difficulty

Drug Interactions

Metabolism/Transport Effects Substrate of COMT

Avoid Concomitant Use

Avoid concomitant use of Norepinephrine with any of the following: Ergot Derivatives; Inhalational Anesthetics; Iobenguane I 123

Increased Effect/Toxicity

Norepinephrine may increase the levels/effects of: Droxidopa; Sympathomimetics

The levels/effects of Norepinephrine may be increased by: AtoMOXetine; Beta-Blockers; Cannabinoid-Containing Products; COMT Inhibitors; Ergot Derivatives; Hyaluronidase; Inhalational Anesthetics; Linezolid; MAO Inhibitors; Serotonin/Norepinephrine Reuptake Inhibitors; Tedizolid; Tricyclic Antidepressants

Decreased Effect

Norepinephrine may decrease the levels/effects of: Benzylpenicilloyl Polylysine; Iobenguane I 123; Ioflupane I 123

The levels/effects of Norepinephrine may be decreased by: Alpha1-Blockers; Spironolactone

Preparation for Administration Dilute with D_5W, D_5NS, or NS; dilution in NS is not recommended by the manufacturer; however, stability in NS has been demonstrated (Tremblay, 2008).

Storage/Stability Readily oxidized. Protect from light. Do not use if brown coloration. Stability of parenteral admixture at room temperature (25°C) is 24 hours.

Mechanism of Action Stimulates $beta_1$-adrenergic receptors and alpha-adrenergic receptors causing increased contractility and heart rate as well as vasoconstriction, thereby increasing systemic blood pressure and coronary blood flow; clinically, alpha effects (vasoconstriction) are greater than beta effects (inotropic and chronotropic effects)

Pharmacodynamics/Kinetics

Onset of action: IV: Very rapid-acting
Duration: vasopressor: 1-2 minutes
Metabolism: Via catechol-o-methyltransferase (COMT) and monoamine oxidase (MAO)
Excretion: Urine (84% to 96% as inactive metabolites)

Dosage Administration requires the use of an infusion pump.

Note: Norepinephrine dosage is stated in terms of norepinephrine base.

Continuous IV infusion:

Children: Initial: 0.05-0.1 mcg/kg/minute; titrate to desired effect; maximum dose: 2 mcg/kg/minute (AHA, 2010; Kleinman, 2007)

Adults: Initial: 8-12 mcg/minute; titrate to desired response. Usual maintenance range: 2-4 mcg/minute; dosage range varies greatly depending on clinical situation. If patient remains hypotensive despite large doses, evaluate for occult hypovolemia and provide fluid resuscitation as appropriate.

ACLS dosing range (weight-based dosing): Post cardiac arrest care: Initial: 0.1-0.5 mcg/**kg**/minute (7-35 mcg/minute in a 70 kg patient); titrate to desired response (AHA, 2010)

Sepsis and septic shock (weight-based dosing): Range from clinical trials: 0.01-3 mcg/**kg**/minute (0.7-210 mcg/minute in a 70 kg patient) (Hollenberg, 2004)

Dosage adjustment in renal impairment: No dosage adjustment provided in manufacturer's labeling.

Dosage adjustment in hepatic impairment: No dosage adjustment provided in manufacturer's labeling.

Usual Infusion Concentrations: Pediatric IV infusion: 8 **mcg**/mL **or** 16 **mcg**/mL

Usual Infusion Concentrations: Adult IV infusion: 4 mg in 250 mL (concentration: 16 **mcg**/mL) **or** 8 mg in 250 mL (concentration: 32 **mcg**/mL) of D_5W or NS

Administration Administer as a continuous infusion with the use of an infusion pump. Dilute prior to use. Administration via central line recommended (may cause severe ischemic necrosis if extravasated). Do not administer sodium bicarbonate (or any alkaline solution) through an IV line containing norepinephrine; inactivation of norepinephrine may occur.

Vesicant; ensure proper needle or catheter placement prior to and during infusion; avoid extravasation.

Extravasation management: If extravasation occurs, stop infusion immediately and disconnect (leave cannula/needle in place); gently aspirate extravasated solution (do **NOT** flush the line); remove needle/cannula; elevate extremity. Initiate phentolamine (or alternative) antidote. Apply dry warm compresses (Hurst, 2004).

Phentolamine: Dilute 5-10 mg in 10-15 mL NS and administer into extravasation site as soon as possible after extravasation (Peberdy, 2010) **or** dilute 5-10 mg in 10 mL NS and administer into extravasation area (within 12 hours of extravasation).

Alternatives to phentolamine (due to shortage):

Nitroglycerin topical 2% ointment (based on limited case reports in neonates/infants): Apply 4 mm/kg as a thin ribbon to the affected areas; may repeat after 8 hours if needed (Wong, 1992) **or** apply a 1-inch strip on the affected site (Denkler, 1989).

Terbutaline (based on limited case reports): Infiltrate extravasation area using a solution of terbutaline 1 mg diluted to 10 mL in NS (large extravasation site; administration volume varied from 3-10 mL) **or** 1 mg diluted in 1 mL NS (small/distal extravasation site; administration volume varied from 0.5-1 mL) (Stier, 1999).

Monitoring Parameters Blood pressure (or mean arterial pressure), heart rate; cardiac output (as appropriate), intravascular volume status, pulmonary capillary wedge pressure (as appropriate); monitor infusion site closely

Consult individual institutional policies and procedures.

Additional Information Norepinephrine dosage is stated in terms of norepinephrine base. Although the intravenous product vial designates the contents as norepinephrine bitartrate, the actual concentration shown is in terms of norepinephrine base 1 mg/mL.

Dosage Forms

Solution, Injection:

Levophed: 1 mg/mL (4 mL)

Generic: 1 mg/mL (4 mL)

Solution, Injection [preservative free]:

Generic: 1 mg/mL (4 mL)

◆ **Norepinephrine Bitartrate** *see* Norepinephrine *on page 1472*

Norethindrone (nor ETH in drone)

Brand Names: U.S. Aygestin; Camila; Deblitane; Errin; Heather; Jencycla; Jolivette; Lyza; Nor-QD; Nora-BE; Norlyroc; Ortho Micronor; Sharobel

Brand Names: Canada Micronor®; Norlutate®

Index Terms Norethindrone Acetate; Norethisterone

Pharmacologic Category Contraceptive; Progestin

Use Treatment of amenorrhea; abnormal uterine bleeding; endometriosis; prevention of pregnancy

Pregnancy Risk Factor X

Pregnancy Considerations First trimester exposure may cause genital abnormalities including hypospadias in male infants and mild virilization of external female genitalia. Significant adverse events related to growth and development have not been observed (limited studies). Use is contraindicated during pregnancy. May be started immediately postpartum if not breast-feeding.

Breast-Feeding Considerations Small amounts of progestins are found in breast milk (1% to 6% of maternal serum concentration). Norethindrone can cause changes in milk production in the mother. When used for contraception, may start 3 weeks after delivery in women who are partially breast-feeding, or 6 weeks after delivery in women who are fully breast-feeding.

Contraindications Hypersensitivity to norethindrone or any component of the formulation; history of or current thrombophlebitis or venous thromboembolic disorders (including DVT, PE); hepatic dysfunction or tumor; known or suspected breast carcinoma; undiagnosed vaginal bleeding; pregnancy; missed abortion or as a diagnostic test for pregnancy

Warnings/Precautions Hazardous agent - use appropriate precautions for handling and disposal (NIOSH 2014 [group 2]).

Progestin only contraceptives do not protect against HIV infection or other sexually-transmitted diseases. Irregular menstrual bleeding patterns are common with progestin-only contraceptives; nonpharmacologic causes of abnormal bleeding should be ruled out. Progestin use has been associated with retinal vascular lesions; discontinue pending examination in case of sudden vision loss, complete loss of vision, sudden onset of proptosis, diplopia or migraine. May have adverse effects on glucose tolerance; use caution in women with diabetes. May have adverse effects on lipid metabolism; use caution in women with hyperlipidemias. Use with caution in patients with depression.

Use with caution in patients with diseases which may be exacerbated by fluid retention, including asthma, epilepsy, migraine, cardiac or renal dysfunction. Use caution in patients at increased risk of thromboembolism; includes elective surgery associated with an increased risk of thromboembolism or during periods of prolonged immobilization. The use of combination hormonal contraceptives has been associated with a slight increase in the frequency of breast cancer, however studies are not consistent. Data is insufficient to determine if progestin-only contraceptives also increase this risk. The risk of cardiovascular side effects increases in women using estrogen containing combined hormonal contraceptives and who smoke cigarettes, especially those who are >35 years of age. This risk relative to progestin-only contraceptives has not been established. Extremely rare hepatic adenomas and focal nodular hyperplasia resulting in fatal intra-abdominal hemorrhage have been reported in association with long-term combination oral contraceptive use. Data is insufficient to determine if progestin-only contraceptives also increase this risk. Not for use prior to menarche.

The use of estrogens and/or progestins may change the results of some laboratory tests (eg, coagulation factors, lipids, glucose tolerance, binding proteins). The dose, route, and the specific estrogen/progestin influences these changes. In addition, personal risk factors (eg, cardiovascular disease, smoking, diabetes, age) also contribute to adverse events; use of specific products may be contraindicated in women with certain risk factors.

Adverse Reactions

Cardiovascular: Cerebral embolism, cerebral thrombosis, deep vein thrombosis, edema, pulmonary embolism, retinal thrombosis

Central nervous system: Depression, dizziness, fatigue, headache, insomnia, migraine, emotional lability, nervousness

Dermatologic: Acne vulgaris, alopecia, chloasma, pruritus, skin rash, urticaria

Endocrine & metabolic: Amenorrhea, hirsutism, hypermenorrhea, menstrual disease, weight gain

Gastrointestinal: Abdominal pain, nausea, vomiting

Genitourinary: Breakthrough bleeding, breast hypertrophy, breast tenderness, cervical erosion, change in cervical secretions, decreased lactation, genital discharge, mastalgia, spotting, vaginal hemorrhage

Hypersensitivity: Anaphylaxis, hypersensitivity

Hepatic: Cholestatic jaundice, hepatitis, abnormal hepatic function tests

Neuromuscular & skeletal: Arm pain, leg pain

Ophthalmic: Optic neuritis (with or without vision loss)

Drug Interactions

Metabolism/Transport Effects Substrate of CYP3A4 (major); **Note:** Assignment of Major/Minor substrate status based on clinically relevant drug interaction potential; **Induces** CYP2C19 (moderate)

Avoid Concomitant Use

Avoid concomitant use of Norethindrone with any of the following: Griseofulvin; Tranexamic Acid; Ulipristal

Increased Effect/Toxicity

Norethindrone may increase the levels/effects of: C1 inhibitors; Selegiline; Thalidomide; Tranexamic Acid; Voriconazole

The levels/effects of Norethindrone may be increased by: Atazanavir; Boceprevir; Cobicistat; Herbs (Progestogenic Properties); Lopinavir; Metreleptin; Mifepristone; Tipranavir; Voriconazole

Decreased Effect

Norethindrone may decrease the levels/effects of: Anticoagulants; Fosamprenavir; Vitamin K Antagonists

The levels/effects of Norethindrone may be decreased by: Acitretin; Aminoglutethimide; Aprepitant; Artemether; Barbiturates; Bexarotene (Systemic); Bile Acid Sequestrants; Bosentan; CarBAMazepine; CloBAZam; Colesevelam; CYP3A4 Inducers (Moderate); CYP3A4 Inducers (Strong); Dabrafenib; Darunavir; Deferasirox; Efavirenz; Eslicarbazepine; Exenatide; Felbamate; Fosamprenavir; Fosaprepitant; Fosphenytoin; Griseofulvin; LamoTRIgine; Lopinavir; Metreleptin; Mifepristone; Mitotane; Mycophenolate; Nelfinavir; Nevirapine; OXcarbazepine; Perampanel; Phenytoin; Primidone; Prucalopride; Retinoic Acid Derivatives; Rifamycin Derivatives; Rufinamide; Saquinavir; Siltuximab; St Johns Wort; Sugammadex; Telaprevir; Tocilizumab; Topiramate; Ulipristal

Storage/Stability Store at controlled room temperature of 25°C (77°F).

Mechanism of Action Inhibits secretion of pituitary gonadotropin (LH) which prevents follicular maturation and ovulation

Pharmacodynamics/Kinetics

Absorption: Oral: Rapidly absorbed

Distribution: V_d: 4 L/kg

Protein binding: 61% to albumin; 36% to sex hormone-binding globulin (SHBG); SHBG capacity affected by plasma ethinyl estradiol levels

Metabolism: Oral: Hepatic via reduction and conjugation; first-pass effect

Bioavailability: 64%

Half-life elimination: ~8 hours

Time to peak: 1-2 hours

Excretion: Urine (>50% as metabolites); feces (20% to 40% as metabolites)

Dosage Oral: Adolescents and Adults: Females:

Contraception: Progesterone only: Norethindrone 0.35 mg every day (no missed days)

Initial dose: Start on first day of menstrual period or the day after a miscarriage or abortion. If switching from a combined oral contraceptive, begin the day after finishing the last active combined tablet.

Missed dose: Take as soon as remembered. A back up method of contraception should be used for 48 hours if dose is taken ≥3 hours late.

Amenorrhea and abnormal uterine bleeding: Norethindrone acetate: 2.5-10 mg/day for 5-10 days during the second half of the menstrual cycle

Endometriosis: Norethindrone acetate: 5 mg/day for 14 days; increase at increments of 2.5 mg/day every 2 weeks to reach 15 mg/day; continue for 6-9 months or until breakthrough bleeding demands temporary termination

Dosage adjustment in renal impairment: No dosage adjustment provided in manufacturer's labeling.

Dosage adjustment in hepatic impairment: No dosage adjustment provided in manufacturer's labeling. However, contraindicated in patients with hepatic tumors or impairment.

Dietary Considerations Should be taken at same time each day.

Administration Administer at the same time each day. When used for the prevention of pregnancy, a back up method of contraception should be used for 48 hours if dose is missed or taken ≥3 hours late.

Hazardous agent; use appropriate precautions for handling and disposal (NIOSH 2014 [group 2]).

Monitoring Parameters Contraception: Before starting therapy, a physical exam with reference to the breasts and pelvis are recommended, including a Papanicolaou smear. Exam may be deferred if appropriate; pregnancy should be ruled out prior to use. Monitor patient closely for loss of vision, sudden onset of proptosis, diplopia, migraine; blood pressure; signs and symptoms of thromboembolic disorders; signs or symptoms of depression; glycemic control in patients with diabetes; lipid profiles in patients being treated for hyperlipidemias. Adequate diagnostic measures, including endometrial sampling, if indicated, should be performed to rule out malignancy in all cases of undiagnosed abnormal vaginal bleeding.

Dosage Forms

Tablet, Oral:

Aygestin: 5 mg

Camila: 0.35 mg

Deblitane: 0.35 mg

Errin: 0.35 mg

Heather: 0.35 mg

Jencycla: 0.35 mg

Jolivette: 0.35 mg
Lyza: 0.35 mg
Nor-QD: 0.35 mg
Nora-BE: 0.35 mg
Norlyroc: 0.35 mg
Ortho Micronor: 0.35 mg
Sharobel: 0.35 mg
Generic: 0.35 mg, 5 mg

◆ **Norethindrone Acetate** *see* Norethindrone *on page 1473*

◆ **Norethindrone Acetate and Ethinyl Estradiol** *see* Ethinyl Estradiol and Norethindrone *on page 808*

◆ **Norethindrone and Estradiol** *see* Estradiol and Norethindrone *on page 781*

◆ **Norethindrone and Leuprolide** *see* Leuprolide and Norethindrone *on page 1189*

Norethindrone and Mestranol

(nor eth IN drone & MES tra nole)

Brand Names: U.S. Necon® 1/50; Norinyl® 1+50

Brand Names: Canada Ortho-Novum® 1/50

Index Terms Mestranol and Norethindrone; Ortho Novum 1/50

Pharmacologic Category Contraceptive; Estrogen and Progestin Combination

Use Prevention of pregnancy

Pregnancy Risk Factor X

Dosage Oral: Adults: Females: Contraception:

Schedule 1 (Sunday starter): Dose begins on first Sunday after onset of menstruation; if the menstrual period starts on Sunday, take first tablet that very same day. **With a Sunday start, an additional method of contraception should be used until after the first 7 days of consecutive administration.**

For 21-tablet package: Dosage is 1 tablet daily for 21 consecutive days, followed by 7 days off of the medication; a new course begins on the 8th day after the last tablet is taken.

For 28-tablet package: Dosage is 1 tablet daily without interruption.

Schedule 2 (Day 1 starter): Dose starts on first day of menstrual cycle taking 1 tablet daily.

For 21-tablet package: Dosage is 1 tablet daily for 21 consecutive days, followed by 7 days off of the medication; a new course begins on the 8th day after the last tablet is taken.

For 28-tablet package: Dosage is 1 tablet daily without interruption.

If all doses have been taken on schedule and one menstrual period is missed, continue dosing cycle. If two consecutive menstrual periods are missed, pregnancy test is required before new dosing cycle is started.

Missed doses **monophasic formulations** (refer to package insert for complete information):

One dose missed: Take as soon as remembered or take 2 tablets next day

Two consecutive doses missed in the first 2 weeks: Take 2 tablets as soon as remembered or 2 tablets next 2 days. **An additional method of contraception should be used for 7 days after missed dose.**

Two consecutive doses missed in week 3 or three consecutive doses missed at any time: **An additional method of contraception must be used for 7 days after a missed dose:**

Schedule 1 (Sunday starter): Continue dose of 1 tablet daily until Sunday, then discard the rest of the pack, and a new pack should be started that same day.

Schedule 2 (Day 1 starter): Current pack should be discarded, and a new pack should be started that same day.

Dosage adjustment in renal impairment: No dosage adjustment provided in manufacturer's labeling. Use with caution and monitor blood pressure closely. Consider other forms of contraception.

Dosage adjustment in hepatic impairment: No dosage adjustment provided in manufacturer's labeling. However, contraindicated in patients with hepatic tumors or impairment.

Additional Information Complete prescribing information should be consulted for additional detail.

Dosage Forms

Tablet, monophasic formulations:

Necon® 1/50: Norethindrone 1 mg and mestranol 0.05 mg [21 light blue tablets and 7 white inactive tablets] (28s)

Norinyl® 1+50: Norethindrone 1 mg and mestranol 0.05 mg [21 white tablets and 7 orange inactive tablets] (28s)

◆ **Norethisterone** *see* Norethindrone *on page 1473*

◆ **Norflex** *see* Orphenadrine *on page 1522*

◆ **Norflex™ (Can)** *see* Orphenadrine *on page 1522*

Norfloxacin (nor FLOKS a sin)

Brand Names: U.S. Noroxin [DSC]

Brand Names: Canada Apo-Norflox®; CO Norfloxacin; Norfloxacine®; Novo-Norfloxacin; PMS-Norfloxacin; Riva-Norfloxacin

Pharmacologic Category Antibiotic, Fluoroquinolone

Use Uncomplicated and complicated urinary tract infections caused by susceptible gram-negative and gram-positive bacteria; sexually-transmitted disease (eg, uncomplicated urethral and cervical gonorrhea) caused by *N. gonorrhoeae*; prostatitis due to *E. coli*

Note: As of April 2007, the CDC no longer recommends the use of fluoroquinolones for the treatment of gonococcal disease.

Pregnancy Risk Factor C

Dosage

Usual dosage range:

Adults: Oral: 400 mg every 12 hours (maximum: 800 mg/day)

Indication-specific dosing:

Adults: Oral:

Dysenteric enterocolitis *(Shigella)* (off-label use): 400 mg twice daily for 3 days (IDSA, 2001)

Prostatitis: 400 mg every 12 hours for 4-6 weeks

Traveler's diarrhea (off-label use): 400 mg twice daily for 3 days (Mattila, 1993), single dose may also be effective

Uncomplicated gonorrhea: 800 mg as a single dose.

Note: As of April 2007, the CDC no longer recommends the use of fluoroquinolones for the treatment of uncomplicated gonococcal disease.

Urinary tract infections:

Uncomplicated due to *E. coli, K. pneumoniae, P. mirabilis*: 400 mg twice daily for 3 days

Uncomplicated due to other organisms: 400 mg twice daily for 7-10 days

Complicated: 400 mg twice daily for 10-21 days

Dosage adjustment in renal impairment: CrCl ≤30 mL/minute/1.73 m^2: 400 mg once daily

Dosage adjustment in hepatic impairment: No dosage adjustment provided in manufacturer's labeling.

Additional Information Complete prescribing information should be consulted for additional detail.

◆ **Norfloxacine® (Can)** *see* Norfloxacin *on page 1475*

◆ **Norgesic** *see* Orphenadrine, Aspirin, and Caffeine *on page 1522*

- **Norgestimate and Ethinyl Estradiol** *see* Ethinyl Estradiol and Norgestimate *on page 810*
- **Norgestrel and Ethinyl Estradiol** *see* Ethinyl Estradiol and Norgestrel *on page 812*
- **Norinyl 1+35** *see* Ethinyl Estradiol and Norethindrone *on page 808*
- **Norinyl® 1+50** *see* Norethindrone and Mestranol *on page 1475*
- **Noritate** *see* MetroNIDAZOLE (Topical) *on page 1357*
- **NorLevo (Can)** *see* Levonorgestrel *on page 1201*
- **Norlutate® (Can)** *see* Norethindrone *on page 1473*
- **Norlyroc** *see* Norethindrone *on page 1473*
- **Normal Human Serum Albumin** *see* Albumin *on page 67*
- **Normal Immunoglobulin** *see* Immune Globulin *on page 1056*
- **Normal Saline** *see* Sodium Chloride *on page 1902*
- **Normal Serum Albumin (Human)** *see* Albumin *on page 67*
- **Normocarb HF® 25** *see* Electrolyte Solution, Renal Replacement *on page 710*
- **Normocarb HF® 35** *see* Electrolyte Solution, Renal Replacement *on page 710*
- **Normodyne (Can)** *see* Labetalol *on page 1151*
- **Noroxin [DSC]** *see* Norfloxacin *on page 1475*
- **Norpace** *see* Disopyramide *on page 653*
- **Norpace CR** *see* Disopyramide *on page 653*
- **Norpramin** *see* Desipramine *on page 593*
- **Norprolac (Can)** *see* Quinagolide [CAN/INT] *on page 1755*
- **Nor-QD** *see* Norethindrone *on page 1473*
- **Nortemp Children's [OTC]** *see* Acetaminophen *on page 32*
- **Nortrel 0.5/35** *see* Ethinyl Estradiol and Norethindrone *on page 808*
- **Nortrel 1/35** *see* Ethinyl Estradiol and Norethindrone *on page 808*
- **Nortrel 7/7/7** *see* Ethinyl Estradiol and Norethindrone *on page 808*

Nortriptyline (nor TRIP ti leen)

Brand Names: U.S. Pamelor

Brand Names: Canada Apo-Nortriptyline; Ava-Nortriptyline; Aventyl; Dom-Nortriptyline; Norventyl; Nu-Nortriptyline; PMS-Nortriptyline; Teva-Nortriptyline

Index Terms Nortriptyline Hydrochloride

Pharmacologic Category Antidepressant, Tricyclic (Secondary Amine)

Additional Appendix Information

Beers Criteria – Potentially Inappropriate Medications for Geriatrics *on page 2271*

Use Treatment of symptoms of depression

Pregnancy Considerations Animal reproduction studies are inconclusive. Nortriptyline and its metabolites cross the human placenta and can be detected in cord blood (Loughhead, 2006). Tricyclic antidepressants may be associated with irritability, jitteriness, and convulsions (rare) in the neonate (Yonkers, 2009).

The ACOG recommends that therapy for depression during pregnancy be individualized; treatment should incorporate the clinical expertise of the mental health clinician, obstetrician, primary healthcare provider, and pediatrician (ACOG, 2008). According to the American Psychiatric Association (APA), the risks of medication treatment should be weighed against other treatment options and untreated depression. For women who discontinue antidepressant medications during pregnancy and who may be at high risk for postpartum depression, the medications can be restarted following delivery (APA, 2010). Treatment algorithms have been developed by the ACOG and the APA for the management of depression in women prior to conception and during pregnancy (Yonkers, 2009).

Breast-Feeding Considerations Nortriptyline is excreted into breast milk and the M/P ratio ranged from 0.87 to 3.71 in one case report (Matheson, 1988). Based on available information, nortriptyline has not been detected in the serum of nursing infants; however, low levels of the active metabolite E-10-hydroxynortriptyline have been detected in the serum of newborns following breast-feeding (Wisner, 1991). Based on information from one mother-infant pair, following maternal use of nortriptyline 125 mg/day, the estimated exposure to the breast-feeding infant would be 0.6% to 3% of the weight-adjusted maternal dose. Adverse events have not been reported in nursing infants. Infants should be monitored for signs of adverse events; routine monitoring of infant serum concentrations is not recommended (Fortinguerra, 2009).

Contraindications Hypersensitivity to nortriptyline and similar chemical class, or any component of the formulation; use in a patient during the acute recovery phase of MI; use of MAO inhibitors intended to treat psychiatric disorders (concurrently or within 14 days of discontinuing either nortriptyline or the MAO inhibitor); initiation of nortriptyline in a patient receiving linezolid or intravenous methylene blue

Warnings/Precautions [U.S. Boxed Warning]: Antidepressants increase the risk of suicidal thinking and behavior in children, adolescents, and young adults (18-24 years of age) with major depressive disorder (MDD) and other psychiatric disorders; consider risk prior to prescribing. Short-term studies did not show an increased risk in patients >24 years of age and showed a decreased risk in patients ≥65 years. Closely monitor for clinical worsening, suicidality, or unusual changes in behavior, particularly during the initial 1-2 months of therapy or during periods of dosage adjustments (increases or decreases); the patient's family or caregiver should be instructed to closely observe the patient and communicate condition with healthcare provider. A medication guide should be dispensed with each prescription. **Nortriptyline is not FDA approved for use in children.**

The possibility of a suicide attempt is inherent in major depression and may persist until remission occurs. Use caution in high-risk patients. Worsening depression and severe abrupt suicidality that are not part of the presenting symptoms may require discontinuation or modification of drug therapy. The patient's family or caregiver should be alerted to monitor patients for the emergence of suicidality and associated behaviors (such as agitation, irritability, hostility, impulsivity, and hypomania) and call healthcare provider.

May worsen psychosis in some patients or precipitate a shift to mania or hypomania in patients with bipolar disorder. Patients presenting with depressive symptoms should be screened for bipolar disorder. Monotherapy in patients with bipolar disorder should be avoided. **Nortriptyline is not FDA approved for the treatment of bipolar depression.**

Potentially life-threatening serotonin syndrome (SS) has occurred with serotonergic agents (eg, SSRIs, SNRIs), particularly when used in combination with other serotonergic agents (eg, triptans, TCAs, fentanyl, lithium, tramadol, buspirone, St John's wort, tryptophan) or agents that impair metabolism of serotonin (eg, MAO inhibitors intended to treat psychiatric disorders, other MAO

inhibitors [ie, linezolid and intravenous methylene blue]). Discontinue treatment (and any concomitant serotonergic agent) immediately if signs/symptoms arise. TCAs may rarely cause bone marrow suppression; monitor for any signs of infection and obtain CBC if symptoms (eg, fever, sore throat) evident. The risk of sedation and orthostatic effects are low relative to other antidepressants. However, nortriptyline may result in impaired performance of tasks requiring alertness (eg, operating machinery or driving). The degree of anticholinergic blockade produced by this agent is moderate relative to other cyclic antidepressants, however, caution should still be used in patients with urinary retention, benign prostatic hyperplasia, narrow-angle glaucoma, xerostomia, visual problems, constipation, or history of bowel obstruction. May cause orthostatic hypotension (risk is low relative to other antidepressants) or conduction disturbances. Use with caution in patients with a history of cardiovascular disease (including previous MI, stroke, tachycardia, or conduction abnormalities). The risk conduction abnormalities with this agent is moderate relative to other antidepressants. CNS effects may be potentiated when used with other sedative drugs or ethanol.

Recommended by the manufacturer to discontinue prior to elective surgery; risks exist for drug interactions with anesthesia and for cardiac arrhythmias. However, definitive drug interactions have not been widely reported in the literature and continuation of tricyclic antidepressants is generally recommended as long as precautions are taken to reduce the significance of any adverse events that may occur (Pass, 2004). May alter glucose regulation - use caution in patients with diabetes. Use caution in patients with a previous seizure disorder or condition predisposing to seizures such as brain damage, alcoholism, or concurrent therapy with other drugs which lower the seizure threshold. May increase the risks associated with electroconvulsive therapy. Bone fractures have been associated with antidepressant treatment. Consider the possibility of a fragility fracture if an antidepressant-treated patient presents with unexplained bone pain, point tenderness, swelling, or bruising (Rabenda, 2013; Rizzoli, 2012). Use with caution in patients with hepatic or renal dysfunction.

Use caution in elderly patients; may cause or exacerbate syndrome of inappropriate antidiuretic hormone secretion or hyponatremia; monitor sodium closely with initiation or dosage adjustments in older adults. May be inappropriate in older adults depending on comorbidities (eg, dementia, delirium) or in patients with a history of falls and fractures due to its potent anticholinergic effects (Beers Criteria).

Benzyl alcohol and derivatives: Some dosage forms may contain sodium benzoate/benzoic acid; benzoic acid (benzoate) is a metabolite of benzyl alcohol; large amounts of benzyl alcohol (≥99 mg/kg/day) have been associated with a potentially fatal toxicity ("gasping syndrome") in neonates; the "gasping syndrome" consists of metabolic acidosis, respiratory distress, gasping respirations, CNS dysfunction (including convulsions, intracranial hemorrhage), hypotension, and cardiovascular collapse (AAP, 1997; CDC, 1982); some data suggests that benzoate displaces bilirubin from protein binding sites (Ahlfors, 2001); avoid or use dosage forms containing benzyl alcohol derivative with caution in neonates. See manufacturer's labeling.

Abrupt discontinuation or interruption of antidepressant therapy has been associated with a discontinuation syndrome. Symptoms arising may vary with antidepressant however commonly include nausea, vomiting, diarrhea, headaches, lightheadedness, dizziness, diminished appetite, sweating, chills, tremors, paresthesias, fatigue, somnolence, and sleep disturbances (eg, vivid dreams, insomnia). Greater risks for developing a discontinuation syndrome have been associated with antidepressants with shorter half-lives, longer durations of treatment, and abrupt discontinuation. For antidepressants of short or intermediate half-lives, symptoms may emerge within 2-5 days after treatment discontinuation and last 7-14 days (APA, 2010; Fava, 2006; Haddad, 2001; Shelton, 2001; Warner, 2006).

Adverse Reactions Some reactions listed are based on reports for other agents in this same pharmacologic class and may not be specifically reported for nortriptyline.

Cardiovascular: Cardiac arrhythmia, cerebrovascular accident, edema, flushing, heart block, hypertension, hypotension, myocardial infarction, palpitations, tachycardia

Central nervous system: Agitation, anxiety, ataxia, confusion, delusions, disorientation, dizziness, drowsiness, drug fever, EEG pattern changes, extrapyramidal reaction, fatigue, hallucination, headache, hypomania, insomnia, nightmares, numbness, panic, peripheral neuropathy, psychosis (exacerbation), restlessness, seizure, tingling of extremities, tingling sensation, withdrawal symptoms

Dermatologic: Alopecia, diaphoresis (excessive), pruritus, skin photosensitivity, skin rash, urticaria

Endocrine & metabolic: Decreased libido, decreased serum glucose, galactorrhea, gynecomastia, increased libido, increased serum glucose, SIADH, weight gain, weight loss

Gastrointestinal: Abdominal cramps, anorexia, constipation, diarrhea, epigastric distress, melanoglossia, nausea, paralytic ileus, parotid gland enlargement, stomatitis, sublingual adenitis, unpleasant taste, vomiting, xerostomia

Genitourinary: Breast hypertrophy, impotence, nocturia, testicular swelling, urinary hesitance, urinary retention, urinary tract dilation

Hematologic & oncologic: Agranulocytosis, eosinophilia, petechia, purpura, thrombocytopenia

Hepatic: Abnormal hepatic function tests, cholestatic jaundice

Neuromuscular & skeletal: Tremor, weakness

Ophthalmic: Accommodation disturbance, blurred vision, eye pain, mydriasis

Otic: Tinnitus

Renal: Polyuria

Rare but important or life-threatening: Angle-closure glaucoma, serotonin syndrome, suicidal ideation

Drug Interactions

Metabolism/Transport Effects Substrate of CYP1A2 (minor), CYP2C19 (minor), CYP2D6 (major), CYP3A4 (minor); **Note:** Assignment of Major/Minor substrate status based on clinically relevant drug interaction potential; **Inhibits** CYP2D6 (weak), CYP2E1 (weak)

Avoid Concomitant Use

Avoid concomitant use of Nortriptyline with any of the following: Aclidinium; Azelastine (Nasal); Dapoxetine; Glucagon; Iobenguane I 123; Ipratropium (Oral Inhalation); Linezolid; MAO Inhibitors; Methylene Blue; Moxonidine; Orphenadrine; Paraldehyde; Potassium Chloride; Thalidomide; Tiotropium; Umeclidinium

Increased Effect/Toxicity

Nortriptyline may increase the levels/effects of: AbobotulinumtoxinA; Alcohol (Ethyl); Alpha-/Beta-Agonists (Direct-Acting); Alpha1-Agonists; Amphetamines; Analgesics (Opioid); Anticholinergic Agents; Antipsychotic Agents; ARIPiprazole; Azelastine (Nasal); Beta2-Agonists; Buprenorphine; Citalopram; CNS Depressants; Desmopressin; Escitalopram; Glucagon; Highest Risk QTc-Prolonging Agents; Hydrocodone; Methotrimeprazine; Methylene Blue; Metyrosine; Mirabegron; Moderate Risk QTc-Prolonging Agents; Nicorandil; OnabotulinumtoxinA; Orphenadrine; Paraldehyde; Potassium Chloride; Pramipexole; QuiNIDine; RimabotulinumtoxinB; ROPINIRole; Rotigotine; Serotonin Modulators; Sodium Phosphates; Sulfonylureas; Suvorexant; Thalidomide;

Thiazide Diuretics; Tiotropium; Topiramate; TraMADol; Vitamin K Antagonists; Yohimbine; Zolpidem

The levels/effects of Nortriptyline may be increased by: Abiraterone Acetate; Aclidinium; Altretamine; Antiemetics (5HT3 Antagonists); Antipsychotic Agents; Brimonidine (Topical); BuPROPion; Cannabis; Cimetidine; Cinacalcet; Citalopram; Cobicistat; CYP2D6 Inhibitors (Moderate); CYP2D6 Inhibitors (Strong); Dapoxetine; Darunavir; Dexmethylphenidate; Doxylamine; Dronabinol; Droperidol; DULoxetine; Escitalopram; FLUoxetine; FluvoxaMINE; HydrOXYzine; Ipratropium (Oral Inhalation); Kava Kava; Linezolid; Lithium; Magnesium Sulfate; MAO Inhibitors; Methotrimeprazine; Methylphenidate; Metoclopramide; Metyrosine; Mianserin; Mifepristone; Nabilone; PARoxetine; Peginterferon Alfa-2b; Perampanel; Pramlintide; Protease Inhibitors; QuiNIDine; Rufinamide; Sertraline; Sodium Oxybate; Tapentadol; Tedizolid; Terbinafine (Systemic); Tetrahydrocannabinol; Thyroid Products; TraMADol; Umeclidinium; Valproic Acid and Derivatives

Decreased Effect

Nortriptyline may decrease the levels/effects of: Acetylcholinesterase Inhibitors; Alpha1-Agonists; Alpha2-Agonists; Alpha2-Agonists (Ophthalmic); Iobenguane I 123; Itopride; Moxonidine; Secretin

The levels/effects of Nortriptyline may be decreased by: Acetylcholinesterase Inhibitors; Barbiturates; CarBAMazepine; Peginterferon Alfa-2b; St Johns Wort

Storage/Stability Store at 20°C to 25°C (68°F to 77°F). Protect from light.

Mechanism of Action Traditionally believed to increase the synaptic concentration of serotonin and/or norepinephrine in the central nervous system by inhibition of their reuptake by the presynaptic neuronal membrane. However, additional receptor effects have been found including desensitization of adenyl cyclase, down regulation of beta-adrenergic receptors, and down regulation of serotonin receptors.

Pharmacodynamics/Kinetics

Onset of action: Therapeutic: 1-3 weeks
Distribution: V_d: 21 L/kg
Protein binding: 93% to 95%
Metabolism: Primarily hepatic; extensive first-pass effect
Half-life elimination: 28-31 hours
Time to peak, serum: 7-8.5 hours
Excretion: Urine (as metabolites and small amounts of unchanged drug); feces (small amounts)

Dosage Oral:

Nocturnal enuresis: Children (off-label use): 10-20 mg/day; titrate to a maximum of 40 mg/day

Depression: Children (off-label use): 1-3 mg/kg/day

Depression:

Adults: 25 mg 3-4 times/day up to 150 mg/day; doses may be given once daily

Elderly: Initial: 30-50 mg/day, given as a single daily dose or in divided doses. **Note:** Nortriptyline is one of the best tolerated TCAs in the elderly.

Myofascial pain, neuralgia, burning mouth syndrome (off-label uses): Adults: Initial: 10-25 mg at bedtime; dosage may be increased by 25 mg/day weekly, if tolerated; usual maintenance dose: 75 mg as a single bedtime dose or 2 divided doses

Chronic urticaria, angioedema, nocturnal pruritus (off-label use): Adults: Oral: 75 mg/day

Smoking cessation (off-label use; Fiore, 2008): Adults: Initial: 25 mg/day; titrate dose to 75-100 mg/day 10-28 days prior to selected "quit" date; continue therapy for ≥12 weeks after "quit" day

Discontinuation of therapy: Upon discontinuation of antidepressant therapy, gradually taper the dose to minimize the incidence of withdrawal symptoms and allow for the detection of re-emerging symptoms. Evidence supporting ideal taper rates is limited. APA and NICE guidelines suggest tapering therapy over at least several weeks with consideration to the half-life of the antidepressant; antidepressants with a shorter half-life may need to be tapered more conservatively. In addition for long-term treated patients, WFSBP guidelines recommend tapering over 4-6 months. If intolerable withdrawal symptoms occur following a dose reduction, consider resuming the previously prescribed dose and/or decrease dose at a more gradual rate (APA, 2010; Bauer, 2002; Haddad, 2001; NCCMH, 2010; Schatzberg, 2006; Shelton, 2001; Warner, 2006).

MAO inhibitor recommendations:

Switching to or from an MAO inhibitor intended to treat psychiatric disorders:

Allow 14 days to elapse between discontinuing an MAO inhibitor intended to treat psychiatric disorders and initiation of nortriptyline.

Allow 14 days to elapse between discontinuing nortriptyline and initiation of an MAO inhibitor intended to treat psychiatric disorders.

Use with other MAO inhibitors (linezolid or IV methylene blue):

Do not initiate nortriptyline in patients receiving linezolid or IV methylene blue; consider other interventions for psychiatric condition.

If urgent treatment with linezolid or IV methylene blue is required in a patient already receiving nortriptyline and potential benefits outweigh potential risks, discontinue nortriptyline promptly and administer linezolid or IV methylene blue. Monitor for serotonin syndrome for 2 weeks or until 24 hours after the last dose of linezolid or IV methylene blue, whichever comes first. May resume nortriptyline 24 hours after the last dose of linezolid or IV methylene blue.

Dosage adjustment in renal impairment: No dosage adjustment provided in manufacturer's labeling.

Dosage adjustment in hepatic impairment: Lower doses and slower titration dependent on individualization of dosage is recommended

Monitoring Parameters Blood pressure and pulse rate (ECG, cardiac monitoring) prior to and during initial therapy in older adults; weight; blood levels are useful for therapeutic monitoring; suicide ideation (especially at the beginning of therapy or when doses are increased or decreased); signs/symptoms of serotonin syndrome

Reference Range

Plasma levels do not always correlate with clinical effectiveness
Therapeutic: 50-150 ng/mL (SI: 190-570 nmol/L)
Toxic: >500 ng/mL (SI: >1900 nmol/L)

Additional Information The maximum antidepressant effect of nortriptyline may not be seen for ≥2 weeks after initiation of therapy.

Dosage Forms

Capsule, Oral:

Pamelor: 10 mg, 25 mg, 50 mg, 75 mg
Generic: 10 mg, 25 mg, 50 mg, 75 mg

Solution, Oral:

Generic: 10 mg/5 mL (473 mL)

◆ **Nortriptyline Hydrochloride** *see* Nortriptyline *on page 1476*

◆ **Norvasc** *see* AmLODIPine *on page 123*

◆ **Norventyl (Can)** *see* Nortriptyline *on page 1476*

◆ **Norvir** *see* Ritonavir *on page 1822*

◆ **Norvir SEC (Can)** *see* Ritonavir *on page 1822*

◆ **NovaFerrum 50 [OTC]** *see* Polysaccharide-Iron Complex *on page 1677*

- ◆ **NovaFerrum Pediatric Drops [OTC]** *see* Polysaccharide-Iron Complex *on page 1677*
- ◆ **Novahistex® DM Decongestant (Can)** *see* Pseudoephedrine and Dextromethorphan *on page 1743*
- ◆ **Novahistex® Expectorant with Decongestant (Can)** *see* Guaifenesin and Pseudoephedrine *on page 989*
- ◆ **Novahistine DH [DSC]** *see* Dihydrocodeine, Chlorpheniramine, and Phenylephrine *on page 633*
- ◆ **Novahistine® DM Decongestant (Can)** *see* Pseudoephedrine and Dextromethorphan *on page 1743*
- ◆ **Novamoxin® (Can)** *see* Amoxicillin *on page 130*
- ◆ **Novantrone** *see* MitoXANtrone *on page 1382*
- ◆ **Novarel** *see* Chorionic Gonadotropin (Human) *on page 431*
- ◆ **Novasen (Can)** *see* Aspirin *on page 180*
- ◆ **Novel Erythropoiesis-Stimulating Protein** *see* Darbepoetin Alfa *on page 565*
- ◆ **Novo-5 ASA (Can)** *see* Mesalamine *on page 1301*
- ◆ **Novo-Ampicillin (Can)** *see* Ampicillin *on page 141*
- ◆ **Novo-Atorvastatin (Can)** *see* AtorvaSTATin *on page 194*
- ◆ **Novo-Azithromycin (Can)** *see* Azithromycin (Systemic) *on page 216*
- ◆ **Novo-AZT (Can)** *see* Zidovudine *on page 2196*
- ◆ **Novo-Baclofen (Can)** *see* Baclofen *on page 223*
- ◆ **Novo-Benzydamine (Can)** *see* Benzydamine [CAN/INT] *on page 249*
- ◆ **Novo-Bicalutamide (Can)** *see* Bicalutamide *on page 262*
- ◆ **Novo-Bisoprolol (Can)** *see* Bisoprolol *on page 266*
- ◆ **Novo-Bromazepam (Can)** *see* Bromazepam [CAN/INT] *on page 290*
- ◆ **Novo-Bupropion SR (Can)** *see* BuPROPion *on page 305*
- ◆ **Novo-Buspirone (Can)** *see* BusPIRone *on page 311*
- ◆ **Novo-Carvedilol (Can)** *see* Carvedilol *on page 367*
- ◆ **Novo-Cefaclor (Can)** *see* Cefaclor *on page 372*
- ◆ **Novo-Chloroquine (Can)** *see* Chloroquine *on page 424*
- ◆ **Novo-Cholamine (Can)** *see* Cholestyramine Resin *on page 431*
- ◆ **Novo-Cholamine Light (Can)** *see* Cholestyramine Resin *on page 431*
- ◆ **Novo-Cilazapril (Can)** *see* Cilazapril [CAN/INT] *on page 434*
- ◆ **Novo-Cilazapril/HCTZ (Can)** *see* Cilazapril and Hydrochlorothiazide [CAN/INT] *on page 436*
- ◆ **Novo-Cimetidine (Can)** *see* Cimetidine *on page 438*
- ◆ **Novo-Ciprofloxacin (Can)** *see* Ciprofloxacin (Systemic) *on page 441*
- ◆ **Novo-Clavamoxin (Can)** *see* Amoxicillin and Clavulanate *on page 133*
- ◆ **Novo-Clobazam (Can)** *see* CloBAZam *on page 465*
- ◆ **Novo-Clobetasol (Can)** *see* Clobetasol *on page 468*
- ◆ **Novo-Clomipramine (Can)** *see* ClomiPRAMINE *on page 475*
- ◆ **Novo-Clonidine (Can)** *see* CloNIDine *on page 480*
- ◆ **Novo-Clopate (Can)** *see* Clorazepate *on page 487*
- ◆ **Novo-Cloxin (Can)** *see* Cloxacillin [CAN/INT] *on page 488*
- ◆ **Novo-Cycloprine (Can)** *see* Cyclobenzaprine *on page 516*
- ◆ **Novo-Cyproterone (Can)** *see* Cyproterone [CAN/INT] *on page 530*
- ◆ **Novo-Cyproterone/Ethinyl Estradiol (Can)** *see* Cyproterone and Ethinyl Estradiol [CAN/INT] *on page 532*
- ◆ **Novo-Desipramine (Can)** *see* Desipramine *on page 593*
- ◆ **Novo-Desmopressin (Can)** *see* Desmopressin *on page 594*
- ◆ **Novo-Diflunisal (Can)** *see* Diflunisal *on page 626*
- ◆ **Novo-Dimenate [OTC] (Can)** *see* DimenhyDRINATE *on page 637*
- ◆ **Novo-Dipam (Can)** *see* Diazepam *on page 613*
- ◆ **Novo-Divalproex (Can)** *see* Valproic Acid and Derivatives *on page 2123*
- ◆ **Novo-Docusate Calcium [OTC] (Can)** *see* Docusate *on page 661*
- ◆ **Novo-Docusate Sodium [OTC] (Can)** *see* Docusate *on page 661*
- ◆ **Novo-Doxepin (Can)** *see* Doxepin (Systemic) *on page 676*
- ◆ **Novoeight** *see* Antihemophilic Factor (Recombinant) *on page 152*
- ◆ **Novo-Enalapril/Hctz (Can)** *see* Enalapril and Hydrochlorothiazide *on page 725*
- ◆ **Novo-Etidronatecal (Can)** *see* Etidronate and Calcium Carbonate [CAN/INT] *on page 814*
- ◆ **Novo-Fenofibrate Micronized (Can)** *see* Fenofibrate and Derivatives *on page 852*
- ◆ **Novo-Ferrogluc (Can)** *see* Ferrous Gluconate *on page 870*
- ◆ **Novo-Fluconazole (Can)** *see* Fluconazole *on page 885*
- ◆ **Novo-Flunarizine (Can)** *see* Flunarizine [CAN/INT] *on page 892*
- ◆ **Novo-Fluoxetine (Can)** *see* FLUoxetine *on page 899*
- ◆ **Novo-Flurprofen (Can)** *see* Flurbiprofen (Systemic) *on page 906*
- ◆ **Novo-Fluvoxamine (Can)** *see* FluvoxaMINE *on page 916*
- ◆ **Novo-Furantoin (Can)** *see* Nitrofurantoin *on page 1463*
- ◆ **Novo-Gemfibrozil (Can)** *see* Gemfibrozil *on page 956*
- ◆ **Novo-Gesic (Can)** *see* Acetaminophen *on page 32*
- ◆ **Novo-Glimepiride (Can)** *see* Glimepiride *on page 966*
- ◆ **Novo-Hydroxyzin (Can)** *see* HydrOXYzine *on page 1024*
- ◆ **Novo-Hylazin (Can)** *see* HydrALAZINE *on page 1007*
- ◆ **Novo-Indapamide (Can)** *see* Indapamide *on page 1065*
- ◆ **Novo-Ipramide (Can)** *see* Ipratropium (Systemic) *on page 1108*
- ◆ **Novo-Ketorolac (Can)** *see* Ketorolac (Systemic) *on page 1146*
- ◆ **Novo-Ketotifen (Can)** *see* Ketotifen (Systemic) [CAN/INT] *on page 1149*
- ◆ **Novo-Levobunolol (Can)** *see* Levobunolol *on page 1194*
- ◆ **Novo-Levofloxacin (Can)** *see* Levofloxacin (Systemic) *on page 1197*
- ◆ **NovoLIN® 70/30** *see* Insulin NPH and Insulin Regular *on page 1090*
- ◆ **Novolin® ge 30/70 (Can)** *see* Insulin NPH and Insulin Regular *on page 1090*
- ◆ **Novolin® ge 40/60 (Can)** *see* Insulin NPH and Insulin Regular *on page 1090*
- ◆ **Novolin® ge 50/50 (Can)** *see* Insulin NPH and Insulin Regular *on page 1090*
- ◆ **Novolin® ge NPH (Can)** *see* Insulin NPH *on page 1089*

- **Novolin ge Toronto (Can)** *see* Insulin Regular *on page 1091*
- **NovoLIN N [OTC]** *see* Insulin NPH *on page 1089*
- **NovoLIN N ReliOn [OTC]** *see* Insulin NPH *on page 1089*
- **NovoLIN R [OTC]** *see* Insulin Regular *on page 1091*
- **NovoLIN R ReliOn [OTC]** *see* Insulin Regular *on page 1091*
- **NovoLOG** *see* Insulin Aspart *on page 1083*
- **NovoLog 70/30** *see* Insulin Aspart Protamine and Insulin Aspart *on page 1084*
- **NovoLOG FlexPen** *see* Insulin Aspart *on page 1083*
- **NovoLOG® Mix 70/30** *see* Insulin Aspart Protamine and Insulin Aspart *on page 1084*
- **NovoLOG® Mix 70/30 FlexPen®** *see* Insulin Aspart Protamine and Insulin Aspart *on page 1084*
- **NovoLOG PenFill** *see* Insulin Aspart *on page 1083*
- **Novo-Loperamide (Can)** *see* Loperamide *on page 1236*
- **Novo-Medopa (Can)** *see* Methyldopa *on page 1332*
- **Novo-Medrone (Can)** *see* MedroxyPROGESTERone *on page 1277*
- **Novo-Meprazine (Can)** *see* Methotrimeprazine [CAN/INT] *on page 1329*
- **Novo-Metformin (Can)** *see* MetFORMIN *on page 1307*
- **Novo-Methacin (Can)** *see* Indomethacin *on page 1067*
- **Novo-Mexiletine (Can)** *see* Mexiletine *on page 1359*
- **Novo-Minocycline (Can)** *see* Minocycline *on page 1371*
- **Novo-Misoprostol (Can)** *see* Misoprostol *on page 1379*
- **NovoMix® 30 (Can)** *see* Insulin Aspart Protamine and Insulin Aspart *on page 1084*
- **Novo-Moclobemide (Can)** *see* Moclobemide [CAN/INT] *on page 1384*
- **Novo-Morphine SR (Can)** *see* Morphine (Systemic) *on page 1394*
- **Novo-Mycophenolate (Can)** *see* Mycophenolate *on page 1405*
- **Novo-Nabumetone (Can)** *see* Nabumetone *on page 1411*
- **Novo-Nidazol (Can)** *see* MetroNIDAZOLE (Systemic) *on page 1353*
- **Novo-Nizatidine (Can)** *see* Nizatidine *on page 1471*
- **Novo-Norfloxacin (Can)** *see* Norfloxacin *on page 1475*
- **Novo-Ofloxacin (Can)** *see* Ofloxacin (Systemic) *on page 1490*
- **Novo-Oxybutynin (Can)** *see* Oxybutynin *on page 1536*
- **Novo-Paroxetine (Can)** *see* PARoxetine *on page 1579*
- **Novo-Pen-VK (Can)** *see* Penicillin V Potassium *on page 1614*
- **Novo-Peridol (Can)** *see* Haloperidol *on page 993*
- **Novo-Phenytoin (Can)** *see* Phenytoin *on page 1640*
- **Novo-Pirocam (Can)** *see* Piroxicam *on page 1662*
- **Novo-Pramine (Can)** *see* Imipramine *on page 1054*
- **Novo-Pranol (Can)** *see* Propranolol *on page 1731*
- **Novo-Prazin (Can)** *see* Prazosin *on page 1703*
- **Novo-Prednisolone (Can)** *see* PrednisoLONE (Systemic) *on page 1703*
- **Novo-Prednisone (Can)** *see* PredniSONE *on page 1706*
- **Novo-Profen (Can)** *see* Ibuprofen *on page 1032*
- **Novo-Purol (Can)** *see* Allopurinol *on page 90*
- **Novo-Quinidin (Can)** *see* QuiNIDine *on page 1759*
- **Novo-Quinine (Can)** *see* QuiNINE *on page 1761*
- **NovoRapid® (Can)** *see* Insulin Aspart *on page 1083*
- **Novo-Risedronate (Can)** *see* Risedronate *on page 1816*
- **Novo-Rivastigmine (Can)** *see* Rivastigmine *on page 1833*
- **Novo-Rythro Estolate (Can)** *see* Erythromycin (Systemic) *on page 762*
- **Novo-Rythro Ethylsuccinate (Can)** *see* Erythromycin (Systemic) *on page 762*
- **Novo-Salbutamol HFA (Can)** *see* Albuterol *on page 69*
- **Novo-Selegiline (Can)** *see* Selegiline *on page 1873*
- **Novo-Semide (Can)** *see* Furosemide *on page 940*
- **NovoSeven RT** *see* Factor VIIa (Recombinant) *on page 836*
- **Novo-Sorbide (Can)** *see* Isosorbide Dinitrate *on page 1124*
- **Novo-Sotalol (Can)** *see* Sotalol *on page 1927*
- **Novo-Sucralate (Can)** *see* Sucralfate *on page 1940*
- **Novo-Temazepam (Can)** *see* Temazepam *on page 1990*
- **Novo-Theophyl SR (Can)** *see* Theophylline *on page 2026*
- **Novo-Ticlopidine (Can)** *see* Ticlopidine *on page 2040*
- **Novo-Timol (Can)** *see* Timolol (Ophthalmic) *on page 2043*
- **Novo-Trazodone (Can)** *see* TraZODone *on page 2091*
- **Novo-Trifluzine (Can)** *see* Trifluoperazine *on page 2102*
- **Novo-Triptyn (Can)** *see* Amitriptyline *on page 119*
- **Novo-Valproic (Can)** *see* Valproic Acid and Derivatives *on page 2123*
- **Novo-Veramil (Can)** *see* Verapamil *on page 2154*
- **Novo-Veramil SR (Can)** *see* Verapamil *on page 2154*
- **Novo-Warfarin (Can)** *see* Warfarin *on page 2186*
- **Novoxapram® (Can)** *see* Oxazepam *on page 1532*
- **Novo-Zopiclone (Can)** *see* Zopiclone [CAN/INT] *on page 2217*
- **Noxafil** *see* Posaconazole *on page 1683*
- **Nozinan (Can)** *see* Methotrimeprazine [CAN/INT] *on page 1329*
- **NPH Insulin** *see* Insulin NPH *on page 1089*
- **NPH Insulin and Regular Insulin** *see* Insulin NPH and Insulin Regular *on page 1090*
- **Nplate** *see* RomiPLOStim *on page 1842*
- **NP Thyroid** *see* Thyroid, Desiccated *on page 2031*
- **NRP104** *see* Lisdexamfetamine *on page 1224*
- **NSC-14106** *see* Clofazimine [INT] *on page 473*
- **NTBC** *see* Nitisinone *on page 1461*
- **NTG** *see* Nitroglycerin *on page 1465*
- **NTP-Alprazolam (Can)** *see* ALPRAZolam *on page 94*
- **NTP-Amoxicillin (Can)** *see* Amoxicillin *on page 130*
- **NTP-Furosemide (Can)** *see* Furosemide *on page 940*
- ***N*-trifluoroacetyladriamycin-14-valerate** *see* Valrubicin *on page 2127*
- **NTZ** *see* Nitazoxanide *on page 1461*
- **Nu-Acebutolol (Can)** *see* Acebutolol *on page 29*
- **Nu-Acyclovir (Can)** *see* Acyclovir (Systemic) *on page 47*
- **Nu-Alpraz (Can)** *see* ALPRAZolam *on page 94*
- **Nu-Amoxi (Can)** *see* Amoxicillin *on page 130*
- **Nu-Ampi (Can)** *see* Ampicillin *on page 141*
- **Nuartez** *see* Artesunate *on page 178*
- **Nu-Atenol (Can)** *see* Atenolol *on page 189*
- **Nubain** *see* Nalbuphine *on page 1416*

- ◆ **Nu-Bromazepam (Can)** *see* Bromazepam [CAN/INT] *on page 290*
- ◆ **Nu-Carbamazepine (Can)** *see* CarBAMazepine *on page 346*
- ◆ **Nu-Cefaclor (Can)** *see* Cefaclor *on page 372*
- ◆ **Nu-Cimet (Can)** *see* Cimetidine *on page 438*
- ◆ **Nu-Cloxi (Can)** *see* Cloxacillin [CAN/INT] *on page 488*
- ◆ **Nu-COPD [OTC]** *see* Guaifenesin and Phenylephrine *on page 988*
- ◆ **NuCort** *see* Hydrocortisone (Topical) *on page 1014*
- ◆ **Nucynta** *see* Tapentadol *on page 1975*
- ◆ **Nucynta ER** *see* Tapentadol *on page 1975*
- ◆ **Nucynta IR (Can)** *see* Tapentadol *on page 1975*
- ◆ **Nu-Desipramine (Can)** *see* Desipramine *on page 593*
- ◆ **Nuedexta™** *see* Dextromethorphan and Quinidine *on page 611*
- ◆ **Nu-Erythromycin-S (Can)** *see* Erythromycin (Systemic) *on page 762*
- ◆ **Nu-Fluoxetine (Can)** *see* FLUoxetine *on page 899*
- ◆ **Nu-Flurprofen (Can)** *see* Flurbiprofen (Systemic) *on page 906*
- ◆ **Nu-Furosemide (Can)** *see* Furosemide *on page 940*
- ◆ **Nu-Gemfibrozil (Can)** *see* Gemfibrozil *on page 956*
- ◆ **Nu-Hydral (Can)** *see* HydrALAZINE *on page 1007*
- ◆ **Nu-Hydroxyzine (Can)** *see* HydrOXYzine *on page 1024*
- ◆ **Nu-Ipratropium (Can)** *see* Ipratropium (Systemic) *on page 1108*
- ◆ **Nu-Iron [OTC]** *see* Polysaccharide-Iron Complex *on page 1677*
- ◆ **Nu-Ketotifen® (Can)** *see* Ketotifen (Systemic) [CAN/INT] *on page 1149*
- ◆ **NuLev** *see* Hyoscyamine *on page 1026*
- ◆ **Nulojix** *see* Belatacept *on page 233*
- ◆ **NuLYTELY** *see* Polyethylene Glycol-Electrolyte Solution *on page 1674*
- ◆ **Nu-Metoclopramide (Can)** *see* Metoclopramide *on page 1345*
- ◆ **Nu-Metop (Can)** *see* Metoprolol *on page 1350*
- ◆ **Nu-Moclobemide (Can)** *see* Moclobemide [CAN/INT] *on page 1384*
- ◆ **Nu-Nizatidine (Can)** *see* Nizatidine *on page 1471*
- ◆ **Nu-Nortriptyline (Can)** *see* Nortriptyline *on page 1476*
- ◆ **Nu-Oxybutyn (Can)** *see* Oxybutynin *on page 1536*
- ◆ **Nu-Pen-VK (Can)** *see* Penicillin V Potassium *on page 1614*
- ◆ **Nu-Prazo (Can)** *see* Prazosin *on page 1703*
- ◆ **Nu-Prochlor (Can)** *see* Prochlorperazine *on page 1718*
- ◆ **Nu-Propranolol (Can)** *see* Propranolol *on page 1731*
- ◆ **Nuquin HP** *see* Hydroquinone *on page 1020*
- ◆ **Nu-Selegiline (Can)** *see* Selegiline *on page 1873*
- ◆ **Nu-Sotalol (Can)** *see* Sotalol *on page 1927*
- ◆ **Nu-Sucralate (Can)** *see* Sucralfate *on page 1940*
- ◆ **Nu-Terazosin (Can)** *see* Terazosin *on page 2001*
- ◆ **Nu-Tetra (Can)** *see* Tetracycline *on page 2017*
- ◆ **Nu-Ticlopidine (Can)** *see* Ticlopidine *on page 2040*
- ◆ **Nu-Timolol (Can)** *see* Timolol (Systemic) *on page 2042*
- ◆ **Nutracort** *see* Hydrocortisone (Topical) *on page 1014*
- ◆ **Nutraplus [OTC]** *see* Urea *on page 2114*
- ◆ **Nu-Trazodone (Can)** *see* TraZODone *on page 2091*
- ◆ **Nu-Trazodone D (Can)** *see* TraZODone *on page 2091*
- ◆ **Nutr-E-Sol [OTC]** *see* Vitamin E *on page 2174*
- ◆ **NutreStore** *see* Glutamine *on page 971*
- ◆ **Nutrilipid** *see* Fat Emulsion (Plant Based) *on page 848*
- ◆ **Nutropin [DSC]** *see* Somatropin *on page 1918*
- ◆ **Nutropin AQ NuSpin (Can)** *see* Somatropin *on page 1918*
- ◆ **Nutropin AQ NuSpin 5** *see* Somatropin *on page 1918*
- ◆ **Nutropin AQ NuSpin 10** *see* Somatropin *on page 1918*
- ◆ **Nutropin AQ NuSpin 20** *see* Somatropin *on page 1918*
- ◆ **Nutropin AQ Pen** *see* Somatropin *on page 1918*
- ◆ **NuvaRing®** *see* Ethinyl Estradiol and Etonogestrel *on page 802*
- ◆ **Nu-Verap (Can)** *see* Verapamil *on page 2154*
- ◆ **Nu-Verap SR (Can)** *see* Verapamil *on page 2154*
- ◆ **Nuvigil** *see* Armodafinil *on page 175*
- ◆ **NuZon [DSC]** *see* Hydrocortisone (Topical) *on page 1014*
- ◆ **NVA237** *see* Glycopyrrolate *on page 975*
- ◆ **NVP** *see* Nevirapine *on page 1440*
- ◆ **Nyaderm (Can)** *see* Nystatin (Topical) *on page 1482*
- ◆ **Nyamyc** *see* Nystatin (Topical) *on page 1482*
- ◆ **Nymalize** *see* NiMODipine *on page 1456*

Nystatin (Oral) (nye STAT in)

Brand Names: U.S. Bio-Statin
Brand Names: Canada PMS-Nystatin
Pharmacologic Category Antifungal Agent, Oral Nonabsorbed
Use Treatment of susceptible cutaneous, mucocutaneous, and oral cavity fungal infections normally caused by the *Candida* species
Pregnancy Risk Factor C
Dosage Oral:

Oral candidiasis:

Suspension:

Premature infants: 100,000 units 4 times/day; paint suspension into recesses of the mouth

Infants: 200,000 units 4 times/day or 100,000 units to each side of mouth 4 times/day; paint suspension into recesses of the mouth

Children and Adults: 400,000-600,000 units 4 times/day; swish in the mouth and retain for as long as possible (several minutes) before swallowing

Powder for compounding: Children and Adults: 1/8 teaspoon (500,000 units) to equal approximately 1/2 cup of water; give 4 times/day

Intestinal infections: Adults: 500,000-1,000,000 units every 8 hours

Dosage adjustment in renal impairment: No dosage adjustment provided in manufacturer's labeling.

Dosage adjustment in hepatic impairment: No dosage adjustment provided in manufacturer's labeling.

Additional Information Complete prescribing information should be consulted for additional detail.

Dosage Forms

Capsule, Oral [preservative free]:
Bio-Statin: 500,000 units, 1,000,000 units

Powder, Oral:
Bio-Statin: (1 ea)
Generic: (1 ea)

Suspension, Mouth/Throat:
Generic: 100,000 units/mL (5 mL, 60 mL, 473 mL, 480 mL)

Tablet, Oral:
Generic: 500,000 units

Nystatin (Topical) (nye STAT in)

Brand Names: U.S. Nyamyc; Nystop; Pedi-Dri [DSC]; Pediaderm AF Complete

Brand Names: Canada Candistatin; Nyaderm

Pharmacologic Category Antifungal Agent, Topical

Use Treatment of susceptible cutaneous and mucocutaneous fungal infections normally caused by the *Candida* species

Pregnancy Risk Factor C

Dosage Mucocutaneous infections: Children and Adults: Topical: Apply 2-3 times/day to affected areas; very moist topical lesions are treated best with powder

Additional Information Complete prescribing information should be consulted for additional detail.

Dosage Forms

Cream, External:

Generic: 100,000 units/g (15 g, 30 g)

Kit, External:

Pediaderm AF Complete: 100,000 units/g

Ointment, External:

Generic: 100,000 units/g (15 g, 30 g)

Powder, External:

Nyamyc: 100,000 units/g (15 g, 30 g, 60 g)

Nystop: 100,000 units/g (15 g, 30 g, 60 g)

Generic: 100,000 units/g (15 g, 30 g, 60 g)

◆ **Nystatin and Metronidazole** *see* Metronidazole and Nystatin [CAN/INT] *on page 1358*

Nystatin and Triamcinolone

(nye STAT in & trye am SIN oh lone)

Index Terms Triamcinolone and Nystatin

Pharmacologic Category Antifungal Agent, Topical; Corticosteroid, Topical

Use Treatment of cutaneous candidiasis

Pregnancy Risk Factor C

Dosage Children and Adults: Topical: Apply sparingly to affected area(s) twice daily. Therapy should be discontinued when control is achieved or if symptoms persist for >25 days of therapy.

Additional Information Complete prescribing information should be consulted for additional detail.

Dosage Forms

Cream: Nystatin 100,000 units and triamcinolone 0.1% (15 g, 30 g, 60 g)

Ointment: Nystatin 100,000 units and triamcinolone 0.1% (15 g, 30 g, 60 g)

◆ **Nystop** *see* Nystatin (Topical) *on page 1482*

◆ **Nytol [OTC]** *see* DiphenhydrAMINE (Systemic) *on page 641*

◆ **Nytol (Can)** *see* DiphenhydrAMINE (Systemic) *on page 641*

◆ **Nytol Extra Strength (Can)** *see* DiphenhydrAMINE (Systemic) *on page 641*

◆ **Nytol Maximum Strength [OTC]** *see* DiphenhydrAMINE (Systemic) *on page 641*

Obinutuzumab (oh bi nue TOOZ ue mab)

Brand Names: U.S. Gazyva

Brand Names: Canada Gazyva

Index Terms GA101; R05072759; R7159

Pharmacologic Category Antineoplastic Agent, Anti-CD20; Antineoplastic Agent, Monoclonal Antibody

Use Chronic lymphocytic leukemia: Treatment of patients with previously untreated chronic lymphocytic leukemia (CLL) in combination with chlorambucil

Pregnancy Risk Factor C

Pregnancy Considerations Teratogenic effects were not observed in animal reproduction studies. However based on animal data, if exposure occurs during pregnancy, B-cell counts and immunologic function may be affected in the neonate after birth. The U.S. labeling recommends that women of child bearing potential use effective contraception during therapy and for 12 months after treatment. The Canadian labeling recommends that women of child bearing potential use effective contraception during therapy and for 18 months after the last treatment.

Breast-Feeding Considerations It is not known if obinutuzumab is excreted into breast milk. However, human immunoglobulin can be detected in milk. Due to the potential for serious adverse reactions in the nursing infant, the U.S. labeling recommends a decision be made to discontinue nursing or to discontinue the drug, taking into account the importance of treatment to the mother. The Canadian labeling recommends discontinuing nursing during therapy and for 18 months after the last treatment.

Contraindications

U.S. labeling: There are no contraindications listed in the manufacturer's labeling.

Canadian labeling: Known hypersensitivity (IgE mediated) to obinutuzumab or any component of the formulation.

Warnings/Precautions [U.S. Boxed Warning]: Hepatitis B virus (HBV) reactivation may occur with use of CD20-directed cytolytic antibodies (including obinutuzumab) and may result in fulminant hepatitis, hepatic failure, and death. Screen all patients for HBV infection by measuring hepatitis B surface antigen (HBsAg) and hepatitis B core antibody (anti-HBc) prior to therapy initiation; monitor patients for clinical and laboratory signs of hepatitis or HBV during and for several months after treatment. Discontinue obinutuzumab (and concomitant chemotherapy) if viral hepatitis develops and initiate appropriate antiviral therapy. Reactivation has occurred in patients who are HBsAg positive as well as in those who are HBsAg negative but are anti-HBc positive; HBV reactivation has also been observed in patients who had previously resolved HBV infection. HBV reactivation has been reported for other CD20-directed antibodies after therapy discontinuation. Reactivation of HBV replication is often followed by hepatitis. Use cautiously in patients who show evidence of prior HBV infection (eg, HBsAg positive [regardless of antibody status] or HBsAG negative but anti-HBc positive); consult with appropriate clinicians regarding monitoring and consideration of antiviral therapy before and/or during obinutuzumab treatment. The safety of resuming obinutuzumab treatment following HBV reactivation is not known; discuss reinitiation of therapy in patients with resolved HBV reactivation with physicians experienced in HBV management. **[U.S. Boxed Warning]: Progressive multifocal leukoencephalopathy (PML) resulting in death may occur with treatment.** PML is due to JC virus infection. Consider PML in any patient with new onset or worsening neurological symptoms and if PML is suspected, discontinue obinutuzumab (consider discontinuation or dose reduction of any concomitant chemotherapy or immunosuppressive therapy) and evaluate promptly.

May cause severe and life-threatening infusion reactions; reactions may include bronchospasm, dyspnea, tachycardia, larynx and throat irritation, wheezing, laryngeal edema, flushing, hypertension, hypotension, fever, nausea, vomiting, diarrhea, headache and/or chills. Infusion reactions occur more frequently with the first 1,000 mg infused. Delayed reactions (up to 24 hours later) and reactions with subsequent infusions have occurred. Premedicate with acetaminophen, an antihistamine, and a glucocorticoid prior to infusion; may require rate reduction, interruption of therapy, or treatment discontinuation.

Monitor during the entire infusion; monitor patients with preexisting cardiac or pulmonary conditions closely. Due to the risk for hypotension, consider temporarily withholding antihypertensive therapies for 12 hours prior to, during, and for 1 hour after administration. Administer in a facility with immediate access to resuscitative measures (eg, glucocorticoids, epinephrine, bronchodilators, and/or oxygen). Serious cardiovascular events (some fatal) have been reported.

In clinical trials, grade 3 and 4 neutropenia and thrombocytopenia occurred when used in combination with chlorambucil. Neutropenia may have a late onset (>28 days after therapy completion) and/or be prolonged (duration >28 days). Monitor for signs/symptoms of infection; antimicrobial prophylaxis is recommended in neutropenic patients. Antiviral and/or antifungal prophylaxis may also be considered. In a small percentage of patients, thrombocytopenia occurred acutely (within 24 hours) after obinutuzumab administration; platelet transfusions may be necessary. Fatal hemorrhagic events during the first cycle have been reported; monitor frequently for thrombocytopenia and bleeding episodes, particularly during the initial cycle. Thrombocytopenia may require dose delays of obinutuzumab and chlorambucil and/or dose reductions of chlorambucil. Consider withholding platelet inhibitors, anticoagulants, or other medications which may increase bleeding risk (especially during the first cycle). Leukopenia and lymphopenia commonly occur. Monitor blood counts frequently throughout therapy. Bacterial, fungal, and new or reactivated viral infections may occur during and/or following therapy; fatal infections have been reported. Do not administer to patients with an active infection. Patients with a history of recurrent or chronic infections may be at increased risk. Tumor lysis syndrome may occur within 12 to 24 hours following the first dose. Acute renal failure, hyperkalemia, hypocalcemia, hyperuricemia, and/or hyperphosphatemia may occur. Administer prophylaxis (antihyperuricemic therapy, hydration) in patients at high risk (high numbers of circulating malignant cells ≥25,000/mm^3 or high tumor burden). Correct electrolyte abnormalities; monitor renal function and hydration status. Administration of live virus vaccines during treatment (and until B-cell recovery) is not recommended; the safety and efficacy of immunization with live or attenuated viral vaccines during or after obinutuzumab therapy has not been determined. If obinutuzumab exposure occurs during pregnancy, the safety and timing of live virus vaccinations for the infant should be evaluated. Potentially significant drug-drug interactions may exist, requiring dose or frequency adjustment, additional monitoring, and/or selection of alternative therapy.

Adverse Reactions Adverse reactions reported in combination with chlorambucil.

Cardiovascular: Exacerbation of cardiac disease

Central nervous system: Progressive multifocal leukoencephalopathy

Endocrine & metabolic: Hyperkalemia, hypoalbuminemia, hypocalcemia, hypokalemia, hyponatremia

Hematologic & oncologic: Anemia, leukopenia, lymphocytopenia, neutropenia, thrombocytopenia, tumor lysis syndrome

Hepatic: Increased serum alkaline phosphatase, increased serum ALT, increased serum AST

Immunologic: Antibody development

Infection: Infection, reactivation of HBV

Neuromuscular & skeletal: Musculoskeletal signs and symptoms

Renal: Increased serum creatinine

Respiratory: Cough

Miscellaneous: Fever, infusion related reaction

Drug Interactions

Metabolism/Transport Effects None known.

Avoid Concomitant Use

Avoid concomitant use of Obinutuzumab with any of the following: BCG; Belimumab; CloZAPine; Dipyrone; Natalizumab; Pimecrolimus; Tacrolimus (Topical); Tofacitinib; Vaccines (Live)

Increased Effect/Toxicity

Obinutuzumab may increase the levels/effects of: Belimumab; CloZAPine; Leflunomide; Natalizumab; Tofacitinib; Vaccines (Live)

The levels/effects of Obinutuzumab may be increased by: Agents with Antiplatelet Properties; Anticoagulants; Antihypertensives; Denosumab; Dipyrone; Pimecrolimus; Roflumilast; Tacrolimus (Topical); Trastuzumab

Decreased Effect

Obinutuzumab may decrease the levels/effects of: BCG; Coccidioides immitis Skin Test; Sipuleucel-T; Vaccines (Inactivated); Vaccines (Live)

The levels/effects of Obinutuzumab may be decreased by: Echinacea

Preparation for Administration

Cycle 1, day 1 and 2 doses (100 mg and 900 mg, respectively): Withdraw 40 mL of obinutuzumab solution from vial. Dilute 4 mL into a 100 mL infusion bag of NS (100 mg dose; use immediately). Dilute remaining 36 mL into a 250 mL NS infusion bag (900 mg dose, for use on day 2); store at 2°C to 8°C (36°F to 46°F) for up to 24 hours; use immediately after reaching room temperature. Gently invert to mix; do not shake or freeze.

Cycle 1 (day 8 and 15 doses) and cycles 2 through 6 (1000 mg): Withdraw 40 mL of obinutuzumab solution from vial. Dilute into a 250 mL NS infusion bag. Gently invert to mix; do not shake or freeze.

Do not use other diluents (eg, dextrose) to prepare the infusion. Final concentration for administration should be 0.4 to 4 mg/mL. May use PVC or non-PVC infusion bags.

Storage/Stability Store intact vials at 2°C to 8°C (36°F to 46°F); do not freeze or shake. Protect from light. Diluted solutions for infusion should be used immediately. If not used immediately, the diluted solutions may be stored up to 24 hours at 2°C to 8°C (36°F to 46°F) followed by 48 hours (including infusion time) at room temperature of ≤30°C (≤86°F).

Mechanism of Action Obinutuzumab is a glycoengineered type II anti-CD20 monoclonal antibody. The CD20 antigen is expressed on the surface of pre B- and mature B-lymphocytes; upon binding to CD20, obinutuzumab activates complement-dependent cytotoxicity, antibody-dependent cellular cytotoxicity and antibody-dependent cellular phagocytosis, resulting in cell death (Sehn, 2012).

Pharmacodynamics/Kinetics

Distribution: V_d: ~3.9 L

Half-life elimination: ~29.7 days

Dosage Note: Premedication with acetaminophen, an antihistamine, and a glucocorticoid 30 to 60 minutes prior to treatment may be necessary (see Administration). Antihyperuricemic prophylaxis and adequate hydration are recommended for patients with a high tumor burden and/or high circulating absolute lymphocyte count. Antimicrobial, antiviral, and antifungal prophylaxis may be considered in certain patients.

Chronic lymphocytic leukemia (CLL): Adults: IV:

Cycle 1: 100 mg on day 1, followed by 900 mg on day 2, followed by 1000 mg weekly for 2 doses (days 8 and 15)

Cycles 2 through 6: 1000 mg on day 1 every 28 days for 5 doses

Missed doses: Administer the missed dose as soon as possible; adjust dosing schedule accordingly. In some cases, patients who do not complete the day 1 cycle 1 dose may proceed to the day 2 cycle 1 treatment (if appropriate).

Dosage adjustment for toxicity:

Hematologic: Grade 3 or 4 cytopenias: Consider treatment interruption

Infusion reactions:

Mild-to-moderate (Grades 1 and 2): Reduce infusion rate or interrupt infusion and manage symptoms as appropriate. Upon symptom resolution, continue or resume infusion. If no further infusion reaction symptoms occur, may resume infusion rate escalation as appropriate for the treatment cycle dose. Day 1 (cycle 1) infusion rate may be increased back up to a maximum of 25 mg/hour after 1 hour.

Severe (Grade 3): Interrupt therapy; manage symptoms as appropriate. Upon symptom resolution, may reinitiate infusion at no more than 50% of the rate at which the reaction occurred. If no further infusion reaction symptoms occur, may resume infusion rate escalation as appropriate for the treatment cycle dose. Day 1 (cycle 1) infusion rate may be increased back up to a maximum of 25 mg/hour after 1 hour. Permanently discontinue if ≥ grade 3 toxicity occurs upon rechallenge.

Life-threatening (Grade 4): Discontinue infusion immediately; permanently discontinue therapy.

Infection: Consider treatment interruption.

Other toxicity: Consider treatment interruption for ≥ grade 2 nonhematologic toxicity.

Dosage adjustment for renal impairment:

CrCl ≥30 mL/minute: There are no dosage adjustments provided in the U.S. manufacturer's labeling; however, pharmacokinetics are not affected (based on pharmacokinetic analysis). The Canadian labeling recommends that no dosage adjustment is necessary.

CrCl <30 mL/minute: There are no dosage adjustments provided in the manufacturer's labeling (has not been studied).

Dosage adjustment for hepatic impairment: There are no dosage adjustments provided in the manufacturer's labeling (has not been studied).

Administration For IV infusion only. Do not administer IV push or as a bolus. Premedication with acetaminophen, an antihistamine, and a glucocorticoid (eg, dexamethasone or methylprednisolone) may be required (see below). Do not mix with or infuse with other medications. May use PVC or non-PVC administration sets.

Premedication:

Cycle 1 (days 1 and 2): All patients should receive acetaminophen (650 to 1000 mg) and an antihistamine (eg, diphenhydramine 50 mg) at least 30 minutes prior to infusion. In addition, an IV glucocorticoid (eg, dexamethasone 20 mg or methylprednisolone 80 mg) should be administered at least 1 hour prior to infusion.

Cycle 1 (days 8 and 15), and cycles 2 through 6: All patients should receive acetaminophen 650 to 1000 mg at least 30 minutes prior to infusion.

If patients experienced grade 1 or higher infusion-related reaction with previous infusion: Administer an antihistamine (eg, diphenhydramine 50 mg) in addition to acetaminophen at least 30 minutes prior to infusion.

If patients experienced a grade 3 infusion-related reaction with previous infusion **or** have a lymphocyte count >25,000 cells/mm^3 prior to next treatment: Administer an IV glucocorticoid (eg, dexamethasone 20 mg or methylprednisolone 80 mg) at least 1 hour prior to infusion, in addition to acetaminophen and an antihistamine at least 30 minutes prior to infusion.

Infusion rate:

Cycle 1 (day 1): Infuse at 25 mg/hour over 4 hours; do not increase the infusion rate

Cycle 1 (day 2): If no reaction to previous infusion, initiate infusion at 50 mg/hour for 30 minutes; if tolerated, may escalate rate in increments of 50 mg/hour every 30 minutes to a maximum rate of 400 mg/hour.

Cycle 1 (days 8 and 15), and cycles 2 through 6: If no reaction to previous infusion, initiate infusion at 100 mg/hour for 30 minutes; if tolerated, may escalate infusion rate in increments of 100 mg/hour every 30 minutes to a maximum rate of 400 mg/hour.

Monitoring Parameters CBC with differential (at regular intervals), hepatitis B screening in all patients (HBsAG and anti-HBc measurements) prior to therapy initiation; renal function, electrolytes; signs of active hepatitis B infection (during and for several months after therapy completion); signs or symptoms of infusion reaction; signs of infection; fluid status; signs/symptoms of progressive multifocal leukoencephalopathy (PML; focal neurologic deficits, which may present as hemiparesis, visual field deficits, cognitive impairment, aphasia, ataxia, and/or cranial nerve deficits); evaluate for PML with brain MRI, lumbar puncture, and neurologist consultation.

Dosage Forms

Solution, Intravenous [preservative free]:

Gazyva: 1000 mg/40 mL (40 mL)

◆ **Obizur** *see* Antihemophilic Factor (Recombinant [Porcine Sequence]) *on page 153*

◆ **OCBZ** *see* OXcarbazepine *on page 1532*

◆ **Ocean Complete Sinus Rinse [OTC]** *see* Sodium Chloride *on page 1902*

◆ **Ocean for Kids [OTC]** *see* Sodium Chloride *on page 1902*

◆ **Oceanic Selenium [OTC]** *see* Selenium *on page 1876*

◆ **Ocean Nasal Spray [OTC]** *see* Sodium Chloride *on page 1902*

◆ **Ocean Ultra Saline Mist [OTC]** *see* Sodium Chloride *on page 1902*

◆ **Ocella** *see* Ethinyl Estradiol and Drospirenone *on page 801*

◆ **Ocphyl (Can)** *see* Octreotide *on page 1485*

Ocriplasmin (ok ri PLAZ min)

Brand Names: U.S. Jetrea

Brand Names: Canada Jetrea

Pharmacologic Category Ophthalmic Agent; Vitreolytic

Use Vitreomacular adhesion: Treatment of symptomatic vitreomacular adhesion (VMA)

Pregnancy Risk Factor C

Dosage Vitreomacular adhesion: Adults: Intravitreal: 0.125 mg once (as a single dose to the affected eye)

Dosage adjustment in renal impairment: There are no dosage adjustments provided in the manufacturer's labeling. However, dosage adjustment unlikely due to low systemic absorption.

Dosage adjustment in hepatic impairment: There are no dosage adjustments provided in the manufacturer's labeling. However, dosage adjustment unlikely due to low systemic absorption.

Additional Information Complete prescribing information should be consulted for additional detail.

Dosage Forms

Solution, Intraocular [preservative free]:

Jetrea: 0.5 mg/0.2 mL (0.2 mL)

◆ **Octacog Alfa** *see* Antihemophilic Factor (Recombinant) *on page 152*

◆ **Octagam** *see* Immune Globulin *on page 1056*

◆ **Octagam 10%** *see* Immune Globulin *on page 1056*

◆ **Octaplex (Can)** *see* Prothrombin Complex Concentrate (Human) [(Factors II, VII, IX, X), Protein C, and Protein S] *on page 1738*

◆ **Octostim (Can)** *see* Desmopressin *on page 594*

Octreotide (ok TREE oh tide)

Brand Names: U.S. SandoSTATIN; SandoSTATIN LAR Depot

Brand Names: Canada Ocphyl; Octreotide Acetate Omega; Octreotide Injection; Sandostatin; Sandostatin LAR

Index Terms Longastatin; Octreotide Acetate

Pharmacologic Category Antidiarrheal; Antidote; Somatostatin Analog

Use Control of symptoms (diarrhea and flushing) in patients with metastatic carcinoid tumors; treatment of watery diarrhea associated with vasoactive intestinal peptide-secreting tumors (VIPomas); treatment of acromegaly

Pregnancy Risk Factor B

Pregnancy Considerations Adverse effects were not observed in animal reproduction studies. Octreotide crosses the placenta and can be detected in the newborn at delivery (Caron, 1995; Fassnacht, 2001; Maffei, 2010); data concerning use in pregnancy is limited. In case reports of acromegalic women who received normal doses of octreotide during pregnancy, no congenital malformations were reported. Because normalization of IGF-1 and GH may restore fertility in women with acromegaly, women of childbearing potential should use adequate contraception during treatment. Long-acting formulations should be discontinued 2 to 3 months prior to a planned pregnancy when possible; however, octreotide therapy may be resumed in pregnant women with worsening symptoms if needed (Katznelson, 2011).

Breast-Feeding Considerations Octreotide is excreted in breast milk. In a case report, a woman was taking octreotide SubQ in doses up to 2400 mcg/day prior to and throughout pregnancy. Octreotide was measurable in the colostrum in concentrations similar to those in the maternal serum (Maffei, 2010); however, oral absorption of octreotide is considered to be poor (Battershill, 1989). The manufacturer recommends that caution be exercised when administering octreotide to nursing women.

Contraindications Hypersensitivity to octreotide or any component of the formulation

Warnings/Precautions May impair gallbladder function; monitor patients for cholelithiasis. The incidence of gallbladder stone or biliary sludge increases with a duration of therapy of ≥12 months. In patients with neuroendocrine tumors, the NCCN guidelines (v.1.2011) recommend considering prophylactic cholecystectomy in patients undergoing abdominal surgery if octreotide treatment is planned. Use with caution in patients with renal and/or hepatic impairment; dosage adjustment may be required in patients receiving dialysis and in patients with established cirrhosis. Somatostatin analogs may affect glucose regulation. In type I diabetes, severe hypoglycemia may occur; in type II diabetes or patients without diabetes, hyperglycemia may occur. Insulin and other hypoglycemic medication requirements may change. Octreotide may worsen hypoglycemia in patients with insulinomas; use with caution. Do not use depot formulation for the treatment of sulfonylurea-induced hypoglycemia. Bradycardia, conduction abnormalities, and arrhythmia have been observed in acromegalic and carcinoid syndrome patients; use caution with CHF or concomitant medications that alter heart rate or rhythm. Cardiovascular medication requirements may change. Octreotide may enhance the adverse/toxic effects of other QTc-prolonging agents. May alter absorption of dietary fats; monitor for pancreatitis. May reduce excessive fluid loss in patients with conditions that cause such loss; monitor for elevations in zinc levels in such patients that are maintained on total parenteral nutrition (TPN). Chronic treatment has been associated with abnormal Schillings test; monitor vitamin B_{12} levels. Suppresses secretion of TSH; monitor for hypothyroidism.

Postmarketing cases of serious and fatal events, including hypoxia and necrotizing enterocolitis, have been reported with octreotide use in children (usually with serious underlying conditions), particularly in children <2 years of age. In studies with octreotide depot, the incidence of cholelithiasis in children is higher than the reported incidences for adults and efficacy was not demonstrated. Therapy may restore fertility; females of childbearing potential should use adequate contraception. Dosage adjustment may be necessary in the elderly; significant increases in elimination half-life have been observed in older adults. Vehicle used in depot injection (polylactide-co-glycolide microspheres) has rarely been associated with retinal artery occlusion in patients with abnormal arteriovenous anastomosis.

Adverse Reactions Adverse reactions vary by route of administration or dosage form.

Cardiovascular: Angina, arrhythmia, cardiac failure, chest pain (non-depot formulations), conduction abnormalities, edema, flushing, hematoma, hypertension, palpitation, peripheral edema, phlebitis, sinus bradycardia

Central nervous system: Abnormal gait, amnesia, anxiety, confusion, depression, dizziness, dysphonia, fatigue, fever, hallucinations, headache, hypoesthesia, insomnia, malaise, nervousness, neuralgia, neuropathy, pain, somnolence, tremor, vertigo

Dermatologic: Acne, alopecia, bruising, cellulitis, pruritus, rash (depot formulation)

Endocrine & metabolic: Breast pain, cachexia, goiter (non-depot formulations), gout, hyper-/hypoglycemia, hypokalemia, hypoproteinemia, hypothyroidism (non-depot formulations), impotence

Gastrointestinal: Abdominal pain, anorexia, biliary duct dilatation, biliary sludge (length of therapy dependent), cholelithiasis (length of therapy dependent), colitis, constipation, cramping, dehydration, diarrhea, diverticulitis, dyspepsia, dysphagia, fat malabsorption, feces discoloration, flatulence, gastritis, gastroenteritis, gingivitis, glossitis, loose stools, melena, nausea, steatorrhea, stomatitis, taste perversion, tenesmus, vomiting, xerostomia

Genitourinary: Incontinence, pollakiuria (non-depot formulations), urinary tract infection

Hematologic: Anemia (more common with depot formulations)

Local: Injection site hematoma/pain (dose and formulation related)

Neuromuscular & skeletal: Arthralgia, arthropathy, back pain, hyperkinesia, hypertonia, joint pain, myalgia, neuropathy, paresthesia, rigors, tremor, weakness

Ocular: Blurred vision, visual disturbance

Otic: Earache, tinnitus

Renal: Albuminuria, renal abscess, renal calculus

Respiratory: Bronchitis, cough, dyspnea (non-depot formulations), epistaxis, pharyngitis, rhinitis, sinusitis, upper respiratory infection

Miscellaneous: Allergy, antibodies to octreotide, bacterial infection, cold symptoms, diaphoresis, flu symptoms, moniliasis

Rare but important or life-threatening: Amenorrhea, anaphylactic shock, anaphylactoid reactions, aneurysm, aphasia, appendicitis, arthritis, ascending cholangitis, ascites, atrial fibrillation, basal cell carcinoma, Bell's palsy, biliary obstruction, breast carcinoma, cardiac arrest, cerebral vascular disorder, CHF, cholecystitis, cholestatic hepatitis, CK increased, deafness, diabetes insipidus, diabetes mellitus, fatty liver, galactorrhea, gallbladder polyp, GI bleeding, GI hemorrhage, GI ulcer, glaucoma, gynecomastia, hematuria, hepatitis, hypoadrenalism, hypoxia (children), intestinal obstruction, intracranial hemorrhage, intraocular pressure increased, ischemia, joint effusion, malignant hyperpyrexia, MI, migraine, necrotizing enterocolitis (neonates), nephrolithiasis, neuritis, oligomenorrhea, orthostatic hypotension, pancreatitis, pancytopenia, paresis, pituitary apoplexy, pleural effusion, pneumonia, pneumothorax, polymenorrhea, pulmonary embolism, pulmonary hypertension, pulmonary nodule, Raynaud's syndrome, renal failure, renal insufficiency, retinal vein thrombosis, seizures, status asthmaticus, suicide attempt, syncope, tachycardia, thrombocytopenia, thrombophlebitis, thrombosis, weight loss

Drug Interactions

Metabolism/Transport Effects None known.

Avoid Concomitant Use

Avoid concomitant use of Octreotide with any of the following: Ceritinib

Increased Effect/Toxicity

Octreotide may increase the levels/effects of: Bradycardia-Causing Agents; Bromocriptine; Ceritinib; Codeine; Highest Risk QTc-Prolonging Agents; Hypoglycemic Agents; Lacosamide; Moderate Risk QTc-Prolonging Agents; Pegvisomant

The levels/effects of Octreotide may be increased by: Bretylium; Herbs (Hypoglycemic Properties); MAO Inhibitors; Mifepristone; Salicylates; Selective Serotonin Reuptake Inhibitors; SGLT2 Inhibitors; Tofacitinib

Decreased Effect

Octreotide may decrease the levels/effects of: CycloSPORINE (Systemic)

The levels/effects of Octreotide may be decreased by: Loop Diuretics

Food Interactions Octreotide may alter absorption of dietary fats. Management: Administer injections between meals to decrease GI effects.

Storage/Stability

Solution: Octreotide is a clear solution and should be stored at refrigerated temperatures between 2°C and 8°C (36°F and 46°F). Protect from light. May be stored at room temperature of 20°C to 30°C (68°F and 86°F) for up to 14 days when protected from light. Stable as a parenteral admixture in NS for 96 hours at room temperature (25°C) and in D_5W for 24 hours. Stable for up to 7 days in a polypropylene syringe. Discard multidose vials within 14 days after initial entry.

Suspension: Prior to dilution, store at refrigerated temperatures between 2°C and 8°C (36°F and 46°F). Protect from light. Additionally, the manufacturer reports that octreotide suspension may be stored at room temperature of 20°C to 25°C (68°F and 77°F) for up to 10 days when protected from light (data on file [Novartis, 2011]). Depot drug product kit may be at room temperature for 30 to 60 minutes prior to use. Use suspension immediately after preparation.

Mechanism of Action Mimics natural somatostatin by inhibiting serotonin release, and the secretion of gastrin, VIP, insulin, glucagon, secretin, motilin, and pancreatic polypeptide. Decreases growth hormone and IGF-1 in acromegaly. Octreotide provides more potent inhibition of growth hormone, glucagon, and insulin as compared to endogenous somatostatin. Also suppresses LH response to GnRH, secretion of thyroid-stimulating hormone and decreases splanchnic blood flow.

Pharmacodynamics/Kinetics

Duration: SubQ: 6 to 12 hours

Absorption: SubQ: Rapid and complete; IM (depot formulation): Released slowly (via microsphere degradation in the muscle)

Distribution: V_d: 14 L (13 to 30 L in acromegaly)

Protein binding: 65%, primarily to lipoprotein (41% in acromegaly)

Metabolism: Extensively hepatic

Bioavailability: SubQ: 100%; IM: 60% to 63% of SubQ dose

Half-life elimination: 1.7 to 1.9 hours; Increased in elderly patients; Cirrhosis: Up to 3.7 hours; Fatty liver disease: Up to 3.4 hours; Renal impairment: Up to 3.1 hours

Time to peak, plasma: SubQ: 0.4 hours (0.7 hours acromegaly); IM: 1 hour

Excretion: Urine (32% as unchanged drug)

Dosage

Acromegaly: Adults:

SubQ, IV: Initial: 50 mcg 3 times/day; titrate to achieve growth hormone levels <5 ng/mL or IGF-I (somatomedin C) levels <1.9 units/mL in males and <2.2 units/mL in females. Usual effective dose 100 to 200 mcg 3 times/day; range: 300 to 1500 mcg/day. **Note:** Should be withdrawn yearly for a 4-week interval (8 weeks for depot injection) in patients who have received irradiation. Resume if levels increase and signs/symptoms recur.

IM depot injection: Patients must be stabilized on subcutaneous octreotide for at least 2 weeks before switching to the long-acting depot. Upon switch: 20 mg IM intragluteally every 4 weeks for 3 months, then the dose may be modified based upon response.

Dosage adjustment for acromegaly: After 3 months of depot injections, the dosage may be continued or modified as follows:

GH ≤1 ng/mL, IGF-1 normal, and symptoms controlled: Reduce octreotide depot to 10 mg IM every 4 weeks

GH ≤2.5 ng/mL, IGF-1 normal, and symptoms controlled: Maintain octreotide depot at 20 mg IM every 4 weeks

GH >2.5 ng/mL, IGF-1 elevated, and/or symptoms uncontrolled: Increase octreotide depot to 30 mg IM every 4 weeks

Note: Patients not adequately controlled at a dose of 30 mg may increase dose to 40 mg every 4 weeks. Dosages >40 mg are not recommended.

Carcinoid tumors: Adults:

Manufacturer labeling:

SubQ, IV: Initial 2 weeks: 100 to 600 mcg/day in 2 to 4 divided doses; usual range: 50 to 750 mcg/day (some patients may require up to 1500 mcg/day)

IM depot injection: Patients must be stabilized on subcutaneous octreotide for at least 2 weeks before switching to the long-acting depot. Upon switch: 20 mg IM intragluteally every 4 weeks for 2 months, then the dose may be modified based upon response.

NCCN guidelines (Neuroendocrine Tumor, v.1.2011):

SubQ: 150 to 250 mcg 3 times/day; dose and frequency may be increased if needed for symptom control

IM depot injection: 20 to 30 mg every 4 weeks; dose and frequency may be increased if needed for symptom control; SubQ octreotide may be used for breakthrough symptoms

Note: Patients should continue to receive their SubQ injections for the first 2 weeks at the same dose in order to maintain therapeutic levels (some patients may require 3 to 4 weeks of continued SubQ injections). Patients who experience periodic exacerbations of symptoms may require temporary SubQ injections in addition to depot injections (at their previous SubQ dosing regimen) until symptoms have resolved.

Dosage adjustment for carcinoid tumors: After 2 months of depot injections, the dosage may be continued or modified as follows:

Increase to 30 mg IM every 4 weeks if symptoms are inadequately controlled

Decrease to 10 mg IM every 4 weeks, for a trial period, if initially responsive to 20 mg dose

Dosage >30 mg is not recommended

VIPomas:

Manufacturer labeling:

SubQ, IV: Initial 2 weeks: 200 to 300 mcg/day in 2 to 4 divided doses; titrate dose based on response/tolerance. Range: 150 to 750 mcg/day (doses >450 mcg/day are rarely required)

IM depot injection: Patients must be stabilized on subcutaneous octreotide for at least 2 weeks before switching to the long-acting depot. Upon switch: 20 mg IM intragluteally every 4 weeks for 2 months, then the dose may be modified based upon response.

NCCN guidelines (Neuroendocrine Tumor, v.1.2011):

SubQ: 150 to 250 mcg 3 times/day; dose and frequency may be increased if needed for symptom control

IM depot injection: 20 to 30 mg every 4 weeks dose and frequency may be increased if needed for symptom control; SubQ octreotide may be used for breakthrough symptoms

Note: Patients receiving depot injection should continue to receive their SubQ injections for the first 2 weeks at the same dose in order to maintain therapeutic levels (some patients may require 3 to 4 weeks of continued SubQ injections). Patients who experience periodic exacerbations of symptoms may require temporary SubQ injections in addition to depot injections (at their previous SubQ dosing regimen) until symptoms have resolved.

Dosage adjustment for VIPomas: After 2 months of depot injections, the dosage may be continued or modified as follows:

Increase to 30 mg IM every 4 weeks if symptoms are inadequately controlled

Decrease to 10 mg IM every 4 weeks, for a trial period, if initially responsive to 20 mg dose

Dosage >30 mg is not recommended

Congenital hyperinsulinism (off-label use): Infants and Children: SubQ: Initial: 2 to 10 mcg/kg/day; up to 40 mcg/kg/day have been used (Stanley, 1997)

Diarrhea (off-label use):

Infants and Children: IV, SubQ: Doses of 1 to 10 mcg/kg every 12 hours have been used in children beginning at the low end of the range and increasing by 0.3 mcg/kg/dose at 3-day intervals. Suppression of growth hormone (animal data) is of concern when used as long-term therapy.

Adults: IV: Initial: 50 to 100 mcg every 8 hours; increase by 100 mcg/dose at 48-hour intervals; maximum dose: 500 mcg every 8 hours

Diarrhea associated with chemotherapy (off-label use):

Low grade or uncomplicated: SubQ: 100 to 150 mcg every 8 hours (Benson, 2004; Kornblau, 2000)

Severe: Initial: SubQ: 100 to 150 mcg every 8 hours; may increase to 500 to 1500 mcg IV or SubQ every 8 hours (Kornblau, 2000)

Complicated: IV, SubQ: Initial: 100 to 150 mcg 3 times/day or IV Infusion: 25 to 50 mcg/hour; may escalate to 500 mcg 3 times/day until controlled (Benson, 2004)

Diarrhea associated with GVHD (off-label use): IV: 500 mcg every 8 hours; discontinue within 24 hours of resolution; Maximum duration of therapy if diarrhea is not resolved: 7 days (Kornblau, 2000)

Esophageal varices bleeding (off-label use): Adults: IV bolus: 25 to 100 mcg (usual bolus dose: 50 mcg) followed by continuous IV infusion of 25 to 50 mcg/hour for 2 to 5 days; may repeat bolus in first hour if hemorrhage not controlled (Corley, 2001; Erstad, 2001; Garcia-Tsao, 2010)

Islet cell tumors (off-label use): SubQ: 150 to 250 mcg 3 times/day or IM (depot): 20 to 30 mg every 4 weeks dose and frequency may be increased if needed for symptom control; SubQ octreotide may be used for breakthrough symptoms (NCCN Neuroendocrine Tumor guidelines v.1.2011)

Malignant bowel obstruction (off-label use):

SubQ: 100 to 300 mcg 2 to 3 times/day (Mercadante, 2007; NCCN Palliative Care guidelines v.2.2011)

Continuous SubQ/IV infusion: 10 to 40 mcg/hour (NCCN Palliative Care guidelines v.2.2011)

Sulfonylurea-induced hypoglycemia (off-label use): **Note:** Although octreotide use has been advocated as a first line therapy, indications and dosing for octreotide are not firmly established (Glatstein, 2012). Octreotide may reduce the incidence of recurrent hypoglycemia seen with dextrose-alone therapy (Fasano, 2008). In addition, although subcutaneous administration is the preferred route, administration via intravenous bolus and intravenous infusion have also been described in the literature (Barkin, 2013; Braatvedt, 1997; Carr, 2002; Crawford, 2004; Dougherty, 2010; Dougherty, 2013; Fasano, 2008; Graudins, 1997; Green, 2003; Hung, 1997; McLaughlin, 2000; Mordel, 1998). Optimal care decisions should be made based upon patient-specific details. Repeat dosing, dose escalation, or initiation of a continuous infusion may be required in patients who experience recurrent hypoglycemia. Duration of treatment may exceed 24 hours.

Children and Adolescents: SubQ: 1 to 1.25 mcg/kg; repeat in 6 hours as needed based upon blood glucose concentrations (Howland, 2011). Children generally need only a single dose (Dougherty, 2013).

Adults:

SubQ: 50 to 75 mcg; repeat every 6 hours as needed based upon blood glucose concentrations (Fasano, 2008; Howland, 2011)

IV: Doses up to 125 mcg/hour have been used successfully (McLaughlin, 2000)

Elderly: Elimination half-life is increased by 46% and clearance is decreased by 26%; dose adjustment may be required. Dosing should generally begin at the lower end of dosing range.

Dosage adjustment in renal impairment:

Regular injection:

Mild to severe impairment: No dosage adjustment provided in manufacturer's labeling.

Dialysis-dependent impairment: No specific dosage adjustment provided in manufacturer's labeling; however, a dosage adjustment may be needed since clearance is reduced by ~50%.

Depot injection:

Mild to severe impairment: No dosage adjustment necessary.

Dialysis-dependent impairment: Initial dose: 10 mg IM every 4 weeks; titrate based upon response (clearance is reduced by ~50%).

Dosage adjustment in hepatic impairment:

Regular injection: No dosage adjustment provided in manufacturer's labeling. Half-life is prolonged and total body clearance is decreased in patients with cirrhosis and fatty liver disease.

Depot injection: Patients with established cirrhosis of the liver: Initial dose: 10 mg IM every 4 weeks; titrate based upon response.

Dietary Considerations Schedule injections between meals to decrease GI effects. May alter absorption of dietary fats.

Usual Infusion Concentrations: Adult IV infusion: 500 mcg in 250 mL (concentration: 2 **mcg**/mL) of D_5W or NS

Administration

Regular injection formulation (do not use if solution contains particles or is discolored): Administer SubQ or IV; IV administration may be IV push (undiluted over 3 minutes), intermittent IV infusion (over 15 to 30 minutes), or continuous IV infusion (off-label route).

SubQ: Use the concentration with smallest volume to deliver dose to reduce injection site pain. Rotate injection site; may bring to room temperature prior to injection.

Depot formulation: Administer IM intragluteal (avoid deltoid administration); alternate gluteal injection sites to avoid irritation. **Do not** administer Sandostatin LAR® intravenously or subcutaneously; must be administered immediately after mixing.

Monitoring Parameters

Acromegaly: Growth hormone, somatomedin C (IGF-1)

Carcinoid: 5-HIAA, plasma serotonin and plasma substance P

VIPomas: Vasoactive intestinal peptide

Chronic therapy: Thyroid function (baseline and periodic), vitamin B_{12} level, blood glucose, glycemic control and antidiabetic regimen (patients with diabetes mellitus), cardiac function (heart rate, ECG), zinc level (patients with excessive fluid loss maintained on TPN)

Reference Range Vasoactive intestinal peptide: <75 ng/L; levels vary considerably between laboratories

Dosage Forms

Kit, Intramuscular:

SandoSTATIN LAR Depot: 10 mg, 20 mg, 30 mg

Solution, Injection:

SandoSTATIN: 50 mcg/mL (1 mL); 100 mcg/mL (1 mL); 200 mcg/mL (5 mL); 500 mcg/mL (1 mL); 1000 mcg/mL (5 mL)

Generic: 50 mcg/mL (1 mL); 100 mcg/mL (1 mL); 200 mcg/mL (5 mL); 1000 mcg/5 mL (5 mL); 500 mcg/mL (1 mL); 1000 mcg/mL (5 mL)

Solution, Injection [preservative free]:

Generic: 100 mcg/mL (1 mL); 500 mcg/mL (1 mL)

- ◆ **Octreotide Acetate** *see* Octreotide *on page 1485*
- ◆ **Octreotide Acetate Omega (Can)** *see* Octreotide *on page 1485*
- ◆ **Octreotide Injection (Can)** *see* Octreotide *on page 1485*
- ◆ **Ocudox** *see* Doxycycline *on page 689*
- ◆ **Ocufen** *see* Flurbiprofen (Ophthalmic) *on page 906*
- ◆ **Ocuflox** *see* Ofloxacin (Ophthalmic) *on page 1491*
- ◆ **Ocuflox® (Can)** *see* Ofloxacin (Ophthalmic) *on page 1491*
- ◆ **O-desmethylvenlafaxine** *see* Desvenlafaxine *on page 598*
- ◆ **ODV** *see* Desvenlafaxine *on page 598*
- ◆ **Oesclim (Can)** *see* Estradiol (Systemic) *on page 775*

Ofatumumab (oh fa TOOM yoo mab)

Brand Names: U.S. Arzerra

Brand Names: Canada Arzerra

Index Terms HuMax-CD20

Pharmacologic Category Antineoplastic Agent, Anti-CD20; Antineoplastic Agent, Monoclonal Antibody

Use

Chronic lymphocytic leukemia (CLL), previously untreated: Treatment of previously untreated CLL (in combination with chlorambucil) when fludarabine-based therapy is considered inappropriate

Chronic lymphocytic leukemia (CLL), refractory: Treatment of CLL refractory to fludarabine and alemtuzumab

Pregnancy Risk Factor C

Pregnancy Considerations Teratogenicity was not observed in animal reproduction studies, although prolonged depletion of circulating B cells was observed in animal offspring. The Canadian labeling recommends women of childbearing potential avoid pregnancy during and for 6 months after the last treatment.

Breast-Feeding Considerations It is not known if ofatumumab is excreted in human milk. However, human IgG is excreted in breast milk, and therefore, ofatumumab may also be excreted in milk. The effects of local GI and systemic exposure are unknown, therefore caution should be used in nursing women receiving ofatumumab.

Contraindications

U.S. labeling: There are no contraindications listed in the manufacturer's labeling.

Canadian labeling: Hypersensitivity to ofatumumab or any component of the formulation; presence or history of progressive multifocal leukoencephalopathy.

Warnings/Precautions [U.S. Boxed Warning]: Hepatitis B virus (HBV) reactivation may occur in patients receiving CD20-directed antibody treatment, including ofatumumab; may result in fulminant hepatitis, hepatic failure, and death. Fatal cases of HBV have also occurred in patients not previously infected with HBV. Prior to initiating therapy, obtain hepatitis B surface antigen (HBsAg) and hepatitis B core antibody (anti-HBc) measurements in all patients; monitor for clinical and laboratory signs of hepatitis or HBV during and for several months after treatment. HBV reactivation has been reported up to 12 months after therapy discontinuation. Discontinue ofatumumab (and concomitant medications) if viral hepatitis develops and initiate appropriate antiviral therapy. Reactivation has occurred in patients who are HBsAg positive as well as in those who are HBsAg negative but are anti-HBc positive; HBV reactivation has also been observed in patients who had previously resolved HBV infection. Use cautiously in patients who show evidence of prior HBV infection (eg, HBsAg positive [regardless of antibody status] or HBsAG negative but anti-HBc positive); consult with appropriate clinicians regarding monitoring and consideration of antiviral therapy before and/or during ofatumumab treatment. The safety of resuming ofatumumab treatment following HBV reactivation is not known; discuss reinitiation of therapy in patients with resolved HBV reactivation with physicians experienced in HBV management. Bacterial, fungal, and other new or reactivated viral infections may occur during and/or following therapy; monitor closely for signs/symptoms of infection. Discontinue therapy for serious infections and treat appropriately.

May cause serious infusion reaction (some fatal); reactions may include bronchospasm, dyspnea, laryngeal edema, pulmonary edema, flushing, hypertension, hypotension, syncope, cardiac ischemia/infarction, acute coronary syndrome, arrhythmia, bradycardia, back pain, abdominal pain, fever, rash, urticaria, angioedema, cytokine release syndrome, and/or anaphylactoid/anaphylactic reactions. Infusion reactions occur more frequently with the first 2 infusions and may occur despite premedication. Premedicate prior to infusion with acetaminophen, an antihistamine, and a corticosteroid. Interrupt infusion for reaction of any severity and institute appropriate treatment; may require subsequent rate modification. Discontinue immediately and permanently if anaphylactic reaction occurs. Bowel obstruction and abdominal pain have been reported; patients presenting with abdominal pain should be assessed for presence of obstruction and treated appropriately.

[U.S. Boxed Warning]: Progressive multifocal leukoencephalopathy (PML) resulting in death may occur with CD20-directed antibody treatment, including ofatumumab. Consider PML in any patient with new onset or worsening neurological symptoms, and if suspected, discontinue ofatumumab and evaluate promptly. Severe and prolonged (≥1 week) cytopenias (neutropenia, thrombocytopenia, and anemia) may occur. Grade 3 or 4 late-onset neutropenia (onset ≥42 days after last treatment dose) and/or prolonged neutropenia (not resolved 24 to 42 days after last dose) has been reported. Pancytopenia, agranulocytosis, and fatal neutropenic sepsis have occurred when used in combination with chlorambucil. Monitor blood counts regularly during and after treatment; more frequently if grade 3 or 4 cytopenias develop. Tumor lysis syndrome (TLS) has occurred in patients receiving ofatumumab; patients with a high tumor burden and/or high circulating lymphocyte counts (>25,000/mm^3) are at increased risk for TLS. Administer prophylactic antihyperuricemic therapy and aggressive hydration beginning 12 to 24 hours prior to ofatumumab treatment. Correct electrolyte abnormalities; monitor renal function and hydration status.

Potentially significant drug-drug interactions may exist, requiring dose or frequency adjustment, additional monitoring, and/or selection of alternative therapy. Live vaccines should not be given to patients who have recently received ofatumumab; there is no data concerning secondary transmission; the ability to generate an immune response to any vaccine following treatment is unknown. Patients ≥65 years experienced a higher incidence of adverse reactions (compared with younger patients).

Adverse Reactions

Cardiovascular: Hypertension, hypotension, peripheral edema, tachycardia

Central nervous system: Chills, fatigue, headache, insomnia

Dermatologic: Hyperhidrosis, skin rash, urticaria

Gastrointestinal: Diarrhea, nausea

Hematologic & oncologic: Anemia, neutropenia (may be prolonged >2 weeks)

Infection: Herpes zoster, infection (includes bacterial, fungal, or viral), sepsis

Neuromuscular & skeletal: Back pain, muscle spasm

Respiratory: Bronchitis, cough, dyspnea, nasopharyngitis, pneumonia, sinusitis, upper respiratory tract infection

Miscellaneous: Fever, infusion related reaction

Rare but important or life-threatening: Angina pectoris, bacteremia, hemolytic anemia, hepatitis B (new onset or reactivation), hepatitis (cytolytic), hypoxia, interstitial pulmonary disease (infectious), intestinal obstruction, peritonitis, progressive multifocal leukoencephalopathy (PML), rigors, sepsis (neutropenic), septic shock, thrombocytopenia

Drug Interactions

Metabolism/Transport Effects None known.

Avoid Concomitant Use

Avoid concomitant use of Ofatumumab with any of the following: BCG; Belimumab; Natalizumab; Pimecrolimus; Tacrolimus (Topical); Tofacitinib; Vaccines (Live)

Increased Effect/Toxicity

Ofatumumab may increase the levels/effects of: Belimumab; Leflunomide; Natalizumab; Tofacitinib; Vaccines (Live)

The levels/effects of Ofatumumab may be increased by: Denosumab; Pimecrolimus; Roflumilast; Tacrolimus (Topical); Trastuzumab

Decreased Effect

Ofatumumab may decrease the levels/effects of: BCG; Coccidioides immitis Skin Test; Sipuleucel-T; Vaccines (Inactivated); Vaccines (Live)

The levels/effects of Ofatumumab may be decreased by: Echinacea

Preparation for Administration Prepare all doses in 1000 mL NS. Begin infusion within 12 hours of preparation.

300 mg dose: Withdraw 15 mL from a 1000 mL NS bag. Add contents of 3 ofatumumab 100 mg vials to NS bag. Gently invert to mix; do not shake.

1000 mg dose: Withdraw 50 mL from a 1000 mL NS bag. Add contents of 1 ofatumumab 1000 mg vial. Gently invert to mix; do not shake.

2000 mg dose: Withdraw 100 mL from a 1000 mL NS bag. Add contents of 2 ofatumumab 1000 mg vials to NS bag. Gently invert to mix; do not shake.

Storage/Stability Store intact vials at 2°C to 8°C (36°F to 46°F); do not freeze. Protect from light. Diluted solutions for infusion must be started within 12 hours of preparation (may store at 2°C to 8°C [36°F to 46°F] if not used immediately); discard any remaining solution 24 hours after preparation.

Mechanism of Action Ofatumumab is a monoclonal antibody which binds specifically the extracellular (large and small) loops of the CD20 molecule (which is expressed on normal B lymphocytes and in B-cell CLL) resulting in potent complement-dependent cell lysis and antibody-dependent cell-mediated toxicity in cells that overexpress CD20.

Pharmacodynamics/Kinetics

Distribution: V_{dss}: 5.7 L (following repeated infusions)

Half-life elimination: 15.6 days (following repeated infusions)

Dosage Note: Premedicate with acetaminophen, an antihistamine, and a corticosteroid 30 to 120 minutes prior to treatment (see Administration).

Chronic lymphocytic leukemia (CLL), previously untreated: Adults: IV: Cycle 1 (cycle is 28 days): 300 mg on day 1, followed by 1000 mg on day 8; Subsequent cycles: 1000 mg on day 1 every 28 days; continue for at least 3 cycles until best response or a maximum of 12 cycles (in combination with chlorambucil)

CLL, refractory: Adults: IV: Initial dose: 300 mg week 1, followed 1 week later by 2000 mg once weekly for 7 doses (doses 2 to 8), followed 4 weeks later by 2000 mg once every 4 weeks for 4 doses (doses 9 to 12; for a total of 12 doses)

Dosage adjustment for toxicity:

Infusion reaction: Interrupt infusion for infusion reaction (any severity). If the reaction resolves or remains at ≤ grade 2, resume with the following modifications (based on the grade of the initial reaction):

Grade 1 or 2 infusion reaction:

U.S. labeling: Resume at one-half of the previous rate; may increase (see Administration) based on patient tolerance

Canadian labeling: Resume at one-half of the previous rate; may increase (see Administration) based on patient tolerance. If the infusion rate had not been increased above 12 mL/hour prior to interrupting therapy, resume infusion at 12 mL/hour; may then increase based on patient tolerance.

Grade 3 or 4 infusion reaction: Resume infusion at 12 mL/hour; may increase (see Administration) based on patient tolerance

If reaction severity does not resolve to ≤ grade 2 despite management: Consider permanent discontinuation

Anaphylactic reaction: Discontinue permanently

Dosage adjustment in renal impairment:

Mild or moderate impairment: There are no dosage adjustments provided in the U.S. manufacturer's labeling; however, there were no clinically relevant pharmacokinetic effects observed in patients with baseline CrCl ≥30 mL/minute. The Canadian labeling recommends that no dosage adjustment is necessary for CrCl >30 mL/minute.

Severe impairment: There are no dosage adjustments provided in the manufacturer's labeling.

Dosage adjustment in hepatic impairment: There are no dosage adjustments provided in the manufacturer's labeling (has not been studied).

Administration Do not administer IV push, IV bolus, or as a subcutaneous injection. Premedicate with acetaminophen, an antihistamine, and a corticosteroid 30 to 120 minutes prior to administration. Infuse in an environment equipped to monitor for and manage infusion reactions. Administer with infusion pump and administration set. Do not exceed infusion rates below. Do not mix with or infuse with other medications. Flush line before and after infusion with NS. Begin infusion within 12 hours of preparation. Interrupt infusion for any severity of infusion reaction; if the reaction resolves or remains at ≤ grade 2, may resume infusion (see Dosage adjustment for toxicity).

Previously untreated chronic lymphocytic leukemia:

Premedication: Premedicate with oral acetaminophen (1000 mg) or equivalent, an oral or IV antihistamine (eg, diphenhydramine 50 mg or cetirizine 10 mg orally or equivalent), and an IV corticosteroid (prednisolone 50 mg or equivalent). Full dose corticosteroid is recommended for the first 2 infusions; in the absence of infusion reaction ≥ grade 3, may gradually reduce or omit corticosteroid dose for subsequent infusions.

Cycle 1, day 1: Initiate infusion at 12 mL/hour for 30 minutes, if tolerated (no infusion reaction) increase to 25 mL/hour for 30 minutes, if tolerated, increase to 50 mL/hour for 30 minutes, if tolerated, increase to 100 mL/hour for 30 minutes, if tolerated, increase to 200 mL/hour for 30 minutes, if tolerated increase to 300 mL/hour for 30 minutes, if tolerated, increase to 400 mL/hour for remainder of infusion. Median duration of infusion: 5.2 hours.

Cycle 1, day 8 and cycles 2 to 12 (if no reaction to previous infusion): Initiate infusion at 25 mL/hour for 30 minutes, if tolerated (no infusion reaction) increase to 50 mL/hour for 30 minutes, if tolerated, increase to 100 mL/hour for 30 minutes, if tolerated, increase to 200 mL/hour for 30 minutes, if tolerated, increase to 400 mL/hour for remainder of infusion. Median duration of infusion: 4.2 to 4.4 hours.

Refractory chronic lymphocytic leukemia:

Premedication: Premedicate with oral acetaminophen (1000 mg) or equivalent, an oral or IV antihistamine (eg, diphenhydramine 50 mg or cetirizine 10 mg orally or equivalent), and an IV corticosteroid (prednisolone 100 mg or equivalent). Full dose corticosteroid is recommended for doses 1, 2, and 9; in the absence of infusion reaction ≥ grade 3, may gradually reduce or omit corticosteroid dose for doses 3 to 8; administer full or half corticosteroid dose with doses 10 to 12 if ≥ grade 3 reaction did not occur with dose 9.

Doses 1 and 2: Initiate infusion at 12 mL/hour for 30 minutes, if tolerated (no infusion reaction) increase to 25 mL/hour for 30 minutes, if tolerated, increase to 50 mL/hour for 30 minutes, if tolerated, increase to 100 mL/hour for 30 minutes, if tolerated, increase to 200 mL/hour for remainder of infusion. Median duration of infusion: 6.8 hours.

Doses 3 to 12: Initiate infusion at 25 mL/hour for 30 minutes, if tolerated (no infusion reaction) increase to 50 mL/hour for 30 minutes, if tolerated, increase to 100 mL/hour for 30 minutes, if tolerated, increase to 200 mL/hour for 30 minutes, if tolerated, increase to 400 mL/hour for remainder of infusion. Median duration of infusion: 4.2 to 4.4 hours.

Monitoring Parameters CBC with differential, hepatitis B screening in all patients (HBsAG and anti-HBc measurements) prior to therapy initiation; renal function, electrolytes; signs of active hepatitis B infection (during and for up to 12 months after therapy completion); signs or symptoms of infusion reaction; signs of infection; fluid status; signs/symptoms of intestinal obstruction (eg, abdominal pain, repeated vomiting); signs/symptoms of progressive multifocal leukoencephalopathy (focal neurologic deficits, which may present as hemiparesis, visual field deficits, cognitive impairment, aphasia, ataxia, and/or cranial nerve deficits).

Dosage Forms

Concentrate, Intravenous [preservative free]:

Arzerra: 100 mg/5 mL (5 mL); 1000 mg/50 mL (50 mL)

◆ **Ofev** *see* Nintedanib *on page 1458*

◆ **Ofirmev** *see* Acetaminophen *on page 32*

Ofloxacin (Systemic) (oh FLOKS a sin)

Brand Names: Canada Apo-Oflox; Novo-Ofloxacin

Pharmacologic Category Antibiotic, Fluoroquinolone

Use Quinolone antibiotic for the treatment of acute exacerbations of chronic bronchitis, community-acquired pneumonia, skin and skin structure infections (uncomplicated), urethral and cervical gonorrhea (acute, uncomplicated), urethritis and cervicitis (nongonococcal), mixed infections of the urethra and cervix, pelvic inflammatory disease (acute), cystitis (uncomplicated), urinary tract infections (complicated), prostatitis

Note: As of April 2007, the CDC no longer recommends the use of fluoroquinolones for the treatment of gonococcal disease.

Pregnancy Risk Factor C

Dosage

Usual dosage range: Adults: Oral: 200 to 400 mg every 12 hours

Indication-specific dosing: Adults: Oral:

Cervicitis/urethritis:

Nongonococcal: 300 mg every 12 hours for 7 days

Gonococcal (acute, uncomplicated): 400 mg as a single dose; **Note:** As of April 2007, the CDC no longer recommends the use of fluoroquinolones for the treatment of uncomplicated gonococcal disease.

Chronic bronchitis (acute exacerbation), community-acquired pneumonia, skin and skin structure infections (uncomplicated): 400 mg every 12 hours for 10 days

Epididymitis, nongonococcal (off-label use): 300 mg twice daily for 10 days (CDC, 2010); 200 mg twice daily for 14 days (Canadian STI Guidelines, 2008)

Leprosy (off-label use): 400 mg once daily

Pelvic inflammatory disease (acute): 400 mg every 12 hours for 10 to 14 days with or without metronidazole; **Note:** The CDC recommends use only if standard cephalosporin therapy is not feasible and community prevalence of quinolone-resistant gonococcal organisms is low. Culture sensitivity must be confirmed.

Prostatitis:

Acute: 400 mg for 1 dose, then 300 mg twice daily for 10 days

Chronic: 200 mg every 12 hours for 6 weeks

Traveler's diarrhea (off-label use): 200 mg twice daily for 3 days (Hill 2006)

UTI:

Uncomplicated: 200 mg every 12 hours for 3 to 7 days

Complicated: 200 mg every 12 hours for 10 days

Dosing adjustment/interval in renal impairment: Adults:

Oral: After a normal initial dose, adjust as follows:

CrCl 20 to 50 mL/minute: Administer usual dose every 24 hours

CrCl <20 mL/minute: Administer half the usual dose every 24 hours

Continuous arteriovenous or venovenous hemodiafiltration effects: Administer 300 mg every 24 hours

Dosing adjustment in hepatic impairment: Severe impairment: Maximum dose: 400 mg/day

Additional Information Complete prescribing information should be consulted for additional detail.

Dosage Forms

Tablet, Oral:

Generic: 300 mg, 400 mg

Ofloxacin (Ophthalmic) (oh FLOKS a sin)

Brand Names: U.S. Ocuflox

Brand Names: Canada Ocuflox®

Pharmacologic Category Antibiotic, Fluoroquinolone; Antibiotic, Ophthalmic

Use Treatment of superficial ocular infections involving the conjunctiva or cornea due to strains of susceptible organisms

Pregnancy Risk Factor C

Dosage

Usual dosage range: Ophthalmic:

Children >1 year: 1-2 drops every 30 minutes to 4 hours initially, decreasing to every 4-6 hours

Adults: 1-2 drops every 30 minutes to 4 hours initially, decreasing to every 4-6 hours

Indication-specific dosing: Children >1 year and Adults: Ophthalmic:

Conjunctivitis: Instill 1-2 drops in affected eye(s) every 2-4 hours for the first 2 days, then use 4 times/day for an additional 5 days

Corneal ulcer: Instill 1-2 drops every 30 minutes while awake and every 4-6 hours after retiring for the first 2 days; beginning on day 3, instill 1-2 drops every hour while awake for 4-6 additional days; thereafter, 1-2 drops 4 times/day until clinical cure.

Dosage adjustment in renal impairment: No dosage adjustment provided in manufacturer's labeling. However, dosage adjustment unlikely due to low systemic absorption.

Dosage adjustment in hepatic impairment: No dosage adjustment provided in manufacturer's labeling. However, dosage adjustment unlikely due to low systemic absorption.

Additional Information Complete prescribing information should be consulted for additional detail.

Dosage Forms

Solution, Ophthalmic:

Ocuflox: 0.3% (5 mL)

Generic: 0.3% (5 mL, 10 mL)

Ofloxacin (Otic) (oh FLOKS a sin)

Index Terms Floxin Otic Singles

Pharmacologic Category Antibiotic, Fluoroquinolone; Antibiotic, Otic

Use Otitis externa, chronic suppurative otitis media, acute otitis media

Pregnancy Risk Factor C

Dosage

Usual dosage range: Otic:

Children ≥6 months: 5 drops daily

Children >12 years: 10 drops once or twice daily

Adults: 10 drops once or twice daily

Indication-specific dosing: Otic:

Children 6 months to 13 years: **Otitis externa:** Instill 5 drops (or the contents of 1 single-dose container) into affected ear(s) once daily for 7 days

Children 1-12 years: **Acute otitis media with tympanostomy tubes:** Instill 5 drops (or the contents of 1 single-dose container) into affected ear(s) twice daily for 10 days

Children >12 years and Adults: **Otitis media, chronic suppurative with perforated tympanic membranes:** Instill 10 drops (or the contents of 2 single-dose containers) into affected ear twice daily for 14 days

Children ≥13 years and Adults: **Otitis externa:** Instill 10 drops (or the contents of 2 single-dose containers) into affected ear(s) once daily for 7 days

Dosage adjustment in renal impairment: No dosage adjustment provided in manufacturer's labeling. However, dosage adjustment unlikely due to low systemic absorption.

Dosage adjustment in hepatic impairment: No dosage adjustment provided in manufacturer's labeling. However, dosage adjustment unlikely due to low systemic absorption.

Additional Information Complete prescribing information should be consulted for additional detail.

Dosage Forms

Solution, Otic:

Generic: 0.3% (5 mL, 10 mL)

- **Ogen (Can)** *see* Estropipate *on page 793*
- **Ogestrel** *see* Ethinyl Estradiol and Norgestrel *on page 812*
- **OGMT** *see* Metyrosine *on page 1359*
- **OGT-918** *see* Miglustat *on page 1367*
- **17OHPC** *see* Hydroxyprogesterone Caproate *on page 1021*
- **9-OH-risperidone** *see* Paliperidone *on page 1556*

OLANZapine (oh LAN za peen)

Brand Names: U.S. ZyPREXA; ZyPREXA Relprevv; ZyPREXA Zydis

Brand Names: Canada Abbott-Olanzapine ODT; ACT Olanzapine; Apo-Olanzapine; Apo-Olanzapine ODT; CO Olanzapine ODT; JAMP-Olanzapine ODT; Mar-Olanzapine; Mar-Olanzapine ODT; Mylan-Olanzapine; Mylan-Olanzapine ODT; Olanzapine for injection; Olanzapine ODT; PHL-Olanzapine; PHL-Olanzapine ODT; PMS-Olanzapine; PMS-Olanzapine ODT; RAN-Olanzapine; RAN-Olanzapine ODT; Riva-Olanzapine; Riva-Olanzapine ODT; Sandoz-Olanzapine; Sandoz-Olanzapine ODT; Teva-Olanzapine; Teva-Olanzapine OD; Zyprexa; Zyprexa Intramuscular; Zyprexa Zydis

Index Terms LY170053; Olanzapine Pamoate; Zyprexa Zydis

Pharmacologic Category Antimanic Agent; Second Generation (Atypical) Antipsychotic

Additional Appendix Information

Beers Criteria – Potentially Inappropriate Medications for Geriatrics *on page 2271*

Use

Oral: Treatment of the manifestations of schizophrenia; treatment of acute or mixed mania episodes associated with bipolar I disorder (as monotherapy or in combination with lithium or valproate); maintenance treatment of bipolar I disorder; in combination with fluoxetine for treatment-resistant or bipolar I depression

IM, extended-release (Zyprexa Relprevv): Treatment of schizophrenia

IM, short-acting (Zyprexa IntraMuscular): Treatment of acute agitation associated with schizophrenia and bipolar I mania

Pregnancy Risk Factor C

Pregnancy Considerations Adverse events were observed in animal reproduction studies. Olanzapine crosses the placenta and can be detected in cord blood at birth (Newport, 2007). Information related to olanzapine use in pregnancy is limited (Goldstein, 2000). Antipsychotic use during the third trimester of pregnancy has a risk for abnormal muscle movements (extrapyramidal symptoms [EPS]) and/or withdrawal symptoms in newborns following delivery. Symptoms in the newborn may include agitation, feeding disorder, hypertonia, hypotonia, respiratory distress, somnolence, and tremor; these effects may be self-limiting or require hospitalization. Olanzapine may cause hyperprolactinemia, which may decrease reproductive function in both males and females.

The ACOG recommends that therapy during pregnancy be individualized; treatment with psychiatric medications during pregnancy should incorporate the clinical expertise of the mental health clinician, obstetrician, primary healthcare provider, and pediatrician. Safety data related to atypical antipsychotics during pregnancy is limited and routine use is not recommended. However, if a woman is inadvertently exposed to an atypical antipsychotic while pregnant, continuing therapy may be preferable to switching to a typical antipsychotic that the fetus has not yet been exposed to; consider risk:benefit (ACOG, 2008). Evaluate risk factors for gestational diabetes and weight gain if considering use of olanzapine in a pregnant woman (NICE, 2007).

Healthcare providers are encouraged to enroll women 18-45 years of age exposed to olanzapine during pregnancy in the Atypical Antipsychotics Pregnancy Registry (1-866-961-2388 or http://www.womensmentalhealth.org/pregnancyregistry).

Breast-Feeding Considerations Olanzapine is excreted into breast milk. At steady-state concentrations, it is estimated that a breast-fed infant may be exposed to ~2% of the maternal dose. In one study, the median time to peak milk concentration was ~5 hours after the maternal dose and serum concentrations in the nursing infants were low (<5 ng/mL; n=5) (Gardiner, 2003). An increased risk of adverse events in nursing infants has not been reported (Gardiner, 2003; Gilad, 2011). Breast-feeding is not recommended by the manufacturer.

Contraindications There are no contraindications listed in the manufacturer's labeling.

Canadian labeling: Hypersensitivity to olanzapine or any component of the formulation

Warnings/Precautions [U.S. Boxed Warning]: Elderly patients with dementia-related psychosis treated with antipsychotics are at an increased risk of death compared with placebo. Most deaths appeared to be either cardiovascular (eg, heart failure, sudden death) or infectious (eg, pneumonia) in nature. In addition, an increased incidence of cerebrovascular effects (eg, transient ischemic attack, stroke) has been reported in studies of placebo-controlled trials of olanzapine in elderly patients with dementia-related psychosis. Olanzapine is not approved for the treatment of dementia-related psychosis.

May cause CNS depression, which impair physical and mental abilities; patients must be cautioned about performing tasks that require mental alertness (eg, operating machinery, driving). May be moderate to highly sedating in comparison with other antipsychotics (APA [Lehman, 2004]); dose-related effects have been observed. Use caution in patients with cardiac disease. Use with caution in Parkinson disease, predisposition to seizures, or severe hepatic or renal disease. Life-threatening arrhythmias have occurred with therapeutic doses of some neuroleptics. May induce orthostatic hypotension; use caution with history of cardiovascular disease, hemodynamic instability, prior myocardial infarction, or ischemic heart disease. Dose-related increases in cholesterol and triglycerides have been noted. Use with caution in patients with preexisting abnormal lipid profile. Esophageal dysmotility and aspiration have been associated with antipsychotic use; use with caution in patients at risk of aspiration pneumonia. May cause dose-related increases in prolactin levels; clinical significance of hyperprolactinemia in patients with breast cancer or other prolactin-dependent tumors is unknown. Clinical manifestations of increased prolactin levels included menstrual-, sexual- and breast-related events. Significant dose-related weight gain (>7% of baseline weight) may occur; monitor waist circumference and BMI. Impaired core body temperature regulation may occur; caution with strenuous exercise, heat exposure, dehydration, and concomitant medication possessing anticholinergic effects.

Leukopenia, neutropenia, and agranulocytosis (sometimes fatal) have been reported in clinical trials and postmarketing reports with antipsychotic use; presence of risk factors (eg, preexisting low WBC or history of drug-induced leuko-/neutropenia) should prompt periodic blood count assessment. Discontinue therapy at first signs of blood dyscrasias or if absolute neutrophil count <1,000/mm^3.

May cause anticholinergic effects; use with caution in patients with decreased gastrointestinal motility, urinary retention, BPH, xerostomia, or narrow-angle glaucoma. Relative to other neuroleptics, olanzapine has a moderate potency of cholinergic blockade. May cause extrapyramidal symptoms (EPS), although risk of these reactions is lower relative to other neuroleptics. Risk of dystonia (and probably other EPS) may be greater with increased doses, use of conventional antipsychotics, males, and younger patients. May be associated with neuroleptic malignant syndrome (NMS). May cause extreme and life-threatening hyperglycemia; use with caution in patients with diabetes or other disorders of glucose regulation; monitor. Olanzapine levels may be lower in patients who smoke. Smokers may require a daily dose 30% higher than nonsmokers in order to obtain an equivalent olanzapine concentration (Tsuda, 2014); however, the manufacturer does not routinely recommend dosage adjustments.

Use in adolescent patients ≥13 years of age may result in increased weight gain and sedation, as well as greater increases in LDL cholesterol, total cholesterol, triglycerides, prolactin, and liver transaminase levels when compared with adults. Adolescent patients should be maintained on the lowest dose necessary. Use in elderly patients with dementia is associated with an increased risk of mortality and cerebrovascular accidents; avoid antipsychotic use for behavioral problems associated with dementia unless alternative nonpharmacologic therapies have failed and patient may harm self or others. In addition, use may cause or exacerbate syndrome of inappropriate antidiuretic hormone secretion or hyponatremia; monitor sodium closely with initiation or dosage adjustments in older adults. May also be inappropriate in older adults depending on comorbidities (eg, dementia, delirium) due to its potent anticholinergic effects (Beers Criteria).

The possibility of a suicide attempt is inherent in psychotic illness or bipolar disorder; use caution in high-risk patients during initiation of therapy. Prescriptions should be written for the smallest quantity consistent with good patient care.

Some dosage forms may contain polysorbate 80 (also known as Tweens). Hypersensitivity reactions, usually a delayed reaction, have been reported following exposure to pharmaceutical products containing polysorbate 80 in certain individuals (Isaksson, 2002; Lucente 2000; Shelley, 1995). Thrombocytopenia, ascites, pulmonary deterioration, and renal and hepatic failure have been reported in premature neonates after receiving parenteral products containing polysorbate 80 (Alade, 1986; CDC, 1984). See manufacturer's labeling.

There are two Zyprexa formulations for intramuscular injection: Zyprexa Relprevv is an extended-release formulation and Zyprexa Intramuscular is short-acting:

Extended-release IM injection (Zyprexa Relprevv): **[U.S. Boxed Warning]: Sedation (including coma) and delirium (including agitation, anxiety, confusion, disorientation) have been observed following use of *Zyprexa Relprevv*.** Administer at a registered health care facility where patients should be continuously monitored (≥3 hours) for symptoms of olanzapine overdose; symptom development highest in first hour but may occur within or after 3 hours; risk of syndrome is cumulative with each injection; recovery expected by 72 hours. Upon determining alert status, patient should be escorted to their destination and not drive or operate heavy machinery for the remainder of the day.

Two unexplained deaths in patients who received *Zyprexa Relprevv* have been reported. The patients died 3 to 4 days after receiving an appropriate dose of the drug. Both patients were found to have high blood concentrations of olanzapine postmortem. It is unclear if these deaths were the result of postinjection delirium sedation syndrome (PDSS) (FDA Safety Communication, 2013).

Zyprexa Relprevv is only available under a restricted distribution program. Only prescribers, health care facilities, and pharmacies registered with the program are able to prescribe, distribute, or dispense *Zyprexa Relprevv* for patients who are enrolled in and meet all conditions of the program.

Short-acting IM injection (Zyprexa IntraMuscular): Patients should remain recumbent if drowsy/dizzy until hypotension, bradycardia, and/or hypoventilation have been ruled out. Concurrent use of IM/IV benzodiazepines is not recommended (fatalities have been reported, though causality not determined).

Adverse Reactions

Oral: Unless otherwise noted, adverse events are reported for placebo-controlled trials in adult patients on monotherapy:

Cardiovascular: Chest pain, hypertension, orthostatic hypotension, peripheral edema, tachycardia

Central nervous system: Abnormal gait, akathisia, articulation impairment, dizziness (more common in adults), drowsiness (dose dependent; adolescents and adults), extrapyramidal reaction (dose dependent; more common in adults), falling, fatigue (dose dependent; adolescents and adults), headache (adolescents), hypertonia, insomnia, personality changes, restlessness (adolescents)

Endocrine & metabolic: Breast changes ([adolescents] discharge, enlargement, galactorrhea, gynecomastia, lactation disorder), increased gamma-glutamyl transferase (adolescents), increased serum prolactin (more common in adolescents), menstrual disease (amenorrhea, hypomenorrhea, delayed menstruation, oligomenorrhea), weight gain (adolescents and adults)

Gastrointestinal: Abdominal pain (adolescents), constipation (adolescents and adults), diarrhea (adolescents), dyspepsia (more common in adults), flatulence, increased appetite (more common in adolescents), nausea (dose dependent), vomiting, xerostomia (dose dependent; more common in adults)

Genitourinary: Incontinence, sexual disorder (anorgasmia, delayed ejaculation, erectile dysfunction, changes in libido, abnormal orgasm, sexual dysfunction), urinary tract infection

Hematologic & oncologic: Bruise

Hepatic: Decreased serum bilirubin (adolescents), increased liver enzyme (adolescents), increased serum ALT (adolescents and adults), increased serum AST (adolescents)

Neuromuscular & skeletal: Arthralgia (adolescents and adults), back pain, limb pain (adolescents and adults), muscle rigidity (adolescents), tremor (dose dependent), weakness (dose dependent)

Ophthalmic: Amblyopia

Respiratory: Cough, epistaxis (adolescents), nasopharyngitis (adolescents), pharyngitis, respiratory tract infection (adolescents), rhinitis, sinusitis (adolescents)

Miscellaneous: Accidental injury, fever

Rare but important or life-threatening: Accommodation disturbance, acidosis, agranulocytosis, akinesia, albuminuria, alopecia, anaphylactoid reaction, angioedema, apnea, arteritis, asthma, ataxia, atelectasis, atrial fibrillation, brain disease, cardiac arrest, cardiac failure, cerebrovascular accident, coma, confusion, deafness, diabetes mellitus, diabetic ketoacidosis, diabetic coma, dysarthria, dyskinesia, dysphagia, dystonia, dysuria, facial paralysis, glaucoma, heart failure, hematuria, hemoptysis, hemorrhage (eye, rectal, subarachnoid, vaginal), hepatic injury (cholestatic or mixed), hepatitis, hypercholesterolemia, hyperglycemia, hyperkalemia, hyperlipidemia, hypernatremia, hypertriglyceridemia, hyperuricemia, hyperventilation, hypoesthesia, hypoglycemia, hypokalemia, hypokinesia, hyponatremia, hypoproteinemia, hypoventilation, hypoxia, intestinal obstruction, jaundice, ketosis, leukocytosis (eosinophilia), leukopenia, liver steatosis, lymphadenopathy, migraine, myasthenia, myopathy, neuralgia, neuroleptic malignant syndrome, neuropathy, neutropenia, osteoporosis, pancreatitis, paralysis, priapism, pruritus, pulmonary edema, pulmonary embolism, rhabdomyolysis, seizure, skin rash, stridor, suicidal tendencies, syncope, tardive dyskinesia, thrombocythemia, thrombocytopenia, tongue edema, transient ischemic attacks, urticaria, venous thrombosis, withdrawal syndrome

Injection: Unless otherwise noted, adverse events are reported for placebo-controlled trials in adult patients on extended release IM injection (Zyprexa Relprevv). Also refer to adverse reactions noted with oral therapy.

Cardiovascular: Hypertension, hypotension (short-acting), orthostatic hypotension (short-acting), prolonged Q-T interval on ECG

Central nervous system: Abnormal dreams, abnormality in thinking, auditory hallucination, dizziness, drowsiness, dysarthria, extrapyramidal reaction, fatigue, headache, pain, restlessness, sedation

Dermatologic: Acne vulgaris

Endocrine & metabolic: Weight gain

Gastrointestinal: Abdominal pain, diarrhea, flatulence, increased appetite, nausea, toothache, vomiting, xerostomia

Genitourinary: Vaginal discharge

Hepatic: Increased liver enzymes

Infection: Tooth infection, viral infection

Local: Pain at injection site

Neuromuscular & skeletal: Arthralgia, back pain, muscle spasm, stiffness, tremor, weakness (short-acting)

Otic: Otalgia

Respiratory: Cough, nasal congestion, nasopharyngitis, pharyngolaryngeal pain, sneezing, upper respiratory tract infection

Miscellaneous: Fever

Rare but important or life-threatening: Increased creatine phosphokinase, postinjection delirium/sedation syndrome, syncope (short-acting)

Drug Interactions

Metabolism/Transport Effects **Substrate** of CYP1A2 (major), CYP2D6 (minor); **Note:** Assignment of Major/Minor substrate status based on clinically relevant drug interaction potential; **Inhibits** CYP1A2 (weak), CYP2C19 (weak), CYP2C9 (weak), CYP2D6 (weak), CYP3A4 (weak)

Avoid Concomitant Use

Avoid concomitant use of OLANZapine with any of the following: Aclidinium; Amisulpride; Azelastine (Nasal); Benzodiazepines; Glucagon; Ipratropium (Oral Inhalation); Metoclopramide; Orphenadrine; Paraldehyde; Pimozide; Potassium Chloride; Sulpiride; Thalidomide; Tiotropium; Umeclidinium

Increased Effect/Toxicity

OLANZapine may increase the levels/effects of: AbobotulinumtoxinA; Alcohol (Ethyl); Amisulpride; Analgesics (Opioid); Anticholinergic Agents; ARIPiprazole; Azelastine (Nasal); Benzodiazepines; Buprenorphine; CNS Depressants; Glucagon; Highest Risk QTc-Prolonging Agents; Hydrocodone; Lomitapide; Methotrimeprazine; Methylphenidate; Metyrosine; Mirabegron; Mirtazapine; Moderate Risk QTc-Prolonging Agents; OnabotulinumtoxinA; Orphenadrine; Paraldehyde; Pimozide; Potassium Chloride; RimabotulinumtoxinB; Selective Serotonin Reuptake Inhibitors; Serotonin Modulators; Sulpiride; Suvorexant; Thalidomide; Thiazide Diuretics; Tiotropium; Topiramate; Zolpidem

The levels/effects of OLANZapine may be increased by: Abiraterone Acetate; Acetylcholinesterase Inhibitors (Central); Aclidinium; Brimonidine (Topical); Cannabis; CYP1A2 Inhibitors (Moderate); CYP1A2 Inhibitors (Strong); Deferasirox; Doxylamine; Dronabinol; Droperidol; FluvoxaMINE; HydrOXYzine; Ipratropium (Oral Inhalation); Kava Kava; LamoTRIgine; Lithium; Magnesium Sulfate; Methotrimeprazine; Methylphenidate; Metoclopramide; Metyrosine; Mianserin; Mifepristone; Nabilone; Peginterferon Alfa-2b; Perampanel; Pramlintide; Rufinamide; Serotonin Modulators; Sodium Oxybate; Tapentadol; Tetrahydrocannabinol; Umeclidinium; Vemurafenib

Decreased Effect

OLANZapine may decrease the levels/effects of: Acetylcholinesterase Inhibitors; Amphetamines; Anti-Parkinson's Agents (Dopamine Agonist); Itopride; Quinagolide; Secretin

The levels/effects of OLANZapine may be decreased by: Acetylcholinesterase Inhibitors; Cannabis; CYP1A2 Inducers (Strong); Cyproterone; Lithium; Teriflunomide; Valproic Acid and Derivatives

Preparation for Administration

Injection, extended-release: Dilute as directed to final concentration of 150 mg/mL. Shake vigorously to mix; will form yellow, opaque suspension. Following reconstitution, suspension may be stored at room temperature and used within 24 hours. Shake vigorously to resuspend prior to administration. Use immediately once suspension is in syringe. Suspension may be irritating to skin; wear gloves during reconstitution. Do not mix diazepam, lorazepam, or haloperidol in the same syringe.

Injection, short-acting: Reconstitute 10 mg vial with 2.1 mL SWFI. Resulting solution is ~5 mg/mL. Use immediately (within 1 hour) following reconstitution. Discard any unused portion.

Storage/Stability

Injection, extended-release: Store at controlled room temperature, not to exceed 30°C (86°F).

Injection, short-acting: Store at 20°C to 25°C (68°F to 77°F); excursions permitted to 15°C to 30°C (59°F to 86°F); do not freeze. Protect from light.

Tablet and orally disintegrating tablet: Store at 20°C to 25°C (68°F to 77°F); excursions permitted to 15°C to 30°C (59°F to 86°F). Protect from light and moisture.

Mechanism of Action Olanzapine is a second generation thienobenzodiazepine antipsychotic which displays potent antagonism of serotonin 5-HT_{2A} and 5-HT_{2C}, dopamine D_{1-4}, histamine H_1, and alpha$_1$-adrenergic receptors. Olanzapine shows moderate antagonism of 5-HT_3 and muscarinic M_{1-5} receptors, and weak binding to GABA-A, BZD, and beta-adrenergic receptors. Although the precise mechanism of action in schizophrenia and bipolar disorder is not known, the efficacy of olanzapine is thought to be mediated through combined antagonism of dopamine and serotonin type 2 receptor sites.

Pharmacodynamics/Kinetics

Absorption:

Oral: Well absorbed; not affected by food; tablets and orally disintegrating tablets are bioequivalent

Short-acting injection: Rapidly absorbed

Distribution: V_d: Extensive, 1000 L

Protein binding, plasma: 93% bound to albumin and alpha$_1$-glycoprotein

Metabolism: Highly metabolized via direct glucuronidation and cytochrome P450 mediated oxidation (CYP1A2, CYP2D6); 40% removed via first pass metabolism

Half-life elimination: 21 to 54 hours; ~1.5 times greater in elderly; Extended-release injection: ~30 days

Time to peak, plasma: Maximum plasma concentrations after IM administration are 5 times higher than maximum plasma concentrations produced by an oral dose.

Extended-release injection: ~7 days

Short-acting injection: 15 to 45 minutes

Oral: ~6 hours

Excretion: Urine (57%, 7% as unchanged drug); feces (30%)

Clearance: 40% increase in olanzapine clearance in smokers; 30% decrease in females

Dosage

Children and Adolescents 10 to 17 years: Depression associated with bipolar I disorder (in combination with fluoxetine): Oral: Initial: 2.5 mg once daily in the evening (in combination with fluoxetine); adjust dose, if needed, as tolerated; safety of doses >12 mg of olanzapine in combination with fluoxetine doses >50 mg has not been studied in pediatrics. See **"Note"** below for olanzapine/fluoxetine combination (Symbyax).

Adolescents ≥13 years:

Bipolar I (acute mixed or manic episodes): Oral: Initial: 2.5 to 5 mg once daily; adjust by 2.5 to 5 mg daily to target dose of 10 mg daily; dosing range: 2.5 to 20 mg daily

Schizophrenia: Oral: Initial: 2.5 to 5 mg once daily; adjust by 2.5 to 5 mg daily to target dose of 10 mg daily; dosing range: 2.5 to 20 mg daily

Adults:

Agitation (acute, associated with bipolar I mania or schizophrenia): Short-acting IM injection: Initial dose: 10 mg (a lower dose of 5 to 7.5 mg may be considered when clinical factors warrant); additional doses (up to 10 mg) may be considered, however, 2 hours after the initial dose and 4 hours after the second dose should be allowed between doses to evaluate response (maximum total daily dose: 30 mg)

Special risk patients: Consider a lower dose of 2.5 mg in patients who are debilitated, who have a predisposition to hypotensive reactions, or who may be more pharmacodynamically sensitive to olanzapine.

Bipolar I (acute mixed or manic episodes): Oral:

Monotherapy: Initial: 10 to 15 mg once daily; increase by 5 mg daily at intervals of not less than 24 hours. Maintenance: 5 to 20 mg daily; recommended maximum dose: 20 mg daily.

Combination therapy (with lithium or valproate): Initial: 10 mg once daily; dosing range: 5 to 20 mg daily; recommended maximum dose: 20 mg daily.

Depression:

Depression associated with bipolar disorder (in combination with fluoxetine): Oral: Initial: 5 mg in the evening; adjust as tolerated to usual range of 5 to 12.5 mg daily. See **"Note"**

Treatment-resistant depression (in combination with fluoxetine): Oral: Initial: 5 mg in the evening; adjust as tolerated to range of 5 to 20 mg daily. See **"Note"**

Note (olanzapine/fluoxetine combination [Symbyax]):

When using individual components of fluoxetine with olanzapine rather than fixed dose combination product (Symbyax), approximate dosage correspondence is as follows:

Olanzapine 2.5 mg + fluoxetine 20 mg = Symbyax 3/25

Olanzapine 5 mg + fluoxetine 20 mg = Symbyax 6/25

Olanzapine 12.5 mg + fluoxetine 20 mg = Symbyax 12/25

Olanzapine 5 mg + fluoxetine 50 mg = Symbyax 6/50

Olanzapine 12.5 mg + fluoxetine 50 mg = Symbyax 12/50

Special risk patients: Initial: 2.5 to 5 mg once daily is recommended in patients who have a predisposition to hypotensive reactions, who have hepatic impairment, who exhibit a combination of factors that may result in slower metabolism of olanzapine (eg, female, elderly, nonsmoking status), or who may be more pharmacodynamically sensitive to olanzapine; increase dose with caution as clinically indicated.

Schizophrenia:

Oral: Initial: 5 to 10 mg once daily (increase to 10 mg once daily within 5 to 7 days); thereafter, adjust by 5 mg daily at 1-week intervals, up to a recommended maximum of 20 mg daily. Maintenance: 10 to 20 mg once daily. Doses up to 60 mg daily have been used in treatment-resistant schizophrenia; however, supporting evidence is limited (APA [Lehman, 2004]).

Special risk patients: Initial: 5 mg once daily is recommended in patients who are debilitated, who have a predisposition to hypotensive reactions, who exhibit a combination of factors that may result in slower metabolism of olanzapine (eg, nonsmoking female patients ≥65 years), or who may be more pharmacodynamically sensitive to olanzapine; increase dose with caution as clinically indicated.

Extended-release IM injection: **Note:** Establish tolerance to oral olanzapine prior to changing to extended-release IM injection. Maximum dose: 300 mg/2 weeks or 405 mg/4 weeks

Patients established on oral olanzapine 10 mg daily: Initial dose: 210 mg every 2 weeks for 4 doses or 405 mg every 4 weeks for 2 doses; Maintenance dose: 150 mg every 2 weeks or 300 mg every 4 weeks

Patients established on oral olanzapine 15 mg daily: Initial dose: 300 mg every 2 weeks for 4 doses; Maintenance dose: 210 mg every 2 weeks or 405 mg every 4 weeks

Patients established on oral olanzapine 20 mg daily: Initial and maintenance dose: 300 mg every 2 weeks

Special risk patients: Initial: 150 mg every 4 weeks is recommended in patients who are debilitated, who have a predisposition to hypotensive reactions, who exhibit a combination of factors that may result in slower metabolism of olanzapine (eg, nonsmoking female patients ≥65 years), or who may be more pharmacodynamically sensitive to olanzapine; increase dose with caution as clinically indicated.

Delirium (off-label use): Oral: 5 mg daily for up to 5 days (NICE, 2010)

Prevention of chemotherapy-associated delayed nausea or vomiting (off-label use; in combination with a corticosteroid and serotonin [5-HT_3] antagonist): Oral: 10 mg once daily for 3 to 5 days, beginning on day 1 of chemotherapy **or** 5 mg once daily for 2 days before chemotherapy, followed by 10 mg once daily (beginning on the day of chemotherapy) for 3 to 8 days

Elderly:

Short-acting IM, Oral: Consider lower starting dose of 2.5 to 5 mg daily for elderly patients; may increase as clinically indicated and tolerated with close monitoring of orthostatic blood pressure

Extended release IM: Consider lower starting dose of 150 mg every 4 weeks for elderly patients; increase dose with caution as clinically indicated.

Delirium (off-label use): Patients >60 years: 2.5 mg daily for up to 5 days (NICE, 2010)

Psychosis/agitation related to Alzheimer dementia (off-label use): Oral: Initial: 2.5 to 5 mg daily (Sultzer, 2008)

Dosage adjustment in renal impairment: No dosage adjustment necessary. Not removed by dialysis.

Dosage adjustment in hepatic impairment: There are no dosage adjustments provided in the manufacturer's labeling except when used in combination with fluoxetine (as separate components) the initial olanzapine dose should be limited to 2.5 to 5 mg daily. Use with caution (cases of hepatitis and liver injury have been reported with olanzapine use).

Dietary Considerations Tablets may be taken without regard to meals. Some products may contain phenylalanine.

Administration

Short-acting IM injection: **For IM administration only**; do not administer injection intravenously or subcutaneously; inject slowly, deep into muscle. If dizziness and/or drowsiness are noted, patient should remain recumbent until examination indicates postural hypotension and/or bradycardia are not a problem.

Extended-release IM injection: **For IM gluteal injection only**; do not administer IV or subcutaneously. After needle insertion into muscle, aspirate to verify that no blood appears. Do not massage injection site. Use diluent, syringes, and needles provided in convenience kit; obtain a new kit if aspiration of blood occurs.

Tablet: May be administered without regard to meals.

Orally-disintegrating: Remove from foil blister by peeling back (do not push tablet through the foil); place tablet in mouth immediately upon removal; tablet dissolves rapidly in saliva and may be swallowed with or without liquid. May be administered with or without food/meals.

Monitoring Parameters Mental status; vital signs (as clinically indicated); blood pressure (baseline; repeat 3 months after antipsychotic initiation, then yearly); weight, height, BMI, waist circumference (baseline; repeat at 4, 8, and 12 weeks after initiating or changing therapy, then quarterly; consider switching to a different antipsychotic for a weight gain ≥5% of initial weight); CBC (as clinically indicated; monitor frequently during the first few months of therapy in patients with preexisting low WBC or history of drug-induced leukopenia/neutropenia); electrolytes and liver function (annually and as clinically indicated); personal and family history of obesity, diabetes, dyslipidemia, hypertension, or cardiovascular disease (baseline; repeat annually); fasting plasma glucose level/HbA_{1c} (baseline; repeat 3 months after starting antipsychotic, then yearly); fasting lipid panel (baseline; repeat 3 months after initiation of antipsychotic; if LDL level is normal repeat at 2-5 year intervals or more frequently if clinical indicated); changes in menstruation, libido, development of galactorrhea, erectile and ejaculatory function (at each visit for the first 12 weeks after the antipsychotic is initiated or until the dose is stable, then yearly); abnormal involuntary movements or parkinsonian signs (baseline; repeat weekly until dose stabilized for at least 2 weeks after introduction and for 2 weeks after any significant dose increase); tardive dyskinesia (every 12 months; high-risk patients every 6 months); ocular examination (yearly in patients >40 years; every 2 years in younger patients) (ADA, 2004; Lehman, 2004; Marder, 2004)

Extended-release IM injection: Sedation/delirium for 3 hours after each dose

Dosage Forms

Solution Reconstituted, Intramuscular:
ZyPREXA: 10 mg (1 ea)
Generic: 10 mg (1 ea)

Suspension Reconstituted, Intramuscular:
ZyPREXA Relprevv: 210 mg (1 ea); 300 mg (1 ea); 405 mg (1 ea)

Tablet, Oral:
ZyPREXA: 2.5 mg, 5 mg, 7.5 mg, 10 mg, 15 mg, 20 mg
Generic: 2.5 mg, 5 mg, 7.5 mg, 10 mg, 15 mg, 20 mg

Tablet Dispersible, Oral:
ZyPREXA Zydis: 5 mg, 10 mg, 15 mg, 20 mg
Generic: 5 mg, 10 mg, 15 mg, 20 mg

Dosage Forms: Canada Note: Refer to Dosage Forms. ZyPREXA Relprevv is not available in Canada.

◆ **Olanzapine for injection (Can)** *see* OLANZapine *on page 1491*
◆ **Olanzapine ODT (Can)** *see* OLANZapine *on page 1491*
◆ **Olanzapine Pamoate** *see* OLANZapine *on page 1491*
◆ **Oleovitamin A** *see* Vitamin A *on page 2173*
◆ **Oleptro** *see* TraZODone *on page 2091*
◆ **Olestyr (Can)** *see* Cholestyramine Resin *on page 431*
◆ **Olex (Can)** *see* Omeprazole *on page 1508*

Olmesartan (ole me SAR tan)

Brand Names: U.S. Benicar

Brand Names: Canada Olmetec

Index Terms Olmesartan Medoxomil

Pharmacologic Category Angiotensin II Receptor Blocker; Antihypertensive

Use Hypertension: Treatment of hypertension with or without concurrent use of other antihypertensive agents

The 2014 guideline for the management of high blood pressure in adults (Eighth Joint National Committee [JNC 8; James, 2013]) recommends initiation of pharmacologic treatment to lower blood pressure for the following patients:

- Patients ≥60 years of age with systolic blood pressure (SBP) ≥150 mm Hg or diastolic blood pressure (DBP) ≥90 mm Hg. Goal of therapy is SBP <150 mm Hg and DBP <90 mm Hg.
- Patients <60 years of age with SBP ≥140 mm Hg or DBP ≥90 mm Hg. Goal of therapy is SBP <140 mm Hg and DBP <90 mm Hg.
- Patients ≥18 years of age with diabetes and SBP ≥140 mm Hg or DBP ≥90 mm Hg. Goal of therapy is SBP <140 mm Hg and DBP <90 mm Hg.
- Patients ≥18 years of age with chronic kidney disease (CKD) and SBP ≥140 mm Hg or DBP ≥90 mm Hg. Goal of therapy is SBP <140 mm Hg and DBP <90 mm Hg.

In patients with CKD, regardless of race or diabetes status, the use of an ACE inhibitor (ACEI) or angiotensin receptor blocker (ARB) as initial therapy is recommended to improve kidney outcomes. In the general nonblack population (without CKD), including those with diabetes, initial antihypertensive treatment should consist of a thiazide-type diuretic, calcium channel blocker, ACEI, or ARB. In the general black population (without CKD), including those with diabetes, initial antihypertensive treatment should consist of a thiazide-type diuretic or a calcium channel blocker instead of an ACEI or ARB.

Pregnancy Risk Factor D

Pregnancy Considerations [U.S. Boxed Warning]: Drugs that act on the renin-angiotensin system can cause injury and death to the developing fetus. Discontinue as soon as possible once pregnancy is detected. The use of drugs which act on the renin-angiotensin system are associated with oligohydramnios. Oligohydramnios, due to decreased fetal renal function, may lead to fetal lung hypoplasia and skeletal malformations. Use is also associated with anuria, hypotension, renal failure, skull hypoplasia, and death in the fetus/neonate. The exposed fetus should be monitored for fetal growth, amniotic fluid volume, and organ formation. Infants exposed *in utero* should be monitored for hyperkalemia, hypotension, and oliguria (exchange transfusions or dialysis may be needed). These adverse events are generally associated with maternal use in the second and third trimesters.

Untreated chronic maternal hypertension is also associated with adverse events in the fetus, infant, and mother. The use of angiotensin II receptor blockers is not recommended to treat chronic uncomplicated hypertension in pregnant women and should generally be avoided in women of reproductive potential (ACOG, 2013).

Breast-Feeding Considerations It is not known if olmesartan is excreted into breast milk. Due to the potential for serious adverse reactions in the nursing infant, the manufacturer recommends a decision be made whether to discontinue nursing or to discontinue the drug, taking into account the importance of treatment to the mother.

Contraindications Concomitant use with aliskiren in patients with diabetes mellitus

Canadian labeling: Additional contraindications (not in U.S. labeling): Hypersensitivity to olmesartan or any component of the formulation; concomitant use with aliskiren in patients with moderate to severe renal impairment (GFR <60 mL/minute/1.73 m^2)

Documentation of allergenic cross-reactivity for angiotensin II receptor blockers is limited. However, because of similarities in chemical structure and/or pharmacologic actions, the possibility of cross-sensitivity cannot be ruled out with certainty.

Warnings/Precautions [U.S. Boxed Warning]: Drugs that act on the renin-angiotensin system can cause injury and death to the developing fetus. Discontinue as soon as possible once pregnancy is detected. May cause hyperkalemia; avoid potassium supplementation unless specifically required by healthcare provider. Avoid use or use a smaller dose in patients who are volume depleted; correct depletion first. May be associated with deterioration of renal function and/or increases in serum creatinine, particularly in patients with low renal blood flow (eg, renal artery stenosis, heart failure) whose glomerular filtration rate (GFR) is dependent on efferent arteriolar vasoconstriction by angiotensin II. Use with caution in unstented unilateral/bilateral renal artery stenosis. When unstented bilateral renal artery stenosis is present, use is generally avoided due to the elevated risk of deterioration in renal function unless possible benefits outweigh risks. Use with caution with preexisting renal insufficiency; significant aortic/mitral stenosis. Potentially significant drug-drug interactions may exist, requiring dose or frequency adjustment, additional monitoring, and/or selection of alternative therapy. In surgical patients on chronic angiotensin receptor blocker (ARB) therapy, intraoperative hypotension may occur with induction and maintenance of general anesthesia.

Symptoms of sprue-like enteropathy (ie, severe, chronic diarrhea with significant weight loss) has been reported; may develop months to years after treatment initiation with villous atrophy commonly found on intestinal biopsy. Once other etiologies have been excluded, discontinue treatment and consider other antihypertensive treatment. Clinical and histologic improvement was noted after treatment was discontinued in a case series of 22 patients (Ianiro, 2014; Rubio-Tapia, 2012).

Angioedema has been reported rarely with some angiotensin II receptor antagonists (ARBs) and may occur at any time during treatment (especially following first dose). It may involve the head and neck (potentially compromising airway) or the intestine (presenting with abdominal pain). Patients with idiopathic or hereditary angioedema or previous angioedema associated with ACE-inhibitor therapy may be at an increased risk. Prolonged frequent monitoring may be required, especially if tongue, glottis, or larynx are involved, as they are associated with airway obstruction. Patients with a history of airway surgery may have a higher risk of airway obstruction. Discontinue therapy immediately if angioedema occurs. Aggressive early management is critical. Intramuscular (IM) administration of epinephrine may be necessary. Do not readminister to patients who have had angioedema with ARBs.

Olmesartan has not been shown to be effective for hypertension in children younger than 6 years. Children younger than 1 year must not receive olmesartan for hypertension. The renin-angiotensin-aldosterone system plays a critical role in kidney development. Administering drugs that act directly on the renin-angiotensin-aldosterone system can have effects on the development of immature kidneys and alter normal renal development.

Adverse Reactions

Central nervous system: Dizziness, headache
Endocrine & metabolic: Hyperglycemia, hypertriglyceridemia
Gastrointestinal: Diarrhea
Neuromuscular & skeletal: Back pain, CPK increased
Renal: Hematuria
Respiratory: Bronchitis, pharyngitis, rhinitis, sinusitis
Miscellaneous: Flu-like syndrome
Rare but important or life-threatening: Acute renal failure, alopecia, anaphylaxis, angioedema, arthritis, gastroenteritis, hypercholesterolemia, hyperkalemia, hyperlipidemia, hyperuricemia, liver enzymes increased, peripheral edema, rhabdomyolysis, serum creatinine increased, sprue-like symptoms, tachycardia

Drug Interactions

Metabolism/Transport Effects Substrate of SLCO1B1

Avoid Concomitant Use There are no known interactions where it is recommended to avoid concomitant use.

Increased Effect/Toxicity

Olmesartan may increase the levels/effects of: ACE Inhibitors; Amifostine; Antihypertensives; CycloSPORINE (Systemic); DULoxetine; Hypotensive Agents; Levodopa; Lithium; Nonsteroidal Anti-Inflammatory Agents; Obinutuzumab; Potassium-Sparing Diuretics; RisperiDONE; RiTUXimab; Sodium Phosphates

The levels/effects of Olmesartan may be increased by: Alfuzosin; Aliskiren; Barbiturates; Brimonidine (Topical); Canagliflozin; Dapoxetine; Diazoxide; Eltrombopag; Eplerenone; Heparin; Heparin (Low Molecular Weight); Herbs (Hypotensive Properties); MAO Inhibitors; Nicorandil; Pentoxifylline; Phosphodiesterase 5 Inhibitors; Potassium Salts; Prostacyclin Analogues; Teriflunomide; Tolvaptan; Trimethoprim

Decreased Effect

The levels/effects of Olmesartan may be decreased by: Colesevelam; Herbs (Hypertensive Properties); Methylphenidate; Nonsteroidal Anti-Inflammatory Agents; Yohimbine

Storage/Stability Store at 20°C to 25°C (68°F to 77°F).

Mechanism of Action As a selective and competitive, nonpeptide angiotensin II receptor antagonist, olmesartan blocks the vasoconstrictor and aldosterone-secreting effects of angiotensin II; olmesartan interacts reversibly at the AT1 and AT2 receptors of many tissues and has slow dissociation kinetics; its affinity for the AT1 receptor is 12,500 times greater than the AT2 receptor. Angiotensin II receptor antagonists may induce a more complete inhibition of the renin-angiotensin system than ACE inhibitors, they do not affect the response to bradykinin, and are less likely to be associated with nonrenin-angiotensin effects (eg, cough and angioedema). Olmesartan increases urinary flow rate and, in addition to being natriuretic and kaliuretic, increases excretion of chloride, magnesium, uric acid, calcium, and phosphate.

Pharmacodynamics/Kinetics

Distribution: 17 L; does not cross the blood-brain barrier (animal studies)
Protein binding: 99%
Metabolism: Olmesartan medoxomil is hydrolyzed in the GI tract to active olmesartan. No further metabolism occurs.
Bioavailability: 26%
Half-life elimination: Terminal: 13 hours
Time to peak: 1 to 2 hours
Excretion: All as unchanged drug: Feces (50% to 65%); urine (35% to 50%)

Dosage Hypertension:

Children 6 to 16 years: Oral:
- 20 kg to <35 kg: Initial: 10 mg once daily; if initial response inadequate after 2 weeks, dose may be increased (maximum: 20 mg once daily)
- ≥35 kg: Initial: 20 mg once daily; if initial response inadequate after 2 weeks, dose may be increased (maximum: 40 mg once daily)

Adults: Oral: Initial: 20 mg once daily; if initial response is inadequate, may be increased to 40 mg once daily after 2 weeks. Usual dosage range (ASH/ISH [Weber, 2014]): 20 to 40 mg daily. May administer with other antihypertensive agents if blood pressure inadequately controlled with olmesartan. Consider lower starting dose in patients with possible depletion of intravascular volume (eg, patients receiving diuretics).

Elderly: Oral: No initial dosage adjustment is necessary per labeling; however, may consider starting at 5 to 10 mg once daily (due to concomitant disease or age changes).

Dosage adjustment in renal impairment:

U.S. labeling: Initial: No dosage adjustment is necessary for patients with moderate to severe renal impairment (creatinine clearance <40 mL/minute). However, AUC increased 3-fold in patients with CrCl <20 mL/minute; use with caution.

Canadian labeling:
- Mild to moderate impairment: Maximum dose: 20 mg once daily
- Severe impairment: There are no dosage adjustments provided in the manufacturer's labeling; use is not recommended.

Dosage adjustment in hepatic impairment:

U.S. labeling: Initial: No dosage adjustment is necessary for patients with moderate to severe hepatic dysfunction. Total drug exposure increased 60% in patients with moderate impairment.

Canadian labeling:

Mild impairment: No dosage adjustment necessary.

Moderate impairment: Initial: Lower starting dose is recommended (maximum: 20 mg once daily)

Severe impairment: There are no dosage adjustments provided in the manufacturer's labeling; use is not recommended.

Dietary Considerations May be taken with or without food.

Administration May be administered with or without food.

Monitoring Parameters Blood pressure, electrolytes, serum creatinine, BUN, urinalysis

Dosage Forms

Tablet, Oral:

Benicar: 5 mg, 20 mg, 40 mg

Extemporaneous Preparations A 2 mg/mL oral suspension may be made with olmesartan tablets. Combine 50 mL purified water and twenty 20 mg tablets in an 8-ounce amber bottle and allow to stand for ≥5 minutes. Shake well for ≥1 minute, then allow to stand for ≥1 minute. Repeat shaking and standing process four additional times. Add 100 mL Ora-Sweet® and 50 mL Ora-Plus® to the suspension and shake well for ≥1 minute. Label "shake well" and "refrigerate". Stable for 28 days refrigerated.

Benicar® prescribing information, Daiichi Sankyo, Inc, Parsippany, NJ, 2010.

Olmesartan, Amlodipine, and Hydrochlorothiazide

(ole me SAR tan, am LOE di peen, & hye droe klor oh THYE a zide)

Brand Names: U.S. Tribenzor™

Index Terms Amlodipine Besylate, Olmesartan Medoxomil, and Hydrochlorothiazide; Amlodipine, Hydrochlorothiazide, and Olmesartan; Hydrochlorothiazide, Olmesartan, and Amlodipine; Olmesartan, Hydrochlorothiazide, and Amlodipine

Pharmacologic Category Angiotensin II Receptor Blocker; Antianginal Agent; Antihypertensive; Calcium Channel Blocker; Calcium Channel Blocker, Dihydropyridine; Diuretic, Thiazide

Use Treatment of hypertension (not for initial therapy)

Pregnancy Risk Factor D

Dosage Oral: **Note:** Not for initial therapy. Dose is individualized; combination product may be substituted for individual components in patients currently maintained on all 3 agents separately or in patients not adequately controlled with any 2 of the following antihypertensive classes: Calcium channel blockers, angiotensin II receptor blockers, and diuretics.

Adults: Hypertension: Add-on/switch/replacement therapy: Amlodipine 5-10 mg, olmesartan 20-40 mg, and hydrochlorothiazide 12.5-25 mg once daily; dose may be titrated after 2 weeks of therapy. Maximum recommended daily dose: Amlodipine 10 mg/olmesartan 40 mg/hydrochlorothiazide 25 mg

Elderly: Patients ≥75 years of age should start amlodipine at 2.5 mg (combination product dosage form not available in this strength)

Dosage adjustment in renal impairment:

CrCl >30 mL/minute: No dosage adjustment necessary.

CrCl ≤30 mL/minute: Use of combination not recommended; contraindicated in patients with anuria

Dosage adjustment in hepatic impairment:

Mild-to-moderate hepatic impairment: No dosage adjustment provided in manufacturer's labeling. Use with caution.

Severe hepatic impairment: Use not recommended; initial daily dose of amlodipine is 2.5 mg (this dose of amlodipine is not available as a combination product).

Additional Information Complete prescribing information should be consulted for additional detail.

Dosage Forms

Tablet, oral:

Tribenzor™: Olmesartan medoxomil 40 mg, amlodipine 5 mg, and hydrochlorothiazide 25 mg, olmesartan medoxomil 40 mg, amlodipine 10 mg, and hydrochlorothiazide 25 mg, olmesartan medoxomil 20 mg, amlodipine 5 mg, and hydrochlorothiazide 12.5 mg, olmesartan medoxomil 40 mg, amlodipine 5 mg, and hydrochlorothiazide 12.5 mg, olmesartan medoxomil 40 mg, amlodipine 10 mg, and hydrochlorothiazide 12.5 mg

◆ **Olmesartan and Amlodipine** *see* Amlodipine and Olmesartan *on page 126*

Olmesartan and Hydrochlorothiazide

(ole me SAR tan & hye droe klor oh THYE a zide)

Brand Names: U.S. Benicar HCT

Brand Names: Canada Olmetec Plus

Index Terms Hydrochlorothiazide and Olmesartan Medoxomil; Olmesartan Medoxomil and Hydrochlorothiazide

Pharmacologic Category Angiotensin II Receptor Blocker; Diuretic, Thiazide

Use Treatment of hypertension (not recommended for initial treatment)

Pregnancy Risk Factor D

Dosage Hypertension: Adults: Oral: One tablet daily; dosage must be individualized. May be titrated at 2- to 4-week intervals.

Replacement therapy: May be substituted for previously titrated dosages of the individual components.

Patients not controlled with single-agent therapy: Initiate by adding the lowest available dose of the alternative component (hydrochlorothiazide 12.5 mg or olmesartan 20 mg). Titrate to effect (maximum daily hydrochlorothiazide dose: 25 mg; maximum daily olmesartan dose: 40 mg).

Dosage adjustment in renal impairment:

CrCl >30 mL/minute: No dosage adjustment necessary.

CrCl ≤30 mL/minute: Use not recommended.

Dosage adjustment in hepatic impairment: No dosage adjustment necessary.

Additional Information Complete prescribing information should be consulted for additional detail.

Dosage Forms

Tablet:

Benicar HCT®: 20/12.5: Olmesartan 20 mg and hydrochlorothiazide 12.5 mg; 40/12.5: Olmesartan 40 mg and hydrochlorothiazide 12.5 mg; 40/25: Olmesartan 40 mg and hydrochlorothiazide 25 mg

◆ **Olmesartan, Hydrochlorothiazide, and Amlodipine** *see* Olmesartan, Amlodipine, and Hydrochlorothiazide *on page 1498*

◆ **Olmesartan Medoxomil** *see* Olmesartan *on page 1496*

◆ **Olmesartan Medoxomil and Hydrochlorothiazide** *see* Olmesartan and Hydrochlorothiazide *on page 1498*

◆ **Olmetec (Can)** *see* Olmesartan *on page 1496*

◆ **Olmetec Plus (Can)** *see* Olmesartan and Hydrochlorothiazide *on page 1498*

Olodaterol (oh loe DA ter ol)

Brand Names: U.S. Striverdi Respimat

Index Terms Olodaterol Hydrochloride

Pharmacologic Category $Beta_2$ Agonist; $Beta_2$-Adrenergic Agonist, Long-Acting

Use Chronic obstructive pulmonary disease: Long-term maintenance treatment of airflow obstruction in chronic obstructive pulmonary disease (COPD), including chronic bronchitis and/or emphysema

Pregnancy Risk Factor C

Pregnancy Considerations Adverse events were observed in some animal reproduction studies. Beta-agonists have the potential to affect uterine contractility if administered during labor.

Breast-Feeding Considerations Excretion of olodaterol into breast milk is unknown but likely. The manufacturer recommends that caution be used if administered to a nursing woman. The use of $beta_2$-receptor agonists are not considered a contraindication to breast-feeding (NAEPP, 2005).

Contraindications Monotherapy in the treatment of asthma (ie, use without a concomitant long-term asthma control medication). **Note:** Olodaterol is not FDA approved for treatment of asthma.

Documentation of allergenic cross-reactivity for sympathomimetics is limited. However, because of similarities in chemical structure and/or pharmacologic actions, the possibility of cross-sensitivity cannot be ruled out with certainty.

Warnings/Precautions [U.S. Boxed Warning]: Long-acting $beta_2$-agonists (LABAs) increase the risk of asthma-related deaths. The safety and efficacy of olodaterol in the treatment of asthma have not been established. In a large, randomized, placebo-controlled U.S. clinical trial (SMART, 2006), salmeterol was associated with an increase in asthma-related deaths (when added to usual asthma therapy); risk is considered a class effect among all LABAs. It is unknown if olodaterol increases asthma-related deaths. No data exist associating LABA use with an increased risk of death in patients with COPD. Rarely, paradoxical, life-threatening bronchospasm may occur with use of inhaled $beta_2$-agonists; distinguish from inadequate response, discontinue medication immediately, institute alternative therapy. Do **not** use for acute bronchospastic episodes of COPD; always prescribe olodaterol with an inhaled short-acting $beta_2$-agonist and educate patient on appropriate use. Do not initiate in patients with significantly worsening or acutely deteriorating COPD. Do not increase the olodaterol dose or frequency beyond what is recommended. Hypersensitivity reactions, including angioedema, may occur; discontinue therapy if patient develops an allergic reaction. Use with caution in patients with cardiovascular disease (arrhythmia, coronary insufficiency, hypertension, or HF); beta-agonists may cause elevation in blood pressure and heart rate. $Beta_2$-agonists may also produce electrocardiogram (ECG) changes (eg, T-wave flattening, QTc prolongation, ST segment depression). Use with caution in patients with diabetes mellitus; $beta_2$-agonists may increase serum glucose. Use with caution in patients with hyperthyroidism; may stimulate thyroid activity. Use with caution in patients with hypokalemia; $beta_2$-agonists may decrease serum potassium. Use with caution in patients with seizure disorders; $beta_2$-agonists may result in CNS stimulation/excitation. Potentially significant drug-drug interactions may exist, requiring dose or frequency adjustment, additional monitoring, and/or selection of alternative therapy. Do not use with other long-acting $beta_2$-agonists; deaths and significant cardiovascular effects have been reported with excessive sympathomimetic use.

Adverse Reactions

Dermatologic: Skin rash

Genitourinary: Urinary tract infection

Neuromuscular & skeletal: Arthralgia, back pain

Respiratory: Bronchitis, nasopharyngitis

Rare but important or life-threatening: Asthma-related death, depression of ST segment on ECG, flattened T wave on ECG, hypersensitivity reaction (includes angioedema), hypokalemia (transient), increased serum glucose (high doses), increased diastolic blood pressure, increased pulse, increased systolic blood pressure, malignant neoplasm of lung, paradoxical bronchospasm, pneumonia, prolonged Q-T interval on ECG

Drug Interactions

Metabolism/Transport Effects Substrate of CYP2C8 (minor), CYP2C9 (minor), CYP3A4 (minor), UGT1A1, UGT1A7, UGT1A9, UGT2B7; **Note:** Assignment of Major/Minor substrate status based on clinically relevant drug interaction potential

Avoid Concomitant Use

Avoid concomitant use of Olodaterol with any of the following: Beta-Blockers (Nonselective); Iobenguane I 123; Long-Acting Beta2-Agonists

Increased Effect/Toxicity

Olodaterol may increase the levels/effects of: Atosiban; Highest Risk QTc-Prolonging Agents; Long-Acting Beta2-Agonists; Loop Diuretics; Moderate Risk QTc-Prolonging Agents; Sympathomimetics; Thiazide Diuretics

The levels/effects of Olodaterol may be increased by: AtoMOXetine; Caffeine and Caffeine Containing Products; Cannabinoid-Containing Products; Linezolid; MAO Inhibitors; Mifepristone; Tedizolid; Theophylline Derivatives; Tricyclic Antidepressants

Decreased Effect

Olodaterol may decrease the levels/effects of: Iobenguane I 123

The levels/effects of Olodaterol may be decreased by: Beta-Blockers (Beta1 Selective); Beta-Blockers (Nonselective); Betahistine

Storage/Stability Store at 25°C (77°F); excursions are permitted between 15°C and 30°C (59°F and 86°F). Avoid freezing. Discard 3 months after cartridge is inserted into inhaler.

Mechanism of Action Long acting $beta_2$-receptor agonist; activates $beta_2$ airway receptors, resulting in the stimulation of intracellular adenyl cyclase and a subsequent increase in the synthesis of cyclic-3',5' adenosine monophosphate (cAMP). Elevated cAMP levels induce bronchodilation by relaxation of airway smooth muscle cells. Has much greater affinity for $beta_2$-receptors than for $beta_1$- or $beta_3$-receptors.

Pharmacodynamics/Kinetics

Onset of action: 5 minutes

Duration: 24 hours

Distribution: V_d: 1110 L

Protein binding: ~60%

Metabolism: Direct glucuronidation (UGT2B7, UGT1A1, 1A7, and 1A9) and O-demethylation (primarily CYP2C9 and 2C8)

Bioavailability: 30% (inhalation)

Half-life elimination: 7.5 hours

Time to peak: 10 to 20 minutes

Excretion: Urine (5% to 7% unchanged); feces

Dosage COPD: Adults: Inhalation: Two inhalations once daily (maximum: 2 inhalations per day)

Dosing adjustment in renal impairment: No dosage adjustment necessary.

Dosing adjustment in hepatic impairment:

Mild to moderate impairment: No dosage adjustment necessary.

Severe impairment: There are no dosage adjustments provided in the manufacturer's labeling (has not been studied).

Administration For oral inhalation only. Prime inhaler prior to initial use or if not used for >21 days by pointing inhaler towards ground and actuating until aerosol cloud is seen, then repeat 3 additional times before use. If not used for >3 days (but ≤21 days), actuate once before use. To prepare inhaler for use after priming, refer to manufacturer labeling. When dose is ready to be administered, breathe in slowly through the mouth and press the dose release button; continue to breathe in slowly as long as possible, then hold breath for 10 seconds or for as long as comfortable. Repeat for second inhalation.

Monitoring Parameters FEV_1, FVC, and/or other pulmonary function tests; serum potassium, serum glucose; blood pressure, heart rate; CNS stimulation. Monitor for increased use of short-acting $beta_2$-agonist inhalers; may be marker of a deteriorating condition.

Dosage Forms

Aerosol Solution, Inhalation:

Striverdi Respimat: 2.5 mcg/actuation (4 g)

◆ **Olodaterol Hydrochloride** *see* Olodaterol *on page 1498*

Olopatadine (Nasal) (oh la PAT a deen)

Brand Names: U.S. Patanase

Index Terms Olopatadine Hydrochloride

Pharmacologic Category Histamine H_1 Antagonist; Histamine H_1 Antagonist, Second Generation; Piperidine Derivative

Use Treatment of the symptoms of seasonal allergic rhinitis

Pregnancy Risk Factor C

Dosage Intranasal:

Children 6-11 years: 1 spray into each nostril twice daily

Children ≥12 years, Adolescents, and Adults: 2 sprays into each nostril twice daily

Dosage adjustment in renal impairment: No dosage adjustment necessary.

Dosage adjustment in hepatic impairment: No dosage adjustment necessary.

Additional Information Complete prescribing information should be consulted for additional detail.

Dosage Forms Considerations

Patanase 30.5 g bottles contain 240 sprays.

Dosage Forms

Solution, Nasal:

Patanase: 0.6% (30.5 g)

Generic: 0.6% (30.5 g)

Olopatadine (Ophthalmic) (oh la PAT a deen)

Brand Names: U.S. Pataday; Patanol

Brand Names: Canada ACT-Olopatadine; Apo-Olopatadine; CO Olopatadine; Pataday; Patanol; Sandoz-Olopatadine

Index Terms Olopatadine Hydrochloride

Pharmacologic Category Histamine H_1 Antagonist; Histamine H_1 Antagonist, Second Generation; Piperidine Derivative

Use Treatment of the signs and symptoms of allergic conjunctivitis

Pregnancy Risk Factor C

Dosage Ophthalmic:

Children ≥3 years, Adolescents, and Adults: Patanol®: Instill 1 drop into each affected eye twice daily (allowing 6-8 hours between doses); results from an environmental study demonstrated that olopatadine was effective when dosed twice daily for up to 6 weeks

Children ≥2 years, Adolescents, and Adults: Pataday™: Instill 1 drop into each affected eye once daily

Dosage adjustment in renal impairment: No dosage adjustment provided in manufacturer's labeling. However, dosage adjustment unlikely due to low systemic absorption.

Dosage adjustment in hepatic impairment: No dosage adjustment provided in manufacturer's labeling. However, dosage adjustment unlikely due to low systemic absorption.

Additional Information Complete prescribing information should be consulted for additional detail.

Product Availability

Pazeo (olopatadine 0.7% solution): FDA approved February 2015. Availability anticipated in March 2015. Consult prescribing information for additional information.

Dosage Forms

Solution, Ophthalmic:

Pataday: 0.2% (2.5 mL)

Patanol: 0.1% (5 mL)

◆ **Olopatadine Hydrochloride** *see* Olopatadine (Nasal) *on page 1500*

◆ **Olopatadine Hydrochloride** *see* Olopatadine (Ophthalmic) *on page 1500*

Olsalazine (ole SAL a zeen)

Brand Names: U.S. Dipentum

Brand Names: Canada Dipentum®

Index Terms Olsalazine Sodium

Pharmacologic Category 5-Aminosalicylic Acid Derivative

Use Maintenance of remission of ulcerative colitis in patients intolerant to sulfasalazine

Pregnancy Risk Factor C

Pregnancy Considerations Animal studies have demonstrated fetal developmental toxicities. There are no well-controlled studies in pregnant women. Use during pregnancy only if clearly necessary.

Breast-Feeding Considerations The active metabolite, 5-aminosalicylic acid may pass into breast milk. Diarrhea has been reported in breast-fed infants whose mothers took olsalazine.

Contraindications Hypersensitivity to olsalazine, salicylates, or any component of the formulation

Warnings/Precautions Diarrhea is a common adverse effect of olsalazine. May exacerbate symptoms of colitis. Use with caution in patients with renal or hepatic impairment. Use with caution in elderly patients. Use with caution in patients with severe allergies or asthma.

Adverse Reactions

Central nervous system: Depression, dizziness, vertigo

Dermatologic: Pruritus, rash

Gastrointestinal: Abdominal pain/cramps, bloating, diarrhea (dose related), nausea, stomatitis, vomiting

Neuromuscular & skeletal: Arthralgia

Respiratory: Upper respiratory infection

Rare but important or life-threatening: Alkaline phosphatase increased, Alopecia, ALT increased, anemia, angioedema, aplastic anemia, AST increased, bilirubin increased, blood in stool, blurred vision, bronchospasm, cholestatic hepatitis, cholestatic jaundice, chest pain, chills, cirrhosis, dehydration, dry eyes, dyspnea, dysuria, eosinophilia, epigastric discomfort, erythema, erythema nodosum, fever, flare of symptoms, flatulence, GGT increased, heart block (second degree), hematuria, hemolytic anemia, hepatitis, hepatic failure, hepatic necrosis, hot flashes, hypertension, impotence, insomnia, interstitial nephritis, interstitial pneumonia, irritability, jaundice, Kawasaki-like syndrome, LDH increased, leukopenia, lymphopenia, menorrhagia, mood swings, muscle cramps, myalgia, myocarditis, nephrotic syndrome, neutropenia, orthostatic hypotension, palpitation, pancreatitis, pancytopenia, paresthesia, pericarditis, peripheral edema, peripheral neuropathy, photosensitivity, proteinuria, rectal bleeding, rectal discomfort, reticulocytosis, rigors, tachycardia, thrombocytopenia, tinnitus, tremor, urinary frequency, watery eyes, xerostomia

Drug Interactions

Metabolism/Transport Effects None known.

Avoid Concomitant Use There are no known interactions where it is recommended to avoid concomitant use.

Increased Effect/Toxicity

Olsalazine may increase the levels/effects of: Heparin; Heparin (Low Molecular Weight); Thiopurine Analogs; Varicella Virus-Containing Vaccines

The levels/effects of Olsalazine may be increased by: Nonsteroidal Anti-Inflammatory Agents

Decreased Effect

Olsalazine may decrease the levels/effects of: Cardiac Glycosides

Storage/Stability Store at 20°C to 25°C (77°F); excursions permitted to 15°C to 30°C (59°F to 86°F).

Mechanism of Action Mesalamine (5-aminosalicylic acid) is the active component of olsalazine; the specific mechanism of action of mesalamine is unknown; however, it is thought that it modulates local chemical mediators of the inflammatory response, especially leukotrienes, and is also postulated to be a free radical scavenger or an inhibitor of tumor necrosis factor (TNF); action appears topical rather than systemic.

Pharmacodynamics/Kinetics

Absorption: <3%; very little intact olsalazine is systemically absorbed

Protein binding, plasma: >99%

Metabolism: Primarily via colonic bacteria to active drug, 5-aminosalicylic acid (5-ASA)

Half-life elimination: 54 minutes

Time to peak: ~1 hour

Excretion: Primarily feces; urine (<1%)

Dosage Adults: Oral: 1 g/day in 2 divided doses

Dosage adjustment in renal impairment: No dosage adjustment provided in manufacturer's labeling. Monitor patients with impaired renal function.

Dosage adjustment in hepatic impairment: No dosage adjustment provided in manufacturer's labeling. Monitor patients with impaired hepatic function.

Dietary Considerations Take with food.

Administration Administer with food in evenly divided doses.

Monitoring Parameters CBC, hepatic function, renal function; stool frequency

Dosage Forms

Capsule, Oral:

Dipentum: 250 mg

◆ **Olsalazine Sodium** *see* Olsalazine *on page* 1500

◆ **Olux** *see* Clobetasol *on page* 468

◆ **Olux-E** *see* Clobetasol *on page* 468

◆ **Olysio** *see* Simeprevir *on page* 1887

Omacetaxine (oh ma se TAX een)

Brand Names: U.S. Synribo

Index Terms CGX-625; HHT; Homoharringtonine; Omacetaxine Mepesuccinate

Pharmacologic Category Antineoplastic Agent, Cephalotaxine; Antineoplastic Agent, Protein Synthesis Inhibitor

Use Chronic myeloid leukemia: Treatment of chronic or accelerated phase chronic myeloid leukemia (CML) in adult patients resistant and/or intolerant to ≥2 tyrosine kinase inhibitors

Pregnancy Risk Factor D

Pregnancy Considerations Adverse events were observed in animal reproduction studies at doses less than the equivalent human dose (based on BSA). Based on the mechanism of action, omacetaxine may cause fetal harm if administered during pregnancy. Women of reproductive potential should avoid pregnancy during therapy. Omacetaxine may impair fertility in males.

Breast-Feeding Considerations It is not known if omacetaxine is excreted in breast milk. Due to the potential for serious adverse reactions in the nursing infant, the decision to discontinue omacetaxine or to discontinue breast-feeding should take into account the importance of treatment to the mother.

Contraindications There are no contraindications listed in the manufacturer's labeling.

Warnings/Precautions Hazardous agent: Use appropriate precautions for handling and disposal (NIOSH 2014 [group 1]). Grade 3/4 neutropenia, thrombocytopenia, and anemia commonly occur; generally reversible, although may require treatment delay and/or a reduction in the number of treatment days with future cycles. Myelosuppression may rarely be fatal. Monitor blood counts (in induction and maintenance cycles). Neutropenia may increase the risk for infection. Thrombocytopenia may increase the risk of bleeding; cerebrovascular hemorrhages have been reported (some fatal); gastrointestinal hemorrhages have occurred. Due to the increased risk of bleeding, avoid the use of anticoagulants, aspirin, and NSAIDs when the platelet count is <50,000/mm³. Patients ≥65 years of age are more likely to experience hematologic toxicity. Omacetaxine may induce glucose intolerance; hyperglycemia has been observed; hyperosmolar nonketotic hyperglycemia has been reported (case report). Monitor blood glucose frequently, especially in patients with diabetes or with risk factors for diabetes. Avoid use in patients with poorly controlled diabetes; may initiate after glycemic control has been established. Potentially significant interactions may exist, requiring dose or frequency adjustment, additional monitoring, and/or selection of alternative therapy.

Adverse Reactions

Cardiovascular: Acute coronary syndrome, angina pectoris, arrhythmia, bradycardia, cerebral hemorrhage, chest pain, edema, hypertension, hypotension, palpitations, peripheral edema, tachycardia, ventricular extrasystoles

Central nervous system: Agitation, anxiety, chills, confusion, depression, dizziness, dysphonia, fatigue, headache, hyperthermia, hypoesthesia, insomnia, lethargy, malaise, mental status change, pain, seizures

Dermatologic: Alopecia, bruising, burning sensation, dry skin, erythema, hyperhidrosis, hyperpigmentation, petechiae, pruritus, purpura, skin exfoliation, skin lesions, skin rash, skin ulceration

Endocrine & metabolic: Dehydration, diabetes mellitus, glucose decreased, gout, hot flashes, hyperglycemia (including hyperosmolar nonketotic hyperglycemia), uric acid increased

Gastrointestinal: Abdominal distension, abdominal pain, abnormal taste, anal fissure, anorexia, aphthous stomatitis, appetite decreased, constipation, diarrhea, dyspepsia, dysphagia, gastritis, gastroesophageal reflux disease, GI bleeding, gingival bleeding, gingival pain, gingivitis, hemorrhoids, melena, mouth ulceration, mouth hemorrhage, mucosal inflammation, nausea, oral pain, stomatitis, vomiting, xerostomia

Genitourinary: Dysuria

Hematologic: Anemia, bone marrow failure, hematoma, leukocytes decreased, lymphopenia, neutropenia, neutropenic fever, thrombocytopenia

Hepatic: ALT increased, bilirubin increased

Local: Injection site reactions (includes infusion related reaction, erythema, hematoma, hemorrhage, hypersensitivity, induration, inflammation, irritation, mass, edema, pruritus, and rash)
Neuromuscular & skeletal: Arthralgia, back pain, bone pain, limb pain, muscle spasms, muscle weakness, musculoskeletal chest pain, musculoskeletal discomfort, musculoskeletal pain, myalgia, paresthesia, sciatica, stiffness, tremor, weakness
Ocular: Blurred vision, cataract, conjunctival hemorrhage, conjunctivitis, diplopia, dry eyes, eye pain, eyelid edema, lacrimation increased
Otic: Ear hemorrhage, ear pain, tinnitus
Renal: Creatinine increased
Respiratory: Cough, dyspnea, epistaxis, hemoptysis, nasal congestion, pharyngolaryngeal pain, rales, rhinorrhea, sinus congestion
Miscellaneous: Fever, flu-like syndrome, hypersensitivity reactions, infection, night sweats, transfusion reaction

Drug Interactions

Metabolism/Transport Effects Substrate of P-glycoprotein

Avoid Concomitant Use

Avoid concomitant use of Omacetaxine with any of the following: Anticoagulants; Aspirin; BCG; Natalizumab; Nonsteroidal Anti-Inflammatory Agents; Pimecrolimus; Tacrolimus (Topical); Tofacitinib; Vaccines (Live)

Increased Effect/Toxicity

Omacetaxine may increase the levels/effects of: Leflunomide; Natalizumab; Tofacitinib; Vaccines (Live)

The levels/effects of Omacetaxine may be increased by: Anticoagulants; Aspirin; Denosumab; Nonsteroidal Anti-Inflammatory Agents; Pimecrolimus; Roflumilast; Tacrolimus (Topical); Trastuzumab

Decreased Effect

Omacetaxine may decrease the levels/effects of: BCG; Coccidioides immitis Skin Test; Sipuleucel-T; Vaccines (Inactivated); Vaccines (Live)

The levels/effects of Omacetaxine may be decreased by: Echinacea

Preparation for Administration Hazardous agent: Use appropriate precautions for handling and disposal (NIOSH 2014 [group 1]). Avoid skin and eye contact; wear protective eyewear and gloves during handling and administration. Reconstitute each 3.5 mg vial with sodium chloride 0.9% (NS) 1 mL, resulting in a concentration of 3.5 mg/mL. Gently swirl until solution is clear (lyophilized powder dissolves completely in <1 minute).

Storage/Stability Store intact vials at 20°C to 25°C (68°F to 77°F); excursions are permitted between15°C and 30°C (59°F and 86°F). Protect from light (intact vial and reconstituted solutions). Reconstituted solution should be used within 12 hours if stored at room temperature or within 6 days (144 hours) if refrigerated at 2°C to 8°C (36°F to 46°F).

Mechanism of Action Omacetaxine is a reversible protein synthesis inhibitor which binds to the A-site cleft of the ribosomal subunit to interfere with chain elongation and inhibit protein synthesis. It acts independently of BCR-ABL1 kinase-binding activity, and has demonstrated activity against tyrosine kinase inhibitor-resistant BCR-ABL mutations.

Pharmacodynamics/Kinetics

Onset:
Chronic phase CML: Mean time to major cytogenetic response: 3.5 months
Accelerated phase CML: Mean time to response: 2.3 months

Duration:
Chronic phase CML: Median duration of major cytogenetic response: 12.5 months
Accelerated phase CML: Median duration of major hematologic response: 4.7 months

Absorption: SubQ: Rapid (Nemunaitis, 2013)
Distribution: V_{dss}: 141 ± 93 L
Protein binding: ≤50%
Metabolism: Hydrolyzed by plasma esterases to 4'-DMHHT; minimal hepatic metabolism
Half-life elimination: ~6 hours
Time to peak: SubQ: ~30 minutes
Excretion: Urine (<15%)

Dosage Chronic myeloid leukemia (CML), chronic or accelerated phase: Adults: SubQ:

Induction: 1.25 mg/m^2 twice daily for 14 consecutive days of a 28-day treatment cycle; continue until hematologic response is achieved
Maintenance: 1.25 mg/m^2 twice daily for 7 consecutive days of a 28-day treatment cycle; continue until no longer achieving clinical treatment benefit
Missed doses: If a dose is missed, skip that dose and resume with the next regularly scheduled dose. Do not administer 2 doses at the same time to make up for a missed dose.

Dosing adjustment for toxicity:

Hematologic toxicity: May delay treatment cycles and/or reduce the number of treatment days during a cycle for hematologic toxicities.
Neutropenia grade 4 (ANC <500/mm^3) or thrombocytopenia ≥ grade 3 (platelets <50,000/mm^3) during a cycle: Delay the start of the next cycle until ANC ≥1000/mm^3 and platelets ≥50,000/mm^3 **AND** reduce the number of treatment days by 2 days (eg, reduce from 14 days to 12 days or reduce from 7 days to 5 days)
Nonhematologic toxicity: Manage symptomatically; interrupt and/or delay treatment until toxicity resolves.

Dosage adjustment in renal impairment: There are no dosage adjustments provided in the manufacturer's labeling (has not been studied). Based on the minimal amount of unchanged drug excreted in the urine, dosage adjustment is not likely necessary (Nemunaitis, 2013).

Dosage adjustment in hepatic impairment: There are no dosage adjustments provided in the manufacturer's labeling (has not been studied).

Dosing in obesity: *ASCO Guidelines for appropriate chemotherapy dosing in obese adults with cancer:* Utilize patient's actual body weight (full weight) for calculation of body surface area- or weight-based dosing, particularly when the intent of therapy is curative; manage regimen-related toxicities in the same manner as for nonobese patients; if a dose reduction is utilized due to toxicity, consider resumption of full weight-based dosing with subsequent cycles, especially if cause of toxicity (eg, hepatic or renal impairment) is resolved (Griggs, 2012).

Administration Administer subcutaneously at approximately 12 hour intervals. If home administration is to occur, advise patient on proper handling, storage conditions, administration, disposal, and clean-up of accidental spillage; ensure that the patient or patient's caregiver is an appropriate candidate for home administration.

Hazardous agent: Use appropriate precautions for handling and disposal (NIOSH 2014 [group 1]). Avoid skin and eye contact; wear protective eyewear and gloves during handling and administration.

Monitoring Parameters CBC with differential and platelets (weekly during induction and initial maintenance cycles, then every 2 weeks or as clinically indicated after initial maintenance cycles); blood glucose (frequently); signs/symptoms of infection; signs of bleeding

Dosage Forms

Solution Reconstituted, Subcutaneous [preservative free]:

Synribo: 3.5 mg (1 ea)

◆ **Omacetaxine Mepesuccinate** *see* Omacetaxine *on page 1501*

Omalizumab (oh mah lye ZOO mab)

Brand Names: U.S. Xolair

Brand Names: Canada Xolair

Index Terms rhuMAb-E25

Pharmacologic Category Monoclonal Antibody, Anti-Asthmatic

Use

Asthma: Treatment of moderate to severe persistent asthma in adults and adolescents 12 years and older who have a positive skin test or *in vitro* reactivity to a perennial aeroallergen and whose symptoms are inadequately controlled with inhaled corticosteroids.

Chronic idiopathic urticaria: Treatment of chronic idiopathic urticaria in adults and adolescents 12 years and older who remain symptomatic despite H_1 antihistamine treatment.

Pregnancy Risk Factor B

Pregnancy Considerations Adverse events have not been observed in animal reproduction studies. IgG molecules are known to cross the placenta. A registry has been established to monitor outcomes of women exposed to omalizumab during pregnancy or within 8 weeks prior to pregnancy (http://www.xolairpregnancyregistry.com or 866-496-5247).

Breast-Feeding Considerations It is not known if omalizumab is excreted in breast milk; however, IgG is excreted in human milk and excretion of omalizumab is expected. The manufacturer recommends that caution be exercised when administering omalizumab to breast-feeding women.

Contraindications Severe hypersensitivity reaction to omalizumab or any component of the formulation

Warnings/Precautions [U.S. Boxed Warning]: Anaphylaxis, including delayed-onset anaphylaxis, has been reported following administration; anaphylaxis may present as bronchospasm, hypotension, syncope, urticaria, and/or angioedema of the throat or tongue. Anaphylaxis has occurred after the first dose and in some cases >1 year after initiation of regular treatment. Due to the risk, patients should be observed closely for an appropriate time period after administration and should receive treatment only under direct medical supervision. Healthcare providers should be prepared to administer appropriate therapy for managing potentially life-threatening anaphylaxis. Patients should be instructed on identifying signs/symptoms of anaphylaxis and to seek immediate care if they arise. In postmarketing reports, anaphylaxis usually occurred with the first or second dose and with a time to onset of ≤60 minutes; however, reactions have been reported with subsequent doses (after 39 doses) and with a time to onset of up to 4 days after administration. Discontinue therapy following any severe reaction.

In rare cases, patients may present with systemic eosinophilia, sometimes presenting with clinical features of vasculitis consistent with Churg-Strauss syndrome, a condition which is often treated with systemic corticosteroid therapy. Healthcare providers should be alert to eosinophilia, vasculitic rash, worsening pulmonary symptoms, cardiac complications, and/or neuropathy presenting in their patients. A causal association between omalizumab and these underlying conditions has not been established. Reports of a constellation of symptoms including fever, arthritis or arthralgia, rash, and lymphadenopathy have been reported with postmarketing use (symptoms resemble those seen in patients experiencing serum sickness, although circulating immune complexes or a skin biopsy consistent with a Type III hypersensitivity reaction were not seen with these cases). Onset of symptoms generally occurred 1-5 days following the first or subsequent doses. Discontinue therapy in any patient reporting this constellation of signs/symptoms. Malignant neoplasms have been reported rarely with use in short-term studies; impact of long-term use is not known. Use caution with and monitor patients at high risk for parasitic (helminth) infections (risk of infection may be increased).

Therapy has not been shown to alleviate acute asthma exacerbations; do not use to treat acute bronchospasm or status asthmaticus. Do not use to treat forms of urticaria other than chronic idiopathic urticaria. Dosing for allergic asthma is based on body weight and pretreatment total IgE serum levels. IgE levels remain elevated up to 1 year following treatment; therefore, levels taken during treatment or for up to 1 year following treatment cannot and should not be used as a dosage guide. Dosing in chronic idiopathic urticaria is not dependent on serum IgE (free or total) level or body weight. Gradually taper systemic or inhaled corticosteroid therapy; do not discontinue corticosteroids abruptly following initiation of omalizumab therapy. The combined use of omalizumab and corticosteroids in patients with chronic idiopathic urticaria has not been evaluated. Potentially significant drug-drug interactions may exist, requiring dose or frequency adjustment, additional monitoring, and/or selection of alternative therapy.

Adverse Reactions

Asthma:

Cardiovascular: Myocardial infarction, pulmonary embolism, unstable angina pectoris, venous thrombosis

Central nervous system: Dizziness, fatigue, pain

Dermatologic: Dermatitis, pruritus

Local: Injection site reaction (includes bruising, redness, warmth, burning, stinging, itching, hive formation, pain, indurations, mass, and inflammation; most reactions occurred within 1 hour, lasted <8 days, and decreased in frequency with additional dosing)

Neuromuscular & skeletal: Arm pain, arthralgia, bone fracture, leg pain

Otic: Otalgia

Rare but important or life-threatening: Alopecia, anaphylaxis, antibody development, arthritis, lymphadenopathy, malignant neoplasm, syncope, thrombocytopenia

Chronic idiopathic urticaria:

Cardiovascular: Peripheral edema

Central nervous system: Anxiety, headache, migraine

Dermatologic: Alopecia

Gastrointestinal: Toothache

Genitourinary: Urinary tract infection

Infection: Fungal infection

Local: Injection site reaction

Neuromuscular & skeletal: Arthralgia, limb pain, musculoskeletal pain, myalgia

Respiratory: Asthma, cough, nasopharyngitis, oropharyngeal pain, sinus headache, sinusitis, upper respiratory tract infection, viral upper respiratory tract infection

Miscellaneous: Fever

All indications: Rare but important or life-threatening: Alopecia, anaphylaxis, antibody development, arthritis, chest tightness, Churg-Strauss syndrome, lymphadenopathy, malignant neoplasm, pulmonary hypertension, syncope, thrombocytopenia, transient ischemic attacks

Drug Interactions

Metabolism/Transport Effects None known.

Avoid Concomitant Use

Avoid concomitant use of Omalizumab with any of the following: Belimumab

Increased Effect/Toxicity

Omalizumab may increase the levels/effects of: Belimumab

Decreased Effect There are no known significant interactions involving a decrease in effect.

Preparation for Administration Reconstitute using SWFI only; add SWFI 1.4 mL to upright vial using a 1-inch, 18-gauge needle on a 3 mL syringe and swirl gently for ~1 minute to evenly wet the powder; do not shake. Then gently swirl the upright vial for 5-10 seconds approximately every 5 minutes until dissolved; generally takes 15-20 minutes to dissolve completely. If it takes >20 minutes to dissolve completely, continue to swirl the upright vial for 5-10 seconds every 5 minutes until no gel-like particles are visible in the solution; do not use if contents are not completely dissolved after 40 minutes. Resulting solution is 150 mg/1.2 mL. Invert the vial for 15 seconds so the solution drains toward the stopper. Remove all of the solution by inserting a new 3 mL syringe with a 1-inch, 18-gauge needle into the inverted vial. Replace the 18-gauge needle with a 25-gauge needle for subcutaneous injection, and expel any air, bubbles, or excess solution to obtain the 1.2 mL dose.

Storage/Stability Prior to reconstitution, store under refrigeration at 2°C to 8°C (36°F to 46°F); product may be shipped at room temperature. Following reconstitution, protect from direct sunlight. May be stored for up to 8 hours if refrigerated or 4 hours if stored at room temperature.

Mechanism of Action

Asthma: Omalizumab is an IgG monoclonal antibody (recombinant DNA derived) which inhibits IgE binding to the high-affinity IgE receptor on mast cells and basophils. By decreasing bound IgE, the activation and release of mediators in the allergic response (early and late phase) is limited. Serum free IgE levels and the number of high-affinity IgE receptors are decreased. Long-term treatment in patients with allergic asthma showed a decrease in asthma exacerbations and corticosteroid usage.

Chronic idiopathic urticaria: Omalizumab binds to IgE and lowers free IgE levels. Subsequently, IgE receptors (FcεRI) on cells down-regulate. The mechanism by which these effects of omalizumab result in an improvement of chronic idiopathic urticaria symptoms is unknown.

Pharmacodynamics/Kinetics

Absorption: Slow following SubQ injection

Distribution: V_d: 78 ± 32 mL/kg

Metabolism: Degradation of IgG and omalizumab:IgE complexes by reticuloendothelial system and endothelial cells in the liver

Bioavailability: 62%

Half-life elimination: 26 days (asthma patients); 24 days (chronic idiopathic urticaria patients)

Time to peak: 7-8 days

Excretion: Primarily via hepatic degradation; intact IgG may be secreted in bile

Dosage

Asthma: Adolescents ≥12 years and Adults: SubQ: Dose and frequency based on body weight and **pretreatment** total IgE serum levels. Dosing should be adjusted during therapy for significant changes in body weight. Dosing should **not** be adjusted based on total IgE levels taken during treatment or <1 year following interruption of therapy. If therapy has been interrupted for ≥1 year, total IgE levels may be re-evaluated for dosage determination.

Pretreatment serum IgE ≥30 to 100 units/mL:
- U.S. labeling:
  - 30 to 90 kg: 150 mg every 4 weeks
  - >90 to 150 kg: 300 mg every 4 weeks
- Canadian labeling:
  - >20 to 90 kg: 150 mg every 4 weeks
  - >90 to 150 kg: 300 mg every 4 weeks

Pretreatment serum IgE >100 to 200 units/mL:
- U.S. labeling:
  - 30 to 90 kg: 300 mg every 4 weeks
  - >90 to 150 kg: 225 mg every 2 weeks
- Canadian labeling:
  - >20 to 40 kg: 150 mg every 4 weeks
  - >40 to 90 kg: 300 mg every 4 weeks
  - >90 to 125 kg: 225 mg every 2 weeks
  - >125 to 150 kg: 300 mg every 2 weeks

Pretreatment serum IgE >200 to 300 units/mL:
- U.S. labeling:
  - 30 to 60 kg: 300 mg every 4 weeks
  - >60 to 90 kg: 225 mg every 2 weeks
  - >90 to 150 kg: 300 mg every 2 weeks
- Canadian labeling:
  - >20 to 30 kg: 150 mg every 4 weeks
  - >30 to 60 kg: 300 mg every 4 weeks
  - >60 to 90 kg: 225 mg every 2 weeks
  - >90 to 125 kg: 300 mg every 2 weeks
  - >125 to 150 kg: 375 mg every 2 weeks

Pretreatment serum IgE >300 to 400 units/mL:
- U.S. labeling:
  - 30 to 70 kg: 225 mg every 2 weeks
  - >70 to 90 kg: 300 mg every 2 weeks
  - >90 kg: Do not administer dose
- Canadian labeling:
  - >20 to 40 kg: 300 mg every 4 weeks
  - >40 to 70 kg: 225 mg every 2 weeks
  - >70 to 90 kg: 300 mg every 2 weeks
  - >90 kg: Do not administer dose

Pretreatment serum IgE >400 to 500 units/mL:
- U.S. labeling:
  - 30 to 70 kg: 300 mg every 2 weeks
  - >70 to 90 kg: 375 mg every 2 weeks
  - >90 kg: Do not administer dose
- Canadian labeling:
  - >20 to 30 kg: 300 mg every 4 weeks
  - >30 to 50 kg: 225 mg every 2 weeks
  - >50 to 70 kg: 300 mg every 2 weeks
  - >70 to 90 kg: 375 mg every 2 weeks
  - >90 kg: Do not administer dose

Pretreatment serum IgE >500 to 600 units/mL:
- U.S. labeling:
  - 30 to 60 kg: 300 mg every 2 weeks
  - >60 to 70 kg: 375 mg every 2 weeks
  - >70 kg: Do not administer dose
- Canadian labeling:
  - >20 to 30 kg: 300 mg every 4 weeks
  - >30 to 40 kg: 225 mg every 2 weeks
  - >40 to 60 kg: 300 mg every 2 weeks
  - >60 to 70 kg: 375 mg every 2 weeks
  - >70 kg: Do not administer dose

Pretreatment serum IgE >600 to 700 units/mL:
- U.S. labeling:
  - 30 to 60 kg: 375 mg every 2 weeks
  - >60 kg: Do not administer dose
- Canadian labeling:
  - >20 to 40 kg: 225 mg every 2 weeks
  - >40 to 50 kg: 300 mg every 2 weeks
  - >50 to 60 kg: 375 mg every 2 weeks
  - >60 kg: Do not administer dose

Chronic idiopathic urticaria: Adolescents ≥12 years and Adults: SubQ: 150 or 300 mg every 4 weeks. Dosing is not dependent on serum IgE (free or total) level or body weight.

Dosage adjustment for toxicity:

Severe hypersensitivity reaction or anaphylaxis: Discontinue treatment.

Fever, arthralgia, and rash: Discontinue treatment if this constellation of symptoms occurs.

Dosage adjustment in renal impairment: There are no dosage adjustments provided in manufacturer's labeling.

Dosage adjustment in hepatic impairment: There are no dosage adjustments provided in manufacturer's labeling.

Administration For SubQ injection only; doses >150 mg should be divided over more than one injection site (eg, 225 mg or 300 mg administered as two injections, 375 mg administered as three injections). Injections may take 5 to 10 seconds to administer (solution is slightly viscous). Administer only under direct medical supervision and observe patient for a minimum of 2 hours following administration of any dose given.

Monitoring Parameters Anaphylactic/hypersensitivity reactions, baseline serum total IgE; FEV_1, peak flow, and/or other pulmonary function tests; monitor for signs of infection

Dosage Forms

Solution Reconstituted, Subcutaneous [preservative free]:

Xolair: 150 mg (1 ea)

Ombitasvir, Paritaprevir, Ritonavir, and Dasabuvir

(om BIT as vir, par i TA pre vir, ri TOE na vir, & da SA bue vir)

Brand Names: U.S. Viekira Pak

Brand Names: Canada Holkira Pak

Index Terms Dasabuvir, Ombitasvir, Paritaprevir, and Ritonavir; Paritaprevir, Ombitasvir, Ritonavir, and Dasabuvir; Ritonavir, Ombitasvir, Paritaprevir, and Dasabuvir

Pharmacologic Category Antihepaciviral, NS5A Inhibitor; Antihepaciviral, Polymerase Inhibitor (Anti-HCV); Antihepaciviral, Protease Inhibitor (Anti-HCV); Cytochrome P-450 Inhibitor

Use

Chronic hepatitis C: Treatment of genotype 1 chronic hepatitis C virus infection, with or without ribavirin, including those with compensated cirrhosis.

Limitations of use: Not recommended for use in patients with decompensated liver disease.

Pregnancy Risk Factor B

Pregnancy Considerations Adverse events were not observed in animal reproduction studies. This combination product is contraindicated for use with ribavirin in pregnant women. Health care providers are encouraged to enroll pregnant women exposed to antiretroviral medications in the Antiretroviral Pregnancy Registry (1-800-258-4263 or http://www.APRegistry.com).

Breast-Feeding Considerations It is not known if the components of this combination are excreted into breast milk. According to the manufacturer, the decision to breast-feed during therapy should take into account the risk of exposure to the infant and the benefits of treatment to the mother. Mothers coinfected with HIV are discouraged from breast-feeding to decrease potential transmission of HIV (DHHS [perinatal], 2014).

Contraindications Hypersensitivity to any component of the formulation, including to ritonavir (eg, toxic epidermal necrolysis, Stevens-Johnson syndrome); severe hepatic impairment (Child-Pugh class C); concurrent use of drugs that are highly dependent on CYP3A4 for clearance and for which elevated plasma concentrations are associated with serious and/or life-threatening events; concurrent use of strong inducers of CYP3A and CYP2C8 or strong inhibitors of CYP2C8. Concurrent use of drugs that are contraindicated include, but are not necessarily limited to: alfuzosin, carbamazepine, ergot derivatives (ergonovine, ergotamine, dihydroergotamine, methylergonovine), ethinyl estradiol-containing products, efavirenz, gemfibrozil, lovastatin, midazolam (oral), phenobarbital, phenytoin, pimozide, rifampin, sildenafil (when used for the treatment of pulmonary arterial hypertension [eg, Revatio]), simvastatin, St John's wort, triazolam. If used with ribavirin, contraindications of ribavirin also apply. See ribavirin prescribing information.

Warnings/Precautions Elevations of hepatic enzymes (eg, ALT >5 times ULN) have been reported. Elevations are usually asymptomatic, occur within 4 weeks of treatment initiation, and decline within 2 to 8 weeks with continued dosing. Female patients taking ethinyl estradiol products are at increased risk. For management of women taking concomitant estrogen products, refer to Special populations below. No dosage adjustment is required in mild (Child-Pugh class A) hepatic impairment. Use is not recommended in moderate hepatic impairment (Child-Pugh class B); use is contraindicated in severe hepatic impairment (Child-Pugh class C). If used with concomitant ribavirin, contraindications of ribavirin, particularly pregnancy avoidance warnings, also apply (see ribavirin prescribing information). Potentially significant interactions may exist, requiring dose or frequency adjustment, additional monitoring, and/or selection of alternative therapy. Concomitant use of ethinyl estradiol-containing products is contraindicated; these products may be restarted 2 weeks following completion of HCV therapy. Alternative methods of contraception (eg, nonhormonal methods, progestin only contraception) are recommended during therapy. Women using other estrogens (eg, estradiol, conjugated estrogens) should have hepatic enzymes tested during the first 4 weeks of treatment and as clinically indicated thereafter. If ALT is elevated, repeat testing and continue to monitor closely; patients should contact their health care professional immediately if they experience onset of fatigue, weakness, lack of appetite, nausea and vomiting, jaundice or discolored feces. Consider discontinuation if ALT remains persistently >10 x ULN. Discontinue if ALT increase is accompanied by signs of hepatic inflammation, elevated conjugated bilirubin, alkaline phosphatase, or INR. Ritonavir, a component of the product, is also an HIV-1 protease inhibitor. In HCV/HIV coinfected patients, ritonavir can select for HIV-1 protease inhibitor resistance-associated substitutions. Any HCV/HIV-1 coinfected patients should also be taking a suppressive antiretroviral regimen to reduce resistance risk.

Adverse Reactions

Central nervous system: Fatigue (more common in liver transplant recipients and patients with HCV/HIV-1 co-infection), headache (more common in liver transplant recipients than in patients with HCV/HIV-1 co-infection), insomnia, irritability (patients with HCV/HIV-1 co-infection)

Dermatologic: Dermatological reaction (may include allergic dermatitis, contact dermatitis, dermal ulcer, dermatitis, desquamation, eczema, erythema, erythematous rash, exfoliative dermatitis, macular rash, maculopapular rash, papular rash, pruritic rash, psoriasis, skin photosensitivity, skin rash, urticaria), pruritus

Gastrointestinal: Diarrhea (liver transplant recipients), nausea

Hematologic & oncologic: Decreased hemoglobin (decrease to <10 g/dL: More common in liver transplant recipients than in patients with HCV/HIV-1 co-infection)

Hepatic: increased serum ALT (>5 x ULN; more common in women taking concomitant ethinyl estradiol than in women taking concomitant estrogens other than ethinyl estradiol; increased serum bilirubin (>2 x ULN; more common in patients with HCV/HIV-1 co-infection)

Neuromuscular & skeletal: Muscle spasm (liver transplant recipients), weakness (more common in liver transplant recipients)

Ophthalmic: Scleral icterus (patients with HCV/HIV-1 co-infection)

Respiratory: Cough (more common in liver transplant recipients than in patients with HCV/HIV-1 co-infection), dyspnea

Drug Interactions

Metabolism/Transport Effects Refer to individual components.

Avoid Concomitant Use

Avoid concomitant use of Ombitasvir, Paritaprevir, Ritonavir, and Dasabuvir with any of the following: Ado-Trastuzumab Emtansine; Alfuzosin; Amiodarone; Apixaban; Astemizole; Atovaquone; Avanafil; Axitinib; Bosutinib; Cabozantinib; Ceritinib; Cisapride; Conivaptan; Crizotinib; CYP2C8 Inhibitors (Strong); CYP3A4 Inducers (Strong); Dapoxetine; Dasabuvir; Disulfiram; Dronedarone; Efavirenz; Enzalutamide; Eplerenone; Ergot Derivatives; Ethinyl Estradiol; Etravirine; Everolimus; Flecainide; Fluticasone (Nasal); Fusidic Acid (Systemic); Halofantrine; Ibrutinib; Idelalisib; Irinotecan; Ivabradine; Lapatinib; Lercanidipine; Lomitapide; Lovastatin; Lurasidone; Macitentan; Midazolam; Naloxegol; Nilotinib; Nisoldipine; Olaparib; PAZOPanib; Pimozide; Propafenone; QuiNIDine; QuiNINE; Ranolazine; Red Yeast Rice; Regorafenib; Rifampin; Rivaroxaban; Salmeterol; Silodosin; Simeprevir; Simvastatin; St Johns Wort; Suvorexant; Tamoxifen; Tamsulosin; Terfenadine; Thioridazine; Ticagrelor; Tolvaptan; Topotecan; Toremifene; Trabectedin; Triazolam; Ulipristal; Vemurafenib; VinCRIStine (Liposomal); Vorapaxar; Voriconazole

Increased Effect/Toxicity

Ombitasvir, Paritaprevir, Ritonavir, and Dasabuvir may increase the levels/effects of: Ado-Trastuzumab Emtansine; Afatinib; Alfuzosin; Almotriptan; Alosetron; ALPRAZolam; Amiodarone; Apixaban; ARIPiprazole; Astemizole; AtoMOXetine; AtorvaSTATin; Avanafil; Axitinib; Bedaquiline; Bortezomib; Bosentan; Bosutinib; Brentuximab Vedotin; Brinzolamide; Budesonide (Nasal); Budesonide (Systemic, Oral Inhalation); Cabazitaxel; Cabozantinib; Calcium Channel Blockers (Dihydropyridine); Calcium Channel Blockers (Nondihydropyridine); Cannabis; Ceritinib; Cisapride; Clarithromycin; Clorazepate; Colchicine; Conivaptan; Corticosteroids (Orally Inhaled); Corticosteroids (Systemic); Crizotinib; Cyclophosphamide; CycloSPORINE (Systemic); CYP2C8 Substrates; CYP2D6 Substrates; CYP3A4 Substrates; Dabigatran Etexilate; Dapoxetine; Dasabuvir; Dasatinib; Diazepam; Dienogest; Digoxin; DOXOrubicin (Conventional); Dronabinol; Dronedarone; Dutasteride; Edoxaban; Eliglustat; Enfuvirtide; Enzalutamide; Eplerenone; Ergot Derivatives; Erlotinib; Estazolam; Etizolam; Everolimus; FentaNYL; Fesoterodine; Flecainide; Flurazepam; Fluticasone (Nasal); Fluticasone (Oral Inhalation); Fluvastatin; Fusidic Acid (Systemic); GuanFACINE; Halofantrine; Highest Risk QTc-Prolonging Agents; Hydrocodone; Ibrutinib; Iloperidone; Imatinib; Imidafenacin; Irinotecan; Itraconazole; Ivabradine; Ivacaftor; Ixabepilone; Ketoconazole (Systemic); Lacosamide; Lapatinib; Ledipasvir; Lercanidipine; Levobupivacaine; Levomilnacipran; Linagliptin; Lomitapide; Lovastatin; Lurasidone; Macitentan; Maraviroc; Meperidine; MethylPREDNISolone; Metoprolol; Midazolam; Mifepristone; Moderate Risk QTc-Prolonging Agents; Naloxegol; Nebivolol; Nefazodone; Nilotinib; Nintedanib; Nisoldipine; Olaparib; Ospemifene; OxyCODONE; Paricalcitol; PAZOPanib; P-glycoprotein/ABCB1 Substrates; Pimecrolimus; Pimozide; Pioglitazone; Pitavastatin; PONATinib; Pranlukast; Pravastatin; PrednisoLONE (Systemic); PredniSONE; Propafenone; Protease Inhibitors; Prucalopride; QUEtiapine; QuiNIDine; QuiNINE; Ranolazine; Red Yeast Rice; Regorafenib; Retapamulin; Rifaximin; Rilpivirine; Riociguat; Rivaroxaban; RomiDEPsin; Rosuvastatin; Ruxolitinib; Salmeterol; Saxagliptin; Sildenafil; Silodosin; Simeprevir; Simvastatin; SORAfenib; Suvorexant; Tacrolimus (Systemic); Tacrolimus (Topical); Tadalafil; Tamsulosin; Temsirolimus; Terfenadine; Tetrabenazine; Tetrahydrocannabinol; Thioridazine; Ticagrelor; Tofacitinib; Tolterodine; Tolvaptan; Topotecan; Toremifene; Trabectedin; TraZODone; Treprostinil; Triamcinolone (Systemic); Triazolam; Ulipristal; Vardenafil; Vemurafenib; Vilazodone; VinBLAStine; VinCRIStine; VinCRIStine (Liposomal); Vorapaxar; Vortioxetine; Zopiclone; Zuclopenthixol

The levels/effects of Ombitasvir, Paritaprevir, Ritonavir, and Dasabuvir may be increased by: ARIPiprazole; Clarithromycin; Conivaptan; CYP2C8 Inhibitors (Moderate); CYP2C8 Inhibitors (Strong); CYP3A4 Inhibitors (Moderate); CYP3A4 Inhibitors (Strong); Delavirdine; Disulfiram; Efavirenz; Enfuvirtide; Ethinyl Estradiol; Fusidic Acid (Systemic); Idelalisib; Luliconazole; Mifepristone; Netupitant; P-glycoprotein/ABCB1 Inhibitors; QuiNINE; Simeprevir

Decreased Effect

Ombitasvir, Paritaprevir, Ritonavir, and Dasabuvir may decrease the levels/effects of: Abacavir; Atovaquone; BuPROPion; Canagliflozin; Clarithromycin; Codeine; Contraceptives (Estrogens); Deferasirox; Delavirdine; Etravirine; Hydrocodone; Ifosfamide; Iloperidone; LamoTRIgine; Meperidine; Methadone; Prasugrel; Proguanil; QuiNINE; Tamoxifen; Ticagrelor; Valproic Acid and Derivatives; Voriconazole; Warfarin; Zidovudine

The levels/effects of Ombitasvir, Paritaprevir, Ritonavir, and Dasabuvir may be decreased by: Antacids; CYP2C8 Inducers (Strong); CYP3A4 Inducers (Moderate); CYP3A4 Inducers (Strong); Dabrafenib; Efavirenz; Garlic; P-glycoprotein/ABCB1 Inducers; Rifampin; Siltuximab; St Johns Wort; Tocilizumab

Storage/Stability Store at or below 30°C (86°F). Dispense in original carton.

Mechanism of Action Combines 3 direct-acting hepatitis C virus antiviral agents with distinct mechanisms of action. Ombitasvir inhibits HCV NS5A, and interferes with viral RNA replication and virion assembly. Paritaprevir inhibits HCV NS3/4A protease and interferes with HCV coded polyprotein cleavage necessary for viral replication. Dasabuvir inhibits HCV RNA-dependent RNA polymerase (encoded by the NS5B gene) which is also necessary for viral replication.

Ritonavir is not active against HCV. Ritonavir is a potent CYP3A inhibitor that increases peak and trough plasma drug concentrations of paritaprevir and overall drug exposure (ie, AUC).

Pharmacodynamics/Kinetics

Absorption: Dasabuvir: ~70%; Ombitasvir, paritaprevir, ritonavir: Not evaluated

Distribution:

Ombitasvir: V_d: 50.1 L

Paritaprevir: V_d: 16.7 L

Ritonavir: V_d: 21.5 L

Dasabuvir: V_d: 396 L

Protein binding: Ombitasvir: 99.9%; Paritaprevir: ~98%; Ritonavir: >99%; Dasabuvir: >99%

Metabolism:

Ombitasvir: Metabolized by amide hydrolysis and oxidative metabolism

Paritaprevir: Metabolized by CYP3A4 and to a lesser extent CYP3A5

Ritonavir: Metabolized by CYP3A and to a lesser extent CYP2D6

Dasabuvir: Metabolized by CYP2C8 and to a lesser extent CYP3A

Half-life elimination: Ombitasvir: 21 to 25 hours; Paritaprevir: 5.5 hours; Ritonavir: 4 hours; Dasabuvir 5.5 to 6 hours

Time to peak: Ombitasvir, paritaprevir, ritonavir, dasabuvir: 4 to 5 hours

Excretion:
Ombitasvir: Feces (~90%, mainly as unchanged drug) and urine (<2%, mainly as unchanged drug)
Paritaprevir: Feces (~88%, mainly as metabolites) and urine (~9%, mainly as metabolites)
Ritonavir: Feces (~86%) and urine (~11%)
Dasabuvir: Feces (~94%, mainly as metabolites) and urine (~2%, mainly as metabolites)

Dosage Chronic hepatitis C: Adults: Oral: **Note:** Regimen is a copackaged product; ombitasvir, paritaprevir, and ritonavir are a fixed-dose combination tablet; dasabuvir is an individual tablet

Genotype 1a, without cirrhosis (used with concomitant ribavirin):
Ombitasvir/paritaprevir/ritonavir tablet: Two tablets every morning for 12 weeks
Dasabuvir: 250 mg twice daily for 12 weeks

Genotype 1a, with cirrhosis (used with concomitant ribavirin): **Note:** Based on prior treatment history, some patients may be considered for a duration of therapy of 12 weeks.
Ombitasvir/paritaprevir/ritonavir tablet: Two tablets every morning for 24 weeks
Dasabuvir: 250 mg twice daily for 24 weeks

Genotype 1b, without cirrhosis:
Ombitasvir/paritaprevir/ritonavir tablet: Two tablets every morning for 12 weeks
Dasabuvir: 250 mg twice daily for 12 weeks

Genotype 1b, with cirrhosis (used with concomitant ribavirin):
Ombitasvir/paritaprevir/ritonavir tablet: Two tablets every morning for 12 weeks
Dasabuvir: 250 mg twice daily for 12 weeks

Genotype 1 (unknown subtype) or Genotype 1 (mixed infection) without cirrhosis (used with concomitant ribavirin):
Ombitasvir/paritaprevir/ritonavir tablet: Two tablets every morning for 12 weeks
Dasabuvir: 250 mg twice daily for 12 weeks

Genotype 1 (unknown subtype) or Genotype 1 (mixed infection) with cirrhosis (used with concomitant ribavirin):
Ombitasvir/paritaprevir/ritonavir tablet: Two tablets every morning for 24 weeks
Dasabuvir: 250 mg twice daily for 24 weeks

Genotype 1, liver transplant recipients, Metavir fibrosis score ≤2 (normal hepatic function, mild fibrosis) (regardless of genotype 1 subtype; used with concomitant ribavirin): **Note:** If calcineurin inhibitor used concomitantly, calcineurin inhibitor dosage adjustment is needed.
Ombitasvir/paritaprevir/ritonavir tablet: Two tablets every morning for 24 weeks
Dasabuvir: 250 mg twice daily for 24 weeks

Dosage adjustment for renal impairment:
Mild to severe impairment: No dosage adjustment necessary.
End stage renal disease (ESRD) on dialysis: There are no dosage adjustments provided in the manufacturer's labeling (has not been studied).

Dosage adjustment for hepatic impairment:
Mild impairment (Child-Pugh class A): No dosage adjustment necessary.
Moderate impairment (Child-Pugh class B): Use is not recommended.
Severe impairment (Child-Pugh class C): Use is contraindicated.

Dietary Considerations Take with a meal.

Administration Oral: Administer with a meal.

Monitoring Parameters Baseline hepatic function tests and periodically during therapy, especially in women taking concomitant estrogen products; serum HCV-RNA at baseline and at the end of treatment, during treatment follow-up, and when clinically indicated.

Dosage Forms
Combination package:
Viekira Pak [28 day supply]:
Tablet, oral: Ombitasvir 12.5 mg, paritaprevir 75 mg, and ritonavir 50 mg (56s)
Tablet, oral: Dasabuvir 250 mg (56s)

◆ **Omeclamox-Pak®** *see* Omeprazole, Clarithromycin, and Amoxicillin *on page 1511*

◆ **Omega 3** *see* Omega-3 Fatty Acids *on page 1507*

◆ **Omega-3 2100 [OTC]** *see* Omega-3 Fatty Acids *on page 1507*

◆ **Omega-3-Acid Ethyl Esters** *see* Omega-3 Fatty Acids *on page 1507*

◆ **Omega-3 Fish Oil Ex St [OTC]** *see* Omega-3 Fatty Acids *on page 1507*

Omega-3 Fatty Acids (oh MEG a three FAT tee AS ids)

Brand Names: U.S. Dialyvite Omega-3 Concentrate [OTC]; Fish Oil Ultra [OTC]; High Potency Fish Oil [OTC] [DSC]; Lovaza; Marine Lipid Concentrate [OTC]; MaxEPA [OTC]; MiniCaps Omega-3 [OTC]; Omega-3 2100 [OTC]; Omega-3 Fish Oil Ex St [OTC]; Sea-Omega 50 [OTC]; Systane Omega-3 Healthy Tears [OTC]; Vascepa

Index Terms AMR101; Docosahexaenoic Acid; Eicosapentaenoic Acid; Ethyl Eicosapentaenoate; Ethyl Esters of Omega-3 Fatty Acids; Ethyl Icosapentate; Ethyl-Eicosapentaenoic Acid; Ethyl-EPA; Fish Oil; Icosapent Ethyl; Omega 3; Omega-3-Acid Ethyl Esters; P-OM3

Pharmacologic Category Antilipemic Agent, Omega-3 Fatty Acids

Use
Dietary supplement: As dietary supplements for patients at early risk of coronary artery disease primarily because of effects on platelets and lipids.
Note: The American Heart Association recommends that consumers without documented coronary heart disease eat a variety of fish, preferably oily fish (eg, salmon), at least twice a week. Fish oil supplements should only be considered for individuals with heart disease or high triglyceride levels in consultation with a physician (AHA, 2014).

Hypertriglyceridemia (Lovaza, Omtryg, Epanova, and Vascepa): As an adjunct to diet to reduce triglyceride levels in adults with severe (≥500 mg/dL) hypertriglyceridemia.
Note: The Endocrine Society recommends that omega-3 fatty acids may be considered for triglyceride levels >1000 mg/dL and may be used alone or in combination with HMG-CoA reductase inhibitors (Berglund, 2012). A number of OTC formulations containing omega-3 fatty acids are marketed as nutritional supplements; these do not have FDA-approved indications and may not contain the same amounts of the active ingredient.

Pregnancy Risk Factor C

Dosage Oral: Adults:
Hypertriglyceridemia:
Epanova: 2 g (2 capsules) or 4 g (4 capsules) once daily
Lovaza: 4 g (4 capsules) once daily or 2 g (2 capsules) twice daily
Omtryg: 4.8 g (4 capsules) once daily with meals or 2.4 g (2 capsules) twice daily with meals
Vascepa: 2 g (2 capsules) twice daily with or following meals
Treatment of IgA nephropathy (off-label use): Lovaza: 4 g (4 capsules) daily (Donadio, 2001)

Dosage adjustment in renal impairment: There are no dosage adjustments provided in the manufacturer's labeling (has not been studied). EPA and DHA are not renally eliminated.

Dosage adjustment in hepatic impairment: There are no dosage adjustments provided in the manufacturer's labeling (has not been studied). Periodic monitoring of ALT and AST is recommended in patients with hepatic impairment.

Additional Information Complete prescribing information should be consulted for additional detail.

Product Availability

Epanova: FDA approved May 2014; availability anticipated in the 4th quarter of 2014.

Omtryg: FDA approved April 2014; anticipated availability is currently unknown.

Dosage Forms Considerations

Epanova: Each 1 g capsule contains at least 850 mg of polyunsaturated fatty acids, including multiple omega-3 fatty acids (EPA and DHA being the most abundant).

Lovaza, Omtryg: Each 1 g (Lovaza) or 1.2 g (Omtryg) capsule contains the combination of eicosapentaenoic acid (EPA; ~465 mg) and docosahexaenoic acid (DHA; ~375 mg) ethyl esters.

Vascepa: Icosapent ethyl contains ethyl esters of an omega-3 fatty acid, eicosapentaenoic acid (EPA), obtained from fish oil. It contains ≥96% EPA and does **not** contain docosahexaenoic acid (DHA). Historically, mixtures containing both EPA and DHA have increased LDL cholesterol in patients with severe hypertriglyceridemia. However, studies have suggested that icosapent ethyl has not caused significant increases in LDL cholesterol while significantly decreasing triglyceride levels (Bays, 2011; Miller, 2011).

Dosage Forms

Capsule, Oral:

Dialyvite Omega-3 Concentrate [OTC]: 600 mg
Fish Oil Ultra [OTC]: 1000 mg
Lovaza: 1 g
Marine Lipid Concentrate [OTC]: 240 mg, 360 mg, 5 units
MaxEPA [OTC]: 1000 mg
MiniCaps Omega-3 [OTC]: 350 mg
Omega-3 2100 [OTC]: 1050 mg
Vascepa: 1 g
Generic: 300 mg, 500 mg, 1000 mg, 1 g

Capsule, Oral [preservative free]:

Omega-3 Fish Oil Ex St [OTC]: 880 mg
Sea-Omega 50 [OTC]: 1000 mg
Generic: 1000 mg, 1200 mg

Capsule Delayed Release, Oral:

Systane Omega-3 Healthy Tears [OTC]: 500 mg

Omeprazole (oh MEP ra zole)

Brand Names: U.S. First-Omeprazole; Omeprazole+Syrspend SF Alka; PriLOSEC; PriLOSEC OTC [OTC]

Brand Names: Canada Apo-Omeprazole; Auro-Omeprazole; Ava-Omeprazole; Dom-Omeprazole DR; JAMP-Omeprazole DR; Losec; Mylan-Omeprazole; Olex; PMS-Omeprazole; PMS-Omeprazole DR; Q-Omeprazole; RAN-Omeprazole; ratio-Omeprazole; Riva-Omeprazole DR; Sandoz-Omeprazole; Teva-Omeprazole

Index Terms Omeprazole Magnesium

Pharmacologic Category Proton Pump Inhibitor; Substituted Benzimidazole

Use Short-term (4-8 weeks) treatment of active duodenal ulcer disease or active benign gastric ulcer; treatment of heartburn and other symptoms associated with gastroesophageal reflux disease (GERD); short-term (4-8 weeks) treatment of endoscopically-diagnosed erosive esophagitis; maintenance healing of erosive esophagitis; long-term treatment of pathological hypersecretory conditions (eg, Zollinger-Ellison syndrome); as part of a multidrug regimen for *H. pylori* eradication to reduce the risk of duodenal ulcer recurrence

OTC labeling: Short-term treatment of frequent, uncomplicated heartburn occurring ≥2 days/week

Pregnancy Risk Factor C

Pregnancy Considerations Adverse events were observed in some animal reproduction studies. An increased risk of hypospadias was reported following maternal use of proton pump inhibitors (PPIs) during pregnancy (Anderka, 2012), but this was based on a small number of exposures and the same association was not found in another study (Erichsen, 2012). Most available studies have not shown an increased risk of major birth defects following maternal use of omeprazole during pregnancy (Diav-Citrin, 2005; Källén, 2001; Lalkin, 1998; Matok, 2012; Pasternak, 2010). When treating GERD in pregnancy, PPIs may be used when clinically indicated (Katz, 2013).

Breast-Feeding Considerations Omeprazole is excreted into breast milk. Milk concentrations of omeprazole were studied in a breast-feeding woman at 3 weeks postpartum. The mother had taken omeprazole 20 mg daily starting her 29th week of gestation and continued after delivery. Following administration of omeprazole 20 mg, peak concentrations in the maternal serum occurred 240 minutes after the dose and peak concentrations in the breast milk were 180 minutes after the dose. The concentrations of omeprazole detected in the breast milk were <7% of the highest maternal serum concentration (Marshall, 1998).The manufacturer recommends caution be used if administered to a nursing woman. The acidic content of the nursing infants' stomach may potentially inactivate any ingested omeprazole (Marshall, 1998).

Contraindications Hypersensitivity to omeprazole, other substituted benzimidazole proton pump inhibitors, or any component of the formulation

Warnings/Precautions Use of proton pump inhibitors (PPIs) may increase the risk of gastrointestinal infections (eg, *Salmonella, Campylobacter*). Relief of symptoms does not preclude the presence of a gastric malignancy. Atrophic gastritis (by biopsy) has been noted with long-term omeprazole therapy. In long-term (2-year) studies in rats, omeprazole produced a dose-related increase in gastric carcinoid tumors. While available endoscopic evaluations and histologic examinations of biopsy specimens from human stomachs have not detected a risk from short-term exposure to omeprazole, further human data on the effect of sustained hypochlorhydria and hypergastrinemia are needed to rule out the possibility of an increased risk for the development of tumors in humans receiving long-term therapy. Use of PPIs may increase risk of *Clostridium difficile*-associated diarrhea (CDAD), especially in hospitalized patients; consider CDAD diagnosis in patients with persistent diarrhea that does not improve. Use the lowest dose and shortest duration of PPI therapy appropriate for the condition being treated.

PPIs may diminish the therapeutic effect of clopidogrel, thought to be due to reduced formation of the active metabolite of clopidogrel. The manufacturer of clopidogrel recommends either avoidance both omeprazole (even when scheduled 12 hours apart) and esomeprazole or use of a PPI with comparatively less effect on the active metabolite of clopidogrel (eg, pantoprazole). In contrast to these warnings, others have recommended the continued use of PPIs, regardless of the degree of inhibition, in patients with a history of GI bleeding or multiple risk factors for GI bleeding who are also receiving clopidogrel since no evidence has established clinically meaningful differences in outcome; however, a clinically significant interaction cannot be excluded in those who are poor metabolizers of clopidogrel (Abraham, 2010; Levine, 2011). Additionally, concomitant use of omeprazole with some drugs may require cautious use, may not be recommended, or may require dosage adjustments.

Increased incidence of osteoporosis-related bone fractures of the hip, spine, or wrist may occur with PPI therapy. Patients on high-dose (multiple daily doses) or long-term (≥1 year) therapy should be monitored. Use the lowest effective dose for the shortest duration of time, use vitamin D and calcium supplementation, and follow appropriate guidelines to reduce risk of fractures in patients at risk.

Hypomagnesemia, reported rarely, usually with prolonged PPI use of >3 months (most cases >1 year of therapy); may be symptomatic or asymptomatic; severe cases may cause tetany, seizures, and cardiac arrhythmias. Consider obtaining serum magnesium concentrations prior to beginning long-term therapy, especially if taking concomitant digoxin, diuretics, or other drugs known to cause hypomagnesemia; and periodically thereafter. Hypomagnesemia may be corrected by magnesium supplementation, although discontinuation of omeprazole may be necessary; magnesium levels typically return to normal within 1 week of stopping. Serum chromogranin A levels may be increased if assessed while patient on omeprazole; may lead to diagnostic errors related to neuroendocrine tumors.

Serum chromogranin A (CgA) levels increase secondary to drug-induced decreases in gastric acid. May cause false-positive results in diagnostic investigations for neuroendocrine tumors. Temporarily stop omeprazole treatment ≥14 days before CgA test; if CgA level high, repeat test to confirm. Use same commercial lab for testing to prevent variable results.

Prolonged treatment (≥2 years) may lead to vitamin B_{12} malabsorption and subsequent vitamin B_{12} deficiency. The magnitude of the deficiency is dose-related and the association is stronger in females and those younger in age (<30 years); prevalence is decreased after discontinuation of therapy (Lam, 2013).

Decreased *H. pylori* eradication rates have been observed with short-term (≤7 days) combination therapy. The American College of Gastroenterology recommends 10 to 14 days of therapy (triple or quadruple) for eradication of *H. pylori* (Chey, 2007). Bioavailability may be increased in Asian populations and patients with hepatic dysfunction; consider dosage reductions, especially for maintenance healing of erosive esophagitis. Bioavailability may be increased in the elderly. When used for self-medication (OTC), do not use for >14 days.

Benzyl alcohol and derivatives: Some dosage forms may contain benzyl alcohol; large amounts of benzyl alcohol (≥99 mg/kg/day) have been associated with a potentially fatal toxicity ("gasping syndrome") in neonates; the "gasping syndrome" consists of metabolic acidosis, respiratory distress, gasping respirations, CNS dysfunction (including convulsions, intracranial hemorrhage), hypotension, and cardiovascular collapse (AAP, 1997; CDC, 1982); some data suggests that benzoate displaces bilirubin from protein binding sites (Ahlfors, 2001); avoid or use dosage forms containing benzyl alcohol with caution in neonates. See manufacturer's labeling.

Adverse Reactions

Central nervous system: Dizziness, headache
Dermatologic: Skin rash
Gastrointestinal: Abdominal pain, acid regurgitation, constipation, diarrhea, flatulence, nausea, vomiting
Neuromuscular & skeletal: Back pain, weakness
Respiratory: Cough, upper respiratory infection
Rare but important or life-threatening: Abdominal swelling, abnormal dreams, aggression, agranulocytosis, allergic reactions, alopecia, anaphylaxis, anemia, angina pectoris, angioedema, anorexia, apathy, arthralgia, atrophic gastritis, benign gastric polyps, blurred vision, bone fracture, bradycardia, bronchospasm, chest pain, cholestatic hepatitis, *Clostridium difficile*-associated diarrhea (CDAD), confusion, depression, dermatitis, diplopia, drowsiness, epistaxis, erythema multiforme, esophageal candidiasis, fecal discoloration, gastroduodenal carcinoids, glycosuria, gynecomastia, hallucinations, hematuria, hemolytic anemia, hepatic disease (hepatocellular, cholestatic, mixed), hepatic encephalopathy, hepatic failure, hepatic necrosis, hepatitis, hepatocellular hepatitis, hyperhidrosis, hypersensitivity, hypertension, hypocalcemia, hypoglycemia, hypokalemia, hypomagnesemia, hyponatremia, increased gamma glutamyl transferase, increased serum alkaline phosphatase, increased serum bilirubin, increased serum creatinine, increased serum transaminases, insomnia, interstitial nephritis, irritable bowel syndrome, jaundice, leg pain, leukocytosis, leukopenia, malaise, microscopic colitis, microscopic pyuria, mucosal atrophy (tongue), muscle cramps, myalgia, myasthenia, nervousness, neutropenia, ocular irritation, optic atrophy, optic neuritis, optic neuropathy (anterior ischemic), osteoporosis-related fracture, pain, palpitation, pancreatitis, pancytopenia, paresthesia, peripheral edema, petechiae, photophobia, pneumonia, proteinuria, pruritus, psychiatric disturbance, purpura, sleep disturbance, sore throat, Stevens-Johnson syndrome, stomatitis, tachycardia, testicular pain, thrombocytopenia, toxic epidermal necrolysis, tremor, urinary tract infection, urticaria, weight gain, xeroderma, xerophthalmia, xerostomia

Drug Interactions

Metabolism/Transport Effects **Substrate** of CYP2A6 (minor), CYP2C19 (major), CYP2C9 (minor), CYP2D6 (minor), CYP3A4 (minor); **Note:** Assignment of Major/Minor substrate status based on clinically relevant drug interaction potential; **Inhibits** CYP1A2 (weak), CYP2C19 (moderate), CYP2C9 (moderate), CYP2D6 (weak), CYP3A4 (weak); **Induces** CYP1A2 (moderate)

Avoid Concomitant Use

Avoid concomitant use of Omeprazole with any of the following: Clopidogrel; Dasatinib; Delavirdine; Erlotinib; Nelfinavir; PAZOPanib; Pimozide; Rifampin; Rilpivirine; Risedronate; St Johns Wort

Increased Effect/Toxicity

Omeprazole may increase the levels/effects of: Amphetamine; ARIPiprazole; Bosentan; Cannabis; Carvedilol; Cilostazol; Citalopram; CloZAPine; CycloSPORINE (Systemic); CYP2C19 Substrates; CYP2C9 Substrates; Dexmethylphenidate; Dextroamphetamine; Dofetilide; Dronabinol; Escitalopram; Fosphenytoin; Hydrocodone; Lomitapide; Methotrexate; Methylphenidate; Phenytoin; Pimozide; Raltegravir; Risedronate; Saquinavir; Tacrolimus (Systemic); Tetrahydrocannabinol; Vitamin K Antagonists; Voriconazole

The levels/effects of Omeprazole may be increased by: Fluconazole; Ketoconazole (Systemic); Voriconazole

Decreased Effect

Omeprazole may decrease the levels/effects of: Atazanavir; Bisphosphonate Derivatives; Bosutinib; Cefditoren; Clopidogrel; CloZAPine; Dabigatran Etexilate; Dabrafenib; Dasatinib; Delavirdine; Erlotinib; Gefitinib; Indinavir; Iron Salts; Itraconazole; Ketoconazole (Systemic); Ledipasvir; Mesalamine; Multivitamins/Minerals (with ADEK, Folate, Iron); Mycophenolate; Nelfinavir; Nilotinib; PAZOPanib; Posaconazole; Rilpivirine; Riociguat; Risedronate; Vismodegib

The levels/effects of Omeprazole may be decreased by: CYP2C19 Inducers (Strong); Dabrafenib; Fosphenytoin; Phenytoin; Rifampin; St Johns Wort; Tipranavir

Food Interactions Prolonged treatment (≥2 years) may lead to malabsorption of dietary vitamin B_{12} and subsequent vitamin B_{12} deficiency (Lam, 2013).

Preparation for Administration Granules for oral suspension: For oral administration, empty the contents of the 2.5 mg packet into 5 mL of water (10 mg packet into 15 mL of water); stir. For NG administration, add 5 mL of water into a catheter-tipped syringe, and then add the contents of a 2.5 mg packet (15 mL water for the 10 mg packet); shake. **Note:** Regardless of the route of administration, the suspension should be left to thicken for 2-3 minutes prior to administration.

Storage/Stability

Capsules, tablets: Store at 15°C to 30°C (59°F to 86°F). Protect from light and moisture.

Granules for oral suspension: Store at 25°C (77°F); excursions permitted to 15°C to 30°C (59°F to 86°F).

Powder for suspension (compounding kit): Prior to compounding, store at 15°C to 30°C (59°F to 86°F). Once compounded, the product is stable for 30 days under refrigeration [2°C to 8°C (36°F to 46°F)]; protect from light; protect from freezing.

OTC capsules: Store at 20°C to 25°C (68°F to 77°F); protect from moisture.

Mechanism of Action Proton pump inhibitor; suppresses gastric basal and stimulated acid secretion by inhibiting the parietal cell H+/K+ ATP pump

Pharmacodynamics/Kinetics

Onset of action: Antisecretory: ~1 hour

Peak effect: Within 2 hours

Duration: Up to 72 hours; 50% of maximum effect at 24 hours; after stopping treatment, secretory activity gradually returns over 3-5 days

Absorption: Rapid

Protein binding: ~95%

Metabolism: Hepatic via CYP2C19 primarily and (to a lesser extent) via 3A4 to hydroxy, desmethyl, and sulfone metabolites (all inactive); saturable first-pass effect

Bioavailability: Oral: ~30% to 40%; Hepatic dysfunction: ~100%; Asians: AUC increased up to fourfold compared to Caucasians

Half-life elimination: 0.5-1 hour; hepatic impairment: ~3 hours

Time to peak, plasma: 0.5-3.5 hours

Excretion: Urine (~77% as metabolites, very small amount as unchanged drug); feces

Dosage

Children 1-16 years: Oral: GERD or other acid-related disorders:

5 kg to <10 kg: 5 mg once daily

10 kg to <20 kg: 10 mg once daily

≥20 kg: 20 mg once daily

Adults: Oral:

Active duodenal ulcer: 20 mg once daily for 4-8 weeks

Gastric ulcers: 40 mg once daily for 4-8 weeks

Symptomatic GERD (without esophageal lesions): 20 mg once daily for up to 4 weeks

Erosive esophagitis: 20 mg once daily for 4-8 weeks; maintenance of healing: 20 mg once daily for up to 12 months total therapy (including treatment period of 4-8 weeks)

Helicobacter pylori eradication: Dose varies with regimen:

Manufacturer labeling: 40 mg once daily administered with clarithromycin 500 mg 3 times daily for 14 days **or** 20 mg twice daily administered with amoxicillin 1000 mg *and* clarithromycin 500 mg twice daily for 10 days. **Note:** Presence of ulcer at time of therapy initiation may necessitate an additional 14-18 days of omeprazole 20 mg daily (monotherapy) after completion of combination therapy.

American College of Gastroenterology guidelines (Chey, 2007):

Nonpenicillin allergy: 20 mg twice daily administered with amoxicillin 1000 mg *and* clarithromycin 500 mg twice daily for 10-14 days

Penicillin allergy: 20 mg twice daily administered with clarithromycin 500 mg *and* metronidazole 500 mg twice daily for 10-14 days **or** 20 mg once or twice daily administered with bismuth subsalicylate 525 mg *and* metronidazole 250 mg *plus* tetracycline 500 mg 4 times daily for 10-14 days

Pathological hypersecretory conditions: Initial: 60 mg once daily; doses up to 120 mg 3 times daily have been administered; administer daily doses >80 mg in divided doses

NSAID-induced ulcer treatment (off-label use): 20 mg once daily for 4-8 weeks; Maintenance: 20 mg once daily for up to 6 months (Hawkey, 1998)

NSAID-induced ulcer prophylaxis (off-label use): 20 mg once daily for up to 6 months (Cullen, 1998)

Stress ulcer prophylaxis, ICU patients (off-label use): 40 mg once daily (Levy, 1997) or may administer 40 mg loading dose followed by 20-40 mg once daily (ASHP, 1999). **Note:** Intended for patients with associated risk factors (eg, coagulopathy, mechanical ventilation for ≥48 hours, severe sepsis); discontinue use once risk factors have resolved (Dellinger, 2013). Omeprazole 20 mg via NG tube once daily may be less effective in some critically ill populations compared to 40 mg via NG tube once daily (Balaban, 1997).

Frequent heartburn (OTC labeling): 20 mg once daily for 14 days; treatment may be repeated after 4 months if needed

Dosage adjustment in renal impairment: No dosage adjustment necessary.

Dosage adjustment in hepatic impairment: No dosage adjustment provided in manufacturer's labeling. However, based on increased bioavailability, a dosage reduction should be considered, especially for maintenance of healing of erosive esophagitis.

Dietary Considerations Should be taken on an empty stomach; best if taken before breakfast.

Administration

Oral: Best if administered before breakfast.

Capsule: Should be swallowed whole; do not chew or crush. Delayed release capsule may be opened and contents added to 1 tablespoon of applesauce (use immediately after adding to applesauce); mixture should not be chewed or warmed.

Oral suspension: Following reconstitution, the suspension should be left to thicken for 2-3 minutes and administered within 30 minutes. If any material remains after administration, add more water, stir, and administer immediately.

Tablet: Should be swallowed whole; do not crush or chew.

Nasogastric/orogastric (NG/OG) tube administration:

Oral suspension (using packets): After removing a catheter-tip syringe plunger, add 5 mL of water to the syringe and the contents of a 2.5 mg packet (or 15 mL of water for the 10 mg packet). Immediately shake syringe and leave to thicken for 2-3 minutes; shake syringe again and within 30 minutes administer via NG or gastric tube (French size 6 or larger). Refill syringe with an equal amount of water, shake, and flush remaining contents through NG or gastric tube

Oral suspension (using capsules): The manufacturer of Prilosec® does not give recommendations for extemporaneous preparation of omeprazole capsules for NG/OG administration. Consider using the packets for oral suspension. If packets are unavailable, methods of preparation of capsules for NG/OG administration have been described (Balaban, 1997; Phillips, 1996). An extemporaneously prepared suspension with extended stability may also be used (DiGiacinto, 2000; Quercia, 1997; Sharma, 1999).

Monitoring Parameters Susceptibility testing is recommended in patients who fail *H. pylori*-eradication regimen.

Dosage Forms

Capsule Delayed Release, Oral:
PriLOSEC: 10 mg, 20 mg, 40 mg
Generic: 10 mg, 20 mg, 40 mg, 20 mg

Packet, Oral:
PriLOSEC: 2.5 mg (30 ea); 10 mg (30 ea)

Suspension, Oral:
First-Omeprazole: 2 mg/mL (90 mL, 150 mL, 300 mL)
Omeprazole+Syrspend SF Alka: 2 mg/mL (100 mL)

Tablet Delayed Release, Oral:
PriLOSEC OTC [OTC]: 20 mg
Generic: 20 mg

Extemporaneous Preparations Note: More palatable omeprazole (2 mg/mL) suspensions are commercially available as compounding kits (First-Omeprazole, Omeprazole+Syrspend SF Alka Cherry Kit).

A 2 mg/mL oral omeprazole solution (Simplified Omeprazole Solution) may be made with five omeprazole 20 mg delayed release capsules and 50 mL sodium bicarbonate 8.4%. Empty capsules into beaker. Add sodium bicarbonate solution. Gently stir (about 15 minutes) until a white suspension forms. Transfer to amber-colored syringe or bottle. Stable for 14 days at room temperature or for 30 days refrigerated.

DiGiacinto JL, Olsen KM, Bergman KL, et al, "Stability of Suspension Formulations of Lansoprazole and Omeprazole Stored in Amber-Colored Plastic Oral Syringes," *Ann Pharmacother*, 2000, 34 (5):600-5.

Quercia R, Fan C, Liu X, et al, "Stability of Omeprazole in an Extemporaneously Prepared Oral Liquid," *Am J Health Syst Pharm*, 1997, 54(16):1833-6.

Sharma V, "Comparison of 24-hour Intragastric pH Using Four Liquid Formulations of Lansoprazole and Omeprazole," *Am J Health Syst Pharm*, 1999, 56(23 Suppl 4):18-21.

◆ **Omeprazole, Amoxicillin, and Clarithromycin** *see* Omeprazole, Clarithromycin, and Amoxicillin *on page 1511*

Omeprazole and Sodium Bicarbonate

(oh MEP ra zole & SOW dee um bye KAR bun ate)

Brand Names: U.S. Zegerid; Zegerid OTC [OTC]

Index Terms Sodium Bicarbonate and Omeprazole

Pharmacologic Category Proton Pump Inhibitor; Substituted Benzimidazole

Use Short-term (4-8 weeks) treatment of active duodenal ulcer or active benign gastric ulcer; treatment of heartburn and other symptoms associated with gastroesophageal reflux disease (GERD); short-term (4-8 weeks) treatment of endoscopically-diagnosed erosive esophagitis; maintenance healing of erosive esophagitis; reduction of risk of upper gastrointestinal bleeding in critically-ill patients

OTC labeling: Short-term (2 weeks) treatment of frequent (2 days/week), uncomplicated heartburn

Pregnancy Risk Factor C

Dosage Note: Both strengths of Zegerid® capsule and powder for oral suspension have identical sodium bicarbonate content, respectively. Do not substitute two 20 mg capsules/packets for one 40 mg dose.

Oral: Adults:

Active duodenal ulcer: 20 mg once daily for 4-8 weeks

Gastric ulcers: 40 mg once daily for 4-8 weeks

Symptomatic GERD: 20 mg once daily for up to 4 weeks

Erosive esophagitis: 20 mg once daily for 4-8 weeks; maintenance of healing: 20 mg once daily for up to 12 months total therapy (including treatment period of 4-8 weeks)

Heartburn (OTC labeling): 20 mg once daily for 14 days. Do not take for >14 days or more often than every 4 months, unless instructed by healthcare provider.

Risk reduction of upper GI bleeding in critically-ill patients (Zegerid® powder for oral suspension):

Loading dose: Day 1: 40 mg every 6-8 hours for two doses

Maintenance dose: 40 mg daily for up to 14 days; therapy >14 days has not been evaluated

Dosage adjustment in renal impairment: No dosage adjustment necessary.

Dosage adjustment in hepatic impairment: No dosage adjustment provided in manufacturer's labeling. However, based on increased bioavailability, a dosage reduction should be considered, especially for maintenance of healing of erosive esophagitis.

Additional Information Complete prescribing information should be consulted for additional detail.

Dosage Forms

Capsule, oral: Omeprazole 20 mg [immediate release] and sodium bicarbonate 1100 mg; omeprazole 40 mg [immediate release] and sodium bicarbonate 1100 mg
Zegerid®: Omeprazole 20 mg [immediate release] and sodium bicarbonate 1100 mg
Zegerid®: Omeprazole 40 mg [immediate release] and sodium bicarbonate 1100 mg
Zegerid OTC™ [OTC]: Omeprazole 20 mg [immediate release] and sodium bicarbonate 1100 mg

Powder for suspension, oral:
Zegerid®: Omeprazole 20 mg and sodium bicarbonate 1680 mg per packet
Zegerid®: Omeprazole 40 mg and sodium bicarbonate 1680 mg per packet

Omeprazole, Clarithromycin, and Amoxicillin

(oh MEP ra zole, kla RITH roe mye sin, & a moks i SIL in)

Brand Names: U.S. Omeclamox-Pak®

Index Terms Amoxicillin, Clarithromycin, and Omeprazole; Clarithromycin, Amoxicillin, and Omeprazole; Omeprazole, Amoxicillin, and Clarithromycin

Pharmacologic Category Antibiotic, Macrolide Combination; Antibiotic, Penicillin; Gastrointestinal Agent, Miscellaneous; Proton Pump Inhibitor; Substituted Benzimidazole

Use Eradication of *H. pylori* infection in patients with duodenal ulcer disease (active or a history of up to 1 year)

Pregnancy Risk Factor C

Dosage Oral: Adults: Omeprazole 20 mg (one capsule), clarithromycin 500 mg (one tablet), and amoxicillin 1000 mg (two capsules) twice daily for 10 days. **Note:** If patient has an active duodenal ulcer at therapy initiation, an additional 18 days of omeprazole 20 mg once daily is recommended.

Dosage adjustment in renal impairment: Amoxicillin and clarithromycin pharmacokinetics are altered in renal impairment. The manufacturer's labeling suggests that prolonged dosing intervals for clarithromycin may be appropriate in severe renal impairment, but provides no recommendation in regards to amoxicillin.

Dosage adjustment in hepatic impairment: Avoid use in hepatic impairment.

Additional Information Complete prescribing information should be consulted for additional detail.

Dosage Forms

Combination package, oral [each administration card contains]:
Omeclamox-Pak™:
Capsule, delayed release: Omeprazole: 20 mg (2s)
Tablet: Clarithromycin: 500 mg (2s)
Capsule: Amoxicillin: 500 mg (4s) [contains sodium ≤0.0052 mEq (0.119 mg)/capsule]

◆ **Omeprazole Magnesium** *see* Omeprazole *on page 1508*

◆ **Omeprazole+Syrspend SF Alka** *see* Omeprazole *on page 1508*

◆ **Omnaris** *see* Ciclesonide (Nasal) *on page 432*

◆ **Omnaris HFA (Can)** *see* Ciclesonide (Nasal) *on page 432*

◆ **Omnicef** *see* Cefdinir *on page 376*

◆ **Omni Gel [OTC]** *see* Fluoride *on page 895*

◆ **Omnipred** *see* PrednisoLONE (Ophthalmic) *on page 1706*

◆ **Omnitarg** *see* Pertuzumab *on page 1627*

◆ **Omnitrope** *see* Somatropin *on page 1918*

Omoconazole [INT] (oh moh KON a zole)

International Brand Names Afongan (AR, GR); Fongamil (FR, GR, PT); Mikogal (HU, RU)

Index Terms Omoconazole Nitrate

Pharmacologic Category Antifungal Agent, Imidazole Derivative

Reported Use Treatment of topical fungal skin infections or vaginal candidiasis

Dosage Range Adults:

Topical: Apply once daily

Vaginal: 1 suppository/day

Product Availability Product available in various countries; not currently available in the U.S.

Dosage Forms

Cream: 1% (15 g, 30 g)

Suppository, vaginal: 300 mg

◆ **Omoconazole Nitrate** *see* Omoconazole [INT] *on page 1512*

OnabotulinumtoxinA

(oh nuh BOT yoo lin num TOKS in aye)

Brand Names: U.S. Botox; Botox Cosmetic

Brand Names: Canada Botox; Botox Cosmetic

Index Terms Botulinum Toxin Type A; BTX-A

Pharmacologic Category Neuromuscular Blocker Agent, Toxin; Ophthalmic Agent, Toxin

Use Treatment of strabismus and blepharospasm associated with dystonia (including benign essential blepharospasm or VII nerve disorders) in patients ≥12 years of age; treatment of cervical dystonia (spasmodic torticollis) in patients ≥16 years of age; temporary improvement in the appearance of lines/wrinkles of the face (moderate-to-severe glabellar lines associated with corrugator and/or procerus muscle activity; moderate to severe lateral canthal lines associated with orbicularis oculi activity) in adult patients; treatment of severe primary axillary hyperhidrosis in adults not adequately controlled with topical treatments; treatment of focal spasticity (specifically upper limb spasticity) in adults; prophylaxis of chronic migraine headache (≥15 days/month with ≥4 hours/day headache duration) in adults; treatment of urinary incontinence due to detrusor overactivity associated with neurologic conditions in adults; treatment of overactive bladder (with symptoms of urge urinary incontinence, urgency, and frequency) in adults with an inadequate response or intolerance to anticholinergic medication.

Canadian labeling: Additional use (not in U.S. labeling): Dynamic equinus foot deformity in pediatric cerebral palsy patients; treatment of forehead lines in adults

Pregnancy Risk Factor C

Dosage Note: The lowest recommended dose should be used when initiating treatment (regardless of indication). In adults treated for more than one indication, the maximum cumulative dose should be ≤360 units/3 months. Canadian labeling recommends a maximum cumulative dose of 6 units/kg (adults up to 360 units; children up to 200 units) over 3 months in patients receiving additional treatment for noncosmetic indications.

Bladder dysfunction: Adults: Intradetrusor: **Note:** Prophylactic antimicrobial therapy (excluding aminoglycosides) should be administered 1-3 days prior to, on the day of, and for 1-3 days following onabotulinumtoxinA administration to decrease risk of UTI. Discontinue antiplatelet therapy at least 3 days prior to administration.

Detrusor overactivity associated with neurologic condition: 30 injections of 1 mL (recommended concentration: ~6.7 units/mL) for a total dose of 200 units/30 mL (maximum: 200 units); for the final injection, ~1 mL of sterile NS should be injected to ensure that the remaining medication in the needle is delivered to the bladder; may consider retreatment with diminishing effect but no sooner than 12 weeks from previous administration (median time until second treatment in studies: 42-48 weeks).

Overactive bladder: 20 injections of 0.5 mL (recommended concentration: 10 units/mL) for a total dose of 100 units/10 mL (maximum: 100 units); for the final injection, ~1 mL of sterile NS should be injected to ensure that the remaining medication in the needle is delivered to the bladder; may consider retreatment with diminishing effect but no sooner than 12 weeks from the previous administration (median time until second treatment in studies: ~24 weeks)

Blepharospasm:

Botox: Children ≥12 years and Adults: IM: Initial dose: 1.25-2.5 units injected into the medial and lateral pretarsal orbicularis oculi of the upper lid and lateral pretarsal orbicularis oculi of lower lid

Dose may be increased up to twice the previous dose if the response from the initial dose lasted ≤2 months; maximum dose per site: 5 units. Tolerance may occur if treatments are given more often than every 3 months, but the effect is not usually permanent. Cumulative dose:

U.S. labeling: ≤200 units in 30-day period

Canadian labeling (not in U.S. labeling): Botox: ≤200 units in 2-month period

Cervical dystonia:

Children ≥16 years and Adults: IM: For dosing guidance, the mean dose is 236 units (25th to 75th percentile range 198-300 units) divided among the affected muscles in patients previously treated with botulinum toxin (maximum: ≤50 units/site). Initial dose in previously untreated patients should be lower. Sequential dosing should be based on the patient's head and neck position, localization of pain, muscle hypertrophy, patient response, and previous adverse reactions. The total dose injected into the sternocleidomastoid muscles should be ≤100 units to decrease the occurrence of dysphagia.

Canadian labeling (not in U.S. labeling): Botox: Children ≥16 years and Adults: IM: Effective range of 200-360 units has been used in clinical practice; administer no more frequently than every 2 months

Chronic migraine: Adults: IM: Administer 5 units/0.1 mL per site. Recommended total dose is 155 units once every 12 weeks. Each 155 unit dose should be equally divided and administered bilaterally, into 31 total sites as described below (refer to prescribing information for specific diagrams of recommended injection sites):

Corrugator: 5 units to each side (2 sites)

Procerus: 5 units (1 site only)

Frontalis: 10 units to each side (divided into 2 sites/side)
Temporalis: 20 units to each side (divided into 4 sites/side)
Occipitalis: 15 units to each side (divided into 3 sites/side)
Cervical paraspinal: 10 units to each side (divided into 2 sites/side)
Trapezius: 15 units to each side (divided into 3 sites/side)

Strabismus: Children ≥12 years and Adults: IM: **Note:** Several minutes prior to injection, administration of local anesthetic and ocular decongestant drops are recommended.

Initial dose:

Vertical muscles and for horizontal strabismus <20 prism diopters: 1.25-2.5 units in any one muscle

Horizontal strabismus of 20-50 prism diopters: 2.5-5 units in any one muscle

Persistent VI nerve palsy ≥1 month: 1.25-2.5 units in the medial rectus muscle

Re-examine patients 7-14 days after each injection to assess the effect of that dose. Subsequent doses for patients experiencing incomplete paralysis of the target may be increased up to twice the previous administered dose. The maximum recommended dose as a single injection for any one muscle is 25 units. Do not administer subsequent injections until the effects of the previous dose are gone.

Primary axillary hyperhidrosis: Adults ≥18 years: Intradermal: 50 units/axilla. Injection area should be defined by standard staining techniques. Injections should be evenly distributed into multiple sites (10-15), administered in 0.1-0.2 mL aliquots, ~1-2 cm apart. May repeat when clinical effect diminishes.

Spasticity (cerebral palsy related [dynamic equinus foot deformity]: Canadian labeling [not approved in U.S. labeling]): Children ≥2 years: IM: 4 units/kg (total dose) divided into two injections into medial and lateral heads of the gastrocnemius of affected leg; if clinically indicated, may repeat every 2 months (maximum dose: 200 units); in diplegia, the recommended dose is 6 units/kg (total dose) divided between affected limbs

Spasticity (focal): Adults ≥18 years: IM: Individualize dose based on patient size, extent, and location of muscle involvement, degree of spasticity, local muscle weakness, and response to prior treatment. In clinical trials used to support the FDA-approved labeling, total doses up to 360 units (Botox) were administered as separate injections typically divided among selected muscles; may repeat therapy at ≥3 months with appropriate dosage based upon the clinical condition of patient at time of retreatment. Single session doses of ≤1200 units (off-label dose) have been reported; however, safety and efficacy of routine use of doses >500 units has not been evaluated (Francisco, 2004). Single site doses of ≤400 units (off-label dose) in a lower limb (off-label use) have been reported (Nalysnyk, 2013).

Suggested guidelines for the treatment of upper limb spasticity. The lowest recommended starting dose should be used and ≤50 units/site should be administered. **Note:** Dose listed is total dose administered as individual or separate intramuscular injection(s):

Biceps brachii: 100-200 units (divided into 4 sites)
Flexor digitorum profundus: 30-50 units (1 site)
Flexor digitorum sublimes: 30-50 units (1 site)
Flexor carpi radialis: 12.5-50 units (1 site)
Flexor carpi ulnaris: 12.5-50 units (1 site)

Suggested guidelines for the treatment of stroke-related upper limb spasticity: Canadian labeling: **Note:** Dose listed is total dose administered as individual or separate intramuscular injection(s):

Biceps brachii: 100-200 units (up to 4 sites)
Flexor digitorum profundus: 15-50 units (1-2 sites)
Flexor digitorum sublimes: 15-50 units (1-2 sites)
Flexor carpi radialis: 15-60 units (1-2 sites)
Flexor carpi ulnaris: 10-50 units (1-2 sites)
Adductor pollicis: 20 units (1-2 sites)
Flexor pollicis longus: 20 units (1-2 sites)

Cosmetic uses:

Reduction of glabellar lines: Adults: IM: An effective dose is determined by gross observation of the patient's ability to activate the superficial muscles injected. The location, size and use of muscles may vary markedly among individuals. Inject 0.1 mL (4 units) dose into each of five sites, two in each corrugator muscle and one in the procerus muscle for a total dose 0.5 mL (20 units) administered no more frequently than every 3-4 months. **Note:** Treatment of adults >65 years is approved in the Canadian labeling.

Reduction of lateral canthus lines:

U.S. labeling: Adults: IM: Inject 0.1 mL (4 units) into 3 injection sites per side (6 total injection points) in the lateral orbicularis oculi muscle for a total dose of 0.6 mL (24 units) administered no more frequently than every 3 months.

Canadian labeling: Adults: IM: Inject 2-6 units into each of 1-3 injection sites, lateral to the lateral orbital rim.

Reduction of forehead lines (Canadian labeling; not in U.S. labeling): Adults: IM: Inject 2-6 units into each of four sites in the frontalis muscle every 1-2 cm along either side of forehead crease and 2-3 cm above eyebrows for total dose of 24 units.

Elderly: No specific adjustment recommended; initiate therapy at lowest recommended dose

Dosage adjustment in renal impairment: No dosage adjustment provided in manufacturer's labeling.

Dosage adjustment in hepatic impairment: No dosage adjustment provided in manufacturer's labeling.

Additional Information Complete prescribing information should be consulted for additional detail.

Dosage Forms

Solution Reconstituted, Injection:
Botox: 100 units (1 ea)

Solution Reconstituted, Injection [preservative free]:
Botox: 200 units (1 ea)

Solution Reconstituted, Intramuscular:
Botox Cosmetic: 100 units (1 ea)

Solution Reconstituted, Intramuscular [preservative free]:
Botox Cosmetic: 50 units (1 ea)

Dosage Forms: Canada

Injection, powder for reconstitution [preservative free]:
Botox: Botulinum toxin A 50 units, 100 units, 200 units
Botox Cosmetic: Botulinum toxin A 50 unit, 100 units, 200 units

◆ **Onbrez® Breezhaler® (Can)** *see* Indacaterol *on page 1063*

◆ **Oncaspar** *see* Pegaspargase *on page 1588*

◆ **Oncotice (Can)** *see* BCG *on page 229*

◆ **Oncovin** *see* VinCRIStine *on page 2163*

Ondansetron (on DAN se tron)

Brand Names: U.S. Zofran; Zofran ODT; Zuplenz

Brand Names: Canada Apo-Ondansetron; Ava-Ondansetron; CO Ondansetron; Dom-Ondansetron; JAMP-Ondansetron; Mar-Ondansetron; Mint-Ondansetron; Mylan-Ondansetron; Ondansetron Injection; Ondansetron Injection USP; Ondansetron-Odan; Ondansetron-Omega; Ondissolve ODF; PHL-Ondansetron; PMS-Ondansetron; RAN-Ondansetron; ratio-Ondansetron; Riva-Ondansetron; Sandoz-Ondansetron; Septa-Ondansetron; Teva-Ondansetron; Zofran; Zofran ODT

Index Terms GR38032R; Ondansetron Hydrochloride

Pharmacologic Category Antiemetic; Selective 5-HT_3 Receptor Antagonist

Use

Cancer chemotherapy-induced nausea and vomiting:

IV: Prevention of nausea and vomiting associated with initial and repeat courses of emetogenic cancer chemotherapy (including high-dose cisplatin)

Oral:

Prevention of nausea and vomiting associated with highly emetogenic cancer chemotherapy (including cisplatin ≥50 mg/m^2).

Prevention of nausea and vomiting associated with initial and repeat courses of moderately emetogenic cancer chemotherapy.

Radiotherapy-associated nausea and vomiting: Oral: Prevention of nausea and vomiting associated with radiotherapy in patients receiving either total body irradiation, single high-dose fraction to the abdomen, or daily fractions to the abdomen.

Postoperative nausea and/or vomiting: IV and Oral: Prevention of postoperative nausea and/or vomiting (PONV). If nausea/vomiting occur in a patient who had not received prophylactic ondansetron, IV ondansetron may be administered to prevent further episodes.

Limitations of use: Routine prophylaxis for PONV in patients with minimal expectation of nausea and/or vomiting is not recommended, although use is recommended in patients when nausea and vomiting must be avoided in the postoperative period, even if the incidence of PONV is low.

Canadian labeling: Additional use (not in U.S. labeling): IV: Treatment of PONV

Pregnancy Risk Factor B

Pregnancy Considerations Teratogenic effects were not observed in animal reproduction studies. Ondansetron readily crosses the human placenta in the first trimester of pregnancy and can be detected in fetal tissue (Siu, 2006). The use of ondansetron for the treatment of nausea and vomiting of pregnancy (NVP) has been evaluated. Although a significant increase in birth defects has not been described in case reports and some studies (Ferreira, 2012; Pasternak, 2013), other studies have shown a possible association with ondansetron exposure and adverse fetal events (Anderka, 2012; Einarson, 2004). Additional studies are needed to determine safety to the fetus, particularly during the first trimester. Based on available data, use is generally reserved for severe NVP (hyperemesis gravidarum) or when conventional treatments are not effective (ACOG, 2004; Koren, 2012; Levicheck, 2002; Tan, 2011). Because a dose-dependent QT-interval prolongation occurs with use, the manufacturer recommends ECG monitoring in patients with electrolyte abnormalities (which can be associated with some cases of NVP; Koren, 2012). An international consensus panel recommends that 5-HT_3 antagonists (including ondansetron) should not be withheld in pregnant patients receiving chemotherapy for the treatment of gynecologic cancers, when chemotherapy is given according to general recommendations for chemotherapy use during pregnancy (Amant, 2010).

Breast-Feeding Considerations It is not known if ondansetron is excreted into breast milk. The U.S. manufacturer labeling recommends caution be used if administered to nursing women. The Canadian labeling recommends avoiding nursing during ondansetron treatment.

Contraindications Hypersensitivity to ondansetron or any component of the formulation; concomitant use of apomorphine

Warnings/Precautions Antiemetics are most effective when used prophylactically (Roila, 2010). If emesis occurs despite optimal antiemetic prophylaxis, reevaluate emetic risk, disease, concurrent morbidities and medications to assure antiemetic regimen is optimized (Basch, 2011). Does not stimulate gastric or intestinal peristalsis; may mask progressive ileus and/or gastric distension. Use with caution in patients allergic to other 5-HT_3 receptor antagonists; cross-reactivity has been reported.

Dose-dependent QT interval prolongation occurs with ondansetron use. Cases of torsade de pointes have also been reported to the manufacturer. Selective 5-HT_3 antagonists, including ondansetron, have been associated with a number of dose-dependent increases in ECG intervals (eg, PR, QRS duration, QT/QTc, JT), usually occurring 1 to 2 hours after IV administration. Single doses >16 mg ondansetron IV are no longer recommended due to the potential for an increased risk of QT prolongation. In most patients, these changes are not clinically relevant; however, when used in conjunction with other agents that prolong these intervals or in those at risk for QT prolongation, arrhythmia may occur. When used with agents that prolong the QT interval (eg, Class I and III antiarrhythmics) or in patients with cardiovascular disease, clinically relevant QT interval prolongation may occur resulting in torsade de pointes. Avoid ondansetron use in patients with congenital long QT syndrome. Use caution and monitor ECG in patients with other risk factors for QT prolongation (eg, medications known to prolong QT interval, electrolyte abnormalities [hypokalemia or hypomagnesemia], heart failure, bradyarrhythmias, and cumulative high-dose anthracycline therapy). IV formulations of 5-HT_3 antagonists have more association with ECG interval changes, compared to oral formulations. Dose limitations are recommended for patients with severe hepatic impairment (Child-Pugh class C); use with caution in mild-moderate hepatic impairment; clearance is decreased and half-life increased in hepatic impairment.

Serotonin syndrome has been reported with 5-HT_3 receptor antagonists, predominantly when used in combination with other serotonergic agents (eg, SSRIs, SNRIs, MAOIs, mirtazapine, fentanyl, lithium, tramadol, and/or methylene blue). Some of the cases have been fatal. The majority of serotonin syndrome reports due to 5-HT_3 receptor antagonist have occurred in a postanesthesia setting or in an infusion center. Serotonin syndrome has also been reported following overdose of ondansetron. Monitor patients for signs of serotonin syndrome, including mental status changes (eg, agitation, hallucinations, delirium, coma); autonomic instability (eg, tachycardia, labile blood pressure, diaphoresis, dizziness, flushing, hyperthermia); neuromuscular changes (eg, tremor, rigidity, myoclonus, hyperreflexia, incoordination); gastrointestinal symptoms (eg, nausea, vomiting, diarrhea); and/or seizures. If serotonin syndrome occurs, discontinue 5-HT_3 receptor antagonist treatment and begin supportive management. Potentially significant drug-drug interactions may exist, requiring dose or frequency adjustment, additional monitoring, and/or selection of alternative therapy. Orally disintegrating tablets contain phenylalanine.

Benzyl alcohol and derivatives: Some dosage forms may contain sodium benzoate/benzoic acid; benzoic acid (benzoate) is a metabolite of benzyl alcohol; large amounts of benzyl alcohol (≥99 mg/kg/day) have been associated with a potentially fatal toxicity ("gasping syndrome") in neonates; the "gasping syndrome" consists of metabolic acidosis, respiratory distress, gasping respirations, CNS dysfunction (including convulsions, intracranial hemorrhage), hypotension, and cardiovascular collapse (AAP, 1997; CDC, 1982); some data suggests that benzoate displaces bilirubin from protein binding sites (Ahlfors,

2001); avoid or use dosage forms containing benzyl alcohol derivative with caution in neonates. See manufacturer's labeling.

Adverse Reactions

Central nervous system: Agitation (oral), anxiety (oral), dizziness, drowsiness (IV), fatigue (oral), headache (more common in oral), malaise (oral), paresthesia (IV), sedation (IV), sensation of cold (IV)

Dermatologic: Pruritus, skin rash

Gastrointestinal: Constipation, diarrhea (more common in oral)

Genitourinary: Gynecologic disease (oral), urinary retention (oral)

Hepatic: Increased serum ALT (>2 times ULN; transient), increased serum AST (>2 times ULN; transient)

Local: Injection site reaction (IV, includes burning sensation at injection site, erythema at injection site, injection site pain)

Respiratory: Hypoxia (oral)

Miscellaneous: Fever

Rare but important or life-threatening: Abdominal pain, accommodation disturbance, atrial fibrillation, cardiorespiratory arrest (IV), depression of ST segment on ECG, dyspnea, extrapyramidal reaction (IV), flushing, hepatic failure (when used with other hepatotoxic medications), hiccups, hypersensitivity reaction, hypokalemia, hypotension, laryngospasm (IV), liver enzyme disorder, mucosal tissue reaction, myocardial infarction, neuroleptic malignant syndrome, positive lymphocyte transformation test, prolonged Q-T interval on ECG (dose dependent), second-degree atrioventricular block, serotonin syndrome, shock (IV), Stevens-Johnson syndrome, supraventricular tachycardia, syncope, tachycardia, tonic-clonic seizures, torsades de pointes, transient blindness (lasted ≤48 hours), transient blurred vision (following infusion), vascular occlusive events, ventricular premature contractions, ventricular tachycardia, weakness

Drug Interactions

Metabolism/Transport Effects **Substrate** of CYP1A2 (minor), CYP2C9 (minor), CYP2D6 (minor), CYP2E1 (minor), CYP3A4 (major), P-glycoprotein; **Note:** Assignment of Major/Minor substrate status based on clinically relevant drug interaction potential; **Inhibits** CYP1A2 (weak), CYP2C9 (weak), CYP2D6 (weak)

Avoid Concomitant Use

Avoid concomitant use of Ondansetron with any of the following: Apomorphine; Highest Risk QTc-Prolonging Agents; Ivabradine; Mifepristone

Increased Effect/Toxicity

Ondansetron may increase the levels/effects of: Apomorphine; ARIPiprazole; Highest Risk QTc-Prolonging Agents; Moderate Risk QTc-Prolonging Agents; Serotonin Modulators

The levels/effects of Ondansetron may be increased by: Ivabradine; Mifepristone; P-glycoprotein/ABCB1 Inhibitors; QTc-Prolonging Agents (Indeterminate Risk and Risk Modifying)

Decreased Effect

Ondansetron may decrease the levels/effects of: Tapentadol; TraMADol

The levels/effects of Ondansetron may be decreased by: Bosentan; CYP3A4 Inducers (Moderate); CYP3A4 Inducers (Strong); Dabrafenib; Deferasirox; Mitotane; P-glycoprotein/ABCB1 Inducers; Siltuximab; St Johns Wort; Tocilizumab

Food Interactions Tablet: Food slightly increases the extent of absorption. Management: Administer without regard to meals.

Preparation for Administration Prior to IV infusion, dilute in 50 mL D_5W or NS.

Storage/Stability

Oral soluble film: Store between 20°C and 25°C (68°F and 77°F). Store pouches in cartons; keep film in individual pouch until ready to use.

Oral solution: Store between 15°C and 30°C (59°F and 86°F). Protect from light.

Tablet: Store between 2°C and 30°C (36°F and 86°F).

Vial: Store between 2°C and 30°C (36°F and 86°F). Protect from light. Stable when mixed in D_5W or NS for 48 hours at room temperature.

Premixed bag in D5W: Store at 20°C to 25°C (68°F to 77°F), excursions permitted from 15°C to 30°C (59°F to 86°F); may refrigerate; avoid freezing and excessive heat; protect from light.

Mechanism of Action Selective 5-HT_3-receptor antagonist, blocking serotonin, both peripherally on vagal nerve terminals and centrally in the chemoreceptor trigger zone

Pharmacodynamics/Kinetics

Onset of action: ~30 minutes

Absorption: Oral: Well absorbed from GI tract

Distribution: V_d: Children: 1.9 to 3.7 L/kg

Protein binding, plasma: 70% to 76%

Metabolism: Extensively hepatic via hydroxylation, followed by glucuronide or sulfate conjugation; CYP1A2, CYP2D6, and CYP3A4 substrate; some demethylation occurs

Bioavailability: Oral: ~56% (some first pass metabolism)

Half-life elimination: Children <15 years: 2 to 7 hours; Adults: 3 to 6 hours

Mild-to-moderate hepatic impairment (Child-Pugh classes A and B): Adults: 12 hours

Severe hepatic impairment (Child-Pugh class C): Adults: 20 hours

Time to peak: Oral: ~2 hours; Oral soluble film: ~1 hour

Excretion: Urine (44% to 60% as metabolites, ~5% as unchanged drug); feces (~25%)

Dosage

Children:

Prevention of chemotherapy-induced nausea and vomiting:

U.S. labeling:

Prevention of nausea and vomiting associated with emetogenic chemotherapy: Infants ≥6 months, Children, and Adolescents: IV: 0.15 mg/kg/dose (maximum: 16 mg/dose) over 15 minutes for 3 doses, beginning 30 minutes prior to chemotherapy, followed by subsequent doses administered 4 and 8 hours after the first dose

Prevention of nausea and vomiting associated with moderately-emetogenic chemotherapy: Oral:

Children 4 to 11 years: 4 mg 30 minutes before chemotherapy; repeat 4 and 8 hours after initial dose, then 4 mg every 8 hours for 1 to 2 days after chemotherapy completed

Children ≥12 years: Refer to adult dosing.

Canadian labeling:

Prevention of nausea and vomiting associated with emetogenic chemotherapy: Children 4 to 12 years:

IV: 3 to 5 mg/m^2 over 15 minutes at least 30 minutes prior to chemotherapy, then convert to oral therapy; continue for up to 5 days following chemotherapy

Oral: 4 mg every 8 hours for up to 5 days following chemotherapy; oral therapy is started after an IV dose is given prior to chemotherapy

Pediatric guideline recommendations:

Prevention of chemotherapy-induced nausea and vomiting (off-label dosing; Dupuis, 2013):

Highly emetogenic chemotherapy: Infants ≥1 month and Children <12 years: IV, Oral: 0.15 mg/kg/dose (5 mg/m^2/dose) prior to chemotherapy and then every 8 hours; maximum recommended IV dose: 16 mg. Antiemetic regimen also includes dexamethasone

Highly emetogenic chemotherapy: Children ≥12 years and Adolescents: IV, Oral: 0.15 mg/kg/dose (5 mg/m²/dose) prior to chemotherapy and then every 8 hours; maximum recommended IV dose: 16 mg. Antiemetic regimen includes dexamethasone and if no known or suspected drug interactions, aprepitant.

Moderately emetogenic chemotherapy: Infants ≥1 month, Children, and Adolescents: IV, Oral: 0.15 mg/kg/dose (5 mg/m²/dose; maximum: 8 mg dose); prior to chemotherapy and then every 12 hours. Antiemetic regimen also includes dexamethasone.

Low emetogenicity chemotherapy: Infants ≥1 month, Children, and Adolescents: IV, Oral: 0.3 mg/kg/dose (10 mg/m²/dose; maximum IV dose: 16 mg) prior to chemotherapy

Prevention of postoperative nausea and vomiting (PONV): *U.S. labeling:* Infants ≥1 month and Children ≤12 years: IV:

≤40 kg: 0.1 mg/kg as a single dose over 2 to 5 minutes

>40 kg: 4 mg as a single dose over 2 to 5 minutes

Adults:

Prevention of chemotherapy-induced nausea and vomiting:

U.S. labeling:

Prevention of nausea and vomiting associated with emetogenic chemotherapy: IV: 0.15 mg/kg/dose (maximum: 16 mg/dose) administered over 15 minutes for 3 doses, beginning 30 minutes prior to chemotherapy, followed by subsequent doses 4 and 8 hours after the first dose

Prevention of nausea and vomiting associated with highly emetogenic chemotherapy: Oral: 24 mg 30 minutes prior to the start of single-day chemotherapy

Prevention of nausea and vomiting associated with moderately emetogenic chemotherapy: Oral: 8 mg beginning 30 minutes before chemotherapy; repeat dose 8 hours after initial dose, then 8 mg every 12 hours for 1 to 2 days after chemotherapy completed

Canadian labeling:

Prevention of nausea and vomiting associated with highly emetogenic chemotherapy:

IV: 8 to 16 mg (maximum: 16 mg/dose) administered over 15 minutes at least 30 minutes prior to chemotherapy; may administer an additional 8 mg dose at 4 and 8 hours after the initial dose. May convert to oral therapy after the first 24 hours.

Oral: 8 mg every 8 hours for up to 5 days following chemotherapy; oral therapy is initiated after receiving 24 hours of IV ondansetron.

Prevention of nausea and vomiting associated with less emetogenic chemotherapy:

IV: 8 mg administered over 15 minutes at least 30 minutes prior to chemotherapy; may convert to oral therapy twice daily

Oral: 8 mg administered 1-2 hours prior to chemotherapy, followed by 8 mg orally twice daily for up to 5 days following chemotherapy

Guideline recommendations: Prevention of chemotherapy-induced nausea and vomiting:

American Society of Clinical Oncology (ASCO; Basch, 2011):

High emetic risk: Day(s) chemotherapy is administered (antiemetic regimen also includes dexamethasone and aprepitant or fosaprepitant):

IV: 8 mg or 0.15 mg/kg. **Note:** Single IV doses >16 mg are no longer recommended by the manufacturer due to the potential for QT prolongation.

Oral: 8 mg twice daily

Multinational Association of Supportive Care in Cancer (MASCC) and European Society of Medical Oncology (ESMO) (Roila, 2010):

Highly emetic chemotherapy (antiemetic regimen includes dexamethasone and aprepitant/fosaprepitant):

IV: 8 mg or 0.15 mg/kg as a single dose prior to chemotherapy. **Note:** Single IV doses >16 mg are no longer recommended by the manufacturer due to the potential for QT prolongation

Oral: 24 mg as a single dose prior to chemotherapy

Moderately emetic chemotherapy (antiemetic regimen includes dexamethasone [and aprepitant/fosaprepitant for AC chemotherapy regimen]):

IV: 8 mg or 0.15 mg/kg as a single dose prior to chemotherapy. **Note:** Single IV doses >16 mg are no longer recommended by the manufacturer due to the potential for QT prolongation.

Oral: 16 mg (as 8 mg twice daily)

Low emetic risk: Ondansetron (dose not specified) prior to chemotherapy on day 1

Prevention of radiation therapy-induced nausea and vomiting:

U.S. labeling:

Total body irradiation: Oral: 8 mg administered 1 to 2 hours before each daily fraction of radiotherapy

Single high-dose fraction radiotherapy to abdomen: Oral: 8 mg administered 1-2 hours before irradiation, then 8 mg every 8 hours after first dose for 1 to 2 days after completion of radiotherapy

Daily fractionated radiotherapy to abdomen: Oral: 8 mg administered 1-2 hours before irradiation, then 8 mg every 8 hours after first dose for each day of radiotherapy

Canadian labeling: Oral: 8 mg 1-2 hours prior to radiation followed by 8 mg every 8 hours for up to 5 days after a course of treatment

American Society of Clinical Oncology Antiemetic Guideline recommendations (Basch, 2011): Give before each fraction throughout radiation therapy for high emetic risk (continue for at least 24 hours after completion) and for moderate emetic risk. For low emetic risk, may give either as prevention or rescue; for minimal emetic risk, give as rescue (if rescue used for either low or minimal emetic risk, then prophylaxis should be given until the end of radiation therapy).

IV (off-label route/dosing): 8 mg or 0.15 mg/kg. **Note:** Single IV doses >16 mg are no longer recommended by the manufacturer due to the potential for QT prolongation.

Prevention of postoperative nausea and vomiting (PONV):

IM, IV (U.S. labeling) or IV (Canadian labeling): 4 mg as a single dose (over 2 to 5 minutes if giving IV) administered ~30 minutes before the end of anesthesia (see **Note** below) or as treatment if vomiting occurs after surgery (Gan, 2007).

Note: The manufacturer recommends administration immediately before induction of anesthesia; however, this has been shown not to be as effective as administration at the end of surgery (Sun, 1997). Repeat doses given in response to inadequate control of nausea/vomiting from preoperative doses are generally ineffective.

Oral: 16 mg administered 1 hour prior to induction of anesthesia

Treatment of postoperative nausea and vomiting: *Canadian labeling:* IV: 4 mg as a single dose (preferably over 2 to 5 minutes, but not less than 30 seconds)

Treatment of severe or refractory hyperemesis gravidum (off-label use):
IV: 8 mg administered over 15 minutes every 12 hours (ACOG, 2004)
Oral: 8 mg every 12 hours (Levichek, 2002)

Elderly:
U.S. labeling: IV, Oral: No dosing adjustment required; refer to adult dosing.
Canadian labeling: ≥75 years: IV: In the prevention of nausea and vomiting associated with emetogenic chemotherapy, the initial dose should not exceed 8 mg; refer to adult dosing. May give 2 additional IV doses at least 4 hours apart (if third dose is needed, consider ECG monitoring).

Dosage adjustment in renal impairment: No dosage adjustment necessary (there is no experience for oral ondansetron beyond day 1)
Dosage adjustment in hepatic impairment:
U.S. labeling:
Mild to moderate impairment: No dosage adjustment necessary.
Severe liver impairment (Child-Pugh class C):
IV: Day 1: Maximum daily dose: 8 mg (there is no experience beyond day 1)
Oral: Maximum daily dose: 8 mg
Canadian labeling:
Mild impairment: No dosage adjustment necessary.
Moderate to severe impairment: Maximum daily dose: 8 mg

Dietary Considerations Some products may contain phenylalanine.

Administration
Oral: Oral dosage forms should be administered 30 minutes prior to chemotherapy; 1 to 2 hours before radiotherapy; 1 hour prior to the induction of anesthesia
Orally-disintegrating tablets: Do not remove from blister until needed. Peel backing off the blister, do not push tablet through. Using dry hands, place tablet on tongue and allow to dissolve. Swallow with saliva.
Oral soluble film: Do not remove from pouch until immediately before use. Using dry hands, place film on top of tongue and allow to dissolve (4 to 20 seconds). Swallow with or without liquid. If using more than one film, each film should be allowed to dissolve completely before administering the next film.
IM: Should be administered undiluted.
IV:
IVPB: Infuse diluted solution over 15 to 30 minutes; 24-hour continuous infusions have been reported, but are rarely used.
Chemotherapy-induced nausea and vomiting: Give first dose 30 minutes prior to beginning chemotherapy.
IV push: Prevention of postoperative nausea and vomiting: Single doses may be administered IV injection as undiluted solution over at least 30 seconds but preferably over 2 to 5 minutes

Monitoring Parameters ECG (if applicable in high-risk or elderly patients); potassium, magnesium

Dosage Forms
Film, Oral:
Zuplenz: 4 mg (1 ea, 10 ea); 8 mg (1 ea, 10 ea)
Solution, Injection:
Zofran: 40 mg/20 mL (20 mL)
Generic: 4 mg/2 mL (2 mL); 40 mg/20 mL (20 mL)
Solution, Injection [preservative free]:
Generic: 4 mg/2 mL (2 mL)
Solution, Oral:
Zofran: 4 mg/5 mL (50 mL)
Generic: 4 mg/5 mL (50 mL)
Tablet, Oral:
Zofran: 4 mg, 8 mg
Generic: 4 mg, 8 mg, 24 mg
Tablet Dispersible, Oral:
Zofran ODT: 4 mg, 8 mg
Generic: 4 mg, 8 mg

Dosage Forms: Canada Refer to Dosage Forms. **Note:** Oral Film is not available in Canada.

Extemporaneous Preparations Note: Commercial oral solution is available (0.8 mg/mL)

If commercial oral solution is unavailable, a 0.8 mg/mL syrup may be made with ondansetron tablets, Ora-Plus® (Paddock), and any of the the following syrups: Cherry syrup USP, Syrpalta® (HUMCO), Ora-Sweet® (Paddock), or Ora-Sweet® Sugar-Free (Paddock). Crush ten 8 mg tablets in a mortar and reduce to a fine powder (flaking of the tablet coating occurs). Add 50 mL Ora-Plus® in 5 mL increments, mixing thoroughly; mix while adding the chosen syrup in incremental proportions to **almost** 100 mL; transfer to a calibrated bottle, rinse mortar with syrup, and add sufficient quantity of syrup to make 100 mL. Label "shake well" and "refrigerate". Stable for 42 days refrigerated (Trissel, 1996).

Rectal suppositories: Calibrate a suppository mold for the base being used. Determine the displacement factor (DF) for ondansetron for the base being used (Fattibase® = 1.1; Polybase® = 0.6). Weigh the ondansetron tablet(s). Divide the tablet weight by the DF; this result is the weight of base displaced by the drug. Subtract the weight of base displaced from the calculated weight of base required for each suppository. Grind the ondansetron tablets in a mortar and reduce to a fine powder. Weigh out the appropriate weight of suppository base. Melt the base over a water bath (<55°C). Add the ondansetron powder to the suppository base and mix well. Pour the mixture into the suppository mold and cool. Stable for at least 30 days refrigerated (Tenjarla, 1998).

Tenjarla SN, Ward ES, and Fox JL, "Ondansetron Suppositories: Extemporaneous Preparation, Drug Release, Stability and Flux Through Rabbit Rectal Membrane," *Int J Pharm Compound*, 1998, 2(1):83-8.
Trissel LA, *Trissel's Stability of Compounded Formulations*, Washington, DC: American Pharmaceutical Association, 1996.

◆ **Ondansetron Hydrochloride** *see* Ondansetron *on page 1513*
◆ **Ondansetron Injection (Can)** *see* Ondansetron *on page 1513*
◆ **Ondansetron Injection USP (Can)** *see* Ondansetron *on page 1513*
◆ **Ondansetron-Odan (Can)** *see* Ondansetron *on page 1513*
◆ **Ondansetron-Omega (Can)** *see* Ondansetron *on page 1513*
◆ **Ondissolve ODF (Can)** *see* Ondansetron *on page 1513*
◆ **One-Alpha® (Can)** *see* Alfacalcidol [CAN/INT] *on page 82*
◆ **OneTab™ Congestion & Cold [OTC]** *see* Guaifenesin and Phenylephrine *on page 988*
◆ **Onfi** *see* CloBAZam *on page 465*
◆ **Onglyza** *see* Saxagliptin *on page 1867*
◆ **Onmel** *see* Itraconazole *on page 1130*
◆ **ONO-4538** *see* Nivolumab *on page 1469*
◆ **Onsolis** *see* FentaNYL *on page 857*
◆ **Onxyl** *see* PACLitaxel (Conventional) *on page 1550*
◆ **Opana** *see* Oxymorphone *on page 1546*
◆ **Opana ER** *see* Oxymorphone *on page 1546*
◆ **OPC-13013** *see* Cilostazol *on page 437*
◆ **OPC-14597** *see* ARIPiprazole *on page 171*
◆ **OPC-41061** *see* Tolvaptan *on page 2064*

- ◆ **Opcicon One-Step [OTC]** *see* Levonorgestrel *on page 1201*
- ◆ **Opcon-A [OTC]** *see* Naphazoline and Pheniramine *on page 1426*
- ◆ **o,p'-DDD** *see* Mitotane *on page 1382*
- ◆ **Opdivo** *see* Nivolumab *on page 1469*
- ◆ **Ophtho-Dipivefrin™ (Can)** *see* Dipivefrin *on page 651*
- ◆ **Opium and Belladonna** *see* Belladonna and Opium *on page 238*

Opium Tincture (OH pee um TING chur)

Index Terms Deodorized Tincture of Opium (error-prone synonym); DTO (error-prone abbreviation); Opium Tincture, Deodorized; Tincture of Opium

Pharmacologic Category Analgesic, Opioid; Antidiarrheal

Use Diarrhea: Treatment of diarrhea in adults

Pregnancy Risk Factor C

Pregnancy Considerations Animal reproduction studies have not been conducted. Opium tincture contains morphine; refer to the Morphine (Systemic) monograph for additional information. In addition, this preparation contains large amounts of alcohol (19%).

Breast-Feeding Considerations Opium tincture contains morphine, which is excreted into breast milk; refer to the Morphine (Systemic) monograph for additional information. In addition, this preparation contains large amounts of alcohol (19%). The manufacturer recommends that caution be used if administered to a nursing woman.

Contraindications

Use in children; diarrhea caused by poisoning until the toxic material is eliminated from the GI tract

Documentation of allergenic cross-reactivity for opioids is limited. However, because of similarities in chemical structure and/or pharmacologic actions, the possibility of cross-sensitivity cannot be ruled out with certainty.

Warnings/Precautions May cause CNS depression, which may impair physical or mental abilities; patients must be cautioned about performing tasks which require mental alertness (eg, operating machinery or driving). Use with caution in patients with morbid obesity, adrenal insufficiency, hepatic impairment, biliary tract impairment, pancreatitis, head trauma, GI hemorrhage, thyroid dysfunction, prostatic hyperplasia/urinary stricture, respiratory disease, or a history of drug abuse. Avoid use in patients with CNS depression or coma as these patients are susceptible to intracranial effects of CO_2 retention. May cause hypotension; use with caution in patients with hypovolemia, cardiovascular disease (including acute MI), or with drugs which may exaggerate hypotensive effects (including phenothiazines or general anesthetics). May obscure diagnosis or clinical course of patients with acute abdominal conditions. Concurrent use of agonist/antagonist analgesics may precipitate withdrawal symptoms and/or reduced analgesic efficacy in patients following prolonged therapy with mu opioid agonists. Abrupt discontinuation following prolonged use may also lead to withdrawal symptoms. Use with caution in the elderly and debilitated patients; may be more sensitive to adverse effects. Potentially significant interactions may exist, requiring dose or frequency adjustment, additional monitoring, and/or selection of alternative therapy.

Do not confuse opium tincture with paregoric; opium tincture is 25 times more potent than paregoric; opium shares the toxic potential of opioid agonists, usual precautions of opioid agonist therapy should be observed; abrupt discontinuation after prolonged use may result in withdrawal symptoms. Infants <3 months of age are more susceptible to respiratory depression; if used (off-label), diluted doses are recommended and use with caution. Contraindicated for use in children according to the manufacturer. Opium tincture is not routinely used as a source of morphine to treat neonatal abstinence syndrome in infants exposed to chronic opioids *in utero*. If used, then dilution is necessary. In addition, use for this purpose may increase the risk of drug error and morphine overdose in the infant (AAP, 1998; Dow, 2012; Hudack, 2012).

Adverse Reactions

Cardiovascular: Bradycardia, hypotension, palpitations, peripheral vasodilation

Central nervous system: Central nervous system depression, depression, dizziness, drowsiness, drug dependence, headache, increased intracranial pressure, insomnia, malaise, restlessness

Gastrointestinal: Anorexia, biliary tract spasm, constipation, nausea, stomach cramps, vomiting

Genitourinary: Decreased urine output, genitourinary tract spasm

Hypersensitivity: Histamine release

Neuromuscular & skeletal: Weakness

Ophthalmic: Miosis

Respiratory: Respiratory depression

Rare but important or life-threatening: Hypogonadism (Brennan, 2013; Debono, 2011)

Drug Interactions

Metabolism/Transport Effects None known.

Avoid Concomitant Use

Avoid concomitant use of Opium Tincture with any of the following: Azelastine (Nasal); Orphenadrine; Paraldehyde; Thalidomide

Increased Effect/Toxicity

Opium Tincture may increase the levels/effects of: Alcohol (Ethyl); Alvimopan; Azelastine (Nasal); Buprenorphine; CNS Depressants; Desmopressin; Diuretics; Hydrocodone; Methotrimeprazine; Metyrosine; Mirtazapine; Orphenadrine; Paraldehyde; Pramipexole; ROPINIRole; Rotigotine; Selective Serotonin Reuptake Inhibitors; Suvorexant; Thalidomide; Zolpidem

The levels/effects of Opium Tincture may be increased by: Amphetamines; Anticholinergic Agents; Antipsychotic Agents (Phenothiazines); Brimonidine (Topical); Cannabis; Doxylamine; Dronabinol; Droperidol; HydrOXYzine; Kava Kava; Magnesium Sulfate; Methotrimeprazine; Nabilone; Perampanel; Rufinamide; Sodium Oxybate; Succinylcholine; Tapentadol; Tetrahydrocannabinol

Decreased Effect

Opium Tincture may decrease the levels/effects of: Pegvisomant

The levels/effects of Opium Tincture may be decreased by: Ammonium Chloride; Mixed Agonist / Antagonist Opioids; Naltrexone

Storage/Stability Store at 68°F to 77°F (20°C to 25°C). Protect from light.

Mechanism of Action Contains many opioid alkaloids including morphine; its mechanism for gastric motility inhibition is primarily due to this morphine content; it results in a decrease in digestive secretions, an increase in GI muscle tone, and therefore a reduction in GI propulsion

Pharmacodynamics/Kinetics

Absorption: Variable

Metabolism: Hepatic

Excretion: Urine

Dosage Oral: **Note:** Opium tincture contains morphine 10 mg/mL. Use caution in ordering, dispensing, and/or administering. The following doses are expressed in **mg** (milligram) dosing units of morphine.

Adults: Diarrhea: 6 **mg** of undiluted opium tincture (10 mg/mL) 4 times daily

Dosage adjustment in renal impairment: There are no dosage adjustments provided in the manufacturer's labeling.

Dosage adjustment in hepatic impairment: There are no dosage adjustments provided in the manufacturer's labeling; use with caution.

Monitoring Parameters Observe patient for excessive sedation, respiratory depression, implement safety measures, assist with ambulation; signs or symptoms of hypogonadism or hypoadrenalism (Brennan, 2013)

Dosage Forms

Tincture, Oral:

Generic: 10 mg/mL (1%) (118 mL, 473 mL)

- **Opium Tincture, Deodorized** *see* Opium Tincture *on page 1518*

Oprelvekin (oh PREL ve kin)

Brand Names: U.S. Neumega

Index Terms IL-11; Interleukin-11; Recombinant Human Interleukin-11; Recombinant Interleukin-11; rhIL-11

Pharmacologic Category Biological Response Modulator; Human Growth Factor

Use Prevention of severe thrombocytopenia; reduce the need for platelet transfusions following myelosuppressive chemotherapy for nonmyeloid malignancy

Pregnancy Risk Factor C

Dosage SubQ: Administer first dose ~6-24 hours after the end of chemotherapy. Discontinue at least 48 hours before beginning the next cycle of chemotherapy.

Adults: 50 mcg/kg once daily for ~10-21 days (until postnadir platelet count ≥50,000/mm^3)

Dosage adjustment in renal impairment:

CrCl ≥30 mL/minute: No dosage adjustment necessary.

CrCl <30 mL/minute: 25 mcg/kg once daily for ~10-21 days (until postnadir platelet count ≥50,000/mm^3)

Dosage adjustment in hepatic impairment: No dosage adjustment provided in manufacturer's labeling.

Additional Information Complete prescribing information should be consulted for additional detail.

Dosage Forms

Solution Reconstituted, Subcutaneous [preservative free]:

Neumega: 5 mg (1 ea)

- **OPT-80** *see* Fidaxomicin *on page 875*
- **Opticrom® (Can)** *see* Cromolyn (Ophthalmic) *on page 514*
- **Optimyxin® (Can)** *see* Bacitracin and Polymyxin B *on page 222*
- **Optimyxin Plus® (Can)** *see* Neomycin, Polymyxin B, and Gramicidin *on page 1437*
- **Option 2 (Can)** *see* Levonorgestrel *on page 1201*
- **Optivar [DSC]** *see* Azelastine (Ophthalmic) *on page 213*
- **Oracea** *see* Doxycycline *on page 689*
- **Oracit®** *see* Sodium Citrate and Citric Acid *on page 1905*
- **Oracort (Can)** *see* Triamcinolone (Topical) *on page 2100*
- **Ora-film [OTC]** *see* Benzocaine *on page 246*
- **Oral Cholera Vaccine** *see* Travelers' Diarrhea and Cholera Vaccine [CAN/INT] *on page 2088*
- **Oralone** *see* Triamcinolone (Topical) *on page 2100*
- **Oral Pain Relief Max St [OTC]** *see* Benzocaine *on page 246*
- **Oral Purgative (Can)** *see* Sodium Picosulfate, Magnesium Oxide, and Citric Acid *on page 1911*
- **Orap** *see* Pimozide *on page 1651*
- **Orap® (Can)** *see* Pimozide *on page 1651*
- **Orapred [DSC]** *see* PrednisoLONE (Systemic) *on page 1703*
- **Orapred ODT** *see* PrednisoLONE (Systemic) *on page 1703*
- **Oraqix®** *see* Lidocaine and Prilocaine *on page 1213*
- **OraVerse** *see* Phentolamine *on page 1636*
- **Orazinc [OTC]** *see* Zinc Sulfate *on page 2200*
- **Orbactiv** *see* Oritavancin *on page 1519*
- **Orciprenaline Sulfate** *see* Metaproterenol *on page 1307*
- **Orencia** *see* Abatacept *on page 23*
- **Orenitram** *see* Treprostinil *on page 2093*
- **Orfadin** *see* Nitisinone *on page 1461*
- **ORG 9426** *see* Rocuronium *on page 1838*
- **Orgalutran® (Can)** *see* Ganirelix *on page 949*
- **Organ-I NR [OTC]** *see* GuaiFENesin *on page 986*
- **Orgaran® (Can)** *see* Danaparoid [CAN/INT] *on page 556*
- **ORG NC 45** *see* Vecuronium *on page 2144*
- **Orinase** *see* TOLBUTamide *on page 2062*

Oritavancin (or it a VAN sin)

Brand Names: U.S. Orbactiv

Index Terms LY333328; Oritavancin Diphosphate

Pharmacologic Category Glycopeptide

Use Acute bacterial skin and skin structure infections: Treatment of adult patients with acute bacterial skin and skin structure infections (ABSSSI) caused by susceptible isolates of the following gram-positive microorganisms: *Staphylococcus aureus* (including methicillin-susceptible and methicillin-resistant isolates); *Streptococcus pyogenes; Streptococcus agalactiae; Streptococcus dysgalactiae, Streptococcus anginosus* group (including *S. anginosus, S. intermedius, S. constellatus*); and *Enterococcus faecalis* (vancomycin-susceptible isolates only)

Pregnancy Risk Factor C

Pregnancy Considerations Adverse events were not observed in animal reproduction studies.

Breast-Feeding Considerations It is not known if oritavancin is excreted into breast milk. The manufacturer recommends that caution be used if administered to a nursing woman.

Contraindications Hypersensitivity to oritavancin or any component of the formulation; use of intravenous unfractionated heparin for 48 hours after oritavancin administration (oritavancin falsely elevates aPTT for ~48 hours after administration)

Warnings/Precautions Serious hypersensitivity reactions have been reported (median onset in studies ~1.2 days). If an acute reaction occurs, discontinue infusion immediately and institute appropriate supportive care (median resolution ~2.4 days) Inquire about previous hypersensitivity reactions to glycopeptides; carefully monitor patients with a history of glycopeptide allergy. Infusion related reactions (pruritus, urticaria, flushing) have been reported. If reactions occur, consider slowing or interrupting infusion. In clinical trials, more cases of osteomyelitis were noted in patients treated with oritavancin. Monitor for signs and symptoms of osteomyelitis and institute appropriate alternate antibacterial therapy if warranted. Use may result in fungal or bacterial superinfection, including *C. difficile*-associated diarrhea (CDAD) and pseudomembranous colitis; CDAD has been observed >2 months postantibiotic treatment. Coadministration with warfarin may increase bleeding risk Use in patients on chronic warfarin therapy only when benefit is expected to outweigh risk; monitor frequently for signs of bleeding. Oritavancin has no independent coagulation system effects but artificially prolongs coagulation tests due to reagent reactions; use caution when interpreting results. Potentially significant drug-drug interactions may exist, requiring dose or frequency adjustment, additional monitoring, and/or selection of alternative therapy.

Adverse Reactions

Cardiovascular: Hypersensitivity angiitis, peripheral edema, tachycardia

Central nervous system: Dizziness, headache

Dermatologic: Erythema multiforme, pruritus, skin rash, urticaria

Endocrine & metabolic: Hyperuricemia, hypoglycemia

Gastrointestinal: Diarrhea, nausea, vomiting

Hematologic & oncologic: Anemia, eosinophilia

Hepatic: Increased serum ALT, increased serum AST, increased total serum bilirubin

Hypersensitivity: Angioedema

Infection: Limb abscess, subcutaneous abscess

Local: Erythema at injection site, extravasation, induration at injection site, injection site phlebitis, injection site reaction

Neuromuscular & skeletal: Myalgia, osteomyelitis, tenosynovitis

Respiratory: Bronchospasm, wheezing

Rare but important or life-threatening: *Clostridium difficile*-associated diarrhea, hypersensitivity reaction, INR abnormal, prolonged partial thromboplastin time, prolonged prothrombin time

Drug Interactions

Metabolism/Transport Effects Inhibits CYP2C19 (weak), CYP2C9 (weak); **Induces** CYP3A4 (weak)

Avoid Concomitant Use

Avoid concomitant use of Oritavancin with any of the following: BCG; Heparin

Increased Effect/Toxicity

Oritavancin may increase the levels/effects of: Vitamin K Antagonists

Decreased Effect

Oritavancin may decrease the levels/effects of: ARIPiprazole; BCG; Heparin; Hydrocodone; Saxagliptin; Sodium Picosulfate; Typhoid Vaccine

Preparation for Administration Reconstitute each 400 mg vial with 40 mL of SWFI. Swirl gently to avoid foaming. The reconstituted vial contains 10 mg/mL oritavancin as a clear, colorless to pale yellow solution. Withdraw and discard 120 mL of fluid from a D_5W 1000 mL bag; withdraw 40 mL from each of 3 reconstituted vials and add to D_5W to bring the total bag volume to 1000 mL. (final solution concentration 1.2 mg/mL).

Storage/Stability Store intact vials at 20°C to 25°C (68°F to 77°F); excursions are permitted between 15°C and 30°C (59°F and 86°F). Reconstituted vials and diluted solution may be stored refrigerated at 2°C to 8°C (36°F to 46°F) for 12 hours or at room temperature 20°C to 25°C (68°F to 77°F) for 6 hours. The total time from reconstitution and dilution to completed administration should be ≤6 hours at room temperature or ≤12 hours if refrigerated.

Mechanism of Action Oritavancin is a lipoglycopeptide with concentration-dependent bactericidal activity. It inhibits cell wall biosynthesis by inhibiting the polymerization step by binding to stem peptides of peptidoglycan precursors, by inhibiting crosslinking by binding to bridging segments, and by disrupting bacterial membrane integrity, leading to cell death.

Pharmacodynamics/Kinetics

Distribution: V_d: 87.6 L

Protein binding: 85%

Metabolism: Not metabolized

Half-life elimination: 245 hours

Excretion: Feces and urine as unchanged drug (less than 1% and 5% in feces and urine, respectively, over two weeks postadministration)

Dosage

Usual dosage: Adults: IV: 1200 mg as a single dose

Indication-specific dosing: *Acute bacterial skin and skin structure infections (ABSSI):* Adults: IV: 1200 mg as a single dose

Dosage adjustment in renal impairment:

CrCl ≥30 mL/minute: No dosage adjustment necessary.

CrCl <30 mL/minute: There are no dosage adjustments provided in the manufacturer's labeling (has not been studied); use with caution.

ESRD requiring hemodialysis: There are no dosage adjustments provided in the manufacturer's labeling (has not been studied); use with caution; not removed by hemodialysis.

Dosage in hepatic impairment:

Mild to moderate hepatic impairment (Child-Pugh class A or B): No dosage adjustment necessary.

Severe hepatic impairment (Child-Pugh class C): There are no dosage adjustments provided in the manufacturer's labeling (has not been studied); use with caution.

Administration IV: Infuse over 3 hours. If a common IV line is being used to administer other drugs in addition to oritavancin, the line should be flushed before and after each infusion with D_5W. If infusion-related reaction (pruritus, urticaria, flushing) occurs, consider slowing or interrupting infusion.

Monitoring Parameters Baseline serum urea nitrogen, serum creatinine, and liver function tests (AST, ALT, bilirubin). Monitor patients for any kind of infusion-related reactions (pruritus, urticaria, flushing), hypersensitivity reactions (especially in patients with reported glycopeptide allergy) and signs and symptoms of osteomyelitis.

Dosage Forms

Solution Reconstituted, Intravenous:

Orbactiv: 400 mg (1 ea, 3 ea)

◆ **Oritavancin Diphosphate** *see* Oritavancin *on page 1519*

Orlistat (OR li stat)

Brand Names: U.S. Alli [OTC]; Xenical

Brand Names: Canada Xenical

Pharmacologic Category Lipase Inhibitor

Use Obesity management:

OTC: For weight loss in overweight adults when used along with a reduced-calorie and low-fat diet.

Rx: For obesity management, including weight loss and weight maintenance, when used in conjunction with a reduced-calorie diet; to reduce the risk for weight regain after prior weight loss.

Limitations of use: Orlistat is indicated for obese patients with an initial body mass index of ≥30 kg/m^2 or ≥27 kg/m^2 in the presence of other risk factors (eg, hypertension, diabetes, dyslipidemia).

Pregnancy Risk Factor X

Pregnancy Considerations Adverse events were not observed in animal reproduction studies. Although orlistat is minimally absorbed, weight-loss therapy is not recommended for pregnant women. Obese and overweight women should be encouraged to participate in weight reduction programs prior to attempting pregnancy; weight gain during pregnancy should be determined by their prepregnancy BMI and current guidelines (ADA, 2009; IOM, 2009). Use of orlistat is contraindicated in pregnant women.

Breast-Feeding Considerations Weight-loss therapy is generally not recommended for lactating women. Weight-loss programs which include physical activity and nutrition components should be discussed at the 6-week postpartum visit (ADA, 2009; IOM, 2009).

Contraindications Pregnancy; chronic malabsorption syndrome; cholestasis; hypersensitivity to orlistat or to any component of the formulation

Warnings/Precautions Prior to use other causes for obesity (eg, hypothyroidism) should be ruled out. Cases of severe liver injury (some fatal) with hepatocellular necrosis or acute hepatic failure have been reported; liver transplantation has been required in some patients. Patients should be instructed to report any symptoms of hepatic dysfunction (eg, anorexia, pruritus, jaundice, dark urine, light colored stools, right upper quadrant pain); discontinue therapy and obtain liver function test immediately if symptoms occur. Advise patients to adhere to dietary guidelines; if taken with a diet high in fat (>30% total daily calories from fat) gastrointestinal adverse events may increase. Distribute daily fat intake over 3 main meals. If taken with any 1 meal very high in fat, the possibility of gastrointestinal effects increases. Counsel patients to take a multivitamin supplement that contains fat-soluble vitamins ≥2 hours before or after orlistat administration to ensure adequate nutrition; orlistat has been shown to reduce the absorption of some fat-soluble vitamins and beta-carotene. Increased levels of urinary oxalate following treatment may occur in some patients; cases of oxalate nephrolithiasis and oxalate nephropathy with renal failure have been reported. Monitor renal function in patients at risk for renal impairment; use with caution in patients with a history of hyperoxaluria or calcium oxalate nephrolithiasis. The potential exists for misuse in inappropriate patient populations (eg, patients with anorexia nervosa or bulimia) similar to any weight loss agent. In general, substantial weight loss may increase the risk of cholelithiasis. Potentially significant interactions may exist, requiring dose or frequency adjustment, additional monitoring, and/or selection of alternative therapy.

Self-medication (OTC use): Prior to use, patients should contact their healthcare provider if they have ever had kidney stones, gall bladder disease, or pancreatitis. Patients taking medications for diabetes or thyroid disease, seizures, anticoagulants, or other weight-loss products should consult their healthcare provider or pharmacist before use. Patients who have had an organ transplant should not use orlistat. If severe and/or continuous abdominal pain, itching, yellowing of the eyes or skin, dark urine, or loss of appetite occurs, or seizure worsens, use should be discontinued and healthcare provider consulted.

Adverse Reactions

Cardiovascular: Pedal edema

Central nervous system: Anxiety, fatigue, headache, sleep disorder

Dermatologic: Dry skin

Endocrine & metabolic: Menstrual irregularities

Gastrointestinal: Abdominal pain/discomfort, fatty/oily stool, fecal incontinence, fecal urgency, flatus with discharge, defecation increased, infectious diarrhea, gingival disorder, nausea, oily evacuation, oily spotting, rectal pain/discomfort, tooth disorder

Genitourinary: Urinary tract infection, vaginitis

Neuromuscular & skeletal: Arthritis, back pain, myalgia

Otic: Otitis

Respiratory: Lower/upper respiratory infection

Miscellaneous: Influenza

Rare but important or life-threatening: Abdominal distension (in patients with diabetes), alkaline phosphatase increased, anaphylaxis, angioedema, bronchospasm, bullous eruption, cholelithiasis (may be caused by weight loss), coagulation parameters altered (concurrent use with warfarin), hepatic failure, hepatitis, hypersensitivity, hypoglycemia (in patients with diabetes), hypothyroidism (concurrent use with levothyroxine), kidney injury (acute), pancreatitis, pruritus, rash, transaminases increased, urinary oxalate levels increased, urticaria

Drug Interactions

Metabolism/Transport Effects None known.

Avoid Concomitant Use There are no known interactions where it is recommended to avoid concomitant use.

Increased Effect/Toxicity

Orlistat may increase the levels/effects of: Warfarin

Decreased Effect

Orlistat may decrease the levels/effects of: Amiodarone; Anticonvulsants; CycloSPORINE (Systemic); Levothyroxine; Multivitamins/Fluoride (with ADE); Multivitamins/Minerals (with ADEK, Folate, Iron); Multivitamins/Minerals (with AE, No Iron); Paricalcitol; Propafenone; Vitamin D Analogs; Vitamins (Fat Soluble)

Storage/Stability Store at 25°C (77°F); excursions permitted to 15°C to 30°C (59°F to 86°F).

Mechanism of Action A reversible inhibitor of gastric and pancreatic lipases, thus inhibiting absorption of dietary fats by 30%.

Pharmacodynamics/Kinetics

Onset of action: 24-48 hours

Duration: 48-72 hours

Absorption: Minimal

Protein binding: >99% (lipoproteins and albumin)

Metabolism: Metabolized within the gastrointestinal wall; forms inactive metabolites

Half-life elimination: 1-2 hours

Time to peak, serum: ~8 hours

Excretion: Feces (~97%, 83% as unchanged drug); urine (<2%)

Dosage Obesity management:

Children ≥12 years, Adolescents, and Adults (Xenical): Oral: 120 mg 3 times daily with each main meal containing fat (during or up to 1 hour after the meal); omit dose if meal is occasionally missed or contains no fat.

Adults (Alli): OTC labeling: Oral: 60 mg 3 times daily with each main meal containing fat (maximum dose: 180 mg daily).

Dosing adjustment with concomitant therapy:

Cyclosporine: Administer cyclosporine 3 hours after orlistat.

Levothyroxine: Administer levothyroxine and orlistat at least 4 hours apart and monitor for changes in thyroid function.

Dosage adjustment in renal impairment: There are no dosage adjustments provided in the manufacturer's labeling (has not been studied). However, dosage adjustment unlikely due to low systemic absorption.

Dosage adjustment in hepatic impairment: There are no dosage adjustments provided in the manufacturer's labeling (has not been studied). However, dosage adjustment unlikely due to low systemic absorption.

Dietary Considerations Multivitamin supplements that contain fat-soluble vitamins should be taken once daily at least 2 hours before or after the administration of orlistat (ie, bedtime). Gastrointestinal effects of orlistat may increase if taken with any one meal very high in fat. Distribute daily intake of carbohydrates, fat (~30% of daily calories), and protein over three main meals.

Administration Administer during or up to 1 hour after each main meal containing fat; separate dose by at least 2 hours from multivitamin daily supplement. Omit dose if a meal is missed or contains no fat.

Monitoring Parameters BMI; diet (calorie and fat intake); serum glucose in patients with diabetes; thyroid function in patient with thyroid disease; liver function tests in patients exhibiting symptoms of hepatic dysfunction

Dosage Forms

Capsule, Oral:

Alli [OTC]: 60 mg

Xenical: 120 mg

Ornidazole [INT] (or NI da zole)

International Brand Names Ao Bo Lin (CN); Aurnida (IN); Betiral (GR); Imidakin (TW); Invigan (EC); Pusili (CN); Qi Ke (CN); Tiberal (AE, BE, CH, EC, FR, QA, RU, SA); Tomizol (KR)

Pharmacologic Category Antiprotozoal

Reported Use Treatment of parasitic infections, including amebiasis, giardiasis, and *Trichomonas vaginalis*; treatment of infections due to susceptible strains of anaerobic bacteria

Dosage Range

Oral: Children >35 kg and Adults:

Trichomonas: 1.5 g single dose for one day; alternatively, 0.5 g twice daily for 5 days

Amebiasis (with amebic dysentery): 1.5 g as a single dose for 3 days; patients >60 kg should take 1 g twice daily for 3 days

Giardiasis: 1.5 g as a single dose for 1-2 days

IV: Adults:

Anaerobic bacterial infection: Initially infusion of 0.5-1 g followed by 0.5 g every 12 hours for 5-10 days; oral therapy substituted at the earliest opportunity

Amebic liver abscess and severe amebic dysentery: 0.5-1 g, followed by 0.5 g every 12 hours for 3-6 days

Product Availability Product available in various countries; not currently available in the U.S.

Dosage Forms

Infusion: 500 mg/100 mL

Tablet: 250 mg, 500 mg

Ornipressin [INT] (or ni PRES in)

International Brand Names POR 8 Sandoz (AU); Por-8 (DE, HR, HU, LU); POR-8 (NZ, ZA); POR-8 Ferring (AT, CH)

Index Terms 8-Ornithine-Vasopressin

Pharmacologic Category Vasoconstrictor

Reported Use Used topically/locally to induce ischemia and hemostasis; used systemically for the treatment of bleeding esophageal varices

Dosage Range Adults:

Local tissue infiltration: 1-5 int. units

Topical: 5 int. units

IV: 20 int. units over 48 hours

Product Availability Product available in various countries; not currently available in the U.S.

Dosage Forms

Injection, solution: 5 int. units/mL (1 mL)

◆ **8-Ornithine-Vasopressin** *see* Ornipressin [INT] *on page 1522*

◆ **ORO-Clense (Can)** *see* Chlorhexidine Gluconate *on page 422*

◆ **Orphenace® (Can)** *see* Orphenadrine *on page 1522*

Orphenadrine (or FEN a dreen)

Brand Names: U.S. Norflex

Brand Names: Canada Norflex™; Orphenace®; Rhoxal-orphendrine

Index Terms Orphenadrine Citrate

Pharmacologic Category Skeletal Muscle Relaxant

Additional Appendix Information

Beers Criteria – Potentially Inappropriate Medications for Geriatrics *on page 2271*

Use Treatment of muscle spasm associated with acute painful musculoskeletal conditions

Pregnancy Risk Factor C

Dosage

Adults:

Oral: 100 mg twice daily

IM, IV: 60 mg every 12 hours

Elderly: Use caution; generally not recommended for use in the elderly

Dosage adjustment in renal impairment: No dosage adjustment provided in manufacturer's labeling.

Dosage adjustment in hepatic impairment: No dosage adjustment provided in manufacturer's labeling.

Additional Information Complete prescribing information should be consulted for additional detail.

Dosage Forms

Solution, Injection:

Norflex: 30 mg/mL (2 mL)

Generic: 30 mg/mL (2 mL)

Solution, Injection [preservative free]:

Generic: 30 mg/mL (2 mL)

Tablet Extended Release 12 Hour, Oral:

Generic: 100 mg

Orphenadrine, Aspirin, and Caffeine
(or FEN a dreen, AS pir in, & KAF een)

Index Terms Aspirin, Caffeine, and Orphenadrine; Aspirin, Orphenadrine, and Caffeine; Caffeine, Orphenadrine, and Aspirin; Norgesic

Pharmacologic Category Skeletal Muscle Relaxant

Use Relief of discomfort associated with skeletal muscular conditions

Dosage Oral: 1-2 tablets 3-4 times/day

Dosage adjustment in renal impairment: No dosage adjustment provided in manufacturer's labeling.

Dosage adjustment in hepatic impairment: No dosage adjustment provided in manufacturer's labeling.

Additional Information Complete prescribing information should be consulted for additional detail.

Dosage Forms

Tablet: Orphenadrine 25 mg, aspirin 385 mg, and caffeine 30 mg; orphenadrine 50 mg, aspirin 770 mg, and caffeine 60 mg

◆ **Orphenadrine Citrate** *see* Orphenadrine *on page 1522*

◆ **Orsythia** *see* Ethinyl Estradiol and Levonorgestrel *on page 803*

◆ **Ortho 0.5/35 (Can)** *see* Ethinyl Estradiol and Norethindrone *on page 808*

◆ **Ortho 1/35 (Can)** *see* Ethinyl Estradiol and Norethindrone *on page 808*

◆ **Ortho 7/7/7 (Can)** *see* Ethinyl Estradiol and Norethindrone *on page 808*

◆ **Ortho Cept** *see* Ethinyl Estradiol and Desogestrel *on page 799*

◆ **Ortho-Cept** *see* Ethinyl Estradiol and Desogestrel *on page 799*

◆ **Ortho-CS 250** *see* Ascorbic Acid *on page 178*

◆ **Ortho Cyclen** *see* Ethinyl Estradiol and Norgestimate *on page 810*

◆ **Ortho-Cyclen** *see* Ethinyl Estradiol and Norgestimate *on page 810*

◆ **Ortho Est** *see* Estropipate *on page 793*

◆ **Ortho-Est 0.625** *see* Estropipate *on page 793*

◆ **Ortho-Est 1.25** *see* Estropipate *on page 793*

◆ **Ortho-Evra** *see* Ethinyl Estradiol and Norelgestromin *on page 807*

◆ **Ortho Evra®** *see* Ethinyl Estradiol and Norelgestromin *on page 807*

- ◆ **Ortho Micronor** *see* Norethindrone *on page 1473*
- ◆ **Ortho Novum** *see* Ethinyl Estradiol and Norethindrone *on page 808*
- ◆ **Ortho-Novum 1/35** *see* Ethinyl Estradiol and Norethindrone *on page 808*
- ◆ **Ortho Novum 1/50** *see* Norethindrone and Mestranol *on page 1475*
- ◆ **Ortho-Novum® 1/50 (Can)** *see* Norethindrone and Mestranol *on page 1475*
- ◆ **Ortho-Novum 7/7/7** *see* Ethinyl Estradiol and Norethindrone *on page 808*
- ◆ **Ortho,para-DDD** *see* Mitotane *on page 1382*
- ◆ **Ortho Tri Cyclen** *see* Ethinyl Estradiol and Norgestimate *on page 810*
- ◆ **Ortho Tri-Cyclen** *see* Ethinyl Estradiol and Norgestimate *on page 810*
- ◆ **Ortho Tri-Cyclen Lo** *see* Ethinyl Estradiol and Norgestimate *on page 810*
- ◆ **Orthovisc** *see* Hyaluronate and Derivatives *on page 1006*
- ◆ **OrthoVisc (Can)** *see* Hyaluronate and Derivatives *on page 1006*
- ◆ **OrthoWash** *see* Fluoride *on page 895*
- ◆ **Orviban CF** *see* Butalbital and Acetaminophen *on page 314*
- ◆ **Oscal** *see* Calcium Carbonate *on page 327*
- ◆ **Os-Cal [OTC] [DSC]** *see* Calcium Carbonate *on page 327*
- ◆ **Os-Cal (Can)** *see* Calcium Carbonate *on page 327*
- ◆ **Os-Cal 500+D [OTC]** *see* Calcium and Vitamin D *on page 326*
- ◆ **Oscimin** *see* Hyoscyamine *on page 1026*
- ◆ **Oscimin SR** *see* Hyoscyamine *on page 1026*

Oseltamivir (oh sel TAM i vir)

Brand Names: U.S. Tamiflu

Brand Names: Canada Tamiflu

Pharmacologic Category Antiviral Agent; Neuraminidase Inhibitor

Use

Prophylaxis of influenza: Prophylaxis of influenza (A or B) infection in children ≥1 year of age and adults.

Treatment of influenza: Treatment of uncomplicated acute illness due to influenza (A or B) infection in children ≥2 weeks of age and adults who have been symptomatic for no more than 2 days.

The Advisory Committee on Immunization Practices (ACIP) recommends that **treatment** be considered for the following:

- Persons with severe, complicated or progressive illness
- Hospitalized persons
- Persons at higher risk for influenza complications:
  - Children <2 years of age (highest risk in children <6 months of age)
  - Adults ≥65 years of age
  - Persons with chronic disorders of the pulmonary (including asthma) or cardiovascular systems (except hypertension)
  - Persons with chronic metabolic diseases (including diabetes mellitus), hepatic disease, renal dysfunction, hematologic disorders (including sickle cell disease), or immunosuppression (including immunosuppression caused by medications or HIV)
  - Persons with neurologic/neuromuscular conditions (including conditions such as spinal cord injuries, seizure disorders, cerebral palsy, stroke, mental retardation, moderate to severe developmental delay, or muscular dystrophy) which may compromise respiratory function, the handling of respiratory secretions, or that can increase the risk of aspiration
  - Pregnant or postpartum women (≤2 weeks after delivery)
  - Persons <19 years of age on long-term aspirin therapy
  - American Indians and Alaskan Natives
  - Persons who are morbidly obese (BMI ≥40)
  - Residents of nursing homes or other chronic care facilities
- Use may also be considered for previously healthy, nonhigh-risk outpatients with confirmed or suspected influenza based on clinical judgment when treatment can be started within 48 hours of illness onset.

The ACIP recommends that **prophylaxis** be considered for the following:

- Postexposure prophylaxis may be considered for family or close contacts of suspected or confirmed cases, who are at higher risk of influenza complications, and who have not been vaccinated against the circulating strain at the time of the exposure.
- Postexposure prophylaxis may be considered for unvaccinated healthcare workers who had occupational exposure without protective equipment.
- Pre-exposure prophylaxis should only be used for persons at very high risk of influenza complications who cannot be otherwise protected at times of high risk for exposure.
- Prophylaxis should also be administered to all eligible residents of institutions that house patients at high risk when needed to control outbreaks.

The ACIP recommends that treatment and prophylaxis be given to children <1 year of age when indicated.

Pregnancy Risk Factor C

Pregnancy Considerations Adverse events were observed in some animal reproduction studies. Oseltamivir phosphate and its active metabolite oseltamivir carboxylate cross the placenta (Meijer, 2012). An increased risk of adverse neonatal or maternal outcomes has generally not been observed following maternal use of oseltamivir during pregnancy (CDC, 60[1], 2011; CDC, March 13, 2014).

Untreated influenza infection is associated with an increased risk of adverse events to the fetus and an increased risk of complications or death to the mother. Neuraminidase inhibitors are currently recommended for the treatment or prophylaxis of influenza in pregnant women and women up to 2 weeks postpartum (CDC 60 [1], 2011; CDC March 13, 2014; January 2015).

Breast-Feeding Considerations Low concentrations of oseltamivir and oseltamivir carboxylate (OC) have been detected in breast milk; levels are unlikely to lead to toxicity in a breast-fed infant. The manufacturer recommends that caution be used if administered to a nursing woman.

Influenza may cause serious illness in postpartum women and prompt evaluation for febrile respiratory illnesses is recommended (Louie, 2011).

Contraindications Hypersensitivity to oseltamivir or any component of the formulation

Warnings/Precautions Oseltamivir is not a substitute for the influenza virus vaccine. It has not been shown to prevent primary or concomitant bacterial infections that may occur with influenza virus. Use caution with renal impairment; dosage adjustment is required. Safety and efficacy for use in patients with chronic cardiac and/or kidney disease, severe hepatic impairment, or for treatment or prophylaxis in immunocompromised patients have not been established. Rare but severe hypersensitivity ▶

reactions, including anaphylaxis and severe dermatologic reactions (eg, Stevens-Johnson syndrome, erythema multiforme), have been associated with use. Discontinue use immediately if hypersensitivity occurs or is suspected and treat appropriately. Rare occurrences of neuropsychiatric events (including confusion, delirium, hallucinations, and/or self-injury) have been reported from postmarketing surveillance (primarily in pediatric patients); direct causation is difficult to establish (influenza infection may also be associated with behavioral and neurologic changes). Monitor closely for signs of any unusual behavior.

Antiviral treatment should begin within 48 hours of symptom onset. However, the CDC recommends that treatment may still be beneficial and should be started in hospitalized patients with severe, complicated or progressive illness if >48 hours. Treatment should not be delayed while awaiting results of laboratory tests for influenza. Nonhospitalized persons who are not at high risk for developing severe or complicated illness and who have a mild disease are not likely to benefit if treatment is started >48 hours after symptom onset. Nonhospitalized persons who are already beginning to recover do not need treatment. Oral suspension contains sorbitol (delivers ~2 g sorbitol per 75 mg dose) which is greater than the maximum daily limit for some patients; may cause diarrhea and dyspepsia; use with caution in patients with hereditary fructose intolerance. The Canadian labeling does not approve of use (treatment or prophylaxis) in infants <1 year of age.

Benzyl alcohol and derivatives: Some dosage forms may contain sodium benzoate/benzoic acid; benzoic acid (benzoate) is a metabolite of benzyl alcohol; large amounts of benzyl alcohol (≥99 mg/kg/day) have been associated with a potentially fatal toxicity ("gasping syndrome") in neonates; the "gasping syndrome" consists of metabolic acidosis, respiratory distress, gasping respirations, CNS dysfunction (including convulsions, intracranial hemorrhage), hypotension, and cardiovascular collapse (AAP, 1997; CDC, 1982); some data suggests that benzoate displaces bilirubin from protein binding sites (Ahlfors, 2001); avoid or use dosage forms containing benzyl alcohol derivative with caution in neonates. See manufacturer's labeling.

Adverse Reactions

Gastrointestinal: Abdominal pain, diarrhea, nausea, vomiting

Ocular: Conjunctivitis

Respiratory: Epistaxis

Rare but important or life-threatening: Allergy, anaphylactic/anaphylactoid reaction, angina, arrhythmia, confusion, erythema multiforme, fracture, gastrointestinal bleeding, hemorrhagic colitis, hepatitis, liver function tests abnormal, neuropsychiatric events, pseudomembranous colitis, pyrexia, seizure, Stevens-Johnson syndrome, swelling of face or tongue, toxic epidermal necrolysis

Drug Interactions

Metabolism/Transport Effects None known.

Avoid Concomitant Use There are no known interactions where it is recommended to avoid concomitant use.

Increased Effect/Toxicity

The levels/effects of Oseltamivir may be increased by: Probenecid

Decreased Effect

Oseltamivir may decrease the levels/effects of: Influenza Virus Vaccine (Live/Attenuated)

Preparation for Administration Oral suspension: Reconstitute with 55 mL of water to a final concentration of 6 mg/mL (to make 60 mL total suspension).

Storage/Stability

Capsules: Store at 25°C (77°F); excursions permitted to 15°C to 30°C (59°F to 86°F).

Oral suspension: Store powder for suspension at 25°C (77°F); excursions permitted to 15°C to 30°C (59°F to 86°F). Once reconstituted, store suspension under refrigeration at 2°C to 8°C (36°F to 46°F) or at room temperature; do not freeze. Use within 10 days of preparation if stored at room temperature or within 17 days of preparation if stored under refrigeration.

Mechanism of Action Oseltamivir, a prodrug, is hydrolyzed to the active form, oseltamivir carboxylate (OC). OC inhibits influenza virus neuraminidase, an enzyme known to cleave the budding viral progeny from its cellular envelope attachment point (neuraminic acid) just prior to release.

Pharmacodynamics/Kinetics Note: Concurrent use of extracorporeal membrane oxygenation (ECMO): When used alone, ECMO has been shown not to impact oseltamivir carboxylate C_{max} and AUC in 2 small studies (Lemaitre, 2012; Mulla, 2013).

Absorption: Well absorbed

Distribution: V_d: 23 to 26 L (oseltamivir carboxylate); may be significantly increased in patients receiving ECMO (Lemaitre, 2012; Mulla, 2013)

Protein binding, plasma: Oseltamivir carboxylate: 3%; Oseltamivir: 42%

Metabolism: Hepatic (90%) to oseltamivir carboxylate; neither the parent drug nor active metabolite has any effect on the cytochrome P450 system

Bioavailability: 75% as oseltamivir carboxylate

Half-life elimination: Oseltamivir: 1 to 3 hours; Oseltamivir carboxylate: 6 to 10 hours

Excretion: Urine (>90% as oseltamivir carboxylate); feces

Dosage Oral:

Influenza prophylaxis: Initiate prophylaxis within 48 hours of contact with an infected individual

Manufacturer's recommendation:

Children: 1 to 12 years:

≤15 kg: 30 mg once daily

>15 kg to ≤23 kg: 45 mg once daily

>23 kg to ≤40 kg: 60 mg once daily

>40 kg: 75 mg once daily

Adolescents ≥13 years and Adults: 75 mg once daily

Alternate recommendations:

American Academy of Pediatrics: Infants 0 to 11 months (off-label dosing; AAP, 2013): **Note:** Do not exceed maximum dose of weight-based dosing; see manufacturer's recommendation. Prophylaxis is not recommended for infants <3 months of age unless clinically critical.

0 to 8 months: 3 mg/kg/dose once daily

9 to 11 months: 3.5 mg/kg/dose once daily

Centers for Disease Control: Infants <12 months (off-label dosing; CDC, 2012): 3 mg/kg/dose once daily: **Note:** Do not exceed maximum dose of weight-based dosing; see manufacturer's recommendation. The current CDC weight-based dosing recommendation is not intended for premature neonates. Prophylaxis is not recommended for infants <3 months of age unless clinically critical.

Infectious Disease Society of America/Pediatric Infectious Disease Society (IDSA/PIDS): Infants and Children 3 to 23 months (off-label dosing; Bradley, 2011): **Note:** Do not exceed maximum dose of weight-based dosing; see manufacturer's recommendation.

3 to 8 months: 3 mg/kg/dose once daily

9 to 23 months: 3.5 mg/kg/dose once daily

Prophylaxis duration:

Individual/household exposure:

Manufacturer recommendation: 10 days

Alternate recommendations: 7 days (CDC, 2012); 10 days (AAP, 2013)

Community/institutional outbreak:

Manufacturer recommendation: May be used for up to 6 weeks

Alternate recommendations: Continue for ≥2 weeks and until ~7 days after identification of illness onset in the last patient (CDC, 2012) or until influenza activity in community subsides or immunity obtained from immunization (IDSA/PIDS, 2011). During community outbreaks, duration of protection lasts for length of dosing period; safety and efficacy have been demonstrated for use up to 6 weeks in immunocompetent patients and safety has been demonstrated for use up to 12 weeks in patients who are immunocompromised.

Influenza treatment: Initiate treatment within 48 hours of onset of symptoms; usual duration of treatment is 5 days. However, optimal duration is uncertain for severe or complicated influenza. Consider longer duration (eg, >5 days) of therapy in severely ill patients who remain severely ill after 5 days of therapy. Data suggest that increased doses (>150 mg daily) in critically ill patients is not necessary since blood concentrations of oseltamivir were comparable or higher compared to ambulatory patients given similar dosing regimens (Ariano, 2010; CDC [Influenza Antiviral Medications], 2014). Initiate as early as possible in any hospitalized patient with suspected/confirmed influenza regardless of the time of presentation from symptom onset (even if >48 hours) (CDC [Influenza Antiviral Medications], 2014); may be administered via naso- or orogastric tube in mechanically-ventilated patients (Taylor, 2008).

U.S. manufacturer's recommendation: **Note:** The following dosing is also supported by some clinicians (Bradley, 2011):

Infants ≥2 weeks: 3 mg/kg/dose twice daily

Children: 1 to 12 years:

≤15 kg: 30 mg twice daily

>15 kg to ≤23 kg: 45 mg twice daily

>23 kg to ≤40 kg: 60 mg twice daily

>40 kg: 75 mg twice daily

Adolescents ≥13 years and Adults: 75 mg twice daily

Critically ill: Concurrent use of extracorporeal membrane oxygenation (ECMO) alone: No dosage adjustment necessary (Lemaitre, 2012; Mulla, 2013).

Alternate recommendations:

American Academy of Pediatrics: Infants <12 months (off-label dosing; AAP, 2013):

Infants, premature: **Note:** Age defined as postmenstrual age (first day of mother's last period to birth plus the time elapsed after birth). Weight-based dosing recommendations for premature infants are lower than for term infants. Do not exceed maximum dose of weight-based dosing; see manufacturer's recommendation.

<38 weeks: 1 mg/kg/dose twice daily

38 to 40 weeks: 1.5 mg/kg/dose twice daily

>40 weeks: 3 mg/kg/dose twice daily

Infants, term:

0 to 8 months: 3 mg/kg/dose twice daily

9 to 11 months: 3.5 mg/kg/dose twice daily

Centers for Disease Control: Infants <2 weeks (off-label dosing; CDC, 2012): 3 mg/kg/dose twice daily. **Note:** Do not exceed maximum dose of weight-based dosing; see manufacturer's recommendation. The current CDC weight-based dosing recommendation is not intended for premature neonates.

Infectious Disease Society of America/Pediatric Infectious Disease Society: Infants and Children <24 months (off-label dosing; Bradley, 2011): **Note:** Do not exceed maximum dose of weight-based dosing; see manufacturer's recommendation.

Infants, premature: 1 mg/kg/dose twice daily

0 to 8 months: 3 mg/kg/dose twice daily

9 to 23 months: 3.5 mg/kg/dose twice daily

Dosage adjustment in renal impairment:

Treatment: Adults:

CrCl >60 mL/minute: No dosage adjustment necessary.

CrCl >30 to 60 mL/minute: 30 mg twice daily for 5 days

CrCl >10 to 30 mL/minute: 30 mg once daily for 5 days

End-stage renal disease (ESRD) not undergoing dialysis: Use is not recommended (has not been studied).

Prophylaxis: Adults:

U.S. labeling:

CrCl >60 mL/minute: No dosage adjustment necessary.

CrCl >30 to 60 mL/minute: 30 mg once daily

CrCl >10 to 30 mL/minute: 30 mg every other day

ESRD not undergoing dialysis: Use is not recommended (has not been studied).

Canadian labeling:

CrCl >60 mL/minute: No dosage adjustment necessary.

CrCl >30 to 60 mL/minute: 30 mg once daily for 10-14 days

CrCl 10 to 30 mL/minute: 30 mg every other day for 10-14 days

Intermittent hemodialysis (IHD) (CrCl ≤10 mL/minute):

Children >1 year (off-label dose; Schreuder, 2010): Treatment:

≤15 kg: 7.5 mg after each hemodialysis session

>15 kg to ≤23 kg: 10 mg after each hemodialysis session

>23 kg to ≤40 kg: 15 mg after each hemodialysis session

>40 kg: 30 mg after each hemodialysis session

Adults:

Treatment: 30 mg after every hemodialysis session for 5 days. **Note:** Assumes 3 hemodialysis sessions in the 5-day period. Treatment may be initiated immediately if influenza symptoms develop during the 48 hours between hemodialysis sessions; however the post-hemodialysis dose should still be administered independently of the time of the initial dose administration.

Alternative recommendations: Treatment (AMMI Canada [Aoki, 2012]):

Low-flux hemodialysis: 30 mg after each dialysis session for 5 days

High-flux hemodialysis: 75 mg after each dialysis session for 5 days

Prophylaxis:

U.S. labeling: 30 mg after every other hemodialysis sessions for the recommended prophylaxis duration. **Note:** An initial dose may be administered prior to the start of dialysis.

Canadian labeling: An initial 30 mg dose may be given prior to dialysis if exposed during the 48 hours between dialysis sessions. To maintain therapeutic concentrations, administer 30 mg after every other dialysis session over a period of 10 to 14 days.

CAPD: Adults:

U.S. labeling: CrCl ≤10 mL/minute:

Treatment: 30 mg for one dose to provide a 5-day duration. Administer immediately after a dialysis exchange.

Prophylaxis: 30 mg once weekly for the recommended prophylaxis duration. Administer immediately after a dialysis exchange.

Canadian labeling:

Treatment: 30 mg once (prior to the start of dialysis) to provide a 5-day duration. Dose should be administered as soon as the determination has been made that treatment is necessary, regardless of when dialysis is scheduled.

Prophylaxis: 30 mg prior to start of dialysis, then 30 mg every 7 days for 10 to 14 days. Initial dose should be administered as soon as the determination has been made that prophylaxis is necessary, regardless of when dialysis is scheduled.

Continuous renal replacement therapy (CRRT) (high-flux):

Treatment (off-label dose; limited data): 30 mg once daily for 5 days or 75 mg every 48 hours to provide a 5-day duration (AMMI Canada [Aoki, 2012]; Ariano, 2010)

Prophylaxis (off-label): No data (AMMI Canada [Aoki, 2012])

Continuous veno-venous hemodialysis (CVVHD):

Adults: **Note:** Limited information available; optimal dosing has not been established: 150 mg twice daily administered via nasogastric or postpyloric feeding tube for suspected or confirmed H1N1 influenza demonstrated supratherapeutic oseltamivir carboxylate concentrations at effluent rates of 3,300 ± 919 mL/hour; the authors determined that the manufacturer recommended dosage of 75 mg once daily for patients with CrCl 10 to 30 mL/minute will likely achieve concentrations necessary to inhibit viral neuraminidase activity at these effluent rates; however, doses greater than 75 mg once daily may be required when using higher effluent rates (Eyler, 2012).

CVVHD and concurrent use of ECMO: Adults: Lower oseltamivir carboxylate concentrations (~981 ng/mL) were observed as compared to those with the use of CVVHD alone (~2,760 ng/mL) when patients were administered 150 mg twice daily for suspected or confirmed H1N1 influenza (n=4; Eyler, 2012).

Dosage adjustment in hepatic impairment:

Mild-to-moderate impairment (Child-Pugh score ≤9): No dosage adjustment necessary.

Severe impairment: No dosage adjustment provided in manufacturer's labeling (has not been studied).

Dosing in obesity: In adult morbidly obese patients (BMI >40 kg/m^2), systemic exposure of oseltamivir carboxylate was not reduced; therefore, no dosage adjustment is necessary (Thorne-Humphrey, 2011; CDC 2014).

Dietary Considerations Take without regard to meals; take with food to improve tolerance.

Administration May be administered without regard to meals; take with food to improve tolerance.

Capsules may be opened and mixed with sweetened liquid (eg, chocolate syrup, corn syrup, caramel topping, light brown sugar dissolved in water). Administer oral suspension using the supplied oral syringe (exception: for children <1 year, a smaller volume [ie, <10 mL] oral syringe should be used in place of the supplied oral syringe to ensure accurate dosing); shake well before each use. If oral suspension is not available and/or appropriate strength of capsules are not available to mix with sweetened liquids, an extemporaneous preparation may be prepared (refer to Extemporaneous Preparations for further details).

Mechanically ventilated critically ill patients: May administer via naso- or orogastric (NG/OG) tube. Dissolve powder from capsules in 20 mL of sterile water and inject down the NG/OG tube; follow with a 10 mL sterile water flush (Taylor, 2008).

Monitoring Parameters Signs or symptoms of unusual behavior, including attempts at self-injury, confusion, and/or delirium

Critically-ill patients: Repeat rRT-PCR or viral culture may help to determine on-going viral replication

Additional Information In clinical studies of the influenza virus, 1.3% of post-treatment isolates in adults and adolescents and 8.6% of isolates in children had decreased neuraminidase susceptibility *in vitro* to oseltamivir carboxylate.

The absence of symptoms does not rule out viral influenza infection and clinical judgment should guide the decision for therapy. Treatment should not be delayed while waiting for the results of diagnostic tests. Treatment should be considered for high-risk patients with symptoms despite a negative rapid influenza test when the illness cannot be contributed to another cause. Use of oseltamivir is not a substitute for vaccination (when available); susceptibility to influenza infection returns once therapy is discontinued.

Dosage Forms

Capsule, Oral:

Tamiflu: 30 mg, 45 mg, 75 mg

Suspension Reconstituted, Oral:

Tamiflu: 6 mg/mL (60 mL)

Extemporaneous Preparations

If the commercially prepared oral suspension is not available, the manufacturer provides the following compounding information to prepare a **6 mg/mL** suspension in emergency situations.

1. Place the specified amount of water into a polyethyleneterephthalate (PET) or glass bottle.
2. Carefully separate the capsule body and cap and pour the contents of the required number of 75 mg capsules into the PET or glass bottle.
3. Gently swirl the suspension to ensure adequate wetting of the powder for at least 2 minutes.
4. Slowly add the specified amount of vehicle to the bottle.
5. Close the bottle using a child-resistant cap and shake well for 30 seconds to completely dissolve the active drug.
6. Label "Shake Well Before Use."

Stable for 35 days at 2°C to 8°C (36°F to 46°F) or 5 days at 25°C (77°F). The Canadian labeling suggests that preparations made with water containing preservative (ie, 0.05% sodium benzoate) are stable for 49 days at 2°C to 8°C (36°F to 46°F) and 10 days at 25°C (77°F). Shake gently prior to use. Do **not** dispense with dosing device provided with commercially-available product.

Preparation of Oseltamivir 6 mg/mL Suspension

Body Weight	Total Volume per Patient[1]	# of 75 mg Capsules[2]	Required Volume of Water	Required Volume of Vehicle[2,3]	Treatment Dose (wt based)[4]	Prophylactic Dose (wt based)[4]
≤15 kg	75 mL	6	5 mL	69 mL	5 mL (30 mg) twice daily for 5 days	5 mL (30 mg) once daily for 10 days
16-23 kg	100 mL	8	7 mL	91 mL	7.5 mL (45 mg) twice daily for 5 days	7.5 mL (45 mg) once daily for 10 days
24-40 kg	125 mL	10	8 mL	115 mL	10 mL (60 mg) twice daily for 5 days	10 mL (60 mg) once daily for 10 days
≥41 kg	150 mL	12	10 mL	137 mL	12.5 mL (75 mg) twice daily for 5 days	12.5 mL (75 mg) once daily for 10 days

[1]Entire course of therapy.

[2]Based on total volume per patient.

[3]Acceptable vehicles are cherry syrup (Humco®), Ora-Sweet® SF, or simple syrup.

[4]Using 6 mg/mL suspension.

◆ **OSI-774** *see* Erlotinib *on page 756*

◆ **Osmitrol** *see* Mannitol *on page 1269*

Dosage adjustment in hepatic impairment:
Mild or moderate impairment (Child-Pugh class A or B): No dosage adjustment necessary.
Severe impairment (Child-Pugh class C): No dosage adjustment provided in manufacturer's labeling (has not been studied). Use is not recommended.

Administration Administer with food. Hazardous agent: Use appropriate precautions for handling and disposal (meets NIOSH 2014 criteria).

Monitoring Parameters Monitor for signs of endometrial cancer in female patients with uterus. Adequate diagnostic measures, including endometrial sampling, if indicated, should be performed to rule out malignancy in all cases of undiagnosed abnormal vaginal bleeding. Assess need for therapy at regular intervals. Monitor for signs/symptoms of stroke and VTE.

Dosage Forms
Tablet, Oral:
Osphena: 60 mg

- ◆ **Osphena** *see* Ospemifene *on page* *1527*
- ◆ **Osteocit® (Can)** *see* Calcium Citrate *on page* *330*
- ◆ **Otezla** *see* Apremilast *on page* *165*
- ◆ **OTFC (Oral Transmucosal Fentanyl Citrate)** *see* FentaNYL *on page* *857*
- ◆ **Otrexup** *see* Methotrexate *on page* *1322*
- ◆ **Ovace Plus** *see* Sulfacetamide (Topical) *on page* *1943*
- ◆ **Ovace Plus Wash** *see* Sulfacetamide (Topical) *on page* *1943*
- ◆ **Ovace Wash** *see* Sulfacetamide (Topical) *on page* *1943*
- ◆ **Ovcon 35** *see* Ethinyl Estradiol and Norethindrone *on page* *808*
- ◆ **Ovide** *see* Malathion *on page* *1268*
- ◆ **Ovidrel** *see* Chorionic Gonadotropin (Recombinant) *on page* *432*
- ◆ **Ovidrel® (Can)** *see* Chorionic Gonadotropin (Recombinant) *on page* *432*
- ◆ **Ovine Corticotrophin-Releasing Hormone (oCRH)** *see* Corticorelin *on page* *509*
- ◆ **Ovral® (Can)** *see* Ethinyl Estradiol and Norgestrel *on page* *812*

Oxacillin (oks a SIL in)

Brand Names: U.S. Bactocill in Dextrose

Index Terms Methylphenyl Isoxazolyl Penicillin; Oxacillin Sodium

Pharmacologic Category Antibiotic, Penicillin

Use
Staphylococcal infections: In the treatment of infections caused by penicillinase-producing staphylococci that have demonstrated susceptibility to the drug; to initiate therapy in suspected cases of resistant staphylococcal infections prior to the availability of laboratory test results.
Oxacillin should not be used in infections caused by organisms susceptible to penicillin G. Oxacillin should be used only to treat or prevent infections that are proven or strongly suspected to be caused by susceptible bacteria. If the susceptibility test results indicate a non-penicillinase-producing staphylococcus, discontinue treatment. In the absence of such data, local epidemiology and susceptibility patterns may contribute to the empiric selection of therapy.

Pregnancy Risk Factor B

Dosage Note: Oxacillin contains 57.3 mg (2.5 mEq) of sodium per gram.
Usual dosage range:
Infants and Children: IM, IV: 50-200 mg/kg/day in divided doses every 6 hours (maximum: 12 g daily)
Adults: IM, IV: 250-2000 mg every 4-6 hours
Indication-specific dosing:
Infants >3 months and Children:
Community-acquired pneumonia (CAP) (IDSA/PIDS, 2011), moderate-to-severe infection, *S. aureus* (methicillin-susceptible) (preferred): IV: 150-200 mg/kg/day divided every 6-8 hours
Children:
Mild-to-moderate infections: IM, IV: 50 mg/kg/day in divided doses every 6 hours (maximum: 4 g daily)
Severe infections: Infants and Children: IM, IV: 100 mg/kg/day in divided doses every 4-6 hours (maximum: 12 g daily)
Adults:
Endocarditis: IV: 2 g every 4 hours with gentamicin
Mild-to-moderate infections: IM, IV: 250-500 mg every 4-6 hours
Prosthetic joint infection: IV: 2 g every 4 hours with rifampin
Severe infections: IM, IV: 1 g every 4-6 hours
***Staphylococcus aureus*, methicillin-susceptible infections, including brain abscess, bursitis, erysipelas, mastitis, mastoiditis, osteomyelitis, perinephric abscess, pneumonia, pyomyositis, scalded skin syndrome, toxic shock syndrome:** IV: 2 g every 4 hours
Dosage adjustment in renal impairment: No dosage adjustment provided in manufacturer's labeling.
Intermittent hemodialysis: Not dialyzable (0% to 5%)
Dosage adjustment in hepatic impairment: No dosage adjustment provided in manufacturer's labeling.

Additional Information Complete prescribing information should be consulted for additional detail.

Dosage Forms
Solution, Intravenous:
Bactocill in Dextrose: 1 g/50 mL (50 mL); 2 g/50 mL (50 mL)
Solution Reconstituted, Injection:
Generic: 1 g (1 ea); 2 g (1 ea); 10 g (1 ea)
Solution Reconstituted, Injection [preservative free]:
Generic: 1 g (1 ea); 2 g (1 ea); 10 g (1 ea)

- ◆ **Oxacillin Sodium** *see* Oxacillin *on page* *1528*
- ◆ **Oxalatoplatin** *see* Oxaliplatin *on page* *1528*
- ◆ **Oxalatoplatinum** *see* Oxaliplatin *on page* *1528*

Oxaliplatin (ox AL i pla tin)

Brand Names: U.S. Eloxatin

Brand Names: Canada Eloxatin

Index Terms Diaminocyclohexane Oxalatoplatinum; L-OHP; Oxalatoplatin; Oxalatoplatinum

Pharmacologic Category Antineoplastic Agent, Alkylating Agent; Antineoplastic Agent, Platinum Analog

Use
Colon cancer: Adjuvant treatment of stage III colon cancer (in combination with fluorouracil and leucovorin) after complete resection of primary tumor
Colorectal cancer, advanced: Treatment of advanced colorectal cancer (in combination with fluorouracil and leucovorin)

Pregnancy Risk Factor D

◆ **Osmitrol® (Can)** *see* Mannitol *on page 1269*

◆ **OsmoPrep** *see* Sodium Phosphates *on page 1909*

Ospemifene (os PEM i feen)

Brand Names: U.S. Osphena

Index Terms FC1271a

Pharmacologic Category Selective Estrogen Receptor Modulator (SERM)

Use Treatment of moderate-to-severe dyspareunia due to vulvar and vaginal atrophy (VVA) of menopause

Pregnancy Risk Factor X

Pregnancy Considerations Adverse events were observed in animal reproduction studies. Use is contraindicated in women who are or may become pregnant. Ospemifene is currently approved only for the treatment of moderate-to-severe dyspareunia due to vulvar and vaginal atrophy (VVA) of menopause.

Breast-Feeding Considerations It is not known if ospemifene is excreted into breast milk.

Contraindications Undiagnosed abnormal vaginal bleeding; DVT or PE (current or history of); active or history of arterial thromboembolic disease (eg, stroke, MI); estrogen-dependent tumor (known or suspected); women who are or may become pregnant

Warnings/Precautions Hazardous agent: Use appropriate precautions for handling and disposal (meets NIOSH 2014 criteria). **[U.S. Boxed Warning]: The use of unopposed estrogen in women with an intact uterus is associated with an increased risk of endometrial cancer. The addition of a progestin to estrogen therapy may decrease the risk of endometrial hyperplasia, a precursor to endometrial cancer. Adequate diagnostic measures, including endometrial sampling if indicated, should be performed to rule out malignancy in postmenopausal women with undiagnosed abnormal vaginal bleeding. Ospemifene is an estrogen agonist/antagonist with agonistic effects on the endometrium.** For women with an intact uterus using an estrogen without a progestin, the risk of endometrial cancer is dependent upon dose and duration of therapy. Endometrial cancer was not reported in clinical studies of ospemifene (duration ≤52 weeks) and the use of progestins was not evaluated. Ospemifene was not studied in women with breast cancer. Use is not currently recommended in women with carcinoma of the breast (known, suspected or history of) and use is contraindicated with an estrogen-dependent tumor.

[U.S. Boxed Warning]: Using data from the Women's Health Initiative (WHI) studies, an increased risk of deep vein thrombosis (DVT) and stroke has been reported with oral conjugated estrogens. The following were reported with ospemifene in clinical trials lasting ≤15 months duration: thromboembolic stroke 0.72/1000 women (placebo 1.04/1000 women); hemorrhagic stroke 1.45/1000 women (placebo 0/1000 women); DVT 1.45/1000 women (placebo 1.04/1000 women). Risk factors for cardiovascular disorders, arterial vascular disorders and /or venous thromboembolism (VTE) should be managed appropriately. Risk factors include diabetes mellitus, hypercholesterolemia, hypertension, SLE, obesity, tobacco use, and/or history of VTE. Discontinue immediately if a VTE, thromboembolic or hemorrhagic stroke occur or are suspected.

[U.S. Boxed Warning]: Ospemifene should be used for the shortest duration possible consistent with treatment goals and risks for the individual woman.

Ospemifene has not been studied in patients with severe hepatic impairment; use is not recommended. Potentially significant interactions may exist, requiring dose or frequency adjustment, additional monitoring, and/or selection of alternative therapy. Consult drug interactions database for more detailed information. Whenever possible, discontinue at least 4-6 weeks prior to elective surgery associated with an increased risk of thromboembolism or during periods of prolonged immobilization.

Adverse Reactions

Dermatologic: Hyperhidrosis

Endocrine & metabolic: Hot flashes

Genitourinary: Genital discharge, vaginal discharge

Neuromuscular & skeletal: Muscle spasm

Rare but important or life-threatening: DVT, hemorrhagic stroke, thromboembolic stroke

Drug Interactions

Metabolism/Transport Effects Substrate of CYP2C19 (minor), CYP2C9 (major), CYP3A4 (major); **Note:** Assignment of Major/Minor substrate status based on clinically relevant drug interaction potential; **Inhibits** CYP2B6 (weak), CYP2C19 (weak), CYP2C8 (weak), CYP2C9 (weak), CYP2D6 (weak), CYP3A4 (weak)

Avoid Concomitant Use

Avoid concomitant use of Ospemifene with any of the following: Estrogen Derivatives; Fluconazole; Pimozide; Selective Estrogen Receptor Modulators

Increased Effect/Toxicity

Ospemifene may increase the levels/effects of: ARIPiprazole; Dofetilide; Hydrocodone; Lomitapide; Pimozide

The levels/effects of Ospemifene may be increased by: CYP2C9 Inhibitors (Strong); CYP3A4 Inhibitors (Strong); Estrogen Derivatives; Fluconazole; Selective Estrogen Receptor Modulators

Decreased Effect

The levels/effects of Ospemifene may be decreased by: Bosentan; CYP2C9 Inducers (Strong); CYP3A4 Inducers (Moderate); CYP3A4 Inducers (Strong); Dabrafenib; Deferasirox; Estrogen Derivatives; Mitotane; Selective Estrogen Receptor Modulators; Siltuximab; St Johns Wort; Tocilizumab

Storage/Stability Store at controlled room temperature of 20°C to 25°C (68°F to 77°F); excursions permitted to 15°C to 30°C (59°F to 86°F).

Mechanism of Action Ospemifene is a selective estrogen receptor modulator (SERM); it activates estrogen pathways in some tissues and blocks estrogen pathways in others, and specifically has agonistic effects on the endometrium. In women with VVA, ospemifene was shown to improve vaginal changes associated with the decrease in natural estrogen production associated with menopause (improves vaginal maturation index, decreases vaginal pH) and significantly decreased the most bothersome moderate-to-severe subjective findings reported by women (vaginal dryness and dyspareunia) after 12 weeks of therapy (Bachmann, 2010).

Pharmacodynamics/Kinetics

Onset of action: A significant decrease in vaginal dryness and dyspareunia were observed after 12 weeks of therapy (Bachmann, 2010).

Distribution: V_d: 448 L

Protein binding: >99% bound to serum proteins

Metabolism: Hepatic via CYP3A4, 2C9, and 2C19; forms a metabolite (4-hydroxyospemifene)

Bioavailability: Increased approximately two- to threefold by food

Half-life elimination: ~26 hours

Time to peak: ~2 hours (range: 1-8 hours)

Excretion: Feces (75%); urine (7%; <0.2% as unchanged drug)

Dosage Dyspareunia, moderate-to-severe: Postmenopausal females: Oral: 60 mg once daily

Dosage adjustment in renal impairment: No dosage adjustment necessary.

Pregnancy Considerations Adverse events were observed in animal reproduction studies at one-tenth the equivalent human dose. Women of childbearing potential should be advised to avoid pregnancy and use effective contraception during treatment.

Canadian labeling: Use in pregnant women is contraindicated in the Canadian labeling. Males should be advised not to father children during and for up to 6 months following therapy. May cause permanent infertility in males. Prior to initiating therapy, advise males desiring to father children, to seek counseling on sperm storage.

Breast-Feeding Considerations It is not known if oxaliplatin is excreted in breast milk. Due to the potential for serious adverse reactions in the nursing infant, the decision to discontinue breast-feeding or to discontinue oxaliplatin should take into account the benefits of treatment to the mother.

Contraindications Hypersensitivity to oxaliplatin, other platinum-containing compounds, or any component of the formulation

Canadian labeling: Additional contraindications (not in U.S. labeling): Pregnancy, breast-feeding; severe renal impairment (CrCl <30 mL/minute)

Warnings/Precautions Hazardous agent - use appropriate precautions for handling and disposal (NIOSH 2014 [group 1]). **[U.S. Boxed Warning]: Anaphylactic/anaphylactoid reactions have been reported with oxaliplatin (may occur within minutes of administration); symptoms may be managed with epinephrine, corticosteroids, antihistamines,** and discontinuation; oxygen and bronchodilators have also been used (Kim, 2009). Grade 3 or 4 hypersensitivity has been observed. Allergic reactions are similar to reactions reported with other platinum analogs, and may occur with any cycle. Reactions typically occur after multiple cycles; in retrospective reviews, reaction occurred at a median of 7 to 9 cycles, with an onset of 5 to 70 minutes (Kim, 2009; Polyzos, 2009). Symptoms may include bronchospasm (rare), erythema, hypotension (rare), pruritus, rash, and/or urticaria; previously-untreated patients have also experienced flushing, diaphoresis, diarrhea, shortness of breath, chest pain, hypotension, syncope, and disorientation. According to the manufacturer, rechallenge is contraindicated (deaths due to anaphylaxis have been associated with platinum derivatives). In patients rechallenged after mild hypersensitivity, reaction recurred at a higher level of severity; for patients with severe hypersensitivity, rechallenge (with 2 to 3 days of antihistamine and corticosteroid premedication, and prolongation of infusion time) allowed for 2 to 4 additional oxaliplatin cycles; however, rechallenge was not feasible in nearly two-thirds of patients due to the severity of the initial reaction (Polyzos, 2009).

Two different types of peripheral sensory neuropathy may occur: First, an acute (within hours to 1 to 2 days), reversible (resolves within 14 days), with primarily peripheral symptoms that are often exacerbated by cold (may include pharyngolaryngeal dysesthesia); commonly recur with subsequent doses; avoid mucositis prophylaxis with ice chips during oxaliplatin infusion. Cold-triggered neuropathy may last up to 7 days after oxaliplatin administration (Grothey, 2011). Secondly, a more persistent (>14 days) presentation that often interferes with daily activities (eg, writing, buttoning, swallowing), these symptoms may improve in some patients upon discontinuing treatment. In a retrospective evaluation of patients treated with oxaliplatin for colorectal cancer, the incidence of peripheral sensory neuropathy was similar between diabetic and nondiabetic patients (Ramanathan, 2010). Several retrospective studies (as well as a small, underpowered randomized trial) have suggested calcium and magnesium infusions before and after oxaliplatin administration may reduce incidence of cumulative sensory neuropathy; however, a recent abstract of an ongoing randomized, placebo-controlled, double-blind study in patients with colorectal cancer suggests there is no benefit of calcium and magnesium in preventing sensory neuropathy or in decreasing oxaliplatin discontinuation rates (Loprinzi, 2013).

Oxaliplatin is associated with a moderate emetic potential; antiemetics are recommended to prevent nausea and vomiting (Basch, 2011; Dupuis, 2011; Roila, 2010). Cases of reversible posterior leukoencephalopathy syndrome (RPLS) have been reported. Signs/symptoms include headache, mental status changes, seizure, blurred vision, blindness and/or other vision changes; may be associated with hypertension; diagnosis is confirmed with brain imaging. May cause pulmonary fibrosis; withhold treatment for unexplained pulmonary symptoms (eg, crackles, dyspnea, nonproductive cough, pulmonary infiltrates) until interstitial lung disease or pulmonary fibrosis are excluded. Hepatotoxicity (including rare cases of hepatitis and hepatic failure) has been reported. Liver biopsy has revealed peliosis, nodular regenerative hyperplasia, sinusoidal alterations, perisinusoidal fibrosis, and veno-occlusive lesions; the presence of hepatic vascular disorders (including veno-occlusive disease) should be considered, especially in individuals developing portal hypertension or who present with increased liver function tests. Use caution with renal dysfunction; increased toxicity may occur; reduce initial dose in severe impairment. Potentially significant drug-drug interactions may exist, requiring dose or frequency adjustment, additional monitoring, and/or selection of alternative therapy. Elderly patients are more sensitive to some adverse events including diarrhea, dehydration, hypokalemia, leukopenia, fatigue and syncope. Oxaliplatin is an irritant with vesicant-like properties; ensure proper needle or catheter placement prior to and during infusion; avoid extravasation.

Adverse Reactions

Cardiovascular: Chest pain, edema, flushing, peripheral edema, thromboembolism

Central nervous system: Dizziness, fatigue, fever, headache, insomnia, pain, peripheral neuropathy (may be dose limiting), rigors

Dermatologic: Alopecia, palmar-plantar erythrodysesthesia, skin rash

Endocrine & metabolic: Dehydration, hypokalemia

Gastrointestinal: Abdominal pain, anorexia, constipation, diarrhea, hiccups, palmar-plantar erythrodysesthesia, dyspepsia, dysphagia, flatulence, gastroesophageal reflux, mucositis, nausea, stomatitis, vomiting

Genitourinary: Dysuria

Hematologic & oncologic: Anemia, leukopenia, neutropenia, thrombocytopenia

Hepatic: Increased serum ALT, increased serum AST, increased serum bilirubin

Hypersensitivity: Hypersensitivity reaction (includes urticaria, pruritus, facial flushing, shortness of breath, bronchospasm, diaphoresis, hypotension, syncope)

Local: Injection site reaction (redness/swelling/pain)

Neuromuscular & skeletal: Arthralgia, back pain

Ocular: Abnormal lacrimation

Renal: Increased serum creatinine

Respiratory: Cough, dyspnea, epistaxis, pharyngitis, pharyngolaryngeal dysesthesia, rhinitis, upper respiratory tract infection

Miscellaneous: Fever

Rare but important or life-threatening (reported with mono- and combination therapy): Abnormal gait, acute renal failure, anaphylaxis, anaphylactic shock, anaphylactoid reaction, angioedema, aphonia, ataxia, blepharoptosis, cerebral hemorrhage, colitis, cranial nerve palsy, decreased deep tendon reflex, deafness, decreased visual acuity, diplopia, dysarthria, eosinophilic pneumonitis, fasciculations, febrile neutropenia,hematuria, hemolysis, hemolytic anemia (immuno-allergic), hemolytic-uremic syndrome, hemorrhage, hepatic failure, hepatic sinusoidal obstruction syndrome (SOS; veno-occlusive disease), hepatitis, hepatotoxicity, hypertension, hypomagnesemia, hypoxia, idiopathic noncirrhotic portal hypertension (nodular regenerative hyperplasia), increased INR, increased serum alkaline phosphatase, infusion related reaction (extravasation [including necrosis]), interstitial nephritis (acute), interstitial pulmonary disease, intestinal obstruction, laryngospasm, Lhermittes' sign, metabolic acidosis, muscle spasm, myoclonus, neutropenic enterocolitis, neutropenic infection (sepsis), optic neuritis, pancreatitis, prolonged prothrombin time, purpura, rectal hemorrhage, renal tubular necrosis, reversible posterior leukoencephalopathy syndrome (RPLS), rhabdomyolysis, seizure, sepsis, temporary vision loss, thrombocytopenia (immuno-allergic), trigeminal neuralgia, visual field loss, voice disorder

Drug Interactions

Metabolism/Transport Effects Substrate of OCT2

Avoid Concomitant Use

Avoid concomitant use of Oxaliplatin with any of the following: BCG; CloZAPine; Dipyrone; Natalizumab; Pimecrolimus; Tacrolimus (Topical); Tofacitinib; Vaccines (Live)

Increased Effect/Toxicity

Oxaliplatin may increase the levels/effects of: CloZAPine; Leflunomide; Natalizumab; Taxane Derivatives; Tofacitinib; Topotecan; Vaccines (Live)

The levels/effects of Oxaliplatin may be increased by: BuPROPion; Denosumab; Dipyrone; Pimecrolimus; Roflumilast; Tacrolimus (Topical); Trastuzumab

Decreased Effect

Oxaliplatin may decrease the levels/effects of: BCG; Coccidioides immitis Skin Test; Fosphenytoin-Phenytoin; Sipuleucel-T; Vaccines (Inactivated); Vaccines (Live)

The levels/effects of Oxaliplatin may be decreased by: Echinacea

Preparation for Administration Hazardous agent; use appropriate precautions for handling and disposal (NIOSH 2014 [group 1]).

Do not prepare using a chloride-containing solution such as NaCl due to rapid conversion to monochloroplatinum, dichloroplatinum, and diaquoplatinum; all highly reactive in sodium chloride (Takimoto, 2007). Do not use needles or administration sets containing aluminum during preparation.

Aqueous solution: Dilution with D_5W (250 or 500 mL) is required prior to administration.

Lyophilized powder: Use only SWFI or D_5W to reconstitute powder. To obtain final concentration of 5 mg/mL add 10 mL of diluent to 50 mg vial or 20 mL diluent to 100 mg vial. Gently swirl vial to dissolve powder. Dilution with D_5W (250 or 500 mL) is required prior to administration. Discard unused portion of vial.

Storage/Stability Store intact vials at room temperature of 25°C (77°F); excursions permitted to 15°C to 30°C (59°F to 86°F); do not freeze. Protect concentrated solution from light (store in original outer carton). According to the manufacturer, solutions diluted for infusion are stable up to 6 hours at room temperature of 20°C to 25°C (68°F to 77°F) or up to 24 hours under refrigeration at 2°C to 8°C (36°F to 46°F). Oxaliplatin solution diluted with D_5W to a final concentration of 0.7 mg/mL (polyolefin container) has been shown to retain >90% of the original concentration for up to 30 days when stored at room temperature or refrigerated; artificial light did not affect the concentration (Andre, 2007). As this study did not examine sterility, refrigeration would be preferred to limit microbial growth. Solutions diluted for infusion do not require protection from light.

Mechanism of Action Oxaliplatin, a platinum derivative, is an alkylating agent. Following intracellular hydrolysis, the platinum compound binds to DNA forming cross-links which inhibit DNA replication and transcription, resulting in cell death. Cytotoxicity is cell-cycle nonspecific.

Pharmacodynamics/Kinetics

Distribution: V_d: 440 L

Protein binding: >90% primarily albumin and gamma globulin (irreversible binding to platinum)

Metabolism: Nonenzymatic (rapid and extensive), forms active and inactive derivatives

Half-life elimination: Terminal: 391 hours

Excretion: Urine (~54%); feces (~2%)

Dosage Note: Oxaliplatin is associated with a moderate emetic potential; antiemetics are recommended to prevent nausea and vomiting (Basch, 2011; Dupuis, 2011; Roila, 2010).

Advanced colorectal cancer: Adults: IV: 85 mg/m^2 every 2 weeks until disease progression or unacceptable toxicity (in combination with fluorouracil/leucovorin)

Stage III colon cancer (adjuvant): Adults: IV: 85 mg/m^2 every 2 weeks for a total of 6 months (12 cycles; in combination with fluorouracil/leucovorin)

Colon/colorectal cancer (off-label doses or combinations): Adults: IV: 85 mg/m^2/dose on days 1, 15, and 29 of an 8-week treatment cycle in combination with fluorouracil/leucovorin (Kuebler, 2007) **or** 85 mg/m^2 every 2 weeks in combination with fluorouracil/leucovorin/irinotecan (Falcone, 2007) **or** 130 mg/m^2 every 3 weeks in combination with capecitabine (Cassidy, 2008; Haller, 2011)

Biliary adenocarcinoma, advanced (off-label use): Adults: IV:

GEMOX regimen: 100 mg/m^2 on day 2 every 2 weeks (in combination with gemcitabine) until disease progression or unacceptable toxicity (Andre, 2004) **or**

CAPOX regimen: 130 mg/m^2 on day 1 every 3 weeks (in combination with capecitabine) until disease progression or unacceptable toxicity (Nehls, 2008)

Chronic lymphocytic leukemia, fludarabine-refractory (off-label use): Adults: IV: OFAR regimen: 25 mg/m^2/day for 4 days every 4 weeks (in combination with fludarabine, cytarabine, and rituximab) for up to 6 cycles (Tsimberidou, 2008)

Esophageal/gastric cancers (off-label use): Adults: IV: 130 mg/m^2 on day 1 every 3 weeks (in combination with epirubicin and either capecitabine or fluorouracil) for up to 8 cycles (Cunningham, 2008) **or** 85 mg/m^2 on day 1 every 2 weeks (in combination with docetaxel, leucovorin, and fluorouracil) for up to 8 cycles (Al-Batran, 2008) **or** 85 mg/m^2 on day 1 every 2 weeks (in combination with leucovorin and fluorouracil; FOLFOX4) for 6 cycles (Conroy, 2010)

or

Gastric cancer: Adults: IV: 130 mg/m^2 on day 1 every 3 weeks (in combination with capecitabine) for 8 cycles (Bang, 2012) **or** 100 mg/m^2 on day 1 every 2 weeks (in combination with leucovorin and fluorouracil) for at least 6 cycles (Louvet, 2002)

Non-Hodgkin lymphoma, relapsed/refractory (off-label use): Adults: IV: 100 mg/m^2 on day 1 every 3 weeks (in combination with gemcitabine and rituximab) (Lopez, 2008; Rodriguez, 2007) **or** 130 mg/m^2 on day 1 every 3 weeks (in combination with cytarabine and dexamethasone) (Chau, 2001)

Ovarian cancer, advanced (off-label use): Adults: IV: 130 mg/m^2 once every 3 weeks until disease progression or unacceptable toxicity (Dieras, 2002; Piccart, 2000)

Pancreatic cancer, advanced (off-label use): Adults: IV: 85 mg/m^2 every 2 weeks (in combination with fluorouracil, leucovorin, and irinotecan; FOLFIRINOX regimen) for up to 6 months (Conroy, 2011) **or** 110 to 130 mg/m^2 on day 1 every 3 weeks (in combination with capecitabine) until disease progression or unacceptable toxicity (Xiong, 2008)

Testicular cancer, refractory (off-label use): Adults: IV: 130 mg/m^2 every 3 weeks in combination with gemcitabine (De Georgi, 2006; Kollmannsberger, 2004; Pectasides, 2004) **or** 130 mg/m^2 on day 1 every 3 weeks (in combination with gemcitabine and paclitaxel) for up to 8 cycles (Bokemeyer, 2008)

Elderly: No dosage adjustment recommended; refer to adult dosing.

Dosage adjustments for toxicity: Acute toxicities: Longer infusion time (6 hours) may mitigate acute toxicities (eg, pharyngolaryngeal dysesthesia).

Neurosensory events:

Persistent (>7 days) grade 2 neurosensory events:

Adjuvant treatment of stage III colon cancer: Reduce dose to 75 mg/m^2

Advanced colorectal cancer: Reduce dose to 65 mg/m^2

Consider withholding oxaliplatin for grade 2 neuropathy lasting >7 days despite dose reduction.

Persistent (>7 days) grade 3 neurosensory events:

U.S. labeling: Consider discontinuing oxaliplatin.

Canadian labeling:

Adjuvant treatment of stage III colon cancer: Discontinue oxaliplatin.

Advanced colorectal cancer: Reduce dose to 65 mg/m^2; if not resolved prior to next cycle, then discontinue.

Gastrointestinal toxicity (grade 3/4):

Adjuvant treatment of stage III colon cancer: Delay next dose until recovery from toxicity, then reduce dose to 75 mg/m^2.

Advanced colorectal cancer: Delay next dose until recovery from toxicity, then reduce dose to 65 mg/m^2.

Hematologic toxicity (grade 4 neutropenia or grade 3/4 thrombocytopenia):

Adjuvant treatment of stage III colon cancer: Delay next dose until neutrophils recover to ≥1,500/mm^3 and platelets recover to ≥75,000/mm^3, then reduce dose to 75 mg/m^2.

Advanced colorectal cancer: Delay next dose until neutrophils recover to ≥1,500/mm^3 and platelets recover to ≥75,000/mm^3, then reduce dose to 65 mg/m^2.

Pulmonary toxicity (unexplained respiratory symptoms including nonproductive cough, dyspnea, crackles, pulmonary infiltrates): Discontinue until interstitial lung disease or pulmonary fibrosis have been excluded.

Dosage adjustment in renal impairment:

Manufacturer's recommendations:

U.S. labeling:

CrCl ≥30 mL/minute: No dosage adjustment necessary.

CrCl <30 mL/minute: Reduce dose from 85 mg/m^2 to 65 mg/m^2.

Canadian labeling: CrCl <30 mL/minute: Use is contraindicated.

Alternate recommendations: CrCl ≥20 mL/minute: In a study with a limited number of patients with mild to moderate impairment, defined by the authors as CrCl 20 to 59 mL/minute (determined using 24-hour urine collection), oxaliplatin was well tolerated, suggesting a dose reduction may not be necessary in patients with CrCl ≥20 mL/minute receiving every-3-week dosing (dose range: 80 to 130 mg/m^2 every 3 weeks) (Takimoto, 2003).

Dosage adjustment in hepatic impairment: Mild, moderate, or severe impairment: No dosage adjustment necessary (Doroshow, 2003; Synold, 2007).

Dosing in obesity: *ASCO Guidelines for appropriate chemotherapy dosing in obese adults with cancer:* Utilize patient's actual body weight (full weight) for calculation of body surface area- or weight-based dosing, particularly when the intent of therapy is curative; manage regimen-related toxicities in the same manner as for nonobese patients; if a dose reduction is utilized due to toxicity, consider resumption of full weight-based dosing with subsequent cycles, especially if cause of toxicity (eg, hepatic or renal impairment) is resolved (Griggs, 2012).

Administration Administer as IV infusion over 2 hours; extend infusion time to 6 hours for acute toxicities. Flush infusion line with D_5W prior to administration of any concomitant medication. Avoid mucositis prophylaxis with ice chips during oxaliplatin infusion (may exacerbate acute neurological symptoms). Do not use needles or administration sets containing aluminum.

Oxaliplatin is associated with a moderate emetic potential; antiemetics are recommended to prevent nausea and vomiting (Basch, 2011; Dupuis, 2011; Roila, 2010).

Irritant with vesicant-like properties; ensure proper needle or catheter placement prior to and during infusion. Avoid extravasation; monitor IV site for redness, swelling, or pain.

Extravasation management: If extravasation occurs, stop infusion immediately and disconnect (leave cannula/needle in place); gently aspirate extravasated solution (do **NOT** flush the line); remove needle/cannula; elevate extremity. Information conflicts regarding use of warm or cold compresses. Cold compresses could potentially precipitate or exacerbate peripheral neuropathy (de Lemos, 2005).

Hazardous agent; use appropriate precautions for handling and disposal (NIOSH 2014 [group 1]).

Monitoring Parameters CBC with differential, blood chemistries (including serum creatinine, ALT, AST, and bilirubin); INR and prothrombin time (in patients on oral anticoagulant therapy); signs of neuropathy, hypersensitivity, respiratory effects, and/or RPLS

Dosage Forms

Solution, Intravenous [preservative free]:

Eloxatin: 50 mg/10 mL (10 mL); 100 mg/20 mL (20 mL); 200 mg/40 mL (40 mL)

Generic: 50 mg/10 mL (10 mL); 100 mg/20 mL (20 mL)

Solution Reconstituted, Intravenous [preservative free]:

Generic: 50 mg (1 ea); 100 mg (1 ea)

◆ **Oxandrin** *see* Oxandrolone *on page* 1531

Oxandrolone (oks AN droe lone)

Brand Names: U.S. Oxandrin

Pharmacologic Category Androgen

Use Adjunctive therapy to promote weight gain after weight loss following extensive surgery, chronic infections, or severe trauma, and in some patients who, without definite pathophysiologic reasons, fail to gain or to maintain normal weight; to offset protein catabolism with prolonged corticosteroid administration; relief of bone pain associated with osteoporosis

Pregnancy Risk Factor X

Dosage

Children: Total daily dose: ≤0.1 mg/kg; may be repeated intermittently as needed

Adults: 2.5-20 mg in divided doses 2-4 times daily based on individual response; a course of therapy of 2-4 weeks is usually adequate. This may be repeated intermittently as needed.
Elderly: 5 mg twice daily

Dosing adjustment in renal impairment: No dosage adjustment provided in manufacturer's labeling; use with caution due to propensity to cause edema.
Dosing adjustment in hepatic impairment: No dosage adjustment provided in manufacturer's labeling; use with caution.

Additional Information Complete prescribing information should be consulted for additional detail.

Dosage Forms
Tablet, Oral:
Oxandrin: 2.5 mg, 10 mg
Generic: 2.5 mg, 10 mg

Oxaprozin (oks a PROE zin)

Brand Names: U.S. Daypro
Brand Names: Canada Apo-Oxaprozin
Pharmacologic Category Nonsteroidal Anti-inflammatory Drug (NSAID), Oral
Additional Appendix Information
Beers Criteria – Potentially Inappropriate Medications for Geriatrics *on page 2271*
Use Management of signs and symptoms of osteoarthritis, rheumatoid arthritis, and juvenile idiopathic arthritis (JIA)
Pregnancy Risk Factor C
Dosage Oral: **Note:** Individualize dosage to lowest effective dose for the shortest duration to minimize adverse effects.
Children 6-16 years: Juvenile idiopathic arthritis (JIA):
22-31 kg: 600 mg once daily
32-54 kg: 900 mg once daily
≥55 kg: 1200 mg once daily
Adults: Osteoarthritis, rheumatoid arthritis: 1200 mg once daily. **Note:** Patients with low body weight should start with 600 mg daily. A one-time loading dose of 1200-1800 mg (≤26 mg/kg) may be used when a quick onset of action is desired.
Maximum doses:
Patient <50 kg: Maximum: 1200 mg daily
Patient >50 kg with normal renal/hepatic function and low risk of peptic ulcer: Maximum: 1800 mg daily or 26 mg/kg/day (whichever is lower) in divided doses

Dosing adjustment in renal impairment: In general, NSAIDs are not recommended for use in patients with advanced renal disease but the manufacturer of oxaprozin does provide some guidelines for adjustment in renal dysfunction.
Severe renal impairment or on dialysis: 600 mg once daily; may increase cautiously to 1200 mg daily with close monitoring
Dosing adjustment in hepatic impairment: Use caution in patients with severe hepatic impairment.

Additional Information Complete prescribing information should be consulted for additional detail.

Dosage Forms
Tablet, Oral:
Daypro: 600 mg
Generic: 600 mg

Oxatomide [INT] (oks A toe mide)

International Brand Names Atoxan (PK); Celtect (JP); Cenacert (AR); Cobiona (ES); Danoprox (DE); Dasten (AR); Fensedyl (AR); Oxatadine (KR); Oxatokey (ES); Oxetal (HR); Oxleti (ES); Oxtin (ID); Quoxol (ES); Tanzal (ES); Tinseet (UY); Tinset (AR, AT, BE, CZ, DE, FR, GB, GR, HU, ID, IT, LU, MX, NL, PT, TH, ZA); Tinset Gel (IT)
Index Terms Oxatomide Monohydrate
Pharmacologic Category Antihistamine
Reported Use Symptomatic treatment of allergic rhinitis, chronic urticaria, and conjunctivitis
Dosage Range Adults: Oral: 30 mg twice daily
Product Availability Product available in various countries; not currently available in the U.S.
Dosage Forms
Suspension, oral: 2.5 mg/mL (100 mL)
Tablet: 30 mg

◆ **Oxatomide Monohydrate** *see* Oxatomide [INT] *on page 1532*

Oxazepam (oks A ze pam)

Brand Names: Canada Apo-Oxazepam®; Bio-Oxazepam; Novoxapram®; Oxpam®; Oxpram®; PMS-Oxazepam; Riva-Oxazepam
Index Terms Serax
Pharmacologic Category Benzodiazepine
Additional Appendix Information
Beers Criteria – Potentially Inappropriate Medications for Geriatrics *on page 2271*
Use Management of anxiety disorders, including anxiety associated with depression; management of ethanol withdrawal
Dosage Oral:
Children >12 years, Adolescents, and Adults:
Anxiety, mild-to-moderate: 10-15 mg 3-4 times daily
Anxiety, severe or associated with depression: 15-30 mg 3-4 times daily
Ethanol withdrawal: 15-30 mg 3-4 times daily
Elderly: Anxiety: Initial: 10 mg 3 times daily. If necessary, increase cautiously to 15 mg 3-4 times daily. Dose titration should be slow to evaluate sensitivity.

Dosage adjustment in renal impairment: No dosage adjustment provided in manufacturer's labeling
Hemodialysis: Not dialyzable (0% to 5%) (Greenblatt, 1981; Mokhlesi, 2003)
Dosage adjustment in hepatic impairment: No dosage adjustment provided in manufacturer's labeling; however, pharmacokinetic studies have shown that hepatic dysfunction is not expected to significantly decrease clearance (Furlan, 1999; Greenblatt, 1981).

Additional Information Complete prescribing information should be consulted for additional detail.

Dosage Forms
Capsule, Oral:
Generic: 10 mg, 15 mg, 30 mg

OXcarbazepine (ox car BAZ e peen)

Brand Names: U.S. Oxtellar XR; Trileptal
Brand Names: Canada Apo-Oxcarbazepine; Trileptal
Index Terms GP 47680; OCBZ
Pharmacologic Category Anticonvulsant, Miscellaneous
Use Partial seizures:
Immediate-release:
U.S labeling: Monotherapy or adjunctive therapy in the treatment of partial seizures in adults, as monotherapy in the treatment of partial seizures in children 4 years and older with epilepsy, and as adjunctive therapy in children 2 years and older with partial seizures.
Canadian labeling: Monotherapy or adjunctive therapy in the treatment of partial seizures in patients 6 years and older.
Extended-release: Adjunctive therapy in the treatment of partial seizures in adults and in children 6 to 17 years of age.
Pregnancy Risk Factor C

Pregnancy Considerations Adverse events have been observed in animal reproduction studies; therefore, the manufacturer classifies oxcarbazepine as pregnancy category C. Oxcarbazepine, the active metabolite MHD and the inactive metabolite DHD, crosses the placenta and can be detected in the newborn. An increased risk in the overall rate of major congenital malformations has not been observed following maternal use of oxcarbazepine. Available studies have not been large enough to determine if there is an increased risk of specific defects. In general, the risk of teratogenic effects is higher with AED polytherapy than monotherapy. Plasma concentrations of MHD gradually decrease due to physiologic changes which occur during pregnancy; patients should be monitored during pregnancy and postpartum. Oxcarbazepine may decrease plasma concentrations of hormonal contraceptives.

Patients exposed to oxcarbazepine during pregnancy are encouraged to enroll themselves into the NAAED Pregnancy Registry by calling 1-888-233-2334. Additional information is available at www.aedpregnancyregistry.org.

Breast-Feeding Considerations Oxcarbazepine and the active 10-hydroxy metabolite (MHD) are found in breast milk (small amounts). According to the manufacturer, the decision to continue or discontinue breast-feeding during therapy should take into account the risk of exposure to the infant and the benefits of treatment to the mother.

Contraindications Hypersensitivity to oxcarbazepine or any component of the formulation

Warnings/Precautions Hazardous agent - use appropriate precautions for handling and disposal (NIOSH 2014 [group 2]).

Antiepileptics are associated with an increased risk of suicidal behavior/thoughts with use (regardless of indication); patients should be monitored for signs/symptoms of depression, suicidal tendencies, and other unusual behavior changes during therapy and instructed to inform their healthcare provider immediately if symptoms occur.

Clinically-significant hyponatremia (serum sodium <125 mmol/L) may develop during oxcarbazepine use. Rare cases of anaphylaxis and angioedema have been reported, even after initial dosing; permanently discontinue should symptoms occur. Use caution in patients with previous hypersensitivity to carbamazepine (cross-sensitivity occurs in 25% to 30% of patients). Potentially serious, sometimes fatal, dermatologic reactions (eg, Stevens-Johnson, toxic epidermal necrolysis) and drug reaction with eosinophilia and systemic symptoms (DRESS) also known as multiorgan hypersensitivity reactions have been reported in adults and children; monitor for signs and symptoms of skin reactions and possible disparate manifestations associated with lymphatic, hepatic, renal, cardiovascular, and/or hematologic organ systems; discontinuation and conversion to alternate therapy may be required. Considering screening patients of Asian descent for the variant human leukocyte antigen (HLA) allele B*1502 prior to initiating therapy. This genetic variant has been associated with a significantly increased risk of developing Stevens-Johnson syndrome and/or toxic epidermal necrolysis in patients receiving carbamazepine. Structural similarity of oxcarbazepine to carbamazepine, available clinical evidence, and data from nonclinical studies showing a direct interaction of oxcarbazepine with the HLA-B*1502 protein suggest patients receiving oxcarbazepine may be at a similar risk. Consider avoiding use of oxcarbazepine in patients with a positive result. Screening is not recommending in low-risk populations or in current oxcarbazepine patients (risk usually during first few months of therapy). Clinical trials excluded patients with significant cardiovascular disease or ECG abnormalities; Canadian labeling recommends using caution with cardiac conduction abnormalities or concomitant drugs that depress atrioventricular (AV) conduction and to avoid use in patients with AV block. Monitor body weight/fluid retention in patients with HF; evaluate serum sodium with worsening cardiac function or fluid retention.

Hepatitis and hepatic failure have been reported rarely (Hsu, 2010; Trileptal Canadian product monograph, 2013). Promptly evaluate any symptoms of hepatic dysfunction (eg, anorexia, nausea/vomiting, right upper quadrant pain, pruritus) and discontinue therapy immediately if significant abnormalities are confirmed. Agranulocytosis, leukopenia, and pancytopenia have been reported rarely. Discontinuation and conversion to alternate therapy may be required. Long term use has been associated with decreased bone mineral density, osteopenia, osteoporosis, and fractures.

As with all antiepileptic drugs, oxcarbazepine should be withdrawn gradually to minimize the potential of increased seizure frequency. Use of oxcarbazepine has been associated with CNS-related adverse events, most significant of these were cognitive symptoms including psychomotor slowing, difficulty with concentration, speech or language problems, somnolence or fatigue, and coordination abnormalities, including ataxia and gait disturbances. Single-dose studies show that half-life of the primary active metabolite is prolonged 3- to 4-fold and AUC is doubled in patients with CrCl <30 mL/minute; dose adjustment required in these patients. Potentially significant drug-drug interactions may exist, requiring dose or frequency adjustment, additional monitoring, and/or selection of alternative therapy. Oral suspension contains sorbitol; Canadian labeling recommends avoiding use in patients with fructose intolerance

Adverse Reactions

Cardiovascular: Bradycardia, cardiac failure, flushing, hypertension, hypotension, lower extremity edema, orthostatic hypotension, palpitations, syncope, tachycardia

Central nervous system: Abnormal gait, abnormal electroencephalogram, abnormality in thinking, aggressive behavior, agitation, amnesia, anxiety, apathy, aphasia, ataxia, aura, cerebral hemorrhage, confusion, convulsions, delirium, delusion, depression, dizziness, drowsiness, dysmetria, dystonia, emotional lability, equilibrium disturbance, euphoria extrapyramidal reaction, falling, fatigue, feeling abnormal, headache, hemiplegia, hyperkinesia, hyperreflexia, hypertonia, hypokinesia, hyporeflexia, hypotonia, hysteria, impaired consciousness, insomnia, intoxicated feeling, lack of concentration, malaise, manic behavior, migraine, myasthenia, nervousness, neuralgia, nightmares, oculogyric crisis, panic disorder, paralysis, personality disorder, precordial pain, psychosis, rigors, seizure (aggravated), speech disorder, stupor, vertigo, voice disorder

Dermatologic: Acne vulgaris, alopecia, contact dermatitis, diaphoresis, eczema, erythematosus rash, facial rash, folliculitis, genital pruritus, maculopapular rash, miliaria, psoriasis, skin photosensitivity, skin rash, urticaria, vitiligo

Endocrine & metabolic: Change in libido, decreased serum sodium (<135 mEq/L), hyponatremia, hot flash, hyperglycemia, hypermenorrhea, hypocalcemia, hypoglycemia, hypokalemia, increased gamma-glutamyl transferase, intermenstrual bleeding, weight gain, weight loss

Gastrointestinal: Aphthous stomatitis, biliary colic, bloody stools, cholelithiasis, colitis, constipation, diarrhea, duodenal ulcer, dysgeusia,dyspepsia, dysphagia, enteritis, eructation, esophagitis, flatulence, gastric ulcer, gastritis, gingival hemorrhage, gingival hyperplasia, hematemesis, hemorrhoids, hiccups, increased appetite, retching, sialadenitis, stomatitis, upper abdominal pain, xerostomia

Gastrointestinal: Abdominal pain, nausea, vomiting

Genitourinary: Dysuria, hematuria, leukorrhea, priapism, urinary frequency, urinary tract pain

Hematologic & oncologic: Bruise, purpura, rectal hemorrhage, thrombocytopenia

Hepatic: Increased liver enzymes

Hypersensitivity: Angioedema, hypersensitivity reaction

Neuromuscular & skeletal: Back pain, muscle spasm right hypochondrium pain, sprain, systemic lupus erythematosus, tetany, tremor, weakness

Ophthalmic: Accommodation disturbance, blepharoptosis, blurred vision, cataract, conjunctival hemorrhage, diplopia, hemianopia, mydriasis, nystagmus, ocular edema, photophobia, scotoma, visual disturbance, xerophthalmia

Otic: Otitis externa, tinnitus

Renal: Nephrolithiasis, polyuria, renal pain

Respiratory: asthma, dyspnea, epistaxis, laryngismus, nasopharyngitis, pleurisy, pneumonia, pulmonary infection, rhinitis, sinusitis, upper respiratory tract infection

Miscellaneous: Fever

Rare but important or life-threatening: Abnormal thyroid function test (decreased total T_4 and/or free T_4), acute generalized exanthematous pustulosis, agranulocytosis, anaphylaxis, aplastic anemia, bone fracture (long-term therapy), decreased bone mineral density (long-term therapy), DRESS syndrome, erythema multiforme, folate deficiency, hepatic failure, hepatitis (Hsu, 2010), hypersensitivity reaction, hypothyroidism, increased serum amylase, increased serum lipase, leukopenia, multiorgan hypersensitivity (eosinophilia, arthralgia, rash, fever, lymphadenopathy), osteopenia (long-term therapy), osteoporosis (long-term therapy), pancreatitis, pancytopenia, Stevens-Johnson syndrome, suicidal ideation, suicidal tendencies, toxic epidermal necrolysis

Drug Interactions

Metabolism/Transport Effects **Induces** CYP3A4 (weak)

Avoid Concomitant Use

Avoid concomitant use of OXcarbazepine with any of the following: Dolutegravir; Eslicarbazepine; Ledipasvir; Rilpivirine; Selegiline; Sofosbuvir; Ulipristal

Increased Effect/Toxicity

OXcarbazepine may increase the levels/effects of: Fosphenytoin-Phenytoin; PHENobarbital; Selegiline

The levels/effects of OXcarbazepine may be increased by: Alcohol (Ethyl); Eslicarbazepine; Perampanel; Thiazide Diuretics

Decreased Effect

OXcarbazepine may decrease the levels/effects of: ARIPiprazole; Cobicistat; Contraceptives (Estrogens); Contraceptives (Progestins); Dolutegravir; Elvitegravir; Hydrocodone; Ledipasvir; Perampanel; Rilpivirine; Saxagliptin; Sofosbuvir; Ulipristal

The levels/effects of OXcarbazepine may be decreased by: CarBAMazepine; Fosphenytoin-Phenytoin; Mefloquine; Mianserin; Orlistat; PHENobarbital; Valproic Acid and Derivatives

Storage/Stability Store tablets and suspension at 25°C (77°F); excursions permitted to 15°C to 30°C (59°F to 86°F). Store suspension in the original container; use within 7 weeks of first opening container.

Mechanism of Action Pharmacological activity results from both oxcarbazepine and its monohydroxy metabolite (MHD). Precise mechanism of anticonvulsant effect has not been defined. Oxcarbazepine and MHD block voltage-sensitive sodium channels, stabilizing hyperexcited neuronal membranes, inhibiting repetitive firing, and decreasing the propagation of synaptic impulses. These actions are believed to prevent the spread of seizures. Oxcarbazepine and MHD also increase potassium conductance and modulate the activity of high-voltage activated calcium channels.

Pharmacodynamics/Kinetics

Absorption: Complete

Distribution: MHD: V_d: 49 L

Protein binding, serum: MHD: ~40% (primarily to albumin)

Metabolism: Extensive to 10-monohydroxy metabolite (MHD; active); MHD is further glucuronidated or oxidized to a 10,11-dihydroxy metabolite (DHD; inactive)

Bioavailability: Immediate release: Decreased in children <8 years; increased in elderly >60 years

Half-life elimination: Immediate release: Parent drug: 2 hours; MHD: 9 hours; renal impairment (CrCl 30 mL/minute): MHD: 19 hours; Extended release: Parent drug: 7 to 11 hours; MHD: 9 to 11 hours

Clearance of MHD is increased in younger children (~80% in children 2-4 years of age) and approaches that of adults by ~13 years of age

Time to peak, serum (median): Immediate release: Tablets: 4.5 hours; Oral suspension: 6 hours

Excretion: Urine (95%, <1% as unchanged oxcarbazepine, 27% as unchanged MHD, 49% as MHD glucuronides); feces (<4%)

Dosage Adjunctive therapy, partial seizures (epilepsy): Oral:

Children 2 to 3 years (U.S. labeling): Immediate release (Trileptal):

Initial: 8 to 10 mg/kg/day, not to exceed 600 mg daily, given in 2 divided daily doses

Maintenance: The target maintenance dose should be achieved over 2 to 4 weeks, and is dependent upon patient weight (should not exceed 60 mg/kg/day given in 2 divided daily doses).

<20 kg: Consider initiating dose at 16 to 20 mg/kg/day; maximum maintenance dose should be achieved over 2 to 4 weeks and should not exceed 60 mg/kg/day

Children 4 to 16 years (U.S. labeling) or 6 to 16 years (Canadian labeling): Immediate release (Trileptal):

Initial: 8 to 10 mg/kg/day, not to exceed 600 mg daily, given in 2 divided daily doses

Maintenance: The target maintenance dose should be achieved over 2 weeks, and is dependent upon patient weight, according to the following:

20 to 29 kg: 900 mg daily in 2 divided doses

29.1 to 39 kg: 1200 mg daily in 2 divided doses

>39 kg: 1800 mg daily in 2 divided doses

Children 6 to 17 years: Extended release (Oxtellar XR):

Initial: 8 to 10 mg/kg once daily (not to exceed 600 mg daily in the first week)

Maintenance: The target maintenance dose should be achieved over 2 to 3 weeks with dose increases of 8 to 10 mg/kg/day increments at weekly intervals (maximum dosage incremental increase: 600 mg). Target maintenance dose depends on weight:

20 to 29 kg: 900 mg once daily

29.1 to 39 kg: 1200 mg once daily

>39 kg: 1800 mg once daily

Adults:

Immediate release (Trileptal): Initial: 600 mg daily in 2 divided doses; dose may be increased by as much as 600 mg/day increments at weekly intervals; recommended daily dose: 1200 mg daily in 2 divided doses. Although daily doses >1200 mg daily were somewhat more efficacious, most patients were unable to tolerate 2400 mg daily (due to CNS effects).

Extended release (Oxtellar XR): Initial: 600 mg once daily; dosage may be increased by 600 mg/day increments at weekly intervals. Recommended daily dose is 1200 to 2400 mg once daily. Although daily doses >1200 mg daily were somewhat more efficacious, most patients were unable to tolerate 2400 mg daily (due to CNS effects).

Elderly: Extended release (Oxtellar XR): Initial: 300 mg or 450 mg once daily should be considered; dosage may be increased by 300 to 450 mg daily increments at weekly intervals to desired clinical response.

Conversion to monotherapy, partial seizures (epilepsy): Patients receiving concomitant antiepileptic drugs (AEDs):

Children 4 to 16 years (U.S. labeling) or 6 to 16 years (Canadian labeling): Immediate release (Trileptal): Initial: 8 to 10 mg/kg/day in twice daily divided doses, while simultaneously initiating the dose reduction of concomitant antiepileptic drugs; the concomitant drugs should be withdrawn over 3 to 6 weeks. Oxcarbazepine dose may be increased by a maximum of 10 mg/kg/day at weekly intervals. See below for recommended total daily dose by weight.

Adults: Immediate release (Trileptal): Initial: 600 mg daily in 2 divided doses while simultaneously reducing the dose of concomitant AEDs. Withdraw concomitant AEDs completely over 3 to 6 weeks, while increasing the oxcarbazepine dose in increments of 600 mg daily at weekly intervals, reaching the maximum oxcarbazepine dose (2400 mg daily) in about 2 to 4 weeks (lower doses have been effective in patients in whom monotherapy has been initiated).

Initiation of monotherapy, partial seizures (epilepsy): Patients not receiving prior AEDs:

Children 4 to 16 years (U.S. labeling) or 6 to 16 years (Canadian labeling): Immediate release (Trileptal): Initial: 8 to 10 mg/kg/day in twice daily divided doses; doses may be titrated by 5 mg/kg/day every third day. See below for recommended total daily dose by weight.

Range of maintenance doses by weight during monotherapy:

20 kg: 600 to 900 mg daily
25 to 30 kg: 900 to 1200 mg daily
35 to 40 kg: 900 to 1500 mg daily
45 kg: 1200 to 1500 mg daily
50 to 55 kg: 1200 to 1800 mg daily
60 to 65 kg: 1200 to 2100 mg daily
70 kg: 1500 to 2100 mg daily

Adults: Immediate release (Trileptal): Initial: 600 mg daily in 2 divided doses. Increase dose by 300 mg daily every third day to a dose of 1200 mg daily. Higher dosages (2400 mg daily) have been shown to be effective in patients converted to monotherapy from other AEDs.

Conversion from immediate release (Trileptal) to extended release (Oxtellar XR): Children ≥6 years, Adolescents, and Adults: Higher doses of Oxtellar XR may be necessary.

Dosage adjustment with concomitant antiepileptic drugs (AEDs): Children ≥6 years, Adolescents, and Adults: Extended release (Oxtellar XR): Concomitant use with enzyme-inducing antiepileptic drugs (eg, carbamazepine, phenobarbital, phenytoin): Consider initiating dose at 900 mg once daily.

Dosing adjustment in renal impairment:

Mild-to-moderate impairment: There are no dosage adjustments provided in the manufacturer's labeling.

Severe impairment (CrCl <30 mL/minute): Immediate release (Trileptal), Extended release (Oxtellar XR): Therapy should be initiated at one-half the usual starting dose (300 mg daily in adults) and increased slowly to achieve desired clinical response (eg, 300 to 450 mg daily at weekly intervals).

ESRD (on dialysis): Immediate release formulations should be used instead of extended release formulation.

Dosing adjustment in hepatic impairment:

Mild-to-moderate impairment: No dosage adjustments necessary.

Severe impairment:

Immediate release (Trileptal): There are no dosage adjustments provided in the manufacturer's labeling; Use caution (has not been studied).

Extended release (Oxtellar XR): There are no dosage adjustments provided in the manufacturer's labeling; use is not recommended (has not been studied).

Administration

Immediate release: Administer twice daily without regard to meals.

Suspension: Prior to using for the first time, firmly insert the plastic adapter provided with the bottle. Cover adapter with child-resistant cap when not in use. Shake bottle for at least 10 seconds, remove child-resistant cap, and insert the oral dosing syringe provided to withdraw appropriate dose. Dose may be taken directly from oral syringe or may be mixed in a small glass of water immediately prior to swallowing. Rinse syringe with warm water after use and allow to dry thoroughly. Discard any unused portion after 7 weeks of first opening bottle.

Extended release: Administer once daily on an empty stomach at least 1 hour before or 2 hours after food. Swallow whole; do not cut, crush, or chew the tablets.

Hazardous agent; use appropriate precautions for handling and disposal (NIOSH 2014 [group 2]).

Monitoring Parameters Seizure frequency; serum sodium as deemed necessary (particularly during first 3 months of therapy); symptoms of CNS depression (dizziness, headache, somnolence); hypersensitivity reactions. Additional serum sodium monitoring recommended during maintenance treatment in patients receiving other medications known to decrease sodium levels, in patients with signs/symptoms of hyponatremia, and in patients with an increase in seizure frequency or severity. Periodic thyroid function tests (particularly pediatric patients) and CBC. Monitor for suicidality (eg, suicidal thoughts, depression, behavioral changes). Serum levels of concomitant antiepileptic drugs during titration as necessary.

Reference Range The metabolite of oxcarbazepine, 10-monohydroxy metabolite (MHD), is considered the active entity primarily responsible for the therapeutic effects. A number of studies have suggested optimal MHD concentrations for efficacy may range from 2 to 55 mcg/mL and some experts suggest a target range of 8 to 35 mcg/mL based on clinical experience; however, a clear correlation between plasma concentrations and therapeutic response has not been demonstrated. Therapeutic drug monitoring of MHD is not routinely warranted; however, it may be beneficial in optimizing seizure control in the following situations: Extremes of age, during pregnancy, to investigate the correlation between drug concentrations and toxicity especially with concurrent disease states such as renal impairment, to identify potential drug interactions, to assess reasons for therapeutic failure, or to rule out noncompliance (Bring, 2008; May 2003).

Additional Information At steady state, the extended release product administered once daily is not bioequivalent to the same daily dose of the immediate release formulation administered twice daily.

Dosage Forms

Suspension, Oral:

Trileptal: 300 mg/5 mL (250 mL)
Generic: 300 mg/5 mL (250 mL)

Tablet, Oral:

Trileptal: 150 mg, 300 mg, 600 mg
Generic: 150 mg, 300 mg, 600 mg

Tablet Extended Release 24 Hour, Oral:

Oxtellar XR: 150 mg, 300 mg, 600 mg

◆ **Oxecta** *see* OxyCODONE *on page 1538*
◆ **Oxecta [DSC]** *see* OxyCODONE *on page 1538*
◆ **Oxeze Turbuhaler (Can)** *see* Formoterol *on page 926*

Oxiconazole (oks i KON a zole)

Brand Names: U.S. Oxistat
Brand Names: Canada Oxistat®
Index Terms Oxiconazole Nitrate
Pharmacologic Category Antifungal Agent, Imidazole Derivative; Antifungal Agent, Topical
Use
Cream: Treatment of tinea pedis (athlete's foot), tinea cruris (jock itch), tinea corporis (ringworm), and tinea (pityriasis) versicolor
Lotion: Treatment of tinea pedis (athlete's foot), tinea cruris (jock itch), tinea corporis (ringworm)
Pregnancy Risk Factor B
Dosage Topical: Children ≥12 years, Adolescents, and Adults:
Tinea corporis/tinea cruris: Cream, lotion: Apply to affected areas 1-2 times daily for 2 weeks
Tinea pedis: Cream, lotion: Apply to affected areas 1-2 times daily for 1 month
Tinea versicolor: Cream: Apply to affected areas once daily for 2 weeks
Additional Information Complete prescribing information should be consulted for additional detail.
Dosage Forms
Cream, External:
Oxistat: 1% (30 g, 60 g, 90 g)
Lotion, External:
Oxistat: 1% (30 mL, 60 mL)

◆ **Oxiconazole Nitrate** *see* Oxiconazole *on page 1536*
◆ **Oxilapine Succinate** *see* Loxapine *on page 1255*
◆ **Oxistat** *see* Oxiconazole *on page 1536*
◆ **Oxistat® (Can)** *see* Oxiconazole *on page 1536*

Oxitropium [INT] (oks i TROE pe um)

International Brand Names Oxivent (BE, CH, DE, GB, IE, IT, LU); Tersigan (JP); Tersigat (DE, FR); Ventilat (DE); Ventox (FI)
Index Terms Oxitropium Bromide
Pharmacologic Category Anticholinergic Agent
Reported Use Treatment of bronchospasm associated with chronic obstructive pulmonary disease (COPD)
Dosage Range Adults: Inhalation: 100-200 mcg (2 puffs) 2-3 times/day
Product Availability Product available in various countries; not currently available in the U.S.
Dosage Forms
Aerosal for oral inhalation, as bromide: 100 mcg/metered inhalation

◆ **Oxitropium Bromide** *see* Oxitropium [INT] *on page 1536*
◆ **Oxpam® (Can)** *see* Oxazepam *on page 1532*
◆ **Oxpentifylline** *see* Pentoxifylline *on page 1618*
◆ **Oxpram® (Can)** *see* Oxazepam *on page 1532*
◆ **Oxsoralen** *see* Methoxsalen (Topical) *on page 1331*
◆ **Oxsoralen Ultra** *see* Methoxsalen (Systemic) *on page 1330*
◆ **Oxtellar XR** *see* OXcarbazepine *on page 1532*
◆ **Oxybate** *see* Sodium Oxybate *on page 1908*
◆ **Oxybutyn (Can)** *see* Oxybutynin *on page 1536*

Oxybutynin (oks i BYOO ti nin)

Brand Names: U.S. Ditropan XL; Gelnique; Oxytrol; Oxytrol For Women [OTC]
Brand Names: Canada Apo-Oxybutynin; Ditropan XL; Dom-Oxybutynin; Gelnique; Mylan-Oxybutynin; Novo-Oxybutynin; Nu-Oxybutyn; Oxybutyn; Oxybutynine; Oxytrol; PHL-Oxybutynin; PMS-Oxybutynin; Riva-Oxybutynin; Uromax
Index Terms Ditropan; Oxybutynin Chloride
Pharmacologic Category Antispasmodic Agent, Urinary
Additional Appendix Information
Beers Criteria - Potentially Inappropriate Medications for Geriatrics *on page 2271*
Use Treatment of symptoms associated with overactive uninhibited neurogenic or reflex neurogenic bladder (eg, urgency, frequency, leakage, urge incontinence, dysuria); treatment of symptoms associated with detrusor overactivity due to a neurological condition (eg, spina bifida) (extended release tablet only)
Pregnancy Risk Factor B
Pregnancy Considerations Adverse events were not observed in animal reproduction studies.
Breast-Feeding Considerations It is not known if oxybutynin is excreted into breast milk. The manufacturer recommends that caution be used if administered to a nursing woman. Suppression of lactation has been reported.
Contraindications Hypersensitivity to oxybutynin or any component of the formulation; patients with or at risk for uncontrolled narrow-angle glaucoma, urinary retention, gastric retention or conditions with severely decreased GI motility

OTC labeling: When used for self-medication, do not use if you have pain or burning when urinating, blood in urine, unexplained lower back or side pain, cloudy or foul-smelling urine; in males; age <18 years; only experience accidental urine loss when cough, sneeze, or laugh; diagnosis of urinary or gastric retention; glaucoma; hypersensitivity to oxybutynin.
Warnings/Precautions Cases of angioedema involving the face, lips, tongue, and/or larynx have been reported with oral oxybutynin; some cases have occurred after a single dose. Discontinue immediately if tongue, hypopharynx, or larynx is involved; promptly initiate appropriate management. Use with caution in patients with bladder outflow obstruction (may increase the risk of urinary retention), treated angle-closure glaucoma (use is contraindicated in uncontrolled narrow-angle glaucoma), hyperthyroidism, coronary artery disease, heart failure, hypertension, cardiac arrhythmias, hepatic or renal impairment, prostatic hyperplasia (may cause urinary retention), hiatal hernia, myasthenia gravis, dementia. Use with caution in patients with decreased GI motility or gastrointestinal obstructive disorders (eg, ulcerative colitis, intestinal atony, pyloric stenosis); may increase the risk of gastric retention. In patients with ulcerative colitis, use may decrease gastric motility to the point of increasing the risk of paralytic ileus or toxic megacolon. Use with caution in patients with gastroesophageal reflux or with medications that may exacerbate esophagitis (eg, bisphosphonates). May increase the risk of heat prostration. Anticholinergics may cause agitation, confusion, drowsiness, dizziness, hallucinations, headache, and/or blurred vision, which may impair physical or mental abilities; patients must be cautioned about performing tasks which require mental alertness (eg, operating machinery or driving). Dose reduction or discontinuation should be considered if CNS effects occur. Effects may be potentiated when used with other sedative drugs or ethanol.

Potentially significant drug-drug interactions may exist, requiring dose or frequency adjustment, additional monitoring, and/or selection of alternative therapy. This medication is associated with potent anticholinergic properties which may be inappropriate in older adults depending on comorbidities (eg, dementia, delirium) (Beers Criteria).

The extended release formulation consists of drug within a nondeformable matrix; following drug release/absorption, the matrix/shell is expelled in the stool. The use of nondeformable products in patients with known stricture/narrowing of the GI tract has been associated with symptoms of obstruction. Transdermal patch may contain conducting metal (eg, aluminum); remove patch prior to MRI. When using the topical gel, cover treatment area with clothing after gel has dried to minimize transferring medication to others. Discontinue gel if skin irritation occurs. Gel contains ethanol; do not expose to open flame or smoking until gel has dried.

When used for self-medication (OTC), other causes of frequent urination (UTI, diabetes, early pregnancy, other serious conditions) may need to be considered prior to use. Patients should contact a health care provider if symptoms do not improve within 2 weeks of initial use or for new or worsening symptoms.

Adverse Reactions

Oral:

Cardiovascular: Cardiac arrhythmia (sinus), decreased blood pressure, chest pain, edema, flushing, hypertension, palpitations, peripheral edema

Central nervous system: Confusion, depression, dizziness, drowsiness, fatigue, headache, insomnia, nervousness, pain

Dermatologic: Pruritus, xeroderma

Endocrine & metabolic: Fluid retention, hyperglycemia

Gastrointestinal: Abdominal pain, constipation, diarrhea, dry throat, dyspepsia, dysphagia, eructation, flatulence, gastroesophageal reflux disease, nausea, unpleasant taste, vomiting, xerostomia

Genitourinary: Cystitis, dysuria, pollakiuria, urinary hesitancy, urinary retention, urinary tract infection

Infection: Fungal infection

Neuromuscular & skeletal: Arthralgia, back pain, flank pain, limb pain, weakness

Ophthalmic: Blurred vision, eye irritation, keratoconjunctivitis sicca, xerophthalmia

Respiratory: Asthma, bronchitis, cough, dry nose, dry throat, hoarseness, nasal congestion, nasal dryness, nasopharyngitis, pharyngolaryngeal pain, sinus congestion, upper respiratory tract infection

Miscellaneous: Increased thirst

Rare but important or life-threatening: Anaphylaxis, anorexia, cycloplegia, decreased gastrointestinal motility, glaucoma, hallucination, hypersensitivity reaction, impotence, suppressed lactation, memory impairment, mydriasis, psychotic reaction, prolonged Q-T interval on ECG, seizure, tachycardia

Topical gel:

Central nervous system: Dizziness, fatigue, headache

Dermatologic: Pruritus

Gastrointestinal: Constipation, gastroenteritis, xerostomia

Genitourinary: Urinary tract infection

Local: Application site reaction (includes anesthesia, dermatitis, erythema, irritation, pain, papules, pruritus, rash)

Ophthalmic: Blurred vision, conjunctivitis, xerophthalmia

Respiratory: Nasopharyngitis, upper respiratory tract infection

Transdermal:

Gastrointestinal: Constipation, diarrhea, xerostomia

Genitourinary: Dysuria

Local: Erythema, localized vesiculation, macular eruption, pruritus, skin rash

Ophthalmic: Visual disturbance

Rare but important or life-threatening: Dizziness, drowsiness

Drug Interactions

Metabolism/Transport Effects **Substrate** of CYP3A4 (minor); **Note:** Assignment of Major/Minor substrate status based on clinically relevant drug interaction potential; **Inhibits** CYP2C8 (weak), CYP2D6 (weak), CYP3A4 (weak)

Avoid Concomitant Use

Avoid concomitant use of Oxybutynin with any of the following: Aclidinium; Glucagon; Ipratropium (Oral Inhalation); Pimozide; Potassium Chloride; Tiotropium; Umeclidinium

Increased Effect/Toxicity

Oxybutynin may increase the levels/effects of: AbobotulinumtoxinA; Analgesics (Opioid); Anticholinergic Agents; ARIPiprazole; Cannabinoid-Containing Products; Dofetilide; Glucagon; Hydrocodone; Lomitapide; Mirabegron; OnabotulinumtoxinA; Pimozide; Potassium Chloride; RimabotulinumtoxinB; Thiazide Diuretics; Tiotropium; Topiramate

The levels/effects of Oxybutynin may be increased by: Aclidinium; Alcohol (Ethyl); Ipratropium (Oral Inhalation); Mianserin; Pramlintide; Umeclidinium

Decreased Effect

Oxybutynin may decrease the levels/effects of: Acetylcholinesterase Inhibitors; Itopride; Secretin

The levels/effects of Oxybutynin may be decreased by: Acetylcholinesterase Inhibitors

Storage/Stability

Immediate release tablet and syrup: Store at 20°C to 25°C (68°F to 77°F). Protect from light.

Extended release tablet: Store at 25°C (77°F); excursions permitted to 15°C to 30°C (59°F to 86°F). Protect from moisture and humidity.

Topical gel (pump or sachets): Store at 25°C (77°F); excursions permitted to 15°C to 30°C (59°F to 86°F). Protect from moisture and humidity. Keep gel away from open flame. Do not store sachets outside the sealed pouch; apply immediately after removal from the protective pouch. Discard used sachets such that accidental application or ingestion by children, pets, or others is avoided.

Transdermal patch: Store at 20°C to 25°C (68°F to 77°F). Protect from moisture and humidity. Do not store outside the sealed pouch; apply immediately after removal from the protective pouch. Discard used patches such that accidental application or ingestion by children, pets, or others is avoided.

Mechanism of Action Direct antispasmodic effect on smooth muscle, also inhibits the action of acetylcholine on smooth muscle (exhibits 1/5 the anticholinergic activity of atropine, but has 4-10 times the antispasmodic activity); does not block effects at skeletal muscle or at autonomic ganglia; increases bladder capacity, decreases uninhibited contractions, and delays desire to void, therefore, decreases urgency and frequency

Pharmacodynamics/Kinetics

Onset of action: Oral: Immediate release: 30-60 minutes

Peak effect: 3-6 hours

Duration: Oral: Immediate release: 6-10 hours; Extended release: Up to 24 hours

Absorption: Oral: Rapid and well absorbed; Transdermal: High

Distribution: IV: V_d: 193 L

Protein binding: >99% primarily to alpha$_1$-acid glycoprotein

Metabolism: Hepatic via CYP3A4; Oral: High first-pass metabolism; forms active and inactive metabolites

Bioavailability: Oral: ~6%

Half-life elimination: IV: ~2 hours (parent drug), 7-8 hours (metabolites); Oral: Immediate release: ~2-3 hours; Extended release: ~13 hours; Transdermal: 30-64 hours

Time to peak, serum: Oral: Immediate release: ~60 minutes; Extended release: 4-6 hours; Transdermal: 24-48 hours

Excretion: Urine, as metabolites and unchanged drug (<0.1%)

Dosage Overactive bladder:

Oral:

Children: >5 years: Immediate release: 5 mg twice daily; maximum: 5 mg 3 times daily

Children ≥6 years: Extended release: 5 mg once daily; adjust dose in 5 mg increments; maximum: 20 mg once daily

Adults:

Immediate release: 5 mg 2-3 times daily; maximum: 5 mg 4 times daily

Extended release: Initial: 5-10 mg once daily, adjust dose in 5 mg increments at weekly intervals; maximum: 30 mg once daily

Elderly: Immediate release: Initial: 2.5 mg 2-3 times daily; increase cautiously

Topical gel: Adults:

Gelnique 3%: Apply 3 pumps (84 mg) once daily

Gelnique 10%: Apply contents of 1 sachet (100 mg/g) once daily

Transdermal: Adults: Apply one 3.9 mg/day patch twice weekly (every 3-4 days)

Dosage adjustment in renal impairment: No dosage adjustment provided in the manufacturer's labeling (not studied); use with caution.

Dosage adjustment in hepatic impairment: No dosage adjustment provided in the manufacturer's labeling (not studied); use with caution.

Dietary Considerations Food causes a slight delay in the absorption of the oral solution and bioavailability is increased by ~25%. Absorption of the extended release tablet is not affected by food. May be taken without regard to meals.

Administration

Oral: Administer without regard to meals. Extended release tablets must be swallowed whole with liquid; do not crush, divide, or chew; take at approximately the same time each day.

Topical gel: For topical use only. Apply to clean, dry, intact skin on abdomen, thighs, or upper arms/shoulders. Wash hands after use. Cover treated area with clothing after gel has dried to prevent transfer of medication to others. Do not bathe, shower, or swim until 1 hour after gel applied. Do not apply to recently shaved skin.

Gelnique 3%: Prior to initial use, press pump 4 times to prime pump; discard any gel dispensed from pump during priming. Rotate application sites to avoid skin irritation.

Gelnique 10%: Rotate site; do not apply to same site on consecutive days.

Transdermal: Apply to clean, dry skin on abdomen, hip, or buttock. Select a new site for each new system (avoid reapplication to same site within 7 days). Wear patch under clothing; do not expose to sunlight.

Monitoring Parameters Incontinence episodes, postvoid residual (PVR)

Dosage Forms

Gel, Transdermal:

Gelnique: 10% (1 g); 3% (92 g)

Patch Twice Weekly, Transdermal:

Oxytrol: 3.9 mg/24 hr (1 ea, 2 ea, 4 ea, 8 ea)

Oxytrol For Women [OTC]: 3.9 mg/24 hr (8 ea); 3.9 mg/24hr (4 ea)

Syrup, Oral:

Generic: 5 mg/5 mL (473 mL)

Tablet, Oral:

Generic: 5 mg

Tablet Extended Release 24 Hour, Oral:

Ditropan XL: 5 mg, 10 mg, 15 mg

Generic: 5 mg, 10 mg, 15 mg

◆ **Oxybutynin Chloride** *see* Oxybutynin *on page* 1536

◆ **Oxybutynine (Can)** *see* Oxybutynin *on page* 1536

◆ **Oxycodan® (Can)** *see* Oxycodone and Aspirin *on page* 1542

OxyCODONE (oks i KOE done)

Brand Names: U.S. Oxecta [DSC]; OxyCONTIN; Roxicodone

Brand Names: Canada ACT Oxycodone CR; Apo-Oxycodone CR; CO Oxycodone CR; Oxy.IR; OxyContin; Oxy-NEO; PMS-Oxycodone; PMS-Oxycodone CR; Supeudol

Index Terms Dihydrohydroxycodeinone; Oxecta; Oxycodone Hydrochloride

Pharmacologic Category Analgesic, Opioid

Additional Appendix Information

Opioid Conversion Table *on page* 2232

Use

Immediate release formulations: Management of moderate to severe pain, normally used in combination with non-opioid analgesics

Extended release formulation: Management of pain severe enough to require daily, around-the-clock, long-term opioid treatment and for which alternative treatment options are inadequate.

Limitations of use: Because of the risks of addiction, abuse, and misuse with opioids, even at recommended doses, and because of the greater risks of overdose and death with extended-release opioid formulations, reserve oxycodone ER for use in patients for whom alternative treatment options (eg, nonopioid analgesics, immediate-release opioids) are ineffective, not tolerated, or would be otherwise inadequate to provide sufficient management of pain. Oxycodone ER is not indicated as an as-needed analgesic.

Pregnancy Risk Factor B/C (manufacturer specific)

Pregnancy Considerations Adverse events were observed in some animal reproduction studies. Opioids cross the placenta. Oxycodone should not be used immediately prior to or during labor.

[U.S. Boxed Warning]: Prolonged maternal use of opioids during pregnancy can cause neonatal withdrawal syndrome in the newborn which may be life-threatening if not recognized and treated according to protocols developed by neonatology experts. If prolonged opioid therapy is required in a pregnant woman, ensure treatment is available and warn patient of risk to the neonate. If chronic opioid exposure occurs in pregnancy, adverse events in the newborn (including withdrawal) may occur; monitoring of the neonate is recommended. The minimum effective dose should be used if opioids are needed (Chou, 2009). Neonatal abstinence syndrome following opioid exposure may present with autonomic (eg, fever, temperature instability), gastrointestinal (eg, diarrhea, vomiting, poor feeding/weight gain), or neurologic (eg, high-pitched crying, increased muscle tone, irritability, seizure, tremor) symptoms (Dow, 2012; Hudak, 2012).

Long-term opioid use may cause secondary hypogonadism, which may lead to sexual dysfunction or infertility (Brennan, 2013).

Breast-Feeding Considerations Oxycodone is excreted into breast milk. Breast-feeding is not recommended by the manufacturer. Sedation and/or respiratory depression may occur in the infant; symptoms of opioid withdrawal may occur following the cessation of breast-feeding. Nursing infants exposed to large doses of opioids should be monitored for apnea and sedation. Use caution in a woman who may be an ultrarapid metabolizer; oxycodone is a substrate for CYP2D6 and their nursing infants may be at higher risk for adverse events (Montgomery, 2012).

Contraindications Hypersensitivity to oxycodone or any component of the formulation; significant respiratory depression; hypercarbia; acute or severe bronchial asthma; paralytic ileus (known or suspected); GI obstruction

Warnings/Precautions May cause CNS depression, which may impair physical or mental abilities; patients must be cautioned about performing tasks which require mental alertness (eg, operating machinery or driving). Potentially significant drug interactions may exist, requiring dose or frequency adjustment, additional monitoring, and/or selection of alternative therapy. Effects may be potentiated when used with other CNS depressants (eg, sedatives, anxiolytics, hypnotics, neuroleptics, other opioids). Use with caution in patients with hypersensitivity reactions to other phenanthrene derivative opioid agonists (morphine, hydrocodone, hydromorphone, levorphanol, oxymorphone). Use with caution in pancreatitis or biliary tract disease, acute alcoholism (including delirium tremens), morbid obesity, adrenocortical insufficiency, history of seizure disorders, hypothyroidism (including myxedema), prostatic hyperplasia, urethral stricture, and toxic psychosis. Use with caution and monitor for respiratory depression in patients with significant chronic obstructive pulmonary disease or cor pulmonale, and patients having a substantially decreased respiratory reserve, hypoxia, hypercarbia, or preexisting respiratory depression, particularly when initiating therapy and titrating with oxycodone; even therapeutic doses may decrease respiratory drive to the point of apnea. Consider the use of alternative nonopioid analgesics in these patients. May obscure diagnosis or clinical course of patients with acute abdominal conditions. Avoid use in patients with CNS depression/coma as these patients are susceptible to intracranial effects of CO_2 retention.

Use with caution in the elderly, debilitated, or cachectic patients, and hepatic or renal dysfunction. Hemodynamic effects (hypotension, orthostasis) may be exaggerated in patients with hypovolemia, concurrent vasodilating drugs, or in patients with head injury. Monitor for symptoms of hypotension following initiation or dose titration. Respiratory depressant effects and capacity to elevate CSF pressure may be exaggerated in presence of head injury, other intracranial lesion, or preexisting intracranial pressure. May cause constipation which may be problematic in patients with unstable angina and patients post-myocardial infarction. Concurrent use of mixed agonist/antagonist analgesics (eg, pentazocine, nalbuphine, butorphanol) or partial agonist (eg, buprenorphine) analgesics may precipitate withdrawal symptoms and/or reduced analgesic efficacy in patients following prolonged therapy with mu opioid agonists. Taper dose gradually when discontinuing. Potentially significant interactions may exist, requiring dose or frequency adjustment, additional monitoring, and/or selection of alternative therapy.

Extended release tablets: Therapy should only be prescribed by healthcare professionals familiar with the use of potent opioids for chronic pain. **[U.S. Boxed Warning]: May cause serious, life-threatening, or fatal respiratory depression. Monitor closely for respiratory depression, especially during initiation or dose escalation. Patients should swallow tablets whole; crushing, chewing, or dissolving can cause rapid release and a potentially fatal dose.** Carbon dioxide retention from opioid-induced respiratory depression can exacerbate the sedating effects of opioids. **[U.S. Boxed Warning]: Use with all CYP3A4 inhibitors may result in increased effects and potentially fatal respiratory depression. In addition, discontinuation of a concomitant CYP 3A4 inducer may result in increased oxycodone concentrations. Monitor patients receiving any CYP 3A4 inhibitor or inducer.** Tablets may be difficult to swallow and could become lodged in throat; patients with swallowing difficulties may be at increased risk. Cases of intestinal obstruction or diverticulitis exacerbation have also been reported, including cases requiring medical intervention to remove the tablet; patients with an underlying GI disease (eg, esophageal cancer, colon cancer) may be at increased risk. **[U.S. Boxed Warning]: Users are exposed to the risks of addiction, abuse, and misuse, potentially leading to overdose and death. Assess each patient's risk prior to prescribing; monitor all patients regularly for development of these behaviors or conditions.** Risk of opioid abuse is increased in patients with a history or family history of alcohol or drug abuse or mental illness. **[U.S. Boxed Warning]: Accidental ingestion of even one dose, especially in children, can result in a fatal overdose of oxycodone. [U.S. Boxed Warning]: Prolonged maternal use of opioids during pregnancy can cause neonatal withdrawal syndrome in the newborn which may be life-threatening if not recognized and treated according to protocols developed by neonatology experts. If prolonged opioid therapy is required in a pregnant woman, ensure treatment is available and warn patient of risk to the neonate.** Signs and symptoms include irritability, hyperactivity and abnormal sleep pattern, high pitched cry, tremor, vomiting, diarrhea and failure to gain weight. Onset, duration and severity depend on the drug used, duration of use, maternal dose, and rate of drug elimination by the newborn.

Oral solutions: **[U.S. Boxed Warning]: Highly concentrated oral solution (20 mg/mL) should only be used in opioid tolerant patients (taking ≥30 mg/day of oxycodone or equivalent for ≥1 week). [U.S. Boxed Warning]: Orders for oxycodone oral solutions (20 mg/mL or 5 mg/5 mL) should be clearly written to include the intended dose (in mg vs mL) and the intended product concentration to be dispensed to avoid potential dosing errors. Products should be stored out of reach of children; seek immediate medical care in the event of accidental ingestion.**

Benzyl alcohol and derivatives: Some dosage forms may contain sodium benzoate/benzoic acid; benzoic acid (benzoate) is a metabolite of benzyl alcohol; large amounts of benzyl alcohol (≥99 mg/kg/day) have been associated with a potentially fatal toxicity ("gasping syndrome") in neonates; the "gasping syndrome" consists of metabolic acidosis, respiratory distress, gasping respirations, CNS dysfunction (including convulsions, intracranial hemorrhage), hypotension, and cardiovascular collapse (AAP, 1997; CDC, 1982); some data suggests that benzoate displaces bilirubin from protein binding sites (Ahlfors, 2001); avoid or use dosage forms containing benzyl alcohol derivative with caution in neonates. See manufacturer's labeling.

Adverse Reactions

Cardiovascular: Orthostatic hypotension

Central nervous system: Abnormal dreams, abnormality in thinking, anxiety, chills, confusion, dizziness, drowsiness, dysphoria, euphoria, headache, insomnia, nervousness, twitching

Dermatologic: Diaphoresis, pruritus, skin rash

Gastrointestinal: Abdominal pain, anorexia, constipation, diarrhea, dyspepsie, gastritis, hiccups, nausea, xerostomia, vomiting

Miscellaneous: Fever

Neuromuscular & skeletal: Weakness

Respiratory: Dyspnea

Rare but important or life-threatening: Abnormal stools (tablet in stool [some controlled release dosage forms]), agitation, amnesia, anaphylactoid reaction, anaphylaxis, chest pain, dehydration, depression, depression of ST segment on ECG, diverticulitis (exacerbation), dysphagia (or other swallowing difficulties due to properties of controlled release tablets), dysuria, edema (including facial and peripheral), emotional lability, eructation, hallucination, hematuria, histamine release, hyperalgesia, hyperkinesia, hypoesthesia, hypogonadism (Brennan, 2013; Debono, 2011), hyponatremia, hypotonia, increased intracranial pressure, intestinal obstruction, malaise, paresthesia, seizure, SIADH, speech disturbance, stomatitis, stupor, syncope, tremor, urinary retention, vertigo, withdrawal syndrome

Drug Interactions

Metabolism/Transport Effects Substrate of CYP2D6 (minor), CYP3A4 (major); **Note:** Assignment of Major/Minor substrate status based on clinically relevant drug interaction potential

Avoid Concomitant Use

Avoid concomitant use of OxyCODONE with any of the following: Azelastine (Nasal); Conivaptan; Fusidic Acid (Systemic); Idelalisib; Orphenadrine; Paraldehyde; Thalidomide

Increased Effect/Toxicity

OxyCODONE may increase the levels/effects of: Alcohol (Ethyl); Alvimopan; Azelastine (Nasal); Buprenorphine; CNS Depressants; Desmopressin; Diuretics; Hydrocodone; Methotrimeprazine; Metyrosine; Mirtazapine; Orphenadrine; Paraldehyde; Pramipexole; ROPINIRole; Rotigotine; Selective Serotonin Reuptake Inhibitors; Suvorexant; Thalidomide; Zolpidem

The levels/effects of OxyCODONE may be increased by: Amphetamines; Anticholinergic Agents; Antipsychotic Agents (Phenothiazines); Brimonidine (Topical); Cannabis; Conivaptan; CYP3A4 Inhibitors (Moderate); CYP3A4 Inhibitors (Strong); Dasatinib; Doxylamine; Dronabinol; Droperidol; Fusidic Acid (Systemic); HydrOXYzine; Idelalisib; Ivacaftor; Kava Kava; Luliconazole; Magnesium Sulfate; MAO Inhibitors; Methotrimeprazine; Mifepristone; Nabilone; Perampanel; Rufinamide; Simeprevir; Sodium Oxybate; Stiripentol; Succinylcholine; Tapentadol; Tetrahydrocannabinol; Voriconazole

Decreased Effect

OxyCODONE may decrease the levels/effects of: Pegvisomant

The levels/effects of OxyCODONE may be decreased by: Ammonium Chloride; Bosentan; CYP3A4 Inducers (Moderate); CYP3A4 Inducers (Strong); Dabrafenib; Deferasirox; Mitotane; Mixed Agonist / Antagonist Opioids; Naltrexone; Rifampin; Siltuximab; St Johns Wort; Tocilizumab

Storage/Stability Store at 25°C (77°F); excursions permitted between 15°C to 30°C (59°F to 86°F). Protect from light.

Mechanism of Action Binds to opiate receptors in the CNS, causing inhibition of ascending pain pathways, altering the perception of and response to pain; produces generalized CNS depression

Pharmacodynamics/Kinetics

Onset of action: Pain relief: Immediate release: 10 to 15 minutes

Peak effect: Immediate release: 0.5 to 1 hour

Duration: Immediate release: 3 to 6 hours; Extended release: ≤12 hours

Distribution: V_d: 2.6 L/kg; distributed to skeletal muscle, liver, intestinal tract, lungs, spleen, and brain

Protein binding: ~45%

Metabolism: Hepatically via CYP3A4 to noroxycodone (has weak analgesic), noroxymorphone, and alpha- and beta-noroxycodol. CYP2D6 mediated metabolism produces oxymorphone (has analgesic activity; low plasma concentrations), alpha- and beta-oxymorphol.

Bioavailability: Extended release, immediate release: 60% to 87%

Half-life elimination: Immediate release: 2 to 4 hours; Extended release: ~5 hours

Time to peak, plasma: Immediate release: 1.2 to 1.9 hours; Extended release: 4 to 5 hours

Excretion: Urine (~19% as parent; >64% as metabolites)

Dosage Oral: **Note:** All doses should be titrated to appropriate effect:

Children (off-label use): Immediate release, initial dose: 0.1 to 0.2 mg/kg/dose (moderate pain) or 0.2 mg/kg/dose (severe pain) (APS 6th edition). For severe chronic pain, administer on a regularly scheduled basis, every 4 to 6 hours, at the lowest dose that will achieve adequate analgesia.

Adults:

Immediate release: Initial: 5 to 15 mg every 4 to 6 hours as needed; dosing range: 5 to 20 mg per dose (APS 6th edition). For severe chronic pain, administer on a regularly scheduled basis, every 4 to 6 hours, at the lowest dose that will achieve adequate analgesia.

Extended release: **Note:** Oxycodone ER 60 mg and 80 mg strengths, a single dose >40 mg, or a total dose of >80 mg daily are for use only in opioid-tolerant patients. Opioid tolerance is defined as: Patients already taking at least 60 mg of oral morphine daily, 25 mcg of transdermal fentanyl per hour, 30 mg of oral oxycodone daily, 8 mg oral hydromorphone daily, or an equivalent dose of another opioid for at least 1 week.

Opioid naive (use as the first opioid analgesic or use in patients who are **not** opioid tolerant): Initial: 10 mg every 12 hours

Conversion from other oral oxycodone formulations to extended release oxycodone: Initiate extended release oxycodone with one-half (1/2) the total daily oral oxycodone daily dose (mg/day) administered every 12 hours.

Conversion from other opioids to extended release oxycodone: Discontinue all other around-the-clock opioids when extended release oxycodone is initiated. Initiate with 10 mg every 12 hours. Substantial interpatient variability exists in relative potency. Therefore, it is safer to underestimate a patient's daily oral oxycodone requirement and provide breakthrough pain relief with rescue medication (eg, immediate release opioid) than to overestimate requirements.

Conversion from transdermal fentanyl to extended release oxycodone: For each 25 mcg/hour transdermal dose, substitute 10 mg extended release oxycodone every 12 hours; should be initiated 18 hours after the removal of the transdermal fentanyl patch.

Conversion from methadone to extended release oxycodone: Close monitoring is required when converting methadone to another opioid. Ratio between methadone and other opioid agonists varies widely according to previous dose exposure. Methadone has a long half-life and can accumulate in the plasma.

Concurrent CNS depressants: Reduce usual initial oxycodone dose by one-third (1/3) to one-half (1/2)

Dose adjustment: Doses may be adjusted every 1 to 2 days; the total daily oxycodone dose may be increased by 25% to 50%.

Discontinuation of therapy: Gradually titrate dose downward to prevent withdrawal signs/symptoms. Do not abruptly discontinue.

Dosage adjustment in renal impairment: Serum concentrations are increased ~50% in patients with CrCl <60 mL/minute; adjust dose based on clinical situation.

Dosage adjustment in hepatic impairment:

Immediate release: Reduced initial doses may be necessary (use a conservative approach to initial dosing); adjust dose based on clinical situation.

Extended release: Decrease initial dose to one-third (1/3) to one-half (1/2) the usual starting dose; titrate carefully.

Dietary Considerations Instruct patient to avoid high-fat meals when taking some products (food has no effect on the reformulated OxyContin).

Administration

Extended release: Swallow tablet whole. Do not moisten, dissolve, cut, crush, break, or chew extended release tablets. Extended release tablets are not indicated for rectal administration; increased risk of adverse events due to better rectal absorption. Extended release tablets should be administered one at a time and each followed with water immediately after placing in the mouth.

Immediate release (Oxecta): Must be swallowed whole with enough water to ensure complete swallowing immediately after placing in the mouth. The tablet should not be wet prior to placing in the mouth. Do not crush, chew, or dissolve the tablets. Do not administer via feeding tubes (eg, gastric, NG) due to potential for obstruction. The formulation uses technology designed to discourage common methods of tampering to prevent misuse/abuse.

Appropriate laxatives should be administered to avoid the constipating side effects associated with use. Antiemetics may be needed for persistent nausea.

Monitoring Parameters Pain relief, respiratory and mental status, blood pressure; signs of misuse, abuse, and addiction; signs or symptoms of hypogonadism or hypoadrenalism (Brennan, 2013)

Additional Information Oxecta utilizes Acura Pharmaceutical's Aversion® technology which may help discourage misuse and abuse potential. Reduced abuse potential of Oxecta compared to other immediate-release oxycodone tablet formulations has not been proven; the FDA is requiring Pfizer to complete a post-approval epidemiological study to determine whether the formulation actually results in a decrease of misuse/abuse. In one clinical trial in nondependent recreational opioid users, the "drug-liking" responses and safety of crushed Oxecta tablets were compared to crushed immediate-release oxycodone tablets following the self-administered intranasal use. A small difference in "drug-liking" scores was observed, with lower scores reported in the crushed Oxecta group. In regards to safety, there was an increased incidence of nasopharyngeal and facial adverse events in the Oxecta group. In addition, there was decreased ability in the Oxecta group to completely administer the two crushed Oxecta tablets intranasally within a set time period. However, whether these differences translate into a significant clinical difference is unknown. Of note, pharmacokinetic studies showed that Oxecta is bioequivalent with oxycodone immediate-release tablets with no differences in T_{max} and half-life when administered in the fasted state.

Dosage Forms

Capsule, Oral:

Generic: 5 mg

Concentrate, Oral:

Generic: 100 mg/5 mL (15 mL, 30 mL)

Solution, Oral:

Generic: 5 mg/5 mL (5 mL, 15 mL, 500 mL)

Tablet, Oral:

Roxicodone: 5 mg, 15 mg, 30 mg

Generic: 5 mg, 10 mg, 15 mg, 20 mg, 30 mg

Tablet ER 12 Hour Abuse-Deterrent, Oral:

OxyCONTIN: 10 mg, 15 mg, 20 mg, 30 mg, 40 mg, 60 mg, 80 mg

Generic: 10 mg, 20 mg, 40 mg, 80 mg

Oxycodone and Acetaminophen

(oks i KOE done & a seet a MIN oh fen)

Brand Names: U.S. Endocet; Percocet; Primlev; Roxicet; Xartemis XR; Xolox [DSC]

Brand Names: Canada Apo-Oxycodone/Acet; Endocet; Percocet; Percocet-Demi; PMS-Oxycodone-Acetaminophen; Ratio-Oxycocet; Rivacocet; Sandoz-Oxycodone/Acetaminophen

Index Terms Acetaminophen and Oxycodone; Tylox

Pharmacologic Category Analgesic Combination (Opioid); Analgesic, Opioid

Use

Acute pain (extended-release): Management of acute pain severe enough to require opioid treatment and for which alternative treatment options are inadequate.

Limitations of use: Because of the risks of addiction, abuse, misuse, overdose, and death with opioids, even at recommended doses, reserve extended-release (ER) for use in patients for whom alternative treatment options (eg, nonopioid analgesics) are ineffective, not tolerated, or would be otherwise inadequate.

Moderate to moderately severe pain (immediate release): Management of moderate to moderately-severe pain

Pregnancy Risk Factor C

Dosage Oral: Doses should be titrated to appropriate analgesic effects. **Note:** Initial dose is based on the **oxycodone** content; however, the maximum daily dose is based on the **acetaminophen** content.

Children and Adolescents (off-label; American Pain Society [APS], 2008): **Immediate-release:**

Moderate pain: Initial dose, **based on oxycodone content**: 0.1-0.2 mg/kg/dose. Doses typically given every 4-6 hours as needed; manufacturer's labeling recommends every 6 hours as needed; maxi mum initial oxycodone dose: 5 mg/dose. Do not exceed maximum daily acetaminophen dose: Children <45 kg: 90 mg/kg/day; Children ≥45 kg: 4000 mg daily

Severe pain: Initial dose, **based on oxycodone content**: 0.2 mg/kg/dose. Doses typically given every 4-6 hours as needed; manufacturer's labeling recommends every 6 hours as needed; maximum initial oxycodone dose: 10 mg. Do not exceed maximum daily acetaminophen dose: Children <45 kg: 90 mg/kg/day; Children ≥45 kg: 4000 mg daily

Adults:

Manufacturer's labeling:

Extended-release: Acute pain: Usual dose: 2 tablets every 12 hours; the second initial dose may be administered as early as 8 hours after the first initial dose if needed; subsequent doses are to be administered 2 tablets every 12 hours. Do not exceed acetaminophen 4 g daily. **NOTE:** Oxycodone/acetaminophen ER is not interchangeable with other oxycodone/acetaminophen products because of differing pharmacokinetic profiles that affect the frequency of administration.

Discontinuation: Do not stop abruptly in patients who may be physically dependent; gradually decrease the dose by 50% every 2 to 4 days to prevent signs and symptoms of withdrawal.

Immediate-release: Moderate to moderately severe pain: Initial dose, **based on oxycodone content**: 2.5-10 mg every 6 hours as needed. Titrate according to pain severity and individual response. Do not exceed acetaminophen 4 g daily.

Alternate recommendations (APS, 2008): **Immediate-release:**

Moderate pain (off-label): Initial dose, **based on oxycodone content**: 5 mg. Doses typically given every 4-6 hours as needed; manufacturer's labeling recommends every 6 hours as needed. Do not exceed acetaminophen 4 g daily.

Severe pain (off-label): Initial dose, **based on oxycodone content**: 10-20 mg. Doses typically given every 4-6 hours as needed; manufacturer's labeling recommends every 6 hours as needed. Do not exceed acetaminophen 4 g daily.

Elderly: No dosage adjustment provided in manufacturer's labeling; however, use with caution and consider decreasing the initial dose and/or increasing the frequency.

Severe pain (off-label dosing): **Immediate-release:** Elderly >70 years: Consider decreasing the initial dose **(based on oxycodone content)** by 25% to 50%, then titrating the dose upward or downward as needed; monitor frequently during titration. Do not exceed acetaminophen 4 g daily (APS, 2008).

Dosage adjustment in renal impairment:

Extended-release: Initial dose: One tablet every 12 hours; adjust dose as needed.

Immediate-release: There are no dosage adjustments provided in manufacturer's labeling. Use with caution; reduced clearance in severe impairment may require dosage adjustment.

Dosage adjustment in hepatic impairment:

Extended-release: Initial dose: One tablet every 12 hours; adjust dose as needed.

Immediate-release: There are no dosage adjustments provided in manufacturer's labeling. Use with caution; reduced clearance in severe impairment may require dosage adjustment.

Additional Information Complete prescribing information should be consulted for additional detail.

Dosage Forms

Solution, Oral: Oxycodone 5 mg and acetaminophen 325 mg per 5 mL

Roxicet: Oxycodone 5 mg and acetaminophen 325 mg per 5 mL

Tablet, Oral: 2.5/325: Oxycodone hydrochloride 2.5 mg and acetaminophen 325 mg; 5/325: Oxycodone hydrochloride 5 mg and acetaminophen 325 mg; 7.5/325: Oxycodone hydrochloride 7.5 mg and acetaminophen 325 mg; 10/325: Oxycodone hydrochloride 10 mg and acetaminophen 325 mg

Endocet 2.5/325: Oxycodone 2.5 mg and acetaminophen 325 mg

Endocet 5/325 [scored]: Oxycodone 5 mg and acetaminophen 325 mg

Endocet 7.5/325: Oxycodone 7.5 mg and acetaminophen 325 mg

Endocet 10/325: Oxycodone 10 mg and acetaminophen 325 mg

Percocet 2.5/325: Oxycodone 2.5 mg and acetaminophen 325 mg

Percocet 5/325 [scored]: Oxycodone 5 mg and acetaminophen 325 mg

Percocet 7.5/325: Oxycodone 7.5 mg and acetaminophen 325 mg

Percocet 10/325: Oxycodone 10 mg and acetaminophen 325 mg

Primlev 5/300: Oxycodone 5 mg and acetaminophen 300 mg

Primlev 7.5/300: Oxycodone 7.5 mg and acetaminophen 300 mg

Primlev 10/300: Oxycodone 10 mg and acetaminophen 300 mg

Roxicet [scored]: Oxycodone 5 mg and acetaminophen 325 mg

Tablet, Extended Release, Oral:

Xartemis XR: Oxycodone hydrochloride 7.5 mg and acetaminophen 325 mg

Oxycodone and Aspirin (oks i KOE done & AS pir in)

Brand Names: U.S. Endodan®; Percodan®

Brand Names: Canada Endodan®; Oxycodan®; Percodan®

Index Terms Aspirin and Oxycodone

Pharmacologic Category Analgesic Combination (Opioid); Analgesic, Opioid

Use Management of moderate- to moderately-severe pain

Pregnancy Risk Factor B (oxycodone); D (aspirin)

Dosage Oral:

Children (dose based on total oxycodone content): Oxycodone 0.1-0.2 mg/kg/dose (maximum oxycodone: 5 mg/dose; maximum aspirin: 4 g/day). Doses should be given every 4-6 hours as needed (American Pain Society, 2008)

Adults: One tablet every 6 hours as needed for pain; maximum aspirin dose should not exceed 4 g/day

Dosing adjustment in renal impairment: Use with caution. Avoid use of aspirin in patients with CrCl <10 mL/minute.

Dosing adjustment in hepatic impairment: Use with caution. Avoid use of aspirin-containing products in severe impairment.

Additional Information Complete prescribing information should be consulted for additional detail.

Dosage Forms

Tablet: Oxycodone hydrochloride 4.8355 mg and aspirin 325 mg

Endodan®, Percodan®: Oxycodone hydrochloride 4.8355 mg and aspirin 325 mg

Oxycodone and Ibuprofen
(oks i KOE done & eye byoo PROE fen)

Index Terms Ibuprofen and Oxycodone

Pharmacologic Category Analgesic Combination (Opioid); Analgesic, Opioid; Nonsteroidal Anti-inflammatory Drug (NSAID), Oral

Use Pain: Short-term (≤7 days) management of acute, moderate-to-severe pain

Pregnancy Risk Factor C/D ≥30 weeks gestation

Dosage Oral: Adolescents ≥14 years and Adults: Pain: One oxycodone 5 mg/ibuprofen 400 mg tablet as needed (maximum: oxycodone 20 mg/ibuprofen 1600 mg per 24 hours); do not take for longer than 7 days

Dosage adjustment in renal impairment: There are no dosage adjustments provided in the manufacturer's labeling (has not been studied). Not recommended in advanced renal disease.

Dosage adjustment in hepatic impairment: There are no dosage adjustments provided in the manufacturer's labeling (has not been studied).

Additional Information Complete prescribing information should be consulted for additional detail.

Dosage Forms

Tablet: Oxycodone 5 mg and ibuprofen 400 mg

Oxycodone and Naloxone
(oks i KOE done & nal OKS one)

Brand Names: Canada Targin

Index Terms Naloxone and Oxycodone; Oxycodone Hydrochloride and Naloxone Hydrochloride; Targiniq ER

Pharmacologic Category Analgesic, Opioid; Opioid Antagonist

Use

Pain: Management of moderate to severe pain requiring daily, around-the-clock, long-term opioid treatment and for which alternative treatment options are inadequate

Limitations of use: Reserve for use in patients whom alternative treatment options (eg, nonopioid analgesics or immediate-release opioids) are ineffective, not tolerated, or would be otherwise inadequate to provide sufficient management of pain. Not indicated as an as-needed analgesic; do not exceed recommended doses because higher doses may be associated with symptoms of opioid withdrawal or decreased analgesia.

Canadian labeling: Additional uses (not in U.S. labeling): Relief of opioid-induced constipation in patients who require an opioid

Pregnancy Risk Factor C

Pregnancy Considerations Animal reproduction studies have not been conducted with this combination. The Canadian labeling contraindicates use of this combination product during pregnancy and during labor and delivery. Also see individual agents.

Breast-Feeding Considerations Oxycodone is excreted in breast milk; it is not known if naloxone is excreted in breast milk. Breast feeding is not recommended by the manufacturer. The Canadian labeling contraindicates use of this combination product in nursing women. Also see individual agents.

Contraindications

Hypersensitivity to oxycodone, naloxone, or any component of the formulation; significant respiratory depression; acute or severe bronchial asthma in an unmonitored setting or in the absence of resuscitative equipment; known or suspected paralytic ileus and GI obstruction; moderate-to-severe hepatic impairment

Canadian labeling: Additional contraindications (not in U.S. labeling): Hypersensitivity to other opioids; rectal administration; suspected surgical abdomen (eg, acute appendicitis or pancreatitis); mild, intermittent, or short duration pain that can be managed with other pain medications; management of acute pain, including use in outpatient or day surgeries; management of perioperative pain; cor pulmonale; acute alcoholism, delirium tremens, and convulsive disorders; severe CNS depression, increased cerebrospinal or intracranial pressure, and head injury; concurrent use or use within 14 days of monoamine oxidase (MAO) inhibitors; opioid-dependent patients and for narcotic withdrawal treatment; use in women who are breast-feeding, pregnant, or during labor and delivery

Warnings/Precautions [U.S. Boxed Warning]: Serious, life-threatening, or fatal respiratory depression may occur with use of oxycodone/naloxone ER. Monitor for respiratory depression, especially during initiation of therapy or following a dose increase. To reduce the risk of respiratory depression, proper dosing and titration is essential. Overestimating the oxycodone/naloxone ER dose when converting patients from another opioid product can result in fatal overdose with the first dose.

[U.S. Boxed Warning]: Accidental ingestion of even one dose of oxycodone/naloxone ER, especially in children, can result in a fatal overdose of oxycodone.

[U.S. Boxed Warning]: Oxycodone/naloxone ER exposes patients and other users to the risks of opioid addiction, abuse, and misuse, which can lead to overdose and death. Assess each patient's risk prior to prescribing oxycodone/naloxone ER, and monitor all patients regularly for the development of these behaviors or conditions. Crushing, chewing, or dissolving the product can cause rapid release and absorption of a potentially fatal dose of oxycodone. Use with caution in patients with a history of drug abuse, acute alcoholism, or mental illness (eg, major depression); potential for drug dependency exists. Tolerance, psychological, and physical dependence may occur with prolonged use.

[U.S. Boxed Warning]: Concomitant use of oxycodone/naloxone ER with CYP450 3A4 inhibitors may result in an increase in oxycodone plasma concentrations, which could increase or prolong adverse drug effects and may cause potentially fatal respiratory depression. In addition, discontinuation of a concomitantly used CYP450 3A4 inducer may result in an increase in oxycodone plasma concentration. Monitor patients receiving oxycodone/naloxone ER and any CYP3A4 inhibitor or inducer. Potentially significant interactions may exist requiring dose or frequency adjustment, additional monitoring, and/or selection of alternative therapy.

[U.S. Boxed Warning]: Prolonged use of oxycodone/naloxone ER during pregnancy can result in neonatal opioid withdrawal syndrome, which may be life-threatening if not recognized and requires management according to protocols developed by neonatology experts. If opioid use is required for a prolonged period in a pregnant woman, advise the patient of the risk of neonatal opioid withdrawal syndrome and ensure appropriate treatment will be available.

Tablets must be swallowed whole; tablets that are broken, crushed, chewed, or dissolved may result in a rapid release and absorption of a potentially fatal dose of oxycodone. Do not exceed maximum recommended doses and limit use to patients in whom alternative treatment options (eg, nonopioid analgesics or immediate-release opioids) are ineffective, not tolerated, or otherwise inadequate to provide sufficient pain relief. Not indicated as an as-needed analgesic. Limit use of the 40 mg/20 mg tablet dosage form to patients with established tolerance to an opioid of comparable potency **(single doses >40 mg or daily doses >80 mg of oxycodone may cause fatal respiratory depression in patients who are not tolerant to the respiratory depressant effects of opioids)**. The Canadian labeling contraindicates rectal administration of this combination product and also does not indicate use in patients with cancer associated with peritoneal carcinomatosis or with sub-occlusive syndrome in advanced stages of pelvic and digestive cancer (not studied).

May cause CNS depression, which may impair physical or mental abilities; patients must be cautioned about performing tasks which require mental alertness (eg, operating machinery or driving). Use with extreme caution in patients with head injury, intracranial lesions, or elevated intracranial pressure; exaggerated elevation of ICP may occur. Avoid use in patients with impaired consciousness or coma.

May cause severe hypotension (including orthostatic hypotension and syncope); use with caution in patients with hypovolemia, cardiovascular disease (including acute MI), or drugs which may exaggerate hypotensive effects (including phenothiazines or general anesthetics). Monitor for symptoms of hypotension following initiation or dose titration; dose adjustment may be warranted. Avoid use in patients with circulatory shock.

Use with caution in patients with adrenocortical insufficiency, biliary tract impairment, pancreatitis, prostatic hyperplasia and/or urinary stricture, history of seizure disorders, thyroid dysfunction, toxic psychosis, and those who are morbidly obese. Use with caution in patients with preexisting respiratory compromise (hypoxia and/or hypercapnia), COPD or other obstructive pulmonary disease, and kyphoscoliosis or other skeletal disorder which may alter respiratory function; critical respiratory depression may occur, even at therapeutic dosages. Use with caution in debilitated patients and in the elderly; there is a greater potential for respiratory depression, even at therapeutic dosages.

Use with caution in patients with mild hepatic dysfunction; use is contraindicated with moderate-to-severe hepatic impairment. Use with caution in patients with renal dysfunction. May obscure diagnosis or clinical course of patients with acute abdominal conditions. Naloxone may cause diarrhea; patients should be instructed to report severe or persistent diarrhea lasting >3 days.

Opioids decrease bowel motility; monitor for decrease bowel motility in postoperative patients receiving opioids. The Canadian labeling contraindicates perioperative use (24 hours before or after surgery) of oxycodone/naloxone ER. Patients interrupting therapy to undergo pain-relieving procedures (eg, chordotomy) may require a dosage adjustment when resuming therapy after the postoperative recovery period.

Concurrent use of agonist/antagonist analgesics may precipitate withdrawal symptoms and/or reduced analgesic efficacy in patients following prolonged therapy with mu opioid agonists. Abrupt discontinuation following prolonged use may also lead to withdrawal symptoms. Do not abruptly stop oxycodone/naloxone ER; gradually decrease dose to prevent signs and symptoms of withdrawal.

Adverse Reactions

Cardiovascular: Peripheral edema

Central nervous system: Depression, dizziness, drowsiness, fatigue, headache, migraine, withdrawal syndrome

Dermatologic: Hyperhidrosis, skin rash

Endocrine & metabolic: Hyperglycemia, hyperlipidemia, hyperuricemia, increased gamma-glutamyl transferase, increased serum glucose

Gastrointestinal: Abdominal distention, abdominal pain, anorexia, constipation, diarrhea, gastroenteritis, nausea, vomiting, xerostomia

Genitourinary: Urinary tract infection

Hematologic & oncologic: Anemia, decreased hemoglobin

Infection: Influenza, viral infection

Neuromuscular & skeletal: Osteoarthritis, tremor, weakness

Respiratory: Bronchitis, sinusitis

Rare but important or life-threatening: Anal fissure, angina pectoris, anxiety, biliary obstruction, candidiasis, chest pain, cholelithiasis, deafness (unilateral), decreased platelet count, diverticulitis, eczema, ECG abnormality, erectile dysfunction, falling, first degree atrioventricular block, gastritis, gastroesophageal reflux disease, gastrointestinal hemorrhage, gout, hallucination, hemoptysis, hypersensitivity, hypertensive crisis, hypogonadism (Brennan, 2013; Debono, 2011), hyponatremia, hypophosphatemia, hypotension, increased blood pressure, increased heart rate, increased lactate dehydrogenase, increased liver enzymes, lipoma, loss of libido, memory impairment, neuromuscular blockade, nightmares, otitis externa, panic attack, paresthesia, periodontitis, photopsia, pneumonia, pollakiuria, polyneuropathy, respiratory depression, restless leg syndrome, right bundle branch block, stasis dermatitis, syncope, tenosynovitis, thrombophlebitis, thrombosis, tinnitus, tonic-clonic seizures, urinary incontinence, urinary retention, vaginal hemorrhage, weight loss

Drug Interactions

Metabolism/Transport Effects Refer to individual components.

Avoid Concomitant Use

Avoid concomitant use of Oxycodone and Naloxone with any of the following: Azelastine (Nasal); Conivaptan; Fusidic Acid (Systemic); Idelalisib; Methylnaltrexone; Naloxegol; Orphenadrine; Paraldehyde; Thalidomide

Increased Effect/Toxicity

Oxycodone and Naloxone may increase the levels/effects of: Alcohol (Ethyl); Alvimopan; Azelastine (Nasal); Buprenorphine; CNS Depressants; Desmopressin; Diuretics; Hydrocodone; Methotrimeprazine; Metyrosine; Mirtazapine; Naloxegol; Orphenadrine; Paraldehyde; Pramipexole; ROPINIRole; Rotigotine; Selective Serotonin Reuptake Inhibitors; Suvorexant; Thalidomide; Zolpidem

The levels/effects of Oxycodone and Naloxone may be increased by: Amphetamines; Anticholinergic Agents; Antipsychotic Agents (Phenothiazines); Brimonidine (Topical); Cannabis; Conivaptan; CYP3A4 Inhibitors (Moderate); CYP3A4 Inhibitors (Strong); Dasatinib; Doxylamine; Dronabinol; Droperidol; Fusidic Acid (Systemic); HydrOXYzine; Idelalisib; Ivacaftor; Kava Kava; Luliconazole; Magnesium Sulfate; MAO Inhibitors; Methotrimeprazine; Methylnaltrexone; Mifepristone; Nabilone; Perampanel; Rufinamide; Simeprevir; Sodium Oxybate; Stiripentol; Succinylcholine; Tapentadol; Tetrahydrocannabinol; Voriconazole

Decreased Effect

Oxycodone and Naloxone may decrease the levels/effects of: Pegvisomant

The levels/effects of Oxycodone and Naloxone may be decreased by: Ammonium Chloride; Bosentan; CYP3A4 Inducers (Moderate); CYP3A4 Inducers (Strong); Dabrafenib; Deferasirox; Mitotane; Mixed Agonist / Antagonist Opioids; Naltrexone; Rifampin; Siltuximab; St Johns Wort; Tocilizumab

Storage/Stability Store at 15°C to 30°C (59°F to 86°F). Protect from light and moisture.

Mechanism of Action

Oxycodone binds to opiate receptors in the CNS, causing inhibition of ascending pain pathways, altering the perception of and response to pain; produces generalized CNS depression; also binds to opiate receptors in peripheral organs including the gut to induce constipation.

Naloxone is a pure opioid antagonist that competes and displaces narcotics at opioid receptor sites, including gut opioid receptors, which counteracts opioid-induced constipation.

Pharmacodynamics/Kinetics Note: Pharmacokinetic parameters observed with oxycodone/naloxone controlled release formulation were similar to those observed with separate administration of controlled-release formulations of each agent (Smith, 2008).

Naloxone:

Bioavailability: Oral: <3%

Metabolism: Primarily hepatic via glucuronidation

Half-life elimination: ~4 to 17 hours

Excretion: Urine (as metabolites)

Oxycodone (controlled release):

Duration: ≤12 hours

Distribution: V_d: 2.6 L/kg; distributed to skeletal muscle, liver, intestinal tract, lungs, spleen, and brain

Protein binding: ~45% (Targin Canadian product monograph, 2013)

Metabolism: Hepatically via CYP3A4 to noroxycodone (has weak analgesic activity), noroxymorphone, and alpha- and beta-noroxycodol. CYP2D6 mediated metabolism produces oxymorphone (has analgesic activity; low plasma concentrations), alpha- and beta-oxymorphol. Analgesic activity of metabolites may be of little clinical significance

Bioavailability: 60% to 87% (**Note:** Proportional bioavailability of oxycodone 5 mg/naloxone 2.5 mg tablets to other tablet strengths has not been established)

Half-life elimination: ~4 to 5 hours

Time to peak, plasma: 3 to 4 hours

Excretion: Urine and feces (as parent drug and metabolites)

Dosage

Moderate-to-severe pain: Adults: Oral:

U.S. labeling: **Note:** Oxycodone 40 mg/naloxone 20 mg tablets should only be used in opioid-tolerant patients. Do not exceed oxycodone 80 mg/naloxone 40 mg daily. Opioid tolerance is defined as: Patients already taking at least 60 mg of oral morphine daily, 25 mcg of transdermal fentanyl per hour, 30 mg of oral oxycodone daily, 8 mg oral hydromorphone daily, or an equivalent dose of another opioid for at least 1 week.

Opioid-naive or not opioid tolerant: Initial: Oxycodone 10 mg/naloxone 5 mg every 12 hours

Converting from other opioids:

Currently on other oral oxycodone formulations: Administer 50% of the patient's total daily oral oxycodone dose as oxycodone/naloxone every 12 hours.

Currently on other oral opioids: Discontinue all other around-the-clock opioids; convert the patient's current total daily opioid dose(s) to an equivalent daily oral morphine dose (see manufacturer's labeling for conversion instructions). After equivalent daily oral morphine dose is determined, initiate oxycodone/naloxone as follows:

Oxycodone 10 mg/naloxone 5 mg every 12 hours (for patients with an equivalent daily oral morphine dose of 20 to <70 mg)

Oxycodone 20 mg/naloxone 10 mg every 12 hours (for patients with an equivalent daily oral morphine dose of 70 to <110 mg)

Oxycodone 30 mg/naloxone 15 mg every 12 hours (for patients with an equivalent daily oral morphine dose of 110 to <150 mg)

Oxycodone 40 mg/naloxone 20 mg every 12 hours (for patients with an equivalent daily oral morphine dose of 150 to 160 mg)

Currently on transdermal fentanyl: Initial: Oxycodone 10 mg/naloxone 5 mg every 12 hours substituted for each 25 mcg/hour fentanyl transdermal patch beginning 18 hours after removal of the transdermal fentanyl patch. Monitor closely during conversion.

Currently on transdermal buprenorphine: Initial: Oxycodone 10 mg/naloxone 5 mg every 12 hours for patients receiving transdermal buprenorphine (≤20 mcg/hour). Monitor closely during conversion.

Canadian labeling: **Note:** Oxycodone 5 mg/naloxone 2.5 mg tablets are intended for use in titration or dose adjustments. Multiple oxycodone 5 mg/naloxone 2.5 mg tablets should not be substituted for other tablet strengths. Oxycodone 40 mg/naloxone 20 mg tablets should only be used in opioid-tolerant patients. Do not exceed oxycodone 40 mg/naloxone 20 mg (single dose) or oxycodone 80 mg/naloxone 40 mg (daily dose).

Opioid-naive: Initial: Oxycodone 10 mg/naloxone 5 mg every 12 hours

Opioid-experienced:

Currently on other oral oxycodone formulations: Discontinue other oral oxycodone formulations and initiate oxycodone/naloxone at equivalent total daily dose of oxycodone administered in 2 equally divided doses every 12 hours

Currently on other opioids: Discontinue all other around-the-clock opioids. Initiate oxycodone/naloxone at the lowest available strength every 12 hours. Titrate dose as necessary to achieve adequate pain control with acceptable side effects. Adequate rescue medication should be available.

Dose adjustment:

U.S. labeling: Dose is individualized; titrate dose cautiously in increments of oxycodone 10 mg/naloxone 5 mg every 12 hours every 1 to 2 days until satisfactory response and acceptable adverse effects. Repeated pain at the end of the dosing interval may indicate the need for a dose adjustment rather than adjusting the dosing interval.

Canadian labeling: Dose is individualized; titrate dose cautiously every 1 to 2 days until satisfactory response and acceptable adverse effects. Repeated pain at the end of the dosing interval may indicate the need for a dose adjustment rather than adjusting the dosing interval.

Patients requiring rescue medication: Patients who experience breakthrough pain may require a rescue medication with an appropriate dose of an immediate-release analgesic. **Note:** Rescue medications used in clinical trials were immediate release oxycodone or combination products containing codeine.

U.S. labeling: No specific recommendations are made in the manufacturer's labeling.

Canadian labeling: Administer 1 dose of an immediate release opioid ~1/6 of the equivalent daily dose of oxycodone. Patients requiring >2 doses daily of rescue medication should have oxycodone/naloxone dose titrated upward every 1 to 2 days until satisfactory response is achieved (not to exceed recommended maximum dosing). Dosing interval (every 12 hours) should not be adjusted.

Discontinuation of therapy: Dose should be gradually tapered when no longer required in order to prevent withdrawal; do not abruptly discontinue.

U.S. labeling: See manufacturer's labeling for detailed instruction.

Canadian labeling: Decrease controlled release oxycodone dose by 50% of the previous daily dose (administered in 2 divided doses every 12 hours) for first 2 days, then reduce daily dose by 25% every 2 days.

Elderly: Initiate therapy at low end of dosing range; titrate dose cautiously to lowest dose that provides adequate pain relief with acceptable side effects.

Dosage adjustment in renal impairment:

U.S. labeling: Reduce dose to 50% the usual starting dose; titrate cautiously; consider use of alternative treatments without naloxone in patients with severe renal impairment.

Canadian labeling: There are no specific dosage adjustments provided in the manufacturer's labeling; however, a reduced dose is recommended; use with caution.

Dosage adjustment in hepatic impairment:

Mild impairment:

U.S. labeling: Initial: Reduce dose to 33% to 50% the usual starting dose; titrate cautiously.

Canadian labeling: There are no specific dosage adjustments provided in the manufacturer's labeling; however, a reduced dose is recommended; use with caution.

Moderate-to-severe impairment: Use is contraindicated.

Administration Oral: Administer with or without food. Swallow tablets whole one tablet at a time; do not break, crush, cut, chew, dissolve, or split. Breaking, chewing, crushing, cutting, dissolving, or splitting ER tablets will result in uncontrolled delivery of oxycodone and can lead to overdose or death. Tablets are not indicated for rectal administration; increased risk of adverse events due to enhanced rectal absorption.

Monitoring Parameters Pain relief; respiratory and mental status, blood pressure; constipation; signs of misuse, abuse, and addiction; signs or symptoms of hypogonadism or hypoadrenalism (Brennan, 2013)

Additional Information Compared to controlled release oxycodone, improved bowel function and similar efficacy in terms of pain relief have been observed with a controlled release formulation of oxycodone/naloxone (Ahmedzai, 2012; Löwenstein, 2010; Vondrackova, 2008).

Product Availability Targiniq ER: FDA approved July 2014; anticipated availability is currently unknown.

Dosage Forms: Canada

Tablet, controlled release, oral:

Targin:

Oxycodone 5 mg and naloxone 2.5 mg
Oxycodone 10 mg and naloxone 5 mg
Oxycodone 20 mg and naloxone 10 mg
Oxycodone 40 mg and naloxone 20 mg

◆ **Oxycodone Hydrochloride** *see* OxyCODONE *on page 1538*

◆ **Oxycodone Hydrochloride and Naloxone Hydrochloride** *see* Oxycodone and Naloxone *on page 1542*

◆ **OxyCONTIN** *see* OxyCODONE *on page 1538*

◆ **OxyContin (Can)** *see* OxyCODONE *on page 1538*

◆ **Oxy.IR (Can)** *see* OxyCODONE *on page 1538*

Oxymetholone (oks i METH oh lone)

Brand Names: U.S. Anadrol-50

Pharmacologic Category Anabolic Steroid

Use Treatment of anemias caused by deficient red cell production

Pregnancy Risk Factor X

Dosage Note: The National Kidney Foundation does not recommend the use of androgens as an adjuvant to ESA treatment in anemic patients with chronic kidney disease (KDOQI, 2006).

Oral: Children and Adults: Erythropoietic effects: 1-5 mg/kg/day once daily; usual effective dose: 1-2 mg/kg/day; give for a minimum trial of 3-6 months because response may be delayed

Dosage adjustment in renal impairment: No dosage adjustment provided in manufacturer's labeling. Use with caution due to risk of edema in patients with renal impairment.

Dosage adjustment in hepatic impairment:

Mild to moderate impairment: There are no dosage adjustments provided in the manufacturer's labeling.

Severe impairment: Use is contraindicated.

Additional Information Complete prescribing information should be consulted for additional detail.

Dosage Forms

Tablet, Oral:

Anadrol-50: 50 mg

Oxymorphone (oks i MOR fone)

Brand Names: U.S. Opana; Opana ER

Index Terms Oxymorphone Hydrochloride

Pharmacologic Category Analgesic, Opioid

Additional Appendix Information

Opioid Conversion Table *on page 2232*

Use Pain management:

Parenteral: Management of moderate-to-severe acute pain; analgesia during labor; preoperative medication; anesthesia support; relief of anxiety in patients with dyspnea associated with pulmonary edema secondary to acute left ventricular failure

Oral, regular release: Management of moderate-to-severe acute pain

Oral, extended release: Management of pain severe enough to require daily, around-the-clock, long-term opioid treatment and for which alternative treatment options are inadequate

Limitations of use: Because of the risks of addiction, abuse, and misuse with opioids, even at recommended doses, and because of the greater risks of overdose and death with ER opioid formulations, reserve oxymorphone ER for use in patients for whom alternative treatment options (eg, nonopioid analgesics, immediate-release opioids) are ineffective, not tolerated, or would be otherwise inadequate to provide sufficient pain management. Not indicated as an as-needed analgesic.

Pregnancy Risk Factor C

Pregnancy Considerations Adverse events were observed in some animal reproduction studies. Opioids cross the placenta. When used for pain relief during labor, opioids may temporarily affect the heart rate of the fetus (ACOG, 2002). Oxymorphone injection is indicated for analgesia during labor. Neonates should be monitored for respiratory depression.

[U.S. Boxed Warning]: Prolonged maternal use of opioids during pregnancy can cause neonatal withdrawal syndrome in the newborn which may be life-threatening if not recognized and treated according to protocols developed by neonatology experts. If prolonged opioid therapy is required in a pregnant woman, ensure treatment is available and warn patient of risk to the neonate. If chronic opioid exposure occurs in pregnancy, adverse events in the newborn (including withdrawal) may occur; monitoring of the neonate is recommended. The minimum effective dose should be used if opioids are needed (Chou, 2009). Neonatal abstinence syndrome following opioid exposure may present with autonomic (eg, fever, temperature instability), gastrointestinal (eg, diarrhea, vomiting, poor feeding/weight gain), or neurologic (eg, high-pitched crying, increased muscle tone, irritability, seizure, tremor) symptoms (Dow, 2012; Hudak, 2012).

Long-term opioid use may cause secondary hypogonadism, which may lead to sexual dysfunction or infertility (Brennan, 2013).

Breast-Feeding Considerations Some opioids can be found in breast milk. Withdrawal symptoms may be observed in breast-feeding infants when opioid analgesics are discontinued. The manufacturer recommends that caution be used if administered to a nursing woman. Nursing infants exposed to large doses of opioids should be monitored for apnea and sedation (Montgomery, 2012).

Contraindications Hypersensitivity to oxymorphone, other morphine analogs (phenanthrene derivatives), or any component of the formulation; paralytic ileus (known or suspected); moderate-to-severe hepatic impairment; severe respiratory depression (unless using immediate release or parenteral formulation in monitored setting with resuscitative equipment); acute/severe bronchial asthma; hypercarbia

Note: Parenteral formulation is also contraindicated in the treatment of upper airway obstruction and pulmonary edema due to a chemical respiratory irritant.

Warnings/Precautions An opioid-containing analgesic regimen should be tailored to each patient's needs and based upon the type of pain being treated (acute versus chronic), the route of administration, degree of tolerance for opioids (naive versus chronic user), age, weight, and patient comorbidities. The optimal analgesic dose varies widely among patients. Doses should be titrated to pain relief/prevention.

May cause CNS depression, which may impair physical or mental abilities; patients must be cautioned about performing tasks which require mental alertness (eg, operating machinery or driving). Potentially significant drug interactions may exist, requiring dose or frequency adjustment, additional monitoring, and/or selection of alternative therapy. Effects may be potentiated when used with other CNS depressants (eg, sedatives, anxiolytics, hypnotics, neuroleptics, other opioids). Use not recommended within 14 days of MAO inhibitors. Due to structural similarities, hypersensitivity to other phenanthrene-derivative opioid agonists (codeine, hydrocodone, hydromorphone, levorphanol, morphine) may result in similar hypersensitivity reaction if oxymorphone is used; therefore, the use of oxymorphone is contraindicated in patients with previous hypersensitivity to other phenanthrene derivatives. May cause respiratory depression. Use with caution and monitor for respiratory depression in patients with significant chronic obstructive pulmonary disease or cor pulmonale, and patients having a substantially decreased respiratory reserve, hypoxia, hypercarbia, or preexisting respiratory depression, particularly when initiating therapy and titrating with oxymorphone; even therapeutic doses may decrease respiratory drive to the point of apnea. Consider the use of alternative non-opioid analgesics in these patients. Use with caution in patients (particularly elderly, cachectic, or debilitated) with impaired respiratory function, adrenal disease, morbid obesity, seizure disorders, toxic psychosis, thyroid dysfunction, prostatic hyperplasia, or renal impairment. Use caution in mild hepatic dysfunction; use is contraindicated in moderate-to-severe hepatic impairment. Avoid use in patients with CNS depression or coma as these patients are susceptible to intracranial effects of CO_2 retention. Use only with extreme caution (if at all) in patients with head injury or increased intracranial pressure (ICP); potential to elevate ICP and/or blunt papillary response may be greatly exaggerated in these patients. Use with caution in patients with biliary tract dysfunction including acute pancreatitis; may cause constriction of sphincter of Oddi. May obscure diagnosis or clinical course of patients with acute abdominal conditions. May cause constipation which may be problematic in patients with unstable angina and patients post-myocardial infarction.

Oxymorphone shares the toxic potential of opioid agonists and usual precautions of opioid agonist therapy should be observed; may cause hypotension in patients with acute myocardial infarction, volume depletion, or concurrent drug therapy which may exaggerate vasodilation. The elderly may be particularly susceptible to adverse effects of opioids.

Concurrent use of mixed agonist/antagonist analgesics (eg, pentazocine, nalbuphine, butorphanol) or partial agonist (eg, buprenorphine) analgesics may precipitate withdrawal symptoms and/or reduced analgesic efficacy in patients following prolonged therapy with mu opioid agonists. Taper dose gradually when discontinuing.

Extended release tablets: **[U.S. Boxed Warning]: May cause serious, life-threatening, or fatal respiratory depression. Monitor closely for respiratory depression, especially during initiation or dose escalation. Patients should swallow tablets whole; crushing, chewing, or dissolving can cause rapid release and a potentially fatal dose.** Carbon dioxide retention from opioid-induced respiratory depression can exacerbate the sedating effects of opioids. Therapy should only be prescribed by healthcare professionals familiar with the use of potent opioids for chronic pain. **[U.S. Boxed Warning]: Users are exposed to the risks of addiction, abuse, and misuse, potentially leading to overdose and death. Assess each patient's risk prior to prescribing; monitor all patients regularly for development of these behaviors or conditions. Risk of opioid abuse is increased in patients with a history or family history of alcohol or drug abuse or mental illness.** Cases of thrombotic thrombocytopenic purpura (TTP) resulting in kidney failure (requiring dialysis) and death have been reported as a result of misuse by drug abusers injecting the extended-release tablets intravenously; tablets are intended for oral administration only. **[U.S. Boxed Warning]: Patients should not consume alcoholic beverages or medication containing ethanol while taking oxymorphone ER; ethanol may increase oxymorphone plasma levels resulting in a potentially fatal overdose. [U.S. Boxed Warning]: Accidental ingestion of even one dose, especially in children, can result in a fatal overdose of oxymorphone. [U.S. Boxed Warning]: Prolonged maternal use of opioids during pregnancy can cause neonatal withdrawal syndrome in the newborn which may be life-threatening if not recognized and treated according to protocols developed by neonatology experts. If prolonged opioid therapy is required in a pregnant woman**, ensure treatment is available and warn patient of risk to the neonate. Signs and symptoms include irritability, hyperactivity and abnormal sleep pattern, high pitched cry, tremor, vomiting, diarrhea and failure to gain weight. Onset, duration and severity depend on the drug used, duration of use, maternal dose, and rate of drug elimination by the newborn.

Adverse Reactions

Cardiovascular: Edema, flushing, hypertension, hypotension, tachycardia

Central nervous system: Anxiety, confusion, depression, disorientation, dizziness, drowsiness, fatigue, headache, insomnia, lethargy, nervousness, restlessness, sedation

Dermatologic: Diaphoresis, pruritus

Endocrine & metabolic: Dehydration, weight loss

Gastrointestinal: Abdominal distention, abdominal pain, constipation, decreased appetite, diarrhea, dyspepsia, flatulence, nausea, vomiting, xerostomia

Neuromuscular & skeletal: Weakness

Ophthalmic: Blurred vision

Respiratory: Dyspnea, hypoxia

Miscellaneous: Fever

Rare but important or life-threatening: Agitation, apnea (injection), atelectasis (injection), biliary colic, bradycardia, bronchospasm (injection), cold and clammy skin, dermatitis, difficulty in micturition, diplopia (injection), drug dependence, dysphoria, euphoria, hallucination, hot flash, hypersensitivity, hypersensitivity reaction, hypogonadism (Brennan, 2013; Debono, 2011), injection site reaction, intestinal obstruction, miosis, oliguria (injection), orthostatic hypotension, palpitations, respiratory depression, syncope, thrombotic thrombocytopenic purpura (inappropriate injection of ER tablet), ureteral spasm (injection), urinary retention, urticaria

Drug Interactions

Metabolism/Transport Effects None known.

Avoid Concomitant Use

Avoid concomitant use of Oxymorphone with any of the following: Azelastine (Nasal); MAO Inhibitors; Orphenadrine; Paraldehyde; Thalidomide

Increased Effect/Toxicity

Oxymorphone may increase the levels/effects of: Alcohol (Ethyl); Alvimopan; Azelastine (Nasal); Buprenorphine; CNS Depressants; Desmopressin; Diuretics; Hydrocodone; MAO Inhibitors; Methotrimeprazine; Metyrosine; Mirtazapine; Orphenadrine; Paraldehyde; Pramipexole; ROPINIRole; Rotigotine; Selective Serotonin Reuptake Inhibitors; Suvorexant; Thalidomide; Zolpidem

The levels/effects of Oxymorphone may be increased by: Amphetamines; Anticholinergic Agents; Antipsychotic Agents (Phenothiazines); Brimonidine (Topical); Cannabis; Doxylamine; Dronabinol; Droperidol; HydrOXYzine;

Kava Kava; Magnesium Sulfate; Methotrimeprazine; Nabilone; Perampanel; Rufinamide; Sodium Oxybate; Succinylcholine; Tapentadol; Tetrahydrocannabinol

Decreased Effect

Oxymorphone may decrease the levels/effects of: Pegvisomant

The levels/effects of Oxymorphone may be decreased by: Ammonium Chloride; Mixed Agonist / Antagonist Opioids; Naltrexone

Food Interactions

Ethanol: Ethanol ingestion with extended-release tablets is specifically contraindicated due to possible accelerated release and potentially fatal overdose. Management: Avoid ethanol.

Food: When taken orally with a high-fat meal, peak concentration is 38% to 50% greater. Management: Both immediate-release and extended-release tablets should be taken 1 hour before or 2 hours after eating.

Storage/Stability Injection solution, tablet: Store at 25°C (77°F); excursions permitted to 15°C to 30°C (59°F to 86°F). Protect injection from light.

Mechanism of Action Oxymorphone hydrochloride is a potent opioid analgesic with uses similar to those of morphine. The drug is a semisynthetic derivative of morphine (phenanthrene derivative) and is closely related to hydromorphone chemically (Dilaudid®).

Pharmacodynamics/Kinetics

Onset of action: Parenteral: 5-10 minutes

Duration: Analgesic: Parenteral: 3-6 hours

Distribution: V_d: IV: 1.94-4.22 L/kg

Protein binding: 10% to 12%

Metabolism: Hepatic via glucuronidation to active and inactive metabolites

Bioavailability: Oral: ~10%

Half-life elimination: Oral: Immediate release: 7-9 hours; Extended release: 9-11 hours

Excretion: Urine (<1% as unchanged drug); feces

Dosage Adults: **Note:** Dosage must be individualized.

IM, SubQ: Initial: 1 to 1.5 mg; may repeat every 4 to 6 hours as needed

Labor analgesia: IM: 0.5 to 1 mg

IV: Initial: 0.5 mg

Oral:

Immediate release: Acute pain:

Opioid-naive: Initial: 5 to 10 mg every 4 to 6 hours as needed (American Pain Society [Miaskowski, 2008]). Dosage adjustment should be based on level of analgesia, side effects, pain intensity, and patient comorbidities.

Currently on stable dose of parenteral oxymorphone: Approximately 10 times the total daily parenteral requirement. The calculated total oral daily amount should be given in 4 to 6 equally divided doses.

Currently on other opioids: Use standard conversion chart to convert total daily dose of current opioid to oxymorphone equivalent. Generally start with one-half (1/2) the calculated total daily oxymorphone dosage and administer in divided doses every 4 to 6 hours.

Extended release: Chronic pain:

Opioid-naive (use as the first opioid analgesic or in patients who are not opioid tolerant): Initial: 5 mg every 12 hours.

Note: Opioid tolerance is defined as: Patients already taking at least 60 mg of oral morphine daily, 25 mcg of transdermal fentanyl per hour, 30 mg of oral oxycodone daily, 8 mg oral hydromorphone daily, 25 mg oral oxymorphone daily, or an equivalent dose of another opioid for at least 1 week.

Conversion from stable dose of parenteral oxymorphone to extended-release oxymorphone: Approximately 10 times the total daily parenteral requirement should be given in 2 divided doses as oxymorphone extended-release tablets (eg, [IV dose x 10] divided by 2). Due to patient variability, closely monitor patient for analgesia and adverse reactions upon conversion.

Conversion of stable dose of immediate-release oxymorphone to extended-release oxymorphone: Use same total daily dose. Administer one-half (1/2) of the daily dose of immediate-release oxymorphone as the extended-release formulation every 12 hours

Conversion from other oral opioids to extended-release oxymorphone: Discontinue all other around-the-clock opioids when extended release oxymorphone is initiated. Substantial interpatient variability exists in relative potency of opioids. Therefore, it is safer to underestimate a patient's daily oral oxymorphone requirement and provide breakthrough pain relief with rescue medication (eg, immediate release opioid) than to overestimate requirements. The conversion factors, per the manufacturer, in the chart (see table) provide an estimate to convert the daily dose of current opioid to an oxymorphone equivalent. Select the prior oral opioid, sum the current total daily dose, multiply by the conversion factor on the table to calculate the approximate oral oxymorphone daily dose, then divide daily dose by 2 to administer every 12 hours as oxymorphone extended release. Round down, if necessary, to the nearest strength available. For patients on a regimen of more than one opioid, calculate the approximate oral oxymorphone dose for each opioid and sum the totals to obtain the approximate total oxymorphone daily dose. For patients on a regimen of fixed-ratio opioid/nonopioid analgesic medications, only the opioid component of these medications should be used in the conversion. **Note:** The conversion factors in this conversion table are only to be used for the conversion from current opioid therapy to oxymorphone ER. Conversion factors in this table cannot be used to convert from oxymorphone ER to another opioid (doing so may lead to fatal overdose due to overestimation of the new opioid). This is not a table of equianalgesic doses. When converting from methadone to extended release oxymorphone, close monitoring is required. Ratio between methadone and other opioid agonists varies widely according to previous dose exposure. Methadone has a long half-life and can accumulate in the plasma.

Conversion Factors to Oxymorphone ER

Prior Oral Opioid	Approximate Oral Conversion Factor
Oxymorphone	1
Hydrocodone	0.5
Oxycodone	0.5
Methadone	0.5
Morphine	0.333

Titration and maintenance: Adjust therapy incrementally by 5 to 10 mg every 12 hours at intervals of every 3 to 7 days. Breakthrough pain may require a dose increase or rescue medication with an immediate-release analgesic.

Discontinuation of therapy: Gradually titrate dose downward every 2 to 4 days to prevent withdrawal signs/ symptoms. Do not abruptly discontinue.

Elderly: Initiate dosing at the lower end of the dosage range

Dosage adjustment in renal impairment: CrCl <50 mL/minute: Reduce initial dosage of oral and parenteral formulations (bioavailability increased 57% to 65%). Begin therapy at lowest dose and titrate slowly with careful monitoring.

Dosage adjustment in hepatic impairment:

Mild impairment: Initiate with lowest possible dose and titrate slowly with careful monitoring.

Moderate to severe impairment: Use is contraindicated.

Dietary Considerations Immediate release and extended release tablets should be taken 1 hour before or 2 hours after eating.

Administration Oral: Administer immediate release and extended release tablets 1 hour before or 2 hours after eating. ER tablet should be swallowed whole; do not break, crush, dissolve, or chew.

Monitoring Parameters Respiratory rate, heart rate, blood pressure, CNS activity; signs or symptoms of hypogonadism or hypoadrenalism (Brennan, 2013)

Dosage Forms

Solution, Injection:

Opana: 1 mg/mL (1 mL)

Tablet, Oral:

Opana: 5 mg, 10 mg

Generic: 5 mg, 10 mg

Tablet ER 12 Hour Abuse-Deterrent, Oral:

Opana ER: 5 mg, 7.5 mg, 10 mg, 15 mg, 20 mg, 30 mg, 40 mg

Tablet Extended Release 12 Hour, Oral:

Generic: 5 mg, 7.5 mg, 10 mg, 15 mg, 20 mg, 30 mg, 40 mg

◆ **Oxymorphone Hydrochloride** *see* Oxymorphone *on page 1546*

◆ **OxyNEO (Can)** *see* OxyCODONE *on page 1538*

Oxytocin (oks i TOE sin)

Brand Names: U.S. Pitocin

Brand Names: Canada Oxytocin for injection

Index Terms Pit

Pharmacologic Category Oxytocic Agent

Use

Antepartum: Induction of labor in patients with a medical indication (eg, Rh problems, maternal diabetes, preeclampsia, at or near term); stimulation or reinforcement of labor (as in selected cases of uterine inertia); adjunctive therapy in management of incomplete or inevitable abortion

Postpartum: To produce uterine contractions during the third stage of labor and to control postpartum bleeding or hemorrhage.

Pregnancy Risk Factor C (manufacturer specific)

Pregnancy Considerations [U.S. Boxed Warning]: To be used for medical rather than elective induction of labor. Animal reproduction studies have not been conducted. When used as indicated, teratogenic effects would not be expected. Nonteratogenic adverse reactions are reported in the neonate as well as the mother.

Breast-Feeding Considerations Endogenous levels of oxytocin naturally increase during breast-feeding.

Contraindications Hypersensitivity to oxytocin or any component of the formulation; significant cephalopelvic disproportion; unfavorable fetal positions or presentations (such as transverse lies); fetal distress when delivery is not imminent; hypertonic or hyperactive uterus; contraindicated vaginal delivery (invasive cervical cancer, active genital herpes, prolapse of the cord, cord presentation, total placenta previa, or vasa previa); obstetrical emergencies where surgical intervention is favored; where adequate uterine activity fails to achieve satisfactory progress

Warnings/Precautions Hazardous agent - use appropriate precautions for handling and disposal (NIOSH 2014 [group 3]). **[U.S. Boxed Warning]: To be used for medical rather than elective induction of labor.** Oxytocin is used to initiate or improve uterine contractions in order to achieve a vaginal delivery; it should only be used when medically needed for fetal or maternal reasons. Medical indications for labor induction may include Rh problems, maternal diabetes, preeclampsia at or near term, when delivery is in the best interest of mother or fetus, or premature rupture of membranes when delivery is indicated. Use is generally not recommended in the following conditions: Fetal distress, hydramnios, partial placenta previa, prematurity, borderline cephalopelvic disproportion, or conditions where there is a predisposition for uterine rupture (eg, previous major surgery on cervix or uterus, cesarean section, overdistention of the uterus, grand multiparity, past history of uterine sepsis or traumatic delivery). May produce intrinsic antidiuretic effect (ie, water intoxication). Severe water intoxication with convulsions, coma, and death may occur, particularly with large doses (40 to 50 milliunits/minute) or when given as a slow infusion over 24 hours and if the patient is receiving fluids by mouth. High doses or hypersensitivity to oxytocin may cause uterine hypertonicity, spasm, tetanic contraction, or rupture of the uterus. Intravenous preparations should be administered by adequately trained individuals familiar with its use and able to identify complications; continuous observation is necessary for all patients. Maternal deaths caused by hypertensive episodes, subarachnoid hemorrhage, or rupture of the uterus and fetal deaths have occurred with oxytocic medications when used for induction of labor or for augmentation in the first and second stages of labor.

Adverse Reactions

Fetus or neonate:

Cardiovascular: Arrhythmias (including premature ventricular contractions), bradycardia

Central nervous system: Brain or CNS damage (permanent), neonatal seizure

Hepatic: Neonatal jaundice

Ocular: Neonatal retinal hemorrhage

Miscellaneous: Fetal death, low Apgar score (5 minute)

Mother:

Cardiovascular: Arrhythmias (including premature ventricular contractions), hypertensive episodes

Gastrointestinal: Nausea, vomiting

Genitourinary: Pelvic hematoma, postpartum hemorrhage, tetanic contraction of the uterus, uterine hypertonicity, uterine rupture, uterine spasm

Hematologic: Afibrinogenemia (fatal)

Miscellaneous: Anaphylactic reaction, subarachnoid hemorrhage; severe water intoxication with convulsions, coma, and death is associated with a slow oxytocin infusion over 24 hours

Drug Interactions

Metabolism/Transport Effects None known.

Avoid Concomitant Use

Avoid concomitant use of Oxytocin with any of the following: Carboprost Tromethamine

Increased Effect/Toxicity

Oxytocin may increase the levels/effects of: Highest Risk QTc-Prolonging Agents; Moderate Risk QTc-Prolonging Agents

The levels/effects of Oxytocin may be increased by: Carboprost Tromethamine; Dinoprostone; Mifepristone; Misoprostol

Decreased Effect There are no known significant interactions involving a decrease in effect.

Preparation for Administration Hazardous agent; use appropriate precautions for handling and disposal (NIOSH 2014 [group 3]).

IV:
Induction or stimulation of labor: Add oxytocin 10 units to NS or LR 1,000 mL to yield a solution containing oxytocin 10 milliunits/mL. Rotate solution to mix.
Postpartum uterine bleeding: Add oxytocin 10 to 40 units to running IV infusion; maximum: 40 units to 1,000 mL.
Adjunctive management of abortion: Add oxytocin 10 units to 500 mL of a physiologic saline solution or D_5W.

Storage/Stability Store at 20°C to 25°C (68°F to 77°F).

Mechanism of Action Oxytocin stimulates uterine contraction by activating G-protein-coupled receptors that trigger increases in intracellular calcium levels in uterine myofibrils. Oxytocin also increases local prostaglandin production, further stimulating uterine contraction.

Pharmacodynamics/Kinetics
Onset of action: Uterine contractions: IM: 3 to 5 minutes; IV: ~1 minute
Duration: IM: 2 to 3 hours; IV: 1 hour
Half-life elimination: 1 to 6 minutes; decreased in late pregnancy and during lactation
Excretion: Urine (small amount unchanged)

Dosage Adults: **Note:** IV administration requires the use of an infusion pump
Induction or stimulation of labor: IV: Initial: 0.5 to 1 milliunits/minute; gradually increase dose in increments of 1 to 2 milliunits/minute every 30 to 60 minutes until desired contraction pattern is established; dose may be decreased by similar increments after desired frequency of contractions is reached and labor has progressed to 5 to 6 cm dilation. Infusion rates up to 6 milliunits/minute provide oxytocin levels similar to those with spontaneous labor; rates >9 to 10 milliunits/minute are rarely required. Higher dose regimens (eg, initial dose 2 to 6 milliunits/minute) with larger incremental dose increases (eg, 1 to 6 milliunits/minute) have also been proposed; decrease or discontinue dose for abnormal or excessive uterine contractions (ACOG, 2009).
Note: Discontinue the oxytocin infusion immediately in the event of uterine hyperactivity and/or fetal distress. If uterine contractions become too powerful, the infusion can be stopped abruptly.
Postpartum uterine bleeding:
IM: 10 units after delivery of the placenta
IV: 10 to 40 units added to a running infusion solution depending on amount of infusion fluid remaining (maximum: 40 units in 1,000 mL of IV fluid); adjust infusion rate to sustain uterine contraction and control uterine atony
Adjunctive treatment of abortion: IV:
Incomplete, inevitable, or elective abortion: 10 units as an IV infusion after suction or a sharp curettage (used to help contract the uterus)
Midtrimester elective abortion: 10 to 20 **milli**units/minute; maximum total dose: 30 units/12 hours (may decrease injection to abortion time)

Dosage adjustment in renal impairment: There are no dosage adjustments provided in the manufacturer's labeling.
Dosage adjustment in hepatic impairment: There are no dosage adjustments provided in the manufacturer's labeling.

Administration
Induction or stimulation of labor: Administer as an IV infusion (drip method) by use of an infusion pump; accurate control of the rate of infusion flow is essential.
Incomplete or inevitable abortion: Administer by IV infusion
Postpartum uterine bleeding: Administer by IV infusion or IM.
Hazardous agent; use appropriate precautions for handling and disposal (NIOSH 2014 [group 3]).

Monitoring Parameters Fluid intake and output during administration, uterine activity, blood pressure; electronic fetal monitoring

Dosage Forms
Solution, Injection:
Pitocin: 10 units/mL (1 mL, 10 mL, 50 mL)
Generic: 10 units/mL (1 mL, 10 mL, 30 mL)

Oxytocin and Ergometrine Maleate [INT]
(oks i TOE sin & er GOT a meen MAL ee ate)

International Brand Names Syntometrine (AU, NZ)
Pharmacologic Category Ergot Derivative; Oxytocic Agent
Reported Use Active management of the third stage of labor; treatment and prevention of postpartum hemorrhage associated with uterine atony
Dosage Range IM: Adults:
Active management of the third stage of labor: Ergometrine maleate 0.5 mg and oxytocin 5 units after delivery of anterior shoulder or immediately after full delivery
Treatment or prevention of postpartum hemorrhage: Initial: Ergometrine maleate 0.5 mg and oxytocin 5 units following placental expulsion or when bleeding occurs. If necessary, may repeat dose after ≥2 hours; maximum: 3 doses (ergometrine 1.5 mg and oxytocin 15 units) in 24 hours.
Dosage adjustment in renal impairment:
Mild-to-moderate impairment: No dosage adjustment provided in manufacturer's labeling; use with caution
Severe impairment: Use is contraindicated
Dosage adjustment in hepatic impairment:
Mild-to-moderate impairment: No dosage adjustment provided in manufacturer's labeling; use with caution
Severe impairment: Use is contraindicated
Product Availability Product available in various countries; not currently available in the U.S.
Dosage Forms
Injection, solution: Oxytocin 5 units/mL and ergometrine 0.5 mg/mL (1 mL)

- ◆ **Oxytocin for injection (Can)** *see* Oxytocin *on page 1549*
- ◆ **Oxytrol** *see* Oxybutynin *on page 1536*
- ◆ **Oxytrol For Women [OTC]** *see* Oxybutynin *on page 1536*
- ◆ **Oysco D [OTC]** *see* Calcium and Vitamin D *on page 326*
- ◆ **Oysco 500 [OTC]** *see* Calcium Carbonate *on page 327*
- ◆ **Oysco 500+D [OTC]** *see* Calcium and Vitamin D *on page 326*
- ◆ **Ozurdex** *see* Dexamethasone (Ophthalmic) *on page 602*
- ◆ **P01BE03** *see* Artesunate *on page 178*
- ◆ **P-071** *see* Cetirizine *on page 411*
- ◆ **P-1202** *see* Methyl Aminolevulinate *on page 1332*
- ◆ **PA21** *see* Sucroferric Oxyhydroxide *on page 1941*
- ◆ **Pacerone** *see* Amiodarone *on page 114*

PACLitaxel (Conventional)
(pac li TAKS el con VEN sha nal)

Brand Names: Canada Apo-Paclitaxel; Paclitaxel for Injection; Paclitaxel Injection USP
Index Terms Conventional Paclitaxel; Onxyl; Taxol
Pharmacologic Category Antineoplastic Agent, Antimicrotubular; Antineoplastic Agent, Taxane Derivative

Use

Breast cancer: Adjuvant treatment of node-positive breast cancer; treatment of metastatic breast cancer after failure of combination chemotherapy or relapse within 6 months of adjuvant chemotherapy (prior therapy should have included an anthracycline)

Kaposi sarcoma (AIDS-related): Second-line treatment of AIDS-related Kaposi sarcoma

Non-small cell lung cancer: First-line treatment of non-small cell lung cancer (in combination with cisplatin) in patients who are not candidates for potentially curative surgery and/or radiation therapy

Ovarian cancer: Subsequent therapy for treatment of advanced ovarian cancer; first-line therapy of ovarian cancer (in combination with cisplatin)

Pregnancy Risk Factor D

Pregnancy Considerations Adverse events (embryotoxicity, fetal toxicity, and maternal toxicity) have been observed in animal reproduction studies at doses less than the recommended human dose. An *ex vivo* human placenta perfusion model illustrated that paclitaxel crossed the placenta at term. Placental transfer was low and affected by the presence of albumin; higher albumin concentrations resulted in lower paclitaxel placental transfer (Berveiller, 2012). Some pharmacokinetic properties of paclitaxel may be altered in pregnant women (van Hasselt, 2014). Women of childbearing potential should be advised to avoid becoming pregnant. A pregnancy registry is available for all cancers diagnosed during pregnancy at Cooper Health (877-635-4499).

Breast-Feeding Considerations Paclitaxel is excreted in breast milk (case report). The mother (3 months postpartum) was treated with paclitaxel 30 mg/m^2 (56.1 mg) and carboplatin once weekly for papillary thyroid cancer. Milk samples were obtained 4-316 hours after the infusion given at the sixth and final week of therapy. The average paclitaxel milk concentration over the testing interval was 0.78 mg/L. Although maternal serum concentrations were not noted in the report, the relative infant dose to a nursing infant was calculated to be ~17% of the maternal dose. Paclitaxel continued to be detected in breast milk when sampled at 172 hours after the dose and was below the limit of detection when sampled at 316 hours after the infusion (Griffin, 2012). Due to the potential for serious adverse reactions in a nursing infant, breast-feeding is not recommended.

Contraindications Hypersensitivity to paclitaxel, Cremophor EL (polyoxyethylated castor oil), or any component of the formulation; treatment of solid tumors in patients with baseline neutrophil counts <1,500/mm^3; treatment of Kaposi sarcoma in patients with baseline neutrophil counts <1,000/mm^3.

Warnings/Precautions Hazardous agent - use appropriate precautions for handling and disposal (NIOSH 2014 [group 1]). **[U.S. Boxed Warning]: Anaphylaxis and severe hypersensitivity reactions (dyspnea requiring bronchodilators, hypotension requiring treatment, angioedema, and/or generalized urticaria) have occurred in 2% to 4% of patients in clinical studies; premedicate with corticosteroids, diphenhydramine, and H_2 antagonists prior to infusion. Some reactions have been fatal despite premedication. If severe hypersensitivity occurs, stop infusion and do not rechallenge.** Minor hypersensitivity reactions (flushing, skin reactions, dyspnea, hypotension, or tachycardia) do not require interruption of treatment. Infusion-related hypotension, bradycardia, and/or hypertension may occur; frequent monitoring of vital signs is recommended, especially during the first hour of the infusion. Conventional paclitaxel formulations contain polyoxyethylated castor oil (Cremophor El) which is associated with hypersensitivity reactions. Formulations also contain dehydrated alcohol which may cause adverse CNS effects.

[U.S. Boxed Warning]: Bone marrow suppression (primarily neutropenia; may be severe or result in infection) may occur. Monitor blood counts frequently. Do not administer if baseline neutrophil count is <1,500/mm^3 (for solid tumors) or <1,000/mm^3 (for patients with AIDS-related Kaposi sarcoma). Bone marrow suppression (usually neutropenia) is dose-dependent and is the dose-limiting toxicity; neutrophil nadir is usually at a median of 11 days. Subsequent cycles should not be administered until neutrophils are >1,500/mm^3 (for solid tumors) and 1,000/mm^3 (for Kaposi sarcoma); platelets should recover to 100,000/mm^3. Reduce future doses by 20% for severe neutropenia (<500/mm^3 for 7 days or more) and consider the use of supportive therapy, including growth factor treatment.

Use extreme caution with hepatic dysfunction (myelotoxicity may be worsened in patients with total bilirubin >2 times ULN); dose reductions are recommended. Peripheral neuropathy may commonly occur; patients with preexisting neuropathies from prior chemotherapy or coexisting conditions (eg, diabetes mellitus) may be at a higher risk; reduce dose by 20% for severe neuropathy. Rare but severe conduction abnormalities have been reported; conduct continuous cardiac monitoring during subsequent infusions for these patients. Elderly patients have an increased risk of toxicity (neutropenia, neuropathy, and cardiovascular events); use with caution. Intraperitoneal administration of paclitaxel is associated with a higher incidence of chemotherapy-related toxicity (Armstrong, 2006).

Paclitaxel is an irritant with vesicant-like properties; ensure proper needle or catheter placement prior to and during infusion; avoid extravasation. Injection site reactions are generally mild (skin discoloration, tenderness, erythema, or swelling) and occur more commonly with an extended infusion duration (eg, 24 hours); injection site reactions may be delayed (7 to 10 days). More severe reactions (phlebitis, cellulitis, skin exfoliation, necrosis, fibrosis, and induration) have also been reported. Recall skin reactions may occur despite administering through a different IV site. **[U.S. Boxed Warning]: Should be administered under the supervision of an experienced cancer chemotherapy physician; administer in a facility sufficient to appropriately diagnose and manage complications.** Potentially significant drug-drug interactions may exist, requiring dose or frequency adjustment, additional monitoring, and/or selection of alternative therapy.

Adverse Reactions Myelosuppression is dose related, schedule related, and infusion-rate dependent (increased incidences with higher doses, more frequent doses, and longer infusion times) and, in general, rapidly reversible upon discontinuation.

Cardiovascular: Bradycardia, ECG abnormal, edema, flushing, hyper-/hypotension, rhythm abnormalities, syncope, tachycardia, venous thrombosis

Dermatologic: Alopecia, nail changes, rash

Gastrointestinal: Abdominal pain (with intraperitoneal paclitaxel), diarrhea, mucositis, nausea/vomiting, stomatitis

Hematologic: Anemia, bleeding, febrile neutropenia, leukopenia; neutropenia (onset 8-10 days, median nadir 11 days, recovery 15-21 days); thrombocytopenia

Hepatic: Alkaline phosphatase increased, AST increased, bilirubin increased

Local: Injection site reaction (erythema, tenderness, skin discoloration, swelling)

Neuromuscular & skeletal: Arthralgia/myalgia, peripheral neuropathy, weakness

Renal: Creatinine increased (observed in KS patients only)

Miscellaneous: Hypersensitivity reaction, infection

Rare but important or life-threatening: Anaphylaxis, arrhythmia, ataxia, atrial fibrillation, AV block, back pain, cardiac conduction abnormalities, cellulitis, CHF, chills, conjunctivitis, dehydration, enterocolitis, extravasation recall, hepatic encephalopathy, hepatic necrosis, induration, intestinal obstruction, intestinal perforation, interstitial pneumonia, ischemic colitis, lacrimation increased, maculopapular rash, malaise, MI, myocardial ischemia, necrotic changes and ulceration following extravasation, neuroencephalopathy, neutropenic enterocolitis, neutropenic typhlitis, ototoxicity (tinnitus and hearing loss), pancreatitis, paralytic ileus, phlebitis, pneumonitis, pruritus, pulmonary embolism, pulmonary fibrosis, radiation recall, radiation pneumonitis, renal insufficiency, seizure, skin exfoliation, skin fibrosis, skin necrosis, Stevens-Johnson syndrome, supraventricular tachycardia, toxic epidermal necrolysis, ventricular tachycardia (asymptomatic), visual disturbances (scintillating scotomata)

Drug Interactions

Metabolism/Transport Effects Substrate of CYP2C8 (major), CYP3A4 (major), P-glycoprotein; **Note:** Assignment of Major/Minor substrate status based on clinically relevant drug interaction potential; **Induces** CYP3A4 (weak)

Avoid Concomitant Use

Avoid concomitant use of PACLitaxel with any of the following: Atazanavir; BCG; CloZAPine; Conivaptan; Dipyrone; Fusidic Acid (Systemic); Idelalisib; Natalizumab; Pimecrolimus; SORAfenib; Tacrolimus (Topical); Tofacitinib; Vaccines (Live)

Increased Effect/Toxicity

PACLitaxel may increase the levels/effects of: Antineoplastic Agents (Anthracycline, Systemic); Bexarotene (Systemic); CloZAPine; DOXOrubicin (Conventional); Leflunomide; Natalizumab; Tofacitinib; Trastuzumab; Vaccines (Live); Vinorelbine

The levels/effects of PACLitaxel may be increased by: Aprepitant; Atazanavir; Ceritinib; Conivaptan; CYP2C8 Inhibitors (Moderate); CYP2C8 Inhibitors (Strong); CYP3A4 Inhibitors (Moderate); CYP3A4 Inhibitors (Strong); Dasatinib; Deferasirox; Denosumab; Dipyrone; Fosaprepitant; Fusidic Acid (Systemic); Idelalisib; Ivacaftor; Luliconazole; Mifepristone; Netupitant; P-glycoprotein/ABCB1 Inhibitors; Pimecrolimus; Platinum Derivatives; Roflumilast; Simeprevir; SORAfenib; Stiripentol; Tacrolimus (Topical)

Decreased Effect

PACLitaxel may decrease the levels/effects of: ARIPiprazole; BCG; Coccidioides immitis Skin Test; Hydrocodone; Saxagliptin; Sipuleucel-T; Vaccines (Inactivated); Vaccines (Live)

The levels/effects of PACLitaxel may be decreased by: Bexarotene (Systemic); Bosentan; CYP2C8 Inducers (Strong); CYP3A4 Inducers (Moderate); CYP3A4 Inducers (Strong); Dabrafenib; Deferasirox; Echinacea; Mitotane; P-glycoprotein/ABCB1 Inducers; Siltuximab; St Johns Wort; Tocilizumab; Trastuzumab

Preparation for Administration Hazardous agent; use appropriate precautions for handling and disposal (NIOSH 2014 [group 1]). Dilute for infusion in 250 to 1,000 mL D_5W, D_5LR, D_5NS, or NS to a concentration of 0.3 to 1.2 mg/mL, use a non-PVC container (glass or polyethylene). Chemotherapy dispensing devices (eg, Chemo Dispensing Pin) should not be used to withdraw paclitaxel from the vial; closed system transfer devices may not be compatible with undiluted paclitaxel.

Storage/Stability Store intact vials at room temperature of 20°C to 25°C (68°F to 77°F). Protect from light. Solutions diluted for infusion in D_5W and NS are stable for up to 27 hours at ambient temperature (~25°C). **Paclitaxel** should be dispensed in either glass or non-PVC containers (eg, Excel/PAB). Use **nonpolyvinyl** (non-PVC) tubing (eg, polyethylene) to minimize leaching. Formulated in a vehicle known as Cremophor EL (polyoxyethylated castor oil). Cremophor EL has been found to leach the plasticizer DEHP from polyvinyl chloride infusion bags or administration sets. Contact of the undiluted concentrate with plasticized polyvinyl chloride (PVC) equipment or devices is not recommended.

Mechanism of Action Paclitaxel promotes microtubule assembly by enhancing the action of tubulin dimers, stabilizing existing microtubules, and inhibiting their disassembly, interfering with the late G_2 mitotic phase, and inhibiting cell replication. In addition, the drug can distort mitotic spindles, resulting in the breakage of chromosomes. Paclitaxel may also suppress cell proliferation and modulate immune response.

Pharmacodynamics/Kinetics

V_{dss}: 24-hour infusion: 227 to 688 L/m^2; widely distributed into body fluids and tissues; affected by dose and duration of infusion

Protein binding: 89% to 98%

Metabolism: Hepatic via CYP2C8 and 3A4; forms metabolites (primarily 6α-hydroxypaclitaxel)

Half-life elimination:

3-hour infusion: Mean (terminal): ~13 to 20 hours

24-hour infusion: Mean (terminal): ~16 to 53 hours

Excretion: Feces (~71%; ~5% as unchanged drug); urine (~14%)

Dosage Note: Premedication with dexamethasone (20 mg orally 12 and 6 hours prior to the dose [reduce dexamethasone dose to 10 mg orally with advanced HIV disease]), diphenhydramine (50 mg IV 30 to 60 minutes prior to the dose), and cimetidine, famotidine, or ranitidine (IV 30 to 60 minutes prior to the dose) is recommended.

Breast cancer, adjuvant treatment: Adults: IV: 175 mg/m^2 over 3 hours every 3 weeks for 4 cycles (administer sequentially following an anthracycline-containing regimen)

Breast cancer, metastatic or relapsed: Adults: IV: 175 mg/m^2 over 3 hours every 3 weeks

Non-small cell lung cancer: Adults: IV: 135 mg/m^2 over 24 hours every 3 weeks (in combination with cisplatin)

Ovarian cancer, advanced: Adults:

Previously treated: IV: 135 or 175 mg/m^2 over 3 hours every 3 weeks

Previously untreated: IV: 175 mg/m^2 over 3 hours every 3 weeks (in combination with cisplatin) or 135 mg/m^2 over 24 hours administered every 3 weeks (in combination with cisplatin)

Intraperitoneal (off-label route): 60 mg/m^2 on day 8 of a 21-day treatment cycle for 6 cycles, in combination with IV paclitaxel (135 mg/m^2 over 24 hours on day 1) and intraperitoneal cisplatin (Armstrong, 2006). **Note:** Administration of intraperitoneal paclitaxel should include the standard paclitaxel premedication regimen.

Kaposi sarcoma, AIDS-related: Adults: IV: 135 mg/m^2 over 3 hours every 3 weeks or 100 mg/m^2 over 3 hours every 2 weeks (due to dose-related toxicity, the 100 mg/m^2 dose should be used for patients with a lower performance status). **Note:** Reduce the dexamethasone premedication dose to 10 mg.

Bladder cancer, advanced or metastatic (off-label use): Adults: IV: 150 mg/m^2 every 2 weeks (in combination with gemcitabine) (Sternberg, 2001) **or** 200 mg/m^2 over 1 hour every 3 weeks (in combination with gemcitabine) for 6 cycles (Meluch, 2001)

Cervical cancer, advanced (off-label use): Adults: IV: 135 or 175 mg/m^2 every 3 weeks (in combination with bevacizumab and cisplatin) until disease progression or unacceptable toxicity (Tewari, 2014) **or** 175 mg/m^2 every 3 weeks (in combination with bevacizumab and topotecan) until disease progression or unacceptable toxicity

(Tewari, 2014) **or** 135 mg/m² over 24 hours every 3 weeks (in combination with cisplatin) for 6 cycles (Monk, 2009; Moore, 2006).

Esophageal/gastric cancer, preoperative chemoradiation (off-label use): Adults: IV: 50 mg/m² on days 1, 8, 15, 22, and 29 (in combination with carboplatin and radiation therapy) followed by surgery within 4 to 6 weeks (van Hagen, 2012)

Head and neck cancers, advanced (off-label use): IV: 175 mg/m² over 3 hours every 3 weeks (in combination with cisplatin) for at least 6 cycles (Gibson, 2005)

Penile cancer, metastatic (off-label use): Adults: IV: 175 mg/m² over 3 hours every 3 to 4 weeks (in combination with ifosfamide and cisplatin) for 4 cycles (Pagliaro, 2010)

Small cell lung cancer, relapsed/refractory (off-label use): Adults: IV: 175 mg/m² over 3 hours every 3 weeks (as a single agent) for up to 5 cycles (Smit, 1998) **or** 80 mg/m² over 1 hour weekly for 6 weeks of an 8-week treatment cycle (as a single agent) until disease progression or unacceptable toxicity (Yamamoto, 2006)

Soft tissue sarcoma (angiosarcoma), advanced/unresectable (off-label use): Adults: IV: 80 mg/m² over 1 hour on days 1, 8, and 15 of a 4-week treatment cycle (as a single agent) for up to 6 cycles (Penel, 2008) **or** 135 to 175 mg/m² over 3 hours every 3 weeks (as a single agent) (Schlemmer, 2008) **or** 75 to 100 mg/m² once weekly (as a single agent) (Schlemmer, 2008)

Testicular germ cell tumors, relapsed/refractory (off-label use): Adults: IV: 80 mg/m² over 1 hour on days 1 and 8 of a 3-week treatment cycle (in combination with gemcitabine and oxaliplatin) for 2 cycles beyond best response up to a maximum of 8 cycles (Bokemeyer, 2008) **or** 250 mg/m² over 24 hours on day 1 of a 3-week treatment cycle (in combination with ifosfamide, mesna, cisplatin, and filgrastim) for 4 cycles (Kondagunta, 2005) **or** 100 mg/m² over 1 hour on days 1, 8, and 15 of a 4-week treatment cycle (in combination with gemcitabine) for up to 6 cycles (Einhorn, 2007)

Thymoma/thymic carcinoma, advanced (off-label use): Adults: IV: 225 mg/m² over 3 hours every 3 weeks (in combination with carboplatin) for up to 6 cycles (Lemma, 2011)

Unknown primary adenocarcinoma (off-label use): Adults: IV: 200 mg/m² over 3 hours every 3 weeks (in combination with carboplatin) for 6 to 8 cycles (Briasoulis, 2000) **or** 200 mg/m² over 1 hour every 3 weeks (in combination with carboplatin and etoposide) for 4 to 8 cycles (Greco, 2000)

Dosage modification for toxicity (solid tumors, including ovary, breast, and lung carcinoma): Courses of paclitaxel should not be repeated until the neutrophil count is ≥1,500/mm³ and the platelet count is ≥100,000/mm³; reduce dosage by 20% for patients experiencing severe peripheral neuropathy or severe neutropenia (neutrophil <500/mm³ for a week or longer)

Dosage modification for immunosuppression in advanced HIV disease: Paclitaxel should not be given to patients with HIV if the baseline or subsequent neutrophil count is <1,000/mm³. Additional modifications include: Reduce dosage of dexamethasone in premedication to 10 mg orally; reduce dosage by 20% in patients experiencing severe peripheral neuropathy or severe neutropenia (neutrophil <500/mm³ for a week or longer); initiate concurrent hematopoietic growth factor (G-CSF) as clinically indicated

Dosage adjustment in renal impairment: There are no dosage adjustments provided in the manufacturer's labeling. Aronoff (2007) recommends no dosage adjustment necessary for adults with CrCl <50 mL/minute.

Dosage adjustment in hepatic impairment: Note: The manufacturer's labeling recommendations are based upon the patient's first course of therapy where the usual dose would be 135 mg/m² dose over 24 hours or the 175 mg/m² dose over 3 hours in patients with normal hepatic function. Dosage in subsequent courses should be based upon individual tolerance. Adjustments for other regimens are not available.

24-hour infusion:

- Transaminases <2 times upper limit of normal (ULN) and bilirubin level ≤1.5 mg/dL: 135 mg/m²
- Transaminases 2 to <10 times ULN and bilirubin level ≤1.5 mg/dL: 100 mg/m²
- Transaminases <10 times ULN and bilirubin level 1.6 to 7.5 mg/dL: 50 mg/m²
- Transaminases ≥10 times ULN **or** bilirubin level >7.5 mg/dL: Avoid use

3-hour infusion:

- Transaminases <10 times ULN and bilirubin level ≤1.25 times ULN: 175 mg/m²
- Transaminases <10 times ULN and bilirubin level 1.26 to 2 times ULN: 135 mg/m²
- Transaminases <10 times ULN and bilirubin level 2.01 to 5 times ULN: 90 mg/m²
- Transaminases ≥10 times ULN **or** bilirubin level >5 times ULN: Avoid use

Dosing in obesity: *ASCO Guidelines for appropriate chemotherapy dosing in obese adults with cancer:* Utilize patient's actual body weight (full weight) for calculation of body surface area- or weight-based dosing, particularly when the intent of therapy is curative; manage regimen-related toxicities in the same manner as for nonobese patients; if a dose reduction is utilized due to toxicity, consider resumption of full weight-based dosing with subsequent cycles, especially if cause of toxicity (eg, hepatic or renal impairment) is resolved (Griggs, 2012).

Administration

IV: Infuse over 3 or 24 hours (depending on indication/protocol); some off-label protocols use a 1-hour infusion. Infuse through a 0.22-micron in-line filter and polyethylene-lined (non-PVC) administration set. When administered as a part of a combination chemotherapy regimen, sequence of administration may vary by regimen; refer to specific protocol for sequence recommendation.

Premedication with dexamethasone (20 mg orally or IV at 12 and 6 hours before the dose; reduce to 10 mg with advanced HIV disease), diphenhydramine (50 mg IV 30 to 60 minutes prior to the dose), and cimetidine 300 mg, famotidine 20 mg, or ranitidine 50 mg (IV 30 to 60 minutes prior to the dose) is recommended.

Irritant with vesicant-like properties; avoid extravasation. Ensure proper needle or catheter position prior to administration.

Extravasation management: If extravasation occurs, stop infusion immediately and disconnect (leave cannula/needle in place); gently aspirate extravasated solution (do **NOT** flush the line); remove needle/cannula; initiate antidote (hyaluronidase); remove needle/cannula; elevate extremity. Information conflicts regarding the use of warm or cold compresses (Perez Fidalgo, 2012; Polovich, 2009).

Hyaluronidase: If needle/cannula still in place: Administer 1-6 mL (150 units/mL) into existing IV line; usual dose is 1 mL for each 1 mL of extravasated drug; if needle/cannula has been removed, inject subcutaneously in a clockwise manner around area of extravasation; may repeat several times over the next 3 to 4 hours (Ener, 2004).

Intraperitoneal (off-label route): Solution was prepared in warmed saline and infused as rapidly as possible through an implantable intraperitoneal catheter (Armstrong, 2006).

Hazardous agent; use appropriate precautions for handling and disposal (NIOSH 2014 [group 1]).

Monitoring Parameters CBC with differential and platelet count, liver and kidney function; monitor for hypersensitivity reactions, vital signs (frequently during the first hour of infusion), continuous cardiac monitoring (patients with conduction abnormalities)

Dosage Forms Considerations Paclitaxel injection contains Cremophor EL

Dosage Forms

Concentrate, Intravenous:

Generic: 100 mg/16.7 mL (16.7 mL); 30 mg/5 mL (5 mL); 150 mg/25 mL (25 mL); 300 mg/50 mL (50 mL)

Concentrate, Intravenous [preservative free]:

Generic: 100 mg/16.7 mL (16.7 mL); 30 mg/5 mL (5 mL); 300 mg/50 mL (50 mL)

PACLitaxel (Protein Bound)

(pac li TAKS el PROE teen bownd)

Brand Names: U.S. Abraxane

Brand Names: Canada Abraxane for Injectable Suspension

Index Terms ABI-007; Albumin-Bound Paclitaxel; Albumin-Stabilized Nanoparticle Paclitaxel; nab-Paclitaxel; Nanoparticle Albumin-Bound Paclitaxel; Paclitaxel (Nanoparticle Albumin Bound); Paclitaxel, Albumin-Bound; Protein-Bound Paclitaxel

Pharmacologic Category Antineoplastic Agent, Antimicrotubular; Antineoplastic Agent, Taxane Derivative

Use

Breast cancer, metastatic: Treatment of refractory (metastatic) or relapsed (within 6 months of adjuvant therapy) breast cancer after failure of combination chemotherapy (including anthracycline-based therapy unless clinically contraindicated)

Non-small cell lung cancer (NSCLC): First-line treatment of locally advanced or metastatic NSCLC (in combination with carboplatin) in patients ineligible for curative surgery or radiation therapy

Pancreatic adenocarcinoma: First-line treatment of metastatic adenocarcinoma of the pancreas (in combination with gemcitabine)

Pregnancy Risk Factor D

Dosage Note: When administered as part of a combination chemotherapy regimen, sequence of administration may vary by regimen; refer to specific protocol for sequence of administration. Premedication is not generally necessary prior to paclitaxel (protein bound), but may be needed in patients with prior mild-to-moderate hypersensitivity reactions.

Breast cancer, metastatic: Adults: IV: 260 mg/m^2 every 3 weeks (Gradishar, 2005)

Off-label dosing: Adults: IV: 100 to 150 mg/m^2 on days 1, 8, and 15 of a 28-day cycle (Gradishar, 2009)

Non-small cell lung cancer (NSCLC), locally advanced or metastatic: Adults: IV: 100 mg/m^2 on days 1, 8, and 15 of each 21-day cycle (in combination with carboplatin) (Socinski, 2012)

Pancreatic adenocarcinoma, metastatic: Adults: IV: 125 mg/m^2 on days 1, 8, and 15 of a 28-day cycle (in combination with gemcitabine) (Von Hoff, 2013)

Melanoma, metastatic (off-label use): Adults: IV:

Previously treated patients: 100 mg/m^2 on days 1, 8, and 15 of a 28-day cycle; if tolerated, may increase dose by 25 mg/m^2 in cycle 2 and beyond (Hersh, 2010)

Previously untreated patients: 150 mg/m^2 on days 1, 8, and 15 of a 28-day cycle (Hersh, 2010)

Ovarian, fallopian tube, or primary peritoneal cancer, recurrent (off-label use): Adults: IV: 260 mg/m^2 on day 1 of a 21-day cycle for 6 to 8 cycles (Teneriello, 2009) **or** 100 mg/m^2 on days 1, 8, and 15 of a 28-day cycle until disease progression or unacceptable toxicity (Coleman, 2011)

Dosage adjustment for toxicity:

Breast cancer (every 3 week regimen):

Severe neutropenia (<500 cells/mm^3) ≥1 week: Reduce dose to 220 mg/m^2 for subsequent courses

Recurrent severe neutropenia: Reduce dose to 180 mg/m^2 for subsequent courses

Sensory neuropathy

Grade 1 or 2: Dosage adjustment generally not required

Grade 3: Hold treatment until resolved to grade 1 or 2, then resume with reduced dose for all subsequent cycles

Severe sensory neuropathy: Reduce dose to 220 mg/m^2 for subsequent courses

Recurrent severe sensory neuropathy: Reduce dose to 180 mg/m^2 for subsequent courses

Non-small cell lung cancer (NSCLC):

Neutropenia: ANC <1500 cells/mm^3: Withhold therapy until ANC is ≥1500 cells/mm^3 on day 1 or ≥500 cells/mm^3 on days 8 or 15. Reduce dose upon therapy reinitiation if:

Neutropenic fever (ANC <500 cells/mm^3 with fever >38°C) **or** delay of next cycle by >7 days due to ANC <1500 cells/mm^3 **or** ANC <500 cells/mm^3 for >7 days:

First occurrence: Permanently reduce dose to 75 mg/m^2

Second occurrence: Permanently reduce dose to 50 mg/m^2

Third occurrence: Discontinue therapy.

Thrombocytopenia: Platelet count <100,000 cells/mm^3: Withhold therapy until platelet count is ≥100,000 cells/mm^3 on day 1 or ≥50,000 cells/mm^3 on days 8 or 15. Reduce dose upon therapy reinitiation if:

Platelet count <50,000 cells/mm^3:

First occurrence: Permanently reduce dose to 75 mg/m^2

Second occurrence: Discontinue therapy.

Sensory neuropathy: Withhold therapy for grade 3 or 4 peripheral neuropathy. Resume therapy at reduced doses when neuropathy completely resolves or improves to grade 1:

First occurrence: Permanently reduce dose to 75 mg/m^2

Second occurrence: Permanently reduce dose to 50 mg/m^2

Third occurrence: Discontinue therapy.

Pancreatic adenocarcinoma:

Note: Dose level reductions for toxicity:

Full dose: 125 mg/m^2

First dose reduction: 100 mg/m^2

Second dose reduction: 75 mg/m^2

If additional dose reduction is necessary: Discontinue.

Hematologic toxicity (neutropenia and/or thrombocytopenia):

Day 1: If ANC is <1500 cells/mm^3 **or** platelet count is <100,000 cells/mm^3: Withhold therapy until ANC is ≥1500 cells/mm^3 and platelet count is ≥100,000 cells/mm^3

Day 8:

If ANC is 500 to <1000 cells/mm^3 **or** platelet count is 50,000 to <75,000 cells/mm^3: Reduce 1 dose level

If ANC is <500 cells/mm^3 **or** platelet count is <50,000 cells/mm^3: Withhold day 8 dose

Day 15 (if day 8 doses were reduced or given without modification):

If ANC is 500 to <1000 cells/mm^3 **or** platelet count is 50,000 to <75,000 cells/mm^3: Reduce 1 dose level from day 8

If ANC is <500 cells/mm^3 **or** platelet count is <50,000 cells/mm^3: Withhold day 15 dose

Day 15 (if day 8 doses were withheld):

If ANC is ≥1000 cells/mm^3 or platelet count is ≥75,000 cells/mm^3: Reduce 1 dose level from day 1

If ANC is 500 to <1000 cells/mm^3 or platelet count is 50,000 to <75,000 cells/mm^3: Reduce 2 dose levels from day 1

If ANC is <500 cells/mm^3 **or** platelet count is <50,000 cells/mm^3: Withhold day 15 dose

Neutropenic fever: Withhold therapy for grade 3 or 4 fever. Resume therapy at next lower dose level when fever resolves and ANC is ≥1500 cells/mm^3.

Peripheral neuropathy: Withhold therapy for grade 3 or 4 peripheral neuropathy. Resume therapy at next lower dose level when neuropathy improves to ≤ grade 1.

Dermatologic toxicity: For grade 2 or 3 toxicity, reduce dose to next lower dose level; if toxicity persists, discontinue.

Gastrointestinal toxicity: Withhold therapy for grade 3 mucositis or diarrhea. Resume therapy at next lower dose level when improves to ≤ grade 1.

Dosage adjustment in renal impairment: There are no dosage adjustments provided in the manufacturer's labeling (has not been studied).

Dosage adjustment in hepatic impairment:

Dosage adjustment for hepatic impairment at treatment initiation:

Breast cancer (every 3 week regimen):

Mild impairment (AST ≤10 times ULN and bilirubin >1 to ≤1.5 times ULN): No dosage adjustment is necessary.

Moderate impairment (AST ≤10 times ULN and bilirubin >1.5 to ≤3 times ULN): Reduce dose to 200 mg/m^2; may increase up to 260 mg/m^2 if the reduced dose is tolerated for 2 cycles

Severe impairment:

AST ≤10 times ULN and bilirubin >3 to ≤5 times ULN: Reduce dose to 200 mg/m^2; may increase up to 260 mg/m^2 in subsequent cycles if the reduced dose is tolerated for 2 cycles

AST >10 times ULN or bilirubin >5 times ULN: Use is not recommended

Non-small cell lung cancer (NSCLC) regimen:

Mild impairment (AST ≤10 times ULN and bilirubin >1 to ≤1.5 times ULN): No dosage adjustment is necessary.

Moderate impairment (AST ≤10 times ULN and bilirubin >1.5 to ≤3 times ULN): Reduce dose to 80 mg/m^2; may increase up to 100 mg/m^2 in subsequent cycles if the reduced dose is tolerated for 2 cycles

Severe impairment:

AST ≤10 times ULN and bilirubin >3 to ≤5 times ULN: Reduce dose to 80 mg/m^2; may increase up to 100 mg/m^2 in subsequent cycles if the reduced dose is tolerated for 2 cycles

AST >10 times ULN or bilirubin >5 times ULN: Use is not recommended.

Pancreatic adenocarcinoma:

Mild impairment (AST ≤10 times ULN and bilirubin >1 to ≤1.5 times ULN): No dosage adjustment is necessary.

Moderate impairment (AST ≤10 times ULN and bilirubin >1.5 to ≤3 times ULN): Use is not recommended.

Severe impairment:

AST ≤10 times ULN and bilirubin >3 to ≤5 times ULN: Use is not recommended.

AST >10 times ULN or bilirubin >5 times ULN: Use is not recommended.

Dosage adjustment for hepatic impairment during treatment: AST >10 times ULN or bilirubin >5 times ULN: Withhold treatment

Dosing in obesity: *ASCO Guidelines for appropriate chemotherapy dosing in obese adults with cancer:* Utilize patient's actual body weight (full weight) for calculation of body surface area- or weight-based dosing, particularly when the intent of therapy is curative; manage regimen-related toxicities in the same manner as for nonobese patients; if a dose reduction is utilized due to toxicity, consider resumption of full weight-based dosing with subsequent cycles, especially if cause of toxicity (eg, hepatic or renal impairment) is resolved (Griggs, 2012).

Additional Information Complete prescribing information should be consulted for additional detail.

Dosage Forms

Suspension Reconstituted, Intravenous:

Abraxane: 100 mg (1 ea)

- **Paclitaxel, Albumin-Bound** *see* PACLitaxel (Protein Bound) *on page 1554*
- **Paclitaxel for Injection (Can)** *see* PACLitaxel (Conventional) *on page 1550*
- **Paclitaxel Injection USP (Can)** *see* PACLitaxel (Conventional) *on page 1550*
- **Paclitaxel (Nanoparticle Albumin Bound)** *see* PACLitaxel (Protein Bound) *on page 1554*
- **Pain Eze [OTC]** *see* Acetaminophen *on page 32*
- **Pain & Fever Children's [OTC]** *see* Acetaminophen *on page 32*
- **Pain-Off [OTC]** *see* Acetaminophen, Aspirin, and Caffeine *on page 37*
- **Palafer® (Can)** *see* Ferrous Fumarate *on page 870*
- **Palgic [DSC]** *see* Carbinoxamine *on page 356*

Palifermin (pal ee FER min)

Brand Names: U.S. Kepivance

Brand Names: Canada Kepivance®

Index Terms AMJ 9701; Keratinocyte Growth Factor, Recombinant Human; rhKGF; rhu Keratinocyte Growth Factor; rHu-KGF

Pharmacologic Category Chemoprotective Agent; Keratinocyte Growth Factor

Use Decrease the incidence and duration of severe oral mucositis associated with hematologic malignancies in patients receiving myelotoxic therapy requiring hematopoietic stem cell support (when the preparative regimen is expected to result in mucositis ≥ grade 3 in most patients)

Note: Use (safety and efficacy) is not established for nonhematologic malignancies; use is not recommended with conditioning regimens containing melphalan 200 mg/m^2

Pregnancy Risk Factor C

Dosage IV: Adults: Oral mucositis associated with hematopoietic stem cell transplant (HSCT) conditioning regimens: 60 mcg/kg/day for 3 consecutive days before and 3 consecutive days after myelotoxic therapy; total of 6 doses (Spielberger, 2004)

Note: Administer first 3 doses prior to myelotoxic therapy, with the 3rd dose given 24-48 hours before beginning the myelotoxic conditioning regimen. Administer the last 3 doses after completion of the conditioning regimen, with the first of these doses after but on the same day as HSCT infusion and at least 4 days after the most recent dose of palifermin.

Dosage adjustment in renal impairment: No dosage adjustment necessary.

Dosage adjustment in hepatic impairment: No dosage adjustment provided in the manufacturer's labeling (has not been studied).

Additional Information Complete prescribing information should be consulted for additional detail.

Dosage Forms

Solution Reconstituted, Intravenous [preservative free]: Kepivance: 6.25 mg (1 ea)

Paliperidone (pal ee PER i done)

Brand Names: U.S. Invega; Invega Sustenna

Brand Names: Canada Invega; Invega Sustenna

Index Terms 9-hydroxy-risperidone; 9-OH-risperidone; Paliperidone Palmitate

Pharmacologic Category Second Generation (Atypical) Antipsychotic

Additional Appendix Information

Beers Criteria - Potentially Inappropriate Medications for Geriatrics *on page 2271*

Use

Schizophrenia: Treatment of schizophrenia

Schizoaffective disorder: Treatment of schizoaffective disorder as monotherapy and as an adjunct to mood stabilizers or antidepressants

Pregnancy Risk Factor C

Pregnancy Considerations Adverse events were not observed in animal reproduction studies. Antipsychotic use during the third trimester of pregnancy has a risk for extrapyramidal symptoms (EPS) and/or withdrawal symptoms in newborns following delivery. Symptoms in the newborn may include agitation, feeding disorder, hypertonia, hypotonia, respiratory distress, somnolence, and tremor. These effects may be self-limiting and allow recovery within hours or days with no specific treatment, or they may be severe requiring prolonged hospitalization.

Paliperidone may cause hyperprolactinemia, which may decrease reproductive function in both males and females. Paliperidone is the active metabolite of risperidone; refer to Risperidone monograph for additional information.

The ACOG recommends that therapy during pregnancy be individualized; treatment with psychiatric medications during pregnancy should incorporate the clinical expertise of the mental health clinician, obstetrician, primary healthcare provider, and pediatrician. Safety data related to atypical antipsychotics during pregnancy is limited and routine use is not recommended. However, if a woman is inadvertently exposed to an atypical antipsychotic while pregnant, continuing therapy may be preferable to switching to a typical antipsychotic that the fetus has not yet been exposed to; consider risk:benefit (ACOG, 2008).

Healthcare providers are encouraged to enroll women 18 to 45 years of age exposed to paliperidone during pregnancy in the Atypical Antipsychotics Pregnancy Registry (1-866-961-2388 or http://www.womensmentalhealth.org/pregnancyregistry).

Breast-Feeding Considerations Paliperidone is excreted into breast milk. According to the manufacturer, the decision to continue or discontinue breast-feeding during therapy should take into account the risk of exposure to the infant and the benefits of treatment to the mother.

Contraindications Hypersensitivity to paliperidone, risperidone, or any component of the formulation

Warnings/Precautions [U.S. Boxed Warning]: Elderly patients with dementia-related psychosis treated with antipsychotics are at an increased risk of death compared to placebo. Most deaths appeared to be either cardiovascular (eg, heart failure, sudden death) or infectious (eg, pneumonia) in nature. In addition, an increased incidence of cerebrovascular adverse effects (eg, transient ischemic attack, cerebrovascular accidents) has been reported in studies of placebo-controlled trials of risperidone (paliperidone is the primary active metabolite of risperidone) in elderly patients with dementia-related psychosis. Paliperidone is not approved for the treatment of dementia-related psychosis. In addition, patients with Lewy body dementia (LBD) may be more sensitive to CNS-related and extrapyramidal effects.

Compared with risperidone, paliperidone is low to moderately sedating; use with caution in disorders where CNS depression is a feature. Use caution in patients with predisposition to seizures. Use with caution in mild renal dysfunction; dose reduction recommended. Not recommended in patients with moderate-to-severe impairment. Esophageal dysmotility and aspiration have been associated with antipsychotic use; use with caution in patients at risk of aspiration pneumonia (eg, Alzheimer's disease).

Leukopenia, neutropenia, and agranulocytosis (sometimes fatal) have been reported in clinical trials and postmarketing reports with antipsychotic use; presence of risk factors (eg, preexisting low WBC or history of drug-induced leuko-/neutropenia) should prompt periodic blood count assessment. Discontinue therapy at first signs of blood dyscrasias or if absolute neutrophil count <1000/mm^3.

Paliperidone is associated with increased prolactin levels; clinical significance of hyperprolactinemia in patients with breast cancer or other prolactin-dependent tumors is unknown. May alter temperature regulation. May mask toxicity of other drugs or conditions (eg, intestinal obstruction, Reye's syndrome, brain tumor) due to antiemetic effects. Priapism has been reported rarely with use.

May cause orthostasis and syncope. Use with caution in patients with cardiovascular diseases (eg, heart failure, history of myocardial infarction or ischemia, cerebrovascular disease, conduction abnormalities). Use caution in patients receiving medications for hypertension (orthostatic effects may be exacerbated) or in patients with hypovolemia or dehydration. May alter cardiac conduction; life-threatening arrhythmias have occurred with therapeutic doses of neuroleptics. Avoid use in combination with QTc-prolonging drugs. Avoid use in patients with congenital long QT syndrome and in patients with history of cardiac arrhythmia.

May cause extrapyramidal symptoms (EPS), including pseudoparkinsonism, acute dystonic reactions, akathisia, and tardive dyskinesia (risk of these reactions is low relative to other neuroleptics, and is dose dependent). Risk of dystonia (and probably other EPS) may be greater with increased doses, use of conventional antipsychotics, males, and younger patients. Risk of neuroleptic malignant syndrome (NMS) may be increased in patients with Parkinson's disease or Lewy body dementia; monitor for symptoms of confusion, obtundation, postural instability and extrapyramidal symptoms. May cause hyperglycemia; in some cases may be extreme and associated with ketoacidosis, hyperosmolar coma, or death. Use with caution in patients with diabetes (or risk factors) or other disorders of glucose regulation; monitor for worsening of glucose control. Significant weight gain has been observed with antipsychotic therapy; incidence varies with product. Monitor waist circumference and BMI. May cause lipid abnormalities (LDL and triglycerides increased; HDL decreased). Few case reports describe intraoperative floppy iris syndrome (IFIS) in patients receiving risperidone and undergoing cataract surgery (Ford, 2011). IFIS has not been reported with paliperidone but caution is advised since it is the active metabolite of risperidone. Prior to cataract surgery, evaluate for prior or current paliperidone or risperidone use. The benefits or risks of interrupting paliperidone or risperidone prior to surgery have not been established; clinicians are advised to proceed with surgery cautiously.

The possibility of a suicide attempt is inherent in psychotic illness or bipolar disorder; use caution in high-risk patients during initiation of therapy. Prescriptions should be written for the smallest quantity consistent with good patient care.

Use in elderly patients with dementia is associated with an increased risk of mortality and cerebrovascular accidents; avoid antipsychotic use for behavioral problems associated with dementia unless alternative nonpharmacologic therapies have failed and patient may harm self or others. In addition, use may cause or exacerbate syndrome of inappropriate antidiuretic hormone secretion or hyponatremia; monitor sodium closely with initiation or dosage adjustments in older adults (Beers Criteria).

The tablet formulation consists of drug within a nonabsorbable shell that is expelled and may be visible in the stool. Use is not recommended in patients with preexisting severe gastrointestinal narrowing disorders. Patients with upper GI tract alterations in transit time may have increased or decreased bioavailability of paliperidone. Do not use in patients unable to swallow the tablet whole.

Adverse Reactions Unless otherwise noted, frequency of adverse effects is reported for the oral/IM formulation in adults.

Cardiovascular: Bundle branch block, orthostatic hypotension (dose dependent), tachycardia (adolescents and adults)

Central nervous system: Agitation, akathisia (adolescents and adults; dose dependent), anxiety (adolescents and adults), dizziness (adolescents and adults), drowsiness (more common in adolescents; dose dependent), dysarthria (dose dependent), dystonia (adolescents and adults; dose dependent), extrapyramidal reaction (more common in adolescents; dose dependent), fatigue (adolescents and adults), headache (adolescents and adults), lethargy (adolescents and adults), parkinsonian-like syndrome (adolescents and adults; dose dependent), sleep disorder

Endocrine & metabolic: Abnormal triglycerides (adolescents and adults), altered serum glucose (adolescents and adults), amenorrhea (adolescents and adults), blood cholesterol abnormal (adolescents and adults), galactorrhea (adolescents and adults), gynecomastia (adolescents and adults), weight gain (adolescents and adults; dose dependent)

Gastrointestinal: Abdominal pain, constipation, diarrhea, dyspepsia, increased appetite, nausea, sialorrhea (adolescents and adults; dose dependent), swollen tongue (adolescents and adults), toothache, vomiting (adolescents and adults), xerostomia (adolescents and adults)

Hematologic & oncologic: Change in HDL (adolescents and adults), change in LDL (adolescents and adults)

Local: IM formulation: Injection site reaction

Neuromuscular & skeletal: Back pain, dyskinesia (adolescents and adults), hyperkinesia (adolescents and adults; dose dependent), limb pain, myalgia (dose dependent), tongue paralysis (adolescents), tremor (adolescents and adults), weakness (adolescents and adults)

Ophthalmic: Blurred vision (adolescents and adults)

Respiratory: cough (dose dependent), nasopharyngitis (adolescents and adults; dose dependent), rhinitis (dose dependent), upper respiratory tract infection

Rare but important or life-threatening: Agranulocytosis, alopecia, anaphylaxis, antiemetic effect, aspiration pneumonia, atrial fibrillation, cerebrovascular accident, deep vein thrombosis, diabetes mellitus, diabetic ketoacidosis, edema, epistaxis, erectile dysfunction, first degree atrioventricular block, hyperprolactinemia, hypertension, hypertonia, hypothermia, increased serum ALT, increased serum AST, insomnia, intestinal obstruction, intraoperative floppy iris syndrome, ischemia, jaundice, mania, neuroleptic malignant syndrome, orthostatic dizziness, pancreatitis, postural orthostatic tachycardia, priapism, psychomotor agitation, pulmonary embolism, retrograde ejaculation, seizure, SIADH, sleep apnea, suicidal ideation, syncope, tardive dyskinesia, thrombocytopenia, thrombotic thrombocytopenic purpura, trismus, urinary incontinence, urinary retention, venous thromboembolism

Drug Interactions

Metabolism/Transport Effects **Substrate** of P-glycoprotein

Avoid Concomitant Use

Avoid concomitant use of Paliperidone with any of the following: Amisulpride; Azelastine (Nasal); Highest Risk QTc-Prolonging Agents; Ivabradine; Metoclopramide; Mifepristone; Moderate Risk QTc-Prolonging Agents; Orphenadrine; Paraldehyde; Sulpiride; Thalidomide

Increased Effect/Toxicity

Paliperidone may increase the levels/effects of: Alcohol (Ethyl); Amisulpride; Azelastine (Nasal); Buprenorphine; CNS Depressants; Highest Risk QTc-Prolonging Agents; Hydrocodone; Methotrimeprazine; Methylphenidate; Metyrosine; Orphenadrine; Paraldehyde; Selective Serotonin Reuptake Inhibitors; Serotonin Modulators; Sulpiride; Suvorexant; Thalidomide; Zolpidem

The levels/effects of Paliperidone may be increased by: Acetylcholinesterase Inhibitors (Central); Brimonidine (Topical); Cannabis; Doxylamine; Dronabinol; Itraconazole; Ivabradine; Kava Kava; Magnesium Sulfate; Methotrimeprazine; Methylphenidate; Metoclopramide; Metyrosine; Mifepristone; Moderate Risk QTc-Prolonging Agents; Nabilone; Perampanel; P-glycoprotein/ABCB1 Inhibitors; QTc-Prolonging Agents (Indeterminate Risk and Risk Modifying); RisperiDONE; Rufinamide; Serotonin Modulators; Sodium Oxybate; Tapentadol; Tetrahydrocannabinol; Valproic Acid and Derivatives

Decreased Effect

Paliperidone may decrease the levels/effects of: Amphetamines; Anti-Parkinson's Agents (Dopamine Agonist); Quinagolide

The levels/effects of Paliperidone may be decreased by: CarBAMazepine; P-glycoprotein/ABCB1 Inducers

Storage/Stability Store at controlled room temperature of ≤25°C (77°F); excursions permitted to 15°C to 30°C (59°F to 86°F). Protect tablets from moisture.

Mechanism of Action Paliperidone is considered a benzisoxazole atypical antipsychotic as it is the primary active metabolite of risperidone. As with other atypical antipsychotics, its therapeutic efficacy is believed to result from mixed central serotonergic and dopaminergic antagonism. The addition of serotonin antagonism to dopamine antagonism (classic neuroleptic mechanism) is thought to improve negative symptoms of psychoses and reduce the incidence of extrapyramidal side effects. Similar to risperidone, paliperidone demonstrates high affinity to α_1, D_2, H_1, and 5-HT_{2C} receptors, and low affinity for muscarinic and 5-HT_{1A} receptors. In contrast to risperidone, paliperidone displays nearly 10-fold lower affinity for α_2 and 5-HT_{2A} receptors, and nearly three- to fivefold less affinity for 5-HT_{1A} and 5-HT_{1D}, respectively.

Pharmacodynamics/Kinetics

Absorption: IM: Slow release (begins on day 1 and continues up to 126 days)

Distribution: V_d: 391 to 487 L

Protein binding: 74%

Metabolism: Hepatic via CYP2D6 and 3A4 (limited role in elimination); minor metabolism (<10% each) via dealkylation, hydroxylation, dehydrogenation, and benzisoxazole scission

Bioavailability: 28%

Half-life elimination:

Oral: 23 hours; 24 to 51 hours with renal impairment (CrCl <80 mL/minute)

IM (following a single-dose administration): Range: 25 to 49 days

Time to peak, plasma: Oral: ~24 hours; IM: 13 days

Excretion: Urine (80%); feces (11%)

Dosage

U.S. labeling:

Schizoaffective disorder: Adults:

Oral: Usual: 6 mg once daily in the morning; titration not required, though some may benefit from lower or higher doses (range: 3 to 12 mg daily). If exceeding 6 mg daily, increases of 3 mg daily are recommended no more frequently than every 4 days, up to a maximum of 12 mg daily.

IM: **Note:** Prior to initiation of IM therapy, tolerability should be established with oral paliperidone or oral risperidone. Previous oral antipsychotics can be discontinued at the time of initiation of IM therapy. **Dosing based on paliperidone palmitate.**

Initiation of therapy:

Initial: 234 mg on treatment day 1 followed by 156 mg 1 week later with both doses administered in the deltoid muscle. The second dose may be administered 4 days before or after the weekly time point.

Maintenance: Following the 1-week initiation regimen, adjust the dose based on response and tolerability and begin a maintenance dose of 78 to 234 mg every month administered in either the deltoid or gluteal muscle (the 39 mg strength was not studied in schizoaffective disorder trials). The monthly maintenance dose may be administered 7 days before or after the monthly time point.

Conversion from oral paliperidone to IM paliperidone: Initiate IM therapy as described using the 1-week initiation regimen. Patients previously stabilized on oral doses can expect similar steady state exposure during maintenance treatment with IM therapy using the following conversion:

Oral extended release dose of 12 mg daily, then IM maintenance dose of 234 mg monthly

Oral extended release dose of 6 mg daily, then IM maintenance dose of 117 mg monthly

Oral extended release dose of 3 mg daily, then IM maintenance dose of 39 to 78 mg monthly

Switching from other long-acting injectable antipsychotics to IM paliperidone: Initiate IM paliperidone in the place of the next scheduled injection and continue at monthly intervals. The 1-week initiation regimen is not required in these patients.

Dosage adjustments: Adjustments may be made monthly (full effect from adjustments may not be seen for several months)

Missed second initiation dose:

If <4 weeks have elapsed since the first injection: Administer the missed dose (156 mg) in the deltoid as soon as possible, followed by a third dose of 117 mg in either the deltoid or gluteal muscle 5 weeks after the first injection (regardless of when the second injection was administered), then begin normal monthly maintenance dosing.

If ≥4 weeks and ≤7 weeks have elapsed since the first injection: Administer a dose of 156 mg in the deltoid as soon as possible, followed by another 156 mg dose in the deltoid 1 week later, then begin normal monthly maintenance dosing.

If >7 weeks have elapsed since the first injection: Therapy must be reinitiated following dosing recommendations for initiation of therapy.

Missed maintenance dose:

If ≥4 weeks and ≤6 weeks have elapsed since the last monthly injection: Administer the missed dose as soon as possible and continue therapy at monthly intervals.

If >6 weeks and ≤6 months have elapsed since the last monthly injection:

If the maintenance dose was <234 mg: Administer the same dose the patient was previously stabilized on in the deltoid as soon as possible, followed by a second equivalent dose in the deltoid 1 week later, then resume maintenance dose at monthly intervals.

If the maintenance dose was 234 mg: Administer a 156 mg dose in the deltoid as soon as possible, followed by a second dose of 156 mg in the deltoid 1 week later, then resume maintenance dose at monthly intervals.

If >6 months have elapsed since last monthly maintenance injection: Therapy must be reinitiated following dosing recommendations for initiation of therapy.

Schizophrenia:

Adolescents 12 to 17 years: Oral: Initial: 3 mg once daily; titration not required (no known benefit to efficacy from higher doses [ie, 6 mg daily for patients <51 kg and 12 mg daily for patients ≥51 kg]). If exceeding 3 mg daily, increases of 3 mg daily are recommended no more frequently than every 5 days.

Adults:

Oral: Usual: 6 mg once daily in the morning; titration not required, though some may benefit from lower or higher doses (range: 3 to 12 mg daily). If exceeding 6 mg daily, increases of 3 mg daily are recommended no more frequently than every 5 days, up to a maximum of 12 mg daily.

IM: **Note:** Prior to initiation of IM therapy, tolerability should be established with oral paliperidone or oral risperidone. Previous oral antipsychotics can be discontinued at the time of initiation of IM therapy. **Dosing based on paliperidone palmitate.**

Initiation of therapy:

Initial: 234 mg on treatment day 1 followed by 156 mg 1 week later with both doses administered in the deltoid muscle. The second dose may be administered 4 days before or after the weekly time point.

Maintenance: Following the 1-week initiation regimen, begin a maintenance dose of 117 mg every month administered in either the deltoid or gluteal muscle. Some patients may benefit from higher or lower monthly maintenance doses (monthly maintenance dosage range: 39 to 234 mg). The monthly maintenance dose may be administered 7 days before or after the monthly time point.

Conversion from oral paliperidone to IM paliperidone: Initiate IM therapy as described using the 1-week initiation regimen. Patients previously stabilized on oral doses can expect similar steady state exposure during maintenance treatment with IM therapy using the following conversion:

Oral extended release dose of 12 mg daily, then IM maintenance dose of 234 mg monthly

Oral extended release dose of 6 mg daily, then IM maintenance dose of 117 mg monthly

Oral extended release dose of 3 mg daily, then IM maintenance dose of 39 to 78 mg monthly

Switching from other long-acting injectable antipsychotics to IM paliperidone: Initiate IM paliperidone in the place of the next scheduled injection and continue at monthly intervals. The 1-week initiation regimen is not required in these patients.

Dosage adjustments: Adjustments may be made monthly (full effect from adjustments may not be seen for several months)

Missed second initiation dose:

If <4 weeks have elapsed since the first injection: Administer the missed dose (156 mg) in the deltoid as soon as possible, followed by a third dose of 117 mg in either the deltoid or gluteal muscle 5 weeks after the first injection (regardless of when the second injection was administered), then begin normal monthly maintenance dosing.

If ≥4 weeks and ≤7 weeks have elapsed since the first injection: Administer a dose of 156 mg in the deltoid as soon as possible, followed by another 156 mg dose in the deltoid 1 week later, then begin normal monthly maintenance dosing.

If >7 weeks has elapsed since the first injection: Therapy must be reinitiated following dosing recommendations for initiation of therapy.

Missed maintenance dose:

If ≥4 weeks and ≤6 weeks have elapsed since the last monthly injection: Administer the missed dose as soon as possible and continue therapy at monthly intervals.

If >6 weeks and ≤6 months have elapsed since the last monthly injection:

If the maintenance dose was <234 mg: Administer the same dose the patient was previously stabilized on in the deltoid as soon as possible, followed by a second equivalent dose in the deltoid 1 week later, then resume maintenance dose at monthly intervals.

If the maintenance dose was 234 mg: Administer a 156 mg dose in the deltoid as soon as possible, followed by a second dose of 156 mg in the deltoid 1 week later, then resume maintenance dose at monthly intervals.

If >6 months have elapsed since last monthly maintenance injection: Therapy must be reinitiated following dosing recommendations for initiation of therapy.

Canadian labeling:

Schizophrenia: Adults:

Oral: Usual: 6 mg once daily in the morning; titration not required, though some may benefit from lower or higher doses (range: 3 to 12 mg daily). If exceeding 6 mg daily, increases of 3 mg daily are recommended no more frequently than every 5 days in schizophrenia, up to a maximum of 12 mg daily.

IM: **Note:** Prior to initiation of IM therapy, tolerability should be established with oral paliperidone or oral risperidone. Previous oral antipsychotics can be discontinued at the time of initiation of IM therapy. **Dosing based on paliperidone.**

Initiation of therapy:

Initial: 150 mg on treatment day 1 followed by 100 mg 1 week later (day 8) with both doses administered in the deltoid. The second dose may be administered up to 4 days before or after the weekly time point.

Maintenance: Following the 1-week initiation regimen, begin a maintenance dose of 75 mg every month administered in either the deltoid or gluteal muscle. Some patients may benefit from higher or lower monthly maintenance doses (monthly maintenance dosage range: 50 to 150 mg). The monthly maintenance dose may be administered 7 days before or after the monthly time point.

Conversion from oral paliperidone to IM paliperidone: Initiate IM therapy as described using the 1-week initiation regimen. Patients previously stabilized on oral doses can expect similar steady state exposure during maintenance treatment with IM therapy using the following conversion:

Oral extended release dose of 12 mg daily, then IM maintenance dose of 150 mg monthly

Oral extended release dose of 6 mg daily, then IM maintenance dose of 75 mg monthly

Oral extended release dose of 3 mg daily, then IM maintenance dose of 50 mg monthly

Switching from other long-acting injectable antipsychotics (eg, Risperdal® Consta®) to IM paliperidone: Initiate IM paliperidone in the place of the next scheduled injection and continue at monthly intervals. The 1-week initiation regimen is not required in these patients.

Switching from injectable risperidone (Risperdal Consta) to IM paliperidone:

Risperdal® Consta® dose of 25 mg every 2 weeks, then IM paliperidone maintenance dose of 50 mg monthly

Risperdal® Consta® dose of 37.5 mg every 2 weeks, then IM paliperidone maintenance dose of 75 mg monthly

Risperdal® Consta® dose of 50 mg every 2 weeks, then IM paliperidone maintenance dose of 100 mg monthly

Dosage adjustments: Adjustments may be made monthly (full effect from adjustments may not be seen for several months)

Missed second initiation dose:

If <4 weeks has elapsed since first injection: Administer the missed dose (100 mg) in the deltoid as soon as possible followed by a third dose of 75 mg in either the deltoid or gluteal muscle 5 weeks after the first injection (regardless of the when the second injection was administered), then begin normal monthly maintenance dosing.

If 4 to 7 weeks have elapsed since first injection: Administer a dose of 100 mg in the deltoid as soon as possible, followed by another 100 mg dose in the deltoid 1 week later, then begin normal monthly maintenance dosing.

If >7 weeks has elapsed since the first injection: Therapy must be reinitiated following dosing recommendations for initiation of therapy.

Missed maintenance dose:

If <6 weeks have elapsed since the last monthly injection: Administer the missed dose as soon as possible and continue therapy at monthly intervals.

If >6 weeks and ≤6 months have elapsed since the last monthly injection: Therapy may be resumed at same dose (50 to 100 mg) the patient was previously stabilized on and then repeated 1 week later (day 8) with both doses administered in the deltoid. Resume usual monthly maintenance dosing cycle thereafter. If the dose was 150 mg, administer a 100 mg dose as soon as possible and repeat 1 week later (day 8) with both doses administered in the deltoid, then resume usual monthly maintenance dosing cycle 50 to 150 mg.

If >6 months have elapsed since last monthly maintenance injection: Therapy must be reinitiated following dosing recommendations for initiation of therapy.

Dosage adjustment in renal impairment: Clearance is decreased in renal impairment; adjust dose according to renal function:

Oral:

Mild impairment (CrCl 50 to 79 mL/minute): Initial dose: 3 mg once daily; maximum dose: 6 mg once daily

Moderate-to-severe impairment (CrCl 10 to 49 mL/minute): Initial dose: 1.5 mg once daily; maximum dose: 3 mg once daily

Severe impairment (CrCl <10 mL/minute): Use not recommended (has not been studied).

IM:

US labeling:

Mild impairment (CrCl 50 to 79 mL/minute): Initiation of therapy: 156 mg on treatment day 1, followed by 117 mg 1 week later with both doses administered in the deltoid, followed by a maintenance dose of 78 mg every month (administered in the deltoid or gluteal muscle)

Moderate-to-severe impairment (CrCl <50 mL/minute): Use not recommended

Canadian labeling:

Mild impairment (CrCl 50 to 79 mL/minute): Initiation of therapy: 100 mg on treatment day 1, followed by 75 mg 1 week later with both doses administered in the deltoid, followed by a maintenance dose of 50 mg every month (administered in the deltoid or gluteal muscle). Based on tolerability and/or response, maintenance dose may be adjusted within range of 50 to 100 mg.

Moderate-to-severe impairment (CrCl <50 mL/minute): Use not recommended

Dosage adjustment in hepatic impairment: Oral, IM:

Mild to moderate impairment (Child-Pugh class A or B): No dosage adjustment necessary.

Severe impairment: There are no dosage adjustments provided in the manufacturer's labeling (has not been studied).

Dietary Considerations May be taken without regard to meals.

Administration

Oral: Administer in the morning without regard to meals. Extended release tablets should be swallowed whole with liquids; do not crush, chew, or divide.

Injection: Invega Sustenna should be administered by IM route only as a single injection (do not divide); do not administer by any other route. Avoid inadvertent injection into vasculature. Prior to injection, shake syringe for at least 10 seconds to ensure a homogenous suspension. The 2 initial injections should be administered in the deltoid muscle using a 1½ inch, 22-gauge needle for patients ≥90 kg, and a 1 inch, 23-gauge needle for patients <90 kg. The 2 initial deltoid intramuscular injections help attain therapeutic concentrations rapidly. Alternate deltoid injections (right and left deltoid muscle). The second dose may be administered 4 days before or after the weekly time point. Monthly maintenance doses can be administered in either the deltoid or gluteal muscle. Administer injections in the gluteal muscle using a 1½ inch, 22-gauge needle (regardless of patient weight) in the upper-outer quadrant of the gluteal area. Alternate gluteal injections (right and left gluteal muscle). The monthly maintenance dose may be administered 7 days before or after the monthly time point.

Monitoring Parameters Mental status; vital signs (as clinically indicated); blood pressure (baseline; repeat 3 months after antipsychotic initiation, then yearly); weight, height, BMI, waist circumference (baseline; repeat at 4, 8, and 12 weeks after initiating or changing therapy, then quarterly; consider switching to a different antipsychotic for a weight gain ≥5% of initial weight); CBC (as clinically indicated; monitor frequently during the first few months of therapy in patients with preexisting low WBC or history of drug-induced leukopenia/neutropenia); electrolytes, renal and liver function (annually and as clinically indicated); personal and family history of obesity, diabetes, dyslipidemia, hypertension, or cardiovascular disease (baseline; repeat annually); fasting plasma glucose level/HbA_{1c} (baseline; repeat 3 months after starting antipsychotic, then yearly); fasting lipid panel (baseline; repeat 3 months after initiation of antipsychotic; if LDL level is normal repeat at 2-5 year intervals or more frequently if clinical indicated); changes in menstruation, libido, development of galactorrhea, erectile and ejaculatory function (at each visit for the first 12 weeks after the antipsychotic is initiated or until the dose is stable, then yearly); abnormal involuntary movements or parkinsonian signs (baseline; repeat weekly until dose stabilized for at least 2 weeks after introduction and for 2 weeks after any significant dose increase); tardive dyskinesia (every 12 months; high-risk patients every 6 months); ocular examination (yearly in patients >40 years; every 2 years in younger patients) (ADA, 2004; Lehman, 2004; Marder, 2004).

Additional Information Invega® is an extended release tablet based on the OROS® osmotic delivery system. Water from the GI tract enters through a semipermeable membrane coating the tablet, solubilizing the drug into a gelatinous form which, through hydrophilic expansion, is then expelled through laser-drilled holes in the coating.

Dosage Forms

Suspension, Intramuscular:

Invega Sustenna: 39 mg/0.25 mL (0.25 mL); 78 mg/0.5 mL (0.5 mL); 117 mg/0.75 mL (0.75 mL); 156 mg/mL (1 mL); 234 mg/1.5 mL (1.5 mL)

Tablet Extended Release 24 Hour, Oral:

Invega: 1.5 mg, 3 mg, 6 mg, 9 mg

Dosage Forms: Canada Note: Refer also to Dosage Forms.

Suspension, Intramuscular

Invega Sustenna: 25 mg/0.25 mL, 50 mg/0.5 mL, 75 mg/0.75 mL, 100mg/1 mL, and 150 mg/1.5 mL

◆ **Paliperidone Palmitate** *see* Paliperidone *on page* 1556

Palivizumab (pah li VIZ u mab)

Brand Names: U.S. Synagis

Brand Names: Canada Synagis

Pharmacologic Category Monoclonal Antibody

Use Respiratory syncytial virus prophylaxis: Prevention of serious lower respiratory tract disease caused by respiratory syncytial virus (RSV) in pediatric patients at high risk of RSV disease. Safety and efficacy were established in infants with bronchopulmonary dysplasia (BPD), infants with a history of premature birth (≤35 weeks gestational age), and children with hemodynamically significant congenital heart disease (CHD).

The American Academy of Pediatrics (AAP, 2014) recommends RSV prophylaxis with palivizumab during RSV season for:

Infants born at ≤28 weeks 6 days gestational age and <12 months at the start of RSV season

Infants <12 months of age with chronic lung disease (CLD) of prematurity

Infants ≤12 months of age with hemodynamically significant congenital heart disease (CHD)

Infants and children <24 months of age with CLD of prematurity necessitating medical therapy (eg, supplemental oxygen, bronchodilator, diuretic, or chronic steroid therapy) within 6 months prior to the beginning of RSV season

AAP also suggests that palivizumab prophylaxis may be considered in the following circumstances:

Infants <12 months of age with congenital airway abnormality or neuromuscular disorder that decreases the ability to manage airway secretions

Infants <12 months of age with cystic fibrosis with clinical evidence of CLD and/or nutritional compromise

Children <24 months with cystic fibrosis with severe lung disease (previous hospitalization for pulmonary exacerbation in the first year of life or abnormalities on chest radiography or chest computed tomography that persist when stable) or weight for length less than the 10th percentile

Infants and children <24 months who are profoundly immunocompromised

Infants and children <24 months undergoing cardiac transplantation during RSV season

Limitations of use: Safety and efficacy have not been established for treatment of RSV disease.

Pregnancy Risk Factor C

Pregnancy Considerations Not for adult use; reproduction studies have not been conducted

Contraindications Significant prior hypersensitivity reaction to palivizumab or any component of the formulation

Warnings/Precautions Very rare cases of anaphylaxis, some fatal, have been observed following palivizumab. Rare cases of severe acute hypersensitivity reactions have also been reported. Use with caution after mild hypersensitivity reaction; permanently discontinue for severe hypersensitivity reaction. Safety and efficacy of palivizumab have not been demonstrated in the treatment of established RSV disease. Palivizumab is not recommended for the prevention of health care-associated RSV disease (AAP, 2014). Use with caution in patients with thrombocytopenia or any coagulation disorder; bleeding/hematoma may occur from IM administration.

Adverse Reactions

Central nervous system: Fever

Dermatologic: Rash

Miscellaneous: Antibody formation

Rare but important or life-threatening: Anaphylaxis (very rare - includes angioedema, dyspnea, hypotonia, pruritus, respiratory failure, unresponsiveness, urticaria); hypersensitivity reactions, injection site reactions, thrombocytopenia

Drug Interactions

Metabolism/Transport Effects None known.

Avoid Concomitant Use

Avoid concomitant use of Palivizumab with any of the following: Belimumab

Increased Effect/Toxicity

Palivizumab may increase the levels/effects of: Belimumab

Decreased Effect There are no known significant interactions involving a decrease in effect.

Preparation for Administration Do not shake, vigorously agitate, or dilute the solution. Administer immediately after withdrawal from the vial; discard unused portion.

Storage/Stability Store between 2°C and 8°C (36°F and 46°F) in original container; do not freeze. Extended storage information may be available; contact product manufacturer to obtain current recommendations.

Mechanism of Action Exhibits neutralizing and fusion-inhibitory activity against RSV; these activities inhibit RSV replication in laboratory and clinical studies

Pharmacodynamics/Kinetics

Bioavailability: 70%

Half-life elimination: 24.5 days

Dosage IM: Infants and Children <2 years:

Prevention of RSV: 15 mg/kg of body weight, monthly throughout RSV season (first dose administered prior to commencement of RSV season)

Note: The American Academy of Pediatrics (AAP) recommends a maximum of 5 doses per season; if hospitalization occurs for breakthrough RSV infection, monthly prophylaxis should be discontinued for the remainder of that season (AAP, 2014).

Cardiopulmonary bypass patients: Administer an additional dose as soon as possible after cardiopulmonary bypass procedure or at the conclusion of extracorporeal membrane oxygenation, even if <1 month from previous dose (AAP, 2014).

Dosage adjustment in renal impairment: There are no dosage adjustments provided in the manufacturer's labeling.

Dosage adjustment in hepatic impairment: There are no dosage adjustments provided in the manufacturer's labeling.

Administration IM injection should (preferably) be in the anterolateral aspect of the thigh; gluteal muscle should not be used routinely because of risk of damage to the sciatic nerve. Injection volumes over 1 mL should be administered as divided doses.

Monitoring Parameters Monitor for anaphylaxis or acute hypersensitivity reactions

Dosage Forms

Solution, Intramuscular [preservative free]:

Synagis: 50 mg/0.5 mL (0.5 mL); 100 mg/mL (1 mL)

Palonosetron (pal oh NOE se tron)

Brand Names: U.S. Aloxi

Index Terms Palonosetron Hydrochloride; RS-25259; RS-25259-197

Pharmacologic Category Antiemetic; Selective 5-HT_3 Receptor Antagonist

Use

Chemotherapy-induced nausea and vomiting: Prevention of acute and delayed nausea and vomiting associated with initial and repeat courses in patients treated with moderately emetogenic cancer chemotherapy in adults; prevention of acute nausea and vomiting associated with initial and repeat courses in patients treated with highly emetogenic cancer chemotherapy in adults; prevention of acute nausea and vomiting associated with initial and repeat courses of emetogenic cancer chemotherapy (including highly emetogenic chemotherapy) in pediatric patients 1 month to <17 years.

Postoperative nausea and vomiting: Prevention of postoperative nausea and vomiting (PONV) for up to 24 hours following surgery in adults.

Limitations of use: Routine prophylaxis for PONV in patients with minimal expectation of nausea and/or vomiting is not recommended, although use is recommended in patients when nausea and vomiting must be avoided in the postoperative period, even if the incidence of PONV is low.

Pregnancy Risk Factor B

Pregnancy Considerations Adverse events have not been observed in animal reproduction studies. Use during pregnancy only if clearly needed.

Breast-Feeding Considerations It is not known if palonosetron is excreted in breast milk. Due to the potential for adverse reactions in the nursing infant, the manufacturer recommends a decision be made whether to discontinue nursing or to discontinue palonosetron, taking into account the importance of treatment to the mother.

Contraindications Hypersensitivity to palonosetron or any component of the formulation

Warnings/Precautions Hypersensitivity (including anaphylaxis) has been reported in patients with or without known hypersensitivity to other 5-HT_3 receptor antagonists. Serotonin syndrome has been reported with 5-HT_3 receptor antagonists, predominantly when used in combination with other serotonergic agents (eg, SSRIs, SNRIs, MAOIs, mirtazapine, fentanyl, lithium, tramadol, and/or methylene blue). Some of the cases have been fatal. The majority of serotonin syndrome reports due to 5-HT_3 receptor antagonists have occurred in a post-anesthesia setting or in an infusion center. Serotonin syndrome has also been reported following overdose of another 5-HT_3 receptor antagonist. Monitor patients for signs of serotonin syndrome, including mental status changes (eg, agitation, hallucinations, delirium, coma); autonomic instability (eg, tachycardia, labile blood pressure, diaphoresis, dizziness, flushing, hyperthermia); neuromuscular changes (eg, tremor, rigidity, myoclonus, hyperreflexia, incoordination); gastrointestinal symptoms (eg, nausea, vomiting, diarrhea); and/or seizures. If serotonin syndrome occurs, discontinue 5-HT_3 receptor antagonist treatment and begin supportive management.

Although other selective 5-HT_3 receptor antagonists have been associated with dose-dependent increases in ECG intervals (eg, PR, QRS duration, QT/QTc, JT), palonosetron has not been shown to significantly affect the QT/QTc interval (Gonullu, 2012; Morganroth, 2008). Reduction in heart rate may occur with the 5-HT_3 antagonists, including palonosetron (Gonullu, 2012). Antiemetics are most effective when used prophylactically (Roila, 2010). Potentially significant drug-drug interactions may exist, requiring dose or frequency adjustment, additional monitoring, and/or selection of alternative therapy. If emesis occurs despite optimal antiemetic prophylaxis, re-evaluate emetic risk, disease, concurrent morbidities and medications to assure antiemetic regimen is optimized (Basch, 2011). For postoperative nausea and vomiting (PONV), may use for low expectation of PONV if it is essential to avoid nausea and vomiting in the postoperative period; use is not recommended if there is little expectation of nausea and vomiting.

Adverse Reactions Adverse events reported for adults unless otherwise noted.

Cardiovascular: Bradycardia (chemotherapy-associated), prolonged Q-T interval on ECG (more common in PONV), sinus bradycardia (PONV), tachycardia (may be nonsustained), hypotension

Central nervous system: Anxiety (chemotherapy-associated), dizziness (infants, children, adolescents, and adults), headache (chemotherapy-associated; more common in adults)

Dermatologic: Pruritus (PONV)

Endocrine & metabolic: Hyperkalemia (chemotherapy-associated)

Gastrointestinal: Constipation (chemotherapy-associated), diarrhea, flatulence

Genitourinary: Urinary retention

Hepatic: Increased serum ALT (may be transient), increased serum AST (may be transient)

Neuromuscular & skeletal: Weakness (chemotherapy-associated)

Rare but important or life-threatening: Amblyopia, anasarca, anemia, anorexia, arthralgia, chills, decreased appetite, decreased blood pressure, decreased gastrointestinal motility, decreased platelet count, dermatological disease (infants, children, and adolescents), distended vein, drowsiness, dyskinesia (infants, children, and adolescents), dyspepsia, epistaxis, erythema, euphoria, extrasystoles, eye irritation, flattened T wave on ECG, flu-like symptoms, hiccups, hot flash, hyperglycemia, hypersensitivity (very rare), hypertension, hypokalemia, hypoventilation, increased bilirubin (transient), increased liver enzymes, infusion site pain (infants, children, and adolescents), injection site reaction (very rare; includes burning sensation at injection site, discomfort at injection site, induration at injection site, pain at injection site), insomnia, ischemic heart disease, limb pain, metabolic acidosis, motion sickness, paresthesia, serotonin syndrome, sialorrhea, sinus arrhythmia, sinus tachycardia, supraventricular extrasystole, tinnitus, vein discoloration, ventricular premature contractions

Drug Interactions

Metabolism/Transport Effects **Substrate** of CYP1A2 (minor), CYP2D6 (minor), CYP3A4 (minor); **Note:** Assignment of Major/Minor substrate status based on clinically relevant drug interaction potential

Avoid Concomitant Use

Avoid concomitant use of Palonosetron with any of the following: Apomorphine

Increased Effect/Toxicity

Palonosetron may increase the levels/effects of: Apomorphine; Serotonin Modulators

Decreased Effect

Palonosetron may decrease the levels/effects of: Tapentadol; TraMADol

Storage/Stability Store intact vials at 20°C to 25°C (68°F to 77°F); excursions permitted to 15°C to 30°C (59°F to 86°F). Do not freeze. Protect from light. Solutions of 5 mcg/mL and 30 mcg/mL in NS, D_5W, $D_5{}^1/_2NS$, and D_5LR injection are stable for 48 hours at room temperature and 14 days under refrigeration (Trissel, 2004a).

Mechanism of Action Selective 5-HT_3 receptor antagonist, blocking serotonin, both on vagal nerve terminals in the periphery and centrally in the chemoreceptor trigger zone

Pharmacodynamics/Kinetics

Distribution: V_d: 8.3 ± 2.5 L/kg

Protein binding: ~62%

Metabolism: ~50% metabolized via CYP enzymes (and likely other pathways) to relatively inactive metabolites (N-oxide-palonosetron and 6-S-hydroxy-palonosetron); CYP1A2, 2D6, and 3A4 contribute to its metabolism

Half-life elimination: IV: Adults: ~40 hours; Children: ~20 to 30 hours

Excretion: Urine (80%; 40% as unchanged drug)

Dosage

Prevention of chemotherapy-induced nausea and vomiting:

Infants ≥1 month, Children, and Adolescents <17 years: IV: 20 **mcg**/kg (maximum dose: 1.5 **mg**) beginning ~30 minutes prior to the start of chemotherapy

Adults: IV: 0.25 mg beginning ~30 minutes prior to the start of chemotherapy

Prevention of postoperative nausea and vomiting: Adults: IV: 0.075 mg immediately prior to anesthesia induction

Elderly: No dosage adjustment necessary; refer to adult dosing

Dosage adjustment in renal impairment: No dosage adjustment is necessary

Dosage adjustment in hepatic impairment: No dosage adjustment is necessary

Administration Flush IV line with NS prior to and following administration.

Prevention of chemotherapy-induced nausea and vomiting:

Children: Infuse over 15 minutes, beginning ~30 minutes prior to the start of chemotherapy

Adults: Infuse over 30 seconds, beginning ~30 minutes prior to the start of chemotherapy

Prevention of postoperative nausea and vomiting: Infuse over 10 seconds immediately prior to anesthesia induction

Dosage Forms

Solution, Intravenous:

Aloxi: 0.25 mg/5 mL (5 mL)

◆ **Palonosetron and Netupitant** *see* Netupitant and Palonosetron *on page 1440*

- **Palonosetron Hydrochloride** *see* Palonosetron *on page 1561*
- **Pal-Tizanidine (Can)** *see* TiZANidine *on page 2051*
- **2-PAM** *see* Pralidoxime *on page 1694*

Pamabrom (PAM a brom)

Pharmacologic Category Diuretic

Use Temporary relief of symptoms associated with premenstrual and menstrual periods (eg, bloating, water-weight gain, swelling, full feeling)

Dosage Oral: Adults: 50 mg after breakfast and then every 6 hours as needed (maximum: 200 mg/24 hours); should be taken 5-6 days prior to onset of menstrual period and continued until desired relief or end of period

Additional Information Complete prescribing information should be consulted for additional detail.

- **Pamelor** *see* Nortriptyline *on page 1476*

Pamidronate (pa mi DROE nate)

Brand Names: Canada Aredia; Pamidronate Disodium; Pamidronate Disodium Omega; PMS-Pamidronate

Index Terms Pamidronate Disodium

Pharmacologic Category Bisphosphonate Derivative

Use

Hypercalcemia of malignancy: Treatment of moderate or severe hypercalcemia associated with malignancy, with or without bone metastases, in conjunction with adequate hydration.

Osteolytic bone metastases of breast cancer and osteolytic lesions of multiple myeloma: Treatment of osteolytic bone metastases of breast cancer and osteolytic lesions of multiple myeloma in conjunction with standard antineoplastic therapy.

Paget disease: Treatment of patients with moderate to severe Paget disease of bone.

Pregnancy Risk Factor D

Pregnancy Considerations Adverse events were observed in animal reproduction studies. It is not known if bisphosphonates cross the placenta, but fetal exposure is expected (Djokanovic, 2008; Stathopoulos, 2011). Bisphosphonates are incorporated into the bone matrix and gradually released over time. The amount available in the systemic circulation varies by dose and duration of therapy. Theoretically, there may be a risk of fetal harm when pregnancy follows the completion of therapy; however, available data have not shown that exposure to bisphosphonates during pregnancy significantly increases the risk of adverse fetal events (Djokanovic, 2008; Levy, 2009; Stathopoulos, 2011). Until additional data is available, most sources recommend discontinuing bisphosphonate therapy in women of reproductive potential as early as possible prior to a planned pregnancy; use in premenopausal women should be reserved for special circumstances when rapid bone loss is occurring (Bhalla, 2010; Pereira, 2012; Stathopoulos, 2011). Because hypocalcemia has been described following *in utero* bisphosphonate exposure, exposed infants should be monitored for hypocalcemia after birth (Djokanovic, 2008; Stathopoulos, 2011).

Breast-Feeding Considerations It is not known if pamidronate is excreted in breast milk. Pamidronate was not detected in the milk of a nursing woman receiving pamidronate 30 mg IV monthly (therapy started ~6 months postpartum). Following the first infusion, milk was pumped and collected for 0-24 hours and 25-48 hours, and each day pooled for analysis. Pamidronate readings were below the limit of quantification (<0.4 micromole/L). During therapy, breast milk was pumped and discarded for the first 48 hours following each infusion prior to resuming nursing. The infant was breast-fed >80% of the time; adverse events were not observed in the nursing infant (Simonoski, 2000). Monitoring the serum calcium concentrations of nursing infants is recommended (Stathopoulos, 2011). Due to the potential for serious adverse reactions in the nursing infant, the manufacturer recommends a decision be made whether to discontinue nursing or to discontinue the drug, taking into account the importance of treatment to the mother.

Contraindications Hypersensitivity to pamidronate, other bisphosphonates, or any component of the formulation

Warnings/Precautions Hazardous agent - use appropriate precautions for handling and disposal (meets NIOSH 2014 criteria). Osteonecrosis of the jaw (ONJ) has been reported in patients receiving bisphosphonates. Risk factors include invasive dental procedures (eg, tooth extraction, dental implants, boney surgery); a diagnosis of cancer, with concomitant chemotherapy, radiotherapy, or corticosteroids; poor oral hygiene, ill-fitting dentures; and comorbid disorders (anemia, coagulopathy, infection, preexisting dental disease). Most reported cases occurred after IV bisphosphonate therapy; however, cases have been reported following oral therapy. A dental exam and preventive dentistry should be performed prior to placing patients with risk factors on chronic bisphosphonate therapy. There is no evidence that discontinuing therapy reduces the risk of developing ONJ (Assael, 2009). The benefit/risk must be assessed by the treating physician and/or dentist/surgeon prior to any invasive dental procedure. Patients developing ONJ while on bisphosphonates should receive care by an oral surgeon.

Atypical femur fractures (after minimal or no trauma) have been reported. The fractures include subtrochanteric femur (bone just below the hip joint) and diaphyseal femur (long segment of the thigh bone). Some patients experience prodromal pain weeks or months before the fracture occurs. It is unclear if bisphosphonate therapy is the cause for these fractures. Patients receiving long-term (>3 to 5 years) bisphosphonate therapy may be at an increased risk. Consider discontinuing pamidronate in patients with a suspected femoral shaft fracture. Patients who present with thigh or groin pain in the absence of trauma should be evaluated. Infrequently, severe (and occasionally debilitating) musculoskeletal (bone, joint, and/or muscle) pain have been reported during bisphosphonate treatment. The onset of pain ranged from a single day to several months. Consider discontinuing therapy in patients who experience severe symptoms; symptoms usually resolve upon discontinuation. Some patients experienced recurrence when rechallenged with same drug or another bisphosphonate; avoid use in patients with a history of these symptoms in association with bisphosphonate therapy.

Initial or single doses have been associated with renal deterioration, progressing to renal failure and dialysis. Withhold pamidronate treatment (until renal function returns to baseline) in patients with evidence of renal deterioration. Glomerulosclerosis (focal segmental) with or without nephrotic syndrome has also been reported. Longer infusion times (>2 hours) may reduce the risk for renal toxicity, especially in patients with preexisting renal insufficiency. Single pamidronate doses should not exceed 90 mg. Patients with serum creatinine >3 mg/dL were not studied in clinical trials; limited data are available in patients with CrCl <30 mL/minute. Evaluate serum creatinine prior to each treatment. For the treatment of bone metastases, use is not recommended in patients with severe renal impairment; for renal impairment in indications other than bone metastases, use clinical judgment to determine if benefits outweigh potential risks.

Use has been associated with asymptomatic electrolyte abnormalities (including hypophosphatemia, hypokalemia, hypomagnesemia, and hypocalcemia). Rare cases of symptomatic hypocalcemia, including tetany have been reported. Patients with a history of thyroid surgery may have relative hypoparathyroidism; predisposing them to pamidronate-related hypocalcemia. Patients with preexisting anemia, leukopenia, or thrombocytopenia should be closely monitored during the first 2 weeks of treatment.

Hypercalcemia of malignancy (HCM): Adequate hydration is required during treatment (urine output ~2 L/day); avoid overhydration, especially in patients with heart failure.

Multiple myeloma: Patients with Bence-Jones proteinuria and dehydration should be adequately hydrated prior to therapy. The American Society of Clinical Oncology (ASCO) has also published guidelines on bisphosphonates use for prevention and treatment of bone disease in multiple myeloma (Kyle, 2007). Bisphosphonate (pamidronate or zoledronic acid) use is recommended in multiple myeloma patients with lytic bone destruction or compression spine fracture from osteopenia. Bisphosphonates may also be considered in patients with pain secondary to osteolytic disease, adjunct therapy to stabilize fractures or impending fractures, and for multiple myeloma patients with osteopenia but no radiographic evidence of lytic bone disease. Bisphosphonates are not recommended in patients with solitary plasmacytoma, smoldering (asymptomatic) or indolent myeloma, or monoclonal gammopathy of undetermined significance. The guidelines recommend monthly treatment for a period of 2 years. At that time, consider discontinuing in responsive and stable patients, and reinitiate if a new-onset skeletal-related event occurs. The ASCO guidelines are in alignment with the prescribing information for dosing, renal dose adjustments, infusion times, prevention and management of osteonecrosis of the jaw, and monitoring of laboratory parameter recommendations. According to the guidelines, in patients with extensive bone disease with existing severe renal disease (a serum creatinine >3 mg/dL or CrCl <30 mL/minute) pamidronate at a dose of 90 mg over 4 to 6 hours should be used (unless preexisting renal disease in which case a reduced initial dose should be considered). Monitor for albuminuria every 3 to 6 months; in patients with unexplained albuminuria >500 mg/24 hours, withhold the dose until level returns to baseline, then recheck every 3 to 4 weeks. Pamidronate may be reinitiated at a dose not to exceed 90 mg every 4 weeks with a longer infusion time of at least 4 hours.

Breast cancer (metastatic): The American Society of Clinical Oncology (ASCO) updated guidelines on the role of bone-modifying agents (BMAs) in the prevention and treatment of skeletal-related events for metastatic breast cancer patients (Van Poznak, 2011). The guidelines recommend initiating a BMA (denosumab, pamidronate, zoledronic acid) in patients with metastatic breast cancer to the bone. There is currently no literature indicating the superiority of one particular BMA. Optimal duration is not yet defined; however, the guidelines recommend continuing therapy until substantial decline in patient's performance status. The ASCO guidelines are in alignment with prescribing information for dosing, renal dose adjustments, infusion times, prevention and management of osteonecrosis of the jaw, and monitoring of laboratory parameter recommendations. BMAs are not the first-line therapy for pain. BMAs are to be used as adjunctive therapy for cancer-related bone pain associated with bone metastasis, demonstrating a modest pain control benefit. BMAs should be used in conjunction with agents such as NSAIDS, opioid and nonopioid analgesics, corticosteroids, radiation/surgery, and interventional procedures.

Adverse Reactions

Cardiovascular: Atrial fibrillation, atrial flutter, cardiac failure, edema, hypertension, syncope, tachycardia

Central nervous system: Drowsiness, fatigue, headache, insomnia, psychosis, seizure

Endocrine & metabolic: Hypocalcemia, hypokalemia, hypomagnesemia, hypophosphatemia, hypothyroidism

Gastrointestinal: Abdominal pain, anorexia, constipation, diarrhea, dyspepsia, gastrointestinal hemorrhage, nausea, stomatitis, vomiting

Genitourinary: Uremia, urinary tract infection

Hematologic & oncologic: Anemia, granulocytopenia, leukopenia, metastases, neutropenia, thrombocytopenia

Infection: Candidiasis

Local: Infusion site reaction (includes induration, pain, redness, and swelling)

Neuromuscular & skeletal: Arthralgia, back pain, myalgia, ostealgia, osteonecrosis of the jaw, weakness

Renal: Increased serum creatinine

Respiratory: Cough, dyspnea, pleural effusion, rales, rhinitis, sinusitis, upper respiratory tract infection

Miscellaneous: Fever

Rare but important or life-threatening: Acute renal failure, anaphylactic shock, angioedema, cardiac failure, confusion, episcleritis, focal segmental glomerulosclerosis (including collapsing variant), hallucination (visual), hematuria, herpes virus infection (reactivation), hyperkalemia, hypernatremia, hypersensitivity reaction, hypervolemia, hypotension, inflammation at injection site, injection site phlebitis, iridocyclitis, iritis, left heart failure, lymphocytopenia, nephrotic syndrome, osteonecrosis (other than jaw), renal failure, renal insufficiency, scleritis, uveitis, xanthopsia

Drug Interactions

Metabolism/Transport Effects None known.

Avoid Concomitant Use There are no known interactions where it is recommended to avoid concomitant use.

Increased Effect/Toxicity

Pamidronate may increase the levels/effects of: Deferasirox; Phosphate Supplements

The levels/effects of Pamidronate may be increased by: Aminoglycosides; Nonsteroidal Anti-Inflammatory Agents; Systemic Angiogenesis Inhibitors; Thalidomide

Decreased Effect

The levels/effects of Pamidronate may be decreased by: Proton Pump Inhibitors

Preparation for Administration Hazardous agent; use appropriate precautions for handling and disposal (meets NIOSH 2014 criteria).

Powder for injection: Reconstitute by adding 10 mL of SWFI to each vial of lyophilized powder, the resulting solution will be 30 mg/10 mL or 90 mg/10 mL.

Pamidronate may be further diluted in 250 to 1000 mL of 0.45% or 0.9% sodium chloride or 5% dextrose. (The manufacturers recommend dilution in 1000 mL for hypercalcemia of malignancy, 500 mL for Paget's disease and bone metastases of myeloma, and 250 mL for bone metastases of breast cancer.)

Storage/Stability

Powder for reconstitution: Store at 20°C to 25°C (68°F to 77°F). The reconstituted solution is stable for 24 hours stored under refrigeration at 2°C to 8°C (36°F to 46°F). The diluted solution for infusion is stable at room temperature for up to 24 hours.

Solution for injection: Store at 20°C to 25°C (68°F to 77°F). The diluted solution for infusion is stable at room temperature for up to 24 hours.

Mechanism of Action Nitrogen-containing bisphosphonate; inhibits bone resorption and decreases mineralization by disrupting osteoclast activity (Gralow, 2009; Rogers, 2011)

Pharmacodynamics/Kinetics

Onset of action:

Hypercalcemia of malignancy (HCM): ≤24 hours for decrease in albumin-corrected serum calcium; maximum effect: ≤7 days

Paget disease: ~1 month for ≥50% decrease in serum alkaline phosphatase

Duration: HCM: 7 to 14 days; Paget disease: 1 to 372 days

Distribution: 38% to 70% over 120 hours

Metabolism: Not metabolized

Half-life elimination: 21 to 35 hours

Excretion: Biphasic; urine (30% to 62% as unchanged drug; lower in patients with renal dysfunction) within 120 hours

Dosage Note: Single doses should not exceed 90 mg.

Hypercalcemia of malignancy: Adults: IV:

Moderate cancer-related hypercalcemia (corrected serum calcium: 12 to 13.5 mg/dL): 60 to 90 mg, as a single dose over 2 to 24 hours

Severe cancer-related hypercalcemia (corrected serum calcium: >13.5 mg/dL): 90 mg, as a single dose over 2 to 24 hours

Retreatment in patients who show an initial complete or partial response (allow at least 7 days to elapse prior to retreatment): May retreat at the same dose if serum calcium does not return to normal or does not remain normal after initial treatment.

Multiple myeloma, osteolytic bone lesions: Adults: IV: 90 mg over 4 hours once monthly:

Lytic disease: American Society of Clinical Oncology (ASCO) guidelines: 90 mg over at least 2 hours once every 3-4 weeks for 2 years; discontinue after 2 years in patients with responsive and/or stable disease; resume therapy with new-onset skeletal-related events (Kyle, 2007)

Newly-diagnosed, symptomatic (off-label dose): 30 mg over 2.5 hours once monthly for at least 3 years (Gimsing, 2010)

Breast cancer, osteolytic bone metastases: Adults: IV: 90 mg over 2 hours once every 3 to 4 weeks

Paget's disease (moderate-to-severe): Adults: IV: 30 mg over 4 hours once daily for 3 consecutive days (total dose = 90 mg); may retreat at initial dose if clinically indicated

Prevention of androgen deprivation-induced osteoporosis (off-label use): Adults: Males: IV: 60 mg over 2 hours once every 3 months (Smith, 2001)

Elderly: Begin at lower end of adult dosing range.

Dosage adjustment in renal impairment: Patients with serum creatinine >3 mg/dL were excluded from clinical trials; there are only limited pharmacokinetic data in patients with CrCl <30 mL/minute.

Manufacturer recommends the following guidelines:

Treatment of bone metastases: Use is not recommended in patients with severe renal impairment.

Renal impairment in indications other than bone metastases: Use clinical judgment to determine if benefits outweigh potential risks.

Multiple myeloma: American Society of Clinical Oncology (ASCO) guidelines (Kyle, 2007):

Severe renal impairment (serum creatinine >3 mg/dL **or** CrCl <30 mL/minute) and extensive bone disease: 90 mg over 4 to 6 hours. However, a reduced initial dose should be considered if renal impairment was preexisting.

Albuminuria >500 mg/24 hours (unexplained): Withhold dose until returns to baseline, then recheck every 3 to 4 weeks; consider reinitiating at a dose not to exceed 90 mg every 4 weeks and with a longer infusion time of at least 4 hours

Dosage adjustment in renal toxicity: In patients with bone metastases, treatment should be withheld for deterioration in renal function (increase of serum creatinine ≥0.5 mg/dL in patients with normal baseline [serum creatinine <1.4 mg/dL] or ≥1 mg/dL in patients with abnormal baseline [serum creatinine ≥1.4 mg/dL]). Resumption of therapy may be considered when serum creatinine returns to within 10% of baseline.

Dosage adjustment in hepatic impairment:

Mild to moderate impairment: No dosage adjustment necessary.

Severe impairment: There are no dosage adjustments provided in the manufacturer's labeling (has not been studied).

Dietary Considerations Multiple myeloma or metastatic bone lesions from solid tumors or Paget's disease: Take adequate daily calcium and vitamin D supplement (if patient is not hypercalcemic).

Administration IV: Infusion rate varies by indication. Longer infusion times (>2 hours) may reduce the risk for renal toxicity, especially in patients with preexisting renal insufficiency. The manufacturer recommends infusing over 2 to 24 hours for hypercalcemia of malignancy; over 2 hours for osteolytic bone lesions with metastatic breast cancer; and over 4 hours for Paget's disease and for osteolytic bone lesions with multiple myeloma. The ASCO guidelines for bisphosphonate use in multiple myeloma recommend infusing pamidronate over at least 2 hours; if therapy is withheld due to renal toxicity, infuse over at least 4 hours upon reintroduction of treatment after renal recovery (Kyle, 2007).

Hazardous agent; use appropriate precautions for handling and disposal (meets NIOSH 2014 criteria).

Monitoring Parameters Serum creatinine (prior to each treatment); serum electrolytes, including calcium, phosphate, magnesium, and potassium; CBC with differential; monitor for hypocalcemia for at least 2 weeks after therapy; dental exam and preventive dentistry prior to therapy for patients at risk of osteonecrosis, including all cancer patients; patients with preexisting anemia, leukopenia, or thrombocytopenia should be closely monitored during the first 2 weeks of treatment; in addition, monitor urine albumin every 3 to 6 months in multiple myeloma patients

Reference Range Calcium (total): Adults: 9 to 11 mg/dL (SI: 2.05 to 2.54 mmol/L), may slightly decrease with aging; Phosphorus: 2.5 to 4.5 mg/dL (SI: 0.81 to 1.45 mmol/L)

Dosage Forms

Solution, Intravenous:

Generic: 30 mg/10 mL (10 mL); 90 mg/10 mL (10 mL)

Solution, Intravenous [preservative free]:

Generic: 30 mg/10 mL (10 mL); 6 mg/mL (10 mL); 90 mg/10 mL (10 mL)

Solution Reconstituted, Intravenous:

Generic: 30 mg (1 ea); 90 mg (1 ea)

- ◆ **Pamidronate Disodium** *see* Pamidronate *on page 1563*
- ◆ **Pamidronate Disodium Omega (Can)** *see* Pamidronate *on page 1563*
- ◆ **p-amino-benzenesulfonamide** *see* Sulfanilamide *on page 1950*
- ◆ **p-Aminoclonidine** *see* Apraclonidine *on page 165*
- ◆ **Pamix [OTC]** *see* Pyrantel Pamoate *on page 1744*
- ◆ **Pamprin Ibuprofen Formula (Can)** *see* Ibuprofen *on page 1032*
- ◆ **Pancrease MT (Can)** *see* Pancrelipase *on page 1566*
- ◆ **Pancreatic Enzymes** *see* Pancrelipase *on page 1566*
- ◆ **Pancreaze** *see* Pancrelipase *on page 1566*

Pancrelipase (pan kre LYE pase)

Brand Names: U.S. Creon; Pancreaze; Pancrelipase (Lip-Prot-Amyl); Pertzye; Ultresa; Viokace; Zenpep

Brand Names: Canada Cotazym; Creon; Pancrease MT; Ultrase; Ultrase MT; Viokase

Index Terms Amylase, Lipase, and Protease; Digestive Enzyme; Lipancreatin; Lipase, Protease, and Amylase; Pancreatic Enzymes; Protease, Lipase, and Amylase

Pharmacologic Category Enzyme

Use

Pancreatic insufficiency (exocrine): Treatment of exocrine pancreatic insufficiency caused by cystic fibrosis or other conditions. Creon is also approved for patients with chronic pancreatitis or pancreatectomy. Viokace, in combination with a proton-pump inhibitor, is approved for use in adults with exocrine pancreatic insufficiency caused by chronic pancreatitis or pancreatectomy.

Note: Viokace must be administered with a proton pump inhibitor (PPI) since it is not enteric coated.

Pregnancy Risk Factor C

Dosage Note: Dosing should not exceed recommended maximum dosage set forth by the Cystic Fibrosis Foundation Consensus Conferences Guidelines. Adjust dose based on body weight, clinical symptoms, and stool fat content. Allow several days between dose adjustments. Total daily dose reflects ~3 meals per day and 2 to 3 snacks per day, with half the mealtime dose given with a snack. Doses of lipase >2,500 units/kg/meal, lipase >10,000 units/kg/**day**, or lipase >4,000 units/g fat daily should be used with caution and only with documentation of 3-day fecal fat measures. Doses of lipase >6,000 units/kg/meal are associated with colonic stricture and should be decreased.

Pancreatic insufficiency due to conditions such as cystic fibrosis:

Infants, Children, and Adolescents: Oral:

≤1 year (Creon, Pancreaze, Pancrelipase, Ultresa, Zenpep): Manufacturer's labeling: Lipase 2,000 to 4,000 units per 120 mL of formula or per breast-feeding based on available dosage form:

Creon 3,000 units per 120 mL formula or per breast-feeding

Pancreaze 2,600 units per 120 mL or per breast-feeding

Pancrelipase 2000 to 4,000 per 120 mL or per breast-feeding

Ultresa 4,000 per 120 mL or per breast-feeding

Zenpep: 3,000 units per 120 mL or per breast-feeding

Note: CF Guidelines recommend a dose of 2,000 to 5,000 units per feeding of formula, breast milk, or per breast-feeding (even if volume is <120 mL) for up to 2 years of age. Maximum daily dose: 10,000 lipase units/kg/day (Borowitz, 2009; Borowitz 2013).

>1 and <4 years (Pertzye [and weight ≥8 kg], Ultresa, Creon, Pancreaze, Zenpep): Initial: Lipase 1,000 units/kg/meal. Dosage range: Lipase 1,000 to 2,500 units/kg/meal. Maximum: Lipase ≤2,500 units/kg/**meal or** lipase ≤10,000 units/kg/**day or** lipase <4,000 units/g of fat daily

≥4 years (Pertzye [and weight ≥16 kg], Ultresa, Creon, Pancreaze, Zenpep): Refer to adult dosing.

Adults (Creon, Pancreaze, Pertzye, Ultresa, Zenpep): Oral: Initial: Lipase 500 units/kg/meal. Dosage range: Lipase 500 to 2,500 units/kg/meal. Maximum: Lipase ≤2,500 units/kg/**meal or** lipase ≤10,000 units/kg/**day or** lipase <4,000 units/g of fat daily

Pancreatic insufficiency due to chronic pancreatitis or pancreatectomy:

Adults: Oral:

Creon: Initial: Lipase 500 units/kg/meal with individualized dosage titrations. In one clinical trial, 72,000 units/meal while consuming ≥100 g of fat daily was used. Usually, half the prescribed dose for an individualized full meal should be given with each snack. Maximum: Lipase ≤2,500 units/kg/**meal or** lipase ≤10,000 units/kg/**day or** lipase <4,000 units/g of fat daily.

Viokace (administer in combination with a proton pump inhibitor): Initial: Lipase 500 units/kg/meal with individualized dosage titration. In one clinical trial,125,280 units/meal while consuming ≥100 g of fat daily was used. Usually, half the prescribed dose for an individualized full meal should be given with each snack. Maximum: Lipase ≤2,500 units/kg/**meal or** lipase ≤10,000 units/kg/**day or** lipase <4,000 units/g of fat daily.

Dosage adjustment in renal impairment: There are no dosage adjustments provided in manufacturer's labeling. Use with caution.

Dosage adjustment in hepatic impairment: There are no dosage adjustments provided in manufacturer's labeling.

Additional Information Complete prescribing information should be consulted for additional detail.

Product Availability Ultresa (Lipase 4,000 USP units, protease 8,000 USP units, and amylase 8,000 USP units) capsules: FDA approved October 2014; availability anticipated in mid-2015. Consult prescribing information for additional information.

Dosage Forms

Capsule, delayed release, bicarbonate buffered enteric coated microspheres, oral [porcine derived]:

Pertzye: Lipase 8,000 USP units, protease 28,750 USP units, and amylase 30,250 USP units

Pertzye: Lipase 16,000 USP units, protease 57,500 USP units, and amylase 60,500 USP units

Capsule, delayed release, enteric coated beads, oral [porcine derived]:

Pancrelipase (Lip-Prot-Amyl): Lipase 5000 USP units, protease 17,000 USP units, and amylase 27,000 USP units

Zenpep: Lipase 3000 USP units, protease 10,000 USP units, and amylase 16,000 USP units

Zenpep: Lipase 5000 USP units, protease 17,000 USP units, and amylase 27,000 USP units

Zenpep: Lipase 10,000 USP units, protease 34,000 USP units, and amylase 55,000 USP units

Zenpep: Lipase 15,000 USP units, protease 51,000 USP units, and amylase 82,000 USP units

Zenpep: Lipase 20,000 USP units, protease 68,000 USP units, and amylase 109,000 USP units

Zenpep: Lipase 25,000 USP units, protease 85,000 USP units, and amylase 136,000 USP units

Zenpep: Lipase 40,000 USP units, protease 136,000 USP units, and amylase 218,000 USP units

Capsule, delayed release, enteric coated microspheres, oral [porcine derived]:

Creon: Lipase 3000 USP units, protease 9500 USP units, and amylase 15,000 USP units

Creon: Lipase 6000 USP units, protease 19,000 USP units, and amylase 30,000 USP units

Creon: Lipase 12,000 USP units, protease 38,000 USP units, and amylase 60,000 USP units

Creon: Lipase 24,000 USP units, protease 76,000 USP units, and amylase 120,000 USP units

Creon: Lipase 36,000 USP units, protease 114,000 USP units, and amylase 180,000 USP units

Capsule, delayed release, enteric coated microtablets, oral [porcine derived]:
Pancreaze: Lipase 4200 USP units, protease 10,000 USP units, and amylase 17,500 USP units
Pancreaze: Lipase 10,500 USP units, protease 25,000 USP units, and amylase 43,750 USP units
Pancreaze: Lipase 16,800 USP units, protease 40,000 USP units, and amylase 70,000 USP units
Pancreaze: Lipase 21,000 USP units, protease 37,000 USP units, and amylase 61,000 USP units

Capsule, delayed release, enteric coated minitablets, oral [porcine derived]:
Ultresa: Lipase 13,800 USP units, protease 27,600 USP units, and amylase 27,600 USP units
Ultresa: Lipase 20,700 USP units, protease 41,400 USP units, and amylase 41,400 USP units
Ultresa: Lipase 23,000 USP units, protease 46,000 USP units, and amylase 46,000 USP units

Tablet, oral [porcine derived]:
Viokace: Lipase 10,440 USP units, protease 39,150 USP units, and amylase 39,150 USP units
Viokace: Lipase 20,880 USP units, protease 78,300 USP units, and amylase 78,300 USP units

◆ **Pancrelipase (Lip-Prot-Amyl)** *see* Pancrelipase *on page 1566*

Pancuronium (pan kyoo ROE nee um)

Brand Names: Canada Pancuronium Bromide®

Index Terms Pancuronium Bromide; Pavulon [DSC]

Pharmacologic Category Neuromuscular Blocker Agent, Nondepolarizing

Use Facilitation of endotracheal intubation and relaxation of skeletal muscles during surgery; facilitation of mechanical ventilation in ICU patients; does not relieve pain or produce sedation

Pregnancy Risk Factor C

Pregnancy Considerations Animal reproduction studies have not been conducted. Small amounts of pancuronium cross the placenta (Daily, 1984). May be used short-term in cesarean section; reduced doses recommended in patients also receiving magnesium sulfate due to enhanced effects.

Contraindications Hypersensitivity to pancuronium, bromide, or any component of the formulation

Warnings/Precautions Ventilation must be supported during neuromuscular blockade; use with caution in patients with renal and/or hepatic impairment (adjust dose appropriately); certain clinical conditions may result in potentiation or antagonism of neuromuscular blockade:

Potentiation: Electrolyte abnormalities, severe hyponatremia, severe hypocalcemia, severe hypokalemia, hypermagnesemia, neuromuscular diseases, acidosis, acute intermittent porphyria, renal failure, hepatic failure

Antagonism: Alkalosis, hypercalcemia, demyelinating lesions, peripheral neuropathies, diabetes mellitus

Increased sensitivity in patients with myasthenia gravis, Eaton-Lambert syndrome; resistance in burn patients (>30% of body) for period of 5-70 days postinjury; resistance in patients with muscle trauma, denervation, immobilization, infection. Cross-sensitivity with other neuromuscular-blocking agents may occur; use extreme caution in patients with previous anaphylactic reactions. Use caution in the elderly. **[U.S. Boxed Warning]: Should be administered by adequately trained individuals familiar with its use.**

Benzyl alcohol and derivatives: Some dosage forms may contain benzyl alcohol; large amounts of benzyl alcohol (≥99 mg/kg/day) have been associated with a potentially fatal toxicity ("gasping syndrome") in neonates; the "gasping syndrome" consists of metabolic acidosis, respiratory distress, gasping respirations, CNS dysfunction (including convulsions, intracranial hemorrhage), hypotension, and cardiovascular collapse (AAP, 1997; CDC, 1982); some data suggests that benzoate displaces bilirubin from protein binding sites (Ahlfors, 2001); avoid or use dosage forms containing benzyl alcohol with caution in neonates. See manufacturer's labeling.

Adverse Reactions

Cardiovascular: Circulatory collapse, edema, elevated blood pressure and cardiac output, elevation in pulse rate, skin flushing, tachycardia

Dermatologic: Burning sensation along the vein, erythema, itching, rash

Gastrointestinal: Excessive salivation

Neuromuscular & skeletal: Profound muscle weakness

Respiratory: Bronchospasm, wheezing

Miscellaneous: Hypersensitivity reaction

Postmarketing and/or case reports: Acute quadriplegic myopathy syndrome (prolonged use), anaphylactoid reactions, anaphylaxis, myositis ossificans (prolonged use)

Drug Interactions

Metabolism/Transport Effects None known.

Avoid Concomitant Use

Avoid concomitant use of Pancuronium with any of the following: QuiNINE

Increased Effect/Toxicity

Pancuronium may increase the levels/effects of: Cardiac Glycosides; Corticosteroids (Systemic); OnabotulinumtoxinA; RimabotulinumtoxinB

The levels/effects of Pancuronium may be increased by: AbobotulinumtoxinA; Aminoglycosides; Calcium Channel Blockers; Capreomycin; Clindamycin (Topical); Colistimethate; CycloSPORINE (Systemic); Fosphenytoin-Phenytoin; Inhalational Anesthetics; Ketorolac (Nasal); Ketorolac (Systemic); Lincosamide Antibiotics; Lithium; Loop Diuretics; Magnesium Salts; Polymyxin B; Procainamide; QuiNIDine; QuiNINE; Spironolactone; Tetracycline Derivatives; Theophylline Derivatives; Vancomycin

Decreased Effect

The levels/effects of Pancuronium may be decreased by: Acetylcholinesterase Inhibitors; Fosphenytoin-Phenytoin; Loop Diuretics; Theophylline Derivatives

Storage/Stability Refrigerate; however, stable for up to 6 months at room temperature.

Mechanism of Action Blocks neural transmission at the myoneural junction by binding with cholinergic receptor sites

Pharmacodynamics/Kinetics

Onset of effect: Peak effect: IV: 2-3 minutes

Duration (dose dependent): 60-100 minutes

Metabolism: Hepatic (30% to 45%); active metabolite 3-hydroxypancuronium (1/3 to 1/2 the activity of parent drug)

Half-life elimination: 110 minutes

Excretion: Urine (55% to 70% as unchanged drug)

Dosage Administer IV; dose to effect; doses will vary due to interpatient variability

Surgery:

Infants >1 month, Children, and Adults: Initial: 0.06-0.1 mg/kg or 0.05 mg/kg after initial dose of succinylcholine for intubation; maintenance dose: 0.01 mg/kg administered 60-100 minutes after initial dose and then 0.01 mg/kg every 25-60 minutes

Pretreatment/priming: 10% of intubating dose given 3-5 minutes before intubating dose

ICU paralysis (eg, facilitate mechanical ventilation) in select adequately sedated patients: 0.06-0.1 mg/kg bolus followed by either:

Continuous infusion: 1-2 **mcg**/kg/**minute** (0.06-0.12 **mg**/kg/**hour**) (Murray, 2002) **or** 0.8-1.7 **mcg**/kg/**minute** (0.048-0.102 **mg**/kg/**hour**) (Greenberg, 2013)

or

Intermittent bolus: 0.1-0.2 mg/kg every 1-3 hours

Dosage adjustment in renal impairment: Elimination half-life is doubled, plasma clearance is reduced and rate of recovery is sometimes much slower. No dosage adjustment provided in manufacturer's labeling; however, the following adjustments have been recommended (Aronoff 2007):

CrCl >50 mL/minute: No dosage adjustment necessary.

CrCl 10-50 mL/minute: Administer 50% of normal dose

CrCl <10 mL/minute: Avoid use.

Hemodialysis/peritoneal dialysis: Avoid use.

CRRT: Administer 50% of normal dose.

Dosage adjustment in hepatic impairment: Elimination half-life is doubled, plasma clearance is reduced, recovery time is prolonged, volume of distribution is increased (50%) and results in a slower onset, higher total initial dosage, and prolongation of neuromuscular blockade. Patients with liver disease may develop slow resistance to nondepolarizing muscle relaxant. Large doses may be required and problems may arise in antagonism

Dosing in obesity: Use ideal body weight for obese patients.

Administration May be administered undiluted by rapid IV injection

Monitoring Parameters Heart rate, blood pressure, assisted ventilation status; cardiac monitor, blood pressure monitor, and ventilator required

Additional Information Pancuronium is classified as a long-duration neuromuscular-blocking agent. Neuromuscular blockade will be prolonged in patients with decreased renal function. Pancuronium does not relieve pain or produce sedation. It may produce cumulative effect on duration of blockade. It produces tachycardia secondary to vagolytic activity and sympathetic stimulation.

Dosage Forms

Solution, Intravenous:

Generic: 1 mg/mL (10 mL); 2 mg/mL (2 mL, 5 mL)

◆ **Pancuronium Bromide** *see* Pancuronium *on page 1567*

◆ **Pancuronium Bromide® (Can)** *see* Pancuronium *on page 1567*

◆ **Pandel** *see* Hydrocortisone (Topical) *on page 1014*

◆ **Panglobulin** *see* Immune Globulin *on page 1056*

Panitumumab (pan i TOOM yoo mab)

Brand Names: U.S. Vectibix

Brand Names: Canada Vectibix

Index Terms ABX-EGF; MOAB ABX-EGF; Monoclonal Antibody ABX-EGF; rHuMAb-EGFr

Pharmacologic Category Antineoplastic Agent, Epidermal Growth Factor Receptor (EGFR) Inhibitor; Antineoplastic Agent, Monoclonal Antibody

Use

Colorectal cancer: Treatment of patients with wild-type *KRAS* (exon 2 in codons 12 or 13) metastatic colorectal cancer (mCRC), either as first-line therapy in combination with FOLFOX (fluorouracil, leucovorin, and oxaliplatin) or as a single agent following disease progression after prior treatment with fluoropyrimidine-, oxaliplatin-, and irinotecan-containing chemotherapy regimens

Limitations of use: Panitumumab is not indicated for the treatment of patients with *KRAS* mutation-positive mCRC or for whom *KRAS* mCRC status is unknown. Panitumumab in combination with oxaliplatin-based chemotherapy is not indicated for the treatment of patients with *RAS*-mutant mCRC or for whom *RAS* mutation status is unknown.

Pregnancy Risk Factor C

Pregnancy Considerations Animal reproduction studies have demonstrated adverse fetal effects. Based on animal studies, panitumumab may disrupt normal menstrual cycles. IgG is known to cross the placenta; therefore, it is possible the developing fetus may be exposed to panitumumab. Because panitumumab inhibits epidermal growth factor (EGF), a component of fetal development, adverse effects on pregnancy would be expected. Men and women of childbearing potential should use effective contraception during and for 6 months after treatment. Women who become pregnant during panitumumab treatment are encouraged to enroll in Amgen's Pregnancy Surveillance Program (1-800-772-6436).

Breast-Feeding Considerations It is not known if panitumumab is excreted in breast milk. The decision to discontinue panitumumab or discontinue breast-feeding should take into account the benefits of treatment to the mother. If breast-feeding is interrupted for panitumumab treatment, based on the half-life, breast-feeding should not be resumed for at least 2 months following the last dose. Women who nurse during panitumumab treatment are encouraged to enroll in Amgen's Lactation Surveillance Program (1-800-772-6436).

Contraindications There are no contraindications listed in the manufacturer's labeling.

Warnings/Precautions [U.S. Boxed Warning]: Dermatologic toxicities have been reported in 90% of patients receiving single agent panitumumab and were severe (grade 3 or higher) in 15% of patients); may include dermatitis acneiform, pruritus, erythema, rash, skin exfoliation, paronychia, dry skin, and skin fissures. Severe skin toxicities may be complicated by infection, sepsis, necrotizing fasciitis, or abscesses. The median time to development of skin (or ocular) toxicity was 2 weeks, with resolution ~12 weeks after discontinuation. Monitor all dermatologic toxicities for development of inflammation or infection. Rare cases of Stevens-Johnson syndrome and toxic epidermal necrolysis have been reported; bullous mucocutaneous disease (life-threatening/fatal) have been observed. Withhold treatment for severe or life-threatening dermatologic or soft tissue toxicities associated with severe/life-threatening inflammatory or infectious complications; dermatologic toxicity may require dose reduction or permanent discontinuation. The severity of dermatologic toxicity is predictive for response; grades 2-4 skin toxicity correlates with improved progression free survival and overall survival, compared to grade 1 skin toxicity (Peeters, 2009; Van Cutsem, 2007). Patients should minimize sunlight exposure; may exacerbate skin reactions. Keratitis and ulcerative keratitis (known risk factors for corneal perforation) have occurred. Monitor for evidence of ocular toxicity; interrupt or discontinue treatment for acute or worsening keratitis. Gastric mucosal and nail toxicities have also been reported.

Severe infusion reactions (bronchospasm, dyspnea, fever, chills, and hypotension) have been reported in ~1% of patients; fatal infusion reactions have been reported with postmarketing surveillance. Discontinue infusion for severe reactions; permanently discontinue in patients with persistent severe infusion reactions. Appropriate medical support for the management of infusion reactions should be readily available. Mild-to-moderate infusion reactions are managed by slowing the infusion rate.

Pulmonary fibrosis and interstitial lung disease have been observed (rarely) in clinical trials; fatalities have been reported. Interrupt treatment for acute onset or worsening of pulmonary symptoms; permanently discontinue treatment if interstitial lung disease is confirmed. Patients with a history of or evidence of interstitial pneumonitis or pulmonary fibrosis were excluded from most clinical trials; consider the benefits of therapy versus the risk of pulmonary complications in such patients. May cause diarrhea; the incidence and severity of chemotherapy-induced diarrhea and other toxicities (rash, electrolyte abnormalities, stomatitis) is increased with combination chemotherapy; severe diarrhea and dehydration (which may lead to acute renal failure) has been observed with panitumumab in combination with chemotherapy. In a study of bevacizumab with combination chemotherapy ± panitumumab, the use of panitumumab resulted in decreased progression-free and overall survival and significantly increased toxicity compared to regimens without panitumumab (Hecht, 2009). Toxicities included rash, diarrhea/dehydration, electrolyte disturbances, stomatitis, infection, and an increased incidence of pulmonary embolism. Magnesium and/or calcium depletion may occur during treatment (may be delayed; hypomagnesemia occurred ≥8 weeks after completion of panitumumab) and after treatment is discontinued; electrolyte repletion may be necessary; monitor for hypomagnesemia and hypocalcemia during treatment and for at least 8 weeks after completion. Hypokalemia has also been reported. Patients >65 years of age receiving panitumumab plus FOLFOX experienced a higher incidence of serious adverse events including serious diarrhea.

Patients with colorectal cancer with tumors with a codon 12 or 13 (exon 2) *KRAS* mutation are unlikely to benefit from EGFR inhibitor therapy. Panitumumab is not indicated patients with *KRAS* mutation-positive metastatic colorectal cancer or patients in which *KRAS* mutation status is unknown. In a study of FOLFOX4 (fluorouracil, leucovorin and oxaliplatin) ± panitumumab, patients with a *KRAS* mutation who received panitumumab with FOLFOX4 experienced a significantly shortened progression-free survival (Douillard, 2010). In addition, a subset analysis of patients with wild-type *KRAS* identified additional *RAS* (*KRAS* [exons 3 and 4] or *NRAS* [exons 2, 3, 4]) mutations; progression-free survival and overall survival were significantly shortened in patients with *RAS* mutations who received FOLFOX4 in combination with panitumumab (Douillard, 2013). Panitumumab should not be used in combination with oxaliplatin-based regimens in patients with RAS (KRAS or NRAS) mutations or if mutation status is unknown. Panitumumab is also reported to be ineffective in patients with BRAF V600E mutation (Di Nicolantonio, 2008). According to the manufacturer, evidence of EGFR expression and *KRAS* and *RAS* mutation status is necessary to determine patient selection.

Adverse Reactions

Monotherapy:

Cardiovascular: Pulmonary embolism

Central nervous system: Chills, fatigue

Dermatologic: Acneiform eruption, acne vulgaris, dermal ulcer, desquamation, erythema, exfoliative dermatitis, nail toxicity, papular rash, paronychia, pruritus, pustular rash, rash, skin fissure, skin toxicity, xeroderma

Endocrine & metabolic: Dehydration, hypomagnesemia

Gastrointestinal: Diarrhea, mucositis, nausea, stomatitis, vomiting, xerostomia

Immunologic: Antibody formation

Ophthalmic: Abnormal eyelash growth, conjunctivitis

Respiratory: Cough, dyspnea, epistaxis, interstitial pulmonary disease

Miscellaneous: Fever, infusion related reaction

Rare but important or life-threatening: Hypersensitivity reaction, pulmonary fibrosis

Combination therapy with FOLFOX:

Cardiovascular: Deep vein thrombosis

Central nervous system: Fatigue, paresthesia

Dermatologic: Acneiform eruption, acne vulgaris, alopecia, cellulitis, erythema, nail disorder, palmar-plantar erythrodysesthesia, paronychia, pruritus, skin fissure, skin rash, xeroderma

Endocrine & metabolic: dehydration, hypocalcemia, hypokalemia, hypomagnesemia, weight loss

Gastrointestinal: Abdominal pain, anorexia, diarrhea, mucosal inflammation, stomatitis

Hypersensitivity: Hypersensitivity

Local: Localized infection

Neuromuscular & skeletal: Weakness

Ophthalmic: Conjunctivitis

Respiratory: Epistaxis

Rare but important or life-threatening: Antibody development

Rare but important or life-threatening (mono- and combination therapy): Abscess, angioedema, bullous skin disease (mucocutaneous), corneal ulcer, keratitis, necrotizing fasciitis, sepsis, skin necrosis, Stevens-Johnson syndrome, toxic epidermal necrolysis

Drug Interactions

Metabolism/Transport Effects None known.

Avoid Concomitant Use There are no known interactions where it is recommended to avoid concomitant use.

Increased Effect/Toxicity

Panitumumab may increase the levels/effects of: Porfimer; Verteporfin

Decreased Effect There are no known significant interactions involving a decrease in effect.

Preparation for Administration Inspect vial prior to use; solution is colorless but may contain a small amount of translucent-to-white amorphous panitumumab protein particles (will be removed with administration filter). Dilute in 100 mL (for doses ≤1000 mg) or 150 mL (doses >1000 mg) of normal saline to a final concentration of ≤10 mg/mL. Gently invert to mix; do not shake. Discard any unused portion remaining in the vial.

Storage/Stability Store vials in the original cartons under refrigeration at 2°C to 8°C (36°F to 46°F) until the time of use. Do not freeze; do not shake; protect from direct sunlight. Solution diluted for infusion should be used within 6 hours of preparation if stored at room temperature or within 24 hours of dilution if stored at 2°C to 8°C (36°F to 46°F); do not freeze.

Mechanism of Action Recombinant human IgG2 monoclonal antibody which binds specifically to the epidermal growth factor receptor (EGFR, HER1, c-ErbB-1) and competitively inhibits the binding of epidermal growth factor (EGF) and other ligands. Binding to the EGFR blocks phosphorylation and activation of intracellular tyrosine kinases, resulting in inhibition of cell survival, growth, proliferation and transformation. EGFR signal transduction results in *KRAS* wild-type activation; cells with *KRAS* mutations appear to be unaffected by EGFR inhibition.

Pharmacodynamics/Kinetics Half-life elimination: ~7.5 days (range: 4 to 11 days)

Dosage

Colorectal cancer, metastatic, *KRAS* mutation-negative: Adults: IV: 6 mg/kg every 14 days as a single agent (Van Cutsem, 2007) or in combination with FOLFOX (fluorouracil, leucovorin, and oxaliplatin) (Douillard, 2010; Douillard, 2013); continue until disease progression or unacceptable toxicity (Douillard, 2010; Van Cutsem, 2007)

Colorectal cancer, metastatic (*KRAS* wild-type), in combination with FOLFIRI (fluorouracil, leucovorin, and irinotecan; off-label combination): Adults: IV: 6 mg/kg every 14 days; continue until disease progression or unacceptable toxicity (Peeters, 2010)

Dosing adjustment for toxicity:

Infusion reactions, mild-to-moderate (grade 1 or 2): Reduce the infusion rate by 50% for the duration of infusion.

Infusion reactions, severe (grade 3 or 4): Stop infusion; consider permanent discontinuation (depending on severity or persistence of reaction).

Dermatologic toxicity

Grade 3 toxicity (first occurrence): Withhold 1 to 2 doses; if reaction improves to < grade 3, resume therapy at the initial dose.

Grade 3 toxicity (second occurrence): Withhold 1 to 2 doses; if reaction improves to < grade 3, resume therapy at 80% of the initial dose.

Grade 3 toxicity (third occurrence): Withhold 1 to 2 doses; if reaction improves to < grade 3, resume therapy at 60% of the initial dose.

Grade 3 toxicity (fourth occurrence), grade 3 toxicity that does not recover to < grade 3 after withholding 1 or 2 doses, or grade 4 toxicity: Permanently discontinue.

Ocular toxicity (acute or worsening keratitis): Interrupt or discontinue treatment.

Pulmonary toxicity:

Acute onset or worsening pulmonary symptoms: Interrupt treatment.

Interstitial lung disease: Permanently discontinue treatment.

Dosage adjustment in renal impairment: There are no dosage adjustments provided in the manufacturer's labeling (has not been studied).

Dosage adjustment in hepatic impairment: There are no dosage adjustments provided in the manufacturer's labeling (has not been studied).

Administration IV: Administer via infusion pump; do not administer IV push or as a bolus. Doses ≤1000 mg, infuse over 1 hour; if first infusion is tolerated, subsequent doses may be administered over 30 to 60 minutes. Doses >1000 mg, infuse over 90 minutes. Administer through a low protein-binding 0.2 or 0.22 micrometer in-line filter. Flush line with NS before and after infusion; do not mix or administer with other medications. Reduce infusion rate by 50% for mild-to-moderate infusion reactions (grades 1 and 2); stop infusion for severe infusion reactions (grades 3 and 4) and consider permanent discontinuation. Appropriate medical support for the management of infusion reactions should be readily available.

Monitoring Parameters *KRAS* genotyping of tumor tissue. Monitor serum electrolytes, including magnesium and calcium (periodically during and for at least 8 weeks after therapy), and potassium. Monitor vital signs and temperature before, during, and after infusion. Monitor for skin toxicity, for evidence of ocular toxicity, and for acute onset or worsening pulmonary symptoms.

Additional Information Oncology Comment: The American Society of Clinical Oncology (ASCO) provisional clinical opinion (Allegra, 2009) recommends genotyping tumor tissue for *KRAS* mutation in all patients with metastatic colorectal cancer (genotyping may be done on archived specimens). Patients with known codon 12 or 13 *KRAS* gene mutations are unlikely to respond to EGFR inhibitors and should not receive panitumumab. Favorable progression-free survival and higher response rates have been demonstrated with panitumumab in patients with *KRAS* wild-type; patients with the *KRAS* mutation did not respond to panitumumab (Amado, 2008). Panitumumab is also reported to be ineffective in patients with BRAF V600E mutation (Di Nicolantonio, 2008). Severity of dermatologic toxicity associated with panitumumab is predictive for response; grades 2-4 skin toxicity correlates with improved progression free survival and overall survival, compared to patients with grade 1 skin toxicity (Peeters, 2009; Van Cutsem, 2007). The association between dermatologic toxicity and progression free survival was not noted in patients with *KRAS* mutation (Peeters, 2009).

Dosage Forms

Solution, Intravenous [preservative free]:

Vectibix: 100 mg/5 mL (5 mL); 400 mg/20 mL (20 mL)

◆ **Panto I.V. (Can)** *see* Pantoprazole *on page 1570*

◆ **Pantoloc (Can)** *see* Pantoprazole *on page 1570*

Pantoprazole (pan TOE pra zole)

Brand Names: U.S. Protonix

Brand Names: Canada Abbott-Pantoprazole; ACT Pantoprazole; Apo-Pantoprazole; Ava-Pantoprazole; Dom-Pantoprazole; JAMP-Pantoprazole; Mint-Pantoprazole; Mylan-Pantoprazole; Panto I.V.; Pantoloc; Pantoprazole for Injection; Pantoprazole Sodium for Injection; PMS-Pantoprazole; Q-Pantoprazole; RAN-Pantoprazole; ratio-Pantoprazole; Riva-Pantoprazole; Sandoz-Pantoprazole; Tecta; Teva-Pantoprazole

Index Terms Pantoprazole Magnesium; Pantoprazole Sodium

Pharmacologic Category Proton Pump Inhibitor; Substituted Benzimidazole

Use

Oral: Short-term (up to 8 weeks) treatment and maintenance of healing of erosive esophagitis associated with GERD; reduction in relapse rates of daytime and nighttime heartburn symptoms in GERD; hypersecretory disorders associated with Zollinger-Ellison syndrome or other GI hypersecretory disorders

IV: Short-term treatment (7-10 days) of patients with gastroesophageal reflux disease (GERD) and a history of erosive esophagitis; hypersecretory disorders associated with Zollinger-Ellison syndrome or other GI hypersecretory disorders

Canadian labeling: Additional use (not in U.S. labeling): Oral: Peptic ulcer disease (eg, duodenal or gastric ulcer); adjunct treatment with antibiotics for *Helicobacter pylori* eradication; NSAID-induced ulcer prophylaxis (Pantoloc)

Pregnancy Risk Factor B

Pregnancy Considerations Adverse events were not observed in animal reproduction studies. Most available studies have not shown an increased risk of major birth defects following maternal use of proton pump inhibitors during pregnancy (Diav-Citrin, 2005; Erichsen, 2012; Matok, 2012; Pasternak, 2010). When treating GERD in pregnancy, PPIs may be used when clinically indicated (Katz, 2013).

Breast-Feeding Considerations Pantoprazole is excreted into breast milk. The excretion of pantoprazole into breast milk was studied in a nursing woman, 10 months postpartum. Following a single dose of pantoprazole 40 mg, maternal milk and serum samples were obtained over 24 hours. Peak concentrations appeared in both the plasma and milk 2 hours after the dose. Pantoprazole concentrations in breast milk were below the limits of detection during most of the study period. Based on this single dose study, the authors calculated the expected exposure to a nursing infant to be 0.14% of the weight-adjusted maternal dose (Plante, 2004). Due to the potential for serious adverse reactions in the nursing infant, the manufacturer recommends a decision be made whether to discontinue nursing or to discontinue the drug, taking into account the importance of treatment to the mother; however, the acidic content of the nursing infants' stomach may potentially inactivate any ingested pantoprazole (Plante, 2004).

Contraindications Hypersensitivity to pantoprazole, substituted benzimidazole proton pump inhibitors, or any component of the formulation

Warnings/Precautions Use of proton pump inhibitors (PPIs) may increase the risk of gastrointestinal infections (eg, *Salmonella, Campylobacter*). Relief of symptoms does not preclude the presence of a gastric malignancy. Long-term pantoprazole therapy (especially in patients who were *H. pylori* positive) has caused biopsy-proven atrophic gastritis. Benign and malignant neoplasia has been observed in long-term rodent studies; while not reported in humans, the relevance of these findings in regards to tumorigenicity in humans is not known. Use of PPIs may increase risk of *Clostridium difficile*-associated diarrhea (CDAD), especially in hospitalized patients; consider CDAD diagnosis in patients with persistent diarrhea that does not improve. Use the lowest dose and shortest duration of PPI therapy appropriate for the condition being treated. Prolonged treatment (≥2 years) may lead to vitamin B_{12} malabsorption and subsequent vitamin B_{12} deficiency. The magnitude of the deficiency is dose-related and the association is stronger in females and those younger in age (<30 years); prevalence is decreased after discontinuation of therapy (Lam, 2013).

Intravenous preparation contains edetate sodium (EDTA); use caution in patients who are at risk for zinc deficiency if other EDTA-containing solutions are coadministered. Some dosage forms may contain polysorbate 80 (also known as Tweens). Hypersensitivity reactions, usually a delayed reaction, have been reported following exposure to pharmaceutical products containing polysorbate 80 in certain individuals (Isaksson, 2002; Lucente 2000; Shelley, 1995). Thrombocytopenia, ascites, pulmonary deterioration, and renal and hepatic failure have been reported in premature neonates after receiving parenteral products containing polysorbate 80 (Alade, 1986; CDC, 1984). See manufacturer's labeling. Decreased *H. pylori* eradication rates have been observed with short-term (≤7 days) combination therapy. The American College of Gastroenterology recommends 10-14 days of therapy (triple or quadruple) for eradication of *H. pylori* (Chey, 2007).

PPIs may diminish the therapeutic effect of clopidogrel, thought to be due to reduced formation of the active metabolite of clopidogrel. The manufacturer of clopidogrel recommends either avoidance of both omeprazole (even when scheduled 12 hours apart) and esomeprazole or use of a PPI with comparatively less effect on the active metabolite of clopidogrel. Of the PPIs, pantoprazole has the lowest degree of CYP2C19 inhibition *in vitro* (Li, 2004) and has been shown to have less effect on conversion of clopidogrel to its active metabolite compared to omeprazole (Angiolillo, 2011). In contrast to these warnings, others have recommended the continued use of PPIs, regardless of the degree of inhibition, in patients with a history of GI bleeding or multiple risk factors for GI bleeding who are also receiving clopidogrel since no evidence has established clinically meaningful differences in outcome; however, a clinically-significant interaction cannot be excluded in those who are poor metabolizers of clopidogrel (Abraham, 2010; Levine, 2011). Concomitant use of pantoprazole with some drugs may require cautious use, may not be recommended, or may require dosage adjustments.

Increased incidence of osteoporosis-related bone fractures of the hip, spine, or wrist may occur with PPI therapy. Patients on high-dose or long-term therapy (≥1 year) should be monitored. Use the lowest effective dose for the shortest duration of time, use vitamin D and calcium supplementation, and follow appropriate guidelines to reduce risk of fractures in patients at risk. Thrombophlebitis and hypersensitivity reactions including anaphylaxis, Stevens-Johnson syndrome, and toxic epidermal necrolysis have been reported with IV administration.

Hypomagnesemia, reported rarely, usually with prolonged PPI use of >3 months (most cases >1 year of therapy); may be symptomatic or asymptomatic; severe cases may cause tetany, seizures, and cardiac arrhythmias. Consider obtaining serum magnesium concentrations prior to beginning long-term therapy, especially if taking concomitant digoxin, diuretics, or other drugs known to cause hypomagnesemia; and periodically thereafter. Hypomagnesemia may be corrected by magnesium supplementation, although discontinuation of pantoprazole may be necessary; magnesium levels typically return to normal within 2 weeks of stopping.

Some dosage forms may contain polysorbate 80 (also known as Tweens). Hypersensitivity reactions, usually a delayed reaction, have been reported following exposure to pharmaceutical products containing polysorbate 80 in certain individuals (Isaksson, 2002; Lucente 2000; Shelley, 1995). Thrombocytopenia, ascites, pulmonary deterioration, and renal and hepatic failure have been reported in premature neonates after receiving parenteral products containing polysorbate 80 (Alade, 1986; CDC, 1984). See manufacturer's labeling.

Adverse Reactions

Cardiovascular: Facial edema, generalized edema

Central nervous system: Depression, dizziness, fever, headache, vertigo

Dermatologic: Photosensitivity, pruritus, rash, urticaria

Endocrine & metabolic: Triglycerides increased

Gastrointestinal: Abdominal pain, constipation, diarrhea, flatulence, nausea, vomiting, xerostomia

Genitourinary: Urinary frequency, UTI

Hematologic: Leukopenia, thrombocytopenia

Hepatic: Hepatitis, liver function tests abnormal

Local: Injection site reaction (thrombophlebitis)

Neuromuscular & skeletal: Arthralgia, CPK increased, myalgia

Ocular: Blurred vision

Respiratory: Upper respiratory tract infection

Miscellaneous: Allergic reaction

Rare but important or life-threatening: Ageusia, agranulocytosis, albuminuria, alkaline phosphatase increased, anaphylaxis (including anaphylactic shock), anemia, angioedema, angina pectoris, aphthous stomatitis, arrhythmia, asthma exacerbation, atrial fibrillation/flutter, atrophic gastritis, biliary pain, bone pain, breast pain, bursitis, cataract, CHF, cholecystitis, cholelithiasis, *Clostridium difficile*-associate diarrhea (CDAD), colitis, contact dermatitis, creatinine increased, cystitis, deafness, dehydration, diabetes mellitus, diplopia, duodenitis, dysmenorrhea, dysphagia, dysuria, ecchymosis, ECG abnormality, eosinophilia, epididymitis, epistaxis, erythema multiforme, extraocular palsy, fracture, fungal dermatitis, gastrointestinal carcinoma, gastrointestinal hemorrhage, gastrointestinal moniliasis, GGT increased, gingivitis, glaucoma, glossitis, glycosuria, goiter, gout, hallucinations, hematemesis, hematuria, hemorrhage, hepatic failure, hernia, hyperbilirubinemia, hyperesthesia, hyper-/hypotension, hyperkinesia, hyperuricemia, hypokinesia, hypomagnesemia, hyponatremia, impotence, interstitial nephritis, jaundice, kidney calculus, kidney pain, leukocytosis, lichenoid dermatitis, maculopapular rash, melena, mouth ulceration, myocardial infarction, myocardial ischemia, neoplasm, neuralgia, neuritis, optic neuropathy (including anterior ischemic), palpitation, pancreatitis, pancytopenia, paresthesia, periodontitis, pneumonia, pyelonephritis, rectal hemorrhage, retinal vascular disorder, rhabdomyolysis, scrotal edema, seizure, Stevens-Johnson syndrome, stomach ulcer, stomatitis, syncope, tachycardia, tenosynovitis, thrombosis, tinnitus, tongue discoloration, toxic epidermal necrolysis, urethritis, vision abnormal

Drug Interactions

Metabolism/Transport Effects Substrate of CYP2C19 (major), CYP2D6 (minor), CYP3A4 (minor); **Note:** Assignment of Major/Minor substrate status based on clinically relevant drug interaction potential; **Inhibits** BCRP, CYP2C19 (weak); **Induces** CYP1A2 (moderate)

Avoid Concomitant Use

Avoid concomitant use of Pantoprazole with any of the following: Dasatinib; Delavirdine; Erlotinib; Nelfinavir; PAZOPanib; Rilpivirine; Risedronate

Increased Effect/Toxicity

Pantoprazole may increase the levels/effects of: Amphetamine; Dexmethylphenidate; Dextroamphetamine; Methotrexate; Methylphenidate; PAZOPanib; Raltegravir; Risedronate; Saquinavir; Topotecan; Voriconazole

The levels/effects of Pantoprazole may be increased by: Fluconazole; Ketoconazole (Systemic); Voriconazole

Decreased Effect

Pantoprazole may decrease the levels/effects of: Atazanavir; Bisphosphonate Derivatives; Bosutinib; Cefditoren; Clopidogrel; Dabigatran Etexilate; Dabrafenib; Dasatinib; Delavirdine; Erlotinib; Gefitinib; Indinavir; Iron Salts; Itraconazole; Ketoconazole (Systemic); Ledipasvir; Mesalamine; Multivitamins/Minerals (with ADEK, Folate, Iron); Mycophenolate; Nelfinavir; Nilotinib; PAZOPanib; Posaconazole; Rilpivirine; Riociguat; Risedronate; Vismodegib

The levels/effects of Pantoprazole may be decreased by: CYP2C19 Inducers (Strong); Dabrafenib; Tipranavir

Food Interactions Prolonged treatment (≥2 years) may lead to malabsorption of dietary vitamin B_{12} and subsequent vitamin B_{12} deficiency (Lam, 2013).

Preparation for Administration Reconstitute with 10 mL NS (final concentration 4 mg/mL). When administering by IV infusion, reconstituted solution may be added to 100 mL D_5W, NS, or LR.

Storage/Stability

Oral: Store tablet and oral suspension at controlled room temperature of 20°C to 25°C (68°F to 77°F); excursions permitted to 15°C to 30°C (59°F to 86°F).

IV: Prior to reconstitution, store at controlled room temperature of 20°C to 25°C (68°F to 77°F); excursions permitted to 15°C to 30°C (59°F to 86°F). Do not freeze. Protect from light prior to reconstitution; upon reconstitution, protection from light is not required. Per manufacturer's labeling, reconstituted solution is stable at room temperature for 6 hours; further diluted (admixed) solution should be stored at room temperature and used within 24 hours from the time of initial reconstitution. However, studies have shown that reconstituted solution (4 mg/mL) in polypropylene syringes is stable up to 96 hours at room temperature (Johnson, 2005). Upon further dilution, the admixed solution should be used within 96 hours from the time of initial reconstitution. The preparation should be stored at 3°C to 5°C (37°F to 41°F) if it is stored beyond 48 hours to minimize discoloration.

Mechanism of Action Suppresses gastric acid secretion by inhibiting the parietal cell H^+/K^+ ATP pump

Pharmacodynamics/Kinetics

Absorption: Rapid, well absorbed

Distribution: V_d: 11-24 L

Protein binding: 98%, primarily to albumin

Metabolism: Extensively hepatic; CYP2C19 (demethylation), CYP3A4; no evidence that metabolites have pharmacologic activity

Bioavailability: ~77%

Half-life elimination: 1 hour; increased to 3.5-10 hours with CYP2C19 deficiency

Time to peak: Oral: 2.5 hours

Excretion: Urine (71%); feces (18%)

Dosage

Oral:

Children ≥5 years: Erosive esophagitis associated with GERD:

≥15 to <40 kg: 20 mg once daily for up to 8 weeks

≥40 kg: 40 mg once daily for up to 8 weeks

Adults:

Erosive esophagitis associated with GERD:

Treatment: 40 mg once daily for up to 8 weeks; an additional 8 weeks may be used in patients who have not healed after an 8 week course. **Note:** Canadian labeling recommends initial treatment for up to 4 weeks and an additional 4 weeks in patients who have not healed after the initial 4-week course. Lower doses (20 mg once daily) have been used successfully in mild GERD treatment (Dettmer, 1998).

Maintenance of healing: 40 mg once daily (U.S. labeling) or 20 to 40 mg once daily (Canadian labeling); 20 mg once daily has been used successfully in maintenance of healing (Escourrou, 1999). **Note:** Has not been studied beyond 12 months.

Hypersecretory disorders (including Zollinger-Ellison): Initial: 40 mg twice daily; adjust dose based on patient needs; doses up to 240 mg daily have been administered

Helicobacter pylori eradication (off-label use in U.S.):

American College of Gastroenterology guidelines (Chey, 2007):

Nonpenicillin allergy: 40 mg twice daily administered with amoxicillin 1000 mg *and* clarithromycin 500 mg twice daily for 10 to 14 days

Penicillin allergy: 40 mg twice daily administered with clarithromycin 500 mg *and* metronidazole 500 mg twice daily for 10 to 14 days **or** 40 mg once or twice daily administered with bismuth subsalicylate 525 mg *and* metronidazole 250 mg *plus* tetracycline 500 mg 4 times daily for 10 to 14 days

Canadian labeling: 40 mg twice daily administered with clarithromycin 500 mg twice daily *and* either metronidazole 500 mg **or** amoxicillin 1000 mg twice daily for 7 days

Peptic ulcer disease (Canadian labeling): Treatment: 40 mg once daily for 2 weeks (duodenal ulcer) or 4 weeks (gastric ulcer); may extend therapy for an additional 2 or 4 weeks (based on indication) for inadequate healing

NSAID-induced ulcer prophylaxis (Canadian labeling): 20 mg once daily

Symptomatic GERD (Canadian labeling): Treatment: 40 mg once daily for up to 4 weeks; failure to achieve adequate symptom relief after the initial 4 weeks of therapy warrants further evaluation

IV:

Erosive esophagitis associated with GERD: 40 mg once daily for 7 to 10 days

Hypersecretory disorders: 80 mg every 12 hours; adjust dose based on acid output measurements; 160 to 240 mg daily in divided doses has been used for a limited period (up to 7 days)

Prevention of rebleeding in peptic ulcer bleed (off-label use):

Continuous infusion: Loading dose of 80 mg followed by 8 mg/hour infusion for 72 hours (Barkun, 2010; Zargar, 2006).

Intermittent dosing: Loading dose of 80 mg followed by either 40 mg every 12 hours for 72 hours (Hung, 2007; Yamada, 2012) **or** 40 mg every 6 hours for 72 hours (Hsu, 2009). May also administer 40 mg every 12 hours for 72 hours without a loading dose (Yuksel, 2008).

Note: After completion, continue therapy with a single daily-dose oral PPI for a duration dictated by the underlying etiology (Barkun, 2010).

Elderly: Dosage adjustment not required

Dosage adjustment in renal impairment: No dosage adjustment necessary; pantoprazole is not removed by hemodialysis. Canadian labeling does not recommend use in combination therapy of *Helicobacter pylori* in patients with severe renal impairment (has not been studied).

Dosage adjustment in hepatic impairment:

U.S. labeling: No dosage adjustment necessary; doses >40 mg daily have not been evaluated in patients with hepatic impairment.

Canadian labeling:

Mild-moderate impairment: No dosage adjustment necessary.

Severe impairment: IV, Oral: Manufacturer labeling suggests a maximum dose of 20 mg daily. Use in combination therapy of *Helicobacter pylori* is not recommended in patients with severe hepatic impairment (has not been studied).

Dietary Considerations

Oral: May be taken with or without food; best if taken before breakfast.

IV: Due to EDTA in preparation, zinc supplementation may be needed in patients prone to zinc deficiency.

Usual Infusion Concentrations: Adult IV infusion: 80 mg in 100 mL (concentration: 0.8 mg/mL) of D_5W or NS

Administration

IV: Flush IV line before and after administration. In-line filter not required.

2-minute infusion: The volume of reconstituted solution (4 mg/mL) to be injected may be administered intravenously over at least 2 minutes.

15-minute infusion: Infuse over 15 minutes at a rate not to exceed 7 mL/minute (3 mg/minute).

Continuous infusion: May also be administered as a continuous infusion for the prevention of rebleeding with in peptic ulcer bleed (off-label use).

Oral:

Tablet: Should be swallowed whole, do not crush or chew. Best if taken before breakfast.

Delayed-release oral suspension: Should only be administered in apple juice or applesauce and taken ~30 minutes before a meal. Do not administer with any other liquid (eg, water) or foods.

Oral administration in **applesauce**: Sprinkle intact granules on 1 tablespoon of applesauce and swallow within 10 minutes of preparation.

Oral administration in **apple juice**: Empty intact granules into 5 mL of apple juice, stir for 5 seconds, and swallow immediately after preparation. Rinse container once or twice with apple juice and swallow immediately.

Nasogastric tube administration: Separate the plunger from the barrel of a 60 mL catheter tip syringe and connect to a ≥16 French nasogastric tube. Holding the syringe attached to the tubing as high as possible, empty the contents of the packet into barrel of the syringe, add 10 mL of apple juice and gently tap/shake the barrel of the syringe to help empty the syringe. Add an additional 10 mL of apple juice and gently tap/shake the barrel to help rinse. Repeat rinse with at least 2-10 mL aliquots of apple juice. No granules should remain in the syringe.

Monitoring Parameters Hypersecretory disorders: Acid output measurements, target level <10 mEq/hour (<5 mEq/hour if prior gastric acid-reducing surgery)

Dosage Forms

Packet, Oral:

Protonix: 40 mg (1 ea, 30 ea)

Solution Reconstituted, Intravenous:

Protonix: 40 mg (1 ea)

Generic: 40 mg (1 ea)

Tablet Delayed Release, Oral:

Protonix: 20 mg, 40 mg

Generic: 20 mg, 40 mg

Dosage Forms: Canada Refer also to Dosage Forms.

Note: Oral packets are not available in Canada.

Solution Reconstituted, Intravenous:

Panto IV: 40 mg

Tablet Enteric Coated, Oral, as sodium:

Pantoloc 20 mg. 40 mg

Tablet Enteric Coated, Oral, as magnesium:

Tecta: 40 mg

Extemporaneous Preparations A 2 mg/mL pantoprazole oral suspension may be made with pantoprazole tablets, sterile water, and sodium bicarbonate powder. Remove the Protonix® imprint from twenty 40 mg tablets with a paper towel dampened with ethanol (improves the look of product). Let tablets air dry. Crush the tablets in a mortar and reduce to a fine powder. Transfer to a 600 mL beaker, and add 340 mL sterile water. Place beaker on a magnetic stirrer. Add 16.8 g of sodium bicarbonate powder and stir for about 20 minutes until the tablet remnants have disintegrated. While stirring, add another 16.8 g of sodium bicarbonate powder and stir for about 5 minutes until powder has dissolved. Add enough sterile water for irrigation to bring the final volume to 400 mL. Mix well. Transfer to amber-colored bottle. Label "shake well" and "refrigerate". Stable for 62 days refrigerated.

Dentinger PJ, Swenson CF, and Anaizi NH, "Stability of Pantoprazole in an Extemporaneously Compounded Oral Liquid," *Am J Health Syst Pharm*, 2002, 59(10):953-6.

◆ **Pantoprazole for Injection (Can)** *see* Pantoprazole *on page 1570*

◆ **Pantoprazole Magnesium** *see* Pantoprazole *on page 1570*

◆ **Pantoprazole Sodium** *see* Pantoprazole *on page 1570*

◆ **Pantoprazole Sodium for Injection (Can)** *see* Pantoprazole *on page 1570*

◆ **Pantothenyl Alcohol** *see* Dexpanthenol *on page 606*

Papaverine (pa PAV er een)

Index Terms Papaverine Hydrochloride; Pavabid

Pharmacologic Category Vasodilator

Use Various vascular spasms associated with smooth muscle spasms as in myocardial infarction, angina, peripheral and pulmonary embolism, peripheral vascular disease; cerebral angiospastic states; visceral spasms (ureteral, biliary, and GI colic). **Note:** Labeled uses have fallen out of favor; safer and more effective alternatives are available.

Pregnancy Risk Factor C

Dosage Note: Labeled uses have fallen out of favor; safer and more effective alternatives are available. The manufacturer's labeling recommends the following dosing:

Arterial spasm: Adults: IM, IV: 30-120 mg; may repeat dose every 3 hours; if cardiac extrasystole occurs during use, may administer 2 doses 10 minutes apart

Dosage adjustment in renal impairment: No dosage adjustment provided in the manufacturer's labeling.

Dosage adjustment in hepatic impairment: No dosage adjustment provided in the manufacturer's labeling.

Additional Information Complete prescribing information should be consulted for additional detail.

Dosage Forms

Solution, Injection:

Generic: 30 mg/mL (2 mL, 10 mL)

◆ **Papaverine Hydrochloride** *see* Papaverine *on page 1573*

Papillomavirus (Types 6, 11, 16, 18) Vaccine (Human, Recombinant)

(pap ih LO ma VYE rus typs six e LEV en SIX teen AYE teen vak SEEN YU man ree KOM be nant)

Brand Names: U.S. Gardasil

Brand Names: Canada Gardasil

Index Terms HPV Vaccine (Quadrivalent); HPV4; Human Papillomavirus Vaccine (Quadrivalent); Papillomavirus Vaccine, Recombinant; Quadrivalent Human Papillomavirus Vaccine

Pharmacologic Category Vaccine, Inactivated (Viral)

Additional Appendix Information

Immunization Administration Recommendations *on page 2250*

Immunization Recommendations *on page 2255*

Use

Prevention of human papillomavirus:

U.S. labeling:

Females 9 to 26 years of age:

For the prevention of the following diseases: cervical, vulvar, vaginal, and anal cancer caused by HPV types 16 and 18; genital warts (condyloma acuminatum) caused by HPV types 6 and 11;

For the prevention of the following precancerous or dysplastic lesions caused by HPV types 6, 11, 16, and 18: cervical intraepithelial neoplasia (CIN) grade 2/3 and cervical adenocarcinoma in situ; CIN grade 1; vulvar intraepithelial neoplasia grade 2 and 3; vaginal intraepithelial neoplasia grade 2 and 3; and anal intraepithelial neoplasia grades 1, 2, and 3.

Males 9 through 26 years of age:

For the prevention of the following diseases: anal cancer caused by HPV types 16 and 18; genital warts (condyloma acuminata) caused by HPV types 6 and 11;

For the prevention of anal intraepithelial neoplasia grades 1, 2, and 3 caused by HPV types 6, 11, 16, and 18.

Limitations of use: Does not provide protection against vaccine HPV types to which a person has already been previously exposed, or HPV types not contained in the vaccine; does not prevent CIN grade 2/3 or worse in women >26 years of age. Not intended for the treatment of active external genital lesions or cervical, vulvar, vaginal, and anal cancers.

Canadian labeling:

Females ≥9 years and ≤26 years of age: Prevention of anal cancer caused by HPV types 16 and 18; anal intraepithelial neoplasia caused by HPV types 6, 11, 16, and 18

Females ≥9 years and ≤45 years of age: Prevention of cervical, vulvar, and vaginal cancer caused by HPV types 16 and 18; genital warts caused by HPV types 6 and 11; cervical adenocarcinoma *in situ*, vulvar, vaginal, or cervical intraepithelial neoplasia caused by HPV types 6, 11, 16, and 18

Males ≥9 years and ≤26 years of age: Prevention of anal cancer caused by HPV types 16 and 18; anal intraepithelial neoplasia caused by HPV types 6, 11, 16, and 18; genital warts caused by HPV types 6 and 11

The Advisory Committee on Immunization Practices (ACIP) recommends routine vaccination for females and males 11 to 12 years of age; can be administered as young as 9 years; catch-up vaccination is recommended for females 13 to 26 years of age and males 13 to 21 years of age. Vaccination for males through 26 years of age is recommended if immunocompromised (including HIV) and for men who have sex with men and may be considered for any other male in this age group (CDC/ACIP [Markowitz, 2014]).

Pregnancy Risk Factor B

Dosage

Immunization: IM:

U.S. labeling: Children ≥9 years, Adolescents, and Adults ≤26 years: 0.5 mL at 0, 2, and 6 months

Canadian labeling: Children ≥9 years, Adolescents, and Adults ≤45 years: 0.5 mL at 0, 2, and 6 months

CDC/ACIP recommended immunization schedule: Typically administer first dose at age 11 to 12 years but may administer as young as 9 years; begin series in females ages 13 to 26 years or males 13 to 21 years if not previously vaccinated or who have not completed the 3-dose series. Males may also be vaccinated through 26 years of age. If a patient reaches 27 years of age before the vaccination series is complete, the remaining doses can be administered after age 26 years. Administer the second and third doses at 1 to 2 months and 6 months, respectively, after the first dose. Minimum interval between first and second doses is 4 weeks; the minimum interval between the second and third dose is 12 weeks; the minimum interval between first and third doses is 24 weeks. Inadequate doses or doses received following a shorter than recommended dosing interval should be repeated. Second and third doses may be given after age 26 years to complete a previously initiated series. The HPV vaccine series should be completed with the same product whenever possible (CDC/ACIP [Markowitz, 2014]).

Dosage adjustment in renal impairment: There are no dosage adjustments provided in the manufacturer's labeling.

Dosage adjustment in hepatic impairment: There are no dosage adjustments provided in the manufacturer's labeling.

Additional Information Complete prescribing information should be consulted for additional detail.

Dosage Forms

Injection, suspension [preservative free]:

Gardasil: HPV 6 L1 protein 20 mcg, HPV 11 L1 protein 40 mcg, HPV 16 L1 protein 40 mcg, and HPV 18 L1 protein 20 mcg per 0.5 mL (0.5 mL)

Papillomavirus (Types 16, 18) Vaccine (Human, Recombinant)

(pap ih LO ma VYE rus typs SIX teen AYE teen vak SEEN YU man ree KOM be nant)

Brand Names: U.S. Cervarix

Brand Names: Canada Cervarix

Index Terms Bivalent Human Papillomavirus Vaccine; GSK-580299; HPV 16/18 L1 VLP/AS04 VAC; HPV Vaccine (Bivalent); HPV2; Human Papillomavirus Vaccine (Bivalent); Papillomavirus Vaccine, Recombinant

Pharmacologic Category Vaccine, Inactivated (Viral)

Additional Appendix Information

Immunization Administration Recommendations *on page 2250*

Immunization Recommendations *on page 2255*

Use

Prevention of human papillomavirus:

U.S. labeling: Prevention in females 9 to 25 years of age of the following diseases caused by oncogenic HPV types 16 and 18: Cervical cancer, cervical intraepithelial neoplasia (CIN) grade 2 or higher and adenocarcinoma in situ, and CIN grade 1.

The Advisory Committee on Immunization Practices (ACIP) recommends routine vaccination for females 11 to 12 years of age; can be administered as young as 9 years; catch-up vaccination is recommended for females 13 to 26 years of age (CDC/ACIP [Markowitz, 2014]).

Canadian labeling: Females 9 through 45 years of age: Prevention of cervical cancer, cervical adenocarcinoma *in situ*, and cervical intraepithelial neoplasia caused by human papillomavirus (HPV) types 16, 18

The National Advisory Committee on Immunization (NACI) recommends routine vaccination for females between 9 and 26 years of age. It should not be administered in females <9 years but may be administered to females >26 years who are at ongoing risk of exposure (NACI [CCDR, 2012]).

Pregnancy Risk Factor B

Dosage Immunization: IM:

U.S. labeling: Children ≥9 years, Adolescents, and Adults ≤25 years: Females: 0.5 mL at 0, 1, and 6 months

CDC/ACIP recommended immunization schedule: Typically administer first dose to females at age 11 to 12 years but may administer as young as 9 years; begin series in females ages 13 to 26 years if not previously vaccinated or who have not completed the 3-dose series. If a female reaches 27 years of age before the vaccination series is complete, the remaining doses can be administered after age 26 years. Administer the second and third doses at 1 to 2 months and 6 months after the first dose, respectively. Minimum interval between first and second doses is 4 weeks; the minimum interval between the second and third dose is 12 weeks; the minimum interval between first and third doses is 24 weeks. Inadequate doses or doses received following a shorter than recommended dosing interval should be repeated. The HPV vaccine series should be completed with the same product whenever possible.

Canadian labeling: Children ≥9 years, Adolescents, and Adults ≤45 years: Females: 0.5 mL at 0, 1, and 6 months; if necessary, may administer the second and third doses at 1 to 2.5 months and 5 to 12 months respectively after the initial dose.

Dosage adjustment in renal impairment: There are no dosage adjustments provided in the manufacturer's labeling.

Dosage adjustment in hepatic impairment: There are no dosage adjustments provided in the manufacturer's labeling.

Additional Information Complete prescribing information should be consulted for additional detail.

Dosage Forms

Injection, suspension [preservative free]:

Cervarix: HPV 16 L1 protein 20 mcg and HPV 18 L1 protein 20 mcg per 0.5 mL (0.5 mL)

◆ **Papillomavirus Vaccine, Recombinant** *see* Papillomavirus (Types 6, 11, 16, 18) Vaccine (Human, Recombinant) *on page 1574*

◆ **Papillomavirus Vaccine, Recombinant** *see* Papillomavirus (Types 16, 18) Vaccine (Human, Recombinant) *on page 1574*

◆ **PAR-101** *see* Fidaxomicin *on page 875*

◆ **Paracetamol** *see* Acetaminophen *on page 32*

◆ **Parafon Forte DSC** *see* Chlorzoxazone *on page 430*

◆ **Paraldahyde Injection BP (Can)** *see* Paraldehyde [CAN/INT] *on page 1575*

Paraldehyde [CAN/INT] (par AL de hyde)

Brand Names: Canada Paraldahyde Injection BP

Pharmacologic Category Anticonvulsant, Miscellaneous; Anxiolytics, Sedatives, and Hypnotics, Miscellaneous

Use Note: Not approved in U.S.

Alternative agent (only when conventional treatment is ineffective, inappropriate, or unavailable) in the treatment of convulsive seizure episodes associated with status epilepticus, tetanus, and convulsant drug toxicity. Historically, has also been used as a sedative/hypnotic, as an anxiolytic during withdrawal from opioids or barbiturates, and in the management of acute agitation or delirium due to alcohol withdrawal; however, these uses are not recommended due to the availability of safer and more efficacious agents

Pregnancy Considerations Paraldehyde crosses the placenta; use in pregnancy is contraindicated. Use in obstetric anesthesia is not appropriate due to potential respiratory depression in neonates. Pregnancy should be excluded prior to initiating in females of childbearing potential.

Breast-Feeding Considerations Due to the potential for serious adverse reactions in the nursing infant, breastfeeding is not recommended.

Contraindications Hypersensitivity to paraldehyde or any component of the formulation; severe hepatic insufficiency; bronchopulmonary disease; pregnancy

Warnings/Precautions Hazardous agent; use appropriate precautions for handling and disposal (EPA, U-listed). Not appropriate as a first-line agent for any indication. Limited published information exists for paraldehyde use compared to more conventional agents with more published safety and efficacy data. If used as a hypnotic/sedative agent, therapy should be limited to short-term use.

May cause CNS depression, which may impair physical or mental abilities; patients must be cautioned about performing tasks which require mental alertness (eg, operating machinery or driving). Effects with other sedative drugs or ethanol may be potentiated. Toxic hepatitis, metabolic acidosis, and nephrosis have been reported following prolonged use. Avoid or use with caution in patients with cardiovascular disease. Use with extreme caution in hepatic impairment and monitor closely for toxicity; large portions of the dose are metabolized via the liver (use is contraindicated in severe hepatic impairment). The lungs are responsible for a significant portion of elimination of unchanged paraldehyde; avoid or use caution in patients with respiratory disease (use is contraindicated in patients with bronchopulmonary disease). Use with caution in patients with a history of drug abuse or acute alcoholism; potential for drug dependency exists. Tolerance, psychological and physical dependence may occur with prolonged use. Use caution when withdrawing therapy after prolonged use in physically dependent patients; decrease slowly and monitor for withdrawal symptoms.

Per Canadian manufacturer's labeling, product is intended for IM administration only; avoid injecting IM near nerve trucks due to potential for severe and permanent nerve damage. IM administration is associated with severe pain and may also cause skin reactions (eg, sterile skin abscesses, skin sloughing), fat necrosis, and muscle irritation. Subcutaneous injections are **not** recommended; paraldehyde is a tissue irritant. In addition, do **not** inject intravenously due to potential for thrombophlebitis, pulmonary edema and hemorrhage, respiratory distress, cyanosis, hypotension and cardiac dilatation, and circulatory collapse. Paraldehyde decomposes when opened; prepare using only freshly opened vials. Use of partly decomposed paraldehyde is hazardous and may result in metabolic acidosis; use of decomposed paraldehyde has resulted in death from corrosive poisoning. If solution is a brownish color or smells of acetic acid, it should **not** be used. Avoid contact with skin, eyes, and clothing. Since paraldehyde is a solvent, contact with plastic (eg, plastic syringes) or rubber should be avoided.

Adverse Reactions

Central nervous system: Drowsiness, dizziness
Dermatologic: Rash
Endocrine & metabolic: Metabolic acidosis
Gastrointestinal: Strong, unpleasant breath odor
Hepatic: Hepatitis (toxic)
Local: Injection site pain, injection site reactions (sterile skin abscesses, skin sloughing, fat necrosis, muscle irritation, nerve damage [including permanent damage])
Neuromuscular & skeletal: Muscle cramps, trembling
Renal: Nephrosis
Miscellaneous: Diaphoresis, psychological and physical dependence with prolonged use

Drug Interactions

Metabolism/Transport Effects None known.

Avoid Concomitant Use

Avoid concomitant use of Paraldehyde with any of the following: Alcohol (Ethyl); Azelastine (Nasal); CNS Depressants; Disulfiram; Orphenadrine; Thalidomide

Increased Effect/Toxicity

Paraldehyde may increase the levels/effects of: Azelastine (Nasal); Metyrosine; Orphenadrine; Pramipexole; ROPINIRole; Rotigotine; Selective Serotonin Reuptake Inhibitors; Thalidomide

The levels/effects of Paraldehyde may be increased by: Alcohol (Ethyl); Brimonidine (Topical); Cannabis; CNS Depressants; Disulfiram; Dronabinol; Kava Kava; Magnesium Sulfate; Nabilone; Rufinamide; Tetrahydrocannabinol

Decreased Effect There are no known significant interactions involving a decrease in effect.

Preparation for Administration Use immediately after opening vial; paraldehyde decomposes to acetaldehyde and then to acetic acid, causing toxicity. Do not use if solution is brownish or has an odor of acetic acid. Paraldehyde is not compatible with plastics or rubber. Do not use plastic syringes for preparation or administration; glass syringes are recommended (needles with plastic hubs, polypropylene syringes with rubber tipped plastic plungers, or glass syringes with natural rubber tipped plastic plungers are permissible **ONLY** for immediate administration or for measurement of doses).

Avoid contact with skin, eyes, and clothing.

Hazardous agent; use appropriate precautions for handling and disposal (EPA, U-listed).

Storage/Stability Store intact vials at <25°C (77°F); do not refrigerate. Crystallization occurs at ~12°C (54°F); warm gently if crystallization occurs. Must store in tightly closed containers and protect from light.

Mechanism of Action Paraldehyde, a cyclic trimer of acetaldehyde, has an unknown mechanism of action; causes CNS depression, including the ascending reticular activating system to provide sedation/hypnosis and anticonvulsant activity (at slightly lower doses than those required to produce hypnosis). It has no analgesic properties at sub-anesthetic doses and may cause excitement or delirium in the presence of pain.

Pharmacodynamics/Kinetics

Onset of sedation/hypnosis: IM: 5-15 minutes
Duration: 8 hours
Absorption: IM: Rapid
Distribution: Tissue distribution not extensively studied; diffuses into CSF with concentrations in CSF ~25% to 30% lower than that of serum concentrations
Metabolism: ~80% to 90% of the dose metabolized in the liver to acetaldehyde, then oxidized via aldehyde dehydrogenase to acetic acid, and further metabolized to carbon dioxide and water
Half-life elimination: Adults: ~3.5-9.5 hours (mean: 7.5 hours [in patients with normal hepatic function])
Time to peak: IM: Serum: 20-60 minutes; CSF: 30-60 minutes
Excretion: Significant portion excreted as unchanged drug in expired air via the lungs; trace amounts excreted in urine unchanged

Dosage IM: Canadian labeling: **Note:** Do not administer >5 mL per injection site.

Children: Second- or third-line therapy:
Hypnotic: 0.3 mL/kg/daily
Sedative: 0.15 mL/kg/daily
Seizure associated with status epilepticus: 0.1-0.15 mL/kg/dose every 4-8 hours

Adults: Second- or third-line therapy:
Alcohol withdrawal: 5 mL every 4-6 hours for 24 hours (maximum: 30 mL on day 1), followed by every 6 hours (maximum: 20 mL/day)
Hypnotic: 10 mL
Sedative: 5 mL
Seizure associated with status epilepticus, tetanus, or poisoning: 5-10 mL

Dosing adjustment in renal impairment: No dosage adjustment provided in manufacturer's labeling.

Dosing adjustment in hepatic impairment:

Mild-to-moderate impairment: No dosage adjustment provided in manufacturer's labeling; however, undergoes extensive hepatic metabolism and should be used with extreme caution. Consider dose reductions.
Severe impairment: Use contraindicated

Administration

Administer by IM injection only; avoid injecting near nerve trunks (permanent nerve damage may occur). IM injection is associated with extreme pain and serious injection site reactions.

Do **not** administer intravenously (life-threatening effects may result) or SubQ.

Do **not** use any use plastic syringes or rubber for administration; glass syringes are recommended for administration.

Do **not** use if solution is brownish or has an odor of acetic acid. Use immediately after opening vial (paraldehyde decomposes to acetic acid causing toxicity).

Hazardous agent; use appropriate precautions for handling and disposal (EPA, U-listed).

Additional Information In the literature, paraldehyde has been given rectally (off-label route) in situations where other preferred agents have failed; one advantage of rectal administration reportedly is the limited respiratory depression produced with this method (NICE guidelines, 2012). If given rectally, paraldehyde should be diluted before use. In one study, a 1:1 preparation of paraldehyde with olive oil was used (Rowland, 2009).

Product Availability Not available in the U.S.

◆ **Paraplatin** *see* CARBOplatin *on page 357*

◆ **Parathyroid Hormone (1-34)** *see* Teriparatide *on page 2008*

◆ **Parcaine** *see* Proparacaine *on page 1728*

◆ **Parcopa [DSC]** *see* Carbidopa and Levodopa *on page 351*

Parecoxib [INT] (pa re KOX ib)

International Brand Names Bextra (BR); Dynastat (AE, AT, AU, BE, BH, CN, CY, CZ, DE, DK, EE, FI, FR, GB, GR, HK, HR, ID, IE, IS, IT, KW, LT, MY, NL, NO, NZ, PE, PH,

PL, PT, QA, RO, RU, SE, SG, SI, SK, TH, TR, TW); Pro-Bextra IM/IV (CL); Rayzon (ZA); Superin (IN); Valdure IM (BZ, CR, DO, GT, HN, NI, PA, SV)

Index Terms Parecoxib Sodium

Pharmacologic Category Analgesic, Nonsteroidal Anti-inflammatory Drug; Nonsteroidal Anti-inflammatory Drug (NSAID), COX-2 Selective

Reported Use For the management of postoperative pain

Dosage Range IM, IV: Adults ≥18 years: 40 mg, followed by 20-40 mg every 6-12 hours; maximum daily dose: 80 mg

Dosage adjustment in hepatic impairment:
Mild (Child-Pugh score 5-6): No dosage adjustment
Moderate (Child-Pugh score 7-9): 20 mg, followed by 20 mg every 6-12 hours; maximum daily dose: 40 mg
Severe (Child-Pugh score >9): Not recommended

Product Availability Product available in various countries; not currently available in the U.S.

Dosage Forms
Injection, powder for reconstitution as sodium: 40 mg [package with diluent; strength expressed as base]

◆ **Parecoxib Sodium** *see* Parecoxib [INT] *on page 1576*

Paregoric (par e GOR ik)

Index Terms Camphorated Tincture of Opium (error-prone synonym)

Pharmacologic Category Analgesic, Opioid; Antidiarrheal

Use Diarrhea: Treatment of diarrhea

Pregnancy Risk Factor C

Dosage Diarrhea: Oral: **Note:** Paregoric oral liquid contains morphine 2 mg/5 mL (0.4 mg/mL)
Children and Adolescents: 0.25 to 0.5 mL/kg 1 to 4 times daily
Adults: 5 to 10 mL 1 to 4 times daily

Dosage adjustment in renal impairment: There are no dosage adjustments provided in the manufacturer's labeling. Use with caution in severe impairment.

Dosage adjustment in hepatic impairment: There are no dosage adjustments provided in the manufacturer's labeling. Use with caution in severe impairment.

Additional Information Complete prescribing information should be consulted for additional detail.

Dosage Forms
Tincture, Oral:
Generic: 2 mg/5 mL (473 mL)

◆ **Parenteral Nutrition** *see* Total Parenteral Nutrition *on page 2073*

Paricalcitol (pah ri KAL si tole)

Brand Names: U.S. Zemplar

Brand Names: Canada Zemplar

Pharmacologic Category Vitamin D Analog

Use
IV: Prevention and treatment of secondary hyperparathyroidism associated with stage 5 chronic kidney disease (CKD)
Oral: Prevention and treatment of secondary hyperparathyroidism associated with stage 3 and 4 CKD and stage 5 CKD patients on hemodialysis or peritoneal dialysis

Pregnancy Risk Factor C

Pregnancy Considerations Adverse events were observed in some animal reproduction studies.

Breast-Feeding Considerations It is not known if paricalcitol is excreted in breast milk. Due to the potential for serious adverse reactions in the nursing infant, a decision should be made whether to discontinue nursing or to discontinue the drug, taking into account the importance of treatment to the mother.

Contraindications Hypersensitivity to paricalcitol or any component of the formulation; patients with evidence of vitamin D toxicity; hypercalcemia

Warnings/Precautions Excessive administration may lead to over suppression of PTH, hypercalcemia, hypercalciuria, hyperphosphatemia and adynamic bone disease. Acute hypercalcemia may increase risk of cardiac arrhythmias and seizures; use caution with cardiac glycosides as digitalis toxicity may be increased. Chronic hypercalcemia may lead to generalized vascular and other soft-tissue calcification. Phosphate and vitamin D (and its derivatives) should be withheld during therapy to avoid hypercalcemia. Risk of hypercalcemia may be increased by concomitant use of calcium-containing supplements and/or medications that increase serum calcium (eg, thiazide diuretics). Avoid regular administration of aluminum-containing preparations (eg, antacids, phosphate binders) to prevent aluminum overload and bone toxicity. Dialysate concentration of aluminum should be maintained at <10 mcg/L.

Adverse Reactions
Cardiovascular: Chest pain, edema, hypertension, hypotension, palpitations, peripheral edema, syncope
Central nervous system: Anxiety, chills, depression, dizziness, fatigue, headache, insomnia, malaise, pain, vertigo
Dermatologic: Dermal ulcer, ecchymoses, skin rash
Endocrine & metabolic: Dehydration, hypervolemia, hypoglycemia
Gastrointestinal: Abdominal pain, constipation, diarrhea, dyspepsia, gastrointestinal hemorrhage, nausea, peritonitis, vomiting, xerostomia
Genitourinary: Uremia, urinary tract infection
Hypersensitivity: Hypersensitivity reaction
Infection: Infection (bacterial, fungal, viral), influenza, sepsis
Neuromuscular & skeletal: Arthralgia, arthritis, back pain, leg cramps, muscle spasm, weakness
Respiratory: Bronchitis, cough, nasopharyngitis, oropharyngeal pain, pneumonia, rhinitis, sinusitis
Miscellaneous: Fever
Rare but important or life-threatening:Abnormal gait, abnormal hepatic function tests, anemia, angioedema (including laryngeal edema), atrial flutter, burning sensation of skin, cardiac arrest, cardiac arrhythmia, cerebrovascular accident, confusion, conjunctivitis, delirium, dysphagia, erectile dysfunction, extravasation reactions, gastritis, gastroesophageal reflux disease, glaucoma, hirsutism, hypercalciuria, hypercalcemia, hyperparathyroidism, hyperkalemia, hyperphosphatemia, hypocalcemia, hypoparathyroidism, increased serum creatinine, ischemic bowel disease, lymphadenopathy, malignant neoplasm of breast, myalgia, myoclonus, night sweats, ocular hyperemia, orthopnea, paresthesia, prolonged bleeding time, pruritus, pulmonary edema, rectal hemorrhage, upper respiratory tract infection, urticaria, vaginal infection, weight loss, wheezing

Drug Interactions

Metabolism/Transport Effects Substrate of CYP3A4 (minor); **Note:** Assignment of Major/Minor substrate status based on clinically relevant drug interaction potential

Avoid Concomitant Use
Avoid concomitant use of Paricalcitol with any of the following: Aluminum Hydroxide; Multivitamins/Fluoride (with ADE); Multivitamins/Minerals (with ADEK, Folate, Iron); Sucralfate; Vitamin D Analogs

Increased Effect/Toxicity
Paricalcitol may increase the levels/effects of: Aluminum Hydroxide; Cardiac Glycosides; Digoxin; Sucralfate; Vitamin D Analogs

The levels/effects of Paricalcitol may be increased by: Calcium Salts; CYP3A4 Inhibitors (Strong); Danazol; Multivitamins/Fluoride (with ADE); Multivitamins/Minerals (with ADEK, Folate, Iron); Thiazide Diuretics

Decreased Effect

The levels/effects of Paricalcitol may be decreased by: Bile Acid Sequestrants; Mineral Oil; Orlistat

Storage/Stability Store at 25°C (77°F); excursions permitted between 15°C to 30°C (59°F to 86°F).

Mechanism of Action Decreased renal conversion of vitamin D to its primary active metabolite (1,25-hydroxyvitamin D) in chronic renal failure leads to reduced activation of vitamin D receptor (VDR), which subsequently removes inhibitory suppression of parathyroid hormone (PTH) release; increased serum PTH (secondary hyperparathyroidism) reduces calcium excretion and enhances bone resorption. Paricalcitol is a synthetic vitamin D analog which binds to and activates the VDR in kidney, parathyroid gland, intestine and bone, thus reducing PTH levels and improving calcium and phosphate homeostasis.

Pharmacodynamics/Kinetics

Distribution: V_d:

Healthy subjects: Oral: 34 L; IV: 24 L

Stage 3 and 4 CKD: Oral: 44 to 46 L

Stage 5 CKD: Oral: 38 to 49 L; IV: 31 to 35 L

Protein binding: >99%

Metabolism: Hydroxylation and glucuronidation via hepatic and nonhepatic enzymes, including CYP24, CYP3A4, UGT1A4; forms metabolites (at least one active)

Bioavailability: Oral: 72% to 86% in healthy subjects

Half-life elimination:

Healthy subjects: Oral: 4 to 6 hours; IV: 5 to 7 hours

Stage 3 and 4 CKD: Oral: 17 to 20 hours

Stage 5 CKD (on HD or PD): Oral: 14 to 18 hours; IV: 14 to 15 hours

Time to peak, plasma: 3 hours: Delayed by food

Excretion: Healthy subjects: Feces (oral: 70%; IV: 63%); urine (oral: 18%, IV: 19%)

Dosage Note: In stage 3 to 5 CKD maintain calcium phosphorus product (Ca x P) <55 mg^2/dL^2, reduce or interrupt dosing if recommended Ca x P is exceeded or hypercalcemia is observed (K/DOQI Clinical Practice Guidelines, 2003).

Secondary hyperparathyroidism associated with chronic renal failure (stage 5 CKD):

Children ≥5 years and Adults: IV: 0.04 to 0.1 mcg/kg (2.8 to 7 mcg) given as a bolus dose no more frequently than every other day at any time during dialysis; dose may be increased by 2 to 4 mcg every 2 to 4 weeks; doses as high as 0.24 mcg/kg (16.8 mcg) have been administered safely; the dose of paricalcitol should be adjusted based on serum intact PTH (iPTH) levels, as follows:

Same or increasing iPTH level: Increase paricalcitol dose

iPTH level decreased by <30%: Increase paricalcitol dose

iPTH level decreased by >30% and <60%: Maintain paricalcitol dose

iPTH level decrease by >60%: Decrease paricalcitol dose

iPTH level 1.5 to 3 times upper limit of normal: Maintain paricalcitol dose

Adults: Oral: Initial dose, in mcg, based on baseline iPTH level divided by 80. Administered 3 times weekly, no more frequently than every other day. **Note:** To reduce the risk of hypercalcemia initiate only after baseline serum calcium has been adjusted to ≤9.5 mg/dL.

Dose titration:

Titration dose (mcg) = Most recent iPTH level (pg/mL) divided by 80

Note: In situations where monitoring of iPTH, calcium, and phosphorus occurs less frequently than once per week, a more modest initial and dose titration rate may be warranted:

Modest titration dose (mcg) = Most recent iPTH level (pg/mL) divided by 100

Dosage adjustment for hypercalcemia or elevated Ca x P: Decrease calculated dose by 2 to 4 mcg. If further adjustment is required, dose should be reduced or interrupted until these parameters are normalized. If applicable, phosphate binder dosing may also be adjusted or withheld, or switched to a noncalcium-based phosphate binder

Secondary hyperparathyroidism associated with stage 3 and 4 CKD: Adults: Oral: Initial dose based on baseline serum iPTH:

iPTH ≤500 pg/mL: 1 mcg/day or 2 mcg 3 times/week

iPTH >500 pg/mL: 2 mcg/day or 4 mcg 3 times/week

Dosage adjustment based on iPTH level relative to baseline, adjust dose at 2- to 4-week intervals:

iPTH same or increased: Increase paricalcitol dose by 1 mcg/day or 2 mcg 3 times/week

iPTH decreased by <30%: Increase paricalcitol dose by 1 mcg/day or 2 mcg 3 times/week

iPTH decreased by ≥30% and ≤60%: Maintain paricalcitol dose

iPTH decreased by >60%: Decrease paricalcitol dose by 1 mcg/day* or 2 mcg 3 times/week

iPTH <60 pg/mL: Decrease paricalcitol dose by 1 mcg/day* or 2 mcg 3 times/week

*If patient is taking the lowest dose on a once-daily regimen, but further dose reduction is needed, decrease dose to 1 mcg 3 times/week. If further dose reduction is required, withhold drug as needed and restart at a lower dose and frequency. If applicable, calcium-phosphate binder dosing may also be adjusted or withheld, or switched to noncalcium-based binder.

Dosage adjustment in renal impairment: No dosage adjustment necessary.

Dosage adjustment in hepatic impairment:

Mild to moderate impairment: No dosage adjustment necessary.

Severe impairment: No dosage adjustment provided in manufacturer's labeling (has not been studied).

Dietary Considerations May be taken with or without food. Some products may contain coconut or palm kernel oil.

Administration

Oral: May be administered with or without food. With the 3 times/week dosing schedule, doses should not be given more frequently than every other day.

IV: Administered as a bolus dose at anytime during dialysis. Doses should not be administered more often than every other day.

Monitoring Parameters

Signs and symptoms of vitamin D intoxication; signs and symptoms of hypercalcemia (eg, feeling tired, difficulty thinking clearly, loss of appetite, nausea, vomiting, constipation, increased thirst, increased urination, weight loss).

Serum calcium and phosphorus (closely monitor levels during dosage titration and after initiation of a strong CYP3A4 inhibitor):

IV: Twice weekly during initial phase, then at least monthly once dose established

Oral: At least every 2 weeks for initial 3 months or following dose adjustment, then monthly for 3 months, then every 3 months

Serum or plasma intact PTH (iPTH):

IV: Every 3 months

Oral: At least every 2 weeks for 3 months or following dose adjustment, then monthly for 3 months, then every 3 months

Reference Range

Corrected total serum calcium (K/DOQI, 2003): CKD stages 3 and 4: 8.4 to 10.2 mg/dL (2.1 to 2.6 mmol/L); CKD stage 5: 8.4 to 9.5 mg/dL (2.1 to 2.37 mmol/L); KDIGO guidelines recommend maintaining normal ranges for all stages of CKD (3 to 5D) (KDIGO, 2009)

Phosphorus (K/DOQI, 2003):

CKD stages 3 and 4: 2.7 to 4.6 mg/dL (0.87 to 1.48 mmol/L) (adults); maintain within age-appropriate limits (children)

CKD stage 5 (including those treated with dialysis): 3.5 to 5.5 mg/dL (1.13 to 1.78 mmol/L) (children >12 years and adults); 4 to 6 mg/dL (1.29 to 1.94 mmol/L) (children 1 to 12 years)

KDIGO guidelines recommend maintaining normal ranges for CKD stages 3 to 5 and lowering elevated phosphorus levels toward the normal range for CKD stage 5D (KDIGO, 2009)

Serum calcium-phosphorus product (K/DOQI, 2003): CKD stage 3 to 5: <55 mg^2/dL^2 (children >12 years and adults); <65 mg^2/dL^2 (children ≤12 years)

PTH: Whole molecule, immunochemiluminometric assay (ICMA): 1.0 to 5.2 pmol/L; whole molecule, radioimmunoassay (RIA): 10.0 to 65.0 pg/mL; whole molecule, immunoradiometric, double antibody (IRMA): 1.0 to 6.0 pmol/L

Target ranges by stage of chronic kidney disease (KDIGO, 2009): CKD stage 3 to 5: Optimal iPTH is unknown; maintain normal range (assay-dependent); CKD stage 5D: Maintain iPTH within 2 to 9 times the upper limit of normal for the assay used

Dosage Forms

Capsule, Oral:

Zemplar: 1 mcg, 2 mcg, 4 mcg

Generic: 1 mcg, 2 mcg, 4 mcg

Solution, Intravenous:

Zemplar: 2 mcg/mL (1 mL); 5 mcg/mL (1 mL, 2 mL)

Generic: 2 mcg/mL (1 mL); 5 mcg/mL (1 mL, 2 mL)

◆ **Pariet (Can)** *see* RABEprazole *on page* 1762

◆ **Pariprazole** *see* RABEprazole *on page* 1762

◆ **Paritaprevir, Ombitasvir, Ritonavir, and Dasabuvir** *see* Ombitasvir, Paritaprevir, Ritonavir, and Dasabuvir *on page* 1505

◆ **Parlodel** *see* Bromocriptine *on page* 291

◆ **Parnate** *see* Tranylcypromine *on page* 2083

◆ **Parnate® (Can)** *see* Tranylcypromine *on page* 2083

◆ **Paroex** *see* Chlorhexidine Gluconate *on page* 422

Paromomycin (par oh moe MYE sin)

Brand Names: Canada Humatin

Index Terms Paromomycin Sulfate

Pharmacologic Category Amebicide

Use

Intestinal amebiasis: Treatment of acute and chronic intestinal amebiasis (not effective for extraintestinal amebiasis).

Hepatic coma: Management (adjunctive) of hepatic coma.

Pregnancy Considerations Paromomycin is poorly absorbed when given orally. Information related to the use of paromomycin in pregnancy is limited (Kreutner, 1981). Use may be considered for the treatment of giardiasis throughout pregnancy (Gardner, 2001) or cryptosporidiosis after the first trimester (DHHS, 2013) in pregnant women.

Breast-Feeding Considerations Paromomycin is poorly absorbed when given orally. Available information suggests that paromomycin may be used in nursing women when renal function is normal in both the mother and infant (Davidson, 2009).

Contraindications Hypersensitivity to paromomycin or any component of the formulation; intestinal obstruction

Warnings/Precautions Use with caution in patients with impaired renal function or ulcerative bowel lesions (may lead to renal toxicity due to inadvertent absorption). Prolonged use may result in fungal or bacterial superinfection, including *C. difficile*-associated diarrhea (CDAD) and pseudomembranous colitis; CDAD has been observed >2 months postantibiotic treatment. Use in the absence of proven (or strongly suspected) susceptible infection is unlikely to provide benefit and may increase the risk for drug-resistance.

Adverse Reactions

Gastrointestinal: Abdominal cramps, diarrhea, heartburn, nausea, vomiting

Rare but important or life-threatening: Enterocolitis (secondary), eosinophilia, ototoxicity, pruritus, rash, steatorrhea

Drug Interactions

Metabolism/Transport Effects None known.

Avoid Concomitant Use There are no known interactions where it is recommended to avoid concomitant use.

Increased Effect/Toxicity There are no known significant interactions involving an increase in effect.

Decreased Effect There are no known significant interactions involving a decrease in effect.

Storage/Stability Store at 20°C to 25°C (68°F to 77°F). Protect from moisture.

Mechanism of Action Acts directly on ameba; has antibacterial activity against normal and pathogenic organisms in the GI tract; interferes with bacterial protein synthesis by binding to 30S ribosomal subunits

Pharmacodynamics/Kinetics

Absorption: Poor oral absorption

Excretion: Feces (~100% as unchanged drug)

Dosage

Intestinal amebiasis (acute and chronic): Children, Adolescents, and Adults: Oral: 25-35 mg/kg/day in 3 divided doses for 5-10 days

Hepatic coma: Adults: Oral: 4 g daily in divided doses (at regular intervals) for 5-6 days

Cryptosporidiosis (off-label use): Adults with AIDS: Oral: 500 mg 4 times daily for 14-21 days (with optimized ATR; DHHS, 2013)

Dientamoeba fragilis (off-label use): Children, Adolescents, and Adults: Oral: 25-35 mg/kg/day in 3 divided doses for 7 days (CDC, 2012; Vandenberg, 2006)

Dosage adjustment in renal impairment: No dosage adjustment provided in the manufacturer's labeling (has not been studied).

Dosage adjustment in hepatic impairment: No dosage adjustment provided in the manufacturer's labeling (has not been studied).

Administration Administer orally with meals.

Dosage Forms

Capsule, Oral:

Generic: 250 mg

◆ **Paromomycin Sulfate** *see* Paromomycin *on page* 1579

PARoxetine (pa ROKS e teen)

Brand Names: U.S. Brisdelle; Paxil; Paxil CR; Pexeva

Brand Names: Canada Apo-Paroxetine; Auro-Paroxetine; CO Paroxetine; Dom-Paroxetine; JAMP-Paroxetine;

Mylan-Paroxetine; Novo-Paroxetine; Paxil; Paxil CR; PHL-Paroxetine; PMS-Paroxetine; Q-Paroxetine; ratio-Paroxetine; Riva-Paroxetine; Sandoz-Paroxetine; Teva-Paroxetine

Index Terms Brisdelle; Paroxetine Hydrochloride; Paroxetine Mesylate

Pharmacologic Category Antidepressant, Selective Serotonin Reuptake Inhibitor

Additional Appendix Information

Beers Criteria – Potentially Inappropriate Medications for Geriatrics *on page 2271*

Use

Generalized anxiety disorder (immediate release): For the treatment of generalized anxiety disorder (GAD)

Major depressive disorder (immediate and controlled release): For the treatment of major depressive disorder (MDD)

Obsessive-compulsive disorder (immediate release): For the treatment of obsessions and compulsions in patients with obsessive-compulsive disorder (OCD)

Panic disorder (immediate and controlled release): For the treatment of panic disorder, with or without agoraphobia

Post-traumatic stress disorder (immediate release): For the treatment of post-traumatic stress disorder (PTSD)

Premenstrual dysphoric disorder (controlled release): For the treatment of premenstrual dysphoric disorder (PMDD)

Social anxiety disorder (immediate and controlled release): For the treatment of social anxiety disorder, also known as social phobia

Vasomotor symptoms of menopause (Brisdelle only): For the treatment of moderate to severe vasomotor symptoms associated with menopause

Pregnancy Risk Factor D//X (product specific)

Pregnancy Considerations Studies in pregnant women have demonstrated a risk to the fetus. Paroxetine crosses the placenta. An increased risk of teratogenic effects, including cardiovascular defects, may be associated with maternal use of paroxetine or other SSRIs; however, available information is conflicting. Nonteratogenic effects in the newborn following SSRI/SNRI exposure late in the third trimester include respiratory distress, cyanosis, apnea, seizures, temperature instability, feeding difficulty, vomiting, hypoglycemia, hypo- or hypertonia, hyperreflexia, jitteriness, irritability, constant crying, and tremor. Symptoms may be due to the toxicity of the SSRIs/SNRIs or a discontinuation syndrome and may be consistent with serotonin syndrome associated with SSRI treatment. Persistent pulmonary hypertension of the newborn (PPHN) has also been reported with SSRI exposure. The long-term effects of *in utero* SSRI exposure on infant development and behavior are not known.

Due to pregnancy-induced physiologic changes, some pharmacokinetic parameters of paroxetine may be altered. The maternal CYP2D6 genotype also influences paroxetine plasma concentrations during pregnancy.

The manufacturer suggests discontinuing paroxetine or switching to another antidepressant unless the benefits of therapy justify continuing treatment during pregnancy; consider other treatment options for women who are planning to become pregnant. The ACOG recommends that therapy with SSRIs or SNRIs during pregnancy be individualized; treatment of depression during pregnancy should incorporate the clinical expertise of the mental health clinician, obstetrician, primary healthcare provider, and pediatrician. The ACOG also recommends that therapy with paroxetine be avoided during pregnancy if possible and that fetuses exposed in early pregnancy be assessed with a fetal echocardiography. According to the American Psychiatric Association (APA), the risks of medication treatment should be weighed against other treatment options and untreated depression. The use of paroxetine is not recommended as first line therapy during pregnancy. For women who discontinue antidepressant medications during pregnancy and who may be at high risk for postpartum depression, the medications can be restarted following delivery. Treatment algorithms have been developed by the ACOG and the APA for the management of depression in women prior to conception and during pregnancy. Menopausal vasomotor symptoms do not occur during pregnancy; therefore, the use of paroxetine for the treatment of menopausal vasomotor symptoms is contraindicated in pregnant women.

Breast-Feeding Considerations Paroxetine is excreted in breast milk and concentrations in the hindmilk are higher than in foremilk. Paroxetine has not been detected in the serum of nursing infants. Adverse reactions have been reported in nursing infants exposed to some SSRIs. The manufacturer recommends that caution be exercised when administering paroxetine to nursing women. Maternal use of an SSRI during pregnancy may cause delayed milk secretion. The American Academy of Breast-feeding Medicine suggests that paroxetine may be considered for the treatment of postpartum depression in appropriately selected women who are nursing. Mothers should be monitored for changes in symptoms and infants should be monitored for growth. The long-term effects on development and behavior have not been studied.

Contraindications Concurrent use with or within 14 days of MAOIs intended to treat psychiatric disorders; initiation in patients being treated with linezolid or methylene blue IV; concomitant use with pimozide or thioridazine; hypersensitivity to paroxetine or any of its inactive ingredients; pregnancy (Brisdelle only).

Warnings/Precautions Hazardous agent - use appropriate precautions for handling and disposal (NIOSH 2014 [group 3]). **[U.S. Boxed Warning]: Antidepressants increase the risk of suicidal thinking and behavior in children, adolescents, and young adults (18 to 24 years of age) with major depressive disorder (MDD) and other psychiatric disorders;** consider risk prior to prescribing. Short-term studies did not show an increased risk in patients >24 years of age and showed a decreased risk in patients ≥65 years. Closely monitor patients for clinical worsening, suicidality, or unusual changes in behavior, particularly during the initial 1 to 2 months of therapy or during periods of dosage adjustments (increases or decreases); the patient's family or caregiver should be instructed to closely observe the patient and communicate condition with healthcare provider. A medication guide concerning the use of antidepressants should be dispensed with each prescription. **Paroxetine is not FDA approved for use in children.**

The possibility of a suicide attempt is inherent in major depression and may persist until remission occurs. Use caution in high-risk patients. Worsening depression and severe abrupt suicidality that are not part of the presenting symptoms may require discontinuation or modification of drug therapy. The patient's family or caregiver should be alerted to monitor patients for the emergence of suicidality and associated behaviors (such as agitation, irritability, hostility, impulsivity, and hypomania) and call health care provider.

May worsen psychosis in some patients or precipitate a shift to mania or hypomania in patients with bipolar disorder. Patients presenting with depressive symptoms should be screened for bipolar disorder. Monotherapy in patients with bipolar disorder should be avoided. **Paroxetine is not FDA approved for the treatment of bipolar depression.**

Potentially life-threatening serotonin syndrome (SS) has occurred with serotonergic agents (eg, SSRIs, SNRIs), particularly when used in combination with other serotonergic agents (eg, triptans, TCAs, fentanyl, lithium, tramadol, buspirone, St John's wort, tryptophan) or agents that impair metabolism of serotonin (eg, MAO inhibitors intended to treat psychiatric disorders, other MAO inhibitors [ie, linezolid and intravenous methylene blue]). Discontinue treatment (and any concomitant serotonergic agent) immediately if signs/symptoms arise.

Paroxetine may increase the risks associated with electroconvulsive therapy. Has a low potential to impair cognitive or motor performance - use caution when operating hazardous machinery or driving. Symptoms of agitation and/or restlessness may occur during initial few weeks of therapy. Low potential for sedation or anticholinergic effects relative to cyclic antidepressants. Bone fractures have been associated with SSRI treatment. Consider the possibility of a fragility fracture if an SSRI-treated patient presents with unexplained bone pain, point tenderness, swelling, or bruising.

Use caution in elderly patients; may be potentially inappropriate in patients with a history of falls or fractures, and may cause or exacerbate syndrome of inappropriate antidiuretic hormone secretion or hyponatremia; monitor sodium closely with initiation or dosage adjustments in older adults. Medication associated with potent anticholinergic properties which may be inappropriate in older adults depending on comorbidities (eg, dementia, delirium) (Beers Criteria).

Use caution in patients with a previous seizure disorder or condition predisposing to seizures such as brain damage or alcoholism. Use with caution in patients with hepatic dysfunction. May cause SIADH; volume depletion and/or diuretics may increase risk. Potentially significant drug-drug interactions may exist, requiring dose or frequency adjustment, additional monitoring, and/or selection of alternative therapy. Use with caution in patients with renal insufficiency or other concurrent illness (due to limited experience); dose reduction recommended with severe renal impairment. May cause or exacerbate sexual dysfunction. May cause mild pupillary dilation, which can lead to an episode of narrow-angle glaucoma in susceptible individuals. Consider evaluating patients who have not had an iridectomy for narrow-angle glaucoma risk factors. Avoid use in the first trimester of pregnancy. Menopausal vasomotor symptoms do not occur during pregnancy; therefore, the use of paroxetine for the treatment of menopausal vasomotor symptoms is contraindicated in pregnant women.

Brisdelle contains a lower dose than what is required for the treatment of psychiatric conditions. Patients who require paroxetine for the treatment of psychiatric conditions should discontinue Brisdelle and begin treatment with a paroxetine-containing medication which provides an adequate dosage.

Abrupt discontinuation or interruption of antidepressant therapy has been associated with a discontinuation syndrome. Symptoms arising may vary with antidepressant however commonly include nausea, vomiting, diarrhea, headaches, lightheadedness, dizziness, diminished appetite, sweating, chills, tremors, paresthesias, fatigue, somnolence, and sleep disturbances (eg, vivid dreams, insomnia). Greater risks for developing a discontinuation syndrome have been associated with antidepressants with shorter half-lives, longer durations of treatment, and abrupt discontinuation. For antidepressants of short or intermediate half-lives, symptoms may emerge within 2 to 5 days after treatment discontinuation and last 7 to 14 days (APA, 2010; Fava, 2006; Haddod, 2001; Shelton, 2001; Warner, 2006).

Adverse Reactions

Cardiovascular: Chest pain, hypertension, palpitations, tachycardia, vasodilatation

Central nervous system: Abnormal dreams, agitation, amnesia, anxiety, chills, confusion, depersonalization, dizziness, drowsiness, emotional lability, fatigue, headache, insomnia, lack of concentration, myasthenia, myoclonus, nervousness, paresthesia, vertigo, yawning

Dermatologic: Diaphoresis, pruritus, skin rash

Endocrine & metabolic: Decreased libido, dysmenorrhea, orgasm disturbance, weight gain

Gastrointestinal: Abdominal pain, constipation, decreased appetite, diarrhea, dysgeusia, dyspepsia, flatulence, increased appetite, nausea, vomiting, xerostomia

Genitourinary: Ejaculatory disorder, female genital tract disease, impotence, male genital disease, urinary frequency, urinary tract infection

Infection: Infection

Neuromuscular & skeletal: Arthralgia, back pain, myalgia, myopathy, tremor, weakness

Ophthalmic: Blurred vision, visual disturbance

Otic: Tinnitus

Respiratory: Dyspnea, pharyngitis, rhinitis, sinusitis

Rare but important or life-threatening: Abnormal hepatic function tests, acute angle-closure glaucoma, acute renal failure, adrenergic syndrome, agranulocytosis, akathisia, akinesia, anaphylactoid reaction, anaphylaxis, anemia (various), angina pectoris, angioedema, aphasia, aphthous stomatitis, aplastic anemia, asthma, atrial arrhythmia, atrial fibrillation, bilirubinemia, bloody diarrhea, bone marrow aplasia, bradycardia, bronchitis, bulimia nervosa, bundle branch block, cardiac failure, cataract, cellulitis, cerebral ischemia, cerebrovascular accident, change in platelet count, cholelithiasis, colitis, deafness, dehydration, delirium, depression, diabetes mellitus, disorientation, drug dependence, dyskinesia, dysphagia, dystonia, eclampsia, electrolyte disturbance, emphysema, esophageal achalasia, exfoliative dermatitis, extrapyramidal reaction, fecal impaction, fungal skin infection, gastroenteritis, glaucoma, goiter, Guillain-Barre syndrome, hallucination, hematemesis, hematologic abnormality, hematologic disease, hematoma, hemoptysis, hemorrhage, hemorrhagic pancreatitis, hepatic failure, hepatic necrosis, hepatitis, hepatotoxicity, homicidal ideation, hypercholesteremia, hypergammaglobulinemia, hyperglycemia, hyperhidrosis, hypersensitivity reaction, hyperthyroidism, hypoglycemia, hyponatremia, hypotension, hypothyroidism, immune thrombocytopenia, increased blood urea nitrogen, increased creatine phosphokinase, increased lactate dehydrogenase, increased serum alkaline phosphatase, intestinal obstruction, ischemic heart disease, jaundice, ketosis, low cardiac output, lymphadenopathy, meningitis, migraine, mydriasis, myelitis, myocardial infarction, neuroleptic malignant syndrome, neuropathy, osteoarthritis, osteoporosis, pancreatitis, pancytopenia, paralytic ileus, peptic ulcer, peritonitis, phlebitis, pneumonia, prolonged bleeding time, pulmonary edema, pulmonary embolism, pulmonary fibrosis, pulmonary hypertension, restlessness, seizure, sepsis, serotonin syndrome, spermatozoa disorder (activity altered, DNA fragmentation [abnormal] increased), status epilepticus, Stevens-Johnson syndrome, suicidal ideation, suicidal tendencies, syncope, tetany, thrombophlebitis, thrombosis, torsades de pointes, toxic epidermal necrolysis, uncontrolled diabetes mellitus, vasculitis, ventricular arrhythmia, ventricular fibrillation, ventricular tachycardia, withdrawal syndrome (including increased dreaming/nightmares, muscle cramps/spasms/twitching, headache, nervousness/anxiety, fatigue/tiredness, restless feeling in legs, and trouble sleeping/insomnia)

Drug Interactions

Metabolism/Transport Effects Substrate of CYP2D6 (major); **Note:** Assignment of Major/Minor substrate status based on clinically relevant drug interaction potential; **Inhibits** CYP1A2 (weak), CYP2B6 (moderate), CYP2C19 (weak), CYP2C9 (weak), CYP2D6 (strong), CYP3A4 (weak)

Avoid Concomitant Use

Avoid concomitant use of PARoxetine with any of the following: Dapoxetine; Dosulepin; Iobenguane I 123; Linezolid; MAO Inhibitors; Methylene Blue; Pimozide; Tamoxifen; Thioridazine; Tryptophan; Urokinase

Increased Effect/Toxicity

PARoxetine may increase the levels/effects of: Agents with Antiplatelet Properties; Anticoagulants; Antidepressants (Serotonin Reuptake Inhibitor/Antagonist); Antipsychotic Agents; Apixaban; ARIPiprazole; Asenapine; Aspirin; AtoMOXetine; Beta-Blockers; BusPIRone; CarBAMazepine; CloZAPine; Collagenase (Systemic); CYP2B6 Substrates; CYP2D6 Substrates; Dabigatran Etexilate; Desmopressin; Dextromethorphan; Dosulepin; DOXOrubicin (Conventional); DULoxetine; Eliglustat; Fesoterodine; Galantamine; Highest Risk QTc-Prolonging Agents; Hydrocodone; Hypoglycemic Agents; Ibritumomab; Iloperidone; Lomitapide; Methadone; Methylene Blue; Metoprolol; Mexiletine; Moderate Risk QTc-Prolonging Agents; Nebivolol; NSAID (COX-2 Inhibitor); NSAID (Nonselective); Obinutuzumab; Pimozide; Propafenone; Rivaroxaban; Salicylates; Serotonin Modulators; Tetrabenazine; Thiazide Diuretics; Thioridazine; Thrombolytic Agents; Tositumomab and Iodine I 131 Tositumomab; TraMADol; Tricyclic Antidepressants; Urokinase; Vitamin K Antagonists; Vortioxetine

The levels/effects of PARoxetine may be increased by: Abiraterone Acetate; Alcohol (Ethyl); Analgesics (Opioid); Antiemetics (5HT3 Antagonists); Antipsychotic Agents; ARIPiprazole; Asenapine; BuPROPion; BusPIRone; Cimetidine; CNS Depressants; Cobicistat; CYP2D6 Inhibitors (Moderate); CYP2D6 Inhibitors (Strong); Dapoxetine; Dasatinib; DULoxetine; Glucosamine; Herbs (Anticoagulant/Antiplatelet Properties); Ibrutinib; Limaprost; Linezolid; Lithium; MAO Inhibitors; Metoclopramide; Metyrosine; Mifepristone; Multivitamins/Fluoride (with ADE); Multivitamins/Minerals (with ADEK, Folate, Iron); Multivitamins/Minerals (with AE, No Iron); Omega-3 Fatty Acids; Peginterferon Alfa-2b; Pentosan Polysulfate Sodium; Pentoxifylline; Pravastatin; Prostacyclin Analogues; Tedizolid; TraMADol; Tryptophan; Vitamin E

Decreased Effect

PARoxetine may decrease the levels/effects of: Aprepitant; Codeine; Fosaprepitant; Iloperidone; Iobenguane I 123; Ioflupane I 123; Tamoxifen; Thyroid Products

The levels/effects of PARoxetine may be decreased by: Aprepitant; CarBAMazepine; Cyproheptadine; Darunavir; Fosamprenavir; Fosaprepitant; NSAID (COX-2 Inhibitor); NSAID (Nonselective); Peginterferon Alfa-2b

Food Interactions Peak concentration is increased, but bioavailability is not significantly altered by food. Management: Administer without regard to meals.

Storage/Stability

Capsules: Store between 20°C and 25°C (68°F and 77°F); excursions permitted between 15°C and 30°C (59°F and 86°F). Protect from light and humidity.

Tablets: Store immediate-release tablets between 15°C and 30°C (59°F and 86°F) and controlled-release tablets at or below 25°C (77°F).

Suspension: Store at or below 25°C (77°F).

Mechanism of Action Paroxetine is a selective serotonin reuptake inhibitor, chemically unrelated to tricyclic, tetracyclic, or other antidepressants; presumably, the inhibition of serotonin reuptake from brain synapse stimulated serotonin activity in the brain

Pharmacodynamics/Kinetics

Onset of action: Depression: The onset of action is within a week; however, individual response varies greatly and full response may not be seen until 8-12 weeks after initiation of treatment.

Absorption: Completely absorbed following oral administration

Distribution: V_d: 8.7 L/kg (3-28 L/kg)

Protein binding: 93% to 95%

Metabolism: Extensively hepatic via CYP2D6 enzymes; primary metabolites are formed via oxidation and methylation of parent drug, with subsequent glucuronide/sulfate conjugation; nonlinear pharmacokinetics (via 2D6 saturation) may be seen with higher doses and longer duration of therapy. Metabolites exhibit ~2% potency of parent compound. C_{min} concentrations are 70% to 80% greater in the elderly compared to nonelderly patients; clearance is also decreased.

Half-life elimination: 21 hours (3-65 hours)

Time to peak:

Capsules: 3-8 hours

Tablets, oral suspension: Immediate release: 5.2-8.1 hours

Tablets: Controlled release: 6-10 hours

Excretion: Urine (64%, 2% as unchanged drug); feces (36% primarily via bile, <1% as unchanged drug)

Dosage Oral:

Children and Adolescents:

Obsessive-compulsive disorder (OCD; off-label use): 7-17 years: Initial: 10 mg daily; titrate every 7-14 days in increments of 10 mg daily as necessary to a maximum of 60 mg daily; trials have typically continued for a 10- to 12-week treatment course (Geller, 2004; Rosenberg, 1999)

Social anxiety disorder (off-label use): 8-17 years: Initial: 10 mg once daily; titrate at intervals of at least 7 days in increments of 10 mg daily; maximum daily dose: 50 mg daily; trials have typically continued for a 16-week treatment course (Wagner, 2004)

Adults:

Major depressive disorder (MDD):

Paxil, Pexeva: Initial: 20 mg once daily, preferably in the morning; increase if needed by 10 mg/day increments at intervals of at least 1 week; maximum dose: 50 mg/day

Paxil CR: Initial: 25 mg once daily; increase if needed by 12.5 mg/day increments at intervals of at least 1 week; maximum dose: 62.5 mg/day

Generalized anxiety disorder (GAD) (Paxil, Pexeva): Initial: 20 mg once daily, preferably in the morning (if dose is increased, adjust in increments of 10 mg/day at 1-week intervals); doses of 20-50 mg/day were used in clinical trials, however, no greater benefit was seen with doses >20 mg.

Obsessive-compulsive disorder (OCD) (Paxil, Pexeva): Initial: 20 mg once daily, preferably in the morning; increase if needed by 10 mg/day increments at intervals of at least 1 week; recommended dose: 40 mg/day; range: 20-60 mg/day; maximum dose: 60 mg/day

Panic disorder:

Paxil, Pexeva: Initial: 10 mg once daily, preferably in the morning; increase if needed by 10 mg/day increments at intervals of at least 1 week; recommended dose: 40 mg/day; range: 10-60 mg/day; maximum dose: 60 mg/day

Paxil CR: Initial: 12.5 mg once daily; increase if needed by 12.5 mg/day at intervals of at least 1 week; maximum dose: 75 mg/day

Premenstrual dysphoric disorder (PMDD) (Paxil CR): Initial: 12.5 mg once daily in the morning; may be increased to 25 mg/day; dosing changes should occur at intervals of at least 1 week. May be given daily throughout the menstrual cycle or limited to the luteal phase.

Post-traumatic stress disorder (PTSD) (Paxil): Initial: 20 mg once daily, preferably in the morning; increase if needed by 10 mg/day increments at intervals of at least 1 week; range: 20-50 mg. Limited data suggest doses of 40 mg/day were not more efficacious than 20 mg/day.

Social anxiety disorder:

Paxil: Initial: 20 mg once daily, preferably in the morning; recommended dose: 20 mg/day; range: 20-60 mg/day; doses >20 mg may not have additional benefit

Paxil CR: Initial: 12.5 mg once daily, preferably in the morning; may be increased by 12.5 mg/day at intervals of at least 1 week; maximum dose: 37.5 mg/day

Vasomotor symptoms of menopause:

Brisdelle: 7.5 mg once daily at bedtime

Paxil CR (off-label use): 12.5-25 mg once daily (Stearns, 2003)

Elderly:

Paxil, Pexeva: Initial: 10 mg/day; increase if needed by 10 mg/day increments at intervals of at least 1 week; maximum dose: 40 mg/day

Paxil CR: Initial: 12.5 mg/day; increase if needed by 12.5 mg/day increments at intervals of at least 1 week; maximum dose: 50 mg/day

Discontinuation of therapy: Upon discontinuation of antidepressant therapy, gradually taper the dose to minimize the incidence of withdrawal symptoms and allow for the detection of re-emerging symptoms. Evidence supporting ideal taper rates is limited. APA and NICE guidelines suggest tapering therapy over at least several weeks with consideration to the half-life of the antidepressant; antidepressants with a shorter half-life may need to be tapered more conservatively. In addition for long-term treated patients, WFSBP guidelines recommend tapering over 4-6 months. If intolerable withdrawal symptoms occur following a dose reduction, consider resuming the previously prescribed dose and/or decrease dose at a more gradual rate (APA, 2010; Bauer, 2002; Haddod, 2001; NCCMH, 2010; Schatzberg, 2006; Shelton, 2001; Warner, 2006).

MAO inhibitor recommendations:

Switching to or from an MAO inhibitor intended to treat psychiatric disorders:

Allow 14 days to elapse between discontinuing an MAO inhibitor intended to treat psychiatric disorders and initiation of paroxetine.

Allow 14 days to elapse between discontinuing paroxetine and initiation of an MAO inhibitor intended to treat psychiatric disorders.

Use with other MAO inhibitors (linezolid or IV methylene blue):

Do not initiate paroxetine in patients receiving linezolid or IV methylene blue; consider other interventions for psychiatric condition.

If urgent treatment with linezolid or IV methylene blue is required in a patient already receiving paroxetine and potential benefits outweigh potential risks, discontinue paroxetine promptly and administer linezolid or IV methylene blue. Monitor for serotonin syndrome for 2 weeks or until 24 hours after the last dose of linezolid or IV methylene blue, whichever comes first. May resume paroxetine 24 hours after the last dose of linezolid or IV methylene blue.

Dosage adjustment in renal impairment: Adults:

Brisdelle: No dosage adjustment necessary.

Paxil, Paxil CR, Pexeva:

CrCl 30-60 mL/minute: Plasma concentration is 2 times that seen in normal function. There are no dosage adjustments provided in manufacturer's labeling.

Severe impairment (CrCl <30 mL/minute): Mean plasma concentration is ~4 times that seen in normal function.

Paxil, Pexeva: Initial: 10 mg/day; increase if needed by 10 mg/day increments at intervals of at least 1 week; maximum dose: 40 mg/day

Paxil CR: Initial: 12.5 mg/day; increase if needed by 12.5 mg/day increments at intervals of at least 1 week; maximum dose: 50 mg/day

Dosage adjustment in hepatic impairment: Adults: In hepatic dysfunction, plasma concentration is 2 times that seen in normal function.

Brisdelle: No dosage adjustment necessary.

Paxil, Paxil CR, Pexeva:

Mild-to-moderate impairment: There are no dosage adjustments provided in manufacturer's labeling.

Severe impairment:

Paxil, Pexeva: Initial: 10 mg/day; increase if needed by 10 mg/day increments at intervals of at least 1 week; maximum dose: 40 mg/day

Paxil CR: Initial: 12.5 mg/day; increase if needed by 12.5 mg/day increments at intervals of at least 1 week; maximum dose: 50 mg/day

Dietary Considerations May be taken without regard to meals.

Administration May be administered without regard to meals. Paxil, Paxil CR, and Pexeva should preferentially be administered in the morning; whereas Brisdelle is recommended to be administered at bedtime. Do not crush, break, or chew controlled-release tablets or Pexeva tablets (film-coated).

Hazardous agent; use appropriate precautions for handling and disposal (NIOSH 2014 [group 3]).

Monitoring Parameters Mental status for depression, suicide ideation (especially at the beginning of therapy or when doses are increased or decreased), anxiety, social functioning, mania, panic attacks; signs/symptoms of serotonin syndrome; akathisia

Additional Information Paxil CR incorporates a degradable polymeric matrix (Geomatrix) to control dissolution rate over a period of 4-5 hours. An enteric coating delays the start of drug release until tablets have left the stomach.

Dosage Forms

Capsule, Oral:

Brisdelle: 7.5 mg

Suspension, Oral:

Paxil: 10 mg/5 mL (250 mL)

Tablet, Oral:

Paxil: 10 mg, 20 mg, 30 mg, 40 mg

Pexeva: 10 mg, 20 mg, 30 mg, 40 mg

Generic: 10 mg, 20 mg, 30 mg, 40 mg

Tablet Extended Release 24 Hour, Oral:

Paxil CR: 12.5 mg, 25 mg, 37.5 mg

Generic: 12.5 mg, 25 mg, 37.5 mg

Dosage Forms: Canada Note: Refer to Dosage Forms. Capsule, oral suspension, and tablet (as mesylate) are not available in Canada.

◆ **Paroxetine Hydrochloride** *see* PARoxetine *on page 1579*

◆ **Paroxetine Mesylate** *see* PARoxetine *on page 1579*

◆ **Parvolex® (Can)** *see* Acetylcysteine *on page 40*

Pasireotide (pas i REE oh tide)

Brand Names: U.S. Signifor

Brand Names: Canada Signifor

Index Terms Pasireotide Diaspartate; Signifor LAR; SOM230

Pharmacologic Category Somatostatin Analog

Use

Acromegaly (Signifor LAR): Treatment of patients with acromegaly who have had an inadequate response to surgery and/or for whom surgery is not an option.

Cushing disease (Signifor): Treatment of Cushing disease in patients for whom pituitary surgery is not an option or has not been curative

Pregnancy Risk Factor C

Dosage

Acromegaly (Signifor LAR): Adults: IM: Initial: 40 mg once every 28 days; for patients who have not normalized GH and/or IGF-1 levels after 3 months, increase to a maximum of 60 mg. If adverse reactions occur or IFG-1 level decreases to less than lower limit of normal, decrease dosage (temporarily or permanently) by 20 mg decrements.

Missed dose: If a dose is missed, dose may be given up to but no later than 14 days prior to the next dose.

Cushing disease (Signifor): Adults: SubQ:

Initial:

U.S. labeling: 0.6 mg or 0.9 mg twice daily.

Canadian labeling: 0.6 mg twice daily.

Titrate based on response and tolerability. If adverse reactions occur, temporarily decrease dose by 0.3 mg increments. Recommended dosage range: 0.3-0.9 mg twice daily. **Note:** Maximum urinary free cortisol reductions are usually observed by 2 months of treatment. The Canadian labeling recommends to consider discontinuation if clinical improvement is not observed after 2 months of therapy.

Dosage adjustment in renal impairment: No dosage adjustment necessary.

Dosage adjustment in hepatic impairment:

Acromegaly (Signifor LAR):

Mild impairment (Child-Pugh class A): No dosage adjustment necessary.

Moderate hepatic impairment (Child-Pugh class B): Initial: 20 mg every 28 days (maximum: 40 mg every 28 days).

Severe hepatic impairment (Child-Pugh class C): Avoid use.

Cushing disease (Signifor):

Prior to initiation:

U.S. labeling:

Mild impairment (Child-Pugh class A): No dosage adjustment necessary.

Moderate impairment (Child-Pugh class B): Initial: 0.3 mg twice daily (maximum: 0.6 mg twice daily)

Severe impairment (Child-Pugh class C): Use not recommended.

Canadian labeling:

Mild impairment (Child-Pugh class A): No dosage adjustment necessary.

Moderate or severe impairment (Child-Pugh class B or C): Use is contraindicated.

During therapy:

U.S. labeling:

If ALT increases >3 times ULN or baseline value: Recheck ALT during recommended timeframe per recommendations in manufacturer's labeling for confirmation. If ALT level confirmed or increasing, interrupt therapy and investigate potential cause.

If any liver test ≥5 times ULN (with a normal baseline) **OR** >5 times the baseline value (with an abnormal baseline): Interrupt therapy and monitor liver tests more frequently per recommendations in manufacturer's labeling. If values return to normal or near normal, therapy may be reinitiated with extreme caution/monitoring only if another likely cause for hepatic effects discovered.

Canadian labeling:

If ALT increases >3 times ULN to <5 times ULN: Recheck ALT in 48 hours and if value remains <5 times ULN, continue monitoring ALT every 48 hours. If levels increase >5 times ULN, discontinue therapy and do not reinitiate.

If ALT increases >5 times ULN or if ALT or AST increase >3 times ULN concurrently with an increased bilirubin >2 times ULN or if jaundice or other signs of clinically significant hepatic impairment: Discontinue therapy and investigate potential cause. Do not reinitiate therapy.

Additional Information Complete prescribing information should be consulted for additional detail.

Product Availability

Signifor LAR: FDA approved December 2014; anticipated availability is currently unknown.

Signifor LAR is indicated for the treatment of patients with acromegaly who have had an inadequate response to surgery and/or for whom surgery is not an option.

Dosage Forms

Solution, Subcutaneous:

Signifor: 0.3 mg/mL (1 mL); 0.6 mg/mL (1 mL); 0.9 mg/mL (1 mL)

- ◆ **Pasireotide Diaspartate** *see* Pasireotide *on page 1583*
- ◆ **Pataday** *see* Olopatadine (Ophthalmic) *on page 1500*
- ◆ **Patanase** *see* Olopatadine (Nasal) *on page 1500*
- ◆ **Patanol** *see* Olopatadine (Ophthalmic) *on page 1500*
- ◆ **PAT-Galantamine ER (Can)** *see* Galantamine *on page 946*
- ◆ **Pat-Rabeprazole (Can)** *see* RABEprazole *on page 1762*
- ◆ **Pat-Tramadol/Acet (Can)** *see* Acetaminophen and Tramadol *on page 37*
- ◆ **Pavabid** *see* Papaverine *on page 1573*
- ◆ **Pavulon [DSC]** *see* Pancuronium *on page 1567*
- ◆ **Paxil** *see* PARoxetine *on page 1579*
- ◆ **Paxil CR** *see* PARoxetine *on page 1579*

PAZOPanib (paz OH pa nib)

Brand Names: U.S. Votrient

Brand Names: Canada Votrient

Index Terms GW786034; Pazopanib Hydrochloride

Pharmacologic Category Antineoplastic Agent, Tyrosine Kinase Inhibitor; Antineoplastic Agent, Vascular Endothelial Growth Factor (VEGF) Inhibitor

Use

Renal cell carcinoma: Treatment of advanced renal cell carcinoma

Soft tissue sarcoma: Treatment of advanced soft tissue sarcoma (in patients who have received prior chemotherapy)

Limitations of use: The efficacy of pazopanib for the treatment of adipocytic soft tissue sarcoma or gastrointestinal stromal tumors has not been demonstrated.

Pregnancy Risk Factor D

Pregnancy Considerations Adverse effects were observed in animal reproduction studies. Based on its mechanism of action, pazopanib would be expected to cause fetal harm if administered to a pregnant woman. Women of childbearing potential should avoid becoming pregnant during treatment.

Breast-Feeding Considerations It is not known if pazopanib is excreted in breast milk. According to the manufacturer, the decision to continue or discontinue breast-feeding during therapy should take into account the risk of exposure to the infant and the benefits of treatment to the mother.

Contraindications

There are no contraindications listed in the manufacturer's U.S. labeling.

Canadian labeling: Hypersensitivity to pazopanib or any component of the formulation; use in pediatric patients <2 years of age (due to the antiangiogenic effects)

Warnings/Precautions Hazardous agent - use appropriate precautions for handling and disposal (NIOSH 2014 [group 1]). **[U.S. Boxed Warning]: Severe and fatal hepatotoxicity (transaminase and bilirubin elevations) has been observed in studies. Monitor hepatic function and interrupt treatment, reduce dose, or discontinue as recommended.** Liver function testes should be monitored at baseline; at weeks 3, 5, 7, and 9; at months 3 and 4; and as clinically necessary, then periodically (after month 4). Transaminase elevations usually occur early in the treatment course. Use is not recommended in patients with preexisting severe hepatic impairment (bilirubin >3 times ULN with any ALT level); dosage reductions is recommended for preexisting moderate hepatic impairment (bilirubin >1.5-3 times ULN). Mild indirect (unconjugated) hyperbilirubinemia may occur in patients with Gilbert's syndrome; for patients with known Gilbert syndrome (only a mild indirect bilirubin elevation) and ALT >3 times ULN, follow isolated ALT elevation dosage modification recommendations.

Venous and arterial thromboembolism have been reported. DVT, pulmonary embolism, angina, transient ischemic attack, MI, and ischemic stroke were observed more frequently in the pazopanib group (versus placebo) in clinical trials. Fatalities were observed. Monitor for signs/symptoms of venous thrombotic events and pulmonary embolism. Use with caution in patients with a history of or an increased risk for these events. Use in patients with recent arteriothrombotic event (within 6 months) has not been studied and is not recommended. Thrombotic microangiopathy (TMA), including thrombotic thrombocytopenic purpura (TTP) and hemolytic uremic syndrome (HUS), has been observed in clinical studies. TMA has occurred with pazopanib monotherapy or when used in combination with bevacizumab or topotecan (off-label use); it typically occurs within 90 days of treatment initiation. Monitor for signs/symptoms and permanently discontinue in patients who develop TMA. Hemorrhagic events (including fatal events) have been reported. In clinical studies, the most common events in renal cell carcinoma patients were hematuria, epistaxis, hemoptysis, and rectal hemorrhage. Epistaxis, mouth hemorrhage, and anal hemorrhage were most common in soft tissue sarcoma patients. Use is not recommended in patients with a history of hemoptysis, cerebral hemorrhage or clinically significant gastrointestinal hemorrhage within 6 months (these populations were excluded from clinical trials).

May cause and/or worsen hypertension (hypertensive crisis has been observed); monitor frequently; blood pressure should be controlled prior to treatment initiation; antihypertensive therapy should be used if needed. Hypertension usually occurs early in the treatment course. Dosage reduction may be necessary for persistent hypertension (despite antihypertensive therapy); discontinue for hypertensive crisis, or for severe and persistent hypertension which is refractory to dose reduction and antihypertensive therapy. May cause new-onset or worsening of existing heart failure; baseline and periodic LVEF monitoring is recommended in patients at increased risk of heart failure (eg, prior anthracycline treatment). Concurrent hypertension may increase the risk for cardiac dysfunction. QTc prolongation, including torsade de pointes, has been observed; use caution in patients with a history of QTc prolongation, with medications known to prolong the QT interval, or with preexisting cardiac disease. Obtain baseline and periodic ECGs; correct electrolyte (potassium, calcium, and magnesium) abnormalities prior to and during treatment.

Gastrointestinal perforation and fistula (including fatal events) have been reported; monitor for symptoms of gastrointestinal perforation and fistula. Proteinuria has been reported with use. Obtain baseline and periodic urinalysis and 24-hour urine protein when clinically indicated. Dosage reduction may be necessary for significant proteinuria (≥3 g/24 hours); discontinue for recurrent proteinuria. Hypothyroidism has been reported with use; monitor thyroid function tests. Vascular endothelial growth factor (VEGF) receptor inhibitors are associated with impaired wound healing. Discontinue treatment at least 7 days prior to scheduled surgery; treatment reinitiation should be guided by clinical judgment. Discontinue if wound dehiscence occurs.

Patients with mild-to-moderate renal impairment (CrCl ≥30 mL/minute) were included in trials. There are no pharmacokinetic data in patients with severe renal impairment undergoing dialysis (peritoneal and hemodialysis); however, renal impairment is not expected to significantly influence pazopanib pharmacokinetics or exposure. Potentially significant drug-drug interactions may exist, requiring dose or frequency adjustment, additional monitoring, and/or selection of alternative therapy. Avoid use with strong CYP3A4 inhibitors or inducers. If pazopanib must be administered concomitantly with a potent enzyme inhibitor, dose reductions are recommended. Use is not recommended in situations where the chronic use of a strong CYP3A4 inducer is required. Pazopanib inhibits UGT1A1 and OATP1B1; pazopanib may increase concentration of drugs eliminated by UGT1A1 and OATP1B1. Pazopanib is a P-glycoprotein (P-gp) and breast cancer resistance protein (BCRP) substrate. Avoid concomitant administration with strong P-gp or BCRP inhibitors; may increase exposure to pazopanib. Increased toxicity and mortality has been observed in trials evaluating concurrent use of pazopanib with other chemotherapeutic agents (pemetrexed, lapatinib). Pazopanib is not approved for use in combination with other chemotherapy. Avoid concomitant use of drugs that raise gastric pH (may decrease exposure); if needed, short-acting antacids should be used and dosing should be separated by several hours.

Reversible posterior leukoencephalopathy syndrome (RPLS) has been reported (rarely); may be fatal. Monitor for neurological changes or symptoms (blindness, confusion, headache, lethargy, seizure, visual or neurologic disturbances); permanently discontinue pazopanib in patients who develop RPLS. Serious, including fatal, infections have been reported; monitor for signs and symptoms of infection. Temporarily or permanently discontinue therapy for serious infections as clinically indicated. Patients >60 years of age may be at greater risk for transaminase elevations (ALT >3 time ULN). Patients ≥65 years of age experienced increased incidences of grade 3 or 4 fatigue, hypertension, decreased appetite, and transaminase elevations. Pazopanib is not approved for use in pediatric patients. Based on its mechanism of action, organ growth and maturation during early postnatal development may be affected. May potentially cause serious adverse effects on organ development, particularly in children <2 years of age.

Adverse Reactions

Cardiovascular: Bradycardia, chest pain, facial edema, hypertension, ischemic heart disease or myocardial infarction, left ventricular systolic dysfunction, peripheral edema, prolonged QT interval on ECG, transient ischemic attacks, venous thrombosis

Central nervous system: Chills, dizziness, fatigue, headache, insomnia, voice disorder

Dermatologic: Alopecia, hair discoloration, nail disease, palmar-plantar erythrodysesthesia, skin depigmentation, skin rash, xeroderma

Endocrine & metabolic: Hyperglycemia, hyperkalemia, hypoglycemia, hypomagnesemia, hyponatremia, hypophosphatemia, hypothyroidism, increased thyroid-stimulating hormone (TSH)

Gastrointestinal: Abdominal pain, anorexia, diarrhea, dysgeusia, dyspepsia, increased serum lipase, mucositis, nausea, oral hemorrhage, rectal hemorrhage, stomatitis, vomiting, weight loss

Hematologic & Oncologic: Leukopenia, lymphocytopenia, neutropenia, thrombocytopenia,

Hepatic: Decreased serum albumin, increased serum alkaline phosphatase, increased serum ALT, increased serum AST, increased serum bilirubin

Miscellaneous: Tumor pain

Neuromuscular & skeletal: Musculoskeletal pain, myalgia, weakness

Ophthalmic: Blurred vision

Renal: Hematuria, proteinuria

Respiratory: Cough, dyspnea, epistaxis, hemoptysis, pneumothorax, pulmonary embolism (fatal)

Rare but important or life-threatening: Cardiac disease, cerebral hemorrhage, cerebrovascular accident, congestive heart failure, gastrointestinal fistula, gastrointestinal perforation (including fistulas), hemolytic uremic syndrome, hepatotoxicity, hypertensive crisis, intracranial hemorrhage, nephrotic syndrome, pancreatitis, reversible posterior leukoencephalopathy syndrome (RPLS), thrombotic thrombocytopenic purpura, torsade de pointes

Drug Interactions

Metabolism/Transport Effects **Substrate** of BCRP, CYP1A2 (minor), CYP2C8 (minor), CYP3A4 (major), P-glycoprotein; **Note:** Assignment of Major/Minor substrate status based on clinically relevant drug interaction potential; **Inhibits** CYP2C8 (weak), CYP2D6 (weak), CYP3A4 (weak), SLCO1B1, UGT1A1

Avoid Concomitant Use

Avoid concomitant use of PAZOPanib with any of the following: BCG; BCRP/ABCG2 Inhibitors; Conivaptan; CYP3A4 Inducers (Strong); Fusidic Acid (Systemic); Grapefruit Juice; H2-Antagonists; Highest Risk QTc-Prolonging Agents; Idelalisib; Ivabradine; Lapatinib; Mifepristone; Natalizumab; P-glycoprotein/ABCB1 Inhibitors; Pimecrolimus; Pimozide; Proton Pump Inhibitors; Tacrolimus (Topical); Tofacitinib; Vaccines (Live)

Increased Effect/Toxicity

PAZOPanib may increase the levels/effects of: ARIPiprazole; Bisphosphonate Derivatives; Highest Risk QTc-Prolonging Agents; Hydrocodone; Leflunomide; Moderate Risk QTc-Prolonging Agents; Natalizumab; Pimozide; Tofacitinib; Vaccines (Live)

The levels/effects of PAZOPanib may be increased by: Aprepitant; BCRP/ABCG2 Inhibitors; Conivaptan; CYP3A4 Inhibitors (Moderate); CYP3A4 Inhibitors (Strong); Dasatinib; Denosumab; Fosaprepitant; Fusidic Acid (Systemic); Grapefruit Juice; HMG-CoA Reductase Inhibitors; Idelalisib; Ivabradine; Lapatinib; Luliconazole; Mifepristone; Netupitant; P-glycoprotein/ABCB1 Inhibitors; Pimecrolimus; QTc-Prolonging Agents (Indeterminate Risk and Risk Modifying); Roflumilast; Stiripentol; Tacrolimus (Topical); Trastuzumab

Decreased Effect

PAZOPanib may decrease the levels/effects of: BCG; Coccidioides immitis Skin Test; Sipuleucel-T; Vaccines (Inactivated); Vaccines (Live)

The levels/effects of PAZOPanib may be decreased by: Antacids; Bosentan; CYP3A4 Inducers (Moderate); CYP3A4 Inducers (Strong); Deferasirox; Echinacea; H2-Antagonists; P-glycoprotein/ABCB1 Inducers; Proton Pump Inhibitors; Siltuximab; St Johns Wort; Tocilizumab

Food Interactions Systemic exposure of pazopanib is increased when administered with food (AUC twofold higher with a meal). Grapefruit juice may increase the levels/effects of pazopanib. Management: Take on an empty stomach 1 hour before or 2 hours after a meal. Maintain adequate nutrition and hydration, unless instructed to restrict fluid intake. Avoid grapefruit/grapefruit juice.

Storage/Stability Store at 20°C to 25°C (68°F to 77°F); excursions are permitted between 15°C and 30°C (59°F and 86°F).

Mechanism of Action Tyrosine kinase (multikinase) inhibitor; limits tumor growth via inhibition of angiogenesis by inhibiting cell surface vascular endothelial growth factor receptors (VEGFR-1, VEGFR-2, VEGFR-3), platelet-derived growth factor receptors (PDGFR-alpha and -beta), fibroblast growth factor receptor (FGFR-1 and -3), cytokine receptor (cKIT), interleukin-2 receptor inducible T-cell kinase, leukocyte-specific protein tyrosine kinase (Lck), and transmembrane glycoprotein receptor tyrosine kinase (c-Fms)

Pharmacodynamics/Kinetics

Protein binding: >99%

Metabolism: Hepatic; primarily via CYP3A4, minor metabolism via CYP1A2 and CYP2C8

Bioavailability: Rate and extent of bioavailability are increased with food and increased if tablets are crushed (do not crush tablets)

Half-life elimination: ~31 hours

Time to peak, plasma: 2-4 hours

Excretion: Feces (primarily); urine (<4%)

Dosage

Renal cell carcinoma (RCC), advanced: Adults: Oral: 800 mg once daily (Sternberg, 2010)

Soft tissue sarcoma (STS), advanced refractory: Adults: Oral: 800 mg once daily (Van Der Graaf, 2012)

Thyroid cancer, advanced differentiated (off-label use): Adults: Oral: 800 mg once daily until disease progression or unacceptable toxicity (Bible, 2010)

Missed doses: If a dose is missed, do not take if <12 hours until the next dose.

Dosage adjustment for toxicity:

Initial dosage reduction: **Note:** Prior to dose reduction, temporarily discontinue therapy if 24-hour urine protein ≥3 g or for other toxicities when clinically indicated.
RCC: Reduce to 400 mg once daily
STS: Reduce to 600 mg once daily

Further modification: RCC, STS: Adjust dose in 200 mg increments or decrements based on individual tolerance; maximum dose: 800 mg

Hypertension: Manage as appropriate with antihypertensive therapy and interrupt treatment or reduce dose as clinically warranted.

Hypertension (severe, persistent, and refractory to antihypertensives and dose reduction) or evidence of hypertensive crisis: Discontinue treatment.

Infection, serious: Consider treatment interruption or discontinuation.

Proteinuria, initial (24-hour urine protein ≥3 g): Interrupt treatment and reduce the dose.

Proteinuria (recurrent 24-hour urine protein ≥3 g refractory to dose reduction): Discontinue treatment.

Reversible posterior leukoencephalopathy syndrome (RPLS): Permanently discontinue.

Thrombotic microangiopathy (TMA): Permanently discontinue.

Wound dehiscence: Discontinue treatment.

Concomitant CYP3A4 inhibitors/inducers:

CYP3A4 inhibitors: Avoid concomitant strong CYP3A4 inhibitors (may increase pazopanib concentrations). If pazopanib must be administered concomitantly with a potent enzyme inhibitor, reduce pazopanib to 400 mg once daily with careful monitoring; further dosage reductions may be needed if adverse events occur.

CYP3A4 inducers: Avoid concomitant strong CYP3A4 inducers (may decrease pazopanib concentrations); use of pazopanib is not recommended in situations where the chronic use of a strong CYP3A4 inducer is required.

Dosage adjustment in renal impairment: No dosage adjustment necessary.

Dosage adjustment in hepatic impairment:

Preexisting impairment:

Mild (bilirubin ≤1.5 times ULN or ALT >ULN): No dosage adjustment required (Shibata, 2013).

Moderate (bilirubin >1.5-3 times ULN): Consider alternative therapy or reduce to 200 mg once daily (maximum tolerated dose in patients with moderate hepatic impairment) (Shibata, 2013).

Severe (bilirubin >3 times ULN with any ALT level): Use is not recommended.

During treatment:

Isolated ALT elevations 3-8 times ULN: Continue treatment, monitor liver function weekly until ALT returns to grade 1 or baseline.

Isolated ALT elevations >8 times ULN: Interrupt treatment until ALT returns to grade 1 or baseline. If therapy benefit is greater than the risk of hepatotoxicity, may reinitiate treatment at ≤400 mg once daily (with liver function monitored weekly for 8 weeks); permanently discontinue if ALT >3 times ULN occurs with reinitiation.

ALT >3 times ULN concurrently with bilirubin >2 times ULN: Permanently discontinue; monitor until resolution.

Gilbert syndrome with mild indirect bilirubin elevation and ALT >3 times ULN: Refer to isolated ALT elevations dosage recommendations above.

Dietary Considerations Avoid grapefruit juice.

Administration Administer on an empty stomach, 1 hour before or 2 hours after a meal. Do not crush tablet (rate of absorption may be increased; may affect systemic exposure).

Hazardous agent; use appropriate precautions for handling and disposal (NIOSH 2014 [group 1]).

Monitoring Parameters Monitor liver function tests at baseline; at weeks 3, 5, 7, and 9; at months 3 and 4; and as clinically necessary, then periodically after month 4 (U.S. labeling) or at weeks 2, 4, 6, and 8 (Canadian labeling); months 3 and 4, and periodically thereafter (monitor more frequently if clinically indicated); serum electrolytes (eg, calcium, magnesium, potassium); urinalysis (for proteinuria; baseline and periodic), 24-hour urine protein (if clinically indicated); thyroid function (TSH and T_4 at baseline and TSH every 6-8 weeks during treatment [Appleby, 2011]); blood pressure; ECG (baseline and periodic); LVEF (if at risk for cardiac dysfunction; baseline and periodic); signs/symptoms of gastrointestinal perforation or fistula, venous thrombotic events, pulmonary embolism, infection, heart failure, or neurological changes.

Additional Information Hand-foot skin reaction (Appleby, 2011): Hand-foot skin reaction (HFSR) observed with tyrosine kinase inhibitors (TKIs) is distinct from hand-foot syndrome (palmar-plantar erythrodysesthesia) associated with traditional chemotherapy agents. HFSR due to TKIs is localized with defined hyperkeratotic lesions; symptoms include burning, dysesthesia, paresthesia, or tingling of the palms/soles, and generally occur within the first 2-4 weeks of treatment. Pressure and flexor areas may develop blisters (callus-like), dry/cracked skin, edema, erythema, desquamation, or hyperkeratosis. The incidence of hand-foot skin reaction (HFSR) is lower with pazopanib (compared to other tyrosine kinase inhibitors). Examine skin at baseline (remove calluses with pedicure prior to treatment) and with each visit; apply an emollient based moisturizer twice daily during treatment. If HSFR develops, consider changing moisturizer to a urea-based product; topical steroids may be utilized for the anti-inflammatory effect; avoid excessive friction or pressure to affected areas and avoid restrictive footwear. Temporary dose reduction or treatment interruption may be necessary.

Dosage Forms

Tablet, Oral:

Votrient: 200 mg

- **Pazopanib Hydrochloride** *see* PAZOPanib *on page 1584*
- **PCA (error-prone abbreviation)** *see* Procainamide *on page 1716*
- **PCB** *see* Procarbazine *on page 1717*
- **PCC (Caution: Confusion-prone synonym)** *see* Factor IX Complex (Human) [(Factors II, IX, X)] *on page 838*
- **PCC (Caution: Confusion-prone synonym)** *see* Prothrombin Complex Concentrate (Human) [(Factors II, VII, IX, X), Protein C, and Protein S] *on page 1738*
- **PCE** *see* Erythromycin (Systemic) *on page 762*
- **PCEC** *see* Rabies Vaccine *on page 1764*
- **PCI-32765** *see* Ibrutinib *on page 1030*
- **PCV13** *see* Pneumococcal Conjugate Vaccine (13-Valent) *on page 1670*
- **PCZ** *see* Procarbazine *on page 1717*
- **PDP-Desonide (Can)** *see* Desonide *on page 597*
- **PDP-Isoniazid (Can)** *see* Isoniazid *on page 1120*
- **PDX** *see* PRALAtrexate *on page 1693*
- **PediaCare Childrens Allergy [OTC]** *see* DiphenhydrAMINE (Systemic) *on page 641*
- **PediaCare® Children's Multi-Symptom Cold [OTC]** *see* Dextromethorphan and Phenylephrine *on page 611*
- **Pediacel® (Can)** *see* Diphtheria and Tetanus Toxoids, Acellular Pertussis, Poliovirus and *Haemophilus* b Conjugate Vaccine *on page 648*
- **Pediaderm AF Complete** *see* Nystatin (Topical) *on page 1482*
- **Pediaderm HC** *see* Hydrocortisone (Topical) *on page 1014*
- **Pediaderm TA** *see* Triamcinolone (Topical) *on page 2100*
- **Pedia-Lax [OTC]** *see* Docusate *on page 661*
- **Pedia-Lax [OTC]** *see* Magnesium Hydroxide *on page 1263*
- **Pediapharm Naproxen Suspension (Can)** *see* Naproxen *on page 1427*
- **Pediapred** *see* PrednisoLONE (Systemic) *on page 1703*
- **Pedia Relief Cough and Cold [OTC]** *see* Pseudoephedrine and Dextromethorphan *on page 1743*
- **Pedia Relief™ Cough-Cold [OTC]** *see* Chlorpheniramine, Pseudoephedrine, and Dextromethorphan *on page 428*

◆ **Pediarix®** *see* Diphtheria, Tetanus Toxoids, Acellular Pertussis, Hepatitis B (Recombinant), and Poliovirus (Inactivated) Vaccine *on page 651*

◆ **Pediatex TD [DSC]** *see* Triprolidine and Pseudoephedrine *on page 2105*

◆ **Pediatric Cough & Cold [OTC]** *see* Chlorpheniramine, Pseudoephedrine, and Dextromethorphan *on page 428*

◆ **Pediatric Digoxin CSD (Can)** *see* Digoxin *on page 627*

◆ **Pediatrix (Can)** *see* Acetaminophen *on page 32*

◆ **Pediazole® (Can)** *see* Erythromycin and Sulfisoxazole *on page 765*

◆ **Pedi-Dri [DSC]** *see* Nystatin (Topical) *on page 1482*

◆ **Pedipirox-4 Nail [DSC]** *see* Ciclopirox *on page 433*

◆ **PedvaxHIB** *see Haemophilus* b Conjugate Vaccine *on page 991*

Pefloxacin [INT] (pe FLOKS a sin)

International Brand Names Abaktal (BG, CZ, HN, PL, RU, SI, SK); Dexaflox (ID); Felox (ID); Floxin (VN); Kicindal (KR); Noflexin (ID); Oxaflox (ID); P-Cin (IN); Pebact (PK); Pef (IN); Pefaxin (TW); Pefcin (IN); Peflacin (EG, HU, IT, NZ); Peflacine (AE, FR, GR, ID, LB, PT, SA, TR, VN); Peloxin (TW); Pemax (SG); Peraxin (PH); Perti (VE); Pexacin (TW); Praloxin (KR); Quilaxin (MY); Vancor (AE); Zeflomed (PK)

Index Terms Pefloxacin Mesylate Dihydrate

Pharmacologic Category Antibiotic, Quinolone

Reported Use Treatment of bacterial infections caused by susceptible strains; use limited to serious infections

Dosage Range Adults:

Oral: 400 mg twice daily; taken with food

Ophthalmic: 1-2 drops in affected eye(s) 2-6 times/day, depending on severity of infection

IV: 400 mg twice daily given by slow infusion over 1 hour

Product Availability Product available in various countries; not currently available in the U.S.

Dosage Forms

Infusion [premixed]: 400 mg

Injection, solution: 80 mg/mL (5 mL)

Solution, ophthalmic: 0.3% (5 mL)

Tablet: 400 mg

◆ **Pefloxacin Mesylate Dihydrate** *see* Pefloxacin [INT] *on page 1588*

◆ **PEG** *see* Polyethylene Glycol 3350 *on page 1674*

◆ **PEG-L-asparaginase** *see* Pegaspargase *on page 1588*

◆ **Peg 3350 (Can)** *see* Polyethylene Glycol 3350 *on page 1674*

Pegademase Bovine (peg A de mase BOE vine)

Brand Names: U.S. Adagen

Brand Names: Canada Adagen

Pharmacologic Category Enzyme

Use Adenosine deaminase deficiency: For enzyme replacement therapy for adenosine deaminase (ADA) deficiency in infants to children of any age with severe combined immunodeficiency disease who are not suitable candidates for or who have failed bone marrow transplantation.

Pregnancy Risk Factor C

Dosage Adenosine deaminase deficiency (enzyme replacement therapy): Infants, Children, and Adolescents: IM: Initial dosage: 10 units/kg for the first dose, 15 units/kg for the second dose, and 20 units/kg for the third dose; administer dose every 7 days; maintenance dose: 20 units/kg/week; increase by 5 units/kg/week if necessary; maximum single dose: 30 units/kg

Note: Dose should be individualized based on monitoring of plasma ADA activity levels and dATP content.

Dosage adjustment in renal impairment: There are no dosage adjustments provided in the manufacturer's labeling.

Dosage adjustment in hepatic impairment: There are no dosage adjustments provided in the manufacturer's labeling.

Additional Information Complete prescribing information should be consulted for additional detail.

Dosage Forms

Solution, Intramuscular:

Adagen: 250 units/mL (1.5 mL)

◆ **Pegalax (Can)** *see* Polyethylene Glycol 3350 *on page 1674*

Pegaptanib (peg AP ta nib)

Brand Names: U.S. Macugen

Brand Names: Canada Macugen

Index Terms EYE001; Pegaptanib Sodium

Pharmacologic Category Ophthalmic Agent; Vascular Endothelial Growth Factor (VEGF) Inhibitor

Use Macular degeneration: Treatment of neovascular (wet) age-related macular degeneration (AMD)

Pregnancy Risk Factor B

Dosage Age-related macular degeneration (AMD): Adults: Intravitreous injection: 0.3 mg into affected eye once every 6 weeks

Dosage adjustment in renal impairment:

U.S. labeling: No dosage adjustment provided in manufacturer's labeling.

Canadian labeling:

CrCl ≥30 mL/minute: No dosage adjustment necessary.

CrCl <20 mL/minute: No dosage adjustment provided in manufacturer's labeling (has not been studied).

ESRD requiring hemodialysis: No dosage adjustment provided in manufacturer's labeling (has not been studied).

Dosage adjustment in hepatic impairment:

U.S. labeling: No dosage adjustment provided in manufacturer's labeling.

Canadian labeling: Use has not been studied in patients with hepatic impairment.

Additional Information Complete prescribing information should be consulted for additional detail.

Dosage Forms

Solution, Intraocular [preservative free]:

Macugen: 0.3 mg (0.09 mL)

◆ **Pegaptanib Sodium** *see* Pegaptanib *on page 1588*

◆ **PEG-ASP** *see* Pegaspargase *on page 1588*

◆ **PEG-asparaginase** *see* Pegaspargase *on page 1588*

Pegaspargase (peg AS par jase)

Brand Names: U.S. Oncaspar

Index Terms L-asparaginase with Polyethylene Glycol; PEG-ASP; PEG-asparaginase; PEG-L-asparaginase; PEGLA; Polyethylene Glycol-L-asparaginase

Pharmacologic Category Antineoplastic Agent, Enzyme; Antineoplastic Agent, Miscellaneous

Use

Acute lymphoblastic leukemia and hypersensitivity to asparaginase: Treatment of acute lymphoblastic leukemia (ALL) in patients with hypersensitivity to native forms of L-asparaginase (as a component of a multiagent chemotherapy regimen)

Acute lymphoblastic leukemia, first-line: First-line treatment of ALL (as a component of a multiagent chemotherapy regimen)

Pregnancy Risk Factor C

Dosage Acute lymphoblastic leukemia (ALL): Children, Adolescents, and Adults: IM, IV: 2500 units/m^2 (as part of a combination chemotherapy regimen), do not administer more frequently than every 14 days

Dosage adjustment in renal impairment: There are no dosage adjustments provided in the manufacturer's labeling.

Dosage adjustment in hepatic impairment: There are no dosage adjustments provided in the manufacturer's labeling.

Dosing in obesity: *ASCO Guidelines for appropriate chemotherapy dosing in obese adults with cancer:* Utilize patient's actual body weight (full weight) for calculation of body surface area- or weight-based dosing, particularly when the intent of therapy is curative; manage regimen-related toxicities in the same manner as for nonobese patients; if a dose reduction is utilized due to toxicity, consider resumption of full weight-based dosing with subsequent cycles, especially if cause of toxicity (eg, hepatic or renal impairment) is resolved (Griggs, 2012).

Additional Information Complete prescribing information should be consulted for additional detail.

Dosage Forms

Solution, Injection [preservative free]:
Oncaspar: 750 units/mL (5 mL)

- ◆ **Pegasys** *see* Peginterferon Alfa-2a *on page 1590*
- ◆ **Pegasys ProClick** *see* Peginterferon Alfa-2a *on page 1590*
- ◆ **Pegasys RBV (Can)** *see* Peginterferon Alfa-2a and Ribavirin [CAN/INT] *on page 1592*
- ◆ **Pegetron® (Can)** *see* Peginterferon Alfa-2b and Ribavirin [CAN/INT] *on page 1598*
- ◆ **Pegetron® RediPen® (Can)** *see* Peginterferon Alfa-2b and Ribavirin [CAN/INT] *on page 1598*

Pegfilgrastim (peg fil GRA stim)

Brand Names: U.S. Neulasta; Neulasta Delivery Kit

Brand Names: Canada Neulasta

Index Terms G-CSF (PEG Conjugate); Granulocyte Colony Stimulating Factor (PEG Conjugate); Pegylated G-CSF; SD/01

Pharmacologic Category Colony Stimulating Factor; Hematopoietic Agent

Use

Prevention of chemotherapy-induced neutropenia: To decrease the incidence of infection (as manifested by febrile neutropenia), in patients with nonmyeloid malignancies receiving myelosuppressive cancer chemotherapy associated with a clinically significant incidence of febrile neutropenia.

Limitation of use: Pegfilgrastim is not indicated for mobilization of peripheral blood progenitor cells for hematopoietic stem cell transplant.

Pregnancy Risk Factor C

Pregnancy Considerations Adverse events were observed in some animal reproduction studies.

Women who are exposed to Neulasta during pregnancy are encouraged to enroll in the Amgen Pregnancy Surveillance Program (800-772-6436).

Breast-Feeding Considerations It is not known if pegfilgrastim is excreted in breast milk. The manufacturer recommends that caution be exercised when administering pegfilgrastim to nursing women.

Contraindications Hypersensitivity (serious allergic reaction) to pegfilgrastim, filgrastim, or any component of the formulation

Warnings/Precautions Do not use pegfilgrastim in the period 14 days before to 24 hours after administration of cytotoxic chemotherapy because of the potential sensitivity of rapidly dividing myeloid cells to cytotoxic chemotherapy. Safety and efficacy have not been established with dose-dense chemotherapy regimens (Smith, 2006). Not indicated for peripheral blood progenitor cell (PBPC) mobilization for hematopoietic stem cell transplantation.

Serious allergic reactions (including anaphylaxis) may occur, usually with the initial dose; may recur within days after discontinuation of initial antiallergic treatment. Permanently discontinue for severe reactions. Do not administer in patients with a history of serious allergic reaction to pegfilgrastim or filgrastim. Acute respiratory distress syndrome (ARDS) has been reported with use; evaluate patients with pulmonary symptoms such as fever, pulmonary infiltrates, or respiratory distress for ARDS. Discontinue pegfilgrastim if ARDS occurs. Rare cases of splenic rupture have been reported; patients must be instructed to report left upper abdominal pain or shoulder pain. May precipitate sickle cell crises in patients with sickle cell disorders (severe and sometimes fatal sickle cell crises have occurred with filgrastim). The granulocyte-colony stimulating factor (G-CSF) receptor through which pegfilgrastim (and filgrastim) work has been located on tumor cell lines. May potentially act as a growth factor for any tumor type, including myeloid malignancies and myelodysplasia (pegfilgrastim is not approved for myeloid malignancies).

The On-body injector contains an acrylic adhesive; may result in a significant reaction in patients who react to acrylic adhesives. A health care provider must fill the On-body injector prior to applying to the patient's skin. The On-body delivery system may be applied on the same day as chemotherapy administration as long as pegfilgrastim is delivered no less than 24 hours after chemotherapy is administered. The prefilled syringe provided in the On-body kit contains overfill to compensate for loss during delivery; do not use for manual subcutaneous injection (will result in higher than recommended dose). Do not use prefilled syringe intended for manual injection to fill the On-body injector; may result in lower than intended dose. The On-body injector is only for use with pegfilgrastim; do not use to deliver other medications. Do not expose the On-body injector to oxygen-rich environments (eg, hyperbaric chambers), MRI, x-ray (including airport x-ray), CT scan, or ultrasound (may damage injector system). Keep the On-body injector at least 4 inches away from electrical equipment, including cell phones, cordless phones, microwaves, and other common appliances (injector may not work properly).

The 6 mg fixed dose should not be used in infants, children, and adolescents weighing <45 kg (Smith, 2006). The packaging (needle cover) contains latex.

Adverse Reactions

Cardiovascular: Peripheral edema

Central nervous system: Headache

Gastrointestinal: Constipation, vomiting

Neuromuscular & skeletal: Arthralgia, bone pain, myalgia, weakness

Miscellaneous: Antibody formation

Rare but important or life-threatening: Acute respiratory distress syndrome (ARDS), allergic reaction, anaphylaxis, cutaneous vasculitis, erythema, fever, flushing, hyperleukocytosis, hypoxia, injection site reactions (erythema, induration, pain), leukocytosis, rash, sickle cell crisis, splenic rupture, Sweet's syndrome (acute febrile dermatosis), urticaria. Cytopenias resulting from an antibody response to exogenous growth factors have been reported on rare occasions in patients treated with other recombinant growth factors.

Drug Interactions

Metabolism/Transport Effects None known.

Avoid Concomitant Use There are no known interactions where it is recommended to avoid concomitant use.

Increased Effect/Toxicity There are no known significant interactions involving an increase in effect.

Decreased Effect

The levels/effects of Pegfilgrastim may be decreased by: Pegloticase

Preparation for Administration

On-body injector: A health care provider must fill the On-body injector prior to applying to the patient's skin. The On-body delivery system may be applied on the same day as chemotherapy administration as long as pegfilgrastim is delivered no less than 24 hours after chemotherapy is administered.

The prefilled syringe provided in the On-body kit contains overfill to compensate for loss during delivery; do not use for manual subcutaneous injection (will result in higher than recommended dose). Do not use prefilled syringe intended for manual injection to fill the On-body injector; may result in lower than intended dose.

Storage/Stability Store under refrigeration at 2°C to 8°C (36°F to 46°F); do not freeze. If syringe for manual injection is inadvertently frozen, allow to thaw in refrigerator; discard if frozen more than one time. Protect from light. Do not shake. Allow to reach room temperature prior to injection. Prefilled syringe for manual injection may be kept at room temperature for up to 48 hours. The On-body injector kit should not be held at room temperature for longer than 12 hours prior to use (discard if stored at room temperature for >12 hours).

Mechanism of Action Stimulates the production, maturation, and activation of neutrophils, pegfilgrastim activates neutrophils to increase both their migration and cytotoxicity. Pegfilgrastim has a prolonged duration of effect relative to filgrastim and a reduced renal clearance.

Pharmacodynamics/Kinetics Half-life elimination: SubQ: Adults: 15 to 80 hours; Children (100 mcg/kg dose): ~20 to 30 hours. Pharmacokinetics were comparable between manual subcutaneous injection and the On-body injector system.

Dosage Note: Do not administer in the period between 14 days before and 24 hours after administration of cytotoxic chemotherapy.

Prevention of chemotherapy-induced neutropenia:

Children and Adolescents (off-label use): SubQ: 100 mcg/kg (maximum dose: 6 mg) once per chemotherapy cycle, beginning 24 to 72 hours after completion of chemotherapy (Andre, 2007; Borinstein, 2009)

Adults: SubQ: 6 mg once per chemotherapy cycle, beginning at least 24 hours after completion of chemotherapy

Dosage adjustment in renal impairment: No dosage adjustment necessary.

Dosage adjustment in hepatic impairment: There are no dosage adjustments provided in the manufacturer's labeling (has not been studied).

Administration Administer subcutaneously. Do not use 6 mg fixed dose in infants, children, or adolescents <45 kg (Smith, 2006). Pegfilgrastim is available in prefilled syringes for manual subcutaneous administration or as a kit for use with the On-body injector.

Manual subcutaneous administration: Administer to outer upper arms, abdomen (except within 2 inches of navel), front middle thigh, or upper outer buttocks. Engage/activate needle guard following use to prevent accidental needlesticks

On-body injector: A health care provider must fill the On-body injector prior to applying to the patient's skin. Apply to intact, nonirritated skin on the back of the arm or abdomen (only use the back of the arm if caregiver is available to monitor On-body injection status). The On-body injector system will deliver pegfilgrastim over ~45 minutes approximately 27 hours after application. The On-body delivery system may be applied on the same day as chemotherapy administration as long as pegfilgrastim is delivered at least 24 hours after chemotherapy is administered. Keep the On-body injector dry for ~3 hours before dose delivery. A missed dose may occur if the On-body injector fails or leaks; if a dose is missed, administer a new dose by manual subcutaneous injection as soon as possible after discovery of missed dose. Do not expose the On-body injector to oxygen-rich environments (eg, hyperbaric chambers), MRI, x-ray (including airport x-ray), CT-scan, or ultrasound (may damage injector system). Keep the On-body injector at least 4 inches away from electrical equipment, including cell phones, cordless phones, microwaves, and other common appliances (injector may not work properly).

The prefilled syringe provided in the On-body kit contains overfill to compensate for loss during delivery; do not use for manual subcutaneous injection (will result in higher than recommended dose). Do not use prefilled syringe intended for manual injection to fill the On-body injector; may result in lower than intended dose. The On-body injector is only for use with pegfilgrastim; do not use to deliver other medications.

Monitoring Parameters Complete blood count (with differential) and platelet count should be obtained prior to chemotherapy. Leukocytosis (white blood cell counts 100,000/mm^3) has been observed in <1% of patients receiving pegfilgrastim. Monitor platelets and hematocrit regularly. Evaluate fever, pulmonary infiltrates, and respiratory distress; evaluate for left upper abdominal pain, shoulder tip pain, or splenomegaly. Monitor for sickle cell crisis (in patients with sickle cell anemia).

Dosage Forms

Solution, Subcutaneous [preservative free]:

Neulasta: 6 mg/0.6 mL (0.6 mL)

Neulasta Delivery Kit: 6 mg/0.6 mL (0.6 mL)

◆ **PEG-IFN Alfa-2a** *see* Peginterferon Alfa-2a *on page 1590*

◆ **PEG-IFN Alfa-2b** *see* Peginterferon Alfa-2b *on page 1596*

Peginterferon Alfa-2a

(peg in ter FEER on AL fa too aye)

Brand Names: U.S. Pegasys; Pegasys ProClick

Brand Names: Canada Pegasys

Index Terms Interferon Alfa-2a (PEG Conjugate); PEG-IFN Alfa-2a; Pegylated Interferon Alfa-2a

Pharmacologic Category Interferon

Use

Chronic hepatitis B: Treatment of adults with hepatitis B e antigen (HBeAg)-positive and HBeAG-negative chronic hepatitis B virus (HBV) infection who have compensated liver disease and evidence of viral replication and liver inflammation

Chronic hepatitis C:

Combination therapy: Treatment of adults with chronic hepatitis C (CHC) with compensated liver disease as part of a combination regiment with other hepatitis C virus (HCV) antiviral drugs; treatment of pediatric patients 5 years and older with CHC and compensated liver disease in combination with ribavirin

Monotherapy (for patients with contraindications or who are intolerant to other HCV antiviral drugs): Treatment (as a single agent) of chronic hepatitis C in patients with compensated liver disease in patients with contraindications or significant intolerance to other HCV antiviral drugs

Limitations of use: Peginterferon alfa-2a alone or in combination with ribavirin without additional HCV antiviral drugs is not recommended for treatment of patients with chronic HCV who previously failed therapy with an interferon alfa. Peginterferon alfa-2a is not recommended for treatment of patients with CHC who have had solid organ transplantation.

Pregnancy Risk Factor C / X in combination with ribavirin

Dosage

Chronic hepatitis C: Children ≥5 years and Adolescents: SubQ: 180 mcg/1.73 m^2 x body surface area (BSA) once weekly (maximum dose: 180 mcg) with ribavirin (Copegus). **Note:** Children who reach their 18th birthday during treatment should remain on the pediatric regimen until completion of therapy.

Duration of therapy (based on genotype):

Genotypes 1, 4, 5, 6: 48 weeks

Genotypes 2, 3: 24 weeks

Chronic hepatitis C (monoinfection or coinfection with HIV): Adults: SubQ:

Manufacturer's labeling: 180 mcg once weekly for 48 weeks as monotherapy or in combination with ribavirin (Copegus). **Note:** Discontinue in patients with HCV (genotype 1) after 12 weeks if HCV RNA does not decrease by at least 2 log (compared to pretreatment) or if detectable HCV RNA present at 24 weeks.

Duration of combination therapy: Monoinfection (based on genotype):

Genotypes 1, 2: Refer to the individual agents of HCV antiviral drugs

Genotypes 3: 24 weeks if peg interferon and ribavirin are used without other HCV antiviral drugs

Genotypes 4: 48 weeks if peginterferon and ribavirin are used without other HCV antiviral drugs

Genotypes 5, 6: No dosing recommendations provided; data insufficient

Duration of therapy: Coinfection with HIV: 48 weeks regardless of HCV genotype (if used without other HCV antiviral drugs). When used in combination with other antiviral drugs, refer to individual agents for duration of therapy.

Alternative dosing:

Chronic hepatitis C (off-label uses; recommended regimens, AASLD/IDSA, 2014): Treatment naïve patients:

Genotype 1, 4, 5, or 6: Interferon eligible patients: 180 mcg once weekly in combination with sofosbuvir 400 mg once daily and ribavirin for 12 weeks:

<75 kg: Ribavirin 1000 mg daily

≥75 kg: Ribavirin 1200 mg daily

Chronic hepatitis C (off-label uses; recommended regimens, AASLD/IDSA, 2014): Treatment of **relapser** patients (non responders to a previous regimen of ribavirin and peginterferon **without** an HCV protease inhibitor):

Genotype 4, 5, or 6: Interferon eligible patients: 180 mcg once weekly in combination with sofosbuvir 400 mg once daily and ribavirin for 12 weeks

<75 kg: Ribavirin 1000 mg daily

≥75 kg: Ribavirin 1200 mg daily

Chronic hepatitis C (off-label uses; recommended regimen, AASLD/IDSA, 2014): Treatment of **relapser** patients (non responders to a previous regimen of ribavirin and peginterferon **with or without** an HCV protease inhibitor):

Genotype 1: Interferon eligible patients: 180 mcg once weekly in combination with ribavirin for 12-24 weeks total and sofosbuvir 400 mg once daily for the first 12 weeks only

<75 kg: Ribavirin 1000 mg daily

≥75 kg: Ribavirin 1200 mg daily

Chronic hepatitis B: Adults: SubQ: 180 mcg once weekly for 48 weeks

Dose modifications for adverse reactions/toxicity:

Children ≥5 years and Adolescents: HCV:

For moderate-to-severe adverse reactions: Decrease to 135 mcg/1.73 m^2 x BSA once weekly for initial dose reduction; further dose reductions to 90 mcg/1.73 m^2 x BSA once weekly or 45 mcg/1.73 m^2 x BSA once weekly may be necessary in some cases if reaction persists or recurs. Up to 3 dosing adjustments for toxicity may be made before discontinuation is considered.

Based on hematologic parameters:

ANC 750 to 999/mm^3: Week 1 to 2: 135 mcg/1.73 m^2 x BSA once weekly; Weeks 3-48: No modification

ANC 500 to 749/mm^3: Week 1 to 2: Delay or hold dose until ANC >750/mm^3 then resume dose with 135 mcg/1.73 m^2 x BSA once weekly. Assess WBC weekly for 3 weeks to verify ANC >750/mm^3; Weeks 3 to 48: 135 mcg/1.73 m^2 x BSA once weekly

ANC 250 to 499/mm^3: Week 1 to 2: Delay or hold dose until ANC >750/mm^3 then resume dose with 90 mcg/1.73 m^2 x BSA once weekly; Weeks 3 to 48: Delay or hold dose until ANC >750/mm^3 then resume dose with 135 mcg/1.73 m^2 x BSA once weekly

ANC <250/mm^3 (or febrile neutropenia): Discontinue treatment.

Platelet count <50,000/mm^3: 90 mcg/1.73 m^2 x BSA once weekly

Depression (severity based on DSM-IV criteria [similar to adult dosing adjustment recommendations]):

Mild depression: No dosage adjustment required; evaluate once weekly by visit/phone call. If depression remains stable, continue weekly visits. If depression improves, resume normal visit schedule. For worsening depression, discontinue or reduce dosage to 90 mcg/1.73 m^2 x BSA or 135 mcg/1.73 m^2 x BSA once weekly. Consider psychiatric consultation.

Moderate depression: Decrease to 90 mcg/1.73 m^2 x BSA or 135 mcg/1.73 m^2 x BSA once weekly; evaluate once weekly with an office visit at least every other week. If depression remains stable, consider psychiatric evaluation and continue reduced dosing. If symptoms improve and remain stable for 4 weeks, resume normal visit schedule; continue reduced dosing or return to normal dose. For worsening depression, discontinue interferon permanently and obtain immediate psychiatric consultation.

Severe depression: Discontinue permanently. Obtain immediate psychiatric consultation. Utilize follow-up psychiatric therapy as needed.

Adults: HCV, HBV:

Based on hematologic parameters:

ANC <750/mm^3: 135 mcg once weekly

ANC <500/mm^3: Suspend therapy until ANC >1,000/mm^3, then restart at 90 mcg once weekly; monitor ANC

Platelet count <50,000/mm^3: 90 mcg once weekly

Platelet count <25,000/mm^3: Discontinue therapy

Depression (severity based on DSM-IV criteria):

Mild depression: No dosage adjustment required; evaluate once weekly by visit/phone call. If depression remains stable, continue weekly visits. If depression improves, resume normal visit schedule. For worsening depression, discontinue or reduce dosage to 90 mcg or 135 mcg once weekly. Consider psychiatric consultation.

Moderate depression: Decrease to 90 mcg or 135 mcg once weekly; evaluate once weekly with an office visit at least every other week. If depression remains stable, consider psychiatric evaluation and continue with reduced dosing. If symptoms improve and remain stable for 4 weeks, resume normal visit schedule; continue reduced dosing or return to normal dose. For worsening depression, discontinue interferon permanently and obtain immediate psychiatric consultation.

Severe depression: Discontinue permanently. Obtain immediate psychiatric consultation. Utilize follow-up psychiatric therapy as needed.

Dosage adjustment in renal impairment:

Children: There are no dosage adjustments provided in the manufacturer's labeling (has not been studied).

Adults:

CrCl ≥30 mL/minute: No dosage adjustment required.

CrCl <30 mL/minute: 135 mcg once weekly; monitor for toxicity

End-stage renal disease (ESRD) requiring hemodialysis: 135 mcg once weekly; monitor for toxicity. If severe adverse reactions or laboratory abnormalities occur, may reduce dose to 90 mcg once weekly until adverse reactions resolve; if intolerance persists after dosage adjustment, discontinue

Dosage adjustment in hepatic impairment:

Hepatic impairment prior to initiation: Contraindicated in autoimmune hepatitis, hepatic decompensation (Child-Pugh >6 [class B and C]) in cirrhotic patients before treatment, and hepatic decompensation with Child-Pugh ≥6 in cirrhotic HCV patients coinfected with HIV before treatment.

Hepatic impairment during treatment:

Children: HCV: **Note:** Immediately discontinue therapy if hepatic decompensation (Child-Pugh ≥6 [class B and C]) is observed.

ALT ≥5 but <10 x ULN: Decrease interferon dose to 135 mcg/1.73 m^2 x BSA once weekly. Monitor weekly; further modify dose if needed until ALT stabilizes or decreases.

ALT ≥10 x ULN (persistent): Discontinue treatment.

Adults: **Note:** Immediately discontinue therapy if hepatic decompensation (Child-Pugh ≥6 [class B and C]) is observed.

HCV: ALT progressively rising above baseline: Decrease dose to 135 mcg once weekly **and** monitor LFTs more frequently. If ALT continues to rise despite dose reduction or ALT increase is accompanied by increased bilirubin or hepatic decompensation, discontinue therapy immediately. Therapy may resume after ALT flare subsides.

HBV:

ALT >5 x ULN: Consider decreasing dose to 135 mcg once weekly or temporarily discontinuing **and** monitor LFTs more frequently. If ALT continues to rise despite dose reduction or ALT increase is accompanied by increased bilirubin or hepatic decompensation, discontinue therapy immediately. Therapy may resume after ALT flare subsides.

ALT >10 x ULN: Consider discontinuing.

Additional Information Complete prescribing information should be consulted for additional detail.

Dosage Forms

Kit, Subcutaneous [preservative free]:

Pegasys: 180 mcg/0.5 mL

Solution, Subcutaneous [preservative free]:

Pegasys: 180 mcg/mL (1 mL); 180 mcg/0.5 mL (0.5 mL)

Pegasys ProClick: 135 mcg/0.5 mL (0.5 mL); 180 mcg/0.5 mL (0.5 mL)

Peginterferon Alfa-2a and Ribavirin [CAN/INT]

(peg in ter FEER on AL fa too aye & rye ba VYE rin)

Brand Names: Canada Pegasys RBV

Index Terms Ribavirin and Peginterferon Alfa-2a

Pharmacologic Category Antihepaciviral, Nucleoside (Anti-HCV); Interferon

Use Note: Not approved in U.S.

Hepatitis C: Combination therapy for the treatment of chronic hepatitis C (HCV) in patients without cirrhosis and patients with compensated cirrhosis; includes patients coinfected with stable HIV disease

Pregnancy Considerations Use during pregnancy is contraindicated. Abortifacient and teratogenic effects have been reported in women receiving interferons. Negative pregnancy test is required before initiation and monthly thereafter. Avoid pregnancy in female patients and female partners of male patients during therapy by using two effective forms of contraception; continue contraceptive measures for at least 6 months after completion of therapy. If female patients or female partners of male patients become pregnant during treatment, she should be counseled about potential risks of exposure.

Breast-Feeding Considerations See individual agents.

Contraindications Hypersensitivity to alfa interferons, ribavirin, *E. coli*-derived products, polyethylene glycol (PEG), or any component of the formulation; decompensated cirrhosis; autoimmune hepatitis or history of autoimmune disease; HCV-HIV coinfection with cirrhosis and baseline Child-Pugh score ≥6 (unless score is induced by drugs known to cause indirect hyperbilirubinemia and patient is without evidence of clinical hepatic decompensation); hemoglobinopathies; history of or preexisting severe psychiatric disorder; uncontrolled thyroid dysfunction; neonates and infants (due to benzyl alcohol component); males with a pregnant female partner; pregnancy; breast-feeding

Warnings/Precautions Hazardous agent (ribavirin); use appropriate precautions for handling and disposal (NIOSH 2014 [group 3]).

[Canadian Boxed Warning]: Alfa interferons (including peginterferon alfa-2a) may aggravate or cause fatal or life-threatening neuropsychiatric disorders. Monitor patients closely and discontinue use for persistently severe or worsening symptoms. Resolution occurs in many but not all cases after discontinuation. Use in patients with preexisting or history of severe psychiatric disorders is contraindicated. Use with extreme caution in patients with preexisting depression; monitor all patients for evidence of depressive symptoms. Severe psychiatric adverse events may occur in patients with and without previous psychiatric symptoms; if severe symptoms persist, psychiatric consult should be obtained.

[Canadian Boxed Warning]: Alfa interferons (including peginterferon alfa-2a) may aggravate or cause life-threatening autoimmune disorders. Monitor patients closely and discontinue use for persistently severe or worsening symptoms. Resolution occurs in many but not all cases after discontinuation. Use is contraindicated in patients with a history of autoimmune disease. Exacerbation of myositis, thyroiditis, immune thrombocytopenia (ITP), rheumatoid arthritis, interstitial nephritis, systemic lupus erythematosus, and psoriasis have been reported with interferon therapy; consider therapy discontinuation with appearance of psoriatic lesions and sarcoidosis. **[Canadian Boxed Warning]: Alfa interferons (including peginterferon alfa-2a) may aggravate or cause fatal or life-threatening infectious disorders. Monitor patients closely and discontinue use for**

persistently severe or worsening symptoms. Resolution occurs in many but not all cases after discontinuation.

[Canadian Boxed Warning]: Alfa interferons (including peginterferon alfa-2a) may aggravate or cause life-threatening ischemic disorders. Monitor patients closely and discontinue use for persistently severe or worsening symptoms. Resolution occurs in many but not all cases after discontinuation. Cerebrovascular events (ischemic and hemorrhagic) have been observed in patients receiving alfa interferon therapy, including younger patients (ie, <45 years of age) and those without risk factors. May cause bone marrow suppression, and rarely pancytopenia. Monitor blood counts closely. Use with caution if baseline ANC <1.5 x 10^9/L, platelets <90 x 10^9/L, or hemoglobin <10 g/dL. Temporarily suspend or discontinue therapy for ANC <0.5 x 10^9/L or platelets <25 x 10^9/L. Dosage reduction required if ANC <0.75 x 10^9/L or platelets <50 x 10^9/L. Hemolytic anemia is a significant toxicity, usually occurring within 1 to 2 weeks. Suspend or discontinue ribavirin therapy for any deterioration in hemoglobin levels. Use caution with concomitant use of other myelosuppressive agents.

Use peginterferon alfa-2a with caution in patients with cardiac disease. ECG prior to initiation and during therapy is recommended. Avoid use of ribavirin in patients with unstable or severe cardiac disease within previous 6 months; anemia associated with ribavirin may worsen underlying cardiac disease. Suspend or discontinuation of therapy may be indicated with worsening cardiovascular status. Use with caution in patients with endocrine disorders; hyper-/hypothyroid, diabetes mellitus and/or loss of glucose control have been observed with use of peginterferon alfa-2a. Avoid initiating therapy or discontinue existing therapy in patients whose endocrine disorder is uncontrolled. Monitor TSH and glucose; dosage adjustments of antidiabetic therapy may be necessary.

May cause colitis (ischemic, ulcerative), pancreatitis, or hypertriglyceridemia. Suspend therapy for suspected pancreatitis. Discontinue therapy with confirmed pancreatitis or colitis. Use with caution in patients with hepatic disease (use is contraindicated in decompensated hepatic disease or in [HIV/HCV] coinfection with cirrhosis and baseline Child-Pugh score ≥6 unless score is induced by drugs known to cause indirect hyperbilirubinemia and without evidence of clinical hepatic decompensation). Use with caution in HIV/HCV coinfected patients or with mild-to-moderate hepatic impairment; monitor closely for hepatic decompensation. Discontinue treatment immediately with worsening hepatic function or signs/symptoms of hepatic failure. Elevated ALT may occur during therapy, including patients with a virological response; discontinue for progressive elevations in ALT despite dose reduction or if accompanied by increased bilirubin. Evaluate renal function prior to initiating therapy; use with caution in patients with renal impairment and only if considered essential; avoid use if serum creatinine >2 mg/dL (SI: 177 micromole/L) or CrCl <50 mL/minute; monitor for signs/symptoms of toxicity (therapy discontinuation may be required if toxicity occurs). Maintain adequate hydration as hypotension associated with dehydration has been observed. Use of ribavirin may increase uric acid levels (due to hemolysis); monitor for signs/symptoms of gout (particularly in predisposed patients).

Interferon therapy is commonly associated with flu-like symptoms, including fever. Therapy has been associated with immune-mediated dermatologic reactions including erythema multiforme, SJS, and TEN. Use with caution in psoriasis (exacerbation reported). Rarely, ophthalmologic disorders (including retinal hemorrhages, cotton wool spots, and retinal artery or vein obstruction) have occurred in patients using peginterferon alfa-2a. Visual exams are recommended at baseline for all patients and periodically during therapy for patients with preexisting ophthalmologic disorders (eg, diabetic or hypertensive retinopathy). Use with caution in the elderly. May cause hearing impairment and/or loss. May cause CNS depression (somnolence, fatigue), which may impair physical or mental abilities; patients must be cautioned about performing tasks which require mental alertness (eg, operating machinery or driving).

Negative pregnancy test is required before initiation and monthly thereafter. Avoid pregnancy in female patients and female partners of patients during therapy by using two effective forms of contraception; continue contraceptive measures for at least 6 months after completion of therapy. If patient or female partner becomes pregnant during treatment, she should be counseled about potential risks of exposure. Safety and efficacy have not been established in patients who have failed other alfa interferon therapy, organ transplant patients, hepatitis B virus infection, or pediatric patients. Ribavirin monotherapy is not effective and must be used in combination therapy. Acute hypersensitivity (eg, anaphylaxis, angioedema, bronchoconstriction) has been observed rarely. Due to differences in dosage, patients should not change brands of interferons. Potentially significant drug-drug interactions may exist, requiring dose or frequency adjustment, additional monitoring, and/or selection of alternative therapy.

In combination therapy with alfa interferons, ribavirin may cause a reduction in growth velocity in pediatric patients for the length of treatment. Following treatment, rebound growth and weight gain occurred in most patients; however, a small percentage did not. Long-term data indicate that combination therapy may inhibit growth resulting in reduced adult height. Use in patients <18 years is not recommended.

Hazardous agent (ribavirin); use appropriate precautions for handling and disposal (NIOSH 2014 [group 3]).

Adverse Reactions

Cardiovascular: Chest pain, flushing, hypertension, palpitations, peripheral edema, syncope, tachycardia

Central nervous system: Aggressive behavior, anxiety, apathy, confusion, depression, dizziness, drowsiness, drug abuse, emotional disturbance, emotional lability, fatigue, headache, hyperesthesia, hypoesthesia, insomnia, irritability, lack of concentration, lethargy, malaise, memory impairment, migraine, mood changes, myasthenia, nervousness, nightmares, pain, paresthesia, rigors, suicidal ideation, vertigo

Dermatologic: Alopecia, cheilitis, dermatitis, dermatological reaction, diaphoresis, eczema, night sweats, pruritus, psoriasis, skin photosensitivity, skin rash, urticaria, xeroderma

Endocrine & metabolic: Decreased libido, dehydration, hot flash, hyperthyroidism, hypothyroidism, increased thirst, lactic acidosis, lipodystrophy, weight loss

Gastrointestinal: Abdominal pain, anorexia, constipation, decreased appetite, dental bleeding, diarrhea, dysgeusia, dyspepsia, dysphagia, flatulence, glossitis, nausea, nausea and vomiting, oral candidiasis, oral mucosa ulcer, sore throat, stomatitis, xerostomia

Genitourinary: Impotence, urine discoloration

Hematologic & oncologic: Hemolytic anemia, lymphadenopathy, neutropenia, thrombocytopenia

Infection: Herpes virus infection, influenza

Local: Injection site reaction

Neuromuscular & skeletal: Arthralgia, arthritis, back pain, muscle cramps, musculoskeletal pain, myalgia, neck pain, ostealgia, tremor, weakness

Ophthalmic: Blurred vision, eye pain, uveitis, xerophthalmia

Otic: Otalgia, tinnitus

Respiratory: Bronchitis, cough, dyspnea, dyspnea on exertion, epistaxis, flu-like symptoms, nasal congestion, nasopharyngitis, pharyngolaryngeal pain, pneumonia, rhinitis, sinus congestion, upper respiratory tract infection

Miscellaneous: Fever

Rare but important or life-threatening (reported with other interferon preparations and/or ribavirin): Abdominal distention, acute psychosis, anaphylaxis, angioedema, aplastic anemia (rare), atrial fibrillation, bacterial infection (including sepsis), Bell's palsy, brain disease, bronchoconstriction, cardiac arrhythmia, cardiomyopathy, cerebral hemorrhage, cerebral ischemia, cerebrovascular hemorrhage, cholangitis, coma, congestive heart failure, corneal ulcer, deafness (rare), decreased platelet count, decreased white blood cell count, dental disorders, diabetes mellitus, endocarditis, erythema multiforme, fungal infection, gastrointestinal hemorrhage, gout, hallucination, hepatic insufficiency, hepatitis, hepatotoxicity, homicidal ideation, hyperglycemia, hypersensitivity reaction, hypertriglyceridemia, hypoglycemia, increased serum ALT, increased uric acid, interstitial nephritis, interstitial pneumonitis, ischemic colitis, ischemic heart disease, leukopenia, liver steatosis, macular edema, malignant neoplasm (hepatic), myocardial infarction, myositis, nephrotic syndrome, obtundation, optic neuritis, otitis externa, pancreatitis, pancytopenia, panic attack, papilledema, peptic ulcer, pericarditis, periodontal disease, peripheral neuropathy, pneumonitis, psychiatric signs and symptoms, pulmonary embolism, pulmonary infiltrates, pure red cell aplasia, renal failure, renal insufficiency, retinal blood vessel occlusion, retinal cotton-wool spot, retinal detachment, retinal hemorrhage, rhabdomyolysis, sarcoidosis (including exacerbation), seizure, skin infection, Stevens-Johnson syndrome, suicidal tendencies, thrombotic thrombocytopenic purpura, thyroid dysfunction, thyroiditis, tissue necrosis at injection site, toxic epidermal necrolysis, ulcerative colitis, viral infection

Use of alfa interferons has been associated with rare cases of autoimmune disease, including immune thrombocytopenia (ITP), thyroiditis, rheumatoid arthritis, systemic lupus erythematosus, vasculitis, and Vogt-Koyanagi-Harada syndrome

Drug Interactions

Metabolism/Transport Effects Peginterferon Alfa-2a: **Inhibits** CYP1A2 (weak)

Avoid Concomitant Use

Avoid concomitant use of Peginterferon Alfa-2a and Ribavirin with any of the following: Didanosine

Increased Effect/Toxicity

Peginterferon Alfa-2a and Ribavirin may increase the levels/effects of: Aldesleukin; Didanosine; Reverse Transcriptase Inhibitors (Nucleoside); Ribavirin; Telbivudine; Theophylline Derivatives; Zidovudine

The levels/effects of Peginterferon Alfa-2a and Ribavirin may be increased by: Interferons (Alfa)

Decreased Effect

Peginterferon Alfa-2a and Ribavirin may decrease the levels/effects of: Influenza Virus Vaccine

Storage/Stability

Pegasys RBV combination package: Store under refrigeration between 2°C and 8°C (36°F and 46°F); do not freeze. Protect from light. Do not shake. When the package is separated:

Copegus tablets: Store under refrigeration or below 30°C (86°F).

Pegasys prefilled syringes/vials: Store under refrigeration between 2°C and 8°C (36°F and 46°F); do not freeze. Protect from light. Do not shake.

Mechanism of Action

Peginterferon Alfa-2a: Alpha interferons are a family of proteins, produced by nucleated cells that have antiviral, antiproliferative, and immune-regulating activity. There are 16 known subtypes of alpha interferons. Interferons interact with cells through high affinity cell surface receptors. Following activation, multiple effects can be detected including induction of gene transcription. Inhibits cellular growth, alters the state of cellular differentiation, interferes with oncogene expression, alters cell surface antigen expression, increases phagocytic activity of macrophages, and augments cytotoxicity of lymphocytes for target cells.

Ribavirin: Inhibits replication of RNA and DNA viruses; inhibits influenza virus RNA polymerase activity and inhibits the initiation and elongation of RNA fragments resulting in inhibition of viral protein synthesis.

Pharmacodynamics/Kinetics See individual agents.

Dosage Adults:

Chronic hepatitis C (HCV) monoinfection:

Genotypes 1,4:

<75 kg: Peginterferon alfa-2a (SubQ): 180 mcg once weekly **and** ribavirin (oral) 1000 mg daily (divided into 2 doses) for 48 weeks

≥75 kg: Peginterferon alfa-2a (SubQ): 180 mcg once weekly **and** ribavirin (oral) 1200 mg daily (divided into 2 doses) for 48 weeks

Genotypes 2,3: Peginterferon alfa-2a (SubQ): 180 mcg once weekly **and** ribavirin (oral) 800 mg daily (divided into 2 doses) for 24 weeks

HIV-HCV coinfection: HCV genotypes 1,2,3,4: Peginterferon alfa-2a (SubQ): 180 mcg once weekly **and** ribavirin (oral) 800 mg daily (divided into 2 doses) for 48 weeks

Treatment duration (Canadian Consensus Guidelines [Meyers, 2012]):

HCV genotype 1:

Treatment-naive:

Without cirrhosis:

Receiving concomitant telaprevir: If undetectable HCV RNA at weeks 4 and 12 discontinue telaprevir after week 12 and continue peginterferon alfa-2a/ribavirin for 12 weeks (total of 24 weeks); if HCV RNA detectable at weeks 4 or 12 discontinue telaprevir at week 12 and continue peginterferon alfa-2a/ribavirin for 36 weeks (total: 48 weeks).

Receiving concomitant boceprevir (initiated after 4 weeks of peginterferon alfa-2a/ribavirin therapy): If undetectable HCV RNA at weeks 8 through 24 continue triple therapy for total of 28 weeks; if HCV RNA detectable at week 8 continue triple therapy through week 28 then discontinue boceprevir and continue peginterferon alfa-2a/ribavirin for 20 weeks (total: 48 weeks).

With cirrhosis (compensated):

Receiving concomitant telaprevir: Discontinue telaprevir after week 12 and continue peginterferon alfa-2a/ribavirin for 36 weeks (total: 48 weeks)

Receiving concomitant boceprevir (initiated after 4 weeks of peginterferon alfa-2a/ribavirin therapy): Peginterferon alfa-2a/ribavirin for 4 weeks then initiate triple therapy for 44 weeks (total: 48 weeks)

Patients with <1 log_{10} decrease in HCV RNA after 4 weeks of peginterferon alfa-2a/ribavirin: Triple therapy with boceprevir should be continued for 44 weeks (total: 48 weeks)

Previously-treated patients (relapsers, partial responders, null responders):

Without cirrhosis:

Receiving concomitant telaprevir: Relapsers achieving undetectable HCV RNA at weeks 4 and 12, may discontinue telaprevir after week 12 and continue peginterferon alfa-2a/ribavirin for 12 weeks (total 24 weeks). Relapsers with HCV RNA detectable at weeks 4 and/or 12 and previous partial responders or null responders should discontinue telaprevir after week 12 and continue peginterferon alfa-2a/ribavirin for 36 weeks (total: 48 weeks)

Receiving concomitant boceprevir (initiated after 4 weeks of peginterferon alfa-2a/ribavirin therapy): Relapsers and partial responders achieving undetectable HCV RNA at weeks 8 through 24, may discontinue therapy at 36 week. Relapsers with HCV RNA detectable at week 8 and undetectable at week 24 discontinue boceprevir at 36 weeks and continue peginterferon alfa-2a/ribavirin through week 48. Prior null responders should receive triple therapy for 44 weeks (total therapy: 48 weeks)

With cirrhosis (compensated): Peginterferon alfa-2a/ribavirin are recommended for 48 weeks as part of triple therapy with either boceprevir (weeks 5 to 48) or telaprevir (first 12 weeks)

HCV genotypes 2,3:

Treatment-naive: Treatment recommended for 24 weeks; discontinue therapy in patients failing to achieve early virological response (EVR) at 12 weeks. Full treatment course should be used in patients with cofactors that reduce the likelihood of success (eg, advanced fibrosis, black race, metabolic syndrome/insulin resistance, obesity) even if rapid virological response (RVR) is achieved. May consider abbreviated therapy (12 or 16 weeks) in patients without these cofactors who achieve a RVR with weight-based ribavirin dosing. If relapse occurs following abbreviated therapy, consider retreatment for 24 weeks.

Genotype 3 patients who do not achieve an RVR but have an EVR may be considered for extended treatment (36 to 48 weeks) especially if the patient has cofactors that reduce the likelihood of success (eg, advanced fibrosis, black race, metabolic syndrome/insulin resistance, obesity).

Treatment of relapser patients: May consider retreatment for 48 weeks in patients with ≥ stage 2 fibrosis who have failed a previous 24-week course of therapy

HCV genotype 4,5, and 6: Treatment recommended for 48 weeks; discontinue therapy in patients failing to achieve EVR at 12 weeks or with detectable HCV RNA at 24 weeks. Patients with genotype 4 who have low baseline viral loads <800,000 units/mL and mild fibrosis (METAVIR score ≤F2) may be treated for 36 weeks.

Treatment futility Discontinue all treatment if HCV RNA ≥1000 units/mL at weeks 4 or 12 or detectable at week 24 (with concomitant telaprevir) or if HCV RNA ≥100 units/mL at week 12 or detectable at week 24 (with concomitant boceprevir)

Dosing adjustment for toxicity: Note: Recommendations (per manufacturer labeling - also refer to Dosing in renal and hepatic impairment):

Adverse events/toxicity: For moderate-to-severe adverse reactions (clinical and/or laboratory): Reduce peginterferon alfa-2a dose to 90 to 135 mcg once weekly

Depression:

Mild depression: No dosage adjustment required; monitor closely

Moderate depression: Decrease peginterferon alfa-2a dose to 90 to 135 mcg once weekly; monitor closely

Severe depression: Discontinue combination therapy; obtain immediate psychiatric consultation

Hemoglobin (patients without cardiac disease):

Hemoglobin <10 g/dL: Decrease ribavirin dose to 600 mg daily

Hemoglobin <8.5 g/dL: Discontinue ribavirin; upon resolution of decreased hemoglobin, may reinitiate ribavirin therapy at 600 mg daily with subsequent increase to 800 mg daily as tolerated; higher doses are not recommended

Hemoglobin (patients with stable cardiac disease):

Hemoglobin decrease >2 g/dL in any 4-week period: Permanently decrease ribavirin dose to 600 mg daily

Hemoglobin <12 g/dL after ribavirin dose is decreased for 4 weeks: Discontinue ribavirin; upon resolution of decreased hemoglobin, may reinitiate ribavirin therapy at 600 mg daily with subsequent increase to 800 mg daily as tolerated; higher doses are not recommended

Neutrophils:

Neutrophils <0.75 x 10^9/L: Decrease peginterferon alfa-2a dose to 135 mcg weekly

Neutrophils <0.5 x 10^9/L: Interrupt peginterferon alfa-2a therapy; may reinitiate therapy at 90 mcg weekly when ANC >1 x 10^9/L

Platelets:

Platelet count <50 x 10^9/L: Decrease peginterferon alfa-2a dose to 90 mcg weekly

Platelet count <25 x 10^9/L: Permanently discontinue peginterferon alfa-2a and ribavirin

Dosage adjustment in renal impairment:

Peginterferon alfa-2a: SubQ:

CrCl >20 mL/minute: No dosage adjustment necessary. Monitor closely as dose reduction may be warranted with onset of adverse events.

End-stage renal disease requiring hemodialysis: Reduce initial dosage to 135 mcg once weekly

Ribavirin: Oral: Serum creatinine >2 mg/dL (SI: 177 micromole/L) or CrCl <50 mL/minute. Use is not recommended.

Dosage adjustment in hepatic impairment: Avoid use in decompensated hepatic disease (eg, Child-Pugh class B or C). Use is contraindicated in HCV-HIV coinfected patients with cirrhosis and baseline Child-Pugh score ≥6 (unless score is induced by drugs known to cause indirect hyperbilirubinemia and without evidence of clinical hepatic decompensation).

Peginterferon alfa-2a: SubQ: Reduce dose to 90 mcg/once weekly in the presence of progressive ALT increases greater than baseline. Therapy discontinuation may be necessary for persistently marked ALT elevations despite dose reduction and/or with accompanying elevated bilirubin or with evidence of hepatic decompensation.

Ribavirin: Oral: Dosage adjustments are not required in patients with compensated hepatic impairment

Dietary Considerations Take ribavirin with food.

Administration See individual agents.

Hazardous agent (ribavirin); use appropriate precautions for handling and disposal (NIOSH 2014 [group 3]).

Monitoring Parameters Obtain pretreatment CBC, liver function tests, renal function, lipids, TSH, and electrolytes, then monitor CBC routinely throughout therapy at 2- and 4 weeks (more frequently if indicated) and other tests every 4 weeks (more frequently if indicated).Pretreatment and monthly pregnancy test (up to 6 months following therapy discontinuation) for women of childbearing age. Baseline chest x-ray, ECG, weight; patients with preexisting cardiac abnormalities should have an ECG before and during treatment; glucose (diabetic or symptomatic patients), I & O; dental exams; neuropsychiatric monitoring; vision (pretreatment and periodic during therapy).

Serum HCV RNA levels (pretreatment, 4-, 12-, and 24 weeks after therapy initiation, 24 weeks after completion of therapy)

In addition, the following baseline values were used as entrance criteria in clinical trials:

Platelet count ≥90 x 10^9/L (as low as 75 x 10^9/L in patients with cirrhosis or transition to cirrhosis)

ANC ≥1.5 x 10^9/L

Serum creatinine <1.5 times ULN

TSH and T_4 within normal limits or adequately controlled

$CD4^+$ cell count ≥200 cells/microL or $CD4^+$ cell count ≥100 cells/microL, but <200 cells/microL and HIV-1 RNA <5000 copies/mL in CHC-HIV coinfected patients

Reference Range Canadian consensus guidelines (Myers, 2012): **Note:** Response to peginterferon and ribavirin therapy unless otherwise noted.

Rapid virological response (RVR): Undetectable HCV RNA at week 4 of treatment

Extended RVR: Undetectable HCV RNA at 4 and 12 weeks of treatment (patients treated with telaprevir-based triple therapy)

Early virological response (EVR): ≥2 $\log_{10}$ decrease in HCV RNA at 12 weeks of treatment compared to baseline

Partial virological response (PVR): HCV RNA positive but ≥2 $\log_{10}$ decrease in HCV RNA at 12 weeks of treatment

Sustained virological response (SVR): Absence of HCV RNA at least 24 weeks following completion of treatment

End-of-treatment virological response: Undetectable HCV RNA following completion of treatment.

Null response: <2 $\log_{10}$ decrease in HCV RNA at 12 weeks of treatment compared to baseline

Relapse: Reappearance of HCV RNA following treatment discontinuation after an end of treatment virological response has been achieved

Product Availability Not available in U.S.

Dosage Forms: Canada

Combination package:

Pegasys RBV [1-week package]:

Tablet, oral: Ribavirin 200 mg (28s)
Injection, solution: Peginterferon alfa-2a: 180 mcg/0.5 mL (0.5 mL) (1s)

Tablet, oral: Ribavirin 200 mg (35s)
Injection, solution: Peginterferon alfa-2a: 180 mcg/0.5 mL (0.5 mL) (1s)

Tablet, oral: Ribavirin 200 mg (42s)
Injection, solution: Peginterferon alfa-2a: 180 mcg/0.5 mL (0.5 mL) (1s)

Pegasys RBV [1-week package]:

Tablet, oral: Ribavirin 200 mg (28s)
Injection, solution: Peginterferon alfa-2a: 180 mcg/mL (1 mL) (1s)

Tablet, oral: Ribavirin 200 mg (35s)
Injection, solution: Peginterferon alfa-2a: 180 mcg/mL (1 mL) (1s)

Tablet, oral: Ribavirin 200 mg (42s)
Injection, solution: Peginterferon alfa-2a: 180 mcg/mL (1 mL) (1s)

Pegasys RBV [4-week package]:

Tablet, oral: Ribavirin 200 mg (112s)
Injection, solution: Peginterferon alfa-2a: 180 mcg/0.5 mL (0.5 mL) (4s)

Tablet, oral: Ribavirin 200 mg (140s)
Injection, solution: Peginterferon alfa-2a: 180 mcg/0.5 mL (0.5 mL) (4s)

Tablet, oral: Ribavirin 200 mg (168s)
Injection, solution: Peginterferon alfa-2a: 180 mcg/0.5 mL (0.5 mL) (4s)

Tablet, oral: Ribavirin 200 mg (168s + 28s)
Injection, solution: Peginterferon alfa-2a: 180 mcg/0.5 mL (0.5 mL) (4s)

Pegasys RBV [4-week package]:

Tablet, oral: Ribavirin 200 mg (112s)
Injection, solution: Peginterferon alfa-2a: 180 mcg/mL (1 mL) (4s)

Tablet, oral: Ribavirin 200 mg (140s)
Injection, solution: Peginterferon alfa-2a: 180 mcg/mL (1 mL) (4s)

Tablet, oral: Ribavirin 200 mg (168s)
Injection, solution: Peginterferon alfa-2a: 180 mcg/mL (1 mL) (4s)

Peginterferon Alfa-2b

(peg in ter FEER on AL fa too bee)

Brand Names: U.S. Peg-Intron; Peg-Intron Redipen; Peg-Intron Redipen Pak 4; PegIntron; Sylatron

Brand Names: Canada PegIntron

Index Terms Interferon Alfa-2b (PEG Conjugate); PEG-IFN Alfa-2b; Pegylated Interferon Alfa-2b; Polyethylene Glycol Interferon Alfa-2b

Pharmacologic Category Antineoplastic Agent, Biological Response Modulator; Biological Response Modulator; Immunomodulator, Systemic; Interferon

Use

Chronic hepatitis C (CHC): Peg-Intron: Treatment of chronic hepatitis C (CHC) in compensated liver disease:

Combination therapy with ribavirin and an approved hepatitis C virus [HCV] NS3/4A protease inhibitor in adult patients with HCV genotype 1 infection.

Combination therapy with ribavirin in adult patients with HCV genotypes other than 1, in pediatric patients (3 to 17 years), or in patients with HCV genotype 1 with contraindications or intolerance to HCV NS3/4A protease inhibitor use.

Monotherapy in adult patients with contraindications or significant intolerance to ribavirin if previously untreated.

Limitations of use: Combination therapy with ribavirin provides substantially better response rates than monotherapy

Melanoma: Sylatron: Adjuvant treatment of melanoma (with microscopic or gross nodal involvement within 84 days of definitive surgical resection, including complete lymphadenectomy)

Pregnancy Risk Factor C / X in combination with ribavirin

Dosage

Chronic hepatitis C (CHC): Children 3 to 17 years: SubQ:

Manufacturer's labeling: Combination therapy with ribavirin: 60 mcg/m^2 once weekly; **Note:** Children who reach their 18th birthday during treatment should remain on the pediatric regimen. Treatment duration is 48 weeks for genotype 1, 24 weeks for genotypes 2 and 3. Discontinue combination therapy in patients with HCV (genotype 1) at 12 weeks if HCV-RNA does not decrease by at least 2 log (compared to pretreatment) or if detectable HCV-RNA present at 24 weeks.

American Association for the Study of Liver Diseases (AASLD) guideline recommendations (Ghany, 2009): Children 2 to 17 years: Treatment of choice: **Peginterferon alfa-2b** 60 mcg/m^2 once weekly in combination with oral ribavirin 15 mg/kg/day for 48 weeks

Melanoma: Adults: SubQ: Initial: 6 mcg/kg/week for 8 doses; Maintenance: 3 mcg/kg/week for up to 5 years. **Note:** Premedicate with acetaminophen (500 to 1000 mg orally) 30 minutes prior to the first dose and as needed for subsequent doses thereafter.

CHC: Adults: SubQ:

Manufacturer's labeling: **Note:** Discontinue in patients with HCV (genotype 1) after 12 weeks if HCV RNA does not decrease by at least 2 log (compared to pretreatment) or if detectable HCV RNA present at 24 weeks. Discontinuation is also recommended in patients who previously failed therapy (regardless of genotype) if detectable HCV RNA present at 12 or 24 weeks.

Combination therapy with ribavirin(treatment duration is 48 weeks for genotype 1, 24 weeks for genotypes 2 and 3, or 48 weeks for patients who previously failed therapy [regardless of genotype]): Initial dose (based on an average weekly dose of 1.5 mcg/kg):

- <40 kg: 50 mcg once weekly (with ribavirin 800 mg/day)
- 40 to 50 kg: 64 mcg once weekly (with ribavirin 800 mg/day)
- 51 to 60 kg: 80 mcg once weekly (with ribavirin 800 mg/day)
- 61 to 65 kg: 96 mcg once weekly (with ribavirin 800 mg/day)
- 66 to 75 kg: 96 mcg once weekly (with ribavirin 1000 mg/day)
- 76 to 80 kg: 120 mcg once weekly (with ribavirin 1000 mg/day)
- 81 to 85 kg: 120 mcg once weekly (with ribavirin 1200 mg/day)
- 86 to 105 kg: 150 mcg once weekly (with ribavirin 1200 mg/day)
- >105 kg: 1.5 mcg/kg once weekly (with ribavirin 1400 mg/day)

Monotherapy (duration of treatment is 1 year): Initial dose (based on average weekly dose of 1 mcg/kg):

- ≤45 kg: 40 mcg once weekly
- 46-56 kg: 50 mcg once weekly
- 57 to 72 kg: 64 mcg once weekly
- 73 to 88 kg: 80 mcg once weekly
- 89 to 106 kg: 96 mcg once weekly
- 107 to 136 kg: 120 mcg once weekly
- 137 to 160 kg: 150 mcg once weekly

Alternative dosing: **Note:** Current AASLD/IDSA recommendations do not specify a particular peginterferon (eg, 2a or 2b); however, guideline recommendations are based on clinical trials that used peginterferon alfa-2a. It is not known whether peginterferon alfa 2b could be used interchangeably. Please refer to http://www.hcvguidelines.org for additional information.

Elderly: Refer to adult dosing.

Dosage adjustment for toxicity:

Melanoma:

Discontinue for any of the following: Persistent or worsening severe neuropsychiatric disorders (depression, psychosis, encephalopathy), grade 4 nonhematologic toxicity, new or worsening retinopathy, new-onset ventricular arrhythmia or cardiovascular decompensation, evidence of hepatic injury (severe) or hepatic decompensation (Child-Pugh score >6 [Class B or C]), development of hyper- or hypothyroidism or diabetes that cannot be effectively managed with medication, or inability to tolerate a dose of 1 mcg/kg/week

Temporarily withhold for any of the following: ANC <500/mm^3, platelets <50,000/mm^3, ECOG performance status (PS) ≥2, nonhematologic toxicity ≥ grade 3. May reinitiate at a reduced dose once ANC ≥500/mm^3, platelets ≥50,000/mm^3, ECOG PS at 0 to 1, and nonhematologic toxicity completely resolved or improved to grade 1.

Reduced dose schedule, Weeks 1 to 8:

- First dose reduction (if prior dose 6 mcg/kg/week): 3 mcg/kg/week
- Second dose reduction (if prior dose 3 mcg/kg/week): 2 mcg/kg/week
- Third dose reduction (if prior dose 2 mcg/kg/week): 1 mcg/kg/week
- Discontinue permanently if unable to tolerate 1 mcg/kg/week

Reduced dose schedule, Weeks 9 to 260:

- First dose reduction (if prior dose 3 mcg/kg/week): 2 mcg/kg/week
- Second dose reduction (if prior dose 2 mcg/kg/week): 1 mcg/kg/week
- Discontinue permanently if unable to tolerate 1 mcg/kg/week

***Chronic hepatitis C:* Dosage adjustment for depression (severity based upon DSM-IV criteria):**

Mild depression: No dosage adjustment required; evaluate once weekly by visit/phone call. If depression remains stable, continue weekly visits. If depression improves, resume normal visit schedule. For worsening depression, see "Moderate depression" or "Severe depression" below.

Moderate depression: **Note:** Evaluate once weekly (visit or phone) with an office visit at least every other week. If depression remains stable, consider psychiatric evaluation and continue with reduced dosing. If symptoms improve and remain stable for 4 weeks, resume normal visit schedule; continue reduced dosing or return to normal dose. For worsening depression, see "Severe depression" below.

Children: Decrease peginterferon alfa-2b dose to 40 mcg/m^2/week, may further decrease to 20 mcg/m^2/week if needed

Adults:

- Peginterferon alfa-2b monotherapy: Refer to adult weight-based dosage reduction with monotherapy for depression below
- Peginterferon alfa-2b combination therapy: Refer to adult weight-based dosage reduction with combination therapy for depression below

Severe depression: Discontinue peginterferon alfa-2b and ribavirin permanently. Obtain immediate psychiatric consultation. Utilize follow-up psychiatric therapy as needed.

***Chronic hepatitis C:* Dosage adjustment in hematologic toxicity:**

Children:

- Hemoglobin decrease ≥2 g/dL in any 4-week period and stable cardiac disease: Decrease peginterferon alfa-2b dose by 50%; decrease ribavirin dose by 200 mg daily (regardless of the patient's initial dose); monitor and evaluate weekly. If hemoglobin <8.5 g/dL any time after dose reduction or <12 g/dL after 4 weeks of dose reduction, permanently discontinue both peginterferon alfa-2b and ribavirin.
- Hemoglobin 8.5 to <10 g/dL and no history of cardiac disease: Decrease ribavirin dose to 12 mg/kg/day; may further reduce to 8 mg/kg/day; no dosage adjustment necessary for peginterferon alfa-2b.
- WBC 1000 to <1500/mm^3, neutrophils 500 to <750/mm^3, or platelets 50,000 to <70,000/mm^3: Reduce peginterferon alfa-2b dose to 40 mcg/m^2/week; may further reduce to 20 mcg/m^2/week
- Hemoglobin <8.5 g/dL, WBC <1000/mm^3, neutrophils <500/mm^3, or platelets <50,000/mm^3: Permanently discontinue peginterferon alfa-2b and ribavirin.

Adults:

- Hemoglobin decrease ≥2 g/dL in any 4-week period and stable cardiac disease: Decrease peginterferon alfa-2b dose by 50%; decrease ribavirin dose by 200 mg daily. If hemoglobin <8.5 g/dL any time after dose reduction or <12 g/dL after 4 weeks of dose reduction, permanently discontinue both peginterferon alfa-2b and ribavirin.

Hemoglobin 8.5 to <10 g/dL and no history of cardiac disease: Decrease ribavirin dose by 200 mg daily (patients receiving 1400 mg daily should decrease dose by 400 mg daily [ie, first dose reduction to 1000 mg daily]); may further reduce ribavirin dose by additional 200 mg daily if needed. No dosage adjustment necessary for peginterferon alfa-2b.

WBC 1000 to <1500/mm^3, neutrophils 500 to <750/mm^3, or platelets 25,000 to <50,000/mm^3:

Peginterferon alfa-2b monotherapy: Refer to adult weight-based dosage reduction monotherapy for hematologic toxicity below.

Peginterferon alfa-2b combination therapy: Refer to adult weight-based dosage reduction with combination therapy for hematologic toxicity below.

Hemoglobin <8.5 g/dL, WBC <1000/mm^3, neutrophils <500/mm^3, or platelets <25,000/mm^3: Permanently discontinue peginterferon alfa-2b and ribavirin.

***Chronic hepatitis C:* Adult weight-based dosage reduction for depression or hematologic toxicity:**

Peginterferon alfa-2b combination therapy: Initially reduce to average weekly dose of 1 mcg/kg; may further reduce to average weekly dose of 0.5 mcg/kg if needed as follows:

<40 kg: 35 mcg once weekly; may further reduce to 20 mcg once weekly if needed

40 to 50 kg: 45 mcg once weekly; may further reduce to 25 mcg once weekly if needed

51 to 60 kg: 50 mcg once weekly; may further reduce to 30 mcg once weekly if needed

61 to 75 kg: 64 mcg once weekly; may further reduce to 35 mcg once weekly if needed

76 to 85 kg: 80 mcg once weekly; may further reduce to 45 mcg once weekly if needed

86 to 104 kg: 96 mcg once weekly; may further reduce to 50 mcg once weekly if needed

105 to 125 kg: 108 mcg once weekly; may further reduce to 64 mcg once weekly if needed

>125 kg: 135 mcg once weekly; may further reduce to 72 mcg once weekly if needed

Peginterferon alfa-2b monotherapy: Reduce to average weekly dose of 0.5 mcg/kg as follows:

≤45 kg: 20 mcg once weekly

46 to 56 kg: 25 mcg once weekly

57 to 72 kg: 30 mcg once weekly

73 to 88 kg: 40 mcg once weekly

89 to 106 kg: 50 mcg once weekly

107 to 136 kg: 64 mcg once weekly

≥137 kg: 80 mcg once weekly

Dosage adjustment in renal impairment:

Chronic hepatitis C:

Peginterferon alfa-2b combination with ribavirin:

Children: Serum creatinine >2 mg/dL: Discontinue treatment

Adults: CrCl <50 mL/minute: Combination therapy with ribavirin is not recommended

Peginterferon alfa-2b monotherapy:

CrCl 30 to 50 mL/minute: Reduce dose by 25%

CrCl 10 to 29 mL/minute: Reduce dose by 50%

Hemodialysis: Reduce dose by 50%

Discontinue use if renal function declines during treatment.

Melanoma:

CrCl >50 mL/minute/1.73 m^2: No dosage adjustment is necessary.

CrCl 30 to 50 mL/minute/1.73 m^2: Reduce initial dose to 4.5 mcg/kg/week; reduce maintenance dose to 2.25 mcg/kg/week

CrCl <30 mL/minute/1.73 m^2 and ESRD on dialysis: Reduce initial dose to 3 mcg/kg/week; reduce maintenance dose to 1.5 mcg/kg/week

Hemodialysis: Following a single 1 mcg/kg/ dose, no clinically meaningful amount of peginterferon alfa-2b was removed during hemodialysis.

Dosage adjustment in hepatic impairment:

Decompensated liver disease or autoimmune hepatitis: Use is contraindicated.

Hepatic decompensation or severe hepatic injury during treatment (Child-Pugh score >6 [class B or C]): Discontinue immediately.

Additional Information Complete prescribing information should be consulted for additional detail.

Dosage Forms

Kit, Subcutaneous:

Sylatron: 4 x 296 mcg, 4 x 444 mcg

Kit, Subcutaneous [preservative free]:

Peg-Intron: 50 mcg/0.5 mL, 80 mcg/0.5 mL, 120 mcg/0.5 mL, 150 mcg/0.5 mL

Peg-Intron Redipen: 50 mcg/0.5 mL, 80 mcg/0.5 mL, 120 mcg/0.5 mL, 150 mcg/0.5 mL

Peg-Intron Redipen Pak 4: 50 mcg/0.5 mL, 80 mcg/0.5 mL, 120 mcg/0.5 mL, 150 mcg/0.5 mL

PegIntron: 50 mcg/0.5 mL, 80 mcg/0.5 mL, 120 mcg/0.5 mL, 150 mcg/0.5 mL

Sylatron: 296 mcg, 444 mcg, 888 mcg

Peginterferon Alfa-2b and Ribavirin [CAN/INT]

(peg in ter FEER on AL fa too bee & rye ba VYE rin)

Brand Names: Canada Pegetron®; Pegetron® RediPen®

Index Terms Ribavirin and Peginterferon Alfa-2b

Pharmacologic Category Antihepaciviral, Nucleoside (Anti-HCV); Interferon

Use Note: Not approved in U.S.

Combination therapy for the treatment of chronic hepatitis C in patients with compensated liver disease, including treatment-naive patients and those who have failed prior treatment with pegylated or nonpegylated interferon alpha and ribavirin combination therapy

Pregnancy Considerations Use during pregnancy is contraindicated. Abortifacient and/or teratogenic effects have been reported in animal studies with interferons and ribavirin. Women of childbearing potential should not be treated unless two reliable forms of contraception are used. In addition, male patients and their female partners must also use two reliable forms of contraception. Pregnancy must be avoided during treatment and for 6 months following therapy.

Contraindications Hypersensitivity to polyethylene glycol (PEG), interferons, ribavirin, or any component of the formulation; autoimmune hepatitis or history of autoimmune disease; decompensated liver disease; history of or preexisting severe psychiatric disorder; uncontrolled thyroid dysfunction; epilepsy; severe renal dysfunction (CrCl <50 mL/minute); males with a pregnant female partner; pregnancy

Warnings/Precautions Hazardous agent (ribavirin); use appropriate precautions for handling and disposal (NIOSH 2014 [group 3]).

[Canadian Boxed Warning]: Alpha interferons cause or aggravate fatal or life-threatening autoimmune disorders. Patients predisposed to developing autoimmune disorders may be at greater risk (use is contraindicated in patients with history of autoimmune disease). **[Canadian Boxed Warning]: Alpha interferons cause or aggravate fatal or life-threatening infectious disorders. [Canadian Boxed Warning]: Alpha interferons cause or aggravate fatal or life-threatening ischemic disorders.**

[Canadian Boxed Warning]: Life-threatening or fatal psychiatric adverse events (psychosis, aggressive behavior, severe depression, suicidal behavior/ideation and suicide) have been reported in patients with and without previous psychiatric symptoms. Additional CNS adverse effects (confusion, mental status changes) have also been reported. Use with extreme caution in patients with a history of preexisting psychiatric disorders who report a history of **severe** depression. Use in patients with preexisting or a history of severe psychiatric disorders is contraindicated. Onset of psychiatric or CNS adverse effects (including clinical depression) warrants careful neuropsychiatric monitoring during and for 6 months following discontinuation of therapy.

Monitor patients closely for onset or worsening of autoimmune, infectious, ischemic, or psychiatric disorders. Discontinue therapy for persistently severe or worsening symptoms. Symptom resolution generally occurs upon discontinuation of therapy in most cases, but not all cases.

Use is contraindicated in patients with decompensated liver disease, epilepsy, and uncontrolled thyroid dysfunction. Avoid use with severe cardiac disease within previous 6 months, hemoglobinopathies (eg, sickle-cell anemia, thalassemia), or severe debilitating medical conditions. Avoid use in patients with chronic obstructive pulmonary disease (COPD). Pulmonary effects (eg, pneumonitis, pulmonary infiltrates, pulmonary hypertension), sometimes fatal, have been reported; symptomatic patients should receive a chest x-ray. Concomitant use of the herbal product Shosaikoto has been associated with increased reports of pulmonary symptoms.

Use with caution in patients with prior cardiovascular disease, endocrine disorders, or hepatic disease. Treatment should be discontinued in patients with worsening of cardiovascular status or hepatic function.

May cause anemia and severe cytopenias, including aplastic anemia (rarely).Use caution in patients with low peripheral blood counts or myelosuppression, including concurrent use of myelosuppressive therapy. Reduce dose with decreased neutrophil or platelet count and discontinue therapy if significant decreases in neutrophil (<0.5 x 10^9/L), platelet counts (<25 x 10^9/L), or hemoglobin <8.5 g/dL. Ischemic and hemorrhagic cerebrovascular events have been observed with use including patients without risk factors. Maintain adequate hydration as hypotension associated with dehydration has been observed.

Use in severe renal dysfunction (CrCl <50 mL/minute) is contraindicated and use in moderate renal impairment is not recommended. Patients with renal dysfunction should be monitored for signs/symptoms of toxicity (dosage adjustment required if toxicity occurs). Discontinue therapy if serum creatinine >2 mg/dL. Use of ribavirin may increase uric acid levels (due to hemolysis); monitor for signs/symptoms of gout (particularly in predisposed patients). May cause colitis (ischemic, ulcerative), pancreatitis, or hypertriglyceridemia. Discontinue therapy in suspected/confirmed colitis or pancreatitis. Therapy has been associated with immune-mediated dermatologic reactions including erythema multiforme, SJS, and TEN.

Use with caution in sarcoidosis or psoriasis (exacerbation reported). Rarely, ophthalmologic disorders (including retinal hemorrhages, cotton wool spots, and retinal artery or vein obstruction) have occurred in patients using peginterferon alfa-2b. Visual exams are recommended at baseline for all patients and periodically during therapy for patients at risk for retinopathy (eg, diabetes mellitus, hypertension). Consider discontinuation of therapy with new or worsening ophthalmologic disorders. May cause hearing impairment and/or loss. Dental and periodontal disorders have been reported with ribavirin and peginterferon therapy.

Use caution in the elderly. May cause CNS depression (somnolence, fatigue), which may impair physical or mental abilities; patients must be cautioned about performing tasks which require mental alertness (eg, operating machinery or driving). High-dose peginterferon alfa-2b has been associated with significant obtundation and coma, including cases of encephalopathy (usually elderly patients), and rarely seizures.

Use in pregnancy is contraindicated. Negative pregnancy test is required before initiation and monthly thereafter. Avoid pregnancy in female patients and female partners of patients during therapy by using two effective forms of contraception; continue contraceptive measures for at least 6 months after completion of therapy. If patient or female partner becomes pregnant during treatment, she should be counseled about potential risks of exposure. Safety and efficacy have not been established in organ transplant patients, concurrent hepatitis B virus or HIV exposure. Acute hypersensitivity (eg, anaphylaxis, angioedema, bronchoconstriction) has been observed rarely. Ribavirin monotherapy is not effective and must be used with interferon. Use caution in patients receiving concurrent medications which may cause lactic acidosis (eg, nucleoside analogues).

Adverse Reactions

Cardiovascular: Chest pain, flushing, hyper/hypotension, palpitation, peripheral edema, syncope, tachycardia

Central nervous system: Aggression, agitation, amnesia, anger, anxiety, apathy, chills, confusion, crying, depression, dizziness, emotional lability, fatigue, fever, headache, hyper/hypoesthesia, impaired concentration, insomnia, irritability, lethargy, malaise, memory impairment, migraine, nervousness, pain, restlessness, rigors, sleep disturbances, somnolence, tremor, vertigo; **Note:** Life-threatening psychiatric events (suicidal ideation, suicide attempt, suicide [completed], psychosis including hallucinations and aggressive behavior) have been reported in up to 1.2% of patients.

Dermatologic: Alopecia, cellulitis, cheilitis, dermatitis, dry skin, eczema, erythema, hair texture abnormal, hyperhidrosis, photosensitivity, pruritus, psoriasis, rash (including erythematous and maculopapular), scaling

Endocrine & metabolic: Amenorrhea, dehydration, hyperuricemia, lacrimal gland disorder, libido decreased, menorrhagia, menstrual disorder, thyroid abnormalities (hyper-/hypothyroidism), TSH increased

Gastrointestinal: Abdominal distension, abdominal pain, anorexia, appetite decreased, bleeding gums, burning mouth, constipation, diarrhea, dyspepsia, flatulence, gastritis, GERD, glossitis, herpes labialis, loose stools, mouth ulcerations, nausea, right upper quadrant pain, serum amylase increased, stomach discomfort, stomatitis (including aphthous and ulcerative), taste perversion, vomiting, weight loss, xerostomia

Genitourinary: Erectile dysfunction, polyuria, prostatitis

Hematologic: Anemia (including hemolytic), leukopenia, lymphopenia, neutropenia, thrombocytopenia

Hepatic: Hyperbilirubinemia

Local: Injection site reactions (including erythema, inflammation, pain, pruritus, rash)

Neuromuscular & skeletal: Arthralgia, back pain, bone pain, hypertonia, limb pain, muscle spasms, musculoskeletal pain, myalgia, neck pain, paresthesia, weakness

Ocular: Conjunctivitis, dry eyes, eye pain, photophobia, retinal exudates, vision blurred, visual disturbances

Otic: Hearing impaired/loss, otitis media, tinnitus

Respiratory: Bronchitis, cough, dyspnea, epistaxis, exertional dyspnea, nasal congestion, nasal dryness, nonproductive cough, pharyngitis, pharyngolaryngeal pain, postnasal drip, respiratory disorder, rhinitis, rhinorrhea, sinusitis, upper respiratory tract infection

Miscellaneous: Diaphoresis, flu-like syndrome, fungal infection, herpes simplex, lymphadenopathy, night sweats, sensitivity to temperature extremes, thirst, viral infection

Rare but important or life-threatening (reported with other interferon preparations and/or ribavirin): Anaphylaxis, angioedema, aplastic anemia, arrhythmia, arthritis (including rheumatoid), bacterial infection (including sepsis), bipolar disorder, cardiac ischemia, cardiomyopathy, cerebrovascular hemorrhage, cerebrovascular ischemia, colitis (ischemic, ulcerative), coma, diabetes mellitus, diabetic ketoacidosis, DVT, encephalopathy, erythema multiforme, facial palsy, hepatotoxic reactions, homicidal ideation, hypersensitivity reactions, injection site necrosis, lower respiratory tract infection, macular edema, MI, myositis, nephrotic syndrome, optic neuritis, pancreatitis, papilledema, parosmia, pericarditis, peripheral neuropathy, pneumonia, pneumonitis, pulmonary infiltrates, pure red cell aplasia, rectal bleeding, renal failure, renal insufficiency, restless leg syndrome, retinal hemorrhages, retinal artery or vein obstruction, retinopathy, rhabdomyolysis, sarcoidosis (including exacerbation), seizures, Stevens-Johnson syndrome, toxic epidermal necrolysis

Use of alfa interferons has been associated with rare cases of autoimmune diseases including vasculitis, systemic lupus erythematosus, thrombocytopenic purpura (idiopathic and thrombotic), and Vogt-Koyanagi-Harada syndrome; altered lipid metabolism (including hypercholesterolemia and hyperlipemia), and pulmonary hypertension

Drug Interactions

Metabolism/Transport Effects Refer to individual components.

Avoid Concomitant Use

Avoid concomitant use of Peginterferon Alfa-2b and Ribavirin with any of the following: CloZAPine; Didanosine; Dipyrone; Telbivudine

Increased Effect/Toxicity

Peginterferon Alfa-2b and Ribavirin may increase the levels/effects of: Aldesleukin; ARIPiprazole; AzaTHIOprine; CloZAPine; CYP1A2 Substrates; CYP2D6 Substrates; Didanosine; Methadone; Reverse Transcriptase Inhibitors (Nucleoside); Ribavirin; Telbivudine

The levels/effects of Peginterferon Alfa-2b and Ribavirin may be increased by: Dipyrone; Interferons (Alfa); Zidovudine

Decreased Effect

Peginterferon Alfa-2b and Ribavirin may decrease the levels/effects of: CYP2D6 Substrates; FLUoxetine; Influenza Virus Vaccine (Live/Attenuated)

The levels/effects of Peginterferon Alfa-2b and Ribavirin may be decreased by: Pegloticase

Preparation for Administration Peginterferon alfa-2b injection:

Vials: Peginterferon alfa-2b powder for injection should be reconstituted with 0.7 mL of SWFI (sterile water for injection) (provided). Roll gentle to form solution; do not shake. Vials are calibrated to provide appropriate dose in a volume of 0.5 mL of resulting solution.

Redipen®: Reconstitute with SWFI (provided). Allow solution to form. Gently turn upside down twice; do not shake. Pen provides appropriate dose in a volume of 0.5 mL of resulting solution.

Hazardous agent (ribavirin); use appropriate precautions for handling and disposal (NIOSH 2014 [group 3]).

Storage/Stability Pegetron® capsule/peginterferon alfa-2b injection combination package: Store under refrigeration between 2°C and 8°C (36°F and 46°F).

When the package is separated:

Pegetron® capsules: Store under refrigeration between 2°C and 8°C (36°F and 46°F) or at room temperature between 15°C to 30°C (59°F to 86°F).

Peginterferon alfa-2b injection:

Vials: Store vial/carton under refrigeration between 2°C and 8°C (36°F and 46°F). Use within 3 hours of reconstitution.

Redipen®: Store under refrigeration between 2°C and 8°C (36°F and 46°F). Immediate use after reconstitution is recommended; however, may be stored up to 24 hours under refrigeration between 2°C and 8°C (36°F and 46°F).

Mechanism of Action

Peginterferon Alfa-2b: Alpha interferons are a family of proteins, produced by nucleated cells that have antiviral, antiproliferative, and immune-regulating activity. There are 16 known subtypes of alpha interferons. Interferons interact with cells through high affinity cell surface receptors. Following activation, multiple effects can be detected including induction of gene transcription. Inhibits cellular growth, alters the state of cellular differentiation, interferes with oncogene expression, alters cell surface antigen expression, increases phagocytic activity of macrophages, and augments cytotoxicity of lymphocytes for target cells.

Ribavirin: Inhibits replication of RNA and DNA viruses; inhibits influenza virus RNA polymerase activity and inhibits the initiation and elongation of RNA fragments resulting in inhibition of viral protein synthesis.

Pharmacodynamics/Kinetics See individual agents.

Dosage Adults: **Note:** Canadian Consensus Guidelines recommend peginterferon plus ribavirin as treatment of choice for chronic hepatitis C (HCV) (Sherman, 2007). American Association for the Study of Liver Diseases (AASLD) practice guidelines also recommend the use of boceprevir or telaprevir in combination with peginterferon plus ribavirin for chronic HCV patients with genotype 1 (Ghany, 2011). Administration of acetaminophen 30 minutes prior to therapy may help reduce fever and headache associated with peginterferon.

Chronic hepatitis C:

Pegetron® peginterferon alfa-2b component: SubQ: 1.5 mcg/kg/week

and

Pegetron® ribavirin component: Oral:

HCV genotype 1 (treatment-naive):

≤65 kg: 800 mg/day (two 200 mg capsules in the morning and two 200 mg capsules in the evening)

66-80 kg: 1000 mg/day (two 200 mg capsules in the morning and three 200 mg capsules in the evening)

81-105 kg: 1200 mg/day (three 200 mg capsules in the morning and three 200 mg capsules in the evening)

>105 kg: 1400 mg/day (three 200 mg capsules in the morning and four 200 mg capsules in the evening)

HCV nongenotype 1 (treatment-naive):

≤65 kg: 800 mg/day (two 200 mg capsules in the morning and two 200 mg capsules in the evening)

66-85 kg: 1000 mg/day (two 200 mg capsules in the morning and three 200 mg capsules in the evening)

>85 kg: 1200 mg/day (three 200 mg capsules in the morning and three 200 mg capsules in the evening)

Retreatment (relapser or nonresponder): Any HCV genotype:

≤65 kg: 800 mg/day (two 200 mg capsules in the morning and two 200 mg capsules in the evening)

66-85 kg: 1000 mg/day (two 200 mg capsules in the morning and three 200 mg capsules in the evening)

86-105 kg: 1200 mg/day (three 200 mg capsules in the morning and three 200 mg capsules in the evening)

>105 kg: 1400 mg/day (three 200 mg capsules in the morning and four 200 mg capsules in the evening)

Treatment duration: Canadian consensus guidelines (Sherman, 2007):

HCV genotype 1: Treatment recommended for 48 weeks or may consider extended therapy up to 72 weeks in slow responders; may reduce treatment to 24 weeks in patients achieving RVR at 4 weeks **and** without poor response predictors (eg, high viral load, advanced fibrosis, elderly); discontinue therapy in patients failing to achieve EVR at 12 weeks or with detectable HCV RNA at 24 weeks; retreatment for 48 weeks is required in patients who relapse after discontinuing abbreviated therapy (24 weeks).

HCV genotypes 2,3: Treatment recommended for 24 weeks; may consider abbreviated therapy (12 or 16 weeks) in patients with weight-based ribavirin dosing and RVR; if relapse occurs following abbreviated therapy, retreat for 24 weeks

HCV genotype 4,5, and 6: Treatment recommended for 48 weeks; discontinue therapy in patients failing to achieve EVR at 12 weeks or with detectable HCV RNA at 24 weeks

Relapsing or nonresponding patients (regardless of genotype): Peginterferon/ribavirin therapy may be considered in patients that have relapsed or were nonresponsive to prior interferon monotherapy or interferon/ribavirin combination therapy; discontinue therapy if EVR not achieved after 12 weeks.

Dosing adjustment in renal impairment:

CrCl ≥50 mL/minute: No dosage adjustment provided in manufacturer's labeling; however, use caution and monitor closely for signs/symptoms of toxicity.

CrCl <50 mL/minute: Use is contraindicated.

Serum creatinine >2 mg/dL: Permanently discontinue therapy in any patient.

Dosing adjustment in hepatic impairment:

Mild or moderate impairment (Child-Pugh class A or B): No dosage adjustment provided in manufacturer's labeling; however, limited data shows C_{max} increases with increasing severity of hepatic impairment.

Severe impairment (Child-Pugh class C): Avoid use.

Indirect bilirubin >5 mg/dL:

HCV genotype 1 (treatment-naive): Continue current peginterferon alfa-2b dose; decrease ribavirin by 200 mg/day if receiving ≤1200 mg/day or by 400 mg/day if receiving 1400 mg/day (first reduction), and by an additional 200 mg/day (second reduction) if necessary.

HCV nongenotype 1 (treatment-naive): Continue current peginterferon alfa-2b dose; decrease ribavirin dose to 600 mg/day.

Relapser or nonresponder (any HCV genotype): Continue current peginterferon alfa-2b dose; decrease ribavirin dose by 200 mg/day if receiving ≤1000 mg/day or by 400 mg/day if receiving ≥1200 mg/day (first reduction), and by an additional 200 mg/day (second reduction) if necessary.

Direct bilirubin >2.5 times ULN or indirect bilirubin >4 mg/dL (for >4 weeks): Permanently discontinue both peginterferon alfa-2b and ribavirin in any patient.

AST/ALT 2 times baseline **and** >10 times ULN: Permanently discontinue both peginterferon alfa-2b and ribavirin in any patient.

Dosing adjustment for toxicity: Note: Recommendations (per manufacturer labeling - also refer to Dosing in renal and hepatic impairment):

Hemoglobin:

HCV genotype 1 (treatment-naive):

Hemoglobin <10 g/dL: Continue current peginterferon alfa-2b dose; decrease ribavirin dose by 200 mg/day if receiving ≤1200 mg/day or by 400 mg/day if receiving 1400 mg/day (first reduction), and by an additional 200 mg/day (second reduction) if necessary.

Hemoglobin decrease ≥2 g/dL in any 4-week period and stable cardiac disease: Decrease peginterferon alfa-2b dose in increments of 0.5 mcg/kg/week; decrease ribavirin dose by 200 mg/day if receiving ≤1200 mg/day or by 400 mg/day if receiving 1400 mg/day (first reduction), and by an additional 200 mg/day (second reduction) if necessary.

Hemoglobin <8.5 g/dL **or** <12 g/dL after ribavirin dose is decreased for 4 weeks and stable cardiac disease: Permanently discontinue both peginterferon alfa-2b and ribavirin.

HCV nongenotype 1 (treatment-naive):

Hemoglobin <10 g/dL: Continue current peginterferon alfa-2b dose; decrease ribavirin dose to 600 mg/day

Hemoglobin decrease ≥2 g/dL in any 4-week period and stable cardiac disease: Decrease peginterferon alfa-2b dose by one-half; decrease ribavirin dose to 600 mg/day

Hemoglobin <8.5 g/dL **or** <12 g/dL after ribavirin dose is decreased for 4 weeks and stable cardiac disease: Permanently discontinue both peginterferon alfa-2b and ribavirin

Relapser or nonresponder (any HCV genotype):

Hemoglobin <10 g/dL: Continue current peginterferon alfa-2b dose; decrease ribavirin dose by 200 mg/day if receiving ≤1000 mg/day or by 400 mg/day if receiving ≥1200 mg/day (first reduction), and by an additional 200 mg/day (second reduction) if necessary.

Hemoglobin decrease ≥2 g/dL in any 4-week period and stable cardiac disease: Decrease peginterferon alfa-2b dose in increments of 0.5 mcg/kg/week; decrease ribavirin dose by 200 mg/day if receiving ≤1000 mg/day or by 400 mg/day if receiving ≥1200 mg/day (first reduction), and by an additional 200 mg/day (second reduction) if necessary.

Hemoglobin <8.5 g/dL **or** <12 g/dL after ribavirin dose is decreased for 4 weeks and stable cardiac disease: Permanently discontinue both peginterferon alfa-2b and ribavirin.

White blood cells:

HCV genotype 1 (treatment-naive) or relapser/nonresponder (any HCV genotype): WBC <1.5 x 10^9/L: Decrease peginterferon alfa-2b dose in increments of 0.5 mcg/kg/week.

HCV nongenotype 1 (treatment-naive): WBC <1.5 x 10^9/L: Decrease peginterferon alfa2b-dose by one-half.

Any patient with WBC <1.0 x 10^9/L: Permanently discontinue peginterferon alfa-2b and ribavirin.

Neutrophils:

HCV genotype 1 (treatment-naive) or relapser/nonresponder (any HCV genotype): Neutrophils <0.75 x 10^9/L: Decrease peginterferon alfa-2b dose in increments of 0.5 mcg/kg/week.

HCV nongenotype 1 (treatment-naive): Neutrophils <0.75 x 10^9/L: Decrease peginterferon alfa-2b dose by one-half.

Any patient with neutrophils <0.5 x 10^9/L: Permanently discontinue peginterferon alfa-2b and ribavirin.

Platelets:

HCV genotype 1 (treatment-naive) or relapser/nonresponder (any HCV genotype):

Platelet count <50 x 10^9/L: Decrease peginterferon alfa-2b dose in increments of 0.5 mcg/kg/week.

Platelet count <25 x 10^9/L: Permanently discontinue peginterferon alfa-2b and ribavirin.

HCV nongenotype 1 (treatment-naive):

Platelet count <80 x 10^9/L: Decrease peginterferon alfa-2b dose by one-half.

Platelet count <50 x 10^9/L: Permanently discontinue peginterferon alfa-2b and ribavirin.

Dietary Considerations Take oral formulation without regard to meals, but always in a consistent manner with respect to food intake (ie, always take with food or always take on an empty stomach).

Administration See individual agents.

Hazardous agent (ribavirin); use appropriate precautions for handling and disposal (NIOSH 2014 [group 3]).

Monitoring Parameters CBC (pretreatment, at weeks 2 and 4 [or more frequently if indicated], and routinely during therapy), renal and liver function tests (pretreatment and routinely during therapy), lipids, TSH, and electrolytes; glucose (diabetic or symptomatic patients); uric acid (patients predisposed to gout); ECG (at baseline and during therapy) in patients with preexisting cardiac disease; pretreatment and monthly pregnancy test for women of childbearing age; dental exams; neuropsychiatric monitoring during and for 6 months after discontinuing therapy (patients developing psychiatric or CNS problems); vision and hearing evaluations

Serum HCV RNA levels (pretreatment, 4-,12-, and 24 weeks after therapy initiation, 24 weeks after completion of therapy)

Reference Range Canadian consensus guidelines (Sherman, 2007):

Rapid virological response (RVR): HCV RNA negative (<50 units/mL) after 4 weeks of treatment

Early virological response (EVR):

Early virological clearance (EVC): HCV RNA negative (<50 units/mL) after 12 weeks of treatment **or**

Partial virological response (PVR): ≥2-log decrease in HCV RNA but still positive for HCV RNA after 12 weeks of treatment

Sustained virological response (SVR): Absence of HCV RNA in the serum 6 months following completion of full treatment course

Product Availability Not available in U.S.

Dosage Forms: Canada

Combination package:

Pegetron®:
Capsule: Ribavirin 200 mg (56s)
Injection, powder for reconstitution: Peginterferon alfa-2b: 50 mcg

Pegetron®:
Capsule: Ribavirin 200 mg (56s)
Injection, powder for reconstitution: Peginterferon alfa-2b: 80 mcg

Pegetron®:
Capsule: Ribavirin 200 mg (56s)
Injection, powder for reconstitution: Peginterferon alfa-2b: 100 mcg

Pegetron®:
Capsule: Ribavirin 200 mg (70s)
Injection, powder for reconstitution: Peginterferon alfa-2b: 120 mcg

Pegetron®:
Capsule: Ribavirin 200 mg (84s, 98s)
Injection, powder for reconstitution: Peginterferon alfa-2b: 150 mcg

Peginterferon Beta-1a

(peg inter FEER on BAY ta wun ay)

Brand Names: U.S. Plegridy; Plegridy Starter Pack

Pharmacologic Category Biological Response Modulator; Immunomodulator, Systemic; Interferon

Use Multiple sclerosis: Treatment of patients with relapsing forms of multiple sclerosis

Pregnancy Risk Factor C

Dosage Multiple sclerosis: Adults: SubQ: Initial: 63 mcg on day 1; 94 mcg on day 15. Maintenance: 125 mcg every 14 days beginning on day 29. **Note:** Analgesics and/or antipyretics may help decrease flu-like symptoms during treatment.

Dosage adjustment in renal impairment: There are no dosage adjustments provided in the manufacturer's labeling; use with caution in severe renal impairment (CrCl <30 mL/minute).

Dosage adjustment in hepatic impairment: There are no dosage adjustments provided in the manufacturer's labeling.

Additional Information Complete prescribing information should be consulted for additional detail.

Dosage Forms

Solution Pen-injector, Subcutaneous:
Plegridy: 125 mcg/0.5 mL (0.5 mL)
Plegridy Starter Pack: 63 mcg/0.5 mL & 95 mcg/0.5 mL (1 mL)

Solution Prefilled Syringe, Subcutaneous:
Plegridy: 125 mcg/0.5 mL (0.5 mL)
Plegridy Starter Pack: 63 mcg/0.5 mL & 95 mcg/0.5 mL (1 mL)

◆ **Peg-Intron** *see* Peginterferon Alfa-2b *on page* 1596

◆ **PegIntron (Can)** *see* Peginterferon Alfa-2b *on page* 1596

◆ **Peg-Intron Redipen** *see* Peginterferon Alfa-2b *on page* 1596

◆ **Peg-Intron Redipen Pak 4** *see* Peginterferon Alfa-2b *on page* 1596

◆ **PEGLA** *see* Pegaspargase *on page* 1588

Pegloticase (peg LOE ti kase)

Brand Names: U.S. Krystexxa

Index Terms PEG-Uricase; Pegylated Urate Oxidase; Polyethylene Glycol-Conjugated Uricase; Recombinant Urate Oxidase, Pegylated; Urate Oxidase, Pegylated

Pharmacologic Category Enzyme; Enzyme, Urate-Oxidase (Recombinant)

Use Treatment of chronic gout refractory to conventional therapy

Pregnancy Risk Factor C

Pregnancy Considerations Adequate animal reproduction studies have not been conducted. There are no adequate and well-controlled studies in pregnant women. Use during pregnancy only if the benefit to the mother outweigh the potential risk to the fetus.

Breast-Feeding Considerations Due to the potential for serious adverse reactions in the nursing infant, breast-feeding is not recommended.

Contraindications Glucose-6-phosphate dehydrogenase (G6PD) deficiency

Warnings/Precautions [U.S. Boxed Warning]: Anaphylaxis and infusion reactions have been reported during and after administration; patients should be closely monitored during infusion and for an appropriate period of time after the infusion. Therapy should be administered in a healthcare facility by skilled medical personnel prepared for the immediate treatment of anaphylaxis. All patients should be premedicated with antihistamines and corticosteroids. Anaphylaxis may occur at any time during treatment (including the initial dose). **Reactions generally occur within 2 hours of administration; however, delayed hypersensitivity reactions have also been reported.** Infusion reactions are varied; symptoms range from chest pain, pruritus/urticaria, or dyspnea to a clinical presentation of anaphylaxis (eg, hemodynamic instability, perioral or lingual edema). If a less severe (nonanaphylactic) infusion reaction occurs, the infusion may be slowed, or stopped and restarted at a slower rate, at the physician's discretion. **Risk of an infusion reaction is increased in patients whose uric acid is >6 mg/dL; therefore, monitor serum uric acid concentrations prior to infusion and consider discontinuing treatment if concentrations exceed 6 mg/dL, particularly in the event of 2 consecutive concentrations >6 mg/dL.** Concurrent use with oral antihyperuricemic agents may delay interpretations of ineffective pegloticase treatment (ie, serum uric acid >6 mg/dL) and ultimately increase risk for anaphylactoid and/or infusion reactions. Discontinue use of oral antihyperuricemic agents prior to and do not initiate during the course of pegloticase therapy.

Therapy with antihyperuricemic agents commonly results in gout flare, particularly upon initiation due to rapid lowering of urate concentrations; gout flare-ups during treatment do not warrant discontinuation of therapy. Gout flare prophylaxis is recommended, using nonsteroidal anti-inflammatory agents (NSAID) or colchicines, unless contraindicated, beginning ≥1 week before initiation of pegloticase and continuing for at least 6 months. Exacerbation of heart failure has been observed in clinical trials; use caution in patients with preexisting heart failure. Due to the risk for hemolysis and methemoglobinemia, pegloticase is contraindicated in patients with G6PD deficiency. Patients at higher risk for G6PD deficiency (eg, African, Mediterranean) should be screened prior to therapy. Therapy is not appropriate for the treatment of asymptomatic hyperuricemia. Potential for immunogenicity exists with the use of therapeutic proteins. Antipegloticase antibodies and antiPEG antibodies commonly occurred during clinical trials in pegloticase-treated patients. High antipegloticase antibody titers were associated with failure to maintain uric acid normalization and were also associated with a higher incidence of infusion reactions. Due to potential for immunogenicity, closely monitor patients who reinitiate therapy after discontinuing treatment for >4 weeks; patients may be at increased risk for anaphylaxis and infusion reactions.

Adverse Reactions

Cardiovascular: Chest pain
Central nervous system: Headache
Dermatologic: Bruising, erythema, pruritus, urticaria
Gastrointestinal: Constipation, diarrhea, nausea, vomiting
Hematologic: Anemia
Neuromuscular & skeletal: Muscle spasms
Renal: Nephrolithiasis
Respiratory: Dyspnea, nasopharyngitis
Miscellaneous: Anaphylaxis, antibody formation, gout flare, infusion reactions

Drug Interactions

Metabolism/Transport Effects None known.

Avoid Concomitant Use

Avoid concomitant use of Pegloticase with any of the following: Allopurinol; Febuxostat; Probenecid

Increased Effect/Toxicity

The levels/effects of Pegloticase may be increased by: Allopurinol; Febuxostat; Probenecid

Decreased Effect

Pegloticase may decrease the levels/effects of: Certolizumab Pegol; Pegademase Bovine; Pegaptanib; Pegaspargase; Pegfilgrastim; Peginterferon Alfa-2a; Peginterferon Alfa-2b; Pegvisomant

Preparation for Administration To prepare solution for administration, withdraw 1 mL (8 mg) and add to a 250 mL bag of NS or 1/2NS; invert bag several times to mix thoroughly (do **not** shake). Do not use vial if particulate matter is present or if solution is discolored (solution should be a clear and colorless). After withdrawal, discard any unused portion of the product remaining in the vial.

Storage/Stability Prior to use, vials must be stored in the carton to protect from light and kept under refrigeration between 2°C to 8°C (36°F to 46°F) at all times. Do **not** shake or freeze.

Diluted solution may be stored up to 4 hours at 2°C to 8°C (36°F to 46°F). Diluted solution is also stable for 4 hours at room temperature of 20°C to 25°C (68°F to 77°F); however, refrigeration is preferred. The diluted solution should be protected from light, not frozen, and used within 4 hours of dilution. Prior to administration, allow the diluted solution to reach room temperature; do not warm to room temperature using any form of artificial heating such as a microwave or warm water bath.

Mechanism of Action Pegloticase is a pegylated recombinant form of urate-oxidase enzyme, also known as uricase (an enzyme normally absent in humans and high primates), which converts uric acid to allantoin (an inactive and water soluble metabolite of uric acid); it does not inhibit the formation of uric acid.

Pharmacodynamics/Kinetics

Onset of action: ~24 hours following the first dose, serum uric acid concentrations decreased
Duration: >300 hours (12.5 days)
Half-life elimination: Median: ~14 days

Dosage Note: Discontinue use of oral antihyperuricemic agents prior to initiating pegloticase and do not initiate during the course of therapy. Premedicate with antihistamines and corticosteroids. Gout flare prophylaxis with either NSAIDs or colchicine is also recommended, beginning at least 1 week prior to initiation and continuing for at least 6 months.

IV: Adults: Refractory gout: 8 mg every 2 weeks

Dosage adjustment in renal impairment: No dosage adjustment necessary.

Dosage adjustment in hepatic impairment: No dosage adjustment provided in manufacturer's labeling (has not been studied).

Administration Administer diluted solution by IV infusion over ≥120 minutes via gravity feed or an infusion pump or syringe-type pump. Do **not** administer by IV push or bolus. Administer in a healthcare setting by healthcare providers prepared to manage potential anaphylaxis. Monitor closely for infusion reactions during infusion and for an appropriate period of time after the infusion (anaphylaxis has been reported within 2 hours of the infusion). In the event or a less severe infusion reaction, infusion may be slowed, or stopped and restarted at a slower rate, based on the discretion of the physician.

Monitoring Parameters Serum uric acid levels (prior to infusions; consider discontinuation if levels increase to >6 mg/dL, especially if two consecutive levels of >6 mg/dL are observed); infusion reactions and anaphylaxis (during infusion and post-infusion), G6PD deficiency screening (in patients at high risk for deficiency)

Reference Range

Uric acid, serum: An increase occurs during childhood
Adults:
Males: 3.4-7 mg/dL or slightly more
Females: 2.4-6 mg/dL or slightly more
Values >7 mg/dL are sometimes arbitrarily regarded as hyperuricemia, but there is no sharp line between normals on the one hand, and the serum uric acid of those with clinical gout. Normal ranges cannot be adjusted for purine ingestion, but high purine diet increases uric acid. Uric acid may be increased with body size, exercise, and stress.

Dosage Forms

Solution, Intravenous:
Krystexxa: 8 mg/mL (1 mL)

◆ **PegLyte (Can)** *see* Polyethylene Glycol-Electrolyte Solution *on page 1674*

◆ **PEG-Uricase** *see* Pegloticase *on page 1602*

Pegvisomant (peg VI soe mant)

Brand Names: U.S. Somavert
Brand Names: Canada Somavert
Index Terms B2036-PEG
Pharmacologic Category Growth Hormone Receptor Antagonist
Use Acromegaly: Treatment of acromegaly in patients who have had an inadequate response to surgery or radiation therapy, or for whom these therapies are not appropriate.
Pregnancy Risk Factor C
Dosage Acromegaly: Adults: SubQ: Initial loading dose: 40 mg; maintenance dose: 10 mg once daily following initial loading dose; doses may be adjusted by 5 mg increments or decrements in 4- to 6-week intervals based on IGF-I concentrations (maximum maintenance dose: 30 mg daily)

Dosage adjustment in renal impairment: There are no dosage adjustments provided in the manufacturer's labeling (has not been studied).

Dosage adjustment in hepatic impairment:

At initiation of therapy:

Normal liver function test (LFT): Initiate therapy; monitor LFT monthly for first 6 months, quarterly for next 6 months, then biannually the following year.

Baseline LFT elevated but ≤3 x ULN: May initiate therapy with monthly evaluation of LFT for 1 year then biannually the following year.

Baseline LFT >3 x ULN: Do not initiate treatment without comprehensive work-up to determine cause; monitor closely if treatment is started.

With ongoing therapy:

LFT ≥3 x but <5 x ULN without signs/symptoms of hepatitis, hepatic injury, or increase in total bilirubin: Continue treatment, but monitor LFT weekly for further increases; perform comprehensive hepatic work-up to rule out alternative cause of hepatic dysfunction

LFT ≥5 x ULN or transaminase ≥3 x ULN associated with any increase in total bilirubin (with or without signs/symptoms of hepatitis or other liver injury): Discontinue immediately and perform comprehensive hepatic work-up. If LFTs return to normal, may cautiously consider restarting therapy with frequent LFT monitoring.

Signs or symptoms of hepatitis or hepatic injury: Perform comprehensive hepatic work-up; discontinue permanently if liver injury is confirmed.

Additional Information Complete prescribing information should be consulted for additional detail.

Dosage Forms

Solution Reconstituted, Subcutaneous:

Somavert: 10 mg (1 ea); 15 mg (1 ea); 20 mg (1 ea); 25 mg (1 ea); 30 mg (1 ea)

◆ **Pegylated DOXOrubicin Liposomal** *see* DOXOrubicin (Liposomal) *on page 684*

◆ **Pegylated G-CSF** *see* Pegfilgrastim *on page 1589*

◆ **Pegylated Interferon Alfa-2a** *see* Peginterferon Alfa-2a *on page 1590*

◆ **Pegylated Interferon Alfa-2b** *see* Peginterferon Alfa-2b *on page 1596*

◆ **Pegylated Liposomal DOXOrubicin** *see* DOXOrubicin (Liposomal) *on page 684*

◆ **Pegylated Liposomal DOXOrubicin Hydrochloride (Doxil®, Caelyx®)** *see* DOXOrubicin (Liposomal) *on page 684*

◆ **Pegylated Urate Oxidase** *see* Pegloticase *on page 1602*

◆ **PEGyLAX** *see* Polyethylene Glycol 3350 *on page 1674*

◆ **PE-Hist-DM [OTC]** *see* Chlorpheniramine, Phenylephrine, and Dextromethorphan *on page 428*

Pembrolizumab (pem broe LIZ ue mab)

Brand Names: U.S. Keytruda
Index Terms Anti-PD-1 Monoclonal Antibody MK-3475; Lambrolizumab; MK-3475; SCH 90045
Pharmacologic Category Antineoplastic Agent, Anti-PD-1 Monoclonal Antibody; Antineoplastic Agent, Monoclonal Antibody
Use Melanoma: Treatment of unresectable or metastatic melanoma with disease progression following ipilimumab and a BRAF inhibitor (if BRAF V600 mutation positive).
Pregnancy Risk Factor D
Pregnancy Considerations Animal reproduction studies have not been conducted. Immunoglobulins are known to cross the placenta; therefore fetal exposure to pembrolizumab is expected. Based on the mechanism of action, pembrolizumab may cause fetal harm if administered during pregnancy; an alteration in the immune response or immune mediated disorders may develop following in utero exposure. Women of reproductive potential should use highly effective contraception during therapy and for four months after treatment is complete.
Breast-Feeding Considerations It is not known if pembrolizumab is excreted into breast milk. The manufacturer recommends that nursing be discontinued during therapy. Immunoglobulins are excreted in breast milk; therefore pembrolizimab may be expected to appear in breast milk.
Contraindications There are no contraindications listed in the manufacturer's labeling.
Warnings/Precautions Immune-mediated pneumonitis has been observed, including cases which were grade 2 and 3. The median time to development was 5 months (range: ~2 days to ~10 months) and the median duration was ~5 months (range: 1 week to 14.4 months). Some patients required initial management with high-dose systemic corticosteroids (median initial prednisone dose of 63.4 mg/day or equivalent), the median duration of initial corticosteroid therapy was 3 days (range: 1 to 34 days) followed by a corticosteroid taper. Most patients with grade 2 or 3 pneumonitis had complete resolution. May require treatment interruption, corticosteroid therapy, or permanent discontinuation. Monitor for signs and symptoms of pneumonitis; if pneumonitis is suspected, evaluate with radiographic imaging and administer systemic corticosteroids for grade 2 or higher pneumonitis.

Immune-mediated colitis (including microscopic colitis) has occurred, including cases of grade 2 or 3 colitis. The median time to onset of colitis was 6.5 months (range: ~2 to 10 months) and the mediation duration was 2.6 months (range: 4 days to 3.6 months). Grade 2 or 3 colitis was managed with high-dose systemic corticosteroids (prednisone ≥40 mg/day [median initial dose 70 mg/day] or equivalent) with a median duration of initial corticosteroid therapy of 7 days (range: 4 to 41 days), followed by a corticosteroid taper. Patients with colitis experienced complete resolution. May require treatment interruption, systemic corticosteroid therapy, or permanent discontinuation. Monitor for signs and symptoms of colitis; administer systemic corticosteroids for grade 2 or higher colitis.

Hepatitis, including autoimmune hepatitis, occurred (case reports, including 1 case of grade 4 hepatitis). The median onset for grade 4 hepatitis was 22 days; the duration was 1.1 months. Grade 4 hepatitis was managed with high-dose systemic corticosteroids (prednisone ≥40 mg/day or equivalent), followed a corticosteroid taper. Monitor for liver function changes. May require treatment interruption, systemic corticosteroids (for grade 2 or higher toxicity), or permanent discontinuation.

Immune-mediated hypophysitis occurred (1 case of grade 2 and one case of grade 4). The time to onset was 1.3 and 1.7 months, respectively. Hypophysitis was managed with high-dose systemic corticosteroids (prednisone ≥40 mg/day or equivalent), followed by a corticosteroid taper. Patients then remained on physiologic corticosteroid replacement. Monitor for signs/symptoms of hypophysitis. May require treatment interruption, systemic corticosteroids (for grade 2 or higher toxicity), or permanent discontinuation.

Nephritis, including autoimmune nephritis (1 case) and interstitial nephritis with renal failure (2 cases), has occurred. The onset for autoimmune nephritis was 11.6 months after the first dose and 5 months after the last dose, and duration was 3.2 months. Acute interstitial nephritis was confirmed by renal biopsy in 2 patients with grades 3/4 renal failure. These cases were managed with high-dose systemic corticosteroids (prednisone ≥40 mg/day or equivalent, followed by a corticosteroid taper), with full recovery. Monitor for renal function changes. May require treatment interruption, systemic corticosteroids (for grade 2 or higher toxicity), or permanent discontinuation.

Immune-mediated hyperthyroidism and hypothyroidism have occurred. The median onset for hyperthyroidism was 1.5 months (range: 2 to 8 weeks), and the median duration was 2.8 months (range: 1 to 6 months). May require management with high-dose systemic corticosteroids (prednisone ≥40 mg/day or equivalent), followed by a corticosteroid taper. Hyperthyroidism resolved in all cases observed in the clinical trial. Hypothyroidism occurred with a median onset of 3.5 months (range: 5 days to 19 months). Hypothyroidism was generally managed with long-term thyroid hormone replacement therapy, although some patients only required short-term replacement therapy. Hypothyroidism did not require systemic corticosteroid therapy or discontinuation. Thyroid disorders may occur at any point in pembrolizumab therapy. Monitor for changes in thyroid function (at baseline, periodically during treatment and as clinically indicated). Administer systemic corticosteroids (for grade 3 or higher hyperthyroidism); may require treatment interruption or permanent discontinuation. Isolated hypothyroidism may be managed with replacement therapy (without corticosteroids and treatment interruption).

Other clinically relevant immune-mediated disorders have been observed, including exfoliative dermatitis, uveitis, arthritis, myositis, pancreatitis, hemolytic anemia, partial seizure (in a patient with inflammatory foci in brain parenchyma), and adrenal insufficiency. Myasthenic syndrome, optic neuritis, and rhabdomyolysis have also been observed in patients receiving pembrolizumab. If an immune-mediated adverse event is suspected, evaluate appropriately; withhold treatment and administer systemic corticosteroids based on severity of reaction. Upon resolution to grade 0 or 1, initiate corticosteroid taper (continue tapering over at least 1 month). If reaction remains at grade 1 or less during taper may reinitiate pembrolizumab. Discontinue permanently for severe or grade 3 immune-mediated adverse event that is recurrent or life-threatening.

Adverse Reactions

Cardiovascular: Peripheral edema

Central nervous system: Chills, dizziness, fatigue, headache, insomnia

Dermatologic: Cellulitis, pruritus, skin rash, vitiligo

Endocrine & metabolic: Hyperglycemia, hyperthyroidism (immune-mediated), hypertriglyceridemia, hypoalbuminemia, hypocalcemia, hyponatremia, hypothyroidism (immune-mediated)

Gastrointestinal: Abdominal pain, colitis (including microscopic colitis), constipation, decreased appetite, diarrhea, nausea, vomiting

Hematologic & oncologic: Anemia

Hepatic: Increased serum AST

Infection: Sepsis

Neuromuscular & skeletal: Arthralgia, back pain, limb pain, myalgia

Renal: Renal failure

Respiratory: Cough, dyspnea, pneumonia, pneumonitis, upper respiratory tract infection

Miscellaneous: Fever

Rare but important or life-threatening: Adrenocortical insufficiency (immune-mediated), arthritis (immune-mediated), exfoliative dermatitis (immune-mediated), hemolytic anemia (immune-mediated), hepatitis (including autoimmune hepatitis; grade 4: <1%), hypophysitis (grade 2: <1%; grade 4: <1%), interstitial nephritis (with renal failure; grade 3: <1%; grade 4: <1%), Lambert-Eaton syndrome (immune-mediated), myositis (immune-mediated), nephritis (grade 2 autoimmune: <1%), optic neuritis (immune-mediated), pancreatitis (immune-mediated), partial epilepsy (immune-mediated; in a patient with inflammatory foci in brain parenchyma), rhabdomyolysis (immune-mediated), uveitis (immune-mediated)

Drug Interactions

Metabolism/Transport Effects None known.

Avoid Concomitant Use There are no known interactions where it is recommended to avoid concomitant use.

Increased Effect/Toxicity There are no known significant interactions involving an increase in effect.

Decreased Effect There are no known significant interactions involving a decrease in effect.

Preparation for Administration

Injection solution (100 mg/4 mL vial): Withdraw appropriate volume from vial and transfer to IV bag containing 0.9% sodium chloride or D_5W; final concentration should be between 1 to 10 mg/mL. Mix by gently inverting bag. Discard unused portion of the vial.

Lyophilized powder (50 mg vial): Reconstitute by adding 2.3 mL SWFI along the vial wall (do not add directly to lyophilized powder); resulting vial concentration is 25 mg/mL. Slowly swirl vial; do not shake. Allow up to 5 minutes for bubbles to dissipate. Reconstituted solution is a clear to slightly opalescent and colorless to slightly yellow solution; discard if visible particles present. Withdraw appropriate volume from vial and transfer to IV bag containing 0.9% sodium chloride or D_5W final concentration should be between 1 to 10 mg/mL. Mix by gently inverting bag. Discard unused portion of the vial.

Storage/Stability Lyophilized powder (50 mg vial) and injection solution (100 mg/4 mL vial): Store intact vials refrigerated at 2°C to 8°C (36°F to 46°F); protect injection solution vials from light and do not shake or freeze. Reconstituted solutions and solutions diluted for infusion may be stored at room temperature for up to 6 hours (infusion must be completed within 6 hours of reconstitution) or refrigerated at 2°C to 8°C (36°F to 46°F) for no more than 24 hours from the time of reconstitution. Do not freeze. If refrigerated, allow to reach room temperature prior to administration.

Mechanism of Action Highly selective anti-PD-1 humanized monoclonal antibody which inhibits programmed cell death-1 (PD-1) activity by binding to the PD-1 receptor on T-cells to block PD-1 ligands (PD-L1 and PD-L2) from binding. Blocking the PD-1 pathway inhibits the negative immune regulation caused by PD-1 receptor signaling (Hamid, 2013). Anti-PD-1 antibodies (including pembrolizumab) reverse T-cell suppression and induce antitumor responses (Robert, 2014).

Pharmacodynamics/Kinetics Half-life elimination: 26 days

Dosage Melanoma, unresectable or metastatic: Adults: IV: 2 mg/kg once every 3 weeks until disease progression or unacceptable toxicity.

Dosage adjustment for toxicity: Note: High-dose systemic corticosteroid therapy refers to ≥40 mg/day of prednisone or equivalent.

Withhold treatment for any of the following (may resume upon recovery to grade 0 or 1 toxicity):

Colitis, moderate (grade 2) or severe (grade 3); also administer high-dose systemic corticosteroids (followed by a taper).

Hyperthyroidism, severe (grade 3); also administer high-dose systemic corticosteroids (followed by a taper).

Hypophysitis, grade 2 (symptomatic); also administer high-dose systemic corticosteroids (followed by a taper).

Nephritis, grade 2; also administer high-dose systemic corticosteroids (followed by a taper).

Pneumonitis, grade 2; also administer high-dose systemic corticosteroids (followed by a taper).

Other treatment-related toxicity, severe or grade 3; may require high-dose systemic corticosteroids (based on severity). Upon improvement to grade 0 or 1, initiate corticosteroid taper and continue to taper over at least 1 month. Restart pembrolizumab if the adverse reaction remains at grade 0 or 1.

Withhold (may resume upon recovery to grade 0 or 1 toxicity) or discontinue for: Hypophysitis, severe (grade 3); also administer high-dose systemic corticosteroids

Permanently discontinue for:

Adverse reactions that are life-threatening, persistent grade 2 or 3 adverse reaction that does not recover to grade 0 or 1 within 12 weeks after the last pembrolizumab dose, or any recurrent severe or grade 3 treatment-related adverse reaction. Also administer high-dose systemic corticosteroids.

Colitis, life-threatening (grade 4); also administer high-dose systemic corticosteroids.

Hyperthyroidism, life-threatening (grade 4); also administer high-dose systemic corticosteroids.

Hypophysitis, life-threatening (grade 4); also administer high-dose systemic corticosteroids.

Immune mediated adverse reactions: Discontinue permanently if unable to reduce corticosteroid dose to prednisone ≤10 mg/day (or equivalent) within 12 weeks.

Infusion-related reaction, grade 3 or 4.

Nephritis, severe (grade 3) or life-threatening (grade 4); also administer high-dose systemic corticosteroids.

Pneumonitis, severe (grade 3) or life-threatening (grade 4); also administer high-dose systemic corticosteroids.

Dosage adjustment in renal impairment: No dosage adjustment necessary. In a pharmacokinetic study, no difference in clearance was noted for patients with mild, moderate, or severe impairment (eGFR ≥15 mL/minute to 89 mL/minute) when compared to patients with normal renal function (eGFR ≥90 mL/minute); patients with eGFR <15 mL/minute were not studied.

Dosage adjustment in hepatic impairment:

*Hepatic impairment **prior** to treatment initiation:*

Mild impairment (total bilirubin ≤ULN and AST >ULN or total bilirubin >1 to 1.5 times ULN and any AST): No dosage adjustment is necessary.

Moderate (total bilirubin >1.5 to 3 times ULN and any AST) to severe (total bilirubin >3 times ULN and any AST) impairment: There are no dosage adjustments provided in the manufacturer's labeling (has not been studied).

*Hepatotoxicity **during** treatment (administer high-dose systemic corticosteroids in addition to withholding or discontinuing treatment):* **Note:** For patients with baseline grade 2 ALT or AST abnormalities due to liver metastases, permanently discontinue if AST or ALT increases by ≥50% (relative to baseline) and persists at least 1 week.

AST or ALT >3 to 5 times ULN or total bilirubin >1.5 to 3 times ULN: Withhold treatment; may resume therapy upon recovery to grade 0 or 1 toxicity.

AST or ALT >5 times ULN or total bilirubin >3 times ULN: Permanently discontinue.

Administration IV: Infuse over 30 minutes through a 0.2 to 5 micron sterile, nonpyrogenic, low-protein binding inline or add-on filter. Do not infuse other medications through the same infusion line.

Monitoring Parameters Liver function tests (AST, ALT, and total bilirubin; monitor for changes in liver function); monitor for renal function changes; monitor for changes in thyroid function (at baseline, periodically during treatment and as clinically indicated). Monitor for signs/symptoms of colitis, hypophysitis, pneumonitis, infusion reactions.

Dosage Forms

Solution, Intravenous [preservative free]:

Keytruda: 100 mg/4 mL (4 mL)

Solution Reconstituted, Intravenous [preservative free]:

Keytruda: 50 mg (1 ea)

PEMEtrexed (pem e TREKS ed)

Brand Names: U.S. Alimta

Brand Names: Canada Alimta

Index Terms LY231514; Pemetrexed Disodium

Pharmacologic Category Antineoplastic Agent, Antimetabolite; Antineoplastic Agent, Antimetabolite (Antifolate)

Use

Mesothelioma: Treatment of unresectable malignant pleural mesothelioma (in combination with cisplatin)

Non-small cell lung cancer (NSCLC), nonsquamous: Treatment of locally advanced or metastatic **non**squamous NSCLC (as initial treatment in combination with cisplatin, as single-agent maintenance treatment after 4 cycles of initial platinum-based double therapy, and single-agent treatment after prior chemotherapy)

Limitation of use: Not indicated for the treatment of **squamous** cell NSCLC

Pregnancy Risk Factor D

Pregnancy Considerations Adverse effects (embryotoxicity, fetotoxicity and teratogenicity) were observed in animal reproduction studies. Based on the mechanism of action, may cause fetal harm if administered to a pregnant woman. Women of childbearing potential should have a negative serum pregnancy test prior to treatment and should use effective contraceptive measures to avoid becoming pregnant during treatment. Irreversible infertility has been reported in males; prior to receiving treatment, males should be counseled on sperm storage. The Canadian labeling recommends that males receiving therapy use effective contraceptive measures and not father a child during, and for up to 6 months after therapy.

Breast-Feeding Considerations According to the manufacturer, the decision to continue or discontinue breastfeeding during therapy should take into account the risk of exposure to the infant and the benefits of treatment to the mother.

Contraindications Severe hypersensitivity to pemetrexed or any component of the formulation

Canadian labeling (additional contraindications; not in U.S. labeling): Concomitant yellow fever vaccine

Warnings/Precautions Hazardous agent - use appropriate precautions for handling and disposal (NIOSH 2014 [group 1]). Hypersensitivity (including anaphylaxis) has been reported with use. May cause bone marrow suppression (anemia, neutropenia, thrombocytopenia and/or pancytopenia); frequent laboratory monitoring is necessary

(myelosuppression is often dose-limiting). Dose reductions in subsequent cycles may be required. Prophylactic folic acid and vitamin B_{12} supplements are necessary to reduce hematologic and gastrointestinal toxicity and infection; initiate supplementation 1 week before the first dose of pemetrexed. Pretreatment with dexamethasone is necessary to reduce the incidence and severity of cutaneous reactions. Rarely, Stevens-Johnson syndrome and toxic epidermal necrolysis have been reported. Although the effect of third space fluid is not fully defined, studies have determined pemetrexed concentrations in patients with mild-to-moderate ascites/pleural effusions were similar to concentrations in trials of patients without third space fluid accumulation. Drainage of fluid from ascites/effusions may be considered, but is not likely necessary. Use caution with hepatic dysfunction not due to metastases; may require dose adjustment. Interstitial pneumonitis with respiratory insufficiency has been observed with use; interrupt therapy and evaluate promptly with progressive dyspnea and cough.

The manufacturer does not recommend use in patients with CrCl <45 mL/minute. Decreased renal function results in increased toxicity. Potentially significant drug-drug interactions may exist, requiring dose or frequency adjustment, additional monitoring, and/or selection of alternative therapy. Use caution in patients receiving concurrent nephrotoxins; may result in delayed pemetrexed clearance. NSAIDs may reduce the clearance of pemetrexed. In patients with CrCl 45-79 mL/minute, interruption of NSAID therapy may be necessary prior to, during, and immediately after pemetrexed therapy. Not indicated for use in patients with squamous cell NSCLC.

Adverse Reactions

Cardiovascular: Edema

Central nervous system: Fatigue (dose-limiting), fever

Dermatologic: Alopecia, erythema multiforme, pruritus, rash/desquamation

Gastrointestinal: Abdominal pain, anorexia, constipation, diarrhea, nausea, stomatitis, vomiting, weight loss

Hematologic: Anemia, febrile neutropenia, leukopenia, neutropenia (dose-limiting; nadir: 8-10 days; recovery: 4-8 days after nadir), thrombocytopenia (dose-limiting)

Hepatic: ALT increased, AST increased

Neuromuscular & skeletal: Neuropathy (sensory and motor)

Ocular: Conjunctivitis, lacrimation increased

Renal: Creatinine clearance decreased, creatinine increased

Respiratory: Pharyngitis

Miscellaneous: Allergic reaction/hypersensitivity, infection, sepsis

Rare but important or life-threatening: Arrhythmia, colitis, dehydration, esophagitis, gastrointestinal obstruction, hemolytic anemia, hepatobiliary failure, hypertension, interstitial pneumonitis, pancreatitis, pancytopenia, peripheral ischemia, pulmonary embolism, radiation recall (median onset: 6 days; range: 1-35 days), renal failure, Stevens-Johnson syndrome, supraventricular arrhythmia, syncope, thrombosis/embolism, toxic epidermal necrolysis, ventricular tachycardia

Drug Interactions

Metabolism/Transport Effects None known.

Avoid Concomitant Use

Avoid concomitant use of PEMEtrexed with any of the following: BCG; CloZAPine; Dipyrone; Natalizumab; Pimecrolimus; Tacrolimus (Topical); Tofacitinib; Vaccines (Live)

Increased Effect/Toxicity

PEMEtrexed may increase the levels/effects of: CloZAPine; Leflunomide; Natalizumab; Tofacitinib; Vaccines (Live)

The levels/effects of PEMEtrexed may be increased by: Denosumab; Dipyrone; NSAID (Nonselective); Pimecrolimus; Roflumilast; Tacrolimus (Topical); Trastuzumab

Decreased Effect

PEMEtrexed may decrease the levels/effects of: BCG; Coccidioides immitis Skin Test; Sipuleucel-T; Vaccines (Inactivated); Vaccines (Live)

The levels/effects of PEMEtrexed may be decreased by: Echinacea

Preparation for Administration Hazardous agent; use appropriate precautions for handling and disposal (NIOSH 2014 [group 1]). Reconstitute with NS (preservative free); add 4.2 mL to the 100 mg vial and 20 mL to the 500 mg vial, resulting in a 25 mg/mL concentration. Gently swirl. Solution may be colorless to green-yellow. Further dilute in 100 mL NS prior to infusion (the manufacturer recommends a total volume of 100 mL); may also dilute in D_5W (Zhang, 2006), although the manufacturer recommends NS.

Storage/Stability Store intact vials at room temperature of 25°C (77°F); excursions permitted to 15°C to 30°C (59°F to 86°F). Reconstituted solution in NS and infusion solutions (in D_5W or NS) are stable for 24 hours when refrigerated at 2°C to 8°C (36°F to 46°F). Concentrations at 25 mg/mL are stable in polypropylene syringes for 2 days at room temperature (23°C) (Zhang, 2005).

Mechanism of Action Antifolate; disrupts folate-dependent metabolic processes essential for cell replication. Inhibits thymidylate synthase (TS), dihydrofolate reductase (DHFR), glycinamide ribonucleotide formyltransferase (GARFT), and aminoimidazole carboxamide ribonucleotide formyltransferase (AICARFT), the enzymes involved in folate metabolism and DNA synthesis, resulting in inhibition of purine and thymidine nucleotide and protein synthesis.

Pharmacodynamics/Kinetics

Distribution: V_{dss}: 16.1 L

Protein binding: ~73% to 81%

Metabolism: Minimal

Half-life elimination: Normal renal function: 3.5 hours; CrCl 40 to 59 mL/minute: 5.3 to 5.8 hours

Excretion: Urine (70% to 90% as unchanged drug)

Dosage Note: Start vitamin supplements 1 week before initial pemetrexed dose: Folic acid 400 to 1000 mcg daily orally (begin 7 days prior to treatment initiation; continue daily during treatment and for 21 days after last pemetrexed dose) and vitamin B_{12} 1000 mcg IM 7 days prior to treatment initiation and then every 3 cycles. Give dexamethasone 4 mg orally twice daily for 3 days, beginning the day before treatment to minimize cutaneous reactions. New treatment cycles should not begin unless ANC ≥1500/mm^3, platelets ≥100,000/mm^3, and CrCl ≥45 mL/minute.

Malignant pleural mesothelioma: Adults: IV: 500 mg/m^2 on day 1 of each 21-day cycle (in combination with cisplatin) **or** (off-label) in combination with carboplatin (Castagneto, 2008; Ceresoli, 2006) **or** (off-label) as single-agent therapy (Jassem, 2008; Taylor, 2008)

Non-small cell lung cancer, nonsquamous: Adults: IV:

Initial treatment: 500 mg/m^2 on day 1 of each 21-day cycle (in combination with cisplatin)

Maintenance or second-line treatment: 500 mg/m^2 on day 1 of each 21-day cycle (as a single-agent)

Bladder cancer, metastatic (off-label use): Adults: IV: 500 mg/m^2 on day 1 of each 21-day cycle until disease progression or unacceptable toxicity (Sweeney, 2006)

Cervical cancer, persistent or recurrent (off-label use): Adults: IV: 500 mg/m^2 on day 1 of each 21-day cycle until disease progression or unacceptable toxicity occurs (Lorusso, 2010) **or** 900 mg/m^2 on day 1 of each 21-day cycle (Miller, 2008)

Ovarian cancer, platinum-resistant (off-label use): Adults: IV: 500 mg/m^2 on day 1 of each 21-day cycle (Vergote, 2009)

Thymic malignancies, metastatic (off-label use): Adults: IV: 500 mg/m^2 on day 1 of each 21-day cycle for 6 cycles or until disease progression or unacceptable toxicity occurs (Loehrer, 2006)

Dosage adjustments for toxicities:

Toxicity: Discontinue if patient develops grade 3 or 4 toxicity after two dose reductions or immediately if grade 3 or 4 neurotoxicity develops

Hematologic toxicity: Upon recovery, reinitiate therapy

Nadir ANC <500/mm^3 and nadir platelets ≥50,000/mm^3: Reduce dose to 75% of previous dose of pemetrexed (and cisplatin)

Nadir platelets <50,000/mm^3 **without bleeding** (regardless of nadir ANC): Reduce dose to 75% of previous dose of pemetrexed (and cisplatin)

Nadir platelets <50,000/mm^3 **with bleeding** (regardless of nadir ANC): Reduce dose to 50% of previous dose of pemetrexed (and cisplatin)

Nonhematologic toxicity ≥ grade 3 (excluding neurotoxicity): Withhold treatment until recovery to baseline; upon recovery, reinitiate therapy as follows:

Grade 3 or 4 toxicity (excluding mucositis): Reduce dose to 75% of previous dose of pemetrexed (and cisplatin)

Grade 3 or 4 diarrhea or any diarrhea requiring hospitalization: Reduce dose to 75% of previous dose of pemetrexed (and cisplatin)

Grade 3 or 4 mucositis: Reduce pemetrexed dose to 50% of previous dose (continue cisplatin at 100% of previous dose)

Neurotoxicity:

Grade 0 to 1: Continue pemetrexed at 100% of previous dose (and cisplatin)

Grade 2: Continue pemetrexed at 100% of previous dose; reduce cisplatin dose to 50% of previous dose

Dosage adjustment in renal impairment: Renal function may be estimated using the Cockcroft-Gault formula (using actual body weight) or glomerular filtration rate (GFR) measured by Tc99m-DPTA serum clearance.

CrCl ≥45 mL/minute: No dosage adjustment necessary.

CrCl <45 mL/minute: Use is not recommended (an insufficient number of patients have been studied for dosage recommendations).

Concomitant NSAID use with renal dysfunction:

CrCl ≥80 mL/minute: No dosage adjustment necessary.

CrCl 45 to 79 mL/minute and NSAIDs with short half-lives (eg, ibuprofen, indomethacin, ketoprofen, ketorolac): Avoid NSAID for 2 days before, the day of, and for 2 days following a dose of pemetrexed

Any creatinine clearance and NSAIDs with long half-lives (eg, nabumetone, naproxen, oxaprozin, piroxicam): Avoid NSAID for 5 days before, the day of, and 2 days following a dose of pemetrexed

Dosage adjustment in hepatic impairment: Grade 3 (5.1 to 20 times ULN) **or** 4 (>20 times ULN) transaminase elevation during treatment: Reduce pemetrexed dose to 75% of previous dose (and cisplatin)

Dosing in obesity: *ASCO Guidelines for appropriate chemotherapy dosing in obese adults with cancer:* Utilize patient's actual body weight (full weight) for calculation of body surface area- or weight-based dosing, particularly when the intent of therapy is curative; manage regimen-related toxicities in the same manner as for nonobese patients; if a dose reduction is utilized due to toxicity, consider resumption of full weight-based dosing with subsequent cycles, especially if cause of toxicity (eg, hepatic or renal impairment) is resolved (Griggs, 2012).

Dietary Considerations Initiate folic acid supplementation 1 week before first dose of pemetrexed, continue for full course of therapy, and for 21 days after last dose. Institute vitamin B_{12} 1 week before the first dose; administer every 9 weeks thereafter.

Administration IV: Infuse over 10 minutes. Hazardous agent; use appropriate precautions for handling and disposal (NIOSH 2014 [group 1]).

Monitoring Parameters CBC with differential and platelets (before each dose; monitor for nadir and recovery); serum creatinine, creatinine clearance, BUN, total bilirubin, ALT, AST (periodic); signs/symptoms of mucositis and diarrhea

Dosage Forms

Solution Reconstituted, Intravenous:

Alimta: 100 mg (1 ea); 500 mg (1 ea)

◆ **Pemetrexed Disodium** *see* PEMEtrexed *on page* 1606

Penciclovir (pen SYE kloe veer)

Brand Names: U.S. Denavir

Pharmacologic Category Antiviral Agent

Use Topical treatment of recurrent herpes simplex labialis (cold sores)

Pregnancy Risk Factor B

Dosage Children ≥12 years and Adults: Topical: Apply cream at the first sign or symptom of cold sore (eg, tingling, swelling); apply every 2 hours during waking hours for 4 days

Additional Information Complete prescribing information should be consulted for additional detail.

Dosage Forms

Cream, External:

Denavir: 1% (5 g)

PenicillAMINE (pen i SIL a meen)

Brand Names: U.S. Cuprimine; Depen Titratabs

Brand Names: Canada Cuprimine®

Index Terms D-3-Mercaptovaline; D-Penicillamine; β,β-Dimethylcysteine

Pharmacologic Category Chelating Agent

Use Treatment of Wilson's disease, cystinuria; adjunctive treatment of severe, active rheumatoid arthritis

Canadian labeling: Additional use (not in U.S. labeling): Treatment of chronic lead poisoning

Pregnancy Risk Factor D

Dosage Oral: **Note:** Dose reduction to 250 mg/day may be considered prior to surgical procedures. May resume normal recommended dosing postoperatively once wound healing is complete.

Cystinuria: **Note:** Adjust dose to limit cystine excretion to 100-200 mg/day (<100 mg/day with history of stone formation)

Children: 30 mg/kg/day in 4 divided doses

Adults: 1-4 g/day in 4 divided doses; usual dose: 2 g/day; initiation of therapy at 250 mg/day with gradual upward titration may reduce the risk of unwanted effects

Lead poisoning:

Canadian labeling:

Children: 30-40 mg/kg/day or 600-750 mg/m^2/day in 1-2 divided doses (maximum dose: 750 mg/day); treat until blood lead concentrations <40 mcg/dL for 2 consecutive months and at least 1 of the following: Decrease in erythrocyte protoporphyrin level to <3-5 times the average normal level or the excretion of coproporphyrin or delta-aminolevulinic acid decreases to the upper limit of normal. **Note:** Manufacturer labeling recommends initiating therapy only in children who meet the following criteria: Asymptomatic, blood lead concentrations of 50-80 mcg/dL, erythrocyte protoporphyrin level >400-500 mcg/dL erythrocytes, excessive excretion of delta-aminolevulinic acid and/or coproporphyrin.

Adults: 900-1500 mg/day in 3 divided doses for 1-2 weeks, then 750 mg/day in divided doses until blood lead concentrations <60 mcg/dL or urinary lead excretion <500 mcg/L for 2 consecutive months

Alternate recommendations (off-label dosing): **Note:** The American Academy of Pediatrics (AAP) considers penicillamine a third-line agent for the management of lead poisoning (AAP, 2005; Chandran, 2010): Children: 10-15 mg/kg/day for 4-12 weeks (Chandran, 2010). **Note:** The CDC recommends chelation treatment when blood lead concentrations are >45 mcg/dL (CDC, 2002). Children with blood lead concentrations >70 mcg/dL or symptomatic lead poisoning should be treated with parenteral agents (AAP, 2005).

Rheumatoid arthritis:

Children (off-label use): Initial: 3 mg/kg/day (≤250 mg/day) for 3 months, then 6 mg/kg/day (≤500 mg/day) in divided doses twice daily for 3 months to a maximum of 10 mg/kg/day in 3-4 divided doses; maximum dose: 750 mg/day (Rosenberg, 1989)

Adults: Initial: 125-250 mg/day, may increase dose by 125-250 mg/day at 1- to 3-month intervals up to 1-1.5 g/day; discontinue in patients failing to improve after 3-4 months at these doses

Elderly: Therapy should be initiated at low end of dosing range and titrated upward cautiously.

Wilson's disease: **Note:** Dose that results in an initial 24-hour urinary copper excretion >2 mg/day should be continued for ~3 months; maintenance dose defined by amount resulting in <10 mcg serum free copper/dL.

Manufacturer labeling recommendations:

Adults: 750-1500 mg/day in divided doses; maximum dose: 2000 mg/day. **Note:** Limit daily dose to 750 mg/day (U.S. labeling) or 1000 mg/day (Canadian labeling) in pregnant women; if planned caesarian, limit dose to 250 mg/day during the last 6 weeks of pregnancy and postoperatively until wound healing is complete.

Elderly: Therapy should be initiated at low end of dosing range and titrated upward cautiously.

Alternate recommendations (off-label dosing): American Association for the Study of Liver Diseases (AASLD) guidelines (Roberts, 2008):

Children: 20 mg/kg/day in 2-3 divided doses, round off to the nearest 250 mg dose

Adults: To increase tolerability, therapy may be initiated at 250-500 mg/day then titrated upward in 250 mg increments every 4-7 days; usual maintenance dose: 750-1000 mg/day in 2 divided doses; maximum: 1000-1500 mg/day in 2-4 divided doses

Dosing adjustment in renal impairment:

Manufacturer labeling recommendations: No dosage adjustment provided in manufacturer's labeling; however, the manufacturer labeling does suggest a cautious approach to dosing as this drug undergoes mainly renal elimination.

Alternate recommendations:

CrCl <50 mL/minute: Avoid use (Aronoff, 2007)

Hemodialysis: Dialyzable; Administer 33% of usual dose (Aronoff, 2007); a dosing decrease from 250 mg/day to 250 mg 3 times/week after dialysis has been suggested in the treatment of rheumatoid arthritis (Swarup, 2004).

Dosage adjustment in hepatic impairment: No dosage adjustment provided in manufacturer's labeling; however, only a small fraction is metabolized hepatically.

Additional Information Complete prescribing information should be consulted for additional detail.

Dosage Forms

Capsule, Oral:

Cuprimine: 250 mg

Tablet, Oral:

Depen Titratabs: 250 mg

Penicillin G Benzathine

(pen i SIL in jee BENZ a theen)

Brand Names: U.S. Bicillin L-A

Brand Names: Canada Bicillin L-A

Index Terms Benzathine Benzylpenicillin; Benzathine Penicillin G; Benzylpenicillin Benzathine

Pharmacologic Category Antibiotic, Penicillin

Use Acute glomerulonephritis: Prophylaxis (secondary) in patients with a history of acute glomerulonephritis

Respiratory tract infections: Treatment of mild to moderate upper respiratory tract infections caused by streptococci susceptible to low, prolonged serum concentrations of penicillin G

Rheumatic fever and chorea: Prophylaxis (secondary) of rheumatic fever and/or chorea

Rheumatic heart disease: Prophylaxis (secondary) in patients with rheumatic heart disease

Syphilis and other venereal diseases: Treatment of syphilis, yaws, bejel, and pinta

Pregnancy Risk Factor B

Pregnancy Considerations Adverse events have not been observed in animal reproduction studies. Penicillin crosses the placenta and distributes into amniotic fluid. Maternal use of penicillins has generally not resulted in an increased risk of adverse fetal effects. Penicillin G is the drug of choice for treatment of syphilis during pregnancy.

Breast-Feeding Considerations Penicillins are excreted in breast milk. The manufacturer recommends that caution be exercised when administering penicillin to nursing women. Nondose-related effects could include modification of bowel flora and allergic sensitization.

Contraindications Hypersensitivity to penicillin(s) or any component of the formulation

Warnings/Precautions Use with caution in patients with impaired renal function, seizure disorder, or history of hypersensitivity to other beta-lactams. Serious anaphylactic reactions require immediate emergency treatment with epinephrine, oxygen, intravenous steroids and airway management (including intubation) as indicated. CDC and AAP do not currently recommend the use of penicillin G benzathine to treat congenital syphilis or neurosyphilis due to reported treatment failures and lack of published clinical data on its efficacy. Use only for infections susceptible to the low and very prolonged serum concentrations of benzathine penicillin G. Prolonged use may result in fungal or bacterial superinfection, including *C. difficile*-associated diarrhea (CDAD) and pseudomembranous colitis; CDAD has been observed >2 months postantibiotic treatment. **[U.S. Boxed Warning]: Not for intravenous use; cardiopulmonary arrest and death have occurred from inadvertent IV administration;** administer by deep IM injection only; injection into or near an artery or nerve could result in severe neurovascular damage or permanent neurological damage. Quadriceps femoris fibrosis and atrophy have been reported after repeated IM injections of penicillin preparations into the anterolateral thigh. Extended duration of therapy or use associated with high serum concentrations may be associated with an increased risk for some adverse reactions.

Adverse Reactions

Cardiovascular: Cardiac arrest, cerebral vascular accident, cyanosis, gangrene, hypotension, pallor, palpitations, syncope, tachycardia, vasodilation, vasospasm, vasovagal reaction

Central nervous system: Anxiety, coma, confusion, dizziness, euphoria, fatigue, headache, nervousness, pain, seizure, somnolence

In addition, a syndrome of CNS symptoms has been reported which includes: Severe agitation with confusion, hallucinations (auditory and visual), and fear of death (Hoigne's syndrome); other symptoms include cyanosis, dizziness, palpitations, psychosis, seizures, tachycardia, taste disturbance, tinnitus

Gastrointestinal: Bloody stool, intestinal necrosis, nausea, vomiting

Genitourinary: Impotence, priapism

Hepatic: AST increased

Local: Injection site reactions: Abscess, atrophy, bruising, cellulitis, edema, hemorrhage, inflammation, lump, necrosis, pain, skin ulcer

Neuromuscular & skeletal: Arthritis exacerbation, joint disorder, neurovascular damage, numbness, periostitis, rhabdomyolysis, transverse myelitis, tremor, weakness

Ocular: Blindness, blurred vision

Renal: BUN increased, creatinine increased, hematuria, myoglobinuria, neurogenic bladder, proteinuria, renal failure

Miscellaneous: Diaphoresis, hypersensitivity reactions, Jarisch-Herxheimer reaction, lymphadenopathy, mottling, warmth

Drug Interactions

Metabolism/Transport Effects **Substrate** of OAT3

Avoid Concomitant Use

Avoid concomitant use of Penicillin G Benzathine with any of the following: BCG; Probenecid

Increased Effect/Toxicity

Penicillin G Benzathine may increase the levels/effects of: Methotrexate; Vitamin K Antagonists

The levels/effects of Penicillin G Benzathine may be increased by: Probenecid; Teriflunomide

Decreased Effect

Penicillin G Benzathine may decrease the levels/effects of: BCG; Mycophenolate; Sodium Picosulfate; Typhoid Vaccine

The levels/effects of Penicillin G Benzathine may be decreased by: Tetracycline Derivatives

Storage/Stability Store at 2°C to 8°C (36°F to 46°F); do not freeze. The following stability information has also been reported: May be stored at 25°C (77°F) for 7 days (Cohen, 2007).

Mechanism of Action Interferes with bacterial cell wall synthesis during active multiplication, causing cell wall death and resultant bactericidal activity against susceptible bacteria

Pharmacodynamics/Kinetics

Duration: 1 to 4 weeks (dose dependent); larger doses result in more sustained levels

Distribution: Highest levels in the kidney; lesser amounts in liver, skin, intestines

Protein Binding: ~60%

Absorption: IM: Slow

Excretion: Urine

Dosage Note: Administer undiluted injection; higher doses result in more sustained rather than higher levels. Use a penicillin G benzathine-penicillin G procaine combination to achieve early peak levels in acute infections.

Usual dosage range:

Children: IM: 50,000 units/kg as a single dose (maximum: 2.4 million units)

Adults: IM: 1.2 to 2.4 million units as a single dose

Indication-specific dosing:

Infants and Children: IM:

Upper respiratory infection, group A streptococci (eg, pharyngitis): Manufacturer's recommendations: <27.3 kg: 300,000 to 600,000 units as a single dose. Manufacturer labeling does not provide specific recommendation for children ≥27.3 kg.

For older children, a dose of 900,000 units as a single dose is recommended.

Primary prevention of rheumatic fever: ≤27 kg: 600,000 units as a single dose; >27 kg: 1.2 million units as a single dose (Gerber, 2009)

Secondary prevention of rheumatic fever: ≤27 kg: 600,000 units every 3-4 weeks; >27 kg: 1.2 million units every 3 to 4 weeks (Gerber, 2009)

Pharyngitis, group A streptococci (IDSA guidelines):

Acute treatment: <27 kg: 600,000 units as a single dose; ≥27 kg: 1.2 million units as a single dose (Shulman, 2012)

Chronic carrier treatment: <27 kg: 600,000 units as a single dose (in combination with oral rifampin); ≥27 kg: 1.2 million units as a single dose (in combination with oral rifampin) (Shulman, 2012)

Syphilis (CDC, 2010):

Primary, Secondary, Early Latent (<1 year duration): Infants and Children: IM: 50,000 units/kg as a single injection (maximum: 2.4 million units)

Late Latent, Latent with unknown duration: Children: IM: 50,000 units/kg every week for 3 doses (maximum: 2.4 million units/dose)

Adults: IM:

Upper respiratory infection, group A streptococci: 1.2 million units as a single dose

Secondary prevention of glomerulonephritis: 1.2 million units every 4 weeks or 600,000 units twice monthly

Secondary prevention of rheumatic fever: 1.2 million units every 3 to 4 weeks or 600,000 units twice monthly (Gerber, 2009)

Pharyngitis, group A streptococci (IDSA guidelines):

Acute treatment: 1.2 million units as a single dose (Shulman, 2012)

Chronic carrier treatment: 1.2 million units as a single dose in combination with oral rifampin (Shulman, 2012)

Syphilis (CDC, 2010):

Primary, Secondary, Early Latent (<1 year duration): 2.4 million units as a single dose

Late Latent, Latent with unknown duration: 2.4 million units once weekly for 3 doses

Neurosyphilis: Not indicated as single-drug therapy, but may be given once weekly for 3 weeks following IV treatment; refer to Penicillin G (Parenteral/Aqueous) monograph for dosing

Yaws, bejel, and pinta: 1.2 million units IM as a single dose

Dosage adjustment in renal impairment: There are no dosage adjustments provided in the manufacturer's labeling; use with caution.

Dosage adjustment in hepatic impairment: There are no dosage adjustments provided in the manufacturer's labeling.

Administration IM: Warm to room temperature before administration to lessen the pain associated with injection. Administer by deep IM injection in the upper outer quadrant of the buttock; in children <2 years of age, IM injections should be made into the midlateral muscle of the thigh, not the gluteal region. Do not inject near an artery or a nerve; permanent neurological damage or gangrene may result. When doses are repeated, rotate the injection site. **Do not administer IV, intra-arterially, or SubQ.**

Monitoring Parameters Observe for signs and symptoms of anaphylaxis during first dose

Dosage Forms

Suspension, Intramuscular:

Bicillin L-A: 600,000 units/mL (1 mL); 1,200,000 units/2 mL (2 mL); 2,400,000 units/4 mL (4 mL)

Penicillin G Benzathine and Penicillin G Procaine

(pen i SIL in jee BENZ a theen & pen i SIL in jee PROE kane)

Brand Names: U.S. Bicillin® C-R; Bicillin® C-R 900/300

Index Terms Penicillin G Procaine and Benzathine Combined

Pharmacologic Category Antibiotic, Penicillin

Use May be used in specific situations in the treatment of streptococcal infections; primary prevention of rheumatic fever

Pregnancy Risk Factor B

Dosage

Usual dosage range and indication-specific dosing:

Streptococcal infections:

Children: IM:

<14 kg: 600,000 units in a single dose

14-27 kg: 900,000 units to 1.2 million units in a single dose

Children >27 kg and Adults: 2.4 million units in a single dose

Rheumatic fever, primary prevention (Bicillin® C-R 900/300): Children 6 months to 12 years: 1.2 million units as a single dose (Bass, 1976; Gerber, 2009). **Note:** The efficacy of this regimen for heavier patients is unknown.

Dosage adjustment in renal impairment: No dosage adjustment provided in manufacturer's labeling.

Dosage adjustment in hepatic impairment: No dosage adjustment provided in manufacturer's labeling.

Additional Information Complete prescribing information should be consulted for additional detail.

Dosage Forms

Injection, suspension [prefilled syringe]:

Bicillin® C-R: 1,200,000 units: Penicillin G benzathine 600,000 units and penicillin G procaine 600,000 units per 2 mL (2 mL)

Bicillin® C-R 900/300: 1,200,000 units: Penicillin G benzathine 900,000 units and penicillin G procaine 300,000 units per 2 mL (2 mL)

Penicillin G (Parenteral/Aqueous)

(pen i SIL in jee, pa REN ter al, AYE kwee us)

Brand Names: U.S. Pfizerpen-G

Brand Names: Canada Crystapen®

Index Terms Benzylpenicillin Potassium; Benzylpenicillin Sodium; Crystalline Penicillin; Penicillin G Potassium; Penicillin G Sodium

Pharmacologic Category Antibiotic, Penicillin

Use Treatment of infections (including sepsis, pneumonia, pericarditis, endocarditis, meningitis, anthrax) caused by susceptible organisms; active against some gram-positive organisms, generally not *Staphylococcus aureus*; some gram-negative organisms such as *Neisseria gonorrhoeae*, and some anaerobes and spirochetes

Pregnancy Risk Factor B

Pregnancy Considerations Adverse events have not been observed in animal reproduction studies. Penicillin crosses the placenta and distributes into amniotic fluid. Maternal use of penicillins has generally not resulted in an increased risk of adverse fetal effects. Penicillin G is the drug of choice for treatment of syphilis during pregnancy and penicillin G (parenteral/aqueous) is the drug of choice for the prevention of early-onset Group B Streptococcal (GBS) disease in newborns (consult current guidelines).

Breast-Feeding Considerations Very small amounts of penicillin G transfer into breast milk. Peak milk concentrations occur at approximately 1 hour after an IM dose and are higher if multiple doses are given. The manufacturer recommends that caution be exercised when administering penicillin to nursing women. Nondose-related effects could include modification of bowel flora and allergic sensitization.

Contraindications Hypersensitivity to penicillin or any component of the formulation

Warnings/Precautions Avoid intra-arterial administration or injection into or near major peripheral nerves or blood vessels since such injections may cause severe and/or permanent neurovascular damage; use with caution in patients with renal impairment (dosage reduction required), concomitant renal and hepatic impairment (further dosage adjustment may be required), preexisting seizure disorders, or with a history of hypersensitivity to cephalosporins. Prolonged use may result in fungal or bacterial superinfection, including *C. difficile*-associated diarrhea (CDAD) and pseudomembranous colitis; CDAD has been observed >2 months postantibiotic treatment. Serious and occasionally severe or fatal hypersensitivity (anaphylactoid) reactions have been reported in patients on penicillin therapy, especially with a history of beta-lactam hypersensitivity, history of sensitivity to multiple allergens, or previous IgE-mediated reactions (eg, anaphylaxis, angioedema, urticaria). Use with caution in asthmatic patients. Extended duration of therapy or use associated with high serum concentrations may be associated with an increased risk for some adverse reactions. Neonates may have decreased renal clearance of penicillin and require frequent dosage adjustments depending on age. Product contains sodium and potassium; high doses of IV therapy may alter serum levels.

Adverse Reactions

Cardiovascular: Localized phlebitis, local thrombophlebitis

Central nervous system: Coma (high doses), hyperreflexia (high doses), myoclonus (high doses), seizure (high doses)

Dermatologic: Contact dermatitis, skin rash

Endocrine & metabolic: Electrolyte disturbance (high doses)

Gastrointestinal: Pseudomembranous colitis

Hematologic & oncologic: Neutropenia, positive direct Coombs test (rare, high doses)

Hypersensitivity: Anaphylaxis, hypersensitivity reaction (immediate and delayed), serum sickness

Immunologic: Jarisch-Herxheimer reaction

Local: Injection site reaction

Renal: Acute interstitial nephritis (high doses), renal tubular disease (high doses)

Drug Interactions

Metabolism/Transport Effects **Substrate** of OAT3

Avoid Concomitant Use

Avoid concomitant use of Penicillin G (Parenteral/Aqueous) with any of the following: BCG; Probenecid

Increased Effect/Toxicity

Penicillin G (Parenteral/Aqueous) may increase the levels/effects of: Methotrexate; Vitamin K Antagonists

The levels/effects of Penicillin G (Parenteral/Aqueous) may be increased by: Probenecid; Teriflunomide

Decreased Effect

Penicillin G (Parenteral/Aqueous) may decrease the levels/effects of: BCG; Mycophenolate; Sodium Picosulfate; Typhoid Vaccine

The levels/effects of Penicillin G (Parenteral/Aqueous) may be decreased by: Tetracycline Derivatives

Preparation for Administration

Intermittent IV: 5 million unit vial: Add 8.2 mL for a final concentration of 500,000 units/mL; add 3.2 mL for a final concentration of 1,000,000 units/mL. Dilute further to 50,000-145,000 units/mL prior to infusion.

Continuous IV infusion: 20 million unit vial: Add 11.5 mL for a final concentration of 1,000,000 units/mL. Dilute further in 1-2 L of infusion solution and administer over a 24-hour period.

Storage/Stability

Penicillin G potassium powder for injection should be stored below 86°F (30°C). Following reconstitution, solution may be stored for up to 7 days under refrigeration. Premixed bags for infusion should be stored in the freezer (-20°C or -4°F); frozen bags may be thawed at room temperature or in refrigerator. Once thawed, solution is stable for 14 days if stored in refrigerator or for 24 hours when stored at room temperature. Do not refreeze once thawed.

Penicillin G sodium powder for injection should be stored at controlled room temperature. Reconstituted solution may be stored under refrigeration for up to 3 days.

Mechanism of Action Interferes with bacterial cell wall synthesis during active multiplication, causing cell wall death and resultant bactericidal activity against susceptible bacteria

Pharmacodynamics/Kinetics

Distribution: Poor penetration across blood-brain barrier, despite inflamed meninges

- Relative diffusion from blood into CSF: Poor unless meninges inflamed (exceeds usual MICs)
- CSF:blood level ratio: Normal meninges: <1%; Inflamed meninges: 2% to 6%

Protein binding: 65%

Metabolism: Hepatic (30%) to penicilloic acid

Half-life elimination:

- Neonates: <6 days old: 3.2-3.4 hours; 7-13 days old: 1.2-2.2 hours; >14 days old: 0.9-1.9 hours
- Children and Adults: Normal renal function: 30-50 minutes
- End-stage renal disease: 3.3-5.1 hours

Time to peak, serum: IM: ~30 minutes; IV: ~1 hour

Excretion: Urine (58% to 85% as unchanged drug)

Dosage

Usual dosage range:

Infants ≥1 month and Children: IM, IV: 100,000-400,000 units/kg/day in divided doses every 4-6 hours (maximum dose: 24 million units/day)

Adults: IM, IV: 2-30 million units/day in divided doses every 4-6 hours depending on sensitivity of the organism and severity of the infection

Indication-specific dosing:

Infants ≥1 month and Children:

Community-acquired pneumonia (CAP) (IDSA/PIDS, 2011): IV: Infants >3 months and Children: **Note:** May consider addition of vancomycin or clindamycin to empiric therapy if community-acquired MRSA suspected. In children ≥5 years, a macrolide antibiotic should be added if atypical pneumonia cannot be ruled out.

Empiric treatment or *S. pneumoniae* (moderate-to-severe; MICs to penicillin ≤2.0 mcg/mL) (preferred): 200,000-250,000 units/kg/day divided every 4-6 hours

Group A *Streptococcus* (moderate-to-severe) (preferred): 100,000-250,000 units/kg/day divided every 4-6 hours

***Meningitis* (gonococcal):** IV: 250,000 units/kg/day in 4 divided doses

Moderate infections: IM, IV: 100,000-250,000 units/kg/day in 4 divided doses

Neurosyphilis: IV: 200,000-300,000 units/kg/day divided every 4-6 hours for 10-14 days (maximum dose: 24 million units/day)

Severe infections: IM, IV: 250,000-400,000 units/kg/day in divided doses every 4-6 hours (maximum dose: 24 million units/day)

Syphilis (congenital): IV:

Infants: 50,000 units/kg every 12 hours for first 7 days of life, then every 8 hours for a total of 10 days (CDC, 2010)

Children: 50,000 units/kg every 4-6 hours for 10 days (CDC, 2010)

Adults:

***Actinomyces* species:** IV: 10-20 million units/day in divided doses every 4-6 hours for 4-6 weeks

Clostridium perfringens: IV: 24 million units/day in divided doses every 4-6 hours with clindamycin

Corynebacterium diphtheriae: IV: 2-3 million units/day in divided doses every 4-6 hours for 10-12 days

Erysipelas: IV: 1-2 million units every 4-6 hours

Erysipelothrix: IV: 2-4 million units every 4 hours

Fascial space infections: IV: 2-4 million units every 4-6 hours with metronidazole

Leptospirosis: IV: 1.5 million units every 6 hours for 7 days

Listeria: IV: 15-20 million units/day in divided doses every 4-6 hours for 2 weeks (meningitis) or 4 weeks (endocarditis)

Lyme disease (meningitis): IV: 20 million units/day in divided doses

Neurosyphilis: IV: 18-24 million units/day in divided doses every 4 hours (or by continuous infusion) for 10-14 days (CDC, 2006; CDC, 2009; CDC, 2010)

Prosthetic joint infection: IV:

Enterococcus spp (penicillin-susceptible), streptococci (beta-hemolytic): 20-24 million units daily continuous infusion every 24 hours or in divided doses every 4 hours for 4-6 weeks (Osmon, 2013); **Note:** For penicillin-susceptible *Enterococcus* spp, consider addition of aminoglycoside.

Propionibacterium acnes: 20 million units daily continuous infusion every 24 hours or in divided doses every 4 hours for 4-6 weeks (Osmon, 2013)

Streptococcus:

Brain abscess: IV: 18-24 million units/day in divided doses every 4 hours with metronidazole

Endocarditis or osteomyelitis: IV: 3-4 million units every 4 hours for at least 4 weeks

Group B streptococcus (neonatal prophylaxis): IV: 5 million units x 1 dose, then 2.5-3.0 million units every 4 hours until delivery (CDC, 2010)

Skin and soft tissue: IV: 3-4 million units every 4 hours for 10 days

Toxic shock: IV: 24 million units/day in divided doses with clindamycin

Streptococcal pneumonia: IV: 2-3 million units every 4 hours

Whipple's disease: IV: 2 million units every 4 hours for 2 weeks, followed by oral trimethoprim/sulfamethoxazole or doxycycline for 1 year

Relapse or CNS involvement: 4 million units every 4 hours for 4 weeks

Dosing adjustment in renal impairment:

Manufacturer's recommendation:

Uremic patients with CrCl >10 mL/minute/1.73 m^2: Administer a normal dose followed by 50% of the normal dose every 4-5 hours

CrCl <10 mL/minute/1.73 m^2: Administer a normal dose followed by 50% of the normal dose every 8-10 hours

Alternate recommendation:

GFR >50 mL/minute: No dosage adjustments are necessary (Aronoff, 2007).

GFR 10-50 mL/minute: Administer 75% of the normal dose (Aronoff, 2007).

GFR <10 mL/minute: Administer 20% to 50% of the normal dose (Aronoff, 2007).

Intermittent hemodialysis (IHD) (administer after hemodialysis on dialysis days) (Heintz, 2009): Administer a normal dose followed by either 25% to 50% of normal dose every 4-6 hours **or** 50% to 100% of normal dose every 8-12 hours. For *mild-to-moderate* infections, administer 0.5-1 million units every 4-6 hours **or** 1-2 million units every 8-12 hours. For *neurosyphilis, endocarditis, or serious infections*, administer up to 2 million units every 4-6 hours; administer after dialysis on dialysis days **or** supplement with 500,000 units after dialysis. **Note:** Dosing dependent on the assumption of 3 times weekly, complete IHD sessions.

Continuous renal replacement therapy (CRRT) (Heintz, 2009; Trotman, 2005): Drug clearance is highly dependent on the method of renal replacement, filter type, and flow rate. Appropriate dosing requires close monitoring of pharmacologic response, signs of adverse reactions due to drug accumulation, as well as drug concentrations in relation to target trough (if appropriate). The following are general recommendations only (based on dialysate flow/ultrafiltration rates of 1-2 L/hour and minimal residual renal function) and should not supersede clinical judgment:

CVVH: Loading dose of 4 million units, followed by 2 million units every 4-6 hours

CVVHD: Loading dose of 4 million units, followed by 2-3 million units every 4-6 hours

CVVHDF: Loading dose of 4 million units, followed by 2-4 million units every 4-6 hours

Dosing adjustment in hepatic impairment: No dosage adjustment provided in manufacturer's labeling. However, the manufacturer's labeling recommends further adjustment of doses adjusted for renal impairment in patients with both renal and hepatic impairment.

Dietary Considerations Some products may contain potassium and/or sodium.

Administration

IM; Administer IM by deep injection in the upper outer quadrant of the buttock

IV: **Note:** The 20 million unit dosage form may be administered by continuous IV infusion only.

Intermittent IV: May be dissolved in small amounts of SWFI, NS, D_5W and administered peripherally as a 50,000-100,000 unit/mL solution. In fluid-restricted patients, 146,000 units/mL in SW results in a maximum recommended osmolality for peripheral infusion. Infuse over 15-30 minutes.

Continuous IV infusion: Determine the volume of fluid and rate of its administration required by the patient in a 24-hour period. Add the appropriate daily dosage of penicillin to this fluid. For example, if the daily dose is 10 million units and 2 L of fluid/day is required, add 5 million units to 1 L and adjust the rate of flow so the liter will be infused over 12 hours (83 mL/hour). Repeat steps (5 million units/L at 83 mL/hour) for the remaining 12 hours.

Monitoring Parameters Periodic electrolyte, hepatic, renal, cardiac and hematologic function tests during prolonged/high-dose therapy; observe for signs and symptoms of anaphylaxis during first dose

Additional Information 1 million units is approximately equal to 625 mg.

Dosage Forms

Solution, Intravenous:

Generic: 20,000 units/mL (50 mL); 40,000 units/mL (50 mL); 60,000 units/mL (50 mL)

Solution Reconstituted, Injection:

Pfizerpen-G: 5,000,000 units (1 ea); 20,000,000 units (1 ea)

Generic: 5,000,000 units (1 ea); 20,000,000 units (1 ea)

Solution Reconstituted, Injection [preservative free]:

Generic: 20,000,000 units (1 ea)

◆ **Penicillin G Potassium** *see* Penicillin G (Parenteral/Aqueous) *on page 1611*

Penicillin G Procaine (pen i SIL in jee PROE kane)

Brand Names: Canada Pfizerpen-AS®; Wycillin®

Index Terms APPG; Aqueous Procaine Penicillin G; Procaine Benzylpenicillin; Procaine Penicillin G; Wycillin

Pharmacologic Category Antibiotic, Penicillin

Use Treatment of moderately-severe infections due to *Treponema pallidum* and other penicillin G-sensitive microorganisms that are susceptible to low, but prolonged serum penicillin concentrations; anthrax due to *Bacillus anthracis* (postexposure) to reduce the incidence or progression of disease following exposure to aerolized *Bacillus anthracis*

Pregnancy Risk Factor B

Pregnancy Considerations Adverse events have not been observed in animal reproduction studies. Penicillin crosses the placenta and distributes into amniotic fluid. Maternal use of penicillins has generally not resulted in an increased risk of adverse fetal effects.

Breast-Feeding Considerations Penicillins are excreted in breast milk. The manufacturer recommends that caution be used when administering penicillin to nursing women. Nondose-related effects could include modification of bowel flora and allergic sensitization.

Contraindications Hypersensitivity to penicillin, procaine, or any component of the formulation

Warnings/Precautions May need to modify dosage in patients with severe renal impairment or seizure disorders; avoid IV, intravascular, or intra-arterial administration of penicillin G procaine since severe and/or permanent neurovascular damage may occur. Serious and occasionally severe or fatal hypersensitivity (anaphylactoid) reactions have been reported in patients on penicillin therapy, especially with a history of beta-lactam hypersensitivity, history of sensitivity to multiple allergens, or previous IgE-mediated reactions (eg, anaphylaxis, angioedema, urticaria). Use with caution in asthmatic patients. Extended duration of therapy or use associated with high serum concentrations may be associated with an increased risk for some adverse reactions. Prolonged use may result in fungal or bacterial superinfection, including *C. difficile*-associated diarrhea (CDAD) and pseudomembranous colitis; CDAD has been observed >2 months postantibiotic treatment.

Adverse Reactions

Cardiovascular: Conduction disturbances, myocardial depression, vasodilation

Central nervous system: CNS stimulation, confusion, drowsiness, myoclonus, seizure

Hematologic: Hemolytic anemia, neutropenia, positive Coombs' reaction

Local: Pain at injection site, sterile abscess at injection site, thrombophlebitis

Renal: Interstitial nephritis

Miscellaneous: Hypersensitivity reactions, Jarisch-Herxheimer reaction, pseudoanaphylactic reactions, serum sickness

Drug Interactions

Metabolism/Transport Effects Substrate of OAT3

Avoid Concomitant Use

Avoid concomitant use of Penicillin G Procaine with any of the following: BCG; Probenecid

Increased Effect/Toxicity

Penicillin G Procaine may increase the levels/effects of: Methotrexate; Vitamin K Antagonists

The levels/effects of Penicillin G Procaine may be increased by: Probenecid; Teriflunomide

Decreased Effect

Penicillin G Procaine may decrease the levels/effects of: BCG; Mycophenolate; Sodium Picosulfate; Typhoid Vaccine

The levels/effects of Penicillin G Procaine may be decreased by: Tetracycline Derivatives

Storage/Stability Refrigerate

Mechanism of Action Inhibits bacterial cell wall synthesis by binding to one or more of the penicillin-binding proteins (PBPs); which in turn inhibits the final transpeptidation step of peptidoglycan synthesis in bacterial cell walls, thus inhibiting cell wall biosynthesis. Bacteria eventually lyse due to ongoing activity of cell wall autolytic enzymes (autolysins and murein hydrolases) while cell wall assembly is arrested.

Pharmacodynamics/Kinetics

Duration: Therapeutic: 15-24 hours

Absorption: IM: Slow

Distribution: Penetration across the blood-brain barrier is poor, despite inflamed meninges

Protein binding: 65%

Metabolism: ~30% hepatically inactivated

Time to peak, serum: 1-4 hours

Excretion: Urine (60% to 90% as unchanged drug)

Clearance: Renal: Delayed in neonates, young infants, and with impaired renal function

Dosage

Usual dosage range:

Infants and Children: IM: 25,000-50,000 units/kg/day in divided doses 1-2 times/day (maximum: 4.8 million units/day)

Adults: IM: 0.6-4.8 million units/day in divided doses every 12-24 hours

Indication-specific dosing:

Children: IM:

Anthrax, inhalational (postexposure prophylaxis): 25,000 units/kg every 12 hours (maximum: 1,200,000 units every 12 hours); see **"Note"** in adult dosing

Syphilis (congenital): 50,000 units/kg/day for 10 days; if more than 1 day of therapy is missed, the entire course should be restarted

Adults: IM:

Anthrax:

Inhalational (postexposure prophylaxis): 1,200,000 units every 12 hours

Note: Overall treatment duration should be 60 days. Available safety data suggest continued administration of penicillin G procaine for longer than 2 weeks may incur additional risk for adverse reactions. Clinicians may consider switching to effective alternative treatment for completion of therapy beyond 2 weeks.

Cutaneous (treatment): 600,000-1,200,000 units/day; alternative therapy is recommended in severe cutaneous or other forms of anthrax infection

Endocarditis caused by susceptible viridans *Streptococcus* (when used in conjunction with an aminoglycoside): 1.2 million units every 6 hours for 2-4 weeks

Neurosyphilis: 2.4 million units/day with 500 mg probenecid by mouth 4 times/day for 10-14 days; **Note: Penicillin G aqueous IV is the preferred agent**

Whipple's disease: 1.2 million units/day (with streptomycin) for 10-14 days, followed by oral trimethoprim/ sulfamethoxazole or doxycycline for 1 year

Dosage adjustment in renal impairment:

CrCl 10-30 mL/minute: Administer every 8-12 hours.

CrCl <10 mL/minute: Administer every 12-18 hours.

Hemodialysis: Moderately dialyzable (20% to 50%)

Dosage adjustment in hepatic impairment: No dosage adjustment provided in manufacturer's labeling.

Administration Procaine suspension for deep IM injection only; do not inject in gluteal muscle in children <2 years of age; rotate the injection site; avoid IV, intravascular, or intra-arterial administration of penicillin G procaine since severe and/or permanent neurovascular damage may occur

Monitoring Parameters Periodic renal and hematologic function tests with prolonged therapy; fever, mental status, WBC count

Dosage Forms

Suspension, Intramuscular:

Generic: 600,000 units/mL (1 mL, 2 mL)

◆ **Penicillin G Procaine and Benzathine Combined** *see* Penicillin G Benzathine and Penicillin G Procaine *on page 1611*

◆ **Penicillin G Sodium** *see* Penicillin G (Parenteral/Aqueous) *on page 1611*

Penicillin V Potassium

(pen i SIL in vee poe TASS ee um)

Brand Names: Canada Apo-Pen VK; Novo-Pen-VK; Nu-Pen-VK

Index Terms Pen VK; Phenoxymethyl Penicillin

Pharmacologic Category Antibiotic, Penicillin

Use Treatment of infections caused by susceptible organisms involving the respiratory tract, otitis media, sinusitis, skin, and soft tissues; prophylaxis in rheumatic fever

Pregnancy Considerations Penicillin crosses the placenta and distributes into amniotic fluid. Maternal use of penicillins has generally not resulted in an increased risk of adverse fetal effects. Due to pregnancy-induced physiologic changes, some pharmacokinetic parameters of penicillin V may be altered in the second and third trimester. Higher doses or increased dosing frequency may be required.

Breast-Feeding Considerations Penicillin V is excreted into breast milk (low concentrations) and may be detected in the urine of some breast-feeding infants. Loose stools and rash have been reported in nursing infants.

Contraindications Hypersensitivity to penicillin or any component of the formulation

Warnings/Precautions Use with caution in patients with severe renal impairment or history of seizures. Serious and occasionally severe or fatal hypersensitivity (anaphylactoid) reactions have been reported in patients on penicillin therapy, especially with a history of beta-lactam hypersensitivity, history of sensitivity to multiple allergens, or previous IgE-mediated reactions (eg, anaphylaxis, angioedema, urticaria). Use with caution in asthmatic patients. Extended duration of therapy or use associated with high serum concentrations may be associated with an increased risk for some adverse reactions. Prolonged use may result in fungal or bacterial superinfection, including *C. difficile*-associated diarrhea (CDAD) and pseudomembranous colitis; CDAD has been observed >2 months postantibiotic treatment.

Benzyl alcohol and derivatives: Some dosage forms may contain sodium benzoate/benzoic acid; benzoic acid (benzoate) is a metabolite of benzyl alcohol; large amounts of benzyl alcohol (≥99 mg/kg/day) have been associated with a potentially fatal toxicity ("gasping syndrome") in neonates; the "gasping syndrome" consists of metabolic acidosis, respiratory distress, gasping respirations, CNS dysfunction (including convulsions, intracranial hemorrhage), hypotension, and cardiovascular collapse (AAP, 1997; CDC, 1982); some data suggests that benzoate displaces bilirubin from protein binding sites (Ahlfors, 2001); avoid or use dosage forms containing benzyl alcohol derivative with caution in neonates. See manufacturer's labeling.

Adverse Reactions

Gastrointestinal: Melanoglossia, mild diarrhea, nausea, oral candidiasis, vomiting

Rare but important or life-threatening: Acute interstitial nephritis, convulsions, exfoliative dermatitis, hemolytic anemia, hypersensitivity reaction, positive Coombs' reaction, serum-sickness like reactions

Drug Interactions

Metabolism/Transport Effects None known.

Avoid Concomitant Use

Avoid concomitant use of Penicillin V Potassium with any of the following: BCG; Probenecid

Increased Effect/Toxicity

Penicillin V Potassium may increase the levels/effects of: Methotrexate; Vitamin K Antagonists

The levels/effects of Penicillin V Potassium may be increased by: Probenecid

Decreased Effect

Penicillin V Potassium may decrease the levels/effects of: BCG; Mycophenolate; Sodium Picosulfate; Typhoid Vaccine

The levels/effects of Penicillin V Potassium may be decreased by: Tetracycline Derivatives

Food Interactions Food decreases drug absorption rate; decreases drug serum concentration. Management: Take on an empty stomach 1 hour before or 2 hours after meals around-the-clock to promote less variation in peak and trough serum levels.

Storage/Stability Refrigerate suspension after reconstitution; discard after 14 days.

Mechanism of Action Inhibits bacterial cell wall synthesis by binding to one or more of the penicillin-binding proteins (PBPs); which in turn inhibits the final transpeptidation step of peptidoglycan synthesis in bacterial cell walls, thus inhibiting cell wall biosynthesis. Bacteria eventually lyse due to ongoing activity of cell wall autolytic enzymes (autolysins and murein hydrolases) while cell wall assembly is arrested.

Pharmacodynamics/Kinetics

Absorption: 60% to 73%

Distribution: Widely distributed to kidneys, liver, skin, tonsils, and into synovial, pleural, and pericardial fluids

Protein binding, plasma: 80%

Half-life elimination: 30 minutes; prolonged with renal impairment

Time to peak, serum: 0.5-1 hour

Excretion: Urine (as unchanged drug and metabolites)

Dosage

Usual dosage range:

Children <12 years: Oral: 25-50 mg/kg/day in divided doses every 6-8 hours (maximum dose: 3000 mg daily)

Children ≥12 years and Adults: Oral: 125-500 mg every 6-8 hours

Indication-specific dosing:

Infants >3 months and Children: Oral: **Community-acquired pneumonia (CAP) due to group A *Streptococcus*, mild infection or step-down therapy (preferred) (IDSA/PIDS, 2011):** 50-75 mg/kg/day in 3-4 divided doses

Infants and Children: Oral: **Pneumococcal infection prophylaxis for anatomic or functional asplenia (eg, sickle cell disease [SCD]) (AAP, 2000; AAP, 2002; Kavanagh, 2011; NHLBI, 2002):**

Before 2 months of age (or as soon as SCD diagnosed or asplenia occurs) to 3 years of age: 125 mg twice daily

>3 years: 250 mg twice daily; the decision to discontinue penicillin prophylaxis after 5 years of age in children who have not experienced invasive pneumococcal infection and have received recommended pneumococcal immunizations is patient and clinician dependent; **Note:** Some clinicians recommend in patients <5 years, a lower dose of 125 mg twice daily (*Red Book*, 2012)

Children: Oral:

Community-acquired cutaneous anthrax (off-label use): 25-50 mg/kg/day in divided doses 2-4 times daily (maximum single dose: 500 mg) for 5-9 days (Stevens, 2005)

Pharyngitis (streptococcal) (IDSA guidelines):

Acute treatment: 250 mg 2-3 times daily for 10 days

Chronic carrier treatment, group A streptococci: 50 mg/kg/day in 4 divided doses (maximum: 2000 mg daily) for 10 days in combination with oral rifampin (Shulman, 2012)

Prophylaxis of recurrent rheumatic fever: Refer to adult dosing.

Children ≥ 12 years and Adolescents: Oral:

Fusospirochetosis (Vincent infection): Refer to adult dosing.

Adolescents: Oral:

Pharyngitis (streptococcal), acute treatment (IDSA guidelines): Refer to adult dosing.

Adults: Oral:

Actinomycosis:

Mild: 2000-4000 mg daily in 4 divided doses for 8 weeks

Surgical: 2000-4000 mg in 4 divided doses for 6-12 months (after IV penicillin G therapy of 4-6 weeks)

Erysipelas: 500 mg 4 times daily

Fusospirochetosis (Vincent infection): 250-500 mg 3-4 times daily

Cutaneous anthrax, community-acquired (off-label use): 250-500 mg 4 times daily for 5-9 days (Stevens, 2005)

Cutaneous erysipeloid (off-label use): 500 mg 4 times daily for 7-10 days (Stevens, 2005)

Periodontal infections: 250-500 mg every 6 hours for 5-7 days

Note: Efficacy of antimicrobial therapy in periapical abscess is questionable; the American Academy of Periodontology recommends use of antibiotic therapy only when systemic symptoms (eg, fever, lymphadenopathy) are present or in immunocompromised patients.

Pharyngitis (streptococcal):

Manufacturer's labeling: 500 mg 3-4 times daily for 10 days

Acute treatment, group A streptococci (IDSA guidelines): 250 mg 4 times daily or 500 mg twice daily for 10 days (Shulman, 2012)

Chronic carrier treatment, group A streptococcal (IDSA guidelines): 500 mg 4 times daily (maximum: 2000 mg daily) for 10 days in combination with oral rifampin (Shulman, 2012)

Prophylaxis of recurrent rheumatic fever infections: 250 mg twice daily (Gerber, 2009)

Prosthetic joint infection (off-label use): *Chronic oral antimicrobial suppression (Enterococcus spp [penicillin-susceptible], streptococci [beta-hemolytic], Propionibacterium spp):* 500 mg 2-4 times daily (Osmon, 2013)

Dosage adjustment in renal impairment: No dosage adjustment provided in manufacturer's labeling. Use with caution; excretion is prolonged in patients with renal impairment.

Dosage adjustment in hepatic impairment: No dosage adjustment provided in manufacturer's labeling.

Dietary Considerations Take on an empty stomach 1 hour before or 2 hours after meals.

Administration Administer on an empty stomach to increase oral absorption

Monitoring Parameters Periodic renal and hematologic function tests during prolonged therapy; monitor for signs of anaphylaxis during first dose

Additional Information 0.7 mEq of potassium per 250 mg penicillin V; 250 mg equals 400,000 units of penicillin

Dosage Forms

Solution Reconstituted, Oral:

Generic: 125 mg/5 mL (100 mL, 200 mL); 250 mg/5 mL (100 mL, 200 mL)

Tablet, Oral:

Generic: 250 mg, 500 mg

- ◆ **Penlac** *see* Ciclopirox *on page* *433*
- ◆ **Pentacel®** *see* Diphtheria and Tetanus Toxoids, Acellular Pertussis, Poliovirus and *Haemophilus* b Conjugate Vaccine *on page* *648*
- ◆ **Pentahydrate** *see* Sodium Thiosulfate *on page* *1915*
- ◆ **Pentam** *see* Pentamidine *on page* *1616*

Pentamidine (pen TAM i deen)

Brand Names: U.S. Nebupent; Pentam

Index Terms Pentamidine Isethionate

Pharmacologic Category Antifungal Agent; Antiprotozoal

Use

IM, IV: Treatment of pneumonia caused by *Pneumocystis jirovecii* pneumonia (PCP)

Inhalation: Prevention of PCP in high-risk, HIV-infected patients either with a history of PCP or with a CD4+ count ≤200/mm^3

Pregnancy Risk Factor C

Dosage

Children:

PCP:

FDA-approved labeling: Children >4 months: Treatment: IM, IV: 4 mg/kg once daily for 14-21 days

CDC recommendation:

Prevention (children ≥5 years): Inhalation: 300 mg/dose monthly via Respirgard® II nebulizer

Treatment: IV: 3-4 mg/kg once daily for 21 days

AIDS*info* guidelines (2009):

Prevention: Children ≥5 years: Inhalation: 300 mg/dose monthly via Respirgard® II nebulizer

Treatment: IV: 4 mg/kg once daily, if clinical improvement may change to atovaquone after 7-10 days

PCP prevention in pediatric oncology patients (age <5 years, intolerant to trimethoprim-sulfamethoxazole; off-label use): 4 mg/kg IV once monthly (Kim, 2008; Prasad, 2007)

Cutaneous leishmaniasis (off-label use; CDC recommendation): IM, IV: 2-3 mg/kg once daily or every second day for 4-7 doses

Trypanosomiasis (off-label use; CDC recommendation): IM: 4 mg/kg once daily for 7 days

Adults:

PCP:

FDA-approved labeling:

Prevention: Inhalation: 300 mg every 4 weeks via Respirgard® II nebulizer

Treatment: IM, IV: 4 mg/kg once daily for 14-21 days

CDC recommendation:

Prevention: Inhalation: 300 mg monthly via Respirgard® II nebulizer

Treatment: IV: 3-4 mg/kg once daily for 21 days

AIDS*info* guidelines (2009):

Prevention: Inhalation: 300 mg/dose monthly via Respirgard® II nebulizer

Treatment: IV: 4 mg/kg once daily, 3 mg/kg may be used by some clinicians

Cutaneous leishmaniasis (off-label use; CDC recommendation): IM, IV: 2-3 mg/kg once daily or every second day for 4-7 doses

Trypanosomiasis (off-label use; CDC recommendation): IM: 4 mg/kg once daily for 7 days

Dosing adjustment in renal impairment: IV: The FDA-approved labeling recommends that caution should be used in patients with renal impairment; however, no specific dosage adjustment guidelines are available. The following guidelines have been used by some clinicians (Aronoff, 2007):

Children:

CrCl >30 mL/minute: No dosage adjustment necessary.

CrCl 10-30 mL/minute: Administer 4 mg/kg every 36 hours

CrCl <10 mL/minute and peritoneal dialysis: Administer 4 mg/kg every 48 hours

Hemodialysis: Administer 4 mg/kg every 48 hours, after dialysis on dialysis days

Adults:

CrCl ≥10 mL/minute: No dosage adjustment necessary.

CrCl <10 mL/minute: Administer 4 mg/kg every 24-36 hours

Dosage adjustment in hepatic impairment: No dosage adjustment provided in manufacturer's labeling (has not been studied). Use with caution.

Additional Information Complete prescribing information should be consulted for additional detail.

Dosage Forms

Solution Reconstituted, Inhalation:

Nebupent: 300 mg (1 ea)

Solution Reconstituted, Injection:

Pentam: 300 mg (1 ea)

- ◆ **Pentamidine Isethionate** *see* Pentamidine *on page* *1616*
- ◆ **Pentamycetin® (Can)** *see* Chloramphenicol *on page* *421*
- ◆ **Pentasa** *see* Mesalamine *on page* *1301*
- ◆ **Pentasodium Colistin Methanesulfonate** *see* Colistimethate *on page* *504*
- ◆ **Pentavalent Human-Bovine Reassortant Rotavirus Vaccine (PRV)** *see* Rotavirus Vaccine *on page* *1851*

Pentazocine (pen TAZ oh seen)

Brand Names: U.S. Talwin

Brand Names: Canada Talwin

Index Terms Pentazocine Lactate

Pharmacologic Category Analgesic, Opioid; Analgesic, Opioid Partial Agonist

Additional Appendix Information

Beers Criteria - Potentially Inappropriate Medications for Geriatrics *on page 2271*

Opioid Conversion Table *on page 2232*

Use Relief of moderate-to-severe pain; has also been used as a sedative prior to surgery and as a supplement to surgical anesthesia

Pregnancy Risk Factor C

Dosage

Preoperative/preanesthetic: Children 1-16 years: IM: 0.5 mg/kg

Analgesia:

Children (off-label use): IM:

5-8 years: 15 mg

9-14 years: 30 mg

Adults:

IM, SubQ: 30-60 mg every 3-4 hours; do not exceed 60 mg/dose (maximum: 360 mg/day)

IV: 30 mg every 3-4 hours; do not exceed 30 mg/dose (maximum: 360 mg/day)

Labor pain: Adults:

IM: 30 mg once

IV: 20 mg every 2-3 hours as needed (maximum total dose: 60 mg)

Elderly: Elderly patients may be more sensitive to the analgesic and sedating effects. The elderly may also have impaired renal function. If needed, dosing should be started at the lower end of dosing range and adjust dose for renal function.

Dosing adjustment in renal impairment: No dosage adjustment provided in manufacturer's labeling. Use with caution. The following guidelines have been used by some clinicians (Aronoff, 2007):

CrCl ≥50 mL/minute: No dosage adjustment necessary.

CrCl 10-50 mL/minute: Administer 75% of normal dose.

CrCl <10 mL/minute: Administer 50% of normal dose.

Dosing adjustment in hepatic impairment: No dosage adjustment provided in manufacturer's labeling. However, dosage adjustment may be necessary due to decreased metabolism and predisposition to adverse effects. Use with caution.

Additional Information Complete prescribing information should be consulted for additional detail.

Dosage Forms

Solution, Injection:

Talwin: 30 mg/mL (1 mL, 10 mL)

◆ **Pentazocine Lactate** *see* Pentazocine *on page 1616*

PENTobarbital (pen toe BAR bi tal)

Brand Names: U.S. Nembutal

Brand Names: Canada Nembutal® Sodium

Index Terms Pentobarbital Sodium

Pharmacologic Category Anticonvulsant, Barbiturate; Barbiturate

Additional Appendix Information

Beers Criteria - Potentially Inappropriate Medications for Geriatrics *on page 2271*

Use Sedative/hypnotic; refractory status epilepticus

Pregnancy Risk Factor D

Dosage Note: Adjust dose based on patients age, weight, and condition.

Children:

Hypnotic/sedative:

IM: 2-6 mg/kg; maximum: 100 mg/dose

IV: 1-6 mg/kg titrated in 1-2 mg/kg increments every 3-5 minutes to desired effect (Krauss, 2006)

Refractory status epilepticus: IV: **Note:** Intubation required; adjust dose based on hemodynamics, seizure activity, and EEG. Various regimens available (Abend, 2008; Hanhan, 2001; Holmes, 1999; Kim, 2001):

Loading dose: 5-15 mg/kg given slowly over 1 hour; maintenance infusion: 0.5-5 mg/kg/hour to maintain burst suppression; continue for 12-48 hours of no seizure activity; may taper infusion rate by 0.5 mg/kg/hour every 12 hours

Adults:

Hypnotic/sedative:

IM: 150-200 mg

IV: Initial: 100 mg; decrease dose for elderly or debilitated patients. If needed, may administer additional increments after at least 1 minute, up to a total dose of 200-500 mg

Barbiturate coma in severe brain injury patients/elevated intracranial pressure (off-label use; Bratton, 2007): IV: Loading dose: 10 mg/kg given over 30 minutes (or ≤25 mg/minute), followed by 5 mg/kg every hour for 3 doses; monitor blood pressure and respiratory rate. Maintenance infusion: Initial: 1 mg/kg/hour; may increase to 2-4 mg/kg/hour; maintain burst suppression on EEG.

Refractory status epilepticus: IV: **Note:** Intubation required; adjust dose based on hemodynamics, seizure activity, and EEG. Various regimens available (Abou Khaled, 2008; Millikan, 2009; Mirski, 2008; Yaffe, 1993):

Loading dose: 10-15 mg/kg (5-10 mg/kg in patients with preexisting hypotension) administer slowly over 1 hour; initial maintenance infusion: 0.5-1 mg/kg/hour; adjust to maintain burst suppression pattern on EEG; maintenance infusion dose range: 0.5-10 mg/kg/hour

Note: During active seizure activity when increasing maintenance infusion rate, some experts suggest administration of an additional 5 mg/kg bolus given the long half-life of pentobarbital.

Elderly: Not recommended for use in the elderly; decrease dose if use becomes necessary

Dosing adjustment in renal impairment: No dosage adjustment provided in manufacturer's labeling. However, a reduced dosage in patients with renal dysfunction is recommended.

Dosing adjustment in hepatic impairment: No dosage adjustment provided in manufacturer's labeling. However, a reduced dosage in patients with liver dysfunction is recommended.

Additional Information Complete prescribing information should be consulted for additional detail.

Dosage Forms

Solution, Injection:

Nembutal: 50 mg/mL (20 mL, 50 mL)

◆ **Pentobarbital Sodium** *see* PENTobarbital *on page 1617*

Pentosan Polysulfate Sodium

(PEN toe san pol i SUL fate SOW dee um)

Brand Names: U.S. Elmiron

Brand Names: Canada Elmiron®

Index Terms PPS

Pharmacologic Category Analgesic, Urinary

Use Relief of bladder pain or discomfort due to interstitial cystitis

Pregnancy Risk Factor B

Dosage Children ≥16 years and Adults: Oral: 100 mg 3 times/day taken with water 1 hour before or 2 hours after meals

Note: Patients should be evaluated at 3 months and may be continued an additional 3 months if there has been no improvement and if there are no therapy-limiting side effects. **The risks and benefits of continued use**

beyond 6 months in patients who have not responded is not yet known.

Dosing adjustment in renal impairment: No dosage adjustment provided in manufacturer's labeling (has not been studied).

Dosing adjustment in hepatic impairment: No dosage adjustment provided in manufacturer's labeling (has not been studied). However, dosage adjustment may be necessary due to hepatic impairment impact on pharmacokinetics. Use with caution.

Additional Information Complete prescribing information should be consulted for additional detail.

Dosage Forms

Capsule, Oral:

Elmiron: 100 mg

Pentostatin (pen toe STAT in)

Brand Names: U.S. Nipent

Brand Names: Canada Nipent

Index Terms 2′-Deoxycoformycin; Co-Vidarabine; dCF; Deoxycoformycin

Pharmacologic Category Antineoplastic Agent, Antimetabolite; Antineoplastic Agent, Antimetabolite (Purine Analog)

Use Hairy cell leukemia: Treatment (as a single-agent) of untreated and interferon-refractory hairy cell leukemia in patients with active disease (clinically significant anemia, neutropenia, thrombocytopenia, or disease-related symptoms)

Pregnancy Risk Factor D

Dosage

Hairy cell leukemia: Adults: IV: 4 mg/m^2 every 2 weeks. **Note:** The optimal duration has not been determined; in the absence of unacceptable toxicity, may continue until complete response is achieved or until 2 doses after complete response. Discontinue after 6 months if partial or complete response is not achieved.

Acute graft-versus-host disease (off-label use): Adults: IV:

Initial therapy: 1.5 mg/m^2 days 1 to 3 and days 15 to 17 (in combination with corticosteroids) (Alousi, 2009)

Steroid-refractory disease: 1.5 mg/m^2 daily for 3 days; may repeat after 2 weeks if needed (Bolanos-Meade, 2005)

Chronic graft-versus-host disease, steroid-refractory (off-label use): Pediatrics and Adults: IV: 4 mg/m^2 once every 2 weeks; discontinue after 6 months for sustained objective response, or continue every 2 to 4 weeks for up to 12 months if still improving (Jacobsohn, 2007; Jacobsohn, 2009) **or** 4 mg/m^2 once every 2 weeks for 3 months (Wolff, 2011)

Chronic lymphocytic leukemia (off-label use): Adults: IV:

Previously treated: 4 mg/m^2 once every 3 weeks (in combination with cyclophosphamide and rituximab) for 6 cycles (Lamanna, 2006)

Previously untreated: 2 mg/m^2 once every 3 weeks (in combination with cyclophosphamide and rituximab) for 6 cycles (Kay, 2007)

Cutaneous T-cell lymphomas, mycosis fungoides/Sezary syndrome (off-label use): Adults: IV: 4 mg/m^2 once weekly for 3 weeks, then every 2 weeks for 6 weeks, then once monthly for a maximum of 6 months (Ho, 1999)

T-cell prolymphocytic leukemia, refractory (off-label use): Adults: IV: 4 mg/m^2 once weekly for 4 weeks then every 2 weeks until optimum response is achieved (Mercieca, 1994) **or** 4 mg/m^2 once weekly for 4 weeks then every 2 weeks (in combination with alemtuzumab) until complete or best response or up to a total of 14 doses (Ravandi, 2009)

Dosage adjustment for toxicity:

ANC <200/mm^3 (with baseline ANC >500/mm^3): Temporarily interrupt treatment until ANC returns to pre-dose levels.

CNS toxicity: Withhold treatment or discontinue.

Infection, active: Interrupt treatment until infection is controlled.

Rash: Severe rashes may require treatment interruption or discontinuation.

Other severe adverse reactions: Withhold treatment or discontinue.

Dosage adjustment in renal impairment: There are no dosage adjustments provided in the manufacturer's labeling; although not adequately studied, two patients with CrCl 50 to 60 mL/minute achieved responses when treated with 2 mg/m^2/dose. For renal toxicity *during* treatment, withhold for elevated serum creatinine and determine creatinine clearance. The following adjustments have been recommended:

Kintzel, 1995:

CrCl 46 to 60 mL/minute: Administer 70% of dose

CrCl 31 to 45 mL/minute: Administer 60% of dose

CrCl <30 mL/minute: Consider use of alternative drug

Lathia, 2002:

CrCl ≥60 mL/minute: Administer 4 mg/m^2/dose

CrCl 40 to 59 mL/minute: Administer 3 mg/m^2/dose

CrCl 20 to 39 mL/minute: Administer 2 mg/m^2/dose

Alousi, 2009; Jacobsohn, 2009; Poi, 2013 (for acute GVHD treatment):

CrCl 30 to 50 mL/minute/1.73 m^2: Reduce dose by 50%

CrCl <30 mL/minute/1.73 m^2: Removed from study protocol

Lamanna, 2006 (for previously treated CLL): Serum creatinine >2 mg/dL or 20% above patient's baseline: Withhold treatment until serum creatinine ≤2 mg/dL or returns to baseline, or until CrCl ≥50 mL/minute

Dosage adjustment in hepatic impairment: There are no dosage adjustments provided in the manufacturer's labeling.

Dosing in obesity:

American Society of Clinical Oncology (ASCO) Guidelines for appropriate chemotherapy dosing in obese adults with cancer: Utilize patient's actual body weight (full weight) for calculation of body surface area- or weight-based dosing, particularly when the intent of therapy is curative; manage regimen-related toxicities in the same manner as for nonobese patients; if a dose reduction is utilized due to toxicity, consider resumption of full weight-based dosing with subsequent cycles, especially if cause of toxicity (eg, hepatic or renal impairment) is resolved (Griggs, 2012).

American Society for Blood and Marrow Transplantation (ASBMT) practice guideline committee position statement on chemotherapy dosing in obesity: Utilize actual body weight (full weight) for calculation of body surface area in pentostatin dosing for hematopoietic stem cell transplant conditioning regimens in adults (Bubalo, 2014).

Additional Information Complete prescribing information should be consulted for additional detail.

Dosage Forms

Solution Reconstituted, Intravenous:

Nipent: 10 mg (1 ea)

Pentoxifylline (pen toks IF i lin)

Brand Names: U.S. TRENtal [DSC]

Brand Names: Canada Pentoxifylline SR

Index Terms Oxpentifylline

Pharmacologic Category Blood Viscosity Reducer Agent

Use

Intermittent claudication: Treatment of intermittent claudication on the basis of chronic occlusive arterial disease of the limbs.

Limitations of use: May improve function and symptoms, but not intended to replace more definitive therapy. **Note:** The American College of Chest Physicians (ACCP) discourages the use of pentoxifylline for the treatment of intermittent claudication refractory to exercise therapy (and smoking cessation) (Guyatt, 2012).

Pregnancy Risk Factor C

Dosage Oral:

Adults:

Intermittent claudication: 400 mg 3 times daily; maximal therapeutic benefit may take 2 to 4 weeks to develop; recommended to maintain therapy for at least 8 weeks. May reduce to 400 mg twice daily if GI or CNS side effects occur; discontinue if side effects persist.

Note: Use for the treatment of intermittent claudication refractory to exercise therapy (and smoking cessation) has been discouraged by The American College of Chest Physicians (ACCP) (Guyatt, 2012).

Severe alcoholic hepatitis (Maddrey Discriminant Function [MDF] score ≥32, especially when corticosteroids contraindicated) (off-label use): 400 mg 3 times daily for 4 weeks (O'Shea, 2010)

Venous leg ulcer (off-label use): 400 mg 3 times daily (with compression therapy) (Jull, 2002; Robson, 2006)

Dosage adjustment in renal impairment:

Manufacturer's labeling: CrCl <30 mL/minute: 400 mg once daily

The following guidelines have been used by some clinicians:

Aronoff, 2007: Adults:

CrCl >50 mL/minute: 400 mg every 8 to 12 hours

CrCl 10-50 mL/minute: 400 mg every 12 to 24 hours

CrCl <10 mL minute: 400 mg every 24 hours

Hemodialysis: supplemental postdialysis dose is not necessary

Peritoneal dialysis: 400 mg every 24 hours

Paap, 1996: Adults:

Moderate renal impairment (CrCl ~60 mL/minute): 400 mg twice daily

Severe renal impairment (CrCl ~20 mL/minute): 400 mg once daily; further reduction may be required; Paap suggests 200 mg once daily, but with current products (extended or controlled release; unscored) may require adaptation to 400 mg once every other day

Dosage adjustment in hepatic impairment: There are no dosage adjustments provided in the manufacturer's labeling; use with caution.

Additional Information Complete prescribing information should be consulted for additional detail.

Dosage Forms

Tablet Extended Release, Oral:

Generic: 400 mg

- ◆ **Pentoxifylline SR (Can)** *see* Pentoxifylline *on page 1618*
- ◆ **Pen VK** *see* Penicillin V Potassium *on page 1614*
- ◆ **PEP005** *see* Ingenol Mebutate *on page 1083*
- ◆ **Pepcid** *see* Famotidine *on page 845*
- ◆ **Pepcid AC (Can)** *see* Famotidine *on page 845*
- ◆ **Pepcid Complete (Can)** *see* Famotidine *on page 845*
- ◆ **Peptic guard (Can)** *see* Famotidine *on page 845*
- ◆ **Peptic Relief [OTC]** *see* Bismuth *on page 265*
- ◆ **Pepto-Bismol [OTC]** *see* Bismuth *on page 265*
- ◆ **Pepto-Bismol To-Go [OTC]** *see* Bismuth *on page 265*

Peramivir (pe RA mi veer)

Brand Names: U.S. Rapivab

Index Terms BCX-1812; Rapivab; RWJ-270201

Pharmacologic Category Antiviral Agent; Neuraminidase Inhibitor

Use

Influenza: Treatment of acute, uncomplicated influenza in adults who have been symptomatic ≤2 days.

Limitations of use:

Efficacy has not been established for patients with serious influenza requiring hospitalization.

Efficacy is based on clinical trials in which influenza A was the predominant virus; a limited number of subjects with influenza B have been studied.

Pregnancy Risk Factor C

Pregnancy Considerations Adverse events were observed in some animal reproduction studies. Information related to the use of peramivir in pregnancy is limited (Hernandez 2011; Sorbello 2012). Based on information from one case, the pharmacokinetics of peramivir may be changed with pregnancy (Clay 2011).

Untreated influenza infection is associated with an increased risk of adverse events to the fetus and an increased risk of complications or death to the mother (CDC 62[07], 2013). Neuraminidase inhibitors are currently recommended for the treatment or prophylaxis of influenza in pregnant women and women up to 2 weeks postpartum (CDC 60[1], 2011; CDC March 13, 2014; CDC January 2015).

Breast-Feeding Considerations It is not known if peramivir is excreted into breast milk. According to the manufacturer, the decision to breast-feed during therapy should take into account the risk of exposure to the infant and the benefits of treatment to the mother. Influenza may cause serious illness in postpartum women and prompt evaluation for febrile respiratory illnesses is recommended (Louie 2011).

Contraindications There are no contraindications listed in the manufacturer's labeling.

Warnings/Precautions Rare serious skin reactions (eg, erythema multiforme, Stevens-Johnson syndrome)) have been reported. If skin reactions are suspected or occur, institute appropriate supportive treatment. Serious hypersensitivity reactions (eg, anaphylaxis, urticaria, angioedema) have been reported with other neuraminidase inhibitors. Although these reactions have not yet been observed with peramivir, discontinue infusion immediately and treat reaction if hypersensitivity is suspected. Rare occurrences of neuropsychiatric events (including abnormal behavior, delirium, and hallucinations), including fatalities, have been reported, primarily among pediatric patients. Onset is often abrupt and subsequent resolution is rapid. These events may occur in patients with encephalitis, encephalopathy, or in uncomplicated influenza. Closely monitor for signs of abnormal behavior. Emergence of resistance substitutions or other factors (eg, viral virulence) could decrease drug effectiveness. Consider available information on influenza drug susceptibility patterns/treatment effects when using; efficacy in patients with serious influenza requiring hospitalization has not been established. Elimination is primarily renal; dosage adjustment is required in renal impairment. Potentially significant drug-drug interactions may exist, requiring dose or frequency adjustment, additional monitoring, and/or selection of alternative therapy.

Adverse Reactions

Cardiovascular: Hypertension

Central nervous system: Insomnia

Endocrine: Increased serum glucose

Gastrointestinal: Constipation, diarrhea

Hematologic and oncologic: Neutropenia
Hepatic: Increased serum ALT, increased serum AST
Neuromuscular & skeletal: Increased creatine phosphokinase
Rare but important or life-threatening: Abnormal behavior, delirium, erythema multiforme, exfoliative dermatitis, hallucination, skin rash, Stevens-Johnson syndrome

Drug Interactions

Metabolism/Transport Effects None known.

Avoid Concomitant Use There are no known interactions where it is recommended to avoid concomitant use.

Increased Effect/Toxicity There are no known significant interactions involving an increase in effect.

Decreased Effect

Peramivir may decrease the levels/effects of: Influenza Virus Vaccine (Live/Attenuated)

Preparation for Administration Dilute solution for injection in a compatible vehicle to a maximum volume of 100 mL. Administer immediately or store at 2°C to 8°C (36°F to 46°F) for up to 24 hours.

Storage/Stability Store intact vials at 20°C to 25°C (68°F to 77°F); excursions are permitted between 15°C and 30°C (59°F and 86°F).

Mechanism of Action Peramivir, a cyclopentane analogue, selectively inhibits the influenza virus neuraminidase enzyme, preventing the release of viral particles from infected cells.

Pharmacodynamics/Kinetics

Distribution: V_d: 12.56 L
Protein binding: <30%
Metabolism: Not significantly metabolized
Half-life elimination: ~20 hours
Excretion: Urine (~90% as unchanged drug)

Dosage Influenza (acute [≤2 days], uncomplicated): Adults: IV: 600 mg as a single dose.
Elderly: Refer to adult dosing.

Dosage adjustment in renal impairment: Note: Renal function may be estimated using the Cockcroft-Gault formula.
CrCl ≥50 mL/minute: No dosage adjustment necessary.
CrCl 30 to 49 mL/minute: 200 mg as a single dose
CrCl 10 to 29 mL/minute: 100 mg as a single dose
End-stage renal disease requiring (ESRD) intermittent hemodialysis (IHD): 100 mg as a single dose, administered after dialysis

Dosage adjustment in hepatic impairment: There are no dosage adjustments provided in the manufacturer's labeling (has not been studied); however, not significantly metabolized hepatically.

Administration Administer as an intravenous infusion over 15 to 30 minutes.

Monitoring Parameters Baseline BUN and serum creatinine, neurologic abnormalities (eg, abnormal behavior), rash after administration.

Dosage Forms

Solution, Intravenous [preservative free]:
Rapivab: 200 mg/20 mL (20 mL)

Perampanel (per AM pa nel)

Brand Names: U.S. Fycompa

Pharmacologic Category AMPA Glutamate Receptor Antagonist; Anticonvulsant, Miscellaneous

Use Partial-onset seizures: As adjunctive therapy for the treatment of partial-onset seizures with or without secondarily generalized seizures in patients with epilepsy who are 12 years and older.

Pregnancy Risk Factor C

Pregnancy Considerations Adverse events were observed in animal reproduction studies at doses equivalent to the human dose (based on BSA). Contraceptives containing levonorgestrel may be less effective; additional nonhormonal forms of contraception are recommended during perampanel therapy.

Patients exposed to perampanel during pregnancy are encouraged to enroll in the North American Antiepileptic Drug (NAAED) Pregnancy Registry by calling 1-888-233-2334. Additional information is available at www.aedpregnancyregistry.org.

Breast-Feeding Considerations It is not known if perampanel is excreted in breast milk. The manufacturer recommends that caution be exercised when administering perampanel to nursing women.

Contraindications There are no contraindications listed in manufacturer's labeling.

Warnings/Precautions **[U.S. Boxed Warning]: Dose-related serious and/or life-threatening neuropsychiatric events (including aggression, anger, homicidal thoughts, hostility, and irritability) have been reported most often occurring in first 6 weeks of therapy in patients with or without preexisting psychiatric disease; monitor patients closely especially during dosage adjustments and when receiving higher doses. Adjust dose or immediately discontinue use if severe or worsening symptoms occur. Inform patients and caregivers to contact their healthcare provider immediately if they experience any atypical behavioral and/or mood changes.** Pooled analysis of trials involving various antiepileptics (regardless of indication) showed an increased risk of suicidal thoughts/behavior (incidence rate: 0.43% treated patients compared to 0.24% of patients receiving placebo); risk observed as early as 1 week after initiation and continued through duration of trials (most trials ≤24 weeks). Monitor all patients for notable changes in behavior that might indicate suicidal thoughts or depression; notify healthcare provider immediately if symptoms occur. Dizziness, fatigue (including lethargy and weakness), gait disturbances (including abnormal coordination, ataxia, and balance disorder), and somnolence may occur during therapy; patients should be cautioned about performing tasks which require alertness (eg, operating machinery or driving). Concomitant use with CNS depressant (including alcohol) may increase the risk of CNS depression. Use caution if a CNS depressant must be used concurrently with perampanel. Not recommended for use in patients with severe hepatic impairment, renal impairment, or on hemodialysis; dosage adjustment recommended for mild-to-moderate hepatic impairment. Use with extreme caution in patients who are at risk of falls (including head injuries and bone fracture); perampanel has been associated with falls and traumatic injury. Anticonvulsants should not be discontinued abruptly because of the possibility of increasing seizure frequency; therapy should be withdrawn gradually (≥1 week) to minimize the potential of increased seizure frequency, unless safety concerns require a more rapid withdrawal. Use caution in elderly due to increased risk of dizziness, gait or coordination disturbances, somnolence, fatigue-related events, and falls; proceed slowly with dosing titration in patients ≥65 years of age. Potentially significant drug-drug interactions may exist, requiring dose or frequency adjustment, additional monitoring, and/or selection of alternative therapy.

Adverse Reactions

Cardiovascular: Peripheral edema
Central nervous system: Aggression, anger, anxiety, ataxia, balance impaired, confusion, coordination impaired, dizziness, euphoria, fatigue, gait disturbance, headache, hypersomnia, hypoesthesia, irritability, memory impaired, mood changes, somnolence, vertigo
Dermatologic: Bruising, skin laceration
Endocrine & metabolic: Hyponatremia

Gastrointestinal: Constipation, nausea, vomiting, weight gain
Neuromuscular & skeletal: Arthralgia, back pain, dysarthria, falling, limb injury, limb pain, musculoskeletal pain, myalgia, paresthesia, weakness
Ocular: Blurred vision, diplopia
Respiratory: Cough, oropharyngeal pain, upper respiratory tract infection
Miscellaneous: Head injury

Drug Interactions

Metabolism/Transport Effects Substrate of CYP1A2 (minor), CYP2B6 (minor), CYP3A4 (major); **Note:** Assignment of Major/Minor substrate status based on clinically relevant drug interaction potential; **Induces** CYP3A4 (weak)

Avoid Concomitant Use

Avoid concomitant use of Perampanel with any of the following: Alcohol (Ethyl); Azelastine (Nasal); CYP3A4 Inducers (Strong); Orphenadrine; Paraldehyde; St Johns Wort; Thalidomide

Increased Effect/Toxicity

Perampanel may increase the levels/effects of: Alcohol (Ethyl); Azelastine (Nasal); Buprenorphine; CNS Depressants; Hydrocodone; Methotrimeprazine; Metyrosine; Orphenadrine; OXcarbazepine; Paraldehyde; Pramipexole; ROPINIRole; Rotigotine; Selective Serotonin Reuptake Inhibitors; Suvorexant; Thalidomide; Zolpidem

The levels/effects of Perampanel may be increased by: Brimonidine (Topical); Cannabis; Dronabinol; Droperidol; Kava Kava; Magnesium Sulfate; Methotrimeprazine; Nabilone; Rufinamide; Sodium Oxybate; Tapentadol; Tetrahydrocannabinol

Decreased Effect

Perampanel may decrease the levels/effects of: ARIPiprazole; Contraceptives (Progestins); Saxagliptin

The levels/effects of Perampanel may be decreased by: Bosentan; CarBAMazepine; CYP3A4 Inducers (Moderate); CYP3A4 Inducers (Strong); Dabrafenib; Deferasirox; Fosphenytoin; Mefloquine; Orlistat; OXcarbazepine; Phenytoin; Siltuximab; St Johns Wort; Tocilizumab

Storage/Stability Store at 25°C (77°F); excursions permitted between 15°C to 30°C (59°F to 86°F).

Mechanism of Action The exact mechanism by which perampanel exerts antiseizure activity is not definitively known; it is a noncompetitive antagonist of the ionotropic alpha-amino-3-hydroxy-5-methyl-4-isoxazolepropionic acid (AMPA) glutamate receptor on postsynaptic neurons. Glutamate is a primary excitatory neurotransmitter in the central nervous center causing many neurological disorders from neuronal over excitation.

Pharmacodynamics/Kinetics

Absorption: Rapid and complete
Protein binding: 95% to 96%; primarily albumin and alpha$_1$-acid glycoprotein
Metabolism: Extensive via primary oxidation mediated by CYP3A4 and/or CYP3A5, and to a lesser extent by CYP1A2 and CYP2B6, and sequential glucuronidation
Half-life elimination: 105 hours
Time to peak: 0.5-2.5 hours
Excretion: Feces (48%); urine (22%)

Dosage Partial seizures (adjunct): Children ≥12 years, Adolescents, and Adults: Oral:

Patients **not** receiving enzyme-inducing AED regimens: Initial: 2 mg once daily at bedtime; may increase daily dose by 2 mg at weekly intervals based on response and tolerability. Recommended dose: 8 to 12 mg once daily at bedtime (maximum dose: 12 mg once daily).

Patients receiving enzyme-inducing AED regimens (eg, phenytoin, carbamazepine, oxcarbazepine): Initial: 4 mg once daily at bedtime; may increase daily dose by 2 mg at weekly intervals based on response and tolerability. Recommended dose: 8 to 12 mg once daily at bedtime (maximum dose: 12 mg once daily).

Elderly: Refer to adult dosing. Increase dose no more frequently than every 2 weeks.

Dosage adjustment in renal impairment:

CrCl ≥50 mL/minute: No dosage adjustment necessary.
CrCl 30 to 49 mL/minute: No dosage adjustment necessary; monitor closely and consider slower titration based on response and tolerability.
CrCl <30 mL/minute: Use not recommended (has not been studied).
Hemodialysis: Use not recommended (has not been studied).

Dosage adjustment in hepatic impairment:

Mild impairment (Child-Pugh class A): Initial: 2 mg once daily; may increase daily dose by 2 mg every 2 weeks based on response and tolerability. Maximum: 6 mg once daily
Moderate impairment (Child-Pugh class B): Initial: 2 mg once daily; may increase daily dose by 2 mg every 2 weeks based on response and tolerability. Maximum: 4 mg once daily
Severe impairment (Child-Pugh class C): Use not recommended (has not been studied).

Dietary Considerations May be taken without regard to meals.

Administration Administer at bedtime. May be administered without regard to meals.

Monitoring Parameters Seizure frequency/duration; suicidality (eg, suicidal thoughts, depression, behavioral changes); weight

Dosage Forms

Tablet, Oral:

Fycompa: 2 mg, 4 mg, 6 mg, 8 mg, 10 mg, 12 mg

◆ **Percocet** *see* Oxycodone and Acetaminophen *on page 1541*

◆ **Percocet-Demi (Can)** *see* Oxycodone and Acetaminophen *on page 1541*

◆ **Percodan®** *see* Oxycodone and Aspirin *on page 1542*

◆ **Percogesic® Extra Strength [OTC]** *see* Acetaminophen and Diphenhydramine *on page 36*

◆ **Perforomist** *see* Formoterol *on page 926*

Perhexiline [INT] (per HEKS i leen)

International Brand Names Corzepin (ES); Pexid (AU, BE, ES, FR, LU); Pexsig (AU)

Index Terms Perhexiline Maleate

Pharmacologic Category Antianginal Agent

Reported Use Reduce the frequency of moderate-to-severe attacks of angina pectoris

Dosage Range Adults: Oral: Initial: 100 mg/day; dose may be adjusted at 2-4 week intervals; maximum dose: 300-400 mg/day

Product Availability Product available in various countries; not currently available in the U.S.

Dosage Forms

Tablet: 100 mg

◆ **Perhexiline Maleate** *see* Perhexiline [INT] *on page 1621*

◆ **Periactin** *see* Cyproheptadine *on page 529*

◆ **Perichlor (Can)** *see* Chlorhexidine Gluconate *on page 422*

Periciazine [CAN/INT] (per ee CYE ah zeen)

Brand Names: Canada Neuleptil®

Index Terms Pericyazine

Pharmacologic Category First Generation (Typical) Antipsychotic

Use Note: Not approved in U.S.

Adjunctive therapy in selected psychotic patients to control prevailing hostility, impulsivity, or aggression

Pregnancy Considerations Teratogenic effects were observed in some animal studies. Use of antipsychotic agents during the third trimester may increase the risk of extrapyramidal and/or withdrawal symptoms (eg, agitation, feeding disorder, hypertonia, hypotonia, respiratory distress, somnolence, and tremor) in newborns. Reported adverse events have ranged from self-limiting to severe.

Contraindications Hypersensitivity to periciazine, phenothiazine derivatives, or any component of the formulation; altered states of consciousness or comatose states particularly when due to intoxication with CNS depressant medications; hepatic dysfunction; circulatory collapse; blood dyscrasias; patients receiving spinal or regional anesthesia

Warnings/Precautions Use caution in cardiovascular disease. May alter cardiac conduction (life-threatening arrhythmias have occurred with therapeutic doses of phenothiazines); QT prolongation has been reported rarely with periciazine. Use with caution in patients with electrolyte abnormalities (eg, hypokalemia, hypomagnesemia), hypothyroidism, familial long QT syndrome, concomitant medications which may augment QT prolongation, or any underlying cardiac abnormality which may also potentiate risk. May cause orthostatic hypotension; use with caution in patients at risk of this effect or those who would not tolerate transient hypotensive episodes (cerebrovascular disease, cardiovascular disease, or other medications which may predispose). Phenothiazines have been associated with worsening of pheochromocytoma; use caution.

Elderly patients with dementia-related psychosis treated with antipsychotics are at an increased risk of death compared to placebo. Most deaths appeared to be either cardiovascular (eg, heart failure, sudden death) or infectious (eg, pneumonia) in nature. An increased incidence of cerebrovascular adverse events (including fatalities) has been reported in elderly patients with dementia-related psychosis. Periciazine is not approved for use in elderly patients with dementia. Use with caution in Parkinson's disease (may be more sensitive to adverse effects), hemodynamic instability, and predisposition to seizures. Esophageal dysmotility and aspiration have been associated with antipsychotic use; use with caution in patients at risk of pneumonia (eg, Alzheimer's disease). May cause extrapyramidal symptoms, including pseudoparkinsonism, acute dystonic reactions, akathisia, and tardive dyskinesia. Risk of dystonia (and possibly other EPS) may be greater with increased doses, use of conventional antipsychotics, males, and younger patients. Risk of tardive dyskinesia and potential for irreversibility may be increased in elderly patients (particularly women), prolonged therapy, and higher total cumulative dose. May be associated with neuroleptic malignant syndrome (NMS); monitor for mental status changes, fever, muscle rigidity, and/or autonomic instability (risk may be increased in patients with Parkinson's disease or Lewy body dementia). Discontinue treatment immediately with onset of NMS; recurrence has been reported in patients rechallenged with antipsychotic therapy.

Use associated with increased prolactin levels; clinical significance of hyperprolactinemia in patients with breast cancer or other prolactin-dependent tumors is unknown. Phenothiazines may cause anticholinergic effects (confusion, agitation, constipation, xerostomia, blurred vision, urinary retention); therefore, use with caution in patients with decreased gastrointestinal motility, paralytic ileus, urinary retention, BPH, xerostomia, visual problems, or narrow-angle glaucoma (screening is recommended). May alter temperature regulation; use caution with strenuous exercise, heat exposure, dehydration, and concomitant medication possessing anticholinergic effects. May mask toxicity of other drugs or conditions (eg, intestinal obstruction, Reye's syndrome, brain tumor) due to antiemetic effects.

Check blood counts periodically and discontinue at first signs of blood dyscrasias; use is contraindicated in patients with blood dyscrasias. May be sedating; use with caution in disorders where CNS depression is a feature (risk may be lower than with other phenothiazines); caution patients about performing tasks which require mental alertness. Cigarette smoking may decrease the serum concentrations of periciazine.

Prolonged therapy may cause pigmentary retinopathy, corneal deposits, and/or changes in skin pigmentation. Patients experiencing hypersensitivity to phenothiazines in general should not be rechallenged unless deemed clinically necessary.

Adverse Reactions Listing includes adverse reactions reported with other agents from the phenothiazine class.

Cardiovascular: Arrhythmias, AV block, cardiac arrest, ECG changes, edema, hypotension, orthostatic hypotension, paroxysmal tachycardia, QTc prolongation, syncope, tachycardia, ventricular fibrillation

Central nervous system: Aggressive behavior, agitation, anxiety, bizarre dreams, cerebral edema, depression, dizziness, drowsiness, EEG changes, excitement; extrapyramidal symptoms (tremor, akathisia, dystonia, dyskinesia, oculogyric, opisthotonos, hyper-reflexia, pseudo-Parkinsonism, rigidity, sialorrhea); fatigue, fever, headache, insomnia, NMS, paradoxical psychosis, restlessness, seizure, sleep disturbance, tardive dyskinesia, temperature regulation impaired

Dermatologic: Angioedema, dermatitis, eczema, epithelial keratopathy, erythema, exfoliative dermatitis, photosensitivity, pruritus, rash, seborrhea, skin pigmentation (prolonged therapy), urticaria

Endocrine & metabolic: Delayed ovulation, galactorrhea, gynecomastia, hyperglycemia, libido changes, menstrual irregularities, thirst

Gastrointestinal: Adynamic ileus, anorexia, appetite increased, constipation, diarrhea, fecal impaction, nausea, paralytic ileus, salivation, vomiting, weight changes, xerostomia

Genitourinary: Bladder paralysis, ejaculation disturbance, impotence, incontinence, polyuria, priapism, urinary retention

Hematologic: Agranulocytosis, anemia, eosinophilia, granulocytopenia, leukopenia, neutropenia, pancytopenia, thrombocytopenia

Hepatic: Cholestasis, cholestatic jaundice, jaundice

Ocular: Blurred vision, corneal deposits (prolonged therapy), glaucoma, lenticular deposits, pigmentary retinopathy (prolonged therapy)

Respiratory: Asthma, laryngeal edema, nasal congestion, pneumonia, pneumonitis

Miscellaneous: Diaphoresis increased, lupus-like syndrome

Drug Interactions

Metabolism/Transport Effects None known.

Avoid Concomitant Use

Avoid concomitant use of Periciazine with any of the following: Aclidinium; Amisulpride; Azelastine (Nasal); Glucagon; Ipratropium (Oral Inhalation); Metoclopramide; Orphenadrine; Paraldehyde; Potassium Chloride; Sulpiride; Thalidomide; Tiotropium; Umeclidinium

Increased Effect/Toxicity

Periciazine may increase the levels/effects of: AbobotulinumtoxinA; Alcohol (Ethyl); Amisulpride; Analgesics (Opioid); Anticholinergic Agents; Antidepressants (Serotonin Reuptake Inhibitor/Antagonist); Azelastine (Nasal);

Beta-Blockers; Buprenorphine; CNS Depressants; Glucagon; Highest Risk QTc-Prolonging Agents; Hydrocodone; Methotrimeprazine; Methylphenidate; Metyrosine; Mirabegron; Mirtazapine; Moderate Risk QTc-Prolonging Agents; OnabotulinumtoxinA; Orphenadrine; Paraldehyde; Porfimer; Potassium Chloride; RimabotulinumtoxinB; Selective Serotonin Reuptake Inhibitors; Serotonin Modulators; Sulpiride; Suvorexant; Thalidomide; Thiazide Diuretics; Thiopental; Tiotropium; Topiramate; Verteporfin; Zolpidem

The levels/effects of Periciazine may be increased by: Acetylcholinesterase Inhibitors (Central); Aclidinium; Antidepressants (Serotonin Reuptake Inhibitor/Antagonist); Antimalarial Agents; Beta-Blockers; Brimonidine (Topical); Cannabis; Doxylamine; Dronabinol; Droperidol; HydrOXYzine; Ipratropium (Oral Inhalation); Kava Kava; Lithium; Magnesium Sulfate; Methotrimeprazine; Methylphenidate; Metoclopramide; Metyrosine; Mianserin; Mifepristone; Nabilone; Perampanel; Pramlintide; Rufinamide; Serotonin Modulators; Sodium Oxybate; Tapentadol; Tetrahydrocannabinol; Umeclidinium

Decreased Effect

Periciazine may decrease the levels/effects of: Acetylcholinesterase Inhibitors; Amphetamines; Anti-Parkinson's Agents (Dopamine Agonist); Itopride; Quinagolide; Secretin

The levels/effects of Periciazine may be decreased by: Acetylcholinesterase Inhibitors; Antacids; Anti-Parkinson's Agents (Dopamine Agonist); Lithium

Storage/Stability Store at room temperature of 15°C to 30°C (59°F to 86°F). Protect from light.

Mechanism of Action Blocks postsynaptic mesolimbic dopaminergic receptors in the brain; depresses the release of hypothalamic and hypophyseal hormones.

Dosage Oral:

Children ≥5 years: Psychosis: Initial: 2.5-10 mg in the morning, followed by 5-30 mg in the evening. In general, lower dosage should be used on initiation and gradually increased based on effect and tolerance.

Adults: Psychosis: Initial: 5-20 mg in the morning, followed by 10-40 mg in the evening. Maintenance: Decrease dose to lowest effective dose. **Note:** Reduced doses (2.5-15 mg in the morning and 5-30 mg in the evening) may be considered. In general, lower dosage should be used on initiation and gradually increased based on effect and tolerance.

Elderly: Initial: ~5 mg/day; may increase dose gradually based on effect and tolerance. Doses >30 mg/day are rarely needed. Also see adult dosing.

Dosage adjustment in renal impairment: No dosage adjustment provided in manufacturer's labeling.

Dosage adjustment in hepatic impairment: No dosage adjustment provided in manufacturer's labeling.

Administration To minimize or avoid excessive drowsiness, administer in divided doses with larger dose in the evening.

Monitoring Parameters Vital signs; CBC (at baseline and then periodically thereafter), serum potassium and magnesium, lipid profile; fasting blood glucose/HbA_{1c}; waist circumference, BMI; mental status, abnormal involuntary movement scale (AIMS); periodic eye exam and evaluation of renal and liver function tests (long-term therapy)

Based on experience with other piperidine phenothiazines: Consider baseline and periodic ECG

Product Availability Not available in U.S.

Dosage Forms: Canada

Capsule, oral:

Neuleptil®: 5 mg, 10 mg, 20 mg

Solution, oral [drops]:

Neuleptil®: 10 mg/mL

- ◆ **Peri-Colace [OTC]** *see* Docusate and Senna *on page 662*
- ◆ **Pericyazine** *see* Periciazine [CAN/INT] *on page 1621*
- ◆ **Peridex** *see* Chlorhexidine Gluconate *on page 422*
- ◆ **Peridex Oral Rinse (Can)** *see* Chlorhexidine Gluconate *on page 422*

Perindopril (per IN doe pril)

Brand Names: U.S. Aceon

Brand Names: Canada Coversyl

Index Terms Perindopril Erbumine

Pharmacologic Category Angiotensin-Converting Enzyme (ACE) Inhibitor; Antihypertensive

Use Treatment of hypertension; reduction of cardiovascular mortality or nonfatal myocardial infarction in patients with stable coronary artery disease

The 2014 guideline for the management of high blood pressure in adults (Eighth Joint National Committee [JNC 8]) recommends initiation of pharmacologic treatment to lower blood pressure for the following patients:

- Patients ≥60 years of age with systolic blood pressure (SBP) ≥150 mm Hg or diastolic blood pressure (DBP) ≥ 90 mm Hg. Goal of therapy is SBP <150 mm Hg and DBP <90 mm Hg.
- Patients <60 years of age with SBP ≥140 mm Hg or DBP is ≥90 mm Hg. Goal of therapy is SBP <140 mm Hg and DBP <90 mm Hg.
- Patients ≥18 years of age with diabetes and SBP ≥140 mm Hg or DBP ≥90 mm Hg. Goal of therapy is SBP <140 mm Hg and DBP <90 mm Hg.
- Patients ≥18 years of age with chronic kidney disease (CKD) and SBP ≥140 mm Hg or DBP ≥90 mm Hg. Goal of therapy is SBP <140 mm Hg and DBP <90 mm Hg.

In patients with CKD, regardless of race or diabetes status, the use of an ACE inhibitor (ACEI) or angiotensin receptor blocker (ARB) as initial therapy is recommended to improve kidney outcomes. In the general nonblack population (without CKD) including those with diabetes, initial antihypertensive treatment should consist of a thiazide-type diuretic, calcium channel blocker, ACEI, or ARB. In the general black population (without CKD) including those with diabetes, initial antihypertensive treatment should consist of a thiazide-type diuretic or a calcium channel blocker **instead of** an ACEI or ARB.

Note: The ACCF/AHA 2013 heart failure guidelines recommend the use of ACE inhibitors, along with other guideline-directed medical therapies, to prevent HF in patients with a reduced ejection fraction who have a history of MI (stage B HF), to prevent HF in any patient with a reduced ejection fraction (stage B HF), or to treat those with HF and reduced ejection fraction (stage C HFrEF) (ACCF/AHA [Yancy, 2013])

Canadian labeling: Additional use (off-label use in U.S.): Treatment of mild-moderate (NYHA I-III) heart failure (HF)

Pregnancy Risk Factor D

Pregnancy Considerations [U.S. Boxed Warning]: Drugs that act on the renin-angiotensin system can cause injury and death to the developing fetus. Discontinue as soon as possible once pregnancy is detected. Perindopril crosses the placenta; teratogenic effects may occur following maternal use during pregnancy. Drugs that act on the renin-angiotensin system are associated with oligohydramnios. Oligohydramnios, due to decreased fetal renal function, may lead to fetal lung hypoplasia and skeletal malformations. Their use in pregnancy is also associated with anuria, hypotension, renal failure, skull hypoplasia, and death in the fetus/neonate. Chronic maternal hypertension itself is also associated with adverse events in the fetus/infant. ACE inhibitors are not recommended during pregnancy to treat maternal hypertension or heart failure. Use of an ACE inhibitor should also be avoided in any woman of reproductive age. Women who are planning a pregnancy should be considered for other medication options if an ACE inhibitor is currently prescribed or the ACE inhibitor should be discontinued as soon as possible once pregnancy is detected. The exposed fetus should be monitored for fetal growth, amniotic fluid volume, and organ formation. Infants exposed to an ACE inhibitor *in utero* should be monitored for hyperkalemia, hypotension, and oliguria (exchange transfusions or dialysis may be needed). These adverse events are generally associated with maternal use in the second and third trimesters.

Untreated chronic maternal hypertension is also associated with adverse events in the fetus, infant, and mother. The use of ACE inhibitors is not recommended to treat chronic uncomplicated hypertension in pregnant women and should generally be avoided in women of reproductive potential (ACOG, 2013).

Breast-Feeding Considerations It is not known if perindopril is excreted in human breast milk. The U.S. labeling recommends that caution be exercised when administering perindopril to nursing women. The Canadian labeling contraindicates use in nursing women.

Contraindications

Hypersensitivity to perindopril, any other ACE inhibitor, or any component of the formulation; angioedema related to previous treatment with an ACE inhibitor; history of hereditary/idiopathic angioedema; concomitant use with aliskiren in patients with diabetes mellitus

Canadian labeling: Additional contraindications (not in U.S. labeling): Concomitant use with aliskiren in patients with moderate-to-severe renal impairment (GFR <60 mL/minute/1.73 m^2); women who are pregnant, planning to become pregnant, or nursing; hereditary problems of galactose intolerance, glucose-galactose malabsorption, or the Lapp lactase deficiency (formulation contains lactose)

Warnings/Precautions Anaphylactic reactions may occur rarely with ACE inhibitors. At any time during treatment (especially following first dose), angioedema may occur rarely with ACE inhibitors; it may involve the head and neck (potentially compromising airway) or the intestine (presenting with abdominal pain). African-Americans and patients with idiopathic or hereditary angioedema may be at an increased risk. Prolonged frequent monitoring may be required especially if tongue, glottis, or larynx are involved as they are associated with airway obstruction. Patients with a history of airway surgery may have a higher risk of airway obstruction. Aggressive early and appropriate management is critical. Use in patients with previous angioedema associated with ACE inhibitor therapy is contraindicated. Severe anaphylactoid reactions may be seen during hemodialysis (eg, CVVHD) with high-flux dialysis membranes (eg, AN69), and rarely, during low density lipoprotein apheresis with dextran sulfate cellulose. Rare cases of anaphylactoid reactions have been reported in patients undergoing sensitization treatment with hymenoptera (bee, wasp) venom while receiving ACE inhibitors.

Symptomatic hypotension with or without syncope can occur with ACE inhibitors (usually with the first several doses); effects are most often observed in volume-depleted patients; correct volume depletion prior to initiation; close monitoring of patient is required especially with initial dosing and dosing increases; blood pressure must be lowered at a rate appropriate for the patient's clinical condition. Initiation of therapy in patients with ischemic heart disease or cerebrovascular disease warrants close observation due to the potential consequences posed by falling blood pressure (eg, MI, stroke). Use with caution in hypertrophic cardiomyopathy with outflow tract obstruction, severe aortic stenosis, or before, during, or immediately after major surgery. **[U.S. Boxed Warning]: Drugs that act on the renin-angiotensin system can cause injury and death to the developing fetus. Discontinue as soon as possible once pregnancy is detected.**

Hyperkalemia may occur with ACE inhibitors; risk factors include renal dysfunction, diabetes mellitus, concomitant use of potassium-sparing diuretics, potassium supplements, and/or potassium-containing salts. Use cautiously, if at all, with these agents and monitor potassium closely. Cough may occur with ACE inhibitors. Other causes of cough should be considered (eg, pulmonary congestion in patients with heart failure) and excluded prior to discontinuation.

May be associated with deterioration of renal function and/or increases in serum creatinine, particularly in patients with low renal blood flow (eg, renal artery stenosis, heart failure) whose glomerular filtration rate (GFR) is dependent on efferent arteriolar vasoconstriction by angiotensin II; deterioration may result in oliguria, acute renal failure, and progressive azotemia. Small increases in serum creatinine may occur following initiation; consider discontinuation only in patients with progressive and/or significant deterioration in renal function. Use with caution in patients with unstented unilateral/bilateral renal artery stenosis. When unstented bilateral renal artery stenosis is present, use is generally avoided due to the elevated risk of deterioration in renal function unless possible benefits outweigh risks. Potentially significant drug-drug interactions may exist, requiring dose or frequency adjustment, additional monitoring, and/or selection of alternative therapy.

Rare toxicities associated with ACE inhibitors include cholestatic jaundice (which may progress to fulminant hepatic necrosis), agranulocytosis, neutropenia or leukopenia with myeloid hypoplasia. Patients with collagen vascular diseases (especially with concomitant renal impairment) or renal impairment alone may be at increased risk for hematologic toxicity; periodically monitor CBC with differential in these patients.

Adverse Reactions

Cardiovascular: Chest pain, edema

Central nervous system: Depression, dizziness, fever, headache, nervousness, sleep disorders

Dermatologic: Rash

Endocrine & metabolic: Hyperkalemia, increased triglycerides

Gastrointestinal: Abdominal pain, diarrhea, dyspepsia, flatulence, nausea, vomiting

Genitourinary: Sexual dysfunction

Hepatic: Increased ALT

Neuromuscular & skeletal: Arthritis, back pain, joint pain, lower extremity pain, myalgia, paresthesia, upper extremity pain, weakness

Renal: Proteinuria

Respiratory: Cough (incidence is higher in women, 3:1), pharyngitis, rhinitis, sinusitis

Otic: Tinnitus

Miscellaneous: Seasonal allergy, viral infection

Rare but important or life-threatening: Amnesia, anaphylaxis, angioedema, anxiety, AST increased, dyspnea, erythema, fluid retention, gout, leukopenia, migraine, MI, nephrolithiasis, neutropenia, orthostatic hypotension, pruritus, psychosocial disorder, pulmonary fibrosis, purpura, stroke, syncope, urinary retention, vertigo, visual hallucinations (Doane, 2013)

Additional adverse effects that have been reported with **ACE inhibitors** include agranulocytosis (especially in patients with renal impairment or collagen vascular disease), neutropenia, anemia, bullous pemphigoid, cardiac arrest, eosinophilic pneumonitis, exfoliative dermatitis, falls, hepatic failure, hyponatremia, jaundice, pancreatitis (acute), pancytopenia, pemphigus, psoriasis, thrombocytopenia; decreases in creatinine clearance in some elderly hypertensive patients or those with chronic renal failure, and worsening of renal function in patients with bilateral renal artery stenosis or hypovolemic patients (diuretic therapy). In addition, a syndrome which may include fever, myalgia, arthralgia, interstitial nephritis, vasculitis, rash, eosinophilia and positive ANA, and elevated ESR has been reported with ACE inhibitors.

Drug Interactions

Metabolism/Transport Effects None known.

Avoid Concomitant Use There are no known interactions where it is recommended to avoid concomitant use.

Increased Effect/Toxicity

Perindopril may increase the levels/effects of: Allopurinol; Amifostine; Antihypertensives; AzaTHIOprine; DULoxetine; Ferric Gluconate; Gold Sodium Thiomalate; Grass Pollen Allergen Extract (5 Grass Extract); Hypotensive Agents; Iron Dextran Complex; Levodopa; Lithium; Nonsteroidal Anti-Inflammatory Agents; Obinutuzumab; RisperiDONE; RiTUXimab; Sodium Phosphates

The levels/effects of Perindopril may be increased by: Alfuzosin; Aliskiren; Angiotensin II Receptor Blockers; Barbiturates; Brimonidine (Topical); Canagliflozin; Dapoxetine; Diazoxide; DPP-IV Inhibitors; Eplerenone; Everolimus; Heparin; Heparin (Low Molecular Weight); Herbs (Hypotensive Properties); Loop Diuretics; MAO Inhibitors; Nicorandil; Pentoxifylline; Phosphodiesterase 5 Inhibitors; Potassium Salts; Potassium-Sparing Diuretics; Prostacyclin Analogues; Sirolimus; Temsirolimus; Thiazide Diuretics; TiZANidine; Tolvaptan; Trimethoprim

Decreased Effect

The levels/effects of Perindopril may be decreased by: Aprotinin; Herbs (Hypertensive Properties); Icatibant; Lanthanum; Methylphenidate; Nonsteroidal Anti-Inflammatory Agents; Salicylates; Yohimbine

Food Interactions Perindopril active metabolite concentrations may be lowered if taken with food. Management: Administer prior to a meal.

Storage/Stability Store at room temperature of 20°C to 25°C (68°F to 77°F). Protect from moisture.

Mechanism of Action Perindopril is a prodrug for perindoprilat, which acts as a competitive inhibitor of angiotensin-converting enzyme (ACE); prevents conversion of angiotensin I to angiotensin II, a potent vasoconstrictor; results in lower levels of angiotensin II which, in turn, causes an increase in plasma renin activity and a reduction in aldosterone secretion

Pharmacodynamics/Kinetics

Onset of action: Peak effect: 1-2 hours

Protein binding: Perindopril: 60%; Perindoprilat: 10% to 20%

Metabolism: Hepatically hydrolyzed to active metabolite, perindoprilat (~17% to 20% of a dose) and other inactive metabolites

Bioavailability: Perindopril: 75%; Perindoprilat ~25% (~16% with food)

Half-life elimination: Parent drug: 1.5-3 hours; Metabolite: Effective: 3-10 hours, Terminal: 30-120 hours

Time to peak: Chronic therapy: Perindopril: 1 hour; Perindoprilat: 3-7 hours (maximum perindoprilat serum levels are 2-3 times higher and T_{max} is shorter following chronic therapy); CHF: Perindoprilat: 6 hours

Excretion: Urine (75%, 4% to 12% as unchanged drug)

Dosage Oral:

Adults:

Heart failure (Canadian labeling; off-label use in U.S.): Initial: 2 mg once daily; if necessary, may titrate over 2-4 weeks to 4 mg once daily. The ACCF/AHA 2013 heart failure guidelines recommend an initial dose of 2 mg once daily with gradual dose titration to a target dose of 8-16 mg once daily (Yancy, 2013).

Hypertension: Initial: 4 mg/day but may be titrated to response; usual range: 4-8 mg/day (may be given in 2 divided doses); increase at 1- to 2-week intervals (maximum: 16 mg/day). **Note:** The Canadian labeling recommended maximum dose is 8 mg/day.

Concomitant therapy with diuretics: To reduce the risk of hypotension, discontinue diuretic, if possible, 2-3 days prior to initiating perindopril. If unable to stop diuretic, initiate perindopril at 2-4 mg/day (given in 1-2 divided doses) and monitor blood pressure closely for the first 2 weeks of therapy, and after any dose adjustment of perindopril or diuretic.

Stable coronary artery disease: Initial: 4 mg once daily for 2 weeks; then increase as tolerated to 8 mg once daily.

Elderly:

Hypertension: >65 years:

U.S. labeling: Initial: 4 mg/day; maintenance: 8 mg/day; experience with doses >8 mg/day is limited; may be given in 1-2 divided doses

Canadian labeling: Initial: 2 mg/day; if necessary may increase dose after 4 weeks to 4 mg/day; then to 8 mg/day (based on renal function); may be given in 1 or 2 divided doses.

ACCF/AHA Expert Consensus recommendations: Consider lower initial doses and titrating to response (Aronow, 2011)

Stable coronary artery disease: >70 years: Initial: 2 mg/day for 1 week; then increase as tolerated to 4 mg/day for 1 week; then increase as tolerated to 8 mg/day.

Dosage adjustment in renal impairment:

U.S. labeling:

CrCl >30 mL/minute: Initial: 2 mg/day; maintenance dosing not to exceed 8 mg/day.

CrCl <30 mL/minute: Safety and efficacy not established.

Hemodialysis: Perindopril and its metabolites are dialyzable.

Canadian labeling:

CrCl ≥60 mL/minute: Initial: 4 mg/day; maintenance dosing not to exceed 8 mg/day

CrCl 30-60 mL/minute: 2 mg/day

CrCl 15-30 mL/minute: 2 mg every other day

Hemodialysis (CrCl <15 mL/minute): 2 mg on dialysis days (given after dialysis)

Dosage adjustment in hepatic impairment: No dosage adjustment provided in manufacturer's labeling. However, perindoprilat bioavailability is increased with hepatic impairment.

Administration Administer prior to a meal.

Monitoring Parameters Blood pressure; serum creatinine and potassium; if patient has collagen vascular disease and/or renal impairment, periodically monitor CBC with differential

2013 ACCF/AHA Heart Failure guideline recommendations: Within 1-2 weeks after initiation and periodically thereafter, reassess renal function and serum potassium especially in patients with preexisting hypotension, hyponatremia, diabetes mellitus, azotemia, or those taking potassium supplements (ACCF/AHA [Yancy, 2013]).

Additional Information *International considerations:* International products may be available as either the erbumine/tert-butylamine or arginine salt; dosages are expressed as salt strength: perindopril erbumine/tert-butylamine 4 mg is approximately equivalent to perindopril arginine 5 mg.

Dosage Forms

Tablet, Oral:

Aceon: 4 mg, 8 mg

Generic: 2 mg, 4 mg, 8 mg

Dosage Forms: Canada

Tablet, Oral:

Coversyl: 2 mg, 4 mg, 8 mg

Perindopril and Indapamide [CAN/INT]

(per IN doe pril & in DAP a mide)

Brand Names: Canada Coversyl Plus; Coversyl Plus HD; Coversyl Plus LD

Index Terms Indapamide and Perindopril; Perindopril Erbumine and Indapamide

Pharmacologic Category Angiotensin-Converting Enzyme (ACE) Inhibitor; Antihypertensive; Diuretic, Thiazide-Related

Use Note: Not approved in U.S.

Treatment of hypertension. Coversyl Plus LD may be used as initial treatment. Coversyl Plus and Coversyl Plus HD are not indicated for initial treatment of hypertension

Pregnancy Considerations [Canadian Boxed Warning]: Drugs that act on the renin-angiotensin system can cause injury and death to the developing fetus. Discontinue as soon as possible once pregnancy is detected. Use is contraindicated during the second and third trimesters of pregnancy. Also see individual agents.

Breast-Feeding Considerations Use is contraindicated in breast-feeding women.

Contraindications Hypersensitivity to perindopril, indapamide, any other component of the formulation, or sulfonamide-derived drugs; hereditary/idiopathic angioedema or history of angioedema related to previous treatment with an ACE inhibitor; hypokalemia; severe hepatic impairment; hepatic encephalopathy; second and third trimesters of pregnancy; breast-feeding; concomitant therapy with non-antiarrhythmic agents causing torsade de pointes; concomitant use with aliskiren-containing drugs in patients with diabetes mellitus (type 1 or type 2) or moderate-to-severe renal impairment (GFR <60 mL/minute/1.73 m^2); severe renal impairment (CrCl <30 mL/minute); **Note:** Coversyl Plus HD is also contraindicated in moderate renal impairment (CrCl 30-60 mL/minute)

Warnings/Precautions See individual agents.

Adverse Reactions Note: Observed with perindopril/indapamide; also see individual agents.

Central nervous system: Dizziness

Endocrine & metabolic: Hyper-/hypokalemia

Gastrointestinal: Dyspepsia, nausea, vomiting

Renal: BUN increased

Respiratory: Cough, upper respiratory infection

Rare but important or life-threatening: Agranulocytosis, angina, angioedema, arrhythmias, colitis, creatinine increased, CVA, dermatitis, depression, ECG abnormal, edema, eosinophilic pneumonia, epidermal necrolysis, epistaxis, erythema multiforme, erythroderma purpura, fever, flushing, gout, hemoglobin decreased, hepatitis, hyperbilirubinemia, hyper-/hypotension, hypersensitivity, hyponatremia, impotence, interstitial nephritis, metabolic alkalosis, neutropenia, oliguria, optic neuritis, orthostatic hypotension, palpitation, pancreatitis, photosensitivity, pruritus, rash, renal impairment, respiratory insufficiency, rhabdomyolysis, Stevens-Johnson syndrome, syncope, tachycardia, tetany, thrombocytopenia, tinnitus, torsade de pointes, transaminases increased, uric acid increased, ventricular arrhythmia, visual disturbance

Drug Interactions

Metabolism/Transport Effects None known.

Avoid Concomitant Use

Avoid concomitant use of Perindopril and Indapamide with any of the following: Dofetilide

Increased Effect/Toxicity

Perindopril and Indapamide may increase the levels/effects of: ACE Inhibitors; Allopurinol; Amifostine; Antihypertensives; AzaTHIOprine; Calcium Salts; CarBAMazepine; Cardiac Glycosides; Cyclophosphamide; Diazoxide; Dofetilide; DULoxetine; Ferric Gluconate; Gold Sodium Thiomalate; Grass Pollen Allergen Extract (5 Grass Extract); Highest Risk QTc-Prolonging Agents; Hypotensive Agents; Iron Dextran Complex; Levodopa; Lithium; Moderate Risk QTc-Prolonging Agents; Multivitamins/Minerals (with ADEK, Folate, Iron); Multivitamins/Minerals (with AE, No Iron); Nonsteroidal Anti-Inflammatory Agents; Obinutuzumab; OXcarbazepine; Porfimer; RisperiDONE; RiTUXimab; Sodium Phosphates; Topiramate; Verteporfin; Vitamin D Analogs

The levels/effects of Perindopril and Indapamide may be increased by: Alcohol (Ethyl); Alfuzosin; Aliskiren; Analgesics (Opioid); Angiotensin II Receptor Blockers; Anticholinergic Agents; Barbiturates; Beta2-Agonists; Brimonidine (Topical); Canagliflozin; Corticosteroids (Orally Inhaled); Corticosteroids (Systemic); Dapoxetine; Dexketoprofen; Diazoxide; DPP-IV Inhibitors; Eplerenone; Everolimus; Heparin; Heparin (Low Molecular Weight); Herbs (Hypotensive Properties); Licorice; Loop Diuretics; MAO Inhibitors; Mifepristone; Multivitamins/Fluoride (with ADE); Nicorandil; Pentoxifylline; Phosphodiesterase 5 Inhibitors; Potassium Salts; Potassium-Sparing Diuretics; Prostacyclin Analogues; Selective Serotonin Reuptake Inhibitors; Sirolimus; Temsirolimus; Thiazide Diuretics; TiZANidine; Tolvaptan; Trimethoprim

Decreased Effect

Perindopril and Indapamide may decrease the levels/effects of: Antidiabetic Agents

The levels/effects of Perindopril and Indapamide may be decreased by: Aprotinin; Bile Acid Sequestrants; Herbs (Hypertensive Properties); Icatibant; Lanthanum; Methylphenidate; Nonsteroidal Anti-Inflammatory Agents; Salicylates; Yohimbine

Food Interactions Bioavailability of perindoprilat (active metabolite of perindopril) is reduced ~35% by food. Management: Administer prior to a meal.

Storage/Stability Store at room temperature of 15°C to 30°C (59°F to 86°F).

Mechanism of Action See individual agents.

Pharmacodynamics/Kinetics See individual agents.

Dosage Note: Dosing is individualized. Coversyl® Plus and Coversyl® Plus HD are not indicated for initial treatment of hypertension. Titration of individual components to an appropriate clinical response is required prior to converting to an equivalent dose of Coversyl® Plus or Coversyl® Plus HD.

Hypertension: Oral:

Adults:

Initial: Perindopril 2 mg/indapamide 0.625 mg once daily; may increase as necessary to perindopril 4 mg/indapamide 1.25 mg once daily.

Maintenance dose: Perindopril 2-8 mg/indapamide 0.625-2.5 mg once daily.

Elderly: Use with caution. Dosage adjustments may be necessary; however, specific recommendations are not provided in the approved labeling.

Dosage adjustment in renal impairment:

CrCl >60 mL/minute: No dosage adjustment necessary.

CrCl ≥30-60 mL/minute: No specific dosing guidelines for the combination product are provided with the approved labeling; use lower doses with caution due to perindopril component. Dosing of perindopril 8 mg/indapamide 2.5 mg is contraindicated.

CrCl <30 mL/minute: Use is contraindicated.

Dosage adjustment in hepatic impairment: No dosage adjustment provided in manufacturer's labeling. Use is contraindicated in patients with severe hepatic impairment or hepatic encephalopathy.

Dietary Considerations Take without food.

Administration Administer early in the day to avoid nocturia. Food may decrease the bioavailability of perindoprilat (active metabolite of perindopril). Administer prior to a meal.

Monitoring Parameters Blood pressure; BUN, serum creatinine, uric acid (as appropriate), glucose (as appropriate), and electrolytes; if patient has collagen vascular disease and/or renal impairment, periodically monitor CBC with differential

Product Availability Not available in U.S.

Dosage Forms: Canada

Tablet, oral:

Coversyl® Plus: Perindopril erbumine 4 mg and indapamide 1.25 mg

Coversyl® Plus HD: Perindopril erbumine 8 mg and indapamide 2.5 mg

Coversyl® Plus LD: Perindopril erbumine 2 mg and indapamide 0.625 mg

- ◆ **Perindopril Erbumine** *see* Perindopril *on page* 1623
- ◆ **Perindopril Erbumine and Indapamide** *see* Perindopril and Indapamide [CAN/INT] *on page* 1626
- ◆ **Periogard** *see* Chlorhexidine Gluconate *on page* 422
- ◆ **PerioMed** *see* Fluoride *on page* 895
- ◆ **Periostat (Can)** *see* Doxycycline *on page* 689
- ◆ **Perjeta** *see* Pertuzumab *on page* 1627
- ◆ **Perlane** *see* Hyaluronate and Derivatives *on page* 1006
- ◆ **Perlane-L** *see* Hyaluronate and Derivatives *on page* 1006

Permethrin (per METH rin)

Brand Names: U.S. Acticin; Elimite

Brand Names: Canada Kwellada-P [OTC]; Nix [OTC]

Index Terms Elimite

Pharmacologic Category Antiparasitic Agent, Topical; Pediculocide; Scabicidal Agent

Use Single-application treatment of infestation with *Pediculus humanus capitis* (head louse) and its nits or *Sarcoptes scabiei* (scabies); indicated for prophylactic use during epidemics of lice

Pregnancy Risk Factor B

Dosage Topical:

Head lice: Children >2 months and Adults: After hair has been washed with shampoo, rinsed with water, and towel dried, apply a sufficient volume of topical liquid (lotion or cream rinse) to saturate the hair and scalp. Leave on hair for 10 minutes before rinsing off with water; remove remaining nits; may repeat in 1 week if lice or nits still present.

Scabies: Apply cream from head to toe; leave on for 8-14 hours before washing off with water; for infants, also apply on the hairline, neck, scalp, temple, and forehead; may reapply in 1 week if live mites appear

Additional Information Complete prescribing information should be consulted for additional detail.

Dosage Forms

Cream, External:

Acticin: 5% (60 g)

Elimite: 5% (60 g)

Generic: 5% (60 g)

Lotion, External:

Generic: 1% (59 mL)

Perphenazine (per FEN a zeen)

Brand Names: Canada Apo-Perphenazine®

Index Terms Trilafon

Pharmacologic Category Antiemetic; First Generation (Typical) Antipsychotic

Additional Appendix Information

Beers Criteria – Potentially Inappropriate Medications for Geriatrics *on page* 2271

Use Treatment of schizophrenia; severe nausea and vomiting

Dosage Oral:

Adults:

Schizophrenia:

Nonhospitalized: Initial: 4-8 mg 3 times/day; reduce dose as soon as possible to minimum effective dosage (maximum: 24 mg/day)

Hospitalized: 8-16 mg 2-4 times/day (maximum: 64 mg/day)

Nausea/vomiting: 8-16 mg/day in divided doses; reduce dose as soon as possible to minimum effective dosage (maximum: 24 mg/day)

Elderly: No dosage adjustment provided in manufacturer's labeling; however, initiate dosing at the lower end of the dosing range. Refer to adult dosing.

Dosing adjustment in renal impairment: 0% to 5% removed by hemodialysis (HD); no dosage adjustment provided in manufacturer's labeling.

Dosing adjustment in hepatic impairment: No dosage adjustment provided in manufacturer's labeling.

Additional Information Complete prescribing information should be consulted for additional detail.

Dosage Forms

Tablet, Oral:

Generic: 2 mg, 4 mg, 8 mg, 16 mg

- ◆ **Perphenazine and Amitriptyline Hydrochloride** *see* Amitriptyline and Perphenazine *on page* 122
- ◆ **Persantine** *see* Dipyridamole *on page* 652
- ◆ **Persantine® (Can)** *see* Dipyridamole *on page* 652
- ◆ **Pertussis, Acellular (Adsorbed)** *see* Diphtheria and Tetanus Toxoids, Acellular Pertussis, Poliovirus and *Haemophilus* b Conjugate Vaccine *on page* 648

Pertuzumab (per TU zoo mab)

Brand Names: U.S. Perjeta

Brand Names: Canada Perjeta

Index Terms 2C4 Antibody; MOAB 2C4; Monoclonal Antibody 2C4; Omnitarg; rhuMAb-2C4

Pharmacologic Category Antineoplastic Agent, Anti-HER2; Antineoplastic Agent, Monoclonal Antibody

Use

Breast cancer, metastatic: Treatment of human epidermal growth factor receptor 2 (HER2)-positive metastatic breast cancer (in combination with trastuzumab and docetaxel) in patients who have not received prior anti-HER2 therapy or chemotherapy to treat metastatic disease

Breast cancer, neoadjuvant treatment: Neoadjuvant treatment of locally advanced, inflammatory, or early stage HER2-positive, breast cancer (either greater than 2 cm in diameter or node positive) in combination with trastuzumab and docetaxel (as part of a complete treatment regimen for early breast cancer).

Pregnancy Risk Factor D

Pregnancy Considerations May cause fetal harm if administered during pregnancy. **[U.S. Boxed Warning]: Pertuzumab exposure during pregnancy may result in embryo-fetal mortality and birth defects. Oligohydramnios, delayed fetal kidney development, and embryo-fetal death have been observed in animal reproduction studies. Advise patients of the risks and the need for effective contraception.** Verify pregnancy status prior to treatment initiation. Effective contraception should be used during therapy and for 6 months after treatment. Advise patients to immediately report to healthcare provider if pregnancy is suspected during treatment. Effects during pregnancy are likely to occur in all 3 trimesters. If administered during pregnancy, monitor for oligohydramnios (if oligohydramnios occurs, fetal testing is indicated). Report pregnancies exposed to pertuzumab to the Genentech Adverse Event Line (1-888-835-2555). Women exposed to pertuzumab during pregnancy are encouraged to enroll in MotHER (the Pregnancy Registry; 1-800-690-6720).

Breast-Feeding Considerations It is not known if pertuzumab is excreted in human milk. Because many immunoglobulins are excreted in human milk, and the potential for serious adverse reactions in the nursing infant exists, the decision to discontinue breast-feeding or to discontinue pertuzumab should take into account the benefits of treatment to the mother. The extended half-life should be considered for decisions regarding breast-feeding after treatment is completed.

Contraindications Hypersensitivity to pertuzumab or any component of the formulation

Warnings/Precautions Hazardous agent - use appropriate precautions for handling and disposal (meets NIOSH 2014 criteria). **[U.S. Boxed Warning]: May result in cardiac failure (clinical and subclinical). Assess left ventricular ejection fraction (LVEF) in all patients at baseline and during treatment. Discontinue for confirmed clinically significant decline in left ventricular function.** Decreases in LVEF are associated with HER-2 inhibitors, including pertuzumab. Patients who received prior anthracycline therapy or chest irradiation may be at an increased risk for cardiotoxicity. In studies of pertuzumab (versus placebo) in combination with trastuzumab and docetaxel for the treatment of metastatic breast cancer, the rate of cardiotoxicity (LVEF decline or symptomatic LV systolic dysfunction) was not increased in the pertuzumab group when compared to placebo. In the neoadjuvant setting, the incidence of LV dysfunction was higher in patients treated with pertuzumab. In a study of pertuzumab, trastuzumab and docetaxel, compared with trastuzumab and docetaxel, the incidence of LVEF decline (of >10% decrease from baseline or to <50%) was 8.4% and 1.9%., respectively; LVEF recovered to ≥50% in all patients. In another neoadjuvant study, LVEF declines (of >10% decrease from baseline or to <50%) were noted in 6.9% to 16% of patients receiving various combinations and sequences of pertuzumab plus trastuzumab with FEC (fluorouracil, epirubicin, and cyclophosphamide), docetaxel, and/or carboplatin; LVEF recovered to ≥50% in most patients. Of note, patients with pretreatment LVEF ≤50%, CHF, LVEF decreases to <50% during prior trastuzumab treatment, or conditions which could impair LV function (eg, uncontrolled hypertension, recent MI, serious arrhythmia requiring treatment, or cumulative lifetime anthracycline exposure >360 mg/m^2 doxorubicin or its equivalent) were excluded from studies. Assess LVEF at baseline, every 3 months during treatment (metastatic patients) or every 6 weeks during treatment (neoadjuvant setting), and every 6 months after therapy discontinuation up to 24 months after the last dose of pertuzumab and/or trastuzumab. Withhold pertuzumab and trastuzumab if LVEF <45% **or** 45% to 49% with a ≥10% absolute decline from baseline; repeat LVEF assessment in ~3 weeks; discontinue if LVEF has not improved or has declined further (unless potential benefits outweigh risks).

Infusion reactions (either during or on the day of infusion) have been associated with pertuzumab; commonly described as fever, chills, fatigue, headache, weakness, myalgia, hypersensitivity, abnormal taste or vomiting. The incidence of hypersensitivity/anaphylaxis was slightly higher in the group receiving pertuzumab (compared to placebo) in combination with trastuzumab and docetaxel. Monitor for 1 hour after the first infusion and for 30 minutes after subsequent infusions. For significant infusion reactions, interrupt or slow infusion rate; for severe infusion reactions, consider permanently discontinuing. Medications and equipment for the treatment of hypersensitivity should be available for immediate use during infusion. May cause fetal harm is administered during pregnancy. **[U.S. Boxed Warning]: Pertuzumab exposure during pregnancy may result in embryo-fetal mortality and birth defects. Oligohydramnios, delayed fetal kidney development, and embryo-fetal death have been observed in animal reproduction studies. Advise patients of the risks and the need for effective contraception.** Verify pregnancy status prior to treatment initiation. Effective contraception should be used by all patients receiving pertuzumab during therapy and for 6 months after treatment. Effects during pregnancy are likely to occur in any trimester.

Establish HER2 status prior to treatment; has only been studied in patients with evidence of HER2 overexpression, either as 3+ IHC (Dako Herceptest™) or FISH amplification ratio ≥2 (Dako *HER2* FISH pharmDx™ test). Safety of combination or sequential therapy with doxorubicin-containing regimens has not been established. For early breast cancer, the safety of treatment beyond 6 cycles has not been determined.

Adverse Reactions Note: Reactions reported in combination therapy with trastuzumab and docetaxel unless otherwise noted.

Cardiovascular: Left ventricular dysfunction, peripheral edema

Central nervous system: Decreased left ventricular ejection fraction, dizziness, fatigue, headache, insomnia, peripheral neuropathy, peripheral sensory neuropathy

Dermatologic: Alopecia, nail disease, palmar-plantar erythrodysesthesia, paronychia, pruritus, skin rash, xeroderma

Gastrointestinal: Abdominal pain (monotherapy), anorexia (monotherapy), constipation, decreased appetite, diarrhea, dysgeusia, dyspepsia, mucositis, nausea (monotherapy), stomatitis, vomiting (monotherapy)

Hematologic & oncologic: Anemia, febrile neutropenia, leukopenia, neutropenia, thrombocytopenia

Hepatic: Increased serum ALT

Hypersensitivity: Hypersensitivity

Neuromuscular & skeletal: Arthralgia, myalgia, weakness

Ophthalmic: Increased lacrimation

Respiratory: Cough, dyspnea, epistaxis, nasopharyngitis, oropharyngeal pain, upper respiratory tract infection

Miscellaneous: Fever, infusion reactions

Rare but important or life-threatening: Heart failure, pleural effusion, sepsis

Drug Interactions

Metabolism/Transport Effects None known.

Avoid Concomitant Use

Avoid concomitant use of Pertuzumab with any of the following: Belimumab

Increased Effect/Toxicity

Pertuzumab may increase the levels/effects of: Belimumab

Decreased Effect There are no known significant interactions involving a decrease in effect.

Preparation for Administration Hazardous agent; use appropriate precautions for handling and disposal (meets NIOSH 2014 criteria). Dilute in 250 mL NS only (do not use dextrose 5% solutions) in PVC or non-PVC (polyolefin) bags. Gently invert to mix; do not shake. Do not mix with other medications.

Storage/Stability Store intact vials at 2°C to 8°C (36°F to 46°F) until time of use. Protect from light. Do not freeze. Do not shake. Solutions diluted for infusion should be used immediately; if not used immediately, maybe stored at 2°C to 8°C (36°F to 46°F) for up to 24 hours.

Mechanism of Action Pertuzumab is a recombinant humanized monoclonal antibody which targets the extracellular human epidermal growth factor receptor 2 protein (HER2) dimerization domain. Inhibits HER2 dimerization and blocks HER downstream signaling halting cell growth and initiating apoptosis. Pertuzumab binds to a different HER2 epitope than trastuzumab so that when pertuzumab is combined with trastuzumab, a more complete inhibition of HER2 signaling occurs (Baselga, 2012).

Pharmacodynamics/Kinetics

Distribution: V_d: 5.12 L (Gianni, 2010)

Half-life elimination: Terminal: 18 days

Dosage Note: For pertuzumab, trastuzumab, and docetaxel combination regimens, pertuzumab and trastuzumab may be administered in any order; however, docetaxel should be given after pertuzumab and trastuzumab. Observe patients for 30-60 minutes after each pertuzumab infusion and before subsequent infusions of trastuzumab or docetaxel.

Breast cancer, metastatic HER2+: Adults: IV: 840 mg over 60 minutes followed by a maintenance dose of 420 mg over 30-60 minutes every 3 weeks until disease progression or unacceptable toxicity (in combination with trastuzumab and docetaxel) (Baselga, 2012).

Breast cancer, neoadjuvant treatment HER2+: Adults: IV: 840 mg over 60 minutes followed by a maintenance dose of 420 mg over 30-60 minutes every 3 weeks for 3-6 cycles; may be administered as one of the regimens below. Post-operatively, continue trastuzumab to complete 1 year of treatment.

Four preoperative cycles of pertuzumab, trastuzumab, and docetaxel, followed by 3 postoperative cycles of fluorouracil, epirubicin, and cyclophosphamide (FEC) (Gianni, 2012) **or**

Three preoperative cycles of FEC (alone) followed by 3 preoperative cycles of pertuzumab, trastuzumab, and docetaxel (Schneeweiss, 2013) **or**

Six preoperative cycles of pertuzumab, trastuzumab, docetaxel, and carboplatin (Schneeweiss, 2013)

Missed doses or delays: If <6 weeks has elapsed, administer the 420 mg maintenance dose; do not wait until the next planned dose. If ≥6 weeks has elapsed, readminister the 840 mg initial dose (over 60 minutes), and then follow with a maintenance dose of 420 mg (over 30-60 minutes) every 3 weeks.

Dosage adjustment for toxicity: Note: Dose reductions are not recommended for pertuzumab; if trastuzumab is withheld, pertuzumab should also be withheld; if trastuzumab is discontinued, pertuzumab should be discontinued; pertuzumab and trastuzumab may be continued if docetaxel is discontinued.

Infusion-related reaction: Slow or interrupt the infusion

Serious hypersensitivity: Discontinue immediately

Cardiotoxicity: Left ventricular ejection fraction (LVEF) declines to <45% **or** LVEF between 45% to 49% with ≥10% absolute decrease below pretreatment values: Withhold treatment (pertuzumab and trastuzumab) for at least 3 weeks; may resume if LVEF returns to >49% **or** to 45% to 49% with <10% absolute decrease below pretreatment values. If after a repeat assessment within ~3 weeks, LVEF has not improved (or has declined further), discontinue pertuzumab and trastuzumab (unless the benefit of treatment outweighs risks).

Dosage adjustment in renal impairment:

CrCl ≥30 mL/minute: No dosage adjustment necessary.

CrCl <30 mL/minute: There are no dosage adjustments provided in the manufacturer's labeling (has not been studied).

Dosage adjustment in hepatic impairment: There are no dosage adjustments provided in the manufacturer's labeling (has not been studied).

Administration For IV infusion only, as a short infusion; infuse initial dose (840 mg) over 60 minutes; infuse maintenance dose (420 mg) over 30-60 minutes. Do not administer IV push or as a rapid bolus. Do not mix with other medications. For pertuzumab, trastuzumab, and docetaxel combination regimens, pertuzumab and trastuzumab may be administered in any order; however, docetaxel should be given after pertuzumab and trastuzumab. Observe patients for 30-60 minutes after each pertuzumab infusion and before subsequent infusions of trastuzumab or docetaxel.

Hazardous agent; use appropriate precautions for handling and disposal (meets NIOSH 2014 criteria).

Monitoring Parameters HER2 expression (either as 3+ IHC [Dako Herceptest™] or FISH amplification ratio ≥2 [Dako *HER2* FISH pharmDx™ test]); pregnancy test; assess LVEF at baseline, every 3 months during treatment (more frequently for declines) in metastatic treatment and every 6 weeks for neoadjuvant treatment, and every 6 months following discontinuation for up to 24 months from the last dose of pertuzumab and/or trastuzumab); monitor for infusion reaction and hypersensitivity

Dosage Forms

Solution, Intravenous [preservative free]:

Perjeta: 420 mg/14 mL (14 mL)

- ◆ **Pertzye** *see* Pancrelipase *on page 1566*
- ◆ **Pethidine Hydrochloride** *see* Meperidine *on page 1293*
- ◆ **Pexeva** *see* PARoxetine *on page 1579*
- ◆ **PF-02341066** *see* Crizotinib *on page 511*
- ◆ **PFA** *see* Foscarnet *on page 931*
- ◆ **Pfizerpen-AS® (Can)** *see* Penicillin G Procaine *on page 1613*
- ◆ **Pfizerpen-G** *see* Penicillin G (Parenteral/Aqueous) *on page 1611*
- ◆ **pFVIII** *see* Antihemophilic Factor (Recombinant [Porcine Sequence]) *on page 153*
- ◆ **PGE_1** *see* Alprostadil *on page 96*
- ◆ **PGE_2** *see* Dinoprostone *on page 640*
- ◆ **PGI_2** *see* Epoprostenol *on page 746*
- ◆ **PGX** *see* Epoprostenol *on page 746*
- ◆ **Pharbedryl** *see* DiphenhydrAMINE (Systemic) *on page 641*
- ◆ **Pharbetol [OTC]** *see* Acetaminophen *on page 32*
- ◆ **Pharbetol Extra Strength [OTC]** *see* Acetaminophen *on page 32*
- ◆ **Pharixia (Can)** *see* Benzydamine [CAN/INT] *on page 249*
- ◆ **Pharmorubicin® (Can)** *see* Epirubicin *on page 739*
- ◆ **Phenadoz** *see* Promethazine *on page 1723*

Phenazopyridine (fen az oh PEER i deen)

Brand Names: U.S. Azo-Gesic [OTC]; Baridium [OTC]; Pyridium; Urinary Pain Relief [OTC]

Index Terms Phenazopyridine Hydrochloride; Phenylazo Diamino Pyridine Hydrochloride

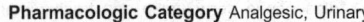

Pharmacologic Category Analgesic, Urinary

Use Symptomatic relief of urinary burning, itching, frequency, and urgency in association with urinary tract infection or following urologic procedures

Pregnancy Risk Factor B

Dosage Oral:

Children: 12 mg/kg/day in 3 divided doses administered after meals for 2 days

Adults: 100-200 mg 3 times/day after meals for 2 days when used concomitantly with an antibacterial agent

Dosage adjustment in renal impairment: Use is contraindicated in renal impairment.

Dosage adjustment in hepatic impairment: No dosage adjustment provided in manufacturer's labeling.

Additional Information Complete prescribing information should be consulted for additional detail.

Dosage Forms

Tablet, Oral:

Azo-Gesic [OTC]: 95 mg

Baridium [OTC]: 97.2 mg

Pyridium: 100 mg, 200 mg

Urinary Pain Relief [OTC]: 95 mg

Generic: 95 mg, 100 mg, 200 mg

◆ **Phenazopyridine Hydrochloride** *see* Phenazopyridine *on page 1629*

Phenelzine (FEN el zeen)

Brand Names: U.S. Nardil

Brand Names: Canada Nardil®

Index Terms Phenelzine Sulfate

Pharmacologic Category Antidepressant, Monoamine Oxidase Inhibitor

Use Symptomatic treatment of atypical, nonendogenous, or neurotic depression

Pregnancy Risk Factor C

Pregnancy Considerations Safe use during pregnancy has not been established; use only if benefits outweigh the risks.

Breast-Feeding Considerations Safe use during breast-feeding has not been established; use only if benefits outweigh the risks.

Contraindications Hypersensitivity to phenelzine or any component of the formulation; congestive heart failure; pheochromocytoma; abnormal liver function tests or history of hepatic disease; renal disease or severe renal disease/impairment

Concurrent use of sympathomimetics (including amphetamines, cocaine, dopamine, epinephrine, methylphenidate, norepinephrine, or phenylephrine) and related compounds (methyldopa, levodopa, phenylalanine, tryptophan, or tyrosine), ophthalmic alpha$_2$-agonists (apraclonidine, brimonidine), CNS depressants, cyclobenzaprine, dextromethorphan, ethanol, meperidine, bupropion, or buspirone

At least 2 weeks should elapse between the discontinuation of serotoninergic agents (including SNRIs, SSRIs, and tricyclics) and other MAO inhibitors and the initiation of phenelzine. At least 5 weeks should elapse between the discontinuation of fluoxetine and the initiation of phenelzine. In all cases, a sufficient amount of time must be allowed for the clearance of the serotoninergic agent and any active metabolites prior to the initiation of phenelzine.

At least 2 weeks should elapse between the discontinuation of phenelzine and the initiation of the following agents: Serotoninergic agents (including SNRIs, SSRIs, fluoxetine, and tricyclics), bupropion, buspirone, and other antidepressants.

General anesthesia, spinal anesthesia (hypotension may be exaggerated). Use caution with local anesthetics containing sympathomimetic agents. Phenelzine should be discontinued ≥10 days prior to elective surgery.

Foods high in tyramine or dopamine content; foods and/or supplements containing tyrosine, phenylalanine, tryptophan, or caffeine

Warnings/Precautions [U.S. Boxed Warning]: Antidepressants increase the risk of suicidal thinking and behavior in children, adolescents, and young adults (18-24 years of age) with major depressive disorder (MDD) and other psychiatric disorders; consider risk prior to prescribing. Short-term studies did not show an increased risk in patients >24 years of age and showed a decreased risk in patients ≥65 years. Closely monitor for clinical worsening, suicidality, or unusual changes in behavior; the patient's family or caregiver should be instructed to closely observe the patient and communicate condition with healthcare provider. Such observation would generally include at least weekly face-to-face contact with patients or their family members or caregivers during the first 4 weeks of treatment, then every other week visits for the next 4 weeks, then at 12 weeks, and as clinically indicated beyond 12 weeks. Additional contact by telephone may be appropriate between face-to-face visits. Adults treated with antidepressants should be observed similarly for clinical worsening and suicidality, especially during the initial few months of a course of drug therapy, or at times of dose changes, either increases or decreases. A medication guide should be dispensed with each prescription. Phenelzine is not generally considered a first-line agent for the treatment of depression; phenelzine is typically used in patients who have failed to respond to other treatments. **Phenelzine is not FDA approved for the treatment of depression in children ≤16 years of age.**

The possibility of a suicide attempt is inherent in major depression and may persist until remission occurs. Monitor for worsening of depression or suicidality, especially during initiation of therapy (generally first 1-2 months) or with dose increases or decreases. Worsening depression and severe abrupt suicidality that are not part of the presenting symptoms may require discontinuation or modification of drug therapy. Use caution in high-risk patients during initiation of therapy. Prescriptions should be written for the smallest quantity consistent with good patient care. The patient's family or caregiver should be alerted to monitor patients for the emergence of suicidality and associated behaviors such as anxiety, agitation, panic attacks, insomnia, irritability, hostility, impulsivity, akathisia, hypomania, and mania; patients should be instructed to notify their healthcare provider if any of these symptoms or worsening depression occur.

May worsen psychosis in some patients or precipitate a shift to mania or hypomania in patients with bipolar disorder. Monotherapy in patients with bipolar disorder should be avoided. Patients presenting with depressive symptoms should be screened for bipolar disorder. Phenelzine is not FDA approved for the treatment of bipolar depression.

Sensitization to the effects of insulin may occur; monitor blood glucose closely in patients with diabetes. Use with caution in patients who have glaucoma, or hyperthyroidism. Cases of hypertensive crisis (sometimes fatal) have occurred; symptoms include: severe headache, nausea/vomiting, neck stiffness/soreness, photophobia, and sweating. Monitor blood pressure closely in all patients. Hypertensive crisis may occur with tyramine-, tryptophan-, or dopamine-containing foods. Phentolamine is recommended for the treatment of hypertensive crisis. Do not use with other MAO inhibitors or antidepressants. Do not use within 5 weeks of fluoxetine discontinuation or 2 weeks of other antidepressant discontinuation. Avoid products containing sympathomimetic stimulants or dextromethorphan. Concurrent use with antihypertensive agents may lead to exaggeration of hypotensive effects. May cause orthostatic hypotension; use with caution in patients with hypotension or patients who would not tolerate transient hypotensive episodes (cardiovascular or cerebrovascular disease); effects may be additive with other agents which cause orthostasis. Use with caution in patients at risk of seizures, or in patients receiving other drugs which may lower seizure threshold. Discontinue at least 48 hours prior to myelography. May increase the risks associated with electroconvulsive therapy. Pyridoxine deficiency has occurred; symptoms include numbness and edema of hands; may respond to supplementation. Effects may be potentiated when used with other sedative drugs or ethanol.

Abrupt discontinuation or interruption of antidepressant therapy has been associated with a discontinuation syndrome. Symptoms arising may vary with antidepressant however commonly include nausea, vomiting, diarrhea, headaches, lightheadedness, dizziness, diminished appetite, sweating, chills, tremors, paresthesias, fatigue, somnolence, and sleep disturbances (eg, vivid dreams, insomnia). Greater risks for developing a discontinuation syndrome have been associated with antidepressants with shorter half-lives, longer durations of treatment, and abrupt discontinuation. More severe symptoms have also been associated with MAO inhibitors. For antidepressants of short or intermediate half-lives, symptoms may emerge within 2-5 days after treatment discontinuation and last 7-14 days (APA, 2010; Fava, 2006; Haddad, 2001; Shelton, 2001; Warner, 2006).

Adverse Reactions

Cardiovascular: Edema, orthostatic hypotension

Central nervous system: Anxiety (acute), ataxia, coma, delirium, dizziness, drowsiness, euphoria, fatigue, fever, headache, hyper-reflexia, hypersomnia, insomnia, mania, schizophrenia, seizure, twitching

Dermatologic: Pruritus, rash

Endocrine & metabolic: Decreased sexual ability (anorgasmia, ejaculatory disturbances, impotence), hypermetabolic syndrome, hypernatremia

Gastrointestinal: Constipation, weight gain, xerostomia

Genitourinary: Urinary retention

Hematologic: Leukopenia

Hepatic: Jaundice, necrotizing hepatocellular necrosis (rare), transaminases increased

Neuromuscular & skeletal: Myoclonia, paresthesia, tremor, weakness

Ocular: Blurred vision, glaucoma, nystagmus

Respiratory: Edema (glottis)

Miscellaneous: Diaphoresis, lupus-like syndrome, transient cardiac or respiratory depression (following ECT), withdrawal syndrome (nausea, vomiting, malaise)

Drug Interactions

Metabolism/Transport Effects **Inhibits** Monoamine Oxidase

Avoid Concomitant Use

Avoid concomitant use of Phenelzine with any of the following: Aclidinium; Alcohol (Ethyl); Alpha-/Beta-Agonists (Indirect-Acting); Alpha1-Agonists; Amphetamines; Anilidopiperidine Opioids; Antidepressants (Serotonin Reuptake Inhibitor/Antagonist); Apraclonidine; AtoMOXetine; Bezafibrate; Buprenorphine; BuPROPion; BusPIRone; CarBAMazepine; Cyclobenzaprine; Cyproheptadine; Dapoxetine; Dexmethylphenidate; Dextromethorphan; Diethylpropion; Glucagon; Hydrocodone; HYDROmorphone; Ipratropium (Oral Inhalation); Isometheptene; Levonordefrin; Linezolid; Maprotiline; Meperidine; Methyldopa; Methylene Blue; Methylphenidate; Mianserin; Mirtazapine; Morphine (Liposomal); Morphine (Systemic); Oxymorphone; Pholcodine; Pizotifen; Potassium Chloride; Selective Serotonin Reuptake Inhibitors; Serotonin 5-HT1D Receptor Agonists; Serotonin/Norepinephrine Reuptake Inhibitors; Tapentadol; Tetrabenazine; Tetrahydrozoline (Nasal); Tiotropium; Tricyclic Antidepressants; Tryptophan; Umeclidinium

Increased Effect/Toxicity

Phenelzine may increase the levels/effects of: AbobotulinumtoxinA; Alpha-/Beta-Agonists (Indirect-Acting); Alpha1-Agonists; Amphetamines; Analgesics (Opioid); Anticholinergic Agents; Antidepressants (Serotonin Reuptake Inhibitor/Antagonist); Antihypertensives; Antipsychotic Agents; Apraclonidine; AtoMOXetine; Beta2-Agonists; Betahistine; Bezafibrate; Brimonidine (Ophthalmic); Brimonidine (Topical); BuPROPion; Cannabinoid-Containing Products; Cyproheptadine; Dexmethylphenidate; Dextromethorphan; Diethylpropion; Domperidone; Doxapram; Doxylamine; EPINEPHrine (Nasal); Epinephrine (Racemic); EPINEPHrine (Systemic, Oral Inhalation); Glucagon; Hydrocodone; HYDROmorphone; Hypoglycemic Agents; Isometheptene; Levonordefrin; Linezolid; Lithium; Meperidine; Methadone; Methyldopa; Methylene Blue; Methylphenidate; Metoclopramide; Mianserin; Mirabegron; Mirtazapine; Morphine (Liposomal); Morphine (Systemic); Norepinephrine; OnabotulinumtoxinA; Orthostatic Hypotension Producing Agents; OxyCODONE; Pizotifen; Potassium Chloride; Reserpine; RimabotulinumtoxinB; Selective Serotonin Reuptake Inhibitors; Serotonin 5-HT1D Receptor Agonists; Serotonin Modulators; Serotonin/Norepinephrine Reuptake Inhibitors; Succinylcholine; Tetrahydrozoline (Nasal); Thiazide Diuretics; Tiotropium; Topiramate; Tricyclic Antidepressants

The levels/effects of Phenelzine may be increased by: Aclidinium; Alcohol (Ethyl); Altretamine; Anilidopiperidine Opioids; Antiemetics (5HT3 Antagonists); Antipsychotic Agents; Buprenorphine; BusPIRone; CarBAMazepine; COMT Inhibitors; Cyclobenzaprine; Dapoxetine; Ipratropium (Oral Inhalation); Levodopa; MAO Inhibitors; Maprotiline; Oxymorphone; Pholcodine; Pramlintide; Tapentadol; Tedizolid; Tetrabenazine; TraMADol; Tryptophan; Umeclidinium

Decreased Effect

Phenelzine may decrease the levels/effects of: Acetylcholinesterase Inhibitors; Domperidone; Itopride; Secretin

The levels/effects of Phenelzine may be decreased by: Acetylcholinesterase Inhibitors; Cyproheptadine; Domperidone

Food Interactions Concurrent ingestion of foods rich in tyramine, dopamine, tyrosine, phenylalanine, tryptophan, or caffeine may cause sudden and severe high blood pressure (hypertensive crisis or serotonin syndrome). Beverages containing tyramine (eg, hearty red wine and beer) may increase toxic effects. Management: Avoid tyramine-containing foods (aged or matured cheese, air-dried or cured meats including sausages and salamis; fava or broad bean pods, tap/draft beers, Marmite concentrate, sauerkraut, soy sauce, and other soybean condiments). Food's freshness is also an important concern; improperly stored or spoiled food can create an environment in which tyramine concentrations may increase. Avoid foods containing dopamine, tyrosine, phenylalanine, tryptophan, or caffeine. Avoid beverages containing tyramine.

Storage/Stability Store at 20°C to 25°C (68°F to 77°F). Protect from heat and light.

Mechanism of Action Thought to act by increasing endogenous concentrations of norepinephrine, dopamine, and serotonin through inhibition of the enzyme (monoamine oxidase) responsible for the breakdown of these neurotransmitters

Pharmacodynamics/Kinetics

Onset of action: Therapeutic: 2-4 weeks; geriatric patients receiving an average of 55 mg/day developed a mean platelet MAO activity inhibition of about 85%.

Duration: May continue to have a therapeutic effect and interactions 2 weeks after discontinuing therapy

Absorption: Well absorbed

Metabolism: Oxidized via monoamine oxidase (primary pathway) and acetylation (minor pathway)

Half-life elimination: 12 hours

Excretion: Urine (73% as metabolites)

Dosage Note: 45 mg phenelzine = 40 mg of isocarboxazid = 20 mg of tranylcypromine (Sheehan 1980). Oral:

Adults: Depression: Initial: 15 mg 3 times/day

Early phase: Increase rapidly, based on patient tolerance, to 60-90 mg/day (may take 4 weeks of 60 mg/day therapy before clinical response)

Maintenance: After maximum benefit is obtained, slowly reduce dose over several weeks; dose may be as low as 15 mg/day to 15 mg every other day

Elderly: Depression: Select dose with caution; generally initiating at the lower end of the dosing range; some clinicians recommend an initial dose of 7.5 mg, with dose increases of 7.5 mg/day every 4-8 days as tolerated to a usual therapeutic dose of 22.5-60 mg/day in older adults (Alexopoulos, 2004).

Discontinuation of therapy: Upon discontinuation of antidepressant therapy, gradually taper the dose to minimize the incidence of withdrawal symptoms and allow for the detection of re-emerging symptoms. Evidence supporting ideal taper rates is limited. APA and NICE guidelines suggest tapering therapy over at least several weeks with consideration to the half-life of the antidepressant; antidepressants with a shorter half-life and MAO inhibitors may need to be tapered more conservatively. In addition for long-term treated patients, WFSBP guidelines recommend tapering over 4-6 months. If intolerable withdrawal symptoms occur following a dose reduction, consider resuming the previously prescribed dose and/or decrease dose at a more gradual rate (APA, 2010; Bauer, 2002; Haddad, 2001; NCCMH, 2010; Schatzberg, 2006; Shelton, 2001; Warner, 2006).

MAO inhibitor recommendations:

Switching to or from an MAO inhibitor intended to treat psychiatric disorders:

Allow 14 days to elapse between discontinuing an alternative antidepressant without long half-life metabolites (eg, TCAs, paroxetine, fluvoxamine, venlafaxine) or MAO inhibitor intended to treat psychiatric disorders and initiation of phenelzine.

Allow 5 weeks to elapse between discontinuing fluoxetine (with long half-life metabolites) intended to treat psychiatric disorders and initiation of phenelzine.

Allow 14 days to elapse between discontinuing phenelzine and initiation of an alternative antidepressant or MAO inhibitor intended to treat psychiatric disorders.

Use with other MAO inhibitors (such as linezolid or IV methylene blue):

Do not initiate phenelzine in patients receiving linezolid or IV methylene blue; consider other interventions for psychiatric condition.

If urgent treatment with linezolid or IV methylene blue is required in a patient already receiving phenelzine and potential benefits outweigh potential risks, discontinue phenelzine promptly and administer linezolid or IV methylene blue. Monitor for serotonin syndrome for 2 weeks or until 24 hours after the last dose of linezolid or IV methylene blue, whichever comes first. May resume phenelzine 24 hours after the last dose of linezolid or IV methylene blue.

Dosage adjustment in renal impairment:

Mild to moderate impairment: No dosage adjustment provided in manufacturer's labeling.

Severe impairment: Use is contraindicated.

Dosage adjustment in hepatic impairment: Use is contraindicated.

Dietary Considerations Avoid tyramine-containing foods/beverages. Some examples include aged or matured cheese, air-dried or cured meats (including sausages and salamis), fava or broad bean pods, tap/draft beers, Marmite concentrate, sauerkraut, soy sauce and other soybean condiments. Food's freshness is also an important concern; improperly stored or spoiled food can create an environment where tyramine concentrations may increase.

Monitoring Parameters Blood pressure, heart rate; diet, weight; mood (if depressive symptoms), suicide ideation (especially during the initial months of therapy or when doses are increased or decreased)

Dosage Forms

Tablet, Oral:

Nardil: 15 mg

Generic: 15 mg

◆ **Phenelzine Sulfate** *see* Phenelzine *on page 1630*

◆ **Phenergan** *see* Promethazine *on page 1723*

◆ **Pheniramine and Naphazoline** *see* Naphazoline and Pheniramine *on page 1426*

PHENobarbital (fee noe BAR bi tal)

Brand Names: Canada PMS-Phenobarbital

Index Terms Luminal Sodium; Phenobarbital Sodium; Phenobarbitone; Phenylethylmalonylurea

Pharmacologic Category Anticonvulsant, Barbiturate; Barbiturate

Additional Appendix Information

Beers Criteria – Potentially Inappropriate Medications for Geriatrics *on page 2271*

Use Management of generalized tonic-clonic (grand mal), status epilepticus, and partial seizures; sedative/hypnotic

Note: Use to treat insomnia is not recommended (Schutte-Rodin, 2008)

Pregnancy Risk Factor B/D (manufacturer dependent)

Pregnancy Considerations Barbiturates can be detected in the placenta, fetal liver, and fetal brain. Fetal and maternal blood concentrations may be similar following parenteral administration. An increased incidence of fetal abnormalities may occur following maternal use. The use of folic acid throughout pregnancy and vitamin K during the last month of pregnancy is recommended; epilepsy itself, number of medications, genetic factors, or a combination of these probably influence the teratogenicity of anticonvulsant therapy. When used during the third trimester of pregnancy, withdrawal symptoms may occur in the neonate, including seizures and hyperirritability; symptoms of withdrawal may be delayed in the neonate up to 14 days after birth. Use during labor does not impair uterine activity; however, respiratory depression may occur in the newborn; resuscitation equipment should be available, especially for premature infants.

Breast-Feeding Considerations Phenobarbital is excreted into breast milk. Infantile spasms and other withdrawal symptoms have been reported following the abrupt discontinuation of breast-feeding.

Contraindications Hypersensitivity to barbiturates or any component of the formulation; marked hepatic impairment; dyspnea or airway obstruction; porphyria (manifest and latent); intra-arterial administration, subcutaneous administration (not recommended); use in patients with a history of sedative/hypnotic addiction; nephritic patients (large doses)

Warnings/Precautions Potential for drug dependency exists, abrupt cessation may precipitate withdrawal, including status epilepticus in epileptic patients. Do not administer to patients in acute pain. Use caution in debilitated, renal or hepatic dysfunction, and pediatric patients. May cause paradoxical responses, including agitation and hyperactivity, particularly in acute pain and pediatric patients. Avoid use in the elderly due to risk of overdose with low dosages, tolerance to sleep effects, and increased risk of physical dependence (Beers Criteria). Use with caution in patients with depression or suicidal tendencies, or in patients with a history of drug abuse. Tolerance, psychological and physical dependence may occur with prolonged use. May cause CNS depression, which may impair physical or mental abilities. Effects with other sedative drugs or ethanol may be potentiated. May cause respiratory depression or hypotension, particularly when administered intravenously. Use with caution in hemodynamically unstable patients (hypovolemic shock, CHF) or patients with respiratory disease. Due to its long half-life and risk of dependence, phenobarbital is not recommended as a sedative in the elderly. Phenobarbital has been associated with cognitive deficits in children receiving chronic therapy for febrile seizures. Use with caution in patients with hypoadrenalism. Intra-arterial administration may cause reactions ranging from transient pain to gangrene and is contraindicated. Subcutaneous administration may cause tissue irritation (eg, redness, tenderness, necrosis) and is not recommended.

Adverse Reactions

Cardiovascular: Bradycardia, hypotension, syncope

Central nervous system: Agitation, anxiety, ataxia, CNS excitation or depression, confusion, dizziness drowsiness, hallucinations, "hangover" effect, headache, hyperkinesia, impaired judgment, insomnia, lethargy, nervousness, nightmares, somnolence

Dermatologic: Exfoliative dermatitis, rash, Stevens-Johnson syndrome

Gastrointestinal: Constipation, nausea, vomiting

Hematologic: Agranulocytosis, megaloblastic anemia, thrombocytopenia

Local: Pain at injection site, thrombophlebitis with IV use

Renal: Oliguria

Respiratory: Apnea (especially with rapid IV use), hypoventilation, laryngospasm, respiratory depression

Miscellaneous: Gangrene with inadvertent intra-arterial injection

Drug Interactions

Metabolism/Transport Effects **Substrate** of CYP2C19 (major), CYP2C9 (minor), CYP2E1 (minor); **Note:** Assignment of Major/Minor substrate status based on clinically relevant drug interaction potential; **Induces** CYP1A2 (strong), CYP2A6 (strong), CYP2B6 (strong), CYP2C8 (strong), CYP2C9 (strong), CYP3A4 (strong), P-glycoprotein

Avoid Concomitant Use

Avoid concomitant use of PHENobarbital with any of the following: Abiraterone Acetate; Apixaban; Apremilast; Artemether; Axitinib; Azelastine (Nasal); Bedaquiline; Boceprevir; Bortezomib; Bosutinib; Cabozantinib; Ceritinib; CloZAPine; Crizotinib; Dabigatran Etexilate; Dasabuvir; Dienogest; Dolutegravir; Dronedarone; Eliglustat; Enzalutamide; Etravirine; Everolimus; Ibrutinib; Idelalisib; Irinotecan; Itraconazole; Ivacaftor; Lapatinib; Ledipasvir; Lumefantrine; Lurasidone; Macitentan; Mianserin; Mifepristone; Naloxegol; Netupitant; NIFEdipine; Nilotinib; Nintedanib; Nisoldipine; Olaparib; Ombitasvir; Orphenadrine; Paraldehyde; Paritaprevir; PAZOPanib; Perampanel; Pirfenidone; Pomalidomide; PONATinib; Praziquantel; Ranolazine; Regorafenib; Rilpivirine; Rivaroxaban; Roflumilast; RomiDEPsin; Simeprevir; Sofosbuvir; Somatostatin Acetate; SORAfenib; Stiripentol; Suvorexant; Tasimelteon; Telaprevir; Thalidomide; Ticagrelor; Tofacitinib; Tolvaptan; Toremifene; Trabectedin; Ulipristal; Vandetanib; Vemurafenib; VinCRIStine (Liposomal); Vorapaxar; Voriconazole

Increased Effect/Toxicity

PHENobarbital may increase the levels/effects of: Alcohol (Ethyl); Azelastine (Nasal); Buprenorphine; Clarithromycin; CNS Depressants; Hydrocodone; Hypotensive Agents; Meperidine; Methotrimeprazine; Metyrosine; Orphenadrine; Paraldehyde; Pramipexole; Prilocaine; QuiNIDine; Rotigotine; Selective Serotonin Reuptake Inhibitors; Sodium Nitrite; Thalidomide; Thiazide Diuretics; Zolpidem

The levels/effects of PHENobarbital may be increased by: Brimonidine (Topical); Cannabis; Chloramphenicol; Clarithromycin; Cosyntropin; CYP2C19 Inhibitors (Moderate); CYP2C19 Inhibitors (Strong); Dexmethylphenidate; Doxylamine; Dronabinol; Droperidol; Felbamate; Fosphenytoin; HydrOXYzine; Kava Kava; Luliconazole; Magnesium Sulfate; Methotrimeprazine; Methylphenidate; Mianserin; Nabilone; Nitric Oxide; OXcarbazepine; Phenytoin; Primidone; QuiNINE; Rufinamide; Sodium Oxybate; Somatostatin Acetate; Tapentadol; Tetrahydrocannabinol; Valproic Acid and Derivatives

Decreased Effect

PHENobarbital may decrease the levels/effects of: Abiraterone Acetate; Acetaminophen; Afatinib; Albendazole; Apixaban; Apremilast; ARIPiprazole; Artemether; Axitinib; Bazedoxifene; Bedaquiline; Bendamustine; Beta-Blockers; Boceprevir; Bortezomib; Bosutinib; Brentuximab Vedotin; Cabozantinib; Calcium Channel Blockers; Canagliflozin; Cannabidiol; Cannabis; Ceritinib; Chloramphenicol; Clarithromycin; CloZAPine; Cobicistat; Contraceptives (Estrogens); Contraceptives (Progestins); Corticosteroids (Systemic); Crizotinib; CycloSPORINE (Systemic); CYP1A2 Substrates; CYP2A6 Substrates; CYP2B6 Substrates; CYP2C8 Substrates; CYP2C9 Substrates; CYP3A4 Substrates; Dabigatran Etexilate; Dasabuvir; Dasatinib; Deferasirox; Diclofenac (Systemic); Dienogest; Disopyramide; Dolutegravir; DOXOrubicin (Conventional); Doxycycline; Dronabinol; Dronedarone; Eliglustat; Elvitegravir; Enzalutamide; Erlotinib; Eslicarbazepine; Etoposide; Etravirine; Everolimus; Exemestane; Felbamate; FentaNYL; Fosphenytoin; Gefitinib; Griseofulvin; GuanFACINE; Ibrutinib; Idelalisib; Imatinib; Irinotecan; Itraconazole; Ivacaftor; Ixabepilone; Lacosamide; LamoTRIgine; Lapatinib; Ledipasvir; Linagliptin; Lopinavir; Lumefantrine; Lurasidone; Macitentan; Maraviroc; Methadone; MetroNIDAZOLE (Systemic); Mianserin; Mifepristone; Naloxegol; Netupitant; NIFEdipine; Nilotinib; Nintedanib; Nisoldipine; Olaparib; Ombitasvir; OXcarbazepine; Paritaprevir; PAZOPanib; Perampanel; P-glycoprotein/ABCB1 Substrates; Phenytoin; Pirfenidone; Pomalidomide; PONATinib; Praziquantel; Propafenone; QUEtiapine; QuiNIDine; QuiNINE; Ranolazine; Regorafenib; Rilpivirine; Rivaroxaban; Roflumilast; RomiDEPsin; Rufinamide; Saxagliptin; Simeprevir; Sofosbuvir; SORAfenib; Stiripentol; SUNItinib; Suvorexant; Tadalafil; Tasimelteon; Telaprevir; Teniposide; Tetrahydrocannabinol; Ticagrelor; Tipranavir; Tofacitinib; Tolvaptan; Toremifene; Trabectedin; Treprostinil; Tricyclic Antidepressants; Ulipristal; Valproic Acid and Derivatives; Vandetanib; Vemurafenib; Vilazodone; VinCRIStine (Liposomal); Vitamin K Antagonists; Vorapaxar; Voriconazole; Vortioxetine; Zonisamide; Zuclopenthixol

The levels/effects of PHENobarbital may be decreased by: Amphetamines; Cholestyramine Resin; CYP2C19 Inducers (Strong); Dabrafenib; Darunavir; Folic Acid; Leucovorin Calcium-Levoleucovorin; Levomefolate; Mefloquine; Methylfolate; Mianserin; Multivitamins/Minerals (with ADEK, Folate, Iron); Orlistat; Pyridoxine; Rifamycin Derivatives; Tipranavir

Food Interactions May cause decrease in vitamin D and calcium.

Storage/Stability

Elixir: Protect from light.

Injection: Protect from light. Not stable in aqueous solutions; use only clear solutions. Do not add to acidic solutions; precipitation may occur.

Mechanism of Action Long-acting barbiturate with sedative, hypnotic, and anticonvulsant properties. Barbiturates depress the sensory cortex, decrease motor activity, alter cerebellar function, and produce drowsiness, sedation, and hypnosis. In high doses, barbiturates exhibit anticonvulsant activity; barbiturates produce dose-dependent respiratory depression.

Pharmacodynamics/Kinetics

Onset of action: Oral: Hypnosis: 20 to 60 minutes; IV: ~5 minutes

Peak effect: IV: ~30 minutes

Duration: Oral: 6 to 10 hours; IV: 4 to 10 hours

Absorption: Oral: 70% to 90%

Protein binding: 20% to 45%; decreased in neonates

Metabolism: Hepatic via hydroxylation and glucuronide conjugation

Half-life elimination: Neonates: 45 to 500 hours; Infants: 20 to 133 hours; Children: 37 to 73 hours; Adults: 53 to 140 hours

Time to peak, serum: Oral: 1 to 6 hours

Excretion: Urine (20% to 50% as unchanged drug)

Dosage

Sedation:

Children: Oral: 2 mg/kg/**dose** 3 times daily; maximum dose: 40 mg

Alternative dosing (limited data available): IM, Oral: 2 to 3 mg/kg/day in divided doses every 8 to 12 hours (Nelson, 1996)

Adults:

IM, IV: 100 to 320 mg; larger doses may occasionally be necessary in persons with psychoses, and pronounced excitement, and in mental patients with insomnia. The effect of large doses must be closely watched. Maximum: 600 mg daily.

Oral: 30 to 120 mg daily in 2 to 3 divided doses; maximum: 400 mg daily

Status epilepticus: Initial: IV:

Infants, Children, and Adolescents: 15 to 20 mg/kg; maximum dose: 1000 mg; may repeat once after 10 to 15 minutes if needed; maximum total dose: 40 mg/kg (Brophy, 2012; Hegenbarth, 2008).

Adults: 20 mg/kg (infused at 50 mg/minute); may repeat with an additional 5 to 10 mg/kg (Brophy, 2012; Meierkord, 2010)

Alternative dosing: Up to 50 mg/minute; may give an additional dose 10 minutes after initial infusion (Brophy, 2012)

Note: Additional respiratory support may be required particularly when maximizing loading dose or if concurrent sedative therapy. Repeat doses administered sooner than 10 to 15 minutes may not allow adequate time for peak CNS concentrations to be achieved and may lead to CNS depression.

Seizures: Maintenance dose:

Manufacturer's labeling:

Infants, Children, and Adolescents: Oral: 3 to 6 mg/kg/day

Adults: Oral:

Elixir, oral solution: 60 to 200 mg daily

Tablets: 50 to 100 mg 2 or 3 times daily

Alternative dosing (limited data available) (Geurinni, 2006; Kliegman, 2011):

Initial: Oral, IV:

Infants and Children ≤5 years: 3 to 5 mg/kg/day in 1 to 2 divided doses

Children >5 years: 2 to 3 mg/kg/day in 1 to 2 divided doses

Adolescents: 1 to 3 mg/kg/day in 1 to 2 divided doses (Nelson, 1996)

Usual dosing range: Oral, IV: **Note:** Dosage should be individualized based upon clinical response and serum concentration; once daily doses usually administered at bedtime in children and adolescents. Some centers have used:

Infants: 5 to 6 mg/kg/day in 1 to 2 divided doses

Children:

1 to 5 years: 6 to 8 mg/kg/day in 1 to 2 divided doses

5 to 12 years: 4 to 6 mg/kg/day in 1 to 2 divided doses

Adolescents and Adults: 1 to 3 mg/kg/day in 1 to 2 divided doses or 50 to 100 mg 2 to 3 times daily

Sedative/hypnotic withdrawal (off-label use): Oral: Initial daily requirement is determined by substituting phenobarbital 30 mg for every 100 mg pentobarbital used during tolerance testing; then daily requirement is decreased by 10% of initial dose (Perry, 1981)

Elderly or debilitated: Initiate at the lowest recommended dose.

Dosage adjustment in renal impairment: No specific dosage adjustment provided in manufacturer's labeling; reduced doses are recommended. The following guidelines have been used by some clinicians (Aronoff, 2007):

Infants, Children, and Adolescents: **Note:** Renally adjusted dose recommendations are based on doses of 3 to 7 mg/kg/day every 12 to 24 hours

GFR ≥10 mL/minute/1.73 m^2: No dosage adjustment necessary.

GFR <10 mL/minute/1.73 m^2: Decrease normal dose by 50% and administer every 24 hours

Intermittent hemodialysis [moderately dialyzable (20% to 50%)]: Supplemental dose may be needed during and after dialysis depending on individual seizure threshold

Peritoneal dialysis (PD): 40% to 50% removed; amount varies depending on number of cycles

Continuous renal replacement therapy (CRRT): Monitor serum concentrations; a case report suggests that clearance and volume of distribution increased with CVVH; more frequent and higher dosing may be necessary in some cases (Pasko, 2004)

Adults:

CrCl ≥10 mL/minute: No dosage adjustment necessary.

CrCl <10 mL/minute: Administer every 12 to 16 hours.

Hemodialysis (moderately dialyzable [20% to 50%]): Administer dose before dialysis and 50% of dose after dialysis.

Peritoneal dialysis: Administer 50% of normal dose.

CRRT: Administer normal dose and monitor levels.

Dosage adjustment in hepatic impairment: There are no dosage adjustments provided in manufacturer's labeling; reduced doses are recommended. Phenobarbital exposure is increased with hepatic impairment; use with caution.

Dietary Considerations Vitamin D: Loss in vitamin D due to malabsorption; increase intake of foods rich in vitamin D. Supplementation of vitamin D and/or calcium may be necessary. Injection may contain sodium.

Administration May be administered IV, IM or orally. Avoid rapid IV administration >60 mg/minute in adults and >30 mg/minute in children; intra-arterial injection is contraindicated; avoid subcutaneous administration; parenteral solutions are highly alkaline; avoid extravasation. For IM administration, inject deep into muscle. Do not exceed 5 mL per injection site due to potential for tissue irritation

Monitoring Parameters Phenobarbital serum concentrations, mental status, CBC, LFTs, seizure activity

Reference Range

Therapeutic:

Infants and Children: 15 to 40 mcg/mL (SI: 65 to 172 micromole/L)

Adults: 20 to 40 mcg/mL (SI: 86 to 172 micromole/L)

Toxic: >40 mcg/mL (SI: >172 micromole/L)

Toxic concentration: Slowness, ataxia, nystagmus: 35 to 80 mcg/mL (SI: 150 to 344 micromole/L)

Coma with reflexes: 65 to 117 mcg/mL (SI: 279 to 502 micromole/L)

Coma without reflexes: >100 mcg/mL (SI: >430 micromole/L)

Additional Information Injectable solutions contain propylene glycol.

Phenobarbital tablets are also available from some generic manufacturers in strengths that are exactly equivalent to fractional grain strengths: 16.2 mg (1/4 grain), 32.4 mg (1/2 grain), 64.8 mg (1 grain). To avoid medication errors, do not prescribe phenobarbital in grains.

Dosage Forms

Elixir, Oral:

Generic: 20 mg/5 mL (473 mL)

Solution, Injection:

Generic: 65 mg/mL (1 mL); 130 mg/mL (1 mL)

Solution, Oral:

Generic: 20 mg/5 mL (473 mL)

Tablet, Oral:

Generic: 15 mg, 16.2 mg, 30 mg, 32.4 mg, 60 mg, 64.8 mg, 97.2 mg, 100 mg

Extemporaneous Preparations An alcohol-free 10 mg/mL phenobarbital oral suspension may be made from tablets and one of two different vehicles (a 1:1 mixture of Ora-Plus® and Ora-Sweet® or a 1:1 mixture of Ora-Plus® and Ora-Sweet® SF). Crush ten phenobarbital 60 mg tablets in a glass mortar and reduce to a fine powder. Mix 30 mL of Ora-Plus® and 30 mL of either Ora-Sweet® or Ora-Sweet® SF; stir vigorously. Add 15 mL of the vehicle to the powder and mix to a uniform paste. Transfer the mixture to a 2 ounce amber plastic prescription bottle. Rinse mortar and pestle with 15 mL of the vehicle; transfer to bottle. Repeat, then add quantity of vehicle sufficient to make 60 mL. Label "shake well." May mix dose with chocolate syrup (1:1 volume) immediately before administration to mask the bitter aftertaste. Stable for 115 days when stored in amber plastic prescription bottles at room temperature.

Cober M and Johnson CE, "Stability of an Extemporaneously Prepared Alcohol-Free Phenobarbital Suspension," *Am J Health Syst Pharm*, 2007, 64(6):644-6.

◆ **Phenobarbital, Hyoscyamine, Atropine, and Scopolamine** *see* Hyoscyamine, Atropine, Scopolamine, and Phenobarbital *on page 1027*

◆ **Phenobarbital Sodium** *see* PHENobarbital *on page 1632*

◆ **Phenobarbitone** *see* PHENobarbital *on page 1632*

◆ **Phenoptin** *see* Sapropterin *on page 1864*

Phenoxybenzamine (fen oks ee BEN za meen)

Brand Names: U.S. Dibenzyline

Index Terms Phenoxybenzamine Hydrochloride

Pharmacologic Category Alpha$_1$ Blocker; Antidote

Use Symptomatic management of pheochromocytoma

Pregnancy Risk Factor C

Dosage Oral:

Children (off-label use): Initial: 0.25-1 mg/kg/day (maximum: 10 mg); increase slowly to blood pressure control

Adults:

Pheochromocytoma, hypertension: Initial: 10 mg twice daily; increase by 10 mg every other day until optimal blood pressure response is achieved; usual range: 20-40 mg 2-3 times/day. Doses up to 240 mg/day have been reported (Kinney, 2000).

Micturition disorders (off-label use): 10-20 mg 1-2 times/day

Dosage adjustment in renal impairment: No dosage adjustment provided in manufacturer's labeling. Use with caution.

Dosage adjustment in hepatic impairment: No dosage adjustment provided in manufacturer's labeling.

Additional Information Complete prescribing information should be consulted for additional detail.

Dosage Forms

Capsule, Oral:

Dibenzyline: 10 mg

◆ **Phenoxybenzamine Hydrochloride** *see* Phenoxybenzamine *on page 1635*

◆ **Phenoxymethyl Penicillin** *see* Penicillin V Potassium *on page 1614*

◆ **Phenprocoumarol** *see* Phenprocoumon [INT] *on page 1635*

◆ **Phenprocoumarole** *see* Phenprocoumon [INT] *on page 1635*

Phenprocoumon [INT] (fen proe KOO mon)

International Brand Names Falithrom (DE); Marcoumar (AT, BE, BR, DK, DE, NL, CH); Marcumar (DE); Marcuphen (DE); Phenpro Abz (DE); Phenprogamma (DE)

Index Terms Fenprocumone; Phenprocoumarol; Phenprocoumarole; Phenprocoumone; Phenprocumone

Pharmacologic Category Anticoagulant, Coumarin Derivative; Vitamin K Antagonist

Dosage Range Adults: Oral: Usual dose: 6-9 mg once on day 1, followed by 6 mg on day 2; beginning on day 3: 1.5-4.5 mg once daily depending on achievement of target INR

Product Availability Product available in various countries; not currently available in the U.S.

Dosage Forms

Tablet: 3 mg

◆ **Phenprocoumone** *see* Phenprocoumon [INT] *on page 1635*

◆ **Phenprocumone** *see* Phenprocoumon [INT] *on page 1635*

Phentermine (FEN ter meen)

Brand Names: U.S. Adipex-P; Suprenza

Index Terms Phentermine Hydrochloride

Pharmacologic Category Anorexiant; Central Nervous System Stimulant; Sympathomimetic

Use Short-term (few weeks) adjunct therapy in obese patients with an initial body mass index (BMI) ≥30 kg/m^2 or ≥27 kg/m^2 in the presence of other risk factors (eg, diabetes, hyperlipidemia, controlled hypertension); therapy should be used in conjunction with a comprehensive weight management program.

Pregnancy Risk Factor X

Dosage Note: Dosing is presented in terms of the salt, phentermine hydrochloride (not as phentermine base).

Oral: Children >16 years and Adults: Obesity:

Capsule, tablet: 15-37.5 mg daily given in 1-2 divided doses. Individualize to achieve adequate response with lowest effective dose.

Orally disintegrating tablet (ODT): One tablet (15-37.5 mg daily) every morning. Individualize to achieve adequate response with lowest effective dose.

Dosing adjustment in renal impairment: No dosage adjustment provided in manufacturer's labeling (has not been studied). Phentermine is excreted in the urine and systemic exposure may be increased in renal impairment; use with caution.

Dosing adjustment in hepatic impairment: No dosage adjustment provided in manufacturer's labeling (has not been studied).

Additional Information Complete prescribing information should be consulted for additional detail.

Dosage Forms

Capsule, Oral:
Adipex-P: 37.5 mg
Generic: 15 mg, 30 mg, 37.5 mg

Tablet, Oral:
Adipex-P: 37.5 mg
Generic: 37.5 mg

Tablet Dispersible, Oral:
Suprenza: 15 mg, 30 mg, 37.5 mg

◆ **Phentermine Hydrochloride** *see* Phentermine *on page* 1635

Phentolamine (fen TOLE a meen)

Brand Names: U.S. OraVerse

Brand Names: Canada OraVerse; Rogitine

Index Terms Phentolamine Mesylate; Regitine [DSC]

Pharmacologic Category $Alpha_1$ Blocker; Antidote, Extravasation; Antihypertensive

Use Diagnosis of pheochromocytoma via the phentolamine-blocking test (see **"Note"**); prevention and management of hypertensive episodes associated with pheochromocytoma resulting from stress or manipulation during the perioperative period; prevention and treatment of dermal necrosis/sloughing after extravasation of norepinephrine

OraVerse: Reversal of soft tissue anesthesia and the associated functional deficits resulting from a local dental anesthetic containing a vasoconstrictor

Note: The phentolamine-blocking test for the diagnosis of pheochromocytoma has largely been supplanted by the measurement of catecholamine concentrations and catecholamine metabolites (eg, metanephrine) in the plasma and urine; reserve phentolamine for cases when additional confirmation is necessary to determine diagnosis.

Pregnancy Risk Factor C

Pregnancy Considerations Adverse events were observed in some oral animal reproduction studies. Diagnosing and treating pheochromocytoma is critical for favorable maternal and fetal outcomes (Schenker, 1971; Schenker, 1982).

Breast-Feeding Considerations It is not known if phentolamine is excreted in breast milk. Due to the potential for serious adverse reaction in the nursing infant, the decision to discontinue phentolamine or discontinue breast-feeding during treatment should take in account the benefits of treatment to the mother.

Contraindications

Hypersensitivity to phentolamine, any component of the formulation, or related compounds; MI (or history of MI), coronary insufficiency, angina, or other evidence suggestive of coronary artery disease

Canadian labeling: Additional contraindications (not in U.S. labeling): Hypotension

OraVerse:

U.S. labeling: There are no contraindications listed in the manufacturer's labeling.

Canadian labeling: Hypersensitivity to phentolamine or any component of the formulation.

Warnings/Precautions MI, cerebrovascular spasm, and cerebrovascular occlusion have been reported following administration, usually associated with hypotensive episodes. Tachycardia and cardiac arrhythmias may occur. Discontinue if symptoms of angina occur or worsen. The use of phentolamine as a blocking agent in the screening of patients with hypertension has predominantly been replaced with urinary/biochemical assays; phentolamine use should be reserved for situations where additional confirmation is necessary and after risks associated with use have been considered. Use with caution in patients with gastritis or peptic ulcer disease. Use with caution in patients with renal impairment; primarily eliminated by the kidneys. Potentially significant drug-drug interactions may exist, requiring dose or frequency adjustment, additional monitoring, and/or selection of alternative therapy.

Adverse Reactions

Cardiovascular: Bradycardia (OraVerse), cerebrovascular occlusion, hypertension (OraVerse), hypotension, myocardial infarction, tachycardia (OraVerse)

Central nervous system: Cerebrovascular spasm, headache (OraVerse), mouth pain (OraVerse), paresthesia (OraVerse; mild, transient)

Dermatologic: Facial swelling (OraVerse), pruritus (OraVerse)

Gastrointestinal: Diarrhea (OraVerse), nausea, upper abdominal pain (OraVerse), vomiting (OraVerse)

Local: Pain at injection site (OraVerse)

Rare but important or life-threatening: Cardiac arrhythmia, orthostatic hypotension

Drug Interactions

Metabolism/Transport Effects None known.

Avoid Concomitant Use

Avoid concomitant use of Phentolamine with any of the following: Alpha1-Blockers

Increased Effect/Toxicity

Phentolamine may increase the levels/effects of: Alpha1-Blockers; Amifostine; Antihypertensives; Calcium Channel Blockers; Obinutuzumab; RiTUXimab

The levels/effects of Phentolamine may be increased by: Beta-Blockers; Brimonidine (Topical); Dapoxetine; Diazoxide; Herbs (Hypotensive Properties); MAO Inhibitors; Pentoxifylline; Phosphodiesterase 5 Inhibitors; Prostacyclin Analogues

Decreased Effect

Phentolamine may decrease the levels/effects of: Alpha-/Beta-Agonists; Alpha1-Agonists

The levels/effects of Phentolamine may be decreased by: Herbs (Hypertensive Properties); Methylphenidate; Yohimbine

Preparation for Administration Powder for injection: Reconstitute 5 mg vial with 1 mL sterile water for injection. For treatment of extravasation, further dilute 5-10 mg in 10 mL of normal saline (manufacturer's recommendation) or in 10-15 mL of saline (Peberdy, 2010).

Storage/Stability

Powder for injection: Store intact vials at room temperature of 15°C to 30°C (59°F to 86°F). Reconstituted solution should be used immediately after preparation (per manufacturer).

Solution for injection (OraVerse): Store at 20°C to 25°C (68°F to 77°F); brief excursions permitted between 15°C to 30°C (59°F to 86°F). Protect from heat and light. Do not freeze.

Mechanism of Action Competitively blocks alpha-adrenergic receptors (nonselective) to produce brief antagonism of circulating epinephrine and norepinephrine to reduce hypertension caused by alpha effects of these catecholamines and minimizes tissue injury due to extravasation of these and other sympathomimetic vasoconstrictors (eg, dopamine, phenylephrine); also has a positive inotropic and chronotropic effect on the heart thought to be due to presynaptic alpha-2 receptor blockade which results in release of presynaptic norepinephrine (Hoffman, 1980)

OraVerse: Causes vasodilation and increased blood flow in injection area via alpha-adrenergic blockade to accelerate reversal of soft tissue anesthesia

Pharmacodynamics/Kinetics

Onset of action: IM: 15-20 minutes; IV: 1-2 minutes (Chobanian, 2003)

Peak effect: OraVerse: 10-20 minutes

Duration: IM: 30-45 minutes; IV: 10-30 minutes (Chobanian, 2003)

Metabolism: Hepatic

Half-life elimination: IV: 19 minutes

Excretion: Urine (~13% as unchanged drug)

Dosage

Extravasation of norepinephrine, management: Children and Adults (manufacturer's labeling): Local infiltration: Inject 5-10 mg (diluted in 10 mL 0.9% sodium chloride) into extravasation area (as soon as extravasation is noted but within 12 hours of extravasation)

Extravasation of sympathomimetic vasopressors, management (off-label use): Infiltrate extravasation site with 5-10 mg diluted in 10-15 mL 0.9% sodium chloride as soon as possible after extravasation (Peberdy, 2010).

Diagnosis of pheochromocytoma (phentolamine-blocking test): **Note:** The phentolamine-blocking test for the diagnosis of pheochromocytoma has largely been supplanted by the measurement of catecholamine concentrations and catecholamine metabolites (eg, metanephrine) in the plasma and urine; reserve phentolamine for cases when additional confirmation is necessary to determine diagnosis.

Children:

IM: 3 mg

IV: 1 mg

Adults: IM, IV: 5 mg

Hypertensive episodes associated with pheochromocytoma, prevention and management: **Note:** In the perioperative period, the use of other agents may be preferred due to slow onset of action and prolonged duration of phentolamine in comparison to the other agents (eg, nitroprusside) (Miller, 2010)

Children:

Preoperative: IM, IV: 1 mg given 1-2 hours before surgery and repeat if needed

Intraoperative: IV: Administer 1 mg as indicated to prevent or control paroxysms of hypertension, tachycardia, respiratory depression, seizure, or other effects associated with epinephrine intoxication resulting from tumor manipulation or other stressor (eg, intubation) (Miller, 2010).

Adults:

Preoperative: IM, IV: 5 mg given 1-2 hours before surgery and repeat if needed

Intraoperative: IV: Administer 5 mg as indicated to prevent or control paroxysms of hypertension, tachycardia, respiratory depression, seizure, or other effects associated with epinephrine intoxication resulting from tumor manipulation or other stressor (eg, intubation) (Miller, 2010).

Hypertensive crisis (off-label use): Adults: **Note:** Generally used in the setting of catecholamine excess (eg, pheochromocytoma) (Marik, 2007): IV: 1-5 mg bolus; maximum single dose: 15 mg. A continuous infusion may be administered after initial bolus dosing (eg, 1 mg/hour titrated to blood pressure response) to a maximum infusion rate of 40 mg/hour (McMillian, 2011)

Reversal of oral soft tissue (lip, tongue) anesthesia (OraVerse): Infiltration or block technique: Submucosal oral injection:

Children: 15-30 kg: 0.2 mg maximum dose

Children >30 kg and <12 years: 0.4 mg maximum dose

Adults: **Note:** Dose is based upon the number of cartridges of local anesthetic administered. Infiltration or block injection:

0.2 mg if one-half cartridge of anesthesia was administered

0.4 mg if 1 cartridge of anesthesia was administered

0.8 mg if 2 cartridges of anesthesia were administered

Dosage adjustment in renal impairment: No dosage adjustment provided in manufacturer's labeling.

Dosage adjustment in hepatic impairment: No dosage adjustment provided in manufacturer's labeling.

Administration

Extravasation management (treatment), sympathomimetic vasopressors: Stop vesicant infusion immediately and disconnect IV line (leave needle/cannula in place); gently aspirate extravasated solution from the IV line (do **NOT** flush the line); remove needle/cannula; elevate extremity. Inject phentolamine 5-10 mg/10 mL saline into extravasation site (as soon as possible but within 12 hours of extravasation). AHA recommends diluting 5-10 mg in 10-15 mL saline and administering into the site (Peberdy, 2010).

Pheochromocytoma diagnosis: Patient should be supine throughout test, preferable in a quiet, dark room. Blood pressure should be monitored every 10 minutes for at least 30 minutes, delay phentolamine administration until after blood pressure is stable (at an untreated, hypertensive level). A drop in blood pressure >35 mm Hg (systolic) and >25 mm Hg (diastolic) is considered a positive response. If blood pressure is elevated, unchanged, or decrease is <35 mm Hg (systolic) and <25 mm Hg (diastolic), then response is negative. Confirm positive response with other diagnostic measure. Negative responses do not exclude a pheochromocytoma diagnosis, particularly in patients with paroxysmal hypertension where an incidence of false negatives is high.

IM: After IM injection, monitor blood pressure every 5 minutes for 35-40 minutes. Blood pressure drops to above parameters within 20 minutes are considered positive.

IV: Inject rapidly (after venous response to venipuncture has subsided); then monitor blood pressure immediately after injection, every 30 seconds for 3 minutes, then every minute for 7 minutes. Maximum response is generally achieved within 2 minutes; duration may last 15-30 minutes (although return to prior blood pressure may be sooner).

Pheochromocytoma-associated hypertensive episode: Administer IM or IV 1-2 hours prior to surgery and repeat during surgery (IV) if necessary.

Reversal of oral soft tissue (lip, tongue) anesthesia (OraVerse): Submucosal oral injection: Use the same location and dental technique employed for administration of the local anesthetic.

Hypertensive crisis (off-label use): Administer as an IV bolus (Marik, 2007); may follow with a continuous IV infusion (McMillian, 2011).

Monitoring Parameters Blood pressure, heart rate; monitor and document extravasation site; monitor patient for orthostasis; assist patient with ambulation

Dosage Forms

Solution, Injection:

Generic: 5 mg/mL (1 mL)

◆ **Phentolamine Mesylate** *see* Phentolamine *on page 1636*

◆ **Phenylalanine Mustard** *see* Melphalan *on page 1283*

◆ **Phenylazo Diamino Pyridine Hydrochloride** *see* Phenazopyridine *on page 1629*

Phenylephrine (Systemic) (fen il EF rin)

Brand Names: U.S. Little Colds Decongestant [OTC]; Medi-Phenyl [OTC]; Nasal Decongestant PE Max St [OTC]; Nasal Decongestant [OTC]; Non-Pseudo Sinus Decongestant [OTC]; Sudafed PE Childrens [OTC]; Sudafed PE Maximum Strength [OTC]; Sudogest PE [OTC]; Vazculep

Index Terms Phenylephrine Hydrochloride

Pharmacologic Category Alpha-Adrenergic Agonist

Use Treatment of hypotension, vascular failure in shock (see **"Note"**); as a vasoconstrictor in regional analgesia; supraventricular tachycardia (see **"Note"**); as a decongestant [OTC]

Note: Not recommended for routine use in the treatment of septic shock or supraventricular tachycardias.

Pregnancy Risk Factor C

Pregnancy Considerations Animal reproduction studies have not been conducted; therefore, the manufacturer classifies phenylephrine as pregnancy category C. Phenylephrine crosses the placenta at term. Maternal use of phenylephrine during the first trimester of pregnancy is not strongly associated with an increased risk of fetal malformations; maternal dose and duration of therapy were not reported in available publications. Phenylephrine is available over-the-counter (OTC) for the symptomatic relief of nasal congestion. Decongestants are not the preferred agents for the treatment of rhinitis during pregnancy. Oral phenylephrine should be avoided during the first trimester of pregnancy; short-term use (<3 days) of intranasal phenylephrine may be beneficial to some patients although its safety during pregnancy has not been studied. Phenylephrine injection is used at delivery for the prevention and/or treatment of maternal hypotension associated with spinal anesthesia in women undergoing cesarean section. Phenylephrine may be associated with a more favorable fetal acid base status than ephedrine; however, overall fetal outcomes appear to be similar. Nausea or vomiting may be less with phenylephrine than ephedrine but is also dependent upon blood pressure control. Phenylephrine may be preferred in the absence of maternal bradycardia.

Breast-Feeding Considerations It is not known if phenylephrine is excreted into breast milk. The manufacturer recommends that caution be exercised when administering phenylephrine to nursing women.

Contraindications Hypersensitivity to phenylephrine or any component of the formulation

Injection: Severe hypertension; ventricular tachycardia

Vazculep: There are no contraindications listed in the manufacturer's labeling.

OTC labeling (Oral): When used for self-medication: Use with or within 14 days of MAO inhibitor therapy

Warnings/Precautions Some products contain sulfites which may cause allergic reactions in susceptible individuals. Use with extreme caution in patients taking MAO inhibitors. Use with caution in patients with hyperthyroidism.

Intravenous: Phenylephrine may cause severe bradycardia (likely baroreflex mediated) and reduced cardiac output due to an increase in cardiac afterload especially in patients with preexisting cardiac dysfunction (Goertz, 1993; Yamazaki, 1982). May also precipitate angina in patients with severe coronary artery disease and increase pulmonary arterial pressure. Use with caution in patients with preexisting bradycardia, partial heart block, myocardial disease, or severe coronary artery disease. Avoid or use with extreme caution in patients with heart failure or cardiogenic shock; increased systemic vascular resistance may significantly reduce cardiac output. Avoid use in patients with hypertension (contraindicated in severe hypertension); monitor blood pressure closely and adjust infusion rate. Assure adequate circulatory volume to minimize need for vasoconstrictors. Vesicant; ensure proper needle or catheter placement prior to and during infusion; avoid extravasation. **[U.S. Boxed Warning]: Should be administered by adequately trained individuals familiar with its use.** Acidosis may reduce the efficacy of phenylephrine; correct acidosis prior to or during use of phenylephrine. Patients with autonomic dysfunction (eg, spinal cord injury) may exhibit an exaggerated increase in blood pressure response to phenylephrine.

Oral: When used for self-medication (OTC), use caution with asthma, bowel obstruction/narrowing, hyperthyroidism, diabetes mellitus, cardiovascular disease, ischemic heart disease, hypertension, increased intraocular pressure, prostatic hyperplasia or in the elderly. Notify healthcare provider if symptoms do not improve within 7 days or are accompanied by fever. Discontinue and contact healthcare provider if nervousness, dizziness, or sleeplessness occur.

Benzyl alcohol and derivatives: Some dosage forms may contain sodium benzoate/benzoic acid; benzoic acid (benzoate) is a metabolite of benzyl alcohol; large amounts of benzyl alcohol (≥99 mg/kg/day) have been associated with a potentially fatal toxicity ("gasping syndrome") in neonates; the "gasping syndrome" consists of metabolic acidosis, respiratory distress, gasping respirations, CNS dysfunction (including convulsions, intracranial hemorrhage), hypotension, and cardiovascular collapse (AAP, 1997; CDC, 1982); some data suggests that benzoate displaces bilirubin from protein binding sites (Ahlfors, 2001); avoid or use dosage forms containing benzyl alcohol derivative with caution in neonates. See manufacturer's labeling.

Adverse Reactions

Injection:

Cardiovascular: Cardiac arrhythmia (rare), exacerbation of angina, hypertension, hypertensive crisis, ischemia, localized blanching, low cardiac output, peripheral vasoconstriction (severe), reflex bradycardia, visceral vasoconstriction (severe), worsening of heart failure

Central nervous system: Anxiety, dizziness, excitability, headache, insomnia, nervousness, paresthesia, precordial pain (or discomfort), restlessness

Dermatologic: Pallor, piloerection, pruritus

Endocrine & metabolic: Metabolic acidosis

Gastrointestinal: Epigastric pain, gastric irritation, nausea, vomiting

Genitourinary: Decreased renal blood flow, decreased urine output

Hypersensitivity: Hypersensitivity reaction (including skin rash, urticaria, leukopenia, agranulocytosis, thrombocytopenia)
Local: Extravasation which may lead to necrosis and sloughing of surrounding tissue
Neuromuscular & skeletal: Neck pain, tremor, weakness
Ophthalmic: Blurred vision
Respiratory: Dyspnea, exacerbation of pulmonary arterial hypertension, respiratory distress

Oral: Central nervous system: Anxiety, dizziness, excitability, headache, insomnia, nervousness, restlessness

Drug Interactions

Metabolism/Transport Effects None known.

Avoid Concomitant Use

Avoid concomitant use of Phenylephrine (Systemic) with any of the following: Ergot Derivatives; Hyaluronidase; Iobenguane I 123; MAO Inhibitors

Increased Effect/Toxicity

Phenylephrine (Systemic) may increase the levels/effects of: Sympathomimetics

The levels/effects of Phenylephrine (Systemic) may be increased by: Acetaminophen; AtoMOXetine; Cannabinoid-Containing Products; Ergot Derivatives; Hyaluronidase; Linezolid; MAO Inhibitors; Tedizolid; Tricyclic Antidepressants

Decreased Effect

Phenylephrine (Systemic) may decrease the levels/effects of: Benzylpenicilloyl Polylysine; FentaNYL; Iobenguane I 123; Ioflupane I 123

The levels/effects of Phenylephrine (Systemic) may be decreased by: Alpha1-Blockers; Tricyclic Antidepressants

Preparation for Administration Solution for injection:

IV infusion: May dilute 10 mg in 500 mL NS or D_5W. May also dilute 50 mg in 500 mL NS or 100 mg in 500 mL NS; both concentrations are stable for at least 14 days at room temperature of 25°C (77°F) (Gupta, 2004). Dilution of 1250 mg in 500 mL NS retained potency for at least 24 hours at 22°C (Weber, 1970).

IV injection: May dilute with SWFI, NS, or D_5W to a concentration of 1 mg/mL. May also prepare a 100 mcg/mL solution for bolus administration.

Stability in syringes (Kiser, 2007): Concentration of 0.1 mg/mL in NS (polypropylene syringes) is stable for at least 30 days at -20°C (-4°F), 3°C to 5°C (37°F to 41°F), or 23°C to 25°C (73.4°F to 77°F).

Storage/Stability

Solution for injection: Store vials at controlled room temperature of 15°C to 25°C (59°F to 77°F). Protect from light. Do not use solution if brown or contains a precipitate.

Oral: Store at controlled room temperature of 15°C to 25°C (59°F to 77°F). Protect from light.

Mechanism of Action Potent, direct-acting alpha-adrenergic agonist with virtually no beta-adrenergic activity; produces systemic arterial vasoconstriction. Such increases in systemic vascular resistance result in dose dependent increases in systolic and diastolic blood pressure and reductions in heart rate and cardiac output especially in patients with heart failure.

Pharmacodynamics/Kinetics

Onset of action:
Blood pressure increase/vasoconstriction: IM, SubQ: 10 to 15 minutes; IV: Immediate
Nasal decongestant: Oral: 15 to 30 minutes (Kollar, 2007)

Duration:
Blood pressure increase/vasoconstriction: IM: 1 to 2 hours; IV: ~15 to 20 minutes; SubQ: 50 minutes
Nasal decongestant: Oral: ≤4 hours (Kollar, 2007)

Absorption: Oral: Rapid and complete (Kanfer, 1993)

Distribution: V_d: Initial: 26 to 61 L; V_{dss}: 184 to 543 L (mean: 340 L) (Hengstmann, 1982)

Metabolism: Hepatic via oxidative deamination (Oral: 24%; IV: 50%); Undergoes sulfation (Oral [mostly within gut wall]: 46%; IV: 8%) and some glucuronidation; forms inactive metabolites (Kanfer, 1993)

Bioavailability: Oral: ≤38% (Hengstmann, 1982; Kanfer, 1993)

Half-life elimination: Alpha phase: ~5 minutes; Terminal phase: 2 to 3 hours (Hengstmann, 1982; Kanfer, 1993)

Time to peak: Oral: 0.75 to 2 hours (Kanfer, 1993)

Excretion: Urine (mostly as inactive metabolites)

Dosage

Hypotension/shock: **Note:** The Society of Critical Care Medicine (SCCM) does not recommend phenylephrine for septic shock except in the following circumstances: Norepinephrine (preferred first-line agent) is associated with serious arrhythmias, cardiac output is known to be high and blood pressure persistently low, or when the combination of inotrope/vasopressor and low-dose vasopressin failed to achieve target mean arterial pressure and phenylephrine is used as salvage therapy (SCCM [Dellinger, 2013]).

Children:
IV bolus: 5 to 20 mcg/kg/dose every 10 to 15 minutes as needed
IV infusion: 0.1 to 0.5 mcg/kg/minute

Adults:
IV bolus: 100 to 500 mcg/dose every 10 to 15 minutes as needed (initial dose should not exceed 500 mcg)
IV infusion: Initial dose: 100 to 180 mcg/minute, **or alternatively**, 0.5 mcg/kg/minute; titrate to desired response. Dosing ranges between 0.4 to 9.1 mcg/kg/minute have been reported when treating septic shock (Gregory, 1991).
ACLS guideline recommendations (to treat severe hypotension [eg, systolic blood pressure <70 mm Hg] and low total peripheral resistance): Initial dose: 0.5 to 2 mcg/kg/minute; titrate to effect (AHA [Peberdy, 2010]).

Hypotension during anesthesia: Adults:
IV bolus: 40 to 100 mcg/dose every 1 to 2 minutes as needed (total dose should not exceed 200 mcg)
IV infusion: Initial dose: 10 to 35 mcg/minute adjusted according to blood pressure goal (not to exceed 200 mcg/minute)

Nasal decongestant: Oral: OTC labeling:
Children:
4 to <6 years: 2.5 mg every 4 hours as needed for ≤7 days (maximum: 15 mg/24 hours)
6 to <12 years: 5 mg every 4 hours as needed for ≤7 days (maximum: 30 mg/24 hours)
Children ≥12 years and Adults: 10 mg every 4 hours as needed for ≤7 days (maximum: 60 mg/24 hours)

Paroxysmal supraventricular tachycardia (**Note:** Not recommended for routine use in treatment of supraventricular tachycardias): IV:
Children: 5 to 10 mcg/kg/dose over 20 to 30 seconds
Adults: 250 to 500 mcg/dose over 20 to 30 seconds

Dietary Considerations Some products may contain phenylalanine and/or sodium.

Usual Infusion Concentrations: Pediatric IV infusion: 20 **mcg**/mL, 40 **mcg**/mL, or 60 **mcg**/mL

Usual Infusion Concentrations: Adult IV infusion: 10 mg in 500 mL (concentration: 20 **mcg**/mL) of D_5W or NS, 50 mg in 500 mL (concentration: 100 **mcg**/mL) of NS, **or** 100 mg in 500 mL (concentration: 200 **mcg**/mL) of NS

Other institutions may use concentrations of 40 **mcg**/mL **or** 160 **mcg**/mL; however, stability information is not available for these concentrations.

Administration IV: Administer by slow injection or as a continuous infusion (after diluting); when administering as a continuous infusion, central line administration is preferred. IV infusions require an infusion pump.

Vesicant; ensure proper needle or catheter placement prior to and during infusion; avoid extravasation.

Extravasation management: If extravasation occurs, stop infusion immediately and disconnect (leave cannula/needle in place); gently aspirate extravasated solution (do **NOT** flush the line); remove needle/cannula; elevate extremity. Initiate phentolamine (or alternative antidote). Apply dry warm compresses (Hurst, 2004).

Phentolamine: Dilute 5 to 10 mg in 10 to 15 mL NS and administer into extravasation site as soon as possible after extravasation (AHA [Peberdy, 2010]).

Alternatives to phentolamine (due to shortage):

Nitroglycerin topical 2% ointment (based on limited case reports in neonates/infants): Apply 4 mm/kg as a thin ribbon to the affected areas; may repeat after 8 hours if needed (Wong, 1992) **or** apply a 1-inch strip on the affected site (Denkler, 1989).

Terbutaline (based on limited case reports): Infiltrate extravasation area using a solution of terbutaline 1 mg diluted to 10 mL in NS (large extravasation site; administration volume varied from 3 to 10 mL) **or** 1 mg diluted in 1 mL NS (small/distal extravasation site; administration volume varied from 0.5 to 1 mL) (Stier, 1999).

Monitoring Parameters Blood pressure (or mean arterial pressure), heart rate; cardiac output (as appropriate), intravascular volume status, pulmonary capillary wedge pressure (as appropriate); monitor infusion site closely

Consult individual institutional policies and procedures.

Product Availability

Vazculep (10 mg/mL injection): FDA approved July 2014; anticipated availability is currently unknown.

Vazculep is indicated for the treatment of clinically important hypotension resulting primarily from vasodilation in the setting of anesthesia.

Dosage Forms

Liquid, Oral:

Little Colds Decongestant [OTC]: 2.5 mg/mL (30 mL)

Solution, Injection:

Generic: 10 mg/mL (1 mL, 5 mL, 10 mL)

Solution, Intravenous:

Vazculep: 10 mg/mL (1 mL, 5 mL, 10 mL)

Solution, Oral:

Sudafed PE Childrens [OTC]: 2.5 mg/5 mL (118 mL)

Tablet, Oral:

Medi-Phenyl [OTC]: 5 mg
Nasal Decongestant [OTC]: 10 mg
Nasal Decongestant PE Max St [OTC]: 10 mg
Non-Pseudo Sinus Decongestant [OTC]: 10 mg
Sudafed PE Maximum Strength [OTC]: 10 mg
Sudogest PE [OTC]: 10 mg

◆ **Phenylephrine and Chlorpheniramine** *see* Chlorpheniramine and Phenylephrine *on page* 426

◆ **Phenylephrine and Cyclopentolate** *see* Cyclopentolate and Phenylephrine *on page* 517

◆ **Phenylephrine and Dextromethorphan** *see* Dextromethorphan and Phenylephrine *on page* 611

◆ **Phenylephrine and Diphenhydramine** *see* Diphenhydramine and Phenylephrine *on page* 644

Phenylephrine and Zinc Sulfate [CAN/INT] (fen il EF rin & zingk SUL fate)

Brand Names: Canada Zincfrin

Index Terms Zinc Sulfate and Phenylephrine

Pharmacologic Category Adrenergic Agonist Agent

Use Note: Not approved in U.S.

Soothe, moisturize, and remove redness due to minor eye irritation

Contraindications Hypersensitivity to phenylephrine, zinc sulfate, or any component of the formulation

Drug Interactions

Metabolism/Transport Effects None known.

Avoid Concomitant Use

Avoid concomitant use of Phenylephrine and Zinc Sulfate with any of the following: Ergot Derivatives; Iobenguane I 123; MAO Inhibitors

Increased Effect/Toxicity

Phenylephrine and Zinc Sulfate may increase the levels/effects of: Sympathomimetics

The levels/effects of Phenylephrine and Zinc Sulfate may be increased by: AtoMOXetine; Cannabinoid-Containing Products; Ergot Derivatives; Linezolid; MAO Inhibitors; Tedizolid; Tricyclic Antidepressants

Decreased Effect

Phenylephrine and Zinc Sulfate may decrease the levels/effects of: Iobenguane I 123

The levels/effects of Phenylephrine and Zinc Sulfate may be decreased by: Alpha1-Blockers; Tricyclic Antidepressants

Pharmacodynamics/Kinetics See individual agents.

Dosage Ophthalmic: Instill 1-2 drops in eye(s) 2-4 times/day as needed

Product Availability Not available in U.S.

Dosage Forms: Canada

Solution, ophthalmic:

Zincfrin® [OTC]: Phenylephrine 0.12% and zinc sulfate 0.25% (15 mL)

◆ **Phenylephrine, Chlorpheniramine, and Dextromethorphan** *see* Chlorpheniramine, Phenylephrine, and Dextromethorphan *on page* 428

◆ **Phenylephrine, Chlorpheniramine, and Dihydrocodeine** *see* Dihydrocodeine, Chlorpheniramine, and Phenylephrine *on page* 633

◆ **Phenylephrine Hydrochloride** *see* Phenylephrine (Systemic) *on page* 1638

◆ **Phenylephrine Hydrochloride and Diphenhydramine Hydrochloride** *see* Diphenhydramine and Phenylephrine *on page* 644

◆ **Phenylephrine Hydrochloride and Guaifenesin** *see* Guaifenesin and Phenylephrine *on page* 988

◆ **Phenylephrine Tannate and Diphenhydramine Tannate** *see* Diphenhydramine and Phenylephrine *on page* 644

◆ **Phenylethylmalonylurea** *see* PHENobarbital *on page* 1632

◆ **Phenyl Salicylate, Methenamine, Methylene Blue, Benzoic Acid, and Hyoscyamine** *see* Methenamine, Phenyl Salicylate, Methylene Blue, Benzoic Acid, and Hyoscyamine *on page* 1318

◆ **Phenyl Salicylate, Methenamine, Methylene Blue, Sodium Biphosphate, and Hyoscyamine** *see* Methenamine, Sodium Phosphate Monobasic, Phenyl Salicylate, Methylene Blue, and Hyoscyamine *on page* 1318

◆ **Phenytek** *see* Phenytoin *on page* 1640

Phenytoin (FEN i toyn)

Brand Names: U.S. Dilantin; Dilantin Infatabs; Phenytek; Phenytoin Infatabs

Brand Names: Canada Dilantin; Novo-Phenytoin; Taro-Phenytoin; Tremytoine Inj

Index Terms Diphenylhydantoin; DPH; Phenytoin Sodium; Phenytoin Sodium, Extended; Phenytoin Sodium, Prompt

Pharmacologic Category Anticonvulsant, Hydantoin

Use Management of generalized tonic-clonic (grand mal), complex partial seizures; prevention of seizures following neurosurgery

Pregnancy Risk Factor D

Pregnancy Considerations Phenytoin crosses the placenta (Harden and Pennell, 2009). An increased risk of congenital malformations and adverse outcomes may occur following *in utero* phenytoin exposure. Reported malformations include orofacial clefts, cardiac defects, dysmorphic facial features, nail/digit hypoplasia, growth abnormalities including microcephaly, and mental deficiency. Isolated cases of malignancies (including neuroblastoma) and coagulation defects in the neonate (may be life threatening) following delivery have also been reported. Maternal use of phenytoin should be avoided when possible to decrease the risk of cleft palate and poor cognitive outcomes. Polytherapy may also increase the risk of congenital malformations; monotherapy is recommended (Harden and Meader, 2009). The maternal use of folic acid throughout pregnancy is recommended to reduce the risk of major congenital malformations (Harden and Pennell, 2009).

Total plasma concentrations of phenytoin are decreased in the mother during pregnancy; unbound plasma (free) concentrations are also decreased and plasma clearance is increased. Due to pregnancy-induced physiologic changes, women who are pregnant may require dose adjustments of phenytoin in order to maintain clinical response; monitoring during pregnancy should be considered (Harden and Pennell, 2009). For women with epilepsy who are planning a pregnancy in advance, baseline serum concentrations should be measured once or twice prior to pregnancy during a period when seizure control is optimal. Monitoring can then be continued once each trimester during pregnancy and postpartum; more frequent monitoring may be needed in some patients. Monitoring of unbound plasma concentrations is recommended (Patsalos, 2008). In women taking phenytoin who are trying to avoid pregnancy, potentially significant interactions may exist with hormone-containing contraceptives; consult drug interactions database for more detailed information.

Patients exposed to phenytoin during pregnancy are encouraged to enroll themselves into the North American Antiepileptic Drug (NAAED) Pregnancy Registry by calling 1-888-233-2334. Additional information is available at https:\\aedpregnancyregistry.org.

Breast-Feeding Considerations Phenytoin is excreted in breast milk; however, the amount to which the infant is exposed is considered small. The manufacturers of phenytoin do not recommend breast-feeding during therapy.

Contraindications Hypersensitivity to phenytoin, other hydantoins, or any component of the formulation; concurrent use of delavirdine (due to loss of virologic response and possible resistance to delavirdine or other non-nucleoside reverse transcriptase inhibitors [NNRTIs])

IV: Sinus bradycardia, sinoatrial block, second- and third-degree heart block, Adams-Stokes syndrome

Warnings/Precautions Hazardous agent - use appropriate precautions for handling and disposal (NIOSH 2014 [group 2]).

Antiepileptics are associated with an increased risk of suicidal behavior/thoughts with use (regardless of indication); patients should be monitored for signs/symptoms of depression, suicidal tendencies, and other unusual behavior changes during therapy and instructed to inform their healthcare provider immediately if symptoms occur.

[U.S. Boxed Warning]: Phenytoin must be administered slowly. Intravenous administration should not exceed 50 mg/minute in adult patients. In pediatric patients, intravenous administration rate should not exceed 1-3 mg/kg/minute or 50 mg/minute whichever is slower. Hypotension and severe cardiac arrhythmias (eg, heart block, ventricular tachycardia, ventricular fibrillation) may occur with rapid administration; adverse cardiac events have been reported at or below the recommended infusion rate. Cardiac monitoring is necessary during and after administration of intravenous phenytoin; reduction in rate of administration or discontinuation of infusion may be necessary. For nonemergency use, intravenous phenytoin should be administered more slowly; the use of oral phenytoin should be used whenever possible. Vesicant (intravenous administration); ensure proper catheter or needle position prior to and during infusion; avoid extravasation; IV form may cause soft tissue irritation and inflammation, and skin necrosis at IV site; avoid IV administration in small veins. The "purple glove syndrome" (ie, discoloration with edema and pain of distal limb) may occur following peripheral IV administration of phenytoin; may or may not be associated with drug extravasation; symptoms may resolve spontaneously; however, skin necrosis and limb ischemia may occur; interventions such as fasciotomies, skin grafts, and amputation (rare) may be required. May increase frequency of petit mal seizures; use with caution in patients with porphyria; discontinue if rash or lymphadenopathy occurs; a spectrum of hematologic effects have been reported with use (eg, agranulocytosis, neutropenia, leukopenia, thrombocytopenia, pancytopenia, and anemias); use with caution in patients with hepatic dysfunction, hypothyroidism, or underlying cardiac disease; IV use is contraindicated in patients with sinus bradycardia, sinoatrial block, or second- and third-degree heart block; use with caution in elderly or debilitated patients, or in any condition associated with low serum albumin levels, which will increase the free fraction of phenytoin in the serum and, therefore, the pharmacologic response. Sedation, confusional states, or cerebellar dysfunction (loss of motor coordination) may occur at higher total serum concentrations, or at lower total serum concentrations when the free fraction of phenytoin is increased. Effects with other sedative drugs or ethanol may be potentiated. Abrupt withdrawal may precipitate status epilepticus. Severe reactions, including toxic epidermal necrolysis and Stevens-Johnson syndromes, although rarely reported, have resulted in fatalities; drug should be discontinued if there are any signs of rash and evaluate for signs and symptoms of drug reaction with eosinophilia and systemic symptoms (DRESS). Preliminary data suggests that patients testing positive for the human leukocyte antigen (HLA) allele HLA-B*1502 have an increased risk of developing Stevens-Johnson syndrome (SJS) and/or toxic epidermal necrolysis (TEN). The risk appears to be highest in the early months of therapy initiation. The presence of this genetic variant exists in up to 15% of people of Asian descent in China, Thailand, Malaysia, Indonesia, Taiwan, and the Philippines, and may vary from <1% in Japanese and Koreans, to 2% to 4% of South Asians and Indians; this variant is virtually absent in those of Caucasian, African-American, Hispanic, or European ancestry; consider avoiding phenytoin use in patients HLA-B*1502 allele positive if other therapeutic options available. Carbamazepine, another antiepileptic with a chemical structure similar to phenytoin, includes in the manufacturer labeling a recommendation to screen patients of Asian descent for the HLA-B*1502 allele prior to initiating therapy; this is not a current recommendation in the phenytoin manufacturer labeling. Chronic use of phenytoin has been associated with decreased bone mineral density (osteopenia, osteoporosis, and osteomalacia) and bone fractures. Chronic use may result in decreased vitamin D concentrations due to hepatic enzyme induction and may lead to hypocalcemia and hypophosphatemia; monitor as appropriate and consider implementing vitamin D and calcium supplementation.

Benzyl alcohol and derivatives: Some dosage forms may contain sodium benzoate/benzoic acid; benzoic acid (benzoate) is a metabolite of benzyl alcohol; large amounts of benzyl alcohol (≥99 mg/kg/day) have been associated with a potentially fatal toxicity ("gasping syndrome") in neonates; the "gasping syndrome" consists of metabolic acidosis, respiratory distress, gasping respirations, CNS dysfunction (including convulsions, intracranial hemorrhage), hypotension, and cardiovascular collapse (AAP, 1997; CDC, 1982); some data suggests that benzoate displaces bilirubin from protein binding sites (Ahlfors, 2001); avoid or use dosage forms containing benzyl alcohol derivative with caution in neonates. See manufacturer's labeling.

Adverse Reactions IV effects: Bradycardia, cardiac arrhythmia, cardiovascular collapse (especially with rapid IV use), hypotension, thrombophlebitis, venous irritation and pain

Effects not related to plasma phenytoin concentrations: Carbohydrate intolerance, folic acid deficiency, gingival hypertrophy, hypertrichosis, osteomalacia, peripheral neuropathy, systemic lupus erythematosus, thickening of facial features, vitamin D deficiency

Concentration-related effects: Ataxia, blurred vision, coma, confusion, diplopia, dizziness, drowsiness, fever, folic acid depletion, gum tenderness, hyperglycemia, lethargy, mood changes, nausea, nystagmus, osteomalacia, rash, slurred speech, vomiting

Related to elevated concentrations:

>20 mcg/mL (SI: >79 micromole/L): Far lateral nystagmus

>30 mcg/mL (SI: >119 micromole/L): 45° lateral gaze nystagmus and ataxia

>40 mcg/mL (SI: >158 micromole/L): Decreased mentation

>100 mcg/mL (SI: >396 micromole/L): Death

Cardiovascular: Bradycardia, cardiac arrhythmia, cardiovascular collapse, hypotension

Central nervous system: Dizziness, drowsiness, headache, insomnia, psychiatric changes, slurred speech, vertigo

Dermatologic: Rash

Gastrointestinal: Constipation, enlargement of lips, gingival hyperplasia, hepatic injury, nausea, taste disturbance, vomiting

Genitourinary: Peyronie's disease

Hematologic: Agranulocytosis, granulocytopenia, leukopenia, pancytopenia, thrombocytopenia

Hepatic: Acute hepatic failure, hepatitis, toxic hepatitis

Local: IV administration: Inflammation, irritation, necrosis, sloughing, tenderness, thrombophlebitis

Neuromuscular & skeletal: Paresthesia, peripheral neuropathy, tremor

Ocular: Blurred vision, diplopia, nystagmus

Rare but important or life-threatening: Anaphylaxis, blood dyscrasias, coarsening of facial features, drug rash with eosinophilia and systemic symptoms (DRESS), dyskinesias, hepatitis, Hodgkin lymphoma, hypertrichosis, immunoglobulin abnormalities, lymphadenopathy, lymphoma, macrocytosis, megaloblastic anemia, periarteritis nodosa, pseudolymphoma, systemic lupus erythematosus-like syndrome, Stevens-Johnson syndrome, toxic epidermal necrolysis, venous irritation and pain

Drug Interactions

Metabolism/Transport Effects Substrate of CYP2C19 (major), CYP2C9 (major), CYP3A4 (minor); **Note:** Assignment of Major/Minor substrate status based on clinically relevant drug interaction potential; **Induces** CYP2B6 (strong), CYP2C19 (strong), CYP2C8 (strong), CYP2C9 (strong), CYP3A4 (strong), P-glycoprotein

Avoid Concomitant Use

Avoid concomitant use of Phenytoin with any of the following: Abiraterone Acetate; Apixaban; Apremilast; Artemether; Axitinib; Azelastine (Nasal); Bedaquiline; Boceprevir; Bortezomib; Bosutinib; Cabozantinib; Ceritinib; CloZAPine; Crizotinib; Dabigatran Etexilate; Dasabuvir; Delavirdine; Dienogest; Dolutegravir; Dronedarone; Eliglustat; Enzalutamide; Etravirine; Everolimus; Ibrutinib; Idelalisib; Irinotecan; Itraconazole; Ivacaftor; Lapatinib; Ledipasvir; Lumefantrine; Lurasidone; Macitentan; Mifepristone; Naloxegol; Netupitant; NIFEdipine; Nilotinib; Nintedanib; Nisoldipine; Olaparib; Ombitasvir; Orphenadrine; Paraldehyde; Paritaprevir; PAZOPanib; PONATinib; Praziquantel; Ranolazine; Regorafenib; Rilpivirine; Rivaroxaban; Roflumilast; RomiDEPsin; Simeprevir; Sofosbuvir; SORAfenib; Stiripentol; Suvorexant; Tasimelteon; Telaprevir; Thalidomide; Ticagrelor; Tofacitinib; Tolvaptan; Toremifene; Trabectedin; Ulipristal; Vandetanib; Vemurafenib; VinCRIStine (Liposomal); Vorapaxar

Increased Effect/Toxicity

Phenytoin may increase the levels/effects of: Azelastine (Nasal); Buprenorphine; Clarithromycin; CNS Depressants; Fosamprenavir; Hydrocodone; Lithium; Methotrexate; Methotrimeprazine; Metyrosine; Neuromuscular-Blocking Agents (Nondepolarizing); Orphenadrine; Paraldehyde; PHENobarbital; Pramipexole; Prilocaine; ROPINIRole; Rotigotine; Selective Serotonin Reuptake Inhibitors; Sodium Nitrite; Thalidomide; Vitamin K Antagonists; Zolpidem

The levels/effects of Phenytoin may be increased by: Alcohol (Ethyl); Amiodarone; Antifungal Agents (Azole Derivatives, Systemic); Benzodiazepines; Brimonidine (Topical); Calcium Channel Blockers; Cannabis; Capecitabine; CarBAMazepine; Carbonic Anhydrase Inhibitors; CeFAZolin; Cimetidine; Clarithromycin; Cosyntropin; CYP2C19 Inhibitors (Moderate); CYP2C19 Inhibitors (Strong); CYP2C9 Inhibitors (Moderate); CYP2C9 Inhibitors (Strong); Delavirdine; Dexketoprofen; Dexmethylphenidate; Disulfiram; Doxylamine; Dronabinol; Droperidol; Efavirenz; Eslicarbazepine; Ethosuximide; Felbamate; Floxuridine; Fluconazole; Fluorouracil (Systemic); Fluorouracil (Topical); FLUoxetine; FluvoxaMINE; Halothane; HydrOXYzine; Isoniazid; Kava Kava; Luliconazole; Magnesium Sulfate; Methotrimeprazine; Methylphenidate; MetroNIDAZOLE (Systemic); Miconazole (Oral); Nabilone; Nitric Oxide; Omeprazole; OXcarbazepine; Rufinamide; Sertraline; Sodium Oxybate; Tacrolimus (Systemic); Tapentadol; Tegafur; Telaprevir; Tetrahydrocannabinol; Ticlopidine; Topiramate; TraZODone; Trimethoprim; Vitamin K Antagonists

Decreased Effect

Phenytoin may decrease the levels/effects of: Abiraterone Acetate; Acetaminophen; Afatinib; Albendazole; Amiodarone; Antifungal Agents (Azole Derivatives, Systemic); Apixaban; Apremilast; ARIPiprazole; Artemether; Axitinib; Bazedoxifene; Bedaquiline; Boceprevir; Bortezomib; Bosutinib; Brentuximab Vedotin; Busulfan; Cabozantinib; Canagliflozin; Cannabidiol; Cannabis; CarBAMazepine; Caspofungin; Ceritinib; Clarithromycin; CloZAPine; Cobicistat; Contraceptives (Estrogens); Contraceptives (Progestins); Crizotinib; CycloSPORINE (Systemic); CYP2B6 Substrates; CYP2C19 Substrates; CYP2C8 Substrates; CYP2C9 Substrates; CYP3A4 Substrates; Dabigatran Etexilate; Dasabuvir; Dasatinib; Deferasirox; Delavirdine; Diclofenac (Systemic); Dienogest; Disopyramide; Dolutegravir; DOXOrubicin (Conventional); Doxycycline; Dronabinol; Dronedarone; Efavirenz; Eliglustat; Elvitegravir; Enzalutamide; Erlotinib; Eslicarbazepine; Ethosuximide; Etoposide; Etoposide

Phosphate; Etravirine; Everolimus; Exemestane; Ezogabine; Felbamate; FentaNYL; Flunarizine; Gefitinib; GuanFACINE; HMG-CoA Reductase Inhibitors; Ibrutinib; Idelalisib; Imatinib; Irinotecan; Itraconazole; Ivacaftor; Ixabepilone; Lacosamide; LamoTRIgine; Lapatinib; Ledipasvir; Levodopa; Linagliptin; Loop Diuretics; Lopinavir; Lumefantrine; Lurasidone; Macitentan; Maraviroc; Mebendazole; Meperidine; Methadone; MethylPREDNISolone; MetroNIDAZOLE (Systemic); Metyrapone; Mexiletine; Mianserin; Mifepristone; Naloxegol; Nelfinavir; Netupitant; Neuromuscular-Blocking Agents (Nondepolarizing); NIFEdipine; Nilotinib; Nintedanib; Nisoldipine; Olaparib; Ombitasvir; Omeprazole; OXcarbazepine; Paritaprevir; PAZOPanib; Perampanel; P-glycoprotein/ABCB1 Substrates; PONATinib; Praziquantel; PrednisoLONE (Systemic); PredniSONE; Primidone; QUEtiapine; QuiNIDine; QuiNINE; Ranolazine; Regorafenib; Rilpivirine; Ritonavir; Rivaroxaban; Roflumilast; RomiDEPsin; Rufinamide; Saxagliptin; Sertraline; Simeprevir; Sirolimus; Sofosbuvir; SORAfenib; SUNItinib; Suvorexant; Tacrolimus (Systemic); Tadalafil; Tasimelteon; Telaprevir; Temsirolimus; Teniposide; Tetrahydrocannabinol; Theophylline Derivatives; Thyroid Products; Ticagrelor; Tipranavir; Tofacitinib; Tolvaptan; Topiramate; Topotecan; Toremifene; Trabectedin; TraZODone; Treprostinil; Trimethoprim; Ulipristal; Valproic Acid and Derivatives; Vandetanib; Vemurafenib; Vilazodone; VinCRIStine; VinCRIStine (Liposomal); Vorapaxar; Vortioxetine; Zonisamide; Zuclopenthixol

The levels/effects of Phenytoin may be decreased by: Alcohol (Ethyl); Amphetamines; Bleomycin; CarBAMazepine; Ciprofloxacin (Systemic); Colesevelam; CYP2C19 Inducers (Strong); CYP2C9 Inducers (Strong); Dabrafenib; Darunavir; Diazoxide; Enzalutamide; Folic Acid; Fosamprenavir; Leucovorin Calcium-Levoleucovorin; Levomefolate; Lopinavir; Mefloquine; Methotrexate; Methylfolate; Mianserin; Multivitamins/Minerals (with ADEK, Folate, Iron); Nelfinavir; Orlistat; PHENobarbital; Platinum Derivatives; Pyridoxine; Rifampin; Ritonavir; Stiripentol; Theophylline Derivatives; Tipranavir; Valproic Acid and Derivatives; Vigabatrin; VinCRIStine

Food Interactions

Ethanol:

Acute use: Ethanol inhibits metabolism of phenytoin and may also increase CNS depression. Management: Monitor patients. Caution patients about effects.

Chronic use: Ethanol stimulates metabolism of phenytoin. Management: Monitor patients.

Food: Phenytoin serum concentrations may be altered if taken with food. If taken with enteral nutrition, phenytoin serum concentrations may be decreased. Tube feedings decrease bioavailability. Phenytoin may decrease calcium, folic acid, and vitamin D levels. Supplementing folic acid may lower the seizure threshold. Management: Hold tube feedings 1-2 hours before and 1-2 hours after phenytoin administration. Do not supplement folic acid. Consider vitamin D supplementation. Take preferably on an empty stomach.

Preparation for Administration Hazardous agent; use appropriate precautions for handling and disposal (NIOSH 2014 [group 2]).

IV: May be further diluted in NS to a final concentration ≥5 mg/mL; infusion must be completed within 4 hours after preparation. Do not refrigerate.

Storage/Stability

Capsule, tablet: Store at 20°C to 25°C (68°F to 77°F). Protect capsules from light. Protect capsules and tablets from moisture.

Oral suspension: Store at room temperature of 20°C to 25°C (68°F to 77°F); do not freeze. Protect from light.

Solution for injection: Store at room temperature of 15°C to 30°C (59°F to 86°F). Use only clear solutions free of precipitate and haziness; slightly yellow solutions may be used. Precipitation may occur if solution is refrigerated and may dissolve at room temperature.

Mechanism of Action Stabilizes neuronal membranes and decreases seizure activity by increasing efflux or decreasing influx of sodium ions across cell membranes in the motor cortex during generation of nerve impulses; prolongs effective refractory period and suppresses ventricular pacemaker automaticity, shortens action potential in the heart

Pharmacodynamics/Kinetics

Onset of action: IV: ~0.5-1 hour

Absorption: Oral: Slow

Distribution: V_d:

Neonates: Premature: 1-1.2 L/kg; Full-term: 0.8-0.9 L/kg

Infants: 0.7-0.8 L/kg

Children: 0.7 L/kg

Adults: 0.6-0.7 L/kg

Protein binding:

Neonates: ≥80% (≤20% free)

Infants: ≥85% (≤15% free)

Adults: 90% to 95%

Others: Decreased protein binding

Disease states resulting in a decrease in serum albumin concentration: Burns, hepatic cirrhosis, nephrotic syndrome, pregnancy, cystic fibrosis

Disease states resulting in an apparent decrease in affinity of phenytoin for serum albumin: Renal failure, jaundice (severe), other drugs (displacers), hyperbilirubinemia (total bilirubin >15 mg/dL), CrCl <25 mL/minute (unbound fraction is increased two- to threefold in uremia)

Metabolism: Follows dose-dependent capacity-limited (Michaelis-Menten) pharmacokinetics with increased V_{max} (ie, metabolic capacity) in infants >6 months of age and children versus adults; major metabolite (via oxidation), HPPA, undergoes enterohepatic recirculation

Bioavailability: Formulation dependent

Half-life elimination: Range: 7-42 hours; **Note:** Elimination is not first-order (ie, follows Michaelis-Menten pharmacokinetics); half-life increases with increasing phenytoin concentrations; best described using parameters such as V_{max} (metabolic capacity) and Km (constant equal to the concentration at which the rate of metabolism is 1/2 of V_{max}).

Time to peak, serum (formulation dependent): Oral: Extended-release capsule: 4-12 hours; Immediate release preparation: 2-3 hours

Excretion: Urine (<5% as unchanged drug); as glucuronides

Clearance: Highly variable, dependent upon intrinsic hepatic function and dose administered; increased clearance and decreased serum concentrations with febrile illness

Dosage Note: Phenytoin base (eg, oral suspension, chewable tablets) contains ~8% more drug than phenytoin sodium (~92 mg base is equivalent to 100 mg phenytoin sodium). Dosage adjustments and closer serum monitoring may be necessary when switching dosage forms.

Status epilepticus: IV:

Infants and Children: Loading dose: 15-20 mg/kg, then begin maintenance therapy usually 12 hours after loading dose

Adolescents and Adults: Loading dose: Manufacturer recommends 10-15 mg/kg; however, 15-20 mg/kg at a maximum rate of 50 mg/minute is generally recommended (Kalvianines, 2007; Lowenstein, 2005); initial maintenance dose: IV or Oral: 100 mg every 6-8 hours

Anticonvulsant (nonemergent use): Oral:

Loading dose: Children, Adolescents, and Adults: 15-20 mg/kg; consider prior phenytoin serum concentrations and/or recent dosing history if available; administer oral loading dose in 3 divided doses given every 2-4 hours to decrease GI adverse effects and to ensure complete oral absorption

Maintenance dose:

Infants and Children: Initial maintenance dose: 5 mg/kg/day in 2-3 divided doses; usual maintenance dose range: 4-8 mg/kg/day; maximum daily dose: 300 mg. Some experts suggest higher maintenance doses may be necessary in infant and young children (range: 8-10 mg/kg/day in divided doses).

Adolescents and Adults: Initial maintenance dose: 300 mg daily in 3 divided doses; may also administer in 1-2 divided doses using extended release formulation; adjust dosage based on individual requirements; usual maintenance dose range: 300-600 mg daily

Dosing adjustment in renal impairment: No dosage adjustment provided in manufacturer's labeling; <5% excreted as unchanged drug. Serum concentration may be difficult to interpret in renal failure. Monitoring of free (unbound) concentrations or adjustment to allow interpretation is recommended.

Dosage adjustment in hepatic impairment: No dosage adjustment provided in manufacturer's labeling; undergoes hepatic metabolism and clearance may be decreased. Monitor free phenytoin levels closely. Dosage adjustments may be necessary.

Dosage in obesity: Adults: Loading dose: Use adjusted body weight (AdjBW) correction based on a pharmacokinetic study of phenytoin loading doses in obese patients (Abernethy, 1985). The larger correction factor (ie, 1.33) is due to a doubling of V_d estimated in these obese patients.

AdjBW = [(Actual body weight – IBW) x 1.33] + IBW

Maintenance doses should be based on ideal body weight, conventional daily doses with adjustments based upon therapeutic drug monitoring and clinical effectiveness. (Abernethy, 1985; Erstad, 2002; Erstad, 2004)

Dietary Considerations

Folic acid: Phenytoin may decrease mucosal uptake of folic acid; to avoid folic acid deficiency and megaloblastic anemia, some clinicians recommend giving patients on anticonvulsants prophylactic doses of folic acid and cyanocobalamin. Folic acid 0.5 mg/day has been shown to reduce the incidence of phenytoin-induced gingival overgrowth in children (Arya, 2011). However, folate supplementation may increase seizures in some patients (dose dependent). Discuss with healthcare provider prior to using any supplements.

Calcium: Hypocalcemia has been reported in patients taking prolonged high-dose therapy with an anticonvulsant. Some clinicians have given an additional 4000 units/week of vitamin D (especially in those receiving poor nutrition and getting no sun exposure) to prevent hypocalcemia.

Vitamin D: Phenytoin interferes with vitamin D metabolism and osteomalacia may result; may need to supplement with vitamin D

Tube feedings: Tube feedings decrease phenytoin absorption. To avoid decreased serum levels with continuous NG feeds, hold feedings for 1-2 hours prior to and 1-2 hours after phenytoin administration, if possible. There is a variety of opinions on how to administer phenytoin with enteral feedings. Be **consistent** throughout therapy.

Injection may contain sodium.

Administration

Oral: Suspension: Shake well prior to use. Absorption is impaired when phenytoin suspension is given concurrently to patients who are receiving continuous nasogastric feedings. A method to resolve this interaction is to divide the daily dose of phenytoin and withhold the administration of nutritional supplements for 1-2 hours before and after each phenytoin dose.

IM: **Avoid** IM administration due to severe risk of local tissue destruction and necrosis; use **fos**phenytoin if IM administration necessary (Boucher, 1996; Meek, 1999). The manufacturer's labeling includes IM administration; however, in general the IM route should be avoided and should **NOT** be used for status epilepticus.

IV: Fosphenytoin may be considered for loading in patients who are in status epilepticus, hemodynamically unstable, or develop hypotension/bradycardia with IV administration of phenytoin. Although, phenytoin may be administered by direct IV injection, it is preferable that phenytoin be administered via infusion pump either undiluted or diluted in normal saline as an IV piggyback (IVPB) to prevent exceeding the maximum infusion rate (monitor closely for extravasation during infusion). The maximum rate of IV administration is 50 mg/minute in adults. Highly sensitive patients (eg, elderly, patients with preexisting cardiovascular conditions) should receive phenytoin more slowly (eg, 20 mg/minute) (Meek, 1999). In neonates, the manufacturer recommends a maximum rate of 1-3 mg/kg/minute; however, a lower maximum rate of 0.5-1 mg/kg/minute is used clinically (Sankar, 2010; Shields, 1989). An in-line 0.22-0.55 micron filter is recommended for IVPB solutions due to the potential for precipitation of the solution. Following IV administration, NS should be injected through the same needle or IV catheter to prevent irritation.

Vesicant; ensure proper needle or catheter placement prior to and during IV infusion. Avoid extravasation.

Extravasation management: If extravasation occurs, stop infusion immediately and disconnect (leave needle/cannula in place); gently aspirate extravasated solution (do **NOT** flush the line); remove needle/cannula; elevate extremity. There is conflicting information regarding an antidote; some sources recommend not to use an antidote (Montgomery, 1999 [pediatric reference]), while other sources recommend hyaluronidase.

Hyaluronidase (if appropriate): SubQ: Administer four separate 0.2 mL injections of a 15 units/mL solution (using a 25-gauge needle) into area of extravasation (Sokol, 1998)

SubQ: SubQ administration is not recommended because of the possibility of local tissue damage (due to high pH).

Hazardous agent; use appropriate precautions for handling and disposal (NIOSH 2014 [group 2]).

Monitoring Parameters CBC, liver function; suicidality (eg, suicidal thoughts, depression, behavioral changes); plasma phenytoin concentrations (if available, free phenytoin concentrations should be obtained in patients with renal impairment and/or hypoalbuminemia; if free phenytoin concentrations are unavailable, the adjusted total concentration may be determined based upon equations in adult patients). Trough concentrations are generally recommended for routine monitoring.

Additional monitoring with IV use: Continuous cardiac monitoring (rate, rhythm, blood pressure) and observation during administration recommended; blood pressure and pulse should be monitored every 15 minutes for 1 hour after administration (Meek, 1999); infusion site reactions

Consult individual institutional policies and procedures.

Reference Range Timing of serum samples: Because it is slowly absorbed, peak blood levels may occur 4-8 hours after ingestion of an oral dose. The serum half-life varies with the dosage and the drug follows Michaelis-Menten kinetics. The average adult half-life is about 24 hours. Steady-state concentrations are reached in 5-10 days.

Children and Adults: Toxicity is measured clinically, and some patients require levels outside the suggested therapeutic range

Therapeutic range:

Total phenytoin: 10-20 mcg/mL (SI: 40-79 micromole/L) (children and adults), 8-15 mcg/mL (SI: 32-59 micromole/L) (neonates)

Concentrations of 5-10 mcg/mL (SI: 20-40 micromole/L) may be therapeutic for some patients but concentrations <5 mcg/mL (SI: <20 micromole/L) are not likely to be effective

50% of patients show decreased frequency of seizures at concentrations >10 mcg/mL (SI: >40 micromole/L)

86% of patients show decreased frequency of seizures at concentrations >15 mcg/mL (SI: >59 micromole/L)

Add another anticonvulsant if satisfactory therapeutic response is not achieved with a phenytoin concentration of 20 mcg/mL (SI: 79 micromole/L)

Free phenytoin: 1-2.5 mcg/mL (SI: 4-10 micromole/L)

Total phenytoin:

Toxic: >30 mcg/mL (SI: >119 micromole/L)

Lethal: >100 mcg/mL (SI: >396 micromole/L)

When to draw levels (Winter, 2010):

Key points: Time of sampling is dependent on the disease state being treated and the clinical condition of the patient. Trough concentrations are generally recommended for routine monitoring. However, timing of sampling is not as critical in patients receiving the extended-release dosage form because the slow absorption minimizes the fluctuations between peak and trough concentrations.

After a loading dose:

First concentration: It is prudent to draw within 2-3 days of therapy initiation to ensure that the patient's metabolism is not remarkably altered. Alternatively, if rapid therapeutic levels are needed, a level may be drawn 2 hours after completion of an IV loading dose (Meek, 1999) or 24 hours after administration of an oral loading dose (Osborn, 1987) to aid in determining maintenance dose or need to reload.

Second concentration: Draw within 5-8 days of therapy initiation with subsequent doses of phenytoin adjusted accordingly

If plasma concentrations have not changed over a 3- to 5-day period, monitoring interval may be increased to once weekly in the acute clinical setting. In stable patients requiring long-term therapy, generally monitor levels at 3- to 12-month intervals

Adjustment of serum concentration: See tables.

Note: Although it is ideal to obtain free phenytoin concentrations to assess serum concentrations in patients with hypoalbuminemia or renal failure (CrCl ≤10 mL/minute), it may not always be possible. If free phenytoin concentrations are unavailable, the following equations may be utilized in adult patients.

Adjustment of Serum Concentration in Adults With Low Serum Albumin

Measured Total Phenytoin Concentration mcg/mL (micromole/L)	Patient's Serum Albumin (g/dL)			
	3.5	3	2.5	2
	Adjusted Total Phenytoin Concentration mcg/mL[1] (micromole/L)			
5 (20)	6 (24)	7 (28)	8 (32)	10 (40)
10 (40)	13 (51.5)	14 (55)	17 (67)	20 (79)
15 (59)	19 (75)	21 (83)	25 (99)	30 (119)

[1]Adjusted concentration = measured total concentration divided by [(0.2 x albumin) + 0.1].

Adjustment of Serum Concentration in Adults With Renal Failure (CrCl ≤10 mL/min)

Measured Total Phenytoin Concentration mcg/mL (micromole/L)	Patient's Serum Albumin (g/dL)				
	4	3.5	3	2.5	2
	Adjusted Total Phenytoin Concentration mcg/mL[1] (micromole/L)				
5 (20)	10 (40)	11 (44)	13 (51.5)	14 (55)	17 (67)
10 (40)	20 (79)	22 (87)	25 (99)	29 (115)	33 (131)
15 (59)	30 (119)	33 (131)	38 (150)	43 (170)	50 (198)

[1]Adjusted concentration = measured total concentration divided by [(0.1 x albumin) + 0.1].

Dosage Forms Considerations The capsule dosage form represents *Extended Phenytoin Sodium Capsules,* USP, a designation differentiating the drug from *Prompt Phenytoin Sodium Capsules,* USP (no longer available) as the extended form was characterized by a slow and extended rate of absorption when the two were compared.

Dosage Forms

Capsule, Oral:

Dilantin: 30 mg, 100 mg

Phenytek: 200 mg, 300 mg

Generic: 100 mg, 200 mg, 300 mg

Solution, Injection:

Generic: 50 mg/mL (2 mL, 5 mL)

Suspension, Oral:

Dilantin: 125 mg/5 mL (237 mL)

Generic: 125 mg/5 mL (4 mL, 237 mL)

Tablet Chewable, Oral:

Dilantin Infatabs: 50 mg

Phenytoin Infatabs: 50 mg

Generic: 50 mg

◆ **Phenytoin Infatabs** *see* Phenytoin *on page* *1640*

◆ **Phenytoin Sodium** *see* Phenytoin *on page* *1640*

◆ **Phenytoin Sodium, Extended** *see* Phenytoin *on page* *1640*

◆ **Phenytoin Sodium, Prompt** *see* Phenytoin *on page* *1640*

◆ **PHiD-CV** *see* Pneumococcal Conjugate Vaccine (10-Valent) [CAN/INT] *on page* *1668*

◆ **Philith** *see* Ethinyl Estradiol and Norethindrone *on page* *808*

◆ **Phillips'® M-O [OTC]** *see* Magnesium Hydroxide and Mineral Oil *on page* *1264*

◆ **PHL-Alendronate (Can)** *see* Alendronate *on page* *79*

◆ **PHL-Amantadine (Can)** *see* Amantadine *on page* *105*

◆ **PHL-Amiodarone (Can)** *see* Amiodarone *on page* *114*

◆ **PHL-Amlodipine (Can)** *see* AmLODIPine *on page* *123*

◆ **PHL-Amoxicillin (Can)** *see* Amoxicillin *on page* *130*

◆ **PHL-Azithromycin (Can)** *see* Azithromycin (Systemic) *on page* *216*

- ◆ **PHL-Baclofen (Can)** *see* Baclofen *on page 223*
- ◆ **PHL-Bethanechol (Can)** *see* Bethanechol *on page 257*
- ◆ **PHL-Bicalutamide (Can)** *see* Bicalutamide *on page 262*
- ◆ **PHL-Bisoprolol (Can)** *see* Bisoprolol *on page 266*
- ◆ **PHL-Cilazapril (Can)** *see* Cilazapril [CAN/INT] *on page 434*
- ◆ **PHL-Ciprofloxacin (Can)** *see* Ciprofloxacin (Systemic) *on page 441*
- ◆ **PHL-Citalopram (Can)** *see* Citalopram *on page 451*
- ◆ **PHL-Clonazepam (Can)** *see* ClonazePAM *on page 478*
- ◆ **PHL-Clonazepam-R (Can)** *see* ClonazePAM *on page 478*
- ◆ **PHL-Cyclobenzaprine (Can)** *see* Cyclobenzaprine *on page 516*
- ◆ **PHL-Dexamethasone (Can)** *see* Dexamethasone (Systemic) *on page 599*
- ◆ **PHL-Divalproex (Can)** *see* Valproic Acid and Derivatives *on page 2123*
- ◆ **PHL-Docusate Sodium [OTC] (Can)** *see* Docusate *on page 661*
- ◆ **PHL-Doxycycline (Can)** *see* Doxycycline *on page 689*
- ◆ **PHL-Fenofibrate Micro (Can)** *see* Fenofibrate and Derivatives *on page 852*
- ◆ **PHL-Fluconazole (Can)** *see* Fluconazole *on page 885*
- ◆ **PHL-Fluoxetine (Can)** *see* FLUoxetine *on page 899*
- ◆ **PHL-Fluvoxamine (Can)** *see* FluvoxaMINE *on page 916*
- ◆ **PHL-Gabapentin (Can)** *see* Gabapentin *on page 943*
- ◆ **PHL-Indapamide (Can)** *see* Indapamide *on page 1065*
- ◆ **PHL-Leflunomide (Can)** *see* Leflunomide *on page 1174*
- ◆ **PHL-Levetiracetam (Can)** *see* LevETIRAcetam *on page 1191*
- ◆ **PHL-Lorazepam (Can)** *see* LORazepam *on page 1243*
- ◆ **PHL-Lovastatin (Can)** *see* Lovastatin *on page 1252*
- ◆ **PHL-Loxapine (Can)** *see* Loxapine *on page 1255*
- ◆ **PHL-Meloxicam (Can)** *see* Meloxicam *on page 1283*
- ◆ **PHL-Metformin (Can)** *see* MetFORMIN *on page 1307*
- ◆ **PHL-Methimazole (Can)** *see* Methimazole *on page 1319*
- ◆ **PHL-Methylphenidate (Can)** *see* Methylphenidate *on page 1336*
- ◆ **PHL-Minocycline (Can)** *see* Minocycline *on page 1371*
- ◆ **PHL-Olanzapine (Can)** *see* OLANZapine *on page 1491*
- ◆ **PHL-Olanzapine ODT (Can)** *see* OLANZapine *on page 1491*
- ◆ **PHL-Ondansetron (Can)** *see* Ondansetron *on page 1513*
- ◆ **PHL-Oxybutynin (Can)** *see* Oxybutynin *on page 1536*
- ◆ **PHL-Paroxetine (Can)** *see* PARoxetine *on page 1579*
- ◆ **PHL-Pioglitazone (Can)** *see* Pioglitazone *on page 1654*
- ◆ **PHL-Pravastatin (Can)** *see* Pravastatin *on page 1700*
- ◆ **PHL-Procyclidine (Can)** *see* Procyclidine [CAN/INT] *on page 1721*
- ◆ **PHL-Quetiapine (Can)** *see* QUEtiapine *on page 1751*
- ◆ **PHL-Ranitidine (Can)** *see* Ranitidine *on page 1777*
- ◆ **PHL-Risperidone (Can)** *see* RisperiDONE *on page 1818*
- ◆ **PHL-Salbutamol (Can)** *see* Albuterol *on page 69*
- ◆ **PHL-Sertraline (Can)** *see* Sertraline *on page 1878*
- ◆ **PHL-Simvastatin (Can)** *see* Simvastatin *on page 1890*
- ◆ **PHL-Sotalol (Can)** *see* Sotalol *on page 1927*
- ◆ **PHL-Sumatriptan (Can)** *see* SUMAtriptan *on page 1953*
- ◆ **PHL-Temazepam (Can)** *see* Temazepam *on page 1990*
- ◆ **PHL-Terazosin (Can)** *see* Terazosin *on page 2001*
- ◆ **PHL-Terbinafine (Can)** *see* Terbinafine (Systemic) *on page 2002*
- ◆ **PHL-Topiramate (Can)** *see* Topiramate *on page 2065*
- ◆ **PHL-Trazodone (Can)** *see* TraZODone *on page 2091*
- ◆ **PHL-Ursodiol C (Can)** *see* Ursodiol *on page 2116*
- ◆ **PHL-Valacyclovir (Can)** *see* ValACYclovir *on page 2119*
- ◆ **PHL-Valproic Acid (Can)** *see* Valproic Acid and Derivatives *on page 2123*
- ◆ **PHL-Valproic Acid E.C. (Can)** *see* Valproic Acid and Derivatives *on page 2123*
- ◆ **PHL-Verapamil SR (Can)** *see* Verapamil *on page 2154*
- ◆ **PHL-Zopiclone (Can)** *see* Zopiclone [CAN/INT] *on page 2217*

Pholcodine [INT] (FOL co deen)

International Brand Names Actuss (AU); Amcal Dry Cough Forte (AU); Biocalyptol (FR); Codisol (DK); Codotussyl toux seche (FR); Codral Dry Cough Liquid (AU); Ducodine (MY); Duro-Tuss (AU, HK, MY, SG); Galenphol (GB); Homocodeina (ES); Humex Fournier (FR); Linctus Tussinol (AU); Pavacol-D (GB); Pectolin (AU); Pholcodin (HR); Pholcodine Linctus (GB); Pholcolin (IE); Pholcotussin (CN); Pholtex Forte (AU); Pholtrate (AU); Respilene (FR); Sedlingtus (AU); Sirop des Vosges (FR); Trophires (ES); Tuxi (NO); Uni-Pholco (HK); Weifacodine (NO)

Pharmacologic Category Antitussive

Reported Use Treatment of cough

Dosage Range Oral:

Children 5-12 years: 2.5-5 mg 3-4 times/day
Adults: 5-10 mg 3-4 times/day

Product Availability Product available in various countries; not currently available in the U.S.

Dosage Forms

Syrup: 2 mg/5 mL (90 mL); 5 mg/5 mL (100 mL); 10 mg/5 mL (100 mL)

- ◆ **Phos-Flur** *see* Fluoride *on page 895*
- ◆ **Phos-Flur Rinse [OTC]** *see* Fluoride *on page 895*
- ◆ **PhosLo** *see* Calcium Acetate *on page 326*
- ◆ **PhosLo® (Can)** *see* Calcium Acetate *on page 326*
- ◆ **Phoslyra** *see* Calcium Acetate *on page 326*
- ◆ **Phos-NaK** *see* Potassium Phosphate and Sodium Phosphate *on page 1692*
- ◆ **Phospha 250 Neutral** *see* Potassium Phosphate and Sodium Phosphate *on page 1692*
- ◆ **Phosphasal** *see* Methenamine, Sodium Phosphate Monobasic, Phenyl Salicylate, Methylene Blue, and Hyoscyamine *on page 1318*
- ◆ **Phosphate, Potassium** *see* Potassium Phosphate *on page 1691*
- ◆ **Phosphates, Sodium** *see* Sodium Phosphates *on page 1909*
- ◆ **Phospholine Iodide** *see* Echothiophate Iodide *on page 703*
- ◆ **Phosphonoformate** *see* Foscarnet *on page 931*
- ◆ **Phosphonoformic Acid** *see* Foscarnet *on page 931*
- ◆ **Photofrin** *see* Porfimer *on page 1682*
- ◆ **Photofrin® (Can)** *see* Porfimer *on page 1682*
- ◆ **Phrenilin Forte** *see* Butalbital and Acetaminophen *on page 314*
- ◆ ***p*-Hydroxyampicillin** *see* Amoxicillin *on page 130*
- ◆ **Phylloquinone** *see* Phytonadione *on page 1647*

◆ **Physicians EZ Use B-12** *see* Cyanocobalamin *on page 515*

◆ **Physicians EZ Use Flu** *see* Influenza Virus Vaccine (Inactivated) *on page 1075*

Physostigmine (fye zoe STIG meen)

Index Terms Eserine Salicylate; Physostigmine Salicylate; Physostigmine Sulfate

Pharmacologic Category Acetylcholinesterase Inhibitor; Antidote

Use Reversal of central nervous system anticholinergic syndrome

Note: Physostigmine should only be used to reverse toxic, life-threatening delirium caused by pure anticholinergic agents (ie, atropine, diphenhydramine, dimenhydrinate, *Atropa belladonna* [deadly nightshade], or jimson weed [*Datura* spp]). Consultation with a clinical toxicologist or poison control center is recommended in patients who require physostigmine administration.

Dosage Reversal of toxic anticholinergic effects:

Children: **Note:** Reserve for life-threatening situations only. When administering by IV injection, administer no faster than 0.5 mg/minute to prevent bradycardia, respiratory distress, and seizures from too rapid administration.

IM, IV: Initial: 0.02 mg/kg; may repeat every 5-10 minutes until response occurs (maximum total dose: 2 mg)

Adults: **Note:** When administering by IV injection, administer no faster than 1 mg/minute to prevent bradycardia, respiratory distress, and seizures from too rapid administration.

IM, IV: Initial: 0.5-2 mg; may repeat every 10-30 minutes until response occurs. Subsequent doses may be required to manage life-threatening anticholinergic effects (Krenzelok, 2010).

Dosage adjustment in renal impairment: No dosage adjustment provided in manufacturer's labeling.

Dosage adjustment in hepatic impairment: No dosage adjustment provided in manufacturer's labeling.

Additional Information Complete prescribing information should be consulted for additional detail.

Dosage Forms

Solution, Injection:

Generic: 1 mg/mL (2 mL)

◆ **Physostigmine Salicylate** *see* Physostigmine *on page 1647*

◆ **Physostigmine Sulfate** *see* Physostigmine *on page 1647*

◆ **Phytomenadione** *see* Phytonadione *on page 1647*

Phytonadione (fye toe na DYE one)

Brand Names: U.S. Mephyton®

Brand Names: Canada AquaMEPHYTON®; Konakion; Mephyton®

Index Terms Methylphytyl Napthoquinone; Phylloquinone; Phytomenadione; Vitamin K; Vitamin K_1

Pharmacologic Category Vitamin, Fat Soluble

Additional Appendix Information

Reversal of Oral Anticoagulants *on page 2235*

Use Prevention and treatment of hypoprothrombinemia caused by vitamin K antagonist (VKA)-induced (eg, warfarin-induced) or other drug-induced vitamin K deficiency, altered activity, or altered metabolism; hypoprothrombinemia caused by malabsorption or inability to synthesize vitamin K; prophylaxis and treatment of hemorrhagic disease of the newborn

Pregnancy Risk Factor C

Pregnancy Considerations Animal reproduction studies have not been conducted. Phytonadione crosses the placenta in limited concentrations (Kazzi, 1990). The dietary requirements of vitamin K are the same in pregnant and nonpregnant women (IOM, 2000). In general, medications used as antidotes should take into consideration the health and prognosis of the mother; antidotes should be administered to pregnant women if there is a clear indication for use and should not be withheld because of fears of teratogenicity (Bailey, 2003).

Breast-Feeding Considerations Small amounts of dietary vitamin K can be detected in breast milk and the dietary requirements of vitamin K are the same in nursing and non-nursing women (IOM, 2000). Information following the use of phytonadione has not been located. The manufacturer recommends caution be used if phytonadione is administered to a nursing woman.

Contraindications Hypersensitivity to phytonadione or any component of the formulation

Warnings/Precautions [U.S. Boxed Warning]: Severe reactions resembling hypersensitivity reactions (eg, anaphylaxis) have occurred rarely during or immediately after IV administration (even with proper dilution and rate of administration); some patients had no previous exposure to phytonadione. Anaphylactoid reactions typically occurred when patients received large IV doses administered rapidly with formulations containing polyethoxylated castor oil; proper dosing, dilution, and administration will minimize risk (Ageno, 2012; Riegert-Johnson, 2002). Limit IV administration to situations where an alternative route of administration is not feasible and the benefit of therapy outweighs the risk of hypersensitivity reactions. Allergic reactions have also occurred with IM and SubQ injections, albeit less frequently. In obstructive jaundice or with biliary fistulas concurrent administration of bile salts is necessary. Manufacturers recommend the SubQ route over other parenteral routes. SubQ is less predictable when compared to the oral route. The American College of Chest Physicians recommends the IV route in patients with major bleeding secondary to warfarin. The IV route should be restricted to emergency situations where oral phytonadione cannot be used. Efficacy is delayed regardless of route of administration; patient management may require other treatments in the interim. In patients receiving a therapeutic vitamin K antagonist (VKA) (eg, warfarin), administer a dose of phytonadione that will quickly lower the INR into a safe range without causing resistance to warfarin. High phytonadione doses may lead to warfarin resistance for at least one week. Patients with LAAR-induced coagulopathy require much larger doses and longer treatment durations (up to months) after exposure compared to that needed to reverse VKA-induced coagulopathy. Use with caution in neonates, especially premature infants; severe hemolytic anemia, jaundice, and hyperbilirubinemia have been reported with larger than recommended doses (10 to 20 mg). In liver disease, if initial doses do not reverse coagulopathy then higher doses are unlikely to have any effect. Ineffective in hereditary hypoprothrombinemia.

Benzyl alcohol and derivatives: Some dosage forms may contain benzyl alcohol; large amounts of benzyl alcohol (≥99 mg/kg/day) have been associated with a potentially fatal toxicity ("gasping syndrome") in neonates; the "gasping syndrome" consists of metabolic acidosis, respiratory distress, gasping respirations, CNS dysfunction (including convulsions, intracranial hemorrhage), hypotension, and cardiovascular collapse (AAP, 1997; CDC, 1982); some data suggests that benzoate displaces bilirubin from protein binding sites (Ahlfors, 2001); avoid or use dosage forms containing benzyl alcohol with caution in neonates. See manufacturer's labeling.

Injectable products may contain aluminum; may result in toxic levels following prolonged administration.

Product may contain polysorbate 80.

Some dosage forms contain Cremophor EL which has been associated with anaphylactoid reactions; use these formulations with caution.

Adverse Reactions

Cardiovascular: Cyanosis, flushing, hyper-/hypotension

Central nervous system: Dizziness

Dermatologic: Erythematous skin eruptions, pruritus, scleroderma-like lesions

Endocrine & metabolic: Hyperbilirubinemia (newborn; greater than recommended doses)

Gastrointestinal: Abnormal taste

Local: Injection site reactions

Respiratory: Dyspnea

Miscellaneous: Diaphoresis, hypersensitivity reactions, nonimmunologic anaphylaxis (formerly known as anaphylactoid reaction), sweating

Drug Interactions

Metabolism/Transport Effects None known.

Avoid Concomitant Use There are no known interactions where it is recommended to avoid concomitant use.

Increased Effect/Toxicity There are no known significant interactions involving an increase in effect.

Decreased Effect

Phytonadione may decrease the levels/effects of: Vitamin K Antagonists

The levels/effects of Phytonadione may be decreased by: Mineral Oil; Orlistat

Preparation for Administration Dilute injection solution in preservative-free NS, D_5W, or D_5NS. To reduce the incidence of anaphylactoid reaction upon IV administration, dilute dose in a minimum of 50 mL of compatible solution and administer using an infusion pump over at least 20 minutes (Ageno, 2012).

Storage/Stability

Injection: Store at 15°C to 30°C (59°F to 86°F). Protect from light. **Note:** Store Hospira product at 20°C to 25°C (68°F to 77°F).

Oral: Store tablets at 15°C to 30°C (59°F to 86°F). Protect from light.

Mechanism of Action Promotes liver synthesis of clotting factors (II, VII, IX, X); however, the exact mechanism as to this stimulation is unknown. Menadiol is a water soluble form of vitamin K; phytonadione has a more rapid and prolonged effect than menadione; menadiol sodium diphosphate (K_4) is half as potent as menadione (K_3).

Pharmacodynamics/Kinetics

Onset of action: Increased coagulation factors: Oral: 6-10 hours; IV: 1-2 hours

Peak effect: INR values return to normal: Oral: 24-48 hours; IV: 12-14 hours

Absorption: Oral: From intestines in presence of bile; SubQ: Variable

Metabolism: Rapidly hepatic

Excretion: Urine and feces

Dosage Note: According to the manufacturer, SubQ is the preferred parenteral route; IM route should be avoided due to the risk of hematoma formation; IV route should be restricted for emergency use only. The American College of Chest Physicians (ACCP) recommends the IV route in patients with major bleeding secondary to use of vitamin K antagonists (VKAs).

Adequate intake (AI): Oral:

Infants:

0-6 months: 2 **mcg**/day

7-12 months: 2.5 **mcg**/day

Children:

1-3 years: 30 **mcg**/day

4-8 years: 55 **mcg**/day

9-13 years: 60 **mcg**/day

14-18 years: 75 **mcg**/day

Adults: Males: 120 **mcg**/day; Females: 90 **mcg**/day

Hemorrhagic disease of the newborn:

Prophylaxis: IM: 0.5-1 mg within 1 hour of birth

Treatment: IM, SubQ: 1 mg/dose/day; higher doses may be necessary if mother has been receiving oral anticoagulants

Hypoprothrombinemia due to drugs (other than coumarin derivatives) or factors limiting absorption or synthesis: Adults: Oral, SubQ, IM, IV: Initial: 2.5-25 mg (rarely up to 50 mg)

Vitamin K deficiency (supratherapeutic INR) secondary to VKAs (eg, warfarin):

Infants and Children (off-label use): ***Excessively prolonged INR (usually INR >8; no significant bleeding):*** **Note:** Limited data available: IV: 0.03 mg/kg/dose; maximum dose: 1 mg (Bolton-Maggs, 2002); if significant bleeding, consider use of fresh frozen plasma, prothrombin complex concentrates, or recombinant factor VIIa (Monagle, 2012).

Adults (off-label dose):

If INR above therapeutic range to <4.5 (no evidence of bleeding): Lower or hold next VKA dose and monitor frequently; when INR approaches desired range, resume VKA dosing with a lower dose (Patriquin, 2011).

If INR 4.5-10 (no evidence of bleeding): The 2012 ACCP guidelines recommend against routine phytonadione (aka, vitamin K) administration in this setting (Guyatt, 2012). Previously, the 2008 ACCP guidelines recommended if no risk factors for bleeding exist, to omit next 1 or 2 VKA doses, monitor INR more frequently, and resume with an appropriately adjusted VKA dose when INR in desired range; may consider administering vitamin K orally 1-2.5 mg if other risk factors for bleeding exist (Hirsh, 2008). Others have recommended consideration of vitamin K 1 mg orally or 0.5 mg IV (Patriquin, 2011).

If INR >10 (no evidence of bleeding): The 2012 ACCP guidelines recommend administration of oral vitamin K (dose not specified) in this setting (Guyatt, 2012). Previously, the 2008 ACCP guidelines recommended to hold warfarin, administer vitamin K orally 2.5-5 mg, expect INR to be reduced within 24-48 hours, monitor INR more frequently and give additional vitamin K at an appropriate dose if necessary; resume warfarin at an appropriately adjusted dose when INR is in desired range (Hirsh, 2008). Others have recommended consideration of vitamin K 2-2.5 mg orally or 0.5-1 mg IV (Patriquin, 2011).

If minor bleeding at any INR elevation: Hold warfarin, may administer vitamin K orally 2.5-5 mg, monitor INR more frequently, may repeat dose after 24 hours if INR correction incomplete; resume warfarin at an appropriately adjusted dose when INR is in desired range (Patriquin, 2011).

If major bleeding at any INR elevation: The 2012 ACCP guidelines recommend administration of four-factor prothrombin complex concentrate (PCC) and IV vitamin K 5-10 mg in this setting (Guyatt, 2012). The only available four-factor PCC in the U.S. is Kcentra. Other four-factor PCCs **not** available in the U.S. include Beriplex P/N, Cofact, Konyne, and Octaplex. Bebulin VH and Profilnine SD **do not** contain adequate levels of factor VII and are considered **three**-factor PCCs. Previously, the 2008 ACCP guidelines recommended to hold warfarin, administer vitamin K 10 mg by slow IV infusion and supplement with PCC depending on the urgency of the situation; IV vitamin K may be repeated every 12 hours (Hirsh, 2008).

Note: Use of high doses of vitamin K (eg, 10-15 mg) may cause warfarin resistance for ≥1 week. During this period of resistance, heparin or low-molecular-weight heparin (LMWH) may be given until INR responds (Ansell, 2008).

Preprocedural/surgical INR normalization in patients receiving warfarin (routine use): Adults: Oral: 1-2.5 mg once administered on the day before surgery; recheck INR on day of procedure/surgery (Douketis, 2012). Others have recommended the use of vitamin K 1 mg orally for mild INR elevations (ie, INR 3.0-4.5) (Patriquin, 2011).

Dosage adjustment in renal impairment: No dosage adjustment provided in manufacturer's labeling.

Dosage adjustment in hepatic impairment: No dosage adjustment provided in manufacturer's labeling.

Administration

IV administration: Infuse slowly; rate of infusion should not exceed 1 mg/minute (3 mg/m^2/minute in children and infants). Alternatively, dilute dose in a minimum of 50 mL of compatible solution and administer using an infusion pump over at least 20 minutes (Ageno, 2012). The injectable route should be used only if the oral route is not feasible or there is a greater urgency to reverse anticoagulation.

Oral: The parenteral formulation may also be used for small oral doses (eg, 1 mg) or situations in which tablets cannot be swallowed (Crowther, 2000; O'Connor, 1986).

Monitoring Parameters PT, INR

Dosage Forms Considerations Injectable products may contain benzyl alcohol, polysorbate 80, propylene glycol, or castor derivatives.

Dosage Forms

Injection, aqueous colloidal: 1 mg/0.5 mL (0.5 mL); 10 mg/mL (1 mL)

Injection, aqueous colloidal [preservative free]: 1 mg/0.5 mL (0.5 mL)

Tablet, oral: 100 mcg

Mephyton®: 5 mg

Extemporaneous Preparations A 1 mg/mL oral suspension may be made with tablets. Crush six 5 mg tablets in a mortar and reduce to a fine powder. Add 5 mL each of water and methylcellulose 1% and mix to a uniform paste. Mix while adding sorbitol in incremental proportions to **almost** 30 mL; transfer to a calibrated bottle, rinse mortar with sorbitol, and add quantity of sorbitol sufficient to make 30 mL. Label "shake well" and "refrigerate". Stable for 3 days.

Nahata MC and Hipple TF, *Pediatric Drug Formulations*, 3rd ed, Cincinnati, OH: Harvey Whitney Books Co, 1997.

Note: The parenteral formulation may also be used for small oral doses (eg, 1 mg) or situations in which tablets cannot be swallowed (Crowther, 2000; O'Connor, 1986).

◆ **PI$_3$K Delta Inhibitor CAL-101** *see* Idelalisib *on page 1038*

◆ **PIC 200 [OTC]** *see* Polysaccharide-Iron Complex *on page 1677*

◆ **Picato** *see* Ingenol Mebutate *on page 1083*

◆ **Picodan (Can)** *see* Sodium Picosulfate, Magnesium Oxide, and Citric Acid *on page 1911*

◆ **Picoflo (Can)** *see* Sodium Picosulfate, Magnesium Oxide, and Citric Acid *on page 1911*

◆ **Pico-Salax® (Can)** *see* Sodium Picosulfate, Magnesium Oxide, and Citric Acid *on page 1911*

◆ **Pidorubicin** *see* Epirubicin *on page 739*

◆ **Pidorubicin Hydrochloride** *see* Epirubicin *on page 739*

Pilocarpine (Systemic) (pye loe KAR peen)

Brand Names: U.S. Salagen

Brand Names: Canada Salagen®

Index Terms Pilocarpine Hydrochloride

Pharmacologic Category Cholinergic Agonist

Use Symptomatic treatment of xerostomia caused by salivary gland hypofunction resulting from radiotherapy for cancer of the head and neck or Sjögren's syndrome

Pregnancy Risk Factor C

Dosage Oral: Adults: Xerostomia:

Following head and neck cancer: 5 mg 3 times daily, titration up to 10 mg 3 times daily may be considered for patients who have not responded adequately; do not exceed 2 tablets per dose

Sjögren's syndrome: 5 mg 4 times daily

Dosage adjustment in renal impairment: No dosage adjustment necessary.

Dosage adjustment in hepatic impairment:

Mild impairment (Child-Pugh score 5-6): No dosage adjustment necessary.

Moderate impairment (Child-Pugh score 7-9): 5 mg twice daily regardless of indication; adjust dose based on response and tolerability

Severe impairment (Child-Pugh score >10): Not recommended.

Additional Information Complete prescribing information should be consulted for additional detail.

Dosage Forms

Tablet, Oral:

Salagen: 5 mg, 7.5 mg

Generic: 5 mg, 7.5 mg

Pilocarpine (Ophthalmic) (pye loe KAR peen)

Brand Names: U.S. Isopto Carpine; Pilopine HS

Brand Names: Canada Diocarpine; Isopto® Carpine; Pilopine HS®

Index Terms Pilocarpine Hydrochloride

Pharmacologic Category Ophthalmic Agent, Antiglaucoma; Ophthalmic Agent, Miotic

Use Management of chronic simple glaucoma, chronic and acute angle-closure glaucoma

Pregnancy Risk Factor C

Dosage Ophthalmic: Adults:

Glaucoma:

Solution: Instill 1-2 drops up to 6 times/day; adjust the concentration and frequency as required to control elevated intraocular pressure

Gel: Instill 0.5" ribbon into lower conjunctival sac once daily at bedtime

To counteract the mydriatic effects of sympathomimetic agents (off-label use): Solution: Instill 1 drop of a 1% solution in the affected eye

Dosage adjustment in renal impairment: No dosage adjustment provided in manufacturer's labeling.

Dosage adjustment in hepatic impairment: No dosage adjustment provided in manufacturer's labeling.

Additional Information Complete prescribing information should be consulted for additional detail.

Dosage Forms

Gel, Ophthalmic:

Pilopine HS: 4% (4 g)

Solution, Ophthalmic:

Isopto Carpine: 1% (15 mL); 2% (15 mL); 4% (15 mL)

Generic: 1% (15 mL); 2% (15 mL); 4% (15 mL)

◆ **Pilocarpine Hydrochloride** *see* Pilocarpine (Ophthalmic) *on page 1649*

◆ **Pilocarpine Hydrochloride** *see* Pilocarpine (Systemic) *on page 1649*

◆ **Pilopine HS** *see* Pilocarpine (Ophthalmic) *on page 1649*

◆ **Pilopine HS® (Can)** *see* Pilocarpine (Ophthalmic) *on page 1649*

◆ **Pimaricin** *see* Natamycin *on page 1432*

Pimecrolimus (pim e KROE li mus)

Brand Names: U.S. Elidel

Brand Names: Canada Elidel

Pharmacologic Category Calcineurin Inhibitor; Immunosuppressant Agent; Topical Skin Product

Use Atopic dermatitis: Second-line therapy for short-term and noncontinuous long-term treatment of mild to moderate atopic dermatitis in nonimmunocompromised patients 2 years and older who have failed to respond adequately to other topical prescription treatments, or when those treatments are not advisable.

Pregnancy Risk Factor C

Pregnancy Considerations Adverse events were not observed in animal reproduction studies following topical application.

Breast-Feeding Considerations It is not known if pimecrolimus is excreted in breast milk. Due to the potential for serious adverse reactions in the nursing infant, the manufacturer recommends a decision be made whether to discontinue nursing or to discontinue the drug, taking into account the importance of treatment to the mother.

Contraindications Hypersensitivity to pimecrolimus or any component of the formulation

Warnings/Precautions Hazardous agent; use appropriate precautions for handling and disposal (meets NIOSH 2014 criteria). **[U.S. Boxed Warning]: Topical calcineurin inhibitors (including pimecrolimus) have been associated with rare cases of lymphoma and skin malignancy.** Avoid use on malignant or premalignant skin conditions (eg, cutaneous T-cell lymphoma). **[U.S. Boxed Warning]: Continuous long-term use of calcineurin inhibitors (including pimecrolimus) should be avoided and application of cream should be limited to areas of involvement with atopic dermatitis. Safety of intermittent use for >1 year has not been established.** Diagnosis should be reconfirmed if sign/symptoms do not improve within 6 weeks of treatment.

May cause local symptoms (eg, burning, pruritus, soreness, stinging) during first few days of treatment; usually self-resolving as atopic dermatitis lesions heal. Should not be used in immunocompromised patients, including patients on concomitant systemic immunosuppressive therapy. Patients with atopic dermatitis are predisposed to skin infections; therapy has been associated with an increased risk of developing eczema herpeticum, varicella zoster, and herpes simplex. Do not apply to areas of active bacterial or viral infection; local infections at the treatment site should be resolved prior to therapy. Skin papilloma (warts) have been observed with use; discontinue use if there is worsening of skin papillomas or they do not respond to conventional treatment. Pimecrolimus may be associated with development of lymphadenopathy; possible infectious causes should be investigated. Discontinue use in patients with unknown cause of lymphadenopathy or acute infectious mononucleosis. Not recommended for use in patients with skin disease which may increase the potential for systemic absorption (eg, Netherton's syndrome). Avoid artificial or natural sunlight exposure, even when pimecrolimus is not on the skin. Safety not established in patients with generalized erythroderma. **[U.S. Boxed Warning]: The use of pimecrolimus in children <2 years of age is not recommended,** particularly since the effect on immune system development is unknown.

Benzyl alcohol and derivatives: Some dosage forms may contain benzyl alcohol; large amounts of benzyl alcohol (≥99 mg/kg/day) have been associated with a potentially fatal toxicity ("gasping syndrome") in neonates; the "gasping syndrome" consists of metabolic acidosis, respiratory distress, gasping respirations, CNS dysfunction (including convulsions, intracranial hemorrhage), hypotension, and cardiovascular collapse (AAP, 1997; CDC, 1982); some data suggests that benzoate displaces bilirubin from protein binding sites (Ahlfors, 2001); avoid or use dosage forms containing benzyl alcohol with caution in neonates. See manufacturer's labeling.

Adverse Reactions

Central nervous system: Fever (more common in children and adolescents), headache (more common in children and adolescents)

Dermatologic: Acne vulgaris, folliculitis (more common in adults), herpes simplex dermatitis, impetigo, molluscum contagiosum (children and adolescents), skin infection, urticaria, warts (children and adolescents)

Gastrointestinal: Abdominal pain, constipation (children and adolescents), diarrhea (more common in children and adolescents), gastroenteritis (more common in children and adolescents), nausea, toothache, vomiting

Genitourinary: Dysmenorrhea

Hypersensitivity: Hypersensitivity

Infection: Bacterial infection, herpes simplex infection, influenza, staphylococcal infection, varicella, viral infection (children and adolescents)

Local: Application site reaction (more common in adults), local burning (more common in adults; tends to resolve/improve as lesions resolve), local irritation (more common in adults), localized erythema, local pruritus

Neuromuscular & skeletal: Arthralgia, back pain

Ocular: Conjunctivitis, eye infection

Otic: Otic infection, otitis media

Respiratory: Asthma, asthma aggravated (children and adolescents), bronchitis (more common in children and adolescents), cough (more common in children and adolescents), dyspnea, epistaxis, flu-like symptoms, nasal congestion, nasopharyngitis (more common in infants, children, and adolescents), pharyngitis (more common in children and adolescents), pneumonia, rhinitis, rhinorrhea (children and adolescents), sinusitis, sore throat, streptococcal pharyngitis (children and adolescents), tonsillitis (more common in children and adolescents), upper respiratory tract infection (more common in children and adolescents), viral upper respiratory tract infection, wheezing (children and adolescents)

Miscellaneous: Laceration (children and adolescents)

Rare but important or life-threatening: Anaphylaxis, angioedema, eczema (herpeticum), lymphadenopathy, malignant neoplasm (basal cell carcinoma, squamous cell carcinoma, malignant melanoma, malignant lymphoma), skin discoloration

Drug Interactions

Metabolism/Transport Effects Substrate of CYP3A4 (minor); **Note:** Assignment of Major/Minor substrate status based on clinically relevant drug interaction potential

Avoid Concomitant Use

Avoid concomitant use of Pimecrolimus with any of the following: Immunosuppressants

Increased Effect/Toxicity

Pimecrolimus may increase the levels/effects of: Immunosuppressants

The levels/effects of Pimecrolimus may be increased by: CYP3A4 Inhibitors (Moderate); CYP3A4 Inhibitors (Strong)

Decreased Effect There are no known significant interactions involving a decrease in effect.

Storage/Stability Store at 25°C (77°F); excursions permitted to 15°C to 30°C (59°F to 86°F); do not freeze.

Mechanism of Action Penetrates inflamed epidermis to inhibit T cell activation by blocking transcription of proinflammatory cytokine genes such as interleukin-2, interferon gamma (Th1-type), interleukin-4, and interleukin-10 (Th2-type). Pimecrolimus binds to the intracellular protein FKBP-12, inhibiting calcineurin, which blocks cytokine transcription and inhibits T-cell activation. Prevents release of inflammatory cytokines and mediators from mast cells *in vitro* after stimulation by antigen/IgE.

Pharmacodynamics/Kinetics Absorption: Poor when applied to 13% to 62% body surface area in adults treated for atopic dermatitis for up to a year; detectable blood levels were observed in a higher proportion of children, as compared to adults. Does not penetrate psoriatic plaque (Menter, 2009)

Dosage

Atopic dermatitis (mild-to-moderate): Children ≥2 years, Adolescents, and Adults: Topical: Apply thin layer to affected area twice daily. **Note:** Limit application to involved areas. Discontinue use when symptoms have resolved; re-evaluate if symptoms persist >6 weeks.

Oral lichen planus (off-label use): Adults: Topical: Apply twice daily for 1 month (Passeron, 2007; Volz, 2008)

Psoriasis (off-label use): Adults: Topical: Apply twice daily (Gribetz, 2004; Menter, 2009)

Administration Apply a thin layer to affected skin. Limit application to areas of involvement. Do not use with occlusive dressings. Burning at the application site is most common in first few days; improves as atopic dermatitis improves. Discontinue use when symptoms have resolved; re-evaluate if symptoms persist >6 weeks. Moisturizers may be applied after use of pimecrolimus cream. Wash hands after use.

Oral lichen planus (off-label use): Apply to affected oral mucosa, cover with a thin layer of gauze to delay dilution with saliva (Volz, 2008). Eating, drinking or chewing gum was not allowed for 30 minutes after application (Passeron, 2007).

Hazardous agent; use appropriate precautions for handling and disposal (meets NIOSH 2014 criteria).

Dosage Forms

Cream, External:

Elidel: 1% (30 g, 60 g, 100 g)

Pimozide (PI moe zide)

Brand Names: U.S. Orap

Brand Names: Canada Apo-Pimozide®; Orap®; PMS-Pimozide

Pharmacologic Category First Generation (Typical) Antipsychotic

Additional Appendix Information

Beers Criteria - Potentially Inappropriate Medications for Geriatrics *on page 2271*

Use Suppression of severe motor and phonic tics in patients with Tourette's disorder who have failed to respond satisfactorily to standard treatment

Pregnancy Risk Factor C

Dosage Oral: **Note:** An ECG should be performed baseline and periodically thereafter, especially during dosage adjustment:

Children 2-12 years: Tourette's disorder: Initial: 0.05 mg/kg preferably once at bedtime; may be increased every third day to a maximum of 0.2 mg/kg/day (do not exceed 10 mg/day); usual range: 2-4 mg/day. **Note:** If therapy requires exceeding dose of 0.05 mg/kg/day, CYP2D6 geno-/phenotyping should be performed; CYP2D6 poor metabolizers should be dose titrated in ≥14-day increments and should not receive doses in excess of 0.05 mg/kg/day.

Children >12 years and Adults: Tourette's disorder: Initial: 1-2 mg/day in divided doses, then increase dosage as needed every other day; maximum dose: 10 mg/day or 0.2 mg/kg/day (whichever is less); **Note:** If therapy requires exceeding dose of 4 mg/day, CYP2D6 geno-/phenotyping should be performed; CYP2D6 poor metabolizers should be dose titrated in ≥14-day increments and should not receive doses in excess of 4 mg/day.

Elderly: Recommend initial dose of 1 mg/day; periodically attempt gradual reduction of dose to determine if tic persists; follow up for 1-2 weeks before concluding the tic is a persistent disease phenomenon and not a manifestation of drug withdrawal. **Note:** An ECG should be performed baseline and periodically thereafter, especially during dosage adjustment.

Dosage adjustment for toxicity:

ECG changes:

Children: QTc prolongation >0.47 seconds or >25% above baseline: Decrease dose

Adults: QTc prolongation >0.52 seconds or >25% above baseline: Decrease dose

NMS syndrome: Discontinue (monitor carefully if therapy is reinitiated)

Tardive dyskinesia signs/symptoms: Consider discontinuing.

Dosage adjustment in renal impairment: No dosage adjustment provided in manufacturer's labeling. Use with caution.

Dosage adjustment in hepatic impairment: No dosage adjustment provided in manufacturer's labeling. Use with caution.

Additional Information Complete prescribing information should be consulted for additional detail.

Dosage Forms

Tablet, Oral:

Orap: 1 mg, 2 mg

Dosage Forms: Canada Tablet, Oral: 2 mg, 4 mg [scored]

◆ **Pimtrea** *see* Ethinyl Estradiol and Desogestrel *on page 799*

◆ **Pin-X [OTC]** *see* Pyrantel Pamoate *on page 1744*

Pinaverium [CAN/INT] (pin ah VEER ee um)

Brand Names: Canada Dicetel

Index Terms Pinaverium Bromide

Pharmacologic Category Calcium Channel Antagonist, Gastrointestinal

Use Note: Not approved in U.S.

Treatment and relief of symptoms associated with irritable bowel syndrome (IBS); treatment of symptoms related to functional disorders of the biliary tract

Pregnancy Considerations Animal reproduction studies are insufficient and information from human pregnancies is not available. The presence of bromine in the formulation poses a theoretical risk of causing neurologic effects (sedation, hypotony) to newborns if pinaverium is used late in pregnancy, though no such cases have been reported.

Breast-Feeding Considerations Manufacturer advises against administration in breast-feeding women.

Contraindications Hypersensitivity to pinaverium or any component of the formulation

Warnings/Precautions May cause esophageal irritation; minimize risk by administering with a full glass of water with a meal/snack (do not crush/chew tablets). Avoid use in patients with possible gastroesophageal reflux or hiatal hernia. Should not be used to treat motility dysfunction associated with underlying disease states. Patients must be advised not to take medication when lying down or at bedtime. Contains lactose; avoid use in patients with hereditary problems of galactose intolerance, Lapp lactase deficiency, or glucose-galactose malabsorption.

Adverse Reactions Rare but important or life-threatening: Abdominal distension, anaphylactic shock, angioedema, constipation, diarrhea, drowsiness, dyspepsia, epigastric pain, headache, nausea, rash, vertigo, xerostomia

Drug Interactions

Metabolism/Transport Effects None known.

Avoid Concomitant Use There are no known interactions where it is recommended to avoid concomitant use.

Increased Effect/Toxicity There are no known significant interactions involving an increase in effect.

Decreased Effect There are no known significant interactions involving a decrease in effect.

Storage/Stability Store at 15°C to 30°C (59°F to 86°F). Protect from light.

Mechanism of Action Blocks influx of calcium via voltage-sensitive channels within smooth muscle cells of the gastrointestinal tract resulting in a spasmolytic effect in the gut.

Pharmacodynamics/Kinetics

Absorption: Poor

Protein binding: 97%

Metabolism: Hepatic via demethylation, hydroxylation

Bioavailability: <1%

Half-life elimination: ~1.5 hours

Time to peak: 1 hour

Excretion: Feces

Dosage Oral: Adults: Initial: 50 mg 3 times daily; dose may be increased up to 100 mg 3 times daily (maximum dose: 300 mg daily)

Dosage adjustment in renal impairment: No dosage adjustment provided in manufacturer's labeling. However, dosage adjustment unlikely due to very low systemic absorption.

Dosage adjustment in hepatic impairment: No dosage adjustment provided in manufacturer's labeling. However, dosage adjustment unlikely due to very low systemic absorption.

Dietary Considerations Should be taken with a full glass of water during a meal/snack.

Administration Do not crush or chew tablet. Should be taken with a glass of water during meals or snacks. The tablet should **not** be swallowed when in the lying position or just before bedtime.

Product Availability Not available in U.S.

Dosage Forms: Canada

Tablet, oral:

Dicetel®: 50 mg, 100 mg

◆ **Pinaverium Bromide** *see* Pinaverium [CAN/INT] *on page 1651*

Pinazepam [INT] (pin AZ e pam)

International Brand Names Domar (HK, IT, SG, TH); Duna (ES); Yunir (MX)

Pharmacologic Category Benzodiazepine

Reported Use Treatment of anxiety, insomnia, convulsions, and skeletal muscle spasms; aid with acute alcohol withdrawal; premedication prior to surgery

Dosage Range Adults: Oral:

Anxiety disorders: 5-20 mg/day

Insomnia: 2.5-5 mg at bedtime

Product Availability Product available in various countries; not currently available in the U.S.

Dosage Forms

Capsule: 5 mg

Pindolol (PIN doe lole)

Brand Names: Canada Apo-Pindol; Dom-Pindolol; PMS-Pindolol; Sandoz-Pindolol; Teva-Pindolol; Visken

Pharmacologic Category Antihypertensive; Beta-Blocker With Intrinsic Sympathomimetic Activity

Use

U.S. labeling: **Hypertension:** Treatment of hypertension, alone or in combination with other agents

The 2014 guideline for the management of high blood pressure in adults (Eighth Joint National Committee [JNC 8]) recommends initiation of pharmacologic treatment to lower blood pressure for the following patients:

- Patients ≥60 years of age with systolic blood pressure (SBP) ≥150 mm Hg or diastolic blood pressure (DBP) ≥90 mm Hg. Goal of therapy is SBP <150 mm Hg and DBP <90 mm Hg.
- Patients <60 years of age with SBP ≥140 mm Hg or DBP ≥90 mm Hg. Goal of therapy is SBP <140 mm Hg and DBP <90 mm Hg.
- Patients ≥18 years of age with diabetes and SBP ≥140 mm Hg or DBP ≥90 mm Hg. Goal of therapy is SBP <140 mm Hg and DBP <90 mm Hg.
- Patients ≥18 years of age with chronic kidney disease (CKD) and SBP ≥140 mm Hg or DBP ≥90 mm Hg. Goal of therapy is SBP <140 mm Hg and DBP <90 mm Hg.

In patients with CKD, regardless of race or diabetes status, the use of an ACE inhibitor (ACEI) or angiotensin receptor blocker (ARB) as initial therapy is recommended to improve kidney outcomes. In the general nonblack population (without CKD) including those with diabetes, initial antihypertensive treatment should consist of a thiazide-type diuretic, calcium channel blocker, ACEI, or ARB. In the general black population (without CKD) including those with diabetes, initial antihypertensive treatment should consist of a thiazide-type diuretic or a calcium channel blocker **instead of** an ACEI or ARB.

Canadian labeling:

Angina pectoris: Prophylaxis of angina pectoris

Hypertension: Treatment of hypertension, alone or in combination with other agents

Pregnancy Risk Factor B

Dosage

U.S. labeling: Hypertension: Adults: Oral: Initial: 5 mg twice daily; increase as necessary by 10 mg daily every 3 to 4 weeks (maximum daily dose: 60 mg).

Canadian labeling:

Angina pectoris: Adults: Oral: Initial: 5 mg 3 times daily; increase as necessary every 1 to 2 weeks. Usual maintenance dose: 15 to 40 mg daily in 3 or 4 divided doses (maximum daily dose: 40 mg)

Hypertension: Adults: Oral: Initial: 5 mg twice daily; increase as necessary by 10 mg daily every 1 to 2 weeks. Usual maintenance dose: 15 to 45 mg daily (maximum daily dose: 45 mg). If daily maintenance dose is ≤20 mg daily, may give as single dose in the morning; if >30 mg daily, administer in 3 divided doses.

Off-label use: Antidepressant augmentation: 2.5 mg 3 times daily (Geretsegger, 2008)

Elderly: Refer to adult dosing. Use with caution.

Dosage adjustment in renal impairment:

U.S. labeling: There are no dosage adjustments provided in the manufacturer's labeling. In uremic patients, use with caution due to significantly decreased clearance.

Canadian labeling: No dosage adjustment necessary in mild or moderate impairment; manufacturer suggests that a reduced dose may be necessary in severe impairment but does not provide specific dosing recommendations.

Dosage adjustment in hepatic impairment:

U.S. labeling: There are no dosage adjustments provided in the manufacturer's labeling. In cirrhotic patients, use with caution due to significantly prolonged elimination half-life (may be 10 times as long compared to normal patients).

Canadian labeling: No dosage adjustment necessary in mild or moderate impairment; manufacturer suggests that a reduced dose may be necessary in severe impairment but does not provide specific dosing recommendations.

Additional Information Complete prescribing information should be consulted for additional detail.

Dosage Forms

Tablet, Oral:

Generic: 5 mg, 10 mg

Dosage Forms: Canada

Tablet, Oral:

Generic: 5 mg, 10 mg, 15 mg

Pindolol and Hydrochlorothiazide [CAN/INT] (PIN doe lole & hye droe klor oh THYE a zide)

Brand Names: Canada Viskazide

Index Terms Hydrochlorothiazide and Pindolol

Pharmacologic Category Antihypertensive; Beta-Blocker With Intrinsic Sympathomimetic Activity; Diuretic, Thiazide

Use Note: Not approved in U.S.

Treatment of hypertension; not for initial therapy

Pregnancy Considerations Reproduction studies have not been conducted with this combination product. See individual agents.

Breast-Feeding Considerations Pindolol and thiazide diuretics are found in breast milk. Breast-feeding is not recommended by the manufacturer. See individual agents.

Contraindications Hypersensitivity to pindolol, hydrochlorothiazide, any other component of the formulation, or sulfonamide-derived drugs; decompensated heart failure, right ventricular failure secondary to pulmonary hypertension, significant cardiomegaly, sinus bradycardia, second/third degree atrioventricular (AV) block; cardiogenic shock; bronchospasm (including bronchial asthma) or severe chronic obstructive pulmonary disease (COPD); anesthetic agents producing myocardial depression; anuria

Warnings/Precautions See individual agents.

Adverse Reactions See individual agents.

Drug Interactions

Metabolism/Transport Effects Refer to individual components.

Avoid Concomitant Use

Avoid concomitant use of Pindolol and Hydrochlorothiazide with any of the following: Beta2-Agonists; Ceritinib; Dofetilide; Floctafenine; Methacholine

Increased Effect/Toxicity

Pindolol and Hydrochlorothiazide may increase the levels/effects of: ACE Inhibitors; Allopurinol; Alpha-/Beta-Agonists (Direct-Acting); Alpha1-Blockers; Alpha2-Agonists; Amifostine; Antihypertensives; Antipsychotic Agents (Phenothiazines); ARIPiprazole; Benazepril; Bradycardia-Causing Agents; Bupivacaine; Calcium Salts; CarBAMazepine; Cardiac Glycosides; Ceritinib; Cholinergic Agonists; Cyclophosphamide; Diazoxide; Disopyramide; Dofetilide; DULoxetine; Ergot Derivatives; Fingolimod; Grass Pollen Allergen Extract (5 Grass Extract); Hypotensive Agents; Insulin; Ivabradine; Lacosamide; Levodopa; Lidocaine (Systemic); Lidocaine (Topical); Lithium; Mepivacaine; Methacholine; Midodrine; Multivitamins/Minerals (with ADEK, Folate, Iron); Multivitamins/Minerals (with AE, No Iron); Obinutuzumab; OXcarbazepine; Porfimer; RisperiDONE; RiTUXimab; Sodium Phosphates; Sulfonylureas; Topiramate; Toremifene; Valsartan; Verteporfin; Vitamin D Analogs

The levels/effects of Pindolol and Hydrochlorothiazide may be increased by: Acetylcholinesterase Inhibitors; Alcohol (Ethyl); Alpha2-Agonists; Aminoquinolines (Antimalarial); Amiodarone; Analgesics (Opioid); Anilidopiperidine Opioids; Anticholinergic Agents; Antipsychotic Agents (Phenothiazines); Barbiturates; Bretylium; Brimonidine (Topical); BuPROPion; Calcium Channel Blockers (Dihydropyridine); Calcium Channel Blockers (Nondihydropyridine); Corticosteroids (Orally Inhaled); Corticosteroids (Systemic); Dexketoprofen; Diazoxide; Dipyridamole; Disopyramide; Dronedarone; Floctafenine; Herbs (Hypotensive Properties); Licorice; MAO Inhibitors; Multivitamins/Fluoride (with ADE); Nicorandil; Pentoxifylline; Phosphodiesterase 5 Inhibitors; Propafenone; Prostacyclin Analogues; Regorafenib; Reserpine; Selective Serotonin Reuptake Inhibitors; Tofacitinib; Valsartan

Decreased Effect

Pindolol and Hydrochlorothiazide may decrease the levels/effects of: Antidiabetic Agents; Beta2-Agonists; Theophylline Derivatives

The levels/effects of Pindolol and Hydrochlorothiazide may be decreased by: Barbiturates; Benazepril; Bile Acid Sequestrants; Herbs (Hypertensive Properties); Methylphenidate; Nonsteroidal Anti-Inflammatory Agents; Rifamycin Derivatives; Yohimbine

Food Interactions See individual agents.

Storage/Stability Store between 15°C to 30°C (59°F to 86°F).

Mechanism of Action

Pindolol: Blocks both $beta_1$- and $beta_2$-receptors and has mild intrinsic sympathomimetic activity; has negative inotropic and chronotropic effects and can significantly slow AV nodal conduction. Augmentive action of antidepressants thought to be mediated via a serotonin 1A autoreceptor antagonism.

Hydrochlorothiazide: Inhibits sodium reabsorption in the distal tubules causing increased excretion of sodium and water as well as potassium and hydrogen ions

Pharmacodynamics/Kinetics See individual agents.

Dosage Oral: Adults: Hypertension: Dosage should be determined by titration of the individual agents and the combination product substituted based upon the daily requirements

Usual dose: Pindolol 10-20 mg and hydrochlorothiazide 25-100 mg once daily. Maximum daily dose: Pindolol: 20 mg/hydrochlorothiazide: 100 mg

Note: When higher doses or dosage adjustments are needed, use individual agents.

Dosing adjustment in renal impairment:

Mild to moderate impairment: No dosage adjustment necessary. Use with caution.

Severe impairment: No dosage adjustment provided in manufacturer's labeling. However, dosage reduction may be necessary; use with caution. Contraindicated with anuria.

Dosing adjustment in hepatic impairment:

Mild to moderate impairment: No dosage adjustment necessary. Use with caution.

Severe impairment: No dosage adjustment provided in manufacturer's labeling. However, dosage reduction may be necessary; use with caution.

Dietary Considerations May be taken with food or milk.

Administration May be administered with food or milk. Take early in day to avoid nocturia.

Monitoring Parameters Blood pressure, heart rate; serum electrolytes, BUN, creatinine

Product Availability Not available in U.S.

Dosage Forms: Canada

Tablet, oral:

Viskazide® 10/25: Pindolol 10 mg and hydrochlorothiazide 25 mg

Viskazide® 10/50: Pindolol 10 mg and hydrochlorothiazide 50 mg

- ◆ **Pink Bismuth** *see* Bismuth *on page 265*
- ◆ **Pink Bismuth [OTC]** *see* Bismuth *on page 265*
- ◆ **Pinnacaine Otic** *see* Benzocaine *on page 246*

Pioglitazone (pye oh GLI ta zone)

Brand Names: U.S. Actos

Brand Names: Canada Accel-Pioglitazone; ACH-Pioglitazone; Actos; Apo-Pioglitazone; Auro-Pioglitazone; CO Pioglitazone; Dom-Pioglitazone; JAMP-Pioglitazone; Mint-Pioglitazone; Mylan-Pioglitazone; PHL-Pioglitazone; PMS-Pioglitazone; PRO-Pioglitazone; RAN-Pioglitazone; ratio-Pioglitazone; Sandoz-Pioglitazone; Teva-Pioglitazone

Pharmacologic Category Antidiabetic Agent, Thiazolidinedione

Use Type 2 diabetes mellitus (noninsulin dependent, NIDDM), monotherapy or combination therapy: Adjunct to diet and exercise, to improve glycemic control

Pregnancy Risk Factor C

Dosage Type 2 diabetes: Adults: Oral:

Initial:

U.S. labeling: Monotherapy or combination therapy: 15-30 mg once daily

Patients with heart failure (NYHA Class I or II): Monotherapy or combination therapy: 15 mg once daily

Note: Not recommended in patients with symptomatic heart failure

Canadian labeling: Monotherapy or combination therapy (with a sulfonylurea or metformin): 15-30 mg once daily

Dosage titration: If response is inadequate based on HbA_{1c}, the dosage may be increased in 15 mg increments with careful monitoring of adverse effects (eg, weight gain, edema, signs/symptoms of heart failure); maximum recommended dose: 45 mg once daily

Dosage adjustment for hypoglycemia with combination therapy:

With an insulin secretagogue (eg, sulfonylurea): Decrease the insulin secretagogue dose.

With insulin: Decrease insulin dose by 10% to 25%

Dosage adjustment with strong CYP2C8 inhibitors (eg, gemfibrozil): Maximum recommended dose: 15 mg once daily

Dosage adjustment in renal impairment: No dosage adjustment necessary.

Dosage adjustment in hepatic impairment: No dosage adjustment necessary (mean AUC values are unaffected in Child-Pugh grade B/C compared to healthy subjects); however, liver injury has been associated with use.

U.S. labeling:

Prior to initiation: Evaluate liver tests (ALT, AST, alkaline phosphatase, total bilirubin) and if abnormal, initiate with caution.

During therapy: If liver injury is suspected (eg, fatigue, jaundice, dark urine): Interrupt therapy, measure serum liver tests, and investigate possible etiologies:

If ALT >3 x ULN **and** without alternative etiologies: Do not reinitiate therapy.

If ALT >3 x ULN **and** total bilirubin >2 x ULN **and** without alternative etiologies: Do not reinitiate therapy (these patients are at increased risk for severe drug-induced hepatotoxicity).

If ALT elevated (but <3 x ULN) **or** total bilirubin elevated (but <2 x ULN) **and** with an alternative etiology: May reinitiate with caution.

Canadian labeling:

Severe hepatic impairment: Use is contraindicated.

Prior to initiation:

If ALT >2.5 x ULN or clinical evidence of active liver disease: Do not initiate therapy.

If ALT 1-2.5 x ULN: Initiate therapy with caution and investigate etiology of liver enzyme elevation.

During therapy:

If ALT levels >3 x ULN: Recheck levels immediately and if ALT elevation >3 x ULN persists, discontinue therapy.

If ALT 1-2.5 x ULN: Continue therapy with caution and investigate etiology of liver enzyme elevation.

Additional Information Complete prescribing information should be consulted for additional detail.

Dosage Forms

Tablet, Oral:

Actos: 15 mg, 30 mg, 45 mg

Generic: 15 mg, 30 mg, 45 mg

Pioglitazone and Glimepiride
(pye oh GLI ta zone & GLYE me pye ride)

Brand Names: U.S. Duetact™

Index Terms Glimepiride and Pioglitazone; Glimepiride and Pioglitazone Hydrochloride

Pharmacologic Category Antidiabetic Agent, Sulfonylurea; Antidiabetic Agent, Thiazolidinedione

Use Management of type 2 diabetes mellitus (noninsulin dependent, NIDDM) as an adjunct to diet and exercise in patients already treated with a thiazolidinedione and a sulfonylurea or who have inadequate control on either agent alone

Pregnancy Risk Factor C

Dosage Oral: Type 2 diabetes mellitus:

Adults: Initial dose should be based on current dose of pioglitazone and/or sulfonylurea.

Patients inadequately controlled on **glimepiride** alone: Initial dose: 30 mg/2 mg or 30 mg/4 mg once daily

Patients inadequately controlled on **pioglitazone** alone: Initial dose: 30 mg/2 mg once daily

Patients with systolic dysfunction (eg, NYHA Class I and II): Initiate only after patient has been safely titrated to 30 mg of pioglitazone. Initial dose: 30 mg/2 mg or 30 mg/4 mg once daily.

Note: No exact dosing relationship exists between glimepiride and other sulfonlyureas. Dosing should be limited to less than or equal to the maximum initial dose of glimepiride (2 mg). When converting patients from other sulfonylureas with longer half-lives (eg, chlorpropamide) to glimepiride, observe patient carefully for 1-2 weeks due to overlapping hypoglycemic effects.

Dosing adjustment: Dosage may be increased up to max dose and formulation strengths available; tablet should not be given more than once daily; see individual agents for frequency of adjustments. Dosage adjustments in patients with systolic dysfunction should be done carefully and patient monitored for symptoms of worsening heart failure.

Maximum dose: Pioglitazone 45 mg/glimepiride 8 mg daily

Elderly: Initial: Glimepiride 1 mg/day prior to initiating Duetact™; dose titration and maintenance dosing should be conservative to avoid hypoglycemia

Dosage adjustment in renal impairment: CrCl <22 mL/minute: Initial dose should be 1 mg of glimepiride and dosage increments should be based on fasting blood glucose levels

Dosage adjustment in hepatic impairment: Do not initiate treatment with active liver disease or ALT >2.5 times ULN. During treatment, if ALT levels elevate >3 times ULN, the test should be repeated as soon as possible. If ALT levels remain >3 times ULN or if the patient is jaundiced, Duetact™ should be discontinued.

Additional Information Complete prescribing information should be consulted for additional detail.

Dosage Forms

Tablet: 30/2: Pioglitazone 30 mg and glimepiride 2 mg; 30/4: Pioglitazone 30 mg and glimepiride 4 mg

Duetact™: 30 mg/2 mg: Pioglitazone 30 mg and glimepiride 2 mg; 30 mg/4 mg: Pioglitazone 30 mg and glimepiride 4 mg

Pioglitazone and Metformin

(pye oh GLI ta zone & met FOR min)

Brand Names: U.S. Actoplus Met; Actoplus Met XR

Index Terms Metformin Hydrochloride and Pioglitazone Hydrochloride

Pharmacologic Category Antidiabetic Agent, Biguanide; Antidiabetic Agent, Thiazolidinedione

Use Type 2 diabetes mellitus: As an adjunct to diet and exercise to improve glycemic control in adults with type 2 diabetes mellitus when treatment with both pioglitazone and metformin is appropriate.

Pregnancy Risk Factor C

Dosage Type 2 diabetes mellitus:

Adults: Oral:

Immediate-release tablet:

Initial: Pioglitazone 15 mg/metformin 500 mg twice daily **or** pioglitazone 15 mg/metformin 850 mg tablets once daily

Patients with heart failure (NYHA Class I or II): Initial: Pioglitazone 15 mg/metformin 500 mg once daily **or** pioglitazone 15 mg/metformin 850 mg once daily. **Note:** Not recommended in patients with symptomatic heart failure.

Inadequately controlled on metformin monotherapy: Pioglitazone 15 mg/metformin 500 mg twice daily or pioglitazone 15 mg/metformin 850 mg once or twice daily (depending on the dose of metformin already being taken).

Inadequately controlled on pioglitazone monotherapy: Pioglitazone 15 mg/metformin 500 twice daily or pioglitazone 15 mg/metformin 850 mg once daily.

Dose titration: If necessary, may titrate gradually with careful monitoring of adverse effects (eg, weight gain, edema, signs/symptoms of heart failure). Maximum daily dose: Pioglitazone 45 mg/metformin 2,550 mg. **Note:** Metformin daily doses >2,000 mg may be better tolerated if given 3 times daily.

Extended-release tablet: Initial (includes patients with NYHA Class I or II heart failure): Pioglitazone 15 to 30 mg/metformin 1,000 mg once daily. If necessary, titrate gradually with careful monitoring of adverse effects (eg, weight gain, edema, signs/symptoms of heart failure). Maximum daily dose: Pioglitazone 45 mg/metformin 2,000 mg.

Inadequately controlled on metformin or pioglitazone monotherapy: Pioglitazone 15 mg/metformin 1,000 mg twice daily or pioglitazone 30 mg/metformin 1,000 mg once daily.

Elderly: *Immediate-release or extended-release tablet:* The initial and maintenance dosing should be conservative, due to the potential for decreased renal function (monitor). Generally, elderly patients should not be titrated to the maximum; do not use in patients ≥80 years of age unless normal renal function has been established.

Dosage adjustment for hypoglycemia with combination therapy:

With an insulin secretagogue (eg, sulfonylurea): Decrease the insulin secretagogue dose.

With insulin: Decrease insulin dose by 10% to 25%.

Dosage adjustment with strong CYP2C8 inhibitors (eg, gemfibrozil): Maximum recommended dose: Pioglitazone 15 mg and metformin 850 mg daily (immediate release) or pioglitazone 15 mg and metformin 1,000 mg daily (extended release).

Dosage adjustment in renal impairment: *Immediate-release or extended-release tablet:* Contraindicated in patients with renal impairment (serum creatinine ≥1.5 mg/dL in males or ≥1.4 mg/dL in females or abnormal creatinine clearance).

Dosage adjustment in hepatic impairment: *Immediate-release or extended-release tablet:* Not recommended in hepatic impairment due to potential for lactic acidosis associated with metformin component.

Additional Information Complete prescribing information should be consulted for additional detail.

Dosage Forms

Tablet, oral: 15/500: Pioglitazone 15 mg and metformin hydrochloride 500 mg; 15/850: Pioglitazone 15 mg and metformin hydrochloride 850 mg

Actoplus Met: 15/500: Pioglitazone 15 mg and metformin 500 mg; 15/850: Pioglitazone 15 mg and metformin 850 mg

Tablet, variable release, oral:

Actoplus Met XR: 15/1000: Pioglitazone 15 mg and metformin 1000 mg; 30/1000: Pioglitazone 30 mg and metformin 1000 mg

Pipamperone [INT] (pi PAM pe rone)

International Brand Names Dipiperon (BE, CH, DE, DK, FR, GR, LU, NL); Pipamperon-neuraxpharm (DE); Piperonil (IT)

Index Terms Pipamperone Hydrochloride

Pharmacologic Category Antipsychotic Agent, Butyrophenone

Reported Use Treatment of chronic psychoses and states of aggressiveness of various origins

Dosage Range Adults: Oral: 40 mg 2-3 times/day; doses ≥360 mg/day have been given in divided doses

Product Availability Product available in various countries; not currently available in the U.S.

Dosage Forms

Solution, oral: 40 mg/mL (30 mL)

Tablet: 40 mg

◆ **Pipamperone Hydrochloride** *see* Pipamperone [INT] *on page 1655*

Pipemidic Acid [INT] (pi pe MI dik AS id)

International Brand Names Balurol (BR); Biosoviran (IT); Cistomid (IT); Deblaston (AT, DE, ZA); Diperpen (IT); Dolcol (JP); Elofuran (BR); Faremid (IT); Finuret (AR); Galusan (ES); Memento (AR); Mixato (CO); Nuril (ES); Palin (PL, RU); Pimidel (RU); Pipeacid (IT); Pipedac (IT); Pipefort (IT); Pipemid (IT, UY); Pipram (BR, FR, GR, IT, NL, UY); Pipurin (IT); Pipurol (BR); Pixelon (UY); Priper (AR, PY); Purid (CL); Septidron (ZA); Uribac (MX); Uriken (MX); Uripiser (MX); Urisan (ES); Urixin (MY); Uro Cefasabal (PE); Uroden (IT); Uronovag (MX); Uropimide (CL, IT, PY); Uropipedil (ES); Uropipemid (MX); Urosan (IT); Urosetic (IT); Urotractin (HK, ID, IT, MY, SG, TH); Uroxina (BR)

Index Terms Pipemidic Acid Trihydrate

Pharmacologic Category Antimicrobial Agent

Reported Use Treatment of acute, chronic, and recurrent urinary tract infections (cystitis, urethritis, prostatitis, pyleonephritis) by sensitive organisms such as *Pseudomonas aeruginosa*, *E. coli*, *Proteus*, *Klebsiella*, *Enterobacter*, and *Citrobacter*

Dosage Range Adults: Oral: Usual dose: 400 mg twice daily after meals; maximum duration of treatment: 10 days

Product Availability Product available in various countries; not currently available in the U.S.

Dosage Forms

Capsule: 200 mg

◆ **Pipemidic Acid Trihydrate** *see* Pipemidic Acid [INT] *on page 1655*

Piperacillin [CAN/INT] (pi PER a sil in)

Brand Names: Canada Piperacillin for Injection, USP

Index Terms Piperacillin Sodium

Pharmacologic Category Antibiotic, Penicillin

Use Note: Not approved in U.S.

Infection: Treatment of infection caused by susceptible gram-negative/gram-positive aerobic and anaerobic bacteria including intra-abdominal infections, septicemia, lower respiratory tract infections, skin and soft tissue infections, bone and joint infections, gynecological infections, urinary tract infections (complicated and uncomplicated), and urethritis (uncomplicated); may also be used to treat mixed infections due to susceptible streptococci

Pregnancy Considerations Adverse events have not been observed in animal reproduction studies. Piperacillin crosses the placenta and distributes into the amniotic fluid (Brown, 1990; Heikkilä, 1991). Due to pregnancy-induced physiologic changes, some pharmacokinetic parameters of piperacillin may be altered. At term, the apparent volume of distribution of piperacillin is increased and peak concentrations are significantly lower. Total clearance is normal to increased at term (Heikkilä, 1991; Voight, 1985). These changes continue into the early postpartum period (Charles, 1985; Martens, 1987).

Breast-Feeding Considerations Small amounts of piperacillin are excreted in breast milk. The manufacturer recommends that caution be exercised when administering piperacillin to nursing women. Nondose-related effects could include modification of bowel flora.

Contraindications Hypersensitivity to any of the penicillins and/or cephalosporins or any component of the formulation; hypersensitivity to local anesthetics of the amide type (when reconstituted with lidocaine for IM use)

Warnings/Precautions Serious and occasionally severe or fatal hypersensitivity (anaphylactoid) reactions have been reported in patients on penicillin therapy, especially with a history of beta-lactam hypersensitivity, history of sensitivity to multiple allergens, or previous IgE-mediated reactions (eg, anaphylaxis, angioedema, urticaria). Use with caution in asthmatic patients. Discontinue if hypersensitivity occurs; initiate appropriate rescue treatment for serious hypersensitivity reactions. Patients with infectious mononucleosis have developed rash during therapy with other penicillins (eg, ampicillin, amoxicillin).

Bleeding disorders have been observed, particularly in patients with renal impairment; discontinue if thrombocytopenia or bleeding occurs. Leukopenia and neutropenia have been reported (during prolonged therapy). Use caution with prolonged therapy in patients with cardiovascular disease and/or those who are sodium-restricted; formulation contains 42.5 mg of sodium per gram. Monitor electrolyte status and cardiac function with prolonged therapy. Due to sodium load and adverse effects (hematologic, neuropsychological changes), use with caution and modify dosage in patients with renal impairment.

Use caution in patients with history of seizure activity. An increased frequency of fever and rash has been reported in patients with cystic fibrosis. Prolonged use may result in fungal or bacterial superinfection, including *C. difficile*-associated diarrhea (CDAD) and pseudomembranous colitis; CDAD has been observed >2 months postantibiotic treatment. Symptoms of syphilis may be masked or delayed in patients receiving high-dose antimicrobial treatment of gonorrhea; patients with gonorrhea should be evaluated for syphilis prior to initiating antimicrobial treatment and if suspected continue serologic testing monthly for at least 4 months.

Adverse Reactions

Central nervous system: Confusion, convulsions, drowsiness, fever, Jarisch-Herxheimer reaction

Dermatologic: Rash, toxic epidermal necrolysis, urticaria

Endocrine & metabolic: Electrolyte imbalance, hypokalemia

Hematologic: Abnormal platelet aggregation and prolonged PT (high doses), agranulocytosis, Coombs' reaction (positive), hemolytic anemia, pancytopenia

Local: Thrombophlebitis

Neuromuscular & skeletal: Myoclonus

Renal: Acute interstitial nephritis, acute renal failure

Miscellaneous: Anaphylaxis, hypersensitivity reactions

Drug Interactions

Metabolism/Transport Effects None known.

Avoid Concomitant Use

Avoid concomitant use of Piperacillin with any of the following: BCG; Probenecid

Increased Effect/Toxicity

Piperacillin may increase the levels/effects of: Flucloxacillin; Methotrexate; Vancomycin; Vecuronium; Vitamin K Antagonists

The levels/effects of Piperacillin may be increased by: Probenecid

Decreased Effect

Piperacillin may decrease the levels/effects of: Aminoglycosides; BCG; Mycophenolate; Sodium Picosulfate; Typhoid Vaccine

The levels/effects of Piperacillin may be decreased by: Tetracycline Derivatives

Storage/Stability Prior to reconstitution store vials at 15°C to 30°C (59°F to 86°F). Protect from light. Reconstituted solution is stable up to 24 hours at room temperature and up to 72 hours when refrigerated. Upon further dilution, the manufacturer labeling recommends storing solution up to 24 hours at room temperature or up to 72 hours when refrigerated.

Mechanism of Action Inhibits bacterial cell wall synthesis by binding to one or more of the penicillin-binding proteins (PBPs); which in turn inhibit the final transpeptidation step of peptidoglycan synthesis in bacterial cell walls, thus inhibiting cell wall biosynthesis. Bacteria eventually lyse due to ongoing activity of cell wall autolytic enzymes (autolysins and murein hydrolases) while cell wall assembly is arrested.

Pharmacodynamics/Kinetics

Absorption: IM: Rapid

Protein binding: ~16%

Half-life elimination (dose dependent; prolonged with renal impairment): Adults: ~1 hour (decreased in patients with cystic fibrosis)

Time to peak, serum: IM: 30 minutes

Excretion: Primarily urine; partially feces

Dosage Children ≥12 years, Adolescents, and Adults: **Note:** Average duration of treatment ranges from 7-10 days (3-10 days for gynecologic infection) depending on severity of infection and clinical response. Treatment of acute infection should extend 48-72 hours beyond resolution of symptoms. Treat Group A beta-hemolytic streptococcal infections for at least 10 days to reduce the risk of rheumatic fever or glomerulonephritis. Significantly longer periods of treatment may be necessary for some severe infections (eg, osteomyelitis).

Community-acquired pneumonia: IM, IV: Usual dosage: 6-8 g daily (100-125 mg/kg daily) in divided doses every 6-12 hours

Severe infections (eg, gynecologic, intra-abdominal, nosocomial pneumonia, septicemia, skin/soft tissue): IV: Usual dosage: 12-18 g daily (200-300 mg/kg daily) in divided doses every 4-6 hours (maximum: 24 g daily)

Urethritis (gonococcal, uncomplicated): IM: 2 g once (**Note:** Administer probenecid 30 minutes prior to piperacillin)

Urinary tract infection (complicated): IV: Usual dosage: 8-16 g daily (125-200 mg/kg daily) in divided doses every 6-8 hours

Urinary tract infection (uncomplicated): IM, IV: Usual dosage: 6-8 g daily (100-125 mg/kg daily) in divided doses every 6-12 hours

Dosage adjustment in renal impairment: Adults: IV:

CrCl >40 mL/minute or serum creatinine 1.5-3 mg/dL: No dosage adjustment necessary.

CrCl 20-40 mL/minute or serum creatinine 3.1-5 mg/dL:

Urinary tract infection (uncomplicated): No dosage adjustment necessary.

Urinary tract infection (complicated): 3 g every 8 hours

Severe systemic infection: 4 g every 8 hours

CrCl <20 mL/minute or serum creatinine >5 mg/dL:

Urinary tract infection (complicated/uncomplicated): 3 g every 12 hours

Severe systemic infection: 4 g every 12 hours

Hemodialysis: Severe systemic infection: 2 g every 8 hours; administer 1 g supplemental dose after each dialysis session; Dialyzable (30% to 50%)

Dosage adjustment in hepatic impairment: No dosage adjustment provided in manufacturer's labeling.

Dietary Considerations Sodium content of 1 g: 1.85 mEq (42.5 mg)

Administration Administer around-the-clock to promote less variation in peak and trough serum levels. Give at least 1 hour apart from aminoglycosides. Rapid administration can lead to seizures. Administer by IV injection over 3-5 minutes or by intermittent infusion over 20-30 minutes. IM injection should be administered into the upper outer quadrant of the buttocks. Do not administer more than 2 g per IM injection site.

Monitoring Parameters Observe for signs and symptoms of anaphylaxis during first dose; with extended therapy consider monitoring of electrolytes and cardiac status (patients with impaired cardiac function), serum creatinine, BUN, hepatic function, and CBC.

Product Availability Not available in the U.S.

Piperacillin and Tazobactam

(pi PER a sil in & ta zoe BAK tam)

Brand Names: U.S. Zosyn

Brand Names: Canada AJ-PIP/TAZ; Piperacillin and Tazobactam for Injection; Tazocin

Index Terms Piperacillin and Tazobactam Sodium; Piperacillin Sodium and Tazobactam Sodium; Tazobactam and Piperacillin

Pharmacologic Category Antibiotic, Penicillin

Use

Moderate to severe bacterial infections: For the treatment of patients with moderate to severe infections caused by susceptible isolates of the designated bacteria in the following conditions.

Community-acquired pneumonia: Treatment of moderate severity community-acquired pneumonia (CAP) caused by beta-lactamase-producing strains of *Haemophilus influenzae*. IDSA/ATS guidelines only recommend piperacillin/tazobactam for CAP caused by *P. aeruginosa* or due to aspiration (Mandell, 2007).

Intra-abdominal infections: Treatment of appendicitis complicated by rupture or abscess and peritonitis caused by beta-lactamase-producing strains of *Escherichia coli*, *Bacteroides fragilis*, *Bacteroides ovatus*, *Bacteroides thetaiotaomicron*, or *Bacteroides vulgatus*.

Nosocomial pneumonia: Treatment of moderate to severe nosocomial pneumonia caused by beta-lactamase-producing strains of *Staphylococcus aureus* and by piperacillin/tazobactam-susceptible *Acinetobacter baumanii*, *H. influenzae*, *Klebsiella pneumoniae*, and *Pseudomonas aeruginosa* (nosocomial pneumonia caused by *P. aeruginosa* should be treated in combination with an aminoglycoside).

Pelvic infections: Treatment of postpartum endometriosis or pelvic inflammatory disease caused by beta-lactamase-producing strains of *E. coli*.

Skin and skin structure infections: Treatment of skin and skin structure infections, including cellulitis, cutaneous abscesses, and ischemic/diabetic foot infections caused by beta-lactamase-producing strains of *S. aureus*.

Pregnancy Risk Factor B

Pregnancy Considerations Adverse events have not been observed in animal reproduction studies. Piperacillin and tazobactam both cross the placenta and are found in the fetal serum, placenta, amniotic fluid, and fetal urine. When used during pregnancy, the clearance and volume of distribution of piperacillin/tazobactam are increased; half-life and AUC are decreased (Bourget, 1998). Piperacillin/tazobactam is approved for the treatment of postpartum gynecologic infections, including endometritis or pelvic inflammatory disease, caused by susceptible organisms.

Breast-Feeding Considerations Low concentrations of piperacillin are excreted in breast milk; information for tazobactam is not available. The manufacturer recommends that caution be used when administering piperacillin/tazobactam to nursing women. Nondose-related effects could include modification of bowel flora.

Contraindications Hypersensitivity to penicillins, cephalosporins, beta-lactamase inhibitors, or any component of the formulation

Warnings/Precautions Serious and occasionally severe or fatal hypersensitivity (anaphylactic/anaphylactoid) reactions have been reported in patients on penicillin therapy, especially with a history of beta-lactam hypersensitivity, history of sensitivity to multiple allergens, or previous IgE-mediated reactions (eg, anaphylaxis, angioedema, urticaria). Serious skin reactions, including toxic epidermal necrolysis (TEN) and Stevens-Johnson syndrome (SJS), have been reported. If a skin rash develops, monitor closely. Discontinue if lesions progress.

Bleeding disorders have been observed, particularly in patients with renal impairment; discontinue if thrombocytopenia or bleeding occurs. Leukopenia/neutropenia may occur; appears to be reversible and most frequently associated with prolonged administration. Assess hematologic parameters periodically, especially with prolonged (≥21 days) use.

Assess electrolytes periodically in patients with low potassium reserves, especially those receiving cytotoxic therapy or diuretics. Due to sodium load and to the adverse effects of high serum concentrations of penicillins, dosage modification is required in patients with impaired or underdeveloped renal function; use with caution in patients with seizures or in patients with history of beta-lactam allergy; associated with an increased incidence of rash and fever in cystic fibrosis patients. Use may result in fungal or bacterial superinfection, including *C. difficile*-associated diarrhea (CDAD) and pseudomembranous colitis; CDAD has been observed >2 months postantibiotic treatment.

Potentially significant drug-drug interactions may exist, requiring dose or frequency adjustment, additional monitoring, and/or selection of alternative therapy.

Adverse Reactions

Cardiovascular: Chest pain, edema, hypertension, phlebitis

Central nervous system: Agitation, anxiety, dizziness, headache, insomnia, pain

Dermatologic: Pruritus, skin rash

Gastrointestinal: Abdominal pain, change in stool, constipation, diarrhea, dyspepsia, nausea, oral candidiasis, vomiting

Hepatic: Increased serum AST

Local: Local irritation

Infection: Abscess, candidiasis, infection, sepsis

Respiratory: Dyspnea, pharyngitis, rhinitis

Miscellaneous: Fever

Rare but important or life-threatening: Agranulocytosis, anaphylactoid reaction, anaphylaxis, anemia, aphthous stomatitis, atrial fibrillation, bradycardia, cardiac arrest, cardiac arrhythmia, cardiac failure, change in platelet count, cholestatic jaundice, circulatory arrest, *Clostridium difficile* associated diarrhea, confusion, convulsions, decreased hematocrit, decreased hemoglobin, decreased serum albumin, depression, dysgeusia, dysuria, electrolyte disturbance, eosinophilia, epistaxis, erythema multiforme, gastritis, genital pruritus, hallucination, hematuria, hemolytic anemia, hemorrhage, hepatitis, hiccups, hyperglycemia, hypersensitivity reaction, hypoglycemia, increased blood glucose, increased blood urea nitrogen, increased gamma-glutamyl transferase, increased serum alkaline phosphatase, increased serum ALT, increased serum AST, increased serum bilirubin, increased serum creatinine, increased thirst, inflammation, interstitial nephritis, intestinal obstruction, leukopenia, leukorrhea, melena, mesenteric embolism, myalgia, myocardial infarction, neutropenia, oliguria, pancytopenia, photophobia, positive direct Coombs test, prolonged partial thromboplastin time, prolonged prothrombin time, pulmonary edema, pulmonary embolism, purpura, renal failure, rigors, Stevens-Johnson syndrome, supraventricular tachycardia, syncope, thrombocythemia, thrombocytopenia, thrombophlebitis, toxic epidermal necrolysis, urinary incontinence, urinary retention, vaginitis, ventricular fibrillation, ventricular tachycardia

Drug Interactions

Metabolism/Transport Effects None known.

Avoid Concomitant Use

Avoid concomitant use of Piperacillin and Tazobactam with any of the following: BCG; Probenecid

Increased Effect/Toxicity

Piperacillin and Tazobactam may increase the levels/effects of: Flucloxacillin; Methotrexate; Vancomycin; Vecuronium; Vitamin K Antagonists

The levels/effects of Piperacillin and Tazobactam may be increased by: Probenecid

Decreased Effect

Piperacillin and Tazobactam may decrease the levels/effects of: Aminoglycosides; BCG; Mycophenolate; Sodium Picosulfate; Typhoid Vaccine

The levels/effects of Piperacillin and Tazobactam may be decreased by: Tetracycline Derivatives

Preparation for Administration Reconstitute single-dose vials with 5 mL of diluent per 1 g of piperacillin and then further dilute to a volume of 50-150 mL. Reconstitute pharmacy bulk vials with 152 mL of diluent to yield a concentration of piperacillin 200 mg/mL and tazobactam 25 mg/mL; transfer reconstituted solution and further dilute to a volume of 50-150 mL for administration.

Storage/Stability

Vials: Store at 20°C to 25°C (68°F to 77°F) prior to reconstitution. Use single-dose or bulk vials immediately after reconstitution. Discard any unused portion after 24 hours if stored at 20°C to 25°C (68°F to 77°F) or after 48 hours if stored refrigerated (2°C to 8°C [36°F to 46°F]). Do not freeze vials after reconstitution. Stability in IV bags has been demonstrated for up to 24 hours at room temperature and up to 1 week at refrigerated temperature. Stability in an ambulatory IV infusion pump has been demonstrated for a period of 12 hours at room temperature.

Galaxy containers: Store at or below -20°C (-4°F). The thawed solution is stable for 14 days under refrigeration (2°C to 8°C [36°F to 46°F]) or 24 hours at 20°C to 25°C (68°F to 77°F). Do not refreeze.

Mechanism of Action Piperacillin inhibits bacterial cell wall synthesis by binding to one or more of the penicillin-binding proteins (PBPs); which in turn inhibits the final transpeptidation step of peptidoglycan synthesis in bacterial cell walls, thus inhibiting cell wall biosynthesis. Bacteria eventually lyse due to ongoing activity of cell wall autolytic enzymes (autolysins and murein hydrolases) while cell wall assembly is arrested. Piperacillin exhibits time-dependent killing. Tazobactam inhibits many beta-lactamases, including staphylococcal penicillinase and Richmond-Sykes types 2, 3, 4, and 5, including extended spectrum enzymes; it has only limited activity against class 1 beta-lactamases other than class 1C types.

Pharmacodynamics/Kinetics

Distribution: Well into lungs, intestinal mucosa, uterus, ovary, fallopian tube, interstitial fluid, gallbladder, and bile; penetration into CSF is low in subjects with noninflamed meninges

Protein binding: Piperacillin and tazobactam: ~30%

Metabolism:

Piperacillin: Desethyl metabolite (weak activity)

Tazobactam: Inactive metabolite

Half-life elimination: Piperacillin and tazobactam: 0.7-1.2 hours (unaffected by dose or duration of infusion)

Time to peak, plasma: Immediately following completion of 30-minute infusion

Excretion: Clearance of both piperacillin and tazobactam are directly proportional to renal function

Piperacillin: Urine (68% as unchanged drug); feces (10% to 20%)

Tazobactam: Urine (80% as unchanged drug; remainder as inactive metabolite)

Dialysis: Hemodialysis removes 30% to 40% of a piperacillin/tazobactam dose; peritoneal dialysis removes 6% of piperacillin and 21% of tazobactam

Dosage Note: Dosing presented is based on traditional infusion method (IV infusion over 30 minutes) unless otherwise specified as the extended infusion method (IV infusion over 4 hours [off-label method]).

Usual dosage range: IV:

Infants 2-8 months: 80 mg of piperacillin component/kg every 8 hours

Infants and Children ≥9 months and ≤40 kg: 100 mg of piperacillin component/kg every 8 hours

Children and Adolescents >40 kg: Refer to adult dosing.

Adults: IV: 3.375 g every 6 hours **or** 4.5 g every 6 hours; maximum: 18 g daily

Extended infusion method (off-label dosing): 3.375-4.5 g IV over 4 hours every 8 hours (Kim, 2007; Shea, 2009); an alternative regimen of 4.5 g IV over 3 hours every 6 hours has also been described (Kim, 2007).

Indication-specific dosing: IV:

Children:

Appendicitis, peritonitis:

Infants 2-8 months: 80 mg/kg of piperacillin component every 8 hours

Infants and Children ≥9 months and ≤40 kg: 100 mg/kg of piperacillin component every 8 hours

Children and Adolescents >40 kg: Refer to adult dosing.

Cystic fibrosis, pseudomonal infections (off-label use): IV: 240-400 mg/kg/day of piperacillin component divided every 8 hours; in some cases, higher doses may be necessary: 450-600 mg/kg/day divided every 4-6 hours (Zobell, 2013)

Intra-abdominal infection, complicated (off-label use): 200-300 mg/kg/day of piperacillin component divided every 6-8 hours (Solomkin, 2010).

Surgical (perioperative) prophylaxis (off-label use): Note: Doses may be repeated in 2 hours if procedure is lengthy or if there is excessive blood loss (Bratzler, 2013):

Infants 2-9 months: 80 mg/kg of piperacillin component within 60 minutes prior to surgical incision (maximum: 3 g piperacillin component).

Infants and Children >9 months and ≤40 kg: 100 mg/kg of piperacillin component within 60 minutes prior to surgical incision (maximum: 3 g piperacillin component).

Children and Adolescents >40 kg: Refer to adult dosing.

Adults:

Diverticulitis, intra-abdominal abscess, peritonitis: IV: 3.375 g every 6 hours for 7-10 days.

Pneumonia:

Community-acquired pneumonia (CAP): IV: 3.375 g every 6 hours for 7-10 days. **Note:** IDSA/ATS guidelines only recommend piperacillin/tazobactam for CAP caused by *P. aeruginosa* or due to aspiration (Mandell, 2007).

Nosocomial pneumonia: IV: 4.5 g every 6 hours for 7-14 days (when used empirically, combination with an aminoglycoside or antipseudomonal fluoroquinolone is recommended; consider discontinuation of additional agent if *P. aeruginosa* is not isolated) (ATS, 2005).

Skin and soft tissue infection: IV: 3.375 g every 6-8 hours for 7-14 days. **Notes:** When used for necrotizing infection of skin, fascia, or muscle, combination with clindamycin and ciprofloxacin is recommended (Stevens, 2005); for severe diabetic foot infections, recommended treatment duration is up to 4 weeks depending on severity of infection and response to therapy (Lipsky, 2012).

Surgical (perioperative) prophylaxis (off-label use): IV: 3.375 g within 60 minutes prior to surgical incision. Doses may be repeated in 2 hours if procedure is lengthy or if there is excessive blood loss (Bratzler, 2013).

Intra-abdominal infection, complicated (off-label use): IV: 3.375 g every 6 hours for 4-7 days (provided source controlled). **Note:** Increase to 3.375 g every 4 hours or 4.5 g every 6 hours if *P. aeruginosa* is suspected. Not recommended for mild-to-moderate, community-acquired intra-abdominal infections due to risk of toxicity and the development of resistant organisms (Solomkin, 2010).

Dosing interval in renal impairment:

Traditional infusion method (ie, IV infusion over 30 minutes): Manufacturer's labeling:

CrCl >40 mL/minute: No dosage adjustment required

CrCl 20-40 mL/minute: Administer 2.25 g every 6 hours (3.375 g every 6 hours for nosocomial pneumonia)

CrCl <20 mL/minute: Administer 2.25 g every 8 hours (2.25 g every 6 hours for nosocomial pneumonia)

Note: Some clinicians suggest adjusting the dose at CrCl ≤20 mL/minute (rather than CrCl <40 mL/minute) in patients receiving either traditional or extended-infusion methods, particularly if treating serious gram-negative infections (empirically or definitively) (Patel, 2010).

Extended infusion method (off-label dosing): CrCl ≤20 mL/minute: 3.375 g IV over 4 hours every 12 hours (Patel, 2010)

Intermittent hemodialysis (IHD)/peritoneal dialysis (PD): 2.25 g every 12 hours (2.25 g every 8 hours for nosocomial pneumonia). **Note:** Dosing dependent on the assumption of 3 times/week, complete IHD sessions. Administer scheduled doses after hemodialysis on dialysis days; if next regularly scheduled dose is not due right after dialysis session, administer an additional dose of 0.75 g after the dialysis session.

Continuous renal replacement therapy (CRRT) (Heintz, 2009; Trotman, 2005): Drug clearance is highly dependent on the method of renal replacement, filter type, and flow rate. Appropriate dosing requires close monitoring of pharmacologic response, signs of adverse reactions due to drug accumulation, as well as drug concentrations in relation to target trough (if appropriate). The following are general recommendations only (based on dialysate flow/ultrafiltration rates of 1-2 L/hour and minimal residual renal function) and should not supersede clinical judgment (Trotman, 2005):

CVVH: 2.25-3.375 g every 6-8 hours

CVVHD: 2.25-3.375 g every 6 hours

CVVHDF: 3.375 g every 6 hours

Note: Higher dose of 3.375 g should be considered when treating resistant pathogens (especially *Pseudomonas* spp); alternative recommendations suggest dosing of 4.5 g every 8 hours (Valtonen, 2001); regardless of regimen, there is some concern of tazobactam (TAZ) accumulation, given its lower clearance relative to piperacillin (PIP). Some clinicians advocate dosing with PIP to alternate with PIP/TAZ, particularly in CVVH-dependent patients, to lessen this concern.

Dosage adjustment in hepatic impairment: No dosage adjustment necessary.

Dietary Considerations Some products may contain sodium.

Administration Administer by IV infusion over 30 minutes. For extended infusion administration (off-label dosing), administer over 3-4 hours (Kim 2007; Shea, 2009).

Some penicillins (eg, carbenicillin, ticarcillin, and piperacillin) have been shown to inactivate aminoglycosides *in vitro*. This has been observed to a greater extent with tobramycin and gentamicin, while amikacin has shown greater stability against inactivation. Concurrent use of these agents may pose a risk of reduced antibacterial efficacy *in vivo*, particularly in the setting of profound renal impairment. However, definitive clinical evidence is lacking. If combination penicillin/aminoglycoside therapy is desired in a patient with renal dysfunction, separation of doses (if feasible), and routine monitoring of aminoglycoside levels, CBC, and clinical response should be considered. **Note:** Reformulated Zosyn® containing EDTA has been shown to be compatible *in vitro* for Y-site infusion with amikacin and gentamicin diluted in NS or D_5W (applies **only** to specific concentrations and varies by product; consult manufacturer's labeling). Reformulated Zosyn® containing EDTA is **not** compatible with tobramycin.

Monitoring Parameters Creatinine, BUN, CBC with differential, PT, PTT, serum electrolytes, LFTs, urinalysis; signs of bleeding; monitor for signs of anaphylaxis during first dose

Dosage Forms 8:1 ratio of piperacillin sodium/tazobactam sodium

Infusion [premixed iso-osmotic solution, frozen]:

Zosyn®:

2.25 g: Piperacillin 2 g and tazobactam 0.25 g (50 mL)

3.375 g: Piperacillin 3 g and tazobactam 0.375 g (50 mL)

4.5 g: Piperacillin 4 g and tazobactam 0.5 g (100 mL)

Injection, powder for reconstitution: 2.25 g: Piperacillin 2 g and tazobactam 0.25 g; 3.375 g: Piperacillin 3 g and tazobactam 0.375 g; 4.5 g: Piperacillin 4 g and tazobactam 0.5 g; 40.5 g: Piperacillin 36 g and tazobactam 4.5 g

Zosyn®:

2.25 g: Piperacillin 2 g and tazobactam 0.25 g

3.375 g: Piperacillin 3 g and tazobactam 0.375 g

4.5 g: Piperacillin 4 g and tazobactam 0.5 g

40.5 g: Piperacillin 36 g and tazobactam 4.5 g

- ◆ **Piperacillin and Tazobactam for Injection (Can)** *see* Piperacillin and Tazobactam *on page 1657*
- ◆ **Piperacillin and Tazobactam Sodium** *see* Piperacillin and Tazobactam *on page 1657*
- ◆ **Piperacillin for Injection, USP (Can)** *see* Piperacillin [CAN/INT] *on page 1656*
- ◆ **Piperacillin Sodium** *see* Piperacillin [CAN/INT] *on page 1656*
- ◆ **Piperacillin Sodium and Tazobactam Sodium** *see* Piperacillin and Tazobactam *on page 1657*
- ◆ **Piperazine Estrone Sulfate** *see* Estropipate *on page 793*
- ◆ **Piperonyl Butoxide and Pyrethrins** *see* Pyrethrins and Piperonyl Butoxide *on page 1746*
- ◆ **Piportil L_4 (Can)** *see* Pipotiazine [CAN/INT] *on page 1660*
- ◆ **Pipothiazine** *see* Pipotiazine [CAN/INT] *on page 1660*

Pipotiazine [CAN/INT] (pip oh TYE a zeen)

Brand Names: Canada Piportil L_4

Index Terms Pipothiazine; Pipotiazine Palmitate

Pharmacologic Category First Generation (Typical) Antipsychotic

Use Note: Not approved in U.S.

Maintenance treatment of schizophrenia

Pregnancy Considerations Antipsychotic use during the third trimester of pregnancy has a risk for abnormal muscle movements (extrapyramidal symptoms [EPS]) and withdrawal symptoms in newborns following delivery. Symptoms in the newborn may include agitation, feeding disorder, hypertonia, hypotonia, respiratory distress, somnolence, and tremor; these effects may be self-limiting or require hospitalization.

Contraindications Hypersensitivity to pipotiazine, phenothiazine derivatives, or any component of the formulation (cross-reactivity between phenothiazines may occur); severe CNS depression; suspected or established subcortical brain damage; psychoneurotic patients or geriatric patients with confusion and/or agitation; hepatic or renal dysfunction; circulatory collapse; severe cardiovascular disorder; severely depressed patients; high doses of hypnotics; blood dyscrasias; altered states of consciousness or coma (particularly when due to intoxication with CNS depressant drugs [eg, hypnotics, opioids, ethanol]); pheochromocytoma; use in children

Warnings/Precautions Antipsychotics increase the risk of death in elderly patients with dementia-related psychosis. Most deaths appeared to be either cardiovascular (eg, heart failure, sudden death) or infectious (eg, pneumonia) in nature. Pipotiazine is not approved for the treatment of dementia or dementia-related psychosis in elderly patients. Use is contraindicated in patients with blood dyscrasias; monitor blood counts periodically and discontinue at first signs of blood dyscrasias.

May be sedating, use with caution in disorders where CNS depression is a feature (risk may be lower than with other phenothiazines). Use with caution in Parkinson's disease; hemodynamic instability; bone marrow suppression; predisposition to seizures; respiratory disease; patients with or at risk of diabetes, or at risk of thromboembolism or stroke. Esophageal dysmotility and aspiration have been associated with antipsychotic use; use with caution in patients at risk of pneumonia (eg, Alzheimer's disease). Caution in breast cancer or other prolactin-dependent tumors (may elevate prolactin levels). May alter temperature regulation or mask toxicity of other drugs due to antiemetic effects.

Use with caution in patients with cardiovascular disease. May alter cardiac conduction and prolong QT interval. Use with caution or avoid use in patients with electrolyte abnormalities (eg, hypokalemia, hypomagnesemia), hypothyroidism, familial long QT syndrome, concomitant medications which may augment QT prolongation, or any underlying cardiac abnormality which may also potentiate risk. May cause orthostatic hypotension (risk may be low relative to other phenothiazines); use with caution in patients at risk of this effect or those who would not tolerate transient hypotensive episodes (cerebrovascular disease, cardiovascular disease, or other medications which may predispose).

Phenothiazines may cause anticholinergic effects (confusion, agitation, constipation, xerostomia, blurred vision, urinary retention); therefore, they should be used with caution in patients with decreased gastrointestinal motility, urinary retention, BPH, xerostomia, visual problems, or narrow-angle glaucoma (screening is recommended).

May cause extrapyramidal symptoms, including pseudoparkinsonism, acute dystonic reactions, akathisia, and tardive dyskinesia. May be associated with neuroleptic malignant syndrome (NMS). Prolonged therapy may cause pigmentary retinopathy, corneal deposits, and/or changes in skin pigmentation. Adverse effects of depot injections may be prolonged. Use with caution in the elderly. Avoid use in patients with known allergy to sesame oil or similar compounds.

Adverse Reactions

Cardiovascular: Cardiac arrest, ECG changes, edema, hypotension, QTc prolongation, syncope, tachycardia, venous thromboembolism

Central nervous system: Agitation, anxiety, bizarre dreams, cerebral edema, depression, dizziness, drowsiness, EEG changes, excitement, extrapyramidal symptoms (akathisia, dyskinesia, dystonia, hyper-reflexia, oculogyric crisis, opisthotonos, pseudoparkinsonism, rigidity, sialorrhea, tremor), fatigue, fever, headache, insomnia, paradoxical psychosis, restlessness, seizure, sleep disturbance, tardive dyskinesia

Dermatologic: Angioedema, eczema, epithelial keratopathy erythema, exfoliative dermatitis, dermatitis, photosensitivity, pruritus, rash, seborrhea, skin pigmentation (prolonged therapy), urticaria

Endocrine & metabolic: Galactorrhea, glucose intolerance, gynecomastia, hyperglycemia, libido (changes in), menstrual irregularities, thirst

Gastrointestinal: Adynamic ileus, anorexia, appetite increased, constipation, fecal impaction, nausea, salivation, vomiting, weight changes, xerostomia

Genitourinary: Bladder paralysis, impotence, incontinence, polyuria, priapism, urinary retention

Hematologic: Agranulocytosis, anemia, eosinophilia, leukopenia, pancytopenia, thrombocytopenia

Hepatic: Biliary stasis, cholestatic jaundice

Ocular: Blurred vision, corneal deposits (prolonged therapy), glaucoma, lenticular deposits, pigmentary retinopathy (prolonged therapy)

Respiratory: Nasal congestion, pneumonia, pneumonitis, pulmonary embolism

Miscellaneous: Diaphoresis increased, lupus-like syndrome

Drug Interactions

Metabolism/Transport Effects Substrate of CYP2D6 (major), CYP3A4 (major); **Note:** Assignment of Major/Minor substrate status based on clinically relevant drug interaction potential

Avoid Concomitant Use

Avoid concomitant use of Pipotiazine with any of the following: Azelastine (Nasal); Conivaptan; Fusidic Acid (Systemic); Idelalisib; Orphenadrine; Paraldehyde; Thalidomide

Increased Effect/Toxicity

Pipotiazine may increase the levels/effects of: Alcohol (Ethyl); Analgesics (Opioid); Antidepressants (Serotonin Reuptake Inhibitor/Antagonist); Azelastine (Nasal); Beta-Blockers; Buprenorphine; CNS Depressants; Hydrocodone; Methotrimeprazine; Metyrosine; Mirtazapine; Orphenadrine; Paraldehyde; Porfimer; Pramipexole; ROPINIRole; Rotigotine; Selective Serotonin Reuptake Inhibitors; Suvorexant; Thalidomide; Thiopental; Verteporfin; Zolpidem

The levels/effects of Pipotiazine may be increased by: Abiraterone Acetate; Antidepressants (Serotonin Reuptake Inhibitor/Antagonist); Antimalarial Agents; Aprepitant; Beta-Blockers; Brimonidine (Topical); Cannabis; Ceritinib; Conivaptan; CYP2D6 Inhibitors (Moderate); CYP2D6 Inhibitors (Strong); CYP3A4 Inhibitors (Moderate); CYP3A4 Inhibitors (Strong); Dasatinib; Doxylamine; Dronabinol; Droperidol; Fosaprepitant; Fusidic Acid (Systemic); HydrOXYzine; Idelalisib; Ivacaftor; Kava Kava; Luliconazole; Magnesium Sulfate; Methotrimeprazine; Mifepristone; Nabilone; Netupitant; Peginterferon Alfa-2b; Perampanel; Rufinamide; Simeprevir; Sodium Oxybate; Stiripentol; Tapentadol; Tetrahydrocannabinol

Decreased Effect

The levels/effects of Pipotiazine may be decreased by: Antacids; Bosentan; CYP3A4 Inducers (Moderate); CYP3A4 Inducers (Strong); Dabrafenib; Deferasirox; Mitotane; Peginterferon Alfa-2b; Siltuximab; St Johns Wort; Tocilizumab

Storage/Stability Store at room temperature of 15°C to 30°C (59°F to 86°F). Protect from light.

Mechanism of Action Blocks postsynaptic mesolimbic dopaminergic receptors in the brain; depresses the release of hypothalamic and hypophyseal hormones. Relative to other piperidine phenothiazines, pipotiazine appears to be less sedating, with less potential to potentiate other CNS depressants, and may possess a lower propensity to cause hypotension. However, it has a relatively high propensity for cause extrapyramidal reactions. Pipotiazine palmitate is an ester of pipotiazine with a prolonged duration of action.

Pharmacodynamics/Kinetics

Onset of action: IM: 2 to 3 days

Duration: 3 to 6 weeks

Time to peak, serum: 1 day (Spanaerello 2014)

Dosage IM: Adults: Initial (dosage must be individualized): 50-100 mg; may be increased in 25 mg increments every 2-3 weeks. Optimal dosage and interval must be determined by individual response. Usual maintenance dose: 75-150 mg every 4 weeks; range: 25-250 mg every 3-4 weeks. A lower dose at a shorter interval (eg, every 3 weeks) may be beneficial in some patients compared to higher doses every 4 weeks.

Elderly >50 years: Initial dosage <50 mg is recommended

Dosage adjustment in renal impairment: Use is contraindicated.

Dosage adjustment in hepatic impairment: Use is contraindicated.

Administration Administer in the gluteal muscle by deep intramuscular injection (Gillespie 2013) using at least a 21-gauge needle for injection. Use a dry syringe and needle for administration; a wet needle/syringe may cause the solution to become cloudy.

Monitoring Parameters Vital signs; liver function test and CBC with differential (at baseline and then periodically during therapy, particularly during the first 2-3 months of therapy); electrolytes; renal function (with long-term therapy); serum potassium and magnesium, fasting blood glucose/HbA_{1c}; waist circumference, BMI; mental status, abnormal involuntary movement scale (AIMS); periodic eye exam

Based on experience with other piperidine phenothiazines: consider baseline and periodic ECG, do not initiate if QTc >450 msec

Product Availability Not available in U.S.

Dosage Forms: Canada

Injection, oil:

Piportil L_4: 25 mg/mL (1 mL); 50 mg/mL (1 mL, 2 mL)

◆ **Pipotiazine Palmitate** *see* Pipotiazine [CAN/INT] *on page 1660*

Piracetam [INT] (pi RA se tam)

International Brand Names Acetar (PT); Alcetam (IN); Antikun (ID); Avigilen (DE); Axonyl (FR); Braintop (BE, LU); Breinox (EC, VE); Ceact (IN); Cebrotonin (DE, EC, MY, SG); Celebral (GR); Cerebroforte (DE); Cerebrol (EC); Cerebropan (IT); Cerebrosteril (DE); Cerebryl (AT, HU); Ceremin (PK); Cerepar N (DE); Cetam (IT, SG); Ciclofalina (ES); Cintilan (BR); Cleveral (IT); Cuxabrain (DE); Cytropil (ID); Dinagen (MX); Docpirace (BE); Embol (TH); Encefalux (ES); Encetrop (CH, DE); Flavis (IT); Gabacet (FR); Genogris (ES); Geram (FR); Geratam (BE, CZ, LU, SE); Huberdasen (ES); Inteluz (PY, UY); Irahex (MY, PH); Jiesilin (CN); Kalicor (CZ); Kang Ling (CN); Ke Jie (CN); Latys (GR); Lucetam (BG, HU, PL, RO, RU); Lytenur (DE); Memoril (PY); Memotal (JO, RO); Memotropil (PL); Memozet (MY); Mempil (TH); Mencetam (TH); Merapiran (AR); Neu-Stam (VN); Neurocetam (MY, SG); Neuronova (ES); Noodis (BE, HU, LU); Noostan (AR, BE, PT); Nootron (BR); Nootrop (BE, DE, SE); Nootropicon (AR); Nootropil (AE, AT, BE, BG, BH, BR, CH, CY, CZ, DE, EC, EE, EG, ES, FI, GB, HK, HU, ID, IN, IT, KW, LB, LT, LU, MX, MY, NL, NO, PE, PH, PK, PL, PT, QA, RO, RU, SA, SE, SG, SI, SK, TH, TR, UY, ZA); Nootropyl (CL, FR, VN); Noottropil (JO); Norcetam (JO); Normabrain (DE, IN, PH); Norzetam (IT); Novocephal (AT); Nupic (IN); Oikamid (CZ, HR); Picetam (SG); Pirabene (AT, DE, HU); Piracas (IN); Piracebral (BG, DE, LU); Piracemed (BE); Piracetam AbZ (DE); Piracetam AL (DE); Piracetam EG (BE); Piracetam Faro (AT); Piracetam Heumann (DE); Piracetam Interpharm (AT); Piracetam Prodes (ES); Piracetam Stada (DE); Piracetam Verla (DE); piracetam von ct (DE); Piracetam-Elbe-Med (DE); Piracetam-Farmatrading (PT); Piracetam-neuraxpharm (DE); Piracetam-ratiopharm (DE, LU, PT); Piracetam-RPh (DE); Piracetan (PY); Piracetop (BE); Piracetrop (DE); Piratam (SG); Piratin (HK); Piratropil (RU); Pirax (CH); Pirazetam-Eurogenerics (LU); Pracetam (VN); Primodex (UY); Psycoton (IT); Pyramen (BG, HU); Pyraminol (GB); Qing Da (CN); Racetam (SG); Resibron (ID); Scarda (TH); Si Tai (CN); Sinapsan (DE); Sotropil (ID); Stammin (GR); Stimubral (PT); Ucetam (PK); YiTing (CN); Zetam (IN); Zetropil (ID); Zynootrop (PH)

Pharmacologic Category Antimyoclonic, Miscellaneous; Nootropic

Reported Use Symptomatic treatment of cognitive/intellectual or memory deficits (excluding Alzheimer disease and other dementias); adjunctive treatment of cortical myoclonus; treatment of dyslexia in combination with speech therapy in children with learning difficulties related to written words that are not explained by general intellectual deficits or educational/environmental factors; vertigo

Dosage Range

Children ≥8 years and Adolescents: Oral: Dyslexia, in combination with speech therapy: 3.2-3.3 g daily in 2 divided doses

Adults: Oral, I.V.:

Cognitive disorders: 1.2-4.8 g daily in 2-3 divided doses

Cortical myoclonus, adjunctive: Initial: 7.2 g daily administered in 2-3 divided doses; may increase total daily dose by 4.8 g every 3-4 days if needed (maximum daily dose: 24 g)

Vertigo: 2.4-4.8 g daily in 2-3 divided doses

Dosage adjustment in renal impairment:

CrCl 50-80 mL/minute: Initial and maximum dose: Decrease to 2/3 of the normal daily dose administered in 2-3 divided doses.

CrCl 30 to <50 mL/minute: Initial and maximum dose: Decrease to 1/3 of the normal daily dose administered in 2 divided doses.

CrCl 20 to <30 mL/minute: Decrease to 1/6 of the normal daily dose administered once daily.

CrCl <20 mL/minute: Use is contraindicated.

Product Availability Product available in various countries; not currently available in the U.S.

Dosage Forms

Capsule, Oral: 400 mg

Granules, Oral: 1200 mg, 2400 mg

Solution, Injection: 200 mg/mL

Solution, Oral: 200 mg/mL, 330 mg/mL

Tablet, Oral: 800 mg, 1200 mg

Pirbuterol (peer BYOO ter ole)

Brand Names: U.S. Maxair Autohaler [DSC]

Index Terms Pirbuterol Acetate

Pharmacologic Category $Beta_2$ Agonist

Use Prevention and treatment of reversible bronchospasm including asthma

Pregnancy Risk Factor C

Dosage Bronchospasm, prevention and treatment: Children ≥12 years, Adolescents, and Adults: Inhalation: 1-2 inhalations every 4-6 hours; not to exceed 12 inhalations daily. Patients should be advised to promptly consult healthcare provider or seek medical attention if no relief from acute treatment

Dosage adjustment in renal impairment: No dosage adjustment provided in manufacturer's labeling. However, dosage adjustment unlikely due to low systemic absorption.

Dosage adjustment in hepatic impairment: No dosage adjustment provided in manufacturer's labeling. However, dosage adjustment unlikely due to low systemic absorption.

Additional Information Complete prescribing information should be consulted for additional detail.

Dosage Forms Considerations

Maxair Autohaler 14 g canisters contain 400 inhalations.

Maxair Autohaler contains chlorofluorocarbons

◆ **Pirbuterol Acetate** *see* Pirbuterol *on page 1662*

Pirenzepine [INT] (pir EN ze peen)

International Brand Names Droxol (AR); Gastropiron (IT); Gastrozepin (AT, AU, CZ, DE, GR, JP, NL, RU, SI); Gastrozepina (PT)

Index Terms Pirenzepine Hydrochloride

Pharmacologic Category Anticholinergic Agent

Reported Use Treatment of peptic ulcer

Dosage Range Children >12 years and Adults: Oral: 50 mg twice daily 1 hour before meals; may increase to 3 times/day

Product Availability Product available in various countries; not currently available in the U.S.

Dosage Forms

Tablet: 50 mg

◆ **Pirenzepine Hydrochloride** *see* Pirenzepine [INT] *on page 1662*

Piribedil [INT] (pye RIB ee dil)

International Brand Names Clarium (DE); Pronoran (BG, PL, RU); Trastal (CN); Trastoner (AR); Travastal (AR, BR, DE, EG, FR, GR, IN, MY, PT, SG, TH); Travastal Retard (EG); Travastan (IT); Trivastal (PH, PY, QA, TR, VE); Trivastal Retard (AE, KW, SA, VN)

Pharmacologic Category Anti-Parkinson's Agent, Dopamine Agonist

Reported Use Treatment of Parkinson's disease, either as monotherapy without levodopa or in combination with levodopa therapy; pathological cognitive deficits in the elderly

Dosage Range Adults: Oral: Parkinson's disease:

Initial: 50 mg/day for 1 week

Dose adjustment: Dosage may be increased weekly:

Monotherapy: 150-250 mg/day in 3-5 divided doses with meals

Combination with levodopa: 50-150 mg in divided doses with meals

Product Availability Product available in various countries; not currently available in the U.S.

Dosage Forms

Tablet, sustained release: 50 mg

◆ **Pirmella 1/35** *see* Ethinyl Estradiol and Norethindrone *on page 808*

◆ **Pirmella 7/7/7** *see* Ethinyl Estradiol and Norethindrone *on page 808*

Piroxicam (peer OKS i kam)

Brand Names: U.S. Feldene

Brand Names: Canada Apo-Piroxicam; Dom-Piroxicam; Novo-Pirocam; PMS-Piroxicam

Pharmacologic Category Nonsteroidal Anti-inflammatory Drug (NSAID), Oral

Additional Appendix Information

Beers Criteria – Potentially Inappropriate Medications for Geriatrics *on page 2271*

Use Symptomatic treatment of acute and chronic rheumatoid arthritis and osteoarthritis

Canadian labeling: Additional use (not in U.S. labeling): Symptomatic treatment of ankylosing spondylitis

Pregnancy Risk Factor C

Dosage

Osteoarthritis, rheumatoid arthritis: Adults: Oral, Rectal suppository [Canadian product]: 10-20 mg daily in 1-2 divided doses (maximum dose: 20 mg daily)

Ankylosing spondylitis (Canadian labeling; not an approved use in U.S. labeling): Adults: Oral, Rectal suppository [Canadian product]: 10-20 mg daily in 1-2 divided doses (maximum dose: 20 mg daily)

Elderly: Refer to adult dosing. Initiate therapy cautiously at low end of dosing range.

Dosing adjustment in renal impairment:
Mild-to-moderate impairment:
U.S. labeling: No dosage adjustment provided in manufacturer's labeling.
Canadian labeling: No specific dosage adjustment provided in manufacturer's labeling; however, a dosage reduction is recommended. Caution and close monitoring is advised for patients with CrCl <60 mL/minute. Use is contraindicated in patients with deteriorating renal disease.
Severe impairment:
U.S. labeling: Use is not recommended (has not been studied); if therapy must be initiated, close monitoring is recommended.
Canadian labeling: Use is contraindicated in severe impairment (CrCl <30 mL/minute) or in patients with deteriorating renal disease.

Dosing adjustment in hepatic impairment: No specific dosage adjustment provided in manufacturer's labeling; however, a dosage reduction is recommended. **Note:** Canadian labeling contraindicates use in severe impairment or in patients with active liver disease.

Additional Information Complete prescribing information should be consulted for additional detail.

Dosage Forms
Capsule, Oral:
Feldene: 10 mg, 20 mg
Generic: 10 mg, 20 mg

Dosage Forms: Canada Note: Refer also to Dosage Forms.
Suppository, Rectal: 10 mg, 20 mg

- ◆ ***p*-Isobutylhydratropic Acid** *see* Ibuprofen *on page 1032*
- ◆ **Pit** *see* Oxytocin *on page 1549*

Pitavastatin (pi TA va sta tin)

Brand Names: U.S. Livalo

Index Terms Pitavastatin Calcium

Pharmacologic Category Antilipemic Agent, HMG-CoA Reductase Inhibitor

Use Adjunct to dietary therapy to reduce elevations in total cholesterol (TC), LDL-C, apolipoprotein B (Apo B), and triglycerides (TG), and to increase low HDL-C in patients with primary hyperlipidemia and mixed dyslipidemia

Pregnancy Risk Factor X

Dosage Note: Doses should be individualized according to the baseline LDL-cholesterol levels, the recommended goal of therapy, and patient response; adjustments should be made at intervals of 4 weeks.

Primary hyperlipidemia and mixed dyslipidemia: Adults: Oral: Initial: 2 mg once daily; may be increased to maximum 4 mg once daily

ACC/AHA Blood Cholesterol Guideline recommendations to reduce the risk of atherosclerotic cardiovascular disease (ASCVD) (off-label use; Stone, 2013): Adults ≥21 years: Oral:
Primary prevention:
LDL-C ≥190 mg/dL: High intensity therapy necessary; use alternate statin therapy (eg, atorvastatin or rosuvastatin)
Type 1 or 2 diabetes and age 40-75 years: Moderate intensity therapy: 2-4 mg once daily
Type 1 or 2 diabetes, age 40-75 years, and an estimated 10-year ASCVD risk ≥7.5%: High intensity therapy necessary; use alternate statin therapy (eg, atorvastatin or rosuvastatin)
Age 40-75 years and an estimated 10-year ASCVD risk ≥7.5%: Moderate to high intensity therapy: 2-4 mg once daily or consider using high intensity statin therapy (eg, atorvastatin or rosuvastatin)
Secondary prevention:
Patient has clinical ASCVD (eg, coronary heart disease, stroke/TIA, or peripheral arterial disease presumed to be of atherosclerotic origin) **and:**
Age ≤75 years: High intensity therapy necessary; use alternate statin therapy (eg, atorvastatin or rosuvastatin)
Age >75 years or not a candidate for high intensity therapy: Moderate intensity therapy: 2-4 mg once daily

Dosage adjustment with concomitant medications:
Erythromycin: Pitavastatin dose should not exceed 1 mg once daily
Rifampin: Pitavastatin dose should not exceed 2 mg once daily

Dosing adjustment for toxicity:
Severe muscle symptoms or fatigue: Promptly discontinue use; evaluate CPK, creatinine, and urinalysis for myoglobinuria (Stone, 2013).
Mild to moderate muscle symptoms: Discontinue use until symptoms can be evaluated; evaluate patient for conditions that may increase the risk for muscle symptoms (eg, hypothyroidism, reduced renal or hepatic function, rheumatologic disorders such as polymyalgia rheumatica, steroid myopathy, vitamin D deficiency, or primary muscle diseases). Upon resolution, resume the original or lower dose of atorvastatin. If muscle symptoms recur, discontinue atorvastatin use. After muscle symptom resolution, may then use a low dose of a different statin; gradually increase if tolerated. In the absence of continued statin use, if muscle symptoms or elevated CPK continues after 2 months, consider other causes of muscle symptoms. If determined to be due to another condition aside from statin use, may resume statin therapy at the original dose (Stone, 2013).

Dosage adjustment in renal impairment:
CrCl 15-60 mL/minute/1.73 m^2 (not receiving hemodialysis): Initial: 1 mg once daily; maximum: 2 mg once daily
ESRD: Initial: 1 mg once daily; maximum: 2 mg once daily

Dosage adjustment in hepatic impairment: Contraindicated in active liver disease or in patients with unexplained persistent elevations of serum transaminases

Additional Information Complete prescribing information should be consulted for additional detail.

Dosage Forms
Tablet, Oral:
Livalo: 1 mg, 2 mg, 4 mg

- ◆ **Pitavastatin Calcium** *see* Pitavastatin *on page 1663*
- ◆ **Pitocin** *see* Oxytocin *on page 1549*
- ◆ **Pitressin Synthetic [DSC]** *see* Vasopressin *on page 2142*
- ◆ **Pitrex (Can)** *see* Tolnaftate *on page 2063*

Pivmecillinam [INT] (piv me SIL e nam)

Index Terms Amdinocillin; Pivmecillinam Hydrochloride

Pharmacologic Category Antibiotic, Penicillin

Reported Use Treatment of bacterial infections caused by susceptible gram-negative organisms

Dosage Range Adults: Oral: 200-400 mg 3 times/day

Product Availability Product available in various countries; not currently available in the U.S.

Dosage Forms

Tablet: 200 mg

◆ **Pivmecillinam Hydrochloride** *see* Pivmecillinam [INT] *on page 1663*

Pizotifen [CAN/INT] (pi ZOE ti fen)

Brand Names: Canada Sandomigran; Sandomigran DS

Index Terms Pizotifen Malate

Pharmacologic Category Serotonin and Histamine Antagonist

Use Note: Not approved in U.S.

Migraine prophylaxis

Pregnancy Considerations Adverse events were not observed in animal reproduction studies. If possible, drug therapy for migraine prophylaxis should be avoided during pregnancy. If therapy is needed, other agents are preferred (Pringsheim, 2012).

Breast-Feeding Considerations The concentration of pizotifen measured in the milk of nursing mothers is unlikely to affect a nursing infant; however, the manufacturer does not recommend use in nursing mothers. If possible, drug therapy for migraine prophylaxis should be avoided in nursing women. If therapy is needed, other agents are preferred (Pringsheim, 2012).

Contraindications Hypersensitivity to pizotifen or any component of the formulation; concurrent use of MAO inhibitors; gastric outlet obstruction (pyloroduodenal obstruction, stenosing pyloric ulcer); use in children <12 years of age

Warnings/Precautions Not for use in acute treatment of migraine attacks. Not considered first-line agent for migraine prophylaxis, but may be considered when other therapies have failed (Pringsheim, 2012). May cause sedation; effects may be additive with other CNS depressants or ethanol. Gradual titration of dose may help minimize sedative effects (eg, drowsiness). Patients must be cautioned to avoid operating machinery or driving until effects are known. Although anticholinergic effects are limited, use with caution in patients intolerant to anticholinergic agents, including tricyclic antidepressants, phenothiazines, or cyproheptadine. Use with caution in patients with myasthenia gravis, bladder outlet obstruction (BPH), or other disorders in which anticholinergic effects may be poorly tolerated. Use caution in renal or hepatic disease/insufficiency, diabetes, cardiovascular disease, or epilepsy (seizure reported rarely with use).

Hepatotoxic effects may occur with prolonged used; periodic evaluation of liver function is recommended during therapy. Discontinue use for signs/symptoms of hepatic dysfunction and do not resume therapy until etiology of hepatic dysfunction is identified. Use with caution in patients with narrow angle glaucoma or other vision problems. Use has been associated with increased intraocular pressure, diplopia, and pupil dilation; limited number of patients experienced lens opacities but effect was not considered drug-related. Instruct patients to report visual disturbances during therapy. Increased appetite and weight gain are common adverse effects; patients may experience rapid weight loss upon discontinuation. Use with caution in obese or other patients who may be vulnerable to these effects.

Therapeutic response may require several weeks of therapy. Some patients may experience a decrease in therapeutic response over time. Avoid abrupt discontinuation which may cause acute withdrawal reactions (eg, depression, dizziness, anxiety, loss of consciousness, anorexia and rapid weight loss); taper dosage over 2 weeks prior to discontinuation. Tolerance may develop in some patients; effect may be overcome by dose increases (not to exceed maximum dosage). Consider drug-free period after several months of treatment. May contain lactose; avoid use in patients with galactose or fructose intolerance, lactase deficiency, sucrose-isomaltase insufficiency, or glucose-galactose malabsorption.

Adverse Reactions

Central nervous system: Dizziness, drowsiness (including fatigue, somnolence)

Gastrointestinal: Appetite increased, nausea, weight gain, xerostomia

Rare but important or life-threatening: Agitation/aggression (children), amenorrhea, anorexia, anxiety, arthralgia, breast enlargement, breast pain, constipation, depression, diplopia, facial edema, fulminant hepatitis, hallucination, hepatitis, hepatic enzymes increased, hypersensitivity reactions, insomnia, intraocular pressure increased, jaundice, loss of consciousness, muscle cramps, myalgia, nonpuerperal lactation, paresthesia, pupil dilation, rash, sedation, seizure, sleep disorder, tremor, urticaria, weight loss (rapid), withdrawal (following abrupt cessation of therapy)

Drug Interactions

Metabolism/Transport Effects None known.

Avoid Concomitant Use

Avoid concomitant use of Pizotifen with any of the following: Aclidinium; Azelastine (Nasal); Glucagon; Ipratropium (Oral Inhalation); MAO Inhibitors; Orphenadrine; Paraldehyde; Potassium Chloride; Thalidomide; Tiotropium; Umeclidinium

Increased Effect/Toxicity

Pizotifen may increase the levels/effects of: AbobotulinumtoxinA; Alcohol (Ethyl); Analgesics (Opioid); Anticholinergic Agents; Azelastine (Nasal); Buprenorphine; CNS Depressants; Glucagon; Hydrocodone; Methotrimeprazine; Metyrosine; Mirabegron; Mirtazapine; OnabotulinumtoxinA; Orphenadrine; Paraldehyde; Potassium Chloride; Pramipexole; RimabotulinumtoxinB; ROPINIRole; Rotigotine; Selective Serotonin Reuptake Inhibitors; Suvorexant; Thalidomide; Thiazide Diuretics; Tiotropium; Topiramate; Zolpidem

The levels/effects of Pizotifen may be increased by: Aclidinium; Brimonidine (Topical); Cannabis; Doxylamine; Dronabinol; Droperidol; HydrOXYzine; Ipratropium (Oral Inhalation); Kava Kava; Magnesium Sulfate; MAO Inhibitors; Methotrimeprazine; Mianserin; Nabilone; Perampanel; Pramlintide; Rufinamide; Sodium Oxybate; Tapentadol; Tetrahydrocannabinol; Umeclidinium

Decreased Effect

Pizotifen may decrease the levels/effects of: Acetylcholinesterase Inhibitors; Benzylpenicilloyl Polylysine; Betahistine; Hyaluronidase; Itopride; Secretin

The levels/effects of Pizotifen may be decreased by: Acetylcholinesterase Inhibitors; Amphetamines

Storage/Stability Store at 15°C to 30°C (59°F to 86°F). Protect from light and moisture.

Mechanism of Action Pizotifen is a strong serotonin antagonist and has weak antihistamine, anticholinergic and antikinin effects; also has appetite-stimulating and sedative properties. The mechanism of action in migraine prophylaxis has not been fully elucidated; may alter pain thresholds by inhibiting the permeability increasing effect of serotonin and histamine to control movement of plasma kinin across cranial vessel membranes. Inhibits serotonin reuptake by platelets, affecting tonicity and reducing passive distension of extracranial arteries.

Pharmacodynamics/Kinetics

Onset of action: May require several weeks of therapy

Distribution: V_d: Parent drug: 833 L; N-glucuronide metabolite: 70 L

Protein binding: >90%

Metabolism: Hepatic (mainly by glucuronidation)

Bioavailability: 78%

Half-life elimination: ~23 hours

Time to peak: 5 hours

Excretion: Feces (~33% of dose); urine (55% as metabolites, <1% as unchanged drug)

Dosage Migraine prophylaxis: Oral: **Note:** Therapeutic response may require several weeks of therapy. Drug holidays are recommended periodically to assess the need for ongoing therapy. Do not discontinue abruptly (reduce gradually over 2-week period).

Adolescents ≥12 years: Initial: 0.5 mg at bedtime; may increase dose gradually up to maximum of 1.5 mg daily. Doses >1 mg should be administered in divided doses.

Adults: Initial: 0.5 mg at bedtime; may increase dose gradually to 1.5 mg daily administered as single dose or in 3 divided doses; average maintenance dose: 1.5 mg daily; usual dosage range: 1-6 mg daily. Doses >3 mg should be administered in divided doses.

Elderly (>65 years): Use with caution; refer to adult dosing.

Dosage adjustment in renal impairment: No dosage adjustment provided in manufacturer's labeling. However, dosage adjustment may be necessary. Use with caution.

Dosage adjustment in hepatic impairment: No dosage adjustment provided in manufacturer's labeling. However, dosage adjustment may be necessary. Use with caution.

Monitoring Parameters Hepatic function tests (prolonged use); weight gain; blood pressure

Product Availability Not available in U.S.

Dosage Forms: Canada

Tablet:

Sandomigran®: 0.5 mg

Tablet, double strength:

Sandomigran® DS: 1 mg

- ◆ **Pizotifen Malate** *see* Pizotifen [CAN/INT] *on page 1664*
- ◆ **PLA** *see* Poly-L-Lactic Acid *on page 1676*
- ◆ **Plan B** *see* Levonorgestrel *on page 1201*
- ◆ **Plan B** *see* Levonorgestrel *on page 1201*
- ◆ **Plan B One-Step** *see* Levonorgestrel *on page 1201*
- ◆ **Plantago Seed** *see* Psyllium *on page 1744*
- ◆ **Plantain Seed** *see* Psyllium *on page 1744*
- ◆ **Plaquenil** *see* Hydroxychloroquine *on page 1021*
- ◆ **Plasbumin-5** *see* Albumin *on page 67*
- ◆ **Plasbumin-25** *see* Albumin *on page 67*
- ◆ **Platinol** *see* CISplatin *on page 448*
- ◆ **Platinol-AQ** *see* CISplatin *on page 448*
- ◆ **Plavix** *see* Clopidogrel *on page 484*
- ◆ **Plegridy** *see* Peginterferon Beta-1a *on page 1602*
- ◆ **Plegridy Starter Pack** *see* Peginterferon Beta-1a *on page 1602*
- ◆ **Plendil** *see* Felodipine *on page 850*

Plerixafor (pler IX a fore)

Brand Names: U.S. Mozobil

Brand Names: Canada Mozobil

Index Terms AMD3100; LM3100

Pharmacologic Category Hematopoietic Agent; Hematopoietic Stem Cell Mobilizer

Use Peripheral stem cell mobilization: Mobilization of hematopoietic stem cells (HSC) for collection and subsequent autologous transplantation (in combination with filgrastim) in patients with non-Hodgkin lymphoma (NHL) and multiple myeloma (MM)

Pregnancy Risk Factor D

Dosage Note: Dosing is based on actual body weight. Begin plerixafor after patient has received filgrastim (10 mcg/kg once daily) for 4 days; plerixafor, filgrastim, and apheresis should be continued daily until sufficient cell collection up to a maximum of 4 days.

Hematopoietic stem cell mobilization (in non-Hodgkin lymphoma and multiple myeloma): Adults: SubQ: 0.24 mg/kg once daily (~11 hours prior to apheresis) for up to 4 consecutive days; maximum dose: 40 mg daily

Dosage adjustment in renal impairment: Note: Creatinine clearance estimate based on Cockcroft-Gault formula:

CrCl >50 mL/minute: No dosage adjustment necessary.

CrCl ≤50 mL/minute: 0.16 mg/kg; maximum dose: 27 mg daily

Hemodialysis: No dosage adjustment provided in manufacturer's labeling (has not been studied).

Dosage adjustment in hepatic impairment: No dosage adjustment provided in manufacturer's labeling.

Dosing in obesity: The manufacturer recommends calculating the dose based on actual weight for patients weighing up to 175% of ideal body weight (maximum dose: 40 mg daily). Dosing in patients >175% of ideal body weight has not been studied.

Additional Information Complete prescribing information should be consulted for additional detail.

Dosage Forms

Solution, Subcutaneous [preservative free]:

Mozobil: 24 mg/1.2 mL (1.2 mL)

- ◆ **Pletal** *see* Cilostazol *on page 437*
- ◆ **Plexion** *see* Sulfur and Sulfacetamide *on page 1953*
- ◆ **Pliaglis** *see* Lidocaine and Tetracaine *on page 1214*
- ◆ **PLX4032** *see* Vemurafenib *on page 2148*
- ◆ **PMPA** *see* Tenofovir *on page 1998*
- ◆ **PMS-Adenosine (Can)** *see* Adenosine *on page 55*
- ◆ **PMS-Alendronate (Can)** *see* Alendronate *on page 79*
- ◆ **PMS-Alendronate-FC (Can)** *see* Alendronate *on page 79*
- ◆ **PMS-Amantadine (Can)** *see* Amantadine *on page 105*
- ◆ **PMS-Amiodarone (Can)** *see* Amiodarone *on page 114*
- ◆ **PMS-Amitriptyline (Can)** *see* Amitriptyline *on page 119*
- ◆ **PMS-Amlodipine (Can)** *see* AmLODIPine *on page 123*
- ◆ **PMS-Amoxicillin (Can)** *see* Amoxicillin *on page 130*
- ◆ **PMS-Anagrelide (Can)** *see* Anagrelide *on page 147*
- ◆ **PMS-Anastrozole (Can)** *see* Anastrozole *on page 148*
- ◆ **PMS-Atenolol (Can)** *see* Atenolol *on page 189*
- ◆ **PMS-Atomoxetine (Can)** *see* AtoMOXetine *on page 191*
- ◆ **PMS-Atorvastatin (Can)** *see* AtorvaSTATin *on page 194*
- ◆ **PMS-Azithromycin (Can)** *see* Azithromycin (Systemic) *on page 216*
- ◆ **PMS-Baclofen (Can)** *see* Baclofen *on page 223*
- ◆ **PMS-Benztropine (Can)** *see* Benztropine *on page 248*
- ◆ **PMS-Bethanechol (Can)** *see* Bethanechol *on page 257*
- ◆ **PMS-Bicalutamide (Can)** *see* Bicalutamide *on page 262*
- ◆ **PMS-Bisacodyl [OTC] (Can)** *see* Bisacodyl *on page 265*
- ◆ **PMS-Bisoprolol (Can)** *see* Bisoprolol *on page 266*
- ◆ **PMS-Bosentan (Can)** *see* Bosentan *on page 280*

- ◆ **PMS-Brimonidine Tartrate (Can)** *see* Brimonidine (Ophthalmic) *on page* 288
- ◆ **PMS-Bromocriptine (Can)** *see* Bromocriptine *on page* 291
- ◆ **PMS-Bupropion SR (Can)** *see* BuPROPion *on page* 305
- ◆ **PMS-Buspirone (Can)** *see* BusPIRone *on page* 311
- ◆ **PMS-Butorphanol (Can)** *see* Butorphanol *on page* 314
- ◆ **PMS-Candesartan (Can)** *see* Candesartan *on page* 335
- ◆ **PMS-Candesartan HCTZ (Can)** *see* Candesartan and Hydrochlorothiazide *on page* 338
- ◆ **PMS-Captopril (Can)** *see* Captopril *on page* 342
- ◆ **PMS-Carbamazepine (Can)** *see* CarBAMazepine *on page* 346
- ◆ **PMS-Carvedilol (Can)** *see* Carvedilol *on page* 367
- ◆ **PMS-Cefaclor (Can)** *see* Cefaclor *on page* 372
- ◆ **PMS-Cephalexin (Can)** *see* Cephalexin *on page* 405
- ◆ **PMS-Cetirizine (Can)** *see* Cetirizine *on page* 411
- ◆ **PMS-Chloral Hydrate (Can)** *see* Chloral Hydrate [CAN/INT] *on page* 418
- ◆ **PMS-Cholestyramine (Can)** *see* Cholestyramine Resin *on page* 431
- ◆ **PMS-Ciclopirox (Can)** *see* Ciclopirox *on page* 433
- ◆ **PMS-Cilazapril (Can)** *see* Cilazapril [CAN/INT] *on page* 434
- ◆ **PMS-Cimetidine (Can)** *see* Cimetidine *on page* 438
- ◆ **PMS-Ciprofloxacin (Can)** *see* Ciprofloxacin (Systemic) *on page* 441
- ◆ **PMS-Ciprofloxacin XL (Can)** *see* Ciprofloxacin (Systemic) *on page* 441
- ◆ **PMS-Citalopram (Can)** *see* Citalopram *on page* 451
- ◆ **PMS-Clarithromycin (Can)** *see* Clarithromycin *on page* 456
- ◆ **PMS-Clindamycin (Can)** *see* Clindamycin (Systemic) *on page* 460
- ◆ **PMS-Clobazam (Can)** *see* CloBAZam *on page* 465
- ◆ **PMS-Clobetasol (Can)** *see* Clobetasol *on page* 468
- ◆ **PMS-Clonazepam (Can)** *see* ClonazePAM *on page* 478
- ◆ **PMS-Clonazepam-R (Can)** *see* ClonazePAM *on page* 478
- ◆ **PMS-Clopidogrel (Can)** *see* Clopidogrel *on page* 484
- ◆ **PMS-Codeine (Can)** *see* Codeine *on page* 497
- ◆ **PMS-Colchicine (Can)** *see* Colchicine *on page* 500
- ◆ **PMS-Conjugated Estrogens C.S.D. (Can)** *see* Estrogens (Conjugated/Equine, Systemic) *on page* 787
- ◆ **PMS-Cyclobenzaprine (Can)** *see* Cyclobenzaprine *on page* 516
- ◆ **PMS-Cyclopentolate (Can)** *see* Cyclopentolate *on page* 517
- ◆ **PMS-Cyproheptadine (Can)** *see* Cyproheptadine *on page* 529
- ◆ **PMS-Deferoxamine (Can)** *see* Deferoxamine *on page* 586
- ◆ **PMS-Desipramine (Can)** *see* Desipramine *on page* 593
- ◆ **PMS-Desmopressin (Can)** *see* Desmopressin *on page* 594
- ◆ **PMS-Dexamethasone (Can)** *see* Dexamethasone (Systemic) *on page* 599
- ◆ **PMS-Diazepam (Can)** *see* Diazepam *on page* 613
- ◆ **PMS-Dicitrate (Can)** *see* Sodium Citrate and Citric Acid *on page* 1905
- ◆ **PMS-Diclofenac (Can)** *see* Diclofenac (Systemic) *on page* 617
- ◆ **PMS-Diclofenac K (Can)** *see* Diclofenac (Systemic) *on page* 617
- ◆ **PMS-Diclofenac-SR (Can)** *see* Diclofenac (Systemic) *on page* 617
- ◆ **PMS-Digoxin (Can)** *see* Digoxin *on page* 627
- ◆ **PMS-Diltiazem CD (Can)** *see* Diltiazem *on page* 634
- ◆ **PMS-Dimenhydrinate [OTC] (Can)** *see* DimenhyDRINATE *on page* 637
- ◆ **PMS-Diphenhydramine (Can)** *see* DiphenhydrAMINE (Systemic) *on page* 641
- ◆ **PMS-Dipivefrin (Can)** *see* Dipivefrin *on page* 651
- ◆ **PMS-Divalproex (Can)** *see* Valproic Acid and Derivatives *on page* 2123
- ◆ **PMS-Docusate Calcium [OTC] (Can)** *see* Docusate *on page* 661
- ◆ **PMS-Docusate Sodium [OTC] (Can)** *see* Docusate *on page* 661
- ◆ **PMS-Domperidone (Can)** *see* Domperidone [CAN/INT] *on page* 666
- ◆ **PMS-Donepezil (Can)** *see* Donepezil *on page* 668
- ◆ **PMS-Doxazosin (Can)** *see* Doxazosin *on page* 674
- ◆ **PMS-Doxycycline (Can)** *see* Doxycycline *on page* 689
- ◆ **PMS-Dutasteride (Can)** *see* Dutasteride *on page* 702
- ◆ **PMS-Enalapril (Can)** *see* Enalapril *on page* 722
- ◆ **PMS-Entecavir (Can)** *see* Entecavir *on page* 731
- ◆ **PMS-Erythromycin (Can)** *see* Erythromycin (Ophthalmic) *on page* 764
- ◆ **PMS-Escitalopram (Can)** *see* Escitalopram *on page* 765
- ◆ **PMS-Esomeprazole DR (Can)** *see* Esomeprazole *on page* 771
- ◆ **PMS-Ezetimibe (Can)** *see* Ezetimibe *on page* 832
- ◆ **PMS-Famciclovir (Can)** *see* Famciclovir *on page* 843
- ◆ **PMS-Fenofibrate Micro (Can)** *see* Fenofibrate and Derivatives *on page* 852
- ◆ **PMS-Fentanyl MTX (Can)** *see* FentaNYL *on page* 857
- ◆ **PMS-Finasteride (Can)** *see* Finasteride *on page* 878
- ◆ **PMS-Fluconazole (Can)** *see* Fluconazole *on page* 885
- ◆ **PMS-Fluorometholone (Can)** *see* Fluorometholone *on page* 896
- ◆ **PMS-Fluoxetine (Can)** *see* FLUoxetine *on page* 899
- ◆ **PMS-Fluphenazine Decanoate (Can)** *see* FluPHENAZine *on page* 905
- ◆ **PMS-Flurazepam (Can)** *see* Flurazepam *on page* 906
- ◆ **PMS-Flutamide (Can)** *see* Flutamide *on page* 907
- ◆ **PMS-Fluvoxamine (Can)** *see* FluvoxaMINE *on page* 916
- ◆ **PMS-Fosinopril (Can)** *see* Fosinopril *on page* 932
- ◆ **PMS-Furosemide (Can)** *see* Furosemide *on page* 940
- ◆ **PMS-Gabapentin (Can)** *see* Gabapentin *on page* 943
- ◆ **PMS-Galantamine ER (Can)** *see* Galantamine *on page* 946
- ◆ **PMS-Gemfibrozil (Can)** *see* Gemfibrozil *on page* 956
- ◆ **PMS-Gentamicin (Can)** *see* Gentamicin (Ophthalmic) *on page* 962
- ◆ **PMS-Gliclazide (Can)** *see* Gliclazide [CAN/INT] *on page* 964
- ◆ **PMS-Glimepiride (Can)** *see* Glimepiride *on page* 966
- ◆ **PMS-Glyburide (Can)** *see* GlyBURIDE *on page* 972
- ◆ **PMS-Haloperidol (Can)** *see* Haloperidol *on page* 993
- ◆ **PMS-Haloperidol LA (Can)** *see* Haloperidol *on page* 993
- ◆ **PMS-Hydrochlorothiazide (Can)** *see* Hydrochlorothiazide *on page* 1009

- **PMS-Hydromorphone (Can)** *see* HYDROmorphone *on page 1016*
- **PMS-Hydroxyzine (Can)** *see* HydrOXYzine *on page 1024*
- **PMS-Ibuprofen (Can)** *see* Ibuprofen *on page 1032*
- **PMS Imipramine (Can)** *see* Imipramine *on page 1054*
- **PMS-Indapamide (Can)** *see* Indapamide *on page 1065*
- **PMS-Ipratropium (Can)** *see* Ipratropium (Systemic) *on page 1108*
- **PMS-Irbesartan (Can)** *see* Irbesartan *on page 1110*
- **PMS-Irbesartan HCTZ (Can)** *see* Irbesartan and Hydrochlorothiazide *on page 1112*
- **PMS-ISMN (Can)** *see* Isosorbide Mononitrate *on page 1126*
- **PMS-Isosorbide (Can)** *see* Isosorbide Dinitrate *on page 1124*
- **PMS-Ketoprofen (Can)** *see* Ketoprofen *on page 1145*
- **PMS-Ketoprofen-E (Can)** *see* Ketoprofen *on page 1145*
- **PMS-Ketotifen (Can)** *see* Ketotifen (Systemic) [CAN/INT] *on page 1149*
- **PMS-Lactulose (Can)** *see* Lactulose *on page 1156*
- **PMS-Lamotrigine (Can)** *see* LamoTRIgine *on page 1160*
- **PMS-Lansoprazole (Can)** *see* Lansoprazole *on page 1166*
- **PMS-Leflunomide (Can)** *see* Leflunomide *on page 1174*
- **PMS-Letrozole (Can)** *see* Letrozole *on page 1181*
- **PMS-Levazine (Can)** *see* Amitriptyline and Perphenazine *on page 122*
- **PMS-Levetiracetam (Can)** *see* LevETIRAcetam *on page 1191*
- **PMS-Levobunolol (Can)** *see* Levobunolol *on page 1194*
- **PMS-Levocarb CR (Can)** *see* Carbidopa and Levodopa *on page 351*
- **PMS-Levofloxacin (Can)** *see* Levofloxacin (Systemic) *on page 1197*
- **PMS-Lisinopril (Can)** *see* Lisinopril *on page 1226*
- **PMS-Lithium Carbonate (Can)** *see* Lithium *on page 1230*
- **PMS-Lithium Citrate (Can)** *see* Lithium *on page 1230*
- **PMS-Loperamine (Can)** *see* Loperamide *on page 1236*
- **PMS-Lorazepam (Can)** *see* LORazepam *on page 1243*
- **PMS-Losartan (Can)** *see* Losartan *on page 1248*
- **PMS-Losartan/HCTZ (Can)** *see* Losartan and Hydrochlorothiazide *on page 1250*
- **PMS-Lovastatin (Can)** *see* Lovastatin *on page 1252*
- **PMS-Medroxyprogesterone (Can)** *see* MedroxyPROGESTERone *on page 1277*
- **PMS-Mefenamic Acid (Can)** *see* Mefenamic Acid *on page 1280*
- **PMS-Meloxicam (Can)** *see* Meloxicam *on page 1283*
- **PMS-Memantine (Can)** *see* Memantine *on page 1286*
- **PMS-Metformin (Can)** *see* MetFORMIN *on page 1307*
- **PMS-Methotrimeprazine (Can)** *see* Methotrimeprazine [CAN/INT] *on page 1329*
- **PMS-Methylphenidate (Can)** *see* Methylphenidate *on page 1336*
- **PMS-Metoclopramide (Can)** *see* Metoclopramide *on page 1345*
- **PMS-Metoprolol-L (Can)** *see* Metoprolol *on page 1350*
- **PMS-Metoprolol-B (Can)** *see* Metoprolol *on page 1350*
- **PMS-Metronidazole (Can)** *see* MetroNIDAZOLE (Systemic) *on page 1353*
- **PMS-Minocycline (Can)** *see* Minocycline *on page 1371*
- **PMS-Mirtazapine (Can)** *see* Mirtazapine *on page 1376*
- **PMS-Misoprostol (Can)** *see* Misoprostol *on page 1379*
- **PMS-Moclobemide (Can)** *see* Moclobemide [CAN/INT] *on page 1384*
- **PMS-Mometasone (Can)** *see* Mometasone (Topical) *on page 1391*
- **PMS-Montelukast (Can)** *see* Montelukast *on page 1392*
- **PMS-Montelukast FC (Can)** *see* Montelukast *on page 1392*
- **PMS-Morphine Sulfate SR (Can)** *see* Morphine (Systemic) *on page 1394*
- **PMS-Naproxen (Can)** *see* Naproxen *on page 1427*
- **PMS-Naproxen EC (Can)** *see* Naproxen *on page 1427*
- **PMS-Nifedipine (Can)** *see* NIFEdipine *on page 1451*
- **PMS-Nizatidine (Can)** *see* Nizatidine *on page 1471*
- **PMS-Norfloxacin (Can)** *see* Norfloxacin *on page 1475*
- **PMS-Nortriptyline (Can)** *see* Nortriptyline *on page 1476*
- **PMS-Nystatin (Can)** *see* Nystatin (Oral) *on page 1481*
- **PMS-Olanzapine (Can)** *see* OLANZapine *on page 1491*
- **PMS-Olanzapine ODT (Can)** *see* OLANZapine *on page 1491*
- **PMS-Omeprazole (Can)** *see* Omeprazole *on page 1508*
- **PMS-Omeprazole DR (Can)** *see* Omeprazole *on page 1508*
- **PMS-Ondansetron (Can)** *see* Ondansetron *on page 1513*
- **PMS-Oxazepam (Can)** *see* Oxazepam *on page 1532*
- **PMS-Oxybutynin (Can)** *see* Oxybutynin *on page 1536*
- **PMS-Oxycodone (Can)** *see* OxyCODONE *on page 1538*
- **PMS-Oxycodone-Acetaminophen (Can)** *see* Oxycodone and Acetaminophen *on page 1541*
- **PMS-Oxycodone CR (Can)** *see* OxyCODONE *on page 1538*
- **PMS-Pamidronate (Can)** *see* Pamidronate *on page 1563*
- **PMS-Pantoprazole (Can)** *see* Pantoprazole *on page 1570*
- **PMS-Paroxetine (Can)** *see* PARoxetine *on page 1579*
- **PMS-Phenobarbital (Can)** *see* PHENobarbital *on page 1632*
- **PMS-Pimozide (Can)** *see* Pimozide *on page 1651*
- **PMS-Pindolol (Can)** *see* Pindolol *on page 1652*
- **PMS-Pioglitazone (Can)** *see* Pioglitazone *on page 1654*
- **PMS-Piroxicam (Can)** *see* Piroxicam *on page 1662*
- **PMS-Polytrimethoprim (Can)** *see* Trimethoprim and Polymyxin B *on page 2105*
- **PMS-Pramipexole (Can)** *see* Pramipexole *on page 1695*
- **PMS-Pravastatin (Can)** *see* Pravastatin *on page 1700*
- **PMS-Prednisolone Sodium Phosphate Forte (Can)** *see* PrednisoLONE (Ophthalmic) *on page 1706*
- **PMS-Pregabalin (Can)** *see* Pregabalin *on page 1710*
- **PMS-Prochlorperazine (Can)** *see* Prochlorperazine *on page 1718*
- **PMS-Procyclidine (Can)** *see* Procyclidine [CAN/INT] *on page 1721*
- **PMS-Promethazine (Can)** *see* Promethazine *on page 1723*

- **PMS-Propafenone (Can)** *see* Propafenone *on page 1725*
- **PMS-Propofol (Can)** *see* Propofol *on page 1728*
- **PMS-Propranolol (Can)** *see* Propranolol *on page 1731*
- **PMS-Pseudoephedrine (Can)** *see* Pseudoephedrine *on page 1742*
- **PMS-Quetiapine (Can)** *see* QUEtiapine *on page 1751*
- **PMS-Quinapril (Can)** *see* Quinapril *on page 1756*
- **PMS-Rabeprazole EC (Can)** *see* RABEprazole *on page 1762*
- **PMS-Raloxifene (Can)** *see* Raloxifene *on page 1765*
- **PMS-Ramipril (Can)** *see* Ramipril *on page 1771*
- **PMS-Ramipril HCTZ (Can)** *see* Ramipril and Hydrochlorothiazide [CAN/INT] *on page 1773*
- **PMS-Ranitidine (Can)** *see* Ranitidine *on page 1777*
- **PMS-Repaglinide (Can)** *see* Repaglinide *on page 1791*
- **PMS-Risedronate (Can)** *see* Risedronate *on page 1816*
- **PMS-Risperidone (Can)** *see* RisperiDONE *on page 1818*
- **PMS-Risperidone ODT (Can)** *see* RisperiDONE *on page 1818*
- **PMS-Rivastigmine (Can)** *see* Rivastigmine *on page 1833*
- **PMS-Rizatriptan RDT (Can)** *see* Rizatriptan *on page 1836*
- **PMS-Ropinirole (Can)** *see* ROPINIRole *on page 1844*
- **PMS-Rosuvastatin (Can)** *see* Rosuvastatin *on page 1848*
- **PMS-Salbutamol (Can)** *see* Albuterol *on page 69*
- **PMS-Sertraline (Can)** *see* Sertraline *on page 1878*
- **PMS-Sildenafil (Can)** *see* Sildenafil *on page 1882*
- **PMS-Simvastatin (Can)** *see* Simvastatin *on page 1890*
- **PMS-Sodium Polystyrene Sulfonate (Can)** *see* Sodium Polystyrene Sulfonate *on page 1912*
- **PMS-Sotalol (Can)** *see* Sotalol *on page 1927*
- **PMS-Sucralate (Can)** *see* Sucralfate *on page 1940*
- **PMS-Sulfacetamide (Can)** *see* Sulfacetamide (Ophthalmic) *on page 1943*
- **PMS-Sulfasalazine (Can)** *see* SulfaSALAzine *on page 1950*
- **PMS-Sumatriptan (Can)** *see* SUMAtriptan *on page 1953*
- **PMS-Tamoxifen (Can)** *see* Tamoxifen *on page 1971*
- **PMS-Telmisartan (Can)** *see* Telmisartan *on page 1988*
- **PMS-Telmisartan HCTZ (Can)** *see* Telmisartan and Hydrochlorothiazide *on page 1990*
- **PMS-Temazepam (Can)** *see* Temazepam *on page 1990*
- **PMS-Terazosin (Can)** *see* Terazosin *on page 2001*
- **PMS-Terbinafine (Can)** *see* Terbinafine (Systemic) *on page 2002*
- **PMS-Testosterone (Can)** *see* Testosterone *on page 2010*
- **PMS-Tetrabenazine (Can)** *see* Tetrabenazine *on page 2016*
- **PMS-Theophylline (Can)** *see* Theophylline *on page 2026*
- **PMS-Tiaprofenic (Can)** *see* Tiaprofenic Acid [CAN/INT] *on page 2034*
- **PMS-Ticlopidine (Can)** *see* Ticlopidine *on page 2040*
- **PMS-Timolol (Can)** *see* Timolol (Ophthalmic) *on page 2043*
- **PMS-Tobramycin (Can)** *see* Tobramycin (Ophthalmic) *on page 2056*
- **PMS-Topiramate (Can)** *see* Topiramate *on page 2065*
- **PMS-Tramadol/Acet (Can)** *see* Acetaminophen and Tramadol *on page 37*
- **PMS-Trazodone (Can)** *see* TraZODone *on page 2091*
- **PMS-Trifluoperazine (Can)** *see* Trifluoperazine *on page 2102*
- **PMS-Trihexyphenidyl (Can)** *see* Trihexyphenidyl *on page 2103*
- **PMS-Ursodiol C (Can)** *see* Ursodiol *on page 2116*
- **PMS-Valacyclovir (Can)** *see* ValACYclovir *on page 2119*
- **PMS-Valproic Acid (Can)** *see* Valproic Acid and Derivatives *on page 2123*
- **PMS-Valproic Acid E.C. (Can)** *see* Valproic Acid and Derivatives *on page 2123*
- **PMS-Valsartan (Can)** *see* Valsartan *on page 2127*
- **PMS-Vancomycin (Can)** *see* Vancomycin *on page 2130*
- **PMS-Venlafaxine XR (Can)** *see* Venlafaxine *on page 2150*
- **PMS-Verapamil SR (Can)** *see* Verapamil *on page 2154*
- **PMS-Zolmitriptan (Can)** *see* ZOLMitriptan *on page 2210*
- **PMS-Zolmitriptan ODT (Can)** *see* ZOLMitriptan *on page 2210*
- **PMS-Zopiclone (Can)** *see* Zopiclone [CAN/INT] *on page 2217*
- **PN** *see* Total Parenteral Nutrition *on page 2073*
- **PN401** *see* Uridine Triacetate *on page 2116*

Pneumococcal Conjugate Vaccine (10-Valent) [CAN/INT]

(noo moe KOK al KON ju gate vak SEEN, ten vay lent)

Brand Names: Canada Synflorix

Index Terms 10-Valent Pneumococcal Nontypeable *Haemophilus influenzae* Protein D Conjugate Vaccine; PHiD-CV; Pneumococcal Conjugate Vaccine (Nontypeable *Haemophilus influenzae* [NTHi] Protein D, Diphtheria or Tetanus Toxoid Conjugates) Adsorbed

Pharmacologic Category Vaccine, Inactivated (Bacterial)

Use Note: Not approved in U.S.

Immunization of infants and children against *Streptococcus pneumoniae* infection and invasive diseases caused by serotypes included in the vaccine

Pregnancy Considerations Animal reproduction studies have not been conducted. Inactivated vaccines have not been shown to cause increased risks to the fetus (CDC, 2011). This product is indicated for use in infants and toddlers.

Breast-Feeding Considerations Inactivated vaccines do not affect the safety of breast-feeding for the mother or the infant. Breast-feeding infants should be vaccinated according to the recommended schedules (CDC, 2011).

Contraindications Hypersensitivity to any component of the vaccine

Warnings/Precautions Immediate treatment (including epinephrine 1:1000) for anaphylactoid and/or hypersensitivity reactions should be available during vaccine use. Packaging may contain natural latex rubber. Apnea has been reported following IM vaccine administration in premature infants; consider risk versus benefit in infants born prematurely. Infants born ≤28 weeks gestation, particularly those with a prior history of respiratory immaturity, may require respiratory function monitoring for 2-3 days after administration. Syncope has been reported with use of injectable vaccines and may be accompanied by transient visual disturbances, weakness, or tonic-clonic movements.

Procedures should be in place to avoid injuries from falling and to restore cerebral perfusion if syncope occurs.

Not to be used to treat pneumococcal infections. Safety and efficacy in children at increased risk for pneumococcal infection (eg, sickle cell disease, splenic dysfunction, HIV infection, malignancy, nephrotic syndrome) has not been established. Use with caution in severely immunocompromised patients (eg, HIV, patients receiving chemo/radiation therapy, or other immunosuppressive therapy including high-dose corticosteroids); may have a reduced response to vaccination. In general, inactivated vaccines should be administered ≥2 weeks prior to planned immunosuppression when feasible (Rubin, 2014). Use with caution in patients with a history of bleeding disorders (including thrombocytopenia) and/or patients on anticoagulant therapy; bleeding/hematoma may occur from IM administration.

Antibody response is provided only against pneumococcal serotypes included in the vaccine. Antibody response may also be observed to diphtheria toxoid, tetanus toxoid, and protein D (derived from nontypeable *Haemophilus influenzae*); however, recommended routine administration schedules for diphtheria, tetanus or *H. influenzae* type b vaccines should still be followed. In order to maximize vaccination rates, the Canadian National Advisory Committee on Immunization (NACI) recommends simultaneous administration of all age-appropriate vaccines (live or inactivated) for which a person is eligible at a single clinic visit, unless contraindications exist. The decision to administer or delay vaccination because of current or recent febrile illness depends on the severity of symptoms and the etiology of the disease. Immunization should be delayed during the course of an acute severe febrile illness; may administer to patients with mild acute illness. Vaccination may not result in effective immunity in all patients. Response depends upon multiple factors (eg, type of vaccine, age of patient) and may be improved by administering the vaccine at the recommended dose, route, and interval. Vaccines may not be effective if administered during periods of altered immune competence (CDC, 2011).

Administration of acetaminophen prior to or immediately following vaccination may reduce incidence and severity of vaccine related fever, although it has been reported that routine prophylactic administration of acetaminophen to prevent fever prior to vaccination, decreased the immune response of some vaccines; the clinical significance of this reduction in immune response has not been established (Prymula, 2009).

Adverse Reactions In Canada, adverse reactions may be reported to local provincial/territorial health agencies or to the Vaccine Safety Section at Public Health Agency of Canada (1-866-844-0018).

Central nervous system: Drowsiness, fever (≥38°C rectally ages <2-5 years), headache, irritability

Gastrointestinal: Loss of appetite

Local: Injection site reactions: Induration, pain, redness, swelling

Rare but important or life-threatening: Abnormal crying; allergic reactions (allergic dermatitis, atopic dermatitis, eczema); apnea in premature infants ≤28 weeks gestation, diarrhea, fever (>39°C rectally age 2-5 years; >40°C rectally age <2 years), injection site hematoma, injection site hemorrhage, injection site nodule, rash, seizure (febrile and nonfebrile), urticaria, vomiting

Drug Interactions

Metabolism/Transport Effects None known.

Avoid Concomitant Use There are no known interactions where it is recommended to avoid concomitant use.

Increased Effect/Toxicity There are no known significant interactions involving an increase in effect.

Decreased Effect

The levels/effects of Pneumococcal Conjugate Vaccine (10-Valent) may be decreased by: Belimumab; Immunosuppressants

Storage/Stability Store at 2°C to 8°C (36°F to 46°F) and in original packaging to protect from light. Do not freeze; discard the vaccine if frozen or exposed to temperatures >37°C (>99°F). Vaccine should be administered upon removal from refrigeration; however, the manufacturer labeling states the vaccine may be administered if left outside of refrigeration for ≤3 days at 8°C to 25°C (46°F to 77°F) or if left outside of refrigeration for ≤1 day at 25°C to 37°C (77°F to 99°F).

Mechanism of Action Promotes active immunization against invasive disease caused by *S. pneumoniae* capsular serotypes 1, 4, 5, 6B, 7F, 9V, 14, 18C, 19F, and 23F, all which are individually conjugated to a carrier protein (protein D, tetanus toxoid, or diphtheria toxoid); the aluminum salt, a mineral adjuvant, enhances the antibody response.

Dosage IM:

Infants and Children:

Primary immunization: Infants 6 weeks to 6 months:

Three-dose primary series: 0.5 mL/dose for 3 doses, followed by a booster dose (for a total of 4 doses). The first dose may be given as young as 6 weeks of age, but is typically given at 2 months of age. The second and third doses should be administered at 4- and 6 months of age. The booster dose should be administered at 12-15 months; allow a minimum interval of 1 month between each of the first 3 doses, and 6 months between dose 3 and the booster dose.

Two-dose primary series: 0.5 mL/dose for 2 doses, followed by a booster dose (for a total of 3 doses). The first dose may be given as young as 6 weeks of age, but is typically given at 2 months of age. The second dose should be administered at 4 months of age. The booster dose should be administered at 11-12 months; allow a minimum interval of 2 months between doses 1 and 2, and 6 months between doses 2 and the booster dose. **Note:** May not provide optimal protection particularly in infants at high risk for pneumococcal disease (eg, asplenia, sickle-cell disease, immunosuppressed).

Previously unvaccinated Older Infants and Children:

Children 7-11 months: 0.5 mL/dose for a total of 3 doses; 2 doses administered at least 1 month apart, followed by a third dose administered after 1 year of age, separated from the second dose by at least 2 months

Children 12-23 months: 0.5 mL/dose for a total of 2 doses, administered at least 2 months apart (manufacturer labeling suggests that a booster dose may be necessary for optimal protection). **Note:** Two-dose regimen in children 12-23 months of age at high risk for pneumococcal disease (eg, asplenia, sickle-cell disease, immunosuppressed) may not provide optimal protection.

Children ≥24 months to <6 years: 0.5 mL/dose for a total of 2 doses, administered at least 2 months apart

Dosage adjustment in renal impairment: No dosage adjustment provided in manufacturer's labeling.

Dosage adjustment in hepatic impairment: No dosage adjustment provided in manufacturer's labeling.

Administration Shake well before use. Administer by IM injection only, preferably into the anterolateral aspect of the thigh in infants and into the deltoid in children. Do not administer intravenously or intradermally. Subcutaneous administration has not been studied.

Rule out bleeding disorders in patients <2 years of age prior to immunization. NACI recommends that patients with bleeding disorders receive all routine recommended vaccinations according to schedule. Bleeding disorders should be corrected prior to immunization (when possible) or immunization should be scheduled shortly after antihemophilia or other similar therapy. In patients with bleeding disorder that cannot be corrected, IM gluteal injections should be avoided (if possible). When immunizing patients with bleeding disorders, a fine-gauge needle of the appropriate length can be used for the vaccination and firm pressure applied to the site (without rubbing) for at least 5 minutes. The patient should be instructed concerning the risk of hematoma from the injection. Patients on anticoagulant therapy (eg, aspirin, warfarin, heparin) may be immunized via intramuscular injection without discontinuation of their anticoagulant therapy (NACI, 2006).

Simultaneous administration of vaccines helps ensure the patients will be fully vaccinated by the appropriate age. Simultaneous administration of vaccines is defined as administering >1 vaccine on the same day at different anatomic sites. Separate vaccines should not be combined in the same syringe unless indicated by product specific labeling.

Monitoring Parameters Consider respiratory monitoring for 48-72 hours in premature infants (born ≤28 weeks gestation) due to risk of apnea. Monitor for syncope for 15 minutes following administration. If seizure-like activity associated with syncope occurs, maintain patient in supine or Trendelenburg position to reestablish adequate cerebral perfusion.

Product Availability Not available in the U.S.

Dosage Forms: Canada

Injection, suspension:

Synflorix™: 1 mcg of each capsular saccharide for serotypes 1, 5, 6B, 7F, 9V, 14, and 23F, and 3 mcg each of serotypes 4, 18C, and 19F (bound to protein D [from nontypeable *H. Influenzae*], tetanus toxoid, or diphtheria toxoid) per 0.5 mL (0.5 mL)

Pneumococcal Conjugate Vaccine (13-Valent)

(noo moe KOK al KON ju gate vak SEEN, thur TEEN vay lent)

Brand Names: U.S. Prevnar 13

Brand Names: Canada Prevnar 13

Index Terms PCV13; Pneumococcal 13-Valent Conjugate Vaccine

Pharmacologic Category Vaccine, Inactivated (Bacterial)

Additional Appendix Information

Immunization Administration Recommendations *on page 2250*

Immunization Recommendations *on page 2255*

Use

U.S. labeling:

Immunization of children 6 weeks through 17 years of age against *Streptococcus pneumoniae* infection caused by serotypes included in the vaccine

Immunization of children 6 weeks through 5 years of age against otitis media caused by *Streptococcus pneumoniae* serotypes 4, 6B, 9V, 14, 18C, 19F, and 23F

Immunization of adults ≥50 years against pneumococcal pneumonia and invasive disease caused by *Streptococcus pneumoniae* serotypes included in the vaccine

Canadian labeling:

Immunization of children 6 weeks through 17 years of age against *Streptococcus pneumoniae* infection caused by serotypes included in the vaccine

Immunization of adults ≥50 years against pneumococcal pneumonia and invasive disease caused by *Streptococcus pneumoniae* serotypes included in the vaccine

The Advisory Committee on Immunization Practices (ACIP) recommends routine vaccination for the following (CDC/ACIP [Nuorti, 2010]):

All children age 2 to 59 months

Children 60 to 71 months with underlying medical conditions including:

Immunocompetent children with chronic heart disease (particularly cyanotic congenital heart disease and heart failure), chronic lung disease (including asthma if treated with high dose corticosteroids), diabetes, cerebrospinal fluid leaks, or cochlear implants

Children with functional or anatomic asplenia, including sickle cell disease or other hemoglobinopathies, congenital or acquired asplenia, or splenic dysfunction.

Children with immunocompromising conditions including congenital immunodeficiency (includes B or T cell deficiency, compliment deficiencies and phagocytic disorders; excludes chronic granulomatous disease), HIV infection, chronic renal failure, nephrotic syndrome, leukemia, lymphoma, Hodgkin disease, generalized malignancies, solid organ transplant, or other diseases requiring immunosuppressive drugs (including long term systemic corticosteroids and radiation therapy)

Children who received ≥1 dose of PCV7

Note: Routine use is not recommended for healthy children ≥5 years of age.

Children ≥6 years and Adolescents ≤18 years of age (CDC/ACIP, 62[25], 2013), and Adults ≥19 years of age (CDC/ACIP, 61[40], 2012): The ACIP also recommends routine vaccination for persons with the following underlying medical conditions:

Immunocompetent persons with cerebrospinal fluid leaks or cochlear implants

Persons with functional or anatomic asplenia, including sickle cell disease or other hemoglobinopathies, congenital or acquired asplenia

Persons with immunocompromising conditions including congenital or acquired immunodeficiency (includes B or T cell deficiency, compliment deficiencies and phagocytic disorders; excludes chronic granulomatous disease), HIV infection, chronic renal failure, nephrotic syndrome, leukemia, lymphoma, Hodgkin disease, generalized malignancies, solid organ transplant, multiple myeloma, or other diseases requiring immunosuppressive drugs (including long term systemic corticosteroids and radiation therapy)

All adults ≥65 years (CDC/ACIP [Tomczyk, 2014])

Pregnancy Risk Factor B

Dosage

Infants, Children, and Adolescents:

Primary immunization: *Infants and Children 6 weeks to 59 months:* IM: 0.5 mL/dose for a total of 4 doses. The first dose may be given as young as 6 weeks of age, but is typically given at 8 weeks (2 months of age). The 3 remaining doses are usually given at 4, 6, and 12-15 months of age. The recommended dosing interval is 4-8 weeks. The minimum interval between doses in children <1 year of age is 1 month. The minimum interval between the third and fourth dose is 8 weeks.

Immunization: *Older Infants, Children, and Adolescents:*

Children 7-11 months (previously unvaccinated): IM: 0.5 mL for a total of 3 doses; 2 doses at least 4 weeks apart, followed by a third dose after the 1-year birthday (12-15 months), separated from the second dose by at least 8 weeks

Children 12-23 months (previously unvaccinated): IM: 0.5 mL for a total of 2 doses, separated by at least 8 weeks

Healthy Children 24-59 months (previously unvaccinated): IM: 0.5 mL as a single dose

Children 24-71 months with an underlying medical condition (previously unvaccinated): IM: 0.5 mL for a total of 2 doses, separated by 8 weeks (CDC/ACIP [Nuorti, 2010])

Children 6 through 17 years: IM: 0.5 mL as a single dose. If PCV7 was previously administered, give PCV13 ≥8 weeks after that dose

Previously vaccinated with PCV7 and/or PCV13, and with a lapse in vaccine administration (CDC/ACIP [Nuorti, 2010]):

Children 7-11 months: Previously received 1 or 2 doses: IM: 0.5 mL dose at 7-11 months of age, followed by a second dose ≥8 weeks later at 12-15 months of age

Children 12-23 months:

Previously received 1 dose <12 months of age: IM: 0.5 mL dose, followed by a second dose ≥8 weeks later

Previously received 1 dose at ≥12 months of age: IM: 0.5 mL dose ≥8 weeks after the most recent dose

Previously received 2 or 3 doses before age 12 months: IM: 0.5 mL dose ≥8 weeks after the most recent dose

Healthy Children 24-59 months with any incomplete schedule: IM: 0.5 mL dose ≥ 8 weeks after the most recent dose

Children 24-71 months with an underlying medical condition:

Previously received <3 doses: IM: 0.5 mL dose ≥8 weeks after the most recent dose, followed by a second dose ≥8 weeks later

Previously received 3 doses: IM: 0.5 mL as a single dose ≥8 weeks after the most recent dose

Previously vaccinated with PCV7 and completed vaccination series of 4 doses (CDC/ACIP [Nuorti, 2010]):

Children 14-59 months: IM: 0.5 mL as a single supplemental dose ≥8 weeks after the most recent dose

Children 60-71 months with an underlying medical condition: IM: 0.5 mL as a single supplemental dose ≥8 weeks after the most recent dose of PCV7 or PPSV23

Children ≥6 years and Adolescents ≤18 years with specified underlying medical conditions (CDC 62 [25], 2013):

Pneumococcal vaccine-naïve (no previous PCV13 or PPSV23 vaccine): IM: Administer PCV13 0.5 mL as a single dose, followed by 1 dose of PPSV23 ≥8-weeks later

Previously vaccinated with PPSV23: If PCV13 has never been administered, give PCV13 0.5 mL IM as a single dose ≥8 weeks after the last dose of PPSV23. PCV13 should be administered even if the child had received PCV7.

Adults: **Immunization:**

Adults ≥19 years with specified underlying medical conditions (CDC 61[40], 2012): Eligible adults should be vaccinated at their next pneumococcal vaccination opportunity

Pneumococcal vaccine naïve (no previous PCV13 or PPSV23 vaccine): IM: Administer PCV13 0.5 mL as a single dose followed by 1 dose of PPSV23 8 weeks later

Previously vaccinated with PPSV23: IM: PCV13 0.5 mL as a single dose ≥1 year after the last dose of PPSV23. **Note:** Although the ACIP recommends waiting at least one year, immunogenicity of PCV13 administered <5 years after PPSV23 is unknown

Adults ≥50 years (manufacturers labeling): 0.5 mL as a single dose

Adults ≥65 years: **Note:** All patients should receive both pneumococcal conjugate vaccine (PCV13) and pneumococcal polysaccharide vaccine (PPSV23) (CDC/ACIP [Tomczyk, 2014]):

Pneumococcal vaccine-naïve: IM: Administer PCV13 0.5 ml as a single dose, followed by PPSV23 6 to 12 months later (minimum interval of 8 weeks)

Previously received pneumococcal polysaccharide vaccine (PPSV23):

Received at age <65 years: IM: Administer PCV13 0.5 mL as a single dose ≥1 year after the last dose of PPSV23, followed by PPSV23 at least 6 to 12 months after the PCV13 dose and at least 5 years after the last dose of PPSV23

Received at age ≥65 years: IM: Administer PCV13 0.5 mL as a single dose ≥1 year after the last dose of PPSV23; no additional doses of PPSV23 are needed for routine vaccination

Dosage adjustment in renal impairment: There are no dosage adjustments provided in the manufacturer's labeling.

Dosage adjustment in hepatic impairment: There are no dosage adjustments provided in the manufacturer's labeling.

Additional Information Complete prescribing information should be consulted for additional detail.

Dosage Forms

Injection, suspension:

Prevnar 13: 2 mcg of each capsular saccharide for serotypes 1, 3, 4, 5, 6A, 7F, 9V, 14, 18C, 19A, 19F, and 23F, and 4 mcg of serotype 6B [bound to diphtheria CRM_{197} protein ~34 mcg] per 0.5 mL (0.5 mL)

◆ **Pneumococcal Conjugate Vaccine (Nontypeable *Haemophilus influenzae* [NTHi] Protein D, Diphtheria or Tetanus Toxoid Conjugates) Adsorbed** *see* Pneumococcal Conjugate Vaccine (10-Valent) [CAN/INT] *on page* 1668

◆ **Pneumococcal 13-Valent Conjugate Vaccine** *see* Pneumococcal Conjugate Vaccine (13-Valent) *on page* 1670

◆ **Pneumo 23 (Can)** *see* Pneumococcal Polysaccharide Vaccine (23-Valent) *on page* 1671

Pneumococcal Polysaccharide Vaccine (23-Valent)

(noo moe KOK al pol i SAK a ride vak SEEN, TWEN tee three VAY lent)

Brand Names: U.S. Pneumovax 23

Brand Names: Canada Pneumo 23; Pneumovax 23

Index Terms 23-Valent Pneumococcal Polysaccharide Vaccine; 23PS; Pneumococcal Polysaccharide Vaccine (Polyvalent); PPSV; PPSV23; PPV23

Pharmacologic Category Vaccine, Inactivated (Bacterial)

Additional Appendix Information

Immunization Administration Recommendations *on page* 2250

Immunization Recommendations *on page* 2255

Use

Pneumococcal disease prevention: Active immunization of children ≥2 years and persons ≥50 years who are at increased risk for pneumococcal disease caused by the 23 serotypes included in the vaccine.

The Advisory Committee on Immunization Practices (ACIP) recommends routine vaccination for patients with the following underlying medical conditions (CDC 59[34], 2010; CDC/ACIP 61[40], 2012]; CDC/ACIP [Nuorti, 2010]; CDC/ACIP [Tomczyk 2014]):

Children ≥2 years of age, adolescents, and adults 19 to 64 years with functional or anatomic asplenia, including sickle cell disease or other hemoglobinopathies, congenital or acquired asplenia, splenic dysfunction, or splenectomy

Immunocompetent children ≥2 years of age and adolescents with chronic heart disease (particularly cyanotic congenital heart disease and heart failure), chronic lung disease (including asthma if treated with high dose corticosteroids), diabetes, cerebrospinal fluid leaks, or cochlear implants

Immunocompetent adults 19 to 64 years with chronic heart disease (including heart failure and cardiomyopathies; excluding hypertension), chronic lung disease (including COPD, emphysema, and asthma), diabetes, cerebrospinal fluid leaks, cochlear implants, alcoholism, chronic liver disease, cirrhosis, and cigarette smokers

Immunocompromised children ≥2 years of age, adolescents, and adults 19 to 64 years with congenital or acquired immunodeficiency (includes B or T cell deficiency, compliment deficiencies and phagocytic disorders; excludes chronic granulomatous disease), HIV infection, chronic renal failure, nephrotic syndrome, leukemia, lymphoma, Hodgkin disease, generalized malignancies, solid organ transplant, multiple myeloma, or other diseases requiring immunosuppressive drugs (including long-term systemic corticosteroids and radiation therapy)

All adults ≥65 years of age

Pregnancy Risk Factor C

Dosage

Children ≥2 years: IM, SubQ: 0.5 mL as a single dose

Primary vaccination: Children with specified underlying medical conditions: One dose of PPSV23 should be given at ≥2 years of age. Immunization with PCV13 should be completed prior to PPSV23 as recommended. The minimum interval between the last dose of PCV13 and PPSV23 is 8 weeks (CDC/ACIP [Nuorti, 2010]).

Revaccination: Children with functional or anatomic asplenia, or who are immunocompromised: One revaccination dose ≥5 years after the first dose of PPSV23. Revaccination of immunocompetent individuals is generally not recommended (CDC/ACIP [Nuorti, 2010]).

Adults 19 to <65 years: IM, SubQ: 0.5 mL as a single dose

Primary vaccination: Adults 19 to 64 years with specified underlying medical conditions and all patients at 65 years of age without previous PPSV23 vaccination should receive one dose of PPSV23 (CDC 59[34], 2010). In patients with specified underlying medical conditions who are pneumococcal vaccine naïve (no previous PCV13 or PPSV23 vaccine), administer a single dose of PCV13 followed by 1 dose of PPSV23 8 weeks later (CDC 61[40], 2012).

Revaccination: Adults 19 to 64 years with functional or anatomic asplenia, chronic renal failure or nephrotic syndrome, or who are immunocompromised: One revaccination dose ≥5 years after first dose of PPSV23 (CDC 59[34], 2010) and ≥8 weeks after PCV13 (CDC 61[40], 2012)

Adults ≥65 years: IM, SubQ: 0.5 mL as a single dose

Note: All patients should receive both pneumococcal conjugate vaccine (PCV 13) and pneumococcal polysaccharide vaccine (PPSV23) (CDC/ACIP [Tomczyk 2014]):

Pneumococcal vaccine-naive or vaccination status unknown: Administer PCV13 followed by PPSV23 6 to 12 months later (minimum interval of 8 weeks)

Previously received pneumococcal polysaccharide vaccine (PPSV23):

Received at age <65 years: Administer PCV13 ≥1 year after the last dose of PPSV23, followed by PPSV23 6 to 12 months later (and ≥5 years after the last dose of PPSV23)

Received at age ≥65 years: Administer PCV13 ≥1 year after the last dose of PPSV23; no additional PPSV23 doses are needed for routine vaccination

Dosage adjustment in renal impairment: There are no dosage adjustments provided in the manufacturer's labeling.

Dosage adjustment in hepatic impairment: There are no dosage adjustments provided in the manufacturer's labeling.

Additional Information Complete prescribing information should be consulted for additional detail.

Dosage Forms

Injection, solution:

Pneumovax 23: 25 mcg each of 23 capsular polysaccharide isolates/0.5 mL (0.5 mL, 2.5 mL)

◆ **Pneumococcal Polysaccharide Vaccine (Polyvalent)** *see* Pneumococcal Polysaccharide Vaccine (23-Valent) *on page 1671*

◆ **Pneumovax 23** *see* Pneumococcal Polysaccharide Vaccine (23-Valent) *on page 1671*

◆ **PNU-140690E** *see* Tipranavir *on page 2047*

◆ **Podactin [OTC]** *see* Miconazole (Topical) *on page 1360*

◆ **Podactin [OTC]** *see* Tolnaftate *on page 2063*

◆ **Podocon** *see* Podophyllum Resin *on page 1672*

◆ **Podofilm® (Can)** *see* Podophyllum Resin *on page 1672*

◆ **Podophyllin** *see* Podophyllum Resin *on page 1672*

Podophyllum Resin (po DOF fil um REZ in)

Brand Names: U.S. Podocon

Brand Names: Canada Podofilm®

Index Terms Mandrake; May Apple; Podophyllin

Pharmacologic Category Keratolytic Agent

Use Topical treatment of soft external genital (venereal) warts (condylomata acuminata); compound benzoin tincture generally is used as the medium for topical application

Dosage Topical: Children and Adults: Condylomata acuminatum: Applied by physician only.

Additional Information Complete prescribing information should be consulted for additional detail.

Dosage Forms

Solution, External:

Podocon: 25% (15 mL)

Polidocanol (pol i DOE kuh nol)

Brand Names: U.S. Asclera; Varithena

Pharmacologic Category Sclerosing Agent

Use Varicose veins:

Asclera: To treat uncomplicated spider veins (varicose veins 1 mm or less in diameter) and uncomplicated reticular veins (varicose veins 1 to 3 mm in diameter) in the lower extremity.

Varithena: To treat incompetent great saphenous veins, accessory saphenous veins, and visible varicosities of the great saphenous vein system above and below the knee.

Pregnancy Risk Factor C

Dosage IV: Adults: Varicose veins:

Asclera:

Reticular veins (1 to 3 mm diameter): 0.1 to 0.3 mL of 1% solution per injection (maximum: 10 mL per session); may repeat in 7 to 14 days

Spider veins (≤1 mm diameter): 0.1 to 0.3 mL of 0.5% solution per injection (maximum: 10 mL per session); may repeat in 7 to 14 days

Varithena: *Great saphenous veins and accessory saphenous veins:* 5 mL of 1% solution per injection (maximum: 15 mL per session); may repeat in ≥5 days

Dosage adjustment in renal impairment: There are no dosage adjustments provided in manufacturer's labeling.

Dosage adjustment in hepatic impairment: There are no dosage adjustments provided in manufacturer's labeling.

Additional Information Complete prescribing information should be consulted for additional detail.

Dosage Forms

Foam, Intravenous:

Varithena: 180 mg/18 mL (45 mL)

Solution, Intravenous [preservative free]:

Asclera: 0.5% (2 mL); 1% (2 mL)

◆ **Polio Vaccine** *see* Poliovirus Vaccine (Inactivated) *on page 1673*

◆ **Poliovirus, Inactivated (IPV)** *see* Diphtheria and Tetanus Toxoids, Acellular Pertussis, and Poliovirus Vaccine *on page 646*

◆ **Poliovirus, Inactivated (IPV)** *see* Diphtheria and Tetanus Toxoids, Acellular Pertussis, Poliovirus and *Haemophilus* b Conjugate Vaccine *on page 648*

Poliovirus Vaccine (Inactivated)

(POE lee oh VYE rus vak SEEN, in ak ti VAY ted)

Brand Names: U.S. IPOL

Brand Names: Canada Imovax Polio

Index Terms Enhanced-Potency Inactivated Poliovirus Vaccine; IPV; Polio Vaccine; Salk Vaccine

Pharmacologic Category Vaccine, Inactivated (Viral)

Additional Appendix Information

Immunization Administration Recommendations *on page 2250*

Immunization Recommendations *on page 2255*

Use Active immunization against poliomyelitis caused by poliovirus types 1, 2, and 3. **Note:** Combination products containing polio vaccine are also available and may be preferred in certain age groups if recipients are likely to be susceptible to the agents contained within each vaccine.

The Advisory Committee on Immunization Practices (ACIP) recommends routine vaccination for the following:

- All infants and children (first dose given at 2 months of age) (CDC, 58[30], 2009)

Routine immunization of adults in the United States is generally not recommended. Adults with previous wild poliovirus disease, who have never been immunized, or those who are incompletely immunized may receive inactivated poliovirus vaccine if they fall into one of the following categories (CDC/ACIP [Prevots, 2000]):

- Travelers to regions or countries where poliomyelitis is endemic or epidemic
- Healthcare workers in close contact with patients who may be excreting poliovirus
- Laboratory workers handling specimens that may contain poliovirus
- Members of communities or specific population groups with diseases caused by wild poliovirus
- Incompletely vaccinated or unvaccinated adults in a household or with other close contact with children receiving oral poliovirus (may be at increased risk of vaccine associated paralytic poliomyelitis)

Pregnancy Risk Factor C

Dosage IM, SubQ:

Children:

Primary immunization: Administer three 0.5 mL doses, at 2, 4, and 6 to 18 months of age; do not administer more frequently than 4 weeks apart (preferably given more than 8 weeks apart)

Booster dose: 0.5 mL at 4 to 6 years of age; Minimum interval between booster and previous dose is 6 months. The final (booster) dose should be given at ≥4 years of age, regardless of the number of previous doses. If the final dose is not given at 4 to 6 years of age, it should be given as soon as feasible.

Note: Use of the minimum age and minimum intervals during the first 6 months of life should only be done when the vaccine recipient is at risk for imminent exposure to circulating poliovirus (shorter intervals and earlier start dates may lead to lower seroconversion).

Adults:

Previously unvaccinated: Two 0.5 mL doses administered at 1- to 2-month intervals, followed by a third dose to 12 months later. If <3 months, but at least 2 months are available before protection is needed, 3 doses may be administered at least 1 month apart. If administration must be completed within 1 to 2 months, give 2 doses at least 1 month apart. If <1 month is available, give 1 dose.

Incompletely vaccinated: Adults with at least 1 previous dose of OPV, <3 doses of IPV, or a combination of OPV and IPV equaling <3 doses, administer at least one 0.5 mL dose of IPV. Additional doses to complete the series may be given if time permits.

Completely vaccinated and at increased risk of exposure: One 0.5 mL dose

Dosage adjustment in renal impairment: There are no dosage adjustments provided in the manufacturer's labeling.

Dosage adjustment in hepatic impairment: There are no dosage adjustments provided in the manufacturer's labeling.

Additional Information Complete prescribing information should be consulted for additional detail.

Dosage Forms

Injection, suspension:

IPOL: Type 1 poliovirus 40 D-antigen units, type 2 poliovirus 8 D-antigen units, and type 3 poliovirus 32 D-antigen units per 0.5 mL (0.5 mL, 5 mL)

◆ **Polocaine** *see* Mepivacaine *on page 1295*

◆ **Polocaine® (Can)** *see* Mepivacaine *on page 1295*

◆ **Polocaine-MPF** *see* Mepivacaine *on page 1295*

◆ **Polycin™** *see* Bacitracin and Polymyxin B *on page 222*

◆ **Polycitra** *see* Citric Acid, Sodium Citrate, and Potassium Citrate *on page 455*

◆ **Polycitra K** *see* Potassium Citrate and Citric Acid *on page 1689*

Polyestradiol [INT] (pol i es tra DYE ole)

International Brand Names Estradurin (CH, DE, DK, ES, FI, NL, NO, SE)

Index Terms Polyestradiol Phosphate

Pharmacologic Category Antineoplastic Agent, Miscellaneous; Estrogen Derivative

Reported Use Palliative treatment of advanced, inoperable carcinoma of the prostate

Dosage Range Adults: Deep I.M.: 80-160 mg every 4 weeks for 2-3 months, followed by 40-80 mg every 4 weeks

Product Availability Product available in various countries; not currently available in the U.S.

Dosage Forms

Powder for injection, as phosphate: 40 mg

◆ **Polyestradiol Phosphate** *see* Polyestradiol [INT] *on page 1673*

◆ **Polyethylene Glycol-L-asparaginase** *see* Pegaspargase *on page 1588*

Polyethylene Glycol 3350

(pol i ETH i leen GLY kol 3350)

Brand Names: U.S. GaviLAX [OTC]; GlycoLax [OTC]; HealthyLax [OTC]; MiraLax [OTC]; PEGyLAX

Brand Names: Canada Peg 3350; Pegalax; Relaxa

Index Terms Macrogol; PEG

Pharmacologic Category Laxative, Osmotic

Use Treatment of occasional constipation in adults

Dosage Oral:

Children ≥6 months: Occasional constipation (off-label use): 0.5-1.5 g/kg daily (initial dose: 0.5-1 g/kg; titrate to effect); not to exceed 17 g/day; do not use for >2 weeks (Bell, 2004; Loening-Baucke, 2005; Michail, 2004; Voskuijl, 2004)

Adults:

Occasional constipation: 17 g of powder (~1 heaping tablespoon) dissolved in 4-8 ounces of beverage, once daily; do not use for >1 week unless directed by healthcare provider

Bowel preparation before colonoscopy (off-label use): Mix 17 g of powder (~1 heaping tablespoon) in 8 ounces of clear liquid and administer the entire mixture every 10 minutes until 2 L are consumed (start within 6 hours after administering 20 mg bisacodyl delayed-release tablets) (Wexner, 2006)

Additional Information Complete prescribing information should be consulted for additional detail.

Dosage Forms

Packet, Oral:

HealthyLax [OTC]: (1 ea, 14 ea)
MiraLax [OTC]: (1 ea, 10 ea, 12 ea, 24 ea)
Generic: (1 ea, 14 ea, 30 ea, 100 ea)

Powder, Oral:

GaviLAX [OTC]: (238 g, 510 g)
GlycoLax [OTC]: (119 g, 255 g, 527 g)
MiraLax [OTC]: (1 ea, 119 g, 238 g, 510 g)
PEGyLAX: (527 g)
Generic: 17 g/dose (119 g, 238 g, 510 g); (119 g, 238 g, 250 g, 255 g, 500 g, 510 g, 527 g, 850 g)

Dosage Forms: Canada

Powder, Oral: 17 g/dose (238 g, 510 g)
Sachet, Oral:17 g/sachet (4 ea, 14 ea)

◆ **Polyethylene Glycol-Conjugated Uricase** *see* Pegloticase *on page 1602*

Polyethylene Glycol-Electrolyte Solution

(pol i ETH i leen GLY kol ee LEK troe lite soe LOO shun)

Brand Names: U.S. Colyte; GaviLyte-C; GaviLyte-G; GaviLyte-N; GoLYTELY; MoviPrep; NuLYTELY; TriLyte

Brand Names: Canada Colyte; Klean-Prep; PegLyte

Index Terms Electrolyte Lavage Solution

Pharmacologic Category Laxative, Osmotic

Use Bowel cleansing prior to colonoscopy or barium enema X-ray examination

Pregnancy Risk Factor C

Pregnancy Considerations Animal reproduction studies have not been conducted. Information related to the use of polyethylene glycol-electrolyte solution in pregnancy is limited (Neri, 2004). Colonoscopy in pregnant women is generally reserved for strong indications or life-threatening emergencies; until additional safety data for polyethylene glycol-electrolyte solution is available, other agents may be preferred for this purpose (Siddiqui, 2006; Wexner, 2006).

Breast-Feeding Considerations It is not known if polyethylene glycol-electrolyte solution is excreted into breast milk. Significant changes in the mother's fluid or electrolyte balance would not be expected with most products.

Contraindications Hypersensitivity to polyethylene glycol or any component of the formulation; ileus, gastrointestinal obstruction, gastric retention, bowel perforation, toxic colitis, toxic megacolon

Warnings/Precautions Evaluate patients with symptoms of bowel obstruction or perforation (nausea, vomiting, abdominal pain or distension) prior to use; if a patient develops severe bloating, distention or abdominal pain during administration, slow the rate of administration or temporarily discontinue use until the symptoms subside. Correct electrolyte abnormalities in patients prior to use. No additional ingredients or flavors (other than the flavor packets provided) should be added to the polyethylene glycol-electrolyte solution.

Fluid and electrolyte disturbances can lead to arrhythmias, seizures, and renal impairment. Advise patients to maintain adequate hydration before, during, and after treatment. If patient becomes dehydrated or experiences significant vomiting after treatment, consider post-colonoscopy lab tests (electrolytes, creatinine, and BUN). Serious arrhythmias have been reported (rarely) with the use of ionic osmotic laxative products. Use with caution in patients who may be at risk of cardiac arrhythmias (eg, patients with a history of prolonged QT, uncontrolled arrhythmias, recent MI, unstable angina, CHF, or cardiomyopathy). Consider pre-dose and post-colonoscopy ECGs in these patients. Generalized tonic-clonic seizures and/or loss of consciousness have occurred rarely in patients with no prior history of seizures. Seizures resolved with the correction of fluid and electrolyte abnormalities. Use with caution in patients with a history of seizures or who are at an increased risk of seizures (eg, concomitant administration of medications that lower the seizures threshold, patients withdrawing from alcohol or benzodiazepines) and in patients with known or suspected hyponatremia or low serum osmolality.

Cases of ischemic colitis have been reported; concomitant use of stimulant laxatives may increase the risk and is not recommended. The potential for mucosal aphthous ulcerations as a result of the bowel preparation should be considered, especially when evaluating colonoscopy results in patients with known or suspected inflammatory bowel disease. Use with caution in patients with severe ulcerative colitis. Use with caution in patients with renal impairment and/or in patients taking medications that may adversely affect renal function (eg, diuretics, NSAIDs, ACE inhibitors, ARBs). Patients with impaired renal function should be instructed to remain adequately hydrated; consider pre-dose and post-colonoscopy lab tests (electrolytes, creatinine, BUN) in these patients. Observe unconscious or semiconscious patients with impaired gag reflex or those who are otherwise prone to regurgitation or aspiration during administration; use with caution.

MoviPrep: Use with caution in patients with G6PD deficiency (especially patients with an active infection, history of hemolysis, or taking concomitant medications known to precipitate hemolytic reactions) due to the presence of sodium ascorbate and ascorbic acid in the formulation. Contains phenylalanine.

Use in patients <2 years of age may result in hypoglycemia, dehydration, and hypokalemia; use with caution and monitor closely. Use with caution in patients >60 years of age; serious adverse events have been reported (eg, asystole, esophageal perforation, chest infiltration following vomiting and aspiration, Mallory-Weiss tear with GI bleeding, pulmonary edema with sudden dyspnea).

Adverse Reactions

Central nervous system: Dizziness, headache, malaise, rigors, sleep disorder

Endocrine & metabolic: Increased thirst

Gastrointestinal: Abdominal distention, abdominal pain, anorectal pain, bloating, dyspepsia, hunger, nausea, vomiting

Rare but important or life-threatening: Anaphylaxis, angioedema, aspiration, asystole (older adults >60 years), chest tightness, esophageal perforation (older adults >60 years), hypersensitivity reaction, ischemic colitis, Mallory-Weiss syndrome (older adults >60 years), pulmonary edema (older adults >60 years), rhinorrhea, seizure, shock, tightness in chest and throat, upper gastrointestinal hemorrhage (older adults >60 years), urticaria

Drug Interactions

Metabolism/Transport Effects None known.

Avoid Concomitant Use There are no known interactions where it is recommended to avoid concomitant use.

Increased Effect/Toxicity There are no known significant interactions involving an increase in effect.

Decreased Effect There are no known significant interactions involving a decrease in effect.

Preparation for Administration

CoLyte, GaviLyte-C, GaviLyte-G, GaviLyte-N, GoLYTELY, NuLYTELY, TriLyte: Using the container provided, add lukewarm water (may use tap water) up to the 4 L water mark; shake vigorously several times to ensure dissolution of the powder. No additional ingredients or flavors should be added to the solution (other than the flavor packets provided).

MoviPrep: Mix the contents of pouch A and pouch B (one each) in container provided. Add lukewarm water to fill line (~1 L); mix the solution until dissolved. No additional ingredients or flavors should be added to the solution.

Concentrations for reconstituted solutions:

CoLyte, GaviLyte-C: When dissolved in sufficient water to make 4 L, the final solution contains PEG-3350 18 mmol/L, sodium 125 mmol/L, sulfate 80 mmol/L, chloride 35 mmol/L, bicarbonate 20 mmol/L, and potassium 10 mmol/L

GaviLyte-G, GoLYTELY: When dissolved in sufficient water to make 4 L, the final solution contains PEG-3350 17.6 mmol/L, sodium 125 mmol/L, sulfate 40 mmol/L, chloride 35 mmol/L, bicarbonate 20 mmol/L, and potassium 10 mmol/L

GaviLyte-N, NuLYTELY, TriLyte: When dissolved in sufficient water to make 4 L, the final solution contains PEG-3350 31.3 mmol/L, sodium 65 mmol/L, chloride 53 mmol/L, bicarbonate 17 mmol/L, and potassium 5 mmol/L.

Storage/Stability

CoLyte, GaviLyte-C, GaviLyte-G, GaviLyte-N, GoLYTELY, NuLYTELY, TriLyte: Prior to reconstitution, store at 25°C (77°F); excursions permitted to 15°C to 30°C (59°F to 86°F). Refrigerate reconstituted solution. Use within 48 hours of preparation; discard any unused portion.

MoviPrep: Prior to reconstitution, store at 20°C to 25°C (68°F to 77°F); excursions permitted to 15°C to 30°C (59°F to 86°F). Refrigerate reconstituted solution in an upright position. Use within 24 hours of preparation; discard any unused portion.

Mechanism of Action Induces catharsis by strong electrolyte and osmotic effects

Pharmacodynamics/Kinetics Onset of effect: Oral: ~1 hour

Dosage

Bowel cleansing:

Infants ≥6 months, Children, and Adolescents: GaviLyte-N, NuLYTELY, TriLyte: Oral, Nasogastric: 25 mL/kg/hour until the rectal effluent is clear (maximum total dose: 4 L)

Adults:

CoLyte, GaviLyte-C, GaviLyte-G, GaviLyte-N, GoLYTELY, NuLYTELY, TriLyte:

Oral: 240 mL (8 oz) every 10 minutes until 4 L are consumed or the rectal effluent is clear; rapid drinking of each portion is preferred to drinking small amounts continuously

Nasogastric: 20-30 mL/minute until 4 L are administered or the rectal effluent is clear

MoviPrep: Oral: Administer 2 L total with an additional 1 L of clear fluid prior to colonoscopy as follows:

Split dose (2 day regimen) (preferred method):

Dose 1: Evening before colonoscopy (10-12 hours before dose 2): 240 mL (8 oz) every 15 minutes until 1 L (entire contents of container) is consumed. Then fill container with 480 mL (16 oz) of clear liquid and consume prior to going to bed.

Dose 2: On the morning of the colonoscopy (beginning at least 3.5 hours prior to procedure): 240 mL (8 oz) every 15 minutes until 1 L (entire contents of container) is consumed. Then fill container with 480 mL (16 oz) of clear liquid and consume at least 2 hours before the procedure.

Evening only dose (1 day regimen) (alternate method):

Dose 1: Evening before colonoscopy (at least 3.5 hours before bedtime): 240 mL (8 oz) every 15 minutes until 1 L (entire contents of container) is consumed

Dose 2: ~90 minutes after starting dose 1: 240 mL (8 oz) every 15 minutes until 1 L (entire contents of container) is consumed. Then fill container with 1 L (32 oz) of clear liquid and consume all of the liquid prior to going to bed.

Whole bowel irrigation (off-label use; AACT, 2004): Nasogastric:

Infants ≥9 months and Children <6 years: 500 mL/hour until the rectal effluent is clear

Children ≥6 years: 1000 mL/hour until the rectal effluent is clear

Adolescents and Adults: 1500-2000 mL/hour until the rectal effluent is clear

Note: Continue treatment at least until the rectal effluent is clear; treatment duration may be extended based on corroborative evidence of continued presence of poisons in the GI tract as determined by radiographic means or the presence of the poison in the effluent.

Dosage adjustment in renal impairment: No dosage adjustment provided in manufacturer's labeling. Use with caution due to risks of fluid and electrolyte abnormalities.

Dosage adjustment in hepatic impairment: No dosage adjustment provided in manufacturer's labeling (has not been studied).

Dietary Considerations

CoLyte, GaviLyte-C, GaviLyte-G, GaviLyte-N, GoLYTELY, NuLYTELY, TriLyte: Ideally, the patient should fast for ~3-4 hours prior to administration, but in no case should solid food be given for at least 2 hours before the solution is given. Some products contain aspartame which is metabolized to phenylalanine.

MoviPrep: Patient should not eat solid food from start of solution administration until after colonoscopy. Patient may have clear liquid soup/plain yogurt for dinner; finish at least 1 hour before start of colon prep. MoviPrep contains phenylalanine.

Administration

Oral: Rapid drinking of each portion is preferred to drinking small amounts continuously. No additional ingredients or flavors (other than the flavor packets provided) should be added to the polyethylene glycol-electrolyte solution. Chilling the solution may improve palatability; administration of a chilled solution is **not** recommended in infants. Oral medications should not be administered within 1 hour of start of therapy.

Nasogastric administration: CoLyte, GaviLyte-C, GaviLyte-G, GaviLyte-N, GoLYTELY, NuLYTELY, TriLyte: The solution may be administered via nasogastric tube for bowel cleansing and whole bowel irrigation (preferred route; off-label use) in patients who are unwilling or unable to drink the solution.

Monitoring Parameters Electrolytes, serum glucose, BUN, urine osmolality; children <2 years of age should be monitored for hypoglycemia, dehydration, hypokalemia

Whole bowel irrigation (off-label use; AACT, 2004): Rectal effluent (continue until clear or the poison is completely removed)

Dosage Forms

Powder, for solution, oral: PEG 3350 240 g, sodium sulfate 22.72 g, sodium bicarbonate 6.72 g, sodium chloride 5.84 g, and potassium 2.98 g (4000 mL); PEG 3350 236 g, sodium sulfate 22.74 g, sodium bicarbonate 6.74 g, sodium chloride 5.86 g, and potassium chloride 2.97 g (4000 mL); PEG 3350 240 g, sodium bicarbonate 5.72 g, sodium chloride 11.2 g, and potassium chloride 1.48 g (4000 mL); PEG 3350 420 g, sodium bicarbonate 5.72 g, sodium chloride 11.2 g, and potassium chloride 1.48 g (4000 mL)

Colyte: PEG 3350 227.1 g, sodium sulfate 21.5 g, sodium bicarbonate 6.36 g, sodium chloride 5.53 g, and potassium chloride 2.82 g (3785 mL)

Colyte: PEG 3350 240 g, sodium sulfate 22.72 g, sodium bicarbonate 6.72 g, sodium chloride 5.84 g, and potassium 2.98 g (4000 mL)

GaviLyte-C: PEG 3350 240 g, sodium sulfate 22.72 g, sodium bicarbonate 6.72 g, sodium chloride 5.84 g, and potassium chloride 2.98 g (4000 mL)

GaviLyte-G: PEG 3350 236 g, sodium sulfate 22.74 g, sodium bicarbonate 6.74 g, sodium chloride 5.86 g, and potassium chloride 2.97 g (4000 mL)

GaviLyte-N: PEG 3350 420 g, sodium bicarbonate 5.72 g, sodium chloride 11.2 g, and potassium chloride 1.48 g (4000 mL)

GoLYTELY: PEG 3350 227.1 g, sodium sulfate 21.5 g, sodium bicarbonate 6.36 g, sodium chloride 5.53 g, and potassium 2.82 g per packet (1s)

GoLYTELY: PEG 3350 236 g, sodium sulfate 22.74 g, sodium bicarbonate 6.74 g, sodium chloride 5.86 g, and potassium 2.97 g (4000 mL)

MoviPrep: Pouch A: PEG 3350 100g, sodium sulfate 7.5 g, sodium chloride 2.69 g, potassium chloride 1.015 g; Pouch B: Ascorbic acid 4.7 g, sodium ascorbate 5.9 g

NuLYTELY: PEG 3350 420 g, sodium bicarbonate 5.72 g, sodium chloride 11.2 g, and potassium 1.48 g

TriLyte: PEG 3350 420 g, sodium bicarbonate 5.72 g, sodium chloride 11.2 g, and potassium 1.48 g

◆ **Polyethylene Glycol Interferon Alfa-2b** *see* Peginterferon Alfa-2b *on page 1596*

◆ **Poly-Iron 150 [OTC]** *see* Polysaccharide-Iron Complex *on page 1677*

Poly-L-Lactic Acid (POL i el LAK tik AS id)

Brand Names: U.S. Sculptra®; Sculptra® Aesthetic

Index Terms New-Fill®; PLA

Pharmacologic Category Cosmetic Agent, Implant

Use Restoration and/or correction of facial lipoatrophy in patients with HIV; correction of shallow to deep nasolabial fold contour deficiencies and other facial wrinkles in immunocompetent patients

Dosage Adults:

Facial wrinkles (Sculptra® Aesthetic): Intradermal: 0.1-0.2 mL per individual injection to a maximum of 2.5 mL per nasolabial fold as a single treatment; may repeat treatment at ≥3 week intervals up to 4 times

Lipoatrophy (Sculptra®): Intradermal or SubQ: ~0.05-0.2 mL per individual injection depending on technique used; ~20 injections may be needed per cheek. Treatment should be individualized. Separate treatments by ≥2 weeks. Typical course involves 3-6 treatments. Supplemental injections may be needed. Do not overfill contour deficiency. For patients with severe facial fat loss, the average treatment requires ~1 vial per cheek area per treatment.

Additional Information Complete prescribing information should be consulted for additional detail.

Dosage Forms

Injection, powder for suspension:

Sculptra®, Sculptra® Aesthetic: Poly-L-lactic acid USP

Polymyxin B (pol i MIKS in bee)

Index Terms Polymyxin B Sulfate

Pharmacologic Category Antibiotic, Irrigation; Antibiotic, Miscellaneous

Use Treatment of acute infections caused by susceptible strains of *Pseudomonas aeruginosa*; parenteral use of polymyxin B has mainly been replaced by less toxic antibiotics, reserved for life-threatening infections caused by organisms resistant to the preferred drugs (eg, pseudomonal meningitis - intrathecal administration)

Dosage

Infants and Children <2 years:

IM: Up to 40,000 units/kg/day divided every 6 hours (not routinely recommended due to pain at injection sites)

IV: Up to 40,000 units/kg/day divided every 12 hours

Intrathecal: 20,000 units daily for 3-4 days, then 25,000 units every other day for at least 2 weeks after CSF cultures are negative and CSF (glucose) has returned to within normal limits

Children ≥2 years, Adolescents, and Adults:

IM: 25,000-30,000 units/kg/day divided every 4-6 hours (not routinely recommended due to pain at injection sites)

IV: 15,000-25,000 units/kg/day divided every 12 hours

Intrathecal: 50,000 units daily for 3-4 days, then every other day for at least 2 weeks after CSF cultures are negative and CSF (glucose) has returned to within normal limits

Total daily dose should not exceed 2,000,000 units

Irrigation:

Bladder irrigation: Continuous irrigant or rinse in the urinary bladder for up to 10 days using 20 mg (equal to 200,000 units) added to 1 L of normal saline; usually no more than 1 L of irrigant is used per day unless urine flow rate is high; administration rate is adjusted to patient's urine output

Topical irrigation or topical solution: 500,000 units/L of normal saline; maximum total daily dose should not exceed 2 million units in adults

Ophthalmic: A concentration of 0.1% to 0.25% is administered as 1-3 drops to the affected eye(s) every hour, then increasing the interval as response indicates to 1-3 drops 4-6 times daily

Oral: Selective gastrointestinal tract decontamination (off-label use): 1,000,000 units orally 4 times daily, starting 2 days prior to surgery through post-operative day 3 in combination with tobramycin and amphotericin B (Roos, 2011).

Otic (in combination with other drugs): 1-2 drops, 3-4 times daily; should be used sparingly to avoid accumulation of excess debris

Dosage adjustment in renal impairment:

For individuals with renal impairment, the manufacturer's labeling recommends a dosage reduction so that the dose does not exceed 15,000 units/kg/day.

The following adjustments have been used by some clinicians (modified from Hoeprich, 1970): IV, IM:

Loading dose (first day of therapy): CrCl <80 mL/minute: 25,000 units/kg in 2 equally divided doses every 12 hours

Subsequent dosage:

CrCl 30-80 mL/minute: 10,000-15,000 units/kg in 2 equally divided doses every 12 hours

CrCl <30 mL/minute: 10,000-15,000 units/kg every 2-3 days

Anuric patients: 10,000 units/kg every 5-7 days

Hemodialysis, peritoneal dialysis (Cunha, 1988): Adults: IM: 250,000 units every 24 hours; no supplemental dose necessary.

Note: Some data suggest that renal adjustment may not be necessary since total body clearance of polymyxin B is not altered in the setting of renal impairment and nonrenal pathways are primarily responsible for elimination (Zavascki, 2008). These authors suggest that renal dosage adjustment recommendations should await further data from larger clinical trials.

Dosage adjustment in hepatic impairment: No dosage adjustment provided in manufacturer's labeling.

Additional Information Complete prescribing information should be consulted for additional detail.

Dosage Forms

Solution Reconstituted, Injection:

Generic: 500,000 units (1 ea)

Solution Reconstituted, Injection [preservative free]:

Generic: 500,000 units (1 ea)

◆ **Polymyxin B and Bacitracin** *see* Bacitracin and Polymyxin B *on page 222*

◆ **Polymyxin B and Neomycin** *see* Neomycin and Polymyxin B *on page 1437*

◆ **Polymyxin B and Trimethoprim** *see* Trimethoprim and Polymyxin B *on page 2105*

◆ **Polymyxin B, Bacitracin, and Neomycin** *see* Bacitracin, Neomycin, and Polymyxin B *on page 223*

◆ **Polymyxin B, Bacitracin, Neomycin, and Hydrocortisone** *see* Bacitracin, Neomycin, Polymyxin B, and Hydrocortisone *on page 223*

◆ **Polymyxin B, Neomycin, and Dexamethasone** *see* Neomycin, Polymyxin B, and Dexamethasone *on page 1437*

◆ **Polymyxin B, Neomycin, and Gramicidin** *see* Neomycin, Polymyxin B, and Gramicidin *on page 1437*

◆ **Polymyxin B, Neomycin, and Hydrocortisone** *see* Neomycin, Polymyxin B, and Hydrocortisone *on page 1438*

◆ **Polymyxin B Sulfate** *see* Polymyxin B *on page 1676*

◆ **Polymyxin E** *see* Colistimethate *on page 504*

◆ **Polynuclear Iron (III)-Oxyhydroxide (pn-FeOOH)** *see* Sucroferric Oxyhydroxide *on page 1941*

Polysaccharide-Iron Complex

(pol i SAK a ride-EYE ern KOM pleks)

Brand Names: U.S. EZFE 200 [OTC]; Ferrex 150 [OTC]; Ferric x-150 [OTC]; FerUS [OTC] [DSC]; iFerex 150 [OTC]; Myferon 150 [OTC]; NovaFerrum 50 [OTC]; NovaFerrum Pediatric Drops [OTC]; Nu-Iron [OTC]; PIC 200 [OTC]; Poly-Iron 150 [OTC]

Index Terms Iron-Polysaccharide Complex

Pharmacologic Category Iron Salt

Use Iron deficiency anemia: Management (prevention and treatment) of iron deficiency anemia

Dosage

Dietary Reference Intake: Dose is RDA presented as elemental iron unless otherwise noted (IOM, 2001):

0-6 months: 0.27 mg daily (adequate intake)

7-12 months: 11 mg daily

1-3 years: 7 mg daily

4-8 years: 10 mg daily

9-13 years: 8 mg daily

14-18 years: Males: 11 mg daily; Females: 15 mg daily; Pregnant females: 27 mg daily; Lactating females: 10 mg daily

19-50 years: Males: 8 mg daily; Females: 18 mg daily; Pregnant females: 27 mg daily; Lactating females: 9 mg daily

≥50 years: 8 mg daily

Iron deficiency anemia: Oral:

Infants and Children <4 years: 15 mg daily

Children ≥12 years: 50 mg daily

Adults: 150-300 mg daily

Additional Information Complete prescribing information should be consulted for additional detail.

Dosage Forms

Capsule, Oral:

EZFE 200 [OTC]: 200 mg

Ferrex 150 [OTC]: 150 mg

Ferric x-150 [OTC]: 150 mg

iFerex 150 [OTC]: 150 mg

Myferon 150 [OTC]: 150 mg

NovaFerrum 50 [OTC]: 50 mg

Nu-Iron [OTC]: 150 mg

PIC 200 [OTC]: 200 mg

Poly-Iron 150 [OTC]: 150 mg

Liquid, Oral:

NovaFerrum Pediatric Drops [OTC]: 15 mg/mL (120 mL)

◆ **Polysporin® [OTC]** *see* Bacitracin and Polymyxin B *on page 222*

◆ **Polystyrene Sulfonate Calcium** *see* Calcium Polystyrene Sulfonate [CAN/INT] *on page 333*

◆ **Polytrim®** *see* Trimethoprim and Polymyxin B *on page 2105*

◆ **Polytrim™ (Can)** *see* Trimethoprim and Polymyxin B *on page 2105*

◆ **P-OM3** *see* Omega-3 Fatty Acids *on page 1507*

Pomalidomide (poe ma LID oh mide)

Brand Names: U.S. Pomalyst

Brand Names: Canada Pomalyst

Index Terms CC-4047

Pharmacologic Category Angiogenesis Inhibitor; Antineoplastic Agent; Immunomodulator, Systemic

Use Multiple myeloma: Treatment of multiple myeloma in patients who have received at least 2 prior therapies (including lenalidomide and bortezomib) and have demonstrated disease progression on or within 60 days of completion of the last therapy.

Pregnancy Risk Factor X

Pregnancy Considerations [U.S. Boxed Warning]: Pomalidomide is an analogue of thalidomide (a known human teratogen) and may cause severe birth defects or embryo-fetal death if taken during pregnancy. Pomalidomide cannot be used in women who are pregnant or may become pregnant during therapy. Obtain 2 negative pregnancy tests prior to initiation of treatment; 2 forms of contraception (or abstain from heterosexual intercourse) must be used at least 4 weeks prior to, during, and for ≥4 weeks after pomalidomide treatment (and during treatment interruptions) in females of reproductive potential. In order to decrease the risk of embryo-fetal exposure, pomalidomide is available only through a restricted distribution program (Pomalyst REMS). In Canada, distribution is restricted to physicians, pharmacists, and patients registered with the RevAid program.

Studies in animals have shown evidence of fetal abnormalities and use is contraindicated in women who are or may become pregnant. Women of childbearing potential should be treated only if they are able to comply with the conditions of the Pomalyst REMS Program (U.S.) or RevAid program (Canada). Reliable contraception is required even with a history of infertility (unless due to hysterectomy or if ≥24 consecutive months postmenopausal (natural). Reliable methods of birth control include one highly effective method (eg, tubal ligation, IUD, hormonal [birth control pills, injections, hormonal patches, vaginal rings, or implants], or partner's vasectomy) and one additional effective method (eg, male latex or synthetic condom, diaphragm, or cervical cap). Pregnancy tests should be performed 10-14 (U.S. labeling) or 7-14 days (Canadian labeling) and 24 hours prior to beginning therapy; weekly for the first 4 weeks and then every 4 weeks (every 2 weeks if menstrual cycle irregular) thereafter and during therapy interruptions. The Canadian labeling also recommends pregnancy testing 4 weeks after discontinuation. Pomalidomide must be immediately discontinued for a missed period, abnormal pregnancy test or abnormal menstrual bleeding; refer patient to a reproductive toxicity specialist if pregnancy occurs during treatment. Pomalidomide is present in the semen of males taking this medication. Males (including those vasectomized) should use a latex or synthetic condom during any sexual contact with women of childbearing age during treatment, during treatment interruptions, and for 28 days after discontinuation. Male patients should not donate sperm. Any suspected fetal exposure should be reported in the U.S. to the FDA via the MedWatch program (1-800-332-1088) and to Celgene Corporation (1-888-423-5436) and in Canada to Celgene (1-888-738-2341).

Breast-Feeding Considerations It is not known if pomalidomide is excreted into breast milk. Due to the potential for serious adverse reactions in the nursing infant, a decision should be made to discontinue nursing or to discontinue treatment with pomalidomide, taking into account the importance of treatment to the mother.

Contraindications Pregnancy

Canadian labeling: Additional contraindications (not in U.S. labeling): Hypersensitivity to pomalidomide, thalidomide, lenalidomide, or any component of the formulation; breast-feeding; women of childbearing potential not using 2 effective means of contraception; male patients unable to comply with required contraceptive measures

Warnings/Precautions Hazardous agent - use appropriate precautions for handling and disposal (meets NIOSH 2014 criteria). Due to the embryo-fetal risk, pomalidomide is only available through a restricted program under the Pomalyst REMS program. Pomalidomide should only be prescribed to patients who can understand and comply with the conditions of the Pomalyst REMS program. Prescribers and pharmacies must be certified with the REMS program. In Canada, pomalidomide is only available through the restricted RevAid program. Prescribers and pharmacists must be registered with the program to prescribe and dispense pomalidomide; patients must also be registered and meet all conditions of the program.

[U.S. Boxed Warning]: Pomalidomide is a thalidomide (human teratogen) analog and may cause severe life-threatening birth defects or embryo-fetal deaths; use is contraindicated in pregnancy. Pregnancy must be excluded prior to therapy initiation with 2 negative pregnancy tests; prevent pregnancy during therapy with 2 reliable forms of contraception (or abstain from heterosexual intercourse) beginning 4 weeks prior to, during and for 4 weeks after pomalidomide therapy (and during treatment interruptions) in females of reproductive potential. In order to decrease the risk of embryo-fetal exposure, pomalidomide is available only through a restricted distribution program (Pomalyst REMS). Reliable methods of birth control include one highly effective method (eg, tubal ligation, IUD, hormonal [birth control pills, injections, hormonal patches, vaginal rings, or implants], or partner's vasectomy) and one additional effective method (eg, male latex or synthetic condom, diaphragm, or cervical cap). Males taking pomalidomide must use a latex or synthetic condom during any sexual contact with a woman of childbearing potential during therapy and for up to 28 days after treatment discontinuation, even if successfully vasectomized. Patients should not donate blood during pomalidomide treatment and for 1 month after therapy discontinuation; male patients receiving pomalidomide must not donate sperm.

Neutropenia, anemia, and thrombocytopenia were frequently reported in clinical trials. Monitor complete blood counts weekly for the first 8 weeks of therapy and monthly or as clinically indicated thereafter; may require therapy interruption, reduction and/or discontinuation. Acute myelogenous leukemia (AML) as a secondary malignancy has been reported in patients receiving pomalidomide in the investigational treatment of condition(s) other than multiple myeloma. **[U.S. Boxed Warning]: Venous thromboembolic events such as deep vein thrombosis (DVT) and pulmonary embolism (PE) have occurred during pomalidomide therapy. Clinical trials utilized antithrombotic prophylaxis and/or treatment; consider individualized anticoagulation prophylaxis based on patient risk factors.** Monitor for signs/symptoms of thromboembolism (shortness of breath, chest pain, or arm or leg swelling) and advise patients to promptly seek medical attention should symptoms occur. May cause dizziness and/or confusion; caution patients about performing tasks that require mental alertness (eg, operating machinery or driving). Avoid concomitant medications which may exacerbate dizziness and confusion. Use with caution in patients with a prior history of serious hypersensitivity reactions to thalidomide or lenalidomide; such patients were excluded from pomalidomide clinical trials and may therefore be at risk for hypersensitivity reactions when administered pomalidomide. Peripheral and sensory neuropathy occurred in clinical trials, but no cases of grade 3 or higher neuropathy were observed. Monitor closely for signs/symptoms of neuropathy; may require therapy interruption, dose modification and/or discontinuation.

Safety and efficacy have not been evaluated in patients with renal or hepatic impairment. Pomalidomide is hepatically metabolized; avoid use in patients with serum bilirubin >2 mg/dL and AST/ALT >3 times ULN (has not been studied). Pomalidomide and its metabolites are excreted by the kidneys; avoid use in patients with serum creatinine >3 mg/dL (has not been studied). The Canadian labeling recommends avoiding use if CrCl <45 mL/minute.

Potentially significant drug-drug interactions may exist, requiring dose or frequency adjustment, additional monitoring, and/or selection of alternative therapy. Cigarette smoking may induce CYP1A2 mediated metabolism of pomalidomide, potentially reducing its systemic exposure and efficacy.

Adverse Reactions

Cardiovascular: Atrial fibrillation, peripheral edema, thrombosis (venous thrombosis, pulmonary embolism)

Central nervous system: Anxiety, chills, confusion, dizziness, fatigue, fever, headache, insomnia, neuropathy, pain, peripheral neuropathy, vertigo

Dermatologic: Hyperhidrosis, pruritus, skin rash, xeroderma

Endocrine & metabolic: Dehydration, hypercalcemia, hyperglycemia, hyperkalemia, hypocalcemia, hypokalemia, hyponatremia

Gastrointestinal: Constipation, decreased appetite, diarrhea, nausea, vomiting, weight gain, weight loss

Genitourinary: Pelvic pain, urinary retention, urinary tract infection

Hematologic & oncologic: Acute myelocytic leukemia, anemia, febrile neutropenia, leukopenia, lymphocytopenia, neutropenia, thrombocytopenia

Hepatic: Hyperbilirubinemia, increased serum ALT

Infection: Sepsis

Neuromuscular & skeletal: Arthralgia, back pain, limb pain, muscle spasm, musculoskeletal chest pain, musculoskeletal pain, myasthenia, ostealgia, tremor

Renal: Increased serum creatinine, renal failure

Respiratory: Cough, dyspnea, epistaxis, interstitial pulmonary disease, *Pneumocystis jiroveci* pneumonia, pneumonia, respiratory syncytial virus infection, upper respiratory tract infection

Miscellaneous: Neutropenic sepsis, night sweats

Drug Interactions

Metabolism/Transport Effects Substrate of CYP1A2 (major), CYP2C19 (minor), CYP2D6 (minor), CYP3A4 (major), P-glycoprotein; **Note:** Assignment of Major/Minor substrate status based on clinically relevant drug interaction potential

Avoid Concomitant Use

Avoid concomitant use of Pomalidomide with any of the following: Abatacept; Anakinra; Azelastine (Nasal); BCG; Canakinumab; Certolizumab Pegol; CloZAPine; Conivaptan; CYP1A2 Inducers (Strong); CYP1A2 Inhibitors (Strong); Dipyrone; Fusidic Acid (Systemic); Idelalisib; Natalizumab; Orphenadrine; Paraldehyde; Pimecrolimus; Rilonacept; Tacrolimus (Topical); Thalidomide; Tocilizumab; Tofacitinib; Vaccines (Live); Vedolizumab

Increased Effect/Toxicity

Pomalidomide may increase the levels/effects of: Abatacept; Alcohol (Ethyl); Anakinra; Azelastine (Nasal); Bisphosphonate Derivatives; Buprenorphine; Canakinumab; Certolizumab Pegol; CloZAPine; CNS Depressants; Hydrocodone; Leflunomide; Methotrimeprazine; Metyrosine; Mirtazapine; Natalizumab; Orphenadrine; Paraldehyde; Pramipexole; Rilonacept; ROPINIRole; Rotigotine; Selective Serotonin Reuptake Inhibitors; Suvorexant; Thalidomide; Tofacitinib; Vaccines (Live); Vedolizumab; Zolpidem

The levels/effects of Pomalidomide may be increased by: Abiraterone Acetate; Aprepitant; Brimonidine (Topical); Cannabis; Ceritinib; Conivaptan; CYP1A2 Inhibitors (Moderate); CYP1A2 Inhibitors (Strong); CYP3A4 Inhibitors (Moderate); CYP3A4 Inhibitors (Strong); Dasatinib; Deferasirox; Denosumab; Dipyrone; Doxylamine; Dronabinol; Droperidol; Fosaprepitant; Fusidic Acid (Systemic); HydrOXYzine; Idelalisib; Ivacaftor; Kava Kava; Luliconazole; Magnesium Sulfate; Methotrimeprazine; Mifepristone; Nabilone; Netupitant; Peginterferon Alfa-2b; Perampanel; P-glycoprotein/ABCB1 Inhibitors; Pimecrolimus; Roflumilast; Rufinamide; Simeprevir; Sodium Oxybate; Tacrolimus (Topical); Tapentadol; Tetrahydrocannabinol; Tocilizumab; Trastuzumab; Vemurafenib

Decreased Effect

Pomalidomide may decrease the levels/effects of: BCG; Coccidioides immitis Skin Test; Sipuleucel-T; Vaccines (Inactivated); Vaccines (Live)

The levels/effects of Pomalidomide may be decreased by: Bosentan; Cannabis; CYP1A2 Inducers (Strong); CYP3A4 Inducers (Moderate); CYP3A4 Inducers (Strong); Cyproterone; Dabrafenib; Deferasirox; Echinacea; Mitotane; P-glycoprotein/ABCB1 Inducers; Siltuximab; St Johns Wort; Teriflunomide

Storage/Stability Store at 20°C to 25°C (68°F to 77°F); excursions permitted to 15°C to 30°C (59°F to 86°F).

Mechanism of Action Induces cell cycle arrest and apoptosis directly in multiple myeloma cells; enhances T cell- and natural killer (NK) cell-mediated cytotoxicity; inhibits production of proinflammatory cytokines tumor necrosis factor-α (TNF-α), IL-1, IL-6, and IL-12; inhibits angiogenesis (Zhu, 2013)

Pharmacodynamics/Kinetics

Absorption: Rapid; slowed by food. Canadian labeling suggests that the overall effect of food on extent of absorption is minimal (AUC decreased 8%).

Distribution: V_{dss}: 62 to 138 L; semen distribution is ~67% of plasma levels

Protein binding: 12% to 44%

Metabolism: Hepatic via CYP1A2 and CYP3A4 (major); CYP2C19 and CYP2D6 (minor)

Half-life elimination: ~9.5 hours (healthy subjects); ~7.5 hours (multiple myeloma patients)

Time to peak: 2 to 3 hours

Excretion: Urine (73%; 2% as unchanged drug); feces (15%; 8% as unchanged drug)

Dosage Note: ANC should be ≥500 cells/mm^3 (U.S. labeling) or ≥1000 cells/mm^3 (Canadian labeling) and platelets ≥50,000 cells/mm^3 prior to initiating new cycles of therapy.

Multiple myeloma, relapsed/refractory: Adults: Oral:

U.S. labeling: 4 mg once daily on days 1 to 21 of 28-day cycles (may be given in combination with dexamethasone); continue until disease progression or unacceptable toxicity.

Canadian labeling: 4 mg once daily on days 1 to 21 of 28-day cycles (in combination with dexamethasone); continue until disease progression or unacceptable toxicity.

Dosage adjustment for concomitant therapy with strong CYP1A2 inhibitors: Avoid concomitant use of strong CYP1A2 inhibitors. If concomitant use cannot be avoided in the presence of strong CYP3A4 and P-gp inhibitors, reduce the pomalidomide dose by 50%.

Dosage adjustment for toxicity:

Hematologic:

If ANC <500 cells/mm^3 (or ANC <1000 cells/mm^3 with fever ≥38.5°C) and/or platelets <25,000 cells/mm^3: Interrupt therapy and follow weekly CBCs. When ANC ≥500 cells/mm^3 (U.S. labeling) or ≥1000 cells/mm^3 (Canadian labeling) and/or platelets ≥50,000 cells/mm^3: Resume dosing at 3 mg once daily.

For each subsequent drop of ANC <500 cells/mm^3 and/or platelets <25,000 cells/mm^3: Interrupt therapy. When ANC ≥500 cells/mm^3 (U.S. labeling) or ≥1000 cells/mm^3 (Canadian labeling) and/or platelets ≥50,000 cells/mm^3: Resume dosing at 1 mg less than the previous dose. If toxicities occur at 1 mg daily dose, discontinue treatment.

Nonhematologic: If grade 3 or 4 toxicity occurs, interrupt therapy until resolved to ≤ grade 2; if appropriate, may restart therapy at 1 mg less than the previous dose. If toxicities occur at 1 mg daily dose, discontinue treatment.

Dosage adjustment for renal impairment: Serum creatinine >3 mg/dL (U.S. labeling) or CrCl <45 mL/minute (Canadian labeling): Avoid use (has not been studied).

Dosage adjustment for hepatic impairment: Bilirubin >2 mg/dL and AST/ALT >3 times ULN: Avoid use (has not been studied).

Administration U.S. labeling recommends administering on an empty stomach with water (at least 2 hours before or 2 hours after a meal). Canadian labeling recommends administering without regard to meals. Should be swallowed whole; do not break, chew, or open the capsules. May administer a missed dose if within 12 hours of usual dosing time. If >12 hours, skip the dose for that day and resume usual dosing the following day. Do not take 2 doses to make up for a skipped dose.

Hazardous agent; use appropriate precautions for handling and disposal (meets NIOSH 2014 criteria).

Monitoring Parameters CBC with differential and platelets weekly for the first 8 weeks and monthly or as clinically necessary thereafter; renal function (ie, serum creatinine, creatinine clearance); liver function tests; monitor for signs/symptoms of thromboembolism and neuropathy. Consider thyroid function tests (TSH recommended at baseline and every 2-3 months during treatment for structurally similar medications [Hamnvik, 2011]).

Women of childbearing potential: Pregnancy test 10-14 days (U.S. labeling) or 7-14 days (Canadian labeling) **and** 24 hours prior to initiating therapy, weekly during the first month, then monthly thereafter in women with regular menstrual cycles or every 2 weeks in women with irregular menstrual cycles. Canadian labeling also recommends a pregnancy test 4 weeks after discontinuation.

Dosage Forms

Capsule, Oral:

Pomalyst: 1 mg, 2 mg, 3 mg, 4 mg

◆ **Pomalyst** *see* Pomalidomide *on page 1677*

PONATinib (poe NA ti nib)

Brand Names: U.S. Iclusig

Index Terms AP24534; Ponatinib Hydrochloride

Pharmacologic Category Antineoplastic Agent, BCR-ABL Tyrosine Kinase Inhibitor; Antineoplastic Agent, Tyrosine Kinase Inhibitor

Use

Acute lymphoblastic leukemia: Treatment of Philadelphia chromosome-positive acute lymphoblastic leukemia (Ph+ ALL) for whom no other tyrosine kinase inhibitor therapy is indicated or who are T315I positive

Chronic myeloid leukemia: Treatment of chronic myeloid leukemia (CML) in chronic, accelerated, or blast phase for whom no other tyrosine kinase inhibitor therapy is indicated or who are T315I positive

Pregnancy Risk Factor D

Pregnancy Considerations Adverse events were observed in animal reproduction studies when administered in doses lower than or equivalent to the normal human dose. Based on its mechanism of action, adverse effects on pregnancy would be expected. Women of childbearing potential should be advised to avoid pregnancy during therapy.

Breast-Feeding Considerations It is not known if ponatinib is excreted in breast milk. Due to the potential for serious adverse reactions in the nursing infant, a decision should be made whether to discontinue nursing or to discontinue the drug, taking into account the importance of treatment to the mother.

Contraindications There are no contraindications listed in the manufacturer's labeling.

Warnings/Precautions Hazardous agent - use appropriate precautions for handling and disposal (meets NIOSH 2014 criteria). **[U.S. Boxed Warning]: Arterial and venous thrombosis and occlusions have occurred in ponatinib-treated patients. Events included fatal myocardial infarction (MI), stroke, stenosis of large arterial vessels of the brain, severe peripheral vascular disease, and the need for urgent revascularization procedures; incidents were observed in patients with and without cardiovascular risk factors (including patients ≤50 years of age). Monitor closely for thromboembolism/vascular occlusion; interrupt or discontinue therapy immediately for vascular occlusion. Consider benefit/risk ratio when deciding to restart therapy.** Fatal and life-threatening vascular occlusion may occur within 2 weeks of therapy initiation and is not dose dependent (events have occurred at doses as low as 15 mg daily), and may cause recurrent or multisite occlusion. Increasing age and a prior history of ischemia, hypertension, diabetes, or hyperlipidemia are risk factors for development of ponatinib-associated vascular occlusion. Many patients required a revascularization procedure (cerebrovascular, coronary, and peripheral arterial) due to serious arterial thrombosis/occlusion. MI and coronary artery occlusion may result in heart failure due to myocardial ischemia. Peripheral arterial occlusive events, including fatal mesenteric artery occlusion and life-threatening peripheral arterial disease, have occurred. Some patients have required amputation due to digital or distal extremity necrosis. Venous thromboembolism, including deep vein thrombosis, pulmonary embolism, superficial thrombophlebitis, and retinal vein thrombosis, have been reported. May require dosage adjustment or discontinuation. Monitor for signs/symptoms of arterial or venous thromboembolism.

[U.S. Boxed Warning]: Serious heart failure (HF) or left ventricular dysfunction, including fatalities, were reported in clinical trials. Monitor for signs/symptoms of HF; interrupt or discontinue ponatinib therapy for new or worsening HF. Treat as clinically warranted if HF develops. Consider ponatinib discontinuation in the event of serious HF. Cardiac arrhythmias (bradyarrhythmias and tachyarrhythmias) have also been reported. Symptomatic bradyarrhythmia which required pacemaker implantation occurred in a few patients; other rhythms identified were complete heart block, sick sinus syndrome, and atrial fibrillation with bradycardia and pauses. Tachyarrhythmias reported include atrial fibrillation (most common), atrial flutter, supraventricular tachycardia, and atrial tachycardia; some events required hospitalization. Monitor for sign/symptoms of bradycardia (fainting, dizziness, chest pain) and tachycardia (palpitations, dizziness). May require therapy interruption. Treatment-emergent hypertension developed in over half of ponatinib-treated patients; symptomatic hypertension or hypertensive crisis were reported in several patients, requiring urgent intervention. Blood pressure may worsen in patients with preexisting hypertension. Monitor blood pressure closely, and manage elevated pressures as clinically indicated. May require therapy interruption, dosage reduction, or discontinuation if hypertension is resistant to medical management.

[U.S. Boxed Warning]: Liver failure and death resulting from ponatinib-induced hepatotoxicity were observed; monitor liver function prior to and at least monthly (or as clinically indicated) during treatment. Hepatotoxicity may require treatment interruption (followed by dose reduction) or discontinuation. One case of fulminant hepatic failure leading to death occurred within 1 week of therapy initiation; acute liver failure has also occurred. Treatment may result in ALT and/or AST elevations, and may be irreversible. A single-dose (30 mg) pharmacokinetic study found that ponatinib exposure was not increased in patients with hepatic impairment (Child-Pugh class A, B, or C) as compared to patients with normal hepatic function. While generally well tolerated, patients with hepatic impairment did have an increased overall incidence of adverse reactions (eg, gastrointestinal disorders, pancreatitis). Monitor closely when administering to patients with impaired hepatic function. The starting dose should be reduced in patients with hepatic impairment.

Severe myelosuppression (grade 3 or 4) was commonly observed in clinical trials, and the incidence was greater in patients with accelerated or blast phase CML and Ph+ ALL. Monitor blood counts closely; may require therapy interruption and/or dosage reduction. Hemorrhagic events occurred commonly in ponatinib-treated patients, including serious events such as cerebral and gastrointestinal hemorrhages; fatalities were reported. Serious bleeding episodes occurred more frequently in patients with accelerated or blast phase CML, and Ph+ ALL; most patients had grade 4 thrombocytopenia. Monitor platelet levels closely and for signs/symptoms of bleeding, and interrupt therapy if necessary.

Treatment-related lipase elevations and clinical pancreatitis occurred in clinical studies; the majority of cases resolved within 2 weeks of therapy interruption or dose reduction. Monitor serum lipase every 2 weeks for the first 2 months and monthly thereafter or as clinically indicated; more frequent monitoring may be considered in patients with a history of pancreatitis or alcohol abuse. Monitor for clinical signs of pancreatitis, such as abdominal symptoms; interrupt therapy if necessary. Do not reinitiate treatment until complete resolution of symptoms and lipase level is <1.5 times ULN. Serious gastrointestinal perforation (fistula) occurred very rarely; monitor for signs/symptoms of perforation and/or fistula. Serious fluid retention events, including fatality due to brain edema (very rare), were observed in ponatinib-treated patients. Peripheral edema, pleural effusions, and pericardial effusions were commonly seen; effusions and ascites were less common. Monitor patients for fluid retention; may require therapy interruption, dosage reduction, or discontinuation.

Peripheral and cranial neuropathy have been reported. Peripheral neuropathy, paresthesia, hypoesthesia, and hyperesthesia occurred most frequently; cranial neuropathy occurred rarely. In one-third of patients who experienced symptoms, neuropathy developed during the first month of therapy. Monitor for signs/symptoms of neuropathy; consider interrupting treatment if neuropathy develops. Serious ocular events such as blindness and blurred vision have occurred with ponatinib use. Macular edema, retinal vein occlusion, and retinal hemorrhage have been reported in a small percentage of patients; conjunctival or corneal irritation, dry eye, or eye pain occurred more frequently. Other toxicities include cataracts, glaucoma, iritis, iridocyclitis, and ulcerative keratitis. Perform comprehensive ophthalmic exams prior to therapy initiation and periodically during treatment.

Hyperuricemia and serious tumor lysis syndrome (rare) were reported. Patients should receive adequate hydration and be monitored for elevated uric acid levels and/or the development of tumor lysis syndrome. Correct elevated uric acid levels prior to initiating therapy. As ponatinib inhibits VEGF activity, therapy may impair wound healing. Hold therapy for at least 1 week prior to major surgery; resume therapy post procedure based on clinical judgment of appropriate wound healing. Potentially significant drug-drug interactions may exist, requiring dose or frequency adjustment, additional monitoring, and/or selection of alternative therapy. Patients ≥65 years of age may be more likely to experience weakness, decreased appetite, dyspnea, increased lipase, muscle spasms, peripheral edema, and thrombocytopenia; monitor closely. Cautious dose selection is recommended based on greater frequency of decreased hepatic, renal, or cardiac function, and of concomitant disease or other drug therapy.

Adverse Reactions

Cardiovascular: Arterial ischemia (including cardiac, cerebrovascular, and peripheral-vascular ischemia), atrial fibrillation, bradycardia (symptomatic), cardiac failure (including congestive heart failure, reduced ejection fraction, pulmonary edema, cardiogenic shock, cardiorespiratory arrest, right ventricular failure), cerebral hemorrhage, cerebrovascular accident, hypertension, myocardial infarction, pericardial effusion, peripheral edema, peripheral ischemia, supraventricular tachycardia, venous thromboembolism

Central nervous system: Chills, dizziness, fatigue, headache, insomnia, pain, weakness

Dermatologic: Cellulitis, skin rash, xeroderma

Endocrine & metabolic: Decreased serum bicarbonate, decreased serum calcium, decreased serum glucose, decreased serum phosphate, decreased serum potassium, decreased serum sodium, hyperuricemia, increased serum calcium, increased serum glucose, increased serum potassium, increased serum sodium, increased serum triglycerides

Gastrointestinal: Abdominal pain, constipation, decreased appetite, diarrhea, gastrointestinal hemorrhage, increased serum amylase, increased serum lipase, mouth pain, nausea, oral mucosa ulcer, oropharyngeal pain, pancreatitis, stomatitis, throat ulcer, tongue ulcer, vomiting, weight loss

Genitourinary: Urinary tract infection

Hematologic & oncologic: Anemia, bone marrow depression, febrile neutropenia, hemorrhage (including cerebral hemorrhage and gastrointestinal hemorrhage), leukopenia, lymphocytopenia, neutropenia, thrombocytopenia

Hepatic: Decreased serum albumin, increased serum alkaline phosphatase, increased serum ALT, increased serum AST, increased serum bilirubin

Infection: Sepsis

Miscellaneous: Fever

Neuromuscular & skeletal: Arthralgia, back pain, limb pain, muscle spasm, myalgia, ostealgia, peripheral neuropathy (including burning sensation)

Ophthalmic: Blurred vision, cataract, conjunctival irritation, corneal ulcer, dry eye syndrome, eye pain, glaucoma, iridocyclitis, iritis, keratitis, retinal toxicity (including macular edema, retinal vein occlusion, retinal hemorrhage)

Renal: Increased serum creatinine

Respiratory: Cough, dyspnea, nasopharyngitis, pleural effusion, pneumonia, upper respiratory tract infection

Rare but important or life-threatening: Acute hepatic failure, ascites, atrial flutter, atrial tachycardia, cerebral edema, complete atrioventricular block, gastrointestinal fistula, gastrointestinal perforation, mesenteric artery occlusion, pulmonary embolism, retinal vein thrombosis, sick sinus syndrome, tumor lysis syndrome (serious)

Drug Interactions

Metabolism/Transport Effects Substrate of BCRP, CYP2C8 (minor), CYP2D6 (minor), CYP3A4 (minor), P-glycoprotein; **Note:** Assignment of Major/Minor substrate status based on clinically relevant drug interaction potential; **Inhibits** BCRP, P-glycoprotein

Avoid Concomitant Use

Avoid concomitant use of PONATinib with any of the following: CloZAPine; CYP3A4 Inducers (Strong); Dipyrone; St Johns Wort

Increased Effect/Toxicity

PONATinib may increase the levels/effects of: CloZAPine

The levels/effects of PONATinib may be increased by: CYP3A4 Inhibitors (Strong); Dipyrone; Grapefruit Juice

Decreased Effect

The levels/effects of PONATinib may be decreased by: CYP3A4 Inducers (Strong); St Johns Wort

Storage/Stability Store at 20°C to 25°C (68°F to 77°F); excursions permitted between 15°C to 30°C (59°F to 86°F).

Mechanism of Action Ponatinib is a pan-BCR-ABL tyrosine kinase inhibitor with *in vitro* activity against cells expressing native or mutant BCR-ABL (including T315I); it also inhibits VEGFR, FGFR, PDGFR, EPH, and SRC kinases, as well as KIT, RET, TIE2, and FLT3.

Pharmacodynamics/Kinetics

Absorption: Plasma concentrations not affected by food

Distribution: V_d: 1223 L

Protein binding: >99% to plasma proteins

Metabolism: Primarily hepatic through CYP3A4; CYP2C8, CYP2D6, and CYP3A5 are also involved in metabolism. Phase II metabolism occurs via esterases and/or amidases.

Half-life elimination: ~24 hours (range: 12 to 66 hours)

Time to peak: ≤6 hours

Excretion: Feces (~87%); urine (~5%)

Dosage Note: The optimal ponatinib dose has not been identified. Consider discontinuing therapy if no response has occurred by 3 months of therapy.

Acute lymphoblastic leukemia (ALL), Philadelphia chromosome-positive (Ph+), in patients for whom no other tyrosine kinase inhibitor therapy is indicated or who are T315I-positive: Adults: Oral: Initial: 45 mg once daily

Chronic myeloid leukemia (CML; chronic, accelerated, or blast phase), in patients for whom no other tyrosine kinase inhibitor therapy is indicated or who are T315I-positive: Adults: Oral: Initial: 45 mg once daily; consider reducing the dose for patients in chronic or accelerated phase who have achieved a major cytogenetic response

Dosage adjustment for strong CYP3A inhibitors: Reduce ponatinib dose to 30 mg once daily when administered with concomitant strong CYP3A inhibitors (eg, boceprevir, clarithromycin, conivaptan, grapefruit juice, indinavir, itraconazole, ketoconazole, lopinavir/ritonavir, nefazodone, nelfinavir, posaconazole, ritonavir, saquinavir, telaprevir, telithromycin, voriconazole).

Dosage adjustment for toxicity:

Hematologic: ANC <1000/mm^3 or platelets <50,000/mm^3:

First occurrence: Interrupt therapy; upon recovery of ANC to ≥1500/mm^3 and platelets to ≥75,000/mm^3, resume therapy at 45 mg daily.

Second occurrence: Interrupt therapy; upon recovery of ANC to ≥1500/mm^3 and platelets to ≥75,000/mm^3, resume therapy at a reduced dose of 30 mg daily.

Third occurrence: Interrupt therapy; upon recovery of ANC to ≥1500/mm^3 and platelets to ≥75,000/mm^3, resume therapy at a reduced dose of 15 mg daily.

Nonhematologic toxicity:

Arterial or venous occlusive reactions: Interrupt therapy; do not resume ponatinib in the event of serious occlusive events unless the potential benefit of therapy outweighs the risk of recurrent occlusions and other treatment options are not available.

Pancreatitis and lipase elevations:

Asymptomatic grade 1 or 2 serum lipase elevation: Consider interrupting therapy or dose reduction.

Asymptomatic grade 3 or 4 serum lipase elevation (>2 times ULN) or asymptomatic radiologic pancreatitis (grade 2): If toxicity occurs at a dose of 45 mg daily, interrupt therapy; upon recovery to ≤ grade 1 (<1.5 times ULN), resume therapy at a reduced dose of 30 mg daily. If toxicity occurs at a dose of 30 mg daily, interrupt therapy; upon recovery to ≤ grade 1, resume therapy at a reduced dose of 15 mg daily. If toxicity occurs at a dose of 15 mg daily, discontinue therapy.

Symptomatic grade 3 pancreatitis: If toxicity occurs at a dose of 45 mg daily, interrupt therapy; upon recovery of serum lipase elevation to ≤ grade 1 and complete symptom resolution, resume therapy at a reduced dose of 30 mg daily. If toxicity occurs at a dose of 30 mg daily, interrupt therapy; upon recovery of serum lipase elevation to ≤ grade 1 and complete symptom resolution, resume therapy at a reduced dose of 15 mg daily. If toxicity occurs at a dose of 15 mg daily, discontinue therapy.

Grade 4 pancreatitis: Discontinue therapy.

Other nonhematologic toxicities: For serious reactions (other than arterial or venous occlusion), do not restart therapy until symptom resolution or unless the benefit of therapy outweighs the risk of recurrent toxicity.

Dosage adjustment for renal impairment: There are no dosage adjustments provided in the manufacturer's labeling (has not been studied); although renal excretion is not a major excretion route for ponatinib.

Dosage adjustment for hepatic impairment:

Hepatic impairment prior to treatment initiation: Mild-to-severe impairment (Child-Pugh class A, B, or C): Initial: 30 mg once daily; monitor closely for toxicity

Hepatotoxicity during treatment:

AST or ALT >3 times ULN (≥ grade 2): If toxicity occurs at a dose of 45 mg daily, interrupt therapy; upon recovery to ≤ grade 1 (<3 times ULN), resume therapy at 30 mg daily. If toxicity occurs at a dose of 30 mg daily, interrupt therapy; upon recovery to ≤ grade 1, resume therapy at 15 mg daily. If toxicity occurs at a dose of 15 mg daily, discontinue therapy.

ALT or AST ≥3 times ULN with bilirubin >2 times ULN and alkaline phosphatase <2 times ULN: Discontinue therapy.

Dietary Considerations May be taken without regard to food. Avoid grapefruit juice.

Administration Administer with or without food. Swallow tablets whole (do not crush or dissolve). Hazardous agent; use appropriate precautions for handling and disposal (meets NIOSH 2014 criteria).

Monitoring Parameters CBC with differential and platelets every 2 weeks for the first 3 months, then monthly or as clinically needed; liver function tests at baseline and at least monthly thereafter or more frequently if clinically warranted; serum lipase every 2 weeks for the first 2 months and monthly thereafter (more frequently in patients with a history of pancreatitis or alcohol abuse); serum electrolytes and uric acid; monitor cardiac function, blood pressure, signs/symptoms of arterial/venous occlusion or thromboembolism, hemorrhage, fluid retention, pancreatitis (clinical signs), gastrointestinal perforation/fistula, hepatotoxicity (jaundice, anorexia, bleeding, bruising); comprehensive ocular exam at baseline and periodically; signs/symptoms of neuropathy

Dosage Forms

Tablet, Oral:

Iclusig: 15 mg, 45 mg

- ◆ **Ponatinib Hydrochloride** *see* PONATinib *on page 1680*
- ◆ **Ponstan (Can)** *see* Mefenamic Acid *on page 1280*
- ◆ **Ponstel** *see* Mefenamic Acid *on page 1280*
- ◆ **Pontocaine (Can)** *see* Tetracaine (Systemic) *on page 2017*
- ◆ **Pontocaine (Can)** *see* Tetracaine (Topical) *on page 2017*

Porfimer (POR fi mer)

Brand Names: U.S. Photofrin

Brand Names: Canada Photofrin®

Index Terms CL-184116; Dihematoporphyrin Ether; Porfimer Sodium

Pharmacologic Category Antineoplastic Agent, Miscellaneous

Use Palliation in patients with obstructing (partial or complete) esophageal cancer; treatment of microinvasive endobronchial non-small cell lung cancer (NSCLC); reduction of obstruction and palliation in patients with obstructing (partial or complete) NSCLC; ablation of high-grade dysplasia in Barrett's esophagus

Canadian labeling: Additional use (not in U.S. labeling): Second-line treatment of recurrent, superficial papillary bladder cancer

Pregnancy Risk Factor C

Dosage IV: Adults:

Photodynamic therapy in esophageal cancer or endobronchial non-small cell lung cancer: 2 mg/kg, followed by endoscopic exposure to the appropriate laser light and debridement; repeat courses must be separated by at least 30 days (delay subsequent treatment for insufficient healing) for a maximum of 3 courses

Photodynamic therapy in Barrett's esophagus dysplasia: 2 mg/kg, followed by endoscopic exposure to the appropriate laser light; repeat courses must be separated by at least 90 days (delay subsequent treatment for insufficient healing) for a maximum of 3 courses

Photodynamic therapy in papillary bladder cancer (Canadian labeling; not in U.S. labeling): 2 mg/kg, followed by cystoscopic exposure to the appropriate laser light. **Note:** Repeat dosing is not recommended due to increased risk of bladder contracture.

Dosage adjustment in renal impairment: No dosage adjustment provided in manufacturer's labeling.

Dosage adjustment in hepatic impairment: No dosage adjustment provided in manufacturer's labeling (has not been studied).

Additional Information Complete prescribing information should be consulted for additional detail.

Dosage Forms

Solution Reconstituted, Intravenous [preservative free]:
Photofrin: 75 mg (1 ea)

Dosage Forms: Canada

Injection, powder for reconstitution, as sodium:
Photofrin®: 15 mg

◆ **Porfimer Sodium** *see* Porfimer *on page 1682*

◆ **Portia** *see* Ethinyl Estradiol and Levonorgestrel *on page 803*

Posaconazole (poe sa KON a zole)

Brand Names: U.S. Noxafil

Brand Names: Canada Posanol

Index Terms SCH 56592

Pharmacologic Category Antifungal Agent, Oral

Additional Appendix Information

Oral Dosages That Should Not Be Crushed *on page 2276*

Use

U.S. labeling:

Invasive *Aspergillus* and *Candida* infections: Suspension and delayed-release tablets (13 years and older) and injection (18 years and older): Prophylaxis of invasive *Aspergillus* and *Candida* infections in patients who are at high risk of developing these infections due to being severely immunocompromised (eg, hematopoietic stem cell transplant [HSCT] recipients with graft-versus-host disease [GVHD] or those with prolonged neutropenia secondary to chemotherapy for hematologic malignancies).

Oropharyngeal candidiasis: Suspension (13 years and older): Treatment of oropharyngeal candidiasis (including patients refractory to itraconazole and/or fluconazole)

Canadian labeling:

Invasive *Aspergillus* and *Candida* infections: Prophylaxis of invasive *Aspergillus* and *Candida* infections in severely-immunocompromised patients (eg, hematopoietic stem cell transplant [HSCT] recipients with graft-versus-host disease [GVHD] or those with prolonged neutropenia); treatment of invasive aspergillosis in patients refractory to or intolerant of itraconazole or amphotericin B; treatment of oropharyngeal candidiasis

Pregnancy Risk Factor C

Pregnancy Considerations Posaconazole has been shown to be teratogenic in animal studies. There are no adequate and well-controlled studies in pregnant women. Use only if the benefit to the mother justifies potential risk to the fetus.

Breast-Feeding Considerations Excretion in breast milk has not been investigated; use only if the benefit to the mother justifies potential risk to the fetus.

Contraindications Coadministration with sirolimus, ergot alkaloids (eg, ergotamine, dihydroergotamine), HMG-CoA reductase inhibitors that are primarily metabolized through CYP3A4 (eg, atorvastatin, lovastatin, simvastatin), or CYP3A4 substrates that prolong the QT interval (eg, pimozide, quinidine); hypersensitivity to posaconazole, other azole antifungal agents, or any component of the formulation.

Warnings/Precautions The delayed-release tablet and oral suspension are not to be used interchangeably due to dosing differences for each formulation. Hepatic dysfunction has occurred, ranging from mild/moderate increases of ALT, AST, alkaline phosphatase, total bilirubin, and/or clinical hepatitis to severe reactions (cholestasis, hepatic failure including death). Consider discontinuation of therapy in patients who develop clinical evidence of liver disease that may be secondary to posaconazole. Elevations in liver function tests have been generally reversible after posaconazole has been discontinued; some cases resolved without drug interruption. More severe reactions have been observed in patients with underlying serious medical conditions (eg, hematologic malignancy) and primarily with suspension total daily doses of 800 mg. Monitor liver function tests at baseline and periodically during therapy. If increases occur, monitor for severe hepatic injury development. Use caution in patients with an increased risk of arrhythmia (long QT syndrome, concurrent QTc-prolonging drugs, drugs metabolized through CYP3A4, hypokalemia). Correct electrolyte abnormalities (eg, potassium, magnesium, and calcium) before initiating therapy. Potentially significant drug-drug interactions may exist, requiring dose or frequency adjustment, additional monitoring, and/or selection of alternative therapy. Concurrent use with midazolam may increase midazolam concentrations and potentiate midazolam-related adverse effects.

U.S. labeling contraindicates use in patients with hypersensitivity to other azole antifungal agents; Canadian labeling does not contraindicate use, but recommends using caution in hypersensitivity with other azole antifungal agents; cross-reaction may occur, but has not been established. Consider alternative therapy or closely monitor for breakthrough fungal infections in patients receiving drugs that decrease absorption or increase the metabolism of posaconazole or in any patient unable to eat or tolerate an oral liquid nutritional supplement. Do not give IV formulation as an intravenous bolus injection. Avoid/limit use of IV formulation in patients with eGFR <50 mL/minute/1.73 m^2; injection contains excipient betadex sulfobutyl ether sodium (SBECD), which may accumulate; consider using oral posaconazole in these patients unless benefit of injection outweighs the risk. Evaluate renal function (particularly serum creatinine) at baseline and periodically during therapy. If increases occur, consider oral therapy. ▶

Monitor for breakthrough fungal infections. Patients weighing >120 kg may have lower plasma drug exposure; monitor closely for breakthrough fungal infections.

Benzyl alcohol and derivatives: Some dosage forms may contain sodium benzoate/benzoic acid; benzoic acid (benzoate) is a metabolite of benzyl alcohol; large amounts of benzyl alcohol (≥99 mg/kg/day) have been associated with a potentially fatal toxicity ("gasping syndrome") in neonates; the "gasping syndrome" consists of metabolic acidosis, respiratory distress, gasping respirations, CNS dysfunction (including convulsions, intracranial hemorrhage), hypotension, and cardiovascular collapse (AAP, 1997; CDC, 1982); some data suggests that benzoate displaces bilirubin from protein binding sites (Ahlfors, 2001); avoid or use dosage forms containing benzyl alcohol derivative with caution in neonates. See manufacturer's labeling.

Adverse Reactions Note: Unless otherwise specified, adverse reactions are identified with oral formulations and reflect data from use in comparator trials with multiple concomitant conditions and medications; some adverse reactions may be due to underlying condition(s). Systemic includes oral and intravenous routes.

Cardiovascular: Edema, hypertension (systemic), hypotension, peripheral edema (systemic), pulmonary embolism, tachycardia, thrombophlebitis (intravenous via peripheral venous catheter), torsades de pointes

Central nervous system: Anxiety, chills (systemic), dizziness, fatigue (systemic), headache (systemic), insomnia, lower extremity edema, pain, paresthesia, rigors

Dermatologic: Diaphoresis, pruritus, skin rash (systemic)

Endocrine & metabolic: Adrenocortical insufficiency, dehydration, hyperglycemia, hypocalcemia, hypokalemia (systemic), hypomagnesemia (systemic), weight loss

Gastrointestinal: Abdominal pain (systemic), anorexia, constipation (systemic), decreased appetite (systemic), diarrhea (systemic), dyspepsia, mucositis, nausea (systemic), oral candidiasis, stomatitis, upper abdominal pain (systemic), vomiting (systemic)

Genitourinary: Vaginal hemorrhage

Hematologic & oncologic: Anemia (systemic), febrile neutropenia, hemolytic-uremic syndrome, neutropenia, petechia (systemic), thrombocytopenia (systemic), thrombotic thrombocytopenic purpura

Hepatic: Hepatic failure, hepatitis, hepatomegaly, hyperbilirubinemia, increased liver enzymes, increased serum alkaline phosphatase, increased serum ALT, increased serum AST, jaundice

Hypersensitivity: Hypersensitivity reaction

Infection: Bacteremia, cytomegalovirus disease, herpes simplex infection

Neuromuscular & skeletal: Arthralgia, back pain, musculoskeletal pain, weakness

Renal: Acute renal failure

Respiratory: Cough (systemic), dyspnea (systemic), epistaxis (systemic), pharyngitis, pneumonia, upper respiratory tract infection

Miscellaneous: Fever (systemic)

Rare but important or life-threatening: Atrial fibrillation, cholestasis, hypersensitivity, prolonged Q-T interval on ECG, reduced ejection fraction, syncope

Drug Interactions

Metabolism/Transport Effects Inhibits CYP3A4 (strong)

Avoid Concomitant Use

Avoid concomitant use of Posaconazole with any of the following: Ado-Trastuzumab Emtansine; Alfuzosin; Apixaban; Astemizole; AtorvaSTATin; Avanafil; Axitinib; Bosutinib; Cabozantinib; Ceritinib; Cisapride; Conivaptan; Crizotinib; Dapoxetine; Dihydroergotamine; Dofetilide; Dronedarone; Efavirenz; Eletriptan; Eplerenone; Ergoloid Mesylates; Ergonovine; Ergotamine; Everolimus; Halofantrine; Ibrutinib; Irinotecan; Ivabradine; Lapatinib; Lercanidipine; Lomitapide; Lovastatin; Lurasidone; Macitentan; Methadone; Methylergonovine; Naloxegol; Nilotinib; Nisoldipine; Olaparib; Pimozide; QuiNIDine; Ranolazine; Red Yeast Rice; Regorafenib; Rivaroxaban; Saccharomyces boulardii; Salmeterol; Silodosin; Simeprevir; Simvastatin; Sirolimus; Suvorexant; Tamsulosin; Terfenadine; Ticagrelor; Tolvaptan; Toremifene; Trabectedin; Ulipristal; Vemurafenib; VinCRIStine (Liposomal); Vorapaxar

Increased Effect/Toxicity

Posaconazole may increase the levels/effects of: Ado-Trastuzumab Emtansine; Alfuzosin; Almotriptan; Alosetron; Antineoplastic Agents (Vinca Alkaloids); Apixaban; ARIPiprazole; Astemizole; Atazanavir; AtorvaSTATin; Avanafil; Axitinib; Bedaquiline; Boceprevir; Bortezomib; Bosentan; Bosutinib; Brentuximab Vedotin; Brinzolamide; Budesonide (Nasal); Budesonide (Systemic, Oral Inhalation); BusPIRone; Busulfan; Cabazitaxel; Cabozantinib; Calcium Channel Blockers; Cannabis; Ceritinib; Cilostazol; Cisapride; Colchicine; Conivaptan; Corticosteroids (Orally Inhaled); Corticosteroids (Systemic); Crizotinib; CycloSPORINE (Systemic); CYP3A4 Substrates; Dapoxetine; Dasatinib; Dienogest; Digoxin; Dihydroergotamine; DOCEtaxel; Dofetilide; DOXOrubicin (Conventional); Dronabinol; Dronedarone; Dutasteride; Eletriptan; Eliglustat; Enzalutamide; Eplerenone; Ergoloid Mesylates; Ergonovine; Ergotamine; Erlotinib; Etizolam; Etravirine; Everolimus; FentaNYL; Fesoterodine; Fluticasone (Nasal); Fluticasone (Oral Inhalation); Fosamprenavir; Fosphenytoin; GlipiZIDE; GuanFACINE; Halofantrine; Highest Risk QTc-Prolonging Agents; Hydrocodone; Ibrutinib; Idelalisib; Iloperidone; Imatinib; Imidafenacin; Irinotecan; Ivabradine; Ivacaftor; Ixabepilone; Lacosamide; Lapatinib; Lercanidipine; Levobupivacaine; Levomilnacipran; Lomitapide; Losartan; Lovastatin; Lurasidone; Macitentan; Macrolide Antibiotics; Maraviroc; Methadone; Methylergonovine; MethylPREDNISolone; Mifepristone; Moderate Risk QTc-Prolonging Agents; Naloxegol; Nilotinib; Nisoldipine; Olaparib; Ospemifene; OxyCODONE; Paricalcitol; PAZOPanib; Phenytoin; Pimecrolimus; Pimozide; PONATinib; Pranlukast; PrednisoLONE (Systemic); PredniSONE; Propafenone; QUEtiapine; QuiNIDine; Ranolazine; Red Yeast Rice; Regorafenib; Repaglinide; Retapamulin; Rifamycin Derivatives; Rilpivirine; Ritonavir; Rivaroxaban; RomiDEPsin; Ruxolitinib; Salmeterol; Saxagliptin; Sildenafil; Silodosin; Simeprevir; Simvastatin; Sirolimus; Solifenacin; SORAfenib; SUNItinib; Suvorexant; Tacrolimus (Systemic); Tacrolimus (Topical); Tadalafil; Tamsulosin; Telaprevir; Temsirolimus; Terfenadine; Tetrahydrocannabinol; Ticagrelor; Tofacitinib; Tolterodine; Tolvaptan; Toremifene; Trabectedin; Ulipristal; Vardenafil; Vemurafenib; Vilazodone; VinCRIStine (Liposomal); Vitamin K Antagonists; Vorapaxar; Zolpidem; Zopiclone; Zuclopenthixol

The levels/effects of Posaconazole may be increased by: Boceprevir; Etravirine; Macrolide Antibiotics; Mifepristone; Telaprevir

Decreased Effect

Posaconazole may decrease the levels/effects of: Amphotericin B; Ifosfamide; Prasugrel; Saccharomyces boulardii; Ticagrelor

The levels/effects of Posaconazole may be decreased by: Didanosine; Efavirenz; Etravirine; Fosamprenavir; Fosphenytoin; H2-Antagonists; Metoclopramide; Phenytoin; Proton Pump Inhibitors; Rifamycin Derivatives; Sucralfate

Food Interactions Bioavailability increased ~3 times when posaconazole suspension was administered with a nonfat meal or an oral liquid nutritional supplement; increased ~4 times when administered with a high-fat meal. Following administration of posaconazole delayed-release tablets, the AUC increased 51% when given with a high-fat meal compared with a fasted state. Management: Suspension must be administered with or within 20 minutes of a full meal or an oral liquid nutritional supplement, or may be administered with an acidic carbonated beverage (eg, ginger ale). Take tablet with food. Consider alternative antifungal therapy in patients with inadequate oral intake or severe diarrhea/vomiting.

Preparation for Administration IV: Equilibrate the refrigerated vial to room temperature. Contents of vial should be withdrawn and admixed with D_5W or NS 150 mL. The admixed solution may be colorless to yellow. Color variations in this range do not affect potency. Admixture should be used immediately; may be stored for up to 24 hours between 2°C and 8°C (36°F and 46°F).

Storage/Stability

Suspension: Store at 25°C (77°F); excursions are permitted between 15°C and 30°C (59°F and 86°F). Do not freeze.

Tablets: Store between 20°C and 25°C (68°F and 77°F); excursions are permitted between 15°C and 30°C (59°F and 86°F).

Injection: Store at 2°C to 8°C (36°F to 46°F).

Mechanism of Action Interferes with fungal cytochrome P450 (latosterol-14α-demethylase) activity, decreasing ergosterol synthesis (principal sterol in fungal cell membrane) and inhibiting fungal cell membrane formation.

Pharmacodynamics/Kinetics

Absorption: Coadministration of the tablets or oral suspension with food or coadministration of the oral suspension with liquid nutritional supplements and/or acidic carbonated beverages (eg, ginger ale) increases absorption; fasting states do not provide sufficient absorption to ensure adequate plasma concentrations.

Distribution: V_d: Oral: 287 L; Injection: ~261 L

Protein binding: >98%; predominantly bound to albumin

Metabolism: Not significantly metabolized; ~15% to 17% undergoes non-CYP-mediated metabolism, primarily via hepatic glucuronidation into metabolites

Half-life elimination: Suspension: 35 hours (range: 20 to 66 hours); Tablets: 26 to 31 hours; Injection: ~27 hours

Time to peak, plasma: Suspension: ~3 to 5 hours; Tablets: ~4 to 5 hours

Excretion: Feces 71% to 77% (~66% of the total dose as unchanged drug); urine 13% to 14% (<0.2% of the total dose as unchanged drug)

Dosage Note: The delayed-release tablet and oral suspension are not to be used interchangeably due to dosing differences for each formulation.

Aspergillosis, invasive:

Prophylaxis:

Adolescents ≥13 years and Adults: Oral:

Tablets (delayed release): Initial: 300 mg twice daily on day 1; Maintenance dose: 300 mg once daily on day 2 and thereafter. Duration is based on recovery from neutropenia or immunosuppression; initiate posaconazole in patients with acute myelogenous leukemia (AML) or myelodysplastic syndromes (MDS) several days before the anticipated onset of neutropenia (eg, at the time of chemotherapy initiation) and discontinue once neutropenia is resolved (Cornely, 2007; NCCN, 2009).

Missed doses: Take as soon as remembered. If it is <12 hours until the next dose, skip the missed does and return to the regular schedule. Do not double doses.

Suspension: 200 mg 3 times daily; duration of therapy is based on recovery from neutropenia or immunosuppression; initiate posaconazole in patients with acute myelogenous leukemia (AML) or myelodysplastic syndromes (MDS) several days before the anticipated onset of neutropenia (eg, at the time of chemotherapy initiation) and discontinue once neutropenia is resolved (Cornely, 2007; NCCN, 2009).

Adults ≥18 years: IV: Loading dose: 300 mg twice daily on day 1; Maintenance dose: 300 mg once daily on day 2 and thereafter. Duration of therapy is based on recovery from neutropenia or immunosuppression

Treatment (refractory to or intolerant of conventional therapy):

U.S. off-label use: Adults: Oral: Suspension: 200 mg 4 times daily initially; after disease stabilization, may decrease frequency to 400 mg twice daily (Walsh, 2007). **Note:** Duration of therapy should be a minimum of 6 to 12 weeks or throughout period of immunosuppression and until lesions have resolved (Walsh, 2008).

Canadian labeling: Adolescents ≥13 years and Adults: Oral: 400 mg twice daily; in patients unable to tolerate food or nutritional supplement, administer 200 mg 4 times daily; duration of therapy is based on severity of underlying disease, recovery from immunosuppression, and clinical response.

Candidal infections:

U.S. labeling: Adolescents ≥13 years and Adults:

Prophylaxis:

Tablets (delayed release): Oral: Initial: 300 mg twice daily on day 1; Maintenance dose: 300 mg once daily on day 2 and thereafter; duration of therapy is based on recovery from neutropenia or immunosuppression.

Missed doses: Take as soon as remembered. If it is <12 hours until the next dose, skip the missed does and return to the regular schedule. Do not double doses.

Suspension: Oral: 200 mg 3 times daily; duration of therapy is based on recovery from neutropenia or immunosuppression

Injection: IV: Initial: 300 mg twice daily on day 1; Maintenance dose: 300 mg once daily on day 2 and thereafter; duration of therapy is based on recovery from neutropenia or immunosuppression.

Treatment: Suspension: Oral:

Oropharyngeal infection: Initial: 100 mg twice daily on day 1; Maintenance: 100 mg once daily on day 2 and thereafter for 13 days

Refractory oropharyngeal infection: 400 mg twice daily; duration of therapy is based on underlying disease and clinical response

Esophageal infection, azole refractory (HIV-exposed/positive patients) (off-label use): Adolescents and Adults: 400 mg twice daily for 28 days. **Note:** If patient has frequent or severe recurrences, may continue for suppressive therapy; consider discontinuing when CD_4 >200/mm^3 (DHHS [adult], 2014).

Canadian labeling: Suspension: Oral:

Prophylaxis: 200 mg 3 times daily; duration of therapy is based on recovery from neutropenia or immunosuppression

Treatment: Oropharyngeal infection: Initial: 100 mg twice daily for 1 day; Maintenance: 100 mg once daily for 13 days

Mucormycosis (off-label use): Adults: Oral: Suspension: 800 mg daily in 2 or 4 divided doses; duration of therapy is based on response and risk of relapse due to immunosuppression (Greenburg, 2006)

Cryptococcal infections: Adults: Oral: Suspension:
Pulmonary, nonimmunosuppressed (off-label use): 400 mg twice daily. **Note:** Fluconazole is considered first-line treatment (Perfect, 2010).
Salvage treatment of relapsed infection (off-label use): 400 mg twice daily (or 200 mg 4 times daily) for 10 to 12 weeks. **Note:** Salvage treatment should only be started after an appropriate course of an induction regimen (Perfect, 2010).

Primary antifungal prophylaxis in allogeneic HSCT with grades 2 to 4 acute graft-versus-host-disease (GVHD) or chronic extensive GVHD (pediatric guideline recommendation): Adolescents ≥13 years: Oral: Suspension: 200 mg 3 times daily beginning with GVHD diagnosis, continue until GVHD resolves (Science, 2014)

Primary antifungal prophylaxis in AML or MDS in centers with a high local incidence of mold infections (alternative to fluconazole; guideline recommendation): Adolescents ≥13 years: Oral: Suspension: 200 mg 3 times daily during chemotherapy-associated neutropenia (Science, 2014)

Dosage adjustment in renal impairment:
Delayed-release tablets and oral suspension:
eGFR 20 to 80 mL/minute/1.73 m^2: No dosage adjustment necessary.
eGFR <20 mL/minute/1.73 m^2: No dosage adjustment necessary; however, monitor for breakthrough fungal infections due to variability in posaconazole exposure.
Intravenous infusion:
eGFR ≥50 mL/minute/1.73 m^2: No dosage adjustment recommended
eGFR <50 mL/minute/1.73 m^2: Avoid use unless risk/benefit has been assessed; intravenous vehicle may accumulate. Monitor serum creatinine levels; if increases occur, consider oral therapy

Dosage adjustment in hepatic impairment: Mild-to-severe insufficiency (Child-Pugh class A, B, or C): No dosage adjustment necessary. **Note:** if patient shows clinical signs and symptoms of liver disease due to posaconazole, consider discontinuing therapy. Hepatic impairment studies were only conducted with oral suspension; however, recommendations also apply to patients receiving injection or delayed-release tablets.

Dietary Considerations
Tablets (delayed release): Take with food.
Suspension: Give during or within 20 minutes following a full meal or liquid nutritional supplement; alternatively, posaconazole may be administered with an acidic carbonated beverage (eg, ginger ale).
Consider alternative antifungal therapy in patients with inadequate oral intake or severe diarrhea/vomiting; if alternative therapy is not an option, closely monitoring for breakthrough fungal infections.
Adequate posaconazole absorption from GI tract and subsequent plasma concentrations are dependent on food for efficacy. Lower average plasma concentrations have been associated with an increased risk of treatment failure.

Administration
Suspension: Oral: Shake well before use. Must be administered during or within 20 minutes following a full meal or an oral liquid nutritional supplement; alternatively, posaconazole may be administered with an acidic carbonated beverage (eg, ginger ale). In patients able to swallow, administer oral suspension using dosing spoon provided by the manufacturer; spoon should be rinsed clean with water after each use and before storage. The oral suspension and delayed-release tablet are not to be used interchangeably due to dosing differences for each formulation.
Tablets (delayed release): Oral: Swallow tablets whole; do not divide, crush, dissolve, or chew. Administer with food. The delayed-release tablet and oral suspension are not to be used interchangeably due to dosing differences for each formulation.
Consider alternative antifungal therapy in patients with inadequate oral intake or severe diarrhea/vomiting; if alternative therapy is not an option, closely monitoring for breakthrough fungal infections. Adequate posaconazole absorption from GI tract and subsequent plasma concentrations are dependent on food. Lower average plasma concentrations have been associated with an increased risk of treatment failure.
Injection: Infuse over 90 minutes via a central venous line. Do not administer IV push or bolus. Must be infused through an in-line filter (0.22-micron polyethersulfone [PES] or polyvinylidene difluoride [PVDF]). Infusion through a peripheral line should only be used as a one-time infusion over 30 minutes in a patient who will be receiving a central venous line for subsequent doses, or to bridge a period during which a central venous line is to be replaced or is in use for another infusion. Note: In clinical trials, multiple peripheral infusions given through the same vein resulted in infusion-site reactions.

Monitoring Parameters Hepatic function (eg, AST/ALT, alkaline phosphatase and bilirubin) prior to initiation and during treatment; renal function, especially in patients on IV therapy if eGFR <50 mL/minute/1.73 m^2; electrolyte disturbances (eg, calcium, magnesium, potassium); CBC; breakthrough fungal infections; adequate oral intake

Dosage Forms
Solution, Intravenous:
Noxafil: 300 mg/16.7 mL (16.7 mL)
Suspension, Oral:
Noxafil: 40 mg/mL (105 mL)
Tablet Delayed Release, Oral:
Noxafil: 100 mg

◆ **Posanol (Can)** *see* Posaconazole *on page* 1683

Potassium Acetate (poe TASS ee um AS e tate)

Pharmacologic Category Electrolyte Supplement, Parenteral

Use Potassium deficiency; to avoid chloride when high concentration of potassium is needed, source of bicarbonate

Pregnancy Risk Factor C

Dosage IV doses should be incorporated into the patient's maintenance IV fluids, intermittent IV potassium administration should be reserved for severe depletion situations and requires ECG monitoring; doses listed as mEq of potassium

Children:
Treatment of hypokalemia: IV: 2-5 mEq/kg/day
IV intermittent infusion (must be diluted prior to administration): 0.5-1 mEq/kg/dose (maximum: 30 mEq/dose) to infuse at 0.3-0.5 mEq/kg/hour (maximum: 1 mEq/kg/hour)
Note: Use caution in premature neonates; potassium acetate for injection contains aluminum.

Adults:
Treatment of hypokalemia: IV: 40-100 mEq/day
IV intermittent infusion (must be diluted prior to administration): 5-10 mEq/dose (maximum: 40 mEq/dose) to infuse over 2-3 hours (maximum: 40 mEq over 1 hour)

Note: Continuous cardiac monitor recommended for rates >0.5 mEq/kg/hour

Potassium dosage/rate of infusion guidelines:
Serum potassium >2.5 mEq/L: Maximum infusion rate: 10 mEq/hour; maximum concentration: 40 mEq/L; maximum 24-hour dose: 200 mEq

Serum potassium <2.5 mEq/L: Maximum infusion rate: 40 mEq/hour; maximum concentration: 80 mEq/L; maximum 24-hour dose: 400 mEq

Dosage adjustment in renal impairment: No dosage adjustment provided in manufacturer's labeling. Use caution; potassium acetate injection may increase serum aluminum and/or potassium.

Dosage adjustment in hepatic impairment: No dosage adjustment provided in manufacturer's labeling. Use with caution.

Additional Information Complete prescribing information should be consulted for additional detail.

Dosage Forms

Solution, Intravenous:

Generic: 2 mEq/mL (20 mL, 50 mL, 100 mL); 4 mEq/mL (50 mL)

Potassium Acid Phosphate
(poe TASS ee um AS id FOS fate)

Brand Names: U.S. K-Phos

Index Terms Potassium Phosphate Monobasic

Pharmacologic Category Urinary Acidifying Agent

Use To acidify the urine to lower urinary calcium concentrations; reduce odor and rash caused by ammonia in urine; to increase the antibacterial activity of methenamine

Pregnancy Risk Factor C

Dosage Adults: Oral: 1000 mg 4 times daily

Dosage adjustment in renal impairment: No dosage adjustment provided in manufacturer's labeling. Use with caution. Contraindicated in patients with severe impairment (<30% of normal function) or with hyperphosphatemia or hyperkalemia.

Dosage adjustment in hepatic impairment: No dosage adjustment provided in manufacturer's labeling. Use with caution.

Additional Information Complete prescribing information should be consulted for additional detail.

Dosage Forms Considerations

500 mg of potassium acid phosphate = elemental potassium 144 mg = potassium 3.7 mEq = potassium 3.7 mmol

500 mg of potassium acid phosphate = elemental phosphorus 114 mg = phosphorus 3.7 mmol

Dosage Forms

Tablet, Oral:

K-Phos: 500 mg

Potassium Bicarbonate and Potassium Chloride
(poe TASS ee um bye KAR bun ate & poe TASS ee um KLOR ide)

Index Terms K-Lyte/Cl; Potassium Bicarbonate and Potassium Chloride (Effervescent)

Pharmacologic Category Electrolyte Supplement, Oral

Use Treatment or prevention of hypokalemia

Pregnancy Risk Factor C

Dosage Oral:

Children: 1-4 mEq/kg/24 hours in divided doses as required to maintain normal serum potassium

Adults:

Prevention: 16-24 mEq/day in 2-4 divided doses

Treatment: 40-100 mEq/day in 2-4 divided doses

Dosage adjustment in renal impairment: No dosage adjustment provided in manufacturer's labeling. However, patients with chronic renal failure require serum potassium monitoring and appropriate dosage adjustment.

Dosage adjustment in hepatic impairment: No dosage adjustment provided in manufacturer's labeling.

Additional Information Complete prescribing information should be consulted for additional detail.

Dosage Forms

Tablet for solution, oral [effervescent]: Potassium chloride 25 mEq

◆ **Potassium Bicarbonate and Potassium Chloride (Effervescent)** *see* Potassium Bicarbonate and Potassium Chloride *on page 1687*

Potassium Bicarbonate and Potassium Citrate
(poe TASS ee um bye KAR bun ate & poe TASS ee um SIT rate)

Brand Names: U.S. Effer-K; K-Effervescent; K-Prime; K-Vescent; Klor-Con/EF

Index Terms Potassium Bicarbonate and Potassium Citrate (Effervescent)

Pharmacologic Category Electrolyte Supplement, Oral

Use Treatment or prevention of hypokalemia, particularly when it is necessary to avoid chloride or the acid/base status requires bicarbonate

Pregnancy Risk Factor C

Dosage Note: Doses expressed as mEq of potassium.

Normal daily requirement: Adults: 40-100 mEq/day or 1-2 mEq/kg/day (off-label dose; Mirtallo, 2004)

Hypokalemia: Adults: Oral:

Prevention: 10-80 mEq/day in 1-4 divided doses

Treatment: 40-100 mEq/day in 2-4 divided doses. **Note:** For asymptomatic mild hypokalemia, generally recommended to limit doses to 20-25 mEq/dose to avoid GI discomfort.

Dosage adjustment in renal impairment: No dosage adjustment provided in manufacturer's labeling. However, patients with chronic renal failure require serum potassium monitoring and appropriate dosage adjustment.

Dosage adjustment in hepatic impairment: No dosage adjustment provided in manufacturer's labeling.

Additional Information Complete prescribing information should be consulted for additional detail.

Dosage Forms Considerations

Strength expressed in terms of mEqs of potassium

Dosage Forms

Tablet Effervescent, Oral:

Effer-K: 10 mEq, 20 mEq, 25 mEq

K-Effervescent: 25 mEq

K-Prime: 25 mEq

K-Vescent: 25 mEq

Klor-Con/EF: 25 mEq

Generic: 25 mEq

◆ **Potassium Bicarbonate and Potassium Citrate (Effervescent)** *see* Potassium Bicarbonate and Potassium Citrate *on page 1687*

Potassium Chloride (poe TASS ee um KLOR ide)

Brand Names: U.S. K-Sol; K-Tab; K-Vescent; Klor-Con; Klor-Con 10; Klor-Con M10; Klor-Con M15; Klor-Con M20; Micro-K

Brand Names: Canada Apo-K; K-10; K-Dur; Micro-K Extencaps; Roychlor; Slo-Pot; Slow-K

Index Terms KCl; Kdur

Pharmacologic Category Electrolyte Supplement, Oral; Electrolyte Supplement, Parenteral

Use Treatment or prevention of hypokalemia

Pregnancy Risk Factor C

Pregnancy Considerations Reproduction studies have not been conducted. Potassium requirements are the same in pregnant and nonpregnant women. Adverse events have not been observed following use of potassium supplements in healthy women with normal pregnancies. Use caution in pregnant women with other medical conditions (eg, pre-eclampsia; may be more likely to develop hyperkalemia) (IOM, 2004). Potassium supplementation (that does not cause maternal hyperkalemia) would not be expected to cause adverse fetal events.

Breast-Feeding Considerations Potassium is excreted into breast milk (IOM, 2004). The normal content of potassium in human milk is ~13 mEq/L. Supplementation (that does not cause maternal hyperkalemia) would not be expected to affect normal concentrations.

Contraindications Hypersensitivity to any component of the formulation; hyperkalemia. In addition, solid oral dosage forms are contraindicated in patients in whom there is a structural, pathological, and/or pharmacologic cause for delay or arrest in passage through the GI tract.

Warnings/Precautions Close monitoring of serum potassium concentrations is needed to avoid hyperkalemia. Use with caution in patients with renal impairment, cardiac disease, acid/base disorders, or potassium-altering conditions/disorders. Use with caution in digitalized patients or patients receiving concomitant medications or therapies that increase potassium (eg, ACEI, potassium-sparing diuretics, potassium containing salt substitutes). Do **NOT** administer undiluted or IV push; inappropriate parenteral administration may be fatal. Always administer potassium further diluted; refer to appropriate dilution and administration rate recommendations. Vesicant/irritant (at concentrations >0.1 mEq/mL); ensure proper catheter or needle position prior to and during infusion; avoid extravasation. Pain and phlebitis may occur during parenteral infusion requiring a decrease in infusion rate or potassium concentration. Avoid administering potassium diluted in dextrose solutions during initial therapy; potential for transient decreases in serum potassium due to intracellular shift of potassium from dextrose-stimulated insulin release. May cause GI upset (eg, nausea, vomiting, diarrhea, abdominal pain, discomfort) and lead to GI ulceration, bleeding, perforation, and/or obstruction. Oral liquid preparations (not solid) should be used in patients with esophageal compression or delayed gastric emptying.

Adverse Reactions

Dermatologic: Rash

Endocrine & metabolic: Hyperkalemia

Gastrointestinal: Abdominal pain/discomfort, diarrhea, flatulence, GI bleeding (oral), GI obstruction (oral), GI perforation (oral), nausea, vomiting

Drug Interactions

Metabolism/Transport Effects None known.

Avoid Concomitant Use

Avoid concomitant use of Potassium Chloride with any of the following: Anticholinergic Agents; Glycopyrrolate

Increased Effect/Toxicity

Potassium Chloride may increase the levels/effects of: ACE Inhibitors; Aliskiren; Angiotensin II Receptor Blockers; Potassium-Sparing Diuretics

The levels/effects of Potassium Chloride may be increased by: Anticholinergic Agents; Eplerenone; Glycopyrrolate; Heparin; Heparin (Low Molecular Weight); Nicorandil

Decreased Effect There are no known significant interactions involving a decrease in effect.

Preparation for Administration Parenteral: Potassium must be diluted prior to parenteral administration. The concentration of infusion may be dependent on patient condition and specific institution policy. Some clinicians recommend that the maximum concentration for peripheral infusion is 10 mEq/100 mL and 20-40 mEq/100 mL for central infusions.

Storage/Stability

Capsule: MicroK®: Store between 20°C to 25°C (68°F to 77°F).

Powder for oral solution: Klor-Con®: Store at room temperature of 15°C to 30°C (59°F to 86°F).

Solution for injection: Store at room temperature; do not freeze. Use only clear solutions. Use admixtures within 24 hours.

Tablet: K-Tab®: Store below 30°C (86°F).

Mechanism of Action Potassium is the major cation of intracellular fluid and is essential for the conduction of nerve impulses in heart, brain, and skeletal muscle; contraction of cardiac, skeletal and smooth muscles; maintenance of normal renal function, acid-base balance, carbohydrate metabolism, and gastric secretion

Pharmacodynamics/Kinetics

Absorption: Well absorbed from upper GI tract

Distribution: Enters cells via active transport from extracellular fluid

Excretion: Primarily urine; skin and feces (small amounts); most intestinal potassium reabsorbed

Dosage IV doses should be incorporated into the patient's maintenance IV fluids; intermittent IV potassium administration should be reserved for severe depletion situations in patients undergoing ECG monitoring. Doses expressed as mEq of potassium.

Normal daily requirements: Oral, IV:
- Children: 1-2 mEq/kg/day
- Adults: 40-80 mEq/day

Prevention of hypokalemia: Oral:
- Children: 1-2 mEq/kg/day in 1-2 divided doses
- Adults: 20-40 mEq/day in 1-2 divided doses

Treatment of hypokalemia: Children:
- Oral: 1-2 mEq/kg initially, then as needed based on frequently obtained lab values. If deficits are severe or ongoing losses are great, IV route should be considered.
- IV intermittent infusion: 0.5-1 mEq/kg/dose (maximum dose: 40 mEq). If infusion exceeds 0.5 mEq/kg/hour, physician should be at bedside and patient should have continuous ECG monitoring; repeat as needed based on frequently obtained lab values.

Treatment of hypokalemia: Adults:
- Oral:
  - Asymptomatic, mild hypokalemia: Usual dosage range: 40-100 mEq/day divided in 2-5 doses; generally recommended to limit doses to 20-25 mEq/dose to avoid GI discomfort.
  - Mild-to-moderate hypokalemia: Some clinicians may administer up to 120-240 mEq/day divided in 3-4 doses; generally recommended to limit doses to 40-60 mEq/dose. If deficits are severe or ongoing losses are great, IV route should be considered.
- IV intermittent infusion: Peripheral or central line: ≤10 mEq/hour; repeat as needed based on frequently obtained lab values; central line infusion and continuous ECG monitoring highly recommended for infusions >10 mEq/hour.
  - Potassium dosage/rate of infusion general guidelines (per product labeling): **Note:** High variability exists in dosing/infusion rate recommendations; therapy guided by patient condition and specific institutional guidelines.

Serum potassium >2.5-3.5 mEq/L: Maximum infusion rate: 10 mEq/hour; maximum concentration: 40 mEq/L; maximum 24-hour dose: 200 mEq

Serum potassium <2.5 mEq/L or symptomatic hypokalemia (excluding emergency treatment of cardiac arrest): Maximum infusion rate (central line only): 40 mEq/hour in presence of continuous ECG monitoring and frequent lab monitoring; In selected situations, patients may require up to 400 mEq/24 hours.

Dosage adjustment in renal impairment: No dosage adjustment provided in manufacturer's labeling. Use caution; potassium acetate injection may increase serum aluminum and/or potassium.

Dosage adjustment in hepatic impairment: No dosage adjustment provided in manufacturer's labeling.

Dietary Considerations Administer with plenty of fluid to decrease stomach irritation and discomfort. Some dietary sources of potassium include leafy green vegetables (eg, spinach, cabbage), tomatoes, cucumbers, zucchini, fruits (eg, apples, oranges, and bananas), root vegetables (eg, carrots, radishes), beans, and peas.

Administration

Parenteral: Potassium must be diluted prior to parenteral administration. Do not administer IV push. In general, the dose, concentration of infusion and rate of administration may be dependent on patient condition and specific institution policy. Some clinicians recommend that the maximum concentration for peripheral infusion is 10 mEq/100 mL and maximum rate of administration for peripheral infusion is 10 mEq/hour (Kraft, 2005). ECG monitoring is recommended for peripheral or central infusions >10 mEq/hour in adults (Kraft, 2005). Concentrations and rates of infusion may be greater with central line administration. Concentrations of 20 to 40 mEq/100 mL at a maximum rate of 40 mEq/hour via central line have been safely administered (Hamill, 1991; Kruse, 1990)

Vesicant/irritant (at concentrations >0.1 mEq/mL); ensure proper needle or catheter placement prior to and during IV infusion. Avoid extravasation.

Extravasation management: If extravasation occurs, stop infusion immediately and disconnect (leave needle/cannula in place); gently aspirate extravasated solution (do **NOT** flush the line); initiate hyaluronidase antidote; remove needle/cannula; apply dry cold compresses (Hurst, 2004); elevate extremity.

Hyaluronidase: Intradermal or SubQ: Inject a total of 1 mL (15 units/mL) as five separate 0.2 mL injections (using a 25-gauge needle) into area of extravasation at the leading edge in a clockwise manner (MacCara, 1983; Zenk, 1981).

Oral: Oral dosage forms should be taken with meals and a full glass of water or other liquid to minimize the risk of GI irritation. Prescribing information for the various oral preparations recommend that no more than 20 mEq or 25 mEq should be given as single dose.

Capsule: MicroK: Swallow whole, do not chew. Capsules may also be opened and contents sprinkled on a spoonful of applesauce or pudding and should be swallowed immediately without chewing.

Powder: Klor-Con: Dissolve one packet in 4-5 ounces of water or other beverage prior to administration.

Tablet:

K-Tab, Kaon-Cl, Klor-Con: Swallow tablets whole; do not crush, chew, or suck on tablet.

Klor-Con M: Swallow tablets whole; do not crush, chew, or suck on tablet. Tablet may also be broken in half and each half swallowed separately; the whole tablet may be dissolved in ~4 ounces of water (allow ~2 minutes to dissolve, stir well and drink immediately)

Monitoring Parameters Serum potassium, chloride, magnesium (to facilitate potassium repletion), cardiac monitor (if intermittent infusion or potassium infusion rates 0.5 mEq/kg/hour in children or >10 mEq/hour in adults); to assess adequate replacement, repeat serum potassium level 2-4 hours after dose

Reference Range Note: Reference ranges may vary depending on the laboratory

Serum potassium: 3.5-5.2 mEq/L

Dosage Forms Considerations 750 mg potassium chloride = elemental potassium 390 mg = potassium 10 mEq = potassium 10 mmol

Dosage Forms

Capsule Extended Release, Oral:

Micro-K: 8 mEq, 10 mEq

Generic: 8 mEq, 10 mEq

Liquid, Oral:

Generic: 20 mEq/15 mL (10%) (473 mL); 40 mEq/15 mL (20%) (473 mL)

Packet, Oral:

K-Vescent: 20 mEq (100 ea)

Klor-Con: 20 mEq (1 ea, 30 ea, 100 ea); 25 mEq (30 ea, 100 ea)

Generic: 20 mEq (30 ea, 100 ea)

Solution, Intravenous:

Generic: 5 mEq (250 mL); 10 mEq (500 mL, 1000 mL); 20 mEq (1000 mL); 30 mEq (1000 mL); 40 mEq (1000 mL); 0.4 mEq/mL (50 mL); 10 mEq/100 mL (100 mL); 10 mEq/50 mL (50 mL); 20 mEq/100 mL (100 mL); 20 mEq/50 mL (50 mL); 40 mEq/100 mL (100 mL); 2 mEq/mL (5 mL, 10 mL, 15 mL, 20 mL, 30 mL, 250 mL); 20 mEq/L (1000 mL); 40 mEq/L (1000 mL)

Solution, Oral:

K-Sol: 20 mEq/15 mL (10%) (473 mL); 40 mEq/15 mL (20%) (473 mL)

Generic: 20 mEq/15 mL (10%) (15 mL, 30 mL, 473 mL)

Tablet Extended Release, Oral:

K-Tab: 10 mEq, 20 mEq

Klor-Con: 8 mEq

Klor-Con 10: 10 mEq

Klor-Con M10: 10 mEq

Klor-Con M15: 15 mEq

Klor-Con M20: 20 mEq

Generic: 8 mEq, 10 mEq, 20 mEq

Potassium Citrate and Citric Acid

(poe TASS ee um SIT rate & SI trik AS id)

Brand Names: U.S. Cytra-K

Index Terms Citric Acid and Potassium Citrate; Polycitra K

Pharmacologic Category Alkalinizing Agent, Oral

Use Treatment of metabolic acidosis; alkalinizing agent in conditions where long-term maintenance of an alkaline urine is desirable

Dosage Urine alkalizing agent:

Children: Solution: 5-15 mL after meals and at bedtime; adjust dose based on urinary pH

Adults:

Powder: One packet dissolved in water after meals and at bedtime; adjust dose to urinary pH

Solution: 15-30 mL after meals and at bedtime; adjust dose based on urinary pH

Dosage adjustment in renal impairment: No dosage adjustment provided in manufacturer's labeling. Use is contraindicated in patients with severe renal impairment with oliguria or azotemia.

Dosage adjustment in hepatic impairment: No dosage adjustment provided in manufacturer's labeling.

Additional Information Complete prescribing information should be consulted for additional detail.

Dosage Forms

Powder for solution, oral:

Cytra-K: Potassium citrate monohydrate 3300 mg and citric acid monohydrate 1002 mg per packet (100s) [sugar free; fruit-punch flavor; each packet contains potassium 30 mEq equivalent to bicarbonate 30 mEq]

Solution, oral:

Cytra-K: Potassium citrate monohydrate 1100 mg and citric acid monohydrate 334 mg per 5 mL (480 mL) [ethanol free, sugar free; contains propylene glycol; cherry flavor; contains potassium 2 mEq/mL equivalent to bicarbonate 2 mEq /mL]

◆ **Potassium Citrate, Citric Acid, and Sodium Citrate** *see* Citric Acid, Sodium Citrate, and Potassium Citrate *on page* 455

Potassium Gluconate

(poe TASS ee um GLOO coe nate)

Brand Names: U.S. K-99 [OTC]

Pharmacologic Category Electrolyte Supplement, Oral

Use Dietary supplement

Dosage Oral: Adults: One tablet daily as dietary supplement

Dosage adjustment in renal impairment: No dosage adjustment provided in manufacturer's labeling.

Dosage adjustment in hepatic impairment: No dosage adjustment provided in manufacturer's labeling.

Additional Information Complete prescribing information should be consulted for additional detail.

Dosage Forms Considerations 1 g potassium gluconate = elemental potassium 167 mg = potassium 4.3 mEq = potassium 4.3 mmol

Dosage Forms

Capsule, Oral [preservative free]:

K-99 [OTC]: 595 mg

Tablet, Oral:

Generic: 80 mg, 2 mEq, 2.5 mEq

Potassium Iodide (poe TASS ee um EYE oh dide)

Brand Names: U.S. SSKI; ThyroShield [OTC]

Index Terms KI; Saturated Potassium Iodide Solution; Saturated Solution of Potassium Iodide

Pharmacologic Category Antidote; Antithyroid Agent; Expectorant

Use Expectorant for the symptomatic treatment of chronic pulmonary diseases complicated by mucous; block thyroidal uptake of radioactive isotopes of iodine in a nuclear radiation emergency

Pregnancy Risk Factor D

Dosage

RDA: Adults: 150 mcg (iodine)

Expectorant (SSKI®): Adults: Oral: 300-600 mg (0.3-0.6 mL) 3-4 times daily

Thyroid block following nuclear radiation emergency (iOSAT™, ThyroSafe®, ThyroShield®): Dosing should continue for 10-14 days or as directed by public officials (until risk of exposure has passed or other measures are implemented): Oral:

Infants ≤1 month: 16.25 mg once daily

Infants >1 month to Children ≤3 years: 32.5 mg once daily

Children >3 to ≤12 years: 65 mg once daily

Children >12-18 years weighing <68 kg: 65 mg once daily

Children >12-18 years weighing ≥68 kg and Adults (including pregnant/lactating women): 130 mg once daily

Thyroidectomy preparation (off-label use): Oral:

Children: 150-350 mg (3-7 drops **or** 0.15-0.35 mL SSKI®) 3 times daily; administer for 10 days before surgery; if not euthyroid prior to surgery, consider concurrent beta-blockade (eg, propranolol) in the immediate preoperative period to reduce the risk of thyroid storm (Bahn, 2011)

Adults: 50-100 mg (1-2 drops **or** 0.05-0.1 mL SSKI®) 3 times daily; administer for 10 days before surgery; if not euthyroid prior to surgery, consider concurrent beta-blockade (eg, propranolol) in the immediate preoperative period to reduce the risk of thyroid storm (Bahn, 2011)

Thyroid gland protection during radiopharmaceutical use (off-label use): Oral:

Note: Begin at 1-48 hours prior to exposure. Continue potassium iodide after radiopharmaceutical administration until risk of exposure has diminished (treatment duration and time of initiation is dependent on the radiopharmaceutical, consult specific protocol).

Children (Giammarile, 2008; Olivier, 2003):

Infants <5 kg: 16 mg once daily

1 month to 3 years or 5-15 kg: 32 mg once daily

3-13 years or 15-50 kg: 65 mg once daily

>13 years or >50 kg: 130 mg once daily

Adults: Tablet: 130 mg once daily **or** Solution (SSKI®): 4 drops 3 times daily (Bexxar® prescribing information, 2012)

Thyrotoxic crisis/thyroid storm (off-label use): Oral: **Note:** Administer at least 1-2 hours after antithyroid drug administration:

Infants: 100 mg (2 drops **or** 0.1 mL SSKI®) 4 times daily (Eyal, 2008)

Children: 250 mg (5 drops **or** 0.25 mL SSKI®) 2-4 times daily (Eyal, 2008)

Adults: 250 mg (5 drops **or** 0.25 mL SSKI®) every 6 hours (Bahn, 2011)

Sporotrichosis (cutaneous, lymphocutaneous; off-label use) (SSKI®): Adults: Oral: Initial: 5 drops 3 times daily; increase to 40-50 drops 3 times daily as tolerated until 2-4 weeks after lesions have resolved (usual duration 3-6 months) (Kauffman, 2007)

Dosage adjustment in renal impairment: No dosage adjustment provided in the manufacturer's labeling.

Dosage adjustment in hepatic impairment: No dosage adjustment provided in the manufacturer's labeling.

Additional Information Complete prescribing information should be consulted for additional detail.

Dosage Forms

Solution, Oral:

SSKI: 1 g/mL (30 mL, 237 mL)

ThyroShield [OTC]: 65 mg/mL (30 mL)

Potassium Iodide and Iodine

(poe TASS ee um EYE oh dide & EYE oh dine)

Index Terms Iodine and Potassium Iodide; Lugol's Solution; Strong Iodine Solution

Pharmacologic Category Antiseptic, Topical; Antithyroid Agent

Use Topical antiseptic

Pregnancy Risk Factor D (potassium iodide)

Dosage

Topical: Adults: Antiseptic: Apply directly to area(s) requiring antiseptic.

Oral:

Children and Adults:

Thyrotoxic crisis (off-label use):

Children: 4-8 drops 3 times daily; begin therapy preferably 2 hours following the initial dose of propylthiouracil or alternatively, methimazole (Eyal, 2008)

Adults: 4-8 drops every 6-8 hours; begin administration ≥1 hour following the initial dose of either propylthiouracil or methimazole (Nayak, 2006)

Adults:

RDA: 150 mcg (iodine)

Preparation for thyroidectomy (off-label use): 5-7 drops (0.25-0.35 mL) 3 times daily; administer for 10 days before surgery; if not euthyroid prior to surgery, consider concurrent beta-blockade (eg, propranolol) in the immediate preoperative period to reduce the risk of thyroid storm (Bahn, 2011)

Thyroid gland protection during radiopharmaceutical use (off-label use): 20 drops 3 times daily has been recommended (Bexxar® prescribing information, 2012)

Note: Initiate 1-48 hours prior to radiopharmaceutical exposure and continue after radiopharmaceutical administration until risk of exposure has diminished (treatment initiation time and duration is dependent on the radiopharmaceutical agent used, consult specific protocol or labeling.

Dosage adjustment in renal impairment: No dosage adjustment provided in manufacturer's labeling.

Dosage adjustment in hepatic impairment: No dosage adjustment provided in manufacturer's labeling.

Additional Information Complete prescribing information should be consulted for additional detail.

Dosage Forms

Solution, oral: Potassium iodide 100 mg/mL and iodine 50 mg/mL (473 mL)

Solution, topical: Potassium iodide 100 mg/mL and iodine 50 mg/mL (8 mL)

Potassium Phosphate (poe TASS ee um FOS fate)

Brand Names: U.S. Neutra-Phos®-K [OTC] [DSC]

Index Terms Phosphate, Potassium

Pharmacologic Category Electrolyte Supplement, Parenteral

Use Treatment and prevention of hypophosphatemia; **Note:** The concomitant amount of potassium must be calculated into the total electrolyte content. For each 1 mmol of phosphate, ~1.5 mEq of potassium will be administered. Therefore, if ordering 30 mmol of potassium phosphate, the patient will receive ~45 mEq of potassium.

Pregnancy Risk Factor C

Pregnancy Considerations Reproduction studies have not been conducted. Phosphorus requirements are the same in pregnant and nonpregnant women (IOM, 1997). Although this product is not used for potassium supplementation, adverse events have not been observed following use of potassium supplements in healthy women with normal pregnancies. Use caution in pregnant women with other medical conditions (eg, pre-eclampsia; may be more likely to develop hyperkalemia) (IOM, 2004).

Breast-Feeding Considerations Phosphorus, sodium, and potassium are normal constituents of human milk.

Contraindications Hyperphosphatemia, hyperkalemia, hypocalcemia

Warnings/Precautions Close monitoring of serum potassium concentrations is needed to avoid hyperkalemia. Use with caution in patients with renal insufficiency, cardiac disease, metabolic alkalosis. Use with caution in digitalized patients and patients receiving concomitant potassium-altering therapies. Parenteral potassium may cause pain and phlebitis, requiring a decrease in infusion rate or potassium concentration. Solutions for injection may contain aluminum; toxic levels may occur following prolonged administration in premature neonates or patients with renal impairment.

Adverse Reactions

Cardiovascular: Arrhythmia, bradycardia, chest pain, ECG changes, edema, heart block, hypotension

Central nervous system: Listlessness, mental confusion, tetany (with large doses of phosphate)

Endocrine & metabolic: Hyperkalemia

Gastrointestinal: Diarrhea, nausea, stomach pain, vomiting

Genitourinary: Urine output decreased

Local: Phlebitis

Neuromuscular & skeletal: Paralysis, paresthesia, weakness

Renal: Acute renal failure

Respiratory: Dyspnea

Drug Interactions

Metabolism/Transport Effects None known.

Avoid Concomitant Use There are no known interactions where it is recommended to avoid concomitant use.

Increased Effect/Toxicity

Potassium Phosphate may increase the levels/effects of: ACE Inhibitors; Aliskiren; Angiotensin II Receptor Blockers; Potassium-Sparing Diuretics

The levels/effects of Potassium Phosphate may be increased by: Bisphosphonate Derivatives; Eplerenone; Heparin; Heparin (Low Molecular Weight); Nicorandil

Decreased Effect

The levels/effects of Potassium Phosphate may be decreased by: Antacids; Calcium Salts; Iron Salts; Magnesium Salts; Multivitamins/Minerals (with ADEK, Folate, Iron); Sucralfate

Food Interactions Avoid administering with oxalate (berries, nuts, chocolate, beans, celery, tomato) or phytate-containing foods (bran, whole wheat).

Preparation for Administration In general, the dose, concentration of infusion, and rate of administration may be dependent on patient condition and specific institution policy. Intermittent infusion doses of potassium phosphate are typically prepared in 100-250 mL of NS or D_5W (usual phosphate concentration range: 0.15-0.6 mmol/mL) (Charron, 2003; Rosen, 1995). Suggested maximum concentrations:

Central line administration: 26.8 mmoL potassium phosphate/100 mL (40 mEq potassium/100 mL)

Peripheral line administration: 6.7 mmoL potassium phosphate/100 mL (10 mEq potassium/100 mL)

Observe the vial for the presence of translucent visible particles. Do not use vial if particles are present. Dilute in a compatible IV fluid. **Note:** Due to the potential presence of particulates, American Regent, Inc recommends the use of a 5 micron filter when preparing IV potassium phosphate-containing solutions (Important Drug Administration Information, American Regent, 2011); a similar recommendation has not been noted by other manufacturers.

Storage/Stability Store intact vials at 20°C to 25°C (68°F to 77°F); excursions permitted between 15°C and 30°C (59°F and 86°F).

Mechanism of Action

Phosphorus in the form of organic and inorganic phosphate has a variety of important biochemical functions in the body and is involved in many significant metabolic and enzymatic reactions in almost all organs and tissues. It exerts a modifying influence on the steady state of calcium levels, a buffering effect on acid-base equilibrium and a primary role in the renal excretion of hydrogen ion.

Potassium is the major cation of intracellular fluid and is essential for the conduction of nerve impulses in heart, brain, and skeletal muscle; contraction of cardiac, skeletal and smooth muscles; maintenance of normal renal function, acid-base balance, carbohydrate metabolism, and gastric secretion.

Dosage Note: If phosphate repletion is required and a phosphate product is not available at your institution, consider the use of sodium glycerophosphate pentahydrate (Glycophos) as a suitable substitute. Concentration and dosing are different from FDA-approved products; use caution when switching between products. Refer to Sodium Glycerophosphate Pentahydrate monograph.

IV: **Caution: The concomitant amount of potassium must be calculated into the total electrolyte content. For each 1 mmol of phosphate, ~1.5 mEq of potassium will be administered. Therefore, if ordering 30 mmol of potassium phosphate, the patient will receive ~45 mEq of potassium. With orders for IV phosphate, there is considerable confusion associated with the use of millimoles (mmol) versus milliequivalents (mEq) to express the phosphate requirement.** The most reliable method of ordering IV phosphate is by millimoles, then specifying the potassium or sodium salt. Doses listed as mmol of phosphate.

Acute treatment of hypophosphatemia: Repletion of severe hypophosphatemia should be done IV because large doses of oral phosphate may cause diarrhea and intestinal absorption may be unreliable. Reserve intermittent IV infusion for severe depletion situations; may require continuous cardiac monitoring depending on potassium administration rate. Guidelines differ based on degree of illness, need/use of parenteral nutrition, and severity of hypophosphatemia. If potassium >4.0 mEq/L consider phosphate replacement strategy without potassium (eg, sodium phosphates). Patients with severe renal impairment were excluded from phosphate supplement trials. **Note:** 1 mmol phosphate = 31 mg phosphorus; 1 mg phosphorus = 0.032 mmol phosphate.

Children and Adults: **Note:** There are no prospective studies of parenteral phosphate replacement in children. The following weight-based guidelines for adult dosing may be cautiously employed in pediatric patients.

General replacement guidelines (Lentz, 1978):

Low dose, if serum phosphate losses are recent and uncomplicated: Initial: 0.08 mmol/kg over 6 hours

Intermediate dose, if serum phosphorus level <1 mg/dL (<0.32 mmol/L): Initial: 0.16 mmol/kg per dose over 6 hours

Note: The initial dose may be increased by 25% to 50% if the patient is symptomatic secondary to hypophosphatemia and lowered by 25% to 50% if the patient is hypercalcemic. Do not exceed the maximum dose of 0.24 mmol/kg/dose (or 16.9 mmol for a 70-kg patient).

Critically-ill adult patients receiving concurrent enteral/parenteral nutrition (Brown, 2006; Clark, 1995): Note: Round doses to the nearest 7.5 mmol for ease of preparation. If administering with phosphate-containing parenteral nutrition, do not exceed 15 mmol/L within parenteral nutrition.

Low dose, serum phosphorus level 2.3-3 mg/dL (0.74-0.96 mmol/L): 0.16-0.32 mmol/kg over 4-6 hours

Intermediate dose, serum phosphorus level 1.6-2.2 mg/dL (0.51-0.71 mmol/L): 0.32-0.64 mmol/kg over 4-6 hours

High dose, serum phosphorus <1.5 mg/dL (<0.5 mmol/L): 0.64-1 mmol/kg over 8-12 hours

Obesity: May use adjusted body weight for patients weighing >130% of ideal body weight (and BMI <40 kg/m^2) by using [IBW + 0.25 (actual body weight - IBW)].

Parenteral nutrition:

Infants and Children: 0.5-2 mmol/kg/24 hours (Mirtallo, 2004 [ASPEN guidelines])

Children >50 kg and Adolescents: 10-40 mmol/24 hours (Mirtallo, 2004 [ASPEN guidelines])

Adults: 10-15 mmol/1000 kcal (Hicks, 2001) **or** 20-40 mmol/24 hours (Mirtallo, 2004 [ASPEN guidelines])

Administration Injection must be diluted in appropriate IV solution and volume prior to administration. In general, the dose, concentration of infusion, and rate of administration may be dependent on patient condition and specific institution policy. Must consider administration precautions for phosphate and potassium when prescribing. **Note:** Due to the potential presence of translucent visible particles, American Regent, Inc recommends the use of a 0.22 micron in-line filter for IV administration (1.2 micron filter if admixture contains lipids) (Important Drug Administration Information, American Regent, 2011); a similar recommendation has not been noted by other manufacturers.

For adult patients with severe symptomatic hypophosphatemia (ie, <1.5 mg/dL), may administer at rates up to 15 mmol phosphate/hour (this rate will deliver potassium at 22.5 mEq/hour) (Charron, 2003; Rosen, 1995). Potassium infusion rates >10 mEq/hour should be administered via central line (minimizes burning and phlebitis). ECG monitoring is recommended for potassium infusions >10 mEq/hour in adults or >0.5 mEq/kg/hour in children. In patients with renal dysfunction and/or less severe hypophosphatemia, slower administration rates (eg, over 4-6 hours) or oral repletion is recommended.

Monitoring Parameters Serum potassium, calcium, phosphorus, magnesium (to facilitate potassium repletion); cardiac monitor (if intermittent infusion or potassium infusion rates >0.5 mEq/kg/hour in children or >10 mEq/hour in adults); to assess adequate replacement, repeat serum potassium and phosphorus levels 2-4 hours after dose

Reference Range Note: Reference ranges may vary depending on the laboratory

Serum calcium: 8.4-10.2 mg/dL

Serum phosphorus: Both low and high ends of the normal range are higher in children than in adults.

Infants: 4.5-7.5 mg/dL (1.45-2.42 mmol/L)

Children: ~4-6 mg/dL (1.29-1.94 mmol/L)

Adults: 2.5-4.5 mg/dL (0.81-1.45 mmol/L)

Serum potassium: 3.5-5.2 mEq/L

Dosage Forms Considerations

Potassium 4.4 mEq is equivalent to potassium 170 mg

Phosphorous 3 mmol is equivalent to phosphorus 93 mg

Dosage Forms

Injection, solution: Potassium 4.4 mEq and phosphorus 3 mmol per mL (5 mL, 15 mL, 50 mL)

Potassium Phosphate and Sodium Phosphate

(poe TASS ee um FOS fate & SOW dee um FOS fate)

Brand Names: U.S. K-Phos Neutral; K-Phos No. 2; Phos-NaK; Phospha 250 Neutral; Virt-Phos 250 Neutral

Index Terms Neutra-Phos; Sodium Phosphate and Potassium Phosphate

Pharmacologic Category Electrolyte Supplement, Oral

Use Phosphorus supplement; to increase urinary phosphate and pyrophosphate; to acidify the urine to lower calcium concentrations; to increase the antibacterial activity of methenamine; reduce odor and rash caused by ammonia in urine

Pregnancy Risk Factor C

Dosage Oral: **Note:** Dosage expressed in terms of **elemental phosphorus**.

Children ≥4 years and Adolescents: Phosphate supplement: 250 mg 4 times daily

Adults:
Phosphate supplement: 250-500 mg 4 times daily
Urinary acidification: 250 mg 4 times daily; may be increased to 250 mg every 2 hours when the urine is difficult to acidify (maximum daily dose: 2000 mg)

Dosage adjustment in renal impairment: No dosage adjustment provided in manufacturer's labeling. Use with caution. Contraindicated in patients with severe impairment (<30% of normal function).

Dosage adjustment in hepatic impairment: No dosage adjustment provided in manufacturer's labeling. Use with caution.

Additional Information Complete prescribing information should be consulted for additional detail.

Dosage Forms

Powder for solution, oral:

Phos-NaK: Dibasic potassium phosphate, monobasic potassium phosphate, dibasic sodium phosphate, and monobasic sodium phosphate per packet (100s)

Tablet, oral:

K-Phos Neutral: Monobasic potassium phosphate 155 mg, dibasic sodium phosphate 852 mg, and monobasic sodium phosphate 130 mg

K-Phos No. 2: Potassium phosphate 305 mg and sodium phosphate 700 mg

Phospha 250 Neutral: Monobasic potassium phosphate 155 mg, dibasic sodium phosphate 852 mg, and monobasic sodium phosphate 130 mg

Virt-Phos 250 Neutral: Monobasic potassium phosphate 155 mg, dibasic sodium phosphate 852 mg, and monobasic sodium phosphate 130 mg

- ◆ **Potassium Phosphate Monobasic** *see* Potassium Acid Phosphate *on page* *1687*
- ◆ **Potassium Sulfate, Magnesium Sulfate, and Sodium Sulfate** *see* Sodium Sulfate, Potassium Sulfate, and Magnesium Sulfate *on page* *1914*
- ◆ **Potassium Sulfate, Sodium Sulfate, and Magnesium Sulfate** *see* Sodium Sulfate, Potassium Sulfate, and Magnesium Sulfate *on page* *1914*
- ◆ **Potiga** *see* Ezogabine *on page* *835*
- ◆ **PPD** *see* Tuberculin Tests *on page* *2110*
- ◆ **PPI-0903** *see* Ceftaroline Fosamil *on page* *391*
- ◆ **PPI-0903M** *see* Ceftaroline Fosamil *on page* *391*
- ◆ **PPS** *see* Pentosan Polysulfate Sodium *on page* *1617*
- ◆ **PPSV** *see* Pneumococcal Polysaccharide Vaccine (23-Valent) *on page* *1671*
- ◆ **PPSV23** *see* Pneumococcal Polysaccharide Vaccine (23-Valent) *on page* *1671*
- ◆ **PPV23** *see* Pneumococcal Polysaccharide Vaccine (23-Valent) *on page* *1671*
- ◆ **PR-171** *see* Carfilzomib *on page* *361*
- ◆ **Pradaxa** *see* Dabigatran Etexilate *on page* *542*

PRALAtrexate (pral a TREX ate)

Brand Names: U.S. Folotyn

Index Terms PDX

Pharmacologic Category Antineoplastic Agent, Antimetabolite; Antineoplastic Agent, Antimetabolite (Antifolate)

Use Treatment of relapsed or refractory peripheral T-cell lymphoma (PTCL)

Pregnancy Risk Factor D

Pregnancy Considerations Adverse effects were observed in animal reproduction studies. May cause fetal harm if administered to a pregnant woman.

Breast-Feeding Considerations Due to the potential for serious adverse reactions in the nursing infant, the decision to discontinue breast-feeding or to discontinue pralatrexate should take into account the benefits of treatment to the mother.

Contraindications There are no contraindications listed within the manufacturer's labeling.

Warnings/Precautions Hazardous agent - use appropriate precautions for handling and disposal (NIOSH 2014 [group 1]). May cause bone marrow suppression (thrombocytopenia, neutropenia and anemia); may require dosage modification; monitor blood counts. Mucositis, including stomatitis or mucosal inflammation of gastrointestinal and genitourinary tracts, may occur; monitor weekly; may require dosage modification. Prophylactic folic acid and vitamin B_{12} supplements are necessary to reduce hematologic toxicity and treatment-related mucositis. Severe and potentially fatal dermatologic reactions, including skin exfoliation, ulceration, and toxic epidermal necrolysis (TEN) have been reported. Skin reaction may be progressive; severity may increase with continued treatment; may also involve skin and subcutaneous tissues which are affected by lymphoma; monitor all dermatologic reactions closely; withhold or discontinue treatment for severe dermatologic reaction.

Pralatrexate may cause tumor lysis syndrome (TLS); monitor closely, if TLS develops, treat for associated complications. Use with caution in patients with moderate-to-severe renal impairment (has not been studied in patients with renal impairment); monitor renal function and for systemic toxicity due to increased exposure. Concurrent use with drugs with substantial renal clearance (eg, NSAIDs, sulfamethoxazole/trimethoprim) may result in delayed pralatrexate clearance. Liver function test abnormalities have been observed with use; monitor liver function; persistent abnormalities may indicate hepatotoxicity and may require dosage modification.

Patients with moderate-to-severe renal impairment are at risk for increased exposure and toxicity. Avoid use in patients with end-stage renal disease (ESRD), including patients undergoing dialysis (unless the potential benefit outweighs potential risks); serious adverse reactions, including toxic epidermal necrolysis and mucositis were reported in patients with ESRD undergoing dialysis. Monitor renal function and for systemic toxicity due to increased exposure.

Adverse Reactions

Cardiovascular: Edema, tachycardia
Central nervous system: Fatigue, fever
Dermatologic: Pruritus, rash
Endocrine & metabolic: Dehydration, hypokalemia
Gastrointestinal: Abdominal pain, anorexia, constipation, diarrhea, mucositis, nausea, vomiting
Hematologic: Anemia, leukopenia, neutropenia, neutropenic fever, thrombocytopenia
Hepatic: Transaminases increased
Neuromuscular & skeletal: Back pain, limb pain, weakness
Respiratory: Cough, dyspnea, epistaxis, pharyngolaryngeal pain, upper respiratory infection
Miscellaneous: Infection, night sweats, sepsis
Rare but important or life-threatening: Bowel obstruction, cardiopulmonary arrest, lymphopenia, odynophagia, pancytopenia, skin exfoliation, skin ulceration, toxic epidermal necrolysis (TEN), tumor lysis syndrome (TLS)

Drug Interactions

Metabolism/Transport Effects Substrate of BCRP

Avoid Concomitant Use

Avoid concomitant use of PRALAtrexate with any of the following: BCG; Natalizumab; Pimecrolimus; Tacrolimus (Topical); Tofacitinib; Vaccines (Live)

Increased Effect/Toxicity

PRALAtrexate may increase the levels/effects of: Leflunomide; Natalizumab; Tofacitinib; Vaccines (Live)

The levels/effects of PRALAtrexate may be increased by: Denosumab; Nonsteroidal Anti-Inflammatory Agents; Pimecrolimus; Probenecid; Roflumilast; Salicylates; Sulfamethoxazole; Tacrolimus (Topical); Trastuzumab; Trimethoprim

Decreased Effect

PRALAtrexate may decrease the levels/effects of: BCG; Coccidioides immitis Skin Test; Sapropterin; Sipuleucel-T; Vaccines (Inactivated); Vaccines (Live)

The levels/effects of PRALAtrexate may be decreased by: Echinacea

Preparation for Administration Hazardous agent; use appropriate precautions for handling and disposal (NIOSH 2014 [group 1]). Withdraw into syringe for administration; do not dilute (manufacturer recommends immediate use after placing in syringe). Discard unused portion in the vial.

Storage/Stability Store intact vials refrigerated at 2°C to 8°C (36°F to 46°F). Store in original carton to protect from light until use. Unopened vials (stored in the original carton) are stable for up to 72 hours at room temperature (discard after 72 hours).

Mechanism of Action Antifolate analog; inhibits DNA, RNA, and protein synthesis by selectively entering cells expressing reduced folate carrier (RFC-1), is polyglutamylated by folylpolyglutamate synthetase (FPGS) and then competes for the DHFR-folate binding site to inhibit dihydrofolate reductase (DHFR)

Pharmacodynamics/Kinetics

Distribution: *S*-diastereomer: 105 L; *R*-diastereomer: 37 L
Protein binding: ~67%
Half-life elimination: 12-18 hours
Excretion: Urine (~34% as unchanged drug)

Dosage Note: Initite vitamin supplements before initial pralatrexate dose: Folic acid 1-1.25 mg/day orally beginning 10 days prior to initial pralatrexate dose; continue during treatment and for 30 days after last pralatrexate dose; vitamin B_{12} 1000 mcg IM within 10 weeks prior to initial pralatrexate dose and every 8-10 weeks thereafter (after initial dose, B_{12} may be administered on the same day as pralatrexate).

Prior to administering any dose, mucositis should be ≤ grade 1 and absolute neutrophil count (ANC) should be ≥1000/mm^3; platelets should be ≥100,000/mm^3 for the first dose and ≥50,000/mm^3 for subsequent doses

IV: Adults:

Peripheral T-cell lymphoma (PTCL), relapsed or refractory: 30 mg/m^2 once weekly for 6 weeks of a 7-week treatment cycle; continue until disease progression or unacceptable toxicity (O'Connor, 2011)

Cutaneous T-cell lymphoma, relapsed or refractory (off-label use): 15 mg/m^2 once weekly for 3 weeks of a 4-week treatment cycle (Horwitz, 2012)

Dosage adjustment for toxicity: Severe or intolerable adverse events may require dose omission, reduction or interruption. Do not make up omitted doses at the end of a cycle; do not re-escalate dose after a reduction due to toxicity.

Hematologic toxicity:

Platelets:

<50,000/mm^3 (for 1-week duration): Omit dose; continue at previous dose if platelets recover within 1 week

<50,000/mm^3 (for 2-week duration): Omit dose; decrease to 20 mg/m^2 if platelets recover within 2 weeks

<50,000/mm^3 (for 3-week duration): Discontinue treatment

ANC:

500-1000/mm^3 without fever (for 1-week duration): Omit dose; continue at previous dose if ANC recovers within 1 week

500-1000/mm^3 with fever **or** ANC <500/mm^3 (for 1-week duration): Omit dose, give filgrastim or sargramostim support; continue at previous dose (with growth factor support) if ANC recovers within 1 week

500-1000/mm^3 with fever **or** ANC <500/mm^3 (recurrent or for 2-week duration): Omit dose and give filgrastim or sargramostim support; decrease to 20 mg/m^2 (with growth factor support) if ANC recovers within 2 weeks

500-1000/mm^3 with fever **or** ANC <500/mm^3 (second recurrence or for 3-week duration): Discontinue treatment

Nonhematologic toxicity: Mucositis (on day of treatment):

Grade 2: Omit dose; continue at previous dose when recovers to ≤ grade 1

Grade 3 or recurrent grade 2: Omit dose and decrease to 20 mg/m^2 when recovers to ≤ grade 1

Grade 4: Discontinue treatment

Nonhematologic toxicity (other than mucositis):

Grade 3: Omit dose; decrease to 20 mg/m^2 when recovers to ≤ grade 2

Grade 4: Discontinue treatment

Dosage adjustment in renal impairment:

Moderate-to-severe renal impairment: Exposure and toxicities may be increased; monitor for toxicities and adjust dose accordingly.

End-stage renal disease (ESRD), including dialysis-dependent: Avoid use (unless the potential benefit outweighs risks).

Dosage adjustment in hepatic impairment: Patients with total bilirubin >1.5 mg/dL, AST or ALT >2.5 times the upper limit of normal (ULN), or ALT or AST >5 times ULN if documented hepatic lymphoma involvement were excluded from clinical trials. Persistent abnormalities may indicate hepatotoxicity requiring dosage modification:

Grade 3 (AST or ALT >5-20 times ULN or bilirubin >3-10 times ULN): Omit dose; decrease to 20 mg/m^2 when recovers to ≤ grade 2

Grade 4 (AST or ALT >20 times ULN or bilirubin >10 times ULN): Discontinue treatment.

Dosing in obesity: *ASCO Guidelines for appropriate chemotherapy dosing in obese adults with cancer:* Utilize patient's actual body weight (full weight) for calculation of body surface area- or weight-based dosing, particularly when the intent of therapy is curative; manage regimen-related toxicities in the same manner as for nonobese patients; if a dose reduction is utilized due to toxicity, consider resumption of full weight-based dosing with subsequent cycles, especially if cause of toxicity (eg, hepatic or renal impairment) is resolved (Griggs, 2012).

Administration Administer IV push (undiluted) over 3-5 minutes into the line of a free-flowing normal saline IV

Hazardous agent; use appropriate precautions for handling and disposal (NIOSH 2014 [group 1]).

Monitoring Parameters CBC with differential (baseline and weekly), serum chemistries, including renal and liver function tests (prior to the first and fourth doses in each cycle); mucositis severity (baseline and weekly); monitor for signs of tumor lysis syndrome

Dosage Forms

Solution, Intravenous [preservative free]:
Folotyn: 20 mg/mL (1 mL); 40 mg/2 mL (2 mL)

Pralidoxime (pra li DOKS eem)

Brand Names: U.S. Protopam Chloride

Index Terms 2-PAM; 2-Pyridine Aldoxime Methochloride; 2PAM; Pralidoxime Chloride

Pharmacologic Category Antidote

Use Treatment of muscle weakness and/or respiratory depression secondary to poisoning due to organophosphate anticholinesterase pesticides and chemicals (eg, nerve agents); control of overdose of anticholinesterase medications used to treat myasthenia gravis (ambenonium, neostigmine, pyridostigmine)

Pregnancy Risk Factor C

Dosage

IV:

Anticholinesterase overdose (eg, neostigmine, pyridostigmine): Adults: 1000-2000 mg; followed by increments of 250 mg every 5 minutes as needed

Organophosphate poisoning: **Note:** Use in conjunction with atropine; a response to atropine should be established before pralidoxime is administered. IM or SubQ administration should be considered when IV administration is not feasible:

Children and Adolescents ≤16 years: Loading dose: 20-50 mg/kg (maximum: 2000 mg/dose); Maintenance infusion: 10-20 mg/kg/hour; alternatively, a repeat bolus of 20-50 mg/kg (maximum: 2000 mg/dose) may be administered after 1 hour and repeated every 10-12 hours thereafter, as needed

Adolescents >16 years and Adults: Loading dose: 1000-2000 mg; Maintenance: Repeat bolus of 1000-2000 mg after 1 hour and repeated every 10-12 hours thereafter, as needed. Alternatively, administer a loading dose of 30 mg/kg followed by a maintenance infusion of 8 mg/kg/hour (off-label dose; Roberts, 2007).

IM: Organophosphate poisoning: **Note:** Use in conjunction with atropine; a response to atropine should be established before pralidoxime is administered. IM or SubQ administration should be considered when IV administration is not feasible:

Children <40 kg:

Mild symptoms: 15 mg/kg; repeat as needed for persistent mild symptoms every 15 minutes to a maximum total dose of 45 mg/kg; may administer doses in rapid succession if severe symptoms develop

Severe symptoms: 15 mg/kg; repeat twice in rapid succession to deliver a total dose of 45 mg/kg

Persistent symptoms: May repeat the entire series (45 mg/kg) beginning ~1 hour after administration of the last injection

Children ≥40 kg, Adolescents, and Adults:

Mild symptoms: 600 mg; repeat as needed for persistent mild symptoms every 15 minutes to a maximum total dose of 1800 mg; may administer doses in rapid succession if severe symptoms develop

Severe symptoms: 600 mg; repeat twice in rapid succession to deliver a total dose of 1800 mg

Persistent symptoms: May repeat the entire series (1800 mg) beginning ~1 hour after administration of the last injection

Elderly: Refer to adult dosing.

Dosing adjustment in renal impairment: No specific dosage adjustment provided in manufacturer's labeling; however, because pralidoxime is excreted in the urine, dosage reduction is recommended in patients with renal impairment.

Dosage adjustment in hepatic impairment: No dosage adjustment provided in the manufacturer's labeling; undergoes hepatic metabolism.

Additional Information Complete prescribing information should be consulted for additional detail.

Dosage Forms

Solution Auto-injector, Intramuscular:

Generic: 600 mg/2 mL (2 mL)

Solution Reconstituted, Intravenous:

Protopam Chloride: 1 g (1 ea)

◆ **Pralidoxime and Atropine** *see* Atropine and Pralidoxime *on page 203*

◆ **Pralidoxime Chloride** *see* Pralidoxime *on page 1694*

◆ **PramCort** *see* Pramoxine and Hydrocortisone *on page 1698*

Pramipexole (pra mi PEKS ole)

Brand Names: U.S. Mirapex; Mirapex ER

Brand Names: Canada ACT-Pramipexole; Apo-Pramipexole; Auro-Pramipexole; Ava-Pramipexole; Dom-Pramipexole; Mirapex; Mylan-Pramipexole; PMS-Pramipexole; Sandoz-Pramipexole; Teva-Pramipexole

Index Terms Pramipexole Dihydrochloride Monohydrate

Pharmacologic Category Anti-Parkinson's Agent, Dopamine Agonist

Use

Parkinson disease: Treatment of the signs and symptoms of idiopathic Parkinson disease.

Restless legs syndrome (immediate release only): Treatment of moderate to severe primary restless legs syndrome (RLS).

Pregnancy Risk Factor C

Pregnancy Considerations Adverse events were observed in animal reproduction studies. Information related to the use of pramipexole for the treatment of Parkinson's disease (Benbir, 2013; Mucchiut 2004) or restless legs syndrome (RLS) (Dostal, 2013) in pregnant women is limited. Current guidelines note that the available information is insufficient to make a recommendation for the treatment of RLS in pregnant women (Aurora, 2012).

Breast-Feeding Considerations It is not known if pramipexole is excreted into breast milk; however, pramipexole inhibits prolactin secretion in humans and may potentially inhibit lactation. Due to the potential for serious adverse reactions in the nursing infant, the manufacturer recommends a decision be made whether to discontinue nursing or to discontinue the drug, taking into account the importance of treatment to the mother.

Contraindications There are no contraindications listed in the manufacturer's labeling.

Warnings/Precautions Caution should be taken in patients with renal impairment; dose adjustment may be necessary. Extended-release tablets are not recommended for use in patients with CrCl <30 mL/minute or ESRD requiring hemodialysis. May cause or exacerbate dyskinesias; use caution in patients with preexisting dyskinesias. May cause orthostatic hypotension; Parkinson disease patients appear to have an impaired capacity to respond to a postural challenge. Use with caution in patients at risk of hypotension or where transient hypotensive episodes would be poorly tolerated. Parkinson's patients being treated with dopaminergic agonists ordinarily require careful monitoring for signs and symptoms of postural hypotension, especially during dose escalation. May cause hallucinations.

Dopamine agonists have been associated with compulsive behaviors and/or loss of impulse control, which has manifested as pathological gambling, compulsive buying, libido increases (hypersexuality), binge eating, and/or other intense urges. Causality has not been established, and controversy exists as to whether this phenomenon is related to the underlying disease, prior behaviors/addictions and/or drug therapy. Dose reduction or discontinuation of therapy has been reported to reverse these behaviors in some, but not all cases. Risk for melanoma development is increased in Parkinson disease patients; drug causation or factors contributing to risk have not been established. Patients should be monitored closely and periodic skin examinations should be performed.

Taper gradually when discontinuing therapy in Parkinson disease; dopaminergic agents have been associated with a syndrome resembling neuroleptic malignant syndrome on abrupt withdrawal or significant dosage reduction after long-term use. Ergot-derived dopamine agonists have been associated with fibrotic complications (eg, retroperitoneal fibrosis, pleural effusion, pleural thickening, pulmonary infiltrates, cardiac valvulopathy). Although pramipexole is not an ergot, there have been postmarketing reports of possible fibrotic complications (peritoneal, pleural, pulmonary) with pramipexole; monitor closely for signs and symptoms of fibrosis. Discontinuation of therapy may resolve complications, but not in all cases.

Pramipexole has been associated with somnolence, particularly at higher dosages (>1.5 mg/day). In addition, patients have reported falling asleep while engaging in activities of daily living; this has been reported to occur without significant warning signs; some of these events had been reported one year after the initiation of therapy. Before initiating treatment, advise patients of the potential to develop drowsiness, and inquire about factors that may increase the risk (eg, concomitant sedating medications and/or alcohol, presence of sleep disorders, concomitant medications that increase pramipexole plasma levels). Patients must be cautioned about performing tasks which require mental alertness (eg, operating machinery or driving). Monitor for daytime somnolence or preexisting sleep disorder; discontinue if significant daytime sleepiness or episodes of falling asleep occur; if a decision is made to continue therapy, advise patients not to drive and to avoid other potentially dangerous activities. Pramipexole has been associated with somnolence. Use caution in elderly patients because they may be more sensitive to these adverse drug reactions.

Pathologic degenerative changes were observed in the retinas of albino rats during studies with this agent, but were not observed in the retinas of albino mice or in other species. The significance of these data for humans remains uncertain. Augmentation (earlier onset of symptoms in the evening/afternoon, increase and/or spread of symptoms to other extremities) or rebound (worsening of symptoms following treatment cessation with greater intensity than before treatment initiation) may occur in some RLS patients. Potentially significant interactions may exist, requiring dose or frequency adjustment, additional monitoring, and/or selection of alternative therapy.

Adverse Reactions

Parkinson's disease:

Cardiovascular: Chest pain, edema, orthostatic hypotension (dose related)

Central nervous system: Abnormal dreams, abnormal thinking, akathisia, amnesia (dose related), confusion, delusions, depression, dizziness, dystonia, extrapyramidal syndrome, fatigue, fever, hallucinations, headache, hypesthesia, insomnia, malaise, myoclonus, paranoia, sleep disorder, somnolence (dose related), sudden onset of sleep, vertigo

Endocrine & metabolic: Libido decreased

Gastrointestinal: Abdominal discomfort/pain, anorexia, appetite increased, constipation, diarrhea, dyspepsia, dysphagia, nausea (dose related), salivary hypersecretion, vomiting, weight loss, xerostomia

Genitourinary: Impotence, urinary frequency, urinary incontinence, urinary tract infection

Neuromuscular & skeletal: Arthritis, back pain, balance abnormalities, bursitis, CPK increased, dyskinesia, falls, gait abnormalities, hypertonia, muscle spasm, muscle twitching, myasthenia, tremor, weakness

Ocular: Accommodation abnormalities, diplopia, vision abnormalities

Respiratory: Cough, dyspnea, pneumonia, rhinitis

Miscellaneous: Accidental injury

Rare but important or life-threatening: Blackouts, heart failure, impulsive/compulsive behaviors (eg, binge eating, hypersexuality, pathological gambling, shopping), libido increased, pruritus, rhabdomyolysis, SIADH, syncope

Restless legs syndrome:

Central nervous system: Abnormal dreams, fatigue, headache, insomnia, somnolence

Gastrointestinal: Constipation, diarrhea, nausea, xerostomia

Neuromuscular & skeletal: Limb pain

Respiratory: Nasal congestion

Miscellaneous: Influenza

Rare but important or life-threatening: Augmentation (~20% but similar to placebo), blackouts, hallucinations, hypotension, impulsive/compulsive behaviors (eg, binge eating, hypersexuality, pathological gambling, shopping), libido changes, pruritus, rebound, tolerance, syncope

Drug Interactions

Metabolism/Transport Effects None known.

Avoid Concomitant Use

Avoid concomitant use of Pramipexole with any of the following: Amisulpride; Sulpiride

Increased Effect/Toxicity

Pramipexole may increase the levels/effects of: BuPROPion

The levels/effects of Pramipexole may be increased by: Alcohol (Ethyl); Cimetidine; CNS Depressants; MAO Inhibitors; Methylphenidate

Decreased Effect

Pramipexole may decrease the levels/effects of: Amisulpride; Antipsychotic Agents (First Generation [Typical]); Sulpiride

The levels/effects of Pramipexole may be decreased by: Amisulpride; Antipsychotic Agents (First Generation [Typical]); Antipsychotic Agents (Second Generation [Atypical]); Metoclopramide; Sulpiride

Food Interactions Food intake does not affect the extent of drug absorption although the time to maximal plasma concentration is delayed when taken with a meal. Management: Administer without regard to meals.

Storage/Stability Store at 25°C (77°F); excursions permitted to 15°C to 30°C (59°F to 86°F). Protect from light and high humidity.

Mechanism of Action Pramipexole is a nonergot dopamine agonist with specificity for the D_2 subfamily dopamine receptor, and has also been shown to bind to D_3 and D_4 receptors. By binding to these receptors, it is thought that pramipexole can stimulate dopamine activity on the nerves of the striatum and substantia nigra.

Pharmacodynamics/Kinetics

Absorption: Rapid

Distribution: V_d: 500 L

Protein binding: ~15%

Metabolism: Negligible (<10%)

Bioavailability: Immediate release: >90%; Extended release (as compared to immediate release): 100%

Half-life elimination: 8.5 hours; Elderly: 12 hours

Time to peak, serum: Immediate release: ~2 hours; Extended release: 6 hours

Excretion: Urine (90% as unchanged drug)

Dosage Oral: Adults: **Note:** Retitration of dose should be considered for any significant interruption in therapy.

Immediate release:

Parkinson disease: Initial: 0.125 mg 3 times daily, increase gradually every 5 to 7 days; maintenance (usual): 0.5 to 1.5 mg 3 times daily

Discontinuation of therapy: Reduce dose by 0.75 mg per day until daily dose is equivalent to 0.75 mg once daily, then reduce by 0.375 mg per day thereafter

Restless legs syndrome: Initial: 0.125 mg once daily 2 to 3 hours before bedtime. Dose may be doubled every 4 to 7 days up to 0.5 mg once daily. **Note:** If augmentation occurs, dose earlier in the day.

Discontinuation of therapy: No gradual dose reduction recommended in manufacturer's labeling; however, worsening of symptoms may occur with abrupt discontinuation.

Depression (off-label use): Initial: 0.25 to 0.375 mg daily given in 2 to 3 divided doses with a gradual titration; mean dose: 1.6 to 1.7 mg daily (Aiken, 2007; Goldberg, 2004)

Fibromyalgia (off-label use): Initial: 0.25 mg once daily at bedtime; may be increased weekly by 0.25 mg/day increments up to 4.5 mg daily (Holman, 2005)

Extended release: Parkinson disease: Initial: 0.375 mg once daily; increase gradually not more frequently than every 5 to 7 days to 0.75 mg once daily and then (if necessary), by 0.75 mg per dose; maximum: 4.5 mg once daily.

Discontinuation of therapy: Reduce dose by 0.75 mg per day until daily dose is equivalent to 0.75 mg once daily, then reduce by 0.375 mg per day thereafter.

Converting from immediate release to extended release: May initiate extended-release tablet the morning after the last immediate-release evening tablet is taken. The total daily dose should remain the same.

Dosage adjustment in renal impairment:

Parkinson disease: Immediate release:

CrCl >50 mL/minute: No dosage adjustment necessary.

CrCl 30 to 50 mL/minute: Initial: 0.125 mg twice daily (maximum: 0.75 mg 3 times daily)

CrCl 15 to 29 mL/minute: Initial: 0.125 mg once daily (maximum: 1.5 mg once daily)

CrCl <15 mL/minute: There are no dosage adjustments provided in the manufacturer's labeling (has not been studied).

ESRD requiring hemodialysis: There are no dosage adjustments provided in the manufacturer's labeling (has not been studied).

Parkinson disease: Extended release:

CrCl >50 mL/minute: No dosage adjustment necessary.

CrCl 30 to 50 mL/minute: Initial: 0.375 mg every other day; may increase to 0.375 mg once daily no sooner than 1 week after initiation. If necessary, may increase by 0.375 mg per dose not more frequently than every 7 days; maximum: 2.25 mg once daily

CrCl <30 mL/minute: Use not recommended.

ESRD requiring hemodialysis: Use not recommended.

Restless legs syndrome: Immediate release:

CrCl >60 mL/minute: No dosage adjustment necessary.

CrCl 20 to 60 mL/minute: No dosage adjustment necessary; however, duration between titration should be increased to 14 days.

CrCl <20 mL/minute: There are no dosage adjustments provided in the manufacturer's labeling (has not been studied).

Dosage adjustment in hepatic impairment: Immediate release and extended release: There are no dosage adjustments provided in the manufacturer's labeling (has not been studied); however, no adjustment expected since undergoes minimal hepatic metabolism.

Dietary Considerations May be taken with or without food. May be taken with food to decrease nausea.

Administration Doses should be titrated gradually to avoid the onset of intolerable side effects. The dosage should be increased to achieve a maximum therapeutic effect, balanced against the side effects of dyskinesia, hallucinations, somnolence, and dry mouth. Administer with or without food; administer with food to decrease nausea. Extended-release tablets should be swallowed whole and not chewed, crushed, or divided. For RLS, administer 2 to 3 hours before bedtime; if augmentation occurs, dose earlier in the day.

Monitoring Parameters Blood pressure, heart rate (especially during dose escalation); body weight changes; CNS depression, fall risk, behavior changes (eg, compulsive behaviors); periodic skin examinations.

Dosage Forms

Tablet, Oral:

Mirapex: 0.125 mg, 0.25 mg, 0.5 mg, 0.75 mg, 1 mg, 1.5 mg

Generic: 0.125 mg, 0.25 mg, 0.5 mg, 0.75 mg, 1 mg, 1.5 mg

Tablet Extended Release 24 Hour, Oral:

Mirapex ER: 0.375 mg, 0.75 mg, 1.5 mg, 2.25 mg, 3 mg, 3.75 mg, 4.5 mg

◆ **Pramipexole Dihydrochloride Monohydrate** *see* Pramipexole *on page 1695*

Pramlintide (PRAM lin tide)

Brand Names: U.S. SymlinPen 120; SymlinPen 60

Index Terms Pramlintide Acetate

Pharmacologic Category Amylinomimetic; Antidiabetic Agent

Use Type 1 and type 2 diabetes: Adjunct treatment in patients with type 1 or type 2 diabetes who use mealtime insulin therapy and who have failed to achieve desired glucose control despite optimal insulin therapy.

Pregnancy Risk Factor C

Pregnancy Considerations Adverse events have been observed in animal reproduction studies. Based on *in vitro* data, pramlintide has a low potential to cross the placenta.

In women with diabetes, maternal hyperglycemia can be associated with congenital malformations as well as adverse effects in the fetus, neonate, and the mother (ACOG, 2005; ADA, 2014; Kitzmiller, 2008; Metzger, 2007). To prevent adverse outcomes, prior to conception and throughout pregnancy maternal blood glucose and HbA_{1c} should be kept as close to normal as possible but without causing significant hypoglycemia (ACOG, 2013; ADA, 2014; Blumer, 2013; Kitzmiller, 2008). Prior to pregnancy, effective contraception should be used until glycemic control is achieved (ADA, 2014; Kitzmiller, 2008). Other agents are currently recommended to treat diabetes in pregnant women (ACOG, 2013; Blumer, 2013).

Breast-Feeding Considerations It is not known if pramlintide is excreted in breast milk. The manufacturer recommends that pramlintide be used in nursing women only when the potential benefit to the mother outweighs the possible risk to the infant.

Contraindications Serious hypersensitivity to pramlintide or any component of the formulation; confirmed diagnosis of gastroparesis; hypoglycemia unawareness

Warnings/Precautions [U.S. Boxed Warning]: Coadministration with insulin may induce severe hypoglycemia (usually within 3 hours following administration); coadministration with insulin therapy is an approved indication but does require an initial dosage reduction of insulin and frequent pre and post blood glucose monitoring to reduce risk of severe hypoglycemia. Concurrent use of other glucose-lowering agents may increase risk of hypoglycemia. Avoid use in patients with poor compliance with their insulin regimen and/or blood glucose monitoring. Do not use in patients with HbA_{1c} levels more than 9%, recurrent episodes of severe hypoglycemia requiring assistance during the past 6 months, or hypoglycemia unawareness; obtain detailed history of glucose control (eg, HbA_{1c}, incidence of hypoglycemia, glucose monitoring, and medication compliance) and body weight before initiating therapy. Use caution in patients with visual or dexterity impairment. Use caution when driving or ▶

operating heavy machinery until effects on blood sugar are known. Potentially significant drug-drug interactions may exist, requiring dose or frequency adjustment, additional monitoring, and/or selection of alternative therapy. Avoid use in patients with conditions or concurrent medications likely to impair gastric motility (eg, anticholinergics); do not use in patients requiring medication(s) to stimulate gastric emptying. Injection site reactions, including erythema, edema, or pruritus, may occur; usually resolve in a few days to weeks. According to the manufacturer and the Centers for Disease Control and Prevention (CDC), pen-shaped injection devices should never be used for more than one person (even when the needle is changed) because of the risk of transmission of blood-borne pathogens. The injection device should be clearly labeled with individual patient information to ensure that the correct pen is used (CDC, 2012).

Adverse Reactions

Central nervous system: Dizziness, fatigue, headache
Endocrine & metabolic: Severe hypoglycemia
Gastrointestinal: Anorexia, nausea, vomiting
Gastrointestinal: Abdominal pain
Hypersensitivity: Hypersensitivity reaction
Neuromuscular & skeletal: Arthralgia
Respiratory: Cough, pharyngitis
Miscellaneous: Accidental injury
Rare but important or life-threatening: Injection site reaction, pancreatitis

Drug Interactions

Metabolism/Transport Effects None known.

Avoid Concomitant Use There are no known interactions where it is recommended to avoid concomitant use.

Increased Effect/Toxicity

Pramlintide may increase the levels/effects of: Anticholinergic Agents; Insulin

Decreased Effect There are no known significant interactions involving a decrease in effect.

Storage/Stability Store at 2°C to 8°C (36°F to 46°F); do not freeze. After initial use, may be kept refrigerated or at room temperature ≤30°C (≤86°F); discard after 30 days. Protect from light.

Mechanism of Action Synthetic analog of human amylin cosecreted with insulin by pancreatic beta cells; reduces postprandial glucose increases via the following mechanisms: 1) prolongation of gastric emptying time, 2) reduction of postprandial glucagon secretion, and 3) reduction of caloric intake through centrally-mediated appetite suppression

Pharmacodynamics/Kinetics

Duration: ~3 hours
Protein binding: ~60%
Metabolism: Primarily renal to des-lys[1] pramlintide (active metabolite)
Bioavailability: ~30% to 40%
Half-life elimination: ~48 minutes
Time to peak, plasma: 20 minutes
Excretion: Primarily urine

Dosage SubQ: Adults: **Note:** When initiating pramlintide, reduce current mealtime insulin dose (including premixed preparations) by 50% to avoid hypoglycemia. If pramlintide is discontinued for any reason, restart therapy with same initial titration protocol. If a dose is missed, wait until the next scheduled dose and administer the usual amount.

Type 1 diabetes mellitus: Initial: 15 mcg immediately prior to major meals; titrate in 15 mcg increments every 3 days (if no significant nausea occurs) to target dose of 30 to 60 mcg prior to major meals (consider discontinuation if intolerant of 30 mcg dose)

Type 2 diabetes mellitus: Initial: 60 mcg immediately prior to major meals; after 3 days, increase to 120 mcg prior to each major meal if no significant nausea occurs (if nausea occurs at 120 mcg dose, reduce to 60 mcg)

Dosage adjustment in renal impairment:

CrCl ≥15 mL/minute: No dosage adjustment necessary.

End-stage renal disease [ESRD]: There are no dosage adjustments provided in the manufacturer's labeling (has not been studied).

Dosage adjustment in hepatic impairment: There are no dosage adjustments provided in the manufacturer's labeling (has not been studied); however, need for adjustment not likely since undergoes minimal hepatic metabolism.

Dietary Considerations Dietary modification based on ADA recommendations is a part of therapy; pramlintide to be administered prior to major meals consisting of ≥250 Kcal or ≥30 g carbohydrates

Administration Subcutaneous: Do not mix with insulins; administer subcutaneously into abdominal or thigh areas at sites distinct from concomitant insulin injections (do not administer into arm due to variable absorption); rotate injection sites frequently. Allow solution to reach room temperature before administering; may reduce injection site reactions. For oral medications in which a rapid onset of action is desired, administer 1 hour before, or 2 hours after pramlintide, if possible.

Monitoring Parameters Prior to initiating therapy: HbA_{1c}, hypoglycemic history, body weight. During therapy: Pre- and postprandial and bedtime serum glucose, HbA_{1c}, signs and symptoms of hypoglycemia

Reference Range

Recommendations for glycemic control in nonpregnant adults with diabetes (ADA, 2015):

HbA_{1c}: <7% (a more aggressive [<6.5%] or less aggressive [<8%] HbA_{1c} goal may be targeted based on patient-specific characteristics)

Preprandial capillary plasma glucose: 80 to 130 mg/dL

Peak postprandial capillary blood glucose: <180 mg/dL

Recommendations for glycemic control in pediatric (all age groups) patients with type 1 diabetes (ADA, 2015):

HbA_{1c}: <7.5% (individualization may be appropriate based on patient-specific characteristics; <7% is reasonable if it can be achieved without excessive hypoglycemia)

Preprandial capillary plasma glucose: 90 to 130 mg/dL

Bedtime and overnight capillary blood glucose: 90 to 150 mg/dL

Dosage Forms

Solution Pen-injector, Subcutaneous:

SymlinPen 60: 1500 mcg/1.5 mL (1.5 mL)
SymlinPen 120: 2700 mcg/2.7 mL (2.7 mL)

- ◆ **Pramlintide Acetate** *see* Pramlintide *on page 1697*
- ◆ **Pramosone®** *see* Pramoxine and Hydrocortisone *on page 1698*
- ◆ **Pramosone E™** *see* Pramoxine and Hydrocortisone *on page 1698*
- ◆ **Pramox® HC (Can)** *see* Pramoxine and Hydrocortisone *on page 1698*

Pramoxine and Hydrocortisone

(pra MOKS een & hye droe KOR ti sone)

Brand Names: U.S. Analpram E™; Analpram HC®; Epifoam®; PramCort; Pramosone E™; Pramosone®; ProCort®; ProctoFoam® HC; Zypram™

Brand Names: Canada Pramox® HC; Proctofoam™-HC

Index Terms Hydrocortisone and Pramoxine; Pramoxine Hydrochloride and Hydrocortisone Acetate

Pharmacologic Category Anesthetic/Corticosteroid

Use Relief of inflammatory and pruritic manifestations of corticosteroid-responsive dermatoses

Pregnancy Risk Factor C

Dosage Topical/rectal: Apply to affected areas 3-4 times/day. If clinical improvement is not seen within 2-3 weeks after initiating treatment or if condition worsens, product should be discontinued.

Additional Information Complete prescribing information should be consulted for additional detail.

Dosage Forms

Aerosol, foam, rectal:

ProctoFoam® HC: Pramoxine 1% and hydrocortisone 1% (10 g)

Aerosol, foam, topical:

Epifoam®: Pramoxine 1% and hydrocortisone 1% (10 g)

Cream, topical: Pramoxine 1% and hydrocortisone 1% (30 g); pramoxine 1% and hydrocortisone 2.5% (4 g, 30 g)

Analpram Advanced™ Kit: Pramoxine 1% and hydrocortisone 2.5% (1s) [kit includes Analpram HC® cream (4 g x 30), diosmiplex (Vasculera™) tablets, AloeClean™ wipes, and applicators]

Analpram Advanced™ Kit: Pramoxine 1% and hydrocortisone 2.5% (1s) [kit includes Analpram HC® cream (30 g), diosmiplex (Vasculera™) tablets, AloeClean™ wipes, and applicator]

Analpram E™: Pramoxine 1% and hydrocortisone 2.5% (4 g, 30 g)

Analpram HC®: Pramoxine 1% and hydrocortisone 1% (4 g, 30 g); pramoxine 1% and hydrocortisone 2.5% (4 g, 30 g)

PramCort: Pramoxine 1% and hydrocortisone 1% (30 g)

Pramosone®: Pramoxine 1% and hydrocortisone 1% (30 g, 60 g); pramoxine 1% and hydrocortisone 2.5% (30 g, 60 g)

Pramosone E™: Pramoxine 1% and hydrocortisone 2.5% (30 g, 60 g)

ProCort®: Pramoxine 1.15% and hydrocortisone 1.85% (60 g)

Zypram™: Pramoxine 1% and hydrocortisone 2.35% (30 g)

Lotion, topical:

Analpram HC®: Pramoxine 1% and hydrocortisone 2.5% (60 mL)

Pramosone®: Pramoxine 1% and hydrocortisone 1% (60 mL, 120 mL, 240 mL); pramoxine 1% and hydrocortisone 2.5% (60 mL, 120 mL)

Ointment, topical:

Pramosone®: Pramoxine 1% and hydrocortisone 1% (30 g); pramoxine 1% and hydrocortisone 2.5% (30 g)

◆ **Pramoxine Hydrochloride and Hydrocortisone Acetate** *see* Pramoxine and Hydrocortisone *on page 1698*

◆ **PrandiMet** *see* Repaglinide and Metformin *on page 1792*

◆ **Prandin** *see* Repaglinide *on page 1791*

◆ **Prascion** *see* Sulfur and Sulfacetamide *on page 1953*

◆ **Prascion FC** *see* Sulfur and Sulfacetamide *on page 1953*

◆ **Prascion RA** *see* Sulfur and Sulfacetamide *on page 1953*

Prasugrel (PRA soo grel)

Brand Names: U.S. Effient

Brand Names: Canada Effient

Index Terms CS-747; LY-640315; Prasugrel Hydrochloride

Pharmacologic Category Antiplatelet Agent; Antiplatelet Agent, Thienopyridine

Additional Appendix Information

Beers Criteria - Potentially Inappropriate Medications for Geriatrics *on page 2271*

Oral Antiplatelet Comparison Chart *on page 2239*

Use Acute coronary syndrome to be managed with percutaneous coronary intervention (PCI): To reduce the rate of thrombotic cardiovascular events (including stent thrombosis) in patients who are to be managed with PCI for unstable angina (UA), non-ST-segment elevation MI (NSTEMI), or ST-elevation MI (STEMI).

Pregnancy Risk Factor B

Dosage Oral:

Adults: Acute coronary syndrome (ACS): Oral:

Percutaneous coronary intervention (PCI) for ACS: Loading dose: 60 mg administered promptly (as soon as coronary anatomy is known or before if risk for bleeding is low and need for CABG considered unlikely) and no later than 1 hour after PCI; Maintenance dose: 10 mg once daily (in combination with aspirin 75-325 mg/day; 81 mg/day recommended [Levine, 2011]). For patients with STEMI, a loading dose may also be administered if PCI is performed >24 hours after treatment with a fibrin-specific thrombolytic (ie, alteplase, reteplase, tenecteplase) (ACCF/AHA [O'Gara, 2013]).

Duration of prasugrel (in combination with aspirin) after stent placement: **Premature interruption of therapy may result in stent thrombosis, MI, and death.** According to the ACCF/AHA/SCAI PCI guidelines, those with ACS receiving either stent type (bare metal [BMS] or drug-eluting stent [DES]) or those receiving a DES for a non-ACS indication, prasugrel for at least 12 months is recommended (ACCF/AHA/SCAI [Levine, 2011]). The ACCF/AHA guidelines for the management of UA/NSTEMI recommend up to 12 months of prasugrel in patients with ACS who receive a BMS (ACCF/AHA [Anderson, 2013]). A duration >12 months may be considered in patients with DES placement. Recent data has demonstrated that continued dual antiplatelet therapy for a total of 30 months (compared to 12 months) significantly reduced the risk of stent thrombosis and major adverse cardiovascular/cerebrovascular events but was associated with a higher risk of bleeding (Mauri, 2014). Those receiving a BMS for a non-ACS indication should be given at least 1 month and ideally up to 12 months; if patient is at increased risk of bleeding, give for a minimum of 2 weeks (ACCF/AHA/SCAI [Levine, 2011]).

Maintenance dosing in low body weight (ie, <60 kg) individuals: Due to a higher incidence of bleeding in patients weighing <60 kg, a maintenance dose of 5 mg once daily may be considered. In aspirin-treated patients weighing <60 kg (mean: 56.4 ± 3.7 kg) with stable coronary artery disease, the use of prasugrel 5 mg once daily was shown to reduce platelet reactivity to a similar extent as prasugrel 10 mg administered once daily to patients >60 kg (mean: 84.7 ± 14.9 kg); clinical events were not evaluated (Erlinge, 2012). In patients with ACS (medically managed) treated with aspirin, a 5 mg daily maintenance dose (after a 30 mg loading dose) in patients <60 kg did not demonstrate a significant difference in the composite primary end point of death from cardiovascular causes, MI, or stroke compared to patients >60 kg treated with a 10 mg maintenance dose; bleeding risk was not increased (Roe, 2012).

Conversion from clopidogrel to prasugrel: Beginning 24 hours after the last clopidogrel dose (loading or maintenance), may initiate prasugrel 10 mg once daily or a 60 mg loading dose followed in 24 hours with 10 mg once daily (Angiolillo, 2010; Payne, 2008; Wiviott, 2007).

Elderly: Refer to adult dosing. Patients ≥75 years: Use not recommended; may be considered in high-risk situations (eg, patients with diabetes or history of MI)

Dosing adjustment in renal impairment: No dosage adjustment necessary

Dosing adjustment in hepatic impairment:

Mild to moderate hepatic impairment (Child-Pugh class A and B): No dosage adjustment necessary

Severe hepatic impairment (Child-Pugh class C): No dosage adjustment provided in manufacturer's labeling (has not been studied).

Additional Information Complete prescribing information should be consulted for additional detail.

Dosage Forms

Tablet, Oral:

Effient: 5 mg, 10 mg

◆ **Prasugrel Hydrochloride** *see* Prasugrel *on page 1699*

◆ **Pravachol** *see* Pravastatin *on page 1700*

Pravastatin (prav a STAT in)

Brand Names: U.S. Pravachol

Brand Names: Canada ACT Pravastatin; Apo-Pravastatin; Dom-Pravastatin; JAMP-Pravastatin; Mint-Pravastatin; Mylan-Pravastatin; PHL-Pravastatin; PMS-Pravastatin; Pravachol; RAN-Pravastatin; Riva-Pravastatin; Sandoz-Pravastatin; Teva-Pravastatin

Index Terms Pravastatin Sodium

Pharmacologic Category Antilipemic Agent, HMG-CoA Reductase Inhibitor

Use Use with dietary therapy for the following:

Primary prevention of coronary events: In hypercholesterolemic patients without established coronary heart disease to reduce cardiovascular morbidity (myocardial infarction, coronary revascularization procedures) and mortality.

Secondary prevention of cardiovascular events in patients with established coronary heart disease: To slow the progression of coronary atherosclerosis; to reduce cardiovascular morbidity (myocardial infarction, coronary vascular procedures) and to reduce mortality; to reduce the risk of stroke and transient ischemic attacks

Primary and secondary prevention of atherosclerotic cardiovascular disease (ASCVD) according to the American College of Cardiology/American Heart Association: To reduce the risk of ASCVD in patients with clinical ASCVD (eg, coronary heart disease, stroke/TIA, or peripheral arterial disease presumed to be of atherosclerotic origin) who are greater than 75 years of age or not a candidate for high-intensity statin therapy; in patients without clinical ASCVD if LDL-C is 190 mg/dL or greater and not a candidate for high-intensity statin therapy; in patients without clinical ASCVD who have type 1 or type 2 diabetes and are between 40 and 75 years of age; in patients with an estimated 10-year ASCVD risk 7.5% or greater and who are between 40 and 75 years of age. Specific recommendations from the Kidney Disease: Improving Global Outcomes (KDIGO) organization have also been released for patients with chronic kidney disease (KDIGO [Tonelli, 2013]).

Hyperlipidemias: Reduce elevations in total cholesterol, LDL-C, apolipoprotein B, and triglycerides (elevations of 1 or more components are present in Fredrickson type IIa, IIb, III, and IV hyperlipidemias)

Heterozygous familial hypercholesterolemia (HeFH): In pediatric patients, 8-18 years of age, with HeFH having LDL-C ≥190 mg/dL **or** LDL ≥160 mg/dL with positive family history of premature cardiovascular disease (CVD) or 2 or more CVD risk factors in the pediatric patient

Pregnancy Risk Factor X

Pregnancy Considerations Adverse events were observed in some animal reproduction studies. Pravastatin was found to cross the placenta in an *ex vivo* study using term human placentas (Nanovskaya, 2013). There are reports of congenital anomalies following maternal use of HMG-CoA reductase Inhibitors in pregnancy; however, maternal disease, differences in specific agents used, and the low rates of exposure limit the interpretation of the available data (Godfrey, 2012; Lecarpentier, 2012). Cholesterol biosynthesis may be important in fetal development; serum cholesterol and triglycerides increase normally during pregnancy. The discontinuation of lipid lowering medications temporarily during pregnancy is not expected to have significant impact on the long term outcomes of primary hypercholesterolemia treatment.

Use of pravastatin is contraindicated in pregnancy. HMG-CoA reductase Inhibitors should be discontinued prior to pregnancy (ADA, 2013). If treatment of dyslipidemias is needed in pregnant women or in women of reproductive age, other agents are preferred (Berglund, 2012; Stone, 2013). The manufacturer recommends administration to women of childbearing potential only when conception is highly unlikely and patients have been informed of potential hazards.

Breast-Feeding Considerations A small amount of pravastatin is excreted into breast milk. Data is available from eight lactating females administered pravastatin 20 mg twice daily for 2.5 days. After the fifth dose, maximum maternal serum concentrations were ~40 ng/mL (pravastatin) and ~26 ng/mL (metabolite) and maximum milk concentrations were ~3.9 ng/mL (pravastatin) and ~2.1 ng/mL (metabolite). Maximum milk concentrations were detected ~3 hours after the dose (Pan, 1988). Due to the potential for serious adverse reactions in a nursing infant, use while breast-feeding is contraindicated by the manufacturer.

Contraindications Hypersensitivity to pravastatin or any component of the formulation; active liver disease; unexplained persistent elevations of serum transaminases; pregnancy; breast-feeding

Warnings/Precautions Secondary causes of hyperlipidemia should be ruled out prior to therapy. Liver function must be monitored by periodic laboratory assessment. Rhabdomyolysis with acute renal failure has occurred. Risk may be increased with concurrent use of other drugs which may cause rhabdomyolysis (including colchicine, gemfibrozil, fibric acid derivatives, or niacin at doses ≥1 g/day). Discontinue in any patient in which CPK levels are markedly elevated (>10 times ULN) or if myopathy is suspected/diagnosed. Immune-mediated necrotizing myopathy (IMNM), an autoimmune-mediated myopathy, has been reported (rarely) with HMG-CoA reductase inhibitor therapy. IMNM presents as proximal muscle weakness with elevated CPK levels, which persists despite discontinuation of HMG-CoA reductase inhibitor therapy; additionally, muscle biopsy may show necrotizing myopathy with limited inflammation; immunosuppressive therapy (eg, corticosteroids, azathioprine) may be used for treatment. The manufacturer recommends temporary discontinuation for elective major surgery, acute medical or surgical conditions, or in any patient experiencing an acute or serious condition predisposing to renal failure (eg, sepsis, hypotension, trauma, uncontrolled seizures). However, based upon current evidence, HMG-CoA reductase inhibitor therapy should be continued in the perioperative period unless risk outweighs cardioprotective benefit. Use with caution in patients with advanced age, these patients are predisposed to myopathy. Use caution in patients with previous liver disease or heavy ethanol use. If serious hepatotoxicity with clinical symptoms and/or hyperbilirubinemia or jaundice occurs during treatment, interrupt therapy. If an alternate etiology is not identified, do not restart pravastatin. Liver enzyme tests should be obtained at baseline and as clinically indicated; routine periodic monitoring of liver enzymes is not necessary. Increases in HbA_{1c} and fasting blood glucose have been reported with HMG-CoA reductase inhibitors; however, the benefits of statin therapy far outweigh the risk of dysglycemia. Treatment in patients <8 years of age is not recommended.

Adverse Reactions

Cardiovascular: Chest pain

Central nervous system: Dizziness, fatigue, headache

Dermatologic: Rash

Gastrointestinal: Diarrhea, heartburn, nausea, vomiting

Hepatic: Transaminases increased

Neuromuscular & skeletal: Myalgia

Respiratory: Cough

Miscellaneous: Influenza

Rare but important or life-threatening: Allergy, amnesia (reversible), anaphylaxis, angioedema, cholestatic jaundice, cirrhosis, cognitive impairment (reversible), confusion (reversible), cranial nerve dysfunction, dermatomyositis, erythema multiforme, ESR increase, fulminant hepatic necrosis, gynecomastia, hemolytic anemia, hepatitis, hepatoma, lens opacity, libido change, lupus erythematosus-like syndrome, memory disturbance (reversible), memory impairment (reversible), muscle weakness, myopathy, neuropathy, pancreatitis, paresthesia, peripheral nerve palsy, polymyalgia rheumatica, positive ANA, purpura, rhabdomyolysis, Stevens-Johnson syndrome, taste disturbance, tremor, vasculitis, vertigo

Additional class-related events or case reports (not necessarily reported with pravastatin therapy): Angioedema, blood glucose increased, cataracts, depression, diabetes mellitus (new onset), dyspnea, eosinophilia, erectile dysfunction, facial paresis, glycosylated hemoglobin (Hb A_{1c}) increased, hypersensitivity reaction, immune-mediated necrotizing myopathy (IMNM), impaired extraocular muscle movement, impotence, interstitial lung disease, leukopenia, malaise, memory loss, ophthalmoplegia, paresthesia, peripheral neuropathy, photosensitivity, psychic disturbance, skin discoloration, thrombocytopenia, thyroid dysfunction, toxic epidermal necrolysis, transaminases increased, vomiting

Drug Interactions

Metabolism/Transport Effects Substrate of CYP3A4 (minor), P-glycoprotein, SLCO1B1; **Note:** Assignment of Major/Minor substrate status based on clinically relevant drug interaction potential; **Inhibits** CYP2C9 (weak), CYP2D6 (weak), CYP3A4 (weak)

Avoid Concomitant Use

Avoid concomitant use of Pravastatin with any of the following: Fusidic Acid (Systemic); Gemfibrozil; Pimozide; Red Yeast Rice

Increased Effect/Toxicity

Pravastatin may increase the levels/effects of: ARIPiprazole; CycloSPORINE (Systemic); DAPTOmycin; Dofetilide; Hydrocodone; Lomitapide; PARoxetine; PAZOPanib; Pimozide; Trabectedin; Vitamin K Antagonists

The levels/effects of Pravastatin may be increased by: Acipimox; Bezafibrate; Boceprevir; Ciprofibrate; Clarithromycin; Colchicine; CycloSPORINE (Systemic); Darunavir; Eltrombopag; Erythromycin (Systemic); Fenofibrate and Derivatives; Fusidic Acid (Systemic); Gemfibrozil; Itraconazole; Niacin; Niacinamide; Paritaprevir; P-glycoprotein/ABCB1 Inhibitors; Raltegravir; Red Yeast Rice; Simeprevir; Telaprevir; Telithromycin; Teriflunomide

Decreased Effect

Pravastatin may decrease the levels/effects of: Lanthanum

The levels/effects of Pravastatin may be decreased by: Antacids; Bile Acid Sequestrants; Efavirenz; Fosphenytoin; Nelfinavir; P-glycoprotein/ABCB1 Inducers; Phenytoin; Rifamycin Derivatives; Saquinavir

Storage/Stability Store at 25°C (77°F); excursions permitted to 15°C to 30°C (59°F to 86°F). Protect from moisture and light.

Mechanism of Action Pravastatin is a competitive inhibitor of 3-hydroxy-3-methylglutaryl coenzyme A (HMG-CoA) reductase, which is the rate-limiting enzyme involved in *de novo* cholesterol synthesis.

Pharmacodynamics/Kinetics

Onset of action: Several days

Peak effect: 4 weeks

Absorption: Rapidly absorbed; average absorption 34%

Protein binding: 50%

Metabolism: Hepatic multiple metabolites; primary metabolite is 3α-hydroxy-iso-pravastatin (2.5% to 10% activity of parent drug)

Bioavailability: 17%

Half-life elimination: 77 hours (including all metabolites); pravastatin: ~2-3 hours (Pan, 1990); 3α-hydroxy-iso-pravastatin: ~1.5 hours (Gustavson, 2005)

Time to peak, serum: 1-1.5 hours

Excretion: Feces (70%); urine (≤20%, 8% as unchanged drug)

Dosage Note: Doses should be individualized according to the baseline LDL-cholesterol levels, the recommended goal of therapy, and patient response; adjustments should be made at intervals of 4 weeks or more; doses may need adjusted based on concomitant medications

Heterozygous familial hypercholesterolemia (HeFH): Oral:

Children 8-13 years: 20 mg/day

Adolescents 14-18 years: 40 mg/day

Dosage adjustment for pravastatin with concomitant medications (clarithromycin, cyclosporine): Refer to adult dosing.

Hyperlipidemias, primary prevention of coronary events, secondary prevention of cardiovascular events (also see ACC/AHA Blood Cholesterol Guideline recommendations): Adults: Oral: Initial: 40 mg once daily; titrate dosage to response; usual range: 10-80 mg; (maximum dose: 80 mg once daily)

ACC/AHA Blood Cholesterol Guideline recommendations to reduce the risk of atherosclerotic cardiovascular disease (ASCVD) (Stone, 2013): Adults ≥21 years: Oral:

Primary prevention:

LDL-C ≥190 mg/dL: High intensity therapy necessary; use alternate statin therapy (eg, atorvastatin or rosuvastatin)

Type 1 or 2 diabetes and age 40-75 years: Moderate intensity therapy: 40-80 mg once daily

Type 1 or 2 diabetes, age 40-75 years, and an estimated 10-year ASCVD risk ≥7.5%: High intensity therapy necessary; use alternate statin therapy (eg, atorvastatin or rosuvastatin)

Age 40-75 years and an estimated 10-year ASCVD risk ≥7.5%: Moderate to high intensity therapy: 40-80 mg once daily or consider using high intensity statin therapy (eg, atorvastatin or rosuvastatin)

Secondary prevention:

Patient has clinical ASCVD (eg, coronary heart disease, stroke/TIA, or peripheral arterial disease presumed to be of atherosclerotic origin) **and**:

Age ≤75 years: High intensity therapy necessary; use alternate statin therapy (eg, atorvastatin or rosuvastatin)

Age >75 years or not a candidate for high intensity therapy: Moderate intensity therapy: 40-80 mg once daily

Dosage adjustment for pravastatin with concomitant medications:

Clarithromycin: Limit daily pravastatin dose to 40 mg/day

Cyclosporine: Initial: 10 mg pravastatin daily, titrate with caution (maximum dose: 20 mg/day)

Elderly: No specific dosage recommendations. Clearance is reduced in the elderly, resulting in an increase in AUC between 25% to 50%. However, substantial accumulation is not expected.

Dosing adjustment for toxicity:

Severe muscle symptoms or fatigue: Promptly discontinue use; evaluate CPK, creatinine, and urinalysis for myoglobinuria (Stone, 2013).

Mild to moderate muscle symptoms: Discontinue use until symptoms can be evaluated; evaluate patient for conditions that may increase the risk for muscle symptoms (eg, hypothyroidism, reduced renal or hepatic function, rheumatologic disorders such as polymyalgia rheumatica, steroid myopathy, vitamin D deficiency, primary muscle diseases). Upon resolution, resume the original or lower dose of pravastatin. If muscle symptoms recur, discontinue pravastatin use. After muscle symptom resolution, may then use a low dose of a different statin; gradually increase if tolerated. In the absence of continued statin use, if muscle symptoms or elevated CPK continues after 2 months, consider other causes of muscle symptoms. If determined to be due to another condition aside from statin use, may resume statin therapy at the original dose (Stone, 2013).

Dosage adjustment in renal impairment: Significant impairment: Initial dose: 10 mg/day

Dosage adjustment in hepatic impairment: Contraindicated in active liver disease or in patients with unexplained persistent elevations of serum transaminases

Dietary Considerations May be taken without regard to meals. Before initiation of therapy, patients should be placed on a standard cholesterol-lowering diet for 6 weeks and the diet should be continued during drug therapy.

Red yeast rice contains variable amounts of several compounds that are structurally similar to HMG-CoA reductase inhibitors, primarily monacolin K (or mevinolin) which is structurally identical to lovastatin; concurrent use of red yeast rice with HMG-CoA reductase inhibitors may increase the incidence of adverse and toxic effects (Lapi, 2008; Smith, 2003).

Administration May be administered without regard to meals.

Monitoring Parameters

2013 ACC/AHA Blood Cholesterol Guideline recommendations (Stone, 2013):

Lipid panel (total cholesterol, HDL, LDL, triglycerides): Baseline lipid panel; fasting lipid profile within 4-12 weeks after initiation or dose adjustment and every 3-12 months (as clinically indicated) thereafter. If 2 consecutive LDL levels are <40 mg/dL, consider decreasing the dose.

Hepatic transaminase levels: Baseline measurement of hepatic transaminase levels (ie, ALT); measure hepatic function if symptoms suggest hepatotoxicity (eg, unusual fatigue or weakness, loss of appetite, abdominal pain, dark-colored urine or yellowing of skin or sclera) during therapy.

CPK: CPK should not be routinely measured. Baseline CPK measurement is reasonable for some individuals (eg, family history of statin intolerance or muscle disease, clinical presentation, concomitant drug therapy that may increase risk of myopathy). May measure CPK in any patient with symptoms suggestive of myopathy (pain, tenderness, stiffness, cramping, weakness, or generalized fatigue).

Evaluate for new-onset diabetes mellitus during therapy; if diabetes develops, continue statin therapy and encourage adherence to a heart-healthy diet, physical activity, a healthy body weight, and tobacco cessation.

If patient develops a confusional state or memory impairment, may evaluate patient for nonstatin causes (eg, exposure to other drugs), systemic and neuropsychiatric causes, and the possibility of adverse effects associated with statin therapy.

Manufacturer recommendations: Liver enzyme tests at baseline and repeated when clinically indicated. **Upon initiation or titration, lipid panel should be analyzed at intervals of 4 weeks or more.**

Dosage Forms

Tablet, Oral:

Pravachol: 20 mg, 40 mg, 80 mg

Generic: 10 mg, 20 mg, 40 mg, 80 mg

- **Pravastatin Sodium** *see* Pravastatin *on page 1700*
- **Praxis ASA EC 81 Mg Daily Dose (Can)** *see* Aspirin *on page 180*

Prazepam [INT] (PRA ze pam)

International Brand Names Centrac (GR); Centrax (IE); Demetrin (AT, CH, CZ, DE, ES, HR, PT, QA); Equipaz (AR); Lysanxia (BE, FR, LU); Mono Demetrin (DE); Pozapam (TH); Prazene (IT); Reapam (NL); Verstran (PK)

Pharmacologic Category Benzodiazepine

Reported Use Treatment of anxiety

Dosage Range Adults: Oral: 30 mg/day in divided doses, may increase gradually to a maximum of 60 mg/day

Product Availability Product available in various countries; not currently available in the U.S.

Dosage Forms

Capsule: 5 mg, 10 mg, 20 mg

Tablet: 5 mg, 10 mg

Praziquantel (pray zi KWON tel)

Brand Names: U.S. Biltricide

Brand Names: Canada Biltricide

Pharmacologic Category Anthelmintic

Use Helminths: Treatment of infections caused by the following: All species of *Schistosoma* (eg, *Schistosoma mekongi*, *S. japonicum*, *S. mansoni*, *S. hematobium*) and the liver flukes *Clonorchis sinensis*/*Opisthorchis viverrini*

Pregnancy Risk Factor B

Dosage Oral: Children ≥4 years, Adolescents, and Adults:

Schistosomiasis: 20 mg/kg/dose 3 times daily at 4- to 6-hour intervals for 1 day

Clonorchiasis/opisthorchiasis: 25 mg/kg/dose 3 times daily at 4- to 6-hour intervals for 1 day

Cysticercosis (off-label use): 50 mg/kg/day divided every 8 hours for 14 days (Takayanagui, 2004)

Tapeworms (off-label use): 5-10 mg/kg as a single dose (25 mg/kg for *Hymenolepis nana*) (Liu, 1996)

Dosage adjustment in renal impairment: No dosage adjustment necessary.

Dosage adjustment in hepatic impairment: There are no dosage adjustments provided in manufacturer's labeling. However, total drug exposure in moderate-to-severe impairment is increased.

Additional Information Complete prescribing information should be consulted for additional detail.

Dosage Forms

Tablet, Oral:

Biltricide: 600 mg

Prazosin (PRAZ oh sin)

Brand Names: U.S. Minipress

Brand Names: Canada Apo-Prazo; Minipress; Novo-Prazin; Nu-Prazo; Teva-Prazosin

Index Terms Furazosin; Prazosin Hydrochloride

Pharmacologic Category Alpha$_1$ Blocker; Antihypertensive

Additional Appendix Information

Beers Criteria – Potentially Inappropriate Medications for Geriatrics *on page 2271*

Use

Hypertension: Treatment of hypertension

Note: The 2014 guideline for the management of high blood pressure in adults (Eighth Joint National Committee [JNC 8]) does **not** recommend the use of prazosin in the treatment of hypertension (James, 2013).

Pregnancy Risk Factor C

Dosage Oral:

Children: Hypertension (off-label use): Initial: 0.05-0.1 mg/kg/day in 3 divided doses; maximum: 0.5 mg/kg/day (not to exceed 20 mg) (NHBPEP, Fourth Report)

Adults:

Hypertension: Initial: 1 mg/dose 2-3 times/day; usual dosage range (ASH/ISH [Weber, 2014]): 1 to 5 mg twice daily; maximum daily dose: 20 mg

PTSD-related nightmares and sleep disruption (off-label use): Initial: 1 mg at bedtime (Raskind, 2002; Raskind, 2007); titrate as tolerated to 2-15 mg at bedtime (Benedek, 2009)

Raynaud's (off-label use): Dosage range: 1-5 mg twice daily (Bakst, 2008)

Benign prostatic hyperplasia (off-label use): Initial: 0.5 mg twice daily; titrate as tolerated to 2 mg twice daily (Moran, 2001)

Elderly: Hypertension: Consider lower initial doses and titrate to response (Aronow, 2011)

Dosage adjustment in renal impairment: No dosage adjustment provided in manufacturer's labeling.

Dosage adjustment in hepatic impairment: No dosage adjustment provided in manufacturer's labeling.

Additional Information Complete prescribing information should be consulted for additional detail.

Dosage Forms

Capsule, Oral:

Minipress: 1 mg, 2 mg, 5 mg

Generic: 1 mg, 2 mg, 5 mg

- **Prazosin Hydrochloride** *see* Prazosin *on page 1703*
- **Precedex** *see* Dexmedetomidine *on page 604*
- **Precise [OTC]** *see* Methyl Salicylate and Menthol *on page 1344*
- **Precose** *see* Acarbose *on page 29*
- **Predator [OTC]** *see* Lidocaine (Topical) *on page 1211*
- **Pred Forte** *see* PrednisoLONE (Ophthalmic) *on page 1706*
- **Pred-G** *see* Prednisolone and Gentamicin *on page 1706*
- **Pred Mild** *see* PrednisoLONE (Ophthalmic) *on page 1706*

Prednicarbate (pred ni KAR bate)

Brand Names: U.S. Dermatop

Brand Names: Canada Dermatop®

Pharmacologic Category Corticosteroid, Topical

Additional Appendix Information

Topical Corticosteroids *on page 2230*

Use Relief of the inflammatory and pruritic manifestations of corticosteroid-responsive dermatoses (medium potency topical corticosteroid)

Pregnancy Risk Factor C

Dosage Note: Therapy should be discontinued when control is achieved; if no improvement is seen within 2 weeks, reassessment of diagnosis may be necessary.

Cream: Children ≥1 year and Adults: Topical: Apply a thin film to affected area twice daily

Ointment: Children ≥10 year and Adults: Topical: Apply a thin film to affected area twice daily

Additional Information Complete prescribing information should be consulted for additional detail.

Dosage Forms

Cream, External:

Dermatop: 0.1% (60 g)

Generic: 0.1% (15 g, 60 g)

Ointment, External:

Dermatop: 0.1% (60 g)

Generic: 0.1% (15 g, 60 g)

PrednisoLONE (Systemic) (pred NISS oh lone)

Brand Names: U.S. Flo-Pred; Millipred; Millipred DP; Millipred DP 12-Day; Orapred ODT; Orapred [DSC]; Pediapred; Prelone; Veripred 20

Brand Names: Canada Hydeltra T.B.A.; Novo-Prednisolone; Pediapred

Index Terms Prednisolone Sodium Phosphate

Pharmacologic Category Corticosteroid, Systemic

Additional Appendix Information

Corticosteroids Systemic Equivalencies *on page 2228*

Use Treatment of endocrine disorders, rheumatic disorders, collagen diseases, allergic states, respiratory diseases, hematologic disorders, neoplastic diseases, edematous states, and gastrointestinal diseases; resolution of acute exacerbations of multiple sclerosis; management of fulminating or disseminated tuberculosis and trichinosis; acute or chronic solid organ rejection

Pregnancy Risk Factor C/D (manufacturer specific)

Pregnancy Considerations Adverse events have been observed with corticosteroids in animal reproduction studies. Prednisolone crosses the placenta; prior to reaching the fetus, prednisolone is converted by placental enzymes to prednisone. As a result, the amount of prednisolone reaching the fetus is ~8-10 times lower than the maternal serum concentration (healthy women at term; similar results observed with preterm pregnancies complicated by HELLP syndrome) (Beitins, 1972; van Runnard Heimel, 2005). Some studies have shown an association between first trimester systemic corticosteroid use and oral clefts (Park-Wyllie, 2000; Pradat, 2003). Systemic corticosteroids may also influence fetal growth (decreased birth weight); however, information is conflicting (Lunghi, 2010). Hypoadrenalism may occur in newborns following maternal use of corticosteroids in pregnancy; monitor.

When systemic corticosteroids are needed in pregnancy, it is generally recommended to use the lowest effective dose for the shortest duration of time, avoiding high doses during the first trimester (Leachman, 2006; Lunghi, 2010; Makol, 2011; Østensen, 2009). Inhaled corticosteroids are preferred for the treatment of asthma during pregnancy. Oral corticosteroids, such as prednisolone, may be used for the treatment of severe persistent asthma if needed; the lowest dose administered on alternate days (if possible) should be used (NAEPP, 2005). Prednisolone may be used to treat women during pregnancy who require therapy for congenital adrenal hyperplasia (Speiser, 2010). Topical agents are preferred for managing atopic dermatitis in pregnancy; for severe symptomatic or recalcitrant atopic dermatitis, a short course of prednisolone may be used during the third trimester (Koutroulis, 2011).

Women exposed to prednisolone during pregnancy for the treatment of an autoimmune disease may contact the OTIS Autoimmune Diseases Study at 877-311-8972.

Breast-Feeding Considerations Prednisolone is excreted into breast milk. In one study (n=6), milk concentrations were 5% to 25% of the maternal serum concentration with peak concentrations occurring ~1 hour after the maternal dose. The milk/plasma ratio was found to be 0.2 with doses ≥30 mg/day and 0.1 with doses <30 mg/day. Following a maternal dose of prednisolone 80 mg/day, it was calculated that a breast-feeding infant would ingest <0.1% of the maternal dose (Ost, 1985). One manufacturer notes that when used systemically, maternal use of corticosteroids have the potential to cause adverse events in a nursing infant (eg, growth suppression, interfere with endogenous corticosteroid production) and therefore caution should be used when administered to nursing women. In order to decrease potential exposure to a nursing infant, one manufacturer recommends administering the dose after nursing, at the time of day with the longest interval between feeds. Other sources recommend waiting 4 hours after the maternal dose before breast-feeding (Bae, 2012; Leachman, 2006; Makol, 2011; Ost, 1985). Other guidelines note that maternal use of systemic corticosteroids is not a contraindication to breast-feeding (NAEPP, 2005).

Contraindications Hypersensitivity to prednisolone or any component of the formulation; acute superficial herpes simplex keratitis; live or attenuated virus vaccines (with immunosuppressive doses of corticosteroids); systemic fungal infections; varicella

Warnings/Precautions May cause hypercorticism or suppression of hypothalamic-pituitary-adrenal (HPA) axis, particularly in younger children or in patients receiving high doses for prolonged periods. HPA axis suppression may lead to adrenal crisis. Withdrawal and discontinuation of a corticosteroid should be done slowly and carefully. Particular care is required when patients are transferred from systemic corticosteroids to inhaled products due to possible adrenal insufficiency or withdrawal from steroids, including an increase in allergic symptoms. Patients receiving >20 mg per day of prednisone (or equivalent) may be most susceptible. Fatalities have occurred due to adrenal insufficiency in asthmatic patients during and after transfer from systemic corticosteroids to aerosol steroids; aerosol steroids do **not** provide the systemic steroid needed to treat patients having trauma, surgery, or infections.

Acute myopathy has been reported with high dose corticosteroids, usually in patients with neuromuscular transmission disorders; may involve ocular and/or respiratory muscles; monitor creatine kinase; recovery may be delayed. Corticosteroid use may cause psychiatric disturbances, including depression, euphoria, insomnia, mood swings, and personality changes. Preexisting psychiatric conditions may be exacerbated by corticosteroid use. Prolonged use of corticosteroids may also increase the incidence of secondary infection, mask acute infection (including fungal infections), prolong or exacerbate viral infections, or limit response to vaccines. Exposure to chickenpox should be avoided; corticosteroids should not be used to treat ocular herpes simplex. Corticosteroids should not be used for cerebral malaria or viral hepatitis. Close observation is required in patients with latent tuberculosis and/or TB reactivity; restrict use in active TB (only in conjunction with antituberculosis treatment). Prolonged use of corticosteroids may result in glaucoma; cataract formation may occur. Prolonged treatment with corticosteroids has been associated with the development of Kaposi's sarcoma (case reports); if noted, discontinuation of therapy should be considered.

Use with caution in patients with thyroid disease, hepatic impairment, renal impairment, cardiovascular disease, diabetes, glaucoma, cataracts, myasthenia gravis, patients at risk for osteoporosis, patients at risk for seizures, or GI diseases (diverticulitis, peptic ulcer, ulcerative colitis) due to perforation risk. Avoid ethanol may enhance gastric mucosal irritation. Use caution following acute MI (corticosteroids have been associated with myocardial rupture). Because of the risk of adverse effects, systemic corticosteroids should be used cautiously in the elderly in the smallest possible effective dose for the shortest duration. Withdraw therapy with gradual tapering of dose. May affect growth velocity; growth should be routinely monitored in pediatric patients. Potentially significant drug-drug interactions may exist, requiring dose or frequency adjustment, additional monitoring, and/or selection of alternative therapy.

Benzyl alcohol and derivatives: Some dosage forms may contain sodium benzoate/benzoic acid; benzoic acid (benzoate) is a metabolite of benzyl alcohol; large amounts of benzyl alcohol (≥99 mg/kg/day) have been associated with a potentially fatal toxicity ("gasping syndrome") in neonates; the "gasping syndrome" consists of metabolic acidosis, respiratory distress, gasping respirations, CNS dysfunction (including convulsions, intracranial hemorrhage), hypotension, and cardiovascular collapse (AAP, 1997; CDC, 1982); some data suggests that benzoate displaces bilirubin from protein binding sites (Ahlfors, 2001); avoid or use dosage forms containing benzyl alcohol derivative with caution in neonates. See manufacturer's labeling.

Adverse Reactions

Cardiovascular: Cardiomyopathy, CHF, edema, facial edema, hypertension

Central nervous system: Headache, insomnia, malaise, nervousness, pseudotumor cerebri, psychic disorders, seizure, vertigo

Dermatologic: Bruising, facial erythema, hirsutism, petechiae, skin test reaction suppression, thin fragile skin, urticaria

Endocrine & metabolic: Carbohydrate tolerance decreased, Cushing's syndrome, diabetes mellitus, growth suppression, hyperglycemia, hypernatremia, hypokalemia, hypokalemic alkalosis, menstrual irregularities, negative nitrogen balance, pituitary adrenal axis suppression

Gastrointestinal: Abdominal distention, increased appetite, indigestion, nausea, pancreatitis, peptic ulcer, ulcerative esophagitis, weight gain

Hepatic: LFTs increased (usually reversible)

Neuromuscular & skeletal: Arthralgia, aseptic necrosis (humeral/femoral heads), fractures, muscle mass decreased, muscle weakness, osteoporosis, steroid myopathy, tendon rupture, weakness

Ocular: Cataracts, exophthalmus, eyelid edema, glaucoma, intraocular pressure increased, irritation

Respiratory: Epistaxis

Miscellaneous: Diaphoresis increased, impaired wound healing

Rare but important or life-threatening: Venous thrombosis (Johannesdottir, 2013)

Drug Interactions

Metabolism/Transport Effects Substrate of CYP3A4 (minor); **Note:** Assignment of Major/Minor substrate status based on clinically relevant drug interaction potential; **Inhibits** CYP3A4 (weak)

Avoid Concomitant Use

Avoid concomitant use of PrednisoLONE (Systemic) with any of the following: Aldesleukin; BCG; Indium 111 Capromab Pendetide; Mifepristone; Natalizumab; Pimecrolimus; Pimozide; Tacrolimus (Topical); Tofacitinib

Increased Effect/Toxicity

PrednisoLONE (Systemic) may increase the levels/effects of: Acetylcholinesterase Inhibitors; Amphotericin B; Androgens; ARIPiprazole; Ceritinib; CycloSPORINE (Systemic); Deferasirox; Dofetilide; Hydrocodone; Leflunomide; Lomitapide; Loop Diuretics; Natalizumab; Nicorandil; NSAID (COX-2 Inhibitor); NSAID (Nonselective); Pimozide; Quinolone Antibiotics; Thiazide Diuretics; Tofacitinib; Vaccines (Live); Warfarin

The levels/effects of PrednisoLONE (Systemic) may be increased by: Aprepitant; Boceprevir; CycloSPORINE (Systemic); CYP3A4 Inhibitors (Strong); Denosumab; Estrogen Derivatives; Fosaprepitant; Indacaterol; Mifepristone; Neuromuscular-Blocking Agents (Nondepolarizing); Pimecrolimus; Ritonavir; Roflumilast; Salicylates; Tacrolimus (Topical); Telaprevir; Trastuzumab

Decreased Effect

PrednisoLONE (Systemic) may decrease the levels/effects of: Aldesleukin; Antidiabetic Agents; BCG; Calcitriol; Coccidioides immitis Skin Test; Corticorelin; CycloSPORINE (Systemic); Hyaluronidase; Indium 111 Capromab Pendetide; Isoniazid; Salicylates; Sipuleucel-T; Telaprevir; Urea Cycle Disorder Agents; Vaccines (Inactivated)

The levels/effects of PrednisoLONE (Systemic) may be decreased by: Aminoglutethimide; Antacids; Barbiturates; Bile Acid Sequestrants; Carbimazole; Echinacea; Fosphenytoin; Methimazole; Mifepristone; Mitotane; Phenytoin; Primidone; Rifamycin Derivatives

Storage/Stability

Flo-Pred™: Store at 20°C to 25°C (68°F to 77°F). Flo-Pred™ should be dispensed in the original container (to avoid loss of formulation during transfer).

Millipred™: Store at 20°C to 25°C (68°F to 77°F).

Orapred ODT®: Store at 20°C to 25°C (68°F to 77°F) in blister pack. Protect from moisture.

Orapred®, Veripred™ 20: 2°C to 8°C (36°F to 46°F).

Pediapred®: 4°C to 25°C (39°F to 77°F); may be refrigerated.

Mechanism of Action Decreases inflammation by suppression of migration of polymorphonuclear leukocytes and reversal of increased capillary permeability; suppresses the immune system by reducing activity and volume of the lymphatic system

Pharmacodynamics/Kinetics

Duration: 18-36 hours

Protein binding (concentration dependent): 65% to 91%; decreased in elderly

Metabolism: Primarily hepatic, but also metabolized in most tissues, to inactive compounds

Half-life elimination: 3.6 hours; End-stage renal disease: 3-5 hours

Excretion: Primarily urine (as glucuronides, sulfates, and unconjugated metabolites)

Dosage Dose depends upon condition being treated and response of patient; dosage for infants and children should be based on severity of the disease and response of the patient rather than on strict adherence to dosage indicated by age, weight, or body surface area. Oral dosage expressed in terms of prednisolone base. Consider alternate day therapy for long-term therapy. Discontinuation of long-term therapy requires gradual withdrawal by tapering the dose. Patients undergoing unusual stress while receiving corticosteroids should receive increased doses prior to, during, and after the stressful situation.

Children: Oral:

Acute asthma: 1-2 mg/kg/day in divided doses 1-2 times daily for 3-5 days

Anti-inflammatory or immunosuppressive dose: 0.1-2 mg/kg/day in divided doses 1-4 times daily

Nephrotic syndrome:

Initial (first 3 episodes): 2 mg/kg/day **or** 60 mg/m^2/day (maximum: 80 mg daily) in divided doses 3-4 times daily until urine is protein free for 3 consecutive days (maximum: 28 days); followed by 1-1.5 mg/kg/dose **or** 40 mg/m^2/dose given every other day for 4 weeks

Maintenance (long-term maintenance dose for frequent relapses): 0.5-1 mg/kg/dose given every other day for 3-6 months

Adolescents ≥16 years: Oral: Bell's palsy (off-label use): 50 mg daily (in 1 or 2 divided doses) for 10 days; treatment should begin within 72 hours of onset of symptoms (Baugh, 2013; Sullivan, 2007)

Adults: Oral:

Usual range: 5-60 mg daily

Multiple sclerosis: 200 mg daily for 1 week followed by 80 mg every other day for 1 month

Rheumatoid arthritis: Initial: 5-7.5 mg daily; adjust dose as necessary

Acute exacerbations of chronic obstructive pulmonary disease (COPD) (off-label use): 30-40 mg daily for 10-14 days (GOLD guidelines, 2013)

Bell's palsy (off-label use): 60 mg once daily for 5 days, then taper dose downward by 10 mg daily for 5 days (total treatment duration: 10 days) (Engstrom, 2008; Berg, 2012) **or** 50 mg daily (in 1 or 2 divided doses) for 10 days (begin within 72 hours of onset of symptoms) (Baugh, 2013; Sullivan, 2007)

Severe alcoholic hepatitis (Maddrey Discriminant Function [MDF] score ≥32) (off-label use): 40 mg daily for 28 days, followed by a 2-week taper (O'Shea, 2010)

Elderly: Use lowest effective dose

Dosing adjustment in hyperthyroidism: Prednisolone dose may need to be increased to achieve adequate therapeutic effects

Dosage adjustment in renal impairment: No dosage adjustment provided in manufacturer's labeling. Use with caution.

Hemodialysis: Slightly dialyzable (5% to 20%); administer dose posthemodialysis

Peritoneal dialysis: Supplemental dose is not necessary

Dosage adjustment in hepatic impairment: No dosage adjustment provided in manufacturer's labeling.

Dietary Considerations Should be taken after meals or with food or milk to decrease GI effects; increase dietary intake of pyridoxine, vitamin C, vitamin D, folate, calcium, and phosphorus.

Administration Administer oral formulation with food or milk to decrease GI effects.

Flo-Pred: Administer using the provided calibrated syringe (supplied by manufacturer) to accurately measure the dose. Syringe should be washed prior to next use.

Orapred ODT: Do not break or use partial tablet. Remove tablet from blister pack just prior to use. May swallow whole or allow to dissolve on tongue.

Monitoring Parameters Blood pressure; blood glucose, electrolytes; intraocular pressure (use >6 weeks); bone mineral density; growth in children

Dosage Forms

Solution, Oral:

Millipred: 10 mg/5 mL (237 mL)

Pediapred: 5 mg/5 mL (120 mL)

Veripred 20: 20 mg/5 mL (237 mL)

Generic: 15 mg/5 mL (237 mL, 240 mL, 480 mL); 25 mg/5 mL (237 mL); 5 mg/5 mL (120 mL)

Suspension, Oral:

Flo-Pred: 15 mg/5 mL (30 mL)

Syrup, Oral:
Prelone: 15 mg/5 mL (240 mL)
Generic: 15 mg/5 mL (240 mL, 480 mL)

Tablet, Oral:
Millipred: 5 mg
Millipred DP: 5 mg
Millipred DP 12-Day: 5 mg

Tablet Dispersible, Oral:
Orapred ODT: 10 mg, 15 mg, 30 mg
Generic: 10 mg, 15 mg, 30 mg

PrednisoLONE (Ophthalmic) (pred NISS oh lone)

Brand Names: U.S. Omnipred; Pred Forte; Pred Mild

Brand Names: Canada Minims Prednisolone Sodium Phosphate; PMS-Prednisolone Sodium Phosphate Forte; Pred Forte; Pred Mild; Ratio-Prednisolone; Sandoz Prednisolone

Index Terms Econopred; Prednisolone Acetate, Ophthalmic; Prednisolone Sodium Phosphate, Ophthalmic

Pharmacologic Category Corticosteroid, Ophthalmic

Use

Corneal injury: Treatment of corneal injury from chemical or thermal burns (excluding Pred Forte) or to radiation burns or penetration of foreign bodies (excluding Pred Forte, Pred Mild).

Ophthalmic inflammatory conditions: Treatment of steroid-responsive inflammatory conditions of the palpebral and bulbar conjunctiva, cornea, and anterior segment of the globe such as acne rosacea, allergic conjunctivitis, cyclitis, herpes zoster keratitis, iritis, superficial punctate keratitis, and selected infective conjunctivitis.

Pregnancy Risk Factor C

Dosage

Ophthalmic inflammation, treatment: Children and Adolescents (off-label use): Ophthalmic: Prednisolone acetate 1%: Limited data available: Instill 1 to 2 drops into conjunctival sac 3 to 6 times daily. If signs and symptoms fail to improve after 2 days, re-evaluate. Initiate with more frequent dosing, and decrease as clinically indicated. If signs and symptoms fail to improve after 2 days, re-evaluate (Wilson, 2009).

Ophthalmic inflammatory conditions/corneal injury: Adults: Ophthalmic:

Prednisolone acetate: Instill 1 to 2 drops in the affected eye(s) 2 to 4 times daily. During the initial 24 to 48 hours, the dosing frequency may be increased if necessary. If signs and symptoms fail to improve after 2 days, re-evaluate. Do not discontinue therapy prematurely; withdraw therapy with gradual tapering of dose in chronic conditions.

Prednisolone sodium phosphate: Instill 1 to 2 drops into conjunctival sac every hour during the day and every 2 hours at night until satisfactory response is obtained, then use 1 drop every 4 hours; subsequent reduction to 1 drop 3 to 4 times daily may be adequate. Do not discontinue therapy prematurely; withdraw therapy with gradual tapering of dose in chronic conditions.

Dosage adjustment in renal impairment: There are no dosage adjustments provided in the manufacturer's labeling.

Dosage adjustment in hepatic impairment: There are no dosage adjustments provided in the manufacturer's labeling.

Additional Information Complete prescribing information should be consulted for additional detail.

Dosage Forms

Solution, Ophthalmic:
Generic: 1% (10 mL)

Suspension, Ophthalmic:
Omnipred: 1% (5 mL, 10 mL)
Pred Forte: 1% (1 mL, 5 mL, 10 mL, 15 mL)
Pred Mild: 0.12% (5 mL, 10 mL)
Generic: 1% (5 mL, 10 mL, 15 mL)

◆ **Prednisolone Acetate, Ophthalmic** *see* PrednisoLONE (Ophthalmic) *on page 1706*

Prednisolone and Gentamicin

(pred NIS oh lone & jen ta MYE sin)

Brand Names: U.S. Pred-G

Index Terms Gentamicin and Prednisolone

Pharmacologic Category Antibiotic/Corticosteroid, Ophthalmic

Use Inflammatory ocular conditions and superficial ocular infections: Treatment of steroid responsive inflammatory ocular conditions where either a superficial bacterial ocular infection or the risk of bacterial ocular infection exists

Pregnancy Risk Factor C

Dosage Inflammatory ocular conditions and superficial ocular infections: Adults: Ophthalmic:

Ointment: Apply 1/2 inch ribbon into the conjunctival sac of the affected eye(s) 1 to 3 times per day

Suspension: Instill 1 drop into the conjunctival sac of the affected eye(s) 2 to 4 times per day; during the initial 24 to 48 hours, the dosing frequency may be increased if necessary up to 1 drop every hour

Note: If signs and symptoms do not improve after 2 days of treatment, the patient should be re-evaluated.

Dosage adjustment for renal impairment: There are no dosage adjustments provided in the manufacturer's labeling.

Dosage adjustment for hepatic impairment: There are no dosage adjustments provided in the manufacturer's labeling.

Additional Information Complete prescribing information should be consulted for additional detail.

Dosage Forms

Ointment, ophthalmic:
Pred-G: Prednisolone 0.6% and gentamicin 0.3% (3.5 g)

Suspension, ophthalmic:
Pred-G: Prednisolone 1% and gentamicin 0.3% (5 mL)

◆ **Prednisolone and Sulfacetamide** *see* Sulfacetamide and Prednisolone *on page 1944*

◆ **Prednisolone Sodium Phosphate** *see* PrednisoLONE (Systemic) *on page 1703*

◆ **Prednisolone Sodium Phosphate, Ophthalmic** *see* PrednisoLONE (Ophthalmic) *on page 1706*

PredniSONE (PRED ni sone)

Brand Names: U.S. PredniSONE Intensol; Rayos

Brand Names: Canada Apo-Prednisone; Novo-Prednisone; Winpred

Index Terms Deltacortisone; Deltadehydrocortisone

Pharmacologic Category Corticosteroid, Systemic

Additional Appendix Information

Corticosteroids Systemic Equivalencies *on page 2228*

Use Treatment of a variety of diseases, including:

Allergic conditions: Atopic dermatitis, drug hypersensitivity reactions, allergic rhinitis, serum sickness, adjunctive treatment of anaphylaxis

Dermatologic diseases: Bullous dermatitis herpetiformis, contact dermatitis, exfoliative erythroderma, mycosis fungoides, pemphigus, severe erythema multiforme (Stevens-Johnson syndrome), severe seborrheic dermatitis (immediate release only)

Endocrine conditions: Congenital adrenal hyperplasia, hypercalcemia of malignancy, nonsuppurative thyroiditis, adrenocortical insufficiency

Gastrointestinal diseases: Crohn disease, ulcerative colitis

Hematologic diseases: Acquired (autoimmune) hemolytic anemia, Diamond-Blackfan anemia, immune thrombocytopenia (ITP), pure red cell aplasia, secondary thrombocytopenia

Infectious diseases: Trichinosis with neurologic or myocardial involvement, tuberculosis meningitis with subarachnoid block or impending block

Neoplastic conditions: Acute leukemia, aggressive lymphomas

Nervous system conditions (delayed release only): Acute exacerbations of multiple sclerosis, cerebral edema associated with primary or metastatic brain tumor, craniotomy or head injury

Ophthalmic conditions:

Immediate release only: Allergic conjunctivitis, keratitis, allergic corneal marginal ulcers, herpes zoster ophthalmicus, iritis and iridocyclitis, chorioretinitis, anterior segment inflammation, diffuse posterior uveitis and choroiditis, optic neuritis

Delayed release only: Uveitis, and ocular inflammatory conditions

Organ transplantation-related conditions (delayed release only): Solid organ rejection

Pulmonary diseases: Aspiration pneumonitis, asthma, pulmonary tuberculosis, symptomatic sarcoidosis

Immediate release only: Loeffler's syndrome not manageable by other means, berylliosis

Delayed release only: Acute exacerbations of chronic obstructive pulmonary disease (COPD), allergic bronchopulmonary aspergillosis, hypersensitivity pneumonitis, idiopathic bronchiolitis obliterans with organizing pneumonia, idiopathic eosinophilic pneumonias, idiopathic pulmonary fibrosis, *Pneumocystis jiroveci* (formerly *carinii*) pneumonia (PCP)

Renal conditions: Nephrotic syndrome (idiopathic or related to lupus erythematosus), without uremia

Rheumatologic conditions, short-term therapy: Psoriatic arthritis, rheumatoid and juvenile arthritis, ankylosing spondylitis, acute gouty arthritis, systemic lupus erythematosus, dermatomyositis/polymyositis

Immediate release only: Bursitis, tenosynovitis, posttraumatic osteoarthritis, synovitis of osteoarthritis, epicondylitis, acute rheumatic carditis

Delayed release only: Polymyalgia rheumatica, relapsing polychondritis, Sjogren's syndrome, vasculitis

Rheumatologic conditions, maintenance therapy: Rheumatoid and juvenile arthritis, systemic lupus erythematosus, dermatomyositis/polymyositis

Immediate release only: Acute rheumatic carditis

Delayed release only: Ankylosing spondylitis, polymyalgia rheumatic, psoriatic arthritis, relapsing polychondritis, Sjogren's syndrome, vasculitis

Pregnancy Risk Factor C/D (product specific)

Pregnancy Considerations Adverse events have been observed with corticosteroids in animal reproduction studies. Prednisone and its metabolite, prednisolone, cross the human placenta. In the mother, prednisone is converted to the active metabolite prednisolone by the liver. Prior to reaching the fetus, prednisolone is converted by placental enzymes back to prednisone. As a result, the level of prednisone remaining in the maternal serum and reaching the fetus are similar; however, the amount of prednisolone reaching the fetus is ~8-10 times lower than the maternal serum concentration (healthy women at term) (Beitins, 1972). Some studies have shown an association between first trimester systemic corticosteroid use and oral clefts (Park-Wyllie, 2000; Pradat, 2003). Systemic corticosteroids may also influence fetal growth (decreased birth weight); however, information is conflicting (Lunghi, 2010). Hypoadrenalism may occur in newborns following maternal use of corticosteroids in pregnancy; monitor.

When systemic corticosteroids are needed in pregnancy, it is generally recommended to use the lowest effective dose for the shortest duration of time, avoiding high doses during the first trimester (Leachman, 2006; Lunghi, 2010; Makol, 2011; Østensen, 2009). Inhaled corticosteroids are preferred for the treatment of asthma during pregnancy. Oral corticosteroids, such as prednisone, may be used for the treatment of severe persistent asthma if needed; the lowest dose administered on alternate days (if possible) should be used (NAEPP, 2005). Prednisone may be used to treat lupus nephritis in pregnant women who have active nephritis or substantial extrarenal disease activity (Hahn, 2012).

Pregnant women exposed to prednisone for antirejection therapy following a transplant may contact the National Transplantation Pregnancy Registry (NTPR) at 215-955-4820. Women exposed to prednisone during pregnancy for the treatment of an autoimmune disease (eg, rheumatoid arthritis) may contact the OTIS Autoimmune Diseases Study at 877-311-8972.

Breast-Feeding Considerations Prednisone and its metabolite, prednisolone, are found in low concentrations in breast milk. Following a maternal dose of 10 mg (n=1), milk concentrations were measured ~2 hours after the maternal dose (prednisone 0.0016 mcg/mL; prednisolone 0.0267 mcg/mL) (Katz, 1975). In a study which included six mother/infant pairs, adverse events were not observed in nursing infants (maternal prednisone dose not provided) (Ito, 1993).

The manufacturer notes that when used systemically, maternal use of corticosteroids have the potential to cause adverse events in a nursing infant (eg, growth suppression, interfere with endogenous corticosteroid production) and therefore, a decision should be made whether to discontinue nursing or to discontinue the drug, taking into account the importance of treatment to the mother. If there is concern about exposure to the infant, some guidelines recommend waiting 4 hours after the maternal dose of an oral systemic corticosteroid before breast-feeding in order to decrease potential exposure to the nursing infant (based on a study using prednisolone) (Bae, 2011; Leachman, 2006; Makol, 2011; Ost, 1985). Other guidelines note that maternal use of prednisone is not a contraindication to breast-feeding (NAEPP, 2005).

Contraindications Hypersensitivity to any component of the formulation; systemic fungal infections; administration of live or live attenuated vaccines with immunosuppressive doses of prednisone

Warnings/Precautions May cause hypercorticism or suppression of hypothalamic-pituitary-adrenal (HPA) axis, particularly in younger children or in patients receiving high doses for prolonged periods. HPA axis suppression may lead to adrenal crisis. Withdrawal and discontinuation of a corticosteroid should be done slowly and carefully. Particular care is required when patients are transferred from systemic corticosteroids to inhaled products due to possible adrenal insufficiency or withdrawal from steroids, including an increase in allergic symptoms. Patients receiving >20 mg per day of prednisone (or equivalent) may be most susceptible. Fatalities have occurred due to adrenal insufficiency in asthmatic patients during and after transfer from systemic corticosteroids to aerosol steroids; aerosol steroids do **not** provide the systemic steroid needed to treat patients having trauma, surgery, or infections.

Acute myopathy has been reported with high dose corticosteroids, usually in patients with neuromuscular transmission disorders; may involve ocular and/or respiratory muscles; monitor creatine kinase; recovery may be delayed. Prolonged use of corticosteroids may increase the incidence of secondary infection, mask acute infection (including fungal infections), prolong or exacerbate viral infections, or limit response to vaccines. Exposure to chickenpox should be avoided. Corticosteroids should not be used to treat ocular herpes simplex or cerebral malaria. Close observation is required in patients with latent tuberculosis and/or TB reactivity; restrict use in active TB (only in conjunction with antituberculosis treatment). Prolonged treatment with corticosteroids has been associated with the development of Kaposi's sarcoma (case reports); if noted, discontinuation of therapy should be considered. Prolonged use may cause posterior subcapsular cataracts, glaucoma (with possible nerve damage) and may increase the risk for ocular infections. Corticosteroid use may cause psychiatric disturbances, including depression, euphoria, insomnia, mood swings, and personality changes. Preexisting psychiatric conditions may be exacerbated by corticosteroid use.

Use with caution in patients with HF, diabetes, GI diseases (diverticulitis, peptic ulcer, ulcerative colitis; due to risk of perforation), hepatic impairment, myasthenia gravis, MI, patients with or who are at risk for osteoporosis, seizure disorders or thyroid disease. Avoid ethanol may enhance gastric mucosal irritation. May affect growth velocity; growth should be routinely monitored in pediatric patients.

Prior to use, the dose and duration of treatment should be based on the risk versus benefit for each individual patient. In general, use the smallest effective dose for the shortest duration of time to minimize adverse events. A gradual tapering of dose may be required prior to discontinuing therapy. Potentially significant drug-drug interactions may exist, requiring dose or frequency adjustment, additional monitoring, and/or selection of alternative therapy.

Benzyl alcohol and derivatives: Some dosage forms may contain sodium benzoate/benzoic acid; benzoic acid (benzoate) is a metabolite of benzyl alcohol; large amounts of benzyl alcohol (≥99 mg/kg/day) have been associated with a potentially fatal toxicity ("gasping syndrome") in neonates; the "gasping syndrome" consists of metabolic acidosis, respiratory distress, gasping respirations, CNS dysfunction (including convulsions, intracranial hemorrhage), hypotension, and cardiovascular collapse (AAP, 1997; CDC, 1982); some data suggests that benzoate displaces bilirubin from protein binding sites (Ahlfors, 2001); avoid or use dosage forms containing benzyl alcohol derivative with caution in neonates. See manufacturer's labeling.

Adverse Reactions

Cardiovascular: Congestive heart failure (in susceptible patients), hypertension

Central nervous system: Emotional instability, headache, intracranial pressure increased (with papilledema), psychic derangements (including euphoria, insomnia, mood swings, personality changes, severe depression), seizure, vertigo

Dermatologic: Bruising, facial erythema, petechiae, thin fragile skin, urticaria, wound healing impaired

Endocrine & metabolic: Adrenocortical and pituitary unresponsiveness (in times of stress), carbohydrate intolerance, Cushing's syndrome, diabetes mellitus, fluid retention, growth suppression (in children), hypokalemic alkalosis, hypothyroidism enhanced, menstrual irregularities, negative nitrogen balance due to protein catabolism, potassium loss, sodium retention

Gastrointestinal: Abdominal distension, pancreatitis, peptic ulcer (with possible perforation and hemorrhage), ulcerative esophagitis

Hepatic: ALT increased, AST increased, alkaline phosphatase increased

Neuromuscular & skeletal: Aseptic necrosis of femoral and humeral heads, muscle mass loss, muscle weakness, osteoporosis, pathologic fracture of long bones, steroid myopathy, tendon rupture (particularly Achilles tendon), vertebral compression fractures

Ocular: Exophthalmos, glaucoma, intraocular pressure increased, posterior subcapsular cataracts

Miscellaneous: Allergic reactions, anaphylactic reactions, diaphoresis, hypersensitivity reactions, infections, Kaposi's sarcoma

Rare but important or life-threatening: Venous thrombosis (Johannesdottir, 2013)

Drug Interactions

Metabolism/Transport Effects Substrate of CYP3A4 (minor); **Note:** Assignment of Major/Minor substrate status based on clinically relevant drug interaction potential; **Induces** CYP2C19 (moderate), CYP3A4 (weak)

Avoid Concomitant Use

Avoid concomitant use of PredniSONE with any of the following: Aldesleukin; BCG; Indium 111 Capromab Pendetide; Mifepristone; Natalizumab; Pimecrolimus; Tacrolimus (Topical); Tofacitinib

Increased Effect/Toxicity

PredniSONE may increase the levels/effects of: Acetylcholinesterase Inhibitors; Amphotericin B; Androgens; Ceritinib; CycloSPORINE (Systemic); Deferasirox; Leflunomide; Loop Diuretics; Natalizumab; Nicorandil; NSAID (COX-2 Inhibitor); NSAID (Nonselective); Quinolone Antibiotics; Thiazide Diuretics; Tofacitinib; Vaccines (Live); Warfarin

The levels/effects of PredniSONE may be increased by: Aprepitant; Boceprevir; CycloSPORINE (Systemic); CYP3A4 Inhibitors (Strong); Denosumab; Estrogen Derivatives; Fluconazole; Fosaprepitant; Indacaterol; Mifepristone; Neuromuscular-Blocking Agents (Nondepolarizing); Pimecrolimus; Ritonavir; Roflumilast; Salicylates; Tacrolimus (Topical); Telaprevir; Trastuzumab

Decreased Effect

PredniSONE may decrease the levels/effects of: Aldesleukin; Antidiabetic Agents; ARIPiprazole; BCG; Calcitriol; Coccidioides immitis Skin Test; Corticorelin; CycloSPORINE (Systemic); Hyaluronidase; Hydrocodone; Indium 111 Capromab Pendetide; Isoniazid; Salicylates; Saxagliptin; Sipuleucel-T; Telaprevir; Urea Cycle Disorder Agents; Vaccines (Inactivated)

The levels/effects of PredniSONE may be decreased by: Aminoglutethimide; Antacids; Barbiturates; Bile Acid Sequestrants; Echinacea; Fosphenytoin; Mifepristone; Mitotane; Phenytoin; Primidone; Rifamycin Derivatives; Somatropin; Tesamorelin

Mechanism of Action Decreases inflammation by suppression of migration of polymorphonuclear leukocytes and reversal of increased capillary permeability; suppresses the immune system by reducing activity and volume of the lymphatic system; suppresses adrenal function at high doses. Antitumor effects may be related to inhibition of glucose transport, phosphorylation, or induction of cell death in immature lymphocytes. Antiemetic effects are thought to occur due to blockade of cerebral innervation of the emetic center via inhibition of prostaglandin synthesis.

Pharmacodynamics/Kinetics

Absorption: 50% to 90% (may be altered in IBS or hyperthyroidism)

Protein binding (concentration dependent): 65% to 91%

Metabolism: Hepatically converted from prednisone (inactive) to prednisolone (active); may be impaired with hepatic dysfunction

Half-life elimination: Normal renal function: ~3.5 hours

Time to peak: Oral:

Immediate release tablet: 2 hours; Delayed release tablet (Rayos®): 6-6.5 hours

Excretion: Urine (small portion)

Dosage Oral:

General dosing range: Children and Adults: Initial: 5 to 60 mg daily: **Note:** Dose depends upon condition being treated and response of patient; dosage for infants and children should be based on severity of the disease and response of the patient rather than on strict adherence to dosage indicated by age, weight, or body surface area. Consider alternate day therapy for long-term therapy. Discontinuation of long-term therapy requires gradual withdrawal by tapering the dose.

Prednisone taper (other regimens also available):

Day 1: 30 mg divided as 10 mg before breakfast, 5 mg at lunch, 5 mg at dinner, 10 mg at bedtime

Day 2: 5 mg at breakfast, 5 mg at lunch, 5 mg at dinner, 10 mg at bedtime

Day 3: 5 mg 4 times daily (with meals and at bedtime)

Day 4: 5 mg 3 times daily (breakfast, lunch, bedtime)

Day 5: 5 mg 2 times daily (breakfast, bedtime)

Day 6: 5 mg before breakfast

Indication-specific dosing:

Children:

Acute asthma (NAEPP, 2007):

0 to 11 years 1 to 2 mg/kg/day for 3 to 10 days (maximum: 60 mg daily)

≥12 years: Refer to Adults dosing

Autoimmune hepatitis (off-label use; Czaja, 2002): Initial treatment: 2 mg/kg/day for 2 weeks (maximum: 60 mg daily), followed by a taper over 6 to 8 weeks to a dose of 0.1 to 0.2 mg/kg/day or 5 mg daily

Nephrotic syndrome (Pediatric Nephrology Panel recommendations [Hogg, 2000]): Initial: 2 mg/kg/day or 60 mg/m^2/day given every day in 1 to 3 divided doses (maximum: 80 mg daily) until urine is protein free or for 4 to 6 weeks; followed by maintenance dose: 2 mg/kg/dose or 40 mg/m^2/dose given every other day in the morning; gradually taper and discontinue after 4 to 6 weeks. **Note:** No definitive treatment guidelines exist. Dosing is dependent on institution protocols and individual response.

PCP pneumonia (AIDS*info* guidelines, 2008): 1 mg/kg twice daily for 5 days, *followed by* 0.5 to 1 mg/kg twice daily for 5 days, *followed by* 0.5 mg/kg once daily for 11 to 21 days

Adolescents and Adults:

Bell palsy (off-label use): Adolescents ≥16 years and Adults: Oral: 60 mg daily for 5 days, followed by a 5-day taper. Treatment should begin within 72 hours of onset of symptoms (Baugh, 2013).

PCP pneumonia (AIDS*info* guidelines, 2008): Note: Begin within 72 hours of PCP therapy: 40 mg twice daily for 5 days, *followed by* 40 mg once daily for 5 days, *followed by* 20 mg once daily for 11 days or until antimicrobial regimen is completed

Adults:

Acute asthma (NAEPP, 2007): 40 to 60 mg daily for 3 to 10 days; administer as single or 2 divided doses

Acute exacerbations of chronic obstructive pulmonary disease (COPD) (off-label use for immediate release products; off-label dose): 40 mg once daily for 5 days (GOLD, 2014).

Acute gout (ACR guidelines [Khanna, 2012]): Initial: ≥0.5 mg/kg for 5 to 10 days

Anaphylaxis, adjunctive treatment (Lieberman, 2005): 0.5 mg/kg

Antineoplastic: Usual range: 10 mg daily to 100 mg/m^2/day (depending on indication). **Note:** Details concerning dosing in combination regimens should also be consulted.

Autoimmune hepatitis (off-label use; Czaja, 2002): Initial treatment: 60 mg daily for 1 week, *followed by* 40 mg daily for 1 week, *then* 30 mg daily for 2 weeks, *then* 20 mg daily. Half this dose should be given when used in combination with azathioprine

Crohn disease, moderate/severe (off-label use): 40 to 60 mg daily until resolution of symptoms and resumption of weight gain (usual duration: 7 to 28 days) (Lichtenstein, 2009)

Dermatomyositis/polymyositis: Oral: 1 mg/kg daily (range: 0.5 to 1.5 mg/kg/day), often in conjunction with steroid-sparing therapies; depending on response/tolerance, consider slow tapering after 2 to 8 weeks depending on response; taper regimens vary widely, but often involve 5 to 10 mg decrements per week and may require 6 to 12 months to reach a low once-daily or every-other-day dose to prevent disease flare (Briemberg, 2003; Hengstman, 2009; Iorizzo, 2008; Wiendl, 2008)

Giant cell arteritis (off-label use): Oral: Initial: 40 to 60 mg daily; typically requires 1 to 2 years of treatment, but may begin to taper after 2 to 3 months; alternative dosing of 30 to 40 mg daily has demonstrated similar efficacy (Hiratzka, 2010)

Graves ophthalmopathy prophylaxis (off-label use): 0.4 to 0.5 mg/kg/day, starting 1 to 3 days after radioactive iodine treatment, and continued for 1 month, then gradually taper over 2 months (Bahn, 2011)

Herpes zoster (off-label use; Dworkin, 2007): 60 mg daily for 7 days, *followed by* 30 mg daily for 7 days, *then* 15 mg daily for 7 days

Immune thrombocytopenia (ITP) (American Society of Hematology, 1997): 1 to 2 mg/kg/day

Lupus nephritis, induction (Hahn, 2012): Oral:

Class III-IV lupus nephritis: 0.5 to 1 mg/kg/day (after glucocorticoid pulse) tapered after a few weeks to lowest effective dose, in combination with an immunosuppressive agent

Class V lupus nephritis: 0.5 mg/kg/day for 6 months in combination mycophenolate mofetil; if not improved after 6 months, use 0.5 to 1 mg/kg/day (after a glucocorticoid pulse) for an additional 6 months in combination with cyclophosphamide

Rheumatoid arthritis (American College of Rheumatology, 2002): ≤10 mg daily

Subacute thyroiditis (off-label use): 40 mg daily for 1 to 2 weeks; gradually taper over 2 to 4 weeks or longer depending on clinical response. **Note:** NSAIDs should be considered first-line therapy in such patients (Bahn, 2011).

Takayasu arteritis (off-label use): Oral: Initial: 40 to 60 mg daily; taper to lowest effective dose when ESR and CRP levels are normal; usual duration: 1 to 2 years (Hiratzka, 2010)

Thyrotoxicosis (type II amiodarone-induced; off-label use): 40 mg daily for 14 to 28 days; gradually taper over 2 to 3 months depending on clinical response (Bahn, 2011)

Tuberculosis, severe, paradoxical reactions (off-label dose, AIDS*info* guidelines, 2008): 1 mg/kg/day, gradually reduce after 1 to 2 weeks

Elderly: Use the lowest effective dose

Dosing adjustment in renal impairment: No dosage adjustment provided in manufacturer's labeling. Use with caution.

Hemodialysis effects: Supplemental dose is not necessary.

Dosing adjustment in hepatic impairment: No dosage adjustment provided in manufacturer's labeling. Prednisone is inactive and must be metabolized by the liver to prednisolone. This conversion may be impaired in patients with liver disease, however, prednisolone levels are observed to be higher in patients with severe liver failure than in normal patients. Therefore, compensation for the inadequate conversion of prednisone to prednisolone occurs.

Dosing adjustment in hyperthyroidism: Prednisone dose may need to be increased to achieve adequate therapeutic effects.

Dietary Considerations Should be taken after meals or with food or milk; may require increased dietary intake of pyridoxine, vitamin C, vitamin D, folate, calcium, and phosphorus; may require decreased dietary intake of sodium

Administration Administer with food to decrease GI upset. Delayed release tablet (Rayos®) should be swallowed whole; do not crush or chew.

Monitoring Parameters Blood pressure, blood glucose, electrolytes

Following prolonged use: Bone mass density, growth in children, signs and symptoms of infection, cataract formation, intraocular pressure (use >6 weeks)

Additional Information Tapering of corticosteroids after a short course of therapy (<7-10 days) is generally not required unless the disease/inflammatory process is slow to respond. Tapering after prolonged exposure is dependent upon the individual patient, duration of corticosteroid treatments, and size of steroid dose. Recovery of the HPA axis may require several months. Subtle but important HPA axis suppression may be present for as long as several months after a course of as few as 10-14 days duration. Testing of HPA axis (cosyntropin) may be required, and signs/symptoms of adrenal insufficiency should be monitored in patients with a history of use.

Dosage Forms

Concentrate, Oral:
PredniSONE Intensol: 5 mg/mL (30 mL)

Solution, Oral:
Generic: 5 mg/5 mL (5 mL, 120 mL, 500 mL)

Tablet, Oral:
Generic: 1 mg, 2.5 mg, 5 mg, 10 mg, 20 mg, 50 mg

Tablet Delayed Release, Oral:
Rayos: 1 mg, 2 mg, 5 mg

◆ **PredniSONE Intensol** *see* PredniSONE *on page 1706*

Pregabalin (pre GAB a lin)

Brand Names: U.S. Lyrica

Brand Names: Canada Apo-Pregabalin; CO Pregabalin; Dom-Pregabalin; GD-Pregabalin; Lyrica; Mint-Pregabalin; MYL Pregabalin; PMS-Pregabalin; RAN-Pregabalin; Riva-Pregabalin; Sandoz-Pregabalin; Teva-Pregabalin

Index Terms CI-1008; S-(+)-3-isobutylgaba

Pharmacologic Category Analgesic, Miscellaneous; Anticonvulsant, Miscellaneous

Use Management of neuropathic pain associated with diabetic peripheral neuropathy or with spinal cord injury; management of postherpetic neuralgia; adjunctive therapy for partial-onset seizure disorder; management of fibromyalgia

Pregnancy Risk Factor C

Pregnancy Considerations Adverse events were observed in animal reproduction studies. In addition, male-mediated teratogenicity has been observed in animal reproduction studies; implications in humans are not defined. Impaired male and female fertility has been noted in animal studies.

Patients exposed to pregabalin during pregnancy are encouraged to enroll themselves into the North American Antiepileptic Drug (NAAED) Pregnancy Registry by calling 1-888-233-2334. Additional information is available at www.aedpregnancyregistry.org.

Breast-Feeding Considerations It is not known if pregabalin is excreted in breast milk. Due to the potential for serious adverse reactions in the nursing infant, a decision should be made whether to discontinue nursing or to discontinue the drug, taking into account the importance of treatment to the mother.

Contraindications Hypersensitivity to pregabalin or any component of the formulation

Warnings/Precautions Antiepileptics are associated with an increased risk of suicidal behavior/thoughts with use (regardless of indication); patients should be monitored for signs/symptoms of depression, suicidal tendencies, and other unusual behavior changes during therapy and instructed to inform their healthcare provider immediately if symptoms occur.

Angioedema has been reported; may be life threatening; use with caution in patients with a history of angioedema episodes. Concurrent use with other drugs known to cause angioedema (eg, ACE inhibitors) may increase risk. Hypersensitivity reactions, including skin redness, blistering, hives, rash, dyspnea, and wheezing have been reported; discontinue treatment of hypersensitivity occurs. Dizziness and somnolence are commonly reported; effects generally occur shortly after initiation and occur more frequently at higher doses. Patients must be cautioned about performing tasks which require mental alertness (eg, operating machinery or driving). Visual disturbances (blurred vision, decreased acuity and visual field changes) have been associated with pregabalin therapy; patients should be instructed to notify their physician if these effects are noted.

Pregabalin has been associated with increases in CPK and rare cases of rhabdomyolysis. Patients should be instructed to notify their prescriber if unexplained muscle pain, tenderness, or weakness, particularly if fever and/or malaise are associated with these symptoms. Use may cause peripheral edema or weight gain; use with caution in patients with heart failure (NYHA Class III or IV) due to limited data in this patient population. In addition, effect on weight gain/edema may be additive with the thiazolidinedione class of antidiabetic agents; use caution when coadministering these agents, particularly in patients with prior cardiovascular disease. May decrease platelet count or prolong PR interval.

Has been noted to be tumorigenic (increased incidence of hemangiosarcoma) in animal studies; significance of these findings in humans is unknown. Pregabalin has been associated with discontinuation symptoms following abrupt cessation, and increases in seizure frequency (when used as an antiepileptic) may occur. Should not be discontinued abruptly; dosage tapering over at least 1 week is recommended. Use caution in renal impairment; dosage adjustment required.

Adverse Reactions

Cardiovascular: Chest pain, edema, hyper-/hypotension, peripheral edema

Central nervous system: Amnesia, anxiety, ataxia, attention disturbance, confusion, depersonalization, disorientation, dizziness, drunk feeling, euphoria, fatigue, feeling abnormal, fever, headache, hypoesthesia, incoordination, insomnia, lethargy, memory impaired, nervousness, neuropathy, pain, somnolence, speech disorder, stupor, thinking abnormal, vertigo

Dermatologic: Bruising, decubitus ulcer, facial edema, pruritus

Endocrine & metabolic: Fluid retention, hypoglycemia, libido decreased

Gastrointestinal: Abdominal distension, abdominal pain, pain, appetite increased, constipation, flatulence, gastroenteritis, nausea, vomiting, weight gain, xerostomia

Genitourinary: Anorgasmia, impotence, incontinence, urinary frequency

Hematologic: Thrombocytopenia

Neuromuscular & skeletal: Abnormal gait, arthralgia, back pain, balance disorder, CPK increased, joint swelling, leg cramps, muscle spasm, myalgia, myasthenia, myoclonus, neck pain, pain in extremity, paresthesia, tremor, twitching, weakness

Ocular: Blurred vision, conjunctivitis, diplopia, eye disorder, nystagmus, visual abnormalities

Otic: Otitis media, tinnitus

Respiratory: Bronchitis, nasopharyngitis, pharyngolaryngeal pain, sinusitis

Miscellaneous: Accidental injury, allergic reaction, flu-like syndrome, infection

Rare but important or life-threatening): Abnormal ejaculation, abscess, acute renal failure, addiction, agitation, albuminuria, alopecia, amenorrhea, anaphylactoid reaction, anemia, angioedema, anisocoria, apathy, aphasia, aphthous stomatitis, apnea, arthrosis, ascites, atelectasis, bladder cancer, blepharitis, blindness, bronchiolitis, cellulitis, cerebellar syndrome, cervicitis, chills, cholecystitis, cholelithiasis, chondrodystrophy, circumoral paresthesia, cogwheel rigidity, colitis, coma, corneal ulcer, crystalluria (urate), delirium, delusions, diarrhea, dry eyes, dysarthria, dysautonomia, dyskinesia, dysmenorrhea, dysphagia, dyspareunia, dystonia, dysuria, eczema, encephalopathy, eosinophilia, epididymitis, esophageal ulcer, esophagitis, exfoliative dermatitis, exophthalmos, extraocular palsy, extrapyramidal syndrome, eye hemorrhage, female lactation, gastritis, GI hemorrhage, glomerulitis, glucose tolerance decreased, granuloma, Guillain-Barré syndrome, gynecomastia, hallucinations, heart failure, hematuria, hirsutism, hostility, hyperacusis, hyperalgesia, hyperesthesia, hyper-/hypokinesia; hypersensitivity (including skin redness, blistering, hives, rash, dyspnea, and wheezing); hypotonia, intracranial hypertension, iritis, keratitis, keratoconjunctivitis, libido increased, laryngismus, leukopenia, leukorrhea, leukocytosis, lichenoid dermatitis, lung edema, lung fibrosis, lymphadenopathy, malaise, manic reaction, melanosis, melena, miosis, mouth ulcer, mydriasis, myelofibrosis, neck rigidity, nephritis, neuralgia, night blindness, ocular hemorrhage, oliguria, ophthalmoplegia, optic atrophy, pancreatitis, papilledema, paranoid reaction, parosmia, pelvic pain, periodontal abscess, peripheral neuritis, personality disorder, photophobia, photosensitivity, polycythemia, postural hypotension, prothrombin decreased, psychotic depression, ptosis, pulmonary edema, pulmonary fibrosis, purpura, pyelonephritis, rash (vesiculobullous, petechial, purpuric, pustular); rectal hemorrhage, renal calculus, retinal edema, retinal vascular disorder, retroperitoneal fibrosis, rhabdomyolysis, schizophrenic reaction, shock, skin atrophy, skin necrosis, skin nodule, skin ulcer, ST depression, Stevens-Johnson syndrome, subcutaneous nodule, suicide, suicide attempt, syncope, taste loss, taste perversion, thrombocythemia, thrombophlebitis, tongue edema, torticollis, trismus, urinary retention, urticaria, uveitis, ventricular fibrillation

Drug Interactions

Metabolism/Transport Effects None known.

Avoid Concomitant Use

Avoid concomitant use of Pregabalin with any of the following: Azelastine (Nasal); Orphenadrine; Paraldehyde; Thalidomide

Increased Effect/Toxicity

Pregabalin may increase the levels/effects of: Alcohol (Ethyl); Antidiabetic Agents (Thiazolidinedione); Azelastine (Nasal); Buprenorphine; CNS Depressants; Hydrocodone; Methotrimeprazine; Metyrosine; Mirtazapine; Orphenadrine; Paraldehyde; Pramipexole; ROPINIRole; Rotigotine; Selective Serotonin Reuptake Inhibitors; Suvorexant; Thalidomide; Zolpidem

The levels/effects of Pregabalin may be increased by: Brimonidine (Topical); Cannabis; Doxylamine; Dronabinol; Droperidol; HydrOXYzine; Kava Kava; Magnesium Sulfate; Methotrimeprazine; Nabilone; Perampanel; Rufinamide; Sodium Oxybate; Tapentadol; Tetrahydrocannabinol

Decreased Effect

The levels/effects of Pregabalin may be decreased by: Mefloquine; Mianserin; Orlistat

Storage/Stability Store at 25°C (77°F); excursions permitted to 15°C to 30°C (59°F to 86°F).

Mechanism of Action Binds to alpha$_2$-delta subunit of voltage-gated calcium channels within the CNS and modulates calcium influx at the nerve terminals, thereby inhibiting excitatory neurotransmitter release including glutamate, norepinephrine (noradrenaline), serotonin, dopamine, substance P, and calcitonin gene-related peptide (Gajraj, 2007; McKeage, 2009). Although structurally related to GABA, it does not bind to GABA or benzodiazepine receptors. Exerts antinociceptive and anticonvulsant activity. Pregabalin may also affect descending noradrenergic and serotonergic pain transmission pathways from the brainstem to the spinal cord.

Pharmacodynamics/Kinetics

Onset of action: Pain management: Effects may be noted as early as the first week of therapy.

Distribution: V_d: 0.5 L/kg

Protein binding: 0%

Metabolism: Negligible

Bioavailability: >90%

Half-life elimination: 6.3 hours

Time to peak, plasma: 1.5 hours (3 hours with food)

Excretion: Urine (90% as unchanged drug; minor metabolites)

Dosage Oral: Adults: **Note:** When discontinuing, taper off gradually over at least 1 week.

Fibromyalgia:

U.S. labeling: Initial: 150 mg daily in divided doses (75 mg twice daily); may be increased to 300 mg daily (150 mg twice daily) within 1 week based on tolerability and effect; may be further increased to 450 mg daily (225 mg twice daily). Maximum dose: 450 mg daily (dosages up to 600 mg daily were evaluated with no significant additional benefit and an increase in adverse effects)

Canadian labeling: Initial: 150 mg daily in divided doses (75 mg twice daily); may be increased to 300 mg daily (150 mg twice daily) after 1 week based on tolerability and effect; may be further increased to 450 mg daily (225 mg twice daily). The manufacturer labeling suggests that patients with severe ongoing symptoms may receive up to a maximum of 600 mg daily (300 mg twice daily). However, dosages up to 600 mg daily have been evaluated with no significant additional benefit and an increase in adverse effects.

Neuropathic pain, diabetes-associated:

U.S. labeling: Initial: 150 mg daily in divided doses (50 mg 3 times daily); may be increased within 1 week based on tolerability and effect; maximum dose: 300 mg daily in 3 divided doses (dosages up to 600 mg daily were evaluated with no significant additional benefit and an increase in adverse effects)

Canadian labeling: Initial: 150 mg daily in divided doses (50 mg 3 times daily or 75 mg twice daily); may be increased after 1 week based on tolerability and effect to 300 mg daily (150 mg twice daily). The manufacturer labeling suggests that patients with severe ongoing symptoms may receive up to a maximum of 600 mg daily (300 mg twice daily). However, dosages up to 600 mg daily have been evaluated with no significant additional benefit and an increase in adverse effects.

Neuropathic pain, spinal cord injury associated: Initial: 150 mg daily in divided doses (75 mg twice daily); may be increased to 300 mg daily (150 mg twice daily) within 1 week based on tolerability and effect; further titration to 600 mg daily (300 mg twice daily) after 2-3 weeks may be considered in patients who do not experience sufficient relief of pain provided they are able to tolerate pregabalin. Maximum dose: 600 mg daily

Partial-onset seizures (adjunctive therapy): Initial: 150 mg daily in divided doses (75 mg twice daily or 50 mg 3 times daily); may be increased based on tolerability and effect (optimal titration schedule has not been defined). Maximum dose: 600 mg daily

Postherpetic neuralgia: Initial: 150 mg daily in divided doses (75 mg twice daily or 50 mg 3 times daily); may be increased to 300 mg daily within 1 week based on tolerability and effect; further titration (to 600 mg daily) after 2-4 weeks may be considered in patients who do not experience sufficient relief of pain provided they are able to tolerate pregabalin. Maximum dose: 600 mg daily

Dosage adjustment in renal impairment: Renal function may be estimated using the Cockcroft-Gault formula. Then determine recommended dosage regimen based on the indication-specific total daily dose for normal renal function (CrCl ≥60 mL/minute). For example, if the indication-specific daily dose is 450 mg daily for normal renal function, the daily dose should be reduced to 225 mg daily (in 2-3 divided doses) for a creatinine clearance of 30-60 mL/minute (see table).

Pregabalin Renal Impairment Dosing

CrCl (mL/minute)	Total Pregabalin Daily Dose (mg/day)				Dosing Frequency
≥60 (normal renal function)	150	300	450	600	2-3 divided doses
30-60	75	150	225	300	2-3 divided doses
15-30	25-50	75	100-150	150	1-2 divided doses
<15	25	25-50	50-75	75	Single daily dose

Posthemodialysis supplementary dosage (as a single additional dose):
25 mg/day schedule: Single supplementary dose of 25 mg **or** 50 mg
25-50 mg/day schedule: Single supplementary dose of 50 mg **or** 75 mg
50-75 mg/day schedule: Single supplementary dose of 75 mg **or** 100 mg
75 mg/day schedule: Single supplementary dose of 100 mg **or** 150 mg

Dosage adjustment in hepatic impairment: No dosage adjustment provided in manufacturer's labeling. However, no adjustment expected since undergoes minimal hepatic metabolism.

Dietary Considerations May be taken with or without food.

Administration May be administered with or without food.

Monitoring Parameters Measures of efficacy (pain intensity/seizure frequency); degree of sedation; symptoms of myopathy or ocular disturbance; weight gain/edema; skin integrity (in patients with diabetes); suicidality (eg, suicidal thoughts, depression, behavioral changes)

Dosage Forms

Capsule, Oral:

Lyrica: 25 mg, 50 mg, 75 mg, 100 mg, 150 mg, 200 mg, 225 mg, 300 mg

Solution, Oral:

Lyrica: 20 mg/mL (473 mL)

- ◆ **Pregnenedione** *see* Progesterone *on page 1722*
- ◆ **Pregnyl** *see* Chorionic Gonadotropin (Human) *on page 431*
- ◆ **Pregnyl® (Can)** *see* Chorionic Gonadotropin (Human) *on page 431*
- ◆ **Prelone** *see* PrednisoLONE (Systemic) *on page 1703*
- ◆ **Premarin** *see* Estrogens (Conjugated/Equine, Systemic) *on page 787*
- ◆ **Premarin** *see* Estrogens (Conjugated/Equine, Topical) *on page 790*
- ◆ **Premarin® (Can)** *see* Estrogens (Conjugated/Equine, Systemic) *on page 787*
- ◆ **Premarin® (Can)** *see* Estrogens (Conjugated/Equine, Topical) *on page 790*
- ◆ **Premium Activated Charcoal [OTC] (Can)** *see* Charcoal, Activated *on page 416*
- ◆ **Preparation H Hydrocortisone [OTC]** *see* Hydrocortisone (Topical) *on page 1014*
- ◆ **Prepidil** *see* Dinoprostone *on page 640*
- ◆ **Prepidil® (Can)** *see* Dinoprostone *on page 640*
- ◆ **Prepopik™** *see* Sodium Picosulfate, Magnesium Oxide, and Citric Acid *on page 1911*
- ◆ **Prepopik™** *see* Sodium Picosulfate, Magnesium Oxide, and Citric Acid *on page 1911*
- ◆ **Pressyn (Can)** *see* Vasopressin *on page 2142*
- ◆ **Pressyn AR (Can)** *see* Vasopressin *on page 2142*
- ◆ **Pretz [OTC]** *see* Sodium Chloride *on page 1902*
- ◆ **Pretz Irrigation [OTC]** *see* Sodium Chloride *on page 1902*
- ◆ **Prevacid** *see* Lansoprazole *on page 1166*
- ◆ **Prevacid 24HR [OTC]** *see* Lansoprazole *on page 1166*
- ◆ **Prevacid FasTab (Can)** *see* Lansoprazole *on page 1166*
- ◆ **Prevacid SoluTab** *see* Lansoprazole *on page 1166*
- ◆ **Prevalite** *see* Cholestyramine Resin *on page 431*
- ◆ **Prevex B (Can)** *see* Betamethasone (Topical) *on page 255*
- ◆ **Prevex® HC (Can)** *see* Hydrocortisone (Topical) *on page 1014*
- ◆ **PreviDent** *see* Fluoride *on page 895*
- ◆ **PreviDent 5000 Booster** *see* Fluoride *on page 895*
- ◆ **PreviDent 5000 Booster Plus** *see* Fluoride *on page 895*
- ◆ **PreviDent 5000 Dry Mouth** *see* Fluoride *on page 895*
- ◆ **PreviDent 5000 Plus** *see* Fluoride *on page 895*
- ◆ **Previfem** *see* Ethinyl Estradiol and Norgestimate *on page 810*
- ◆ **Prevnar 13** *see* Pneumococcal Conjugate Vaccine (13-Valent) *on page 1670*
- ◆ **Prevpac®** *see* Lansoprazole, Amoxicillin, and Clarithromycin *on page 1169*
- ◆ **Prezcobix** *see* Darunavir and Cobicistat *on page 572*
- ◆ **Prezista** *see* Darunavir *on page 569*
- ◆ **Prialt** *see* Ziconotide *on page 2196*

Prifinium [INT] (pri FIN ne um)

International Brand Names Padrin (JP); Prifinial (AT, CH, FR); Riabal (FR, IT)

Index Terms Prifinium Bromide

Pharmacologic Category Anticholinergic Agent; Antispasmodic Agent, Gastrointestinal

Reported Use Treatment of gastrointestinal spasms

Dosage Range Adults:
Oral: 30-60 mg 3 times/day
I.M., I.V., SubQ: 15 mg 2-4 times/day

Product Availability Product available in various countries; not currently available in the U.S.

Dosage Forms
Injection, solution: 7.5 mg/mL (2 mL)
Syrup: 7.5 mg/5 mL (60 mL)
Tablet: 15 mg, 30 mg

- ◆ **Prifinium Bromide** *see* Prifinium [INT] *on page 1712*
- ◆ **Priftin** *see* Rifapentine *on page 1807*
- ◆ **Prilocaine and Lidocaine** *see* Lidocaine and Prilocaine *on page 1213*
- ◆ **PriLOSEC** *see* Omeprazole *on page 1508*
- ◆ **PriLOSEC OTC [OTC]** *see* Omeprazole *on page 1508*
- ◆ **Primaclone** *see* Primidone *on page 1714*

Primaquine (PRIM a kween)

Index Terms Primaquine Phosphate; Prymaccone

Pharmacologic Category Aminoquinoline (Antimalarial)

Use Prevention of relapse of *P. vivax* malaria

Pregnancy Considerations Animal reproduction studies have not been conducted. Primaquine use is not recommended in pregnant women per CDC Guidelines. Consult current CDC guidelines for the treatment of malaria during pregnancy.

Breast-Feeding Considerations It is not known if primaquine is excreted in breast milk. If therapy is needed, the mother and infant should be tested for G6PD deficiency; primaquine before primaquine is given to a woman who is breast-feeding. It may be used in breast-feeding mothers and infants with normal G6PD levelsconcentrations (CDC, 2012).

Contraindications Use in acutely-ill patients who have a tendency to develop granulocytopenia (eg, rheumatoid arthritis, SLE); concurrent use with other medications causing hemolytic anemia or myeloid bone marrow suppression; concurrent use with or recent use of quinacrine

Warnings/Precautions Use with caution in patients with G6PD deficiency (hemolytic anemia may occur), NADH methemoglobin reductase deficiency (methemoglobinemia may occur); do not exceed recommended dosage and duration. Moderate-to-severe hemolytic reactions may occur in individuals with G6PD deficiency and personal or familial history of favism. Geographic regions with a high prevalence of G6PD deficiency (eg, Africa, southern Europe, Mediterranean region, Middle East, southeast Asia, Oceania) are associated with a higher incidence of hemolytic anemia. Promptly discontinue with signs of hemolytic anemia (darkening of urine, marked fall in hemoglobin or erythrocyte count). The CDC recommends screening for G6PD deficiency prior to therapy initiation. Anemia, methemoglobinemia, and leukopenia have been associated with primaquine use; monitor during treatment. **[U.S. Boxed Warning]: Should be prescribed only by physicians familiar with its use.**

Adverse Reactions
Cardiovascular: Arrhythmias (rare)
Central nervous system: Headache
Dermatologic: Pruritus
Gastrointestinal: Abdominal cramps, dyspepsia, nausea, vomiting
Hematologic: Agranulocytosis, anemia, hemolytic anemia (in patients with G6PD deficiency), leukopenia, leukocytosis, methemoglobinemia (in NADH-methemoglobin reductase-deficient individuals)
Ocular: Interference with visual accommodation

Drug Interactions

Metabolism/Transport Effects **Substrate** of CYP2D6 (major), CYP3A4 (major); **Note:** Assignment of Major/Minor substrate status based on clinically relevant drug interaction potential; **Inhibits** CYP1A2 (strong), CYP2D6 (weak), CYP3A4 (weak); **Induces** CYP1A2 (moderate)

Avoid Concomitant Use

Avoid concomitant use of Primaquine with any of the following: Agomelatine; Artemether; DULoxetine; Lumefantrine; Mefloquine; Pimozide; Pomalidomide; Tasimelteon

Increased Effect/Toxicity

Primaquine may increase the levels/effects of: Agomelatine; Antipsychotic Agents (Phenothiazines); ARIPiprazole; Bendamustine; Beta-Blockers; Cardiac Glycosides; CloZAPine; CYP1A2 Substrates; Dapsone (Systemic); Dapsone (Topical); Dofetilide; DULoxetine; Hydrocodone; Lomitapide; Lumefantrine; Mefloquine; Pimozide; Pirfenidone; Pomalidomide; Prilocaine; Sodium Nitrite; Tasimelteon

The levels/effects of Primaquine may be increased by: Abiraterone Acetate; Artemether; Cobicistat; CYP2D6 Inhibitors (Moderate); CYP2D6 Inhibitors (Strong); Dapsone (Systemic); Darunavir; Mefloquine; Nitric Oxide; Peginterferon Alfa-2b

Decreased Effect

Primaquine may decrease the levels/effects of: Anthelmintics

The levels/effects of Primaquine may be decreased by: Bosentan; CYP3A4 Inducers (Moderate); CYP3A4 Inducers (Strong); Dabrafenib; Deferasirox; Mitotane; Peginterferon Alfa-2b; Siltuximab; St Johns Wort; Tocilizumab

Storage/Stability Store at 25°C (77°F); excursions permitted to 15°C to 30°C (59°F to 86°F). Protect from light.

Mechanism of Action Eliminates the primary tissue exoerythrocytic forms of *P. ovale* and *P. vivax*; disrupts mitochondria and binds to DNA

Pharmacodynamics/Kinetics
Absorption: Well absorbed
Metabolism: Hepatic to carboxyprimaquine (active)
Half-life elimination: 3.7-9.6 hours
Time to peak, serum: 1-2 hours
Excretion: Urine (small amounts as unchanged drug)

Dosage Oral: Dosage expressed as mg of base (15 mg base = 26.3 mg primaquine phosphate). **Note:** The CDC requires screening for G6PD deficiency prior to initiating treatment with primaquine.

Malaria:

Treatment or prevention of relapse of *P. vivax* malaria:
Adults: 30 mg once daily for 14 days

Treatment of uncomplicated *P. vivax* and *P. ovale* malaria (off-label use):
Children: 0.5 mg /kg (maximum: 30 mg/day) daily for 14 days with chloroquine or hydroxychloroquine (CDC, 2011)
Adults: 30 mg once daily for 14 days with chloroquine or hydroxychloroquine; alternative regimen (for mild G6PD deficiency or as an alternative to daily regimen): 45 mg once weekly for 8 weeks (use only after consultation with an infectious disease/tropical medicine expert) (CDC, 2011)

Chemoprophylaxis (off-label use):
Children: 0.5 mg/kg once daily (maximum dose: 30 mg/day); start 1-2 days prior to travel and continue for 7 days after departure from malaria-endemic area (CDC, 2012)
Adults: 30 mg once daily; start 1-2 days prior to travel and continue for 7 days after departure from malaria-endemic area (CDC, 2012)

Presumptive antirelapse therapy for *P. vivax* and *P. ovale* malaria (off-label use):

Children: 0.5 mg/kg (maximum dose: 30 mg/day) once daily for 14 days after departure from malaria-endemic area (CDC, 2012)

Adults: 30 mg once daily for 14 days after departure from malaria-endemic area (CDC, 2012)

***Pneumocystis jirovecii* pneumonia treatment (off-label use):** CDC recommendation (as alternative):

Children: 0.3 mg/kg once daily for 21 days (in combination with clindamycin)

Adults: 30 mg once daily for 21 days (in combination with clindamycin)

Dosage adjustment in renal impairment: No dosage adjustment provided in manufacturer's labeling.

Dosage adjustment in hepatic impairment: No dosage adjustment provided in manufacturer's labeling.

Administration Take with meals to decrease adverse GI effects. Drug has a bitter taste.

Monitoring Parameters Periodic CBC, visual color check of urine, glucose, electrolytes; if hemolysis suspected, monitor CBC, haptoglobin, peripheral smear, urinalysis dipstick for occult blood, G6PD deficiency screening (prior to initiating treatment; CDC recommendation)

Dosage Forms

Tablet, Oral:

Generic: 26.3 mg

Extemporaneous Preparations A 6 mg base/5 mL oral suspension may be made using tablets. Crush ten 15 mg base tablets and reduce to a fine powder. In small amounts, add a total of 10 mL Carboxymethylcellulose 1.5% and mix to a uniform paste; mix while adding Simple Syrup, NF to **almost** 125 mL; transfer to a calibrated bottle, rinse mortar with vehicle, and add quantity of vehicle sufficient to make 125 mL. Label "shake well" and "refrigerate". Stable 7 days.

Nahata MC, Pai VB, and Hipple TF, *Pediatric Drug Formulations*, 5th ed, Cincinnati, OH: Harvey Whitney Books Co, 2004.

- **Primaquine Phosphate** *see* Primaquine *on page 1713*
- **Primaxin I.M. [DSC]** *see* Imipenem and Cilastatin *on page 1051*
- **Primaxin® I.V.** *see* Imipenem and Cilastatin *on page 1051*
- **Primaxin I.V. Infusion (Can)** *see* Imipenem and Cilastatin *on page 1051*

Primidone (PRI mi done)

Brand Names: U.S. Mysoline

Brand Names: Canada Apo-Primidone®

Index Terms Desoxyphenobarbital; Primaclone

Pharmacologic Category Anticonvulsant, Miscellaneous; Barbiturate

Use Management of grand mal, psychomotor, and focal seizures

Pregnancy Considerations Primidone and its metabolites (PEMA, phenobarbital, and p-hydroxyphenobarbital) cross the placenta; neonatal serum concentrations at birth are similar to those in the mother. Withdrawal symptoms may occur in the neonate and may be delayed due to the long half-life of primidone and its metabolites. Use may be associated with birth defects and adverse events; the use of folic acid throughout pregnancy and vitamin K during the last month of pregnancy is recommended. Epilepsy itself, number of medications, genetic factors, or a combination of these probably influence the teratogenicity of anticonvulsant therapy.

Patients exposed to primidone during pregnancy are encouraged to enroll themselves into the NAAED Pregnancy Registry by calling 1-888-233-2334. Additional information is available at www.aedpregnancyregistry.org.

Breast-Feeding Considerations Primidone and its metabolites (PEMA, phenobarbital, and p-hydroxyphenobarbital) are found in breast milk (variable concentrations). The manufacturer recommends discontinuing breast-feeding if undue drowsiness and somnolence occur in the newborn.

Contraindications Hypersensitivity to phenobarbital; porphyria

Warnings/Precautions Antiepileptics are associated with an increased risk of suicidal behavior/thoughts with use (regardless of indication); patients should be monitored for signs/symptoms of depression, suicidal tendencies, and other unusual behavior changes during therapy and instructed to inform their healthcare provider immediately if symptoms occur.

Use with caution in patients with renal or hepatic impairment, pulmonary insufficiency; abrupt withdrawal may precipitate status epilepticus. Potential for drug dependency exists. Do not administer to patients in acute pain. Use caution in elderly, debilitated, or pediatric patients - may cause paradoxical responses. May cause CNS depression, which may impair physical or mental abilities. Patients must cautioned about performing tasks which require mental alertness (eg, operating machinery or driving). Effects with other sedative drugs or ethanol may be potentiated. Use with caution in patients with depression or suicidal tendencies, or in patients with a history of drug abuse. Tolerance or psychological and physical dependence may occur with prolonged use. Primidone's active metabolite, phenobarbital, has been associated with cognitive deficits in children receiving chronic therapy for febrile seizures. Use with caution in patients with hypoadrenalism.

Benzyl alcohol and derivatives: Some dosage forms may contain sodium benzoate/benzoic acid; benzoic acid (benzoate) is a metabolite of benzyl alcohol; large amounts of benzyl alcohol (≥99 mg/kg/day) have been associated with a potentially fatal toxicity ("gasping syndrome") in neonates; the "gasping syndrome" consists of metabolic acidosis, respiratory distress, gasping respirations, CNS dysfunction (including convulsions, intracranial hemorrhage), hypotension, and cardiovascular collapse (AAP, 1997; CDC, 1982); some data suggests that benzoate displaces bilirubin from protein binding sites (Ahlfors, 2001); avoid or use dosage forms containing benzyl alcohol derivative with caution in neonates. See manufacturer's labeling.

Adverse Reactions

Central nervous system: Ataxia, drowsiness, emotional disturbances, fatigue, hyperirritability, suicidal ideation, vertigo

Dermatologic: Morbilliform skin eruptions

Gastrointestinal: Anorexia, nausea, vomiting

Genitourinary: Impotence

Hematologic: Agranulocytosis, granulocytopenia, megaloblastic anemia (idiosyncratic), red cell aplasia/hypoplasia

Ocular: Diplopia, nystagmus

Drug Interactions

Metabolism/Transport Effects Induces CYP1A2 (strong), CYP2B6 (strong), CYP2C8 (strong), CYP2C9 (strong), CYP3A4 (strong), P-glycoprotein

Avoid Concomitant Use

Avoid concomitant use of Primidone with any of the following: Abiraterone Acetate; Apixaban; Apremilast; Artemether; Axitinib; Azelastine (Nasal); Bedaquiline; Boceprevir; Bortezomib; Bosutinib; Cabozantinib; Ceritinib; CloZAPine; Crizotinib; Dabigatran Etexilate; Dasabuvir; Dienogest; Dolutegravir; Dronedarone; Eliglustat;

Enzalutamide; Etravirine; Everolimus; Ibrutinib; Idelalisib; Irinotecan; Itraconazole; Ivacaftor; Lapatinib; Ledipasvir; Lumefantrine; Lurasidone; Macitentan; Mifepristone; Naloxegol; Netupitant; NIFEdipine; Nilotinib; Nintedanib; Nisoldipine; Olaparib; Ombitasvir; Orphenadrine; Paraldehyde; Paritaprevir; PAZOPanib; Perampanel; Pirfenidone; Pomalidomide; PONATinib; Praziquantel; Ranolazine; Regorafenib; Rilpivirine; Rivaroxaban; Roflumilast; RomiDEPsin; Simeprevir; Sofosbuvir; SORAfenib; Suvorexant; Tasimelteon; Telaprevir; Thalidomide; Ticagrelor; Tofacitinib; Tolvaptan; Toremifene; Trabectedin; Ulipristal; Vandetanib; Vemurafenib; VinCRIStine (Liposomal); Vorapaxar

Increased Effect/Toxicity

Primidone may increase the levels/effects of: Alcohol (Ethyl); Azelastine (Nasal); Barbiturates; Buprenorphine; Clarithromycin; CNS Depressants; Hydrocodone; Methotrimeprazine; Metyrosine; Orphenadrine; Paraldehyde; Pramipexole; Rotigotine; Selective Serotonin Reuptake Inhibitors; Thalidomide; Valproic Acid and Derivatives; Zolpidem

The levels/effects of Primidone may be increased by: Brimonidine (Topical); Cannabis; Carbonic Anhydrase Inhibitors; Clarithromycin; Cosyntropin; Dexmethylphenidate; Doxylamine; Dronabinol; Droperidol; Felbamate; HydrOXYzine; Kava Kava; Magnesium Sulfate; Methotrimeprazine; Methylphenidate; Nabilone; Sodium Oxybate; Tapentadol; Tetrahydrocannabinol; Valproic Acid and Derivatives

Decreased Effect

Primidone may decrease the levels/effects of: Abiraterone Acetate; Afatinib; Apixaban; Apremilast; ARIPiprazole; Artemether; Axitinib; Bazedoxifene; Bedaquiline; Bendamustine; Boceprevir; Bortezomib; Bosutinib; Brentuximab Vedotin; Cabozantinib; Canagliflozin; Cannabidiol; Cannabis; Ceritinib; Clarithromycin; CloZAPine; Contraceptives (Progestins); Corticosteroids (Systemic); Crizotinib; CYP1A2 Substrates; CYP2B6 Substrates; CYP2C8 Substrates; CYP2C9 Substrates; CYP3A4 Substrates; Dabigatran Etexilate; Dasabuvir; Dasatinib; Diclofenac (Systemic); Dienogest; Dolutegravir; DOXOrubicin (Conventional); Dronabinol; Dronedarone; Eliglustat; Enzalutamide; Erlotinib; Eslicarbazepine; Etravirine; Everolimus; Exemestane; Felbamate; FentaNYL; Gefitinib; GuanFACINE; Ibrutinib; Idelalisib; Imatinib; Irinotecan; Itraconazole; Ivacaftor; Ixabepilone; LamoTRIgine; Lapatinib; Ledipasvir; Linagliptin; Lumefantrine; Lurasidone; Macitentan; Maraviroc; Methadone; MetroNIDAZOLE (Systemic); Mifepristone; Naloxegol; Netupitant; NIFEdipine; Nilotinib; Nintedanib; Nisoldipine; Olaparib; Ombitasvir; Paritaprevir; PAZOPanib; Perampanel; P-glycoprotein/ABCB1 Substrates; Pirfenidone; Pomalidomide; PONATinib; Praziquantel; QUEtiapine; QuiNIDine; Ranolazine; Regorafenib; Rilpivirine; Rivaroxaban; Roflumilast; RomiDEPsin; Rufinamide; Saxagliptin; Simeprevir; Sofosbuvir; SORAfenib; SUNItinib; Suvorexant; Tadalafil; Tasimelteon; Telaprevir; Tetrahydrocannabinol; Ticagrelor; Tofacitinib; Tolvaptan; Toremifene; Trabectedin; Treprostinil; Ulipristal; Vandetanib; Vemurafenib; Vilazodone; VinCRIStine (Liposomal); Vorapaxar; Vortioxetine; Zuclopenthixol

The levels/effects of Primidone may be decreased by: Carbonic Anhydrase Inhibitors; Folic Acid; Fosphenytoin; Leucovorin Calcium-Levoleucovorin; Levomefolate; Mefloquine; Methylfolate; Orlistat; Phenytoin

Food Interactions Protein-deficient diets increase duration of action of primidone.

Storage/Stability Store at 20°C to 25°C (68°F to 77°F).

Mechanism of Action Decreases neuron excitability, raises seizure threshold similar to phenobarbital; primidone has two active metabolites, phenobarbital and phenylethylmalonamide (PEMA); PEMA may enhance the activity of phenobarbital

Pharmacodynamics/Kinetics

Absorption: 60% to 80%

Distribution: Adults: V_d: 0.6 L/kg

Protein binding: 30%

Metabolism: Hepatic to phenobarbital (active) by oxidation and to phenylethylmalonamide (PEMA; active) by scission of the heterocyclic ring

Half-life elimination (age dependent): Primidone: Mean: 5-15 hours (variable); PEMA: 16 hours (variable)

Time to peak, serum: ~3 hours (variable)

Excretion: Urine (40% as unchanged drug; the remainder is unconjugated PEMA, phenobarbital and its metabolites)

Dosage Oral:

Seizure disorders:

Children <8 years: Initial: Days 1-3: 50 mg/day given at bedtime; days 4-6: 50 mg twice daily; days 7-9: 100 mg twice daily; usual dose: 375-750 mg/day in 3-4 divided doses (10-25 mg/kg/day)

Children ≥8 years and Adults: Days 1-3: 100-125 mg/day at bedtime; days 4-6: 100-125 twice daily; days 7-9: 100-125 mg 3 times daily; usual dose: 750-1500 mg/day in divided doses 3-4 times/day with maximum dosage of 2 g/day

Patients already receiving other anticonvulsants: Initial: 100-125 mg at bedtime; gradually increase to maintenance dose as other drug is gradually decreased, continue until desired level obtained or other drug completely withdrawn. If goal is monotherapy, conversion should be completed over ≥2 weeks.

Essential tremor (off-label use): Adults: Initial 12.5-25 mg/day at bedtime; titrate up to 250 mg/day in 1-2 divided doses; doses up to 750 mg/day may be beneficial

Dosage adjustment in renal impairment: Adults: No dosage adjustment provided in manufacturer's labeling. However, the following guidelines have been used by some clinicians (Aronoff, 2007): **Note:** Avoid in renal failure if possible; due to active metabolites with long half-lives and complex kinetics:

CrCl ≥50 mL/minute: Administer every 12 hours

CrCl 10-50 mL/minute: Administer every 12-24 hours

CrCl <10 mL/minute: Administer every 24 hours

Hemodialysis: Administer dose postdialysis

Dosage adjustment in hepatic impairment: No dosage adjustment provided in manufacturer's labeling. However, increased side effects may occur in severe liver disease; monitor plasma levels and adjust dose accordingly.

Dietary Considerations Folic acid: Low erythrocyte and CSF folate concentrations. Megaloblastic anemia has been reported. To avoid folic acid deficiency and megaloblastic anemia, some clinicians recommend giving patients on anticonvulsants prophylactic doses of folic acid and cyanocobalamin.

Monitoring Parameters Serum primidone and phenobarbital concentration, neurological status. Due to CNS effects, monitor closely when initiating drug in elderly. Monitor CBC and sequential multiple analysis-12 (SMA-12) at 6-month intervals to compare with baseline obtained at start of therapy. Monitor for suicidality (eg, suicidal thoughts, depression, behavioral changes). Since elderly metabolize phenobarbital at a slower rate than younger adults, it is suggested to measure both primidone and phenobarbital levels together.

Reference Range Therapeutic: Children <5 years: 7-10 mcg/mL (SI: 32-46 micromole/L); Adults: 5-12 mcg/mL (SI: 23-55 micromole/L); toxic effects rarely present with levels <10 mcg/mL (SI: 46 micromole/L) if phenobarbital concentrations are low. Dosage of primidone is adjusted with reference mostly to the phenobarbital level; Toxic: >15 mcg/mL (SI: >69 micromole/L)

Dosage Forms

Tablet, Oral:

Mysoline: 50 mg, 250 mg

Generic: 50 mg, 250 mg

Dosage Forms: Canada

Tablet:

Apo-Primidone®: 125 mg, 250 mg

◆ **Primlev** *see* Oxycodone and Acetaminophen *on page 1541*

◆ **Primsol** *see* Trimethoprim *on page 2104*

◆ **Prinivil** *see* Lisinopril *on page 1226*

◆ **Prinzide** *see* Lisinopril and Hydrochlorothiazide *on page 1229*

◆ **Priorix (Can)** *see* Measles, Mumps, and Rubella Virus Vaccine *on page 1273*

◆ **Priorix-Tetra (Can)** *see* Measles, Mumps, Rubella, and Varicella Virus Vaccine *on page 1274*

◆ **PrismaSol** *see* Electrolyte Solution, Renal Replacement *on page 710*

◆ **Pristiq** *see* Desvenlafaxine *on page 598*

◆ **Priva-Escitalopram (Can)** *see* Escitalopram *on page 765*

◆ **Priva-Ezetimibe (Can)** *see* Ezetimibe *on page 832*

◆ **Priva-Tramadol/Acet (Can)** *see* Acetaminophen and Tramadol *on page 37*

◆ **Privigen** *see* Immune Globulin *on page 1056*

◆ **Privine® [OTC]** *see* Naphazoline (Nasal) *on page 1426*

◆ **Pro-AAS EC-80 (Can)** *see* Aspirin *on page 180*

◆ **ProAir HFA** *see* Albuterol *on page 69*

◆ **ProAmatine** *see* Midodrine *on page 1365*

◆ **PRO-Amiodarone (Can)** *see* Amiodarone *on page 114*

◆ **Pro-Amox-250 (Can)** *see* Amoxicillin *on page 130*

◆ **Pro-Amox-500 (Can)** *see* Amoxicillin *on page 130*

◆ **PRO-Azithromycine (Can)** *see* Azithromycin (Systemic) *on page 216*

Probenecid (proe BEN e sid)

Brand Names: Canada Benuryl

Index Terms Benemid [DSC]

Pharmacologic Category Uricosuric Agent

Use Treatment of hyperuricemia associated with gout or gouty arthritis; prolongation and elevation of beta-lactam plasma levels (eg, uncomplicated gonococcal infection)

Dosage Oral:

Children:

<2 years: Contraindicated

2-14 years: Prolong penicillin serum levels: Initial: 25 mg/kg, then 40 mg/kg/day in 4 divided doses (maximum: 500 mg/dose)

Gonorrhea: >50 kg: Refer to adult dosing.

Adults:

Hyperuricemia with gout: 250 mg twice daily for 1 week; may increase to 500 mg twice daily; if needed, may increase to a maximum of 2 g/day (increase dosage in 500 mg increments every 4 weeks). If serum uric acid levels are within normal limits and gout attacks have been absent for 6 months, daily dosage may be reduced by 500 mg every 6 months.

Prolong penicillin serum levels: 500 mg 4 times/day. **Note:** Dosing per manufacturer, see indication-specific dosing.

Gonorrhea, uncomplicated infections of cervix, urethra, and rectum: Oral: 1 g once with cefoxitin 2 g IM (CDC, 2010)

Pelvic inflammatory disease (off-label use): Oral: 1 g once with cefoxitin 2 g IM plus doxycycline (CDC, 2010)

Neurosyphilis (off-label use): Oral: 500 mg 4 times/day with procaine penicillin 2.4 million units/day IM for 10-14 days (CDC, 2010). **Note:** Penicillin G aqueous IV is the preferred agent.

Dosing adjustment in renal impairment: CrCl <30 mL/minute: Avoid use.

Dosing adjustment in hepatic impairment: No dosage adjustment provided in manufacturer's labeling.

Additional Information Complete prescribing information should be consulted for additional detail.

Dosage Forms

Tablet, Oral:

Generic: 500 mg

◆ **Probenecid and Colchicine** *see* Colchicine and Probenecid *on page 503*

◆ **PRO-Bicalutamide (Can)** *see* Bicalutamide *on page 262*

◆ **PRO-Bisoprolol (Can)** *see* Bisoprolol *on page 266*

Procainamide (pro KANE a mide)

Brand Names: Canada Apo-Procainamide; Procainamide Hydrochloride Injection, USP; Procan SR

Index Terms PCA (error-prone abbreviation); Procainamide Hydrochloride; Procaine Amide Hydrochloride; Procanbid; Pronestyl

Pharmacologic Category Antiarrhythmic Agent, Class Ia

Additional Appendix Information

Beers Criteria – Potentially Inappropriate Medications for Geriatrics *on page 2271*

Use

Intravenous: Treatment of life-threatening ventricular arrhythmias

Oral [Canadian product]: Treatment of supraventricular arrhythmias. **Note:** In the treatment of atrial fibrillation, use only when preferred treatment is ineffective or cannot be used. Use in paroxysmal atrial tachycardia when reflex stimulation or other measures are ineffective.

Pregnancy Risk Factor C

Dosage Must be titrated to patient's response

Children:

IM: 20 to 30 mg/kg/day divided every 4 to 6 hours; maximum: 4 g/day

IV:

Load: 3 to 6 mg/kg/dose over 5 minutes not to exceed 100 mg/dose; may repeat every 5 to 10 minutes to maximum of 15 mg/kg/load

Maintenance as continuous IV infusion: 20 to 80 mcg/kg/minute; maximum: 2 g/24 hours

Possible VT (PALS, 2010): IV; I.O.: 15 mg/kg over 30 to 60 minutes

Adults:

IM: 50 mg/kg/day divided every 3 to 6 hours **or** 0.5 to 1 g every 4 to 8 hours (Koch-Weser, 1971)

IV:

Loading dose: 15 to 18 mg/kg administered as slow infusion over 25 to 30 minutes **or** 100 mg/dose at a rate not to exceed 50 mg/minute repeated every 5 minutes as needed to a total dose of 1 g.

Hemodynamically stable monomorphic VT or pre-excited atrial fibrillation (ACLS, 2010): Loading dose: Infuse 20 to 50 mg/minute **or** 100 mg every 5 minutes until arrhythmia controlled, hypotension occurs, QRS complex widens by 50% of its original width, or total of 17 mg/kg is given. Follow with a continuous infusion of 1 to 4 mg/minute. **Note:** Not recommended for use in ongoing ventricular fibrillation (VF) or pulseless ventricular tachycardia (VT) due to prolonged administration time and uncertain efficacy.

Maintenance dose: 1 to 4 mg/minute by continuous infusion. Maintenance infusions should be reduced by one-third in patients with moderate renal or cardiac impairment and by two-thirds in patients with severe renal or cardiac impairment.

Oral [Canadian product]: Sustained release formulation (Procan SR®): Maintenance: 50 mg/kg/24 hours given in divided doses every 6 hours

Suggested Procan SR® maintenance dose:
- <55 kg: 500 mg every 6 hours
- 55 to 91 kg: 750 mg every 6 hours
- >91 kg: 1000 mg every 6 hours

Elderly: Initiate doses at lower end of dosage range.

Dosage adjustment in renal impairment:

Oral [Canadian product]:

Manufacturer's labeling: Manufacturer recommends increasing dosing interval; specific interval increase not described

Alternate dosing:
- CrCl >50 mL/minute: No dosage adjustment necessary (Bauer, 2008)
- CrCl 10 to 50 mL/minute: Reduce initial daily dose by 25% to 50% (Bauer, 2008)
- CrCl <10 mL/minute: Reduce initial daily dose by 50% to 75% (Bauer, 2008)

IV:

Manufacturer's labeling: Manufacturer recommends dosage reduction; specific dosage reduction not described; however, close monitoring of procainamide and NAPA concentrations and clinical effectiveness recommended.

Alternate dosing:
- CrCl >50 mL/minute: No dosage adjustment necessary (Bauer, 2008)
- CrCl 10–50 mL/minute: Reduce continuous infusion dose by 25% to 50% (Bauer, 2008)
- CrCl <10 mL/minute: Reduce continuous infusion dose by 50% to 75% (Bauer, 2008). Monitor procainamide/NAPA concentrations closely

Dialysis:

Procainamide: Moderately hemodialyzable (20% to 50%); NAPA: Not dialyzable (0% to 5%): Monitor procainamide/N-acetylprocainamide (NAPA) concentrations; supplementation may be necessary (Aronoff, 2007)

Procainamide/NAPA: Not peritoneal dialyzable (0% to 5%) (Aronoff, 2007)

Continuous renal replacement therapy (CRRT): In patients with chronic kidney disease receiving CRRT, reduce maintenance dose by 50%. In patients with anuria receiving CRRT, further dosage reduction may be required; use of an initial 1 mg/minute continuous infusion dose has been suggested. Monitor procainamide/NAPA concentrations closely (Mohamed, 2013).

Dosing adjustment in hepatic impairment:

Manufacturer's labeling: Manufacturer recommends reduction in frequency of administration; specific frequency reduction not described; however, close monitoring of procainamide and NAPA concentrations and clinical effectiveness recommended.

Alternate dosing (Bauer, 2008):

Oral [Canadian product]:
- Child-Pugh score 8-10: Reduce initial daily dose by 25%. Monitor procainamide/NAPA concentrations closely.
- Child-Pugh score >10: Reduce initial daily dose by 50%. Monitor procainamide/NAPA concentrations closely.

IV:
- Child-Pugh score 8-10: Reduce continuous infusion dose by 25%. Monitor procainamide/NAPA concentrations closely.
- Child-Pugh score >10: Reduce continuous infusion dose by 50%. Monitor procainamide/NAPA concentrations closely.

Additional Information Complete prescribing information should be consulted for additional detail.

Dosage Forms

Solution, Injection:

Generic: 100 mg/mL (10 mL); 500 mg/mL (2 mL)

Dosage Forms: Canada

Tablet, sustained release, oral:

Procan SR®: 250 mg, 500 mg, 750 mg

- ◆ **Procainamide Hydrochloride** *see* Procainamide *on page 1716*
- ◆ **Procainamide Hydrochloride Injection, USP (Can)** *see* Procainamide *on page 1716*
- ◆ **Procaine Amide Hydrochloride** *see* Procainamide *on page 1716*
- ◆ **Procaine Benzylpenicillin** *see* Penicillin G Procaine *on page 1613*
- ◆ **Procaine Penicillin G** *see* Penicillin G Procaine *on page 1613*
- ◆ **Procanbid** *see* Procainamide *on page 1716*
- ◆ **Procan SR (Can)** *see* Procainamide *on page 1716*

Procarbazine (proe KAR ba zeen)

Brand Names: U.S. Matulane

Brand Names: Canada Matulane; Natulan

Index Terms Benzmethyzin; Ibenzmethyzin; N-Methylhydrazine; PCB; PCZ; Procarbazine Hydrochloride

Pharmacologic Category Antineoplastic Agent, Alkylating Agent

Use Treatment of Hodgkin lymphoma

Pregnancy Risk Factor D

Dosage Note: Procarbazine is associated with a high emetic potential; antiemetics are recommended to prevent nausea and vomiting (Dupuis, 2011; Roila, 2010). The manufacturer suggests that an estimated lean body mass be used in obese patients and patients with rapid weight gain due to edema, ascites, or abnormal fluid retention.

Hodgkin lymphoma:

Children and Adults: MOPP regimen: While procarbazine is approved as part of the MOPP regimen, the MOPP regimen is generally no longer used due to improved toxicity profiles with other combination regimens used in the treatment of Hodgkin lymphoma.

Children: BEACOPP regimen (off-label dosing): Oral: 100 mg/m^2 days 0 to 6 of a 21-day treatment cycle (in combination with bleomycin, etoposide, doxorubicin, cyclophosphamide, vincristine, and prednisone) for 4 cycles (Kelley, 2011).

Adults: BEACOPP, standard or escalated regimen (off-label dosing): Oral: 100 mg/m^2 days 1 to 7 every 21 days (in combination with bleomycin, etoposide, doxorubicin, cyclophosphamide, vincristine, and prednisone) for 8 cycles (Diehl, 2003)

Non-Hodgkin lymphomas (NHL; off-label use): Adults:
CEPP regimen: Oral: 60 mg/m^2 days 1 to 10 every 28 days (in combination with cyclophosphamide, etoposide and prednisone) (Chao, 1990)
PEP-C regimen: Oral: 50 mg daily at bedtime (length of induction cycle depends on phase of treatment and blood counts; frequency may vary based on tolerance in maintenance cycle; in combination with prednisone, etoposide, and cyclophosphamide) (Coleman, 2008)
CNS tumors, anaplastic oligodendroglioma/oligoastrocytoma (off-label use): Adults: PCV regimen: Oral: 60 mg/m^2 days 8 to 21 every 6 weeks (in combination with lomustine and vincristine) for 6 cycles (van den Bent, 2006) **or** 75 mg/m^2 days 8 to 21 every 6 weeks (in combination with lomustine and vincristine) for up to 4 cycles (Cairncross, 2006).
Primary CNS lymphoma (off-label use): Adults: Oral: 100 mg/m^2 for 7 days in cycles 1, 3, and 5 (in combination with methotrexate [high-dose], vincristine, methotrexate [intrathecal], leucovorin, dexamethasone, cytarabine [high-dose], and whole brain radiation) (DeAngelis, 2002).

Dosage adjustment for toxicity: Withhold treatment (promptly) for any of the following: CNS toxicity (eg, paresthesia, confusion, neuropathy), hematologic toxicity (WBC <4000/mm^3 or platelets <100,000/mm^3), hypersensitivity, gastrointestinal toxicities (stomatisis, diarrhea), and hemorrhage or bleeding.

Dosage adjustment in renal impairment: No dosage adjustment provided in manufacturer's labeling; use with caution; may result in increased toxicity. However, because predominantly inactive metabolites are excreted via the kidneys, dosage adjustment is not necessary (Kintzel, 1995).

Dosage adjustment in hepatic impairment: No dosage adjustment provided in manufacturer's labeling; use with caution; may result in increased toxicity. The following adjustments have been reported in literature:
Floyd, 2006:
Transaminases 1.6 to 6 times ULN: Administer 75% of dose
Transaminases >6 times ULN: Use clinical judgment
Serum bilirubin >5 mg/dL or transaminases >3 times ULN: Avoid use
King, 2001: Serum bilirubin >5 mg/dL or transaminases >180 units/L: Avoid use

Dosing in obesity: *ASCO Guidelines for appropriate chemotherapy dosing in obese adults with cancer:* Utilize patient's actual body weight (full weight) for calculation of body surface area- or weight-based dosing, particularly when the intent of therapy is curative; manage regimen-related toxicities in the same manner as for nonobese patients; if a dose reduction is utilized due to toxicity, consider resumption of full weight-based dosing with subsequent cycles, especially if cause of toxicity (eg, hepatic or renal impairment) is resolved (Griggs, 2012). **Note:** The manufacturer suggests that an estimated lean body mass be used in obese patients and patients with rapid weight gain due to edema, ascites, or abnormal fluid retention.

Additional Information Complete prescribing information should be consulted for additional detail.

Dosage Forms
Capsule, Oral:
Matulane: 50 mg

◆ **Procarbazine Hydrochloride** *see* Procarbazine *on page 1717*
◆ **Procardia** *see* NIFEdipine *on page 1451*
◆ **Procardia XL** *see* NIFEdipine *on page 1451*
◆ **PRO-Cefadroxil (Can)** *see* Cefadroxil *on page 372*
◆ **PRO-Cefuroxime (Can)** *see* Cefuroxime *on page 399*
◆ **ProCentra** *see* Dextroamphetamine *on page 607*
◆ **Procetofene** *see* Fenofibrate and Derivatives *on page 852*

Prochlorperazine (proe klor PER a zeen)

Brand Names: U.S. Compazine; Compro
Brand Names: Canada Apo-Prochlorperazine; Nu-Prochlor; PMS-Prochlorperazine; Sandoz-Prochlorperazine
Index Terms Chlormeprazine; Prochlorperazine Edisylate; Prochlorperazine Maleate; Prochlorperazine Mesylate
Pharmacologic Category Antiemetic; First Generation (Typical) Antipsychotic
Additional Appendix Information
Beers Criteria – Potentially Inappropriate Medications for Geriatrics *on page 2271*

Use Management of nausea and vomiting; psychotic disorders, including schizophrenia and anxiety (**Note:** Not a recommended therapy by schizophrenia treatment guidelines [Lehman, 2004; Hasan, 2012]); nonpsychotic anxiety

Pregnancy Considerations Jaundice or hyper-/hyporeflexia have been reported in newborn infants following maternal use of phenothiazines. Antipsychotic use during the third trimester of pregnancy has a risk for abnormal muscle movements (extrapyramidal symptoms [EPS]) and withdrawal symptoms in newborns following delivery. Symptoms in the newborn may include agitation, feeding disorder, hypertonia, hypotonia, respiratory distress, somnolence, and tremor; these effects may be self-limiting or require hospitalization. Use may interfere with pregnancy tests, causing false positive results. Prochlorperazine has been used for the treatment of nausea and vomiting associated with pregnancy (Levicheck, 2002; Mahadevan, 2006); however, other agents may be preferred (ACOG, 2004).

Breast-Feeding Considerations Other phenothiazines are excreted in human milk; excretion of prochlorperazine is not known.

Contraindications Hypersensitivity to prochlorperazine or any component of the formulation (cross-reactivity between phenothiazines may occur); coma or presence of large amounts of CNS depressants (eg, alcohol, opioids, barbiturates); postoperative management of nausea/vomiting following pediatric surgery; use in infants and children <2 years or <9 kg; pediatric conditions for which dosing not described

Canadian labeling: Additional contraindications (not in U.S. labeling): Presence of circulatory collapse; severe cardiovascular disorders; altered state of consciousness; concomitant use of high dose hypnotics; severe depression; presence of blood dyscrasias, hepatic or renal impairment, or pheochromocytoma; suspected or established subcortical brain damage with or without hypothalamic damage

Warnings/Precautions [U.S. Boxed Warning]: Elderly patients with dementia-related psychosis treated with antipsychotics are at an increased risk of death compared to placebo. Most deaths appeared to be either cardiovascular (eg, heart failure, sudden death) or infectious (eg, pneumonia) in nature. Prochlorperazine is not approved for the treatment of dementia-related psychosis. May cause extrapyramidal symptoms (EPS), including pseudoparkinsonism, acute dystonic reactions, akathisia, and tardive dyskinesia. Risk of dystonia (and possibly other EPS) may be greater with increased doses, use of conventional antipsychotics, males, and younger patients. Risk of tardive dyskinesia and potential for irreversibility often associated with total cumulative dose and therapy duration and may also be increased in elderly patients (particularly elderly women); antipsychotics may also mask signs/symptoms of tardive dyskinesia. Consider therapy discontinuation with signs/symptoms of tardive dyskinesia. Antipsychotic use has been associated with esophageal dysmotility and aspiration; use with caution in patients at risk of pneumonia (ie, Alzheimer's disease).

May be sedating and impair physical or mental abilities; use with caution in disorders where CNS depression is a feature. Effects with other sedative drugs or ethanol may be potentiated. Use with caution in Parkinson's disease; hemodynamic instability; predisposition to seizures; subcortical brain damage; and in severe cardiac, hepatic, or renal disease. Canadian labeling contraindicates use in patients with severe cardiac disease, hepatic or renal impairment, subcortical brain damage, and circulatory collapse. May alter temperature regulation, obscure intestinal obstruction or brain tumor or mask toxicity of other drugs. May alter cardiac conduction. Hypotension may occur following administration, particularly when parenteral form is used or in high dosages. May cause orthostatic hypotension; use with caution in patients at risk of this effect or in those who would not tolerate transient hypotensive episodes (cerebrovascular disease, cardiovascular disease, hypovolemia, or concurrent medication use which may predispose to hypotension/bradycardia).

Leukopenia, neutropenia, and agranulocytosis (sometimes fatal) have been reported in clinical trials and postmarketing reports with antipsychotic use; presence of risk factors (eg, preexisting low WBC or history of drug-induced leuko-/neutropenia) should prompt periodic blood count assessment. Discontinue therapy at first signs of blood dyscrasias or if absolute neutrophil count <1000/mm^3.

Due to its potent anticholinergic effects, may be inappropriate in older adults depending on comorbidities (eg, dementia, delirium) (Beers Criteria). Use with caution in patients with decreased gastrointestinal motility, urinary retention, BPH, xerostomia, visual problems, or narrow-angle glaucoma (screening is recommended). Use caution with exposure to heat. May cause pigmentary retinopathy, and lenticular and corneal deposits, particularly with prolonged therapy. Use associated with increased prolactin levels; clinical significance of hyperprolactinemia in patients with breast cancer or other prolactin-dependent tumors is unknown. Avoid use in patients with signs/symptoms suggestive of Reye's syndrome. Children with acute illness or dehydration are more susceptible to neuromuscular reactions; use cautiously. May be associated with neuroleptic malignant syndrome (NMS). Some dosage forms may contain sodium sulfite.

Benzyl alcohol and derivatives: Some dosage forms may contain benzyl alcohol; large amounts of benzyl alcohol (≥99 mg/kg/day) have been associated with a potentially fatal toxicity ("gasping syndrome") in neonates; the "gasping syndrome" consists of metabolic acidosis, respiratory distress, gasping respirations, CNS dysfunction (including convulsions, intracranial hemorrhage), hypotension, and cardiovascular collapse (AAP, 1997; CDC, 1982); some data suggests that benzoate displaces bilirubin from protein binding sites (Ahlfors, 2001); avoid or use dosage forms containing benzyl alcohol with caution in neonates. See manufacturer's labeling.

Adverse Reactions Reported with prochlorperazine or other phenothiazines.

Cardiovascular: Cardiac arrest, cerebral edema, hypotension, peripheral edema, Q-wave distortions, sudden death, T-wave distortions

Central nervous system: Agitation, altered cerebrospinal fluid proteins, catatonia, coma, cough reflex suppressed, dizziness, drowsiness, fever (mild [IM]), headache, hyperpyrexia, impairment of temperature regulation, insomnia, neuroleptic malignant syndrome (NMS), oculogyric crisis, opisthotonos, restlessness, seizure, somnolence, tremulousness

Dermatologic: Angioedema, contact dermatitis, epithelial keratopathy, erythema, eczema, exfoliative dermatitis, itching, photosensitivity, skin pigmentation, urticaria

Endocrine & metabolic: Amenorrhea, galactorrhea, gynecomastia, glucosuria, hyper-/hypoglycemia, lactation, libido (changes in), menstrual irregularity

Gastrointestinal: Appetite increased, atonic colon, constipation, ileus, nausea, obstipation, vomiting, weight gain, xerostomia

Genitourinary: Ejaculating dysfunction, ejaculatory disturbances, impotence, priapism, urinary retention

Hematologic: Agranulocytosis, aplastic anemia, eosinophilia, hemolytic anemia, leukopenia, pancytopenia, thrombocytopenic purpura

Hepatic: Biliary stasis, cholestatic jaundice, hepatotoxicity

Neuromuscular & skeletal: Dystonias (torticollis, carpopedal spasm, trismus, protrusion of tongue); extrapyramidal symptoms (pseudoparkinsonism, akathisia, dystonias, tardive dyskinesia, hyperreflexia); SLE-like syndrome, tremor

Ocular: Blurred vision, lenticular/corneal deposits, miosis, mydriasis, pigmentary retinopathy

Respiratory: Asthma, laryngeal edema, nasal congestion

Miscellaneous: Allergic reactions, asphyxia, diaphoresis

Drug Interactions

Metabolism/Transport Effects None known.

Avoid Concomitant Use

Avoid concomitant use of Prochlorperazine with any of the following: Aclidinium; Amisulpride; Azelastine (Nasal); Dofetilide; Glucagon; Ipratropium (Oral Inhalation); Metoclopramide; Orphenadrine; Paraldehyde; Potassium Chloride; Sulpiride; Thalidomide; Tiotropium; Umeclidinium

Increased Effect/Toxicity

Prochlorperazine may increase the levels/effects of: AbobotulinumtoxinA; Alcohol (Ethyl); Amisulpride; Analgesics (Opioid); Anticholinergic Agents; Antidepressants (Serotonin Reuptake Inhibitor/Antagonist); Azelastine (Nasal); Beta-Blockers; Buprenorphine; CNS Depressants; Dofetilide; Glucagon; Hydrocodone; Methotrimeprazine; Methylphenidate; Metyrosine; Mirabegron; Mirtazapine; OnabotulinumtoxinA; Orphenadrine; Paraldehyde; Porfimer; Potassium Chloride; RimabotulinumtoxinB; Selective Serotonin Reuptake Inhibitors; Serotonin Modulators; Sulpiride; Suvorexant; Thalidomide; Thiazide Diuretics; Thiopental; Tiotropium; Topiramate; Verteporfin; Zolpidem

The levels/effects of Prochlorperazine may be increased by: Acetylcholinesterase Inhibitors (Central); Aclidinium; Antidepressants (Serotonin Reuptake Inhibitor/Antagonist); Antimalarial Agents; Beta-Blockers; Brimonidine (Topical); Cannabis; Deferoxamine; Doxylamine; Dronabinol; Droperidol; HydrOXYzine; Ipratropium (Oral Inhalation); Kava Kava; Lithium; Magnesium Sulfate; Methotrimeprazine; Methylphenidate; Metoclopramide; Metyrosine; Mianserin; Nabilone; Perampanel; Pramlintide; Rufinamide; Serotonin Modulators; Sodium Oxybate; Tapentadol; Tetrabenazine; Tetrahydrocannabinol; Umeclidinium

Decreased Effect

Prochlorperazine may decrease the levels/effects of: Acetylcholinesterase Inhibitors; Amphetamines; Anti-Parkinson's Agents (Dopamine Agonist); Itopride; Quinagolide; Secretin

The levels/effects of Prochlorperazine may be decreased by: Acetylcholinesterase Inhibitors; Antacids; Anti-Parkinson's Agents (Dopamine Agonist); Lithium

Storage/Stability

Injection:

Edisylate: Store at 20°C to 25°C (68°F to 77°F); do not freeze. Protect from light. Clear or slightly yellow solutions may be used.

Mesylate (Canadian availability; not available in U.S.): Store at 15°C to 30°C (59°F to 86°F). Protect from light. Do not use if solution is discolored or hazy.

IV infusion: Injection may be diluted in 50-100 mL NS or D_5W.

Suppository: Store at 20°C to 25°C (68°F to 77°F). Protect from light.

Tablet: Store at 20°C to 25°C (68°F to 77°F). Protect from light.

Mechanism of Action Prochlorperazine is a piperazine phenothiazine antipsychotic which blocks postsynaptic mesolimbic dopaminergic D_1 and D_2 receptors in the brain, including the chemoreceptor trigger zone; exhibits a strong alpha-adrenergic and anticholinergic blocking effect and depresses the release of hypothalamic and hypophyseal hormones; believed to depress the reticular activating system, thus affecting basal metabolism, body temperature, wakefulness, vasomotor tone and emesis

Pharmacodynamics/Kinetics

Onset of action: Oral: 30-40 minutes; IM: 10-20 minutes; Rectal: ~60 minutes

Peak antiemetic effect: IV: 30-60 minutes

Duration: Rectal: 3-12 hours; IM, Oral: 3-4 hours

Distribution: V_d: 1400-1548 L (Taylor, 1987)

Metabolism: Primarily hepatic; N-desmethyl prochlorperazine (major active metabolite)

Bioavailability: Oral: 12.5% (Isah, 1991)

Half-life elimination: Oral: 6-10 hours (single dose), 14-22 hours (repeated dosing) (Isah, 1991); IV: 6-10 hours (Isah, 1991; Taylor, 1987)

Excretion: Mainly in feces

Dosage Note: Injection solution mesylate formulation has Canadian availability (not available in U.S.).

Antiemetic: Children (therapy >1 day usually not required): **Note:** Use is contraindicated in children <9 kg or <2 years:

Oral, rectal:

9-13 kg: 2.5 mg 1-2 times/day as needed (maximum: 7.5 mg/day)

>13-18 kg: 2.5 mg 2-3 times/day as needed (maximum: 10 mg/day)

>18-39 kg: 2.5 mg 3 times/day or 5 mg 2 times/day as needed (maximum: 15 mg/day)

IM (as edisylate): 0.13 mg/kg/dose; convert to oral therapy as soon as possible\

IM (as mesylate): 0.14 mg/kg/dose; convert to oral therapy at equivalent or greater dose (if necessary) as soon as possible

Antiemetic: Adults:

Oral (tablet): 5-10 mg 3-4 times/day; usual maximum: 40 mg/day; larger doses may rarely be required

IM (as edisylate): 5-10 mg every 3-4 hours; usual maximum: 40 mg/day

IM (as mesylate): 5-10 mg 2-3 times/day; usual maximum: 40 mg/day

IV (as edisylate): 2.5-10 mg; maximum: 10 mg/dose or 40 mg/day; may repeat dose every 3-4 hours as needed

Rectal:

U.S. labeling: 25 mg twice daily

Canadian labeling: 5-10 mg 3-4 times/day

Surgical nausea/vomiting: Adults: **Note:** Should not exceed 40 mg/day

IM (as edisylate): 5-10 mg 1-2 hours before anesthesia induction or to control symptoms during or after surgery; may repeat once if necessary

IM (as mesylate): 5-10 mg 1-2 hours before anesthesia induction; may repeat once if needed during surgery; postoperatively: 5-10 mg every 3-4 hours as needed up to maximum of 40 mg daily

IV (as edisylate): 5-10 mg 15-30 minutes before anesthesia induction or to control symptoms during or after surgery; may repeat once if necessary

IV (as mesylate): 20 mg/L of IV solution during surgery or postoperatively; usual maximum: 30 mg daily

Rectal (off-label use; Golembiewski, 2005): 25 mg

Antipsychotic:

Children 2-12 years (contraindicated in children <9 kg or <2 years):

Oral, rectal: 2.5 mg 2-3 times/day; do not give more than 10 mg the first day; increase dosage as needed to maximum daily dose of 20 mg for 2-5 years and 25 mg for 6-12 years

IM (as edisylate): 0.13 mg/kg/dose; convert to oral therapy as soon as possible

IM (as mesylate): 0.14 mg/kg/dose; convert to oral therapy at equivalent or greater dose (if necessary) as soon as possible

Adults:

Oral: 5-10 mg 3-4 times/day; titrate dose slowly every 2-3 days; doses up to 150 mg/day may be required in some patients for treatment of severe disturbances

IM (as edisylate): Initial: 10-20 mg; if necessary repeat initial dose every 2-4 hours to gain control; more than 3-4 doses are rarely needed. If parenteral administration is still required; give 10-20 mg every 4-6 hours; convert to oral therapy as soon as possible

IM (as mesylate): Initial: 10-20 mg; if necessary repeat initial dose every 2-4 hours to gain control; more than 3-4 doses are rarely needed; convert to oral therapy as soon as possible

Nonpsychotic anxiety: Oral (tablet): Adults: Usual dose: 5 mg 3-4 times/day; do not exceed 20 mg/day or administer >12 weeks

Elderly: Initiate at lower end of dosage range; titrate slowly and cautiously. Refer to adult dosing.

Dosage adjustment in renal impairment:

U.S. labeling: No dosage adjustment provided in manufacturer's labeling.

Canadian labeling: Use is contraindicated.

Dosage adjustment in hepatic impairment:

U.S. labeling: No dosage adjustment provided in manufacturer's labeling; systemic exposure may be increased as drug undergoes hepatic metabolism.

Canadian labeling: Use is contraindicated.

Dietary Considerations Increase dietary intake of riboflavin; should be administered with food or water. Rectal suppositories may contain coconut and palm oil.

Administration

IM: Inject by deep IM into outer quadrant of buttocks.

IV: May be administered by slow IV push at a rate not exceeding 5 mg/minute or by IV infusion. Do not administer as a bolus injection. To reduce the risk of hypotension, patients receiving IV prochlorperazine must remain lying down and be observed for at least 30 minutes following administration. Avoid skin contact with injection solution, contact dermatitis has occurred. Do not dilute with any diluent containing parabens as a preservative.

Oral: Administer tablet without regard to meals.

Monitoring Parameters Mental status; vital signs (as clinically indicated); weight, height, BMI, waist circumference (baseline; at every visit for the first 6 months; quarterly with stable antipsychotic dose); CBC (as clinically indicated; monitor frequently during the first few months of therapy in patients with preexisting low WBC or history of drug-induced leukopenia/neutropenia); electrolytes and liver function (annually and as clinically indicated); fasting plasma glucose level/HbA_{1c} (baseline, then yearly; in patients with diabetes risk factors or if gaining weight repeat 4 months after starting antipsychotic, then yearly); lipid panel (baseline; repeat every 2 years if LDL level is normal; repeat every 6 months if LDL level is >130 mg/dL); changes in menstruation, libido, development of galactorrhea, erectile and ejaculatory function (at each visit for the first 12 weeks after the antipsychotic is initiated or until the dose is stable, then yearly); abnormal involuntary movements or parkinsonian signs (baseline; repeat weekly until dose stabilized for at least 2 weeks after introduction and for 2 weeks after any significant dose increase); tardive dyskinesia (every 6 months; high-risk patients every 3 months); visual changes (inquire yearly); ocular examination (yearly in patients >40 years; every 2 years in younger patients) (ADA, 2004; Lehman, 2004; Marder, 2004).

Additional Information Not recommended as an antipsychotic due to inferior efficacy compared to other phenothiazines.

Dosage Forms

Solution, Injection:
Generic: 5 mg/mL (2 mL, 10 mL)

Suppository, Rectal:
Compazine: 25 mg (12 ea)
Compro: 25 mg (12 ea)
Generic: 25 mg (12 ea, 1000 ea)

Tablet, Oral:
Compazine: 5 mg, 10 mg
Generic: 5 mg, 10 mg

Dosage Forms: Canada

Injection, solution 5 mg/mL (2 mL)
Suppository, rectal: 10 mg (10s)

- ◆ **Prochlorperazine Edisylate** *see* Prochlorperazine *on page 1718*
- ◆ **Prochlorperazine Maleate** *see* Prochlorperazine *on page 1718*
- ◆ **Prochlorperazine Mesylate** *see* Prochlorperazine *on page 1718*
- ◆ **PRO-Ciprofloxacin (Can)** *see* Ciprofloxacin (Systemic) *on page 441*
- ◆ **PRO-Clonazepam (Can)** *see* ClonazePAM *on page 478*
- ◆ **ProCort®** *see* Pramoxine and Hydrocortisone *on page 1698*
- ◆ **Procrit** *see* Epoetin Alfa *on page 742*
- ◆ **Proctocort** *see* Hydrocortisone (Topical) *on page 1014*
- ◆ **Proctofene** *see* Fenofibrate and Derivatives *on page 852*
- ◆ **ProctoFoam® HC** *see* Pramoxine and Hydrocortisone *on page 1698*
- ◆ **Proctofoam™-HC (Can)** *see* Pramoxine and Hydrocortisone *on page 1698*
- ◆ **Procto-Pak** *see* Hydrocortisone (Topical) *on page 1014*
- ◆ **Proctosol HC** *see* Hydrocortisone (Topical) *on page 1014*
- ◆ **Proctozone-HC** *see* Hydrocortisone (Topical) *on page 1014*

Procyclidine [CAN/INT] (proe SYE kli deen)

Brand Names: Canada PHL-Procyclidine; PMS-Procyclidine

Index Terms Procyclidine Hydrochloride

Pharmacologic Category Anti-Parkinson's Agent, Anticholinergic; Anticholinergic Agent

Use Note: Not approved in U.S.
Relieves symptoms of parkinsonian syndrome and drug-induced extrapyramidal symptoms

Pregnancy Considerations Safe use during pregnancy has not been established. Potential benefits of therapy should be weighed against potential risks to fetus.

Contraindications Angle-closure glaucoma; myasthenia gravis

Warnings/Precautions Use with caution in hot weather or during exercise. Elderly patients frequently develop increased sensitivity and require strict dosage regulation - side effects may be more severe in elderly patients with atherosclerotic changes. Use with caution in patients with tachycardia, cardiac arrhythmias, hypertension, hypotension, prostatic hyperplasia (especially in the elderly) or any tendency toward urinary retention, liver or kidney disorders and obstructive disease of the GI or GU tract. When given in large doses or to susceptible patients, may cause weakness and inability to move particular muscle groups. May be associated with confusion or hallucinations (generally at higher dosages); intensification of symptoms or toxic psychosis may occur in patients with mental disorders. May cause CNS depression, which may impair physical or mental abilities; patients must be cautioned about performing tasks which require mental alertness (eg, operating machinery or driving). Effects may be potentiated when used with other sedative drugs or ethanol.

Adverse Reactions

Cardiovascular: Tachycardia

Central nervous system: Acute toxic psychosis, agitation, concentration impaired, confusion, disorientation, giddiness, hallucinations, lightheadedness, memory impaired, restlessness, slurred speech

Dermatologic: Rash

Gastrointestinal: Constipation, epigastric distress, nausea, parotitis (secondary to xerostomia), vomiting, xerostomia

Genitourinary: Dysuria

Neuromuscular & skeletal: Weakness

Ocular: Blurred vision, mydriasis

Miscellaneous: Allergic reaction

Drug Interactions

Metabolism/Transport Effects None known.

Avoid Concomitant Use

Avoid concomitant use of Procyclidine with any of the following: Aclidinium; Glucagon; Ipratropium (Oral Inhalation); Potassium Chloride; Tiotropium; Umeclidinium

Increased Effect/Toxicity

Procyclidine may increase the levels/effects of: AbobotulinumtoxinA; Analgesics (Opioid); Anticholinergic Agents; Cannabinoid-Containing Products; Glucagon; Mirabegron; OnabotulinumtoxinA; Potassium Chloride; RimabotulinumtoxinB; Thiazide Diuretics; Tiotropium; Topiramate

The levels/effects of Procyclidine may be increased by: Aclidinium; Ipratropium (Oral Inhalation); Mianserin; Pramlintide; Umeclidinium

Decreased Effect

Procyclidine may decrease the levels/effects of: Acetylcholinesterase Inhibitors; Itopride; Secretin

The levels/effects of Procyclidine may be decreased by: Acetylcholinesterase Inhibitors

Food Interactions Ethanol: Avoid ethanol (may potentiate CNS effects).

Storage/Stability Store at 15°C to 30°C (59°F to 86°F). Protect from moisture.

Mechanism of Action Thought to act by blocking excess acetylcholine at cerebral synapses; many of its effects are due to its pharmacologic similarities with atropine; it exerts an antispasmodic effect on smooth muscle, is a potent mydriatic; inhibits salivation

Pharmacodynamics/Kinetics

Onset of action: 45-60 minutes

Duration: Significant autonomic effects have been observed up to 12 hours

Distribution: V_d: 1 L/kg

Metabolism: Hepatic

Bioavailability: ~75%

Half-life elimination: ~12.5 hours

Time to peak: ~1 hour

Excretion: Urine (predominantly as metabolites)

Dosage Oral:

Adults: Initial: 2.5 mg 3 times/day after meals; if tolerated, gradually increase dose as needed; maximum: 30 mg/day (given in 3 or 4 divided doses)

Elderly: Initial: 2.5 mg once or twice daily (use lowest dose possible), gradually increasing as necessary. Avoid use if possible.

Dosage adjustment in renal impairment: No dosage adjustment provided in manufacturer's labeling. Use with caution.

Dosage adjustment in hepatic impairment: No dosage adjustment provided in manufacturer's labeling. Use with caution.

Dietary Considerations Should be taken after meals to minimize stomach upset.

Administration Should be administered after meals to minimize stomach upset.

Monitoring Parameters Symptoms of EPS or Parkinson's disease, pulse, anticholinergic effects (ie, CNS, bowel and bladder function)

Product Availability Not available in U.S.

Dosage Forms: Canada

Tablet, oral: 2.5 mg, 5 mg

Elixir, oral: 2.5 mg/5 mL

- ◆ **Procyclidine Hydrochloride** *see* Procyclidine [CAN/INT] *on page 1721*
- ◆ **Procysbi™** *see* Cysteamine (Systemic) *on page 534*
- ◆ **Procysbi** *see* Cysteamine (Systemic) *on page 534*
- ◆ **Procytox (Can)** *see* Cyclophosphamide *on page 517*
- ◆ **PRO-Dexamethasone (Can)** *see* Dexamethasone (Systemic) *on page 599*
- ◆ **PRO-Diclo-Rapide (Can)** *see* Diclofenac (Systemic) *on page 617*
- ◆ **PRO-Doc Limitee Bromazepam (Can)** *see* Bromazepam [CAN/INT] *on page 290*
- ◆ **PRO-Enalapril (Can)** *see* Enalapril *on page 722*
- ◆ **PRO-Feno-Super (Can)** *see* Fenofibrate and Derivatives *on page 852*
- ◆ **Profilnine SD** *see* Factor IX Complex (Human) [(Factors II, IX, X)] *on page 838*
- ◆ **PRO-Fluconazole (Can)** *see* Fluconazole *on page 885*
- ◆ **PRO-Fluoxetine (Can)** *see* FLUoxetine *on page 899*
- ◆ **PRO-Gabapentin (Can)** *see* Gabapentin *on page 943*

Progesterone (proe JES ter one)

Brand Names: U.S. Crinone; Endometrin; First-Progesterone VGS 100; First-Progesterone VGS 200; First-Progesterone VGS 25; First-Progesterone VGS 400; First-Progesterone VGS 50; Prometrium

Brand Names: Canada Crinone; Endometrin; Prometrium

Index Terms Pregnenedione; Progestin

Pharmacologic Category Progestin

Use

Oral: Prevention of endometrial hyperplasia in nonhysterectomized, postmenopausal women who are receiving conjugated estrogen tablets; secondary amenorrhea

IM: Amenorrhea; abnormal uterine bleeding due to hormonal imbalance

Intravaginal gel: Part of assisted reproductive technology (ART) for infertile women with progesterone deficiency; secondary amenorrhea

Vaginal insert: Part of ART for infertile women with progesterone deficiency

Pregnancy Risk Factor B (oral)

Dosage Adults:

IM: Females:

Amenorrhea: 5 to 10 mg/day for 6 to 8 consecutive days

Functional uterine bleeding: 5 to 10 mg/day for 6 doses

Oral: Females:

Prevention of endometrial hyperplasia (in postmenopausal women with a uterus who are receiving daily conjugated estrogen tablets): 200 mg as a single daily dose every evening for 12 days sequentially per 28-day cycle

Amenorrhea: 400 mg every evening for 10 days

Intravaginal gel: Females:

ART in women who require progesterone supplementation: 90 mg (8% gel) once daily; if pregnancy occurs, may continue treatment for up to 10 to 12 weeks

ART in women with partial or complete ovarian failure: 90 mg (8% gel) intravaginally twice daily; if pregnancy occurs, may continue up to 10 to 12 weeks

Secondary amenorrhea: 45 mg (4% gel) intravaginally every other day for up to 6 doses; women who fail to respond may be increased to 90 mg (8% gel) every other day for up to 6 doses

Reduce the risk of spontaneous preterm delivery (singleton pregnancy and short cervix) (off-label use): 90 mg (8% gel) once daily (Hassan, 2011; O'Brien, 2009). Treatment initiation is recommended before or at gestational week 24 (ACOG, 2012).

Intravaginal insert: Females: ART: 100 mg 2 to 3 times daily starting at oocyte retrieval and continuing for up to 10 weeks.

Dosage adjustment in renal impairment:

Injection, oral: There are no dosage adjustments provided in the manufacturer's labeling (has not been studied). Use with caution.

Intravaginal gel, insert: There are no dosage adjustments provided in the manufacturer's labeling.

Dosage adjustment in hepatic impairment: Use is contraindicated in liver dysfunction or disease.

Additional Information Complete prescribing information should be consulted for additional detail.

Dosage Forms Considerations

Progesterone cream 10% is a compounding kit. Refer to manufacturer's labeling for compounding instructions.

Dosage Forms

Capsule, Oral:

Prometrium: 100 mg, 200 mg

Generic: 100 mg, 200 mg

Cream, Transdermal:

Generic: 10% (60 g)

Gel, Vaginal:

Crinone: 4% (1.125 g); 8% (1.125 g)

Insert, Vaginal:

Endometrin: 100 mg (21 ea)

Oil, Intramuscular:

Generic: 50 mg/mL (10 mL)

Suppository, Vaginal:

First-Progesterone VGS 25: 25 mg (30 ea)
First-Progesterone VGS 50: 50 mg (30 ea)
First-Progesterone VGS 100: 100 mg (30 ea)
First-Progesterone VGS 200: 200 mg (30 ea)
First-Progesterone VGS 400: 400 mg (30 ea)

- ◆ **Progestin** *see* Progesterone *on page 1722*
- ◆ **PRO-Glyburide (Can)** *see* GlyBURIDE *on page 972*
- ◆ **Proglycem** *see* Diazoxide *on page 616*
- ◆ **Proglycem® (Can)** *see* Diazoxide *on page 616*
- ◆ **Prograf** *see* Tacrolimus (Systemic) *on page 1962*
- ◆ **Proguanil and Atovaquone** *see* Atovaquone and Proguanil *on page 198*
- ◆ **Proguanil Hydrochloride and Atovaquone** *see* Atovaquone and Proguanil *on page 198*
- ◆ **PRO-Hydroxyquine (Can)** *see* Hydroxychloroquine *on page 1021*
- ◆ **PRO-Indapamide (Can)** *see* Indapamide *on page 1065*

- ◆ **Pro-Indo (Can)** *see* Indomethacin *on page 1067*
- ◆ **PRO-ISMN (Can)** *see* Isosorbide Mononitrate *on page 1126*
- ◆ **Prokine** *see* Sargramostim *on page 1865*
- ◆ **Prolensa** *see* Bromfenac *on page 291*
- ◆ **Proleukin** *see* Aldesleukin *on page 72*
- ◆ **PRO-Levetiracetam (Can)** *see* LevETIRAcetam *on page 1191*
- ◆ **PRO-Levocarb (Can)** *see* Carbidopa and Levodopa *on page 351*
- ◆ **Prolia** *see* Denosumab *on page 589*
- ◆ **PRO-Lisinopril (Can)** *see* Lisinopril *on page 1226*
- ◆ **Prolopa® (Can)** *see* Benserazide and Levodopa [CAN/INT] *on page 244*
- ◆ **PRO-Lorazepam (Can)** *see* LORazepam *on page 1243*
- ◆ **PRO-Lovastatin (Can)** *see* Lovastatin *on page 1252*
- ◆ **Promacet** *see* Butalbital and Acetaminophen *on page 314*
- ◆ **Promacta** *see* Eltrombopag *on page 714*
- ◆ **PRO-Metformin (Can)** *see* MetFORMIN *on page 1307*

Promethazine (proe METH a zeen)

Brand Names: U.S. Phenadoz; Phenergan; Promethegan

Brand Names: Canada Bioniche Promethazine; Histantil; Phenergan; PMS-Promethazine

Index Terms Promethazine Hydrochloride

Pharmacologic Category Antiemetic; Histamine H_1 Antagonist; Histamine H_1 Antagonist, First Generation; Phenothiazine Derivative

Additional Appendix Information

Beers Criteria – Potentially Inappropriate Medications for Geriatrics *on page 2271*

Use Symptomatic treatment of various allergic conditions; antiemetic; motion sickness; sedative; adjunct to postoperative analgesia and anesthesia

Pregnancy Risk Factor C

Pregnancy Considerations Teratogenic effects were not observed in animal reproduction studies. Promethazine crosses the placenta. Maternal promethazine use has generally not resulted in an increased risk of birth defects. Platelet aggregation may be inhibited in newborns following maternal use of promethazine within 2 weeks of delivery. Promethazine is used for the treatment of nausea and vomiting of pregnancy (refer to current guidelines). Promethazine is also indicated for use during labor for obstetric sedation and may be used alone or as an adjunct to opioid analgesics.

Breast-Feeding Considerations It is not known if promethazine is excreted in breast milk. According to the manufacturer, the decision to continue or discontinue breast-feeding during therapy should take into account the risk of exposure to the infant and the benefits of treatment to the mother. Antihistamines may decrease maternal serum prolactin concentrations when administered prior to the establishment of nursing.

Contraindications Hypersensitivity to promethazine or any component of the formulation (cross-reactivity between phenothiazines may occur); coma; treatment of lower respiratory tract symptoms, including asthma; children <2 years of age; intra-arterial or subcutaneous administration

Warnings/Precautions [U.S. Boxed Warning]: Respiratory fatalities have been reported in children <2 years of age. Contraindicated in children <2 years of age. In children ≥2 years, use the lowest possible dose; other drugs with respiratory depressant effects should be avoided.

[U.S. Boxed Warning]: Promethazine injection can cause severe tissue injury (including gangrene) regardless of the route of administration. Tissue irritation and damage may result from perivascular extravasation, unintentional intra-arterial administration, and intraneuronal or perineuronal infiltration. In addition to gangrene, adverse events reported include tissue necrosis, abscesses, burning, pain, erythema, edema, paralysis, severe spasm of distal vessels, phlebitis, thrombophlebitis, venous thrombosis, sensory loss, paralysis, and palsies. Surgical intervention including fasciotomy, skin graft, and/or amputation have been necessary in some cases. The preferred route of administration is by deep intramuscular (IM) injection. Subcutaneous administration is contraindicated. Discontinue intravenous injection immediately with onset of pain and evaluate for arterial injection or perivascular extravasation. Although there is no proven successful management of unintentional intra-arterial injection or perivascular extravasation, sympathetic block and heparinization have been used in the acute management of unintentional intra-arterial injection based on results from animal studies. Vesicant; for IV administration (**not** the preferred route of administration), ensure proper needle or catheter placement prior to and during administration; avoid extravasation.

May be sedating; use with caution in disorders where CNS depression is a feature. May impair physical or mental abilities; patients must be cautioned about performing tasks which require mental alertness. Use with caution in hemodynamic instability; bone marrow suppression; subcortical brain damage; and in severe cardiac, hepatic or respiratory disease. Avoid use in Reye's syndrome. May lower seizure threshold; use caution in persons with seizure disorders or in persons using opioids or local anesthetics which may also affect seizure threshold. May alter temperature regulation or mask toxicity of other drugs due to antiemetic effects. May alter cardiac conduction (life-threatening arrhythmias have occurred with therapeutic doses of phenothiazines). May cause orthostatic hypotension; use with caution in patients at risk of hypotension or where transient hypotensive episodes would be poorly tolerated (cardiovascular disease or cerebrovascular disease).

Phenothiazines may cause anticholinergic effects; therefore, they should be used with caution in patients with decreased gastrointestinal motility, GI or GU obstruction, urinary retention, BPH, xerostomia, or visual problems. Conditions which also may be exacerbated by cholinergic blockade include narrow-angle glaucoma (screening is recommended) and worsening of myasthenia gravis. Use with caution in Parkinson's disease. May cause extrapyramidal symptoms, including pseudoparkinsonism, acute dystonic reactions, akathisia, and tardive dyskinesia. May be associated with neuroleptic malignant syndrome (NMS). May cause photosensitivity. In the elderly, avoid use of this potent anticholinergic agent due to increased risk of confusion, dry mouth, constipation, and other anticholinergic effects; clearance decreases in patients of advanced age (Beers Criteria). Injection may contain sodium metabisulfite.

Adverse Reactions

Cardiovascular: Bradycardia, hyper-/hypotension, nonspecific QT changes, orthostatic hypotension, tachycardia,

Central nervous system: Agitation akathisia, catatonic states, confusion, delirium, disorientation, dizziness, drowsiness, dystonias, euphoria, excitation, extrapyramidal symptoms, faintness, fatigue, hallucinations, hysteria, insomnia, lassitude, pseudoparkinsonism, tardive dyskinesia, nervousness, neuroleptic malignant syndrome, nightmares, sedation, seizure, somnolence

Dermatologic: Angioneurotic edema, dermatitis, photosensitivity, skin pigmentation (slate gray), urticaria
Endocrine & metabolic: Amenorrhea, breast engorgement, gynecomastia, hyperglycemia, lactation
Gastrointestinal: Constipation, nausea, vomiting, xerostomia
Genitourinary: Ejaculatory disorder, impotence, urinary retention
Hematologic: Agranulocytosis, leukopenia, thrombocytopenia, thrombocytopenic purpura
Hepatic: Jaundice
Local: Abscess, distal vessel spasm, gangrene, injection site reactions (burning, edema, erythema, pain), palsies, paralysis, phlebitis, sensory loss, thrombophlebitis, tissue necrosis, venous thrombosis
Neuromuscular & skeletal: Incoordination, tremor
Ocular: Blurred vision, corneal and lenticular changes, diplopia, epithelial keratopathy, pigmentary retinopathy
Otic: Tinnitus
Respiratory: Apnea, asthma, nasal congestion, respiratory depression

Drug Interactions

Metabolism/Transport Effects **Substrate** of CYP2B6 (major), CYP2D6 (major); **Note:** Assignment of Major/Minor substrate status based on clinically relevant drug interaction potential; **Inhibits** CYP2D6 (weak)

Avoid Concomitant Use

Avoid concomitant use of Promethazine with any of the following: Aclidinium; Azelastine (Nasal); Dapoxetine; Glucagon; Ipratropium (Oral Inhalation); Metoclopramide; Orphenadrine; Paraldehyde; Potassium Chloride; Thalidomide; Tiotropium; Umeclidinium

Increased Effect/Toxicity

Promethazine may increase the levels/effects of: AbobotulinumtoxinA; Alcohol (Ethyl); Analgesics (Opioid); Anticholinergic Agents; Antipsychotic Agents; ARIPiprazole; Azelastine (Nasal); Buprenorphine; CNS Depressants; Glucagon; Highest Risk QTc-Prolonging Agents; Hydrocodone; Methotrimeprazine; Mirabegron; Moderate Risk QTc-Prolonging Agents; OnabotulinumtoxinA; Orphenadrine; Paraldehyde; Potassium Chloride; Pramipexole; RimabotulinumtoxinB; ROPINIRole; Rotigotine; Serotonin Modulators; Suvorexant; Thalidomide; Thiazide Diuretics; Tiotropium; Topiramate; Zolpidem

The levels/effects of Promethazine may be increased by: Abiraterone Acetate; Aclidinium; Antiemetics (5HT3 Antagonists); Antipsychotic Agents; Brimonidine (Topical); Cannabis; Cobicistat; CYP2B6 Inhibitors (Moderate); CYP2D6 Inhibitors (Moderate); CYP2D6 Inhibitors (Strong); Dapoxetine; Darunavir; Doxylamine; Dronabinol; Droperidol; HydrOXYzine; Ipratropium (Oral Inhalation); Kava Kava; Magnesium Sulfate; MAO Inhibitors; Methotrimeprazine; Metoclopramide; Metyrosine; Mianserin; Mifepristone; Nabilone; Peginterferon Alfa-2b; Perampanel; Pramlintide; Quazepam; Rufinamide; Sodium Oxybate; Tapentadol; Tedizolid; Tetrahydrocannabinol; Umeclidinium

Decreased Effect

Promethazine may decrease the levels/effects of: Acetylcholinesterase Inhibitors; EPINEPHrine (Nasal); Epinephrine (Racemic); EPINEPHrine (Systemic, Oral Inhalation); Itopride; Secretin

The levels/effects of Promethazine may be decreased by: Acetylcholinesterase Inhibitors; CYP2B6 Inducers (Strong); Dabrafenib; Peginterferon Alfa-2b

Storage/Stability

Injection: Prior to dilution, store at 20°C to 25°C (68°F to 77°F). Protect from light. Solutions in NS or D_5W are stable for 24 hours at room temperature.
Oral solution: Store at 15°C to 25°C (59°F to 77°F). Protect from light.
Suppositories: Store refrigerated at 2°C to 8°C (36°F to 46°F).
Tablets: Store at 20°C to 25°C (68°F to 77°F). Protect from light.

Mechanism of Action Phenothiazine derivative; blocks postsynaptic mesolimbic dopaminergic receptors in the brain; exhibits a strong alpha-adrenergic blocking effect and depresses the release of hypothalamic and hypophyseal hormones; competes with histamine for the H_1-receptor; muscarinic-blocking effect may be responsible for antiemetic activity; reduces stimuli to the brainstem reticular system

Pharmacodynamics/Kinetics

Onset of action: Oral, IM: ~20 minutes; IV: ~5 minutes
Duration: Usually 4-6 hours (up to 12 hours)
Absorption: Oral: Rapid and complete; large first pass effect limits systemic bioavailability (Sharma, 2003)
Distribution: V_d: Syrup: 98 L/kg (range: 17-277 L/kg) (Strenkoski-Nox, 2000)
Metabolism: Hepatic; hydroxylation via CYP2D6 and N-demethylation via CYP2B6; significant first-pass effect (Sharma, 2003)
Bioavailability: Oral: ~25% (Sharma, 2003)
Half-life elimination: IM: ~10 hours; IV: 9-16 hours; Suppositories, syrup: 16-19 hours (range: 4-34 hours) (Strenkoski-Nox, 2000)
Time to maximum serum concentration: Suppositories: 6.7-8.6 hours; Syrup: 4.4 hours (Strenkoski-Nox, 2000)
Excretion: Urine

Dosage

Children ≥2 years:
Allergic conditions: Oral, rectal: 0.1 mg/kg/dose (maximum: 12.5 mg) every 6 hours during the day and 0.5 mg/kg/dose (maximum: 25 mg) at bedtime as needed
Antiemetic: Oral, IM, IV, rectal: 0.25-1 mg/kg 4-6 times/day as needed (maximum: 25 mg/dose)
Motion sickness: Oral, rectal: 0.5 mg/kg/dose 30 minutes to 1 hour before departure, then every 12 hours as needed (maximum dose: 25 mg twice daily)
Preoperative analgesia/hypnotic adjunct: IM, IV: 1.1 mg/kg in combination with an analgesic or hypnotic (at reduced doses) and an atropine-like agent. **Note:** Dose should not exceed half of suggested adult dose.
Sedation: Oral, IM, IV, rectal: 12.5-25 mg at bedtime or preoperatively (maximum: 25 mg/dose)

Adults:
Allergic conditions (including allergic reactions to blood or plasma):
Oral, rectal: 25 mg at bedtime **or** 12.5 mg before meals and at bedtime (range: 6.25-12.5 mg 3 times/day)
IM, IV: 25 mg, may repeat in 2 hours when necessary; switch to oral route as soon as feasible
Antiemetic: Oral, IM, IV, rectal: 12.5-25 mg every 4-6 hours as needed
Motion sickness: Oral, rectal: 25 mg 30-60 minutes before departure, then every 12 hours as needed
Obstetrics (labor) as adjunct to analgesia: IM, IV: Early labor: 50 mg; Established labor: 25-75 mg; may repeat every 4 hours for up to 2 additional doses (maximum: 100 mg/day while in labor). **Note:** Dosage of concomitant analgesic should be reduced.
Pre-/postoperative analgesia/hypnotic adjunct: IM, IV: 25-50 mg in combination with analgesic or hypnotic (at reduced dosage)
Sedation: Oral, IM, IV, rectal: 12.5-50 mg/dose

Dosage adjustment in renal impairment: No dosage adjustment provided in manufacturer's labeling.

Dosage adjustment in hepatic impairment:

Children ≥2 years: No dosage adjustment provided in manufacturer's labeling; however, avoid use in patients with signs of hepatic disease (adverse reactions caused by promethazine may be confused with signs of hepatic disease).

Adults: No dosage adjustment provided in manufacturer's labeling; use with caution (cholestatic jaundice has been reported with use).

Dietary Considerations Increase dietary intake of riboflavin.

Administration Formulations available for oral, rectal, IM/IV; not for SubQ administration. Administer IM into deep muscle (preferred route of administration). IV administration is **not** the preferred route; severe tissue damage may occur. Solution for injection should be administered in a maximum concentration of 25 mg/mL (more dilute solutions are recommended). Administer via running IV line at port farthest from patient's vein, or through a large bore vein (not hand or wrist). Consider administering over 10-15 minutes (maximum: 25 mg/minute).

Vesicant; ensure proper needle or catheter placement prior to and during infusion; avoid extravasation. Discontinue immediately if burning or pain occurs with administration; evaluate for inadvertent arterial injection or extravasation.

Extravasation management: If extravasation occurs, stop infusion immediately and disconnect (leave cannula/needle in place); gently aspirate extravasated solution (do **NOT** flush the line); remove needle/cannula; elevate extremity. Apply dry cold compresses (Hurst, 2004).

Monitoring Parameters Relief of symptoms, mental status; signs and symptoms of tissue injury (burning or pain at injection site, phlebitis, edema) with IV administration

Dosage Forms

Solution, Injection:

Phenergan: 25 mg/mL (1 mL); 50 mg/mL (1 mL)

Generic: 25 mg/mL (1 mL); 50 mg/mL (1 mL)

Solution, Oral:

Generic: 6.25 mg/5 mL (118 mL, 473 mL)

Suppository, Rectal:

Phenadoz: 12.5 mg (12 ea); 25 mg (12 ea)

Phenergan: 12.5 mg (12 ea); 25 mg (12 ea); 50 mg (12 ea)

Promethegan: 12.5 mg (12 ea); 25 mg (12 ea, 1000 ea); 50 mg (12 ea)

Generic: 12.5 mg (1 ea, 12 ea); 25 mg (1 ea, 12 ea); 50 mg (12 ea)

Syrup, Oral:

Generic: 6.25 mg/5 mL (118 mL, 473 mL)

Tablet, Oral:

Generic: 12.5 mg, 25 mg, 50 mg

Promethazine and Codeine

(proe METH a zeen & KOE deen)

Index Terms Codeine and Promethazine

Pharmacologic Category Analgesic, Opioid; Antitussive; Histamine H_1 Antagonist; Histamine H_1 Antagonist, First Generation; Phenothiazine Derivative

Use Temporary relief of coughs and upper respiratory symptoms associated with allergy or the common cold

Pregnancy Risk Factor C

Dosage Oral:

Children:

<6 years: **Note:** Use of promethazine/codeine combination is contraindicated in children <6 years of age

6-11 years: 2.5-5 mL every 4-6 hours (maximum: 30 mL per 24 hours)

Children ≥12 years and Adults: 5 mL every 4-6 hours (maximum: 30 mL per 24 hours)

Elderly: Use with caution; consider decreased dose

Dosage adjustment in renal/hepatic impairment: Use with caution; consider decreased dose

Additional Information Complete prescribing information should be consulted for additional detail.

Dosage Forms

Syrup, oral: Promethazine 6.25 mg and codeine 10 mg per 5 mL

Promethazine and Dextromethorphan

(proe METH a zeen & deks troe meth OR fan)

Index Terms Dextromethorphan and Promethazine

Pharmacologic Category Antitussive; Histamine H_1 Antagonist; Histamine H_1 Antagonist, First Generation; Phenothiazine Derivative

Use Temporary relief of coughs and upper respiratory symptoms associated with allergy or the common cold

Pregnancy Risk Factor C

Dosage Oral:

Children:

<2 years: Use of promethazine is contraindicated

2-6 years: 1.25-2.5 mL every 4-6 hours up to 10 mL in 24 hours

6-12 years: 2.5-5 mL every 4-6 hours up to 20 mL in 24 hours

Adults: 5 mL every 4-6 hours up to 30 mL in 24 hours

Dosage adjustment in renal impairment: No dosage adjustment provided in manufacturer's labeling.

Dosage adjustment in hepatic impairment:

Children: No dosage adjustment provided in manufacturer's labeling; however, avoid use in patients with signs of hepatic disease (adverse reactions caused by promethazine may be confused with signs of hepatic disease).

Adults: No dosage adjustment provided in manufacturer's labeling; use with caution.

Additional Information Complete prescribing information should be consulted for additional detail.

Dosage Forms

Syrup: Promethazine 6.25 mg and dextromethorphan 15 mg per 5 mL

- ◆ **Promethazine Hydrochloride** *see* Promethazine *on page 1723*
- ◆ **Promethegan** *see* Promethazine *on page 1723*
- ◆ **Prometrium** *see* Progesterone *on page 1722*
- ◆ **PRO-Mirtazapine (Can)** *see* Mirtazapine *on page 1376*
- ◆ **Promolaxin [OTC]** *see* Docusate *on page 661*
- ◆ **PRO-Naproxen EC (Can)** *see* Naproxen *on page 1427*
- ◆ **Pronestyl** *see* Procainamide *on page 1716*
- ◆ **Pronto Complete Lice Removal System [OTC]** *see* Pyrethrins and Piperonyl Butoxide *on page 1746*
- ◆ **Pronto Lice Control (Can)** *see* Pyrethrins and Piperonyl Butoxide *on page 1746*
- ◆ **Pronto Plus Lice Killing Mousse Plus Vitamin E [OTC]** *see* Pyrethrins and Piperonyl Butoxide *on page 1746*
- ◆ **Pronto Plus Lice Killing Mousse Shampoo Plus Natural Extracts and Oils [OTC]** *see* Pyrethrins and Piperonyl Butoxide *on page 1746*
- ◆ **Pronto Plus Warm Oil Treatment and Conditioner [OTC]** *see* Pyrethrins and Piperonyl Butoxide *on page 1746*

Propafenone (pro PAF en one)

Brand Names: U.S. Rythmol; Rythmol SR

Brand Names: Canada Apo-Propafenone; Mylan-Propafenone; PMS-Propafenone; Rythmol Gen-Propafenone

Index Terms Propafenone Hydrochloride

Pharmacologic Category Antiarrhythmic Agent, Class Ic

Additional Appendix Information

Beers Criteria - Potentially Inappropriate Medications for Geriatrics *on page 2271*

Use Treatment of life-threatening ventricular arrhythmias; treatment of paroxysmal atrial fibrillation/flutter (PAF) or paroxysmal supraventricular tachycardia (PSVT) in patients with disabling symptoms and without structural heart disease

Extended release capsule: Prolong the time to recurrence of symptomatic atrial fibrillation in patients without structural heart disease

Note: According to the American Heart Association/American College of Cardiology/Heart Rhythm Society guidelines for the management of atrial fibrillation, propafenone may be used to convert atrial fibrillation/flutter to sinus rhythm. Immediate release propafenone ("pill-in-the-pocket") in addition to a beta blocker or nondihydropyridine calcium channel blocker may also be used to terminate atrial fibrillation outside of the hospital when it is demonstrated to be safe in a monitored setting for selected patients (AHA/ACC/HRS [January, 2014]).

Pregnancy Risk Factor C

Pregnancy Considerations Adverse events were observed in some animal reproduction studies.

Breast-Feeding Considerations Propafenone is excreted in breast milk. Due to the potential for serious adverse reactions in the nursing infant, the manufacturer recommends a decision be made whether to discontinue nursing or to discontinue the drug, taking into account the importance of treatment to the mother.

Contraindications Hypersensitivity to propafenone or any component of the formulation; sinoatrial, AV, and intraventricular disorders of impulse generation and/or conduction (except in patients with a functioning artificial pacemaker); Brugada syndrome, sinus bradycardia; cardiogenic shock; uncompensated cardiac failure; marked hypotension; bronchospastic disorders or severe obstructive pulmonary disease; uncorrected electrolyte abnormalities

Warnings/Precautions **[U.S. Boxed Warning]: In the Cardiac Arrhythmia Suppression Trial (CAST), recent (>6 days but <2 years ago) myocardial infarction patients with asymptomatic, non-life-threatening ventricular arrhythmias did not benefit and may have been harmed by attempts to suppress the arrhythmia with flecainide or encainide.** An increased mortality or nonfatal cardiac arrest rate (7.7%) was seen in the active treatment group compared with patients in the placebo group (3%). The applicability of the CAST results to other populations is unknown. Antiarrhythmic agents should be reserved for patients with life-threatening ventricular arrhythmias.

Can cause life-threatening drug-induced arrhythmias, including ventricular fibrillation, ventricular tachycardia, asystole, and torsade de pointes (Hii, 1991). The manufacturer notes that propafenone may increase the QT interval; however, due to QRS prolongation; changes in the QT interval are difficult to interpret. In an evaluation of propafenone (450 mg/day) in healthy individuals compared to other selected antiarrhythmic agents, propafenone did not affect repolarization time (eg, QT, QTc, JT, JTc) only depolarization time (ie, QRS interval) (Sarubbi, 1998). Monitor for proarrhythmic effects, and when necessary, adjust dose to prevent QTc prolongation. Initiation of propafenone may unmask Brugada syndrome; obtain ECG after treatment initiation and discontinue if ECG indicative of Brugada syndrome.

In the treatment of atrial fibrillation in the elderly, avoid antiarrhythmics as first-line treatment. In older adults, data suggests rate control may provide more benefits than risks compared to rhythm control for most patients (Beers Criteria).

Concurrent use of propafenone with QT-prolonging agents has not been extensively evaluated. The manufacturer recommends withholding Class Ia or Class III antiarrhythmics for at least 5 half-lives prior to starting propafenone. Slows atrioventricular conduction, potentially leading to first degree AV block; degree of PR interval prolongation and increased QRS duration are dose and concentration related. Avoid in patients with conduction disturbances (unless functioning pacemaker present).

May alter pacing and sensing thresholds of artificial pacemakers. Propafenone use may be considered in patients with obstructive lung disease who do not have bronchospasm (AHA/ACC/HRS [January, 2014]). Use in patients with bronchospastic disease or severe obstructive lung disease is contraindicated.

Avoid use in patients with heart failure; similar agents have been shown to increase mortality in this population; may precipitate or exacerbate condition. Correct electrolyte disturbances, especially hypokalemia or hypomagnesemia, prior to use and throughout therapy. Administer cautiously in significant hepatic or renal dysfunction. Use with caution in patients with myasthenia gravis; may exacerbate condition. Avoid the concurrent use of a CYP2D6 inhibitor and CYP3A4 inhibitor; may result in an increased risk of proarrhythmia or exaggerated beta-adrenergic blocking activity Agranulocytosis has been reported; generally occurring within the first 2 months of therapy. Upon therapy discontinuation, WBC usually normalized by 14 days. Positive ANA titers have been reported. Titers have decreased with and without propafenone discontinuation. Positive titers have not usually been associated with clinical symptoms, although at least one case of drug induced lupus erythematosus has been reported. Consider therapy discontinuation in symptomatic patients with positive ANA titers.

Adverse Reactions

Cardiovascular: Angina, atrial fibrillation, AV block (first-degree), bradycardia, bundle branch block, chest pain, CHF, edema, hypotension, increased QRS interval, intraventricular conduction delay, new or worsened arrhythmia (proarrhythmic effect), palpitation, PVCs, syncope, ventricular tachycardia

Central nervous system: Anxiety, ataxia, dizziness, drowsiness, fatigue, headache, insomnia

Dermatologic: Rash

Gastrointestinal: Abdominal pain, anorexia, constipation, diarrhea, dyspepsia, flatulence, nausea, unusual taste, vomiting, xerostomia

Neuromuscular & skeletal: Arthralgia, tremor, weakness

Ocular: Blurred vision

Respiratory: Dyspnea

Miscellaneous: Diaphoresis

Rare but important or life-threatening: Agranulocytosis, alopecia, amnesia, anemia, apnea, AV block (second or third degree), asystole, AV dissociation, cardiac arrest, cholestasis (0.1%), coma, confusion, CHF, depression, granulocytopenia, hepatitis (0.03%), hyperglycemia, impotence, increased bleeding time, leukopenia, lupus erythematosus, mania, memory loss, nephrotic syndrome, paresthesia, peripheral neuropathy, pruritus, psychosis, purpura, renal failure, seizure (0.3%), SIADH, sinus node dysfunction, thrombocytopenia, tinnitus, torsade de pointes, ventricular fibrillation, vertigo

Drug Interactions

Metabolism/Transport Effects Substrate of CYP1A2 (minor), CYP2D6 (minor), CYP3A4 (minor); **Note:** Assignment of Major/Minor substrate status based on clinically relevant drug interaction potential; **Inhibits** CYP1A2 (weak), CYP2D6 (weak)

Avoid Concomitant Use

Avoid concomitant use of Propafenone with any of the following: Amiodarone; Antiarrhythmic Agents (Class Ia); Antiarrhythmic Agents (Class III); Ceritinib; FLUoxetine; Fosamprenavir; Highest Risk QTc-Prolonging Agents; Ivabradine; Mifepristone; QuiNIDine; Ritonavir; Saquinavir; Tipranavir

Increased Effect/Toxicity

Propafenone may increase the levels/effects of: Antiarrhythmic Agents (Class Ia); Antiarrhythmic Agents (Class III); ARIPiprazole; Beta-Blockers; Bradycardia-Causing Agents; Cardiac Glycosides; Ceritinib; CYP2D6 Inhibitors (Moderate); FLUoxetine; Highest Risk QTc-Prolonging Agents; Lacosamide; Moderate Risk QTc-Prolonging Agents; Propranolol; Theophylline Derivatives; Venlafaxine; Vitamin K Antagonists

The levels/effects of Propafenone may be increased by: Amiodarone; Boceprevir; Bretylium; Cimetidine; CYP2D6 Inhibitors (Strong); CYP3A4 Inhibitors (Moderate); CYP3A4 Inhibitors (Strong); FLUoxetine; FluvoxaMINE; Fosamprenavir; Ivabradine; Mifepristone; Mirabegron; PARoxetine; QTc-Prolonging Agents (Indeterminate Risk and Risk Modifying); QuiNIDine; Ritonavir; Saquinavir; Sertraline; Telaprevir; Tipranavir; Tofacitinib

Decreased Effect

The levels/effects of Propafenone may be decreased by: Barbiturates; Etravirine; Orlistat; Rifamycin Derivatives

Food Interactions Propafenone serum concentrations may be increased if taken with food. Management: Administer without regard to meals.

Storage/Stability Store at 25°C (77°F); excursions permitted to 15°C to 30°C (59°F to 86°F).

Mechanism of Action Propafenone is a class 1c antiarrhythmic agent which possesses local anesthetic properties, blocks the fast inward sodium current, and slows the rate of increase of the action potential. Prolongs conduction and refractoriness in all areas of the myocardium, with a slightly more pronounced effect on intraventricular conduction; it prolongs effective refractory period, reduces spontaneous automaticity and exhibits some beta-blockade activity.

Pharmacodynamics/Kinetics

Absorption: Well absorbed

Distribution: V_d: Adults: 252 L

Protein binding: 95% to $alpha_1$-acid glycoprotein

Metabolism: Hepatic via CYP2D6, CYP3A4 and CYP1A2 to two active metabolites (5-hydroxypropafenone and N-depropylpropafenone) then ultimately to glucuronide or sulfate conjugates. Two genetically determined metabolism groups exist (extensive and poor metabolizers); 10% of Caucasians are poor metabolizers. Exhibits nonlinear pharmacokinetics; when dose is increased from 300-900 mg/day, serum concentrations increase tenfold; this nonlinearity is thought to be due to saturable first-pass effect.

Bioavailability: Immediate release (IR): 150 mg: 3.4%; 300 mg: 10.6%; relative bioavailability of extended release (ER) capsule is less than IR tablet; the bioavailability of an ER capsule regimen of 325 mg twice-daily regimen approximates an IR tablet regimen of 150 mg 3 times/day.

Half-life elimination: Extensive metabolizers: 2-10 hours; Poor metabolizers: 10-32 hours

Time to peak, serum: IR: 3.5 hours; ER: 3-8 hours

Excretion: Urine (<1% unchanged; remainder as glucuronide or sulfate conjugates); feces

Dosage Oral: Adults: **Note:** Patients who exhibit significant widening of QRS complex or second- or third-degree AV block may need dose reduction.

Atrial fibrillation (to prevent recurrence):

Extended release capsule: Initial: 225 mg every 12 hours; dosage increase may be made at a minimum of 5-day intervals; may increase to 325 mg every 12 hours; if further increase is necessary, may increase to 425 mg every 12 hours

Immediate release tablet: Initial: 150 mg every 8 hours; dosage increase may be made at minimum of 3- to 4-day intervals, may increase to 225 mg every 8 hours; if further increase is necessary, may increase to 300 mg every 8 hours

Paroxysmal supraventricular tachycardia, ventricular arrhythmias: Immediate release tablet: Initial: 150 mg every 8 hours; dosage increase may be made at minimum of 3- to 4-day intervals, may increase to 225 mg every 8 hours; if further increase is necessary, may increase to 300 mg every 8 hours

Paroxysmal atrial fibrillation, pharmacologic cardioversion (off-label dose): Immediate release tablet: Outpatient: "Pill-in-the-pocket" dose: 450 mg (weight <70 kg), 600 mg (weight ≥70 kg). May not repeat in ≤24 hours (Alboni, 2004; AHA/ACC/HRS [January, 2014]). **Note:** An initial inpatient cardioversion trial should have been successful before sending patient home on this approach. Patient must be taking an AV nodal-blocking agent (eg, beta-blocker, nondihydropyridine calcium channel blocker) prior to initiation of antiarrhythmic

Dosage adjustment in renal impairment: No dosage adjustments provided in manufacturer's labeling; however, 50% of propafenone metabolites (some active) are excreted in the urine; some data suggest that no dosage adjustment is necessary (Burgess, 1989; Fromm, 1994); however, use with caution.

Hemodialysis/CVVH: Minimally dialyzable (Burgess, 1989; Seto, 1999); supplemental dose not necessary

Dosing adjustment in hepatic impairment: No dosage adjustment provided in manufacturer's labeling; however, dosage reduction should be considered as drug undergoes hepatic metabolism. Use with caution.

Dietary Considerations Capsule: May be taken without regard to meals.

Administration Capsules should be swallowed whole; do not crush or chew; may be taken without regard to meals.

Monitoring Parameters ECG, blood pressure, pulse (particularly at initiation of therapy)

Dosage Forms

Capsule Extended Release 12 Hour, Oral:

Rythmol SR: 225 mg, 325 mg, 425 mg

Generic: 225 mg, 325 mg, 425 mg

Tablet, Oral:

Rythmol: 150 mg, 225 mg

Generic: 150 mg, 225 mg, 300 mg

◆ **Propafenone Hydrochloride** *see* Propafenone *on page 1725*

Propantheline (proe PAN the leen)

Index Terms Propantheline Bromide

Pharmacologic Category Anticholinergic Agent

Additional Appendix Information

Beers Criteria – Potentially Inappropriate Medications for Geriatrics *on page 2271*

Use Adjunctive treatment of peptic ulcer

Pregnancy Risk Factor C

Dosage Oral:

Antisecretory (off-label use):

Children: 1-2 mg/kg/day in 3-4 divided doses

Adults: 15 mg 3 times/day before meals or food and 30 mg at bedtime

Elderly: 7.5 mg 3 times/day before meals and at bedtime

Antispasmodic:

Children: 2-3 mg/kg/day in divided doses every 4-6 hours and at bedtime

Adults: 15 mg 3 times/day before meals or food and 30 mg at bedtime

Dosage adjustment in renal impairment: No dosage adjustment provided in manufacturer's labeling.

Dosage adjustment in hepatic impairment: No dosage adjustment provided in manufacturer's labeling.

Additional Information Complete prescribing information should be consulted for additional detail.

Dosage Forms

Tablet, Oral:

Generic: 15 mg

◆ **Propantheline Bromide** *see* Propantheline *on page 1727*

Proparacaine (proe PAR a kane)

Brand Names: U.S. Alcaine; Parcaine

Brand Names: Canada Alcaine®; Diocaine®

Index Terms Proparacaine Hydrochloride; Proxymetacaine

Pharmacologic Category Local Anesthetic, Ophthalmic

Use Topical anesthesia for tonometry, gonioscopy; suture removal from cornea; removal of corneal foreign body; short operative procedure involving the cornea and conjunctiva

Pregnancy Risk Factor C

Dosage Ophthalmic: Children, Adolescents, and Adults:

Short corneal and conjunctival procedures: Instill 1 drop in eye(s) every 5-10 minutes for 5-7 doses

Tonometry, gonioscopy, suture removal: Instill 1-2 drops in eye(s) just prior to procedure

Dosage adjustment in renal impairment: No dosage adjustment provided in manufacturer's labeling.

Dosage adjustment in hepatic impairment: No dosage adjustment provided in manufacturer's labeling.

Additional Information Complete prescribing information should be consulted for additional detail.

Dosage Forms

Solution, Ophthalmic:

Alcaine: 0.5% (15 mL)

Parcaine: 0.5% (15 mL)

Generic: 0.5% (15 mL)

Proparacaine and Fluorescein

(proe PAR a kane & FLURE e seen)

Brand Names: U.S. Flucaine

Index Terms Fluorescein and Proparacaine

Pharmacologic Category Diagnostic Agent; Local Anesthetic

Use For use in ophthalmic procedures when a topical disclosing agent is needed along with an anesthetic

Dosage

Short corneal and conjunctival surgical procedures requiring deep ophthalmic anesthesia: Adults: Ophthalmic: Instill 1 drop in each eye every 5-10 minutes for 5-7 doses

Tonometry, gonioscopy, foreign body or suture removal: Adults: Ophthalmic: Instill 1-2 drops in each eye just prior to procedure

Dosage adjustment in renal impairment: No dosage adjustment provided in manufacturer's labeling.

Dosage adjustment in hepatic impairment: No dosage adjustment provided in manufacturer's labeling.

Additional Information Complete prescribing information should be consulted for additional detail.

Dosage Forms

Solution, ophthalmic: Proparacaine 0.5% and fluorescein 0.25% (5 mL)

Flucaine: Proparacaine 0.5% and fluorescein 0.25% (5 mL)

◆ **Proparacaine Hydrochloride** *see* Proparacaine *on page 1728*

◆ **Propecia** *see* Finasteride *on page 878*

◆ **Propine® (Can)** *see* Dipivefrin *on page 651*

◆ **PRO-Pioglitazone (Can)** *see* Pioglitazone *on page 1654*

Propiverine [INT] (pro PIV e reen)

International Brand Names Bearverin (VN); Detrunorm (GB, HR, ZA); Detrunorm XL (GB); Detrunorm XR (HR); Mictonetten (DE); Mictonorm (AE, BE, CZ, DE, GR, HK, ID, PH, PT, SG, SI, SK, TR); Propinorm (IE); Urostop (KR); Urotrol (TW); Uroverine (KR)

Index Terms Propiverine Hel

Pharmacologic Category Anticholinergic Agent

Reported Use Management of urinary frequency, urgency, and incontinence in neurogenic bladder disorders in idiopathic detrusor instability

Dosage Range Adults: Oral: Usual dosage: 15 mg 2-3 times/day; may increase dose to 4 times/day, some patients may respond to 15 mg/day

Product Availability Product available in various countries; not currently available in the U.S.

Dosage Forms

Tablet: 15 mg

◆ **Propiverine Hel** *see* Propiverine [INT] *on page 1728*

Propofol (PROE po fole)

Brand Names: U.S. Diprivan; Fresenius Propoven

Brand Names: Canada Diprivan; PMS-Propofol; Propofol Injection

Pharmacologic Category General Anesthetic

Use Induction of anesthesia in patients ≥3 years of age; maintenance of anesthesia in patients >2 months of age; in adults, for monitored anesthesia care sedation during procedures; in adults, for sedation in intubated, mechanically-ventilated ICU patients

Note: Consult local regulations and individual institutional policies and procedures.

Pregnancy Risk Factor B

Pregnancy Considerations Propofol crosses the placenta and may be associated with neonatal CNS and respiratory depression. Propofol is not recommended by the manufacturer for obstetrics, including cesarean section deliveries.

Breast-Feeding Considerations Propofol is excreted in breast milk. Breast-feeding is not recommended by the manufacturer. A green discoloration to the breast milk was noted in a woman following administration of propofol during surgery for removal of an ectopic pregnancy. Although other medications were also administered, propofol was detected in the milk and assumed to be the cause; resolution of this effect occurred within 48 hours after surgery (Birkholz, 2009).

Contraindications Hypersensitivity to propofol or any component of the formulation; hypersensitivity to eggs, egg products, soybeans, or soy products; when general anesthesia or sedation is contraindicated

Note: Fresenius Propoven is also contraindicated in patients who are hypersensitive to peanuts. In July 2012, the FDA initiated temporary importation of Fresenius

Propoven 1% (propofol) injection into the U.S. market to address a propofol shortage.

Warnings/Precautions May rarely cause hypersensitivity, anaphylaxis, anaphylactoid reactions, angioedema, bronchospasm, and erythema; medications for the treatment of hypersensitivity reactions should be available for immediate use. Use with caution in patients with history of hypersensitivity/anaphylactic reaction to peanuts; a low risk of crossreactivity between soy and peanuts may exist. Use is contraindicated in patients who are hypersensitive to eggs, egg products, soybeans, or soy products. The major cardiovascular effect of propofol is hypotension especially if patient is hypovolemic or if bolus dosing is used; use with caution in patients who are hemodynamically unstable, hypovolemic, or have abnormally low vascular tone (eg, sepsis). Use requires careful patient monitoring, should only be used by experienced personnel who are not actively engaged in the procedure or surgery. If used in a nonintubated and/or nonmechanically-ventilated patient, qualified personnel and appropriate equipment for rapid institution of respiratory and/or cardiovascular support must be immediately available. Use to induce moderate (conscious) sedation in patients warrants monitoring equivalent to that seen with deep anesthesia. Consult local regulations and individual institutional policies and procedures.

Use a lower induction dose, a slower maintenance rate of administration, and avoid rapidly administered boluses in the elderly, debilitated, or ASA-PS (American Society of Anesthesiologists - Physical Status) 3/4 patients to reduce the incidence of unwanted cardiorespiratory depressive events. Use caution in patients with severe cardiac disease (ejection fraction <50%) or respiratory disease; may have more profound adverse cardiovascular responses to propofol. Use caution in patients with a history of epilepsy or seizures; seizure may occur during recovery phase. Use caution in patients with increased intracranial pressure or impaired cerebral circulation; substantial decreases in mean arterial pressure and subsequent decreases in cerebral perfusion pressure may occur; consider continuous infusion or administer as a slow bolus.

Propofol-related infusion syndrome (PRIS) is a serious side effect with a high mortality rate (up to 33%) characterized by dysrhythmia (eg, bradycardia or tachycardia), heart failure, hyperkalemia, lipemia, metabolic acidosis, and/or rhabdomyolysis or myoglobinuria with subsequent renal failure. Risk factors include poor oxygen delivery, sepsis, serious cerebral injury, and the administration of high doses of propofol (usually doses >83 mcg/kg/minute or >5 mg/kg/hour for >48 hours), but has also been reported following large dose, short term infusions during surgical anesthesia. PRIS has also been reported with lower-dose infusions (Chukwuemeka, 2006; Merz, 2006). The onset of the syndrome is rapid, occurring within 4 days of initiation. Alternate sedative therapy should be considered for patients with escalating doses of vasopressors or inotropes, when cardiac failure occurs during high-dose propofol infusion, when metabolic acidosis is observed, or in whom lengthy and/or high-dose sedation is needed (Barr, 2013; Corbett, 2008).

Because propofol is formulated within a 10% fat emulsion, hypertriglyceridemia is an expected side effect. Patients who develop hypertriglyceridemia (eg, >500 mg/dL) are at risk of developing pancreatitis. An alternative sedative agent should be employed if significant hypertriglyceridemia occurs. Use with caution in patients with preexisting pancreatitis; use of propofol may exacerbate this condition. Use caution in patients with preexisting hyperlipidemia as evidenced by increased serum triglyceride levels or serum turbidity. Transient local pain may occur during IV injection; perioperative myoclonia has occurred. Propofol should only be used in pregnancy if clearly needed. Not recommended for use in obstetrics, including cesarean section deliveries. Safety and efficacy in pediatric intensive care unit patients have not been established. Concurrent use of fentanyl and propofol in pediatric patients may result in bradycardia.

Concomitant use with opioids may lead to increased sedative or anesthetic effects of propofol, more pronounced decreases in systolic, diastolic, and mean arterial pressures and cardiac output; lower doses of propofol may be needed. In addition, fentanyl may cause serious bradycardia when used with propofol in pediatric patients. Alfentanil use with propofol has precipitated seizure activity in patients without any history of epilepsy. Discontinue opioids and paralytic agents prior to weaning. Avoid abrupt discontinuation prior to weaning or daily wake up assessments. Abrupt discontinuation can result in rapid awakening, anxiety, agitation, and resistance to mechanical ventilation; wean the infusion rate so the patient awakens slowly. Propofol lacks analgesic properties; pain management requires specific use of analgesic agents, at effective dosages, propofol must be titrated separately from the analgesic agent.

Propofol vials and prefilled syringes have the potential to support the growth of various microorganisms despite product additives intended to suppress microbial growth. To limit the potential for contamination, recommendations in product labeling for handling and administering propofol should be strictly adhered to. Some formulations may contain edetate disodium which may lead to decreased zinc levels in patients with prolonged therapy (>5 days) or a predisposition to zinc deficiency (eg, burns, diarrhea, or sepsis). A holiday from propofol infusion should take place after 5 days of therapy to allow for evaluation and necessary replacement of zinc. Some formulations may contain sulfites.

Benzyl alcohol and derivatives: Some dosage forms may contain benzyl alcohol; large amounts of benzyl alcohol (≥99 mg/kg/day) have been associated with a potentially fatal toxicity ("gasping syndrome") in neonates; the "gasping syndrome" consists of metabolic acidosis, respiratory distress, gasping respirations, CNS dysfunction (including convulsions, intracranial hemorrhage), hypotension, and cardiovascular collapse (AAP, 1997; CDC, 1982); some data suggests that benzoate displaces bilirubin from protein binding sites (Ahlfors, 2001); avoid or use dosage forms containing benzyl alcohol with caution in neonates. See manufacturer's labeling.

Adverse Reactions

Cardiovascular: Arrhythmia, bradycardia, cardiac output decreased, hyper-/hypotension, tachycardia

Central nervous system: Movement

Dermatologic: Pruritus, rash

Endocrine & metabolic: Hypertriglyceridemia

Local: Injection site burning, stinging, or pain

Respiratory: Apnea, respiratory acidosis during weaning

Rare but important or life-threatening: Agitation, amblyopia, anaphylaxis, anaphylactoid reaction, anticholinergic syndrome, asystole, atrial arrhythmia, bigeminy, cardiac arrest, chills, cough, dizziness, delirium, discoloration (green [urine, hair, or nailbeds]), extremity pain, fever, flushing, hemorrhage, hypersalivation, hypertonia, hypomagnesemia, hypoxia, infusion site reactions (including pain, swelling, blisters and/or tissue necrosis following accidental extravasation); laryngospasm, leukocytosis, lung function decreased, myalgia, myoclonia (rarely including convulsions and opisthotonos), nausea, pancreatitis, paresthesia, phlebitis, postoperative unconsciousness with or without increase in muscle tone, premature atrial contractions, premature ventricular contractions, pulmonary edema, propofol-related infusion syndrome, rhabdomyolysis, somnolence, syncope, thrombosis, urine cloudy, vision abnormality, wheezing

Drug Interactions

Metabolism/Transport Effects Substrate of CYP1A2 (minor), CYP2A6 (minor), CYP2B6 (major), CYP2C19 (minor), CYP2C9 (minor), CYP2D6 (minor), CYP2E1 (minor), CYP3A4 (minor); **Note:** Assignment of Major/Minor substrate status based on clinically relevant drug interaction potential; **Inhibits** CYP1A2 (weak), CYP2C9 (weak), CYP2D6 (weak), CYP2E1 (weak), CYP3A4 (weak)

Avoid Concomitant Use

Avoid concomitant use of Propofol with any of the following: Azelastine (Nasal); Orphenadrine; Paraldehyde; Pimozide; Thalidomide

Increased Effect/Toxicity

Propofol may increase the levels/effects of: Alcohol (Ethyl); ARIPiprazole; Azelastine (Nasal); Buprenorphine; CNS Depressants; Dofetilide; Hydrocodone; Lomitapide; Methotrimeprazine; Metyrosine; Midazolam; Mirtazapine; Orphenadrine; Paraldehyde; Pimozide; Pramipexole; ROPINIRole; Ropivacaine; Rotigotine; Selective Serotonin Reuptake Inhibitors; Suvorexant; Thalidomide; Zolpidem

The levels/effects of Propofol may be increased by: Alfentanil; Brimonidine (Topical); Cannabis; CYP2B6 Inhibitors (Moderate); Doxylamine; Dronabinol; Droperidol; HydrOXYzine; Kava Kava; Magnesium Sulfate; Methotrimeprazine; Midazolam; Nabilone; Perampanel; Quazepam; Rifampin; Rufinamide; Sodium Oxybate; Tapentadol; Tetrahydrocannabinol

Decreased Effect There are no known significant interactions involving a decrease in effect.

Food Interactions Edetate disodium, an ingredient of propofol emulsion, may lead to decreased zinc levels in patients on prolonged therapy (>5 days) or those predisposed to deficiency (burns, diarrhea, and/or major sepsis). Management: Zinc replacement therapy may be needed.

Preparation for Administration Does not need to be diluted; however, propofol may be further diluted in 5% dextrose in water to a concentration of ≥2 mg/mL.

Storage/Stability Store between 4°C to 22°C (40°F to 72°F); refrigeration is not required. Do not freeze. If transferred to a syringe or other container prior to administration, use within 6 hours. If used directly from vial/prefilled syringe, use within 12 hours. If diluted in 5% dextrose stable for 8 hours at room temperature. Shake well before use. Do not use if there is evidence of separation of phases of emulsion.

Mechanism of Action Propofol is a short-acting, lipophilic intravenous general anesthetic. The drug is unrelated to any of the currently used barbiturate, opioid, benzodiazepine, arylcyclohexylamine, or imidazole intravenous anesthetic agents. Propofol causes global CNS depression, presumably through agonism of $GABA_A$ receptors and perhaps reduced glutamatergic activity through NMDA receptor blockade.

Pharmacodynamics/Kinetics

Onset of action: Anesthetic: Bolus infusion (dose dependent): 9-51 seconds (average 30 seconds)

Duration (dose and rate dependent): 3-10 minutes

Distribution: V_d: 2-10 L/kg; after a 10-day infusion, V_d approaches 60 L/kg; decreased in the elderly

Protein binding: 97% to 99%

Metabolism: Hepatic to water-soluble sulfate and glucuronide conjugates (~50%)

Half-life elimination: Biphasic: Initial: 40 minutes; Terminal: 4-7 hours (after 10-day infusion, may be up to 1-3 days)

Excretion: Urine (~88% as metabolites, 40% as glucuronide metabolite); feces (<2%)

Dosage Consult local regulations and individual institutional policies and procedures. Dosage must be individualized based on total body weight and titrated to the desired clinical effect. Wait at least 3-5 minutes between dosage adjustments to clinically assess drug effects. Smaller doses are required when used with opioids; the following are general dosing guidelines:

General anesthesia: Note: Increase dose in patients with chronic alcoholism (Fassoulaki, 1993); decrease dose with acutely intoxicated (alcoholic) patients.

Induction of general anesthesia: IV:

Children (healthy) 3-16 years, ASA-PS 1 or 2: 2.5-3.5 mg/kg over 20-30 seconds; use a lower dose for children ASA-PS 3 or 4

Adults (healthy), ASA-PS 1 or 2, <55 years: 2-2.5 mg/kg (~40 mg every 10 seconds until onset of induction)

Elderly, debilitated, or ASA-PS 3 or 4: 1-1.5 mg/kg (~20 mg every 10 seconds until onset of induction)

Maintenance of general anesthesia: IV infusion:

Children (healthy) 2 months to 16 years, ASA-PS 1 or 2: 125-300 mcg/kg/minute (or 7.5-18 mg/kg/**hour**); after 30 minutes, if clinical signs of light anesthesia are absent, decrease the infusion rate. Children ≤5 years may require larger infusion rates compared to older children.

Adults (healthy), ASA-PS 1 or 2, <55 years: Initial: 100-200 mcg/kg/minute (or 6-12 mg/kg/**hour**) for 10-15 minutes; usual maintenance infusion rate: 50-100 mcg/kg/minute (or 3-6 mg/kg/**hour**) to optimize recovery time

Elderly, debilitated, ASA-PS 3 or 4: 50-100 mcg/kg/minute (or 3-6 mg/kg/**hour**)

Maintenance of general anesthesia: IV intermittent bolus:

Adults (healthy), ASA-PS 1 or 2, <55 years: 25-50 mg increments as needed

Monitored anesthesia care sedation:

Adults (healthy), ASA-PS 1 or 2, <55 years: Slow IV infusion: 100-150 mcg/kg/minute (or 6-9 mg/kg/**hour**) for 3-5 minutes **or** slow injection: 0.5 mg/kg over 3-5 minutes followed by IV infusion of 25-75 mcg/kg/minute (or 1.5-4.5 mg/kg/**hour**) **or** incremental bolus doses: 10 mg or 20 mg

Elderly, debilitated, or ASA-PS 3 or 4 patients: Use 80% of healthy adult dose

ICU sedation in intubated mechanically-ventilated patients: Avoid rapid bolus injection; individualize dose and titrate to response.

Adults: Continuous infusion: Initial: 5 mcg/kg/minute (or 0.3 mg/kg/**hour**); increase by 5-10 mcg/kg/minute (or 0.3-0.6 mg/kg/**hour**) every 5-10 minutes until desired sedation level is achieved; usual maintenance: 5-50 mcg/kg/minute (or 0.3-3 mg/kg/**hour**); reduce dose after adequate sedation established and adjust to response (eg, evaluate frequently to use minimum dose for sedation). Daily interruption with retitration or a light target level of sedation is recommended to minimize prolonged sedative effects (Barr, 2013).

Elderly, debilitated, ASA-PS 3 or 4: Continuous infusion: Use 80% of healthy adult dose; reduce dose after adequate sedation established and adjust to response (eg, evaluate frequently to use minimum dose for sedation). Daily interruption with retitration or a light target level of sedation is recommended to minimize prolonged sedative effects (Barr, 2013).

Postoperative nausea and vomiting (PONV), rescue therapy (off-label use; Gan, 2007; Unlugenc, 2004):

Adults: IV: 20 mg, may be repeated

Refractory status epilepticus (off-label use): Adults: 1-2 mg/kg bolus (optional), then 33-167 mcg/kg/minute (or 2-10 mg/kg/**hour**) (Claassen, 2002; Kälviäinen, 2007; Meierkord, 2010; Rossetti, 2004); titrate to desired effect (eg, burst suppression on EEG). **Note:** Doses >83 mcg/kg/minute (or >5 mg/kg/**hour**) may increase the risk of hypotension and propofol-related infusion syndrome (PRIS) especially if used for >48 hours; consider alternative therapies to avoid the risk of PRIS in longer term propofol infusions.

Dosing adjustment in renal impairment: No dosage adjustment necessary.

Dosing adjustment in hepatic impairment: No dosage adjustment necessary.

Dietary Considerations Propofol is formulated in an oil-in-water emulsion. If on parenteral nutrition, may need to adjust the amount of lipid infused. Propofol emulsion contains 1.1 kcal/mL. Soybean fat emulsion is used as a vehicle for propofol. Formulations also contain egg phosphatide and glycerol.

Administration Consult local regulations and individual institutional policies and procedures. Strict aseptic technique must be maintained in handling although a preservative has been added. Do not use if contamination is suspected. Do not administer through the same IV catheter with blood or plasma. Tubing and any unused portions of propofol vials should be discarded after 12 hours.

To reduce pain associated with injection, use larger veins of forearm or antecubital fossa; lidocaine IV (1 mL of a 1% solution) may also be used prior to administration or it may be added to propofol immediately before administration in a quantity not to exceed 20 mg lidocaine per 200 mg propofol. Do not use filter <5 micron for administration.

Monitoring Parameters Cardiac monitor, blood pressure, oxygen saturation (during monitored anesthesia care sedation), arterial blood gas (with prolonged infusions). With prolonged infusions (eg, ICU sedation), monitor for metabolic acidosis, hyperkalemia, rhabdomyolysis or elevated CPK, hepatomegaly, and progression of cardiac and renal failure.

ICU sedation: Assess and adjust sedation according to scoring system (Richmond Agitation-Sedation Scale [RASS] or Sedation-Agitation Scale [SAS]) (Barr, 2013); assess CNS function daily. Serum triglyceride levels should be obtained prior to initiation of therapy and every 3-7 days thereafter, especially if receiving for >48 hours with doses exceeding 50 mcg/kg/minute (Devlin, 2005); use intravenous port opposite propofol infusion or temporarily suspend infusion and flush port prior to blood draw.

Diprivan®: Monitor zinc levels in patients predisposed to deficiency (burns, diarrhea, major sepsis) or after 5 days of treatment.

Dosage Forms

Emulsion, Intravenous:

Diprivan: 10 mg/mL (10 mL, 20 mL, 50 mL, 100 mL)

Generic: 10 mg/mL (20 mL, 50 mL, 100 mL)

Emulsion, Intravenous [preservative free]:

Fresenius Propoven: 10 mg/mL (20 mL, 50 mL, 100 mL)

Generic: 10 mg/mL (20 mL, 50 mL, 100 mL)

◆ **Propofol Injection (Can)** *see* Propofol *on page 1728*

Propranolol (proe PRAN oh lole)

Brand Names: U.S. Hemangeol; Inderal LA; Inderal XL; InnoPran XL

Brand Names: Canada Apo-Propranolol; Dom-Propranolol; Inderal; Inderal LA; Novo-Pranol; Nu-Propranolol; PMS-Propranolol; Propranolol Hydrochloride Injection, USP; Teva-Propranolol

Index Terms Hemangeol; Propranolol Hydrochloride

Pharmacologic Category Antianginal Agent; Antiarrhythmic Agent, Class II; Antihypertensive; Beta-Adrenergic Blocker, Nonselective

Use Management of hypertension; angina pectoris; pheochromocytoma; essential tremor; supraventricular arrhythmias (such as atrial fibrillation and flutter, AV nodal reentrant tachycardias), ventricular tachycardias (catecholamine-induced arrhythmias, digoxin toxicity); prevention of myocardial infarction; migraine headache prophylaxis; symptomatic treatment of hypertrophic subaortic stenosis (hypertrophic obstructive cardiomyopathy); treatment of proliferating infantile hemangioma requiring systemic therapy (Hemangeol only)

The 2014 guideline for the management of high blood pressure in adults (JNC 8) recommends initiation of pharmacologic treatment to lower blood pressure for the following patients (JNC8 [James, 2013]):

- Patients ≥ 60 years of age, with systolic blood pressure (SBP) ≥150 mm Hg or diastolic blood pressure (DBP) ≥90 mm Hg. Goal of therapy is SBP <150 mm Hg and DBP <90 mm Hg.
- Patients <60 years of age, with SBP ≥140 mm Hg or DBP ≥90 mm Hg. Goal of therapy is SBP <140 mm Hg and DBP <90 mm Hg.
- Patients ≥18 years of age with diabetes, with SBP ≥140 mm Hg or DBP ≥90 mm Hg. Goal of therapy is SBP <140 mm Hg and DBP <90 mm Hg.
- Patients ≥18 years of age with chronic kidney disease (CKD), with SBP ≥140 mm Hg or DBP ≥90 mm Hg. Goal of therapy is SBP <140 mm Hg and DBP <90 mm Hg.

In patients with chronic kidney disease (CKD), regardless of race or diabetes status, the use of an ACE inhibitor (ACEI) or angiotensin receptor blocker (ARB) as initial therapy is recommended to improve kidney outcomes. In the general nonblack population (without CKD) including those with diabetes, initial antihypertensive treatment should consist of a thiazide-type diuretic, calcium channel blocker, ACEI, or ARB. In the general black population (without CKD) including those with diabetes, initial antihypertensive treatment should consist of a thiazide-type diuretic or a calcium channel blocker **instead of** an ACEI or ARB.

Pregnancy Risk Factor C

Pregnancy Considerations Adverse events have been observed in some animal reproduction studies; therefore, the manufacturer classifies propranolol as pregnancy category C. Propranolol crosses the placenta and is measurable in the newborn serum following maternal use during pregnancy. In a cohort study, an increased risk of cardiovascular defects was observed following maternal use of beta-blockers during pregnancy. Intrauterine growth restriction (IUGR), small placentas, as well as fetal/neonatal bradycardia, hypoglycemia, and/or respiratory depression have been observed following *in utero* exposure to beta-blockers as a class. Adequate facilities for monitoring infants at birth should be available. Untreated chronic maternal hypertension and pre-eclampsia are also associated with adverse events in the fetus, infant, and mother. The peak maternal serum concentrations of propranolol and the active metabolite 4-hydroxypropranolol do not change during pregnancy; peak serum concentrations of naphthoxylactic acid are lower in the third trimester when compared to postpartum. Propranolol is recommended for use in the management of thyrotoxicosis in pregnancy. Propranolol has been evaluated for the treatment of hypertension in pregnancy, but other agents may be more appropriate for use. Propranolol has also been used in the management of hypertrophic obstructive cardiomyopathy in pregnancy and has been studied for use ▶

as an adjunctive agent in the management of dysfunctional labor (dystocia).

Breast-Feeding Considerations Propranolol is excreted into breast milk with peak concentrations occurring ~2-3 hours after an oral dose. The inactive metabolites of propranolol have also been detected in breast milk. The manufacturer recommends that caution be exercised when administering propranolol to nursing women. Due to immature hepatic metabolism in newborns, breast-feeding infants should be monitored for adverse events.

Contraindications

Hypersensitivity to propranolol, beta-blockers, or any component of the formulation; uncompensated congestive heart failure (unless the failure is due to tachyarrhythmias being treated with propranolol), cardiogenic shock; severe sinus bradycardia, sick sinus syndrome, or heart block greater than first-degree (except in patients with a functioning artificial pacemaker); bronchial asthma

Hemangeol (additional contraindications): Premature infants with corrected age <5 weeks; infants weighing <2 kg; heart rate <80 bpm; blood pressure <50/30 mm Hg; pheochromocytoma; history of bronchospasm

Warnings/Precautions Consider preexisting conditions such as sick sinus syndrome before initiating. Administer cautiously in compensated heart failure and monitor for a worsening of the condition (efficacy of propranolol in HF has not been demonstrated). **[U.S. Boxed Warning]: Beta-blocker therapy should not be withdrawn abruptly (particularly in patients with CAD), but gradually tapered to avoid acute tachycardia, hypertension, and/or ischemia.** Beta-blockers without alpha1-adrenergic receptor blocking activity should be avoided in patients with Prinzmetal variant angina (Mayer, 1998). Chronic beta-blocker therapy should not be routinely withdrawn prior to major surgery. May precipitate or aggravate symptoms of arterial insufficiency in patients with PVD and Raynaud's disease; use with caution and monitor for progression of arterial obstruction. Bradycardia may be observed more frequently in elderly patients (>65 years of age); dosage reductions may be necessary. Potentially significant drug-drug interactions may exist, requiring dose or frequency adjustment, additional monitoring, and/or selection of alternative therapy. Cigarette smoking may decrease plasma levels of propranolol by increasing metabolism. Patients should be advised to avoid smoking.

Use cautiously in patients with diabetes because it can mask prominent hypoglycemic symptoms. May mask signs of hyperthyroidism (eg, tachycardia); if hyperthyroidism is suspected, carefully manage and monitor; abrupt withdrawal may exacerbate symptoms of hyperthyroidism or precipitate thyroid storm. May alter thyroid-function tests. Use with caution in myasthenia gravis or psychiatric disease (may cause CNS depression). Use cautiously in renal and hepatic dysfunction; dosage adjustment may be required in hepatic impairment. In general, patients with bronchospastic disease should not receive beta-blockers; if used at all, should be used cautiously with close monitoring. Adequate alpha-blockade is required prior to use of any beta-blocker for patients with untreated pheochromocytoma. May induce or exacerbate psoriasis. Use caution with history of severe anaphylaxis to allergens; patients taking beta-blockers may become more sensitive to repeated challenges. Treatment of anaphylaxis (eg, epinephrine) in patients taking beta-blockers may be ineffective or promote undesirable effects.

Considerations when treating infantile hemangioma: Bradycardia and/or hypotension may occur or be worsened; monitor heart rate and blood pressure after propranolol initiation or increase in dose; discontinue treatment if severe (<80 bpm) or symptomatic bradycardia or hypotension (systolic blood pressure <50 mm Hg) occurs. Infants with large facial infantile hemangioma should be investigated for potential arteriopathy associated with PHACE syndrome prior to propranolol therapy; decreases in blood pressure caused by propranolol may increase risk of stroke in PHACE syndrome patients with cerebrovascular anomalies. May potentiate hypoglycemia and/or mask signs and symptoms. Withhold the dose in infants or children who are not feeding regularly or who are vomiting; discontinue therapy and seek immediate treatment if hypoglycemia occurs. May cause bronchospasm. Interrupt therapy in infants or children with lower respiratory tract infection associated with dyspnea or wheezing.

Adverse Reactions

Cardiovascular: Angina pectoris, atrioventricular conduction disturbance, bradycardia, cardiogenic shock, cold extremities, congestive heart failure, hypotension, ineffective myocardial contractions, syncope

Central nervous system: Agitation, amnesia, carpal tunnel syndrome, catatonia, cognitive dysfunction, confusion, dizziness, drowsiness, fatigue, hypersomnia, irritability, lethargy, nightmares, paresthesia, psychosis, sleep disorder, vertigo

Dermatologic: Changes in nails, contact dermatitis, dermal ulcer, eczematous rash, erosive lichen planus, hyperkeratosis, pruritus, skin rash

Endocrine & metabolic: Hyperglycemia, hyperkalemia, hyperlipidemia, hypoglycemia

Gastrointestinal: Abdominal pain, anorexia, constipation, decreased appetite, diarrhea, stomach discomfort

Genitourinary: Oliguria, proteinuria

Hematologic & oncologic: Immune thrombocytopenia, thrombocytopenia

Hepatic: Increased serum alkaline phosphatase, increased serum transaminases

Neuromuscular & skeletal: Arthropathy, oculomucocutaneous syndrome, polyarthritis

Ophthalmic: Conjunctival hyperemia, decreased visual acuity, mydriasis

Renal: Increased blood urea nitrogen, interstitial nephritis (rare)

Respiratory: Bronchiolitis (infants; associated with cough, fever, diarrhea, and vomiting), bronchitis (infants; associated with cough, fever, diarrhea, and vomiting), bronchospasm, dyspnea, pulmonary edema, wheezing

Miscellaneous: Ulcer

Rare but important or life-threatening: Agranulocytosis, alopecia, arterial insufficiency, arterial mesenteric thrombosis, decreased heart rate (infants), decreased serum glucose (infants), depression, emotional lability, epigastric distress, erythema multiforme, fever combined with generalized ache, sore throat, laryngospasm, and respiratory distress), hallucination, hypersensitivity reaction (including anaphylaxis, anaphylactoid reaction), impotence, insomnia, ischemic colitis, lupus-like syndrome, myotonia, myopathy, nonthrombocytopenic purpura, peripheral arterial disease (exacerbation), Peyronie's disease, pharyngitis, psoriasiform eruption, purpura, Raynaud's phenomenon, second degree atrioventricular block (infants; in a patient with an underlying conduction disorder), slightly clouded sensorium, Stevens-Johnson syndrome, systemic lupus erythematosus, temporary amnesia, tingling of extremities (hands), toxic epidermal necrolysis, urticaria, visual disturbance, weakness, xerophthalmia

Drug Interactions

Metabolism/Transport Effects Substrate of CYP1A2 (major), CYP2C19 (minor), CYP2D6 (major), CYP3A4 (minor); **Note:** Assignment of Major/Minor substrate status based on clinically relevant drug interaction potential; **Inhibits** CYP1A2 (weak), CYP2D6 (weak), P-glycoprotein

Avoid Concomitant Use

Avoid concomitant use of Propranolol with any of the following: Beta2-Agonists; Bosutinib; Ceritinib; Floctafenine; Methacholine; PAZOPanib; Silodosin; Topotecan; VinCRIStine (Liposomal)

Increased Effect/Toxicity

Propranolol may increase the levels/effects of: Afatinib; Alpha-/Beta-Agonists (Direct-Acting); Alpha1-Blockers; Alpha2-Agonists; Amifostine; Antihypertensives; Antipsychotic Agents (Phenothiazines); ARIPiprazole; Bosutinib; Bradycardia-Causing Agents; Brentuximab Vedotin; Bupivacaine; Cardiac Glycosides; Ceritinib; Cholinergic Agonists; Colchicine; Dabigatran Etexilate; Disopyramide; DOXOrubicin (Conventional); DULoxetine; Edoxaban; Ergot Derivatives; Everolimus; Fingolimod; Grass Pollen Allergen Extract (5 Grass Extract); Hypotensive Agents; Insulin; Lacosamide; Ledipasvir; Levodopa; Lidocaine (Systemic); Lidocaine (Topical); Mepivacaine; Methacholine; Midodrine; Naloxegol; Obinutuzumab; PAZOPanib; P-glycoprotein/ABCB1 Substrates; Prucalopride; Rifaximin; RisperiDONE; RiTUXimab; Rivaroxaban; Rizatriptan; Silodosin; Sulfonylureas; Topotecan; VinCRIStine (Liposomal); ZOLMitriptan

The levels/effects of Propranolol may be increased by: Abiraterone Acetate; Acetylcholinesterase Inhibitors; Alcohol (Ethyl); Alpha2-Agonists; Aminoquinolines (Antimalarial); Amiodarone; Anilidopiperidine Opioids; Antipsychotic Agents (Phenothiazines); Barbiturates; Bretylium; Brimonidine (Topical); Calcium Channel Blockers (Dihydropyridine); Calcium Channel Blockers (Nondihydropyridine); Cobicistat; CYP1A2 Inhibitors (Moderate); CYP1A2 Inhibitors (Strong); CYP2D6 Inhibitors (Moderate); CYP2D6 Inhibitors (Strong); Darunavir; Deferasirox; Diazoxide; Dipyridamole; Disopyramide; Dronedarone; Floctafenine; FluvoxaMINE; Herbs (Hypotensive Properties); Lacidipine; MAO Inhibitors; NiCARdipine; Nicorandil; Peginterferon Alfa-2b; Pentoxifylline; Phosphodiesterase 5 Inhibitors; Propafenone; Prostacyclin Analogues; QuiNIDine; Regorafenib; Reserpine; Selective Serotonin Reuptake Inhibitors; Tofacitinib; Vemurafenib; Zileuton

Decreased Effect

Propranolol may decrease the levels/effects of: Beta2-Agonists; Lacidipine; Theophylline Derivatives

The levels/effects of Propranolol may be decreased by: Alcohol (Ethyl); Barbiturates; Bile Acid Sequestrants; Cannabis; CYP1A2 Inducers (Strong); Cyproterone; Herbs (Hypertensive Properties); Methylphenidate; Nonsteroidal Anti-Inflammatory Agents; Peginterferon Alfa-2b; Rifamycin Derivatives; Teriflunomide; Yohimbine

Food Interactions

Ethanol: Ethanol may increase or decrease plasma levels of propranolol. Reports are variable and have shown both enhanced as well as inhibited hepatic metabolism (of propranolol). Management: Caution advised with consumption of ethanol and monitor for heart rate and/or blood pressure changes.

Food: Propranolol serum levels may be increased if taken with food. Protein-rich foods may increase bioavailability; a change in diet from high carbohydrate/low protein to low carbohydrate/high protein may result in increased oral clearance. Management: Tablets (immediate release) should be taken on an empty stomach. Capsules (extended release) may be taken with or without food, but be consistent with regard to food.

Storage/Stability

Injection: Store at 20°C to 25°C (68°F to 77°F); protect from freezing or excessive heat. Once diluted, propranolol is stable for 24 hours at room temperature in D_5W or NS. Protect from light. Solution has a maximum stability at pH of 3 and decomposes rapidly in alkaline pH.

Capsule, tablet, oral solution: Store at controlled room temperature; protect from freezing or excessive heat. Protect from light and moisture. Dispense Hemangeol in original container; discard 2 months after first opening.

Mechanism of Action Nonselective beta-adrenergic blocker (class II antiarrhythmic); competitively blocks response to $beta_1$- and $beta_2$-adrenergic stimulation which results in decreases in heart rate, myocardial contractility, blood pressure, and myocardial oxygen demand. Nonselective beta-adrenergic blockers (propranolol, nadolol) reduce portal pressure by producing splanchnic vasoconstriction ($beta_2$ effect) thereby reducing portal blood flow.

Pharmacodynamics/Kinetics

Onset of action: Beta-blockade: Oral: 1 to 2 hours

Duration: Immediate release: 6 to 12 hours; Extended-release formulations: ~24 to 27 hours

Absorption: Oral: Rapid and complete

Distribution: V_d: 4 L/kg (adults)

Protein binding: Newborns: 68%; Adults: ~90% (S-isomer primarily to $alpha_1$-acid glycoprotein; R-isomer primarily to albumin)

Metabolism: Hepatic via CYP2D6, and CYP1A2 to 4-hydroxypropranolol (active) and inactive compounds; extensive first-pass effect

Bioavailability: ~25% reaches systemic circulation due to high first-pass metabolism; protein-rich foods increase bioavailability by ~50%

Half-life elimination: Infants: ~3.5 hours (Hemangeol); Children: 3.9 to 6.4 hours; Adults: Immediate release formulation: 3 to 6 hours; Extended-release formulations: 8 to 10 hours

Time to peak: Immediate release: Adults: 1 to 4 hours; Infants: ≤2 hours (Hemangeol); Extended-release formulations: ~6 to 14 hours

Excretion: Metabolites are excreted primarily in urine (96% to 99%); <1% excreted in urine as unchanged drug

Dosage

Akathisia (off-label use): Oral: Adults: 30 to 120 mg/day in 2 to 3 divided doses

Essential tremor: Oral: Adults: 40 mg twice daily initially; maintenance doses: Usually 120 to 320 mg/day

Hypertension:

- Oral:
  - Children (off-label use): Initial: 0.5 to 1 mg/kg/day in divided doses every 6 to 12 hours; increase gradually every 5 to 7 days; maximum: 16 mg/kg/24 hours
  - Adults: Initial: 40 mg twice daily; increase dosage every 3 to 7 days; usual dose: 120 to 240 mg divided in 2 to 3 doses/day; maximum daily dose: 640 mg; usual dosage range (ASH/ISH [Weber, 2014]): 40 to 160 mg twice daily
    - Extended release formulations:
      - Inderal LA: Initial: 80 mg once daily; usual maintenance: 120 to 160 mg once daily; maximum daily dose: 640 mg
      - Inderal XL, InnoPran XL: Initial: 80 mg once daily at bedtime; if initial response is inadequate, may be increased at 2- to 3-week intervals to a maximum daily dose of 120 mg
  - Elderly: Consider lower initial doses and titrate to response (Aronow, 2011)

Hypertrophic subaortic stenosis: Oral: Adults: 20 to 40 mg 3 to 4 times/day

Inderal LA: 80 to 160 mg once daily

Migraine headache prophylaxis: Oral:

Children (off-label use): Initial: 2 to 4 mg/kg/day **or**

≤35 kg: 10 to 20 mg 3 times/day

>35 kg: 20 to 40 mg 3 times/day

Adults: Initial: 80 mg/day divided every 6 to 8 hours; increase by 20 to 40 mg/dose every 3 to 4 weeks to a maximum of 160 to 240 mg/day given in divided doses every 6 to 8 hours; if satisfactory response not achieved within 6 weeks of starting therapy, drug should be withdrawn gradually over several weeks

Inderal LA: Initial: 80 mg once daily; effective dose range: 160 to 240 mg once daily

Post-MI mortality reduction: Oral: Adults: Initial: 40 mg 3 times/day; usual dosage range: 180 to 240 mg/day in 3 to 4 divided doses

Pheochromocytoma: Oral: Adults: 30 to 60 mg/day in divided doses

Proliferating infantile hemangioma (Hemangeol): Oral: Infants ≥2 kg: **Note:** Initiate treatment at age 5 weeks to 5 months; doses should be administered at least 9 hours apart. Refer to product labeling for detailed weight-based dosing tabulation.

Week 1: 0.15 mL/kg (~0.6 mg/kg) twice daily

Week 2: 0.3 mL/kg (~1.1 mg/kg) twice daily

Week 3 (maintenance): 0.4 mL/kg (~1.7 mg/kg) twice daily; maintain this dose for 6 months. Readjust dose periodically as the child's weight increases. Treatment may be reinitiated if hemangiomas recur.

Stable angina: Oral: Adults: 80 to 320 mg/day in doses divided 2 to 4 times/day

Inderal LA: Initial: 80 mg once daily; maximum dose: 320 mg once daily

Tachyarrhythmias:

Oral:

Children (off-label use): Initial: 0.5 to 1 mg/kg/day in divided doses every 6 to 8 hours; titrate dosage upward every 3 to 7 days; usual dose: 2 to 6 mg/kg/day; higher doses may be needed; do not exceed 16 mg/kg/day or 60 mg/day

Adults: 10 to 30 mg/dose every 6 to 8 hours or a usual maintenance dose of 10 to 40 mg three or four times daily for rate control in patients with atrial fibrillation (AHA/ACC/HRS [January, 2014]).

Elderly: Initial: 10 mg twice daily; increase dosage every 3 to 7 days; usual dosage range: 10 to 320 mg given in 2 divided doses

IV:

Children (off-label use): 0.01 to 0.1 mg/kg/dose slow IVP over 10 minutes; maximum dose: 1 mg for infants; 3 mg for children

Adults: 1 to 3 mg/dose slow IVP; repeat every 2 to 5 minutes up to a total of 5 mg; titrate initial dose to desired response. **Note:** Once response achieved or maximum dose administered, additional doses should not be given for at least 4 hours.

or

0.5 to 1 mg over 1 minute; may repeat, if necessary, up to a total maximum dose of 0.1 mg/kg (ACLS guidelines, 2010)

or

1 mg over 1 minute; may be repeated every 2 minutes up to 3 doses for rate control in patients with atrial fibrillation (AHA/ACC/HRS [January, 2014]).

Elderly: Use caution; initiate at lower end of the dosing range.

Hypercyanotic spells (TOF) (off-label use): Children:

Oral: Palliation: Initial: 1 mg/kg/day every 6 hours; if ineffective, may increase dose after 1 week by 1 mg/kg/day to a maximum of 5 mg/kg/day; if patient becomes refractory, may increase slowly to a maximum of 10 to 15 mg/kg/day. Allow 24 hours between dosing changes.

IV: 0.01 to 0.2 mg/kg/dose infused over 10 minutes; maximum dose: 5 mg

Thyroid storm (off-label use):

Children: 0.5 mg/kg/dose every 4 to 8 hours; titrate to effective dose (Eyal, 2008)

Adults:

Oral: 60 to 80 mg every 4 hours; may consider the use of an intravenous shorter-acting beta-blocker (ie, esmolol) (Bahn, 2011)

IV: 0.5 to 1 mg administered over 10 minutes every 3 hours (Gardner, 2011)

Thyrotoxicosis (off-label use): Oral:

Children: 10 to 40 mg every 6 hours; titrate to effective dose (Eyal, 2008)

Adolescents and Adults: Oral: 10 to 40 mg/dose every 6 to 8 hours; may also consider administering extended or sustained release formulations (Bahn, 2011)

Variceal hemorrhage prophylaxis (off-label use; Garcia-Tsao, 2007): Oral: Adults:

Primary prophylaxis: Initial: 20 mg twice daily; adjust to maximal tolerated dose. **Note:** Risk factors for hemorrhage include Child-Pugh class B/C or variceal red wale markings on endoscopy.

Secondary prophylaxis: Initial: 20 mg twice daily; adjust to maximal tolerated dose

Dosage adjustment in renal impairment: There are no dosage adjustments provided in the manufacturer's labeling. However, renal impairment increases systemic exposure to propranolol. Use with caution.

Not dialyzable (0% to 5%); supplemental dose is not necessary.

Peritoneal dialysis effects: Supplemental dose is not necessary.

Dosage adjustment in hepatic disease: There are no dosage adjustments provided in the manufacturer's labeling. However, hepatic impairment increases systemic exposure to propranolol. Use with caution.

Dietary Considerations Tablets (immediate release) should be taken on an empty stomach; capsules (extended release) may be taken with or without food, but should always be taken consistently (with food or on an empty stomach). Hemangeol should be administered during or right after a feeding to reduce the risk of hypoglycemia; skip dose if child is not eating or is vomiting.

Administration

IV: IV dose is much smaller than oral dose. When administered acutely for cardiac treatment, monitor ECG and blood pressure. May administer by rapid infusion (IV push) at a rate of 1 mg/minute or by slow infusion over ~30 minutes. Necessary monitoring for surgical patients who are unable to take oral beta-blockers (prolonged ileus) has not been defined. Some institutions require monitoring of baseline and postinfusion heart rate and blood pressure when a patient's response to beta-blockade has not been characterized (ie, the patient's initial dose or following a change in dose). Consult individual institutional policies and procedures. Do not crush long-acting oral forms.

Oral: Tablets (immediate release) should be taken on an empty stomach; capsules (extended release) may be taken with or without food, but should always be taken consistently (with food or on an empty stomach). Do not crush long-acting oral forms.

Hemangeol should be administered during or right after a feeding to reduce the risk of hypoglycemia; skip dose if child is not eating or is vomiting. Administer doses at least 9 hours apart. Do not shake Hemangeol before use. Administer Hemangeol directly into the child's mouth using the supplied oral dosing syringe; if needed, may be diluted with a small quantity of milk or fruit juice and given in a baby's bottle.

Monitoring Parameters Acute cardiac treatment: Monitor ECG, heart rate, and blood pressure with IV administration; heart rate and blood pressure with oral administration

Consult individual institutional policies and procedures.

Hemangeol: Monitor heart rate and blood pressure for 2 hours after initiation or dose increases.

Reference Range Therapeutic: 50 to 100 ng/mL (SI: 190 to 390 nmol/L) at end of dose interval

Dosage Forms

Capsule Extended Release 24 Hour, Oral:
Inderal LA: 60 mg, 80 mg, 120 mg, 160 mg
Inderal XL: 80 mg, 120 mg
InnoPran XL: 80 mg, 120 mg
Generic: 60 mg, 80 mg, 120 mg, 160 mg

Solution, Intravenous:
Generic: 1 mg/mL (1 mL)

Solution, Oral:
Hemangeol: 4.28 mg/mL (120 mL)
Generic: 20 mg/5 mL (500 mL); 40 mg/5 mL (500 mL)

Tablet, Oral:
Generic: 10 mg, 20 mg, 40 mg, 60 mg, 80 mg

- **Propranolol Hydrochloride** *see* Propranolol *on page 1731*
- **Propranolol Hydrochloride Injection, USP (Can)** *see* Propranolol *on page 1731*
- **Proprinal® Cold and Sinus [OTC]** *see* Pseudoephedrine and Ibuprofen *on page 1743*
- **Propylene Glycol Diacetate, Acetic Acid, and Hydrocortisone** *see* Acetic Acid, Propylene Glycol Diacetate, and Hydrocortisone *on page 40*
- **2-Propylpentanoic Acid** *see* Valproic Acid and Derivatives *on page 2123*

Propylthiouracil (proe pil thye oh YOOR a sil)

Brand Names: Canada Propyl-Thyracil®

Index Terms PTU (error-prone abbreviation)

Pharmacologic Category Antithyroid Agent; Thioamide

Use Adjunctive therapy in patients intolerant of methimazole to ameliorate hyperthyroidism symptoms in preparation for surgical treatment or radioactive iodine therapy; treatment of hyperthyroidism in patients intolerant of methimazole and not candidates for surgical/radiotherapy

Pregnancy Risk Factor D

Pregnancy Considerations Propylthiouracil has been found to readily cross the placenta. Teratogenic effects have not been observed; however, nonteratogenic adverse effects, including fetal and neonatal hypothyroidism, goiter, and hyperthyroidism, have been reported following maternal propylthiouracil use. The transfer of thyroid-stimulating immunoglobulins can stimulate the fetal thyroid *in utero* and transiently after delivery and may increase the risk of fetal or neonatal hyperthyroidism.

Uncontrolled maternal hyperthyroidism may result in adverse neonatal outcomes (eg, prematurity, low birth weight) and adverse maternal outcomes (eg, pre-eclampsia, congestive heart failure, stillbirth, and abortion). To prevent adverse fetal and maternal events, normal maternal thyroid function should be maintained prior to conception and throughout pregnancy. Antithyroid treatment is recommended for the control of hyperthyroidism during pregnancy. Propylthiouracil is considered first-line therapy, especially during the first trimester. Due to an increased risk of liver toxicity, use of methimazole may be preferred during the second and third trimesters. If drug therapy is changed, maternal thyroid function should be monitored after 2 weeks and then every 2-4 weeks. Propylthiouracil, along with other medications, is used for the treatment of thyroid storm in pregnant women; alternative therapy is recommended if oral administration is not possible.

The pharmacokinetics of propylthiouracil are not significantly changed during pregnancy; however, the severity of hyperthyroidism may fluctuate throughout pregnancy. Doses of propylthiouracil may be decreased as pregnancy progresses and discontinued weeks to months prior to delivery.

Breast-Feeding Considerations Propylthiouracil is excreted in human breast milk; however, the infant dose is considered low and unlikely to affect infant thyroid hormones. The American Thyroid Association considers doses <300 mg/day to be safe during breast-feeding (Stagnaro-Green, 2011).

Contraindications Hypersensitivity to propylthiouracil or any component of the formulation

Warnings/Precautions Hazardous agent - use appropriate precautions for handling and disposal (NIOSH 2014 [group 2]).

[U.S. Boxed Warning]: Severe liver injury (some fatal) and acute liver failure (some cases requiring transplantation) have been reported. Patients should be counseled to recognize and report symptoms suggestive of hepatic dysfunction (especially in first 6 months of treatment), which should prompt immediate discontinuation. Routine liver function test monitoring may not reduce risk due to unpredictable and rapid onset.

Has been associated with significant bone marrow depression. The most severe manifestation is agranulocytosis (commonly within first 3 months of therapy). Aplastic anemia, thrombocytopenia, and leukopenia may also occur. Use with caution in patients receiving other drugs known to cause myelosuppression particularly agranulocytosis. Discontinue if significant bone marrow suppression occurs, particularly agranulocytosis or aplastic anemia.

Rare hypersensitivity reactions have been reported, including the development of ANCA-positive vasculitis, drug fever, interstitial pneumonitis, exfoliative dermatitis, glomerulonephritis, leukocytoclastic vasculitis, and a lupus-like syndrome; prompt discontinuation is warranted in patients who develop symptoms consistent with a form of autoimmunity or other hypersensitivity during therapy. May cause hypoprothrombinemia and bleeding.

Adverse Reactions

Cardiovascular: Periarteritis, vasculitis (ANCA-positive, cutaneous, leukocytoclastic)

Central nervous system: Drowsiness, drug fever, fever, headache, neuritis, vertigo

Dermatologic: Alopecia, erythema nodosum, exfoliative dermatitis, pruritus, skin pigmentation, skin rash, skin ulcers, urticaria

Endocrine & metabolic: Goiter, weight gain

Gastrointestinal: Constipation, loss of taste, nausea, sialoadenopathy, splenomegaly, stomach pain, taste perversion, vomiting

Hematologic: Agranulocytosis, aplastic anemia, bleeding, granulopenia, hypoprothrombinemia, leukopenia, thrombocytopenia

Hepatic: Acute liver failure, cholestatic jaundice, hepatitis

Neuromuscular & skeletal: Arthralgia, myalgia, paresthesia

Renal: Acute renal failure, glomerulonephritis, nephritis

Respiratory: Alveolar hemorrhage, interstitial pneumonitis

Miscellaneous: Lymphadenopathy, SLE-like syndrome

Drug Interactions

Metabolism/Transport Effects None known.

Avoid Concomitant Use

Avoid concomitant use of Propylthiouracil with any of the following: CloZAPine; Dipyrone; Sodium Iodide I131

Increased Effect/Toxicity

Propylthiouracil may increase the levels/effects of: Cardiac Glycosides; CloZAPine; Theophylline Derivatives

The levels/effects of Propylthiouracil may be increased by: Dipyrone

Decreased Effect

Propylthiouracil may decrease the levels/effects of: Sodium Iodide I131; Vitamin K Antagonists

Food Interactions Propylthiouracil serum levels may be altered if taken with food. Management: Administer at the same time in relation to meals each day, either always with meals or always between meals.

Storage/Stability Store at 25°C (77°F); excursions permitted to 15°C to 30°C (59°F to 86°F).

Mechanism of Action Inhibits the synthesis of thyroid hormones by blocking the oxidation of iodine in the thyroid gland; blocks synthesis of thyroxine and triiodothyronine

Pharmacodynamics/Kinetics

Duration: 12-24 hours
Distribution: Concentrated in the thyroid gland
Protein binding: 80% to 85%
Metabolism: Hepatic
Bioavailability: 53% to 88%
Half-life elimination: ~1 hour
Time to peak, serum: 1-2 hours
Excretion: Urine (35%; primarily as metabolites)

Dosage Oral: Administer in equally divided doses every 8 hours. Adjust dosage to maintain T_3, T_4, and TSH levels in normal range; elevated T_3 may be sole indicator of inadequate treatment. Elevated TSH indicates excessive antithyroid treatment.

Children: Initial: 5-7 mg/kg/day **or** 150-200 mg/m^2/day in divided doses every 8 hours

or

Manufacturer's recommendations:
6-10 years: 50-150 mg/day
>10 years: 150-300 mg/day

Adults:

Hyperthyroidism: Initial: 300 mg/day in 3 divided doses; 400 mg/day in patients with severe hyperthyroidism and/or very large goiters; an occasional patient will require 600-900 mg/day; usual maintenance: 100-150 mg/day

Graves' disease (off-label use): Initial: 50-150 mg (depending on severity) 3 times daily to restore euthyroidism; maintenance: 50 mg 2-3 times daily for a total of 12-18 months, then tapered or discontinued if TSH is normal at that time (Bahn, 2011)

Thyrotoxic crisis/thyroid storm (off-label use): **Note:** Recommendations vary widely and have not been evaluated in comparative trials. Typical dosing is 800-1200 mg/day given as 200-300 mg every 4-6 hours; some clinicians advocate an initial loading dose of 600-1000 mg. After initial response, dose may be reduced gradually to a maintenance dosage (100-600 mg/day in divided doses) (Goldberg, 2003; Nayak, 2006). The American Thyroid Association and the American Association of Clinical Endocrinologists recommend 500-1000 mg loading dose followed by 250 mg every 4 hours (Bahn, 2011).

Duration of therapy: Clinical improvement generally occurs in 1-3 months, after which dosage reduction may be employed (to prevent hypothyroidism), with discontinuation considered after 12-18 months of therapy. Thyroid function should be monitored every 2 months thereafter for 6 months until remission is confirmed, followed by annual evaluations (Cooper, 2005).

Dosage adjustment in renal impairment: No dosage adjustment provided in manufacturer's labeling.

Dosage adjustment in hepatic impairment: No dosage adjustment provided in manufacturer's labeling.

Dietary Considerations Take at the same time in relation to meals each day, either always with meals or always between meals.

Administration Administer at the same time in relation to meals each day, either always with meals or always between meals.

Hazardous agent; use appropriate precautions for handling and disposal (NIOSH 2014 [group 2]).

Monitoring Parameters CBC with differential, prothrombin time, liver function tests (bilirubin, alkaline phosphatase, transaminases), and thyroid function tests (TSH, T_3, T_4) every 4-6 weeks until euthyroid; periodic blood counts are recommended for chronic therapy

Reference Range Normal laboratory values:

Total T_4: 5-12 mcg/dL
Serum T_3: 90-185 ng/dL
Free thyroxine index (FT_4 I): 6-10.5
TSH: 0.5-4.0 microunits/mL

Additional Information Preferred over methimazole in thyroid storm due to inhibition of peripheral conversion as well as synthesis of thyroid hormone.

Graves' hyperthyroidism: Elevated T_3 may be the sole indicator of inadequate treatment. Elevated TSH indicates excessive antithyroid treatment. Monitoring of TSH is a poor indicator of treatment effectiveness, as levels may remain suppressed for months, despite euthyroid state (Cooper, 2005).

A potency ratio of methimazole to propylthiouracil of at least 20-30:1 is recommended when changing from one drug to another (eg, 300 mg of propylthiouracil would be roughly equivalent to 10-15 mg of methimazole) (Bahn, 2011).

Dosage Forms

Tablet, Oral:

Generic: 50 mg

Extemporaneous Preparations Hazardous agent; use appropriate precautions for handling and disposal (NIOSH 2014 [group 2]).

A 5 mg/mL oral suspension may be made with tablets and a 1:1 mixture of Ora-Plus® and Ora-Sweet®. Crush twenty 50 mg propylthiouracil tablets in a mortar and reduce to a fine powder. Add small portions of vehicle and mix to a uniform paste; mix while adding vehicle in incremental proportions to **almost** 200 mL; transfer to a calibrated bottle, rinse mortar with vehicle, and add quantity of vehicle sufficient to make 200 mL. Label "shake well" and "refrigerate". Stable for 91 days refrigerated (preferred) and 70 days at room temperature.

Nahata MC, Pai VB, and Hipple TF, *Pediatric Drug Formulations*, 5th ed, Cincinnati, OH: Harvey Whitney Books Co, 2004.

- **Propyl-Thyracil® (Can)** *see* Propylthiouracil *on page 1735*
- **2-Propylvaleric Acid** *see* Valproic Acid and Derivatives *on page 2123*
- **ProQuad** *see* Measles, Mumps, Rubella, and Varicella Virus Vaccine *on page 1274*
- **PRO-Quetiapine (Can)** *see* QUEtiapine *on page 1751*
- **PRO-Rabeprazole (Can)** *see* RABEprazole *on page 1762*
- **Pro-Ramipril (Can)** *see* Ramipril *on page 1771*
- **PRO-Risperidone (Can)** *see* RisperiDONE *on page 1818*
- **Proscar** *see* Finasteride *on page 878*
- **Prosed®/DS** *see* Methenamine, Phenyl Salicylate, Methylene Blue, Benzoic Acid, and Hyoscyamine *on page 1318*
- **ProSom** *see* Estazolam *on page 775*

- ◆ **PRO-Sotalol (Can)** *see* Sotalol *on page 1927*
- ◆ **Prostacyclin** *see* Epoprostenol *on page 746*
- ◆ **Prostacyclin PGI_2** *see* Iloprost *on page 1046*
- ◆ **Prostaglandin E_1** *see* Alprostadil *on page 96*
- ◆ **Prostaglandin E_2** *see* Dinoprostone *on page 640*
- ◆ **Prostaglandin F_2 Alpha Analog** *see* Carboprost Tromethamine *on page 360*
- ◆ **Prostaglandin F_2 Analog** *see* Carboprost Tromethamine *on page 360*
- ◆ **Prostate Cancer Vaccine, Cell-Based** *see* Sipuleucel-T *on page 1893*
- ◆ **Prostigmin** *see* Neostigmine *on page 1438*
- ◆ **Prostin E2** *see* Dinoprostone *on page 640*
- ◆ **Prostin E_2® (Can)** *see* Dinoprostone *on page 640*
- ◆ **Prostin VR** *see* Alprostadil *on page 96*

Protamine (PROE ta meen)

Index Terms Protamine Sulfate

Pharmacologic Category Antidote

Additional Appendix Information

Reversal of Oral Anticoagulants *on page 2235*

Use Treatment of heparin overdosage; neutralize heparin during surgery or dialysis procedures

Pregnancy Risk Factor C

Pregnancy Considerations Animal reproduction studies have not been conducted. In general, medications used as antidotes should take into consideration the health and prognosis of the mother; antidotes should be administered to pregnant women if there is a clear indication for use and should not be withheld because of fears of teratogenicity (Bailey, 2003). Protamine sulfate may be used during delivery to reduce the risk of bleeding following maternal use of heparin or low molecular weight heparin (LMWH) (Bates, 2012).

Breast-Feeding Considerations It is not known if protamine is excreted in breast milk. The manufacturer recommends that caution be exercised when administering protamine to nursing women.

Contraindications Hypersensitivity to protamine or any component of the formulation

Warnings/Precautions May not be totally effective in some patients following cardiac surgery despite adequate doses. May cause hypersensitivity reaction in patients (have epinephrine 1:1000 and resuscitation equipment available). **[U.S. Boxed Warning]: Hypotension, cardiovascular collapse, noncardiogenic pulmonary edema, pulmonary vasoconstriction, and pulmonary hypertension may occur. Risk factors for such events include: use of high doses or overdose, repeated doses, previous protamine administration (including protamine-containing drugs), fish allergy, vasectomy, severe left ventricular dysfunction, abnormal preoperative pulmonary hemodynamics.** Too rapid administration can cause severe hypotensive and anaphylactoid-like reactions. Heparin rebound associated with anticoagulation and bleeding has been reported to occur occasionally; symptoms typically occur 8-9 hours after protamine administration, but may occur as long as 18 hours later.

Adverse Reactions

Cardiovascular: Bradycardia, flushing, hypotension, sudden fall in blood pressure

Central nervous system: Lassitude

Gastrointestinal: Nausea, vomiting

Hematologic: Hemorrhage

Respiratory: Dyspnea, pulmonary hypertension

Miscellaneous: Hypersensitivity reactions

Drug Interactions

Metabolism/Transport Effects None known.

Avoid Concomitant Use There are no known interactions where it is recommended to avoid concomitant use.

Increased Effect/Toxicity There are no known significant interactions involving an increase in effect.

Decreased Effect There are no known significant interactions involving a decrease in effect.

Storage/Stability Refrigerate; do not freeze. Stable for at least 2 weeks at room temperature. Preservative-free formulation does not require refrigeration.

Mechanism of Action Combines with strongly acidic heparin to form a stable complex (salt) neutralizing the anticoagulant activity of both drugs

Pharmacodynamics/Kinetics

Onset of action: IV: Heparin neutralization: ~5 minutes

Half-life elimination: ~7 minutes

Dosage

Heparin neutralization: IV: Protamine dosage is determined by the dosage of heparin; 1 mg of protamine neutralizes ~100 units of heparin; maximum dose: 50 mg

Note: When heparin is given as a continuous IV infusion, only heparin given in the preceding several hours should be considered when administering protamine. For example, a patient receiving heparin at 1250 units/hour will require ~30 mg of protamine for reversal of heparin given in the last 2-2.5 hours (Garcia, 2012).

Heparin overdosage, following intravenous administration: IV: Since blood heparin concentrations decrease rapidly **after** administration, adjust the protamine dosage depending upon the duration of time since heparin administration as follows: See table.

Time Elapsed	Dose of Protamine (mg) to Neutralize 100 units of Heparin
Immediate	1-1.5
30-60 min	0.5-0.75
>2 h	0.25-0.375

Heparin overdosage, following SubQ injection: IV: 1-1.5 mg protamine per 100 units heparin; this may be done by a portion of the dose (eg, 25-50 mg) given slowly IV followed by the remaining portion as a continuous infusion over 8-16 hours (the expected absorption time of the SubQ heparin dose)

LMWH overdose (off-label use): IV: **Note:** Anti-Xa activity is never completely neutralized (maximum: ~60% to 75%). Excessive protamine doses may worsen bleeding potential.

Enoxaparin (Lovenox® prescribing information, 2011):

Enoxaparin administered in ≤8 hours: Dose of protamine should equal the dose of enoxaparin administered. Therefore, 1 mg of protamine sulfate neutralizes 1 mg of enoxaparin.

Enoxaparin administered in >8 hours or if it has been determined that a second dose of protamine is required (eg, if aPTT measured 2-4 hours after the first dose remains prolonged or if bleeding continues): 0.5 mg of protamine sulfate for every 1 mg of enoxaparin administered

Dalteparin or tinzaparin (Fragmin® prescribing information, 2010; Innohep® prescribing information, 2010): 1 mg protamine for each 100 anti-Xa units of dalteparin or tinzaparin; if PTT prolonged 2-4 hours after first dose (or if bleeding continues), consider additional dose of 0.5 mg for each 100 anti-Xa units of dalteparin or tinzaparin.

Dosage adjustment in renal impairment: No dosage adjustment provided in manufacturer's labeling.

Dosage adjustment in hepatic impairment: No dosage adjustment provided in manufacturer's labeling.

Administration For IV use only; **incompatible** with cephalosporins and penicillins; administer slow IVP (50 mg over 10 minutes); rapid IV infusion causes hypotension; inject without further dilution over 1-3 minutes; maximum of 50 mg in any 10-minute period

Monitoring Parameters Coagulation test, aPTT or ACT, cardiac monitor and blood pressure monitor required during administration

Dosage Forms

Solution, Intravenous:
Generic: 10 mg/mL (5 mL, 25 mL)

Solution, Intravenous [preservative free]:
Generic: 10 mg/mL (5 mL, 25 mL)

◆ **Protamine Sulfate** *see* Protamine *on page 1737*

◆ **Protease, Lipase, and Amylase** *see* Pancrelipase *on page 1566*

◆ **Protein C** *see* Protein C Concentrate (Human) *on page 1738*

◆ **Protein-Bound Paclitaxel** *see* PACLitaxel (Protein Bound) *on page 1554*

Protein C Concentrate (Human)

(PROE teen cee KON suhn trate HYU man)

Brand Names: U.S. Ceprotin

Index Terms Protein C

Pharmacologic Category Blood Product Derivative; Enzyme; Protein C

Use Replacement therapy for severe congenital protein C deficiency for the prevention and/or treatment of venous thromboembolism and purpura fulminans

Pregnancy Risk Factor C

Dosage Patient variables (including age, clinical condition, and plasma levels of protein C) will influence dosing and duration of therapy. Individualize dosing based on protein C activity and patient pharmacokinetic profile. Dosing is dependent on the severity of protein C deficiency, age of patient, clinical condition, and patient's level of protein C. The frequency, duration, and dose should be individualized.

IV: Children and Adults: Severe congenital protein C deficiency:

Acute episode/short-term prophylaxis: Initial dose: 100-120 units/kg (for determination of recovery and half-life)

Subsequent 3 doses: 60-80 units/kg every 6 hours (adjust to maintain peak protein C activity of 100%)

Maintenance dose: 45-60 units/kg every 6 or 12 hours (adjust to maintain recommended maintenance trough protein C activity levels >25%)

Long-term prophylaxis: Maintenance dose: 45-60 units/kg every 12 hours (recommended maintenance trough protein C activity levels >25%)

Note: Maintain target peak protein C activity of 100% during acute episodes and short-term prophylaxis. Maintain trough levels of protein C activity >25%. Higher peak levels of protein C may be necessary in prophylactic therapy of patients at increased risk for thrombosis (eg, infection, trauma, surgical intervention).

Dosage adjustment in renal impairment: No dosage adjustment provided in manufacturer's labeling (has not been studied). Patients with renal impairment should be monitored more closely for sodium overload.

Dosage adjustment in hepatic impairment: No dosage adjustment provided in manufacturer's labeling (has not been studied).

Additional Information Complete prescribing information should be consulted for additional detail.

Dosage Forms

Solution Reconstituted, Intravenous [preservative free]:
Ceprotin: 500 units (1 ea); 1000 units (1 ea)

◆ **Prothrombin Complex Concentrate (Caution: Confusion-prone synonym)** *see* Factor IX Complex (Human) [(Factors II, IX, X)] *on page 838*

◆ **Prothrombin Complex Concentrate (Caution: Confusion-prone synonym)** *see* Prothrombin Complex Concentrate (Human) [(Factors II, VII, IX, X), Protein C, and Protein S] *on page 1738*

Prothrombin Complex Concentrate (Human) [(Factors II, VII, IX, X), Protein C, and Protein S]

(PRO throm bin KOM pleks KON cen trate HYU man FAK ters too SEV en nyne ten PROE teen cee & PROE teen ess)

Brand Names: U.S. Kcentra

Brand Names: Canada Octaplex

Index Terms 4 Factor PCC; 4-Factor PCC; Beriplex P/N; Confidex; Four-Factor PCC; PCC (Caution: Confusion-prone synonym); Prothrombin Complex Concentrate (Caution: Confusion-prone synonym)

Pharmacologic Category Blood Product Derivative; Hemostatic Agent; Prothrombin Complex Concentrate (PCC)

Additional Appendix Information

Reversal of Oral Anticoagulants *on page 2235*

Use

Kcentra: Urgent reversal of acquired coagulation factor deficiency induced by vitamin K antagonist (VKA, eg, warfarin) therapy in patients with acute major bleeding or a need for an urgent surgery/invasive procedure

Octaplex (Canadian availability; not available in the U.S.): Prophylaxis (perioperative) and treatment of bleeding due to acquired deficiency (eg, treatment or overdose of VKA) of one or more of the prothrombin complex coagulation factors II, VII, IX, and X, when rapid correction of factor deficiency is necessary

Pregnancy Risk Factor C

Pregnancy Considerations Animal reproduction studies have not been conducted. Parvovirus B19 or hepatitis A, which may be present in plasma-derived products, may affect a pregnant woman more seriously than a nonpregnant woman.

Breast-Feeding Considerations It is not known if prothrombin complex concentrate is excreted in breast milk. The manufacturer recommends that PCC be administered only if clearly needed when treating a nursing woman.

Contraindications

Kcentra: Hypersensitivity (ie, anaphylaxis or severe systemic reaction) to prothrombin complex concentrate (PCC) or any component of the formulation including factors II, VII, IX, X, protein C and S, antithrombin III and human albumin; disseminated intravascular coagulation (DIC); known heparin-induced thrombocytopenia (product contains heparin).

Octaplex (Canadian availability; not available in the U.S.): Hypersensitivity to prothrombin complex concentrate (PCC) or any component of the formulation; heparin-induced thrombocytopenia type II or known allergy to heparin (product contains heparin); non-life-threatening bleeding episodes in individuals with recent myocardial infarction, high risk of thrombosis, or angina pectoris; non-life-threatening bleeding episodes in individuals with untreated disseminated intravascular coagulation (DIC) who can be given fresh frozen plasma (FFP); coagulation disorders due to chronic liver disease or liver transplantation; bleeding associated with hepatic parenchyme disorders, esophageal varices, or major hepatic surgery;

immunoglobulin A (IgA) deficiency, with known antibodies against IgA

Warnings/Precautions [U.S. Boxed Warning]: Because patients being treated with vitamin K antagonist (VKA) therapy have an underlying risk of or a diagnosed thromboembolic disease state, administration of prothrombin complex concentrate (PCC) may predispose the patient to a thromboembolic complication. Benefits of reversing VKA therapy should be weighed against the potential risk of a thromboembolic event. Resumption of anticoagulation should occur once the risk of thromboembolism outweighs the risk of acute bleeding. Fatal and nonfatal arterial and venous thromboembolic complications and DIC have been reported; closely monitor for thromboembolic events during and after administration. Use has not been evaluated in patients who have experienced a thromboembolic event, MI, DIC, CVA, TIA, unstable angina, or severe peripheral vascular disease within the prior 3 months. Administration of PCC may exacerbate underlying hypercoagulable states in recipients of vitamin K antagonists.

Prothrombin complex concentrate (Human) [(Factors II, VII, IX, X), Protein C, Protein S] (Kcentra, Octaplex) contains therapeutic levels of factor VII component and should not be confused with Factor IX complex (Human) [Factors II, IX, X] (Bebulin, Profilnine) which contains low or nontherapeutic levels of factor VII. Hypersensitivity reaction (eg, angioedema, bronchospasm, dyspnea, flushing, hypotension, nausea/vomiting, pulmonary edema, urticaria, tachycardia, tachypnea) may occur; if serious reaction occurs, discontinue administration and begin appropriate treatment. Since severe hypersensitivity and anaphylactic reactions may rarely occur with use; immediate medical treatment (including epinephrine 1:1000) should be readily available in the event of a severe reaction. May consider prophylactic treatment (eg, antihistamines, glucocorticoids) in patients predisposed to allergies. Formulations contain heparin.

Product of human plasma; may potentially contain infectious agents which could transmit disease. Screening of donors, as well as testing and/or inactivation or removal of certain viruses, reduces the risk. Infections thought to be transmitted by this product should be reported to the manufacturer. Octaplex (Canadian availability; not available in the U.S.) labeling recommends hepatitis B vaccination for all patients and hepatitis A vaccination for seronegative patients.

Hepatic synthesis of the prothrombin complex (Factors II, VII, IX and X) coagulation factors is vitamin K dependent. Severe hepatic dysfunction, inadequate absorption of vitamin K (eg, pancreatic disorders, diarrhea) or vitamin K antagonist therapy or overdose may lead to coagulation factor deficiencies. In patients with an acquired deficiency of the vitamin K-dependent coagulation factors, administer PCC only if a rapid correction (eg, emergency surgery, major bleeding) is necessary. If not indicated and caused by Vitamin K antagonist therapy, coagulation factor deficiencies may be managed by reducing or discontinuing therapy of the vitamin K antagonist and/or administration of vitamin K.

Octaplex (Canadian labeling): Development of antibodies to one or more of the human prothrombin factors may occur rarely, resulting in an inadequate clinical response; monitor for signs of antibody formation. Product labeling recommends monitoring antithrombin (AT) levels in patients being treated for bleeding as a result of chronic liver disease or liver transplantation. If AT levels are deficient, AT should be administered concomitantly with PCC. No clinical data are available for use of PCC to treat bleeding due to liver parenchyme disorders, major liver surgery, or esophageal varices; use of PCC for these indications is contraindicated and the preferred method of treatment is fresh frozen plasma (FFP).

Adverse Reactions

Cardiovascular: Arteriovenous fistula site complication (clot), atrial fibrillation, cerebrovascular accident, chest pain, deep vein thrombosis, hypertension, hypotension, pulmonary edema, pulmonary embolism, tachycardia, thrombosis (microthrombosis of toes), venous thrombosis (calf, radial vein)

Central nervous system: Headache, insomnia, intracranial hemorrhage, mental status changes

Endocrine & metabolic: Hypervolemia, hypokalemia

Gastrointestinal: Constipation, diarrhea, nausea and vomiting

Hematologic and oncologic: Anemia, prolonged bleeding time (skin laceration, contusion, subcutaneous hematoma)

Hepatic: Increased serum transaminases

Immunologic: Antibody development (parvovirus B19 seropositive)

Local: Burning sensation at injection site

Neuromuscular & skeletal: Arthralgia

Respiratory: Pleural effusion, rales, respiratory distress

Rare but important or life-threatening: Angioedema, arterial thrombosis, bronchospasm, disseminated intravascular coagulation, hypersensitivity reaction, myocardial infarction, peripheral ischemia, thromboembolic complications, thrombosis, transient ischemic attacks, venous insufficiency

Preparation for Administration Kcentra or Octaplex: Prior to reconstitution, allow diluent (SWFI) and prothrombin complex concentrate (PCC) vials to warm to room temperature. Aseptically push the plastic spike at the blue end of the Mix2Vial transfer set through the center of the stopper of the diluent vial. After carefully removing only the clear package from the Mix2Vial transfer set, invert the diluent vial with the transfer set still attached and push the plastic spike through the center of the stopper of PCC vial; diluent will automatically transfer. While still attached, gently swirl PCC vial to ensure product is dissolved; do not shake. Disconnect the 2 vials; contents of PCC vial are now available for removal by screwing a syringe onto the transfer set. Inject appropriate amount of air into vial, invert vial, and withdraw amount needed. Remove syringe from transfer set and attach an administration set to the syringe.

Note: Kcentra vials: Kcentra vials may contain differing amounts of factor IX units per vial. The exact amount of factor IX units in each vial should be used when calculating and preparing the total dose to be administered. Overdosage errors have occurred when the dose has been improperly calculated. (ISMP, 2014)

Storage/Stability

Kcentra: Store at 2°C to 25°C (36°F to 77°F); do not freeze. Protect from light. Reconstituted product may be stored at 2°C to 25°C (36°F to 77°F) and used within 4 hours following reconstitution. If cooled, warm to 20°C to 25°C (68°F to 77°F) prior to administration.

Octaplex (Canadian product labeling): Store at 2°C to 25°C (36°F to 77°F); do not freeze. Protect from light. Reconstituted solution should be administered immediately, but may be stored for up to 8 hours at 2°C to 25°C (36°F to 77°F) if sterility is maintained.

Mechanism of Action Prothrombin complex concentrate provides an increase in the levels of the vitamin K-dependent coagulation factors (II, VII, IX, and X) with the addition of protein C and protein S. Coagulation factors II, IX, and X are part of the intrinsic coagulation pathway, while factor VII is part of the extrinsic coagulation pathway. In the *extrinsic* pathway, damaged blood vessels release endothelial tissue factor (TF) which complexes with factor VII to form TF-factor VIIa. Within the *intrinsic* pathway, factor IX is converted to IXa. Factor IXa (as well as TF-factor VIIa) converts factor X to factor Xa in the final common pathway of coagulation. Factor Xa activates prothrombin (factor II) into thrombin (IIa) which converts fibrinogen into fibrin resulting in clot formation. Proteins C and S are vitamin K-dependent inhibiting enzymes involved in regulating the coagulation process. Protein S serves as a cofactor for protein C which is converted to activated protein C (APC). APC is a serine protease which inactivates factors Va and VIIIa, limiting thrombotic formation.

Pharmacodynamics/Kinetics

Onset of action: Rapid; significant INR decline within 10 minutes

Duration: ~6-8 hours

Distribution: V_{dss}: Factor II: 71.4 mL/kg; Factor VII: 45 mL/kg; Factor IX: 114.3 mL/kg; Factor X: 55.5 mL/kg; Protein C: 62.2 mL/kg; Protein S: 78.8 mL/kg

Half-life elimination: Factor II: 48–60 hours; Factor VII: 1.5-6 hours; Factor IX: 20-24 hours; Factor X: 24-48 hours; Protein C: 1.5–6 hours; Protein S: 24-48 hours

Note: Half-lives may be significantly reduced in severe hepatocellular damage, DIC, or extended catabolic metabolism.

Dosage Note: Prothrombin complex concentrate (Human) [(Factors II, VII, IX, X), Protein C, Protein S] (Kcentra, Octaplex) contains therapeutic levels of factor VII component and should not be confused with Factor IX complex (Human) [Factors II, IX, X] (Bebulin, Profilnine) which contains low or nontherapeutic levels of factor VII.

Kcentra: Vitamin K antagonist (VKA) reversal in patients with acute major bleeding or need for an urgent surgery/invasive procedure: Adults: IV: Individualize dosing based on current pre-dose INR. Dosage is expressed in units of factor IX activity. Administer with vitamin K concurrently. Repeat dosing is not recommended (has not been studied).

Pretreatment INR: 2 to <4: Administer 25 units/kg (maximum dose: 2500 units)

Pretreatment INR: 4-6: Administer 35 units/kg (maximum dose: 3500 units)

Pretreatment INR: >6: Administer 50 units/kg (maximum dose: 5000 units)

Octaplex (Canadian product labeling): Bleeding/perioperative prophylaxis of bleeding during vitamin K antagonist therapy: Individualize dosing based on severity of disorder, extent and location of bleeding, and clinical status of patient. Adolescents ≥17 years and Adults: IV: Approximate doses required for normalization of INR (≤1.2 within 1 hour):

Pretreatment INR: 2-2.5: Administer 22.5-32.5 units/kg (or 0.9-1.3 **mL**/kg)

Pretreatment INR: 2.5-3: Administer 32.5-40 units/kg (or 1.3-1.6 **mL**/kg)

Pretreatment INR: 3-3.5: Administer 40-47.5 units/kg (or 1.6-1.9 **mL**/kg)

Pretreatment INR: >3.5: Administer >47.5 units/kg (or >1.9 **mL**/kg)

Maximum dose: 3000 units (or 120 mL)

With the correction of vitamin K antagonist-induced impairment of hemostasis in patients who have been treated concomitantly with an appropriate vitamin K dose, repeat dosing with PCC is usually not necessary.

Dosing in obesity: Kcentra: In patients weighing >100 kg, do not exceed maximum dose.

Dosage adjustment in renal impairment: No dosage adjustment provided in manufacturer's labeling.

Dosage adjustment in hepatic impairment: No dosage adjustment provided in manufacturer's labeling.

Administration

Kcentra: IV: Administer at room temperature at a rate of 0.12 mL/kg/minute (~3 **units**/kg/minute); do **not** exceed 8.4 mL/minute (~210 **units**/minute). Do not allow blood to enter into syringe; since fibrin clot formation may occur.

Octaplex (Canadian product labeling): IV: Administer at a rate of 1 mL/minute initially, followed by 2-3 mL/minute. Reduce infusion rate or interrupt infusion if patient's pulse rate increases significantly.

Monitoring Parameters

Kcentra: INR (baseline and at 30 minutes post dose); clinical response during and after treatment

Octaplex (Canadian product labeling): Coagulation factor assays, protein C, protein S, aPTT, PT, INR, CBC, AT, D-dimer, fibrinogen; transaminases; development of circulating coagulation factor antibodies (inhibitors); heart rate (before and during administration)

Additional Information

Kcentra: Composition per 500-unit vial (exact potency of active and inactive components is listed on each container):

Factor II: 380-800 units
Factor VII: 200-500 units
Factor IX: 400-620 units
Factor X: 500-1020 units
Protein C: 420-820 units
Protein S: 240-680 units

Octaplex Composition per 500-unit vial (exact potency of active and inactive components is listed on each container):

Factor II: 280-760 units
Factor VII: 180-480 units
Factor IX: 500 units
Factor X: 360-600 units
Protein C: 140-620 units
Protein S: 140-640 units

Dosage Forms Considerations Kcentra strengths are expressed in terms of Factor IX activity units with nominal strength values of 500 units and 1000 units. Consult individual vial labels for exact potency within each vial.

Dosage Forms

Kit, Intravenous [preservative free]:

Kcentra: ~500 units, ~1000 units

Dosage Forms: Canada

Injection, powder for reconstitution:

Octaplex: Human coagulation factor II: 11-38 units/mL; factor VII: 9-24 units/mL; factor IX: 20-31 units/mL; factor X: 18-30 units/mL: protein C: 7-31 units/mL; protein S: 7-32 units/mL (20 mL)

- **Protonix** *see* Pantoprazole *on page 1570*
- **Protopam Chloride** *see* Pralidoxime *on page 1694*
- **Protopic** *see* Tacrolimus (Topical) *on page 1968*
- **Protopic® (Can)** *see* Tacrolimus (Topical) *on page 1968*
- **PRO-Topiramate (Can)** *see* Topiramate *on page 2065*
- **Pro-Triazide (Can)** *see* Hydrochlorothiazide and Triamterene *on page 1012*
- **Protrin DF (Can)** *see* Sulfamethoxazole and Trimethoprim *on page 1946*

Protriptyline (proe TRIP ti leen)

Brand Names: U.S. Vivactil [DSC]

Index Terms Protriptyline Hydrochloride

Pharmacologic Category Antidepressant, Tricyclic (Secondary Amine)

Additional Appendix Information

Beers Criteria – Potentially Inappropriate Medications for Geriatrics *on page 2271*

Use Depression: Treatment of depression

Dosage Depression:

Adolescents: Oral: Initial: 15 mg daily in 3 divided doses; gradually increase based on response and tolerability; maximum 60 mg/day. **Note:** Controlled clinical trials have not shown tricyclic antidepressants to be superior to placebo for the treatment of children and adolescents; not recommended as a first-line medication (Dopheide, 2006; Wagner, 2005)

Adults: Oral: Initial: 10 to 20 mg daily divided in 3 to 4 doses; gradually increase based on response and tolerability to a usual dose of 20 to 60 mg/day in 3 to 4 divided doses; maximum 60 mg/day (APA, 2010; Bauer 2013)

Elderly: Oral: Initial: 15 mg daily in 3 divided doses; gradually increase based on response and tolerability; maximum 60 mg/day. **Note:** Monitor cardiovascular system closely if daily dose exceeds 20 mg

Discontinuation of therapy: Upon discontinuation of antidepressant therapy, gradually taper the dose to minimize the incidence of withdrawal symptoms and allow for the detection of re-emerging symptoms. Evidence supporting ideal taper rates is limited. APA and NICE guidelines suggest tapering therapy over at least several weeks with consideration to the half-life of the antidepressant; antidepressants with a shorter half-life may need to be tapered more conservatively. In addition for long-term treated patients, WFSBP guidelines recommend tapering over 4-6 months. If intolerable withdrawal symptoms occur following a dose reduction, consider resuming the previously prescribed dose and/or decrease dose at a more gradual rate (APA, 2010; Bauer, 2002; Haddad, 2001; NCCMH, 2010; Schatzberg, 2006; Shelton, 2001; Warner, 2006).

MAO inhibitor recommendations:

Switching to or from an MAO inhibitor intended to treat psychiatric disorders:

Allow 14 days to elapse between discontinuing an MAO inhibitor intended to treat psychiatric disorders and initiation of protriptyline.

Allow 14 days to elapse between discontinuing protriptyline and initiation of an MAO inhibitor intended to treat psychiatric disorders.

Use with other MAO inhibitors (such as linezolid or IV methylene blue):

Do not initiate protriptyline in patients receiving linezolid or IV methylene blue; consider other interventions for psychiatric condition.

If urgent treatment with linezolid or IV methylene blue is required in a patient already receiving protriptyline and potential benefits outweigh potential risks, discontinue protriptyline promptly and administer linezolid or IV methylene blue. Monitor for serotonin syndrome for 2 weeks or until 24 hours after the last dose of linezolid or IV methylene blue, whichever comes first. May resume protriptyline 24 hours after the last dose of linezolid or IV methylene blue.

Dosage adjustment in renal impairment: There are no dosage adjustments provided in the manufacturer's labeling.

Dosage adjustment in hepatic impairment: There are no dosage adjustments provided in the manufacturer's labeling.

Additional Information Complete prescribing information should be consulted for additional detail.

Dosage Forms

Tablet, Oral:

Generic: 5 mg, 10 mg

- ◆ **Protriptyline Hydrochloride** *see* Protriptyline *on page 1740*
- ◆ **Protylol (Can)** *see* Dicyclomine *on page 622*
- ◆ **PRO-Valacyclovir (Can)** *see* ValACYclovir *on page 2119*
- ◆ **Provenge** *see* Sipuleucel-T *on page 1893*
- ◆ **Proventil HFA** *see* Albuterol *on page 69*
- ◆ **Provera** *see* MedroxyPROGESTERone *on page 1277*
- ◆ **Provera-Pak (Can)** *see* MedroxyPROGESTERone *on page 1277*
- ◆ **PRO-Verapamil SR (Can)** *see* Verapamil *on page 2154*
- ◆ **Provigil** *see* Modafinil *on page 1386*
- ◆ **Provil [OTC]** *see* Ibuprofen *on page 1032*
- ◆ **Provir** *see* Crofelemer *on page 514*
- ◆ **Provisc** *see* Hyaluronate and Derivatives *on page 1006*
- ◆ **Provocholine** *see* Methacholine *on page 1310*
- ◆ **Provocholine® (Can)** *see* Methacholine *on page 1310*
- ◆ **Proxymetacaine** *see* Proparacaine *on page 1728*
- ◆ **PROzac** *see* FLUoxetine *on page 899*
- ◆ **Prozac (Can)** *see* FLUoxetine *on page 899*
- ◆ **PROzac Weekly** *see* FLUoxetine *on page 899*
- ◆ **PRO-Zopiclone (Can)** *see* Zopiclone [CAN/INT] *on page 2217*
- ◆ **PRP-OMP (PedvaxHIB)** *see Haemophilus* b Conjugate Vaccine *on page 991*
- ◆ **PRP-T (ActHIB)** *see Haemophilus* b Conjugate Vaccine *on page 991*
- ◆ **PRP-T (Hiberix)** *see Haemophilus* b Conjugate Vaccine *on page 991*

Prucalopride [CAN/INT] (proo KAL oh pride)

Brand Names: Canada Resotran

Index Terms Prucalopride Succinate; R093877; R108512

Pharmacologic Category Serotonin 5-HT_4 Receptor Agonist

Use Note: Not approved in U.S.

Treatment of chronic idiopathic constipation in adult females with inadequate response to laxatives

Pregnancy Considerations Reproductive animal studies did not demonstrate adverse effects. Spontaneous abortion has been observed in pregnant women during clinical trials, although a causal association with prucalopride has not been established. Use during pregnancy is not recommended. Women of childbearing potential should employ effective contraception during therapy. An additional method of contraception is recommended for patients experiencing severe diarrhea and receiving oral contraceptives due to the potential for decreased efficacy of the oral contraceptive; cases of unintended pregnancies have been reported with prucalopride.

Breast-Feeding Considerations Prucalopride is excreted into breast milk. Breast-feeding is not recommended by the manufacturer.

Contraindications Hypersensitivity to prucalopride or any component of the formulation; renal impairment requiring dialysis; intestinal perforation or obstruction due to structural or functional disorder of the gut wall, obstructive ileus, severe inflammatory conditions of the GI tract (eg, Crohn disease, ulcerative colitis, toxic megacolon).

Warnings/Precautions Use with caution in patients with a history of arrhythmias, ischemic cardiovascular disease, pre-excitation syndromes (eg, Wolff-Parkinson-White syndrome), or A-V nodal rhythm disorders. Slight increases in heart rate and shortened PR intervals were observed in healthy subjects during clinical trials; treatment-related effects on QRS duration or QTc interval were not observed. Palpitations have also been observed; monitoring of cardiovascular status is recommended. Instruct patients to report severe or persistent palpitations.

Use with caution in renal impairment; manufacturer's labeling recommends a dose reduction in severe impairment; contraindicated in patients requiring dialysis. Use with caution in patients with severe and unstable concomitant disease (eg, cancer, AIDS, psychiatric, hepatic, pulmonary, insulin-dependent diabetes mellitus); has not been studied. Patients with severe or persistent diarrhea should discontinue therapy and consult healthcare provider. Ischemic colitis has not observed during clinical trials but is a potential concern with treatment; instruct patients with onset of severe or worsening GI symptoms, bloody diarrhea or rectal bleeding to discontinue treatment and consult healthcare provider.

Dizziness and fatigue have been observed with initiation of therapy (generally the first day of therapy); caution patients in regards to operating dangerous machinery or driving. May contain lactose; do not use in patients with galactose intolerance, Lapp lactase deficiency, or glucose-galactose malabsorption syndromes. Use with caution in the elderly (limited data); dose reductions may be necessary. Efficacy not established in males. Women of childbearing potential should use effective contraceptive methods during treatment. An additional method of contraception is recommended in patients receiving oral contraceptives who experience severe diarrhea (potential decreased efficacy of the oral contraceptive). Cases of unintended pregnancies have been reported with prucalopride. Use is not recommended in children <18 years of age.

Adverse Reactions

Cardiovascular: Palpitation (similar to placebo)

Central nervous system: Dizziness, fatigue, fever, headache, malaise

Gastrointestinal: Abdominal pain, diarrhea, nausea

Genitourinary: Pollakiuria

Gastrointestinal: Anorexia, bowel sounds abnormal, dyspepsia, flatulence, gastroenteritis, upper abdominal pain, vomiting

Neuromuscular & skeletal: Muscle spasms

Rare but important or life-threatening: Abdominoplasty, angina pectoris, anxiety, arrhythmias, atrial arrhythmias, bronchitis, chest pain, cholecystectomy, cholecystitis, cholelithiasis, colectomy, confusion, constipation, depression, dyspnea, hyperhidrosis, hysterectomy, MI, migraine, ovarian cyst, pancreatitis, pneumonia, pregnancy, sinusitis, spontaneous abortion, stomach discomfort, supraventricular tachycardia, syncope, tremor, urinary incontinence, urinary tract infection, vaginal hemorrhage

Drug Interactions

Metabolism/Transport Effects Substrate of P-glycoprotein

Avoid Concomitant Use There are no known interactions where it is recommended to avoid concomitant use.

Increased Effect/Toxicity

The levels/effects of Prucalopride may be increased by: P-glycoprotein/ABCB1 Inhibitors

Decreased Effect

Prucalopride may decrease the levels/effects of: Contraceptives (Estrogens); Contraceptives (Progestins)

Storage/Stability Store at 15°C to 30°C (59°F to 86°F). Store in original container to protect from moisture.

Mechanism of Action Prucalopride is a selective, high affinity 5-HT_4 receptor agonist whose action at the receptor site promotes cholinergic and nonadrenergic, noncholinergic neurotransmission by enteric neurons leading to stimulation of the peristaltic reflex, intestinal secretions, and gastrointestinal motility.

Pharmacodynamics/Kinetics

Absorption: Rapid

Distribution: V_d: 567 L

Protein binding: ~30%

Metabolism: Minor route of elimination; 8 metabolites produced (*in vitro* data suggest that 4 of 8 metabolites have lower or similar affinity to prucalopride for 5-HT_4 receptor)

Bioavailability: >90%

Half-life elimination: ~24 hours; terminal half-life increases to 34, 43, and 47 hours in mild, moderate, and severe renal impairment, respectively

Time to peak: 2-3 hours

Excretion: Primarily as unchanged drug: Urine (55% to 74%); feces (4% to 8%)

Dosage Oral:

Adults: Females (≥18 years): 2 mg once daily; **Note:** If no bowel movement within 3-4 days, consider adjunctive laxative therapy for acute treatment. Discontinue use if therapy is not effective within 4 weeks of initiation.

Elderly: Females (>65 years): Initial: 1 mg once daily; may increase to 2 mg once daily if necessary

Dosage adjustment in renal impairment:

Mild-moderate impairment: No dosage adjustment necessary

Severe impairment (GFR <30 mL/minute/1.73 m^2): 1 mg once daily

Dialysis: Use is contraindicated

Dosage adjustment in hepatic impairment: No dosage adjustment necessary.

Administration May administer without regard to meals. If a dose is missed, do not double to make up for a missed dose.

Monitoring Parameters Cardiovascular symptoms (eg, palpitations) particularly in patients with cardiovascular disease; frequency of bowel movements

Product Availability Not available in U.S.

Dosage Forms: Canada

Tablet, oral:

Resotran™: 1 mg, 2 mg [contains lactose]

◆ **Prucalopride Succinate** *see* Prucalopride [CAN/INT] *on page 1741*

◆ **Prudoxin** *see* Doxepin (Topical) *on page 678*

Prulifloxacin [INT] (pru li FLOKS a sin)

International Brand Names Aifude (CN); Chinoplus (PL); Darflox (TH); Glimbax (GR); Keraflox (IT, PT); Oliflox (PT); Prixina (PL); Prulif (IN); Puribact (IN); Unidrox (AT, CZ, HK, HU, IT); Xun Ao (CN)

Pharmacologic Category Antibiotic, Quinolone

Reported Use Treatment of complicated and uncomplicated urinary tract infections; chronic bronchitis

Dosage Range Adults: Oral:

Chronic bronchitis: 600 mg daily up to 10 days

Urinary Tract Infection:

Complicated: 600 mg daily up to 10 days

Uncomplicated: 600 mg daily

Product Availability Product available in various countries; not currently available in the U.S.

Dosage Forms

Tablet: 600 mg

◆ **Prussian Blue** *see* Ferric Hexacyanoferrate *on page 870*

◆ **Prymaccone** *see* Primaquine *on page 1713*

◆ **23PS** *see* Pneumococcal Polysaccharide Vaccine (23-Valent) *on page 1671*

◆ **PS-341** *see* Bortezomib *on page 276*

Pseudoephedrine (soo doe e FED rin)

Brand Names: U.S. Childrens Silfedrine [OTC]; Decongestant 12Hour Max St [OTC]; ElixSure Congestion [OTC]; Genaphed [OTC]; Nasal Decongestant [OTC]; Nexafed [OTC]; Psudatabs [OTC]; Shopko Nasal Decongestant

Max [OTC]; Shopko Nasal Decongestant [OTC]; Simply Stuffy [OTC]; Sudafed 12 Hour [OTC]; Sudafed 24 Hour [OTC]; Sudafed Childrens [OTC]; Sudafed [OTC]; Sudanyl [OTC]; SudoGest 12 Hour [OTC]; SudoGest [OTC]; Suphedrine [OTC]; Zephrex-D [OTC]

Brand Names: Canada Balminil Decongestant; Benylin® D for Infants; Contac® Cold 12 Hour Relief Non Drowsy; Drixoral® ND; Eltor®; PMS-Pseudoephedrine; Pseudofrin; Robidrine®; Sudafed® Decongestant

Index Terms *d*-Isoephedrine Hydrochloride; Pseudoephedrine Hydrochloride; Pseudoephedrine Sulfate; Sudafed

Pharmacologic Category Alpha/Beta Agonist; Decongestant

Use Temporary symptomatic relief of nasal congestion due to common cold, upper respiratory allergies, and sinusitis; also promotes nasal or sinus drainage

Dosage Oral: General dosing guidelines:

Children:

4-5 years: 15 mg every 4-6 hours: maximum: 60 mg/24 hours

6-12 years: 30 mg every 4-6 hours; maximum: 120 mg/24 hours

Children >12 years and Adults: Immediate release: 60 mg every 4-6 hours; Extended release: 120 mg every 12 hours **or** 240 mg every 24 hours; maximum: 240 mg/24 hours

Dosage adjustment in renal impairment: No dosage adjustment provided in manufacturer's labeling.

Dosage adjustment in hepatic impairment: No dosage adjustment provided in manufacturer's labeling.

Additional Information Complete prescribing information should be consulted for additional detail.

Dosage Forms

Gel, Oral:

ElixSure Congestion [OTC]: 15 mg/5 mL (120 mL)

Liquid, Oral:

Childrens Silfedrine [OTC]: 15 mg/5 mL (118 mL, 237 mL)

Nasal Decongestant [OTC]: 30 mg/5 mL (118 mL)

Sudafed Childrens [OTC]: 15 mg/5 mL (118 mL)

Syrup, Oral:

Nasal Decongestant [OTC]: 30 mg/5 mL (473 mL)

Tablet, Oral:

Genaphed [OTC]: 30 mg

Nasal Decongestant [OTC]: 30 mg

Psudatabs [OTC]: 30 mg

Shopko Nasal Decongestant Max [OTC]: 30 mg

Simply Stuffy [OTC]: 30 mg

Sudafed [OTC]: 30 mg

Sudanyl [OTC]: 30 mg

SudoGest [OTC]: 30 mg, 60 mg

Suphedrine [OTC]: 30 mg

Generic: 30 mg, 60 mg

Tablet Abuse-Deterrent, Oral:

Nexafed [OTC]: 30 mg

Zephrex-D [OTC]: 30 mg

Tablet Extended Release 12 Hour, Oral:

Decongestant 12Hour Max St [OTC]: 120 mg

Shopko Nasal Decongestant [OTC]: 120 mg

Sudafed 12 Hour [OTC]: 120 mg

SudoGest 12 Hour [OTC]: 120 mg

Generic: 120 mg

Tablet Extended Release 24 Hour, Oral:

Sudafed 24 Hour [OTC]: 240 mg

◆ **Pseudoephedrine and Chlorpheniramine** *see* Chlorpheniramine and Pseudoephedrine *on page* 427

◆ **Pseudoephedrine and Desloratadine** *see* Desloratadine and Pseudoephedrine *on page* 594

Pseudoephedrine and Dextromethorphan

(soo doe e FED rin & deks troe meth OR fan)

Brand Names: U.S. Pedia Relief Cough and Cold [OTC]; Sudafed® Children's Cold & Cough [OTC]

Brand Names: Canada Balminil DM D; Benylin® DM-D; Koffex DM-D; Novahistex® DM Decongestant; Novahistine® DM Decongestant; Robitussin® Childrens Cough & Cold

Index Terms Dextromethorphan and Pseudoephedrine

Pharmacologic Category Antitussive/Decongestant

Use Temporary symptomatic relief of nasal congestion and cough due to common cold, hay fever, upper respiratory allergies

Dosage Relief of nasal congestion and cough: Oral:

General dosing guidelines base on pseudoephedrine component:

Children 2-6 years: 15 mg every 4-6 hours (maximum: 60 mg/24 hours)

Children 6-12 years: 30 mg every 4-6 hours (maximum: 120 mg/24 hours)

Children ≥12 years and Adults: 60 mg every 4-6 hours (maximum: 240 mg/24 hours)

Product-specific dosing:

Children 2-6 years (Sudafed® Children's Cold & Cough): 5 mL every 4 hours (maximum: 20 mL/24 hours)

Children 6-12 years (Sudafed® Children's Cold & Cough): 10 mL every 4 hours (maximum: 40 mL/24 hours)

Children ≥12 years and Adults (Sudafed® Children's Cold & Cough): 20 mL every 4 hours (maximum: 80 mL/24 hours)

Additional Information Complete prescribing information should be consulted for additional detail.

Dosage Forms

Liquid:

Sudafed® Children's Cold & Cough [OTC]: Pseudoephedrine 15 mg and dextromethorphan 5 mg per 5 mL

Syrup:

Pedia Relief Cough and Cold [OTC]: Pseudoephedrine 15 mg and dextromethorphan 7.5 mg per 5 mL

◆ **Pseudoephedrine and Fexofenadine** *see* Fexofenadine and Pseudoephedrine *on page* 874

◆ **Pseudoephedrine and Guaifenesin** *see* Guaifenesin and Pseudoephedrine *on page* 989

Pseudoephedrine and Ibuprofen

(soo doe e FED rin & eye byoo PROE fen)

Brand Names: U.S. Advil® Cold & Sinus [OTC]; Proprinal® Cold and Sinus [OTC]

Brand Names: Canada Advil® Cold & Sinus; Advil® Cold & Sinus Daytime; Children's Advil® Cold; Sudafed® Sinus Advance

Index Terms Ibuprofen and Pseudoephedrine

Pharmacologic Category Decongestant/Analgesic

Use For temporary relief of cold, sinus, and flu symptoms (including nasal congestion, sinus pressure, headache, minor body aches and pains, and fever)

Dosage OTC labeling: Oral: Children ≥12 years and Adults: Ibuprofen 200 mg and pseudoephedrine 30 mg per dose: One dose every 4-6 hours as needed; may increase to 2 doses if necessary (maximum: 6 doses/24 hours). Contact healthcare provider if symptoms have not improved within 7 days when treating cold symptoms or within 3 days when treating fever.

Additional Information Complete prescribing information should be consulted for additional detail.

Dosage Forms

Caplet:

Advil® Cold & Sinus [OTC], Proprinal® Cold and Sinus [OTC]: Pseudoephedrine 30 mg and ibuprofen 200 mg

Capsule, liquid filled:

Advil® Cold & Sinus [OTC]: Pseudoephedrine 30 mg and ibuprofen 200 mg

◆ **Pseudoephedrine and Loratadine** *see* Loratadine and Pseudoephedrine *on page* 1242

◆ **Pseudoephedrine and Triprolidine** *see* Triprolidine and Pseudoephedrine *on page* 2105

◆ **Pseudoephedrine, Chlorpheniramine, and Dextromethorphan** *see* Chlorpheniramine, Pseudoephedrine, and Dextromethorphan *on page* 428

◆ **Pseudoephedrine, Codeine, and Triprolidine** *see* Triprolidine, Pseudoephedrine, and Codeine [CAN/INT] *on page* 2105

◆ **Pseudoephedrine, Dextromethorphan, and Guaifenesin** *see* Guaifenesin, Pseudoephedrine, and Dextromethorphan *on page* 989

◆ **Pseudoephedrine, Guaifenesin, and Codeine** *see* Guaifenesin, Pseudoephedrine, and Codeine *on page* 989

◆ **Pseudoephedrine Hydrochloride** *see* Pseudoephedrine *on page* 1742

◆ **Pseudoephedrine Hydrochloride and Acrivastine** *see* Acrivastine and Pseudoephedrine *on page* 46

◆ **Pseudoephedrine Sulfate** *see* Pseudoephedrine *on page* 1742

◆ **Pseudoephedrine, Triprolidine, and Codeine** *see* Triprolidine, Pseudoephedrine, and Codeine [CAN/INT] *on page* 2105

◆ **Pseudofrin (Can)** *see* Pseudoephedrine *on page* 1742

◆ **Pseudomonic Acid A** *see* Mupirocin *on page* 1404

◆ **Psudatabs [OTC]** *see* Pseudoephedrine *on page* 1742

Psyllium (SIL i yum)

Brand Names: U.S. Dietary Fiber Laxative [OTC]; Evac [OTC]; Fiber Therapy [OTC]; Geri-Mucil [OTC]; Konsyl [OTC]; Konsyl-D [OTC]; Metamucil MultiHealth Fiber [OTC]; Natural Fiber Therapy [OTC]; Natural Psyllium Seed [OTC]; Natural Vegetable Fiber [OTC]; Reguloid [OTC]; Sorbulax [OTC]

Brand Names: Canada Metamucil®

Index Terms Plantago Seed; Plantain Seed; Psyllium Husk; Psyllium Hydrophilic Mucilloid

Pharmacologic Category Antidiarrheal; Fiber Supplement; Laxative, Bulk-Producing

Use OTC labeling: Dietary fiber supplement; treatment of occasional constipation; reduce risk of coronary heart disease (CHD)

Dosage Oral: General dosing guidelines; consult specific product labeling.

Adequate intake for total fiber: Note: The definition of "fiber" varies; however, the soluble fiber in psyllium is only one type of fiber which makes up the daily recommended intake of total fiber.

Children 1-3 years: 19 g/day
Children 4-8 years: 25 g/day
Children 9-13 years: Males: 31 g/day; Females: 26 g/day
Children 14-18 years: Males: 38 g/day; Females: 26 g/day
Adults 19-50 years: Males: 38 g/day; Females: 25 g/day
Adults ≥51 years: Males: 30 g/day; Females: 21 g/day
Pregnancy: 28 g/day
Lactation: 29 g/day

Constipation:

Children 6-11 years: Psyllium: 1.25-15 g per day in divided doses
Children ≥12 years and Adults: Psyllium: 2.5-30 g per day in divided doses

Reduce risk of CHD: Children ≥12 years and Adults: Soluble fiber ≥7 g (psyllium seed husk ≥10.2 g) per day (DHHS, 1998)

Additional Information Complete prescribing information should be consulted for additional detail.

Dosage Forms Considerations Psyllium hydrophilic mucilloid 3.4 g is equivalent to 2 g Soluble fiber

Dosage Forms

Capsule, Oral:

Konsyl [OTC]: 520 mg
Reguloid [OTC]: 0.52 g

Packet, Oral:

Konsyl [OTC]: 28.3% (1 ea, 30 ea); 60.3% (1 ea, 30 ea); 100% (1 ea, 30 ea, 100 ea)

Powder, Oral:

Dietary Fiber Laxative [OTC]: 28.3% (283 g, 300 g, 425 g, 660 g)
Fiber Therapy [OTC]: 58.6% (283 g)
Geri-Mucil [OTC]: 68% (283 g, 284 g, 368 g)
Konsyl [OTC]: 28.3% (538 g); 30.9% (397 g); 60.3% (283 g, 450 g); 71.67% (300 g); 100% (300 g, 450 g)
Konsyl-D [OTC]: 52.3% (397 g)
Metamucil MultiHealth Fiber [OTC]: 58.6% (425 g); 63% (660 g)
Natural Fiber Therapy [OTC]: 30.9% (368 g, 539 g); 48.57% (368 g, 538 g)
Natural Psyllium Seed [OTC]: 100% (480 g)
Natural Vegetable Fiber [OTC]: 48.57% (368 g)
Reguloid [OTC]: 48.57% (369 g, 540 g); 58.6% (284 g, 426 g); 28.3% (369 g, 540 g)
Sorbulax [OTC]: 100% (420 g)

Powder, Oral [preservative free]:

Evac [OTC]: (480 g)

◆ **Psyllium Husk** *see* Psyllium *on page* 1744

◆ **Psyllium Hydrophilic Mucilloid** *see* Psyllium *on page* 1744

◆ **Pteroylglutamic Acid** *see* Folic Acid *on page* 919

◆ **PTG** *see* Teniposide *on page* 1997

◆ **PTU (error-prone abbreviation)** *see* Propylthiouracil *on page* 1735

◆ **Pulmicort** *see* Budesonide (Systemic) *on page* 293

◆ **Pulmicort Flexhaler** *see* Budesonide (Systemic) *on page* 293

◆ **Pulmicort Turbuhaler (Can)** *see* Budesonide (Systemic) *on page* 293

◆ **Pulmophylline (Can)** *see* Theophylline *on page* 2026

◆ **PulmoSal** *see* Sodium Chloride *on page* 1902

◆ **Pulmozyme** *see* Dornase Alfa *on page* 672

◆ **Puregon (Can)** *see* Follitropin Beta *on page* 921

◆ **Purg-Odan™ (Can)** *see* Sodium Picosulfate, Magnesium Oxide, and Citric Acid *on page* 1911

◆ **Purified Chick Embryo Cell** *see* Rabies Vaccine *on page* 1764

◆ **Purinethol** *see* Mercaptopurine *on page* 1296

◆ **Purixan** *see* Mercaptopurine *on page* 1296

◆ **PXD101** *see* Belinostat *on page* 236

Pyrantel Pamoate (pi RAN tel PAM oh ate)

Brand Names: U.S. Pamix [OTC]; Pin-X [OTC]; Reeses Pinworm Medicine [OTC]

Brand Names: Canada Combantrin

Pharmacologic Category Anthelmintic

Use Pinworms: Treatment of pinworms caused by *Enterobius vermicularis* (alternative agent; not preferred therapy)

Dosage Oral: Children ≥2 years, Adolescents, and Adults:

Note: Dose is expressed as pyrantel base; not preferred therapy since newer treatments are available.

Enterobius vermicularis (pinworm): 11 mg/kg administered as a single dose; maximum: 1 g per dose

Ancylostoma caninum (hookworm) (off-label use): 11 mg/kg (maximum: 1 g per dose) administered once daily for 3 days

Ancylostoma duodenale (hookworm), *Ascariasis lumbricoides* (roundworm), *Necator americanus* (hookworm) (off-label use): 11 mg/kg (maximum: 1 g/dose) administered once daily for 3 days (Kappagoda, 2011)

Moniliformis (off-label use): 11 mg/kg administered as a single dose; repeat twice 2 weeks apart

Trichostrongylus (off-label use): 11 mg/kg administered as a single dose; maximum: 1 g per dose

Dosage adjustment in renal impairment: There are no dosage adjustments provided in the manufacturer's labeling.

Dosage adjustment in hepatic impairment: There are no dosage adjustments provided in the manufacturer's labeling; use with caution.

Additional Information Complete prescribing information should be consulted for additional detail.

Dosage Forms

Suspension, Oral:

Pamix [OTC]: 50 mg/mL (30 mL, 60 mL, 240 mL)

Pin-X [OTC]: 50 mg/mL (30 mL, 60 mL)

Reeses Pinworm Medicine [OTC]: 50 mg/mL (30 mL)

Tablet, Oral:

Reeses Pinworm Medicine [OTC]: 62.5 mg

Tablet Chewable, Oral:

Pin-X [OTC]: 250 mg

Pyrazinamide (peer a ZIN a mide)

Brand Names: Canada Tebrazid™

Index Terms Pyrazinoic Acid Amide

Pharmacologic Category Antitubercular Agent

Use Adjunctive treatment of tuberculosis in combination with other antituberculosis agents

Pregnancy Risk Factor C

Pregnancy Considerations Teratogenic effects have not been observed in animal reproduction studies. Due to the risk of tuberculosis to the fetus, treatment is recommended when the probability of maternal disease is moderate to high. Although not recommended as the initial treatment regimen, the use of pyrazinamide during pregnancy is recommended by The World Health Organization (Blumberg, 2003).

Breast-Feeding Considerations Low concentrations of pyrazinamide have been detected in breast milk; concentrations are less than maternal plasma concentration (Holdiness, 1984). The amount of drug in breast milk is considered insufficient for the treatment of tuberculosis in breast-fed infants.

Contraindications Hypersensitivity to pyrazinamide or any component of the formulation; acute gout; severe hepatic damage

Warnings/Precautions Use with caution in patients with a history of alcoholism, renal failure, chronic gout, diabetes mellitus, or porphyria. Dose-related hepatotoxicity ranging from transient ALT/AST elevations to jaundice, hepatitis and/or liver atrophy (rare) has occurred. Use with caution in patients receiving concurrent medications associated with hepatotoxicity (particularly with rifampin). The 2-month rifampin-pyrazinamide regimen for the treatment of latent tuberculosis infection (LTBI) has been associated with severe and fatal liver injuries; incidence increased with pyrazinamide doses >30 mg/kg/day. The Infectious Diseases Society of America and Centers for Disease Control and Prevention recommend that the 2-month rifampin-pyrazinamide regimen should not generally be used in patients with LTBI.

Adverse Reactions

Central nervous system: Malaise

Gastrointestinal: Anorexia, nausea, vomiting

Neuromuscular & skeletal: Arthralgia, myalgia

Rare but important or life-threatening: Acne, angioedema (rare), anticoagulant effect, dysuria, fever, gout, hepatotoxicity, interstitial nephritis, itching, photosensitivity, porphyria, rash, sideroblastic anemia, thrombocytopenia, urticaria

Drug Interactions

Metabolism/Transport Effects None known.

Avoid Concomitant Use There are no known interactions where it is recommended to avoid concomitant use.

Increased Effect/Toxicity

Pyrazinamide may increase the levels/effects of: CycloSPORINE (Systemic); Rifampin

Decreased Effect There are no known significant interactions involving a decrease in effect.

Storage/Stability Store at controlled room temperature of 15°C to 30°C (59°F to 86°F).

Mechanism of Action Converted to pyrazinoic acid in susceptible strains of *Mycobacterium* which lowers the pH of the environment; exact mechanism of action has not been elucidated

Pharmacodynamics/Kinetics Bacteriostatic or bactericidal depending on drug's concentration at infection site

Absorption: Well absorbed

Distribution: Widely into body tissues and fluids including liver, lung, and CSF

Relative diffusion from blood into CSF: Adequate with or without inflammation (exceeds usual MICs)

CSF:blood level ratio: Inflamed meninges: 100%

Protein binding: 50%

Metabolism: Hepatic

Half-life elimination: 9-10 hours

Time to peak, serum: Within 2 hours

Excretion: Urine (4% as unchanged drug)

Dosage Oral: Treatment of tuberculosis:

Note: Used as part of a multidrug regimen. Treatment regimens consist of an initial 2-month phase, followed by a continuation phase of 4 or 7 additional months; pyrazinamide is administered in the initial phase of treatment.

Children:

HIV negative (CDC, 2003):

Daily therapy: 15-30 mg/kg/day (maximum: 2 g/day)

Twice weekly directly observed therapy (DOT): 50 mg/kg/dose (maximum: 2 g/dose)

HIV-exposed/-infected: Daily therapy: 20-40 mg/kg/dose once daily (maximum: 2 g/day) (CDC, 2009)

Adults: Suggested dosing based on lean body weight (Blumberg, 2003; CDC, 2003):

Daily therapy:

40-55 kg: 1000 mg

56-75 kg: 1500 mg

76-90 kg: 2000 mg (maximum dose regardless of weight)

Twice weekly directly observed therapy (DOT):

40-55 kg: 2000 mg

56-75 kg: 3000 mg

76-90 kg: 4000 mg (maximum dose regardless of weight)

Three times/week DOT:
40-55 kg: 1500 mg
56-75 kg: 2500 mg
76-90 kg: 3000 mg (maximum dose regardless of weight)

Dosage adjustment in renal impairment: Adults: CrCl <30 mL/minute or receiving hemodialysis: Treatment of TB: 25-35 mg/kg/dose 3 times per week administered after dialysis (Blumberg, 2003; CDC, 2003)

Dosage adjustment in hepatic impairment: No dosage adjustment provided in manufacturer's labeling. Use is contraindicated in cases of severe hepatic impairment.

Monitoring Parameters Periodic liver function tests, serum uric acid, sputum culture, chest x-ray 2-3 months into treatment and at completion

Dosage Forms

Tablet, Oral:
Generic: 500 mg

Extemporaneous Preparations A 100 mg/mL oral suspension may be made with tablets. Crush two-hundred pyrazinamide 500 mg tablets and mix with a suspension containing 500 mL methylcellulose 1% and 500 mL simple syrup. Add to this a suspension containing one-hundred forty crushed pyrazinamide tablets in 350 mL methylcellulose 1% and 350 mL simple syrup to make 1.7 L suspension. Label "shake well" and "refrigerate". Stable for 60 days refrigerated (preferred) and 45 days at room temperature.

Nahata MC, Morosco RS, and Peritre SP, "Stability of Pyrazinamide in Two Suspensions," *Am J Health Syst Pharm*, 1995, 52(14):1558-60.

◆ **Pyrazinoic Acid Amide** *see* Pyrazinamide *on page 1745*

Pyrethrins and Piperonyl Butoxide
(pye RE thrins & pi PER oh nil byo TOKS ide)

Brand Names: U.S. A-200 Lice Treatment Kit [OTC]; A-200 Maximum Strength [OTC]; LiceMD [OTC]; Licide [OTC]; Pronto Complete Lice Removal System [OTC]; Pronto Plus Lice Killing Mousse Plus Vitamin E [OTC]; Pronto Plus Lice Killing Mousse Shampoo Plus Natural Extracts and Oils [OTC]; Pronto Plus Warm Oil Treatment and Conditioner [OTC]; RID Maximum Strength [OTC]

Brand Names: Canada Pronto Lice Control; R & C II; R & C Shampoo/Conditioner; RID Mousse

Index Terms Piperonyl Butoxide and Pyrethrins

Pharmacologic Category Antiparasitic Agent, Topical; Pediculocide; Shampoo, Pediculocide

Use *Pediculus humanus* infestations: Treatment of *Pediculus humanus* infestations (head lice, body lice, pubic lice, and their eggs)

Dosage Treatment of *Pediculus humanus* infestations: Children ≥2 years, Adolescents, and Adults: Topical: Apply to dry hair and/or other infested area; allow to remain on area for 10 minutes and then wash and rinse; repeat treatment in 7 to 10 days.

Dosage adjustment in renal impairment: There are no dosage adjustments provided in the manufacturer's labeling.

Dosage adjustment in hepatic impairment: There are no dosage adjustments provided in the manufacturer's labeling.

Additional Information Complete prescribing information should be consulted for additional detail.

Dosage Forms

Kit:

A-200 Lice Treatment Kit [OTC]:
Shampoo: Pyrethrins 0.33% and piperonyl butoxide 4% (120 mL)
Solution: Permethrin 0.5% (180 mL)

LiceMD [OTC]:
Gel: Pyrethrins 0.33% and piperonyl butoxide 4% (118 mL)

Pronto Complete Lice Removal System [OTC]:
Shampoo: Pyrethrins 0.33% and piperonyl butoxide 4% (60 mL)
Solution, topical: Benzalkonium chloride 0.1% (60 mL)

Oil, topical:

Pronto Plus Warm Oil Treatment and Conditioner [OTC]: Pyrethrins 0.33% and piperonyl butoxide 4% (36 mL)

Shampoo:

A-200 Maximum Strength [OTC]: Pyrethrins 0.33% and piperonyl butoxide 4% (60 mL, 120 mL)

Licide [OTC], Pronto Plus Lice Killing Mousse Shampoo Plus Vitamin E [OTC]: Pyrethrins 0.33% and piperonyl butoxide 4% (120 mL)

Pronto Plus Lice Killing Mousse Shampoo Plus Natural Extracts and Oils [OTC]: Pyrethrins 0.33% and piperonyl butoxide 4% (60 mL)

Pronto Plus Lice Killing Mousse Shampoo Plus Vitamin E [OTC]: Pyrethrins 0.33% and piperonyl butoxide 4% (120 mL)

RID Maximum Strength [OTC]: Pyrethrins 0.33% and piperonyl butoxide 4% (60 mL, 120 mL, 180 mL, 240 mL)

◆ **Pyri 500 [OTC]** *see* Pyridoxine *on page 1747*

◆ **2-Pyridine Aldoxime Methochloride** *see* Pralidoxime *on page 1694*

◆ **Pyridium** *see* Phenazopyridine *on page 1629*

Pyridostigmine (peer id oh STIG meen)

Brand Names: U.S. Mestinon; Regonol

Brand Names: Canada Mestinon®; Mestinon®-SR

Index Terms Pyridostigmine Bromide

Pharmacologic Category Acetylcholinesterase Inhibitor

Use Symptomatic treatment of myasthenia gravis; antagonism of nondepolarizing neuromuscular blockers

Military use: Pretreatment for Soman nerve gas exposure

Pregnancy Risk Factor B

Pregnancy Considerations Safety has not been established for use during pregnancy. The potential benefit to the mother should outweigh the potential risk to the fetus. When pyridostigmine is needed in myasthenic mothers, giving dose parenterally 1 hour before completion of the second stage of labor may facilitate delivery and protect the neonate during the immediate postnatal state.

Breast-Feeding Considerations Neonates of myasthenia gravis mothers may have difficulty in sucking and swallowing (as well as breathing). Neonatal pyridostigmine may be indicated by symptoms (confirmed by edrophonium test).

Contraindications Hypersensitivity to pyridostigmine, bromides, or any component of the formulation; GI or GU obstruction

Warnings/Precautions Use with caution in patients with epilepsy, bradycardia, hyperthyroidism, cardiac arrhythmias, or peptic ulcer; use with extreme caution in patients with asthma or bronchospastic disease; adequate facilities should be available for cardiopulmonary resuscitation when testing and adjusting dose for myasthenia gravis; have atropine and epinephrine ready to treat hypersensitivity reactions; overdosage may result in cholinergic crisis, this must be distinguished from myasthenic crisis; anticholinesterase insensitivity can develop for brief or prolonged periods. Regonol injection must be administered by trained personnel.

Benzyl alcohol and derivatives: Some dosage forms may contain benzyl alcohol; large amounts of benzyl alcohol (≥99 mg/kg/day) have been associated with a potentially fatal toxicity ("gasping syndrome") in neonates; the "gasping syndrome" consists of metabolic acidosis, respiratory distress, gasping respirations, CNS dysfunction (including convulsions, intracranial hemorrhage), hypotension, and cardiovascular collapse (AAP, 1997; CDC, 1982); some data suggests that benzoate displaces bilirubin from protein binding sites (Ahlfors, 2001); avoid or use dosage forms containing benzyl alcohol with caution in neonates. See manufacturer's labeling.

Adverse Reactions

Cardiovascular: Arrhythmias (especially bradycardia), AV block, cardiac arrest, decreased carbon monoxide, flushing, hypotension, nodal rhythm, nonspecific ECG changes, syncope, tachycardia

Central nervous system: Convulsions, dizziness, drowsiness, dysphonia, headache, loss of consciousness

Dermatologic: Skin rash, thrombophlebitis (IV), urticaria

Gastrointestinal: Abdominal pain, diarrhea, dysphagia, flatulence, hyperperistalsis, nausea, salivation, stomach cramps, vomiting

Genitourinary: Urinary urgency

Neuromuscular & skeletal: Arthralgia, dysarthria, fasciculations, muscle cramps, myalgia, spasms, weakness

Ocular: Amblyopia, lacrimation, small pupils

Respiratory: Bronchial secretions increased, bronchiolar constriction, bronchospasm, dyspnea, laryngospasm, respiratory arrest, respiratory depression, respiratory muscle paralysis

Miscellaneous: Allergic reactions, anaphylaxis, diaphoresis increased

Drug Interactions

Metabolism/Transport Effects None known.

Avoid Concomitant Use There are no known interactions where it is recommended to avoid concomitant use.

Increased Effect/Toxicity

Pyridostigmine may increase the levels/effects of: Beta-Blockers; Cholinergic Agonists; Succinylcholine

The levels/effects of Pyridostigmine may be increased by: Corticosteroids (Systemic)

Decreased Effect

Pyridostigmine may decrease the levels/effects of: Anticholinergic Agents; Neuromuscular-Blocking Agents (Nondepolarizing)

The levels/effects of Pyridostigmine may be decreased by: Anticholinergic Agents; Dipyridamole; Methocarbamol

Storage/Stability

Injection: Protect from light.

Tablet:

30 mg: Store under refrigeration at 2°C to 8°C (36°F to 46°F). Protect from light. Stable at room temperature for up to 3 months.

Mestinon®: Store at 25°C (77°F). Protect from moisture.

Mechanism of Action Inhibits destruction of acetylcholine by acetylcholinesterase which facilitates transmission of impulses across myoneural junction

Pharmacodynamics/Kinetics

Onset of action: Oral, IM: 15-30 minutes; IV injection: 2-5 minutes

Duration: Oral: Up to 6-8 hours (due to slow absorption); IV: 2-3 hours

Absorption: Oral: Very poor

Distribution: 19 ± 12 L

Metabolism: Hepatic

Bioavailability: 10% to 20%

Half-life elimination: 1-2 hours; Renal failure: ≤6 hours

Excretion: Urine (80% to 90% as unchanged drug)

Dosage

Myasthenia gravis:

Oral:

Children: 7 mg/kg/24 hours divided into 5-6 doses

Adults: Highly individualized dosing ranges: 60-1500 mg/day, usually 600 mg/day divided into 5-6 doses, spaced to provide maximum relief

Sustained release formulation: Highly individualized dosing ranges: 180-540 mg once or twice daily (doses separated by at least 6 hours); **Note:** Most clinicians reserve sustained release dosage form for bedtime dose only.

IM, slow IV push:

Children: 0.05-0.15 mg/kg/dose

Adults: To supplement oral dosage pre- and postoperatively during labor and postpartum, during myasthenic crisis, or when oral therapy is impractical: ~1/30th of oral dose; observe patient closely for cholinergic reactions

or

IV infusion: Initial: 2 mg/hour with gradual titration in increments of 0.5-1 mg/hour, up to a maximum rate of 4 mg/hour

Reversal of nondepolarizing muscle relaxants: **Note:** Atropine sulfate (0.6-1.2 mg) IV immediately prior to pyridostigmine to minimize side effects: IV:

Children: Dosing range: 0.1-0.25 mg/kg/dose*

Adults: 0.1-0.25 mg/kg/dose; 10-20 mg is usually sufficient*

*Full recovery usually occurs ≤15 minutes, but ≥30 minutes may be required

Pretreatment for Soman nerve gas exposure (military use): Oral: Adults: 30 mg every 8 hours beginning several hours prior to exposure; discontinue at first sign of nerve agent exposure, then begin atropine and pralidoxime

Dosage adjustment in renal impairment: No dosage adjustment provided in manufacturer's labeling. However, lower dosages may be required due to prolonged elimination in renal impairment.

Dosage adjustment in hepatic impairment: No dosage adjustment provided in manufacturer's labeling.

Administration Do **not** crush sustained release tablet.

Monitoring Parameters Observe for cholinergic reactions, particularly when administered IV; consult individual institutional policies and procedures

Dosage Forms

Solution, Injection:

Regonol: 5 mg/mL (2 mL)

Syrup, Oral:

Mestinon: 60 mg/5 mL (473 mL)

Tablet, Oral:

Mestinon: 60 mg

Generic: 60 mg

Tablet Extended Release, Oral:

Mestinon: 180 mg

◆ **Pyridostigmine Bromide** *see* Pyridostigmine *on page 1746*

Pyridoxine (peer i DOKS een)

Brand Names: U.S. Neuro-K-250 T.D. [OTC]; Neuro-K-250 Vitamin B6 [OTC]; Neuro-K-50 [OTC]; Neuro-K-500 [OTC]; Pyri 500 [OTC]

Index Terms B6; B_6; Pyridoxine Hydrochloride; Vitamin B_6

Pharmacologic Category Vitamin, Water Soluble

Use Prevention and treatment of vitamin B_6 deficiency

Pregnancy Risk Factor A

Pregnancy Considerations Water soluble vitamins cross the placenta. Maternal pyridoxine plasma concentrations may decrease as pregnancy progresses and requirements may be increased in pregnant women (IOM, 1998). Pyridoxine is used to treat nausea and vomiting of pregnancy (Neibyl, 2010). In general, medications used as antidotes should take into consideration the health and prognosis of the mother; antidotes should be administered to pregnant women if there is a clear indication for use and should not be withheld because of fears of teratogenicity (Bailey, 2003).

Breast-Feeding Considerations Pyridoxine is found in breast milk and concentrations vary by maternal intake. Pyridoxine requirements are increased in nursing women compared to non-nursing women (IOM, 1998). Possible inhibition of lactation at doses >600 mg/day when taken immediately postpartum (Foukas, 1973).

Contraindications Hypersensitivity to pyridoxine or any component of the formulation

Warnings/Precautions Severe, permanent peripheral neuropathies have been reported; neurotoxicity is more common with long-term administration of large doses (>2 g/day). Dependence and withdrawal may occur with doses >200 mg/day. Single vitamin deficiency is rare; evaluate for other deficiencies. Some parenteral products contain aluminum; use caution in patients with impaired renal function and neonates.

Pharmacy supply of emergency antidotes: Guidelines suggest that at least 8-24 g be stocked. This is enough to treat 1 patient weighing 100 kg for an initial 8- to 24-hour period. In areas where tuberculosis is common, hospitals should consider stocking 24 g. This is enough to treat 1 patient for 24 hours (Dart, 2009).

Adverse Reactions

Central nervous system: Headache, seizure (following very large IV doses), somnolence
Endocrine & metabolic: Acidosis, folic acid decreased
Gastrointestinal: Nausea
Hepatic: AST increased
Neuromuscular & skeletal: Neuropathy, paresthesia
Miscellaneous: Allergic reactions

Drug Interactions

Metabolism/Transport Effects None known.

Avoid Concomitant Use There are no known interactions where it is recommended to avoid concomitant use.

Increased Effect/Toxicity There are no known significant interactions involving an increase in effect.

Decreased Effect

Pyridoxine may decrease the levels/effects of: Altretamine; Barbiturates; Fosphenytoin; Levodopa; Phenytoin

Storage/Stability Injection: Store at 20°C to 25°C (68°F to 77°F). Protect from light.

Mechanism of Action Precursor to pyridoxal, which functions in the metabolism of proteins, carbohydrates, and fats; pyridoxal also aids in the release of liver and muscle-stored glycogen and in the synthesis of GABA (within the central nervous system) and heme

Pharmacodynamics/Kinetics

Absorption: Enteral, parenteral: Well absorbed
Metabolism: Hepatic to pyridoxal phosphate and pyridoxamine phosphate (active forms)
Half-life elimination: Biologic: 15-20 days
Excretion: Urine

Dosage

Oral:

Adequate intake (AI) (IOM, 1998):
Infants:
1-6 months: 0.1 mg/day
7-12 months: 0.3 mg/day

Recommended daily allowance (RDA) (IOM, 1998):
Children:
1-3 years: 0.5 mg
4-8 years: 0.6 mg
9-13 years: 1 mg
14-18 years:
Females: 1.2 mg
Males: 1.3 mg
Adults:
19-50 years: 1.3 mg
≥51 years:
Females: 1.5 mg
Males: 1.7 mg
Pregnancy: 1.9 mg
Lactation: 2 mg

Prevention of peripheral neuropathy associated with isoniazid therapy for *Mycobacterium tuberculosis:*
Adults: 25-50 mg/day (CDC, 2009)

Treatment of nausea and vomiting of pregnancy (off-label use): 10 to 25 mg every 8 hours (Neibyl, 2010)

IM, IV: Dietary deficiency: Adults: 10-20 mg/day for 3 weeks, followed by oral therapy. Doses up to 600 mg/day may be needed with pyridoxine dependency syndrome.

IV:

Treatment of isoniazid-induced seizures and/or coma (off-label use):

Children:

Acute ingestion of known amount: Initial: A total dose of pyridoxine equal to the amount of isoniazid ingested (maximum dose: 70 mg/kg, up to 5 g); administer at a rate of 0.5-1 g/minute until seizures stop or the maximum initial dose has been administered; may repeat every 5-10 minutes as needed to control persistent seizure activity and/or CNS toxicity. If seizures stop prior to the administration of the calculated initial dose, infuse the remaining pyridoxine over 4-6 hours (Howland, 2006; Morrow, 2006).

Acute ingestion of unknown amount: Initial: 70 mg/kg (maximum dose: 5 g); administer at a rate of 0.5-1 g/minute; may repeat every 5-10 minutes as needed to control persistent seizure activity and/or CNS toxicity (Howland, 2006; Morrow, 2006; Santucci, 1999)

Adults:

Acute ingestion of known amount: Initial: A total dose of pyridoxine equal to the amount of isoniazid ingested (maximum dose: 5 g); administer at a rate of 0.5-1 g/minute until seizures stop or the maximum initial dose has been administered; may repeat every 5-10 minutes as needed to control persistent seizure activity and/or CNS toxicity. If seizures stop prior to the administration of the calculated initial dose, infuse the remaining pyridoxine over 4-6 hours (Howland, 2006; Morrow, 2006).

Acute ingestion of unknown amount: Initial: 5 g; administer at a rate of 0.5-1 g/minute; may repeat every 5-10 minutes as needed to control persistent seizure activity and/or CNS toxicity (Howland, 2006; Morrow, 2006)

Prevention of isoniazid-induced seizures and/or coma (off-label use): Children and Adults: Asymptomatic patients who present within 2 hours of ingesting a potentially toxic amount of isoniazid should receive a prophylactic dose of pyridoxine (Boyer, 2006). Dosing recommendations are the same as for the treatment of symptomatic patients.

Treatment of seizures from acute Gyromitrin-containing mushroom toxicity (off-label use): Children and Adults: 25 mg/kg over 15-30 minutes; repeat dose as needed to control seizures (Diaz, 2005)

Administration Burning may occur at the injection site after IM administration; seizures have occurred following IV administration of very large doses.

Isoniazid toxicity (off-label use): Initial doses should be administered at a rate of 0.5-1 g/minute. If the parenteral formulation is not available, anecdotal reports suggest that pyridoxine tablets may be crushed and made into a slurry and given at the same dose orally or via nasogastric (NG) tube (Boyer, 2006). Oral administration is not recommended for acutely poisoned patients with seizure activity.

Monitoring Parameters For treatment of isoniazid or Gyromitrin-containing mushroom toxicity: Anion gap, arterial blood gases, electrolytes, neurological exam, seizure activity

Reference Range Over 50 ng/mL (SI: 243 nmol/L) (varies considerably with method). A broad range is ~25-80 ng/mL (SI: 122-389 nmol/L). HPLC method for pyridoxal phosphate has normal range of 3.5-18 ng/mL (SI: 17-88 nmol/L).

Dosage Forms

Capsule, Oral:

Neuro-K-250 T.D. [OTC]: 250 mg

Solution, Injection:

Generic: 100 mg/mL (1 mL)

Tablet, Oral:

Neuro-K-50 [OTC]: 50 mg

Neuro-K-500 [OTC]: 500 mg

Neuro-K-250 Vitamin B6 [OTC]: 250 mg

Pyri 500 [OTC]: 500 mg

Generic: 25 mg, 50 mg, 100 mg, 250 mg

Tablet, Oral [preservative free]:

Generic: 25 mg, 50 mg, 100 mg

Tablet Extended Release, Oral:

Generic: 200 mg

Extemporaneous Preparations A 1 mg/mL oral solution may be made using pyridoxine injection. Withdraw 100 mg (1 mL of a 100 mg/mL injection) from a vial with a needle and syringe; add to 99 mL simple syrup in an amber bottle. Label "refrigerate". Stable for 30 days refrigerated.

Nahata MC, Pai VB, and Hipple TF, *Pediatric Drug Formulations*, 5th ed, Cincinnati, OH: Harvey Whitney Books Co, 2004.

◆ **Pyridoxine and Doxylamine** *see* Doxylamine and Pyridoxine *on page 693*

◆ **Pyridoxine, Folic Acid, and Cyanocobalamin** *see* Folic Acid, Cyanocobalamin, and Pyridoxine *on page 921*

◆ **Pyridoxine Hydrochloride** *see* Pyridoxine *on page 1747*

Pyrimethamine (peer i METH a meen)

Brand Names: U.S. Daraprim

Brand Names: Canada Daraprim [DSC]

Pharmacologic Category Antimalarial Agent

Use Prophylaxis of malaria due to susceptible strains of plasmodia; used in conjunction with a sulfonamide for the treatment of uncomplicated malaria due to susceptible strains of plasmodia (alternative agent; not preferred therapy); synergistic combination with sulfonamide in treatment of toxoplasmosis

Pregnancy Risk Factor C

Pregnancy Considerations Teratogenic effects have been observed in animal reproduction studies. If administered during pregnancy (ie, for toxoplasmosis), supplementation of folate is strongly recommended. Pregnancy should be avoided during therapy.

Breast-Feeding Considerations Pyrimethamine enters breast milk and may result in significant systemic concentrations in breast-fed infants. The effect of concurrent therapy with sulfonamide or dapsone (frequently used with pyrimethamine as combination treatment) must be considered.

Contraindications Hypersensitivity to pyrimethamine or any component of the formulation; megaloblastic anemia secondary to folate deficiency

Warnings/Precautions When used for more than 3-4 days, it may be advisable to administer leucovorin calcium to prevent hematologic complications due to pyrimethamine-induced folic acid deficiency-state; continue leucovorin during therapy and for 1 week after therapy is discontinued (to account for the long half-life of pyrimethamine) (DHHS [pediatric], 2013). Monitor CBC and platelet counts every 2 weeks in patients receiving high-dose therapy (eg, when used for toxoplasmosis treatment). Use with caution in patients with impaired renal or hepatic function or with possible G6PD. Use caution in patients with seizure disorders or possible folate deficiency (eg, malabsorption syndrome, pregnancy, alcoholism).

Adverse Reactions

Cardiovascular: Arrhythmias (large doses)

Dermatologic: Erythema multiforme, rash, Stevens-Johnson syndrome, toxic epidermal necrolysis

Gastrointestinal: Anorexia, atrophic glossitis, vomiting

Hematologic: Leukopenia, megaloblastic anemia, pancytopenia, pulmonary eosinophilia, thrombocytopenia

Genitourinary: Hematuria

Miscellaneous: Anaphylaxis

Drug Interactions

Metabolism/Transport Effects **Inhibits** CYP2C9 (moderate)

Avoid Concomitant Use

Avoid concomitant use of Pyrimethamine with any of the following: Artemether; Lumefantrine

Increased Effect/Toxicity

Pyrimethamine may increase the levels/effects of: Antipsychotic Agents (Phenothiazines); Bosentan; Cannabis; Carvedilol; CYP2C9 Substrates; Dapsone (Systemic); Dapsone (Topical); Dronabinol; Lumefantrine; Tetrahydrocannabinol

The levels/effects of Pyrimethamine may be increased by: Artemether; Dapsone (Systemic)

Decreased Effect

The levels/effects of Pyrimethamine may be decreased by: Methylfolate

Storage/Stability Store at 15°C to 25°C (59°F to 77°F). Protect from light.

Mechanism of Action Inhibits parasitic dihydrofolate reductase, resulting in inhibition of vital tetrahydrofolic acid synthesis

Pharmacodynamics/Kinetics

Onset of action: ~1 hour

Absorption: Well absorbed

Distribution: Widely, mainly in blood cells, kidneys, lungs, liver, and spleen; crosses into CSF

Protein binding: 80% to 87%

Metabolism: Hepatic

Half-life elimination: 80-95 hours

Time to peak, serum: 1.5-8 hours

Excretion: Urine (20% to 30% as unchanged drug)

Dosage Oral:

Isosporiasis (*Isospora belli* infection) in HIV-positive patients (off-label use; CDC, 2009): Adults:

Treatment (alternative to trimethoprim-sulfamethoxazole): 50-75 mg once daily in combination with leucovorin calcium

Chronic maintenance (secondary prophylaxis): 25 mg once daily in combination with leucovorin calcium

Malaria chemoprophylaxis: Begin prophylaxis before entering endemic area: **Note:** Current CDC recommendations for malaria prophylaxis do not include the use of pyrimethamine; resistance to pyrimethamine is prevalent worldwide.

Manufacturer's labeling:

Children <4 years: 6.25 mg once weekly

Children 4-10 years: 12.5 mg once weekly

Children >10 years and Adults: 25 mg once weekly

Malaria treatment (non-*falciparum* malaria; use in conjunction with a sulfonamide [eg, sulfadoxine]): Note: Current CDC recommendations for the malaria treatment do not include the use of pyrimethamine; resistance to pyrimethamine is prevalent worldwide.

Manufacturer's labeling:

Children 4-10 years: 25 mg daily for 2 days; following clinical cure, administer a once weekly chemoprophylaxis regimen for ≥10 weeks

Children >10 years and Adults: 25 mg daily for 2 days; following clinical cure, administer a once weekly chemoprophylaxis regimen for ≥10 weeks

Note: Pyrimethamine use alone is **not** recommended; if circumstances arise where it must be used alone in semi-immune patients, give adults 50 mg daily for 2 days (children receive 25 mg daily for 2 days), then (following clinical cure) administer a once-weekly chemoprophylaxis regimen for ≥10 weeks.

***Pneumocystis jirovecii* pneumonia (PCP) in HIV-positive patients (off-label use; CDC, 2009):** Adults:

Prophylaxis (alternative to trimethoprim-sulfamethoxazole): 50 mg once weekly in combination with dapsone and leucovorin calcium; **or** 25 mg once daily with atovaquone in combination with oral leucovorin calcium

Chronic maintenance (secondary prophylaxis; alternative to trimethoprim-sulfamethoxazole): 50-75 mg once weekly in combination with dapsone and leucovorin calcium; **or** 25 mg once daily with atovaquone in combination with leucovorin calcium

Toxoplasmosis treatment: *Manufacturer's labeling:*

Children: Loading dose: 1 mg/kg/day divided into 2 equal daily doses for 2-4 days, then may decrease dose to 0.5 mg/kg/day divided into 2 doses for 4 weeks; use with a sulfonamide in combination with leucovorin calcium

Adults: 50-75 mg/day for 1-3 weeks depending on patient's tolerance and response, then may reduce dose by 50% and continue for 4-5 weeks; use with a sulfonamide in combination with leucovorin calcium

Toxoplasmosis prophylaxis and treatment in HIV-positive patients (off-label; CDC, 2009):

Prophylaxis for first episode of Toxoplasma gondii:

Children ≥1 month of age: 1 mg/kg/day (or 15 mg/m^2) once daily (maximum: 25 mg), with dapsone or atovaquone in combination with leucovorin calcium

Adolescents and Adults (alternative to trimethoprim sulfamethoxazole): 50 mg or 75 mg once weekly with dapsone in combination with leucovorin calcium; **or** 25 mg once daily with atovaquone in combination with leucovorin calcium

Prophylaxis to prevent recurrence of Toxoplasma gondii:

Children ≥1 month of age: 1 mg/kg/day (or 15 mg/m^2) once daily (maximum: 25 mg) given with sulfadiazine (or atovaquone or clindamycin) in combination with leucovorin calcium

Adolescents and Adults: 25-50 mg once daily with sulfadiazine in combination with leucovorin calcium (preferred); **or** 25-50 mg once daily with clindamycin in combination with leucovorin calcium; **or** 25 mg once daily with atovaquone in combination with leucovorin calcium

Treatment of congenital toxoplasmosis: Infants and Children: Loading dose: 2 mg/kg/day once daily for 2 days, then 1 mg/kg/day once daily for 2-6 months, followed by 1 mg/kg administered 3 times weekly, with sulfadiazine or clindamycin in combination with leucovorin calcium (treatment duration: 12 months)

Treatment of acquired toxoplasmosis: Infants and Children: Acute induction: Loading dose: 2 mg/kg once daily (maximum: 50 mg/day) for 3 days, then 1 mg/kg/day once daily (maximum: 25 mg/day), with sulfadiazine or clindamycin in combination with leucovorin calcium (treatment duration: ≥6 weeks)

Treatment of Toxoplasma gondii encephalitis: Adolescents and Adults: 200 mg as a single dose, followed by 50 mg (<60 kg) or 75 mg (≥60 kg) daily, with sulfadiazine in combination with leucovorin calcium for at least 6 weeks (preferred); **or** 200 mg as a single dose, followed by 50 mg (<60 kg) or 75 mg (≥60 kg) daily, with clindamycin, atovaquone, or azithromycin in combination with leucovorin calcium

Dosage adjustment in renal impairment: No dosage adjustment provided in manufacturer's labeling. Use with caution.

Dosage adjustment in hepatic impairment: No dosage adjustment provided in manufacturer's labeling. Use with caution.

Dietary Considerations Take with meals to minimize GI distress.

Administration Administer with meals to minimize GI distress.

Monitoring Parameters CBC, including platelet counts twice weekly with high-dose therapy (eg, when used for toxoplasmosis treatment; frequency not defined for lower doses); liver and renal function

Dosage Forms

Tablet, Oral:

Daraprim: 25 mg

Extemporaneous Preparations A 2 mg/mL oral suspension may be made with tablets and a 1:1 mixture of Simple Syrup, NF and methylcellulose 1%. Crush forty 25 mg tablets in a mortar and reduce to a fine powder. Add small portions of vehicle and mix to a uniform paste; mix while adding vehicle in incremental proportions to **almost** 500 mL; transfer to a calibrated bottle, rinse mortar with vehicle, and add quantity of vehicle sufficient to make 500 mL. Label "shake well" and "refrigerate". Stable for 91 days.

Nahata MC, Pai VB, and Hipple TF, *Pediatric Drug Formulations*, 5th ed, Cincinnati, OH: Harvey Whitney Books Co, 2004.

- ◆ **Pyrimethamine and Sulfadoxine** *see* Sulfadoxine and Pyrimethamine [INT] *on page 1946*
- ◆ **QAB149** *see* Indacaterol *on page 1063*
- ◆ **Q-Alendronate (Can)** *see* Alendronate *on page 79*
- ◆ **Q-Amlodipine (Can)** *see* AmLODIPine *on page 123*
- ◆ **Q-Citalopram (Can)** *see* Citalopram *on page 451*
- ◆ **Q-Cyclobenzaprine (Can)** *see* Cyclobenzaprine *on page 516*
- ◆ **Q-Dryl [OTC]** *see* DiphenhydrAMINE (Systemic) *on page 641*
- ◆ **Q-Fenofibrate Micro (Can)** *see* Fenofibrate and Derivatives *on page 852*
- ◆ **Q-Fluoxetine (Can)** *see* FLUoxetine *on page 899*
- ◆ **Qinghao Derivative** *see* Artesunate *on page 178*
- ◆ **Qinghaosu Derivative** *see* Artesunate *on page 178*
- ◆ **Q-Lansoprazole (Can)** *see* Lansoprazole *on page 1166*
- ◆ **QlearQuil 24 Hour Relief [OTC]** *see* Loratadine *on page 1241*
- ◆ **Q-Metformin (Can)** *see* MetFORMIN *on page 1307*
- ◆ **Qnasl** *see* Beclomethasone (Nasal) *on page 232*
- ◆ **Qnasl Childrens** *see* Beclomethasone (Nasal) *on page 232*
- ◆ **Q-Omeprazole (Can)** *see* Omeprazole *on page 1508*
- ◆ **Q-Pan H5N1 Influenza Vaccine** *see* Influenza A Virus Vaccine (H5N1) *on page 1074*
- ◆ **Q-Pantoprazole (Can)** *see* Pantoprazole *on page 1570*
- ◆ **Q-Pap [OTC]** *see* Acetaminophen *on page 32*
- ◆ **Q-Pap Children's [OTC]** *see* Acetaminophen *on page 32*
- ◆ **Q-Pap Extra Strength [OTC]** *see* Acetaminophen *on page 32*
- ◆ **Q-Pap Infant's [OTC]** *see* Acetaminophen *on page 32*
- ◆ **Q-Paroxetine (Can)** *see* PARoxetine *on page 1579*
- ◆ **Q-Sertraline (Can)** *see* Sertraline *on page 1878*
- ◆ **Q-Simvastatin (Can)** *see* Simvastatin *on page 1890*
- ◆ **Q-Terbinafine (Can)** *see* Terbinafine (Systemic) *on page 2002*
- ◆ **Q-Topiramate (Can)** *see* Topiramate *on page 2065*

- ◆ **Q-Tussin [OTC]** *see* GuaiFENesin *on page 986*
- ◆ **Q-Tussin DM [OTC]** *see* Guaifenesin and Dextromethorphan *on page 987*
- ◆ **Quad Pill** *see* Elvitegravir, Cobicistat, Emtricitabine, and Tenofovir *on page 718*
- ◆ **Quadrivalent Human Papillomavirus Vaccine** *see* Papillomavirus (Types 6, 11, 16, 18) Vaccine (Human, Recombinant) *on page 1574*
- ◆ **Qualaquin** *see* QuiNINE *on page 1761*
- ◆ **Quartette** *see* Ethinyl Estradiol and Levonorgestrel *on page 803*
- ◆ **Quasense** *see* Ethinyl Estradiol and Levonorgestrel *on page 803*
- ◆ **Quaternium-18 Bentonite** *see* Bentoquatam *on page 246*

Quazepam (KWAZ e pam)

Brand Names: U.S. Doral
Brand Names: Canada Doral
Pharmacologic Category Benzodiazepine
Additional Appendix Information

Beers Criteria – Potentially Inappropriate Medications for Geriatrics *on page 2271*

Use Insomnia: For the treatment of insomnia characterized by difficulty in falling asleep, frequent nocturnal awakenings, and/or early morning

Pregnancy Risk Factor C

Dosage

Adults: Oral: Initial: 7.5 mg at bedtime; in some patients, the dose may be increased to 15 mg if necessary for efficacy.

Elderly: Dosing should be cautious; begin at lower end of dosing range (ie, 7.5 mg)

Dosing adjustment in renal impairment: No dosage adjustment provided in manufacturer's labeling.

Dosing adjustment in hepatic impairment: No dosage adjustment provided in manufacturer's labeling.

Additional Information Complete prescribing information should be consulted for additional detail.

Dosage Forms

Tablet, Oral:
Doral: 15 mg
Generic: 15 mg

- ◆ **Qudexy XR** *see* Topiramate *on page 2065*
- ◆ **Quelicin** *see* Succinylcholine *on page 1939*
- ◆ **Quelicin® (Can)** *see* Succinylcholine *on page 1939*
- ◆ **Quelicin-1000** *see* Succinylcholine *on page 1939*
- ◆ **Quenalin [OTC]** *see* DiphenhydrAMINE (Systemic) *on page 641*
- ◆ **Questran** *see* Cholestyramine Resin *on page 431*
- ◆ **Questran Light** *see* Cholestyramine Resin *on page 431*
- ◆ **Questran Light Sugar Free (Can)** *see* Cholestyramine Resin *on page 431*

QUEtiapine (kwe TYE a peen)

Brand Names: U.S. SEROquel; SEROquel XR
Brand Names: Canada Apo-Quetiapine; Auro-Quetiapine; Ava-Quetiapine; CO Quetiapine; Dom-Quetiapine; JAMP-Quetiapine; Mar-Quetiapine; Mylan-Quetiapine; PHL-Quetiapine; PMS-Quetiapine; PRO-Quetiapine; Quetiapine XR; RAN-Quetiapine; ratio-Quetiapine; Riva-Quetiapine; Sandoz-Quetiapine; Sandoz-Quetiapine XRT; Seroquel; Seroquel XR; Teva-Quetiapine; Teva-Quetiapine XR
Index Terms Quetiapine Fumarate
Pharmacologic Category Second Generation (Atypical) Antipsychotic
Additional Appendix Information

Beers Criteria – Potentially Inappropriate Medications for Geriatrics *on page 2271*

Use

Bipolar disorder: Acute treatment of manic (both immediate release and extended release [ER]) or mixed (ER only) episodes associated with bipolar I disorder, both as monotherapy and as an adjunct to lithium or divalproex; maintenance treatment of bipolar I disorder, as an adjunct to lithium or divalproex; acute treatment of depressive episodes associated with bipolar disorder

Major depressive disorder (ER only): Adjunctive therapy to antidepressants for the treatment of major depressive disorder.

Schizophrenia: Treatment of schizophrenia.

Pregnancy Risk Factor C

Pregnancy Considerations Adverse events were observed in animal reproduction studies. Quetiapine crosses the placenta and can be detected in cord blood (Newport, 2007). Congenital malformations have not been observed in humans (based on limited data). Antipsychotic use during the third trimester of pregnancy has a risk for abnormal muscle movements (extrapyramidal symptoms [EPS]) and/or withdrawal symptoms in newborns following delivery. Symptoms in the newborn may include agitation, feeding disorder, hypertonia, hypotonia, respiratory distress, somnolence, and tremor; these effects may be self-limiting or require hospitalization. Quetiapine may cause hyperprolactinemia, which may decrease reproductive function in both males and females.

Treatment algorithms have been developed by the ACOG and the APA for the management of depression in women prior to conception and during pregnancy (Yonkers, 2009). The ACOG recommends that therapy during pregnancy be individualized; treatment with psychiatric medications during pregnancy should incorporate the clinical expertise of the mental health clinician, obstetrician, primary healthcare provider, and pediatrician. Safety data related to atypical antipsychotics during pregnancy is limited and routine use is not recommended. However, if a woman is inadvertently exposed to an atypical antipsychotic while pregnant, continuing therapy may be preferable to switching to a typical antipsychotic that the fetus has not yet been exposed to; consider risk:benefit (ACOG, 2008).

Healthcare providers are encouraged to enroll women 18-45 years of age exposed to quetiapine during pregnancy in the Atypical Antipsychotics Pregnancy Registry (1-866-961-2388 or http://www.womensmentalhealth.org/pregnancyregistry).

Breast-Feeding Considerations Quetiapine is excreted into breast milk. Based on information from 8 mother-infant pairs, concentrations of quetiapine in breast milk have been reported from undetectable to 170 mcg/L. The estimated exposure to the breast-feeding infant would be up to 0.1 mg/kg/day (relative infant dose up to 0.43% based on a weight adjusted maternal dose of 400 mg/day). Due to the potential for serious adverse reactions in the nursing infant, the manufacturer recommends a decision be made whether to discontinue nursing or to discontinue the drug, taking into account the importance of treatment to the mother.

Contraindications Hypersensitivity to quetiapine or any component of the formulation

Warnings/Precautions [U.S. Boxed Warning]: Antidepressants increase the risk of suicidal thinking and behavior in children, adolescents, and young adults (18-24 years of age) with major depressive disorder (MDD) and other psychiatric disorders; consider risk prior to prescribing. Short-term studies did not show an increased risk in patients >24 years of age and showed a decreased risk in patients ≥65 years. Closely monitor all patients for clinical worsening, suicidality, or unusual changes in behavior; particularly during the initial 1-2 months of therapy or during periods of dosage adjustments (increased or decreases); the patient's family or caregiver should be instructed to closely observe the patient and communicate condition with healthcare provider. A medication guide concerning the use of antidepressants should be dispensed with each prescription. **Quetiapine is not approved in the U.S. for use in children <10 years of age.**

May precipitate a shift to mania or hypomania in patients with bipolar disorder. Patients presenting with depressive symptoms should be screened for bipolar disorder; the screening should include a detailed psychiatric history covering a family history of suicide, bipolar disorder, and depression. Quetiapine is approved in the U.S. for the treatment of bipolar depression. Pharmacologic treatment for pediatric bipolar I disorder or schizophrenia should be initiated only after thorough diagnostic evaluation and a careful consideration of potential risks vs benefits. If a pharmacologic agent is initiated, it should be a component of a total treatment program including psychological, educational and social interventions. Increased blood pressure (including hypertensive crisis) has been reported in children and adolescents; monitor blood pressure at baseline and periodically during use.

Leukopenia, neutropenia, and agranulocytosis (sometimes fatal) have been reported with antipsychotic use; presence of risk factors (eg, preexisting low WBC or history of drug-induced leuko-/neutropenia) should prompt periodic blood count assessment. Discontinue therapy at first signs of blood dyscrasias or if absolute neutrophil count <1000/mm^3.

May cause orthostatic hypotension; use with caution in patients at risk of this effect or in those who would not tolerate transient hypotensive episodes (cerebrovascular disease, cardiovascular disease, dehydration, hypovolemia, or concurrent medication use which may predispose to hypotension/bradycardia) especially during the initial dose titration period. Use has been associated with QT prolongation; postmarketing reports have occurred in patients with concomitant illness, quetiapine overdose, or who were receiving concomitant therapy known to increase QT interval or cause electrolyte imbalance. Avoid use in patients at increased risk of torsade de pointes/sudden death (eg, hypokalemia, hypomagnesemia, history of cardiac arrhythmias, congenital prolongation of QT interval, concomitant medications with QTc interval-prolonging properties). Use with caution in patients at increased risk of QT prolongation (eg, cardiovascular disease, heart failure, cardiac hypertrophy, elderly, family history of QT prolongation). May cause hyperglycemia; in some cases may be extreme and associated with ketoacidosis, hyperosmolar coma, or death. All patients should be monitored for symptoms of hyperglycemia (eg, polydipsia, polyuria, polyphagia, weakness) and undergo a fasting blood glucose test if symptoms develop during treatment. Patients with risk factors for diabetes (eg, obesity or family history) should have a baseline fasting blood sugar (FBS) and periodically during treatment. Use with caution in patients with preexisting abnormal lipid profile. Significant weight gain has been observed with antipsychotic therapy; incidence varies with product. Monitor waist circumference and BMI.

[U.S. Boxed Warning]: Elderly patients with dementia-related psychosis treated with antipsychotics are at an increased risk of death compared to placebo. Most deaths appeared to be either cardiovascular (eg, heart failure, sudden death) or infectious (eg, pneumonia) in nature. Quetiapine is not approved for the treatment of dementia-related psychosis. Avoid antipsychotic use for behavioral problems associated with dementia unless alternative nonpharmacologic therapies have failed and patient may harm self or others. In addition, use may cause or exacerbate syndrome of inappropriate antidiuretic hormone secretion or hyponatremia; monitor sodium closely with initiation or dosage adjustments in older adults (Beers Criteria).

May cause dose-related decreases in thyroid levels, including cases requiring thyroid replacement therapy. Measure both TSH and free T_4, along with clinical assessment, at baseline and follow-up to determine thyroid status; measurement of TSH alone may not be accurate (exact mechanism of quetiapine's effect on the thyroid axis is unknown). Due to anticholinergic effects, use with caution in patients with decreased gastrointestinal motility, urinary retention, BPH, xerostomia, visual problems, and narrow-angle glaucoma. Relative to other antipsychotics, quetiapine has a moderate potency of cholinergic blockade. May cause extrapyramidal symptoms (EPS) and/or tardive dyskinesia. Risk of dystonia (and probably other EPS) may be greater with increased doses, use of conventional antipsychotics, males, and younger patients. Impaired core body temperature regulation may occur; caution with strenuous exercise, heat exposure, dehydration, and concomitant medication possessing anticholinergic effects. Use may be associated with neuroleptic malignant syndrome (NMS); monitor for mental status changes, fever, muscle rigidity and/or autonomic instability. Rare cases have been reported with quetiapine. Esophageal dysmotility and aspiration have been associated with antipsychotic use; use with caution in patients at risk of aspiration pneumonia (eg, Alzheimer disease). Development of cataracts has been observed in animal studies; lens changes have been observed in humans during long-term treatment. Lens examination, such as a slit-lamp exam, on initiation of therapy and every 6 months thereafter is recommended by manufacturer. Use caution with Parkinson disease, history of seizures, and renal impairment. Use caution with hepatic impairment; may cause elevations of liver enzymes. May cause CNS depression, which may impair physical or mental abilities; patients must be cautioned about performing tasks that require mental alertness (eg, operating machinery or driving). Effects with other sedative drugs or ethanol may be potentiated. Anaphylactic reactions have been reported with use. May increase prolactin levels; clinical significance of hyperprolactinemia in patients with breast cancer or other prolactin-dependent tumors is unknown. Potentially significant drug-drug interactions may exist, requiring dose or frequency adjustment, additional monitoring, and/or selection of alternative therapy. May cause withdrawal symptoms (rare) with abrupt cessation; gradually taper dose during discontinuation.

Adverse Reactions Actual frequency may be dependent upon dose and/or indication.

Cardiovascular: Hypertension (diastolic; children and adolescents), hypertension (systolic; children and adolescents), hypotension, increased heart rate, orthostatic hypotension (more common in adults), palpitations, peripheral edema, syncope, tachycardia

Central nervous system: Abnormal dreams, abnormality in thinking, aggressive behavior (children and adolescents), agitation, akathisia, anxiety, ataxia, confusion, decreased mental acuity, depression, disorientation, disturbance in attention, dizziness, drowsiness, drug-induced Parkinson's disease, dysarthria, dystonic reaction, extrapyramidal reaction, falling, fatigue, headache, hypersomnia, hypertonia, hypoesthesia, irritability, lack of concentration, lethargy, migraine, pain, paresthesia, restless leg syndrome, restlessness, twitching, vertigo

Dermatologic: Acne vulgaris (children and adolescents), diaphoresis, pallor (children and adolescents), skin rash
Endocrine & metabolic: Decreased HDL cholesterol (≤40 mg/dL), decreased libido, hyperglycemia (≥200 mg/dL post glucose challenge or fasting glucose ≥126 mg/dL), hyperprolactinemia, hypothyroidism, increased LDL cholesterol (≥160 mg/dL), increased serum triglycerides (≥200 mg/dL), increased thirst (children and adolescents), total cholesterol increased (≥240 mg/dL), weight gain (dose related)
Gastrointestinal: Abdominal pain, anorexia, constipation, decreased appetite, dyspepsia (dose related), dysphagia, flatulence, gastroenteritis, gastroesophageal reflux disease, increased appetite, nausea, periodontal abscess (adolescents), toothache, vomiting, xerostomia (more common in adults)
Genitourinary: Pollakiuria, urinary tract infection
Hematologic & oncologic: Leukopenia, neutropenia
Hepatic: Increased serum transaminases
Hypersensitivity: Seasonal allergy
Neuromuscular & skeletal: Arthralgia, back pain, dyskinesia, limb pain, muscle rigidity, muscle spasm, myalgia, neck pain, stiffness (children and adolescents), tremor, weakness
Ophthalmic: Amblyopia, blurred vision
Otic: Otalgia
Respiratory: Cough, dyspnea, epistaxis (adolescents), influenza, nasal congestion, pharyngitis, rhinitis, sinus congestion, sinus headache, sinusitis, upper respiratory tract infection
Miscellaneous: Fever
Rare but important or life-threatening: Abnormality of blepharitis, abnormal T waves on ECG, accommodation, acute hepatic failure, acute renal failure, agranulocytosis, alcohol intolerance, amenorrhea, amnesia, anemia, angina pectoris, apathy, aphasia, arthritis, atrial arrhythmia, atrial fibrillation, atrioventricular block, bone pain, bruxism, buccoglossal syndrome, bundle branch block, cardiac failure, cardiomyopathy, cataract, catatonic reaction, cerebrovascular accident, choreoathetosis, cyanosis, cystitis, deafness, deep vein thrombophlebitis, dehydration, dehydration, delirium, delusions, depersonalization, diabetes mellitus, dysmenorrhea, dysuria, ecchymosis, eosinophilia, facial edema, first degree atrioventricular block, flattened T wave on ECG, galactorrhea, glossitis, glycosuria, hemiplegia, hemolysis, hyperkinesia, hyperlipemia, hypersensitivity, hyperthyroidism, hyperventilation, hypochromic anemia, hypoglycemia, increased cough, increased creatinine phosphokinase, increased gamma-glutamyl transferase, increased libido, increased QRS duration, increased salivation, increased serum alkaline phosphatase, increased ST segment on ECG, intestinal obstruction, irregular pulse, leukocytosis, leukorrhea, lymphadenopathy, malaise, manic reaction, melena, myasthenia, myocarditis, myoclonus, neuralgia, neuroleptic malignant syndrome, orchitis, pancreatitis, paranoid reaction, pathological fracture, pelvic pain, pneumonia, polyuria, priapism, prolonged Q-T interval on ECG, pruritus, psoriasis, psychosis, rectal hemorrhage, rhabdomyolysis, seborrhea, seizure, SIADH, stomatitis, ST segment changes on ECG, stupor, subdural hematoma, suicidal ideation, tardive dyskinesia, thrombocytopenia, thrombophlebitis, tongue edema, uterine hemorrhage, vaginal hemorrhage, vaginitis, vasodilation, vulvovaginal moniliasis, vulvovaginitis, water intoxication, widened QRS complex on ECG

Drug Interactions

Metabolism/Transport Effects **Substrate** of CYP2D6 (minor), CYP3A4 (major); **Note:** Assignment of Major/Minor substrate status based on clinically relevant drug interaction potential

Avoid Concomitant Use

Avoid concomitant use of QUEtiapine with any of the following: Aclidinium; Amisulpride; Azelastine (Nasal); Conivaptan; Fusidic Acid (Systemic); Glucagon; Highest Risk QTc-Prolonging Agents; Idelalisib; Ipratropium (Oral Inhalation); Ivabradine; Metoclopramide; Mifepristone; Moderate Risk QTc-Prolonging Agents; Orphenadrine; Paraldehyde; Potassium Chloride; Sulpiride; Thalidomide; Tiotropium; Umeclidinium

Increased Effect/Toxicity

QUEtiapine may increase the levels/effects of: AbobotulinumtoxinA; Alcohol (Ethyl); Amisulpride; Analgesics (Opioid); Anticholinergic Agents; Azelastine (Nasal); Buprenorphine; CarBAMazepine; CNS Depressants; DULoxetine; Glucagon; Highest Risk QTc-Prolonging Agents; Hydrocodone; Hypotensive Agents; Methotrimeprazine; Methylphenidate; Metyrosine; OnabotulinumtoxinA; Orphenadrine; Paraldehyde; Potassium Chloride; RimabotulinumtoxinB; Selective Serotonin Reuptake Inhibitors; Serotonin Modulators; St Johns Wort; Sulpiride; Suvorexant; Thalidomide; Thiazide Diuretics; Tiotropium; Topiramate; Zolpidem

The levels/effects of QUEtiapine may be increased by: Acetylcholinesterase Inhibitors (Central); Aclidinium; Aprepitant; Barbiturates; Brimonidine (Topical); Cannabis; Conivaptan; CYP3A4 Inhibitors (Moderate); CYP3A4 Inhibitors (Strong); Doxylamine; Dronabinol; Fosaprepitant; Fusidic Acid (Systemic); Idelalisib; Ipratropium (Oral Inhalation); Ivabradine; Ivacaftor; Kava Kava; Luliconazole; Magnesium Sulfate; Methotrimeprazine; Methylphenidate; Metoclopramide; Metyrosine; Mifepristone; Moderate Risk QTc-Prolonging Agents; Nabilone; Netupitant; Nicorandil; Perampanel; Pramlintide; QTc-Prolonging Agents (Indeterminate Risk and Risk Modifying); Rufinamide; Serotonin Modulators; Simeprevir; Sodium Oxybate; Stiripentol; Tapentadol; Tetrahydrocannabinol; Umeclidinium

Decreased Effect

QUEtiapine may decrease the levels/effects of: Acetylcholinesterase Inhibitors; Amphetamines; Anti-Parkinson's Agents (Dopamine Agonist); Itopride; Quinagolide; Secretin

The levels/effects of QUEtiapine may be decreased by: Acetylcholinesterase Inhibitors; Bosentan; CarBAMazepine; CYP3A4 Inducers (Moderate); CYP3A4 Inducers (Strong); Dabrafenib; Deferasirox; Mitotane; Siltuximab; St Johns Wort; Tocilizumab

Food Interactions In healthy volunteers, administration of quetiapine (immediate release) with food resulted in an increase in the peak serum concentration and AUC by 25% and 15%, respectively, compared to the fasting state. Administration of the extended release formulation with a high-fat meal (~800-1000 calories) resulted in an increase in peak serum concentration by 44% to 52% and AUC by 20% to 22% for the 50 mg and 300 mg tablets; administration with a light meal (≤300 calories) had no significant effect on the C_{max} or AUC. Management: Administer without food or with a light meal (≤300 calories).

Storage/Stability Store at 25°C (77°F); excursions permitted between 15°C and 30°C (59°F and 86°F).

Mechanism of Action Quetiapine is a dibenzothiazepine atypical antipsychotic. It has been proposed that this drug's antipsychotic activity is mediated through a combination of dopamine type 2 (D_2) and serotonin type 2 ($5\text{-}HT_2$) antagonism. It is an antagonist at multiple neurotransmitter receptors in the brain: Serotonin $5\text{-}HT_{1A}$ and $5\text{-}HT_2$, dopamine D_1 and D_2, histamine H_1, and adrenergic $alpha_1$- and $alpha_2$-receptors; but appears to have no appreciable affinity at cholinergic muscarinic and benzodiazepine receptors. Norquetiapine, an active metabolite, differs from its parent molecule by exhibiting high affinity for muscarinic M1 receptors.

Antagonism at receptors other than dopamine and 5-HT_2 with similar receptor affinities may explain some of the other effects of quetiapine. The drug's antagonism of histamine H_1-receptors may explain the somnolence observed. The drug's antagonism of adrenergic alpha$_1$-receptors may explain the orthostatic hypotension observed.

Pharmacodynamics/Kinetics

Absorption: Rapidly absorbed following oral administration; high-fat meals (800-1000 calories) increase C_{max} 8% and AUC 2% of quetiapine XR; light meals (300 calories) had no effect.

Distribution: V_d: 6-14 L/kg

Protein binding, plasma: 83%

Metabolism: Primarily hepatic; via CYP3A4; forms the metabolite N-desalkyl quetiapine (active) and two inactive metabolites

Bioavailability: 100% (relative to oral solution)

Half-life elimination:

Mean: Terminal: Quetiapine: ~6 hours; Extended release: ~7 hours

Metabolite: N-desalkyl quetiapine: 12 hours

Time to peak, plasma: Immediate release: 1.5 hours; Extended release: 6 hours

Excretion: Urine (73% as metabolites, <1% of total dose as unchanged drug); feces (20%)

Dosage

Bipolar disorder: Oral:

Children ≥10 years and Adolescents ≤17 years: *Mania (monotherapy):*

Immediate release: Initial: 25 mg twice daily on day 1; increase to 50 mg twice daily on day 2, then increase by 100 mg daily (administered twice daily) each day until 200 mg twice day is reached on day 5. May further increase up to 600 mg daily in increments of ≤100 mg daily. Usual dosage range: 400-600 mg daily; maximum: 600 mg daily. **Note:** Total daily doses may also be divided into 3 doses per day, based on response and tolerability.

Extended release: Initial: 50 mg once daily on day 1; increase to 100 mg once daily on day 2, further increase by 100 mg once daily until 400 mg once daily is reached on day 5. Usual dosage range: 400-600 mg once daily; maximum dose: 600 mg once daily.

Adults:

Depressive episodes:

Immediate release: Initial: 50 mg once daily at bedtime on day 1; increase to 100 mg once daily on day 2, further increase by 100 mg daily each day until 300 mg once daily is reached by day 4. Usual dose: 300 mg once daily; maximum dose: 300 mg once daily.

Extended release: Initial: 50 mg once daily on day 1; increase to 100 mg once daily on day 2, further increase by 100 mg once daily until 300 mg once daily is reached by day 4. Usual dose: 300 mg once daily; maximum dose: 300 mg once daily.

Mania (monotherapy or as an adjunct to lithium or divalproex): Immediate release: Initial: 50 mg twice daily on day 1, further increase by 100 mg daily (administered twice daily) until 200 mg twice daily is reached by day 4; may further increase to 800 mg daily by day 6 in increments of ≤200 mg daily. Usual dosage range: 400-800 mg daily; maximum dose: 800 mg daily.

Manic or mixed (monotherapy or as an adjunct to lithium or divalproex): Extended release: Initial: 300 mg once daily on day 1; increase to 600 mg once daily on day 2 and increase dose to between 400-800 mg once daily on day 3; usual dosage range: 400-800 mg once daily; maximum dose: 800 mg once daily.

Maintenance therapy (adjunct to lithium or divalproex): Immediate release or extended release: Usual dosage range: 400-800 mg daily; maximum dose: 800 mg daily. **Note:** In the maintenance phase, patients generally continue on the same dose on which they were stabilized. Average time of stabilization was 15 weeks in clinical trials. During maintenance treatment, periodically reassess need for continued therapy and the appropriate dose.

Elderly: Immediate release and extended-release: Initial: 50 mg daily; may increase in increments of 50 mg daily to an effective dose, based on individual clinical response and tolerability

Major depressive disorder (adjunct to antidepressants): Oral:

Adults: Extended release: Initial: 50 mg once daily on days 1 and 2; increase to 150 mg once daily on day 3. Usual dosage range: 150-300 mg daily; maximum dose: 300 mg once daily.

Elderly: Extended release: 50 mg once daily; may increase by 50 mg once daily to an effective dose, based on individual clinical response and tolerability.

Schizophrenia: Oral:

Adolescents 13 to ≤17 years:

Immediate release: Initial: 25 mg twice daily on day 1; increase to 50 mg twice daily on day 2, further increase by 100 mg daily each day (divided twice daily) until 400 mg twice daily is reached on day 5. May further increase up to 800 mg daily in increments of ≤100 mg daily. Usual dosage range: 400-800 mg daily; maximum dose: 800 mg daily. **Note:** Total daily doses may also be divided into 3 doses per day, based on response and tolerability.

Extended release: Initial: 50 mg once daily on day 1; increase to 100 mg once daily on day 2, further increase by 100 mg once daily until 400 mg once daily is reached on day 5. Usual dosage range: 400-800 mg once daily; maximum dose: 800 mg once daily.

Adults:

Immediate release: Initial: 25 mg twice daily; increase in increments of 25-50 mg divided 2-3 times daily on days 2 and 3 to a range of 300-400 mg daily in 2-3 divided doses by day 4. Further adjustments as needed at intervals of at least 2 days in increments of 25-50 mg twice daily. Usual dosage range: 150-750 mg daily; maximum dose: 750 mg daily.

Extended release: Initial: 300 mg once daily; increase in increments of up to 300 mg once daily (in intervals of ≥1 day). Usual dosage range: 400-800 mg once daily; maximum dose: 800 mg once daily.

Maintenance therapy (monotherapy): Extended release: Usual dosage range: 400-800 mg once daily; maximum dose: 800 mg once daily. **Note:** During maintenance treatment, periodically reassess need for continued therapy and the appropriate dose.

Elderly: Immediate release and extended release: Initial: 50 mg daily; may increase in increments of 50 mg daily to an effective dose, based on individual clinical response and tolerability

ICU delirium (off-label use): Oral: Adults: Immediate release: Initial: 50 mg twice daily; may increase as necessary on a daily basis in increments of 50 mg twice daily to a maximum dose of 400 mg daily (Devlin, 2010)

Obsessive-compulsive disorder, treatment-resistant (augmentation; off-label use): Oral: Adults: Immediate release: Initial: 50 mg once daily on day 1; increase to 100 mg once daily on day 2. Further increase as tolerated based on response every 2 weeks at 100 mg increments. Usual dosage range: 50-300 mg daily (Atmaca 2002; Denys 2004).

Psychosis/agitation related to Alzheimer's dementia (off-label use): Oral: Elderly: Initial: 12.5-50 mg daily; if necessary, gradually increase as tolerated not to exceed 200-300 mg daily (Rabins, 2007)

Switching from immediate release to extended release: Children ≥10 years, Adolescents, Adults, and Elderly: May convert patients from immediate release to extended release tablets at the equivalent total daily dose and administer once daily; individual dosage adjustments may be necessary.

Reinitiation of treatment: Patients who have discontinued therapy for >1 week should generally be retitrated following reinitiation of therapy; patients who have discontinued <1 week, can generally be reinitiated on their previous maintenance dose.

Dosage adjustment for concomitant therapy: Children ≥10 years, Adolescents, Adults, and Elderly:

Concomitant use with a strong CYP3A4 inhibitor (eg, ketoconazole, itraconazole, indinavir, ritonavir, nefazodone): Immediate release or extended release: Decrease quetiapine to one-sixth of the original dose; when strong CYP3A4 inhibitor is discontinued, increase quetiapine by sixfold.

Concomitant use with a strong CYP3A4 inducer (eg, phenytoin, carbamazepine, rifampin, St John's wort): Immediate release or extended release: Increase quetiapine up to fivefold of the original dose when combined with chronic treatment (>7-14 days) of a strong CYP3A4 inducer; titrate based on clinical response and tolerance; when the strong CYP3A4 inducer is discontinued, decrease quetiapine to the original dose within 7-14 days.

Dosage adjustment in renal impairment: No dosage adjustment necessary.

Dosage adjustment in hepatic impairment:

Immediate release tablet: Initial: 25 mg daily, increase dose by 25-50 mg daily to effective dose, based on individual clinical response and tolerability

Extended release tablet: Initial: 50 mg once daily; increase dose by 50 mg once daily to effective dose, based on individual clinical response and tolerability

Dietary Considerations Administer extended release tablet without food or with a light meal (≤300 calories).

Administration

Oral:

Immediate release tablet: Administer with or without food.

Extended release tablet: Administer without food or with a light meal (≤300 calories), preferably in the evening. Swallow tablet whole; do not break, crush, or chew.

Nasogastric/enteral tube (off-label route): Hold tube feeds for 30 minutes before administration; flush with 25 mL of sterile water. Crush dose using immediate-release formulation, mix in 10 mL water and administer via NG/enteral tube; follow with a 50 mL flush of sterile water (Devlin, 2010).

Monitoring Parameters Mental status; vital signs (as clinically indicated); blood pressure (baseline; repeat 3 months after antipsychotic initiation, then yearly, particularly in children and adolescents); weight, height, BMI, waist circumference (baseline; repeat at 4, 8, and 12 weeks after initiating or changing therapy, then quarterly; consider switching to a different antipsychotic for a weight gain ≥5% of initial weight); CBC (as clinically indicated; monitor frequently during the first few months of therapy in patients with preexisting low WBC or history of drug-induced leukopenia/neutropenia); electrolytes and liver function (annually and as clinically indicated); TSH, free T_4, and thyroid clinical assessment (baseline and follow-up); fasting plasma glucose level/HbA_{1c} (baseline; repeat 3 months after starting antipsychotic, then yearly); fasting lipid panel (baseline; repeat 3 months after initiation of antipsychotic; if LDL level is normal, repeat at 2-5 year intervals or more frequently if clinically indicated); changes in menstruation, libido, development of galactorrhea, erectile and ejaculatory function (at each visit for the first 12 weeks after the antipsychotic is initiated or until the dose is stable, then yearly); abnormal involuntary movements or parkinsonian signs (baseline; repeat weekly until dose stabilized for at least 2 weeks after introduction and for 2 weeks after any significant dose increase); tardive dyskinesia (every 12 months; high-risk patients every 6 months); lens examination, such as a slit-lamp exam, on initiation of therapy and every 6 months is recommended by manufacturer; alternatively, experts suggest it may be reasonable to inquire yearly about visual changes and perform ocular examinations yearly in patients >40 years or every 2 years in younger patients (ADA, 2004; Lehman, 2004; Marder, 2004).

Dosage Forms

Tablet, Oral:

SEROquel: 25 mg, 50 mg, 100 mg, 200 mg, 300 mg, 400 mg

Generic: 25 mg, 50 mg, 100 mg, 200 mg, 300 mg, 400 mg

Tablet Extended Release 24 Hour, Oral:

SEROquel XR: 50 mg, 150 mg, 200 mg, 300 mg, 400 mg

◆ **Quetiapine Fumarate** *see* QUEtiapine *on page 1751*

◆ **Quetiapine XR (Can)** *see* QUEtiapine *on page 1751*

◆ **Quillivant XR** *see* Methylphenidate *on page 1336*

Quinagolide [CAN/INT] (kwin AG o lide)

Brand Names: Canada Norprolac

Index Terms Quinagolide Hydrochloride

Pharmacologic Category Hyperprolactinemia Agent, Dopamine (D_2) Agonist

Use Note: Not approved in U.S.

Treatment of hyperprolactinemia due to prolactin-secreting pituitary tumors (microadenoma or macroadenoma) or idiopathic in nature

Pregnancy Considerations Animal studies revealed no embryotoxic or teratogenic effects. Fertility may be restored with treatment. Discontinue use with confirmed pregnancy unless medically necessary to continue. No increase in the incidence of abortion has been seen with a discontinuation of the drug during pregnancy. The reinstitution of therapy may be necessary in patients who display symptoms of tumor enlargement (headaches, visual field changes).

Breast-Feeding Considerations By inhibiting prolactin secretion, quinagolide suppresses lactation.

Contraindications Hypersensitivity to quinagolide or any component of the formulation; hepatic or renal impairment

Warnings/Precautions Use caution in patients with a history of psychosis. Although rare, treatment has been associated with the onset of acute psychosis (reversible). Use in patients with pituitary adenomas may not eliminate the need for radiation and/or surgical therapy. Sudden sleep onset and somnolence have been reported with use especially in individuals with Parkinson's disease. Concurrent use with other agents known to induce somnolence or sleep may be expected to potentiate these risks. Hypotensive episodes and syncope may be observed early in therapy. Patients should be cautioned about performing dangerous tasks such as operating heavy machinery or driving. Use may be associated with the restoration of fertility; women wanting to avoid conception should implement a reliable method of birth control. Transient nausea and vomiting are common with the onset of therapy but may be alleviated by premedication with a peripheral dopamine antagonist. Ethanol may reduce tolerability of quinagolide.

Adverse Reactions

Cardiovascular: Edema, flushing, hypotension, palpitation, syncope

Central nervous system: Concentration decreased, dizziness, fatigue, headache, insomnia, malaise, mood lability, sedation

Gastrointestinal: Abdominal pain/discomfort, anorexia, constipation, diarrhea, dyspepsia, nausea, vomiting, weight gain

Endocrine & metabolic: Breast pain

Neuromuscular & skeletal: Extremity pain, weakness

Respiratory: Nasal congestion

Rare but important or life-threatening: Acute psychosis, bilirubin increased, creatine phosphokinase increased, hematocrit decreased, hemoglobin decreased, neutropenia, potassium increased, somnolence, transaminases increased, triglycerides increased

Drug Interactions

Metabolism/Transport Effects None known.

Avoid Concomitant Use

Avoid concomitant use of Quinagolide with any of the following: Amisulpride; Pipamperone [INT]; Sulpiride

Increased Effect/Toxicity There are no known significant interactions involving an increase in effect.

Decreased Effect

Quinagolide may decrease the levels/effects of: Amisulpride; Pipamperone [INT]; Sulpiride

The levels/effects of Quinagolide may be decreased by: Amisulpride; Antipsychotic Agents; Metoclopramide; Pipamperone [INT]; Sulpiride

Storage/Stability Store at 15°C to 30°C (59°F to 86°F). Protect from light and humidity.

Mechanism of Action Selective dopamine D_2 receptor agonist that exerts a direct inhibitory effect on cells (lactotrophs) in the anterior pituitary gland which synthesize and secrete prolactin; not an ergot alkaloid

Pharmacodynamics/Kinetics

Onset of action: 2 hours; maximum effect: 4-6 hours

Duration: >24 hours

Absorption: Rapid

Distribution: V_d: 100 L

Protein binding: 90%

Metabolism: Hepatic; via conjugation (glucuronide and sulfate)

Bioavailability: 4%

Half-life elimination: 11.5 hours; steady state: 17 hours

Time to peak, serum: 30-60 minutes

Excretion: Urine (50%); feces (40%); >95% as metabolites

Dosage Oral: Adults: Hyperprolactinemia:

Initial: 0.025 mg/day for 3 days followed by 0.05 mg/day for 3 days (starter pack)

Maintenance (beginning on day 7): 0.075 mg/day; if needed, a further stepwise titration of dose may occur with intervals of at least 1 week minimum; usual maintenance range: 0.075-0.15 mg/day

Maximum dose: Titrate by increasing dose by 0.075-0.15 mg/day no more frequently than every 4 weeks, up to 0.9 mg/day

Dosage adjustment in renal impairment: Use is contraindicated

Dosage adjustment in hepatic impairment: Use is contraindicated

Administration Administer with snack at bedtime. Nausea and vomiting may be alleviated by premedicating with a peripheral dopamine antagonist.

Monitoring Parameters CBC, basic metabolic panel, transaminases, triglycerides, prolactin levels; blood pressure; sedation, mental changes

Product Availability Not available in U.S.

Dosage Forms: Canada

Combination package:

Norprolac® [starter pack]:

Tablet: 0.025 mg (3s)

Tablet: 0.05 mg (3s)

Tablet: 0.075 mg (3s)

Tablet:

Norprolac®: 0.075 mg, 0.15 mg

◆ **Quinagolide Hydrochloride** *see* Quinagolide [CAN/INT] *on page 1755*

◆ **Quinalbarbitone Sodium** *see* Secobarbital *on page 1872*

Quinapril (KWIN a pril)

Brand Names: U.S. Accupril

Brand Names: Canada Accupril; Apo-Quinapril; GD-Quinapril; PMS-Quinapril

Index Terms Quinapril Hydrochloride

Pharmacologic Category Angiotensin-Converting Enzyme (ACE) Inhibitor; Antihypertensive

Use

Heart failure: Adjunctive treatment of heart failure (HF)

Note: The ACCF/AHA 2013 heart failure guidelines recommend the use of ACE inhibitors, along with other guideline directed medical therapies, to prevent HF in patients with a reduced ejection fraction who have a history of MI (stage B HF), to prevent HF in any patient with a reduced ejection fraction (stage B HF), or to treat those with HF and reduced ejection fraction (stage C HFrEF) (ACCF/AHA [Yancy, 2013]).

Hypertension: Treatment of hypertension

The 2014 guideline for the management of high blood pressure in adults (Eighth Joint National Committee [JNC 8]) recommends initiation of pharmacologic treatment to lower blood pressure for the following patients:

- Patients ≥60 years of age with systolic blood pressure (SBP) ≥150 mm Hg or diastolic blood pressure (DBP) ≥ 90 mm Hg. Goal of therapy is SBP <150 mm Hg and DBP <90 mm Hg.
- Patients <60 years of age with SBP ≥140 mm Hg or DBP is ≥90 mm Hg. Goal of therapy is SBP <140 mm Hg and DBP <90 mm Hg.
- Patients ≥18 years of age with diabetes and SBP ≥140 mm Hg or DBP ≥90 mm Hg. Goal of therapy is SBP <140 mm Hg and DBP <90 mm Hg.
- Patients ≥18 years of age with chronic kidney disease (CKD) and SBP ≥140 mm Hg or DBP ≥90 mm Hg. Goal of therapy is SBP <140 mm Hg and DBP <90 mm Hg.

In patients with CKD, regardless of race or diabetes status, the use of an ACE inhibitor (ACEI) or angiotensin receptor blocker (ARB) as initial therapy is recommended to improve kidney outcomes. In the general nonblack population (without CKD) including those with diabetes, initial antihypertensive treatment should consist of a thiazide-type diuretic, calcium channel blocker, ACEI, or ARB. In the general black population (without CKD) including those with diabetes, initial antihypertensive treatment should consist of a thiazide-type diuretic or a calcium channel blocker **instead of** an ACEI or ARB.

Pregnancy Risk Factor D

Pregnancy Considerations [U.S. Boxed Warning]: Drugs that act on the renin-angiotensin system can cause injury and death to the developing fetus. Discontinue as soon as possible once pregnancy is detected. Quinapril crosses the placenta; teratogenic effects may occur following maternal use during pregnancy. Drugs that act on the renin-angiotensin system are associated with oligohydramnios. Oligohydramnios, due to decreased fetal renal function, may lead to fetal lung hypoplasia and skeletal malformations. Their use in pregnancy is also associated with anuria, hypotension, renal failure, skull hypoplasia, and death in the fetus/neonate. Chronic maternal hypertension itself is also associated with adverse events in the fetus/infant. ACE inhibitors are not recommended during pregnancy to treat maternal hypertension or heart failure. Use of an ACE inhibitor should also be avoided in any woman of reproductive age. Women who are planning a pregnancy should be considered for other medication options if an ACE inhibitor is currently prescribed or the ACE inhibitor should be discontinued as soon as possible once pregnancy is detected. The exposed fetus should be monitored for fetal growth, amniotic fluid volume, and organ formation. Infants exposed to an ACE inhibitor *in utero* should be monitored for hyperkalemia, hypotension, and oliguria (exchange transfusions or dialysis may be needed). These adverse events are generally associated with maternal use in the second and third trimesters.

Untreated chronic maternal hypertension is also associated with adverse events in the fetus, infant, and mother. The use of ACE inhibitors is not recommended to treat chronic uncomplicated hypertension in pregnant women and should generally be avoided in women of reproductive potential (ACOG, 2013).

Breast-Feeding Considerations Quinapril is excreted in breast milk. The manufacturer recommends that caution be exercised when administering quinapril to nursing women. The Canadian labeling contraindicates use in nursing women.

Contraindications

Hypersensitivity to quinapril or any component of the formulation; angioedema related to previous treatment with an ACE inhibitor; concomitant use with aliskiren in patients with diabetes mellitus.

Documentation of allergenic cross-reactivity for ACE inhibitors is limited. However, because of similarities in chemical structure and/or pharmacologic actions, the possibility of cross-sensitivity cannot be ruled out with certainty.

Canadian labeling: Additional contraindications (not in U.S. labeling): Women who are pregnant, intend to become pregnant, or of childbearing potential and not using adequate contraception; breast-feeding; concomitant use with aliskiren, angiotensin receptor blockers (ARBs), or other ACE inhibitors in patients with moderate-to-severe renal impairment (GFR <60 mL/minute/1.73 m^2), hyperkalemia (>5 mmol/L), or congestive heart failure who are hypotensive; concomitant use with angiotensin receptor blockers (ARBs) or other ACE inhibitors in diabetic patients with end organ damage; hereditary problems of galactose intolerance, glucose-galactose malabsorption or Lapp lactase deficiency

Warnings/Precautions Anaphylactic reactions may occur rarely with ACE inhibitors. At any time during treatment (especially following first dose) angioedema may occur rarely with ACE inhibitors; it may involve the head and neck (potentially compromising airway) or the intestine (presenting with abdominal pain). African-Americans and patients with idiopathic or hereditary angioedema may be at an increased risk. Prolonged frequent monitoring may be required especially if tongue, glottis, or larynx are involved as they are associated with airway obstruction. Patients with a history of airway surgery may have a higher risk of airway obstruction. Aggressive early and appropriate management is critical. Use in patients with previous angioedema associated with ACE inhibitor therapy is contraindicated. Severe anaphylactoid reactions may be seen during hemodialysis (eg, CVVHD) with high-flux dialysis membranes (eg, AN69), and rarely, during low density lipoprotein apheresis with dextran sulfate cellulose. Rare cases of anaphylactoid reactions have been reported in patients undergoing sensitization treatment with hymenoptera (bee, wasp) venom while receiving ACE inhibitors. Formulation may contain lactose.

Symptomatic hypotension with or without syncope can occur with ACE inhibitors (usually with the first several doses); effects are most often observed in volume-depleted patients; close monitoring of patient is required especially with initial dosing and dosing increases; blood pressure must be lowered at a rate appropriate for the patient's clinical condition. Initiation of therapy in patients with ischemic heart disease or cerebrovascular disease warrants close observation due to the potential consequences posed by falling blood pressure (eg, MI, stroke). Use with caution in hypertrophic cardiomyopathy with outflow tract obstruction, severe aortic stenosis, or before, during, or immediately after major surgery. **[U.S. Boxed Warning]: Drugs that act on the renin-angiotensin system can cause injury and death to the developing fetus. Discontinue as soon as possible once pregnancy is detected.**

Hyperkalemia may occur with ACE inhibitors; risk factors include renal dysfunction, diabetes mellitus, concomitant use of potassium-sparing diuretics, potassium supplements, and/or potassium-containing salts. Use cautiously, if at all, with these agents and monitor potassium closely. Cough may occur with ACE inhibitors. Other causes of cough should be considered (eg, pulmonary congestion in patients with heart failure) and excluded prior to discontinuation.

May be associated with deterioration of renal function and/or increases in serum creatinine, particularly in patients with low renal blood flow (eg, renal artery stenosis, heart failure) whose glomerular filtration rate (GFR) is dependent on efferent arteriolar vasoconstriction by angiotensin II; deterioration may result in oliguria, acute renal failure, and progressive azotemia. Small increases in serum creatinine may occur following initiation; consider discontinuation only in patients with progressive and/or significant deterioration in renal function. Use with caution in patients with unstented unilateral/bilateral renal artery stenosis. When unstented bilateral renal artery stenosis is present, use is generally avoided due to the elevated risk of deterioration in renal function unless possible benefits outweigh risks. Potentially significant drug-drug interactions may exist, requiring dose or frequency adjustment, additional monitoring, and/or selection of alternative therapy.

Rare toxicities associated with ACE inhibitors include cholestatic jaundice (which may progress to fulminant hepatic necrosis), agranulocytosis, neutropenia, or leukopenia with myeloid hypoplasia. Patients with collagen vascular diseases (especially with concomitant renal impairment) or renal impairment alone may be at increased risk for hematologic toxicity; periodically monitor CBC with differential in these patients.

Adverse Reactions

Cardiovascular: Chest pain, first-dose hypotension, hypotension

Central nervous system: Dizziness, fatigue, headache

Dermatologic: Rash

Endocrine & metabolic: Hyperkalemia

Gastrointestinal: Diarrhea, nausea, vomiting

Neuromuscular & skeletal: Back pain, myalgia

Renal: BUN/serum creatinine increased, worsening of renal function (in patients with bilateral renal artery stenosis or hypovolemia)

Respiratory: Cough, dyspnea, upper respiratory symptoms

Rare but important or life-threatening: Acute renal failure, agranulocytosis, alopecia, amblyopia, anaphylactoid reaction, angina, angioedema, arrhythmia, cerebrovascular accident, depression, dermatopolymyositis, eosinophilic pneumonitis, exfoliative dermatitis, gastrointestinal hemorrhage, heart failure, hemolytic anemia, hepatitis, hyperkalemia, hypertensive crisis, impotence, insomnia, MI, orthostatic hypotension, pancreatitis, pemphigus, photosensitivity, shock, stroke, syncope, thrombocytopenia, viral infection, visual hallucinations (Doane, 2013)

A syndrome which may include arthralgia, elevated ESR, eosinophilia and positive ANA, fever, interstitial nephritis, myalgia, rash, and vasculitis has been reported with ACE inhibitors. In addition, hepatic necrosis, neutropenia, pancreatitis, and/or agranulocytosis (particularly in patients with collagen-vascular disease or renal impairment) have been associated with many ACE inhibitors.

Drug Interactions

Metabolism/Transport Effects None known.

Avoid Concomitant Use There are no known interactions where it is recommended to avoid concomitant use.

Increased Effect/Toxicity

Quinapril may increase the levels/effects of: Allopurinol; Amifostine; Antihypertensives; AzaTHIOprine; DULoxetine; Ferric Gluconate; Gold Sodium Thiomalate; Grass Pollen Allergen Extract (5 Grass Extract); Hypotensive Agents; Iron Dextran Complex; Levodopa; Lithium; Nonsteroidal Anti-Inflammatory Agents; Obinutuzumab; RisperiDONE; RiTUXimab; Sodium Phosphates

The levels/effects of Quinapril may be increased by: Alfuzosin; Aliskiren; Angiotensin II Receptor Blockers; Barbiturates; Brimonidine (Topical); Canagliflozin; Dapoxetine; Diazoxide; DPP-IV Inhibitors; Eplerenone; Everolimus; Heparin; Heparin (Low Molecular Weight); Herbs (Hypotensive Properties); Loop Diuretics; MAO Inhibitors; Nicorandil; Pentoxifylline; Phosphodiesterase 5 Inhibitors; Potassium Salts; Potassium-Sparing Diuretics; Prostacyclin Analogues; Sirolimus; Temsirolimus; Thiazide Diuretics; TiZANidine; Tolvaptan; Trimethoprim

Decreased Effect

Quinapril may decrease the levels/effects of: Quinolone Antibiotics; Tetracycline Derivatives

The levels/effects of Quinapril may be decreased by: Aprotinin; Herbs (Hypertensive Properties); Icatibant; Lanthanum; Methylphenidate; Nonsteroidal Anti-Inflammatory Agents; Salicylates; Yohimbine

Storage/Stability Store at 15°C to 30°C (59°F to 86°F). Protect from light.

Mechanism of Action Competitive inhibitor of angiotensin-converting enzyme (ACE); prevents conversion of angiotensin I to angiotensin II, a potent vasoconstrictor; results in lower levels of angiotensin II which causes an increase in plasma renin activity and a reduction in aldosterone secretion; a CNS mechanism may also be involved in hypotensive effect as angiotensin II increases adrenergic outflow from CNS; vasoactive kallikreins may be decreased in conversion to active hormones by ACE inhibitors, thus reducing blood pressure

Pharmacodynamics/Kinetics

Onset of action: 1 hour

Duration: 24 hours

Absorption: Quinapril: ≥60%

Protein binding: Quinapril: 97%; Quinaprilat: 97%

Metabolism: Rapidly hydrolyzed to quinaprilat, the active metabolite

Half-life elimination: Quinapril: 0.8 hours; Quinaprilat: 3 hours; increases as CrCl decreases

Time to peak, serum: Quinapril: 1 hour; Quinaprilat: ~2 hours

Excretion: Urine (50% to 60% primarily as quinaprilat)

Dosage

Children and Adolescents (off-label use): Hypertension: Oral: Initial 5 to 10 mg once daily; maximum: 80 mg daily (National High Blood Pressure Education Program Working Group on High Blood Pressure in Children and Adolescents, 2004)

Adults:

Heart failure: Oral: Initial: 5 mg twice daily, titrated at weekly intervals to 20 to 40 mg daily in 2 divided doses; target dose: 20 mg twice daily (ACCF/AHA [Yancy, 2013])

Canadian labeling: Oral: Initial: 5 mg once daily; as tolerated, may double daily dose (eg, 10 mg once daily) at weekly intervals to a maximum of 40 mg daily given in 2 divided doses.

Hypertension: Oral: Initial: 10 to 20 mg once daily in patients not on diuretics, adjust according to blood pressure response at peak (2 to 6 hours post-dose) and trough blood levels; initial dose may be reduced to 5 mg in patients receiving diuretics if the diuretic is continued. Usual dose range (ASH/ISH [Weber, 2014]): 10 to 40 mg once daily. **Note:** The Canadian labeling recommends a maximum dose of 40 mg daily.

Elderly:

Heart failure: Refer to adult dosing.

Hypertension: Oral: Initial: 10 mg once daily; titrate to optimal response.

Dosage adjustment in renal impairment: Lower initial doses should be used; after initial dose (if tolerated), administer initial dose twice daily; may be increased at weekly intervals to optimal response:

Heart failure: Initial:

CrCl >30 mL/minute: Administer 5 mg daily

CrCl 10 to 30 mL/minute: Administer 2.5 mg daily

CrCl <10 mL/minute: There are no dosage adjustments provided in manufacturer's labeling.

Hypertension: Initial:

CrCl >60 mL/minute: Administer 10 mg daily

CrCl 30 to 60 mL/minute: Administer 5 mg daily

CrCl 10 to 30 mL/minute: Administer 2.5 mg daily

CrCl <10 mL/minute: There are no dosage adjustments provided in manufacturer's labeling.

Dosage adjustment in hepatic impairment: There are no dosage adjustments provided in manufacturer's labeling (has not been studied).

Administration Administer without regard to meals.

Monitoring Parameters Blood pressure; serum creatinine and potassium; if patient has collagen vascular disease and/or renal impairment, periodically monitor CBC with differential

2013 ACCF/AHA Heart Failure guideline recommendations: Within 1-2 weeks after initiation and periodically thereafter, reassess renal function and serum potassium especially in patients with preexisting hypotension, hyponatremia, diabetes mellitus, azotemia, or those taking potassium supplements (ACCF/AHA [Yancy, 2013]).

Dosage Forms

Tablet, Oral:

Accupril: 5 mg, 10 mg, 20 mg, 40 mg

Generic: 5 mg, 10 mg, 20 mg, 40 mg

Extemporaneous Preparations A 1 mg/mL quinapril oral suspension may be made with tablets, K-Phos® Neutral (equivalent to 250 mg elemental phosphorus, 13 mEq sodium, and 1.1 mEq potassium per tablet), Bicitra®, and Ora-Sweet SF™. Place ten quinapril 20 mg tablets in an amber plastic prescription bottle (eg, 240 mL). In a separate container, prepare a buffer solution by crushing one K-Phos® Neutral tablet and dissolving it in 100 mL sterile water for irrigation. Add 30 mL of the prepared K-Phos® buffer solution to the quinapril tablets. Shake for at least 2 minutes, then remove cap and allow the concentrate to stand for 15 minutes, then shake the concentrate again for an additional minute. Add 30 mL of Bicitra® and shake for 2 minutes. Add quantity sufficient of Ora-Sweet SF® (~140 mL) to make 200 mL and shake the suspension. Store in amber plastic prescription bottles; label "shake well" and "refrigerate." Stable for 28 days refrigerated (Freed, 2005).

Freed A, Silbering SB, Kolodsick KJ, et al, "The Development and Stability Assessment of Extemporaneous Pediatric Formulations of Accupril," *Int J Pharm*, 2005, 304(1-2):135-44.

◆ **Quinapril Hydrochloride** *see* Quinapril *on page 1756*

◆ **Quinate (Can)** *see* QuiNIDine *on page 1759*

QuiNIDine (KWIN i deen)

Brand Names: Canada Apo-Quinidine; BioQuin Durules; Novo-Quinidin; Quinate

Index Terms Quinidine Gluconate; Quinidine Polygalacturonate; Quinidine Sulfate

Pharmacologic Category Antiarrhythmic Agent, Class Ia; Antimalarial Agent

Additional Appendix Information

Beers Criteria - Potentially Inappropriate Medications for Geriatrics *on page 2271*

Use

Quinidine gluconate and sulfate salts: Conversion and prevention of relapse into atrial fibrillation and/or flutter; suppression of ventricular arrhythmias. **Note:** Due to proarrhythmic effects, use should be reserved for life-threatening arrhythmias. Moreover, the use of quinidine has largely been replaced by more effective/safer antiarrhythmic agents and/or nonpharmacologic therapies (eg, radiofrequency ablation).

Quinidine gluconate (IV formulation): Conversion of atrial fibrillation/flutter and ventricular tachycardia. **Note:** The use of IV quinidine gluconate for these indications has been replaced by more effective/safer antiarrhythmic agents (eg, amiodarone and procainamide).

Quinidine gluconate (IV formulation) and quinidine sulfate: Treatment of malaria (*Plasmodium falciparum*)

Pregnancy Risk Factor C

Pregnancy Considerations Animal reproduction studies have not been conducted. Quinidine crosses the placenta and can be detected in the amniotic fluid, cord blood, and neonatal serum. Quinidine is indicated for use in the treatment of severe malaria infection in pregnant women (CDC, 2011; Smereck, 2011) and has also been used to treat arrhythmias in pregnancy when other agents are ineffective (European Society of Cardiology, 2003).

Breast-Feeding Considerations Quinidine can be detected in breast milk at concentrations slightly lower than those in the maternal serum. The manufacturer recommends avoiding use in nursing women.

Contraindications Hypersensitivity to quinidine or any component of the formulation; thrombocytopenia; thrombocytopenic purpura; myasthenia gravis; heart block greater than first degree; idioventricular conduction delays (except in patients with a functioning artificial pacemaker); those adversely affected by anticholinergic activity; concurrent use of quinolone antibiotics which prolong QT interval, cisapride, amprenavir, or ritonavir

Warnings/Precautions Watch for proarrhythmic effects; may cause QT prolongation and subsequent torsade de pointes. Monitor and adjust dose to prevent QTc prolongation. Avoid use in patients with diagnosed or suspected congenital long QT syndrome. Correct hypokalemia before initiating therapy. Hypokalemia may worsen toxicity. **[U.S. Boxed Warning]: Antiarrhythmic drugs have not been shown to enhance survival in non-life-threatening ventricular arrhythmias and may increase mortality; the risk is greatest with structural heart disease. Quinidine may increase mortality in treatment of atrial fibrillation/flutter.** May precipitate or exacerbate HF. Reduce dosage in hepatic impairment. Use may cause digoxin-induced toxicity (adjust digoxin's dose). Use caution with concurrent use of other antiarrhythmics. Hypersensitivity reactions can occur. Can unmask sick sinus syndrome (causes bradycardia); use with caution in patients with heart block. In the treatment of atrial fibrillation in the elderly, avoid antiarrhythmics as first-line treatment. In older adults, data suggests rate control may provide more benefits than risks compared to rhythm control for most patients (Beers Criteria).

Has been associated with severe hepatotoxic reactions, including granulomatous hepatitis. Hemolysis may occur in patients with G6PD (glucose-6-phosphate dehydrogenase) deficiency. Different salt products are not interchangeable.

Adverse Reactions

Cardiovascular: Angina, new or worsened arrhythmia (proarrhythmic effect), hypotension, palpitation, QTc prolongation (modest prolongation is common, however, excessive prolongation is rare and indicates toxicity), syncope

Central nervous system: Fatigue, headache, incoordination, lightheadedness, nervousness, sleep disturbance, syncope, tremor

Dermatologic: Rash

Gastrointestinal: Anorexia, bitter taste, diarrhea, nausea, stomach cramping, upper GI distress, vomiting

Neuromuscular & skeletal: Weakness

Ocular: Blurred vision

Otic: Tinnitus

Respiratory: Wheezing

Rare but important or life-threatening: Abnormal pigmentation, acute psychotic reactions, agranulocytosis, angioedema, arthralgia, bronchospasm, cerebral hypoperfusion (possibly resulting in ataxia, apprehension, and seizure), cholestasis, confusion, CPK increased, delirium, depression, drug-induced lupus-like syndrome, eczematous dermatitis, esophagitis, exacerbated bradycardia (in sick sinus syndrome), exfoliative rash, fever, flushing, granulomatous hepatitis, hallucinations, hearing impaired, heart block, hemolytic anemia, hepatotoxic reaction (rare), lichen planus, livedo reticularis, lymphadenopathy, melanin pigmentation of the hard palate, myalgia, mydriasis, nephropathy, optic neuritis, pancytopenia, paradoxical increase in ventricular rate during atrial fibrillation/flutter, photosensitivity, pneumonitis, pruritus, psoriaform rash, QTc prolongation (excessive), respiratory depression, sicca syndrome, tachycardia, thrombocytopenia, thrombocytopenic purpura, torsade de pointes, urticaria, uveitis, vascular collapse, vasculitis, ventricular fibrillation, ventricular tachycardia, vertigo, visual field loss

Note: Cinchonism, a syndrome which may include tinnitus, high-frequency hearing loss, deafness, vertigo, blurred vision, diplopia, photophobia, headache, confusion, and delirium has been associated with quinidine use. Usually associated with chronic toxicity, this syndrome has also been described after brief exposure to a moderate dose in sensitive patients. Vomiting and diarrhea may also occur as isolated reactions to therapeutic quinidine levels.

Drug Interactions

Metabolism/Transport Effects Substrate of CYP2C9 (minor), CYP2E1 (minor), CYP3A4 (major), P-glycoprotein; **Note:** Assignment of Major/Minor substrate status based on clinically relevant drug interaction potential; **Inhibits** CYP2C9 (weak), CYP2D6 (strong), CYP3A4 (weak), P-glycoprotein

Avoid Concomitant Use

Avoid concomitant use of QuiNIDine with any of the following: Amiodarone; Antifungal Agents (Azole Derivatives, Systemic); Bosutinib; Conivaptan; Crizotinib; Enzalutamide; Fingolimod; Fusidic Acid (Systemic); Haloperidol; Highest Risk QTc-Prolonging Agents; Idelalisib; Ivabradine; Macrolide Antibiotics; Mefloquine; Mifepristone; Moderate Risk QTc-Prolonging Agents; PAZOPanib; Pimozide; Propafenone; Protease Inhibitors; Silodosin; Tamoxifen; Thioridazine; Topotecan; VinCRIStine (Liposomal)

Increased Effect/Toxicity

QuiNIDine may increase the levels/effects of: Afatinib; ARIPiprazole; AtoMOXetine; Bosutinib; Brentuximab Vedotin; Calcium Channel Blockers (Dihydropyridine); Cardiac Glycosides; Colchicine; CYP2D6 Substrates; Dabigatran Etexilate; Dalfampridine; Dextromethorphan; DOXOrubicin (Conventional); Edoxaban; Everolimus; Fesoterodine; FluvoxaMINE; Haloperidol; Highest Risk QTc-Prolonging Agents; Ledipasvir; Lomitapide; Mefloquine; Metoprolol; Naloxegol; Nebivolol; Neuromuscular-Blocking Agents; PAZOPanib; P-glycoprotein/ABCB1 Substrates; Pimozide; Propafenone; Propranolol; Prucalopride; Rifaximin; Rivaroxaban; Silodosin; Thioridazine; Topotecan; Tricyclic Antidepressants; Verapamil; VinCRIStine (Liposomal); Vitamin K Antagonists; Vortioxetine

The levels/effects of QuiNIDine may be increased by: Amiodarone; Antacids; Antifungal Agents (Azole Derivatives, Systemic); Aprepitant; Boceprevir; Calcium Channel Blockers (Dihydropyridine); Carbonic Anhydrase Inhibitors; Cimetidine; Conivaptan; Crizotinib; CYP3A4 Inhibitors (Moderate); CYP3A4 Inhibitors (Strong); Diltiazem; Fingolimod; FluvoxaMINE; Fosaprepitant; Fosphenytoin; Fusidic Acid (Systemic); Haloperidol; Idelalisib; Ivabradine; Ivacaftor; Luliconazole; Lurasidone; Macrolide Antibiotics; Mifepristone; Moderate Risk QTc-Prolonging Agents; Netupitant; P-glycoprotein/ABCB1 Inhibitors; PHENobarbital; Protease Inhibitors; QTc-Prolonging Agents (Indeterminate Risk and Risk Modifying); Reserpine; Simeprevir; Stiripentol; Telaprevir; Tricyclic Antidepressants; Verapamil

Decreased Effect

QuiNIDine may decrease the levels/effects of: Codeine; Dihydrocodeine; Hydrocodone; Tamoxifen; TraMADol

The levels/effects of QuiNIDine may be decreased by: Bosentan; Calcium Channel Blockers (Dihydropyridine); CYP3A4 Inducers (Moderate); CYP3A4 Inducers (Strong); Dabrafenib; Deferasirox; Enzalutamide; Etravirine; Fosphenytoin; Kaolin; Mitotane; P-glycoprotein/ABCB1 Inducers; PHENobarbital; Phenytoin; Potassium-Sparing Diuretics; Primidone; Rifamycin Derivatives; Siltuximab; St Johns Wort; Sucralfate; Tocilizumab

Food Interactions Changes in dietary salt intake may alter the rate and extent of quinidine absorption. Quinidine serum levels may be increased if taken with food. Food has a variable effect on absorption of sustained release formulation. The rate of absorption of quinidine may be decreased following the ingestion of grapefruit juice. Excessive intake of fruit juice or vitamin C may decrease urine pH and result in increased clearance of quinidine with decreased serum concentration. Alkaline foods may result in increased quinidine serum concentrations. Management: Avoid changes in dietary salt intake. Grapefruit juice should be avoided. Take around-the-clock to avoid variation in serum levels and with food or milk to avoid GI irritation.

Storage/Stability

Solution for injection: Store at room temperature of 25°C (77°F).

Tablets: Store at controlled room temperature of 20°C to 25°C (68°F to 77°F). Protect from light.

Mechanism of Action Class Ia antiarrhythmic agent; depresses phase O of the action potential; decreases myocardial excitability and conduction velocity, and myocardial contractility by decreasing sodium influx during depolarization and potassium efflux in repolarization; also reduces calcium transport across cell membrane

Pharmacodynamics/Kinetics

Distribution: V_d: Adults: 2 to 3 L/kg, decreased with congestive heart failure (0.5 L/kg), malaria; increased with cirrhosis

Protein binding: Newborns: 50% to 70%; Adults: 80% to 88%

Binds mainly to $alpha_1$-acid glycoprotein and to a lesser extent albumin; protein-binding changes may occur in periods of stress due to increased $alpha_1$-acid glycoprotein concentrations (eg, acute myocardial infarction) or in certain disease states due to decreased $alpha_1$-acid glycoprotein concentrations (eg, cirrhosis,hyperthyroidism, malnutrition)

Metabolism: Extensively hepatic (50% to 90%) to inactive compounds

Bioavailability: Sulfate: ~70% with wide variability between patients (45% to 100%); Gluconate: 70% to 80%

Half-life elimination, plasma: Children: 3 to 4 hours; Adults: 6 to 8 hours; prolonged with elderly, cirrhosis, and congestive heart failure

Time to peak, serum: Sulfate: 2 hours; Gluconate: 3 to 6 hours

Excretion: Urine (15% to 25% as unchanged drug)

Dosage Note: Dosage expressed in terms of the salt: 267 mg of quinidine gluconate = 200 mg of quinidine sulfate.

Atrial fibrillation/flutter (pharmacological conversion): Adults: Oral: **Note:** Discontinue use if at any time during therapy, the QRS complex widens to 130% of its pretreatment duration, the QTc interval widens to 130% of its pretreatment duration and is >500 msecs, P waves disappear, or the patient develops significant tachycardia, symptomatic bradycardia, or hypotension; consider other means of cardioversion (eg, direct current cardioversion).

Immediate release formulations: Quinidine sulfate: Initial: 400 mg every 6 hours; if after 4 or 5 doses there is no conversion, may increase cautiously to desired effect.

Extended release formulations:

Quinidine sulfate: Initial: 300 mg every 8 to 12 hours; the dose may be increased cautiously to desired effect

Quinidine gluconate: Initial: 648 mg every 8 hours; if after 3 or 4 doses there is no conversion, may increase cautiously to desired effect.

or

Initial: 324 mg every 8 hours for 2 days; then 648 mg every 12 hours for 2 days; then 648 mg every 8 hours for up to 4 days. The 4 day stretch may come at one of the lower doses if a lower dose is the highest tolerated dosing regimen.

Maintenance of sinus rhythm in patients with paroxysmal atrial fibrillation/flutter or life-threatening ventricular arrhythmias: Adults: Oral: Note: Dosing regimens for suppression of life-threatening ventricular arrhythmias have not been adequately studied. Reduce total daily dose if at any time during therapy, the QRS complex widens to 130% of its pretreatment duration, the QTc interval widens to 130% of its pretreatment duration and is >500 msecs, P waves disappear, or the patient develops significant tachycardia, symptomatic bradycardia, or hypotension.

Immediate release formulations: Quinidine sulfate: Initial: 200 mg every 6 hours; the dose may be increased cautiously to desired effect.

Extended release formulations:

Quinidine sulfate: Initial: 300 mg every 8 to 12 hours; the dose may be increased cautiously to desired effect.

Quinidine gluconate: Initial: 324 mg every 8 to 12 hours; the dose may be increased cautiously to desired effect. Usual dose range according to the AHA/ACC/HRS guidelines for management of atrial fibrillation: 324 to 648 mg every 8 hours (AHA/ACC/HRS [January, 2014]).

Severe malaria, treatment: Children and Adults: IV (quinidine gluconate): 10 mg/kg infused over 60 to 120 minutes followed by 0.02 mg/kg/minute continuous infusion for ≥24 hours; alternatively, may administer 24 mg/kg loading dose over 4 hours, followed by 12 mg/kg over 4 hours every 8 hours (beginning 8 hours after initiation of the loading dose); complete treatment with oral quinine once parasite density <1% and patient can receive oral medication; total duration of treatment (quinidine/quinine): 3 days (Africa or South America) or 7 days (Southeast Asia); use in combination with doxycycline, tetracycline or clindamycin (CDC malaria guidelines, 2009). **Note:** Close monitoring, including telemetry, required.

Dosing adjustment in renal impairment: No dosage adjustment provided in manufacturer's labeling. Use with caution. The following guidelines have been used by some clinicians (Aronoff, 2007): Oral:

CrCl ≥10 mL/minute: No dosage adjustment necessary.

CrCl <10 mL/minute: Administer 75% of normal dose.

Hemodialysis: Dose following hemodialysis

Peritoneal dialysis: Supplemental dose is not necessary

CRRT: No dosage adjustment required; monitor serum concentrations

Dosing adjustment/comments in hepatic impairment: No dosage adjustment provided in manufacturer's labeling. Use with caution due to reduced clearance.

Dietary Considerations Administer with food or milk to decrease gastrointestinal irritation. Avoid changes in dietary salt intake.

Usual Infusion Concentrations: Adult IV infusion: Quinidine gluconate: 800 mg in 50 mL (concentration: 16 mg/mL) of D_5W

Administration Administer around-the-clock to promote less variation in peak and trough serum levels

Oral: Do not crush, chew, or break sustained release dosage forms. Some preparations of quinidine gluconate extended release tablets may be split in half to facilitate dosage titration; tablets are not scored.

Parenteral: Minimize use of PVC tubing to enhance bioavailability; shorter tubing lengths are recommended by the manufacturer

Monitoring Parameters Cardiac monitor required during IV administration; CBC, liver and renal function tests, should be routinely performed during long-term administration

Consult individual institutional policies and procedures.

Reference Range Therapeutic: 2 to 5 mcg/mL (SI: 6.2 to 15.4 micromole/L). Patient-dependent therapeutic response occurs at levels of 3 to 6 mcg/mL (SI: 9.2 to 18.5 micromole/L). Optimal therapeutic level is method dependent; >6 mcg/mL (SI: >18 micromole/L).

Dosage Forms

Solution, Injection:

Generic: 80 mg/mL (10 mL)

Tablet, Oral:

Generic: 200 mg, 300 mg

Tablet Extended Release, Oral:

Generic: 300 mg, 324 mg

Extemporaneous Preparations A 10 mg/mL oral liquid preparation may be made with tablets and one of three different vehicles (cherry syrup, a 1:1 mixture of Ora-Sweet® and Ora-Plus®, or a 1:1 mixture of Ora-Sweet® SF and Ora-Plus®). Crush six 200 mg tablets in a mortar and reduce to a fine powder. Add 15 mL of the chosen vehicle and mix to a uniform paste; mix while adding vehicle in incremental proportions to **almost** 120 mL; transfer to a calibrated bottle, rinse mortar with vehicle, and add quantity of vehicle sufficient to make 120 mL. Label "shake well" and "protect from light". Stable for 60 days when stored in amber plastic prescription bottles in the dark at room temperature or refrigerated.

Allen LV and Erickson MA, "Stability of Bethanechol Chloride, Pyrazinamide, Quinidine Sulfate, Rifampin, and Tetracycline in Extemporaneously Compounded Oral Liquids," *Am J Health Syst Pharm*, 1998, 55(17):1804-9.

◆ **Quinidine and Dextromethorphan** *see* Dextromethorphan and Quinidine *on page 611*

◆ **Quinidine Gluconate** *see* QuiNIDine *on page 1759*

◆ **Quinidine Polygalacturonate** *see* QuiNIDine *on page 1759*

◆ **Quinidine Sulfate** *see* QuiNIDine *on page 1759*

QuiNINE (KWYE nine)

Brand Names: U.S. Qualaquin

Brand Names: Canada Apo-Quinine®; Novo-Quinine; Quinine-Odan

Index Terms Quinine Sulfate

Pharmacologic Category Antimalarial Agent

Use In conjunction with other antimalarial agents, treatment of uncomplicated chloroquine-resistant *P. falciparum* malaria

Pregnancy Risk Factor C

Dosage Note: Actual duration of quinine treatment for malaria may be dependent upon the geographic region or pathogen. Dosage expressed in terms of the salt; 1 capsule Qualaquin® = 324 mg of quinine sulfate = 269 mg of base.

Children: Oral:

Treatment of uncomplicated chloroquine-resistant *P. falciparum* malaria (CDC guidelines): 30 mg/kg/day in divided doses every 8 hours for 3-7 days. Tetracycline, doxycycline, or clindamycin (consider risk versus benefit of using tetracycline or doxycycline in children <8 years) should also be given.

Treatment of uncomplicated chloroquine-resistant *P. vivax* malaria (off-label use; CDC guidelines): 30 mg/kg/day in divided doses every 8 hours for 3-7 days. Tetracycline or doxycycline (consider risk versus benefit of using tetracycline or doxycycline in children <8 years) plus primaquine should also be given.

Adults: Oral:

Treatment of uncomplicated chloroquine-resistant *P. falciparum* malaria (CDC guidelines): 648 mg every 8 hours for 3-7 days. Tetracycline, doxycycline, or clindamycin should also be given.

Treatment of uncomplicated chloroquine-resistant *P. vivax* malaria (off-label use; CDC guidelines): 648 mg every 8 hours for 3-7 days. Tetracycline or doxycycline plus primaquine should also be given.

Babesiosis (off-label use): 650 mg every 6-8 hours for 7-10 days with clindamycin (Wormser, 2006; Vannier, 2012). **Note:** Relapsing infection may require at least 6 weeks of therapy (Vannier, 2012).

Dosing interval/adjustment in renal impairment:

CrCl 10-50 mL/minute: Administer every 8-12 hours

CrCl <10 mL/minute: Administer every 24 hours

Severe chronic renal failure not on dialysis: Initial dose: 648 mg followed by 324 mg every 12 hours

Dialysis: Administer dose after dialysis. **Note:** Clearance of ~6.5% achieved with 1 hour of hemodialysis.

Peritoneal dialysis: Dose as for CrCl <10 mL/minute

Continuous arteriovenous or hemodialysis: Dose as for CrCl 10-50 mL/minute

Dosing adjustment in hepatic impairment:
Mild-to-moderate impairment (Child-Pugh classes A and B): No dosing adjustment required; monitor closely.
Severe impairment (Child-Pugh class C): Avoid use.

Additional Information Complete prescribing information should be consulted for additional detail.

Dosage Forms
Capsule, Oral:
Qualaquin: 324 mg
Generic: 324 mg

◆ **Quinine-Odan (Can)** *see* QuiNINE *on page 1761*
◆ **Quinine Sulfate** *see* QuiNINE *on page 1761*
◆ **Quinol** *see* Hydroquinone *on page 1020*

Quinupristin and Dalfopristin
(kwi NYOO pris tin & dal FOE pris tin)

Brand Names: U.S. Synercid®
Brand Names: Canada Synercid®
Index Terms Dalfopristin and Quinupristin; RP-59500
Pharmacologic Category Antibiotic, Streptogramin
Use Treatment of complicated skin and skin structure infections caused by methicillin-susceptible *Staphylococcus aureus* or *Streptococcus pyogenes*
Pregnancy Risk Factor B
Dosage IV: Children ≥12 years and Adults:
Complicated skin and skin structure infection: 7.5 mg/kg every 12 hours for at least 7 days
Bacteremia, MRSA (persistent, vancomycin failure) (off-label use): 7.5 mg/kg every 8 hours (Liu, 2011)

Dosage adjustment in renal impairment: No dosage adjustment necessary.
Dosage adjustment in hepatic impairment: No dosage adjustment provided in manufacturer's labeling. However, pharmacokinetic data suggest dosage adjustment may be necessary.

Additional Information Complete prescribing information should be consulted for additional detail.

Dosage Forms
Injection, powder for reconstitution:
Synercid®: 500 mg: Quinupristin 150 mg and dalfopristin 350 mg

◆ **QVA149** *see* Indacaterol and Glycopyrronium [CAN/INT] *on page 1063*
◆ **Qvar** *see* Beclomethasone (Systemic) *on page 230*
◆ **QVAR (Can)** *see* Beclomethasone (Systemic) *on page 230*
◆ **Q-Zopiclone (Can)** *see* Zopiclone [CAN/INT] *on page 2217*
◆ **R & C II (Can)** *see* Pyrethrins and Piperonyl Butoxide *on page 1746*
◆ **R & C Shampoo/Conditioner (Can)** *see* Pyrethrins and Piperonyl Butoxide *on page 1746*
◆ **R-1569** *see* Tocilizumab *on page 2057*
◆ **R7159** *see* Obinutuzumab *on page 1482*
◆ **R093877** *see* Prucalopride [CAN/INT] *on page 1741*
◆ **R108512** *see* Prucalopride [CAN/INT] *on page 1741*
◆ **R207910** *see* Bedaquiline *on page 233*
◆ **R05072759** *see* Obinutuzumab *on page 1482*
◆ **RabAvert** *see* Rabies Vaccine *on page 1764*

RABEprazole (ra BEP ra zole)

Brand Names: U.S. Aciphex; AcipHex Sprinkle
Brand Names: Canada Apo-Rabeprazole; Pariet; Pat-Rabeprazole; PMS-Rabeprazole EC; PRO-Rabeprazole; Rabeprazole EC; RAN-Rabeprazole; Riva-Rabeprazole EC; Sandoz-Rabeprazole; Teva-Rabeprazole EC
Index Terms Pariprazole
Pharmacologic Category Proton Pump Inhibitor; Substituted Benzimidazole
Use
Duodenal ulcers: Short-term (4 weeks or fewer) treatment in the healing and symptomatic relief of duodenal ulcers in adults.
Gastroesophageal reflux disease:
Erosive or ulcerative: Short-term (4 to 8 weeks) treatment in the healing and symptomatic relief of erosive or ulcerative gastroesophageal reflux disease (GERD) in adults; for maintaining healing and reduction in relapse rates of heartburn symptoms in adults with erosive or ulcerative GERD.
Symptomatic: Treatment of symptomatic GERD in adults and pediatric patients 1 year and older.
***Helicobacter pylori* eradication:** In combination with amoxicillin and clarithromycin as a 3-drug regimen for the treatment of adults with *H. pylori* infection and duodenal ulcer disease (active or history of within the past 5 years) to eradicate *H. pylori*.
Pathological hypersecretory conditions: Long-term treatment of pathological hypersecretory conditions, including Zollinger-Ellison syndrome in adults.

Canadian labeling: Additional uses (not in U.S. labeling): Treatment of nonerosive reflux disease (NERD); treatment of gastric ulcers

Pregnancy Risk Factor C
Pregnancy Considerations Adverse events were not observed in animal reproduction studies. Available studies have not shown an increased risk of major birth defects following maternal use of proton pump inhibitors during pregnancy; however, information specific to rabeprazole is limited (Pasternak, 2010); most information available for omeprazole. When treating GERD in pregnancy, PPIs may be used when clinically indicated (Katz, 2013).
Breast-Feeding Considerations It is not known if rabeprazole is excreted in breast milk. The manufacturer recommends that caution be exercised when administering rabeprazole to nursing women.
Contraindications Hypersensitivity to rabeprazole, substituted benzimidazoles, or any component of the formulation
Warnings/Precautions Use of proton pump inhibitors (PPIs) may increase the risk of gastrointestinal infections (eg, *Salmonella, Campylobacter*). Use caution in severe hepatic impairment. Relief of symptoms with rabeprazole does not preclude the presence of a gastric malignancy. Use of PPIs may increase risk of *Clostridium difficile*-associated diarrhea (CDAD), especially in hospitalized patients; consider CDAD diagnosis in patients with persistent diarrhea that does not improve. Use the lowest dose and shortest duration of PPI therapy appropriate for the condition being treated. Decreased *H. pylori* eradication rates have been observed with short-term (≤7 days) combination therapy. The American College of Gastroenterology recommends 10 to 14 days of therapy (triple or quadruple) for eradication of *H. pylori* (Chey, 2007).

PPIs may diminish the therapeutic effect of clopidogrel, thought to be due to reduced formation of the active metabolite of clopidogrel. The manufacturer of clopidogrel recommends either avoidance of both omeprazole (even when scheduled 12 hours apart) and esomeprazole or use of a PPI with comparatively less effect on the active metabolite of clopidogrel. Avoidance of rabeprazole appears prudent due to potent *in vitro* CYP2C19 inhibition (Li, 2004) and lack of sufficient comparative *in vivo* studies with other PPIs. In contrast to these warnings, others have recommended the continued use of PPIs, regardless of the degree of inhibition, in patients with a history of GI bleeding or multiple risk factors for GI bleeding who are also receiving clopidogrel since no evidence has established clinically meaningful differences in outcome; however, a clinically-significant interaction cannot be excluded in those who are poor metabolizers of clopidogrel (Abraham, 2010; Levine, 2011). Potentially significant drug-drug interactions may exist, requiring dose or frequency adjustment, additional monitoring, and/or selection of alternative therapy.

Increased incidence of osteoporosis-related bone fractures of the hip, spine, or wrist may occur with PPI therapy. Patients on high-dose (multiple daily doses) or long-term therapy (≥1 year) should be monitored. Use the lowest effective dose for the shortest duration of time, use vitamin D and calcium supplementation, and follow appropriate guidelines to reduce risk of fractures in patients at risk.

Hypomagnesemia, reported rarely, usually with prolonged PPI use of >3 months (most cases >1 year of therapy); may be symptomatic or asymptomatic; severe cases may cause tetany, seizures, and cardiac arrhythmias. Consider obtaining serum magnesium concentrations prior to beginning long-term therapy, especially if taking concomitant digoxin, diuretics, or other drugs known to cause hypomagnesemia; and periodically thereafter. Hypomagnesemia may be corrected by magnesium supplementation, although discontinuation of rabeprazole may be necessary; magnesium levels typically return to normal within 1 week of stopping.

Prolonged treatment (≥2 years) may lead to vitamin B_{12} malabsorption and subsequent vitamin B_{12} deficiency. The magnitude of the deficiency is dose-related and the association is stronger in females and those younger in age (<30 years); prevalence is decreased after discontinuation of therapy (Lam, 2013).

Adverse Reactions

Cardiovascular: Peripheral edema

Central nervous system: Dizziness, headache, pain

Gastrointestinal: Abdominal pain, constipation, diarrhea, flatulence, nausea, vomiting, xerostomia

Hepatic: Hepatic encephalopathy, hepatitis, increased liver enzymes

Infection: Increased susceptibility to infection

Neuromuscular & skeletal: Arthralgia, myalgia

Respiratory: Pharyngitis

Rare but important or life-threatening: Agranulocytosis, albuminuria, alopecia, amblyopia, anaphylaxis, anemia, angioedema, bone fracture, bullous rash, cholecystitis, cholelithiasis, *Clostridium difficile* associated diarrhea (CDAD), colitis, coma, delirium, disorientation, erythema multiforme, gynecomastia, hematuria, hemolytic anemia, hyperammonemia, hypersensitivity reaction, hypertension, hypokalemia, hypomagnesemia, hyponatremia, increased thyroid stimulating hormone level, interstitial nephritis, jaundice, leukocytosis, leukopenia, melena, migraine, neutropenia, osteoporosis, palpitation, pancreatitis, pancytopenia, pathological fracture due to osteoporosis, pneumonia, rhabdomyolysis, sinus bradycardia, Stevens-Johnson syndrome, thrombocytopenia, toxic epidermal necrolysis

Drug Interactions

Metabolism/Transport Effects **Substrate** of CYP2C19 (major), CYP3A4 (major); **Note:** Assignment of Major/Minor substrate status based on clinically relevant drug interaction potential; **Inhibits** CYP2C19 (weak), CYP2C8 (moderate), CYP2D6 (weak), CYP3A4 (weak)

Avoid Concomitant Use

Avoid concomitant use of RABEprazole with any of the following: Dasatinib; Delavirdine; Erlotinib; Nelfinavir; PAZOPanib; Pimozide; Rilpivirine; Risedronate

Increased Effect/Toxicity

RABEprazole may increase the levels/effects of: Amphetamine; ARIPiprazole; CYP2C8 Substrates; Dexmethylphenidate; Dextroamphetamine; Dofetilide; Hydrocodone; Lomitapide; Methotrexate; Methylphenidate; Pimozide; Raltegravir; Risedronate; Saquinavir; Tacrolimus (Systemic); Voriconazole

The levels/effects of RABEprazole may be increased by: Fluconazole; Ketoconazole (Systemic); Voriconazole

Decreased Effect

RABEprazole may decrease the levels/effects of: Atazanavir; Bisphosphonate Derivatives; Bosutinib; Cefditoren; Clopidogrel; Dabigatran Etexilate; Dabrafenib; Dasatinib; Delavirdine; Erlotinib; Gefitinib; Indinavir; Iron Salts; Itraconazole; Ketoconazole (Systemic); Ledipasvir; Mesalamine; Multivitamins/Minerals (with ADEK, Folate, Iron); Mycophenolate; Nelfinavir; Nilotinib; PAZOPanib; Posaconazole; Rilpivirine; Riociguat; Risedronate; Vismodegib

The levels/effects of RABEprazole may be decreased by: Bosentan; CYP2C19 Inducers (Strong); CYP3A4 Inducers (Moderate); CYP3A4 Inducers (Strong); Dabrafenib; Deferasirox; Mitotane; Siltuximab; St Johns Wort; Tipranavir; Tocilizumab

Food Interactions Prolonged treatment (≥2 years) may lead to malabsorption of dietary vitamin B_{12} and subsequent vitamin B_{12} deficiency (Lam, 2013).

Storage/Stability Store at 25°C (77°F); excursions are permitted between 15°C and 30°C (59°F and 86°F). Protect from moisture.

Mechanism of Action Potent proton pump inhibitor; suppresses gastric acid secretion by inhibiting the parietal cell H+/K+ ATP pump

Pharmacodynamics/Kinetics

Onset of action: Within 1 hour

Duration: 24 hours

Absorption: Oral: Well absorbed within 1 hour

Protein binding, serum: ~96%

Metabolism: Hepatic via CYP3A and 2C19 to inactive metabolites

Bioavailability: Tablet: ~52%

Half-life elimination (dose dependent): 1 to 2 hours

Time to peak, plasma: Tablet: 2 to 5 hours; Capsule: 1 to 6.5 hours

Excretion: Urine (90% primarily as thioether carboxylic acid metabolites); remainder in feces

Dosage

Duodenal ulcer: Adults: Oral: 20 mg once daily for ≤4 weeks; additional therapy may be required for some patients

Gastric ulcers: *Canadian labeling:* Adults: Oral: 20 mg once daily up to 6 weeks; additional therapy may be required for some patients

Gastroesophageal reflux disease (GERD):

Children 1 to 11 years: Oral:

<15 kg: 5 mg once daily for ≤12 weeks; if inadequate response may increase to 10 mg once daily

≥15 kg: 10 mg once daily for ≤12 weeks

Children ≥12 years and Adolescents: Oral: 20 mg once daily for ≤8 weeks

Adults: Oral:

Erosive or ulcerative GERD: Treatment: 20 mg once daily for 4 to 8 weeks; if inadequate response, may repeat up to an additional 8 weeks; maintenance: 20 mg once daily

Canadian labeling: 20 mg once daily for 4 weeks; if inadequate response, may repeat for an additional 4 weeks (lack of symptom control after 4 weeks warrants further evaluation); maintenance: 10 mg once daily (maximum: 20 mg once daily).

Symptomatic GERD: Treatment: 20 mg once daily for 4 weeks; if inadequate response, may repeat for an additional 4 weeks.

Canadian labeling: 10 mg once daily (maximum: 20 mg once daily) for 4 weeks; lack of symptom control after 4 weeks warrants further evaluation

***Helicobacter pylori* eradication:** Adults: Oral:

Manufacturer labeling: 20 mg twice daily administered with amoxicillin 1000 mg *and* clarithromycin 500 mg twice daily for 7 days

American College of Gastroenterology guidelines (Chey, 2007):

Nonpenicillin allergy: 20 mg twice daily administered with amoxicillin 1000 mg *and* clarithromycin 500 mg twice daily for 10 to 14 days

Penicillin allergy: 20 mg twice daily administered with clarithromycin 500 mg *and* metronidazole 500 mg twice daily for 10 to 14 days **or** 20 mg once or twice daily administered with bismuth subsalicylate 525 mg *and* metronidazole 250 mg *plus* tetracycline 500 mg 4 times daily for 10 to 14 days

Hypersecretory conditions: Adults: Oral: 60 mg once daily; dose may need to be adjusted as necessary. Doses as high as 100 mg once daily and 60 mg twice daily have been used, and continued as long as necessary (up to 1 year in some patients).

Nonerosive reflux disease (NERD): *Canadian labeling:* Adults: Oral: Treatment: 10 mg (maximum: 20 mg once daily) for 4 weeks; lack of symptom control after 4 weeks warrants further evaluation

Dosage adjustment in renal impairment: No dosage adjustment necessary

Dosage adjustment in hepatic impairment:

Mild-to-moderate: No dosage adjustment necessary.

Severe: No dosage adjustment provided in manufacturer's labeling (has not been studied). Use with caution.

Dietary Considerations

Capsules: Take 30 minutes before a meal.

Tablets: May be taken with or without food. However, when used for the healing of duodenal ulcers, it is best if taken after breakfast. When used for the eradication of *Helicobacter pylori*, take with the morning and evening meals.

Administration May be administered with an antacid.

Capsules: Administer 30 minutes before a meal. Open capsule and sprinkle contents on a small amount of soft food (eg, applesauce, fruit or vegetable based baby food, yogurt) or empty contents into a small amount of liquid (eg, infant formula, apple juice, pediatric electrolyte solution); food or liquid should be at or below room temperature. Do not chew or crush granules; administer whole dose within 15 minutes of preparation (do not store for future use).

Tablets: May be administered with or without food. However, when used for the healing of duodenal ulcers, administration after breakfast is recommended. When used for the eradication of *H. pylori*, administration with the morning and evening meals is recommended. Swallow tablets whole; do not crush, split, or chew.

Monitoring Parameters Magnesium levels in patients on long-term treatment or those taking digoxin, diuretics, or other drugs that cause hypomagnesemia; susceptibility testing recommended in patients who fail *H. pylori* eradication regimen.

Dosage Forms

Capsule Sprinkle, Oral:

AcipHex Sprinkle: 5 mg, 10 mg

Tablet Delayed Release, Oral:

Aciphex: 20 mg

Generic: 20 mg

Dosage Forms: Canada

Tablet, delayed release, enteric coated:

Pariet: 10 mg, 20 mg

◆ **Rabeprazole EC (Can)** *see* RABEprazole *on page* 1762

Rabies Immune Globulin (Human)

(RAY beez i MYUN GLOB yoo lin, HYU man)

Brand Names: U.S. HyperRAB S/D; Imogam Rabies-HT

Brand Names: Canada HyperRAB S/D; Imogam Rabies Pasteurized

Index Terms HRIG; RIG

Pharmacologic Category Blood Product Derivative; Immune Globulin

Additional Appendix Information

Immunization Administration Recommendations *on page* 2250

Immunization Recommendations *on page* 2255

Use

Rabies exposure: Part of postexposure prophylaxis of persons with suspected rabies exposure. Provides passive immunity until active immunity with rabies vaccine is established. Not for use in persons with a history of vaccination (preexposure or postexposure prophylaxis) and documentation of antibody response. Each exposure to possible rabies infection should be individually evaluated.

Factors to consider include: species of biting animal, circumstances of biting incident (provoked vs unprovoked bite), type of exposure to rabies infection (bite vs nonbite), vaccination status of biting animal, presence of rabies in the region. See product information for additional details.

Pregnancy Risk Factor C

Dosage Infants, Children, Adolescents, and Adults: Postexposure prophylaxis: Local wound infiltration/IM: 20 units/kg in a single dose, RIG administered as soon as possible after exposure; should always be administered as part of rabies vaccine regimen. Do not exceed recommended dose since passive antibody can interfere with response to rabies vaccine. If anatomically feasible, the full rabies immune globulin dose should be infiltrated around and into the wound(s); remaining volume should be administered IM at a site distant from the vaccine administration site. If rabies vaccine was initiated without rabies immune globulin, rabies immune globulin may be administered through the seventh day after the administration of the first dose of the vaccine (day 0). Administration of RIG is not recommended after the seventh day post vaccine since an antibody response to the vaccine is expected during this time period.

Note: Not recommended for use in persons with a history of rabies vaccination (preexposure or postexposure prophylaxis) and documentation of antibody response.

Dosage adjustment in renal impairment: There are no dosage adjustments provided in manufacturer's labeling.

Dosage adjustment in hepatic impairment: There are no dosage adjustments provided in manufacturer's labeling.

Additional Information Complete prescribing information should be consulted for additional detail.

Dosage Forms

Injectable, Intramuscular:

Imogam Rabies-HT: 150 units/mL (2 mL, 10 mL)

Injectable, Intramuscular [preservative free]:

HyperRAB S/D: 150 units/mL (2 mL, 10 mL)

Rabies Vaccine (RAY beez vak SEEN)

Brand Names: U.S. Imovax Rabies; RabAvert

Brand Names: Canada Imovax Rabies; RabAvert

Index Terms HDCV; Human Diploid Cell Cultures Rabies Vaccine; PCEC; Purified Chick Embryo Cell

Pharmacologic Category Vaccine, Inactivated (Viral)

Additional Appendix Information

Immunization Administration Recommendations *on page 2250*

Immunization Recommendations *on page 2255*

Use Pre-exposure and postexposure vaccination against rabies

The Advisory Committee on Immunization Practices (ACIP) recommends a primary course of prophylactic immunization (pre-exposure vaccination) for the following:

- Persons with continuous risk of infection, including rabies research laboratory and biologics production workers
- Persons with frequent risk of infection in areas where rabies is enzootic, including rabies diagnostic laboratory workers, cavers, veterinarians and their staff, and animal control and wildlife workers; persons who frequently handle bats
- Persons with infrequent risk of infection, including veterinarians and animal control staff with terrestrial animals in areas where rabies infection is rare, veterinary students, and travelers visiting areas where rabies is enzootic and immediate access to medical care and biologicals is limited

The ACIP recommends the use of postexposure vaccination for a particular person be assessed by the severity and likelihood versus the actual risk of acquiring rabies. Consideration should include the type of exposure, epidemiology of rabies in the area, species of the animal, circumstances of the incident, and the availability of the exposing animal for observation or rabies testing. Postexposure vaccination is used in both previously vaccinated and previously unvaccinated individuals.

Pregnancy Risk Factor C

Dosage

Pre-exposure vaccination: IM: A total of 3 doses, 1 mL each, on days 0, 7, and 21-28. **Note:** Prolonging the interval between doses does not interfere with immunity achieved after the concluding dose of the basic series.

Postexposure vaccination: All postexposure treatment should begin with immediate cleansing of the wound with soap and water

Persons not previously immunized as above: IM: 5 doses (1 mL each) on days 0, 3, 7, 14, 28. In addition, patients should also receive rabies immune globulin with the first dose (day 0). **Note:** A regimen of 4 doses (1 mL each) on days 0, 3, 7, 14 may be used in persons who are not immunosuppressed (ACIP recommendations, 2010).

Persons who have previously received postexposure prophylaxis with rabies vaccine, received a recommended IM pre-exposure series of rabies vaccine or have a previously documented rabies antibody titer considered adequate: IM: Two doses (1 mL each) on days 0 and 3; do not administer rabies immune globulin

Booster (for persons with continuous or frequent risk of infection): 1 mL IM based on antibody titers

Dosage adjustment in renal impairment: No dosage adjustment provided in manufacturer's labeling.

Dosage adjustment in hepatic impairment: No dosage adjustment provided in manufacturer's labeling.

Additional Information Complete prescribing information should be consulted for additional detail.

Dosage Forms

Injectable, Intramuscular [preservative free]:
Imovax Rabies: 2.5 units/mL (1 ea)

Suspension Reconstituted, Intramuscular:
RabAvert: (1 ea)

Racecadotril [INT] (race ca DO til)

International Brand Names Aquasec (IN); Cadotril (PE); Feloact (PH); Hidrasec (CL, CN, CO, CR, CZ, DO, EC, EE, FI, GB, GR, GT, HK, HN, HR, MX, MY, NI, PA, PH, PY, RO, SE, SG, TH, VE, VN); Hidratan (PY); Mo Ni Ka (CN); Race-F (IN); Raceca (VN); Resorcal (CL); Tiorfan (BR, DE, ES, FR, PT); Tiorfix (BE, IT); Zedott (IN)

Pharmacologic Category Enkephalinase Inhibitor

Reported Use Treatment of acute diarrhea

Dosage Range Adults: Oral: Initial: 100 mg, may repeat every 8 hours as needed until diarrhea stops for up to 7 days

Product Availability Product available in various countries; not currently available in the U.S.

Dosage Forms

Capsule: 100 mg

- ◆ **Racemic Epinephrine** *see* EPINEPHrine (Systemic, Oral Inhalation) *on page 735*
- ◆ **Racepinephrine** *see* EPINEPHrine (Systemic, Oral Inhalation) *on page 735*
- ◆ **RAD001** *see* Everolimus *on page 822*
- ◆ **Radiogardase** *see* Ferric Hexacyanoferrate *on page 870*
- ◆ **rAHF** *see* Antihemophilic Factor (Recombinant) *on page 152*
- ◆ **rAHF** *see* Antihemophilic Factor (Recombinant [Porcine Sequence]) *on page 153*
- ◆ **RAL** *see* Raltegravir *on page 1767*
- ◆ **R-albuterol** *see* Levalbuterol *on page 1189*
- ◆ **Ralivia (Can)** *see* TraMADol *on page 2074*

Raloxifene (ral OKS i feen)

Brand Names: U.S. Evista

Brand Names: Canada ACT Raloxifene; Apo-Raloxifene; Evista; PMS-Raloxifene; Teva-Raloxifene

Index Terms Keoxifene Hydrochloride; Raloxifene Hydrochloride

Pharmacologic Category Selective Estrogen Receptor Modulator (SERM)

Use Prevention and treatment of osteoporosis in postmenopausal women; risk reduction for invasive breast cancer in postmenopausal women with osteoporosis and in postmenopausal women with high risk for invasive breast cancer

Pregnancy Risk Factor X

Pregnancy Considerations Adverse events were observed in in animal reproduction studies. Raloxifene is contraindicated for use in women who are or may become pregnant.

Breast-Feeding Considerations It is not known if raloxifene is excreted into breast milk. Breast-feeding is contraindicated by the manufacturer.

Contraindications History of or current venous thromboembolic disorders (including DVT, PE, and retinal vein thrombosis); pregnancy or women who could become pregnant; breast-feeding

Warnings/Precautions Hazardous agent - use appropriate precautions for handling and disposal (NIOSH 2014 [group 2]).

[U.S. Boxed Warning]: May increase the risk for DVT or PE; use contraindicated in patients with history of or current venous thromboembolic disorders. Use with caution in patients at high risk for venous thromboembolism; the risk for DVT and PE are higher in the first 4 months of treatment. Discontinue at least 72 hours prior to and during prolonged immobilization (postoperative recovery or prolonged bedrest). **[U.S. Boxed Warning]: The risk of death due to stroke may be increased in women with coronary heart disease or in women at risk for coronary events;** use with caution in patients with cardiovascular disease. Not be used for the prevention of cardiovascular disease. Use caution with moderate-to-severe renal dysfunction, hepatic impairment, unexplained uterine bleeding, and in women with a history of elevated triglycerides in response to treatment with oral estrogens (or estrogen/progestin). Safety with concomitant estrogen therapy has not been established. Safety and efficacy in premenopausal women or men have not been established. Not indicated for treatment of invasive breast cancer, to reduce the risk of recurrence of invasive breast cancer or to reduce the risk of noninvasive breast cancer. The efficacy (for breast cancer risk reduction) in women with inherited BRCA1 and BRCA1 mutations has not been established.

Adverse Reactions Note: Raloxifene has been associated with increased risk of thromboembolism (DVT, PE) and superficial thrombophlebitis; risk is similar to reported risk of HRT

Cardiovascular: Chest pain, peripheral edema, venous thromboembolism

Central nervous system: Insomnia

Dermatologic: Rash

Endocrine & metabolic: Breast pain, hot flashes

Gastrointestinal: Abdominal pain, cholelithiasis, flatulence, gastroenteritis, vomiting, weight gain

Genitourinary: Endometrial disorder, leukorrhea, urinary tract disorder, uterine disorder, vaginal bleeding, vaginal hemorrhage

Neuromuscular & skeletal: Arthralgia, leg cramps/muscle spasm, myalgia, tendon disorder

Respiratory: Bronchitis, laryngitis, pharyngitis, pneumonia, sinusitis

Miscellaneous: Diaphoresis, flu-like syndrome, infection

Rare but important or life-threatening: Apolipoprotein A-1 increased, apolipoprotein B decreased, death related to VTE, fibrinogen decreased, hypertriglyceridemia (in women with a history of increased triglycerides in response to oral estrogens), intermittent claudication, LDL cholesterol decreased, lipoprotein decreased, retinal vein occlusion, stroke related to VTE, superficial thrombophlebitis, total serum cholesterol decreased

Drug Interactions

Metabolism/Transport Effects None known.

Avoid Concomitant Use

Avoid concomitant use of Raloxifene with any of the following: Ospemifene

Increased Effect/Toxicity

Raloxifene may increase the levels/effects of: Ospemifene

Decreased Effect

Raloxifene may decrease the levels/effects of: Levothyroxine; Ospemifene

The levels/effects of Raloxifene may be decreased by: Bile Acid Sequestrants

Storage/Stability Store at controlled room temperature of 20°C to 25°C (68°F to 77°F); excursions permitted to 15°C to 30°C (59°F to 86°F).

Mechanism of Action A selective estrogen receptor modulator (SERM), meaning that it affects some of the same receptors that estrogen does, but not all, and in some instances, it antagonizes or blocks estrogen; it acts like estrogen to prevent bone loss and has the potential to block some estrogen effects in the breast and uterine tissues. Raloxifene decreases bone resorption, increasing bone mineral density and decreasing fracture incidence.

Pharmacodynamics/Kinetics

Onset of action: 8 weeks

Absorption: Rapid; ~60%

Distribution: 2348 L/kg

Protein binding: >95% to albumin and α-glycoprotein; does not bind to sex-hormone-binding globulin

Metabolism: Hepatic, extensive first-pass effect; metabolized to glucuronide conjugates

Bioavailability: ~2%

Half-life elimination: 28-33 hours

Excretion: Primarily feces; urine (<0.2% as unchanged drug; <6% as glucuronide conjugates)

Dosage Adults: Females: Oral:

Osteoporosis: 60 mg once daily

Invasive breast cancer risk reduction: 60 mg once daily for 5 years per ASCO guidelines (Visvanathan, 2009)

Dosage adjustment in renal impairment: No dosage adjustment provided in manufacturer's labeling. Use caution in moderate-to-severe impairment.

Dosage adjustment in hepatic impairment: No dosage adjustment provided in manufacturer's labeling (has not been studied). Use with caution.

Dietary Considerations May be taken without regard to meals. Osteoporosis prevention or treatment: Ensure adequate calcium and vitamin D intake; if dietary intake is inadequate, dietary supplementation is recommended. Women and men should consume:

Calcium: 1000 mg/day (men: 50-70 years) **or** 1200 mg/day (women ≥51 years and men ≥71 years) (IOM, 2011; NOF, 2013)

Vitamin D: 800-1000 IU/day (men and women ≥50 years) (NOF, 2013). Recommended Dietary Allowance (RDA): 600 IU/day (men and women ≤70 years) **or** 800 IU/day (men and women ≥71 years) (IOM, 2011).

Administration May be administered without regard to meals.

Hazardous agent; use appropriate precautions for handling and disposal (NIOSH 2014 [group 2]).

Monitoring Parameters Lipid profile; adequate diagnostic measures, including endometrial sampling, if indicated, should be performed to rule out malignancy in all cases of undiagnosed abnormal vaginal bleeding

Osteoporosis: Bone mineral density (BMD) should be re-evaluated every 2 years (or more frequently) after initiating therapy (NOF, 2013); annual measurements of height and weight; serum calcium and 25(OH)D; may consider monitoring biochemical markers of bone turnover

Reference Range

Calcium (total): Adults: 9.0-11.0 mg/dL (2.05-2.54 mmol/L), may slightly decrease with aging

Phosphorus: 2.5-4.5 mg/dL (0.81-1.45 mmol/L)

Vitamin D: There is no clear consensus on a reference range for total serum 25(OH)D concentrations or the validity of this level as it relates clinically to bone health. In addition, there is significant variability in the reporting of serum 25(OH)D levels as a result of different assay types in use; however, the following ranges have been suggested:

Adults (IOM, 2011): Sufficient levels in practically all persons: ≥20 ng/mL (50 nmol/L); concern for risk of toxicity: >50 ng/mL (125 nmol/L)

Osteoporosis patients (NOF, 2013): Recommended level to reach and maintain: ~30 ng/mL (75 nmol/L)

Additional Information The decrease in estrogen-related adverse effects with the selective estrogen-receptor modulators in general and raloxifene in particular should improve compliance and decrease the incidence of cardiovascular events and fractures while not increasing breast cancer.

Oncology Comment: The American Society of Clinical Oncology (ASCO) guidelines for breast cancer risk reduction (Visvanathan, 2009) recommend raloxifene (for 5 years) as an option to reduce the risk of ER-positive invasive breast cancer in postmenopausal women with a

5-year projected risk (based on NCI trial model) of ≥1.66%, or with lobular carcinoma *in situ*. Raloxifene should not be used in premenopausal women. Women with osteoporosis may use raloxifene beyond 5 years of treatment. According to the NCCN breast cancer risk reduction guidelines (v.2.2009), raloxifene is only recommended for postmenopausal women (≥35 years of age), and is equivalent to tamoxifen although, raloxifene has a better adverse event profile; however, tamoxifen is superior in reducing the risk on noninvasive breast cancer.

Dosage Forms

Tablet, Oral:

Evista: 60 mg

Generic: 60 mg

◆ **Raloxifene Hydrochloride** *see* Raloxifene *on page 1765*

Raltegravir (ral TEG ra vir)

Brand Names: U.S. Isentress

Brand Names: Canada Isentress

Index Terms MK-0518; RAL

Pharmacologic Category Antiretroviral, Integrase Inhibitor (Anti-HIV)

Use HIV infection:

U.S. labeling: Treatment of HIV-1 infection in combination with other antiretroviral agents in patients 4 weeks and older and weighing at least 3 kg

Canadian labeling: Treatment of HIV-1 infection in combination with other antiretroviral agents in patients ≥2 years of age

Pregnancy Risk Factor C

Pregnancy Considerations Adverse events were observed in some animal reproduction studies. Raltegravir has high transfer across the human placenta and can be detected in neonatal serum after delivery. Standard doses appear to be appropriate in pregnant women. The DHHS Perinatal HIV Guidelines consider raltegravir to be an alternative for use in antiretroviral-naïve pregnant patients when drug interactions with protease inhibitors are a concern. Because of its ability to rapidly suppress viral load, some experts have suggested using raltegravir in late pregnancy in women who have high viral loads; however, this use is not routinely recommended at this time. Reversible elevation of liver enzymes occurred in a patient who initiated raltegravir late in pregnancy; monitor liver enzymes if used during pregnancy.

Regardless of CD4 count or HIV RNA copy number, all HIV-infected pregnant women should receive a combination antiretroviral (ARV) drug regimen. A combination of antepartum, intrapartum, and infant ARV prophylaxis is recommended. ARV therapy should be started as soon as possible in women with symptomatic infection. Although earlier initiation may be more effective in reducing the perinatal transmission of HIV, initiation may be delayed until after 12 weeks gestation in women who do not require immediate treatment after careful consideration of maternal conditions (eg, nausea and vomiting) and the potential risks of first trimester fetal exposure for specific agents. A scheduled cesarean delivery at 38 weeks gestation is recommended for all women with HIV RNA >1000 copies/mL or unknown concentrations near delivery in order to decrease transmission. If ARV therapy must be interrupted for <24 hours during the peripartum period, stop then restart all medications simultaneously in order to decrease the chance of developing resistance. Long-term follow-up is recommended for all infants exposed to ARV medications. In couples who want to conceive, the HIV-infected partner should attain maximum viral suppression prior to conception.

Health care providers are encouraged to enroll pregnant women exposed to antiretroviral medications in the Antiretroviral Pregnancy Registry (1-800-258-4263 or www.-APRegistry.com). Health care providers caring for HIV-infected women and their infants may contact the National Perinatal HIV Hotline (888-448-8765) for clinical consultation (HHS [perinatal], 2014).

Breast-Feeding Considerations It is not known if raltegravir is excreted into breast milk. Maternal or infant antiretroviral therapy does not completely eliminate the risk of postnatal HIV transmission. In addition, multiclass-resistant virus has been detected in breast-feeding infants despite maternal therapy. Therefore, in the United States, where formula is accessible, affordable, safe, and sustainable, and the risk of infant mortality due to diarrhea and respiratory infections is low, complete avoidance of breast-feeding by HIV-infected women is recommended to decrease potential transmission of HIV (HHS [perinatal], 2014).

Contraindications

There are no contraindications listed in the manufacturer's labeling.

Canadian labeling: Hypersensitivity to raltegravir or any other component of the formulation

Warnings/Precautions Patients may develop immune reconstitution syndrome resulting in the occurrence of an inflammatory response to an indolent or residual opportunistic infection during initial HIV treatment or activation of autoimmune disorders (eg, Graves' disease, polymyositis, Guillain-Barré syndrome) later in therapy; further evaluation and treatment may be required. Severe, life-threatening or fatal cases of Stevens-Johnson syndrome and toxic epidermal necrolysis have been reported. Hypersensitivity reactions (rash [may occur with fever, fatigue, malaise, conjunctivitis, or other constitutional symptoms], organ dysfunction and/or hepatic failure) have also been reported. Discontinue immediately if a severe skin reaction or hypersensitivity symptoms develop. Monitor liver transaminases and start supportive therapy. Myopathy and rhabdomyolysis have been reported; use caution in patients with risk factors for CK elevations and/or skeletal muscle abnormalities. Potentially significant drug-drug interactions may exist, requiring dose or frequency adjustment, additional monitoring, and/or selection of alternative therapy. Avoid use as a boosted PI replacement in antiretroviral experienced patients with documented resistance to nucleoside reverse transcriptase inhibitors. Chewable tablet contains phenylalanine. Raltegravir film-coated tablets and chewable tablets or oral suspension are not bioequivalent and are not substitutable on a mg/mg basis.

Adverse Reactions

Central nervous system: Dizziness, fatigue, headache, insomnia

Endocrine & metabolic: Increased serum glucose

Gastrointestinal: Increased serum amylase, increased serum lipase, nausea

Hematologic: Abnormal absolute neutrophil count, thrombocytopenia

Hepatic: Hyperbilirubinemia, increased serum alkaline phosphatase, increased serum ALT (incidence higher with hepatitis B and/or C coinfection), increased serum AST (incidence higher with hepatitis B and/or C coinfection)

Neuromuscular & skeletal: Increased creatine phosphokinase

Rare but important or life-threatening: Anemia, cerebellar ataxia, depression (particularly in subjects with a preexisting history of psychiatric illness), drug rash with eosinophilia and systemic symptoms (DRESS; Perry, 2013), gastritis, hepatic failure, hepatitis, hypersensitivity, myopathy, nephrolithiasis, psychomotor agitation (children;

grade 3), renal failure, rhabdomyolysis, Stevens-Johnson syndrome, suicidal ideation, toxic epidermal necrolysis

Drug Interactions

Metabolism/Transport Effects None known.

Avoid Concomitant Use

Avoid concomitant use of Raltegravir with any of the following: Aluminum Hydroxide; Magnesium Salts

Increased Effect/Toxicity

Raltegravir may increase the levels/effects of: Fibric Acid Derivatives; HMG-CoA Reductase Inhibitors; Zidovudine

The levels/effects of Raltegravir may be increased by: Proton Pump Inhibitors

Decreased Effect

Raltegravir may decrease the levels/effects of: Fosamprenavir

The levels/effects of Raltegravir may be decreased by: Aluminum Hydroxide; Efavirenz; Fosamprenavir; Magnesium Salts; Rifabutin; Rifampin; Tipranavir

Food Interactions Variable absorption depending upon meal type (low- vs high-fat meal) and dosage form. Management: Raltegravir was administered without regard to meals in clinical trials.

Storage/Stability

Store at 20°C to 25°C (68°F to 77°F); excursions are permitted between 15°C and 30°C (59°F and 86°F).

Chewable tablets: Store in the original package; keep desiccant in the bottle to protect from moisture.

Oral suspension: Store in the original container; do not open foil packet until ready for reconstitution and use.

Mechanism of Action Incorporation of viral DNA into the host cell's genome is required to produce a self-replicating provirus and propagation of infectious virion particles. The viral cDNA strand produced by reverse transcriptase is subsequently processed and inserted into the human genome by the enzyme HIV-1 integrase (encoded by the pol gene of HIV). Raltegravir inhibits the catalytic activity of integrase, thus preventing integration of the proviral gene into human DNA.

Pharmacodynamics/Kinetics

Absorption: Film-coated tablet: AUC increased twofold with high-fat meal; Chewable tablet: AUC decreased by ~6% with high-fat meal (not clinically significant); Oral suspension: The effect of food was not studied

Protein binding: ~83%

Metabolism: Primarily hepatic glucuronidation mediated by UGT1A1

Bioavailability: Film-coated tablet: Not established; however, chewable tablet and oral suspension have higher bioavailability compared to film-coated tablet

Half-life elimination: ~9 hours

Time to peak, plasma: Film-coated tablet: ~3 hours

Excretion: Feces (~51%, as unchanged drug); urine (~32%; 9% as unchanged drug)

Dosage

HIV treatment: Oral:

Note: Raltegravir film-coated tablets and chewable tablets or oral suspension are not bioequivalent and are not substitutable on a mg/mg basis

U.S. labeling:

Infants ≥4 weeks and Children (≥3 to <25 kg): Weight-based dosing based on ~6 mg/kg/dose twice daily (maximum dose: 600 mg/day [chewable tablet]; 200 mg/day [oral suspension]).

3 to <4 kg: 20 mg twice daily (oral suspension)
4 to <6 kg: 30 mg twice daily (oral suspension)
6 to <8 kg: 40 mg twice daily (oral suspension)
8 to <11 kg: 60 mg twice daily (oral suspension)
11 to <14 kg: 80 mg twice daily (oral suspension) or 75 mg twice daily (chewable tablet) (see **"Note"**)
14 to <20 kg: 100 mg twice daily (oral suspension or chewable tablet) (see **"Note"**)
20 to <25 kg: 150 mg twice daily (chewable tablet)

Note: Infants and Children ≥4 weeks who are between 11 and <20 kg may use either the chewable tablet or the oral suspension. Patients can remain on the oral suspension as long as their weight is <20 kg.

Children and Adolescents ≥25 kg: **Note:** If unable to swallow a tablet, chewable tablets may be used.

Film-coated tablet: 400 mg twice daily.

Chewable tablet: Weight-based dosing based on ~6 mg/kg/dose twice daily (maximum dose: 600 mg daily).

25 to <28 kg: 150 mg twice daily (see **"Note"**)
28 to <40 kg: 200 mg twice daily (see **"Note"**)
≥40 kg: 300 mg twice daily (see **"Note"**)

Note: May use either weight-based dosing (chewable tablet) or adult dosing (film-coated tablet).

Children ≥12 years, Adolescents, and Adults: Film-coated tablet: 400 mg twice daily. **Note:** Raltegravir is a component of a recommended regimen with emtricitabine/tenofovir in antiretroviral-naive naive patients (DHHS [INSTI], 2013; HHS [adult], 2014).

Canadian labeling: Chewable tablet: Children 2 to <12 years (maximum dose: 600 mg/day):

7 to <10 kg: 50 mg twice daily
10 to <14 kg: 75 mg twice daily
14 to <20 kg: 100 mg twice daily
20 to <28 kg: 150 mg twice daily
28 to <40 kg: 200 mg twice daily
≥40 kg: 300 mg twice daily

Occupational HIV postexposure, prophylaxis (off-label use): Adults: Oral: Film-coated tablet: 400 mg twice daily for 4 weeks with concomitant emtricitabine/tenofovir. Recommended as preferred therapy (Kuhar, 2013).

Dosage adjustment for rifampin coadministration: 800 mg twice daily. There are no data to guide dose adjustment in patients <18 years of age.

Dosage adjustment in renal impairment:

Mild, moderate, and severe impairment: No dosage adjustment necessary.

End-stage renal disease (ESRD) on intermittent hemodialysis (IHD): Dose after dialysis on dialysis days.

Dosage adjustment in hepatic impairment:

Mild to moderate impairment: No dosage adjustment necessary.

Severe impairment: There are no dosage adjustments provided in manufacturer's labeling (has not been studied).

Dietary Considerations Some products may contain phenylalanine.

Administration May be administered without regard to meals.

Chewable tablets: May be chewed or swallowed whole; the 100 mg chewable tablet may be divided into equal halves.

Film-coated tablets: Must be swallowed whole.

Oral suspension: Open foil packet of drug (100 mg). Measure 5 mL water in provided mixing cup. Pour packet contents into 5 mL water, close lid and swirl for 30-60 seconds. Do not turn the mixing cup upside down. Once mixed, measure recommended suspension dose with an oral syringe. Administer within 30 minutes of mixing with water. Discard any remaining suspension in the trash.

Monitoring Parameters Viral load, CD4 count, lipid profile

HIV occupational postexposure prophylaxis (PEP) (Kuhar, 2013): Documented HIV test (at baseline and 6 weeks, 12 weeks and 6 months after exposure); if confirmation that a fourth generation HIV p2 antigen-HIV antibody test is being used, monitor at baseline, 6 weeks and 4 months after exposure. CBC, renal and hepatic function assessments at baseline and 2 weeks after exposure (minimum recommendations, others dictated by clinical assessment)

Dosage Forms

Packet, Oral:

Isentress: 100 mg (60 ea)

Tablet, Oral:

Isentress: 400 mg

Tablet Chewable, Oral:

Isentress: 25 mg, 100 mg

Raltitrexed [CAN/INT] (ral ti TREX ed)

Brand Names: Canada Tomudex

Index Terms D1694; ICI-D1694; Raltitrexed Disodium; TDX; ZD1694

Pharmacologic Category Antineoplastic Agent, Antimetabolite; Antineoplastic Agent, Antimetabolite (Antifolate)

Use Note: Not approved in U.S.

Treatment of advanced colorectal cancer

Pregnancy Considerations Use is contraindicated in women who are or may become pregnant during treatment. Pregnancy should be excluded prior to treatment, and should be avoided during treatment and for 6 months following treatment (including women with male partners receiving treatment). Pregnant women should not handle this medication.

Breast-Feeding Considerations Use in nursing women is contraindicated by the manufacturer.

Contraindications Hypersensitivity to raltitrexed or any component of the formulation; severe renal or hepatic impairment; pregnancy or breast-feeding

Warnings/Precautions Hazardous agent - use appropriate precautions for handling and disposal (meets NIOSH 2014 criteria). Neutropenia, leukopenia, anemia, and thrombocytopenia may occur. Use with caution in patients with preexisting marrow suppression. Nausea, vomiting and diarrhea are common; mucositis and stomatitis may also occur. Severe diarrhea with concomitant hematologic toxicity (neutropenia) may be life-threatening and may require discontinuation or subsequent dose reduction.

Use caution in elderly, mild-to-moderate hepatic or renal dysfunction (use in severe hepatic or renal impairment is contraindicated). Use is not recommended in clinical jaundice or decompensated hepatic disease. Therapy interruption is required in patients with hepatotoxicity; may reintroduce therapy only with decrease in hepatic enzymes to grade 2. Asymptomatic and self-limiting increases (reversible) in ALT and AST may occur. Use caution in patients who have received prior radiation therapy.

Folinic acid (leucovorin calcium), folic acid, or folate-containing medications (eg, multivitamins) may interfere with raltitrexed; do not administer immediately prior to or concurrently with raltitrexed. May cause malaise/weakness (caution patients concerning operation of machinery/driving). Use in pediatric patients is not recommended by the manufacturer.

Adverse Reactions

Cardiovascular: Arrhythmias, CHF, peripheral edema

Central nervous system: Chills, depression, dizziness, fever, headache, insomnia, malaise, pain

Dermatologic: Alopecia, cellulitis, exfoliative eruptions, pruritus, rash

Endocrine & metabolic: Dehydration, hypokalemia

Gastrointestinal: Abdominal pain, anorexia, constipation, diarrhea, dyspepsia, flatulence, mucositis, nausea, stomatitis, taste perversion, vomiting, weight loss, xerostomia

Genitourinary: Urinary tract infection

Hematologic: Anemia, leukopenia, thrombocytopenia

Hepatic: Alkaline phosphatase increased, bilirubin increased, transaminases increased

Neuromuscular & skeletal: Arthralgia, hypotonia, myalgia, paresthesia, weakness

Ocular: Conjunctivitis

Renal: Creatinine increased (serum)

Respiratory: Cough, dyspnea, pharyngitis

Miscellaneous: Diaphoresis, flu-like syndrome, infection, sepsis

Rare but important or life-threatening: Desquamation

Drug Interactions

Metabolism/Transport Effects None known.

Avoid Concomitant Use

Avoid concomitant use of Raltitrexed with any of the following: CloZAPine; Dipyrone; Folic Acid; Leucovorin Calcium-Levoleucovorin; Levomefolate; Methylfolate; Multivitamins/Minerals (with ADEK, Folate, Iron)

Increased Effect/Toxicity

Raltitrexed may increase the levels/effects of: CloZAPine

The levels/effects of Raltitrexed may be increased by: Dipyrone

Decreased Effect

The levels/effects of Raltitrexed may be decreased by: Folic Acid; Leucovorin Calcium-Levoleucovorin; Levomefolate; Methylfolate; Multivitamins/Minerals (with ADEK, Folate, Iron)

Preparation for Administration Hazardous agent; use appropriate precautions for handling and disposal (meets NIOSH 2014 criteria). Reconstitute 2 mg vial with 4 mL SWFI to produce 0.5 mg/mL solution; volume required for dose should be further diluted by adding to 50-250 mL NS or D_5W.

Storage/Stability Intact vials should be refrigerated at 2°C to 25°C (36°F to 77°F). Protect from light. Reconstituted and subsequent IV admixture solutions (saline or dextrose) are stable for up to 24 hours under refrigeration at 2°C to 8°C (36°F to 46°F), although the manufacturer recommends use as soon as possible after preparation.

Mechanism of Action Raltitrexed is a folate analogue that inhibits thymidylate synthase, blocking purine synthesis. This results in an overall inhibition of DNA synthesis.

Pharmacodynamics/Kinetics

Distribution: V_{ss}: 548 L

Protein binding: 93%

Metabolism: Undergoes extensive intracellular metabolism to active polyglutamate forms; appears to be little or no systemic metabolism of the drug

Half-life elimination: Triphasic; Beta: 2 hours; Terminal: 198 hours

Excretion: Urine (~50% as unchanged drug); feces (~15%)

Dosage Note: Treatment should be administered only if WBC >4000/mm^3, ANC >2000/mm^3, and platelets >100,000/mm^3

IV: Adults:

Colorectal cancer, advanced: 3 mg/m^2 every 3 weeks

Malignant pleural mesothelioma (off-label use): 3 mg/m^2 every 3 weeks (in combination with cisplatin) (van Meerbeeck, 2005)

Dosage adjustment for toxicity: Delay dose in subsequent cycles until recovery from toxicity.

Grade 4 gastrointestinal toxicity (diarrhea or mucositis) or grade 3 gastrointestinal toxicity in combination with grade 4 hematologic toxicity: Discontinue therapy and manage with supportive measures.

Grade 3 hematologic toxicity (neutropenia or thrombocytopenia) or grade 2 gastrointestinal toxicity (diarrhea or mucositis): Reduce dose by 25%

Grade 4 hematologic toxicity (neutropenia or thrombocytopenia) or grade 3 gastrointestinal toxicity (diarrhea or mucositis): Reduce dose by 50%

Dosage adjustment in renal impairment:

CrCl >65 mL/minute: No dosage adjustment necessary.

CrCl 55-65 mL/minute: Administer 75% of dose every 4 weeks

CrCl 25-54 mL/minute: Administer percentage of dose equivalent to CrCl every 4 weeks (eg, 25% of dose for CrCl of 25 mL/minute)

CrCl <25 mL/minute: Do not administer (use is contraindicated in severe renal impairment)

Dosage adjustment for hepatic impairment: Use is not recommended in clinical jaundice or decompensated liver disease. Patients who develop hepatic toxicity should have treatment held until returns to grade 2.

Mild-to-moderate impairment: No dosage adjustment necessary.

Severe impairment: Use is contraindicated.

Dosing in obesity: *ASCO Guidelines for appropriate chemotherapy dosing in obese adults with cancer:* Utilize patient's actual body weight (full weight) for calculation of body surface area- or weight-based dosing, particularly when the intent of therapy is curative; manage regimen-related toxicities in the same manner as for nonobese patients; if a dose reduction is utilized due to toxicity, consider resumption of full weight-based dosing with subsequent cycles, especially if cause of toxicity (eg, hepatic or renal impairment) is resolved (Griggs, 2012).

Dietary Considerations Avoid folic acid, folinic acid (leucovorin calcium), and multivitamins with folic acid close to and during administration.

Administration Administer via IV infusion over 15 minutes. Hazardous agent; use appropriate precautions for handling and disposal (meets NIOSH 2014 criteria).

Monitoring Parameters CBC with differential (at baseline, prior to each treatment, or weekly if GI toxicity observed); hepatic function tests and serum creatinine (at baseline and prior to each treatment); signs of GI toxicity

Product Availability Not available in U.S.

Dosage Forms: Canada

Injection, powder for reconstitution, as disodium:

Tomudex®: 2 mg

◆ **Raltitrexed Disodium** *see* Raltitrexed [CAN/INT] *on page 1769*

Ramelteon (ra MEL tee on)

Brand Names: U.S. Rozerem

Index Terms TAK-375

Pharmacologic Category Hypnotic, Miscellaneous; Melatonin Receptor Agonist

Use Treatment of insomnia characterized by difficulty with sleep onset

Pregnancy Risk Factor C

Pregnancy Considerations Animal studies have demonstrated teratogenic effects. May cause disturbances of reproductive hormonal regulation (eg, disruption of menses or decreased libido). There are no adequate and well-controlled studies in pregnant women.

Breast-Feeding Considerations It is not known if ramelteon is excreted in breast milk. The manufacturer recommends that caution be exercised when administering ramelteon to nursing women.

Contraindications History of angioedema with previous ramelteon therapy (do not rechallenge); concurrent use with fluvoxamine

Warnings/Precautions Symptomatic treatment of insomnia should be initiated only after careful evaluation of potential causes of sleep disturbance. Failure of sleep disturbance to resolve after a reasonable period of treatment may indicate psychiatric and/or medical illness. Because of the rapid onset of action, administer immediately prior to bedtime or after the patient has gone to bed and is having difficulty falling asleep. Hypnotics/sedatives have been associated with abnormal thinking and behavior changes including decreased inhibition, aggression, bizarre behavior, agitation, hallucinations, and depersonalization. These changes may occur unpredictably and may indicate previously unrecognized psychiatric disorders; evaluate appropriately. Postmarketing studies have indicated that the use of hypnotic/sedative agents (including ramelteon) for sleep has been associated with hypersensitivity reactions including anaphylaxis as well as angioedema. Do not rechallenge patients who have developed angioedema with ramelteon therapy. An increased risk for hazardous sleep-related activities such as sleep-driving; cooking and eating food, and making phone calls while asleep have also been noted. Use caution with preexisting depression or other psychiatric conditions. Caution when using with other CNS depressants; avoid engaging in hazardous activities or activities requiring mental alertness. Not recommended for use in patients with severe sleep apnea or COPD. Use caution with moderate hepatic impairment; not recommended in patients with severe impairment. May cause disturbances of hormonal regulation. Use caution when administered concomitantly with strong CYP1A2 inhibitors.

Adverse Reactions

Central nervous system: Depression, dizziness, fatigue, insomnia worsened, somnolence

Endocrine & metabolic: Serum cortisol decreased

Gastrointestinal: Nausea, taste perversion

Neuromuscular & skeletal: Arthralgia, myalgia

Respiratory: Upper respiratory infection

Miscellaneous: Influenza

Postmarketing and/or case reports: Anaphylaxis, angioedema, complex sleep-related behavior (sleep-driving, cooking or eating food, making phone calls), prolactin levels increased, testosterone levels decreased

Drug Interactions

Metabolism/Transport Effects Substrate of CYP1A2 (major), CYP2C19 (minor), CYP3A4 (minor); **Note:** Assignment of Major/Minor substrate status based on clinically relevant drug interaction potential

Avoid Concomitant Use

Avoid concomitant use of Ramelteon with any of the following: Azelastine (Nasal); FluvoxaMINE; Orphenadrine; Paraldehyde; Sodium Oxybate; Thalidomide

Increased Effect/Toxicity

Ramelteon may increase the levels/effects of: Alcohol (Ethyl); Azelastine (Nasal); Buprenorphine; CNS Depressants; Hydrocodone; Methotrimeprazine; Metyrosine; Mirtazapine; Orphenadrine; Paraldehyde; Pramipexole; ROPINIRole; Rotigotine; Selective Serotonin Reuptake Inhibitors; Sodium Oxybate; Suvorexant; Thalidomide; Zolpidem

The levels/effects of Ramelteon may be increased by: Abiraterone Acetate; Brimonidine (Topical); Cannabis; CYP1A2 Inhibitors (Moderate); CYP1A2 Inhibitors (Strong); Deferasirox; Doxylamine; Dronabinol; Droperidol; Fluconazole; FluvoxaMINE; HydrOXYzine; Kava Kava; Ketoconazole (Systemic); Magnesium Sulfate; Methotrimeprazine; Nabilone; Peginterferon Alfa-2b; Perampanel; Rufinamide; Tapentadol; Tetrahydrocannabinol; Vemurafenib

Decreased Effect

The levels/effects of Ramelteon may be decreased by: Rifamycin Derivatives

Food Interactions Taking with high-fat meal delays T_{max} and increases AUC (~31%). Management: Do not take with a high-fat meal.

Storage/Stability Store at 25°C (77°F); excursions permitted to 15°C to 30°C (59°F to 86°F). Protect from moisture.

Mechanism of Action Potent, selective agonist of melatonin receptors MT_1 and MT_2 (with little affinity for MT_3) within the suprachiasmic nucleus of the hypothalamus, an area responsible for determination of circadian rhythms and synchronization of the sleep-wake cycle. Agonism of MT_1 is thought to preferentially induce sleepiness, while MT_2 receptor activation preferentially influences regulation of circadian rhythms. Ramelteon is eightfold more selective for MT_1 than MT_2 and exhibits nearly sixfold higher affinity for MT_1 than melatonin, presumably allowing for enhanced effects on sleep induction.

Pharmacodynamics/Kinetics

Onset of action: 30 minutes

Absorption: Rapid; high-fat meal delays T_{max} and increases AUC (~31%)

Distribution: 74 L

Protein binding: ~82%

Metabolism: Extensive first-pass effect; oxidative metabolism primarily through CYP1A2 and to a lesser extent through CYP2C and CYP3A4; forms active metabolite (M-II)

Bioavailability: Absolute: 1.8%

Half-life elimination: Ramelteon: 1-2.6 hours; M-II: 2-5 hours

Time to peak, plasma: Median: 0.5-1.5 hours

Excretion: Primarily as metabolites: Urine (84%); feces (4%)

Dosage Oral: Adults: One 8 mg tablet within 30 minutes of bedtime

Dosage adjustment in renal impairment: No dosage adjustment necessary.

Dosage adjustment in hepatic impairment:

Mild-to-moderate impairment: No dosage adjustment necessary. Use with caution.

Severe impairment: Use is not recommended.

Dietary Considerations Do not take with high-fat meal.

Administration Do not administer with a high-fat meal. Swallow tablet whole; do not break.

Dosage Forms

Tablet, Oral:

Rozerem: 8 mg

Ramipril (RA mi pril)

Brand Names: U.S. Altace

Brand Names: Canada ACT Ramipril; Altace; Apo-Ramipril; Auro-Ramipri; Dom-Ramipril; JAMP-Ramipril; Mar-Ramipril; Mint-Ramipril; Mylan-Ramipril; PMS-Ramipril; Pro-Ramipril; RAN-Ramipril; ratio-Ramipril; Sandoz-Ramipril; Teva-Ramipril

Pharmacologic Category Angiotensin-Converting Enzyme (ACE) Inhibitor; Antihypertensive

Use

Heart failure post-myocardial infarction: Treatment of heart failure (HF) after myocardial infarction (MI)

The 2013 American College of Cardiology Foundation/American Heart Association (ACCF/AHA) heart failure guidelines recommend the use of ACE inhibitors, along with other guideline-directed medical therapies, to prevent HF in patients with a reduced ejection fraction who have a history of MI (stage B HF), to prevent HF in any patient with a reduced ejection fraction (stage B HF), or to treat those with HF and reduced ejection fraction (stage C HFrEF) (Yancy, 2013)

The 2013 ACCF/AHA guidelines for the management of patients with ST-elevation myocardial infarction (STEMI) state that an ACE inhibitor should be initiated within the first 24 hours after STEMI in patients with anterior MI, heart failure, or left ventricular ejection fraction (LVEF) ≤0.4. It is also reasonable to initiate an ACE inhibitor in all patients with STEMI (O'Gara, 2013)

Hypertension: Treatment of hypertension, alone or in combination with thiazide diuretics

The 2014 guideline for the management of high blood pressure in adults (Eighth Joint National Committee [JNC 8]) recommends initiation of pharmacologic treatment to lower blood pressure for the following patients:

- Patients ≥60 years of age with systolic blood pressure (SBP) ≥150 mm Hg or diastolic blood pressure (DBP) ≥ 90 mm Hg. Goal of therapy is SBP <150 mm Hg and DBP <90 mm Hg.
- Patients <60 years of age with SBP ≥140 mm Hg or DBP is ≥90 mm Hg. Goal of therapy is SBP <140 mm Hg and DBP <90 mm Hg.
- Patients ≥18 years of age with diabetes and SBP ≥140 mm Hg or DBP ≥90 mm Hg. Goal of therapy is SBP <140 mm Hg and DBP <90 mm Hg.
- Patients ≥18 years of age with chronic kidney disease (CKD) and SBP ≥140 mm Hg or DBP ≥90 mm Hg. Goal of therapy is SBP <140 mm Hg and DBP <90 mm Hg.

In patients with CKD, regardless of race or diabetes status, the use of an ACE inhibitor (ACEI) or angiotensin receptor blocker (ARB) as initial therapy is recommended to improve kidney outcomes. In the general nonblack population (without CKD) including those with diabetes, initial antihypertensive treatment should consist of a thiazide-type diuretic, calcium channel blocker, ACEI, or ARB. In the general black population (without CKD) including those with diabetes, initial antihypertensive treatment should consist of a thiazide-type diuretic or a calcium channel blocker **instead of** an ACEI or ARB.

Reduction in risk of MI, stroke, and death from cardiovascular causes: To reduce the risk of MI, stroke, and death in patients ≥55 years of age at high risk of developing major cardiovascular events

Pregnancy Risk Factor D

Pregnancy Considerations **[U.S. Boxed Warning]: Drugs that act on the renin-angiotensin system can cause injury and death to the developing fetus. Discontinue as soon as possible once pregnancy is detected.** Ramipril crosses the placenta; teratogenic effects may occur following maternal use during pregnancy. Drugs that act on the renin-angiotensin system are associated with oligohydramnios. Oligohydramnios, due to decreased fetal renal function, may lead to fetal lung hypoplasia and skeletal malformations. Their use in pregnancy is also associated with anuria, hypotension, renal failure, skull hypoplasia, and death in the fetus/neonate. Chronic maternal hypertension itself is also associated with adverse events in the fetus/infant. ACE inhibitors are not recommended during pregnancy to treat maternal hypertension or heart failure. Use of an ACE inhibitor should also be avoided in any woman of reproductive age. Women who are planning a pregnancy should be considered for other medication options if an ACE inhibitor is currently prescribed or the ACE inhibitor should be discontinued as soon as possible once pregnancy is detected. The exposed fetus should be monitored for fetal growth, amniotic fluid volume, and organ formation. Infants exposed to an ACE inhibitor in utero should be monitored for hyperkalemia, hypotension, and oliguria (exchange transfusions or dialysis may be needed). These adverse events are generally associated with maternal use in the second and third trimesters.

Untreated chronic maternal hypertension is also associated with adverse events in the fetus, infant, and mother.

The use of ACE inhibitors is not recommended to treat chronic uncomplicated hypertension in pregnant women and should generally be avoided in women of reproductive potential (ACOG, 2013).

Breast-Feeding Considerations Ramipril and its metabolites were not detected in breast milk following a single oral dose of 10 mg. It is not known if multiple doses will produce detectable levels. Breast-feeding is not recommended by the manufacturer.

Contraindications Hypersensitivity to ramipril or any component of the formulation; prior hypersensitivity (including angioedema) to ACE inhibitors; concomitant use with aliskiren in patients with diabetes mellitus

Warnings/Precautions Anaphylactic reactions may occur rarely with ACE inhibitors. At any time during treatment (especially following first dose) angioedema may occur rarely with ACE inhibitors; it may involve the head and neck (potentially compromising airway) or the intestine (presenting with abdominal pain). African-Americans and patients with idiopathic or hereditary angioedema may be at an increased risk. Prolonged frequent monitoring may be required especially if tongue, glottis, or larynx are involved as they are associated with airway obstruction. Patients with a history of airway surgery may have a higher risk of airway obstruction. Aggressive early and appropriate management is critical. Use in patients with previous angioedema associated with ACE inhibitor therapy is contraindicated. Severe anaphylactoid reactions may be seen during hemodialysis (eg, CVVHD) with high-flux dialysis membranes (eg, AN69), and rarely, during low density lipoprotein apheresis with dextran sulfate cellulose. Rare cases of anaphylactoid reactions have been reported in patients undergoing sensitization treatment with hymenoptera (bee, wasp) venom while receiving ACE inhibitors.

Symptomatic hypotension with or without syncope can occur with ACE inhibitors (usually with the first several doses); effects are most often observed in volume-depleted patients; close monitoring of patient is required especially with initial dosing and dosing increases; blood pressure must be lowered at a rate appropriate for the patient's clinical condition. Initiation of therapy in patients with ischemic heart disease or cerebrovascular disease warrants close observation due to the potential consequences posed by falling blood pressure (eg, MI, stroke). Use with caution in hypertrophic cardiomyopathy with outflow tract obstruction, severe aortic stenosis, or before, during, or immediately after major surgery. **[U.S. Boxed Warning]: Drugs that act on the renin-angiotensin system can cause injury and death to the developing fetus. Discontinue as soon as possible once pregnancy is detected.**

Hyperkalemia may occur with ACE inhibitors; risk factors include renal dysfunction, diabetes mellitus, concomitant use of potassium-sparing diuretics, potassium supplements, and/or potassium containing salts. Use cautiously, if at all, with these agents and monitor potassium closely. Cough may occur with ACE inhibitors. Other causes of cough should be considered (eg, pulmonary congestion in patients with heart failure) and excluded prior to discontinuation.

May be associated with deterioration of renal function and/or increases in serum creatinine, particularly in patients with low renal blood flow (eg, renal artery stenosis, heart failure) whose glomerular filtration rate (GFR) is dependent on efferent arteriolar vasoconstriction by angiotensin II; deterioration may result in oliguria, acute renal failure, and progressive azotemia. Small increases in serum creatinine may occur following initiation; consider discontinuation only in patients with progressive and/or significant deterioration in renal function. Use with caution in patients with unstented unilateral/bilateral renal artery stenosis. When unstented bilateral renal artery stenosis is present, use is generally avoided due to the elevated risk of deterioration in renal function unless possible benefits outweigh risks. Potentially significant drug-drug interactions may exist, requiring dose or frequency adjustment, additional monitoring, and/or selection of alternative therapy.

Rare toxicities associated with ACE inhibitors include cholestatic jaundice (which may progress to fulminant hepatic necrosis), agranulocytosis, neutropenia, or leukopenia with myeloid hypoplasia. Patients with collagen vascular diseases (especially with concomitant renal impairment) or renal impairment alone may be at increased risk for hematologic toxicity; periodically monitor CBC with differential in these patients.

Adverse Reactions

Cardiovascular: Angina, hypotension, orthostatic hypotension, syncope

Central nervous system: Dizziness, fatigue, headache, vertigo

Endocrine & metabolic: Hyperkalemia

Gastrointestinal: Nausea, vomiting

Neuromuscular & skeletal: Chest pain (noncardiac)

Renal: Increased BUN or serum creatinine (transient elevations of creatinine and/or BUN may occur more frequently), renal dysfunction

Respiratory: Cough increased

Rare but important or life-threatening: Agranulocytosis, amnesia, anaphylactoid reaction, angioedema, arrhythmia, bone marrow depression, convulsions, depression, dysphagia, eosinophilia, erythema multiforme, hearing loss, hemolytic anemia, hepatitis, hypersensitivity reactions (urticaria, rash, fever), impotence, insomnia, MI, neuropathy, onycholysis, pancreatitis, pancytopenia, pemphigoid, pemphigus, photosensitivity, proteinuria, Stevens-Johnson syndrome, symptomatic hypotension, thrombocytopenia, toxic epidermal necrolysis, visual hallucinations (Doane, 2013)

Worsening of renal function may occur in patients with bilateral renal artery stenosis or in hypovolemia. In addition, a syndrome which may include fever, myalgia, arthralgia, interstitial nephritis, vasculitis, rash, eosinophilia and positive ANA, and elevated ESR has been reported with ACE inhibitors. Risk of pancreatitis and/or agranulocytosis may be increased in patients with collagen vascular disease or renal impairment.

Drug Interactions

Metabolism/Transport Effects None known.

Avoid Concomitant Use

Avoid concomitant use of Ramipril with any of the following: Telmisartan

Increased Effect/Toxicity

Ramipril may increase the levels/effects of: Allopurinol; Amifostine; Antihypertensives; AzaTHIOprine; DULoxetine; Ferric Gluconate; Gold Sodium Thiomalate; Grass Pollen Allergen Extract (5 Grass Extract); Hypotensive Agents; Iron Dextran Complex; Levodopa; Lithium; Nonsteroidal Anti-Inflammatory Agents; Obinutuzumab; RisperiDONE; RiTUXimab; Sodium Phosphates

The levels/effects of Ramipril may be increased by: Alfuzosin; Aliskiren; Angiotensin II Receptor Blockers; Barbiturates; Brimonidine (Topical); Canagliflozin; Dapoxetine; Diazoxide; DPP-IV Inhibitors; Eplerenone; Everolimus; Heparin; Heparin (Low Molecular Weight); Herbs (Hypotensive Properties); Loop Diuretics; MAO Inhibitors; Nicorandil; Pentoxifylline; Phosphodiesterase 5 Inhibitors; Potassium Salts; Potassium-Sparing Diuretics; Prostacyclin Analogues; Sirolimus; Telmisartan; Temsirolimus; Thiazide Diuretics; TiZANidine; Tolvaptan; Trimethoprim

Decreased Effect

The levels/effects of Ramipril may be decreased by: Aprotinin; Herbs (Hypertensive Properties); Icatibant; Lanthanum; Methylphenidate; Nonsteroidal Anti-Inflammatory Agents; Salicylates; Yohimbine

Storage/Stability Store at 15°C to 30°C (59°F to 86°F). Ramipril mixed with applesauce, apple juice, or water may be stored at room temperature for up to 24 hours or for up to 48 hours under refrigeration.

Mechanism of Action Ramipril is an ACE inhibitor which prevents the formation of angiotensin II from angiotensin I and exhibits pharmacologic effects that are similar to captopril. Ramipril must undergo enzymatic saponification by esterases in the liver to its biologically active metabolite, ramiprilat. The pharmacodynamic effects of ramipril result from the high-affinity, competitive, reversible binding of ramiprilat to angiotensin-converting enzyme, thus preventing the formation of the potent vasoconstrictor angiotensin II. This isomerized enzyme-inhibitor complex has a slow rate of dissociation, which results in high potency and a long duration of action; a CNS mechanism may also be involved in the hypotensive effect as angiotensin II increases adrenergic outflow from CNS; vasoactive kallikreins may be decreased in conversion to active hormones by ACE inhibitors, thus reducing blood pressure

Pharmacodynamics/Kinetics

Onset of action: 1-2 hours

Duration: 24 hours

Absorption: Well absorbed (50% to 60%)

Distribution: Plasma levels decline in a triphasic fashion; rapid decline is a distribution phase to peripheral compartment, plasma protein and tissue ACE (half-life: 2-4 hours); second phase is an apparent elimination phase representing the clearance of free ramiprilat (half-life: 9-18 hours); and final phase is the terminal elimination phase representing the equilibrium phase between tissue binding and dissociation

Protein binding: Ramipril: 73%; Ramiprilat: 56%

Metabolism: Hepatic to the active form, ramiprilat

Bioavailability: Ramipril: 28%; Ramiprilat: 44%

Half-life elimination: Ramiprilat: Effective: 13-17 hours; Terminal: >50 hours

Time to peak, serum: Ramipril: ~1 hour; Ramiprilat: 2-4 hours

Excretion: Urine (60%) and feces (40%) as parent drug and metabolites

Dosage

Adults: Oral: **Note:** Consider discontinuation or dose reduction of concomitant diuretic when initiating ramipril. If diuretic cannot be discontinued or dose reduced, consider reduced initial ramipril dose. Monitor blood pressure closely until stabilized.

Heart failure post-myocardial infarction: Initial: 2.5 mg twice daily (patient should be monitored for at least 2 hours after initial dose and for at least an additional hour after blood pressure has stabilized); may reduce dose to 1.25 mg twice daily for hypotension. Reduce the dose of any concomitant diuretics, if possible. Continue initial dose for one week then titrate upward every 3 weeks as tolerated to target dose of 5 mg twice daily

Heart failure (off-label use): Initial: 1.25 to 2.5 mg once daily; target dose: 10 mg once daily (ACCF/AHA [Yancy, 2013])

Hypertension: Initial dose in patients not receiving a diuretic is 2.5 mg once daily; titrate to effect. Usual maintenance (per the manufacturer): 2.5 to 20 mg daily in 1 or 2 divided doses (consider twice daily administration for patients unable to maintain adequate blood pressure control with once daily administration). Usual dosage range (ASH/ISH [Weber, 2014]): 5 to 10 mg daily

Reduction in risk of MI, stroke, and death from cardiovascular causes: Initial: 2.5 mg once daily for 1 week, then 5 mg once daily for the next 3 weeks, then increase as tolerated to 10 mg once daily (may be given as divided dose in hypertensive or recently post-MI patients)

Elderly: Oral: Adjust for renal function for elderly since glomerular filtration rates are decreased; may see exaggerated hypotensive effects if renal clearance is not considered. In the management of hypertension, consider lower initial doses and titrate to response (Aronow, 2011).

Dosage adjustment for patients with volume depletion: Initial: Administer 1.25 mg once daily; titrate as tolerated to effect.

Dosage adjustment in renal impairment:

CrCl >40 mL/minute: No dosage adjustment necessary.

CrCl <40 mL/minute: Administer 25% of normal dose.

Renal artery stenosis: Initial: 1.25 mg once daily; titrate as tolerated to effect

Renal failure and heart failure post-MI: Initial: 1.25 mg once daily, may increase to 1.25 mg twice daily and then up to 2.5 mg twice daily as tolerated

Renal failure and hypertension: Initial: 1.25 mg once daily, titrated as tolerated to effect; maximum: 5 mg daily

Dosage adjustment in hepatic impairment: No dosage adjustment provided in manufacturer's labeling; discontinue use for jaundice or marked elevation of hepatic enzymes.

Administration Swallow capsule whole; may open the capsule and the mix contents with 120 mL of water, apple juice, or applesauce.

Monitoring Parameters Blood pressure; serum creatinine and potassium; if patient has collagen vascular disease and/or renal impairment, periodically monitor CBC with differential

2013 ACCF/AHA Heart Failure guideline recommendations: Within 1-2 weeks after initiation and periodically thereafter, reassess renal function and serum potassium especially in patients with preexisting hypotension, hyponatremia, diabetes mellitus, azotemia, or those taking potassium supplements (ACCF/AHA [Yancy, 2013]).

Dosage Forms

Capsule, Oral:

Altace: 1.25 mg, 2.5 mg, 5 mg, 10 mg

Generic: 1.25 mg, 2.5 mg, 5 mg, 10 mg

Dosage Forms: Canada Note: Also refer to Dosage Forms.

Capsule, Oral:

Altace:15 mg

Ramipril and Hydrochlorothiazide [CAN/INT] (RA mi pril & hye droe klor oh THYE a zide)

Brand Names: Canada Altace HCT; PMS-Ramipril HCTZ

Index Terms Hydrochlorothiazide and Ramipril

Pharmacologic Category Angiotensin-Converting Enzyme (ACE) Inhibitor; Antihypertensive; Diuretic, Thiazide

Use Note: Not approved in U.S.

Treatment of primary hypertension (not for initial therapy)

Pregnancy Considerations Drugs that act on the renin-angiotensin system can cause injury and death to the developing fetus. Discontinue as soon as possible once pregnancy is detected. Use is contraindicated in pregnant women. See individual agents.

Breast-Feeding Considerations Ramipril and thiazide diuretics are found in breast milk. Use in breast-feeding women is contraindicated. See individual agents.

Contraindications Hypersensitivity to ramipril, hydrochlorothiazide, other ACE inhibitors or thiazides, sulfonamide-derived drugs, or any other component of the formulation; angioedema related to previous treatment with an ACE inhibitor; patients with idiopathic or hereditary angioedema; anuria; hemodynamically relevant bilateral or unilateral renal artery stenosis; hypotensive states; pregnancy; breast-feeding

Warnings/Precautions See individual agents.

Adverse Reactions Note: Observed with ramipril/hydrochlorothiazide. Also see individual agents.

Central nervous system: Dizziness, headache

Neuromuscular & skeletal: Back pain, neuralgia, weakness

Respiratory: Bronchitis, cough increased, upper respiratory infection

Miscellaneous: Infection

Rare but important or life-threatening: Acute liver failure, acute renal failure, agranulocytosis, allergic reactions, anaphylactoid reaction, angina, angioedema, arrhythmia, arthralgia, auditory disturbance, bilirubin increased, bone marrow depression, bronchospasm, BUN increased, creatinine (serum) increased, dyspnea, eosinophilia, erythema multiforme, exanthema, gastroenteritis, gout, hemolytic anemia, hypercalcemia, hypercholesterolemia, hyperglycemia, hyper-/hypokalemia, hypertriglyceridemia, hyperuricemia, hypochloremia, hypomagnesemia, hyponatremia, hypotension, impotence, interstitial nephritis, ischemic stroke, jaundice, leukopenia, liver function test abnormalities, maculopapular rash, magnesium increased (serum), metabolic alkalosis, MI, myalgia, orthostatic hypotension, palpitation, pancreatitis, pancytopenia, paresthesia, pemphigus, peripheral edema, photosensitivity, polydipsia, psoriasis, rash, renal failure, shock, Stevens-Johnson syndrome, syncope, tachycardia, thrombocytopenia, toxic epidermal necrolysis, tinnitus, tremor, transaminases increased, urticaria, vasculitis, visual disturbances

Drug Interactions

Metabolism/Transport Effects None known.

Avoid Concomitant Use

Avoid concomitant use of Ramipril and Hydrochlorothiazide with any of the following: Dofetilide; Telmisartan

Increased Effect/Toxicity

Ramipril and Hydrochlorothiazide may increase the levels/effects of: ACE Inhibitors; Allopurinol; Amifostine; Antihypertensives; AzaTHIOprine; Benazepril; Calcium Salts; CarBAMazepine; Cardiac Glycosides; Cyclophosphamide; Diazoxide; Dofetilide; DULoxetine; Ferric Gluconate; Gold Sodium Thiomalate; Grass Pollen Allergen Extract (5 Grass Extract); Hypotensive Agents; Iron Dextran Complex; Ivabradine; Levodopa; Lithium; Multivitamins/Minerals (with ADEK, Folate, Iron); Multivitamins/Minerals (with AE, No Iron); Nonsteroidal Anti-Inflammatory Agents; Obinutuzumab; OXcarbazepine; Porfimer; RisperiDONE; RiTUXimab; Sodium Phosphates; Topiramate; Toremifene; Verteporfin; Vitamin D Analogs

The levels/effects of Ramipril and Hydrochlorothiazide may be increased by: Alcohol (Ethyl); Alfuzosin; Aliskiren; Analgesics (Opioid); Angiotensin II Receptor Blockers; Anticholinergic Agents; Barbiturates; Beta2-Agonists; Brimonidine (Topical); Canagliflozin; Corticosteroids (Orally Inhaled); Corticosteroids (Systemic); Dapoxetine; Dexketoprofen; Diazoxide; DPP-IV Inhibitors; Eplerenone; Everolimus; Heparin; Heparin (Low Molecular Weight); Herbs (Hypotensive Properties); Licorice; Loop Diuretics; MAO Inhibitors; Multivitamins/Fluoride (with ADE); Nicorandil; Pentoxifylline; Phosphodiesterase 5 Inhibitors; Potassium Salts; Potassium-Sparing Diuretics; Prostacyclin Analogues; Selective Serotonin Reuptake Inhibitors; Sirolimus; Telmisartan; Temsirolimus; Thiazide Diuretics; TiZANidine; Tolvaptan; Trimethoprim

Decreased Effect

Ramipril and Hydrochlorothiazide may decrease the levels/effects of: Antidiabetic Agents

The levels/effects of Ramipril and Hydrochlorothiazide may be decreased by: Aprotinin; Benazepril; Bile Acid Sequestrants; Herbs (Hypertensive Properties); Icatibant; Lanthanum; Methylphenidate; Nonsteroidal Anti-Inflammatory Agents; Salicylates; Yohimbine

Food Interactions See individual agents.

Storage/Stability Store at 15°C to 30°C (59°F to 86°F).

Pharmacodynamics/Kinetics See individual agents.

Dosage Note: Not for initial therapy. Dose is individualized; may be substituted for individual components in patients currently maintained on both agents separately or in patients not controlled with monotherapy.

Oral: Adults: Hypertension: Usual dosage: Ramipril 2.5 mg/hydrochlorothiazide 12.5 mg once daily; titrate to maximum ramipril 10 mg/hydrochlorothiazide 50 mg once daily

Dosage adjustment in renal impairment:

CrCl 30-60 mL/minute/1.73 m^2: Initial dose: Ramipril 2.5 mg/hydrochlorothiazide 12.5 mg once daily; Maximum dose: Ramipril 5 mg/hydrochlorothiazide 25 mg once daily

CrCl <30 mL/minute/1.73 m^2: Use is contraindicated.

Dosage adjustment in hepatic impairment:

Mild-to-moderate impairment: Maximum dose: 2.5 mg of ramipril/12.5 mg hydrochlorothiazide once daily. Initiate treatment under close medical supervision.

Severe impairment: Use is contraindicated.

Dietary Considerations May be taken without regard to meals.

Administration Administer in the morning without regard to meals. Administer with 1/2 glass of water. Do not chew or crush tablets.

Monitoring Parameters Blood pressure; BUN, serum creatinine, and electrolytes; if patient has collagen vascular disease and/or renal impairment, periodically monitor CBC with differential

Product Availability Not available in U.S.

Dosage Forms: Canada

Tablet, oral:

Altace® HCT: 2.5/12.5: Ramipril 2.5 mg and hydrochlorothiazide 12.5 mg; 5/12.5: Ramipril 5 mg and hydrochlorothiazide 12.5 mg; 5/25: Ramipril 5 mg and hydrochlorothiazide 25 mg; 10/12.5: Ramipril 10 mg and hydrochlorothiazide 12.5 mg;10/25: Ramipril 10 mg and hydrochlorothiazide 25 mg

Ramosetron [INT] (ra MOS e tron)

International Brand Names Irribow (JP, KR, TH); Nasea (ID, JP, KR, PH, TH); Naseron OD (PH); Ramset (KR); Ramset OD (KR); Setoral (TW)

Index Terms Ramosetron Hydrochloride

Pharmacologic Category 5-HT_3 Receptor Antagonist

Reported Use Antiemetic for the management of nausea and vomiting due to cancer chemotherapy

Dosage Range Adults:

Oral: 100 mcg/day

IV: 300 mcg/day

Product Availability Product available in various countries; not currently available in the U.S.

Dosage Forms

Injection: 300 mcg/mL (2 mL)

Tablet, orally disintegrating: 100 mcg

◆ **Ramosetron Hydrochloride** *see* Ramosetron [INT] *on page 1774*

Ramucirumab (ra mue SIR ue mab)

Brand Names: U.S. Cyramza

Index Terms IMC-1121B

Pharmacologic Category Antineoplastic Agent, Monoclonal Antibody; Antineoplastic Agent, Vascular Endothelial Growth Factor (VEGF) Inhibitor; Antineoplastic Agent, Vascular Endothelial Growth Factor Receptor 2 (VEGFR2) Inhibitor

Use

Gastric cancer, advanced or metastatic: Treatment (single-agent or in combination with paclitaxel) of advanced or metastatic gastric or gastroesophageal junction adenocarcinoma with disease progression on or following fluoropyrimidine- or platinum-containing chemotherapy

Non-small cell lung cancer: Treatment (in combination with docetaxel) of metastatic non-small cell lung cancer (NSCLC) in patients with disease progression on or after platinum-based chemotherapy. Patients with EGFR or ALK genomic tumor aberrations should have disease progression on FDA-approved therapy for these aberrations prior to receiving ramucirumab.

Pregnancy Risk Factor C

Pregnancy Considerations Animal reproduction studies have not been conducted. Ramucirumab inhibits angiogenesis, which is of critical importance to human fetal development. Based on the mechanism of action, ramucirumab may cause fetal harm if administered during pregnancy. Women of reproductive potential should avoid becoming pregnant during and for at least 3 months after the last ramucirumab dose. Ramucirumab may impair fertility in women.

Breast-Feeding Considerations It is not known if ramucirumab is excreted in breast milk. Immunoglobulins are excreted in breast milk, and it is assumed that ramucirumab may appear in breast milk. Because of the potential for serious adverse reactions in the nursing infant, the manufacturer recommends a decision be made whether to discontinue nursing or the drug, taking into account the importance of treatment to the mother.

Contraindications There are no contraindications listed in the manufacturer's labeling.

Warnings/Precautions **[U.S. Boxed Warning]: Ramucirumab is associated with an increased risk of hemorrhage, which may be severe or sometimes fatal. Discontinue ramucirumab permanently in patients who experience serious bleeding.** Patients receiving NSAIDs were excluded from some clinical trials; the risk of gastric hemorrhage in patients with gastric tumors receiving NSAIDs is not known. Gastrointestinal hemorrhages have been reported. In addition, NSCLC patients receiving therapeutic anticoagulation or chronic NSAID or other antiplatelet therapy (other than aspirin), or with radiograph evidence of major airway or blood vessel involvement or intratumor cavitation were also excluded from the clinical study; the risk of pulmonary hemorrhage in such patients is not known. Serious and fatal arterial thrombotic events, including MI, cardiac arrest, cerebrovascular accident, and cerebral ischemia, have occurred with ramucirumab. Discontinue permanently in patients who experience serious arterial thrombotic events.

Ramucirumab is associated with infusion-related reactions (may be severe), generally occurring with the first or second dose. Symptoms of infusion reactions have included chills, flushing, hypotension, bronchospasm, dyspnea, hypoxia, wheezing, chest pain/tightness, supraventricular tachycardia, back pain/spasms, rigors/tremors, and/or paresthesia. Monitor for infusion reaction symptoms during infusion; discontinue immediately and permanently for grade 3 or 4 reactions. Administer in a facility equipped to manage infusion reactions. May cause and/or worsen hypertension; the incidence of severe hypertension is increased with ramucirumab. Blood pressure should be controlled prior to treatment initiation. Monitor BP every 2 weeks (more frequently if indicated) during treatment. If severe hypertension occurs, temporarily withhold until medically controlled. Discontinue permanently if medically significant hypertension cannot be controlled with antihypertensive therapy or in patients with hypertensive crisis or hypertensive encephalopathy.

Antiangiogenic therapy, including ramucirumab, is associated with gastrointestinal perforation (sometimes fatal). Discontinue permanently in patients who experience gastrointestinal perforation. Cases of reversible posterior leukoencephalopathy syndrome (RPLS) have been reported (may be fatal). Symptoms of RPLS include headache, seizure, confusion, lethargy, blindness and/or other vision, or neurologic disturbances. Confirm diagnosis of RPLS with MRI; discontinue ramucirumab with confirmed RPLS diagnosis. Resolution of symptoms may occur within days after discontinuation, although neurologic sequelae may remain in some patients. Antiangiogenic therapy is associated with impairment of wound healing. Ramucirumab was not studied in patients with serious or nonhealing wounds. Withhold treatment prior to surgery; after surgery, use clinical judgment to resume based on adequate wound healing. If wound healing complications develop during treatment, withhold ramucirumab until wound is fully healed. New onset or worsening encephalopathy, ascites, or hepatorenal syndrome have been reported in patients with Child-Pugh class B or C cirrhosis receiving ramucirumab. Use in patients with Child-Pugh class B or C impairment only if the potential benefits outweigh the potential risks.

Adverse Reactions As reported with monotherapy.

Cardiovascular: Hypertension, arterial thrombosis (including myocardial infarction, cardiac arrest, cerebrovascular accident, and cerebral ischemia)

Central nervous system: Headache

Dermatologic: Skin rash

Endocrine & metabolic: Hyponatremia

Gastrointestinal: Diarrhea, intestinal obstruction

Genitourinary: Proteinuria

Hematologic & oncologic: Decreased red blood cells (requiring transfusion), neutropenia, anemia, hemorrhage

Immunologic: Antibody development

Respiratory: Epistaxis

Miscellaneous: Infusion related reaction (reactions minimized with premedications)

Rare but important or life-threatening: Gastrointestinal perforation, reversible posterior leukoencephalopathy syndrome

Drug Interactions

Metabolism/Transport Effects None known.

Avoid Concomitant Use

Avoid concomitant use of Ramucirumab with any of the following: Belimumab

Increased Effect/Toxicity

Ramucirumab may increase the levels/effects of: Belimumab; Bisphosphonate Derivatives

Decreased Effect There are no known significant interactions involving a decrease in effect.

Preparation for Administration Dilute total dose in NS 250 mL prior to administration (the manufacturer recommends a final volume of 250 mL). Do not use dextrose containing solutions. Invert gently to mix thoroughly; do not shake. Discard unused portion of the vial.

Storage/Stability Store intact vials at 2°C to 8°C (36°F to 46°F); do not freeze. Retain in original carton to protect from light. Do not shake. Solutions diluted for infusion may be stored at 2°C to 8°C (36°F to 46°F) for no longer than 24 hours (do not freeze) or may be stored for 4 hours at room temperature (below 25°C [77°F]); do not shake diluted product.

Mechanism of Action Ramucirumab is a recombinant monoclonal antibody which inhibits vascular endothelial growth factor receptor 2 (VEGFR2). Ramucirumab has a high affinity for VEGFR2 (Spratlin, 2010), binding to it and blocking binding of VEGFR ligands, VEGF-A, VEGF-C, and VEGF-D to inhibit activation of VEGFR2, thereby inhibiting ligand-induced proliferation and migration of endothelial cells. VEGFR2 inhibition results in reduced tumor vascularity and growth (Fuchs, 2014).

Pharmacodynamics/Kinetics

Distribution: V_d: 5.5 to 7.1 L

Half-life elimination: 15 to 23 days

Dosage Note: Premedicate prior to infusion with an IV H_1 antagonist (for patients who experienced a grade 1 or 2 infusion reaction with a prior infusion, also premedicate with dexamethasone or equivalent and acetaminophen).

Gastric cancer, advanced or metastatic: Adults: IV: 8 mg/kg every 2 weeks as a single agent or in combination with paclitaxel; continue until disease progression or unacceptable toxicity.

Non-small cell lung cancer, metastatic: Adults: IV: 10 mg/kg on day 1 every 21 days in combination with docetaxel; continue until disease progression or unacceptable toxicity.

Dosage adjustment for toxicity:

Infusion-related reaction:

Grade 1 or 2: Reduce infusion rate by 50%

Grade 3 or 4: Permanently discontinue

Hypertension:

Severe hypertension: Interrupt infusion until controlled with medical management

Severe hypertension, uncontrolled: Permanently discontinue

Proteinuria:

Urine protein ≥2 g/24 hours (first dose reduction): Withhold treatment; when urine protein returns to <2 g/24 hours, reinitiate at a reduced dose of 6 mg/kg every 2 weeks (gastric cancer) or 8 mg/kg every 3 weeks (non-small cell lung cancer)

Recurrent urine protein ≥2 g/24 hours (second dose reduction): Withhold treatment; when urine protein returns to <2 g/24 hours, reinitiate at a reduced dose of 5 mg/kg every 2 weeks (gastric cancer) or 6 mg/kg every 3 weeks (non-small cell lung cancer)

Urine protein >3 g/24 hours: Discontinue permanently

Nephrotic syndrome: Discontinue permanently

Arterial thrombotic events: Discontinue permanently

Bleeding, grade 3 or 4: Discontinue permanently

Gastrointestinal perforation: Discontinue permanently

Reversible posterior leukoencephalopathy syndrome (RPLS): Discontinue permanently for confirmed diagnosis

Wound healing complications: Withhold treatment prior to surgery; do not reinitiate until the surgical wound is fully healed.

Dosage adjustment in renal impairment: No dosage adjustment necessary.

Dosage adjustment in hepatic impairment:

Mild impairment (normal bilirubin with AST > ULN **or** total bilirubin >1 to 1.5 times ULN and any AST): No dosage adjustment necessary.

Moderate to severe impairment (Child-Pugh class B or C): There are no dosage adjustments provided in the manufacturer's labeling. However, new onset or worsening encephalopathy, ascites, or hepatorenal syndrome have been reported in patients with Child-Pugh class B or C cirrhosis receiving ramucirumab. Use in patients with Child-Pugh class B or C impairment only if the potential benefits outweigh the potential risks.

Administration Premedicate prior to infusion with an IV H_1 antagonist; for patients who experienced a grade 1 or 2 infusion reaction with a prior infusion, also premedicate with dexamethasone (or equivalent) and acetaminophen.

Infuse over 60 minutes through a separate infusion line using an infusion pump; the use of a 0.22 micron protein sparing filter is recommended. Do not administer as an IV push or bolus. Flush the line with NS after infusion is complete. Do not infuse in the same IV line with electrolytes or other medications. Administer ramucirumab prior to docetaxel or paclitaxel when giving in combination. Monitor for infusion reaction; reduce infusion rate (by 50%) for grade 1 or 2 infusion reaction; discontinue permanently for grade 3 or 4 infusion reaction.

Monitoring Parameters Blood pressure (every 2 weeks; more frequently if indicated); liver function tests; urine protein; signs/symptoms of infusion-related reactions (during infusion); signs/symptoms of arterial thromboembolic events, hemorrhage, gastrointestinal perforation, wound healing impairment, and reversible posterior leukoencephalopathy syndrome

Dosage Forms

Solution, Intravenous [preservative free]:

Cyramza: 100 mg/10 mL (10 mL); 500 mg/50 mL (50 mL)

- ◆ **Ran-Alendronate (Can)** *see* Alendronate *on page* 79
- ◆ **RAN-Amlodipine (Can)** *see* AmLODIPine *on page* 123
- ◆ **RAN-Anastrozole (Can)** *see* Anastrozole *on page* 148
- ◆ **RAN-Atenolol (Can)** *see* Atenolol *on page* 189
- ◆ **RAN-Atorvastatin (Can)** *see* AtorvaSTATin *on page* 194
- ◆ **RAN-Bicalutamide (Can)** *see* Bicalutamide *on page* 262
- ◆ **Ran-Candesartan (Can)** *see* Candesartan *on page* 335
- ◆ **RAN-Carvedilol (Can)** *see* Carvedilol *on page* 367
- ◆ **RAN™-Cefprozil (Can)** *see* Cefprozil *on page* 389
- ◆ **RAN-Ciproflox (Can)** *see* Ciprofloxacin (Systemic) *on page* 441
- ◆ **RAN-Citalo (Can)** *see* Citalopram *on page* 451
- ◆ **RAN-Clarithromycin (Can)** *see* Clarithromycin *on page* 456
- ◆ **RAN-Clopidogrel (Can)** *see* Clopidogrel *on page* 484
- ◆ **RAN-Domperidone (Can)** *see* Domperidone [CAN/INT] *on page* 666
- ◆ **RAN-Donepezil (Can)** *see* Donepezil *on page* 668
- ◆ **RAN-Enalapril (Can)** *see* Enalapril *on page* 722
- ◆ **RAN-Escitalopram (Can)** *see* Escitalopram *on page* 765
- ◆ **Ranexa** *see* Ranolazine *on page* 1779
- ◆ **RAN-Ezetimibe (Can)** *see* Ezetimibe *on page* 832
- ◆ **RAN-Fentanyl Matrix Patch (Can)** *see* FentaNYL *on page* 857
- ◆ **RAN-Finasteride (Can)** *see* Finasteride *on page* 878
- ◆ **RAN-Fosinopril (Can)** *see* Fosinopril *on page* 932
- ◆ **RAN-Gabapentin (Can)** *see* Gabapentin *on page* 943

Ranibizumab (ra ni BIZ oo mab)

Brand Names: U.S. Lucentis

Brand Names: Canada Lucentis

Index Terms rhuFabV2

Pharmacologic Category Angiogenesis Inhibitor; Monoclonal Antibody; Ophthalmic Agent; Vascular Endothelial Growth Factor (VEGF) Inhibitor

Use

Macular degeneration: Treatment of neovascular (wet) age-related macular degeneration (AMD)

Macular edema: Treatment of macular edema following retinal vein occlusion (RVO); diabetic macular edema (DME)

Choroidal neovascularization secondary to pathologic myopia: Canadian labeling: Additional use (not in U.S. labeling): Treatment of visual impairment due to choroidal neovascularization (CNV) secondary to pathologic myopia

Pregnancy Risk Factor C

Dosage

Age-related macular degeneration (AMD): Adults: Intravitreal:

U.S. labeling: 0.5 mg once a month. Frequency may be reduced (eg, 4-5 injections over 9 months) after the first 3 injections or may be reduced after the first 4 injections to once every 3 months if monthly injections are not feasible.

Canadian labeling: 0.5 mg once a month. Frequency may be reduced after the first 3 injections to once every 3 months if monthly injections are not feasible.

Note: A regimen averaging 4-5 doses over 9 months is expected to maintain visual acuity and an every-3-month dosing regimen has reportedly resulted in a ~5 letter (1 line) loss of visual acuity over 9 months, as compared to monthly dosing which may result in an additional ~1-2 letter gain.

Choroidal neovascularization secondary to pathologic myopia: Adults: Intravitreal: *Canadian labeling:* Initial: 0.5 mg; may repeat 0.5 mg dose at monthly intervals if clinically indicated.

Diabetic macular edema (DME): Adults: Intravitreal:

U.S. labeling: 0.3 mg once a month

Canadian labeling: 0.5 mg once a month until achievement of stable visual acuity for 3 consecutive months. Upon discontinuation, may resume monthly therapy if monitoring identifies a loss of visual acuity.

Macular edema following retinal vein occlusion (RVO): Adults: Intravitreal: 0.5 mg once a month. **Note:** Canadian labeling recommends continuing therapy until achievement of stable visual acuity for 3 consecutive months; upon discontinuation, may resume monthly therapy if monitoring identifies a loss of visual acuity.

Dosage adjustment in renal impairment: No dosage adjustment necessary.

Dosage adjustment in hepatic impairment: There are no dosage adjustments provided in the manufacturer's labeling. However, significant systemic exposure is not expected.

Additional Information Complete prescribing information should be consulted for additional detail.

Dosage Forms

Solution, Intraocular [preservative free]:

Lucentis: 0.3 mg/0.05 mL (0.05 mL); 0.5 mg/0.05 mL (0.05 mL)

Dosage Forms: Canada

Solution, intraocular [preservative free]:

Lucentis: 10 mg/mL (0.23 mL)

◆ **RAN-Imipenem-Cilastatin (Can)** *see* Imipenem and Cilastatin *on page 1051*

◆ **RAN-Irbesartan (Can)** *see* Irbesartan *on page 1110*

◆ **Ran-Irbesartan HCTZ (Can)** *see* Irbesartan and Hydrochlorothiazide *on page 1112*

Ranitidine (ra NI ti deen)

Brand Names: U.S. Acid Reducer Maximum Strength [OTC] [DSC]; Acid Reducer [OTC]; Deprizine FusePaq; GoodSense Acid Reducer [OTC]; Ranitidine Acid Reducer [OTC]; Zantac; Zantac 150 Maximum Strength [OTC]; Zantac 75 [OTC]

Brand Names: Canada Acid Reducer; ACT Ranitidine; Apo-Ranitidine; Dom-Ranitidine; Myl-Ranitidine; Mylan-Ranitidine; PHL-Ranitidine; PMS-Ranitidine; RAN-Ranitidine; Ranitidine Injection, USP; ratio-Ranitidine; Riva-Ranitidine; Sandoz-Ranitidine; ScheinPharm Ranitidine; Teva-Ranitidine; Zantac; Zantac 75; Zantac Maximum Strength Non-Prescription

Index Terms Ranitidine Hydrochloride

Pharmacologic Category Histamine H_2 Antagonist

Use

Zantac: Short-term and maintenance therapy of duodenal ulcer, gastric ulcer, gastroesophageal reflux disease (GERD), active benign ulcer, erosive esophagitis, and pathological hypersecretory conditions; as part of a multi-drug regimen for *H. pylori* eradication to reduce the risk of duodenal ulcer recurrence

Zantac 75 [OTC]: Relief of heartburn, acid indigestion, and sour stomach

Pregnancy Risk Factor B

Pregnancy Considerations Adverse events were not observed in animal studies; therefore, ranitidine is classified as pregnancy category B. Ranitidine crosses the placenta. An increased risk of congenital malformations or adverse events in the newborn has generally not been observed following maternal use of ranitidine during pregnancy. Histamine H_2 antagonists have been evaluated for the treatment of gastroesophageal reflux disease (GERD) as well as gastric and duodenal ulcers during pregnancy. If needed, ranitidine is the agent of choice. Histamine H_2 antagonists may be used for aspiration prophylaxis prior to cesarean delivery.

Breast-Feeding Considerations Ranitidine is excreted into breast milk. The manufacturer recommends that caution be exercised when administering ranitidine to nursing women. Peak milk concentrations of ranitidine occur ~5.5 hours after the dose (case report).

Contraindications Hypersensitivity to ranitidine or any component of the formulation

Warnings/Precautions Ranitidine has been associated with confusional states (rare). Use with caution in patients with hepatic impairment; use with caution in renal impairment, dosage modification required. Avoid use in patients with history of acute porphyria (may precipitate attacks). Prolonged treatment (≥2 years) may lead to vitamin B_{12} malabsorption and subsequent vitamin B_{12} deficiency. The magnitude of the deficiency is dose-related and the association is stronger in females and those younger in age (<30 years); prevalence is decreased after discontinuation of therapy (Lam, 2013). Symptoms of GI distress may be associated with a variety of conditions; symptomatic response to H_2 antagonists does not rule out the potential for significant pathology (eg, malignancy).

Adverse Reactions

Cardiovascular: Asystole, atrioventricular block, bradycardia (with rapid IV administration), premature ventricular beats, tachycardia, vasculitis

Central nervous system: Agitation, dizziness, depression, hallucinations, headache, insomnia, malaise, mental confusion, somnolence, vertigo

Dermatologic: Alopecia, erythema multiforme, rash

Endocrine & metabolic: Prolactin levels increased

Gastrointestinal: Abdominal discomfort/pain, constipation, diarrhea, nausea, necrotizing enterocolitis (VLBW neonates; Guillet, 2006), pancreatitis, vomiting

Hematologic: Acquired immune hemolytic anemia, acute porphyritic attack, agranulocytosis, aplastic anemia, granulocytopenia, leukopenia, pancytopenia, thrombocytopenia

Hepatic: Cholestatic hepatitis, hepatic failure, hepatitis, jaundice

Local: Transient pain, burning or itching at the injection site
Neuromuscular & skeletal: Arthralgia, involuntary motor disturbance, myalgia
Ocular: Blurred vision
Renal: Acute interstitial nephritis, serum creatinine increased
Respiratory: Pneumonia (causal relationship not established)
Miscellaneous: Anaphylaxis, angioneurotic edema, hypersensitivity reactions (eg, bronchospasm, fever, eosinophilia)

Drug Interactions

Metabolism/Transport Effects Substrate of CYP1A2 (minor), CYP2C19 (minor), CYP2D6 (minor), OCT2, P-glycoprotein; **Note:** Assignment of Major/Minor substrate status based on clinically relevant drug interaction potential; **Inhibits** CYP1A2 (weak), CYP2D6 (weak)

Avoid Concomitant Use

Avoid concomitant use of Ranitidine with any of the following: Dasatinib; Delavirdine; PAZOPanib; Risedronate

Increased Effect/Toxicity

Ranitidine may increase the levels/effects of: ARIPiprazole; Dexmethylphenidate; Methylphenidate; Procainamide; Risedronate; Saquinavir; Sulfonylureas; Varenicline; Warfarin

The levels/effects of Ranitidine may be increased by: BuPROPion; P-glycoprotein/ABCB1 Inhibitors

Decreased Effect

Ranitidine may decrease the levels/effects of: Atazanavir; Bosutinib; Cefditoren; Cefpodoxime; Cefuroxime; Dabrafenib; Dasatinib; Delavirdine; Erlotinib; Fosamprenavir; Gefitinib; Indinavir; Iron Salts; Itraconazole; Ketoconazole (Systemic); Ledipasvir; Mesalamine; Multivitamins/Minerals (with ADEK, Folate, Iron); Nelfinavir; Nilotinib; PAZOPanib; Posaconazole; Prasugrel; Rilpivirine; Vismodegib

The levels/effects of Ranitidine may be decreased by: P-glycoprotein/ABCB1 Inducers

Food Interactions Prolonged treatment (≥2 years) may lead to malabsorption of dietary vitamin B_{12} and subsequent vitamin B_{12} deficiency (Lam, 2013).

Preparation for Administration Vials can be mixed with NS or D_5W.
Intermittent bolus injection, continuous infusion: Dilute to maximum of 2.5 mg/mL.
Intermittent infusion: Dilute to maximum of 0.5 mg/mL.

Storage/Stability

Injection: Vials: Store between 4°C to 25°C (39°F to 77°F); excursion permitted to 30°C (86°F). Protect from light. Solution is a clear, colorless to yellow solution; slight darkening does not affect potency. Vials mixed with NS or D_5W are stable for 48 hours at room temperature.
Syrup: Store between 4°C to 25°C (39°F to 77°F). Protect from light.
Tablets: Store in dry place, between 15°C to 30°C (59°F to 86°F). Protect from light.

Mechanism of Action Competitive inhibition of histamine at H_2-receptors of the gastric parietal cells, which inhibits gastric acid secretion, gastric volume, and hydrogen ion concentration are reduced. Does not affect pepsin secretion, pentagastrin-stimulated intrinsic factor secretion, or serum gastrin.

Pharmacodynamics/Kinetics

Absorption: Oral: 50%
Distribution: Normal renal function: V_d: ~1.4 L/kg; CrCl 25-35 mL/minute: 1.76 L/kg minimally penetrates the blood-brain barrier
Protein binding: 15%
Metabolism: Hepatic to N-oxide, S-oxide, and N-desmethyl metabolites
Bioavailability: Oral: 48% to 50%; IM: 90% to 100%
Half-life elimination:
Oral: Normal renal function: 2.5-3 hours
IV: Normal renal function: 2-2.5 hours; CrCl 25-35 mL/minute: 4.8 hours
Time to peak, serum: Oral: 2-3 hours; IM: ≤15 minutes
Excretion: Urine: Oral: 30%, IV: 70% (as unchanged drug); feces (as metabolites)

Dosage

Children 1 month to 16 years:
Duodenal and gastric ulcer:
Oral:
Treatment: 4-8 mg/kg/day divided twice daily; maximum: 300 mg/day
Maintenance: 2-4 mg/kg/day once daily; maximum: 150 mg/day
IV: 2-4 mg/kg/day divided every 6-8 hours; maximum: 200 mg/day
GERD and erosive esophagitis:
Oral: 5-10 mg/kg/day divided twice daily; maximum: GERD: 300 mg/day, erosive esophagitis: 600 mg/day
IV (off-label): 2-4 mg/kg/day divided every 6-8 hours; maximum: 200 mg/day **or as an alternative**
Continuous infusion: Initial: 1 mg/kg/dose for one dose followed by infusion of 0.08-0.17 mg/kg/hour or 2-4 mg/kg/day
Children ≥12 years: Prevention of heartburn: Oral: Zantac 75 [OTC]: 75 mg 30-60 minutes before eating food or drinking beverages which cause heartburn; maximum: 150 mg/24 hours; do not use for more than 14 days

Adults:
Duodenal ulcer: Oral: Treatment: 150 mg twice daily, or 300 mg once daily after the evening meal or at bedtime; maintenance: 150 mg once daily at bedtime
Helicobacter pylori eradication: 150 mg twice daily; requires combination therapy
Pathological hypersecretory conditions:
Oral: 150 mg twice daily; adjust dose or frequency as clinically indicated; doses of up to 6 g/day have been used
IV: Continuous infusion for Zollinger-Ellison: Initial: 1 mg/kg/hour; measure gastric acid output at 4 hours, if >10 mEq or if patient is symptomatic, increase dose in increments of 0.5 mg/kg/hour; doses of up to 2.5 mg/kg/hour (or 220 mg/hour) have been used
Gastric ulcer, benign: Oral: 150 mg twice daily; maintenance: 150 mg once daily at bedtime
GERD: Oral: 150 mg twice daily
Erosive esophagitis: Oral: Treatment: 150 mg 4 times/day; maintenance: 150 mg twice daily
Prevention of heartburn: Oral: Zantac 75 [OTC]: 75 mg 30-60 minutes before eating food or drinking beverages which cause heartburn; maximum: 150 mg in 24 hours; do not use for more than 14 days
Stress ulcer prophylaxis, ICU patients (off-label use; ASHP, 1999): **Note:** Intended for patients with associated risk factors (eg, coagulopathy, mechanical ventilation for >48 hours, severe sepsis); discontinue use once risk factors have resolved. The Surviving Sepsis Campaign guidelines suggest the use of proton pump inhibitors rather than H_2 antagonist therapy (Dellinger, 2013).
Oral, nasogastric (NG) tube: 150 mg twice daily; may administer a 300 mg loading dose prior to maintenance dosing (Pemberton, 1993)
IV: Intermittent bolus: 50 mg every 6-8 hours (Cook, 1998; Geus 1993)
Patients not able to take oral medication:
IM: 50 mg every 6-8 hours
IV: Intermittent bolus or infusion: 50 mg every 6-8 hours
Continuous IV infusion: 6.25 mg/hour

Elderly: Ulcer healing rates and incidence of adverse effects are similar in the elderly, when compared to younger patients; dosing adjustments not necessary based on age alone

Dosage adjustment in renal impairment: Adults:

CrCl <50 mL/minute:

Oral: 150 mg every 24 hours; adjust dose cautiously if needed

IV: 50 mg every 18-24 hours; adjust dose cautiously if needed

Hemodialysis: Adjust dosing schedule so that dose coincides with the end of hemodialysis

Stress ulcer prophylaxis (ASHP, 1999): CrCl <50 mL/minute:

Oral, nasogastric (NG) tube: 150 mg 1-2 times daily

IV: Intermittent bolus: 50 mg every 12-24 hours

Dosage adjustment in hepatic disease: No dosage adjustment provided in manufacturer's labeling. However, no adjustment expected since undergoes minimal hepatic metabolism.

Dietary Considerations Some products may contain phenylalanine and/or sodium. Oral dosage forms may be taken with or without food.

Usual Infusion Concentrations: Pediatric Note: Premixed solutions available

IV infusion: 0.5 mg/mL

Usual Infusion Concentrations: Adult Note: Premixed solutions available

IV infusion: 50 mg in 50 mL (concentration: 1 mg/mL) **or** 500 mg in 250 mL (concentration: 2 mg/mL) of D_5W or NS

Administration

Ranitidine injection may be administered IM or IV:

IM: Injection is administered undiluted

IV: Must be diluted; may be administered IV push, intermittent IV infusion, or continuous IV infusion

IV push: Manufacturer recommends a maximum rate of administration of 10 mg/minute (or over 5 minutes); however, may also be administered at a maximum rate of 25 mg/minute (or over 2 minutes) if necessary (Coursin, 1988; Goelzer, 1988; Smith, 1987).

Intermittent IV infusion: Administer over 15-20 minutes

Continuous IV infusion: Titrate dosage based on gastric pH.

Monitoring Parameters AST, ALT, serum creatinine; when used to prevent stress-related GI bleeding, measure the intragastric pH and try to maintain pH >4; signs and symptoms of peptic ulcer disease, occult blood with GI bleeding, monitor renal function to correct dose

Dosage Forms Considerations

Deprizine FusePaq is a compounding kit for the preparation of an oral suspension. Refer to manufacturer's labeling for compounding instructions.

Dosage Forms

Capsule, Oral:

Generic: 150 mg, 300 mg

Solution, Injection:

Zantac: 50 mg/2 mL (2 mL); 150 mg/6 mL (6 mL); 1000 mg/40 mL (40 mL)

Generic: 50 mg/2 mL (2 mL); 150 mg/6 mL (6 mL); 1000 mg/40 mL (40 mL)

Suspension Reconstituted, Oral:

Deprizine FusePaq: 22.4 mg/mL (250 mL)

Syrup, Oral:

Generic: 15 mg/mL (10 mL, 473 mL, 474 mL, 480 mL); 75 mg/5 mL (473 mL, 480 mL); 150 mg/10 mL (10 mL)

Tablet, Oral:

Acid Reducer [OTC]: 75 mg, 150 mg

GoodSense Acid Reducer [OTC]: 75 mg

Ranitidine Acid Reducer [OTC]: 75 mg

Zantac 75 [OTC]: 75 mg

Zantac: 150 mg, 300 mg

Zantac 150 Maximum Strength [OTC]: 150 mg

Generic: 75 mg, 150 mg, 300 mg

- **Ranitidine Acid Reducer [OTC]** *see* Ranitidine *on page 1777*
- **Ranitidine Hydrochloride** *see* Ranitidine *on page 1777*
- **Ranitidine Injection, USP (Can)** *see* Ranitidine *on page 1777*
- **RAN-Lansoprazole (Can)** *see* Lansoprazole *on page 1166*
- **RAN-Letrozole (Can)** *see* Letrozole *on page 1181*
- **RAN-Levetiracetam (Can)** *see* LevETIRAcetam *on page 1191*
- **RAN-Lisinopril (Can)** *see* Lisinopril *on page 1226*
- **RAN-Losartan (Can)** *see* Losartan *on page 1248*
- **RAN-Memantine (Can)** *see* Memantine *on page 1286*
- **RAN™-Metformin (Can)** *see* MetFORMIN *on page 1307*
- **RAN-Montelukast (Can)** *see* Montelukast *on page 1392*
- **RAN-Olanzapine (Can)** *see* OLANZapine *on page 1491*
- **RAN-Olanzapine ODT (Can)** *see* OLANZapine *on page 1491*

Ranolazine (ra NOE la zeen)

Brand Names: U.S. Ranexa

Pharmacologic Category Antianginal Agent; Cardiovascular Agent, Miscellaneous

Use Chronic angina: Treatment of chronic angina

Note: According to the 2012 ACCF/AHA/ACP/AATS/PCNA/SCAI/STS guidelines for patients with stable ischemic heart disease, ranolazine may be useful when prescribed as a substitute for beta blockers for relief of symptoms if initial treatment with beta blockers leads to unacceptable side effects, is less effective, or if initial treatment with beta blockers is contraindicated. May also be used in combination with beta blockers, for relief of symptoms when initial treatment with beta blockers is not successful (Fihn, 2012).

Pregnancy Risk Factor C

Pregnancy Considerations Adverse events have been observed in animal reproduction studies.

Breast-Feeding Considerations It is not known if ranolazine is excreted into breast milk. Due to the potential for serious adverse reactions in the nursing infant, the manufacturer recommends a decision be made whether to discontinue nursing or to discontinue the drug, taking into account the importance of treatment to the mother.

Contraindications Hepatic cirrhosis; concurrent strong CYP3A inhibitors; concurrent CYP3A inducers

Warnings/Precautions Ranolazine has been shown to prolong QT interval in a dose/plasma concentration-related manner. Cirrhotic patients with mild to moderate hepatic impairment demonstrated a 3-fold increase in QT prolongation. The incidence of symptomatic arrhythmias was similar to placebo in one trial (Morrow, 2007). Risk versus benefit should be assessed in patient maintained on a higher dose (>2000 mg/day) or exposure, concurrent use of other QT-prolonging drugs, potassium-channel variants known to cause QT prolongation, family history of or congenital long QT syndrome, or known acquired QT interval prolongation. Use is contraindicated in patients with hepatic cirrhosis. Ranolazine plasma levels increase in patients with mild and moderate hepatic impairment. Acute renal failure has been observed in some patients with severe renal impairment (CrCl <30 mL/minute); if acute renal failure develops (marked increase in serum creatinine associated with increased BUN), discontinue ranolazine and manage appropriately. Monitor renal function periodically in patients with moderate to severe renal impairment; particularly for increases in serum creatinine accompanied but increased BUN. In a renal impairment study, patients with severe impairment exhibited an initial elevation in diastolic blood pressure (~12-17 mm Hg at day 3), however this diminished to ~4 mm Hg increase by day 5 (Jerling, 2005); consider monitoring blood pressure in patients with renal dysfunction. Ranolazine has not been evaluated in patients requiring dialysis.

Ranolazine will not relieve acute angina episode and has not demonstrated benefit in acute coronary syndrome. Although ranolazine produces small reductions in hemoglobin A_{1c}, it is not a treatment for diabetes. Potentially significant drug-drug interactions may exist, requiring dose or frequency adjustment, additional monitoring, and/or selection of alternative therapy. Use is contraindicated with inducers and strong inhibitors of CYP3A. Use with caution in patients ≥75 years of age; they may experience more adverse events (including serious adverse events) and drug discontinuations due to adverse events.

Adverse Reactions

Cardiovascular: Bradycardia, hypotension, orthostatic hypotension, palpitation, peripheral edema, prolonged QT interval on ECG (>500 msec)

Central nervous system: Confusion, dizziness, headache, syncope, vertigo

Dermatologic: Hyperhidrosis

Gastrointestinal: Abdominal pain, anorexia, constipation, dyspepsia, nausea (dose related), vomiting, xerostomia

Genitourinary: Hematuria

Neuromuscular: Weakness

Ophthalmic: Blurred vision

Otic: Tinnitus

Respiratory: Dyspnea

Rare but important or life-threatening: Angioedema, decreased glycosylated hemoglobin, decreased T-wave amplitude, dysuria, eosinophilia, hallucination, hypoesthesia, increased blood urea nitrogen, increased serum creatinine, leukopenia, pancytopenia, paresthesia, pruritus, pulmonary fibrosis, renal failure, thrombocytopenia, tremor, T-wave changes (notched), torsade de pointes (case report [Morrow, 2007]), urinary retention, urine discoloration

Drug Interactions

Metabolism/Transport Effects Substrate of CYP2D6 (minor), CYP3A4 (major), P-glycoprotein; **Note:** Assignment of Major/Minor substrate status based on clinically relevant drug interaction potential; **Inhibits** CYP2D6 (weak), CYP3A4 (weak), P-glycoprotein

Avoid Concomitant Use

Avoid concomitant use of Ranolazine with any of the following: Antifungal Agents (Azole Derivatives, Systemic); Bosutinib; Conivaptan; CYP3A4 Inducers (Strong); CYP3A4 Inhibitors (Strong); Fusidic Acid (Systemic); Highest Risk QTc-Prolonging Agents; Idelalisib; Ivabradine; Mifepristone; PAZOPanib; Pimozide; Rifampin; Silodosin; St Johns Wort; Topotecan; VinCRIStine (Liposomal)

Increased Effect/Toxicity

Ranolazine may increase the levels/effects of: Afatinib; ARIPiprazole; AtorvaSTATin; Bosutinib; Brentuximab Vedotin; Colchicine; Dabigatran Etexilate; Digoxin; DOXOrubicin (Conventional); Edoxaban; Everolimus; Highest Risk QTc-Prolonging Agents; Hydrocodone; Ledipasvir; Lomitapide; Lovastatin; MetFORMIN; Moderate Risk QTc-Prolonging Agents; Naloxegol; PAZOPanib; P-glycoprotein/ABCB1 Substrates; Pimozide; Prucalopride; Rifaximin; Rivaroxaban; Silodosin; Simvastatin; Tacrolimus (Systemic); Topotecan; VinCRIStine (Liposomal)

The levels/effects of Ranolazine may be increased by: Antifungal Agents (Azole Derivatives, Systemic); Calcium Channel Blockers (Nondihydropyridine); Conivaptan; CYP3A4 Inhibitors (Moderate); CYP3A4 Inhibitors (Strong); Dasatinib; Fusidic Acid (Systemic); Idelalisib; Ivabradine; Ivacaftor; Luliconazole; Mifepristone; P-glycoprotein/ABCB1 Inhibitors; QTc-Prolonging Agents (Indeterminate Risk and Risk Modifying); Simeprevir

Decreased Effect

The levels/effects of Ranolazine may be decreased by: Bosentan; CYP3A4 Inducers (Moderate); CYP3A4 Inducers (Strong); Dabrafenib; Deferasirox; P-glycoprotein/ABCB1 Inducers; Rifampin; Siltuximab; St Johns Wort; Tocilizumab

Food Interactions Grapefruit, grapefruit juice, or grapefruit-containing products may increase the serum concentration of ranolazine. Management: Avoid grapefruit-containing products or dose adjustment of ranolazine may be required.

Storage/Stability Store at 25°C (77°F); excursions permitted to 15°C to 30°C (59°F to 86°F).

Mechanism of Action Ranolazine exerts antianginal and anti-ischemic effects without changing hemodynamic parameters (heart rate or blood pressure). At therapeutic levels, ranolazine inhibits the late phase of the inward sodium channel (late I_{Na}) in ischemic cardiac myocytes during cardiac repolarization reducing intracellular sodium concentrations and thereby reducing calcium influx via Na^+-Ca^{2+} exchange. Decreased intracellular calcium reduces ventricular tension and myocardial oxygen consumption. It is thought that ranolazine produces myocardial relaxation and reduces anginal symptoms through this mechanism although this is uncertain. At higher concentrations, ranolazine inhibits the rapid delayed rectifier potassium current (I_{Kr}) thus prolonging the ventricular action potential duration and subsequent prolongation of the QT interval.

Pharmacodynamics/Kinetics

Absorption: Highly variable

Protein binding: ~62%

Metabolism: Extensive; Hepatic via CYP3A (major) and 2D6 (minor); intestines

Bioavailability: Tablet: 76% (compared to solution)

Half-life elimination: Ranolazine: Terminal: 7 hours; Metabolites (activity undefined): 6-22 hours

Time to peak, plasma: 2-5 hours

Excretion: Primarily urine (75% mostly as metabolites; <5% as unchanged drug); feces (25% mostly as metabolites; <5% as unchanged drug)

Dosage Note: May be used with beta-blockers, nitrates, calcium channel blockers, antiplatelet therapy, lipid-lowering therapy, angiotensin-converting enzyme (ACE) inhibitors, and angiotensin-receptor blockers.

Chronic angina: Oral:

Adults: Initial: 500 mg twice daily; may increase to 1000 mg twice daily as needed (based on symptoms); maximum recommended dose: 1000 mg twice daily

Elderly: Select dose cautiously, starting at the lower end of the dosing range

Missed doses: If a dose is missed, it should be taken at the next scheduled time; the next dose should not be doubled.

Dosage adjustment for ranolazine with concomitant medications:

Diltiazem, erythromycin, fluconazole, verapamil, and other moderate CYP3A inhibitors: Ranolazine dose should not exceed 500 mg twice daily

P-glycoprotein inhibitors (eg, cyclosporine): Titrate ranolazine based on clinical response

Dosage adjustment in renal impairment: No dosage adjustments provided in the manufacturer's labeling. However, plasma ranolazine levels increased ~40% to 50% in patients with varying degrees of renal dysfunction. Discontinue if acute renal failure develops. Ranolazine has not been evaluated in patients requiring dialysis.

Dosage adjustment in hepatic impairment: No dosage adjustment provided in the manufacturer's labeling. Use is contraindicated with hepatic cirrhosis.

Dietary Considerations Limit the use of grapefruit juice; the ranolazine dose should not exceed 500 mg twice daily when taken with grapefruit juice or grapefruit-containing products.

Administration Administer with or without meals. Swallow tablet whole; do not crush, break, or chew.

Monitoring Parameters Baseline and follow up ECG to evaluate QT interval; monitor renal function periodically in patients with moderate to severe renal impairment, particularly for increases in serum creatinine accompanied by increased BUN; consider monitoring blood pressure in patients with renal dysfunction; correct and maintain serum potassium in normal limits

Dosage Forms

Tablet Extended Release 12 Hour, Oral:
Ranexa: 500 mg, 1000 mg

- ◆ **RAN-Omeprazole (Can)** *see* Omeprazole *on page 1508*
- ◆ **RAN-Ondansetron (Can)** *see* Ondansetron *on page 1513*
- ◆ **RAN-Pantoprazole (Can)** *see* Pantoprazole *on page 1570*
- ◆ **RAN-Pioglitazone (Can)** *see* Pioglitazone *on page 1654*
- ◆ **RAN-Pravastatin (Can)** *see* Pravastatin *on page 1700*
- ◆ **RAN-Pregabalin (Can)** *see* Pregabalin *on page 1710*
- ◆ **RAN-Quetiapine (Can)** *see* QUEtiapine *on page 1751*
- ◆ **RAN-Rabeprazole (Can)** *see* RABEprazole *on page 1762*
- ◆ **RAN-Ramipril (Can)** *see* Ramipril *on page 1771*
- ◆ **RAN-Ranitidine (Can)** *see* Ranitidine *on page 1777*
- ◆ **RAN-Risperidone (Can)** *see* RisperiDONE *on page 1818*
- ◆ **RAN-Ropinirole (Can)** *see* ROPINIRole *on page 1844*
- ◆ **RAN-Rosuvastatin (Can)** *see* Rosuvastatin *on page 1848*
- ◆ **Ran-Sertraline (Can)** *see* Sertraline *on page 1878*
- ◆ **RAN-Sildenafil (Can)** *see* Sildenafil *on page 1882*
- ◆ **RAN-Simvastatin (Can)** *see* Simvastatin *on page 1890*
- ◆ **Ran-Telmisartan (Can)** *see* Telmisartan *on page 1988*
- ◆ **RAN-Telmisartan HCTZ (Can)** *see* Telmisartan and Hydrochlorothiazide *on page 1990*
- ◆ **RAN-Topiramate (Can)** *see* Topiramate *on page 2065*
- ◆ **RAN-Tramadol/Acet (Can)** *see* Acetaminophen and Tramadol *on page 37*
- ◆ **Ran-Valsartan (Can)** *see* Valsartan *on page 2127*
- ◆ **Ran-Venlafaxine XR (Can)** *see* Venlafaxine *on page 2150*
- ◆ **RAN-Zopiclone (Can)** *see* Zopiclone [CAN/INT] *on page 2217*
- ◆ **Rapaflo** *see* Silodosin *on page 1885*
- ◆ **Rapaflo® (Can)** *see* Silodosin *on page 1885*
- ◆ **Rapamune** *see* Sirolimus *on page 1893*
- ◆ **Rapamycin** *see* Sirolimus *on page 1893*
- ◆ **RapiMed Children's [OTC]** *see* Acetaminophen *on page 32*
- ◆ **RapiMed Junior [OTC]** *see* Acetaminophen *on page 32*
- ◆ **Rapivab** *see* Peramivir *on page 1619*

- ◆ **Rapivab** *see* Peramivir *on page 1619*

Rasagiline (ra SA ji leen)

Brand Names: U.S. Azilect

Brand Names: Canada Azilect

Index Terms AGN 1135; Rasagiline Mesylate; TVP-1012

Pharmacologic Category Anti-Parkinson's Agent, MAO Type B Inhibitor

Use Parkinson disease: Treatment of Parkinson disease

Pregnancy Risk Factor C

Pregnancy Considerations Adverse effects have been observed in animal reproduction studies.

Breast-Feeding Considerations It is not known if rasagiline is excreted in breast milk. The manufacturer recommends caution be exercised when administering rasagiline to nursing women.

Contraindications Concomitant use of an MAO inhibitor (including selective MAO-B inhibitors), meperidine, methadone, propoxyphene, or tramadol within 14 days of rasagiline; concomitant use with cyclobenzaprine, dextromethorphan, or St John's wort

Warnings/Precautions Hazardous agent - use appropriate precautions for handling and disposal (NIOSH 2014 [group 2]).

May cause exacerbation of hypertension; monitor for new onset hypertension or hypertension not adequately controlled after starting rasagiline. Medication adjustment may be necessary if blood pressure elevation is sustained. In patients taking recommended doses of rasagiline, dietary restriction of most tyramine-containing products is not necessary; however, certain foods (eg, aged cheeses) may contain high amounts (>150 mg) of tyramine and could lead to hypertensive crisis. Avoid concomitant use with foods high in tyramine. Rasagiline is a selective inhibitor of MAO-B at the recommended doses; however, MAO-B selectivity diminishes in a dose-related manner above the recommended daily doses. May cause orthostatic hypotension, particularly in combination with levodopa. Orthostatic hypotension occurs most frequently during the first 2 months of therapy and decreases over time.

Serotonin syndrome (SS) has been reported with concomitant antidepressant (eg, SSRI, SNRI, TCA, tetracyclic and triazolopyridine antidepressants) use; concomitant use is not recommended within 14 days of rasagiline administration (within 5 weeks for antidepressants with long half-lives such as fluoxetine). SS has also been reported with concomitant use of MAO inhibitors (including selective MAO-B inhibitors), meperidine, methadone, propoxyphene, and tramadol; concomitant use within 14 days of rasagiline administration is contraindicated. A symptom complex resembling neuroleptic malignant syndrome (NMS) has been reported in association with rapid dose reduction, withdrawal of, or changes in drugs that increase central dopaminergic tone. Discontinue treatment (and any concomitant antidepressants) immediately if signs/symptoms arise.

Somnolence and falling asleep while engaged in activities of daily living (including operation of motor vehicles) have been reported; some cases reported that there were no warning signs for the onset of symptoms. Symptom onset may occur well after initiation of treatment; some events have occurred >1 year after initiation of rasagiline. Prior to treatment initiation evaluate for factors that may increase these risks such as concomitant sedating medications, the presence of sleep disorders, and concomitant medications that increase rasagiline plasma levels (eg, ciprofloxacin). Monitor for drowsiness or sleepiness. If significant daytime sleepiness or episodes of falling asleep during activities that require active participation occurs (eg, driving, conversations, eating), discontinue rasagiline. There is insufficient information to suggest that dose reductions will eliminate these symptoms. If therapy is continued, advise patient to avoid driving and other potentially dangerous activities.

Dyskinesia, exacerbation of preexisting dyskinesia, or increased dopaminergic side effects may occur when used as an adjunct to levodopa. Decreasing the dose of levodopa may mitigate these side effects. May cause new or worsening mental status and behavioral changes, which may be severe, including paranoid ideation, delusions, hallucinations, confusion, psychotic-like behavior, disorientation, aggressive behavior, agitation, and delirium after starting or increasing the dose of rasagiline. Intense urges to gamble or spend money, increased sexual urges, binge eating, and/or other intense urges, as well as the inability to control these urges have also been reported. Monitor for these symptoms. If symptoms develop, consider dose reduction or discontinue of therapy. Avoidance of use is recommended in patients with major psychotic disorder due to the risk of exacerbating psychosis with an increase in central dopaminergic tone. Many treatments for psychosis that decrease central dopaminergic tone may also decrease the effectiveness of rasagiline.

Risk of melanoma may be increased with rasagiline, although increased risk has been associated with Parkinson's disease itself; patients should have regular and frequent skin examinations. Use with caution in patients with mild hepatic impairment; dose reduction recommended. Avoid use in patients with moderate-to-severe hepatic impairment. Potentially significant drug-drug interactions may exist, requiring dose or frequency adjustment, additional monitoring, and/or selection of alternative therapy. Hazardous agent - use appropriate precautions for handling and disposal (NIOSH, 2012).

Adverse Reactions Unless otherwise noted, the following adverse reactions are as reported for monotherapy. Spectrum of adverse events was generally similar with adjunctive therapy, though the incidence tended to be higher.

Cardiovascular: Angina, bundle branch block, chest pain, hypotension, increased blood pressure, orthostatic hypotension, peripheral edema

Central nervous system: Abnormal dreams (adjunctive therapy), anxiety, ataxia (adjunctive therapy), depression, dizziness, drowsiness (adjunctive therapy), dystonia (adjunctive therapy), falling, hallucinations, headache, insomnia (adjunctive therapy), malaise, myasthenia (adjunctive therapy), paresthesia, vertigo

Dermatologic: Alopecia, diaphoresis (adjunctive therapy), ecchymosis, skin carcinoma, skin rash (adjunctive therapy), vesiculobullous rash

Endocrine & metabolic: Impotence, libido decreased, weight loss (adjunctive therapy; dose-related)

Gastrointestinal: Abdominal pain (adjunctive therapy), anorexia (adjunctive therapy), constipation (adjunctive therapy), diarrhea (adjunctive therapy), dyspepsia, gastroenteritis, gastrointestinal hemorrhage, gingivitis (adjunctive therapy), hernia (adjunctive therapy), nausea (adjunctive therapy), vomiting (adjunctive therapy), xerostomia (adjunctive therapy; dose-related)

Genitourinary: Hematuria, urinary incontinence

Hematologic and oncologic: Hemorrhage (adjunctive therapy), leukopenia

Hepatic: Liver function tests increased

Infection: Infection (adjunctive therapy)

Neuromuscular & skeletal: Abnormal gait, arthralgia, arthritis, back pain (adjunctive therapy), dyskinesia (adjunctive therapy), hyperkinesias, hypertonia, neck pain, neuropathy, tenosynovitis (adjunctive therapy), weakness

Ophthalmic: Conjunctivitis

Renal: Albuminuria

Respiratory: Asthma, cough (adjunctive therapy), dyspnea (adjunctive therapy), flu-like symptoms, rhinitis, upper respiratory tract infection (adjunctive therapy)

Miscellaneous: Allergic reaction, fever, trauma (adjunctive therapy)

Rare but important or life-threatening: Acute kidney failure, aggressive behavior, agitation, amyotrophy, aphasia, apnea, arterial thrombosis, atrial arrhythmia, atrioventricular block, bigeminy, blepharitis, blepharoptosis, blindness, cardiac failure, cerebral hemorrhage, cerebral ischemia, deafness, deep vein thrombophlebitis, delirium, delusions, diplopia, disorientation, dysautonomia, dysesthesia, emphysema, esophageal ulcer, exacerbation of hypertension, excessive daytime sleepiness (including during operation of motor vehicles), exfoliative dermatitis, facial paralysis, gastric ulcer, genitourinary disorders, glaucoma, gynecomastia, hematemesis, hemiplegia, hostility, hypocalcemia, hypotension (while supine), impulse control disorder (pathological gambling, hypersexuality, intense urges to spend money, binge eating, and/or other intense urges and the inability to control the urges), interstitial pneumonitis, intestinal obstruction, intestinal perforation, intestinal stenosis, jaundice, keratitis, large intestine perforation, laryngeal edema, laryngismus, leukoderma, leukorrhea, macrocytic anemia, manic depressive reaction, mania, megacolon, menstrual abnormalities, myelitis, myocardial infarction, nephrolithiasis, neuralgia, neuritis, (a complex resembling) neuroleptic malignant syndrome (associated with rapid dose reduction, withdrawal of or changes in medication; includes autonomic insufficiency, hyperthermia, impaired consciousness, muscle rigidity), nocturia, oral paresthesia, osteonecrosis, paranoia, personality disorder, pleural effusion, pneumothorax, polyuria, psychiatric disturbance (new or worsening mental status and behavioral changes that may be severe, including psychotic-like behavior during or after starting or increasing doses), psychoneurosis, psychotic symptoms, psychotic depression, pulmonary fibrosis, purpura, retinal degeneration, retinal detachment, seizure, strabismus, stupor, thrombocythemia, tongue edema, ventricular fibrillation, ventricular tachycardia, vestibular disturbance, visual field defect, vulvovaginal candidiasis

Drug Interactions

Metabolism/Transport Effects Substrate of CYP1A2 (major); **Note:** Assignment of Major/Minor substrate status based on clinically relevant drug interaction potential; **Inhibits** Monoamine Oxidase

Avoid Concomitant Use

Avoid concomitant use of Rasagiline with any of the following: Alcohol (Ethyl); Alpha-/Beta-Agonists (Indirect-Acting); Alpha1-Agonists; Amphetamines; Anilidopiperidine Opioids; Antidepressants (Serotonin Reuptake Inhibitor/Antagonist); Apraclonidine; AtoMOXetine; Bezafibrate; Buprenorphine; BuPROPion; BusPIRone; CarBAMazepine; Cyclobenzaprine; Cyproheptadine; Dapoxetine; Dexmethylphenidate; Dextromethorphan; Diethylpropion; Hydrocodone; HYDROmorphone; Isometheptene; Levonordefrin; Linezolid; Maprotiline; Meperidine; Methyldopa; Methylene Blue; Methylphenidate; Mianserin; Mirtazapine; Morphine (Liposomal); Morphine (Systemic); Oxymorphone; Pholcodine; Pizotifen; Selective Serotonin Reuptake Inhibitors; Serotonin 5-HT1D Receptor Agonists; Serotonin/Norepinephrine Reuptake Inhibitors; Tapentadol; Tetrabenazine; Tetrahydrozoline (Nasal); Tricyclic Antidepressants; Tryptophan

Increased Effect/Toxicity

Rasagiline may increase the levels/effects of: Alpha-/Beta-Agonists (Indirect-Acting); Alpha1-Agonists; Amphetamines; Antidepressants (Serotonin Reuptake Inhibitor/Antagonist); Antihypertensives; Antipsychotic Agents; Apraclonidine; AtoMOXetine; Beta2-Agonists;

Betahistine; Bezafibrate; Brimonidine (Ophthalmic); Brimonidine (Topical); BuPROPion; Cyproheptadine; Dexmethylphenidate; Dextromethorphan; Diethylpropion; Domperidone; Doxapram; Doxylamine; EPINEPHrine (Nasal); Epinephrine (Racemic); EPINEPHrine (Systemic, Oral Inhalation); Hydrocodone; HYDROmorphone; Hypoglycemic Agents; Isometheptene; Levonordefrin; Linezolid; Lithium; Meperidine; Methadone; Methyldopa; Methylene Blue; Methylphenidate; Metoclopramide; Mianserin; Mirtazapine; Morphine (Liposomal); Morphine (Systemic); Norepinephrine; Orthostatic Hypotension Producing Agents; OxyCODONE; Pizotifen; Reserpine; Selective Serotonin Reuptake Inhibitors; Serotonin 5-HT1D Receptor Agonists; Serotonin Modulators; Serotonin/Norepinephrine Reuptake Inhibitors; Tetrahydrozoline (Nasal); Tricyclic Antidepressants

The levels/effects of Rasagiline may be increased by: Abiraterone Acetate; Alcohol (Ethyl); Altretamine; Anilidopiperidine Opioids; Antiemetics (5HT3 Antagonists); Antipsychotic Agents; Buprenorphine; BusPIRone; CarBAMazepine; COMT Inhibitors; Cyclobenzaprine; CYP1A2 Inhibitors (Moderate); CYP1A2 Inhibitors (Strong); Dapoxetine; Deferasirox; Levodopa; MAO Inhibitors; Maprotiline; Oxymorphone; Peginterferon Alfa-2b; Pholcodine; Tapentadol; Tedizolid; Tetrabenazine; TraMADol; Tryptophan; Vemurafenib

Decreased Effect

Rasagiline may decrease the levels/effects of: Domperidone; Pipamperone [INT]

The levels/effects of Rasagiline may be decreased by: Cannabis; CYP1A2 Inducers (Strong); Cyproheptadine; Cyproterone; Domperidone; Pipamperone [INT]; Teriflunomide

Food Interactions Concurrent ingestion of foods rich in tyramine, dopamine, tyrosine, phenylalanine, tryptophan, or caffeine may cause sudden and severe high blood pressure (hypertensive crisis or serotonin syndrome). Management: Avoid foods containing high amounts (>150 mg) of tyramine (aged or matured cheese, air-dried or cured meats including sausages and salamis; fava or broad bean pods, tap/draft beers, Marmite concentrate, sauerkraut, soy sauce, and other soybean condiments). Food's freshness is also an important concern; improperly stored or spoiled food can create an environment in which tyramine concentrations may increase. Avoid these foods during and for 2 weeks after discontinuation of medication. Avoid foods containing dopamine, tyrosine, phenylalanine, tryptophan, or caffeine.

Storage/Stability Store at 25°C (77°F); excursions permitted to 15°C to 30°C (59°F to 86°F).

Mechanism of Action Potent, irreversible and selective inhibitor of brain monoamine oxidase (MAO) type B, which plays a major role in the catabolism of dopamine. Inhibition of dopamine depletion in the striatal region of the brain reduces the symptomatic motor deficits of Parkinson's disease. There is also experimental evidence of rasagiline conferring neuroprotective effects (antioxidant, antiapoptotic), which may delay onset of symptoms and progression of neuronal deterioration.

Pharmacodynamics/Kinetics

Duration: ~1 week (irreversible inhibition)

Absorption: Rapid

Protein binding: 88% to 94%, primarily to albumin

Metabolism: Hepatic N-dealkylation and/or hydroxylation via CYP1A2 to multiple inactive metabolites

Distribution: V_{dss}: 87 L

Bioavailability: ~36%

Half-life elimination: ~3 hours (no correlation with biologic effect due to irreversible inhibition)

Time to peak, plasma: ~1 hour

Excretion: Urine (62%, <1% of total dose as unchanged drug); feces (7%)

Dosage Oral: Adults: Parkinson disease:

Monotherapy or adjunctive therapy (not including levodopa): 1 mg once daily (maximum: 1 mg once daily).

Adjunctive therapy with levodopa: Initial: 0.5 mg once daily; may increase to 1 mg once daily based on response and tolerability (maximum: 1 mg once daily).

Note: When added to existing levodopa therapy, a dose reduction of levodopa may be required to avoid exacerbation of dyskinesias; typical dose reductions of ~9% to 13% were employed in clinical trials

Dose reduction with concomitant ciprofloxacin or other CYP1A2 inhibitors: Maximum dose: 0.5 mg once daily

Dosage adjustment in renal impairment:

Mild to moderate impairment: No dosage adjustment necessary.

Severe impairment: There are no dosage adjustments provided in the manufacturer's labeling (has not been studied).

Dosage adjustment in hepatic impairment:

Mild impairment (Child-Pugh score 5 to 6): Maximum dose: 0.5 mg once daily

Moderate to severe impairment (Child-Pugh score 7 to 15): Use is not recommended.

Dietary Considerations May be taken without regard to meals. Avoid products containing high amounts of tyramine (>150 mg), such as aged cheeses (eg, Stilton cheese). Restriction of tyramine-containing products with lower amounts (<150 mg) of tyramine is not necessary in patients taking recommended doses. Some examples of tyramine-containing products include aged or matured cheese, air-dried or cured meats (including sausages and salamis), fava or broad bean pods, tap/draft beers, Marmite concentrate, sauerkraut, soy sauce and other soybean condiments. Food's freshness is also an important concern; improperly stored or spoiled food can create an environment where tyramine concentrations may increase.

Administration Administer without regard to meals.

Hazardous agent; use appropriate precautions for handling and disposal (NIOSH 2014 [group 2]).

Monitoring Parameters Blood pressure; symptoms of parkinsonism; new or worsening mental status and behavioral changes; somnolence and falling asleep during activities of daily living; skin examination for presence of melanoma (higher incidence in Parkinson's patients- drug causation not established)

Additional Information When adding rasagiline to levodopa/carbidopa, the dose of the latter can usually be decreased. Studies are investigating the use of rasagiline in early Parkinson's disease to slow the progression of the disease.

Dosage Forms

Tablet, Oral:

Azilect: 0.5 mg, 1 mg

◆ **Rasagiline Mesylate** *see* Rasagiline *on page 1781*

Rasburicase (ras BYOOR i kayse)

Brand Names: U.S. Elitek

Brand Names: Canada Fasturtec®

Index Terms Recombinant Urate Oxidase; Urate Oxidase

Pharmacologic Category Enzyme; Enzyme, Urate-Oxidase (Recombinant)

Use Initial management of uric acid levels in patients with leukemia, lymphoma, and solid tumor malignancies receiving chemotherapy expected to result in tumor lysis and elevation of plasma uric acid

Pregnancy Risk Factor C

Pregnancy Considerations Adverse effects were observed in animal reproduction studies. There are no adequate and well-controlled studies in pregnant women. Use during pregnancy only if the benefit to the mother outweighs the potential risk to the fetus.

Breast-Feeding Considerations Due to the potential for serious adverse reactions in the nursing infant, the decision to discontinue breast-feeding or to discontinue rasburicase should take into account the benefits of treatment to the mother.

Contraindications History of anaphylaxis or severe hypersensitivity to rasburicase or any component of the formulation; history of hemolytic reaction or methemoglobinemia associated with rasburicase; glucose-6-phosphatase dehydrogenase (G6PD) deficiency

Warnings/Precautions [U.S. Boxed Warning]: Severe hypersensitivity reactions (including anaphylaxis) have been reported; immediately and permanently discontinue in patients developing serious hypersensitivity reaction; reactions may occur at any time during treatment, including the initial dose. Signs and symptoms of hypersensitivity may include bronchospasm, chest pain/tightness, dyspnea, hypotension, hypoxia, shock, or urticaria. The safety and efficacy of more than one course of administration has not been established. **[U.S. Boxed Warning]: Due to the risk for hemolysis (<1%), rasburicase is contraindicated in patients with G6PD deficiency; discontinue immediately and permanently in any patient developing hemolysis. Patients at higher risk for G6PD deficiency (eg, African, Mediterranean, or Southeast Asian descent) should be screened prior to therapy;** severe hemolytic reactions occurred within 2-4 days of rasburicase initiation. **[U.S. Boxed Warning]: Methemoglobinemia has been reported (<1%). Discontinue immediately and permanently in any patient developing methemoglobinemia;** initiate appropriate treatment (eg, transfusion, methylene blue) if methemoglobinemia occurs.

[U.S. Boxed Warning]: Enzymatic degradation of uric acid in blood samples will occur if left at room temperature, which may interfere with serum uric acid measurements; specific guidelines for the collection of plasma uric acid samples must be followed, including collection in prechilled tubes with heparin anticoagulant, immediate ice water bath immersion and assay within 4 hours. Patients at risk for tumor lysis syndrome should receive appropriate IV hydration as part of uric acid management; however, alkalinization (with sodium bicarbonate) concurrently with rasburicase is not recommended (Coiffier, 2008). Rasburicase is immunogenic and can elicit an antibody response; efficacy may be reduced with subsequent courses of therapy.

Adverse Reactions

Cardiovascular: Fluid overload, ischemic coronary disease, peripheral edema, supraventricular arrhythmia

Central nervous system: Anxiety, fever, headache,

Dermatologic: Rash

Endocrine & metabolic: Hyper-/hypophosphatemia

Gastrointestinal: Abdominal/gastrointestinal infection, abdominal pain, constipation, diarrhea, mucositis, nausea, vomiting

Hematologic: Neutropenia, neutropenia with fever

Hepatic: ALT increased, hyperbilirubinemia

Respiratory: Pharyngolaryngeal pain, pulmonary hemorrhage, respiratory distress/failure

Miscellaneous: Antibody formation, hypersensitivity, sepsis

Rare but important or life-threatening: Acute renal failure, anaphylaxis, arrhythmia, cardiac arrest, cardiac failure, cellulitis, cerebrovascular disorder, chest pain, cyanosis, dehydration, hemolysis, hemorrhage, hot flashes, ileus, infection, intestinal obstruction, liver enzymes increased, methemoglobinemia, MI, pancytopenia, paresthesia, pneumonia, pulmonary edema, pulmonary hypertension, retinal hemorrhage, rigors, seizure, thrombosis, thrombophlebitis

Drug Interactions

Metabolism/Transport Effects None known.

Avoid Concomitant Use There are no known interactions where it is recommended to avoid concomitant use.

Increased Effect/Toxicity There are no known significant interactions involving an increase in effect.

Decreased Effect There are no known significant interactions involving a decrease in effect.

Preparation for Administration Reconstitute with provided diluent (use 1 mL diluent for the 1.5 mg vial and 5 mL diluent for the 7.5 mg vial). Mix by gently swirling; do **not** shake or vortex. Discard if discolored or containing particulate matter. Total dose should be further diluted in NS to a final volume of 50 mL.

Storage/Stability Prior to reconstitution, store with diluent at 2°C to 8°C (36°F to 46°F); do not freeze. Protect from light. Reconstituted and final solution may be stored up to 24 hours at 2°C to 8°C (36°F to 46°F). Discard unused product.

Mechanism of Action Rasburicase is a recombinant urate-oxidase enzyme, which converts uric acid to allantoin (an inactive and soluble metabolite of uric acid); it does not inhibit the formation of uric acid.

Pharmacodynamics/Kinetics

Onset: Uric acid levels decrease within 4 hours of initial administration

Distribution: Children: 110-127 mL/kg; Adults: 76-138 mL/kg

Half-life elimination: ~16-23 hours

Dosage IV: Hyperuricemia associated with malignancy:

Children: 0.2 mg/kg once daily for up to 5 days (manufacturer-recommended dose) **or**

Alternate dosing (off-label; Coiffier, 2008): 0.05-0.2 mg/kg once daily for 1-7 days (average of 2-3 days) with the duration of treatment dependent on plasma uric acid levels and clinical judgment (patients with significant tumor burden may require an increase to twice daily); the following dose levels are recommended based on risk of tumor lysis syndrome (TLS):

High risk: 0.2 mg/kg once daily (duration is based on plasma uric acid levels)

Intermediate risk: 0.15 mg/kg once daily (duration is based on plasma uric acid levels); may consider managing initially with a single dose

Low risk: 0.1 mg/kg once daily (duration is based on clinical judgment); a dose of 0.05 mg/kg was used effectively in one trial

Single-dose rasburicase (off-label use; based on limited data): 0.15 mg/kg; additional doses may be needed based on serum uric acid levels (Liu, 2005)

Adults: 0.2 mg/kg once daily for up to 5 days (manufacturer-recommended dose) **or**

Alternate dosing (off-label; Coiffier, 2008): 0.05-0.2 mg/kg once daily for 1-7 days (average of 2-3 days) with the duration of treatment dependent on plasma uric acid levels and clinical judgment (patients with significant tumor burden may require an increase to twice daily); the following dose levels are recommended based on risk of tumor lysis syndrome (TLS):

High risk: 0.2 mg/kg once daily (duration is based on plasma uric acid levels)

Intermediate risk: 0.15 mg/kg once daily (duration is based on plasma uric acid levels)

Low risk: 0.1 mg/kg once daily (duration is based on clinical judgment); a dose of 0.05 mg/kg was used effectively in one trial

Single-dose rasburicase (off-label use; based on limited data): 0.15 mg/kg (Campara, 2009; Liu, 2005) **or** 3-7.5 mg as a single dose (Hutcherson, 2006; McDonnell, 2006; Reeves, 2008; Trifilio, 2006); repeat doses (1.5-6 mg) may be needed based on serum uric acid levels

Dosage adjustment in renal impairment: No dosage adjustment provided in manufacturer's labeling.

Dosage adjustment in hepatic impairment: No dosage adjustment provided in manufacturer's labeling.

Administration IV infusion over 30 minutes; do **not** administer as a bolus infusion. Do **not** filter during infusion. If not possible to administer through a separate line, IV line should be flushed with at least 15 mL saline prior to and following rasburicase infusion. The optimal timing of rasburicase administration (with respect to chemotherapy administration) is not specified in the manufacturer's labeling. In some studies, chemotherapy was administered 4-24 hours after the first rasburicase dose (Cortes, 2010; Kikuchi, 2009; Vadhan-Raj, 2012); however, rasburicase generally may be administered irrespective of chemotherapy timing.

Monitoring Parameters Plasma uric acid levels (4 hours after rasburicase administration, then every 6-8 hours until TLS resolution), CBC, G6PD deficiency screening (in patients at high risk for deficiency); monitor for hypersensitivity

Dosage Forms

Solution Reconstituted, Intravenous:

Elitek: 1.5 mg (1 ea); 7.5 mg (1 ea)

- ◆ **Rasilez (Can)** *see* Aliskiren *on page 85*
- ◆ **Rasilez HCT (Can)** *see* Aliskiren and Hydrochlorothiazide *on page 87*
- ◆ **Rasuvo** *see* Methotrexate *on page 1322*
- ◆ **rATG** *see* Antithymocyte Globulin (Rabbit) *on page 158*
- ◆ **ratio-Aclavulanate (Can)** *see* Amoxicillin and Clavulanate *on page 133*
- ◆ **ratio-Acyclovir (Can)** *see* Acyclovir (Systemic) *on page 47*
- ◆ **ratio-Alendronate (Can)** *see* Alendronate *on page 79*
- ◆ **ratio-Amlodipine (Can)** *see* AmLODIPine *on page 123*
- ◆ **ratio-Atenolol (Can)** *see* Atenolol *on page 189*
- ◆ **ratio-Atorvastatin (Can)** *see* AtorvaSTATin *on page 194*
- ◆ **ratio-Baclofen (Can)** *see* Baclofen *on page 223*
- ◆ **ratio-Bisacodyl [OTC] (Can)** *see* Bisacodyl *on page 265*
- ◆ **ratio-Brimonidine (Can)** *see* Brimonidine (Ophthalmic) *on page 288*
- ◆ **ratio-Bupropion SR (Can)** *see* BuPROPion *on page 305*
- ◆ **ratio-Carvedilol (Can)** *see* Carvedilol *on page 367*
- ◆ **ratio-Cefuroxime (Can)** *see* Cefuroxime *on page 399*
- ◆ **ratio-Ciprofloxacin (Can)** *see* Ciprofloxacin (Systemic) *on page 441*
- ◆ **ratio-Clobetasol (Can)** *see* Clobetasol *on page 468*
- ◆ **ratio-Clonazepam (Can)** *see* ClonazePAM *on page 478*
- ◆ **ratio-Codeine (Can)** *see* Codeine *on page 497*
- ◆ **ratio-Cotridin (Can)** *see* Triprolidine, Pseudoephedrine, and Codeine [CAN/INT] *on page 2105*
- ◆ **ratio-Cyclobenzaprine (Can)** *see* Cyclobenzaprine *on page 516*
- ◆ **ratio-Dexamethasone (Can)** *see* Dexamethasone (Systemic) *on page 599*
- ◆ **ratio-Diltiazem CD (Can)** *see* Diltiazem *on page 634*
- ◆ **ratio-Docusate Sodium [OTC] (Can)** *see* Docusate *on page 661*
- ◆ **ratio-Domperidone (Can)** *see* Domperidone [CAN/INT] *on page 666*
- ◆ **ratio-Ectosone (Can)** *see* Betamethasone (Topical) *on page 255*
- ◆ **ratio-Emtec-30 (Can)** *see* Acetaminophen and Codeine *on page 36*
- ◆ **ratio-Fenofibrate MC (Can)** *see* Fenofibrate and Derivatives *on page 852*
- ◆ **ratio-Finasteride (Can)** *see* Finasteride *on page 878*
- ◆ **ratio-Fluoxetine (Can)** *see* FLUoxetine *on page 899*
- ◆ **ratio-Fluticasone (Can)** *see* Fluticasone (Nasal) *on page 910*
- ◆ **ratio-Fluvoxamine (Can)** *see* FluvoxaMINE *on page 916*
- ◆ **ratio-Gabapentin (Can)** *see* Gabapentin *on page 943*
- ◆ **ratio-Glimepiride (Can)** *see* Glimepiride *on page 966*
- ◆ **ratio-Glyburide (Can)** *see* GlyBURIDE *on page 972*
- ◆ **ratio-Indomethacin (Can)** *see* Indomethacin *on page 1067*
- ◆ **ratio-Ipra-Sal (Can)** *see* Albuterol *on page 69*
- ◆ **ratio-Ipra Sal UDV (Can)** *see* Ipratropium and Albuterol *on page 1109*
- ◆ **ratio-Ipratropium UDV (Can)** *see* Ipratropium (Systemic) *on page 1108*
- ◆ **ratio-Irbesartan (Can)** *see* Irbesartan *on page 1110*
- ◆ **ratio-Irbesartan HCTZ (Can)** *see* Irbesartan and Hydrochlorothiazide *on page 1112*
- ◆ **ratio-Ketorolac (Can)** *see* Ketorolac (Ophthalmic) *on page 1149*
- ◆ **Ratio-Lactulose (Can)** *see* Lactulose *on page 1156*
- ◆ **ratio-Lamotrigine (Can)** *see* LamoTRIgine *on page 1160*
- ◆ **ratio-Lenoltec (Can)** *see* Acetaminophen and Codeine *on page 36*
- ◆ **Ratio-Levobunolol (Can)** *see* Levobunolol *on page 1194*
- ◆ **ratio-Meloxicam (Can)** *see* Meloxicam *on page 1283*
- ◆ **ratio-Memantine (Can)** *see* Memantine *on page 1286*
- ◆ **ratio-Metformin (Can)** *see* MetFORMIN *on page 1307*
- ◆ **ratio-Methotrexate Sodium (Can)** *see* Methotrexate *on page 1322*
- ◆ **ratio-Methylphenidate (Can)** *see* Methylphenidate *on page 1336*
- ◆ **ratio-Minocycline (Can)** *see* Minocycline *on page 1371*
- ◆ **ratio-Mirtazapine (Can)** *see* Mirtazapine *on page 1376*
- ◆ **ratio-Mometasone (Can)** *see* Mometasone (Topical) *on page 1391*
- ◆ **ratio-Morphine (Can)** *see* Morphine (Systemic) *on page 1394*
- ◆ **ratio-Morphine SR (Can)** *see* Morphine (Systemic) *on page 1394*
- ◆ **ratio-Omeprazole (Can)** *see* Omeprazole *on page 1508*
- ◆ **ratio-Ondansetron (Can)** *see* Ondansetron *on page 1513*
- ◆ **ratio-Orciprenaline® (Can)** *see* Metaproterenol *on page 1307*
- ◆ **Ratio-Oxycocet (Can)** *see* Oxycodone and Acetaminophen *on page 1541*
- ◆ **ratio-Pantoprazole (Can)** *see* Pantoprazole *on page 1570*
- ◆ **ratio-Paroxetine (Can)** *see* PARoxetine *on page 1579*
- ◆ **ratio-Pioglitazone (Can)** *see* Pioglitazone *on page 1654*
- ◆ **Ratio-Prednisolone (Can)** *see* PrednisoLONE (Ophthalmic) *on page 1706*

- **ratio-Quetiapine (Can)** *see* QUEtiapine *on page 1751*
- **ratio-Ramipril (Can)** *see* Ramipril *on page 1771*
- **ratio-Ranitidine (Can)** *see* Ranitidine *on page 1777*
- **ratio-Risedronate (Can)** *see* Risedronate *on page 1816*
- **ratio-Risperidone (Can)** *see* RisperiDONE *on page 1818*
- **ratio-Rivastigmine (Can)** *see* Rivastigmine *on page 1833*
- **ratio-Salbutamol (Can)** *see* Albuterol *on page 69*
- **ratio-Sertraline (Can)** *see* Sertraline *on page 1878*
- **ratio-Sildenafil R (Can)** *see* Sildenafil *on page 1882*
- **ratio-Simvastatin (Can)** *see* Simvastatin *on page 1890*
- **ratio-Sotalol (Can)** *see* Sotalol *on page 1927*
- **ratio-Tamsulosin (Can)** *see* Tamsulosin *on page 1974*
- **ratio-Temazepam (Can)** *see* Temazepam *on page 1990*
- **ratio-Terazosin (Can)** *see* Terazosin *on page 2001*
- **ratio-Theo-Bronc (Can)** *see* Theophylline *on page 2026*
- **Ratio-Topilene (Can)** *see* Betamethasone (Topical) *on page 255*
- **Ratio-Topisone (Can)** *see* Betamethasone (Topical) *on page 255*
- **ratio-Trazodone (Can)** *see* TraZODone *on page 2091*
- **ratio-Valproic (Can)** *see* Valproic Acid and Derivatives *on page 2123*
- **ratio-Zopiclone (Can)** *see* Zopiclone [CAN/INT] *on page 2217*

Raxibacumab (rax i BAK ue mab)

Index Terms ABthrax

Pharmacologic Category Antidote; Monoclonal Antibody

Use Treatment of inhalational anthrax following exposure to *Bacillus anthracis* in combination with appropriate antimicrobial therapy; prophylaxis of inhalational anthrax when alternative therapies are unavailable or not appropriate

Pregnancy Risk Factor B

Dosage Anthrax, prophylaxis or treatment: Note: Administer diphenhydramine (adult dose: 25-50 mg; in all patients, may administer oral or IV depending on the proximity to start of raxibacumab infusion) ≤1 hour prior to administration of raxibacumab to reduce the risk of infusion reactions. Must be administered in combination with antimicrobial therapy.

Children and Adolescents: IV:

≤15 kg: 80 mg/kg as a single dose

>15 kg to 50 kg: 60 mg/kg as a single dose

>50 kg: 40 mg/kg as a single dose

Adults: IV: 40 mg/kg as a single dose

Dosage adjustment in renal impairment: No dosage adjustment provided in manufacturer's labeling. However, dosage adjustment unlikely as clearance is nonrenal.

Dosage adjustment in hepatic impairment: No dosage adjustment provided in manufacturer's labeling (has not been studied).

Additional Information Complete prescribing information should be consulted for additional detail.

Dosage Forms Injection, solution: 50 mg/mL (34 mL)

- **Rayos** *see* PredniSONE *on page 1706*
- **Razadyne** *see* Galantamine *on page 946*
- **Razadyne ER** *see* Galantamine *on page 946*
- **6R-BH4** *see* Sapropterin *on page 1864*
- **Reactine (Can)** *see* Cetirizine *on page 411*
- **Rea-Lo [OTC]** *see* Urea *on page 2114*
- **Rea Lo 39** *see* Urea *on page 2114*
- **Rea Lo 40** *see* Urea *on page 2114*

Rebamipide [INT] (re BAM e pide)

International Brand Names Becantex (ID); Gastrix (PH); Huining (CN); Mucopide (IN); Mucopro (PH); Mucoprotec (PH); Mucosta (CN, ID, JP, KR, MY, PH, TH, VN); Novepide (ID); Rebagen (IN); Rebis (KR); Recostar (KR); Remide (KR); Repampia (VN); Sysmuco (ID); Unireda (VN)

Pharmacologic Category Cytoprotective Agent

Reported Use Treatment of peptic ulcer disease and gastritis

Dosage Range Adults: Oral: 100 mg 3 times/day

Product Availability Product available in various countries; not currently available in the U.S.

Dosage Forms

Tablet: 100 mg

- **Rebetol** *see* Ribavirin *on page 1797*
- **Rebif** *see* Interferon Beta-1a *on page 1100*
- **Rebif Rebidose** *see* Interferon Beta-1a *on page 1100*
- **Rebif Rebidose Titration Pack** *see* Interferon Beta-1a *on page 1100*
- **Rebif Titration Pack** *see* Interferon Beta-1a *on page 1100*

Reboxetine [INT] (ree BOKS e teen)

International Brand Names Edronax (AE, AT, AU, BE, BG, BH, CH, DE, DK, EE, EG, FI, GB, HN, HR, IE, IL, IS, IT, NO, NZ, PL, PT, QA, SA, SE, SI, TH, TR); Integrex (CO); Narebox (IN); Prolift (BR, CL); Reboot (IN); Reboxxin (IN); Solvex (DE); Yeloshu (CN); Zuolexin (CN)

Pharmacologic Category Norepinephrine Reuptake Inhibitor, Selective

Reported Use Treatment of depression

Dosage Range Oral:

Adults: 4 mg twice daily (8 mg/day). After 3 weeks, the dose can be increased up to 10 mg/day in case of incomplete clinical response.

Elderly: 2 mg twice daily (4 mg/day); may increase dose to 6 mg/day after 3 weeks if needed

Dosing adjustment in hepatic/renal impairment: 2 mg twice daily

Product Availability Product available in various countries; not currently available in the U.S.

Dosage Forms

Tablet: 2 mg, 4 mg

- **Reclast** *see* Zoledronic Acid *on page 2206*
- **Reclipsen** *see* Ethinyl Estradiol and Desogestrel *on page 799*
- **Recombinant α-L-Iduronidase (Glycosaminoglycan α-L-Iduronohydrolase)** *see* Laronidase *on page 1172*
- **Recombinant C1 Inhibitor** *see* C1 Inhibitor (Recombinant) *on page 316*
- **Recombinant Desulfatohirudin** *see* Desirudin *on page 593*
- **Recombinant Granulocyte-Macrophage Colony Stimulating Factor** *see* Sargramostim *on page 1865*
- **Recombinant Hirudin** *see* Desirudin *on page 593*
- **Recombinant Human Deoxyribonuclease** *see* Dornase Alfa *on page 672*
- **Recombinant Human Interleukin-2** *see* Aldesleukin *on page 72*
- **Recombinant Human Interleukin-11** *see* Oprelvekin *on page 1519*

- ◆ **Recombinant Human Luteinizing Hormone** *see* Lutropin Alfa [CAN/INT] *on page 1259*
- ◆ **Recombinant Human Parathyroid Hormone (1-34)** *see* Teriparatide *on page 2008*
- ◆ **Recombinant Human Platelet-Derived Growth Factor B** *see* Becaplermin *on page 230*
- ◆ **Recombinant Human Thyrotropin** *see* Thyrotropin Alfa *on page 2031*
- ◆ **Recombinant Interleukin-11** *see* Oprelvekin *on page 1519*
- ◆ **Recombinant Methionyl-Human Leptin** *see* Metreleptin *on page 1353*
- ◆ **Recombinant Plasminogen Activator** *see* Reteplase *on page 1794*
- ◆ **Recombinant Urate Oxidase** *see* Rasburicase *on page 1783*
- ◆ **Recombinant Urate Oxidase, Pegylated** *see* Pegloticase *on page 1602*
- ◆ **Recombinate** *see* Antihemophilic Factor (Recombinant) *on page 152*
- ◆ **Recombivax HB** *see* Hepatitis B Vaccine (Recombinant) *on page 1002*
- ◆ **Recort Plus [OTC]** *see* Hydrocortisone (Topical) *on page 1014*
- ◆ **Rectacort-HC** *see* Hydrocortisone (Topical) *on page 1014*
- ◆ **RectiCare [OTC]** *see* Lidocaine (Topical) *on page 1211*
- ◆ **Rectiv** *see* Nitroglycerin *on page 1465*
- ◆ **Rederm [OTC]** *see* Hydrocortisone (Topical) *on page 1014*
- ◆ **Reeses Pinworm Medicine [OTC]** *see* Pyrantel Pamoate *on page 1744*
- ◆ **Refenesen [OTC]** *see* GuaiFENesin *on page 986*
- ◆ **Refenesen 400 [OTC]** *see* GuaiFENesin *on page 986*
- ◆ **Refenesen DM [OTC]** *see* Guaifenesin and Dextromethorphan *on page 987*
- ◆ **Refenesen™ PE [OTC]** *see* Guaifenesin and Phenylephrine *on page 988*
- ◆ **Refenesen Plus [OTC]** *see* Guaifenesin and Pseudoephedrine *on page 989*
- ◆ **Refissa** *see* Tretinoin (Topical) *on page 2099*
- ◆ **Regitine [DSC]** *see* Phentolamine *on page 1636*
- ◆ **Reglan** *see* Metoclopramide *on page 1345*
- ◆ **Regonol** *see* Pyridostigmine *on page 1746*

Regorafenib (re goe RAF e nib)

Brand Names: U.S. Stivarga

Brand Names: Canada Stivarga

Index Terms BAY 73-4506

Pharmacologic Category Antineoplastic Agent, Tyrosine Kinase Inhibitor; Antineoplastic Agent, Vascular Endothelial Growth Factor (VEGF) Inhibitor

Use

Gastrointestinal stromal tumors: Treatment of locally-advanced, unresectable, or metastatic gastrointestinal stromal tumor (GIST) in patients previously treated with imatinib and sunitinib

Metastatic colorectal cancer: Treatment of metastatic colorectal cancer in patients previously treated with fluoropyrimidine-, oxaliplatin-, and irinotecan-based chemotherapy, anti-VEGF therapy, or anti-EGFR therapy (if *KRAS* wild type)

Pregnancy Risk Factor D

Pregnancy Considerations In animal reproduction studies, teratogenic effects were observed with doses less than the equivalent human dose. Patients (male and female) should use effective contraception during therapy and for at least 2 months following treatment.

Breast-Feeding Considerations It is not known if regorafenib is excreted into breast milk. According to the manufacturer, the decision to discontinue regorafenib or to discontinue breast-feeding during therapy should take into account the benefits of treatment to the mother.

Contraindications There are no contraindications listed in the manufacturer's U.S. product labeling.

Canadian labeling: Hypersensitivity to regorafenib, any component of the formulation, or sorafenib.

Warnings/Precautions Hazardous agent - use appropriate precautions for handling and disposal (meets NIOSH 2014 criteria). Myocardial ischemia and infarction were observed at a higher incidence than placebo in a clinical trial. Interrupt therapy in patients who develop new or acute onset ischemia or infarction; resume only if the benefit of therapy outweighs the cardiovascular risk. Hand-foot skin reaction (HFSR), also known as palmar-plantar erythrodysesthesia (PPE), and rash were commonly seen in clinical trials; erythema multiforme and Stevens Johnson syndrome were also observed more frequently in regorafenib-treated patients. Toxic epidermal necrolysis occurred rarely. Onset of dermatologic toxicity typically occurs in the first cycle of treatment. Therapy interruptions, dosage reductions, and/or discontinuation may be necessary depending on the severity and persistence. Supportive treatment may be of benefit for symptomatic relief. Gastrointestinal perforation or fistula has occurred in a small number of patients treated with regorafenib; some cases were fatal. Monitor for signs/symptoms of perforation (fever, abdominal pain with constipation, and/or nausea/vomiting); permanently discontinue therapy if perforation or fistula develop. The incidence of hemorrhage was increased with regorafenib. Hemorrhage of the respiratory, gastrointestinal, or genitourinary tracts was observed in trials; some cases were fatal. Permanently discontinue in patients who experience severe or life-threatening bleeding. In patients receiving concomitant warfarin, monitor INR frequently.

[U.S. Boxed Warning]: Severe liver toxicity and hepatic failure (sometimes resulting in death) have been observed in clinical trials; hepatocyte necrosis with lymphocyte infiltration has been demonstrated with liver biopsy. Monitor hepatic function at baseline and during treatment. Interrupt therapy for hepatotoxicity; dose reductions or discontinuation are necessary depending on the severity and persistence.

Elevated blood pressure was observed in clinical trials (onset typically in the first cycle of therapy); ensure blood pressure is adequately controlled prior to initiation. Monitor blood pressure weekly for the first 6 weeks and monthly thereafter or as clinically indicated; if hypertension develops, interrupt therapy or permanently discontinue for severe or uncontrolled hypertension. Hypertensive crisis has occurred in some patients. Reversible posterior leukoencephalopathy syndrome (RPLS) occurred very rarely in regorafenib-treated patients; evaluate promptly if symptoms (eg, seizures, headache, visual disturbances, confusion, or altered mental function) occur. Discontinue if diagnosis is confirmed. Regorafenib inhibits vascular endothelial growth factor, which may lead to impaired wound healing. Stop therapy at least 2 weeks prior to scheduled surgery; resume regorafenib postsurgery based on clinical judgment of wound healing; discontinue therapy if wound dehiscence occurs.

Potentially significant drug-drug or drug-food interactions may exist, requiring dose or frequency adjustment, additional monitoring, and/or selection of alternative therapy.

Adverse Reactions

Cardiovascular: Hypertension, myocardial ischemia and infarction

Central nervous system: Dysphonia, fatigue, fever, headache, pain

Dermatologic: Alopecia, palmar-plantar erythrodysesthesia, rash

Endocrine & metabolic: Hypocalcemia, hypokalemia, hyponatremia, hypophosphatemia, hypothyroidism

Gastrointestinal: Amylase increased, appetite decreased, diarrhea, gastroesophageal reflux, lipase increased, mucositis, nausea, taste disturbance, vomiting, weight loss, xerostomia

Hematologic: Anemia, hemorrhage, INR increased, lymphopenia, neutropenia, thrombocytopenia

Hepatic: ALT increased, AST increased, hyperbilirubinemia

Neuromuscular & skeletal: Stiffness, tremor

Renal: Proteinuria

Respiratory: Dyspnea

Miscellaneous: Infection

Rare but important or life-threatening: Bradycardia, erythema multiforme, gastrointestinal fistula, hypertensive crisis, liver injury (severe), liver failure, reversible posterior encephalopathy syndrome (RPLS), skin cancer (keratoacanthoma, squamous cell carcinoma), Stevens-Johnson syndrome, toxic epidermal necrolysis

Drug Interactions

Metabolism/Transport Effects **Substrate** of CYP3A4 (major), UGT1A9; **Note:** Assignment of Major/Minor substrate status based on clinically relevant drug interaction potential; **Inhibits** BCRP, P-glycoprotein, UGT1A1, UGT1A9

Avoid Concomitant Use

Avoid concomitant use of Regorafenib with any of the following: Conivaptan; CYP3A4 Inducers (Strong); CYP3A4 Inhibitors (Strong); Fusidic Acid (Systemic); Grapefruit Juice; Idelalisib; St Johns Wort

Increased Effect/Toxicity

Regorafenib may increase the levels/effects of: Beta-Blockers; Bisphosphonate Derivatives; Calcium Channel Blockers (Nondihydropyridine); Digoxin; Irinotecan; Ivabradine

The levels/effects of Regorafenib may be increased by: Aprepitant; Ceritinib; Conivaptan; CYP3A4 Inhibitors (Moderate); CYP3A4 Inhibitors (Strong); Dasatinib; Fosaprepitant; Fusidic Acid (Systemic); Grapefruit Juice; Idelalisib; Ivacaftor; Luliconazole; Mifepristone; Netupitant; Simeprevir; Warfarin

Decreased Effect

The levels/effects of Regorafenib may be decreased by: Bosentan; CYP3A4 Inducers (Moderate); CYP3A4 Inducers (Strong); Dabrafenib; Deferasirox; Siltuximab; St Johns Wort; Tocilizumab

Food Interactions Regorafenib serum concentrations may be altered when taken with grapefruit or grapefruit juice. Management: Avoid concurrent use.

Storage/Stability Store at 25°C (77°F); excursions permitted to 15°C to 30°C (59°F to 86°F). Store tablets in the original bottle and protect from moisture (do not remove the desiccant); keep container tightly closed. Discard any unused tablets 7 weeks after opening the bottle.

Mechanism of Action Regorafenib is a multikinase inhibitor; it targets kinases involved with tumor angiogenesis, oncogenesis, and maintenance of the tumor microenvironment which results in inhibition of tumor growth. Specifically, it inhibits VEGF receptors 1-3, KIT, PDGFR-alpha, PDGFR-beta, RET, FGFR1 and 2, TIE2, DDR2, TrkA, Eph2A, RAF-1. BRAF, $BRAF^{V600E}$, SAPK2, PTK5, and Abl.

Pharmacodynamics/Kinetics

Absorption: A high-fat meal increased the mean AUC of the parent drug by 48% compared to the fasted state and decreased the mean AUC of the M-2 (N-oxide) and M-5 (N-oxide and N-desmethyl) active metabolites by 20% and 51%, respectively. A low-fat meal increased the mean AUC of regorafenib, M-2, and M-5 by 36%, 40% and 23%, respectively (as compared to the fasted state).

Protein binding: 99.5% (active metabolites M-2 and M-5 are also highly protein bound)

Metabolism: Hepatic via CYP3A4 and UGT1A9, primarily to active metabolites M-2 (N-oxide) and M-5 (N-oxide and N-desmethyl)

Bioavailability: Tablets: 69%; Oral solution: 83%

Half-life elimination: Regorafenib: 28 hours (range: 14-58 hours); M-2 metabolite: 25 hours (range: 14-32 hours); M-5 metabolite: 51 hours (range: 32-70 hours)

Time to peak: 4 hours

Excretion: Feces (71%; 47% as parent compound; 24% as metabolites); Urine (19%)

Dosage

Colorectal cancer, metastatic: Adults: Oral: 160 mg once daily for the first 21 days of each 28-day cycle; continue until disease progression or unacceptable toxicity (Grothey, 2013)

Gastrointestinal stromal tumor (GIST), locally-advanced, unresectable, or metastatic: Adults: Oral: 160 mg once daily for the first 21 days of each 28-day cycle; continue until disease progression or unacceptable toxicity (Demetri, 2013)

Missed doses: Do not administer 2 doses on the same day to make up for a missed dose from the previous day.

Dosage adjustment for toxicity:

Dermatologic:

Grade 2 hand-foot skin reaction (HFSR; palmar-plantar erythrodysesthesia [PPE]) of any duration: Reduce dose to 120 mg once daily for first occurrence. If grade 2 HFSR recurs at this dose, further reduce the dose to 80 mg once daily. Interrupt therapy for grade 2 HFSR that is recurrent or fails to improve within 7 days in spite of dosage reduction.

Grade 3 HFSR: Interrupt therapy for a minimum of 7 days. Upon recovery, reduce dose to 120 mg once daily. If grade 2-3 toxicity recurs at this dose, further reduce dose to 80 mg once daily upon recovery. Interrupt therapy for grade 2-3 HFSR that is recurrent or fails to improve within 7 days in spite of dosage reduction.

Recurrent or persistent HFSR at 80 mg once daily: Discontinue treatment.

Hypertension: Grade 2 (symptomatic): Interrupt therapy.

Other toxicity: Any grade 3 or 4 adverse reaction (other than hepatotoxicity): Interrupt therapy; upon recovery, reduce dose to 120 mg once daily. If any grade 3 or 4 adverse reaction occurs while on this reduced dose, may further reduce dose to 80 mg once daily upon recovery. For any grade 4 adverse reaction, only resume therapy if the benefit outweighs the risk. Permanently discontinue therapy if unable to tolerate 80 mg once daily.

Gastrointestinal perforation/fistula: Discontinue permanently.

Hemorrhage (severe or life-threatening): Discontinue permanently.

Reversible posterior leukoencephalopathy syndrome (RPLS): Discontinue.

Wound dehiscence: Discontinue.

Dosage adjustment for renal impairment:

Preexisting mild impairment (CrCl 60-89 mL/minute): No dosage adjustment necessary.

Preexisting moderate impairment (CrCl 30-59 mL/minute): No dosage adjustment provided in manufacturer's labeling (limited pharmacokinetic data available).
Preexisting severe impairment (CrCl <30 mL/minute): No dosage adjustment provided in manufacturer's labeling (has not been studied).

Dosage adjustment for hepatic impairment:

Preexisting mild or moderate impairment (Child-Pugh Class A or B): No dosage adjustment necessary; closely monitor for adverse effects.
Preexisting severe impairment (Child-Pugh Class C): Use is not recommended (has not been studied).
Hepatotoxicity during treatment:
Grade 3 AST and/or ALT elevation: Withhold dose until recovery. If benefit of treatment outweighs toxicity risk, resume therapy at a reduced dose of 120 mg once daily.
AST or ALT >20 times ULN: Discontinue permanently.
AST or ALT >3 times ULN **and** bilirubin >2 times ULN: Discontinue permanently.
Recurrence of AST or ALT >5 times ULN despite dose reduction to 120 mg: Discontinue permanently.

Dietary Considerations Take with a low-fat breakfast (<30% fat)

Administration Take at the same time each day with a low-fat (<30% fat) breakfast; swallow tablets whole. Hazardous agent; use appropriate precautions for handling and disposal (meets NIOSH 2014 criteria).

Monitoring Parameters Monitor for hand-foot skin reaction (HFSR)/palmar-plantar erythrodysesthesia (PPE); signs/symptoms of cardiac ischemia or infarction; bleeding; signs/symptoms of GI perforation or fistula; signs/symptoms of reversible posterior leukoencephalopathy syndrome (severe headaches, seizure, confusion, or change in vision). Monitor for impaired wound healing. Obtain liver function tests at baseline, every 2 weeks during the first 2 months of treatment, then monthly or more frequently if clinically necessary (weekly until improvement if liver function tests are elevated). Monitor blood pressure weekly for the first 6 weeks of therapy and with every subsequent cycle, or more frequently if indicated. CBC with differential and platelets and serum electrolytes (baseline and periodic). Monitor INR more frequently if receiving warfarin.

Dosage Forms

Tablet, Oral:
Stivarga: 40 mg

- **Regranex** *see* Becaplermin *on page 230*
- **Regular Insulin** *see* Insulin Regular *on page 1091*
- **Reguloid [OTC]** *see* Psyllium *on page 1744*
- **Rejuva-A (Can)** *see* Tretinoin (Topical) *on page 2099*
- **Relafen** *see* Nabumetone *on page 1411*
- **Relaxa (Can)** *see* Polyethylene Glycol 3350 *on page 1674*
- **Relenza® (Can)** *see* Zanamivir *on page 2194*
- **Relenza Diskhaler** *see* Zanamivir *on page 2194*
- **Relistor** *see* Methylnaltrexone *on page 1334*
- **Relpax** *see* Eletriptan *on page 711*
- **Relpax® (Can)** *see* Eletriptan *on page 711*
- **Remedy Antifungal [OTC]** *see* Miconazole (Topical) *on page 1360*
- **Remergent HQ** *see* Hydroquinone *on page 1020*
- **Remeron** *see* Mirtazapine *on page 1376*
- **Remeron RD (Can)** *see* Mirtazapine *on page 1376*
- **Remeron SolTab** *see* Mirtazapine *on page 1376*
- **Remeven** *see* Urea *on page 2114*
- **Remicade** *see* InFLIXimab *on page 1070*

Remifentanil (rem i FEN ta nil)

Brand Names: U.S. Ultiva

Brand Names: Canada Ultiva®

Index Terms GI87084B

Pharmacologic Category Analgesic, Opioid; Anilidopiperidine Opioid

Use Analgesic for use during the induction and maintenance of general anesthesia; for continued analgesia into the immediate postoperative period; analgesic component of monitored anesthesia

Pregnancy Risk Factor C

Pregnancy Considerations Adverse events were not observed in animal reproduction studies. Remifentanil has been shown to cross the placenta; fetal and maternal concentrations may be similar.

Breast-Feeding Considerations It is not known if remifentanil is excreted into breast milk. The manufacturer recommends that caution be used if administered to a nursing woman. Remifentanil has a limited duration of action; use may be appropriate for breast-feeding women undergoing short procedures (Montgomery, 2012).

Contraindications Not for intrathecal or epidural administration, due to the presence of glycine in the formulation; hypersensitivity to remifentanil, fentanyl, or fentanyl analogs, or any component of the formulation

Warnings/Precautions Remifentanil is not recommended as the sole agent for induction of anesthesia, because the loss of consciousness cannot be assured. Due to the high incidence of apnea, hypotension, respiratory depression, tachycardia and muscle rigidity remifentanil should only be administered by individuals specifically trained in the use of anesthetic agents and should not be used in diagnostic or therapeutic procedures outside the monitored anesthesia setting; resuscitative and intubation equipment should be readily available. May cause hypotension; use with caution in patients with hypovolemia, cardiovascular disease (including acute MI), or drugs which may exaggerate hypotensive effects (including phenothiazines or general anesthetics). Shares the toxic potentials of opioid agonists, and precautions of opioid agonist therapy should be observed. In patients <55 years of age, intraoperative awareness has been reported when used with propofol rates of ≤75 mcg/kg/minute.

Rapid IV infusion (single dose >1 mcg/kg over 30-60 seconds and infusion rates >0.1 mcg/kg/minute) should only be used during maintenance of general anesthesia; may result in skeletal muscle and chest wall rigidity, impaired ventilation, or respiratory distress/arrest; nondepolarizing skeletal muscle relaxant may be required. Chest wall rigidity may resolve by decreasing the infusion rate or temporarily stopping the infusion. Inadequate clearing of IV tubing following remifentanil administration could result in chest wall rigidity, respiratory depression, and apnea when another fluid is administered through the same line. Interruption of an infusion will result in offset of effects within 5-10 minutes; the discontinuation of remifentanil infusion should be preceded by the establishment of adequate postoperative analgesia orders, especially for patients in whom postoperative pain is anticipated. Use caution in the morbidly obese. Use with caution in patients with a history of drug abuse or acute alcoholism; potential for drug dependency exists. Tolerance, psychological and physical dependence may occur with prolonged use.

Adverse Reactions

Cardiovascular: Bradycardia (dose dependent), flushing, hypertension (dose dependent), hypotension, tachycardia (dose dependent)
Central nervous system: Agitation, chills, dizziness, fever, headache, postoperative pain
Dermatologic: Pruritus

Gastrointestinal: Nausea, vomiting
Local: Pain at injection site
Neuromuscular & skeletal: Muscle rigidity
Respiratory: Apnea, hypoxia, respiratory depression
Miscellaneous: Diaphoresis, shivering, warm sensation
Rare but important or life-threatening: Abdominal discomfort, amnesia, anaphylaxis, anxiety, arrhythmias, awareness under anesthesia without pain, bronchitis, bronchospasm, chest pain, confusion, constipation, cough, CPK increased, diarrhea, disorientation, dysphagia, dysphoria, dyspnea, dysuria, ECG changes, electrolyte disorders, erythema, gastroesophageal reflux, hallucinations, heart block, heartburn, hiccups, hyperglycemia, ileus, incontinence, involuntary movement, laryngospasm, leukocytosis, liver dysfunction, lymphopenia, nasal congestion, nightmares, nystagmus, oliguria, paresthesia, pharyngitis, pleural effusion, prolonged emergence from anesthesia, pulmonary edema, rales, rapid awakening from anesthesia, rash, rhinorrhea, rhonchi, seizure, sleep disturbance, stridor, syncope, temperature regulation impaired, thrombocytopenia, tremors, twitching, urine retention, urticaria, xerostomia

Drug Interactions

Metabolism/Transport Effects None known.

Avoid Concomitant Use

Avoid concomitant use of Remifentanil with any of the following: Azelastine (Nasal); MAO Inhibitors; Orphenadrine; Paraldehyde; Thalidomide

Increased Effect/Toxicity

Remifentanil may increase the levels/effects of: Alcohol (Ethyl); Alvimopan; Azelastine (Nasal); Beta-Blockers; Buprenorphine; Calcium Channel Blockers (Nondihydropyridine); CNS Depressants; Desmopressin; Diuretics; Hydrocodone; MAO Inhibitors; Methotrimeprazine; Metyrosine; Mirtazapine; Orphenadrine; Paraldehyde; Pramipexole; ROPINIRole; Rotigotine; Selective Serotonin Reuptake Inhibitors; Suvorexant; Thalidomide; Zolpidem

The levels/effects of Remifentanil may be increased by: Amphetamines; Anticholinergic Agents; Antipsychotic Agents (Phenothiazines); Brimonidine (Topical); Cannabis; Doxylamine; Dronabinol; Droperidol; HydrOXYzine; Kava Kava; Magnesium Sulfate; Methotrimeprazine; Nabilone; Perampanel; Rufinamide; Sodium Oxybate; Succinylcholine; Tapentadol; Tetrahydrocannabinol

Decreased Effect

Remifentanil may decrease the levels/effects of: Pegvisomant

The levels/effects of Remifentanil may be decreased by: Ammonium Chloride; Mixed Agonist / Antagonist Opioids; Naltrexone

Preparation for Administration Prepare solution by adding 1 mL of diluent per 1 mg of remifentanil. Shake well. Further dilute to a final concentration of 20, 25, 50, or 250 mcg/mL.

Storage/Stability Prior to reconstitution, store at 2°C to 25°C (36°F to 77°F). Stable for 24 hours at room temperature after reconstitution and further dilution to concentrations of 20-250 mcg/mL (4 hours if diluted with LR).

Mechanism of Action Binds with stereospecific mu-opioid receptors at many sites within the CNS, increases pain threshold, alters pain reception, inhibits ascending pain pathways

Pharmacodynamics/Kinetics

Onset of action: IV: 1-3 minutes
Distribution: V_d: 100 mL/kg; increased in children
Protein binding: ~70% (primarily $alpha_1$ acid glycoprotein)
Metabolism: Rapid via blood and tissue esterases
Half-life elimination (dose dependent): Terminal: 10-20 minutes; effective: 3-10 minutes
Excretion: Urine

Dosage IV continuous infusion:

Children Birth to 2 months: Maintenance of anesthesia with nitrous oxide (70%): 0.4 mcg/kg/minute (range: 0.4-1 mcg/kg/minute); supplemental bolus dose of 1 mcg/kg may be administered, smaller bolus dose may be required with potent inhalation agents, potent neuraxial anesthesia, significant comorbidities, significant fluid shifts, or without atropine pretreatment. Clearance in neonates is highly variable; dose should be carefully titrated.

Children 1-12 years: Maintenance of anesthesia with halothane, sevoflurane, or isoflurane: 0.25 mcg/kg/minute (range: 0.05-1.3 mcg/kg/minute); supplemental bolus dose of 1 mcg/kg may be administered every 2-5 minutes. Consider increasing concomitant anesthetics with infusion rate >1 mcg/kg/minute. Infusion rate can be titrated upward in increments up to 50% or titrated downward in decrements of 25% to 50%. May titrate every 2-5 minutes.

Adults:

Induction of anesthesia: 0.5-1 mcg/kg/minute; if endotracheal intubation is to occur in <8 minutes, an initial dose of 1 mcg/kg may be given over 30-60 seconds
Coronary bypass surgery: 1 mcg/kg/minute

Maintenance of anesthesia: **Note:** Supplemental bolus dose of 1 mcg/kg may be administered every 2-5 minutes. Consider increasing concomitant anesthetics with infusion rate >1 mcg/kg/minute. Infusion rate can be titrated upward in increments of 25% to 100% or downward in decrements of 25% to 50%. May titrate every 2-5 minutes.
With nitrous oxide (66%): 0.4 mcg/kg/minute (range: 0.1-2 mcg/kg/minute)
With isoflurane: 0.25 mcg/kg/minute (range: 0.05-2 mcg/kg/minute)
With propofol: 0.25 mcg/kg/minute (range: 0.05-2 mcg/kg/minute)
Coronary bypass surgery: 1 mcg/kg/minute (range: 0.125-4 mcg/kg/minute); supplemental dose: 0.5-1 mcg/kg

Continuation as an analgesic in immediate postoperative period: 0.1 mcg/kg/minute (range: 0.025-0.2 mcg/kg/minute). Infusion rate may be adjusted every 5 minutes in increments of 0.025 mcg/kg/minute. Bolus doses are not recommended. Infusion rates >0.2 mcg/kg/minute are associated with respiratory depression.
Coronary bypass surgery, continuation as an analgesic into the ICU: 1 mcg/kg/minute (range: 0.05-1 mcg/kg/minute)

Analgesic component of monitored anesthesia care: **Note:** Supplemental oxygen is recommended:
Single IV dose given 90 seconds prior to local anesthetic:
Remifentanil alone: 1 mcg/kg over 30-60 seconds
With midazolam: 0.5 mcg/kg over 30-60 seconds
Continuous infusion beginning 5 minutes prior to local anesthetic:
Remifentanil alone: 0.1 mcg/kg minute
With midazolam: 0.05 mcg/kg/minute
Continuous infusion given after local anesthetic:
Remifentanil alone: 0.05 mcg/kg/minute (range: 0.025-0.2 mcg/kg/minute)
With midazolam: 0.025 mcg/kg/minute (range: 0.025-0.2 mcg/kg/minute)
Note: Following local or anesthetic block, infusion rate should be decreased to 0.05 mcg/kg/minute; rate adjustments of 0.025 mcg/kg/minute may be done at 5-minute intervals

Critically-ill patients (off-label dose): Loading dose: 1.5 mcg/kg; followed by 0.008-0.25 mcg/kg/minute (**or** 0.5-15 mcg/kg/**hour**) (Barr, 2013)

Elderly: Elderly patients have an increased sensitivity to effect of remifentanil; doses should be decreased by 50% and titrated.

Dosage adjustment in renal impairment: No dosage adjustment necessary.

Dosage adjustment in hepatic impairment: No dosage adjustment necessary.

Dosing in obesity: Dose should be based on ideal body weight (IBW) in obese patients (>30% over IBW).

Administration An infusion device should be used to administer continuous infusions. During the maintenance of general anesthesia, IV boluses may be administered over 30-60 seconds. Injections should be given into IV tubing close to the venous cannula; tubing should be cleared after treatment to prevent residual effects when other fluids are administered through the same IV line.

Monitoring Parameters Respiratory and cardiovascular status, blood pressure, heart rate

Additional Information Ultra short-acting opioid that is unique compared to other short-acting opioids. This agent is not considered suitable as the sole agent for induction; remifentanil should be used in combination with other induction agents. Bolus doses are not recommended for sedation cases and in treatment of postoperative pain due to risk of respiratory depression and muscle rigidity. Due to remifentanil's short duration of action, when postoperative pain is anticipated, discontinuation of an infusion of remifentanil should be preceded by an adequate postoperative analgesic (ie, fentanyl, morphine).

Dosage Forms

Solution Reconstituted, Intravenous [preservative free]:
Ultiva: 1 mg (1 ea); 2 mg (1 ea); 5 mg (1 ea)

◆ **Reminyl ER (Can)** *see* Galantamine *on page 946*

◆ **Remodulin** *see* Treprostinil *on page 2093*

◆ **Renagel** *see* Sevelamer *on page 1881*

◆ **Renal Replacement Solution** *see* Electrolyte Solution, Renal Replacement *on page 710*

◆ **Renova** *see* Tretinoin (Topical) *on page 2099*

◆ **Renova Pump** *see* Tretinoin (Topical) *on page 2099*

◆ **Renvela** *see* Sevelamer *on page 1881*

◆ **ReoPro** *see* Abciximab *on page 24*

Repaglinide (re PAG li nide)

Brand Names: U.S. Prandin

Brand Names: Canada ACT-Repaglinide; Apo-Repaglinide; Auro-Repaglinide; CO-Repaglinide; GlucoNorm®; PMS-Repaglinide; Sandoz-Repaglinide

Pharmacologic Category Antidiabetic Agent, Meglitinide Analog

Use Management of type 2 diabetes mellitus (noninsulin dependent, NIDDM) as an adjunct to diet and exercise; may be used in combination with metformin or thiazolidinediones

Pregnancy Risk Factor C

Pregnancy Considerations Adverse events have been observed in some animal reproduction studies. Repaglinide was shown to have a low potential to cross the placenta using an *ex vivo* perfusion model (Tertti, 2011). Information describing the effects of repaglinide on pregnancy outcomes is limited.

In women with diabetes, maternal hyperglycemia can be associated with congenital malformations as well as adverse effects in the fetus, neonate, and the mother (ACOG, 2005; ADA, 2014; Kitzmiller, 2008; Metzger, 2007). To prevent adverse outcomes, prior to conception and throughout pregnancy maternal blood glucose and HbA_{1c} should be kept as close to normal as possible but without causing significant hypoglycemia (ACOG, 2013; ADA, 2014; Blumer, 2013; Kitzmiller, 2008). Prior to pregnancy, effective contraception should be used until glycemic control is achieved (ADA, 2014; Kitzmiller, 2008). Other agents are currently recommended to treat diabetes in pregnant women (ACOG, 2013; Blumer, 2013).

Breast-Feeding Considerations It is not known if repaglinide is excreted in breast milk. Due to the potential for serious adverse reactions in the nursing infant, the manufacturer recommends a decision be made whether to discontinue nursing or to discontinue the drug, taking into account the importance of treatment to the mother.

Contraindications Hypersensitivity to repaglinide or any component of the formulation; diabetic ketoacidosis, with or without coma; type 1 diabetes (insulin dependent, IDDM); concurrent gemfibrozil therapy

Warnings/Precautions Use with caution in patients with hepatic impairment. Use caution in severe renal dysfunction, elderly, malnourished, or patients with adrenal/pituitary dysfunction; may be more susceptible to glucose-lowering effects. May cause hypoglycemia; appropriate patient selection, dosage, and patient education are important to avoid hypoglycemic episodes. Ethanol may increase risk of hypoglycemia; instruct patients to avoid ethanol. It may be necessary to discontinue repaglinide and administer insulin if the patient is exposed to stress (fever, trauma, infection, surgery). Theoretically, repaglinide may increase cardiovascular events as observed in some studies using sulfonylureas, but there are no long-term studies assessing this concern. Not indicated for use in combination with NPH insulin as there have been case reports of myocardial ischemia; further evaluation required to assess the safety of this combination.

Adverse Reactions

Cardiovascular: Chest pain, ischemia

Central nervous system: Headache

Endocrine & metabolic: Hypoglycemia

Gastrointestinal: Constipation, diarrhea

Genitourinary: Urinary tract infection

Neuromuscular & skeletal: Arthralgia, back pain

Respiratory: Bronchitis, sinusitis, upper respiratory tract infection

Miscellaneous: Allergy

Rare but important or life-threatening: Anaphylactoid reaction, arrhythmia, hemolytic anemia, hepatic dysfunction (severe), hepatitis, hypertension, leukopenia, MI, pancreatitis, Stevens-Johnson syndrome, thrombocytopenia, visual disturbances (transient)

Drug Interactions

Metabolism/Transport Effects Substrate of CYP2C8 (major), CYP3A4 (major), SLCO1B1; **Note:** Assignment of Major/Minor substrate status based on clinically relevant drug interaction potential

Avoid Concomitant Use

Avoid concomitant use of Repaglinide with any of the following: Atazanavir; Gemfibrozil

Increased Effect/Toxicity

Repaglinide may increase the levels/effects of: Hypoglycemic Agents

The levels/effects of Repaglinide may be increased by: Androgens; Atazanavir; CycloSPORINE (Systemic); CYP2C8 Inhibitors (Moderate); CYP2C8 Inhibitors (Strong); CYP3A4 Inhibitors (Strong); Deferasirox; Eltrombopag; Gemfibrozil; Herbs (Hypoglycemic Properties); Macrolide Antibiotics; MAO Inhibitors; Mifepristone; Pegvisomant; Salicylates; Selective Serotonin Reuptake Inhibitors; SGLT2 Inhibitors; Telaprevir; Teriflunomide; Trimethoprim

Decreased Effect

The levels/effects of Repaglinide may be decreased by: Bosentan; Corticosteroids (Orally Inhaled); Corticosteroids (Systemic); CYP2C8 Inducers (Strong); CYP3A4 Inducers (Moderate); CYP3A4 Inducers (Strong); Dabrafenib; Danazol; Loop Diuretics; Luteinizing Hormone-Releasing Hormone Analogs; Mitotane; Rifampin; Siltuximab; Somatropin; St Johns Wort; Thiazide Diuretics; Tocilizumab

Food Interactions When given with food, the AUC of repaglinide is decreased. Taking medication without eating may cause hypoglycemia. Management: Administer 15-30 minutes prior to a meal. If a meal is skipped, skip dose for that meal.

Storage/Stability Do not store above 25°C (77°F). Protect from moisture.

Mechanism of Action Nonsulfonylurea hypoglycemic agent which blocks ATP-dependent potassium channels, depolarizing the membrane and facilitating calcium entry through calcium channels. Increased intracellular calcium stimulates insulin release from the pancreatic beta cells. Repaglinide-induced insulin release is glucose-dependent.

Pharmacodynamics/Kinetics

Onset of action: Single dose: Increased insulin levels: ~15-60 minutes

Duration: 4-6 hours

Absorption: Rapid and complete

Distribution: V_d: 31 L

Protein binding, plasma: >98% to albumin

Metabolism: Hepatic via CYP3A4 and CYP2C8 isoenzymes and glucuronidation to inactive metabolites

Bioavailability: ~56%

Half-life elimination: ~1 hour

Time to peak, plasma: ~1 hour

Excretion: Feces (~90%, <2% as unchanged drug); Urine (~8%, 0.1% as unchanged drug)

Dosage Oral: Adults:

Initial: For patients not previously treated or whose HbA_{1c} is <8%, the starting dose is 0.5 mg before each meal. For patients previously treated with blood glucose-lowering agents whose HbA_{1c} is ≥8%, the initial dose is 1 or 2 mg before each meal.

Dose adjustment: Determine dosing adjustments by blood glucose response, usually fasting blood glucose. Double the preprandial dose up to 4 mg until satisfactory blood glucose response is achieved. At least 1 week should elapse to assess response after each dose adjustment.

Dose range: 0.5-4 mg taken with meals. Repaglinide may be dosed preprandially 2, 3, or 4 times/day in response to changes in the patient's meal pattern. Maximum recommended daily dose: 16 mg.

Patients receiving other oral hypoglycemic agents: When repaglinide is used to replace therapy with other oral hypoglycemic agents, it may be started the day after the final dose is given. Observe patients carefully for hypoglycemia because of potential overlapping of drug effects. When transferred from longer half-life sulfonylureas (eg, chlorpropamide), close monitoring may be indicated for up to ≥1 week.

Combination therapy: If repaglinide monotherapy does not result in adequate glycemic control, metformin or a thiazolidinedione may be added. Or, if metformin or thiazolidinedione therapy does not provide adequate control, repaglinide may be added. The starting dose and dose adjustments for combination therapy are the same as repaglinide monotherapy. Carefully adjust the dose of each drug to determine the minimal dose required to achieve the desired pharmacologic effect. Failure to do so could result in an increase in the incidence of hypoglycemic episodes. Use appropriate monitoring of FPG and HbA_{1c} measurements to ensure that the patient is not subjected to excessive drug exposure or increased probability of secondary drug failure. If glucose is not achieved after a suitable trial of combination therapy, consider discontinuing these drugs and using insulin.

Dosage adjustment in renal impairment:

CrCl 40-80 mL/minute (mild-to-moderate renal dysfunction): Initial: No dosage adjustment necessary.

CrCl 20-40 mL/minute (severe renal impairment): Initial: 0.5 mg with meals; titrate carefully.

CrCl <20 mL/minute: No dosage adjustment provided in manufacturer's labeling (has not been studied).

Hemodialysis: No dosage adjustment provided in manufacturer's labeling (has not been studied).

Dosage adjustment in hepatic impairment: No dosage adjustment provided in manufacturer's labeling. Use with caution; use conservative initial and maintenance doses. Use longer intervals between dosage adjustments.

Dietary Considerations Take repaglinide 15-30 minutes before meals. Individualized medical nutrition therapy (MNT) based on ADA recommendations is an integral part of therapy. May cause hypoglycemia. Must be able to recognize symptoms of hypoglycemia (palpitations, tachycardia, sweaty palms, diaphoresis, lightheadedness).

Administration Administer 15 minutes before meals; however, time may vary from immediately preceding a meal to as long as 30 minutes before a meal. If the patient misses a meal or is unable to take anything by mouth, repaglinide should not be administered to avoid hypoglycemia. Patients consuming extra meals should be instructed to add a dose for the extra meal.

Monitoring Parameters Monitor fasting blood glucose (periodically) and glycosylated hemoglobin (HbA_{1c}) levels (every 3 months) with a goal of decreasing these levels towards the normal range. During dose adjustment, fasting glucose can be used to determine response.

Reference Range

Recommendations for glycemic control in nonpregnant adults with diabetes (ADA, 2015):

HbA_{1c}: <7% (a more aggressive [<6.5%] or less aggressive [<8%] HbA_{1c} goal may be targeted based on patient-specific characteristics)

Preprandial capillary plasma glucose: 80 to 130 mg/dL

Peak postprandial capillary blood glucose: <180 mg/dL

Recommendations for glycemic control in pediatric (all age groups) patients with type 1 diabetes (ADA, 2015):

HbA_{1c}: <7.5% (individualization may be appropriate based on patient-specific characteristics; <7% is reasonable if it can be achieved without excessive hypoglycemia)

Preprandial capillary plasma glucose: 90 to 130 mg/dL

Bedtime and overnight capillary blood glucose: 90 to 150 mg/dL

Dosage Forms

Tablet, Oral:

Prandin: 0.5 mg, 1 mg, 2 mg

Generic: 0.5 mg, 1 mg, 2 mg

Repaglinide and Metformin

(re PAG li nide & met FOR min)

Brand Names: U.S. PrandiMet

Index Terms Metformin and Repaglinide; Repaglinide and Metformin Hydrochloride

Pharmacologic Category Antidiabetic Agent, Biguanide; Antidiabetic Agent, Meglitinide Analog

Use Management of type 2 diabetes mellitus (noninsulin dependent, NIDDM), as an adjunct to diet and exercise, in patients currently receiving or not adequately controlled on metformin and/or a meglitinide

Pregnancy Risk Factor C

Dosage Oral: Adults: Type 2 diabetes mellitus: **Note:** Daily doses should be divided and given 2-3 times daily with meals (maximum single dose: 4 mg/dose [repaglinide], 1000 mg/dose [metformin]; maximum daily dose: 10 mg/day [repaglinide], 2500 mg/day [metformin])

Patients currently taking repaglinide and metformin: Initial doses should be based on (but not exceeding) the patient's current doses of repaglinide and metformin; titrate as needed to the maximum daily dose to achieve targeted glycemic control

Patients inadequately controlled on metformin alone: Initial dose: Repaglinide 1 mg/ metformin 500 mg twice daily with meals. Titrate slowly to reduce the risk of repaglinide-induced hypoglycemia.

Patients inadequately controlled on a meglitinide alone: Initial dose: Metformin 500 mg twice daily plus repaglinide at a dose similar to (but not exceeding) the patient's current dose. Titrate slowly to reduce the risk of metformin-induced gastrointestinal adverse effects.

Dosing adjustment in renal impairment: Do not use in renal impairment; metformin use is contraindicated in patients with renal impairment (serum creatinine ≥1.5 mg/dL in males or ≥1.4 mg/dL in females)

Dosing adjustment in hepatic impairment: Avoid use in patients with impaired liver function

Additional Information Complete prescribing information should be consulted for additional detail.

Dosage Forms

Tablet:

PrandiMet®: 1/500: Repaglinide 1 mg and metformin hydrochloride 500 mg; 2/500: Repaglinide 2 mg and metformin hydrochloride 500 mg

◆ **Repaglinide and Metformin Hydrochloride** *see* Repaglinide and Metformin *on page* 1792

◆ **Replagal [DSC] (Can)** *see* Agalsidase Alfa [CAN/INT] *on page* 63

◆ **Reprexain** *see* Hydrocodone and Ibuprofen *on page* 1013

◆ **Repronex** *see* Menotropins *on page* 1292

◆ **Requip** *see* ROPINIRole *on page* 1844

◆ **Requip XL** *see* ROPINIRole *on page* 1844

◆ **Rescon DM [OTC]** *see* Chlorpheniramine, Pseudoephedrine, and Dextromethorphan *on page* 428

◆ **Rescon GG [OTC]** *see* Guaifenesin and Phenylephrine *on page* 988

◆ **Rescriptor** *see* Delavirdine *on page* 587

◆ **Resectisol** *see* Mannitol *on page* 1269

Reserpine (re SER peen)

Pharmacologic Category Central Monoamine-Depleting Agent; Rauwolfia Alkaloid

Additional Appendix Information

Beers Criteria – Potentially Inappropriate Medications for Geriatrics *on page* 2271

Use

Agitated psychotic states: Treatment of agitated psychotic states (schizophrenia)

Hypertension: Management of mild to moderate hypertension

Note: According to the Eighth Joint National Committee (JNC 8) guidelines, reserpine is **not** recommended for the initial treatment of hypertension (James, 2013).

Pregnancy Risk Factor C

Dosage Note: When used for management of hypertension, full antihypertensive effects may take as long as 3 weeks.

Oral:

Children: Hypertension: 0.01-0.02 mg/kg/24 hours divided every 12 hours; maximum dose: 0.25 mg/day (not recommended in children)

Adults:

Hypertension:

Manufacturer's labeling: Initial: 0.5 mg/day for 1-2 weeks; maintenance: 0.1-0.25 mg/day

Note: Clinically, the need for a "loading" period (as recommended by the manufacturer) is not well supported, and alternative dosing is preferred.

Alternative dosing (off-label): Initial: 0.1 mg once daily; adjust as necessary based on response.

Usual dose range (ASH/ISH [Weber, 2014]): 0.1-0.25 mg once daily

Schizophrenia: Dosing recommendations vary; initial dose recommendations generally range from 0.05-0.25 mg (although manufacturer recommends 0.5 mg once daily initially). May be increased in increments of 0.1-0.25 mg.

Elderly: Initial: 0.05 mg once daily, increasing by 0.05 mg every week as necessary (Beers Criteria: Avoid doses >0.25 mg daily)

Dosage adjustment in renal impairment: No dosage adjustment provided in manufacturer's labeling. The following dosing adjustments have been used by some clinicians (Aronoff, 2007):

CrCl <10 mL/minute: Avoid use.

Hemodialysis, peritoneal dialysis: Not removed by hemo- or peritoneal dialysis; supplemental dose is not necessary.

Dosage adjustment in renal impairment: No dosage adjustment provided in manufacturer's labeling.

Additional Information Complete prescribing information should be consulted for additional detail.

Dosage Forms

Tablet, Oral:

Generic: 0.1 mg, 0.25 mg

◆ **Resistant Dextrin** *see* Wheat Dextrin *on page* 2190

◆ **Resistant Maltodextrin** *see* Wheat Dextrin *on page* 2190

◆ **Resonium Calcium® (Can)** *see* Calcium Polystyrene Sulfonate [CAN/INT] *on page* 333

◆ **Resotran (Can)** *see* Prucalopride [CAN/INT] *on page* 1741

◆ **Respa-BR** *see* Brompheniramine *on page* 292

◆ **Restasis** *see* CycloSPORINE (Ophthalmic) *on page* 529

◆ **Restasis® (Can)** *see* CycloSPORINE (Ophthalmic) *on page* 529

◆ **Restoril** *see* Temazepam *on page* 1990

◆ **Restylane** *see* Hyaluronate and Derivatives *on page* 1006

◆ **Restylane-L** *see* Hyaluronate and Derivatives *on page* 1006

◆ **Restylane Silk** *see* Hyaluronate and Derivatives *on page* 1006

Retapamulin (re te PAM ue lin)

Brand Names: U.S. Altabax

Pharmacologic Category Antibiotic, Pleuromutilin; Antibiotic, Topical

Use Treatment of impetigo caused by susceptible strains of *S. pyogenes* or methicillin-susceptible *S. aureus*

Pregnancy Risk Factor B

Dosage Topical: Impetigo:

Children ≥9 months: Apply to affected area twice daily for 5 days. Total treatment area should not exceed 2% of total body surface area.

Adults: Apply to affected area twice daily for 5 days. Total treatment area should not exceed 100 cm^2 total body surface area.

Additional Information Complete prescribing information should be consulted for additional detail.

Dosage Forms

Ointment, External:

Altabax: 1% (15 g, 30 g)

◆ **Retavase [DSC]** *see* Reteplase *on page 1794*

◆ **Retavase® (Can)** *see* Reteplase *on page 1794*

◆ **Retavase Half-Kit [DSC]** *see* Reteplase *on page 1794*

Reteplase (RE ta plase)

Brand Names: U.S. Retavase Half-Kit [DSC]; Retavase [DSC]

Brand Names: Canada Retavase®

Index Terms r-PA; Recombinant Plasminogen Activator

Pharmacologic Category Thrombolytic Agent

Use Management of ST-elevation myocardial infarction (STEMI) for the improvement of ventricular function, the reduction of the incidence of CHF, and the reduction of mortality following STEMI

Recommended criteria for treatment of STEMI (ACCF/AHA; O'Gara, 2013): Ischemic symptoms within 12 hours of treatment or evidence of ongoing ischemia 12-24 hours after symptom onset with a large area of myocardium at risk or hemodynamic instability.

STEMI ECG definition: New ST-segment elevation at the J point in at least 2 contiguous leads of ≥2 mm (0.2 mV) in men or ≥1.5 mm (0.15 mV) in women in leads V_2-V_3 and/or of ≥1 mm (0.1 mV) in other contiguous precordial leads or limb leads on ECG. New or presumably new left bundle branch block (LBBB) may interfere with ST-elevation analysis and should not be considered diagnostic in isolation.

At non-PCI-capable hospitals, the ACCF/AHA recommends thrombolytic therapy administration when the anticipated first medical contact (FMC)-to-device time at a PCI-capable hospital is >120 minutes due to unavoidable delays.

Pregnancy Risk Factor C

Dosage

Children: Not recommended

Adults: 10 units IV over 2 minutes, followed by a second dose 30 minutes later of 10 units IV over 2 minutes; withhold second dose if serious bleeding or anaphylaxis occurs

Note: Thrombolytic should be administered within 30 minutes of hospital arrival. Administer concurrent aspirin, clopidogrel, and anticoagulant therapy (ie, unfractionated heparin, enoxaparin, or fondaparinux) with reteplase (O'Gara, 2013).

Dosage adjustment in renal impairment: No dosage adjustment provided in manufacturer's labeling. However, risks of reteplase therapy may be increased.

Dosage adjustment in hepatic disease: No dosage adjustment provided in manufacturer's labeling. However, risks of reteplase therapy may be increased.

Additional Information Complete prescribing information should be consulted for additional detail.

◆ **Retigabine** *see* Ezogabine *on page 835*

◆ **Retin-A** *see* Tretinoin (Topical) *on page 2099*

◆ **Retin-A Micro** *see* Tretinoin (Topical) *on page 2099*

◆ **Retin-A Micro Pump** *see* Tretinoin (Topical) *on page 2099*

◆ **Retinoic Acid** *see* Tretinoin (Topical) *on page 2099*

◆ **Retinova (Can)** *see* Tretinoin (Topical) *on page 2099*

◆ **Retrovir** *see* Zidovudine *on page 2196*

◆ **Retrovir (AZT) (Can)** *see* Zidovudine *on page 2196*

◆ **Revatio** *see* Sildenafil *on page 1882*

◆ **ReVia** *see* Naltrexone *on page 1422*

◆ **Revlimid** *see* Lenalidomide *on page 1177*

◆ **Revolade** *see* Eltrombopag *on page 714*

◆ **Revonto** *see* Dantrolene *on page 559*

◆ **Reyataz** *see* Atazanavir *on page 185*

◆ **rFSH-alpha** *see* Follitropin Alfa *on page 921*

◆ **rFSH-beta** *see* Follitropin Beta *on page 921*

◆ **rFVIIa** *see* Factor VIIa (Recombinant) *on page 836*

◆ **RG7204** *see* Vemurafenib *on page 2148*

◆ **R-Gene 10** *see* Arginine *on page 171*

◆ **rhAT** *see* Antithrombin *on page 156*

◆ **rhATIII** *see* Antithrombin *on page 156*

◆ **r-hCG** *see* Chorionic Gonadotropin (Recombinant) *on page 432*

◆ **rhDNase** *see* Dornase Alfa *on page 672*

◆ **Rheumatrex** *see* Methotrexate *on page 1322*

◆ **rhFSH-alpha** *see* Follitropin Alfa *on page 921*

◆ **rhFSH-beta** *see* Follitropin Beta *on page 921*

◆ **rhGAA** *see* Alglucosidase Alfa *on page 85*

◆ **r-h α-GAL** *see* Agalsidase Beta *on page 64*

◆ **RhIG** *see* Rh_o(D) Immune Globulin *on page 1794*

◆ **rhIL-11** *see* Oprelvekin *on page 1519*

◆ **Rhinalar® (Can)** *see* Flunisolide (Nasal) *on page 893*

◆ **Rhinaris [OTC]** *see* Sodium Chloride *on page 1902*

◆ **Rhinaris-CS Anti-Allergic Nasal Mist (Can)** *see* Cromolyn (Nasal) *on page 514*

◆ **Rhinocort Aqua** *see* Budesonide (Nasal) *on page 296*

◆ **Rhinocort® Aqua® (Can)** *see* Budesonide (Nasal) *on page 296*

◆ **Rhinocort® Turbuhaler® (Can)** *see* Budesonide (Nasal) *on page 296*

◆ **r-Hirudin** *see* Desirudin *on page 593*

◆ **rhKGF** *see* Palifermin *on page 1555*

◆ **r-hLH** *see* Lutropin Alfa [CAN/INT] *on page 1259*

◆ **Rho(D) Immune Globulin (Human)** *see* Rh_o(D) Immune Globulin *on page 1794*

Rh_o(D) Immune Globulin

(ar aych oh (dee) i MYUN GLOB yoo lin)

Brand Names: U.S. HyperRHO S/D; MICRhoGAM Ultra-Filtered Plus; RhoGAM Ultra-Filtered Plus; Rhophylac; WinRho SDF

Brand Names: Canada WinRho SDF

Index Terms Anti-D Immunoglobulin; RhIG; Rho(D) Immune Globulin (Human); RhoIGIV; RhoIVIM

Pharmacologic Category Blood Product Derivative; Immune Globulin

Use

Immune thrombocytopenia (ITP):

Rhophylac: To increase platelet counts in Rh_o(D) positive nonsplenectomized adults with chronic ITP.

WinRho SDF: To increase platelet counts in Rho (D) positive nonsplenectomized patients with the following conditions: acute ITP (children), chronic ITP (adults and children), or ITP secondary to HIV infection (adults and children).

Pregnancy and other obstetric conditions:

Prevention of rhesus (Rh) isoimmunization in an Rh-incompatible pregnancy. All products are for use in Rh_o(D) negative mothers who are not already sensitized to the Rh_o(D) factor. An Rh-incompatible pregnancy is assumed if the fetus/baby is either Rh_o(D) positive or Rh_o(D) unknown or if the father is either Rh_o (D) positive or Rh_o(D) unknown. Use in not needed if the father or baby is conclusively Rh_o(D) negative. Product specific indications are as follows based on the above criteria:

HyperRHO S/D Full Dose: For antepartum prophylaxis at ~28 weeks gestation; for administration within 72 hours of birth for the prevention of hemolytic disease of the newborn; for administration within 72 hours of spontaneous or induced abortion, ruptured tubal pregnancy, amniocentesis or abdominal trauma.

HyperRHO S/D Mini Dose: For administration within 3 hours (or as soon as possible) of spontaneous or induced abortion up to 12 weeks' gestation.

MICRhoGAM Ultra-Filtered Plus: For administration within 72 hours of actual or threatened termination of pregnancy (spontaneous or induced) up to and including 12 weeks' gestation.

RhoGAM Ultra-Filtered Plus: For antepartum prophylaxis at 26 to 28 weeks' gestation; for administration within 72 hours of birth for prevention of hemolytic disease of the newborn; for administration within 72 hours of amniocentesis, chorionic villus sampling (CVS), percutaneous umbilical blood sampling (PUBS), abdominal trauma or obstetrical manipulation, ectopic pregnancy, threatened pregnancy loss after 12 weeks' gestation (with continuation of pregnancy), pregnancy termination (spontaneous or induced) after 12 weeks' gestation.

Rhophylac: For antepartum prophylaxis at 28 to 30 weeks' gestation; for administration within 72 hours of birth for the prevention of hemolytic disease of the newborn; for administration within 72 hours of obstetric complications including miscarriage, abortion, threatened abortion, ectopic pregnancy or hydatiform mole, transplacental hemorrhage resulting from antepartum hemorrhage; for administration within 72 hours of invasive procedures during pregnancy including amniocentesis, chorionic biopsy, or obstetric manipulative procedures such as external version or abdominal trauma.

WinRho SDF: For antepartum prophylaxis at 28 weeks' gestation; for administration within 72 hours of birth for the prevention of hemolytic disease of the newborn; for administration following obstetric complications including miscarriage, abortion, threatened abortion, ectopic pregnancy or hydatiform mole, transplacental hemorrhage resulting from antepartum hemorrhage; for administration following invasive procedures during pregnancy including amniocentesis, chorionic biopsy, or obstetric manipulative procedures such as external version or abdominal trauma.

Transfusion:

HyperRHO S/D Full Dose, MICRhoGAM Ultra-Filtered Plus, RhoGAM Ultra-Filtered Plus, Rhophylac, and WinRho SDF: To prevent isoimmunization in Rh_o(D) negative individuals who have been transfused with Rh_o(D) positive red blood cells or blood components containing red blood cells.

Pregnancy Risk Factor C

Dosage Note: Rh_o(D) immune globulin 300 mcg has traditionally been referred to as a "full dose". Potency and dosing recommendations may also be expressed in international units by comparison to the WHO anti-Rh_o(D) standard where 1 mcg = 5 international units.

Immune thrombocytopenia (ITP):

Rhophylac: Adults: IV: 50 mcg/kg

WinRho SDF: Children, Adolescents, and Adults: IV:

Initial: 50 mcg/kg as a single injection, or can be given as a divided dose on separate days. If hemoglobin is <10 g/dL: Dose should be reduced to 25 to 40 mcg/kg.

Subsequent dosing: 25 to 60 mcg/kg can be used if required to increase platelet count; frequency of dosing is dependent upon clinical response

Maintenance dosing if patient **did respond** to initial dosing: 25 to 60 mcg/kg based on platelet count and hemoglobin concentration

Maintenance dosing if patient **did not respond** to initial dosing:

Hemoglobin <8 g/dL: Alternative treatment should be used

Hemoglobin 8 to 10 g/dL: Redose between 25 to 40 mcg/kg

Hemoglobin >10 g/dL: Redose between 50 to 60 mcg/kg

Rh_o(D) suppression: Adults: **Note:** In general, a 300 mcg dose will suppress the immune response to a fetal-maternal hemorrhage with ≤15 mL of Rh-positive RBC. If exposure to >15 mL of Rh-positive RBC is suspected, an appropriate dose should be calculated. If the first dose is administered early in pregnancy, additional doses may be needed to ensure adequate levels of passively acquired anti-D at delivery (ACOG, 1999). If delivery occurs within 3 weeks after the last antepartum dose, a postpartum dose may be withheld, but testing for fetal-maternal hemorrhage of >15 mL should be performed (ACOG, 1999).

Pregnancy prophylaxis: Note: if antepartum prophylaxis is indicated, the mother may also need a postpartum dose if the infant is Rh-positive.

Antepartum prophylaxis:

HyperRHO S/D Full Dose: IM: 300 mcg at ~28 weeks' gestation

RhoGAM: IM: 300 mcg at 26 to 28 weeks' gestation; if delivery does not occur within 12 weeks after the dose, a second 300 mcg dose is recommended. If the first dose is prior to 26 weeks' gestation, administer every 12 weeks to ensure adequate levels of passively acquired anti-D. If delivery occurs within 3 weeks after the last antepartum dose, a postpartum dose may be withheld, but testing for fetal-maternal hemorrhage of >15 mL should be performed.

Rhophylac: IM, IV: 300 mcg at 28 to 30 weeks' gestation

WinRho SDF: IM, IV: 300 mcg at 28 weeks' gestation. If the first dose is administered early in pregnancy, administer every 12 weeks to ensure adequate levels of passively acquired anti-D.

Postpartum prophylaxis:

HyperRHO S/D Full Dose: IM: 300 mcg provides sufficient antibody if volume of Rh-positive RBC exposure is ≤15 mL. If exposure to >15 mL of Rh-positive RBC is suspected, an appropriate dose should be calculated (see dosing for excessive fetomaternal hemorrhage). The dose should be administered within 72 hours of delivery, but may provide some benefit if given later.

RhoGAM: IM: 300 mcg provides sufficient antibody if volume of Rh-positive RBC exposure is ≤15 mL. If exposure to >15 mL of Rh-positive RBC is suspected, an appropriate dose should be calculated.

The dose should be administered within 72 hours of delivery.

Rhophylac: IM, IV: 300 mcg provides sufficient antibody if volume of Rh-positive RBC exposure is ≤15 mL. If exposure to >15 mL of Rh-positive RBC is suspected, an appropriate dose should be calculated (see dosing for excessive fetomaternal hemorrhage). The dose should be administered within 72 hours of delivery.

WinRho SDF: IM, IV: 120 mcg. The dose should be administered within 72 hours of delivery but may be given up to 28 days after delivery.

Other pregnancy/obstetric conditions:

Abdominal trauma:

HyperRHO S/D Full Dose: IM: 300 mcg following abdominal trauma in the second or third trimester. If exposure to >15 mL of Rh-positive RBC is suspected, an appropriate dose should be calculated (see dosing for excessive fetomaternal hemorrhage).

RhoGam: IM: 300 mcg within 72 hours following abdominal trauma or obstetrical manipulation occurring at ≥13 weeks' gestation. If exposure to >15 mL of Rh-positive RBC is suspected, an appropriate dose should be calculated.

Rhophylac: IV, IM: 300 mcg within 72 hours of procedure. If exposure to >15 mL of Rh-positive RBC is suspected, an appropriate dose should be calculated (see dosing for excessive fetomaternal hemorrhage).

Amniocentesis:

HyperRHO S/D Full Dose: IM: 300 mcg at 15 to 18 weeks' gestation or during the third trimester. If exposure to >15 mL of Rh-positive RBC is suspected, an appropriate dose should be calculated (see dosing for excessive fetomaternal hemorrhage).

RhoGam: IM: 300 mcg within 72 hours of a procedure occurring at ≥13 weeks' gestation. If exposure to >15 mL of Rh-positive RBC is suspected, an appropriate dose should be calculated.

Rhophylac: IV, IM: 300 mcg within 72 hours of procedure. If exposure to >15 mL of Rh-positive RBC is suspected, an appropriate dose should be calculated (see dosing for excessive fetomaternal hemorrhage).

WinRho SDF: IV, IM: 300 mcg immediately after amniocentesis occurring before 34 weeks' gestation; repeat dose every 12 weeks during pregnancy. Administer 120 mcg within 72 hours of amniocentesis occurring after 34 weeks' gestation.

Ectopic pregnancy:

HyperRHO S/D Full Dose: IM: 300 mcg for complications occurring at ≥13 weeks' gestation. If exposure to >15 mL of Rh-positive RBC is suspected, an appropriate dose should be calculated (see dosing for excessive fetomaternal hemorrhage).

RhoGam: IM: 300 mcg within 72 hours of complications occurring at ≥13 weeks' gestation. If exposure to >15 mL of Rh-positive RBC is suspected, an appropriate dose should be calculated.

Rhophylac: IV, IM: 300 mcg within 72 hours of complication. If exposure to >15 mL of Rh-positive RBC is suspected, an appropriate dose should be calculated (see dosing for excessive fetomaternal hemorrhage).

Termination of pregnancy (spontaneous or induced):

HyperRHO S/D Mini Dose: IM: 50 mcg within 3 hours or as soon as possible following spontaneous or induced abortion occurring <13 weeks' gestation; administer within 72 hours of termination if prompt administration is not possible.

HyperRHO S/D Full Dose: IM: 300 mcg following miscarriage or abortion occurring ≥13 weeks' gestation. If exposure to >15 mL of Rh-positive RBC is suspected, an appropriate dose should be calculated (see dosing for excessive fetomaternal hemorrhage).

MICRhoGAM: IM: 50 mcg within 72 hours of actual or threatened termination occurring <13 weeks' gestation.

RhoGAM: IM: 300 mcg within 72 hours following spontaneous or induced termination occurring ≥13 weeks' gestation. If exposure to >15 mL of Rh-positive RBC is suspected, an appropriate dose should be calculated.

Rhophylac: IV, IM: 300 mcg within 72 hours of miscarriage or abortion. If exposure to >15 mL of Rh-positive RBC is suspected, an appropriate dose should be calculated (see dosing for excessive fetomaternal hemorrhage).

WinRho SDF: IV, IM: 120 mcg within 72 hours of abortion occurring after 34 weeks' gestation.

Threatened pregnancy loss with continuation of pregnancy:

HyperRHO S/D Full Dose: IM: 300 mcg following threatened loss at any time during pregnancy; administer as soon as possible. If exposure to >15 mL of Rh-positive RBC is suspected, an appropriate dose should be calculated (see dosing for excessive fetomaternal hemorrhage).

RhoGAM: I.M.: 300 mcg within 72 hours following threatened loss ≥13 weeks' gestation. If exposure to >15 mL of Rh-positive RBC is suspected, an appropriate dose should be calculated.

Rhophylac: IV, IM: 300 mcg within 72 hours of threatened abortion. If exposure to >15 mL of Rh-positive RBC is suspected, an appropriate dose should be calculated (see dosing for excessive fetomaternal hemorrhage).

WinRho SDF: IV, IM: 300 mcg immediately following a threatened abortion occurring any time during pregnancy

Additional invasive/manipulative procedures or obstetric complications:

RhoGam: IM: 300 mcg within 72 hours of chorionic villus sampling or percutaneous umbilical blood sampling ≥13 weeks' gestation. If exposure to >15 mL of Rh-positive RBC is suspected, an appropriate dose should be calculated.

Rhophylac: IV, IM: 300 mcg within 72 hours of procedures such as chorionic biopsy or external version, or within 72 hours of complications such as hydatidiform mole, or transplacental hemorrhage resulting from antepartum hemorrhage. If exposure to >15 mL of Rh-positive RBC is suspected, an appropriate dose should be calculated (see dosing for excessive fetomaternal hemorrhage).

WinRho SDF: IV, IM: 300 mcg immediately after chorionic villus sampling before 34 weeks' gestation; repeat dose every 12 weeks during pregnancy. Administer 120 mcg within 72 hours of manipulation occurring after 34 weeks' gestation.

Dosing for excessive fetomaternal hemorrhage:

HyperRHO S/D Full Dose: I.M.: When exposure to >15 mL Rh-positive RBC or >30 mL whole blood is suspected, a fetal red cell count should be calculated. The fetal RBC volume is then divided by 15 mL, providing the number of 300 mcg doses (vials/syringes) to administer. If the dose calculated results in a fraction, round up to the next higher whole 300 mcg dose (vial/syringe).

Rhophylac: IV, IM: When exposure to >15 mL Rh-positive RBC, administer 300 mcg; in addition, administer 20 mcg per mL fetal RBC in excess of 15 mL if bleeding can be quantified or an additional 300 mcg if excess bleeding cannot be quantified. Total dose should be administered within 72 hours of complication.

Transfusion: Adults: **Note:** Actual dose is based upon volume of blood/blood product exposure.

WinRho SDF: Administer within 72 hours after exposure of incompatible blood transfusion.

IV: Calculate dose as follows; administer 600 mcg every 8 hours until the total dose is administered:

Exposure to Rh_o(D) positive whole blood: 9 mcg/mL blood

Exposure to Rh_o(D) positive red blood cells: 18 mcg/mL cells

IM: Calculate dose as follows; administer 1,200 mcg every 12 hours until the total dose is administered:

Exposure to Rh_o(D) positive whole blood: 12 mcg/mL blood

Exposure to Rh_o(D) positive red blood cells: 24 mcg/mL cells

HyperRHO S/D Full Dose: IM: Multiply the volume of Rh-positive whole blood administered by the hematocrit of the donor unit to equal the volume of RBCs transfused. The volume of RBCs is then divided by 15 mL, providing the number of 300 mcg doses (vials/syringes) to administer. If the dose calculated results in a fraction, round up to the next higher whole 300 mcg dose (vial/syringe). Administer as soon as possible and within 72 hours after an incompatible transfusion.

MICRhoGAM: IM: <2.5 mL of Rh-positive red blood cell exposure: 50 mcg. Administer within 72 hours after an incompatible transfusion.

RhoGAM: IM:

2.5 to 15 mL Rh-positive red blood cell exposure: 300 mcg. Administer within 72 hours after an incompatible transfusion.

>15 mL Rh-positive red blood cell exposure: 20 mcg per mL of Rh-positive red blood cell exposure. Multiple doses may be given at the same time or spaced at intervals; total dose must be given within 72 hours of exposure.

Rhophylac: IM, IV: 20 mcg per 2 mL transfused blood or 20 mcg per mL erythrocyte concentrate. Administer within 72 hours after an incompatible transfusion.

Elderly: Patients >65 years of age with a concurrent comorbid condition may be at increased risk of developing acute hemolytic reactions. Fatal outcomes associated with IVH have occurred most frequently in those >65 years. Use caution; consider starting at lower doses.

Dosage adjustment in renal impairment: There are no dosage adjustments provided in the manufacturer's labeling.

Dosage adjustment in hepatic disease: There are no dosage adjustments provided in the manufacturer's labeling.

Additional Information Complete prescribing information should be consulted for additional detail.

Dosage Forms

Injectable, Intramuscular [preservative free]:

HyperRHO S/D: 50 mcg (1 ea); 300 mcg (1 ea)

MICRhoGAM Ultra-Filtered Plus: 50 mcg (1 ea)

RhoGAM Ultra-Filtered Plus: 300 mcg (1 ea)

Solution, Injection:

WinRho SDF: 2500 units/2.2 mL (2.2 mL); 5000 units/4.4 mL (4.4 mL); 1500 units/1.3 mL (1.3 mL); 15,000 units/13 mL (13 mL)

Solution, Injection [preservative free]:

Rhophylac: 1500 units/2 mL (2 mL)

WinRho SDF: 2500 units/2.2 mL (2.2 mL); 5000 units/4.4 mL (4.4 mL); 1500 units/1.3 mL (1.3 mL); 15,000 units/13 mL (13 mL)

- ◆ **RhoGAM Ultra-Filtered Plus** *see* Rh_o(D) Immune Globulin *on page 1794*
- ◆ **RhoIGIV** *see* Rh_o(D) Immune Globulin *on page 1794*
- ◆ **RhoIVIM** *see* Rh_o(D) Immune Globulin *on page 1794*
- ◆ **Rho®-Loperamine (Can)** *see* Loperamide *on page 1236*
- ◆ **Rho-Nitro Pump Spray (Can)** *see* Nitroglycerin *on page 1465*
- ◆ **Rhophylac** *see* Rh_o(D) Immune Globulin *on page 1794*
- ◆ **Rhotral (Can)** *see* Acebutolol *on page 29*
- ◆ **Rhovane (Can)** *see* Zopiclone [CAN/INT] *on page 2217*
- ◆ **Rhoxal-loperamide (Can)** *see* Loperamide *on page 1236*
- ◆ **Rhoxal-nabumetone (Can)** *see* Nabumetone *on page 1411*
- ◆ **Rhoxal-orphendrine (Can)** *see* Orphenadrine *on page 1522*
- ◆ **Rhoxal-sotalol (Can)** *see* Sotalol *on page 1927*
- ◆ **rhPTH(1-34)** *see* Teriparatide *on page 2008*
- ◆ **Rh-TSH** *see* Thyrotropin Alfa *on page 2031*
- ◆ **rHuEPO** *see* Epoetin Alfa *on page 742*
- ◆ **rhuFabV2** *see* Ranibizumab *on page 1776*
- ◆ **rHu-GM-CSF** *see* Molgramostim [INT] *on page 1388*
- ◆ **rhuGM-CSF** *see* Sargramostim *on page 1865*
- ◆ **rhu Keratinocyte Growth Factor** *see* Palifermin *on page 1555*
- ◆ **rHu-KGF** *see* Palifermin *on page 1555*
- ◆ **rhuMAb-2C4** *see* Pertuzumab *on page 1627*
- ◆ **rhuMAb-E25** *see* Omalizumab *on page 1503*
- ◆ **rHuMAb-EGFr** *see* Panitumumab *on page 1568*
- ◆ **rhuMAb HER2** *see* Trastuzumab *on page 2085*
- ◆ **rhuMAb-VEGF** *see* Bevacizumab *on page 257*
- ◆ **RiaSTAP®** *see* Fibrinogen Concentrate (Human) *on page 874*
- ◆ **Ribasphere** *see* Ribavirin *on page 1797*
- ◆ **Ribasphere RibaPak** *see* Ribavirin *on page 1797*

Ribavirin (rye ba VYE rin)

Brand Names: U.S. Copegus; Moderiba; Rebetol; Ribasphere; Ribasphere RibaPak; Virazole

Brand Names: Canada Virazole

Index Terms RTCA; Tribavirin

Pharmacologic Category Antihepaciviral, Nucleoside (Anti-HCV)

Use

Inhalation: Treatment of hospitalized infants and young children with respiratory syncytial virus (RSV) infections; specially indicated for treatment of severe lower respiratory tract RSV infections in patients with an underlying compromising condition (prematurity, cardiopulmonary disease, or immunosuppression)

Oral capsule: In combination with interferon alfa 2b (pegylated or nonpegylated) injection for the treatment of chronic hepatitis C in interferon alfa-naive or experienced-patients with compensated liver disease. Patients likely to fail retreatment after a prior failed course include previous nonresponders, those who received previous pegylated interferon treatment, patients who have significant bridging fibrosis or cirrhosis, or those with genotype 1 infection.

Oral solution: In combination with interferon alfa-2b (pegylated or nonpegylated) injection for the treatment of chronic hepatitis C in interferon alfa-naive or experienced patients ≥3 years of age with compensated liver disease. Patients likely to fail retreatment after a prior failed course include previous nonresponders, those who received previous pegylated interferon treatment, patients who have significant bridging fibrosis or cirrhosis, or those with genotype 1 infection.

Oral tablet: In combination with peginterferon alfa-2a for the treatment of adults (Copegus, Moderiba, Ribasphere) and patients ≥5 years of age (Copegus only) with chronic HCV infection who have compensated liver disease and have not previously been treated with interferon alpha, and in adult chronic hepatitis C patients coinfected with HIV

Pregnancy Risk Factor X

Pregnancy Considerations [U.S. Boxed Warning]: Significant teratogenic and/or embryocidal effects have been observed in all animal studies. Use is contraindicated in pregnant women or male partners of pregnant women. Avoid pregnancy in female patients and female partners of male patients during therapy by using two effective forms of contraception; continue contraceptive measures for at least 6 months after completion of therapy. A negative pregnancy test is required immediately before initiation, monthly during therapy, and for 6 months after treatment is discontinued. If patient or female partner becomes pregnant during treatment, she should be counseled about potential risks of exposure. The manufacturer recommends that pregnant health care workers take precautions to limit exposure to ribavirin aerosol; potential occupational exposure may be greatest if administration is via oxygen tent or hood, and lower if administered via mechanical ventilation.

Health care providers and patients are encouraged to enroll women exposed to ribavirin during pregnancy or within 6 months after treatment in the Ribavirin Pregnancy Registry (800-593-2214).

Breast-Feeding Considerations It is not known if ribavirin is excreted into breast milk. Due to the potential for serious adverse reactions in the nursing infant, the manufacturer recommends that a decision be made whether to discontinue nursing or to discontinue the drug, taking into account the importance of treatment to the mother.

Contraindications

Inhalation: Hypersensitivity to ribavirin or any component of the formulation; women who are pregnant or may become pregnant

Oral formulations: Hypersensitivity to ribavirin or any component of the formulation; women who are pregnant or may become pregnant; males whose female partners are pregnant; patients with hemoglobinopathies (eg, thalassemia major, sickle cell anemia); patients with autoimmune hepatitis; concomitant use with didanosine

Ribasphere capsules and Rebetol capsules/solution: Additional contraindications: Patients with a CrCl <50 mL/minute

Oral combination therapy with alfa interferons: Autoimmune hepatitis, hepatic decompensation (Child-Pugh score >6; class B and C) in cirrhotic chronic hepatitis C monoinfected patients prior to treatment, hepatic decompensation (Child-Pugh score ≥6) in cirrhotic chronic hepatitis C patients coinfected with HIV prior to treatment. Also refer to individual monographs for Interferon Alfa-2b (Intron A), Peginterferon Alfa-2b, and Peginterferon Alfa-2a (Pegasys) for additional contraindication information.

Warnings/Precautions Hazardous agent - use appropriate precautions for handling and disposal (NIOSH 2014 [group 3]).

Oral: Safety and efficacy have not been established in patients who have received organ transplants, or been coinfected with hepatitis B or HIV (ribavirin tablets may be used in adult HIV-coinfected patients unless CD4+ cell count is <100 cells/microliter and HIV-1 RNA <5000 cells/mm^3). Hemoglobin at initiation must be ≥12 g/dL (women) or ≥13 g/dL (men) in CHC monoinfected patients and ≥11 g/dL (women) or ≥12 g/dL (men) in CHC and HIV coinfected patients. Oral ribavirin should not be used for adenovirus, RSV, influenza or parainfluenza infections; ribavirin inhalation is approved for severe RSV infection in children.

[U.S. Boxed Warning]: Monotherapy not effective for chronic hepatitis C infection. Severe psychiatric events have occurred including depression and suicidal behavior during combination therapy. Avoid use in patients with a psychiatric history; discontinue if severe psychiatric symptoms occur. Acute hypersensitivity reactions (eg, anaphylaxis, angioedema, bronchoconstriction, and urticaria) have been observed (rarely) with ribavirin and alfa interferon combination therapy. Severe cutaneous reactions, including Stevens-Johnson syndrome and exfoliative dermatitis have been reported (rarely) with ribavirin and alfa interferon combination therapy; discontinue with signs or symptoms of severe skin reactions. Use with caution in patients with renal impairment; dosage adjustment or discontinuation may be required. Elderly patients are more susceptible to adverse effects; use caution.

[U.S. Boxed Warning]: Hemolytic anemia is the primary clinical toxicity of oral therapy; anemia associated with ribavirin may worsen underlying cardiac disease and lead to fatal and nonfatal myocardial infarctions. Avoid use in patients with significant/unstable cardiac disease. Anemia usually occurs within 1 to 2 weeks of therapy initiation; observed in ~10% to 13% of patients when alfa interferons were combined with ribavirin. Assess cardiac function before initiation of therapy. If patient has underlying cardiac disease, assess electrocardiogram prior to and periodically during treatment. If any deterioration in cardiovascular status occurs, discontinue therapy. Use caution in patients with baseline risk of severe anemia. Assess hemoglobin and hematocrit at baseline and, at minimum, weeks 2 and 4 of therapy since initial drop may be significant. Patients with renal dysfunction and/or those >50 years of age should be carefully assessed for development of anemia. Pancytopenia and bone marrow suppression have been reported with the combination of ribavirin, interferon, and azathioprine. Use caution in pulmonary disease; pulmonary symptoms have been associated with administration. Discontinue therapy if evidence of hepatic decompensation is observed. Use caution in patients with sarcoidosis (exacerbation reported). Dental and periodontal disorders have been reported with ribavirin and interferon therapy; patients should be instructed to brush teeth twice daily and have regular dental exams. Serious ophthalmologic disorders have occurred with combination therapy. All patients require an eye exam at baseline; those with preexisting ophthalmologic disorders (eg, diabetic or hypertensive retinopathy) require periodic follow up. Delay in weight and height increases have been noted in children treated with combination therapy for CHC. In clinical studies, decreases were noted in weight and height for age z-scores and normative growth curve percentiles. Following treatment, rebound growth and weight gain occurred in most patients; however, a small percentage did not. Long-term data indicate that combination therapy may inhibit growth resulting in reduced adult height. Growth should be closely monitored in pediatric patients during therapy and post-treatment for growth catch-up.

Inhalation: **[U.S. Boxed Warning]: Use with caution in patients requiring assisted ventilation because precipitation of the drug in the respiratory equipment may interfere with safe and effective patient ventilation; sudden deterioration of respiratory function has been observed;** monitor carefully in patients with COPD and asthma for deterioration of respiratory function. Ribavirin is potentially mutagenic, tumor-promoting, and gonadotoxic. Although anemia has not been reported with inhalation therapy, consider monitoring for anemia 1 to 2 weeks post-treatment. Hazardous agent - use appropriate precautions for handling and disposal.

[U.S. Boxed Warning]: Sudden respiratory deterioration has been observed during the initiation of aerosolized ribavirin in infants; carefully monitor during treatment. If deterioration of respiratory function occurs, stop treatment; reinstitute with extreme caution, continuous monitoring, and consider concomitant administration of bronchodilators.

[U.S. Boxed Warning]: Significant teratogenic and/or embryocidal effects have been observed in all animal studies. Use is contraindicated in pregnant women or male partners of pregnant women. Avoid pregnancy in female patients and female partners of male patients during therapy by using two effective forms of contraception; continue contraceptive measures for at least 6 months after completion of therapy. The manufacturer recommends that pregnant health care workers take precautions to limit exposure to ribavirin aerosol.

Benzyl alcohol and derivatives: Some dosage forms may contain sodium benzoate/benzoic acid; benzoic acid (benzoate) is a metabolite of benzyl alcohol; large amounts of benzyl alcohol (≥99 mg/kg/day) have been associated with a potentially fatal toxicity ("gasping syndrome") in neonates; the "gasping syndrome" consists of metabolic acidosis, respiratory distress, gasping respirations, CNS dysfunction (including convulsions, intracranial hemorrhage), hypotension, and cardiovascular collapse (AAP, 1997; CDC, 1982); some data suggests that benzoate displaces bilirubin from protein binding sites (Ahlfors, 2001); avoid or use dosage forms containing benzyl alcohol derivative with caution in neonates. See manufacturer's labeling.

Adverse Reactions

Inhalation:

Cardiovascular: Cardiac arrest, digitalis toxicity, hypotension

Central nervous system: Fatigue, headache, insomnia

Gastrointestinal: Nausea, anorexia

Hematologic: Anemia

Ocular: Conjunctivitis

Respiratory: Apnea, mild bronchospasm, worsening of respiratory function

Oral (all adverse reactions are documented while receiving combination therapy with alfa interferons; as reported in adults unless noted; most common pediatric adverse reactions were similar to adults):

Cardiovascular: Chest pain, flushing

Central nervous system: Agitation, anxiety, depression, dizziness, emotional lability, fatigue (children and adults), fever, headache, insomnia (children and adults), impaired concentration, irritability, malaise, memory impairment, mood alteration, nervousness, pain, suicidal ideation

Dermatologic: Alopecia (children and adults), dermatitis, dry skin, eczema, pruritus (children and adults), rash

Endocrine & metabolic: Growth suppression (pediatric), hyperuricemia, hypothyroidism, menstrual disorder

Gastrointestinal: Abdominal pain, anorexia, constipation, diarrhea, dyspepsia, nausea (children and adults), RUQ pain, taste perversion, vomiting, weight loss, xerostomia

Hematologic: Anemia, hemoglobin decreased, hemolytic anemia, leukopenia, lymphopenia, neutropenia, thrombocytopenia

Hepatic: Bilirubin increased, hepatic decompensation, hepatomegaly, transaminases increased

Local: Inflammation at injection site, injection site reaction

Neuromuscular & skeletal: Arthralgia, back pain, decreased linear skeletal growth (including lagging weight gain), musculoskeletal pain (children and adults), myalgia (children and adults), rigors, weakness

Ocular: Blurred vision, conjunctivitis

Respiratory: Cough, dyspnea (including exertional), pharyngitis, rhinitis, sinusitis, upper respiratory tract infection (children)

Miscellaneous: Bacterial infection, diaphoresis, flu-like syndrome (children and adults), fungal infection, viral infection

Rare but important or life-threatening: Aggression, angina, aplastic anemia, arrhythmia; autoimmune disorders (systemic lupus erythematosus, rheumatoid arthritis, sarcoidosis); bone marrow suppression, cerebral hemorrhage, cholangitis, colitis, coma, corneal ulcer, dehydration, diabetes mellitus, drug abuse relapse/overdose, exfoliative dermatitis, fatty liver, hearing impairment/loss, gastrointestinal bleeding, gout, hallucination, hepatic dysfunction, hyper-/hypothyroidism, hypersensitivity (including anaphylaxis, angioedema, bronchoconstriction, and urticaria), macular edema, myositis, optic neuritis, papilledema, pancreatitis, peptic ulcer, peripheral neuropathy, pneumonitis, psychosis, psychotic disorder, pulmonary dysfunction, pulmonary embolism, pulmonary infiltrates, pure red cell aplasia, retinal artery/vein thrombosis, retinal detachment, retinal hemorrhage, retinopathy, sarcoidosis exacerbation; skin reactions (erythema multiforme, exfoliative dermatitis, urticaria, vesiculobullous eruptions); Stevens-Johnson syndrome, suicide, thrombotic thrombocytopenic purpura, thyroid function test abnormalities; transplant rejection (kidney, liver); vision loss

Note: Incidence of headache, fever, suicidal ideation, and vomiting are higher in children.

Drug Interactions

Metabolism/Transport Effects None known.

Avoid Concomitant Use

Avoid concomitant use of Ribavirin with any of the following: Didanosine

Increased Effect/Toxicity

Ribavirin may increase the levels/effects of: AzaTHIOprine; Didanosine; Reverse Transcriptase Inhibitors (Nucleoside)

The levels/effects of Ribavirin may be increased by: Interferons (Alfa); Zidovudine

Decreased Effect

Ribavirin may decrease the levels/effects of: Influenza Virus Vaccine (Live/Attenuated)

Food Interactions Oral: High-fat meal increases the AUC and C_{max}. Management: Capsule (in combination with peginterferon alfa-2b) and tablet should be administered with food. Other dosage forms and combinations should be taken consistently in regards to food.

Preparation for Administration Hazardous agent; use appropriate precautions for handling and disposal (NIOSH 2014 [group 3]).

Inhalation: Do not use any water containing an antimicrobial agent to reconstitute drug.

Storage/Stability

Inhalation: Store vials in a dry place at 15°C to 30°C (59°F to 86°F). Reconstituted solution is stable for 24 hours at room temperature.

Oral: Store at controlled room temperature of 25°C (77°F); excursions permitted between 15°C and 30°C (59°F and 86°F). Keep bottle tightly closed. Solution may also be refrigerated at 2°C to 8°C (36°F to 46°F).

Mechanism of Action Inhibits replication of RNA and DNA viruses; inhibits influenza virus RNA polymerase activity and inhibits the initiation and elongation of RNA fragments resulting in inhibition of viral protein synthesis

Pharmacodynamics/Kinetics

Absorption: Inhalation: Systemic; dependent upon respiratory factors and method of drug delivery; maximal absorption occurs with the use of aerosol generator via endotracheal tube; highest concentrations in respiratory tract and erythrocytes

Distribution: Oral capsule: Single dose: V_d: 2825 L; distribution significantly prolonged in the erythrocyte (16 to 40 days), which can be used as a marker for intracellular metabolism

Protein binding: Oral: None

Metabolism: Hepatically and intracellularly (forms active metabolites); may be necessary for drug action

Bioavailability: Oral: 64%

Half-life elimination, plasma:

Children: Inhalation: 6.5 to 11 hours

Adults: Oral:

Capsule, single dose: 24 hours in healthy adults, 44 hours with chronic hepatitis C infection (increases to ~298 hours at steady state)

Tablet, single dose: ~120 to 170 hours

Time to peak, serum: Inhalation: At end of inhalation period; Oral capsule: Multiple doses: 3 hours; Tablet: 2 hours

Excretion: Inhalation: Urine (40% as unchanged drug and metabolites); Oral capsule: Urine (61%), feces (12%)

Dosage

Infants and Children: Aerosol inhalation: RSV infection: Use with small particle aerosol generator (SPAG-2) at a concentration of 20 mg/mL (6 **g** reconstituted with 300 mL of sterile water without preservatives). Continuous aerosol administration: 12 to 18 hours per day for 3 days, up to 7 days in length

Children ≥3 years: Oral capsule or solution (Rebetol, Ribasphere): Chronic hepatitis C monoinfection (in combination with pegylated or nonpegylated interferon alfa-2b): **Note:** Oral solution should be used in children <47 kg, or those unable to swallow capsules. Children who start treatment prior to age 18 years should continue on pediatric dosing regimen through therapy completion. Recommended therapy duration (manufacturer labeling): Genotypes 2,3: 24 weeks; all other genotypes: 48 weeks

Capsule, oral solution dosing recommendations:

<47 kg: 15 mg/kg/day in 2 divided doses (morning and evening) as oral solution

47 to 59 kg: 800 mg daily (400 mg in morning and evening)

60 to 73 kg: 1000 mg daily (400 mg in morning and 600 mg in the evening)

>73 kg: 1200 mg daily (600 mg in morning and evening)

Alternative recommendations: *American Association for the Study of Liver Diseases (AASLD) guidelines:* Children 2 to 17 years with chronic hepatitis C infection (Ghany, 2009): Treatment of choice: Ribavirin 15 mg/kg daily (in combination with weekly SubQ peginterferon alfa-2b) for 48 weeks

Children ≥5 years: Oral tablet (Copegus): Chronic hepatitis C monoinfection (in combination with peginterferon alfa-2a): **Note:** Assess child's ability to swallow tablet; children who start treatment prior to age 18 years should continue on pediatric dosing regimen through therapy completion. Recommended therapy duration (manufacturer labeling): Genotypes 2,3: 24 weeks; all other genotypes: 48 weeks

23 to 33 kg: 400 mg daily (200 mg in the morning and evening)

34 to 46 kg: 600 mg daily (200 mg in the morning and 400 mg in the evening)

47 to 59 kg: 800 mg daily (400 mg in the morning and evening)

60 to 74 kg: 1000 mg daily (400 mg in the morning and 600 mg in the evening)

≥75 kg: 1200 mg daily (600 mg in the morning and evening)

Adults:

Manufacturer's labeling:

Note: Oral solution may be used those unable to swallow capsules.

Oral capsule, oral solution (Rebetol, Ribasphere):

Chronic hepatitis C monoinfection (in combination with peginterferon alfa-2b) (recommended therapy duration [manufacturer labeling]: Genotype 1: 48 weeks; genotypes 2,3: 24 weeks); recommended therapy duration for patients who previously failed therapy: 48 weeks [regardless of genotype])

<66 kg: 800 mg daily (400 mg in the morning and evening)

66 to 80 kg: 1000 mg daily (400 mg in the morning, 600 mg in the evening)

81 to 105 kg: 1200 mg daily (600 mg in the morning, 600 mg in the evening)

>105 kg: 1400 mg daily (600 mg in the morning, 800 mg in the evening)

Chronic hepatitis C monoinfection (in combination with interferon alfa-2b) (individualized therapy duration [manufacturer labeling] 24 to 48 weeks):

≤75 kg: 1000 mg daily (400 mg in the morning, 600 mg in the evening)

>75 kg: 1200 mg daily (600 mg in the morning, 600 mg in the evening)

Oral tablet (Copegus, Moderiba, Ribasphere):

Chronic hepatitis C monoinfection (in combination with peginterferon alfa-2a):

Genotype 1,4:

<75 kg: 1000 mg daily in 2 divided doses for 48 weeks

≥75 kg: 1200 mg daily in 2 divided doses for 48 weeks

Genotype 2,3: 800 mg daily in 2 divided doses for 24 weeks

Chronic hepatitis C coinfection with HIV (in combination with peginterferon alfa-2a): 800 mg daily in 2 divided doses for 48 weeks (regardless of genotype)

Alternative recommendations: Note: *AALSD/IDSA guidelines do not specify which peginterferon is preferred but in clinical trials cited peginterferon alfa 2a was used.*

Chronic hepatitis C (off-label regimens; recommended by AASLD/IDSA, 2014): Treatment-naive patients:

Genotype 1:

Interferon eligible patients: in combination with sofosbuvir and peginterferon alfa

<75 kg: 1000 mg daily in 2 divided doses for 12 weeks

≥75 kg: 1200 mg daily in 2 divided doses for 12 weeks

Interferon-ineligible patients: in combination with sofosbuvir and simeprevir: **Note: Ribavirin therapy is optional** in these patients:

<75 kg: 1000 mg daily in 2 divided doses for 12 weeks

≥75 kg: 1200 mg daily in 2 divided doses for 12 weeks

Genotype 2: Regardless of interferon eligibility: in combination with sofosbuvir

<75 kg: 1000 mg daily in 2 divided doses for 12 weeks

≥75 kg: 1200 mg daily in 2 divided doses for 12 weeks

Genotype 3: Regardless of interferon eligibility: in combination with sofosbuvir
<75 kg: 1000 mg daily in 2 divided doses for 24 weeks
≥75 kg: 1200 mg daily in 2 divided doses for 24 weeks
Genotype 4:
Interferon eligible patients: in combination with sofosbuvir and peginterferon alfa
<75 kg: 1000 mg daily in 2 divided doses for 12 weeks
≥75 kg: 1200 mg daily in 2 divided doses for 12 weeks
Interferon-ineligible patients: in combination with sofosbuvir:
<75 kg: 1000 mg daily in 2 divided doses for 24 weeks
≥75 kg: 1200 mg daily in 2 divided doses for 24 weeks
Genotype 5 or 6: Interferon eligible patients: in combination with sofosbuvir and peginterferon alfa
<75 kg: 1000 mg daily in 2 divided doses for 12 weeks
≥75 kg: 1200 mg daily in 2 divided doses for 12 weeks

Chronic hepatitis C (off-label regimens; recommended by AASLD/IDSA, 2014): Treatment of **relapser** patients (nonresponders to a previous regimen of ribavirin and peginterferon alfa **without** an HCV protease inhibitor):
Genotype 1: Regardless of interferon eligibility: in combination with sofosbuvir and simeprevir:
Ribavirin therapy is optional in these patients:
<75 kg: 1000 mg daily in 2 divided doses for 12 weeks
≥75 kg: 1200 mg daily in 2 divided doses for 12 weeks
Genotype 2: Regardless of interferon eligibility: in combination with sofosbuvir
<75 kg: 1000 mg daily in 2 divided doses for 12 weeks
≥75 kg: 1200 mg daily in 2 divided doses for 12 weeks
Note: Patients with cirrhosis may benefit from extension of treatment to 16 weeks.
Genotype 3: Regardless of interferon eligibility: in combination with sofosbuvir
<75 kg: 1000 mg daily in 2 divided doses for 24 weeks
≥75 kg: 1200 mg daily in 2 divided doses for 24 weeks
Genotype 4: Interferon eligible patients: in combination with sofosbuvir and weekly peginterferon alfa
<75 kg: 1000 mg daily in 2 divided doses for 12 weeks
≥75 kg: 1200 mg daily in 2 divided doses for 12 weeks
Genotype 5 or 6: Interferon eligible patients: in combination with sofosbuvir and weekly peginterferon alfa
<75 kg: 1000 mg daily in 2 divided doses for 12 weeks
≥75 kg: 1200 mg daily in 2 divided doses for 12 weeks

Chronic hepatitis C (off-label regimens; recommended by AASLD/IDSA, 2014): Treatment of **relapser** patients (nonresponders to a previous regimen of ribavirin and peginterferon alfa **with or without** an HCV protease inhibitor):
Genotype 1: **Note:** Alternative regimen (AALSD/IDSA, 2014)
Interferon eligible patients: in combination with sofosbuvir for the first 12 weeks and peginterferon alfa for the entire regimen:
<75 kg: 1000 mg daily in 2 divided doses for 12 to 24 weeks total
≥75 kg: 1200 mg daily in 2 divided doses for 12 to 24 weeks total

Aerosol inhalation: RSV infection in hematopoietic cell or heart/lung transplant recipients (off-label use): 2000 mg (over 2 hours) every 8 hours (Boeckh, 2007; Liu, 2010)
Note: Heart/lung transplant recipients also received IVIG, methylprednisolone and palivizumab. Dosage and protocol may be institution specific. (Boeckh, 2007; Chemaly, 2006; Liu, 2010).

Dosage adjustment for toxicity:
Notes:
Children: Once a laboratory abnormality or clinical adverse event has resolved, the ribavirin dose may be increased, based on clinical judgment, to its original assigned dose. Initiate restart at 50% of the full dose.
Adults: Once ribavirin has been withheld due to clinical adverse event or laboratory abnormality, an attempt can be made to restart ribavirin, in divided doses, at 600 mg daily, with a further ribavirin increase to 800 mg daily. Increasing the ribavirin dose to its original assigned dose (1000 to 1200 mg daily) is not recommended.

Patient **without** cardiac history:
Hemoglobin 8.5 to <10 g/dL:
Children ≥3 years: Oral capsules, oral solution:
First reduction: Decrease to 12 mg/kg/day
Second reduction: Decrease to 8 mg/kg/day
Children ≥5 years: Oral tablets (Copegus):
23 to 33 kg: Decrease dose to 200 mg daily (in the morning)
34 to 59 kg: Decrease dose to 400 mg daily (200 mg in the morning and evening)
≥60 kg: Decrease dose to 600 mg daily (200 mg in the morning and 400 mg in the evening)
Adults:
Oral capsules, oral solution:
First reduction: ≤105 kg: Decrease by 200 mg daily; >105 kg: Decrease by 400 mg daily
Second reduction: Decrease by an additional 200 mg daily (not weight-based)
Oral tablets: Decrease dose to 600 mg daily (200 mg in the morning, 400 mg in the evening)
Hemoglobin <8.5 g/dL: Children and Adults: Oral capsules, solution, tablets: Permanently discontinue treatment.
WBC <1000 mm^3, neutrophils <500 mm^3: Children and Adults: Oral capsules, solution: Permanently discontinue treatment.
Platelets <50 x 10^9/L: Children: Oral capsules, solution: Permanently discontinue treatment.
Platelets <25 x 10^9/L: Adults: Oral capsules, solution: Permanently discontinue treatment.

Patient **with** stable cardiac history:
Hemoglobin has decreased ≥2 g/dL during any 4-week period of treatment:
Children: Oral capsules, solution: Decrease ribavirin by 200 mg daily (regardless of the patient's initial dose); decrease peginterferon alfa-2b dose by 50%; monitor and evaluate weekly. If hemoglobin <8.5 g/dL any time after dose reduction or <12 g/dL after 4 weeks of dose reduction, permanently discontinue treatment.
Children ≥5 years: Oral tablets (Copegus):
23 to 33 kg: Decrease dose to 200 mg daily (in the morning)
34 to 59 kg: Decrease dose to 400 mg daily (200 mg in the morning and evening)
≥60 kg: 600 mg daily (200 mg in the morning, 400 mg in the evening)

Hemoglobin has decreased >2 g/dL during any 4-week period of treatment: Adults:

Oral capsules, solution: Decrease dose by 200 mg daily; decrease peginterferon alfa-2b dose by 50%. If hemoglobin <8.5 g/dL any time after dose reduction or <12 g/dL after 4 weeks of dose reduction, permanently discontinue treatment.

Oral tablets: Decrease dose to 600 mg daily (200 mg in the morning, 400 mg in the evening). If hemoglobin <8.5 g/dL any time after dose reduction or <12 g/dL after 4 weeks of dose reduction, permanently discontinue treatment.

Hemoglobin <8.5 g/dL: Children and Adults: Oral capsules, solution, tablets: Permanently discontinue treatment.

WBC <1000 mm^3, neutrophils <500 mm^3: Children and Adults: Oral capsules, solution: Permanently discontinue treatment.

Platelets <50 x 10^9/L: Children: Oral capsules, solution: Permanently discontinue treatment.

Platelets <25 x 10^9/L: Adults: Oral capsules, solution: Permanently discontinue treatment.

Dosage adjustment in renal impairment: Chronic hepatitis C infection: Oral:

Rebetol capsules/solution, Ribasphere capsules:

Children: Serum creatinine >2 mg/dL: Permanently discontinue treatment.

Adults:

CrCl ≥50 mL/minute: No dosage adjustment necessary.

CrCl <50 mL/minute: Use is contraindicated.

Ribasphere, Moderiba tablets: Adults:

CrCl ≥50 mL/minute: No dosage adjustment necessary.

CrCl <50 mL/minute: Use is not recommended.

Copegus tablets: Adults:

CrCl >50 mL/minute: No dosage adjustment necessary.

CrCl 30 to 50 mL/minute: Alternate 200 mg and 400 mg every other day

CrCl <30 mL/minute: 200 mg once daily

ESRD requiring hemodialysis: 200 mg once daily

Note: The dose of Copegus should not be further modified in patients with renal impairment. If severe adverse reactions or laboratory abnormalities develop it should be discontinued, if appropriate, until the adverse reactions resolve or decrease in severity. If abnormalities persist after restarting, therapy should be discontinued.

Dosage adjustment in hepatic impairment: Chronic hepatitis C infection: Hepatic decompensation (Child-Pugh class B and C): Manufacturer's labeling: Oral tablets: Use contraindicated.

Dietary Considerations Capsules, solution, and tablets should be taken with food.

Administration

Inhalation: Ribavirin should be administered in well-ventilated rooms (at least 6 air changes/hour). In mechanically-ventilated patients, ribavirin can potentially be deposited in the ventilator delivery system depending on temperature, humidity, and electrostatic forces; this deposition can lead to malfunction or obstruction of the expiratory valve, resulting in inadvertently high positive end-expiratory pressures. The use of one-way valves in the inspiratory lines, a breathing circuit filter in the expiratory line, and frequent monitoring and filter replacement have been effective in preventing these problems. Solutions in SPAG-2 unit should be discarded at least every 24 hours and when the liquid level is low before adding newly reconstituted solution. Should not be mixed with other aerosolized medication.

Oral:

Capsule: Administer with food. Capsule should not be opened, crushed, chewed, or broken.

Solution: Administer with food. Use oral solution for children <47 kg, or those who cannot swallow capsules.

Tablet: Administer with food.

Hazardous agent; use appropriate precautions for handling and disposal (NIOSH 2014 [group 3]).

Monitoring Parameters

Inhalation: Respiratory function, hemoglobin, reticulocyte count, CBC with differential, I & O

Oral: Pretreatment hematological and biochemical tests are recommended for all patients; dental exam, ECG (if preexisting cardiac abnormalities or disease) and ophthalmic exam (also periodically during treatment for those with preexisting ophthalmologic disorders) are also recommended. In adults, hematologic tests should be at treatment weeks 2 and 4, biochemical tests at week 4, and TSH at week 12. In pediatric patients, monitor growth closely during and after treatment.

Pregnancy screening (in woman of childbearing age) and pregnancy tests monthly during and for 6 months after treatment discontinuation.

In pediatric clinical studies, hematologic and biochemical assessments were made at weeks 1, 3, 5 and 8, then every 4 weeks thereafter. Growth velocity and weight should also be monitored during and periodically after treatment discontinuation.

Baseline values used in adult clinical trials in combination with alfa interferons:

Platelet count ≥90,000/mm^3 (75,000/mm^3 for cirrhosis or 70,000/mm^3 for coinfection with HIV)

ANC ≥1500/mm^3

Hemoglobin ≥12 g/dL for women and ≥13 g/dL for men (11 g/dL for HIV coinfected women and 12 g/dL for HIV coinfected men)

TSH and T_4 within normal limits or adequately controlled

$CD4^+$ cell count ≥200 cells/microL or $CD4^+$ cell count 100-200 cells/microL and HIV-1 RNA <5000 copies/mL for coinfection with HIV

Serum HCV RNA (pretreatment, week 12 and week 24, and 24 weeks after completion of therapy). **Note:** Discontinuation of therapy may be considered after 12 weeks in patients with HCV (genotypes 1,4) who fail to achieve an early virologic response (EVR) (defined as ≥2-log decrease in HCV RNA compared to pretreatment) or after 24 weeks with detectable HCV RNA. Treat patients with HCV (genotypes 2,3) for 24 weeks (if tolerated) and then evaluate HCV RNA levels (Ghany, 2009).

Reference Range

Rapid virological response (RVR): Absence of detectable HCV RNA after 4 weeks of treatment

Early viral response (EVR): ≥2-log decrease in HCV RNA after 12 weeks of treatment

End of treatment response (ETR): Absence of detectable HCV RNA at end of the recommended treatment period

Sustained treatment response (STR) or sustained virologic response (SVR): Absence of HCV RNA in the serum 6 months following completion of full treatment course

Dosage Forms

Capsule, oral: 200 mg

Rebetol: 200 mg

Ribasphere: 200 mg

Powder for solution, for nebulization:

Virazole: 6 g

Solution, oral:

Rebetol: 40 mg/mL (100 mL)

Tablet, oral: 200 mg

Copegus: 200 mg

Ribasphere: 200 mg, 400 mg, 600 mg

Tablet, oral [dose-pack]:
Moderiba 600 Dose Pack: 200 mg & 400 mg (56s)
Moderiba 800 Dose Pack: 400 mg (56s)
Moderiba 1000 Dose Pack: 400 mg & 600 mg (56s)
Moderiba 1200 Dose Pack: 600 mg (56s)
Ribasphere RibaPak 600: 200 mg AM dose, 400 mg PM dose (14s, 56s)
Ribasphere RibaPak 800: 400 mg AM dose, 400 mg PM dose (14s, 56s)
Ribasphere RibaPak 1000: 600 mg AM dose, 400 mg PM dose (14s, 56s)
Ribasphere RibaPak 1200: 600 mg AM dose, 600 mg PM dose (14s, 56s)

- ◆ **Ribavirin and Peginterferon Alfa-2a** *see* Peginterferon Alfa-2a and Ribavirin [CAN/INT] *on page 1592*
- ◆ **Ribavirin and Peginterferon Alfa-2b** *see* Peginterferon Alfa-2b and Ribavirin [CAN/INT] *on page 1598*

Riboflavin (RYE boe flay vin)

Brand Names: U.S. B-2-400 [OTC]
Index Terms Lactoflavin; Vitamin B_2; Vitamin G
Pharmacologic Category Vitamin, Water Soluble
Use Dietary supplement
Dosage Oral:
Dietary supplement: Adults: 100 mg once or twice daily
Adequate intake:
1-6 months: 0.3 mg/day
7-12 months: 0.4 mg/day
Recommended daily intake:
1-3 years: 0.5 mg
4-8 years: 0.6 mg
9-13 years: 0.9 mg
14-18 years: Females: 1 mg; Males: 1.3 mg
≥19 years: Females: 1.1 mg; Males: 1.3 mg
Pregnancy: 1.4 mg
Lactation 1.6 mg
Additional Information Complete prescribing information should be consulted for additional detail.
Dosage Forms
Capsule, Oral:
B-2-400 [OTC]: 400 mg
Generic: 50 mg
Tablet, Oral:
Generic: 25 mg, 50 mg, 100 mg
Tablet, Oral [preservative free]:
Generic: 100 mg

- ◆ **Ridaura** *see* Auranofin *on page 204*
- ◆ **Ridaura® (Can)** *see* Auranofin *on page 204*
- ◆ **RID Maximum Strength [OTC]** *see* Pyrethrins and Piperonyl Butoxide *on page 1746*
- ◆ **RID Mousse (Can)** *see* Pyrethrins and Piperonyl Butoxide *on page 1746*

Rifabutin (rif a BYOO tin)

Brand Names: U.S. Mycobutin
Brand Names: Canada Mycobutin
Index Terms Ansamycin
Pharmacologic Category Antibiotic, Miscellaneous; Antitubercular Agent
Use Prevention of disseminated *Mycobacterium avium* complex (MAC) in patients with advanced HIV infection
Pregnancy Risk Factor B
Pregnancy Considerations Adverse events were seen in some animal reproduction studies.
Breast-Feeding Considerations In the United States, where formula is accessible, affordable, safe, and sustainable, and the risk of infant mortality due to diarrhea and respiratory infections is low, complete avoidance of breast-feeding by HIV-infected women is recommended to decrease potential transmission of HIV (DHHS [perinatal], 2011).
Contraindications Hypersensitivity to rifabutin, any other rifamycins, or any component of the formulation
Warnings/Precautions Rifabutin must not be administered for MAC prophylaxis to patients with active tuberculosis since its use may lead to the development of tuberculosis that is resistant to both rifabutin and rifampin. Caution that active TB in the HIV-positive patient may present atypically (ie, negative PPD or extrapulmonary manifestations). Uveitis may occur; carefully monitor patients when used in combination with macrolides or azole antifungals. If uveitis is suspected, refer patient to an ophthalmologist and consider temporarily discontinuing treatment. May be associated with neutropenia and/or thrombocytopenia (rarely); consider blood monitoring and discontinue permanently if signs of thrombocytopenia (eg, petechial rash) (DHHS, 2014). Use with caution in patients with renal impairment; dosage reduction recommended in severe renal impairment (CrCl <30 mL/minute). Use with caution in patients with liver impairment; discontinue in patients with AST >3 x ULN (symptomatic) or ≥5 x ULN (regardless of symptoms) or if significant bilirubin and/or alkaline phosphatase elevations occur (DHHS, 2014). Prolonged use may result in fungal or bacterial superinfection, including *C. difficile*-associated diarrhea (CDAD) and pseudomembranous colitis; CDAD has been observed >2 months postantibiotic treatment. May cause brown/orange discoloration of urine, feces, saliva, sweat, tears, and skin. Remove soft contact lenses during therapy since permanent staining may occur. Potentially significant drug-drug interactions may exist, requiring dose or frequency adjustment, additional monitoring, and/or selection of alternative therapy.
Adverse Reactions
Central nervous system: Headache, fever
Dermatologic: Rash
Gastrointestinal: Abdominal pain, dyspepsia, eructation, flatulence, nausea, taste perversion, vomiting
Genitourinary: Discoloration of urine
Hematologic: Leukopenia, neutropenia, thrombocytopenia
Hepatic: ALT increased, AST increased
Neuromuscular & skeletal: Myalgia
Rare but important or life-threatening: Aphasia, arthralgia, chest pain, confusion, dyspnea, flu-like syndrome, hepatitis, hemolysis, myositis, parasthesia, seizures, skin discoloration, T-wave abnormalities, uveitis
Drug Interactions
Metabolism/Transport Effects **Substrate** of CYP1A2 (minor), CYP3A4 (major); **Note:** Assignment of Major/Minor substrate status based on clinically relevant drug interaction potential; **Induces** CYP3A4 (strong)
Avoid Concomitant Use
Avoid concomitant use of Rifabutin with any of the following: Abiraterone Acetate; Apixaban; Apremilast; Artemether; Atovaquone; Axitinib; BCG; Bedaquiline; Boceprevir; Bortezomib; Bosutinib; Cabozantinib; Ceritinib; CloZAPine; Crizotinib; Dasabuvir; Delavirdine; Dienogest; Dronedarone; Eliglustat; Elvitegravir; Enzalutamide; Everolimus; Ibrutinib; Idelalisib; Irinotecan; Itraconazole; Ivacaftor; Lapatinib; Ledipasvir; Lumefantrine; Lurasidone; Macitentan; Mifepristone; Mycophenolate; Naloxegol; Netupitant; NIFEdipine; Nilotinib; Nisoldipine; Olaparib; Ombitasvir; Paritaprevir; PAZOPanib; Perampanel; PONATinib; Praziquantel; Ranolazine; Regorafenib; Rivaroxaban; Roflumilast; RomiDEPsin; Simeprevir; Sofosbuvir; SORAfenib; Suvorexant; Tasimelteon; Telaprevir; Ticagrelor; Tofacitinib; Tolvaptan; Toremifene; Trabectedin; Ulipristal; Vandetanib; Vemurafenib; VinCRIStine (Liposomal); Vorapaxar; Voriconazole

Increased Effect/Toxicity

Rifabutin may increase the levels/effects of: Clarithromycin; Clopidogrel; Darunavir; Fosamprenavir; Ifosfamide; Isoniazid; Lopinavir; Pitavastatin

The levels/effects of Rifabutin may be increased by: Antifungal Agents (Azole Derivatives, Systemic); Atazanavir; Boceprevir; Clarithromycin; Darunavir; Delavirdine; Fosamprenavir; Indinavir; Lopinavir; Macrolide Antibiotics; Nelfinavir; Nevirapine; Ritonavir; Saquinavir; Telaprevir; Tipranavir; Voriconazole

Decreased Effect

Rifabutin may decrease the levels/effects of: Abiraterone Acetate; Alfentanil; Antiemetics (5HT3 Antagonists); Antifungal Agents (Azole Derivatives, Systemic); Apixaban; Apremilast; ARIPiprazole; Artemether; Atovaquone; Axitinib; Barbiturates; BCG; Bedaquiline; Boceprevir; Bortezomib; Bosutinib; Brentuximab Vedotin; BusPIRone; Cabozantinib; Calcium Channel Blockers; Cannabidiol; Cannabis; Ceritinib; Clarithromycin; CloZAPine; Contraceptives (Estrogens); Contraceptives (Progestins); Corticosteroids (Systemic); Crizotinib; CycloSPORINE (Systemic); CYP3A4 Substrates; Dapsone (Systemic); Dasabuvir; Dasatinib; Delavirdine; Dienogest; DOXOrubicin (Conventional); Dronabinol; Dronedarone; Efavirenz; Eliglustat; Elvitegravir; Enzalutamide; Erlotinib; Etravirine; Everolimus; Exemestane; FentaNYL; Gefitinib; GuanFACINE; HMG-CoA Reductase Inhibitors; Hydrocodone; Ibrutinib; Idelalisib; Ifosfamide; Imatinib; Indinavir; Irinotecan; Itraconazole; Ivacaftor; Ixabepilone; Lapatinib; Ledipasvir; Linagliptin; Lumefantrine; Lurasidone; Macitentan; Maraviroc; Mifepristone; Morphine (Systemic); Mycophenolate; Naloxegol; Nelfinavir; Netupitant; Nevirapine; NIFEdipine; Nilotinib; Nisoldipine; Olaparib; Ombitasvir; Paritaprevir; PAZOPanib; Perampanel; PONATinib; Praziquantel; Propafenone; QUEtiapine; QuiNIDine; Raltegravir; Ramelteon; Ranolazine; Regorafenib; Rilpivirine; Rivaroxaban; Roflumilast; RomiDEPsin; Saquinavir; Saxagliptin; Simeprevir; Sodium Picosulfate; Sofosbuvir; SORAfenib; SUNItinib; Suvorexant; Tacrolimus (Systemic); Tadalafil; Tamoxifen; Tasimelteon; Telaprevir; Temsirolimus; Tetrahydrocannabinol; Ticagrelor; Tofacitinib; Tolvaptan; Toremifene; Trabectedin; Typhoid Vaccine; Ulipristal; Vandetanib; Vemurafenib; Vilazodone; VinCRIStine (Liposomal); Vitamin K Antagonists; Vorapaxar; Voriconazole; Vortioxetine; Zaleplon; Zolpidem; Zuclopenthixol

The levels/effects of Rifabutin may be decreased by: Bosentan; CYP3A4 Inducers (Moderate); CYP3A4 Inducers (Strong); Dabrafenib; Deferasirox; Efavirenz; Mitotane; Nevirapine; Siltuximab; St Johns Wort; Tocilizumab

Food Interactions High-fat meal may decrease the rate but not the extent of absorption. Management: May administer with meals.

Storage/Stability Store at 25°C (77°F); excursions permitted to 15°C to 30°C (59°F to 86°F).

Mechanism of Action Inhibits DNA-dependent RNA polymerase at the beta subunit which prevents chain initiation

Pharmacodynamics/Kinetics

Absorption: Readily, 53%

Distribution: V_d: 9.32 L/kg; distributes to body tissues including the lungs, liver, spleen, eyes, and kidneys

Protein binding: 85%

Metabolism: To 5 metabolites; predominantly 25-O-desacetyl-rifabutin (antimicrobial activity equivalent to parent drug; serum AUC 10% of parent drug) and 31-hydroxy-rifabutin (serum AUC 7% of parent drug)

Bioavailability: Absolute: HIV: 20%

Half-life elimination: Terminal: 45 hours (range: 16 to 69 hours)

Time to peak, serum: 2 to 4 hours

Excretion: Urine (53% as metabolites); feces (30%)

Dosage Oral:

Infants and Children:

Prophylaxis for recurrence of *Mycobacterium avium* complex (MAC) in HIV-exposed/-infected patients (off-label use; CDC, 2009): 5 mg/kg (maximum dose: 300 mg) once daily as an optional add-on to primary therapy of clarithromycin and ethambutol

Treatment of active TB (as alternative to rifampin) in HIV-exposed/-infected patients (off-label use; CDC, 2009): 10 to 20 mg/kg (maximum dose: 300 mg) once daily or intermittently 2 to 3 times weekly

Treatment of severe MAC in HIV-exposed/-infected patients (off-label use; CDC, 2009): 10 to 20 mg/kg (maximum dose: 300 mg) once daily, in addition to primary therapy of clarithromycin and ethambutol

Children ≥6 years: Prophylaxis for first episode of MAC in HIV-exposed/-infected patients (off-label use; CDC, 2009): 300 mg once daily

Adolescents and Adults:

Disseminated MAC in advanced HIV infection:

Prophylaxis: 300 mg once daily or 150 mg twice daily to reduce gastrointestinal upset

Treatment (off-label use; AIDS*info* guidelines): 300 mg once daily as an optional add-on to primary therapy of clarithromycin and ethambutol

Tuberculosis (off-label use as alternative to rifampin; AIDS*info* guidelines):

Prophylaxis of LTBI: 300 mg once daily for 4 months

Treatment of active TB: 300 mg once daily or intermittently 2 to 3 times weekly as part of multidrug regimen

Dosage adjustment for concurrent nelfinavir, amprenavir, indinavir: Reduce rifabutin dose to 150 mg/day; no change in dose if administered twice weekly

Dosage adjustment for concurrent efavirenz (no concomitant protease inhibitor): Increase rifabutin dose to 450 to 600 mg daily, or 600 mg 3 times/week

Dosage adjustment in renal impairment:

CrCl ≥30 mL/minute: No dosage adjustment necessary.

CrCl <30 mL/minute: Reduce dose by 50%

Dosage adjustment in hepatic impairment:

Mild impairment: No dosage adjustment necessary.

Moderate to severe impairment: There are no dosage adjustments provided in manufacturer's labeling.

Dietary Considerations May be taken with meals.

Administration May be taken with meals to minimize nausea or vomiting.

Monitoring Parameters Periodic liver function tests, CBC with differential, platelet count, signs/symptoms of uveitis

Dosage Forms

Capsule, Oral:

Mycobutin: 150 mg

Generic: 150 mg

Extemporaneous Preparations A 20 mg/mL rifabutin oral suspension may be made with capsules and a 1:1 mixture of Ora-Sweet® and Ora-Plus®. Empty the the powder from eight 150 mg rifabutin capsules into a glass mortar; add 20 mL of vehicle and mix to a uniform paste. Mix while adding vehicle in incremental proportions to **almost** 60 mL; transfer to a calibrated bottle, rinse mortar with vehicle, and add quantity of vehicle sufficient to make 60 mL. Label "shake well". Stable for 12 weeks at 4°C, 25°C, 30°C, and 40°C.

Haslam JL, Egodage KL, Chen Y, et al, "Stability of Rifabutin in Two Extemporaneously Compounded Oral Liquids," *Am J Health Syst Pharm*, 1999, 56(4):333-6.

◆ **Rifadin** *see* Rifampin *on page 1804*

◆ **Rifampicin** *see* Rifampin *on page 1804*

Rifampin (rif AM pin)

Brand Names: U.S. Rifadin

Brand Names: Canada Rifadin; Rofact

Index Terms Rifampicin

Pharmacologic Category Antibiotic, Miscellaneous; Antitubercular Agent

Use Management of active tuberculosis in combination with other agents; elimination of meningococci from the nasopharynx in asymptomatic carriers

Pregnancy Risk Factor C

Pregnancy Considerations Teratogenic effects have been reported in animal studies. Rifampin crosses the human placenta. Due to the risk of tuberculosis to the fetus, treatment is recommended when the probability of maternal disease is moderate to high. Postnatal hemorrhages have been reported in the infant and mother with isoniazid administration during the last few weeks of pregnancy.

Breast-Feeding Considerations The manufacturer does not recommend breast-feeding due to tumorigenicity observed in animal studies; however, the CDC does not consider rifampin a contraindication to breast-feeding.

Contraindications Hypersensitivity to rifampin, any rifamycins, or any component of the formulation; concurrent use of atazanavir, darunavir, fosamprenavir, ritonavir/saquinavir, ritonavir, or tipranavir

Warnings/Precautions Use with caution and modify dosage in patients with liver impairment; observe for hyperbilirubinemia; discontinue therapy if this in conjunction with clinical symptoms or any signs of significant hepatocellular damage develop. Use with caution in patients receiving concurrent medications associated with hepatotoxicity. Use with caution in patients with a history of alcoholism (even if ethanol consumption is discontinued during therapy). Since rifampin since rifampin has enzyme-inducing properties, porphyria exacerbation is possible; use with caution in patients with porphyria; do not use for meningococcal disease, only for short-term treatment of asymptomatic carrier states

Regimens of >600 mg once or twice weekly in adults have been associated with a high incidence of adverse reactions including a flu-like syndrome, hypersensitivity, thrombocytopenia, leukopenia, and anemia. Urine, feces, saliva, sweat, tears, and CSF may be discolored to red/orange; remove soft contact lenses during therapy since permanent staining may occur. Do not administer IV form via IM or SubQ routes; restart infusion at another site if extravasation occurs. Prolonged use may result in fungal or bacterial superinfection, including *C. difficile*-associated diarrhea (CDAD) and pseudomembranous colitis; CDAD has been observed >2 months postantibiotic treatment. Monitor for compliance in patients on intermittent therapy.

Adverse Reactions

Cardiovascular: Edema, flushing

Central nervous system: Ataxia, behavioral changes, concentration impaired, confusion, dizziness, drowsiness, fatigue, fever, headache, numbness, psychosis

Dermatologic: Pemphigoid reaction, pruritus, rash, urticaria

Endocrine & metabolic: Adrenal insufficiency, menstrual disorders

Gastrointestinal: Anorexia, cramps, diarrhea, epigastric distress, flatulence, heartburn, nausea, pseudomembranous colitis, pancreatitis, vomiting

Hematologic: Agranulocytosis (rare), DIC, eosinophilia, hemoglobin decreased, hemolysis, hemolytic anemia, leukopenia, thrombocytopenia (especially with high-dose therapy)

Hepatic: Hepatitis (rare), jaundice, LFTs increased

Neuromuscular & skeletal: Myalgia, osteomalacia, weakness

Ocular: Exudative conjunctivitis, visual changes

Renal: Acute renal failure, BUN increased, hemoglobinuria, hematuria, interstitial nephritis, uric acid increased

Miscellaneous: Flu-like syndrome

Drug Interactions

Metabolism/Transport Effects **Substrate** of P-glycoprotein, SLCO1B1; **Induces** CYP1A2 (strong), CYP2A6 (strong), CYP2B6 (strong), CYP2C19 (strong), CYP2C8 (strong), CYP2C9 (strong), CYP3A4 (strong), P-glycoprotein

Avoid Concomitant Use

Avoid concomitant use of Rifampin with any of the following: Abiraterone Acetate; Apixaban; Apremilast; Artemether; Atazanavir; Atovaquone; Axitinib; BCG; Bedaquiline; Boceprevir; Bortezomib; Bosutinib; Cabozantinib; Ceritinib; CloZAPine; Cobicistat; Crizotinib; Dabigatran Etexilate; Darunavir; Dasabuvir; Delavirdine; Dienogest; Dronedarone; Edoxaban; Eliglustat; Elvitegravir; Enzalutamide; Esomeprazole; Etravirine; Everolimus; Fosamprenavir; Ibrutinib; Idelalisib; Indinavir; Irinotecan; Itraconazole; Ivacaftor; Lapatinib; Ledipasvir; Lopinavir; Lumefantrine; Lurasidone; Macitentan; Mifepristone; Mycophenolate; Naloxegol; Nelfinavir; Netupitant; NIFEdipine; Nilotinib; Nintedanib; Nisoldipine; Olaparib; Ombitasvir; Omeprazole; Paritaprevir; PAZOPanib; Perampanel; Pirfenidone; Pomalidomide; PONATinib; Praziquantel; QuiNINE; Ranolazine; Regorafenib; Rilpivirine; Ritonavir; Rivaroxaban; Roflumilast; RomiDEPsin; Saquinavir; Simeprevir; Sofosbuvir; SORAfenib; Suvorexant; Tasimelteon; Telaprevir; Ticagrelor; Tipranavir; Tofacitinib; Tolvaptan; Toremifene; Trabectedin; Ulipristal; Vandetanib; Vemurafenib; VinCRIStine (Liposomal); Vorapaxar; Voriconazole

Increased Effect/Toxicity

Rifampin may increase the levels/effects of: Bosentan; Clarithromycin; Clopidogrel; Fexofenadine; Isoniazid; Leflunomide; Lopinavir; Pitavastatin; Propofol; RomiDEPsin; Saquinavir

The levels/effects of Rifampin may be increased by: Antifungal Agents (Azole Derivatives, Systemic); Clarithromycin; Delavirdine; Eltrombopag; Macrolide Antibiotics; P-glycoprotein/ABCB1 Inhibitors; Pyrazinamide; Teriflunomide; Voriconazole

Decreased Effect

Rifampin may decrease the levels/effects of: Abiraterone Acetate; Afatinib; Alfentanil; Amiodarone; Antidiabetic Agents (Thiazolidinedione); Antiemetics (5HT3 Antagonists); Antifungal Agents (Azole Derivatives, Systemic); Apixaban; Apremilast; Aprepitant; ARIPiprazole; Artemether; Atazanavir; Atovaquone; Axitinib; Barbiturates; Bazedoxifene; BCG; Bedaquiline; Bendamustine; Beta-Blockers; Boceprevir; Bortezomib; Bosentan; Bosutinib; Brentuximab Vedotin; BusPIRone; Cabozantinib; Calcium Channel Blockers; Canagliflozin; Cannabidiol; Cannabis; Caspofungin; Ceritinib; Chloramphenicol; Citalopram; Clarithromycin; CloZAPine; Cobicistat; Contraceptives (Estrogens); Contraceptives (Progestins); Corticosteroids (Systemic); Crizotinib; CycloSPORINE (Systemic); CYP1A2 Substrates; CYP2A6 Substrates; CYP2B6 Substrates; CYP2C19 Substrates; CYP2C8 Substrates; CYP2C9 Substrates; CYP3A4 Substrates; Dabigatran Etexilate; Dapsone (Systemic); Darunavir; Dasabuvir; Dasatinib; Deferasirox; Delavirdine; Diclofenac (Systemic); Dienogest; Disopyramide; Dolutegravir; DOXOrubicin (Conventional); Doxycycline; Dronabinol; Dronedarone; Edoxaban; Efavirenz; Eliglustat; Elvitegravir; Enzalutamide; Erlotinib; Esomeprazole; Etravirine; Everolimus; Exemestane; FentaNYL; Fexofenadine; Fosamprenavir; Fosaprepitant; Fosphenytoin; Gefitinib; GuanFACINE; HMG-CoA Reductase Inhibitors; Hydrocodone; Ibrutinib; Idelalisib; Imatinib; Indinavir; Irinotecan; Itraconazole; Ivacaftor; Ixabepilone; LamoTRIgine;

Lapatinib; Ledipasvir; Linagliptin; Lopinavir; Losartan; Lumefantrine; Lurasidone; Macitentan; Maraviroc; Methadone; Mifepristone; Mirabegron; Morphine (Systemic); Mycophenolate; Naloxegol; Nelfinavir; Netupitant; Nevirapine; NIFEdipine; Nilotinib; Nintedanib; Nisoldipine; Nitrazepam; Olaparib; Ombitasvir; Omeprazole; OxyCODONE; Paritaprevir; PAZOPanib; Perampanel; P-glycoprotein/ABCB1 Substrates; Phenytoin; Pirfenidone; Pomalidomide; PONATinib; Prasugrel; Praziquantel; Propafenone; QUEtiapine; QuiNIDine; QuiNINE; Raltegravir; Ramelteon; Ranolazine; Regorafenib; Repaglinide; Rilpivirine; Ritonavir; Rivaroxaban; Roflumilast; Saquinavir; Saxagliptin; Simeprevir; Sirolimus; Sodium Picosulfate; Sofosbuvir; SORAfenib; Sulfonylureas; SUNItinib; Suvorexant; Tacrolimus (Systemic); Tadalafil; Tamoxifen; Tasimelteon; Telaprevir; Temsirolimus; Terbinafine (Systemic); Tetrahydrocannabinol; Thyroid Products; Ticagrelor; Tipranavir; Tofacitinib; Tolvaptan; Toremifene; Trabectedin; Treprostinil; Typhoid Vaccine; Ulipristal; Valproic Acid and Derivatives; Vandetanib; Vemurafenib; Vilazodone; VinCRIStine (Liposomal); Vorapaxar; Voriconazole; Vortioxetine; Zaleplon; Zidovudine; Zolpidem; Zuclopenthixol

The levels/effects of Rifampin may be decreased by: P-glycoprotein/ABCB1 Inducers

Food Interactions Food decreases the extent of absorption; rifampin concentrations may be decreased if taken with food. Management: Administer on an empty stomach with a glass of water (ie, 1 hour prior to, or 2 hours after meals or antacids).

Preparation for Administration Reconstitute vial with 10 mL SWFI. Prior to injection, dilute in appropriate volume of a compatible solution (eg, 100 mL D_5W).

Storage/Stability Store capsules and intact vials at 25°C (77°F); excursions permitted to 15°C to 30°C (59°F to 86°F); avoid excessive heat (>40°C [104°F]). Protect the intact vials from light. Reconstituted vials are stable for 24 hours at room temperature.

Stability of parenteral admixture at room temperature (25°C [77°F]) is 4 hours for D_5W and 24 hours for NS.

Mechanism of Action Inhibits bacterial RNA synthesis by binding to the beta subunit of DNA-dependent RNA polymerase, blocking RNA transcription

Pharmacodynamics/Kinetics

Duration: ≤24 hours

Absorption: Oral: Well absorbed; food may delay or slightly reduce peak

Distribution: Highly lipophilic; crosses blood-brain barrier well

Relative diffusion from blood into CSF: Adequate with or without inflammation (exceeds usual MICs)

CSF:blood level ratio: Inflamed meninges: 25%

Protein binding: 80%

Metabolism: Hepatic; undergoes enterohepatic recirculation

Half-life elimination: 3-4 hours; prolonged with hepatic impairment; End-stage renal disease: 1.8-11 hours

Time to peak, serum: Oral: 2-4 hours

Excretion: Feces (60% to 65%) and urine (~30%) as unchanged drug

Dosage

Usual dosage ranges: *Oral, IV:*

Infants and Children: 10-20 mg/kg/day as a single dose or in 2 divided doses; maximum: 600 mg/day

Adults: 600 mg once or twice daily

Indication-specific dosing: *Oral:*

Pharyngeal chronic carriers of group A streptococci, treatment (off-label use; IDSA guidelines): Children, Adolescents, and Adults: 20 mg/kg/day once daily (maximum: 600 mg daily) for the last 4 days of treatment when combined with oral penicillin V **or** 20 mg/kg/day in 2 divided doses (maximum: 600 mg daily) for 4 days when combined with intramuscular benzathine penicillin G (Shulman, 2012)

Indication-specific dosing: *Oral, IV:*

Endocarditis, prosthetic valve due to MRSA (off-label use): Adults: 300 mg every 8 hours for at least 6 weeks (combine with vancomycin for the entire duration of therapy and gentamicin for the first 2 weeks) (Liu, 2011)

H. influenzae **prophylaxis (off-label use):**

Infants and Children: 20 mg/kg/day every 24 hours for 4 days, not to exceed 600 mg/dose

Adults: 600 mg every 24 hours for 4 days

Leprosy (off-label use): Adults:

Multibacillary: 600 mg once monthly for 24 months in combination with ofloxacin and minocycline

Paucibacillary: 600 mg once monthly for 6 months in combination with dapsone

Single lesion: 600 mg as a single dose in combination with ofloxacin 400 mg and minocycline 100 mg

Meningitis *(Pneumococcus* or *Staphylococcus)* (off-label use): Adults: 600 mg once daily

Note: Recommended only for organisms known to be rifampin-susceptible and highly penicillin- or cephalosporin-resistant. May be used in place of or in addition to vancomycin when dexamethasone therapy employed.

Meningococcal meningitis prophylaxis (off-label use):

Infants <1 month: 10 mg/kg/day in divided doses every 12 hours for 2 days

Infants ≥1 month and Children: 20 mg/kg/day in divided doses every 12 hours for 2 days (maximum: 600 mg/dose)

Adults: 600 mg every 12 hours for 2 days

Nasal carriers of *Staphylococcus aureus* (off-label use): Note: Must use in combination with at least one other systemic antistaphylococcal antibiotic. Not recommended as first-line drug for decolonization; evidence is weak for use in patients with recurrent infections (Liu, 2011).

Children: 15 mg/kg/day divided every 12 hours for 5-10 days in combination with other antibiotics

Adults: 600 mg/day for 5-10 days in combination with other antibiotics

Nontuberculous mycobacterium *(M. kansasii)* (off-label use): Adults: 10 mg/kg/day (maximum: 600 mg/day) for duration to include 12 months of culture-negative sputum; typically used in combination with ethambutol and isoniazid

Prosthetic joint infection (off-label use): *Staphylococci (oxacillin-susceptible or -resistant):* Oral: Adults:

Debridement and prosthesis retention or following 1-stage exchange, acute treatment: 300-450 mg every 12 hours in combination with an IV antistaphylococcal antibiotic for 2-6 weeks (Osmon, 2013)

Debridement and prosthesis retention or following 1-stage exchange, chronic treatment:

Total ankle, elbow, hip, or shoulder arthroplasty: 300-450 mg every 12 hours in combination with an oral antistaphylococcal antibiotic for 3 months (Osmon, 2013)

Total knee arthroplasty: 300-450 mg every 12 hours in combination with an oral antistaphylococcal antibiotic for 6 months (Osmon, 2013)

Following resection arthroplasty with or without planned staged reimplantation: 300-450 mg every 12 hours in combination with an IV antistaphylococcal antibiotics for 4-6 weeks (Osmon, 2013)

Staphylococcus aureus **infections, adjunctive therapy (off-label use):** Adults: 600 mg once daily or 300-450 mg every 12 hours with other antibiotics. **Note:** Must be used in combination with another antistaphylococcal antibiotic to avoid rapid development of resistance (Liu, 2011).

Tuberculosis, active: Note: A four-drug regimen (isoniazid, rifampin, pyrazinamide, and ethambutol) is preferred for the initial, empiric treatment of TB. When the drug susceptibility results are available, the regimen should be altered as appropriate.

Infants and Children <12 years:

Daily therapy: 10-20 mg/kg/day usually as a single dose (maximum: 600 mg/day)

Twice weekly directly observed therapy (DOT): 10-20 mg/kg (maximum: 600 mg)

Adults:

Daily therapy: 10 mg/kg/day (maximum: 600 mg/day)

Directly observed therapy (DOT): 10 mg/kg (maximum: 600 mg) administered 2 or 3 times/week (*MMWR*, 2003)

Tuberculosis, latent infection (LTBI): As an alternative to isoniazid:

Children: 10-20 mg/kg/day (maximum: 600 mg/day) for 6 months

Adults: 10 mg/kg/day (maximum: 600 mg/day) for 4 months. **Note:** Combination with pyrazinamide should not generally be offered (*MMWR*, Aug 8, 2003).

Dosage adjustment in renal impairment: No dosage adjustment necessary.

Poorly dialyzed; no supplemental dose or dosage adjustment necessary, including patients on intermittent hemodialysis, peritoneal dialysis, or continuous renal replacement therapy (eg, CVVHD).

Dosage adjustment in hepatic impairment: No dosage adjustment provided in manufacturer's labeling.

Dietary Considerations Rifampin should be taken on an empty stomach.

Administration

IV: Administer IV preparation by slow IV infusion over 30 minutes to 3 hours at a final concentration not to exceed 6 mg/mL. Do **not** administer IM or SubQ. Avoid extravasation.

Oral: Administer on an empty stomach (ie, 1 hour prior to, or 2 hours after meals or antacids) to increase total absorption. The compounded oral suspension must be shaken well before using. May mix contents of capsule with applesauce or jelly.

Monitoring Parameters Periodic (baseline and every 2-4 weeks during therapy) monitoring of liver function (AST, ALT, bilirubin), CBC, mental status, sputum culture, chest x-ray 2-3 months into treatment

Dosage Forms

Capsule, Oral:

Rifadin: 150 mg, 300 mg

Generic: 150 mg, 300 mg

Solution Reconstituted, Intravenous:

Rifadin: 600 mg (1 ea)

Generic: 600 mg (1 ea)

Extemporaneous Preparations A rifampin 1% w/v suspension (10 mg/mL) may be made with capsules and one of four syrups (Syrup NF, simple syrup, Syrpalta® syrup, or raspberry syrup). Empty the contents of four 300 mg capsules or eight 150 mg capsules onto a piece of weighing paper. If necessary, crush contents to produce a fine powder. Transfer powder to a 4-ounce amber glass or plastic prescription bottle. Rinse paper and spatula with 20 mL of chosen syrup and add the rinse to bottle; shake vigorously. Add 100 mL syrup to the bottle and shake vigorously. Label "shake well". Stable for 4 weeks at room temperature or refrigerated.

A 25 mg/mL oral suspension may be made with capsules and cherry syrup concentrate diluted 1:4 with simple syrup, NF. Empty the contents of ten 300 mg capsules into a mortar and reduce to a fine powder. Add 20 mL of the vehicle and mix to a uniform paste; mix while adding the vehicle in incremental proportions to **almost** 120 mL; transfer to a calibrated bottle, rinse mortar with vehicle, and add quantity of vehicle sufficient to make 120 mL. Label "shake well" and "refrigerate". Stable for 28 days refrigerated (preferred) or at room temperature.

Nahata MC, Pai VB, and Hipple TF, *Pediatric Drug Formulations*, 5th ed, Cincinnati, OH: Harvey Whitney Books Co, 2004.

Rifapentine (rif a PEN teen)

Brand Names: U.S. Priftin

Pharmacologic Category Antitubercular Agent

Use

Active pulmonary tuberculosis: Treatment of active pulmonary tuberculosis caused by *Mycobacterium tuberculosis* in adults and children 12 years and older; must be used in combination with one or more antituberculosis drugs to which the isolate is susceptible.

Limitations of use: Rifapentine should not be used once weekly in the continuation phase regimen in combination with isoniazid in HIV-infected patients with active pulmonary tuberculosis because of a higher rate of failure and/or relapse with rifampin-resistant organisms. Rifapentine has not been studied as part of the initial phase treatment regimen in HIV-infected patients with active pulmonary tuberculosis.

Latent tuberculosis infection: Treatment of latent tuberculosis infection caused by *Mycobacterium tuberculosis*, in combination with isoniazid, in adults and children 2 years and older at high risk of progression to tuberculosis disease. To identify candidates for latent tuberculosis infection treatment, refer to Centers for Disease Control and Prevention (CDC) guidelines for current recommendations.

Limitations of use: Rifapentine in combination with isoniazid is not recommended for individuals presumed to be exposed to rifamycin- or isoniazid-resistant *M. tuberculosis*.

Pregnancy Risk Factor C

Pregnancy Considerations Adverse events have been observed in animal reproduction studies. Postnatal hemorrhages have been reported in the infant and mother with rifampin (another rifamycin) administration during the last few weeks of pregnancy. Due to the risk of tuberculosis to the fetus, treatment is recommended when the probability of maternal disease is moderate to high. The CDC does not recommend rifapentine as part of the treatment regimen due to insufficient data in pregnant women (CDC, 2003).

Breast-Feeding Considerations It is not known if rifapentine is excreted in breast milk. Because of the potential for serious adverse reactions in the nursing infant, the manufacturer recommends a decision be made whether to discontinue nursing or the drug, taking into account the importance of treatment to the mother. Rifapentine may discolor breast milk.

Contraindications Hypersensitivity to rifapentine, other rifamycins, or any component of the formulation

Warnings/Precautions Patients with abnormal liver tests and/or liver disease should only be given rifapentine when absolutely necessary and under strict medical supervision. Monitoring of liver function tests (eg, serum transaminases) should be carried out prior to therapy and then every 2 to 4 weeks during therapy. Combination therapy should be discontinued if ALT is ≥5 times the upper limit of normal (ULN) even in the absence of liver dysfunction symptoms or ≥3 times ULN in the presence of symptoms (CDC, 2012). Use is not recommended in patients with porphyria; exacerbation is possible due to enzyme-inducing properties. Hypersensitivity reactions, including anaphylaxis, may occur. Discontinue therapy and administer supportive measures if hypersensitivity occurs.

Use of rifapentine during the **initial phase** of treatment in HIV-seropositive patients has not been evaluated. Rifapentine should not be used during the **continuation phase** of treatment in HIV-seropositive patients; a higher rate of failure and/ or relapse with rifampin-resistant organisms has been reported. Use with caution in patients with cavitary pulmonary lesions and/or positive sputum cultures after initial treatment phase and patients with bilateral pulmonary disease; higher relapse rates may occur in these patients. Rifapentine may produce a red-orange discoloration of body tissues/fluids including skin, teeth, tongue, urine, feces, saliva, sputum, tears, sweat, and cerebral spinal fluid. Contact lenses may become permanently stained; remove soft contact lenses during therapy. Advise patients with dentures that permanent staining of dentures may occur.

Prolonged use may result in fungal or bacterial superinfection, including *C. difficile*-associated diarrhea (CDAD) and pseudomembranous colitis; CDAD has been observed >2 months postantibiotic treatment. Compliance with dosing regimen is absolutely necessary for successful drug therapy. Potentially significant interactions may exist, requiring dose or frequency adjustment, additional monitoring, and/or selection of alternative therapy.

Adverse Reactions

Hematologic & oncologic: Anemia, lymphocytopenia, neutropenia

Cardiovascular: Chest pain, edema

Central nervous system: Dizziness, fatigue, headache, pain

Dermatologic: Acne vulgaris, diaphoresis, maculopapular rash, pruritus, skin rash

Endocrine & metabolic: Gout, hyperglycemia, hyperphosphatemia, hyperuricemia (most likely due to pyrazinamide from initiation phase), hypoglycemia, increased nonprotein nitrogen

Gastrointestinal: Abdominal pain, anorexia, constipation, diarrhea, dyspepsia, hemorrhoids, nausea, vomiting

Genitourinary: Casts in urine, cystitis, hematuria, pyuria, urinary tract infection

Hematologic & oncologic: Leukocytosis, leukopenia, lymphadenopathy, neutrophilia, polycythemia, thrombocythemia, thrombocytosis

Hepatic: Hepatotoxicity, increased serum ALT, increased serum AST

Hypersensitivity: Hypersensitivity reaction (less common in children and adolescents)

Infection: Herpes zoster, infection, influenza

Neuromuscular & skeletal: Arthralgia, back pain, osteoarthrosis, tremor

Ophthalmic: Conjunctivitis

Respiratory: Bronchitis, cough, epistaxis, hemoptysis, pharyngitis, pleurisy

Miscellaneous: Accidental injury, fever

Rare but important or life-threatening: Ageusia, allergic skin reaction, alopecia, anaphylaxis, asthma, azotemia, confusion, convulsions, depression, diabetes mellitus, disorientation, dysuria, enlargement of salivary glands, erythematous rash, esophagitis, fungal infection, gastritis, hematoma, hepatitis, hepatomegaly, hyperbilirubinemia, hypercalcemia, hyperhidrosis, hyperkalemia, hyperlipidemia, increased blood urea nitrogen, increased serum alkaline phosphatase, jitteriness, laryngeal edema, laryngitis, leukorrhea, lymphocytosis, myalgia, myasthenia, myositis, oropharyngeal pain, orthostatic hypotension, palpitations, pancreatitis, paresthesia, pericarditis, peripheral neuropathy, pneumonitis, pulmonary fibrosis, pulmonary tuberculosis (exacerbation), purpura, pyelonephritis, rhabdomyolysis, seizure, skin discoloration, suicidal ideation, syncope, tachycardia, thrombosis, urinary incontinence, vaginal hemorrhage, vaginitis, viral infection, voice disorder, vulvovaginal candidiasis, weight gain, weight loss

Drug Interactions

Metabolism/Transport Effects Induces CYP2C8 (strong), CYP2C9 (strong), CYP3A4 (strong)

Avoid Concomitant Use

Avoid concomitant use of Rifapentine with any of the following: Abiraterone Acetate; Apixaban; Apremilast; Artemether; Atovaquone; Axitinib; Bedaquiline; Boceprevir; Bortezomib; Bosutinib; Cabozantinib; Ceritinib; CloZAPine; Cobicistat; Crizotinib; Dasabuvir; Delavirdine; Dienogest; Dronedarone; Eliglustat; Elvitegravir; Enzalutamide; Etravirine; Everolimus; Ibrutinib; Idelalisib; Irinotecan; Itraconazole; Ivacaftor; Lapatinib; Ledipasvir; Lumefantrine; Lurasidone; Macitentan; Mifepristone; Mycophenolate; Naloxegol; Netupitant; NIFEdipine; Nilotinib; Nisoldipine; Olaparib; Ombitasvir; Paritaprevir; PAZOPanib; Perampanel; PONATinib; Praziquantel; Ranolazine; Regorafenib; Rilpivirine; Rivaroxaban; Roflumilast; RomiDEPsin; Simeprevir; Sofosbuvir; SORAfenib; Suvorexant; Tasimelteon; Telaprevir; Ticagrelor; Tofacitinib; Tolvaptan; Toremifene; Trabectedin; Ulipristal; Vandetanib; Vemurafenib; VinCRIStine (Liposomal); Vorapaxar; Voriconazole

Increased Effect/Toxicity

Rifapentine may increase the levels/effects of: Clarithromycin; Clopidogrel; Ifosfamide; Isoniazid; Pitavastatin

The levels/effects of Rifapentine may be increased by: Antifungal Agents (Azole Derivatives, Systemic); Clarithromycin; Delavirdine; Voriconazole

Decreased Effect

Rifapentine may decrease the levels/effects of: Abiraterone Acetate; Alfentanil; Antiemetics (5HT3 Antagonists); Antifungal Agents (Azole Derivatives, Systemic); Apixaban; Apremilast; ARIPiprazole; Artemether; Atovaquone; Axitinib; Barbiturates; Bedaquiline; Beta-Blockers; Boceprevir; Bortezomib; Bosutinib; Brentuximab Vedotin; BusPIRone; Cabozantinib; Calcium Channel Blockers; Cannabidiol; Cannabis; Ceritinib; Clarithromycin; CloZAPine; Cobicistat; Contraceptives (Estrogens); Contraceptives (Progestins); Corticosteroids (Systemic); Crizotinib; CycloSPORINE (Systemic); CYP2C8 Substrates; CYP2C9 Substrates; CYP3A4 Substrates; Dapsone (Systemic); Dasabuvir; Dasatinib; Delavirdine; Diclofenac (Systemic); Dienogest; DOXOrubicin (Conventional); Dronabinol; Dronedarone; Eliglustat; Elvitegravir; Enzalutamide; Erlotinib; Etravirine; Everolimus; Exemestane; FentaNYL; Gefitinib; GuanFACINE; HMG-CoA Reductase Inhibitors; Hydrocodone; Ibrutinib; Idelalisib; Ifosfamide; Imatinib; Irinotecan; Itraconazole; Ivacaftor; Ixabepilone; Lapatinib; Ledipasvir; Linagliptin; Lumefantrine; Lurasidone; Macitentan; Maraviroc; Methadone; Mifepristone; Morphine (Systemic); Mycophenolate; Naloxegol; Netupitant; NIFEdipine; Nilotinib; Nisoldipine; Olaparib; Ombitasvir; Paritaprevir; PAZOPanib; Perampanel; PONATinib; Praziquantel; Propafenone; QUEtiapine; QuiNIDine; Ramelteon; Ranolazine; Regorafenib; Rilpivirine; Rivaroxaban; Roflumilast; RomiDEPsin; Saxagliptin; Simeprevir; Sofosbuvir; SORAfenib; SUNItinib; Suvorexant; Tacrolimus (Systemic); Tadalafil; Tamoxifen; Tasimelteon; Telaprevir; Temsirolimus; Tetrahydrocannabinol; Ticagrelor; Tofacitinib; Tolvaptan; Toremifene; Trabectedin; Treprostinil; Ulipristal; Vandetanib; Vemurafenib; Vilazodone; VinCRIStine (Liposomal);

Vorapaxar; Voriconazole; Vortioxetine; Zaleplon; Zidovudine; Zolpidem; Zuclopenthixol

Food Interactions High-fat meals increase AUC and maximum serum concentration by 40% to 50%. Management: Administer with meals.

Storage/Stability Store at 25°C (77°F); excursions permitted to 15°C to 30°C (59°F to 86°F). Protect from excessive heat and humidity.

Mechanism of Action Inhibits DNA-dependent RNA polymerase in susceptible strains of *Mycobacterium tuberculosis* (MTB) (but not in mammalian cells). Rifapentine is bactericidal against both intracellular and extracellular MTB organisms.

Pharmacodynamics/Kinetics

Absorption: High-fat meals increase AUC and C_{max} by 40% to 50%.

Distribution: V_d: ~70 L

Protein binding: Rifapentine: ~98%, primarily to albumin; 25-desacetyl rifapentine: ~93%

Metabolism: Hepatic; hydrolyzed by an esterase enzyme to form the active metabolite 25-desacetyl rifapentine

Bioavailability: 70%

Half-life elimination: Rifapentine: ~17 hours; 25-desacetyl rifapentine: ~24 hours

Time to peak, serum: 3 to 10 hours

Excretion: Feces (70%); urine (17%, primarily as metabolites)

Dosage

Active pulmonary tuberculosis: Children ≥12 years, Adolescents, and Adults: Oral: **Rifapentine should not be used alone**; initial phase should include a 3- to 4-drug regimen

Initial phase: 600 mg twice weekly (with an interval ≥72 hours between doses) by directly observed therapy (DOT) for 2 months

Continuation phase: 600 mg once weekly by DOT for 4 months

Latent tuberculosis infection:

Children ≥2 years, Adolescents, and Adults: Oral: Use once weekly for 3 months; **Note:** Must be administered under DOT and given in combination with isoniazid (maximum dose: 900 mg):

10 to 14 kg: 300 mg

14.1 to 25 kg: 450 mg

25.1 to 32 kg: 600 mg

32.1 to 50 kg: 750 mg

>50 kg: 900 mg

Dosing adjustment in renal impairment: There are no dosage adjustments provided in the manufacturer's labeling (has not been studied).

Dosing adjustment in hepatic impairment: There are no dosage adjustments provided in the manufacturer's labeling; use with caution. Pharmacokinetics in varying degrees of hepatic impairment were similar to those in healthy volunteers.

Dietary Considerations Take with food.

Administration Administer with meals. For patients who cannot swallow tablets, the tablets may be crushed and added to a small amount of semi-solid food and consumed immediately.

Monitoring Parameters Patients with preexisting hepatic problems should have liver function tests monitored (eg, serum transaminases) prior to therapy and then every 2 to 4 weeks during therapy. In treatment of latent infection with rifapentine and isoniazid combination therapy, patients with HIV infection, liver disorders, immediate postpartum (≤3 months after delivery), or regular ethanol use should have liver function (at least alanine aminotransferase [ALT]) monitored prior to therapy and then at subsequent clinical visits whose baseline testing is abnormal or for others at risk for liver disease (CDC, 2012).

Additional Information Rifapentine has been studied in patients with tuberculosis receiving a 6-month short-course intensive regimen approval. Outcomes were based on 6-month follow-up treatment observed in clinical trial 008 as a surrogate for the 2-year follow-up generally accepted as evidence for efficacy in the treatment of pulmonary tuberculosis. In a study of rifapentine and isoniazid given weekly by direct observation therapy for 12 weeks in latent tuberculosis, the regimen was as effective as 36 weeks of daily isoniazid alone and had higher treatment completion rates (Sterling, 2011). CDC recommends the combination of rifapentine and isoniazid once weekly for 12 weeks as an equal alternative to daily isoniazid for 9 months (CDC, 2011).

Dosage Forms

Tablet, Oral:

Priftin: 150 mg

Rifaximin (rif AX i min)

Brand Names: U.S. Xifaxan

Pharmacologic Category Antibiotic, Miscellaneous

Use Treatment of travelers' diarrhea caused by noninvasive strains of *E. coli*; reduction in the risk of overt hepatic encephalopathy (HE) recurrence

Pregnancy Risk Factor C

Pregnancy Considerations Adverse events have been observed in some animal reproduction studies. Due to the limited oral absorption of rifaximin in patients with normal hepatic function, exposure to the fetus is expected to be low.

Breast-Feeding Considerations It is not known if rifaximin is excreted in human milk. Due to the potential for serious adverse reactions in the nursing infant, the manufacturer recommends a decision be made whether to discontinue nursing or to discontinue the drug, taking into account the importance of treatment to the mother. Because of the limited oral absorption of rifaximin in patients with normal hepatic function, exposure to the nursing infant is expected to be low.

Contraindications Hypersensitivity to rifaximin, other rifamycin antibiotics, or any component of the formulation

Warnings/Precautions Efficacy has not been established for the treatment of diarrhea due to pathogens other than *E. coli*, including *C. jejuni*, *Shigella* and *Salmonella*. Consider alternative therapy if symptoms persist or worsen after 24-48 hours of treatment. Not for treatment of systemic infections; <1% is absorbed orally. Prolonged use may result in fungal or bacterial superinfection, including *C. difficile*-associated diarrhea (CDAD) and pseudomembranous colitis; CDAD has been observed >2 months postantibiotic treatment. Use caution in severe hepatic impairment (Child-Pugh class C); efficacy for prevention of encephalopathy has not been established in patients with a Model for End-Stage Liver Disease (MELD) score >25. Potentially significant drug-drug interactions may exist, requiring dose or frequency adjustment, additional monitoring, and/or selection of alternative therapy.

Adverse Reactions

Cardiovascular: Chest pain, edema, hypotension, peripheral edema

Central nervous system: Attention disturbance, amnesia, confusion, depression, dizziness, fatigue, fever, headache, hypoesthesia, pain, tremor, vertigo

Dermatological: Cellulitis, pruritus, rash

Endocrine and metabolism: Hyper-/hypoglycemia, hyperkalemia, hyponatremia

Hepatic: Ascites

Gastrointestinal: Abdominal pain, abdominal tenderness, anorexia, dehydration, esophageal varices, nausea, weight gain, xerostomia

Hematologic: Anemia

Neuromuscular & skeletal: Arthralgia, muscle spasms, myalgia
Respiratory: Dyspnea, epistaxis, nasopharyngitis, pneumonia, rhinitis, upper respiratory tract infection
Miscellaneous: Influenza-like illness

All indications: Rare but important or life-threatening: Abnormal dreams, allergic dermatitis, anaphylaxis, angioneurotic edema, AST increased, choluria, CDAD, dry lips, dysuria, ear pain, exfoliative dermatitis, flushing, gingival disorder, hematuria, hot flashes, hypersensitivity reactions, lymphocytosis, migraine, monocytosis, motion sickness, nasal irritation, nasopharyngitis, neck pain, neutropenia, pharyngitis, pharyngolaryngeal pain, polyuria, proteinuria, sunburn, syncope, taste loss, tinnitus, urticaria, weakness, weight loss

Drug Interactions

Metabolism/Transport Effects **Substrate** of P-glycoprotein

Avoid Concomitant Use

Avoid concomitant use of Rifaximin with any of the following: BCG

Increased Effect/Toxicity

The levels/effects of Rifaximin may be increased by: CycloSPORINE (Systemic); P-glycoprotein/ABCB1 Inhibitors

Decreased Effect

Rifaximin may decrease the levels/effects of: BCG; Sodium Picosulfate

Storage/Stability Store at controlled room temperature of 20°C to 25°C (68°F to 77°F).

Mechanism of Action Rifaximin inhibits bacterial RNA synthesis by binding to bacterial DNA-dependent RNA polymerase.

Pharmacodynamics/Kinetics

Absorption: Oral: Travelers' diarrhea: Low; Increased in prevention of hepatic encephalopathy with Child-Pugh class C having a greater exposure than A
Protein binding: Healthy subjects: ~68%; Hepatic impairment: 62%
Half-life elimination: ~2-5 hours
Time to peak: Hepatic encephalopathy prevention: ~1 hour
Excretion: Feces (~97% as unchanged drug); urine (<1%)

Dosage Oral:

Children ≥12 years and Adults: Travelers' diarrhea: 200 mg 3 times daily for 3 days

Adults:

Hepatic encephalopathy:

Reduction of overt hepatic encephalopathy recurrence: 550 mg 2 times daily. **Note:** Supporting clinical trial evaluated efficacy over 6-month treatment period.

Treatment of hepatic encephalopathy (off-label use): 400 mg every 8 hours for 5 to 10 days (Mas, 2003)

Clostridium difficile-associated diarrhea (off-label use): 200 to 400 mg 2 to 3 times daily for 14 days (Johnson, 2007)

Irritable bowel syndrome (off-label use): 550 mg 3 times daily for 14 days (Pimentel, 2011)

Dosage adjustment in renal impairment: There are no dosage adjustments provided in the manufacturer's labeling (has not been studied).

Dosage adjustment in hepatic impairment: No dosage adjustment necessary. Use with caution in severe impairment (Child-Pugh class C) as systemic absorption does occur and pharmacokinetic parameters are highly variable

Dietary Considerations May be taken with or without food.

Administration May be administered with or without food.

Monitoring Parameters Temperature, blood in stool, change in symptoms; monitor changes in mental status in hepatic encephalopathy

Dosage Forms

Tablet, Oral:

Xifaxan: 200 mg, 550 mg

Extemporaneous Preparations A 20 mg/mL oral suspension may be made using tablets. Crush six 200 mg tablets and reduce to a fine powder. Add 30 mL of a 1:1 mixture of Ora-Sweet® and Ora-Plus® or a 1:1 mixture of Ora-Sweet® SF and Ora-Plus®; mix well while adding the vehicle in geometric proportions to **almost** 60 mL; transfer to a calibrated bottle, rinse mortar with vehicle, and add quantity of vehicle sufficient to make 60 mL. Label "shake well". Stable 60 days at room temperature.

Cober MP, Johnson CE, Lee J, et al, "Stability of Extemporaneously Prepared Rifaximin Oral Suspensions," *Am J Health Syst Pharm*, 2010, 67(4):287-89.

◆ **rIFN beta-1a** *see* Interferon Beta-1a *on page 1100*
◆ **rIFN beta-1b** *see* Interferon Beta-1b *on page 1103*
◆ **RIG** *see* Rabies Immune Globulin (Human) *on page 1764*

Rilonacept (ri LON a sept)

Brand Names: U.S. Arcalyst

Pharmacologic Category Interleukin-1 Inhibitor

Use Treatment of cryopyrin-associated periodic syndromes (CAPS) including familial cold autoinflammatory syndrome (FCAS) and Muckle-Wells syndrome (MWS)

Pregnancy Risk Factor C

Dosage Cryopyrin-associated periodic syndromes: SubQ:

Children ≥12 years: Loading dose 4.4 mg/kg (maximum dose: 320 mg) given as 1-2 separate injections (maximum: 2 mL/injection; administer at 2 different sites if multiple injections are necessary) on the same day, followed by a once-weekly dose of 2.2 mg/kg (maximum dose: 160 mg). **Note:** Do not administer more frequently than once weekly.

Adults: Loading dose 320 mg given as 2 separate injections (160 mg each) on the same day at 2 different sites, followed by a once-weekly dose of 160 mg. **Note:** Do not administer more frequently than once weekly.

Dosage adjustment in renal impairment: No dosage adjustment provided in manufacturer's labeling (has not been studied).

Dosage adjustment in hepatic impairment: No dosage adjustment provided in manufacturer's labeling (has not been studied).

Additional Information Complete prescribing information should be consulted for additional detail.

Dosage Forms

Solution Reconstituted, Subcutaneous [preservative free]:

Arcalyst: 220 mg (1 ea)

Rilpivirine (ril pi VIR een)

Brand Names: U.S. Edurant

Brand Names: Canada Edurant®

Index Terms TMC278

Pharmacologic Category Antiretroviral, Reverse Transcriptase Inhibitor, Non-nucleoside (Anti-HIV)

Use Treatment of HIV-1 infections in treatment-naive patients with HIV-1 RNA ≤100,000 copies/mL in combination with at least 2 other antiretroviral agents

Pregnancy Risk Factor B

Pregnancy Considerations Adverse events have not been observed in animal reproduction studies. Available data in pregnant women are insufficient and the DHHS Perinatal HIV Guidelines do not recommend use unless other alternatives are not available. Hypersensitivity reactions (including hepatic toxicity and rash) are more common in women on NNRTI therapy; it is not known if pregnancy increases this risk.

Regardless of CD4 count or HIV RNA copy number, all HIV-infected pregnant women should receive a combination antiretroviral (ARV) drug regimen. A combination of antepartum, intrapartum, and infant ARV prophylaxis is recommended. ARV therapy should be started as soon as possible in women with symptomatic infection. Although earlier initiation may be more effective in reducing the perinatal transmission of HIV, initiation may be delayed until after 12 weeks gestation in women who do not require immediate treatment after careful consideration of maternal conditions (eg, nausea and vomiting) and the potential risks of first trimester fetal exposure for specific agents. A scheduled cesarean delivery at 38 weeks gestation is recommended for all women with HIV RNA >1000 copies/mL or unknown concentrations near delivery in order to decrease transmission. If ARV therapy must be interrupted for <24 hours during the peripartum period, stop then restart all medications simultaneously in order to decrease the chance of developing resistance. Long-term follow-up is recommended for all infants exposed to ARV medications. In couples who want to conceive, the HIV-infected partner should attain maximum viral suppression prior to conception.

Health care providers are encouraged to enroll pregnant women exposed to antiretroviral medications in the Antiretroviral Pregnancy Registry (1-800-258-4263 or www.APRegistry.com). Health care providers caring for HIV-infected women and their infants may contact the National Perinatal HIV Hotline (888-448-8765) for clinical consultation (HHS [perinatal], 2014).

Breast-Feeding Considerations It is not known if rilpivirine is excreted into breast milk. Maternal or infant antiretroviral therapy does not completely eliminate the risk of postnatal HIV transmission. In addition, multiclass-resistant virus has been detected in breast-feeding infants despite maternal therapy. Therefore, in the United States, where formula is accessible, affordable, safe, and sustainable, and the risk of infant mortality due to diarrhea and respiratory infections is low, complete avoidance of breast-feeding by HIV-infected women is recommended to decrease potential transmission of HIV (HHS [perinatal], 2014).

Contraindications Coadministration with anticonvulsants (carbamazepine, oxcarbazepine, phenobarbital, phenytoin), antimycobacterials (rifampin, rifapentine), proton pump inhibitors (esomeprazole, lansoprazole, omeprazole, pantoprazole, rabeprazole), systemic dexamethasone (more than a single dose), or St John's wort.

Warnings/Precautions Use in treatment-naive patients with HIV-1 RNA ≤100,000 copies/mL; not for use in treatment-experienced patients. May cause depressive disorders (depression, depressed mood, dysphoria, mood changes, negative thoughts, suicide attempts, or suicidal ideation); monitor for changes and need for intervention. Causes hepatotoxicity; patients with significant transaminase elevations or hepatitis B or C prior to treatment may be at greater risk; has occurred in a few patients with no prior hepatic disease or risk factors. Baseline and periodic laboratory LFT evaluation during therapy is recommended. May cause redistribution of fat (eg, buffalo hump, peripheral wasting with increased abdominal girth, cushingoid appearance). Patients may develop immune reconstitution syndrome resulting in the occurrence of an inflammatory response to an indolent or residual opportunistic infection during initial HIV treatment or activation of autoimmune disorders (eg, Graves' disease, polymyositis, Guillain-Barré syndrome) later in therapy; further evaluation and treatment may be required.

Potentially significant interactions may exist, requiring dose or frequency adjustment, additional monitoring, and/or selection of alternative therapy. Doses >25 mg daily (ie, 75 mg daily, 300 mg daily) have been associated with QTc prolongation; use caution when coadministering with a drug with a known risk of torsades de pointes (HHS [adult], 2014).

Adverse Reactions

Central nervous system: Abnormal dreams; depressive disorders (depression, depressed mood, dysphoria, mood changes, negative thoughts, suicide attempts, suicidal ideation); fatigue, headache, insomnia

Dermatologic: Rash

Endocrine & metabolic: Cholesterol increased, LDL increased, triglycerides increased

Gastrointestinal: Abdominal pain

Hepatic: ALT increased, AST increased, total bilirubin increased

Renal: Creatinine increased

Rare but important or life-threatening: Abdominal discomfort, anxiety, appetite decreased, cholecystitis, cholelithiasis, diarrhea, dizziness, glomerulonephritis (membranous and mesangioproliferative), nausea, nephrolithiasis, nephrotic syndrome, sleep disorders, somnolence, vomiting

Drug Interactions

Metabolism/Transport Effects Substrate of CYP3A4 (major); **Note:** Assignment of Major/Minor substrate status based on clinically relevant drug interaction potential

Avoid Concomitant Use

Avoid concomitant use of Rilpivirine with any of the following: CarBAMazepine; Dexamethasone (Systemic); Efavirenz; Etravirine; Fosphenytoin; OXcarbazepine; PHENobarbital; Phenytoin; Primidone; Proton Pump Inhibitors; Reverse Transcriptase Inhibitors (Non-Nucleoside); Rifamycin Derivatives; St Johns Wort

Increased Effect/Toxicity

Rilpivirine may increase the levels/effects of: Efavirenz; Etravirine; Highest Risk QTc-Prolonging Agents; Moderate Risk QTc-Prolonging Agents

The levels/effects of Rilpivirine may be increased by: Boceprevir; CYP3A4 Inhibitors (Strong); Darunavir; Ketoconazole (Systemic); Lopinavir; Macrolide Antibiotics; Mifepristone; Reverse Transcriptase Inhibitors (Non-Nucleoside); Ritonavir; Simeprevir

Decreased Effect

Rilpivirine may decrease the levels/effects of: CarBAMazepine; Didanosine; Efavirenz; Etravirine; Ketoconazole (Systemic); Methadone

The levels/effects of Rilpivirine may be decreased by: Antacids; Bosentan; CarBAMazepine; CYP3A4 Inducers (Moderate); CYP3A4 Inducers (Strong); Dabrafenib; Deferasirox; Dexamethasone (Systemic); Didanosine; Fosphenytoin; H2-Antagonists; Mitotane; OXcarbazepine; PHENobarbital; Phenytoin; Primidone; Proton Pump Inhibitors; Reverse Transcriptase Inhibitors (Non-Nucleoside); Rifabutin; Rifamycin Derivatives; Siltuximab; St Johns Wort; Tocilizumab

Food Interactions Absorption increased by ~40% when taken with a normal- to high-calorie meal. Management: Administer with a normal- to high-calorie meal. Administration with a protein supplement drink alone does not increase absorption.

Storage/Stability Store at 25°C (77°F); excursions permitted to 15°C to 30°C (59°F to 86°F). Keep in original container; protect from light.

Mechanism of Action As a non-nucleoside reverse transcriptase inhibitor, rilpivirine has activity against HIV-1 by binding to reverse transcriptase. It consequently blocks the RNA-dependent and DNA-dependent DNA polymerase activities, including HIV-1 replication. It does not require intracellular phosphorylation for antiviral activity.

Pharmacodynamics/Kinetics

Absorption: Increased 40% with a meal (normal-to-high calorie)

Protein binding: 99.7% (primarily albumin)

Metabolism: Hepatic, primarily by CYP3A4

Half-life elimination: ~50 hours

Time to peak, plasma: 4 to 5 hours

Excretion: Feces (85%, ~25% as unchanged drug); urine (~6%; <1% as unchanged drug)

Dosage HIV-1 infection: Adults: Oral: 25 mg once daily. **Note:** Rilpivirine is a component of a recommended regimen only in antiretroviral treatment-naive patients with HIV-1 RNA ≤100,000 copies/mL and CD4 count >200 cells/mm^3 at the start of therapy (HHS [adult], 2014).

Dosage adjustment for concomitant therapy with rifabutin: Increase to 50 mg once daily in patients on concomitant rifabutin. Decrease to 25 mg once daily when rifabutin is stopped.

Dosage adjustment in renal impairment:

Mild-to-moderate renal impairment: No dosage adjustment necessary

Severe or end-stage renal impairment: Use with caution; no dosage adjustment necessary (HHS [adult], 2014)

Hemodialysis/peritoneal dialysis: Due to extensive protein binding, significant removal by hemodialysis or peritoneal dialysis is unlikely.

Dosage adjustment in hepatic impairment:

Mild-to-moderate impairment (Child-Pugh class A or B): No dosage adjustment necessary

Severe impairment (Child-Pugh class C): There are no dosage adjustments provided in the manufacturer's labeling (has not been studied); DHHS HIV guidelines also have no dosage recommendation (HHS [adult], 2014).

Dietary Considerations Take with a normal- to high-calorie meal. Taking with a protein supplement drink alone does not increase absorption.

Administration Administer with a normal- to high-calorie meal. Taking with a protein supplement drink alone does not increase absorption.

Monitoring Parameters Cholesterol, triglycerides, hepatic transaminases; signs of skin rash, signs and symptoms of infection

Additional Information Rilpivirine has been shown in several studies to be noninferior to efavirenz in treatment-naive HIV-1 patients. Efficacy data in clinical studies exist for up to 96 weeks. Patients with CD4+ counts <200 cells/mm^3 (regardless of HIV-1 RNA at the start of therapy) are more likely to experience virologic failure (defined as HIV-1 RNA ≥50 copies/mL) than patients with CD4+ counts ≥200 cells/mm^3. Additionally, patients with increased HIV-1 viral loads at treatment initiation (HIV-1 RNA >100,000 copies/mL) are more likely to develop virologic failure. Increased viral load patients also are more likely to develop rilpivirine-resistance, tenofovir and emtricitabine/lamivudine resistance and NNRTI class cross-resistance. Rilpivirine resistance patterns are very similar to those of etravirine (including cross resistance with single substitutions at K101P, Y181I, and Y181V) (Azijn, 2010). In rilpivirine-treated patients who experience virologic failure, rilpivirine-resistant mutations are very common (HHS [adult], 2014).

Dosage Forms

Tablet, Oral:

Edurant: 25 mg

◆ **Rilpivirine, Emtricitabine, and Tenofovir** *see* Emtricitabine, Rilpivirine, and Tenofovir *on page 722*

◆ **Rilutek** *see* Riluzole *on page 1812*

◆ **Rilutek® (Can)** *see* Riluzole *on page 1812*

Riluzole (RIL yoo zole)

Brand Names: U.S. Rilutek

Brand Names: Canada Apo-Riluzole®; Mylan-Riluzole; Rilutek®

Index Terms 2-Amino-6-Trifluoromethoxy-benzothiazole; RP-54274

Pharmacologic Category Glutamate Inhibitor

Use Treatment of amyotrophic lateral sclerosis (ALS); riluzole can extend survival or time to tracheostomy

Pregnancy Risk Factor C

Pregnancy Considerations Impaired fertility, decreased implantation, increased intrauterine death, and adverse effects on offspring growth and viability were observed in animal studies. There are no adequate or well-controlled studies in pregnant women.

Breast-Feeding Considerations It is not known if riluzole is excreted in breast milk. Breast-feeding is not recommended by the manufacturer.

Contraindications Severe hypersensitivity reactions to riluzole or any component of the formulation

Warnings/Precautions Among 4000 patients given riluzole for ALS, there were 3 cases of marked neutropenia (ANC <500/mm^3), all seen within the first 2 months of treatment. Interstitial lung disease (primarily hypersensitivity pneumonitis) has occurred, requires prompt evaluation and possible discontinuation. Use with caution in patients with concomitant renal insufficiency. Use with caution in patients with current evidence or history of abnormal liver function; do not administer if baseline liver function tests are elevated. May cause elevations in transaminases (usually transient). May cause elevations in transaminases (usually transient) within first 3 months of therapy; discontinue if ALT levels are ≥5 times upper limit of normal or if jaundice develops. The elderly or female patients may have decreased clearance of riluzole; use with caution. May cause dizziness or somnolence; caution should be used performing tasks which require alertness (operating machinery or driving). Effects may be potentiated when used with other sedative drugs or ethanol.

Adverse Reactions

Cardiovascular: Hypertension, peripheral edema, tachycardia

Central nervous system: Dizziness, malaise, somnolence, vertigo

Dermatologic: Eczema, exfoliative dermatitis, pruritus

Gastrointestinal: Abdominal pain, flatulence, nausea, oral moniliasis, stomatitis, tooth caries, vomiting

Genitourinary: Dysuria, urinary tract infection

Hepatic: Liver function tests increased

Neuromuscular & skeletal: Arthralgia, paresthesia (circumoral), tremor, weakness

Respiratory: Cough increased, lung function decreased

Rare but important or life-threatening: Alkaline phosphatase increased, amblyopia, anaphylactoid reaction, anaphylaxis, angioedema, aplastic anemia, arthrosis, asthma, ataxia, bone necrosis, bradycardia, bundle branch block, cataract, cerebral hemorrhage, deafness, dementia, diabetes mellitus, diabetes insipidus, edema, erythema multiforme, extrapyramidal syndrome, facial paralysis, gastrointestinal hemorrhage, gastrointestinal ulcer, GGT increased, glaucoma, hallucination, heart failure, hematemesis, hematuria, hemoptysis, hepatitis, hypercalcemia, hypokalemia, hypokinesia, hyponatremia, hypotension, hypersensitivity pneumonitis, interstitial lung disease, jaundice, LDH increased, leukocytosis, leukopenia, lymphadenopathy, mania, myoclonus, neutropenia, osteoporosis, pancreatitis, peripheral neuritis, pleural effusion, pseudomembranous colitis, purpura, respiratory acidosis, seizure, subarachnoid hemorrhage, thrombosis, urinary retention, urticaria, uterine hemorrhage, ventricular fibrillation, ventricular tachycardia

Drug Interactions

Metabolism/Transport Effects Substrate of CYP1A2 (major); **Note:** Assignment of Major/Minor substrate status based on clinically relevant drug interaction potential

Avoid Concomitant Use There are no known interactions where it is recommended to avoid concomitant use.

Increased Effect/Toxicity There are no known significant interactions involving an increase in effect.

Decreased Effect

The levels/effects of Riluzole may be decreased by: Cannabis; CYP1A2 Inducers (Strong); Cyproterone; Teriflunomide

Food Interactions A high-fat meal decreases absorption of riluzole (decreasing AUC by 20% and peak blood levels by 45%). Charbroiled food may increase riluzole elimination. Management: Administer at the same time each day, at least 1 hour before or 2 hours after a meal.

Storage/Stability Store at 20°C to 25°C (68°F to 77°F). Protect from bright light.

Mechanism of Action Mechanism of action is not known. Pharmacologic properties include inhibitory effect on glutamate release, inactivation of voltage-dependent sodium channels; and ability to interfere with intracellular events that follow transmitter binding at excitatory amino acid receptors

Pharmacodynamics/Kinetics

Absorption: ~90%; high-fat meal decreases AUC by 20% and peak blood levels by 45%

Protein binding, plasma: 96%, primarily to albumin and lipoproteins

Metabolism: Extensively hepatic to six major and a number of minor metabolites via CYP1A2 dependent hydroxylation and glucuronidation

Bioavailability: Oral: Absolute: ~60%

Half-life elimination: 12 hours

Excretion: Urine (90%; 85% as metabolites, 2% as unchanged drug) and feces (5%) within 7 days

Dosage Adults: Oral: 50 mg every 12 hours; no increased benefit can be expected from higher daily doses, but adverse events are increased

Dosage adjustment in smoking: Cigarette smoking is known to induce CYP1A2; patients who smoke cigarettes would be expected to eliminate riluzole faster. There is no information, however, on the effect of, or need for, dosage adjustment in these patients.

Dosage adjustment in renal impairment: No dosage adjustment provided in manufacturer's labeling. Use with caution.

Dosage adjustment in hepatic impairment: No dosage adjustment provided in manufacturer's labeling. Use with caution.

Dietary Considerations Take at least 1 hour before or 2 hours after a meal.

Administration Administer at the same time each day, at least 1 hour before or 2 hours after a meal.

Monitoring Parameters Monitor serum aminotransferases including ALT levels before and during therapy. Evaluate serum ALT levels every month during the first 3 months of therapy, every 3 months during the remainder of the first year and periodically thereafter. Evaluate ALT levels more frequently in patients who develop elevations. Maximum increases in serum ALT usually occurred within 3 months after the start of therapy and were usually transient when <5 times ULN (upper limits of normal). Discontinue therapy if ALT levels are ≥5 times upper limit of normal or if jaundice develops.

In trials, if ALT levels were <5 times ULN, treatment continued and ALT levels usually returned to below 2 times ULN within 2-6 months. There is no experience with continued treatment of ALS patients once ALT values exceed 5 times ULN.

Dosage Forms

Tablet, Oral:

Rilutek: 50 mg

Generic: 50 mg

RimabotulinumtoxinB
(rime uh BOT yoo lin num TOKS in bee)

Brand Names: U.S. Myobloc

Index Terms Botulinum Toxin Type B

Pharmacologic Category Neuromuscular Blocker Agent, Toxin

Use Treatment of cervical dystonia (spasmodic torticollis)

Pregnancy Risk Factor C (manufacturer)

Dosage

Children: Not established in pediatric patients

Adults: Cervical dystonia: IM: Initial: 2500-5000 units divided among the affected muscles in patients **previously treated** with botulinum toxin; initial dose in **previously untreated** patients should be lower. Subsequent dosing should be optimized according to patient's response.

Elderly: No dosage adjustments required, but limited experience in patients ≥75 years old

Dosage adjustment in renal impairment: No dosage adjustment provided in manufacturer's labeling.

Dosage adjustment in hepatic impairment: No dosage adjustment provided in manufacturer's labeling.

Additional Information Complete prescribing information should be consulted for additional detail.

Dosage Forms

Solution, Intramuscular [preservative free]:

Myobloc: 2500 units/0.5 mL (0.5 mL); 5000 units/mL (1 mL); 10,000 units/2 mL (2 mL)

Rimantadine (ri MAN ta deen)

Brand Names: U.S. Flumadine

Brand Names: Canada Flumadine®

Index Terms Rimantadine Hydrochloride

Pharmacologic Category Antiviral Agent; Antiviral Agent, Adamantane

Use Prophylaxis (adults and children >1 year of age) and treatment (adults) of influenza A viral infection (per manufacturer labeling; also refer to current ACIP guidelines for recommendations during current flu season)

Note: In certain circumstances, the ACIP recommends use of rimantadine in combination with oseltamivir for the treatment or prophylaxis of influenza A infection when resistance to oseltamivir is suspected.

Pregnancy Risk Factor C

Dosage Oral:

Prophylaxis:

Children

1-9 years: 5 mg/kg/day in 1-2 divided doses; maximum: 150 mg/day

≥10 years and <40 kg: 5 mg/kg/day in 2 divided doses (CDC, 2011)

Children ≥10 years (and ≥40 kg) and Adults: 100 mg twice daily

Elderly: 100 mg daily in the elderly (≥65 years), including elderly nursing home patients

Note: Prophylaxis (institutional outbreak): In order to control outbreaks in institutions, if influenza A virus subtyping is unavailable and oseltamivir resistant viruses are circulating, rimantadine may be used in combination with oseltamivir if zanamivir cannot be used. Treatment should continue for ≥2 weeks and until ~10 days after illness onset in the last patient (CDC, 2011; Harper, 2009).

Treatment:
Children ≥17 years and Adults: 100 mg twice daily
Elderly: 100 mg daily in the elderly (≥65 years) or nursing home patients

Dosage adjustment in renal impairment:
CrCl ≥30 mL/minute: No dosage adjustment necessary.
CrCl <30 mL/minute: Maximum: 100 mg daily
Dosage adjustment in hepatic impairment: Severe dysfunction: Maximum: 100 mg daily
Additional Information Complete prescribing information should be consulted for additional detail.
Dosage Forms
Tablet, Oral:
Flumadine: 100 mg
Generic: 100 mg

◆ **Rimantadine Hydrochloride** *see* Rimantadine *on page 1813*

Rimexolone (ri MEKS oh lone)

Brand Names: U.S. Vexol
Brand Names: Canada Vexol®
Pharmacologic Category Corticosteroid, Ophthalmic
Use Treatment of inflammation after ocular surgery and the treatment of anterior uveitis
Pregnancy Risk Factor C
Dosage Ophthalmic: Adults:
Anti-inflammatory: Instill 1-2 drops in conjunctival sac of affected eye 4 times/day beginning 24 hours after surgery and continuing through the first 2 weeks of the postoperative period
Anterior uveitis: Instill 1-2 drops in conjunctival sac of affected eye every hour during waking hours for the first week, then 1 drop every 2 hours during waking hours of the second week, and then taper until uveitis is resolved

Dosage adjustment in renal impairment: No dosage adjustment provided in manufacturer's labeling.
Dosage adjustment in hepatic impairment: No dosage adjustment provided in manufacturer's labeling.
Additional Information Complete prescribing information should be consulted for additional detail.
Dosage Forms
Suspension, Ophthalmic:
Vexol: 1% (5 mL, 10 mL)

Rimonabant [INT] (ri MOE na bant)

International Brand Names Acomplia (AE, BH, IS, LU, MX, SE); Lipocura (PY); Redufast (PY); Ribafit (IN); Rimogras (PY); Rimoslim (IN); Riobant (IN); Riomont (IN); Zimulti (SE)
Pharmacologic Category Endocannabinoid CB1 Receptor Antagonist
Reported Use Adjunct treatment to diet and exercise for obese patients (body mass index >30 kg/m^2) or overweight patients (body mass index >27 kg/m^2) with associated risk factor(s) such as type 2 diabetes mellitus (noninsulin dependent, NIDDM) or dyslipidemia
Dosage Range Adolescents ≥18 years and Adults: Oral: 20 mg/day before breakfast
Product Availability Product available in various countries; not currently available in the U.S.
Dosage Forms
Tablet: 20 mg

Riociguat (rye oh SIG ue at)

Brand Names: U.S. Adempas
Brand Names: Canada Adempas
Index Terms Adempas; BAY 63-2521
Pharmacologic Category Soluble Guanylate Cyclase (sGC) Stimulator
Use
Chronic thromboembolic pulmonary hypertension: Treatment of adults with persistent/recurrent chronic thromboembolic pulmonary hypertension (CTEPH) (WHO group 4) after surgical treatment or inoperable CTEPH to improve exercise capacity and WHO functional class
Pulmonary arterial hypertension: Treatment of adults with pulmonary artery hypertension (PAH) (WHO group 1) to improve exercise capacity, improve WHO functional class and to delay clinical worsening
Pregnancy Risk Factor X
Pregnancy Considerations Reproduction studies in animals have shown evidence of fetal abnormalities and use is contraindicated in women who are or may become pregnant. **[U.S. Boxed Warnings]: Riociguat may cause fetal harm if given to pregnant women. Riociguat is available to females only through the restricted Adempas Risk Evaluation and Mitigation Strategy (REMS) Program. All females of reproductive potential should have a negative pregnancy test prior to beginning therapy and testing should continue monthly during treatment and one month after discontinuing therapy. Females of childbearing potential should not become pregnant during therapy or for 1 month following discontinuation riociguat.** All females regardless of their reproductive potential must be enrolled in the REMS program; prescribers and pharmacies must also be enrolled in the program. Females of reproductive potential must be able to comply with pregnancy testing and contraception requirements of the program. Women may use one highly effective form of contraception (intrauterine device, contraceptive implant, or tubal sterilization) or a combination of methods (hormonal contraceptive with a barrier method or two barrier methods). A hormonal contraceptive or barrier method must be used in addition to a partner's vasectomy, if that method is chosen. Females should be counseled on pregnancy prevention and planning and instructed to notify their prescriber immediately if a pregnancy should occur. Women with pulmonary arterial hypertension (PAH) are encouraged to avoid pregnancy (Badesch, 2007; McLaughlin, 2009).
Breast-Feeding Considerations It is not known if riociguat is excreted into breast milk. Due to the potential for adverse reactions in the nursing infant, the manufacturer recommends a decision be made whether to discontinue nursing or to discontinue the drug, taking into account the importance of treatment to the mother. The Canadian labeling contraindicates use in breast-feeding women.
Contraindications Pregnancy; coadministration with nitrates or nitric oxide donors (eg, amyl nitrite) in any form; concomitant administration with phosphodiesterase (PDE) inhibitors, including specific PDE-5 inhibitors (eg, sildenafil, tadalafil, vardenafil) or nonspecific PDE inhibitors (eg, dipyridamole, theophylline)

Canadian labeling: Additional contraindications (not in U.S. labeling): Hypersensitivity to riociguat or any component of the formulation; breast-feeding
Warnings/Precautions Reduces blood pressure. Use with caution in patients at increased risk for symptomatic hypotension or ischemia (eg, patients with hypovolemia, severe left ventricular outflow obstruction, resting hypotension, autonomic dysfunction) or concurrent use of antihypertensives or strong CYP and P-gp/BCRP inhibitors. Consider initiating at a lower dose for patients at risk of hypotension and/or dose reduction if hypotension develops. The Canadian labeling recommends avoiding use in patients with systolic blood pressure <95 mm Hg at initiation of therapy (has not been studied). Patients must

be cautioned about performing tasks which require mental alertness (eg, operating machinery or driving). Serious bleeding has been observed; consider periodic monitoring for bleeding.

Use is not recommended in patients with pulmonary veno-occlusive disease (PVOD). Discontinue in any patient with pulmonary edema suggestive of PVOD. Use with caution in patients with renal and hepatic impairment. The Canadian labeling does not recommend use in patients with severe hepatic impairment (Child-Pugh class C) and patients with CrCl <15 mL/minute or receiving dialysis (has not been studied).

[U.S. Boxed Warning] May cause fetal harm if given to pregnant women. All females of reproductive potential should have a negative pregnancy test prior to beginning therapy and testing should continue monthly during treatment and one month after discontinuing therapy. Females of childbearing potential should not become pregnant during therapy or for 1 month following discontinuation of riociguat. Women may use one highly effective form of contraception (intrauterine device, contraceptive implant, or tubal sterilization) or a combination of methods (hormonal contraceptive with a barrier method or two barrier methods). A hormonal contraceptive or barrier method must be used in addition to a partner's vasectomy, if that method is chosen. Females should be counseled on pregnancy prevention and planning and instructed to notify their prescriber immediately if a pregnancy should occur. **[U.S. Boxed Warning]: Riociguat is available to females only through the restricted Adempas Risk Evaluation and Mitigation Strategy (REMS) Program.** All females, regardless of their reproductive potential, must be enrolled in the REMS program; prescribers and pharmacies must also be enrolled in the program. Females of reproductive potential must be able to comply with pregnancy testing and contraception requirements of the program. Call 855-4-ADEMPAS or visit www.AdempasREMS.com for more information.

Riociguat concentrations are 50% to 60% lower in patients who smoke compared to nonsmokers; consider titrating dose to >2.5 mg 3 times daily, if tolerated. A decreased dose may be necessary in patients who stop smoking during therapy. Potentially significant drug-drug interactions may exist, requiring dose or frequency adjustment, additional monitoring, and/or selection of alternative therapy.

Adverse Reactions

Cardiovascular: Hypotension, palpitations, peripheral edema

Central nervous system: Dizziness, headache

Gastrointestinal: Abdominal distention, constipation, diarrhea, dyspepsia, dysphagia, gastritis, gastroesophageal reflux disease, nausea, vomiting

Hematologic & oncologic: Anemia, major hemorrhage (including vaginal hemorrhage, catheter site hemorrhage, subdural hematoma, hematemesis, and intra-abdominal hemorrhage)

Respiratory: Epistaxis, hemoptysis, nasal congestion

Drug Interactions

Metabolism/Transport Effects Substrate of BCRP, CYP2C8 (major), CYP3A4 (major), P-glycoprotein; **Note:** Assignment of Major/Minor substrate status based on clinically relevant drug interaction potential

Avoid Concomitant Use

Avoid concomitant use of Riociguat with any of the following: Amyl Nitrite; Dipyridamole; Ibudilast; Phosphodiesterase 5 Inhibitors; Theophylline Derivatives; Vasodilators (Organic Nitrates)

Increased Effect/Toxicity

Riociguat may increase the levels/effects of: DULoxetine; Hypotensive Agents; Levodopa; RisperiDONE

The levels/effects of Riociguat may be increased by: Amyl Nitrite; Anagrelide; Apremilast; Barbiturates; Cilostazol; Cobicistat; Dipyridamole; Ibudilast; Itraconazole; Ketoconazole (Systemic); Milrinone; P-glycoprotein/ABCB1 Inhibitors; Phosphodiesterase 5 Inhibitors; Protease Inhibitors; Roflumilast; Teriflunomide; Theophylline Derivatives; Vasodilators (Organic Nitrates)

Decreased Effect

The levels/effects of Riociguat may be decreased by: Antacids; Bosentan; CYP2C8 Inducers (Strong); CYP3A4 Inducers (Moderate); CYP3A4 Inducers (Strong); Dabrafenib; Deferasirox; Mitotane; P-glycoprotein/ABCB1 Inducers; Proton Pump Inhibitors; Siltuximab; St Johns Wort; Tocilizumab

Storage/Stability Store at 25°C (77°F); excursions are permitted from 15°C to 30°C (59°F to 86°F).

Mechanism of Action Riociguat has a dual mode of action. It sensitizes soluble guanylate cyclase (sGC) to endogenous nitric oxide (NO) by stabilizing the NO-sGC binding. Riociguat also directly stimulates sGC independent of NO. Riociguat stimulates the NO-sGC-cGMP pathway and leads to increased generation of cGMP with subsequent vasodilation.

Pharmacodynamics/Kinetics

Distribution: ~30 L

Protein binding: Plasma: ~95%

Metabolism: Mainly cleared by metabolism by CYP1A1, CYP3A, CYP2C8 and CYP2J2. Formation of the major active metabolite, M1, is catalyzed by CYP1A1, which is inducible by polycyclic aromatic hydrocarbons such as those present in cigarette smoke. M1 is only 1/3 to 1/10 as potent as the parent drug and is further metabolized to the inactive N-glucuronide. Plasma concentrations of M1 in patients with pulmonary arterial hypertension are about half those for riociguat.

Bioavailability: ~94%

Half-life elimination: Patients: 12 hours; Healthy subjects: 7 hours

Time to peak, plasma: 1.5 hours

Excretion: Feces (~53%); urine (~40%)

Dosage Chronic thromboembolic pulmonary hypertension, pulmonary arterial hypertension: Adults: Oral: Initial: 1 mg 3 times daily; may initiate dose at 0.5 mg 3 times daily in patients who may not tolerate the hypotensive effects. If tolerated, may increase the dose by 0.5 mg 3 times daily if systolic blood pressure (SBP) remains >95 mm Hg and the patient has no signs or symptoms of hypotension; increase dose at intervals of ≥2 weeks. Maximum dose: 2.5 mg 3 times daily.

Missed doses: If a dose is missed, continue with the next regularly scheduled dose. If therapy is interrupted for ≥3 days, retitration is required.

Elderly: Refer to adult dosing. Use with caution; riociguat exposure is increased.

Dosage adjustment for concurrent use in patients receiving strong multi-pathway CYP and P-gp/BCRP inhibitors (eg, azole antifungals or protease inhibitors):

U.S. labeling: Consider a starting dose of 0.5 mg 3 times daily.

Canadian labeling: Concomitant use is not recommended

Dosage adjustment for patients who smoke: Dose may be titrated to >2.5 mg 3 times daily, if tolerated. A decreased dose may be necessary in patients who stop smoking during therapy.

Dosage adjustment for toxicity:

Hypotension:

U.S. labeling: Decrease dose by 0.5 mg 3 times daily if hypotensive effects are not tolerated.

Canadian labeling: If SBP <95 mm Hg and no signs/symptoms of hypotension may maintain current dose. If SBP is <95 mm Hg and signs/symptoms of hypotension are present, hold the next 3 doses and if clinically appropriate, resume 24 hours later by decreasing dose by 0.5 mg 3 times daily.

Pulmonary edema: Consider the possibility of pulmonary veno-occlusive disease (PVOD); if confirmed discontinue treatment with riociguat.

Dosage adjustment in renal impairment:

CrCl ≥15 mL/minute: No dosage adjustment provided in manufacturer's labeling.

CrCl <15 mL/minute: No dosage adjustment provided in manufacturer's labeling (has not been studied). Canadian labeling recommends avoiding use.

Dialysis: No dosage adjustment provided in manufacturer's labeling (has not been studied). Canadian labeling recommends avoiding use.

Dosage adjustment in hepatic impairment:

Mild to moderate hepatic impairment (Child-Pugh class A and B): No dosage adjustment provided in manufacturer's labeling.

Severe hepatic impairment (Child-Pugh class C): No dosage adjustment provided in manufacturer's labeling (has not been studied). Canadian labeling recommends avoiding use.

Administration Oral: Administer with or without food.

Monitoring Parameters Monitor blood pressure and signs and symptoms of hypotension. Monitor for significant peripheral edema and improvements in pulmonary function and exercise tolerance. Women of childbearing potential must have a negative pregnancy test prior to the initiation of therapy, monthly during treatment, and 1 month after discontinuation of therapy.

Dosage Forms

Tablet, Oral:

Adempas: 0.5 mg, 1 mg, 1.5 mg, 2 mg, 2.5 mg

◆ **Riomet** *see* MetFORMIN *on page 1307*

◆ **Riopan Plus** *see* Magaldrate and Simethicone *on page 1261*

Risedronate (ris ED roe nate)

Brand Names: U.S. Actonel; Atelvia

Brand Names: Canada Actonel®; Actonel® DR; Apo-Risedronate®; Dom-Risedronate; Novo-Risedronate; PMS-Risedronate; ratio-Risedronate; Riva-Risedronate; Sandoz-Risedronate; Teva-Risedronate

Index Terms Risedronate Sodium

Pharmacologic Category Bisphosphonate Derivative

Use

Actonel®: Treatment of Paget's disease of the bone; treatment and prevention of glucocorticoid-induced osteoporosis; treatment and prevention of osteoporosis in postmenopausal women; treatment of osteoporosis in men

Atelvia™: Treatment of osteoporosis in postmenopausal women

Pregnancy Risk Factor C

Pregnancy Considerations Adverse events were observed in some animal reproduction studies. It is not known if bisphosphonates cross the placenta, but fetal exposure is expected (Djokanovic, 2008; Stathopoulos, 2011). Bisphosphonates are incorporated into the bone matrix and gradually released over time. The amount available in the systemic circulation varies by dose and duration of therapy. Theoretically, there may be a risk of fetal harm when pregnancy follows the completion of therapy; however, available data have not shown that exposure to bisphosphonates during pregnancy significantly increases the risk of adverse fetal events (Djokanovic, 2008; Levy, 2009; Stathopoulos, 2011). Until additional data is available, most sources recommend discontinuing bisphosphonate therapy in women of reproductive potential as early as possible prior to a planned pregnancy; use in premenopausal women should be reserved for special circumstances when rapid bone loss is occurring (Bhalla, 2010; Pereira, 2012; Stathopoulos, 2011). Because hypocalcemia has been described following *in utero* bisphosphonate exposure, exposed infants should be monitored for hypocalcemia after birth (Djokanovic, 2008; Stathopoulos, 2011).

Breast-Feeding Considerations It is not known if risedronate is excreted into breast milk. Due to the potential for serious adverse reactions in the nursing infant, the manufacturer recommends a decision be made whether to discontinue nursing or to discontinue the drug, taking into account the importance of treatment to the mother.

Contraindications Hypersensitivity to risedronate, bisphosphonates, or any component of the formulation; hypocalcemia; inability to stand or sit upright for at least 30 minutes; abnormalities of the esophagus (eg, stricture, achalasia) which delay esophageal emptying

Warnings/Precautions Bisphosphonates may cause upper gastrointestinal disorders such as dysphagia, esophagitis, esophageal ulcer, and gastric ulcer; risk increases in patients unable to comply with dosing instructions. Use with caution in patients with dysphagia, esophageal disease, gastritis, duodenitis, or ulcers (may worsen underlying condition). Discontinue if new or worsening symptoms occur. Use caution in patients with renal impairment (not recommended in patients with a CrCl <30 mL/minute). Hypocalcemia must be corrected before therapy initiation with risedronate. Ensure adequate calcium and vitamin D intake, especially for patients with Paget's disease in whom the pretreatment rate of bone turnover may be greatly elevated.

Bisphosphonate therapy has been associated with osteonecrosis, primarily of the jaw. Risk factors for osteonecrosis of the jaw (ONJ) include invasive dental procedures (eg, tooth extraction, dental implants, boney surgery); a diagnosis of cancer, with concomitant chemotherapy or corticosteroids; poor oral hygiene, ill-fitting dentures; and comorbid disorders (anemia, coagulopathy, infection, preexisting dental disease); risk may increase with duration of bisphosphonate use. Most reported cases occurred after IV bisphosphonate therapy; however, cases have been reported following oral therapy. A dental exam and preventive dentistry should be performed prior to placing patients with risk factors on chronic bisphosphonate therapy. The manufacturer's labeling states that discontinuing bisphosphonates in patients requiring invasive dental procedures may reduce the risk of ONJ. However, other experts suggest that there is no evidence that discontinuing therapy reduces the risk of developing ONJ (Assael, 2009). The benefit/risk must be assessed by the treating physician and/or dentist/surgeon prior to any invasive dental procedure. Patients developing ONJ while on bisphosphonates should receive care by an oral surgeon.

Atypical femur fractures have been reported in patients receiving bisphosphonates for treatment/prevention of osteoporosis. The fractures include subtrochanteric femur (bone just below the hip joint) and diaphyseal femur (long segment of the thigh bone). Some patients experience prodromal pain weeks or months before the fracture occurs. It is unclear if bisphosphonate therapy is the cause for these fractures, although the majority of cases have been reported in patients taking bisphosphonates. Patients receiving long-term (>3-5 years) therapy may be at an increased risk. Discontinue bisphosphonate therapy in patients who develop a femoral shaft fracture.

Infrequently, severe (and occasionally debilitating) bone, joint, and/or muscle pain have been reported during bisphosphonate treatment. The onset of pain ranged from a single day to several months. Consider discontinuing therapy in patients who experience severe symptoms; symptoms usually resolve upon discontinuation. Some patients experienced recurrence when rechallenged with same drug or another bisphosphonate; avoid use in patients with a history of these symptoms in association with bisphosphonate therapy.

In the management of osteoporosis, re-evaluate the need for continued therapy periodically; the optimal duration of treatment has not yet been determined. Consider discontinuing after 3-5 years of use in patients at low-risk for fracture; following discontinuation, re-evaluate fracture risk periodically. When using for glucocorticoid-induced osteoporosis, evaluate sex steroid hormonal status prior to treatment initiation; consider appropriate hormone replacement if necessary. Not approved for use in pediatric patients with osteogenesis imperfecta due to lack of efficacy in reducing the risk of fracture. Potentially significant drug-drug interactions may exist, requiring dose or frequency adjustment, additional monitoring, and/or selection of alternative therapy.

Adverse Reactions

Cardiovascular: Cardiac arrhythmia, chest pain, hypertension, peripheral edema

Central nervous system: Depression, dizziness, headache

Dermatologic: Skin rash

Endocrine & metabolic: Hypocalcemia, hypophosphatemia, increased parathyroid hormone (transient)

Gastrointestinal: Abdominal pain, constipation, diarrhea, duodenitis, dyspepsia, gastritis, glossitis, nausea, vomiting

Genitourinary: Benign prostatic hyperplasia, nephrolithiasis, urinary tract infection

Immunologic: Acute phase reaction (includes fever, influenza-like illness)

Infection: Increased susceptibility to infection

Neuromuscular & skeletal: Arthralgia, back pain, muscle spasm, myalgia, neck pain

Ophthalmic: Cataract

Respiratory: Bronchitis, dyspnea, flu-like symptoms, pharyngitis, rhinitis

Rare but important or life-threatening: Dysphagia, esophageal ulcer, esophagitis, exacerbation of asthma, femur fracture (diaphyseal, subtrochanteric), gastric ulcer, hypersensitivity reaction, malignant neoplasm of esophagus, musculoskeletal pain (rarely severe or incapacitating), osteonecrosis (primarily of the jaw)

Drug Interactions

Metabolism/Transport Effects None known.

Avoid Concomitant Use

Avoid concomitant use of Risedronate with any of the following: H2-Antagonists; Proton Pump Inhibitors

Increased Effect/Toxicity

Risedronate may increase the levels/effects of: Deferasirox; Phosphate Supplements

The levels/effects of Risedronate may be increased by: Aminoglycosides; H2-Antagonists; Nonsteroidal Anti-Inflammatory Agents; Proton Pump Inhibitors; Systemic Angiogenesis Inhibitors

Decreased Effect

The levels/effects of Risedronate may be decreased by: Antacids; Calcium Salts; Iron Salts; Magnesium Salts; Multivitamins/Minerals (with ADEK, Folate, Iron); Multivitamins/Minerals (with AE, No Iron); Proton Pump Inhibitors

Food Interactions Food reduces absorption (similar to other bisphosphonates); mean oral bioavailability is decreased when given with food. Management: Administer immediate release tablet with at least 6 oz of plain water (not mineral water) ≥30 minutes before the first food or drink of the day other than water. Administer delayed release tablet with at least 4 ounces of plain water immediately after breakfast.

Storage/Stability Store at room temperature of 20°C to 25°C (68°F to 77°F).

Mechanism of Action A bisphosphonate which inhibits bone resorption via actions on osteoclasts or on osteoclast precursors; decreases the rate of bone resorption, leading to an indirect increase in bone mineral density. In Paget's disease, characterized by disordered resorption and formation of bone, inhibition of resorption leads to an indirect decrease in bone formation; but the newly-formed bone has a more normal architecture.

Pharmacodynamics/Kinetics

Onset of action: May require weeks

Absorption: Rapid

Distribution: V_d: 13.8 L/kg

Protein binding: ~24%

Metabolism: None

Bioavailability: Poor, ~0.54% to 0.75%

Half-life elimination: Initial: 1.5 hours; Terminal: 480-561 hours

Time to peak, serum: 1-3 hours

Excretion: Urine (up to 85%); feces (as unabsorbed drug)

Dosage Note: Patients should receive supplemental calcium and vitamin D if dietary intake is inadequate. Consider discontinuing after 3-5 years of use for osteoporosis in patients at low-risk for fracture.

Paget's disease of bone: Adults: Oral: *Immediate release tablet:* 30 mg once daily for 2 months

Note: Retreatment may be considered (following post-treatment observation of at least 2 months) if relapse occurs, or if treatment fails to normalize serum alkaline phosphatase. For retreatment, the dose and duration of therapy are the same as for initial treatment. No data are available on more than one course of retreatment.

Osteoporosis (postmenopausal): Adults: Oral:

Immediate release tablet: Prevention and treatment: 5 mg once daily **or** 35 mg once weekly **or** 150 mg once a month

Delayed release tablet: Treatment: 35 mg once weekly

Osteoporosis (males) treatment: Adults: Oral: *Immediate release tablet:* 35 mg once weekly

Osteoporosis (glucocorticoid-induced) prevention and treatment: Adults: Oral: *Immediate release tablet:* 5 mg once daily

Missed doses: Immediate release tablet:

Once-weekly: If a once-weekly dose is missed, it should be given the next morning after remembered; may then return to the original once-weekly schedule (original scheduled day of the week), however, do not give 2 doses on the same day.

Monthly (150 mg once monthly): If 150 mg once-monthly dose is missed, it should be given the next morning after remembered if the next month's scheduled dose is >7 days away. If the next month's scheduled dose is within 7 days, wait until the next month's scheduled dose. For either scenario, may then return to the original monthly schedule (original scheduled day of the month). Do not give >150 mg within 7 days.

Dosage adjustment in renal impairment:

CrCl ≥30 mL/minute: No dosage adjustment necessary.

CrCl <30 mL/minute: Use is not recommended.

Dosage adjustment in hepatic impairment: No dosage adjustment provided in manufacturer's labeling (has not been studied). However, dosage adjustment unlikely because risendronate is not metabolized by the liver.

Dietary Considerations Ensure adequate calcium and vitamin D intake; if dietary intake is inadequate, dietary supplementation is recommended. Women and men should consume:

Calcium: 1000 mg/day (men: 50-70 years) **or** 1200 mg/day (women ≥51 years and men ≥71 years) (IOM, 2011; NOF, 2013)

Vitamin D: 800-1000 IU/day (men and women ≥50 years) (NOF, 2013). Recommended Dietary Allowance (RDA): 600 IU/day (men and women ≤70 years) **or** 800 IU/day (men and women ≥71 years) (IOM, 2011).

Take immediate release tablet with at least 6 oz of **plain water** (not mineral water) ≥30 minutes before the first food or drink of the day other than water. Take delayed release tablet with at least 4 ounces of **plain water** immediately **after** breakfast.

Administration Note: Avoid administration of oral calcium supplements, antacids, magnesium supplements/laxatives, and iron preparations within 30 minutes of risedronate administration.

Immediate release tablet: Risedronate immediate release tablets must be taken on an empty stomach with a full glass (6-8 oz) of **plain water** (not mineral water) at least 30 minutes before any food, drink, or other medications orally to avoid interference with absorption. Patient must remain sitting upright or standing for at least 30 minutes after taking (to reduce esophageal irritation). Tablet should be swallowed whole; do not crush or chew.

Delayed release tablet: Risedronate delayed release tablets must be taken with at least 4 oz of **plain water** (not mineral water) immediately after breakfast. Patient must remain sitting upright or standing for at least 30 minutes after taking (to reduce esophageal irritation). Tablet should be swallowed whole; do not cut, split, crush, or chew.

Monitoring Parameters

Osteoporosis: Bone mineral density (BMD) should be reevaluated every 2 years (or more frequently) after initiating therapy (NOF, 2013); in patients with combined risedronate and glucocorticoid treatment, BMD should be made at initiation and repeated after 6-12 months; annual measurements of height and weight, assessment of chronic back pain; serum calcium and 25(OH)D; consider measuring biochemical markers of bone turnover

Paget's disease: Alkaline phosphatase; pain; serum calcium and 25(OH)D

Reference Range

Calcium (total): Adults: 9.0-11.0 mg/dL (2.05-2.54 mmol/L), may slightly decrease with aging

Phosphorus: 2.5-4.5 mg/dL (0.81-1.45 mmol/L)

Vitamin D: There is no clear consensus on a reference range for total serum 25(OH)D concentrations or the validity of this level as it relates clinically to bone health. In addition, there is significant variability in the reporting of serum 25(OH)D levels as a result of different assay types in use; however, the following ranges have been suggested:

Adults (IOM, 2011): Sufficient levels in practically all persons: ≥20 ng/mL (50 nmol/L); concern for risk of toxicity: >50 ng/mL (125 nmol/L)

Osteoporosis patients (NOF, 2013): Recommended level to reach and maintain: ~30 ng/mL (75 nmol/L)

Dosage Forms

Tablet, Oral:

Actonel: 5 mg, 30 mg, 35 mg, 150 mg

Generic: 150 mg

Tablet Delayed Release, Oral:

Atelvia: 35 mg

◆ **Risedronate Sodium** *see* Risedronate *on page 1816*

◆ **RisperDAL** *see* RisperiDONE *on page 1818*

◆ **Risperdal (Can)** *see* RisperiDONE *on page 1818*

◆ **Risperdal M-Tab** *see* RisperiDONE *on page 1818*

◆ **RisperDAL M-TAB** *see* RisperiDONE *on page 1818*

◆ **RisperDAL Consta** *see* RisperiDONE *on page 1818*

◆ **Risperdal Consta (Can)** *see* RisperiDONE *on page 1818*

RisperiDONE (ris PER i done)

Brand Names: U.S. RisperDAL; RisperDAL Consta; RisperDAL M-TAB; RisperiDONE M-TAB

Brand Names: Canada ACT Risperidone; Apo-Risperidone; Ava-Risperidone; Dom-Risperidone; JAMP-Risperidone; Mar-Risperidone; Mint-Risperidon; Mylan-Risperidone; Mylan-Risperidone ODT; PHL-Risperidone; PMS-Risperidone; PMS-Risperidone ODT; PRO-Risperidone; RAN-Risperidone; ratio-Risperidone; Risperdal; Risperdal Consta; Risperdal M-Tab; Riva-Risperidone; Sandoz-Risperidone; Teva-Risperidone

Index Terms Risperdal M-Tab

Pharmacologic Category Antimanic Agent; Second Generation (Atypical) Antipsychotic

Additional Appendix Information

Beers Criteria – Potentially Inappropriate Medications for Geriatrics *on page 2271*

Use

Oral: Treatment of schizophrenia; treatment of acute mania or mixed episodes associated with bipolar I disorder (as monotherapy in children or adults, or in combination with lithium or valproate in adults); treatment of irritability/aggression associated with autistic disorder

Injection: Treatment of schizophrenia; maintenance treatment of bipolar I disorder in adults as monotherapy or in combination with lithium or valproate

Pregnancy Risk Factor C

Pregnancy Considerations Adverse events were observed in animal reproduction studies. In human studies, risperidone and its metabolite cross the placenta (Newport, 2007). An increased risk of teratogenic effects has not been observed following maternal use of risperidone (limited data) (Coppola, 2007). Agenesis of the corpus callosum has been noted in one case report of an infant exposed *in utero*; relationship to risperidone exposure is not known. Antipsychotic use during the third trimester of pregnancy has a risk for extrapyramidal symptoms (EPS) and/or withdrawal symptoms in newborns following delivery. Symptoms in the newborn may include agitation, feeding disorder, hypertonia, hypotonia, respiratory distress, somnolence, and tremor. These effects may be self-limiting and allow recovery within hours or days with no specific treatment, or they may be severe requiring prolonged hospitalization. When using Risperdal® Consta®, patients should notify healthcare provider if they become or intend to become pregnant during therapy or within 12 weeks of last injection. Risperidone may cause hyperprolactinemia, which may decrease reproductive function in both males and females.

The ACOG recommends that therapy during pregnancy be individualized; treatment with psychiatric medications during pregnancy should incorporate the clinical expertise of the mental health clinician, obstetrician, primary healthcare provider, and pediatrician. Safety data related to atypical antipsychotics during pregnancy is limited and routine use is not recommended. However, if a woman is inadvertently exposed to an atypical antipsychotic while pregnant, continuing therapy may be preferable to switching to a typical antipsychotic that the fetus has not yet been exposed to; consider risk:benefit (ACOG, 2008).

Healthcare providers are encouraged to enroll women 18-45 years of age exposed to risperidone during pregnancy in the Atypical Antipsychotics Pregnancy Registry (1-866-961-2388 or http://www.womensmentalhealth.org/pregnancyregistry).

Breast-Feeding Considerations Risperidone and its metabolite are excreted in breast milk. Due to the potential for serious adverse reactions in the nursing infant, the manufacturer recommends a decision be made whether to discontinue nursing or to discontinue the drug, taking into account the importance of treatment to the mother. It is also recommended that women using Risperdal Consta not breast-feed during therapy or for 12 weeks after the last injection.

Contraindications Hypersensitivity to risperidone or any component of the formulation

Warnings/Precautions Hazardous agent - use appropriate precautions for handling and disposal (NIOSH 2014 [group 2]).

[U.S. Boxed Warning]: Elderly patients with dementia-related psychosis treated with antipsychotics are at an increased risk of death compared to placebo. Most deaths appeared to be either cardiovascular (eg, heart failure, sudden death) or infectious (eg, pneumonia) in nature. In addition, an increased incidence of cerebrovascular effects (eg, transient ischemic attack, cerebrovascular accidents) has been reported in studies of placebo-controlled trials of risperidone in elderly patients with dementia-related psychosis. Risperidone is not approved for the treatment of dementia-related psychosis.

Leukopenia, neutropenia, and agranulocytosis (sometimes fatal) have been reported in clinical trials and postmarketing reports with antipsychotic use; presence of risk factors (eg, preexisting low WBC or history of drug-induced leuko-/neutropenia) should prompt periodic blood count assessment. Discontinue therapy at first signs of blood dyscrasias or if absolute neutrophil count <1000/mm^3.

Low to moderately sedating, use with caution in disorders where CNS depression is a feature. Effects with other sedative drugs or ethanol may be potentiated. Use with caution in Parkinson's disease. Caution in patients with predisposition to seizures. Use with caution in renal or hepatic dysfunction; dose reduction recommended. Esophageal dysmotility and aspiration have been associated with antipsychotic use; use with caution in patients at risk of aspiration pneumonia (ie, Alzheimer's disease). Risperidone is associated with greater increases in prolactin levels as compared to other antipsychotic agents; clinical significance of hyperprolactinemia in patients with breast cancer or other prolactin-dependent tumors is unknown. May alter temperature regulation. May mask toxicity of other drugs or conditions (eg, intestinal obstruction, Reyes syndrome, brain tumor) due to antiemetic effects. Neutropenia has been reported with antipsychotic use, including fatal cases of agranulocytosis. Preexisting myelosuppression (disease or drug-induced) increases risk and these patients should have frequent CBC monitoring; decreased blood counts in absence of other causative factors should prompt discontinuation of therapy.

Use with caution in patients with cardiovascular diseases (eg, heart failure, history of myocardial infarction or ischemia, cerebrovascular disease, conduction abnormalities). May cause orthostatic hypotension; use with caution in patients at risk of this effect (eg, concurrent medication use which may predispose to hypotension/bradycardia or presence of hypovolemia) or in those who would not tolerate transient hypotensive episodes. May alter cardiac conduction (low risk relative to other neuroleptics); life-threatening arrhythmias have occurred with therapeutic doses of neuroleptics.

May cause anticholinergic effects (confusion, agitation, constipation, xerostomia, blurred vision, urinary retention); therefore, they should be used with caution in patients with decreased gastrointestinal motility, urinary retention, BPH, xerostomia, or visual problems (including narrow-angle glaucoma). Relative to other neuroleptics, risperidone has a low potency of cholinergic blockade. Few case reports describe intraoperative floppy iris syndrome (IFIS) in patients receiving risperidone and undergoing cataract surgery (Ford, 2011). Prior to cataract surgery, evaluate for prior or current risperidone use. The benefits or risks of interrupting risperidone prior to surgery have not been established; clinicians are advised to proceed with surgery cautiously.

May cause extrapyramidal symptoms, including pseudoparkinsonism, acute dystonic reactions, akathisia, and tardive dyskinesia. Risk of dystonia (and possibly other EPS) may be greater with increased doses, use of conventional antipsychotics, males, and younger patients. Risk of tardive dyskinesia and potential for irreversibility may be increased in elderly patients (particularly women), prolonged therapy, and higher total cumulative dose. Risk of neuroleptic malignant syndrome (NMS) may be increased in patients with Parkinson's disease or Lewy body dementia; monitor for symptoms of confusion, obtundation, postural instability and extrapyramidal symptoms. May cause hyperglycemia; in some cases may be extreme and associated with ketoacidosis, hyperosmolar coma, or death. Use with caution in patients with diabetes or other disorders of glucose regulation; monitor for worsening of glucose control. Dyslipidemia has been reported with atypical antipsychotics; risk profile may differ between agents. Discrepant results have been reported in clinical trials, regarding lipid changes associated with risperidone (American Diabetes Association, 2004). Significant weight gain has been observed with antipsychotic therapy; incidence varies with product. Monitor waist circumference and BMI. Rare cases of priapism have been reported.

Use in elderly patients with dementia is associated with an increased risk of mortality and cerebrovascular accidents; avoid antipsychotic use for behavioral problems associated with dementia unless alternative nonpharmacologic therapies have failed and patient may harm self or others. In addition, use may cause or exacerbate syndrome of inappropriate antidiuretic hormone secretion or hyponatremia; monitor sodium closely with initiation or dosage adjustments in older adults (Beers Criteria).

The possibility of a suicide attempt is inherent in psychotic illness or bipolar disorder; use caution in high-risk patients during initiation of therapy. Prescriptions should be written for the smallest quantity consistent with good patient care. Long-term effects on growth or sexual maturation have not been evaluated. Vehicle used in injectable (polylactide-co-glycolide microspheres) has rarely been associated with retinal artery occlusion in patients with abnormal arteriovenous anastomosis.

Benzyl alcohol and derivatives: Some dosage forms may contain sodium benzoate/benzoic acid; benzoic acid (benzoate) is a metabolite of benzyl alcohol; large amounts of benzyl alcohol (≥99 mg/kg/day) have been associated with a potentially fatal toxicity ("gasping syndrome") in neonates; the "gasping syndrome" consists of metabolic acidosis, respiratory distress, gasping respirations, CNS dysfunction (including convulsions, intracranial hemorrhage), hypotension, and cardiovascular collapse (AAP, 1997; CDC, 1982); some data suggests that benzoate displaces bilirubin from protein binding sites (Ahlfors, 2001); avoid or use dosage forms containing benzyl alcohol derivative with caution in neonates. See manufacturer's labeling.

Adverse Reactions

Cardiovascular: Bradycardia, bundle branch block, buttock pain, chest pain, ECG changes, facial edema, first degree atrioventricular block, hypertension, hypotension, orthostatic hypotension, palpitations, paresthesia, peripheral edema, prolonged Q-T interval on ECG, syncope, tachycardia (more common in adults)

Central nervous system: Abnormal gait, agitation, akathisia, anxiety, ataxia, decreased attention span, depression, disturbed sleep, dizziness, drooling (more common in children), drowsiness (more common in adults), dystonia, falling, fatigue (more common in children), headache, hypoesthesia, insomnia, lethargy, malaise, nervousness, orthostatic dizziness, pain, parkinsonian-like syndrome (more common in children), sedation (more common in children), seizure, tardive dyskinesia, vertigo

Dermatologic: Acne vulgaris, eczema, pruritus, skin sclerosis, skin rash, xeroderma

Endocrine & metabolic: Amenorrhea, decreased libido, galactorrhea, gynecomastia, hyperglycemia, hyperprolactinemia, increased gamma-glutamyl transferase, increased thirst (more common in children), oligomenorrhea, weight gain (more common in children), weight loss

Gastrointestinal: Abdominal pain (more common in children), anorexia, constipation, decreased appetite, diarrhea, dyspepsia, gastritis, gastroenteritis, increased appetite (more common in children), nausea, sialorrhea, toothache, vomiting (more common in children), xerostomia

Genitourinary: Cystitis, ejaculatory disorder, erectile dysfunction, glycosuria, irregular menses, mastalgia, menstruation, sexual disorder, urinary incontinence (more common in children), urinary tract infection

Hematologic & oncologic: Anemia, neutropenia

Hepatic: Increased serum ALT, increased serum AST

Hypersensitivity: Hypersensitivity

Infection: Infection, influenza, localized infection, subcutaneous abscess, viral infection

Local: Induration at injection site, injection site reaction, pain at injection site, swelling at injection site

Neuromuscular & skeletal: Abnormal posture, akinesia, arthralgia, back pain, dyskinesia (more common in adults), hypokinesia, increased creatine phosphokinase, limb pain, musculoskeletal chest pain, myalgia, neck pain, tremor (more common in adults), weakness

Ophthalmic: Blurred vision, conjunctivitis, reduced visual acuity

Otic: Otalgia, otic infection

Respiratory: bronchitis, cough (more common in children), dyspnea, epistaxis, flu-like symptoms, nasal congestion, nasopharyngitis (more common in children), pharyngitis, pharyngolaryngeal pain, pneumonia, respiratory tract infection, rhinitis, rhinorrhea (more common in children), sinus congestion, sinusitis

Miscellaneous: Fever (more common in children)

Rare but important or life-threatening: Abnormal erythrocytes, abscess at injection site, acariasis, agranulocytosis, alopecia, anaphylaxis, angioedema, apnea, aspiration, atrial fibrillation, atrial premature contractions, cardiorespiratory arrest, cerebral ischemia, cerebrovascular accident, cholestatic hepatitis, cholinergic syndrome, coma, cyst, delirium, depression of ST segment on ECG, dermal ulcer, diabetes mellitus, diabetic coma, diabetic ketoacidosis, disruption of body temperature regulation, diverticulitis, esophageal motility disorder, eye infection, fecal incontinence, fecaloma, glaucoma, granulocytopenia, hematoma, hemorrhage, hepatic failure, hepatic injury, hyperkeratosis, hyperthermia, hypertonia, hypertriglyceridemia, hyperuricemia, hypoglycemia, hypokalemia, hyponatremia, hypothermia, impaired consciousness, increased serum cholesterol, intestinal obstruction, intraoperative floppy iris syndrome, leukocytosis, leukopenia, leukorrhea, lower respiratory tract infection, lymphadenopathy, mania, migraine, myocardial infarction, myocarditis, neuroleptic malignant syndrome, nystagmus, ocular hyperemia, pancreatitis, Pelger-Huët anomaly, phlebitis, pituitary neoplasm, precocious puberty, priapism, pulmonary embolism, renal insufficiency, retinal artery occlusion, retrograde ejaculation, rhabdomyolysis, SIADH, sleep apnea, swelling of eye, synostosis, thrombocytopenia, thrombophlebitis, thrombotic thrombocytopenic purpura, tissue necrosis, tongue paralysis, torticollis, transient ischemic attacks, unresponsive to stimuli, urinary retention, ventricular premature contractions, ventricular tachycardia, water intoxication, withdrawal syndrome

Drug Interactions

Metabolism/Transport Effects Substrate of CYP2D6 (major), CYP3A4 (minor), P-glycoprotein; **Note:** Assignment of Major/Minor substrate status based on clinically relevant drug interaction potential; **Inhibits** CYP2D6 (weak), CYP3A4 (weak)

Avoid Concomitant Use

Avoid concomitant use of RisperiDONE with any of the following: Aclidinium; Amisulpride; Azelastine (Nasal); Glucagon; Ipratropium (Oral Inhalation); Metoclopramide; Orphenadrine; Paraldehyde; Pimozide; Potassium Chloride; Sulpiride; Thalidomide; Tiotropium; Umeclidinium

Increased Effect/Toxicity

RisperiDONE may increase the levels/effects of: AbobotulinumtoxinA; Alcohol (Ethyl); Amisulpride; Analgesics (Opioid); Anticholinergic Agents; ARIPiprazole; Azelastine (Nasal); Buprenorphine; CNS Depressants; Glucagon; Highest Risk QTc-Prolonging Agents; Hydrocodone; Lomitapide; Methotrimeprazine; Methylphenidate; Metyrosine; Mirabegron; Mirtazapine; Moderate Risk QTc-Prolonging Agents; OnabotulinumtoxinA; Orphenadrine; Paliperidone; Paraldehyde; Pimozide; Potassium Chloride; RimabotulinumtoxinB; Selective Serotonin Reuptake Inhibitors; Serotonin Modulators; Sulpiride; Suvorexant; Thalidomide; Tiotropium; Topiramate; Zolpidem

The levels/effects of RisperiDONE may be increased by: Abiraterone Acetate; Acetylcholinesterase Inhibitors (Central); Aclidinium; Brimonidine (Topical); Cannabis; Cobicistat; CYP2D6 Inhibitors (Moderate); CYP2D6 Inhibitors (Strong); Darunavir; Doxylamine; Dronabinol; Droperidol; HydrOXYzine; Hypotensive Agents; Ipratropium (Oral Inhalation); Kava Kava; Lithium; Loop Diuretics; Magnesium Sulfate; Methotrimeprazine; Methylphenidate; Metoclopramide; Metyrosine; Mianserin; Mifepristone; Nabilone; Peginterferon Alfa-2b; Perampanel; P-glycoprotein/ABCB1 Inhibitors; Pramlintide; Rufinamide; Selective Serotonin Reuptake Inhibitors; Serotonin Modulators; Sodium Oxybate; Tapentadol; Tetrahydrocannabinol; Umeclidinium; Valproic Acid and Derivatives; Verapamil

Decreased Effect

RisperiDONE may decrease the levels/effects of: Acetylcholinesterase Inhibitors; Amphetamines; Anti-Parkinson's Agents (Dopamine Agonist); Itopride; Quinagolide; Secretin

The levels/effects of RisperiDONE may be decreased by: Acetylcholinesterase Inhibitors; CarBAMazepine; Lithium; Peginterferon Alfa-2b; P-glycoprotein/ABCB1 Inducers

Food Interactions Oral solution is not compatible with beverages containing tannin or pectinate (cola or tea). Management: Administer oral solution with water, coffee, orange juice, or low-fat milk.

Preparation for Administration Hazardous agent; use appropriate precautions for handling and disposal (NIOSH 2014 [group 2]).

Risperdal® Consta®: Bring to room temperature prior to reconstitution. Reconstitute with provided diluent only. Shake vigorously to mix; will form thick, milky suspension. Following reconstitution, store at room temperature and use within 6 hours. Suspension settles in ~2 minutes; shake vigorously to resuspend prior to administration.

Storage/Stability

Injection: Risperdal® Consta®: Store in refrigerator at 2°C to 8°C (36°F to 46°F) and protect from light. May be stored at room temperature of 25°C (77°F) for up to 7 days prior to administration. Following reconstitution, store at room temperature and use within 6 hours. Suspension settles in ~2 minutes; shake vigorously to resuspend prior to administration.

Oral solution, tablet: Store at 15°C to 25°C (59°F to 77°F). Protect from light and moisture. Keep orally-disintegrating tablets sealed in foil pouch until ready to use. Do not freeze solution.

Mechanism of Action Risperidone is a benzisoxazole atypical antipsychotic with mixed serotonin-dopamine antagonist activity that binds to 5-HT_2-receptors in the CNS and in the periphery with a very high affinity; binds to dopamine-D_2 receptors with less affinity. The binding affinity to the dopamine-D_2 receptor is 20 times lower than the 5-HT_2 affinity. The addition of serotonin antagonism to dopamine antagonism (classic neuroleptic mechanism) is thought to improve negative symptoms of psychoses and reduce the incidence of extrapyramidal side effects. $Alpha_1$, $alpha_2$ adrenergic, and histaminergic receptors are also antagonized with high affinity. Risperidone has low to moderate affinity for 5-HT_{1C}, 5-HT_{1D}, and 5-HT_{1A} receptors, weak affinity for D_1 and no affinity for muscarinics or $beta_1$ and $beta_2$ receptors

Pharmacodynamics/Kinetics

Absorption:

Oral: Rapid and well absorbed; food does not affect rate or extent

Injection: <1% absorbed initially; main release occurs at ~3 weeks and is maintained from 4-6 weeks

Distribution: V_d: 1-2 L/kg

Protein binding, plasma: Risperidone 90%; 9-hydroxyrisperidone: 77%

Metabolism: Extensively hepatic via CYP2D6 to 9-hydroxyrisperidone (similar pharmacological activity as risperidone); *N*-dealkylation is a second minor pathway

Bioavailability: Oral: 70%; Tablet (relative to solution): 94%; orally-disintegrating tablets and oral solution are bioequivalent to tablets

Half-life elimination: Active moiety (risperidone and its active metabolite 9-hydroxyrisperidone)

Oral: 20 hours (mean)

Extensive metabolizers: Risperidone: 3 hours; 9-hydroxyrisperidone: 21 hours

Poor metabolizers: Risperidone: 20 hours; 9-hydroxyrisperidone: 30 hours

Injection: 3-6 days; related to microsphere erosion and subsequent absorption of risperidone

Time to peak, plasma: Oral: Risperidone: Within 1 hour; 9-hydroxyrisperidone: Extensive metabolizers: 3 hours; Poor metabolizers: 17 hours

Excretion: Urine (70%); feces (14%)

Dosage Note: When reinitiating treatment after discontinuation, the initial titration schedule should be followed.

Oral:

Children ≥5 years and Adolescents: Autism:

<15 kg: Use with caution; specific dosing recommendations not available

15 to <20 kg: Initial: 0.25 mg daily; may increase dose to 0.5 mg daily after ≥4 days, maintain dose for ≥14 days. In patients not achieving sufficient clinical response, may increase dose by 0.25 mg daily in ≥2-week intervals. Doses ranging from 0.5-3 mg daily have been evaluated; however, therapeutic effect reached plateau at 1 mg daily in clinical trials. Following clinical response, consider gradually lowering dose. May be administered once daily or in divided doses twice daily.

≥20 kg: Initial: 0.5 mg daily; may increase dose to 1 mg daily after ≥4 days, maintain dose for ≥14 days. In patients not achieving sufficient clinical response, may increase dose by 0.5 mg daily in ≥2-week intervals. Doses ranging from 0.5-3 mg daily have been evaluated; however, therapeutic effect reached plateau at 2.5 mg daily (3 mg daily in children >45 kg) in clinical trials. Following clinical response, consider gradually lowering dose. May be administered once daily or in divided doses twice daily.

Children and Adolescents:

Schizophrenia: Adolescents 13-17 years: Initial: 0.5 mg once daily; dose may be adjusted in increments of 0.5-1 mg daily at intervals ≥24 hours to a dose of 3 mg daily. Doses ranging from 1-6 mg daily have been evaluated, however, doses >3 mg daily do not confer additional benefit and are associated with increased adverse events.

Bipolar mania: Children and Adolescents 10-17 years: Initial: 0.5 mg once daily; dose may be adjusted in increments of 0.5-1 mg daily at intervals ≥24 hours to a dose of 1-2.5 mg daily. Doses ranging from 0.5-6 mg daily have been evaluated; however doses >2.5 mg daily do not confer additional benefit and are associated with increased adverse events.

Maintenance: No dosing recommendation available for treatment >3 weeks duration

Adolescents and Adults: Tourette's syndrome (off-label use): Initial: 0.25 mg once daily for 2 days, then 0.25 mg twice daily for 3 days, then 0.5 mg twice daily for 2 days; titrate slowly thereafter in increments/decrements ≤0.5 mg twice daily and at intervals ≥3 days; maximum dose: 6 mg daily (Dion, 2002)

Adults:

Schizophrenia:

Initial: 2 mg daily in 1-2 divided doses; may be increased by 1-2 mg daily at intervals ≥24 hours to a recommended dosage range of 4-8 mg daily; may be given as a single daily dose once maintenance dose is achieved; daily dosages >6 mg do not appear to confer any additional benefit, and the incidence of extrapyramidal symptoms is higher than with lower doses. Further dose adjustments should be made in increments/decrements of 1-2 mg daily on a weekly basis. Dose range studied in clinical trials: 4-16 mg daily.

Maintenance: Recommended dosage range: 2-8 mg daily

Bipolar mania:

Initial: 2-3 mg once daily; if needed, adjust dose by 1 mg daily in intervals ≥24 hours; dosing range: 1-6 mg daily

Maintenance: No dosing recommendation available for treatment >3 weeks duration.

Post-traumatic stress disorder (PTSD) (off-label use): 0.5-8 mg daily (Bandelow, 2008; Benedek, 2009)

Elderly:

Initial: 0.5 mg twice daily; titration should progress slowly in increments of no more than 0.5 mg twice daily; increases to dosages >1.5 mg twice daily should occur at intervals of ≥1 week.

Note: Additional monitoring of renal function and orthostatic blood pressure may be warranted. If once-a-day dosing in the elderly or debilitated patient is considered, a twice daily regimen should be used to titrate to the target dose, and this dose should be maintained for 2-3 days prior to attempts to switch to a once-daily regimen.

Psychosis/agitation related to Alzheimer's dementia (off-label use): Initial: 0.25-1 mg daily; if necessary, gradually increase as tolerated not to exceed 1.5-2 mg daily; doses >1 mg daily are associated with higher rates of extrapyramidal symptoms (Rabins, 2007)

IM: **Note:** Oral risperidone (or other antipsychotic) should be administered with the initial injection of Risperdal® Consta® and continued for 3 weeks (then discontinued) to maintain adequate therapeutic plasma concentrations prior to main release phase of risperidone from injection site. When switching from depot administration to a short-acting formulation, administer short-acting agent in place of the next regularly-scheduled depot injection.

Adults: Schizophrenia, bipolar I maintenance (Risperdal® Consta®): Initial: 25 mg every 2 weeks; if unresponsive, some may benefit from larger doses (37.5-50 mg); maximum dose: 50 mg every 2 weeks. Dosage adjustments should not be made more frequently than every 4 weeks. A lower initial dose of 12.5 mg may be appropriate in some patients (eg, demonstrated poor tolerability to other psychotropic medications).

Elderly (Risperdal® Consta®): 25 mg every 2 weeks; a lower initial dose of 12.5 mg may be appropriate in some patients

Dosing adjustment in renal impairment: Adults:

Oral: CrCl <30 mL/minute: Starting dose of 0.5 mg twice daily; titration should progress slowly in increments of no more than 0.5 mg twice daily; increases to dosages >1.5 mg twice daily should occur at intervals of ≥1 week. Clearance of the active moiety is decreased by 60% in patients with moderate-to-severe renal disease (CrCl <60 mL/minute) compared to healthy subjects.

IM: Initiate with **oral** dosing (0.5 mg twice daily for 1 week then 2 mg daily for 1 week); if tolerated, begin 25 mg **IM** every 2 weeks; continue oral dosing for 3 weeks after the first IM injection. An initial IM dose of 12.5 mg may also be considered.

Dosing adjustment in hepatic impairment: Adults:

Oral: Child-Pugh class C: Starting dose of 0.5 mg twice daily; titration should progress slowly in increments of no more than 0.5 mg twice daily; increases to dosages >1.5 mg twice daily should occur at intervals of ≥1 week. The mean free fraction of risperidone in plasma was increased by 35% in patients with hepatic impairment compared to healthy subjects.

IM: Initiate with **oral** dosing (0.5 mg twice daily for 1 week then 2 mg daily for 1 week); if tolerated, begin 25 mg **IM** every 2 weeks; continue oral dosing for 3 weeks after the first IM injection. An initial IM dose of 12.5 mg may also be considered.

Dietary Considerations May be taken without regard to meals. Some products may contain phenylalanine.

Administration

Oral: May be administered without regard to meals.

Oral solution can be administered directly from the provided pipette or may be mixed with water, coffee, orange juice, or low-fat milk, but is **not compatible** with cola or tea.

In children or adolescents experiencing somnolence, half the daily dose may be administered twice daily **or** the once-daily dose may be administered at bedtime.

Risperdal® M-Tab® should not be removed from blister pack until administered. Do not push tablet through foil (tablet may become damaged); peel back foil to expose tablet. Using dry hands, place immediately on tongue. Tablet will dissolve within seconds, and may be swallowed with or without liquid. Do not split or chew.

IM: Risperdal® Consta® should be administered into either the deltoid muscle or the upper outer quadrant of the gluteal area. Avoid inadvertent injection into vasculature. Injection should alternate between the two arms or buttocks. Do not combine two different dosage strengths into one single administration. Do not substitute any components of the dose-pack; administer with needle provided (1-inch needle for deltoid administration or 2-inch needle for gluteal administration).

Hazardous agent; use appropriate precautions for handling and disposal (NIOSH 2014 [group 2]).

Monitoring Parameters Mental status; vital signs (as clinically indicated); blood pressure (baseline; repeat 3 months after antipsychotic initiation, then yearly); weight, height, BMI, waist circumference (baseline; repeat at 4, 8, and 12 weeks after initiating or changing therapy, then quarterly; consider switching to a different antipsychotic for a weight gain ≥5% of initial weight); CBC (as clinically indicated; monitor frequently during the first few months of therapy in patients with preexisting low WBC or history of drug-induced leukopenia/neutropenia); electrolytes, renal and liver function (annually and as clinically indicated); personal and family history of obesity, diabetes, dyslipidemia, hypertension, or cardiovascular disease (baseline; repeat annually); fasting plasma glucose level/HbA_{1c} (baseline; repeat 3 months after starting antipsychotic, then yearly); fasting lipid panel (baseline; repeat 3 months after initiation of antipsychotic; if LDL level is normal repeat at 2-5 year intervals or more frequently if clinical indicated); changes in menstruation, libido, development of galactorrhea, erectile and ejaculatory function (at each visit for the first 12 weeks after the antipsychotic is initiated or until the dose is stable, then yearly); abnormal involuntary movements or parkinsonian signs (baseline; repeat weekly until dose stabilized for at least 2 weeks after introduction and for 2 weeks after any significant dose increase); tardive dyskinesia (every 12 months; high-risk patients every 6 months); ocular examination (yearly in patients >40 years; every 2 years in younger patients) (ADA, 2004; Lehman, 2004; Marder, 2004).

Additional Information Risperdal® Consta® is an injectable formulation of risperidone using the extended release Medisorb® drug-delivery system; small polymeric microspheres degrade slowly, releasing the medication at a controlled rate.

Dosage Forms

Solution, Oral:

RisperDAL: 1 mg/mL (30 mL)

Generic: 1 mg/mL (30 mL)

Suspension Reconstituted, Intramuscular:

RisperDAL Consta: 12.5 mg (1 ea); 25 mg (1 ea); 37.5 mg (1 ea); 50 mg (1 ea)

Tablet, Oral:

RisperDAL: 0.25 mg, 0.5 mg, 1 mg, 2 mg, 3 mg, 4 mg

Generic: 0.25 mg, 0.5 mg, 1 mg, 2 mg, 3 mg, 4 mg

Tablet Dispersible, Oral:

RisperDAL M-TAB: 0.5 mg, 1 mg, 2 mg, 3 mg, 4 mg

RisperiDONE M-TAB: 0.5 mg, 1 mg, 2 mg, 3 mg, 4 mg

Generic: 0.25 mg, 0.5 mg, 1 mg, 2 mg, 3 mg, 4 mg

- ◆ **RisperiDONE M-TAB** *see* RisperiDONE *on page 1818*
- ◆ **Ritalin** *see* Methylphenidate *on page 1336*
- ◆ **Ritalin LA** *see* Methylphenidate *on page 1336*
- ◆ **Ritalin SR [DSC]** *see* Methylphenidate *on page 1336*
- ◆ **Ritalin SR (Can)** *see* Methylphenidate *on page 1336*

Ritonavir (ri TOE na veer)

Brand Names: U.S. Norvir

Brand Names: Canada Norvir; Norvir SEC

Pharmacologic Category Antiretroviral, Protease Inhibitor (Anti-HIV)

Use Treatment of HIV infection; should always be used as part of a multidrug regimen

Pregnancy Risk Factor B

Pregnancy Considerations Adverse events were observed in animal reproduction studies only with doses which were also maternally toxic. Ritonavir has a low level of transfer across the human placenta; no increased risk of overall birth defects has been observed following first trimester exposure according to data collected by the antiretroviral pregnancy registry. Early studies have shown lower plasma levels during pregnancy compared to postpartum, however dosage adjustment is not needed when used as a low-dose booster in pregnant women. The DHHS Perinatal HIV Guidelines consider ritonavir to be a preferred protease inhibitor (PI) for use during pregnancy when used as a booster for other Pis (not recommended as a single protease inhibitor in ART naïve pregnant women). The oral solution contains alcohol and therefore may not be the best formulation for use in pregnancy. A small increased risk of preterm birth has been associated with maternal use of protease inhibitor-based combination antiretroviral (ARV) therapy during pregnancy; however, the benefits of use generally outweigh this risk and PIs should not be withheld if otherwise recommended. Hyperglycemia, new onset of diabetes mellitus, or diabetic ketoacidosis have been reported with protease inhibitors; it is not clear if pregnancy increases this risk.

Regardless of CD4 count or HIV RNA copy number, all HIV-infected pregnant women should receive a combination antiretroviral ARV drug regimen. A combination of antepartum, intrapartum, and infant ARV prophylaxis is recommended. ARV therapy should be started as soon as possible in women with symptomatic infection. Although earlier initiation may be more effective in reducing the perinatal transmission of HIV, initiation may be delayed until after 12 weeks gestation in women who do not require immediate treatment after careful consideration of maternal conditions (eg, nausea and vomiting) and the potential risks of first trimester fetal exposure for specific agents. A scheduled cesarean delivery at 38 weeks gestation is recommended for all women with HIV RNA >1000 copies/mL or unknown concentrations near delivery in order to decrease transmission. If ARV therapy must be interrupted for <24 hours during the peripartum period, stop then restart all medications simultaneously in order to decrease the chance of developing resistance. Long-term follow-up is recommended for all infants exposed to ARV medications. In couples who want to conceive, the HIV-infected partner should attain maximum viral suppression prior to conception.

Health care providers are encouraged to enroll pregnant women exposed to antiretroviral medications in the Antiretroviral Pregnancy Registry (1-800-258-4263 or www.APRegistry.com). Health care providers caring for HIV-infected women and their infants may contact the National Perinatal HIV Hotline (888-448-8765) for clinical consultation (HHS [perinatal], 2014).

Breast-Feeding Considerations It is not known if ritonavir is excreted into breast milk; serum concentrations in nursing infants were undetectable at 12 weeks of age. Maternal or infant antiretroviral therapy does not completely eliminate the risk of postnatal HIV transmission. In addition, multiclass-resistant virus has been detected in breast-feeding infants despite maternal therapy. Therefore, in the United States, where formula is accessible, affordable, safe, and sustainable, and the risk of infant mortality due to diarrhea and respiratory infections is low, complete avoidance of breast-feeding by HIV-infected women is recommended to decrease potential transmission of HIV (HHS [perinatal], 2014).

Contraindications Hypersensitivity to ritonavir or any component of the formulation; concurrent alfuzosin, amiodarone, cisapride, dihydroergotamine, ergonovine, ergotamine, flecainide, lovastatin, methylergonovine, midazolam (oral), pimozide, propafenone, quinidine, sildenafil (when used for the treatment of pulmonary arterial hypertension [eg, Revatio®]), simvastatin, St John's wort, triazolam, and voriconazole (when ritonavir ≥800 mg/day)

Canadian labeling: Additional contraindications (not in U.S. labeling): Concurrent use with rivaroxaban, voriconazole (regardless of ritonavir dose), salmeterol, vardenafil, bepridil, astemizole, or terfenadine

Warnings/Precautions **[U.S. Boxed Warning]: Ritonavir may interact with many medications, including antiarrhythmics, ergot alkaloids, and sedatives/hypnotics, resulting in potentially serious and/or life-threatening adverse events.** Some interactions may require dose or frequency adjustment, additional monitoring, and/or selection of alternative therapy. Pancreatitis has been observed (including fatalities); use with caution in patients with increased triglycerides; monitor serum lipase and amylase and for gastrointestinal symptoms. Increases in total cholesterol and triglycerides have been reported; screening should be done prior to therapy and periodically throughout treatment. Temporary or permanent discontinuation may be clinically indicated.

Protease inhibitors have been associated with a variety of hypersensitivity events (some severe), including rash, anaphylaxis (rare), angioedema, bronchospasm, erythema multiforme, toxic epidermal necrolysis, and/or Stevens-Johnson syndrome (rare). It is generally recommended to discontinue treatment if severe rash or moderate symptoms accompanied by other systemic symptoms occur. Use with caution in patients with cardiomyopathy, ischemic heart disease, preexisting conduction abnormalities, or structural heart disease; may be at increased risk of conduction abnormalities (eg, second- or third-degree AV block). Ritonavir has been associated with AV block due to prolongation of PR interval; use caution with drugs that prolong the PR interval. Use with caution in patients with hemophilia A or B; increased bleeding during protease inhibitor therapy has been reported and additional Factor VIII may be needed. Changes in glucose tolerance, hyperglycemia, exacerbation of diabetes, DKA, and new-onset diabetes mellitus have been reported in patients receiving protease inhibitors. May be associated with fat redistribution (buffalo hump, increased abdominal girth, breast engorgement, facial atrophy, and dyslipidemia). Immune reconstitution syndrome may develop resulting in the occurrence of an inflammatory response to an indolent or residual opportunistic infection during initial HIV treatment or activation of autoimmune disorders (eg, Graves' disease, polymyositis, Guillain-Barré syndrome) later in therapy; further evaluation and treatment may be required. May cause hepatitis or exacerbate preexisting hepatic dysfunction (including fatalities); use with caution in patients with hepatitis B or C, cirrhosis, or those with high baseline transaminases; consider increased monitoring of transaminases in these patients. Norvir® tablets are **not** bioequivalent to Norvir® capsules. Gastrointestinal side effects (eg, nausea, vomiting, abdominal pain, diarrhea) or paresthesias may be more common when patients are switching from the capsule to the tablet formulation due to a higher C_{max} (26% increase) observed with the tablet formulation compared to the capsule. These side effects should decrease as therapy is continued.

Oral solution contains ethanol and propylene glycol; healthcare providers should pay special attention to accurate calculation, measurement, and administration of dose; ethanol competitively inhibits propylene glycol metabolism; preterm infants may be at increased risk of toxicity due to decreased ability to metabolize propylene glycol. Postmarketing adverse reactions (cardiac toxicity, lactic acidosis, renal failure, CNS depression, respiratory complications, acute renal failure including fatalities) have been reported in preterm neonates receiving ritonavir-containing solutions. Do not use in neonates with a postmenstrual age (first day of mother's last menstrual period to birth plus elapsed time after birth) <44 weeks, unless benefit outweighs risk and neonate is closely monitored (serum creatinine and osmolality, CNS depression, renal toxicity, lactic acidosis, cardiac conduction abnormalities, hemolysis).

Adverse Reactions

Cardiovascular: Edema (including peripheral edema), flushing, hypertension, syncope, vasodilatation

Central nervous system: Anxiety, confusion, depression, disturbance in attention, dizziness, drowsiness, fatigue, headache, insomnia, malaise, paresthesia, peripheral neuropathy

Dermatologic: Acne vulgaris, diaphoresis, pruritus, skin rash

Endocrine & metabolic: Hypercholesterolemia, increased serum triglycerides, increased uric acid, lipodystrophy (acquired)

Gastrointestinal: Abdominal pain, anorexia, diarrhea, dysgeusia, dyspepsia, flatulence, gastrointestinal hemorrhage, increased serum amylase (pediatric), nausea, throat irritation (local), vomiting

Hematologic & oncologic: Anemia (pediatric), neutropenia (pediatric), thrombocytopenia (pediatric)

Hepatic: Hepatitis, increased gamma-glutamyl transferase, increased serum ALT, increased serum AST

Hypersensitivity: Hypersensitivity reaction

Neuromuscular & skeletal: Increased creatine phosphokinase, musculoskeletal pain (arthralgia and back pain), myalgia, weakness

Ophthalmic: Blurred vision

Renal: Polyuria

Respiratory: Cough, oropharyngeal pain, pharyngitis

Miscellaneous: Fever

Rare but important or life-threatening: Adrenal suppression, adrenocortical cortex insufficiency, anaphylaxis, amnesia, angioedema, aphasia, asthma, atrioventricular block (first, second, or third degree), cachexia, cerebral ischemia, chest pain, cholestatic jaundice, coma, Cushing's syndrome, dementia, depersonalization, diabetes mellitus, diabetic ketoacidosis, esophageal ulcer, gastroenteritis, gastroesophageal reflux disease, gout, hallucination, hematologic disease (myeloproliferative), hemorrhage (in patients with hemophilia A or B), hepatic coma, hepatitis, hepatomegaly, hepatosplenomegaly, hyperglycemia, hypotension, hypothermia, hypoventilation, immune reconstitution syndrome, intestinal obstruction, leukemia (acute myeloblastic), leukopenia, lymphadenopathy, lymphocytosis, malignant melanoma, manic behavior, myocardial infarction, neuropathy, orthostatic hypotension, palpitations, pancreatitis, paralysis, pneumonia, prolongation P-R interval on ECG, prolonged Q-T interval on ECG, pseudomembranous colitis, rectal hemorrhage, redistribution of body fat, renal failure, renal insufficiency, right bundle branch block, seizure, Stevens-Johnson syndrome, subdural hematoma, syncope, tachycardia, torsades de pointes, toxic epidermal necrolysis, ulcerative colitis, vasospasm, venous thrombosis (cerebral)

Drug Interactions

Metabolism/Transport Effects Substrate of CYP1A2 (minor), CYP2B6 (minor), CYP2D6 (minor), CYP3A4 (major), P-glycoprotein; **Note:** Assignment of Major/Minor substrate status based on clinically relevant drug interaction potential; **Inhibits** CYP2C19 (weak), CYP2C8 (strong), CYP2C9 (weak), CYP2D6 (strong), CYP2E1 (weak), CYP3A4 (strong), P-glycoprotein; **Induces** CYP1A2 (moderate), CYP2C9 (moderate), CYP3A4 (weak)

Avoid Concomitant Use

Avoid concomitant use of Ritonavir with any of the following: Ado-Trastuzumab Emtansine; Alfuzosin; Amiodarone; Apixaban; Astemizole; Atovaquone; Avanafil; Axitinib; Bosutinib; Cabozantinib; Ceritinib; Cisapride; Conivaptan; Crizotinib; Dapoxetine; Dasabuvir; Disulfiram; Dronedarone; Enzalutamide; Eplerenone; Ergot Derivatives; Etravirine; Everolimus; Flecainide; Fluticasone (Nasal); Fusidic Acid (Systemic); Halofantrine; Ibrutinib; Irinotecan; Ivabradine; Lapatinib; Lercanidipine; Lomitapide; Lovastatin; Lurasidone; Macitentan; Midazolam; Naloxegol; Nilotinib; Nisoldipine; Olaparib; PAZOPanib; Pimozide; Propafenone; QuiNIDine; QuiNINE; Ranolazine; Red Yeast Rice; Regorafenib; Rifampin; Rivaroxaban; Salmeterol; Silodosin; Simeprevir; Simvastatin; St Johns Wort; Suvorexant; Tamoxifen; Tamsulosin; Terfenadine; Thioridazine; Ticagrelor; Tolvaptan; Topotecan; Toremifene; Trabectedin; Triazolam; Ulipristal; Vemurafenib; VinCRIStine (Liposomal); Vorapaxar; Voriconazole

Increased Effect/Toxicity

Ritonavir may increase the levels/effects of: Ado-Trastuzumab Emtansine; Afatinib; Alfuzosin; Almotriptan; Alosetron; ALPRAZolam; Amiodarone; Apixaban; ARIPiprazole; Astemizole; AtoMOXetine; AtorvaSTATin; Avanafil; Axitinib; Bedaquiline; Bortezomib; Bosentan; Bosutinib; Brentuximab Vedotin; Brinzolamide; Budesonide (Nasal); Budesonide (Systemic, Oral Inhalation); Cabazitaxel; Cabozantinib; Calcium Channel Blockers (Dihydropyridine); Calcium Channel Blockers (Nondihydropyridine); Cannabis; CarBAMazepine; Ceritinib; Cisapride; Clarithromycin; Clorazepate; Colchicine; Conivaptan; Corticosteroids (Orally Inhaled); Corticosteroids (Systemic); Crizotinib; Cyclophosphamide; CycloSPORINE (Systemic); CYP2C8 Substrates; CYP2D6 Substrates; CYP3A4 Substrates; Dabigatran Etexilate; Dapoxetine; Dasabuvir; Dasatinib; Diazepam; Dienogest; Digoxin; DOXOrubicin (Conventional); Dronabinol; Dronedarone; Dutasteride; Edoxaban; Efavirenz; Eliglustat; Enfuvirtide; Enzalutamide; Eplerenone; Ergot Derivatives; Erlotinib; Estazolam; Etizolam; Everolimus; FentaNYL; Fesoterodine; Flecainide; Flurazepam; Fluticasone (Nasal); Fluticasone (Oral Inhalation); Fusidic Acid (Systemic); GuanFACINE; Halofantrine; Highest Risk QTc-Prolonging Agents; Hydrocodone; Ibrutinib; Idelalisib; Iloperidone; Imatinib; Imidafenacin; Irinotecan; Itraconazole; Ivabradine; Ivacaftor; Ixabepilone; Ketoconazole (Systemic); Lacosamide; Lapatinib; Ledipasvir; Lercanidipine; Levobupivacaine; Levomilnacipran; Linagliptin; Lomitapide; Lovastatin; Lurasidone; Macitentan; Maraviroc; Meperidine; MethylPREDNISolone; Metoprolol; Midazolam; Mifepristone; Moderate Risk QTc-Prolonging Agents; Naloxegol; Nebivolol; Nefazodone; Nilotinib; Nintedanib; Nisoldipine; Olaparib; Ospemifene; OxyCODONE; Paricalcitol; PAZOPanib; P-glycoprotein/ABCB1 Substrates; Pimecrolimus; Pimozide; Pioglitazone; PONATinib; Pranlukast; PrednisoLONE (Systemic); PredniSONE; Propafenone; Protease Inhibitors; Prucalopride; QUEtiapine; QuiNIDine; QuiNINE; Ranolazine; Red Yeast Rice; Regorafenib; Retapamulin; Rifabutin; Rifaximin; Rilpivirine; Riociguat; Rivaroxaban; RomiDEPsin; Rosuvastatin; Ruxolitinib; Salmeterol; Saxagliptin; Sildenafil; Silodosin; Simeprevir; Simvastatin; SORAfenib; Suvorexant; Tacrolimus (Systemic); Tacrolimus (Topical); Tadalafil; Tamsulosin; Telaprevir; Temsirolimus; Terfenadine; Tetrabenazine; Tetrahydrocannabinol; Thioridazine; Ticagrelor; Tofacitinib; Tolterodine; Tolvaptan; Topotecan; Toremifene; Trabectedin; TraZODone; Treprostinil; Triamcinolone (Systemic); Triazolam; Ulipristal; Vardenafil; Vemurafenib; Vilazodone; VinBLAStine; VinCRIStine; VinCRIStine (Liposomal); Vorapaxar; Vortioxetine; Zopiclone; Zuclopenthixol

The levels/effects of Ritonavir may be increased by: ARIPiprazole; Clarithromycin; Delavirdine; Disulfiram; Efavirenz; Enfuvirtide; Fusidic Acid (Systemic); Mifepristone; P-glycoprotein/ABCB1 Inhibitors; Posaconazole; QuiNINE; Simeprevir

Decreased Effect

Ritonavir may decrease the levels/effects of: Abacavir; Atovaquone; Boceprevir; BuPROPion; Canagliflozin; Clarithromycin; Codeine; Contraceptives (Estrogens); Deferasirox; Delavirdine; Etravirine; Fosphenytoin; Hydrocodone; Ifosfamide; Iloperidone; LamoTRIgine; Meperidine; Methadone; Phenytoin; Prasugrel; Proguanil; QuiNINE; Tamoxifen; Telaprevir; Ticagrelor; Valproic Acid and Derivatives; Voriconazole; Warfarin; Zidovudine

The levels/effects of Ritonavir may be decreased by: Antacids; Boceprevir; CarBAMazepine; CYP3A4 Inducers (Moderate); CYP3A4 Inducers (Strong); Dabrafenib; Fosphenytoin; Garlic; Mitotane; P-glycoprotein/ABCB1 Inducers; Phenytoin; Rifampin; Siltuximab; St Johns Wort; Tocilizumab

Food Interactions Food enhances absorption. Management: Manufacturer recommends taking with food. Maintain adequate hydration, unless instructed to restrict fluid intake.

Storage/Stability

Capsule: Store under refrigeration at 2°C to 8°C (36°F to 46°F); may be left out at room temperature of <25°C (<77°F) if used within 30 days. Protect from light. Avoid exposure to excessive heat.

Solution: Store at room temperature at 20°C to 25°C (68°F to 77°F); do not refrigerate. Avoid exposure to excessive heat. Keep cap tightly closed.

Tablet: Store at ≤30°C (86°F); exposure to temperatures ≤50°C (122°F) permitted for ≤7 days. Exposure to high humidity outside of the original container (or a USP equivalent container) for >2 weeks is not recommended.

Mechanism of Action Binds to the site of HIV-1 protease activity and inhibits cleavage of viral Gag-Pol polyprotein precursors into individual functional proteins required for infectious HIV. This results in the formation of immature, noninfectious viral particles.

Pharmacodynamics/Kinetics

Absorption: Variable; increased with food; In the fed state, mean C_{max} of the tablet formulation increased by 26% compared to the capsule.

Distribution: High concentrations in serum and lymph nodes; V_d: 0.16 to 0.66 L/kg

Protein binding: 98% to 99%

Metabolism: Hepatic via CYP3A4 and 2D6; five metabolites, low concentration of an active metabolite (M-2) achieved in plasma (oxidative)

Half-life elimination: 3 to 5 hours

Time to peak, plasma: Oral solution: 2 hours (fasted); 4 hours (nonfasted)

Excretion: Urine (~11%, ~4% as unchanged drug); feces (~86%, ~34% as unchanged drug)

Dosage Note: Must be given in combination with other antiretroviral agents. Norvir tablets are **not** bioequivalent to Norvir capsules. Gastrointestinal side effects or paresthesias may be more common initially when patients are switching from the capsule to the tablet formulation.

Treatment of HIV infection: Oral: Manufacturer's labeling:

Infants >1 month and Children: Initiate dose at 250 mg/m²/dose twice daily; titrate dose upward every 2 to 3 days by 50 mg/m² twice daily to recommended dosage of 350 to 400 mg/m²/dose twice daily (maximum dose: 600 mg twice daily). If 400 mg/m²/dose twice daily is not tolerated, the highest tolerated dose may be used for maintenance therapy. **Note:** Oral solution should not be administered to neonates before a postmenstrual age (first day of mother's last period to birth plus the time elapsed after birth) <44 weeks.

Adolescents and Adults (**Note:** Not recommended as the primary protease inhibitor in any regimen (HHS [adult], 2014): Initiate dose at 300 mg twice daily, then increase by 100 mg twice daily every 2 to 3 days to recommended dosage of 600 mg twice daily (maximum: 600 mg twice daily)

Pharmacokinetic "booster" in combination with other protease inhibitors (off-label use): Adults: 100 to 400 mg daily in 1 to 2 divided doses (HHS [adult], 2014)

Note: Used as the "booster" component in the following recommended regimens in all treatment-naive patients: Atazanavir and tenofovir/emtricitabine, or darunavir and tenofovir/emtricitabine; and in patients with pre-ART plasma HIV RNA <100,000 copies/mL who are HLA-B*5701 negative: Atazanavir and abacavir/lamivudine (HHS [adult], 2014). In patients without evidence of PI resistance, once-daily booster-dosing of 100 mg ritonavir may be preferred to 200 mg daily due to less gastrointestinal and metabolic adverse events. Refer to individual protease inhibitor monographs; specific dosage recommendations often require adjustment of both agents.

Dosage adjustment in renal impairment: No dosage adjustment necessary.

Dosage adjustment in hepatic impairment:

Mild-to-moderate impairment (Child-Pugh class A or B): No dosage adjustment necessary; however, ritonavir levels may be decreased in moderate impairment and patient response should be monitored.

Severe impairment (Child-Pugh class C): Not recommended (has not been studied).

Dietary Considerations The manufacturer recommends taking with food. Oral solution contains 43% ethanol by volume.

Administration Administer all formulations with food, per the manufacturer. DHHS guidelines recommend administering the tablets with food and administering capsules or oral solution with food, if possible, to improve tolerability (HHS [adult], 2014). Liquid formulations usually have an unpleasant taste. Consider mixing it with chocolate milk or a liquid nutritional supplement and taking within 60 minutes. Whenever possible, administer oral solution with calibrated dosing syringe. Shake solution well before use. Tablets should be swallowed whole; do not chew, break, or crush.

Monitoring Parameters Triglycerides, cholesterol, CBC, LFTs, CPK, uric acid, basic HIV monitoring, viral load, CD4 count, glucose, serum amylase and lipase

Additional Information Potential compliance problems, frequency of administration and adverse effects should be discussed with patients before initiating therapy to help prevent the emergence of resistance.

Dosage Forms

Capsule, Oral:

Norvir: 100 mg

Solution, Oral:

Norvir: 80 mg/mL (240 mL)

Tablet, Oral:

Norvir: 100 mg

◆ **Ritonavir and Lopinavir** *see* Lopinavir and Ritonavir *on page 1237*

◆ **Ritonavir, Ombitasvir, Paritaprevir, and Dasabuvir** *see* Ombitasvir, Paritaprevir, Ritonavir, and Dasabuvir *on page 1505*

◆ **Rituxan** *see* RiTUXimab *on page 1825*

RiTUXimab (ri TUK si mab)

Brand Names: U.S. Rituxan

Brand Names: Canada Rituxan

Index Terms Anti-CD20 Monoclonal Antibody; C2B8 Monoclonal Antibody; IDEC-C2B8

Pharmacologic Category Antineoplastic Agent, Anti-CD20; Antineoplastic Agent, Monoclonal Antibody; Antirheumatic Miscellaneous; Immunosuppressant Agent; Monoclonal Antibody

Use

Treatment of CD20-positive non-Hodgkin lymphomas (NHL):

- Relapsed or refractory, low-grade or follicular B-cell NHL (as a single agent)
- Follicular B-cell NHL, previously untreated (in combination with first-line chemotherapy, and as single-agent maintenance therapy if response to first-line rituximab with chemotherapy)
- Nonprogressing, low-grade B-cell NHL (as a single agent after first-line CVP treatment)
- Diffuse large B-cell NHL, previously untreated (in combination with CHOP chemotherapy [or other anthracycline-based regimen])

Treatment of CD20-positive chronic lymphocytic leukemia (CLL) (in combination with fludarabine and cyclophosphamide)

Treatment of moderately- to severely-active rheumatoid arthritis (in combination with methotrexate) in adult patients with inadequate response to one or more TNF antagonists

Treatment of granulomatosis with polyangiitis (GPA; Wegener's granulomatosis) (in combination with glucocorticoids)

Treatment of microscopic polyangiitis (MPA) (in combination with glucocorticoids)

Pregnancy Risk Factor C

Pregnancy Considerations Animal reproduction studies have demonstrated adverse effects including decreased (reversible) B-cells and immunosuppression. Rituximab crosses the placenta and can be detected in the newborn. In one infant born at 41 weeks gestation, *in utero* exposure occurred from week 16-37; rituximab concentrations were higher in the neonate at birth (32,095 ng/mL) than the mother (9750 ng/mL) and still measurable at 18 weeks of age (700 ng/mL infant; 500 ng/mL mother) (Friedrichs, 2006).

B-cell lymphocytopenia lasting <6 months may occur in exposed infants. Limited information is available following maternal use of rituximab for the treatment of lymphomas and hematologic disorders (Ton, 2011). Retrospective case reports of inadvertent pregnancy during rituximab treatment collected by the manufacturer (often combined with concomitant teratogenic therapies) describe premature births and infant hematologic abnormalities and infections; no specific pattern of birth defects has been observed (limited data) (Chakravarty, 2010). Use is not recommended to treat non-life-threatening maternal conditions (eg, rheumatoid arthritis) during pregnancy (Makol, 2011; Østensen, 2008) and other agents are preferred for treating lupus nephritis in pregnant women (Hahn, 2012).

Effective contraception should be used during and for 12 months following treatment. Healthcare providers are encouraged to enroll women with rheumatoid arthritis exposed to rituximab during pregnancy in the Mother-ToBabyAutoImmune Diseases Study by contacting the Organization of Teratology Information Specialists (OTIS) (877-311-8972).

Breast-Feeding Considerations It is not known if rituximab is excreted in human milk. However, human IgG is excreted in breast milk, and therefore, rituximab may also be excreted in milk. Although rituximab would not be expected to enter the circulation of a nursing infant in significant amounts, the decision to discontinue rituximab or discontinue breast-feeding should take into account the benefits of treatment to the mother.

Contraindications There are no contraindications listed in the FDA-approved manufacturer's labeling.

Canadian labeling (not in U.S. labeling): Type 1 hypersensitivity or anaphylactic reaction to murine proteins, Chinese Hamster Ovary (CHO) cell proteins, or any component of the formulation; patients who have or have had progressive multifocal leukoencephalopathy (PML)

Warnings/Precautions [U.S. Boxed Warning]: Severe (occasionally fatal) infusion-related reactions have been reported, usually with the first infusion; fatalities have been reported within 24 hours of infusion; monitor closely during infusion; discontinue for severe reactions and provide medical intervention for grades 3 or 4 infusion reactions. Reactions usually occur within 30-120 minutes and may include hypotension, angioedema, bronchospasm, hypoxia, urticaria, and in more severe cases pulmonary infiltrates, acute respiratory distress syndrome, myocardial infarction, ventricular fibrillation, cardiogenic shock and/or anaphylaxis. Risk factors associated with fatal outcomes include chronic lymphocytic leukemia, female gender, mantle cell lymphoma, or pulmonary infiltrates. Closely monitor patients with a history of prior cardiopulmonary reactions or with preexisting cardiac or pulmonary conditions and patients with high numbers of circulating malignant cells (>25,000/mm^3). Prior to infusion, premedicate patients with acetaminophen and an antihistamine (and methylprednisolone for patients with RA). Discontinue infusion for severe reactions; treatment is symptomatic. Medications for the treatment of hypersensitivity reactions (eg, bronchodilators, epinephrine, antihistamines, corticosteroids) should be available for immediate use. Discontinue infusion for serious or life-threatening cardiac arrhythmias. Perform cardiac monitoring during and after the infusion in patients who develop clinically significant arrhythmias or who have a history of arrhythmia or angina. Mild-to-moderate infusion-related reactions (eg, chills, fever, rigors) occur frequently and are typically managed through slowing or interrupting the infusion. Infusion may be resumed at a 50% infusion rate reduction upon resolution of symptoms. Due to the potential for hypotension, consider withholding antihypertensives 12 hours prior to treatment.

[U.S. Boxed Warning]: Hepatitis B virus (HBV) reactivation may occur with use and may result in fulminant hepatitis, hepatic failure, and death. Screen all patients for HBV infection by measuring hepatitis B surface antigen (HBsAG) and hepatitis B core antibody (anti-HBc) prior to therapy initiation; monitor patients for clinical and laboratory signs of hepatitis or HBV during and for several months after treatment. Discontinue rituximab (and concomitant medications) if viral hepatitis develops and initiate appropriate antiviral therapy. Reactivation has occurred in patients who are HBsAg positive as well as in those who are HBsAg negative but are anti-HBc positive; HBV reactivation has also been observed in patients who had previously resolved HBV infection. HBV reactivation has been reported up to 24 months after therapy discontinuation. Use cautiously in patients who show evidence of prior HBV infection (eg, HBsAg positive [regardless of antibody status] or HBsAG negative but anti-HBc positive); consult with appropriate clinicians regarding monitoring and consideration of antiviral therapy before and/or during rituximab treatment. The safety of resuming rituximab treatment following HBV reactivation is not known; discuss reinitiation of therapy in patients with resolved HBV reactivation with physicians experienced in HBV management.

[U.S. Boxed Warning]: Progressive multifocal leukoencephalopathy (PML) due to JC virus infection has been reported with rituximab use; may be fatal. Cases were reported in patients with hematologic malignancies receiving rituximab either with combination chemotherapy, or with hematopoietic stem cell transplant. Cases were also reported in patients receiving rituximab for autoimmune diseases who had received prior or concurrent immunosuppressant therapy. Onset may be delayed, although most cases were diagnosed within 12 months of the last rituximab dose. A retrospective analysis of patients (n=57) diagnosed with PML following rituximab therapy, found a median of 16 months (following rituximab initiation), 5.5 months (following last rituximab dose), and 6 rituximab doses preceded PML diagnosis. Clinical findings included confusion/disorientation, motor weakness/hemiparesis, altered vision/speech, and poor motor coordination with symptoms progressing over weeks to months (Carson, 2009). Promptly evaluate any patient presenting with neurological changes; consider neurology consultation, brain MRI and lumbar puncture for suspected PML. Discontinue rituximab in patients who develop PML; consider reduction/discontinuation of concurrent chemotherapy or immunosuppressants. Avoid use if severe active infection is present. Serious and potentially fatal bacterial, fungal, and either new or reactivated viral infections may occur during treatment and after completing rituximab. Infections have been observed in patients with prolonged hypogammaglobulinemia, defined as hypogammaglobulinemia >11 months after rituximab exposure; monitor immunoglobulin levels as necessary. Associated new or reactivated viral infections have included cytomegalovirus, herpes simplex virus, parvovirus B19, varicella zoster virus, West Nile virus, and hepatitis B and C. Discontinue rituximab in patients who develop other serious infections and initiate appropriate anti-infective treatment.

Tumor lysis syndrome leading to acute renal failure requiring dialysis (some fatal) may occur 12-24 hours following the first dose when used as a single agent in the treatment of NHL. Hyperkalemia, hypocalcemia, hyperuricemia, and/or hyperphosphatemia may occur. Administer prophylaxis (antihyperuricemic therapy, hydration) in patients at high risk (high numbers of circulating malignant cells ≥25,000/mm^3 or high tumor burden). May cause fatal renal toxicity in patients with hematologic malignancies. Patients who received combination therapy with cisplatin and rituximab for NHL experienced renal toxicity during clinical trials; this combination is not an approved treatment regimen. Monitor for signs of renal failure; discontinue rituximab with increasing serum creatinine or oliguria. Correct electrolyte abnormalities; monitor hydration status.

[U.S. Boxed Warning]: Severe and sometimes fatal mucocutaneous reactions (lichenoid dermatitis, paraneoplastic pemphigus, Stevens-Johnson syndrome, toxic epidermal necrolysis and vesiculobullous dermatitis) have been reported; onset has been variable but has occurred as early as the first day of exposure. Discontinue in patients experiencing severe mucocutaneous skin reactions; the safety of re-exposure following mucocutaneous reactions has not been evaluated. Use caution with preexisting cardiac or pulmonary disease, or prior cardiopulmonary events. Rheumatoid arthritis patients are at increased risk for cardiovascular events; monitor closely during and after each infusion. Elderly patients are at higher risk for cardiac (supraventricular arrhythmia) and pulmonary adverse events (pneumonia, pneumonitis). Abdominal pain, bowel obstruction, and perforation (rarely fatal) have been reported with an average onset of symptoms of ~6 days (range: 1-77 days); complaints of abdominal pain or repeated vomiting should be evaluated, especially if early in the treatment course. Live vaccines should not be given concurrently with rituximab; there is no data available concerning secondary transmission of live vaccines with or following rituximab treatment. RA patients should be brought up to date with nonlive immunizations (following current guidelines) at least 4 weeks before initiating therapy; evaluate risks of therapy delay versus benefit (of nonlive vaccines) for NHL patients. Safety and efficacy of rituximab in combination with biologic agents or disease-modifying antirheumatic drugs (DMARDs) other than methotrexate have not been established. Rituximab is not recommended for use in RA patients who have not had prior inadequate response to TNF antagonists. Safety and efficacy of retreatment for RA have not been established. The safety of concomitant immunosuppressants other than corticosteroids has not been evaluated in patients with granulomatosis with polyangiitis (GPA; Wegener's granulomatosis) or microscopic polyangiitis (MPA) after rituximab-induced B-cell depletion. There are only limited data on subsequent courses of rituximab for GPA or MPA; safety and efficacy of retreatment have not been established.

Adverse Reactions Note: Patients treated with rituximab for rheumatoid arthritis (RA) may experience fewer adverse reactions.

Cardiovascular: Flushing, hyper-/hypotension, peripheral edema

Central nervous system: Anxiety, chills, dizziness, fatigue, fever, headache, insomnia, migraine, pain

Dermatologic: Angioedema, pruritus, rash, urticaria

Endocrine & metabolic: Hyperglycemia

Gastrointestinal: Abdominal pain, diarrhea, dyspepsia, nausea, vomiting, weight gain

Hematologic: Anemia, cytopenia, lymphopenia, leukopenia, neutropenia, neutropenic fever, thrombocytopenia

Hepatic: ALT increased

Neuromuscular & skeletal: Arthralgia, back pain, muscle spasm, myalgia, neuropathy, paresthesia, weakness

Respiratory: Bronchospasm, cough, dyspnea, epistaxis, rhinitis, sinusitis, throat irritation, upper respiratory tract infection

Miscellaneous: Infusion-related reactions (may include angioedema, bronchospasm, chills, dizziness, fever, headache, hyper-/hypotension, myalgia, nausea, pruritus, rash, rigors, urticaria, and vomiting); infection (including bacterial, viral, fungal); night sweats; human antichimeric antibody (HACA) positive

Rare but important or life-threatening: Acute renal failure, anaphylactoid reaction/anaphylaxis, angina, aplastic anemia, ARDS, arrhythmia, bowel obstruction/perforation, bronchiolitis obliterans, cardiac failure, cardiogenic shock, encephalomyelitis, fatal infusion-related reactions, fulminant hepatitis, gastrointestinal perforation, hemolytic anemia, hepatic failure, hepatitis, hepatitis B reactivation, hyperviscosity syndrome (in Waldenström's macroglobulinemia), hypogammaglobulinemia (prolonged), hypoxia, interstitial pneumonitis, laryngeal edema, lichenoid dermatitis, lupus-like syndrome, marrow hypoplasia, MI, mucositis, mucocutaneous reaction, neutropenia (late-onset occurring >40 days after last dose), optic neuritis, pancytopenia (prolonged), paraneoplastic pemphigus (uncommon), pleuritis, pneumonia, pneumonitis, polyarticular arthritis, polymyositis, posterior reversible encephalopathy syndrome (PRES), progressive multifocal leukoencephalopathy (PML), pure red cell aplasia, renal toxicity, reversible posterior leukoencephalopathy syndrome (RPLS), serum sickness, Stevens-Johnson syndrome, supraventricular arrhythmia, systemic vasculitis, toxic epidermal necrolysis, tuberculosis reactivation, tumor lysis syndrome, uveitis, vasculitis with rash, ventricular fibrillation, ventricular tachycardia, vesiculobullous dermatitis, viral reactivation (includes JC virus, cytomegalovirus, herpes simplex virus, parvovirus B19, varicella zoster virus, West Nile virus, and hepatitis C), wheezing

Drug Interactions

Metabolism/Transport Effects None known.

Avoid Concomitant Use

Avoid concomitant use of RiTUXimab with any of the following: Abatacept; BCG; Belimumab; Certolizumab Pegol; CloZAPine; Dipyrone; Natalizumab; Pimecrolimus; Tacrolimus (Topical); Tofacitinib; Vaccines (Live)

Increased Effect/Toxicity

RiTUXimab may increase the levels/effects of: Abatacept; Belimumab; Certolizumab Pegol; CloZAPine; Leflunomide; Natalizumab; Tofacitinib; Vaccines (Live)

The levels/effects of RiTUXimab may be increased by: Antihypertensives; Denosumab; Dipyrone; Pimecrolimus; Roflumilast; Tacrolimus (Topical); Trastuzumab

Decreased Effect

RiTUXimab may decrease the levels/effects of: BCG; Coccidioides immitis Skin Test; Sipuleucel-T; Vaccines (Inactivated); Vaccines (Live)

The levels/effects of RiTUXimab may be decreased by: Echinacea

Preparation for Administration Withdraw necessary amount of rituximab and dilute to a final concentration of 1-4 mg/mL with 0.9% sodium chloride or 5% dextrose in water. Gently invert the bag to mix the solution. Do not shake.

Storage/Stability Store intact vials refrigerated at 2°C to 8°C (36°F to 46°F); do not freeze. Do not shake. Protect vials from direct sunlight. Solutions for infusion are stable at 2°C to 8°C (36°F to 46°F) for 24 hours and at room temperature for an additional 24 hours.

Mechanism of Action Rituximab is a monoclonal antibody directed against the CD20 antigen on B-lymphocytes. CD20 regulates cell cycle initiation; and, possibly, functions as a calcium channel. Rituximab binds to the antigen on the cell surface, activating complement-dependent B-cell cytotoxicity; and to human Fc receptors, mediating cell killing through an antibody-dependent cellular toxicity. B-cells are believed to play a role in the development and progression of rheumatoid arthritis. Signs and symptoms of RA are reduced by targeting B-cells and the progression of structural damage is delayed.

Pharmacodynamics/Kinetics

Duration: Detectable in serum 3-6 months after completion of treatment; B-cell recovery begins ~6 months following completion of treatment; median B-cell levels return to normal by 12 months following completion of treatment

Absorption: IV: Immediate and results in a rapid and sustained depletion of circulating and tissue-based B cells

Distribution: RA: 3.1 L; GPA/MPA: 4.5 L

Half-life elimination:

- CLL: Median terminal half-life: 32 days (range: 14-62 days)
- NHL: Median terminal half-life: 22 days (range: 6-52 days)
- RA: Mean terminal half-life: 18 days (range: 5-78 days)
- GPA/MPA: 23 days (range: 9-49 days)

Excretion: Uncertain; may undergo phagocytosis and catabolism in the reticuloendothelial system (RES)

Dosage Note: Details concerning dosing in combination regimens should also be consulted. Pretreatment with acetaminophen and an antihistamine is recommended for all indications. For oncology uses, antihyperuricemic therapy and aggressive hydration are recommended for patients at risk for tumor lysis syndrome (high tumor burden or lymphocytes >25,000/mm^3). In patients with CLL, *Pneumocystis jirovecii* pneumonia (PCP) and antiherpetic viral prophylaxis is recommended during treatment (and for up to 12 months following treatment). In patients with granulomatosis with polyangiitis (GPA) and microscopic polyangiitis (MPA), PCP prophylaxis is recommended during and for 6 months after rituximab treatment. For patients with RA, premedication with methylprednisolone 100 mg IV (or equivalent) is recommended 30 minutes prior to each dose.

Children: IV infusion:

- AIHA (off-label use): 375 mg/m^2 once weekly for 2-4 doses (Zecca, 2003)
- Chronic ITP (off-label use): 375 mg/m^2 once weekly for 4 doses (Parodi, 2009; Wang, 2005)
- Nephrotic syndrome, severe, refractory (off-label use): 375 mg/m^2 once weekly for 1-4 doses has been used in small case series, case reports, and retrospective analyses, including reports of successful remission induction of severe or refractory nephrotic syndromes that are poorly responsive to standard therapies (Dello Strologo, 2009; Fujinaga, 2010; Guigonis, 2008; Prytula, 2010)

Adults: IV infusion:

- CLL: 375 mg/m^2 on the day prior to fludarabine/cyclophosphamide in cycle 1, then 500 mg/m^2 on day 1 (every 28 days) of cycles 2-6
- Granulomatosis with polyangiitis (GPA; Wegener's granulomatosis): 375 mg/m^2 once weekly for 4 doses (in combination with methylprednisolone IV for 1-3 days followed by daily prednisone)
- NHL (relapsed/refractory, low-grade or follicular CD20-positive, B-cell): 375 mg/m^2 once weekly for 4 or 8 doses
  - Retreatment following disease progression: 375 mg/m^2 once weekly for 4 doses
- NHL (diffuse large B-cell): 375 mg/m^2 given on day 1 of each chemotherapy cycle for up to 8 doses
- NHL (follicular, CD20-positive, B-cell, previously untreated): 375 mg/m^2 given on day 1 of each chemotherapy cycle for up to 8 doses
  - Maintenance therapy (as a single agent, in patients with partial or complete response to rituximab plus chemotherapy; begin 8 weeks after completion of combination chemotherapy): 375 mg/m^2 every 8 weeks for 12 doses
- NHL (nonprogressing, low-grade, CD20-positive, B-cell, after 6-8 cycles of first-line CVP are completed): 375 mg/m^2 once weekly for 4 doses every 6 months for a maximum of 16 doses
- NHL: Combination therapy with ibritumomab: 250 mg/m^2 IV day 1; repeat in 7-9 days with ibritumomab
- *Canadian labeling:* NHL, low grade or follicular:
  - Initial: 375 mg/m^2 once weekly for 4 doses (as a single agent) or 375 mg/m^2 on day 1 of each 21-day cycle for 8 cycles (in combination with CVP chemotherapy)
  - Maintenance (responding to induction therapy): 375 mg/m^2 every 3 months until disease progression or up to a maximum of 2 years
- Rheumatoid arthritis: 1000 mg on days 1 and 15 in combination with methotrexate; subsequent courses may be administered every 24 weeks (based on clinical evaluation), if necessary may be repeated no sooner than every 16 weeks
- Microscopic polyangiitis (MPA): 375 mg/m^2 once weekly for 4 doses (in combination with methylprednisolone IV for 1-3 days followed by daily prednisone)
- Chronic GVHD, refractory (off-label use): 375 mg/m^2 once weekly for 4 doses (Cutler, 2006)
- Idiopathic thrombocytopenic purpura (ITP) (off-label use): 375 mg/m^2 once weekly for 4 doses (Arnold, 2007; Godeau, 2008)
- Hodgkin lymphoma (off-label use): 375 mg/m^2 once weekly for 4 weeks (Ekstrand, 2003; Schulz, 2008)

Idiopathic membranous nephropathy (IMN), resistant (off-label use): 375 mg/m^2 once weekly for 4 doses with retreatment at 6 months (Fervenza, 2010) **or** 1000 mg on days 1 and 15 (Fervenza, 2008) **or** 375 mg/m^2 single doses titrated to B cell response (Cravedi, 2007)

Lupus nephritis, refractory (off-label use): 375 mg/m^2 once weekly for 4 doses (Melander, 2009) **or** 500-1000 mg on days 1 and 15 (Vigna-Perez, 2006)

Pemphigus vulgaris, refractory (off-label use): 375 mg/m^2 once weekly of weeks 1, 2, and 3 of a 4-week cycle, repeat for 1 additional cycle, then 1 dose per month for 4 months (total of 10 doses in 6 months) (Ahmed, 2006)

Post-transplant lymphoproliferative disorder (off-label use): 375 mg/m^2 once weekly for 4 doses (Choquet, 2006)

Thrombotic thrombocytopenic purpura (TTP), relapsed/refractory (off-label use): 375 mg/m^2 once weekly for 4 doses (Scully, 2007; Scully, 2011)

Waldenström's macroglobulinemia (off-label use): 375 mg/m^2 once weekly for 4 doses (Dimopoulos, 2002)

Dosage adjustment in renal impairment: No dosage adjustment provided in manufacturer's labeling (has not been studied).

Dosage adjustment in hepatic impairment: No dosage adjustment provided in manufacturer's labeling (has not been studied)

Administration Do **not** administer IV push or bolus. If a reaction occurs, slow or stop the infusion. If the reaction abates, restart infusion at 50% of the previous rate. Discontinue infusion in the event of serious or life-threatening cardiac arrhythmias.

IV: Initial infusion: Start rate of 50 mg/hour; if there is no reaction, increase the rate by 50 mg/hour increments every 30 minutes, to a maximum rate of 400 mg/hour.

Subsequent infusions:

Standard infusion rate: If patient tolerated initial infusion, start at 100 mg/hour; if there is no reaction, increase the rate by 100 mg/hour increments every 30 minutes, to a maximum rate of 400 mg/hour.

Accelerated infusion rate (90 minutes): For patients with previously untreated follicular NHL and diffuse large B-cell NHL who are receiving a corticosteroid as part of their combination chemotherapy regimen, have a circulating lymphocyte count <5000/mm^3, or have no significant cardiovascular disease. After tolerance has been established (no grade 3 or 4 infusion-related event) at the recommended infusion rate in cycle 1, a rapid infusion rate may be used beginning with cycle 2. The daily corticosteroid, acetaminophen, and diphenhydramine are administered prior to treatment, then the rituximab dose is administered over 90 minutes, with 20% of the dose administered over the first 30 minutes and the remaining 80% is given over 60 minutes (Sehn, 2007). If the 90-minute infusion in cycle 2 is tolerated, the same rate may be used for the remainder of the treatment regimen (through cycles 6 or 8).

Monitoring Parameters CBC with differential and platelets (obtain at weekly to monthly intervals and more frequently in patients with cytopenias, or at 2-4 month intervals in rheumatoid arthritis patients, GPA and MPA), peripheral CD20$^+$ cells; HAMA/HACA titers (high levels may increase the risk of allergic reactions); renal function, fluid balance; vital signs; monitor for infusion reactions, cardiac monitoring during and after infusion in rheumatoid arthritis patients and in patients with preexisting cardiac disease or if arrhythmias develop during or after subsequent infusions.

Screen all patients for HBV infection prior to therapy initiation (eg, HBsAG and anti-HBc measurements). In addition, carriers and patients with evidence of current infection or recovery from prior hepatitis B infection should be monitored closely for clinical and laboratory signs of HBV reactivation and/or infection during therapy and for up to 2 years following completion of treatment. High-risk patients should be screened for hepatitis C (per NCCN NHL guidelines v.2.2013).

Complaints of abdominal pain, especially early in the course of treatment, should prompt a thorough diagnostic evaluation and appropriate treatment. Signs or symptoms of progressive multifocal leukoencephalopathy (focal neurologic deficits, which may present as hemiparesis, visual field deficits, cognitive impairment, aphasia, ataxia, and/or cranial nerve deficits). If PML is suspected, obtain brain MRI scan and lumbar puncture.

Dosage Forms

Concentrate, Intravenous [preservative free]:

Rituxan: 10 mg/mL (10 mL, 50 mL)

- ◆ **Riva-Alendronate (Can)** *see* Alendronate *on page* 79
- ◆ **Riva-Amiodarone (Can)** *see* Amiodarone *on page* 114
- ◆ **Riva-Amlodipine (Can)** *see* AmLODIPine *on page* 123
- ◆ **Riva-Anastrozole (Can)** *see* Anastrozole *on page* 148
- ◆ **Riva-Atenolol (Can)** *see* Atenolol *on page* 189
- ◆ **RIVA-Atomoxetine (Can)** *see* AtoMOXetine *on page* 191
- ◆ **Riva-Atorvastatin (Can)** *see* AtorvaSTATin *on page* 194
- ◆ **Riva-Azithromycin (Can)** *see* Azithromycin (Systemic) *on page* 216
- ◆ **Riva-Baclofen (Can)** *see* Baclofen *on page* 223
- ◆ **Riva-Buspirone (Can)** *see* BusPIRone *on page* 311
- ◆ **Riva-Ciprofloxacin (Can)** *see* Ciprofloxacin (Systemic) *on page* 441
- ◆ **Riva-Citalopram (Can)** *see* Citalopram *on page* 451
- ◆ **Riva-Clarithromycin (Can)** *see* Clarithromycin *on page* 456
- ◆ **Riva-Clindamycin (Can)** *see* Clindamycin (Systemic) *on page* 460
- ◆ **Riva-Clonazepam (Can)** *see* ClonazePAM *on page* 478
- ◆ **Rivacocet (Can)** *see* Oxycodone and Acetaminophen *on page* 1541
- ◆ **Riva-Cycloprine (Can)** *see* Cyclobenzaprine *on page* 516
- ◆ **Riva-Dicyclomine (Can)** *see* Dicyclomine *on page* 622
- ◆ **Riva-Donepezil (Can)** *see* Donepezil *on page* 668
- ◆ **Riva-Dutasteride (Can)** *see* Dutasteride *on page* 702
- ◆ **Riva-Enalapril (Can)** *see* Enalapril *on page* 722
- ◆ **Riva-Escitalopram (Can)** *see* Escitalopram *on page* 765
- ◆ **Riva-Ezetimibe (Can)** *see* Ezetimibe *on page* 832
- ◆ **Riva-Fenofibrate Micro (Can)** *see* Fenofibrate and Derivatives *on page* 852
- ◆ **Riva-Fluconazole (Can)** *see* Fluconazole *on page* 885
- ◆ **Riva-Fluoxetine (Can)** *see* FLUoxetine *on page* 899
- ◆ **Riva-Fluvox (Can)** *see* FluvoxaMINE *on page* 916
- ◆ **Riva-Fosinopril (Can)** *see* Fosinopril *on page* 932
- ◆ **Riva-Gabapentin (Can)** *see* Gabapentin *on page* 943
- ◆ **Riva-Glyburide (Can)** *see* GlyBURIDE *on page* 972
- ◆ **Riva-Hydroxyzine (Can)** *see* HydrOXYzine *on page* 1024
- ◆ **Riva-Indapamide (Can)** *see* Indapamide *on page* 1065
- ◆ **Riva-Lansoprazole (Can)** *see* Lansoprazole *on page* 1166
- ◆ **Riva-Letrozole (Can)** *see* Letrozole *on page* 1181
- ◆ **Riva-Lisinopril (Can)** *see* Lisinopril *on page* 1226
- ◆ **Riva-Loperamide (Can)** *see* Loperamide *on page* 1236
- ◆ **Riva-Lovastatin (Can)** *see* Lovastatin *on page* 1252

- **Riva-Memantine (Can)** *see* Memantine *on page 1286*
- **Riva-Metformin (Can)** *see* MetFORMIN *on page 1307*
- **Riva-Metoprolol-L (Can)** *see* Metoprolol *on page 1350*
- **Riva-Minocycline (Can)** *see* Minocycline *on page 1371*
- **Riva-Mirtazapine (Can)** *see* Mirtazapine *on page 1376*
- **Riva-Montelukast FC (Can)** *see* Montelukast *on page 1392*
- **Rivanase AQ (Can)** *see* Beclomethasone (Nasal) *on page 232*
- **Riva-Norfloxacin (Can)** *see* Norfloxacin *on page 1475*
- **Riva-Olanzapine (Can)** *see* OLANZapine *on page 1491*
- **Riva-Olanzapine ODT (Can)** *see* OLANZapine *on page 1491*
- **Riva-Omeprazole DR (Can)** *see* Omeprazole *on page 1508*
- **Riva-Ondansetron (Can)** *see* Ondansetron *on page 1513*
- **Riva-Oxazepam (Can)** *see* Oxazepam *on page 1532*
- **Riva-Oxybutynin (Can)** *see* Oxybutynin *on page 1536*
- **Riva-Pantoprazole (Can)** *see* Pantoprazole *on page 1570*
- **Riva-Paroxetine (Can)** *see* PARoxetine *on page 1579*
- **Riva-Pravastatin (Can)** *see* Pravastatin *on page 1700*
- **Riva-Pregabalin (Can)** *see* Pregabalin *on page 1710*
- **Riva-Quetiapine (Can)** *see* QUEtiapine *on page 1751*
- **Riva-Rabeprazole EC (Can)** *see* RABEprazole *on page 1762*
- **Riva-Ranitidine (Can)** *see* Ranitidine *on page 1777*
- **Riva-Risedronate (Can)** *see* Risedronate *on page 1816*
- **Riva-Risperidone (Can)** *see* RisperiDONE *on page 1818*
- **Riva-Rizatriptan ODT (Can)** *see* Rizatriptan *on page 1836*
- **Riva-Rosuvastatin (Can)** *see* Rosuvastatin *on page 1848*

Rivaroxaban (riv a ROX a ban)

Brand Names: U.S. Xarelto; Xarelto Starter Pack

Brand Names: Canada Xarelto

Index Terms BAY 59-7939

Pharmacologic Category Anticoagulant; Anticoagulant, Factor Xa Inhibitor

Additional Appendix Information

Oral Anticoagulant Comparison Chart *on page 2233*

Reversal of Oral Anticoagulants *on page 2235*

Use

Deep vein thrombosis prophylaxis: Postoperative thrombophylaxis of deep vein thrombosis (DVT) which may lead to pulmonary embolism in patients undergoing knee or hip replacement surgery.

Deep vein thrombosis treatment: Treatment of DVT.

Nonvalvular atrial fibrillation: Prevention of stroke and systemic embolism in patients with nonvalvular atrial fibrillation (AF).

Note: The 2014 American Heart Association/American College of Cardiology/Heart Rhythm Society guidelines for the management of AF recommend oral anticoagulation for patients with nonvalvular AF or atrial flutter with prior stroke, TIA, or a CHA_2DS_2-VASc score ≥2. As an alternative to warfarin, rivaroxaban may also be used for 3 weeks prior and 4 weeks after cardioversion in patients with AF or atrial flutter of ≥48 hours duration or when the duration is unknown. (January, 2014).

Pulmonary embolism treatment: Treatment of pulmonary embolism.

Reduction in the risk (secondary prevention) of recurrent deep vein thrombosis and/or pulmonary embolism: Reduction in the risk of recurrence of DVT and pulmonary embolism following initial 6 months of treatment for DVT and/or pulmonary embolism.

Pregnancy Risk Factor C

Pregnancy Considerations Adverse events were observed in animal reproduction studies. Data are insufficient to evaluate the safety of oral factor Xa inhibitors during pregnancy; use during pregnancy should be avoided (Guyatt, 2012). Use may increase the risk of pregnancy related hemorrhage. Clinicians should note that the anticoagulant effect cannot be easily monitored or readily reversed. Prompt clinical evaluation is warranted with any unexplained decrease in hemoglobin, hematocrit or blood pressure, or fetal distress. Pregnancy planning should be discussed if use is needed in women of reproductive potential. Use during pregnancy is contraindicated in the Canadian labeling.

Breast-Feeding Considerations It is not known if rivaroxaban is excreted into breast milk. Due to the potential for serious adverse reactions in the nursing infant, the decision to discontinue rivaroxaban or to discontinue breastfeeding during therapy should take into account the benefits of treatment to the mother; use of alternative anticoagulants is preferred (Guyatt, 2012). Use in breastfeeding mothers is contraindicated in the Canadian labeling.

Contraindications Severe hypersensitivity to rivaroxaban or any component of the formulation; active pathological bleeding

Canadian labeling: Additional contraindications (not in U.S. labeling): Hepatic disease (including Child-Pugh classes B and C) associated with coagulopathy and clinically relevant bleeding risk; lesions or conditions at increased risk of clinically significant bleeding (eg, hemorrhagic or ischemic cerebral infarction, spontaneous or acquired impairment of hemostasis, active peptic ulcer disease with recent bleeding); concomitant systemic treatment with strong CYP3A4 and P-glycoprotein (P-gp) inhibitors; concomitant use with any other anticoagulant including unfractionated heparin (except at doses used to maintain central venous or arterial catheter patency), low molecular weight heparins (eg, enoxaparin, dalteparin) or heparin derivatives (eg, fondaparinux); concomitant use with warfarin, dabigatran, or apixaban except when switching therapy to or from rivaroxaban; pregnancy; lactation

Warnings/Precautions Most common complication is bleeding; major hemorrhages (eg, intracranial, GI, retinal, epidural hematoma, adrenal bleeding) have been reported. Certain patients are at increased risk of bleeding; risk factors include bacterial endocarditis, congenital or acquired bleeding disorders, thrombocytopenia, recent puncture of large vessels or organ biopsy, stroke, intracerebral surgery, or other neuraxial procedure, severe uncontrolled hypertension, renal impairment, recent major surgery, recent major bleeding (intracranial, GI, intraocular, or pulmonary), concomitant use of drugs that affect hemostasis, and advanced age. Monitor for signs and symptoms of bleeding. Prompt clinical evaluation is warranted with any unexplained decrease in hemoglobin or blood pressure. **Note:** No specific antidote exists for rivaroxaban reversal; not dialyzable due to high plasma protein binding. Protamine sulfate and vitamin K are not expected to affect the anticoagulant activity of rivaroxaban. The use of activated prothrombin complex concentrate (aPCC) or recombinant factor VIIa has not been evaluated. The use of a four-factor PCC (Cofact, not available in the U.S.) in healthy subjects has been shown to reverse the anticoagulant effect (ie, normalize the prothrombin time) of rivaroxaban (Eerenberg, 2011).

[U.S. Boxed Warning]: Spinal or epidural hematomas may occur with neuraxial anesthesia (epidural or spinal anesthesia) or spinal puncture in patients who are anticoagulated; may result in long-term or permanent paralysis. The risk of spinal/epidural hematoma is increased with the use of indwelling epidural catheters, concomitant administration of other drugs that affect hemostasis (eg, NSAIDS, platelet inhibitors, other anticoagulants), in patients with a history of traumatic or repeated epidural or spinal punctures, or a history of spinal deformity or spinal surgery. Monitor for signs of neurologic impairment (eg, midline back pain, numbness/weakness of legs, bowel/ bladder dysfunction); prompt diagnosis and treatment are necessary. In patients who are anticoagulated or pharmacologic thromboprophylaxis is anticipated, assess risks versus benefits prior to neuraxial interventions. The optimal timing between the administration of rivaroxaban and neuraxial procedures is not known. Placement or removal of an epidural catheter or lumbar puncture is best performed when the anticoagulant effect of rivaroxaban is low. European guidelines recommend waiting at least 22-26 hours following the last rivaroxaban dose when using prophylactic dosing (eg, 10 mg once daily) before catheter placement or lumbar puncture (Gogarten, 2010). When higher doses are used (eg, 20 mg once daily), some suggest avoidance of neuraxial procedures for at least 48 hours (Rosencher, 2013). In patients who have received neuraxial anesthesia concurrently with rivaroxaban (usually in patients undergoing knee or hip replacement surgery), avoid removal of epidural catheter for at least 18 hours following the last rivaroxaban dose; avoid rivaroxaban administration for at least 6 hours following epidural catheter removal; if traumatic puncture occurs, avoid rivaroxaban administration for at least 24 hours. In addition to these and other clinical variables, consider renal function and the age of the patient (elderly patients exhibit a prolonged rivaroxaban half-life [11 to 13 hours]) (Kubitza, 2010; Rosencher, 2013). The Canadian labeling recommends avoiding doses >10 mg in patients with a postoperative indwelling epidural catheter.

[U.S. Boxed Warning]: As with any oral anticoagulant in the absence of adequate alternative anticoagulation, an increased risk of thrombotic events (including stroke) may occur with premature discontinuation of rivaroxaban. Consider the addition of alternative anticoagulant therapy when discontinuing rivaroxaban for reasons other than pathological bleeding or completion of a course of therapy. An increased rate of stroke was observed during the transition from rivaroxaban to warfarin in clinical trials in atrial fibrillation patients. In a post-hoc analysis of the ROCKET AF trial, patients who temporarily (>3 days) or permanently discontinued anticoagulation, the risk of stroke or non-CNS embolism was similar with rivaroxaban as compared to warfarin (Patel, 2013).

Avoid use in patients with moderate-to-severe hepatic impairment (Child-Pugh classes B and C) or in patients with any hepatic disease associated with coagulopathy; use in this patient population is contraindicated in the Canadian labeling. Use with caution in patients with moderate renal impairment (CrCl 30-49 mL/minute) when used for postoperative thromboprophylaxis including patients receiving concomitant drug therapy that may increase rivaroxaban systemic exposure and those with deteriorating renal function. Monitor for any signs or symptoms of blood loss. Avoid use in severe renal impairment (DVT/PE, postoperative thromboprophylaxis: CrCl <30 mL/minute; nonvalvular atrial fibrillation: CrCl <15 mL/minute) since rivaroxaban exposure is expected to increase; discontinue use in patients who develop acute renal failure. According to the AHA/ACC/HRS, may consider dose reduction in patients with nonvalvular AF and moderate-to-severe chronic kidney disease (CKD), although safety and efficacy of this approach has not been established (AHA/ ACC/HRS [January, 2014]). Use with caution in the elderly. Elderly patients exhibit higher rivaroxaban concentrations compared to younger patients due primarily to reduced clearance. Overall, efficacy of rivaroxaban in the elderly (age ≥65 years) was similar to that of patients <65 years of age. Both thrombotic and bleeding events were higher in the elderly; however, the risk to benefit profile was favorable among all age groups.

Potentially significant drug-drug interactions may exist, requiring dose or frequency adjustment, additional monitoring, and/or selection of alternative therapy. In patients with renal impairment, concomitant use of rivaroxaban with combined P-gp and weak or moderate CYP3A4 inhibitors should only occur if the potential benefit outweighs the risk of bleeding. Formulation contains lactose; use is not recommended in patients with lactose or galactose intolerance (eg, Lapp lactase deficiency, glucose-galactose malabsorption).

Discontinue rivaroxaban at least 24 hours prior to surgery/ invasive procedures. Some have recommended to discontinue rivaroxaban 3 days prior to a procedure in patients with a CrCl ≥50 mL/minute or 5 days prior in patients with a CrCl <50 mL/minute (Wysokinski, 2012). The risk of bleeding should be weighed against the urgency of the procedure; reinitiate when adequate hemostasis has been achieved unless oral therapy cannot be administered then consider administration of a parenteral anticoagulant. Safety and efficacy have not been established in patients with prosthetic heart valves or significant rheumatic heart disease (eg, mitral stenosis); use is not recommended. Non-valvular atrial fibrillation is defined as atrial fibrillation that occurs in the absence of rheumatic mitral valve disease, mitral valve repair, or prosthetic heart valve (AHA/ACC/HRS [January, 2014]). Rivaroxaban is **not** recommended as an alternative to unfractionated heparin in the treatment of acute pulmonary embolism in hemodynamically unstable patients or patients requiring thrombolysis or pulmonary embolectomy.

Adverse Reactions

Central nervous system: Fatigue, syncope

Dermatologic: Pruritus, skin blister, wound secretion

Gastrointestinal: Abdominal pain, dyspepsia, nausea, toothache

Genitourinary: Urinary tract infection

Hematologic & oncologic: Gastrointestinal hemorrhage, hemorrhage (atrial fibrillation, major; DVT prophylaxis, major; DVT/PE treatment, major), pulmonary hemorrhage (with and without bronchiectasis)

Hepatic: Increased serum transaminases (ULN: 2% [Watkins, 2011])

Neuromuscular & skeletal: Back pain, limb pain, muscle spasm, osteoarthritis

Respiratory: Oropharyngeal pain, sinusitis

Rare but important or life-threatening: Agranulocytosis, cholestasis, decreased hemoglobin (≥2 g/dL), dysuria, ecchymoses, epidural hematoma, hemiparesis, hemophthalmos, hepatic cytolysis, hepatic injury (Liakoni, 2014), hypermenorrhea, hypersensitivity, hypotension, increased amylase, increased blood urea nitrogen, increased lactate dehydrogenase, increased serum alkaline phosphatase, increased serum creatinine, increased serum lipase, intracranial hemorrhage, jaundice, retroperitoneal hemorrhage, Stevens-Johnson syndrome, subdural hematoma, tachycardia, thrombocytopenia (<100,000/mm^3 or <50% baseline)

Drug Interactions

Metabolism/Transport Effects Substrate of CYP2J2 (minor), CYP3A4 (major), P-glycoprotein; **Note:** Assignment of Major/Minor substrate status based on clinically relevant drug interaction potential

Avoid Concomitant Use

Avoid concomitant use of Rivaroxaban with any of the following: Anticoagulants; Apixaban; Conivaptan; CYP3A4 Inducers (Strong); CYP3A4 Inhibitors (Strong); Dabigatran Etexilate; Edoxaban; Idelalisib; Omacetaxine; St Johns Wort; Urokinase; Vorapaxar

Increased Effect/Toxicity

Rivaroxaban may increase the levels/effects of: Collagenase (Systemic); Deferasirox; Ibritumomab; Nintedanib; Obinutuzumab; Omacetaxine; Tositumomab and Iodine I 131 Tositumomab

The levels/effects of Rivaroxaban may be increased by: Agents with Antiplatelet Properties; Anticoagulants; Apixaban; Azithromycin (Systemic); Clarithromycin; Conivaptan; CYP3A4 Inhibitors (Moderate); CYP3A4 Inhibitors (Strong); Dabigatran Etexilate; Dasatinib; Edoxaban; Erythromycin (Systemic); Fusidic Acid (Systemic); Herbs (Anticoagulant/Antiplatelet Properties); Idelalisib; Limaprost; Luliconazole; Mifepristone; Nonsteroidal Anti-Inflammatory Agents; Omega-3 Fatty Acids; Pentosan Polysulfate Sodium; P-glycoprotein/ABCB1 Inhibitors; Prostacyclin Analogues; Salicylates; Sugammadex; Thrombolytic Agents; Tibolone; Tipranavir; Urokinase; Vitamin E; Vorapaxar

Decreased Effect

The levels/effects of Rivaroxaban may be decreased by: Bosentan; CYP3A4 Inducers (Moderate); CYP3A4 Inducers (Strong); Dabrafenib; Deferasirox; Estrogen Derivatives; P-glycoprotein/ABCB1 Inducers; Progestins; Siltuximab; St Johns Wort; Tocilizumab

Food Interactions Grapefruit juice may increase levels/effects of rivaroxaban. Management: Use caution.

Storage/Stability Store at 25°C (77°F); excursions permitted to 15°C to 30°C (59°F to 86°F).

Mechanism of Action Inhibits platelet activation and fibrin clot formation via direct, selective and reversible inhibition of factor Xa (FXa) in both the intrinsic and extrinsic coagulation pathways. FXa, as part of the prothrombinase complex consisting also of factor Va, calcium ions, factor II and phospholipid, catalyzes the conversion of prothrombin to thrombin. Thrombin both activates platelets and catalyzes the conversion of fibrinogen to fibrin.

Pharmacodynamics/Kinetics

Absorption: Rapid

Distribution: V_{dss}: ~50 L

Protein binding: ~92% to 95% (primarily to albumin)

Metabolism: Hepatic via CYP3A4/5 and CYP2J2

Bioavailability: Absolute bioavailability: 10 mg dose: ~80% to 100%; 20 mg dose: ~66% (fasting; increased with food)

Half-life elimination: Terminal: 5-9 hours; Elderly: 11-13 hours

Time to peak, plasma: 2-4 hours

Excretion: Urine (66% primarily via active tubular secretion [36% as unchanged drug; 30% as inactive metabolites]); feces (28% [7% as unchanged drug; 21% as inactive metabolites])

Dosage

Note: Extremes of body weight (<50 kg or >120 kg) do not significantly influence rivaroxaban exposure (Kubitza, 2007).

Deep vein thrombosis (DVT), pulmonary embolism (PE) treatment: Adults: Oral: Initial: 15 mg twice daily with food for 21 days followed by 20 mg once daily with food. **Note:** The American College of Chest Physicians (ACCP) recommends anticoagulant treatment for 3 months in patients with provoked DVT or ≥3 months with unprovoked DVT (duration depends on bleeding risk) (Guyatt, 2012). Canadian labeling recommends continuation of treatment for at least 3 months if first episode of DVT is secondary to transient risk factors (eg, recent trauma, surgery, immobilization) and an extended duration of treatment if patient has permanent risk factors or idiopathic DVT/PE.

Reduction in the risk (secondary prevention) of recurrent DVT/PE after an initial 6 months of treatment: Adults: Oral: 20 mg once daily with food; duration of treatment in the EINSTEIN-Extension Study was 6 to 12 months in addition to the initial treatment duration of 6 to 12 months (EINSTEIN Investigators, 2010).

Postoperative DVT thromboprophylaxis: Adults: Oral: **Note:** Initiate therapy after hemostasis has been established, 6 to 10 hours postoperatively.

Knee replacement: 10 mg once daily; recommended total duration of therapy: 12 to 14 days; ACCP recommendation: Minimum of 10 to 14 days; extended duration of up to 35 days suggested (Guyatt, 2012).

Hip replacement: 10 mg once daily; total duration of therapy: 35 days; ACCP recommendation: Minimum of 10 to 14 days; extended duration of up to 35 days suggested (Guyatt, 2012).

Nonvalvular atrial fibrillation (to prevent stroke and systemic embolism): Adults: Oral: 20 mg once daily with the evening meal.

Conversion *from* warfarin: Discontinue warfarin and initiate rivaroxaban as soon as INR falls to <3.0 (U.S. labeling) or ≤2.5 (Canadian labeling)

Conversion *to* warfarin: **Note:** Rivaroxaban affects INR; therefore, initial INR measurements after initiating warfarin may be unreliable.

U.S. labeling: Discontinue rivaroxaban and initiate both warfarin and a parenteral anticoagulant at the time the next dose of rivaroxaban would have been taken (other approaches to this conversion may be acceptable).

Canadian labeling: Continue rivaroxaban concomitantly with warfarin until INR ≥2.0 and then discontinue rivaroxaban. **Note:** Caution must be employed with this strategy given the lack of an antidote for rivaroxaban reversal. During the first 2 days of concomitant therapy, usual doses of warfarin may be given without INR testing. Thereafter, while on concomitant therapy, measure INR daily just prior to the next scheduled rivaroxaban dose, as appropriate. After rivaroxaban has been discontinued, INR testing may be done at least 24 hours after the last rivaroxaban dose.

Conversion *from* continuous infusion unfractionated heparin: Initiate rivaroxaban at the time of heparin discontinuation

Conversion *to* continuous infusion unfractionated heparin: Discontinue rivaroxaban and initiate continuous infusion unfractionated heparin at the time the next dose of rivaroxaban would have been taken.

Conversion *from* anticoagulants (other than warfarin and continuous infusion unfractionated heparin):

U.S. labeling: Discontinue current anticoagulant and initiate rivaroxaban ≤2 hours prior to the next regularly scheduled evening dose of the discontinued anticoagulant.

Canadian labeling: Discontinue current anticoagulant and initiate rivaroxaban ≤2 hours prior to the next regularly scheduled evening dose of the discontinued anticoagulant; patients previously receiving prophylactic doses of anticoagulant may initiate rivaroxaban ≥6 hours after last prophylactic dose.

Conversion *to* other anticoagulants (other than warfarin): Discontinue rivaroxaban and initiate the anticoagulant at the time the next dose of rivaroxaban would have been taken

Elderly: Refer to adult dosing.

Dosage adjustment in renal impairment: Note: Clinical trials evaluating safety and efficacy utilized the Cockcroft-Gault formula with the use of actual body weight (weight range of patients enrolled in clinical trials: 33 to 209 kg) (data on file; Janssen Pharmaceuticals Inc, 2012).

DVT, PE, reduction of the risk of recurrent DVT/PE:

U.S. labeling:

CrCl ≥30 mL/minute: There are no dosage adjustments provided in manufacturer's labeling.

CrCl <30 mL/minute: Avoid use.

Canadian labeling:

CrCl ≥30 mL/minute: No dosage adjustment necessary.

CrCl <30 mL/minute: Avoid use.

Nonvalvular atrial fibrillation:

U.S. labeling:

CrCl >50 mL/minute: No dosage adjustment necessary.

CrCl 15 to 50 mL/minute: 15 mg once daily with the evening meal. According to the AHA/ACC/HRS, may consider dose reduction in patients with moderate-to-severe chronic kidney disease (CKD), although safety and efficacy of this approach has not been established (AHA/ACC/HRS [January, 2014]).

CrCl <15 mL/minute: Avoid use. **Note:** In patients with severe or end-stage chronic kidney disease, warfarin remains the anticoagulant of choice (AHA/ACC/HRS [January, 2014]).

ESRD requiring hemodialysis: Avoid use. **Note:** In patients with severe or end-stage chronic kidney disease, warfarin remains the anticoagulant of choice (AHA/ACC/HRS [January, 2014]).

Canadian labeling:

CrCl ≥50 mL/minute: No dosage adjustment necessary.

CrCl 30 to 49 mL/minute: 15 mg once daily

CrCl <30 mL/minute: Avoid use.

Postoperative thromboprophylaxis:

CrCl >50 mL/minute: No dosage adjustment necessary.

CrCl 30 to 50 mL/minute: No dosage adjustment necessary; use with caution.

CrCl <30 mL/minute: Avoid use.

ESRD requiring hemodialysis: Avoid use.

Dosage adjustment in hepatic impairment:

Mild hepatic impairment: There are no dosage adjustments provided in manufacturer's labeling. Limited data indicates pharmacokinetics and pharmacodynamic response were similar to healthy subjects.

Moderate-to-severe hepatic impairment (Child-Pugh class B or C) and patients with any hepatic disease associated with coagulopathy: Avoid use. **Note:** The Canadian labeling contraindicates use in these patient populations.

Dosing in obesity: Body weight >120 kg does not significantly influence rivaroxaban exposure (Kubitza, 2007). Clinical outcomes in postoperative thromboprophylaxis trials were also not affected by weight (up to 190 kg) (Turpie, 2011). Therefore, dosage adjustment is not required.

Administration Administer doses ≥15 mg/day with food; dose of 10 mg/day may be administered without regard to meals. For nonvalvular atrial fibrillation, administer with the evening meal. For patients who cannot swallow whole tablets, the tablets (all strengths) may be crushed and mixed with applesauce immediately prior to use; immediately follow administration of the 15 mg and 20 mg tablets with food (10 mg tablets may be administered without regards to food).

For nasogastric/gastric feeding tube administration, the tablets (all strengths) may be crushed and mixed in 50 mL of water; administer the suspension within 4 hours of preparation and follow administration of the 15 mg and 20 mg tablets immediately with enteral feeding (10 mg tablets may be administered without regards to food). Avoid administration distal to the stomach; a decrease in the AUC and C_{max} (29% and 56%, respectively) was observed when rivaroxaban was delivered to the proximal small intestine; further decreases may be seen with delivery to the distal small intestine or ascending colon.

Missed doses: Patients receiving 15 mg twice daily dosing who miss a dose should take a dose immediately to ensure 30 mg of rivaroxaban is administered per day (two 15 mg tablets may be taken together); resume therapy the following day as previously taken. Patients receiving once-daily dosing who miss a dose should take a dose as soon as possible on the same day; resume therapy the following day as previously taken.

Monitoring Parameters Routine monitoring of coagulation tests not required; in major clinical trials, monitoring of coagulation tests (eg, aPTT, PT/INR, or antifactor Xa activity) did not occur. Prothrombin time (PT) or antifactor Xa activity may be used to detect presence of rivaroxaban (neither is intended to be used for dosage adjustment). However, variability exists among PT assays and even more so when converted to INR. Therefore, antifactor Xa activity measurement is the preferred test (Asmis, 2012; Barrett, 2010; Kubitza, 2005). A therapeutic range has not been defined, and dosage adjustment based on results has not been established.

CBC with differential; renal function prior to initiation, when clinically indicated, and at least annually (AHA/ACC/HRS [January, 2014]); hepatic function

Dosage Forms

Tablet, Oral:

Xarelto: 10 mg, 15 mg, 20 mg

Tablet Therapy Pack, Oral:

Xarelto Starter Pack: 15 mg (42s) and 20 mg (9s) (51 ea)

◆ **Riva-Sertraline (Can)** *see* Sertraline *on page 1878*

◆ **Riva-Simvastatin (Can)** *see* Simvastatin *on page 1890*

◆ **Rivasol (Can)** *see* Zinc Sulfate *on page 2200*

◆ **Rivasone (Can)** *see* Betamethasone (Topical) *on page 255*

◆ **Riva-Sotalol (Can)** *see* Sotalol *on page 1927*

Rivastigmine (ri va STIG meen)

Brand Names: U.S. Exelon

Brand Names: Canada Apo-Rivastigmine; Exelon; Mylan-Rivastigmine; Novo-Rivastigmine; PMS-Rivastigmine; ratio-Rivastigmine; Sandoz-Rivastigmine

Index Terms ENA 713; Rivastigmine Tartrate; SDZ ENA 713

Pharmacologic Category Acetylcholinesterase Inhibitor (Central)

Use Dementia associated with Alzheimer's or Parkinson's disease:

U.S. labeling: Treatment of mild, moderate, or severe dementia associated with Alzheimer's disease; treatment of mild-to-moderate dementia associated with Parkinson's disease

Canadian labeling: Treatment of mild-to-moderate dementia associated with Alzheimer's disease; treatment of mild-to-moderate dementia associated with Parkinson's disease

Pregnancy Risk Factor B

Pregnancy Considerations Adverse events were observed in some animal reproduction studies. Use in women of reproductive age is not recommended.

Breast-Feeding Considerations It is not known if rivastigmine is excreted in breast milk. Rivastigmine is not indicated in nursing mothers.

Contraindications Hypersensitivity to rivastigmine, other carbamate derivatives (eg, neostigmine, pyridostigmine, physostigmine), or any component of the formulation; history of application site reactions with rivastigmine patch

Canadian labeling: Additional contraindications (not in U.S. labeling): Severe hepatic impairment

Warnings/Precautions Significant nausea/vomiting/diarrhea or anorexia/weight loss/decreased appetite are associated with use; occurs more frequently in women and during the titration phase. The incidence and severity of these reactions are dose-related. Monitor weight during therapy. Therapy should be initiated at lowest dose and titrated; if treatment is interrupted for >3 days, reinstate at the lowest daily dose. May have vagotonic effects which may cause bradycardia and/or heart block with or without a history of cardiac disease. Alzheimer's treatment guidelines consider bradycardia to be a relative contraindication for use of centrally-active cholinesterase inhibitors. Postmarketing cases of overdose (including fatalities) have been reported in association with medication errors/improper use of rivastigmine transdermal patches. No more than 1 patch should be applied daily and existing patch must be removed prior to applying new patch.

Use of patch may result in allergic contact dermatitis; discontinue therapy if an intense local reaction occurs (eg, increasing erythema, edema, papules, vesicles) and if symptoms do not improve after 48 hours of patch removal. If therapy is still required, oral rivastigmine may be used following negative allergy testing; some patients may not be able to take rivastigmine in any form. Postmarketing reports of disseminated hypersensitivity skin reactions have occurred with use of oral or transdermal products; discontinue use of all rivastigmine therapy in these cases.

Use caution in patients with a history of peptic ulcer disease or concurrent NSAID use; may increase gastric acid secretion. Monitor for active or occult bleeding. Use caution in patients with sick-sinus syndrome, bradycardia or supraventricular conduction conditions, urinary obstruction, seizure disorders, or pulmonary conditions such as asthma or COPD. May exacerbate or induce extrapyramidal symptoms; worsening of symptoms (eg, tremor) in patients with Parkinson's disease has been observed. May cause CNS depression, which may impair physical or mental abilities; patients must be cautioned about performing tasks which require mental alertness (eg, operating machinery or driving). CNS effects may be potentiated when used with other sedative drugs or ethanol. Systemic exposure may be increased in patients <50 kg and decreased in patients >100 kg. Consider dose reduction if toxicities develop in patients <50 kg (oral and transdermal). Consider a dose increase in patients >100 kg (transdermal). Potentially significant drug-drug interactions may exist, requiring dose or frequency adjustment, additional monitoring, and/or selection of alternative therapy. Nicotine increases the clearance of rivastigmine by 23%.

Adverse Reactions

Cardiovascular: Hypertension, syncope

Central nervous system: Abnormal gait, aggressive behavior, agitation, anxiety, cogwheel rigidity, confusion, depression, dizziness, drowsiness, exacerbation of Parkinson's disease, falling, fatigue, hallucinations, headache, insomnia, malaise, paranoia, parkinsonism symptoms worsening, psychomotor agitation, restlessness, vertigo

Dermatologic: Diaphoresis

Endocrine & metabolic: Dehydration, weight loss

Gastrointestinal: Abdominal pain, anorexia, constipation, decreased appetite, diarrhea, dyspepsia, eructation, flatulence, nausea, sialorrhea, upper abdominal pain, vomiting, weight loss

Genitourinary: Urinary incontinence, urinary tract infection

Local: Application site reaction (including erythema, irritation, pruritus, and rash)

Neuromuscular & skeletal: Back pain, bradykinesia, dyskinesia, hypokinesia, tremor, weakness

Respiratory: Flu-like symptoms, rhinitis

Miscellaneous: Accidental injury

Rare but important or life-threatening: Adams-Stokes syndrome, ageusia, anemia, aneurysm, angina pectoris, aphthous stomatitis, apraxia, atrial fibrillation, atrioventricular block, benign prostate adenoma, bradycardia, bundle branch block, cardiac arrest, cardiac failure, cellulitis, cerebrovascular accident, cholecystitis, convulsions, dermal ulcer, diplopia, diverticulitis, duodenal ulcer, endometritis, epilepsy, fecal impaction, gastritis, gastroesophageal reflux, glaucoma, hepatic failure, hepatitis, hematoma, hemiparesis, hernia, hip fracture, hyperglycemia, hypercholesterolemia, hyperlipidemia, hypersensitivity reaction, hypoglycemia, hypothyroidism, ileus, impotence, increased gamma-glutamyl transferase, increased serum alkaline phosphatase, intestinal obstruction, intracranial hemorrhage, laryngitis, mastalgia, mastitis, Meniere's disease, migraine, myocardial infarction, neuralgia, otitis media, pancreatitis, paresis, peripheral ischemia, peripheral neuropathy, pneumonia, psychiatric signs and symptoms (eg, delirium, delusions, dementia, depersonalization, emotional lability, personality disorder, psychosis, suicidal ideation or tendencies), pulmonary embolism, rectal hemorrhage, renal failure, respiratory depression, retinopathy, seizure, sick-sinus syndrome, Stevens-Johnson syndrome, supraventricular tachycardia, thrombocytopenia, thrombophlebitis, thrombosis, transient ischemic attacks, vasodepressor syncope

Drug Interactions

Metabolism/Transport Effects None known.

Avoid Concomitant Use

Avoid concomitant use of Rivastigmine with any of the following: Ceritinib

Increased Effect/Toxicity

Rivastigmine may increase the levels/effects of: Antipsychotic Agents; Beta-Blockers; Bradycardia-Causing Agents; Ceritinib; Cholinergic Agonists; Lacosamide; Succinylcholine

The levels/effects of Rivastigmine may be increased by: Bretylium; Corticosteroids (Systemic); Tofacitinib

Decreased Effect

Rivastigmine may decrease the levels/effects of: Anticholinergic Agents; Neuromuscular-Blocking Agents (Nondepolarizing)

The levels/effects of Rivastigmine may be decreased by: Anticholinergic Agents; Dipyridamole

Food Interactions Food delays absorption by 90 minutes, lowers C_{max} by 30% and increases AUC by 30%. Management: Administer with meals.

Storage/Stability

Oral: Store at 25°C (77°F); excursions permitted between 15°C and 30°C (59°F to 86°F); do not freeze. Store solution in an upright position. Stable at room temperature for up to 4 hours when solution is mixed with cold fruit juice or soda.

Transdermal patch: Store at 25°C (77°F); excursions permitted between 15°C and 30°C (59°F to 86°F). Patches should be kept in sealed pouch until use.

Mechanism of Action A deficiency of cortical acetylcholine is thought to account for some of the symptoms of Alzheimer's disease and the dementia of Parkinson's disease; rivastigmine increases acetylcholine in the central nervous system through reversible inhibition of its hydrolysis by cholinesterase

Pharmacodynamics/Kinetics

Duration: Anticholinesterase activity (CSF): ~10 hours (6 mg oral dose)

Absorption: Oral: Fasting: Rapid and complete within 1 hour; Transdermal patch: Within 30-60 minutes

Distribution: V_d: 1.8-2.7 L/kg; penetrates blood-brain barrier (CSF levels are ~40% of plasma levels following oral administration)

Protein binding: 40%

Metabolism: Extensively via cholinesterase-mediated hydrolysis in the brain; metabolite undergoes N-demethylation and/or sulfate conjugation hepatically; CYP minimally involved; linear kinetics at 3 mg twice daily, but nonlinear at higher doses

Bioavailability: Oral: 36%

Half-life elimination: Oral: 1.5 hours; Transdermal patch: ~3 hours (after removal)

Time to peak: Oral: 1 hour; Transdermal patch: 8-16 hours following first dose

Excretion: Urine (97% as metabolites); feces (0.4%)

Dosage Note: Exelon oral solution and capsules are bioequivalent.

Alzheimer's dementia, mild-to-moderate: Adults:

Oral: Initial: 1.5 mg twice daily; may increase by 3 mg daily (1.5 mg/dose) every 2 weeks based on tolerability (maximum recommended dose: 6 mg twice daily)

Low body weight: Careful titration and monitoring should be performed in patients with low body weight. In patients <50 kg, monitor closely for toxicities (eg, excessive nausea, vomiting) and consider reducing the dose if such toxicities develop.

Note: If GI adverse events occur, discontinue treatment for several doses then restart at the same or next lower dosage level; antiemetics have been used to control GI symptoms. If dosing is interrupted for ≤3 days, restart the treatment at the lowest dose and titrate as previously described.

Transdermal patch:

U.S. labeling: Initial: Apply 4.6 mg/24 hours patch once daily; if well tolerated, may titrate (no sooner than every 4 weeks) to 9.5 mg/24 hours (continue as long as therapeutically beneficial), and then to 13.3 mg/24 hours (maximum dose); doses >13.3 mg/24 hours have not been shown to be more effective and are associated with significant increases in adverse events. Remove old patch and replace with a new patch every 24 hours. Recommended effective dose: Apply 9.5 mg/24 hours or 13.3 mg/24 hours patch once daily; remove old patch and replace with a new patch every 24 hours

Canadian labeling: Initial: Apply 4.6 mg/24 hours patch once daily; if well tolerated, may titrate (no sooner than after 4 weeks) to 9.5 mg/24 hours (maximum recommended dose); continue as long as therapeutically beneficial.

Low body weight: Careful titration and monitoring should be performed in patients with low body weight. In patients <50 kg, monitor closely for toxicities (eg, excessive nausea, vomiting) and consider reducing the maintenance dose to 4.6 mg/24 hour if such toxicities develop. Consider doses >9.5 mg/24 hours in patients >100 kg.

Note: If dosing is interrupted for ≤3 days, restart treatment with the same or a lower strength patch. If interrupted for >3 days, reinitiate at 4.6 mg/24 hours and titrate (no sooner than every 4 weeks) to lowest effective maintenance dose.

Conversion from oral therapy: If oral daily dose <6 mg, switch to 4.6 mg/24 hours patch; if oral daily dose 6-12 mg, switch to 9.5 mg/24 hours patch. Apply patch on the next day following last oral dose.

Alzheimer's dementia, severe: Adults: Transdermal patch: Initial: Apply 4.6 mg/24 hours patch once daily. Titrate dose as recommended for transdermal dosing for mild-to-moderate Alzheimer's dementia. Recommended effective dose: Apply 13.3 mg/24 hours patch once daily; remove old patch and replace with a new patch every 24 hours

Low body weight: Careful titration and monitoring should be performed in patients with low body weight. In patients <50 kg, monitor closely for toxicities (eg, excessive nausea, vomiting) and consider reducing the maintenance dose to 4.6 mg/24 hour if such toxicities develop. Consider doses >9.5 mg/24 hours in patients >100 kg.

Note: If dosing is interrupted for ≤3 days, restart treatment with the same or a lower strength patch. If interrupted for >3 days, reinitiate at 4.6 mg/24 hours and titrate (no sooner than every 4 weeks) to lowest effective maintenance dose.

Parkinson's-related dementia, mild-to-moderate: Adults:

Oral: Initial: 1.5 mg twice daily; may increase by 3 mg daily (1.5 mg per dose) every 4 weeks based on tolerability (maximum recommended dose: 6 mg twice daily)

Low body weight: Careful titration and monitoring should be performed in patients with low body weight. In patients <50 kg, monitor closely for toxicities (eg, excessive nausea, vomiting) and consider reducing the dose if such toxicities develop.

Note: If GI adverse events occur, discontinue treatment for several doses then restart at the same or next lower dosage level; antiemetics have been used to control GI symptoms. If dosing is interrupted for ≤3 days, restart the treatment at the lowest dose and titrate as previously described.

Transdermal patch: Initial: Apply 4.6 mg/24 hours patch once daily. If well tolerated, may titrate (no sooner than every 4 weeks) to 9.5 mg/24 hours (continue as long as therapeutically beneficial), and then to 13.3 mg/24 hours (maximum dose); doses >13.3 mg/24 hours have not been shown to be more effective and are associated with significant increases in adverse events. Recommended effective dose: Apply 9.5 mg/24 hours or 13.3 mg/24 hours patch once daily; remove old patch and replace with a new patch every 24 hours

Low body weight: Careful titration and monitoring should be performed in patients with low body weight. In patients <50 kg, monitor closely for toxicities (eg, excessive nausea, vomiting) and consider reducing the maintenance dose to 4.6 mg/24 hour if such toxicities develop. Consider doses >9.5 mg/24 hours in patients >100 kg.

Note: If dosing is interrupted for ≤3 days, restart treatment with the same or a lower strength patch. If interrupted for >3 days, reinitiate at 4.6 mg/24 hours and titrate (no sooner than every 4 weeks) to lowest effective maintenance dose.

Dementia with Lewy bodies (off-label use): Adults: Oral: Initial: 1.5 mg twice daily; may increase by 3 mg daily (1.5 mg per dose) every 2 weeks based on tolerability up to a maximum of 6 mg twice daily (titration lasted up to 8 weeks); study duration was 23 weeks (McKeith, 2000). An extension study was conducted in a limited number of patients (at the same dose) for up to 96 weeks (Grace, 2001).

Elderly: Following oral administration, clearance is significantly lower in patients >60 years of age, but dosage adjustments are not recommended. Age was not associated with exposure in patients treated transdermally. Titrate dose to individual's tolerance. **Note:** Canadian labeling recommends an initial oral dose of 1.5 mg once daily in patients >85 years of age with low body weight (<50 kg) or serious comorbidities, with a slower titration rate than used for adults.

Dosage adjustment in renal impairment:

U.S. labeling:

Oral: Moderate-to-severe impairment (CrCl ≤50 mL/minute): No dosage adjustment provided in manufacturer's labeling; clearance is reduced and patients may require lower doses.

Transdermal: No dosage adjustment necessary.

Canadian labeling:

Oral: Initial dose: 1.5 mg once daily; titrate dose at a rate slower than recommended for healthy adults

Transdermal: No dosage adjustment provided in manufacturer's labeling (has not been studied); titrate dose cautiously

Dosage adjustment in hepatic impairment:

U.S. labeling:

Oral:

Mild-to-moderate impairment (Child-Pugh class A and B): No dosage adjustment provided in manufacturer's labeling; clearance is reduced and patients may require lower doses.

Severe impairment (Child-Pugh class C): No dosage adjustment provided in manufacturer's labeling (has not been studied).

Transdermal:

Mild-to-moderate impairment (Child-Pugh class A and B): Initial and maximum dose: 4.6 mg/24 hours

Severe impairment (Child-Pugh class C): No dosage adjustment provided in manufacturer's labeling (has not been studied).

Canadian labeling:

Oral:

Mild-to-moderate impairment (Child-Pugh class A and B): Initial dose: 1.5 mg once daily; titrate dose at a rate slower than recommended for healthy adults

Severe impairment (Child-Pugh class C): Use is contraindicated.

Transdermal:

Mild-to-moderate impairment (Child-Pugh class A and B): No dosage adjustment provided in manufacturer's labeling; titrate dose cautiously

Severe impairment (Child-Pugh class C): Use is contraindicated.

Administration

Oral: Administer with meals (breakfast and dinner). Capsule should be swallowed whole. Liquid form, which is available for patients who cannot swallow capsules, can be swallowed directly from syringe or mixed with water, soda, or cold fruit juice. Stir well and drink within 4 hours of mixing.

Topical: Apply transdermal patch to upper or lower back (alternatively, may apply to upper arm or chest). Do not use patch if the pouch seal is broken or if the patch is cut, altered, or damaged. Avoid reapplication to same spot of skin for 14 days (eg, may rotate sections of back). Apply to clean, dry, and hairless skin. Patch should be pressed down firmly by applying pressure with the hand over the entire patch for at least 30 seconds, making sure edges stick well. Do not apply to red, irritated, or broken skin. Avoid areas of recent application of lotion or powder. After removal, fold patch to press adhesive surfaces together, place in previously saved pouch, and discard. Avoid eye contact; wash hands after handling patch. Remove old patch and replace with a new patch every 24 hours (at the same time each day). If a dose is missed or if the patch falls off, apply a new patch immediately and replace the following day at the usual application time. Avoid exposing the patch to external sources of heat (eg, sauna, excessive light) for prolonged periods of time. No more than 1 patch should be applied daily and existing patch must be removed prior to applying new patch.

Monitoring Parameters Cognitive function at periodic intervals, symptoms of GI intolerance, weight

Dosage Forms

Capsule, Oral:

Exelon: 1.5 mg, 3 mg, 4.5 mg, 6 mg

Generic: 1.5 mg, 3 mg, 4.5 mg, 6 mg

Patch 24 Hour, Transdermal:

Exelon: 4.6 mg/24 hr (1 ea, 30 ea); 9.5 mg/24 hr (1 ea, 30 ea); 13.3 mg/24 hr (1 ea, 30 ea)

Dosage Forms: Canada Refer to Dosage Forms. **Note:** Exelon 13.3 mg/24 hour transdermal patch is not available in Canada.

- ◆ **Rivastigmine Tartrate** *see* Rivastigmine *on page 1833*
- ◆ **Riva-Terbinafine (Can)** *see* Terbinafine (Systemic) *on page 2002*
- ◆ **Riva-Valacyclovir (Can)** *see* ValACYclovir *on page 2119*
- ◆ **Riva-Venlafaxine XR (Can)** *see* Venlafaxine *on page 2150*
- ◆ **Riva-Verapamil SR (Can)** *see* Verapamil *on page 2154*
- ◆ **Riva-Zolmitriptan (Can)** *see* ZOLMitriptan *on page 2210*
- ◆ **Riva-Zopiclone (Can)** *see* Zopiclone [CAN/INT] *on page 2217*
- ◆ **Rivotril (Can)** *see* ClonazePAM *on page 478*
- ◆ **Rixubis** *see* Factor IX (Recombinant) *on page 841*

Rizatriptan (rye za TRIP tan)

Brand Names: U.S. Maxalt; Maxalt-MLT

Brand Names: Canada ACT Rizatriptan; ACT Rizatriptan ODT; Apo-Rizatriptan; Apo-Rizatriptan RPD; Dom-Rizatriptan RDT; JAMP-Rizatriptan; JAMP-Rizatriptan IR; Mar-Rizatriptan; Maxalt; Maxalt RPD; Mylan-Rizatriptan ODT; PMS-Rizatriptan RDT; Riva-Rizatriptan ODT; Rizatriptan RDT; Sandoz-Rizatriptan ODT

Index Terms MK462

Pharmacologic Category Antimigraine Agent; Serotonin 5-$HT_{1B, 1D}$ Receptor Agonist

Use Acute treatment of migraine with or without aura

Pregnancy Risk Factor C

Pregnancy Considerations Adverse events were observed in animal reproduction studies. Information related to rizatriptan use in pregnancy is limited (Källén, 2011; Nezvalová-Henriksen, 2010; Nezvalová-Henriksen, 2012).

A pregnancy registry has been established to monitor outcomes of women exposed to rizatriptan during pregnancy (800-986-8999). Preliminary data from the pregnancy registry (prospectively collected from 65 live births 1998-2004) does not show an increased risk of congenital malformations (Fiore, 2005). Until additional information is available, other agents are preferred for the initial treatment of migraine in pregnancy (Da Silva, 2012; MacGregor, 2012; Williams, 2012).

Breast-Feeding Considerations It is not known if rizatriptan is excreted in breast milk. The manufacturer recommends that caution be exercised when administering rizatriptan to nursing women.

Contraindications Hypersensitivity to rizatriptan or any component of the formulation; documented ischemic heart disease or other significant cardiovascular disease; coronary artery vasospasm (including Prinzmetal's angina); history of stroke or transient ischemic attack; peripheral vascular disease; ischemic bowel disease; uncontrolled hypertension; basilar or hemiplegic migraine; during or within 2 weeks of MAO inhibitors; during or within 24 hours of treatment with another 5-HT_1 agonist, or an ergot-containing or ergot-type medication (eg, methysergide, dihydroergotamine)

Warnings/Precautions Only indicated for treatment of acute migraine; not for the prevention of migraines or the treatment of cluster headache. If a patient does not respond to the first dose, the diagnosis of migraine should be reconsidered. Coronary artery vasospasm, transient ischemia, myocardial infarction, ventricular tachycardia/fibrillation, cardiac arrest, and death have been reported with 5-HT_1 agonist administration. Patients who experience sensations of chest pain/pressure/tightness or symptoms suggestive of angina following dosing should be evaluated for coronary artery disease or Prinzmetal's angina before receiving additional doses; if dosing is resumed and similar symptoms recur, monitor with ECG. Should not be given to patients who have risk factors for CAD (eg, hypertension, hypercholesterolemia, smoker, obesity, diabetes, strong family history of CAD, menopause, male >40 years of age) without adequate cardiac evaluation. Patients with suspected CAD should have cardiovascular evaluation to rule out CAD before considering use; if cardiovascular evaluation is "satisfactory," first dose should be given in the healthcare provider's office (consider ECG monitoring). Periodic evaluation of cardiovascular status should be done in all patients. Significant elevation in blood pressure, including hypertensive crisis, has also been reported on rare occasions in patients with and without a history of hypertension. Cerebral/subarachnoid hemorrhage, stroke, peripheral vascular ischemia, gastrointestinal ischemia/infarction, splenic infarction and Raynaud's syndrome have been reported with 5-HT_1 agonist administration. Use is contraindicated in patients with a history of stroke or transient ischemic attack. Rarely, partial vision loss and blindness (transient and permanent) have been reported with 5-HT_1 agonists.

Use with caution in elderly or patients with hepatic or renal impairment (including dialysis patients). Symptoms of agitation, confusion, hallucinations, hyper-reflexia, myoclonus, shivering, and tachycardia may occur with concomitant proserotonergic drugs (eg, SSRIs/SNRIs or triptans) or agents which reduce rizatriptan's metabolism. Concurrent use of serotonin precursors (eg, tryptophan) is not recommended. If concomitant administration with SSRIs is warranted, monitor closely, especially at initiation and with dose increases. Acute migraine agents (eg, triptans, opioids, ergotamine, or a combination of the agents) used for 10 or more days per month may lead to worsening of headaches (medication overuse headache); withdrawal treatment may be necessary in the setting of overuse. Maxalt-MLT tablets contain phenylalanine.

Adverse Reactions

Cardiovascular: Chest pain, flushing, palpitation

Central nervous system: Dizziness, euphoria, fatigue (dose related; more common in adults), headache, hypoesthesia, pain, somnolence

Dermatologic: Skin flushing

Gastrointestinal: Abdominal discomfort, diarrhea, nausea, vomiting, xerostomia

Neuromuscular & skeletal: Neck, throat, and jaw pain/tightness/pressure; paresthesia; tremor; weakness

Respiratory: Dyspnea

Miscellaneous: Feeling of heaviness

Rare but important or life-threatening: Anaphylaxis/anaphylactoid reactions, angina, angioedema, blurred vision, bradycardia, confusion, edema, hallucination (children), hearing impairment, hypertensive crisis, memory impairment, MI, myocardial ischemia, pruritus, seizure, syncope, tachycardia, tinnitus, tongue edema, toxic epidermal necrolysis, vasospasm, vertigo, wheezing

Drug Interactions

Metabolism/Transport Effects None known.

Avoid Concomitant Use

Avoid concomitant use of Rizatriptan with any of the following: Dapoxetine; Ergot Derivatives; MAO Inhibitors

Increased Effect/Toxicity

Rizatriptan may increase the levels/effects of: Antipsychotic Agents; Droxidopa; Ergot Derivatives; Metoclopramide; Serotonin Modulators

The levels/effects of Rizatriptan may be increased by: Antiemetics (5HT3 Antagonists); Antipsychotic Agents; Dapoxetine; Ergot Derivatives; MAO Inhibitors; Propranolol

Decreased Effect There are no known significant interactions involving a decrease in effect.

Food Interactions Food delays absorption. Management: Administer without regard to meals.

Storage/Stability Store at room temperature of 15°C to 30°C (59°F to 86°F); orally disintegrating tablets should be stored in blister pack until administration.

Mechanism of Action Selective agonist for serotonin (5-HT_{1B} and 5-HT_{1D} receptors) in cranial arteries; causes vasoconstriction and reduces sterile inflammation associated with antidromic neuronal transmission correlating with relief of migraine

Pharmacodynamics/Kinetics

Onset of action: Most patients have response to treatment within 2 hours

Distribution: V_d: Females: 110 L; Males 140 L

Protein binding: 14%

Metabolism: Via monoamine oxidase-A; forms metabolites; significant first-pass metabolism

Bioavailability: ~45%

Half-life elimination: 2-3 hours

Time to peak: Maxalt®: 1-1.5 hours (delayed up to 0.7 hour with Maxalt-MLT®)

Excretion: Urine (82%, 14% as unchanged drug); feces (12%)

Dosage Note: In patients with risk factors for coronary artery disease, following adequate evaluation to establish the absence of coronary artery disease, the initial dose should be administered in a setting where response may be evaluated (physician's office or similarly staffed setting). ECG monitoring may be considered.

Children 6-17 years: Oral: **Note:** Safety and efficacy of multiple rizatriptan doses in a 24-hour period have not been established for pediatric patients.

<40 kg: 5 mg as a single dose

≥40 kg: 10 mg as a single dose

Dose adjustment with concomitant propranolol therapy:

<40 kg: Use not recommended

≥40 kg: 5 mg as a single dose (maximum: 5 mg/24 hours)

Adults: Oral: 5-10 mg, repeat after 2 hours if significant relief is not attained; maximum: 30 mg/24 hours

Dose adjustment with concomitant propranolol therapy: 5 mg/dose (maximum: 15 mg/24 hours)

Dosage adjustment in renal impairment: No dosage adjustment provided in manufacturer's labeling; however, the AUC was 44% greater in patients on hemodialysis.

Dosage adjustment in hepatic impairment: No dosage adjustment provided in manufacturer's labeling; however, plasma concentrations are increased by 30% in patients with moderate hepatic dysfunction.

Dietary Considerations Some products may contain phenylalanine.

Administration May be administered with or without food. For orally-disintegrating tablets (Maxalt-MLT®), patient should be instructed to place tablet on tongue and allow to dissolve. Dissolved tablet will be swallowed with saliva.

Monitoring Parameters Headache severity, signs/symptoms suggestive of angina; consider monitoring blood pressure, heart rate, and/or ECG with first dose in patients with likelihood of unrecognized coronary disease, such as patients with significant hypertension, hypercholesterolemia, obese patients, patients with diabetes, smokers with other risk factors or strong family history of coronary artery disease

Dosage Forms

Tablet, Oral:

Maxalt: 5 mg, 10 mg

Generic: 5 mg, 10 mg

Tablet Dispersible, Oral:

Maxalt-MLT: 5 mg, 10 mg

Generic: 5 mg, 10 mg

- ◆ **Rizatriptan RDT (Can)** *see* Rizatriptan *on page 1836*
- ◆ **rLFN-α2** *see* Interferon Alfa-2b *on page 1096*
- ◆ **R-modafinil** *see* Armodafinil *on page 175*
- ◆ **Ro 5488** *see* Tretinoin (Systemic) *on page 2096*
- ◆ **RO5185426** *see* Vemurafenib *on page 2148*
- ◆ **RoActemra** *see* Tocilizumab *on page 2057*
- ◆ **Robafen [OTC]** *see* GuaiFENesin *on page 986*
- ◆ **Robafen AC** *see* Guaifenesin and Codeine *on page 987*
- ◆ **Robafen DM [OTC]** *see* Guaifenesin and Dextromethorphan *on page 987*
- ◆ **Robaxin** *see* Methocarbamol *on page 1320*
- ◆ **Robaxin® (Can)** *see* Methocarbamol *on page 1320*
- ◆ **Robaxin-750** *see* Methocarbamol *on page 1320*
- ◆ **Robidrine® (Can)** *see* Pseudoephedrine *on page 1742*
- ◆ **Robinul** *see* Glycopyrrolate *on page 975*
- ◆ **Robinul-Forte** *see* Glycopyrrolate *on page 975*
- ◆ **Robitussin® (Can)** *see* GuaiFENesin *on page 986*
- ◆ **Robitussin AC** *see* Guaifenesin and Codeine *on page 987*
- ◆ **Robitussin Chest Congestion [OTC]** *see* GuaiFENesin *on page 986*
- ◆ **Robitussin® Childrens Cough & Cold (Can)** *see* Pseudoephedrine and Dextromethorphan *on page 1743*
- ◆ **Robitussin® Children's Cough & Cold Long-Acting [OTC]** *see* Dextromethorphan and Chlorpheniramine *on page 610*
- ◆ **Robitussin Cough & Cold Extra Strength (Can)** *see* Guaifenesin, Pseudoephedrine, and Dextromethorphan *on page 989*
- ◆ **Robitussin Mucus+Chest Congest [OTC]** *see* GuaiFENesin *on page 986*
- ◆ **Robitussin Peak Cold Cough + Chest Congestion DM [OTC]** *see* Guaifenesin and Dextromethorphan *on page 987*
- ◆ **Robitussin Peak Cold Maximum Strength Cough + Chest Congestion DM [OTC]** *see* Guaifenesin and Dextromethorphan *on page 987*
- ◆ **Robitussin Peak Cold Sugar-Free Cough + Chest Congestion DM [OTC]** *see* Guaifenesin and Dextromethorphan *on page 987*
- ◆ **Rocaltrol** *see* Calcitriol *on page 323*
- ◆ **Rocephin** *see* CefTRIAXone *on page 396*

Rocuronium (roe kyoor OH nee um)

Brand Names: U.S. Zemuron

Brand Names: Canada Rocuronium Bromide Injection; Zemuron®

Index Terms ORG 9426; Rocuronium Bromide

Pharmacologic Category Neuromuscular Blocker Agent, Nondepolarizing

Use Facilitate both rapid sequence and routine endotracheal intubation and to relax skeletal muscles during surgery; to facilitate mechanical ventilation in ICU patients

Pregnancy Risk Factor C

Pregnancy Considerations Teratogenic effects were not observed in animal reproduction studies. Rocuronium crosses the placenta; umbilical venous plasma levels are ~18% of the maternal concentration following a maternal dose of 0.6 mg/kg (Abouleish, 1994). The manufacturer does not recommend use for rapid sequence induction during cesarean section.

Breast-Feeding Considerations Information related to rocuronium use and breast-feeding has not been located. If present in breast milk, oral absorption by a nursing infant would be expected to be minimal (Lee, 1993).

Contraindications Hypersensitivity (eg, anaphylaxis) to rocuronium, other neuromuscular-blocking agents, or any component of the formulation

Warnings/Precautions Use with caution in patients with cardiovascular disease and pulmonary disease; ventilation must be supported during neuromuscular blockade; certain clinical conditions may result in potentiation or antagonism of neuromuscular blockade:

Potentiation: Electrolyte abnormalities, severe hyponatremia, severe hypocalcemia, severe hypokalemia, hypermagnesemia, cachexia, neuromuscular diseases, metabolic acidosis, metabolic alkalosis, Eaton-Lambert syndrome, and myasthenia gravis

Antagonism: Respiratory alkalosis, hypercalcemia, demyelinating lesions, peripheral neuropathies, denervation, infection, and muscle trauma

Use with caution in patients with hepatic impairment; clinical duration may be prolonged. Resistance may occur in burn patients (>30% of body) for period of 5-70 days postinjury or in immobilized patients. Cross-sensitivity with other neuromuscular-blocking agents may occur; use is contraindicated in patients with previous anaphylactic reactions to other neuromuscular blockers. Use with caution in patients with pulmonary hypertension or valvular heart disease. Use caution in the elderly. Should be administered by adequately trained individuals familiar with its use. Use appropriate anesthesia, pain control, and sedation. In patients requiring long-term administration in the ICU, use of a peripheral nerve stimulator to monitor drug effects is strongly recommended. Additional doses of rocuronium or any other neuromuscular-blocking agent should be avoided unless definite excessive response to nerve stimulation is present.

Some patients may experience prolonged recovery of neuromuscular function after administration (especially after prolonged use). Patients should be adequately recovered prior to extubation. Other factors associated with prolonged recovery should be considered (eg, corticosteroid use, patient condition). In addition to prolonging recovery from neuromuscular blockade, concomitant use with corticosteroids has been associated with development of acute quadriplegic myopathy syndrome (AQMS). Current guidelines recommend neuromuscular blockers be discontinued as soon as possible in patients receiving corticosteroids or interrupted daily until necessary to restart them based on clinical condition (Murray, 2002). Numerous drugs either *antagonize* (eg, acetylcholinesterase inhibitors) or *potentiate* (eg, calcium channel blockers, certain antimicrobials, inhalation anesthetics, lithium, magnesium salts, procainamide, and quinidine) the effects of neuromuscular blockade; use with caution in patients receiving these agents. Immediate treatment (including epinephrine 1:1000) for anaphylactoid and/or hypersensitivity reactions should be available during use. Not recommended by the manufacturer for rapid sequence intubation in pediatric patients; however, it has been used successfully in clinical trials for this indication. If extravasation occurs, local irritation may ensue; discontinue administration immediately and restart in another vein.

Adverse Reactions

Cardiovascular: Hypertension, hypotension (transient)

Rare but important or life-threatening: Abnormal ECG, anaphylactoid reaction, anaphylaxis, arrhythmia, bronchospasm, injection site edema, hiccups, pruritus, nausea, pulmonary vascular resistance (increased), rash, rhonchi, shock, tachycardia, vomiting, wheezing

Drug Interactions

Metabolism/Transport Effects None known.

Avoid Concomitant Use

Avoid concomitant use of Rocuronium with any of the following: QuiNINE

Increased Effect/Toxicity

Rocuronium may increase the levels/effects of: Cardiac Glycosides; Corticosteroids (Systemic); OnabotulinumtoxinA; RimabotulinumtoxinB

The levels/effects of Rocuronium may be increased by: AbobotulinumtoxinA; Aminoglycosides; Calcium Channel Blockers; Capreomycin; Clindamycin (Topical); Colistimethate; CycloSPORINE (Systemic); Fosphenytoin-Phenytoin; Inhalational Anesthetics; Ketorolac (Nasal); Ketorolac (Systemic); Lincosamide Antibiotics; Lithium; Loop Diuretics; Magnesium Salts; Polymyxin B; Procainamide; QuiNIDine; QuiNINE; Spironolactone; Tetracycline Derivatives; Vancomycin

Decreased Effect

The levels/effects of Rocuronium may be decreased by: Acetylcholinesterase Inhibitors; Fosphenytoin-Phenytoin; Loop Diuretics

Storage/Stability Store unopened/undiluted vials under refrigeration at 2°C to 8°C (36°F to 46°F); do not freeze. When stored at room temperature, it is stable for 60 days; once opened, use within 30 days. Dilutions up to 5 mg/mL in 0.9% sodium chloride, dextrose 5% in water, 5% dextrose in sodium chloride 0.9%, or lactated Ringer's are stable for up to 24 hours at room temperature.

Mechanism of Action Blocks acetylcholine from binding to receptors on motor endplate inhibiting depolarization

Pharmacodynamics/Kinetics

Onset of action: Good intubation conditions within 1-2 minutes (depending on dose administered); maximum neuromuscular blockade within 4 minutes

Duration: ~30 minutes (with standard doses, increases with higher doses and inhalational anesthetic agents; patient age dependent)

Distribution: V_d: ~0.25 L/kg

Protein binding: ~30%

Metabolism: Minimally hepatic; 17-desacetylrocuronium (5% to 10% activity of parent drug)

Half-life elimination: 60-144 minutes

Excretion: Feces (50%); urine (30%)

Dosage Dose to effect; doses will vary due to interpatient variability. Dosing also dependent on anesthetic technique and age of patient.

Infants 28 days to 3 months and Children ≥3 months: **Note:** In general, onset is shortened and duration is prolonged as dose increases. Duration is shortest in children >2 to ≤11 years and longest in neonates and infants.

Rapid sequence intubation (off-label use): IV: 0.9 mg/kg or 1.2 mg/kg. Not recommended, per the manufacturer, for rapid sequence intubation in pediatric patients; however, it has been used successfully in clinical trials for this indication in children >1 year of age (Cheng, 2002; Fuchs-Buder, 1996; Mazurek, 1998; Naguib, 1997).

Tracheal intubation: IV: 0.45 mg/kg or 0.6 mg/kg

Maintenance for continued surgical relaxation: IV: 0.075-0.15 mg/kg; redosing interval is guided by monitoring with a peripheral nerve stimulator **or** 7-12 **mcg**/kg/**minute** (0.42-0.72 **mg**/kg/**hour**) as a continuous infusion; use lower end of the continuous infusion dosing range for neonates and infants up to age 28 days and the upper end for children >2 to ≤11 years of age

Adults:

Rapid sequence intubation: IV: 0.6-1.2 mg/kg

Obesity: In adult patients with morbid obesity (BMI >40 kg/m^2), the use of 1.2 mg/kg using ideal body weight (IBW) provided a short onset of action and excellent or good intubating conditions at 60 seconds in one study (Gaszynski, 2011).

Tracheal intubation: IV:

Initial: 0.45-0.6 mg/kg; administration of 0.3 mg/kg may also provide optimal conditions for tracheal intubation (Barclay, 1997)

Obesity: May use ideal body weight (IBW) for morbidly obese (BMI >40 kg/m^2) adult patients (Leykin, 2004); onset time may be slightly delayed using IBW. The manufacturer recommends dosing based on actual body weight in all obese patients.

Maintenance for continued surgical relaxation: 0.1-0.2 mg/kg; repeat as needed **or** a continuous infusion of 10-12 **mcg**/kg/**minute** (0.6-0.72 **mg**/kg/**hour**) only after recovery of neuromuscular function is evident; infusion rates have ranged from 4-16 **mcg**/kg/**minute** (0.24-0.96 **mg**/kg/**hour**)

Note: Inhaled anesthetic agents prolong the duration of action of rocuronium. Use lower end of the dosing range; redosing interval guided by monitoring with a peripheral nerve stimulator.

Preinduction defasciculating dose: IV: 0.03-0.06 mg/kg given 1.5-3 minutes before administration of succinylcholine (Harvey, 1998; Martin, 1998)

ICU paralysis (eg, facilitate mechanical ventilation) in selected adequately sedated patients (Greenberg, 2013; Murray, 2002; Rudis, 1996; Sparr, 1997; Warr, 2011): Initial bolus dose: 0.6-1 mg/kg, then a continuous IV infusion of 8-12 **mcg**/kg/**minute** (0.48-0.72 **mg**/kg/**hour**); monitor depth of blockade every 2-3 hours initially until stable dose, then every 8-12 hours; adjust rate of administration by 10% increments according to peripheral nerve stimulation response or desired clinical response

Note: When possible, minimize depth and duration of paralysis. Stopping the infusion for some time until forced to restart based on patient condition is recommended to reduce post-paralytic complications (eg, acute quadriplegic myopathy syndrome [AQMS]) (Murray, 2002).

Intermittent dosing has also been described with an initial loading dose of 50 mg followed by 25 mg given when peripheral nerve stimulation returns (Sparr, 1997).

Dosage adjustment in renal impairment: No dosage adjustment necessary. Duration of neuromuscular blockade may vary in patients with renal impairment.

Dosage adjustment in hepatic impairment: No dosage adjustment provided in manufacturer's labeling. However, dosage reductions may be necessary in patients with liver disease; duration of neuromuscular blockade may be prolonged due to increased volume of distribution. When rapid sequence intubation is required in adult patients with ascites, a dose on the higher end of the dosage range may be necessary to achieve adequate neuromuscular blockade.

Administration Administer IV only; may be administered as a bolus injection (undiluted) or via a continuous infusion (diluted to a concentration up to 5 mg/mL)

Monitoring Parameters Peripheral nerve stimulator measuring twitch response, heart rate, blood pressure, assisted ventilation status

Additional Information Rocuronium is classified as an intermediate-duration neuromuscular-blocking agent. Do not mix in the same syringe with barbiturates. Rocuronium does not relieve pain or produce sedation.

Dosage Forms

Solution, Intravenous:

Zemuron: 50 mg/5 mL (5 mL); 100 mg/10 mL (10 mL)

Generic: 50 mg/5 mL (5 mL); 100 mg/10 mL (10 mL)

Solution, Intravenous [preservative free]:

Generic: 50 mg/5 mL (5 mL); 100 mg/10 mL (10 mL)

◆ **Rocuronium Bromide** *see* Rocuronium *on page 1838*

◆ **Rocuronium Bromide Injection (Can)** *see* Rocuronium *on page 1838*

◆ **Rofact (Can)** *see* Rifampin *on page 1804*

Roflumilast (roe FLUE mi last)

Brand Names: U.S. Daliresp

Brand Names: Canada Daxas

Pharmacologic Category Phosphodiesterase-4 Enzyme Inhibitor

Use Chronic obstructive pulmonary disease: To reduce the risk of chronic obstructive pulmonary disease (COPD) exacerbations in patients with severe COPD associated with chronic bronchitis and a history of exacerbations

Pregnancy Risk Factor C

Pregnancy Considerations Adverse events were observed in some animal reproduction studies. The Canadian labeling recommends avoiding use during pregnancy and in women of childbearing potential not using adequate contraception.

Breast-Feeding Considerations It is not known if roflumilast can be detected in breast milk; however, excretion into human breast milk is likely. Breast-feeding is not recommended by the manufacturer.

Contraindications Moderate or severe hepatic impairment (Child-Pugh class B or C)

Canadian labeling: Additional contraindication (not in U.S. labeling): Hypersensitivity to roflumilast or any component of the formulation

Warnings/Precautions Not indicated for relieving acute bronchospasms or for use as monotherapy of COPD; use only as adjunctive therapy to bronchodilator therapy. Neuropsychiatric effects (eg, anxiety, depression) have been reported with use; rarely, suicidal behavior/ ideation and completed suicide were reported. Avoid use in patients with a history of depression with suicidal behavior/ideations; instruct patients/caregivers to report psychiatric symptoms and consider discontinuation of therapy in such patients. Systemic exposure may be increased in patients with mild hepatic impairment; use in moderate to severe impairment is contraindicated.

May cause weight loss and/or diarrhea (sometimes severe); weight loss usually observed within 6 months of initiating therapy and diarrhea within 4 weeks. Instruct patients to monitor weight regularly. Avoid initiation of therapy or discontinue therapy with unexplained/pronounced weight loss. Potentially significant drug-drug interactions may exist, requiring dose or frequency adjustment, additional monitoring, and/or selection of alternative therapy. May contain lactose; the Canadian labeling recommends avoiding use in patients with galactose intolerance, Lapp lactase deficiency, or glucose-galactose malabsorption. The Canadian labeling recommends avoiding use in patients with cancer (excluding basal cell carcinoma), heart failure (NYHA III/IV), severe acute infection, immunosuppression, or immunosuppressive therapy (excludes short-term systemic corticosteroid use for COPD exacerbation).

Adverse Reactions

Central nervous system: Dizziness, headache, insomnia

Endocrine & metabolic: Weight loss

Gastrointestinal: Decreased appetite, diarrhea, nausea

Infection: Influenza

Neuromuscular & skeletal: Back pain

Rare but important or life-threatening: Abdominal pain, anemia, arthritis, atrial fibrillation, depression, dysgeusia, epistaxis, gastritis, gastroesophageal reflux disease, gynecomastia, hematochezia, hypersensitivity, increased gamma-glutamyl transferase, increased lactate dehydrogenase, increased serum AST, lung carcinoma, muscle spasm, myalgia, myasthenia, pancreatitis, paresthesia, prostate carcinoma, renal failure, respiratory tract infection, rhinitis, sinusitis, suicidal ideation, suicidal tendencies, suicide completed, supraventricular cardiac arrhythmia, urinary tract infection

Drug Interactions

Metabolism/Transport Effects Substrate of CYP1A2 (minor), CYP3A4 (major); **Note:** Assignment of Major/ Minor substrate status based on clinically relevant drug interaction potential

Avoid Concomitant Use

Avoid concomitant use of Roflumilast with any of the following: CYP3A4 Inducers (Strong); Rifampin

Increased Effect/Toxicity

Roflumilast may increase the levels/effects of: Immunosuppressants; Riociguat

The levels/effects of Roflumilast may be increased by: Cimetidine; Ciprofloxacin (Systemic); FluvoxaMINE

Decreased Effect

The levels/effects of Roflumilast may be decreased by: Bosentan; CYP3A4 Inducers (Moderate); CYP3A4 Inducers (Strong); Dabrafenib; Deferasirox; Rifampin; St Johns Wort

Storage/Stability Store at 20°C to 25°C (68°F to 77°F), excursions permitted from 15°C to 30°C (59°F to 86°F).

Mechanism of Action Roflumilast and its active N-oxide metabolite selectively inhibit phosphodiesterase-4 (PDE4) leading to an accumulation of cyclic AMP (cAMP) within inflammatory and structural cells important in the pathogenesis of COPD. Anti-inflammatory effects include suppression of cytokine release and inhibition of lung infiltration by neutrophils and other leukocytes. Pulmonary remodeling and mucociliary malfunction are also attenuated.

Pharmacodynamics/Kinetics

Distribution: V_d: 2.9 L/kg

Protein binding: 99%; N-oxide metabolite: 97%

Metabolism: Hepatic via CYP3A4 and CYP1A2 to active N-oxide metabolite; also undergoes conjugation

Bioavailability: ~80%

Half-life elimination: 17 hours; N-oxide metabolite: 30 hours

Time to peak: ~1 hour (delayed by food); N-oxide metabolite: ~8 hours

Excretion: Urine (~70% as metabolites)

Dosage Oral: Adults: COPD: 500 mcg once daily

Dosage adjustment in renal impairment: No dosage adjustment necessary.

Dosage adjustment in hepatic impairment:

Mild impairment (Child-Pugh class A): No dosage adjustment necessary. Use with caution; 500 mcg once daily dose has not been evaluated in mild impairment.

Moderate-to-severe impairment (Child-Pugh class B or C): Use is contraindicated.

Administration Administer without regard to meals.

Monitoring Parameters Liver function tests. Measure weight regularly during therapy

Dosage Forms

Tablet, Oral:

Daliresp: 500 mcg

Dosage Forms: Canada

Tablet, oral:

Daxas: 500 mcg

- ◆ **Rogaine® (Can)** *see* Minoxidil (Topical) *on page 1374*
- ◆ **Rogaine Mens Extra Strength [OTC]** *see* Minoxidil (Topical) *on page 1374*
- ◆ **Rogitine (Can)** *see* Phentolamine *on page 1636*
- ◆ **Rolaids** *see* Calcium Carbonate and Magnesium Hydroxide *on page 328*
- ◆ **Rolene (Can)** *see* Betamethasone (Topical) *on page 255*
- ◆ **Romazicon (Can)** *see* Flumazenil *on page 892*

RomiDEPsin (roe mi DEP sin)

Brand Names: U.S. Istodax

Index Terms Depsipeptide; FK228; FR901228

Pharmacologic Category Antineoplastic Agent, Histone Deacetylase Inhibitor

Use

Cutaneous T-cell lymphoma: Treatment of cutaneous T-cell lymphoma (CTCL) in patients who have received at least one systemic prior therapy

Peripheral T-cell lymphoma: Treatment of peripheral T-cell lymphoma (PTCL) in patients who have received at least one prior therapy

Pregnancy Risk Factor D

Pregnancy Considerations Adverse events were observed in animal reproduction studies. Based on the mechanism of action, romidepsin may cause fetal harm if administered during pregnancy.

Breast-Feeding Considerations It is not known if romidepsin is excreted in breast milk. Due to the potential for serious adverse reactions in the nursing infant, the manufacturer recommends a decision be made whether to discontinue nursing or to discontinue the drug, taking into account the importance of treatment to the mother.

Contraindications There are no contraindications listed in the manufacturer's labeling.

Warnings/Precautions Hazardous agent - use appropriate precautions for handling and disposal (NIOSH 2014 [group 1]). Anemia, leukopenia, neutropenia, lymphopenia and thrombocytopenia may occur; may require dosage modification; monitor blood counts during treatment. Serious infections (occasionally fatal), including pneumonia, sepsis, and viral reactivation (eg, Epstein Barr and hepatitis B) have occurred during or within 30 days of treatment. Monitor patients with a history of hepatitis B infections closely for viral reactivation; consider antiviral prophylaxis. Epstein Barr reactivation leading to liver failure has also been reported, with ganciclovir antiviral prophylaxis failure in one case. The risk of life-threatening infection may be increased in patients who have received prior with antilymphocytic monoclonal antibodies or who have disease involvement in the bone marrow. QTc prolongation has been observed; use caution in patients with a history of QTc prolongation, congenital long QT syndrome, with medications known to prolong the QT interval, or with preexisting cardiac disease. Obtain baseline and periodic ECG (12-lead); monitor and correct electrolyte (potassium, magnesium, and calcium) abnormalities prior to and during treatment. T-wave and ST-segment changes have also been reported. Use with caution in patients with moderate-to-severe hepatic impairment or end-stage renal disease. Tumor lysis syndrome (TLS) has been observed; closely monitor patients with advanced disease and/or with a high tumor burden (risk of TLS may be higher); if TLS occurs, initiate appropriate treatment. Potentially significant drug-drug interactions may exist, requiring dose or frequency adjustment, additional monitoring, and/or selection of alternative therapy.

Adverse Reactions

Cardiovascular: Chest pain, DVT, edema, hypotension, myocardial ischemia, peripheral edema, QT prolongation, ST-T wave changes, supraventricular arrhythmia, syncope, tachycardia, ventricular arrhythmia

Central nervous system: Chills, fatigue, fever, headache,

Dermatologic: Dermatitis/exfoliative dermatitis, pruritus

Endocrine & metabolic: Dehydration, hyperglycemia, hyper-/hypomagnesemia, hyperuricemia, hypoalbuminemia, hypocalcemia, hypokalemia, hypophosphatemia, hyponatremia

Gastrointestinal: Abdominal pain, anorexia, constipation, diarrhea, nausea, stomatitis, taste alteration, vomiting, weight loss

Hematologic: Anemia, leukopenia, lymphopenia, neutropenia, neutropenic fever, thrombocytopenia

Hepatic: ALT increased, AST increased, hyperbilirubinemia

Neuromuscular & skeletal: Weakness

Respiratory: Acute respiratory distress syndrome, cough, dyspnea, hypoxia, pneumonia, pneumonitis, pulmonary embolism

Miscellaneous: Central line infection, hypersensitivity, infection, sepsis, tumor lysis syndrome

Rare but important or life-threatening: Acute renal failure, acute respiratory distress syndrome, atrial fibrillation, bacteremia, candida infection, cardiopulmonary failure, cardiogenic shock, Epstein-Barr virus reactivation, multi-organ failure, septic shock

Drug Interactions

Metabolism/Transport Effects Substrate of CYP3A4 (major), P-glycoprotein; **Note:** Assignment of Major/Minor substrate status based on clinically relevant drug interaction potential

Avoid Concomitant Use

Avoid concomitant use of RomiDEPsin with any of the following: BCG; CloZAPine; CYP3A4 Inducers (Strong); Dexamethasone (Systemic); Dipyrone; Highest Risk QTc-Prolonging Agents; Ivabradine; Mifepristone; Natalizumab; Pimecrolimus; Rifampin; St Johns Wort; Tacrolimus (Topical); Tofacitinib; Vaccines (Live)

Increased Effect/Toxicity

RomiDEPsin may increase the levels/effects of: CloZAPine; Highest Risk QTc-Prolonging Agents; Leflunomide; Moderate Risk QTc-Prolonging Agents; Natalizumab; Tofacitinib; Vaccines (Live); Warfarin

The levels/effects of RomiDEPsin may be increased by: CYP3A4 Inhibitors (Strong); Denosumab; Dipyrone; Ivabradine; Mifepristone; P-glycoprotein/ABCB1 Inhibitors; Pimecrolimus; QTc-Prolonging Agents (Indeterminate Risk and Risk Modifying); Rifampin; Roflumilast; Tacrolimus (Topical); Trastuzumab

Decreased Effect

RomiDEPsin may decrease the levels/effects of: BCG; Coccidioides immitis Skin Test; Sipuleucel-T; Vaccines (Inactivated); Vaccines (Live)

The levels/effects of RomiDEPsin may be decreased by: Bosentan; CYP3A4 Inducers (Moderate); CYP3A4 Inducers (Strong); Dabrafenib; Deferasirox;

Dexamethasone (Systemic); Echinacea; P-glycoprotein/ABCB1 Inducers; Siltuximab; St Johns Wort; Tocilizumab

Food Interactions Grapefruit juice may increase the levels/effects of romidepsin. Management: Avoid grapefruit juice.

Preparation for Administration Hazardous agent; use appropriate precautions for handling and disposal (NIOSH 2014 [group 1]). Reconstitute each 10 mg vial with 2 mL of supplied diluent to a reconstituted concentration of 5 mg/mL; swirl until dissolved. (**Note:** Although the reconstituted vial contains a final volume of 2 mL, due to the viscosity of the reconstituted solution, a total volume <2 mL [usually ~1.6-1.8 mL] can be withdrawn from each vial.) Further dilute in 500 mL normal saline; compatible with polyvinyl chloride (PVC), ethylene vinyl acetate (EVA), polyethylene (PE) and glass infusion containers.

Storage/Stability Store intact vials at room temperature of 20°C to 25°C (68°F to 77°F); excursions are permitted between 15°C and 30°C (59°F and 86°F). The reconstituted solution is stable for 8 hours at room temperature. Solutions diluted for infusion are stable for 24 hours at room temperature; however, the manufacturer recommends use as soon as possible after dilution.

Mechanism of Action Histone deacetylase inhibitor; catalyzes acetyl group removal from protein lysine residues (including histone and transcription factors). Inhibition of histone deacetylase results in accumulation of acetyl groups, leading to alterations in chromatin structure and transcription factor activation causing termination of cell growth (induces arrest in cell cycle at G_1 and G_2/M phases) leading to cell death.

Pharmacodynamics/Kinetics

Protein binding: 92% to 94%; primarily to α_1-acid glycoprotein

Metabolism: Hepatic, primarily via CYP3A4, minor metabolism from CYP3A5, 1A1, 2B6, and 2C19

Half-life elimination: ~3 hours

Dosage

Cutaneous T-cell lymphoma: Adults: IV: 14 mg/m^2 days 1, 8, and 15 of a 28-day treatment cycle; repeat cycle as long as benefit continues and treatment is tolerated

Peripheral T-cell lymphoma: Adults: IV: 14 mg/m^2 days 1, 8, and 15 of a 28-day treatment cycle; repeat cycle as long as benefit continues and treatment is tolerated

Dosage adjustment for toxicity:

Nonhematologic toxicity (excluding alopecia):

Grade 2 or 3: Delay treatment until toxicity returns to ≤ grade 1 or baseline, may restart at 14 mg/m^2

Grade 4 or recurrent grade 3 toxicity: Delay treatment until toxicity returns to ≤ grade 1 or baseline, permanently reduce dose to 10 mg/m^2

Recurrent grade 3 or 4 toxicity despite dosage reduction: Discontinue treatment

Hematologic toxicity:

Grade 3 or 4 neutropenia or thrombocytopenia: Delay treatment until ANC ≥1500/mm^3 and/or platelets ≥75,000/mm^3 or baseline, may restart at 14 mg/m^2

Grade 4 febrile neutropenia (≥38.5°C [101.3°F]) or thrombocytopenia requiring platelet transfusion: Delay treatment until toxicity returns to ≤ grade 1 or baseline, permanently reduce dose to 10 mg/m^2

Dosage adjustment in renal impairment: There are no dosage adjustments provided in the manufacturer's labeling (has not been studied). However, dosage adjustment is not likely necessary since pharmacokinetics are unaffected by renal impairment. Use with caution in patients with end-stage renal disease (has not been studied).

Dosage adjustment in hepatic impairment:

Mild impairment: There are no dosage adjustments provided in the manufacturer's labeling. However, mild hepatic impairment does not significantly influence the pharmacokinetics of romidepsin.

Moderate or severe impairment: There are no dosage adjustments provided in the manufacturer's labeling. Use with caution.

Dosing in obesity: *American Society of Clinical Oncology (ASCO) Guidelines for appropriate chemotherapy dosing in obese adults with cancer:* Utilize patient's actual body weight (full weight) for calculation of body surface area- or weight-based dosing, particularly when the intent of therapy is curative; manage regimen-related toxicities in the same manner as for nonobese patients; if a dose reduction is utilized due to toxicity, consider resumption of full weight-based dosing with subsequent cycles, especially if cause of toxicity (eg, hepatic or renal impairment) is resolved (Griggs, 2012).

Dietary Considerations Avoid grapefruit juice.

Administration Infuse over 4 hours. Although romidepsin has a low emetic potential, antiemetics to prevent nausea and vomiting were used in clinical trials (Piekarz, 2009; Piekarz, 2011).

Hazardous agent; use appropriate precautions for handling and disposal (NIOSH 2014 [group 1]).

Monitoring Parameters Serum electrolytes (baseline and periodic; especially potassium and magnesium); CBC with differential and platelets, ECG (baseline and periodic; in patients with significant cardiovascular disease, congenital long QT syndrome, and in patients taking QT-prolonging medications); signs/symptoms of infection or tumor lysis syndrome

Dosage Forms

Solution Reconstituted, Intravenous:

Istodax: 10 mg (1 ea)

RomiPLOStim (roe mi PLOE stim)

Brand Names: U.S. Nplate

Brand Names: Canada Nplate

Index Terms AMG 531

Pharmacologic Category Colony Stimulating Factor; Hematopoietic Agent; Thrombopoietic Agent

Use

Chronic immune thrombocytopenia: Treatment of thrombocytopenia in patients with chronic immune thrombocytopenia (ITP) who have had insufficient response to corticosteroids, immune globulin, or splenectomy

Limitations of use: Should be used only when the degree of thrombocytopenia and clinical condition increase the risk for bleeding; should not be used in attempt to normalize platelet counts; **not** indicated for the treatment of thrombocytopenia due to myelodysplastic syndrome or any cause of thrombocytopenia other than chronic ITP.

Pregnancy Risk Factor C

Pregnancy Considerations Adverse events have been observed in animal reproduction studies. Use during pregnancy only if the potential benefit to the mother outweighs the potential risk to the fetus.

Women exposed to romiplostim during pregnancy are encouraged to enroll in the Nplate pregnancy (1-800-772-6436).

Breast-Feeding Considerations It is not known if romiplostim is excreted in breast milk. Due to the potential for serious adverse reactions in the nursing infant, the manufacturer recommends a decision be made whether to discontinue breast-feeding or to discontinue romiplostim, taking into account the importance of treatment to the mother.

Contraindications There are no contraindications listed in the manufacturer's labeling.

Warnings/Precautions May increase the risk for bone marrow reticulin formation or progression; this formation may improve upon discontinuation of therapy. Thromboembolism or thrombotic complications may occur with increased platelets; follow dosage adjustment recommendations to minimize the risk for thrombotic or thromboembolic complications; use with caution in patients with a history of cerebrovascular disease. Progression from existing myelodysplastic syndrome (MDS) to acute myeloid leukemia (AML) has been observed in clinical trials studying romiplostim for severe thrombocytopenia associated with MDS (not an approved indication); a higher percentage of patients receiving romiplostim experienced transformation to AML (compared to placebo). An increase in the percentage of circulating myeloblasts in peripheral blood counts was also noted (both in patients who progressed to AML and in those who did not); blast cells decreased to baseline after discontinuation in some patients.

Indicated only when the degree of thrombocytopenia and clinical conditions increase the risk for bleeding; use the lowest dose necessary to achieve and maintain platelet count ≥50,000/mm^3. Do not use to normalize platelet counts. Discontinue if platelet count does not respond to a level to avoid clinically important bleeding after 4 weeks at the maximum recommended dose. May be used in combination with other therapies for ITP, including corticosteroids, danazol, azathioprine, immune globulin, or Rho (D) immune globulin; not indicated for the treatment of thrombocytopenia due to any cause other than chronic ITP. Reduce dose or discontinue ITP medications when platelet count ≥50,000/mm^3. Lack of response or failure to maintain platelet response should trigger investigation in to causative factors, including neutralizing antibodies to romiplostim.

Overdose may result in thrombotic/thromboembolic complications due to excessive platelet levels; underdose may result in lack of platelet response and potential for bleeding. Use caution when calculating dose and appropriate volume for administration (volume may be very small; administer with syringe that allows for 0.01 mL graduations).

Upon discontinuation of therapy, rebound thrombocytopenia and risk of bleeding may develop. Severity may be greater than pretreatment level; monitor CBCs and platelet counts weekly for at least 2 weeks after discontinuation.

Use with caution in patients with chronic liver disease; portal vein thrombosis has been reported in these patients.

Adverse Reactions

Central nervous system: Dizziness, headache, insomnia

Gastrointestinal: Abdominal pain, dyspepsia

Hematologic: AML, bone marrow reticulin formation/deposition, circulating myeloblasts increased, rebound thrombocytopenia

Neuromuscular & skeletal: Arthralgia, limb pain, myalgia, paresthesia, shoulder pain

Miscellaneous: Antibody formation

Rare but important or life-threatening: Angioedema, erythromelalgia, hypersensitivity, marrow fibrosis with collagen, thromboembolism, thrombotic complications

Drug Interactions

Metabolism/Transport Effects None known.

Avoid Concomitant Use There are no known interactions where it is recommended to avoid concomitant use.

Increased Effect/Toxicity There are no known significant interactions involving an increase in effect.

Decreased Effect There are no known significant interactions involving a decrease in effect.

Preparation for Administration Reconstitute with only preservative free SWFI (add 0.72 mL to 250 mcg vial or 1.2 mL to 500 mcg vial). Do not use bacteriostatic water for injection. Gently invert vial and swirl; do not shake. Usually dissolves within 2 minutes.

Storage/Stability Store intact vials refrigerated at 2°C to 8°C (36°F to 46°F); do not freeze. Protect from light. Store in original carton until use. Reconstituted solution may be stored at room temperature of 25°C (77°F) or refrigerated at 2°C to 8°C (36°F to 46°F) for up to 24 hours prior to administration. Protect reconstituted solution from light; discard any unused portion.

Mechanism of Action Thrombopoietin (TPO) peptide mimetic which increases platelet counts in ITP by binding to and activating the human TPO receptor.

Pharmacodynamics/Kinetics

Onset of action: Platelet count increase: SubQ: 4-9 days (Wang, 2004); Peak platelet count increase: Days 12-16 (Wang, 2004)

Duration: Platelet counts return to baseline by day 28 (Wang, 2004)

Absorption: SubQ: Slow (Wang, 2004)

Half-life elimination: Median: 3.5 days (range: 1-34 days)

Time to peak, plasma: SubQ: Median: 14 hours (range: 7-50 hours)

Dosage Note: Initial dose is based on actual body weight. Use the lowest dose sufficient to maintain platelet count ≥50,000/mm^3 as necessary to reduce the risk of bleeding. Adjust dose based on platelet count response; discontinue if platelet count does not respond to a level that avoids clinically important bleeding after 4 weeks at the maximum recommended dose.

Chronic immune thrombocytopenia (ITP): Adults: SubQ: Initial: 1 mcg/kg once weekly; adjust dose by 1 mcg/kg/week increments to achieve platelet count ≥50,000/mm^3 and to reduce the risk of bleeding; Maximum dose: 10 mcg/kg/week (median dose needed to achieve response in clinical trials: 2 mcg/kg)

Dosage adjustment recommendations:

Platelet count <50,000/mm^3: Increase weekly dose by 1 mcg/kg

Platelet count >200,000/mm^3 for 2 consecutive weeks: Reduce weekly dose by 1 mcg/kg

Platelet count >400,000/mm^3: Withhold dose; assess platelet count weekly; when platelet count <200,000/mm^3, resume with the weekly dose reduced by 1 mcg/kg

Dosage adjustment in renal impairment: No dosage adjustment provided in manufacturer's labeling (has not been studied)

Dosage adjustment in hepatic impairment: No dosage adjustment provided in manufacturer's labeling (has not been studied)

Dietary Considerations Some products may contain sucrose.

Administration Administer SubQ. Administration volume may be small; use appropriate syringe (with graduations to 0.01 mL) for administration. Verify calculations, final concentration, and volume drawn up for administration.

Monitoring Parameters CBC with differential and platelets (baseline, during treatment [weekly until platelet response stable for at least 4 weeks then monthly] and weekly for at least 2 weeks following discontinuation or completion of treatment)

Evaluate for neutralizing antibodies in patients with inadequate response (blood samples may be submitted to the manufacturer for assay [1-800-772-6436]).

Reference Range Target platelet count of 50,000-200,000/mm^3; platelet life span: 8-11 days

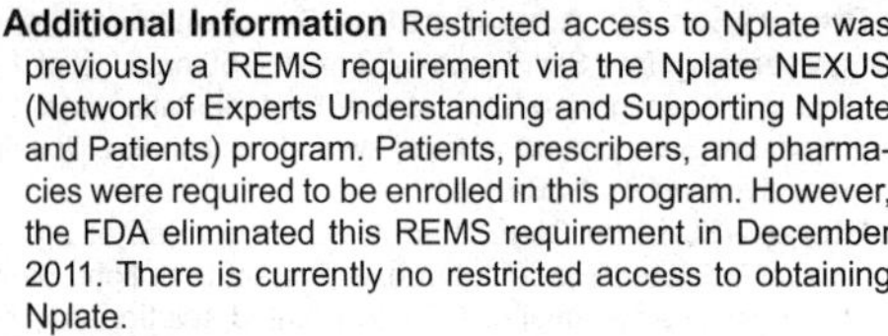

Additional Information Restricted access to Nplate was previously a REMS requirement via the Nplate NEXUS (Network of Experts Understanding and Supporting Nplate and Patients) program. Patients, prescribers, and pharmacies were required to be enrolled in this program. However, the FDA eliminated this REMS requirement in December 2011. There is currently no restricted access to obtaining Nplate.

Dosage Forms

Solution Reconstituted, Subcutaneous [preservative free]:

Nplate: 250 mcg (1 ea); 500 mcg (1 ea)

◆ **Romycin** *see* Erythromycin (Ophthalmic) *on page 764*

ROPINIRole (roe PIN i role)

Brand Names: U.S. Requip; Requip XL

Brand Names: Canada ACT-Ropinirole; JAMP-Ropinirole; PMS-Ropinirole; RAN-Ropinirole; Requip

Index Terms Ropinirole Hydrochloride

Pharmacologic Category Anti-Parkinson's Agent, Dopamine Agonist

Use

Parkinson disease: Treatment of Parkinson disease

Restless legs syndrome (immediate release only): Treatment of moderate to severe primary restless legs syndrome (RLS)

Pregnancy Risk Factor C

Pregnancy Considerations Adverse events have been observed in animal reproduction studies. Information related to the use of ropinirole for the treatment of restless legs syndrome (RLS) in pregnant women is limited. Current guidelines note that the available information is insufficient to make a recommendation for use in pregnant women (Aurora, 2012; Dostal, 2013).

Breast-Feeding Considerations It is not known if ropinirole is excreted into breast milk. Ropinirole inhibits prolactin secretion in humans and may potentially inhibit lactation. The manufacturer recommends that caution be exercised when administering ropinirole to nursing women.

Contraindications Hypersensitivity to ropinirole or any component of the formulation

Warnings/Precautions May cause orthostatic hypotension; Parkinson disease patients appear to have an impaired capacity to respond to a postural challenge. Use with caution in patients at risk of hypotension (such as those receiving antihypertensive or antiarrhythmic drugs) or where transient hypotensive episodes would be poorly tolerated (cardiovascular disease or cerebrovascular disease). Parkinson patients being treated with dopaminergic agonists ordinarily require careful monitoring for signs and symptoms of postural hypotension, especially during dose escalation, and should be informed of this risk. Syncope, sometimes associated with bradycardia, was observed in association with ropinirole in both Parkinson disease patients and patients with RLS.

Use with caution in patients with preexisting dyskinesia, hepatic impairment or ESRD on dialysis (use in patients with severe renal impairment and who are not undergoing regular hemodialysis is not recommended in the Canadian labeling). May cause hallucinations, particularly in older patients. May also cause or exacerbate mental status and behavioral changes, which may be severe, including psychotic-like behavior during treatment or after starting or increasing the dose; manifestations may include paranoid ideation, delusions, hallucinations, confusion, psychotic-like behavior, disorientation, aggressive behavior, agitation, and delirium. Avoid use in patients with a major psychotic disorder; may exacerbate psychosis. Patients have reported falling asleep while engaging in activities of daily living; this has been reported to occur without significant warning signs; some of these events had been reported one year after the initiation of therapy. Ropinirole has also been associated with somnolence. Before initiating treatment, advise patients of the potential to develop drowsiness, and inquire about factors that may increase the risk (eg, concomitant sedating medications and/or alcohol, presence of sleep disorders, concomitant medications that increase pramipexole plasma levels). Patients must be cautioned about performing tasks which require mental alertness (eg, operating machinery or driving). Monitor for daytime somnolence or preexisting sleep disorder; discontinue if significant daytime sleepiness or episodes of falling asleep occur; if a decision is made to continue therapy, advise patients not to drive and to avoid other potentially dangerous activities.

Has been associated with compulsive behaviors and/or loss of impulse control, which has manifested as pathological gambling, libido increases (hypersexuality), compulsive buying, binge or compulsive eating and/or other intense urges. Dose reduction or discontinuation of therapy has been reported to reverse these behaviors in some, but not all cases. Risk for melanoma development is increased in Parkinson disease patients; drug causation or factors contributing to risk have not been established. Patients should be monitored closely and periodic skin examinations should be performed.

Augmentation (earlier onset of symptoms in the evening/afternoon, increase and/or spread of symptoms to other extremities) or rebound (shifting of symptoms to early morning hours) may occur in some RLS patients. Consider dosage adjustment or discontinuation of treatment if augmentation or rebound symptoms occur. Pathologic degenerative changes were observed in the retinas of albino rats during studies with this agent, but were not observed in the retinas of albino mice or in other species. The significance of these data for humans remains uncertain.

Taper gradually when discontinuing therapy in Parkinson disease; dopaminergic agents have been associated with a syndrome resembling neuroleptic malignant syndrome on abrupt withdrawal or significant dosage reduction after long-term use. Ergot-derived dopamine agonists have been associated with fibrotic complications (eg, pericarditis, retroperitoneal fibrosis, pleural effusion, pleural thickening, pulmonary infiltrates, cardiac valvulopathy). Although ropinirole is not an ergot, there have been postmarketing reports of possible fibrotic complications (pleural effusion, pleural fibrosis, interstitial lung disease, and cardiac valvulopathy) with ropinirole; monitor closely for signs and symptoms of fibrosis. Discontinuation of therapy may resolve complications, but not in all cases. The elderly may be prone to an increased risk of adverse drug reactions. Extended release ropinirole is designed to release medication over a 24-hour period; if rapid gastrointestinal transit occurs, there may be risk of incomplete release of medication and medication residue being passed in the stool. Potentially significant drug-drug interactions may exist, requiring dose or frequency adjustment, additional monitoring, and/or selection of alternative therapy.

Adverse Reactions Data inclusive of trials in early Parkinson disease (without levodopa) and Restless Legs Syndrome.

Cardiovascular: Atrial fibrillation, chest pain, dependent edema, extrasystoles, flushing, hypertension, hypotension (including orthostatic), lower extremity edema, palpitations, peripheral edema, peripheral ischemia, syncope, tachycardia

Central nervous system: Amnesia, confusion, drowsiness, dizziness, falling, fatigue (including weakness, malaise), hallucination (dose related), headache (extended release), hypoesthesia, insomnia, lack of concentration, pain, paresthesia, vertigo, yawning

Dermatologic: Diaphoresis, hyperhidrosis

Gastrointestinal: Abdominal pain, anorexia, constipation, diarrhea, dyspepsia, flatulence, nausea (more common in immediate release than extended release), vomiting, xerostomia

Infection: Viral infection

Genitourinary: Impotence, urinary tract infection

Hepatic: Increased serum alkaline

Infection: Influenza

Neuromuscular & skeletal: Arthralgia, hyperkinesia, limb pain, muscle cramps, muscle spasm, myalgia

Ophthalmic: Eye disease, visual disturbance, xerophthalmia

Respiratory: Bronchitis, cough, dyspnea, nasal congestion, nasopharyngitis, pharyngitis, rhinitis, sinusitis

Miscellaneous: Fever

Advanced Parkinson disease (with levodopa):

Cardiovascular: Bradycardia, decreased blood pressure (combined systolic and diastolic; orthostatic; mild to moderate), decreased diastolic blood pressure (orthostatic), decreased heart rate, hypertension (dose related), hypotension (including orthostatic), increased heart rate, peripheral edema, syncope, systolic hypertension (≥40 mm Hg), systolic hypotension (orthostatic; more common when ≥20 mm Hg)

Central nervous system: Abnormal dreams, amnesia, anxiety, confusion, dizziness (more common with immediate release than with extended release), drowsiness (more common with immediate release than with extended release), falling (dose related), hallucination (dose related), headache, nervousness, pain, paresis, paresthesia, vertigo

Dermatologic: Diaphoresis

Endocrine & metabolic: Weight loss

Gastrointestinal: Abdominal pain, constipation, diarrhea, dysphagia, flatulence, nausea (more common with immediate release than with extended release), sialorrhea, vomiting, xerostomia

Genitourinary: Pyuria, urinary incontinence, urinary tract infection

Hematologic& oncologic: Anemia

Infection: Viral infection

Neuromuscular & skeletal: Arthralgia, arthritis, back pain, dyskinesia (more common with immediate release than with extended release; dose related), hypokinesia, tremor

Ophthalmic: Diplopia

Respiratory: Dyspnea, nasopharyngitis, upper respiratory tract infection

Miscellaneous: Increased drug level

Rare but important or life-threatening: Heart valve disease, hypersensitivity reaction (angioedema, pruritus), impulse control disorder (eg, pathological gambling, hypersexuality, binge eating), interstitial pulmonary disease, mental status changes, pleural effusion

Drug Interactions

Metabolism/Transport Effects Substrate of CYP1A2 (major), CYP3A4 (minor); **Note:** Assignment of Major/Minor substrate status based on clinically relevant drug interaction potential; **Inhibits** CYP1A2 (weak), CYP2D6 (weak)

Avoid Concomitant Use

Avoid concomitant use of ROPINIRole with any of the following: Amisulpride; Sulpiride

Increased Effect/Toxicity

ROPINIRole may increase the levels/effects of: BuPROPion

The levels/effects of ROPINIRole may be increased by: Abiraterone Acetate; Alcohol (Ethyl); Ciprofloxacin (Systemic); CNS Depressants; CYP1A2 Inhibitors (Moderate); CYP1A2 Inhibitors (Strong); Deferasirox; Estrogen Derivatives; MAO Inhibitors; Methylphenidate; Peginterferon Alfa-2b; Vemurafenib

Decreased Effect

ROPINIRole may decrease the levels/effects of: Amisulpride; Antipsychotic Agents (First Generation [Typical]); Sulpiride

The levels/effects of ROPINIRole may be decreased by: Amisulpride; Antipsychotic Agents (First Generation [Typical]); Antipsychotic Agents (Second Generation [Atypical]); Cannabis; CYP1A2 Inducers (Strong); Cyproterone; Metoclopramide; Sulpiride; Teriflunomide

Storage/Stability Store at room temperature. Protect from light and moisture.

Mechanism of Action Ropinirole has a high relative *in vitro* specificity and full intrinsic activity at the D_2 and D_3 dopamine receptor subtypes, binding with higher affinity to D_3 than to D_2 or D_4 receptor subtypes; relevance of D_3 receptor binding in Parkinson disease is unknown. Ropinirole has moderate *in vitro* affinity for opioid receptors. Ropinirole and its metabolites have negligible *in vitro* affinity for dopamine D_1, 5-HT_1, 5-HT_2, benzodiazepine, GABA, muscarinic, $alpha_1$-, $alpha_2$-, and beta-adrenoreceptors. Although precise mechanism of action of ropinirole is unknown, it is believed to be due to stimulation of postsynaptic dopamine D_2-type receptors within the caudate putamen in the brain. Ropinirole caused decreases in systolic and diastolic blood pressure at doses >0.25 mg. The mechanism of ropinirole-induced postural hypotension is believed to be due to D_2-mediated blunting of the noradrenergic response to standing and subsequent decrease in peripheral vascular resistance.

Pharmacodynamics/Kinetics

Absorption: Immediate release: Rapid

Distribution: V_d: 7.5 L/kg

Protein binding: 40%

Metabolism: Extensively hepatic via CYP1A2 to inactive metabolites; first-pass effect

Bioavailability: Absolute: 45% to 55%

Half-life elimination: ~6 hours

Time to peak: Immediate release: ~1-2 hours; Extended release: 6-10 hours; T_{max} increased by 2.5-3 hours when taken with a high-fat meal

Excretion: Urine (<10% as unchanged drug, 60% as metabolites)

Dosage

Parkinson disease: Adults: Oral:

Immediate-release tablet: The dosage should be increased to achieve a maximum therapeutic effect, balanced against the principal side effects of nausea, dizziness, somnolence, and dyskinesia. Recommended starting dose is 0.25 mg 3 times/day; based on individual patient response, the dosage should be titrated with weekly increments as described below:

- Week 1: 0.25 mg 3 times/day; total daily dose: 0.75 mg
- Week 2: 0.5 mg 3 times/day; total daily dose: 1.5 mg
- Week 3: 0.75 mg 3 times/day; total daily dose: 2.25 mg
- Week 4: 1 mg 3 times/day; total daily dose: 3 mg

Note: After week 4, if necessary, daily dosage may be increased by 1.5 mg/day on a weekly basis up to a dose of 9 mg/day, and then by up to 3 mg/day weekly to a total of 24 mg/day. If a significant interruption in therapy with ropinirole occurs, retitration may be warranted.

Parkinson disease discontinuation taper: Gradually taper over 7 days as follows: reduce frequency of administration from 3 times daily to twice daily for 4 days, then reduce to once daily for remaining 3 days.

Extended-release tablet: Initial: 2 mg once daily for 1 to 2 weeks, followed by increases of 2 mg/day at weekly or longer intervals based on therapeutic response and tolerability (maximum: 24 mg/day); **Note:** If a significant interruption in therapy with ropinirole occurs, retitration may be warranted. When discontinuing, gradually taper over 7 days.

Restless legs syndrome (RLS): Adults: Oral: Immediate-release tablets: Initial: 0.25 mg once daily 1 to 3 hours before bedtime. Dose may be increased after 2 days to 0.5 mg daily, and after 7 days to 1 mg daily. Dose may be further titrated upward in 0.5 mg increments every week until reaching a daily dose of 3 mg during week 6. Daily dose may be increased to a maximum of 4 mg beginning week 7.

Note: If a significant interruption in therapy with ropinirole occurs, retitration may be warranted. Doses up to 4 mg per day may be discontinued without tapering.

Converting from ropinirole immediate release tablets to ropinirole extended-release tablets: Choose a once daily extended-release dose that most closely matches current immediate-release daily dose.

Elderly: Titrate dose to clinical response. Refer to adult dosing.

Dosage adjustment in renal impairment:

Moderate renal impairment (CrCl 30 to 50 mL/minute): No dosage adjustment necessary.

Severe renal impairment (CrCl <30 mL/minute): There are no dosage adjustments provided in the manufacturer's labeling (has not been studied). Use with caution. **Note:** The Canadian labeling recommends to avoid use in patients with severe renal impairment and who are not undergoing regular hemodialysis.

ESRD requiring hemodialysis:

Immediate release:

Parkinson disease: Initial: 0.25 mg 3 times daily; may titrate dose upward based on tolerability and efficacy (maximum dose: 18 mg daily); postdialysis supplemental doses are not required

Restless legs syndrome: Initial: 0.25 mg once daily; may titrate dose upward based on tolerability and efficacy (maximum dose: 3 mg daily); postdialysis supplemental doses are not required

Extended release: Initial: 2 mg once daily; may titrate dose upward based on tolerability and efficacy (maximum dose: 18 mg daily); postdialysis supplemental doses are not required.

Dosage adjustment in hepatic impairment: There are no dosage adjustments provided in the manufacturer's labeling (has not been studied). Titrate with caution.

Administration Administer without regard to meals. Swallow extended-release tablet whole; do not crush, split, or chew.

Monitoring Parameters Blood pressure (orthostatic); daytime alertness; CNS depression, fall risk, behavior changes (eg, compulsive behaviors); periodic skin examinations

Additional Information If therapy with a drug known to be a potent inhibitor of CYP1A2 is stopped or started during treatment with ropinirole, adjustment of ropinirole dose may be required. Ropinirole binds to melanin-containing tissues (ie, eyes, skin) in pigmented rats. After a single dose, long-term retention of drug was demonstrated, with a half-life in the eye of 20 days; not known if ropinirole accumulates in these tissues over time.

Dosage Forms

Tablet, Oral:

Requip: 0.25 mg, 0.5 mg, 1 mg, 2 mg, 3 mg, 4 mg, 5 mg

Generic: 0.25 mg, 0.5 mg, 1 mg, 2 mg, 3 mg, 4 mg, 5 mg

Tablet Extended Release 24 Hour, Oral:

Requip XL: 2 mg, 4 mg, 6 mg, 8 mg, 12 mg

Generic: 2 mg, 4 mg, 6 mg, 8 mg, 12 mg

◆ **Ropinirole Hydrochloride** *see* ROPINIRole *on page 1844*

Ropivacaine (roe PIV a kane)

Brand Names: U.S. Naropin

Brand Names: Canada Naropin®; Ropivacaine Hydrochloride Injection, USP

Index Terms Ropivacaine Hydrochloride

Pharmacologic Category Local Anesthetic

Use Local anesthetic for use in surgery, postoperative pain management, and obstetrical procedures when local or regional anesthesia is needed

Pregnancy Risk Factor B

Dosage Dose varies with procedure, onset and depth of anesthesia desired, vascularity of tissues, duration of anesthesia, and condition of patient: Adults:

Surgical anesthesia:

Lumbar epidural: 15-30 mL of 0.5% to 1% solution

Lumbar epidural block for cesarean section:

20-30 mL dose of 0.5% solution

15-20 mL dose of 0.75% solution

Thoracic epidural block: 5-15 mL dose of 0.5% or 0.75% solution

Major nerve block:

35-50 mL dose of 0.5% solution (175-250 mg)

10-40 mL dose of 0.75% solution (75-300 mg)

Field block: 1-40 mL dose of 0.5% solution (5-200 mg)

Labor pain management: Lumbar epidural: Initial: 10-20 mL 0.2% solution; continuous infusion dose: 6-14 mL/hour of 0.2% solution with incremental injections of 10-15 mL/hour of 0.2% solution

Postoperative pain management:

Peripheral nerve block: Continuous infusion dose: 5-10 mL/hour of 0.2% solution (Bagry, 2008; Klein, 2000)

Lumbar or thoracic epidural: Continuous infusion dose: 6-14 mL/hour of 0.2% solution

Infiltration/minor nerve block:

1-100 mL dose of 0.2% solution

1-40 mL dose of 0.5% solution

Dosage adjustment in renal impairment: No dosage adjustment provided in manufacturer's labeling. However, ropivacaine and its metabolites are renally excreted, and the risk of toxic reactions may be greater.

Dosage comment in hepatic impairment: No dosage adjustment provided in manufacturer's labeling. Use with caution since patients may be at a greater risk for developing toxic drug levels.

Additional Information Complete prescribing information should be consulted for additional detail.

Dosage Forms

Solution, Injection [preservative free]:

Naropin: 2 mg/mL (10 mL, 20 mL, 100 mL, 200 mL); 5 mg/mL (20 mL, 30 mL, 100 mL, 200 mL); 7.5 mg/mL (20 mL); 10 mg/mL (10 mL, 20 mL)

Generic: 2 mg/mL (10 mL, 20 mL); 5 mg/mL (30 mL); 7.5 mg/mL (20 mL); 10 mg/mL (10 mL, 20 mL)

◆ **Ropivacaine Hydrochloride** *see* Ropivacaine *on page 1846*

◆ **Ropivacaine Hydrochloride Injection, USP (Can)** *see* Ropivacaine *on page 1846*

- **Rosadan** *see* MetroNIDAZOLE (Topical) *on page 1357*
- **Rosanil** *see* Sulfur and Sulfacetamide *on page 1953*
- **Rosasol (Can)** *see* MetroNIDAZOLE (Topical) *on page 1357*

Rosiglitazone (roh si GLI ta zone)

Brand Names: U.S. Avandia

Brand Names: Canada Avandia

Pharmacologic Category Antidiabetic Agent, Thiazolidinedione

Use

Type 2 diabetes: Adjunct to diet and exercise to improve glycemic control in adults with type 2 diabetes mellitus (noninsulin dependent, NIDDM); may be used as monotherapy or in combination with metformin or a sulfonylurea.

Limitations of use: Should not be used in patients with type 1 diabetes mellitus or diabetic ketoacidosis; use with insulin is not recommended.

Pregnancy Risk Factor C

Dosage Type 2 diabetes: Oral: **Note:** All patients should be initiated at the lowest recommended dose.

Adults: Initial: 4 mg daily as a single daily dose or in divided doses twice daily. If response is inadequate after 8-12 weeks of treatment, the dosage may be increased to 8 mg daily (maximum dose) as a single daily dose or in divided doses twice daily. In clinical trials, the 4 mg twice-daily regimen resulted in the greatest reduction in fasting plasma glucose and HbA_{1c}. **Note:** When used in combination therapy with other hypoglycemic agents, a dose reduction of the concurrent agent may be necessary if hypoglycemia occurs. The Canadian labeling recommends a maximum rosiglitazone dose of 4 mg daily when used in combination with a sulfonylurea.

Elderly: Refer to adult dosing. No dosage adjustment is recommended.

Dosage adjustment in renal impairment: No dosage adjustment necessary.

Dosage adjustment in hepatic impairment: There are no dosage adjustments provided in the manufacturer's labeling. Clearance is significantly lower in hepatic impairment; therapy should not be initiated if the patient exhibits active liver disease or increased transaminases (ALT >2.5 times the upper limit of normal) at baseline.

Additional Information Complete prescribing information should be consulted for additional detail.

Dosage Forms

Tablet, Oral:

Avandia: 2 mg, 4 mg, 8 mg

Rosiglitazone and Glimepiride
(roh si GLI ta zone & GLYE me pye ride)

Brand Names: U.S. Avandaryl

Index Terms Glimepiride and Rosiglitazone Maleate

Pharmacologic Category Antidiabetic Agent, Sulfonylurea; Antidiabetic Agent, Thiazolidinedione

Use

Type 2 diabetes: Adjunct to diet and exercise to improve glycemic control in adults with type 2 diabetes mellitus (noninsulin dependent, NIDDM) and in whom dual rosiglitazone/glimepiride therapy is appropriate

Limitations of use: Should not be used in patients with type 1 diabetes mellitus or diabetic ketoacidosis; use with insulin is not recommended.

Pregnancy Risk Factor C

Dosage Type 2 diabetes mellitus: Adults: Oral: **Note:** Rosiglitazone dose should be initiated at the lowest recommended dose.

Initial: Rosiglitazone 4 mg and glimepiride 1 mg once daily **or** rosiglitazone 4 mg and glimepiride 2 mg once daily (for patients previously treated with sulfonylurea or thiazolidinedione monotherapy)

Patients switching from combination therapy of rosiglitazone and glimepiride as separate tablets: Use current dose

Titration:

Dose adjustment in patients previously on sulfonylurea monotherapy: May take 2 weeks to observe decreased blood glucose and 2 to 3 months to see full effects of rosiglitazone component. If not adequately controlled after 8 to 12 weeks, increase daily dose of rosiglitazone component.

Dose adjustment in patients previously on thiazolidinedione monotherapy: If not adequately controlled after 1-2 weeks, increase daily dose of glimepiride component in ≤2 mg increments in 1 to 2 week intervals.

Maximum dose: Rosiglitazone 8 mg and glimepiride 4 mg once daily

Elderly: Rosiglitazone 4 mg and glimepiride 1 mg once daily; carefully titrate dose.

Dosage adjustment in renal impairment: Rosiglitazone 4 mg and glimepiride 1 mg once daily; carefully titrate dose.

Dosage adjustment in hepatic impairment: Rosiglitazone 4 mg and glimepiride 1 mg once daily; carefully titrate dose. Therapy should not be initiated if the patient exhibits symptoms of active liver disease or increased transaminases (ALT >2.5 times the upper limit of normal) at baseline since clearance is significantly lower in hepatic impairment. Discontinue if ALT >3 times ULN or jaundice occurs.

Additional Information Complete prescribing information should be consulted for additional detail.

Dosage Forms

Tablet:

Avandaryl®: 4 mg/1 mg: Rosiglitazone 4 mg and glimepiride 1 mg; 4 mg/2 mg: Rosiglitazone 4 mg and glimepiride 2 mg; 4 mg/4 mg: Rosiglitazone 4 mg and glimepiride 4 mg; 8 mg/2 mg: Rosiglitazone 8 mg and glimepiride 2 mg; 8 mg/4 mg: Rosiglitazone 8 mg and glimepiride 4 mg

Rosiglitazone and Metformin
(roh si GLI ta zone & met FOR min)

Brand Names: U.S. Avandamet

Brand Names: Canada Avandamet

Index Terms Metformin and Rosiglitazone; Metformin Hydrochloride and Rosiglitazone Maleate; Rosiglitazone Maleate and Metformin Hydrochloride

Pharmacologic Category Antidiabetic Agent, Biguanide; Antidiabetic Agent, Thiazolidinedione

Use

Type 2 diabetes: Adjunct to diet and exercise to improve glycemic control in adults with type 2 diabetes mellitus (noninsulin dependent, NIDDM).

Limitations of use: Should not be used in patients with type 1 diabetes mellitus or diabetic ketoacidosis; use with insulin is not recommended.

Pregnancy Risk Factor C

Dosage Type 2 diabetes mellitus: Adults: Oral: **Note:** Daily dose should be divided. Rosiglitazone dose should be initiated at the lowest recommended dose.

Patients inadequately controlled on diet and exercise alone: Initial dose: Rosiglitazone 2 mg and metformin 500 mg once or twice daily. Patients with HbA_{1c} >11% or fasting plasma glucose (FPG) >270 mg/dL: Initial: Rosiglitazone 2 mg and metformin 500 mg twice daily may be considered. If not adequately controlled after 4 weeks, the dose may be increased in increments of rosiglitazone 2 mg and metformin 500 mg per day given in divided doses.

Patients inadequately controlled on **metformin alone**: Initial dose: Rosiglitazone 4 mg daily plus current dose of metformin

Patients inadequately controlled on **rosiglitazone alone**: Initial dose: Metformin 1000 mg daily plus current dose of rosiglitazone

Patients switching from combination therapy of rosiglitazone and metformin as separate tablets: Use current dose.

Titration:

Dose adjustment after rosiglitazone dosage increase: If not adequately controlled after 8 to 12 weeks, increase daily dose of rosiglitazone component in 4 mg increments.

Dose adjustment after metformin dosage increase: If not adequately controlled after 1 to 2 weeks, increase daily dose of metformin component in 500 mg increments.

Maximum daily dose: Rosiglitazone 8 mg/metformin 2000 mg.

Elderly: The initial and maintenance dosing should be conservative, due to the potential for decreased renal function (monitor). Generally, elderly patients should not be titrated to the maximum; do not use in patients ≥80 years unless normal renal function has been established.

Dosage adjustment in renal impairment: Contraindicated in the presence of renal disease or renal dysfunction (serum creatinine ≥1.5 mg/dL [males], ≥1.4 mg/dL [females] or abnormal clearance)

Dosage adjustment in hepatic impairment: There are no dosage adjustments provided in manufacturer's labeling. Do not initiate therapy with active liver disease or ALT >2.5 times the upper limit of normal

Additional Information Complete prescribing information should be consulted for additional detail.

Dosage Forms

Tablet, Oral:

Avandamet: 4/500: Rosiglitazone 4 mg and metformin 500 mg; 2/1000: Rosiglitazone 2 mg and metformin 1000 mg

Dosage Forms: Canada

Tablet, Oral:

Avandamet: 1/500: Rosiglitazone 1 mg and metformin hydrochloride 500 mg

◆ **Rosiglitazone Maleate and Metformin Hydrochloride** *see* Rosiglitazone and Metformin *on page 1847*

◆ **Rosone (Can)** *see* Betamethasone (Topical) *on page 255*

Rosuvastatin (roe soo va STAT in)

Brand Names: U.S. Crestor

Brand Names: Canada Apo-Rosuvastatin; CO Rosuvastatin; Crestor; Dom-Rosuvastatin; Jamp-Rosuvastatin; Med-Rosuvastatin; Mint-Rosuvastatin; Mylan-Rosuvastatin; PMS-Rosuvastatin; RAN-Rosuvastatin; Riva-Rosuvastatin; Sandoz-Rosuvastatin; Teva-Rosuvastatin

Index Terms Rosuvastatin Calcium

Pharmacologic Category Antilipemic Agent, HMG-CoA Reductase Inhibitor

Use

Heterozygous familial hypercholesterolemia in children: Adjunct to diet to reduce total cholesterol, low-density lipoprotein cholesterol (LDL-C), and apolipoprotein B (apo B) levels in adolescent males and females who are at least 1 year postmenarche and are 10-17 years of age with heterozygous familial hypercholesteremia if after an adequate trial of diet therapy the following findings are present: LDL-C more than 190 mg/dL or more than 160 mg/dL and there is a positive family history of premature cardiovascular (CV) disease or 2 or more other CV disease risk factors.

Homozygous familial hypercholesterolemia: To reduce LDL-C, total cholesterol, and apo B in adults with homozygous familial hypercholesterolemia as an adjunct to other lipid-lowering treatments (eg, LDL apheresis) or alone if such treatments are unavailable.

Hyperlipidemia and mixed dyslipidemia: Adjunctive therapy to diet to reduce elevated total cholesterol, LDL-C, apo B, non–high-density lipoprotein cholesterol (non-HDL-C), and triglyceride levels, and to increase HDL-C in patients with primary hyperlipidemia or mixed dyslipidemia.

Hypertriglyceridemia: Adjunct to diet for the treatment of adults with hypertriglyceridemia.

Primary dysbetalipoproteinemia (type III hyperlipoproteinemia): Adjunct to diet for the treatment of patients with primary dysbetalipoproteinemia (type III hyperlipoproteinemia).

Prevention of cardiovascular disease:

Primary prevention: To reduce the risk of stroke, myocardial infarction, or arterial revascularization procedures in patients without clinically evident coronary heart disease or lipid abnormalities but with all of the following: 1) an increased risk of cardiovascular disease based on age ≥50 years old in men and ≥60 years old in women, 2) hsCRP ≥2 mg/L, and 3) the presence of at least one additional cardiovascular disease risk factor such as hypertension, low HDL-C, smoking, or a family history of premature coronary heart disease.

Secondary prevention: Adjunctive therapy to diet to slow the progression of atherosclerosis in adults as part of a treatment strategy to lower total cholesterol and LDL-C to target levels.

Primary and secondary prevention of atherosclerotic cardiovascular disease (ASCVD) according to the American College of Cardiology/American Heart Association: To reduce the risk of ASCVD in patients with clinical ASCVD (eg, coronary heart disease, stroke/TIA, or peripheral arterial disease presumed to be of atherosclerotic origin); in patients without clinical ASCVD if LDL-C is 190 mg/dL or greater; in patients without clinical ASCVD who have type 1 or type 2 diabetes and are between 40 and 75 years of age; in patients with an estimated 10-year ASCVD risk 7.5% or greater and who are between 40 and 75 years of age (Stone, 2013). Specific recommendations from the Kidney Disease: Improving Global Outcomes (KDIGO) organization have also been released for patients with chronic kidney disease (KDIGO [Tonelli, 2013]).

Pregnancy Risk Factor X

Pregnancy Considerations Adverse events were observed in some animal reproduction studies. There are reports of congenital anomalies following maternal use of HMG-CoA reductase inhibitors in pregnancy; however, maternal disease, differences in specific agents used, and the low rates of exposure limit the interpretation of the available data (Godfrey, 2012; Lecarpentier, 2012). Cholesterol biosynthesis may be important in fetal development; serum cholesterol and triglycerides increase normally during pregnancy. The discontinuation of lipid lowering medications temporarily during pregnancy is not expected to have significant impact on the long term outcomes of primary hypercholesterolemia treatment.

Use of rosuvastatin is contraindicated in pregnancy. HMG-CoA reductase inhibitors should be discontinued prior to pregnancy (ADA, 2013). If treatment of dyslipidemias is needed in pregnant women or in women of reproductive age, other agents are preferred (Berglund, 2012; Stone, 2013). The manufacturer recommends administration to women of childbearing potential only when conception is highly unlikely and patients have been informed of potential hazards.

Breast-Feeding Considerations It is not known if rosuvastatin is excreted into breast milk. Due to the potential for serious adverse reactions in a nursing infant, use while breast-feeding is contraindicated by the manufacturer.

Contraindications

Known hypersensitivity to any component of the formulation; active liver disease or unexplained persistent elevations of serum transaminases; pregnancy; breast-feeding.

Canadian labeling: Additional contraindications (not in U.S. labeling): Concomitant administration of cyclosporine; use of 40 mg dose in Asian patients, patients with predisposing risk factors for myopathy/rhabdomyolysis (eg, hereditary muscle disorders, history of myotoxicity with other HMG-CoA reductase inhibitors, concomitant use with fibrates or niacin, severe hepatic impairment, severe renal impairment [CrCl <30 mL/minute/1.73 m^2], hypothyroidism, alcohol abuse)

Warnings/Precautions Secondary causes of hyperlipidemia should be ruled out prior to therapy. Rosuvastatin has not been studied when the primary lipid abnormality is chylomicron elevation (Fredrickson types I and V). Postmarketing reports of fatal and nonfatal hepatic failure are rare. If serious hepatotoxicity with clinical symptoms and/or hyperbilirubinemia or jaundice occurs during treatment, interrupt therapy. If an alternate etiology is not identified, do not restart rosuvastatin. Liver enzyme tests should be obtained at baseline and as clinically indicated; routine periodic monitoring of liver enzymes is not necessary. Use with caution in patients who consume large amounts of ethanol or have a history of liver disease; use is contraindicated with active liver disease or unexplained transaminase elevations. Hematuria (microscopic) and proteinuria have been observed; more commonly reported in adults receiving rosuvastatin 40 mg daily, but typically transient and not associated with a decrease in renal function. Consider dosage reduction if unexplained hematuria and proteinuria persists. HMG-CoA reductase inhibitors may cause rhabdomyolysis with acute renal failure and/or myopathy. Discontinue in any patient in which CPK levels are markedly elevated (>10 times ULN) or if myopathy is suspected/diagnosed. This risk is dose-related and is increased with concurrent use of other lipid-lowering medications (fibric acid derivatives or niacin doses ≥1 g/day), other interacting drugs, drugs associated with myopathy (eg, colchicine), age ≥65 years, female gender, certain subgroups of Asian ancestry, uncontrolled hypothyroidism, and renal dysfunction. Dose reductions may be necessary. Immune-mediated necrotizing myopathy (IMNM), an autoimmune-mediated myopathy, has been reported (rarely) with HMG-CoA reductase inhibitor therapy. IMNM presents as proximal muscle weakness with elevated CPK levels, which persists despite discontinuation of HMG-CoA reductase inhibitor therapy; additionally, muscle biopsy may show necrotizing myopathy with limited inflammation; immunosuppressive therapy (eg, corticosteroids, azathioprine) may be used for treatment.

The manufacturer recommends temporary discontinuation for elective major surgery, acute medical or surgical conditions, or in any patient experiencing an acute or serious condition predisposing to renal failure (eg, sepsis, dehydration, electrolyte disorders, hypotension, trauma, uncontrolled seizures). Based on current research and clinical guidelines (Fleisher, 2009), HMG-CoA reductase inhibitors should be continued in the perioperative period. Patients should be instructed to report unexplained muscle pain, tenderness, weakness, or dark urine; in Canada, concomitant use with cyclosporine or niacin is contraindicated, and rosuvastatin at a dose of 40 mg/day in Asian patients is contraindicated. Small increases in HbA_{1c} (mean: ~0.1%) and fasting blood glucose have been reported with rosuvastatin; however, the benefits of statin therapy far outweigh the risk of dysglycemia.

Potentially significant interactions may exist, requiring dose or frequency adjustment, additional monitoring, and/or selection of alternative therapy. Consult drug interactions database for more detailed information. Dosage adjustment required in patients with a CrCl <30 mL/minute/1.73 m^2 and not receiving hemodialysis (contraindicated in the Canadian labeling. Use with caution in elderly patients as they are more predisposed to myopathy.

Adverse Reactions

Central nervous system: Dizziness, headache

Endocrine & metabolic: Diabetes mellitus (new onset)

Gastrointestinal: Abdominal pain, constipation, nausea

Hepatic: Increased serum ALT (>3 times ULN)

Neuromuscular & skeletal: Arthralgia, increased creatine phosphokinase, myalgia, weakness

Rare but important or life-threatening: Abnormal thyroid function test, cognitive dysfunction (reversible; includes amnesia, confusion, memory impairment), depression, elevated glycosylated hemoglobin (HbA_{1c}), gynecomastia, hematuria (microscopic), hepatic failure, hepatitis, hypersensitivity reaction (including angioedema, pruritus, skin rash, urticaria), immune-mediated necrotizing myopathy, increased gamma-glutamyl transferase, increased serum alkaline phosphatase, increased serum bilirubin, increased serum glucose, increased serum transaminases, jaundice, myoglobinuria, myopathy, myositis, pancreatitis, peripheral neuropathy, proteinuria (dose related), renal failure, rhabdomyolysis, sleep disorder (including insomnia and nightmares), thrombocytopenia

Drug Interactions

Metabolism/Transport Effects **Substrate** of CYP2C9 (minor), CYP3A4 (minor), SLCO1B1; **Note:** Assignment of Major/Minor substrate status based on clinically relevant drug interaction potential

Avoid Concomitant Use

Avoid concomitant use of Rosuvastatin with any of the following: Fusidic Acid (Systemic); Gemfibrozil; Ledipasvir; Red Yeast Rice

Increased Effect/Toxicity

Rosuvastatin may increase the levels/effects of: DAPTOmycin; PAZOPanib; Trabectedin; Vitamin K Antagonists

The levels/effects of Rosuvastatin may be increased by: Acipimox; Amiodarone; Bezafibrate; Boceprevir; Ciprofibrate; Clopidogrel; Colchicine; CycloSPORINE (Systemic); Dronedarone; Eltrombopag; Fenofibrate and Derivatives; Fusidic Acid (Systemic); Gemfibrozil; Itraconazole; Ledipasvir; Niacin; Niacinamide; Paritaprevir; Protease Inhibitors; Raltegravir; Red Yeast Rice; Simeprevir; Telaprevir; Teriflunomide

Decreased Effect

Rosuvastatin may decrease the levels/effects of: Lanthanum

The levels/effects of Rosuvastatin may be decreased by: Antacids; Eslicarbazepine

Storage/Stability Store between 20°C and 25°C (68°F to 77°F). Protect from moisture.

Mechanism of Action Inhibitor of 3-hydroxy-3-methylglutaryl coenzyme A (HMG-CoA) reductase, the rate-limiting enzyme in cholesterol synthesis (reduces the production of mevalonic acid from HMG-CoA); this then results in a compensatory increase in the expression of LDL receptors on hepatocyte membranes and a stimulation of LDL catabolism

Pharmacodynamics/Kinetics

Onset of action: Within 1 week; maximal at 4 weeks

Distribution: V_d: 134 L

Protein binding: 88%

Metabolism: Hepatic (10%), via CYP2C9 (1 active metabolite identified: N-desmethyl rosuvastatin, one-sixth to one-half the HMG-CoA reductase activity of the parent compound)

Bioavailability: 20% (high first-pass extraction by liver)
- Asian patients have been noted to have increased bioavailability.

Half-life elimination: 19 hours

Time to peak, plasma: 3-5 hours

Excretion: Feces (90%), primarily as unchanged drug

Dosage Oral: **Note:** Doses should be individualized according to the baseline LDL-cholesterol levels, the recommended goal of therapy, and patient response; adjustments should be made at intervals of 4 weeks or more

Children and Adolescents 10-17 years (females >1 year postmenarche): Heterozygous familial hypercholesterolemia (HeFH):
- U.S. labeling: 5-20 mg once daily; maximum: 20 mg daily
  - **Dosage adjustment for rosuvastatin with concomitant cyclosporine, gemfibrozil, atazanavir/ritonavir, or lopinavir/ritonavir:** Refer to adult dosing.
- Canadian labeling: 5-10 mg once daily; maximum: 10 mg daily

Adults:
- Hyperlipidemia, mixed dyslipidemia, hypertriglyceridemia, primary dysbetalipoproteinemia, slowing progression of atherosclerosis, primary prevention of cardiovascular disease:
  - Initial dose:
    - General dosing: 10-20 mg once daily; 20 mg once daily may be used in patients with severe hyperlipidemia (LDL >190 mg/dL) and aggressive lipid targets (McKenney, 2009)
    - Conservative dosing: Patients requiring less aggressive treatment or predisposed to myopathy (including patients of Asian descent): 5 mg once daily
  - Titration: After initiation or upon titration, analyze lipid levels within 2-4 weeks (peak, steady-state lowering effects usually seen between 4-6 weeks [McKenney, 2009]) and adjust dose accordingly; dosing range: 5-40 mg daily (maximum dose: 40 mg once daily).
  - **Note:** The 40 mg dose should be reserved for patients who have not achieved goal cholesterol levels on a dose of 20 mg daily, including patients switched from another HMG-CoA reductase inhibitor.
- Homozygous familial hypercholesterolemia (FH): Initial: 20 mg once daily (maximum dose: 40 mg daily)

ACC/AHA Blood Cholesterol Guideline recommendations to reduce the risk of atherosclerotic cardiovascular disease (ASCVD) (Stone, 2013): Adults ≥21 years:

Primary prevention:
- *LDL-C ≥190 mg/dL:* High-intensity therapy: 20-40 mg once daily.
- *Type 1 or 2 diabetes and age 40-75 years:* Moderate-intensity therapy: 5-10 mg once daily.
- *Type 1 or 2 diabetes, age 40-75 years, and an estimated 10-year ASCVD risk ≥7.5%:* High intensity therapy: 20-40 mg once daily
- *Age 40-75 years and an estimated 10-year ASCVD risk ≥7.5%:* Moderate to high intensity therapy: 5-40 mg once daily

Secondary prevention:

Patient has clinical ASCVD (eg, coronary heart disease, stroke/TIA, or peripheral arterial disease presumed to be of atherosclerotic origin) **and**:
- *Age ≤75 years:* High-intensity therapy: 20-40 mg once daily.
- *Age >75 years or not a candidate for high-intensity therapy:* Moderate-intensity therapy: 5-10 mg once daily.

Dosage adjustment for rosuvastatin with concomitant medications:

U.S. labeling:
- Cyclosporine: Rosuvastatin dose should not exceed 5 mg once daily
- Gemfibrozil: Avoid concurrent use; if unable to avoid concurrent use, initiate rosuvastatin at 5 mg once daily; dose should not exceed 10 mg once daily
- Atazanavir/ritonavir or lopinavir/ritonavir: Initiate rosuvastatin at 5 mg once daily; dose should not exceed 10 mg once daily

Canadian labeling:
- Cyclosporine: Concomitant use is contraindicated
- Gemfibrozil: Rosuvastatin dose should not exceed 20 mg daily

Dosage adjustment for toxicity:

Severe muscle symptoms or fatigue: Promptly discontinue use; evaluate CPK, creatinine, and urinalysis for myoglobinuria (Stone, 2013).

Mild to moderate muscle symptoms: Discontinue use until symptoms can be evaluated; evaluate patient for conditions that may increase the risk for muscle symptoms (eg, hypothyroidism, reduced renal or hepatic function, rheumatologic disorders such as polymyalgia rheumatica, steroid myopathy, vitamin D deficiency, or primary muscle diseases). Upon resolution, resume the original or lower dose of rosuvastatin. If muscle symptoms recur, discontinue rosuvastatin use. After muscle symptom resolution, may then use a low dose of a different statin; gradually increase if tolerated. In the absence of continued statin use, if muscle symptoms or elevated CPK continues after 2 months, consider other causes of muscle symptoms. If determined to be due to another condition aside from statin use, may resume statin therapy at the original dose (Stone, 2013).

Dosage adjustment for hematuria and/or persistent, unexplained proteinuria while on 40 mg daily: Reduce dose and evaluate causes

Dosage adjustment in renal impairment:
- CrCl ≥30 mL/minute/1.73 m^2: No dosage adjustment necessary.
- CrCl <30 mL/minute/1.73 m^2: Initial: 5 mg once daily; maximum: 10 mg once daily

Dosage adjustment in hepatic impairment:

U.S. labeling: Manufacturer labeling does not provide specific dosing recommendations; however, systemic exposure may be increased in patients with liver disease (increased AUC and C_{max}); use is contraindicated in active liver disease or unexplained transaminase elevations.

Canadian labeling:
- Active hepatic disease or unexplained persistent transaminase >3 x ULN: Use is contraindicated
- Mild-to-moderate impairment: No dosage adjustment necessary.
- Severe impairment: Initial: 5 mg daily. Maximum: 20 mg once daily

Dietary Considerations Red yeast rice contains variable amounts of several compounds that are structurally similar to HMG-CoA reductase inhibitors, primarily monacolin K (or mevinolin) which is structurally identical to lovastatin; concurrent use of red yeast rice with HMG-CoA reductase inhibitors may increase the incidence of adverse and toxic effects (Lapi, 2008; Smith, 2003).

Administration May be administered with or without food. May be taken at any time of the day.

Monitoring Parameters

2013 ACC/AHA Blood Cholesterol Guideline recommendations (Stone, 2013):

Lipid panel (total cholesterol, HDL, LDL, triglycerides): Baseline lipid panel; fasting lipid profile within 4-12 weeks after initiation or dose adjustment and every 3-12 months (as clinically indicated) thereafter. If 2 consecutive LDL levels are <40 mg/dL, consider decreasing the dose.

Hepatic transaminase levels: Baseline measurement of hepatic transaminase levels (ie, ALT); measure hepatic function if symptoms suggest hepatotoxicity (eg, unusual fatigue or weakness, loss of appetite, abdominal pain, dark-colored urine or yellowing of skin or sclera) during therapy.

CPK: CPK should not be routinely measured. Baseline CPK measurement is reasonable for some individuals (eg, family history of statin intolerance or muscle disease, clinical presentation, concomitant drug therapy that may increase risk of myopathy). May measure CPK in any patient with symptoms suggestive of myopathy (pain, tenderness, stiffness, cramping, weakness, or generalized fatigue).

Evaluate for new-onset diabetes mellitus during therapy; if diabetes develops, continue statin therapy and encourage adherence to a heart-healthy diet, physical activity, a healthy body weight, and tobacco cessation.

If patient develops a confusional state or memory impairment, may evaluate patient for nonstatin causes (eg, exposure to other drugs), systemic and neuropsychiatric causes, and the possibility of adverse effects associated with statin therapy.

Manufacturer recommendations: Liver enzyme tests at baseline and repeated when clinically indicated. Upon initiation or titration, lipid panel should be analyzed within 2-4 weeks.

Dosage Forms

Tablet, Oral:

Crestor: 5 mg, 10 mg, 20 mg, 40 mg

◆ **Rosuvastatin Calcium** *see* Rosuvastatin *on page 1848*

◆ **Rotarix** *see* Rotavirus Vaccine *on page 1851*

◆ **RotaTeq** *see* Rotavirus Vaccine *on page 1851*

Rotavirus Vaccine (ROE ta vye rus vak SEEN)

Brand Names: U.S. Rotarix; RotaTeq

Brand Names: Canada Rotarix; RotaTeq

Index Terms Human Rotavirus Vaccine, Attenuated (HRV); Pentavalent Human-Bovine Reassortant Rotavirus Vaccine (PRV); Rotavirus Vaccine, Pentavalent; RV1 (Rotarix); RV5 (RotaTeq)

Pharmacologic Category Vaccine, Live (Viral)

Additional Appendix Information

Immunization Administration Recommendations *on page 2250*

Immunization Recommendations *on page 2255*

Use

Rotavirus gastroenteritis prevention:

Rotarix: Prevention of rotavirus gastroenteritis in infants 6 to 24 weeks of age caused by the serotypes G1,G3, G4, and G9 when administered as a 2-dose series.

RotaTeq: Prevention of rotavirus gastroenteritis in infants 6 to 32 weeks of age caused by the serotypes G1, G2, G3, and G4 when administered as a 3-dose series.

The Advisory Committee on Immunization Practices (ACIP) recommends routine vaccination of all infants (CDC/ACIP [Cortese, 2009]).

Pregnancy Risk Factor C

Dosage Prevention of rotavirus gastroenteritis: Oral:

Manufacturer's labeling:

Infants 6 to 24 weeks of age: Rotarix: A total of two 1 mL doses (U.S. labeling) or two 1.5 mL doses (Canadian labeling), the first dose given at 6 weeks of age, followed by the second dose given ≥4 weeks later. The 2-dose series should be completed by 24 weeks of age.

Infants 6 to 32 weeks of age: RotaTeq: A total of three 2 mL doses, the first dose given at 6 to 12 weeks of age, followed by subsequent doses at 4- to 10-week intervals. Administer all doses by 32 weeks of age.

ACIP recommendations (CDC/ACIP [Cortese, 2009]): The first dose can be given at 6 to 14 weeks of age. The series should not be started in infants ≥15 weeks. The final dose in the series should be administered by 8 months 0 days of age. The minimum interval between doses is 4 weeks. RotaTeq should be given in 3 doses administered at 2-, 4-, and 6 months of age. Rotarix should be given in 2 doses administered at 2- and 4 months of age. For infants inadvertently administered rotavirus vaccine at ≥15 weeks of age, the vaccine series may be completed according to schedule. The ACIP recommends to complete the vaccine series with the same product whenever possible. If continuing with same product will cause vaccination to be deferred, or if product used previously is unknown, vaccination should be completed with the product available. If RotaTeq was used in any previous doses, or if the specific product used was unknown, a total of 3 doses should be given. Infants who have had rotavirus gastroenteritis before getting the full course of vaccine should still initiate or complete the recommended schedule; initial infection provides only partial immunity.

Dosage adjustment in renal impairment: There are no dosage adjustments provided in the manufacturer's labeling.

Dosage adjustment in hepatic impairment: There are no dosage adjustments provided in the manufacturer's labeling.

Additional Information Complete prescribing information should be consulted for additional detail.

Dosage Forms

Powder, for suspension, oral [preservative free; human derived]:

Rotarix: G1P[8] ≥10^6 $CCID_{50}$ per 1 mL

Solution, oral [preservative free]:

RotaTeq: G1 ≥2.2 x 10^6 infectious units, G2 ≥2.8 x 10^6 infectious units, G3 ≥2.2 x 10^6 infectious units, G4 ≥2 x 10^6 infectious units, and P1A [8] ≥2.3 x 10^6 infectious units per 2 mL (2 mL)

Dosage Forms: Canada

Suspension, oral [human derived]:

Rotarix: ≥10^6 $CCID_{50}$ per 1.5 mL (1.5 mL)

◆ **Rotavirus Vaccine, Pentavalent** *see* Rotavirus Vaccine *on page 1851*

Rotigotine (roe TIG oh teen)

Brand Names: U.S. Neupro

Brand Names: Canada Neupro

Index Terms N-0923

Pharmacologic Category Anti-Parkinson's Agent, Dopamine Agonist

Use Treatment of the signs and symptoms of idiopathic Parkinson's disease (early-stage to advanced-stage disease); treatment of moderate-to-severe primary restless legs syndrome (RLS)

Pregnancy Risk Factor C

Pregnancy Considerations Adverse events were observed in animal reproduction studies. The Canadian labeling does not recommend use in pregnant women.

Breast-Feeding Considerations Prolactin secretion is decreased and lactation may be inhibited. The Canadian labeling recommends discontinuing breast-feeding in women who require therapy.

Contraindications Hypersensitivity to rotigotine or any component of the formulation

Warnings/Precautions Use is commonly associated with somnolence. In addition, falling asleep during activities of daily living, including while driving, has also been reported and may occur without significant warning signs. Monitor for daytime somnolence or preexisting sleep disorder. Patients must be cautioned about performing tasks which require mental alertness (eg, operating machinery or driving). Use with caution in patients receiving other CNS depressants or psychoactive agents; discontinue if significant daytime sleepiness or episodes of falling asleep occur. Effects with other sedative drugs or ethanol may be potentiated.

Dopamine agonists may cause orthostatic hypotension and syncope; Parkinson's disease patients appear to have an impaired capacity to respond to a postural challenge. Use with caution in patients at risk of hypotension (such as those receiving antihypertensive drugs) or where transient hypotensive episodes would be poorly tolerated (cardiovascular disease or cerebrovascular disease). Parkinson's and restless legs syndrome (RLS) patients being treated with dopaminergic agonists ordinarily require careful monitoring for signs and symptoms of postural hypotension, especially during dose escalation, and should be informed of this risk. Weight gain and fluid retention have been reported, primarily associated with development of peripheral edema in Parkinson's disease patients; use caution in patients with heart failure or renal insufficiency. Therapy has also been associated with increases in blood pressure (may be significant), and increased heart rate; use caution in preexisting cardiovascular disease.

Dopamine agonists have been associated with compulsive behaviors and/or loss of impulse control, which has manifested as pathological gambling, libido increases (hypersexuality), and/or binge eating. Causality has not been established, and controversy exists as to whether this phenomenon is related to the underlying disease, prior behaviors/addictions and/or drug therapy. Dose reduction or discontinuation of therapy has been reported to reverse these behaviors in some, but not all cases.

In RLS patents, augmentation (earlier onset of symptoms each day and/or an overall increase in symptom severity) or rebound (considered to be an end of dose effect) may occur.

Use with caution in patients with preexisting dyskinesia; therapy may exacerbate. Therapy may also cause hallucinations (dose-related) and other psychotic like behaviors (eg, agitation, delirium, delusions, aggression); in general, avoid use in patients with preexisting major psychotic disorders. Risk for melanoma development is increased in Parkinson's disease patients; drug causation or factors contributing to risk have not been established. Patients receiving therapy for any indication should be monitored closely and periodic skin examinations should be performed. Other dopaminergic agents have been associated with a syndrome resembling neuroleptic malignant syndrome on withdrawal and/or significant dosage reduction. Taper treatment when discontinuing therapy; do not stop abruptly. Rare cases of pleural effusion, pleural thickening, pulmonary infiltrates, retroperitoneal fibrosis, pericarditis and/or cardiac valvulopathy have been reported in patients treated with ergot-derived dopamine agonists, generally with prolonged use. The potential of rotigotine, a non-ergot-derived dopamine agonist, to cause similar fibrotic complications is unknown.

Patch contains aluminum; remove patch prior to magnetic resonance imaging or cardioversion to avoid skin burns. Patch also contains sodium metabisulfite which may cause allergic reaction in susceptible individuals. Dose-dependent application site reactions, potentially severe, have been observed; daily rotation of application sites has been shown to decrease incidence of reactions. If a generalized (nonapplication site) skin reaction occurs; discontinue therapy. Avoid exposure of application site to any direct external heat sources (eg, hair dryers, heating pads, electric blankets, saunas, hot tubs, direct sunlight); heat exposure has not been studied with the rotigotine patch, but an increase in the rate and extent of absorption has been observed with other transdermal products.

Adverse Reactions

Cardiovascular: Hypertension (dose related), peripheral edema (dose related), syncope, T-wave abnormalities on ECG

Central nervous system: Abnormal dreams (dose related), balance disorder, depression, dizziness, early morning awakening (dose related), fatigue, hallucinations (dose related), headache, insomnia, lethargy, nightmare (dose related), orthostatic hypotension, postural dizziness, sleep attacks (dose related), sleep disorder (disturbance in initiating/maintaining sleep; dose related), somnolence (dose related), vertigo

Dermatologic: Application site reactions (dose related), erythema (dose related), hyperhidrosis (dose related), pruritic rash (dose related), pruritus

Endocrine & metabolic: Hot flash, serum ferritin decreased (dose related), serum glucose decreased

Gastrointestinal: Anorexia, appetite decreased, constipation, diarrhea, dyspepsia (dose related), nausea (dose related), vomiting (dose related), weight gain, weight loss (dose related), xerostomia (dose related)

Genitourinary: Erectile dysfunction (dose related), urinary WBC positive

Hematologic: Contusion (dose related), hemoglobin decreased, hematocrit decreased

Neuromuscular & skeletal: Arthralgia, dyskinesia (dose related), muscle spasms (dose related), musculoskeletal pain, paresthesia (dose related), tremor, weakness

Ocular: Vision changes

Otic: Tinnitus

Renal: BUN increased

Respiratory: Cough, nasal congestion, nasopharyngitis, pharyngolaryngeal pain, sinus congestion, sinusitis (dose related), upper respiratory tract infection

Miscellaneous: Hiccups (dose related)

Rare but important or life-threatening: Agitation, aggression, confusion, delirium, delusions, disorientation, generalized skin reaction, impulsive/compulsive behaviors (eg, binge eating, hypersexuality, pathological gambling, shopping), paranoid ideation, psychotic-like behavior

Drug Interactions

Metabolism/Transport Effects None known.

Avoid Concomitant Use

Avoid concomitant use of Rotigotine with any of the following: Amisulpride

Increased Effect/Toxicity

Rotigotine may increase the levels/effects of: BuPROPion

The levels/effects of Rotigotine may be increased by: Alcohol (Ethyl); CNS Depressants; MAO Inhibitors; Methylphenidate

Decreased Effect

Rotigotine may decrease the levels/effects of: Amisulpride; Antipsychotic Agents (First Generation [Typical])

The levels/effects of Rotigotine may be decreased by: Amisulpride; Antipsychotic Agents (First Generation [Typical]); Antipsychotic Agents (Second Generation [Atypical]); Metoclopramide

Storage/Stability Store at 20°C to 25°C (68°F to 77°F). Store in original pouch until application.

Mechanism of Action Rotigotine is a nonergot dopamine agonist with specificity for D_3-, D_2-, and D_1-dopamine receptors. Although the precise mechanism of action of rotigotine is unknown, it is believed to be due to stimulation of postsynaptic dopamine D_2-type auto receptors within the substantia nigra in the brain, leading to improved dopaminergic transmission in the motor areas of the basal ganglia, notably the caudate nucleus/putamen regions.

Pharmacodynamics/Kinetics

Distribution: V_d: 84 L/kg

Protein binding: ~90%

Metabolism: Extensive via conjugation and N-dealkylation; multiple CYP isoenzymes, sulfotransferases, and two UDP-glucuronosyltransferases involved in catalyzing the metabolism

Half-life elimination: After removal of patch: ~5-7 hours

Time to peak, plasma: 15-18 hours; can occur 4-27 hours post application

Excretion: Urine (~71% as inactive conjugates and metabolites, <1% as unchanged drug); feces (~23%)

Dosage Topical: Transdermal: Adults:

Parkinson disease:

Early-stage: Initial: Apply 2 mg/24 hours patch once daily; may increase by 2 mg/24 hours weekly, based on clinical response and tolerability; lowest effective dose: 4 mg/24 hours (maximum dose: 6 mg/24 hours [U.S. labeling] or 8 mg/24 hours [Canadian labeling])

Advanced-stage: Initial: Apply 4 mg/24 hours patch once daily; may increase by 2 mg/24 hours weekly, based on clinical response and tolerability. Recommended dose: 8 mg/24 hours; in clinical trials maximum doses up to 16 mg/24 hours were used.

Discontinuation of treatment in Parkinson's disease: Decrease by ≤2 mg/24 hours preferably every other day until withdrawal complete

Restless legs syndrome (RLS): Initial: Apply 1 mg/24 hours patch once daily; may increase by 1 mg/24 hours weekly, based on clinical response and tolerability; lowest effective dose: 1 mg/24 hours (maximum dose: 3 mg/24 hours)

Discontinuation of treatment for RLS: Decrease by 1 mg/24 hours preferably every other day until withdrawal complete

Dosage adjustment in renal impairment: Mild-to-severe impairment (CrCl ≥15 mL/minute) including dialysis patients: No dosage adjustment necessary.

Dosage adjustment in hepatic impairment:

Mild-to-moderate hepatic impairment (Child-Pugh class A or B): No dosage adjustment necessary.

Severe hepatic impairment: There are no dosage adjustments provided in manufacturer's labeling (has not been studied).

Administration Transdermal patch: Apply patch to clean, dry, hairless area of intact healthy skin on the front of the abdomen, thigh, hip, flank, shoulder, or upper arm at approximately the same time daily. Remove from pouch immediately before use and press patch firmly in place on skin for 30 seconds. Application sites should be rotated on a daily basis. Do not apply to same application site more than once every 14 days or apply patch to oily, irritated or damaged skin. Avoid exposing patch to external heat sources (eg, heating pad, electric blanket, heat lamp, hot tub, direct sunlight). If applied to hairy area, shave ≥3 days prior to applying patch. If patch falls off, immediately apply a new one to a new site.

Monitoring Parameters Blood pressure (including orthostatic); daytime alertness; periodic skin evaluations (melanoma development)

Additional Information In April 2008, Neupro was removed from the market following a recall due to the formation of rotigotine crystals (resembling snowflakes) on the patch. The crystallization resulted in decreased drug available for absorption and altered efficacy. Reintroduction of a reformulated Neupro into the U.S. market was announced in 2012.

Dosage Forms

Patch 24 Hour, Transdermal:

Neupro: 1 mg/24 hr (30 ea); 2 mg/24 hr (30 ea); 3 mg/24 hr (30 ea); 4 mg/24 hr (30 ea); 6 mg/24 hr (30 ea); 8 mg/24 hr (30 ea)

- **Rovamycine® (Can)** *see* Spiramycin [CAN/INT] *on page 1931*
- **Rowasa** *see* Mesalamine *on page 1301*
- **Roxanol** *see* Morphine (Systemic) *on page 1394*
- **Roxicet** *see* Oxycodone and Acetaminophen *on page 1541*
- **Roxicodone** *see* OxyCODONE *on page 1538*

Roxithromycin [INT] (roks ith roe MYE sin)

International Brand Names Alborina (ES); Anuar (AR); Assoral (IT); Biaxsig (AU); Claramid (BE, FR, LU); Claramida (AR); Delos (AR); Forilin (DK); Forimycin (DK); Herem (AR); Infectoroxit (DE); Klomicina (AR); Macrosil (ES); MTW-Roxithromycin (DE); Overal (IT); Rossitrol (IT); Rotesan (ES); Rotram (BR); Rotramin (ES); Roxi 1A Pharma (DE); Roxi Basics (DE); roxi von ct (DE); Roxipaed 1A Pharma (DE); Roxi-Puren (DE); Roxi-saar (DE); Roxi-Wolff (DE); Roxibeta (DE); Roxibion (FI); Roxid (IN); roxidura (DE); Roxigamma (DE); Roxigrun (DE); Roxihexal (DE); Roxiklinge (DE); Roximol (IN); Roxithro-Lich (DE); Roxithromycin AZU (DE); Roxithromycin Heumann (DE); Roxithromycin Stada (DE); Roxithromycin "UNP" (DK); Roxithromycin-ratiopharm (DE); Roxyrol (IN); Rulid (AR, BE, BR, CH, CZ, DE, FR, HR, HU, IT, JP, LU, MX); Rulide (AT, AU, ES, NL, PT); Surlid (DK, FI, SE)

Pharmacologic Category Antibiotic, Macrolide

Reported Use Treatment of mild to moderately severe bacterial infections caused by susceptible organisms

Dosage Range Oral: Doses should be taken before meals:

Children: 5-8 mg/kg/day; maximum dose: 150 mg twice daily

Adults: 300 mg/day in a single dose or 2 divided doses

Product Availability Product available in various countries; not currently available in the U.S.

Dosage Forms

Drops: 25 mg/mL (10 mL)

Liquid, oral: 50 mg/5 mL (30 mL)

Packets for oral suspension: 50 mg

Tablet: 50 mg, 150 mg, 300 mg

- **Roychlor (Can)** *see* Potassium Chloride *on page 1687*
- **Rozerem** *see* Ramelteon *on page 1770*
- **RP-6976** *see* DOCEtaxel *on page 656*
- **RP-54274** *see* Riluzole *on page 1812*
- **RP-59500** *see* Quinupristin and Dalfopristin *on page 1762*
- **r-PA** *see* Reteplase *on page 1794*
- **rPDGF-BB** *see* Becaplermin *on page 230*

- ◆ **rpFVIII** *see* Antihemophilic Factor (Recombinant [Porcine Sequence]) *on page 153*
- ◆ **RPR-116258A** *see* Cabazitaxel *on page 316*
- ◆ **(R,R)-Formoterol L-Tartrate** *see* Arformoterol *on page 168*
- ◆ **RS-25259** *see* Palonosetron *on page 1561*
- ◆ **RS-25259-197** *see* Palonosetron *on page 1561*
- ◆ **RTCA** *see* Ribavirin *on page 1797*
- ◆ **RTG** *see* Ezogabine *on page 835*
- ◆ **RU 0211** *see* Lubiprostone *on page 1255*
- ◆ **RU-486** *see* Mifepristone *on page 1366*
- ◆ **RU-23908** *see* Nilutamide *on page 1455*
- ◆ **RU-38486** *see* Mifepristone *on page 1366*
- ◆ **Rubella, Measles and Mumps Vaccines** *see* Measles, Mumps, and Rubella Virus Vaccine *on page 1273*
- ◆ **Rubella, Varicella, Measles, and Mumps Vaccine** *see* Measles, Mumps, Rubella, and Varicella Virus Vaccine *on page 1274*
- ◆ **Rubidomycin Hydrochloride** *see* DAUNOrubicin (Conventional) *on page 577*
- ◆ **Ruconest** *see* C1 Inhibitor (Recombinant) *on page 316*
- ◆ **RUF 331** *see* Rufinamide *on page 1854*

Rufinamide (roo FIN a mide)

Brand Names: U.S. Banzel

Brand Names: Canada Banzel

Index Terms CGP 33101; E 2080; RUF 331; Xilep

Pharmacologic Category Anticonvulsant, Triazole Derivative

Use Lennox-Gastaut syndrome: Adjunctive treatment of seizures associated with Lennox-Gastaut syndrome in adults and children 4 years and older

Pregnancy Risk Factor C

Pregnancy Considerations Adverse effects were seen in animal reproduction studies. Hormonal contraceptives may be less effective with concurrent rufinamide use; additional forms of nonhormonal contraceptives should be used.

Patients exposed to rufinamide during pregnancy are encouraged to enroll themselves into the AED Pregnancy Registry by calling 1-888-233-2334. Additional information is available at www.aedpregnancyregistry.org.

Breast-Feeding Considerations Excretion into breast milk is unknown, but may be expected. Due to the potential for serious adverse reactions in the nursing infant, the manufacturer recommends a decision be made whether to discontinue nursing or to discontinue the drug, taking into account the importance of treatment to the mother.

Contraindications Patients with familial short QT syndrome

Canadian labeling: Additional contraindications (not in U.S. labeling): Family history of short QT syndrome; presence or history of short QT interval; hypersensitivity to rufinamide, triazole derivatives, or any component of the formulation

Warnings/Precautions Has been associated with shortening of the QT interval. Use caution in patients receiving concurrent medications that shorten the QT interval. Contraindicated in patients with familial short-QT syndrome (Canadian labeling also contraindicates use in patients with a family history of short QT syndrome or presence or history of short QT interval). Use has been associated with CNS-related adverse events, most significant of these were cognitive symptoms (including somnolence or fatigue) and coordination abnormalities (including ataxia, dizziness, and gait disturbances). Caution patients about performing tasks which require mental alertness (eg, operating machinery or driving).

Potentially serious, sometimes fatal, multiorgan hypersensitivity reactions (also known as drug reaction with eosinophilia and systemic symptoms [DRESS]) have been reported. Monitor for signs and symptoms (eg, fever, rash, lymphadenopathy, eosinophilia) in association with other organ system involvement (eg, hepatitis, nephritis, hematological abnormalities, myocarditis, myositis). Evaluate immediately if signs or symptoms are present. Discontinuation and conversion to alternate therapy may be required. Potentially serious, sometimes fatal, dermatologic reactions including Stevens-Johnson syndrome (SJS) have been reported; monitor for signs and symptoms of skin reactions; discontinuation and conversion to alternate therapy may be required. Potentially significant drug-drug interactions may exist, requiring dose or frequency adjustment, additional monitoring, and/or selection of alternative therapy.

Antiepileptics are associated with an increased risk of suicidal behavior/thoughts with use (regardless of indication); patients should be monitored for signs/symptoms of depression, suicidal tendencies, and other unusual behavior changes during therapy and instructed to inform their healthcare provider immediately if symptoms occur. Use with caution in patients with mild-to-moderate hepatic impairment; use in not recommended in patients with severe hepatic impairment. Anticonvulsants should not be discontinued abruptly because of the possibility of increasing seizure frequency; therapy should be withdrawn gradually to minimize the potential of increased seizure frequency, unless safety concerns require a more rapid withdrawal. Reducing dose by ~25% every two days was effective in trials.

Adverse Reactions

Cardiovascular: QT shortening (dose related)

Central nervous system: Aggression, anxiety, ataxia, attention disturbance, dizziness, fatigue, headache, hyperactivity, seizure, somnolence, status epilepticus, vertigo

Dermatologic: Pruritus, rash

Gastrointestinal: Abdominal pain, appetite decreased/increased, constipation, dyspepsia, nausea, vomiting

Hematologic: Anemia. leukopenia

Neuromuscular & skeletal: Back pain, gait disturbance, tremor

Ocular: Blurred vision, diplopia, nystagmus

Otic: Otitis media

Renal: Pollakiuria

Respiratory: Bronchitis, nasopharyngitis, sinusitis

Miscellaneous: Influenza

Rare but important or life-threatening: Atrioventricular block (first degree), bundle branch block (right), dysuria, enuresis, hematuria; hypersensitivity (multiorgan; includes eosinophilia, facial edema, fever, hepatitis [severe], LFTs increased, rash, stupor, urticaria); incontinence, iron-deficiency anemia, lymphadenopathy, nephrolithiasis, neutropenia, nocturia, polyuria, thrombocytopenia, urinary incontinence

Drug Interactions

Metabolism/Transport Effects Inhibits CYP2E1 (weak); **Induces** CYP3A4 (weak)

Avoid Concomitant Use There are no known interactions where it is recommended to avoid concomitant use.

Increased Effect/Toxicity

Rufinamide may increase the levels/effects of: CNS Depressants; Fosphenytoin; PHENobarbital; Phenytoin

The levels/effects of Rufinamide may be increased by: Alcohol (Ethyl); Valproic Acid and Derivatives

Decreased Effect

Rufinamide may decrease the levels/effects of: ARIPiprazole; CarBAMazepine; Ethinyl Estradiol; Hydrocodone; Norethindrone; Saxagliptin

The levels/effects of Rufinamide may be decreased by: CarBAMazepine; Fosphenytoin; PHENobarbital; Phenytoin; Primidone

Food Interactions Food increases the absorption of rufinamide. Management: Take with food.

Storage/Stability Store at 25°C (77°F); excursions permitted to 15°C to 30°C (59°F to 86°F). Protect tablets from moisture. Discard oral suspension within 90 days after opening; cap of bottle fits over the adapter.

Mechanism of Action A triazole-derivative antiepileptic whose exact mechanism is unknown. *In vitro*, it prolongs the inactive state of the sodium channels, thereby limiting repetitive firing of sodium-dependent action potentials mediating anticonvulsant effects.

Pharmacodynamics/Kinetics

Absorption: Slow; extensive ≥85%; increased with food

Distribution: V_d: ~50 L

Protein binding: 34%, primarily to albumin (27%)

Metabolism: Extensively via carboxylesterase-mediated hydrolysis of the carboxylamide group to CGP 47292 (inactive metabolite); weak inhibitor of CYP2E1 and weak inducer of CYP3A4

Bioavailability: Extent decreased with increased dose; oral tablets and oral suspension are bioequivalent

Half-life elimination: ~6 to 10 hours

Time to peak, plasma: 4 to 6 hours

Excretion: Urine (85%, ~66% as CGP 47292, 2% as unchanged drug)

Dosage Lennox-Gastaut syndrome (adjunctive): Oral:

U.S. labeling:

Children ≥4 years: Initial: 10 mg/kg/day in 2 equally divided doses; increase dose by ~10 mg/kg every other day to a target dose of 45 mg/kg/day **or** 3200 mg/day (whichever is lower) in 2 equally divided doses

Adults: Initial: 400 to 800 mg/day in 2 equally divided doses; increase dose by 400 to 800 mg/day every other day to a maximum dose of 3200 mg/day in 2 equally divided doses

Canadian labeling: Children ≥4 years and Adults:

<30 kg: Initial: 200 mg/day in 2 equally divided doses; increase dose by 5 mg/kg/day every 2 weeks until satisfactory control (maximum dose: 1300 mg/day)

≥30 kg: Initial: 400 mg/day in 2 equally divided doses; increase dose by 5 mg/kg/day every 2 weeks until satisfactory control (maximum dose: 30 to 50 kg: 1800 mg/day; 50.1 to 70 kg: 2400 mg/day; ≥70.1 kg: 3200 mg/day). **Note:** Dose was increased as frequently as every other day in clinical trials.

Elderly: Refer to adult dosing. Initiate at the low end of the dosing range; use with caution.

Note: Discontinue therapy gradually to minimize the potential of increased seizure frequency, unless safety concerns require a more rapid withdrawal. Reducing dose by approximately 25% every 2 days was effective in trials.

Dosage adjustment for concomitant medications: Valproate:

U.S. labeling: Initial rufinamide dose should be <10 mg/kg/day (children) or <400 mg/day (adults)

Canadian labeling: Initial rufinamide dose should be less than the initial daily recommended dosage; however, a specific dosage recommendation is not included in the manufacturer's labeling.

Dosage adjustment in renal impairment:

CrCl <30 mL/minute: No dosage adjustment necessary.

Hemodialysis: There are no dosage adjustments provided in the manufacturer's labeling. However, consider dosage adjustment for loss of drug.

Dosage adjustment in hepatic impairment:

Mild to moderate impairment: Use with caution

Severe impairment: There are no dosage adjustments provided in the manufacturer's labeling (has not been studied); use is not recommended.

Dietary Considerations Take with food.

Administration Administer with food. Tablets may be swallowed whole, split in half, or crushed. Oral suspension should be administered using the provided adapter and calibrated oral syringe; shake well before each dose.

Monitoring Parameters Seizure (frequency and duration); serum levels of concurrent anticonvulsants; suicidality (eg, suicidal thoughts, depression, behavioral changes); rash (may indicate multi-organ hypersensitivity reactions)

Dosage Forms

Suspension, Oral:

Banzel: 40 mg/mL (460 mL)

Tablet, Oral:

Banzel: 200 mg, 400 mg

Dosage Forms: Canada

Tablet, oral:

Banzel: 100 mg

Extemporaneous Preparations A 40 mg/mL oral suspension may be made using tablets. Crush twelve 400 mg tablets (or twenty-four 200 mg tablets) and reduce to a fine powder. Add 60 mL of Ora-Plus® in incremental proportions until a smooth suspension is obtained; then mix well while adding 60 mL of Ora-Sweet® or Ora-Sweet® SF; transfer to a calibrated bottle. Label "shake well". Stable 90 days at room temperature.

Hutchinson DJ, Liou Y, Best R, et al, "Stability of Extemporaneously Prepared Rufinamide Oral Suspensions," *Ann Pharmacother*, 2010, 44(3):462-5.

Rufloxacin [INT] (rue FLOKS a sin)

International Brand Names Kang Zan (CN); Monos (IT); Qari (CN, IT, PK); Ruflam (CO); Tebraxin (IT); Uroclar (PH); Uroflox (MX, TH)

Index Terms Rufloxacin Hydrochloride

Pharmacologic Category Antibiotic, Quinolone

Reported Use Treatment of susceptible infections of the lower urinary tract (cystitis, pyelonephritis, and chronic prostatitis)

Dosage Range Adults: Oral: Usual dose: 400 mg, followed by 200 mg/day; 400 mg/day should be reserved for more severe infections (chronic pyelonephritis); duration: 5-10 days for acute infections, longer for more serious infections (up to 4 weeks for bacterial prostatitis)

Product Availability Product available in various countries; not currently available in the U.S.

Dosage Forms

Tablet: 200 mg

◆ **Rufloxacin Hydrochloride** *see* Rufloxacin [INT] *on page 1855*

◆ **Rulox [OTC]** *see* Aluminum Hydroxide, Magnesium Hydroxide, and Simethicone *on page 104*

Rupatadine [INT] (rue PA ta deen)

International Brand Names Alergoliber (ES); Levostar-R (IN); Ralzal (IN); Repafet (MX); Rinepan (PE); Rinialer (ES, PT); Rupafin (AR, BR, CY, DE, EE, ES, GB, GR, HR, IT, LT, NL, SG, SI, SK, TH, TR); Rupahjist (IN); Rupastar (IN); Rupatal (NZ); Rupatall (BE, SE); Rupax (CR, DO, GT, HN, NI, PA, SV); Rupiz (IN); Tamalis (CZ); Wystamm (FR)

Index Terms Rupatadine Fumarate
Pharmacologic Category Antihistamine
Reported Use Treatment of allergic rhinitis
Dosage Range Children >12 years and Adults: Oral: 10 mg/day
Product Availability Product available in various countries; not currently available in the U.S.
Dosage Forms
Tablet: 10 mg

◆ **Rupatadine Fumarate** *see* Rupatadine [INT] *on page 1855*

Ruxolitinib (rux oh LI ti nib)

Brand Names: U.S. Jakafi
Brand Names: Canada Jakavi
Index Terms INCB 18424; INCB018424; INCB424; Ruxolitinib Phosphate
Pharmacologic Category Antineoplastic Agent, Janus Associated Kinase Inhibitor; Antineoplastic Agent, Tyrosine Kinase Inhibitor; Janus Associated Kinase Inhibitor
Use
Myelofibrosis: Treatment of intermediate or high-risk myelofibrosis, including primary myelofibrosis, post-polycythemia vera (post-PV) myelofibrosis and post-essential thrombocythemia (post-ET) myelofibrosis
Polycythemia vera: Treatment of polycythemia vera with an inadequate response to or intolerance to hydroxyurea
Pregnancy Risk Factor C
Pregnancy Considerations Increased resorptions (late) and reduced fetal weights were observed in animal reproduction studies. Use during human pregnancy only if the potential treatment benefits outweigh risks.
Breast-Feeding Considerations It is not known if ruxolitinib is excreted in breast milk. According to the manufacturer, due to the potential for serious adverse reactions in the nursing infant, a decision should be made to discontinue ruxolitinib or to discontinue breast-feeding during therapy, taking into account the benefits of treatment to the mother.
Contraindications
There are no contraindications listed in the manufacturer's U.S. labeling.
Canadian labeling: Hypersensitivity to ruxolitinib or any component of the formulation or container; history of or current progressive multifocal leukoencephalopathy
Warnings/Precautions Hazardous agent - use appropriate precautions for handling and disposal (meets NIOSH 2014 criteria). Hematologic toxicity, including thrombocytopenia, anemia and neutropenia may occur; may require dosage modification; monitor complete blood counts at baseline, every 2 to 4 weeks during dose stabilization, and then as clinically necessary. Thrombocytopenia is generally reversible with treatment interruption or dose reduction; platelet transfusions may be administered during treatment if clinically indicated. Anemia may require blood transfusion; may consider dose modification. Neutropenia (ANC <500/mm^3) is generally reversible and managed by treatment interruption.

Serious bacterial, mycobacterial (including tuberculosis), fungal, or viral infections have occurred. Active serious infections should be resolved prior to treatment initiation. Monitor for infections (including signs/symptoms of active tuberculosis and herpes zoster) during treatment. Prompt treatment is recommended if symptoms of active tuberculosis and/or herpes zoster infection develop. Evaluate for tuberculosis risk factors prior to treatment initiation; patients at higher risk for tuberculosis (prior residence/travel to countries with a high tuberculosis prevalence, close contacts with active tuberculosis, or history of latent or active tuberculosis where adequate treatment course cannot be confirmed) should be tested for latent infection. For patients with evidence of tuberculosis (active or latent), decide risk-benefit of continuing treatment. Progressive multifocal leukoencephalopathy (PML) has been reported; discontinue and evaluate if suspected. May require initial dosage reduction for hepatic impairment; in patients with myelofibrosis, avoid use if platelets <50,000/mm^3 and with hepatic impairment (any degree). May require initial dosage reduction for renal impairment. Avoid use in patients with ESRD not requiring dialysis; in patients with myelofibrosis, avoid use if platelets <50,000/mm^3 and with moderate-to-severe renal impairment. Ruxolitinib is not removed by dialysis, however, some active metabolites may be removed. On dialysis days, patients are advised to take their dose following dialysis sessions. Potentially significant drug-drug interactions may exist, requiring dose or frequency adjustment, additional monitoring, and/or selection of alternative therapy. Discontinue treatment in myelofibrosis patients after 6 months if no reduction in spleen size or no improvement in symptoms. Consider gradually tapering off if discontinuing for reasons other than thrombocytopenia. Within ~1 week after discontinuation, symptoms of myelofibrosis generally return to pretreatment levels. Acute relapse of myelofibrosis symptoms (eg, fever, respiratory distress, hypotension, DIC, multiorgan failure), splenomegaly, worsening cytopenias, hemodynamic compensation, and septic shock-like syndrome have been reported with treatment tapering or discontinuation (Tefferi, 2011). Symptoms generally return over approximately 1 week. Evaluate and treat any intercurrent illness and consider restarting or increasing dose. Consider gradually tapering off if discontinuing for reasons other than thrombocytopenia or neutropenia. Patients should not interrupt/discontinue treatment without consulting healthcare provider.

Non-melanoma skin cancers (basal cell, squamous cell, and Merkel cell carcinoma) have been reported in patients who have received ruxolitinib; periodic skin examinations should be performed. Use with caution in patients with a history of bradycardia, conduction disturbances, ischemic heart disease, heart failure and/or receiving other drugs that also affect heart rate/conduction; decreased heart rate (mean change 6 to 8 bpm) and prolongation of the PR interval (mean change 6 to 9 msec) and of the QT interval (mean 4 to 5 msec) were observed during some clinical trials. Canadian labeling recommends obtaining an ECG at baseline and periodically; monitor heart rate and blood pressure during treatment.
Adverse Reactions
Cardiovascular: Peripheral edema
Central nervous system: Dizziness, headache, insomnia
Dermatologic: Bruise
Endocrine & metabolic: Increased serum cholesterol, weight gain
Gastrointestinal: Constipation, diarrhea, flatulence, nausea, vomiting
Genitourinary: Urinary tract infection
Hematologic & oncologic: Anemia, neutropenia, thrombocytopenia
Hepatic: Increased serum ALT, increased serum AST
Neuromuscular & skeletal: Limb pain
Respiratory: Dyspnea, nasopharyngitis
Infection: Herpes zoster
Rare but important or life-threatening: Bradycardia, fever, hemorrhagic diathesis, increased systolic blood pressure, progressive multifocal leukoencephalopathy, prolonged Q-T interval on ECG, tuberculosis, withdrawal syndrome (myelofibrosis symptom exacerbation, including fever, respiratory distress, hypotension, disseminated intravascular coagulation, multi-organ failure; upon abrupt discontinuation, dose tapering recommended)

Drug Interactions

Metabolism/Transport Effects Substrate of CYP3A4 (major); **Note:** Assignment of Major/Minor substrate status based on clinically relevant drug interaction potential

Avoid Concomitant Use

Avoid concomitant use of Ruxolitinib with any of the following: BCG; CloZAPine; Conivaptan; Dipyrone; Fusidic Acid (Systemic); Idelalisib; Natalizumab; Pimecrolimus; Tacrolimus (Topical); Tofacitinib; Vaccines (Live)

Increased Effect/Toxicity

Ruxolitinib may increase the levels/effects of: CloZAPine; Leflunomide; Natalizumab; Tofacitinib; Vaccines (Live)

The levels/effects of Ruxolitinib may be increased by: Aprepitant; Ceritinib; Conivaptan; CYP3A4 Inhibitors (Moderate); CYP3A4 Inhibitors (Strong); Dasatinib; Denosumab; Dipyrone; Fluconazole; Fosaprepitant; Fusidic Acid (Systemic); Grapefruit Juice; Idelalisib; Ivacaftor; Luliconazole; Mifepristone; Netupitant; Pimecrolimus; Roflumilast; Simeprevir; Stiripentol; Tacrolimus (Topical); Trastuzumab

Decreased Effect

Ruxolitinib may decrease the levels/effects of: BCG; Coccidioides immitis Skin Test; Sipuleucel-T; Vaccines (Inactivated); Vaccines (Live)

The levels/effects of Ruxolitinib may be decreased by: Bosentan; CYP3A4 Inducers (Moderate); CYP3A4 Inducers (Strong); Dabrafenib; Deferasirox; Echinacea; Mitotane; Siltuximab; St Johns Wort; Tocilizumab

Food Interactions Grapefruit juice may increase the effects of ruxolitinib. Management: Avoid grapefruit juice.

Storage/Stability Store at 20°C to 25°C (68°F to 77°F); excursions are permitted between 15°C and 30°C (59°F and 86°F).

Mechanism of Action Kinase inhibitor which selectively inhibits Janus Associated Kinases (JAKs), JAK1 and JAK2. JAK1 and JAK2 mediate signaling of cytokine and growth factors responsible for hematopoiesis and immune function; JAK mediated signaling involves recruitment of STATs (signal transducers and activators of transcription) to cytokine receptors which leads to modulation of gene expression. In myelofibrosis and polycythemia vera, JAK1/2 activity is dysregulated; ruxolitinib modulates the affected JAK1/2 activity.

Pharmacodynamics/Kinetics

Absorption: Rapid

Distribution: V_d: Myelofibrosis: 72 L; Polycythemia vera: 75 L

Protein binding: ~97%; primarily to albumin

Metabolism: Hepatic, primarily via CYP3A4 (and minimally CYP2C9); forms active metabolites responsible for 20% to 50% of activity

Half-life elimination: Ruxolitinib: 2.8 to 3 hours (hepatic impairment: 4 to 5 hours); Ruxolitinib + metabolites: ~6 hours

Time to peak: Within 1 to 2 hours

Excretion: Urine (74%, <1% as unchanged drug); feces (22%, <1% as unchanged drug)

Dosage Note: Consider gradually tapering off (by 5 mg twice daily each week) if discontinuing for reasons other than thrombocytopenia.

Myelofibrosis: Adults: Oral: Initial dose (based on platelet count, titrate dose thereafter based on efficacy and safety):

U.S. labeling:

Platelets >200,000/mm^3: 20 mg twice daily

Platelets 100,000 to 200,000/mm^3: 15 mg twice daily

Platelets 50,000 to <100,000/mm^3: 5 mg twice daily

Canadian labeling:

Platelets >200,000/mm^3: 20 mg twice daily

Platelets 100,000 to 200,000/mm^3: 15 mg twice daily

Platelets 50,000 to 100,000/ mm^3: Initial dose should not exceed 5 mg twice daily; titrate dose cautiously

Polycythemia vera: Adults: Oral: Initial dose: 10 mg twice daily (titrate dose based on efficacy and safety)

Dose modifications for myelofibrosis:

Dosage modification based on response in patients with baseline platelet count ≥100,000/mm^3 prior to initial treatment with ruxolitinib: For insufficient response (with adequate platelet and neutrophil counts), may increase the dose in 5 mg twice daily increments to a maximum dose of 25 mg twice daily. Do not increase during initial 4 weeks and no more frequently than every 2 weeks. Discontinue treatment after 6 months if no reduction in spleen size or no improvement in symptoms. When discontinuing for reasons other than thrombocytopenia, consider gradually tapering by ~5 mg twice daily per week.

Dose increases may be considered if meet all of the following situations:

- Failure to achieve either a 50% reduction (from baseline) in palpable spleen length or a 35% reduction (from baseline) in spleen volume (measured by CT or MRI)
- Platelet count >125,000/mm^3 at 4 weeks (and never <100,000/mm^3)
- Absolute neutrophil count (ANC) >750/mm^3

Dosage modification based on response in patients with baseline platelet 50,000 to <100,000/mm^3 prior to initial treatment with ruxolitinib: For insufficient response (with adequate platelet and neutrophil counts), may increase the dose in 5 mg daily increments to a maximum dose of 10 mg twice daily. Do not increase during initial 4 weeks and no more frequently than every 2 weeks. Discontinue treatment after 6 months if no reduction in spleen size or no improvement in symptoms.

Dose increases may be considered if meet all of the following situations:

- Platelet count remains ≥40,000/mm^3 and did not decrease more than 20% in prior 4 weeks
- Absolute neutrophil count (ANC) >1,000/mm^3
- No adverse event or hematological toxicity resulting in dose reduction or interruption occurred in prior 4 weeks

Dosage modification for bleeding requiring intervention (regardless of platelet count): Interrupt treatment until bleeding resolved; may consider resuming at the prior dose if the underlying cause of bleeding has resolved or at a reduced dose if the underlying cause of bleeding persists.

Dosage modification for treatment interruption:

U.S. labeling:

If baseline platelet count ≥100,000/mm^3 prior to initial treatment with ruxolitinib and:

Platelets <50,000/mm^3 and ANC <500/mm^3: Interrupt treatment; upon platelet recovery (to ≥50,000/mm^3) or ANC recovery (to ≥750/mm^3), dosing may be restarted or increased based on the following platelet or ANC levels:

Platelets ≥125,000/mm^3: Dose should be at least 5 mg twice daily below the dose at treatment interruption, up to a maximum of 20 mg twice daily

Platelets 100,000 to <125,000/mm^3: Dose should be at least 5 mg twice daily below the dose at treatment interruption, up to a maximum of 15 mg twice daily

Platelets 75,000 to <100,000/mm^3: Dose should be at least 5 mg twice daily below the dose at treatment interruption, up to a maximum of 10 mg twice daily for at least 2 weeks; may increase to 15 mg twice daily if stable

Platelets 50,000 to <75,000/mm^3: 5 mg twice daily for at least 2 weeks; may increase to 10 mg twice daily if stable

Platelets <50,000/mm^3: Continue to withhold treatment

ANC ≥750/mm^3: Resume at 5 mg once daily or 5 mg twice daily below the largest dose in the week prior to treatment interruption, whichever is greater

Note: Long-term maintenance at 5 mg twice daily has not demonstrated responses; limit use of the dose level to patients where the benefits outweigh risks

If baseline platelet count 50,000 to <100,000/mm^3 prior to initial treatment with ruxolitinib and:

Platelets <25,000/mm^3 and ANC <500/mm^3: Interrupt treatment; upon platelet recovery (to ≥35,000/mm^3) or ANC recovery (to ≥750/mm^3), resume at 5 mg once daily or 5 mg twice daily below the largest dose in the week prior to treatment interruption, whichever is greater

Note: Long-term maintenance at 5 mg twice daily has not demonstrated responses; limit use of the dose level to patients where the benefits outweigh risks

Canadian labeling: Platelets <50,000/mm^3 or ANC <500 mm^3: Interrupt treatment; upon recovery of platelets to ≥50,000/mm^3 or ANC to ≥500/mm^3, dosing may be restarted at 5 mg twice daily and then gradually titrated based on blood cell counts.

Dosage reduction for thrombocytopenia in patients with baseline platelet count ≥100,000/mm^3 prior to initial treatment with ruxolitinib:

Platelet Count	Dose at Time of Thrombocytopenia				
	25 mg twice/day	20 mg twice/day	15 mg twice/day	10 mg twice/day	5 mg twice/day
	New Dose	New Dose	New Dose	New Dose	New Dose
100,000 to <125,000/mm^3	20 mg twice/day	15 mg twice/day	No change	No change	No change
75,000 to <100,000/mm^3	10 mg twice/day	10 mg twice/day	10 mg twice/day	No change	No change
50,000 to <75,000/mm^3	5 mg twice/day	5 mg twice/day	5 mg twice/day	5 mg twice/day	No change
<50,000/mm^3	Hold dose	Hold dose	Hold dose	Hold dose	Hold dose

Note: Long-term maintenance at 5 mg twice daily has not demonstrated responses; limit use of the dose level to patients where the benefits outweigh risks

Dosage reduction for thrombocytopenia in patients with baseline platelet 50,000 to <100,000/mm^3 prior to initial treatment with ruxolitinib:

Platelets 25,000 to <35,000/mm^3 **and** platelet count decreased <20% during prior 4 weeks:

If current daily dose >5 mg: Reduce dose by 5 mg once daily

If current dose 5 mg once daily: Continue 5 mg once daily

Platelets 25,000 to <35,000/mm^3 **and** platelet count decreased ≥20% during prior four weeks:

If current daily dose >10 mg: Reduce dose by 5 mg twice daily

If current dose 5 mg twice daily: Reduce dose to 5 mg once daily

If current dose 5 mg once daily: Continue 5 mg once daily

Platelets <25,000 mm^3: Continue to withhold treatment

Note: Long-term maintenance at 5 mg twice daily has not demonstrated responses; limit use of the dose level to patients where the benefits outweigh risks

Dose modifications for polycythemia vera:

Hematologic toxicity:

Hemoglobin ≥12 g/dL AND platelets ≥100,000/mm^3: No dosage adjustment necessary.

Hemoglobin 10 to <12 g/dL AND platelets 75,000 to <100,000/mm^3: Consider dosage adjustment to avoid dose interruptions due to anemia and thrombocytopenia.

Hemoglobin 8 to <10 g/dL OR platelets 50,000 to <75,000/mm^3: Reduce dose by 5 mg twice daily; for patients currently receiving 5 mg twice daily, reduce dose to 5 mg once daily.

Hemoglobin <8 g/dL OR platelets <50,000/mm^3 OR ANC <1,000/mm^3: Interrupt dosing.

Dosage reduction following treatment interruption (use the most severe category of hemoglobin, platelets, or ANC to determine reinitiation dose):

Hemoglobin <8 g/dL OR platelets <50,000/mm^3 OR ANC <1,000/mm^3: Continue to hold.

Hemoglobin 8 to <10 g/dL OR platelets 50,000 to <75,000/mm^3 OR ANC 1,000 to <1500/mm^3: Restart at a maximum of 5 mg twice daily (continue treatment for at least 2 weeks, if stable, then may increase dose by 5 mg twice daily) or no more than 5 mg twice daily less than the dose that resulted in dose interruption

Hemoglobin 10 to <12 g/dL OR platelets 75,000 to <100,000/mm^3 OR ANC 1,500 to <2,000/mm^3: Restart at a maximum of 10 mg twice daily (continue treatment for at least 2 weeks, if stable, then may increase dose by 5 mg twice daily) or no more than 5 mg twice daily less than the dose that resulted in dose interruption

Hemoglobin ≥12 g/dL OR platelets ≥100,000/mm^3 OR ANC ≥2,000/mm^3: Restart at a maximum of 15 mg twice daily (continue treatment for at least 2 weeks, if stable, then may increase dose by 5 mg twice daily) or no more than 5 mg twice daily less than the dose that resulted in dose interruption

Note: If dose interruption was required while receiving 5 mg twice daily, may restart at 5 mg twice daily or 5 mg once daily (but not higher) once hemoglobin is ≥10 g/dL, platelets are ≥75,000/mm^3, and ANC is ≥1,500/mm^3.

Dose management after restarting treatment: After restarting following a dose interruption, the dose may be titrated, although the maximum total daily dose should not exceed 5 mg less than the dose resulting in the interruption (unless dose interruption following phlebotomy-associated anemia, in which case the maximum total daily dose is not limited).

Dose modification due to insufficient response: If response is insufficient and platelet, hemoglobin, and neutrophil counts are adequate, the dose may be increased in 5 mg twice daily increments to a maximum of 25 mg twice daily, Do not increase dose in the first 4 weeks of treatment and not more frequently than every 2 weeks. Consider dose increases in patients who meet all of the following conditions:

- Inadequate efficacy demonstrated by one or more of the following: Continued need for phlebotomy, WBC >ULN of normal range, platelet count >ULN of normal range, or palpable spleen that is reduced by <25% from baseline.
- Platelet count ≥140,000/mm^3
- Hemoglobin ≥12 g/dL
- ANC ≥1,500/mm^3

Dosage adjustment with concomitant strong CYP3A4 inhibitors (eg, azole antifungals, clarithromycin, conivaptin, grapefruit juice, mibefradil, nefazodone, protease inhibitors, telithromycin) and fluconazole (≤200 mg):

U.S. labeling: **Note:** Avoid concomitant use with fluconazole doses >200 mg daily.

Myelofibrosis: Initial dose:

Platelets ≥100,000/mm^3: 10 mg twice daily.

Platelets 50,000/mm^3 to <100,000/mm^3: 5 mg once daily.

Polycythemia vera: Initial dose: 5 mg twice daily

Patients stabilized on ruxolitinib ≥10 mg twice daily: Reduce dose by 50% (rounded up to the closest available tablet strength).

Patients stabilized on ruxolitinib 5 mg twice daily: Reduce dose to 5 mg once daily.

Patients stabilized on ruxolitinib 5 mg once daily: Avoid strong CYP3A4 inhibitors or fluconazole or interrupt treatment for the duration of strong CYP3A4 inhibitor or fluconazole use.

Monitor closely and further adjust dose based on safety and efficacy.

Canadian labeling: Initial dose: 10 mg twice daily (~50% of the dose, rounded to the closest available strength); monitor hematologic parameters more frequently and titrate dose based on safety and efficacy. Avoid concomitant strong CYP3A4 use if platelets <100,000/mm^3.

Dosage adjustment in renal impairment:

U.S. labeling:

Myelofibrosis:

CrCl 15 to 59 mL/minute and platelets >150,000/mm^3: No dosage adjustment is necessary.

CrCl 15 to 59 mL/minute and platelets 100,000 to 150,000/mm^3: Initial dose: 10 mg twice daily; additional dose adjustments should be made with careful monitoring.

CrCl 15 to 59 mL/minute and platelets 50,000 to <100,000/mm^3: Initial dose: 5 mg once daily; additional dose adjustments should be made with careful monitoring.

CrCl 15 to 59 mL/minute and platelets <50,000/mm^3: Avoid use.

End-stage renal disease (ESRD) on dialysis and platelets 100,000 to 200,000/mm^3: Initial dose: 15 mg once after dialysis; administer subsequent doses after dialysis on dialysis days. Additional dose adjustments should be made with frequent monitoring.

ESRD on dialysis and platelets >200,000/mm^3: Initial dose: 20 mg once after dialysis; administer subsequent doses after dialysis on dialysis days. Additional dose adjustments should be made with frequent monitoring.

ESRD not requiring dialysis: Avoid use.

Polycythemia vera:

CrCl 15 to 59 mL/minute and any platelet count: Initial: 5 mg twice daily. Additional dose adjustments should be made with frequent monitoring.

End-stage renal disease (ESRD) on dialysis: Initial dose: 10 mg once after dialysis; additional dose adjustments should be made with careful monitoring

ESRD not requiring dialysis: Avoid use.

Canadian labeling:

CrCl <50 mL/minute and platelets ≥100,000/mm^3: Initial dose: 10 mg twice daily; additional dose adjustments should be made with careful monitoring

CrCl <50 mL/minute and platelets <100,000/mm^3: Avoid use

ESRD on dialysis and platelets 100,000 to 200,000/mm^3: Initial dose: 15 mg; administer subsequent doses after dialysis on dialysis days. Additional dose adjustments should be made with careful monitoring.

ESRD on dialysis and platelets >200,000/mm^3: Initial dose: 20 mg; administer subsequent doses after dialysis on dialysis days. Additional dose adjustments should be made with careful monitoring.

Dosage adjustment in hepatic impairment:

U.S. labeling:

Myelofibrosis:

Mild-to-severe impairment (Child-Pugh class A, B, or C) and platelets >150,000/mm^3: No dosage adjustment is necessary.

Mild-to-severe impairment (Child-Pugh class A, B, or C) and platelets 100,000 to 150,000/mm^3: Initial dose: 10 mg twice daily; additional dose adjustments should be made with careful monitoring.

Mild-to-severe impairment (Child-Pugh class A, B, or C) and platelets 50,000 to <100,000/mm^3: Initial dose: 5 mg once daily; additional dose adjustments should be made with careful monitoring.

Mild-to-severe impairment (Child-Pugh class A, B, or C) and platelets <50,000/mm^3: Avoid use.

Polycythemia vera: Mild-to-severe impairment (Child-Pugh class A, B, or C) and any platelet count: Initial dose: 5 mg twice daily; additional dose adjustments should be made with careful monitoring.

Canadian labeling:

Hepatic impairment and platelets ≥100,000/mm^3: Initial dose: 10 mg twice daily; additional dose adjustments should be made with careful monitoring.

Hepatic impairment and platelets <100,000/mm^3: Avoid use.

Dietary Considerations Avoid grapefruit juice (may increase the effects of ruxolitinib).

Administration May be administered orally with or without food. If a dose is missed, return to the usual dosing schedule and do **not** administer an additional dose.

If unable to ingest tablets, may administer through a nasogastric (NG) tube (≥8 Fr): Suspend 1 tablet in ~40 mL water and stir for ~10 minutes and administer (within 6 hours after dispersion) with appropriate syringe; rinse NG tube with ~75 mL water (effect of enteral tube feeding on ruxolitinib exposure has not been evaluated)

Hazardous agent; use appropriate precautions for handling and disposal (meets NIOSH 2014 criteria).

Monitoring Parameters CBC (baseline, every 2 to 4 weeks until dose stabilized, then as clinically indicated), renal function, hepatic function. Perform periodic skin examinations monitor for signs/symptoms of infection. Canadian labeling recommends obtaining an ECG at baseline and then periodically during therapy; monitor heart rate and blood pressure during therapy

Dosage Forms

Tablet, Oral:

Jakafi: 5 mg, 10 mg, 15 mg, 20 mg, 25 mg

Extemporaneous Preparations Hazardous agent; use appropriate precautions for handling and disposal (meets NIOSH 2014 criteria).

A suspension for nasogastric administration may be prepared with tablets. Place one tablet into ~40 mL water; stir for approximately 10 minutes. Administer within 6 hour after preparation.

Jakafi (ruxolitinib) [prescribing information]. Wilmington, DE: Incyte Corporation; December 2014.

◆ **Ruxolitinib Phosphate** *see* Ruxolitinib *on page 1856*

◆ **RV1 (Rotarix)** *see* Rotavirus Vaccine *on page 1851*

◆ **RV5 (RotaTeq)** *see* Rotavirus Vaccine *on page 1851*

◆ **RWJ-270201** *see* Peramivir *on page 1619*

◆ **Ryanodex** *see* Dantrolene *on page 559*

◆ **Rylosol (Can)** *see* Sotalol *on page 1927*

◆ **Rytary** *see* Carbidopa and Levodopa *on page 351*

◆ **Rytary** *see* Carbidopa and Levodopa *on page 351*

◆ **Rythmodan (Can)** *see* Disopyramide *on page 653*

◆ **Rythmodan-LA (Can)** *see* Disopyramide *on page 653*

◆ **Rythmol** *see* Propafenone *on page 1725*

◆ **Rythmol Gen-Propafenone (Can)** *see* Propafenone *on page 1725*

◆ **Rythmol SR** *see* Propafenone *on page 1725*

◆ **S2 [OTC]** *see* EPINEPHrine (Systemic, Oral Inhalation) *on page 735*

◆ **S2 (Can)** *see* EPINEPHrine (Systemic, Oral Inhalation) *on page 735*

◆ **S-(+)-3-isobutylgaba** *see* Pregabalin *on page 1710*

◆ **S-4661** *see* Doripenem *on page 671*

◆ **Sabril** *see* Vigabatrin *on page 2158*

Sacrosidase (sak ROE si dase)

Brand Names: U.S. Sucraid

Brand Names: Canada Sucraid®

Pharmacologic Category Enzyme, Gastrointestinal

Use Oral replacement therapy in sucrase deficiency, as seen in congenital sucrase-isomaltase deficiency (CSID)

Pregnancy Risk Factor C

Dosage Oral:

Infants ≥5 months and Children ≤15 kg: 8500 units (1 mL) per meal or snack

Children >15 kg, Adolescents, and Adults: 17,000 units (2 mL) per meal or snack

Doses should be diluted with 2-4 oz of cold or room temperature water, milk, or formula. Approximately one-half of the dose should be taken before and the remainder of a dose taken during each meal or snack.

Dosage adjustment in renal impairment: No dosage adjustment provided in manufacturer's labeling.

Dosage adjustment in hepatic impairment: No dosage adjustment provided in manufacturer's labeling.

Additional Information Complete prescribing information should be consulted for additional detail.

Dosage Forms

Solution, Oral:

Sucraid: 8500 units/mL (118 mL)

◆ **Safetussin® CD [OTC]** *see* Dextromethorphan and Phenylephrine *on page 611*

◆ **Safe Tussin DM [OTC]** *see* Guaifenesin and Dextromethorphan *on page 987*

◆ **Safe Wash [OTC]** *see* Sodium Chloride *on page 1902*

◆ **Safyral** *see* Ethinyl Estradiol, Drospirenone, and Levomefolate *on page 812*

◆ **SAHA** *see* Vorinostat *on page 2182*

◆ **Saizen** *see* Somatropin *on page 1918*

◆ **Saizen Click.Easy** *see* Somatropin *on page 1918*

◆ **Salagen** *see* Pilocarpine (Systemic) *on page 1649*

◆ **Salagen® (Can)** *see* Pilocarpine (Systemic) *on page 1649*

◆ **Salazopyrin (Can)** *see* SulfaSALAzine *on page 1950*

◆ **Salazopyrin En-Tabs (Can)** *see* SulfaSALAzine *on page 1950*

◆ **Salbutamol** *see* Albuterol *on page 69*

◆ **Salbutamol and Ipratropium** *see* Ipratropium and Albuterol *on page 1109*

◆ **Salbutamol HFA (Can)** *see* Albuterol *on page 69*

◆ **Salbutamol Sulphate** *see* Albuterol *on page 69*

◆ **Salcatonin** *see* Calcitonin *on page 322*

◆ **Salicylazosulfapyridine** *see* SulfaSALAzine *on page 1950*

◆ **Salicylsalicylic Acid** *see* Salsalate *on page 1862*

◆ **Saline** *see* Sodium Chloride *on page 1902*

◆ **Saline Flush ZR** *see* Sodium Chloride *on page 1902*

◆ **Saline Mist Spray [OTC]** *see* Sodium Chloride *on page 1902*

◆ **Saljet [OTC]** *see* Sodium Chloride *on page 1902*

◆ **Saljet Rinse [OTC]** *see* Sodium Chloride *on page 1902*

◆ **Salk Vaccine** *see* Poliovirus Vaccine (Inactivated) *on page 1673*

Salmeterol (sal ME te role)

Brand Names: U.S. Serevent Diskus

Brand Names: Canada Serevent Diskhaler Disk; Serevent Diskus

Index Terms Salmeterol Xinafoate

Pharmacologic Category $Beta_2$ Agonist; $Beta_2$-Adrenergic Agonist, Long-Acting

Use

Asthma/Bronchospasm: Treatment of asthma and the prevention of bronchospasm (only as concomitant therapy with a long-term asthma control medication, such as an inhaled corticosteroid), in patients 4 years and older with reversible obstructive airway disease, including patients with symptoms of nocturnal asthma.

Chronic obstructive pulmonary disease: Maintenance treatment of bronchospasm associated with chronic obstructive pulmonary disease (COPD) (including emphysema and chronic bronchitis).

Exercise-induced bronchospasm: Prevention of exercise-induced bronchospasm (EIB) in patients 4 years and older (monotherapy may be indicated in patients without persistent asthma).

Limitations of use: Salmeterol is not indicated for the relief of acute bronchospasm.

Pregnancy Risk Factor C

Pregnancy Considerations Adverse events were observed in some animal reproduction studies. Beta-agonists have the potential to affect uterine contractility if administered during labor.

Uncontrolled asthma is associated with adverse events on pregnancy (increased risk of perinatal mortality, pre-eclampsia, preterm birth, low birth weight infants). Although data related to its use in pregnancy is limited, salmeterol may be used when a long-acting beta agonist is needed to treat moderate persistent or severe persistent asthma in pregnant women (NAEPP, 2005).

Breast-Feeding Considerations It is not known if salmeterol is excreted into breast milk. The manufacturer recommends that caution be exercised when administering salmeterol to nursing women. The use of $beta_2$-receptor agonists are not considered a contraindication to breast-feeding (NAEPP, 2005).

Contraindications

Hypersensitivity to salmeterol or any component of the formulation (milk proteins); monotherapy in the treatment of asthma (ie, use without a concomitant long-term asthma control medication, such as an inhaled corticosteroid); treatment of status asthmaticus or other acute episodes of asthma or COPD

Canadian labeling: Additional contraindications (not in U.S. labeling): Presence of tachyarrhythmias

Documentation of allergenic cross-reactivity for sympathomimetics is limited. However, because of similarities in chemical structure and/or pharmacologic actions, the possibility of cross-sensitivity cannot be ruled out with certainty.

Warnings/Precautions Asthma treatment: **[U.S. Boxed Warning]: Long-acting beta$_2$-agonists (LABAs) increase the risk of asthma-related deaths. Salmeterol should only be used in asthma patients as adjuvant therapy in patients who are currently receiving but are not adequately controlled on a long-term asthma control medication (ie, an inhaled corticosteroid).** Monotherapy with an LABA is contraindicated in the treatment of asthma. In a large, randomized, placebo-controlled U.S. clinical trial (SMART, 2006), salmeterol was associated with an increase in asthma-related deaths (when added to usual asthma therapy); risk is considered a class effect among all LABAs. Data are not available to determine if the addition of an inhaled corticosteroid lessens this increased risk of death associated with LABA use. Assess patients at regular intervals once asthma control is maintained on combination therapy to determine if step-down therapy is appropriate and the LABA can be discontinued (without loss of asthma control), and the patient can be maintained on an inhaled corticosteroid. LABAs are not appropriate in patients whose asthma is adequately controlled on low- or medium-dose inhaled corticosteroids. Do **not** use for acute bronchospasm. Short-acting beta$_2$-agonist (eg, albuterol) should be used for acute symptoms and symptoms occurring between treatments. Do **not** initiate in patients with significantly worsening or acutely deteriorating asthma; reports of severe (sometimes fatal) respiratory events have been reported when salmeterol has been initiated in this situation. Corticosteroids should not be stopped or reduced when salmeterol is initiated. During initiation, watch for signs of worsening asthma. Patients must be instructed to use short-acting beta$_2$-agonists (eg, albuterol) for acute asthmatic or COPD symptoms and to seek medical attention in cases where acute symptoms are not relieved or a previous level of response is diminished. The need to increase frequency of use of short-acting beta$_2$-agonist may indicate deterioration of asthma, and treatment must not be delayed. Because LABAs may disguise poorly controlled persistent asthma, frequent or chronic use of LABAs for exercise-induced bronchospasm is discouraged by the NIH Asthma Guidelines (NIH, 2007). Salmeterol should not be used more than twice daily; do not use with other long-acting beta$_2$-agonists. **[U.S. Boxed Warning]: LABAs may increase the risk of asthma-related hospitalization in pediatric and adolescent patients.** In general, a combination product containing a LABA and an inhaled corticosteroid is preferred in patients <18 years of age to ensure compliance.

COPD treatment: Appropriate use: Do **not** use for acute episodes of COPD. Do **not** initiate in patients with significantly worsening or acutely deteriorating COPD. Data are not available to determine if LABA use increases the risk of death in patients with COPD. Canadian labeling suggest concurrent use of oral or inhaled corticosteroids may not be necessary in COPD because the role of inhaled corticosteroids is less well established; concurrent use should be determined by the treating physician.

Use caution in patients with cardiovascular disease (eg, arrhythmia, coronary insufficiency, or hypertension), seizure disorders, diabetes, hyperthyroidism, hepatic impairment, or hypokalemia. Beta-agonists may cause elevation in blood pressure, heart rate, CNS stimulation/excitation, increase serum glucose, decrease serum potassium, increase risk of arrhythmia, and electrocardiogram (ECG) changes, such as flattening of the T wave, prolongation of the QTc interval, and ST segment depression.

Immediate hypersensitivity reactions (urticaria, angioedema, rash, bronchospasm) bronchospasm, hypotension) including anaphylaxis have been reported. There have been reports of laryngeal spasm, irritation, swelling (stridor, choking) with use. Salmeterol should not be used more than twice daily; do not exceed recommended dose; do not use with other long-acting beta$_2$-agonists; serious adverse events have been associated with excessive use of inhaled sympathomimetics. Rarely, paradoxical bronchospasm, which may be life threatening, may occur with use of inhaled bronchodilating agents; this should be distinguished from inadequate response. Potentially significant drug-drug interactions may exist, requiring dose or frequency adjustment, additional monitoring, and/or selection of alternative therapy (consult drug interactions database for more detailed information). Powder for oral inhalation contains lactose; very rare anaphylactic reactions have been reported in patients with severe milk protein allergy.

Adverse Reactions

Cardiovascular: Edema, hypertension, pallor

Central nervous system: Anxiety, dizziness, fever, headache, migraine, sleep disturbance

Dermatologic: Contact dermatitis, eczema, photodermatitis, rash, urticaria

Endocrine & metabolic: Hyperglycemia

Gastrointestinal: Dental pain, dyspepsia, gastrointestinal infection, nausea, oropharyngeal candidiasis, throat irritation, xerostomia

Hepatic: Liver enzymes increased

Neuromuscular & skeletal: Arthralgia, articular rheumatism, joint pain, muscular cramps/spasm/stiffness, pain, paresthesia, rigidity

Ocular: Keratitis/conjunctivitis

Respiratory: Asthma, cough, influenza, nasal congestion, pharyngitis, rhinitis, sinusitis, tracheitis/bronchitis, viral respiratory tract infection

Rare but important or life-threatening: Abdominal pain, agitation, aggression, anaphylactic reaction (some in patients with severe milk allergy [Diskus®]), angioedema, aphonia, arrhythmia, atrial fibrillation, cataracts, chest congestion, chest tightness, choking, contusions, Cushing syndrome, Cushingoid features, depression, dysmenorrhea, dyspnea, earache, ecchymoses, edema (facial, oropharyngeal), eosinophilic conditions, glaucoma, growth velocity reduction in children/adolescents, hypercorticism, hypersensitivity reaction (immediate and delayed), hypokalemia, hypothyroidism, intraocular pressure increased, laryngeal spasm/irritation, irregular menstruation, myositis, oropharyngeal irritation, osteoporosis, pallor, paradoxical bronchospasm, paradoxical tracheitis, paranasal sinus pain, PID, QTc prolongation, restlessness, stridor, supraventricular tachycardia, syncope, tremor, vaginal candidiasis, vaginitis, vulvovaginitis, rare cases of vasculitis (Churg-Strauss syndrome), ventricular tachycardia, weight gain

Drug Interactions

Metabolism/Transport Effects

Substrate of CYP3A4 (major); **Note:** Assignment of Major/Minor substrate status based on clinically relevant drug interaction potential

Avoid Concomitant Use

Avoid concomitant use of Salmeterol with any of the following: Beta-Blockers (Nonselective); Cobicistat; Conivaptan; CYP3A4 Inhibitors (Strong); Fusidic Acid (Systemic); Idelalisib; Iobenguane I 123; Long-Acting Beta2-Agonists; Telaprevir; Tipranavir

Increased Effect/Toxicity

Salmeterol may increase the levels/effects of: Atosiban; Highest Risk QTc-Prolonging Agents; Long-Acting Beta2-Agonists; Loop Diuretics; Moderate Risk QTc-Prolonging Agents; Sympathomimetics; Thiazide Diuretics

The levels/effects of Salmeterol may be increased by: Aprepitant; AtoMOXetine; Cannabinoid-Containing Products; Ceritinib; Cobicistat; Conivaptan; CYP3A4 Inhibitors (Moderate); CYP3A4 Inhibitors (Strong); Dasatinib; Fosaprepitant; Fusidic Acid (Systemic); Idelalisib; Ivacaftor; Linezolid; Luliconazole; MAO Inhibitors; Mifepristone;

Netupitant; Simeprevir; Tedizolid; Telaprevir; Tipranavir; Tricyclic Antidepressants

Decreased Effect

Salmeterol may decrease the levels/effects of: Iobenguane I 123

The levels/effects of Salmeterol may be decreased by: Beta-Blockers (Beta1 Selective); Beta-Blockers (Nonselective); Betahistine

Storage/Stability Store at 68°F and 77°F (20°C and 25°C); excursions are permitted between 59°F and 86°F (15°C and 30°C). Protect from direct heat or sunlight. Store Diskus in the unopened foil pouch and only open when ready for use; stable for 6 weeks after removal from foil pouch.

Mechanism of Action Relaxes bronchial smooth muscle by selective action on $beta_2$-receptors with little effect on heart rate; salmeterol acts locally in the lung.

Pharmacodynamics/Kinetics

Onset of action: Asthma: 30-48 minutes, COPD: 2 hours

Peak effect: Asthma: 3 hours, COPD: 2-5 hours

Duration: 12 hours

Absorption: Systemic: Inhalation: Undetectable to poor

Protein binding: 96%

Metabolism: Hepatic; hydroxylated via CYP3A4

Half-life elimination: 5.5 hours

Time to peak, serum: ~20 minutes

Excretion: Feces (60%); urine (25%)

Dosage Note: Do not use for the relief of acute bronchospasm.

Asthma/Bronchospasm (maintenance and prevention): Children ≥4 years and Adults: Inhalation: One inhalation twice daily (~12 hours apart); maximum: 1 inhalation twice daily. **Note:** For asthma control, long acting $beta_2$-agonists (LABAs) should be used in combination with inhaled corticosteroids and not as monotherapy.

COPD (maintenance): Adults: Inhalation: One inhalation twice daily (~12 hours apart); maximum: 1 inhalation twice daily

Exercise-induced bronchospasm (prevention): Children ≥4 years and Adults: Inhalation: One inhalation at least 30 minutes prior to exercise; additional doses should not be used for 12 hours; should not be used in individuals already receiving salmeterol twice daily. **Note:** Because LABAs may disguise poorly controlled persistent asthma, frequent or chronic use of LABAs for exercise-induced bronchospasm is discouraged by the Asthma Guidelines (NAEPP, 2007).

Dosage adjustment in renal impairment: There are no dosage adjustments provided in the manufacturer's labeling.

Dosage adjustment in hepatic impairment: There are no dosage adjustments provided in the manufacturer's labeling (has not been studied). Use with caution.

Dietary Considerations Some products may contain lactose; very rare anaphylactic reactions have been reported in patients with severe milk protein allergy.

Administration For oral inhalation route only. Before inhaling the dose, breath out fully; do not exhale into the Diskus device; activate and use only in a level, horizontal position. Inhale quickly and deeply through the Diskus; hold breath for about 10 seconds or for as long as comfortable and exhale slowly. Do not use with a spacer device or wash mouthpiece; Diskus should be kept dry. Discard device 6 weeks after removal from foil pouch or when the dose counter reads "0" (whichever comes first).

Monitoring Parameters FEV_1, peak flow, and/or other pulmonary function tests; blood pressure, heart rate; CNS stimulation; serum glucose, serum potassium. Monitor for increased use of short-acting $beta_2$-agonist inhalers; may be marker of a deteriorating asthma condition.

Dosage Forms

Aerosol Powder Breath Activated, Inhalation:

Serevent Diskus: 50 mcg/dose (28 ea, 60 ea)

Dosage Forms: Canada

Powder for oral inhalation:

Serevent Diskhaler Disk: 50 mcg (60s)

- ◆ **Salmeterol and Fluticasone** *see* Fluticasone and Salmeterol *on page* *912*
- ◆ **Salmeterol Xinafoate** *see* Salmeterol *on page* *1860*
- ◆ **Salofalk (Can)** *see* Mesalamine *on page* *1301*
- ◆ **Salonpas Arthritis Pain [OTC]** *see* Methyl Salicylate and Menthol *on page* *1344*
- ◆ **Salonpas Jet Spray [OTC]** *see* Methyl Salicylate and Menthol *on page* *1344*
- ◆ **Salonpas Massage Foam [OTC]** *see* Methyl Salicylate and Menthol *on page* *1344*
- ◆ **Salonpas Pain Relief Patch [OTC]** *see* Methyl Salicylate and Menthol *on page* *1344*

Salsalate (SAL sa late)

Brand Names: U.S. Disalcid

Index Terms Disalicylic Acid; Salicylsalicylic Acid

Pharmacologic Category Salicylate

Use Rheumatic disorders: Treatment of signs and symptoms of osteoarthritis, rheumatoid arthritis, and related rheumatic disorders

Pregnancy Risk Factor C

Dosage Rheumatic disorders: Oral: **Note:** Use the lowest effective dose for the shortest duration; after observing the response to initial therapy, adjust dose as needed.

Adults: Usual dose: 3 g per day in 2 to 3 divided doses

Elderly: May require lower dosage

Dosage adjustment in renal impairment: There are no dosage adjustments provided in the manufacturer's labeling. Use is not recommended in patients with advanced renal disease.

Dosage adjustment in hepatic impairment: There are no dosage adjustments provided in the manufacturer's labeling.

Additional Information Complete prescribing information should be consulted for additional detail.

Dosage Forms

Tablet, Oral:

Disalcid: 500 mg, 750 mg

Generic: 500 mg, 750 mg

- ◆ **Salt** *see* Sodium Chloride *on page* *1902*
- ◆ **Salt Poor Albumin** *see* Albumin *on page* *67*
- ◆ **Samsca** *see* Tolvaptan *on page* *2064*
- ◆ **Samsca™ (Can)** *see* Tolvaptan *on page* *2064*
- ◆ **Sanctura [DSC]** *see* Trospium *on page* *2108*
- ◆ **Sanctura XR [DSC]** *see* Trospium *on page* *2108*
- ◆ **Sanctura® XR (Can)** *see* Trospium *on page* *2108*
- ◆ **Sancuso** *see* Granisetron *on page* *983*
- ◆ **SandIMMUNE** *see* CycloSPORINE (Systemic) *on page* *522*
- ◆ **Sandimmune I.V. (Can)** *see* CycloSPORINE (Systemic) *on page* *522*
- ◆ **Sandomigran (Can)** *see* Pizotifen [CAN/INT] *on page* *1664*
- ◆ **Sandomigran DS (Can)** *see* Pizotifen [CAN/INT] *on page* *1664*
- ◆ **SandoSTATIN** *see* Octreotide *on page* *1485*
- ◆ **Sandostatin (Can)** *see* Octreotide *on page* *1485*
- ◆ **Sandostatin LAR (Can)** *see* Octreotide *on page* *1485*

◆ **SandoSTATIN LAR Depot** *see* Octreotide *on page 1485*
◆ **Sandoz-Acebutolol (Can)** *see* Acebutolol *on page 29*
◆ **Sandoz-Alendronate (Can)** *see* Alendronate *on page 79*
◆ **Sandoz-Alfuzosin (Can)** *see* Alfuzosin *on page 84*
◆ **Sandoz-Almotriptan (Can)** *see* Almotriptan *on page 92*
◆ **Sandoz-Amiodarone (Can)** *see* Amiodarone *on page 114*
◆ **Sandoz Amlodipine (Can)** *see* AmLODIPine *on page 123*
◆ **Sandoz-Anagrelide (Can)** *see* Anagrelide *on page 147*
◆ **Sandoz-Anastrozole (Can)** *see* Anastrozole *on page 148*
◆ **Sandoz-Atenolol (Can)** *see* Atenolol *on page 189*
◆ **Sandoz-Atomoxetine (Can)** *see* AtoMOXetine *on page 191*
◆ **Sandoz-Atorvastatin (Can)** *see* AtorvaSTATin *on page 194*
◆ **Sandoz-Azithromycin (Can)** *see* Azithromycin (Systemic) *on page 216*
◆ **Sandoz-Betaxolol (Can)** *see* Betaxolol (Ophthalmic) *on page 257*
◆ **Sandoz-Bicalutamide (Can)** *see* Bicalutamide *on page 262*
◆ **Sandoz-Bisoprolol (Can)** *see* Bisoprolol *on page 266*
◆ **Sandoz-Bosentan (Can)** *see* Bosentan *on page 280*
◆ **Sandoz-Brimonidine (Can)** *see* Brimonidine (Ophthalmic) *on page 288*
◆ **Sandoz-Bupropion SR (Can)** *see* BuPROPion *on page 305*
◆ **Sandoz-Candesartan (Can)** *see* Candesartan *on page 335*
◆ **Sandoz-Candesartan Plus (Can)** *see* Candesartan and Hydrochlorothiazide *on page 338*
◆ **Sandoz-Carbamazepine (Can)** *see* CarBAMazepine *on page 346*
◆ **Sandoz-Cefprozil (Can)** *see* Cefprozil *on page 389*
◆ **Sandoz-Ciprofloxacin (Can)** *see* Ciprofloxacin (Systemic) *on page 441*
◆ **Sandoz-Citalopram (Can)** *see* Citalopram *on page 451*
◆ **Sandoz-Clarithromycin (Can)** *see* Clarithromycin *on page 456*
◆ **Sandoz-Clonazepam (Can)** *see* ClonazePAM *on page 478*
◆ **Sandoz-Clopidogrel (Can)** *see* Clopidogrel *on page 484*
◆ **Sandoz-Cyclosporine (Can)** *see* CycloSPORINE (Systemic) *on page 522*
◆ **Sandoz-Diclofenac (Can)** *see* Diclofenac (Systemic) *on page 617*
◆ **Sandoz-Diclofenac Rapide (Can)** *see* Diclofenac (Systemic) *on page 617*
◆ **Sandoz-Diclofenac SR (Can)** *see* Diclofenac (Systemic) *on page 617*
◆ **Sandoz-Diltiazem CD (Can)** *see* Diltiazem *on page 634*
◆ **Sandoz-Diltiazem T (Can)** *see* Diltiazem *on page 634*
◆ **Sandoz-Dimenhydrinate [OTC] (Can)** *see* DimenhyDRINATE *on page 637*
◆ **Sandoz-Donepezil (Can)** *see* Donepezil *on page 668*
◆ **Sandoz-Donepezil ODT (Can)** *see* Donepezil *on page 668*
◆ **Sandoz-Dorzolamide (Can)** *see* Dorzolamide *on page 673*
◆ **Sandoz-Dorzolamide/Timolol (Can)** *see* Dorzolamide and Timolol *on page 673*
◆ **Sandoz-Dutasteride (Can)** *see* Dutasteride *on page 702*
◆ **Sandoz-Enalapril (Can)** *see* Enalapril *on page 722*
◆ **Sandoz-Entacapone (Can)** *see* Entacapone *on page 730*
◆ **Sandoz Escitalopram (Can)** *see* Escitalopram *on page 765*
◆ **Sandoz-Estradiol Derm 50 (Can)** *see* Estradiol (Systemic) *on page 775*
◆ **Sandoz-Estradiol Derm 75 (Can)** *see* Estradiol (Systemic) *on page 775*
◆ **Sandoz-Estradiol Derm 100 (Can)** *see* Estradiol (Systemic) *on page 775*
◆ **Sandoz Ezetimibe (Can)** *see* Ezetimibe *on page 832*
◆ **Sandoz-Famciclovir (Can)** *see* Famciclovir *on page 843*
◆ **Sandoz-Felodipine (Can)** *see* Felodipine *on page 850*
◆ **Sandoz-Fenofibrate E (Can)** *see* Fenofibrate and Derivatives *on page 852*
◆ **Sandoz-Fenofibrate S (Can)** *see* Fenofibrate and Derivatives *on page 852*
◆ **Sandoz Fentanyl Patch (Can)** *see* FentaNYL *on page 857*
◆ **Sandoz-Finasteride (Can)** *see* Finasteride *on page 878*
◆ **Sandoz-Finasteride A (Can)** *see* Finasteride *on page 878*
◆ **Sandoz-Fluoxetine (Can)** *see* FLUoxetine *on page 899*
◆ **Sandoz-Fluvoxamine (Can)** *see* FluvoxaMINE *on page 916*
◆ **Sandoz-Glimepiride (Can)** *see* Glimepiride *on page 966*
◆ **Sandoz-Glyburide (Can)** *see* GlyBURIDE *on page 972*
◆ **Sandoz-Indomethacin (Can)** *see* Indomethacin *on page 1067*
◆ **Sandoz-Irbesartan (Can)** *see* Irbesartan *on page 1110*
◆ **Sandoz-Irbesartan HCT (Can)** *see* Irbesartan and Hydrochlorothiazide *on page 1112*
◆ **Sandoz-Lansoprazole (Can)** *see* Lansoprazole *on page 1166*
◆ **Sandoz-Leflunomide (Can)** *see* Leflunomide *on page 1174*
◆ **Sandoz-Letrozole (Can)** *see* Letrozole *on page 1181*
◆ **Sandoz-Levobunolol (Can)** *see* Levobunolol *on page 1194*
◆ **Sandoz-Levofloxacin (Can)** *see* Levofloxacin (Systemic) *on page 1197*
◆ **Sandoz-Linezolid (Can)** *see* Linezolid *on page 1217*
◆ **Sandoz-Lisinopril (Can)** *see* Lisinopril *on page 1226*
◆ **Sandoz-Lisinopril/Hctz (Can)** *see* Lisinopril and Hydrochlorothiazide *on page 1229*
◆ **Sandoz-Loperamide (Can)** *see* Loperamide *on page 1236*
◆ **Sandoz Losartan (Can)** *see* Losartan *on page 1248*
◆ **Sandoz-Losartan HCT (Can)** *see* Losartan and Hydrochlorothiazide *on page 1250*
◆ **Sandoz-Losartan HCT DS (Can)** *see* Losartan and Hydrochlorothiazide *on page 1250*
◆ **Sandoz-Lovastatin (Can)** *see* Lovastatin *on page 1252*
◆ **Sandoz-Memantine (Can)** *see* Memantine *on page 1286*
◆ **Sandoz-Metformin FC (Can)** *see* MetFORMIN *on page 1307*
◆ **Sandoz-Methylphenidate SR (Can)** *see* Methylphenidate *on page 1336*
◆ **Sandoz-Metoprolol SR (Can)** *see* Metoprolol *on page 1350*

- **Sandoz-Metoprolol (Type L) (Can)** *see* Metoprolol *on page 1350*
- **Sandoz-Minocycline (Can)** *see* Minocycline *on page 1371*
- **Sandoz-Mirtazapine (Can)** *see* Mirtazapine *on page 1376*
- **Sandoz-Montelukast (Can)** *see* Montelukast *on page 1392*
- **Sandoz-Montelukast Granules (Can)** *see* Montelukast *on page 1392*
- **Sandoz-Morphine SR (Can)** *see* Morphine (Systemic) *on page 1394*
- **Sandoz-Mycophenolate Mofetil (Can)** *see* Mycophenolate *on page 1405*
- **Sandoz-Nabumetone (Can)** *see* Nabumetone *on page 1411*
- **Sandoz-Naratriptan (Can)** *see* Naratriptan *on page 1430*
- **Sandoz-Nitrazepam (Can)** *see* Nitrazepam [CAN/INT] *on page 1461*
- **Sandoz-Olanzapine (Can)** *see* OLANZapine *on page 1491*
- **Sandoz-Olanzapine ODT (Can)** *see* OLANZapine *on page 1491*
- **Sandoz-Olopatadine (Can)** *see* Olopatadine (Ophthalmic) *on page 1500*
- **Sandoz-Omeprazole (Can)** *see* Omeprazole *on page 1508*
- **Sandoz-Ondansetron (Can)** *see* Ondansetron *on page 1513*
- **Sandoz-Oxycodone/Acetaminophen (Can)** *see* Oxycodone and Acetaminophen *on page 1541*
- **Sandoz-Pantoprazole (Can)** *see* Pantoprazole *on page 1570*
- **Sandoz-Paroxetine (Can)** *see* PARoxetine *on page 1579*
- **Sandoz-Pindolol (Can)** *see* Pindolol *on page 1652*
- **Sandoz-Pioglitazone (Can)** *see* Pioglitazone *on page 1654*
- **Sandoz-Pramipexole (Can)** *see* Pramipexole *on page 1695*
- **Sandoz-Pravastatin (Can)** *see* Pravastatin *on page 1700*
- **Sandoz Prednisolone (Can)** *see* PrednisoLONE (Ophthalmic) *on page 1706*
- **Sandoz-Pregabalin (Can)** *see* Pregabalin *on page 1710*
- **Sandoz-Prochlorperazine (Can)** *see* Prochlorperazine *on page 1718*
- **Sandoz-Quetiapine (Can)** *see* QUEtiapine *on page 1751*
- **Sandoz-Quetiapine XRT (Can)** *see* QUEtiapine *on page 1751*
- **Sandoz-Rabeprazole (Can)** *see* RABEprazole *on page 1762*
- **Sandoz-Ramipril (Can)** *see* Ramipril *on page 1771*
- **Sandoz-Ranitidine (Can)** *see* Ranitidine *on page 1777*
- **Sandoz-Repaglinide (Can)** *see* Repaglinide *on page 1791*
- **Sandoz-Risedronate (Can)** *see* Risedronate *on page 1816*
- **Sandoz-Risperidone (Can)** *see* RisperiDONE *on page 1818*
- **Sandoz-Rivastigmine (Can)** *see* Rivastigmine *on page 1833*
- **Sandoz-Rizatriptan ODT (Can)** *see* Rizatriptan *on page 1836*
- **Sandoz-Rosuvastatin (Can)** *see* Rosuvastatin *on page 1848*
- **Sandoz-Salbutamol (Can)** *see* Albuterol *on page 69*
- **Sandoz-Sertraline (Can)** *see* Sertraline *on page 1878*
- **Sandoz-Sildenafil (Can)** *see* Sildenafil *on page 1882*
- **Sandoz-Simvastatin (Can)** *see* Simvastatin *on page 1890*
- **Sandoz-Sotalol (Can)** *see* Sotalol *on page 1927*
- **Sandoz-Sumatriptan (Can)** *see* SUMAtriptan *on page 1953*
- **Sandoz-Tacrolimus (Can)** *see* Tacrolimus (Systemic) *on page 1962*
- **Sandoz-Tamsulosin (Can)** *see* Tamsulosin *on page 1974*
- **Sandoz-Telmisartan (Can)** *see* Telmisartan *on page 1988*
- **Sandoz-Telmisartan HCT (Can)** *see* Telmisartan and Hydrochlorothiazide *on page 1990*
- **Sandoz-Terbinafine (Can)** *see* Terbinafine (Systemic) *on page 2002*
- **Sandoz-Ticlopidine (Can)** *see* Ticlopidine *on page 2040*
- **Sandoz-Timolol (Can)** *see* Timolol (Ophthalmic) *on page 2043*
- **Sandoz-Tobramycin (Can)** *see* Tobramycin (Ophthalmic) *on page 2056*
- **Sandoz-Topiramate (Can)** *see* Topiramate *on page 2065*
- **Sandoz-Travoprost (Can)** *see* Travoprost *on page 2089*
- **Sandoz-Trifluridine (Can)** *see* Trifluridine *on page 2103*
- **Sandoz-Valproic (Can)** *see* Valproic Acid and Derivatives *on page 2123*
- **Sandoz-Valsartan (Can)** *see* Valsartan *on page 2127*
- **Sandoz Valsartan HCT (Can)** *see* Valsartan and Hydrochlorothiazide *on page 2129*
- **Sandoz-Venlafaxine XR (Can)** *see* Venlafaxine *on page 2150*
- **Sandoz-Voriconazole (Can)** *see* Voriconazole *on page 2176*
- **Sandoz-Zolmitriptan (Can)** *see* ZOLMitriptan *on page 2210*
- **Sandoz-Zolmitriptan ODT (Can)** *see* ZOLMitriptan *on page 2210*
- **Sandoz-Zopiclone (Can)** *see* Zopiclone [CAN/INT] *on page 2217*
- **Santyl** *see* Collagenase (Topical) *on page 507*
- **Santyl® (Can)** *see* Collagenase (Topical) *on page 507*
- **Saphris** *see* Asenapine *on page 179*

Sapropterin (sap roe TER in)

Brand Names: U.S. Kuvan

Brand Names: Canada Kuvan

Index Terms 6R-BH4; Phenoptin; Sapropterin Dihydrochloride; Tetrahydrobiopterin

Pharmacologic Category Enzyme Cofactor

Use Hyperphenylalaninemia: To reduce blood phenylalanine (PHE) levels in patients with hyperphenylalaninemia caused by tetrahydrobiopterin (BH4)-responsive phenylketonuria in conjunction with a PHE-restricted diet.

Pregnancy Risk Factor C

Dosage

Hyperphenylalaninemia:

Infants and Children ≥1 month to 6 years: Oral: Initial: 10 mg/kg once daily

Children ≥7 years, Adolescents, and Adults: Oral: Initial: 10 to 20 mg/kg once daily

Note: Adjust dose after 1 month based on blood phenylalanine levels (if phenylalanine levels do not decrease from baseline after initiating 10 mg/kg, increase dose to 20 mg/kg once daily); discontinue if phenylalanine levels do not decrease after 1 month of treatment at 20 mg/kg/day (nonresponder). Maintenance range: 5 to 20 mg/kg once daily

Missed dose: A missed dose should be taken as soon as possible, but 2 doses should not be taken on the same day.

Dosage adjustment in renal impairment: There are no dosage adjustments provided in manufacturer's labeling (has not been studied). Use with caution.

Dosage adjustment in hepatic impairment: There are no dosage adjustments provided in manufacturer's labeling (has not been studied). Use with caution.

Additional Information Complete prescribing information should be consulted for additional detail.

Dosage Forms

Packet, Oral:

Kuvan: 100 mg (1 ea, 30 ea)

Tablet Soluble, Oral:

Kuvan: 100 mg

◆ **Sapropterin Dihydrochloride** *see* Sapropterin *on page 1864*

Saquinavir (sa KWIN a veer)

Brand Names: U.S. Invirase

Brand Names: Canada Invirase

Index Terms Saquinavir Mesylate; SQV

Pharmacologic Category Antiretroviral, Protease Inhibitor (Anti-HIV)

Use Treatment of HIV infection; used in combination with ritonavir and other antiretroviral agents

Pregnancy Risk Factor B

Dosage Note: ECG should be done prior to starting therapy; do not initiate therapy if pretreatment QT interval >450 msec. Saquinavir should always be used with concomitant ritonavir.

Children ≥2 years and Adolescents <16 years (off-label dosing) (HHS [pediatric], 2014): Oral:

5 kg to <15 kg: Saquinavir 50 mg/kg/dose (maximum single dose: 1000 mg) **plus** ritonavir 3 mg/kg/dose twice daily

15 kg to <40 kg: Saquinavir 50 mg/kg/dose (maximum single dose: 1000 mg) **plus** ritonavir 2.5 mg/kg/dose twice daily

≥40 kg: Saquinavir 1000 mg **plus** ritonavir 100 mg twice daily

Adolescents >16 years and Adults: Oral: 1000 mg twice daily given in combination with ritonavir 100 mg twice daily. This combination should be given together and within 2 hours after a full meal in combination with a nucleoside analog.

Treatment-naive patients: Canadian labeling (not in U.S. labeling): Initial: Saquinavir 500 mg twice daily given in combination with ritonavir 100 mg twice daily for 7 days. Maintenance: Saquinavir 1000 mg twice daily given in combination with ritonavir 100 mg twice daily. Patients with recent exposure (without washout) to a ritonavir or non-nucleoside reverse transcriptase inhibitor based regimen may receive usual initial dosing (ie, saquinavir 1000 mg twice daily in combination with ritonavir 100 mg twice daily).

Dosage adjustments when administered in combination therapy: Saquinavir: 1000 mg twice daily administered with lopinavir 400 mg/ritonavir 100 mg (Kaletra) twice daily; no additional ritonavir is necessary

Elderly: Clinical studies did not include sufficient numbers of patients ≥65 years of age; use caution due to increased frequency of organ dysfunction

Dosage adjustment in renal impairment: No dosage adjustment necessary. However, has not been studied in severe renal impairment or ESRD.

Dosage adjustment in hepatic impairment:

Mild to moderate impairment (Child-Pugh classes A and B): No dosage adjustment necessary.

Severe impairment (Child-Pugh class C): Use is contraindicated when coadministered with ritonavir.

Additional Information Complete prescribing information should be consulted for additional detail.

Dosage Forms

Capsule, Oral:

Invirase: 200 mg

Tablet, Oral:

Invirase: 500 mg

◆ **Saquinavir Mesylate** *see* Saquinavir *on page 1865*

◆ **Sarafem** *see* FLUoxetine *on page 899*

Sargramostim (sar GRAM oh stim)

Brand Names: U.S. Leukine

Brand Names: Canada Leukine

Index Terms GM-CSF; GMCSF; Granulocyte-Macrophage Colony Stimulating Factor; Prokine; Recombinant Granulocyte-Macrophage Colony Stimulating Factor; rhuGM-CSF

Pharmacologic Category Colony Stimulating Factor; Hematopoietic Agent

Use

Acute myeloid leukemia (AML; following induction chemotherapy): To shorten time to neutrophil recovery and to reduce the incidence of severe and life-threatening infections and infections resulting in death following induction chemotherapy in older adults (≥55 years of age)

Bone marrow transplant (allogeneic or autologous) failure or engraftment delay: For graft failure or engraftment delay in patients who have undergone allogeneic or autologous bone marrow transplantation, to prolong survival (survival benefit may be greater in patients with autologous bone marrow transplant failure or engraftment delay, no previous total body irradiation, malignancy other than leukemia, or multiple organ failure score ≤2)

Myeloid reconstitution after allogeneic bone marrow transplantation: To accelerate myeloid recovery in patients undergoing allogeneic bone marrow transplant from HLA-matched related donors (safe and effective in accelerating myeloid engraftment, reducing the incidence of bacteremia and other culture-positive infections, and shortening the median hospitalization duration)

Myeloid reconstitution after autologous bone marrow transplantation: To accelerate myeloid recovery following transplantation in non-Hodgkin lymphoma (NHL), acute lymphoblastic leukemia (ALL), Hodgkin lymphoma patients undergoing autologous bone marrow transplant (safe and effective in accelerating myeloid engraftment, reducing the median duration of antibiotic administration, reducing the median duration of infectious episodes, and shortening the median hospitalization duration)

Peripheral stem cell transplantation (autologous), mobilization and post-transplant: Mobilization of hematopoietic progenitor cells for collection by leukapheresis (increases the number of progenitor cells capable of engraftment and may lead to more rapid engraftment); to accelerate myeloid reconstitution following peripheral blood progenitor cell transplantation

Pregnancy Risk Factor C

Pregnancy Considerations Animal reproduction studies have not been conducted.

Breast-Feeding Considerations It is not known if sargramostim is excreted in breast milk. Breast-feeding is not recommended by the manufacturer.

Contraindications Hypersensitivity to sargramostim, yeast-derived products, or any component of the formulation; concurrent (24 hours preceding/following) use with myelosuppressive chemotherapy or radiation therapy; patients with excessive (≥10%) leukemic myeloid blasts in bone marrow or peripheral blood

Warnings/Precautions Simultaneous administration or administration 24 hours preceding/following cytotoxic chemotherapy or radiotherapy is contraindicated due to the sensitivity of rapidly dividing hematopoietic progenitor cells. If there is a rapid increase in blood counts (ANC >20,000/mm^3, WBC >50,000/mm^3, or platelets >500,000/mm^3), decrease the dose by 50% or discontinue therapy. Excessive blood counts should fall to normal within 3 to 7 days after the discontinuation of therapy. Monitor CBC with differential twice weekly during treatment. Limited response to sargramostim may be seen in patients who have received bone marrow purged by chemical agents which do not preserve an adequate number of responsive hematopoietic progenitors (eg, <1.2 x 10^4/kg progenitors). In patients receiving autologous bone marrow transplant, response to sargramostim may be limited if extensive radiotherapy to the abdomen or chest or multiple myelotoxic agents were administered prior to transplantation. May potentially act as a growth factor for any tumor type, particularly myeloid malignancies; caution should be exercised when using in any malignancy with myeloid characteristics. Discontinue use if disease progression occurs during treatment.

Anaphylaxis or other serious allergic reactions have been reported; discontinue immediately and initiate appropriate therapy if a serious allergic or anaphylactic reaction occurs. A "first-dose effect", characterized by respiratory distress, hypoxia, flushing, hypotension, syncope, and/or tachycardia, may occur (rarely) with the first dose of a cycle and resolve with appropriate symptomatic treatment; symptoms do not usually occur with subsequent doses within that cycle. Sequestration of granulocytes in pulmonary circulation and dyspnea have been reported; monitor respiratory symptoms during and following IV infusion. Decrease infusion rate by 50% if dyspnea occurs; discontinue the infusion if dyspnea persists despite reduction in the rate of administration. Subsequent doses may be administered at the standard rate with careful monitoring. Use with caution in patients with hypoxia or preexisting pulmonary disease. Edema, capillary leak syndrome, pleural and/or pericardial effusion have been reported; fluid retention has been shown to be reversible with dosage reduction or discontinuation of sargramostim with or without concomitant use of diuretics. Use with caution in patients with preexisting fluid retention, pulmonary infiltrates, or congestive heart failure; may exacerbate fluid retention.

Use with caution in patients with preexisting cardiac disease. Reversible transient supraventricular arrhythmias have been reported, especially in patients with a history of arrhythmias. Use with caution in patients with hepatic impairment (hyperbilirubinemia and elevated transaminases have been observed) or renal impairment (serum creatinine elevations have been observed). Monitor hepatic and renal function at least every other week in patients with history of impairment.

Benzyl alcohol and derivatives: Some dosage forms may contain benzyl alcohol; large amounts of benzyl alcohol (≥99 mg/kg/day) have been associated with a potentially fatal toxicity ("gasping syndrome") in neonates; the "gasping syndrome" consists of metabolic acidosis, respiratory distress, gasping respirations, CNS dysfunction (including convulsions, intracranial hemorrhage), hypotension, and cardiovascular collapse (AAP, 1997; CDC, 1982); some data suggests that benzoate displaces bilirubin from protein binding sites (Ahlfors, 2001); avoid or use dosage forms containing benzyl alcohol with caution in neonates. See manufacturer's labeling.

Adverse Reactions

Cardiovascular: Chest pain, edema, hypertension, pericardial effusion, peripheral edema, tachycardia, thrombosis

Central nervous system: Anxiety, chills, headache, insomnia, malaise

Dermatologic: Pruritus, skin rash

Endocrine & metabolic: Hypercholesterolemia, hyperglycemia, hypomagnesemia, weight loss

Gastrointestinal: Abdominal pain, anorexia, diarrhea, dysphagia, gastric ulcer, gastrointestinal hemorrhage, hematemesis, nausea, vomiting

Hepatic: Hyperbilirubinemia

Immunologic: Antibody development

Neuromuscular & skeletal: Arthralgia, myalgia, ostealgia, weakness

Ophthalmic: Retinal hemorrhage

Renal: Increased blood urea nitrogen, increased serum creatinine

Respiratory: Dyspnea, epistaxis, pharyngitis, pleural effusion

Miscellaneous: Fever

Rare but important or life-threatening: Anaphylaxis, capillary leak syndrome, cardiac arrhythmia, eosinophilia, hypoxia, leukocytosis, liver function impairment (transient), pericarditis, prolonged prothrombin time, respiratory distress, rigors, sore throat, supraventricular cardiac arrhythmia, syncope, thrombocythemia, thrombophlebitis

Drug Interactions

Metabolism/Transport Effects None known.

Avoid Concomitant Use There are no known interactions where it is recommended to avoid concomitant use.

Increased Effect/Toxicity

Sargramostim may increase the levels/effects of: Bleomycin

The levels/effects of Sargramostim may be increased by: Cyclophosphamide

Decreased Effect There are no known significant interactions involving a decrease in effect.

Preparation for Administration

Powder for injection: May be reconstituted with 1 mL of preservative free SWFI or bacteriostatic water for injection. Direct the diluent toward the side of the vial and gently swirl to reconstitute; do not shake. Do not mix the contents of vials which have been reconstituted with different diluents.

SubQ: May be administered without further dilution.

IV: Further dilution with NS is required. If the final sargramostim concentration is <10 mcg/mL, 1 mg of human albumin per 1 mL of NS should be added (eg, add 1 mL of 5% human albumin per 50 mL of NS).

Storage/Stability Store intact vials at 2°C to 8°C (36°F to 46°F); do not freeze. Do not shake.

Solution for injection: May be stored for up to 20 days at 2°C to 8°C (36°F to 46°F) once the vial has been entered. Discard remaining solution after 20 days.

Powder for injection: Preparations made with SWFI should be administered as soon as possible, and discarded within 6 hours of reconstitution. Solutions reconstituted with bacteriostatic water may be stored for up to 20 days at 2°C to 8°C (36°F to 46°F); do not freeze. When combining previously reconstituted solutions with freshly reconstituted solutions, administer within 6 hours following preparation; the contents of vials reconstituted with different diluents should not be mixed together.

Mechanism of Action Stimulates proliferation, differentiation and functional activity of neutrophils, eosinophils, monocytes, and macrophages.

Pharmacodynamics/Kinetics

Duration: WBCs return to baseline within 1 to 2 weeks of discontinuing drug

Half-life elimination: IV: ~60 minutes; SubQ: ~2.7 hours

Time to peak, serum: SubQ: 1 to 3 hours

Dosage Note: May round the dose to the nearest vial size (Ozer, 2000).

Acute myeloid leukemia (following induction chemotherapy): Adults ≥55 years: IV: 250 mcg/m^2/day (infused over 4 hours) starting approximately on day 11 or 4 days following the completion of induction chemotherapy (if day 10 bone marrow is hypoplastic with <5% blasts), continue until ANC >1500/mm^3 for 3 consecutive days or a maximum of 42 days. If WBC >50,000/mm^3 and/or ANC >20,000/mm^3, interrupt treatment or reduce the dose by 50%.

If a second cycle of chemotherapy is necessary, administer ~4 days after the completion of chemotherapy if the bone marrow is hypoplastic with <5% blasts

Discontinue sargramostim immediately if leukemic regrowth occurs. If a severe adverse reaction occurs, reduce the dose by 50% or temporarily discontinue the dose until the reaction abates.

Bone marrow transplantation (allogeneic or autologous) failure or engraftment delay: Adults: IV: 250 mcg/m^2/day (infused over 2 hours) for 14 days; If engraftment has not occurred after 7 days off sargramostim, may repeat. If engraftment still has not occurred after 7 days off sargramostim, a third course of 500 mcg/m^2/day for 14 days may be attempted. If there is still no improvement, it is unlikely that further dose escalation will be of benefit.

If a severe adverse reaction occurs, reduce the dose by 50% or temporarily discontinue the dose until the reaction abates

If blast cells appear or disease progression occurs, discontinue treatment

If WBC >50,000/mm^3 and/or ANC >20,000 cells/mm^3, interrupt treatment or reduce the dose by 50%.

Myeloid reconstitution after allogeneic or autologous bone marrow transplantation: Adults: IV: 250 mcg/m^2/day (infused over 2 hours), begin 2 to 4 hours after the marrow infusion and ≥24 hours after chemotherapy or radiotherapy, when the post marrow infusion ANC is <500 /mm^3, and continue until ANC >1500 /mm^3 for 3 consecutive days. If WBC >50,000/mm^3 and/or ANC >20,000/mm^3, interrupt treatment or reduce the dose by 50%.

If a severe adverse reaction occurs, reduce dose by 50% or temporarily discontinue the dose until the reaction abates

If blast cells appear or progression of the underlying disease occurs, discontinue treatment

Peripheral stem cell transplantation (autologous), mobilization: Adults: IV, SubQ: 250 mcg/m^2/day IV (infused over 24 hours) or SubQ once daily; continue the same dose throughout peripheral blood progenitor cell collection. If WBC >50,000/mm^3, reduce the dose by 50%.

Note: The optimal schedule for peripheral blood progenitor cell collection has not been established (usually begun by day 5 and performed daily until protocol specified targets are achieved). If adequate numbers of progenitor cells are not collected, consider other mobilization therapy.

Peripheral stem cell transplantation (autologous) post-transplant: Adults: IV, SubQ: 250 mcg/m^2/day IV (infused over 24 hours) or SubQ once daily beginning immediately following infusion of progenitor cells; continue until ANC is >1500/mm^3 for 3 consecutive days.

Primary prophylaxis of neutropenia in patients receiving chemotherapy (outside transplant and AML) or who are at high risk for neutropenic fever (off-label use): Adults: SubQ: 250 mcg/m^2/day (may round to the nearest vial size [Ozer, 2000]) beginning at least 24 hours after chemotherapy administration; continue until ANC >2000 to 3000/mm^3 (Smith, 2006).

Treatment of radiation-induced myelosuppression of the bone marrow (off-label use): Adults: SubQ: 250 mcg/m^2/day; continue until ANC >1000/mm^3 (Smith, 2006; Waselenko, 2004).

Dosage adjustment in renal impairment: There are no dosage adjustments provided in the manufacturer's labeling.

Dosage adjustment in hepatic impairment: There are no dosage adjustments provided in the manufacturer's labeling.

Administration Sargramostim is administered as a subcutaneous injection or intravenous infusion.

IV: Infuse over 2 hours, 4 hours or 24 hours (indication specific). An in-line membrane filter should **NOT** be used for intravenous administration.

SubQ: Administer undiluted; rotate injection sites, avoiding navel/waistline.

Monitoring Parameters CBC with differential (twice weekly during treatment), renal/liver function tests (at least every 2 weeks in patients displaying renal or hepatic dysfunction prior to treatment initiation); pulmonary function; vital signs; hydration status; weight

Dosage Forms

Solution Reconstituted, Intravenous [preservative free]:
Leukine: 250 mcg (1 ea)

- ◆ **Sarna® HC (Can)** *see* Hydrocortisone (Topical) *on page 1014*
- ◆ **Sarnol-HC [OTC]** *see* Hydrocortisone (Topical) *on page 1014*
- ◆ **Sativex® (Can)** *see* Tetrahydrocannabinol and Cannabidiol [CAN/INT] *on page 2018*
- ◆ **Saturated Potassium Iodide Solution** *see* Potassium Iodide *on page 1690*
- ◆ **Saturated Solution of Potassium Iodide** *see* Potassium Iodide *on page 1690*
- ◆ **Savella** *see* Milnacipran *on page 1368*
- ◆ **Savella Titration Pack** *see* Milnacipran *on page 1368*

Saxagliptin (sax a GLIP tin)

Brand Names: U.S. Onglyza

Brand Names: Canada Onglyza

Index Terms BMS-477118

Pharmacologic Category Antidiabetic Agent, Dipeptidyl Peptidase IV (DPP-IV) Inhibitor

Use Treatment of type 2 diabetes mellitus (noninsulin dependent, NIDDM) as an adjunct to diet and exercise as monotherapy or in combination therapy with other antidiabetic agents to improve glycemic control

Pregnancy Risk Factor B

Pregnancy Considerations Teratogenic effects were not observed in animal reproduction studies.

In women with diabetes, maternal hyperglycemia can be associated with congenital malformations as well as adverse effects in the fetus, neonate, and the mother (ACOG, 2005; ADA, 2014; Kitzmiller, 2008; Metzger, 2007). To prevent adverse outcomes, prior to conception and throughout pregnancy maternal blood glucose and HbA_{1c} should be kept as close to normal as possible but without causing significant hypoglycemia (ACOG, 2013; ADA, 2014; Blumer, 2013; Kitzmiller, 2008). Prior to pregnancy, effective contraception should be used until glycemic control is achieved (ADA, 2014; Kitzmiller, 2008). Other agents are currently recommended to treat diabetes in pregnant women (ACOG, 2013; Blumer, 2013).

Breast-Feeding Considerations It is not known if saxagliptin is excreted in breast milk. The manufacturer recommends that caution be exercised when administering saxagliptin to nursing women.

Contraindications Hypersensitivity to saxagliptin or any component of the formulation

Canadian labeling: Additional contraindications (not in U.S. labeling): Diabetic ketoacidosis, diabetic coma/precoma, type 1 diabetes mellitus

Warnings/Precautions Use with caution in patients with moderate-to-severe renal dysfunction, end-stage renal disease (ESRD) requiring hemodialysis, and in patients taking strong CYP3A4/5 inhibitors (eg, atazanavir, clarithromycin, indinavir, itraconazole, nefazodone, nelfinavir, ritonavir, saquinavir, telithromycin [also see Drug Interactions]); dosing adjustment required. No specific recommendations regarding patients with heart failure are provided in the U.S. manufacturer labeling (Canadian labeling recommends against use in this population). Initial clinical trials included only a limited number of patients with heart failure (HF). However, recent data from a large multicenter, randomized, double-blind, placebo-controlled trial in patients with type 2 diabetes with a history of, or at risk for, cardiovascular events demonstrated an increased risk of hospitalization for HF especially during the first 12 months of therapy for patients with elevated levels of natriuretic peptides, previous HF, or chronic kidney disease (Scirica, 2013; Scirica, 2014).

Use caution when used in conjunction with insulin or insulin secretagogues (eg, sulfonylureas); risk of hypoglycemia is increased. Monitor blood glucose closely; dosage adjustments of insulin or the insulin secretagogue may be necessary. Rare hypersensitivity reactions, including anaphylaxis, angioedema, and/or exfoliative dermatologic reactions have been reported; discontinue if signs/symptoms of severe hypersensitivity reactions occur. Cases of acute pancreatitis have been reported; discontinue immediately if suspected. Contains lactose; Canadian labeling recommends avoiding use in patients with galactose intolerance, Lapp lactase deficiency, or glucose-galactose malabsorption syndromes.

Adverse Reactions Note: Adverse reactions reported with monotherapy unless otherwise noted.

Cardiovascular: Peripheral edema (incidence increased in conjunction with thiazolidinediones)
Central nervous system: Headache
Endocrine & metabolic: Hypoglycemia (incidence increased in conjunction with insulin secretagogues)
Gastrointestinal: Abdominal pain, gastroenteritis, vomiting
Genitourinary: Urinary tract infection
Hematologic: Lymphopenia (dose related)
Respiratory: Sinusitis
Miscellaneous: Hypersensitivity reactions (including urticaria and facial edema)

Rare but important or life-threatening: Angioedema, anaphylaxis, creatinine increased, creatine phosphokinase increased, exfoliative skin reactions, immune thrombocytopenia (ITP), pancreatitis (acute), rash

Drug Interactions

Metabolism/Transport Effects Substrate of CYP3A4 (major), P-glycoprotein; **Note:** Assignment of Major/Minor substrate status based on clinically relevant drug interaction potential

Avoid Concomitant Use

Avoid concomitant use of Saxagliptin with any of the following: Conivaptan; Fusidic Acid (Systemic); Idelalisib

Increased Effect/Toxicity

Saxagliptin may increase the levels/effects of: ACE Inhibitors

The levels/effects of Saxagliptin may be increased by: Androgens; Aprepitant; Ceritinib; Conivaptan; CYP3A4 Inhibitors (Moderate); CYP3A4 Inhibitors (Strong); Dasatinib; Fosaprepitant; Fusidic Acid (Systemic); Idelalisib; Ivacaftor; Luliconazole; Mifepristone; Netupitant; Pegvisomant; P-glycoprotein/ABCB1 Inhibitors; Simeprevir; Stiripentol

Decreased Effect

The levels/effects of Saxagliptin may be decreased by: Corticosteroids (Orally Inhaled); Corticosteroids (Systemic); CYP3A4 Inducers; Danazol; Luteinizing Hormone-Releasing Hormone Analogs; P-glycoprotein/ABCB1 Inducers; Somatropin; Thiazide Diuretics

Storage/Stability Store at 20°C to 25°C (68°F to 77°F); excursions permitted between 15°C to 30°C (59°F to 86°F).

Mechanism of Action Saxagliptin inhibits dipeptidyl peptidase IV (DPP-IV) enzyme resulting in prolonged active incretin levels. Incretin hormones (eg, glucagon-like peptide-1 [GLP-1] and glucose-dependent insulinotropic polypeptide [GIP]) regulate glucose homeostasis by increasing insulin synthesis and release from pancreatic beta cells and decreasing glucagon secretion from pancreatic alpha cells. Decreased glucagon secretion results in decreased hepatic glucose production. Under normal physiologic circumstances, incretin hormones are released by the intestine throughout the day and levels are increased in response to a meal; incretin hormones are rapidly inactivated by the DPP-IV enzyme.

Pharmacodynamics/Kinetics

Duration: 24 hours
Protein binding: Negligible
Metabolism: Hepatic via CYP3A4/5 to 5-hydroxy saxagliptin (active; ~50% potency of the parent compound)
Half-life elimination: Saxagliptin: 2.5 hours; 5-hydroxy saxagliptin: 3.1 hours
Time to peak, plasma: Saxagliptin: 2 hours; 5-hydroxy saxagliptin: 4 hours
Excretion: Urine (75%, 24% of the total dose as saxagliptin, 36% of the total dose as 5-hydroxy saxagliptin); feces (22%)

Dosage Oral: Adults: Type 2 diabetes: 2.5-5 mg once daily

Concomitant use with strong CYP3A4/5 inhibitors: 2.5 mg once daily

Concomitant use with insulin or insulin secretagogues: Reduced dose of insulin or insulin secretagogues (eg, sulfonylureas) may be needed

Dosage adjustment in renal impairment:

Note: Renal function may be estimated using the Cockcroft-Gault formula or the MDRD formula for dosage adjustment purposes.
CrCl >50 mL/minute: No dosage adjustment necessary
CrCl ≤50 mL/minute: 2.5 mg once daily
ESRD requiring hemodialysis:
U.S. labeling: 2.5 mg once daily; administer postdialysis
Canadian labeling: Use is not recommended.

Peritoneal dialysis: There are no dosage adjustments provided in the manufacturer's labeling (has not been studied).

Dosage adjustment in hepatic impairment:

U.S. labeling: Mild-to-severe impairment: No dosage adjustment necessary.

Canadian labeling:

Mild impairment: No dosage adjustment provided in manufacturer's labeling.

Moderate-to-severe impairment: Use is not recommended.

Dietary Considerations May be taken without regard to meals. Individualized medical nutrition therapy (MNT) is an integral part of therapy (ADA, 2013).

Administration May be administered without regard to meals. Swallow whole; do not split or cut tablets.

Monitoring Parameters Plasma glucose, HbA_{1c}, renal function

Reference Range

Recommendations for glycemic control in nonpregnant adults with diabetes (ADA, 2015):

HbA_{1c}: <7% (a more aggressive [<6.5%] or less aggressive [<8%] HbA_{1c} goal may be targeted based on patient-specific characteristics)

Preprandial capillary plasma glucose: 80 to 130 mg/dL

Peak postprandial capillary blood glucose: <180 mg/dL

Recommendations for glycemic control in pediatric (all age groups) patients with type 1 diabetes (ADA, 2015):

HbA_{1c}: <7.5% (individualization may be appropriate based on patient-specific characteristics; <7% is reasonable if it can be achieved without excessive hypoglycemia)

Preprandial capillary plasma glucose: 90 to 130 mg/dL

Bedtime and overnight capillary blood glucose: 90 to 150 mg/dL

Dosage Forms

Tablet, Oral:

Onglyza: 2.5 mg, 5 mg

Saxagliptin and Metformin

(sax a GLIP tin & met FOR min)

Brand Names: U.S. Kombiglyze™ XR

Brand Names: Canada Komboglyze™

Index Terms Metformin and Saxagliptin; Metformin Hydrochloride and Saxagliptin; Saxagliptin and Metformin Hydrochloride

Pharmacologic Category Antidiabetic Agent, Biguanide; Antidiabetic Agent, Dipeptidyl Peptidase IV (DPP-IV) Inhibitor

Use Management of type 2 diabetes mellitus (noninsulin dependent, NIDDM) as an adjunct to diet and exercise when treatment with both saxagliptin and metformin is appropriate

Pregnancy Risk Factor B

Dosage Oral: Type 2 diabetes mellitus:

Adults:

U.S. labeling: Initial doses should be based on current dose of saxagliptin and metformin; daily doses should be given once daily with the evening meal. Maximum: Saxagliptin 5 mg/metformin 2000 mg daily

Patients inadequately controlled on metformin alone: Initial dose: Saxagliptin 2.5-5 mg daily plus current dose of metformin. **Note:** Patients who require saxagliptin 2.5 mg (eg, dose adjusted for concomitant use of strong CYP3A4/5 inhibitors) and metformin >1000 mg should not be switched to the combination product.

Patients inadequately controlled on saxagliptin alone: Initial dose: Metformin 500 mg daily plus saxagliptin 5 mg daily. **Note:** Metformin-naive patients currently receiving saxagliptin 2.5 mg daily (eg, dose adjusted for concomitant use of strong CYP3A4/5 inhibitors) should not be switched to the combination product.

Concomitant use with strong CYP3A4/5 inhibitors: Maximum: Saxagliptin 2.5 mg/metformin 1000 mg daily

Concomitant use with insulin or insulin secretagogues: Reduced dose of insulin or insulin secretagogues (eg, sulfonylureas) may be needed.

Canadian labeling: Initial doses should be based on current dose of saxagliptin and metformin; daily dose should be divided into 2 equal doses given with meals. Maximum: Saxagliptin 5 mg/metformin 2000 mg daily

Patients inadequately controlled on metformin alone: Initial dose: Saxagliptin 2.5 mg twice daily plus current dose of metformin.

Concomitant use with insulin: Reduced dose of insulin may be needed.

Elderly: The initial and maintenance dosing should be conservative, due to the potential for decreased renal function (monitor). Do not use in patients ≥80 years of age unless normal renal function has been established.

Dosage adjustment in renal impairment:

U.S. labeling: Do not use in patients with renal disease or renal dysfunction (serum creatinine ≥1.5 mg/dL [≥136 micromole/L] in males or ≥1.4 mg/dL [≥124 micromole/L] in females or abnormal clearance).

Canadian labeling: Use is contraindicated.

Dosage adjustment in hepatic impairment:

U.S. labeling: Avoid metformin; liver disease is a risk factor for the development of lactic acidosis during metformin therapy.

Canadian labeling: Use is not recommended with clinical or laboratory evidence of disease and contraindicated in the presence of moderate-to-severe impairment.

Additional Information Complete prescribing information should be consulted for additional detail.

Dosage Forms

Tablet, variable release, oral:

Kombiglyze XR 2.5/1000: Saxagliptin 2.5 mg [immediate release] and metformin hydrochloride 1000 mg [extended release]; 5/500: Saxagliptin 5 mg [immediate release] and metformin hydrochloride 500 mg [extended release]; 5/1000: Saxagliptin 5 mg [immediate release] and metformin hydrochloride 1000 mg [extended release]

Dosage Forms: Canada

Tablet, oral:

Komboglyze 2.5/500: Saxagliptin 2.5 mg [immediate release] and metformin hydrochloride 500 mg [immediate release]; 2.5/850: Saxagliptin 5 mg [immediate release] and metformin hydrochloride 850 mg [immediate release]; 2.5/1000: Saxagliptin 2.5 mg [immediate release] and metformin hydrochloride 1000 mg [immediate release]

- ◆ **Saxagliptin and Metformin Hydrochloride** *see* Saxagliptin and Metformin *on page* 1869
- ◆ **Saxenda** *see* Liraglutide *on page* 1222
- ◆ **SB-265805** *see* Gemifloxacin *on page* 957
- ◆ **SB-497115** *see* Eltrombopag *on page* 714
- ◆ **SB-497115-GR** *see* Eltrombopag *on page* 714
- ◆ **SB659746-A** *see* Vilazodone *on page* 2158
- ◆ **(S)-bupivacaine** *see* Levobupivacaine [INT] *on page* 1194
- ◆ **SC 33428** *see* IDArubicin *on page* 1037
- ◆ **Scalacort** *see* Hydrocortisone (Topical) *on page* 1014
- ◆ **Scalacort DK** *see* Hydrocortisone (Topical) *on page* 1014
- ◆ **Scalpicin Maximum Strength [OTC]** *see* Hydrocortisone (Topical) *on page* 1014

- ◆ **S-Carboxymethyl L-Cysteine** *see* Carbocisteine [INT] *on page 357*
- ◆ **S-Carboxymethylcysteine** *see* Carbocisteine [INT] *on page 357*
- ◆ **SCH 13521** *see* Flutamide *on page 907*
- ◆ **SCH 52365** *see* Temozolomide *on page 1991*
- ◆ **SCH 56592** *see* Posaconazole *on page 1683*
- ◆ **SCH 90045** *see* Pembrolizumab *on page 1604*
- ◆ **SCH503034** *see* Boceprevir *on page 273*
- ◆ **SCH530348** *see* Vorapaxar *on page 2175*
- ◆ **ScheinPharm Ranitidine (Can)** *see* Ranitidine *on page 1777*
- ◆ **SCIG** *see* Immune Globulin *on page 1056*
- ◆ **S-Citalopram** *see* Escitalopram *on page 765*
- ◆ **Scleromate** *see* Morrhuate Sodium *on page 1401*
- ◆ **Sclerosol Intrapleural** *see* Talc (Sterile) *on page 1971*
- ◆ **S-CMC** *see* Carbocisteine [INT] *on page 357*

Scopolamine (Systemic) (skoe POL a meen)

Brand Names: U.S. Transderm-Scop

Brand Names: Canada Buscopan; Scopolamine Hydrobromide Injection; Transderm-V

Index Terms Hyoscine Butylbromide; Scopolamine Base; Scopolamine Butylbromide; Scopolamine Hydrobromide

Pharmacologic Category Anticholinergic Agent

Additional Appendix Information

Beers Criteria – Potentially Inappropriate Medications for Geriatrics *on page 2271*

Use

Scopolamine base: Transdermal: Prevention of nausea/vomiting associated with motion sickness and recovery from anesthesia and surgery

Scopolamine hydrobromide: Injection: Preoperative medication to produce amnesia, sedation, tranquilization, antiemetic effects, and decrease salivary and respiratory secretions

Scopolamine butylbromide [Canadian product]: Oral/injection: Treatment of smooth muscle spasm of the genitourinary or gastrointestinal tract; injection may also be used prior to radiological/diagnostic procedures to prevent spasm

Pregnancy Risk Factor C

Pregnancy Considerations Adverse events were observed in some animal reproduction studies. Scopolamine crosses the placenta; may cause respiratory depression and/or neonatal hemorrhage when used during pregnancy. Transdermal scopolamine has been used as an adjunct to epidural anesthesia for cesarean delivery without adverse CNS effects on the newborn. Parenteral administration does not increase the duration of labor or affect uterine contractions. Except when used prior to cesarean section, use during pregnancy only if the benefit to the mother outweighs the potential risk to the fetus.

Breast-Feeding Considerations Scopolamine is excreted into breast milk. The manufacturer recommends caution be used if scopolamine is administered to a nursing woman.

Contraindications

Transdermal, oral: Hypersensitivity to scopolamine, other belladonna alkaloids, or any component of the formulation; narrow-angle glaucoma

Injection: Hypersensitivity to scopolamine, other belladonna alkaloids, or any component of the formulation; narrow-angle glaucoma; chronic lung disease (repeated administration)

Canadian labeling: Additional contraindications (not in U.S. labeling):

Oral: Glaucoma, megacolon, myasthenia gravis, obstructive prostatic hypertrophy

Injection:

Hyoscine butylbromide: Untreated narrow-angle glaucoma; megacolon, prostatic hypertrophy with urinary retention; stenotic lesions of the GI tract; myasthenia gravis; tachycardia, angina, or heart failure; IM administration in patients receiving anticoagulant therapy

Scopolamine hydrobromide: Glaucoma or predisposition to narrow-angle glaucoma; paralytic ileus; prostatic hypertrophy; pyloric obstruction; tachycardia secondary to cardiac insufficiency or thyrotoxicosis

Warnings/Precautions Use with caution in patients with coronary artery disease, tachyarrhythmias, heart failure, hypertension, or hyperthyroidism; evaluate tachycardia prior to administration. Use caution in hepatic or renal impairment; adverse CNS effects occur more often in these patients. Use injectable and transdermal products with caution in patients with prostatic hyperplasia or urinary retention. Discontinue if patient reports unusual visual disturbances or pain within the eye. Use caution in GI obstruction, hiatal hernia, reflux esophagitis, and ulcerative colitis. Use with caution in patients with a history of seizure or psychosis; may exacerbate these conditions.

Anaphylaxis including episodes of shock has been reported following parenteral administration; observe for signs/symptoms of hypersensitivity following parenteral administration. Patients with a history of allergies or asthma may be at increased risk of hypersensitivity reactions. Adverse events (including dizziness, headache, nausea, vomiting) may occur following abrupt discontinuation of large doses or in patients with Parkinson's disease; adverse events may also occur following removal of the transdermal patch although symptoms may not appear until ≥24 hours after removal.

Idiosyncratic reactions may rarely occur; patients may experience acute toxic psychosis, agitation, confusion, delusions, hallucinations, paranoid behavior, and rambling speech. May cause CNS depression, which may impair physical or mental abilities; patients must be cautioned about performing tasks which require mental alertness (eg, operating machinery or driving). Effects with other sedative drugs or ethanol may be potentiated.

Transdermal patch may contain conducting metal (eg, aluminum); remove patch prior to MRI. Use of the transdermal product in patients with open-angle glaucoma may necessitate adjustments in glaucoma therapy.

Scopolamine (hyoscine) hydrobromide should not be interchanged with scopolamine butylbromide formulations; dosages are not equivalent.

Avoid use in the elderly due to potent anticholinergic adverse effects and uncertain effectiveness (Beers Criteria). Use with caution in infants and children since they may be more susceptible to adverse effects of scopolamine. Tablets may contain sucrose; avoid use of tablets in patients who are fructose intolerant.

Adverse Reactions

Cardiovascular: Bradycardia, flushing, orthostatic hypotension, tachycardia

Central nervous system: Acute toxic psychosis (rare), agitation (rare), ataxia, confusion, delusion (rare), disorientation, dizziness, drowsiness, fatigue, hallucination (rare), headache, irritability, loss of memory, paranoid behavior (rare), restlessness, sedation

Dermatologic: Drug eruptions, dry skin, dyshidrosis, erythema, pruritus, rash, urticaria

Endocrine & metabolic: Thirst

Gastrointestinal: Constipation, diarrhea, dry throat, dysphagia, nausea, vomiting, xerostomia
Genitourinary: Dysuria, urinary retention
Neuromuscular & skeletal: Tremor, weakness
Ocular: Accommodation impaired, blurred vision, conjunctival infection, cycloplegia, dryness, glaucoma (narrow-angle), increased intraocular pain, itching, photophobia, pupil dilation, retinal pigmentation
Respiratory: Dry nose, dyspnea
Miscellaneous: Anaphylaxis (rare), anaphylactic shock (rare), angioedema, diaphoresis decreased, heat intolerance, hypersensitivity reactions

Drug Interactions

Metabolism/Transport Effects None known.

Avoid Concomitant Use

Avoid concomitant use of Scopolamine (Systemic) with any of the following: Aclidinium; Azelastine (Nasal); Glucagon; Ipratropium (Oral Inhalation); Orphenadrine; Paraldehyde; Potassium Chloride; Thalidomide; Tiotropium; Umeclidinium

Increased Effect/Toxicity

Scopolamine (Systemic) may increase the levels/effects of: AbobotulinumtoxinA; Alcohol (Ethyl); Analgesics (Opioid); Anticholinergic Agents; Azelastine (Nasal); Buprenorphine; CNS Depressants; Glucagon; Hydrocodone; Methotrimeprazine; Metyrosine; Mirabegron; Mirtazapine; OnabotulinumtoxinA; Orphenadrine; Paraldehyde; Potassium Chloride; Pramipexole; RimabotulinumtoxinB; ROPINIRole; Rotigotine; Selective Serotonin Reuptake Inhibitors; Suvorexant; Thalidomide; Thiazide Diuretics; Tiotropium; Topiramate; Zolpidem

The levels/effects of Scopolamine (Systemic) may be increased by: Aclidinium; Brimonidine (Topical); Cannabis; Doxylamine; Dronabinol; Droperidol; HydrOXYzine; Ipratropium (Oral Inhalation); Kava Kava; Magnesium Sulfate; Methotrimeprazine; Mianserin; Nabilone; Perampanel; Pramlintide; Rufinamide; Sodium Oxybate; Tapentadol; Tetrahydrocannabinol; Umeclidinium

Decreased Effect

Scopolamine (Systemic) may decrease the levels/effects of: Acetylcholinesterase Inhibitors; Itopride; Secretin

The levels/effects of Scopolamine (Systemic) may be decreased by: Acetylcholinesterase Inhibitors

Preparation for Administration Solution for injection:
IM: Butylbromide: No dilution required.
IV:
Butylbromide: No dilution is necessary prior to injection.
Hydrobromide: Dilute with an equal volume of sterile water.

Storage/Stability

Solution for injection:
Butylbromide [Canadian product]: Store at room temperature. Do not freeze. Protect from light and heat. Stable in D_5W, $D_{10}W$, NS, Ringer's solution, and LR for up to 8 hours.
Hydrobromide: Store at room temperature of 20°C to 25°C (68°F to 77°F). Protect from light. Avoid acid solutions; hydrolysis occurs at pH <3.
Tablet [Canadian product]: Store at room temperature. Protect from light and heat.
Transdermal system: Store at 20°C to 25°C (68°F to 77°F).

Mechanism of Action Blocks the action of acetylcholine at parasympathetic sites in smooth muscle, secretory glands and the CNS; increases cardiac output, dries secretions, antagonizes histamine and serotonin

Pharmacodynamics/Kinetics

Onset of action: Oral, IM: 0.5-1 hour; IV: 10 minutes; Transdermal: 6-8 hours
Duration: IM, IV, SubQ: 4 hours
Absorption: IM, SubQ: Rapid; Oral: Quaternary salts (butylbromide) are poorly absorbed (local concentrations in the GI tract following oral dosing may be high)
Distribution: V_d: Butylbromide: 128 L
Protein binding: Butylbromide: ~4% (albumin)
Metabolism: Hepatic
Bioavailability: Oral: 8%
Half-life elimination: Butylbromide: ~5-11 hours; Hydrobromide: ~1-4 hours; Scopolamine base: 9.5 hours
Time to peak: Hydrobromide: IM: ~20 minutes, SubQ: ~15 minutes; Butylbromide: Oral: ~2 hours; Scopolamine base: Transdermal: 24 hours
Excretion: Urine (<10%, as parent drug and metabolites); IV: Butylbromide: Urine (42% to 61% [half as parent drug]), feces (28% to 37%)

Dosage Note: Scopolamine (hyoscine) hydrobromide should not be interchanged with scopolamine butylbromide formulations. Dosages are not equivalent.

Scopolamine base: Transdermal patch: Adults:
Preoperative: Apply 1 patch to hairless area behind ear the night before surgery or 1 hour prior to cesarean section (apply no sooner than 1 hour before surgery to minimize newborn exposure); remove 24 hours after surgery
Motion sickness: Apply 1 patch to hairless area behind the ear at least 4 hours prior to exposure and every 3 days as needed; effective if applied as soon as 2-3 hours before anticipated need, best if 12 hours before
Chemotherapy-induced nausea and vomiting, breakthrough (off-label use): Apply 1 patch every 72 hours (NCCN Antiemesis guidelines v.1.2012)

Scopolamine hydrobromide:
Antiemetic: SubQ:
Children: 0.006 mg/kg
Adults: 0.6-1 mg
Preoperative: IM, IV, SubQ:
Children 6 months to 3 years: 0.1-0.15 mg
Children 3-6 years: 0.2-0.3 mg
Adults: 0.3-0.65 mg
Sedation, tranquilization: IM, IV, SubQ: Adults:
U.S. labeling: 0.6 mg 3-4 times/day
Canadian labeling: 0.3-0.6 mg 3-4 times/day

Scopolamine butylbromide [Canadian product]: Gastrointestinal/genitourinary spasm: Adults:
Oral: Acute therapy: 10-20 mg daily (1-2 tablets); prolonged therapy: 10 mg (1 tablet) 3-5 times/day; maximum: 60 mg/day
IM, IV, SubQ: 10-20 mg; maximum: 100 mg/day

Elderly: Lower dosages may be required. Refer to adult dosing.

Dosage adjustment in renal impairment: No dosage adjustment provided in manufacturer's labeling. However, caution is recommended due to increased risks of adverse effects.

Dosage adjustment in hepatic impairment: No dosage adjustment provided in manufacturer's labeling. However, caution is recommended due to increased risks of adverse effects.

Administration Note: Butylbromide or hydrobromide may be administered by IM, IV, or SubQ injection.
IM: **Butylbromide:** Intramuscular injections should be administered 10-15 minutes prior to radiological/diagnostic procedures.
IV:
Butylbromide: No dilution is necessary prior to injection; inject at a rate of 1 mL/minute
Hydrobromide: Dilute with an equal volume of sterile water and administer by direct IV; inject over 2-3 minutes
Oral: Tablet should be swallowed whole and taken with a full glass of water.

Transdermal: Apply to hairless area of skin behind the ear. Wash hands before and after applying the disc to avoid drug contact with eyes. Do not use any patch that has been damaged, cut, or manipulated in any way. Topical patch is programmed to deliver 1 mg over 3 days. Once applied, do not remove the patch for 3 full days (motion sickness). When used postoperatively for nausea/vomiting, the patch should be removed 24 hours after surgery. If patch becomes displaced, discard and apply a new patch.

Monitoring Parameters Body temperature, heart rate, urinary output, intraocular pressure

Dosage Forms

Patch 72 Hour, Transdermal:

Transderm-Scop: 1.5 mg (1 ea, 4 ea, 10 ea, 24 ea)

Solution, Injection:

Generic: 0.4 mg/mL (1 mL)

Dosage Forms: Canada

Tablet, oral:

Buscopan: 10 mg

Solution, Injection:

Buscopan: 20 mg/mL (1 mL)

- **Scopolamine Base** *see* Scopolamine (Systemic) *on page 1870*
- **Scopolamine Butylbromide** *see* Scopolamine (Systemic) *on page 1870*
- **Scopolamine Hydrobromide** *see* Scopolamine (Systemic) *on page 1870*
- **Scopolamine Hydrobromide Injection (Can)** *see* Scopolamine (Systemic) *on page 1870*
- **Scopolamine, Hyoscyamine, Atropine, and Phenobarbital** *see* Hyoscyamine, Atropine, Scopolamine, and Phenobarbital *on page 1027*
- **Scorpion Antivenin** *see* *Centruroides* Immune F(ab')$_2$ (Equine) *on page 405*
- **Scorpion Antivenom** *see* *Centruroides* Immune F(ab')$_2$ (Equine) *on page 405*
- **Scot-Tussin Allergy Relief [OTC]** *see* DiphenhydrAMINE (Systemic) *on page 641*
- **Scot-Tussin® DM Maximum Strength [OTC]** *see* Dextromethorphan and Chlorpheniramine *on page 610*
- **Scot-Tussin Expectorant [OTC]** *see* GuaiFENesin *on page 986*
- **Scot-Tussin Senior [OTC]** *see* Guaifenesin and Dextromethorphan *on page 987*
- **Sculptra®** *see* Poly-L-Lactic Acid *on page 1676*
- **Sculptra® Aesthetic** *see* Poly-L-Lactic Acid *on page 1676*
- **SD/01** *see* Pegfilgrastim *on page 1589*
- **SDX-105** *see* Bendamustine *on page 241*
- **SDZ ENA 713** *see* Rivastigmine *on page 1833*
- **Se-100 [OTC]** *see* Selenium *on page 1876*
- **Sea-Clens Wound Cleanser [OTC]** *see* Sodium Chloride *on page 1902*
- **Sea-Omega 50 [OTC]** *see* Omega-3 Fatty Acids *on page 1507*
- **Sea Soft Nasal Mist [OTC]** *see* Sodium Chloride *on page 1902*
- **Seasonale (Can)** *see* Ethinyl Estradiol and Levonorgestrel *on page 803*
- **Seasonique** *see* Ethinyl Estradiol and Levonorgestrel *on page 803*
- **Se Aspartate [OTC]** *see* Selenium *on page 1876*
- **Seb-Prev [DSC]** *see* Sulfacetamide (Topical) *on page 1943*
- **Seb-Prev Wash** *see* Sulfacetamide (Topical) *on page 1943*

Secnidazole [INT] (sek NE da zol)

International Brand Names Ambese (VE); Amitab (IN); Bianos (EC, PE); Daksol (CO, VE); Deprozol (BR); Etisec (IN); Flagentyl (KR, PH, PT, TR, VN); Ke Ni (CL); Sabima (MX); Secfar (BR); Secnidal (CO, EC, PE); Secnil (IN); Secnol (FR, VN); Seczol (VE); Sha Ba Ke (CL); Tecnid (BR); You Ke Xin (CL)

Pharmacologic Category Antibiotic, Miscellaneous; Antiprotozoal

Reported Use Treatment of parasitic infections, including amebiasis, giardiasis, and *Trichomonas vaginalis*

Dosage Range Adults: Oral: 2 g single dose; tablets may be given with food to avoid gastrointestinal intolerance

Product Availability Product available in various countries; not currently available in the U.S.

Dosage Forms

Tablet: 500 mg

Secobarbital (see koe BAR bi tal)

Brand Names: U.S. Seconal

Index Terms Quinalbarbitone Sodium; Secobarbital Sodium

Pharmacologic Category Barbiturate

Additional Appendix Information

Beers Criteria – Potentially Inappropriate Medications for Geriatrics *on page 2271*

Use Preanesthetic agent; short-term treatment of insomnia

Pregnancy Risk Factor D

Dosage Oral: Adults:

Insomnia (hypnotic): Usual: 100 mg at bedtime. **Note:** Limit to short-term use only; efficacy for sleep induction and maintenance is lost after 14 days.

Preoperative sedation: 200-300 mg 1-2 hours before procedure

Elderly: Manufacturer's labeling recommends a dose reduction, but does not provide specific dosing recommendations.

Dosage adjustment in renal impairment: No specific dosage adjustment provided in manufacturer's labeling. However, a dosage reduction is recommended. Slightly dialyzable (5% to 20%).

Dosage adjustment in hepatic impairment: No dosage adjustment provided in manufacturer's labeling. However, dosage reduction is recommended.

Additional Information Complete prescribing information should be consulted for additional detail.

Dosage Forms

Capsule, Oral:

Seconal: 100 mg

- **Secobarbital Sodium** *see* Secobarbital *on page 1872*
- **Seconal** *see* Secobarbital *on page 1872*
- **Sectral** *see* Acebutolol *on page 29*
- **Sectral® (Can)** *see* Acebutolol *on page 29*
- **Secura Antifungal [OTC]** *see* Miconazole (Topical) *on page 1360*
- **Secura Antifungal Extra Thick [OTC]** *see* Miconazole (Topical) *on page 1360*
- **Seebri Breezhaler (Can)** *see* Glycopyrrolate *on page 975*
- **Selax [OTC] (Can)** *see* Docusate *on page 661*
- **Select 1/35 (Can)** *see* Ethinyl Estradiol and Norethindrone *on page 808*

Selegiline (se LE ji leen)

Brand Names: U.S. Eldepryl; Emsam; Zelapar

Brand Names: Canada Apo-Selegiline; Gen-Selegiline; Mylan-Selegiline; Novo-Selegiline; Nu-Selegiline

Index Terms Deprenyl; L-Deprenyl; Selegiline Hydrochloride

Pharmacologic Category Anti-Parkinson's Agent, MAO Type B Inhibitor; Antidepressant, Monoamine Oxidase Inhibitor

Use

Parkinson disease: Adjunct in the management of patients with Parkinson disease being treated with levodopa/carbidopa who exhibit deterioration in the quality of their response to therapy (oral products)

Major depressive disorder: Treatment of major depressive disorder (transdermal product)

Pregnancy Risk Factor C

Pregnancy Considerations Adverse events were observed in some animal reproduction studies.

Breast-Feeding Considerations It is not known if selegiline is excreted in breast milk. Due to the potential for serious adverse reactions in the nursing infant, breast-feeding is not recommended by the manufacturer.

Contraindications Hypersensitivity to selegiline or any component of the formulation; concomitant use of meperidine

Orally disintegrating tablet: Additional contraindications: Use with meperidine, methadone, propoxyphene, tramadol, MAO inhibitors (concurrently or within 14 days of discontinuing selegiline or one of these medications); use with St. John's wort, cyclobenzaprine, or dextromethorphan

Transdermal: Additional contraindications: Pheochromocytoma; use of carbamazepine, serotonin reuptake inhibitors (including SSRIs and SNRIs), clomipramine, imipramine, meperidine, tramadol, propoxyphene, methadone, pentazocine, and dextromethorphan (concurrently, within 2 weeks of selegiline discontinuation, or selegiline use within 4 to 5 half-lives (approximately 1 week; 5 weeks for fluoxetine) of discontinuation of the contraindicated drug); patients <12 years of age

Warnings/Precautions **Antidepressants increase the risk of suicidal thinking and behavior in children, adolescents, and young adults in short-term studies. Short-term studies did not show an increased risk in patients >24 years of age and showed a decreased risk in patients ≥65 years. Closely monitor patients for clinical worsening, and emergence of suicidal thoughts and behaviors,** particularly during the initial 1 to 2 months of therapy or during periods of dosage adjustments (increases or decreases); **the patient's family or caregiver should be instructed to closely observe the patient and communicate condition with health care provider.** A medication guide concerning the use of antidepressants should be dispensed with each prescription. **Transdermal selegiline is not FDA approved for use in children <12 years of age.**

The possibility of a suicide attempt is inherent in major depression and may persist until remission occurs. Worsening depression and severe abrupt suicidality that are not part of the presenting symptoms may require discontinuation or modification of drug therapy. Use caution in high-risk patients during initiation of therapy. Prescriptions should be written for the smallest quantity consistent with good patient care. The patient's family or caregiver should be alerted to monitor patients for the emergence of suicidality and associated behaviors such as anxiety, agitation, panic attacks, insomnia, irritability, hostility, impulsivity, akathisia, hypomania, and mania; patients should be instructed to notify their healthcare provider if any of these symptoms or worsening depression or psychosis occur.

Dopaminergic agents used for Parkinson disease or restless legs syndrome have been associated with compulsive behaviors and/or loss of impulse control, which has manifested as pathological gambling, libido increases (hypersexuality), uncontrolled spending of money, binge eating, and/or other intense urges. Causality has not been established, and controversy exists as to whether this phenomenon is related to the underlying disease, prior behaviors/addictions and/or drug therapy. Dose reduction or discontinuation of therapy has been reported to reverse these behaviors in some, but not all cases. The orally disintegrating tablets may cause new or worsening mental status and behavioral changes including hallucinations and psychotic-like behavior with initiation of therapy, after dose increases, or during the course of therapy. Symptoms may consist of paranoid ideation, delusions, hallucinations, confusion, psychotic-like behavior, disorientation, aggressive behavior, agitation, and delirium. Avoid use in patients with a major psychotic disorder. The transdermal product may precipitate a shift to mania or hypomania in patients with bipolar disorder. Monotherapy in patients with bipolar disorder should be avoided. Patients presenting with depressive symptoms should be screened for bipolar disorder, including a family history of suicide, bipolar disorder, and depression. **Selegiline is not FDA approved for the treatment of bipolar depression.** The orally disintegrating tablet may cause somnolence and episodes of sudden sleep onset, which may impair physical or mental abilities. Elderly patients, patients with current sleep disorders, and patients with concomitant sedating medications are at greatest risk. Patients must be cautioned about performing tasks that require mental alertness (eg, operating machinery or driving). Discontinue if significant daytime sleepiness or episodes of falling asleep occur; if a decision is made to continue therapy, advise patients not to drive and to avoid other potentially dangerous activities. The orally disintegrating tablet may potentiate the dopaminergic side effects of levodopa and cause dyskinesia or exacerbate preexisting dyskinesia requiring a reduction of the dose of levodopa.

Orally disintegrating tablet may cause orthostatic hypotension; use with caution in patients at risk of this effect or in those who would not tolerate transient hypotensive episodes (cerebrovascular disease, cardiovascular disease, hypovolemia, or concurrent medication use which may predispose to hypotension/bradycardia). Incidence may also be increased in older adults and when titrating to the 2.5 mg dosage in patients taking the orally disintegrating tablet. Monitor patients for new onset or exacerbation of hypertension. Risk for melanoma development is increased in Parkinson disease patients; drug causation or factors contributing to risk have not been established. Patients should be monitored closely and periodic skin examinations should be performed. Orally disintegrating tablets may cause irritation of buccal mucosa including swallowing pain, mouth pain, discrete areas of focal reddening, multiple foci of reddening, edema, and/or ulceration. Elderly patients have a greater incidence of adverse effects with orally disintegrating products. Use oral products with caution in patients with renal impairment; orally disintegrating tablets are not recommended in patients with severe renal impairment (CrCl <30 mL/minute) and ESRD. Use oral products with caution in patients with hepatic impairment; dosage adjustments may be necessary with orally disintegrating tablets in patients with mild to moderate hepatic impairment (Child-Pugh class A and B); orally disintegrating tablets are not recommended in patients with severe hepatic impairment (Child-Pugh class C).

Potentially life-threatening serotonin syndrome (SS) has occurred with serotonergic agents (eg, SSRIs, SNRIs) when used in combination with other serotonergic agents (eg, triptans, TCAs, fentanyl, lithium, tramadol, buspirone, St John's wort, tryptophan) or agents that impair metabolism of serotonin (eg, MAO inhibitors intended to treat psychiatric disorders, other MAO inhibitors [ie, linezolid and intravenous methylene blue]). Monitor patients closely for signs of SS such as mental status changes (eg, agitation, hallucinations, delirium, coma); autonomic instability (eg, tachycardia, labile blood pressure, diaphoresis); neuromuscular changes (eg, tremor, rigidity, myoclonus); GI symptoms (eg, nausea, vomiting, diarrhea); and/or seizures. Discontinue treatment (and any concomitant serotonergic agent) immediately if signs/symptoms arise. Potentially significant interactions may exist, requiring dose or frequency adjustment, additional monitoring, and/or selection of alternative therapy. Do not use the orally disintegrating product concurrently with other selegiline products; wait at least 14 days from discontinuation before initiating treatment with another selegiline dosage form. Transdermal patches may contain conducting metal (eg, aluminum); remove patch prior to MRI. Avoid exposure of application site and surrounding area to direct external heat sources (eg, heating pads, electric blankets, heat lamps, saunas, hot tubs); may increase drug absorption. Some products may contain phenylalanine.

Nonselective MAO inhibition occurs with transdermal delivery and is necessary for antidepressant efficacy. Hypertensive crisis as a result of ingesting tyramine-rich foods is always a concern with nonselective MAO inhibition. Although transdermal delivery minimizes inhibition of MAO-A in the gut, there is limited data with higher transdermal doses; dietary modifications are recommended with doses >6 mg/24 hours. Discontinue therapy immediately if hypertensive crisis occurs. With the oral product, MAO-B selective inhibition should not pose a problem with tyramine-containing products as long as the typical oral doses are employed, however, rare hypertensive reactions have been reported. Increased risk of nonselective MAO inhibition occurs with oral capsule/tablet doses >10 mg/day or orally disintegrating tablet doses >2.5 mg/day.

Abrupt discontinuation or interruption of antidepressant therapy has been associated with a discontinuation syndrome. Symptoms arising may vary with antidepressant however commonly include nausea, vomiting, diarrhea, headaches, lightheadedness, dizziness, diminished appetite, sweating, chills, tremors, paresthesias, fatigue, somnolence, and sleep disturbances (eg, vivid dreams, insomnia). Less common symptoms include electric shock-like sensations, cardiac arrhythmias (more common with tricyclic antidepressants), myalgias, parkinsonism, arthralgias, and balance difficulties. Psychological symptoms may also emerge such as agitation, anxiety, akathisia, panic attacks, irritability, aggressiveness, worsening of mood, dysphoria, mood lability, hyperactivity, mania/hypomania, depersonalization, decreased concentration, slowed thinking, confusion, and memory or concentration difficulties. Greater risks for developing a discontinuation syndrome have been associated with antidepressants with shorter half-lives, longer durations of treatment, and abrupt discontinuation. More severe symptoms have also been associated with MAO inhibitors. For antidepressants of short or intermediate half-lives, symptoms may emerge within 2 to 5 days after treatment discontinuation and last 7 to 14 days (APA, 2010; Fava, 2006; Haddad, 2001; Shelton, 2001; Warner, 2006).

Adverse Reactions

Cardiovascular: Chest pain, hyper-/hypotension (including postural), palpitation, peripheral edema

Central nervous system: Agitation, amnesia, ataxia, confusion, depression, dizziness, hallucinations, headache, insomnia, lethargy, pain, paresthesia, somnolence, thinking abnormal, vivid dreams

Dermatologic: Acne, bruising, pruritus, rash

Endocrine & metabolic: Hypokalemia, sexual side effects, weight loss

Gastrointestinal: Abdominal pain, anorexia, constipation, diarrhea, dyspepsia, dysphagia, flatulence, gastroenteritis, nausea, stomatitis, taste perversion, dental caries, vomiting

Genitourinary: Dysmenorrhea, metrorrhagia, urinary frequency, urinary retention, UTI

Local: Application site reaction

Neuromuscular & skeletal: Ataxia, back pain, dyskinesia, leg cramps, myalgia, neck pain, tremor

Otic: Tinnitus

Respiratory: Bronchitis, cough, dyspnea, pharyngitis, rhinitis, sinusitis

Miscellaneous: Diaphoresis

Rare but important or life-threatening): Abnormal liver function tests, alkaline phosphatase increased, appetite increased, arrhythmia, asthma, ataxia, atrial fibrillation, bacterial infection, behavior/mood changes, bilirubinemia, bradycardia, bradykinesia, breast neoplasm (female), breast pain, chorea, circumoral paresthesia, colitis, dehydration, delusions, depersonalization, depression, emotional lability, epistaxis, eructation, euphoria, face edema, fever, fungal infection, gastritis, generalized spasm, glossitis, heat stroke, hematuria (female), hernia, hostility, hypercholesterolemia, hyperesthesia, hyperglycemia, hyperkinesias, hypertonia, hypoglycemic reaction, hyponatremia, impulsive/compulsive behaviors (eg, pathological gambling, hypersexuality, binge eating), kidney calculus (female), lactate dehydrogenase increased, laryngismus, leukocytosis, leukopenia, libido increased, loss of balance, lymphadenopathy, maculopapular rash, manic reaction, melena, MI, migraine, moniliasis, myasthenia, myoclonus, neoplasia, neurosis, osteoporosis, otitis external, palpitation, paranoid reaction, parasitic infection, parosmia, pelvic pain, periodontal abscess, peripheral vascular disorder, pneumonia, polyuria (female), prostatic hyperplasia, rectal hemorrhage, salivation increased, skin hypertrophy, skin benign neoplasm, suicide attempt, syncope, tachycardia, tenosynovitis, tongue edema, twitching, urinary retention, urinary urgency (male and female), urination impaired (male), urticaria, vaginal hemorrhage, vaginal moniliasis, vaginitis, vasodilatation, vertigo, vesiculobullous rash, viral infection, visual field defect

Drug Interactions

Metabolism/Transport Effects Substrate of CYP1A2 (minor), CYP2A6 (minor), CYP2B6 (major), CYP2C8 (minor), CYP2D6 (minor), CYP3A4 (minor); **Note:** Assignment of Major/Minor substrate status based on clinically relevant drug interaction potential; **Inhibits** CYP1A2 (weak), CYP2A6 (weak), CYP2C19 (weak), CYP2D6 (weak), CYP2E1 (weak), CYP3A4 (weak), Monoamine Oxidase

Avoid Concomitant Use

Avoid concomitant use of Selegiline with any of the following: Alcohol (Ethyl); Alpha-/Beta-Agonists (Indirect-Acting); Alpha1-Agonists; Amphetamines; Anilidopiperidine Opioids; Antidepressants (Serotonin Reuptake Inhibitor/Antagonist); Apraclonidine; AtoMOXetine; Bezafibrate; Buprenorphine; BuPROPion; BusPIRone; CarBAMazepine; Cyclobenzaprine; Cyproheptadine; Dapoxetine; Dexmethylphenidate; Dextromethorphan; Diethylpropion; Hydrocodone; HYDROmorphone; Isometheptene; Levonordefrin; Linezolid; Maprotiline; Meperidine; Methyldopa; Methylene Blue; Methylphenidate; Mianserin; Mirtazapine; Morphine (Liposomal); Morphine (Systemic); OXcarbazepine; Oxymorphone; Pholcodine;

Pimozide; Pizotifen; Selective Serotonin Reuptake Inhibitors; Serotonin 5-HT1D Receptor Agonists; Serotonin/Norepinephrine Reuptake Inhibitors; Tapentadol; Tetrabenazine; Tetrahydrozoline (Nasal); Tricyclic Antidepressants; Tryptophan

Increased Effect/Toxicity

Selegiline may increase the levels/effects of: Alpha-/Beta-Agonists (Indirect-Acting); Alpha1-Agonists; Amphetamines; Antidepressants (Serotonin Reuptake Inhibitor/Antagonist); Antihypertensives; Antipsychotic Agents; Apraclonidine; ARIPiprazole; AtoMOXetine; Beta2-Agonists; Betahistine; Bezafibrate; Brimonidine (Ophthalmic); Brimonidine (Topical); BuPROPion; Cyproheptadine; Dexmethylphenidate; Dextromethorphan; Diethylpropion; Dofetilide; Domperidone; Doxapram; Doxylamine; EPINEPHrine (Nasal); Epinephrine (Racemic); EPINEPHrine (Systemic, Oral Inhalation); Hydrocodone; HYDROmorphone; Hypoglycemic Agents; Isometheptene; Levonordefrin; Linezolid; Lithium; Lomitapide; Meperidine; Methadone; Methyldopa; Methylene Blue; Methylphenidate; Metoclopramide; Mianserin; Mirtazapine; Morphine (Liposomal); Morphine (Systemic); Norepinephrine; Orthostatic Hypotension Producing Agents; OxyCODONE; Pimozide; Pizotifen; Reserpine; Selective Serotonin Reuptake Inhibitors; Serotonin 5-HT1D Receptor Agonists; Serotonin Modulators; Serotonin/Norepinephrine Reuptake Inhibitors; Tetrahydrozoline (Nasal); Tricyclic Antidepressants

The levels/effects of Selegiline may be increased by: Alcohol (Ethyl); Altretamine; Anilidopiperidine Opioids; Antiemetics (5HT3 Antagonists); Antipsychotic Agents; Buprenorphine; BusPIRone; CarBAMazepine; COMT Inhibitors; Contraceptives (Estrogens); Contraceptives (Progestins); Cyclobenzaprine; CYP2B6 Inhibitors (Moderate); Dapoxetine; Levodopa; MAO Inhibitors; Maprotiline; OXcarbazepine; Oxymorphone; Pholcodine; Quazepam; Tapentadol; Tedizolid; Tetrabenazine; TraMADol; Tryptophan

Decreased Effect

Selegiline may decrease the levels/effects of: Domperidone; Ioflupane I 123; Pipamperone [INT]

The levels/effects of Selegiline may be decreased by: CYP2B6 Inducers (Strong); Cyproheptadine; Dabrafenib; Domperidone; Pipamperone [INT]

Food Interactions Concurrent ingestion of foods rich in tyramine, dopamine, tyrosine, phenylalanine, tryptophan, or caffeine may cause sudden and severe high blood pressure (hypertensive crisis or serotonin syndrome). Beverages containing tyramine (eg, hearty red wine and beer) may increase toxic effects. Management: Avoid tyramine-containing foods (aged or matured cheese, air-dried or cured meats including sausages and salamis; fava or broad bean pods, tap/draft beers, Marmite concentrate, sauerkraut, soy sauce, and other soybean condiments). Food's freshness is also an important concern; improperly stored or spoiled food can create an environment in which tyramine concentrations may increase. Avoid foods containing dopamine, tyrosine, phenylalanine, tryptophan, or caffeine. Avoid beverages containing tyramine.

Storage/Stability

Capsule, tablet, transdermal: Store at 20°C to 25°C (68°F to 77°F). Store patch in sealed pouch and apply immediately after removal.

Orally disintegrating tablet: Store at 25°C (77°F); excursions permitted to 15°C to 30°C (59°F to 86°F). Use within 3 months of opening pouch and immediately after opening individual blister.

Mechanism of Action Potent, irreversible inhibitor of monoamine oxidase (MAO). Plasma concentrations achieved via administration of oral dosage forms in recommended doses confer selective inhibition of MAO type B, which plays a major role in the metabolism of dopamine; selegiline may also increase dopaminergic activity by interfering with dopamine reuptake at the synapse. When administered transdermally in recommended doses, selegiline achieves higher blood levels and effectively inhibits both MAO-A and MAO-B, which blocks catabolism of other centrally active biogenic amine neurotransmitters.

Pharmacodynamics/Kinetics

Onset of action: Therapeutic: Oral: Within 1 hour

Duration: Oral: 24 to 72 hours

Absorption:

Orally disintegrating tablet: Rapid; greater bioavailability than capsule/tablet. Food decreases C_{max} and AUC ~60%.

Transdermal: 25% to 30% (of total selegiline content) over 24 hours

Protein binding: ~90%; up to 85% (orally disintegrating tablet)

Metabolism: Hepatic, primarily via CYP2B6, CYP3A4, and CYP2A6 (minor) to active (N-desmethylselegiline, amphetamine, methamphetamine) and inactive metabolites

Half-life elimination: Oral: 10 hours; Transdermal: 18 to 25 hours

Excretion: Urine (primarily metabolites); feces

Dosage

Parkinson disease:

Adults:

Capsule/tablet: 5 mg twice daily with breakfast and lunch

Orally disintegrating tablet: Initial 1.25 mg once daily for at least 6 weeks; may increase to 2.5 mg once daily based on clinical response and tolerability (maximum: 2.5 mg once daily)

Elderly: Capsule/tablet: ≤5 mg/day (when combined with levodopa) is recommended by some clinicians to decrease the enhanced dopaminergic side effects (Olanow, 2001).

Depression:

Adults: Transdermal: Initial: 6 mg/24 hours once daily; may titrate based on clinical response in increments of 3 mg/day every 2 weeks up to a maximum of 12 mg/24 hours

Elderly: Transdermal: 6 mg/24 hours.

ADHD (off-label use): Children and Adolescents: Capsule/Tablet: Oral: 5 to 15 mg/day (Jankovic, 1993)

Discontinuation of therapy: Upon discontinuation of antidepressant therapy, gradually taper the dose to minimize the incidence of withdrawal symptoms and allow for the detection of re-emerging symptoms. Evidence supporting ideal taper rates is limited. APA and NICE guidelines suggest tapering therapy over at least several weeks with consideration to the half-life of the antidepressant; antidepressants with a shorter half-life and MAO inhibitors may need to be tapered more conservatively. In addition for long-term treated patients, WFSBP guidelines recommend tapering over 4 to 6 months. If intolerable withdrawal symptoms occur following a dose reduction, consider resuming the previously prescribed dose and/or decrease dose at a more gradual rate (APA, 2010; Bauer, 2002; Haddad, 2001; NCCMH, 2010; Schatzberg, 2006; Shelton, 2001; Warner, 2006).

MAO inhibitor recommendations:

Switching to or from an MAO inhibitor intended to treat psychiatric disorders:

Allow 14 days (or a time equal to 4 to 5 half-lives of the drug) to elapse between discontinuing an alternative antidepressant without long half-life metabolites (eg, TCAs, paroxetine, fluvoxamine, venlafaxine) or MAO inhibitor intended to treat psychiatric disorders and initiation of selegiline.

Allow 5 weeks to elapse between discontinuing fluoxetine (with long half-life metabolites) intended to treat psychiatric disorders and initiation of selegiline.

Allow 14 days to elapse between discontinuing selegiline and initiation of an alternative antidepressant or MAO inhibitor intended to treat psychiatric disorders.

Use with other MAO inhibitors (such as linezolid or IV methylene blue):

Do not initiate selegiline in patients receiving linezolid or IV methylene blue; consider other interventions for psychiatric condition.

If urgent treatment with linezolid or IV methylene blue is required in a patient already receiving selegiline and potential benefits outweigh potential risks, discontinue selegiline promptly and administer linezolid or IV methylene blue. Monitor for serotonin syndrome for 2 weeks or until 24 hours after the last dose of linezolid or IV methylene blue, whichever comes first. May resume selegiline 24 hours after the last dose of linezolid or IV methylene blue.

Dosage adjustment in renal impairment:

Oral:

Capsules/tablets: There are no dosage adjustments provided in the manufacturer's labeling (has not been studied). Use with caution.

Orally disintegrating tablet:

Mild to moderate impairment (CrCl 30 to 89 mL/minute): No dosage adjustments necessary.

Severe impairment (CrCl <30 mL/minute): Use is not recommended.

End-stage renal disease: Use is not recommended.

Transdermal:

eGFR ≥15 mL/minute/1.73 m^2: No dosage adjustment necessary.

eGFR <15 mL/minute/1.73 m^2: There are no dosage adjustments provided in the manufacturer's labeling (has not been studied).

ESRD requiring dialysis: There are no dosage adjustments provided in the manufacturer's labeling (has not been studied).

Dosage adjustment in hepatic impairment:

Oral:

Capsules/tablets: There are no dosage adjustments provided in the manufacturer's labeling (has not been studied). Use with caution.

Orally disintegrating tablet:

Mild to moderate impairment (Child-Pugh class A and B): 1.25 mg once daily.

Severe impairment (Child-Pugh class C): Use is not recommended.

Transdermal:

Mild to moderate impairment (Child-Pugh class A and B): No dosage adjustment necessary.

Severe impairment (Child-Pugh class C): There are no dosage adjustments provided in the manufacturer's labeling (has not been studied).

Dietary Considerations Avoid or limit tyramine-containing foods/beverages (product and/or dose-dependent). Some examples include aged or matured cheese, air-dried or cured meats (including sausages and salamis), fava or broad bean pods, tap/draft beers, Marmite concentrate, sauerkraut, soy sauce and other soybean condiments. Food's freshness is also an important concern; improperly stored or spoiled food can create an environment where tyramine concentrations may increase.

Transdermal: 9 mg/24 hours or 12 mg/24 hours: Avoid tyramine-rich foods or beverages beginning the first day of treatment or for 2 weeks after discontinuation or dose reduction to 6 mg/24 hours.

Orally disintegrating tablet: Do not take with food or liquid. Some products may contain phenylalanine.

Administration

Oral: Orally disintegrating tablet: Administer in morning before breakfast; place on top of tongue and allow to dissolve. Avoid food or liquid 5 minutes before and after administration.

Topical: Transdermal: Apply to clean, dry, intact skin to the upper torso (below the neck and above the waist), upper thigh, or outer surface of the upper arm. Avoid exposure of application site to external heat source, which may increase the amount of drug absorbed. Do not apply to skin that is hairy, oily, irritated, broken, scarred, or calloused. Apply at the same time each day and rotate application sites. Wash hands with soap and water after handling. Avoid touching the sticky side of the patch. Avoid tyramine-rich foods and beverages beginning on the first day of 9 mg/24 hours or 12 mg/24 hours doses; avoid tyramine-rich foods and beverages for 2 weeks following a dose reduction to 6 mg/24 hours or discontinuation of 9 mg/24 hours or 12 mg/hours.

Monitoring Parameters Blood pressure; symptoms of parkinsonism; general mood and behavior (increased anxiety, presence of mania or agitation); suicidal ideation (especially at the beginning of therapy or when doses are increased or decreased); periodic skin examinations

Additional Information When adding selegiline to levodopa/carbidopa, the dose of the latter can usually be decreased.

Dosage Forms

Capsule, Oral:

Eldepryl: 5 mg

Generic: 5 mg

Patch 24 Hour, Transdermal:

Emsam: 6 mg/24 hr (30 ea); 9 mg/24 hr (30 ea); 12 mg/24 hr (30 ea)

Tablet, Oral:

Generic: 5 mg

Tablet Dispersible, Oral:

Zelapar: 1.25 mg

Dosage Forms: Canada Note: Refer to Dosage Forms. Capsule, dispersible tablet, and transdermal patch are not available in Canada.

◆ **Selegiline Hydrochloride** *see* Selegiline *on page 1873*

◆ **Selenicaps-200 [OTC]** *see* Selenium *on page 1876*

◆ **Selenimin [OTC]** *see* Selenium *on page 1876*

◆ **Selenimin-200 [OTC]** *see* Selenium *on page 1876*

Selenium (se LEE nee um)

Brand Names: U.S. Aqueous Selenium [OTC]; Oceanic Selenium [OTC]; Se Aspartate [OTC]; Se-100 [OTC]; Se-Plus Protein [OTC]; Selenicaps-200 [OTC]; Selenimin [OTC]; Selenimin-200 [OTC]

Pharmacologic Category Trace Element, Parenteral

Use Trace metal supplement

Pregnancy Risk Factor C

Dosage Nutritional supplement:

Oral:

Adequate intake (AI):

1-6 months: 15 mcg/day

7-12 months: 20 mcg/day

Recommended daily allowance (RDA):

1-3 years: 20 mcg/day

4-8 years: 30 mcg/day

9-13 years 40 mcg/day

≥14 years and Adults: 55 mcg/day

Pregnancy: 60 mcg/day

Lactation: 70 mcg/day

IV in TPN solutions:
  Children: 3 mcg/kg/day
  Adults:
    Metabolically stable: 20-40 mcg/day
    Deficiency from prolonged TPN support: 100 mcg/day

Additional Information Complete prescribing information should be consulted for additional detail.

Dosage Forms

Capsule, Oral:
Selenicaps-200 [OTC]: 200 mcg

Capsule, Oral [preservative free]:
Se-100 [OTC]: 100 mcg

Liquid, Oral:
Aqueous Selenium [OTC]: 95 mcg/drop (15 mL)

Solution, Intravenous:
Generic: 40 mcg/mL (10 mL)

Tablet, Oral:
Oceanic Selenium [OTC]: 50 mcg, 200 mcg
Se Aspartate [OTC]: 50 mcg
Se-Plus Protein [OTC]: 200 mcg
Selenimin [OTC]: 125 mcg
Selenimin-200 [OTC]: 200 mcg
Generic: 50 mcg, 200 mcg

Tablet, Oral [preservative free]:
Generic: 50 mcg, 200 mcg

Tablet Extended Release, Oral [preservative free]:
Generic: 200 mcg

Selenium Sulfide (se LEE nee um SUL fide)

Brand Names: U.S. Anti-Dandruff [OTC]; Dandrex [OTC]; Selsun [DSC]; Tersi

Brand Names: Canada Versel®

Pharmacologic Category Topical Skin Product

Use Treatment of itching and flaking of the scalp associated with dandruff, to control scalp seborrheic dermatitis; treatment of tinea versicolor

Pregnancy Risk Factor C

Dosage Topical: Adults:

Dandruff, seborrhea: Massage 5-10 mL of shampoo into wet scalp, leave on scalp 2-3 minutes, rinse thoroughly. Usually 2 applications each week for 2 weeks will provide control. After this, may repeat at less frequent intervals (eg, once weekly, every 2-4 weeks). Rub foam into affected skin twice daily.

Tinea versicolor: Apply the 2.5% lotion to affected area and lather with small amounts of water; leave on skin for 10 minutes, then rinse thoroughly; apply every day for 7 days; rub foam into affected skin twice daily

Additional Information Complete prescribing information should be consulted for additional detail.

Dosage Forms

Foam, External:
Tersi: 2.25% (70 g)

Lotion, External:
Generic: 2.5% (118 mL, 120 mL)

Shampoo, External:
Anti-Dandruff [OTC]: 1% (207 mL)
Dandrex [OTC]: 1% (240 mL)

- ◆ **Selsun [DSC]** *see* Selenium Sulfide *on page 1877*
- ◆ **Selzentry** *see* Maraviroc *on page 1272*
- ◆ **Semprex®-D** *see* Acrivastine and Pseudoephedrine *on page 46*
- ◆ **Senexon-S [OTC]** *see* Docusate and Senna *on page 662*
- ◆ **Senna and Docusate** *see* Docusate and Senna *on page 662*
- ◆ **SennaLax-S [OTC]** *see* Docusate and Senna *on page 662*
- ◆ **Senna Plus [OTC]** *see* Docusate and Senna *on page 662*
- ◆ **Senna-S** *see* Docusate and Senna *on page 662*
- ◆ **Sennosides and Docusate** *see* Docusate and Senna *on page 662*
- ◆ **Senokot-S [OTC]** *see* Docusate and Senna *on page 662*
- ◆ **SenoSol-SS [OTC]** *see* Docusate and Senna *on page 662*
- ◆ **Sensipar** *see* Cinacalcet *on page 439*
- ◆ **Sensorcaine** *see* Bupivacaine *on page 299*
- ◆ **Sensorcaine® (Can)** *see* Bupivacaine *on page 299*
- ◆ **Sensorcaine-MPF** *see* Bupivacaine *on page 299*
- ◆ **Sensorcaine-MPF Spinal** *see* Bupivacaine *on page 299*
- ◆ **Se-Plus Protein [OTC]** *see* Selenium *on page 1876*
- ◆ **Septa-Amlodipine (Can)** *see* AmLODIPine *on page 123*
- ◆ **Septa-Atenolol (Can)** *see* Atenolol *on page 189*
- ◆ **Septa-Ciprofloxacin (Can)** *see* Ciprofloxacin (Systemic) *on page 441*
- ◆ **Septa-Citalopram (Can)** *see* Citalopram *on page 451*
- ◆ **Septa Losartan (Can)** *see* Losartan *on page 1248*
- ◆ **Septa-Metformin (Can)** *see* MetFORMIN *on page 1307*
- ◆ **Septa-Ondansetron (Can)** *see* Ondansetron *on page 1513*
- ◆ **Septa-Zopiclone (Can)** *see* Zopiclone [CAN/INT] *on page 2217*
- ◆ **Septra** *see* Sulfamethoxazole and Trimethoprim *on page 1946*
- ◆ **Septra DS** *see* Sulfamethoxazole and Trimethoprim *on page 1946*
- ◆ **Septra Injection (Can)** *see* Sulfamethoxazole and Trimethoprim *on page 1946*
- ◆ **Serax** *see* Oxazepam *on page 1532*
- ◆ **Serc (Can)** *see* Betahistine [CAN/INT] *on page 252*
- ◆ **Serevent Diskhaler Disk (Can)** *see* Salmeterol *on page 1860*
- ◆ **Serevent Diskus** *see* Salmeterol *on page 1860*
- ◆ **Serophene** *see* ClomiPHENE *on page 473*
- ◆ **SEROquel** *see* QUEtiapine *on page 1751*
- ◆ **Seroquel (Can)** *see* QUEtiapine *on page 1751*
- ◆ **SEROquel XR** *see* QUEtiapine *on page 1751*
- ◆ **Seroquel XR (Can)** *see* QUEtiapine *on page 1751*
- ◆ **Serostim** *see* Somatropin *on page 1918*

Sertaconazole (ser ta KOE na zole)

Brand Names: U.S. Ertaczo

Index Terms Sertaconazole Nitrate

Pharmacologic Category Antifungal Agent, Imidazole Derivative; Antifungal Agent, Topical

Use Tinea pedis: For the topical treatment of interdigital tinea pedis in immunocompetent patients 12 years of age and older, caused by *Trichophyton rubrum*, *Trichophyton mentagrophytes*, and *Epidermophyton floccosum*.

Pregnancy Risk Factor C

Dosage Topical: Children ≥12 years, Adolescents, and Adults: Tinea pedis: Apply between toes and to surrounding healthy skin twice daily for 4 weeks

Additional Information Complete prescribing information should be consulted for additional detail.

Dosage Forms

Cream, External:
Ertaczo: 2% (60 g)

- ◆ **Sertaconazole Nitrate** *see* Sertaconazole *on page 1877*

Sertindole [INT] (ser TIN dole)

International Brand Names Serdolect (AE, AR, AT, AU, BE, BG, CH, CZ, DE, DK, EE, ES, FI, GR, HR, HU, IE, IL, IS, KW, LB, MY, NL, NO, PH, PL, PT, QA, RO, RU, SE, SK, TR); Serlect (MX)

Pharmacologic Category Antipsychotic Agent, Atypical

Reported Use Treatment of schizophrenia

Dosage Range Adults: Oral: 4-24 mg/day; maximum dose: 24 mg/day

Product Availability Product available in various countries; not currently available in the U.S.

Dosage Forms

Tablet: 4 mg, 12 mg, 16 mg, 20 mg

Sertraline (SER tra leen)

Brand Names: U.S. Zoloft

Brand Names: Canada ACT Sertraline; Apo-Sertraline; Auro-Sertraline; Dom-Sertraline; GD-Sertraline; JAMP-Sertraline; Mar-Sertraline; MINT-Sertraline; Mylan-Sertraline; PHL-Sertraline; PMS-Sertraline; Q-Sertraline; Ran-Sertraline; ratio-Sertraline; Riva-Sertraline; Sandoz-Sertraline; Teva-Sertraline; Zoloft

Index Terms Sertraline Hydrochloride

Pharmacologic Category Antidepressant, Selective Serotonin Reuptake Inhibitor

Use

Major depressive disorder: Treatment of major depressive disorder (MDD) in adults.

Obsessive-compulsive disorder: Treatment of obsessions and compulsions in patients with obsessive-compulsive disorder (OCD).

Panic disorder: Treatment of panic disorder in adults with or without agoraphobia.

Post-traumatic stress disorder: Treatment of post-traumatic stress disorder (PTSD) in adults.

Premenstrual dysphoric disorder: Treatment of premenstrual dysphoric disorder (PMDD) in adults.

Social anxiety disorder: Treatment of social anxiety disorder (social phobia) in adults.

Pregnancy Risk Factor C

Pregnancy Considerations Adverse events have been observed in animal reproduction studies. Sertraline crosses the human placenta. An increased risk of teratogenic effects, including cardiovascular defects, may be associated with maternal use of sertraline or other SSRIs; however, available information is conflicting. Nonteratogenic effects in the newborn following SSRI/SNRI exposure late in the third trimester include respiratory distress, cyanosis, apnea, seizures, temperature instability, feeding difficulty, vomiting, hypoglycemia, hypo- or hypertonia, hyper-reflexia, jitteriness, irritability, constant crying, and tremor. Symptoms may be due to the toxicity of the SSRIs/SNRIs or a discontinuation syndrome and may be consistent with serotonin syndrome associated with SSRI treatment. Persistent pulmonary hypertension of the newborn (PPHN) has also been reported with SSRI exposure. The long-term effects of *in utero* SSRI exposure on infant development and behavior are not known.

Due to pregnancy-induced physiologic changes, women who are pregnant may require adjusted doses of sertraline to achieve euthymia. The ACOG recommends that therapy with SSRIs or SNRIs during pregnancy be individualized; treatment of depression during pregnancy should incorporate the clinical expertise of the mental health clinician, obstetrician, primary healthcare provider, and pediatrician. According to the American Psychiatric Association (APA), the risks of medication treatment should be weighed against other treatment options and untreated depression. For women who discontinue antidepressant medications during pregnancy and who may be at high risk for postpartum depression, the medications can be restarted following delivery. Treatment algorithms have been developed by the ACOG and the APA for the management of depression in women prior to conception and during pregnancy.

Breast-Feeding Considerations Sertraline and desmethylsertraline are excreted in breast milk. Adverse events have been reported in nursing infants exposed to some SSRIs. The American Academy of Breast-feeding Medicine suggests that sertraline may be considered for the treatment of postpartum depression in appropriately selected women who are nursing. Infants exposed to sertraline while breast-feeding generally receive a low relative dose and serum concentrations are not detectable in most infants. Sertraline concentrations in the hindmilk are higher than in foremilk. If the benefits of the mother receiving the sertraline and breast-feeding outweigh the risks, the mother may consider pumping and discarding breast milk with the feeding 7-9 hours after the daily dose to decrease sertraline exposure to the infant. The long-term effects on development and behavior have not been studied. The manufacturer recommends that caution be exercised when administering sertraline to nursing women. Maternal use of an SSRI during pregnancy may cause delayed milk secretion.

Contraindications

Use of MAOIs intended to treat psychiatric disorders (concurrently or within 14 days of stopping an MAOI or sertraline); concurrent use with pimozide; initiation in patients treated with linezolid or methylene blue IV; hypersensitivity to sertraline or any component of the formulation; concurrent use with disulfiram (oral concentrate only).

Documentation of allergenic cross-reactivity for SSRIs is limited. However, because of similarities in chemical structure and/or pharmacologic actions, the possibility of cross-sensitivity cannot be ruled out with certainty.

Warnings/Precautions [U.S. Boxed Warning]: Antidepressants increase the risk of suicidal thinking and behavior in children, adolescents, and young adults (18 to 24 years of age) with major depressive disorder (MDD) and other psychiatric disorders; consider risk prior to prescribing. Short-term studies did not show an increased risk in patients >24 years of age and showed a decreased risk in patients ≥65 years. Closely monitor patients for clinical worsening, suicidality, or unusual changes in behavior, particularly during the initial 1 to 2 months of therapy or during periods of dosage adjustments (increases or decreases); the patient's family or caregiver should be instructed to closely observe the patient and communicate condition with healthcare provider. A medication guide concerning the use of antidepressants should be dispensed with each prescription. **Sertraline is not FDA approved for use in children with major depressive disorder (MDD). However, it is approved for the treatment of obsessive-compulsive disorder (OCD) in children ≥6 years of age.**

The possibility of a suicide attempt is inherent in major depression and may persist until remission occurs. Use caution in high-risk patients. Worsening depression and severe abrupt suicidality that are not part of the presenting symptoms may require discontinuation or modification of drug therapy. The patient's family or caregiver should be alerted to monitor patients for the emergence of suicidality and associated behaviors (such as agitation, irritability, hostility, impulsivity, and hypomania) and call healthcare provider.

May precipitate a mixed/manic episode in patients at risk for bipolar disorder. Use with caution in patients with a family history of bipolar disorder, mania, or hypomania. Patients presenting with depressive symptoms should be screened for bipolar disorder. **Sertraline is not FDA approved for the treatment of bipolar depression.**

Potentially life-threatening serotonin syndrome (SS) has occurred with serotonergic agents (eg, SSRIs, SNRIs), particularly when used in combination with other serotonergic agents (eg, triptans, TCAs, fentanyl, lithium, tramadol, buspirone, St John's wort, tryptophan) or agents that impair metabolism of serotonin (eg, MAO inhibitors intended to treat psychiatric disorders, other MAO inhibitors [ie, linezolid and intravenous methylene blue]). Discontinue treatment (and any concomitant serotonergic agent) immediately if signs/symptoms arise. Has a very low potential to impair cognitive or motor performance. However, caution patients regarding activities requiring alertness until response to sertraline is known. Does not appear to potentiate the effects of alcohol, however, ethanol use is not advised.

Use caution in patients with a previous seizure disorder or condition predisposing to seizures such as brain damage, alcoholism, or concurrent therapy with other drugs which lower the seizure threshold. May increase the risks associated with electroconvulsive therapy. May cause mild pupillary dilation which in susceptible individuals can lead to an episode of narrow-angle glaucoma. Consider evaluating patients who have not had an iridectomy for narrow-angle glaucoma risk factors. Use with caution in patients with hepatic dysfunction and in elderly patients. May cause hyponatremia/SIADH (elderly at increased risk); volume depletion (diuretics may increase risk). Use caution in elderly patients; may be potentially inappropriate in patients with a history of falls or fractures, and may cause or exacerbate syndrome of inappropriate antidiuretic hormone secretion or hyponatremia; monitor sodium closely with initiation or dosage adjustments in older adults (Beers Criteria). Sertraline acts as a mild uricosuric; use with caution in patients at risk of uric acid nephropathy. Use with caution in patients where weight loss is undesirable. May cause or exacerbate sexual dysfunction. Potentially significant drug-drug interactions may exist, requiring dose or frequency adjustment, additional monitoring, and/or selection of alternative therapy.

Use oral concentrate formulation with caution in patients with latex sensitivity; dropper dispenser contains dry natural rubber. Monitor growth in pediatric patients. Given their lower body weight, lower doses are advisable in pediatric patients in order to avoid excessive plasma levels, despite slightly greater metabolism efficiency than adults.

Abrupt discontinuation or interruption of antidepressant therapy has been associated with a discontinuation syndrome. Symptoms arising may vary with antidepressant however commonly include nausea, vomiting, diarrhea, headaches, lightheadedness, dizziness, diminished appetite, sweating, chills, tremors, paresthesias, fatigue, somnolence, and sleep disturbances (eg, vivid dreams, insomnia). Greater risks for developing a discontinuation syndrome have been associated with antidepressants with shorter half-lives, longer durations of treatment, and abrupt discontinuation. For antidepressants of short or intermediate half-lives, symptoms may emerge within 2 to 5 days after treatment discontinuation and last 7 to 14 days (APA, 2010; Fava, 2006; Haddad, 2001; Shelton, 2001; Warner, 2006).

Adverse Reactions

Cardiovascular: Chest pain, palpitations

Central nervous system: Agitation, aggressive behavior (children ≥2%), anxiety, dizziness, drowsiness, fatigue, headache, hypertonia, hypoesthesia, insomnia, malaise, nervousness, pain, paresthesia, yawning

Dermatologic: Diaphoresis, skin rash

Endocrine & metabolic: Decreased libido, weight gain

Gastrointestinal: Abdominal pain, anorexia, constipation, diarrhea, dyspepsia, flatulence, increased appetite, nausea, vomiting, xerostomia

Genitourinary: Ejaculatory disorder, impotence, urinary incontinence (children ≥2%)

Hematologic & oncologic: Purpura (children)

Neuromuscular & skeletal: Back pain (≥1%), hyperkinesia (children ≥2%), myalgia(≥1%), tremor, weakness

Ophthalmic: Visual disturbance

Otic: Tinnitus

Respiratory: Epistaxis (children ≥2%), rhinitis, sinusitis (children ≥2%)

Miscellaneous: Fever (children ≥2%)

Rare but important or life-threatening: Acute renal failure, agranulocytosis, altered platelet function, anaphylactoid reaction, aplastic anemia, apnea, ataxia, atrial arrhythmia, atrioventricular block, bradycardia, cerebrovascular spasm, choreoathetosis, colitis, coma, cystitis, depression, diverticulitis, dystonia, edema, esophagitis, extrapyramidal reaction, hematuria, hemoptysis, hepatic failure, hepatitis, hepatomegaly, hypertension, hypoglycemia, hyponatremia, increased INR, increased serum bilirubin, increased serum transaminases, leukopenia, myocardial infarction, neuroleptic malignant syndrome, oculogyric crisis, orthostatic hypotension, pancreatitis, peptic ulcer bleed, peripheral ischemia, proctitis, prolonged Q-T interval on ECG, pulmonary hypertension, pyelonephritis, rectal hemorrhage, serotonin syndrome, SIADH, Stevens-Johnson syndrome, suicidal ideation, thrombocytopenia, torsades de pointes, ventricular tachycardia, withdrawal syndrome

Drug Interactions

Metabolism/Transport Effects Substrate of CYP2B6 (minor), CYP2C19 (minor), CYP2C9 (minor), CYP2D6 (minor), CYP3A4 (minor); **Note:** Assignment of Major/Minor substrate status based on clinically relevant drug interaction potential; **Inhibits** CYP1A2 (weak), CYP2B6 (moderate), CYP2C19 (moderate), CYP2C8 (weak), CYP2C9 (weak), CYP2D6 (moderate), CYP3A4 (weak)

Avoid Concomitant Use

Avoid concomitant use of Sertraline with any of the following: Dapoxetine; Disulfiram; Dosulepin; Iobenguane I 123; Linezolid; MAO Inhibitors; Methylene Blue; Pimozide; Thioridazine; Tryptophan; Urokinase

Increased Effect/Toxicity

Sertraline may increase the levels/effects of: Agents with Antiplatelet Properties; Anticoagulants; Antidepressants (Serotonin Reuptake Inhibitor/Antagonist); Antipsychotic Agents; Apixaban; ARIPiprazole; Aspirin; Beta-Blockers; BusPIRone; CarBAMazepine; Citalopram; CloZAPine; Collagenase (Systemic); CYP2B6 Substrates; CYP2C19 Substrates; CYP2D6 Substrates; Dabigatran Etexilate; Desmopressin; Dextromethorphan; Dosulepin; DOXOrubicin (Conventional); Eliglustat; Fesoterodine; Fosphenytoin; Galantamine; Highest Risk QTc-Prolonging Agents; Hydrocodone; Hypoglycemic Agents; Ibritumomab; Lomitapide; Methadone; Methylene Blue; Metoprolol; Moderate Risk QTc-Prolonging Agents; Nebivolol; NSAID (COX-2 Inhibitor); NSAID (Nonselective); Obinutuzumab; Phenytoin; Pimozide; Propafenone; RisperiDONE; Rivaroxaban; Salicylates; Serotonin Modulators; Thiazide Diuretics; Thioridazine; Thrombolytic Agents; Tositumomab and Iodine I 131 Tositumomab; TraMADol; Tricyclic Antidepressants; Urokinase; Vitamin K Antagonists

The levels/effects of Sertraline may be increased by: Alcohol (Ethyl); Analgesics (Opioid); Antiemetics (5HT3 Antagonists); Antipsychotic Agents; BusPIRone; Cimetidine; CNS Depressants; Dapoxetine; Dasatinib; Disulfiram; Glucosamine; Grapefruit Juice; Herbs (Anticoagulant/Antiplatelet Properties); Ibrutinib; Limaprost; Linezolid; Lithium; Macrolide Antibiotics; MAO Inhibitors; Metoclopramide; Metyrosine; Mifepristone;

Multivitamins/Fluoride (with ADE); Multivitamins/Minerals (with ADEK, Folate, Iron); Multivitamins/Minerals (with AE, No Iron); Omega-3 Fatty Acids; Pentosan Polysulfate Sodium; Pentoxifylline; Prostacyclin Analogues; Tedizolid; Tipranavir; TraMADol; Tryptophan; Vitamin E

Decreased Effect

Sertraline may decrease the levels/effects of: Clopidogrel; Codeine; Iobenguane I 123; Ioflupane I 123; Tamoxifen; Thyroid Products

The levels/effects of Sertraline may be decreased by: CarBAMazepine; Cyproheptadine; Darunavir; Efavirenz; Fosphenytoin; NSAID (COX-2 Inhibitor); NSAID (Nonselective); Phenytoin

Food Interactions Sertraline average peak serum levels may be increased if taken with food. Management: Administer consistently with or without food.

Preparation for Administration Oral concentrate: Must be diluted before use. **Immediately before administration**, use the dropper provided to measure the required amount of concentrate; mix with 4 ounces (1/2 cup) of water, ginger ale, lemon/lime soda, lemonade, or orange juice only. Do not mix with any other liquids than these. The dose should be taken immediately after mixing; do not mix in advance. A slight haze may appear after mixing; this is normal.

Storage/Stability Store at 25°C (77°F); excursions are permitted between 15°C and 30°C (59°F and 86°F).

Mechanism of Action Antidepressant with selective inhibitory effects on presynaptic serotonin (5-HT) reuptake and only very weak effects on norepinephrine and dopamine neuronal uptake. *In vitro* studies demonstrate no significant affinity for adrenergic, cholinergic, GABA, dopaminergic, histaminergic, serotonergic, or benzodiazepine receptors.

Pharmacodynamics/Kinetics

Onset of action: Depression: The onset of action is within a week, however, individual response varies greatly and full response may not be seen until 8-12 weeks after initiation of treatment.

Absorption: Area under the plasma concentration time curve (AUC) slightly increased and mean peak plasma concentrations (C_{max}) 25% greater when administered with food.

Protein binding: 98%

Metabolism: Hepatic; may involve CYP2C19 and CYP2D6; extensive first pass metabolism; forms metabolite N-desmethylsertraline (APA, 2010)

Bioavailability: Bioavailability of tablets and solution are equivalent

Half-life elimination: Sertraline: 26 hours; N-desmethylsertraline: 66 hours (range: 62-104 hours)

Time to peak, plasma: Sertraline: 4.5-8.4 hours

Excretion: Urine and feces

Dosage

Children 6-12 years: Oral:

Obsessive-compulsive disorder (OCD): Initial: 25 mg once daily. **Note:** May increase daily dose, at intervals of not less than 1 week, to a maximum of 200 mg daily.

Depression (off-label use): Initial: 12.5-25 mg once daily; titrate dose upwards if clinically needed; may increase by 25-50 mg daily increments at intervals of at least 1 week; mean final dose in 21 children (8-18 years of age) was 100 ± 53 mg or 1.6 mg/kg/day (n=11); range: 25-200 mg daily; maximum dose: 200 mg daily (Dopheide, 2006; Tierney, 1995); avoid excessive dosing

Adolescents 13-17 years: Oral:

Obsessive-compulsive disorder (OCD): Initial: 50 mg once daily. **Note:** May increase daily dose, at intervals of not less than 1 week, to a maximum of 200 mg daily.

Depression (off-label use): Initial 25-50 mg once daily; titrate dose upwards if clinically needed; may increase by 50 mg daily increments at intervals of at least 1 week; mean final dose in 13 adolescents was 110 ± 50 mg or about 2 mg/kg/day (McConville, 1996); in another study using a slower titration, the mean dose at week 6 was 93 mg (n=41) and at week 10 was 127 mg (n=34) (Ambrosini, 1999); range: 25-200 mg daily; maximum dose: 200 mg daily (Dopheide, 2006).

Adults: Oral:

Depression/obsessive-compulsive disorder: Initial: 50 mg daily. **Note:** May increase daily dose, at intervals of not less than 1 week, to a maximum of 200 mg daily.

Panic disorder, post-traumatic stress disorder (PTSD), social anxiety disorder: Initial: 25 mg once daily; increase to 50 mg once daily after 1 week; maximum dose: 200 mg daily

Premenstrual dysphoric disorder (PMDD): 50 mg daily either daily throughout menstrual cycle **or** limited to the luteal phase of menstrual cycle. Patients not responding to 50 mg daily may benefit from dose increases (50 mg increments per menstrual cycle) up to 150 mg daily when dosing throughout menstrual cycle **or** up to 100 mg day when dosing during luteal phase only. If a 100 mg daily dose has been established with luteal phase dosing, a 50 mg daily titration step for 3 days should be utilized at the beginning of each luteal phase dosing period.

Binge-eating disorder (off-label use): Initial: 25 mg daily after lunch for 3 days; increase at 25 mg increments every 3 days based on response and tolerability. Usual dose range: 100-200 mg daily. Maximum dose: 200 mg daily (Leombruni P, 2008).

Bulimia nervosa (off-label use): Initial: 50 mg daily; increase at 50 mg increments each week based on response and tolerability. Maximum dose: 200 mg daily (Milano 2004; Sloan 2003).

Generalized anxiety disorder (GAD) (off-label use): Initial dose: 25 mg once daily for 1week; increase based on response and tolerability. Maximum dose: 200 mg daily (Ball 2005; Brawman, 2006; Dahl, 2005).

Discontinuation of therapy: Upon discontinuation of antidepressant therapy, gradually taper the dose to minimize the incidence of withdrawal symptoms and allow for the detection of re-emerging symptoms. Evidence supporting ideal taper rates is limited. APA and NICE guidelines suggest tapering therapy over at least several weeks with consideration to the half-life of the antidepressant; antidepressants with a shorter half-life may need to be tapered more conservatively. In addition for long-term treated patients, WFSBP guidelines recommend tapering over 4-6 months. If intolerable withdrawal symptoms occur following a dose reduction, consider resuming the previously prescribed dose and/or decrease dose at a more gradual rate (APA, 2010; Bauer, 2002; Haddad, 2001; NCCMH, 2010; Schatzberg, 2006; Shelton, 2001; Warner, 2006).

MAO inhibitor recommendations:

Switching to or from an MAO inhibitor intended to treat psychiatric disorders:

Allow 14 days to elapse between discontinuing an MAO inhibitor intended to treat psychiatric disorders and initiation of sertraline.

Allow 14 days to elapse between discontinuing sertraline and initiation of an MAO inhibitor intended to treat psychiatric disorders.

Use with other MAO inhibitors (linezolid or IV methylene blue):

Do not initiate sertraline in patients receiving linezolid or IV methylene blue; consider other interventions for psychiatric condition.

If urgent treatment with linezolid or IV methylene blue is required in a patient already receiving sertraline and potential benefits outweigh potential risks, discontinue sertraline promptly and administer linezolid or IV methylene blue. Monitor for serotonin syndrome for 2 weeks or until 24 hours after the last dose of linezolid or IV methylene blue, whichever comes first. May resume sertraline 24 hours after the last dose of linezolid or IV methylene blue.

Dosage adjustment/comment in renal impairment: No dosage adjustment is provided in manufacturer's labeling; however, sertraline pharmacokinetics does not appear to be affected by renal impairment.

Dosage adjustment/comment in hepatic impairment: No specific dosage adjustment provided in manufacturer's labeling (has not been studied). Use with caution due to extensive hepatic metabolism and risk of increased exposure. A lower dose or less frequent dosing is recommended.

Administration Administer once daily either in the morning or evening; if somnolence is noted, administer at bedtime.

Oral concentrate: Must be diluted immediately before use. **Note:** Use with caution in patients with latex sensitivity; dropper dispenser contains dry natural rubber.

Monitoring Parameters Weight, height, BMI (longitudinal monitoring); mental status for depression, suicide ideation (especially at the beginning of therapy or when doses are increased or decreased), anxiety, social functioning, mania, panic attacks, or other unusual changes in behavior; signs/symptoms of serotonin syndrome.

Dosage Forms

Concentrate, Oral:

Zoloft: 20 mg/mL (60 mL)

Generic: 20 mg/mL (60 mL)

Tablet, Oral:

Zoloft: 25 mg, 50 mg, 100 mg

Generic: 25 mg, 50 mg, 100 mg

Dosage Forms: Canada

Capsule, Oral: 25 mg, 50 mg, 100 mg

◆ **Sertraline Hydrochloride** *see* Sertraline *on page 1878*

◆ **Serzone** *see* Nefazodone *on page 1435*

Sevelamer (se VEL a mer)

Brand Names: U.S. Renagel; Renvela

Brand Names: Canada Renagel; Renvela

Index Terms Sevelamer Carbonate; Sevelamer Hydrochloride

Pharmacologic Category Phosphate Binder

Use Reduction or control of serum phosphorous in patients with chronic kidney disease on hemodialysis

Pregnancy Risk Factor C

Pregnancy Considerations Adverse events were observed in animal reproduction studies. Sevelamer is not absorbed systemically; however, it may cause a reduction in the absorption of some vitamins.

Breast-Feeding Considerations Sevelamer is not absorbed systemically; however, it may cause a reduction in the absorption of some vitamins.

Contraindications Bowel obstruction

Warnings/Precautions Use with caution in patients with gastrointestinal disorders including dysphagia, swallowing disorders, severe gastrointestinal motility disorders (including constipation), or major gastrointestinal surgery. May cause reductions in vitamin D, E, K, or folic acid absorption. May bind to some drugs in the gastrointestinal tract and decrease their absorption; when changes in absorption of oral medications may have significant clinical consequences (such as antiarrhythmic and antiseizure medications), these medications should be taken at least 1 hour before or 3 hours after a dose of sevelamer. Tablets should not be taken apart or chewed; broken or crushed tablets will rapidly expand in water/saliva and may be a choking hazard.

Adverse Reactions

Endocrine & metabolic: Hypercalcemia, metabolic acidosis (more common in children)

Gastrointestinal: Abdominal pain, constipation, diarrhea, dyspepsia, flatulence, nausea, peritonitis (peritoneal dialysis), vomiting

Rare but important or life-threatening: Fecal impaction, intestinal obstruction (rare), intestinal perforation (rare)

Drug Interactions

Metabolism/Transport Effects None known.

Avoid Concomitant Use There are no known interactions where it is recommended to avoid concomitant use.

Increased Effect/Toxicity There are no known significant interactions involving an increase in effect.

Decreased Effect

Sevelamer may decrease the levels/effects of: Calcitriol; CycloSPORINE (Systemic); Levothyroxine; Mycophenolate; Quinolone Antibiotics; Tacrolimus (Systemic)

Food Interactions May cause reductions in vitamin D, E, K, or folic acid absorption. Management: Must be administered with meals. Consider vitamin supplementation.

Preparation for Administration Powder for oral suspension: Mix powder with water prior to administration. The 0.8 g packet should be mixed with 30 mL of water and the 2.4 g packet should be mixed with 60 mL of water (multiple packets may be mixed together using the appropriate amount of water).

Storage/Stability Store at controlled room temperature of 25°C (77°F); excursions permitted to 15°C to 30°C (59°F to 86°F). Protect from moisture.

Mechanism of Action Sevelamer (a polymeric compound) binds phosphate within the intestinal lumen, limiting absorption and decreasing serum phosphate concentrations without altering calcium, aluminum, or bicarbonate concentrations.

Pharmacodynamics/Kinetics

Onset of action: Reduction in serum phosphorus has been demonstrated after 1-2 weeks (Burke, 1997; Chertow, 1997).

Absorption: Not systemically absorbed

Excretion: Feces

Dosage Oral: **Note:** The dosing of sevelamer carbonate and sevelamer hydrochloride are similar; when switching from one product to another, the same dose (on a mg per mg basis) should be utilized.

Children (off-label use): In a pilot study of 17 pediatric patients aged 11.8 ± 3.7 years on hemodialysis (n=3) or peritoneal dialysis (n=14), initial doses of 121 ± 50 mg/kg/day (4.5 ± 5 g/day) were used. Doses were adjusted based on the serum phosphorus with final doses of 163 ± 46 mg/kg (6.7 ± 2.4 g/day) without any adverse effects (Mahdavi, 2003). In a study of 18 patients aged 0.9-18 years with chronic kidney disease, a mean dose of 140 ± 86 mg/kg/day (5.38 ± 3.24 g/day) resulted in good phosphorus control with minimal adverse effects. Initial doses were based on prior phosphate-binder dose and were adjusted based on the serum phosphorus (Pieper, 2006).

Adults: Patients not taking a phosphate binder: 800-1600 mg 3 times/day with meals; the initial dose may be based on serum phosphorous levels:

>5.5 mg/dL to <7.5 mg/dL: 800 mg 3 times/day

≥7.5 mg/dL to <9.0 mg/dL: 1200-1600 mg 3 times/day

≥9.0 mg/dL: 1600 mg 3 times/day

Maintenance dose adjustment based on serum phosphorous concentration (goal range of 3.5-5.5 mg/dL; maximum dose studied was equivalent to 13 g/day [sevelamer hydrochloride] or 14 g/day [sevelamer carbonate]):

>5.5 mg/dL: Increase by 400-800 mg per meal at 2-week intervals

3.5-5.5 mg/dL: Maintain current dose

<3.5 mg/dL: Decrease by 400-800 mg per meal

Dosage adjustment when switching between phosphate-binder products: 667 mg of calcium acetate is equivalent to ~800 mg sevelamer (carbonate or hydrochloride)

Conversion based on dose per meal:

Calcium acetate 667 mg: Convert to 800 mg Renagel/Renvela

Calcium acetate 1334 mg: Convert to 1600 mg as Renagel/Renvela (800 mg tablets x 2) **or** 1200 mg as Renagel (400 mg tablets x 3)

Calcium acetate 2001 mg: Convert to 2400 mg as Renagel/Renvela (800 mg tablets x 3) **or** 2000 mg as Renagel (400 mg tablets x 5)

Dosage adjustment in renal impairment: No dosage adjustment provided in manufacturer's labeling (has not been studied).

Dosage adjustment in hepatic impairment: No dosage adjustment provided in manufacturer's labeling.

Dietary Considerations Take with meals. Reduced levels of folic acid, and vitamins D, E, and K may occur; most hemodialysis patients in clinical trials received vitamin supplementation.

Administration Must be administered with meals.

Powder for oral suspension: Stir vigorously to suspend mixture just prior to drinking; powder does not dissolve. Drink within 30 minutes of preparing and resuspend just prior to drinking.

Tablets: Swallow whole; do not crush, chew, or break.

Monitoring Parameters

Serum chemistries, including bicarbonate and chloride

Serum calcium and phosphorus: Frequency of measurement may be dependent upon the presence and magnitude of abnormalities, the rate of progression of CKD, and the use of treatments for CKD-mineral and bone disorders (KDIGO, 2009):

CKD stage 3: Every 6-12 months

CKD stage 4: Every 3-6 months

CKD stage 5 and 5D: Every 1-3 months

Periodic 24-hour urinary calcium and phosphorus; magnesium; alkaline phosphatase every 12 months or more frequently in the presence of elevated PTH; creatinine, BUN, albumin; intact parathyroid hormone (iPTH) every 3-12 months depending on CKD severity

Reference Range

Corrected total serum calcium (K/DOQI, 2003): CKD stages 3 and 4: 8.4-10.2 mg/dL (2.1-2.6 mmol/L); CKD stage 5: 8.4-9.5 mg/dL (2.1-2.37 mmol/L); KDIGO guidelines recommend maintaining normal ranges for all stages of CKD (3-5D) (KDIGO, 2009)

Phosphorus (K/DOQI, 2003):

CKD stages 3 and 4: 2.7-4.6 mg/dL (0.87-1.48 mmol/L) (adults); maintain within age-appropriate limits (children)

CKD stage 5 (including those treated with dialysis): 3.5-5.5 mg/dL (1.13-1.78 mmol/L) (children >12 years and adults); 4-6 mg/dL (1.29-1.94 mmol/L) (children 1-12 years)

KDIGO guidelines recommend maintaining normal ranges for CKD stages 3-5 and lowering elevated phosphorus levels toward the normal range for CKD stage 5D (KDIGO, 2009)

Serum calcium-phosphorus product (K/DOQI, 2003): CKD stage 3-5: <55 mg^2/dL^2 (children >12 years and adults); <65 mg2/dL2 (children ≤12 years)

PTH: Whole molecule, immunochemiluminometric assay (ICMA): 1.0-5.2 pmol/L; whole molecule, radioimmunoassay (RIA): 10.0-65.0 pg/mL; whole molecule, immunoradiometric, double antibody (IRMA): 1.0-6.0 pmol/L

Target ranges by stage of chronic kidney disease (KDIGO, 2009): CKD stage 3-5: Optimal iPTH is unknown; maintain normal range (assay-dependent); CKD stage 5D: Maintain iPTH within 2-9 times the upper limit of normal for the assay used

Dosage Forms

Packet, Oral:

Renvela: 0.8 g (1 ea, 90 ea); 2.4 g (1 ea, 90 ea)

Tablet, Oral:

Renagel: 400 mg, 800 mg

Renvela: 800 mg

◆ **Sevelamer Carbonate** *see* Sevelamer *on page 1881*

◆ **Sevelamer Hydrochloride** *see* Sevelamer *on page 1881*

◆ **SfRowasa** *see* Mesalamine *on page 1301*

◆ **SGN-35** *see* Brentuximab Vedotin *on page 286*

◆ **SH 714** *see* Cyproterone [CAN/INT] *on page 530*

◆ **Sharobel** *see* Norethindrone *on page 1473*

◆ **Shingles Vaccine** *see* Zoster Vaccine *on page 2218*

◆ **Shohl's Solution (Modified)** *see* Sodium Citrate and Citric Acid *on page 1905*

◆ **Shopko Nasal Decongestant [OTC]** *see* Pseudoephedrine *on page 1742*

◆ **Shopko Nasal Decongestant Max [OTC]** *see* Pseudoephedrine *on page 1742*

◆ **Shur-Seal Contraceptive [OTC]** *see* Nonoxynol 9 *on page 1471*

◆ **Sig-Enalapril (Can)** *see* Enalapril *on page 722*

◆ **Signifor** *see* Pasireotide *on page 1583*

◆ **Signifor LAR** *see* Pasireotide *on page 1583*

◆ **Silace [OTC]** *see* Docusate *on page 661*

◆ **Siladryl Allergy [OTC]** *see* DiphenhydrAMINE (Systemic) *on page 641*

◆ **Silapap Children's [OTC]** *see* Acetaminophen *on page 32*

◆ **Silapap Infant's [OTC]** *see* Acetaminophen *on page 32*

Sildenafil (sil DEN a fil)

Brand Names: U.S. Revatio; Viagra

Brand Names: Canada ACT-Sildenafil; Apo-Sildenafil; GD-Sildenafil; Mint-Sildenafil; MYL-Sildenafil; PMS-Sildenafil; RAN-Sildenafil; ratio-Sildenafil R; Revatio; Sandoz-Sildenafil; Teva-Sildenafil; Viagra

Index Terms Sildenafil Citrate; UK92480

Pharmacologic Category Phosphodiesterase-5 Enzyme Inhibitor

Use

Revatio: Treatment of pulmonary arterial hypertension (PAH) (WHO Group I) in adults to improve exercise ability and delay clinical worsening.

Viagra: Treatment of erectile dysfunction (ED)

Pregnancy Risk Factor B

Pregnancy Considerations Adverse events were not observed in animal reproduction studies. Information related to the use of sildenafil for the treatment of pulmonary arterial hypertension (PAH) in pregnant women is limited (Hsu, 2011). Current guidelines recommend that women with PAH use effective contraception and avoid pregnancy (Badesch, 2007; McLaughlin, 2009). Less than 0.001% appears in the semen.

Breast-Feeding Considerations It is not known if sildenafil is excreted in breast milk. The manufacturer recommends that caution be exercised when administering sildenafil to nursing women.

Contraindications

Hypersensitivity to sildenafil or any component of the formulation; concurrent use (regularly/intermittently) of organic nitrates in any form (eg, nitroglycerin, isosorbide dinitrate).

According to the manufacturers of protease inhibitors (atazanavir, darunavir, fosamprenavir, indinavir, lopinavir/ritonavir, nelfinavir, ritonavir, saquinavir, tipranavir): Concurrent use with a protease inhibitor regimen when sildenafil is used for pulmonary artery hypertension (eg, Revatio).

Warnings/Precautions Decreases in blood pressure may occur due to vasodilator effects; use with caution in patients with left ventricular outflow obstruction (aortic stenosis, hypertrophic obstructive cardiomyopathy), those on antihypertensive therapy, with resting hypotension (BP <90/50 mm Hg), fluid depletion, or autonomic dysfunction; may be more sensitive to hypotensive actions. Patients should be hemodynamically stable prior to initiating therapy at the lowest possible dose. Use with caution in patients with uncontrolled hypertension (>170/110 mm Hg); life-threatening arrhythmias, stroke or MI within the last 6 months; cardiac failure or coronary artery disease causing unstable angina; safety and efficacy have not been studied in these patients. There is a degree of cardiac risk associated with sexual activity; therefore, physicians should consider the cardiovascular status of their patients prior to initiating any treatment for erectile dysfunction. If pulmonary edema occurs when treating pulmonary arterial hypertension (PAH), consider the possibility of pulmonary veno-occlusive disease (PVOD); continued use is not recommended in patient with PVOD. Substantial consumption of ethanol may increase the risk of hypotension and orthostasis. Lower ethanol consumption has not been associated with significant changes in blood pressure or increase in orthostatic symptoms. Have patients avoid or limit ethanol consumption.

Sildenafil should be used with caution in patients with anatomical deformation of the penis (angulation, cavernosal fibrosis, or Peyronie's disease) and in patients who have conditions which may predispose them to priapism (sickle cell anemia, multiple myeloma, leukemia). All patients should be instructed to seek medical attention if erection persists >4 hours. Painful erection >6 hours in duration has been reported rarely.

Vision loss, including permanent loss of vision, may occur and be a sign of nonarteritic anterior ischemic optic neuropathy (NAION). Risk may be increased with history of vision loss. Other risk factors for NAION include low cup-to-disc ratio ("crowded disc"), coronary artery disease, diabetes, hypertension, hyperlipidemia, smoking, and age >50 years. May cause dose-related impairment of color discrimination. Use caution in patients with retinitis pigmentosa; a minority have genetic disorders of retinal phosphodiesterases (no safety information available). Sudden decrease or loss of hearing has been reported; hearing changes may be accompanied by tinnitus and dizziness. A direct relationship between therapy and vision or hearing loss has not been determined.

The potential underlying causes of erectile dysfunction should be evaluated prior to treatment. Potentially significant drug-drug interactions may exist, requiring dose or frequency adjustment, additional monitoring, and/or selection of alternative therapy. Use of sildenafil is contraindicated in patients currently taking nitrate preparations. However, when nitrate administration becomes medically necessary, the ACCF/AHA 2013 guidelines on treatment of ST-segment elevation MI and the ACCF/AHA 2012 guidelines on treatment of unstable angina/non ST-segment elevation MI support administration of nitrates only if 24 hours have elapsed after use of sildenafil (ACCF/AHA [Anderson, 2013]; ACCF/AHA [O'Gara, 2013]). Hypersensitivity reactions, including anaphylactic reaction and anaphylactic shock, have been reported.

Avoid abrupt discontinuation, especially if used as monotherapy in PAH as exacerbation may occur. Use caution in patients with bleeding disorders or with active peptic ulcer disease; safety has not been established. Efficacy has not be established for treatment of pulmonary hypertension associated with sickle cell disease. Use with caution in the elderly, or patients with renal or hepatic dysfunction; dose adjustment may be needed. Use of Revatio, especially chronic use, is not recommended in children. After 2 years of treatment, increased mortality seen in long-term (median treatment exposure: 3.8 years) study at higher doses (20-80 mg [depending upon weight] 3 times/day) (Barst, 2012a; Barst, 2012b).

Benzyl alcohol and derivatives: Some dosage forms may contain sodium benzoate/benzoic acid; benzoic acid (benzoate) is a metabolite of benzyl alcohol; large amounts of benzyl alcohol (≥99 mg/kg/day) have been associated with a potentially fatal toxicity ("gasping syndrome") in neonates; the "gasping syndrome" consists of metabolic acidosis, respiratory distress, gasping respirations, CNS dysfunction (including convulsions, intracranial hemorrhage), hypotension, and cardiovascular collapse (AAP, 1997; CDC, 1982); some data suggests that benzoate displaces bilirubin from protein binding sites (Ahlfors, 2001); avoid or use dosage forms containing benzyl alcohol derivative with caution in neonates. See manufacturer's labeling. Oral suspensions may be available in multiple concentrations (commercially available: 10 mg/mL; extemporaneous preparation: 2.5 mg/mL); dosing should be presented in mg of sildenafil; use extra precaution when verifying product formulation and calculation of dose volumes. The 2 mL oral syringe provided by the manufacturer only provides measurements for fixed doses of 5 mg and 20 mg; for patients not receiving either of these fixed doses, an appropriate-size calibrated oral syringe will need to be dispensed.

Adverse Reactions Based upon normal doses for either indication or route. (Adverse effects such as flushing, diarrhea, myalgia, and visual disturbances may be increased with adult doses >100 mg/24 hours.)

Cardiovascular: Flushing

Central nervous system: Dizziness, headache, insomnia, paresthesia

Dermatologic: Erythema, skin rash

Gastrointestinal: Diarrhea, dyspepsia, gastritis, nausea

Genitourinary: Urinary tract infection

Hepatic: Increased liver enzymes

Neuromuscular & skeletal: Back pain, myalgia

Ophthalmic: Visual disturbance (including vision color changes, blurred vision, and photophobia)

Respiratory: Epistaxis, exacerbation of dyspnea, nasal congestion, rhinitis, sinusitis

Miscellaneous: Fever

Rare but important or life-threatening: Abnormal hepatic function tests, absent reflexes, amnesia (transient global), anemia, anorgasmia, anterior chamber eye hemorrhage, anterior ischemic optic neuropathy, arthritis, auditory impairment, breast hypertrophy, burning sensation of eyes, cardiac failure, cataract, cerebrovascular hemorrhage, colitis, cystitis, depression, diaphoresis, diplopia, dry eye syndrome, dysphagia, ECG abnormality, ejaculatory disorder, exfoliative dermatitis, falling, gastroenteritis, genital edema, gingivitis, glossitis, gout, herpes simplex infection, hyperglycemia, hypernatremia, hypersensitivity reaction, hypertension, hypertonia, hypoglycemia, increased bronchial secretions, increased intraocular pressure, ischemic heart disease, laryngitis, leukopenia, malignant melanoma (Li, 2014), migraine, myasthenia, mydriasis, myocardial infarction, neuralgia, neuropathy, orthostatic hypotension, otalgia, peripheral edema, pharyngitis, photophobia, priapism, prolonged erection, pulmonary hemorrhage, rectal hemorrhage, retinal edema, retinal hemorrhage, retinal vascular disease, rupture of tendon, seizure, severe sickle cell crisis (vaso-occlusive crisis in patients with pulmonary hypertension associated with sickle cell disease), skin photosensitivity, stomatitis, syncope, synovitis, tachycardia, transient ischemic attacks, unstable diabetes, urinary incontinence, ventricular arrhythmia, vitreous detachment, vitreous traction

Drug Interactions

Metabolism/Transport Effects **Substrate** of CYP1A2 (minor), CYP2C19 (minor), CYP2C9 (minor), CYP2D6 (minor), CYP2E1 (minor), CYP3A4 (major); **Note:** Assignment of Major/Minor substrate status based on clinically relevant drug interaction potential; **Inhibits** CYP2C9 (weak), CYP3A4 (weak)

Avoid Concomitant Use

Avoid concomitant use of Sildenafil with any of the following: Alprostadil; Amyl Nitrite; Boceprevir; Cobicistat; Conivaptan; Dapoxetine; Fusidic Acid (Systemic); Idelalisib; Phosphodiesterase 5 Inhibitors; Pimozide; Riociguat; Telaprevir; Vasodilators (Organic Nitrates)

Increased Effect/Toxicity

Sildenafil may increase the levels/effects of: Alpha1-Blockers; Alprostadil; Amyl Nitrite; Antihypertensives; ARIPiprazole; Bosentan; Dofetilide; HMG-CoA Reductase Inhibitors; Hydrocodone; Lomitapide; Phosphodiesterase 5 Inhibitors; Pimozide; Riociguat; Vasodilators (Organic Nitrates)

The levels/effects of Sildenafil may be increased by: Alcohol (Ethyl); Aprepitant; Boceprevir; Ceritinib; Cobicistat; Conivaptan; CYP3A4 Inhibitors (Moderate); CYP3A4 Inhibitors (Strong); Dapoxetine; Dasatinib; Erythromycin (Systemic); Fluconazole; Fosaprepitant; Fusidic Acid (Systemic); Idelalisib; Itraconazole; Ivacaftor; Ketoconazole (Systemic); Lorcaserin; Luliconazole; Mifepristone; Netupitant; Posaconazole; Protease Inhibitors; Sapropterin; Simeprevir; Stiripentol; Telaprevir; Voriconazole

Decreased Effect

The levels/effects of Sildenafil may be decreased by: Bosentan; CYP3A4 Inducers (Moderate); CYP3A4 Inducers (Strong); Dabrafenib; Deferasirox; Etravirine; Mitotane; Siltuximab; St Johns Wort; Tocilizumab

Food Interactions Grapefruit juice may increase serum levels/toxicity of sildenafil. Management: Avoid grapefruit juice.

Storage/Stability

Tablets/injection: Store at 20°C to 25°C (68°F to 77°F); excursions are permitted between 15°C and 30°C (59°F and 86°F).

Oral suspension: Store unreconstituted powder below 30°C (86°F); protect from moisture. Store reconstituted oral suspension below 30°C (86°F) or in refrigerator at 2°C to 8°C (36°F to 46°F). Do not freeze. Discard unused Revatio oral suspension after 60 days.

Mechanism of Action

Erectile dysfunction: Does not directly cause penile erections, but affects the response to sexual stimulation. The physiologic mechanism of erection of the penis involves release of nitric oxide (NO) in the corpus cavernosum during sexual stimulation. NO then activates the enzyme guanylate cyclase, which results in increased levels of cyclic guanosine monophosphate (cGMP), producing smooth muscle relaxation and inflow of blood to the corpus cavernosum. Sildenafil enhances the effect of NO by inhibiting phosphodiesterase type 5 (PDE-5), which is responsible for degradation of cGMP in the corpus cavernosum; when sexual stimulation causes local release of NO, inhibition of PDE-5 by sildenafil causes increased levels of cGMP in the corpus cavernosum, resulting in smooth muscle relaxation and inflow of blood to the corpus cavernosum; at recommended doses, it has no effect in the absence of sexual stimulation.

Pulmonary arterial hypertension (PAH): Inhibits phosphodiesterase type 5 (PDE-5) in smooth muscle of pulmonary vasculature where PDE-5 is responsible for the degradation of cyclic guanosine monophosphate (cGMP). Increased cGMP concentration results in pulmonary vasculature relaxation; vasodilation in the pulmonary bed and the systemic circulation (to a lesser degree) may occur.

Pharmacodynamics/Kinetics

Onset of action: ~60 minutes

Duration: 2-4 hours

Absorption: Rapid; slower with a high-fat meal

Distribution: V_{dss}: 105 L

Protein binding, plasma: ~96%

Metabolism: Hepatic via CYP3A4 (major) and CYP2C9 (minor route); forms N-desmethyl metabolite (active)

Bioavailability: 41% (25% to 63%)

Half-life elimination: ~4 hours; the elderly and those with severe renal impairment have reduced clearance of sildenafil and its active N-desmethyl metabolite

Time to peak: 30-120 minutes; delayed by 60 minutes with a high-fat meal

Excretion: Feces (~80%); urine (~13%)

Dosage

IV: Adults: Pulmonary arterial hypertension (PAH) (Revatio): 2.5 mg or 10 mg 3 times daily

Oral:

Adults:

Erectile dysfunction (Viagra): Usual dose: 50 mg once daily 1 hour (range: 30 minutes to 4 hours) before sexual activity as needed; dosing range: 25-100 mg once daily; maximum recommended dose: 100 mg once daily

PAH (Revatio): 5 mg or 20 mg 3 times daily, administered 4-6 hours apart; maximum recommended dose: 20 mg 3 times daily

Elderly >65 years: Use with caution.

Revatio: Refer to adult dosing.

Viagra: Starting dose of 25 mg should be considered.

Dosage considerations for patients stable on alpha-blockers: Viagra: Initial 25 mg

Dosage adjustment for concomitant use of potent CYP34A inhibitors:

Revatio:

Strong CYP3A inhibitors (eg, itraconazole, ketoconazole): Not recommended

Protease inhibitors: Concurrent use is contraindicated

Viagra:

Strong CYP3A inhibitors (eg, itraconazole, ketoconazole) or erythromycin: Starting dose of 25 mg should be considered

Protease inhibitors: Maximum sildenafil dose: 25 mg every 48 hours

Dosage adjustment in renal impairment:

CrCl ≥30 mL/minute:

Revatio: No dosage adjustment necessary.

Viagra: No dosage adjustment recommended.

CrCl <30 mL/minute:

Revatio: No dosage adjustment necessary.

Viagra: Starting dose of 25 mg should be considered.

Dosage adjustment in hepatic impairment:
Mild to moderate impairment (Child-Pugh classes A and B):
Revatio: No dosage adjustment necessary.
Viagra: Starting dose of 25 mg should be considered.
Severe impairment (Child-Pugh class C):
Revatio: There are no dosage adjustments provided in manufacturer's labeling (has not been studied).
Viagra: Starting dose of 25 mg should be considered.

Dietary Considerations Avoid grapefruit juice.

Administration
Revatio: Administer without regard to meals at least 4-6 hours apart. Shake oral suspension well before administering dose; do not mix with any other medication or additional flavoring agent. Administer injection as an IV bolus.
Viagra: Administer with or without food 30 minutes to 4 hours before sexual activity

Monitoring Parameters PAH: Monitor blood pressure and pulse when used concurrently with medications that lower blood pressure

Additional Information Sildenafil is ~10 times more selective for PDE-5 as compared to PDE6. This enzyme is found in the retina and is involved in phototransduction. At higher plasma levels, interference with PDE6 is believed to be the basis for changes in color vision noted in some patients.

Dosage Forms
Solution, Intravenous:
Revatio: 10 mg/12.5 mL (12.5 mL)
Suspension Reconstituted, Oral:
Revatio: 10 mg/mL (112 mL)
Tablet, Oral:
Revatio: 20 mg
Viagra: 25 mg, 50 mg, 100 mg
Generic: 20 mg

Extemporaneous Preparations A 2.5 mg/mL sildenafil citrate oral suspension may be made with tablets and either a 1:1 mixture of methylcellulose 1% and simple syrup NF or a 1:1 mixture of Ora-Sweet and Ora-Plus. Crush thirty sildenafil 25 mg tablets (Viagra) in a mortar and reduce to a fine powder. Add small portions of chosen vehicle and mix to a uniform paste; mix while adding vehicle in incremental proportions to **almost** 300 mL; transfer to a graduated cylinder, rinse mortar with vehicle, and add quantity of vehicle sufficient to make 300 mL. Store in amber plastic bottles and label "shake well". Stable for 90 days at room temperature or refrigerated.

Nahata MC, Morosco RS, and Brady MT, "Extemporaneous Sildenafil Citrate Oral Suspensions for the Treatment of Pulmonary Hypertension in Children," *Am J Health-Syst Pharm*, 2006, 63(3):254-7.

- **Sildenafil Citrate** *see* Sildenafil *on page 1882*
- **Silenor** *see* Doxepin (Systemic) *on page 676*
- **Silexin [OTC]** *see* Guaifenesin and Dextromethorphan *on page 987*
- **Silkis (Can)** *see* Calcitriol *on page 323*

Silodosin (SI lo doe sin)

Brand Names: U.S. Rapaflo
Brand Names: Canada Rapaflo®
Index Terms KMD 3213
Pharmacologic Category Alpha$_1$ Blocker
Use Treatment of signs and symptoms of benign prostatic hyperplasia (BPH)
Pregnancy Risk Factor B
Dosage Oral: Adults: BPH: 8 mg once daily with a meal
Dosage adjustment in renal impairment:
CrCl >50 mL/minute: No dosage adjustment necessary.
CrCl 30-50 mL/minute: 4 mg once daily
CrCl <30 mL/minute: Use is contraindicated.
Dosage adjustment in hepatic impairment:
Mild-to-moderate impairment (Child-Pugh class A or B): No dosage adjustment necessary.
Severe impairment (Child-Pugh class C): Use is contraindicated (has not been studied).

Additional Information Complete prescribing information should be consulted for additional detail.

Dosage Forms
Capsule, Oral:
Rapaflo: 4 mg, 8 mg

- **Silphen Cough [OTC]** *see* DiphenhydrAMINE (Systemic) *on page 641*
- **Siltussin DAS [OTC]** *see* GuaiFENesin *on page 986*
- **Siltussin DM [OTC]** *see* Guaifenesin and Dextromethorphan *on page 987*
- **Siltussin DM DAS [OTC]** *see* Guaifenesin and Dextromethorphan *on page 987*
- **Siltussin SA [OTC]** *see* GuaiFENesin *on page 986*

Siltuximab (sil TUX i mab)

Brand Names: U.S. Sylvant
Index Terms CNTO 328
Pharmacologic Category Antineoplastic Agent, Monoclonal Antibody; Interleukin-6 Receptor Antagonist

Use
Castleman disease: Treatment of patients with multicentric Castleman disease (MCD) who are human immunodeficiency virus (HIV) negative and human herpesvirus-8 (HHV-8) negative
Limitations of use: Has not been studied in patients with MCD who are HIV positive or HHV-8 positive because in a nonclinical study, siltuximab did not bind to virally produced IL-6

Pregnancy Risk Factor C

Pregnancy Considerations Adverse events were not observed in animal reproduction studies. However, decreased globulin levels were detected in the pregnant animals and their offspring. Infants born to pregnant women treated with siltuximab may be at increased risk for infection. Use during pregnancy only if the potential benefit outweighs the possible risk to the fetus. Women of childbearing potential should use effective contraception during and for 3 months following treatment discontinuation.

Breast-Feeding Considerations It is not known if siltuximab is excreted in breast milk. Because many immunoglobulins are excreted in breast milk and the potential for adverse reactions in the nursing infant exists, the manufacturer recommends a decision be made whether to discontinue nursing or to discontinue the drug, taking into account the importance of treatment to the mother.

Contraindications Severe hypersensitivity to siltuximab or any component of the formulation

Warnings/Precautions Discontinue infusion immediately if signs of anaphylaxis occur; do not reinitiate therapy. If a mild to moderate infusion reaction develops, temporarily discontinue the infusion; if the reaction resolves, may reinitiate at a lower rate. Consider premedication with acetaminophen, antihistamines, and corticosteroids. If infusion-related reactions recur despite appropriate premedication and infusion rate reduction, discontinue therapy. Administer in a setting equipped to provide resuscitation equipment; medications for the treatment of hypersensitivity reactions (eg, bronchodilators, epinephrine, antihistamines, and corticosteroids) should be readily available. Siltuximab may mask signs and symptoms of infection, including signs of acute inflammation (eg, fever, C-reactive protein elevation). Do not administer to patients with severe infections; monitor closely for infections and initiate appropriate antibiotic therapy if needed. If infection develops, withhold therapy until resolved. Siltuximab administration may result in elevated hemoglobin levels in patients with multicentric Castleman disease; monitor blood counts prior to each dose for the first 12 months and every 3 dosing cycles thereafter, or as clinically necessary. May require therapy interruption. Gastrointestinal perforation has been observed in clinical trials. Use with caution in patients at risk for perforation; promptly evaluate concerning symptoms. Do not administer live vaccines to patients receiving siltuximab; IL-6 inhibition may interfere with immune response to vaccination. Approved for use only in patients who are HIV negative and HHV-8 negative. Siltuximab was not studied in patients positive for these disease states due to the lack of drug binding to virally produced IL-6 in a nonclinical study.

Adverse Reactions

Cardiovascular: Hypotension, peripheral edema

Central nervous system: Fatigue (long-term exposure), headache

Dermatologic: Eczema, pruritus, psoriasis, skin hyperpigmentation, skin rash, xeroderma

Endocrine & metabolic: Dehydration, hypercholesterolemia, hypertriglyceridemia, hyperuricemia, weight gain

Gastrointestinal: Abdominal pain, constipation, decreased appetite, diarrhea (long-term exposure)

Hematologic & oncologic: Thrombocytopenia

Neuromuscular & skeletal: Arthralgia (long-term exposure), limb pain (long-term exposure)

Renal: Renal insufficiency

Respiratory: Lower respiratory tract infection, oropharyngeal pain, upper respiratory tract infection (more common with long-term exposure)

Miscellaneous: Infusion related reaction

Drug Interactions

Metabolism/Transport Effects None known.

Avoid Concomitant Use

Avoid concomitant use of Siltuximab with any of the following: BCG; Belimumab; Natalizumab; Pimecrolimus; Tacrolimus (Topical); Tofacitinib; Vaccines (Live)

Increased Effect/Toxicity

Siltuximab may increase the levels/effects of: Belimumab; Leflunomide; Natalizumab; Tofacitinib; Vaccines (Live)

The levels/effects of Siltuximab may be increased by: Denosumab; Pimecrolimus; Roflumilast; Tacrolimus (Topical); Trastuzumab

Decreased Effect

Siltuximab may decrease the levels/effects of: BCG; Coccidioides immitis Skin Test; CYP3A4 Substrates; Sipuleucel-T; Vaccines (Inactivated); Vaccines (Live)

The levels/effects of Siltuximab may be decreased by: Echinacea

Preparation for Administration Allow intact vials to come to room temperature (~30 minutes). Reconstitute with 5.2 mL (100 mg vial) or 20 mL (400 mg vial) SWFI to a final concentration of 20 mg/mL; gently swirl to fully dissolve powder. Do not shake or swirl vigorously. Must further dilute within 2 hours to 250 mL with D_5W (infusion bag must be made of polyvinyl chloride (PVC) with di-[2-ethylhexyl]phthalate (DEHP) or polyolefin). Remove a volume equal to the total calculated dose volume of reconstituted siltuximab from the bag of D_5W; slowly add the appropriate volume of reconstituted siltuximab solution to the infusion bag and gently invert to mix. Complete infusion within 4 hours of dilution of the reconstituted solution to the infusion bag.

Storage/Stability Store intact vials at 2°C to 8°C (36°F to 46°F); protect from light. Reconstituted solution should be further diluted for infusion within 2 hours; complete infusion within 4 hours of dilution of the reconstituted solution to the infusion bag. Discard any unused portion of the reconstituted solution or solution diluted for infusion.

Mechanism of Action Chimeric monoclonal antibody which binds with high affinity and specificity to IL-6; prevents IL-6 from binding to both soluble and membrane-bound IL-6 receptors. Overproduction of IL-6 may lead to systemic manifestations in multicentric Castleman disease (MCD) patients by inducing C-reactive protein (CRP) synthesis (Kurzrock, 2010). Lowering serum IL-6 levels may improve systemic symptoms of Castleman disease.

Pharmacodynamics/Kinetics

Distribution: 4.5 L

Half-life elimination: ~21 days (range: 14.2 to 29.7 days)

Dosage Note: Consider delaying first dose if ANC <1000/mm³, platelets <75,000/mm³, and hemoglobin ≥17 g/dL; subsequent doses may be delayed if ANC <1000/mm³, platelets <50,000/mm³, and hemoglobin ≥17 g/dL. Do not reduce dose.

Castleman disease, multicentric (in patients who are HIV negative and HHV-8 negative): Adults: IV: 11 mg/kg over 1 hour every 3 weeks until treatment failure

Dosage adjustment for toxicity:

Hematologic toxicity: ANC <1000/mm³, platelets <50,000/mm³, and hemoglobin ≥17 g/dL: Consider delaying treatment until ANC ≥1000/mm³, platelets ≥50,000/mm³, and hemoglobin <17 g/dL

Anaphylaxis, cytokine release syndromes, and/or severe infusion-related or allergic reactions: Discontinue permanently.

Infection, severe: Withhold treatment until infection resolves.

Dosage adjustment for renal impairment:

CrCl ≥15 mL/minute: No initial dosage adjustment is necessary.

CrCl <15 mL/minute: There are no dosage adjustments provided in the manufacturer's labeling (has not been studied).

End-stage renal disease (ESRD): There are no dosage adjustments provided in the manufacturer's labeling (has not been studied).

Dosage adjustment for hepatic impairment:

Mild to moderate impairment (Child Pugh class A or B): No initial dosage adjustment is necessary.

Severe impairment (Child Pugh class C): There are no dosage adjustments provided in the manufacturer's labeling (has not been studied).

Administration Administer IV over 1 hour using administration sets lined with polyvinyl chloride (PVC) with di-[2-ethylhexyl]phthalate (DEHP) or polyurethane (PU) which contain a 0.2 micron inline polyethersulfone (PES) filter. Do not infuse in the same line with other medications. Complete infusion within 4 hours of dilution of the reconstituted solution to the infusion bag.

Monitoring Parameters Monitor complete blood count with differential prior to each dose for the first 12 months and every 3 dosing cycles thereafter, or as clinically necessary; monitor for anaphylaxis and signs/symptoms of infusion-related, allergic, or cytokine release reactions; monitor for infection and signs/symptoms of gastrointestinal perforation.

Dosage Forms

Solution Reconstituted, Intravenous [preservative free]: Sylvant: 100 mg (1 ea); 400 mg (1 ea)

◆ **Silvadene** *see* Silver Sulfadiazine *on page 1887*

◆ **Silver Bullet Suppository [OTC] (Can)** *see* Bisacodyl *on page 265*

Silver Nitrate (SIL ver NYE trate)

Index Terms $AgNO_3$

Pharmacologic Category Antibiotic, Topical; Cauterizing Agent, Topical; Topical Skin Product, Antibacterial

Use Astringent, cauterization of wounds, germicidal, removal of granulation tissue, corns, and warts

Dosage Children and Adults:

Sticks: Apply to mucous membranes and other moist skin surfaces only on area to be treated

Topical solution: Usual: Apply a cotton applicator dipped in solution on the affected area 2-3 times/week for 2-3 weeks

Additional Information Complete prescribing information should be consulted for additional detail.

Dosage Forms

Applicator sticks, topical: Silver nitrate 75% and potassium 25%

Solution, topical: 0.5% (960 mL); 10% (30 mL); 25% (30 mL); 50% (30 mL)

Silver Sulfadiazine (SIL ver sul fa DYE a zeen)

Brand Names: U.S. Silvadene; SSD; Thermazene [DSC]

Brand Names: Canada Flamazine®

Pharmacologic Category Antibiotic, Topical

Use Prevention and treatment of infection in second and third degree burns

Pregnancy Risk Factor B

Dosage Children and Adults: Topical: Apply once or twice daily with a sterile-gloved hand; apply to a thickness of 1/16"; burned area should be covered with cream at all times

Additional Information Complete prescribing information should be consulted for additional detail.

Dosage Forms

Cream, External:

Silvadene: 1% (20 g, 50 g, 85 g, 400 g, 1000 g)

SSD: 1% (25 g, 50 g, 85 g, 400 g)

Generic: 1% (20 g, 25 g, 50 g, 85 g, 400 g)

Simeprevir (sim E pre vir)

Brand Names: U.S. Olysio

Brand Names: Canada Galexos

Index Terms TMC435

Pharmacologic Category Antihepaciviral, Protease Inhibitor (Anti-HCV)

Use

Chronic hepatitis C: Treatment of genotype 1 chronic hepatitis C (in combination with other antihepacivirals)

Limitations of use: Not for use as monotherapy; when used in combination with peginterferon alfa and ribavirin, screening patients with HCV genotype 1a infection for the presence of virus with the NS3 Q80k polymorphism is strongly recommended (if detected, consider alternative therapy); not recommended for use in patients who have previously failed a simeprevir-containing regimen or another regimen containing HCV protease inhibitors.

Pregnancy Risk Factor C

Pregnancy Considerations Adverse events were observed in animal reproduction studies. Women of reproductive potential should use effective contraception during therapy. Treatment of HCV is not recommended for women who are already pregnant (AASLD, 2014).

If simeprevir is used in combination with ribavirin all warnings related to the use of ribavirin and pregnancy and/or contraception should be followed. Current guidelines note that ribavirin should not be used in pregnant women and males with female partners who are pregnant. A negative pregnancy test is required before initiation. Female patients (and their male partners) as well as male patients (and their female partners) should use two forms of effective contraception during therapy and for 6 months after therapy is discontinued. Pregnancy testing should be done at appropriate intervals (AASLD, 2014).

Breast-Feeding Considerations It is not known if simeprevir is excreted into breast milk. Due to the potential for serious adverse reactions in the nursing infant, the manufacturer recommends a decision be made whether to discontinue nursing or to discontinue the drug, taking into account the importance of treatment to the mother.

Contraindications

There are no contraindications listed in the manufacturer's labeling, however, all contraindications to other antihepaciviral drugs used in combination with simeprevir for the treatment of chronic hepatitis C infection also apply to their use in a simeprevir-containing regimen; refer to each monograph for individual product contraindications

Canadian labeling: Additional contraindications (not in U.S. labeling): Hypersensitivity to simeprevir or any component of the formulation

Warnings/Precautions Reduced sustained virologic response (SVR) rates of simeprevir in combination with peginterferon alfa and ribavirin were observed in patients infected with hepatitis C genotype 1a with an NS3 Q80K polymorphism at baseline compared to patients without the polymorphism; consider alternative therapy in these patients. Test hepatitis C genotype 1a patients treated with simeprevir in combination with peginterferon alfa and ribavirin prior to treatment initiation for the Q80K polymorphism; consider testing in hepatitis C genotype 1a patients treated with simeprevir in combination with sofosbuvir (AASLD/IDSA, 2014).

Higher simeprevir exposures have been associated with an increased risk of adverse effects (including rash and photosensitivity) in people of East Asian ancestry. An appropriate dose in these patients has not been determined. Use with caution. Rash has been typically observed within first 4 weeks of therapy initiation but may occur at any time. Severe rashes and rash requiring discontinuation have occurred in combination with peginterferon alfa and ribavirin. If a patient experiences a mild to moderate rash, follow for progression and/or development of mucosal signs (eg, oral lesions, conjunctivitis) or systemic symptoms. If rash becomes severe, discontinue simeprevir and monitor for rash resolution. Avoid excessive sunlight, tanning devices, and take precautions to limit exposure (eg, loose fitting clothing, sunscreen); may cause moderate to severe phototoxicity reactions (exaggerated sunburn appearance, burning, erythema, exudation, blistering, and edema). Most reactions have occurred within the first 4 weeks of therapy. Discontinue use if photosensitivity occurs and monitor until the reaction resolves. If therapy is to be continued in a patient who has experienced photosensitivity, expert consultation is advised. Contains a sulfonamide moiety. In patients with a history of sulfa allergy, no increased incidence of rash or photosensitivity has been reported, although the risk of reaction (or potential severity) cannot be excluded. Discontinue if signs of hypersensitivity are noted.

U.S. manufacturer's labeling does not recommend use in severe hepatic impairment (Child-Pugh class C). Do not administer in combination with peginterferon and ribavirin patients with decompensated cirrhosis (moderate to severe hepatic impairment [Child-Pugh class B or C]). Combination therapy with ribavirin may cause birth defects; avoid pregnancy in females and female partners of male patients. Combination therapy with ribavirin is contraindicated in pregnancy. Use 2 effective forms of contraception during treatment and for 6 months after completion of treatment. Do not use as monotherapy. See other agents for additional warnings and precautions associated with their use. Safety and efficacy have not been established in patients who have received liver transplants, who have HCV genotypes other than genotype 1, or who have failed to respond to other HCV direct-acting inhibitors or on repeated courses of simeprevir. Potentially significant drug-drug interactions may exist, requiring dose or frequency adjustments, additional monitoring, and/or selection of alternative therapy.

Adverse Reactions Reported for combination therapy with peginterferon alfa and ribavirin (Peg-IFN-alfa and RBV) unless otherwise noted.

Central nervous system: Dizziness (with sofosbuvir), fatigue (with sofosbuvir), headache (with sofosbuvir), insomnia (with sofosbuvir)

Dermatologic: Pruritus (more common with Peg-IFN-alfa and RBV), skin photosensitivity (slightly more common with sofosbuvir than with Peg-IFN-alfa and RBV), skin rash (with Peg-IFN-alfa and RBV; including erythema, eczema, rash maculopapular, urticaria, toxic skin eruption, dermatitis exfoliative, cutaneous vasculitis, photosensitivity reaction)

Gastrointestinal: Diarrhea (with sofosbuvir), nausea (slightly more common with Peg-IFN-alfa and RBV)

Hepatic: Increased serum alkaline phosphatase, increased serum bilirubin

Neuromuscular & skeletal: Myalgia

Respiratory: Dyspnea

Drug Interactions

Metabolism/Transport Effects Substrate of CYP3A4 (major), P-glycoprotein, SLCO1B1; **Note:** Assignment of Major/Minor substrate status based on clinically relevant drug interaction potential; **Inhibits** CYP1A2 (weak), P-glycoprotein, SLCO1B1

Avoid Concomitant Use

Avoid concomitant use of Simeprevir with any of the following: Bosutinib; Cisapride; Conivaptan; CycloSPORINE (Systemic); CYP3A4 Inducers (Moderate); CYP3A4 Inducers (Strong); CYP3A4 Inhibitors (Moderate); CYP3A4 Inhibitors (Strong); Erythromycin (Systemic); Fusidic Acid (Systemic); Idelalisib; Ledipasvir; Milk Thistle; PAZOPanib; Protease Inhibitors; Silodosin; St Johns Wort; Topotecan; VinCRIStine (Liposomal)

Increased Effect/Toxicity

Simeprevir may increase the levels/effects of: Afatinib; AtorvaSTATin; Bosutinib; Brentuximab Vedotin; Cisapride; Colchicine; CycloSPORINE (Systemic); CYP3A4 Substrates; Dabigatran Etexilate; Digoxin; DOXOrubicin (Conventional); Edoxaban; Everolimus; Ledipasvir; Lovastatin; Midazolam; Naloxegol; PAZOPanib; P-glycoprotein/ABCB1 Substrates; Phosphodiesterase 5 Inhibitors; Pitavastatin; Porfimer; Pravastatin; Protease Inhibitors; Prucalopride; Rifaximin; Rilpivirine; Rivaroxaban; Rosuvastatin; Silodosin; Simvastatin; Tenofovir; Topotecan; Triazolam; Verteporfin; VinCRIStine (Liposomal)

The levels/effects of Simeprevir may be increased by: Conivaptan; CycloSPORINE (Systemic); CYP3A4 Inhibitors (Moderate); CYP3A4 Inhibitors (Strong); Dasatinib; Eltrombopag; Erythromycin (Systemic); Fusidic Acid (Systemic); Idelalisib; Ivacaftor; Ledipasvir; Luliconazole; Mifepristone; Milk Thistle; Protease Inhibitors; Teriflunomide

Decreased Effect

The levels/effects of Simeprevir may be decreased by: CYP3A4 Inducers (Moderate); CYP3A4 Inducers (Strong); Deferasirox; Escitalopram; Siltuximab; St Johns Wort; Tenofovir; Tocilizumab

Storage/Stability Store below 30°C (86°F). Store in the original bottle. Protect from light.

Mechanism of Action Simeprevir is an inhibitor of HCV NS3/4A protease, a protease that is essential for viral replication. It is considered a direct-acting antiviral treatment for HCV, also called a specifically targeted antiviral therapy for HCV (STAT-C).

Pharmacodynamics/Kinetics

Absorption: Food enhances absorption.

Protein binding: >99% (albumin and alpha 1-acid glycoprotein)

Metabolism: Primarily oxidative metabolism by CYP3A4 (and possibly CYP2C8 and CYP2C19) to unchanged drug and metabolites (minor).

Half-life elimination: Plasma: 10 to 13 hours (healthy volunteers); 41 hours (HCV-infected patients)

Time to peak, serum: 4 to 6 hours

Excretion: Feces (~91%); urine (<1%)

Dosage Treatment of chronic hepatitis C (CHC): Adults: Oral: **Note:** If other antihepaciviral treatment (sofosbuvir or peginterferon and ribavirin) is discontinued for any reason, simeprevir must also be discontinued. Do not reduce simeprevir dosage or interrupt therapy; if therapy must be interrupted due to adverse reactions or inadequate response, do not reinitiate.

Manufacturer's labeling: 150 mg once daily (in combination with sofosbuvir or peginterferon alfa and ribavirin). Treatment duration is indication and response-specific.

Missed dose: If a dose is missed within 12 hours of the time it is usually taken, take as soon as possible. If more than 12 hours have passed since the dose is usually taken, do not take the missed dose and the patient should resume the usual schedule.

Treatment-naive or prior relapse patients when used with sofosbuvir: **Note:** No treatment stopping rules apply to the combination of simeprevir with sofosbuvir:

Patients without cirrhosis: Weeks 1 to 12: Dual therapy: Simeprevir 150 mg once daily

Patients with cirrhosis: Weeks 1 to 24: Dual therapy: Simeprevir 150 mg once daily

Treatment-naive or prior relapse patients when used with peginterferon alfa and ribavirin (including those with cirrhosis): **Note:** Prior relapsers include patients with an undetectable HCV-RNA upon completion of treatment (prior interferon-based regimen) but with detectable HCV-RNA during the follow up period.

U.S. labeling:

Weeks 1 to 12: Triple therapy: Simeprevir 150 mg once daily

HCV-RNA **detectable** (level ≥25 units/mL) at week 4: Discontinue simeprevir, peginterferon alfa, and ribavirin (treatment determined to be inadequate).

Weeks 13 to 23 (based on HCV-RNA results at week 12):

HCV-RNA **undetectable** (level <25 units/mL) at week 12: Discontinue simeprevir (treatment completed). Dual therapy: Peginterferon alfa and ribavirin only (through week 24)

HCV-RNA **detectable** (level ≥25 units/mL) at week 12: Discontinue simeprevir (treatment completed), peginterferon alfa, and ribavirin (treatment determined to be inadequate).

Week 24 (based on HCV-RNA results at week 24):

HCV-RNA **undetectable** (level <25 units/mL) at week 24: Dual therapy: Peginterferon alfa and ribavirin only (through week 24)

HCV-RNA **detectable** (level ≥25 units/mL) at week 24: Discontinue peginterferon alfa and ribavirin (treatment determined to be inadequate).

Canadian labeling: **Note:** HCV-RNA assays with a lower limit of HCV-RNA quantification ≥25 units/mL and a lower limit of HCV-RNA detection of ~10 to 15 units/mL are recommended.

Weeks 1 to 12: Triple therapy: Simeprevir 150 mg once daily

HCV-RNA **detectable** (level ≥25 units/mL) at week 4: Discontinue simeprevir, peginterferon alfa, and ribavirin (treatment determined to be inadequate).

Weeks 13 and beyond (based on HCV-RNA results at weeks 12 and 24):

HCV-RNA **undetectable** at week 12: Discontinue simeprevir (treatment completed). Dual therapy: Peginterferon alfa and ribavirin only (through week 24)

HCV-RNA **detectable** but level <25 units/mL or below the lower limit of quantification of the assay used at week 12: Discontinue simeprevir (treatment completed). Continue dual therapy with peginterferon alfa and ribavirin only through week 24, then recheck HCV-RNA levels. If HCV-RNA remains detectable but <25 units/mL or below the lower limit of quantification of the assay used, continue though week 48.

HCV-RNA level **detectable** at week 12: Discontinue simeprevir (treatment completed), peginterferon alfa, and ribavirin (treatment determined to be inadequate).

HCV-RNA level **detectable** at week 24: Discontinue peginterferon alfa and ribavirin (treatment determined to be inadequate).

Previously treated patients (partial response or null responders) including those with cirrhosis when used with peginterferon alfa and ribavirin: **Note:** Partial response includes patients with a ≥2-$\log_{10}$ HCV-RNA decrease at week 12 but detectable HCV-RNA at the end of prior interferon-based therapy. Prior null responders include patients with a <2-$\log_{10}$ HCV-RNA decrease at week 12 during interferon-based therapy.

U.S. labeling:

Weeks 1 to 12: Triple therapy: Simeprevir 150 mg daily

HCV-RNA **detectable** (level ≥25 units/mL) at week 4: Discontinue simeprevir, peginterferon alfa, and ribavirin (treatment determined to be inadequate).

HCV-RNA **undetectable** (level <25 units/mL) at week 12: Discontinue simeprevir (treatment completed). Dual therapy: Peginterferon alfa and ribavirin only (through week 48)

Weeks 13 to 48 (based on HCV-RNA results at weeks 12 and 24):

HCV-RNA **detectable** (level ≥25 units/mL) at week 12: Discontinue simeprevir (treatment completed) and peginterferon alfa and ribavirin (treatment determined to be inadequate).

HCV-RNA **undetectable** (level <25 units/mL) at week 24: Discontinued simeprevir (treatment was completed after week 12). Dual therapy: Peginterferon alfa and ribavirin only (through week 48)

HCV-RNA **detectable** (level ≥25 units/mL) at week 24: Discontinue peginterferon alfa, and ribavirin (treatment determined to be inadequate).

Canadian labeling: **Note:** HCV-RNA assays with a lower limit of HCV-RNA quantification ≥25 units/mL and a lower limit of HCV-RNA detection of ~10 to 15 units/mL are recommended.

Weeks 1 to 12: Triple therapy: Simeprevir 150 mg daily

HCV-RNA **detectable** (level ≥25 units/mL) at week 4: Discontinue simeprevir, peginterferon alfa, and ribavirin (treatment determined to be inadequate).

HCV-RNA **undetectable** or **detectable** but level <25 units/mL or below the lower limit of quantification of the assay used at week 12: Discontinue simeprevir (treatment completed). Dual therapy: Peginterferon alfa and ribavirin only (through week 48).

HCV-RNA **detectable** at week 12: Discontinue simeprevir (treatment completed), peginterferon alfa, and ribavirin (treatment determined to be inadequate).

Weeks 13 and beyond (based on HCV-RNA results at weeks 12 and 24):

HCV-RNA **detectable** but level <25 units/mL or below the lower limit of quantification of the assay used at week 24: Discontinued simeprevir (treatment was completed after week 12). Dual therapy: Peginterferon alfa and ribavirin only (through week 48).

HCV-RNA **detectable** at week 24: Discontinue peginterferon alfa and ribavirin (treatment determined to be inadequate).

Alternative dosing:

Treatment-naive patients:

Patients who can receive interferon: Genotype 4 (off-label use): 150 mg once daily with ribavirin and peginterferon for 12 weeks, then only peginterferon and ribavirin for an additional 12 to 36 weeks. **Note:** A recommended *alternative* regimen (AASLD/IDSA, 2014)

Patients who cannot receive peginterferon: Genotype 1a (off-label regimen): 150 mg once daily with sofosbuvir and with ribavirin for 12 weeks (without cirrhosis) or 24 weeks (with cirrhosis). **Note:** A recommended regimen (AASLD/IDSA, 2014)

Relapsed chronic hepatitis C patients (nonresponders to a previous regimen of ribavirin and peginterferon alfa without an HCV protease inhibitor): Genotype 1 patients: 150 mg once daily with sofosbuvir and with ribavirin for 12 weeks (without cirrhosis) or 24 weeks (with cirrhosis). **Note:** A recommended regimen (AASLD/IDSA, 2014).

Dosage adjustment in renal impairment: No dosage adjustment necessary. Not studied in patients with CrCl ≤30 mL/minute or with end -stage renal disease (ESRD), including those requiring hemodialysis.

Dosage adjustment in hepatic impairment:

U.S. labeling:

Mild impairment (Child-Pugh class A): No dosage adjustment necessary.

Moderate impairment (Child-Pugh class B): There are no dosage adjustments provided in the manufacturer's labeling; use with caution. Do not administer in combination with peginterferon and ribavirin in patients with decompensated cirrhosis (moderate or severe hepatic impairment).

Severe impairment (Child-Pugh class C): Use is not recommended.

Canadian labeling:

Mild or moderate impairment (Child-Pugh class A or B): No dosage adjustment necessary.

Severe impairment (Child-Pugh class C): There are no dosage adjustments provided in the manufacturer's labeling (has not been studied).

Administration Administer orally with food. Administer concurrently with peginterferon alfa and ribavirin or sofosbuvir. Maintain adequate fluid intake/hydration. Swallow capsules whole; do not chew, crush, break, cut, or dissolve the capsule.

Monitoring Parameters

Bilirubin, liver enzymes, and uric acid at baseline and periodically when clinically indicated

Serum HCV-RNA at baseline, weeks 4, 12, and 24, at end of treatment, during treatment follow-up, and when clinically indicated

Pretreatment and monthly pregnancy tests up to 6 months following discontinuation of therapy for women of childbearing age

Dosage Forms

Capsule, Oral:

Olysio: 150 mg

- ◆ **Simethicone, Aluminum Hydroxide, and Magnesium Hydroxide** *see* Aluminum Hydroxide, Magnesium Hydroxide, and Simethicone *on page 104*
- ◆ **Simethicone and Loperamide Hydrochloride** *see* Loperamide and Simethicone *on page 1237*
- ◆ **Simethicone and Magaldrate** *see* Magaldrate and Simethicone *on page 1261*
- ◆ **Simply Allergy [OTC]** *see* DiphenhydrAMINE (Systemic) *on page 641*
- ◆ **Simply Sleep [OTC]** *see* DiphenhydrAMINE (Systemic) *on page 641*
- ◆ **Simply Sleep (Can)** *see* DiphenhydrAMINE (Systemic) *on page 641*
- ◆ **Simply Stuffy [OTC]** *see* Pseudoephedrine *on page 1742*
- ◆ **Simponi** *see* Golimumab *on page 977*
- ◆ **Simponi Aria** *see* Golimumab *on page 977*
- ◆ **Simponi I.V. (Can)** *see* Golimumab *on page 977*
- ◆ **Simulect** *see* Basiliximab *on page 228*

Simvastatin (sim va STAT in)

Brand Names: U.S. Zocor

Brand Names: Canada ACT-Simvastatin; Apo-Simvastatin; Auro-Simvastatin; Ava-Simvastatin; Dom-Simvastatin; JAMP-Simvastatin; Mar-Simvastatin; Mint-Simvastatin; Mylan-Simvastatin; PHL-Simvastatin; PMS-Simvastatin; Q-Simvastatin; RAN-Simvastatin; ratio-Simvastatin; Riva-Simvastatin; Sandoz-Simvastatin; Simvastatin-Odan; Teva-Simvastatin; Zocor

Pharmacologic Category Antilipemic Agent, HMG-CoA Reductase Inhibitor

Use Used with dietary therapy for the following:

Secondary prevention of cardiovascular events in hypercholesterolemic patients with established coronary heart disease (CHD) or at high risk for CHD: To reduce cardiovascular morbidity (myocardial infarction, coronary/noncoronary revascularization procedures) and mortality; to reduce the risk of stroke

Hyperlipidemias: To reduce elevations in total cholesterol (total-C), LDL-C, apolipoprotein B, triglycerides, and VLDL-C, and to increase HDL-C in patients with primary hypercholesterolemia (elevations of 1 or more components are present in Fredrickson type IIa, IIb, III, and IV hyperlipidemias); treatment of homozygous familial hypercholesterolemia

Heterozygous familial hypercholesterolemia (HeFH): In adolescent patients (10-17 years of age, females >1 year postmenarche) with HeFH having LDL-C ≥190 mg/dL **or** LDL-C ≥160 mg/dL with positive family history of premature cardiovascular disease (CVD), or 2 or more CVD risk factors in the adolescent patient

Primary and secondary prevention of atherosclerotic cardiovascular disease (ASCVD) according to the American College of Cardiology/American Heart Association: To reduce the risk of ASCVD in patients with clinical ASCVD (eg, coronary heart disease, stroke/TIA, or peripheral arterial disease presumed to be of atherosclerotic origin) who are greater than 75 years of age or not a candidate for high-intensity statin therapy; in patients without clinical ASCVD if LDL-C is 190 mg/dL or greater and not a candidate for high-intensity statin therapy; in patients without clinical ASCVD who have type 1 or type 2 diabetes and are between 40 and 75 years of age; in patients with an estimated 10-year ASCVD risk 7.5% or greater and who are between 40 and 75 years of age (Stone, 2013). Specific recommendations from the Kidney Disease: Improving Global Outcomes (KDIGO) organization have also been released for patients with chronic kidney disease (KDIGO [Tonelli, 2013]).

Pregnancy Risk Factor X

Pregnancy Considerations Adverse events were not observed in animal reproduction studies. There are reports of congenital anomalies following maternal use of HMG-CoA reductase inhibitors in pregnancy; however, maternal disease, differences in specific agents used, and the low rates of exposure limit the interpretation of the available data (Godfrey, 2012; Lecarpentier, 2012). Cholesterol biosynthesis may be important in fetal development; serum cholesterol and triglycerides increase normally during pregnancy. The discontinuation of lipid lowering medications temporarily during pregnancy is not expected to have significant impact on the long term outcomes of primary hypercholesterolemia treatment.

Use of simvastatin is contraindicated in pregnancy. HMG-CoA reductase inhibitors should be discontinued prior to pregnancy (ADA, 2013). If treatment of dyslipidemias is needed in pregnant women or in women of reproductive age, other agents are preferred (Berglund, 2012; Stone, 2013). The manufacturer recommends administration to women of childbearing potential only when conception is highly unlikely and patients have been informed of potential hazards.

Breast-Feeding Considerations It is not known if simvastatin is excreted into breast milk. Due to the potential for serious adverse reactions in a nursing infant, breast-feeding is contraindicated by the manufacturer.

Contraindications Hypersensitivity to simvastatin or any component of the formulation; active liver disease; unexplained persistent elevations of serum transaminases; concomitant use of strong CYP3A4 inhibitors (eg, clarithromycin, erythromycin, itraconazole, ketoconazole, nefazodone, posaconazole, voriconazole, protease inhibitors [including boceprevir and telaprevir], telithromycin, cobicistat-containing products), cyclosporine, danazol, and gemfibrozil; pregnancy; breast-feeding

Warnings/Precautions Secondary causes of hyperlipidemia should be ruled out prior to therapy. Liver enzyme tests should be obtained at baseline and as clinically indicated; routine periodic monitoring of liver enzymes is not necessary. Use with caution in patients who consume large amounts of ethanol or have a history of liver disease; use is contraindicated with active liver disease and with unexplained transaminase elevations. Rhabdomyolysis with acute renal failure has occurred. Risk of rhabdomyolysis is dose-related and increased with high doses (80 mg), concurrent use of lipid-lowering agents which may also cause rhabdomyolysis (other fibrates or niacin doses ≥1 g/day), or moderate-to-strong CYP3A4 inhibitors (eg, amiodarone, grapefruit juice in large quantities, or verapamil), age ≥65 years, female gender, uncontrolled hypothyroidism, and renal dysfunction. In Chinese patients, do not use high-dose simvastatin (80 mg) if concurrently taking niacin ≥1 g/day; may increase risk of myopathy. Immune-mediated necrotizing myopathy (IMNM), an autoimmune-mediated myopathy, has been reported (rarely) with HMG-CoA reductase inhibitor therapy. IMNM presents as proximal muscle weakness with elevated CPK levels, which persists despite discontinuation of HMG-CoA reductase inhibitor therapy; additionally, muscle biopsy may show necrotizing myopathy with limited inflammation; immunosuppressive therapy (eg, corticosteroids, azathioprine) may be used for treatment. Concomitant use of simvastatin with some drugs may require cautious use, may not be recommended, may require dosage adjustments, or may be contraindicated. If concurrent use of a contraindicated interacting medication is unavoidable, treatment with simvastatin should be suspended during use or consider the use of an alternative HMG-CoA reductase inhibitor void of CYP3A4 metabolism. Monitor closely if used with other drugs associated with myopathy (eg, colchicine). Increases in HbA_{1c} and fasting blood glucose have been reported with HMG-CoA reductase inhibitors; however, the benefits of statin therapy far outweigh the risk of dysglycemia. The manufacturer recommends temporary discontinuation for elective major surgery, acute medical or surgical conditions, or in any patient experiencing an acute or serious condition predisposing to renal failure (eg, sepsis, hypotension, trauma, uncontrolled seizures). Based on current research and clinical guidelines (Fleisher, 2009), HMG-CoA reductase inhibitors should be continued in the perioperative period. Use with caution in patients with severe renal impairment; initial dosage adjustment is necessary; monitor closely.

Adverse Reactions

Cardiovascular: Atrial fibrillation, edema

Central nervous system: Headache, vertigo

Dermatologic: Eczema

Gastrointestinal: Abdominal pain, constipation, gastritis, nausea

Hepatic: Transaminases increased (>3 x ULN)

Neuromuscular & skeletal: CPK increased (>3 x normal), myalgia

Respiratory: Bronchitis, upper respiratory infections

Rare but important or life-threatening: Alkaline phosphatase increased, alopecia, amnesia (reversible), anaphylaxis, anemia, angioedema, arthralgia, arthritis, blood glucose increased, chills, cognitive impairment (reversible), confusion (reversible), depression, dermatomyositis, diabetes mellitus (new onset), diarrhea, dizziness, dryness of skin/mucous membranes, dyspepsia, dyspnea, eosinophilia, erythema multiforme, ESR increased, fever, flatulence, flushing, glycosylated hemoglobin (Hb A_{1c}) increased, GGT increased, hemolytic anemia, hepatic failure, hepatitis, hypersensitivity reaction, jaundice, leukopenia, malaise, memory disturbance (reversible), memory impairment (reversible), muscle cramps, nail changes, nodules, pancreatitis, paresthesia, peripheral neuropathy, photosensitivity, polymyalgia rheumatica, positive ANA, pruritus, purpura, rash, rhabdomyolysis, skin discoloration, Stevens-Johnson syndrome, systemic lupus erythematosus-like syndrome, thrombocytopenia, toxic epidermal necrolysis, urticaria, vasculitis, vomiting, weakness

Additional class-related events or case reports (not necessarily reported with simvastatin therapy): Alteration in taste, anorexia, anxiety, bilirubin increased, cataracts, cholestatic jaundice, cirrhosis, decreased libido, depression, erectile dysfunction/impotence, facial paresis, fatty liver, fulminant hepatic necrosis, gynecomastia, hepatoma, hyperbilirubinemia, immune-mediated necrotizing myopathy (IMNM), impaired extraocular muscle movement, increased CPK (>10 x normal), interstitial lung disease, ophthalmoplegia, peripheral nerve palsy, psychic disturbance, renal failure (secondary to rhabdomyolysis), thyroid dysfunction, tremor, vertigo

Drug Interactions

Metabolism/Transport Effects Substrate of CYP3A4 (major), SLCO1B1; **Note:** Assignment of Major/Minor substrate status based on clinically relevant drug interaction potential; **Inhibits** CYP2C8 (weak), CYP2C9 (weak), CYP2D6 (weak)

Avoid Concomitant Use

Avoid concomitant use of Simvastatin with any of the following: Boceprevir; Clarithromycin; Conivaptan; CycloSPORINE (Systemic); CYP3A4 Inhibitors (Strong); Erythromycin (Systemic); Fusidic Acid (Systemic); Gemfibrozil; Idelalisib; Mifepristone; Protease Inhibitors; Red Yeast Rice; Telaprevir; Telithromycin

Increased Effect/Toxicity

Simvastatin may increase the levels/effects of: ARIPiprazole; DAPTOmycin; Diltiazem; PAZOPanib; Trabectedin; Vitamin K Antagonists

The levels/effects of Simvastatin may be increased by: Acipimox; Amiodarone; AmLODIPine; Aprepitant; Azithromycin (Systemic); Bezafibrate; Boceprevir; Ceritinib; Ciprofibrate; Clarithromycin; Colchicine; Conivaptan; CycloSPORINE (Systemic); CYP3A4 Inhibitors (Moderate); CYP3A4 Inhibitors (Strong); Cyproterone; Danazol; Dasatinib; Diltiazem; Dronedarone; Eltrombopag; Erythromycin (Systemic); Fenofibrate and Derivatives; Fluconazole; Fosaprepitant; Fusidic Acid (Systemic); Gemfibrozil; Grapefruit Juice; Green Tea; Idelalisib; Imatinib; Ivacaftor; Lercanidipine; Lomitapide; Luliconazole; Mifepristone; Netupitant; Niacin; Niacinamide; Protease Inhibitors; QuiNINE; Raltegravir; Ranolazine; Red Yeast Rice; Sildenafil; Simeprevir; Telaprevir; Telithromycin; Teriflunomide; Ticagrelor; Verapamil

Decreased Effect

Simvastatin may decrease the levels/effects of: Lanthanum

The levels/effects of Simvastatin may be decreased by: Antacids; Bosentan; CYP3A4 Inducers (Moderate); CYP3A4 Inducers (Strong); Dabrafenib; Deferasirox; Efavirenz; Eslicarbazepine; Etravirine; Fosphenytoin; Mitotane; Phenytoin; Rifamycin Derivatives; Siltuximab; St Johns Wort; Tocilizumab

Food Interactions Simvastatin serum concentration may be increased when taken with grapefruit juice. Management: Avoid concurrent intake of large quantities of grapefruit juice (>1 quart/day).

Storage/Stability Tablets should be stored in tightly-closed containers at temperatures between 5°C to 30°C (41°F to 86°F).

Mechanism of Action Simvastatin is a methylated derivative of lovastatin that acts by competitively inhibiting 3-hydroxy-3-methylglutaryl-coenzyme A (HMG-CoA) reductase, the enzyme that catalyzes the rate-limiting step in cholesterol biosynthesis

Pharmacodynamics/Kinetics

Onset of action: >3 days

Peak effect: 2 weeks

Absorption: 85%

Protein binding: ~95%

Metabolism: Hepatic via CYP3A4; extensive first-pass effect

Bioavailability: <5%

Half-life elimination: Unknown

Time to peak: 1.3-2.4 hours

Excretion: Feces (60%); urine (13%)

Dosage Oral: **Note:** Doses should be individualized according to the baseline LDL-cholesterol levels, the recommended goal of therapy, and the patient's response; adjustments should be made at intervals of 4 weeks or more; doses may need adjusted based on concomitant medications

Children 10-17 years (females >1 year postmenarche):

HeFH: 10 mg once daily in the evening; range: 10-40 mg/day (maximum: 40 mg/day)

Dosage adjustment for simvastatin with concomitant amiodarone, amlodipine, diltiazem, dronedarone, lomitapide, ranolazine, or verapamil: Refer to drug-specific dosing in adult dosing section

Adults:

Note: Dosing limitation: Simvastatin 80 mg is limited to patients that have been taking this dose for >12 consecutive months without evidence of myopathy and are not currently taking or beginning to take a simvastatin dose-limiting or contraindicated interacting medication. If patient is unable to achieve low-density lipoprotein cholesterol (LDL-C) goal using the 40 mg dose of simvastatin, increasing to 80 mg dose is not recommended. Instead, switch patient to an alternative LDL-C-lowering treatment providing greater LDL-C reduction.

Homozygous familial hypercholesterolemia: 40 mg once daily in the evening

Prevention of cardiovascular events (also see ACC/AHA Blood Cholesterol Guideline recommendations), hyperlipidemias: 10-20 mg once daily in the evening; range: 5-40 mg/day

Patients requiring only moderate reduction of LDL-C may be started at 5-10 mg once daily in the evening; adjust to achieve recommended LDL-C goal

Patients requiring reduction of >40% of LDL-C may be started at 40 mg once daily in the evening; adjust to achieve recommended LDL-C goal

Patients with CHD or at high risk for cardiovascular events (patients with diabetes, PVD, history of stroke or other cerebrovascular disease): Dosing should be started at 40 mg once daily in the evening; start simultaneously with diet therapy.

ACC/AHA Blood Cholesterol Guideline recommendations to reduce the risk of atherosclerotic cardiovascular disease (ASCVD) (Stone, 2013): Adults ≥21 years:

Primary prevention:

LDL-C ≥190 mg/dL: High intensity therapy necessary; use alternate statin therapy (eg, atorvastatin or rosuvastatin)

Type 1 or 2 diabetes and age 40-75 years: Moderate intensity therapy: 20-40 mg once daily

Type 1 or 2 diabetes, age 40-75 years, and an estimated 10-year ASCVD risk ≥7.5%: High intensity therapy necessary; use alternate statin therapy (eg, atorvastatin or rosuvastatin)

Age 40-75 years and an estimated 10-year ASCVD risk ≥7.5%: Moderate to high intensity therapy: 20-40 mg once daily or consider using high intensity statin therapy (eg, atorvastatin or rosuvastatin)

Secondary prevention:

Patient has clinical ASCVD (eg, coronary heart disease, stroke/TIA, or peripheral arterial disease presumed to be of atherosclerotic origin) **and**:

Age ≤75 years: High intensity therapy necessary; use alternate statin therapy (eg, atorvastatin or rosuvastatin)

Age >75 years or not a candidate for high intensity therapy: Moderate intensity therapy: 20-40 mg once daily

Dosage adjustment with concomitant medications: **Note:** Patients currently tolerating and requiring a dose of simvastatin 80 mg who require initiation of an interacting drug with a dose cap for simvastatin should be switched to an alternative statin with less potential for drug-drug interaction.

Amiodarone, amlodipine, or ranolazine: Simvastatin dose should **not** exceed 20 mg/day

Diltiazem, dronedarone, or verapamil: Simvastatin dose should **not** exceed 10 mg/day

Lomitapide: Reduce simvastatin dose by 50% when initiating lomitapide. Simvastatin dose should not exceed 20 mg/day (or 40 mg daily for those who previously tolerated simvastatin 80 mg daily for ≥1 year without evidence of muscle toxicity)

Dosage adjustment in Chinese patients on niacin doses ≥1 g/day: Use caution with simvastatin doses exceeding 20 mg/day; because of an increased risk of myopathy, do not administer simvastatin 80 mg concurrently.

Dosing adjustment for toxicity:

Severe muscle symptoms or fatigue: Promptly discontinue use; evaluate CPK, creatinine, and urinalysis for myoglobinuria (Stone, 2013).

Mild to moderate muscle symptoms: Discontinue use until symptoms can be evaluated; evaluate patient for conditions that may increase the risk for muscle symptoms (eg, hypothyroidism, reduced renal or hepatic function, rheumatologic disorders such as polymyalgia rheumatica, steroid myopathy, vitamin D deficiency, or primary muscle diseases). Upon resolution, resume the original or lower dose of simvastatin. If muscle symptoms recur, discontinue simvastatin use. After muscle symptom resolution, may then use a low dose of a different statin; gradually increase if tolerated. In the absence of continued statin use, if muscle symptoms or elevated CPK continues after 2 months, consider other causes of muscle symptoms. If determined to be due to another condition aside from statin use, may resume statin therapy at the original dose (Stone, 2013).

Dosage adjustment in renal impairment: Manufacturer's recommendations:

Mild to moderate impairment: No dosage adjustment necessary; simvastatin does not undergo significant renal excretion

Severe impairment: CrCl <30 mL/minute: Initial: 5 mg/day with close monitoring.

Dosage adjustment in hepatic impairment: Use is contraindicated in the setting of active liver disease.

Dietary Considerations May be taken without regard to meals. Red yeast rice contains variable amounts of several compounds that are structurally similar to HMG-CoA reductase inhibitors, primarily monacolin K (or mevinolin) which is structurally identical to lovastatin; concurrent use of red yeast rice with HMG-CoA reductase inhibitors may increase the incidence of adverse and toxic effects (Lapi, 2008; Smith, 2003).

Administration May be administered without regard to meals. Administer in the evening for maximal efficacy.

Monitoring Parameters ***2013 ACC/AHA Blood Cholesterol Guideline recommendations (Stone, 2013):***

Lipid panel (total cholesterol, HDL, LDL, triglycerides): Baseline lipid panel; fasting lipid profile within 4-12 weeks after initiation or dose adjustment and every 3-12 months (as clinically indicated) thereafter. If 2 consecutive LDL levels are <40 mg/dL, consider decreasing the dose.v

Hepatic transaminase levels: Baseline measurement of hepatic transaminase levels (ie, ALT); measure hepatic function if symptoms suggest hepatotoxicity (eg, unusual fatigue or weakness, loss of appetite, abdominal pain, dark-colored urine or yellowing of skin or sclera) during therapy.

CPK: CPK should not be routinely measured. Baseline CPK measurement is reasonable for some individuals (eg, family history of statin intolerance or muscle disease, clinical presentation, concomitant drug therapy that may increase risk of myopathy). May measure CPK in any patient with symptoms suggestive of myopathy (pain, tenderness, stiffness, cramping, weakness, or generalized fatigue).

Evaluate for new-onset diabetes mellitus during therapy; if diabetes develops, continue statin therapy and encourage adherence to a heart-healthy diet, physical activity, a healthy body weight, and tobacco cessation.

If patient develops a confusional state or memory impairment, may evaluate patient for nonstatin causes (eg, exposure to other drugs), systemic and neuropsychiatric causes, and the possibility of adverse effects associated with statin therapy.

Manufacturer recommendations: Liver enzyme tests at baseline and repeated when clinically indicated. Measure CPK when myopathy is being considered or may measure CPK periodically in high risk patients (eg, drug-drug interaction). Lipid panel should be analyzed after 4 weeks of therapy and periodically thereafter.

Dosage Forms

Tablet, Oral:

Zocor: 5 mg, 10 mg, 20 mg, 40 mg, 80 mg

Generic: 5 mg, 10 mg, 20 mg, 40 mg, 80 mg

◆ **Simvastatin and Ezetimibe** *see* Ezetimibe and Simvastatin *on page 834*

◆ **Simvastatin and Sitagliptin** *see* Sitagliptin and Simvastatin *on page 1899*

◆ **Simvastatin-Odan (Can)** *see* Simvastatin *on page 1890*

◆ **Sinemet** *see* Carbidopa and Levodopa *on page 351*

◆ **Sinemet CR** *see* Carbidopa and Levodopa *on page 351*

◆ **Sinequan (Can)** *see* Doxepin (Systemic) *on page 676*

◆ **Singulair** *see* Montelukast *on page 1392*

◆ **Sintrom (Can)** *see* Acenocoumarol [CAN/INT] *on page 30*

Sipuleucel-T (si pu LOO sel tee)

Brand Names: U.S. Provenge

Index Terms APC8015; Prostate Cancer Vaccine, Cell-Based

Pharmacologic Category Cellular Immunotherapy, Autologous

Use Treatment of metastatic hormone-refractory prostate cancer in patients who are asymptomatic or minimally symptomatic

Dosage Note: Premedicate with oral acetaminophen 650 mg and an antihistamine (eg, diphenhydramine 50 mg) ~30 minutes prior to infusion. For autologous use only. Do not infuse until confirmation of product release has been received from the company.

IV: Adults: Prostate cancer, metastatic: Each dose contains ≥50 million autologous CD54+ cells (obtained through leukapheresis) activated with PAP-GM-CSF; administer doses at ~2 week intervals for a total of 3 doses (Kantoff, 2010)

Dosage adjustment for toxicity: Acute infusion reaction: Interrupt or slow infusion rate (depending on the severity of infusion reaction); may require acetaminophen, IV H_1 and/or H_2 antagonists, or low-dose meperidine to manage acute symptoms.

Dosage adjustment in renal impairment: No dosage adjustment provided in manufacturer's labeling.

Dosage adjustment in hepatic impairment: No dosage adjustment provided in manufacturer's labeling.

Additional Information Complete prescribing information should be consulted for additional detail.

Dosage Forms

Suspension, Intravenous [preservative free]:

Provenge: (250 mL)

◆ **Sirdalud** *see* TiZANidine *on page 2051*

Sirolimus (sir OH li mus)

Brand Names: U.S. Rapamune

Brand Names: Canada Rapamune

Index Terms Rapamycin

Pharmacologic Category Immunosuppressant Agent; mTOR Kinase Inhibitor

Use Prophylaxis of organ rejection in patients receiving renal transplants

Pregnancy Risk Factor C

Pregnancy Considerations Adverse events have been observed in animal reproduction studies. Effective contraception must be initiated before therapy with sirolimus and continued for 12 weeks after discontinuation.

The National Transplantation Pregnancy Registry (NTPR, Temple University) is a registry for pregnant women taking immunosuppressants following any solid organ transplant. The NTPR encourages reporting of all immunosuppressant exposures during pregnancy in transplant recipients at 877-955-6877.

Breast-Feeding Considerations It is not known if sirolimus is excreted in breast milk. Due to the potential for adverse reactions in the breast-fed infant, including possible immunosuppression, breast-feeding is not recommended.

Contraindications Hypersensitivity to sirolimus or any component of the formulation

Warnings/Precautions Hazardous agent - use appropriate precautions for handling and disposal (NIOSH 2014 [group 2]).

[U.S. Boxed Warning]: Immunosuppressive agents, including sirolimus, increase the risk of infection and may be associated with the development of lymphoma. Immune suppression may also increase the risk of opportunistic infections (including activation of latent viral infections including BK virus-associated nephropathy), fatal infections, and sepsis. Prophylactic treatment for *Pneumocystis jirovecii* pneumonia (PCP) should be administered for 1 year post-transplant; prophylaxis for cytomegalovirus (CMV) should be taken for 3 months post-transplant in patients at risk for CMV. Progressive multifocal leukoencephalopathy (PML), an opportunistic CNS infection caused by reactivation of the JC virus, has been reported in patients receiving immunosuppressive therapy, including sirolimus. Clinical findings of PML include apathy, ataxia, cognitive deficiency, confusion, and hemiparesis; promptly evaluate any patient presenting with neurological changes; consider decreasing the degree of immunosuppression with consideration to the risk of organ rejection in transplant patients.

[U.S. Boxed Warning]: Sirolimus is not recommended for use in liver or lung transplantation. Bronchial anastomotic dehiscence cases have been reported in lung transplant patients when sirolimus was used as part of an immunosuppressive regimen; most of these reactions were fatal. Studies indicate an association with an increased risk of hepatic artery thrombosis (HAT), graft failure, and increased mortality (with evidence of infection) in liver transplant patients when sirolimus is used in combination with cyclosporine and/or tacrolimus. Most cases of HAT occurred within 30 days of transplant.

In renal transplant patients, *de novo* use without cyclosporine has been associated with higher rates of acute rejection. Sirolimus should be used in combination with cyclosporine (and corticosteroids) initially. Cyclosporine may be withdrawn in low-to-moderate immunologic risk patients after 2-4 months, in conjunction with an increase in sirolimus dosage. In high immunologic risk patients, use in combination with cyclosporine and corticosteroids is recommended for the first year. Safety and efficacy of combination therapy with cyclosporine in high immunologic risk patients has not been studied beyond 12 months of treatment; adjustment of immunosuppressive therapy beyond 12 months should be considered based on clinical judgement. Monitor renal function closely when combined with cyclosporine; consider dosage adjustment or discontinue in patients with increasing serum creatinine.

May increase serum creatinine and decrease GFR. Use caution when used concurrently with medications which may alter renal function. May delay recovery of renal function in patients with delayed allograft function. Increased urinary protein excretion has been observed when converting renal transplant patients from calcineurin inhibitors to sirolimus during maintenance therapy. A ▶

higher level of proteinuria prior to sirolimus conversion correlates with a higher degree of proteinuria after conversion. In some patients, proteinuria may reach nephrotic levels; nephrotic syndrome (new onset) has been reported. Increased risk of BK viral-associated nephropathy which may impair renal function and cause graft loss; consider decreasing immunosuppressive burden if evidence of deteriorating renal function.

Use caution with hepatic impairment; a reduction in the maintenance dose is recommended. Has been associated with an increased risk of fluid accumulation and lymphocele; peripheral edema, lymphedema, ascites, and pleural and pericardial effusions (including significant effusions and tamponade) were reported; use with caution in patients in whom fluid accumulation may be poorly tolerated, such as in cardiovascular disease (heart failure or hypertension) and pulmonary disease. Cases of interstitial lung disease (eg, pneumonitis, bronchiolitis obliterans organizing pneumonia [BOOP], pulmonary fibrosis) have been observed; risk may be increased with higher trough levels. Potentially significant drug-drug interactions may exist, requiring dose or frequency adjustment, additional monitoring, and/or selection of alternative therapy. Concurrent use with a calcineurin inhibitor (cyclosporine, tacrolimus) may increase the risk of calcineurin inhibitor-induced hemolytic uremic syndrome/thrombotic thrombocytopenic purpura/thrombotic microangiopathy (HUS/TTP/TMA).

Hypersensitivity reactions, including anaphylactic/anaphylactoid reactions, angioedema, exfoliative dermatitis, and hypersensitivity vasculitis have been reported. Concurrent use with other drugs known to cause angioedema (eg, ACE inhibitors) may increase risk. Immunosuppressant therapy is associated with an increased risk of skin cancer; limit sun and ultraviolet light exposure; use appropriate sun protection. May increase serum lipids (cholesterol and triglycerides); use with caution in patients with hyperlipidemia; monitor cholesterol/lipids; if hyperlipidemia occurs, follow current guidelines for management (diet, exercise, lipid lowering agents); antihyperlipidemic therapy may not be effective in normalizing levels. May be associated with wound dehiscence and impaired healing; use caution in the perioperative period. Patients with a body mass index (BMI) >30 kg/m^2 are at increased risk for abnormal wound healing.

Sirolimus tablets and oral solution are not bioequivalent, due to differences in absorption. Clinical equivalence was seen using 2 mg tablet and 2 mg solution. It is not known if higher doses are also clinically equivalent. Monitor sirolimus levels if changes in dosage forms are made. **[U.S. Boxed Warning]: Should only be used by physicians experienced in immunosuppressive therapy and management of transplant patients. Adequate laboratory and supportive medical resources must be readily available.** Sirolimus concentrations are dependent on the assay method (eg, chromatographic and immunoassay) used; assay methods are not interchangeable. Variations in methods to determine sirolimus whole blood concentrations, as well as interlaboratory variations, may result in improper dosage adjustments, which may lead to subtherapeutic or toxic levels. Determine the assay method used to assure consistency (or accommodations if changes occur), and for monitoring purposes, be aware of alterations to assay method or reference range. The manufacturer recommends high performance liquid chromatography (HPLC) as the reference standard to determine sirolimus trough concentrations.

Adverse Reactions

Cardiovascular: Atrial fibrillation, CHF, DVT, edema, facial edema, hyper-/hypotension, hypervolemia, orthostatic hypotension, palpitation, peripheral edema, peripheral vascular disorder, syncope, tachycardia, thrombosis, vasodilation

Central nervous system: Anxiety, chills, confusion, depression, dizziness, emotional lability, headache, hypoesthesia, insomnia, malaise, neuropathy, pain, somnolence

Dermatologic: Acne, cellulitis, dermal ulcer, dermatitis (fungal), ecchymosis, hirsutism, pruritus, rash, skin carcinoma (includes basal cell carcinoma, squamous cell carcinoma, melanoma), skin hypertrophy, wound healing abnormal

Endocrine & metabolic: Acidosis, Cushing's syndrome, dehydration, diabetes mellitus, glycosuria, hypercalcemia, hypercholesterolemia, hyperglycemia, hyperphosphatemia, hypertriglyceridemia, hypocalcemia, hypoglycemia, hypomagnesemia, hyponatremia

Gastrointestinal: Abdomen enlarged, abdominal pain, anorexia, constipation, diarrhea, dysphagia, eructation, esophagitis, flatulence, gastritis, gastroenteritis, gingival hyperplasia, gingivitis, ileus, mouth ulceration, nausea, oral moniliasis, stomatitis, weight loss

Genitourinary: Amenorrhea, hypermenorrhea, impotence, menstrual disease, ovarian cyst, pelvic pain, scrotal edema, testis disorder, urinary tract infection

Hematologic: Anemia, hemolytic-uremic syndrome, hemorrhage, leukopenia, leukocytosis, polycythemia, thrombocytopenia, TTP

Hepatic: Abnormal liver function tests, alkaline phosphatase increased, ascites, LDH increased

Local: Thrombophlebitis

Neuromuscular & skeletal: Arthralgia, arthrosis, bone necrosis, CPK increased, hyper-/hypotonia, leg cramps, myalgia, osteoporosis, paresthesia, tetany

Renal: Albuminuria, bladder pain, BUN increased, dysuria, hematuria, hydronephrosis, kidney pain, nephropathy (toxic), nocturia, oliguria, pyelonephritis, pyuria, serum creatinine increased, tubular necrosis, urinary frequency, urinary incontinence, urinary retention

Respiratory: Asthma, atelectasis, bronchitis, cough, epistaxis, hypoxia, lung edema, pleural effusion, pneumonia, pulmonary embolism, rhinitis, sinusitis

Ocular: Abnormal vision, cataract, conjunctivitis

Otic: Ear pain, otitis media, tinnitus

Miscellaneous: Abscess, diaphoresis, flu-like syndrome, hernia, herpesvirus infection, infection (including opportunistic), lymphadenopathy, lymphocele, lymphoproliferative disease/lymphoma, peritonitis, sepsis

Rare but important or life-threatening: ALT increased, alveolar proteinosis, anaphylactoid reaction, anaphylaxis, anastomotic disruption, angioedema, ascites, AST increased, azoospermia, *Clostridium difficile* colitis, cytomegalovirus, Epstein-Barr virus, exfoliative dermatitis, fascial dehiscence, focal segmental glomerulosclerosis, hepatic necrosis, hepatotoxicity, hypersensitivity reaction, hypersensitivity vasculitis, hypophosphatemia, incisional hernia; interstitial lung disease (dose-related; includes pneumonitis, pulmonary fibrosis, and bronchiolitis obliterans organizing pneumonia [BOOP] with no identified infectious etiology); joint disorders, lymphedema, myocardial infarction, mycobacterial infection, nephropathy (BK virus-associated), nephrotic syndrome, neutropenia, pancreatitis, pancytopenia, pericardial effusion, *Pneumocystis* pneumonia, progressive multifocal leukoencephalopathy (PML), proteinuria, pulmonary hemorrhage, reversible posterior leukoencephalopathy syndrome (RPLS), tamponade, tuberculosis, wound dehiscence

Note: Hepatic artery thrombosis [HAT] and graft failure have been reported in liver transplant patients (not an approved use); bronchial anastomotic dehiscence has been reported in lung transplant patients (not an approved use).

Drug Interactions

Metabolism/Transport Effects Substrate of CYP3A4 (major), P-glycoprotein; **Note:** Assignment of Major/Minor substrate status based on clinically relevant drug interaction potential; **Inhibits** CYP3A4 (weak)

Avoid Concomitant Use

Avoid concomitant use of Sirolimus with any of the following: BCG; CloZAPine; Conivaptan; Crizotinib; Dipyrone; Enzalutamide; Fusidic Acid (Systemic); Idelalisib; Mifepristone; Natalizumab; Pimecrolimus; Pimozide; Posaconazole; Tacrolimus (Systemic); Tacrolimus (Topical); Tofacitinib; Vaccines (Live); Voriconazole

Increased Effect/Toxicity

Sirolimus may increase the levels/effects of: ACE Inhibitors; ARIPiprazole; CloZAPine; CycloSPORINE (Systemic); Dofetilide; Hydrocodone; Leflunomide; Lomitapide; Natalizumab; Pimozide; Tacrolimus (Systemic); Tacrolimus (Topical); Tofacitinib; Vaccines (Live)

The levels/effects of Sirolimus may be increased by: Aprepitant; Boceprevir; Ceritinib; Clotrimazole (Topical); Conivaptan; Crizotinib; CycloSPORINE (Systemic); CYP3A4 Inhibitors (Moderate); CYP3A4 Inhibitors (Strong); Dasatinib; Denosumab; Dipyrone; Fluconazole; Fosaprepitant; Fusidic Acid (Systemic); Idelalisib; Itraconazole; Ivacaftor; Ketoconazole (Systemic); Luliconazole; Macrolide Antibiotics; Mifepristone; Nelfinavir; Netupitant; P-glycoprotein/ABCB1 Inhibitors; Pimecrolimus; Posaconazole; Roflumilast; Stiripentol; Tacrolimus (Systemic); Tacrolimus (Topical); Telaprevir; Trastuzumab; Voriconazole

Decreased Effect

Sirolimus may decrease the levels/effects of: BCG; Coccidioides immitis Skin Test; Sipuleucel-T; Tacrolimus (Systemic); Vaccines (Inactivated); Vaccines (Live)

The levels/effects of Sirolimus may be decreased by: Bosentan; CYP3A4 Inducers (Moderate); CYP3A4 Inducers (Strong); Dabrafenib; Deferasirox; Echinacea; Efavirenz; Enzalutamide; Fosphenytoin; Mitotane; P-glycoprotein/ABCB1 Inducers; Phenytoin; Rifampin; Siltuximab; St Johns Wort; Tocilizumab

Food Interactions Grapefruit juice may decrease clearance of sirolimus. Ingestion with high-fat meals decreases peak concentrations but increases AUC by 23% to 35%. Management: Avoid grapefruit juice. Take consistently (either with or without food) to minimize variability.

Storage/Stability

Oral solution: Store under refrigeration, 2°C to 8°C (36°F to 46°F). Protect from light. A slight haze may develop in refrigerated solutions, but the quality of the product is not affected. After opening, solution should be used in 1 month. If necessary, may be stored at temperatures up to 25°C (77°F) for ≤15 days after opening. Product may be stored in amber syringe for a maximum of 24 hours (at room temperature or refrigerated). Discard syringe after single use. Solution should be used immediately following dilution.

Tablet: Store at room temperature of 20°C to 25°C (68°F to 77°F). Protect from light.

Mechanism of Action Sirolimus inhibits T-lymphocyte activation and proliferation in response to antigenic and cytokine stimulation and inhibits antibody production. Its mechanism differs from other immunosuppressants. Sirolimus binds to FKBP-12, an intracellular protein, to form an immunosuppressive complex which inhibits the regulatory kinase, mTOR (mechanistic target of rapamycin). This inhibition suppresses cytokine mediated T-cell proliferation, halting progression from the G1 to the S phase of the cell cycle. It inhibits acute rejection of allografts and prolongs graft survival.

Pharmacodynamics/Kinetics

Absorption: Rapid

Distribution: 12 L/kg (range: 4-20 L/kg)

Protein binding: ~92%, primarily to albumin

Metabolism: Extensive; in intestinal wall via P-glycoprotein and hepatic via CYP3A4; to 7 major metabolites

Bioavailability: Oral solution: 14%; Oral tablet: 18%

Half-life elimination: Mean: 62 hours (range: 46-78 hours); extended in hepatic impairment (Child-Pugh class A or B) to 113 hours

Time to peak: Oral solution: 1-3 hours; Tablet: 1-6 hours

Excretion: Feces (91% due to P-glycoprotein-mediated efflux into gut lumen); urine (2%)

Dosage

Low-to-moderate immunologic risk renal transplant patients: Adolescents ≥13 years and Adults: Dosing by body weight: Oral:

<40 kg: Loading dose: 3 mg/m^2 on day 1, followed by maintenance dosing of 1 mg/m^2 once daily

≥40 kg: Loading dose: 6 mg on day 1; maintenance: 2 mg once daily

High immunologic risk renal transplant patients: Adults: Oral: Loading dose: Up to 15 mg on day 1; maintenance: 5 mg/day; obtain trough concentration between days 5-7 and adjust accordingly. Continue concurrent cyclosporine/sirolimus therapy for 1 year following transplantation. Further adjustment of the regimen must be based on clinical status.

Dosage adjustment: Sirolimus dosages should be adjusted to maintain trough concentrations within desired range based on risk and concomitant therapy. Maximum daily dose: 40 mg. Dosage should be adjusted at intervals of 7-14 days to account for the long half-life of sirolimus. In general, dose proportionality may be assumed. New sirolimus dose **equals** current dose **multiplied by** (target concentration **divided by** current concentration). **Note:** If large dose increase is required, consider loading dose calculated as:

Loading dose **equals** (new maintenance dose **minus** current maintenance dose) **multiplied by** 3

Maximum dose in 1 day: 40 mg; if required dose is >40 mg (due to loading dose), divide loading dose over 2 days. Whole blood concentrations should not be used as the sole basis for dosage adjustment (monitor clinical signs/symptoms, tissue biopsy, and laboratory parameters).

Maintenance therapy after withdrawal of cyclosporine: Cyclosporine withdrawal is not recommended in high immunological risk patients. Following 2-4 months of combined therapy, withdrawal of cyclosporine may be considered in low-to-moderate immunologic risk patients. Cyclosporine should be discontinued over 4-8 weeks, and a necessary increase in the dosage of sirolimus (up to fourfold) should be anticipated due to removal of metabolic inhibition by cyclosporine and to maintain adequate immunosuppressive effects. Dose-adjusted trough target concentrations are typically 16-24 ng/mL for the first year post-transplant and 12-20 ng/mL thereafter (measured by chromatographic methodology).

Graft-versus-host disease (GVHD): Adults: Oral:

GVHD prophylaxis (off-label use): 12 mg loading dose on day -3, followed by 4 mg daily (target trough level: 3-12 ng/mL); taper off after 6-9 months (Armand, 2008; Cutler, 2007)

Treatment of refractory acute GVHD (off-label use): 4-5 mg/m^2 for 14 days (no loading dose) (Benito, 2001)

Treatment of chronic GVHD (off-label use): 6 mg loading dose, followed by 2 mg daily (target trough level: 7-12 ng/mL) for 6-9 months (Couriel, 2005)

Heart transplantation (off-label use): Adults: Oral: **Note:** The use of sirolimus in the immediate post-cardiac transplant period (ie, *de novo* heart transplant) as a primary immunosuppressant has fallen out of favor due to adverse effects (eg, impaired wound healing and infection); however, patients may be converted to sirolimus from a calcineurin inhibitor (after at least 6 months from time of transplant [Costanzo, 2010]) or may have sirolimus added to a calcineurin inhibitor to prevent or minimize further transplant related vasculopathy or renal toxicity due to calcineurin inhibitor use.

Conversion from a calcineurin inhibitor (CNI) (ie, cyclosporine, tacrolimus): Reduce cyclosporine by 25 mg twice daily or tacrolimus by 1 mg twice daily followed by initiation of sirolimus 1 mg once daily; adjust sirolimus dose to target trough level of 8-14 ng/mL, withdraw CNI, repeat biopsy 2 weeks after CNI withdrawal (Topilsky, 2012). Alternatively, maintain CNI concentrations and initiate sirolimus 1 mg once daily for 1 week; adjust sirolimus to target trough levels of 10-15 ng/mL over 2 weeks, then reduce CNI to target 50% of therapeutic concentrations and after 2 weeks evaluate for rejection. If no rejection, continue same regimen for an additional month, then reduce CNI to 25% of therapeutic concentrations with repeat biopsy 2 weeks later; if no rejection, may discontinue CNI after 2 weeks and continue to maintain sirolimus trough levels of 10-15 ng/mL (usual doses required to maintain target levels: 1-8 mg daily) (Kushwaha, 2005).

Conversion from antiproliferative drug (ie, azathioprine or mycophenolate) while maintaining calcineurin inhibitor: Upon discontinuation of antiproliferative, administer sirolimus 6 mg loading dose followed by 2 mg once daily titrated to a target trough level of 4-15 ng/mL (Mancini, 2003) or 4-12 ng/mL per ISHLT recommendations (Costanzo, 2010).

Renal angiomyolipoma or lymphangioleiomyomatosis (off-label use): Adults: Oral: Initial: 0.5 mg/m^2 once daily titrated to a target trough level of 3-6 ng/mL (may increase to target trough level of 6-10 ng/mL if <10% reduction in lesion diameters at 2 months) for 2 years (Davies, 2011) **or** Initial: 2 mg once daily titrated to a target trough level of 5-15 ng/mL for 1 year (McCormack, 2011)

Dosage adjustment in renal impairment: No dosage adjustment necessary. However, adjustment of regimen (including discontinuation of therapy) should be considered when used concurrently with cyclosporine and elevated or increasing serum creatinine is noted.

Dosage adjustment in hepatic impairment:

Loading dose: No dosage adjustment necessary.

Maintenance dose:

Mild to moderate impairment (Child-Pugh classes A and B): Reduce maintenance dose by ~33%.

Severe impairment (Child-Pugh class C): Reduce maintenance dose by ~50%.

Dietary Considerations Take consistently (either with or without food) to minimize variability of absorption.

Administration Initial dose should be administered as soon as possible after transplant. Sirolimus should be taken 4 hours after oral cyclosporine (Neoral® or Gengraf®). Should be administered consistently (either with or without food).

Solution: Mix (by stirring vigorously) with at least 2 ounces of water or orange juice. No other liquids should be used for dilution. Patient should drink diluted solution immediately. The cup should then be refilled with an additional 4 ounces of water or orange juice, stirred vigorously, and the patient should drink the contents at once.

Tablet: Do not crush, split, or chew.

Hazardous agent; use appropriate precautions for handling and disposal (NIOSH 2014 [group 2]).

Monitoring Parameters Monitor LFTs and CBC during treatment. Monitor sirolimus levels in all patients (especially in pediatric patients, patients ≥13 years of age weighing <40 kg, patients with hepatic impairment, or on concurrent potent inhibitors or inducers of CYP3A4 or P-gp, and/or if cyclosporine dosing is markedly reduced or discontinued), and when changing dosage forms of sirolimus. Also monitor serum cholesterol and triglycerides, blood pressure, serum creatinine, and urinary protein. Serum drug concentrations should be determined 3-4 days after loading doses and 7-14 days after dosage adjustments; however, these concentrations should not be used as the sole basis for dosage adjustment, especially during withdrawal of cyclosporine (monitor clinical signs/symptoms, tissue biopsy, and laboratory parameters). **Note:** Concentrations and ranges are dependent on and will vary with assay methodology (chromatographic or immunoassay); assay methods are not interchangeable.

Reference Range Note: Sirolimus concentrations are dependent on the assay method (eg, chromatographic and immunoassay) used; assay methods are not interchangeable. Determine the assay method used to assure consistency (or accommodations if changes occur) and for monitoring purposes, be aware of alterations to assay method or reference range.

Serum trough concentration goals for renal transplantation (based on HPLC methods):

Concomitant cyclosporine: 4-12 ng/mL

Low-to-moderate immunologic risk (after cyclosporine withdrawal): 16-24 ng/mL for the first year after transplant; after 1 year: 12-20 ng/mL

High immunologic risk (with cyclosporine): 10-15 ng/mL

Note: Trough concentrations vary based on clinical context and use of additional immunosuppressants. The following represents typical ranges.

When combined with tacrolimus and mycophenolate mofetil (MMF) without steroids: 6-8 ng/mL

As a substitute for tacrolimus (starting 4-8 weeks post-transplant), in combination with MMF and steroids: 8-12 ng/mL

Following conversion from tacrolimus to sirolimus >6 months post-transplant due to chronic allograft nephropathy: 4-6 ng/mL

Serum trough concentrations for heart transplantation (off-label use):

With calcineurin inhibitor (eg, cyclosporine): 4-12 ng/mL (Costanzo, 2010)

Without calcineurin inhibitor: 10-15 ng/mL (Raichlin, 2007a; Raichlin, 2007b)

Following conversion from cyclosporine or tacrolimus to sirolimus: Initial (maintained until completion of conversion [~2 weeks]): 8-14 ng/mL (Topilsky, 2012) **or** 9-15 ng/mL (Zuckermann, 2012); Maintenance: 10-15 ng/mL (Kushwaha, 2005) **or** 7-15 ng/mL (Zuckermann, 2012)

Serum trough concentrations for GVHD prophylaxis in allogeneic stem cell transplant (off-label use): 3-12 ng/mL (Armand, 2008; Cutler, 2007)

Serum trough concentrations for advanced chordoma (off-label use): 15-20 ng/mL (Stacchiotti, 2009)

Serum trough concentrations for renal angiomyolipoma or lymphangioleiomyomatosis (off-label use): 3-6 ng/mL; may increase to 6-10 ng/mL if <10% reduction in lesion diameters at 2 months (Davies, 2011) **or** 5-15 ng/mL (McCormack, 2011)

Additional Information Sirolimus tablets and oral solution are not bioequivalent, due to differences in absorption. Clinical equivalence was seen using 2 mg tablet and 2 mg solution. It is not known if higher doses are also clinically equivalent. Monitor sirolimus levels if changes in dosage forms are made.

Sirolimus solution may cause irritation if administered undiluted.

High-risk renal transplant patients are defined (per the manufacturer's labeling) as African-American transplant recipients and/or repeat renal transplant recipients who lost a previous allograft based on an immunologic process and/or patients with high PRA (panel-reactive antibodies; peak PRA level >80%). Individual transplant centers may have differences in their definitions. For example, some centers would consider a PRA >50% to be at higher risk of rejection.

Dosage Forms

Solution, Oral:

Rapamune: 1 mg/mL (60 mL)

Tablet, Oral:

Rapamune: 0.5 mg, 1 mg, 2 mg

Generic: 0.5 mg, 1 mg, 2 mg

◆ **Sirop Docusate De Sodium [OTC] (Can)** *see* Docusate *on page 661*

◆ **Sirturo** *see* Bedaquiline *on page 233*

SitaGLIPtin (sit a GLIP tin)

Brand Names: U.S. Januvia

Brand Names: Canada Januvia®

Index Terms MK-0431; Sitagliptin Phosphate

Pharmacologic Category Antidiabetic Agent, Dipeptidyl Peptidase IV (DPP-IV) Inhibitor

Use Management of type 2 diabetes mellitus (noninsulin dependent, NIDDM) as an adjunct to diet and exercise as monotherapy or in combination therapy with other antidiabetic agents

Pregnancy Risk Factor B

Pregnancy Considerations Adverse events have not been observed in animal reproduction studies.

In women with diabetes, maternal hyperglycemia can be associated with congenital malformations as well as adverse effects in the fetus, neonate, and the mother (ACOG, 2005; ADA, 2014; Kitzmiller, 2008; Metzger, 2007). To prevent adverse outcomes, prior to conception and throughout pregnancy maternal blood glucose and HbA_{1c} should be kept as close to normal as possible but without causing significant hypoglycemia (ACOG, 2013; ADA, 2014; Blumer, 2013; Kitzmiller, 2008). Prior to pregnancy, effective contraception should be used until glycemic control is achieved (ADA, 2014; Kitzmiller, 2008). Other agents are currently recommended to treat diabetes in pregnant women (ACOG, 2013; Blumer, 2013).

Breast-Feeding Considerations It is not known if sitagliptin is excreted in breast milk. The manufacturer recommends that caution be used if administered to breast-feeding women.

Contraindications Serious hypersensitivity (eg, anaphylaxis, angioedema) to sitagliptin or any component of the formulation

Warnings/Precautions Avoid use in type 1 diabetes mellitus (insulin dependent, IDDM) and diabetic ketoacidosis (DKA) due to lack of efficacy in these populations. Use caution when used in conjunction with insulin or insulin secretagogues; risk of hypoglycemia is increased. Monitor blood glucose closely; dosage adjustments of insulin or insulin secretagogues may be necessary. Use with caution in patients with moderate-to-severe renal dysfunction and end-stage renal disease (ESRD) requiring hemodialysis or peritoneal dialysis; dosing adjustment required. Safety and efficacy have not been established in severe hepatic dysfunction.

Rare hypersensitivity reactions, including anaphylaxis, angioedema, and/or severe dermatologic reactions (such as Stevens-Johnson syndrome), have been reported in postmarketing surveillance; discontinue if signs/symptoms of hypersensitivity reactions occur. Use with caution if patient has experienced angioedema with other DPP-IV inhibitor use. Cases of acute pancreatitis (including hemorrhagic and necrotizing with some fatalities) have been reported with use; monitor for signs/symptoms of pancreatitis. Discontinue use immediately if pancreatitis is suspected and initiate appropriate management. Use with caution in patients with a history of pancreatitis (not known if this population is at greater risk).

Clinical trials included only a limited number of patients with heart failure (HF). No specific recommendations regarding this population are provided in the approved U.S. labeling (Canadian labeling recommends against use in this population). Diabetes self-management education (DSME) is essential to maximize the effectiveness of therapy.

Adverse Reactions As reported with monotherapy:

Cardiovascular: Peripheral edema

Endocrine & metabolic: Hypoglycemia

Gastrointestinal: Constipation, diarrhea, nausea

Neuromuscular & skeletal: Osteoarthritis

Respiratory: Nasopharyngitis, pharyngitis, upper respiratory tract infection (viral)

Rare but important or life-threatening: Acute renal failure (possibly requiring dialysis), anaphylaxis, anemia, angioedema, bundle branch block, depression, erectile dysfunction, exfoliative dermatitis, gastritis (*Helicobacter*), GERD, hepatic steatosis, hyper-/hypotension, hypersensitivity, liver enzymes increased, migraine, orthostasis, pancreatitis (acute cases including hemorrhagic or necrotizing forms with some fatalities), peripheral neuropathy, renal function decreased, rosacea, Stevens-Johnson syndrome

Drug Interactions

Metabolism/Transport Effects **Substrate** of P-glycoprotein

Avoid Concomitant Use There are no known interactions where it is recommended to avoid concomitant use.

Increased Effect/Toxicity

SitaGLIPtin may increase the levels/effects of: ACE Inhibitors; Digoxin

The levels/effects of SitaGLIPtin may be increased by: Androgens; Pegvisomant; P-glycoprotein/ABCB1 Inhibitors

Decreased Effect

The levels/effects of SitaGLIPtin may be decreased by: Corticosteroids (Orally Inhaled); Corticosteroids (Systemic); Danazol; Luteinizing Hormone-Releasing Hormone Analogs; P-glycoprotein/ABCB1 Inducers; Somatropin; Thiazide Diuretics

Storage/Stability Store at 20°C to 25°C (68°F to 77°F); excursions permitted to 15°C to 30°C (59°F to 86°F).

Mechanism of Action Sitagliptin inhibits dipeptidyl peptidase IV (DPP-IV) enzyme resulting in prolonged active incretin levels. Incretin hormones (eg, glucagon-like peptide-1 [GLP-1] and glucose-dependent insulinotropic polypeptide [GIP]) regulate glucose homeostasis by increasing insulin synthesis and release from pancreatic beta cells and decreasing glucagon secretion from pancreatic alpha cells. Decreased glucagon secretion results in decreased hepatic glucose production. Under normal physiologic circumstances, incretin hormones are released by the intestine throughout the day and levels are increased in response to a meal; incretin hormones are rapidly inactivated by the DPP-IV enzyme.

Pharmacodynamics/Kinetics

Absorption: Rapid

Distribution: ~198 L

Protein binding: 38%
Metabolism: Not extensively metabolized; minor metabolism via CYP3A4 and 2C8 to metabolites (inactive) suggested by *in vitro* studies
Bioavailability: ~87%
Half-life elimination: 12 hours
Time to peak, plasma: 1-4 hours
Excretion: Urine 87% (79% as unchanged drug, 16% as metabolites); feces 13%

Dosage Oral: Adults: Type 2 diabetes: 100 mg once daily
Concomitant use with insulin and/or insulin secretagogues (eg, sulfonylureas): Reduced dose of insulin and/or insulin secretagogues may be needed.

Dosage adjustment in renal impairment: Note: Renal function may be estimated using the Cockcroft-Gault formula for dosage adjustment purposes.
CrCl ≥50 mL/minute: No dosage adjustment necessary.
CrCl ≥30 to <50 mL/minute (approximate S_{cr} of >1.7 to ≤3.0 mg/dL [males] or >1.5 to ≤2.5 mg/dL [females]): 50 mg once daily
CrCl <30 mL/minute (approximate S_{cr} of >3.0 mg/dL [males] or >2.5 mg/dL [females]): 25 mg once daily
ESRD requiring hemodialysis or peritoneal dialysis: 25 mg once daily; administered without regard to timing of hemodialysis

Dosage adjustment in hepatic impairment:
Mild to moderate impairment (Child-Pugh classes A and B): No dosage adjustment necessary.
Severe impairment (Child-Pugh class C): No dosage adjustment provided in manufacturer's labeling (has not been studied).

Dietary Considerations May be taken with or without food. Individualized medical nutrition therapy (MNT) based on ADA recommendations is an integral part of therapy.

Administration May be administered with or without food.

Monitoring Parameters HbA_{1c}, serum glucose; renal function prior to initiation and periodically during treatment

Reference Range
Recommendations for glycemic control in nonpregnant adults with diabetes (ADA, 2015):
HbA_{1c}: <7% (a more aggressive [<6.5%] or less aggressive [<8%] HbA_{1c} goal may be targeted based on patient-specific characteristics)
Preprandial capillary plasma glucose: 80 to 130 mg/dL
Peak postprandial capillary blood glucose: <180 mg/dL

Recommendations for glycemic control in pediatric (all age groups) patients with type 1 diabetes (ADA, 2015):
HbA_{1c}: <7.5% (individualization may be appropriate based on patient-specific characteristics; <7% is reasonable if it can be achieved without excessive hypoglycemia)
Preprandial capillary plasma glucose: 90 to 130 mg/dL
Bedtime and overnight capillary blood glucose: 90 to 150 mg/dL

Dosage Forms
Tablet, Oral:
Januvia: 25 mg, 50 mg, 100 mg

Sitagliptin and Metformin

(sit a GLIP tin & met FOR min)

Brand Names: U.S. Janumet; Janumet XR

Brand Names: Canada Janumet; Janumet XR

Index Terms Metformin and Sitagliptin; Sitagliptin Phosphate and Metformin Hydrochloride

Pharmacologic Category Antidiabetic Agent, Biguanide; Antidiabetic Agent, Dipeptidyl Peptidase IV (DPP-IV) Inhibitor

Use Type 2 diabetes mellitus: As an adjunct to diet and exercise to improve glycemic control in adults with type 2 diabetes mellitus when treatment with both sitagliptin and metformin is appropriate

Pregnancy Risk Factor B

Dosage Oral: Type 2 diabetes mellitus: **Note:** Patients receiving concomitant insulin and/or insulin secretagogues (eg, sulfonylureas) may require dosage adjustments of these agents.

Adults: Initial doses should be based on current dose of sitagliptin and metformin.

Patients inadequately controlled on metformin alone: Initial dose:
Immediate release: Sitagliptin 100 mg daily plus current daily dose of metformin given in 2 equally divided doses; maximum: sitagliptin 100 mg/metformin 2000 mg daily. **Note:** The U.S. labeling recommends patients currently receiving metformin 850 mg twice daily receive an initial dose of sitagliptin 50 mg and metformin 1000 mg twice daily.
Extended release: Sitagliptin 100 mg daily plus current daily dose of metformin given once daily; maximum: sitagliptin 100 mg/metformin 2000 mg daily. **Note:** The U.S. labeling recommends patients currently receiving immediate release metformin 850-1000 mg twice daily receive an initial dose of sitagliptin 100 mg and metformin 2000 mg once daily.

Patients inadequately controlled on sitagliptin alone: Initial dose: **Note:** Patients currently receiving a renally-adjusted dose of sitagliptin should not be switched to a combination product.
Immediate release: Metformin 1000 mg daily plus sitagliptin 100 mg daily given in 2 equally divided doses
Extended release: Metformin 1000 mg and sitagliptin 100 mg once daily

Conversion from immediate release to extended release: Convert using same total daily dose (up to the maximum recommended dose), but adjust frequency as indicated for immediate (twice daily) or extended (once daily) release products.

Patients inadequately controlled on combination metformin and either pioglitazone, a sulfonylurea, or insulin: Canadian labeling (not in U.S. labeling): Sitagliptin 100 mg daily plus current daily dose of metformin given in 2 equally divided doses. If taking insulin or a sulfonylurea concomitantly with sitagliptin/metformin, the dosage of insulin or sulfonylurea may need adjusted.

Patients inadequately controlled on combination therapy with sitagliptin and insulin: Canadian labeling (not in U.S. labeling): Sitagliptin 100 mg daily plus metformin (dose based on glycemic control) given in 2 equally divided doses. Insulin dose may need adjusted.

Dosing adjustment: Metformin component may be gradually increased up to the maximum dose. Maximum dose: Sitagliptin 100 mg/metformin 2000 mg daily

Elderly: The initial and maintenance dosing should be conservative, due to the potential for decreased renal function (monitor). Do not use in patients ≥80 years of age unless normal renal function has been established.

Dosage adjustment in renal impairment:
U.S. labeling: Use is contraindicated in patients with renal impairment (eg, serum creatinine ≥1.5 mg/dL in males or ≥1.4 mg/dL in females or abnormal clearance).
Canadian labeling: Use is contraindicated.

Dosage adjustment in hepatic impairment:
U.S. labeling: Avoid metformin; liver disease is a risk factor for the development of lactic acidosis during metformin therapy.
Canadian labeling: Use is not recommended with clinical or laboratory evidence of disease and contraindicated in the presence of severe impairment.

Additional Information Complete prescribing information should be consulted for additional detail.

Dosage Forms

Tablet, oral:

Janumet: 50/500: Sitagliptin 50 mg and metformin 500 mg; 50/1000: Sitagliptin 50 mg and metformin 1000 mg

Tablet, extended release, oral:

Janumet XR: 50/500: Sitagliptin 50 mg and metformin 500 mg

Janumet XR: 50/1000: Sitagliptin 50 mg and metformin 1000 mg

Janumet XR: 100/1000: Sitagliptin 100 mg and metformin 1000 mg

Dosage Forms: Canada

Tablet, oral:

Janumet: 50/850: Sitagliptin 50 mg and metformin 850 mg

Sitagliptin and Simvastatin

(sit a GLIP tin & sim va STAT in)

Brand Names: U.S. Juvisync™ [DSC]

Index Terms Simvastatin and Sitagliptin; Sitagliptin Phosphate and Simvastatin

Pharmacologic Category Antidiabetic Agent, Dipeptidyl Peptidase IV (DPP-IV) Inhibitor; Antilipemic Agent, HMG-CoA Reductase Inhibitor

Use For use when treatment with both sitagliptin and simvastatin is appropriate:

Sitagliptin: Management of type 2 diabetes mellitus (noninsulin dependent, NIDDM) as an adjunct to diet and exercise as monotherapy or in combination therapy with other antidiabetic agents

Simvastatin: Used with dietary therapy for the following:

Secondary prevention of cardiovascular events in hypercholesterolemic patients with established coronary heart disease (CHD) or at high risk for CHD: To reduce cardiovascular morbidity (myocardial infarction, coronary/noncoronary revascularization procedures) and mortality; to reduce the risk of stroke

Hyperlipidemias: To reduce elevations in total cholesterol (total-C), LDL-C, apolipoprotein B, triglycerides, and VLDL-C, and to increase HDL-C in patients with primary hypercholesterolemia (elevations of 1 or more components are present in Fredrickson type IIa, IIb, III, and IV hyperlipidemias); treatment of homozygous familial hypercholesterolemia

Primary and secondary prevention of atherosclerotic cardiovascular disease (ASCVD) according to the American College of Cardiology/American Heart Association: To reduce the risk of ASCVD in patients with clinical ASCVD (eg, coronary heart disease, stroke/TIA, or peripheral arterial disease presumed to be of atherosclerotic origin) who are greater than 75 years of age or not a candidate for high-intensity statin therapy; in patients without clinical ASCVD if LDL-C is 190 mg/dL or greater and not a candidate for high-intensity statin therapy; in patients without clinical ASCVD who have type 1 or type 2 diabetes and are between 40 and 75 years of age; in patients with an estimated 10-year ASCVD risk 7.5% or greater and who are between 40 and 75 years of age (Stone, 2013). Specific recommendations from the Kidney Disease: Improving Global Outcomes (KDIGO) organization have also been released for patients with chronic kidney disease (KDIGO [Tonelli, 2013]).

Pregnancy Risk Factor X

Dosage Hyperlipidemia and type 2 diabetes: Adults: Oral: Initial dose: Sitagliptin 100 mg and simvastatin 40 mg once daily. **Note:** Patients already taking simvastatin <40 mg daily (with or without sitagliptin 100 mg daily) can be converted to the comparable equivalent of the combination product. Dose adjustments should be made at intervals of ≥4 weeks.

Concomitant use with insulin and/or insulin secretagogues (eg, sulfonylureas): Reduced dose of insulin and/or insulin secretagogues may be needed.

Dosage adjustment for simvastatin with concomitant medications:

Amiodarone, amlodipine, or ranolazine: Simvastatin dose should **not** exceed 20 mg daily

Diltiazem, dronedarone, or verapamil: Simvastatin dose should **not** exceed 10 mg daily

Lomitapide: Reduce simvastatin dose by 50% when initiating lomitapide. Simvastatin dose should not exceed 20 mg daily (or 40 mg daily for those who previously tolerated simvastatin 80 mg daily for ≥1 year without evidence of muscle toxicity)

Dosage adjustment for simvastatin in Chinese patients on niacin doses ≥1 g daily: Use caution with simvastatin doses of 40 mg daily because of an increased risk of myopathy

Dosage adjustment in renal impairment: Note: Renal function may be estimated using Cockcroft-Gault formula for dosage adjustment purposes.

CrCl ≥50 mL/minute: No dosage adjustment necessary.

CrCl ≥30 to <50 mL/minute (approximate S_{cr} of >1.7 to ≤3.0 mg/dL [males] or >1.5 to ≤2.5 mg/dL [females]): Initial: Sitagliptin 50 mg and simvastatin 40 mg once daily. **Note:** Patients already taking simvastatin <40 mg daily (with or without sitagliptin 50 mg daily) can be converted to the comparable equivalent of the combination product.

CrCl <30 mL/minute (approximate S_{cr} of >3.0 mg/dL [males] or >2.5 mg/dL [females]): Use is not recommended.

End-stage renal disease (ESRD): Use is not recommended

Dosage adjustment in hepatic impairment: Use is contraindicated

Additional Information Complete prescribing information should be consulted for additional detail.

◆ **Sitagliptin Phosphate** *see* SitaGLIPtin *on page 1897*

◆ **Sitagliptin Phosphate and Metformin Hydrochloride** *see* Sitagliptin and Metformin *on page 1898*

◆ **Sitagliptin Phosphate and Simvastatin** *see* Sitagliptin and Simvastatin *on page 1899*

◆ **Sitavig** *see* Acyclovir (Topical) *on page 51*

◆ **Sivextro** *see* Tedizolid *on page 1981*

◆ **Skelaxin** *see* Metaxalone *on page 1307*

◆ **Skelaxin® (Can)** *see* Metaxalone *on page 1307*

◆ **Skelid** *see* Tiludronate *on page 2042*

◆ **SKF 104864** *see* Topotecan *on page 2069*

◆ **SKF 104864-A** *see* Topotecan *on page 2069*

◆ **SKI-606** *see* Bosutinib *on page 282*

◆ **SKI-2053R** *see* Eptaplatin [INT] *on page 751*

◆ **Skin Bleaching** *see* Hydroquinone *on page 1020*

◆ **Skin Bleaching-Sunscreen** *see* Hydroquinone *on page 1020*

◆ **Sklice** *see* Ivermectin (Topical) *on page 1137*

◆ **Skyla** *see* Levonorgestrel *on page 1201*

◆ **Sleep Tabs [OTC]** *see* DiphenhydrAMINE (Systemic) *on page 641*

◆ **S-leucovorin** *see* LEVOleucovorin *on page 1200*

◆ **6S-leucovorin** *see* LEVOleucovorin *on page 1200*

◆ **Slo-Niacin [OTC]** *see* Niacin *on page 1443*

◆ **Slo-Pot (Can)** *see* Potassium Chloride *on page 1687*

◆ **Slow Fe [OTC]** *see* Ferrous Sulfate *on page 871*

◆ **Slow Iron [OTC]** *see* Ferrous Sulfate *on page 871*

◆ **Slow-K (Can)** *see* Potassium Chloride *on page 1687*

◆ **Slow-Mag [OTC]** *see* Magnesium Chloride *on page 1261*

◆ **Slow Magnesium/Calcium [OTC]** *see* Magnesium Chloride *on page 1261*

◆ **Slow Release Iron [OTC] [DSC]** *see* Ferrous Sulfate *on page 871*

◆ **SM-13496** *see* Lurasidone *on page 1256*

Smallpox Vaccine (SMAL poks vak SEEN)

Brand Names: U.S. ACAM2000®

Index Terms Live Smallpox Vaccine; Vaccinia Vaccine

Pharmacologic Category Vaccine, Live (Viral)

Additional Appendix Information

Immunization Administration Recommendations *on page 2250*

Immunization Recommendations *on page 2255*

Use Smallpox disease prevention: Active immunization against smallpox disease in persons determined to be at high risk for smallpox infection.

The Advisory Committee on Immunization Practices (ACIP) recommends routine vaccination for the following (CDC/ACIP [Rotz, 2001]):

- Laboratory workers at risk of exposure from cultures or contaminated animals which may be a source of vaccinia or related Orthopoxviruses capable of causing infections in humans (eg, monkeypox, cowpox, variola, vaccinia).
- Consideration may also be given for vaccination of healthcare workers having contact with clinical specimens, contaminated material, or patients receiving vaccinia or recombinant vaccinia viruses.

In a Pre-Event Vaccination Program, the ACIP recommends vaccination for the following (CDC/ACIP [Wharton, 2003):

- Persons designated by authorities to investigate smallpox cases with the likelihood of direct patient contact
- Persons responsible for administering smallpox vaccine

In the event of an intentional release of smallpox virus, the ACIP recommends vaccination for the following (CDC/ACIP [Rotz, 2001]):

- Persons exposed to the initial release of the virus
- Persons who had close contact with a confirmed or suspected smallpox patient at any time from the onset of the patient's fever until all scabs have separated
- Healthcare providers involved in evaluation, care, or transport of confirmed or suspected smallpox patients
- Laboratory personnel involved in processing specimens of confirmed or suspected smallpox patients
- Persons likely to have increased contact with infectious materials from smallpox patients

Pregnancy Risk Factor D

Dosage Percutaneous: Not for IM, intradermal, IV, or SubQ injection: Vaccination by scarification (multiple-puncture technique) only: **Note:** A trace of blood should appear at vaccination site after 15-20 seconds; if no trace of blood is visible, an additional 3 insertions should be made using the same needle, without reinserting the needle into the vaccine bottle.

Children ≥12 months (in emergency conditions only), Adolescents, and Adults:

Primary vaccination and revaccination: Use a single drop of vaccine suspension and 15 needle punctures (using the same bifurcated needle) into the superficial skin

Note: According to the manufacturer, revaccination is recommended every 3 years for patients at a continued high risk for smallpox infection. The ACIP recommends routine nonemergency revaccination every 3-10 years, depending on type of exposure (CDC/ACIP [Rotz, 2001]). Additional information can be obtained from the Department of Defense and the CDC.

Dosage adjustment in renal impairment: There are no dosage adjustments provided in the manufacturer's labeling.

Dosage adjustment in hepatic impairment: There are no dosage adjustments provided in the manufacturer's labeling.

Additional Information Complete prescribing information should be consulted for additional detail.

Dosage Forms

Injection, powder for reconstitution [purified monkey cell source]:

ACAM2000: 1-5 x 10^8 plaque-forming units per mL

◆ **SMOFlipid (Can)** *see* Fat Emulsion (Fish Oil Based) [CAN/INT] *on page 847*

◆ **SMX-TMP** *see* Sulfamethoxazole and Trimethoprim *on page 1946*

◆ **SMZ-TMP** *see* Sulfamethoxazole and Trimethoprim *on page 1946*

◆ **(+)-(*S*)-*N*-Methyl-γ-(1-naphthyloxy)-2-thiophenepropylamine Hydrochloride** *see* DULoxetine *on page 698*

◆ **Sochlor [OTC]** *see* Sodium Chloride *on page 1902*

◆ **Sodium 2-Mercaptoethane Sulfonate** *see* Mesna *on page 1305*

◆ **Sodium 4-Hydroxybutyrate** *see* Sodium Oxybate *on page 1908*

◆ **Sodium *L*-Triiodothyronine** *see* Liothyronine *on page 1221*

Sodium Acetate (SOW dee um AS e tate)

Pharmacologic Category Electrolyte Supplement, Parenteral

Use Sodium source in large volume IV fluids to prevent or correct hyponatremia in patients with restricted intake; used to counter acidosis through conversion to bicarbonate

Pregnancy Risk Factor C

Dosage Sodium acetate is metabolized to bicarbonate on an equimolar basis outside the liver; administer in large volume IV fluids as a sodium source. Refer to Sodium Bicarbonate monograph.

Maintenance electrolyte requirements of sodium in parenteral nutrition solutions:

Daily requirements: 3-4 mEq/kg/24 hours or 25-40 mEq/1000 kcal/24 hours

Maximum: 100-150 mEq/24 hours

Dosage adjustment in renal impairment: No dosage adjustment provided in manufacturer's labeling. Use with caution.

Dosage adjustment in hepatic impairment: No dosage adjustment provided in manufacturer's labeling. Use with caution.

Additional Information Complete prescribing information should be consulted for additional detail.

Dosage Forms

Solution, Intravenous:

Generic: 2 mEq/mL (20 mL, 50 mL, 100 mL); 4 mEq/mL (50 mL, 100 mL)

◆ **Sodium Acid Carbonate** *see* Sodium Bicarbonate *on page 1901*

◆ **Sodium Acid Phosphate and Methenamine** *see* Methenamine and Sodium Acid Phosphate *on page 1318*

◆ **Sodium Artesunate** *see* Artesunate *on page 178*

◆ **Sodium Benzoate and Caffeine** *see* Caffeine *on page 319*

◆ **Sodium Benzoate and Sodium Phenylacetate** *see* Sodium Phenylacetate and Sodium Benzoate *on page 1908*

Sodium Bicarbonate (SOW dee um bye KAR bun ate)

Brand Names: U.S. Neut

Index Terms Baking Soda; $NaHCO_3$; Sodium Acid Carbonate; Sodium Hydrogen Carbonate

Pharmacologic Category Alkalinizing Agent; Antacid; Electrolyte Supplement, Oral; Electrolyte Supplement, Parenteral

Use

Management of metabolic acidosis; gastric hyperacidity; as an alkalinization agent for the urine; treatment of hyperkalemia; management of overdose of certain drugs, including tricyclic antidepressants and aspirin

Neutralizing additive (dental use): Improves onset of analgesia and reduces injection site pain by adjusting lidocaine with epinephrine solution to a more physiologic pH.

Pregnancy Risk Factor C

Pregnancy Considerations Animal reproduction studies have not been conducted. The use of sodium bicarbonate in pregnant women for the management of cardiac arrest and metabolic acidosis is the same as in nonpregnant women (Campbell, 2009; Vanden Hoek, 2010). Antacids containing sodium bicarbonate should not be used during pregnancy due to their potential to cause metabolic alkalosis and fluid overload (Mahadevan, 2007).

Breast-Feeding Considerations Sodium is found in breast milk (IOM, 2004).

Contraindications

Alkalosis, hypernatremia, severe pulmonary edema, hypocalcemia, unknown abdominal pain

Neutralizing additive (dental use): Not for use as a systemic alkalizer

Warnings/Precautions Rapid administration in neonates, infants, and children <2 years of age has led to hypernatremia, decreased CSF pressure, and intracranial hemorrhage. **Use of IV $NaHCO_3$ should be reserved for documented metabolic acidosis and for hyperkalemia-induced cardiac arrest.** Routine use in cardiac arrest is not recommended. Vesicant (at concentrations ≥8.4%); ensure proper catheter or needle position prior to and during infusion; avoid extravasation (tissue necrosis may occur due to hypertonicity). May cause sodium retention especially if renal function is impaired; not to be used in treatment of peptic ulcer; use with caution in patients with HF, edema, cirrhosis, or renal failure. Not the antacid of choice for the elderly because of sodium content and potential for systemic alkalosis.

Adverse Reactions

Cardiovascular: Cerebral hemorrhage, CHF (aggravated), edema

Central nervous system: Tetany

Gastrointestinal: Belching, flatulence (with oral), gastric distension

Endocrine & metabolic: Hypernatremia, hyperosmolality, hypocalcemia, hypokalemia, increased affinity of hemoglobin for oxygen-reduced pH in myocardial tissue necrosis when extravasated, intracranial acidosis, metabolic alkalosis, milk-alkali syndrome (especially with renal dysfunction)

Respiratory: Pulmonary edema

Drug Interactions

Metabolism/Transport Effects None known.

Avoid Concomitant Use There are no known interactions where it is recommended to avoid concomitant use.

Increased Effect/Toxicity

Sodium Bicarbonate may increase the levels/effects of: Alpha-/Beta-Agonists (Indirect-Acting); Amphetamines; Calcium Polystyrene Sulfonate; Dexmethylphenidate; Flecainide; Memantine; Methylphenidate; QuiNIDine; QuiNINE

The levels/effects of Sodium Bicarbonate may be increased by: AcetaZOLAMIDE

Decreased Effect

Sodium Bicarbonate may decrease the levels/effects of: Antipsychotic Agents (Phenothiazines); Atazanavir; Bisacodyl; Bosutinib; Captopril; Cefditoren; Cefpodoxime; Cefuroxime; Chloroquine; Corticosteroids (Oral); Dabigatran Etexilate; Dabrafenib; Dasatinib; Delavirdine; Elvitegravir; Erlotinib; Flecainide; Fosinopril; Gabapentin; HMG-CoA Reductase Inhibitors; Hyoscyamine; Iron Salts; Isoniazid; Itraconazole; Ketoconazole (Systemic); Ledipasvir; Lithium; Mesalamine; Methenamine; Multivitamins/Minerals (with ADEK, Folate, Iron); Nilotinib; PAZOPanib; PenicillAMINE; Phosphate Supplements; Potassium Acid Phosphate; Protease Inhibitors; Rilpivirine; Riociguat; Sulpiride; Tetracycline Derivatives; Trientine; Vismodegib

Preparation for Administration

Prevention of contrast-induced nephropathy (off-label use): Remove 154 mL from 1000 mL bag of D_5W; replace with 154 mL of 8.4% sodium bicarbonate; resultant concentration is 154 mEq/L (Merten, 2004); more practically, institutions may remove 150 mL from 1000 mL bag of D_5W and replace with 150 mL of 8.4% sodium bicarbonate; resultant concentration is 150 mEq/L

Neutralizing additive (dental use): Add specified volume of 8.4% sodium bicarbonate directly with lidocaine and epinephrine injection and mix; use immediately after mixing.

Storage/Stability

Store injection at room temperature. Protect from heat and from freezing. Use only clear solutions.

Neutralizing additive (dental use): Store at 20°C to 25°C (68°F to 77°F).

Mechanism of Action

Dissociates to provide bicarbonate ion which neutralizes hydrogen ion concentration and raises blood and urinary pH

Neutralizing additive (dental use): Increases pH of lidocaine and epinephrine solution to improve tolerability and increase tissue uptake

Pharmacodynamics/Kinetics

Onset of action: Oral: Rapid; IV: 15 minutes

Duration: Oral: 8-10 minutes; IV: 1-2 hours

Absorption: Oral: Well absorbed

Excretion: Urine (<1%)

Dosage

Cardiac arrest (ACLS, 2010; PALS, 2010): **Routine use of $NaHCO_3$ is not recommended.** May be considered in the setting of prolonged cardiac arrest only after adequate alveolar ventilation has been established and effective cardiac compressions. **Note:** In some cardiac arrest situations (eg, metabolic acidosis, hyperkalemia, or tricyclic antidepressant overdose), sodium bicarbonate may be beneficial.

Infants and Children: IV, I.O.: 1 mEq/kg/dose; repeat doses should be guided by arterial blood gases; children <2 years of age should receive 4.2% (0.5 mEq/mL) solution. **Note:** If I.O. route is used for administration and is subsequently used to obtain blood samples for acid-base analysis, results will be inaccurate.

Adults: IV: Initial: 1 mEq/kg/dose; repeat doses should be guided by arterial blood gases

Metabolic acidosis: Infants, Children, and Adults: Dosage should be based on the following formula if blood gases and pH measurements are available:

HCO_3^- (mEq) = 0.5 x weight (kg) x [24 - serum HCO_3^-(mEq/L)] **or** HCO_3^-(mEq) = 0.5 x weight (kg) x [desired increase in serum HCO_3^-(mEq/L)]

Administer 1/2 dose initially, then remaining 1/2 dose over the next 24 hours; monitor pH, serum HCO_3^-, and clinical status. **Note:** These equations provide an estimated replacement dose. The underlying cause and degree of acidosis may result in the need for larger or smaller replacement doses. In most cases, the initial goal of therapy is to target a pH of ~7.2 and a plasma bicarbonate level of ~10 mEq/L to prevent overalkalinization.

Note: If acid-base status is not available: Dose for older Children and Adults: 2-5 mEq/kg IV infusion over 4-8 hours; subsequent doses should be based on patient's acid-base status

Chronic renal failure: Oral: Initiate when plasma HCO_3^- <15 mEq/L

Children: 1-3 mEq/kg/day

Adults: Start with 20-36 mEq/day in divided doses, titrate to bicarbonate level of 18-20 mEq/L

Hyperkalemia (ACLS, 2010): Adults: IV: 50 mEq over 5 minutes (as appropriate, consider methods of enhancing potassium removal/excretion)

Renal tubular acidosis: Oral:

Distal:

Children: 2-3 mEq/kg/day

Adults: 0.5-2 mEq/kg/day in 4-5 divided doses

Proximal: Children and Adults: Initial: 5-10 mEq/kg/day; maintenance: Increase as required to maintain serum bicarbonate in the normal range

Urine alkalinization: Oral:

Children: 1-10 mEq (84-840 mg)/kg/day in divided doses every 4-6 hours; dose should be titrated to desired urinary pH

Adults: Initial: 48 mEq (4 g), then 12-24 mEq (1-2 g) every 4 hours; dose should be titrated to desired urinary pH; doses up to 16 g/day (200 mEq) in patients <60 years and 8 g (100 mEq) in patients >60 years

Antacid: Adults: Oral: 325 mg to 2 g 1-4 times/day

Neutralize lidocaine with epinephrine dental anesthetic: Children, Adolescents, and Adults: Neutralizing additive: Mix 10 parts anesthetic (lidocaine with epinephrine) to 1 part 8.4% sodium bicarbonate:

Add 0.18 mL sodium bicarbonate to 1.8 mL cartridge of lidocaine 2% with epinephrine 1:50,000 or 1:100,000

Add 2 mL sodium bicarbonate to 20 mL vial of lidocaine 2% with epinephrine 1:100,000

Add 3 mL sodium bicarbonate to 30 mL vial of lidocaine 2% with epinephrine 1:100,000

Add 5 mL sodium bicarbonate to 50 mL vial of lidocaine 2% with epinephrine 1:100,000

Prevention of contrast-induced nephropathy (off-label use): Adults: IV infusion: 154 mEq/L sodium bicarbonate in D_5W solution: 3 mL/kg/hour for 1 hour immediately before contrast injection, then 1mL/kg/hour during contrast exposure and for 6 hours after procedure

To prepare solution, remove 154 mL from 1000 mL bag of D_5W; replace with 154 mL of 8.4% sodium bicarbonate; resultant concentration is 154 mEq/L (Merten, 2004); more practically, institutions may remove 150 mL from 1000 mL bag of D_5W and replace with 150 mL of 8.4% sodium bicarbonate; resultant concentration is 150 mEq/L

Dietary Considerations Some products may contain sodium. Oral product should be taken 1-3 hours after meals.

Administration For IV administration to infants, use the 0.5 mEq/mL solution or dilute the 1 mEq/mL solution 1:1 with **sterile water**; for direct IV infusion in emergencies, administer slowly (maximum rate in infants: 10 mEq/minute); for infusion, dilute to a maximum concentration of 0.5 mEq/mL in dextrose solution and infuse over 2 hours (maximum rate of administration: 1 mEq/kg/hour).

Vesicant (at concentrations ≥8.4%); ensure proper needle or catheter placement prior to and during IV infusion. Avoid extravasation.

Extravasation management: If extravasation occurs, stop infusion immediately and disconnect (leave needle/cannula in place); gently aspirate extravasated solution (do **NOT** flush the line); initiate hyaluronidase antidote; remove needle/cannula; apply dry cold compresses (Hurst, 2004); elevate extremity.

Hyaluronidase: SubQ: Inject four to five separate 0.2 mL injections of 15 units/mL around area of extravasation (Hurst, 2004).

Oral product should be administered 1-3 hours after meals.

Infiltration (dental use; Onpharma): Add specified volume of 8.4% sodium bicarbonate directly with lidocaine and epinephrine injection and mix; use immediately after mixing.

Dosage Forms Considerations

Sodium bicarbonate solution 4.2% [42 mg/mL] provides 0.5 mEq/mL each of sodium and bicarbonate

Sodium bicarbonate solution 7.5% [75 mg/mL] provides 0.9 mEq/mL each of sodium and bicarbonate

Sodium bicarbonate solution 8.4% [84 mg/mL] provides 1 mEq/mL each of sodium and bicarbonate

Dosage Forms

Powder, Oral:

Generic: (1 g, 120 g, 454 g, 500 g, 1000 g, 2500 g, 12000 g, 25000 g, 45000 g)

Solution, Intravenous:

Neut: 4% (5 mL)

Generic: 4.2% (5 mL, 10 mL); 7.5% (50 mL); 8.4% (10 mL, 50 mL)

Tablet, Oral:

Generic: 325 mg, 650 mg

◆ **Sodium Bicarbonate and Omeprazole** *see* Omeprazole and Sodium Bicarbonate *on page 1511*

Sodium Chloride (SOW dee um KLOR ide)

Brand Names: U.S. 4-Way Saline [OTC]; Afrin Saline Nasal Mist [OTC]; Altachlore [OTC]; Altamist Spray [OTC]; Ayr Nasal Mist Allergy/Sinus [OTC]; Ayr Saline Nasal Drops [OTC]; Ayr Saline Nasal Gel [OTC]; Ayr Saline Nasal No-Drip [OTC]; AYR Saline Nasal Rinse [OTC]; Ayr Saline Nasal [OTC]; Ayr [OTC]; Baby Ayr Saline [OTC]; Broncho Saline [OTC]; Deep Sea Nasal Spray [OTC]; Entsol Nasal Wash [OTC]; Entsol Nasal [OTC]; Entsol [OTC]; Humist [OTC]; HyperSal; Muro 128 [OTC]; Na-Zone [OTC]; Nasal Moist [OTC]; Nebusal; Ocean Complete Sinus Rinse [OTC]; Ocean for Kids [OTC]; Ocean Nasal Spray [OTC]; Ocean Ultra Saline Mist [OTC]; Pretz Irrigation [OTC]; Pretz [OTC]; PulmoSal; Rhinaris [OTC]; Safe Wash [OTC]; Saline Flush ZR; Saline Mist Spray [OTC]; Saljet Rinse [OTC]; Saljet [OTC]; Sea Soft Nasal Mist [OTC]; Sea-Clens Wound Cleanser [OTC]; Sochlor [OTC]; Sodium Chloride Thermoject Sys; Swab-Flush Saline Flush; Wound Wash Saline [OTC]

Index Terms Hypertonic Saline; NaCl; Normal Saline; Saline; Salt

Pharmacologic Category Electrolyte Supplement, Parenteral; Genitourinary Irrigant; Irrigant; Lubricant, Ocular; Sodium Salt

Use

Parenteral: Restores sodium ion in patients with restricted oral intake (especially hyponatremia states or low salt syndrome).

Concentrated sodium chloride: Additive for parenteral fluid therapy
Hypertonic sodium chloride: For severe hyponatremia and hypochloremia
Hypotonic sodium chloride: Hydrating solution
Normal saline: Restores water/sodium losses
Ophthalmic: Reduces corneal edema
Inhalation: Restores moisture to pulmonary system; loosens and thins congestion caused by colds or allergies; diluent for bronchodilator solutions that require dilution before inhalation
Intranasal: Restores moisture to nasal membranes
Irrigation: Wound cleansing, irrigation, and flushing

Pregnancy Risk Factor C

Pregnancy Considerations Animal reproduction studies have not been conducted. Sodium requirements do not change during pregnancy (IOM, 2004). Nasal saline rinses may be used for the treatment of pregnancy rhinitis (Wallace, 2008)

Breast-Feeding Considerations Sodium is found in breast milk. Sodium requirements do not change during lactation (IOM, 2004).

Contraindications Hypersensitivity to sodium chloride or any component of the formulation; hypertonic uterus, hypernatremia, fluid retention

Warnings/Precautions The use of hypotonic saline solutions (eg, 0.225% sodium chloride) may result in hemolysis if administered rapidly and for prolonged periods. If hypotonic saline solutions become necessary, administration as D_5W/0.2% NaCl or 0.45% NaCl is recommended for most patients (eg, those without hyperglycemia). Use with caution in patients with HF, renal insufficiency, liver cirrhosis, hypertension, edema.

Administration of low sodium or sodium-free IV solutions may result in significant hyponatremia or water intoxication; monitor serum sodium concentration closely. In the treatment of acute hypernatremia (ie, development over a couple of hours), serum sodium concentration should be corrected no faster than 1-2 mEq/L per hour. If patient has been chronically hypernatremic, correct serum sodium no faster than 0.5 mEq/L per hour and by no more than 10-12 mEq/L in a given 24-hour period; use extreme caution since rapid correction may result in cerebral edema, herniation, coma, and death (Adrogue, 2000; Kraft, 2005).

When treating hyponatremia, rate of correction is dependent upon whether or not it is acute or chronic. Sodium toxicity (eg, osmotic demyelination syndrome) is almost exclusively related to how fast a sodium deficit is corrected; both rate and magnitude are extremely important. For patients with acute (<24 hours) or chronic (>48 hours), severe (<120 mEq/L) hyponatremia, a serum sodium concentration increase of 4-6 mEq/L within a 24-hour period is sufficient for most patients. In chronic severe hyponatremia, overcorrection risks iatrogenic osmotic demyelination syndrome. For patients with severe symptoms or other need for urgent correction, may increase by 4-6 mEq/L within the first 6 hours and postpone any further correction until the next day at a correction rate of 4-6 mEq/L per day. Choice of infusate sodium concentration is dependent upon the severity of the hyponatremia with more concentrated solutions (eg, 3% NaCl) for more severe cases; monitor serum sodium closely during administration (Sterns, 2013).

Benzyl alcohol and derivatives: Bacteriostatic sodium chloride contains benzyl alcohol; large amounts of benzyl alcohol (≥99 mg/kg/day) have been associated with a potentially fatal toxicity ("gasping syndrome") in neonates; the "gasping syndrome" consists of metabolic acidosis, respiratory distress, gasping respirations, CNS dysfunction (including convulsions, intracranial hemorrhage), hypotension, and cardiovascular collapse (AAP, 1997; CDC, 1982); some data suggests that benzoate displaces bilirubin from protein binding sites (Ahlfors, 2001); avoid or use dosage forms containing benzyl alcohol with caution in neonates. See manufacturer's labeling.

Wound Wash Saline is for single-patient use only.

Irrigants: For external use only; not for parenteral use. Do not use during electrosurgical procedures. Irrigating fluids may be absorbed into systemic circulation; monitor for fluid or solute overload.

Concentrated solutions of sodium chloride (>1%) are vesicants; ensure proper needle or catheter placement prior to and during infusion; avoid extravasation.

Adverse Reactions
Cardiovascular: Congestive heart failure, transient hypotension (especially with adult administration of 23.4% NaCl)
Central nervous system: Central pontine myelinolysis (due to rapid correction of hyponatremia)
Endocrine & metabolic: Dilution of serum electrolytes, extravasation, hypernatremia, hypervolemia, hypokalemia, overhydration
Gastrointestinal: Nausea, vomiting (oral use)
Local: Thrombosis, phlebitis, extravasation
Respiratory: Bronchospasm (inhalation with hypertonic solutions), pulmonary edema

Drug Interactions

Metabolism/Transport Effects None known.

Avoid Concomitant Use

Avoid concomitant use of Sodium Chloride with any of the following: Tolvaptan

Increased Effect/Toxicity

Sodium Chloride may increase the levels/effects of: Tolvaptan

Decreased Effect

Sodium Chloride may decrease the levels/effects of: Lithium

Storage/Stability Store injection at room temperature; do not freeze. Protect from heat. Use only clear solutions.

Mechanism of Action Principal extracellular cation; functions in fluid and electrolyte balance, osmotic pressure control, and water distribution

Pharmacodynamics/Kinetics
Absorption: Oral: Rapid
Distribution: Widely distributed
Excretion: Primarily urine; also sweat, tears, saliva

Dosage
Children: IV: Hypertonic solutions (>0.9%) should only be used for the initial treatment of acute serious symptomatic hyponatremia or increased intracranial pressure in the setting of traumatic brain injury.
Maintenance: 3-4 mEq/kg/day; maximum: 100-150 mEq/day; dosage varies widely depending on clinical condition
Replacement: Determined by laboratory determinations mEq
Sodium deficiency (mEq/kg) = [% dehydration (L/kg)/ 100 x 70 (mEq/L)] + [0.6 (L/kg) x (140 - serum sodium) (mEq/L)]
Hypovolemic septic shock, initial fluid resuscitation (off-label use): IV: Normal saline (0.9% NaCl): Up to 20 mL/kg/dose over 5-10 minutes; titrate to hypotension reversal, increasing urine output, and attainment of normal capillary refill, peripheral pulses, and level of consciousness (Dellinger, 2013)
Increased intracranial pressure (off-label use): Hypertonic saline (3%): 0.1-1 mL/kg/hour continuous infusion titrated to maintain ICP <20 mm Hg (Addleson, 2003)
Children ≥2 years and Adults:
Intranasal: 2-3 sprays in each nostril as needed
Irrigation: Spray affected area

Children and Adults: Inhalation: Bronchodilator diluent: 1-3 sprays (1-3 mL) to dilute bronchodilator solution in nebulizer prior to administration

Adults:

Refractory elevated ICP due to various etiologies (eg, subarachnoid hemorrhage, trauma, neoplasm), transtentorial herniation syndromes (off-label use): IV: Hypertonic saline: 23.4% (30-60 mL) given over 2-20 minutes administered via central venous access only (Koenig, 2008; Suarez, 1998; Ware, 2005)

Severe sepsis, initial fluid resuscitation (off-label use): IV: Normal saline (0.9% NaCl): Minimum of 30 mL/kg. **Note:** Administer within 3 hours of sepsis recognition for hypotension or lactate ≥4 mmol/L (≥36 mg/dL). Some patients may require more rapid administration and/or greater amount of fluid for complete resuscitation (Dellinger, 2013).

Subarachnoid hemorrhage with hyponatremia (ie, ≤135 mEq/L) to enhance cerebral perfusion (off-label use): IV: Hypertonic saline: 3% sodium chloride/acetate (50:50 mixture) 100-200 mL/hour administered via central venous catheter; titrate to clinical response up to a maximum serum sodium between 150-160 mEq/L (achieved at a rate of 0.5-1 mEq/L/hour) (Suarez, 1999)

Traumatic brain injury with elevated ICP (off-label use): IV: Hypertonic saline: **Note:** Optimal dose has not been established; due to insufficient evidence, the Brain Trauma Foundation guidelines (Bratton, 2007) do not make specific recommendations on the use of hypertonic saline for the treatment of traumatic intracranial hypertension. Clinical trials are small; few are prospective. **Some concentrations may not be commercially available; administer via central venous catheter;** protocols include:

3%: 300 mL administered over 20 minutes when ICP values exceed 20 mm Hg (Huang, 2006)

7.2%: 1.5 mL/kg administered over 15 minutes when ICP values exceed 15 mm Hg (Munar, 2000)

7.5%: 2 mL/kg administered over 20 minutes when ICP values exceed 25 mm Hg (Vialet, 2003)

23.4%: 30 mL administered over 2 minutes (Ware, 2005) **or** over >30 minutes when ICP values exceed 20 mm Hg (Kerwin, 2009)

GU irrigant: 1-3 L/day by intermittent irrigation

Replacement IV: Determined by laboratory determinations mEq

Hyponatremia: IV: To correct acute (<24 hours) or chronic (>48 hours), severe (<120 mEq/L) hyponatremia: In general, a serum sodium concentration increase of 4-6 mEq/L within a 24-hour period is sufficient to improve most symptoms of hyponatremia. In chronic severe hyponatremia, overcorrection risks iatrogenic osmotic demyelination syndrome. For patients with severe symptoms or other need for urgent correction, one approach is to increase serum sodium concentration by 4-6 mEq/L within the first 6 hours and postpone any further correction until the next day at a correction rate of 4-6 mEq/L per day. Choice of sodium correction fluid concentration is dependent upon the severity of the hyponatremia with more concentrated solutions (eg, 3% NaCl) for more severe cases; monitor serum sodium closely during administration (Sterns, 2013).

Chloride maintenance electrolyte requirement in parenteral nutrition: IV: As needed to maintain acid-base balance with parenteral nutrition; use equal amounts of chloride and acetate to maintain balance and adjust ratio based on individual patient needs (Mirtallo, 2004).

Sodium maintenance electrolyte requirement in parenteral nutrition: IV: 1-2 mEq/kg/24 hours; customize amounts based on individual patient needs (Mirtallo, 2004).

Ophthalmic:

Ointment: Apply once daily or more often

Solution: Instill 1-2 drops into affected eye(s) every 3-4 hours

Administration

Irrigation solution: Do not warm >66°C (150°F); not for IV use. Wound Wash Saline: Before use, expel a short stream into air to clear nozzle.

IV: >2% solutions: Administration through a central line is recommended due to high osmolarity and tonicity (Mortimer, 2006). Consult individual institutional policies and procedures.

Vesicant at higher concentrations (>1%); ensure proper needle or catheter placement prior to and during infusion; avoid extravasation.

Extravasation management: If extravasation occurs, stop infusion immediately and disconnect (leave cannula/needle in place); gently aspirate extravasated solution (do **NOT** flush the line); remove needle/cannula; elevate extremity. Apply dry warm compresses (Hastings-Tolsma, 1993).

Monitoring Parameters Serum sodium, potassium, chloride, and bicarbonate concentrations; I & O, weight

Reference Range Serum/plasma sodium concentration:

Neonates:

Full-term: 133-142 mEq/L

Premature: 132-140 mEq/L

Children ≥2 months to Adults: 135-145 mEq/L

Additional Information

Normal saline (0.9%) = 154 mEq/L; 3% NaCl = 513 mEq/L; 5% NaCl = 856 mEq/L

Tablet 1g = 17.1 mEq

Dosage Forms Considerations 1 g sodium chloride = elemental sodium 393.3 mg = 17.1 mEq sodium = sodium 17.1 mmol

Dosage Forms

Aerosol Solution, Inhalation:

Broncho Saline [OTC]: 0.9% (90 mL, 240 mL)

Aerosol Solution, Nasal [preservative free]:

Ocean Complete Sinus Rinse [OTC]: (177 mL)

Gel, Nasal:

Ayr Saline Nasal [OTC]: (14.1 g)

Ayr Saline Nasal No-Drip [OTC]: (22 mL)

Entsol Nasal [OTC]: (20 g)

Rhinaris [OTC]: 0.2% (28.4 g)

Liquid, External:

Sea-Clens Wound Cleanser [OTC]: (355 mL)

Nebulization Solution, Inhalation:

Generic: 0.9% (3 mL)

Nebulization Solution, Inhalation [preservative free]:

HyperSal: 3.5% (4 mL); 7% (4 mL)

Nebusal: 3% (4 mL); 6% (4 mL)

PulmoSal: 7% (4 mL)

Generic: 0.9% (3 mL, 5 mL, 15 mL); 3% (4 mL, 15 mL); 7% (4 mL); 10% (4 mL, 15 mL)

Ointment, Ophthalmic:

Altachlore [OTC]: 5% (3.5 g)

Muro 128 [OTC]: 5% (3.5 g)

Generic: 5% (3.5 g)

Packet, Nasal [preservative free]:

AYR Saline Nasal Rinse [OTC]: 1.57 g (50 ea, 100 ea)

Solution, External:

Saljet [OTC]: 0.9% (30 mL)

Wound Wash Saline [OTC]: 0.9% (210 mL)

Solution, External [preservative free]:

Safe Wash [OTC]: 0.9% (210 mL)

Saljet Rinse [OTC]: 0.9% (30 mL)

Solution, Injection:

Sodium Chloride Thermoject Sys: 0.9% (10 mL)

Generic: 0.9% (2 mL, 2.5 mL, 3 mL, 5 mL, 10 mL, 20 mL, 100 mL); 23.4% (20 mL, 40 mL)

Solution, Injection [preservative free]:
Generic: 0.9% (1 mL, 2 mL, 2.5 mL, 3 mL, 5 mL, 10 mL, 20 mL, 50 mL, 125 mL)
Solution, Intravenous:
SwabFlush Saline Flush: 0.9% (10 mL)
Generic: 0.45% (25 mL, 50 mL, 100 mL, 250 mL, 500 mL, 1000 mL); 0.9% (2.5 mL, 3 mL, 10 mL, 25 mL, 50 mL, 100 mL, 150 mL, 250 mL, 500 mL, 1000 mL); 3% (500 mL); 5% (500 mL); 14.6% (30 mL, 100 mL, 200 mL, 250 mL)
Solution, Intravenous [preservative free]:
Saline Flush ZR: 0.9% (2.5 mL, 5 mL, 10 mL)
Generic: 0.9% (1 mL, 2 mL, 2.5 mL, 3 mL, 5 mL, 10 mL, 50 mL, 100 mL, 500 mL, 1000 mL)
Solution, Irrigation:
Generic: 0.9% (250 mL, 500 mL, 1000 mL, 1500 mL, 2000 mL, 3000 mL, 4000 mL, 5000 mL)
Solution, Nasal:
4-Way Saline [OTC]: (29.6 mL)
Afrin Saline Nasal Mist [OTC]: 0.65% (30 mL, 45 mL)
Altamist Spray [OTC]: 0.65% (45 mL, 60 mL)
Ayr [OTC]: 0.65% (50 mL)
Ayr Nasal Mist Allergy/Sinus [OTC]: 2.65% (50 mL)
Ayr Saline Nasal Drops [OTC]: 0.65% (50 mL)
Baby Ayr Saline [OTC]: 0.65% (30 mL)
Deep Sea Nasal Spray [OTC]: 0.65% (44 mL)
Entsol [OTC]: (30 mL)
Humist [OTC]: 0.65% (45 mL)
Na-Zone [OTC]: 0.65% (59 mL)
Nasal Moist [OTC]: 0.65% (15 mL, 45 mL)
Ocean for Kids [OTC]: 0.65% (37.5 mL)
Ocean Nasal Spray [OTC]: 0.65% (45 mL, 66 mL, 104 mL, 480 mL)
Pretz [OTC]: (50 mL, 946 mL)
Pretz Irrigation [OTC]: (237 mL)
Rhinaris [OTC]: 0.2% (30 mL)
Saline Mist Spray [OTC]: 0.65% (45 mL)
Sea Soft Nasal Mist [OTC]: 0.65% (45 mL)
Generic: 0.65% (44 mL, 45 mL)
Solution, Nasal [preservative free]:
Entsol Nasal [OTC]: 3% (100 mL)
Entsol Nasal Wash [OTC]: (237 mL)
Ocean Ultra Saline Mist [OTC]: (90 mL)
Solution, Ophthalmic:
Altachlore [OTC]: 5% (15 mL, 30 mL)
Muro 128 [OTC]: 2% (15 mL); 5% (15 mL, 30 mL)
Sochlor [OTC]: 5% (15 mL)
Generic: 5% (15 mL)
Swab, Nasal:
Ayr Saline Nasal Gel [OTC]: (20 ea)
Tablet, Oral:
Generic: 1 g

◆ **Sodium Chloride Thermoject Sys** *see* Sodium Chloride *on page 1902*

Sodium Chondroitin Sulfate and Sodium Hyaluronate

(SOW de um kon DROY tin SUL fate & SOW de um hye al yoor ON ate)

Brand Names: U.S. DisCoVisc®; Viscoat®
Index Terms Chondroitin Sulfate and Sodium Hyaluronate; Sodium Hyaluronate and Chondroitin Sulfate
Pharmacologic Category Ophthalmic Agent, Viscoelastic
Use Ophthalmic surgical aid in the anterior segment during cataract extraction and intraocular lens implantation
Dosage Ophthalmic: Adults: Carefully introduce (using a 27-gauge cannula) into anterior chamber during surgery

Dosage adjustment in renal impairment: No dosage adjustment provided in manufacturer's labeling.
Dosage adjustment in hepatic impairment: No dosage adjustment provided in manufacturer's labeling.
Additional Information Complete prescribing information should be consulted for additional detail.
Dosage Forms
Injection, solution, intraocular:
DisCoVisc®: Sodium chondroitin sulfate ≤4% and sodium hyaluronate ≤1.7% (0.5 mL, 1 mL)
Viscoat®: Sodium chondroitin sulfate ≤4% and sodium hyaluronate ≤3% (0.5 mL, 0.75 mL)

Sodium Citrate and Citric Acid

(SOW dee um SIT rate & SI trik AS id)

Brand Names: U.S. Cytra-2; Oracit®; Shohl's Solution (Modified)
Brand Names: Canada PMS-Dicitrate
Index Terms Bicitra; Citric Acid and Sodium Citrate; Modified Shohl's Solution
Pharmacologic Category Alkalinizing Agent, Oral
Use Treatment of metabolic acidosis; alkalinizing agent in conditions where long-term maintenance of an alkaline urine is desirable
Pregnancy Risk Factor Not established
Dosage Oral: Systemic alkalization:
Infants and Children: 2-3 mEq/kg/day in divided doses 3-4 times/day **or** 5-15 mL with water after meals and at bedtime
Adults: 10-30 mL with water after meals and at bedtime

Dosage adjustment in renal impairment: Use is contraindicated.
Dosage adjustment in hepatic impairment: No dosage adjustment provided in manufacturer's labeling.
Additional Information Complete prescribing information should be consulted for additional detail.
Dosage Forms Considerations
Each mL provides 1 mEq sodium, and is equivalent to 1 mEq bicarbonate
Dosage Forms
Solution, oral:
Generic: Sodium citrate 500 mg and citric acid 334 mg per 5 mL
Cytra-2: Sodium citrate 500 mg and citric acid 334 mg per 5 mL
Oracit®: Sodium citrate 490 mg and citric acid 640 mg per 5 mL
Shohl's Solution (Modified): Sodium citrate 500 mg and citric acid 300 mg er 5 mL

◆ **Sodium Citrate, Citric Acid, and Potassium Citrate** *see* Citric Acid, Sodium Citrate, and Potassium Citrate *on page 455*

◆ **Sodium Cromoglicate** *see* Cromolyn (Nasal) *on page 514*

◆ **Sodium Cromoglicate** *see* Cromolyn (Ophthalmic) *on page 514*

◆ **Sodium Diuril** *see* Chlorothiazide *on page 426*

◆ **Sodium Edecrin** *see* Ethacrynic Acid *on page 797*

◆ **Sodium Etidronate** *see* Etidronate *on page 813*

◆ **Sodium Ferric Gluconate** *see* Ferric Gluconate *on page 869*

◆ **Sodium Ferric Gluconate Complex** *see* Ferric Gluconate *on page 869*

◆ **Sodium Fluorescein** *see* Fluorescein *on page 894*

◆ **Sodium Fluoride** *see* Fluoride *on page 895*

◆ **Sodium Fusidate** *see* Fusidic Acid (Ophthalmic) [CAN/INT] *on page 942*

◆ **Sodium Fusidate** *see* Fusidic Acid (Systemic) [INT] *on page 942*

◆ **Sodium Fusidate** *see* Fusidic Acid (Topical) [CAN/INT] *on page 943*

Sodium Glycerophosphate Pentahydrate

(SOE dee um glis er oh FOS fate pen ta HYE drate)

Brand Names: U.S. Glycophos

Pharmacologic Category Electrolyte Supplement, Parenteral

Use Supplement in intravenous nutrition to meet the requirements of phosphate

Dosage Note: When converting from inorganic phosphate products (ie, sodium phosphate and potassium phosphate), maintain the same mmol amount of phosphate. Doses are listed as mmol of phosphate. Sodium glycerophosphate pentahydrate 306.1 mg = sodium glycerophosphate 216 mg = phosphate 1 **mmol**. Sodium glycerophosphate pentahydrate will provide 2 mEq of sodium for every 1 mmol of phosphate delivered.

Phosphate replacement, parenteral nutrition: Manufacturer's labeling: IV:

Infants: 1-1.5 mmol/kg per day admixed within parenteral nutrition solution. Dosage should be individualized.

Adults: 10-20 mmol per day admixed within parenteral nutrition solution. Dosage should be individualized.

Phosphate repletion, general (off-label use):

Caution: With orders for IV phosphate, there is considerable confusion associated with the use of millimoles (mmol) versus milliequivalents (mEq) to express the phosphate requirement. The most reliable method of ordering IV phosphate is by millimoles.

Acute treatment of hypophosphatemia: IV: It is difficult to provide concrete guidelines for the treatment of severe hypophosphatemia because the extent of total body deficits and response to therapy are difficult to predict. Aggressive doses of phosphate may result in a transient serum elevation followed by redistribution into intracellular compartments or bone tissue. It is recommended that repletion of severe hypophosphatemia be done IV because large doses of oral phosphate may cause diarrhea and intestinal absorption may be unreliable. Intermittent IV infusion should be reserved for severe depletion situations; requires continuous cardiac monitoring. Guidelines differ based on degree of illness, need/use of TPN, and severity of hypophosphatemia. Obese patients and/or severe renal impairment were excluded from phosphate supplement trials. **Note:** 1 mmol phosphate = 31 mg phosphorus; 1 mg phosphorus = 0.032 mmol phosphate.

There are no prospective studies of parenteral phosphate replacement in children. **The following weight-based guidelines for adult dosing may be cautiously employed in pediatric patients.** Guidelines differ based on degree of illness, use of TPN, and severity of hypophosphatemia.

General replacement guidelines (Lentz, 1978):

Low dose, serum phosphorus losses are recent and uncomplicated: 0.08 mmol/kg over 6 hours

Intermediate dose, serum phosphorus level 0.5-1 mg/dL (0.16-0.32 mmol/L): 0.16-0.24 mmol/kg over 6 hours

Note: The initial dose may be increased by 25% to 50% if the patient is symptomatic secondary to hypophosphatemia, and lowered by 25% to 50% if the patient is hypercalcemic.

Critically-ill adult patients receiving concurrent enteral/parenteral nutrition (Brown, 2006; Clark, 1995): **Note:** Round doses to the nearest 7.5 mmol for ease of preparation. If administering with phosphate-containing parenteral nutrition, do not exceed 15 mmol/L within parenteral nutrition. May use adjusted body weight for patients weighing >130% of ideal body weight (and BMI <40 kg/m^2) by using [IBW + 0.25 (ABW-IBW)]:

Low dose, serum phosphorus level 2.3-3 mg/dL (0.74-0.96 mmol/L): 0.16-0.32 mmol/kg over 4-6 hours

Intermediate dose, serum phosphorus level 1.6-2.2 mg/dL (0.51-0.71 mmol/L): 0.32-0.64 mmol/kg over 4-6 hours

High dose, serum phosphorus <1.5 mg/dL (<0.5 mmol/L): 0.64-1 mmol/kg over 8-12 hours

Parenteral nutrition: IV:

Infants and Children: 0.5-2 mmol/kg/24 hours (Mirtallo, 2004 [ASPEN guidelines])

Children >50 kg and Adolescents: 10-40 mmol/24 hours (Mirtallo, 2004 [ASPEN guidelines])

Adults: 10-15 mmol/1000 kcal (Hicks, 2001) **or** 20-40 mmol/24 hours (Mirtallo, 2004 [ASPEN guidelines])

Dosage adjustment in renal impairment: No dosage adjustment provided in manufacturer's labeling (has not been studied); use with caution since phosphate excretion is primarily renal.

Dosage adjustment in hepatic impairment: No dosage adjustment provided in manufacturer's labeling (has not been studied); however, phosphate excretion is primarily renal

Additional Information Complete prescribing information should be consulted for additional detail.

Dosage Forms

Solution, Intravenous:

Glycophos: 1 mmol/mL (20 mL)

◆ **Sodium Hyaluronate** *see* Hyaluronate and Derivatives *on page 1006*

◆ **Sodium Hyaluronate and Chondroitin Sulfate** *see* Sodium Chondroitin Sulfate and Sodium Hyaluronate *on page 1905*

◆ **Sodium Hydrogen Carbonate** *see* Sodium Bicarbonate *on page 1901*

Sodium Hypochlorite Solution

(SOW dee um hye poe KLOR ite soe LOO shun)

Brand Names: U.S. Di-Dak-Sol [OTC]; H-Chlor 12 [OTC]; HySept [OTC]

Index Terms Modified Dakin's Solution

Pharmacologic Category Disinfectant, Antibacterial (Topical)

Use

Atrapro™ Dermal (0.004%): Management (via debridement) of wounds such as stage I-IV pressure ulcers; partial and full thickness wounds; diabetic foot ulcers; post surgical and donor sites; first- and second-degree burns

Dakin's Solution (0.125%, 0.25%, 0.5%); Di-Dak-Sol (0.0125%): Prevention/treatment of skin and tissue infections, cuts, abrasions, skin ulcers; pre- and postsurgery

Dosage Children and Adults:

Atrapro™ Dermal spray: Apply to affected area 3 times daily.

Dakin's solution, Di-Dak-Sol: Topical via irrigation:

Lightly-to-moderately exudative wounds: Apply once daily.

Highly exudative or contaminated wounds: Apply twice daily.

Additional Information Complete prescribing information should be consulted for additional detail.

Dosage Forms

Solution, External:

Di-Dak-Sol [OTC]: 0.0125% (473 mL)

H-Chlor 12 [OTC]: 0.125% (473 mL)

HySept [OTC]: 0.25% (473 mL); 0.5% (473 mL)

Generic: 0.125% (473 mL); 0.25% (473 mL); 0.5% (473 mL)

◆ **Sodium Hyposulfate** *see* Sodium Thiosulfate *on page 1915*

◆ **Sodium Nafcillin** *see* Nafcillin *on page 1414*

Sodium Nitrite (SOW dee um NYE trite)

Pharmacologic Category Antidote

Use Cyanide poisoning: Treatment of acute, life-threatening cyanide poisoning in combination with sodium thiosulfate. Consider consultation with a poison control center at 1-800-222-1222.

Pregnancy Risk Factor C

Dosage Cyanide poisoning: IV: **Note:** Given in conjunction with sodium thiosulfate. Administer sodium nitrite first, followed immediately by the administration of sodium thiosulfate. Sodium nitrite is generally discontinued for methemoglobin levels >30%.

Children: 6 mg/kg (0.2 mL/kg or 6-8 mL/m^2 of a 3% solution); maximum dose: 300 mg (10 mL of a 3% solution); may repeat at one-half the original dose if symptoms of cyanide toxicity return

Adults: 300 mg (10 mL of a 3% solution); may repeat at one-half the original dose if symptoms of cyanide toxicity return

Alternatively, in patients who are unable to tolerate significant methemoglobinemia (eg, patients with comorbidities that compromise oxygen delivery, such as heart disease, lung disease), dosing may be based on hemoglobin levels (when rapid bedside testing is available) to prevent fatal methemoglobinemia; see table (Berlin, 1970):

Hemoglobin Level (g/dL)	Dose of 3% Sodium Nitrite Solution (maximum dose: 10 mL)
7	0.19 mL/kg
8	0.22 mL/kg
9	0.25 mL/kg
10	0.27 mL/kg
11	0.3 mL/kg
12	0.33 mL/kg
13	0.36 mL/kg
14	0.39 mL/kg

Note: Monitor the patient for 24-48 hours; if symptoms return, repeat sodium nitrite and sodium thiosulfate at one-half the original dose.

Elderly: Refer to adult dosing; use with caution due to the likelihood of decreased renal function

Dosage adjustment in renal impairment: No dosage adjustment provided in the manufacturer's labeling; however, renal elimination of sodium nitrite is significant and risk of adverse effects may be increased in patients with renal impairment.

Dosage adjustment in hepatic impairment: No dosage adjustment provided in manufacturer's labeling (has not been studied).

Additional Information Complete prescribing information should be consulted for additional detail.

Dosage Forms

Solution, Intravenous:

Generic: 30 mg/mL (10 mL)

Sodium Nitrite and Sodium Thiosulfate

(SOW dee um NYE trite & SOW dee um thye oh SUL fate)

Brand Names: U.S. Nithiodote

Index Terms Sodium Thiosulfate and Sodium Nitrite

Pharmacologic Category Antidote

Use Cyanide poisoning: Treatment of acute, life-threatening cyanide poisoning. Consider consultation with a poison control center at 1-800-222-1222.

Pregnancy Risk Factor C

Dosage IV: **Note:** Administer sodium nitrite first, followed immediately by the administration of sodium thiosulfate. Sodium nitrite is generally discontinued for methemoglobin levels >30%.

Sodium nitrite:

Children: 6 mg/kg (0.2 mL/kg or 6-8 mL/m^2 of a 3% solution); maximum dose: 300 mg (10 mL of a 3% solution); may repeat at one-half the original dose if symptoms of cyanide toxicity return

Adults: 300 mg (10 mL of a 3% solution); may repeat at one-half the original dose if symptoms of cyanide toxicity return

Alternatively, in patients who are unable to tolerate significant methemoglobinemia (eg, patients with comorbidities that compromise oxygen delivery, such as heart disease, lung disease), dosing may be based on hemoglobin levels (when rapid bedside testing is available) to prevent fatal methemoglobinemia; see table (Berlin, 1970):

Hemoglobin Level (g/dL)	Dose of 3% Sodium Nitrite Solution (maximum dose: 10 mL)
7	0.19 mL/kg
8	0.22 mL/kg
9	0.25 mL/kg
10	0.27 mL/kg
11	0.3 mL/kg
12	0.33 mL/kg
13	0.36 mL/kg
14	0.39 mL/kg

Sodium thiosulfate:

Children: 250 mg/kg (1 mL/kg or ~30-40 mL/m^2 of a 25% solution) or 500 mg/kg (2 mL/kg of a 25% solution) (Howland, 2011); maximum dose: 12.5 g (50 mL of a 25% solution); may repeat at one-half the original dose if symptoms of cyanide toxicity return

Adults: 12.5 g (50 mL of a 25% solution); may repeat at one-half the original dose if symptoms of cyanide toxicity return

Note: Monitor the patient for 24-48 hours; if symptoms return, repeat both sodium nitrite and sodium thiosulfate at one-half the original doses.

Elderly: Refer to adult dosing; use with caution due to the likelihood of decreased renal function

Dosage adjustment in renal impairment: No dosage adjustment provided in manufacturer's labeling; however, renal elimination of sodium nitrite and sodium thiosulfate is significant and risk of adverse effects may be increased in patients with renal impairment.

Dosage adjustment in hepatic impairment: No dosage adjustment provided in manufacturer's labeling (has not been studied).

Additional Information Complete prescribing information should be consulted for additional detail.

Dosage Forms

Injection, solution [combination package]:

Nithiodote: Sodium nitrite 300 mg/10 mL (10 mL) and sodium thiosulfate 12.5 g/50 mL (50 mL)

◆ **Sodium Nitroferricyanide** *see* Nitroprusside *on page 1467*

◆ **Sodium Nitroprusside** *see* Nitroprusside *on page 1467*

Sodium Oxybate (SOW dee um ox i BATE)

Brand Names: U.S. Xyrem

Brand Names: Canada Xyrem

Index Terms 4-Hydroxybutyrate; Gamma Hydroxybutyric Acid; GHB; Oxybate; Sodium 4-Hydroxybutyrate

Pharmacologic Category Central Nervous System Depressant

Use Excessive daytime sleepiness/cataplexy: Treatment of cataplexy and excessive daytime sleepiness in patients with narcolepsy

Pregnancy Risk Factor C

Dosage Excessive daytime sleepiness/cataplexy: Oral:

Adults: Initial: 2.25 g at bedtime after the patient is in bed, and 2.25 g 2.5 to 4 hours later (4.5 g per night). Titrate to effect; usual effective dosage range: 6 to 9 g per night

Dose titration:

U.S. labeling: Increase dose by 1.5 g per night (0.75 g per dose) in weekly intervals (maximum dose: 9 g per night)

Canadian labeling: Increase dose by 1.5 g per night (0.75 g per dose) at 2-week intervals (maximum dose: 9 g per night). Dosage may be decreased using the same titration schedule.

Elderly: Use with caution; initiate at lower dosage range. Limited studies available in patients >65 years. Refer to adult dosing.

Dosage adjustment for concomitant therapy: Patients stabilized on sodium oxybate should have dose reduced by at least 20% with the addition of divalproex sodium. The sodium oxybate starting dose should be reduced for patients already taking divalproex sodium. Adjust dose as necessary.

Dosage adjustment in renal impairment: There are no dosage adjustments provided in manufacturer's labeling (has not been studied).

Dosage adjustment in hepatic impairment: Initial: ~1.13 g at bedtime after the patient is in bed and ~1.13 g 2.5 to 4 hours later (2.25 g per night)

Additional Information Complete prescribing information should be consulted for additional detail.

Dosage Forms

Solution, Oral:

Xyrem: 500 mg/mL (180 mL)

Sodium Phenylacetate and Sodium Benzoate

(SOW dee um fen il AS e tate & SOW dee um BENZ oh ate)

Brand Names: U.S. Ammonul®

Index Terms NAPA and NABZ; Sodium Benzoate and Sodium Phenylacetate

Pharmacologic Category Antidote; Urea Cycle Disorder (UCD) Treatment Agent

Use Adjunct to treatment of acute hyperammonemia and encephalopathy in patients with urea cycle disorders involving partial or complete deficiencies of carbamyl-phosphate synthetase (CPS), ornithine transcarbamoylase (OTC), argininosuccinate lysase (ASL), or argininosuccinate synthetase (ASS); for use with hemodialysis in acute neonatal hyperammonemic coma, moderate-to-severe hyperammonemic encephalopathy and hyperammonemia which fails to respond to initial therapy

Pregnancy Risk Factor C

Dosage Administer as a loading dose over 90-120 minutes, followed by an equivalent maintenance infusion given over 24 hours. Dosage based on weight and specific enzyme deficiency; therapy should continue until ammonia levels are in normal range. Repeat loading doses are not recommended due to the prolonged plasma levels.

Children ≤20 kg:

CPS and OTC deficiency: Ammonul® 2.5 mL/kg and arginine 10% 2 mL/kg (provides sodium phenylacetate 250 mg/kg, sodium benzoate 250 mg/kg, and arginine hydrochloride 200 mg/kg).

ASS and ASL deficiency: Ammonul® 2.5 mL/kg and arginine 10% 6 mL/kg (provides sodium phenylacetate 250 mg/kg, sodium benzoate 250 mg/kg, and arginine hydrochloride 600 mg/kg)

Note: Pending a specific diagnosis in infants, the bolus and maintenance dose of arginine should be 6 mL/kg. If ASS or ASL are excluded as diagnostic possibilities, reduce dose of arginine to 2 mL/kg/day.

Children >20 kg and Adults:

CPS and OTC deficiency: Ammonul® 55 mL/m^2 and arginine 10% 2 mL/kg (provides sodium phenylacetate 5.5 g/m^2, sodium benzoate 5.5 g/m^2, and arginine hydrochloride 200 mg/kg)

ASS and ASL deficiency: Ammonul® 55 mL/m^2 and arginine 10% 6 mL/kg (provides sodium phenylacetate 5.5 g/m^2, sodium benzoate 5.5 g/m^2, and arginine hydrochloride 600 mg/kg)

Dosage adjustment in renal impairment: No dosage adjustment provided in manufacturer's labeling. However, renal impairment increases systemic exposure to sodium phenylacetate and sodium benzoate..Use with caution; monitor closely.

Dialysis: Ammonia clearance is ~10 times greater with hemodialysis than by peritoneal dialysis or hemofiltration. Exchange transfusion is ineffective.

Dosage adjustment in hepatic impairment: No dosage adjustment provided in manufacturer's labeling. Use with caution.

Additional Information Complete prescribing information should be consulted for additional detail.

Dosage Forms

Injection, solution [concentrate]:

Ammonul®: Sodium phenylacetate 100 mg and sodium benzoate 100 mg per 1 mL (50 mL)

Sodium Phenylbutyrate

(SOW dee um fen il BYOO ti rate)

Brand Names: U.S. Buphenyl

Index Terms Ammonapse

Pharmacologic Category Urea Cycle Disorder (UCD) Treatment Agent

Use Adjunctive therapy in the chronic management of patients with urea cycle disorder involving deficiencies of carbamoylphosphate synthetase, ornithine transcarbamylase, or argininosuccinic acid synthetase

Pregnancy Risk Factor C

Dosage Oral: Management of urea cycle disorders:

Children <20 kg: Powder: 450-600 mg/kg/day, administered in equally divided amounts with each meal or feeding, 3-6 times daily (maximum dose: 20 g/day)

Children ≥20 kg and Adults: Powder or tablet: 9.9-13 g/m²/day, administered in equally divided amounts with each meal or feeding, 3-6 times daily (maximum dose: 20 g/day)

Dosage adjustment in renal impairment: No dosage adjustment provided in manufacturer's labeling. Use with caution.

Dosage adjustment in hepatic impairment: No dosage adjustment provided in manufacturer's labeling. Use with caution.

Additional Information Complete prescribing information should be consulted for additional detail.

Dosage Forms Considerations Powder products: 1 level teaspoon provides 3 g sodium phenylbutyrate, 1 level tablespoon provides 8.6 g sodium phenylbutyrate. Measurers provided with the product.

Dosage Forms

Powder, Oral:

Buphenyl: (250 g)

Generic: (250 g)

Tablet, Oral:

Buphenyl: 500 mg

◆ **Sodium Phosphate and Potassium Phosphate** *see* Potassium Phosphate and Sodium Phosphate *on page 1692*

◆ **Sodium Phosphate Monobasic, Methenamine, Methylene Blue, Phenyl Salicylate, and Hyoscyamine** *see* Methenamine, Sodium Phosphate Monobasic, Phenyl Salicylate, Methylene Blue, and Hyoscyamine *on page 1318*

Sodium Phosphates (SOW dee um FOS fates)

Brand Names: U.S. Fleet Enema Extra [OTC]; Fleet Enema [OTC]; Fleet Pedia-Lax Enema [OTC]; LaCrosse Complete [OTC]; OsmoPrep

Brand Names: Canada Fleet Enema

Index Terms Phosphates, Sodium

Pharmacologic Category Cathartic; Electrolyte Supplement, Parenteral; Laxative, Bowel Evacuant

Use

Oral solution, rectal: Short-term treatment of constipation

Oral tablets: Bowel cleansing prior to colonoscopy

IV: Source of phosphate in large volume IV fluids and parenteral nutrition; treatment and prevention of hypophosphatemia

Pregnancy Risk Factor C

Pregnancy Considerations Reproduction studies have not been conducted with these products. Use with caution in pregnant women.

Breast-Feeding Considerations Phosphorus, sodium, and potassium are normal constituents of human milk.

Contraindications Hypersensitivity to sodium phosphate salts or any component of the formulation; additional contraindications vary by product:

Enema: Ascites, clinically significant renal impairment, heart failure, imperforate anus, known or suspected GI obstruction, megacolon (congenital or acquired)

Intravenous preparation: Diseases with hyperphosphatemia, hypocalcemia, or hypernatremia

Tablets: Acute phosphate nephropathy (biopsy proven), bowel obstruction, bowel perforation, gastric bypass or stapling surgery, toxic colitis, toxic megacolon

OTC labeling (Oral Solution): When used for self-medication: Dehydration, heart failure, renal impairment, electrolyte abnormalities; use for bowel cleansing, use in children <5 years

Warnings/Precautions [U.S. Boxed Warning]: Acute phosphate nephropathy has been reported (rarely) with use of oral products as a colon cleanser prior to colonoscopy. Some cases have resulted in permanent renal impairment (some requiring dialysis). Risk factors for acute phosphate nephropathy may include increased age (>55 years of age), preexisting renal dysfunction, bowel obstruction, active colitis, or dehydration, and the use of medicines that affect renal perfusion or function (eg, ACE inhibitors, angiotensin receptor blockers, diuretics, and possibly NSAIDs), although some cases have been reported in patients without apparent risk factors. Other preventive measures may include avoid exceeding maximum recommended doses and concurrent use of other laxatives containing sodium phosphate; encourage patients to adequately hydrate before, during, and after use; obtain baseline and postprocedure labs in patients at risk; consider hospitalization and intravenous hydration during bowel cleansing for patients unable to hydrate themselves (eg, frail patients). Use is contraindicated in patients with acute phosphate nephropathy (biopsy proven).

Use with caution in patients with impaired renal dysfunction, preexisting electrolyte imbalances, risk of electrolyte disturbance (hypocalcemia, hyperphosphatemia, hypernatremia), or dehydration. If using as a bowel evacuant, correct electrolyte abnormalities before administration. Use caution in patients with unstable angina, history of myocardial infarction arrhythmia, cardiomyopathy; use caution in patients with or at risk for arrhythmias (eg, cardiomyopathy, prolonged QT interval, history of uncontrolled arrhythmias, recent MI) or with concurrent use of other QT-prolonging medications; pre-/postdose ECGs should be considered in high-risk patients.

Use caution in inflammatory bowel disease or severe active ulcerative colitis; may induce colonic aphthous ulceration and ischemic colitis (some requiring hospitalization). Use caution in patients with any of the following: Gastric retention or hypomotility, ileus, severe, chronic constipation, colitis. Use is contraindicated in patients with bowel obstruction (including pseudo) or perforation, congenital megacolon, gastric bypass or bariatric surgery, toxic colitis, or toxic megacolon. Use with caution in patients with impaired gag reflex and those prone to regurgitation or aspiration.

Use with caution in patients with a history of seizures and those at higher risk of seizures. Ensure adequate clear liquid intake prior to and during bowel evacuation regimens; inadequate fluid intake may lead to dehydration. Other oral medications may not be well absorbed when given during bowel evacuation because of rapid intestinal peristalsis. Use with caution in debilitated patients; consider each patient's ability to hydrate properly. Use with caution in geriatric patients. Laxatives and purgatives have the potential for abuse by bulimia nervosa patients. Solutions for injection may contain aluminum; toxic levels may occur following prolonged administration in premature neonates or patients with renal impairment. Enemas and oral solution are available in pediatric and adult sizes; prescribe by "volume" not by "bottle."

Benzyl alcohol and derivatives: Some dosage forms may contain sodium benzoate/benzoic acid; benzoic acid (benzoate) is a metabolite of benzyl alcohol; large amounts of benzyl alcohol (≥99 mg/kg/day) have been associated with a potentially fatal toxicity ("gasping syndrome") in neonates; the "gasping syndrome" consists of metabolic acidosis, respiratory distress, gasping respirations, CNS dysfunction (including convulsions, intracranial hemorrhage), hypotension, and cardiovascular collapse (AAP, 1997; CDC, 1982); some data suggests that benzoate displaces bilirubin from protein binding sites (Ahlfors, 2001); avoid or use dosage forms containing benzyl alcohol derivative with caution in neonates. See manufacturer's labeling.

Adverse Reactions

Central nervous system: Dizziness, headache

Gastrointestinal: Abdominal pain, bloating, mucosal bleeding, nausea, superficial mucosal ulcerations, vomiting

Endocrine & metabolic: Hypernatremia, hyperphosphatemia, hypocalcemia (on colonoscopy day), hypokalemia (on colonoscopy day), hypophosphatemia (2-3 days postcolonoscopy)

Postmarketing and/or case reports: Acute phosphate nephropathy, anaphylaxis, bronchospasm, calcium nephrolithiasis, cardiac arrhythmia, dehydration, dysphagia, dyspnea, facial edema, increased blood urea nitrogen, increased serum creatinine, ischemic colitis, lip edema, paresthesia, pharyngeal edema, pruritus, rectal bleeding, renal failure, renal insufficiency, renal tubular necrosis, seizure, skin rash, tightness in throat, tongue edema, urticaria

Drug Interactions

Metabolism/Transport Effects None known.

Avoid Concomitant Use There are no known interactions where it is recommended to avoid concomitant use.

Increased Effect/Toxicity

Sodium Phosphates may increase the levels/effects of: Nonsteroidal Anti-Inflammatory Agents

The levels/effects of Sodium Phosphates may be increased by: ACE Inhibitors; Angiotensin II Receptor Blockers; Bisphosphonate Derivatives; Diuretics; Tricyclic Antidepressants

Decreased Effect

The levels/effects of Sodium Phosphates may be decreased by: Antacids; Calcium Salts; Iron Salts; Magnesium Salts; Multivitamins/Minerals (with ADEK, Folate, Iron); Sucralfate

Preparation for Administration Solution for injection: In general, the dose, concentration of infusion, and rate of administration may be dependent on patient condition and specific institution policy. Intermittent infusion doses are typically prepared in 100-250 mL of NS or D_5W (usual concentration range: 0.15-0.6 mmol/mL). Observe the vial for the presence of crystals. Do not use vial if crystals are present. **Note:** Due to the potential for solution crystallization, American Regent, Inc recommends the use of a 5 micron filter when preparing IV sodium phosphate containing solutions (Important Drug Safety Information, American Regent, 2013); a similar recommendation has not been noted by other manufacturers.

Storage/Stability

Enema: Store at room temperature.

Oral solution: Store at room temperature.

Solution for injection: Store intact vials at 20°C to 25°C (68°F to 77°F); excursions permitted between 15°C and 30°C (59°F and 86°F).

Tablet: Store at 25°C (77°F); excursions permitted between 15°C and 30°C (59°F and 86°F).

Mechanism of Action As a laxative, exerts osmotic effect in the small intestine by drawing water into the lumen of the gut, producing distention and promoting peristalsis and evacuation of the bowel; phosphorous participates in bone deposition, calcium metabolism, utilization of B complex vitamins, and as a buffer in acid-base equilibrium

Pharmacodynamics/Kinetics

Onset of action: Cathartic: 3-6 hours; Rectal: 2-5 minutes

Absorption: Oral: ~1% to 20%

Excretion: Urine

Dosage Note: If phosphate repletion is required and a phosphate product is not available at your institution, consider the use of sodium glycerophosphate pentahydrate (Glycophos) as a suitable substitute. Concentration and dosing are different from FDA-approved products; use caution when switching between products. Refer to Sodium Glycerophosphate Pentahydrate monograph.

Caution: With orders for IV phosphate, there is considerable confusion associated with the use of millimoles (mmol) versus milliequivalents (mEq) to express the phosphate requirement. The most reliable method of ordering IV phosphate is by millimoles, then specifying the potassium or sodium salt. Intravenous doses listed as mmol of phosphate.

Acute treatment of hypophosphatemia: IV: It is difficult to provide concrete guidelines for the treatment of severe hypophosphatemia because the extent of total body deficits and response to therapy are difficult to predict. Aggressive doses of phosphate may result in a transient serum elevation followed by redistribution into intracellular compartments or bone tissue. It is recommended that repletion of severe hypophosphatemia be done IV because large doses of oral phosphate may cause diarrhea and intestinal absorption may be unreliable. Intermittent IV infusion should be reserved for severe depletion situations; requires continuous cardiac monitoring. Guidelines differ based on degree of illness, need/use of TPN, and severity of hypophosphatemia. If hypokalemia exists (some clinicians recommend threshold of <4 mmol/L), consider phosphate replacement strategy with potassium (eg, potassium phosphates). Obese patients and/or severe renal impairment were excluded from phosphate supplement trials.

Children and Adults: There are no prospective studies of parenteral phosphate replacement in children. The following weight-based guidelines for adult dosing may be cautiously employed in pediatric patients. **Note:** 1 mmol phosphate = 31 mg phosphorus; 1 mg phosphorus = 0.032 mmol phosphate

General replacement guidelines (Lentz, 1978):

Low dose, serum phosphorus losses are recent and uncomplicated: 0.08 mmol/kg over 6 hours

Intermediate dose, serum phosphorus level 0.5-1 mg/dL (0.16-0.32 mmol/L): 0.16-0.24 mmol/kg over 6 hours

Note: The initial dose may be increased by 25% to 50% if the patient is symptomatic secondary to hypophosphatemia and lowered by 25% to 50% if the patient is hypercalcemic.

Critically-ill adult patients receiving concurrent enteral/parenteral nutrition (Brown, 2006; Clark, 1995): **Note:** Round doses to the nearest 7.5 mmol for ease of preparation. If administering with phosphate-containing parenteral nutrition, do not exceed 15 mmol/L within parenteral nutrition. May use adjusted body weight for patients weighing >130% of ideal body weight (and BMI <40 kg/m^2) by using [IBW + 0.25 (ABW-IBW)]:

Low dose, serum phosphorus level 2.3-3 mg/dL (0.74-0.96 mmol/L): 0.16-0.32 mmol/kg over 4-6 hours

Intermediate dose, serum phosphorus level 1.6-2.2 mg/dL (0.51-0.71 mmol/L): 0.32-0.64 mmol/kg over 4-6 hours

High dose, serum phosphorus <1.5 mg/dL (<0.5 mmol/L): 0.64-1 mmol/kg over 8-12 hours

Parenteral nutrition: IV:

Infants and Children: 0.5-2 mmol/kg/24 hours (Mirtallo, 2004 [ASPEN guidelines])

Children >50 kg and Adolescents: 10-40 mmol/24 hours (Mirtallo, 2004 [ASPEN guidelines])

Adults: 10-15 mmol/1000 kcal (Hicks, 2001) **or** 20-40 mmol/24 hours (Mirtallo, 2004 [ASPEN guidelines])

Laxative (Fleet): Rectal:
Children 2-4 years: One-half contents of one 2.25 oz pediatric enema
Children 5-11 years: Contents of one 2.25 oz pediatric enema
Children ≥12 years and Adults: Contents of one 4.5 oz enema as a single dose

Laxative: Oral solution:
Children 5-9 years: 7.5 mL as a single dose; maximum single daily dose: 7.5 mL
Children 10-11 years: 15 mL as a single dose; maximum single daily dose: 15 mL
Children ≥12 years and Adults: 15 mL as a single dose; maximum single daily dose: 45 mL

Bowel cleansing prior to colonoscopy: Oral tablets:
Adults: **Note:** Do not use additional agents, especially other sodium phosphate products.
OsmoPrep: A total of 32 tablets and 2 quarts of clear liquids (8 ounces of clear liquids with each dose) divided as follows:
Evening before colonoscopy: 4 tablets every 15 minutes for 5 doses (total of 20 tablets)
3-5 hours prior to colonoscopy: 4 tablets every 15 minutes for 3 doses (total of 12 tablets)

Elderly: Use with caution due to increased risk of renal impairment in the elderly.

Dosage adjustment in renal impairment: No dosage adjustment provided in manufacturer's labeling. Use with caution; ionized inorganic phosphate is excreted by the kidneys. Oral solution is contraindicated in patients with kidney disease.

Dosage adjustment in hepatic impairment: No dosage adjustment provided in manufacturer's labeling.

Dietary Considerations Bowel cleansing: Should be taken on an empty stomach with clear liquids; a clear liquid diet should be used for 12 hours prior to and during tablet administration. Clear liquids may include water, flavored water, pulp-free lemonade, ginger ale, or apple juice; purple or red colored liquids should be avoided. Some products may contain phenylalanine and/or sodium.

Administration
Intermittent IV infusion; do **not** administer IV push. Must be diluted prior to parenteral administration. In general, the dose, concentration of infusion, and rate of administration may be dependent on patient condition and specific institution policy. For adult patients with severe symptomatic hypophosphatemia (ie, <1.5 mg/dL), may administer at rates up to 15 mmol/hour (Charron, 2003; Rosen, 1995). In patients with renal dysfunction and/or less severe hypophosphatemia, slower administration rates (eg, over 4-6 hours) or oral repletion is recommended. **Note:** Due to the potential for solution crystallization, American Regent, Inc recommends the use of a 0.22 micron in-line filter for IV administration (1.2 micron filter if admixture contains lipids) (Important Drug Safety Information, American Regent, 2013); a similar recommendation has not been noted by other manufacturers.
Bowel cleansing (oral tablets): Have patient drink 8 ounces of clear liquids with each dose of sodium phosphate; have patient rehydrate before and after colonoscopy. Clear liquids may include water, flavored water, pulp-free lemonade, ginger ale, or apple juice; purple or red colored liquids should be avoided.
Constipation (oral solution): Take on an empty stomach; dilute dose with 8 ounces cool water, then follow dose with 8 ounces water; **do not repeat dose within 24 hours**

Monitoring Parameters
IV: Serum calcium, sodium and phosphorus levels; renal function; after IV phosphate repletion, repeat serum phosphorus level should be checked 2-4 hours later
Oral: Bowel cleansing: Baseline and postprocedure labs (electrolytes, calcium, phosphorus, BUN, creatinine) in patients at risk for acute renal nephropathy, seizure, or who have a history of electrolyte abnormality; ECG in patients with risks for prolonged QT or arrhythmias. Ensure euvolemia before initiating bowel preparation.

Reference Range Note: Reference ranges may vary depending on the laboratory
Serum calcium: 8.4-10.2 mg/dL
Serum phosphorus: Both low and high ends of the normal range are higher in children than in adults.
Infants: 4.5-7.5 mg/dL (1.45-2.42 mmol/L)
Children: ~4.0-6.0 mg/dL (1.29-1.94 mmol/L)
Adults: 2.5-4.5 mg/dL (0.81-1.45 mmol/L)

Additional Information Phosphate salts may precipitate when mixed with calcium salts; solubility is improved in amino acid parenteral nutrition solutions; check with a pharmacist to determine compatibility.

Dosage Forms Considerations
Sodium 4 mEq is equivalent to sodium 92 mg
Phosphorous 3 mmol is equivalent to phosphorus 93 mg

Dosage Forms
Injection, solution [concentrate; preservative free]: Phosphorus 3 mmol and sodium 4 mEq per 1 mL (5 mL, 15 mL, 50 mL)
Solution, oral: Monobasic sodium phosphate 2.4 g and dibasic sodium phosphate 0.9 g per 5 mL (45 mL)
Solution, rectal [enema]: Monobasic sodium phosphate 19 g and dibasic sodium phosphate 7 g per 118 mL delivered dose (133 mL)
Fleet Enema [OTC], LaCrosse Complete [OTC]: Monobasic sodium phosphate 19 g and dibasic sodium phosphate 7 g per 118 mL delivered dose (133 mL)
Fleet Enema Extra [OTC]: Monobasic sodium phosphate 19 g and dibasic sodium phosphate 7 g per 197 mL delivered dose (230 mL)
Fleet Pedia-Lax™ Enema [OTC]: Monobasic sodium phosphate 9.5 g and dibasic sodium phosphate 3.5 g per 59 mL delivered dose (66 mL)
Tablet, oral [scored]:
OsmoPrep: Monobasic sodium phosphate 1.102 g and dibasic sodium phosphate 0.398 g

Sodium Picosulfate, Magnesium Oxide, and Citric Acid

(SOW dee um pye ko SUL fate mag NEE zhum OKS ide & SI trik AS id)

Brand Names: U.S. Prepopik™
Brand Names: Canada Oral Purgative; Pico-Salax®; Picodan; Picoflo; Purg-Odan™
Index Terms Citric Acid, Sodium Picosulfate, and Magnesium Oxide; DA-1773; Magnesium Oxide, Sodium Picosulfate, and Citric Acid; Prepopik™; Sodium Picosulphate, Magnesium Oxide, and Citric Acid
Pharmacologic Category Laxative, Osmotic; Laxative, Stimulant
Use Bowel cleansing prior to colonoscopy
Canadian labeling: Additional uses (not in U.S. labeling): Bowel cleansing prior to x-ray examination, endoscopy, or surgery
Pregnancy Risk Factor B
Dosage Bowel cleansing:
Prepopik™: Adults: Oral:
Split-dose regimen (preferred): 150 mL (5 oz) the evening before the colonoscopy (5 PM-9 PM), followed by a second 150 mL (5 oz) dose ~5 hours before the colonoscopy.
Day-before regimen (alternative): 150 mL (5 oz) in the early evening before the colonoscopy (4 PM-6 PM), followed by a second 150 mL (5 oz) dose 6 hours later (10 PM-12 AM) the night before the colonoscopy.

Purg-Odan™ (Canadian availability): Oral:

Children 1-5 years: One-fourth (1/4) of one sachet (mixed and dissolved in water) in the morning (8 AM) the day prior to the procedure, followed by a second dose of one-fourth (1/4) of one sachet in the afternoon (2 PM-4 PM) on the day prior to the procedure.

Children 6-12 years: One-half (1/2) of one sachet (mixed and dissolved in water) in the morning (8 AM) the day prior to the procedure, followed by a second dose of one-half (1/2) of one sachet in the afternoon (2 PM-4 PM) on the day prior to the procedure.

Adults: One sachet (mixed and dissolved in water) in the morning (8 AM) the day prior to the procedure followed by a second dose of one sachet in the afternoon (2 PM-4 PM) on the day prior to the procedure.

Pico-Salax® (Canadian availability): Oral:

Children 1-5 years: One-fourth (1/4) of one sachet (mixed and dissolved in water) in the evening (6 PM) the day prior to the procedure, followed by a second dose of one-fourth (1/4) of one sachet in the morning (8 AM) on the day of the procedure

Children 6-12 years: One-half (1/2) of one sachet (mixed and dissolved in water) in the evening (6 PM) the day prior to the procedure, followed by a second dose of one-half (1/2) of one sachet in the morning (8 AM) on the day of the procedure

Adults:

Early colonoscopy (before 12 PM): One sachet (mixed and dissolved in water) in the evening (5 PM) the day prior to the procedure, followed by a second dose of one sachet 5 hours later (10 PM) the night before the procedure

Late colonoscopy (after 12 PM): One sachet (mixed and dissolved in water) in the late evening (7 PM) the day prior to the procedure, followed by a second dose of one sachet in the morning (6 AM) on the day of the procedure

Additional Information Complete prescribing information should be consulted for additional detail.

Dosage Forms

Powder for solution, oral:

Prepopik™: Sodium picosulfate 10 mg, magnesium oxide 3.5 g, and citric acid 12 g per packet (2s)

Dosage Forms: Canada

Powder for solution, oral [kit]:

Pico-Salax®: Sodium picosulphate 10 mg, magnesium oxide 3.5 g, and citric acid 12 g per sachet (1s, 2s) [orange or cranberry flavor]

Purg-Odan™: Sodium picosulphate 10 mg, magnesium oxide 3.5 g, and citric acid 12 g per sachet (1s, 2s) [orange flavor]

◆ **Sodium Picosulphate, Magnesium Oxide, and Citric Acid** *see* Sodium Picosulfate, Magnesium Oxide, and Citric Acid *on page 1911*

Sodium Polystyrene Sulfonate

(SOW dee um pol ee STYE reen SUL fon ate)

Brand Names: U.S. Kalexate; Kayexalate; Kionex; SPS

Brand Names: Canada Kayexalate®; PMS-Sodium Polystyrene Sulfonate

Pharmacologic Category Antidote

Use Treatment of hyperkalemia

Pregnancy Risk Factor C

Pregnancy Considerations Animal reproduction studies have not been conducted. There are no adequate and well-controlled studies in pregnant women. Use during pregnancy only if benefits outweigh the risks.

Breast-Feeding Considerations It is not known if sodium polystyrene sulfonate is excreted in breast milk. The manufacturer recommends that caution be exercised when administering sodium polystyrene sulfonate to nursing women.

Contraindications Hypersensitivity to sodium polystyrene sulfonate or any component of the formulation; hypokalemia; obstructive bowel disease; neonates with reduced gut motility (postoperatively or drug-induced); oral administration in neonates

Additional contraindications: Sodium polystyrene sulfonate suspension (**with** sorbitol): Rectal administration in neonates (particularly in premature infants); any postoperative patient until normal bowel function resumes

Warnings/Precautions Intestinal necrosis (including fatalities) and other serious gastrointestinal events (eg, bleeding, ischemic colitis, perforation) have been reported, especially when administered with sorbitol. Increased risk may be associated with a history of intestinal disease or surgery, hypovolemia, prematurity, and renal insufficiency or failure; use with sorbitol is not recommended. Avoid use in any postoperative patient until normal bowel function resumes or in patients at risk for constipation or impaction; discontinue use if constipation occurs. Oral or rectal administration of sorbitol-containing sodium polystyrene sulfonate suspensions is contraindicated in neonates (particularly with prematurity). Use with caution in patients with severe HF, hypertension, or edema; sodium load may exacerbate condition. Effective lowering of serum potassium from sodium polystyrene sulfonate may take hours to days after administration; consider alternative measures (eg, dialysis) or concomitant therapy (eg, IV sodium bicarbonate) in situations where rapid correction of severe hyperkalemia is required. Severe hypokalemia may occur; frequent monitoring of serum potassium is recommended within each 24-hour period; ECG monitoring may be appropriate in select patients. In addition to serum potassium-lowering effects, cation-exchange resins may also affect other cation concentrations possibly resulting in decreased serum magnesium and calcium. Large oral doses may cause fecal impaction (especially in elderly).

Concomitant administration of oral sodium polystyrene sulfonate with nonabsorbable cation-donating antacids or laxatives (eg, magnesium hydroxide) may result in systemic alkalosis and may diminish ability to reduce serum potassium concentrations; use with such agents is not recommended. In addition, intestinal obstruction has been reported with concomitant administration of aluminum hydroxide due to concretion formation. Enema will reduce the serum potassium faster than oral administration, but the oral route will result in a greater reduction over several hours. Oral administration in neonates and use in neonates with reduced gut motility (postoperatively or drug-induced) is contraindicated. Oral or rectal administration of sorbitol-containing sodium polystyrene sulfonate suspensions in neonates (particularly with prematurity) is also contraindicated due to propylene glycol content and risk of intestinal necrosis and digestive hemorrhage. Use sodium polystyrene sulfonate (**without** sorbitol) with caution in premature or low-birth-weight infants. Use with caution in children when administering rectally; excessive dosage or inadequate dilution may result in fecal impaction.

Adverse Reactions

Endocrine & metabolic: Hypernatremia, hypocalcemia, hypokalemia, hypomagnesemia, sodium retention

Gastrointestinal: Anorexia, constipation, diarrhea, fecal impaction, intestinal necrosis (rare), intestinal obstruction (due to concretions in association with aluminum hydroxide), nausea, vomiting

Rare but important or life-threatening: Acute bronchitis (rare; associated with inhalation of particles), concretions, gastrointestinal bleeding, gastrointestinal ulceration, intestinal perforation, ischemic colitis

Drug Interactions

Metabolism/Transport Effects None known.

Avoid Concomitant Use

Avoid concomitant use of Sodium Polystyrene Sulfonate with any of the following: Laxatives (Magnesium Containing); Meloxicam; Sorbitol

Increased Effect/Toxicity

Sodium Polystyrene Sulfonate may increase the levels/effects of: Aluminum Hydroxide; Digoxin

The levels/effects of Sodium Polystyrene Sulfonate may be increased by: Antacids; Laxatives (Magnesium Containing); Meloxicam; Sorbitol

Decreased Effect

Sodium Polystyrene Sulfonate may decrease the levels/effects of: Lithium; Thyroid Products

Food Interactions Some liquids may contain potassium: Management: Do not mix in orange juice or in any fruit juice known to contain potassium.

Storage/Stability Store at 25°C (77°F); excursions permitted to 15°C to 30°C (59°F to 86°F). Store repackaged product in refrigerator and use within 14 days. Freshly prepared suspensions should be used within 24 hours. Do not heat resin suspension.

Mechanism of Action Removes potassium by exchanging sodium ions for potassium ions in the intestine (especially the large intestine) before the resin is passed from the body; exchange capacity is 1 mEq/g *in vivo*, and *in vitro* capacity is 3.1 mEq/g, therefore, a wide range of exchange capacity exists such that close monitoring of serum electrolytes is necessary

Pharmacodynamics/Kinetics

Onset of action: 2-24 hours

Absorption: None

Excretion: Completely feces (primarily as potassium polystyrene sulfonate)

Dosage

Children: Hyperkalemia:

Oral: 1 g/kg/dose every 6 hours

Rectal: 1 g/kg/dose every 2-6 hours (In small children and infants, employ lower doses by using the practical exchange ratio of 1 mEq K^+/g of resin as the basis for calculation)

Adults: Hyperkalemia:

Oral: 15 g 1-4 times/day

Rectal: 30-50 g every 6 hours

Dosage adjustment in renal impairment: No dosage adjustment provided in manufacturer's labeling. Use with caution; risks of gastrointestinal adverse effects are greater in patients with renal insufficiency or failure.

Dosage adjustment in hepatic impairment: No dosage adjustment provided in manufacturer's labeling.

Dietary Considerations Do **not** mix in orange juice or in any fruit juice known to contain potassium. Some products may contain sodium.

Administration

Oral: Shake suspension well prior to administration. Administer orally (or via NG tube) as a suspension. **Do not mix in orange juice.** Chilling the oral mixture will increase palatability.

Powder for suspension: For each 1 g of the powdered resin, add 3-4 mL of water or syrup (amount of fluid usually ranges from 20-100 mL)

Rectal: Enema route is less effective than oral administration. Administer cleansing enema first. Each dose of the powder for suspension should be suspended in 100 mL of aqueous vehicle and administered as a warm emulsion (body temperature). The commercially available suspension should also be warmed to body temperature. During administration, the solution should be agitated gently. Retain enema in colon for at least 30-60 minutes and for several hours, if possible. Once retention time is complete, irrigate colon with a non-sodium-containing solution to remove resin.

Monitoring Parameters Serum electrolytes (potassium, sodium, calcium, magnesium); ECG in select patients

Reference Range Serum potassium: Adults: 3.5-5.2 mEq/L

Additional Information 1 g of resin binds approximately 1 mEq of potassium

Historically, sorbitol was often recommended as a cathartic agent to be administered with sodium polystyrene sulfonate (SPS) to prevent SPS-induced fecal impaction. However, SPS, particularly when used with sorbitol, has been associated with cases of intestinal necrosis and other serious GI adverse events. Due to the concern that sorbitol may increase the risk of intestinal necrosis, concomitant use of sorbitol is no longer recommended.

Sodium polystyrene sulfonate is commercially available in a liquid suspension containing 33% sorbitol (~20 g sorbitol per 60 mL suspension).

Dosage Forms

Powder, Oral:

Kalexate: (454 g)

Kayexalate: (453.6 g)

Kionex: (454 g)

Generic: (453.6 g, 454 g)

Suspension, Oral:

Kionex: 15 g/60 mL (60 mL, 473 mL)

SPS: 15 g/60 mL (60 mL, 120 mL, 473 mL)

Generic: 15 g/60 mL (60 mL, 480 mL, 500 mL)

Suspension, Rectal:

Generic: 30 g/120 mL (120 mL); 50 g/200 mL (200 mL)

Sodium Stibogluconate [INT]

(SOW dee um STY oh GLOO koe nate)

International Brand Names Pentostam (AE, EG, GB, IL, KW, QA, SA, SI)

Pharmacologic Category Antiprotozoal

Reported Use Treatment of cutaneous and visceral leishmaniasis

Dosage Range Adults: I.M., I.V.: 20 mg/kg/day for 28 days in visceral leishmaniasis and for 20 days in cutaneous infection

Dosage adjustment in renal impairment: Avoid with significant impairment

Dosage adjustment in hepatic impairment: Use with caution

Product Availability Product available in various countries; not currently available in the U.S.

Dosage Forms

Injection, solution, as sodium: Equivalent to 100 mg of pentavalent antimony/mL (30 mL, 100 mL)

◆ **Sodium Sulamyd (Can)** *see* Sulfacetamide (Ophthalmic) *on page 1943*

◆ **Sodium Sulfacetamide** *see* Sulfacetamide (Ophthalmic) *on page 1943*

◆ **Sodium Sulfacetamide** *see* Sulfacetamide (Topical) *on page 1943*

◆ **Sodium Sulfacetamide and Sulfur** *see* Sulfur and Sulfacetamide *on page 1953*

◆ **Sodium Sulfate, Magnesium Sulfate, and Potassium Sulfate** *see* Sodium Sulfate, Potassium Sulfate, and Magnesium Sulfate *on page 1914*

Sodium Sulfate, Potassium Sulfate, and Magnesium Sulfate

(SOW dee um SUL fate, poe TASS ee um SUL fate, & mag NEE zhum SUL fate)

Brand Names: U.S. Suprep® Bowel Prep Kit

Index Terms Magnesium Sulfate, Potassium Sulfate, and Sodium Sulfate; Magnesium Sulfate, Sodium Sulfate, and Potassium Sulfate; Potassium Sulfate, Magnesium Sulfate, and Sodium Sulfate; Potassium Sulfate, Sodium Sulfate, and Magnesium Sulfate; Sodium Sulfate, Magnesium Sulfate, and Potassium Sulfate

Pharmacologic Category Laxative, Osmotic

Use Bowel cleansing prior to GI examination

Pregnancy Risk Factor C

Dosage Oral: Adults: Bowel cleansing prior to GI exam:

Split-dose regimen: Total volume of liquid consumed over the course of treatment: 2880 mL (96 oz)

Evening before colonoscopy: Drink the entire contents of 1 bottle, diluted to a final volume of 480 mL (16 oz). Then drink 2 additional containers of water each (filled to the 16-ounce line) over the next hour, for an additional volume of 960 mL (32 oz).

Morning of the colonoscopy (10-12 hours after the evening dose): Repeat entire process with the second bottle: Drink entire contents of second bottle diluted to a final volume of 480 mL (16 oz); then drink 2 additional containers of water (each filled to the 16-ounce line) over the next hour, for an additional volume of 960 mL (32 oz). Complete at least 2 hours before the procedure.

Dosage adjustment in renal impairment: No adjustments provided in manufacturer's labeling. Use with caution, ensure adequate hydration, and consider baseline and post-colonoscopy renal function assessment.

Dosage adjustment in hepatic impairment: No dosage adjustment provided in manufacturer's labeling. However, no adjustment expected due to similar disposition to healthy patients in pharmacokinetic studies.

Additional Information Complete prescribing information should be consulted for additional detail.

Dosage Forms

Solution, oral:

Suprep® Bowel Prep Kit: Sodium sulfate 17.5 g, potassium sulfate 3.13 g, and magnesium sulfate 1.6 g per 180 mL (180 mL) [contains sodium benzoate]

◆ **Sodium Sulfate, Potassium Sulfate, Magnesium Sulfate and PEG-Electrolyte Solution** *see* Sodium Sulfate, Potassium Sulfate, Magnesium Sulfate, and Polyethylene Glycol-Electrolyte Solution *on page 1914*

◆ **Sodium Sulfate, Potassium Sulfate, Magnesium Sulfate and PEG Solution** *see* Sodium Sulfate, Potassium Sulfate, Magnesium Sulfate, and Polyethylene Glycol-Electrolyte Solution *on page 1914*

Sodium Sulfate, Potassium Sulfate, Magnesium Sulfate, and Polyethylene Glycol-Electrolyte Solution

(SOW dee um SUL fate, poe TASS ee um SUL fate, mag NEE zhum SUL fate, & pol i ETH i leen GLY kol ee LEK troe lite soe LOO shun)

Brand Names: U.S. Suclear™

Index Terms Sodium Sulfate, Potassium Sulfate, Magnesium Sulfate and PEG Solution; Sodium Sulfate, Potassium Sulfate, Magnesium Sulfate and PEG-Electrolyte Solution

Pharmacologic Category Laxative, Osmotic

Use Bowel cleansing prior to colonoscopy

Pregnancy Risk Factor C

Dosage Bowel cleansing prior to colonoscopy: Adults: Oral: May be administered as the *split-dose (2-day) regimen* (preferred method) or the *day-before (1-day) regimen* (alternative method).

Split-dose (2-day) regimen: Total volume of liquid consumed over the course of treatment: 3440 mL (~115 oz)

Dose 1: Evening before colonoscopy (10-12 hours prior to Dose 2): Dilute the contents of the 6-ounce oral solution bottle to a final volume of 480 mL (16 oz), and drink the contents within 20 minutes. Refill container with 16 ounces of water and drink over the next 2 hours. Refill the container with the second refill of 16 oz of water, and finish drinking before bedtime (2 refills totaling 960 mL [32 oz]). Total volume of liquid consumed with Dose 1: 1440 mL (48 oz).

Dose 2: Morning of the colonoscopy (beginning at least 3.5 hours prior to colonoscopy): Drink the entire contents of the reconstituted powder which has been diluted to a final volume of 2000 mL (2 L [~67 oz]) as follows: Using the 16-ounce container provided, drink at a rate of 480 mL (16 oz) every 20 minutes (four 16-ounce containers over ~1.5 hours). Complete at least 2 hours prior to colonoscopy. Total volume of liquid consumed with Dose 2: 2000 mL (~67 oz)

Day-before (1-day) regimen: Total volume of liquid consumed over the course of treatment: 3440 mL (~115 oz)

Dose 1: Evening before colonoscopy (beginning at least 3.5 hours prior to bedtime): Drink the diluted contents of the 6-ounce oral solution bottle, which has been further diluted to a final volume of 480 mL (16 oz), preferably within 20 minutes. Refill container with 480 mL (16 oz) of water, and drink over the next 2 hours. Total volume of liquid consumed with Dose 1: 960 mL (32 oz).

Dose 2: Evening before colonoscopy (~2 hours after starting Dose 1): Drink the entire contents of the reconstituted powder which has been diluted to a final volume of 2000 mL (2 L [~67 oz]) as follows: Using the 16-ounce container provided, drink at a rate of 480 mL (16 oz) every 20 minutes (four 16-ounce containers over ~1.5 hours). Refill the container with 480 mL (16 oz) of water and finish drinking before bedtime. Total volume of liquid consumed with Dose 2: 2480 mL (~83 oz).

Dosage adjustment in renal impairment: No dosage adjustment provided in manufacturer's labeling (safety has not been adequately studied); however, use caution and ensure adequate hydration in patients with renal impairment or at risk for impairment. Moderate renal impairment (CrCl 30-49 mL/minute) resulted in a 43% higher C_{max} and a 16% lower urinary clearance of serum sulfates compared to healthy patients.

Dosage adjustment in hepatic impairment: No dosage adjustment provided in manufacturer's labeling.

Additional Information Complete prescribing information should be consulted for additional detail.

Dosage Forms

Kit, oral:

Suclear™: Powder for solution, oral: PEG 3350 210 g, sodium bicarbonate 2.86 g, sodium chloride 5.6 g, potassium chloride 0.74 g (2000 mL) [contains cherry, lemon-lime, orange, and pineapple flavor packs] and Solution, oral: Sodium sulfate 17.5 g, potassium sulfate 3.13 g, and magnesium sulfate 1.6 g (177 mL) [contains sodium benzoate]

Sodium Tetradecyl Sulfate

(SOW dee um tetra DEK il SUL fate)

Brand Names: U.S. Sotradecol

Brand Names: Canada Trombovar

Pharmacologic Category Sclerosing Agent

Use Treatment of small, uncomplicated varicose veins of the lower extremities

Pregnancy Risk Factor C

Dosage IV: Test dose: 0.5 mL given several hours prior to administration of larger dose; 0.5-2 mL (preferred maximum: 1 mL) in each vein, maximum: 10 mL per treatment session; 3% solution reserved for large varices

Dosage adjustment in renal impairment: No dosage adjustment provided in manufacturer's labeling.

Dosage adjustment in hepatic impairment: No dosage adjustment provided in manufacturer's labeling.

Additional Information Complete prescribing information should be consulted for additional detail.

Dosage Forms

Solution, Intravenous:

Sotradecol: 1% (2 mL); 3% (2 mL)

Sodium Thiosulfate (SOW dee um thye oh SUL fate)

Index Terms Disodium Thiosulfate Pentahydrate; Pentahydrate; Sodium Hyposulfate; Sodium Thiosulphate; Thiosulfuric Acid Disodium Salt

Pharmacologic Category Antidote; Antidote, Extravasation

Use Cyanide poisoning: Treatment of acute, life-threatening cyanide poisoning in combination with sodium nitrite. Consider consultation with a poison control center at 1-800-222-1222.

Pregnancy Risk Factor C

Dosage

Cyanide poisoning: IV: **Note:** Administer in conjunction with sodium nitrite. Administer sodium nitrite first, followed immediately by the administration of sodium thiosulfate.

Children: 250 mg/kg (1 mL/kg or ~30-40 mL/m^2 of a 25% solution) or 500 mg/kg (2 mL/kg of a 25% solution) (Howland, 2011); maximum dose: 12.5 g (50 mL of a 25% solution); may repeat at one-half the original dose if symptoms of cyanide toxicity return

Adults: 12.5 g (50 mL of a 25% solution); may repeat at one-half the original dose if symptoms of cyanide toxicity return

Note: Monitor the patient for 24-48 hours; if symptoms return, repeat both sodium nitrite and sodium thiosulfate at one-half the original doses.

Extravasation management (off-label use): Adults:

Mechlorethamine: SubQ (off-label route): Inject 2 mL of a 1/6 M (~4%) sodium thiosulfate solution (into the extravasation site) for each mg of mechlorethamine suspected to have extravasated (Pérez Fidalgo, 2012; Polovich, 2009)

Cisplatin, concentrated: Inject 2 mL of a 1/6 M (~4%) sodium thiosulfate solution into existing IV line for each 100 mg of cisplatin extravasated; consider also injecting 1 mL of a 1/6 M (~4%) sodium thiosulfate solution as 0.1 mL subcutaneous injections (clockwise) into the area around the extravasation, may repeat subcutaneous injections several times over the next 3-4 hours (Ener, 2004)

Bendamustine: SubQ: Bendamustine extravasation may be managed with 1/6 M (~4%) sodium thiosulfate solution in the same manner as mechlorethamine extravasation (Schulmeister, 2011)

Elderly: Refer to adult dosing; use with caution due to likelihood of decreased renal function.

Dosage adjustment in renal impairment: No dosage adjustment provided in manufacturer's labeling; however, renal elimination is significant and risk of adverse effects may be increased in patients with renal impairment.

Dosage adjustment in hepatic impairment: No dosage adjustment provided in the manufacturer's labeling (has not been studied).

Additional Information Complete prescribing information should be consulted for additional detail.

Dosage Forms

Injection, solution: 250 mg/mL (50 mL)

Injection, solution [preservative free]: 100 mg/mL (10 mL); 250 mg/mL (50 mL)

- **Sodium Thiosulfate and Sodium Nitrite** *see* Sodium Nitrite and Sodium Thiosulfate *on page 1907*
- **Sodium Thiosulphate** *see* Sodium Thiosulfate *on page 1915*
- **Sof-Lax [OTC]** *see* Docusate *on page 661*
- **Soflax [OTC] (Can)** *see* Docusate *on page 661*
- **Soflax C [OTC] (Can)** *see* Docusate *on page 661*
- **Soflax EX [OTC] (Can)** *see* Bisacodyl *on page 265*
- **Soflax Pediatric Drops [OTC] (Can)** *see* Docusate *on page 661*

Sofosbuvir (soe FOS bue vir)

Brand Names: U.S. Sovaldi

Brand Names: Canada Sovaldi

Index Terms Sovaldi

Pharmacologic Category Antihepaciviral, Polymerase Inhibitor (Anti-HCV)

Use Chronic hepatitis C: Treatment of genotype 1, 2, 3, or 4 chronic hepatitis C (CHC) (in combination with ribavirin or with peginterferon alfa and ribavirin), including patients with hepatocellular carcinoma meeting Milan criteria (awaiting liver transplantation) and those with HCV/HIV-1 coinfection

Pregnancy Risk Factor B (sofosbuvir)/X (in combination with ritonavir or peginterferon alfa/ribavirin)

Pregnancy Considerations Adverse events were not observed in animal reproduction studies using sofosbuvir. However, sofosbuvir is only to be used in combination with ribavirin or peginterferon alfa/ribavirin for the treatment of hepatitis C virus (HCV), therefore use is contraindicated in pregnancy. A negative pregnancy test is required before initiation and monthly thereafter. Avoid pregnancy in female patients and female partners of male patients during therapy by using two effective forms of nonhormonal contraception; continue contraceptive measures for at least 6 months after completion of therapy. Also refer to the Peginterferon Alfa and Ribavirin monographs for additional information.

If pregnancy occurs during use or within 6 months after treatment with ribavirin, report to the ribavirin pregnancy registry (800-593-2214). In addition, because sofosbuvir may be used for the treatment of HCV infection in women coinfected with HIV, inadvertent administration of sofosbuvir in women with HCV/HIV coinfection during pregnancy should also be reported to the Antiretroviral Pregnancy Registry (1-800-258-4263).

Breast-Feeding Considerations It is not known if sofosbuvir is excreted into breast milk. Due to the potential for serious adverse reactions in the nursing infant, the manufacturer recommends a decision be made whether to discontinue nursing or to discontinue the drug, taking into account the importance of treatment to the mother. Breast-feeding is not linked to the spread of hepatitis C virus; however, if nipples are cracked or bleeding, breast-feeding is not recommended (Workowski, 2010). Mothers coinfected with HIV are discouraged from breast-feeding to decrease potential transmission of HIV (DHHS [perinatal], 2012). Also refer to the Peginterferon Alfa and Ribavirin monographs for additional information.

Contraindications

All contraindications also applicable to ribavirin and peginterferon alfa including women who are pregnant or who may become pregnant and use by male partners of pregnant women.

Also refer to Peginterferon Alfa and Ribavirin monographs for individual product contraindications.

Canadian labeling: Additional contraindications (not in U.S. labeling): Hypersensitivity to sofosbuvir or any component of the formulation; males whose female partners may become pregnant

Warnings/Precautions Avoid pregnancy in females and female partners of male patients during therapy and for at least 6 months following treatment since used in combination with ribavirin for all indications; two nonhormonal forms of effective contraception must be used. Combination therapy with ribavirin is contraindicated in pregnancy; ribavirin may cause birth defects and/or death of the exposed fetus. Do not use as monotherapy; use only in combination with ribavirin (with or without peginterferon alfa depending upon the clinical indication). Alternative recommendations also use in combination with simeprevir in select patients (AASLD/IDSA, 2014). Potentially significant drug-drug interactions may exist, requiring dose or frequency adjustment, additional monitoring, and/or selection of alternative therapy, including use with potent P-gp inducers (eg, rifampin, St John's wort).

Adverse Reactions

Central nervous system: Chills, fatigue, headache, insomnia, irritability

Dermatologic: Pruritus, skin rash

Gastrointestinal: Decreased appetite, diarrhea, increased serum lipase, nausea

Hematologic & oncologic: Anemia, decreased hemoglobin, decreased neutrophils, neutropenia, thrombocytopenia

Hepatic: Increased serum bilirubin

Neuromuscular & skeletal: Myalgia, weakness

Renal: Increased creatine kinase

Respiratory: Flu-like symptoms

Miscellaneous: Fever

Rare but important or life-threatening: Pancytopenia, severe depression, suicidal ideation

Drug Interactions

Metabolism/Transport Effects **Substrate** of P-glycoprotein

Avoid Concomitant Use

Avoid concomitant use of Sofosbuvir with any of the following: Modafinil; OXcarbazepine; P-glycoprotein/ABCB1 Inducers; Rifabutin; Rifapentine

Increased Effect/Toxicity

The levels/effects of Sofosbuvir may be increased by: P-glycoprotein/ABCB1 Inhibitors

Decreased Effect

The levels/effects of Sofosbuvir may be decreased by: Modafinil; OXcarbazepine; P-glycoprotein/ABCB1 Inducers; Rifabutin; Rifapentine

Storage/Stability Store at room temperature below 30°C (86°F). Dispense only in original container.

Mechanism of Action Sofosbuvir, a direct-acting antiviral agent against the hepatitis C virus, is a prodrug converted to its pharmacologically active form (GS-461203) via intracellular metabolism. It inhibits HCV NS5B RNA-dependent RNA polymerase, essential for viral replication, and acts as a chain terminator.

Pharmacodynamics/Kinetics

Protein binding: ~61% to 65%

Metabolism: Hepatic; forms pharmacologically active nucleoside (uridine) analog triphosphate GS-461203; dephosphorylation results in the formation of nucleoside inactive metabolite GS-331007

Half-life elimination: 0.4 hours

Time to peak: ~0.5 to 2 hours

Excretion: Urine (80%)

Dosage Adults: Oral: 400 mg once daily with concomitant ribavirin and with or without peginterferon alfa (maximum: 400 mg daily). **Note:** Treatment regimen and duration based on HCV genotype and/or clinical scenario as noted below:

Chronic hepatitis C (CHC) infection in monoinfected (HCV) or coinfected (HCV/HIV-1) patients:

Treatment-naive patients:

Genotype 1:

Patients who can receive interferon: 400 mg once daily with concomitant ribavirin and peginterferon alfa for 12 weeks. **Note:** A recommended regimen (AASLD/IDSA, 2014)

Patients who cannot receive interferon:

Manufacturer's labeling: 400 mg once daily with concomitant ribavirin for 24 weeks. **Note:** A recommended regimen (AASLD/IDSA, 2014)

Alternative dosing (off-label regimen): 400 mg once daily with simeprevir and with or without ribavirin for 12 weeks. **Note:** A recommended regimen (AASLD/IDSA, 2014)

Genotype 2: 400 mg once daily with concomitant ribavirin for 12 weeks. **Note:** A recommended regimen (AASLD/IDSA, 2014)

Genotype 3:

Patients who can receive interferon: 400 mg once daily with concomitant ribavirin and peginterferon alfa for 12 weeks. **Note:** A recommended regimen (AASLD/IDSA, 2014)

Regardless of patient eligibility for peginterferon: 400 mg once daily with concomitant ribavirin for 24 weeks. **Note:** A recommended regimen (AASLD/IDSA, 2014)

Genotype 4:

Patients who can receive interferon: *Manufacturer's labeling:* 400 mg once daily with concomitant ribavirin and peginterferon alfa for 12 weeks. **Note:** A recommended regimen (AASLD/IDSA, 2014)

Patients who cannot receive interferon: *Alternative dosing (off-label regimen):*400 mg once daily with concomitant ribavirin for 24 weeks. **Note:** A recommended regimen (AASLD/IDSA, 2014)

Genotype 5 or 6 (off-label use): Patients who can receive interferon: 400 mg once daily with concomitant ribavirin and peginterferon alfa for 12 weeks. **Note:** A recommended regimen (AASLD/IDSA, 2014)

Relapser patients (nonresponders to a previous regimen of ribavirin and peginterferon alfa **without** an HCV protease inhibitor):

Regardless of patient eligibility for peginterferon:

Genotype 1 (off-label regimen): 400 mg once daily with simeprevir and **with** or **without** ribavirin for 12 weeks. **Note:** A recommended regimen (AASLD/IDSA, 2014)

Relapser patients (nonresponders to a previous regimen of ribavirin and peginterferon alfa **with** or **without** an HCV protease inhibitor):

Patients who can receive interferon:

Genotype 1 (off-label regimen): 400 mg once daily for 12 weeks with ribavirin and peginterferon alfa for 12-24 weeks. **Note:** A recommended regimen (AASLD/IDSA, 2014)

Genotype 4: 400 mg once daily with concomitant ribavirin and peginterferon alfa for 12 weeks. **Note:** A recommended regimen (AASLD/IDSA, 2014)

Genotype 5 or 6 (off-label use): 400 mg once daily with concomitant ribavirin and peginterferon alfa for 12 weeks. Note: A recommended regimen (AASLD/IDSA, 2014)

Regardless of patient eligibility for peginterferon:

Genotype 2 (off-label regimen): 400 mg once daily with concomitant ribavirin for 12 weeks. **Note:** A recommended regimen; also patients with cirrhosis may benefit from a total of 16 weeks of treatment (AASLD/IDSA, 2014)

Genotype 3: 400 mg once daily with concomitant ribavirin for 24 weeks. **Note:** A recommended regimen (AASLD/IDSA, 2014)

Patients with hepatocellular carcinoma awaiting liver transplantation: 400 mg once daily with concomitant ribavirin for 48 weeks or until the time of liver transplantation, whichever occurs first

Missed dose: If a dose is missed within the calendar day it is usually taken, take as soon as possible. If the calendar day when the dose is usually taken has passed, do not take the missed dose and resume the usual dosing schedule. Do not take >400 mg daily. The Canadian labeling recommends that patients who vomit <2 hours after administration take another dose but if >2 hours, take dose at the next regularly scheduled time.

Dosage adjustment for toxicity: Sofosbuvir requires no dosage adjustment; concomitant agents should be adjusted as described below:

Patients with Genotype 1 or 4: Dose reduction dependent upon ribavirin and/or peginterferon doses; refer to individual monographs.

Patients with Genotype 2 or 3 **without** cardiac history:

Hemoglobin 8.5 to <10 g/dL: Decrease ribavirin dose to 600 mg daily in divided doses (eg, 200 mg in the morning, 400 mg in the evening).

Hemoglobin <8.5 g/dL: Permanently discontinue treatment.

Patients with Genotype 2 or 3 **with** stable cardiac history:

Hemoglobin has decreased ≥2 g/dL during any 4-week period of treatment: Decrease ribavirin dose to 600 mg daily in divided doses (eg, 200 mg in the morning, 400 mg in the evening).

Hemoglobin has decreased to <12 g/dL despite 4 weeks at reduced dose: Permanently discontinue treatment.

Note: Once ribavirin has been withheld due to clinical adverse event or laboratory abnormality, an attempt to restart ribavirin at 600 mg daily (in divided doses) can be made, with a further ribavirin increase to 800 mg daily. Increasing the ribavirin dose to its original level (usually 1000-1200 mg daily) is not recommended.

Dosage adjustment in renal impairment:

Sofosbuvir:

CrCl >30 mL/minute: No dosage adjustment necessary.

CrCl ≤30 mL/minute: There are no dosage adjustments provided in the manufacturer's labeling (has not been studied). Predominant metabolite accumulates in impaired renal function.

End stage renal disease (ESRD), including those requiring intermittent hemodialysis (IHD): There are no dosage adjustments provided in manufacturer's labeling (has not been studied). Predominant metabolite accumulates in impaired renal function.

Peginterferon Alfa and Ribavirin: Refer to individual monographs.

Dosage adjustment in hepatic impairment:

Child-Pugh class A, B, or C: No dosage adjustment necessary.

Decompensated cirrhosis: There are no dosage adjustments provided in the manufacturer's labeling (has not been studied).

Peginterferon Alfa and Ribavirin: Refer to individual monographs; peginterferon alfa is contraindicated in hepatic decompensation.

Administration Administer with or without food.

Monitoring Parameters

Bilirubin, liver enzymes, and serum creatinine at baseline and periodically when clinically indicated.

Serum HCV-RNA at baseline, during treatment, at the end of treatment, during treatment follow-up, and when clinically indicated.

Pretreatment and monthly pregnancy tests up to 6 months following discontinuation of therapy for women of childbearing age.

Dosage Forms

Tablet, Oral:

Sovaldi: 400 mg

◆ **Sofosbuvir and Ledipasvir** *see* Ledipasvir and Sofosbuvir *on page 1173*

◆ **Solaquin® (Can)** *see* Hydroquinone *on page 1020*

◆ **Solaquin Forte® (Can)** *see* Hydroquinone *on page 1020*

Solifenacin (sol i FEN a sin)

Brand Names: U.S. VESIcare

Index Terms Solifenacin Succinate; YM905

Pharmacologic Category Anticholinergic Agent

Additional Appendix Information

Beers Criteria – Potentially Inappropriate Medications for Geriatrics *on page 2271*

Use Treatment of overactive bladder with symptoms of urinary frequency, urgency, or urge incontinence

Pregnancy Risk Factor C

Pregnancy Considerations Adverse events were observed in some animal reproduction studies.

Breast-Feeding Considerations It is not known if solifenacin is excreted in breast milk. The manufacturer recommends a decision be made whether to discontinue nursing or to discontinue the drug.

Contraindications Hypersensitivity to solifenacin or any component of the formulation; urinary retention; gastric retention; uncontrolled narrow-angle glaucoma.

Warnings/Precautions Cases of angioedema involving the face, lips, tongue, and/or larynx have been reported during treatment; some cases have occurred after the first dose. Immediately discontinue if tongue, hypopharynx, or larynx is involved. Anaphylactic reactions have been reported rarely with solifenacin; immediately discontinue therapy if anaphylactic reaction develops. Do not use in patients with a known or suspected hypersensitivity. Central nervous system effects have been reported (eg, headache, confusion, hallucinations, somnolence); monitor, particularly at treatment initiation or dose increase, reduce dose or discontinue if necessary. May cause drowsiness and/or blurred vision, which may impair physical or mental abilities; patients must be cautioned about performing tasks which require mental alertness (eg, operating machinery or driving). Heat prostration may occur in the presence of increased environmental temperature; use caution in hot weather and/or exercise. Use with caution in patients with bladder outflow obstruction, gastrointestinal obstructive disorders, and decreased gastrointestinal motility. Use with caution in patients with a known history of QT prolongation or other risk factors for QT prolongation (eg, concomitant use of medications known to prolong QT interval and/or electrolyte abnormalities); the risk for QT prolongation is dose-related. Use with caution in patients with controlled (treated) narrow-angle glaucoma; use is contraindicated with uncontrolled narrow-angle glaucoma. Dosage adjustment is required for patients with severe renal impairment (CrCl <30 mL/minute) or moderate (Child-Pugh class B) hepatic impairment; use is not recommended with severe hepatic impairment (Child-Pugh class C). Patients on potent CYP3A4 inhibitors require the lower dose of solifenacin. This medication is ▶

associated with potent anticholinergic properties which may be inappropriate in older adults depending on comorbidities (eg, dementia, delirium) (Beers Criteria).

Adverse Reactions

Cardiovascular: Edema, hypertension

Central nervous system: Depression, fatigue

Gastrointestinal: Constipation, dyspepsia, nausea, upper abdominal pain, xerostomia

Genitourinary: Urinary retention, urinary tract infection

Ophthalmic: Blurred vision, dry eye syndrome

Respiratory: Cough

Miscellaneous: Influenza

Rare but important or life-threatening: Abnormal hepatic function tests, anaphylaxis, angioedema, atrial fibrillation, confusion, delirium, erythema multiforme, exfoliative dermatitis, fecal impaction, gastroesophageal reflux disease, gastrointestinal obstruction, glaucoma, hallucination, hyperkalemia, hypersensitivity reactions, intestinal obstruction, palpitations, prolonged Q-T interval on ECG, renal insufficiency, tachycardia, torsades de pointes, voice disorder

Drug Interactions

Metabolism/Transport Effects Substrate of CYP3A4 (major); **Note:** Assignment of Major/Minor substrate status based on clinically relevant drug interaction potential

Avoid Concomitant Use

Avoid concomitant use of Solifenacin with any of the following: Aclidinium; Conivaptan; Fusidic Acid (Systemic); Glucagon; Idelalisib; Ipratropium (Oral Inhalation); Potassium Chloride; Tiotropium; Umeclidinium

Increased Effect/Toxicity

Solifenacin may increase the levels/effects of: AbobotulinumtoxinA; Analgesics (Opioid); Anticholinergic Agents; Cannabinoid-Containing Products; Glucagon; Highest Risk QTc-Prolonging Agents; Moderate Risk QTc-Prolonging Agents; OnabotulinumtoxinA; Potassium Chloride; RimabotulinumtoxinB; Thiazide Diuretics; Tiotropium; Topiramate

The levels/effects of Solifenacin may be increased by: Aclidinium; Antifungal Agents (Azole Derivatives, Systemic); Aprepitant; Ceritinib; Conivaptan; CYP3A4 Inhibitors (Moderate); CYP3A4 Inhibitors (Strong); Dasatinib; Fosaprepitant; Fusidic Acid (Systemic); Idelalisib; Ipratropium (Oral Inhalation); Ivacaftor; Luliconazole; Mianserin; Mifepristone; Mirabegron; Netupitant; Pramlintide; Simeprevir; Stiripentol; Umeclidinium

Decreased Effect

Solifenacin may decrease the levels/effects of: Acetylcholinesterase Inhibitors; Itopride; Secretin

The levels/effects of Solifenacin may be decreased by: Acetylcholinesterase Inhibitors; Bosentan; CYP3A4 Inducers (Moderate); CYP3A4 Inducers (Strong); Dabrafenib; Deferasirox; Mitotane; Siltuximab; St Johns Wort; Tocilizumab

Food Interactions Grapefruit juice may increase the serum level effects of solifenacin. Management: Monitor closely with concurrent use.

Storage/Stability Store at controlled room temperature of 25°C (77°F); excursions permitted to 15°C to 30°C (59°F to 86°F).

Mechanism of Action Inhibits muscarinic receptors resulting in decreased urinary bladder contraction, increased residual urine volume, and decreased detrusor muscle pressure.

Pharmacodynamics/Kinetics

Distribution: V_d: ~600 L

Protein binding: ~98% bound primarily to $alpha_1$-acid glycoprotein

Metabolism: Extensively hepatic; via N-oxidation and 4 R-hydroxylation, forms 1 active and 3 inactive metabolites; primary pathway for elimination is via CYP3A4

Bioavailability: ~90%

Half-life elimination: 45-68 hours following chronic dosing; prolonged in severe renal (CrCl <30 mL/minute) or moderate hepatic (Child-Pugh class B) impairment

Time to peak, plasma: 3-8 hours

Excretion: Urine (69%; <15% as unchanged drug); feces (23%)

Dosage Oral: Adults: 5 mg once daily; if tolerated, may increase to 10 mg once daily

Dosage adjustment with concomitant CYP3A4 inhibitors: Maximum solifenacin dose: 5 mg/day

Dosage adjustment in renal impairment: Use with caution in reduced renal function

CrCl <30 mL/minute: Maximum dose: 5 mg/day

Dosage adjustment in hepatic impairment: Use with caution in reduced hepatic function

Moderate (Child-Pugh class B): Maximum dose: 5 mg/day

Severe (Child-Pugh class C): Use is not recommended

Dietary Considerations May be taken without regard to meals.

Administration Swallow tablet whole; administer with liquids; may be administered without regard to meals.

Monitoring Parameters Anticholinergic effects (eg, fixed and dilated pupils, blurred vision, tremors, or dry skin); creatinine clearance (prior to treatment for dosing adjustment); liver function

Dosage Forms

Tablet, Oral:

VESIcare: 5 mg, 10 mg

- **Solifenacin Succinate** *see* Solifenacin *on page 1917*
- **Soliris** *see* Eculizumab *on page 703*
- **Solodyn** *see* Minocycline *on page 1371*
- **Soltamox** *see* Tamoxifen *on page 1971*
- **Soluble Fluorescein** *see* Fluorescein *on page 894*
- **Solu-CORTEF** *see* Hydrocortisone (Systemic) *on page 1013*
- **Solu-Cortef (Can)** *see* Hydrocortisone (Systemic) *on page 1013*
- **Solumedrol** *see* MethylPREDNISolone *on page 1340*
- **Solu-MEDROL** *see* MethylPREDNISolone *on page 1340*
- **Solu-Medrol (Can)** *see* MethylPREDNISolone *on page 1340*
- **Solzira** *see* Gabapentin Enacarbil *on page 946*
- **SOM230** *see* Pasireotide *on page 1583*
- **Soma** *see* Carisoprodol *on page 363*
- **Soma Compound** *see* Carisoprodol and Aspirin *on page 364*
- **Soma Compound w/Codeine** *see* Carisoprodol, Aspirin, and Codeine *on page 364*

Somatropin (soe ma TROE pin)

Brand Names: U.S. Genotropin; Genotropin MiniQuick; Humatrope; Norditropin FlexPro; Norditropin NordiFlex Pen; Nutropin AQ NuSpin 10; Nutropin AQ NuSpin 20; Nutropin AQ NuSpin 5; Nutropin AQ Pen; Nutropin [DSC]; Omnitrope; Saizen; Saizen Click.Easy; Serostim; Tev-Tropin; Zorbtive

Brand Names: Canada Genotropin GoQuick; Genotropin MiniQuick; Humatrope; Norditropin Nordiflex; Norditropin Simplexx; Nutropin AQ NuSpin; Nutropin AQ Pen; Omnitrope; Saizen; Serostim

Index Terms Growth Hormone, Human; hGH; Human Growth Hormone

Pharmacologic Category Growth Hormone

Additional Appendix Information

Beers Criteria – Potentially Inappropriate Medications for Geriatrics *on page 2271*

Use

Children:

Treatment of growth failure due to inadequate endogenous growth hormone secretion (Genotropin, Humatrope, Norditropin, Nutropin, Nutropin AQ, Omnitrope, Saizen, Tev-Tropin)

Treatment of short stature associated with Turner syndrome (Genotropin, Humatrope, Norditropin, Nutropin, Nutropin AQ, Omnitrope)

Treatment of Prader-Willi syndrome (Genotropin, Omnitrope)

Treatment of growth failure associated with chronic renal insufficiency (CRI) up until the time of renal transplantation (Nutropin, Nutropin AQ)

Treatment of growth failure in children born small for gestational age who fail to manifest catch-up growth by 2 years of age (Genotropin, Omnitrope) or by 2-4 years of age (Humatrope, Norditropin)

Treatment of idiopathic short stature (nongrowth hormone-deficient short stature) defined by height standard deviation score (SDS) ≤-2.25 and growth rate not likely to attain normal adult height (Genotropin, Humatrope, Nutropin, Nutropin AQ, Omnitrope)

Treatment of short stature or growth failure associated with short stature homeobox gene (SHOX) deficiency (Humatrope)

Treatment of short stature associated with Noonan syndrome (Norditropin)

Adults:

HIV patients with wasting or cachexia with concomitant antiviral therapy (Serostim)

Replacement of endogenous growth hormone in patients with adult growth hormone deficiency who meet both of the following criteria (Genotropin, Humatrope, Norditropin, Nutropin, Nutropin AQ, Omnitrope, Saizen):

Biochemical diagnosis of adult growth hormone deficiency by means of a subnormal response to a standard growth hormone stimulation test (peak growth hormone ≤5 mcg/L). Confirmatory testing may not be required in patients with congenital/genetic growth hormone deficiency or multiple pituitary hormone deficiencies due to organic diseases.

and

Adult-onset: Patients who have adult growth hormone deficiency whether alone or with multiple hormone deficiencies (hypopituitarism) as a result of pituitary disease, hypothalamic disease, surgery, radiation therapy, or trauma

or

Childhood-onset: Patients who were growth hormone deficient during childhood, confirmed as an adult before replacement therapy is initiated

Treatment of short-bowel syndrome (Zorbtive)

Pregnancy Risk Factor B/C (depending upon manufacturer)

Pregnancy Considerations Teratogenic effects were not observed in animal studies. Reproduction studies have not been conducted with all agents. During normal pregnancy, maternal production of endogenous growth hormone decreases as placental growth hormone production increases. Data with somatropin use during pregnancy is limited.

Breast-Feeding Considerations It is not known if somatropin is excreted in breast milk. The manufacturer recommends that caution be exercised when administering somatropin to nursing women.

Contraindications Hypersensitivity to growth hormone or any component of the formulation; growth promotion in pediatric patients with closed epiphyses; progression or recurrence of any underlying intracranial lesion or actively growing intracranial tumor; acute critical illness due to complications following open heart or abdominal surgery; multiple accidental trauma or acute respiratory failure; evidence of active malignancy; active proliferative or severe nonproliferative diabetic retinopathy; use in patients with Prader-Willi syndrome **without** growth hormone deficiency (except Genotropin) or in patients with Prader-Willi syndrome **with** growth hormone deficiency who are severely obese, have a history of upper airway obstruction or sleep apnea, or have severe respiratory impairment

Warnings/Precautions Initiation of somatropin is contraindicated with acute critical illness due to complications following open heart or abdominal surgery, multiple accidental trauma, or acute respiratory failure; mortality may be increased. The safety of continuing somatropin in patients who develop these illnesses during therapy has not been established; use with caution. Use in contraindicated with active malignancy; monitor patients with preexisting tumors or growth failure secondary to an intracranial lesion for recurrence or progression of underlying disease; discontinue therapy with evidence of recurrence. An increased risk of second neoplasm has been reported in childhood cancer survivors treated with somatropin; the most common second neoplasms were meningiomas in patients treated with radiation to the head for their first neoplasm. Patients with HIV and pediatric patients with short stature (genetic cause) have increased baseline risk of developing malignancies; consider risk/benefits prior to initiation of therapy and monitor these patients carefully. Monitor all patients for any malignant transformation of skin lesions.

Somatropin may decrease insulin sensitivity; use with caution in patients with diabetes or with risk factors for impaired glucose tolerance. Adjustment of antidiabetic medications may be necessary. Pancreatitis has been rarely reported; incidence in children (especially girls) with Turner syndrome may be greater than adults. Monitor for hypersensitivity reactions. Patients with hypoadrenalism may require increased dosages of glucocorticoids (especially cortisone acetate and prednisone) due to somatropin-mediated inhibition of 11 beta-hydroxysteroid dehydrogenase type 1; undiagnosed central hypoadrenalism may be unmasked. Excessive glucocorticoid therapy may inhibit the growth promoting effects of somatropin in children; monitor and adjust glucocorticoids carefully. Untreated/undiagnosed hypothyroidism may decrease response to therapy; monitor thyroid function test periodically and initiate/adjust thyroid replacement therapy as needed. Closely monitor other hormonal replacement treatments in patients with hypopituitarism. Obese patients may experience an increased incidence of adverse events when using a weight-based dosing regimen. Intracranial hypertension (IH) with headache, nausea, papilledema, visual changes, and/or vomiting has been reported with somatropin; funduscopic examination prior to initiation of therapy and periodically thereafter is recommended. Treatment should be discontinued in patients who develop papilledema; resuming treatment at a lower dose may be considered once IH-associated signs and symptoms have resolved. Patients with Turner syndrome, chronic renal failure and Prader-Willi syndrome may be at increased risk for IH. Progression of scoliosis may occur in children experiencing rapid growth. Patients with growth hormone deficiency may develop slipped capital epiphyses more frequently, evaluate any child with new onset of a limp or with complaints of hip or knee pain. Patients with Turner syndrome are at increased risk for otitis media and other ear/hearing disorders, cardiovascular disorders (including stroke, aortic aneurysm, hypertension), and thyroid disease, monitor carefully. Fluid retention may occur frequently in adults during use; manifestations of fluid retention (eg, edema, arthralgia, myalgia, nerve compression syndromes/paresthesias) are generally transient and dose dependent. Potentially significant drug-drug interactions may exist, requiring dose or frequency adjustment, additional monitoring, and/or selection of alternative therapy. Products may contain m-cresol. Not for IV injection. According to the Centers for Disease Control and Prevention (CDC), pen-shaped injection devices should never be used for more than one person (even when the needle is changed) because of the risk of infection. The injection device should be clearly labeled with individual patient information to ensure that the correct pen is used (CDC, 2012).

Benzyl alcohol and derivatives: Diluent may contain benzyl alcohol; large amounts of benzyl alcohol (≥99 mg/kg/day) have been associated with a potentially fatal toxicity ("gasping syndrome") in neonates; the "gasping syndrome" consists of metabolic acidosis, respiratory distress, gasping respirations, CNS dysfunction (including convulsions, intracranial hemorrhage), hypotension, and cardiovascular collapse (AAP, 1997; CDC, 1982); some data suggests that benzoate displaces bilirubin from protein binding sites (Ahlfors, 2001); avoid or use dosage forms containing benzyl alcohol with caution in neonates. See manufacturer's labeling.

Fatalities have been reported in pediatric patients with Prader-Willi syndrome following the use of growth hormone. The reported fatalities occurred in patients with one or more risk factors, including severe obesity, sleep apnea, respiratory impairment, or unidentified respiratory infection; male patients with one or more of these factors may be at greater risk. Treatment interruption is recommended in patients who show signs of upper airway obstruction, including the onset of, or increased, snoring. In addition, evaluation of and/or monitoring for sleep apnea and respiratory infections are recommended.

Patients with HIV infection should be maintained on antiretroviral therapy to prevent the potential increase in viral replication.

Avoid use in the elderly, except as hormone replacement following pituitary gland removal; use results in minimal effect on body composition and is associated with edema, arthralgia, carpal tunnel syndrome, gynecomastia, and impaired fasting glucose (Beers Criteria). Elderly may be more sensitive to the actions of somatropin; consider lower starting doses.

Safety and efficacy have not been established for the treatment of Noonan syndrome in children with significant cardiac disease. Children with epiphyseal closure who are treated for adult GHD need reassessment of therapy and dose. Administration site rotation is necessary to prevent tissue atrophy.

Adverse Reactions

Growth hormone deficiency: Adverse reactions reported with growth hormone deficiency vary greatly by age. Generally, percentages are less in pediatric patients than adults, and many of the reactions reported in adults are dose related. Percentages reported also vary by product. Below is a listing by age group; events reported more commonly overall are noted with an asterisk (*).

Children: Antibodies development, arthralgia, benign intracranial hypertension, edema, eosinophilia, glycosuria, Hb A_{1c} increased, headache, hematoma, hematuria, hyperglycemia (mild), hypertriglyceridemia, hypoglycemia, hypothyroidism, injection site reaction, intracranial tumor, leg pain, lipoatrophy, leukemia, meningioma, muscle pain, papilledema, pseudotumor cerebri, psoriasis exacerbation, rash, scoliosis progression, seizure, slipped capital femoral epiphysis, weakness

Adults: Acne, ALT increased, AST increased, arthralgia*, back pain, bronchitis, carpal tunnel syndrome, chest pain, cough, depression, diabetes mellitus (type 2), diaphoresis, dizziness, edema*, fatigue, flu-like syndrome*, gastritis, glucose intolerance, glucosuria, headache*, hyperglycemia (mild), hypertension, hypoesthesia, hypothyroidism, infection, insomnia, insulin resistance, joint disorder, leg edema, muscle pain, myalgia*, nausea, pain in extremities, paresthesia*, peripheral edema*, pharyngitis, retinopathy, rhinitis, skeletal pain*, stiffness in extremities, surgical procedure, upper respiratory tract infection, weakness

Additional/postmarketing reactions observed with growth hormone deficiency: Gynecomastia, increased growth of preexisting nevi, pancreatitis

HARS: Serostim®: Arthrlagia, blood glucose increased, edema (peripheral), headache, hypoesthesia, myalgia, pain (extremity), paresthesia

Idiopathic short stature: Humatrope®: Arthralgia, arthrosis, gynecomastia, hip pain, hyperlipidemia, hypertension, myalgia, otitis media, scoliosis. Additional adverse reactions listed as reported using other products from ISS NCGS Cohort: Aggressiveness, benign intracranial hypertension, diabetes, edema, hair loss, headache, injection site reaction

Prader-Willi syndrome: Genotropin®: Aggressiveness, arthralgia, edema, hair loss, headache, benign intracranial hypertension, myalgia; fatalities associated with use in this population have been reported

Turner syndrome: Humatrope®: Ear disorders, otitis media, joint pain, respiratory illness, surgical procedures, urinary tract infection

HIV patients with wasting or cachexia: Serostim®: Edema, gynecomastia, headache, hypoesthesial; musculoskeletal disorders (arthralgia, arthrosis, myalgia); nausea, paresthesia, peripheral edema,

Short-bowel syndrome: Zorbtive®: Abdominal pain, arthralgia, chest pain, dehydration, diaphoresis, dizziness, facial edema,flatulence, generalized edema, hearing symptoms, infection, injection site pain, injection site reaction, malaise, moniliasis, myalgia, nausea, pain, peripheral edema,rash, rhinitis, vomiting

SHOX deficiency: Humatrope®: Arthralgia, excessive cutaneous nevi, gynecomastia, scoliosis

Small for gestational age: Genotropin®, Humatrope®: Mild, transient hyperglycemia; benign intracranial hypertension (rare); central precocious puberty; jaw prominence (rare); aggravation of preexisting scoliosis (rare); injection site reactions; progression of pigmented nevi; carpal tunnel syndrome (rare) diabetes mellitus (rare); otitis media; headache; slipped capital femoral epiphysis

Drug Interactions

Metabolism/Transport Effects None known.

Avoid Concomitant Use There are no known interactions where it is recommended to avoid concomitant use.

Increased Effect/Toxicity There are no known significant interactions involving an increase in effect.

Decreased Effect

Somatropin may decrease the levels/effects of: Antidiabetic Agents; Cortisone; PredniSONE

The levels/effects of Somatropin may be decreased by: Estrogen Derivatives

Preparation for Administration

Genotropin: Reconstitute with diluent provided.

Genotropin MiniQuick: Reconstitute with diluent provided. Consult the instructions provided with the reconstitution device.

Humatrope:

Cartridge: Consult HumatroPen User Guide for complete instructions for reconstitution. **Dilute with solution provided with cartridges ONLY; do not use diluent provided with vials.**

Vial: 5 mg: Reconstitute with 1.5-5 mL diluent provided. Swirl gently; do not shake.

Nutropin: Vial:

5 mg: Reconstitute with 1-5 mL bacteriostatic water for injection. Swirl gently, do not shake.

10 mg: Reconstitute with 1-10 mL bacteriostatic water for injection. Swirl gently, do not shake.

Omnitrope powder: Reconstitute with provided diluent. Swirl gently; do not shake.

Saizen: Vial:

5 mg: Reconstitute with 1-3 mL bacteriostatic water for injection or sterile water for injection. Gently swirl; do not shake.

8.8 mg: Reconstitute with 2-3 mL bacteriostatic water for injection or sterile water for injection. Gently swirl; do not shake.

Serostim: Vial: Reconstitute with 0.5-1 mL sterile water for injection.

Tev-Tropin: Reconstitute 5 mg vial with 1 to 5 mL and 10 mg vial with 1 mL of diluent provided. Gently swirl; do not shake. Use preservative-free NS for use in newborns.

Zorbtive: 8.8 mg vial: Reconstitute with 1-2 mL bacteriostatic water for injection. Swirl gently.

Storage/Stability

Genotropin: Store at 2°C to 8°C (36°F to 46°F); do not freeze. Protect from light. Following reconstitution of 5.8 mg and 13.8 mg cartridge, store under refrigeration and use within 28 days.

Genotropin Miniquick: Store in refrigerator prior to dispensing, but may be stored ≤25°C (77°F) for up to 3 months after dispensing. Once reconstituted, solution must be refrigerated and used within 24 hours. Discard unused portion.

Humatrope:

Vial: Before and after reconstitution, store at 2°C to 8°C (36°F to 46°F); do not freeze. When reconstituted with provided diluent or bacteriostatic water for injection, use within 14 days. When reconstituted with sterile water for injection, use within 24 hours and discard unused portion.

Cartridge: Before and after reconstitution, store at 2°C to 8°C (36°F to 46°F); do not freeze. Following reconstitution with provided diluent, stable for 28 days under refrigeration.

Norditropin: Store at 2°C to 8°C (36°F to 46°F); do not freeze. Avoid direct light. When refrigerated, prefilled pen must be used within 4 weeks after initial injection. Orange and blue prefilled pens may also be stored up to 3 weeks at ≤25°C (77°F).

Nutropin: Before and after reconstitution, store at 2°C to 8°C (36°F to 46°F); do not freeze.

Nutropin vial: Use reconstituted vials within 14 days. When reconstituted with sterile water for injection, use immediately and discard unused portion.

Nutropin AQ formulations: Use within 28 days following initial use.

Omnitrope:

Powder for injection: Prior to reconstitution, store under refrigeration at 2°C to 8°C (36°F to 46°F); do not freeze. Protect from light. Reconstitute with provided diluent. Swirl gently; do not shake. Following reconstitution with the provided diluents, the 5.8 mg vial may be stored under refrigeration for up to 3 weeks. Store vial in carton to protect from light.

Solution: Prior to use, store under refrigeration at 2°C to 8°C (36°F to 46°F). Once the cartridge is loaded into the pen delivery system, store under refrigeration for up to 28 days after first use.

Saizen: Prior to reconstitution, store at room temperature 15°C to 30°C (59°F to 86°F). Following reconstitution with bacteriostatic water for injection, reconstituted solution should be refrigerated and used within 14 days. When reconstituted with sterile water for injection, use immediately and discard unused portion. The Saizen easy click cartridge, when reconstituted with the provided bacteriostatic water, should be stored under refrigeration and used within 21 days.

Serostim: Prior to reconstitution, store at room temperature 15°C to 30°C (59°F to 86°F). When reconstituted with sterile water for injection, use immediately and discard unused portion.

Tev-Tropin: Prior to reconstitution, store at 2°C to 8°C (36°F to 46°F). Following reconstitution with the provided diluents, should be refrigerated and used within 14 days (5 mg vial) or 28 days (10 mg vial); do not freeze. Some cloudiness may occur; do not use if cloudiness persists after warming to room temperature.

Zorbtive: Store unopened vials and diluent at room temperature of 15°C to 30°C (59°F to 86°F). Store reconstituted vial under refrigeration at 2°C to 8°C (36°F to 46°F) for up to 14 days; do not freeze.

Mechanism of Action Somatropin is a purified polypeptide hormones of recombinant DNA origin; somatropin contains the identical sequence of amino acids found in human growth hormone; human growth hormone assists growth of linear bone, skeletal muscle, and organs by stimulating chondrocyte proliferation and differentiation, lipolysis, protein synthesis, and hepatic glucose output; stimulates erythropoietin which increases red blood cell mass; exerts both insulin-like and diabetogenic effects; enhances the transmucosal transport of water, electrolytes, and nutrients across the gut

Pharmacodynamics/Kinetics

Duration: Maintains supraphysiologic levels for 18-20 hours

Absorption: IM, SubQ: Well absorbed

Distribution: ~1 L/kg

Metabolism: Hepatic and renal (~90%)

Bioavailability: SubQ: ~70% to 90%; **Note:** Variable; product-dependent

Half-life elimination: Preparation and route of administration dependent; SubQ: ~2-4 hours

Excretion: Urine (small amount)

Note: Patients with chronic renal failure (CRF) and end-stage renal disease ESRD) have decreased clearance compared with healthy individuals.

Dosage

Children (individualize dose):

Chronic renal insufficiency (CRI): Nutropin, Nutropin AQ: SubQ: Weekly dosage: 0.35 mg/kg divided into daily injections; continue until the time of renal transplantation

Dosage recommendations in patients treated for CRI who require dialysis:

Hemodialysis: Administer dose at night prior to bedtime or at least 3-4 hours after hemodialysis to prevent hematoma formation from heparin

CCPD: Administer dose in the morning following dialysis

CAPD: Administer dose in the evening at the time of overnight exchange

Growth hormone deficiency:

Genotropin, Omnitrope: SubQ: Weekly dosage: 0.16-0.24 mg/kg divided into equal doses 6-7 days per week

Humatrope: SubQ: Weekly dosage: 0.18-0.3 mg/kg divided into equal doses 6-7 days per week

Norditropin: SubQ: 0.024-0.034 mg/kg/day, 6-7 days per week

Nutropin, Nutropin AQ: SubQ: Weekly dosage: 0.3 mg/kg divided into equal daily doses; pubertal patients: ≤0.7 mg/kg divided into equal daily doses

Tev-Tropin: SubQ: Up to 0.1 mg/kg/dose administered 3 days per week

Saizen: IM, SubQ: Weekly dosage: 0.18 mg/kg divided into equal daily doses **or** as 0.06 mg/kg/dose administered 3 days per week **or** as 0.03 mg/kg/dose administered 6 days per week

Note: Therapy should be discontinued when patient has reached satisfactory adult height, when epiphyses have fused, or when the patient ceases to respond. Growth of 5 cm/year or more is expected, if growth rate does not exceed 2.5 cm in a 6-month period, double the dose for the next 6 months; if there is still no satisfactory response, discontinue therapy

HIV patients with wasting or cachexia (off-label use): Serostim: SubQ: Limited data; doses of 0.04 mg/kg/day were reported in five children, 6-17 years of age; doses of 0.07 mg/kg/day were reported in six children, 8-14 years of age

Idiopathic short stature:

Genotropin, Omnitrope: SubQ: Weekly dosage: 0.47 mg/kg divided into equal doses 6-7 days per week

Humatrope: SubQ: Weekly dosage: 0.37 mg/kg divided into equal doses 6-7 days per week

Nutropin, Nutropin AQ: SubQ: Weekly dosage: Up to 0.3 mg/kg divided into equal daily doses

Noonan syndrome: Norditropin: SubQ: Up to 0.066 mg/kg/day

Prader-Willi syndrome: Genotropin, Omnitrope: SubQ: Weekly dosage: 0.24 mg/kg divided into equal doses 6-7 days per week

SHOX deficiency: Humatrope: SubQ: Weekly dosage: 0.35 mg/kg divided into equal doses 6-7 days per week

Small for gestational age:

Genotropin, Omnitrope: SubQ: Weekly dosage: 0.48 mg/kg divided into equal doses 6-7 days per week

Humatrope: SubQ: Weekly dosage: 0.47 mg/kg divided into equal doses 6-7 days per week

Norditropin: SubQ: Up to 0.067 mg/kg/day

Alternate dosing (small for gestational age): In older/early pubertal children or children with very short stature, consider initiating therapy at higher doses (0.067 mg/kg/day) and then consider reducing the dose (0.033 mg/kg/day) if substantial catch-up growth observed. In younger children (<4 years) with less severe short stature, consider initiating therapy with lower doses (0.033 mg/kg/day) and then titrating the dose upwards as needed.

Turner syndrome:

Genotropin, Omnitrope: SubQ: Weekly dosage: 0.33 mg/kg divided into equal doses 6-7 days per week

Humatrope: SubQ: Weekly dosage: 0.375 mg/kg divided into equal doses 6-7 days per week

Norditropin: SubQ: Up to 0.067 mg/kg/day

Nutropin, Nutropin AQ: SubQ: Weekly dosage: ≤0.375 mg/kg divided into equal doses 3-7 days per week

Adults:

Growth hormone deficiency: Adjust dose based on individual requirements: To minimize adverse events in older or overweight patients, reduced dosages may be necessary. During therapy, dosage should be decreased if required by the occurrence of side effects or excessive IGF-I levels.

Weight-based dosing:

Norditropin: SubQ: Initial dose ≤0.004 mg/kg/day; after 6 weeks of therapy, may increase dose up to 0.016 mg/kg/day

Nutropin, Nutropin AQ: SubQ: ≤0.006 mg/kg/day; dose may be increased up to a maximum of 0.025 mg/kg/day in patients <35 years of age, or up to a maximum of 0.0125 mg/kg/day in patients ≥35 years of age

Humatrope: SubQ: ≤0.006 mg/kg/day; dose may be increased up to a maximum of 0.0125 mg/kg/day

Genotropin, Omnitrope: SubQ: Weekly dosage: ≤0.04 mg/kg divided into equal doses 6-7 days per week; dose may be increased at 4- to 8-week intervals to a maximum of 0.08 mg/kg/week

Saizen: SubQ: ≤0.005 mg/kg/day; dose may be increased to not more than 0.01 mg/kg/day after 4 weeks

Nonweight-based dosing: SubQ: Initial: 0.2 mg/day (range: 0.15-0.3 mg/day); may increase every 1-2 months by 0.1-0.2 mg/day based on response and/or serum IGF-I levels

Dosage adjustment with estrogen supplementation (growth hormone deficiency): Larger doses of somatropin may be needed for women taking oral estrogen replacement products; dosing not affected by topical products

HIV-associated adipose redistribution syndrome (HARS) (off-label use): Serostim: SubQ: Induction: 4 mg once daily at bedtime for 12 weeks; Maintenance: 2 mg or 4 mg every other day at bedtime for 12-24 weeks. **Note:** Every-other-day dosing during induction has also been studied. Although a greater response was seen with daily dosing, it was associated with an increased incidence of adverse events.

HIV patients with wasting or cachexia: Serostim: SubQ: 0.1 mg/kg once daily at bedtime (maximum: 6 mg/day). Alternately, patients at risk for side effects may be started at 0.1 mg/kg every other day. Patients who continue to lose weight after 12 weeks should be re-evaluated for opportunistic infections or other clinical events; rotate injection sites to avoid lipodystrophy Adjust dose if needed to manage side effects.

Daily dose based on body weight:

<35 kg: 0.1 mg/kg

35-45 kg: 4 mg

45-55 kg: 5 mg

>55 kg: 6 mg

Short-bowel syndrome (Zorbtive): SubQ: 0.1 mg/kg once daily for 4 weeks (maximum: 8 mg/day)

Fluid retention (moderate) or arthralgias: Treat symptomatically or reduce dose by 50%

Severe toxicity: Discontinue therapy for up to 5 days; when symptoms resolve, restart at 50% of dose. If severe toxicity recurs or does not disappear within 5 days after discontinuation, permanently discontinue treatment.

Elderly: Patients ≥65 years of age may be more sensitive to the action of growth hormone and more prone to adverse effects; in general, dosing should be cautious, beginning at low end of dosing range

Dosage adjustment in renal impairment No dosage adjustment provided in manufacturer's labeling (has not been studied).

Dosage adjustment in hepatic impairment: No dosage adjustment provided in manufacturer's labeling (has not been studied).

Dietary Considerations

Prader-Willi syndrome: All patients should have effective weight control (use is contraindicated in severely-obese patients).

Short-bowel syndrome: Intravenous parenteral nutrition requirements may need reassessment as gastrointestinal absorption improves.

Administration Do not shake; administer SubQ or IM (not all products are approved for IM administration). Rotate administration sites to avoid tissue atrophy. When administering to newborns, do not reconstitute with a diluent that contains benzyl alcohol; sterile water for injection may be used as an alternative.

Norditropin cartridge must be administered using the corresponding color-coded NordiPen injection pen.

Omnitrope: Solution in the cartridges must be administered using the Omnitrope pen; when installing a new cartridge, prime pen prior to first use.

Humatrope: When administering for growth hormone deficiency, SubQ route is preferred

Tev-Tropin: SubQ injections of solutions >1 mL not recommended.

Monitoring Parameters Growth curve, Tanner staging (children), periodic thyroid function tests, bone age (annually), periodical urine testing for glucose, somatomedin C (IGF-I) levels; funduscopic examinations at initiation of therapy and periodically during treatment; serum phosphorus, alkaline phosphatase and parathyroid hormone. If growth deceleration is observed in children treated for growth hormone deficiency, and not due to other causes, evaluate for presence of antibody formation. Periodic blood glucose monitoring; strict blood glucose monitoring in patients with diabetes. Progression or recurrence of preexisting tumors or malignant transformation of skin lesions. **Note:** Practice guidelines recommend monitoring for efficacy and adverse effects every 1-2 months during dose titration and semiannually, thereafter (TES, 2006).

CRI: Progression of renal osteodystrophy

Prader-Willi syndrome: Monitor for sleep apnea, respiratory infections, snoring (onset of or increased)

Turner syndrome: Ear disorders including otitis media; cardiovascular disorders

Noonan syndrome: Prior to use, verify short stature syndrome.

Dosage Forms

Solution, Subcutaneous:

Norditropin FlexPro: 5 mg/1.5 mL (1.5 mL); 10 mg/1.5 mL (1.5 mL); 15 mg/1.5 mL (1.5 mL)

Norditropin NordiFlex Pen: 30 mg/3 mL (3 mL)

Nutropin AQ NuSpin 5: 5 mg/2 mL (2 mL)

Nutropin AQ NuSpin 10: 10 mg/2 mL (2 mL)

Nutropin AQ NuSpin 20: 20 mg/2 mL (2 mL)

Nutropin AQ Pen: 10 mg/2 mL (2 mL); 20 mg/2 mL (2 mL)

Omnitrope: 5 mg/1.5 mL (1.5 mL); 10 mg/1.5 mL (1.5 mL)

Solution Reconstituted, Injection:

Humatrope: 5 mg (1 ea); 6 mg (1 ea); 12 mg (1 ea); 24 mg (1 ea)

Saizen: 5 mg (1 ea); 8.8 mg (1 ea)

Saizen Click.Easy: 8.8 mg (1 ea)

Solution Reconstituted, Subcutaneous:

Genotropin: 5 mg (1 ea); 12 mg (1 ea)

Omnitrope: 5.8 mg (1 ea)

Serostim: 4 mg (1 ea); 5 mg (1 ea); 6 mg (1 ea)

Tev-Tropin: 5 mg (1 ea)

Zorbtive: 8.8 mg (1 ea)

Solution Reconstituted, Subcutaneous [preservative free]:

Genotropin MiniQuick: 0.2 mg (1 ea); 0.4 mg (1 ea); 0.6 mg (1 ea); 0.8 mg (1 ea); 1 mg (1 ea); 1.2 mg (1 ea); 1.4 mg (1 ea); 1.6 mg (1 ea); 1.8 mg (1 ea); 2 mg (1 ea)

- ◆ **Somatuline Autogel (Can)** *see* Lanreotide *on page 1165*
- ◆ **Somatuline Depot** *see* Lanreotide *on page 1165*
- ◆ **Somavert** *see* Pegvisomant *on page 1604*
- ◆ **Sominex [OTC]** *see* DiphenhydrAMINE (Systemic) *on page 641*
- ◆ **Sominex (Can)** *see* DiphenhydrAMINE (Systemic) *on page 641*
- ◆ **Sominex Maximum Strength [OTC]** *see* DiphenhydrAMINE (Systemic) *on page 641*
- ◆ **Som Pam (Can)** *see* Flurazepam *on page 906*
- ◆ **Sonata** *see* Zaleplon *on page 2193*
- ◆ **Soolantra** *see* Ivermectin (Topical) *on page 1137*
- ◆ **Soolantra** *see* Ivermectin (Topical) *on page 1137*
- ◆ **Soothe & Cool INZO Antifungal [OTC]** *see* Miconazole (Topical) *on page 1360*

SORAfenib (sor AF e nib)

Brand Names: U.S. NexAVAR

Brand Names: Canada Nexavar

Index Terms BAY 43-9006; Sorafenib Tosylate

Pharmacologic Category Antineoplastic Agent, Tyrosine Kinase Inhibitor; Antineoplastic Agent, Vascular Endothelial Growth Factor (VEGF) Inhibitor

Use

Hepatocellular cancer: Treatment of unresectable hepatocellular cancer (HCC)

Renal cell cancer, advanced: Treatment of advanced renal cell cancer (RCC)

Thyroid cancer, differentiated: Treatment of locally recurrent or metastatic, progressive, differentiated thyroid cancer (refractory to radioactive iodine treatment)

Pregnancy Risk Factor D

Pregnancy Considerations Animal reproduction studies have demonstrated teratogenicity and fetal loss. Based on its mechanism of action and because sorafenib inhibits angiogenesis, a critical component of fetal development, adverse effects on pregnancy would be expected. Women of childbearing potential should be advised to avoid pregnancy. Men and women of reproductive potential should use effective birth control during treatment and for at least 2 weeks after treatment is discontinued.

Breast-Feeding Considerations It is not known if sorafenib is excreted in human milk. Due to the potential for serious adverse reactions in the nursing infant, the decision to discontinue sorafenib or to discontinue breast-feeding during therapy should take into account the benefits of treatment to the mother.

Contraindications Known severe hypersensitivity to sorafenib or any component of the formulation; use in combination with carboplatin and paclitaxel in patients with squamous cell lung cancer

Warnings/Precautions Hazardous agent - use appropriate precautions for handling and disposal (NIOSH 2014 [group 1]). May cause hypertension (generally mild-to-moderate), especially in the first 6 weeks of treatment; monitor; use caution in patients with underlying or poorly-controlled hypertension; consider discontinuing (temporary or permanent) in patients who develop severe or persistent hypertension while on appropriate antihypertensive therapy. May cause cardiac ischemia or infarction; consider discontinuing (temporarily or permanently) in patients who develop these conditions; use in patients with unstable coronary artery disease or recent myocardial infarction has not been studied. QT prolongation has been observed; may increase the risk for ventricular arrhythmia. Avoid use in patients with congenital long QT syndrome; monitor electrolytes and ECG in patients with heart failure, bradyarrhythmias, and concurrent medications known to prolong the QT interval; correct electrolyte (calcium, magnesium, potassium) imbalances; interrupt treatment for QTc interval >500 msec or for ≥60 msec increase from baseline.

Serious bleeding events may occur (consider permanently discontinuing if serious); monitor PT/INR in patients on warfarin therapy. Fatal bleeding events have been reported. Thyroid cancer patients with tracheal, bronchial, and esophageal infiltration should be treated with local therapy prior to administering sorafenib due to the potential bleeding risk. May complicate wound healing; temporarily withhold treatment for patients undergoing major surgical procedures (the appropriate timing for reinitiation after surgical procedures has not been determined). Gastrointestinal perforation has been reported (rare); monitor patients for signs/symptoms (abdominal pain, constipation, or vomiting); discontinue treatment if gastrointestinal perforation occurs. Potentially significant drug-drug interactions may exist, requiring dose or frequency adjustment, additional monitoring, and/or selection of alternative therapy. Avoid concurrent use with strong CYP3A4 inducers (eg, carbamazepine, dexamethasone, phenobarbital, phenytoin, rifampin, St John's wort); may decrease sorafenib levels/effects. Use caution when administering sorafenib with compounds that are metabolized predominantly via UGT1A1 (eg, irinotecan). Use in combination with carboplatin and paclitaxel in patients with squamous cell lung cancer is contraindicated.

Hand-foot skin reaction and rash (generally grades 1 or 2) are the most common drug-related adverse events, and typically appear within the first 6 weeks of treatment; usually managed with topical treatment, treatment delays, and/or dose reductions. Consider permanently discontinuing with severe or persistent dermatological toxicities. The risk for hand-foot skin reaction increased with cumulative doses of sorafenib (Azad, 2009). The incidence of hand-foot syndrome is also increased in patients treated with sorafenib plus bevacizumab in comparison to those treated with sorafenib monotherapy (Azad, 2009). Severe dermatologic toxicities, including Stevens-Johnson syndrome (SJS) and toxic epidermal necrolysis (TEN) have been reported; may be life-threatening; discontinue sorafenib for suspected SJS or TEN.

Sorafenib impairs exogenous thyroid suppression; TSH level elevations were commonly observed in the thyroid cancer study; monitor TSH levels monthly and as clinically necessary, and adjust thyroid replacement as needed. Sorafenib levels in patients with mild-to-moderate hepatic impairment (Child-Pugh classes A and B) were similar to levels observed in patients without hepatic impairment; has not been studied in patients with severe hepatic impairment. In a small study of Asian patients with advanced HCC, sorafenib demonstrated efficacy with adequate tolerability in a hepatitis B-endemic area (Yau, 2009). There have been reports of sorafenib-induced hepatitis (including hepatic failure and death) which is characterized by hepatocellular liver damage and transaminase increases (significant); increased bilirubin and INR may also occur. Monitor hepatic function regularly; discontinue sorafenib for unexplained significant transaminase increases.

Adverse Reactions

Cardiovascular: Cardiac failure (congestive), flushing, hypertension, ischemic heart disease (including myocardial infarction)

Central nervous system: Depression, fatigue, glossalgia, headache, mouth pain, pain, peripheral sensory neuropathy, voice disorder

Dermatologic: Acne vulgaris, alopecia, erythema, exfoliative dermatitis, folliculitis, hyperkeratosis, Palmar-plantar erythrodysesthesia, pruritus, skin rash (including desquamation), xeroderma

Endocrine & metabolic: Hypoalbuminemia, hypocalcemia, hypokalemia, hyponatremia, hypophosphatemia, hypothyroidism, increased amylase (usually transient), increased thyroid stimulating hormone level (due to impairment of exogenous thyroid suppression), weight loss

Gastrointestinal: Abdominal pain, anorexia, constipation, decreased appetite, diarrhea, dysgeusia, dyspepsia, dysphagia, gastroesophageal reflux disease, increased serum lipase (usually transient), mucositis, nausea, stomatitis, vomiting, xerostomia

Genitourinary: Erectile dysfunction, proteinuria

Hematologic & oncologic: Anemia, hemorrhage, increased INR, leukopenia, lymphocytopenia, neutropenia, thrombocytopenia, squamous cell carcinoma of skin

Hepatic: Increased serum ALT, increased serum AST, hepatic insufficiency, increased serum transaminases (transient)

Infection: Infection

Neuromuscular & skeletal: Arthralgia, limb pain, myalgia, muscle spasm, myalgia, weakness

Renal: Renal failure

Respiratory: Cough, dyspnea, epistaxis, flu-like symptoms, hoarseness, rhinorrhea

Miscellaneous: Fever

Rare but important or life-threatening: Acute renal failure, amyotrophy, anaphylaxis, angioedema, aortic dissection, cardiac arrhythmia, cardiac failure, cerebral hemorrhage, cholangitis, cholecystitis, dehydration, eczema, erythema multiforme, gastritis, gastrointestinal hemorrhage, gastrointestinal perforation, gynecomastia, hepatic failure, hepatitis, hypersensitivity reaction (skin reaction, urticaria), hypertensive crisis, hyperthyroidism, increased serum alkaline phosphatase, increased serum bilirubin, interstitial pulmonary disease (acute respiratory distress, interstitial pneumonia, lung inflammation, pneumonitis, pulmonitis, radiation pneumonitis), malignant neoplasm of skin (keratoacanthomas), nephrotic syndrome, ostealgia, osteonecrosis (jaw), pancreatitis, pleural effusion, prolonged QT interval on ECG, respiratory tract hemorrhage, reversible posterior leukoencephalopathy syndrome (RPLS), rhabdomyolysis, Stevens-Johnson syndrome, thromboembolism, toxic epidermal necrolysis (TEN), transient ischemic attacks, tumor lysis syndrome, tumor pain

Drug Interactions

Metabolism/Transport Effects **Substrate** of CYP3A4 (minor), UGT1A9; **Note:** Assignment of Major/Minor substrate status based on clinically relevant drug interaction potential; **Inhibits** CYP2B6 (moderate), CYP2C8 (weak), CYP2C9 (moderate), UGT1A1, UGT1A9

Avoid Concomitant Use

Avoid concomitant use of SORAfenib with any of the following: BCG; CARBOplatin; CloZAPine; CYP3A4 Inducers (Strong); Dipyrone; Highest Risk QTc-Prolonging Agents; Ivabradine; Mifepristone; Natalizumab; PACLitaxel; Pimecrolimus; St Johns Wort; Tacrolimus (Topical); Tofacitinib; Vaccines (Live)

Increased Effect/Toxicity

SORAfenib may increase the levels/effects of: Acetaminophen; Bisphosphonate Derivatives; Bosentan; BuPROPion; Cannabis; CARBOplatin; Carvedilol; CloZAPine; CYP2B6 Substrates; CYP2C9 Substrates; DOCEtaxel; DOXOrubicin (Conventional); Dronabinol; Fluorouracil (Systemic); Fluorouracil (Topical); Highest Risk QTc-Prolonging Agents; Irinotecan; Leflunomide; Moderate Risk QTc-Prolonging Agents; Natalizumab; PACLitaxel; Tetrahydrocannabinol; Tofacitinib; Vaccines (Live); Warfarin

The levels/effects of SORAfenib may be increased by: Acetaminophen; Bevacizumab; CYP3A4 Inhibitors (Strong); Denosumab; Dipyrone; Ivabradine; Mifepristone; Pimecrolimus; QTc-Prolonging Agents (Indeterminate Risk and Risk Modifying); Roflumilast; Tacrolimus (Topical); Trastuzumab

Decreased Effect

SORAfenib may decrease the levels/effects of: BCG; Coccidioides immitis Skin Test; Dacarbazine; Fluorouracil (Systemic); Fluorouracil (Topical); Sipuleucel-T; Vaccines (Inactivated); Vaccines (Live)

The levels/effects of SORAfenib may be decreased by: CYP3A4 Inducers (Strong); Echinacea; Neomycin; St Johns Wort

Food Interactions Bioavailability is decreased 29% with a high-fat meal (bioavailability is similar to fasting state when administered with a moderate-fat meal). Management: Administer on an empty stomach 1 hour before or 2 hours after eating.

Storage/Stability Store at 25°C (77°F); excursions are permitted between 15°C and 30°C (59°F and 86°F). Protect from moisture.

Mechanism of Action Multikinase inhibitor; inhibits tumor growth and angiogenesis by inhibiting intracellular Raf kinases (CRAF, BRAF, and mutant BRAF), and cell surface kinase receptors (VEGFR-1, VEGFR-2, VEGFR-3, PDGFR-beta, cKIT, FLT-3, RET, and RET/PTC)

Pharmacodynamics/Kinetics

Protein binding: 99.5%

Metabolism: Hepatic, via CYP3A4 (primarily oxidated to the pyridine N-oxide; active, minor) and UGT1A9 (glucuronidation)

Bioavailability: 38% to 49%; reduced by 29% when administered with a high-fat meal

Half-life elimination: 25 to 48 hours

Time to peak, plasma: ~3 hours

Excretion: Feces (77%, 51% of dose as unchanged drug); urine (19%, as metabolites)

Dosage Note: Interrupt treatment (temporarily) in patients undergoing major surgical procedures.

Hepatocellular cancer (HCC): Adults: Oral: 400 mg twice daily; continue until no longer clinically benefiting or until unacceptable toxicity occurs (Llovet, 2008)

Renal cell cancer (RCC), advanced: Adults: Oral: 400 mg twice daily; continue until no longer clinically benefiting or until unacceptable toxicity occurs (Escudier, 2007; Escudier, 2009)

Thyroid cancer, differentiated: Adults: Oral: 400 mg twice daily; continue until no longer clinically benefiting or until unacceptable toxicity occurs (Brose, 2013)

Angiosarcoma (off-label use): 400 mg twice daily (Maki, 2009)

GIST (off-label use): 400 mg twice daily (Wiebe, 2008)

Dosage adjustment for toxicity: Temporary interruption and/or dosage reduction may be necessary for management of adverse drug reactions.

Cardiovascular toxicity:

Cardiac ischemia or infarction: Consider temporary interruption or permanent discontinuation.

Hypertension, severe or persistent (despite antihypertensive therapy): Consider temporary interruption or permanent discontinuation.

QT prolongation (QTc interval >500 msec or ≥60 msec increase from baseline): Interrupt treatment.

Gastrointestinal perforation: Permanently discontinue.

Hemorrhage requiring medical intervention: Consider permanent discontinuation.

Dermatologic toxicity: If Stevens-Johnson syndrome or toxic epidermal necrolysis is suspected, discontinue therapy.

U.S. labeling:

RCC and HCC: If dosage reductions are necessary, decrease dose to 400 mg once daily. If further reductions are needed, decrease dose to 400 mg every other day.

Grade 1 (numbness, dysesthesia, paresthesia, tingling, painless swelling, erythema, or discomfort of the hands or feet which do not disrupt normal activities): Continue sorafenib and consider symptomatic treatment with topical therapy.

Grade 2 (painful erythema and swelling of the hands or feet and/or discomfort affecting normal activities):

First occurrence: Continue sorafenib and consider symptomatic treatment with topical therapy. **Note:** If no improvement within 7 days, see dosing for second or third occurrence.

Second or third occurrence (or no improvement after 7 days of 1st occurrence): Hold treatment until resolves to grade 0-1; resume treatment with dose reduced by one dose level (400 mg daily or 400 mg every other day).

Fourth occurrence: Discontinue treatment.

Grade 3 (moist desquamation, ulceration, blistering, or severe pain of the hands or feet or severe discomfort that prevents working or performing daily activities):

First or second occurrence: Hold treatment until resolves to grade 0-1; resume treatment with dose reduced by one dose level (400 mg daily or 400 mg every other day).

Third occurrence: Discontinue treatment.

Thyroid cancer:

First dose level reduction: Reduce to 600 mg daily (in 2 divided doses, as 400 mg and 200 mg, separated by 12 hours).

Second dose level reduction: Reduce dose to 200 mg twice daily.

Third dose level reduction: Reduce dose to 200 mg once daily.

Grade 1 (numbness, dysesthesia, paresthesia, tingling, painless swelling, erythema, or discomfort of the hands or feet which do not disrupt normal activities): Continue sorafenib treatment.

Grade 2 (painful erythema and swelling of the hands or feet and/or discomfort affecting normal activities):

First occurrence: Decrease dose to 600 mg daily (in divided doses). **Note:** If no improvement within 7 days, see dosing for second occurrence.

Second occurrence (or no improvement after 7 days of the reduced dose after 1st occurrence): Hold treatment until resolved or improved to grade 1; if resumed, decrease the dose by 1 dose level.

Third occurrence: Hold treatment until resolved or improved to grade 1; if resumed, decrease the dose by 1 dose level.

Fourth occurrence: Permanently discontinue.

Grade 3 (moist desquamation, ulceration, blistering, or severe pain of the hands or feet or severe discomfort that prevents working or performing daily activities):

First occurrence: Hold treatment until resolved or improved to grade 1; if resumed, decrease by 1 dose level.

Second occurrence: Hold treatment until resolved or improved to grade 1; if resumed, decrease by 2 dose levels.

Third occurrence: Permanently discontinue.

Following improvement of grade 2 or 3 dermatologic toxicity to grade 0 or 1 after at least 28 days of a reduced dose, the sorafenib dose may be increased 1 dose level from the reduced dose (~50% of patients requiring dose reduction for dermatologic toxicity may meet the criteria for increased dosing; and half of those patients may tolerate the increased dose without recurrent grade 2 or higher dermatologic toxicity).

Canadian labeling: RCC and HCC:

Grade 1 (any occurrence): Initiate supportive treatment immediately and continue sorafenib.

Grade 2:

First occurrence: Initiate supportive treatment immediately and consider a dose reduction to 400 mg daily for 28 days. If toxicity resolves to ≤ grade 1 after 28 days with dose reduction, increase dose to 400 mg twice daily. If toxicity does not resolve to ≤ grade 1 despite dose reduction, withhold treatment for a minimum of 7 days until toxicity resolves to ≤ grade 1, then resume treatment at reduced dose of 400 mg daily for 28 days. If toxicity remains ≤ grade 1 at the reduced dose for 28 days, increase dose to 400 mg twice daily.

Second or third occurrence: Follow procedure for first occurrence; however, when resuming treatment, decrease dose to 400 mg daily (indefinitely).

Fourth occurrence: Treatment discontinuation should be considered based on clinical assessment and patient preference.

Grade 3:

First occurrence: Initiate supportive measures immediately and withhold treatment for a minimum of 7 days and until toxicity ≤ grade 1. Resume at reduced dose of 400 mg daily for 28 days. If toxicity remains ≤ grade 1 at the reduced dose for 28 days, increase dose to 400 mg twice daily.

Second occurrence: Follow procedure for first occurrence; however, when resuming treatment, decrease dose to 400 mg daily (indefinitely).

Third occurrence: Treatment discontinuation should be considered based on clinical assessment and patient preference.

Dosage adjustment in renal impairment:

Manufacturer's labeling: No dosage adjustment is necessary for mild, moderate, or severe impairment (not dependent on dialysis); has not been studied in dialysis patients.

The following adjustments have also been reported: Safety and pharmacokinetics were studied in varying degrees of renal dysfunction with the following empiric dose levels recommended based on patient tolerance (Miller, 2009):

Mild renal dysfunction (CrCl 40 to 59 mL/minute): 400 mg twice daily

Moderate renal dysfunction (CrCl 20 to 39 mL/minute): 200 mg twice daily

Severe renal dysfunction (CrCl <20 mL/minute): Data inadequate to define dose

Hemodialysis (any CrCl): 200 mg once daily

Dosage adjustment in hepatic impairment:

Hepatic impairment at baseline:

Manufacturer's labeling:

Mild to moderate (Child-Pugh class A and B) impairment: No dosage adjustment is necessary.

Severe impairment (Child-Pugh class C): There are no dosage adjustments provided in the manufacturer's labeling (has not been studied).

The following adjustments have also been reported: Safety and pharmacokinetics were studied in varying degrees of hepatic dysfunction with the following empiric dose levels recommended based on patient tolerance (Miller, 2009):

Mild hepatic dysfunction (bilirubin >1 to ≤1.5 times ULN and/or AST >ULN): 400 mg twice daily

Moderate hepatic dysfunction (bilirubin >1.5 to ≤3 times ULN; any AST): 200 mg twice daily

Severe hepatic dysfunction:

Bilirubin >3 to 10 x ULN (any AST): 200 mg every 3 days was **not** tolerated

Albumin <2.5 g/dL (any bilirubin and any AST): 200 mg once daily

Drug-induced liver injury during treatment: Unexplained (eg, not due to viral hepatitis or progressive underlying malignancy) significantly increased transaminases: Discontinue treatment.

Administration Administer on an empty stomach (1 hour before or 2 hours after eating).

Hazardous agent; use appropriate precautions for handling and disposal (NIOSH 2014 [group 1]).

Monitoring Parameters

CBC with differential, electrolytes (magnesium, potassium, calcium), phosphorus, lipase and amylase levels; liver function tests; blood pressure (baseline, weekly for the first 6 weeks, then periodic); monitor for hand-foot skin reaction and other dermatologic toxicities; monitor ECG in patients at risk for prolonged QT interval; signs/symptoms of bleeding; signs/symptoms of GI perforation. Additionally the Canadian labeling recommends considering monitoring of left ventricular ejection fraction at baseline and periodically during treatment.

Thyroid function testing:

Patients with differentiated thyroid cancer: Monitor TSH monthly.

Patients with RCC and HCC (Hamnvik, 2011):

Preexisting levothyroxine therapy: Obtain baseline TSH levels, then monitor every 4 weeks until levels and levothyroxine dose are stable, then monitor every 2 months

Without preexisting thyroid hormone replacement: TSH at baseline, then every 4 weeks for 4 months, then every 2 to 3 months

Additional Information Hand-foot skin reaction (HFSR) management (Lacouture, 2008): The following treatments may be used in addition to the recommended dosage modifications. Prior to treatment initiation, a pedicure is recommended to remove hyperkeratotic areas/calluses, which may predispose to HFSR; avoid vigorous exercise/activities which may stress hands or feet. During therapy, patients should reduce exposure to hot water (may exacerbate hand-foot symptoms); avoid constrictive footwear and excessive skin friction. Patients may also wear thick cotton gloves or socks and should wear shoes with padded insoles. Grade 1 HFSR may be relieved with moisturizing creams, cotton gloves and socks (at night) and/or keratolytic creams such as urea (20% to 40%) or salicylic acid (6%). Apply topical steroid (eg, clobetasol ointment) twice daily to erythematous areas of Grade 2 HFSR; topical anesthetics (eg, lidocaine 2%) and then systemic analgesics (if appropriate) may be used for pain control. Resolution of acute erythema may result in keratotic areas which may be softened with keratolytic agents.

Dosage Forms

Tablet, Oral:

NexAVAR: 200 mg

Extemporaneous Preparations Hazardous agent: Use appropriate precautions for handling and disposal (NIOSH 2014 [group 1]).

An oral suspension may be prepared with tablets. Place two 200 mg tablets into a glass containing 60 mL (2 oz) water; let stand 5 minutes before stirring. Stir until tablets are completely disintegrated, forming a uniform suspension. Administer within 1 hour after preparation. Stir suspension again immediately before administration. To ensure the full dose is administered, rinse glass several times with a total of 180 mL (6 oz) water and administer residue. **Note:** Brown tablet coating may initially form a thin film but has no effect on the dosing accuracy.

Nexavar data on file, Bayer Healthcare Pharmaceuticals.

◆ **Sorafenib Tosylate** *see* SORAfenib *on page 1923*

Sorbitol (SOR bi tole)

Brand Names: U.S. SyrSpend SF

Pharmacologic Category Genitourinary Irrigant; Laxative, Osmotic

Use Genitourinary irrigant in transurethral prostatic resection or other transurethral resection or other transurethral surgical procedures; diuretic; humectant; sweetening agent; hyperosmotic laxative; facilitate the passage of sodium polystyrene sulfonate through the intestinal tract

Pregnancy Risk Factor C

Dosage

Hyperosmotic laxative (as single dose, at infrequent intervals):

Children 2-11 years:

Oral: 2 mL/kg (as 70% solution)

Rectal enema: 30-60 mL as 25% to 30% solution

Children >12 years and Adults:

Oral: 30-150 mL (as 70% solution)

Rectal enema: 120 mL as 25% to 30% solution

Adjunct to sodium polystyrene sulfonate: Adults: 15 mL as 70% solution orally until diarrhea occurs (10-20 mL/2 hours) or 20-100 mL as an oral vehicle for the sodium polystyrene sulfonate resin

Transurethral surgical procedures: Adults: Irrigation: Topical: 3% to 3.3% as transurethral surgical procedure irrigation

Additional Information Complete prescribing information should be consulted for additional detail.

Dosage Forms

Liquid, Oral:

SyrSpend SF: (4000 mL)

Solution, Irrigation:

Generic: 3% (3000 mL); 3.3% (2000 mL, 4000 mL)

Solution, Oral:

Generic: 70% (30 mL, 473 mL, 474 mL, 480 mL, 3840 mL)

Solution, Rectal:

Generic: 70% (473 mL)

◆ **Sorbulax [OTC]** *see* Psyllium *on page 1744*

◆ **Sore Throat Relief [OTC]** *see* Benzocaine *on page 246*

◆ **Soriatane** *see* Acitretin *on page 43*

◆ **Sorilux** *see* Calcipotriene *on page 321*

◆ **Sorine** *see* Sotalol *on page 1927*

Sotalol (SOE ta lole)

Brand Names: U.S. Betapace; Betapace AF; Sorine

Brand Names: Canada Apo-Sotalol; CO Sotalol; Dom-Sotalol; Med-Sotalol; Mylan-Sotalol; Novo-Sotalol; Nu-Sotalol; PHL-Sotalol; PMS-Sotalol; PRO-Sotalol; ratio-Sotalol; Rhoxal-sotalol; Riva-Sotalol; Rylosol; Sandoz-Sotalol; ZYM-Sotalol

Index Terms Sotalol Hydrochloride; Sotylize

Pharmacologic Category Antiarrhythmic Agent, Class II; Antiarrhythmic Agent, Class III; Beta-Adrenergic Blocker, Nonselective

Additional Appendix Information

Beers Criteria – Potentially Inappropriate Medications for Geriatrics *on page 2271*

Use

Betapace, Sorine, Sotylize: Treatment of documented ventricular arrhythmias (ie, sustained ventricular tachycardia), that in the judgment of the health care provider are life-threatening

Betapace AF, Sotylize: Maintenance of normal sinus rhythm (delay in time to recurrence of atrial fibrillation/atrial flutter) in patients with symptomatic atrial fibrillation/atrial flutter who are currently in sinus rhythm. Manufacturer states substitutions should not be made for Betapace AF due to significant differences in labeling (ie, patient package insert and safety information)

According to the American Heart Association/American College of Cardiology/Heart Rhythm Society (AHA/ACC/HRS), sotalol is not effective for conversion of atrial fibrillation to sinus rhythm but may be used to prevent atrial fibrillation (AHA/ACC/HRS [January, 2014])

Pregnancy Risk Factor B

Pregnancy Considerations Adverse events were not observed in the initial animal reproduction studies; therefore, the manufacturer classifies sotalol as pregnancy category B. Sotalol crosses the placenta and is found in amniotic fluid. In a cohort study, an increased risk of cardiovascular defects was observed following maternal use of beta-blockers during pregnancy (Lennestål 2009). Intrauterine growth restriction (IUGR), small placentas, as well as fetal/neonatal bradycardia, hypoglycemia, and/or respiratory depression have been observed following *in utero* exposure to beta-blockers as a class. Adequate facilities for monitoring infants at birth should be available. Untreated chronic maternal hypertension and pre-eclampsia are also associated with adverse events in the fetus, infant, and mother; however, sotalol is currently not recommended for the initial treatment of hypertension in pregnancy (ACOG 2013). Because sotalol crosses the placenta in concentrations similar to the maternal serum, it has been used for the treatment of fetal atrial flutter or fetal supraventricular tachycardia without hydrops (Sonesson 1998). The clearance of sotalol is increased during the third trimester of pregnancy, but other pharmacokinetic parameters do not significantly differ from nonpregnant values (O'Hare 1983).

Breast-Feeding Considerations Sotalol is excreted in breast milk in concentrations higher than those found in the maternal serum (O'Hare 1980). Although adverse events in nursing infants have not been observed in case reports, close monitoring for bradycardia, hypotension, respiratory distress, and hypoglycemia is advised. Due to the potential for serious adverse reactions in the nursing infant, the manufacturer recommends a decision be made whether to discontinue nursing or to discontinue the drug, taking into account the importance of treatment to the mother.

Contraindications

Hypersensitivity to sotalol or any component of the formulation; bronchial asthma; sinus bradycardia (<50 bpm during waking hours [Betapace AF, Sotylize]); second- or third-degree AV block (unless a functioning pacemaker is present); congenital or acquired long QT syndromes; cardiogenic shock; uncontrolled heart failure

Additional contraindications (Betapace AF, Sotylize): Baseline QTc interval >450 msec; bronchospastic conditions; CrCl <40 mL/minute; serum potassium <4 mEq/L; sick sinus syndrome

Warnings/Precautions [U.S. Boxed Warning]: Sotalol can cause life-threatening ventricular tachycardia associated with QT interval prolongation (ie, torsades

de pointes). Do not initiate if baseline QTc interval is >450 msec (Betapace AF, Sotylize). If QTc interval prolongs to 500 msec or exceeds 500 msec during therapy, reduce the dose, prolong the interval between doses, or discontinue use (Betapace AF, Sotylize). QTc prolongation is directly related to the concentration of sotalol; reduced creatinine clearance (CrCl), female gender, and large doses increase the risk of QTc prolongation and subsequent torsades de pointes. Manufacturer recommends initiation (or reinitiation) and dose increases be done in a hospital setting with continuous monitoring and staff familiar with the recognition and treatment of life-threatening arrhythmias. Some experts will initiate therapy on an outpatient basis in patients if in sinus rhythm provided the QT interval and serum potassium are normal and the patient is not receiving any other QT-interval prolonging medications but require inpatient hospitalization if patient is in atrial fibrillation (AHA/ACC/HRS [January, 2014]). Calculation of CrCl must occur prior to administration of the first dose. Dosage should be adjusted gradually with 3 days between dosing increments to achieve steady-state concentrations, and to allow time to monitor QT intervals. Monitor and adjust dose to prevent QTc prolongation. Potentially significant drug-drug interactions may exist, requiring dose or frequency adjustment, additional monitoring, and/or selection of alternative therapy.

Correct electrolyte imbalances before initiating (especially hypokalemia and hypomagnesemia) since these conditions increase the risk of torsades de pointes. Consider preexisting conditions such as sick sinus syndrome before initiating. May cause bradycardia (including heart block) and hypotension. Dose adjustments of agents that slow AV nodal conduction may be necessary when sotalol is initiated. Use cautiously within the first 2 weeks post-MI especially in patients with markedly impaired ventricular function (experience limited). Administer cautiously in compensated heart failure and monitor for a worsening of the condition. Use is contraindicated in patients with uncontrolled (or decompensated) heart failure. May precipitate or aggravate symptoms of arterial insufficiency in patients with PVD and Raynaud's disease; use with caution and monitor for progression of arterial obstruction. Bradycardia may be observed more frequently in elderly patients (>65 years of age); dosage reductions may be necessary. In the treatment of atrial fibrillation in the elderly, avoid antiarrhythmics as first-line treatment. In older adults, data suggests rate control may provide more benefits than risks compared to rhythm control for most patients (Beers Criteria). Beta-blocker therapy should not be withdrawn abruptly (particularly in patients with CAD), but gradually tapered to avoid acute tachycardia, hypertension, and/or ischemia. Severe exacerbation of angina, ventricular arrhythmias, and myocardial infarction (MI) have been reported following abrupt withdrawal of beta-blocker therapy. Temporary but prompt resumption of beta-blocker therapy may be indicated with worsening of angina or acute coronary insufficiency. When QTc prolongation occurs, consider weighing the risk of abrupt withdrawal of sotalol with the risk of QTc prolongation. Chronic beta-blocker therapy should not be routinely withdrawn prior to major surgery. Use cautiously in diabetics because it can mask prominent hypoglycemic symptoms. Use with caution in patients with bronchospastic disease, myasthenia gravis, or psychiatric disease. Adequate alpha-blockade is required prior to use of any beta-blocker for patients with untreated pheochromocytoma. May mask signs of hyperthyroidism (eg, tachycardia); if hyperthyroidism is suspected, carefully manage and monitor; abrupt withdrawal may exacerbate symptoms of hyperthyroidism or precipitate thyroid storm. Use caution with history of severe anaphylaxis to allergens; patients taking beta-blockers may become more sensitive to repeated challenges. Treatment of anaphylaxis (eg, epinephrine) in patients taking beta-blockers may be ineffective or promote undesirable effects.

[U.S. Boxed Warning]: Sotalol is indicated for both the treatment of documented life-threatening ventricular arrhythmias (marketed as Betapace, Sorine, and Sotylize) and for the maintenance of normal sinus rhythm in patients with symptomatic atrial fibrillation/flutter who are currently in sinus rhythm (marketed as Betapace AF and Sotylize). Betapace should not be substituted for Betapace AF; Betapace AF is distributed with an educational insert specifically for patients with atrial fibrillation/flutter.

Adverse Reactions

Cardiovascular: Angina pectoris, bradycardia (dose related), cardiac failure, cardiovascular signs and symptoms, cerebrovascular accident, chest pain, ECG abnormality, edema, hypertension, hypotension, palpitations, peripheral vascular disease, presyncope, proarrhythmia, prolonged Q-T interval on ECG (dose related), syncope, torsades de pointes (dose related), vasodilation, worsened ventricular tachycardia

Central nervous system: Anxiety, confusion, depression, dizziness, fatigue (dose related), headache, impaired consciousness, insomnia, mood changes, sensation of cold, sleep disorder

Dermatologic: Diaphoresis, hyperhidrosis, skin rash

Endocrine & metabolic: Sexual disorder, weight changes

Gastrointestinal: Abdominal distention, abdominal pain, change in appetite, colonic disease, decreased appetite, diarrhea, dyspepsia, flatulence, nausea and vomiting, stomach pain

Genitourinary: Genitourinary complaint, impotence

Hematologic & oncologic: Hemorrhage

Infection: Infection, influenza

Local: Local pain

Neuromuscular & skeletal: Back pain, limb pain, musculoskeletal chest pain, musculoskeletal pain, weakness

Ophthalmic: Visual disturbance

Respiratory: Asthma, dyspnea (dose related), pulmonary disease, tracheobronchitis, upper respiratory complaint

Miscellaneous: AICD discharge, fever, laboratory test abnormality

Rare but important or life-threatening: Alopecia, bronchiolitis obliterans organizing pneumonia, crusted skin (red), eosinophilia, hypersensitivity angiitis, increased liver enzymes, increased serum transaminases, leukopenia, paralysis, phlebitis, pruritus, pulmonary edema, Raynaud's phenomenon, retroperitoneal fibrosis, serum transaminases increased, skin necrosis (after extravasation), skin photosensitivity, thrombocytopenia

Drug Interactions

Metabolism/Transport Effects None known.

Avoid Concomitant Use

Avoid concomitant use of Sotalol with any of the following: Beta2-Agonists; Ceritinib; Fingolimod; Floctafenine; Highest Risk QTc-Prolonging Agents; Ivabradine; Methacholine; Mifepristone; Moderate Risk QTc-Prolonging Agents; Propafenone

Increased Effect/Toxicity

Sotalol may increase the levels/effects of: Alpha-/Beta-Agonists (Direct-Acting); Alpha1-Blockers; Alpha2-Agonists; Amifostine; Antihypertensives; Antipsychotic Agents (Phenothiazines); Bradycardia-Causing Agents; Bupivacaine; Cardiac Glycosides; Ceritinib; Cholinergic Agonists; DULoxetine; Ergot Derivatives; Grass Pollen Allergen Extract (5 Grass Extract); Highest Risk QTc-Prolonging Agents; Hypotensive Agents; Insulin; Lacosamide; Levodopa; Lidocaine (Systemic); Lidocaine (Topical); Mepivacaine; Methacholine; Midodrine; Obinutuzumab; RiTUXimab; Sulfonylureas

The levels/effects of Sotalol may be increased by: Acetylcholinesterase Inhibitors; Alpha2-Agonists; Anilidopiperidine Opioids; Antipsychotic Agents (Phenothiazines); Barbiturates; Bretylium; Brimonidine (Topical); Calcium Channel Blockers (Dihydropyridine); Calcium Channel Blockers (Nondihydropyridine); Diazoxide; Dipyridamole; Fingolimod; Floctafenine; Herbs (Hypotensive Properties); Ivabradine; Lidocaine (Topical); MAO Inhibitors; Mifepristone; Moderate Risk QTc-Prolonging Agents; Nicorandil; Pentoxifylline; Phosphodiesterase 5 Inhibitors; Propafenone; Prostacyclin Analogues; QTc-Prolonging Agents (Indeterminate Risk and Risk Modifying); Regorafenib; Reserpine; Tofacitinib

Decreased Effect

Sotalol may decrease the levels/effects of: Beta2-Agonists; Theophylline Derivatives

The levels/effects of Sotalol may be decreased by: Barbiturates; Herbs (Hypertensive Properties); Methylphenidate; Nonsteroidal Anti-Inflammatory Agents; Rifamycin Derivatives; Yohimbine

Food Interactions Sotalol peak serum concentrations may be decreased if taken with food. Management: Administer without regard to meals.

Storage/Stability Store at ~25°C (77°F); excursions are permitted between 15°C and 30°C (59°F and 86°F).

Mechanism of Action

Beta-blocker which contains both beta-adrenoreceptor-blocking (Vaughan Williams Class II) and cardiac action potential duration prolongation (Vaughan Williams Class III) properties

Class II effects: Increased sinus cycle length, slowed heart rate, decreased AV nodal conduction, and increased AV nodal refractoriness Sotalol has both beta$_1$- and beta$_2$-receptor blocking activity. The beta-blocking effect of sotalol is a noncardioselective (half maximal at about 80 mg/day and maximal at doses of 320-640 mg/day). Significant beta-blockade occurs at oral doses as low as 25 mg/day.

Class III effects: Prolongation of the atrial and ventricular monophasic action potentials, and effective refractory prolongation of atrial muscle, ventricular muscle, and atrioventricular accessory pathways in both the antegrade and retrograde directions. Sotalol is a racemic mixture of *d*- and *l*-sotalol; both isomers have similar Class III antiarrhythmic effects while the *l*-isomer is responsible for virtually all of the beta-blocking activity. The Class III effects are seen only at oral doses ≥160 mg/day

Pharmacodynamics/Kinetics

Onset of action: Rapid; at 1 to 2 hours post dosing (steady-state), reductions in heart rate and cardiac index seen (Winters 1993)

Absorption: Well absorbed (Hanyok 1993); decreased ~20% by meals compared to fasting

Distribution: V_d: 1.2 to 2.4 L/kg (Hanyok 1993)

Protein binding: None

Metabolism: None

Bioavailability: 90% to 100%

Half-life elimination: 12 hours; Children: 9.5 hours; terminal half-life decreases with age <2 years (time to steady state may be ≥1 week in neonates); increases with renal dysfunction

Time to peak, serum: 2.5 to 4 hours

Excretion: Urine (as unchanged drug)

Dosage Baseline QTc interval and creatinine clearance must be determined prior to initiation. If CrCl ≤60 mL/minute, dosing interval adjustment is necessary. Sotalol should be initiated and doses increased in a hospital for at least 3 days with facilities for cardiac rhythm monitoring and assessment. Proarrhythmic events can occur after initiation of therapy and with each upward dosage adjustment.

Infants, Children, and Adolescents: Oral: Ventricular arrhythmias and atrial fibrillation/flutter:

Note: Dosing per manufacturer, based on pediatric pharmacokinetic data; wait at least 36 hours between dosage adjustments to allow monitoring of QT intervals

≤2 years: Dosage should be adjusted (decreased) by plotting of the child's age on a logarithmic scale; see graph or refer to manufacturer's package labeling.

Sotalol Age Factor Nomogram for Patients ≤2 Years of Age

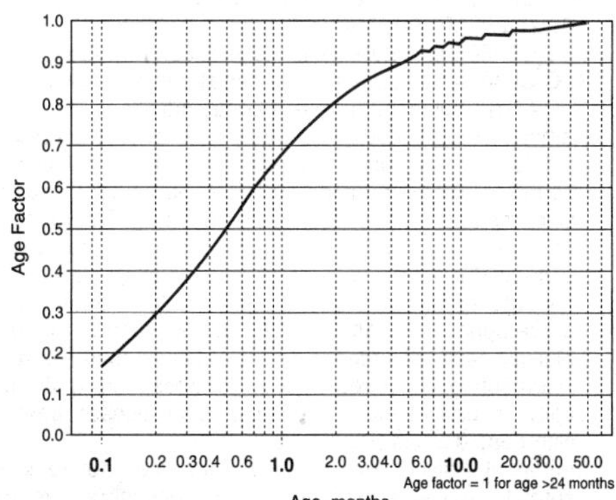

Adapted from U.S. Food and Drug Administration. http://www.fda.gov/cder/foi/label/2001/2115s3lbl.PDF

>2 years: Initial: 90 mg/m^2/day in 3 divided doses; may be incrementally increased to a maximum of 180 mg/m^2/day

Adults: Oral:

Ventricular arrhythmias (Betapace, Sorine, Sotylize):

Initial: 80 mg twice daily; dose may be increased gradually (in increments of 80 mg/day [Sotylize]) to 160 to 320 mg daily; allow 3 days between dosing increments in order to attain steady-state plasma concentrations and to allow for monitoring of QT intervals

Usual range: Most patients respond to a total daily dose of 160 to 320 mg in 2 to 3 divided doses.

Some patients, with life-threatening refractory ventricular arrhythmias, may require total daily doses as high as 480 to 640 mg; however, these doses should only be prescribed when the potential benefit outweighs the increased risk of adverse events.

Atrial fibrillation or atrial flutter (Betapace AF, Sotylize): Initial: 80 mg twice daily. If the frequency of relapse does not reduce and excessive QTc prolongation does not occur after 3 days, the dose may be increased to 120 mg twice daily; may further increase to a maximum dose of 160 mg twice daily if response is inadequate and QTc prolongation is not excessive.

Elderly: Age does not significantly alter the pharmacokinetics of sotalol, but impaired renal function in elderly patients can increase the terminal half-life, resulting in increased drug accumulation

Dosage adjustment for toxicity:

QTc ≥500 msec during initiation period (Betapace AF, Sotylize): Reduce dose, prolong the dosing interval (Sotylize), or discontinue sotalol

QTc ≥520 msec (or JT interval ≥430 msec if the QRS >100 msec) during maintenance therapy (Betapace AF): Reduce dose and carefully monitor QTc until <520 msec. If QTc interval ≥520 msec on the lowest maintenance dose, discontinue sotalol.

QTc ≥550 msec (Betapace, Sorine): Reduce dose or discontinue sotalol.

Dosage adjustment in renal impairment: Adults: Dose escalations in renal impairment should be done after administration of at least 5 to 6 doses at appropriate intervals.

Betapace, Sorine:

CrCl >60 mL/minute: Administer every 12 hours

CrCl 30 to 60 mL/minute: Administer every 24 hours

CrCl 10 to 29 mL/minute: Administer every 36 to 48 hours

CrCl <10 mL/minute: Individualize dose

Betapace AF, Sotylize:

CrCl >60 mL/minute: Administer every 12 hours

CrCl 40 to 60 mL/minute: Administer every 24 hours

CrCl <40 mL/minute: Use is contraindicated

Hemodialysis: Hemodialysis would be expected to reduce sotalol plasma concentrations because sotalol is not bound to plasma proteins and does not undergo extensive metabolism. According to the manufacturers of Betapace and Sorine, extreme caution should be employed if sotalol is used in patients with renal failure undergoing hemodialysis. According to the manufacturer of Betapace AF and Sotylize, use is contraindicated. Multiple cases of torsades de pointes have been reported when sotalol was used even at low dosages (eg, 80 mg daily) in patients with end-stage renal disease treated with hemodialysis (Huynh-Do 1996).

Peritoneal dialysis: Peritoneal dialysis does not remove sotalol; supplemental dose is not necessary (Aronoff 2007). Cases of torsades de pointes have been reported when sotalol was used even at low dosages (eg, 80 mg daily) in patients with end-stage renal disease treated with peritoneal dialysis (Dancey 1997; Tang 1997).

Dosage adjustment in hepatic impairment: There are no dosage adjustments provided in the manufacturer's labeling. However, dosage adjustment unlikely because sotalol is not metabolized by the liver.

Administration Administer without regard to meals.

Monitoring Parameters Serum creatinine (creatinine clearance), magnesium, potassium; heart rate, blood pressure; ECG (eg, QTc interval, PR interval). If baseline QTc >450 msec (or JT interval >330 msec if QRS over 100 msec), sotalol (Betapace AF, Sotylize) is contraindicated.

Betapace AF, Sotylize; During initiation and titration period, monitor QTc interval 2 to 4 hours after each dose. If QTc interval is ≥500 msec, reduce dose, prolong the dosing interval (Sotylize), or discontinue sotalol. If the QTc interval is <500 msec after 3 days (after fifth or sixth dose if patient receiving once-daily dosing), patient may be discharged on current regimen. Monitor QTc interval periodically thereafter.

Consult individual institutional policies and procedures.

Additional Information Pharmacokinetics in children are more relevant for BSA than age.

Product Availability Sotylize (5 mg/mL oral solution): FDA approved October 2014; availability anticipated in the first quarter 2015.

Dosage Forms

Tablet, Oral:

Betapace: 80 mg, 120 mg, 160 mg

Betapace AF: 80 mg, 120 mg, 160 mg

Sorine: 80 mg, 120 mg, 160 mg, 240 mg

Generic: 80 mg, 120 mg, 160 mg, 240 mg

Extemporaneous Preparations

Note: Commercial oral solution is available (5 mg/mL)

A 5 mg/mL sotalol syrup may be made with Betapace, Sorine, or Betapace AF tablets and Simple Syrup containing sodium benzoate 0.1% (Syrup, NF). Place 120 mL Syrup, NF in a 6-ounce amber plastic (polyethylene terephthalate) prescription bottle; add five Betapace, Sorine, or Betapace AF 120 mg tablets and shake the bottle to wet the tablets. Allow tablets to hydrate for at least 2 hours, then shake intermittently over ≥2 hours until the tablets are completely disintegrated; a dispersion of fine particles (water-insoluble inactive ingredients) in syrup should be obtained. **Note:** To simplify the disintegration process, tablets can hydrate overnight; tablets may also be crushed, carefully transferred into the bottle and shaken well until a dispersion of fine particles in syrup is obtained. Label "shake well". Stable for 3 months at 15°C to 30°C (59°F to 86°F) and ambient humidity.

Betapace prescribing information, Bayer HealthCare Pharmaceuticals Inc, Wayne, NJ, 2011.

Betapace AF prescribing information, Bayer HealthCare Pharmaceuticals Inc, Wayne, NJ, 2011.

Sorine prescribing information, Upsher-Smith, Minneapolis, MN, 2012.

◆ **Sotalol Hydrochloride** *see* Sotalol *on page 1927*

◆ **Sotradecol** *see* Sodium Tetradecyl Sulfate *on page 1914*

◆ **Sotylize** *see* Sotalol *on page 1927*

◆ **Sovaldi** *see* Sofosbuvir *on page 1915*

◆ **SP-303** *see* Crofelemer *on page 514*

◆ **SPA** *see* Albumin *on page 67*

Sparfloxacin [INT] (spar FLOKS a sin)

International Brand Names Aspax (VN); Newspar (ID); Resflox (ID); Spara (CN, JP, KR, TW); Spardac (IN); Sparflo (VN); Sparlox (IN); Sparos (ID); Sparx (BF, BJ, CI, ET, GH, GM, GN, KE, LR, MA, ML, MR, MU, MW, NE, NG, SC, SD, SL, SN, TN, TZ, UG, ZA, ZM, ZW); Torospar (IN); Zagam (CH, DE, FR, HK, LU, NZ, PH, PL)

Pharmacologic Category Antibiotic, Quinolone

Reported Use Treatment of adults with community-acquired pneumonia caused by *C. pneumoniae*, *H. influenzae*, *H. parainfluenzae*, *M. catarrhalis*, *M. pneumoniae* or *S. pneumoniae*; treatment of acute bacterial exacerbations of chronic bronchitis caused by *C. pneumoniae*, *E. cloacae*, *H. influenzae*, *H. parainfluenzae*, *K. pneumoniae*, *M. catarrhalis*, *S. aureus* or *S. pneumoniae*

Dosage Range Adults: Oral:

Loading dose: 400 mg on day 1

Maintenance: 200 mg/day for 10 days total therapy

Dosing adjustment in renal impairment: CrCl <50 mL/minute: Administer 400 mg on day 1, then 200 mg every 48 hours for a total of 9 days of therapy (total 6 tablets)

Product Availability Product available in various countries; not currently available in the U.S.

Dosage Forms

Tablet: 200 mg

◆ **SPD417** *see* CarBAMazepine *on page 346*

◆ **Spectracef** *see* Cefditoren *on page 378*

◆ **SPI 0211** *see* Lubiprostone *on page 1255*

Spinosad (SPIN oh sad)

Brand Names: U.S. Natroba

Index Terms NatrOVA

Pharmacologic Category Antiparasitic Agent, Topical; Pediculocide

Use Head lice: Topical treatment of head lice (*Pediculosis capitis*) infestation in adults and children ≥6 months of age

Pregnancy Risk Factor B

Dosage Head lice: Infants ≥6 months, Children, Adolescents, and Adults: Topical: Apply sufficient amount to cover dry scalp and completely cover dry hair; 120 mL may be necessary depending on the length of hair. If live lice are seen 7 days after first treatment, repeat with second application.

Dosage adjustment in renal impairment: There are no dosage adjustments provided in the manufacturer's labeling. However, dosage adjustment unlikely due to low systemic absorption.

Dosage adjustment in hepatic impairment: There are no dosage adjustments provided in the manufacturer's labeling. However, dosage adjustment unlikely due to low systemic absorption.

Additional Information Complete prescribing information should be consulted for additional detail.

Dosage Forms

Suspension, External:

Natroba: 0.9% (120 mL)

Generic: 0.9% (120 mL)

Spiramycin [CAN/INT] (speer a MYE sin)

Brand Names: Canada Rovamycine®

Pharmacologic Category Antibiotic, Macrolide

Use Note: Not approved in U.S.

Treatment of infections of the respiratory tract, buccal cavity, skin and soft tissues due to susceptible organisms. *N. gonorrhoeae*: as an alternate choice of treatment for gonorrhea in patients allergic to the penicillins. Before treatment of gonorrhea, the possibility of concomitant infection due to *T. pallidum* should be excluded

Pregnancy Risk Factor Not assigned (other macrolides rated B); C per expert analysis

Pregnancy Considerations Crosses placenta. Specific safety information is not available. However, spiramycin has been used to treat *Toxoplasma gondii* to prevent transmission from mother to fetus.

Breast-Feeding Considerations Excreted in breast milk in bacteriostatic concentrations.

Contraindications Hypersensitivity to spiramycin, other macrolides (eg, erythromycin) or any component of the formulation

Warnings/Precautions Prolonged use may result in fungal or bacterial superinfection, including *C. difficile*-associated diarrhea (CDAD) and pseudomembranous colitis; CDAD has been observed >2 months postantibiotic treatment. Use with caution in patients with preexisting liver disease; hepatic impairment, including hepatocellular and/or cholestatic hepatitis, with or without jaundice, has been observed. Discontinue if symptoms of malaise, nausea, vomiting, abdominal colic, and fever. Macrolides have been associated with rare QTc prolongation and ventricular arrhythmias, including torsade de pointes; use with caution in patients at risk of prolonged cardiac repolarization.

Adverse Reactions

Dermatologic: Angioedema (rare), pruritus, rash, urticaria

Gastrointestinal: Diarrhea, nausea, pseudomembranous colitis (rare), vomiting

Hepatic: Transaminases increased

Neuromuscular & skeletal: Paresthesia (rare)

Miscellaneous: Anaphylactic shock (rare)

Note: Rare adverse reactions associated with other macrolide antibiotics include life-threatening ventricular arrhythmia, prolongation of QTc, and neuromuscular blockade.

Drug Interactions

Metabolism/Transport Effects Substrate of CYP3A4 (major); **Note:** Assignment of Major/Minor substrate status based on clinically relevant drug interaction potential

Avoid Concomitant Use

Avoid concomitant use of Spiramycin with any of the following: BCG; Conivaptan; Fusidic Acid (Systemic); Idelalisib; QuiNINE; Terfenadine

Increased Effect/Toxicity

Spiramycin may increase the levels/effects of: Antineoplastic Agents (Vinca Alkaloids); Cardiac Glycosides; QuiNINE; Rilpivirine; Terfenadine

The levels/effects of Spiramycin may be increased by: Aprepitant; Ceritinib; Conivaptan; CYP3A4 Inhibitors (Moderate); CYP3A4 Inhibitors (Strong); Dasatinib; Fosaprepitant; Fusidic Acid (Systemic); Idelalisib; Ivacaftor; Luliconazole; Mifepristone; Netupitant; Simeprevir; Stiripentol

Decreased Effect

Spiramycin may decrease the levels/effects of: BCG; Sodium Picosulfate; Typhoid Vaccine

The levels/effects of Spiramycin may be decreased by: Bosentan; CYP3A4 Inducers (Moderate); CYP3A4 Inducers (Strong); Dabrafenib; Deferasirox; Etravirine; Mitotane; Siltuximab; St Johns Wort; Tocilizumab

Storage/Stability Store at 20°C to 25°C (68°F to 77°F).

Mechanism of Action Inhibits growth of susceptible organisms; mechanism not established.

Dosage Oral:

Children: Dosage by body weight; usual dosage 150,000 units/kg; expressed as the number of 750,000 unit (Rovamycine® "250") capsules per day. Daily dose should be administered in 2-3 divided doses.

15 kg = 3 capsules per day

20 kg = 4 capsules per day

30 kg = 6 capsules per day

Note: In severe infections, dosage may be increased by 50%.

Adults:

Mild-to-moderate infections: 6,000,000 to 9,000,000 units (4-6 capsules of Rovamycine® "500" per day) in 2 divided doses

Severe infections: 12,000,000 to 15,000,000 units (8-10 capsules of Rovamycine® "500" per day) in 2 divided doses

Gonorrhea: 12,000,000 to 13,500,000 units (8-9 capsules of Rovamycine® "500") as a single dose

Dosage adjustment in renal impairment: No dosage adjustment required.

Dietary Considerations May be taken without regard to meals. Food may improve gastrointestinal tolerance.

Administration Administer without regard to meals.

Product Availability Not available in U.S.

Dosage Forms: Canada

Capsule, oral:

Rovamycine® "250": 750,000 units

Rovamycine® "500": 1,500,000 units

Spirapril [INT] (SPYE ra pril)

International Brand Names Cardiopril (CH); Quadropril (AT, DE, HU); Renormax (ES, IT); Renpress (ES, NL, NO); Sandopril (AT, LU); Setrilan (IT); Spirapril Sanabo (AT)

Pharmacologic Category Angiotensin-Converting Enzyme (ACE) Inhibitor

Reported Use Management of mild to severe hypertension; treatment of left ventricular dysfunction after myocardial infarction

Dosage Range Adults: Oral: 6 mg once daily

Product Availability Product available in various countries; not currently available in the U.S.

Dosage Forms

Tablet: 3 mg, 6 mg

◆ **Spiriva (Can)** *see* Tiotropium *on page 2046*

◆ **Spiriva HandiHaler** *see* Tiotropium *on page 2046*

◆ **Spiriva Respimat** *see* Tiotropium *on page 2046*

Spironolactone (speer on oh LAK tone)

Brand Names: U.S. Aldactone

Brand Names: Canada Aldactone; Teva-Spironolactone

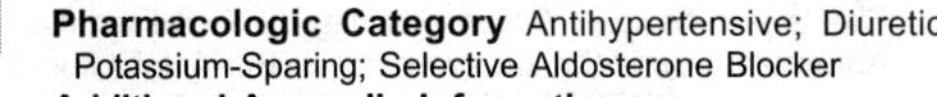

Pharmacologic Category Antihypertensive; Diuretic, Potassium-Sparing; Selective Aldosterone Blocker

Additional Appendix Information

Beers Criteria – Potentially Inappropriate Medications for Geriatrics *on page 2271*

Use Management of edema associated with excessive aldosterone excretion or with congestive heart failure (HF) unresponsive to other therapies; hypertension; primary hyperaldosteronism (establishing diagnosis, short-term preoperative treatment, and long-term maintenance therapy in selected patients); hypokalemia; cirrhosis of liver accompanied by edema or ascites; nephrotic syndrome; severe HF (NYHA class III-IV) to increase survival and reduce hospitalization when added to standard therapy

Note: The ACCF/AHA 2013 heart failure guidelines recommend the use of aldosterone antagonists, along with other guideline-directed medical therapies, to reduce morbidity and mortality in patients with HF (NYHA class III-IV) with LVEF ≤35% (Yancy, 2013).

According to the Eighth Joint National Committee (JNC 8) guidelines, aldosterone antagonists are not recommended for the initial treatment of hypertension (James, 2013).

According to the 2013 ACCF/AHA guidelines for the management of ST-elevation myocardial infarction (STEMI) and the guidelines for the management of unstable angina/non-STEMI, an aldosterone antagonist should be given to patients who are already on an ACE inhibitor and beta-blocker, who have an LVEF ≤40% and either symptomatic HF or diabetes mellitus (ACCF/AHA [Anderson, 2013]; ACCF/AHA [O'Gara, 2013]).

Pregnancy Risk Factor C

Pregnancy Considerations Adverse events were observed in some animal reproduction studies. The antiandrogen effects of spironolactone have been shown to cause feminization of the male fetus in animal studies. Spironolactone crosses the placenta (Regitz-Zagrosek, 2011).

The treatment of heart failure is generally the same in pregnant and nonpregnant women; however, spironolactone should be avoided in the first trimester due to its antiandrogenic effects (Regitz-Zagrosek, 2011). The use of mineralocorticoid receptor antagonists is not recommended to treat chronic uncomplicated hypertension in pregnant women and should generally be avoided in women of reproductive potential. When treatment for hypertension in pregnancy is needed, other agents are preferred (ACOG, 2013). Use of diuretics to treat edema during normal pregnancies is not appropriate; use may be considered when edema is due to pathologic causes (as in the nonpregnant patient); monitor.

Breast-Feeding Considerations The active metabolite of spironolactone (canrenone) has been found in breast milk. Information is available from a case report following maternal use of spironolactone 25 mg twice daily throughout pregnancy, then 4 times daily after delivery. Milk and maternal serum samples were obtained 17 days after birth. Two hours after the maternal dose, canrenone concentrations were ~144 ng/mL (serum) and ~104 ng/mL (milk). When measured 14.5 hours after the dose, canrenone concentrations were ~92 ng/mL (serum) and ~47 ng/mL (milk). The authors calculated the estimated maximum amount of canrenone to the nursing infant to be ~0.2% of the maternal dose (Phelps, 1977). Effects to humans are not known; however, this metabolite was found to be carcinogenic in rats. Diuretics have the potential to decrease milk volume and suppress lactation. According to the manufacturer, the decision to continue or discontinue breast-feeding during therapy should take into account the risk of exposure to the infant and the benefits of treatment to the mother; if use of spironolactone is essential, an alternative method of feeding should be used.

Contraindications

Anuria; acute renal insufficiency; significant impairment of renal excretory function; hyperkalemia; Addison's disease; concomitant use with eplerenone

Canadian labeling: Additional contraindications (not in U.S. labeling): Hypersensitivity to spironolactone or any component of the formulation; concomitant use with heparin or low molecular weight heparin

Warnings/Precautions Hazardous agent - use appropriate precautions for handling and disposal (NIOSH 2014 [group 2]).

[U.S. Boxed Warning]: Shown to be a tumorigen in chronic toxicity animal studies. Avoid unnecessary use.

Monitor closely for hyperkalemia; increases in serum potassium are dose related and rates of hyperkalemia also increase with declining renal function. The concurrent use of larger doses of ACE inhibitors (eg, ≥ lisinopril 10 mg daily in adults) also increases the risk of hyperkalemia (ACCF/AHA [Yancy, 2013]). Dose reduction or interruption of therapy may be necessary with development of hyperkalemia. Use is contraindicated in patients with hyperkalemia; use caution in conditions known to cause hyperkalemia. Risk of hyperkalemia is increased with declining renal function. Use with caution in patients with mild renal impairment; contraindicated with anuria, acute renal insufficiency, or significant impairment of renal excretory function. Potentially significant drug-drug interactions may exist, requiring dose or frequency adjustment, additional monitoring, and/or selection of alternative therapy. Somnolence and dizziness have been reported with use; advise patients to use caution when driving or operating machinery until response to initial treatment has been determined. Concurrent use with ethanol may Increase risk of orthostasis. Excess amounts can lead to profound diuresis with fluid and electrolyte loss; close medical supervision and dose evaluation are required. Watch for and correct electrolyte disturbances; adjust dose to avoid dehydration. In cirrhosis, avoid electrolyte and acid/base imbalances that might lead to hepatic encephalopathy. Gynecomastia is related to dose and duration of therapy; typically is reversible following discontinuation of therapy but may persist (rare). Discontinue use prior to adrenal vein catheterization. When evaluating a heart failure patient for spironolactone treatment, eGFR should be >30 mL/minute/1.73 m^2 or creatinine should be ≤2.5 mg/dL (men) or ≤2 mg/dL (women) with no recent worsening and potassium <5 mEq/L with no history of severe hyperkalemia (ACCF/AHA [Yancy, 2013]). Serum potassium levels require close monitoring and management if elevated. The manufacturer recommends to discontinue or interrupt therapy if serum potassium >5 mEq/L or serum creatinine >4 mg/dL. The ACCF/AHA recommends considering discontinuation upon the development of serum potassium >5.5 mEq/L or worsening renal function with careful evaluation of the entire medical regimen. Avoid routine triple therapy with the combined use of an ACE inhibitor, ARB, and spironolactone. Instruct patients with heart failure to discontinue use during an episode of diarrhea or dehydration or when loop diuretic therapy is interrupted (ACCF/AHA [Yancy, 2013]).

In the elderly, avoid use of doses >25 mg/day in patients with heart failure or with reduced renal function (eg, CrCl <30 mL/minute or eGFR ≤30 mL/minute/1.73 m^2 [Yancy, 2013]); risk of hyperkalemia is increased for heart failure patients receiving >25 mg/day, particularly if taking concomitant medications such as NSAIDS, ACE inhibitor, angiotensin receptor blocker, or potassium supplements (Beers Criteria).

Adverse Reactions

Cardiovascular: Vasculitis

Central nervous system: Ataxia, confusion, drowsiness, headache, lethargy

Dermatologic: Erythematous maculopapular rash, Stevens-Johnson syndrome, toxic epidermal necrolysis, urticaria

Endocrine & metabolic: Amenorrhea, gynecomastia, hyperkalemia

Gastrointestinal: Abdominal cramps, diarrhea, gastritis, gastrointestinal hemorrhage, gastrointestinal ulcer, nausea, vomiting

Genitourinary: Impotence, irregular menses, postmenopausal bleeding

Hematologic & oncologic: Agranulocytosis, malignant neoplasm of breast

Hepatic: Hepatotoxicity

Hypersensitivity: Anaphylaxis

Immunologic: DRESS syndrome

Renal: Increased blood urea nitrogen, renal failure, renal insufficiency

Miscellaneous: Fever

Drug Interactions

Metabolism/Transport Effects None known.

Avoid Concomitant Use

Avoid concomitant use of Spironolactone with any of the following: AMILoride; CycloSPORINE (Systemic); Tacrolimus (Systemic); Triamterene

Increased Effect/Toxicity

Spironolactone may increase the levels/effects of: ACE Inhibitors; Amifostine; Ammonium Chloride; Antihypertensives; Cardiac Glycosides; CycloSPORINE (Systemic); Digoxin; DULoxetine; Hypotensive Agents; Levodopa; Neuromuscular-Blocking Agents (Nondepolarizing); Obinutuzumab; RisperiDONE; RiTUXimab; Sodium Phosphates; Tacrolimus (Systemic)

The levels/effects of Spironolactone may be increased by: Alfuzosin; AMILoride; Analgesics (Opioid); Angiotensin II Receptor Blockers; AtorvaSTATin; Barbiturates; Brimonidine (Topical); Canagliflozin; Cholestyramine Resin; Diazoxide; Drospirenone; Eplerenone; Heparin; Heparin (Low Molecular Weight); Herbs (Hypotensive Properties); MAO Inhibitors; Nicorandil; Nitrofurantoin; Nonsteroidal Anti-Inflammatory Agents; Pentoxifylline; Phosphodiesterase 5 Inhibitors; Potassium Salts; Prostacyclin Analogues; Tolvaptan; Triamterene; Trimethoprim

Decreased Effect

Spironolactone may decrease the levels/effects of: Abiraterone Acetate; Alpha-/Beta-Agonists; Cardiac Glycosides; Mitotane; QuiNIDine

The levels/effects of Spironolactone may be decreased by: Herbs (Hypertensive Properties); Methylphenidate; Nonsteroidal Anti-Inflammatory Agents; Yohimbine

Food Interactions Food increases absorption. Management: Administer with food to increase absorption and decrease GI upset.

Storage/Stability Store below 25°C (77°F).

Mechanism of Action Competes with aldosterone for receptor sites in the distal renal tubules, increasing sodium chloride and water excretion while conserving potassium and hydrogen ions; may block the effect of aldosterone on arteriolar smooth muscle as well

Pharmacodynamics/Kinetics

Duration: 2-3 days

Protein binding: >90%

Metabolism: Hepatic to multiple metabolites, including active metabolites canrenone and 7-alpha-spirolactone

Half-life elimination: Spironolactone: ~1.4 hours; Canrenone: 12-20 hours (Skluth, 1990); 7-alpha-spirolactone: ~13.8 hours

Time to peak, serum: 3-4 hours (primarily as the active metabolite)

Excretion: Urine and feces

Dosage Oral:

Children: Diuretic, hypertension (off-label use): Children 1-17 years: Initial: 1 mg/kg/day divided every 12 to 24 hours (maximum dose: 3.3 mg/kg/day, up to 100 mg daily) (NHBPEP, 2004)

Adults:

Ascites, due to cirrhosis (off-label dose): Initial: 100 mg once daily; titrate every 3 to 5 days as clinically indicated (usual maximum: 400 mg once daily) (Runyon, 2013)

Edema: 25 to 200 mg daily in 1 to 2 divided doses

Hypokalemia: 25 to 100 mg once daily

Hypertension: Initial: 50 to 100 mg in 1 to 2 divided doses; after 2 weeks, may adjust dose. Usual dosage range (ASH/ISH [Weber, 2014]): 25 to 50 mg daily

Diagnosis of primary aldosteronism: Long test: 400 mg once daily for 3 to 4 weeks; short test: 400 mg once daily for 4 days; maintenance until surgical correction: 100 to 400 mg once daily

Heart failure (HF), severe (NYHA class III-IV): Initial: 12.5 to 25 mg once daily; maximum daily dose: 50 mg. If 25 mg once daily not tolerated, may reduce to 25 mg every other day. The ACCF/AHA 2013 HF guidelines also recommend the use of aldosterone receptor antagonists (eg, spironolactone) in patients with NYHA class II HF and LVEF ≤35% who have a history of prior cardiovascular hospitalization or elevated plasma natriuretic peptide levels and postmyocardial infarction patients with LVEF ≤40% who develop HF symptoms or have a history of diabetes mellitus (ACCF/AHA [Yancy, 2013]).

Note: Per the manufacturer, if potassium >5 mEq/L or serum creatinine >4 mg/dL, discontinue or interrupt therapy. Alternatively, the ACCF/AHA 2013 HF guidelines recommend withholding treatment if potassium >5.5 mEq/L or renal function worsens; hold doses until potassium is <5 mEq/L and consider restarting with a reduced dose after confirming resolution of hyperkalemia/renal insufficiency for at least 72 hours (ACCF/AHA [Yancy, 2013]).

Acne in women (off-label use): 50 to 200 mg once daily (Goodfellow, 1984; Muhlemann, 1986)

Hirsutism in women (off-label use): 50 to 200 mg daily in 1 to 2 divided doses (Koulouri, 2008; Martin, 2008)

Elderly:

Hypertension: No initial dosage adjustment necessary (Aronow, 2011).

Heart failure: Avoid using doses >25 mg daily (Beers Criteria); monitor potassium closely/use with caution.

Dosage adjustment in renal impairment: Heart failure (ACCF/AHA [Yancy, 2013]):

eGFR ≥50 mL/minute/1.73 m^2: Initial dose: 12.5 to 25 mg once daily; Maintenance dose (after 4 weeks of treatment with potassium ≤5 mEq/L): 25 mg once or twice daily

eGFR 30-49 mL/minute/1.73 m^2: Initial dose: 12.5 mg once daily or every other day; Maintenance dose (after 4 weeks of treatment with potassium ≤5 mEq/L): 12.5 to 25 mg once daily

eGFR <30 mL/minute/1.73 m^2: Not recommended.

Note: Contraindicated in patients with anuria, acute renal insufficiency, or significant impairment of renal excretory function.

Dosage adjustment in hepatic impairment: There are no dosage adjustments provided in manufacturer's labeling.

Dietary Considerations Should be taken with food to decrease gastrointestinal irritation and to increase absorption. Excessive potassium intake (eg, salt substitutes, low-salt foods, bananas, nuts) should be avoided.

Monitoring Parameters Blood pressure, serum electrolytes (potassium, sodium), renal function, I & O ratios and daily weight throughout therapy

ACCF/AHA heart failure guideline recommendations (ACCF/AHA [Yancy, 2013]): Serum potassium and renal function should be checked in 3 days after initiation, at 1 week after initiation, at least monthly for the first 3 months of therapy, and every 3 months thereafter. If adding or increasing the dose of concomitant ACE inhibitors or ARBs, a new cycle of monitoring should be done. If serum potassium increases to >5.5 mEq/L or renal function worsens, hold doses until potassium is <5 mEq/L and consider restarting with a reduced dose after confirming resolution of hyperkalemia/renal insufficiency for at least 72 hours.

Additional Information Maximum diuretic effect may be delayed 2-3 days and maximum antihypertensive effects may be delayed 2-3 weeks.

Dosage Forms

Tablet, Oral:

Aldactone: 25 mg, 50 mg, 100 mg

Generic: 25 mg, 50 mg, 100 mg

Dosage Forms: Canada Refer to Dosage Forms. **Note:** Aldactone 50 mg tablets are not available in Canada.

Extemporaneous Preparations Hazardous agent; use appropriate precautions for handling and disposal (NIOSH 2014 [group 2]).

A 1 mg/mL oral suspension may be made with tablets. Crush ten 25 mg tablets in a mortar and reduce to a fine powder. Add a small amount of purified water and soak for 5 minutes; add 50 mL 1.5% carboxymethylcellulose, 100 mL syrup NF, and mix to a uniform paste; mix while adding purified water in incremental proportions to **almost** 250 mL; transfer to a calibrated bottle, rinse mortar with purified water, and add quantity of purified water sufficient to make 250 mL. Label "shake well". Stable for 3 months at room temperature or refrigerated (Nahata, 1993).

A 2.5 mg/mL oral suspension may be made with tablets. Crush twelve 25 mg tablets in a mortar and reduce to a fine powder. Add small portions of distilled water or glycerin and mix to a uniform paste; mix while adding cherry syrup to **almost** 120 mL; transfer to a calibrated bottle, rinse mortar with cherry syrup, and add quantity of cherry syrup sufficient to make 120 mL. Label "shake well" and "refrigerate". This method may also be used with twenty-four 25 mg tablets for a 5 mg/mL oral suspension. Both concentrations are stable for 28 days refrigerated (Mathur, 1989).

A 25 mg/mL oral suspension may be made with tablets and either a 1:1 mixture of Ora-Sweet and Ora-Plus or a 1:1 mixture of Ora-Sweet SF and Ora-Plus. Crush one-hundred-twenty 25 mg tablets in a mortar and reduce to a fine powder. Add small portions of chosen vehicle and mix to a uniform paste; mix while adding vehicle in incremental proportions to **almost** 120 mL; transfer to a calibrated bottle, rinse mortar with vehicle, and add quantity of vehicle sufficient to make 120 mL. Store in amber bottles; label "shake well" and "refrigerate". Stable for 60 days refrigerated (Allen, 1996).

Allen LV Jr and Erickson MA 3rd, "Stability of Ketoconazole, Metolazone, Metronidazole, Procainamide Hydrochloride, and Spironolactone in Extemporaneously Compounded Oral Liquids," *Am J Health Syst Pharm*, 1996, 53(17):2073-8.

Mathur LK and Wickman A, "Stability of Extemporaneously Compounded Spironolactone Suspensions," *Am J Hosp Pharm*, 1989, 46(10):2040-2.

Nahata MC, Morosco RS, and Hipple TF, "Stability of Spironolactone in an Extemporaneously Prepared Suspension at Two Temperatures," *Ann Pharmacother*, 1993, 27(10):1198-9.

◆ **SPM 927** *see* Lacosamide *on page 1154*
◆ **Sporanox** *see* Itraconazole *on page 1130*
◆ **Sporanox Pulsepak** *see* Itraconazole *on page 1130*
◆ **SPP100** *see* Aliskiren *on page 85*
◆ **Sprintec** *see* Ethinyl Estradiol and Norgestimate *on page 810*
◆ **Sprix** *see* Ketorolac (Nasal) *on page 1149*
◆ **Sprycel** *see* Dasatinib *on page 574*
◆ **SPS** *see* Sodium Polystyrene Sulfonate *on page 1912*
◆ **SQV** *see* Saquinavir *on page 1865*
◆ **SR33589** *see* Dronedarone *on page 695*
◆ **Sronyx** *see* Ethinyl Estradiol and Levonorgestrel *on page 803*
◆ **SS734** *see* Besifloxacin *on page 251*
◆ **SSD** *see* Silver Sulfadiazine *on page 1887*
◆ **SSKI** *see* Potassium Iodide *on page 1690*
◆ **SSS 10-5** *see* Sulfur and Sulfacetamide *on page 1953*
◆ **Stadol** *see* Butorphanol *on page 314*
◆ **Stagesic [DSC]** *see* Hydrocodone and Acetaminophen *on page 1012*
◆ **Stalevo** *see* Levodopa, Carbidopa, and Entacapone *on page 1196*
◆ **StanGard Perio** *see* Fluoride *on page 895*
◆ **Stannous Fluoride** *see* Fluoride *on page 895*
◆ **Starlix** *see* Nateglinide *on page 1432*
◆ **Statex (Can)** *see* Morphine (Systemic) *on page 1394*

Stavudine (STAV yoo deen)

Brand Names: U.S. Zerit

Brand Names: Canada Zerit

Index Terms d4T

Pharmacologic Category Antiretroviral, Reverse Transcriptase Inhibitor, Nucleoside (Anti-HIV)

Use Treatment of HIV infection in combination with other antiretroviral agents

Pregnancy Risk Factor C

Dosage Oral:

Newborns (Birth to 13 days): 0.5 mg/kg every 12 hours

Children:

≥14 days and <30 kg: 1 mg/kg every 12 hours

≥30 kg: Refer to adult dosing

Adults:

<60 kg: 30 mg every 12 hours

≥60 kg: 40 mg every 12 hours

Note: The World Health Organization recommends 30 mg every 12 hours in all adult and adolescent patients regardless of body weight (HHS [adult], 2014).

Elderly: Older patients should be closely monitored for signs and symptoms of peripheral neuropathy; dosage should be carefully adjusted to renal function

Dosage adjustment in renal impairment:

Children: Specific recommendations not available. Reduction in dose or increase in dosing interval should be considered.

Adults:

CrCl >50 mL/minute:

<60 kg: 30 mg every 12 hours

≥60 kg: 40 mg every 12 hours

CrCl 26-50 mL/minute:

<60 kg: 15 mg every 12 hours

≥60 kg: 20 mg every 12 hours

CrCl 10-25 mL/minute, hemodialysis (administer dose after hemodialysis on day of dialysis):

<60 kg: 15 mg every 24 hours

≥60 kg: 20 mg every 24 hours

Dosage adjustment in hepatic impairment: There are no dosage adjustments provided in the manufacturer's labeling. Use with caution.

Additional Information Complete prescribing information should be consulted for additional detail.

Dosage Forms

Capsule, Oral:

Zerit: 15 mg, 20 mg, 30 mg, 40 mg

Generic: 15 mg, 20 mg, 30 mg, 40 mg

Solution Reconstituted, Oral:

Zerit: 1 mg/mL (200 mL)

Generic: 1 mg/mL (200 mL)

- ◆ **Stavzor** *see* Valproic Acid and Derivatives *on page 2123*
- ◆ **Staxyn** *see* Vardenafil *on page 2138*
- ◆ **Stelara** *see* Ustekinumab *on page 2117*
- ◆ **Stelazine** *see* Trifluoperazine *on page 2102*
- ◆ **Stendra** *see* Avanafil *on page 205*
- ◆ **Sterile Talc** *see* Talc (Sterile) *on page 1971*
- ◆ **Sterile Talc Powder** *see* Talc (Sterile) *on page 1971*
- ◆ **Sterile Vancomycin Hydrochloride, USP (Can)** *see* Vancomycin *on page 2130*
- ◆ **STI-571** *see* Imatinib *on page 1047*
- ◆ **Stieprox (Can)** *see* Ciclopirox *on page 433*
- ◆ **Stieva-A (Can)** *see* Tretinoin (Topical) *on page 2099*
- ◆ **Stimate** *see* Desmopressin *on page 594*
- ◆ **Stimulant Laxative [OTC]** *see* Bisacodyl *on page 265*

Stiripentol [CAN/INT] (stir i PEN tol)

Brand Names: Canada Diacomit

Index Terms BCX 2600; Estiripentol

Pharmacologic Category Anticonvulsant, Miscellaneous

Additional Appendix Information

Oral Dosages That Should Not Be Crushed *on page 2276*

Use Note: Not approved in U.S.

Dravet syndrome: Adjunctive treatment of refractory generalized tonic-clonic seizures in conjunction with clobazam and valproic acid in patients with severe myoclonic epilepsy in infancy (SMEI, Dravet syndrome) and whose seizures are not adequately controlled with clobazam and valproic acid alone

Pregnancy Considerations Adverse effects have not been observed in animal reproduction studies. Use of stiripentol in pregnant women has not been studied; however, infants exposed to antiepileptic drugs in utero are at increased risk for malformations.

Breast-Feeding Considerations It is not known whether stiripentol is excreted into human breast milk. The manufacturer does not recommend use in breast-feeding women.

Contraindications Hypersensitivity to stiripentol or any component of the formulation

Warnings/Precautions [Canadian Boxed Warning]: Delirium and hallucinations have been reported (rarely) in adult patients; closely monitor patients with prior episodes of delirium. Additional psychiatric effects (eg, hyperexcitability, aggressiveness, irritability, insomnia, nightmares) have also been reported. Pooled analysis of trials involving various antiepileptics (regardless of indication) showed an increased risk of suicidal thoughts/behavior (incidence rate: 0.43% treated patients compared to 0.24% of patients receiving placebo); risk observed as early as 1 week after initiation and continued through duration of trials (most trials ≤24 weeks). Monitor all patients for notable changes in behavior that might indicate suicidal thoughts or depression; notify healthcare provider immediately if symptoms occur. May cause CNS depression (eg, drowsiness, sleepiness) and impair physical or mental abilities; patients must be cautioned about performing tasks which require mental alertness (eg, operating machinery or driving). Effects with other sedative drugs or ethanol may be potentiated.

Use with caution in hepatic and/or renal impairment. Loss of appetite and weight loss have been observed in up to 50% and 29% of patients respectively during clinical trials; monitor the growth rate of pediatric patients closely. Valproate dose reduction by 30% may help minimize appetite and weight loss. Equilibrium disorders and movement disorders (eg, dysarthria, ataxia, tremor, hypotonia) have been reported with use. Neutropenia has been observed in clinical trials (Chiron, 2000) and in long-term studies; monitor CBC during therapy.

[Canadian Boxed Warning]: Stiripentol inhibits multiple cytochrome P450 isoenzymes (eg, 2D6, 3A4, 2C8, 1A2, 2C19); concurrent use with drugs metabolized by these isoenzymes may increase their systemic exposure. Concurrent use with carbamazepine, phenobarbital, or phenobarbital is not recommended. Clobazam and valproate dose reductions may be necessary, based on tolerability, during adjunctive therapy with stiripentol. Must be used in conjunction with clobazam and valproate; not approved for use as monotherapy. Efficacy in treating other forms of epilepsy has not been established. Anticonvulsants should not be discontinued abruptly because of the possibility of increasing seizure frequency; therapy should be withdrawn gradually to minimize the potential of increased seizure frequency, unless safety concerns require a more rapid withdrawal.

Systemic exposure is slightly higher with the powder for suspension than that observed with capsules; patient monitoring is recommended when switching between dosage forms.

Adverse Reactions

Central nervous system: Aggressive behavior/irritability, ataxia, drowsiness, dysarthria, equilibrium disturbance, fatigue, hyperexcitability/agitation, hypotonia, insomnia/nightmares, reduced intellectual ability

Dermatologic: Facial erythema, urticaria, xeroderma

Endocrine & metabolic: Weight gain, weight loss

Gastrointestinal: Abdominal pain, anorexia, nausea/vomiting, sialorrhea

Genitourinary: Dysuria

Hematologic & oncologic: Eosinophilia, neutropenia, thrombocytopenia

Hepatic: Increased serum AST

Neuromuscular & skeletal: Tremor

Rare but important or life-threatening: Apathy, coma, convulsions, delirium (rare), esophageal pain, hallucination (rare), hepatitis (cytolytic), hyperthermia, increased creatine phosphokinase, increased gamma-glutamyl transferase, increased serum ALT, increased serum transaminases, infection, muscle spasm (involuntary), movement disorder (including ataxia, hypotonia, physical health deterioration, tremor, hyperkinesia, dysarthria, and equilibrium disorders), pancreatitis, skin rash, Stevens-Johnson syndrome, testicular disease, thyroiditis

Drug Interactions

Metabolism/Transport Effects Substrate of CYP1A2 (major), CYP2C19 (major), CYP3A4 (major); **Note:** Assignment of Major/Minor substrate status based on clinically relevant drug interaction potential; **Inhibits** CYP1A2 (strong), CYP2C19 (strong), CYP2C8 (strong), CYP2D6 (strong), CYP3A4 (strong)

Avoid Concomitant Use

Avoid concomitant use of Stiripentol with any of the following: Ado-Trastuzumab Emtansine; Agomelatine; Alcohol (Ethyl); Alfuzosin; Apixaban; Astemizole; Avanafil; Axitinib; Azelastine (Nasal); Bosutinib; Cabozantinib; Caffeine and Caffeine Containing Products; CarBAMazepine; Ceritinib; Conivaptan; Crizotinib; Dapoxetine; Dasabuvir; Dronedarone; DULoxetine; Enzalutamide; Eplerenone; Everolimus; Fusidic Acid (Systemic); Halofantrine; Ibrutinib; Idelalisib; Irinotecan; Ivabradine; Lapatinib; Lercanidipine; Lomitapide; Lovastatin; Lurasidone; Macitentan; Naloxegol; Nilotinib; Nisoldipine; Olaparib; Orphenadrine; Paraldehyde; PHENobarbital; Phenytoin; Pimozide; Pomalidomide; Ranolazine; Red Yeast Rice; Regorafenib; Rivaroxaban; Salmeterol; Silodosin; Simeprevir; Simvastatin; Suvorexant; Tamoxifen; Tamsulosin; Tasimelteon; Terfenadine; Thalidomide; Theophylline; Thioridazine; Ticagrelor; Tolvaptan; Toremifene; Trabectedin; Ulipristal; Vemurafenib; VinCRIStine (Liposomal); Vorapaxar

Increased Effect/Toxicity

Stiripentol may increase the levels/effects of: Ado-Trastuzumab Emtansine; Agomelatine; Alcohol (Ethyl); Alfuzosin; Almotriptan; Apixaban; ARIPiprazole; Astemizole; AtoMOXetine; Avanafil; Axitinib; Azelastine (Nasal); Bedaquiline; Bendamustine; Bortezomib; Bosentan; Bosutinib; Brentuximab Vedotin; Brinzolamide; Budesonide (Nasal); Budesonide (Systemic, Oral Inhalation); Buprenorphine; Cabazitaxel; Cabozantinib; Caffeine and Caffeine Containing Products; Cannabis; CarBAMazepine; Ceritinib; Citalopram; CloBAZam; CloZAPine; CNS Depressants; Colchicine; Conivaptan; Corticosteroids (Orally Inhaled); Corticosteroids (Systemic); Crizotinib; CYP1A2 Substrates; CYP2C19 Substrates; CYP2C8 Substrates; CYP2D6 Substrates; CYP3A4 Substrates; Dapoxetine; Dasabuvir; Dasatinib; Dienogest; Dofetilide; DOXOrubicin (Conventional); Dronabinol; Dronedarone; DULoxetine; Dutasteride; Eliglustat; Enzalutamide; Eplerenone; Erlotinib; Etizolam; Everolimus; FentaNYL; Fesoterodine; Fluticasone (Nasal); Fluticasone (Oral Inhalation); GuanFACINE; Halofantrine; Hydrocodone; Ibrutinib; Iloperidone; Imatinib; Imidafenacin; Irinotecan; Ivabradine; Ivacaftor; Ixabepilone; Lacosamide; Lapatinib; Lercanidipine; Levobupivacaine; Levomilnacipran; Lomitapide; Lovastatin; Lumefantrine; Lurasidone; Macitentan; Maraviroc; Methotrimeprazine; MethylPREDNISolone; Metoprolol; Metyrosine; Mifepristone; Naloxegol; Nebivolol; Nilotinib; Nisoldipine; Olaparib; Orphenadrine; Ospemifene; OxyCODONE; Paraldehyde; Paricalcitol; PAZOPanib; Pimecrolimus; Pimozide; Pioglitazone; Pirfenidone; Pomalidomide; PONATinib; Pramipexole; Pranlukast; PrednisoLONE (Systemic); PredniSONE; Propafenone; QUEtiapine; Ranolazine; Red Yeast Rice; Regorafenib; Retapamulin; Rilpivirine; Rivaroxaban; RomiDEPsin; Rotigotine; Ruxolitinib; Salmeterol; Saxagliptin; Selective Serotonin Reuptake Inhibitors; Sildenafil; Silodosin; Simeprevir; Simvastatin; SORAfenib; Suvorexant; Tadalafil; Tamsulosin; Tasimelteon; Terfenadine; Tetrabenazine; Tetrahydrocannabinol; Thalidomide; Theophylline; Thioridazine; Ticagrelor; Tofacitinib; Tolterodine; Tolvaptan; Toremifene; Trabectedin; Treprostinil; Ulipristal; Vardenafil; Vemurafenib; Vilazodone; VinCRIStine (Liposomal); Vorapaxar; Vortioxetine; Zolpidem; Zopiclone; Zuclopenthixol

The levels/effects of Stiripentol may be increased by: Abiraterone Acetate; Brimonidine (Topical); Cannabis; CloBAZam; Conivaptan; CYP1A2 Inhibitors (Moderate); CYP1A2 Inhibitors (Strong); CYP2C19 Inhibitors (Moderate); CYP2C19 Inhibitors (Strong); CYP3A4 Inhibitors (Moderate); CYP3A4 Inhibitors (Strong); Deferasirox; Doxylamine; Dronabinol; Droperidol; Fusidic Acid (Systemic); HydrOXYzine; Idelalisib; Kava Kava; Luliconazole; Magnesium Sulfate; Methotrimeprazine; Mifepristone; Nabilone; Netupitant; Peginterferon Alfa-2b; Perampanel; Rufinamide; Sodium Oxybate; Tapentadol; Tetrahydrocannabinol

Decreased Effect

Stiripentol may decrease the levels/effects of: Clopidogrel; Codeine; Ifosfamide; Iloperidone; Phenytoin; Prasugrel; Tamoxifen; Ticagrelor

The levels/effects of Stiripentol may be decreased by: Bosentan; Cannabis; CYP1A2 Inducers (Strong); CYP2C19 Inducers (Strong); CYP3A4 Inducers (Moderate); CYP3A4 Inducers (Strong); Dabrafenib; Deferasirox; Mefloquine; Mianserin; Mitotane; Orlistat; PHENobarbital; Siltuximab; St Johns Wort; Teriflunomide; Tocilizumab

Preparation for Administration Mix powder for suspension with a glass of water.

Storage/Stability Store at 15°C to 30°C (59°F to 86°F). Store in original package. Protect from light. Powder for suspension should be consumed immediately after reconstitution and not stored.

Mechanism of Action Precise mechanism behind anticonvulsant effects is unknown. May enhance GABAergic inhibitory neurotransmission by weak partial agonism and/or positive allosteric modulation of gamma-aminobutyric acid (GABA)-A receptors (Fisher, 2009). Also inhibits multiple cytochrome P450 isoenzymes involved in the metabolism of other anticonvulsants; concurrent use may increase their systemic exposure and efficacy.

Pharmacodynamics/Kinetics

Absorption: Rapid; well absorbed; maximum concentration obtained with powder for suspension is slightly higher than that observed with capsules

Protein binding: ~99% to plasma proteins

Metabolism: Hepatic through demethylenation, primarily by CYP1A2, 2C19, 3A4, and glucuronidation

Half-life elimination: Adults: 4.5-13 hours (dose-dependent); clearance decreases with repeated administration possibly due to inhibition of cytochrome P450 isoenzymes and is markedly decreased at higher doses

Time to peak: 1.5 hours

Excretion: Urine (73% as metabolites); feces (13% to 24% as unchanged drug)

Dosage Note: Use only in conjunction with clobazam and valproate; the dosage of clobazam and valproate may need to be adjusted. Systemic exposure is slightly higher with the powder for suspension than that observed with capsules; patient monitoring is recommended when switching between dosage forms.

Refractory generalized tonic-clonic seizures in Dravet syndrome, adjunctive therapy: Oral:

Infants and Children <3 years: Use is recommended only after clinical confirmation of Dravet syndrome and under close monitoring; the manufacturer labeling does not provide specific dosing recommendations.

Children ≥3 years, Adolescents, and Adults: Oral: Initial: Titrate dose upward over 3 days to 50 mg/kg daily given in 2 or 3 divided doses (maximum daily dose: 50 mg/kg).

Dosage adjustment in renal impairment: No dosage adjustment provided in manufacturer's labeling (has not been studied). Use with caution; metabolites primarily undergo renal elimination.

Dosage adjustment in hepatic impairment: No dosage adjustment provided in manufacturer's labeling (has not been studied). Use with caution; metabolism is primarily hepatic.

Dietary Considerations Must be taken with food; gastric acid in empty stomach promotes rapid degradation. Do not take with milk, dairy products, or fruit juices. Increased dietary intake may be necessary for patients who experience weight loss.

Administration Administer orally in 2 or 3 divided doses daily with a meal. Capsule should be swallowed whole with a glass of water. Do not crush, chew, or open capsule. Powder for suspension should be mixed with a glass of water and consumed immediately.

Monitoring Parameters CBC and hepatic function (prior to initiation and every 6 months or as clinically indicated thereafter); weight; growth rate in children.

Product Availability Not available in the U.S.

Dosage Forms: Canada

Capsule, Oral:

Diacomit: 250 mg, 500 mg

Powder for oral suspension:

Diacomit: 250 mg

- **Stivarga** *see* Regorafenib *on page 1787*
- **St Joseph Adult Aspirin [OTC]** *see* Aspirin *on page 180*
- **Stomach Relief [OTC]** *see* Bismuth *on page 265*
- **Stomach Relief Max St [OTC]** *see* Bismuth *on page 265*
- **Stomach Relief Plus [OTC]** *see* Bismuth *on page 265*
- **Stool Softener [OTC]** *see* Docusate *on page 661*
- **Stool Softener Laxative DC [OTC]** *see* Docusate *on page 661*
- **Stop** *see* Fluoride *on page 895*
- **Strattera** *see* AtoMOXetine *on page 191*

Streptomycin (strep toe MYE sin)

Brand Names: Canada Streptomycin for Injection

Index Terms Streptomycin Sulfate

Pharmacologic Category Antibiotic, Aminoglycoside; Antitubercular Agent

Use Part of combination therapy of active tuberculosis; used in combination with other agents for treatment of bacteremia caused by susceptible gram-negative bacilli, brucellosis, chancroid granuloma inguinale, *H. influenzae* (respiratory, endocardial, meningeal infections), *K. pneumoniae*, plague, streptococcal or enterococcal endocarditis, tularemia, urinary tract infections (caused by *A. aerogenes, E. coli, E. faecalis, K. pneumoniae, Proteus* spp)

Pregnancy Risk Factor D

Pregnancy Considerations Streptomycin crosses the placenta. Many case reports of hearing impairment in children exposed *in utero* have been published. Impairment has ranged from mild hearing loss to bilateral deafness. Because of several reports of total irreversible bilateral congenital deafness in children whose mothers received streptomycin during pregnancy, the manufacturer classifies streptomycin as pregnancy risk factor D.

Breast-Feeding Considerations Streptomycin is excreted into breast milk; however, it is not well absorbed when taken orally. This limited oral absorption may minimize exposure to the nursing infant. Nondose-related effects could include modification of bowel flora. Breast-feeding is not recommended by the manufacturer.

Contraindications Hypersensitivity to streptomycin, other aminoglycosides, or any component of the formulation

Warnings/Precautions [U.S. Boxed Warnings]: May cause neurotoxicity, nephrotoxicity, and/or neuromuscular blockade and respiratory paralysis; usual risk factors include preexisting renal impairment, concomitant neuro-/nephrotoxic medications, advanced age and dehydration. The drug's neurotoxicity can result in respiratory paralysis from neuromuscular blockade, especially when the drug is given soon after anesthesia or muscle relaxants. Use with caution in patients with preexisting vertigo, tinnitus, hearing loss, neuromuscular disorders, or renal impairment; modify dosage in patients with renal impairment; ototoxicity is directly proportional to the amount of drug given and the duration of treatment; tinnitus or vertigo are indications of vestibular injury and impending bilateral irreversible damage; renal damage is usually reversible. Monitor renal function closely; peak serum concentrations should not surpass 20-25 mcg/mL in patients with renal impairment. Formulation contains metabisulfite; may cause allergic reactions in patients with sulfite sensitivity. **[U.S. Boxed Warning]: Parenteral form should be used only where appropriate audiometric and laboratory testing facilities are available.** Prolonged use may result in fungal or bacterial superinfection, including *C. difficile*-associated diarrhea (CDAD) and pseudomembranous colitis; CDAD has been observed >2 months postantibiotic treatment. IM injections should be administered in a large muscle well within the body to avoid peripheral nerve damage and local skin reactions.

Adverse Reactions

Cardiovascular: Hypotension

Central nervous system: Drug fever, headache, neurotoxicity, paresthesia of face

Dermatologic: Angioedema, exfoliative dermatitis, skin rash, urticaria

Gastrointestinal: Nausea, vomiting

Hematologic: Eosinophilia, hemolytic anemia, leukopenia, pancytopenia, thrombocytopenia

Neuromuscular & skeletal: Arthralgia, tremor, weakness

Ocular: Amblyopia

Otic: Ototoxicity (auditory), ototoxicity (vestibular)

Renal: Azotemia, nephrotoxicity

Respiratory: Difficulty in breathing

Miscellaneous: Anaphylaxis

Rare but important or life-threatening: Drug reaction with eosinophilia and systemic symptoms (DRESS), toxic epidermal necrolysis

Drug Interactions

Metabolism/Transport Effects None known.

Avoid Concomitant Use

Avoid concomitant use of Streptomycin with any of the following: Bacitracin (Systemic); BCG; Foscarnet; Mannitol

Increased Effect/Toxicity

Streptomycin may increase the levels/effects of: AbobotulinumtoxinA; Bacitracin (Systemic); Bisphosphonate Derivatives; CARBOplatin; Colistimethate; CycloSPORINE (Systemic); Neuromuscular-Blocking Agents; OnabotulinumtoxinA; RimabotulinumtoxinB; Tenofovir

The levels/effects of Streptomycin may be increased by: Amphotericin B; Capreomycin; Cephalosporins (2nd Generation); Cephalosporins (3rd Generation); Cephalosporins (4th Generation); CISplatin; Foscarnet; Loop Diuretics; Mannitol; Nonsteroidal Anti-Inflammatory Agents; Tenofovir; Vancomycin

Decreased Effect

Streptomycin may decrease the levels/effects of: BCG; Sodium Picosulfate; Typhoid Vaccine

The levels/effects of Streptomycin may be decreased by: Penicillins

Storage/Stability

Lyophilized powder: Store dry powder at controlled room temperature 20°C to 25°C (68°F to 77°F). Protect from light.

Solution: Store in refrigerator at 2°C to 8°C (36°F to 46°F).

Depending upon manufacturer, reconstituted solution remains stable for 24 hours at room temperature. Exposure to light causes darkening of solution without apparent loss of potency.

Mechanism of Action Inhibits bacterial protein synthesis by binding directly to the 30S ribosomal subunits causing faulty peptide sequence to form in the protein chain

Pharmacodynamics/Kinetics

Absorption: Oral: Poorly absorbed; IM: Well absorbed

Distribution: To extracellular fluid including serum, abscesses, ascitic, pericardial, pleural, synovial, lymphatic, and peritoneal fluids; poorly distributed into CSF

Half-life elimination: Adults: ~5 hours

Time to peak: IM: Within 1 hour

Excretion: Urine (29% to 89% as unchanged drug); feces, saliva, sweat, and tears (minimal)

Dosage Note: For IM administration only.

Usual dosage range: IM:

Children: 20-40 mg/kg/day (maximum: 1 g)

Adults: 15-30 mg/kg/day or 1-2 g/day

Indication-specific dosing:

Children: IM:

***Mycobacterium ulcerans* (Buruli ulcers):** 15 mg/kg once daily (maximum: 1 g) for 8 weeks (WHO, 2004)

Plague: 30 mg/kg/day divided every 12 hours for 10 days (WHO, 2010)

Tularemia: 15 mg/kg twice daily (maximum: 2 g) for 10 days (WHO, 2007)

Tuberculosis:

Daily therapy: 20-40 mg/kg/day (maximum: 1 g daily)

Directly observed therapy (DOT), twice weekly: 25-30 mg/kg (maximum: 1.5 g)

Directly observed therapy (DOT), 3 times weekly: 25-30 mg/kg (maximum: 1.5 g)

Adults: IM:

Brucellosis: 1 g daily in 2-4 divided doses for 14-21 days (with doxycycline) (Skalsky, 2008)

Endocarditis:

Enterococcal: 1 g every 12 hours for 2 weeks, 500 mg every 12 hours for 4 weeks in combination with penicillin

Streptococcal: 1 g every 12 hours for 1 week, 500 mg every 12 hours for 1 week in combination with penicillin. **Note:** For patients >60 years, 500 mg every 12 hours for 2 weeks is recommended.

***Mycobacterium avium* complex:** Adjunct therapy (with macrolide, rifamycin, and ethambutol): 8-25 mg/kg 2-3 times weekly for first 2-3 months for severe disease (maximum single dose for age >50 years: 500 mg) (Griffith, 2007)

***Mycobacterium kansasii* disease (rifampin-resistant):** 750 mg to 1 g daily (as part of a three-drug regimen based on susceptibilities) (Campbell, 2000; Griffith, 2007)

***Mycobacterium ulcerans* (Buruli ulcers):** 15 mg/kg once daily for 8 weeks (WHO, 2004)

Plague: 30 mg/kg/day (or 2 g) divided every 12 hours until the patient is afebrile for at least 3 days. **Note:** Full course is considered 10 days (WHO, 2010).

Tuberculosis:

Daily therapy: 15 mg/kg/day (maximum: 1 g)

Directly observed therapy (DOT), twice weekly: 25-30 mg/kg (maximum: 1.5 g)

Directly observed therapy (DOT), 3 times weekly: 25-30 mg/kg (maximum: 1.5 g)

Tularemia:

Manufacturer's labeling: 1-2 g daily in divided doses every 12 hours (maximum: 2 g daily) for 7-14 days until the patients is afebrile for 5-7 days

Alternative regimen: 2 g daily in 2 divided doses (maximum: 2 g daily) for 10 days (WHO, 2007)

Elderly: IM: Manufacturer states dose reductions are necessary in patients >60 years.

Dosage adjustment in renal impairment: The following adjustments have been recommended (Aronoff, 2007):

CrCl 10-50 mL/minute: Administer every 24-72 hours.

CrCl <10 mL/minute: Administer every 72-96 hours.

Intermittent hemodialysis (IHD): One-half the dose administered after hemodialysis on dialysis days. **Note:** Dosing dependent on the assumption of 3 times weekly complete IHD sessions.

Peritoneal dialysis (PD): Administration via PD fluid: 20-40 mg/L (20-40 mcg/mL) of PD fluid

Continuous renal replacement therapy (CRRT): Administer every 24-72 hours; monitor levels. **Note:** Drug clearance is highly dependent on the method of renal replacement, filter type, and flow rate. Appropriate dosing requires close monitoring of pharmacologic response, signs of adverse reactions due to drug accumulation, as well as drug concentrations in relation to target trough (if appropriate).

Dosage adjustment in hepatic impairment: No dosage adjustment provided in manufacturer's labeling.

Administration Inject deep IM into large muscle mass; midlateral thigh muscle (preferred site for children); midlateral thigh muscle or upper buttocks (adults).

Monitoring Parameters Hearing (audiogram), BUN, creatinine; serum concentration of the drug should be monitored in all patients; eighth cranial nerve damage is usually preceded by high-pitched tinnitus, roaring noises, sense of fullness in ears, or impaired hearing and may persist for weeks after drug is discontinued

Reference Range Therapeutic: Peak: 20-30 mcg/mL; Trough: <5 mcg/mL; Toxic: Peak: >50 mcg/mL; Trough: >10 mcg/mL

Dosage Forms

Solution Reconstituted, Intramuscular:

Generic: 1 g (1 ea)

- **Streptomycin for Injection (Can)** *see* Streptomycin *on page 1937*
- **Streptomycin Sulfate** *see* Streptomycin *on page 1937*
- **Striant** *see* Testosterone *on page 2010*
- **Stribild** *see* Elvitegravir, Cobicistat, Emtricitabine, and Tenofovir *on page 718*
- **Striverdi Respimat** *see* Olodaterol *on page 1498*
- **Stromectol** *see* Ivermectin (Systemic) *on page 1136*
- **Strong Iodine Solution** *see* Potassium Iodide and Iodine *on page 1690*

Strontium Ranelate [INT]

(STRON shee um RAN el ate)

International Brand Names Osseor (CN, EE); Prodinam (AR); Protaxos (MY, TH); Protelos (AE, AT, BE, BH, CL, CR, CY, CZ, DE, DK, DO, EE, FR, GB, GR, GT, HN, HR, IE, IL, IT, KW, LT, NI, NL, PA, PE, PL, PT, QA, RO, SA, SE, SI, SK, SV, TR, UY, VN); Protos (AR, AU, BR, CO, HK, ID, NZ, PH, SG, TW); Ranemax (UY); Renelate (IN); Stronat (IN); Troncel (AR)

Pharmacologic Category Strontium Salt

Reported Use Treatment of postmenopausal osteoporosis to reduce the risk of vertebral fractures; treatment of severe osteoporosis in men at increased risk of fracture due to age/bone mineral density (BMD) score

Dosage Range

Adults: 2 g/day dissolved in water, prior to bedtime, 2 hours after eating (preferably)

Dosage adjustment in renal impairment: CrCl <30 mL/minute: Not recommended

Product Availability Product available in various countries; not currently available in the U.S.

Dosage Forms

Granules, oral suspension: 2 g/sachet (7s, 14s, 28s, 56s, 84s, 100s) [contains phenylalanine]

◆ **SU011248** *see* SUNItinib *on page 1957*

◆ **Suberoylanilide Hydroxamic Acid** *see* Vorinostat *on page 2182*

◆ **Sublinox (Can)** *see* Zolpidem *on page 2212*

◆ **Suboxone** *see* Buprenorphine and Naloxone *on page 304*

◆ **Subsys** *see* FentaNYL *on page 857*

Succimer (SUKS si mer)

Brand Names: U.S. Chemet
Brand Names: Canada Chemet
Index Terms DMSA
Pharmacologic Category Antidote
Use Treatment of lead poisoning in children with serum lead levels >45 mcg/dL
Pregnancy Risk Factor C

Dosage Lead poisoning: **Note:** For the treatment of high blood lead levels in children, the CDC recommends chelation treatment when blood lead levels are >45 mcg/dL (CDC, 2002). Children with blood lead levels >70 mcg/dL or symptomatic lead poisoning should be treated with parenteral agents (AAP, 2005). In adults, chelation therapy is recommended with blood lead levels >50 mcg/dL and significant symptoms; chelation therapy may also be indicated with blood lead levels ≥100 mcg/dL and/or symptoms. (Kosnett, 2007).

Children and Adolescents: Oral: 10 mg/kg/dose (or 350 mg/m^2/dose) every 8 hours for 5 days followed by 10 mg/kg/dose (or 350 mg/m^2/dose) every 12 hours for 14 days. Maximum: 500 mg/dose.

Adults (off-label use; Kosnett, 2007): Oral: Consider using labeled dose for children: 10 mg/kg/dose (or 350 mg/m^2/dose) every 8 hours for 5 days, followed by 10 mg/kg/dose (or 350 mg/m^2/dose) every 12 hours for 14 days; Maximum: 500 mg/dose

Note: Treatment courses may be repeated, but 2-week intervals between courses is generally recommended.

Dosage adjustment for toxicity: ANC <1200 mm^3: The manufacturer recommends withholding treatment; treatment may be cautiously resumed when ANC returns to baseline or >1500/mm^3. Consultation with a medical toxicologist to determine the risk versus benefit of withholding treatment is recommended.

Dosage adjustment in renal impairment: No dosage adjustment provided in the manufacturer's labeling; use with caution. Succimer is dialyzable; however, the lead chelates are not.

Dosage adjustment in hepatic impairment: No dosage adjustment provided in the manufacturer's labeling; has not been studied. More frequent monitoring of serum transaminases may be required in patients with a history of liver disease due to the risk of transient increases.

Additional Information Complete prescribing information should be consulted for additional detail.

Dosage Forms

Capsule, Oral:

Chemet: 100 mg

Succinylcholine (suks in il KOE leen)

Brand Names: U.S. Anectine; Quelicin; Quelicin-1000
Brand Names: Canada Quelicin®
Index Terms Succinylcholine Chloride; Suxamethonium Chloride
Pharmacologic Category Neuromuscular Blocker Agent, Depolarizing

Use To facilitate both rapid sequence and routine endotracheal intubation and to relax skeletal muscles during surgery

Note: Does not relieve pain or produce sedation

Pregnancy Risk Factor C

Pregnancy Considerations Reproduction studies have not been conducted. Small amounts cross the placenta. Sensitivity to succinylcholine may be increased due to a ~24% decrease in plasma cholinesterase activity during pregnancy and several days postpartum.

Breast-Feeding Considerations It is not known if succinylcholine is excreted in breast milk. The manufacturer recommends that caution be exercised when administering succinylcholine to nursing women.

Contraindications Hypersensitivity to succinylcholine or any component of the formulation; personal or familial history of malignant hyperthermia; myopathies associated with elevated serum creatine phosphokinase (CPK) values; acute phase of injury following major burns, multiple trauma, extensive denervation of skeletal muscle or upper motor neuron injury

Warnings/Precautions [U.S. Boxed Warning]: Use caution in children and adolescents. Acute rhabdomyolysis with hyperkalemia, ventricular arrhythmias and cardiac arrest have been reported (rarely) in children with undiagnosed skeletal muscle myopathy. Use in children should be reserved for emergency intubation or where immediate airway control is necessary. Use with caution in patients with preexisting hyperkalemia, extensive or severe burns; severe hyperkalemia may develop in patients with chronic abdominal infections, burn injuries, children with skeletal muscle myopathy, subarachnoid hemorrhage, or conditions which cause degeneration of the nervous system. Alkalosis, hypercalcemia, demyelinating lesions, peripheral neuropathies, denervation, infection, muscle trauma, and diabetes mellitus may result in antagonism of neuromuscular blockade. Electrolyte abnormalities, severe hyponatremia, severe hypocalcemia, severe hypokalemia, hypermagnesemia, neuromuscular diseases, acidosis, acute intermittent porphyria, Eaton-Lambert syndrome, myasthenia gravis, renal failure, and hepatic failure may result in potentiation of neuromuscular blockade. May increase vagal tone.

Succinylcholine is metabolized by plasma cholinesterase; use with caution (if at all) in patients suspected of being homozygous for the atypical plasma cholinesterase gene.

Use with caution in patients with extensive or severe burns; risk of hyperkalemia is increased following injury. May increase intraocular pressure; use caution with narrow angle glaucoma or penetrating eye injuries. Risk of bradycardia may be increased with second dose and may occur more in children. Use may be associated with acute onset of malignant hyperthermia; risk may be increased with concomitant administration of volatile anesthetics. Use with caution in the elderly; effects and duration are more variable.

Maintenance of an adequate airway and respiratory support is critical. Should be administered by adequately trained individuals familiar with its use.

Adverse Reactions

Cardiovascular: Arrhythmias, bradycardia (higher with second dose, more frequent in children), cardiac arrest, hyper-/hypotension, tachycardia

Dermatologic: Rash

Endocrine & metabolic: Hyperkalemia

Gastrointestinal: Salivation (excessive)

Neuromuscular & skeletal: Jaw rigidity, muscle fasciculation, postoperative muscle pain, rhabdomyolysis (with possible myoglobinuric acute renal failure)

▶

Ocular: Intraocular pressure increased
Renal: Acute renal failure (secondary to rhabdomyolysis)
Respiratory: Apnea, respiratory depression (prolonged)
Miscellaneous: Anaphylaxis, malignant hyperthermia
Rare but important or life-threatening: Acute quadriplegic myopathy syndrome (prolonged use), myositis ossificans (prolonged use)

Drug Interactions

Metabolism/Transport Effects None known.

Avoid Concomitant Use

Avoid concomitant use of Succinylcholine with any of the following: QuiNINE

Increased Effect/Toxicity

Succinylcholine may increase the levels/effects of: Analgesics (Opioid); Cardiac Glycosides; OnabotulinumtoxinA; RimabotulinumtoxinB

The levels/effects of Succinylcholine may be increased by: AbobotulinumtoxinA; Acetylcholinesterase Inhibitors; Aminoglycosides; Bambuterol; Capreomycin; Clindamycin (Topical); Colistimethate; Cyclophosphamide; CycloSPORINE (Systemic); Echothiophate Iodide; Lincosamide Antibiotics; Lithium; Loop Diuretics; Magnesium Salts; Phenelzine; Polymyxin B; Procainamide; QuiNIDine; QuiNINE; Tetracycline Derivatives; Vancomycin

Decreased Effect

The levels/effects of Succinylcholine may be decreased by: Loop Diuretics

Preparation for Administration May dilute to a final concentration of 1-2 mg/mL. Do not mix with alkaline solutions (pH >8.5).

Storage/Stability Manufacturer recommends refrigeration at 2°C to 8°C (36°F to 46°F) and may be stored at room temperature for 14 days; however, additional testing has demonstrated stability for ≤6 months unrefrigerated (25°C) (Ross, 1988; Roy, 2008). Stability in polypropylene syringes (20 mg/mL) at room temperature (25°C) is 45 days (Storms, 2003). Stability of parenteral admixture (1-2 mg/mL) at refrigeration temperature (4°C) is 24 hours in D_5W or NS.

Mechanism of Action Acts similar to acetylcholine, produces depolarization of the motor endplate at the myoneural junction which causes sustained flaccid skeletal muscle paralysis produced by state of accommodation that develops in adjacent excitable muscle membranes

Pharmacodynamics/Kinetics

Onset of action: IM: 2-3 minutes; IV: Complete muscular relaxation: 30-60 seconds
Duration: IM: 10-30 minutes; IV: 4-6 minutes with single administration
Metabolism: Rapidly hydrolyzed by plasma pseudocholinesterase
Excretion: Urine

Dosage IM, IV: Dose to effect; doses will vary due to interpatient variability. Use carefully and/or consider dose reduction in patients with reduced plasma cholinesterase activity due to genetic abnormalities of plasma cholinesterase or when associated with other conditions (eg, pregnancy, severe liver disease, renal disease); prolonged neuromuscular blockade may occur.

IM: Children and Adults: Up to 3-4 mg/kg, total dose should not exceed 150 mg

IV:

Smaller Children: Intermittent: Initial: 2 mg/kg/dose; maintenance: 0.3-0.6 mg/kg/dose every 5-10 minutes as needed

Older Children and Adolescents: Intermittent: Initial: 1 mg/kg/dose; maintenance: 0.3-0.6 mg/kg every 5-10 minutes as needed

Adults:

Intubation: 0.6 mg/kg (range: 0.3-1.1 mg/kg)
Rapid sequence intubation: 1-1.5 mg/kg (Sluga, 2005; Weiss, 1997)

Note: Initial dose of succinylcholine must be increased when nondepolarizing agent pretreatment used because of the antagonism between succinylcholine and nondepolarizing neuromuscular-blocking agents.

Dosing adjustment in renal impairment: No dosage adjustment provided in manufacturer's labeling.

Dosing adjustment in hepatic impairment: No dosage adjustment provided in manufacturer's labeling.

Dosing in obesity: Use total body weight for obese patients (Bentley, 1982; Brunette, 2004; Rose, 2000).

Administration May be administered by rapid IV injection without further dilution. IM injections should be made deeply, preferably high into deltoid muscle; use only when IV access is not available.

Monitoring Parameters Monitor cardiac, blood pressure, and oxygenation during administration; temperature, serum potassium and calcium, assisted ventilator status; neuromuscular function with a peripheral nerve stimulator

Dosage Forms

Solution, Injection:

Anectine: 20 mg/mL (10 mL)
Quelicin: 20 mg/mL (10 mL)
Quelicin-1000: 100 mg/mL (10 mL)

◆ **Succinylcholine Chloride** *see* Succinylcholine *on page 1939*

◆ **Suclear™** *see* Sodium Sulfate, Potassium Sulfate, Magnesium Sulfate, and Polyethylene Glycol-Electrolyte Solution *on page 1914*

◆ **Sucraid** *see* Sacrosidase *on page 1860*

◆ **Sucraid® (Can)** *see* Sacrosidase *on page 1860*

Sucralfate (soo KRAL fate)

Brand Names: U.S. Carafate

Brand Names: Canada Apo-Sucralfate; Dom-Sucralfate; Novo-Sucralate; Nu-Sucralate; PMS-Sucralate; Sucralfate-1; Sulcrate®; Sulcrate® Suspension Plus; Teva-Sucralfate

Index Terms Aluminum Sucrose Sulfate, Basic

Pharmacologic Category Gastrointestinal Agent, Miscellaneous

Use Short-term (≤8 weeks) management of duodenal ulcers; maintenance therapy for duodenal ulcers

Pregnancy Risk Factor B

Dosage Oral:

Children (off-label use): Doses of 40-80 mg/kg/day divided every 6 hours have been used

Adults: Duodenal ulcer:

Treatment: 1 g 4 times daily on an empty stomach for 4-8 weeks
Maintenance: Prophylaxis: 1 g twice daily

Dosage adjustment in renal impairment: No dosage adjustment provided in manufacturer's labeling. Aluminum salt is minimally absorbed; however, may accumulate in renal impairment; use with caution in patients with chronic renal failure.

Dosage adjustment in hepatic impairment: No dosage adjustment provided in manufacturer's labeling.

Additional Information Complete prescribing information should be consulted for additional detail.

Dosage Forms

Suspension, Oral:

Carafate: 1 g/10 mL (420 mL)

Tablet, Oral:

Carafate: 1 g

Generic: 1 g

- **Sucralfate-1 (Can)** *see* Sucralfate *on page 1940*
- **Sucrets® Children's [OTC]** *see* Dyclonine *on page 702*
- **Sucrets® Maximum Strength [OTC]** *see* Dyclonine *on page 702*
- **Sucrets® Regular Strength [OTC]** *see* Dyclonine *on page 702*

Sucroferric Oxyhydroxide

(soo kroe FER ik ox ee hye DROX ide)

Brand Names: U.S. Velphoro

Index Terms PA21; Polynuclear Iron (III)-Oxyhydroxide (pn-FeOOH)

Pharmacologic Category Phosphate Binder

Use Hyperphosphatemia: For control of serum phosphorus levels in patients with chronic kidney disease (CKD) receiving dialysis

Pregnancy Risk Factor B

Pregnancy Considerations Adverse events were not observed in most animal reproduction studies. Maternal systemic absorption of sucroferric oxyhydroxide is low

Breast-Feeding Considerations It is not known if sucroferric oxyhydroxide is excreted into breast milk; however, because maternal systemic absorption is limited, it is unlikely

Contraindications There are no contraindications listed in the manufacturer's labeling.

Warnings/Precautions Patients with significant gastrointestinal (GI) disorders or hepatic disorders, post major GI surgery, peritonitis during peritoneal dialysis, or with a history of hemochromatosis or other conditions associated with iron accumulation were not included in clinical studies; monitor effect and iron homeostasis in these patients. Chew tablets thoroughly to decrease risk of adverse GI effects; do not swallow whole. Potentially significant interactions may exist, requiring dose or frequency adjustment, additional monitoring, and/or selection of alternative therapy.

Adverse Reactions Gastrointestinal: Darkening of stools, diarrhea, dysgeusia, nausea

Drug Interactions

Metabolism/Transport Effects None known.

Avoid Concomitant Use

Avoid concomitant use of Sucroferric Oxyhydroxide with any of the following: Levothyroxine

Increased Effect/Toxicity There are no known significant interactions involving an increase in effect.

Decreased Effect

Sucroferric Oxyhydroxide may decrease the levels/effects of: Levothyroxine; Tetracycline Derivatives

Storage/Stability Store at 25°C (77°F); excursions are permitted between 15°C and 30°C (59°F and 86°F). Protect from moisture.

Mechanism of Action Binds phosphate in the aqueous environment of the GI tract via ligand exchange between hydroxyl groups and/or water in sucroferric oxyhydroxide and dietary phosphate. Reduced dietary phosphate absorption results in reduced serum phosphorus levels and calcium-phosphorus product levels.

Pharmacodynamics/Kinetics

Absorption: Not systemically absorbed

Metabolism: Not metabolized

Excretion: Feces (as bound phosphate)

Dosage

Oral: Adults: Hyperphosphatemia: Initial: 500 mg iron 3 times daily with meals. May titrate weekly (beginning 1 week after initiation) in increments or decrements of 500 mg iron per day as needed to appropriate serum phosphorus levels (≤5.5 mg/dL); usual maintenance dose: 1.5 to 2 g iron daily; doses of up to 3 g iron daily have been evaluated.

Dosage adjustment in renal impairment: There are no dosage adjustments provided in the manufacturer's labeling; however, not systemically absorbed or metabolized.

Dosage adjustment in hepatic impairment: There are no dosage adjustments provided in the manufacturer's labeling; however, not systemically absorbed or metabolized.

Administration Tablets must be chewed; do not swallow whole. Tablets may be crushed to aid with chewing and swallowing. Must administer with meals. The total daily dose should be divided among meals.

Monitoring Parameters Serum phosphorus levels

Dosage Forms

Tablet Chewable, Oral:

Velphoro: 500 mg

- **Sudafed** *see* Pseudoephedrine *on page 1742*
- **Sudafed [OTC]** *see* Pseudoephedrine *on page 1742*
- **Sudafed 12 Hour [OTC]** *see* Pseudoephedrine *on page 1742*
- **Sudafed 24 Hour [OTC]** *see* Pseudoephedrine *on page 1742*
- **Sudafed Childrens [OTC]** *see* Pseudoephedrine *on page 1742*
- **Sudafed® Children's Cold & Cough [OTC]** *see* Pseudoephedrine and Dextromethorphan *on page 1743*
- **Sudafed® Decongestant (Can)** *see* Pseudoephedrine *on page 1742*
- **Sudafed PE Childrens [OTC]** *see* Phenylephrine (Systemic) *on page 1638*
- **Sudafed PE® Children's Cold & Cough [OTC]** *see* Dextromethorphan and Phenylephrine *on page 611*
- **Sudafed PE Maximum Strength [OTC]** *see* Phenylephrine (Systemic) *on page 1638*
- **Sudafed PE® Non-Drying Sinus [OTC]** *see* Guaifenesin and Phenylephrine *on page 988*
- **Sudafed PE® Sinus + Allergy [OTC]** *see* Chlorpheniramine and Phenylephrine *on page 426*
- **Sudafed® Sinus Advance (Can)** *see* Pseudoephedrine and Ibuprofen *on page 1743*
- **Sudanyl [OTC]** *see* Pseudoephedrine *on page 1742*
- **SudoGest [OTC]** *see* Pseudoephedrine *on page 1742*
- **SudoGest 12 Hour [OTC]** *see* Pseudoephedrine *on page 1742*
- **Sudogest PE [OTC]** *see* Phenylephrine (Systemic) *on page 1638*
- **SudoGest™ Sinus & Allergy [OTC]** *see* Chlorpheniramine and Pseudoephedrine *on page 427*
- **Sufenta** *see* SUFentanil *on page 1941*

SUFentanil (soo FEN ta nil)

Brand Names: U.S. Sufenta

Brand Names: Canada Sufenta; Sufentanil Citrate Injection, USP

Index Terms Sufentanil Citrate

Pharmacologic Category Analgesic, Opioid; Anilidopiperidine Opioid; General Anesthetic

Use

Epidural analgesia: For epidural administration as an analgesic combined with low-dose bupivacaine during labor and vaginal delivery.

Surgical analgesia: Analgesic adjunct for the maintenance of balanced general anesthesia in patients who are intubated and ventilated.

Surgical anesthesia: As a primary anesthetic agent for the induction and maintenance of anesthesia with 100% oxygen in patients undergoing major surgical procedures; in patients who are intubated and ventilated, such as cardiovascular surgery or neurosurgical procedures in the sitting position; to provide favorable myocardial and cerebral oxygen balance or when extended postoperative ventilation is anticipated.

Pregnancy Risk Factor C

Dosage

IV:

Children <12 years: Surgical *anesthesia* (cardiovascular surgery): Induction: 10 to 25 mcg/kg with 100% O_2; Maintenance: Up to 25 to 50 mcg based on response to initial dose and as determined by changes in vital signs indicating surgical stress or lightening of anesthesia.

Adults:

Surgical analgesia (as a component of balanced anesthesia) (surgery expected to last **1 to 2** hours): Total dose: 1 to 2 mcg/kg with N_2O/O_2; ≥75% of total dose may be administered by slow injection or infusion prior to intubation (titrate to individual response)

Maintenance:

Incremental dosing: According to the manufacturer, 10 to 25 mcg may be administered as needed when movement and/or changes in vital signs indicate surgical stress or lightening of analgesia. May also administer doses in the range of 5 to 20 mcg as needed (Barash, 2009) **or** 0.1 to 0.25 mcg/**kg** as needed (Miller, 2010). Total dose should not exceed 1 mcg/kg/hour of expected surgical time.

Continuous infusion: May also be administered as a continuous infusion with the infusion rate based on the induction dose used. Maximum infusion rate according to the manufacturer: 1 mcg/kg/hour. May also administer doses in the range of 0.3 to 0.9 mcg/kg/hour (Barash, 2009) **or** 0.5 to 1.5 mcg/kg/hour (Miller, 2010).

Surgical analgesia (as a component of balanced anesthesia) (surgery expected to last **2 to 8** hours): Total dose: 2 to 8 mcg/kg with N_2O/O_2; ≤75% of total dose may be administered by slow injection or infusion prior to intubation (titrate to individual response).

Maintenance:

Incremental dosing: According to the manufacturer, 10 to 50 mcg may be administered as needed when movement and/or changes in vital signs indicate surgical stress or lightening of analgesia. Total dose should not exceed 1 mcg/kg/hour of expected surgical time.

Continuous infusion: May also be administered as a continuous infusion with the infusion rate based on the induction dose used. Maximum infusion rate according to the manufacturer: 1 mcg/kg/hour. May also administer doses in the range of 0.3 to 0.9 mcg/kg/hour (Barash, 2009) **or** 0.5 to 1.5 mcg/kg/hour (Miller, 2010).

Surgical *anesthesia*: Total dose: 8 to 30 mcg/kg as a slow injection, infusion, or injection followed by infusion; titrate to individual patient response. **Note:** In patients administered high doses of sufentanil, qualified personnel and adequate facilities are necessary to manage the potential for postoperative respiratory depression.

Maintenance:

Incremental dosing: 0.5 to 10 mcg/kg as needed in anticipation of surgical stress

Continuous infusion: Base infusion rate on the induction dose so that the total dose for the procedure does not exceed 30 mcg/kg

Epidural: Analgesia for labor and delivery: Adults: 10 to 15 mcg with bupivacaine 0.125% with/without epinephrine. Dose can be repeated twice (for a total of 3 doses) at not less than 1-hour intervals until delivery.

Elderly: Dosage should be reduced.

Dosing in obesity: IV: In adult obese patients (eg, >20% above ideal body weight), use lean body weight to determine dosage.

Dosage adjustment in renal impairment: There are no dosage adjustments provided in the manufacturer's labeling. Use with caution.

Dosage adjustment in hepatic impairment: There are no dosage adjustments provided in the manufacturer's labeling. Use with caution.

Additional Information Complete prescribing information should be consulted for additional detail.

Dosage Forms

Solution, Intravenous [preservative free]:

Sufenta: 50 mcg/mL (1 mL); 100 mcg/2 mL (2 mL); 250 mcg/5 mL (5 mL)

Generic: 50 mcg/mL (1 mL); 100 mcg/2 mL (2 mL); 250 mcg/5 mL (5 mL)

◆ **Sufentanil Citrate** *see* SUFentanil *on page 1941*

◆ **Sufentanil Citrate Injection, USP (Can)** *see* SUFentanil *on page 1941*

Sugammadex [INT] (soo GAM ma dex)

International Brand Names Bridion (AR, AT, AU, BE, BR, CH, CL, CO, CY, CZ, DK, EE, ES, FR, GB, GR, HR, HU, IL, IS, JP, KR, LB, LT, MX, MY, NL, NO, NZ, PE, PH, PL, PT, RO, RU, SE, SG, SI, SK, TH, TR)

Pharmacologic Category Antidote

Reported Use Reversal of neuromuscular blockade induced by rocuronium or vecuronium

Dosage Range IV:

Children and Adolescents ≥2 to ≤17 years: Routine reversal of rocuronium-induced neuromuscular blockade: 2 mg/kg

Adults ≥18 years:

Reversal of rocuronium- or vecuronium-induced deep blockade: 4 mg/kg

Reversal of rocuronium- or vecuronium-induced moderate blockade: 2 mg/kg; may repeat with 4 mg/kg if reoccurrence of blockade occurs

Immediate reversal of rocuronium-induced blockade: 16 mg/kg

Note: Wait 24 hours before readministering rocuronium or vecuronium after immediate reversal

Dosage adjustment in renal impairment:

CrCl ≥30 to <80 mL/minute: No dosage adjustment necessary

CrCl <30 mL/minute or patients on dialysis: Use not recommended

Dosage adjustment in hepatic impairment:

Mild-to-moderate impairment: No dosage adjustment necessary

Severe impairment: No dosage adjustment provided in manufacturer's labeling (has not been studied)

Product Availability Product available in various countries; not currently available in the U.S.

Dosage Forms

Injection, solution: 100 mg/mL (2 mL, 5 mL)

- ◆ **Sulamyd** *see* Sulfacetamide (Ophthalmic) *on page 1943*
- ◆ **Sulamyd** *see* Sulfacetamide (Topical) *on page 1943*
- ◆ **Sular** *see* Nisoldipine *on page 1459*
- ◆ **Sulbactam and Ampicillin** *see* Ampicillin and Sulbactam *on page 145*
- ◆ **Sulbactam and Cefoperazone** *see* Cefoperazone and Sulbactam [INT] *on page 382*

Sulconazole (sul KON a zole)

Brand Names: U.S. Exelderm

Brand Names: Canada Exelderm®

Index Terms Sulconazole Nitrate

Pharmacologic Category Antifungal Agent, Imidazole Derivative; Antifungal Agent, Topical

Use Treatment of superficial fungal infections of the skin, including tinea cruris (jock itch), tinea corporis (ringworm), tinea versicolor, and tinea pedis (athlete's foot, cream only)

Pregnancy Risk Factor C

Dosage Adults: Topical: Apply a small amount to the affected area and gently massage once or twice daily (tinea pedis apply twice daily) for 3 weeks (tinea cruris, tinea corporis, tinea versicolor) to 4 weeks (tinea pedis).

Additional Information Complete prescribing information should be consulted for additional detail.

Dosage Forms

Cream, External:

Exelderm: 1% (15 g, 30 g, 60 g)

Solution, External:

Exelderm: 1% (30 mL)

- ◆ **Sulconazole Nitrate** *see* Sulconazole *on page 1943*
- ◆ **Sulcrate® (Can)** *see* Sucralfate *on page 1940*
- ◆ **Sulcrate® Suspension Plus (Can)** *see* Sucralfate *on page 1940*

Sulfacetamide (Ophthalmic) (sul fa SEE ta mide)

Brand Names: U.S. Bleph-10

Brand Names: Canada AK Sulf Liq; Bleph 10 DPS; Diosulf; PMS-Sulfacetamide; Sodium Sulamyd

Index Terms Sodium Sulfacetamide; Sulamyd; Sulfacetamide Sodium

Pharmacologic Category Antibiotic, Ophthalmic

Use

Ocular infections: Treatment of conjunctivitis and other superficial ocular infections due to susceptible microorganisms, and as an adjunctive in systemic sulfonamide therapy of trachoma: *Escherichia coli*, *Staphylococcus aureus*, *Streptococcus pneumoniae*, *Streptococcus* (viridans group), *Haemophilus influenzae*, *Klebsiella species*, and *Enterobacter* species.

Limitations of use: Topically applied sulfonamides do not provide adequate coverage against *Neisseria* species, *Serratia marcescens* and *Pseudomonas aeruginosa*. A significant percentage of staphylococcal isolates are also completely resistant to sulfa drugs.

Pregnancy Risk Factor C

Dosage Infants ≥2 months, Children, Adolescents, and Adults: Ophthalmic:

Conjunctivitis, other superficial ocular infections: Instill 1 to 2 drops every 2 to 3 hours; taper by increasing dosage time interval as condition responds. Usual duration of treatment: 7 to 10 days

Trachoma: Instill 2 drops every 2 hours; must be used in conjunction with systemic therapy

Additional Information Complete prescribing information should be consulted for additional detail.

Dosage Forms

Ointment, Ophthalmic:

Generic: 10% (3.5 g)

Solution, Ophthalmic:

Bleph-10: 10% (5 mL)

Generic: 10% (15 mL)

Sulfacetamide (Topical) (sul fa SEE ta mide)

Brand Names: U.S. APOP [DSC]; Klaron; Ovace Plus; Ovace Plus Wash; Ovace Wash; Seb-Prev Wash; Seb-Prev [DSC]

Brand Names: Canada Sulfacet-R

Index Terms Sodium Sulfacetamide; Sulamyd; Sulfacetamide Sodium

Pharmacologic Category Acne Products; Antibiotic, Sulfonamide Derivative; Topical Skin Product, Acne

Use

Acne (Klaron lotion, topical suspension): Treatment of acne vulgaris.

Bacterial infections (cream, wash, Ovace Plus lotion): Treatment of bacterial infections of the skin.

Scaling dermatoses (cream, shampoo, wash, Ovace Plus lotion): Treatment of scaling dermatoses (seborrheic dermatitis and seborrhea sicca [dandruff]).

Pregnancy Risk Factor C

Dosage Topical: Children ≥12 years, Adolescents, and Adults:

Acne: Klaron lotion, topical suspension: Apply thin film to affected area twice daily

Bacterial infections:

Cream, Ovace Plus lotion: Apply to affected areas twice daily for 8 to 10 days.

Wash: Apply to affected areas 1 to 2 times daily for 8 to 10 days.

Scaling dermatoses:

Cream, Ovace Plus lotion: Apply to affected areas twice daily for 8 to 10 days. Dosing interval may be lengthened as eruption subsides. Applications once or twice weekly, or every other week may be used for prevention. If treatment needs to be reinitiated, start therapy as a twice-daily regimen.

Shampoo: Wash hair at least twice weekly.

Wash:

Ovace Plus Wash Liquid, Ovace Plus Wash cleansing gel, Ovace wash: Wash affected areas twice with a 10- to 20-second interval between washings; repeat twice daily for 8 to 10 days. Dosing interval may be lengthened as eruption subsides. Applications once or twice weekly, or every other week may be used for prevention. If treatment needs to be reinitiated, start therapy as a twice-daily regimen.

SEB-Prev: Wash affected areas twice daily for 8 to 10 days. Dosing interval may be lengthened as eruption subsides. Applications once or twice weekly, or every other week may be used for prevention. If treatment needs to be reinitiated, start therapy as a twice-daily regimen.

Additional Information Complete prescribing information should be consulted for additional detail.

Dosage Forms Considerations APOP gel is formulated in a vehicle containing 0.5% bakuchiol, a natural compound extracted from *Psoralea corylifolia* purported to exert antimicrobial and anti-inflammatory activity, as well as reduce scarring from acne lesions.

Dosage Forms

Cream, External:

Ovace Plus: 10% (57 g)

Gel, External:
Ovace Plus Wash: 10% (355 mL)
Generic: 10% (340.2 g); 10% (355 mL)
Liquid, External:
Ovace Plus Wash: 10% (180 mL, 473 mL)
Ovace Wash: 10% (180 mL, 355 mL, 480 mL)
Seb-Prev Wash: 10% (340 mL)
Generic: 10% (177 mL, 354.8 mL, 355 mL, 480 mL)
Lotion, External:
Klaron: 10% (118 mL)
Ovace Plus: 9.8% (57 g)
Generic: 10% (118 mL)
Shampoo, External:
Ovace Plus: 10% (237 mL)
Generic: 10% (237 mL)
Suspension, External:
Generic: 10% (118 mL)

Sulfacetamide and Prednisolone

(sul fa SEE ta mide & pred NIS oh lone)

Brand Names: U.S. Blephamide®
Brand Names: Canada AK Cide Oph; Blephamide®; Dioptimyd®
Index Terms Prednisolone and Sulfacetamide
Pharmacologic Category Antibiotic/Corticosteroid, Ophthalmic
Use Steroid-responsive inflammatory ocular conditions in which a corticosteroid is indicated and where infection is present or there is a risk of infection
Pregnancy Risk Factor C
Dosage Ophthalmic:
Children ≥6 years and Adults:
Ointment: Apply ~1/2 inch ribbon to lower conjunctival sac 3-4 times/day and 1-2 times at night
Solution: Instill 2 drops every 4 hours
Suspension: Instill 2 drops every 4 hours during the day and at bedtime
Additional Information Complete prescribing information should be consulted for additional detail.
Dosage Forms
Ointment, ophthalmic:
Blephamide®: Sulfacetamide 10% and prednisolone 0.2% (3.5 g)
Solution, ophthalmic: Sulfacetamide 10% and prednisolone 0.25% (5 mL, 10 mL)
Suspension, ophthalmic:
Blephamide®: Sulfacetamide 10% and prednisolone 0.2% (5 mL, 10 mL)

◆ **Sulfacetamide and Sulfur** *see* Sulfur and Sulfacetamide *on page 1953*

◆ **Sulfacetamide Sodium** *see* Sulfacetamide (Ophthalmic) *on page 1943*

◆ **Sulfacetamide Sodium** *see* Sulfacetamide (Topical) *on page 1943*

◆ **Sulfacet-R (Can)** *see* Sulfacetamide (Topical) *on page 1943*

◆ **Sulfacet-R (Can)** *see* Sulfur and Sulfacetamide *on page 1953*

◆ **SulfaCleanse 8/4** *see* Sulfur and Sulfacetamide *on page 1953*

SulfADIAZINE

(sul fa DYE a zeen)

Pharmacologic Category Antibiotic, Sulfonamide Derivative
Use Treatment of the following conditions (per product labeling): Chancroid, trachoma, inclusion conjunctivitis, nocardiosis, urinary tract infections, toxoplasmosis encephalitis, malaria, meningococcal meningitis, acute otitis media, rheumatic fever (prophylaxis), meningitis (adjunctive)

Refer to current guidelines for appropriate use.
Pregnancy Risk Factor C
Pregnancy Considerations Adverse events have been observed in animal reproduction studies. Sulfadiazine crosses the placenta (Speert, 1943). Available studies and case reports have failed to show an increased risk for congenital malformations after sulfadiazine use (Heinonen, 1977); however, studies with sulfonamides as a class have shown mixed results (ACOG, 2011).

Sulfadiazine is recommended for use in pregnant women to prevent *T. gondii* infection of the fetus, for the maternal treatment of *Toxoplasmic gondii* encephalitis, and as an alternative agent for the secondary prevention of rheumatic fever (CDC, 2009; DHHS, 2013; Gerber, 2009). Sulfonamides may be used to treat other infections in pregnant women when clinically appropriate for confirmed infections caused by susceptible organisms; use during the first trimester should be limited to situations where no alternative therapies are available (ACOG, 2011). Because safer options are available for the treatment of urinary tract infections in pregnant women, use of sulfonamide-containing products >32 weeks gestation should be avoided (Lee, 2008). Due to the theoretical increased risk for hyperbilirubinemia and kernicterus, sulfadiazine is contraindicated by the manufacturer for use near term. Neonatal healthcare providers should be informed if maternal sulfonamide therapy is used near the time of delivery (DHHS, 2013).
Breast-Feeding Considerations Sulfadiazine distributes into human milk. Sulfonamides should not be used while nursing an infant with G6PD deficiency or hyperbilirubinemia (Della-Giustina, 2003). Per the manufacturer, sulfadiazine is contraindicated in nursing mothers since sulfonamides cross into the milk and may cause kernicterus in the newborn. Nondose-related effects could include modification of bowel flora.
Contraindications Hypersensitivity to any sulfa drug or any component of the formulation; infants <2 months of age unless indicated for the treatment of congenital toxoplasmosis; pregnancy (at term); breast-feeding
Warnings/Precautions Fatalities associated with severe reactions including agranulocytosis, aplastic anemia and other blood dyscrasias, hepatic necrosis, Stevens-Johnson syndrome, and toxic epidermal necrolysis have occurred; discontinue use at first sign of rash or signs of serious adverse reactions. Use with caution in patients with allergies or asthma.

Chemical similarities are present among sulfonamides, sulfonylureas, carbonic anhydrase inhibitors, thiazides, and loop diuretics (except ethacrynic acid). Use in patients with sulfonamide allergy is specifically contraindicated in product labeling; however, a risk of cross-reaction exists in patients with allergy to any of these compounds; avoid use when previous reaction has been severe.

Not for the treatment of group A beta-hemolytic streptococcal infections. Prolonged use may result in fungal or bacterial superinfection, including *C. difficile*-associated diarrhea (CDAD) and pseudomembranous colitis; CDAD has been observed >2 months postantibiotic treatment. Use with caution in patients with G6PD deficiency; hemolysis may occur. Use with caution in patients with hepatic impairment. Use with caution in patients with renal impairment; dosage modification required. Maintain adequate hydration to prevent crystalluria. Sulfa antibiotics have been shown to displace bilirubin from protein binding sites which may potentially lead to hyperbilirubinemia and kernicterus in neonates and young infants; do not use in neonates; avoid use in infants <2 months unless other options are not available.

Benzyl alcohol and derivatives: Some dosage forms may contain sodium benzoate/benzoic acid; benzoic acid (benzoate) is a metabolite of benzyl alcohol; large amounts of benzyl alcohol (≥99 mg/kg/day) have been associated with a potentially fatal toxicity ("gasping syndrome") in neonates; the "gasping syndrome" consists of metabolic acidosis, respiratory distress, gasping respirations, CNS dysfunction (including convulsions, intracranial hemorrhage), hypotension, and cardiovascular collapse (AAP, 1997; CDC, 1982); some data suggests that benzoate displaces bilirubin from protein binding sites (Ahlfors, 2001); avoid or use dosage forms containing benzyl alcohol derivative with caution in neonates. See manufacturer's labeling.

Adverse Reactions

Cardiovascular: Allergic myocarditis, periarteritis nodosa

Central nervous system: Ataxia, chills, convulsions, depression, fever, hallucinations, headache, insomnia, vertigo

Dermatologic: Epidermal necrolysis, erythema multiforme, exfoliative dermatitis, photosensitivity, pruritus, purpura, rash, skin eruptions, Stevens-Johnson syndrome, urticaria

Endocrine & metabolic: Hypoglycemia, thyroid function disturbance

Gastrointestinal: Abdominal pain, anorexia, diarrhea, nausea, pancreatitis, stomatitis, vomiting

Genitourinary: Crystalluria, stone formation, toxic nephrosis with oliguria and anuria

Hematologic: Agranulocytopenia, aplastic anemia, hemolytic anemia, hypoprothrombinemia, leukopenia, methemoglobinemia, thrombocytopenia

Hepatic: Hepatitis

Neuromuscular & skeletal: Arthralgia, peripheral neuritis

Ocular: Conjunctival/scleral injection, periorbital edema

Otic: Tinnitus

Renal: Diuresis

Miscellaneous: Anaphylactoid reactions, lupus erythematosus, serum sickness-like reactions

Drug Interactions

Metabolism/Transport Effects Substrate of CYP2C9 (major), CYP2E1 (minor), CYP3A4 (minor); **Note:** Assignment of Major/Minor substrate status based on clinically relevant drug interaction potential; **Inhibits** CYP2C9 (strong)

Avoid Concomitant Use

Avoid concomitant use of SulfADIAZINE with any of the following: BCG; Methenamine; Potassium P-Aminobenzoate; Procaine

Increased Effect/Toxicity

SulfADIAZINE may increase the levels/effects of: Bosentan; Carvedilol; CycloSPORINE (Systemic); CYP2C9 Substrates; Diclofenac (Systemic); Dronabinol; Lacosamide; Methotrexate; Ospemifene; Porfimer; Prilocaine; Sodium Nitrite; Sulfonylureas; Tetrahydrocannabinol; Verteporfin; Vitamin K Antagonists

The levels/effects of SulfADIAZINE may be increased by: Cannabis; Ceritinib; CYP2C9 Inhibitors (Moderate); CYP2C9 Inhibitors (Strong); Dexketoprofen; Methenamine; Mifepristone; Nitric Oxide

Decreased Effect

SulfADIAZINE may decrease the levels/effects of: BCG; CycloSPORINE (Systemic); Sodium Picosulfate; Typhoid Vaccine

The levels/effects of SulfADIAZINE may be decreased by: CYP2C9 Inducers (Strong); Dabrafenib; Potassium P-Aminobenzoate; Procaine

Food Interactions Vitamin C or acidifying agents (cranberry juice) may cause crystalluria. Management: Avoid large quantities of vitamin C or acidifying agents (cranberry juice).

Storage/Stability Store at controlled room temperature of 20°C to 25°C (68°F to 77°F). Protect from light.

Mechanism of Action Interferes with bacterial growth by inhibiting bacterial folic acid synthesis through competitive antagonism of PABA

Pharmacodynamics/Kinetics

Absorption: Well absorbed

Distribution: Throughout body tissues and fluids including pleural, peritoneal, synovial, and ocular fluids; throughout total body water; readily diffused into CSF

Protein binding: 38% to 48%

Metabolism: Via N-acetylation

Half-life elimination: 10 hours

Time to peak: Within 3-6 hours

Excretion: Urine (43% to 60% as unchanged drug, 15% to 40% as metabolites)

Dosage Oral:

General dosing guidelines:

Children >2 months of age: Initial: 75 mg/kg; Maintenance: 150 mg/kg/day in 4-6 divided doses (maximum: 6 g/24 hours)

Adults: 2-4 g/day in 3-6 divided doses

Rheumatic fever prophylaxis: Children and Adults:

<30 kg: 0.5 g/day

≥30 kg: 1 g/day

Toxoplasmosis (HIV-exposed/-positive patients) (CDC, 2009):

Congenital toxoplasmosis: Infants: 100 mg/kg/day in divided doses every 12 hours for 12 months in combination with pyrimethamine plus leucovorin calcium

Acquired toxoplasmosis: Infants and Children:

Acute induction therapy: 25-50 mg/kg/dose given 4 times/day (maximum: 1-1.5 g/dose) in combination with pyrimethamine and leucovorin calcium. Continue acute induction therapy for ≥6 weeks, then follow with chronic suppressive therapy.

Prophylaxis to prevent recurrence (prior to encephalitis): 85-120 mg/kg/day divided every 6-12 hours (maximum: 2-4 g/day) in combination with pyrimethamine plus leucovorin calcium

Toxoplasma gondii encephalitis: Adolescents and Adults:

Acute therapy (duration of therapy: ≥6 weeks): 1000 mg (<60 kg) or 1500 mg (≥60 kg) every 6 hours in combination with pyrimethamine plus leucovorin calcium (preferred) **or** alternatively, may give 1000-1500 mg every 6 hours in combination with atovaquone

Prophylaxis to prevent recurrence: 2000-4000 mg/day in 2-4 divided doses in combination with pyrimethamine and leucovorin calcium (preferred) **or** alternatively, may give 2000-4000 mg/day in 2-4 divided doses in combination with atovaquone

Dietary Considerations Supplemental leucovorin calcium should be administered to reverse symptoms or prevent problems due to folic acid deficiency.

Administration Administer with at least 8 ounces of water and around-the-clock to promote less variation in peak and trough serum levels. Oral sodium bicarbonate may be used to alkalinize the urine of patients unable to maintain adequate fluid intake (in order to prevent crystalluria, azotemia, oliguria) (Lerner, 1996).

Monitoring Parameters Perform culture and sensitivity testing prior to initiating therapy; frequent CBC and urinalysis during therapy; signs of serious blood disorders (sore throat, fever, pallor, purpura, jaundice); CD4+ count in HIV-exposed/-positive patients treated for toxoplasmosis; sulfonamide blood concentrations may be monitored for severe infections (target: 12-15 mg/100 mL)

Dosage Forms

Tablet, Oral:

Generic: 500 mg

Extemporaneous Preparations A 200 mg/mL oral suspension may be made with sulfadiazine powder and sterile water. Place 50 g sulfadiazine powder in a glass mortar. Add small portions of sterile water and mix to a uniform paste; mix while incrementally adding sterile water to **almost** 250 mL; transfer to a calibrated bottle, rinse mortar with sterile water, and add sufficient quantity of sterile water to make 250 mL. Label "shake well" and "refrigerate". Stable for 3 days refrigerated. **Note:** Suspension may also be prepared by crushing one-hundred 500 mg tablets; however, it is stable for only 2 days.

Pathmanathan U, Halgrain D, Chiadmi F, et al, "Stability of Sulfadiazine Oral Liquids Prepared From Tablets and Powder," *J Pharm Pharm Sci*, 2004, 7(1):84-7.

Sulfadoxine and Pyrimethamine [INT]

(sul fa DOKS een & peer i METH a meen)

International Brand Names Amalar (VN); Croydoxin-FM (IN); Falcistat (TR); Fansidar (AE, AT, AU, BH, BR, CH, CY, EG, FR, GB, GH, GR, ID, IE, IL, IQ, IR, JO, KW, LB, LY, OM, PE, PH, PK, PL, QA, SA, SY, TZ, UG, VN, YE, ZM); Fansitab (AE, BH, CY, EG, IL, IQ, IR, JO, KW, LB, LY, OM, QA, SA, SY, YE); Laridox (IN); Madomine (MY); Malafon (MY); Malerim (AE, BH, CY, EG, IL, IQ, IR, JO, KW, LB, LY, OM, QA, SA, SY, YE); Malocide (IN); Pansida (KR); Plasmodin (ID); Pyralfin (BF, BJ, CI, ET, GH, GM, GN, KE, LR, MA, ML, MR, MU, MW, NE, NG, SC, SD, SL, SN, TN, TZ, UG, ZA, ZM, ZW); Rimodar (IN); Suldox (ID); Vansilar (TH)

Index Terms Pyrimethamine and Sulfadoxine

Pharmacologic Category Antimalarial Agent

Reported Use Treatment or prophylaxis of *Plasmodium falciparum* malaria (wide-spread resistance may require combination therapy with other antimalarial agents).

Dosage Range

Adults: Oral: 3 tablets (total of sulfadoxine 1500 mg and pyrimethamine 75 mg) as a single dose.

Weight-based dosing: Sulfadoxine 25 to 70 mg/kg and pyrimethamine 1.25 to 3.5 mg/kg as a single dose.

Product Availability Product available in various countries; not currently available in the U.S.

Dosage Forms

Tablet, oral: Sulfadoxine 500 mg and pyrimethamine 25 mg

Sulfamethoxazole and Trimethoprim

(sul fa meth OKS a zole & trye METH oh prim)

Brand Names: U.S. Bactrim; Bactrim DS; Septra DS; Sulfatrim

Brand Names: Canada Apo-Sulfatrim; Apo-Sulfatrim DS; Apo-Sulfatrim Pediatric; Protrin DF; Septra Injection; Teva-Trimel; Teva-Trimel DS; Trisulfa; Trisulfa DS; Trisulfa S

Index Terms Co-Trimoxazole; Septra; SMX-TMP; SMZ-TMP; Sulfatrim; TMP-SMX; TMP-SMZ; Trimethoprim and Sulfamethoxazole

Pharmacologic Category Antibiotic, Miscellaneous; Antibiotic, Sulfonamide Derivative

Use

Oral: Treatment of urinary tract infections due to *E. coli, Klebsiella* and *Enterobacter* sp, *M. morganii, P. mirabilis* and *P. vulgaris*; acute otitis media; acute exacerbations of chronic bronchitis due to susceptible strains of *H. influenzae* or *S. pneumoniae*; treatment and prophylaxis of *Pneumocystis jirovecii* pneumonia (PCP); traveler's diarrhea due to enterotoxigenic *E. coli*; treatment of enteritis caused by *Shigella flexneri* or *Shigella sonnei*

IV: Treatment of *Pneumocystis jirovecii* pneumonia (PCP); treatment of enteritis caused by *Shigella flexneri* or *Shigella sonnei*; treatment of severe or complicated urinary tract infections due to *E. coli, Klebsiella* and *Enterobacter* spp, *M. morganii, P. mirabilis,* and *P. vulgaris*

Pregnancy Risk Factor D

Pregnancy Considerations Adverse events have been observed in animal reproduction studies. Trimethoprim-sulfamethoxazole (TMP-SMX) crosses the placenta and distributes to amniotic fluid (Ylikorkala, 1973). An increased risk of congenital malformations (neural tube defects, cardiovascular malformations, urinary tract defects, oral clefts, club foot) following maternal use of TMP-SMX during pregnancy has been observed in some studies. Folic acid supplementation may decrease this risk (Crider, 2009; Czeizel, 2001; Hernandez-Diaz, 2000; Hernandez-Diaz, 2001; Matok, 2009). Due to theoretical concerns that sulfonamides pass the placenta and may cause kernicterus in the newborn, neonatal healthcare providers should be informed if maternal sulfonamide therapy is used near the time of delivery (DHHS, 2013).

The pharmacokinetics of TMP-SMX are similar to non-pregnant values in early pregnancy (Ylikorkala, 1973). TMP-SMX is recommended for the prophylaxis or treatment of *Pneumocystis jirovecii* pneumonia (PCP), prophylaxis of *Toxoplasmic gondii* encephalitis (TE), and for the acute and chronic treatment of Q fever in pregnancy (CDC, 2013; DHHS, 2013). Sulfonamides may also be used to treat other infections in pregnant women when clinically appropriate; use during the first trimester should be limited to situations where no alternative therapies are available (ACOG, 2011). Because safer options are available for the treatment of urinary tract infections in pregnant women, use of TMP-containing products in the first trimester and sulfonamide-containing products >32 weeks gestation should be avoided (Lee, 2008).

Breast-Feeding Considerations Small amounts of TMP and SMX are transferred into breast milk. The manufacturer recommends that caution be used if administered to nursing women, especially if breast-feeding ill, jaundiced, premature, or stressed infants due to the potential risk of bilirubin displacement and kernicterus. Sulfonamides should not be used while nursing an infant with G6PD deficiency or hyperbilirubinemia (Della-Giustina, 2003). Maternal indications for TMP-SMX must also be considered prior to nursing. Nondose-related effects could include modification of bowel flora.

Contraindications Hypersensitivity to any sulfa drug, trimethoprim, or any component of the formulation; history of drug induced-immune thrombocytopenia with use of sulfonamides or trimethoprim; megaloblastic anemia due to folate deficiency; infants <2 months of age (manufacturer's labeling), infants <4 weeks of age (CDC, 2009); marked hepatic damage or severe renal disease (if patient not monitored)

Warnings/Precautions Use with caution in patients with G6PD deficiency, impaired renal or hepatic function or potential folate deficiency (malnourished, chronic anticonvulsant therapy, or elderly); maintain adequate hydration to prevent crystalluria; adjust dosage in patients with renal impairment.

Chemical similarities are present among sulfonamides, sulfonylureas, carbonic anhydrase inhibitors, thiazides, and loop diuretics (except ethacrynic acid). Use in patients with sulfonamide allergy is specifically contraindicated in product labeling, however, a risk of cross-reaction exists in patients with allergy to any of these compounds; avoid use when previous reaction has been severe.

Fatalities associated with severe reactions including Stevens-Johnson syndrome, toxic epidermal necrolysis, hepatic necrosis, agranulocytosis, aplastic anemia, thrombocytopenia and other blood dyscrasias have been reported; discontinue use at first sign of rash or serious adverse reactions. Elderly patients appear at greater risk for more severe adverse reactions. May cause hypoglycemia, particularly in malnourished, or patients with renal or hepatic impairment. Use with caution in patients with porphyria or thyroid dysfunction. Potentially significant interactions may exist, requiring dose or frequency adjustment, additional monitoring, and/or selection of alternative therapy. Slow acetylators may be more prone to adverse reactions. Caution in patients with allergies or asthma. May cause hyperkalemia (associated with high doses of trimethoprim) or hyponatremia. Incidence of adverse effects appears to be increased in patients with AIDS. Prolonged use may result in fungal or bacterial superinfection, including *C. difficile*-associated diarrhea (CDAD) and pseudomembranous colitis; CDAD has been observed >2 months postantibiotic treatment. Avoid concomitant use with leucovorin when treating *Pneumocystis jirovecii* pneumonia (PCP) in HIV patients; may increase risk of treatment failure and death.

When used for uncomplicated urinary tract infections, this combination should not be used if a single agent is effective. Additionally, sulfonamides should not be used to treat group A beta-hemolytic streptococcal infections.

Injection vehicle may contain and sodium metabisulfite.

Benzyl alcohol and derivatives: Some dosage forms may contain benzyl alcohol; large amounts of benzyl alcohol (≥99 mg/kg/day) have been associated with a potentially fatal toxicity ("gasping syndrome") in neonates; the "gasping syndrome" consists of metabolic acidosis, respiratory distress, gasping respirations, CNS dysfunction (including convulsions, intracranial hemorrhage), hypotension, and cardiovascular collapse (AAP, 1997; CDC, 1982); some data suggests that benzoate displaces bilirubin from protein binding sites (Ahlfors, 2001); avoid or use dosage forms containing benzyl alcohol with caution in neonates. See manufacturer's labeling.

Adverse Reactions

Cardiovascular: Allergic myocarditis, periarteritis nodosa (rare)

Central nervous system: Apathy, aseptic meningitis, ataxia, chills, depression, fatigue, hallucination, headache, insomnia, nervousness, peripheral neuritis, seizure, vertigo

Dermatologic: Erythema multiforme (rare), exfoliative dermatitis (rare), pruritus, skin photosensitivity, skin rash, Stevens-Johnson syndrome (rare), toxic epidermal necrolysis (rare), urticaria

Endocrine & metabolic: Hyperkalemia (generally at high dosages), hypoglycemia (rare), hyponatremia

Gastrointestinal: Abdominal pain, anorexia, diarrhea, glottis edema, kernicterus (in neonates), nausea, pancreatitis, pseudomembranous colitis, stomatitis, vomiting

Genitourinary: Crystalluria, diuresis (rare), nephrotoxicity (in association with cyclosporine), toxic nephrosis (with anuria and oliguria)

Hematologic & oncologic: Agranulocytosis, anaphylactoid purpura (IgA vasculitis; rare), aplastic anemia, eosinophilia, hemolysis (with G6PD deficiency), hemolytic anemia, hypoprothrombinemia, leukopenia, megaloblastic anemia, methemoglobinemia, neutropenia, thrombocytopenia

Hepatic: Cholestatic jaundice, hepatotoxicity (including hepatitis, cholestasis, and hepatic necrosis), hyperbilirubinemia, increased transaminases

Hypersensitivity: Anaphylaxis, angioedema, hypersensitivity reaction, serum sickness

Neuromuscular & skeletal: Arthralgia, myalgia, rhabdomyolysis (mainly in AIDS patients), systemic lupus erythematosus (rare), weakness

Ophthalmic: Conjunctival injection, injected sclera

Otic: Tinnitus

Renal: Increased blood urea nitrogen, increased serum creatinine, interstitial nephritis, renal failure

Respiratory: Cough, dyspnea, pulmonary infiltrates

Miscellaneous: Fever

Rare but important or life-threatening: Idiopathic thrombocytopenic purpura, prolonged Q-T interval on ECG, thrombotic thrombocytopenic purpura

Drug Interactions

Metabolism/Transport Effects Refer to individual components.

Avoid Concomitant Use

Avoid concomitant use of Sulfamethoxazole and Trimethoprim with any of the following: BCG; Dofetilide; Leucovorin Calcium-Levoleucovorin; Methenamine; Potassium P-Aminobenzoate; Procaine

Increased Effect/Toxicity

Sulfamethoxazole and Trimethoprim may increase the levels/effects of: ACE Inhibitors; Amantadine; Angiotensin II Receptor Blockers; Antidiabetic Agents (Thiazolidinedione); AzaTHIOprine; Bosentan; Cannabis; Carvedilol; CycloSPORINE (Systemic); CYP2C8 Substrates; CYP2C9 Substrates; Dapsone (Systemic); Dapsone (Topical); Digoxin; Dofetilide; Dronabinol; Eplerenone; Fosphenytoin; Highest Risk QTc-Prolonging Agents; LamiVUDine; Memantine; Mercaptopurine; MetFORMIN; Methotrexate; Moderate Risk QTc-Prolonging Agents; Phenytoin; Porfimer; PRALAtrexate; Prilocaine; Procainamide; Repaglinide; Sodium Nitrite; Spironolactone; Sulfonylureas; Tetrahydrocannabinol; Varenicline; Verteporfin; Vitamin K Antagonists

The levels/effects of Sulfamethoxazole and Trimethoprim may be increased by: Amantadine; Ceritinib; CYP2C9 Inhibitors (Moderate); CYP2C9 Inhibitors (Strong); Dapsone (Systemic); Dexketoprofen; Memantine; Methenamine; Mifepristone; Nitric Oxide

Decreased Effect

Sulfamethoxazole and Trimethoprim may decrease the levels/effects of: BCG; CycloSPORINE (Systemic); Sodium Picosulfate; Typhoid Vaccine

The levels/effects of Sulfamethoxazole and Trimethoprim may be decreased by: Bosentan; CYP2C9 Inducers (Strong); CYP3A4 Inducers (Moderate); CYP3A4 Inducers (Strong); Dabrafenib; Deferasirox; Fosphenytoin; Leucovorin Calcium-Levoleucovorin; Mitotane; Phenytoin; Potassium P-Aminobenzoate; Procaine; Siltuximab; St Johns Wort; Tocilizumab

Preparation for Administration IV: Must dilute well prior to administration (ie, 1:15 to 1:25, which equates to 5 mL of drug solution diluted in 75-125 mL base solution)

Storage/Stability

Injection: Store at room temperature; do not refrigerate. Less soluble in more alkaline pH. Protect from light. Solution must be diluted prior to administration. Following dilution, store at room temperature; do not refrigerate. Manufacturer recommended dilutions and stability of parenteral admixture at room temperature (25°C):

5 mL/125 mL D_5W; stable for 6 hours.

5 mL/100 mL D_5W; stable for 4 hours.

5 mL/75 mL D_5W; stable for 2 hours.

Studies have also confirmed limited stability in NS; detailed references should be consulted.

Suspension, tablet: Store at controlled room temperature of 15°C to 25°C (59°F to 77°F). Protect from light.

Mechanism of Action Sulfamethoxazole interferes with bacterial folic acid synthesis and growth via inhibition of dihydrofolic acid formation from para-aminobenzoic acid; trimethoprim inhibits dihydrofolic acid reduction to tetrahydrofolate resulting in sequential inhibition of enzymes of the folic acid pathway

Pharmacodynamics/Kinetics

Absorption: Oral: Rapid

Distribution: Both SMX and TMP distribute to middle ear fluid, sputum, vaginal fluid; TMP also distributes into bronchial secretions

Protein binding: SMX: ~70%, TMP: ~44%

Metabolism: Hepatic, both to multiple metabolites; SMX to hydroxy (via CYP2C9) and acetyl derivatives, and also conjugated with glucuronide; TMP to oxide and hydroxy derivatives; the free forms of both SMX and TMP are therapeutically active

Half-life elimination: Oral (mean): SMX: 10 hours, TMP: 8-10 hours; both are prolonged in renal failure

Time to peak, serum: Oral: 1-4 hours

Excretion: Both are excreted in urine as metabolites and unchanged drug

Dosage Dosage recommendations are based on the trimethoprim component. Double-strength tablets are equivalent to sulfamethoxazole 800 mg and trimethoprim 160 mg.

Usual dosage ranges:

Children >2 months: Manufacturer's labeling:

Mild-to-moderate infections: Oral: 8 mg TMP/kg/day in divided doses every 12 hours

Serious infection:

Oral: 15-20 mg TMP/kg/day in divided doses every 6 hours

IV: 8-12 mg TMP/kg/day in divided doses every 6-12 hours

Adults:

Oral: 1-2 double-strength tablets (sulfamethoxazole 800 mg; trimethoprim 160 mg) every 12-24 hours

IV: 8-20 mg TMP/kg/day divided every 6-12 hours

Indication-specific dosing:

Children >2 months:

Acute otitis media: Oral: 8 mg TMP/kg/day in divided doses every 12 hours for 10 days. **Note:** Recommended by the American Academy of Pediatrics as an alternative agent in penicillin-allergic patients at a dose of 6-10 mg TMP/kg/day (AOM guidelines, 2004).

Cyclosporiasis (off-label use): Oral, IV: 5 mg TMP/kg twice daily for 7-10 days (*Red Book*, 2009)

Pneumocystis jirovecii:

Treatment: Oral, IV: 15-20 mg TMP/kg/day in divided doses every 6-8 hours for 21 days

Prophylaxis: Oral, 150 mg TMP/m²/day in divided doses every 12 hours and administered for 3 days/week on consecutive or alternate days; an alternative dosing regimen allows for same dose to be administered in 2 divided doses daily (maximum: trimethoprim 320 mg and sulfamethoxazole 1600 mg daily) (CDC, 2009)

Q fever (off-label use): Oral:

Acute: Infants ≥2 months and Children <8 years with mild or uncomplicated illness (if patient remains febrile past 5 days of doxycycline treatment): 4-20 mg TMP/kg/day in divided doses every 12 hours (maximum: trimethoprim 320 mg daily) (CDC, 2013). **Note:** Some clinicians may recommend initial treatment with sulfamethoxazole and trimethoprim for children <8 years with mild or uncomplicated illness (CDC, 2013; Hartzell, 2008).

Chronic: Infectious Disease consult recommended for treatment of chronic Q fever (CDC, 2013)

Shigellosis: Note: Due to reported widespread resistance, empiric therapy with sulfamethoxazole and trimethoprim is not recommended (CDC-NARMS, 2010; WHO, 2005).

Oral:

Manufacturer's recommendation: 8 mg TMP/kg/day in divided doses every 12 hours for 5 days

Alternate recommendations (off-label dose): 10 mg TMP/kg/day in divided doses every 12 hours for 5 days (Ashkenazi, 1993)

IV: 8-10 mg TMP/kg/day in divided doses every 6, 8, or 12 hours for up to 5 days

Skin/soft tissue infection due to community-acquired MRSA (off-label use): Oral: 4-6 mg TMP/kg/dose every 12 hours for 5-10 days (Liu, 2011); **Note:** If beta-hemolytic *Streptococcus* spp are also suspected, a beta-lactam antibiotic should be added to the regimen (Liu, 2011)

Toxoplasmosis primary prophylaxis in HIV-exposed/infected patients (off-label use; CDC, 2009): Oral: 150 mg TMP/m²/day in 2 divided doses (preferred) or 150 mg TMP/m²/day in a single dose 3 times/week on consecutive days; or 150 mg TMP/m²/day in 2 divided doses 3 times/week on alternate days

Urinary tract infection:

Treatment:

Oral: Manufacturer's labeling: 8 mg TMP/kg/day in divided doses every 12 hours for 10 days

IV: Manufacturer's labeling: 8-10 mg TMP/kg/day in divided doses every 6, 8, or 12 hours for up to 14 days with serious infections

Prophylaxis: Oral: 2 mg TMP/kg/dose daily or 5 mg TMP/kg/dose twice weekly

Children, Adolescents, and Adults:

Melioidosis (*Burkholderia pseudomallei*) (off-label use; Lipsitz, 2012): Oral, IV:

Severe, acute phase involving brain, prostate, bone, or joint: Administer as 2 divided doses; given with ceftazidime or a carbapenem for ≥10 days followed by eradication therapy:

Children: 16 mg TMP/kg/day (maximum: 640 mg TMP daily)

Adults <40 kg: 320 mg TMP daily

Adults 40-60 kg: 480 mg TMP daily

Adults >60 kg: 640 mg TMP daily

Eradication therapy: Administer as 2 divided doses for ≥12 weeks:

Children: 16 mg TMP/kg/day (maximum: 640 mg TMP daily)

Adults <40 kg: 320 mg TMP daily

Adults 40-60 kg: 480 mg TMP daily

Adults >60 kg: 640 mg TMP daily

Postexposure prophylaxis: Administer as 2 divided doses for 21 days:

Children: 16 mg TMP/kg/day (maximum: 640 mg TMP daily)

Adults <40 kg: 320 mg TMP daily

Adults 40-60 kg: 480 mg TMP daily

Adults >60 kg: 640 mg TMP daily

Adults:

Chronic bronchitis (acute): Oral: One double-strength tablet every 12 hours for 10-14 days

Cyclosporiasis (off-label use): Oral, IV: 160 mg TMP twice daily for 7-10 days. **Note:** AIDS patients: Oral: One double-strength tablet 2-4 times/day for 10 days, then 1 double-strength tablet 3 times/week for 10 weeks (Pape, 1994; Verdier, 2000)

Granuloma inguinale (donovanosis) (off-label use): Oral: One double-strength tablet every 12 hours for at least 3 weeks and until lesions have healed (CDC, 2010)

Isosporiasis (*Isospora belli* infection) in HIV-positive patients (off-label use; CDC, 2009):
Treatment: Oral, IV: 160 mg TMP 4 times/day for 10 days **or** 160 mg TMP 2 times/day for 7-10 days. May increase dose and/or duration up to 3-4 weeks if symptoms worsen or persist
Secondary prophylaxis (in patients with CD4+ count <200 /microL): Oral: 160 mg TMP 3 times/week (preferred) **or** alternatively, 160 mg TMP daily **or** 320 mg TMP 3 times/week

Meningitis (bacterial): IV: 10-20 mg TMP/kg/day in divided doses every 6-12 hours

Nocardia (off-label use): Oral, IV:
Cutaneous infections: 5-10 mg TMP/kg/day in 2-4 divided doses
Severe infections (pulmonary/cerebral): 15 mg TMP/kg/day in 2-4 divided doses for 3-4 weeks, then 10 mg TMP/kg/day in 2-4 divided doses. Treatment duration is controversial; an average of 7 months has been reported.
Note: Therapy for severe infection may be initiated IV and converted to oral therapy (frequently converted to approximate dosages of oral solid dosage forms: 2 DS tablets every 8-12 hours). Although not widely available, sulfonamide levels should be considered in patients with questionable absorption, at risk for dose-related toxicity, or those with poor therapeutic response.

Osteomyelitis due to MRSA (off-label use): Oral, IV: 3.5-4 mg TMP/kg/dose every 8-12 hours for a minimum of 8 weeks with rifampin 600 mg once daily (Liu, 2011)

***Pneumocystis jirovecii* pneumonia (PCP):** Oral: Manufacturer's labeling:
Prophylaxis: 160 mg TMP daily
Treatment: 15-20 mg TMP/kg/day divided every 6 hours for 14-21 days

***Pneumocystis jirovecii* pneumonia (PCP) prophylaxis and treatment in HIV-positive patients (CDC, 2009):**
Note: Sulfamethoxazole and trimethoprim is the preferred regimen for this indication.
Prophylaxis: Oral: 80-160 mg TMP daily **or** alternatively, 160 mg TMP 3 times/week
Treatment:
Mild-to-moderate: Oral: 15-20 mg TMP/kg/day in 3 divided doses for 21 days **or** alternatively, 320 mg TMP 3 times/day for 21 days
Moderate-to-severe: Oral, IV: 15-20 mg TMP/kg/day in 3-4 divided doses for 21 days

Prosthetic joint infection (off-label use): Oral phase treatment (after completion of pathogen-specific IV therapy) following debridement and prosthesis retention or 1-stage exchange:
Total ankle, elbow, hip, or shoulder arthroplasty: 160 mg TMP 2 times daily for 3 months. **Note:** Must be used in combination with rifampin (Cordero-Ampuero, 2007; Osmon, 2013).
Total knee arthroplasty: Adults: 160 mg TMP 2 times daily for 6 months. **Note:** Must be used in combination with rifampin (Cordero-Ampuero, 2007; Osmon, 2013).

Q fever (off-label use): Oral:
Acute (in pregnant women) (CDC, 2013): 160 mg TMP twice daily throughout pregnancy but not beyond 32 weeks gestation. **Note:** Discontinue therapy for the final 8 weeks of pregnancy due to hyperbilirubinemia risk
Chronic: Infectious Disease consult recommended for treatment of chronic Q fever

Sepsis: IV: 20 mg TMP/kg/day divided every 6 hours

Septic arthritis due to MRSA (off-label use): Oral, IV: 3.5-4 mg TMP/kg/dose every 8-12 hours for 3-4 weeks (some experts combine with rifampin) (Liu, 2011)

Shigellosis: Note: Due to reported widespread resistance, empiric therapy with sulfamethoxazole and trimethoprim is not recommended (CDC-NARMS, 2010; WHO, 2005).
Oral: One double-strength tablet every 12 hours for 5 days
IV: 8-10 mg TMP/kg/day in divided doses every 6, 8, or 12 hours for up to 5 days

Skin/soft tissue infection due to community-acquired MRSA (off-label use): Oral: 1-2 double-strength tablets every 12 hours for 5-10 days (Liu, 2011); **Note:** If beta-hemolytic *Streptococcus* spp are also suspected, a beta-lactam antibiotic should be added to the regimen (Liu, 2011)

***Stenotrophomonas maltophilia* (ventilator-associated pneumonia) (off-label use):** IV: Most clinicians have utilized 12-15 mg TMP/kg/day for the treatment of VAP caused by *Stenotrophomonas maltophilia*. Higher doses (up to 20 mg TMP/kg/day) have been mentioned for treatment of severe infection in patients with normal renal function (Looney, 2009; Vartivarian, 1989; Wood, 2010)

***Toxoplasma gondii* encephalitis (off-label use; CDC, 2009):** Oral:
Primary prophylaxis: Oral: 160 mg TMP daily (preferred) **or** 160 mg TMP 3 times/week **or** 80 mg TMP daily
Treatment (alternative to sulfadiazine, pyrimethamine and leucovorin calcium): Oral, IV: 5 mg/kg TMP twice daily

Travelers' diarrhea: Oral: One double-strength tablet every 12 hours for 5 days

Urinary tract infection:
Oral: One double-strength tablet every 12 hours
Duration of therapy: Uncomplicated: 3-5 days; Complicated: 7-10 days
Pyelonephritis: 14 days
Prostatitis: Acute: 2 weeks; Chronic: 2-3 months
IV: 8-10 mg TMP/kg/day in divided doses every 6, 8, or 12 hours for up to 14 days with severe infections

Dosage adjustment in renal impairment: Oral, IV:
Manufacturer's recommendation: Children and Adults:
CrCl >30 mL/minute: No dosage adjustment required
CrCl 15-30 mL/minute: Administer 50% of recommended dose
CrCl <15 mL/minute: Use is not recommended
Alternate recommendations:
CrCl 15-30 mL/minute:
Treatment: Administer full daily dose (divided every 12 hours) for 24-48 hours, then decrease daily dose by 50% and administer every 24 hours (**Note:** For serious infections including *Pneumocystis jirovecii* pneumonia (PCP), full daily dose is given in divided doses every 6-8 hours for 2 days, followed by reduction to 50% daily dose divided every 12 hours) (Nahata, 1995).
PCP prophylaxis: One-half single-strength tablet (40 mg trimethoprim) daily **or** 1 single-strength tablet (80 mg trimethoprim) daily or 3 times weekly (Masur, 2002).
CrCl <15 mL/minute:
Treatment: Administer full daily dose every 48 hours (Nahata, 1995)
PCP prophylaxis: One-half single-strength tablet (40 mg trimethoprim) daily **or** 1 single-strength tablet (80 mg trimethoprim) 3 times weekly (Masur, 2002). While the guidelines do acknowledge the alternative of giving 1 single-strength tablet daily, this may be inadvisable in the uremic/ESRD patient.
GFR <10 mL/minute/1.73 m^2: Children: Use is not recommended, but if required, administer 5-10 mg trimethoprim/kg every 24 hours (Aronoff, 2007).

Intermittent Hemodialysis (IHD) (administer after hemodialysis on dialysis days):

Children: Use is not recommended, but if required, administer 5-10 mg trimethoprim/kg every 24 hours (Aronoff, 2007).

Adults: 2.5-10 mg/kg trimethoprim every 24 hours or 5-20 mg/kg trimethoprim 3 times weekly after IHD. **Note:** Dosing is highly dependent upon indication for use (eg, treatment of cystitis versus treatment of PCP pneumonia (Heinz, 2009).

PCP prophylaxis: One single-strength tablet (80 mg trimethoprim) after each dialysis session (Masur, 2002)

Note: Dosing dependent on the assumption of 3 times/week, complete IHD sessions.

Peritoneal dialysis (PD):

Use CrCl <15 mL/minute dosing recommendations. Not significantly removed by PD; supplemental dosing is not required (Aronoff, 2007):

GFR <10 mL/minute/1.73 m^2: Children: Use is not recommended, but if required 5-10 mg TMP/kg every 24 hours.

Exit-site and tunnel infections: Oral: One single-strength tablet daily (Li, 2010)

Intraperitoneal: Loading dose: TMP-SMX 320/1600 mg/L; Maintenance: TMP-SMX 80/400 mg/L (Aronoff, 2007; Warady, 2000)

Peritonitis: Oral: One double-strength tablet twice daily (Li, 2010)

Continuous renal replacement therapy (CRRT) (Heintz, 2009; Trotman, 2005): Drug clearance is highly dependent on the method of renal replacement, filter type, and flow rate. Appropriate dosing requires close monitoring of pharmacologic response, signs of adverse reactions due to drug accumulation, as well as drug concentrations in relation to target trough (if appropriate). The following are general recommendations only (based on dialysate flow/ultrafiltration rates of 1-2 L/hour and minimal residual renal function) and should not supersede clinical judgment:

CVVH/CVVHD/CVVHDF: 2.5-7.5 mg/kg of TMP every 12 hours. **Note:** Dosing regimen dependent on clinical indication. Critically-ill patients with *P. jirovecii* pneumonia receiving CVVHDF may require up to 10 mg/kg every 12 hours (Heintz, 2009).

Dosage adjustment in renal impairment: There are no dosage adjustments provided in manufacturer's labeling. Use with caution; use is contraindicated in cases of marked hepatic damage.

Dietary Considerations Should be taken with 8 oz of water. May be taken without regard to meals.

Administration

IV: Infuse diluted solution over 60-90 minutes; not for IM injection

Oral: Administer without regard to meals. Administer with at least 8 ounces of water.

Monitoring Parameters Perform culture and sensitivity testing prior to initiating therapy; CBC, serum potassium, creatinine, BUN

Dosage Forms The 5:1 ratio (SMX:TMP) remains constant in all dosage forms.

Injection, solution: Sulfamethoxazole 80 mg and trimethoprim 16 mg per mL (5 mL, 10 mL, 30 mL)

Suspension, oral: Sulfamethoxazole 200 mg and trimethoprim 40 mg per 5 mL

Sulfatrim: Sulfamethoxazole 200 mg and trimethoprim 40 mg per 5 mL

Tablet, oral: Sulfamethoxazole 400 mg and trimethoprim 80 mg

Bactrim: Sulfamethoxazole 400 mg and trimethoprim 80 mg

Tablet, double-strength, oral: Sulfamethoxazole 800 mg and trimethoprim 160 mg

Bactrim DS, Septra DS: Sulfamethoxazole 800 mg and trimethoprim 160 mg

◆ **Sulfamylon** *see* Mafenide *on page 1261*

Sulfanilamide (sul fa NIL a mide)

Brand Names: U.S. AVC Vaginal

Index Terms p-amino-benzenesulfonamide

Pharmacologic Category Antifungal Agent, Vaginal

Use Vulvovaginitis: Treatment of vulvovaginitis caused by *Candida albicans*

Pregnancy Risk Factor C

Dosage Intravaginal: Adults: Insert one applicatorful intravaginally once or twice daily for 30 days

Dosage adjustment in renal impairment: There are no dosage adjustments provided in the manufacturer's labeling.

Dosage adjustment in hepatic impairment: There are no dosage adjustments provided in the manufacturer's labeling.

Additional Information Complete prescribing information should be consulted for additional detail.

Dosage Forms

Cream, Vaginal:

AVC Vaginal: 15% (120 g)

SulfaSALAzine (sul fa SAL a zeen)

Brand Names: U.S. Azulfidine; Azulfidine EN-tabs; Sulfazine; Sulfazine EC

Brand Names: Canada Apo-Sulfasalazine; PMS-Sulfasalazine; Salazopyrin; Salazopyrin En-Tabs

Index Terms Salicylazosulfapyridine

Pharmacologic Category 5-Aminosalicylic Acid Derivative

Use

U.S. labeling:

Juvenile rheumatoid arthritis: Delayed release: Treatment of pediatric patients with polyarticular-course juvenile rheumatoid arthritis who have responded inadequately to salicylates or other nonsteroidal anti-inflammatory drugs (NSAIDs).

Rheumatoid arthritis: Delayed release: Treatment of patients with rheumatoid arthritis who have responded inadequately to salicylates or other NSAIDs.

Ulcerative colitis: Immediate and delayed release: Treatment of mild to moderate ulcerative colitis; adjunctive therapy in severe ulcerative colitis; prolongation of the remission period between acute attacks of ulcerative colitis.

Canadian labeling: Adjunctive therapy in severe ulcerative colitis, distal ulcerative colitis or proctitis, and Crohn disease; enteric coated tablets are also used for rheumatoid arthritis unsuccessfully treated with first-line therapy

Pregnancy Risk Factor B

Pregnancy Considerations Adverse events have not been observed in animal reproduction studies. Sulfasalazine and sulfapyridine cross the placenta; a potential for kernicterus in the newborn exists. Agranulocytosis was noted in an infant following maternal use of sulfasalazine during pregnancy. Additionally, cases of neural tube defects have been reported (causation undetermined); sulfasalazine is known to inhibit the absorption and metabolism of folic acid and may diminish the effects of folic acid supplementation. Based on available data, an increase in fetal malformations has not been observed following maternal use of sulfasalazine for the treatment of inflammatory bowel disease or ulcerative colitis. When treatment for inflammatory bowel disease is needed during pregnancy, sulfasalazine may be used, although supplementation with folic acid is recommended (Habal, 2012; Mahadevan, 2009; Mottet, 2007).

Breast-Feeding Considerations Sulfasalazine is excreted in breast milk; sulfapyridine concentrations are ~30% to 60% of the maternal serum. Bloody stools or diarrhea have been reported in nursing infants. Although sulfapyridine has poor bilirubin-displacing ability, exposure may cause kernicterus in the newborn. The manufacturer recommends that caution be used in women who are breast-feeding. Other sources consider use of sulfasalazine to be safe while breast-feeding; monitoring of the infant is recommended (Habal, 2012; Mahadevan, 2009; Mottet, 2007).

Contraindications

Hypersensitivity to sulfasalazine, sulfa drugs, salicylates, or any component of the formulation; intestinal or urinary obstruction; porphyria

Canadian labeling: Additional contraindications (not in U.S. labeling): Severe renal impairment (GFR <30 mL/minute/ 1.73 m^2); severe hepatic impairment; use in pediatric patients <2 years of age; patients in whom acute asthmatic attacks, urticaria, rhinitis or other allergic manifestations are precipitated by acetyl salicylic acid (ASA) or other NSAIDs

Warnings/Precautions Use with extreme caution in patients with renal impairment (Canadian labeling contraindicates use in severe impairment [GFR <30 mL/minute/ 1.73 m^2]), impaired hepatic function (Canadian labeling contraindicates use in severe impairment), or blood dyscrasias. Fatalities associated with severe reactions including agranulocytosis, aplastic anemia, and other blood dyscrasias have occurred; discontinue use at first sign of rash or signs of serious adverse reactions. The presence of clinical signs such as sore throat, fever, pallor, or purpura may be indicative of a serious blood disorder; monitor complete blood counts frequently. Serious infections (some fatal), including sepsis and pneumonia, have been reported. Infections may be associated with agranulocytosis, neutropenia, or myelosuppression. Monitor for signs/symptoms of infection during and after sulfasalazine therapy and promptly evaluate if infection occurs; discontinue therapy for serious infections. Use cautiously in patients with a history of recurring or chronic infections or with underlying conditions or concomitant therapy which may predispose them to infectious complications.

Use caution in patients with severe allergies or bronchial asthma. Hemolytic anemia may occur when used in patients with G6PD deficiency; use cautiously. May decrease folic acid absorption. Deaths from irreversible neuromuscular or central nervous system changes, fibrosing alveolitis, agranulocytosis, aplastic anemia, and other blood dyscrasias have been reported. In males, oligospermia (rare) and infertility has been reported. Chemical similarities are present among sulfonamides, sulfonylureas, carbonic anhydrase inhibitors, thiazides, and loop diuretics (except ethacrynic acid). Nausea, vomiting, and abdominal discomfort commonly occur; titration of dose and/or using the enteric coated formulation may decrease GI adverse effects. Use in patients with sulfonamide allergy is specifically contraindicated in product labeling, however, a risk of cross-reaction exists in patients with allergy to any of these compounds; avoid use when previous reaction has been severe. Slow acetylators may be more prone to adverse reactions. Discontinue enteric coated tablets if noted to pass without disintegrating.

Severe skin reactions (some fatal), including Stevens-Johnson syndrome (SJS), exfoliative dermatitis, and toxic epidermal necrolysis (TEN) have occurred with sulfonamides (including sulfasalazine), most commonly during the first month of treatment; discontinue use at first sign of skin rash, mucosal lesions, or any other sign of dermatologic toxicity. Severe and life-threatening hypersensitivity reactions, including drug rash with eosinophilia and systemic symptoms (DRESS) syndrome have been reported. Fever or lymphadenopathy may be present prior to rash development. Other severe hypersensitivity reactions may include internal organ involvement, such as hepatitis, nephritis, myocarditis, mononucleosis-like syndrome, hematologic abnormalities (including hematophagic histiocytosis), and/ or pneumonitis including eosinophilic infiltration. Discontinue treatment for severe reactions and evaluate promptly.

Adverse Reactions

Central nervous system: Dizziness, headache

Dermatologic: Pruritus, skin rash, urticaria

Gastrointestinal: Abdominal pain, anorexia, dyspepsia, gastric distress, nausea, stomatitis, vomiting

Genitourinary: Oligospermia (reversible)

Hematologic & oncologic: Heinz body anemia, hemolytic anemia, leukopenia, thrombocytopenia

Hepatic: Abnormal hepatic function tests

Respiratory: Cyanosis

Miscellaneous: Fever

Rare but important or life-threatening (includes reactions reported with mesalamine or other sulfonamides): Agranulocytosis, alopecia, anaphylaxis, angioedema, aplastic anemia, arthralgia, cauda equina syndrome, cholestatic hepatitis, cholestatic jaundice, conjunctival injection, crystalluria, depression, diarrhea, DRESS syndrome, drowsiness, eosinophilia, exfoliative dermatitis, folate deficiency, fulminant hepatitis, Guillain-Barré syndrome, hallucination, hearing loss, hematologic abnormality, hematologic disease (pseudomononucleosis), hematuria, hemolytic-uremic syndrome, hepatic cirrhosis, hepatic failure, hepatic necrosis, hepatitis, hypoglycemia, hypoprothrombinemia, injected sclera, insomnia, interstitial nephritis, interstitial pulmonary disease, jaundice, Kawasaki syndrome (single case report), lupus-like syndrome, megaloblastic anemia, meningitis, methemoglobinemia, myelitis, myelodysplastic syndrome, myocarditis (allergic), nephritis, nephrolithiasis, nephrotic syndrome, neutropenia (congenital), neutropenic enterocolitis, oropharyngeal pain, pancreatitis, parapsoriasis varioliformis acuta, periarteritis nodosa, pericarditis, periorbital edema, peripheral neuropathy, pleurisy, pneumonia, pneumonitis, proteinuria, pulmonary alveolitis, purpura, renal disease (acute), rhabdomyolysis, seizure, sepsis, serum sickness-like reaction (children with JRA have frequent and severe reaction), skin discoloration, skin photosensitivity, Stevens-Johnson syndrome, thyroid function impairment, toxic epidermal necrolysis, toxic nephrosis, urine discoloration, vasculitis

Drug Interactions

Metabolism/Transport Effects None known.

Avoid Concomitant Use There are no known interactions where it is recommended to avoid concomitant use.

Increased Effect/Toxicity

SulfaSALAzine may increase the levels/effects of: Heparin; Heparin (Low Molecular Weight); Methotrexate; Prilocaine; Sodium Nitrite; Thiopurine Analogs; Varicella Virus-Containing Vaccines

The levels/effects of SulfaSALAzine may be increased by: Nitric Oxide; Nonsteroidal Anti-Inflammatory Agents

Decreased Effect

SulfaSALAzine may decrease the levels/effects of: Cardiac Glycosides; Folic Acid; Methylfolate

Storage/Stability Store at 25°C (77°F); excursions permitted to 15°C to 30°C (59°F to 86°F).

Mechanism of Action 5-aminosalicylic acid (5-ASA) is the active component of sulfasalazine; the specific mechanism of action of 5-ASA is unknown; however, it is thought that it modulates local chemical mediators of the inflammatory response, especially leukotrienes, and is also postulated to be a free radical scavenger or an inhibitor of tumor necrosis factor (TNF); action appears topical rather than systemic

Pharmacodynamics/Kinetics

Absorption: ≤15% as unchanged drug from small intestine

Protein binding: Sulfasalazine: >99% to albumin; Sulfapyridine: ~70% to albumin; Acetylsulfapyridine (AcSP): ~90% to plasma proteins

Distribution: V_d: Sulfasalazine ~7.5 L

Metabolism: Via colonic intestinal flora to sulfapyridine and 5-aminosalicylic acid (5-ASA). Following absorption, sulfapyridine undergoes acetylation to form AcSP and ring hydroxylation while 5-ASA undergoes N-acetylation (non-acetylation phenotype dependent process); rate of metabolism via acetylation dependent on acetylation phenotype

Bioavailability: Sulfasalazine: <15%; Sulfapyridine: ~60%; 5-aminosalicylic acid: ~10% to 30%

Half-life elimination: Sulfasalazine: 5.7-10 hours (prolonged in elderly); Sulfapyridine: 14.8 hours (slow acetylators) and 10.4 hours (fast acetylators)

Time to peak: Sulfasalazine: 3-12 hours (mean: 6 hours); Metabolites: ~10 hours

Excretion: Primarily urine (as unchanged drug, conjugates, and acetylated metabolites); feces (small amounts)

Dosage Oral:

U.S. labeling:

Children ≥6 years:

Juvenile rheumatoid arthritis: Enteric-coated tablet: 30 to 50 mg/kg/day in 2 divided doses; Initial: Begin with 1/4 to 1/3 of expected maintenance dose; increase weekly; maximum: 2 g daily typically

Ulcerative colitis: Initial: 40 to 60 mg/kg/day in 3 to 6 divided doses; maintenance dose: 30 mg/kg/day in 4 divided doses

Adults:

Rheumatoid arthritis: Enteric-coated tablet: Initial: 0.5 to 1 g daily; increase weekly to maintenance dose of 2 g daily in 2 divided doses; maximum: 3 g daily (if response to 2 g daily is inadequate after 12 weeks of treatment)

Ulcerative colitis:

Initial: 3 to 4 g daily in evenly divided doses at ≤8-hour intervals; may initiate therapy with 1 to 2 g daily to reduce GI intolerance. **Note:** American College of Gastroenterology guideline recommendations: Titrate to 4 to 6 g daily in 4 divided doses (Kornbluth, 2010).

Maintenance dose: 2 g daily in evenly divided doses at ≤8-hour intervals; if GI intolerance occurs reduce dosage by 50% and gradually increase to target dose after several days. If GI intolerance persists, stop drug for 5 to 7 days and reintroduce at a lower daily dose.

Crohn disease, active mild/moderate, ileocolonic or colonic disease (off-label use): 3 to 6 g daily in divided doses (Lichtenstein, 2009)

Desensitization regimen: For patients who may be sensitive to treatment, it is suggested to start with a total dose of 50 to 250 mg daily and double it every 4 to 7 days until the desired dose is achieved. Discontinue if symptoms of sensitivity occur. Do not attempt in patients with a history of agranulocytosis or those who have had a previous anaphylactoid reaction on sulfasalazine therapy.

Canadian labeling:

Children: Ulcerative colitis, inflammatory bowel disease, Crohn disease: **Note:** Consider dose reduction or use of enteric-coated tablet in patients experiencing adverse gastrointestinal effects with uncoated tablet.

Acute attacks:

Body weight 25 to <35 kg: 500 mg 3 times daily

Body weight 35 to 50 kg: 1 g 2 to 3 times daily

Maintenance of remission:

Body weight 25 to <35 kg: 500 mg 2 times daily

Body weight 35 to 50 kg: 500 mg 2 to 3 times daily

Adults:

Rheumatoid arthritis: Enteric-coated tablet: Initial: 500 mg daily; increase dose weekly by 500 mg (total daily dose given in 2 divided doses) to maintenance dose of 1 g twice daily; if inadequate response to 1 g twice daily after 2 months, may increase dose to 3 g daily. Clinical improvement usually observed 1 to 2 months after initiating therapy. Concurrent use of analgesics and/or anti-inflammatory agents is recommended until therapeutic effect of sulfasalazine is observed.

Ulcerative colitis, inflammatory bowel disease, Crohn disease: **Note:** Consider dose reduction or use of enteric-coated tablet in patients experiencing adverse gastrointestinal effects with uncoated tablet.

Acute attacks: Severe: 1 to 2 g 3 to 4 times daily; mild to moderate: 1 g 3 to 4 times daily

Maintenance of remission: 1 g 2 to 3 times daily; continue dose indefinitely unless patient experiences adverse effects. In the event patient condition worsens, increase dose to 1 to 2 g 3 to 4 times daily.

Dosage adjustment in renal impairment: There are no dosage adjustments provided in the manufacturer's labeling; use with extreme caution. Canadian labeling contraindicates use in severe impairment (GFR <30 mL/minute/1.73 m^2).

Dosage adjustment in hepatic impairment: There are no dosage adjustments provided in the manufacturer's labeling; use with extreme caution. Canadian labeling contraindicates use in severe impairment.

Dietary Considerations Sulfasalazine impairs folate absorption. Adequate fluid intake is required to prevent crystalluria and stone formation.

Administration Tablets should be administered in evenly divided doses, preferably after meals. Enteric coated tablets should be swallowed whole.

Monitoring Parameters CBC with differential and liver function tests (prior to therapy, then every other week for first 3 months of therapy, followed by every month for the second 3 months, then once every 3 months thereafter or as clinically indicated); periodic urinalysis and renal/liver function tests (Canadian labeling also recommends renal function tests [including urinalysis] prior to therapy and monthly for first 3 months); stool frequency; signs of infection, dermatologic toxicity, or hypersensitivity reactions

Reference Range Sulfapyridine concentrations >50 mcg/mL are associated with increased adverse events.

Dosage Forms

Tablet, Oral:

Azulfidine: 500 mg

Sulfazine: 500 mg

Generic: 500 mg

Tablet Delayed Release, Oral:

Azulfidine EN-tabs: 500 mg

Sulfazine EC: 500 mg

Generic: 500 mg

Extemporaneous Preparations A 100 mg/mL oral suspension may be made with tablets. Place twenty 500 mg tablets in a mortar and add a small amount of a 1:1 mixture of Ora-Sweet® and Ora-Plus® to cover the tablets. Let soak for 20-30 minutes. Crush the tablets and mix to a uniform paste; mix while adding the vehicle in equal proportions to **almost** 100 mL; transfer to a calibrated bottle, rinse mortar with vehicle, and add sufficient quantity of vehicle to make 100 mL. Label "shake well". Stable 91 days under refrigeration or at room temperature.

Lingertat-Walsh K, Walker SE, Law S, et al, "Stability of Sulfasalazine Oral Suspension," *Can J Hosp Pharm*, 2006, 59(4):194-200.

- **Sulfatrim** *see* Sulfamethoxazole and Trimethoprim *on page 1946*
- **Sulfazine** *see* SulfaSALAzine *on page 1950*
- **Sulfazine EC** *see* SulfaSALAzine *on page 1950*
- **Sulfisoxazole and Erythromycin** *see* Erythromycin and Sulfisoxazole *on page 765*

Sulfur and Sulfacetamide

(SUL fur & sul fa SEE ta mide)

Brand Names: U.S. AVAR; AVAR LS; AVAR-e; AVAR-e Green; AVAR-e LS; BP 10-1; BP Cleansing Wash; Clarifoam EF; Claris; Clenia [DSC]; Plexion; Prascion; Prascion FC; Prascion RA; Rosanil; SSS 10-5; SulfaCleanse 8/4; Sumadan; Sumadan XLT; Sumaxin; Sumaxin TS; Verti-sulf; Zencia

Brand Names: Canada Sulfacet-R

Index Terms Sodium Sulfacetamide and Sulfur; Sulfacetamide and Sulfur; Sulfur and Sulfacetamide Sodium

Pharmacologic Category Acne Products; Antibiotic, Sulfonamide Derivative; Antiseborrheic Agent, Topical; Topical Skin Product, Acne

Use Aid in the treatment of acne vulgaris, acne rosacea, and seborrheic dermatitis

Pregnancy Risk Factor C

Dosage Topical: Children ≥12 years and Adults: Apply in a thin film 1-3 times/day. Cleansing products should be used 1-2 times/day.

Dosage adjustment in renal impairment: Use is contraindicated.

Dosage adjustment in hepatic impairment: No dosage adjustment provided in manufacturer's labeling.

Additional Information Complete prescribing information should be consulted for additional detail.

Dosage Forms

Aerosol, foam, topical: Sulfur 5% and sulfacetamide 10% (60 g)

Clarifoam EF: Sulfur 5% and sulfacetamide 10% (60 g, 100 g)

SSS 10-5: Sulfur 5% and sulfacetamide sodium 10% (60 g, 100 g)

Cleanser, topical: Sulfur 2% and sulfacetamide 10% (227 g), Sulfur 4.8% and sulfacetamide sodium 9.8% (285 g), Sulfur 5% and sulfacetamide 10% (170 g, 340 g)

AVAR: Sulfur 5% and sulfacetamide 10% (227 g)

AVAR LS: Sulfur 2% and sulfacetamide 10% (227 g)

Plexion: Sulfur 4.8% and sulfacetamide 9.8% (285 g)

Prascion: Sulfur 5% and sulfacetamide 10% (170 g, 340 g)

Rosanil: Sulfur 5% and sulfacetamide 10% (170 g)

Cream, topical: Sulfur 2% and sulfacetamide sodium 10% (57 g), Sulfur 4.8% and sulfacetamide sodium 9.8% (57 g), Sulfur 5% and sulfacetamide sodium 10% (28 g)

AVAR-e, AVAR-e LS: Sulfur 2% and sulfacetamide 10% (57 g)

AVAR-e Green: Sulfur 5% and sulfacetamide 10% (57 g)

Plexion: Sulfur 4.8% and sulfacetamide 9.8% (57 g)

Prascion RA: Sulfur 5% and sulfacetamide 10% (45 g)

SSS 10-5: Sulfur 5% and sulfacetamide sodium 10% (28 g)

Virti-sulf: Sulfur 5% and sulfacetamide sodium 10% (28 g)

Gel, topical: Sulfur 5% and sulfacetamide 10% (45 g)

Lotion, topical: Sulfur 4.8% and sulfacetamide sodium 9.8% (57 g)

Plexion: Sulfur 4.8% and sulfacetamide 9.8% (57 g)

Pad, topical [cleansing cloth]: Sulfur 4% and sulfacetamide 10% (60s)

Avar: Sulfur 5% and sulfacetamide sodium 9.5% (30s, 60s)

Avar LS: Sulfur 2% and sulfacetamide sodium 10% (30s, 60s)

Plexion: Sulfur 4.8% and sulfacetamide 9.8% (60s)

Prascion FC: Sulfur 5% and sulfacetamide 10% (30s, 60s)

Sumaxin: Sulfur 4% and sulfacetamide 10% (60s)

Suspension, topical: Sulfur 4% and sulfacetamide 8% (473 mL), sulfur 5% and sulfacetamide 10% (30 g)

SulfaCleanse 8/4: Sulfur 4% and sulfacetamide 8% (473 mL)

Sumaxin TS: Sulfur 4% and sulfacetamide 8% (473 mL)

Wash, topical: Sulfur 4% and sulfacetamide 9% (480 mL); Sulfur 4.5% and sulfacetamide 9% (454 g)

BP 10-1: Sulfur 1% and sulfacetamide 10% (170 g)

Sumaxin: Sulfur 4% and sulfacetamide 9% (473 mL)

Zencia: Sulfur 4% and sulfacetamide 9% (480 mL)

Wash, topical [emulsion-based]:

BP Cleansing Wash: Sulfur 4% and sulfacetamide 10% (473 mL)

Claris: Sulfur 4% and sulfacetamide 10% (473 mL)

Sumadan: Sulfur 4.5% and sulfacetamide 9% (454 g)

Sumadan XLT: Sulfur 4.5% and sulfacetamide 9% (454 g)

- **Sulfur and Sulfacetamide Sodium** *see* Sulfur and Sulfacetamide *on page 1953*

Sulindac (SUL in dak)

Brand Names: Canada Apo-Sulin; Teva-Sulindac

Index Terms Clinoril

Pharmacologic Category Nonsteroidal Anti-inflammatory Drug (NSAID), Oral

Additional Appendix Information

Beers Criteria – Potentially Inappropriate Medications for Geriatrics *on page 2271*

Use Management of inflammatory diseases including osteoarthritis, rheumatoid arthritis, acute gouty arthritis, ankylosing spondylitis, acute painful shoulder (bursitis/tendonitis)

Pregnancy Risk Factor C

Dosage Oral:

Children: Dose not established

Adults: **Note:** Maximum daily dose: 400 mg

Osteoarthritis, rheumatoid arthritis, ankylosing spondylitis: 150 mg twice daily

Acute painful shoulder (bursitis/tendonitis): 200 mg twice daily; usual treatment: 7-14 days

Acute gouty arthritis: 200 mg twice daily; usual treatment: 7 days

Dosing adjustment in renal impairment: No dosage adjustment provided in manufacturer's labeling. However, sulindac is not recommended with advanced renal impairment; if required, decrease dose and monitor closely.

Dosing adjustment in hepatic impairment: No dosage adjustment provided in manufacturer's labeling. However, dosage reduction may be necessary; discontinue if abnormal liver function tests occur.

Additional Information Complete prescribing information should be consulted for additional detail.

Dosage Forms

Tablet, Oral:

Generic: 150 mg, 200 mg

- **Sulpyrine** *see* Dipyrone [INT] *on page 653*
- **Sumadan** *see* Sulfur and Sulfacetamide *on page 1953*
- **Sumadan XLT** *see* Sulfur and Sulfacetamide *on page 1953*

SUMAtriptan (soo ma TRIP tan)

Brand Names: U.S. Alsuma; Imitrex; Imitrex STATdose Refill; Imitrex STATdose System; Sumavel DosePro

Brand Names: Canada ACT-Sumatriptan; Apo-Sumatriptan; Ava-Sumatriptan; Dom-Sumatriptan; Imitrex DF; Imitrex Injection; Imitrex Nasal Spray; Mylan-Sumatriptan; PHL-Sumatriptan; PMS-Sumatriptan; Sandoz-Sumatriptan; Sumatriptan DF; Taro-Sumatriptan; Teva-Sumatriptan; Teva-Sumatriptan DF

Index Terms Sumatriptan Succinate; Zecuity

Pharmacologic Category Antimigraine Agent; Serotonin 5-$HT_{1B,\ 1D}$ Receptor Agonist

Use

Migraine: Intranasal, Oral, SubQ, Transdermal: Acute treatment of migraine with or without aura in adults

Cluster headache: SubQ: Acute treatment of cluster headache episodes in adults

Pregnancy Risk Factor C

Pregnancy Considerations Adverse events were observed in animal reproduction studies. In a study using full term healthy human placentas, limited amounts of sumatriptan were found to cross the placenta (Schenker, 1995).

An overall increased risk of major congenital malformations has not been observed following first trimester exposure to sumatriptan in several studies. Pregnancy outcome information for sumatriptan is available from a pregnancy registry sponsored by GlaxoSmithKline. As of October 2008, data was available for 558 infants/fetuses exposed to sumatriptan, and seven exposed to both sumatriptan and naratriptan. The risk of major birth defects following sumatriptan exposure was 4.6% (95% CI: 2.9-7.2) (Cunnington, 2009). The pregnancy registry was closed in January, 2012 and additional information may be obtained from the manufacturer (800-336-2176). An analysis of data collected between 1995-2008 using the Swedish Medical Birth Register reported pregnancy outcomes following 5-$HT_{1B/1D}$ agonist exposure. An increased risk of major congenital malformations was not observed following sumatriptan exposure (2229 exposed during the first trimester) (Källén, 2011). An increased risk of major congenital malformations was not observed in the prospective Norwegian Mother and Child Cohort Study. The study included women with 5-$HT_{1B/1D}$ agonist exposure between 1999-2006 (n=455); of these, 217 were exposed to sumatriptan (Nezvalová-Henriksen, 2010; Nezvalová-Henriksen, 2012).

If treatment for cluster headaches is needed during pregnancy, sumatriptan may be used (Jürgens, 2009). Other agents are preferred for the initial treatment of migraine in pregnancy (Da Silva, 2012; MacGregor, 2012; Williams, 2012); however, sumatriptan may be considered if first-line agents fail (MacGregor, 2012).

Breast-Feeding Considerations The excretion of sumatriptan into breast milk was studied in five lactating women, 10-28 weeks postpartum (mean: 22.2 weeks). Sumatriptan 6 mg SubQ was administered and maternal milk and blood samples were collected over 8 hours after the dose. Sumatriptan was detected in breast milk. Maximum concentrations in the maternal blood (mean: 80.2 mcg/L; 0.25 hours after the dose) and milk (mean: 87.2 mcg/L; 2.5 hours after the dose) were similar. However, the amount of sumatriptan an infant would be exposed to following breast-feeding is considered to be small (although the mean milk-to-plasma ratio is ~4.9, weight-adjusted doses estimates suggest breast-fed infants receive 3.5% of a maternal dose). Expressing and discarding the milk for 8-12 hours after a single dose is suggested to reduce the amount present even further (Wojnar-Horton, 1996). Breast-feeding is not recommended by some manufacturers; however, according to other sources if treatment is needed, breast-feeding does not need to be discontinued (Jürgens, 2009; MacGregor, 2012).

Contraindications Hypersensitivity to sumatriptan or any component of the formulation, including allergic contact dermatitis to the transdermal patch; ischemic heart disease or signs or symptoms of ischemic heart disease (including Prinzmetal's angina, angina pectoris, myocardial infarction, silent myocardial ischemia); cerebrovascular syndromes (including strokes, transient ischemic attacks); peripheral vascular disease (including ischemic bowel disease); uncontrolled hypertension; use within 24 hours of ergotamine derivatives; use within 24 hours of another 5-HT_1 agonist; concurrent administration or within 2 weeks of discontinuing an MAO type A inhibitors; management of hemiplegic or basilar migraine; Wolff-Parkinson-White syndrome or arrhythmias associated with other cardiac accessory conduction pathway disorders; severe hepatic impairment (not Sumavel)

Warnings/Precautions Anaphylactic, anaphylactoid, and hypersensitivity reactions (including angioedema) have been reported; may be life threatening or fatal. Sumatriptan is only indicated for the acute treatment of migraine or cluster headache (product dependent); not indicated for migraine prophylaxis, or for the treatment of hemiplegic or basilar migraine. Acute migraine agents (eg, 5-HT_1 agonists, opioids, ergotamine, or a combination of the agents) used for 10 or more days per month may lead to worsening of headaches (medication overuse headache); withdrawal treatment may be necessary in the setting of overuse. May cause CNS depression, such as dizziness, weakness, or drowsiness, which may impair physical or mental abilities; patients must be cautioned about performing tasks which require mental alertness (eg, operating machinery or driving). If a patient does not respond to the first dose, the diagnosis of migraine or cluster headache should be reconsidered; rule out underlying neurologic disease in patients with atypical headache and in patients with no prior history of migraine or cluster headache. Cardiac events (coronary artery vasospasm, transient ischemia, myocardial infarction, ventricular tachycardia/fibrillation, cardiac arrest and death), cerebral/subarachnoid hemorrhage, and stroke have been reported with 5-HT_1 agonist administration (some occurring within a few hours of administration). Discontinue sumatriptan if these events occur. Patients who experience sensations of chest pain/pressure/tightness or symptoms suggestive of angina following dosing should be evaluated for coronary artery disease or Prinzmetal's angina before receiving additional doses; if dosing is resumed and similar symptoms recur, monitor with ECG. Perform a cardiovascular evaluation in 5-HT_1 agonists-naive patients who have risk factors for CAD prior to initiation of therapy. Patients with suspected CAD should have cardiovascular evaluation to rule out CAD before considering use; if cardiovascular evaluation is "satisfactory," first dose should be given in the health care provider's office (consider ECG monitoring). Periodic evaluation of cardiovascular status should be done in these patients during intermittent long-term use.

Significant elevation in blood pressure, including hypertensive crisis, has been reported on rare occasions in patients with and without a history of hypertension; use is contraindicated in patients with uncontrolled hypertension. Peripheral vascular ischemia, GI vascular ischemia and infarction, splenic infarction, and Raynaud syndrome been reported with 5-HT_1 agonists. Transient and permanent blindness and significant partial vision loss have been very rarely reported. Use with caution in patients with a history of seizure disorder or in patients with a lowered seizure threshold; seizures have been reported after sumatriptan administration in patients with or without a history of seizures. Use the oral formulation with caution (and with dosage limitations) in patients with mild to moderate hepatic impairment where treatment is necessary and advisable. Presystemic clearance of orally administered sumatriptan is reduced in hepatic impairment, leading to increased plasma concentrations; dosage reduction of the oral product is recommended. Non-oral routes of administration (intranasal, subcutaneous) do not undergo similar hepatic first-pass metabolism and are not expected to result in significantly altered pharmacokinetics in patients with hepatic impairment. Use of the oral, intranasal, transdermal, or Imitrex injectable is contraindicated in severe hepatic impairment; Sumavel is not recommended in severe hepatic impairment. Allergic contact dermatitis may occur with use of transdermal patch; erythematous plaque and/or erythemato-vesicular or erythemato-bullous eruptions may develop. Erythema alone is common and not by itself an indication of sensitization. Discontinue use if allergic contact dermatitis is suspected. Patients sensitized from use of transdermal system may develop systemic sensitization or other systemic reactions if sumatriptan-containing products are taken by other routes (oral, subcutaneous); if treatment with sumatriptan by other routes is required, first dose should be taken under close medical supervision. Do not apply transdermal patch in areas near or over electrically-active implantable or body-worn medical devices (eg, implantable cardiac pacemaker, body-worn insulin pump, implantable deep brain stimulator); patch contains metal parts and must be removed before magnetic resonance imaging (MRI) procedures.

Potentially significant drug-drug interactions may exist, requiring dose or frequency adjustment, additional monitoring, and/or selection of alternative therapy. Serotonin syndrome may occur with 5-HT$_1$ agonists, particularly when used concomitantly with other serotonergic drugs; symptoms (eg, mental status changes, tachycardia, hyperthermia, nausea, vomiting, diarrhea, hyperreflexia, incoordination) typically occur minutes to hours after initiation/dose increase of a serotonergic drug. Discontinue use if serotonin syndrome is suspected. Use with caution in the elderly; perform a cardiovascular evaluation prior to initiation of therapy in elderly patients with cardiovascular risk factors (eg, diabetes, hypertension, smoking, obesity, strong family history of coronary artery disease) and periodically during intermittent long-term use.

Adverse Reactions

Injection:

Cardiovascular: Chest discomfort, flushing

Central nervous system: Anxiety, burning sensation, cold sensation, dizziness, drowsiness, feeling of heaviness, feeling of tightness, feeling strange, headache, localized warm feeling, malaise, nasal cavity pain, paresthesia, pressure sensation, tight feeling in head

Dermatologic: Diaphoresis

Gastrointestinal: Abdominal distress, dysphagia, nausea and vomiting, sore throat

Local: Injection site reaction (includes bleeding, bruising, swelling, and erythema)

Neuromuscular & skeletal: Jaw pain, muscle cramps, myalgia, neck pain, numbness, weakness

Ophthalmic: Visual disturbance

Respiratory: Bronchospasm, nasal signs and symptoms, sinus discomfort

Nasal spray:

Central nervous system: Dizziness

Gastrointestinal: Nausea, sore throat, unpleasant taste, vomiting

Respiratory: Nasal signs and symptoms

Tablet:

Cardiovascular: Chest pain, hot and cold flashes, palpitations, syncope

Central nervous system: Burning sensation, dizziness, drowsiness, headache, hyperacusis, malaise, migraine, numbness, pain (nonspecified), paresthesia, sensation of pressure (neck/throat/jaw or nonspecified), sleepiness, vertigo

Gastrointestinal: Diarrhea, nausea, reduced salivation, vomiting

Genitourinary: Hematuria

Hematologic & oncologic: Hemolytic anemia, hemorrhage (ear or nose/throat)

Hypersensitivity: Hypersensitivity reaction

Neuromuscular & skeletal: Myalgia

Otic: Hearing loss, tinnitus

Respiratory: Allergic rhinitis, dyspnea, rhinitis, sinusitis, upper respiratory tract inflammation

Transdermal system:

Central nervous system: Feeling abnormal (paresthesia, warm/cold sensation), localized warm feeling, sensation of pressure (chest/neck/throat/jaw)

Dermatologic: Allergic contact dermatitis, skin discoloration (application site), skin vesicle (application site)

Hematologic & oncologic: Bruise (application site)

Local: Localized irritation, localized pain, localized pruritus

Rare but important or life-threatening: Skin erosion (application site)

Route unspecified: Rare but important or life-threatening: Abdominal aortic aneurysm, abnormal hepatic function tests, accommodation disturbance, acute renal failure, anemia, cardiac arrhythmia, cardiomyopathy, cerebrovascular accident, colonic ischemia, coronary artery vasospasm, cyanosis, deafness, dystonic reaction, giant-cell arteritis, hallucination, hematuria, hemorrhage (nose/throat), hypersensitivity reaction, increased intracranial pressure, increased thyroid stimulating hormone level, intestinal obstruction, myocardial infarction, optic neuropathy (ischemic), pancytopenia, Prinzmetal angina, psychomotor disturbance, pulmonary embolism, Raynaud's phenomenon, retinal blood vessel occlusion (artery), seizure, serotonin syndrome, skin photosensitivity, subarachnoid hemorrhage, thrombosis, vasculitis

Drug Interactions

Metabolism/Transport Effects None known.

Avoid Concomitant Use

Avoid concomitant use of SUMAtriptan with any of the following: Dapoxetine; Ergot Derivatives; MAO Inhibitors

Increased Effect/Toxicity

SUMAtriptan may increase the levels/effects of: Antipsychotic Agents; Droxidopa; Ergot Derivatives; Metoclopramide; Serotonin Modulators

The levels/effects of SUMAtriptan may be increased by: Antiemetics (5HT3 Antagonists); Antipsychotic Agents; Dapoxetine; Ergot Derivatives; MAO Inhibitors

Decreased Effect There are no known significant interactions involving a decrease in effect.

Storage/Stability

Alsuma: Store at 25°C (77°F); excursions are permitted between 15°C and 30°C (59°F and 86°F); do not refrigerate. Protect from light.

Imitrex injectable, tablet, intranasal: Store at 2°C to 30°C (36°F to 86°F). Protect from light.

Sumavel DosePro: Store at 20°C to 25°C (68°F to 77°F); excursions are permitted between 15°C and 30°C (59°F and 86°F); do not freeze. Protect from light.

Zecuity: Store at 20°C to 25°C (68°F to 77°F); excursions are permitted between 15°C and 30°C (59°F and 86°F); do not refrigerate or freeze.

Mechanism of Action Selective agonist for serotonin (5-HT_{1B} and 5-HT_{1D} receptors) on intracranial blood vessels and sensory nerves of the trigeminal system; causes vasoconstriction and reduces neurogenic inflammation associated with antidromic neuronal transmission correlating with relief of migraine

Pharmacodynamics/Kinetics

Onset of action: Oral: ~30 minutes; Intranasal: ~15 to 30 minutes; SubQ: ~10 minutes

Distribution: V_d: 2.4 L/kg

Protein binding: 14% to 21%

Metabolism: Hepatic, primarily via MAO-A isoenzyme; extensive first-pass metabolism following oral administration

Bioavailability: Intranasal: 17% (compared to SubQ); Oral: 15%; SubQ: 97% ± 16%

Half-life elimination: ~2 to 3 hours

Time to peak, serum: Oral: 2 to 2.5 hours; SubQ: 12 minutes (range: 4 to 20 minutes); Transdermal patch: ~1 hour

Excretion:

Intranasal: Urine (42% of total dose as indole acetic acid metabolite; 3% of total dose as unchanged drug)

Oral: Urine (~60% of total dose, mostly as indole acetic acid metabolite; 3% of total dose as unchanged drug); feces (~40%)

SubQ: Urine (38% of total dose as indole acetic acid metabolite; 22% of total dose as unchanged drug)

Transdermal patch: Urine (69% of total dose as indole acetic acid metabolite; 11% of total dose as unchanged drug)

Dosage

Adults:

Oral: A single dose of 25 mg, 50 mg, or 100 mg (taken with fluids). If a satisfactory response has not been obtained at 2 hours, a second dose may be administered. Results from clinical trials show that initial doses of 50 mg and 100 mg are more effective than doses of 25 mg, and that 100 mg doses do not provide a greater effect than 50 mg and may have increased incidence of side effects. Although doses of up to 300 mg/day have been studied, the total daily dose should not exceed 200 mg. The safety of treating an average of >4 headaches in a 30-day period have not been established.

Intranasal: A single dose of 5 mg, 10 mg, or 20 mg administered in one nostril. A 10 mg dose may be achieved by administering a single 5 mg dose in each nostril. If headache returns, the dose may be repeated once after 2 hours, not to exceed a total daily dose of 40 mg. In clinical trials, a greater number of patients responded to initial doses of 20 mg versus 5 or 10 mg. The safety of treating an average of >4 headaches in a 30-day period has not been established.

SubQ:

Cluster headache: Initial: 6 mg; may repeat if needed ≥1 hour after initial dose (maximum: 6 mg per dose; two 6 mg injections per 24-hour period)

Migraine: Initial: Alsuma: 6 mg; Imitrex: 6 mg, if side effects are dose limiting, use lower doses 1 to 5 mg; Sumavel: 6 mg, if side effects are dose limiting, use 4 mg. May repeat if needed ≥1 hour after initial dose (maximum: 6 mg per dose; two 6 mg injections per 24-hour period; or maximum cumulative dose of 12 mg in 24 hours, separated by at least 1 hour). However, controlled clinical trials have failed to document a benefit with administration of a second 6 mg dose in nonresponders.

Transdermal patch: Initial: Apply one patch (provides 6.5 mg per 4 hour); if necessary, may apply a second patch no sooner than 2 hours after activation of the first patch (maximum: 2 patches per 24-hour period). The safety of using >4 transdermal systems in 1 month has not been established.

Elderly: Refer to adult dosing.

Dosage adjustment in renal impairment: There are no dosage adjustments provided in the manufacturer's labeling (has not been studied). However, dosage adjustment not expected due to extensive metabolism to inactive agents.

Dosage adjustment in hepatic impairment:

Mild to moderate hepatic impairment:

Oral: Bioavailability of oral sumatriptan is increased with liver disease. If treatment is needed, do not exceed single doses of 50 mg.

Intranasal: There are no dosage adjustments provided in the manufacturer's labeling (has not been studied). However, because the spray does not undergo first-pass metabolism, levels would not be expected to be altered.

Subcutaneous: No dosage adjustment necessary.

Transdermal patch: There are no dosage adjustments provided in the manufacturer's labeling (has not been studied).

Severe hepatic impairment: Oral, intranasal, subcutaneous (Alsuma and Imitrex injection), and transdermal formulations are contraindicated in severe hepatic impairment. Sumavel is not recommended in severe hepatic impairment.

Administration Administer as soon as symptoms appear.

Intranasal: Each nasal spray unit is preloaded with 1 dose; **do not** test the spray unit before use; remove unit from plastic pack when ready to use; while sitting down, gently blow nose to clear nasal passages; keep head upright and close one nostril gently with index finger; hold container with other hand, with thumb supporting bottom and index and middle fingers on either side of nozzle; insert nozzle into nostril about 1/2 inch; close mouth; take a breath through nose while releasing spray into nostril by pressing firmly on blue plunger; remove nozzle from nostril; keep head level for 10 to 20 seconds and gently breathe in through nose and out through mouth; **do not breathe deeply**

SubQ: Not for IM or IV use. Needle penetrates 1/4 inch of skin; use in areas of the body with adequate skin and subcutaneous thickness (lateral thigh or upper arm).

Needleless administration (Sumavel DosePro): Administer to the abdomen (>2 inches from the navel) or thigh; not for IM or IV administration. Do not administer to other areas of the body (eg, arm). Device is for single use only, discard after use; do not use if the tip of the device is tilted or broken.

Transdermal: Apply transdermal system to dry intact, non-irritated skin on the upper arm or thigh on a site that is relatively hair free and without scars, tattoos, abrasions, or other skin conditions (ie, generalized skin irritation, eczema, psoriasis, melanoma, contact dermatitis); secure with medical tape if needed. Do not apply to a previous application site until the site remains erythema free for at least 3 days. After application, the activation button must be pushed, and the red light emitting diode (LED) will turn on; the system will stop operating when dosing is completed and the LED will turn off, signaling that the system can be removed; if the LED turns off before 4 hours, dosing has stopped and the system can be removed. If headache relief is incomplete, a second system can be applied to a different site, if >2 hours have elapsed since the first system was applied. Patient should not swim, bathe, or shower while wearing patch. After use, fold the system so the adhesive side sticks to itself and discard away from children and pets. The system contains lithium-manganese dioxide batteries; dispose in accordance with state and local regulations.

Monitoring Parameters Headache severity, blood pressure, signs/symptoms suggestive of angina; perform a cardiovascular evaluation prior to initiation of therapy in 5-HT_1 agonist-naive patients who have multiple cardiovascular risk factors (eg, increased age, diabetes, hypertension, smoking, obesity, strong family history of CAD); monitor ECG with first dose in patients with multiple cardiovascular risk factors who have a negative cardiovascular evaluation and consider periodic cardiovascular evaluation in such patients during intermittent long-term use.

Product Availability Zecuity (transdermal system): FDA approved January 2013; anticipated availability is currently unknown. Refer to prescribing information for additional information.

Dosage Forms

Solution, Nasal:
- Imitrex: 5 mg/actuation (1 ea); 20 mg/actuation (1 ea)
- Generic: 5 mg/actuation (1 ea); 20 mg/actuation (1 ea)

Solution, Subcutaneous:
- Alsuma: 6 mg/0.5 mL (0.5 mL)
- Imitrex: 6 mg/0.5 mL (0.5 mL)
- Imitrex STATdose Refill: 4 mg/0.5 mL (0.5 mL)
- Imitrex STATdose System: 4 mg/0.5 mL (0.5 mL)
- Generic: 4 mg/0.5 mL (0.5 mL); 6 mg/0.5 mL (0.5 mL)

Solution, Subcutaneous [preservative free]:
- Generic: 6 mg/0.5 mL (0.5 mL)

Solution Auto-injector, Subcutaneous:
- Imitrex STATdose System: 6 mg/0.5 mL (0.5 mL)
- Generic: 6 mg/0.5 mL (0.5 mL)

Solution Cartridge, Subcutaneous:
- Imitrex STATdose Refill: 6 mg/0.5 mL (0.5 mL)

Solution Jet-injector, Subcutaneous:
- Sumavel DosePro: 4 mg/0.5 mL (0.5 mL); 6 mg/0.5 mL (0.5 mL)

Solution Prefilled Syringe, Subcutaneous [preservative free]:
- Generic: 6 mg/0.5 mL (0.5 mL)

Tablet, Oral:
- Imitrex: 25 mg, 50 mg, 100 mg
- Generic: 25 mg, 50 mg, 100 mg

Extemporaneous Preparations A 5 mg/mL oral liquid preparation made from tablets and one of three different vehicles (Ora-Sweet®, Ora-Sweet® SF, or Syrpalta® syrups). **Note:** Ora-Plus® Suspending Vehicle is used with Ora-Sweet® or Ora-Sweet® SF to facilitate dispersion of the tablets (Ora-Plus® is not necessary if Syrpalta® is the vehicle). Crush nine 100 mg tablets in a mortar and reduce to a fine powder. Add 40 mL of Ora-Plus® in 5 mL increments and mix thoroughly between each addition; rinse mortar and pestle 5 times with 10 mL of Ora-Plus®, pouring into bottle each time, and add quantity of appropriate syrup (Ora-Sweet® or Ora-Sweet® SF) sufficient to make 180 mL. Store in amber glass bottles in the dark; label "shake well", "refrigerate", and "protect from light". Stable for 21 days refrigerated.

Fish DN, Beall HD, Goodwin SD, et al, "Stability of Sumatriptan Succinate in Extemporaneously Prepared Oral Liquids," *Am J Health Syst Pharm*, 1997, 54(14):1619-22.

Sumatriptan and Naproxen

(soo ma TRIP tan & na PROKS en)

Brand Names: U.S. Treximet

Index Terms Naproxen and Sumatriptan; Naproxen Sodium and Sumatriptan; Naproxen Sodium and Sumatriptan Succinate; Sumatriptan Succinate and Naproxen; Sumatriptan Succinate and Naproxen Sodium

Pharmacologic Category Antimigraine Agent; Nonsteroidal Anti-inflammatory Drug (NSAID), Oral; Serotonin 5-$HT_{1B, 1D}$ Receptor Agonist

Use Acute treatment of migraine with or without aura

Pregnancy Risk Factor C

Dosage Oral: Adults: 1 tablet (sumatriptan 85 mg and naproxen 500 mg). If a satisfactory response has not been obtained at 2 hours, a second dose may be administered (maximum: 2 tablets/24 hours). **Note:** The safety of treating an average of >5 migraine headaches in a 30-day period has not been established.

Dosage adjustment in renal impairment:
- CrCl ≥30 mL/minute: No dosage adjustmentprovided in manufacturer's labeling(has not been studied). Use with caution.
- CrCl <30 mL/minute: Use not recommended.

Dosage adjustment in hepatic impairment: Use is contraindicated.

Additional Information Complete prescribing information should be consulted for additional detail.

Dosage Forms

Tablet, oral:
- Treximet® 85/500: Sumatriptan 85 mg and naproxen sodium 500 mg

◆ **Sumatriptan DF (Can)** *see* SUMAtriptan *on page 1953*

◆ **Sumatriptan Succinate** *see* SUMAtriptan *on page 1953*

◆ **Sumatriptan Succinate and Naproxen** *see* Sumatriptan and Naproxen *on page 1957*

◆ **Sumatriptan Succinate and Naproxen Sodium** *see* Sumatriptan and Naproxen *on page 1957*

◆ **Sumavel DosePro** *see* SUMAtriptan *on page 1953*

◆ **Sumaxin** *see* Sulfur and Sulfacetamide *on page 1953*

◆ **Sumaxin TS** *see* Sulfur and Sulfacetamide *on page 1953*

SUNItinib (su NIT e nib)

Brand Names: U.S. Sutent

Brand Names: Canada Sutent

Index Terms SU011248; SU11248; Sunitinib Malate

Pharmacologic Category Antineoplastic Agent, Tyrosine Kinase Inhibitor; Antineoplastic Agent, Vascular Endothelial Growth Factor (VEGF) Inhibitor; Vascular Endothelial Growth Factor (VEGF) Inhibitor

Use

Gastrointestinal stromal tumor: Treatment of gastrointestinal stromal tumor (GIST) after disease progression on or intolerance to imatinib

Pancreatic neuroendocrine tumors, advanced: Treatment of progressive, well-differentiated pancreatic neuroendocrine tumors in patients with unresectable locally advanced or metastatic disease

Renal cell carcinoma, advanced: Treatment of advanced renal cell carcinoma

Pregnancy Risk Factor D

Pregnancy Considerations Animal reproduction studies have demonstrated teratogenicity, embryotoxicity, and fetal loss. Because sunitinib inhibits angiogenesis, a critical component of fetal development, adverse effects on pregnancy would be expected. Women of childbearing potential should be advised to avoid pregnancy if receiving sunitinib.

Breast-Feeding Considerations It is not known if sunitinib is excreted in human milk. Due to the potential for serious adverse reactions in the nursing infant, the decision to discontinue breast-feeding or discontinue sunitinib should take into account the benefits of treatment to the mother.

Contraindications There are no contraindications listed in the manufacturer's labeling.

Canadian labeling: Hypersensitivity to sunitinib or any component of the formulation; pregnancy

Warnings/Precautions Hazardous agent - use appropriate precautions for handling and disposal (NIOSH 2014 [group 1]). **[U.S. Boxed Warning]: Hepatotoxicity, which**

may be severe and/or result in fatal liver failure, has been observed in clinical trials and in postmarketing surveillance. Signs of liver failure include jaundice, elevated transaminases, and/or hyperbilirubinemia, in conjunction with encephalopathy, coagulopathy and/or renal failure. Monitor liver function tests at baseline, with each treatment cycle and if clinically indicated. Withhold treatment for grade 3 or 4 hepatotoxicity; discontinue if hepatotoxicity does not resolve. Do not reinitiate in patients with severe changes in liver function tests or other signs/symptoms of liver failure. Sunitinib has not been studied in patients with ALT or AST >2.5 times ULN (or >5 times ULN if due to liver metastases).

May cause a decrease in left ventricular ejection fraction (LVEF), including grade 3 reductions; consider obtaining LVEF evaluation prior to treatment. Mean onset of symptomatic heart failure (HF) is 22 days from treatment initiation. Interrupt therapy or decrease dose with LVEF <50% or >20% reduction from baseline. Discontinue with clinical signs and symptoms of HF. Cardiovascular events (some fatal), including symptomatic HF, myocardial disorders and cardiomyopathy have been reported with use. QTc prolongation and torsade de pointes have been observed (dose dependent); a baseline and periodic ECG should be obtained; correct electrolyte abnormalities prior to treatment and monitor and correct potassium, calcium and magnesium levels during therapy; use caution in patients with a history of QTc prolongation, with medications known to prolong the QTc interval, or patients with preexisting (relevant) cardiac disease, bradycardia, or electrolyte imbalance. Use with caution in patients with cardiac dysfunction; monitor for clinical signs/symptoms of HF, obtain baseline and periodic LVEF evaluation patients with MI, bypass grafts, symptomatic HF, vascular diseases (including CVA and TIA), and PE were excluded from clinical trials. May cause hypertension; monitor and control with antihypertensives if needed; interrupt therapy until hypertension is controlled for severe hypertension. Use caution and closely monitor in patients with underlying or poorly controlled hypertension. Potentially significant drug-drug interactions may exist, requiring dose or frequency adjustment, additional monitoring, and/or selection of alternative therapy.

Hemorrhagic events have been reported including epistaxis, rectal, gingival, upper GI, urinary tract, genital, brain, wound bleeding, tumor-related, and hemoptysis/pulmonary hemorrhage; may be serious and/or fatal. Proteinuria and (rare) cases of nephrotic syndrome have been reported; some cases have led to renal failure and fatal outcomes. Monitor for new onset or worsening proteinuria with baseline and periodic urinalysis and follow up with 24-hour urine protein if clinically indicated. If urine protein is ≥3 grams/24 hours, interrupt treatment and reduce the dose. Discontinue treatment in patients with nephrotic syndrome or persistent urine protein ≥3 grams/24 hours despite dose reductions. The safety of continuing treatment with sunitinib in patients with moderate to severe proteinuria has not been evaluated. Microangiopathic hemolytic anemia (MAHA) and dose-limiting hypertension have been reported when sunitinib has been used in combination with bevacizumab. Impaired wound healing has been reported with sunitinib; temporarily withhold treatment for patients undergoing major surgical procedures; the optimal time to resume treatment after a procedure has not been determined. Serious and fatal gastrointestinal complications, including gastrointestinal perforation, have occurred (rarely). Pancreatitis has been observed in RCC patients; discontinue sunitinib if symptoms are present. Thyroid dysfunction (eg, hypothyroidism, hyperthyroidism, and thyroiditis) may occur; the risk for hypothyroidism appears to increase with therapy duration; hyperthyroidism, sometimes followed by hypothyroidism has also been reported; monitor thyroid function at baseline. Patients not receiving thyroid hormone replacement therapy at sunitinib initiation should be monitored (TSH) every 4 weeks for 4 months and then every 2 to 3 months; those already receiving levothyroxine prior to initiating sunitinib should have TSH monitored every 4 weeks until levels and levothyroxine dose are stable, then monitor every 2 months (Hamnvik, 2011). Adrenal function abnormalities have been reported; monitor for adrenal insufficiency in patients with stress such as trauma, severe infection, or who are undergoing surgery. Symptomatic hypoglycemia has been associated with sunitinib; may result in loss of consciousness or require hospitalization. Hypoglycemia occurred infrequently in patients with renal cell cancer and gastrointestinal stromal tumors (GIST); however, the incidence is higher (~10%) in patients with pancreatic neuroendocrine tumors (PNET); preexisting glucose homeostasis abnormalities were not always present in hypoglycemic patients with PNET. Blood glucose decreases may be worse in patients with diabetes. Monitor blood glucose levels regularly during and following discontinuation of treatment. Dose modifications of antidiabetic medications may be necessary to minimize the risk of hypoglycemia.

Severe cutaneous reactions, including erythema multiforme (EM), Stevens-Johnson syndrome (SJS), and toxic epidermal necrolysis (TEN) have been reported (some fatal); if signs/symptoms of EM, SJS, or TEN (progressive skin rash, often with blisters or mucosal lesions) are present, discontinue sunitinib. Do not restart treatment if SJS or TEN are suspected. Necrotizing fasciitis (with fatalities) has been reported, including perineum necrotizing fasciitis secondary to fistula formation. Discontinue sunitinib in patients who develop necrotizing fasciitis. Sunitinib may cause skin and/or hair depigmentation or discoloration. Reversible posterior leukoencephalopathy syndrome (RPLS) has been reported (rarely, some fatal); symptoms include confusion, headache, hypertension, lethargy, seizure, blindness and/or other vision, or neurologic disturbances; interrupt treatment and begin hypertension management. Tumor lysis syndrome (TLS), including fatalities, has been reported, predominantly in patients with RCC or GIST; risk for TLS is higher in patients with a high tumor burden prior to treatment; monitor closely; correct clinically significant dehydration and treat high uric acid levels prior to initiation of treatment. An increased incidence of fatigue, thyroid dysfunction and treatment-induced hypertension was reported in patients with renal insufficiency (CrCl ≤60 mL/minute) who received sunitinib for the treatment of renal cell cancer (Gupta, 2011). Osteonecrosis of the jaw (ONJ) has been observed with sunitinib; concurrent bisphosphonate use or dental disease may increase the risk for ONJ. If possible, avoid invasive dental procedures in patients with current or prior bisphosphonate use. Consider a dental exam and appropriate prophylactic dentistry prior to treatment initiation Dosing schedules vary by indication; some treatment regimens are continuous daily dosing; other treatment schedules are daily dosing for 4 weeks of a 6-week cycle (4 weeks on, 2 weeks off).

Adverse Reactions

Cardiovascular: Chest pain, decreased left ventricular ejection fraction, deep vein thrombosis, heart failure, hypertension, peripheral edema, pulmonary embolism, venous thrombosis

Central nervous system: Chills, depression, dizziness, fatigue, glossalgia, headache, insomnia, mouth pain

Dermatologic: Alopecia, erythema, hair discoloration, palmar-plantar erythrodysesthesia, pruritus, skin discoloration, skin rash, xeroderma

Endocrine & metabolic: Hyper-/hypocalcemia, hyper-/hypoglycemia, hyper-/hypokalemia, hyper-/hyponatremia, hyperuricemia, hypoalbuminemia, hypomagnesemia, hypophosphatemia, hypothyroidism

Gastrointestinal: Abdominal pain, anorexia, constipation, diarrhea, dysgeusia, dyspepsia, flatulence, gastroesophageal reflux disease, hemorrhoids, increased serum amylase, increased serum lipase, mucositis, nausea, pancreatitis, vomiting, weight loss, xerostomia

Hematologic & oncologic: Anemia, hemorrhage, leukopenia, lymphocytopenia, neutropenia, thrombocytopenia

Hepatic: Hyperbilirubinemia, increased serum alkaline phosphatase, increased serum ALT, increased serum AST

Neuromuscular & skeletal: Arthralgia, back pain, increased creatine kinase, limb pain, myalgia, weakness

Renal: Increased serum creatinine

Respiratory: Cough, dyspnea, epistaxis, flu-like symptoms, nasopharyngitis, upper respiratory tract infection

Miscellaneous: Fever

Rare but important or life-threatening: Acute renal failure, adrenocortical insufficiency, angioedema, arterial thrombosis, atrial flutter, cardiomyopathy, cerebral hemorrhage, cerebral infarction, cerebrovascular accident, cholecystitis (particularly acalculous), coma, coronary artery dissection (aortic), erythema multiforme, esophagitis, febrile neutropenia, fistula (sometimes associated with tumor necrosis and/or regression), gastrointestinal perforation, glomerulonephritis (segmental glomerular sclerosis), hemorrhage (tumor), hepatic failure, hepatotoxicity, hypersensitivity, hyperthyroidism, hypotension, hypothyroidism (myxedema coma), infection, macrocytosis, hemolytic anemia (microangiopathic; when used in combination with bevacizumab), myocardial infarction, myopathy, necrotizing fasciitis (including of the perineum), nephrotic syndrome, neutropenic infection, osteonecrosis (jaw), pneumonitis (recall), pre-eclampsia, prolonged Q-T interval on ECG, proteinuria, pulmonary hemorrhage, pyoderma gangrenosum (including positive dechallenges), renal impairment, reversible posterior leukoencephalopathy syndrome, rhabdomyolysis, seizure, septic shock, sepsis, skin infection, Stevens-Johnson syndrome, thrombotic microangiopathy, thyroiditis, tissue necrosis (tumor), torsades de pointes, toxic epidermal necrolysis, transient ischemic attacks, tumor lysis syndrome, urinary tract infection, ventricular arrhythmia, wound healing impairment

Drug Interactions

Metabolism/Transport Effects Substrate of CYP3A4 (major); **Note:** Assignment of Major/Minor substrate status based on clinically relevant drug interaction potential; **Inhibits** BCRP, P-glycoprotein

Avoid Concomitant Use

Avoid concomitant use of SUNItinib with any of the following: BCG; Bevacizumab; Bosutinib; Conivaptan; Fusidic Acid (Systemic); Highest Risk QTc-Prolonging Agents; Idelalisib; Ivabradine; Mifepristone; Natalizumab; PAZOPanib; Pimecrolimus; Silodosin; St Johns Wort; Tacrolimus (Topical); Temsirolimus; Tofacitinib; Topotecan; Vaccines (Live); VinCRIStine (Liposomal)

Increased Effect/Toxicity

SUNItinib may increase the levels/effects of: Afatinib; Bevacizumab; Bisphosphonate Derivatives; Bosutinib; Brentuximab Vedotin; Colchicine; Dabigatran Etexilate; DOXOrubicin (Conventional); Edoxaban; Everolimus; Highest Risk QTc-Prolonging Agents; Ledipasvir; Leflunomide; Moderate Risk QTc-Prolonging Agents; Naloxegol; Natalizumab; PAZOPanib; P-glycoprotein/ABCB1 Substrates; Prucalopride; Rifaximin; Rivaroxaban; Silodosin; Tofacitinib; Topotecan; Vaccines (Live); VinCRIStine (Liposomal)

The levels/effects of SUNItinib may be increased by: Antifungal Agents (Azole Derivatives, Systemic); Aprepitant; Bevacizumab; Conivaptan; CYP3A4 Inhibitors (Moderate); CYP3A4 Inhibitors (Strong); Dasatinib; Denosumab; Fosaprepitant; Fusidic Acid (Systemic); Idelalisib; Ivabradine; Ivacaftor; Luliconazole; Mifepristone; Netupitant; Pimecrolimus; QTc-Prolonging Agents (Indeterminate Risk and Risk Modifying); Roflumilast; Simeprevir; Stiripentol; Tacrolimus (Topical); Temsirolimus; Trastuzumab

Decreased Effect

SUNItinib may decrease the levels/effects of: BCG; Coccidioides immitis Skin Test; Sipuleucel-T; Vaccines (Inactivated); Vaccines (Live)

The levels/effects of SUNItinib may be decreased by: Bosentan; CYP3A4 Inducers (Moderate); CYP3A4 Inducers (Strong); Dabrafenib; Deferasirox; Dexamethasone (Systemic); Echinacea; Mitotane; Siltuximab; St Johns Wort; Tocilizumab

Food Interactions Grapefruit juice may increase the levels/effects of sunitinib. Food has no effect on the bioavailability of sunitinib. Management: Avoid grapefruit juice.

Storage/Stability Store at 25°C (77°F); excursions are permitted between 15°C to 30°C (59°F to 86°F).

Mechanism of Action Exhibits antitumor and antiangiogenic properties by inhibiting multiple receptor tyrosine kinases, including platelet-derived growth factors (PDGFRα and PDGFRβ), vascular endothelial growth factors (VEGFR1, VEGFR2, and VEGFR3), FMS-like tyrosine kinase-3 (FLT3), colony-stimulating factor type 1 (CSF-1R), and glial cell-line-derived neurotrophic factor receptor (RET).

Pharmacodynamics/Kinetics

Distribution: V_d/F: 2230 L

Protein binding: Sunitinib: 95%; SU12662: 90%

Metabolism: Hepatic; primarily metabolized by CYP3A4 to the N-desethyl metabolite SU12662 (active)

Half-life elimination: Terminal: Sunitinib: 40 to 60 hours; SU12662: 80 to 110 hours

Time to peak, plasma: 6 to 12 hours

Excretion: Feces (61%); urine (16%)

Dosage Note: Dosage modifications should be done in increments or decrements of 12.5 mg; individualize based on safety and tolerability.

Gastrointestinal stromal tumor (GIST): Adults: Oral: 50 mg once daily for 4 weeks of a 6-week treatment cycle (4 weeks on, 2 weeks off)

GIST off-label dosing: Adults: Oral: 37.5 mg once daily, continuous daily dosing (George, 2009, *EJC*)

Pancreatic neuroendocrine tumors, advanced (PNET): Adults: Oral: 37.5 mg once daily, continuous daily dosing (maximum daily dose used in clinical trials: 50 mg)

Renal cell cancer, advanced (RCC): Adults: Oral: 50 mg once daily for 4 weeks of a 6-week treatment cycle (4 weeks on, 2 weeks off)

Soft tissue sarcoma, non-GIST (off-label use): Adults: Oral: 37.5 mg once daily, continuous daily dosing (George, 2009, *JCO*)

Thyroid cancer, refractory (off-label use): Adults: Oral: 50 mg once daily for 4 weeks of a 6-week treatment cycle (4 weeks on, 2 weeks off) (Cohen, 2008; Ravaud, 2008)

Dosage adjustment with concurrent CYP3A4 inhibitor: Avoid concomitant administration with strong CYP3A4 inhibitors (eg, clarithromycin, erythromycin, itraconazole, ketoconazole, nefazodone, protease inhibitors, telithromycin, voriconazole); if concomitant administration with a strong CYP3A4 inhibitor cannot be avoided, consider a dose reduction to a minimum of 37.5 mg/day (GIST, RCC) or 25 mg/day (PNET).

Dosage adjustment with concurrent CYP3A4 inducer: Avoid concomitant administration with strong CYP3A4 inducers (eg, carbamazepine, dexamethasone, phenobarbital, phenytoin, rifampin, St John's wort); if concomitant administration with a strong CYP3A4 inducer cannot be avoided, consider a dosage increase (with careful monitoring for toxicity) to a maximum of 87.5 mg/day (GIST, RCC) or 62.5 mg/day (PNET).

Dosage adjustment for toxicity: Dosage modifications should be done in increments or decrements of 12.5 mg; individualize based on safety and tolerability.

Cardiac toxicity:

Ejection fraction <50% and >20% below baseline without evidence of CHF: Interrupt treatment and/or reduce dose.

LV dysfunction with CHF clinical manifestations: Discontinue treatment.

Dermatologic toxicity:

Signs/symptoms of erythema multiforme (EM), Stevens-Johnson syndrome (SJS), and toxic epidermal necrolysis (TEN), including progressive skin rash, often with blisters or mucosal lesions: Discontinue sunitinib; do not restart treatment if SJS or TEN are suspected.

Necrotizing fasciitis: Discontinue sunitinib.

Hypertension, severe: Temporarily interrupt treatment until hypertension is controlled.

Nephrotic syndrome: Discontinue treatment.

Pancreatitis: Discontinue treatment.

Proteinuria:

Urine protein ≥3 g/24 hours: Interrupt treatment and reduce the dose.

Persistent urine protein ≥3 g/24 hours despite dose reductions: Discontinue treatment.

Reversible posterior leukoencephalopathy (RPLS): Temporarily withhold treatment; after resolution, may resume with discretion.

Thrombotic microangiopathy: Temporarily withhold treatment; after resolution, may resume with discretion.

Dosage adjustment in renal impairment:

Mild, moderate, or severe impairment: No initial dosage adjustment necessary; subsequent adjustments may be needed based on safety and tolerance.

ESRD on hemodialysis: No initial dosage adjustment necessary; subsequent dosage increases (up to two-fold) may be required due to reduced (47%) exposure.

Dosage adjustment in hepatic impairment:

Preexisting hepatic impairment: No adjustment is necessary with mild-to-moderate (Child-Pugh class A or B) hepatic impairment; not studied in patients with severe (Child-Pugh class C) hepatic impairment. Studies excluded patients with ALT or AST >2.5 x ULN, or if due to liver metastases, ALT or AST >5 x ULN.

Hepatotoxicity during treatment: Hepatic adverse events ≥ grade 3 or 4: Withhold treatment; discontinue if hepatotoxicity does not resolve. Do not reinitiate in patients with severe changes in liver function tests or other signs/symptoms of liver failure.

Dietary Considerations Avoid grapefruit juice.

Administration May be administered with or without food. Hazardous agent; use appropriate precautions for handling and disposal (NIOSH 2014 [group 1]).

Monitoring Parameters LVEF, baseline (and periodic with cardiac risk factors), ECG (12-lead; baseline and periodic), blood pressure; adrenal function CBC with differential and platelets (prior to each treatment cycle), liver function tests (baseline, with each cycle and if clinically indicated), serum chemistries including magnesium, phosphate, and potassium (prior to each treatment cycle), blood glucose levels (regularly during and following discontinuation of treatment), urinalysis (for proteinuria development or worsening); consider dental exam prior to treatment initiation; symptoms of hypothyroidism, hyperthyroidism, or thyroiditis; signs/symptoms of hypoglycemia

Thyroid function testing (Hamnvik, 2011):

Preexisting levothyroxine therapy: Obtain baseline TSH levels, then monitor every 4 weeks until levels and levothyroxine dose are stable, then monitor every 2 months

Without preexisting thyroid hormone replacement: TSH at baseline, then every 4 weeks for 4 months, then every 2-3 months

Additional Information Hand-foot skin reaction (HFSR) observed with tyrosine kinase inhibitors (TKIs) is distinct from hand-foot syndrome (palmar-plantar erythrodysesthesia) associated with traditional chemotherapy agents; HFSR due to TKIs is localized with defined hyperkeratotic lesions; symptoms include burning, dysesthesia, paresthesia, or tingling on the palms/soles, and generally occur within the first 2-4 weeks of treatment; pressure and flexor areas may develop blisters (callus-like), dry/cracked skin, edema, erythema, desquamation, or hyperkeratosis (Appleby, 2011).

HFSR management (Lacouture, 2008): The following treatments may be used in addition to the recommended dosage modifications. Prior to treatment initiation, a pedicure is recommended to remove hyperkeratotic areas/calluses, which may predispose to HFSR; avoid vigorous exercise/activities which may stress hands or feet. During therapy, patients should reduce exposure to hot water (may exacerbate hand-foot symptoms); avoid constrictive footwear and excessive skin friction. Patients may also wear thick cotton gloves or socks and should wear shoes with padded insoles. Grade 1 HFSR may be relieved with moisturizing creams, cotton gloves and socks (at night) and/or keratolytic creams such as urea (20% to 40%) or salicylic acid (6%). Apply topical steroid (eg, clobetasol ointment) twice daily to erythematous areas of Grade 2 HFSR; topical anesthetics (eg, lidocaine 2%) and then systemic analgesics (if appropriate) may be used for pain control. Resolution of acute erythema may result in keratotic areas which may be softened with keratolytic agents.

Dosage Forms

Capsule, Oral:

Sutent: 12.5 mg, 25 mg, 37.5 mg, 50 mg

Extemporaneous Preparations Hazardous agent: Use appropriate precautions for handling and disposal (NIOSH 2014 [group 1]).

A 10 mg/mL sunitinib oral suspension may be made with capsules and a 1:1 mixture of Ora-Sweet and Ora-Plus. Empty the contents of three 50 mg sunitinib capsules into a mortar; add small portions of vehicle and mix to a uniform paste. Mix while adding vehicle in incremental proportions to 15 mL. Transfer to amber plastic bottle and label "shake well". This suspension maintains an average concentration of 96% to 106% (of the original concentration) at room temperature or refrigerated for up to 60 days in plastic amber prescription bottles.

Navid F, Christensen R, Minkin P, et al, "Stability of Sunitinib in Oral Suspension," *Ann Pharmacother*, 2008, 42(7):962-6.

◆ **Sunitinib Malate** *see* SUNItinib *on page 1957*

◆ **Supartz** *see* Hyaluronate and Derivatives *on page 1006*

◆ **Super Strength Motrin IB Liquid Gel Capsules (Can)** *see* Ibuprofen *on page 1032*

◆ **Supeudol (Can)** *see* OxyCODONE *on page 1538*

◆ **Suphedrine [OTC]** *see* Pseudoephedrine *on page 1742*

◆ **Suplasyn (Can)** *see* Hyaluronate and Derivatives *on page 1006*

◆ **Supprelin LA** *see* Histrelin *on page 1005*

◆ **Suprax** *see* Cefixime *on page 380*

◆ **Suprefact (Can)** *see* Buserelin [CAN/INT] *on page 309*

- ◆ **Suprefact Depot (Can)** *see* Buserelin [CAN/INT] *on page 309*
- ◆ **Suprenza** *see* Phentermine *on page 1635*
- ◆ **Suprep® Bowel Prep Kit** *see* Sodium Sulfate, Potassium Sulfate, and Magnesium Sulfate *on page 1914*
- ◆ **Surfaxin** *see* Lucinactant *on page 1256*
- ◆ **Sur-Q-Lax [OTC]** *see* Docusate *on page 661*
- ◆ **Survanta** *see* Beractant *on page 250*
- ◆ **Survanta® (Can)** *see* Beractant *on page 250*
- ◆ **Sustiva** *see* Efavirenz *on page 707*
- ◆ **Sutent** *see* SUNItinib *on page 1957*

Suvorexant (soo voe REX ant)

Brand Names: U.S. Belsomra

Index Terms MK4305

Pharmacologic Category Hypnotic, Miscellaneous; Orexin Receptor Antagonist

Use Insomnia: Treatment of insomnia characterized by difficulties with sleep onset and/or sleep maintenance.

Pregnancy Risk Factor C

Pregnancy Considerations Adverse events have been observed in some animal reproduction studies.

Breast-Feeding Considerations It is not known if suvorexant is excreted into breast milk. The manufacturer recommends that caution be used if administered to a nursing woman.

Contraindications Narcolepsy

Warnings/Precautions Hypnotics have been associated with abnormal thinking and behavior changes (eg, amnesia, anxiety, hallucinations). May cause CNS depression impairing physical and mental capabilities; patients must be cautioned about performing tasks which require mental alertness (operating machinery or driving). Suvorexant should only be administered when the patient is able to stay in bed a full night (≥7 hours) before being active again. Discontinue or decrease the dose in patients who drive if daytime somnolence occurs. Sleep paralysis (inability to move or speak for up to several minutes during sleep-wake transitions), hypnagogic/hypnopompic hallucinations, and mild cataplexy may occur. Cataplexy symptoms may include periods of leg weakness lasting from seconds to a few minutes, can occur both at night and during the day, and may not be associated with a triggering event (eg, laughter, surprise). An increased risk for hazardous sleep-related activities such as sleep-driving; cooking and eating food, making phone calls, or having sex while asleep have also been noted. Discontinue treatment in patients who report any sleep-related episodes. Potentially significant interactions may exist, requiring dose or frequency adjustment, additional monitoring, and/or selection of alternative therapy.

Symptomatic treatment of insomnia should be initiated only after careful evaluation of potential causes of sleep disturbance. Failure of sleep disturbance to resolve after 7 to 10 days may indicate psychiatric and/or medical illness. Use with caution in patients with depression; worsening of depression, including suicide or suicidal ideation has been reported with the use of hypnotics. Intentional overdose may be an issue in this population. The minimum dose that will effectively treat the individual patient should be used. Prescriptions should be written for the smallest quantity consistent with good patient care. Use with caution in patients with a history of drug dependence. Risk of abuse is increased with prolonged use of suvorexant, in patients with a history of drug abuse, or those who use suvorexant in combination with alcohol or other abused drugs. Use with caution in patients with respiratory compromise, COPD, or sleep apnea. Use is not recommended in patients with severe hepatic impairment (has not been studied). Exposure is increased in females compared to males and in obese compared to nonobese patients. Consider the increased risk of exposure-related adverse effects, particularly in obese females, before increasing the dose.

Adverse Reactions

Central nervous system: Abnormal dreams (more common in females), abnormality in thinking, amnesia, anxiety, behavioral changes, central nervous system depression, drowsiness (dose dependent and more common in females), dizziness, drug abuse, drug dependence, exacerbation of depression, hallucination, headache (more common in females), hypnagogic hallucinations, sleep driving, suicidal ideation

Endocrine & metabolic: Increased serum cholesterol

Gastrointestinal: Diarrhea, xerostomia (more common in females)

Neuromuscular & skeletal: Lower extremity weakness, sleep paralysis

Respiratory: Cough (more common in females), upper respiratory tract infection (more common in females)

Drug Interactions

Metabolism/Transport Effects Substrate of CYP2C19 (minor), CYP3A4 (major); **Note:** Assignment of Major/Minor substrate status based on clinically relevant drug interaction potential

Avoid Concomitant Use

Avoid concomitant use of Suvorexant with any of the following: Alcohol (Ethyl); Azelastine (Nasal); Conivaptan; CYP3A4 Inducers (Strong); CYP3A4 Inhibitors (Strong); Fusidic Acid (Systemic); Idelalisib; Orphenadrine; Paraldehyde; Sodium Oxybate; Thalidomide

Increased Effect/Toxicity

Suvorexant may increase the levels/effects of: Azelastine (Nasal); Buprenorphine; Hydrocodone; Methotrimeprazine; Metyrosine; Orphenadrine; Paraldehyde; Pramipexole; ROPINIRole; Rotigotine; Selective Serotonin Reuptake Inhibitors; Sodium Oxybate; Thalidomide; Zolpidem

The levels/effects of Suvorexant may be increased by: Alcohol (Ethyl); Brimonidine (Topical); Cannabis; CNS Depressants; Conivaptan; CYP3A4 Inhibitors (Moderate); CYP3A4 Inhibitors (Strong); Dasatinib; Dronabinol; Droperidol; Fusidic Acid (Systemic); Idelalisib; Ivacaftor; Kava Kava; Luliconazole; Magnesium Sulfate; Methotrimeprazine; Mifepristone; Nabilone; Perampanel; Rufinamide; Simeprevir; Tapentadol; Tetrahydrocannabinol

Decreased Effect

The levels/effects of Suvorexant may be decreased by: Bosentan; CYP3A4 Inducers (Moderate); CYP3A4 Inducers (Strong); Dabrafenib; Deferasirox; Siltuximab; St Johns Wort; Tocilizumab

Storage/Stability Store at 20°C to 25°C (68°F to 77°F); excursions are permitted between 15°C and 30°C (59°F and 86°F). Protect from light and moisture.

Mechanism of Action Suvorexant blocks the binding of wake-promoting neuropeptides orexin A and orexin B to receptors OX1R and OX2R, which is thought to suppress wake drive. Antagonism of orexin receptors may also underlie potential adverse effects such as signs of narcolepsy/cataplexy.

Pharmacodynamics/Kinetics

Onset of action: ~30 minutes

Absorption: Decreased at higher doses

Distribution: V_d: ~49 L

Protein binding: >99%

Metabolism: Primarily hepatic by CYP3A with a minor contribution from CYP2C19; the hydroxy-suvorexant metabolite is inactive.

Bioavailability: 82%

Half-life elimination: ~12 hours

Time to peak: 2 hours (range: 30 minutes to 6 hours); Delayed ~1.5 hours when administered with a meal
Excretion: Feces (~66%); urine (~23%)

Dosage Insomnia: Adults: Oral: **Note:** Use the lowest effective dose for the patient. Usual dose: 10 mg once daily within 30 minutes of bedtime; may increase to a maximum of 20 mg once daily if the 10 mg dose is well tolerated but not effective. Maximum daily dose: 20 mg

Dosage adjustment for concomitant therapy:

Moderate CYP3A inhibitors (eg, amprenavir, aprepitant, atazanavir, ciprofloxacin, diltiazem, erythromycin, fluconazole, fosamprenavir, grapefruit juice, imatinib, verapamil): Usual dose: 5 mg once daily; maximum daily dose: 10 mg

Strong CYP3A inhibitors (eg, ketoconazole, itraconazole, posaconazole, clarithromycin, nefazodone, ritonavir, saquinavir, nelfinavir, indinavir, boceprevir, telaprevir, telithromycin, conivaptan): Use of suvorexant is not recommended.

CNS depressants: Dosage adjustment of suvorexant and/or the other CNS depressant may be necessary.

Dosage adjustment in renal impairment: No dosage adjustment necessary.

Dosage adjustment in hepatic impairment:

Mild or moderate impairment: No dosage adjustment necessary.

Severe impairment: Use is not recommended (has not been studied).

Dosing in obesity: Consider the increased risk of exposure-related adverse effects in obese women before increasing the dose.

Dietary Considerations For faster sleep onset, do no administer with (or immediately after) a meal.

Administration Oral: Administer within 30 minutes of bedtime with at least 7 hours remaining before planned time of awakening. Onset is delayed with food; do not administer with or immediately after a meal.

Monitoring Parameters Daytime alertness; respiratory rate; behavior profile; tolerance, abuse, dependence

Dosage Forms

Tablet, Oral:

Belsomra: 5 mg, 10 mg, 15 mg, 20 mg

- **Suxamethonium Chloride** *see* Succinylcholine *on page 1939*
- **SwabFlush Saline Flush** *see* Sodium Chloride *on page 1902*
- **Sween Cream® [OTC]** *see* Vitamin A and Vitamin D (Topical) *on page 2174*
- **Syeda** *see* Ethinyl Estradiol and Drospirenone *on page 801*
- **Sylatron** *see* Peginterferon Alfa-2b *on page 1596*
- **Sylvant** *see* Siltuximab *on page 1885*
- **Symax Duotab** *see* Hyoscyamine *on page 1026*
- **Symax FasTabs** *see* Hyoscyamine *on page 1026*
- **Symax-SL** *see* Hyoscyamine *on page 1026*
- **Symax-SR** *see* Hyoscyamine *on page 1026*
- **Symbicort** *see* Budesonide and Formoterol *on page 297*
- **SymlinPen 60** *see* Pramlintide *on page 1697*
- **SymlinPen 120** *see* Pramlintide *on page 1697*
- **Symmetrel** *see* Amantadine *on page 105*
- **Sympt-X [OTC]** *see* Glutamine *on page 971*
- **Sympt-X G.I. [OTC]** *see* Glutamine *on page 971*
- **Synacthen** *see* Cosyntropin *on page 510*
- **Synacthen Depot (Can)** *see* Cosyntropin *on page 510*
- **Synagis** *see* Palivizumab *on page 1560*
- **Synalar** *see* Fluocinolone (Topical) *on page 893*
- **Synalar® (Can)** *see* Fluocinolone (Topical) *on page 893*
- **Synalar (Cream)** *see* Fluocinolone (Topical) *on page 893*
- **Synalar (Ointment)** *see* Fluocinolone (Topical) *on page 893*
- **Synalar TS** *see* Fluocinolone (Topical) *on page 893*
- **Synalgos®-DC** *see* Dihydrocodeine, Aspirin, and Caffeine *on page 632*
- **Synapryn FusePaq** *see* TraMADol *on page 2074*
- **Synarel** *see* Nafarelin *on page 1414*
- **Synarel® (Can)** *see* Nafarelin *on page 1414*
- **Synera** *see* Lidocaine and Tetracaine *on page 1214*
- **Synercid®** *see* Quinupristin and Dalfopristin *on page 1762*
- **Synflorix (Can)** *see* Pneumococcal Conjugate Vaccine (10-Valent) [CAN/INT] *on page 1668*
- **Synphasic (Can)** *see* Ethinyl Estradiol and Norethindrone *on page 808*
- **Synribo** *see* Omacetaxine *on page 1501*
- **Synthroid** *see* Levothyroxine *on page 1205*
- **Synvisc** *see* Hyaluronate and Derivatives *on page 1006*
- **Synvisc-One** *see* Hyaluronate and Derivatives *on page 1006*
- **Syprine** *see* Trientine *on page 2102*
- **Syprine® (Can)** *see* Trientine *on page 2102*
- **SyrSpend SF** *see* Sorbitol *on page 1927*
- **Systane Omega-3 Healthy Tears [OTC]** *see* Omega-3 Fatty Acids *on page 1507*
- **T_3 Sodium (error-prone abbreviation)** *see* Liothyronine *on page 1221*
- **T_3/T_4 Liotrix** *see* Liotrix *on page 1221*
- **T_4** *see* Levothyroxine *on page 1205*
- **T-20** *see* Enfuvirtide *on page 726*
- **T-91825** *see* Ceftaroline Fosamil *on page 391*
- **Tabloid** *see* Thioguanine *on page 2029*
- **Taclonex** *see* Calcipotriene and Betamethasone *on page 321*

Tacrolimus (Systemic) (ta KROE li mus)

Brand Names: U.S. Astagraf XL; Hecoria; Prograf

Brand Names: Canada Advagraf; Prograf; Sandoz-Tacrolimus

Index Terms FK506

Pharmacologic Category Calcineurin Inhibitor; Immunosuppressant Agent

Use Organ rejection prophylaxis:

U.S. labeling:

Astagraf XL: Prevention of organ rejection in kidney transplant recipients

Hecoria: Prevention of organ rejection in heart, kidney, and liver transplant recipients

Prograf: Prevention of organ rejection in heart, kidney, and liver transplant recipients

Canadian labeling:

Advagraf: Prevention of organ rejection in kidney and liver transplant recipients

Prograf: Prevention of organ rejection in heart, kidney, or liver transplant recipients; treatment of refractory rejection in kidney or liver transplant recipients; treatment of active rheumatoid arthritis in adult patients nonresponsive to disease-modifying antirheumatic drug (DMARD) therapy or when DMARD therapy is inappropriate

Pregnancy Risk Factor C

Pregnancy Considerations Adverse events were observed in animal reproduction studies. Tacrolimus crosses the human placenta and is measurable in the cord blood, amniotic fluid, and newborn serum. Tacrolimus concentrations in the placenta may be higher than the maternal serum (Jain, 1997). Infants with lower birth weights have been found to have higher tacrolimus concentrations (Bramham, 2013). Transient neonatal hyperkalemia and renal dysfunction have been reported.

Tacrolimus pharmacokinetics are altered during pregnancy. Whole blood concentrations decrease as pregnancy progresses; however, unbound concentrations increase. Measuring unbound concentrations may be preferred, especially in women with anemia or hypoalbuminemia. If unbound concentration measurement is not available, interpretation of whole blood concentrations should account for RBC count and serum albumin concentration (Hebert, 2013; Zheng, 2012).

In general, women who have had a kidney transplant should be instructed that fertility will be restored following the transplant but that pregnancy should be avoided for ~2 years. Tacrolimus may be used as an immunosuppressant during pregnancy. The risk of infection, hypertension, and pre-eclampsia may be increased in pregnant women who have had a kidney transplant (EPBG, 2002).

The National Transplantation Pregnancy Registry (NTPR) is a registry which follows pregnancies which occur in maternal transplant recipients or those fathered by male transplant recipients. The NTPR encourages reporting of pregnancies following solid organ transplant by contacting them at 877-955-6877.

Breast-Feeding Considerations Tacrolimus is excreted into breast milk; concentrations are variable and lower than that of the maternal serum. The low bioavailability of tacrolimus following oral absorption may also decrease the amount of exposure to a nursing infant (Bramham, 2013; French, 2003; Gardiner, 2006). In one study, tacrolimus serum concentrations in the infants did not differ between those who were bottle fed or breast-fed (all infants were exposed to tacrolimus throughout pregnancy) (Bramham, 2013). Available information suggests that tacrolimus exposure to the nursing infant is ≤0.5% of the weight-adjusted maternal dose (Bramham, 2013; French, 2003; Gardiner, 2006). The manufacturer recommends that nursing be discontinued, taking into consideration the importance of the drug to the mother.

Contraindications Hypersensitivity to tacrolimus or any component of the formulation

Warnings/Precautions Hazardous agent - use appropriate precautions for handling and disposal (NIOSH 2014 [group 2]).

[U.S. Boxed Warning]: Risk of developing infections (including bacterial, viral [including CMV], fungal, and protozoal infections [including opportunistic infections]) is increased. Latent viral infections may be activated, including BK virus (associated with polyoma virus-associated nephropathy [PVAN]) and JC virus (associated with progressive multifocal leukoencephalopathy [PML]); may result in serious adverse effects. Immunosuppression increases the risk for CMV viremia and/or CMV disease; the risk of CMV disease is increased for patients who are CMV-seronegative prior to transplant and receive a graft from a CMV-seropositive donor. Consider reduction in immunosuppression if PVAN, PML, CMV viremia and/or CMV disease occurs. **[U.S. Boxed Warning]: Immunosuppressive therapy may result in the development of lymphoma and other malignancies (predominantly skin malignancies).** The risk for new-onset diabetes and insulin-dependent post-transplant diabetes mellitus (PTDM) is increased with tacrolimus use after transplantation, including in patients without pretransplant history of diabetes mellitus; insulin dependence may be reversible; monitor blood glucose frequently; risk is increased in African-American and Hispanic kidney transplant patients. Nephrotoxicity (acute or chronic) has been reported, especially with higher doses; to avoid excess nephrotoxicity do not administer simultaneously with other nephrotoxic drugs (eg, sirolimus, cyclosporine). Neurotoxicity may occur especially when used in high doses; tremor headache, coma and delirium have been reported and are associated with serum concentrations. Seizures may also occur. Posterior reversible encephalopathy syndrome (PRES) has been reported; symptoms (altered mental status, headache, hypertension, seizures, and visual disturbances) are reversible with dose reduction or discontinuation of therapy; stabilize blood pressure and reduce dose with suspected or confirmed PRES diagnosis.

Pure red cell aplasia (PRCA) has been reported in patients receiving tacrolimus. Use with caution in patients with risk factors for PRCA including parvovirus B19 infection, underlying disease, or use of concomitant medications associated with PRCA (eg, mycophenolate). Discontinuation of therapy should be considered with diagnosis of PRCA. Monitoring of serum concentrations (trough for oral therapy) is essential to prevent organ rejection and reduce drug-related toxicity. Use caution in renal or hepatic dysfunction, dosing adjustments may be required. Delay initiation of therapy in kidney transplant patients if postoperative oliguria occurs; begin therapy no sooner than 6 hours and within 24 hours post-transplant, but may be delayed until renal function has recovered. Mild-to-severe hyperkalemia may occur; monitor serum potassium levels. Hypertension may commonly occur; antihypertensive treatment may be necessary; avoid use of potassium-sparing diuretics due to risk of hyperkalemia; concurrent use of calcium channel blockers may require tacrolimus dosage adjustment. Gastrointestinal perforation may occur; all reported cases were considered to be a complication of transplant surgery or accompanied by infection, diverticulum, or malignant neoplasm. Myocardial hypertrophy has been reported (rare). Prolongation of the QT/QTc and torsade de pointes may occur; avoid use in patients with congenital long QT syndrome. Consider obtaining electrocardiograms and monitoring electrolytes (magnesium, potassium, calcium) periodically during treatment in patients with congestive heart failure, bradyarrhythmias, those taking certain antiarrhythmic medications or other medicinal products that lead to QT prolongation, and those with electrolyte disturbances such as hypokalemia, hypocalcemia, or hypomagnesemia. Potentially significant drug-drug/drug-food interactions may exist, requiring dose or frequency adjustment, additional monitoring, and/or selection of alternative therapy. In liver transplantation, the tacrolimus dose and target range should be reduced to minimize the risk of nephrotoxicity when used in combination with everolimus. Extended release tacrolimus in combination with sirolimus is not recommended in renal transplant patients; the safety and efficacy of immediate release tacrolimus in combination with sirolimus has not been established in this patient population. Concomitant use was associated with increased mortality, graft loss, and hepatic artery thrombosis in liver transplant patients, as well as increased risk of renal impairment, wound healing complications, and PTDM in heart transplant recipients.

Immediate release and extended release capsules are NOT interchangeable or substitutable. The extended release formulation is a once daily preparation; and immediate release is intended for twice daily administration. Serious adverse events, including organ rejection may occur if inadvertently substituted. **[U.S. Boxed Warning]: Extended release tacrolimus was associated with increased mortality in female liver transplant**

recipients; the use of extended release tacrolimus is not recommended in liver transplantation. Mortality at 12 months was 18% in females who received extended release tacrolimus compared to 8% for females who received regular release tacrolimus. Each mL of injection contains polyoxyl 60 hydrogenated castor oil (HCO-60) (200 mg) and dehydrated alcohol USP 80% v/v. Anaphylaxis has been reported with the injection, use should be reserved for those patients not able to take oral medications. Patients should not be immunized with live vaccines during or shortly after treatment and should avoid close contact with recently vaccinated (live vaccine) individuals. Oral formulations contain lactose; the Canadian labeling does not recommend use of these products in patients who may be lactose intolerant (eg, Lapp lactase deficiency, glucose-galactose malabsorption, galactose intolerance). **[U.S. Boxed Warning]: Should be administered under the supervision of a physician experienced in immunosuppressive therapy and organ transplantation in a facility appropriate for monitoring and managing therapy.**

Adverse Reactions As reported for kidney, liver, and heart transplantation:

Cardiovascular: Angina pectoris, atrial fibrillation, atrial flutter, bradycardia, cardiac arrest, cardiac arrhythmia, cardiac failure, cardiorespiratory arrest, cerebral infarction, cerebral ischemia, chest pain, decreased heart rate, deep vein thrombophlebitis, deep vein thrombosis, ECG abnormality (QRS or ST segment or T wave), edema, flushing, hemorrhagic stroke, hypertension, hypertrophic cardiomyopathy, hypotension, ischemic heart disease, myocardial infarction, orthostatic hypotension, pericardial effusion (heart transplant), peripheral edema, peripheral vascular disease, phlebitis, syncope, tachycardia, thrombosis, vasodilatation, ventricular premature contractions

Central nervous system: Abnormal dreams, abnormality in thinking, agitation, amnesia, anxiety, aphasia, ataxia, brain disease, carpal tunnel syndrome, chills, confusion, convulsions, depression, dizziness, drowsiness, emotional lability, excessive crying, falling, fatigue, flaccid paralysis, hallucinations, headache, hypertonia, hypoesthesia, insomnia, mental status changes, mood elevation, myasthenia, myoclonus, nervousness, neurotoxicity, nightmares, pain, paresis, paresthesia, peripheral neuropathy, psychosis, seizure, vertigo, voice disorder, writing difficulty

Dermatologic: Acne vulgaris, alopecia, bruise, cellulitis, condyloma acuminatum, dermal ulcer, dermatological reaction, dermatitis (including fungal), diaphoresis, exfoliative dermatitis, hypotrichosis, pruritus, skin discoloration, skin photosensitivity, skin rash

Endocrine & metabolic: Acidosis, albuminuria, alkalosis, anasarca, Cushing's syndrome, decreased serum bicarbonate, decreased serum iron, dehydration, diabetes mellitus (post-transplant), gout, hirsutism, hypercalcemia, hypercholesterolemia, hyperglycemia, hyperkalemia, hyperlipidemia, hypertriglyceridemia, hyperuricemia, hypervolemia, hypocalcemia, hypoglycemia, hypokalemia, hypomagnesemia, hyponatremia, hypophosphatemia, increased gamma-glutamyl transferase, increased lactate dehydrogenase, weight changes

Gastrointestinal: Abdominal pain, anorexia, aphthous stomatitis, cholangitis, colitis, constipation, delayed gastric emptying, diarrhea, duodenitis, dyspepsia, dysphagia, enlargement of abdomen, esophagitis (including ulcerative), flatulence, gastric ulcer, gastritis, gastroenteritis, gastroesophageal reflux disease, gastrointestinal hemorrhage, gastrointestinal perforation, hernia, hiccups, increased appetite, intestinal obstruction, nausea, oral candidiasis, pancreatic disease (pseudocyst), pancreatitis (including hemorrhagic and necrotizing), peritonitis, rectal disease, stomach cramps, stomatitis, vomiting

Genitourinary: Anuria, bladder spasm, cystitis, dysuria, hematuria, nocturia, oliguria, proteinuria, toxic nephrosis, urinary frequency, urinary incontinence, urinary retention, urinary tract infection, urinary urgency, vaginitis

Hematologic & oncologic: Anemia, blood coagulation disorder, decreased prothrombin time, hemolytic anemia, hemorrhage, hypochromic anemia, hypoproteinemia, increased hematocrit, increased INR, Kaposi's sarcoma, leukocytosis, leukopenia, malignant neoplasm of bladder, malignant neoplasm of thyroid (papillary), neutropenia, pancytopenia, polycythemia, skin neoplasm, thrombocytopenia

Hepatic: Abnormal hepatic function tests, ascites, cholestatic jaundice, hepatic injury, hepatitis (including acute, chronic, and granulomatous), hyperbilirubinemia, increased liver enzymes, increased serum alkaline phosphatase, jaundice

Hypersensitivity: Hypersensitivity reaction

Infection: Abscess, bacterial infection, cytomegalovirus disease, Epstein Barr virus infection, herpes simplex infection, infection, polyoma virus infection, sepsis, serious infection, tinea versicolor

Local: Localized phlebitis, postoperative wound complication

Neuromuscular & skeletal: Arthralgia, arthropathy, back pain, leg cramps, muscle spasm, muscle weakness of the extremities, myalgia, neuropathy (including compression), osteopenia, osteoporosis, tremor, weakness

Ophthalmic: Amblyopia, blurred vision, conjunctivitis, visual disturbance

Otic: Hearing loss, otalgia, otitis externa, otitis media, tinnitus

Renal: Acute renal failure, hydronephrosis, increased blood urea nitrogen, increased serum creatinine, renal disease (BK nephropathy), renal function abnormality, renal tubular necrosis

Respiratory: Allergic rhinitis, asthma, atelectasis, bronchitis, cough, dyspnea, emphysema, flu-like symptoms, pharyngitis, pleural effusion, pneumonia, pneumothorax, pulmonary disease, pulmonary edema, pulmonary infiltrates, respiratory depression, respiratory failure, respiratory tract infection, rhinitis, sinusitis

Miscellaneous: Fever, graft complications, postoperative pain, wound healing impairment

Rare but important or life-threatening: Adult respiratory distress syndrome, agranulocytosis, anaphylactoid reaction, anaphylaxis, angioedema, basal cell carcinoma, biliary tract disease (stenosis), blindness, cerebrovascular accident, coma, deafness, decreased serum fibrinogen, delirium, disseminated intravascular coagulation, dysarthria, graft versus host disease (acute and chronic), hemiparesis, hemolytic-uremic syndrome, hemorrhagic cystitis, hepatic cirrhosis, hepatic failure, hepatic necrosis, hepatic veno-occlusive disease, hepatosplenic T-cell lymphomas, hepatotoxicity, hyperpigmentation, interstitial pulmonary disease, leukemia, leukoencephalopathy, liver steatosis, lymphoproliferative disorder (post-transplant or related to EBV), malignant melanoma, multiorgan failure, mutism, optic atrophy, osteomyelitis, photophobia, polyarthritis, progressive multifocal leukoencephalopathy (PML), prolonged partial thromboplastin time, prolonged Q-T interval on ECG, pulmonary hypertension, pure red cell aplasia, quadriplegia, reversible posterior leukoencephalopathy syndrome, rhabdomyolysis, septicemia, squamous cell carcinoma, status epilepticus, Stevens-Johnson syndrome, supraventricular extrasystole, supraventricular tachycardia, thrombocytopenic purpura, thrombotic thrombocytopenic purpura, torsades de pointes, toxic epidermal necrolysis, venous thrombosis, ventricular fibrillation

Note: Calcineurin inhibitor-induced hemolytic uremic syndrome/thrombotic thrombocytopenic purpura/thrombotic microangiopathy (HUS/TTP/TMA) have been reported (with concurrent sirolimus).

Drug Interactions

Metabolism/Transport Effects **Substrate** of CYP3A4 (major), P-glycoprotein; **Note:** Assignment of Major/Minor substrate status based on clinically relevant drug interaction potential; **Inhibits** CYP3A4 (weak), P-glycoprotein

Avoid Concomitant Use

Avoid concomitant use of Tacrolimus (Systemic) with any of the following: BCG; Bosutinib; CloZAPine; Conivaptan; Crizotinib; CycloSPORINE (Systemic); Dipyrone; Enzalutamide; Eplerenone; Foscarnet; Fusidic Acid (Systemic); Grapefruit Juice; Idelalisib; Mifepristone; Natalizumab; PAZOPanib; Pimecrolimus; Pimozide; Potassium-Sparing Diuretics; Silodosin; Sirolimus; Tacrolimus (Topical); Temsirolimus; Tofacitinib; Topotecan; Vaccines (Live); VinCRIStine (Liposomal)

Increased Effect/Toxicity

Tacrolimus (Systemic) may increase the levels/effects of: Afatinib; ARIPiprazole; Bosutinib; Brentuximab Vedotin; CloZAPine; Colchicine; CycloSPORINE (Systemic); Dabigatran Etexilate; DOXOrubicin (Conventional); Dronedarone; Edoxaban; Everolimus; Fenofibrate and Derivatives; Fosphenytoin; Highest Risk QTc-Prolonging Agents; Hydrocodone; Ledipasvir; Leflunomide; Lomitapide; Moderate Risk QTc-Prolonging Agents; Naloxegol; Natalizumab; PAZOPanib; P-glycoprotein/ABCB1 Substrates; Phenytoin; Pimozide; Prucalopride; Rifaximin; Rivaroxaban; Silodosin; Sirolimus; Temsirolimus; Tofacitinib; Topotecan; Vaccines (Live); VinCRIStine (Liposomal)

The levels/effects of Tacrolimus (Systemic) may be increased by: Alcohol (Ethyl); Antidepressants (Serotonin Reuptake Inhibitor/Antagonist); Aprepitant; Boceprevir; Calcium Channel Blockers (Dihydropyridine); Calcium Channel Blockers (Nondihydropyridine); Ceritinib; Chloramphenicol; Clotrimazole (Oral); Clotrimazole (Topical); Conivaptan; Crizotinib; CycloSPORINE (Systemic); CYP3A4 Inhibitors (Moderate); CYP3A4 Inhibitors (Strong); Danazol; Dasatinib; Denosumab; Dipyrone; Dronedarone; Eplerenone; Ertapenem; Fluconazole; Fosaprepitant; Foscarnet; Fusidic Acid (Systemic); Grapefruit Juice; Idelalisib; Itraconazole; Ivacaftor; Ketoconazole (Systemic); Levofloxacin (Systemic); Luliconazole; Macrolide Antibiotics; Mifepristone; Netupitant; Nonsteroidal Anti-Inflammatory Agents; P-glycoprotein/ABCB1 Inhibitors; Pimecrolimus; Posaconazole; Potassium-Sparing Diuretics; Protease Inhibitors; Proton Pump Inhibitors; Ranolazine; Ritonavir; Roflumilast; Sirolimus; Stiripentol; Tacrolimus (Topical); Telaprevir; Temsirolimus; Trastuzumab; Voriconazole

Decreased Effect

Tacrolimus (Systemic) may decrease the levels/effects of: BCG; Coccidioides immitis Skin Test; Sipuleucel-T; Vaccines (Inactivated); Vaccines (Live)

The levels/effects of Tacrolimus (Systemic) may be decreased by: Bosentan; Caspofungin; Cinacalcet; CYP3A4 Inducers (Moderate); CYP3A4 Inducers (Strong); Dabrafenib; Deferasirox; Echinacea; Efavirenz; Enzalutamide; Fosphenytoin; Mitotane; P-glycoprotein/ABCB1 Inducers; Phenytoin; Rifamycin Derivatives; Sevelamer; Siltuximab; Sirolimus; St Johns Wort; Temsirolimus; Tocilizumab

Food Interactions

Ethanol: Alcohol may increase the rate of release of extended-release tacrolimus and adversely affect tacrolimus safety and/or efficacy. Management: Avoid alcohol.

Food: Food decreases rate and extent of absorption. High-fat meals have most pronounced effect (37% and 25% decrease in AUC, respectively, and 77% and 25% decrease in C_{max}, respectively, for immediately release and extended release formulations). Grapefruit juice, a CYP3A4 inhibitor, may increase serum level and/or toxicity of tacrolimus. Management: Administer with or without food (immediate release), but be consistent. Administer extended release on an empty stomach. Avoid concurrent use of grapefruit juice.

Preparation for Administration Hazardous agent; use appropriate precautions for handling and disposal (NIOSH 2014 [group 2]).

Injection: Dilute with 5% dextrose injection or 0.9% sodium chloride injection to a final concentration between 0.004 mg/mL and 0.02 mg/mL.

Storage/Stability

Injection: Prior to dilution, store at 5°C to 25°C (41°F to 77°F). Following dilution, stable for 24 hours in D_5W or NS in glass or polyethylene containers. Do not store in polyvinyl chloride containers since the polyoxyl 60 hydrogenated castor oil injectable vehicle may leach phthalates from polyvinyl chloride containers.

Capsules:

Astagraf XL, Prograf: Store at 25°C (77°F); excursions permitted between 15°C and 30°C (59°F and 86°F).

Hecoria: Store at 20°C to 25°C (68°F to 77°F).

Mechanism of Action Suppresses cellular immunity (inhibits T-lymphocyte activation), by binding to an intracellular protein, FKBP-12 and complexes with calcineurin dependent proteins to inhibit calcineurin phosphatase activity

Pharmacodynamics/Kinetics

Absorption: Better in resected patients with a closed stoma; unlike cyclosporine, clamping of the T-tube in liver transplant patients does not alter trough concentrations or AUC; Oral: Incomplete and variable; the rate and extent of absorption is decreased by food (particularly a high-fat meal). Oral absorption may be variable in stem cell transplant patients with mucositis due to the conditioning regimen.

Distribution: V_d: Children: 0.5 to 4.7 L/kg; Adults: 0.55 to 2.47 L/kg

Protein binding: ~99% primarily to albumin and alpha$_1$-acid glycoprotein glycoprotein

Metabolism: Extensively hepatic via CYP3A4 to eight possible metabolites (major metabolite, 31-demethyl tacrolimus, shows same activity as tacrolimus *in vitro*)

Bioavailability: Oral: Children: 7% to 55%, Adults: 7% to 32%; Absolute: Unknown

Half-life elimination:

Immediate release: Variable, 23 to 46 hours in healthy volunteers; 2.1 to 36 hours in transplant patients

Extended release: 34.5 to 41 hours

Time to peak: 0.5 to 6 hours

Excretion: Feces (~93%); urine (<1% as unchanged drug)

Dosage

Children:

Liver transplant:

Oral: Immediate release: Initial: 0.15 to 0.20 mg/kg/day in 2 divided doses, given every 12 hours (titrate to target trough concentrations)

IV: Initial: 0.03 to 0.05 mg/kg/day as a continuous infusion

Note: The initial postoperative dose of tacrolimus should begin no sooner than 6 hours after liver and heart transplant and within 24 hours of kidney transplant (but may be delayed until renal function has recovered). Adjunctive therapy with corticosteroids is recommended early post-transplant. IV route should only be used in patients not able to take oral medications and continued only until oral medication can be tolerated; anaphylaxis has been reported with IV administration. If switching from IV to oral, the oral dose should be started 8 to 12 hours after stopping the infusion. Patients without pre-existing renal or hepatic dysfunction have required (and tolerated) higher doses than adults to achieve similar blood concentrations. It is recommended that therapy be initiated at the **high end** of the recommended adult IV and oral dosing ranges; dosage adjustments may be required.

Prevention of graft-vs-host disease (GVHD) (off-label use): Oral, IV: Refer to adult dosing.

Adults:

Prevention of organ rejection in transplant recipients:
Note: The initial postoperative dose of tacrolimus (immediate release) should begin no sooner than 6 hours after liver and heart transplant and within 24 hours of kidney transplant (but may be delayed until renal function has recovered); titrate to target trough concentrations. Adjunctive therapy with corticosteroids is recommended early post-transplant. IV route should only be used in patients not able to take oral medications and continued only until oral medication can be tolerated; anaphylaxis has been reported with IV administration. If switching from IV to oral, the oral dose should be started 8 to 12 hours after stopping the infusion.

Liver transplant:
Oral:
Immediate release: Initial: 0.1 to 0.15 mg/kg/day in 2 divided doses, given every 12 hours (titrate to target trough concentrations)
Extended release: Canadian labeling (Advagraf): 0.1 to 0.2 mg/kg once daily in combination with corticosteroids; initiate within 12 to 18 hours of transplantation. Titrate to target trough concentrations.
Conversion from immediate release to extended release: Patients stable on immediate release tacrolimus may be converted to extended release by initiating extended release treatment in a 1:1 ratio (mg:mg) using previously established total daily dose of immediate release product. Administer once daily.
IV: Initial: 0.03 to 0.05 mg/kg/day as a continuous infusion

Heart transplant: Use in combination with azathioprine or mycophenolate mofetil is recommended.
Oral: Immediate release: Initial: 0.075 mg/kg/day in 2 divided doses, given every 12 hours (titrate to target trough concentrations)
IV: Initial: 0.01 mg/kg/day as a continuous infusion

Kidney transplant: Use in combination with azathioprine or mycophenolate mofetil is recommended. **Note:** African-American patients may require larger doses to attain trough concentration.
Oral:
U.S. labeling:
Immediate release (Hecoria, Prograf): Initial: 0.2 mg/kg/day in combination with azathioprine or 0.1 mg/kg/day in combination with mycophenolate mofetil; titrate to target trough concentrations. Administer in 2 divided doses, given every 12 hours.
Extended release (Astagraf XL):
With basiliximab induction (prior to or within 48 hours of transplant completion): 0.15 mg/kg once daily (in combination with corticosteroids and mycophenolate); titrate to target trough concentrations
Without basiliximab induction: Preoperative dose (administer within 12 hours prior to reperfusion): 0.1 mg/kg
Without basiliximab induction: Postoperative dosing (administer at least 4 hours after preoperative dose and within 12 hours of reperfusion): 0.2 mg/kg once daily (in combination with corticosteroids and mycophenolate); titrate to target trough concentrations
Conversion from IV to extended release: Administer the first oral extended release dose 8 to 12 hours after discontinuation of IV tacrolimus
Conversion from immediate release to extended release: Initiate extended release treatment in a 1:1 ratio (mg:mg) using previously established total daily dose of immediate release (Van Hooff, 2012). Administer once daily.
Canadian labeling:
Immediate release (Prograf): Initial: 0.2 to 0.3 mg/kg/day in 2 divided doses, given every 12 hours in combination with corticosteroids and other immunosuppressive agents; titrate to target trough concentrations
Extended release (Advagraf): Initial: 0.15 to 0.2 mg/kg once daily; titrate to target trough concentrations. Administer in combination with corticosteroids and mycophenolate mofetil (MMF) in *de novo* kidney transplant recipients. Antibody induction therapy should also be used.
Conversion from immediate release to extended release: Initiate extended release treatment in a 1:1 ratio (mg:mg) using previously established total daily dose of immediate release. Administer once daily.
IV: Initial: 0.03 to 0.05 mg/kg/day as a continuous infusion

Graft-versus-host disease (GVHD) (off-label use):
Adults:
Prevention:
Oral: Convert from IV to immediate release oral dose (1:4 ratio): Multiply total daily IV dose times 4 and administer in 2 divided oral doses per day, every 12 hours (Uberti, 1999; Yanik, 2000).
IV: Initial: 0.03 mg/kg/day (based on lean body weight) as continuous infusion. Treatment should begin at least 24 hours prior to stem cell infusion and continued only until oral medication can be tolerated (Przepiorka, 1999; Yanik, 2000).
Treatment:
Oral: Immediate release: 0.06 mg/kg twice daily (Furlong, 2000; Przepiorka, 1999)
IV: Initial: 0.03 mg/kg/day (based on lean body weight) as continuous infusion (Furlong, 2000; Przepiorka, 1999)

Rheumatoid arthritis: Canadian labeling (not in U.S. labeling): Oral: Immediate release: 3 mg once daily; carefully monitor serum creatinine during therapy

Dosing adjustment in renal impairment: Systemic therapy: Evidence suggests that lower doses should be used; patients should receive doses at the lowest value of the recommended IV and oral dosing ranges; further reductions in dose below these ranges may be required. May also require dose reductions due to nephrotoxicity.
Kidney transplant: Tacrolimus therapy in patients with postoperative oliguria should begin no sooner than 6 hours and within 24 hours (immediate release) or 48 hours (extended release) post-transplant, but may be delayed until renal function displays evidence of recovery.
Hemodialysis: Not removed by hemodialysis; supplemental dose is not necessary.
Peritoneal dialysis: Significant drug removal is unlikely based on physiochemical characteristics.

Dosing adjustment in hepatic impairment: Systemic therapy: Use of tacrolimus in liver transplant recipients experiencing post-transplant hepatic impairment may be associated with increased risk of developing renal insufficiency related to high whole blood levels of tacrolimus. The presence of moderate-to-severe hepatic dysfunction (serum bilirubin >2 mg/dL; Child-Pugh score ≥10) appears to affect the metabolism of tacrolimus. The half-life of the drug was prolonged and the clearance reduced after IV administration. The bioavailability of tacrolimus was also increased after oral administration. The higher plasma concentrations as determined by ELISA, in patients with severe hepatic dysfunction are probably due to the accumulation of metabolites of lower activity. These patients should be monitored closely and dosage adjustments should be considered. Some evidence indicates that lower doses could be used in these patients.

Dietary Considerations Capsule: Administer immediate release with or without food; be consistent with timing and composition of meals, food decreases bioavailability. Administer extended release on an empty stomach 1 hour before or 2 hours after a meal. Avoid grapefruit juice. Avoid alcohol.

Administration

IV: If IV administration is necessary, administer by continuous infusion only. Do not use PVC tubing when administering diluted solutions. Tacrolimus is usually intended to be administered as a continuous infusion over 24 hours. Do not mix with solutions with a pH ≥9 (eg, acyclovir or ganciclovir) due to chemical degradation of tacrolimus (use different ports in multilumen lines). Do not alter dose with concurrent T-tube clamping. Adsorption of the drug to PVC tubing may become clinically significant with low concentrations.

Oral:

Immediate release: Administer with or without food; be consistent with timing and composition of meals if GI intolerance occurs and administration with food becomes necessary (per manufacturer). If dosed once daily, administer in the morning. If dosed twice daily, doses should be 12 hours apart. If the morning and evening doses differ, the larger dose (differences are never >0.5-1 mg) should be given in the morning. If dosed 3 times daily, separate doses by 8 hours.

Combination therapy with everolimus for liver transplantation: Administer tacrolimus at the same time as everolimus.

Extended release: Administer on an empty stomach at least 1 hour before or 2 hours after a meal. Advagraf [Canadian product] labeling suggests that the capsule may be taken with food if necessary but should be administered consistently with or without food. Swallow whole, do not chew, crush, or divide. Take once daily in the morning at a consistent time each day. Missed doses may be taken up to 14 hours after scheduled time; if >14 hours, resume at next regularly scheduled time; do not double a dose to make up for a missed dose.

Hazardous agent; use appropriate precautions for handling and disposal (NIOSH 2014 [group 2]).

Monitoring Parameters Renal function, hepatic function, serum electrolytes (calcium, magnesium, potassium), glucose and blood pressure, measure 3 times/week for first few weeks, then gradually decrease frequency as patient stabilizes. Whole blood concentrations should be used for monitoring (trough for oral therapy). Signs/symptoms of anaphylactic reactions during IV infusion should also be monitored. Patients should be monitored during the first 30 minutes of the infusion, and frequently thereafter. Monitor for QT prolongation; consider echocardiographic evaluation in patients who develop renal failure, electrolyte abnormalities, or clinical manifestations of ventricular dysfunction.

Tacrolimus serum levels may be falsely elevated in infected liver transplant patients due to interference from β-galactosidase antibodies.

Reference Range

Heart transplant: Typical whole blood trough concentrations:
- Months 1 to 3: 10 to 20 ng/mL
- Months ≥4: 5 to 15 ng/mL

Kidney transplant: Whole blood trough concentrations:
- Immediate release:
  - In combination with azathioprine:
    - Months 1 to 3: 7 to 20 ng/mL
    - Months 4 to 12: 5 to 15 ng/mL
  - In combination with mycophenolate mofetil/IL-2 receptor antagonist (eg, daclizumab): Months 1 to 12: 4 to 11 ng/mL
- Extended release:
  - With basiliximab induction:
    - Days 1 to 60: 5 to 17 ng/mL
    - Month 3 to 12: 4 to 12 ng/mL
  - Without induction:
    - Days 1 to 60: 6 to 20 ng/mL
    - Month 3 to 12: 6 to 14 ng/mL

Liver transplant: Whole blood trough concentrations:
- *U.S. labeling:* Months 1 to 12: 5 to 20 ng/mL
- *Canadian labeling:* Months 1 to 2: 5 to 20 ng/mL; Months 3 to 12: 5 to 15 ng/mL.
- *Recommended therapeutic ranges when administered in combination with everolimus for liver transplant (Zortress product labeling, 2013):* By 3 weeks after first everolimus dose and through month 12 post-transplant: 3 to 5 ng/mL

Prevention of graft-versus-host disease (off-label use): 10 to 20 ng/mL (Uberti, 1999) although some institutions use a lower limit of 5 ng/mL and an upper limit of 15 ng/mL (Przepiorka, 1999; Yanik, 2000)

Dosage Forms

Capsule, Oral:
- Hecoria: 0.5 mg, 1 mg, 5 mg
- Prograf: 0.5 mg, 1 mg, 5 mg
- Generic: 0.5 mg, 1 mg, 5 mg

Capsule Extended Release 24 Hour, Oral:
- Astagraf XL: 0.5 mg, 1 mg, 5 mg

Solution, Intravenous:
- Prograf: 5 mg/mL (1 mL)

Dosage Forms: Canada

Capsule Extended Release 24 Hour, Oral:
- Advagraf: 0.5 mg, 1 mg, 3 mg, 5 mg

Extemporaneous Preparations Hazardous agent; use appropriate precautions for handling and disposal (NIOSH 2014 [group 2]).

A 0.5 mg/mL tacrolimus oral suspension may be made with immediate release capsules and a 1:1 mixture of Ora-Plus® and Simple Syrup, N.F. Mix the contents of six 5 mg tacrolimus capsules with quantity of vehicle sufficient to make 60 mL. Store in glass or plastic amber prescription bottles; label "shake well". Stable for 56 days at room temperature (Esquivel, 1996; Foster, 1996).

A 1 mg/mL tacrolimus oral suspension may be made with immediate release capsules, sterile water, Ora-Plus®, and Ora-Sweet®. Pour the contents of six 5 mg capsules into a plastic amber prescription bottle. Add ~5 mL of sterile water and agitate bottle until drug disperses into a slurry. Add equal parts Ora-Plus® and Ora-Sweet® in sufficient quantity to make 30 mL. Store in plastic amber prescription bottles; label "shake well". Stable for 4 months at room temperature (Elefante, 2006).

Elefante A, Muindi J, West K, et al, "Long-Term Stability of a Patient-Convenient 1 mg/mL Suspension of Tacrolimus for Accurate Maintenance of Stable Therapeutic Levels," *Bone Marrow Transplant*, 2006, 37(8):781-4.

Esquivel C, So S, McDiarmid S, Andrews W, and Colombani PM, "Suggested Guidelines for the Use of Tacrolimus in Pediatric Liver Transplant Patients," *Transplantation*, 1996, 61(5):847-8.

Foster JA, Jacobson PA, Johnson CE, et al, "Stability of Tacrolimus in an Extemporaneously Compounded Oral Liquid (Abstract of Meeting Presentation)," *American Society of Health-System Pharmacists Annual Meeting*, 1996, 53:P-52(E).

Tacrolimus (Topical) (ta KROE li mus)

Brand Names: U.S. Protopic

Brand Names: Canada Protopic®

Pharmacologic Category Calcineurin Inhibitor; Immunosuppressant Agent; Topical Skin Product

Use Moderate-to-severe atopic dermatitis in immunocompetent patients not responsive to conventional therapy or when conventional therapy is not appropriate

Canadian labeling: Additional use (not in U.S. labeling): Maintenance therapy to prevent flares and extend flare-free intervals in patients with moderate-to-severe atopic dermatitis who are responsive to initial therapy and experiencing ≥5 flares per year

Pregnancy Risk Factor C

Dosage Topical: Atopic dermatitis (moderate-to-severe):

Treatment:

Children ≥2-15 years: Apply thin layer of 0.03% ointment to affected area twice daily; rub in gently and completely. Discontinue use when symptoms have cleared. If no improvement within 6 weeks, patients should be re-examined to confirm diagnosis.

Children >15 years and Adults: Apply thin layer of 0.03% or 0.1% ointment to affected area twice daily; rub in gently and completely. Discontinue use when symptoms have cleared. If no improvement within 6 weeks, patients should be re-examined to confirm diagnosis.

Maintenance therapy (Canadian labeling; not in U.S. labeling):

Children ≥2-15 years: Apply one application (thin layer of 0.03% ointment) to areas usually affected twice a week, allowing 2-3 days between applications (eg, one application on Monday and Thursday). Reevaluate after 12 months. Safety of maintenance therapy >12 months has not been established.

Children >15 years and Adults: Apply one application (thin layer of 0.03% or 0.1% ointment) to areas usually affected twice a week, allowing 2-3 days between applications (eg, one application on Monday and Thursday). Re-evaluate after 12 months. Safety of maintenance therapy >12 months has not been established.

Note: Patients experiencing flares should resume twice daily treatment.

Additional Information Complete prescribing information should be consulted for additional detail.

Dosage Forms

Ointment, External:

Protopic: 0.03% (30 g, 60 g, 100 g); 0.1% (30 g, 60 g, 100 g)

Generic: 0.03% (30 g, 60 g, 100 g); 0.1% (30 g, 60 g, 100 g)

◆ **Tactuo™ (Can)** *see* Adapalene and Benzoyl Peroxide *on page 54*

Tadalafil (tah DA la fil)

Brand Names: U.S. Adcirca; Cialis

Brand Names: Canada Adcirca; Cialis

Index Terms GF196960

Pharmacologic Category Phosphodiesterase-5 Enzyme Inhibitor

Use

Benign prostatic hyperplasia (Cialis only): Treatment of the signs and symptoms of benign prostatic hyperplasia (BPH).

Erectile dysfunction (Cialis only): Treatment of erectile dysfunction.

Erectile dysfunction and benign prostatic hyperplasia (Cialis only): Treatment of erectile dysfunction and the signs and symptoms of BPH.

Pulmonary arterial hypertension (Adcirca only): Treatment of pulmonary arterial hypertension (World Health Organization group 1) to improve exercise ability. Studies establishing effectiveness included predominately patients with New York Heart Association (NYHA) functional class II to III symptoms and etiologies of idiopathic or heritable pulmonary arterial hypertension (61%) or pulmonary arterial hypertension associated with connective tissue diseases (23%).

Pregnancy Risk Factor B

Pregnancy Considerations Teratogenic events were not reported in animal reproduction studies. Postnatal development and pup survival was decreased at some doses. There are no adequate and well-controlled studies in pregnant women. Less than 0.0005% is found in the semen of healthy males.

Breast-Feeding Considerations It is not known if tadalafil is excreted in breast milk. The manufacturer recommends that caution be exercised when administering tadalafil to nursing women.

Contraindications Concurrent use of organic nitrate (regularly and/or intermittently); serious hypersensitivity to tadalafil or any component of the formulation

Warnings/Precautions There is a degree of cardiac risk associated with sexual activity; therefore, physicians should consider the cardiovascular status of their patients prior to initiation. Use is not recommended in patients with hypotension (<90/50 mm Hg), uncontrolled hypertension (>170/100 mm Hg), NYHA class II-IV heart failure within the last 6 months, uncontrolled arrhythmias, stroke within the last 6 months, MI within the last 3 months, unstable angina or angina during sexual intercourse; safety and efficacy have not been evaluated in these patients. Safety and efficacy in PAH have not been evaluated in patients with clinically significant aortic and/or mitral valve disease, life-threatening arrhythmias, hypotension (<90/50 mm Hg), uncontrolled hypertension, significant left ventricular dysfunction, pericardial constriction, restrictive or congestive cardiomyopathy, symptomatic coronary artery disease. Use caution in patients with left ventricular outflow obstruction (eg, aortic stenosis, hypertrophic obstructive cardiomyopathy); may be more sensitive to vasodilator effects. Patients experiencing anginal chest pain after tadalafil administration should seek immediate medical attention.

Pulmonary vasodilators may exacerbate the cardiovascular status in patients with pulmonary veno-occlusive disease (PVOD); use is not recommended. In patients with unrecognized PVOD, signs of pulmonary edema should prompt investigation into this diagnosis. Use with caution in patients with mild-to-moderate hepatic impairment; dosage adjustment/limitation is needed. Use is not recommended in patients with severe hepatic impairment or cirrhosis. Use with caution in patients with renal impairment; dosage adjustment/limitation is needed. Use caution in patients with bleeding disorders or peptic ulcer disease due to effect on platelets (bleeding).

When used to treat BPH or erectile dysfunction, potential underlying causes of BPH or erectile dysfunction should be evaluated prior to treatment. Use with caution in patients with anatomical deformation of the penis (angulation, cavernosal fibrosis, or Peyronie's disease), or who have conditions which may predispose them to priapism (sickle cell anemia, multiple myeloma, leukemia). Priapism, painful erection >6 hours in duration has been reported (rarely). Instruct patients to seek immediate medical attention if erection persists >4 hours. Potentially significant drug-drug interactions may exist, requiring dose or frequency adjustment, additional monitoring, and/or selection of alternative therapy. Concomitant use (regularly/intermittently) with all forms of nitrates is contraindicated. Nitrate-mediated vasodilation is markedly exaggerated and prolonged in the presence of PDE-5 inhibitors. When tadalafil is used for BPH, erectile dysfunction, or PAH and nitrate administration is medically necessary (eg, chest pain refractory to other treatments) following the use of tadalafil, at least 48 hours should elapse after the tadalafil dose and nitrate administration. When used for PAH, per the manufacturer, nitrate may be administered within 48 hours of tadalafil. For both situations, administration of nitrates should only be done under close medical supervision with hemodynamic monitoring.

Rare cases of nonarteritic anterior ischemic optic neuropathy (NAION) have been reported; patients who have already experienced NAION are at an increased risk of recurrence. Other risk factors for NAION include heart disease, diabetes, hypertension, smoking, age >50 years, or history of certain eye problems. Use with caution in these patients only when the benefits outweigh the risks. Sudden decrease or loss of hearing has been reported rarely; hearing changes may be accompanied by tinnitus and dizziness. A direct relationship between therapy and vision or hearing loss has not been determined. Instruct patients to seek medical assistance for sudden loss of vision in one or both eyes, sudden decrease in hearing, or sudden loss of hearing.

Patients with genetic retinal disorders (eg, retinitis pigmentosa) were not evaluated in clinical trials; use is not recommended.

Adverse Reactions Based upon usual doses for either indication. For erectile dysfunction, similar adverse events are reported with once-daily versus intermittent dosing, but are generally lower than with doses used intermittently.

Cardiovascular: Flushing, hypertension

Central nervous system: Headache

Gastrointestinal: Abdominal pain, diarrhea, dyspepsia, gastroenteritis (viral), GERD, nausea

Genitourinary: Urinary tract infection

Neuromuscular & skeletal: Back pain, extremity pain, myalgia

Respiratory: Bronchitis, cough, nasal congestion, nasopharyngitis, respiratory tract infection

Miscellaneous: Flu-like syndrome

Rare but important or life-threatening: Amnesia (transient global), angina pectoris, arthralgia, blurred vision, chest pain, color vision decreased, conjunctival hyperemia, conjunctivitis, diaphoresis, dizziness, dysphagia, dyspnea, epistaxis, esophagitis, exfoliative dermatitis, eye pain, eyelid swelling, facial edema, fatigue, gastritis, GGTP increased, hearing decreased, hearing loss, hepatic enzymes increased, hypoesthesia, hypotension, insomnia, lacrimation, migraine, MI, neck pain, nonarteritic ischemic optic neuropathy (NAION), orthostatic hypotension, pain, palpitation, paresthesia, pharyngitis, priapism, pruritus, rash, retinal artery occlusion, retinal vein occlusion, seizure, somnolence, spontaneous penile erection, Stevens-Johnson syndrome, stroke, sudden cardiac death, syncope, tachycardia, tinnitus, urticaria, vertigo, visual field loss, vomiting, weakness, xerostomia

Drug Interactions

Metabolism/Transport Effects Substrate of CYP3A4 (major); **Note:** Assignment of Major/Minor substrate status based on clinically relevant drug interaction potential

Avoid Concomitant Use

Avoid concomitant use of Tadalafil with any of the following: Alprostadil; Amyl Nitrite; Conivaptan; Dapoxetine; Fusidic Acid (Systemic); Idelalisib; Phosphodiesterase 5 Inhibitors; Riociguat; Tipranavir; Vasodilators (Organic Nitrates)

Increased Effect/Toxicity

Tadalafil may increase the levels/effects of: Alpha1-Blockers; Alprostadil; Amyl Nitrite; Antihypertensives; Bosentan; Phosphodiesterase 5 Inhibitors; Riociguat; Vasodilators (Organic Nitrates)

The levels/effects of Tadalafil may be increased by: Alcohol (Ethyl); Aprepitant; Boceprevir; Ceritinib; Cobicistat; Conivaptan; CYP3A4 Inhibitors (Moderate); CYP3A4 Inhibitors (Strong); Dapoxetine; Dasatinib; Fluconazole; Fosaprepitant; Fusidic Acid (Systemic); Idelalisib; Itraconazole; Ivacaftor; Ketoconazole (Systemic); Lorcaserin; Luliconazole; Mifepristone; Netupitant; Posaconazole; Ritonavir; Sapropterin; Simeprevir; Stiripentol; Telaprevir; Tipranavir; Voriconazole

Decreased Effect

The levels/effects of Tadalafil may be decreased by: Bosentan; CYP3A4 Inducers (Strong); Etravirine

Food Interactions Rate and extent of absorption are not affected by food. Grapefruit juice may increase serum levels/toxicity of tadalafil. Management: Use of grapefruit juice should be limited or avoided.

Storage/Stability Store at 25°C (77°F); excursions permitted to 15°C to 30°C (59°F to 86°F).

Mechanism of Action

BPH: Exact mechanism unknown; effects likely due to PDE-5 mediated reduction in smooth muscle and endothelial cell proliferation, decreased nerve activity, and increased smooth muscle relaxation and tissue perfusion of the prostate and bladder

Erectile dysfunction: Does not directly cause penile erections, but affects the response to sexual stimulation. The physiologic mechanism of erection of the penis involves release of nitric oxide (NO) in the corpus cavernosum during sexual stimulation. NO then activates the enzyme guanylate cyclase, which results in increased levels of cyclic guanosine monophosphate (cGMP), producing smooth muscle relaxation and inflow of blood to the corpus cavernosum. Tadalafil enhances the effect of NO by inhibiting phosphodiesterase type 5 (PDE-5), which is responsible for degradation of cGMP in the corpus cavernosum; when sexual stimulation causes local release of NO, inhibition of PDE-5 by tadalafil causes increased levels of cGMP in the corpus cavernosum, resulting in smooth muscle relaxation and inflow of blood to the corpus cavernosum. At recommended doses, it has no effect in the absence of sexual stimulation.

PAH: Inhibits phosphodiesterase type 5 (PDE-5) in smooth muscle of pulmonary vasculature where PDE-5 is responsible for the degradation of cyclic guanosine monophosphate (cGMP). Increased cGMP concentration results in pulmonary vasculature relaxation; vasodilation in the pulmonary bed and the systemic circulation (to a lesser degree) may occur.

Pharmacodynamics/Kinetics

Onset of action: Within 1 hour

Peak effect (pulmonary artery vasodilation): 75 to 90 minutes (Ghofrani, 2004)

Duration: Erectile dysfunction: Up to 36 hours

Distribution: V_d: 63 to 77 L

Protein binding: 94%

Metabolism: Hepatic, via CYP3A4 to metabolites (inactive)

Half-life elimination: 15 to 17.5 hours; Pulmonary hypertension (not receiving bosentan): 35 hours

Time to peak, plasma: ~2 hours (range: 30 minutes to 6 hours)

Excretion: Feces (~61%, predominantly as metabolites); urine (~36%, predominantly as metabolites)

Dosage Oral: Adults:

Benign prostatic hyperplasia (with or without concomitant erectile dysfunction) (Cialis): 5 mg once daily. **Note:** When tadalafil is used with finasteride to initiate BPH therapy, the recommended duration of therapy is ≤26 weeks.

Dosing adjustment with concomitant medications:

$Alpha_1$-blockers: Not recommended for use in combination with alpha-blockers for the treatment of BPH.

CYP3A4 inhibitors (strong): 2.5 mg once daily; maximum: 2.5 mg once daily

Erectile dysfunction (Cialis):

As-needed dosing: 10 mg (U.S. labeling) or 20 mg (Canadian labeling) at least 30 minutes prior to anticipated sexual activity as one single dose and not more than once daily. Dose may be adjusted based on tolerability (dosing range: 5 to 20 mg). **Note:** Erectile function may be improved for up to 36 hours following a single dose.

Once-daily dosing: 2.5 mg once daily (U.S. labeling) or 5 mg once daily (Canadian labeling) at approximately the same time daily without regard to timing of sexual activity. Dose may be adjusted based on tolerability (dosage range: 2.5 to 5 mg/day).

Dosing adjustment with concomitant medications:

U.S. labeling: Alpha$_1$-blockers: Patients should be stable on alpha-blocker therapy prior to initiating tadalafil treatment, and tadalafil should be initiated at the lowest recommended dose.

Canadian labeling: Nonselective alpha-blockers (eg, doxazosin): *As-needed dosing:* 10 mg at least 30 minutes prior to anticipated sexual activity

CYP3A4 inhibitors (strong):

As-needed dosing:

U.S. labeling: Maximum: 10 mg, not more frequently than every 72 hours

Canadian labeling: 10 mg, not more frequently than every 48 hours (maximum: 3 doses/week); may increase to 20 mg if lower dose is tolerated but ineffective. Discontinue use if 10 mg dose is not tolerated.

Once-daily dosing:

U.S. labeling: Maximum: 2.5 mg once daily

Canadian labeling: 2.5 to 5 mg once daily

Pulmonary arterial hypertension (Adcirca): 40 mg once daily

Dosing adjustment with concomitant medications:

Concurrent use with ritonavir:

Initiation of tadalafil in patients currently receiving ritonavir for at least 1 week: Initiate tadalafil at 20 mg once daily; increase to 40 mg once daily based on individual tolerability.

Initiation of ritonavir in patients currently receiving tadalafil: Discontinue tadalafil at least 24 hours prior to the initiation of ritonavir. After at least 1 week of ritonavir, resume tadalafil at 20 mg once daily; increase to 40 mg once daily based on individual tolerability.

Elderly: No dose adjustment for patients >65 years of age in the absence of renal or hepatic impairment

Dosage adjustment in renal impairment:

Benign prostatic hyperplasia (with or without concomitant erectile dysfunction) (Cialis):

CrCl ≥51 mL/minute: No dosage adjustment necessary.

CrCl 30 to 50 mL/minute: Initial: 2.5 mg once daily; maximum: 5 mg once daily

CrCl <30 mL/minute: Use not recommended

ESRD requiring hemodialysis: Use not recommended

Erectile dysfunction (Cialis):

As-needed use:

U.S. labeling:

CrCl ≥51 mL/minute: No dosage adjustment necessary.

CrCl 30 to 50 mL/minute: Initial: 5 mg once daily; maximum: 10 mg (not more frequently than every 48 hours)

CrCl <30 mL/minute: Maximum: 5 mg (not more frequently than every 72 hours)

ESRD requiring hemodialysis: Maximum: 5 mg (not more frequently than every 72 hours)

Canadian labeling:

CrCl >80 mL/minute: No dosage adjustment necessary.

CrCl ≥31 to 80 mL/minute: 10 mg, not more frequently than every 48 hours (maximum: 3 doses/week); may increase to 20 mg if lower dose is tolerated but ineffective. Discontinue use if 10 mg dose is not tolerated.

CrCl <30 mL/minute: Use with extreme caution; has not been adequately studied

ESRD requiring hemodialysis: Use with extreme caution; has not been adequately studied

Once-daily use:

CrCl ≥31 mL/minute: No dosage adjustment necessary.

CrCl <30 mL/minute: Use not recommended

ESRD requiring hemodialysis: Use not recommended

Pulmonary arterial hypertension (Adcirca):

CrCl 31 to 80 mL/minute: Initial: 20 mg once daily; increase to 40 mg once daily based on individual tolerability

CrCl ≤30 mL/minute: Avoid use due to increased tadalafil exposure, limited clinical experience, and lack of ability to influence clearance by dialysis.

ESRD requiring hemodialysis: Avoid use due to increased tadalafil exposure, limited clinical experience, and lack of ability to influence clearance by dialysis.

Dosage adjustment in hepatic impairment:

Benign prostatic hyperplasia (with or without concomitant erectile dysfunction) (Cialis):

Mild-to-moderate impairment (Child-Pugh class A or B): Use with caution; the use of tadalafil for once-daily use has not been extensively evaluated in patients with hepatic impairment.

Severe impairment (Child-Pugh class C): Use is not recommended

Erectile dysfunction (Cialis):

As-needed use:

U.S. labeling:

Mild-to-moderate impairment (Child-Pugh class A or B): Use with caution; dose should not exceed 10 mg once daily. The use of tadalafil once per day has not been evaluated extensively in patients with hepatic impairment.

Severe impairment (Child-Pugh class C): Use is not recommended

Canadian labeling:

Mild-to-moderate impairment (Child-Pugh class A or B): 10 mg, not more frequently than every 48 hours (maximum 3 doses/week); may increase to 20 mg if lower dose is tolerated but ineffective. Discontinue use if 10 mg dose is not tolerated.

Severe impairment (Child-Pugh class C): Use with extreme caution; has not been adequately studied

Once-daily use:

U.S. labeling:

Mild-to-moderate impairment (Child-Pugh class A or B): Use with caution; the use of tadalafil for once-daily use has not been extensively evaluated in patients with hepatic impairment.

Severe impairment (Child-Pugh class C): Use is not recommended

Canadian labeling:

Mild-to-moderate impairment (Child-Pugh class A or B): No dosage adjustment necessary.

Severe impairment (Child-Pugh class C): Use with extreme caution; has not been adequately studied

Pulmonary arterial hypertension (Adcirca):

Mild-to-moderate impairment (Child-Pugh class A or B): Use with caution; consider initial dose of 20 mg once daily

Severe impairment (Child-Pugh class C): Avoid use; has not been studied in patients with severe hepatic cirrhosis.

Administration May be administered with or without food.
Adcirca: Administer daily dose all at once; dividing doses throughout the day is not advised.
Cialis: When used on an as-needed basis, should be taken at least 30 minutes prior to sexual activity. When used on a once-daily basis, should be taken at the same time each day, without regard to timing of sexual activity.

Monitoring Parameters Blood pressure, response and adverse effects; urine flow, PSA

Dosage Forms

Tablet, Oral:
Adcirca: 20 mg
Cialis: 2.5 mg, 5 mg, 10 mg, 20 mg

Extemporaneous Preparations A 5 mg/mL tadalafil oral suspension may be made with tablets in a 1:1 mixture of Ora-Plus® and Ora-Sweet®. Crush fifteen 20 mg tadalafil tablets in a glass mortar and reduce to a fine powder. Prepare the vehicle by mixing 30 mL of Ora-Plus® and 30 mL of Ora-Sweet®; stir vigorously. Add 30 mL of the vehicle in geometric proportions to the powder and mix to form a smooth suspension. Transfer the mixture to a 2 ounce amber plastic prescription bottle. Rinse mortar with a quantity of the vehicle sufficient to make a final volume of 60 mL. Label "shake well." Stable for 91 days when stored in amber plastic prescription bottles at room temperature.
Pettit RS, Johnson CE, and Caruthers RL, "Stability of an Extemporaneously Prepared Tadalafil Suspension," *Am J Health Syst Pharm*, 2012, 69(7):592-4.

- **Tafinlar** *see* Dabrafenib *on page 546*
- **Tagamet HB [OTC]** *see* Cimetidine *on page 438*
- **TAK-375** *see* Ramelteon *on page 1770*
- **TAK-390MR** *see* Dexlansoprazole *on page 603*
- **TAK-599** *see* Ceftaroline Fosamil *on page 391*
- **Take Action [OTC]** *see* Levonorgestrel *on page 1201*
- **Talc** *see* Talc (Sterile) *on page 1971*
- **Talc for Pleurodesis** *see* Talc (Sterile) *on page 1971*

Talc (Sterile) (talk STARE il)

Brand Names: U.S. Sclerosol Intrapleural; Sterile Talc Powder

Index Terms Intrapleural Talc; Sterile Talc; Talc; Talc for Pleurodesis

Pharmacologic Category Sclerosing Agent

Use Pleural effusion, malignant: Sclerosing agent to decrease or prevent the recurrence of malignant pleural effusion in symptomatic patients (following maximal drainage of pleural effusion)

Pregnancy Risk Factor B

Dosage
Pleural effusion, malignant: Adults: Intrapleural aerosol: 4 to 8 g (1 to 2 cans) as a single dose
Pleural effusion: Adults: Intrapleural suspension: 5 g

Dosage adjustment in renal impairment: There are no dosage adjustments provided in the manufacturer's labeling.
Dosage adjustment in hepatic impairment: There are no dosage adjustments provided in the manufacturer's labeling.

Additional Information Complete prescribing information should be consulted for additional detail.

Dosage Forms

Aerosol Powder, Intrapleural:
Sclerosol Intrapleural: 4 g (30 g)

Suspension Reconstituted, Intrapleural:
Sterile Talc Powder: 5 g (1 ea)

Taliglucerase Alfa (tal i GLOO ser ase AL fa)

Brand Names: U.S. Elelyso

Pharmacologic Category Enzyme

Use Gaucher disease: For long-term enzyme replacement therapy for adult and pediatric patients with a confirmed diagnosis of type 1 Gaucher disease.

Pregnancy Risk Factor B

Dosage Note: Pretreatment with antihistamines, antipyretics, and/or corticosteroids can be considered for prevention of subsequent infusion reactions in patients with an infusion reaction requiring symptomatic treatment; during clinical studies, patients were not routinely premedicated prior to infusion.

Gaucher disease (type 1): Children ≥4 years, Adolescents, and Adults: IV: 60 units/kg every 2 weeks; dosing is individualized based on disease severity.
Conversion from imiglucerase: Initiate taliglucerase alfa using the patient's same previous imiglucerase dose and administer every 2 weeks. **Note:** Conversion to taliglucerase alfa is based on a single study of patients stabilized on a biweekly imiglucerase dose for ≥6 months.

Dosage adjustment in renal impairment: There are no dosage adjustments provided in the manufacturer's labeling.
Dosage adjustment in hepatic impairment: There are no dosage adjustments provided in the manufacturer's labeling.

Additional Information Complete prescribing information should be consulted for additional detail.

Dosage Forms

Solution Reconstituted, Intravenous [preservative free]:
Elelyso: 200 units (1 ea)

- **Talwin** *see* Pentazocine *on page 1616*
- **Tambocor [DSC]** *see* Flecainide *on page 882*
- **Tambocor™ (Can)** *see* Flecainide *on page 882*
- **Tamiflu** *see* Oseltamivir *on page 1523*

Tamoxifen (ta MOKS i fen)

Brand Names: U.S. Soltamox

Brand Names: Canada Apo-Tamox; Mylan-Tamoxifen; Nolvadex-D; PMS-Tamoxifen; Teva-Tamoxifen

Index Terms ICI-46474; Nolvadex; Tamoxifen Citras; Tamoxifen Citrate

Pharmacologic Category Antineoplastic Agent, Estrogen Receptor Antagonist; Selective Estrogen Receptor Modulator (SERM)

Use Treatment of metastatic (female and male) breast cancer; adjuvant treatment of breast cancer after primary treatment with surgery and radiation; reduce risk of invasive breast cancer in women with ductal carcinoma *in situ* (DCIS) after surgery and radiation; reduce the incidence of breast cancer in women at high risk

Pregnancy Risk Factor D

Pregnancy Considerations Animal reproduction studies have demonstrated fetal adverse effects and fetal loss. There have been reports of vaginal bleeding, birth defects and fetal loss in pregnant women. Tamoxifen use during pregnancy may have a potential long term risk to the fetus of a DES-like syndrome. For sexually-active women of childbearing age, initiate during menstruation (negative β-hCG immediately prior to initiation in women with irregular cycles). Tamoxifen may induce ovulation. Barrier or nonhormonal contraceptives are recommended. Pregnancy should be avoided during treatment and for 2 months after treatment has been discontinued.

Breast-Feeding Considerations It is not known if tamoxifen is excreted in breast milk, however, it has been shown to inhibit lactation. Due to the potential for adverse reactions, women taking tamoxifen should not breast-feed.

Contraindications Hypersensitivity to tamoxifen or any component of the formulation; concurrent warfarin therapy or history of deep vein thrombosis or pulmonary embolism (when tamoxifen is used for breast cancer risk reduction in women at high risk for breast cancer or with ductal carcinoma *in situ* [DCIS])

Warnings/Precautions Hazardous agent - use appropriate precautions for handling and disposal (NIOSH 2014 [group 1]). **[U.S. Boxed Warning]: Serious and life-threatening events (some fatal), including stroke, pulmonary emboli, and uterine or endometrial malignancies, have occurred at an incidence greater than placebo during use for breast cancer risk reduction in women at high-risk for breast cancer and in women with ductal carcinoma *in situ* (DCIS). In women already diagnosed with breast cancer, the benefits of tamoxifen treatment outweigh risks; evaluate risks versus benefits (and discuss with patients) when used for breast cancer risk reduction.** An increased incidence of thromboembolic events, including DVT and pulmonary embolism, has been associated with use for breast cancer; risk is increased with concomitant chemotherapy; use with caution in individuals with a history of thromboembolic events. Thrombocytopenia and/or leukopenia may occur; neutropenia and pancytopenia have been reported rarely. Although the relationship to tamoxifen therapy is uncertain, rare hemorrhagic episodes have occurred in patients with significant thrombocytopenia. Use with caution in patients with hyperlipidemias; infrequent postmarketing cases of hyperlipidemias have been reported. Decreased visual acuity, retinal vein thrombosis, retinopathy, corneal changes, color perception changes, and increased incidence of cataracts (and the need for cataract surgery), have been reported. Hypercalcemia has occurred in some patients with bone metastasis, usually within a few weeks of therapy initiation; institute appropriate hypercalcemia management; discontinue if severe. Local disease flare and increased bone and tumor pain may occur in patients with metastatic breast cancer; may be associated with (good) tumor response.

Potentially significant drug-drug interactions may exist, requiring dose or frequency adjustment, additional monitoring, and/or selection of alternative therapy. Decreased efficacy and an increased risk of breast cancer recurrence has been reported with concurrent moderate or strong CYP2D6 inhibitors (Aubert, 2009; Dezentje, 2009). Concomitant use with select SSRIs may result in decreased tamoxifen efficacy. Strong CYP2D6 inhibitors (eg, fluoxetine, paroxetine) and moderate CYP2D6 inhibitors (eg, sertraline) are reported to interfere with transformation to the active metabolite endoxifen; when possible, select alternative medications with minimal or no impact on endoxifen levels (NCCN Breast Cancer Risk Reduction Guidelines v.1.2013; Sideras, 2010). Weak CYP2D6 inhibitors (eg, venlafaxine, citalopram) have minimal effect on the conversion to endoxifen (Jin, 2005; NCCN Breast Cancer Risk Reduction Guidelines v.1.2013); escitalopram is also a weak CYP2D6 inhibitor. In a retrospective analysis of breast cancer patients taking tamoxifen and SSRIs, concomitant use of paroxetine and tamoxifen was associated with an increased risk of death due to breast cancer (Kelly, 2010). Lower plasma concentrations of endoxifen have been observed in patients associated with reduced CYP2D6 activity (Jin, 2005; Schroth, 2009) and may be associated with reduced efficacy, although data is conflicting. Routine CYP2D6 testing is not recommended at this time in order to determine optimal endocrine therapy (NCCN Breast Cancer Guidelines v.2.2013; Visvanathan, 2009).

Tamoxifen use may be associated with changes in bone mineral density (BMD) and the effects may be dependent upon menstrual status. In postmenopausal women, tamoxifen use is associated with a protective effect on bone mineral density (BMD), preventing loss of BMD which lasts over the 5-year treatment period. In premenopausal women, a decline (from baseline) in BMD mineral density has been observed in women who continued to menstruate; may be associated with an increased risk of fractures. Liver abnormalities such as cholestasis, fatty liver, hepatitis, and hepatic necrosis have occurred. Hepatocellular carcinomas have been reported in some studies; relationship to treatment is unclear. Tamoxifen is associated with an increased incidence of uterine or endometrial cancers. Endometrial hyperplasia, polyps, endometriosis, uterine fibroids, and ovarian cysts have occurred. Monitor and promptly evaluate any report of abnormal vaginal bleeding. Amenorrhea and menstrual irregularities have been reported with tamoxifen use.

Adverse Reactions

Cardiovascular: Angina, cardiovascular ischemia, chest pain, deep venous thrombus, edema, flushing, hypertension, MI, peripheral edema, vasodilation, venous thrombotic events

Central nervous system: Anxiety, depression, dizziness, fatigue, headache, insomnia, mood changes, pain

Dermatologic: Alopecia, rash, skin changes

Endocrine & metabolic: Altered menses, amenorrhea, breast neoplasm, breast pain, fluid retention, hot flashes, hypercholesterolemia, menstrual disorder, oligomenorrhea

Gastrointestinal: Abdominal cramps, abdominal pain, anorexia, constipation, diarrhea, dyspepsia, nausea, throat irritation (oral solution), vomiting, weight gain/loss

Genitourinary: Leukorrhea, ovarian cyst, urinary tract infection, vaginal bleeding, vaginal discharge, vaginal hemorrhage, vaginitis, vulvovaginitis

Hematologic: Anemia, thrombocytopenia

Hepatic: AST increased, serum bilirubin increased

Neuromuscular & skeletal: Arthralgia, arthritis, arthrosis, back pain, bone pain, fracture, joint disorder, musculoskeletal pain, myalgia, osteoporosis, paresthesia, weakness

Ocular: Cataract

Renal: Serum creatinine increased

Respiratory: Bronchitis, cough, dyspnea, pharyngitis, sinusitis

Miscellaneous: Allergic reaction, cyst, diaphoresis, flu-like syndrome, infection/sepsis, lymphedema, neoplasm

Rare but important or life-threatening: Angioedema, bullous pemphigoid, cholestasis, corneal changes, endometrial cancer, endometrial hyperplasia, endometrial polyps, endometriosis, erythema multiforme, fatty liver, hepatic necrosis, hepatitis, hypercalcemia, hyperlipidemia, hypersensitivity reactions, hypertriglyceridemia, impotence (males), interstitial pneumonitis, loss of libido (males), pancreatitis, phlebitis, pruritus vulvae, pulmonary embolism, retinal vein thrombosis, retinopathy, second primary tumors, Stevens-Johnson syndrome, stroke, tumor pain and local disease flare (including increase in lesion size and erythema) during treatment of metastatic breast cancer (generally resolves with continuation); uterine fibroids, vaginal dryness, visual color perception changes

Drug Interactions

Metabolism/Transport Effects Substrate of CYP2A6 (minor), CYP2B6 (minor), CYP2C9 (major), CYP2D6 (major), CYP2E1 (minor), CYP3A4 (major); **Note:** Assignment of Major/Minor substrate status based on clinically relevant drug interaction potential; **Inhibits**

CYP2B6 (weak), CYP2C8 (moderate), CYP2C9 (weak), CYP3A4 (weak), P-glycoprotein

Avoid Concomitant Use

Avoid concomitant use of Tamoxifen with any of the following: Bosutinib; Conivaptan; CYP2D6 Inhibitors (Strong); Fusidic Acid (Systemic); Idelalisib; Ospemifene; PAZOPanib; Pimozide; Silodosin; Topotecan; VinCRIStine (Liposomal); Vitamin K Antagonists

Increased Effect/Toxicity

Tamoxifen may increase the levels/effects of: Afatinib; ARIPiprazole; Bosutinib; Brentuximab Vedotin; Colchicine; CYP2C8 Substrates; Dabigatran Etexilate; DOXOrubicin (Conventional); Edoxaban; Everolimus; Highest Risk QTc-Prolonging Agents; Hydrocodone; Ledipasvir; Lomitapide; Mipomersen; Moderate Risk QTc-Prolonging Agents; Naloxegol; Ospemifene; PAZOPanib; P-glycoprotein/ABCB1 Substrates; Pimozide; Prucalopride; Rifaximin; Rivaroxaban; Silodosin; Topotecan; VinCRIStine (Liposomal); Vitamin K Antagonists

The levels/effects of Tamoxifen may be increased by: Abiraterone Acetate; Ceritinib; Conivaptan; CYP2C9 Inhibitors (Moderate); CYP2C9 Inhibitors (Strong); CYP3A4 Inhibitors (Moderate); CYP3A4 Inhibitors (Strong); Dasatinib; Fosaprepitant; Fusidic Acid (Systemic); Idelalisib; Ivacaftor; Luliconazole; Mifepristone; Netupitant; Peginterferon Alfa-2b; Simeprevir

Decreased Effect

Tamoxifen may decrease the levels/effects of: Anastrozole; Letrozole; Ospemifene

The levels/effects of Tamoxifen may be decreased by: Aminoglutethimide; Bexarotene (Systemic); Bosentan; CYP2C9 Inducers (Strong); CYP2D6 Inhibitors (Moderate); CYP2D6 Inhibitors (Strong); CYP3A4 Inducers (Moderate); CYP3A4 Inducers (Strong); Dabrafenib; Deferasirox; Mitotane; Peginterferon Alfa-2b; Rifamycin Derivatives; Siltuximab; St Johns Wort; Tocilizumab

Food Interactions Grapefruit juice may decrease the metabolism of tamoxifen. Management: Avoid grapefruit juice.

Storage/Stability

Oral solution: Store at ≤25°C (77°F); do not freeze or refrigerate. Protect from light. Discard opened bottle after 3 months.

Tablets: Store at 20°C to 25°C (68°F to 77°F). Protect from light.

Mechanism of Action Competitively binds to estrogen receptors on tumors and other tissue targets, producing a nuclear complex that decreases DNA synthesis and inhibits estrogen effects; nonsteroidal agent with potent antiestrogenic properties which compete with estrogen for binding sites in breast and other tissues; cells accumulate in the G_0 and G_1 phases; therefore, tamoxifen is cytostatic rather than cytocidal.

Pharmacodynamics/Kinetics

Absorption: Well absorbed

Distribution: High concentrations found in uterus, endometrial and breast tissue

Protein binding: 99%

Metabolism: Hepatic; via CYP2D6 to 4-hydroxytamoxifen and via CYP3A4/5 to N-desmethyl-tamoxifen. Each is then further metabolized into endoxifen (4-hydroxy-tamoxifen via CYP3A4/5 and N-desmethyl-tamoxifen via CYP2D6); both 4-hydroxy-tamoxifen and endoxifen are 30- to 100-fold more potent than tamoxifen

Half-life elimination: Tamoxifen: ~5-7 days; N-desmethyl tamoxifen: ~14 days

Time to peak, serum: ~5 hours

Excretion: Feces (26% to 51%); urine (9% to 13%)

Dosage Oral: **Note:** For the treatment of breast cancer, patients receiving both tamoxifen and chemotherapy should receive treatment sequentially, with tamoxifen following completion of chemotherapy.

Children: Females: Precocious puberty secondary to McCune-Albright syndrome (off-label use): A dose of 20 mg daily has been reported in patients 2-10 years of age; safety and efficacy have not been established for treatment of longer than 1 year duration (Eugster, 2003)

Adults:

Breast cancer treatment:

Adjuvant therapy (females): 20 mg once daily for 5 years

Premenopausal women: Duration of treatment is 5 years (Burstein, 2010; NCCN Breast Cancer guidelines v.2.2013)

Postmenopausal women: Duration of tamoxifen treatment is 2-3 years followed by an aromatase inhibitor (AI) to complete 5 years; may take tamoxifen for the full 5 years (if contraindications or intolerance to AI) or extended therapy: 4.5-6 years of tamoxifen followed by 5 years of an AI (Burstein, 2010; NCCN Breast Cancer guidelines v.2.2013)

ER-positive early breast cancer: Extended duration: Duration of treatment of 10 years demonstrated a reduced risk of recurrence and mortality (Davies, 2012)

Metastatic (males and females): 20-40 mg daily (doses >20 mg should be given in 2 divided doses). **Note:** Although the FDA-approved labeling recommends dosing up to 40 mg daily, clinical benefit has not been demonstrated with doses above 20 mg daily (Bratherton, 1984).

Ductal carcinoma *in situ* (DCIS) (females), to reduce the risk for invasive breast cancer: 20 mg once daily for 5 years

Breast cancer risk reduction (pre- and postmenopausal high-risk females): 20 mg once daily for 5 years

Endometrial carcinoma, recurrent, metastatic, or high-risk (endometrioid histologies only) (off-label use):

Monotherapy: 20 mg twice daily until disease progression or unacceptable toxicity (Thigpen, 2001)

Combination therapy: 20 mg twice daily for 3 weeks (alternating with megestrol acetate every 3 weeks); continue alternating until disease progression or unacceptable toxicity) (Fiorica, 2004)

Induction of ovulation (off-label use): 20 mg once daily (range: 20-80 mg once daily) for 5 days (Steiner, 2005)

Ovarian cancer, advanced and/or recurrent (off-label use): 20 mg twice daily (Hatch, 1991; Markman, 1996)

Paget's disease of the breast (risk reduction; with DCIS or without associated cancer): 20 mg once daily for 5 years (NCCN Breast Cancer Guidelines, v.2.2013)

Dosage adjustment for DVT, pulmonary embolism, cerebrovascular accident, or prolonged immobilization: Discontinue tamoxifen (NCCN Breast Cancer Risk Reduction Guidelines, v.1.2013)

Dosage adjustment in renal impairment: No dosage adjustment provided in manufacturer's labeling.

Chronic dialysis: No dosage adjustment necessary (Janus, 2013).

Dosage adjustment in hepatic impairment: No dosage adjustment provided in manufacturer's labeling (has not been studied).

Dietary Considerations Tablets and oral solution may be taken with or without food. Avoid grapefruit and grapefruit juice.

Administration Administer tablets or oral solution orally with or without food. Use supplied dosing cup for oral solution.

Hazardous agent; use appropriate precautions for handling and disposal (NIOSH 2014 [group 1]).

Monitoring Parameters CBC with platelets, serum calcium, LFTs; triglycerides and cholesterol (in patients with preexisting hyperlipidemias); INR and PT (in patients on vitamin K antagonists); abnormal vaginal bleeding; breast and gynecologic exams (baseline and routine), mammogram (baseline and routine); signs/symptoms of DVT (leg swelling, tenderness) or PE (shortness of breath); ophthalmic exam (if vision problem or cataracts); bone mineral density (premenopausal women)

Additional Information Estrogen receptor status may predict if adjuvant treatment with tamoxifen is of benefit. In metastatic breast cancer, patients with estrogen receptor positive tumors are more likely to benefit from tamoxifen treatment. With tamoxifen use to reduce the incidence of breast cancer in high risk-women, high risk is defined as women ≥35 years of age with a 5 year NCI Gail model predicted risk of breast cancer ≥1.67%.

Oncology Comment: The American Society of Clinical Oncology (ASCO) guidelines for adjuvant endocrine therapy in postmenopausal women with HR-positive breast cancer (Burstein, 2010) recommend considering aromatase inhibitor (AI) therapy at some point in the treatment course (primary, sequentially, or extended). Optimal duration at this time is not known; however, treatment with an AI should not exceed 5 years in primary and extended therapies, and 2-3 years if followed by tamoxifen in sequential therapy (total of 5 years). If initial therapy with AI has been discontinued before the 5 years, consideration should be taken to receive tamoxifen for a total of 5 years. The optimal time to switch to an AI is also not known; but data supports switching after 2-3 years of tamoxifen (sequential) or after 5 years of tamoxifen (extended). If patient becomes intolerant or has poor adherence, consideration should be made to switch to another AI or initiate tamoxifen.

Recent data suggest that continuing tamoxifen for 10 years (rather than stopping after 5 years of therapy) may provide a further reduction in breast cancer recurrence and mortality in women with early stage disease (Davies, 2012). The Adjuvant Tamoxifen: Longer Against Shorter (ATLAS) trial randomized 6846 patients with estrogen receptor positive disease to continue tamoxifen for a total of 10 years of treatment or to stop after 5 years. Breast cancer recurrence was observed in 617 patients in the 10-year arm versus 711 recurrences in the 5-year arm (p=0.002). Breast cancer mortality was significantly reduced with 10 years of tamoxifen therapy versus 5 years (331 deaths vs 397 deaths, respectively; p=0.01) (Davies, 2012).

The adjuvant endocrine therapy of choice is tamoxifen for men with breast cancer and for pre- or perimenopausal women at diagnosis. CYP2D6 genotyping is not recommended, however, due to the potential for drug-drug interactions use caution and consider avoiding concomitant therapy with tamoxifen and known CYP2D6 inhibitors.

Dosage Forms

Solution, Oral:

Soltamox: 10 mg/5 mL (150 mL)

Tablet, Oral:

Generic: 10 mg, 20 mg

Extemporaneous Preparations Hazardous agent: Use appropriate precautions for handling and disposal (NIOSH 2014 [group 1]).

A 0.5 mg/mL oral suspension may be prepared with tablets. Place two 10 mg tablets into 40 mL purified water and let stand ~2-5 minutes. Stir until tablets are completely disintegrated (dispersion time for each 10 mg tablet is ~2-5 minutes). Administer immediately after preparation. To ensure the full dose is administered, rinse glass several times with water and administer residue.

Lam MS, "Extemporaneous Compounding of Oral Liquid Dosage Formulations and Alternative Drug Delivery Methods for Anticancer Drugs," *Pharmacotherapy*, 2011, 31(2):164-92.

◆ **Tamoxifen Citras** *see* Tamoxifen *on page 1971*

◆ **Tamoxifen Citrate** *see* Tamoxifen *on page 1971*

Tamsulosin (tam SOO loe sin)

Brand Names: U.S. Flomax

Brand Names: Canada Apo-Tamsulosin CR; Flomax CR; Mylan-Tamsulosin; ratio-Tamsulosin; Sandoz-Tamsulosin; Tamsulosin CR; Teva-Tamsulosin; Teva-Tamsulosin CR

Index Terms Tamsulosin Hydrochloride

Pharmacologic Category Alpha$_1$ Blocker

Use

Benign prostatic hyperplasia: Treatment of signs and symptoms of benign prostatic hyperplasia (BPH)

Limitations of use: Not indicated for the treatment of hypertension.

Pregnancy Risk Factor B

Pregnancy Considerations Adverse events were not observed in animal reproduction studies. For pregnant women with kidney stones, other treatments such as stents or ureteroscopy, are recommended if stone removal is needed (Preminger, 2007; Tan, 2013).

Contraindications Hypersensitivity to tamsulosin or any component of the formulation

Warnings/Precautions Not intended for use as an antihypertensive drug. May cause significant orthostatic hypotension and syncope, especially with first dose; anticipate a similar effect if therapy is interrupted for a few days, if dosage is rapidly increased, or if another antihypertensive drug (particularly vasodilators) or a PDE-5 inhibitor (eg, sildenafil, tadalafil, vardenafil) is introduced. "First-dose" orthostatic hypotension may occur 4 to 8 hours after dosing; may be dose related. Patients should be cautioned about performing hazardous tasks, driving, or operating heavy machinery when starting new therapy or adjusting dosage upward. Discontinue if symptoms of angina occur or worsen. Rule out prostatic carcinoma with screening before beginning therapy with tamsulosin and then screen at regular intervals.

Intraoperative floppy iris syndrome (IFIS) is characterized by a combination of flaccid iris that billows with intraoperative currents, progressive intraoperative miosis despite dilation, and potential iris prolapse. IFIS has been observed in cataract and glaucoma surgery patients who were on or were previously treated with alpha$_1$-blockers, particularly with tamsulosin use (Abdel-Aziz, 2009); in some cases, patients had discontinued the alpha$_1$-blocker 5 weeks to 9 months prior to the surgery. The benefit of discontinuing alpha-blocker therapy prior to cataract or glaucoma surgery has not been established. IFIS may increase the risk of ocular complications during and after surgery. May require modifications to surgical technique; instruct patients to inform ophthalmologist of current or previous alpha$_1$-blocker use when considering eye surgery. Initiation of tamsulosin therapy in patients with planned cataract or glaucoma surgery is not recommended. Priapism has been associated with use (rarely). Rarely, patients with a sulfa allergy have also developed an allergic reaction to tamsulosin; avoid use when previous reaction has been severe or life-threatening. Potentially significant drug-drug interactions may exist, requiring dose or frequency adjustment, additional monitoring, and/or selection of alternative therapy.

Adverse Reactions

Cardiovascular: Orthostatic hypotension

Central nervous system: Dizziness, drowsiness, headache, insomnia, vertigo

Endocrine & metabolic: Loss of libido

Gastrointestinal: Diarrhea, nausea

Genitourinary: Ejaculation failure

Infection: Infection

Neuromuscular & skeletal: Back pain, weakness

Ophthalmic: Blurred vision

Respiratory: Cough, pharyngitis, rhinitis, sinusitis

Rare but important or life-threatening): Epistaxis, exfoliative dermatitis, hypersensitivity reaction, hypotension, intraoperative floppy iris syndrome, palpitation, priapism, syncope

Drug Interactions

Metabolism/Transport Effects Substrate of CYP2D6 (minor), CYP3A4 (major); **Note:** Assignment of Major/Minor substrate status based on clinically relevant drug interaction potential

Avoid Concomitant Use

Avoid concomitant use of Tamsulosin with any of the following: Alpha1-Blockers; Conivaptan; CYP3A4 Inhibitors (Strong); Fusidic Acid (Systemic); Idelalisib

Increased Effect/Toxicity

Tamsulosin may increase the levels/effects of: Alpha1-Blockers; Calcium Channel Blockers

The levels/effects of Tamsulosin may be increased by: Aprepitant; Beta-Blockers; Ceritinib; Conivaptan; CYP3A4 Inhibitors (Moderate); CYP3A4 Inhibitors (Strong); Dapoxetine; Dasatinib; Fosaprepitant; Fusidic Acid (Systemic); Idelalisib; Ivacaftor; Luliconazole; MAO Inhibitors; Mifepristone; Netupitant; Phosphodiesterase 5 Inhibitors; Simeprevir

Decreased Effect

Tamsulosin may decrease the levels/effects of: Alpha-/Beta-Agonists; Alpha1-Agonists

The levels/effects of Tamsulosin may be decreased by: Bosentan; CYP3A4 Inducers (Moderate); CYP3A4 Inducers (Strong); Dabrafenib; Deferasirox; Mitotane; Siltuximab; St Johns Wort; Tocilizumab

Food Interactions Fasting increases bioavailability by 30% and peak concentration 40% to 70%. Management: Administer 30 minutes after the same meal each day.

Storage/Stability Store at 25°C (77°F); excursions are permitted between 15°C and 30°C (59°F and 86°F).

Mechanism of Action Tamsulosin is an antagonist of $alpha_{1A}$-adrenoreceptors in the prostate. Smooth muscle tone in the prostate is mediated by $alpha_{1A}$-adrenoreceptors; blocking them leads to relaxation of smooth muscle in the bladder neck and prostate causing an improvement of urine flow and decreased symptoms of BPH. Approximately 75% of the $alpha_1$-receptors in the prostate are of the $alpha_{1A}$ subtype.

Pharmacodynamics/Kinetics

Absorption: >90%

Distribution: V_d: 16 L

Protein binding: 94% to 99%, primarily to $alpha_1$ acid glycoprotein (AAG)

Metabolism: Hepatic (extensive) via CYP3A4 and 2D6; metabolites undergo extensive conjugation to glucuronide or sulfate

Bioavailability: Fasting: 30% increase

Steady-state: By the fifth day of once-daily dosing

Half-life elimination: Healthy volunteers: 9 to 13 hours; Target population: 14 to 15 hours

Time to peak: Fasting: 4 to 5 hours; With food: 6 to 7 hours

Excretion: Urine (76%, <10% as unchanged drug); feces (21%)

Dosage Benign prostatic hyperplasia (BPH): Adult males: Oral: 0.4 mg once daily ~30 minutes after the same meal each day; dose may be increased after 2 to 4 weeks to 0.8 mg once daily in patients who fail to respond. If therapy is discontinued or interrupted for several days, restart with 0.4 mg once daily.

Bladder outlet obstruction symptoms (off-label use): Adults: Oral: 0.4 mg once daily (Rossi, 2001)

Ureteral calculi (distal) expulsion (off-label use): Adults: Oral: 0.4 mg once daily, discontinue after successful expulsion (average time to expulsion was 1 to 2 weeks) (Agrawal, 2009; Ahmed, 2010). **Note:** Patients with stones >10 mm were excluded from studies.

Dosage adjustment in renal impairment:

CrCl ≥10 mL/minute: No dosage adjustment necessary.

CrCl <10 mL/minute: There are no dosage adjustments provided in the manufacturer's labeling (has not been studied).

Dosage adjustment in hepatic impairment:

Mild-to-moderate impairment: No dosage adjustment needed

Severe impairment: There are no dosage adjustments provided in the manufacturer's labeling (has not been studied).

Administration Administer 30 minutes after the same mealtime each day. Capsules should be swallowed whole; do not crush, chew, or open.

Monitoring Parameters Blood pressure; urinary symptoms

Dosage Forms

Capsule, Oral:

Flomax: 0.4 mg

Generic: 0.4 mg

◆ **Tamsulosin and Dutasteride** *see* Dutasteride and Tamsulosin *on page 702*

◆ **Tamsulosin CR (Can)** *see* Tamsulosin *on page 1974*

◆ **Tamsulosin Hydrochloride** *see* Tamsulosin *on page 1974*

◆ **Tamsulosin Hydrochloride and Dutasteride** *see* Dutasteride and Tamsulosin *on page 702*

◆ **Tanta-Orciprenaline® (Can)** *see* Metaproterenol *on page 1307*

◆ **Tantum (Can)** *see* Benzydamine [CAN/INT] *on page 249*

◆ **Tanzeum** *see* Albiglutide *on page 66*

◆ **TAP-144** *see* Leuprolide *on page 1186*

◆ **Tapazole** *see* Methimazole *on page 1319*

Tapentadol (ta PEN ta dol)

Brand Names: U.S. Nucynta; Nucynta ER

Brand Names: Canada Nucynta ER; Nucynta IR

Index Terms CG5503; Tapentadol Hydrochloride

Pharmacologic Category Analgesic, Opioid

Use Pain:

Immediate release formulations: Management of moderate-to-severe acute pain in adults

Extended release formulation:

U.S. labeling: Pain or neuropathic pain associated with diabetic peripheral neuropathy (DPN) severe enough to require daily, around-the-clock, long-term opioid analgesia and for which alternative treatments are inadequate.

Canadian labeling: Relief of moderate to moderately severe pain in patients who require continuous treatment for several days or more.

Limitations of use: Because of the risks of addiction, abuse, and misuse with opioids, even at recommended doses, and because of the greater risks of overdose and death with extended-release opioid formulations, reserve tapentadol ER for use in patients for whom alternative treatment options (eg, nonopioid analgesics, immediate-release opioids) are ineffective, not tolerated, or would be otherwise inadequate to provide sufficient management of pain. Tapentadol ER is not indicated as an as-needed analgesic.

Pregnancy Risk Factor C

Pregnancy Considerations Adverse events were observed in animal reproduction studies. Opioids cross the placenta. Tapentadol is not recommended for use during labor and delivery and if exposure occurs the neonate should be monitored for respiratory depression. Use in pregnant women is contraindicated in the Canadian labeling.

U.S. Boxed Warning]: Prolonged maternal use of opioids during pregnancy can cause neonatal withdrawal syndrome in the newborn which may be life-threatening if not recognized and treated according to protocols developed by neonatology experts. If prolonged opioid therapy is required in a pregnant woman, ensure treatment is available and warn patient of risk to the neonate. If chronic opioid exposure occurs in pregnancy, adverse events in the newborn (including withdrawal) may occur; monitoring of the neonate is recommended. The minimum effective dose should be used if opioids are needed (Chou, 2009). Neonatal abstinence syndrome following opioid exposure may present with autonomic (eg, fever, temperature instability), gastrointestinal (eg, diarrhea, vomiting, poor feeding/weight gain), or neurologic (eg, high-pitched crying, increased muscle tone, irritability, seizure, tremor) symptoms (Dow, 2012; Hudak, 2012).

Long-term opioid use may cause secondary hypogonadism, which may lead to sexual dysfunction or infertility (Brennan, 2013).

Breast-Feeding Considerations Limited information is available on the excretion of tapentadol in human milk; however, data suggests it may be excreted in human milk. The possibility of sedation or respiratory depression in the nursing infant should be considered; withdrawal may occur when maternal therapy is stopped. Due to the potential for serious adverse reactions in the nursing infant, the U.S. manufacturer recommends a decision be made whether to discontinue nursing or to discontinue the drug, taking into account the importance of treatment to the mother. Use while breast-feeding is contraindicated in the Canadian labeling.

Contraindications

Hypersensitivity to tapentadol or any component of the formulation; significant respiratory depression; acute or severe asthma or hypercapnia in unmonitored settings or in absence of resuscitative equipment or ventilatory support; known or suspected paralytic ileus; use with or within 14 days of MAO inhibitors

Canadian labeling: Additional contraindications (not in U.S. labeling): Hypersensitivity to opioids; acute respiratory depression, cor pulmonale; obstructive airway; gastrointestinal obstruction or any disease/condition that affects bowel transit (eg, ileus of any type, strictures); severe renal impairment (CrCl <30 mL/minute); severe hepatic impairment (Child-Pugh class C); mild, intermittent, or short-duration pain that can be managed with alternative pain medication; management of perioperative pain (extended-release tablets); acute alcoholism, delirium tremens, and seizure disorders; severe CNS depression, increased cerebrospinal or intracranial pressure or head injury; pregnancy; breast-feeding; use during labor/delivery

Warnings/Precautions Use with caution and monitor for respiratory depression in patients with significant chronic obstructive pulmonary disease or cor pulmonale, and patients having a substantially decreased respiratory reserve, hypoxia, hypercarbia, or preexisting respiratory depression, particularly when initiating therapy and titrating with tapentadol; even therapeutic doses may decrease respiratory drive to the point of apnea. Consider the use of alternative nonopioid analgesics in these patients. Use with caution in debilitated or cachectic patients; there is a greater potential for critical respiratory depression, even at therapeutic dosages. Use with extreme caution in patients with head injury, intracranial lesions, or elevated intracranial pressure (ICP); exaggerated elevation of ICP may occur. Use caution in patients with a history of seizures or conditions predisposing patients to seizures; patients with a history of seizures were excluded in clinical trials of tapentadol. Tramadol, an analgesic with similar pharmacologic properties to tapentadol, has been associated with seizures, particularly in patients with predisposing factors. May cause severe hypotension; use with caution in patients with risk factors (eg, hypovolemia, concomitant use of other hypotensive agents). Avoid use in patients with circulatory shock. Potentially life-threatening serotonin syndrome (SS) has occurred with concomitant use of tapentadol and serotonergic agents (eg, SSRIs, SNRIs, triptans, TCAs, fentanyl, lithium, tramadol, buspirone, St John's wort, tryptophan) or agents that impair metabolism of serotonin (eg, MAO inhibitors intended to treat psychiatric disorders, other MAO inhibitors [ie, linezolid and intravenous methylene blue]). Monitor patients closely for signs of SS such as mental status changes (eg, agitation, hallucinations, delirium, coma); autonomic instability (eg, tachycardia, labile blood pressure, diaphoresis); neuromuscular changes (eg, tremor, rigidity, myoclonus); GI symptoms (eg, nausea, vomiting, diarrhea); and/or seizures. Discontinue treatment (and any concomitant serotonergic agent) immediately if signs/symptoms arise.

Opioids may obscure diagnosis or clinical course of patients with acute abdominal conditions. May cause CNS depression, which may impair physical or mental abilities; patients must be cautioned about performing tasks which require mental alertness (eg, operating machinery or driving). Effects may be potentiated when used with other CNS depressants (eg, sedatives, anxiolytics, hypnotics, neuroleptics, other opioids). Potentially significant drug-drug interactions may exist, requiring dose or frequency adjustment, additional monitoring, and/or selection of alternative therapy.

Use with caution in patients with adrenal insufficiency (including Addison's disease), patients with biliary tract dysfunction or acute pancreatitis (opioids may cause spasm of the sphincter of Oddi), patients with CNS depression (avoid use in patients with impaired consciousness or coma as these patients are susceptible to intracranial effects of CO_2 retention), patients with hypothyroidism, prostatic hyperplasia and/or urinary stricture. Use opioids with caution in the elderly; consider decreasing initial dose. May have a greater potential for critical respiratory depression. Serum concentrations are increased in hepatic impairment; use with caution in patients with moderate hepatic impairment (dosage adjustment required). Not recommended for use in severe hepatic impairment (not studied). Use with caution in patients with mild-to-moderate renal impairment; no dosage adjustments recommended. Not recommended for use in severe renal impairment (not studied). Canadian labeling contraindicates use of the extended-release formulation for perioperative pain relief and also recommends withholding its use for at least 48 hours prior to surgery and during the immediate postoperative period. May resume therapy after the patient recovers from the postoperative period; dosage adjustment may be necessary to provide adequate pain relief (Nucynta ER Canadian product monograph, 2014).

Prolonged use increases risk of abuse, addiction, and withdrawal symptoms. An opioid-containing regimen should be tailored to each patient's needs with respect to degree of tolerance for opioids (naïve versus chronic user), age, weight, and medical condition. Concurrent use of mixed agonist/antagonist analgesics (eg, pentazocine, nalbuphine, butorphanol) or partial agonist (eg, buprenorphine) analgesics may precipitate withdrawal symptoms and/or reduced analgesic efficacy in patients following prolonged therapy with mu opioid agonists. Taper dose gradually when discontinuing. In order to avoid dosing errors, include the dose in mL and mg when writing prescriptions. Instruct patients to always use the enclosed calibrated oral syringe to ensure the dose is measured and administered accurately.

Extended release tablets:

[U.S. Boxed Warning]: May cause serious, life-threatening, or fatal respiratory depression. Monitor closely for respiratory depression, especially during initiation or dose escalation. Patients should swallow tablets whole; crushing, chewing, or dissolving can cause rapid release and a potentially fatal dose. Carbon dioxide retention from opioid-induced respiratory depression can exacerbate the sedating effects of opioids. Therapy should only be prescribed by healthcare professionals familiar with the use of potent opioids for chronic pain. **[U.S. Boxed Warning]: Accidental ingestion of even one dose, especially in children, can result in a fatal overdose of tapentadol.**

[U.S. Boxed Warning]: Patients should not consume alcoholic beverages or medication containing ethanol while taking tapentadol ER; ethanol may increase tapentadol plasma levels resulting in a potentially fatal overdose.

[U.S. Boxed Warning]: Prolonged maternal use of opioids during pregnancy can cause neonatal withdrawal syndrome in the newborn which may be life-threatening if not recognized and treated according to protocols developed by neonatology experts. If prolonged opioid therapy is required in a pregnant woman, ensure treatment is available and warn patient of risk to the neonate. Signs and symptoms include irritability, hyperactivity and abnormal sleep pattern, high pitched cry, tremor, vomiting, diarrhea and failure to gain weight. Onset, duration and severity depend on the drug used, duration of use, maternal dose, and rate of drug elimination by the newborn.

[U.S. Boxed Warning]: Users are exposed to the risks of addiction, abuse, and misuse, potentially leading to overdose and death. Assess each patient's risk prior to prescribing; monitor all patients regularly for development of these behaviors or conditions. Risk of opioid abuse is increased in patients with a history or family history of alcohol or drug abuse or mental illness.

Adverse Reactions

Immediate release:

Central nervous system: Abnormal dreams, anxiety, confusion, dizziness, drowsiness, fatigue, insomnia, lethargy

Dermatologic: Hyperhidrosis, pruritus, skin rash

Endocrine & metabolic: Hot flash

Gastrointestinal: Constipation, decreased appetite, dyspepsia, nausea, vomiting, xerostomia

Genitourinary: Urinary tract infection

Neuromuscular & skeletal: Arthralgia, tremor

Respiratory: Nasopharyngitis, upper respiratory tract infection

Extended release:

Cardiovascular: Hypotension

Central nervous system: Abnormal dreams, anxiety, chills, depression, dizziness, drowsiness, fatigue, headache, hypoesthesia, insomnia, irritability, lack of concentration, lethargy, nervousness, sedation, vertigo, withdrawal syndrome

Dermatologic: Hyperhidrosis, pruritus, skin rash

Endocrine & metabolic: Hot flash

Gastrointestinal: Abdominal distress, constipation, decreased appetite, diarrhea, dyspepsia, nausea, vomiting, xerostomia

Genitourinary: Erectile dysfunction

Neuromuscular & skeletal: Tremor, weakness

Ophthalmic: Blurred vision

Respiratory: Dyspnea

Immediate and/or extended release: Rare but important or life-threatening: Abnormality in thinking, altered mental status, anaphylaxis, angioedema, ataxia, decreased blood pressure, delayed gastric emptying, disorientation, drug withdrawal, dysarthria, euphoria, hallucination, hypersensitivity, hypogonadism (Brennan, 2013; Debono, 2011), impaired consciousness, intoxicated feeling, memory impairment, panic attack, pollakiuria, presyncope, respiratory depression, seizure, syncope, urinary hesitation, visual disturbance

Drug Interactions

Metabolism/Transport Effects Substrate of CYP2C9 (minor), CYP2D6 (minor); **Note:** Assignment of Major/Minor substrate status based on clinically relevant drug interaction potential

Avoid Concomitant Use

Avoid concomitant use of Tapentadol with any of the following: Alcohol (Ethyl); Azelastine (Nasal); Dapoxetine; MAO Inhibitors; Orphenadrine; Paraldehyde; Thalidomide

Increased Effect/Toxicity

Tapentadol may increase the levels/effects of: Alvimopan; Azelastine (Nasal); Buprenorphine; CNS Depressants; Desmopressin; Diuretics; Hydrocodone; MAO Inhibitors; Methotrimeprazine; Metoclopramide; Metyrosine; Orphenadrine; Paraldehyde; Pramipexole; ROPINIRole; Rotigotine; Serotonin Modulators; Suvorexant; Thalidomide; Zolpidem

The levels/effects of Tapentadol may be increased by: Alcohol (Ethyl); Amphetamines; Anticholinergic Agents; Brimonidine (Topical); Cannabis; Dapoxetine; Dronabinol; Droperidol; Kava Kava; Magnesium Sulfate; Methotrimeprazine; Nabilone; Perampanel; Rufinamide; Sodium Oxybate; Succinylcholine; Tetrahydrocannabinol

Decreased Effect

Tapentadol may decrease the levels/effects of: Pegvisomant

The levels/effects of Tapentadol may be decreased by: Ammonium Chloride; Antiemetics (5HT3 Antagonists); Naltrexone

Food Interactions

Ethanol: Concomitant use with alcohol can increase the bioavailability of extended release tablets. Management: Avoid use of alcohol during therapy.

Food: When administered after a high fat/calorie meal, the AUC and C_{max} increased by 25% and 16%, respectively. Management: May administer without regard to meals.

Storage/Stability Store at room temperature up to 25°C (77°F); excursions are permitted between 15°C and 30°C (59°F and 86°F). Protect tablets from moisture.

Mechanism of Action Binds to μ-opiate receptors in the CNS causing inhibition of ascending pain pathways, altering the perception of and response to pain; also inhibits the reuptake of norepinephrine, which also modifies the ascending pain pathway

Pharmacodynamics/Kinetics

Absorption: Rapid and complete

Distribution: V_d: IV: 442-638 L

Protein binding: ~20%

Metabolism: Extensive metabolism, including first pass metabolism; metabolized primarily via phase 2 glucuronidation to glucuronides (major metabolite: tapentadol-O-glucuronide); minimal phase 1 oxidative metabolism; also metabolized to a lesser degree by CYP2C9, CYP2C19, and CYP2D6; all metabolites pharmacologically inactive

Bioavailability: ~32%

Half-life elimination: Immediate release: ~4 hours; Long acting formulations: ~5-6 hours

Time to peak, plasma: Immediate release: 1.25 hours; Long acting formulations: 3-6 hours

Excretion: Urine (99%: 70% conjugated metabolites; 3% unchanged drug)

Dosage Adults: **Note:** Dose and dosage intervals should be individualized according to pain severity with respect to patient's previous experience with similar opioid analgesics. In patients receiving extended release tapentadol, immediate-release opioid or nonopioid medication may be used for rescue relief of breakthrough pain and during dosage adjustments. The Canadian labeling does not recommend use of fentanyl as rescue medication. To reduce the risk of withdrawal symptoms, it is recommended to taper the dose when discontinuing therapy.

Acute moderate-severe pain: Oral: *Immediate release tablets and solution:* Day 1: 50 to 100 mg (2.5 to 5 mL) every 4 to 6 hours as needed; may administer a second dose ≥1 hour after the initial dose (maximum dose on first day: 700 mg daily); Day 2 and subsequent dosing: 50 to 100 mg (2.5 to 5 mL) every 4 to 6 hours as needed (maximum: 600 mg daily)

Chronic pain (U.S. and Canadian labeling), neuropathic pain associated with diabetic peripheral neuropathy (U.S. labeling): Oral: *Extended release:*

Opioid naive (use as the first opioid analgesic or use in patients who are **not** opioid tolerant): Initial: 50 mg twice daily (recommended interval: every 12 hours) **Note:** Opioid tolerance is defined as: Patients already taking at least 60 mg of oral morphine daily, 25 mcg of transdermal fentanyl per hour, 30 mg of oral oxycodone daily, 8 mg oral hydromorphone daily, 25 mg oral oxymorphone daily, or an equivalent dose of another opioid for at least 1 week.

Conversion from other oral opioids to extended release tapentadol: Discontinue all other around-the-clock opioids when extended release tapentadol is initiated. Substantial interpatient variability exists in relative potency. Therefore, it is safer to underestimate a patient's daily oral tapentadol requirement and provide breakthrough pain relief with rescue medication (eg, immediate release opioid) than to overestimate requirements. In general, begin with a dose that is 50% of the estimated daily tapentadol requirement and use immediate release rescue medications to supplement dose. Per the Canadian product labeling, comparable pain relief was observed between tapentadol ER and oxycodone CR at a dose ratio of 5:1 in clinical studies.

Conversion from tapentadol immediate release to extended release: Convert using same total daily dose but divide into 2 equal doses and administer twice daily (recommended interval: ~12 hours) (maximum dose: 500 mg daily).

Conversion from methadone to extended release tapentadol: Close monitoring is required when converting methadone to another opioid. Ratio between methadone and other opioid agonists varies widely according to previous dose exposure. Methadone has a long half-life and can accumulate in the plasma.

Dose titration: Titrate in increments of 50 mg no more frequently than twice daily every 3 days to effective dose (therapeutic range: 100 to 250 mg twice daily) (maximum dose: 500 mg daily)

Discontinuation of therapy: Gradually titrate dose downward to prevent withdrawal signs/symptoms. Do not abruptly discontinue.

Elderly: Initial: Consider initiating at lower range of dosing. Refer to adult dosing.

Dosage adjustment in renal impairment:

CrCl ≥30 mL/minute: No dosage adjustment necessary.

CrCl <30 mL/minute: Use not recommended (not studied); use is contraindicated in the Canadian labeling.

Dosage adjustment in hepatic impairment:

Mild impairment (Child-Pugh class A): No dosage adjustment necessary.

Moderate impairment (Child-Pugh class B):

Immediate release tablets and solution: Initial: 50 mg every 8 hours or longer (maximum: 3 doses/24 hours). Further treatment for maintenance of analgesia may be achieved by either shortening or lengthening the dosing interval.

Extended release: Initial: 50 mg every 24 hours or longer; maximum: 100 mg once daily

Severe impairment (Child-Pugh class C): Use not recommended (not studied); use is contraindicated in the Canadian labeling.

Dietary Considerations May be taken without regard to meals.

Administration Administer orally with or without food.

Tablets: Long acting formulations must be swallowed whole and should **not** be split, crushed, broken, chewed, or dissolved; patients should be instructed to swallow 1 tablet at a time, immediately after placing in mouth. The Canadian labeling recommends that immediate release tablets be swallowed whole.

Oral solution: Always use the enclosed calibrated oral syringe to ensure the dose is measured and administered accurately.

Monitoring Parameters Respiratory and cardiovascular status, blood pressure, heart rate; signs of misuse, abuse, or addiction; signs or symptoms of hypogonadism or hypoadrenalism (Brennan, 2013)

Extended release tablets: Monitor for respiratory depression for 72 hours of initiating dose.

Dosage Forms

Tablet, Oral:

Nucynta: 50 mg, 75 mg, 100 mg

Tablet Extended Release 12 Hour, Oral:

Nucynta ER: 50 mg, 100 mg, 150 mg, 200 mg, 250 mg

Dosage Forms: Canada

Tablet, Oral:

Nucynta IR: 50 mg, 75 mg, 100 mg

Tablet, Controlled Release, Oral, as hydrochloride:

Nucynta ER: 50 mg, 100 mg, 150 mg, 200 mg, 250 mg

- ◆ **Tapentadol Hydrochloride** *see* Tapentadol *on page 1975*
- ◆ **Tarceva** *see* Erlotinib *on page 756*
- ◆ **Targin (Can)** *see* Oxycodone and Naloxone *on page 1542*
- ◆ **Targiniq ER** *see* Oxycodone and Naloxone *on page 1542*
- ◆ **Targretin** *see* Bexarotene (Systemic) *on page 261*
- ◆ **Targretin** *see* Bexarotene (Topical) *on page 261*
- ◆ **Tarina FE 1/20** *see* Ethinyl Estradiol and Norethindrone *on page 808*
- ◆ **Tarka®** *see* Trandolapril and Verapamil *on page 2080*
- ◆ **Taro-Anastrozole (Can)** *see* Anastrozole *on page 148*

- ◆ **Taro-Carbamazepine Chewable (Can)** *see* CarBAMazepine *on page 346*
- ◆ **Taro-Ciclopirox (Can)** *see* Ciclopirox *on page 433*
- ◆ **Taro-Ciprofloxacin (Can)** *see* Ciprofloxacin (Systemic) *on page 441*
- ◆ **Taro-Clindamycin (Can)** *see* Clindamycin (Topical) *on page 464*
- ◆ **Taro-Clobetasol (Can)** *see* Clobetasol *on page 468*
- ◆ **Taro-Docusate [OTC] (Can)** *see* Docusate *on page 661*
- ◆ **Taro-Enalapril (Can)** *see* Enalapril *on page 722*
- ◆ **Taro-Fluconazole (Can)** *see* Fluconazole *on page 885*
- ◆ **Taro-Mometasone (Can)** *see* Mometasone (Topical) *on page 1391*
- ◆ **Taro-Phenytoin (Can)** *see* Phenytoin *on page 1640*
- ◆ **Taro-Sone (Can)** *see* Betamethasone (Topical) *on page 255*
- ◆ **Taro-Sumatriptan (Can)** *see* SUMAtriptan *on page 1953*
- ◆ **Taro-Terconazole (Can)** *see* Terconazole *on page 2006*
- ◆ **Taro-Warfarin (Can)** *see* Warfarin *on page 2186*
- ◆ **Taro-Zoledronic Acid (Can)** *see* Zoledronic Acid *on page 2206*
- ◆ **Taro-Zoledronic Acid Concentrate (Can)** *see* Zoledronic Acid *on page 2206*
- ◆ **Tasigna** *see* Nilotinib *on page 1454*

Tasimelteon (tas i MEL tee on)

Brand Names: U.S. Hetlioz

Index Terms VEC-162

Pharmacologic Category Hypnotic, Miscellaneous; Melatonin Receptor Agonist

Use Non-24-hour sleep-wake disorder: Treatment of non-24-hour sleep-wake disorder (non-24). **Note:** Efficacy was established in totally blind patients with non-24-hour sleep-wake disorder.

Pregnancy Risk Factor C

Pregnancy Considerations Adverse events were observed in some animal reproduction studies.

Breast-Feeding Considerations It is not known if tasimelteon is excreted into breast milk. The manufacturer recommends that caution be used if administered to a breast-feeding woman.

Contraindications There are no contraindications listed in the manufacturer's labeling.

Warnings/Precautions May cause CNS depression impairing physical and mental capabilities; patients must be cautioned about performing tasks, which require mental alertness (operating machinery or driving). Use is not recommended in patients with severe hepatic impairment. Smoking causes induction of CYP1A2 levels; tasimelteon exposure is decreased in smokers compared to non-smokers that may reduce tasimelteon efficacy. Use with caution in the elderly; exposure is increased; may increase the risk of adverse events. Potentially significant drug-drug interactions may exist, requiring dose or frequency adjustment, additional monitoring, and/or selection of alternative therapy.

Adverse Reactions

Central nervous system: Abnormal dreams, headache

Genitourinary: Urinary tract infection

Hepatic: Increased serum ALT

Respiratory: Upper respiratory tract infection

Drug Interactions

Metabolism/Transport Effects Substrate of CYP1A2 (major), CYP3A4 (major); **Note:** Assignment of Major/Minor substrate status based on clinically relevant drug interaction potential

Avoid Concomitant Use

Avoid concomitant use of Tasimelteon with any of the following: Azelastine (Nasal); CYP1A2 Inhibitors (Strong); CYP3A4 Inducers (Strong); Orphenadrine; Paraldehyde; Sodium Oxybate; Thalidomide

Increased Effect/Toxicity

Tasimelteon may increase the levels/effects of: Alcohol (Ethyl); Azelastine (Nasal); Buprenorphine; CNS Depressants; Hydrocodone; Methotrimeprazine; Metyrosine; Mirtazapine; Orphenadrine; Paraldehyde; Pramipexole; ROPINIRole; Rotigotine; Selective Serotonin Reuptake Inhibitors; Sodium Oxybate; Suvorexant; Thalidomide; Zolpidem

The levels/effects of Tasimelteon may be increased by: Abiraterone Acetate; Brimonidine (Topical); Cannabis; CYP1A2 Inhibitors (Moderate); CYP1A2 Inhibitors (Strong); Deferasirox; Doxylamine; Dronabinol; Droperidol; HydrOXYzine; Kava Kava; Magnesium Sulfate; Methotrimeprazine; Nabilone; Peginterferon Alfa-2b; Perampanel; Rufinamide; Tapentadol; Tetrahydrocannabinol; Vemurafenib

Decreased Effect

The levels/effects of Tasimelteon may be decreased by: Bosentan; Cannabis; CYP3A4 Inducers (Moderate); CYP3A4 Inducers (Strong); Cyproterone; Dabrafenib; Deferasirox; Siltuximab; St Johns Wort; Teriflunomide; Tocilizumab

Storage/Stability Store at 25°C (77°F); excursions are permitted between 15°C and 30°C (59°F and 86°F). Protect from light and moisture.

Mechanism of Action Agonist of melatonin receptors MT_1 and MT_2 (greater affinity for the MT_2 receptor than the MT_1 receptor). Agonism of MT_1 is thought to preferentially induce sleepiness, while MT_2 receptor activation preferentially influences regulation of circadian rhythms.

Pharmacodynamics/Kinetics

Onset: Effect may take weeks or months (due to individual differences in circadian rhythms)

Absorption: High-fat meals delayed T_{max} and maximum serum concentration was reduced by 44%

Protein binding: ~90%

Distribution: V_d: ~59 to 126 L

Metabolism: Hepatic (extensive); oxidative metabolism primarily through CYP1A2 and CYP3A4. Phenolic glucuronidation is the major phase II metabolic route.

Bioavailability: ~38%

Half-life elimination: ~1 to 2 hours

Time to peak: Fasting: ~0.5 to 3 hours (increased by ~1.75 hours with a high-fat meal)

Excretion: Urine (80%; <1% as unchanged drug); feces (~4%)

Dosage Note: Effect may not occur for weeks or months due to differences in circadian rhythms.

Non-24-hour sleep-wake disorder: Adults: Oral: 20 mg once daily at the same time each night before bedtime.

Dosage adjustment in renal impairment: No dosage adjustment necessary.

Dosage adjustment in hepatic impairment:

Mild or moderate impairment: No dosage adjustment necessary.

Severe impairment: There are no dosage adjustments provided in manufacturer's labeling (has not been studied). Use is not recommended.

Dietary Considerations Avoid or limit ethanol.

Administration Administer orally without food. Should be taken at the same time every night before bedtime. Swallow capsule whole. After administration, activities should be limited to preparing for sleep. If the dose cannot be taken at approximately the same time on a given night, that dose should be skipped.

Dosage Forms
Capsule, Oral:
Hetlioz: 20 mg

◆ **Tasmar** *see* Tolcapone *on page 2062*

Tavaborole (ta va BOR ole)

Brand Names: U.S. Kerydin
Pharmacologic Category Antifungal Agent, Topical
Use Onychomycosis: Topical treatment of onychomycosis of the toenail(s) due to *Trichophyton rubrum* and *Trichophyton mentagrophytes*
Pregnancy Risk Factor C
Dosage Onychomycosis: Adults: Topical: Apply to affected toenail(s) once daily for 48 weeks.

Dosage adjustment in renal impairment: There are no dosage adjustments provided in the manufacturer's labeling. However, dosage adjustment unlikely due to low systemic absorption.
Dosage adjustment in hepatic impairment: There are no dosage adjustments provided in the manufacturer's labeling. However, dosage adjustment unlikely due to low systemic absorption.
Additional Information Complete prescribing information should be consulted for additional detail.
Dosage Forms
Solution, External:
Kerydin: 5% (4 mL, 10 mL)

◆ **Tavist Allergy [OTC]** *see* Clemastine *on page 459*
◆ **Tavist ND** *see* Loratadine *on page 1241*
◆ **Taxol** *see* PACLitaxel (Conventional) *on page 1550*
◆ **Taxotere** *see* DOCEtaxel *on page 656*

Tazarotene (taz AR oh teen)

Brand Names: U.S. Avage; Fabior; Tazorac
Brand Names: Canada Tazorac
Pharmacologic Category Acne Products; Keratolytic Agent; Topical Skin Product, Acne
Use
Acne (Fabior, Tazorac 0.1% cream, Tazorac 0.1% gel): Topical treatment of acne vulgaris in patients 12 years and older.
Psoriasis:
Tazorac 0.05% and 0.1% cream: Topical treatment of plaque psoriasis in patients 18 years and older.
Tazorac 0.05% and 0.1% gel: Topical treatment of stable plaque psoriasis of up to 20% body surface area involvement in patients 12 years and older.
Wrinkling, hyper- and hypopigmentation, lentigines (Avage): Adjunctive agent for use in the mitigation (palliation) of facial fine wrinkling, facial mottled hyper- and hypopigmentation, and benign facial lentigines in patients 17 years and older who use comprehensive skin care and sunlight avoidance programs.
Limitations of use: Does not eliminate or prevent wrinkles, repair sun-damaged skin, reverse photoaging, or restore more youthful or younger skin. Has not demonstrated a mitigating effect on significant signs of chronic sunlight exposure such as coarse or deep wrinkling, tactile roughness, telangiectasia, skin laxity, keratinocytic atypia, melanocytic atypia, or dermal elastosis. Safety and effectiveness for the prevention or treatment of actinic keratoses, skin neoplasms, or lentigo maligna has not been established. Use for greater than 52 weeks has not been established.
Pregnancy Risk Factor X
Dosage Topical: **Note:** In patients experiencing excessive pruritus, burning, skin redness, or peeling, discontinue until integrity of the skin is restored, or reduce dosing to an interval the patient is able to tolerate.
Children ≥12 years, Adolescents, and Adults:
Acne:
Fabior: Apply a small amount to affected area once daily in the evening.
Tazorac cream/gel 0.1%: Apply a thin film (2 mg/cm^2) to affected area once daily in the evening.
Psoriasis: Tazorac gel: Initial: 0.05%: Apply once daily to psoriatic lesions using enough (2 mg/cm^2) to cover only the lesion with a thin film to no more than 20% of body surface area. May increase strength to 0.1% if tolerated and necessary.
Adolescents ≥17 years and Adults: Palliation of fine facial wrinkles, facial mottled hyper-/hypopigmentation, benign facial lentigines: Avage: Apply a pea-sized amount to entire face once daily at bedtime.
Adults: Psoriasis: Tazorac cream: Initial: 0.05%: Apply once daily to psoriatic lesions using enough (2 mg/cm^2) to cover only the lesion with a thin film. May increase strength to 0.1% if tolerated and necessary.
Additional Information Complete prescribing information should be consulted for additional detail.
Dosage Forms
Cream, External:
Avage: 0.1% (30 g)
Tazorac: 0.05% (30 g, 60 g); 0.1% (30 g, 60 g)
Foam, External:
Fabior: 0.1% (50 g, 100 g)
Gel, External:
Tazorac: 0.05% (30 g, 100 g); 0.1% (30 g, 100 g)

◆ **Tazicef** *see* CefTAZidime *on page 392*
◆ **Tazobactam and Ceftolozane** *see* Ceftolozane and Tazobactam *on page 394*
◆ **Tazobactam and Piperacillin** *see* Piperacillin and Tazobactam *on page 1657*
◆ **Tazocin (Can)** *see* Piperacillin and Tazobactam *on page 1657*
◆ **Tazorac** *see* Tazarotene *on page 1980*
◆ **Taztia XT** *see* Diltiazem *on page 634*
◆ **TBC** *see* Trypsin, Balsam Peru, and Castor Oil *on page 2109*
◆ **Tbo-Filgrastim** *see* Filgrastim *on page 875*
◆ **TB Skin Test** *see* Tuberculin Tests *on page 2110*
◆ **3TC** *see* LamiVUDine *on page 1157*
◆ **3TC, Abacavir, and Zidovudine** *see* Abacavir, Lamivudine, and Zidovudine *on page 22*
◆ **T-Cell Growth Factor** *see* Aldesleukin *on page 72*
◆ **TCGF** *see* Aldesleukin *on page 72*
◆ **TCN** *see* Tetracycline *on page 2017*
◆ **Td** *see* Diphtheria and Tetanus Toxoid *on page 645*
◆ **TD-6424** *see* Telavancin *on page 1986*
◆ **Td Adsorbed (Can)** *see* Diphtheria and Tetanus Toxoid *on page 645*
◆ **Tdap** *see* Diphtheria and Tetanus Toxoids, and Acellular Pertussis Vaccine *on page 649*
◆ **TDF** *see* Tenofovir *on page 1998*
◆ **T-DM1** *see* Ado-Trastuzumab Emtansine *on page 58*
◆ **TDX** *see* Raltitrexed [CAN/INT] *on page 1769*
◆ **Tebrazid™ (Can)** *see* Pyrazinamide *on page 1745*
◆ **Tecfidera** *see* Dimethyl Fumarate *on page 639*
◆ **Tecnu First Aid [OTC]** *see* Lidocaine (Topical) *on page 1211*
◆ **Tecta (Can)** *see* Pantoprazole *on page 1570*

Tedizolid (ted eye ZOE lid)

Brand Names: U.S. Sivextro

Index Terms DA-7157; DA-7158; DA-7218; Tedizolid Phosphate; Torezolid; TR-700; TR-701 FA

Pharmacologic Category Antibiotic, Oxazolidinone

Use Acute bacterial skin and skin structure infections: Treatment of adult patients with acute bacterial skin and skin structure infections (ABSSSI) caused by susceptible isolates of the following gram-positive microorganisms: *Staphylococcus aureus* (including methicillin-resistant [MRSA] and methicillin-susceptible [MSSA] isolates), *Streptococcus pyogenes, Streptococcus agalactiae, Streptococcus anginosus* group (including *Streptococcus anginosus, Streptococcus intermedius,* and *Streptococcus constellatus*), and *Enterococccus faecalis*

Pregnancy Risk Factor C

Pregnancy Considerations Adverse events were observed in animal reproduction studies.

Breast-Feeding Considerations It is not known if tedizolid is excreted into breast milk. The manufacturer recommends that caution be used if administered to a nursing woman.

Contraindications There are no contraindications listed in the manufacturer's labeling.

Warnings/Precautions Not recommended for use in patients with neutrophil counts <1000 cells/mm^3). Alternative therapies should be considered when treating patients with neutropenia and ABSSI. Prolonged use may result in fungal or bacterial superinfection, including *C. difficile*-associated diarrhea (CDAD) and pseudomembranous colitis; CDAD has been observed >2 months postantibiotic treatment.

Adverse Reactions

Cardiovascular: Flushing, hypertension, palpitations, tachycardia

Central nervous system: Dizziness, facial paralysis, headache, hypoesthesia, insomnia, paresthesia, peripheral neuropathy

Dermatologic: Dermatitis, pruritus, urticaria

Gastrointestinal: Diarrhea, nausea, oral candidiasis, pseudomembranous colitis, vomiting

Hematologic & oncologic: Anemia, decreased hemoglobin (males <10.1 g/dL; females <9 g/dL), decreased platelet count (<112,000/mm^3), decreased white blood cell count

Hepatic: Increased serum transaminases

Hypersensitivity: Hypersensitivity

Infection: Fungal infection (vulvovaginal)

Ophthalmic: Asthenopia, blurred vision, visual impairment, vitreous opacity

Miscellaneous: Infusion related reaction

Rare but important or life-threatening: *Clostridium difficile* associated diarrhea, decrease in absolute neutrophil count (<800/mm^3), optic neuropathy

Drug Interactions

Metabolism/Transport Effects Inhibits Monoamine Oxidase

Avoid Concomitant Use

Avoid concomitant use of Tedizolid with any of the following: Alcohol (Ethyl); Anilidopiperidine Opioids; Apraclonidine; AtoMOXetine; BCG; Bezafibrate; Buprenorphine; BuPROPion; BusPIRone; CarBAMazepine; CloZAPine; Cyclobenzaprine; Cyproheptadine; Dapoxetine; Dextromethorphan; Diethylpropion; Dipyrone; Hydrocodone; HYDROmorphone; Isometheptene; Levonordefrin; Linezolid; Maprotiline; Meperidine; Methyldopa; Methylene Blue; Methylphenidate; Mianserin; Morphine (Liposomal); Morphine (Systemic); Oxymorphone; Pholcodine; Pizotifen; Serotonin 5-HT1D Receptor Agonists; Tapentadol; Tetrabenazine; Tetrahydrozoline (Nasal)

Increased Effect/Toxicity

Tedizolid may increase the levels/effects of: Antipsychotic Agents; Apraclonidine; AtoMOXetine; Betahistine; Bezafibrate; Brimonidine (Ophthalmic); Brimonidine (Topical); BuPROPion; CloZAPine; Cyproheptadine; Dextromethorphan; Diethylpropion; Domperidone; Doxylamine; Hydrocodone; HYDROmorphone; Isometheptene; Levonordefrin; Linezolid; Lithium; Meperidine; Methadone; Methyldopa; Methylene Blue; Methylphenidate; Metoclopramide; Mianserin; Morphine (Liposomal); Morphine (Systemic); OxyCODONE; Pizotifen; Reserpine; Serotonin 5-HT1D Receptor Agonists; Serotonin Modulators; Sympathomimetics; Tetrahydrozoline (Nasal)

The levels/effects of Tedizolid may be increased by: Alcohol (Ethyl); Anilidopiperidine Opioids; Antiemetics (5HT3 Antagonists); Antipsychotic Agents; Buprenorphine; BusPIRone; CarBAMazepine; COMT Inhibitors; Cyclobenzaprine; Dapoxetine; Dipyrone; Levodopa; Maprotiline; Oxymorphone; Pholcodine; Tapentadol; Tetrabenazine; TraMADol

Decreased Effect

Tedizolid may decrease the levels/effects of: BCG; Domperidone; Sodium Picosulfate; Typhoid Vaccine

The levels/effects of Tedizolid may be decreased by: Cyproheptadine; Domperidone

Preparation for Administration Reconstitute with 4 mL SWFI. Do **NOT** shake. Gently swirl the contents and let the vial stand until the cake has completely dissolved and any foam disperses. If necessary, invert the vial to dissolve any remaining powder and swirl gently to prevent foaming. The reconstituted solution is clear and colorless to pale-yellow in color; Tilt the upright vial and insert a syringe into the bottom corner of the vial and remove 4 mL of the reconstituted solution. Do **NOT** invert the vial during extraction. The reconstituted solution must be further diluted in 250 mL of NS only. Invert the bag gently to mix. Do not shake the bag (may cause foaming).

Storage/Stability Store at 20°C to 25°C (68°F to 77°F); excursions are permitted between 15°C and 30°C (59°F and 86°F) The total storage time of the reconstituted solution should not exceed 24 hours at either room temperature or under refrigeration at 2°C to 8°C (36°F to 46°F).

Mechanism of Action After conversion from the prodrug, tedizolid phosphate, tedizolid binds to the 50S bacterial ribosomal subunit. This prevents the formation of a functional 70S initiation complex that is essential for the bacterial translation process and subsequently inhibits protein synthesis. Tedizolid is bacteriostatic against enterococci, staphylococci, and streptococci (Kisgen, 2014).

Pharmacodynamics/Kinetics

Absorption: Oral: Well absorbed

Distribution: V_{dss}: 67 to 80 L

Protein binding: 70% to 90%

Metabolism: Tedizolid phosphate is converted by phosphatases to tedizolid (active, parent drug); no other significant circulating metabolites.

Bioavailability: Oral: ~91%

Half-life elimination: ~12 hours

Time to peak: Oral: ~3 hours; IV: 1 to 1.5 hours

Excretion: Feces (82%) and urine (18%), both as inactive sulfate conjugates. Less than 3% excreted in feces or urine as parent drug.

Dosage

Usual dosage range: Adults: Oral, IV: 200 mg once daily

Acute bacterial skin and skin structure infections: Adults: Oral, IV: 200 mg once daily for 6 days

Missed doses: Administer as soon as possible any time up to 8 hours prior to the next scheduled dose; if less than 8 hours remain before the next dose, wait until the next scheduled dose.

Dosage adjustment in renal impairment: No dosage adjustment necessary.

Dosage adjustment in hepatic impairment: No dosage adjustment necessary.

Usual Infusion Concentrations: Adult 200 mg in 250 mL (concentration: 0.8 **mg**/mL) of NS only

Administration

Oral: Administer with or without food.

Intravenous: Administer as an IV infusion over 1 hour; do not administer as an IV push or bolus. Not for intra-arterial, IM, intrathecal, intraperitoneal, or subcutaneous administration. If the same IV line is to be used for sequential infusion of other drugs or solutions, the line should be flushed with NS before and after tedizolid infusion.

Monitoring Parameters Baseline complete blood count (CBC) with differential

Dosage Forms

Solution Reconstituted, Intravenous [preservative free]:
Sivextro: 200 mg (10 ea)

Tablet, Oral:
Sivextro: 200 mg

◆ **Tedizolid Phosphate** *see* Tedizolid *on page 1981*

Teduglutide (te due GLOO tide)

Brand Names: U.S. Gattex

Index Terms ALX-0600; Teduglutide Recombinant; Teduglutide [rDNA origin]

Pharmacologic Category Glucagon-Like Peptide-2 (GLP-2) Analog

Use Short bowel syndrome: Treatment of short bowel syndrome in adults who are dependent on parenteral support.

Pregnancy Risk Factor B

Pregnancy Considerations Adverse events were not observed in animal reproduction studies.

Breast-Feeding Considerations It is not known if teduglutide is excreted into breast milk. Due to the potential for serious adverse reactions in the nursing infant, a decision should be made whether to discontinue nursing or to discontinue the drug, taking into account the importance of treatment to the mother.

Contraindications There are no contraindications listed in the manufacturer's labeling.

Warnings/Precautions Teduglutide may increase the risk of hyperplastic changes, including neoplasia. In patients at increased risk for malignancy, consider treatment only if benefits outweigh the risks. Discontinue treatment in patients with active gastrointestinal malignancy (GI tract, hepatobiliary, pancreatic); evaluate risk versus benefit in patients with active non-GI malignancy. Monitor for small bowel neoplasia; remove any benign neoplasm. Development of colorectal polyps has occurred. Preform a baseline colonoscopy of the entire colon with polyp removal ≤6 months prior to initiation of therapy. Follow-up colonoscopy (or alternative imaging) should be performed at 1 year and at least every 5 years, thereafter. Discontinue teduglutide in patients who develop colorectal cancer.

Intestinal and stomal obstructions have been reported; temporarily discontinue treatment in patients that develop obstruction. Teduglutide may be resumed (if clinically indicated) once the obstruction is resolved. Increased fluid absorption and subsequent fluid overload/congestive heart failure has been reported; consider modification of parenteral support in patients who develop fluid overload, especially in patients with underlying cardiovascular disease; if significant cardiac deterioration develops, reassess the need for continued teduglutide treatment. Cholecystitis, cholangitis, cholelithiasis, and pancreatitis have been reported; monitor serum bilirubin, alkaline phosphatase, lipase, and amylase ≤ 6 month prior to initiation of therapy and at least every 6 months for duration of therapy; if clinically meaningful changes are detected, perform gallbladder/biliary tract/pancreatic imaging and reassess the need for continued teduglutide treatment.

Teduglutide may increase absorption of oral medications; monitor therapy of medications with a narrow therapeutic index. Treatment discontinuation may result in fluid and electrolyte imbalance; carefully monitor fluid/electrolyte status.

Adverse Reactions

Central nervous system: Disturbed sleep, headache

Dermatologic: Dermal hemorrhage

Endocrine & metabolic: Hypervolemia

Gastrointestinal: Abdominal distension, abdominal pain, change in appetite, flatulence, intestinal obstruction, intestinal polyps, nausea, vomiting

Hypersensitivity: Hypersensitivity reaction

Immunologic: Antibody development

Local: Injection site reaction

Respiratory: Cough, upper respiratory tract infection

Miscellaneous: Intestinal stoma complication

Rare but important or life-threatening: Cardiac arrest, cardiac failure, cerebral hemorrhage, cholecystitis, cholelithiasis, cholestasis, congestive heart failure, gallbladder perforation, malignant neoplasm, pancreatic pseudocyst, pancreatitis

Drug Interactions

Metabolism/Transport Effects None known.

Avoid Concomitant Use There are no known interactions where it is recommended to avoid concomitant use.

Increased Effect/Toxicity

Teduglutide may increase the levels/effects of: Benzodiazepines

Decreased Effect There are no known significant interactions involving a decrease in effect.

Preparation for Administration Reconstitute each vial with 0.5 mL of preservative-free SWFI (provided in syringe); let stand for 30 seconds and then roll vial between palms for 15 seconds. Do not shake. Allow vial to stand for an additional ~2 minutes; if undissolved material remains, roll between palms again. If particles are not dissolved after second attempt, discard vial. Once reconstituted, each vial provides 3.8 mg/0.38 mL (concentration is 10 mg/mL).

Storage/Stability Prior to dispensing, store intact vials refrigerated at 2°C to 8°C (36°F to 46°F); do not freeze. The carton of ancillary supplies should be stored at 25°C (77°F). After dispensing, store vials at 25°C (77°F); once dispensed, vials must be used within 90 days. Once reconstituted, use within 3 hours. Discard any unused portion.

Mechanism of Action Teduglutide is an analog of glucagon-like peptide-2 (GLP-2), which is secreted in the distal intestine. Endogenous GLP-2 increases intestinal and portal blood flow while inhibiting gastric acid secretion, thereby reducing intestinal losses and improving intestinal absorption. Teduglutide binds and activates GLP-2 receptors, resulting in release of mediators including insulin-like growth factor (IGF)-1, nitric oxide and keratinocyte growth factor (KGF).

Pharmacodynamics/Kinetics

Distribution: 0.1 L/kg

Metabolism: Similar to endogenous catabolism of GLP-2 but slower due to a single amino acid substitution (Ferrone, 2006)

Bioavailability: SubQ: 88%

Half-life elimination: ~2 hours (healthy patients); 1.3 hours (short bowel syndrome patients)

Time to peak, plasma: 3-5 hours

Excretion: Urine

Dosage Short bowel syndrome: Adults: SubQ: 0.05 mg/kg once daily

Missed doses: If a dose is missed, take as soon as possible on that day; do **NOT** take 2 doses on the same day.

Dosage adjustment in renal impairment:
CrCl ≥50 mL/minute: No dosage adjustment necessary.
CrCl <50 mL/minute: Administer 50% of the usual dose.
ESRD: Administer 50% of the usual dose.

Dosage adjustment in hepatic impairment:
Mild-to-moderate impairment (Child-Pugh class B): No dosage adjustment necessary.
Severe impairment: There are no dosage adjustments provided in the manufacturer's labeling (has not been studied).

Administration SubQ: Rotate injection site between thighs, upper arms, and quadrants of the abdomen. Do not administer IM or IV

Monitoring Parameters Serum bilirubin, alkaline phosphatase, lipase and amylase (baseline [within 6 months prior to initiation] and every 6 months thereafter); colonoscopy of entire colon and removal of polyps (baseline [within 6 months prior to initiation], 1 year, and ≤5 years thereafter if no polyps found); monitor fluid status in patients with cardiovascular disease; signs/symptoms of intestinal obstruction; signs/symptoms suggestive of gall bladder disease or pancreatitis; monitor fluid and electrolyte balance following therapy discontinuation

Dosage Forms
Kit, Subcutaneous [preservative free]:
Gattex: 5 mg

- ◆ **Teduglutide [rDNA origin]** *see* Teduglutide *on page 1982*
- ◆ **Teduglutide Recombinant** *see* Teduglutide *on page 1982*
- ◆ **Teflaro** *see* Ceftaroline Fosamil *on page 391*
- ◆ **Tegaderm CHG Dressing [OTC]** *see* Chlorhexidine Gluconate *on page 422*
- ◆ **TEGretol** *see* CarBAMazepine *on page 346*
- ◆ **Tegretol (Can)** *see* CarBAMazepine *on page 346*
- ◆ **TEGretol-XR** *see* CarBAMazepine *on page 346*
- ◆ **TEI-6720** *see* Febuxostat *on page 848*

Teicoplanin [INT] (tye koe PLAN in)

International Brand Names Tagocin (KR); Tapocin (CN, KR); Targocid (AE, AR, AT, AU, BE, BG, BH, BR, CH, CL, CN, CZ, DE, DK, ES, FI, FR, GB, GR, HK, HN, HR, HU, ID, IE, IL, IN, JO, KR, KW, LB, LU, MX, MY, NL, NO, NZ, PE, PK, PL, PY, QA, RO, SA, SE, SG, SI, SK, TH, TR, TW, UY, VE, VN, ZA); Targoplanin (JO); Targosid (IT, PT); Teicocid (PY, UY); Teicod (TW); Teicoin (TW); Teicon (BR); Teicosin (KR); Teicox (AR); Tigein (TW); Tilatep (VN); Tocopin (VN)

Pharmacologic Category Antibiotic, Miscellaneous

Reported Use Treatment of infections caused by susceptible gram-positive bacteria; peritonitis associated with CAPD; *C. difficile*-associated diarrhea; surgical prophylaxis

Dosage Range
Oral: Adults: 100-200 mg twice daily
Parenteral:
Neonates: I.V.: Initial: 16 mg/kg loading dose followed by 8 mg/kg once daily
Infants >2 months and Children ≤12 years: I.V.: Initial: 10 mg/kg every 12 hours for 3 doses, followed by 6-10 mg/kg once daily
Adolescents, Adults, and Elderly: I.V: Initial: 400-800 mg (6-12 mg/kg) every 12 hours for 3-5 doses; maintenance: I.V. or I.M.: 6-12 mg/kg once daily

Product Availability Product available in various countries; not currently available in the U.S.

Dosage Forms
Injection, powder for reconstitution: 200 mg, 400 mg

- ◆ **Tekturna** *see* Aliskiren *on page 85*
- ◆ **Tekturna HCT** *see* Aliskiren and Hydrochlorothiazide *on page 87*

Telaprevir (tel A pre vir)

Brand Names: U.S. Incivek [DSC]

Brand Names: Canada Incivek™

Index Terms LY570310; MP-424; MP424; VRT111950; VX-950; VX950

Pharmacologic Category Antihepaciviral, Protease Inhibitor (Anti-HCV)

Use Chronic hepatitis C: Treatment of genotype 1 chronic hepatitis C (in combination with peginterferon alfa and ribavirin) in adult patients with compensated liver disease (including cirrhosis) who are treatment naive or who have received previous interferon-based treatment, including null or partial responders, and treatment relapsers.

Pregnancy Risk Factor B / X (in combination with ribavirin)

Pregnancy Considerations Adverse events were not observed in telaprevir animal developmental studies; however, telaprevir must not be used as monotherapy (must be used in combination with peginterferon alfa and ribavirin). Significant ribavirin teratogenic effects have been observed in all animal studies at ~0.01 times the maximum recommended daily human dose. Use of ribavirin is contraindicated in pregnancy. In addition, animal studies with interferons have demonstrated abortifacient effects. Negative pregnancy test is required before initiation and monthly thereafter. Hormonal contraceptive measures may not be effective in patients taking telaprevir or for 2 weeks after discontinuing therapy. Avoid pregnancy in female patients and female partners of male patients during therapy by using two effective nonhormonal forms of contraception; continue contraceptive measures for at least 6 months after completion of therapy. If patient or female partner becomes pregnant during treatment, she should be counseled about potential risks of exposure. If pregnancy occurs during use or within 6 months after treatment, report to the ribavirin pregnancy registry (800-593-2214).

Breast-Feeding Considerations It is not known if telaprevir or ribavirin are excreted into breast milk. The manufacturer recommends that breast-feeding be discontinued prior to the initiation of treatment.

Contraindications
Combination treatment with ribavirin: Pregnancy; male partners of pregnant women
Coadministration with alfuzosin, cisapride, ergot derivatives (eg, dihydroergotamine, ergonovine, ergotamine, methylergonovine), lovastatin, midazolam (oral), pimozide, sildenafil/tadalafil (when used for treatment of pulmonary arterial hypertension), simvastatin, triazolam, rifampin, St John's wort, carbamazepine, phenobarbital, phenytoin
Canadian labeling: Additional contraindications (not in U.S. labeling): Hypersensitivity to telaprevir or any component of the formulation; coadministration with amiodarone, astemizole (not available in Canada), eletriptan, eplerenone, flecainide, propafenone, quinidine, terfenadine (not available in Canada), vardenafil

Also refer to Peginterferon Alfa and Ribavirin monographs for individual product contraindications.

Warnings/Precautions [U.S. Boxed Warning] Serious skin reactions (some fatal) including Stevens-Johnson syndrome (SJS), drug reaction with eosinophilia and

systemic symptoms (DRESS), and toxic epidermal necrolysis (TEN), have been reported with telaprevir combination therapy. Fatal cases have been reported in patients with progressive rash and systemic symptoms who received ongoing therapy after diagnoses of serious skin reactions. Discontinue telaprevir, peginterferon alfa, and ribavirin immediately for serious skin reactions (including rash with systemic symptoms or a progressive severe rash) and refer for immediate medical care. Rash has been typically observed within first 4 weeks of therapy initiation but may occur at any time. Severe rashes (other than DRESS, SJS) are generalized, bullous, vesicular or ulcerative; may also have an eczematous appearance. Discontinue telaprevir (may continue peginterferon alfa and ribavirin) for severe rash or for mild-to-moderate rash that progresses; if no improvement in rash within 1 week of stopping telaprevir, interruption or discontinuation of peginterferon alfa and/or ribavirin should be considered (or sooner if clinically indicated). May use oral antihistamines/topical corticosteroids for rash treatment; do not use systemic corticosteroids. Do not restart telaprevir if discontinued due to any skin reaction.

Telaprevir-containing regimens are not recommended for treatment-naive patients or for prior relapse patients nonresponsive to peginterferon/ribavirin regimens with or without an HCV protease inhibitor (AASLD/IDSA, 2014).

Prerenal azotemia (with or without acute renal failure) and uric acid nephropathy have been reported. Assess serum electrolytes, creatinine, and uric acid pretreatment, at weeks 2, 4, 8, and 12, and when clinically indicated. Maintain adequate hydration. Anemia has been reported with peginterferon alfa and ribavirin; addition of telaprevir is associated with further hemoglobin decreases. Low hemoglobin levels were measured during the first 4 weeks of treatment, and the lowest at the end of telaprevir treatment (week 12). Dose modifications of ribavirin were needed more often in patients also taking telaprevir. Assess hematologic parameters (CBC with differential and platelet count) pretreatment, at weeks 2, 4, 8, and 12, and when clinically indicated. May require ribavirin dose reduction, interruption or discontinuation of treatment; if ribavirin dose reductions are inadequate, may consider discontinuing telaprevir. Do not reduce telaprevir dose. If ribavirin is discontinued, telaprevir must also be discontinued. Do not restart telaprevir if ribavirin therapy is reinitiated.

Avoid pregnancy in female patients and female partners of male patients, during therapy, and for at least 6 months after treatment; two forms of nonhormonal contraception should be used. Hormonal contraceptives may not be effective in patients taking telaprevir or for two weeks after discontinuing therapy. Safety and efficacy have not been established in patients who have uncompensated cirrhosis, received liver transplants, or who have failed to respond to other NS3/4A inhibitors (including repeated courses of telaprevir). Monotherapy is not effective for chronic hepatitis C infection. Not recommended in moderate or severe hepatic impairment (Child-Pugh class B or C) or decompensated hepatic disease. Potentially significant drug-drug interactions may exist, requiring dose or frequency adjustments, additional monitoring, and/or selection of alternative therapy.

Adverse Reactions

Central nervous system: Fatigue
Dermatologic: Rash, pruritus
Endocrine and Metabolic: Hyperuricemia
Gastrointestinal: Abnormal taste, anal pruritus, nausea, diarrhea, vomiting, hemorrhoids, anorectal discomfort
Hematologic: Anemia, lymphopenia, thrombocytopenia
Hepatic: Hyperbilirubinemia

Rare but important or life-threatening: Drug reaction with eosinophilia and systemic symptoms (DRESS), erythema multiforme, prerenal azotemia (with or without acute renal failure/insufficiency), Stevens-Johnson syndrome, toxic epidermal necrolysis, uric acid nephropathy

Drug Interactions

Metabolism/Transport Effects **Substrate** of CYP3A4 (major), P-glycoprotein; **Note:** Assignment of Major/Minor substrate status based on clinically relevant drug interaction potential; **Inhibits** CYP3A4 (strong), P-glycoprotein, SLCO1B1

Avoid Concomitant Use

Avoid concomitant use of Telaprevir with any of the following: Ado-Trastuzumab Emtansine; Alfuzosin; Apixaban; Astemizole; AtorvaSTATin; Avanafil; Axitinib; Bosutinib; Cabozantinib; CarBAMazepine; Ceritinib; Cisapride; Cobicistat; Conivaptan; Crizotinib; CYP3A4 Inducers (Strong); Dapoxetine; Darunavir; Dihydroergotamine; Dronedarone; Eplerenone; Ergoloid Mesylates; Ergonovine; Ergotamine; Everolimus; Fosamprenavir; Fosphenytoin; Fusidic Acid (Systemic); Halofantrine; Ibrutinib; Idelalisib; Irinotecan; Ivabradine; Lapatinib; Lercanidipine; Lomitapide; Lopinavir; Lovastatin; Lurasidone; Macitentan; Methylergonovine; Midazolam; Naloxegol; Nilotinib; Nisoldipine; Olaparib; PAZOPanib; PHENobarbital; Phenytoin; Pimozide; Ranolazine; Red Yeast Rice; Regorafenib; Rifabutin; Rifampin; Rivaroxaban; Salmeterol; Sildenafil; Silodosin; Simeprevir; Simvastatin; St Johns Wort; Suvorexant; Tamsulosin; Terfenadine; Ticagrelor; Tipranavir; Tolvaptan; Topotecan; Toremifene; Trabectedin; Triazolam; Ulipristal; Vemurafenib; VinCRIStine (Liposomal); Vorapaxar

Increased Effect/Toxicity

Telaprevir may increase the levels/effects of: Ado-Trastuzumab Emtansine; Afatinib; Alfuzosin; Almotriptan; Alosetron; ALPRAZolam; Amiodarone; Apixaban; ARIPiprazole; Astemizole; Atazanavir; AtorvaSTATin; Avanafil; Axitinib; Bedaquiline; Bepridil [Off Market]; Bortezomib; Bosentan; Bosutinib; Brentuximab Vedotin; Brinzolamide; Budesonide (Nasal); Budesonide (Systemic, Oral Inhalation); Cabazitaxel; Cabozantinib; Cannabis; CarBAMazepine; Ceritinib; Cisapride; Clarithromycin; Colchicine; Conivaptan; Corticosteroids; Corticosteroids (Systemic); Crizotinib; CycloSPORINE (Systemic); CYP3A4 Substrates; Dabigatran Etexilate; Dapoxetine; Dasatinib; Digoxin; Dihydroergotamine; Dofetilide; DOXOrubicin (Conventional); Dronabinol; Dronedarone; Dutasteride; Edoxaban; Eliglustat; Eplerenone; Ergoloid Mesylates; Ergonovine; Ergotamine; Erlotinib; Erythromycin (Systemic); Etizolam; Everolimus; FentaNYL; Fesoterodine; Flecainide; Fluticasone (Nasal); Fluticasone (Oral Inhalation); Fluvastatin; Fosphenytoin; GuanFACINE; Halofantrine; Hydrocodone; Ibrutinib; Iloperidone; Imatinib; Imidafenacin; Irinotecan; Itraconazole; Ivabradine; Ivacaftor; Ixabepilone; Ketoconazole (Systemic); Lacosamide; Lapatinib; Ledipasvir; Lercanidipine; Levobupivacaine; Levomilnacipran; Lidocaine (Systemic); Lomitapide; Lovastatin; Lumefantrine; Lurasidone; Macitentan; Maraviroc; Methylergonovine; MethylPREDNISolone; Midazolam; Mifepristone; Naloxegol; Nilotinib; Nintedanib; Nisoldipine; Olaparib; Ospemifene; OxyCODONE; Paricalcitol; PAZOPanib; P-glycoprotein/ABCB1 Substrates; Phenytoin; Pimecrolimus; Pimozide; Pitavastatin; PONATinib; Posaconazole; Pranlukast; Pravastatin; Propafenone; Prucalopride; QUEtiapine; QuiNIDine; Ranolazine; Red Yeast Rice; Regorafenib; Repaglinide; Retapamulin; Rifabutin; Rifaximin; Rilpivirine; Rivaroxaban; RomiDEPsin; Rosuvastatin; Ruxolitinib; Salmeterol; Saxagliptin; Sildenafil; Silodosin; Simeprevir; Simvastatin; Sirolimus; SORAfenib; Suvorexant; Tacrolimus (Systemic); Tadalafil; Tamsulosin; Telithromycin; Tenofovir; Terfenadine; Tetrahydrocannabinol; Ticagrelor; Tofacitinib; Tolterodine;

Tolvaptan; Topotecan; Toremifene; Trabectedin; TraZODone; Triazolam; Ulipristal; Vardenafil; Vemurafenib; Vilazodone; VinCRIStine (Liposomal); Vorapaxar; Voriconazole; Warfarin; Zopiclone; Zuclopenthixol

The levels/effects of Telaprevir may be increased by: Clarithromycin; Cobicistat; Conivaptan; CYP3A4 Inhibitors (Moderate); CYP3A4 Inhibitors (Strong); Erythromycin (Systemic); Fusidic Acid (Systemic); Idelalisib; Itraconazole; Ketoconazole (Systemic); Luliconazole; Mifepristone; Netupitant; P-glycoprotein/ABCB1 Inhibitors; Posaconazole; Ritonavir; Stiripentol; Telithromycin; Voriconazole

Decreased Effect

Telaprevir may decrease the levels/effects of: Contraceptives (Estrogens); Contraceptives (Progestins); Darunavir; Efavirenz; Escitalopram; Fosamprenavir; Ifosfamide; Methadone; Prasugrel; Ticagrelor; Voriconazole; Warfarin; Zolpidem

The levels/effects of Telaprevir may be decreased by: Atazanavir; Bosentan; CarBAMazepine; Corticosteroids; Corticosteroids (Systemic); CYP3A4 Inducers (Moderate); CYP3A4 Inducers (Strong); Dabrafenib; Darunavir; Deferasirox; Efavirenz; Etravirine; Fosamprenavir; Fosphenytoin; Lopinavir; PHENobarbital; Phenytoin; Rifabutin; Rifampin; Ritonavir; Siltuximab; St Johns Wort; Tipranavir; Tocilizumab

Storage/Stability Store at 25°C (77°F); excursions permitted to 15°C to 30°C (59°F to 86°F).

Mechanism of Action Binds reversibly to nonstructural protein 3 (NS 3) serine protease and inhibits replication of the hepatitis C virus. Considered a direct-acting antiviral treatment for HCV, also called a specifically targeted antiviral therapy for HCV (STAT-C).

Pharmacodynamics/Kinetics Note: Telaprevir total exposure ($AUC_{24h,ss}$) was similar regardless of whether the total daily dose of 2250 mg was administered as 750 mg every 8 hours or 1125 mg twice daily.

Absorption: Food (not low fat) enhances absorption
Distribution: V_d: ~252 L
Protein binding: 59% to 76%
Metabolism: Primarily hepatic to less active (30x) and inactive metabolites. Some oxidative CYP3A4 metabolism.
Half-life elimination: Plasma: Adults: ~4-5 hours (single dose); steady state: ~9-11 hours
Time to peak, serum: 4-5 hours
Excretion: Feces (82%); urine (1%)

Dosage Oral: Adults: 1125 mg twice daily (in combination with peginterferon alfa and ribavirin).

Treatment-naive or prior relapse patients: **Note:** Relapse includes patients with an undetectable HCV-RNA upon completion of treatment (non-telaprevir based regimen) but with detectable HCV-RNA during the follow up period.

Weeks 1-12: Triple therapy: Telaprevir 1125 mg twice daily in combination with peginterferon alfa and ribavirin

Weeks 13-23 (based on HCV-RNA results at weeks 4 and 12):

HCV-RNA **undetectable** (level less than ~10-15 units/mL) at both weeks 4 and 12 (eRVR): Dual therapy: Peginterferon alfa and ribavirin only (through week 24)

HCV-RNA **detectable** (level greater than ~10-15 units/mL but ≤1000 units/mL) at week 4 and/or week 12: Dual therapy: Peginterferon alfa and ribavirin only (through week 48 discussed below)

HCV-RNA **detectable** (level >1000 units/mL) at week 4 or week 12 (treatment futility): Discontinue telaprevir, peginterferon alfa and ribavirin at week 12

Weeks ≥24 (based on HCV-RNA results at week 24):

HCV-RNA **detectable** (level greater than ~10-15 units/mL but ≤1000 units/mL) at week 4 and/or week 12: Peginterferon alfa with concomitant ribavirin only (through week 48)

HCV-RNA **detectable** (level greater than ~10-15 units/mL) at week 24 (treatment futility): Discontinue peginterferon alfa and concomitant ribavirin

Treatment naïve patients with cirrhosis, compensated:

Weeks 1-12: Triple therapy: Telaprevir 1125 mg twice daily in combination with peginterferon alfa and ribavirin

Weeks 13-24 (based on HCV-RNA results at weeks 4 and 12):

HCV-RNA **undetectable** at both weeks 4 and 12 (eRVR): Dual therapy: Peginterferon alfa and ribavirin only (through week 48 discussed below)

HCV-RNA **detectable** (level greater than ~10-15 units/mL but ≤1000 units/mL) at week 4 and/or week 12: Dual therapy: Peginterferon alfa and ribavirin only (through week 48 discussed below)

HCV-RNA **detectable** (level >1000 units/mL) at week 4 or week 12 (treatment futility): Discontinue telaprevir, peginterferon alfa and ribavirin at week 12

Weeks ≥ 24 (based on HCV-RNA results at week 24):

HCV-RNA **undetectable** at week 24: Peginterferon alfa with concomitant ribavirin only (through week 48)

HCV-RNA **detectable** (level greater than ~10-15 units/mL) at week 24 (treatment futility): Discontinue peginterferon alfa and ribavirin

Previously-treated patients (partial response or null responders): **Note:** Previously treated does not include prior treatment with telaprevir. Partial response includes patients with a >2-log_{10} HCV-RNA decrease by week 12 but a nonsustained virologic response thereafter. Null response includes patients with a <2-log_{10} HCV-RNA decrease at week 12.

Weeks 1-12: Triple therapy: Telaprevir 1125 mg twice daily with peginterferon alfa and ribavirin

Weeks 13-48 (based on HCV-RNA results at weeks 4 and 12):

HCV-RNA **undetectable** (level less than ~10-15 units/mL) or detectable (level ≤1000 units/mL) at both weeks 4 and 12: Dual therapy: Peginterferon alfa and ribavirin only (through week 48)

HCV-RNA **detectable** (level >1000 units/mL) at week 4 or week 12: Discontinue telaprevir, peginterferon alfa, and ribavirin at week 12

HCV-RNA **detectable** (level greater than ~10-15 units/mL) at week 24: Discontinue peginterferon alfa and concomitant ribavirin

Missed dose: If a dose is missed within 6 hours of the time it is usually taken, take as soon as possible. If more than 6 hours have passed since the dose is usually taken, do not take the missed dose and the patient should resume the usual schedule.

Dosage adjustment in renal impairment:

Telaprevir: No dosage adjustment necessary. Not studied in patients with CrCl ≤50 mL/minute or in hemodialysis.

Peginterferon Alfa and Ribavirin: Refer to individual monographs.

Dosage adjustment in hepatic impairment: Telaprevir:

Mild impairment (Child-Pugh class A): No dosage adjustment necessary.

Moderate or severe impairment (Child-Pugh class B or C): Use is not recommended in patients with decompensated liver disease or with moderate or severe hepatic impairment (has not been studied).

Peginterferon Alfa and Ribavirin: Refer to individual monographs.

Dietary Considerations Take with a meal (not low fat).

Administration Administer with a meal (not low fat) within 30 minutes prior to each dose. Doses should be taken approximately every 10-14 hours. Administer concurrently with peginterferon alfa and ribavirin. Maintain adequate fluid intake/hydration. Swallow tablets whole; do not chew, crush, break, cut, or dissolve the tablets. If a dose is missed within 6 hours of the time it is usually taken, take as soon as possible. If more than 6 hours have passed since the dose is usually taken, the missed dose should not be taken and the patient should resume the usual schedule.

Monitoring Parameters

CBC with differential and platelet count, serum electrolytes, serum creatinine, TSH, bilirubin, liver enzymes, and uric acid at baseline and weeks 2, 4, 8 and 12, then periodically (and when clinically indicated)

Serum HCV-RNA at baseline, weeks 4, 8, 12 and 24, end of treatment, during treatment follow up, and when clinically indicated

Pretreatment and monthly pregnancy test up to 6 months following discontinuation of therapy for women of childbearing age

Hydration status, including fluid intake/output, urine output, signs/symptoms of dehydration

Reference Range

Treatment futility: HCV-RNA ≥1000 units/mL at treatment week 4 or 12 or confirmed, detectable HCV-RNA at treatment week 24

Rapid virologic response (RVR): Absence of detectable HCV-RNA after 4 weeks of treatment

Extended rapid virologic response (eRVR): Absence of detectable HCV-RNA after 4 and 12 weeks of treatment

Early virologic response (EVR): Absence of detectable HCV-RNA after 12 weeks of treatment

Sustained virologic response (SVR): Absence of HCV-RNA in the serum 32-78 weeks after completion of a 24 week treatment course or 56-78 weeks after a 48 week treatment course.

Additional Information In clinical studies of treatment-naive patients, a sustained virologic response (SVR) of ~75% (~65% in African-Americans) was observed with peginterferon alfa, ribavirin, and telaprevir versus 46% with peginterferon and ribavirin alone. Adherence to 3 times/day dosing is needed; resistance is increased and efficacy is affected when dosed every 12 hours.

Telavancin (tel a VAN sin)

Brand Names: U.S. Vibativ

Index Terms TD-6424; Telavancin Hydrochloride

Pharmacologic Category Glycopeptide

Use

Complicated skin and skin structure infections: Treatment of complicated skin and skin structure infections caused by susceptible gram-positive organisms including methicillin-susceptible or -resistant *Staphylococcus aureus*, vancomycin-susceptible *Enterococcus faecalis*, and *Streptococcus pyogenes*, *Streptococcus agalactiae*, or *Streptococcus anginosus* group

Hospital-acquired and ventilator-associated bacterial pneumonia (HABP/VABP): Treatment of HABP/VABP caused by susceptible isolates of *Staphylococcus aureus* when alternative treatments are not appropriate

Pregnancy Risk Factor C

Pregnancy Considerations **[U.S. Boxed Warning]: Based on animal data, adverse developmental outcomes have been observed. Prior to use, women of childbearing potential should have a serum pregnancy test. Use of telavancin is not recommended during pregnancy unless the potential benefit to the mother outweighs the possible risk to the fetus.** Telavancin crosses the placenta (Nanovskaya, 2012). In women of childbearing potential, effective contraception should be used during therapy.

Healthcare providers are encouraged to enroll women exposed to telavancin during pregnancy in the Vibativ Pregnancy Registry 855-633-8479).

Breast-Feeding Considerations It is not known if telavancin is excreted in breast milk. The manufacturer recommends that caution be exercised when administering telavancin to nursing women.

Contraindications Hypersensitivity to telavancin or any component of the formulation; concomitant use of intravenous unfractionated heparin

Warnings/Precautions Hazardous agent - use appropriate precautions for handling and disposal (NIOSH 2014 [group 3]). **[U.S. Boxed Warning]: Based on animal data, adverse developmental outcomes have been observed. Prior to use, women of childbearing potential should have a serum pregnancy test. Use of telavancin is not recommended during pregnancy unless the potential benefit outweighs the risk to the fetus. [U.S. Boxed Warning]: New-onset or worsening renal impairment has occurred. Monitor renal function prior to, during (at least every 48 to 72 hours; more frequently if indicated), and following therapy in all patients.** May cause nephrotoxicity; usual risk factors include concomitant nephrotoxic medications or baseline comorbidities associated with decreased renal function (eg, baseline renal dysfunction, diabetes, hypertension, or heart failure). **[U.S. Boxed Warning]: In clinical studies, patients with preexisting moderate-to-severe renal impairment (CrCl ≤50 mL/minute) treated for hospital-acquired/ventilator-associated bacterial pneumonia (HABP/VABP) had increased (all cause) mortality versus vancomycin. Use in HABP/VABP only when benefit outweighs risk.** Serious hypersensitivity reactions, including anaphylaxis, have been reported after first or subsequent doses; some have been fatal. Discontinue if hypersensitivity or rash occurs. Telavancin is a semisynthetic derivative of vancomycin; cross-reactivity rates are unknown. Use with caution in patients with known vancomycin hypersensitivity.

May prolong QTc interval; avoid use in patients with a history of QTc prolongation, uncompensated heart failure, severe left ventricular hypertrophy, or concurrent administration of other medications known to prolong the QT interval. Clinical studies indicate mean maximal QTc prolongation of 12 to 15 msec at the end of 10 mg/kg infusion. Contains solubilizer cyclodextrin (hydroxypropyl-beta-cyclodextrin) which may accumulate in patients with renal dysfunction. Prolonged use may result in fungal or bacterial superinfection, including *C. difficile*-associated diarrhea (CDAD) and pseudomembranous colitis; CDAD has been observed >2 months postantibiotic treatment. Potentially significant drug-drug interactions may exist, requiring dose or frequency adjustment, additional monitoring, and/or selection of alternative therapy.

May interfere with tests used to monitor coagulation (eg, prothrombin time, INR, activated partial thromboplastin time, activated clotting time, coagulation based factor Xa tests) when samples drawn ≤18 hours after drug administration. Blood samples should be collected as close to the next dose of telavancin as possible or a non-phospholipid dependent coagulation test (eg, bleeding time, factor Xa [chromogenic assay], platelet aggregation study, thrombin time) should be used. Consider selecting an alternative anticoagulant not requiring aPTT monitoring; concomitant use of telavancin with IV unfractionated heparin is contraindicated. Rapid IV administration may result in flushing, rash, urticaria, and/or pruritus; slowing or stopping the infusion may alleviate these symptoms. In the elderly, lower doses are often required secondary to age-related decreases in renal function.

Adverse Reactions

Central nervous system: Dizziness, headache, insomnia, local pain, paresthesia, psychiatric disturbance, rigors
Dermatologic: Localized erythema, pruritus, skin rash
Endocrine & metabolic: Albuminuria (micro), hypokalemia
Gastrointestinal: Abdominal pain, decreased appetite, diarrhea, metallic taste, nausea, vomiting
Genitourinary: Acute renal failure, proteinuria
Hematologic & oncologic: Thrombocytopenia
Renal: Increased serum creatinine, renal insufficiency
Respiratory: Dyspnea
Rare but important or life-threatening: *Clostridium difficile* associated diarrhea, hearing loss (transient), hypersensitivity reaction, nephrotoxicity, prolonged Q-T interval on ECG, urticaria

Drug Interactions

Metabolism/Transport Effects None known.

Avoid Concomitant Use

Avoid concomitant use of Telavancin with any of the following: BCG; Heparin; Highest Risk QTc-Prolonging Agents; Ivabradine; Mifepristone

Increased Effect/Toxicity

Telavancin may increase the levels/effects of: Highest Risk QTc-Prolonging Agents; Moderate Risk QTc-Prolonging Agents

The levels/effects of Telavancin may be increased by: Ivabradine; Mifepristone; QTc-Prolonging Agents (Indeterminate Risk and Risk Modifying)

Decreased Effect

Telavancin may decrease the levels/effects of: BCG; Heparin; Sodium Picosulfate; Typhoid Vaccine

Preparation for Administration Hazardous agent; use appropriate precautions for handling and disposal (NIOSH 2014 [group 3]).

Reconstitute 250 mg vial with 15 mL of D_5W, NS, or SWFI to yield 15 mg/mL (total volume of ~17 mL). Reconstitute 750 mg vial with 45 mL of of D_5W, NS, or SWFI to yield 15 mg/mL (total volume of ~50 mL). Allow vacuum to pull the diluent into the vial; discard vial if this did not occur. Reconstitution generally takes <2 minutes, although may take up to 20 minutes. Do not shake the vial or final solution for infusion. Prior to administration, dilute dose in 100-250 mL D_5W, LR, or NS to a final concentration of 0.6-8 mg/mL.

Storage/Stability Store intact vials at 2°C to 8°C (35°F to 46°F); excursions permitted up to 25°C (77°F); avoid excess heat. **Note:** Vials contain no bacteriostatic agent. Reconstituted solution in the vial should be used within 12 hours at room temperature or 7 days refrigerated; solutions admixed for infusion are stable at room temperature for 12 hours or under refrigeration for 7 days. Total time in vial **plus** time in infusion bag should not exceed 12 hours at room temperature or 7 days if refrigerated at 2°C to 8°C (35°F to 46°F). Solutions admixed for infusion can also be stored at -30°C to -10°C (-22°F to 14°F) for ≤32 days.

Mechanism of Action Exerts concentration-dependent bactericidal activity; inhibits bacterial cell wall synthesis by blocking polymerization and cross-linking of peptidoglycan by binding to D-Ala-D-Ala portion of cell wall. Unlike vancomycin, additional mechanism involves disruption of membrane potential and changes cell permeability due to presence of lipophilic side chain moiety.

Pharmacodynamics/Kinetics

Distribution: V_{ss}: 0.13 L/kg
Protein binding: ~90%; primarily to albumin
Half-life elimination: 6.6-9.6 hours
Excretion: Urine (~76%); feces (<1%)

Dosage

Complicated skin and skin structure infection: Adults: IV: 10 mg/kg every 24 hours for 1-2 weeks
Hospital-acquired and ventilator-associated bacterial pneumonia (HABP/VABP): Adults: IV: 10 mg/kg every 24 hours for 1-3 weeks

Dosage adjustment in renal impairment: Note: Renal function may be estimated using the Cockcroft-Gault formula for dosage adjustment purposes.
CrCl >50 mL/minute: No dosage adjustment necessary
CrCl 30-50 mL/minute: 7.5 mg/kg every 24 hours
CrCl 10 to <30 mL/minute: 10 mg/kg every 48 hours
CrCl <10 mL/minute: No dosage adjustment provided in manufacturer's labeling (has not been studied).
ESRD and hemodialysis patients: No dosage adjustment provided in manufacturer's labeling (has not been studied).

Dosage adjustment in hepatic impairment:
Mild-to-moderate hepatic impairment (Child-Pugh class A or B): No dosage adjustment necessary.
Severe hepatic impairment (Child-Pugh class C): No dosage adjustment provided in manufacturer's labeling (has not been studied).

Administration Administer IV over 60 minutes. Other medications should not be infused simultaneously through the same IV line. When the same intravenous line is used for sequential infusion of other medications, flush line with D_5W, LR, or NS before and after infusing telavancin.

Red-man syndrome may occur if the infusion is too rapid. It is not an allergic reaction, but may be characterized by hypotension and/or a maculopapular rash appearing on the face, neck, trunk, and/or upper extremities. If this should occur, discontinuing or slowing the infusion rate may eliminate these reactions.

Hazardous agent; use appropriate precautions for handling and disposal (NIOSH 2014 [group 3]).

Monitoring Parameters Renal function (prior to start, every 48-72 hours; more frequently if indicated, and following therapy), pregnancy test

Dosage Forms

Solution Reconstituted, Intravenous [preservative free]:
Vibativ: 250 mg (1 ea); 750 mg (1 ea)

◆ **Telavancin Hydrochloride** *see* Telavancin *on page 1986*

Telithromycin (tel ith roe MYE sin)

Brand Names: U.S. Ketek

Index Terms HMR 3647

Pharmacologic Category Antibiotic, Ketolide

Use Community-acquired pneumonia: Treatment of mild to moderate community-acquired pneumonia (CAP) due to *Streptococcus pneumoniae* (including multidrug-resistant isolates), *Haemophilus influenzae*, *Moraxella catarrhalis*, *Chlamydophila pneumoniae*, or *Mycoplasma pneumoniae* in patients 18 years and older.

Pregnancy Risk Factor C

Dosage Community-acquired pneumonia (CAP): Adults: Oral: 800 mg once daily for 7-10 days

Dosage adjustment in renal impairment:
CrCl ≥30 mL/minute: No dosage adjustment necessary
CrCl <30 mL/minute: 600 mg once daily;
CrCl <30 mL/minute and concomitant hepatic impairment: 400 mg once daily
Hemodialysis: 600 mg once daily; administer after dialysis on dialysis days

Dosage adjustment in hepatic impairment: No dosage adjustment necessary, unless concurrent renal impairment (eg,CrCl <30 mL/minute) is present

Additional Information Complete prescribing information should be consulted for additional detail.

Dosage Forms

Tablet, Oral:

Ketek: 300 mg, 400 mg

Telmisartan (tel mi SAR tan)

Brand Names: U.S. Micardis

Brand Names: Canada ACT Telmisartan; Micardis; Mylan-Telmisartan; PMS-Telmisartan; Ran-Telmisartan; Sandoz-Telmisartan; Teva-Telmisartan

Pharmacologic Category Angiotensin II Receptor Blocker; Antihypertensive

Use

Cardiovascular risk reduction: Cardiovascular risk reduction in patients ≥55 years of age unable to take ACE inhibitors and who are at high risk of major cardiovascular events (eg, MI, stroke, death)

Hypertension: For the treatment of hypertension, alone or in combination with other antihypertensive agents

The 2014 guideline for the management of high blood pressure in adults (Eighth Joint National Committee [JNC 8; James, 2013]) recommends initiation of pharmacologic treatment to lower blood pressure for the following patients:

- Patients ≥60 years of age with systolic blood pressure (SBP) ≥150 mm Hg or diastolic blood pressure (DBP) ≥90 mm Hg. Goal of therapy is SBP <150 mm Hg and DBP <90 mm Hg.
- Patients <60 years of age with SBP ≥140 mm Hg or DBP ≥90 mm Hg. Goal of therapy is SBP <140 mm Hg and DBP <90 mm Hg.
- Patients ≥18 years of age with diabetes and SBP ≥140 mm Hg or DBP ≥90 mm Hg. Goal of therapy is SBP <140 mm Hg and DBP <90 mm Hg.
- Patients ≥18 years of age with chronic kidney disease (CKD) and SBP ≥140 mm Hg or DBP ≥90 mm Hg. Goal of therapy is SBP <140 mm Hg and DBP <90 mm Hg.

In patients with CKD, regardless of race or diabetes status, the use of an ACE inhibitor (ACEI) or angiotensin receptor blocker (ARB) as initial therapy is recommended to improve kidney outcomes. In the general nonblack population (without CKD), including those with diabetes, initial antihypertensive treatment should consist of a thiazide-type diuretic, calcium channel blocker, ACEI, or ARB. In the general black population (without CKD), including those with diabetes, initial antihypertensive treatment should consist of a thiazide-type diuretic or a calcium channel blocker instead of an ACEI or ARB.

Pregnancy Risk Factor D

Pregnancy Considerations [U.S. Boxed Warning]: Drugs that act on the renin-angiotensin system can cause injury and death to the developing fetus. Discontinue as soon as possible once pregnancy is detected. The use of drugs which act on the renin-angiotensin system are associated with oligohydramnios. Oligohydramnios, due to decreased fetal renal function, may lead to fetal lung hypoplasia and skeletal malformations. Use is also associated with anuria, hypotension, renal failure, skull hypoplasia, and death in the fetus/neonate. The exposed fetus should be monitored for fetal growth, amniotic fluid volume, and organ formation. Infants exposed *in utero* should be monitored for hyperkalemia, hypotension, and oliguria (exchange transfusions or dialysis may be needed). These adverse events are generally associated with maternal use in the second and third trimesters.

Untreated chronic maternal hypertension is also associated with adverse events in the fetus, infant, and mother. The use of angiotensin II receptor blockers is not recommended to treat chronic uncomplicated hypertension in pregnant women and should generally be avoided in women of reproductive potential (ACOG, 2013).

Breast-Feeding Considerations It is not known if telmisartan is excreted in breast milk. Due to the potential for serious adverse reactions in the nursing infant, a decision should be made whether to discontinue nursing or to discontinue the drug, taking into account the importance of treatment to the mother. The Canadian labeling contraindicates use in nursing women.

Contraindications Known hypersensitivity (eg, anaphylaxis, angioedema) to telmisartan or any component of the formulation; concurrent use of aliskiren in patients with diabetes

Canadian labeling: Additional contraindications: Concomitant use with aliskiren in patients with moderate-to-severe renal impairment (GFR <60 mL/min/1.73 m^2); pregnancy; breast-feeding; fructose intolerance

Warnings/Precautions [U.S. Boxed Warning]: Drugs that act on the renin-angiotensin system can cause injury and death to the developing fetus. Discontinue as soon as possible once pregnancy is detected. May cause hyperkalemia; avoid potassium supplementation unless specifically required by healthcare provider. Avoid use or use a smaller dose in patients who are volume depleted; correct depletion first. May be associated with deterioration of renal function and/or increases in serum creatinine, particularly in patients with low renal blood flow (eg, renal artery stenosis, heart failure) whose glomerular filtration rate (GFR) is dependent on efferent arteriolar vasoconstriction by angiotensin II. Use with caution in unstented unilateral/bilateral renal artery stenosis. When unstented bilateral renal artery stenosis is present, use is generally avoided due to the elevated risk of deterioration in renal function unless possible benefits outweigh risks. Use with caution with preexisting renal insufficiency; significant aortic/mitral stenosis. Potentially significant drug-drug interactions may exist, requiring dose or frequency adjustment, additional monitoring, and/or selection of alternative therapy. Use with caution in patients who have biliary obstructive disorders or hepatic dysfunction. In surgical patients on chronic angiotensin receptor blocker (ARB) therapy, intraoperative hypotension may occur with induction and maintenance of general anesthesia. Product contains sorbitol. The Canadian labeling contraindicates use in fructose intolerant patients.

Angioedema has been reported rarely with some angiotensin II receptor antagonists (ARBs) and may occur at any time during treatment (especially following first dose). It may involve the head and neck (potentially compromising airway) or the intestine (presenting with abdominal pain). Patients with idiopathic or hereditary angioedema or previous angioedema associated with ACE-inhibitor therapy may be at an increased risk. Prolonged frequent monitoring may be required, especially if tongue, glottis, or larynx are involved, as they are associated with airway obstruction. Patients with a history of airway surgery may have a higher risk of airway obstruction. Discontinue therapy immediately if angioedema occurs. Aggressive early management is critical. Intramuscular (IM) administration of epinephrine may be necessary. Do not readminister to patients who have had angioedema with ARBs.

Adverse Reactions May be associated with worsening of renal function in patients dependent on renin-angiotensin-aldosterone system.

Cardiovascular: Chest pain, hypertension, intermittent claudication, peripheral edema

Central nervous system: Dizziness, fatigue, headache, pain

Dermatologic: Skin ulcer

Gastrointestinal: Abdominal pain, diarrhea, dyspepsia, nausea

Genitourinary: Urinary tract infection

Neuromuscular & skeletal: Back pain, myalgia

Respiratory: Cough, pharyngitis, sinusitis, upper respiratory infection

Rare but important or life-threatening: Abnormal ECG, abscess, allergic reaction, anaphylaxis, anemia, angina, angioedema, arthritis, asthma, atrial fibrillation, bradycardia, cerebrovascular disorder, CHF, conjunctivitis, creatinine kinase increased, depression, diabetes mellitus, eczema, edema, epistaxis, erectile dysfunction, fixed drug eruption, fungal infection, gastroenteritis, gout, hepatic dysfunction, hypercholesterolemia, hyperkalemia, hypersensitivity, hypoglycemia (diabetic patients), hypotension, impotence, insomnia, MI, migraine, neoplasm, orthostatic hypotension (more frequent in dialysis patients), otitis media, renal failure, rhabdomyolysis, reflux, serum creatinine increased, syncope, tachycardia, tendon pain, thrombocytopenia, uric acid increased

Drug Interactions

Metabolism/Transport Effects Inhibits CYP2C19 (weak)

Avoid Concomitant Use

Avoid concomitant use of Telmisartan with any of the following: Ramipril

Increased Effect/Toxicity

Telmisartan may increase the levels/effects of: ACE Inhibitors; Amifostine; Antihypertensives; Cardiac Glycosides; CycloSPORINE (Systemic); DULoxetine; Hypotensive Agents; Levodopa; Lithium; Nonsteroidal Anti-Inflammatory Agents; Obinutuzumab; Potassium-Sparing Diuretics; Ramipril; RisperiDONE; RiTUXimab; Sodium Phosphates

The levels/effects of Telmisartan may be increased by: Alfuzosin; Aliskiren; Barbiturates; Brimonidine (Topical); Canagliflozin; Dapoxetine; Diazoxide; Eplerenone; Heparin; Heparin (Low Molecular Weight); Herbs (Hypotensive Properties); MAO Inhibitors; Nicorandil; Pentoxifylline; Phosphodiesterase 5 Inhibitors; Potassium Salts; Prostacyclin Analogues; Tolvaptan; Trimethoprim

Decreased Effect

The levels/effects of Telmisartan may be decreased by: Herbs (Hypertensive Properties); Methylphenidate; Nonsteroidal Anti-Inflammatory Agents; Yohimbine

Storage/Stability Store at 25°C (77°F); excursions are permitted between 15°C and 30°C (59°F and 86°F). Tablets should not be removed from blisters until immediately before administration.

Mechanism of Action Angiotensin II acts as a vasoconstrictor. In addition to causing direct vasoconstriction, angiotensin II also stimulates the release of aldosterone. Once aldosterone is released, sodium as well as water is reabsorbed. The end result is an elevation in blood pressure. Telmisartan is a nonpeptide AT1 angiotensin II receptor antagonist. This binding prevents angiotensin II from binding to the receptor thereby blocking the vasoconstriction and the aldosterone secreting effects of angiotensin II.

Pharmacodynamics/Kinetics Orally active, not a prodrug

Onset of action: 1 to 2 hours

Duration: Up to 24 hours

Distribution: V_d: 500 L

Protein binding: >99.5%; primarily to albumin and $alpha_1$-acid glycoprotein

Metabolism: Hepatic via conjugation to inactive metabolites; not metabolized via CYP

Bioavailability (dose dependent): 42% to 58%; Hepatic impairment: Approaches 100%

Half-life elimination: Terminal: 24 hours

Time to peak, plasma: 0.5 to 1 hours

Excretion: Feces (97%)

Clearance: Total body: 800 mL/minute

Dosage

Adults: Oral:

Hypertension: Initial: 40 mg once daily; usual dosage range (ASH/ISH [Weber, 2014]): 40 to 80 mg daily. Patients with volume depletion should be initiated on the lower dosage with close supervision.

Cardiovascular risk reduction: Oral: 80 mg once daily. **Note:** It is unknown whether doses <80 mg daily are associated with a reduction in risk of cardiovascular morbidity or mortality.

Elderly: Refer to adult dosing.

Dosage adjustment in renal impairment: No dosage adjustment necessary; hemodialysis patients are more susceptible to orthostatic hypotension

Dosage adjustment in hepatic impairment: Initiate therapy with low dose; titrate slowly and monitor closely.

Canadian labeling: Recommended initial dose: 40 mg daily

Dietary Considerations May be taken without regard to meals. Product contains sorbitol.

Administration May be administered without regard to meals.

Monitoring Parameters Blood pressure; electrolytes, serum creatinine, BUN

Dosage Forms

Tablet, Oral:

Micardis: 20 mg, 40 mg, 80 mg

Generic: 20 mg, 40 mg, 80 mg

Telmisartan and Amlodipine

(tel mi SAR tan & am LOE di peen)

Brand Names: U.S. Twynsta

Brand Names: Canada Twynsta

Index Terms Amlodipine and Telmisartan; Amlodipine Besylate and Telmisartan

Pharmacologic Category Angiotensin II Receptor Blocker; Antianginal Agent; Antihypertensive; Calcium Channel Blocker; Calcium Channel Blocker, Dihydropyridine

Use Hypertension:

U.S. labeling: Treatment of hypertension, including initial treatment in patients who will require multiple antihypertensives for adequate control

Canadian labeling: Treatment of mild-to-moderate hypertension in patients whom combination therapy is appropriate; not indicated for initial therapy

Pregnancy Risk Factor D

Dosage Oral: Adults: Dose is individualized; combination product may be substituted for individual components in patients currently maintained on both agents separately or in patients not adequately controlled with monotherapy (using one of the agents or an agent within the same antihypertensive class). May also be used as initial therapy in patients who are likely to need >1 antihypertensive to control blood pressure. **Note:** Use as initial therapy is not an approved indication in the Canadian labeling.

Hypertension:

Initial therapy (antihypertensive naive): Telmisartan 40 mg/amlodipine 5 mg once daily; dose may be increased after 2 weeks of therapy. Patients requiring larger blood pressure reductions may be started on telmisartan 80 mg/amlodipine 5 mg once daily. Maximum recommended dose: Telmisartan 80 mg/day, amlodipine 10 mg/day

Add-on/replacement therapy: Telmisartan 40-80 mg and amlodipine 5-10 mg once daily depending upon previous doses, current control, and goals of therapy; dose may be titrated after 2 weeks of therapy. Maximum recommended dose: Telmisartan 80 mg/day; amlodipine 10 mg/day

Elderly: Not recommended for initial therapy in patients ≥75 years of age. For add-on/replacement therapy, initiate amlodipine therapy at 2.5 mg once daily and titrate slowly. **Note:** Use of individual agents may be necessary if the appropriate combination dose is not available.

Dosage adjustment in renal impairment: No dosage adjustment necessary; titrate slowly in severe impairment.

Dosage adjustment in hepatic impairment: Not recommended for initial therapy. For add-on/replacement therapy, initiate amlodipine at 2.5 mg once daily with low-dose telmisartan and titrate slowly; **Note:** Use of individual agents is necessary as the appropriate combination dose is not available. Upon titration to therapeutic dose, may initiate combination dose if available. Canadian labeling contraindicates use in severe hepatic impairment or with biliary obstructive disorders.

Additional Information Complete prescribing information should be consulted for additional detail.

Dosage Forms

Tablet, oral:

Twynsta® 40/5: Telmisartan 40 mg and amlodipine 5 mg; Twynsta® 40/10: telmisartan 40 mg and amlodipine 10 mg; Twynsta® 80/5: telmisartan 80 mg and amlodipine 5 mg; Twynsta® 80/10: telmisartan 80 mg and amlodipine10 mg

Telmisartan and Hydrochlorothiazide

(tel mi SAR tan & hye droe klor oh THYE a zide)

Brand Names: U.S. Micardis HCT

Brand Names: Canada ACH-Telmisartan HCTZ; ACT Telmisartan/HCT; Micardis Plus; Mylan-Telmisartan HCTZ; PMS-Telmisartan HCTZ; RAN-Telmisartan HCTZ; Sandoz-Telmisartan HCT; Telmisartan HCTZ; Teva-Telmisartan HCTZ

Index Terms Hydrochlorothiazide and Telmisartan

Pharmacologic Category Angiotensin II Receptor Blocker; Antihypertensive; Diuretic, Thiazide

Use Hypertension: Treatment of hypertension; **Note:** A fixed-dose combination product should not be used for initial therapy

Pregnancy Risk Factor D

Dosage

Hypertension: Adults: Oral:

Replacement therapy: Combination product can be substituted for individual titrated agents.

Initiation of combination therapy when monotherapy has failed to achieve desired effects:

Patients currently on telmisartan:

U.S. labeling: Initial dose if blood pressure is not currently controlled on monotherapy of 80 mg telmisartan: Telmisartan 80 mg/hydrochlorothiazide 12.5 mg once daily; manufacturer labeling suggests that dose may be titrated up to telmisartan 160 mg/ hydrochlorothiazide 25 mg if needed; however, in mild to moderate hypertension, doses of telmisartan >80 mg were not associated with a greater reduction in blood pressure (Smith, 2000).

Canadian labeling: If blood pressure is not currently controlled on monotherapy of telmisartan 80 mg: Telmisartan 80 mg/hydrochlorothiazide 12.5 mg once daily; may titrate up to telmisartan 80 mg/ hydrochlorothiazide 25 mg if needed.

Patients currently on hydrochlorothiazide:

U.S. labeling: Initial dose if blood pressure is not currently controlled on monotherapy of 25 mg once daily: Telmisartan 80 mg/hydrochlorothiazide 12.5 mg once daily or telmisartan 80 mg/hydrochlorothiazide 25 mg once daily; manufacturer labeling suggests that dose may be titrated up to telmisartan 160 mg/hydrochlorothiazide 25 mg if blood pressure remains uncontrolled after 2-4 weeks of therapy. In mild to moderate hypertension, doses of telmisartan >80 mg were not associated with a greater reduction in blood pressure (Smith, 2000). Patients who develop hypokalemia while on hydrochlorothiazide 25 mg may be switched to telmisartan 80 mg/hydrochlorothiazide 12.5 mg.

Canadian labeling: Specific dosing recommendations for the combination product are not provided by the manufacturer. When possible, discontinue the diuretic 2-3 days prior to initiation of telmisartan monotherapy. If diuretic therapy is necessary, use of individual agents may be necessary to allow for dose titration.

Dosage adjustment in renal impairment:

CrCl >30 mL/minute: No dosage adjustment necessary

CrCl ≤30 mL/minute: Not recommended

Dosage adjustment in hepatic impairment:

Mild to moderate hepatic impairment or biliary obstructive disorders: Initial: Telmisartan 40 mg/hydrochlorothiazide 12.5 mg

Severe hepatic impairment: Not recommended

Additional Information Complete prescribing information should be consulted for additional detail.

Dosage Forms

Tablet, oral:

Micardis® HCT: 40/12.5: Telmisartan 40 mg and hydrochlorothiazide 12.5 mg; 80/12.5: Telmisartan 80 mg and hydrochlorothiazide 12.5 mg; 80/25: Telmisartan 80 mg and hydrochlorothiazide 25 mg

Dosage Forms: Canada

Tablet, oral:

Micardis Plus:

80/12.5: Telmisartan 80 mg and hydrochlorothiazide 12.5 mg

80/25: Telmisartan 80 mg and hydrochlorothiazide 25 mg

◆ **Telmisartan HCTZ (Can)** *see* Telmisartan and Hydrochlorothiazide *on page 1990*

◆ **Telzir (Can)** *see* Fosamprenavir *on page 928*

Temazepam (te MAZ e pam)

Brand Names: U.S. Restoril

Brand Names: Canada Apo-Temazepam; CO Temazepam; Dom-Temazepam; Novo-Temazepam; PHL-Temazepam; PMS-Temazepam; ratio-Temazepam; Restoril; Temazepam-15; Temazepam-30

Pharmacologic Category Benzodiazepine

Additional Appendix Information

Beers Criteria – Potentially Inappropriate Medications for Geriatrics *on page 2271*

Use Insomnia: Short-term treatment of insomnia

Pregnancy Risk Factor X

Dosage Oral:

Adults: Usual dose: 15-30 mg at bedtime; some patients may respond to 7.5 mg in transient insomnia

Elderly or debilitated patients:

U.S. labeling: Initial: 7.5 mg at bedtime.

Canadian labeling: Initial: 15 mg at bedtime.

Dosage adjustment in renal impairment: No dosage adjustment provided in manufacturer's labeling.

Dosage adjustment in hepatic impairment: No dosage adjustment provided in manufacturer's labeling.

Additional Information Complete prescribing information should be consulted for additional detail.

Dosage Forms

Capsule, Oral:

Restoril: 7.5 mg, 15 mg, 22.5 mg, 30 mg

Generic: 7.5 mg, 15 mg, 22.5 mg, 30 mg

Dosage Forms: Canada

Capsule, Oral:

Restoril: 15 mg, 30 mg

- ◆ **Temazepam-15 (Can)** *see* Temazepam *on page 1990*
- ◆ **Temazepam-30 (Can)** *see* Temazepam *on page 1990*

Temocapril [INT] (tem OH ka pril)

International Brand Names Acecol (JP, KR)

Index Terms Temocapril Hydrochloride

Pharmacologic Category Angiotensin-Converting Enzyme (ACE) Inhibitor

Reported Use Hypertension

Dosage Range Adults: Oral: 1-4 mg/day reported in clinical trials

Product Availability Product available in various countries; not currently available in the U.S.

Dosage Forms

Tablet: 1 mg, 2 mg, 4 mg

- ◆ **Temocapril Hydrochloride** *see* Temocapril [INT] *on page 1991*
- ◆ **Temodal (Can)** *see* Temozolomide *on page 1991*
- ◆ **Temodar** *see* Temozolomide *on page 1991*
- ◆ **Temovate** *see* Clobetasol *on page 468*
- ◆ **Temovate E** *see* Clobetasol *on page 468*

Temozolomide (te moe ZOE loe mide)

Brand Names: U.S. Temodar

Brand Names: Canada ACH-Temozolomide; Co-Temozolomide; Temodal

Index Terms SCH 52365; TMZ

Pharmacologic Category Antineoplastic Agent, Alkylating Agent (Triazene)

Use

Anaplastic astrocytoma: Treatment of refractory anaplastic astrocytoma (refractory to a regimen containing a nitrosourea and procarbazine)

Glioblastoma multiforme: Treatment of newly-diagnosed glioblastoma multiforme (initially in combination with radiotherapy, then as maintenance treatment)

Canadian labeling: Treatment of newly-diagnosed glioblastoma multiforme (initially in combination with radiotherapy, then as maintenance treatment), treatment of recurrent or progressive glioblastoma multiforme or anaplastic astrocytoma

Pregnancy Risk Factor D

Pregnancy Considerations Adverse events were observed in animal reproduction studies. May cause fetal harm when administered to pregnant women. Male and female patients should avoid pregnancy while receiving temozolomide.

Breast-Feeding Considerations It is not known if temozolomide is excreted in breast milk. Due to the potential for serious adverse reactions in the nursing infant, a decision should be made to discontinue nursing or to discontinue temozolomide, taking into account the importance of treatment to the mother.

Contraindications Hypersensitivity (eg, allergic reaction, anaphylaxis, urticaria, Stevens-Johnson syndrome, toxic epidermal necrolysis) to temozolomide or any component of the formulation; hypersensitivity to dacarbazine (both drugs are metabolized to MTIC)

Canadian labeling: Additional contraindications (not in U.S. labeling): Not recommended in patients with severe myelosuppression

Warnings/Precautions Hazardous agent - use appropriate precautions for handling and disposal (NIOSH 2014 [group 1]). *Pneumocystis jirovecii* pneumonia (PCP) may occur; risk is increased in those receiving steroids or longer dosing regimens; monitor all patients for development of PCP (particularly if also receiving corticosteroids); PCP prophylaxis is required in patients receiving radiotherapy in combination with the 42-day temozolomide regimen. Myelosuppression may occur; may require treatment interruption, dose reduction, and/or discontinuation; monitor blood counts; an increased incidence has been reported in geriatric and female patients. Prolonged pancytopenia resulting in aplastic anemia has been reported (may be fatal); concurrent use of temozolomide with medications associated with aplastic anemia (eg, carbamazepine, co-trimoxazole, phenytoin) may obscure assessment for development of aplastic anemia. ANC should be ≥1500/mm^3 and platelets ≥100,000/mm^3 prior to treatment. Rare cases of myelodysplastic syndrome and secondary malignancies, including acute myeloid leukemia, have been reported. Use caution in patients with severe hepatic or renal impairment; has not been studied in dialysis patients. Hepatotoxicity has been reported; may be severe or fatal. Monitor liver function tests at baseline, halfway through the first cycle, prior to each subsequent cycle, and at ~2 to 4 weeks after the last dose. Postmarketing reports of hepatotoxicity have included liver function abnormalities, hepatitis, hepatic failure, cholestasis, hepatitis cholestasis, jaundice, cholelithiasis, hepatic steatosis, hepatic necrosis, hepatic lesion, and hepatic encephalopathy (Sarganas, 2012).

Temozolomide is associated with a moderate emetic potential (Dupuis, 2011; Roila, 2010); antiemetics are recommended to prevent nausea and vomiting. Increased MGMT (O-6-methylguanine-DNA methyltransferase) activity/levels within tumor tissue is associated with temozolomide resistance. Glioblastoma patients with decreased levels (due to methylated MGMT promoter) may be more likely to benefit from the combination of radiation therapy and temozolomide (Hegi, 2008; Stupp, 2009). Determination of MGMT status may be predictive for response to alkylating agents. Potentially significant drug-drug interactions may exist, requiring dose or frequency adjustment, additional monitoring, and/or selection of alternative therapy. Bioequivalence has only been established when IV temozolomide is administered over 90 minutes; shorter or longer infusion times may result in suboptimal dosing.

Adverse Reactions

Cardiovascular: Peripheral edema

Central nervous system: Abnormal gait, amnesia, anxiety, ataxia, confusion, convulsions, depression, dizziness, drowsiness, fatigue, headache, hemiparesis, insomnia, memory impairment, paresis, paresthesia

Dermatologic: Alopecia, erythema, pruritus, skin rash, xeroderma

Endocrine & metabolic: Hypercorticoidism, weight gain

Gastrointestinal: Abdominal pain, anorexia, constipation, diarrhea, dysgeusia, dysphagia, nausea (less common in grades 3/4), stomatitis, vomiting (less common in grades 3/4)

Genitourinary: Mastalgia (less common in females), urinary frequency, urinary incontinence, urinary tract infection

Hematologic & oncologic: Anemia (less common in grades 3/4), leukopenia (more common in grades 3/4), lymphocytopenia (more common in grades 3/4), neutropenia (more common in grades 3/4), thrombocytopenia (more common in grades 3/4)

Hypersensitivity: Hypersensitivity reaction

Infection: Viral infection

Neuromuscular & skeletal: Arthralgia, back pain, myalgia, weakness

Ophthalmic: Blurred vision, diplopia, visual disturbance (visual deficit/vision changes)

Respiratory: Cough, dyspnea, pharyngitis, upper respiratory tract infection, sinusitis

Miscellaneous: Fever, radiation injury (less common in maintenance phase after radiotherapy)

Rare by important or life-threatening: Alveolitis, anaphylaxis, aplastic anemia, cytomegalovirus disease (reactivation), diabetes insipidus, emotional lability, erythema multiforme, febrile neutropenia, flu-like symptoms, hallucination, hematoma, hemorrhage, hepatitis, hepatitis B (reactivation), hepatotoxicity, herpes simplex infection, herpes zoster, hyperbilirubinemia, hyperglycemia, hypersensitivity pneumonitis, hypokalemia, metastases (including myeloid leukemia) myelodysplastic syndrome, opportunistic infection (including pneumocystosis), oral candidiasis, pancytopenia (may be prolonged), peripheral neuropathy, petechia, pneumonitis, pulmonary fibrosis, Stevens-Johnson syndrome

Drug Interactions

Metabolism/Transport Effects None known.

Avoid Concomitant Use

Avoid concomitant use of Temozolomide with any of the following: BCG; CloZAPine; Dipyrone; Natalizumab; Pimecrolimus; Tacrolimus (Topical); Tofacitinib; Vaccines (Live)

Increased Effect/Toxicity

Temozolomide may increase the levels/effects of: CloZAPine; Leflunomide; Natalizumab; Tofacitinib; Vaccines (Live)

The levels/effects of Temozolomide may be increased by: Denosumab; Dipyrone; Pimecrolimus; Roflumilast; Tacrolimus (Topical); Trastuzumab; Valproic Acid and Derivatives

Decreased Effect

Temozolomide may decrease the levels/effects of: BCG; Coccidioides immitis Skin Test; Sipuleucel-T; Vaccines (Inactivated); Vaccines (Live)

The levels/effects of Temozolomide may be decreased by: Echinacea

Food Interactions Food reduces rate and extent of absorption. Management: Administer consistently either with food or without food (was administered in studies under fasting and nonfasting conditions).

Preparation for Administration Hazardous agent; use appropriate precautions for handling and disposal (NIOSH 2014 [group 1]). Bring to room temperature prior to reconstitution. Reconstitute each 100 mg vial with 41 mL sterile water for injection to a final concentration of 2.5 mg/mL. Swirl gently; do not shake. Place dose without further dilution into a 250 mL empty sterile infusion bag. Infusion must be completed within 14 hours of reconstitution.

Storage/Stability

Capsule: Store at room temperature of 25°C (77°F); excursions permitted to 15°C to 30°C (59°F to 86°F).

Injection: Store intact vials refrigerated at 2°C to 8°C (36°F to 46°F). Reconstituted vials may be stored for up to 14 hours at room temperature of 25°C (77°F); infusion must be completed within 14 hours of reconstitution.

Mechanism of Action Temozolomide is a prodrug which is rapidly and nonenzymatically converted to the active alkylating metabolite MTIC [(methyl-triazene-1-yl)-imidazole-4-carboxamide]; this conversion is spontaneous, nonenzymatic, and occurs under physiologic conditions in all tissues to which it distributes. The cytotoxic effects of MTIC are manifested through alkylation (methylation) of DNA at the O^6, N^7 guanine positions which lead to DNA double strand breaks and apoptosis. Non-cell cycle specific.

Pharmacodynamics/Kinetics

Absorption: Oral: Rapid and complete

Distribution: V_d: Parent drug: 0.4 L/kg; penetrates blood-brain barrier; CSF levels are ~35% to 39% of plasma levels (Yung, 1999)

Protein binding: 15%

Metabolism: Prodrug, hydrolyzed to the active form, MTIC; MTIC is eventually eliminated as CO_2 and 5-aminoimidazole-4-carboxamide (AIC), a natural constituent in urine; CYP isoenzymes play only a minor role in metabolism (of temozolomide and MTIC)

Bioavailability: Oral: 100% (on a mg-per-mg basis, IV temozolomide, infused over 90 minutes, is bioequivalent to an oral dose)

Half-life elimination: Mean: Parent drug: 1.8 hours

Time to peak: Oral: Empty stomach: 1 hour; with food (high-fat meal): 2.25 hours

Excretion: Urine (~38%; parent drug 6%); feces <1%

Dosage Note: Temozolomide is associated with a moderate emetic potential (Dupuis, 2011; Roila, 2010); antiemetics are recommended to prevent nausea and vomiting. Prior to dosing, ANC should be ≥1500/mm³ and platelets ≥100,000/mm³.

Anaplastic astrocytoma (refractory): Adults: Oral, IV: Initial dose: 150 mg/m² once daily for 5 consecutive days of a 28-day treatment cycle. If ANC ≥1500/mm³ and platelets ≥100,000/mm³, on day 1 of subsequent cycles, may increase to 200 mg/m² once daily for 5 consecutive days of a 28-day treatment cycle. May continue until disease progression.

Dosage modification for toxicity:

ANC <1000/mm³ or platelets <50,000/mm³ on day 22 or day 29 (day 1 of next cycle): Postpone therapy until ANC >1500/mm³ and platelets >100,000/mm³; reduce dose by 50 mg/m²/day (but not below 100 mg/m²) for subsequent cycle

ANC 1000-1500/mm³ or platelets 50,000-100,000/mm³ on day 22 or day 29 (day 1 of next cycle): Postpone therapy until ANC >1500/mm³ and platelets >100,000/mm³; maintain initial dose

Glioblastoma multiforme (newly diagnosed, high-grade glioma): Adults: Oral, IV:

Concomitant phase: 75 mg/m²/day for 42 days with focal radiotherapy (60 Gy administered in 30 fractions). **Note:** PCP prophylaxis is required during concomitant phase and should continue in patients who develop lymphocytopenia until lymphocyte recovery to ≤ grade 1. Obtain weekly CBC.

Continue at 75 mg/m²/day throughout the 42-day concomitant phase (up to 49 days) as long as ANC ≥1500/mm³, platelet count ≥100,000/mm³, and nonhematologic toxicity ≤ grade 1 (excludes alopecia, nausea/vomiting)

Dosage modification for toxicity:

ANC ≥500/mm³ but <1500/mm³ **or** platelet count ≥10,000/mm³ but <100,000/mm³ **or** grade 2 nonhematologic toxicity (excludes alopecia, nausea/vomiting): Interrupt therapy

ANC <500/mm³ **or** platelet count <10,000/mm³ **or** grade 3/4 nonhematologic toxicity (excludes alopecia, nausea/vomiting): Discontinue therapy

Maintenance phase (consists of 6 treatment cycles): Begin 4 weeks after concomitant phase completion. **Note:** Each subsequent cycle is 28 days (consisting of 5 days of drug treatment followed by 23 days without treatment). Draw CBC within 48 hours of day 22; hold next cycle and do weekly CBC until ANC >1500/mm³ and platelet count >100,000/mm³; dosing modification should be based on lowest blood counts and worst nonhematologic toxicity during the previous cycle.

Cycle 1: 150 mg/m² once daily for 5 days of a 28-day treatment cycle

Cycles 2 to 6: May increase to 200 mg/m^2 once daily for 5 days; repeat every 28 days (if ANC ≥1500/mm^3, platelets ≥100,000/mm^3 and nonhematologic toxicities for cycle 1 are ≤ grade 2 [excludes alopecia, nausea/vomiting]); **Note:** If dose was not escalated at the onset of cycle 2, do not increase for cycles 3-6)

Dosage modification (during maintenance phase) for toxicity:

ANC <1000/mm^3, platelet count <50,000/mm^3, or grade 3 nonhematologic toxicity (excludes alopecia, nausea/vomiting) during previous cycle: Decrease dose by 1 dose level (by 50 mg/m^2/day for 5 days), unless dose has already been lowered to 100 mg/m^2/day, then discontinue therapy.

If dose reduction <100 mg/m^2/day is required or grade 4 nonhematologic toxicity (excludes alopecia, nausea/vomiting), or if the same grade 3 nonhematologic toxicity occurs after dose reduction: Discontinue therapy

Glioblastoma multiforme (recurrent glioma): *Canadian labeling (off-label use in the U.S.):* Adults: Oral: 200 mg/m^2/day for 5 days every 28 days; if previously treated with chemotherapy, initiate at 150 mg/m^2/day for 5 days every 28 days and increase to 200 mg/m^2/day for 5 days every 28 days with cycle 2 if no hematologic toxicity (Brada, 2001; Yung, 2000)

Cutaneous T-cell lymphoma, advanced (mycosis fungoides [MF] and Sézary syndrome [SS]; off-label use): Adults: Oral: 200 mg/m^2 once daily for 5 days every 28 days for up to 1 year (Querfeld, 2011)

Ewing's sarcoma, recurrent or progressive (off-label use): Children, Adolescents, and Adults: Oral: 100 mg/m^2/dose days 1 to 5 every 21 days (in combination with irinotecan) (Casey, 2009); however, additional data may be necessary to further define the role of temozolomide in this condition

Melanoma, advanced or metastatic (off-label use): Adults: Oral: 200 mg/m^2/day for 5 days every 28 days (for up to 12 cycles). For subsequent cycles, reduce dose to 75% of the original dose for grade 3/4 hematologic toxicity and reduce the dose to 50% of the original dose for grade 3/4 nonhematologic toxicity (Middleton, 2000).

Neuroblastoma, relapsed or refractory (off-label use):

Children and Adolescents: Oral: 100 mg/m^2/dose days 1-5 every 21 days (in combination with irinotecan) for up to 6 cycles (Bagatell, 2011)

Children ≥6 months and Adolescents: Oral: 150 mg/m^2/dose days 1 to 5 every 28 days (in combination with topotecan) until disease progression or unacceptable toxicity (Di Giannatale, 2014)

Neuroendocrine tumors, advanced (off-label use): Adults: Oral: 150 mg/m^2/day for 7 days every 14 days (in combination with thalidomide) until disease progression (Kulke, 2006) **or** 200 mg/m^2 once daily (at bedtime) days 10 to 14 of a 28-day treatment cycle (in combination with capecitabine) (Strosberg, 2011)

Primary CNS lymphoma, refractory (off-label use): Adults: Oral: 150 mg/m^2/day for 5 days every 28 days, initially in combination with rituximab (for 4 cycles), followed by temozolomide monotherapy: 150 mg/m^2/day for 5 days every 28 days for 8 cycles (Wong, 2004) **or** 150 mg/m^2/day on days 1 to 7 and 15 to 21 every 28 days (initially in combination with rituximab for 1 or 2 cycles), followed by temozolomide maintenance monotherapy: 150 mg/m^2/day for 5 days every 28 days (Enting, 2004). Additional data may be necessary to further define the role of temozolomide in this condition.

Soft tissue sarcoma (off-label use): Adults: Oral:

Soft tissue sarcoma, metastatic or unresectable: 75 mg/m^2/day for 6 weeks (Garcia del Muro, 2005)

Hemangiopericytoma/solitary fibrous tumor: 150 mg/m^2 once daily days 1 to 7 and days 15 to 21 of a 28-day treatment cycle (in combination with bevacizumab) (Park, 2011). Additional data may be necessary to further define the role of temozolomide in this condition

Elderly: Refer to adult dosing. **Note:** Patients ≥70 years of age in the anaplastic astrocytoma study had a higher incidence of grade 4 neutropenia and thrombocytopenia in the first cycle of therapy than patients <70 years of age.

Dosage adjustment in renal impairment: Oral:

CrCl ≥36 mL/minute/m^2: There are no dosage adjustments provided in the manufacturer's labeling; however, dosage adjustment is not likely needed as no effect on temozolomide clearance was demonstrated.

Severe renal impairment (CrCl <36 mL/minute/m^2): There are no dosage adjustments provided in the manufacturer's labeling; use with caution (has not been studied).

Dialysis patients: There are no dosage adjustments provided in the manufacturer's labeling (has not been studied).

Dosage adjustment in hepatic impairment:

Mild-to-moderate impairment: There are no dosage adjustments provided in the manufacturer's labeling; however, pharmacokinetics are similar to patients with normal hepatic function.

Severe hepatic impairment: There are no dosage adjustments provided in the manufacturer's labeling; use with caution (has not been studied).

Dosing in obesity: *ASCO Guidelines for appropriate chemotherapy dosing in obese adults with cancer:* Utilize patient's actual body weight (full weight) for calculation of body surface area- or weight-based dosing, particularly when the intent of therapy is curative; manage regimen-related toxicities in the same manner as for nonobese patients; if a dose reduction is utilized due to toxicity, consider resumption of full weight-based dosing with subsequent cycles, especially if cause of toxicity (eg, hepatic or renal impairment) is resolved (Griggs, 2012).

Dietary Considerations The incidence of nausea/vomiting is decreased when taken on an empty stomach. Take capsules consistently either with food or without food (absorption is affected by food).

Administration Temozolomide is associated with a moderate emetic potential (Dupuis, 2011; Roila, 2010); antiemetics are recommended to prevent nausea and vomiting.

Oral: Swallow capsules whole with a glass of water. Absorption is affected by food; therefore, administer consistently either with food or without food (was administered in studies under fasting and nonfasting conditions). May administer on an empty stomach and/or at bedtime to reduce nausea and vomiting. Do not repeat if vomiting occurs after dose is administered; wait until the next scheduled dose. Do not open or chew capsules; avoid contact with skin or mucous membranes if capsules are accidentally opened or damaged.

IV: Infuse over 90 minutes. Flush line before and after administration. May be administered through the same IV line as sodium chloride 0.9%; do not administer other medications through the same IV line.

Hazardous agent; use appropriate precautions for handling and disposal (NIOSH 2014 [group 1]).

Monitoring Parameters CBC with differential and platelets (prior to each cycle; weekly during glioma concomitant phase treatment; at or within 48 hours of day 22 and weekly until ANC >1500/mm^3 and platelets >100,000/mm^3 for glioma maintenance and astrocytoma treatment). Monitor liver function tests at baseline, halfway through the first cycle, prior to each subsequent cycle, and at ~2 to 4 weeks after the last dose.

Dosage Forms

Capsule, Oral:

Temodar: 5 mg, 20 mg, 100 mg, 140 mg, 180 mg, 250 mg

Generic: 5 mg, 20 mg, 100 mg, 140 mg, 180 mg, 250 mg

Solution Reconstituted, Intravenous:

Temodar: 100 mg (1 ea)

Extemporaneous Preparations Hazardous agent: Use appropriate precautions for handling and disposal (NIOSH 2014 [group 1]).

A 10 mg/mL temozolomide oral suspension may be compounded in a vertical flow hood. Mix the contents of ten 100 mg capsules and 500 mg of povidone K-30 powder in a glass mortar; add 25 mg anhydrous citric acid dissolved in 1.5 mL purified water and mix to a uniform paste; mix while adding 50 mL Ora-Plus® in incremental proportions. Transfer to an amber plastic bottle, rinse mortar 4 times with small portions of either Ora-Sweet® or Ora-Sweet® SF, and add quantity of Ora-Sweet® or Ora-Sweet® SF sufficient to make 100 mL. Store in plastic amber prescription bottles; label "shake well" and "refrigerate"; include the beyond-use date. Stable for 7 days at room temperature or 60 days refrigerated (preferred).

Trissel LA, Yanping Z, and Koontz SE, "Temozolomide Stability in Extemporaneously Compounded Oral Suspension," *Int J Pharm Compound*, 2006, 10(5):396-9.

◆ **Tempra (Can)** *see* Acetaminophen *on page 32*

Temsirolimus (tem sir OH li mus)

Brand Names: U.S. Torisel

Brand Names: Canada Torisel

Index Terms CCI-779

Pharmacologic Category Antineoplastic Agent, mTOR Kinase Inhibitor

Use Renal cell carcinoma, advanced: Treatment of advanced renal cell carcinoma (RCC)

Pregnancy Risk Factor D

Pregnancy Considerations Adverse events have been observed in animal reproduction studies. Based on its mechanism of action, temsirolimus may cause fetal harm if administered to a pregnant woman. Women of childbearing potential should be advised to avoid pregnancy. Men and women should use effective birth control during temsirolimus treatment, and continue for 3 months after temsirolimus discontinuation.

Breast-Feeding Considerations It is not known if temsirolimus is excreted in breast milk. Due to the potential for serious adverse reactions in the nursing infant, a decision should be made to discontinue breast-feeding or to discontinue temsirolimus, taking into account the importance of treatment to the mother.

Contraindications Bilirubin >1.5 times the upper limit of normal (ULN)

Canadian labeling: Additional contraindications (not in U.S. labeling): History of anaphylaxis after exposure to temsirolimus, sirolimus, or any component of the formulation

Warnings/Precautions Hazardous agent - use appropriate precautions for handling and disposal (NIOSH 2014 [group 1]).

Hypersensitivity/infusion reactions (eg, anaphylaxis, apnea, dyspnea, flushing, loss of consciousness, hypotension, and/or chest pain) have been reported. Infusion reaction may occur during the initial infusion (early in infusion) or with subsequent infusions. Premedicate with an antihistamine (H_1 antagonist) prior to infusion; monitor throughout infusion (appropriate supportive care should be available); interrupt infusion for hypersensitivity reaction and observe patient for 30-60 minutes. With discretion, treatment may be resumed at a slower infusion rate; administer an H_1 antagonist (if not given as premedication) and/or an IV H_2 antagonist ~30 minutes prior to resuming infusion. For severe infusion reactions, assess risk versus benefit of continued treatment. Use with caution in patients with hypersensitivity temsirolimus, sirolimus (a metabolite), or polysorbate 80. Angioneurotic edema has been reported; concurrent use with other drugs known to cause angioedema (eg, ACE inhibitors) may increase risk.

Temsirolimus is predominantly cleared by the liver; use with caution and reduce dose in patients with mild hepatic impairment (bilirubin >1 to 1.5 x ULN or AST >ULN with bilirubin ≤ULN). Toxicities were increased in patients with baseline bilirubin >1.5 x ULN. Use is contraindicated in patients with moderate-to-severe hepatic impairment (bilirubin >1.5 x ULN).

Potentially significant interactions may exist, requiring dose or frequency adjustment, additional monitoring, and/or selection of alternative therapy. Avoid concomitant use with strong CYP3A4 inhibitors and strong CYP3A4 inducers; consider alternative agents that avoid or lessen the potential for CYP-mediated interactions. Patients should not be immunized with live, viral vaccines during or shortly after treatment and should avoid close contact with recently vaccinated (live vaccine) individuals. Patients who are receiving anticoagulant therapy or those with CNS tumors/metastases may be at increased risk for developing intracerebral bleeding (may be fatal). Combination therapy with temsirolimus and sunitinib has resulted in dose-limiting toxicities, including grade 3 or 4 rash, gout, and/or cellulitis.

Increases in serum glucose commonly occur during treatment; initiation or alteration of insulin and/or oral hypoglycemic therapy may be required; monitor serum glucose before and during treatment; use with caution in patients with diabetes. Use with caution in patients with hyperlipidemia; may increase serum lipids (cholesterol and triglycerides); initiation or dosage adjustment of antihyperlipidemic agents may be required; monitor cholesterol/triglyceride panel at baseline and periodically during treatment. Treatment may result in immunosuppression, may increase risk of opportunistic infections and/or sepsis. Pneumocystis jiroveci pneumonia (PCP) has been reported; some cases were fatal. Development of PCP may be associated with the use of concomitant corticosteroids or other immunosuppressive agents; consider PCP prophylaxis in patients receiving concomitant immunosuppressive or corticosteroid therapy. Interstitial lung disease (ILD), sometimes fatal, has been reported; symptoms include dyspnea, cough, hypoxia, and/or fever, although asymptomatic or mild cases may present; promptly evaluate worsening respiratory symptoms. If symptoms develop, consider withholding temsirolimus until symptom recovery and radiographic improvement occur. Consider empiric treatment with corticosteroids and/or antibiotic therapy; baseline chest radiographic assessment (CT scan or x-ray) is recommended; follow periodically, even in the absence of clinical pulmonary symptoms. Cases of bowel perforation (fatal) have occurred (usually presenting with abdominal pain, bloody stools, diarrhea, fever, or metabolic acidosis); promptly evaluate any new or worsening abdominal pain or bloody stools. Temsirolimus may be associated with impaired wound healing; use caution in the perioperative period. Cases of acute renal failure with rapid progression have been reported (unrelated to disease progression), including cases unresponsive to dialysis. An increased incidence of rash, infection and dose interruptions have been reported in patients with renal insufficiency (CrCl ≤60 mL/minute) who received mTOR inhibitors for the treatment of renal cell cancer (Gupta, 2011). Elderly patients may be more likely to experience adverse reactions, including diarrhea, edema, and pneumonia.

Adverse Reactions

Cardiovascular: Chest pain, edema, hypertension, peripheral edema, thrombophlebitis, venous thromboembolism (includes DVT and PE)

Central nervous system: Chills, depression, fever, headache, insomnia, pain

Dermatologic: Acne, dry skin, nail disorder/thinning, pruritus, rash, wound healing impaired

Endocrine & metabolic: Hypercholesterolemia, hyperglycemia, hyperlipidemia, hypertriglyceridemia, hypokalemia, hypophosphatemia

Gastrointestinal: Abdominal pain, anorexia, bowel perforation, constipation, diarrhea, mucositis, nausea, stomatitis, taste disturbance, vomiting, weight loss

Genitourinary: Urinary tract infection

Hematologic: Anemia, leukopenia, lymphopenia, neutropenia, thrombocytopenia (dose-limiting toxicity)

Hepatic: Alkaline phosphatase increased, AST increased, hyperbilirubinemia

Neuromuscular & skeletal: Arthralgia, back pain, myalgia, weakness

Ocular: Conjunctivitis

Renal: Creatinine increased

Respiratory: Cough, dyspnea, epistaxis, interstitial lung disease, pharyngitis, pneumonia, rhinitis, upper respiratory tract infection

Miscellaneous: Allergic/hypersensitivity/infusion reaction (includes anaphylaxis, apnea, chest pain, dyspnea, flushing, hypotension, loss of consciousness); infection (includes abscess, bronchitis, cellulitis, herpes simplex, herpes zoster)

Rare but important or life-threatening: Acute renal failure, angioneurotic edema, glucose intolerance, infusion site extravasation (with pain, swelling, warmth, erythema), pericardial effusion, pleural effusion, pneumonitis, reflex sympathetic dystrophy, rhabdomyolysis, seizure, Stevens-Johnson syndrome

Drug Interactions

Metabolism/Transport Effects **Substrate** of CYP3A4 (major), P-glycoprotein; **Note:** Assignment of Major/Minor substrate status based on clinically relevant drug interaction potential; **Inhibits** CYP2D6 (weak), CYP3A4 (weak)

Avoid Concomitant Use

Avoid concomitant use of Temsirolimus with any of the following: BCG; CloZAPine; Conivaptan; Dipyrone; Fusidic Acid (Systemic); Idelalisib; Natalizumab; Pimecrolimus; Pimozide; SUNItinib; Tacrolimus (Systemic); Tacrolimus (Topical); Tofacitinib; Vaccines (Live)

Increased Effect/Toxicity

Temsirolimus may increase the levels/effects of: ACE Inhibitors; ARIPiprazole; CloZAPine; CycloSPORINE (Systemic); Dofetilide; Hydrocodone; Leflunomide; Lomitapide; Natalizumab; Pimozide; SUNItinib; Tacrolimus (Systemic); Tacrolimus (Topical); Tofacitinib; Vaccines (Live)

The levels/effects of Temsirolimus may be increased by: Aprepitant; Ceritinib; Conivaptan; CYP3A4 Inhibitors (Moderate); CYP3A4 Inhibitors (Strong); Dasatinib; Denosumab; Dipyrone; Fluconazole; Fosaprepitant; Fusidic Acid (Systemic); Idelalisib; Itraconazole; Ivacaftor; Ketoconazole (Systemic); Luliconazole; Macrolide Antibiotics; Mifepristone; Netupitant; P-glycoprotein/ABCB1 Inhibitors; Pimecrolimus; Posaconazole; Protease Inhibitors; Roflumilast; Simeprevir; Stiripentol; Tacrolimus (Systemic); Tacrolimus (Topical); Trastuzumab

Decreased Effect

Temsirolimus may decrease the levels/effects of: BCG; Coccidioides immitis Skin Test; Sipuleucel-T; Tacrolimus (Systemic); Vaccines (Inactivated); Vaccines (Live)

The levels/effects of Temsirolimus may be decreased by: Bosentan; CarBAMazepine; CYP3A4 Inducers (Moderate); CYP3A4 Inducers (Strong); Dabrafenib; Deferasirox; Echinacea; Fosphenytoin; Mitotane; P-glycoprotein/ABCB1 Inducers; Phenytoin; Rifamycin Derivatives; Siltuximab; St Johns Wort; Tocilizumab

Food Interactions Grapefruit and grapefruit juice may increase the levels/effects of sirolimus. Management: Avoid grapefruit and grapefruit juice.

Preparation for Administration Hazardous agent; use appropriate precautions for handling and disposal (NIOSH 2014 [group 1]). Preparation requires a two-step dilution process (do not add undiluted temsirolimus to aqueous solution; addition to aqueous solution prior to step 1 will result in precipitation). *Step 1:* Total amount in undiluted vial is 30 mg/1.2 mL (25 mg/mL concentration); contains overfill. Vials should initially be diluted with 1.8 mL of provided diluent to a concentration of 10 mg/mL. Once diluted with provided diluent, mix by inverting vial. *Step 2:* After allowing air bubbles to subside, the intended dose should be withdrawn from the 10 mg/mL diluted vial (ie, 2.5 mL for a 25 mg dose) and further diluted in 250 mL of NS in a non-DEHP/non-PVC container (glass, polyolefin, or polypropylene). Mix by inverting bottle or bag; avoid excessive shaking (may result in foaming).

Storage/Stability Store intact vials refrigerated at 2°C to 8°C (36°F to 46°F). Diluted solution in the vial (10 mg/mL) is stable for 24 hours at room temperature (below 25°C [77°F]). Solutions diluted for infusion (in NS) must be infused within 6 hours of preparation. Protect from light during storage, preparation, and handling.

Mechanism of Action Temsirolimus and its active metabolite, sirolimus, are targeted inhibitors of mTOR (mechanistic target of rapamycin) kinase activity. Temsirolimus (and sirolimus) bind to FKBP-12, an intracellular protein, to form a complex which inhibits mTOR signaling, halting the cell cycle at the G1 phase in tumor cells. Inhibition of mTOR blocks downstream phosphorylation of p70S6k and S6 ribosomal proteins. In renal cell carcinoma, mTOR inhibition also exhibits anti-angiogenesis activity by reducing levels of HIF-1 and HIF-2 alpha (hypoxia inducible factors) and vascular endothelial growth factor (VEGF).

Pharmacodynamics/Kinetics

Distribution: V_{dss}: 172 L

Metabolism: Hepatic; via CYP3A4 to sirolimus (primary active metabolite) and 4 minor metabolites

Half-life elimination: Temsirolimus: ~17 hours; Sirolimus: ~55 hours

Time to peak, plasma: Temsirolimus: At end of infusion; Sirolimus: 0.5 to 2 hours after temsirolimus infusion

Excretion: Feces (78%); urine (<5%)

Dosage Note: For infusion reaction prophylaxis, premedicate with an H_1 antagonist (eg, diphenhydramine 25 to 50 mg IV) ~30 minutes prior to infusion.

Renal cell cancer (RCC), advanced: Adults: IV: 25 mg once weekly; continue until disease progression or unacceptable toxicity

Dosage adjustment for concomitant CYP3A4 inhibitors/inducers:

CYP3A4 inhibitors: Avoid concomitant administration with strong CYP3A4 inhibitors (eg, clarithromycin, itraconazole, ketoconazole, nefazodone, protease inhibitors, telithromycin, voriconazole); if concomitant administration with a strong CYP3A4 inhibitor cannot be avoided, consider a dose reduction to 12.5 mg once weekly. When a strong CYP3A4 inhibitor is discontinued; allow ~1 week to elapse prior to adjusting the temsirolimus upward to the dose used prior to initiation of the CYP3A4 inhibitor.

CYP3A4 inducers: Avoid concomitant administration with strong CYP3A4 inducers (eg, carbamazepine, dexamethasone, phenobarbital, phenytoin, rifabutin, rifampin, St John's wort); if concomitant administration with a strong CYP3A4 inducer cannot be avoided, consider adjusting temsirolimus dose up to 50 mg once weekly. If the strong CYP3A4 enzyme inducer is discontinued, reduce the temsirolimus to the dose used prior to initiation of the CYP3A4 inducer.

Dosage adjustment for toxicity:

Hematologic toxicity: ANC <1000/mm^3 or platelets <75,000/mm^3: Withhold treatment until resolves and reinitiate treatment with the dose reduced by 5 mg weekly; minimum dose: 15 mg weekly if adjustment for toxicity is needed.

Nonhematologic toxicity: Any toxicity ≥ grade 3: Withhold treatment until resolves to ≤ grade 2; reinitiate treatment with the dose reduced by 5 mg weekly; minimum dose: 15 mg weekly if adjustment for toxicity is needed.

Infusion/hypersensitivity reaction: Interrupt infusion and observe for 30 to 60 minutes; treatment may be resumed with discretion at a slower infusion rate (up to 60 minutes); administer an H_1 antagonist (if not given as premedication) and/or an IV H_2 antagonist 30 minutes prior to resuming infusion.

Interstitial lung disease: Consider withholding treatment for clinically significant respiratory symptoms until after recovery of symptoms or radiographic improvement.

Dosage adjustment in renal impairment: No dosage adjustment necessary.

Hemodialysis: There are no dosage adjustments provided in the manufacturer's labeling (has not been studied).

Dosage adjustment in hepatic impairment:

Mild hepatic impairment (bilirubin >1 to 1.5 x ULN or AST >ULN with bilirubin ≤ULN): Reduce dose to 15 mg once weekly

Moderate-to-severe hepatic impairment (bilirubin >1.5 x ULN): Use is contraindicated

Dietary Considerations Avoid grapefruit juice (may increase the levels of the major metabolite, sirolimus).

Administration Infuse over 30 to 60 minutes via an infusion pump (preferred). Use polyethylene-lined non-DEHP administration tubing. Administer through an inline polyethersulfone filter ≤5 micron; if set does not contain an inline filter, a polyethersulfone end filter (0.2 to 5 micron) should be added (do not use both an inline and an end filter). Premedicate with an H_1 antagonist (eg, diphenhydramine 25 to 50 mg IV) ~30 minutes prior to infusion. Monitor during infusion; interrupt infusion for hypersensitivity/infusion reaction; monitor for 30 to 60 minutes; may reinitiate at a reduced infusion rate (over 60 minutes) with discretion, 30 minutes after administration of a histamine H_1 antagonist and/or a histamine H_2 antagonist (eg, famotidine or ranitidine). Administration should be completed within 6 hours of admixture.

Hazardous agent; use appropriate precautions for handling and disposal (NIOSH 2014 [group 1]).

Monitoring Parameters CBC with differential and platelets (weekly), serum chemistries including glucose (baseline and every other week), serum cholesterol and triglycerides (baseline and periodic), liver function (baseline and periodic), renal function tests (baseline and periodic)

Monitor for infusion reactions; infection; symptoms of ILD (or radiographic changes), symptoms of hyperglycemia (excessive thirst, polyuria); symptoms of bowel perforation

Dosage Forms

Solution, Intravenous:

Torisel: 25 mg/mL (1 mL)

Tenecteplase (ten EK te plase)

Brand Names: U.S. TNKase

Brand Names: Canada TNKase®

Pharmacologic Category Thrombolytic Agent

Use Management of ST-elevation myocardial infarction (STEMI) for the lysis of thrombi in the coronary vasculature to restore perfusion and reduce mortality.

Recommended criteria for treatment of STEMI (ACCF/AHA; O'Gara, 2013): Ischemic symptoms within 12 hours of treatment or evidence of ongoing ischemia 12-24 hours after symptom onset with a large area of myocardium at risk or hemodynamic instability.

STEMI ECG definition: New ST-segment elevation at the J point in at least 2 contiguous leads of ≥2 mm (0.2 mV) in men or ≥1.5 mm (0.15 mV) in women in leads V_2-V_3 and/or of ≥1 mm (0.1 mV) in other contiguous precordial leads or limb leads on ECG. New or presumably new left bundle branch block (LBBB) may interfere with ST-elevation analysis and should not be considered diagnostic in isolation.

At non-PCI-capable hospitals, the ACCF/AHA recommends thrombolytic therapy administration when the anticipated first medical contact (FMC)-to-device time at a PCI-capable hospital is >120 minutes due to unavoidable delays.

Pregnancy Risk Factor C

Pregnancy Considerations Adverse events have been observed in some animal reproduction studies. The risk of bleeding may be increased in pregnant women. Administer to pregnant women only if the potential benefits justify the risk to the fetus.

Breast-Feeding Considerations It is not known if tenecteplase is excreted in breast milk. The manufacturer recommends that caution be exercised when administering tenecteplase to nursing women.

Contraindications Active internal bleeding; history of cerebrovascular accident; recent (ie, within 2 months) intracranial/intraspinal surgery or trauma; intracranial neoplasm; arteriovenous malformation or aneurysm; bleeding diathesis; severe uncontrolled hypertension

Additional contraindications (ACCF/AHA; O'Gara, 2013): Ischemic stroke within 3 months; prior intracranial hemorrhage; active bleeding (excluding menses); suspected aortic dissection; significant closed head or facial trauma within 3 months

Warnings/Precautions Use with caution in patients receiving oral anticoagulants; increased risk of bleeding. Adjunctive use of parenteral anticoagulants (eg, enoxaparin, heparin, or fondaparinux) is recommended to improve vessel patency and prevent reocclusion and may also contribute to bleeding; monitor for bleeding (ACCF/AHA; O'Gara, 2013). Stop antiplatelet agents and heparin if serious bleeding occurs. Avoid IM injections and nonessential handling of the patient for a few hours after administration. Monitor for bleeding complications. Venipunctures should be performed carefully and only when necessary. If arterial puncture is necessary, then use an upper extremity that can be easily compressed manually. For the following conditions, the risk of bleeding is higher with use of tenecteplase and the use of tenecteplase should be weighed against the benefits: Recent major surgery, cerebrovascular disease, recent GI or GU bleed, recent trauma, uncontrolled hypertension (systolic BP >180 mm Hg and/or diastolic BP >110 mm Hg), suspected left heart thrombus, acute pericarditis, subacute bacterial endocarditis, hemostatic defects, severe hepatic dysfunction, hemorrhagic diabetic retinopathy or other hemorrhagic ophthalmic conditions, pregnancy, septic thrombophlebitis or occluded arteriovenous cannula at seriously infected site, advanced age, anticoagulants, recent administration of GP IIb/IIIa inhibitors. Use with caution in patients with advanced age; increased risk of bleeding. Mortality and rate of intracranial hemorrhage increases with increasing age >65 years of age; the risks and benefits of use should be weighed carefully in the elderly. Coronary thrombolysis may result in reperfusion arrhythmias. Caution with readministration of tenecteplase.

Adverse Reactions As with all drugs which may affect hemostasis, bleeding is the major adverse effect associated with tenecteplase. Hemorrhage may occur at virtually any site. Risk is dependent on multiple variables, including the dosage administered, concurrent use of multiple agents which alter hemostasis, and patient predisposition. Rapid lysis of coronary artery thrombi by thrombolytic agents may be associated with reperfusion-related arterial and/or ventricular arrhythmia. The incidence of stroke and bleeding increase with age above 65 years.

Central nervous system: Stroke
Gastrointestinal: Epistaxis, GI hemorrhage
Genitourinary: GU bleeding
Hematologic: Bleeding
Local: Bleeding at catheter puncture site, hematoma
Respiratory: Pharyngeal

Rare but important or life-threatening: Anaphylaxis, angioedema, bleeding at catheter puncture site (<1% major), cholesterol embolism (clinical features may include livedo reticularis, "purple toe" syndrome, acute renal failure, gangrenous digits, hypertension, pancreatitis, MI, cerebral infarction, spinal cord infarction, retinal artery occlusion, bowel infarction, rhabdomyolysis), GU bleeding (<1% major), intracranial hemorrhage (0.9%), laryngeal edema, rash, respiratory tract bleeding, retroperitoneal bleeding, urticaria

Additional cardiovascular events associated with use in MI: Arrhythmia, AV block, cardiac arrest, cardiac tamponade, cardiogenic shock, embolism, electromechanical dissociation, fever, heart failure, hypotension, mitral regurgitation, myocardial reinfarction, myocardial rupture, nausea, pericardial effusion, pericarditis, pulmonary edema, recurrent myocardial ischemia, thrombosis, vomiting

Drug Interactions

Metabolism/Transport Effects None known.

Avoid Concomitant Use There are no known interactions where it is recommended to avoid concomitant use.

Increased Effect/Toxicity

Tenecteplase may increase the levels/effects of: Anticoagulants; Dabigatran Etexilate; Prostacyclin Analogues

The levels/effects of Tenecteplase may be increased by: Agents with Antiplatelet Properties; Herbs (Anticoagulant/Antiplatelet Properties); Limaprost; Salicylates

Decreased Effect

The levels/effects of Tenecteplase may be decreased by: Aprotinin

Preparation for Administration Tenecteplase should be reconstituted using the supplied 10 mL syringe with TwinPak™ Dual Cannula Device and 10 mL sterile water for injection. Do not shake when reconstituting. Slight foaming is normal and will dissipate if left standing for several minutes. The reconstituted solution is 5 mg/mL. Any unused solution should be discarded. If reconstituted and not used immediately, store in refrigerator and use within 8 hours.

Storage/Stability Store under refrigeration of 2°C to 8°C (36°F to 46°F) or at room temperature; do not exceed 30°C (86°F). If reconstituted and not used immediately, store in refrigerator and use within 8 hours.

Mechanism of Action Promotes initiation of fibrinolysis by binding to fibrin and converting plasminogen to plasmin. Tenecteplase is essentially alteplase with the exception of 3 point mutations and is more fibrin specific, more resistant to plasminogen activator inhibitor -1 (PAI-1), with a longer duration of action compared to alteplase. Produced by recombinant DNA technology using a mammalian cell line (Chinese hamster ovary cells).

Pharmacodynamics/Kinetics

Distribution: V_d is weight related and approximates plasma volume
Metabolism: Primarily hepatic
Half-life elimination: Biphasic: Initial: 20-24 minutes; Terminal: 90-130 minutes
Excretion: Clearance: Plasma: 99-119 mL/minute

Dosage IV:

Adult: Recommended total dose should not exceed 50 mg and is based on patient's weight; administer as a single bolus over 5 seconds

If patient's weight:
<60 kg: 30 mg
≥60 to <70 kg: 35 mg
≥70 to <80 kg: 40 mg
≥80 to <90 kg: 45 mg
≥90 kg: 50 mg

Note: Thrombolytic should be administered within 30 minutes of hospital arrival. Administer concurrent aspirin, clopidogrel, and anticoagulant therapy (ie, unfractionated heparin, enoxaparin, or fondaparinux) with tenecteplase (O'Gara, 2013).

Elderly: Refer to adult dosing. Although dosage adjustments are not recommended, the elderly have a higher incidence of morbidity and mortality with the use of tenecteplase.

Dosage adjustment in renal impairment: No dosage adjustment necessary.

Dosage adjustment in hepatic impairment:

Mild to moderate impairment: No dosage adjustment provided in manufacturer's labeling.

Severe impairment: No dosage adjustment provided in manufacturer's labeling; weigh the risk of bleeding against the benefits with tenecteplase especially in those with a coagulopathy.

Administration Tenecteplase is **incompatible** with dextrose solutions. Dextrose-containing lines must be flushed with a saline solution before and after administration. Administer as a single IV bolus over 5 seconds. Avoid IM injections and nonessential handling of patient.

Monitoring Parameters CBC, aPTT, signs and symptoms of bleeding, ECG monitoring

Dosage Forms

Kit, Intravenous:
TNKase: 50 mg

◆ **Tenex** *see* GuanFACINE *on page 990*

Teniposide (ten i POE side)

Brand Names: Canada Vumon®

Index Terms EPT; PTG; VM-26

Pharmacologic Category Antineoplastic Agent, Podophyllotoxin Derivative; Antineoplastic Agent, Topoisomerase II Inhibitor

Use Treatment of refractory childhood acute lymphoblastic leukemia (ALL) in combination with other chemotherapy

Pregnancy Risk Factor D

Dosage IV: **Note:** Patients with Down syndrome and leukemia may be more sensitive to the myelosuppressive effects; administer the first course at half the usual dose and adjust dose in subsequent cycles upward based on degree of toxicities (myelosuppression and mucositis) in the previous course(s).

Children: Acute lymphoblastic leukemia (ALL; combination chemotherapy): 165 mg/m^2 twice weekly for 8-9 doses **or** 250 mg/m^2 weekly for 4-8 weeks **or** (off-label dosing) 165 mg/m^2/dose days 1 and 2 of weeks 3, 13, and 23 (Lauer, 2001)

Adults: ALL consolidation treatment (off-label use; combination chemotherapy): 165 mg/m^2/dose days 1, 4, 8, and 11 of alternating consolidation cycles (Linker, 1991)

Dosage adjustment in renal impairment: No dosage adjustment provided in manufacturer's labeling (has not been studied). However, dosage adjustment may be necessary in patient with significant renal impairment.

Dosage adjustment in hepatic impairment: No dosage adjustment provided in manufacturer's labeling (has not been studied). However, dosage adjustment may be necessary in patient with significant hepatic impairment.

Dosing in obesity: *ASCO Guidelines for appropriate chemotherapy dosing in obese adults with cancer:* Utilize patient's actual body weight (full weight) for calculation of body surface area- or weight-based dosing, particularly when the intent of therapy is curative; manage regimen-related toxicities in the same manner as for nonobese patients; if a dose reduction is utilized due to toxicity, consider resumption of full weight-based dosing with subsequent cycles, especially if cause of toxicity (eg, hepatic or renal impairment) is resolved (Griggs, 2012).

Additional Information Complete prescribing information should be consulted for additional detail.

Dosage Forms

Solution, Intravenous:

Generic: 10 mg/mL (5 mL)

◆ **Tenivac** *see* Diphtheria and Tetanus Toxoid *on page 645*

Tenofovir (ten OF oh vir)

Brand Names: U.S. Viread

Brand Names: Canada Viread

Index Terms PMPA; TDF; Tenofovir Disoproxil Fumarate

Pharmacologic Category Antihepadnaviral, Reverse Transcriptase Inhibitor, Nucleotide (Anti-HBV); Antiretroviral, Reverse Transcriptase Inhibitor, Nucleotide (Anti-HIV)

Use

Chronic hepatitis B: Treatment of chronic hepatitis B virus (HBV) in patients ≥12 years of age

HIV infection: In combination with other antiretroviral agents for the treatment of HIV-1 infection in adults and pediatric patients ≥2 years of age

Pregnancy Risk Factor B

Pregnancy Considerations Adverse events were observed in some animal reproduction studies. Tenofovir has a high level of transfer across the human placenta. Intrauterine growth has not been affected in human studies, but one study found lower length and head circumference. Clinical studies in children have shown bone demineralization with chronic use. No increased risk of overall birth defects has been observed following first trimester exposure according to data collected by the antiretroviral pregnancy registry. Limited data indicate decreased maternal bioavailability during the third trimester; dose adjustments are not needed. Cases of lactic acidosis/hepatic steatosis syndrome related to mitochondrial toxicity have been reported in pregnant women with prolonged use of nucleoside analogues. It is not known if pregnancy itself potentiates this known side effect; however, women may be at increased risk of lactic acidosis and liver damage. In addition, these adverse events are similar to other rare but life-threatening syndromes which occur during pregnancy (eg, HELLP syndrome). Hepatic enzymes and electrolytes should be monitored in women receiving nucleoside analogues and clinicians should watch for early signs of the syndrome. In addition, mitochondrial dysfunction may develop in infants following *in utero* exposure. Renal function should also be monitored. The DHHS Perinatal HIV Guidelines consider tenofovir in combination with either emtricitabine or lamivudine to be a preferred NRTI backbone for use in antiretroviral-naïve pregnant women. The DHHS Perinatal HIV Guidelines consider emtricitabine plus tenofovir, or lamivudine plus tenofovir as recommended dual NRTI/NtRTI backbones for HIV/HBV coinfected pregnant women. Hepatitis B flare may occur if tenofovir is discontinued postpartum.

Regardless of CD4 count or HIV RNA copy number, all HIV-infected pregnant women should receive a combination antiretroviral (ARV) drug regimen. A combination of antepartum, intrapartum, and infant ARV prophylaxis is recommended. ARV therapy should be started as soon as possible in women with symptomatic infection. Although earlier initiation may be more effective in reducing the perinatal transmission of HIV, also consider maternal conditions (eg, nausea and vomiting) and the potential risks of first trimester fetal exposure for specific agents. A scheduled cesarean delivery at 38 weeks' gestation is recommended for all women with HIV RNA >1000 copies/mL or unknown concentrations near delivery in order to decrease transmission. If ARV therapy must be interrupted for <24 hours during the peripartum period, stop then restart all medications simultaneously in order to decrease the chance of developing resistance. Long-term follow-up is recommended for all infants exposed to ARV medications. In couples who want to conceive, the HIV-infected partner should attain maximum viral suppression prior to conception.

Health care providers are encouraged to enroll pregnant women exposed to antiretroviral medications in the Antiretroviral Pregnancy Registry (1-800-258-4263 or www.APRegistry.com). Health care providers caring for HIV-infected women and their infants may contact the National Perinatal HIV Hotline (888-448-8765) for clinical consultation (HHS [perinatal], 2014).

Breast-Feeding Considerations Tenofovir is excreted in breast milk. Maternal or infant antiretroviral therapy does not completely eliminate the risk of postnatal HIV transmission. In addition, multiclass-resistant virus has been detected in breast-feeding infants despite maternal therapy. Therefore, in the United States, where formula is accessible, affordable, safe, and sustainable, and the risk of infant mortality due to diarrhea and respiratory infections is low, complete avoidance of breast-feeding by HIV-infected women is recommended to decrease potential transmission of HIV (HHS [perinatal], 2014).

Contraindications

U.S. labeling: There are no contraindications listed in the manufacturer's labeling.

Canadian labeling: Hypersensitivity to tenofovir or any component of the formulation; concurrent use with fixed-dose combination products that contain tenofovir (Truvada, Atripla, Complera, or Stribild); concurrent use with adefovir (Hepsera)

Warnings/Precautions [U.S Boxed Warning]: Lactic acidosis and severe hepatomegaly with steatosis have been reported with tenofovir and other nucleoside analogues, including fatal cases; use with caution in patients with risk factors for liver disease (risk may be increased in obese patients or prolonged exposure) and suspend treatment in any patient who develops clinical or laboratory findings suggestive of lactic acidosis (transaminase elevation may/may not accompany hepatomegaly and steatosis). May cause redistribution of fat (eg, buffalo hump, peripheral wasting with increased abdominal girth, cushingoid appearance). Immune reconstitution syndrome may develop resulting in the occurrence of an inflammatory response to an indolent or residual opportunistic infection during initial HIV treatment or activation of autoimmune disorders (eg, Graves' disease, polymyositis, Guillain-Barré syndrome) later in therapy; further evaluation and treatment may be required. Use caution in hepatic impairment; limited data supporting treatment of chronic hepatitis B in patients with decompensated liver disease; observe for increased adverse reactions, including renal dysfunction.

In clinical trials, use has been associated with decreases in bone mineral density in HIV-1 infected adults and increases in bone metabolism markers. Serum parathyroid hormone and 1,25 vitamin D levels were also higher. Decreases in bone mineral density have also been observed in clinical trials of HIV-1 infected pediatric patients. Observations in chronic hepatitis B infected pediatric patients (aged 12-18 years) were similar. Consider monitoring of bone density in adult and pediatric patients with a history of pathologic fractures or with other risk factors for bone loss or osteoporosis. Consider calcium and vitamin D supplementation for all patients; effect of supplementation has not been studied but may be beneficial. Long-term bone health and fracture risk unknown. Skeletal growth (height) appears to be unaffected in tenofovir-treated children and adolescents.

May cause osteomalacia with proximal renal tubulopathy. Bone pain, extremity pain, fractures, arthralgias, weakness and muscle pain have been reported. In patients at risk for renal dysfunction, persistent or worsening bone or muscle symptoms should be evaluated for hypophosphatemia and osteomalacia.

Do not use as monotherapy in treatment of HIV. Clinical trials in HIV-infected patients whose regimens contained only three nucleoside reverse transcriptase inhibitors (NRTI) show less efficacy, early virologic failure and high rates of resistance substitutions. Use three NRTI regimens with caution and monitor response carefully. Triple drug regimens with two NRTIs in combination with a non-nucleoside reverse transcriptase inhibitor or a HIV-1 protease inhibitor are usually more effective. Treatment of HIV in patients with unrecognized/untreated hepatitis B virus (HBV) may lead to rapid HBV resistance. Patients should be tested for presence of chronic hepatitis B infection prior to initiation of therapy. In patients coinfected with HIV and HBV, an appropriate antiretroviral combination should be selected due to HIV resistance potential; these patients should receive tenofovir dosed for HIV therapy.

Tenofovir is predominately eliminated renally; use caution in renal impairment. May cause acute renal failure or Fanconi syndrome; use caution with other nephrotoxic agents (including high dose or multiple NSAID use or those which compete for active tubular secretion). Acute renal failure has occurred in HIV-infected patients with risk factors for renal impairment who were on a stable tenofovir regimen to which a high dose or multiple NSAID therapy was added. Consider alternatives to NSAIDS in patients taking tenofovir and at risk for renal impairment. Calculate creatinine clearance prior to initiation of therapy and monitor renal function (including recalculation of creatinine clearance and serum phosphorus) during therapy. Dosage adjustment required in patients with CrCl <50 mL/minute. Use caution in patients with low body weight, or concurrent medications which increase tenofovir levels. Use caution in the elderly; dosage adjustment based on renal function may be required. Pancreatitis has been reported; use with caution in patients with a prior history or risk factors for pancreatitis. Discontinue if pancreatitis is suspected.

[U.S. Boxed Warning]: If treating HBV, acute exacerbation of hepatitis B may occur upon discontinuation. Monitor liver function closely for several months after discontinuing treatment; reinitiation of antihepatitis B therapy may be required. Treatment of HBV in patients with unrecognized/untreated HIV may lead to HIV resistance; patients should be tested for presence of HIV infection prior to initiating therapy. Do not use as monotherapy in treatment of HIV. Treatment of HIV in patients with unrecognized/untreated HBV may lead to rapid HBV resistance. Patients should be tested for presence of chronic hepatitis B prior to initiation of therapy. Potentially significant drug-drug interactions may exist, requiring dose or frequency adjustment, additional monitoring, and/or selection of alternative therapy. Do not use concurrently with adefovir or tenofovir combination products.

Adverse Reactions Includes data from both treatment-naive and treatment-experienced HIV patients and in chronic hepatitis B.

Cardiovascular: Chest pain

Central nervous system: Anxiety, depression, dizziness, fatigue, headache, insomnia, pain, peripheral neuropathy

Dermatologic: Diaphoresis, pruritus, skin rash (includes maculopapular, pustular, or vesiculobullous rash; pruritus; or urticaria)

Endocrine & metabolic: Glycosuria, hypercholesterolemia, hyperglycemia, increased serum triglycerides, lipodystrophy, weight loss

Gastrointestinal: Abdominal pain, anorexia, diarrhea, dyspepsia, flatulence, increased serum amylase, nausea, vomiting

Genitourinary: Hematuria

Hematologic & oncologic: Neutropenia

Hepatic: Increased serum alkaline phosphatase, increased serum ALT, increased serum AST, increased serum transaminases

Neuromuscular & skeletal: Arthralgia, back pain, decreased bone mineral density, increased creatine phosphokinase, myalgia, weakness

Renal: Increased serum creatinine, renal failure

Respiratory: Nasopharyngitis, pneumonia, sinusitis, upper respiratory tract infection

Miscellaneous: Fever

Rare but important or life-threatening: Angioedema, exacerbation of hepatitis B (following discontinuation), Fanconi's syndrome, hepatitis, hypersensitivity reaction, hypokalemia, hypophosphatemia, immune reconstitution syndrome, increased gamma-glutamyl transferase, interstitial nephritis, lactic acidosis, myopathy, nephrogenic diabetes insipidus, nephrotoxicity, osteomalacia, pancreatitis, polyuria, proteinuria, proximal tubular nephropathy, renal insufficiency, renal tubular necrosis, rhabdomyolysis, severe hepatomegaly with steatosis

Drug Interactions

Metabolism/Transport Effects Substrate of BCRP, P-glycoprotein; **Inhibits** CYP1A2 (weak); **Induces** P-glycoprotein

Avoid Concomitant Use

Avoid concomitant use of Tenofovir with any of the following: Adefovir; Dabigatran Etexilate; Didanosine; VinCRIStine (Liposomal)

Increased Effect/Toxicity

Tenofovir may increase the levels/effects of: Adefovir; Aminoglycosides; Darunavir; Didanosine; Ganciclovir-Valganciclovir

The levels/effects of Tenofovir may be increased by: Acyclovir-Valacyclovir; Adefovir; Aminoglycosides; Atazanavir; Cidofovir; Cobicistat; Darunavir; Diclofenac (Systemic); Ganciclovir-Valganciclovir; Ledipasvir; Lopinavir; Nonsteroidal Anti-Inflammatory Agents; Simeprevir; Telaprevir

Decreased Effect

Tenofovir may decrease the levels/effects of: Afatinib; Atazanavir; Brentuximab Vedotin; Dabigatran Etexilate; Didanosine; DOXOrubicin (Conventional); Linagliptin; P-glycoprotein/ABCB1 Substrates; Simeprevir; Tipranavir; VinCRIStine (Liposomal)

The levels/effects of Tenofovir may be decreased by: Adefovir; Tipranavir

Food Interactions Fatty meals may increase the bioavailability of tenofovir. Management: May administer with or without food.

Storage/Stability Store at 25°C (77°F); excursions are permitted between 15°C and 30°C (59°F and 86°F). Dispense only in original container.

Mechanism of Action Tenofovir disoproxil fumarate (TDF), a nucleotide reverse transcriptase inhibitor, is an analog of adenosine 5'-monophosphate; it interferes with the HIV viral RNA dependent DNA polymerase resulting in inhibition of viral replication. TDF is first converted intracellularly by hydrolysis to tenofovir and subsequently phosphorylated to the active tenofovir diphosphate. Tenofovir inhibits replication of HBV by inhibiting HBV polymerase.

Pharmacodynamics/Kinetics

Distribution: V_d: 1.2-1.3 L/kg

Protein binding: <7% to serum proteins

Metabolism: Tenofovir disoproxil fumarate (TDF) is converted intracellularly by hydrolysis (by non-CYP enzymes) to tenofovir, then phosphorylated to the active tenofovir diphosphate

Bioavailability: ~25% (fasting); increases ~40% with high-fat meal

Half-life elimination: ~17 hours

Time to peak, serum: Fasting: 36-84 minutes; With high-fat meal: 96-144 minutes

Excretion: Urine (70% to 80%) via filtration and active secretion, primarily as unchanged tenofovir

Dosage Oral: **Note:** Concurrent use with adefovir and/or tenofovir combination products should be avoided. Canadian labeling does not approve of use in children <12 years with HIV or patients <18 years with chronic HBV.

Children 2 to <12 years: HIV infection: 8 mg/kg once daily (maximum: 300 mg once daily) (in combination with other antiretrovirals)

Dosing recommendations based on body weight if using the **oral powder**: **Note:** One level scoop of powder = 40 mg tenofovir

10 to <12 kg: 80 mg once daily
12 to <14 kg: 100 mg once daily
14 to <17 kg: 120 mg once daily
17 to <19 kg: 140 mg once daily
19 to <22 kg: 160 mg once daily
22 to <24 kg: 180 mg once daily
24 to <27 kg: 200 mg once daily
27 to <29 kg: 220 mg once daily
29 to <32 kg: 240 mg once daily
32 to <34 kg: 260 mg once daily
34 to <35 kg: 280 mg once daily
≥35 kg: 300 mg once daily

Dosing recommendations based on body weight if using the **oral tablets**:

17 to <22 kg: 150 mg once daily
22 to <28 kg: 200 mg once daily
28 to <35 kg: 250 mg once daily
≥35 kg: 300 mg once daily

Children ≥12 years (and ≥35 kg), Adolescents, and Adults:

Hepatitis B infection: 300 mg once daily; **Note:** Tenofovir is recommended for first-line treatment of HBV (Lok, 2009)

Treatment duration (AASLD practice guidelines, 2009): **Note:** Patients not achieving <2 log decrease in serum HBV DNA after at least 6 months of therapy should either receive additional treatment or be switched to an alternative therapy (Lok, 2009).

Hepatitis Be antigen (HBeAg) positive chronic hepatitis: Treat ≥1 year until HBeAg seroconversion and undetectable serum HBV DNA; continue therapy for ≥6 months after HBeAg seroconversion

HBeAg negative chronic hepatitis: Treat >1 year until hepatitis B surface antigen (HBsAg) clearance

Decompensated liver disease: Lifelong treatment is recommended

HIV infection: 300 mg once daily (in combination with other antiretrovirals). **Note:** Tenofovir in combination with emtricitabine is a component of initial recommended regimens (with atazanavir/ritonavir, with darunavir/ritonavir, with efavirenz, or with raltegravir) in all treatment-naive patients and a component of a recommended regimen (with rilpivirine and emtricitabine) for treatment-naive patients with a CD4 count >200 cells/mm^3 (HHS [adult], 2014).

Dosage adjustment in renal impairment:

Children: There are no dosage adjustments provided in the manufacturer's labeling (has not been studied).

Adults: **Note:** Use of powder formulation has not been evaluated in renal impairment.

CrCl ≥50 mL/minute: No dosage adjustment necessary
CrCl 30-49 mL/minute: 300 mg every 48 hours
CrCl 10-29 mL/minute: 300 mg every 72-96 hours
CrCl <10 mL/minute without hemodialysis: No dosage adjustment provided in manufacturer's labeling; has not been studied.

Hemodialysis: 300 mg following dialysis every 7 days or after a total of ~12 hours of dialysis (usually once weekly assuming 3 dialysis sessions lasting about 4 hours each)

Dosage adjustment in hepatic impairment: No dosage adjustment necessary.

Dietary Considerations Consider calcium and vitamin D supplementation.

Administration Tablets may be administered without regard to meals. Powder should be mixed with 2-4 ounces of soft food (applesauce, baby food, yogurt) and swallowed immediately (avoids bitter taste); do not mix in liquid (powder may float on top of the liquid even after stirring). Measure powder using only the supplied dosing scoop.

Monitoring Parameters

Patients with HIV: CBC with differential, reticulocyte count, creatine kinase, CD4 count, HIV RNA plasma levels, serum phosphorus; serum creatinine (prior to initiation and as clinically indicated during therapy), urine glucose and urine protein (in patients at risk for renal impairment or who experienced renal impairment while taking adefovir), hepatic function tests, bone density (patients with a history of bone fracture or have risk factors for bone loss); testing for HBV is recommended prior to the initiation of antiretroviral therapy; weight (children)

Patients with HBV: HIV status (prior to initiation of therapy); serum phosphorus; serum creatinine (prior to initiation and as clinically indicated during therapy), urine glucose and urine protein (in patients at risk for renal impairment or who experienced renal impairment while taking adefovir); bone density (patients with a history of bone fracture or have risk factors for bone loss); HBV DNA (every 3-6 months during therapy); HBeAg and anti-HBe; LFTs every 3 months during therapy and for several months following discontinuation of tenofovir; signs/symptoms of HBV relapse/exacerbation following discontinuation of therapy

Patients with HIV and HBV coinfection should be monitored for several months following tenofovir discontinuation.

Dosage Forms

Powder, Oral:

Viread: 40 mg/g (60 g)

Tablet, Oral:

Viread: 150 mg, 200 mg, 250 mg, 300 mg

Dosage Forms: Canada Refer to Dosage Forms. **Note:** Oral powder for reconstitution is not available in Canada.

◆ **Tenofovir and Emtricitabine** *see* Emtricitabine and Tenofovir *on page 721*

◆ **Tenofovir Disoproxil Fumarate** *see* Tenofovir *on page 1998*

◆ **Tenofovir Disoproxil Fumarate, Efavirenz, and Emtricitabine** *see* Efavirenz, Emtricitabine, and Tenofovir *on page 709*

◆ **Tenofovir Disoproxil Fumarate, Rilpivirine, and Emtricitabine** *see* Emtricitabine, Rilpivirine, and Tenofovir *on page 722*

◆ **Tenofovir, Elvitegravir, Cobicistat, and Emtricitabine** *see* Elvitegravir, Cobicistat, Emtricitabine, and Tenofovir *on page 718*

◆ **Tenofovir, Emtricitabine, and Rilpivirine** *see* Emtricitabine, Rilpivirine, and Tenofovir *on page 722*

◆ **Tenormin** *see* Atenolol *on page 189*

Tenoxicam [INT] (ten OKS i kam)

International Brand Names Alganex (SE); Arthirinal (CY); Artriunic (ES); Artrocam (CZ, HR); Bioreucam (PT); Calibral (PT); Dolmen (IT); Doxican (PT); Legil (BR); Liman (AT, DE); Mefenix (AR); Mobiflex (GB, IE); Reutenox (ES); Rexalgan (IT); Tenoxen (BR); Texicam (AR); Tilatil (AR, BR); Tilcotil (AT, AU, BE, CH, CZ, DE, DK, ES, FI, FR, HU, IT, LU, MX, NL, PT); Tilcotil "Roche" (HU); Tobitil (IN)

Pharmacologic Category Analgesic, Nonsteroidal Anti-inflammatory Drug; Nonsteroidal Anti-inflammatory Drug (NSAID), Oral

Reported Use Treatment of rheumatoid arthritis and osteoarthritis; short-term management of acute musculoskeletal disorders

Dosage Range Adults:

Oral: 20 mg daily for 7 days; maximum 14 days

IM, IV: 20 mg daily for 1-2 days

Product Availability Product available in various countries; not currently available in the U.S.

Dosage Forms

Injection, powder for reconstitution: 20 mg

Tablet: 20 mg

◆ **Tensilon® (Can)** *see* Edrophonium *on page 706*

◆ **Tenuate** *see* Diethylpropion *on page 624*

◆ **Tenuate Dospan** *see* Diethylpropion *on page 624*

◆ **Terazol 3** *see* Terconazole *on page 2006*

◆ **Terazol 7** *see* Terconazole *on page 2006*

Terazosin (ter AY zoe sin)

Brand Names: Canada Apo-Terazosin; Dom-Terazosin; Hytrin; Nu-Terazosin; PHL-Terazosin; PMS-Terazosin; ratio-Terazosin; Teva-Terazosin

Index Terms Hytrin

Pharmacologic Category Alpha$_1$ Blocker; Antihypertensive

Additional Appendix Information

Beers Criteria – Potentially Inappropriate Medications for Geriatrics *on page 2271*

Use

Hypertension: Management of mild-to-moderate hypertension; alone or in combination with other agents such as diuretics or beta-blockers

Note: The 2014 guideline for the management of high blood pressure in adults (Eighth Joint National Committee [JNC 8]) does **not** recommend the use of terazosin in the treatment of hypertension (JNC8 [James, 2013]).

Benign prostate hyperplasia: Benign prostate hyperplasia (BPH)

Pregnancy Risk Factor C

Pregnancy Considerations Teratogenic effects have not been observed in animal studies. Decreased fetal weight and increased risk of fetal mortality were noted in some animal reproduction studies. There are no adequate and well-controlled studies in pregnant women. Use only if benefit outweighs risk.

Untreated chronic maternal hypertension is associated with adverse events in the fetus, infant, and mother. If treatment for hypertension during pregnancy is needed, other agents are generally preferred (ACOG, 2013).

Breast-Feeding Considerations It is not known if terazosin is excreted in breast milk. The manufacturer recommends that caution be exercised when administering terazosin to nursing women.

Contraindications Hypersensitivity to terazosin or any component of the formulation

Warnings/Precautions Can cause significant orthostatic hypotension and syncope, especially with first dose; anticipate a similar effect if therapy is interrupted for a few days, if dosage is rapidly increased, or if another antihypertensive drug (particularly vasodilators) or a PDE-5 inhibitor is introduced. Discontinue if symptoms of angina occur or worsen. Patients should be cautioned about performing hazardous tasks when starting new therapy or adjusting dosage upward. Prostate cancer should be ruled out before starting for BPH. Intraoperative floppy iris syndrome has been observed in cataract surgery patients who were on or were previously treated with alpha$_1$-blockers. Causality has not been established and there appears to be no benefit in discontinuing alpha-blocker therapy prior to surgery. Priapism has been associated with use (rarely). In the elderly, avoid use as an antihypertensive due to high risk of orthostatic hypotension; alternative agents preferred due to a more favorable risk/benefit profile (Beers Criteria).

Adverse Reactions

Cardiovascular: Orthostatic hypotension, palpitation, peripheral edema, syncope, tachycardia

Central nervous system: Dizziness, somnolence, vertigo

Gastrointestinal: Nausea, weight gain

Genitourinary: Impotence, libido decreased

Neuromuscular & skeletal: Back pain, extremity pain, muscle weakness, paresthesia

Ocular: Blurred vision

Respiratory: Dyspnea, nasal congestion, sinusitis

Rare but important or life-threatening: Abdominal pain, abnormal vision, allergic reactions, anaphylaxis, anxiety, arrhythmia, arthralgia, arthritis, atrial fibrillation, bronchitis, chest pain, conjunctivitis, constipation, cough, diaphoresis, diarrhea, dyspepsia, epistaxis, facial edema, fever, flatulence, flu-like syndrome, gout, insomnia, intraoperative floppy iris syndrome (IFIS), joint disorder, myalgia, neck pain, pharyngitis, polyuria, priapism, pruritus, rash, rhinitis, shoulder pain, thrombocytopenia, tinnitus, urinary incontinence, urinary tract infection, vasodilation, vomiting, xerostomia

Drug Interactions

Metabolism/Transport Effects None known.

Avoid Concomitant Use

Avoid concomitant use of Terazosin with any of the following: Alpha1-Blockers

Increased Effect/Toxicity

Terazosin may increase the levels/effects of: Alpha1-Blockers; Amifostine; Antihypertensives; Calcium Channel Blockers; DULoxetine; Hypotensive Agents; Levodopa; Obinutuzumab; RisperiDONE; RiTUXimab

The levels/effects of Terazosin may be increased by: Barbiturates; Beta-Blockers; Brimonidine (Topical); Dapoxetine; Diazoxide; Herbs (Hypotensive Properties); MAO Inhibitors; Nicorandil; Pentoxifylline; Phosphodiesterase 5 Inhibitors; Prostacyclin Analogues

Decreased Effect

Terazosin may decrease the levels/effects of: Alpha-/Beta-Agonists; Alpha1-Agonists

The levels/effects of Terazosin may be decreased by: Herbs (Hypertensive Properties); Methylphenidate; Yohimbine

Storage/Stability Store at 20°C to 25°C (68°F to 77°F); protect from light and moisture.

Mechanism of Action $Alpha_1$-specific blocking agent with minimal $alpha_2$ effects; this allows peripheral postsynaptic blockade, with the resultant decrease in arterial tone, while preserving the negative feedback loop which is mediated by the peripheral presynaptic $alpha_2$-receptors; terazosin relaxes the smooth muscle of the bladder neck, thus reducing bladder outlet obstruction

Pharmacodynamics/Kinetics

Onset of action: 1-2 hours

Absorption: Rapid and complete

Protein binding: 90% to 95%

Metabolism: Hepatic; minimal first-pass

Half-life elimination: ~12 hours

Time to peak, serum: ~1 hour

Excretion: Feces (~60%, ~20% as unchanged drug); urine (~40%, ~10% as unchanged drug)

Dosage Oral: **Note:** If drug is discontinued for greater than several days, consider beginning with initial dose and retitrate as needed.

Hypertension:

Children (off-label use): Initial: 1 mg once daily; gradually increase dose as necessary, up to maximum of 20 mg/day

Adults: Initial: 1 mg at bedtime; slowly increase dose to achieve desired blood pressure, up to 20 mg/day; usual dosage range (ASH/ISH [Weber, 2014]: 1-2 mg daily. **Note:** Dosage may be given on a twice daily regimen if response is diminished at 24 hours and hypotension is observed at 2-4 hours following a dose.

Elderly: Consider lower initial doses (eg, immediate release: 0.5 mg once daily) and titrate to response (Aronow, 2011)

Benign prostatic hyperplasia: Adults: Initial: 1 mg at bedtime; thereafter, titrate upwards, if needed, over several weeks, balancing therapeutic benefit with terazosin-induced postural hypotension; most patients require 10 mg day; if no response after 4-6 weeks of 10 mg/day, may increase to 20 mg/day

Dosage adjustment with concurrent medication:

Concurrent use with a diuretic or other antihypertensive agent (especially verapamil): Dosage reduction may be needed when adding

Concurrent use with PDE-5 inhibitors: Initiate PDE-5 inhibitor therapy at the lowest dose due to additive orthostatic and blood pressure lowering effects

Dosage adjustment in renal impairment: No dosage adjustment necessary.

Hemodialysis: No supplemental dose necessary.

Dosage adjustment in hepatic impairment: No dosage adjustment provided in manufacturer's labeling.

Dietary Considerations May be taken without regard to meals at the same time each day.

Administration Administer without regard to meals at the same time each day.

Monitoring Parameters Standing and sitting/supine blood pressure, especially following the initial dose at 2-4 hours following the dose and thereafter at the trough point to ensure adequate control throughout the dosing interval; urinary symptoms

Dosage Forms

Capsule, Oral:

Generic: 1 mg, 2 mg, 5 mg, 10 mg

Dosage Forms: Canada Tablet, Oral: 1 mg, 2 mg, 5 mg, 10 mg

Terbinafine (Systemic) (TER bin a feen)

Brand Names: U.S. LamISIL; Terbinex

Brand Names: Canada Apo-Terbinafine; Auro-Terbinafine; CO Terbinafine; Dom-Terbinafine; GD-Terbinafine; JAMP-Terbinafine; Lamisil; Mylan-Terbinafine; PHL-Terbinafine; PMS-Terbinafine; Q-Terbinafine; Riva-Terbinafine; Sandoz-Terbinafine; Teva-Terbinafine

Index Terms Terbinafine Hydrochloride

Pharmacologic Category Antifungal Agent, Oral

Use

Onychomycosis (tablets only): Treatment of onychomycosis of the toenail or fingernail caused by dermatophytes (tinea unguium).

Tinea capitis (granules only): Treatment of tinea capitis in patients 4 years and older.

Canadian labeling: Additional use (not in U.S. labeling): Severe tineal skin infections (tinea cruris and tinea pedis) unresponsive to topical therapy

Pregnancy Risk Factor B

Pregnancy Considerations Adverse events were not observed in animal reproduction studies. Avoid use in pregnancy since treatment of onychomycosis is postponable.

Breast-Feeding Considerations Terbinafine is excreted in breast milk; the milk/plasma ratio is 7:1. Breast-feeding is not recommended by the manufacturer.

Contraindications Hypersensitivity to terbinafine or any component of the formulation

Warnings/Precautions Due to potential toxicity, confirmation of diagnostic testing of nail or skin specimens prior to treatment of onychomycosis or dermatomycosis is recommended. Use caution in patients sensitive to allylamine antifungals (eg, naftifine, butenafine); cross sensitivity to terbinafine may exist. Transient decreases in absolute lymphocyte counts were observed in clinical trials; severe neutropenia (reversible upon discontinuation) has also been reported. Monitor CBC in patients with preexisting immunosuppression if therapy is to continue >6 weeks and discontinue therapy if ANC ≤1000/mm^3.

Serious skin and hypersensitivity reactions (eg, Stevens-Johnson syndrome, toxic epidermal necrolysis, erythema multiforme, exfoliative dermatitis, bullous dermatitis, drug reaction with eosinophilia and systemic symptoms [DRESS] syndrome) have occurred. If progressive skin rash or signs and symptoms of a hypersensitivity reaction occur, discontinue treatment. Cases of hepatic failure, some leading to liver transplant or death, have been reported; not recommended for use in patients with active or chronic liver disease. If clinical evidence of liver injury develops (eg, nausea, anorexia, fatigue, vomiting, right upper abdominal pain, jaundice, dark urine, pale stools), assess hepatic function immediately; discontinue therapy in cases of elevated liver function tests. Use with caution in patients with renal dysfunction (CrCl ≤50 mL/minute) (per Canadian labeling, not recommended for use); clearance is reduced by ~50%.

Disturbances of taste and/or smell may occur; resolution may be delayed (eg, >1 year) following discontinuation of therapy or in some cases, disturbance may be permanent. Discontinue therapy in patients with symptoms of taste or smell disturbance.

Adverse Reactions Adverse events listed for tablets unless otherwise specified. Granules were studied in patients 4-12 years of age.

Central nervous system: Headache

Dermatologic: Pruritus, skin rash, urticaria

Gastrointestinal: Abdominal pain, diarrhea, dysgeusia, dyspepsia, flatulence, nausea, sore throat (granules), toothache (granules), vomiting

Hepatic: Liver enzyme disorder

Infection: Influenza (granules)

Ophthalmic: Visual disturbance

Respiratory: Cough (granules), nasal congestion (granules), nasopharyngitis (granules), rhinorrhea (granules), upper respiratory tract infection (children, granules)

Miscellaneous: Fever (granules)

Rare but important or life-threatening: Acute generalized exanthematous pustulosis, acute pancreatitis, agranulocytosis, alopecia, altered sense of smell, anaphylaxis, angioedema, depression, DRESS syndrome, exacerbation of psoriasis, exacerbation of systemic lupus erythematosus, hepatic disease, hepatic failure, hypersensitivity reaction, pancytopenia, rhabdomyolysis, severe neutropenia, Stevens-Johnson syndrome, thrombocytopenia, toxic epidermal necrolysis, vasculitis, visual field loss

Drug Interactions

Metabolism/Transport Effects **Substrate** of CYP1A2 (minor), CYP2C19 (minor), CYP2C9 (minor), CYP3A4 (minor); **Note:** Assignment of Major/Minor substrate status based on clinically relevant drug interaction potential; **Inhibits** CYP2D6 (strong); **Induces** CYP3A4 (weak)

Avoid Concomitant Use

Avoid concomitant use of Terbinafine (Systemic) with any of the following: Pimozide; Saccharomyces boulardii; Tamoxifen; Thioridazine

Increased Effect/Toxicity

Terbinafine (Systemic) may increase the levels/effects of: ARIPiprazole; AtoMOXetine; CYP2D6 Substrates; DOXOrubicin (Conventional); Eliglustat; Fesoterodine; Iloperidone; Metoprolol; Nebivolol; Pimozide; Propafenone; Tetrabenazine; Thioridazine; Tricyclic Antidepressants; Vortioxetine

Decreased Effect

Terbinafine (Systemic) may decrease the levels/effects of: ARIPiprazole; Codeine; Hydrocodone; Iloperidone; Saccharomyces boulardii; Saxagliptin; Tamoxifen; TraMADol

The levels/effects of Terbinafine (Systemic) may be decreased by: Rifampin

Storage/Stability

Granules: Store at 25°C (77°F); excursions permitted between 15°C to 30°C (59°F to 86°F).

Tablet: Store below 25°C (77°F). Protect from light.

Mechanism of Action Synthetic allylamine derivative which inhibits squalene epoxidase, a key enzyme in sterol biosynthesis in fungi. This results in a deficiency in ergosterol within the fungal cell wall and results in fungal cell death.

Pharmacodynamics/Kinetics

Absorption: >70%

Distribution: Distributed to sebum and skin predominantly

Protein binding: Plasma: >99%

Metabolism: Hepatic predominantly via CYP1A2, 3A4, 2C8, 2C9, and 2C19 to inactive metabolites

Bioavailability: ~40%; Children 36% to 64%

Half-life elimination: Terminal half-life: 200-400 hours; very slow release of drug from skin and adipose tissues occurs; effective half-life: ~36 hours; Children: 27-31 hours

Time to peak, plasma: Within 2 hours

Excretion: Urine (~70%)

Dosage Oral:

Children ≥4 years, Adolescents, and Adults: Granules:

Tinea capitis:

<25 kg: 125 mg once daily for 6 weeks

25-35 kg: 187.5 mg once daily for 6 weeks

>35 kg: 250 mg once daily for 6 weeks

Children and Adolescents: Tablet: Onychomycosis (off-label use; Gupta, 1997):

10-20 kg: 62.5 mg once daily for 6 weeks (fingernails) **or** 12 weeks (toenails)

20-40 kg: 125 mg once daily for 6 weeks (fingernails) **or** 12 weeks (toenails)

>40 kg: 250 mg once daily for 6 weeks (fingernails) **or** 12 weeks (toenails)

Adults:

Tablet:

U.S. labeling: Onychomycosis: Fingernail: 250 mg once daily for 6 weeks; Toenail: 250 mg once daily for 12 weeks

Missed doses: If a dose is missed, take as soon as remembered, unless it is less than 4 hours before the next dose is due.

Canadian labeling: **Note:** Mycologic cure may precede complete resolution of symptoms by several weeks (skin infections) or by several months (onychomycosis).

Onychomycosis (finger or toenail): 250 mg/day in 1-2 divided doses for 6 weeks to 3 months (≥6 months may be necessary in some patients with infections of the big toenail)

Tinea corporis, tinea cruris: 250 mg/day in 1-2 divided doses for 2-4 weeks

Tinea pedis (interdigital and plantar/moccasin type): 250 mg/day in 1-2 divided doses for 2-6 weeks

Sporotrichosis, lymphocutaneous and cutaneous (off-label use): 500 mg twice daily as alternative therapy; treat for 2-4 weeks after resolution of all lesions (usual duration: 3-6 months) (Kauffman, 2007)

Elderly: Use with caution; refer to adult dosing.

Dosing adjustment in renal impairment:

U.S. labeling: No dosage adjustment provided in manufacturer's labeling (has not been studied); however, clearance is decreased 50% in patients with CrCl ≤50 mL/minute.

Canadian labeling: Use is not recommended in patients with CrCl ≤50 mL/minute.

Dosing adjustment in hepatic impairment: Use is not recommended in chronic or active hepatic disease.

Administration Administer tablets without regard to meals. Administer granules with food; sprinkle granules on a spoonful of pudding or other soft, nonacidic food (eg, mashed potatoes); swallow entire spoonful without chewing; do not mix granules with applesauce or other fruit-based foods.

Monitoring Parameters AST/ALT prior to initiation, repeat if used >6 weeks; CBC; taste and/or smell disturbances

Dosage Forms Considerations

Terbinex Kit contains terbinafine 250 mg tablets and hydroxypropyl-chitosan 1% nail lacquer

Dosage Forms

Kit, Combination:

Terbinex: 250 mg & 1%

Packet, Oral:

LamISIL: 125 mg (1 ea, 14 ea); 187.5 mg (1 ea, 14 ea)

Tablet, Oral:

LamISIL: 250 mg

Generic: 250 mg

Dosage Forms: Canada

Tablet, oral:

LamISIL: 125 mg

Extemporaneous Preparations A 25 mg/mL oral suspension may be made using tablets. Crush twenty 250 mg tablets and reduce to a fine powder. Add small amount of a 1:1 mixture of Ora-Sweet® and Ora-Plus® and mix to a uniform paste; mix while adding the vehicle in geometric proportions to **almost** 200 mL; transfer to a calibrated bottle, rinse mortar with vehicle, and add quantity of vehicle sufficient to make 200 mL. Label "shake well" and "refrigerate". Stable 42 days.

Nahata MC, Pai VB, and Hipple TF, *Pediatric Drug Formulations*, 5th ed, Cincinnati, OH: Harvey Whitney Books Co, 2004.

Terbinafine (Topical) (TER bin a feen)

Brand Names: U.S. LamISIL Advanced [OTC]; LamISIL AT Jock Itch [OTC]; LamISIL AT Spray [OTC]; LamISIL AT [OTC]; LamISIL Spray

Brand Names: Canada Lamisil

Index Terms Terbinafine Hydrochloride

Pharmacologic Category Antifungal Agent, Topical

Use Antifungal for the treatment of tinea pedis (athlete's foot), tinea cruris (jock itch), and tinea corporis (ringworm) [OTC/Canadian prescription formulations]; cutaneous candidiasis and tinea versicolor [Canadian prescription formulations]

Dosage Topical:

Children ≥12 years and Adolescents:

Tinea pedis:

Cream: Apply between the toes to affected area twice daily for at least 1 week [OTC formulations]; apply on the bottom or sides of feet twice daily for 2 weeks [OTC formulations]

Gel: Apply to affected area once daily for at least 1 week [OTC formulations]

Solution: Apply to affected area once daily for at least 1 week [OTC formulations]

Tinea corporis, Tinea cruris:

Cream: Apply to affected area once daily for 1 week [OTC formulations]

Gel: Apply to affected area once daily for 1 week [OTC formulations]

Solution: Apply to affected area once daily for 1 week [OTC formulations]

Adults:

Tinea pedis:

Cream: Apply between the toes to affected area once or twice daily for at least 1 week [OTC/Canadian prescription formulations]; apply on the bottom or sides of feet twice daily for 2 weeks [OTC formulations]

Gel: Apply to affected area once daily for at least 1 week [OTC formulations]

Solution: Apply to affected area once daily for at least 1 week [OTC/Canadian prescription formulations]

Tinea corporis, Tinea cruris:

Cream: Apply to affected area once daily for 1 week [OTC/Canadian prescription formulations]

Gel: Apply to affected area once daily for 1 week [OTC formulations]

Solution: Apply to affected area once daily for 1 week [OTC/Canadian prescription formulations]

Cutaneous candidiasis: Apply to affected area once or twice daily for 1-2 weeks [Canadian prescription formulation]

Tinea versicolor:

Cream: Apply to affected area once or twice daily for 1-2 weeks [Canadian prescription formulation]

Solution: Apply to affected area twice daily for 1 week [Canadian prescription formulation]

Additional Information Complete prescribing information should be consulted for additional detail.

Dosage Forms

Cream, External:

LamISIL AT [OTC]: 1% (12 g, 24 g, 30 g, 36 g, 42 g)

LamISIL AT Jock Itch [OTC]: 1% (12 g)

Generic: 1% (12 g, 15 g, 24 g, 30 g)

Gel, External:

LamISIL Advanced [OTC]: 1% (12 g)

Solution, External:

LamISIL AT Spray [OTC]: 1% (30 mL, 125 mL)

LamISIL Spray: 1% (30 mL)

Dosage Forms: Canada

Cream, topical:

Lamisil®: 1% (15 g, 30 g)

Solution, topical [spray]:

Lamisil®: 1% (30 mL)

◆ **Terbinafine Hydrochloride** *see* Terbinafine (Systemic) *on page 2002*

◆ **Terbinafine Hydrochloride** *see* Terbinafine (Topical) *on page 2004*

◆ **Terbinex** *see* Terbinafine (Systemic) *on page 2002*

Terbutaline (ter BYOO ta leen)

Brand Names: Canada Bricanyl® Turbuhaler®

Index Terms Brethaire; Brethine; Bricanyl; Terbutaline Sulfate

Pharmacologic Category Antidote, Extravasation; Beta$_2$ Agonist

Use Bronchodilator in reversible airway obstruction and bronchial asthma

Pregnancy Risk Factor C

Pregnancy Considerations Adverse events have been observed in animal reproduction studies. Terbutaline crosses the placenta; umbilical cord concentrations are ~11% to 48% of maternal blood levels.

Uncontrolled asthma is associated with adverse events on pregnancy (increased risk of perinatal mortality, preeclampsia, preterm birth, low birth weight infants). Terbutaline is not recommended for the treatment of asthma during pregnancy; inhaled beta$_2$-receptor agonists are preferred (NAEPP, 2005).

[U.S. Boxed Warning]: Terbutaline is not FDA approved for and should not be used for prolonged tocolysis (>48-72 hours). Use for maintenance tocolysis should not be done in the outpatient setting. Adverse events observed in pregnant women include arrhythmias, increased heart rate, hyperglycemia (transient), hypokalemia, myocardial ischemia, and pulmonary edema. Heart rate may be increased in the fetus and hypoglycemia may occur in the neonate. Terbutaline has been used in the management of preterm labor. Tocolytics may be used for the short-term (48 hour) prolongation of pregnancy to allow for the administration of antenatal steroids and should not be used prior to fetal viability or when the risks of use to the fetus or mother are greater than the risk of preterm birth (ACOG, 2012).

Breast-Feeding Considerations Terbutaline is excreted in breast milk; concentrations are similar to or higher than those in the maternal plasma. Based on information from four cases, exposure to the breast-fed infant would be <1% of the weight-adjusted maternal dose. Adverse events were not observed in nursing infants (Boréus, 1982; Lönnerholm, 1982). The manufacturer recommends that terbutaline be used in breast-feeding women only if the potential benefit to the mother outweighs the possible risk to the infant. The use of beta$_2$-receptor agonists are not considered a contraindication to breast-feeding (NAEPP, 2005).

Contraindications

Hypersensitivity to terbutaline, sympathomimetic amines, or any component of the formulation

Injection: Additional contraindications: Prolonged (>72 hours) prevention or management of preterm labor

Oral: Additional contraindications: Prevention or treatment of preterm labor

Warnings/Precautions [U.S. Boxed Warning]: Terbutaline is not FDA approved for and should not be used for prolonged tocolysis (>48-72 hours). Use for maintenance tocolysis should not be done in the outpatient setting. Adverse events observed in pregnant women include arrhythmias, increased heart rate, hyperglycemia (transient), hypokalemia, myocardial ischemia, and pulmonary edema. Heart rate may be increased in the fetus and hypoglycemia may occur in the neonate. Oral terbutaline is contraindicated for acute or chronic use in the management of preterm labor.

Use caution in patients with cardiovascular disease (arrhythmia or hypertension or HF), convulsive disorders, diabetes, glaucoma, hyperthyroidism, or hypokalemia. Beta-agonists may cause elevation in blood pressure, heart rate, and result in CNS stimulation/excitation. $Beta_2$-agonists may increase risk of arrhythmia, increase serum glucose, or decrease serum potassium.

When used as a bronchodilator, optimize anti-inflammatory treatment before initiating maintenance treatment with terbutaline. Do not use as a component of chronic therapy without an anti-inflammatory agent. Only the mildest form of asthma (Step 1 and/or exercise-induced) would not require concurrent use based upon asthma guidelines. Patient must be instructed to seek medical attention in cases where acute symptoms are not relieved or a previous level of response is diminished. The need to increase frequency of use may indicate deterioration of asthma, and treatment must not be delayed.

Immediate hypersensitivity reactions (urticaria, angioedema, rash, bronchospasm) have been reported. Do not exceed recommended dose; serious adverse events including fatalities, have been associated with excessive use of inhaled sympathomimetics. Rarely, paradoxical bronchospasm may occur with use of inhaled bronchodilating agents; this should be distinguished from inadequate response.

Adverse Reactions

Cardiovascular: Hypertension, pounding heartbeat, tachycardia

Central nervous system: Nervousness, restlessness

Endocrine & metabolic: Decreased serum potassium, increased serum glucose

Gastrointestinal: Bad taste in mouth, dry mouth, nausea, vomiting

Neuromuscular & skeletal: Dizziness, drowsiness, headache, insomnia, lightheadedness, muscle cramps, trembling, weakness

Miscellaneous: Diaphoresis

Rare but important or life-threatening: Arrhythmia, cardiac arrest (preterm labor), chest pain, hyperglycemia (preterm labor), hypokalemia (preterm labor), hypotension (preterm labor), paradoxical bronchospasm, myocardial infarction (preterm labor), myocardial ischemia (preterm labor), pulmonary edema (preterm labor)

Drug Interactions

Metabolism/Transport Effects None known.

Avoid Concomitant Use

Avoid concomitant use of Terbutaline with any of the following: Beta-Blockers (Nonselective); Iobenguane I 123

Increased Effect/Toxicity

Terbutaline may increase the levels/effects of: Atosiban; Loop Diuretics; Sympathomimetics; Thiazide Diuretics

The levels/effects of Terbutaline may be increased by: AtoMOXetine; Cannabinoid-Containing Products; Linezolid; MAO Inhibitors; Tedizolid; Tricyclic Antidepressants

Decreased Effect

Terbutaline may decrease the levels/effects of: Iobenguane I 123

The levels/effects of Terbutaline may be decreased by: Beta-Blockers (Beta1 Selective); Beta-Blockers (Nonselective); Betahistine

Preparation for Administration For extravasation management (off-label use): Using vial for injection, dilute 1 mg with 9 mL (total volume: 10 mL) (large extravasation site) **or** 1 mg with 1 mL (total volume: 2 mL) (small/distal extravasation site) of 0.9% sodium chloride (Stier, 1999).

Storage/Stability Store injection at room temperature; do not freeze. Protect from heat and light. Use only clear solutions. Store powder for inhalation (Bricanyl® Turbuhaler [Canadian availability]) at room temperature between 15°C and 30°C (58°F and 86°F).

Mechanism of Action Relaxes bronchial and uterine smooth muscle by action on $beta_2$-receptors with less effect on heart rate

Pharmacodynamics/Kinetics

Onset of action: Oral: 30-45 minutes; SubQ: 6-15 minute; Inhalation: 5 minutes (maximum effect: 15-60 minutes)

Duration: Inhalation: 4-7 hours

Protein binding: 25%

Metabolism: Hepatic to inactive sulfate conjugates

Bioavailability: SubQ doses are more bioavailable than oral

Half-life elimination: 11-16 hours

Excretion: Urine

Dosage

Children <12 years: Bronchoconstriction:

Oral: Initial: 0.05 mg/kg/dose 3 times/day, increased gradually as required; maximum: 0.15 mg/kg/dose 3 to 4 times/day or a total of 5 mg/24 hours

SubQ: 0.005-0.01 mg/kg/dose to a maximum of 0.4 mg/dose every 15 to 20 minutes for 3 doses; may repeat every 2 to 6 hours as needed

Children ≥6 years and Adults: Bronchospasm (acute): Inhalation: Bricanyl Turbuhaler: (Canadian labeling; not available in U.S.): One puff as needed; may repeat with 1 inhalation (after 5 minutes); more than 6 inhalations should not be necessary in any 24-hour period. **Note:** If adequate relief is not obtained with previously effective dose, or if effects of inhalation last <3 hours, patient should be reassessed; may indicate worsening asthma.

Children >12 years and Adults: Bronchoconstriction:

Oral:

12 to 15 years: 2.5 mg every 6 hours 3 times/day; not to exceed 7.5 mg in 24 hours

>15 years: 5 mg/dose every 6 hours 3 times/day; if side effects occur, reduce dose to 2.5 mg every 6 hours; not to exceed 15 mg in 24 hours

SubQ:

Manufacturer's labeling: 0.25 mg/dose; may repeat in 15 to 30 minutes (maximum: 0.5 mg/4-hour period)

Off-label dose: 0.25 mg/dose; may repeat every 20 minutes for 3 doses (maximum: 0.75 mg/1-hour period) (NAEPP, 2007)

Adults: Premature labor (acute; short-term [≤72 hours] tocolysis; off-label use):

IV: 2.5 to 5 mcg/minute; increased gradually every 20 to 30 minutes by 2.5 to 5 mcg/minute; effective maximum dosages from 17.5 to 30 mcg/minute have been used with caution. Duration of infusion is at least 12 hours (Travis, 1993).

SubQ: 0.25 mg every 20 minutes to 3 hours; hold for pulse >120 beats per minute. Terbutaline has not been approved for and should not be used for prolonged tocolysis (beyond 48 to 72 hours) (ACOG, 2012; Hearne, 2000).

Adults: Extravasation management, sympathomimetic vasoconstrictors (off-label use; based on limited case reports): SubQ:

Large extravasations: Infiltrate extravasation area using a solution of 1 mg diluted in 9 mL (total volume: 10 mL) of 0.9% sodium chloride; volume of terbutaline solution administered varied from 3 to 10 mL (Stier, 1999).

Small/distal extravasations: Infiltrate extravasation area using a solution of 1 mg diluted in 1 mL (total volume: 2 mL) of 0.9% sodium chloride; volume of terbutaline solution administered varied from 0.5 to 1 mL (Stier, 1999).

Dosage adjustment in renal impairment: No dosage adjustment provided in manufacturer's labeling.

Dosage adjustment in hepatic impairment: No dosage adjustment provided in manufacturer's labeling.

Administration

IV: Use infusion pump.

Oral: Administer around-the-clock to promote less variation in peak and trough serum levels

Inhalation: Bricanyl® Turbuhaler® (Canadian availability): After removing lid, patient should hold inhaler upright and turn blue grip as far as it will go in one direction then turn it back to original position. Clicking sound indicates that inhaler is ready for use. Patient should exhale fully but not into the inhaler and then place mouthpiece gently between teeth, close lips around inhaler and inhale deeply. Inhaler should be removed from mouth prior to exhaling. Instruct patients to rinse mouth with water after each inhalation as some medication may stick to the inside of the mouth and throat. If inhaler is dropped or shaken, or if patient exhales into the inhaler after a dose is loaded, the dose will be lost and a new dose should be loaded and inhaled. Outside of mouthpiece should be cleaned once weekly with a dry tissue. Instruct patient to keep inhaler dry. First appearance of red mark in dose indicator (window underneath mouthpiece) indicates that 20 doses remain. When red mark reaches bottom of dose indicator no doses remain and Turbuhaler should be discarded.

SubQ: Extravasation management, sympathomimetic vasopressors (off-label use): Stop vesicant infusion immediately and disconnect IV line (leave needle/cannula in place); gently aspirate extravasated solution from the IV line (do **NOT** flush the line); remove needle/cannula; elevate extremity. Infiltrate extravasation area with terbutaline solution 1 mg diluted with 9 mL (large extravasation site) **or** 1 mg diluted with 1 mL (small/distal extravasation site) of 0.9% sodium chloride into extravasation site (Stier, 1999).

Monitoring Parameters Serum potassium, glucose; intake/output; heart rate, blood pressure, respiratory rate; chest pain, shortness of breath; monitor for signs and symptoms of pulmonary edema (when used as a tocolytic); monitor FEV_1, peak flow, and/or other pulmonary function tests (when used as bronchodilator). If used for extravasation management, monitor and document extravasation site.

Dosage Forms

Solution, Injection:

Generic: 1 mg/mL (1 mL)

Tablet, Oral:

Generic: 2.5 mg, 5 mg

Dosage Forms: Canada

Powder for oral inhalation:

Bricanyl® Turbuhaler®: 500 mcg/actuation [100 or 200 metered actuations]

Extemporaneous Preparations A 1 mg/mL oral suspension may be made with tablets. Crush twenty-four 5 mg tablets in a mortar and reduce to a fine powder. Add 5 mL purified water USP and mix to a uniform paste; mix while adding simple syrup, NF in incremental proportions to **almost** 120 mL; transfer to a calibrated bottle, rinse mortar with vehicle, and add quantity of simple syrup, NF sufficient to make 120 mL. Label "shake well" and "refrigerate". Stable for 30 days.

Nahata MC, Pai VB, and Hipple TF, *Pediatric Drug Formulations*, 5th ed, Cincinnati, OH: Harvey Whitney Books Co, 2004.

◆ **Terbutaline Sulfate** *see* Terbutaline *on page 2004*

Terconazole (ter KONE a zole)

Brand Names: U.S. Terazol 3; Terazol 7; Zazole

Brand Names: Canada Taro-Terconazole; Terazol 7

Index Terms Triaconazole

Pharmacologic Category Antifungal Agent, Azole Derivative; Antifungal Agent, Vaginal

Use Candidiasis: For the local treatment of vulvovaginal candidiasis (moniliasis). As terconazole is effective only for vulvovaginitis caused by the genus *Candida*, the diagnosis should be confirmed by KOH smears or cultures.

Pregnancy Risk Factor C

Dosage Intravaginal: Adults: Females:

Vaginal cream 0.4%: Insert 1 applicatorful intravaginally at bedtime for 7 consecutive days

Vaginal cream 0.8%: Insert 1 applicatorful intravaginally at bedtime for 3 consecutive days

Vaginal suppository: Insert 1 suppository intravaginally at bedtime for 3 consecutive days

Additional Information Complete prescribing information should be consulted for additional detail.

Dosage Forms

Cream, Vaginal:

Terazol 7: 0.4% (45 g)

Terazol 3: 0.8% (20 g)

Zazole: 0.4% (45 g); 0.8% (20 g)

Generic: 0.4% (45 g); 0.8% (20 g)

Suppository, Vaginal:

Zazole: 80 mg (3 ea)

Generic: 80 mg (3 ea)

◆ **Terfluzine (Can)** *see* Trifluoperazine *on page 2102*

Teriflunomide (ter i FLOO noh mide)

Brand Names: U.S. Aubagio

Brand Names: Canada Aubagio

Index Terms A771726; HMR1726

Pharmacologic Category Pyrimidine Synthesis Inhibitor

Use Multiple sclerosis: Treatment of patients with relapsing forms of multiple sclerosis.

Pregnancy Risk Factor X

Pregnancy Considerations Adverse events have been observed in animal reproduction studies conducted using doses lower than the expected human exposure. **[U.S. Boxed Warning]: Based on animal data, teriflunomide may cause major birth defects if used in pregnant women. Teriflunomide is contraindicated in pregnant women or women of childbearing potential who are not using reliable contraception. Pregnancy must be avoided during therapy or prior to completing the accelerated elimination treatment protocol.** Pregnancy must be excluded prior to initiating treatment. Women of childbearing potential should not receive therapy until pregnancy has been excluded, they have been counseled concerning fetal risk, and reliable contraceptive measures have been confirmed. Following treatment, pregnancy should be avoided until undetectable serum concentrations (<0.02 mg/L) are verified. This may be accomplished by the use of an enhanced drug elimination procedure using cholestyramine or activated charcoal powder. If pregnancy occurs during treatment, discontinue therapy and initiate the accelerated elimination procedure. Pregnant women exposed to teriflunomide should be registered with the pregnancy registry (800-745-4447, option 2). Teriflunomide is also found in semen. Males and their female partners should use reliable contraception during therapy. Males taking teriflunomide who wish to father a child should consider discontinuing therapy and using the accelerated elimination procedure to decrease the potential risk of fetal exposure. (**Note:** Without use of the accelerated elimination procedure, teriflunomide may remain in the serum for up to 2 years)

Breast-Feeding Considerations It is not known whether teriflunomide is secreted in human milk. Because the potential for serious adverse reactions exists in the nursing infant, a decision should be made whether to discontinue nursing or discontinue the drug, taking into account the importance of the drug to the mother.

Contraindications

Severe hepatic impairment; concomitant use with leflunomide; women of childbearing age who will not use contraception reliably; pregnancy

Canadian labeling: Additional contraindications (not in U.S. labeling): Hypersensitivity to teriflunomide, leflunomide or any component of the formulation; immunodeficiency states (eg, AIDS); impaired bone marrow function or significant anemias, leucopenia, neutropenia, or thrombocytopenia; serious active infections

Warnings/Precautions Hazardous agent; use appropriate precautions for handling and disposal (meets NIOSH 2014 criteria). **[U.S. Boxed Warning]: Use of leflunomide has been associated with reports of hepatotoxicity, hepatic failure, and death, therefore, a similar risk is expected with teriflunomide. Patients with preexisting liver disease (acute or chronic liver disease or ALT >2 x ULN) may be at an increased risk of developing elevated transaminases during therapy; use is contraindicated in patients with severe impairment. Use in patients with concurrent exposure to potentially hepatotoxic drugs may increase the risk of hepatotoxicity. Obtain transaminase and bilirubin levels within 6 months prior to initiation of treatment. Monitor ALT levels at least monthly for first 6 months during therapy; if hepatotoxicity is likely teriflunomide-induced, start drug elimination procedures (eg, cholestyramine, activated charcoal)** and monitor liver function tests weekly until normalized. Discontinuation of therapy may be considered if transaminases increase >3 x ULN.

Use of leflunomide has been associated with interstitial lung disease; discontinue in patients who develop new onset or worsening of pulmonary symptoms. Drug elimination procedures should be considered (eg, cholestyramine, activated charcoal) if evidence of interstitial lung disease; fatal outcomes have been reported. May increase susceptibility to infection, including opportunistic pathogens. Severe infections, sepsis, and fatalities have been reported with leflunomide. One case of fatal sepsis has been reported with teriflunomide. Not recommended in patients with severe immunodeficiency, bone marrow dysplasia, or severe, uncontrolled infections. Caution should be exercised when considering the use in patients with a history of new/recurrent infections, with conditions that predispose them to infections, or with chronic, latent, or localized infections. Patients who develop a new infection while undergoing treatment should be monitored closely; consider suspension or discontinuation of therapy and drug elimination procedures if infection is serious.

Use may affect defenses against malignancies; impact on the development and course of malignancies is not fully defined. As compared to the general population, an increased risk of lymphoma has been noted in clinical trials with use of some immunosuppressive medications. Use with caution in patients with a prior history of significant hematologic abnormalities; avoid use with bone marrow dysplasia. Neutropenia, leukopenia, and thrombocytopenia have been reported in clinical trials. Use of leflunomide has been associated with rare pancytopenia, agranulocytosis, and thrombocytopenia, therefore, a similar risk may be expected with teriflunomide. Monitoring of hematologic function is required; discontinue if evidence of bone marrow suppression and begin drug elimination procedures (eg, cholestyramine, activated charcoal). If coadministered with other potential immunosuppressive agents or switching from teriflunomide to another known immunosuppressant, increased monitoring for hematological adverse effects is necessary. Rare cases of dermatologic reactions (including Stevens-Johnson syndrome and toxic epidermal necrolysis) have been reported with leflunomide, therefore patients taking teriflunomide may also be at risk; discontinue if evidence of severe dermatologic reaction occurs, and begin drug elimination procedures (eg, cholestyramine or activated charcoal). Cases of peripheral neuropathy (including polyneuropathy and mononeuropathy) have been reported; use with caution in patients >60 years of age, receiving concomitant neurotoxic medications, or patients with diabetes; discontinue if evidence of peripheral neuropathy occurs and begin drug elimination procedures (eg, cholestyramine, activated charcoal).

Transient acute renal failure, most likely due to acute uric acid nephropathy has been reported. Increases in blood pressure have been reported; monitor at initiation of therapy and periodically thereafter.

Safety has not been established in patients with latent tuberculosis infection. Patients should be screened for tuberculosis and if necessary, treated prior to initiating therapy. Potentially significant drug-drug interactions may exist, requiring dose or frequency adjustment, additional monitoring, and/or selection of alternative therapy. Patients should be brought up to date with all immunizations before initiating therapy. Live vaccines should not be given concurrently; there is no data available concerning secondary transmission of live vaccines in patients receiving therapy. Due to variations in clearance, it may take up to 2 years to reach low levels of teriflunomide metabolite serum concentrations. A drug elimination procedure using cholestyramine or activated charcoal is recommended when a more rapid elimination is needed. If a response to teriflunomide had already been observed, the use of a rapid elimination procedure may result in the return of disease activity. **[U.S. Boxed Warning]: Based on animal data, teriflunomide may cause major birth defects if used in pregnant women. Teriflunomide is contraindicated in pregnant women or women of childbearing potential who are not using reliable contraception. Pregnancy must be avoided during therapy or prior to completing the accelerated elimination treatment protocol.**

Adverse Reactions

Cardiovascular: Hypertension, palpitations

Central nervous system: Anxiety, burning sensation, headache, parasthesia, sciatica

Dermatologic: Acne vulgaris, alopecia, pruritus

Endocrine & metabolic: Hyperkalemia, hypophosphatemia, increased gamma-glutamyl transferase, weight loss

Gastrointestinal: Abdominal distension, abdominal pain, diarrhea, nausea, viral gastroenteritis

Genitourinary: Cystitis

Hematologic & oncologic: Decreased platelet count, leukopenia, lymphocytopenia, neutropenia
Hepatic: Increased serum ALT, increased serum AST
Hypersensitivity: Seasonal allergy
Infection: Herpes simplex infection, influenza, serious infection
Neuromuscular & skeletal: Arthralgia, carpal tunnel syndrome, musculoskeletal pain, myalgia, peripheral neuropathy
Ophthalmic: Blurred vision, conjunctivitis
Renal: Renal failure (transient)
Respiratory: Bronchitis, sinusitis, upper respiratory tract infection
Rare but important or life-threatening: Cytomegalovirus disease (reactivation), jaundice, increased serum creatinine, infection, myocardial infarction

Drug Interactions

Metabolism/Transport Effects Substrate of BCRP; **Inhibits** BCRP, CYP2C8 (moderate), SLCO1B1; **Induces** CYP1A2 (moderate)

Avoid Concomitant Use

Avoid concomitant use of Teriflunomide with any of the following: BCG; Leflunomide; Natalizumab; PAZOPanib; Pimecrolimus; Tacrolimus (Topical); Tofacitinib; Vaccines (Live)

Increased Effect/Toxicity

Teriflunomide may increase the levels/effects of: BCRP/ABCG2 Substrates; CYP2C8 Substrates; Natalizumab; OAT3 Substrates; OATP1B1/SLCO1B1 Substrates; PAZOPanib; Repaglinide; Rosuvastatin; Tofacitinib; Topotecan; Vaccines (Live)

The levels/effects of Teriflunomide may be increased by: Denosumab; Leflunomide; Pimecrolimus; Roflumilast; Tacrolimus (Topical); Trastuzumab

Decreased Effect

Teriflunomide may decrease the levels/effects of: BCG; Caffeine and Caffeine Containing Products; Coccidioides immitis Skin Test; CYP1A2 Substrates; Sipuleucel-T; Vaccines (Inactivated); Vaccines (Live); Warfarin

The levels/effects of Teriflunomide may be decreased by: Bile Acid Sequestrants; Charcoal, Activated; Echinacea

Storage/Stability Store at 20°C to 25°C (68°F to 77°F); excursions permitted to 15°C to 30°C (59°F to 86°F).

Mechanism of Action Teriflunomide is an immunomodulatory agent that inhibits pyrimidine synthesis, resulting in antiproliferative and anti-inflammatory effects. It may reduce the number of activated lymphocytes in the CNS.

Pharmacodynamics/Kinetics

Distribution: V_d: IV: 11 L
Protein binding: >99%
Metabolism: Primarily by hydrolysis to minor metabolites; secondary pathways include oxidation, conjugation, and N-acetylation
Half-life elimination: Median: 18-19 days; enterohepatic recycling appears to contribute to the long half-life of this agent, since activated charcoal and cholestyramine substantially reduce plasma half-life
Time to peak, plasma: 1-4 hours
Excretion: Feces (~38%); urine (~23%)

Dosage

Multiple sclerosis: Adults: Oral:
U.S. labeling: 7 mg or 14 mg once daily
Canadian labeling: 14 mg once daily

Dosage adjustment in renal impairment:

Mild, moderate, or severe impairment: No dosage adjustment necessary.

Severe impairment requiring dialysis: Data from a small pharmacokinetic study (n=5) suggest that hemodialysis removes a negligible amount of teriflunomide (Bergner, 2013); the Canadian labeling recommends avoiding use in this patient population.

Dosage adjustment in hepatic impairment:

Mild to moderate impairment: No dosage adjustment necessary.

Severe impairment: Use is contraindicated (has not been studied).

Dosage adjustment in hepatic toxicity: ALT elevations >3 times ULN: Discontinue teriflunomide and initiate cholestyramine or activated charcoal to enhance elimination

Drug elimination procedure: To achieve nondetectable serum concentrations (<0.02 mg/L) of teriflunomide administer either of the following:

Cholestyramine: 8 g every 8 hours for 11 days. If not tolerated, may decrease to 4 g every 8 hours for 11 days. The 11 days do not need to be consecutive unless plasma concentrations need to be lowered rapidly.

or

Activated charcoal: 50 g every 12 hours for 11 days. The 11 days do not need to be consecutive unless plasma concentrations need to be lowered rapidly.

Note: Both treatments have successfully lead to >98% decrease in teriflunomide concentrations.

Dietary Considerations May be taken with or without food.

Administration Administer without regard to meals. Hazardous agent; use appropriate precautions for handling and disposal (meets NIOSH 2014 criteria).

Monitoring Parameters CBC within 6 months of initiation and periodically thereafter based on signs/symptoms of infection; serum creatinine; serum transaminase and bilirubin within 6 months of initiation of therapy and monthly during the initial 6 months of treatment. In addition, monitor for signs/symptoms of severe infection, abnormalities in hepatic function tests, symptoms of hepatotoxicity, and blood pressure (baseline and periodically thereafter). Monitor hepatic function tests weekly until normalized in patients with suspected teriflunomide-induced hepatotoxicity. Screen for tuberculosis and pregnancy prior to therapy.

Dosage Forms

Tablet, Oral:

Aubagio: 7 mg, 14 mg

Dosage Forms: Canada

Tablet, Oral:

Aubagio: 14 mg

Teriparatide (ter i PAR a tide)

Brand Names: U.S. Forteo

Brand Names: Canada Forteo®

Index Terms Parathyroid Hormone (1-34); Recombinant Human Parathyroid Hormone (1-34); rhPTH(1-34)

Pharmacologic Category Parathyroid Hormone Analog

Use Treatment of osteoporosis in postmenopausal women at high risk of fracture; treatment of primary or hypogonadal osteoporosis in men at high risk of fracture; treatment of glucocorticoid-induced osteoporosis in men and women at high risk for fracture

Pregnancy Risk Factor C

Pregnancy Considerations Adverse events were observed in animal studies; the effect on human fetal development has not been studied. Teriparatide is not indicated for use in pregnant or premenopausal women.

Breast-Feeding Considerations Indicated for use in postmenopausal women. Studies have not been conducted to determine excretion in breast milk. Not recommended for use in breast-feeding women.

Contraindications Hypersensitivity to teriparatide or any component of the formulation

Canadian labeling: Additional contraindications (not in U.S. labeling): Preexisting hypercalcemia; severe renal impairment; metabolic bone diseases other than primary osteoporosis (including hyperparathyroidism and Paget's disease of the bone); unexplained elevations of alkaline phosphatase; prior external beam or implant radiation therapy involving the skeleton; bone metastases or history of skeletal malignancies; pregnancy; breast-feeding mothers; pediatric patients or young adults with open epiphysis

Warnings/Precautions [U.S. Boxed Warning]: In animal studies, teriparatide has been associated with an increase in osteosarcoma; risk was dependent on both dose and duration. Avoid use in patients with an increased risk of osteosarcoma (including Paget's disease, prior radiation, unexplained elevation of alkaline phosphatase, or in patients with open epiphyses). Do not use in patients with a history of skeletal metastases, hyperparathyroidism, or preexisting hypercalcemia. Not for use in patients with metabolic bone disease other than osteoporosis. Use caution in patients with active or recent urolithiasis. Use caution in patients at risk of orthostasis (including concurrent antihypertensive therapy), or in patients who may not tolerate transient hypotension (cardiovascular or cerebrovascular disease). Use caution in patients with cardiac, renal or hepatic impairment (limited data available concerning safety and efficacy). Use in severe renal impairment is contraindicated in the Canadian labeling. Use of teriparatide for longer than 2 years is not recommended. Not approved for use in pediatric patients.

Adverse Reactions

Cardiovascular: Chest pain, orthostatic hypotension (transient), syncope

Central nervous system: Anxiety, depression, dizziness, insomnia, vertigo

Dermatologic: Rash

Endocrine & metabolic: Hypercalcemia, hyperuricemia

Gastrointestinal: Dyspepsia, gastritis, nausea, vomiting

Neuromuscular & skeletal: Arthralgia, leg cramps, weakness

Respiratory: Dyspnea, pharyngitis, pneumonia, rhinitis

Miscellaneous: Antibodies to teriparatide, herpes zoster

Rare but important or life-threatening: Acute dyspnea, allergic reactions, edema (facial/oral), hypercalcemia >13 mg/dL, injection site reactions (bruising, pain, swelling), muscle spasm, osteosarcoma, urticaria

Drug Interactions

Metabolism/Transport Effects None known.

Avoid Concomitant Use There are no known interactions where it is recommended to avoid concomitant use.

Increased Effect/Toxicity There are no known significant interactions involving an increase in effect.

Decreased Effect There are no known significant interactions involving a decrease in effect.

Storage/Stability Store at 2°C to 8°C (36°F to 46°F); do not freeze. Protect from light. Discard pen 28 days after first injection. Do not use if solution is cloudy, colored, or contains solid particles.

Mechanism of Action Teriparatide is a recombinant formulation of endogenous parathyroid hormone (PTH), containing a 34-amino-acid sequence which is identical to the N-terminal portion of this hormone. The pharmacologic activity of teriparatide, which is similar to the physiologic activity of PTH, includes stimulating osteoblast function, increasing gastrointestinal calcium absorption, and increasing renal tubular reabsorption of calcium. Treatment with teriparatide results in increased bone mineral density, bone mass, and strength. In postmenopausal women, teriparatide has been shown to decrease osteoporosis-related fractures.

Pharmacodynamics/Kinetics

Distribution: V_d: ~0.12 L/kg

Metabolism: Hepatic (nonspecific proteolysis)

Bioavailability: 95%

Half-life elimination: IV: 5 minutes; SubQ: ~1 hour

Time to peak, serum: ~30 minutes

Excretion: Urine (as metabolites)

Dosage SubQ: Adults: 20 mcg once daily; **Note:** Initial administration should occur under circumstances in which the patient may sit or lie down, in the event of orthostasis.

Dosage adjustment in renal impairment: No dosage adjustment necessary. Bioavailability and half-life increase with CrCl <30 mL/minute. Use in severe renal impairment is contraindicated in the Canadian labeling.

Dosage adjustment in hepatic impairment: No dosage adjustment provided in manufacturer's labeling (has not been studied).

Dietary Considerations Ensure adequate calcium and vitamin D intake; if dietary intake is inadequate, dietary supplementation is recommended. Women and men should consume:

Calcium: 1000 mg/day (men: 50-70 years) **or** 1200 mg/day (women ≥51 years and men ≥71 years) (IOM, 2011; NOF, 2013)

Vitamin D: 800-1000 IU/day (men and women ≥50 years) (NOF, 2013). Recommended Dietary Allowance (RDA): 600 IU/day (men and women ≤70 years) **or** 800 IU/day (men and women ≥71 years) (IOM, 2011).

Administration Administer by subcutaneous injection into the thigh or abdominal wall. Initial administration should occur under circumstances in which the patient may sit or lie down, in the event of orthostasis. **Note:** The 3 mL prefilled pen (Canadian availability; not available in U.S.) must be primed prior to each dose.

Monitoring Parameters

Osteoporosis: Bone mineral density (BMD) should be reevaluated every 2 years (or more frequently) after initiating therapy (NOF, 2013); annual measurements of height and weight, assessment of chronic back pain; serum calcium and 25(OH)D; consider measuring biochemical markers of bone turnover

Paget's disease: Alkaline phosphatase; pain; serum calcium and 25(OH)D

Reference Range

Calcium (total): Adults: 9.0-11.0 mg/dL (2.05-2.54 mmol/L), may slightly decrease with aging

Phosphorus: 2.5-4.5 mg/dL (0.81-1.45 mmol/L)

Vitamin D: There is no clear consensus on a reference range for total serum 25(OH)D concentrations or the validity of this level as it relates clinically to bone health. In addition, there is significant variability in the reporting of serum 25(OH)D levels as a result of different assay types in use; however, the following ranges have been suggested:

Adults (IOM, 2011): Sufficient levels in practically all persons: ≥20 ng/mL (50 nmol/L); concern for risk of toxicity: >50 ng/mL (125 nmol/L)

Osteoporosis patients (NOF, 2013): Recommended level to reach and maintain: ~30 ng/mL (75 nmol/L)

Additional Information Teriparatide was formerly marketed as a diagnostic agent (Perithar™); that agent was withdrawn from the market in 1997. Teriparatide (Forteo®) is manufactured through recombinant DNA technology using a strain of *E. coli.*

Patients are encouraged to enroll in the Forteo® Patient Registry which is designed to monitor the potential risk of osteosarcoma and teriparatide treatment. Enrollment information may be found at www.forteoregistry.rti.org or by calling 1-866-382-6813.

Dosage Forms

Solution, Subcutaneous:

Forteo: 600 mcg/2.4 mL (2.4 mL)

Dosage Forms: Canada

Injection, solution:

Forteo®: 250 mcg/mL (3 mL)

Terlipressin [INT] (ter li PRES sin)

International Brand Names Acupressin (IN); Glipressina (IT); Glycylpressin (AT, DE); Glypressin (AR, AU, BE, CH, CN, CY, CZ, DK, EC, EE, EG, ES, FI, GB, GR, HK, HR, HU, IE, IL, IS, JO, KR, LT, LU, MY, NL, NO, NZ, PE, PH, PL, QA, RO, SA, SE, SG, SI, SK, TH, TR, TW, UY, VN); Glypressine (FR, PT); Glyverase (MX); Haemopressin (AT, CH, DE, FR, NL); Lucassin (AU); Novapressin (PK); Remestyp (BG, CZ, IN, KR, PL, RU); Remwestyp (CN); Stemflova (FI, NO); Teripin (KR); Terlissin (TW); Terlistat (IN); Variquel (BE, DK, GB, SE)

Index Terms Triglycyl Lysine Vasopressin

Pharmacologic Category Hormone, Posterior Pituitary

Reported Use Treatment of acute esophageal variceal hemorrhage; treatment of hepatorenal syndrome (type 1) in combination with albumin

Dosage Range Adults: IV: 1-2 mg every 4-8 hours

Product Availability Product available in various countries; not currently available in the U.S.

Dosage Forms

Injection, powder for reconstitution: 1 mg

◆ **Tersi** *see* Selenium Sulfide *on page 1877*

Tesamorelin (tes a moe REL in)

Brand Names: U.S. Egrifta

Index Terms Tesamorelin Acetate; TH9507

Pharmacologic Category Growth Hormone Releasing Factor

Use HIV-associated lipodystrophy: Reduction of excess abdominal fat in HIV-infected patients with lipodystrophy

Pregnancy Risk Factor X

Dosage HIV-associated lipodystrophy: Adults: SubQ: 2 mg once daily

Dosing adjustment for toxicity: Consider discontinuing with persistent elevations of IGF-1 (eg, >3 standard deviation scores). Discontinue if symptoms of hypersensitivity occur.

Dosage adjustment in renal impairment: There are no dosage adjustmentsprovided in the manufacturer's labeling (has not been studied).

Dosage adjustment in hepatic impairment: There are no dosage adjustments provided in the manufacturer's labeling (has not been studied).

Additional Information Complete prescribing information should be consulted for additional detail.

Dosage Forms

Solution Reconstituted, Subcutaneous [preservative free]:

Egrifta: 1 mg (1 ea); 2 mg (1 ea)

◆ **Tesamorelin Acetate** *see* Tesamorelin *on page 2010*

◆ **TESPA** *see* Thiotepa *on page 2030*

◆ **Tessalon Perles** *see* Benzonatate *on page 247*

◆ **Tessalon Perles** *see* Benzonatate *on page 247*

◆ **Testim** *see* Testosterone *on page 2010*

◆ **Testopel** *see* Testosterone *on page 2010*

Testosterone (tes TOS ter one)

Brand Names: U.S. Androderm; AndroGel; AndroGel Pump; Aveed; Axiron; Depo-Testosterone; First-Testosterone; First-Testosterone MC; Fortesta; Striant; Testim; Testopel; Vogelxo; Vogelxo Pump

Brand Names: Canada Andriol; Androderm; AndroGel; Andropository; Axiron; Delatestryl; Depotest 100; Everone 200; PMS-Testosterone; Testim

Index Terms Natesto; Testosterone Cypionate; Testosterone Enanthate; Testosterone Undecanoate

Pharmacologic Category Androgen

Additional Appendix Information

Beers Criteria – Potentially Inappropriate Medications for Geriatrics *on page 2271*

Use

Injection: Androgen replacement therapy in the treatment of delayed male puberty; male hypogonadism (primary or hypogonadotropic); inoperable metastatic female breast cancer (enanthate only)

Pellet: Androgen replacement therapy in the treatment of delayed male puberty; male hypogonadism (primary or hypogonadotropic)

Buccal system, intranasal gel, topical gel, topical solution, transdermal system: Male hypogonadism (primary or hypogonadotropic)

Capsule (not available in U.S.): Conditions associated with a deficiency or absence of endogenous testosterone

Pregnancy Risk Factor X

Pregnancy Considerations Testosterone may cause adverse effects, including masculinization of the female fetus, if used during pregnancy. Females who are or may become pregnant should also avoid skin-to-skin contact to areas where testosterone has been applied topically on another person.

Breast-Feeding Considerations High levels of endogenous maternal testosterone, such as those caused by certain ovarian cysts, suppress milk production. Maternal serum testosterone levels generally fall following pregnancy and return to normal once breast-feeding is stopped. The amount of testosterone present in breast milk or the effect to the nursing infant following maternal supplementation is not known. Some products are contraindicated while breast-feeding. Females who are nursing should avoid skin-to-skin contact to areas where testosterone has been applied topically on another person.

Contraindications

Hypersensitivity to testosterone or any component of the formulation; males with carcinoma of the breast or known or suspected carcinoma of the prostate; women who are breast-feeding, pregnant, or who may become pregnant.

Depo-Testosterone: Also contraindicated in serious hepatic, renal, or cardiac disease

Documentation of allergenic cross-reactivity for androgens is limited. However, because of similarities in chemical structure and/or pharmacologic actions, the possibility of cross-sensitivity cannot be ruled out with certainty.

Warnings/Precautions Hazardous agent; use appropriate precautions for handling and disposal (NIOSH 2014 [group 3]).

When used to treat delayed male puberty, perform radiographic examination of the hand and wrist every 6 months to determine the rate of bone maturation. May cause hypercalcemia in patients with prolonged immobilization or cancer. May accelerate bone maturation without producing compensating gain in linear growth. May decrease glucose levels. May alter serum lipid profile; use caution with history of MI or coronary artery disease. Androgens may worsen BPH; patients may also be at an increased risk of prostate cancer. Use caution in elderly patients or patients with other demographic factors which may increase the risk of prostatic carcinoma; careful monitoring is required. Discontinue therapy if urethral obstruction develops in patients with BPH (use lower dose if restarted). Withhold therapy pending urological evaluation in patients with palpable prostate nodule or induration, PSA >4 ng/mL, or PSA >3 ng/mL in men at high risk of prostate cancer (Bhasin, 2010). Venous thromboembolic events including deep vein thrombosis (DVT) and pulmonary embolism (PE) have been reported with testosterone products. Evaluate patients with symptoms of pain, edema, warmth and erythema in the lower extremity for DVT and those with acute shortness of breath for PE. Discontinue therapy if a venous thromboembolism is suspected. Use with caution in patients with diseases that may be exacerbated by fluid retention including cardiac, hepatic, or renal dysfunction; testosterone may cause fluid retention. May cause gynecomastia. Large doses may suppress spermatogenesis. During treatment for metastatic breast cancer, women should be monitored for signs of virilization; discontinue if mild virilization is present to prevent irreversible symptoms.

May be inappropriate in the elderly due to potential risk of cardiac problems and contraindication for use in men with prostate cancer; in general, avoid use in older adults except in the setting of moderate-to-severe hypogonadism (Beers Criteria). In addition, elderly patients may be at greater risk for prostatic hyperplasia, prostate cancer, fluid retention, and transaminase elevations.

Prolonged use of high doses of oral androgens has been associated with serious hepatic effects (peliosis hepatis, hepatic neoplasms, cholestatic hepatitis, jaundice). Prolonged use of intramuscular testosterone enanthate has been associated with multiple hepatic adenomas. Discontinue therapy if signs or symptoms of hepatic dysfunction (such as jaundice) develop.

May potentiate sleep apnea in some male patients (obesity or chronic lung disease). May increase hematocrit requiring dose adjustment or discontinuation; discontinue therapy if hematocrit exceeds 54%; may reinitiate at lower dose (Bhasin, 2010).

Testosterone undecanoate injection: **[U.S. Boxed Warning]: Serious pulmonary oil microembolism (POME) reactions and anaphylaxis have been reported with testosterone undecanoate injection. Reactions include anaphylaxis, chest pain, urge to cough, dizziness, dyspnea, throat tightening, and syncope; may be life threatening. Reactions may occur after any injection during the course of therapy, including the first dose. Patients must be monitored for 30 minutes after injection. Due to the risk of serious POME reactions, Aveed is only available through the Aveed REMS program.** To minimize risk of adverse reactions, inject deeply into gluteal muscle.

[U.S. Boxed Warning]: Virilization in children has been reported following contact with unwashed or unclothed application sites of men using topical testosterone. Patients should strictly adhere to instructions for use in order to prevent secondary exposure. Virilization of female sexual partners has also been reported with male use of topical testosterone. Symptoms of virilization generally regress following removal of exposure; however, in some children, enlarged genitalia and bone age did not fully return to age appropriate normal. Signs of inappropriate virilization in women or children following secondary exposure to topical testosterone should be brought to the attention of a healthcare provider. Topical testosterone products (gels and solution) may have different doses, strengths, or application instructions that may result in different systemic exposure; these products are not interchangeable. Use of the intranasal gel is not recommended in patients with sinus disease, mucosal inflammatory disorders (eg, Sjogren syndrome), or with a history of nasal disorders, nasal or sinus surgery, nasal fracture within the previous 6 months, or nasal fracture that caused a deviated anterior nasal septum. Safety and efficacy have not been established in males with a BMI >35 kg/m^2. Transdermal patch may contain conducting metal (eg, aluminum); remove patch prior to MRI. Gels, solution, transdermal, and buccal system have not been evaluated in males <18 years of age; safety and efficacy of injection have not been established in males <12 years of age. Some testosterone products may be chemically synthesized from soy. Some products may contain castor oil. Use of Axiron in males with BMI >35 kg/m2 has not been established. Anabolic steroids may be abused; abuse may be associated with adverse physical and psychological effects. Dependance may occur when used outside of approved dosage/indications.

Benzyl alcohol and derivatives: Some dosage forms may contain benzyl alcohol; large amounts of benzyl alcohol (≥99 mg/kg/day) have been associated with a potentially fatal toxicity ("gasping syndrome") in neonates; the "gasping syndrome" consists of metabolic acidosis, respiratory distress, gasping respirations, CNS dysfunction (including convulsions, intracranial hemorrhage), hypotension, and cardiovascular collapse (AAP, 1997; CDC, 1982); some data suggests that benzoate displaces bilirubin from protein binding sites (Ahlfors, 2001); avoid or use dosage forms containing benzyl alcohol with caution in neonates. See manufacturer's labeling.

Adverse Reactions

Cardiovascular: Decreased blood pressure, deep vein thrombosis, edema, hypertension, increased blood pressure, vasodilatation

Central nervous system: Abnormal dreams, aggressive behavior, altered sense of smell, amnesia, anxiety, chills, depression, dizziness, emotional lability, excitement, fatigue, headache, hostility, insomnia, irritability, malaise, mood swings, nervousness, outbursts of anger, paresthesia, seizure, sleep apnea, suicidal ideation, taste disorder

Dermatologic: Acne vulgaris, alopecia, contact dermatitis, diaphoresis, erythema, folliculitis, hair discoloration, hyperhidrosis, pruritus, seborrhea, skin rash, xeroderma

Endocrine & metabolic: Change in libido, decreased gonadotropin, fluid retention, gynecomastia, hirsutism (increase in pubic hair growth), hot flash, hypercalcemia, hyperchloremia, hypercholesterolemia, hyperglycemia, hyperkalemia, hyperlipidemia, hypernatremia, hypoglycemia, hypokalemia, increased plasma estradiol concentration, inorganic phosphate retention, menstrual disease (including amenorrhea), weight gain

Gastrointestinal: Diarrhea, gastroesophageal reflux disease, gastrointestinal hemorrhage, gastrointestinal irritation, increased appetite, nausea, vomiting

Following buccal administration (most common): Dysgeusia, gingival pain, gingival swelling, mouth irritation (including gums), unpleasant taste

Genitourinary: Benign prostatic hypertrophy, difficulty in micturition, ejaculatory disorder, hematuria, impotence, irritable bladder, mastalgia, oligospermia, priapism, prostate induration, prostate specific antigen increase, prostatitis, spontaneous erections, testicular atrophy, urinary tract infection, virilization

Hepatic: Abnormal hepatic function tests, cholestatic hepatitis, cholestatic jaundice, hepatic insufficiency, hepatic necrosis, hepatocellular neoplasms, increased serum bilirubin, peliosis hepatis

Hematologic & oncologic: Anemia, clotting factors suppression, hemorrhage, increased hematocrit, increased hemoglobin, leukopenia, malignant neoplasm of prostate, polycythemia, prostate carcinoma

Hypersensitivity: Anaphylactoid reaction, hypersensitivity reaction (including pulmomary oil microembolism)

Local: Application site reaction (gel, solution), erythema at injection site, inflammation at injection site, pain at injection site

Transdermal system: Application site burning, application site erythema, application site induration, application site pruritus, application site vesicles (including burn-like blisters under system), local allergic contact dermatitis, local skin exfoliation

Neuromuscular & skeletal: Abnormal bone growth (accelerated), arthralgia, back pain, hemarthrosis, hyperkinesia, weakness
Ophthalmic: Increased lacrimation
Renal: Increased serum creatinine, polyuria
Respiratory: Bronchitis (≥3%), nasopharyngitis (≥3%), sinusitis (≥3%), upper respiratory tract infection (≥3%), dyspnea
Rare but important or life-threatening: Injection, gel: Abnormal erythropoiesis, abscess at injection site, anaphylaxis, androgenetic alopecia, asthma, cardiac arrest, cardiac failure, cerebrovascular accident, chronic obstructive pulmonary disease, cognitive dysfunction, diabetes mellitus, epididymitis, hearing loss (sudden), hematoma at injection site, hyperparathyroidism, hypersensitivity angiitis, increased intraocular pressure, Korsakoff's psychosis (nonalcoholic), migraine, myocardial infarction, personality disorder, prolonged prothrombin time, prostatic intraepithelial neoplasia, reversible ischemic neurological deficit, spermatocele, systemic lupus erythematosus, tachycardia, thrombocytopenia, thrombosis, urinary incontinence, venous insufficiency, vesicobullous rash, virilization (of children, following secondary exposure to topical gel [advanced bone age, aggressive behavior, enlargement of clitoris requiring surgery, enlargement of penis, increased erections, increased libido, pubic hair development]), vitreous detachment

Drug Interactions

Metabolism/Transport Effects Substrate of CYP2B6 (minor), CYP2C19 (minor), CYP2C9 (minor), CYP3A4 (minor); **Note:** Assignment of Major/Minor substrate status based on clinically relevant drug interaction potential

Avoid Concomitant Use

Avoid concomitant use of Testosterone with any of the following: Dehydroepiandrosterone

Increased Effect/Toxicity

Testosterone may increase the levels/effects of: Antidiabetic Agents; C1 inhibitors; CycloSPORINE (Systemic); Vitamin K Antagonists

The levels/effects of Testosterone may be increased by: Corticosteroids (Systemic); Dehydroepiandrosterone

Decreased Effect There are no known significant interactions involving a decrease in effect.

Storage/Stability

Androderm: Store at 20°C to 25°C (68°F to 77°F). Do not store outside of pouch. Excessive heat may cause system to burst.
AndroGel 1%, AndroGel 1.62%, Axiron: Store at 25°C (77°F); excursions are permitted between 15°C and 30°C (59°F and 86°F).
Fortesta, Testim: Store at 20°C to 25°C (68°F to 77°F); excursions are permitted between 15°C and 30°C (59°F and 86°F). Do not freeze.
Aveed: Store at 25°C (77°F); excursions are permitted between 15°C and 30°C (59°F and 86°F) Store in original container.
Depo-Testosterone: Store at room temperature. Protect from light.
Natesto: Store at 20°C and 25°C (68°F to 77°F); excursions are permitted between 15°C and 30°C (59°F and 86°F).
Striant: Store at 20°C to 25°C (68°F to 77°F). Protect from heat and moisture.
Testopel: Store in a cool location.

Mechanism of Action Principal endogenous androgen responsible for promoting the growth and development of the male sex organs and maintaining secondary sex characteristics in androgen-deficient males

Pharmacodynamics/Kinetics

Duration (route and ester dependent): IM: Cypionate and enanthate esters have longest duration, ≤2 to 4 weeks; Undecanoate 10 weeks; Gel: 24 to 48 hours; buccal system: 2 to 4 hours after removal
Absorption: Transdermal gel: ~10% of applied dose
Protein binding: 98%; bound to sex hormone-binding globulin (40%) and albumin
Metabolism: Hepatic; forms metabolites, including dihydrotestosterone (DHT) and estradiol (both active)
Half-life elimination: Variable: 10 to 100 minutes
Time to peak: IM undecanoate: 7 days (median; range: 4 to 42 days); Intranasal: ~40 minutes.
Excretion: Urine (90%); feces (6%)

Dosage

Adolescents and Adults: Males:
IM:
Primary hypogonadism or hypogonadotropic hypogonadism: Testosterone enanthate or testosterone cypionate: 50 to 400 mg every 2 to 4 weeks (FDA-approved dosing range); 75 to 100 mg/week or 150 to 200 mg every 2 weeks (Bhasin, 2010)
Delayed puberty: Testosterone enanthate: 50 to 200 mg every 2 to 4 weeks for a limited duration
Pellet (for subcutaneous implantation): Delayed puberty, primary hypogonadism or hypogonadotropic hypogonadism: 150 to 450 mg every 3 to 6 months
Adults:
IM: Females: Inoperable metastatic breast cancer: Testosterone enanthate: 200 to 400 mg every 2 to 4 weeks
IM: Males: Primary hypogonadism or hypogonadotropic hypogonadism: Testosterone undecanoate: Initial dose: 750 mg, followed by 750 mg administered 4 weeks later, then 750 mg administered every 10 weeks thereafter.
Intranasal: Males: Primary hypogonadism or hypogonadotropic hypogonadism: Testosterone gel: 11 mg (2 pump actuations; 1 actuation per nostril) administered intranasally 3 times daily (6 to 8 hours apart)
Oral: Males: Conditions associated with a deficiency or absence of endogenous testosterone: Capsule (Andriol; not available in U.S.): Initial: 120 to 160 mg daily in 2 divided doses for 2 to 3 weeks; adjust according to individual response; usual maintenance dose: 40 to 120 mg daily (in divided doses)
Topical: Primary male hypogonadism **or** hypogonadotropic hypogonadism:
Buccal: 30 mg twice daily (every 12 hours) applied to the gum region above the incisor tooth
Gel: Apply to clean, dry, intact skin. **Do not apply testosterone gel to the genitals**.
AndroGel 1%: 50 mg applied once daily in the morning to the shoulder and upper arms, or abdomen. Dosage may be increased to a maximum of 100 mg daily.
Dose adjustment based on testosterone levels:
Less than normal range: Increase dose from 50 mg to 75 mg or from 75 mg to 100 mg once daily
Greater than normal range: Decrease dose. Discontinue if consistently above normal at 50 mg daily
AndroGel 1.62%: 40.5 mg applied once daily in the morning to the shoulder and upper arms. Dosage may be increased to a maximum of 81 mg daily.
Dose adjustment based on testosterone levels:
>750 ng/dL: Decrease dose by 20.25 mg daily
≥350 ng/dL to ≤750 ng/dL: Maintain current dose
<350 ng/dL: Increase dose by 20.25 mg daily
Fortesta: 40 mg once daily in the morning. Apply to the thighs. Dosing range: 10 to 70 mg daily

Dose adjustment based on serum testosterone levels:

≥2500 ng/dL: Decrease dose by 20 mg daily

≥1250 to <2500 ng/dL: Decrease dose by 10 mg daily

≥500 and <1250 ng/dL: Maintain current dose

<500 ng/dL: Increase dose by 10 mg daily

Testim: 50 mg applied once daily (preferably in the morning) to the shoulder and upper arms. Dosage may be increased to a maximum of 100 mg daily.

Dose adjustment based on testosterone levels:

Less than normal range: Increase dose from 50 mg to 100 mg once daily

Greater than normal range: Decrease dose

Solution: Axiron: 60 mg once daily (dosage range: 30 to 120 mg daily). Apply to the axilla at the same time each morning; do not apply to other parts of the body. Apply to clean, dry, intact skin. **Do not apply testosterone solution to the genitals.**

Dose adjustment based on serum testosterone levels:

>1050 ng/dL: Decrease 60 mg daily dose to 30 mg daily; if levels >1050 ng/dL persist after dose reduction discontinue therapy

<300 ng/dL: Increase 60 mg daily dose to 90 mg daily, or increase 90 mg daily dose to 120 mg daily

Transdermal system (Androderm):

Initial: 4 mg daily (as one 4 mg/day patch; do **not** use two 2 mg/day patches)

Dose adjustment based on testosterone levels:

>930 ng/dL: Decrease dose to 2 mg daily

400 to 930 ng/dL: Continue 4 mg daily

<400 ng/dL: Increase dose to 6 mg daily (as one 4 mg/day and one 2 mg/day patch)

Dosing conversion: The 2.5 mg/day and the 5 mg/day patches have been discontinued in the U.S.; patients may be switched from the 2.5 mg/day patch, 5 mg/day patch, or the combination (ie, 7.5 mg/day) as follows:

From 2.5 mg/day patch to 2 mg/day patch

From 5 mg/day patch to 4 mg/day patch

From 7.5 mg daily (one 2.5 mg/day and one 5 mg/day patch) to 6 mg daily (one 2 mg/day and one 4 mg/day patch)

Note: Patch change should occur at the next scheduled dosing. Measure early morning testosterone concentrations ~2 weeks after switching therapy.

Dosage adjustment in renal impairment: There are no dosage adjustments provided in manufacturer's labeling (has not been studied). Use with caution; may enhance edema formation. Testosterone cypionate is contraindicated in serious renal disease.

Dosage adjustment in hepatic impairment: There are no dosage adjustments provided in manufacturer's labeling (has not been studied). Use with caution; may enhance edema formation. Testosterone cypionate is contraindicated in serious hepatic disease.

Dietary Considerations Testosterone USP may be synthesized from soy. Food and beverages have not been found to interfere with buccal system; ensure system is in place following eating, drinking, or brushing teeth.

Administration

IM: Administer by deep IM injection into the gluteal muscle.

Testosterone enanthate or testosterone cypionate: Warm to room temperature; shaking vial will help redissolve crystals that have formed after storage.

Testosterone undecanoate: Inject into the gluteus medius; avoid intravascular injection; may lead to pulmonary oil microembolism.

Intranasal gel (Natesto): With first time use, invert the pump and prime by depressing the pump 10 times discarding any product dispensed directly into a sink. Administer doses 6 to 8 hours apart, preferably at the same time each day. Insert actuator into nostril until pump reaches base of nose; tilt so the tip is in contact with the lateral wall of nostril. Depress slowly until pump stops, then remove from nose while wiping tip to transfer gel to lateral side of nostril. Following administration, press on the nostrils at a point just below the bridge of the nose and lightly massage. Refrain from blowing nose or sniffing for 1 hour after administration. If gel gets on hands, wash with warm soap and water. Temporarily discontinue with episodes of severe rhinitis; if severe rhinitis symptoms persist consider an alternative therapy.

Oral, buccal application (Striant): One mucoadhesive for buccal application (buccal system) should be applied to a comfortable area above the incisor tooth. Gently push the curved side against the upper gum. Hold buccal system firmly in place by pushing down on outside of the upper lip for 30 seconds to ensure adhesion. The buccal system should adhere to gum until it is removed. Rotate to alternate sides of mouth with each application. If the buccal system falls out, replace with a new system. If the system falls out within the first 8 hours of dosing, replace with a new buccal system and continue for a total of 12 hours from the placement of the first system. If the system falls out of position after 8 hours of dosing, a new buccal system should be applied and it may remain in place for 12 hours, then continue with the next regularly scheduled dosing. System will soften and mold to shape of gum as it absorbs moisture from mouth. Do not chew or swallow the buccal system. The buccal system will not dissolve; gently remove by sliding downwards from gum; avoid scratching gum.

Oral, capsule (Andriol; not available in the U.S.): Should be administered with meals. Should be swallowed whole; do not crush or chew.

Subcutaneous implant (Testopel): Using strict sterile technique, must be surgically implanted.

Transdermal patch (Androderm): Apply patch to clean, dry area of skin on the back, abdomen, upper arms, or thigh. Do not apply to bony areas or parts of the body that are subject to prolonged pressure while sleeping or sitting. **Do not apply to the scrotum.** Avoid showering, washing the site, or swimming for 3 hours after application. Following patch removal, mild skin irritation may be treated with OTC hydrocortisone cream. A small amount of triamcinolone acetonide 0.1% cream may be applied under the system to decrease irritation; do not use ointment. Patch should be applied nightly. Rotate administration sites, allowing 7 days between applying to the same site.

Topical gel and solution: Apply to clean, dry, intact skin. Application sites should be allowed to dry for a few minutes prior to dressing. Hands should be washed with soap and water after application. **Do not apply testosterone gel or solution to the genitals.** Alcohol-based gels and solutions are flammable; avoid fire, flames, or smoking until dry. Testosterone may be transferred to another person following skin-to-skin contact with the application site. Strict adherence to application instructions is needed in order to decrease secondary exposure. Thoroughly wash hands after application and cover application site with clothing (ie, shirt) once gel or solution has dried, or clean application site thoroughly with soap and water prior to contact in order to minimize transfer. In addition to skin-to-skin contact, secondary exposure has also been reported following exposure to secondary items (eg, towel, shirt, sheets). If secondary exposure occurs, the other person should thoroughly wash the skin with soap and water as soon as possible.

AndroGel 1%, AndroGel 1.62%, Testim: Apply (preferably in the morning) to the shoulder and upper arms; AndroGel 1% may also be applied to the abdomen. Do not apply AndroGel 1% to the genitals, chest, axillae, knees, or back; AndroGel 1.62% to the abdomen, genitals, chest, axillae, or knees; or Testim to the genitals or abdomen. Area of application should be limited to what will be covered by a short sleeve t-shirt. Apply at the same time each day. Upon opening the packet(s), the entire contents should be squeezed into the palm of the hand and immediately applied to the application site(s). Alternatively, a portion may be squeezed onto palm of hand and applied, repeating the process at the same or other site until entire packet has been applied. Application site(s) should not be washed for ≥2 hours following application of AndroGel 1.62% or Testim, or >5 hours for AndroGel 1%.

AndroGel 1% multidose pump: Prime pump 3 times (and discard this portion of product) prior to initial use. Each actuation delivers 12.5 mg of testosterone (4 actuations = 50 mg; 6 actuations = 75 mg; 8 actuations = 100 mg); each actuation may be applied individually or all at the same time. Application site should not be washed for >5 hours following application.

AndroGel 1.62% multidose pump: Prime pump 3 times (and discard this portion of product) prior to initial use. Each actuation delivers 20.25 mg of testosterone (2 actuations = 40.5 mg; 3 actuations = 60.75 mg; 4 actuations = 81 mg); each actuation may be applied individually or all at the same time. Avoid washing the site or swimming for ≥2 hours following application.

Axiron: Apply using the applicator to the axilla at the same time each morning. Do not apply to other parts of the body (eg, abdomen, genitals, shoulders, upper arms). Avoid washing the site or swimming for 2 hours after application. Prior to first use, prime the applicator pump by depressing it 3 times (discard this portion of the product). After priming, position the nozzle over the applicator cup and depress pump fully one time; ensure liquid enters cup. Each pump actuation delivers testosterone 30 mg. No more than 30 mg (one pump) should be added to the cup at one time. The total dose should be divided between axilla (example, 30 mg/day: apply to one axilla only; 60 mg/day: apply 30 mg to each axilla; 90 mg/day: apply 30 mg to each axilla, allow to dry, then apply an additional 30 mg to one axilla; etc). To apply dose, keep applicator upright and wipe into the axilla; if solution runs or drips, use cup to wipe. Do not rub into skin with fingers or hand. If more than one 30 mg dose is needed, repeat process. Apply roll-on or stick antiperspirants or deodorants prior to testosterone. Once application site is dry, cover with clothing. After use, rinse applicator under running water and pat dry with a tissue. The application site and dose of this product are not interchangeable with other topical testosterone products.

Fortesta: Apply to skin of front and inner thighs. Do not apply to other parts of the body. Use one finger to rub gel evenly onto skin of each thigh. Avoid showering, washing the site, or swimming for 2 hours after application. Prior to first dose, prime the pump by holding canister upright and fully depressing the pump 8 times (discard this portion of the product). Each pump actuation delivers testosterone 10 mg. The total dose should be divided between thighs (example, 10 mg/day: apply 10 mg to one thigh only; 20 mg/day: apply 10 mg to each thigh; 30 mg/day: apply 20 mg to one thigh and 10 mg to the other thigh; etc). Once application site is dry, cover with clothing. The application site and dose of this product are not interchangeable with other topical testosterone products.

Hazardous agent; use appropriate precautions for handling and disposal (NIOSH 2014 [group 3]).

Monitoring Parameters Periodic liver function tests, lipid panel, hemoglobin and hematocrit (prior to therapy, at 3 to 6 months, then annually); radiologic examination of wrist and hand every 6 months (when using in prepubertal children). Withhold initial treatment with hematocrit >50% (discontinue therapy if hematocrit exceeds 54% [Bhasin, 2010]), hyperviscosity, untreated obstructive sleep apnea, or uncontrolled severe heart failure. Monitor urine and serum calcium and signs of virilization in women treated for breast cancer. Serum glucose (may be decreased by testosterone, monitor patients with diabetes). Evaluate males for response to treatment and adverse events 3 to 6 months after initiation and then annually.

Aveed: Monitor for 30 minutes after injection; appropriate treatment should be available in the event of a serous POME reaction or anaphylaxis.

Bone mineral density: Monitor after 1 to 2 years of therapy in hypogonadal men with osteoporosis or low trauma fracture (Bhasin, 2010)

PSA: In men >40 years of age with baseline PSA >0.6 ng/mL, PSA and prostate exam (prior to therapy, at 3 to 6 months, then as based on current guidelines). Withhold treatment pending urological evaluation in patients with palpable prostate nodule or induration or PSA >4 ng/mL or if PSA >3 ng/mL in men at high risk of prostate cancer (Bhasin, 2010).

Do not treat with severe untreated BPH with IPSS symptom score >19.

Serum testosterone: After initial dose titration (if applicable), monitor 3 to 6 months after initiating treatment, then annually.

Injection:

Testosterone enanthate or cypionate: Measure midway between injections. Adjust dose or frequency if testosterone concentration is <400 ng/dL or >700 ng/dL (Bhasin, 2010).

Testosterone undecanoate: Measure just prior to each subsequent injection and adjust dosing interval to maintain serum testosterone in mid-normal range (Bhasin, 2010).

AndroGel 1%, Testim: Morning serum testosterone levels ~14 days after start of therapy or dose adjustments

AndroGel 1.62%: Morning serum testosterone levels after 14 and 28 days of starting therapy or dose adjustments and periodically thereafter

Androderm: Morning serum testosterone levels (following application the previous evening) ~14 days after start of therapy or dose adjustments

Axiron: Serum testosterone levels can be measured 2 to 8 hours after application and after 14 days of starting therapy or dose adjustments

Fortesta: Serum testosterone levels can be measured 2 hours after application and after 14 and 35 days of starting therapy or dose adjustments

Natesto: Measure total serum testosterone periodically, beginning 1 month after initiating therapy. Discontinue therapy if if the total serum testosterone consistently exceed 1050 ng/dL. If total serum testosterone is consistently <300 ng/dL consider an alternative therapy.

Striant: Examine application area of gums; total serum testosterone 4 to 12 weeks after initiating treatment, prior to morning dose. Discontinue therapy if the total serum testosterone are consistently outside of the normal range (300 to 1050 ng/dL).

Testopel: Measure at the end of the dosing interval (Bhasin, 2010)

Reference Range

Total testosterone, males:

12 to 13 years: <800 ng/dL
14 years: <1200 ng/dL
15 to 16 years: 100 to 1200 ng/dL
17 to 18 years: 300 to 1200 ng/dL
19 to 40 years: 300 to 950 ng/dL
>40 years: 240 to 950 ng/dL

Free testosterone, males: 9 to 30 ng/dL

Product Availability Natesto (testosterone nasal gel): FDA approved May 2014; anticipated availability is currently unknown.

Dosage Forms

Cream, Transdermal:

First-Testosterone MC: 2% (60 g)

Gel, Transdermal:

AndroGel: 25 mg/2.5 g (2.5 g); 50 mg/5 g (5 g); 40.5 mg/2.5 g (1.62%) (2.5 g); 20.25 mg/1.25 g (1.62%) (1.25 g)

AndroGel Pump: 12.5 mg/actuation (1%) (75 g); 20.25 mg/actuation (1.62%) (75 g)

Fortesta: 10 mg/actuation (2%) (60 g)

Testim: 50 mg/5 g (5 g)

Vogelxo: 50 mg/5 g (5 g)

Vogelxo Pump: 12.5 mg/actuation (1%) (75 g)

Generic: 25 mg/2.5 g (2.5 g); 50 mg/5 g (5 g); 10 mg/actuation (2%) (60 g); 12.5 mg/actuation (1%) (75 g)

Miscellaneous, Buccal:

Striant: 30 mg (60 ea)

Ointment, Transdermal:

First-Testosterone: 2% (60 g)

Patch 24 Hour, Transdermal:

Androderm: 2 mg/24 hr (1 ea, 60 ea); 4 mg/24 hr (1 ea, 30 ea)

Pellet, Implant:

Testopel: 75 mg (10 ea, 100 ea)

Solution, Intramuscular:

Aveed: 750 mg/3 mL (3 mL)

Depo-Testosterone: 100 mg/mL (10 mL); 200 mg/mL (1 mL, 10 mL)

Generic: 100 mg/mL (10 mL); 200 mg/mL (1 mL, 5 mL, 10 mL)

Solution, Transdermal:

Axiron: 30 mg/actuation (90 mL)

Dosage Forms: Canada

Capsule, gelatin:

Andriol: 40 mg (10s)

◆ **Testosterone Cypionate** *see* Testosterone *on page 2010*

◆ **Testosterone Enanthate** *see* Testosterone *on page 2010*

◆ **Testosterone Undecanoate** *see* Testosterone *on page 2010*

◆ **Testred** *see* MethylTESTOSTERone *on page 1345*

◆ **Tetanus and Diphtheria Toxoid** *see* Diphtheria and Tetanus Toxoid *on page 645*

Tetanus Immune Globulin (Human)

(TET a nus i MYUN GLOB yoo lin HYU man)

Brand Names: U.S. HyperTET S/D

Brand Names: Canada HyperTET S/D

Index Terms TIG

Pharmacologic Category Blood Product Derivative; Immune Globulin

Additional Appendix Information

Immunization Administration Recommendations *on page 2250*

Immunization Recommendations *on page 2255*

Use

Tetanus prophylaxis: For prophylaxis against tetanus following injury in patients whose immunization is incomplete or uncertain

Tetanus treatment: Treatment of active tetanus

The Advisory Committee on Immunization Practices (ACIP) recommends passive immunization with TIG for the following:

- Persons with a wound that is not clean or minor and who have received ≤2 or an unknown number of adsorbed tetanus toxoid doses (CDC 55[RR3] 2006; CDC 55[RR17] 2006).
- Persons who are wounded in bombings or similar mass casualty events if no reliable history of completed primary vaccination with tetanus exists. In case of shortage, use should be reserved for persons ≥60 years of age and immigrants from regions other than Europe or North America (CDC 57[RR6] 2008).

Pregnancy Risk Factor C

Dosage

Prophylaxis of tetanus:

Children <7 years: IM: 4 units/kg; some recommend administering 250 units to small children

Children ≥7 years, Adolescents, and Adults: IM: 250 units

Tetanus prophylaxis in wound management: Children, Adolescents, and Adults: Tetanus prophylaxis in patients with wounds should be based on if the wound is clean or contaminated and the immunization status of the patient. Wound management includes proper use of tetanus toxoid and/or tetanus immune globulin (TIG), wound cleaning, and (if required) surgical debridement and the proper use of antibiotics. Patients with an uncertain or incomplete tetanus immunization status should have additional follow up to ensure a series is completed. Patients with a history of Arthus reaction following a previous dose of a tetanus toxoid-containing vaccine should not receive a tetanus toxoid-containing vaccine until >10 years after the most recent dose even if they have a wound that is neither clean nor minor. See table. IM:

Tetanus Prophylaxis in Wound Management

History of Tetanus Immunization Doses	Clean, Minor Wounds		All Other Wounds[1]	
	Tetanus Toxoid[2]	TIG	Tetanus Toxoid[2]	TIG
Uncertain or <3 doses	Yes	No	Yes	Yes
3 or more doses	No[3]	No	No[4]	No

[1]Such as, but not limited to, wounds contaminated with dirt, feces, soil, and saliva; puncture wounds; wounds from crushing, tears, burns, and frostbite.

[2]Tetanus toxoid in this chart refers to a tetanus toxoid-containing vaccine. For children <7 years of age, DTaP (DT, if pertussis vaccine contraindicated) is preferred to tetanus toxoid alone. For children ≥7 years, adolescents, and Adults, Td is preferred to tetanus toxoid alone; Tdap may be preferred if the patient has not previously been vaccinated with Tdap.

[3]Yes, if >10 years since last dose.

[4]Yes, if >5 years since last dose.

Adapted from CDC "Pink Book," "Epidemiology and Prevention of Vaccine-Preventable Diseases, Tetanus" (available at http://www.cdc.gov/vaccines/pubs/pinkbook/index.html) and *MMWR* 2006, 55(RR-17).

Abbreviations: **DT** = Diphtheria and Tetanus Toxoids (formulation for age ≤6 years); **DTaP** = Diphtheria and Tetanus Toxoids, and Acellular Pertussis (formulation for age ≤6 years; Daptacel, Infanrix); **Td** = Diphtheria and Tetanus Toxoids (formulation for age ≥7 years; Decavac, Tenivac); **TT**= Tetanus toxoid (adsorbed [formulation for age ≥7 years]); **Tdap** = Diphtheria and Tetanus Toxoids, and Acellular Pertussis (Adacel or Boostrix [formulations for age ≥7 years]); **TIG** = Tetanus Immune Globulin

Treatment of tetanus: Children, Adolescents, and Adults: IM: 500 to 6,000 units. Infiltration of part of the dose around the wound is recommended. The lower dose (500 units) appears to be as effective as higher doses and may cause less discomfort (*Red Book* [AAP, 2012]).

Dosage adjustment in renal impairment: There are no dosage adjustments provided in the manufacturer's labeling.

Dosage adjustment in hepatic impairment: There are no dosage adjustments provided in the manufacturer's labeling.

Additional Information Complete prescribing information should be consulted for additional detail.

Dosage Forms

Injectable, Intramuscular:

HyperTET S/D: 250 units/mL (1 ea)

◆ **Tetanus Toxoid** *see* Diphtheria and Tetanus Toxoids, Acellular Pertussis, Poliovirus and *Haemophilus* b Conjugate Vaccine *on page* 648

Tetanus Toxoid (Adsorbed)

(TET a nus TOKS oyd, ad SORBED)

Index Terms TT

Pharmacologic Category Vaccine, Inactivated (Bacterial)

Additional Appendix Information

Immunization Administration Recommendations *on page* 2250

Immunization Recommendations *on page* 2255

Use Active immunization against tetanus when combination antigen preparations are not indicated; tetanus prophylaxis in wound management. **Note:** Tetanus and diphtheria toxoids for adult use (Td) is the preferred immunizing agent for most adults and for children after their seventh birthday. Young children should receive trivalent DTaP (diphtheria/tetanus/acellular pertussis) as part of their childhood immunization program, unless pertussis is contraindicated, then DT is warranted.

Pregnancy Risk Factor C

Dosage Note: In most patients, Td is the recommended product for primary immunization, booster doses, and tetanus immunization in wound management (refer to Diphtheria and Tetanus Toxoid monograph).

Children ≥7 years and Adults: IM:

Primary immunization: 0.5 mL; repeat 0.5 mL at 4-8 weeks after first dose and at 6-12 months after second dose

Routine booster dose: Recommended every 10 years

Tetanus prophylaxis in wound management: Tetanus prophylaxis in patients with wounds should consider if the wound is clean or contaminated, the immunization status of the patient, proper use of tetanus toxoid and/or tetanus immune globulin (TIG), wound cleaning, and (if required) surgical debridement and the proper use of antibiotics. Patients with an uncertain or incomplete tetanus immunization status should have additional follow up to ensure a series is completed. Patients with a history of Arthus reaction following a previous dose of a tetanus toxoid-containing vaccine should not receive a tetanus toxoid-containing vaccine until >10 years after the most recent dose even if they have a wound that is neither clean nor minor. See table.

Tetanus Prophylaxis in Wound Management

History of Tetanus Immunization Doses	Clean, Minor Wounds		All Other Wounds[1]	
	Tetanus Toxoid[2]	TIG	Tetanus Toxoid[2]	TIG
Uncertain or <3 doses	Yes	No	Yes	Yes
3 or more doses	No[3]	No	No[4]	No

[1]Such as, but not limited to, wounds contaminated with dirt, feces, soil, and saliva; puncture wounds; wounds from crushing, tears, burns, and frostbite.

[2]Tetanus toxoid in this chart refers to a tetanus toxoid-containing vaccine. For children <7 years of age, DTaP (DT, if pertussis vaccine contraindicated) is preferred to tetanus toxoid alone. For children ≥7 years and Adults, Td preferred to tetanus toxoid alone; Tdap may be preferred if the patient has not previously been vaccinated with Tdap.

[3]Yes, if ≥10 years since last dose.

[4]Yes, if ≥5 years since last dose.

Adapted from CDC "Yellow Book" (*Health Information for International Travel 2010*), "Routine Vaccine-Preventable Diseases, Tetanus" (available at http://www.cdc.gov/yellowbook) and *MMWR* 2006, 55 (RR-17).

Abbreviations: **DT** = Diphtheria and Tetanus Toxoids (formulation for age ≤6 years); **DTaP** = Diphtheria and Tetanus Toxoids, and Acellular Pertussis (formulation for age ≤6 years; Daptacel®, Infanrix®); **Td** = Diphtheria and Tetanus Toxoids (formulation for age ≥7 years; Decavac®,Tenivac™); **TT**= Tetanus toxoid (adsorbed [formulation for age ≥7 years]); **Tdap** = Diphtheria and Tetanus Toxoids, and Acellular Pertussis (Adacel® or Boostrix® [formulations for age ≥7 years]); **TIG** = Tetanus Immune Globulin

Additional Information Complete prescribing information should be consulted for additional detail.

◆ **Tetanus Toxoid, Reduced Diphtheria Toxoid, and Acellular Pertussis, Adsorbed** *see* Diphtheria and Tetanus Toxoids, and Acellular Pertussis Vaccine *on page* 649

◆ **Tetcaine** *see* Tetracaine (Ophthalmic) *on page* 2017

Tetrabenazine (tet ra BEN a zeen)

Brand Names: U.S. Xenazine

Brand Names: Canada Nitoman; PMS-Tetrabenazine

Pharmacologic Category Central Monoamine-Depleting Agent

Use Treatment of chorea associated with Huntington's disease

Canadian labeling: Treatment of hyperkinetic movement disorders, including Huntington's chorea, hemiballismus, senile chorea, Tourette syndrome, and tardive dyskinesia

Pregnancy Risk Factor C

Dosage Oral: Dose should be individualized; titrate slowly

Chorea associated with Huntington's disease: Adults:

Initial: 12.5 mg once daily, may increase to 12.5 mg twice daily after 1 week

Maintenance: May be increased by 12.5 mg/day at weekly intervals; doses >37.5 mg/day should be divided into 3 doses (maximum single dose: 25 mg)

Patients requiring doses >50 mg/day: Genotype for CYP2D6:

Extensive/intermediate metabolizers: Maximum: 100 mg/day; 37.5 mg/dose

Poor metabolizers: Maximum: 50 mg/day; 25 mg/dose

Concomitant use with strong CYP2D6 inhibitors (eg, fluoxetine, paroxetine, quinidine): Dose of tetrabenazine should be reduced by 50% in patients receiving strong CYP2D6 inhibitors, follow dosing for poor CYP2D6 metabolizers. Use caution when adding a CYP2D6 inhibitor to patients already taking tetrabenazine.

Note: If treatment is interrupted for >5 days, retitration is recommended. If treatment is interrupted for <5 days resume at previous maintenance dose.

Canadian labeling: Hyperkinetic movement disorders:
Adults: Initial: 12.5 mg twice daily (may be given 3 times/day); may be increased by 12.5 mg/day every 3-5 days; should be titrated slowly to maximal tolerated and effective dose (dose is individualized)
Usual maximum tolerated dosage: 25 mg 3 times/day; maximum recommended dose: 200 mg/day
Note: If there is no improvement at the maximum tolerated dose after 7 days, improvement is unlikely; discontinuation should be considered.
Elderly and/or debilitated patients: Consider initiation at lower doses; must be titrated slowly to individualize dosage

Dosage adjustment for toxicity: For toxicity/adverse reaction, including akathisia, restlessness, parkinsonism, insomnia, depression, suicidality, anxiety, sedation (intolerable): Suspend upward dosage titration and reduce dose; consider discontinuing if adverse reaction does not resolve (may be discontinued without tapering).

Dosage adjustment in renal impairment: No dosage adjustment provided in manufacturer's labeling (has not been studied).
Dosage adjustment in hepatic impairment: Use is contraindicated
Additional Information Complete prescribing information should be consulted for additional detail.
Dosage Forms
Tablet, Oral:
Xenazine: 12.5 mg, 25 mg
Dosage Forms: Canada
Tablet:
Nitoman™: 25 mg

Tetracaine (Systemic) (TET ra kane)

Brand Names: Canada Pontocaine
Index Terms Amethocaine Hydrochloride; Tetracaine Hydrochloride
Pharmacologic Category Local Anesthetic
Use Spinal anesthesia
Pregnancy Risk Factor C
Dosage Injection: Adults: Spinal anesthesia: **Note:** Dosage varies with the anesthetic procedure, the degree of anesthesia required, and the individual patient response; it is administered by subarachnoid injection for spinal anesthesia.
Perineal anesthesia: 5 mg
Perineal and lower extremities: 10 mg
Anesthesia extending up to costal margin: 15 mg; doses up to 20 mg may be given, but are reserved for exceptional cases
Low spinal anesthesia (saddle block): 2-5 mg

Dosage adjustment in renal impairment: No dosage adjustment provided in manufacturer's labeling.
Dosage adjustment in hepatic impairment: No dosage adjustment provided in manufacturer's labeling.
Additional Information Complete prescribing information should be consulted for additional detail.
Dosage Forms
Solution, Injection [preservative free]:
Generic: 1% (2 mL)

Tetracaine (Ophthalmic) (TET ra kane)

Brand Names: U.S. Altacaine; Tetcaine; TetraVisc; TetraVisc Forte
Index Terms Amethocaine Hydrochloride; Tetracaine Hydrochloride
Pharmacologic Category Local Anesthetic
Use Local anesthesia for various ophthalmic procedures of short duration (eg, tonometry, gonioscopy); minor ophthalmic surgical procedures (eg, removal of corneal foreign bodies, suture removal); and for various diagnostic purposes (eg, conjunctival scrapings)
Pregnancy Risk Factor C
Dosage Ophthalmic: Adults:
Short-term (nonsurgical procedures) anesthesia: Instill 1-2 drops into affected eye just prior to evaluation
Minor surgical procedures: Instill 1-2 drops into affected eye every 5-10 minutes for up to 3 doses
Prolonged surgical procedures: Instill 1-2 drops into affected eye every 5-10 minutes for up to 5 doses

Dosage adjustment in renal impairment: No dosage adjustment provided in manufacturer's labeling.
Dosage adjustment in hepatic impairment: No dosage adjustment provided in manufacturer's labeling.
Additional Information Complete prescribing information should be consulted for additional detail.
Dosage Forms
Solution, Ophthalmic:
Altacaine: 0.5% (1 ea, 15 mL, 30 mL)
Tetcaine: 0.5% (15 mL)
TetraVisc: 0.5% (1 ea, 5 mL)
TetraVisc Forte: 0.5% (1 ea, 5 mL)
Generic: 0.5% (1 mL, 2 mL, 15 mL)

Tetracaine (Topical) (TET ra kane)

Brand Names: Canada Ametop; Pontocaine
Index Terms Amethocaine Hydrochloride; Tetracaine Hydrochloride
Pharmacologic Category Local Anesthetic
Use Applied to nose and throat for diagnostic procedures
Pregnancy Risk Factor C
Dosage Adults: Topical mucous membranes (rhinolaryngology): Used as a 0.25% or 0.5% solution by direct application or nebulization; total dose should not exceed 20 mg
Additional Information Complete prescribing information should be consulted for additional detail.

- ◆ **Tetracaine and Lidocaine** *see* Lidocaine and Tetracaine *on page 1214*
- ◆ **Tetracaine, Benzocaine, and Butamben** *see* Benzocaine, Butamben, and Tetracaine *on page 247*
- ◆ **Tetracaine Hydrochloride** *see* Tetracaine (Ophthalmic) *on page 2017*
- ◆ **Tetracaine Hydrochloride** *see* Tetracaine (Systemic) *on page 2017*
- ◆ **Tetracaine Hydrochloride** *see* Tetracaine (Topical) *on page 2017*
- ◆ **Tetracosactide** *see* Cosyntropin *on page 510*

Tetracycline (tet ra SYE kleen)

Brand Names: Canada Apo-Tetra; Nu-Tetra
Index Terms Achromycin; TCN; Tetracycline Hydrochloride
Pharmacologic Category Antibiotic, Tetracycline Derivative
Use Treatment of susceptible bacterial infections of both gram-positive and gram-negative organisms; also infections due to *Mycoplasma*, *Chlamydia*, and *Rickettsia*; indicated for acne, exacerbations of chronic bronchitis, and treatment of gonorrhea and syphilis in patients who are allergic to penicillin; as part of a multidrug regimen for *H. pylori* eradication to reduce the risk of duodenal ulcer recurrence
Pregnancy Risk Factor D

Dosage

Usual dosage range:

Children >8 years: Oral: 25-50 mg/kg/day in divided doses every 6 hours

Adults: Oral: 250-500 mg/dose every 6 hours

Indication-specific dosing:

Children ≥8 years: Oral:

Malaria, severe, treatment (off-label use): 25 mg/kg/day in divided doses every 6 hours (maximum dose: 250 mg every 6 hours) for 7 days with quinidine gluconate. **Note:** Quinidine gluconate duration is region specific; consult CDC for current recommendations (CDC, 2009).

Malaria, uncomplicated, treatment (off-label use): 25 mg/kg/day in divided doses every 6 hours (maximum dose: 250 mg every 6 hours) for 7 days with quinine sulfate. **Note:** Quinine sulfate duration is region specific; consult CDC for current recommendations (CDC, 2009).

Adults: Oral:

Acne: 250-500 twice daily

Chronic bronchitis, acute exacerbation: 500 mg 4 times daily

Erlichiosis: 500 mg 4 times daily for 7-14 days

Malaria, severe, treatment (off-label use): 250 mg 4 times daily for 7 days with quinidine gluconate. **Note:** Quinidine gluconate duration is region specific; consult CDC for current recommendations (CDC, 2009).

Malaria, uncomplicated, treatment (off-label use): 250 mg 4 times daily for 7 days with quinine sulfate. **Note:** Quinine sulfate duration is region specific; consult CDC for current recommendations (CDC, 2009).

Peptic ulcer disease: Eradication of *Helicobacter pylori*: 500 mg 2-4 times daily depending on regimen; requires combination therapy with at least one other antibiotic and an acid-suppressing agent (proton pump inhibitor or H_2 blocker)

Periodontitis (off-label use): 250 mg every 6 hours until improvement (usually 10 days)

Syphilis:

Early syphilis (primary or secondary infection): 500 mg 4 times daily for 14 days. **Note:** Alternative treatment for non-pregnant, penicillin-allergic patients (CDC, 2010).

Latent syphilis (late or of unknown duration): 500 mg 4 times daily for 28 days. **Note:** Alternative treatment for non-pregnant, penicillin-allergic patients. Effectiveness not well documented; close clinical and serologic follow-up recommended (CDC, 2010).

Vibrio cholerae: 500 mg 4 times/day for 3 days

Dosage adjustment in renal impairment:

CrCl 50-80 mL/minute: Administer every 8-12 hours

CrCl 10-50 mL/minute: Administer every 12-24 hours

CrCl <10 mL/minute: Administer every 24 hours

Dialysis: Slightly dialyzable (5% to 20%) via hemo- and peritoneal dialysis or via continuous arteriovenous or venovenous hemofiltration; no supplemental dosage necessary

Dosage adjustment in hepatic impairment: No dosage adjustment necessary. Use with caution.

Additional Information Complete prescribing information should be consulted for additional detail.

Dosage Forms

Capsule, Oral:

Generic: 250 mg, 500 mg

◆ **Tetracycline Hydrochloride** *see* Tetracycline *on page 2017*

◆ **Tetraferric Tricitrate Decahydrate** *see* Ferric Citrate *on page 869*

◆ **Tetra-Formula Nighttime Sleep [OTC]** *see* DiphenhydrAMINE (Systemic) *on page 641*

◆ **Tetrahydrobiopterin** *see* Sapropterin *on page 1864*

◆ **Tetrahydrocannabinol** *see* Dronabinol *on page 694*

Tetrahydrocannabinol and Cannabidiol [CAN/INT]

(TET ra hye droe can NAB e nol & can nab e DYE ol)

Brand Names: Canada Sativex®

Index Terms Cannabidiol and Tetrahydrocannabinol; Delta-9-Tetrahydrocannabinol and Cannabinol; GW-1000-02; Nabiximols; THC and CBD

Pharmacologic Category Analgesic, Miscellaneous

Use Note: Not approved in U.S.

Adjunctive treatment of neuropathic pain or spasticity in multiple sclerosis; adjunctive treatment of moderate-to-severe pain in advanced cancer

Pregnancy Considerations Cannabinoids have been associated with reproductive toxicity. Animal studies indicate possible effects on fetal development and spermatogenesis. Use in pregnancy is contraindicated. Women of childbearing potential and males who are capable of causing pregnancy should use a reliable form of contraception for the duration of treatment and for 3 months following discontinuation.

Contraindications Hypersensitivity to cannabinoids or any component of the formulation; serious cardiovascular disease (including arrhythmias, severe heart failure, poorly controlled hypertension, and ischemic heart disease); history of psychotic disorders (including schizophrenia); women of childbearing potential who are not using a reliable form of contraception; males intending to start a family; children <18 years of age; pregnancy; breast-feeding

Warnings/Precautions [Canadian Boxed Warnings]: May cause physical and psychological dependence in long-term use; avoid use in patients with a history or risk of drug or alcohol dependency. Prescriptions should be written for the minimal amount needed between clinic visits. Use may be associated with changes in mood, cognitive performance, memory, impulsivity, and coordination, as well as an altered perception of reality, particularly with respect to an awareness/sensation of time. May impair physical or mental abilities; patients must be cautioned about performing tasks which require mental alertness (eg, operating machinery or driving). **[Canadian Boxed Warnings]: Use with caution in patients with a history of seizures. Concurrent use of ethanol or other CNS active drugs may be additive.** Dosage must be carefully titrated and monitored, with downward adjustment in patients with unacceptable adverse events. Avoid use in patients with personal or strong familial history of psychosis; suicidal ideation and depression have been reported with use. Discontinue use immediately in patients experiencing psychotic reactions, suicidal ideation, delusions, hallucinations, and/or confusion and monitor until complete resolution of symptoms.

[Canadian Boxed Warning]: May be associated with adverse cardiovascular effects, including tachycardia and alterations in blood pressure (including orthostatic changes). Dosage must be carefully titrated and monitored, with downward adjustment in patients with unacceptable adverse events. Use with caution in the perioperative setting. Use is contraindicated in ischemic heart disease, arrhythmias, poorly-controlled hypertension, and severe heart failure.

Use with caution in severe hepatic and renal dysfunction. Use with caution in elderly patients. May be irritating to the buccal mucosa; avoid administration in an area of soreness or inflammation. Use in cancer patients associated with increased risk of urinary retention and infection.

Formulation contains ethanol; use may be harmful in patients with alcoholism or hepatic dysfunction. Due to accumulation in body fat, cannabinoids may be detectable in the urine and serum for several weeks following drug discontinuation.

Adverse Reactions

Cardiovascular: Hypotension, palpitation, syncope, tachycardia

Central nervous system: Amnesia, attention disturbance, confusion, depression, disorientation, dissociation, dizziness, euphoria, fatigue, feeling abnormal, hallucination, headache, impaired balance, insomnia, lethargy, malaise, memory impairment, panic attack, paranoia, somnolence, suicidal ideation, vertigo

Gastrointestinal: Abdominal pain, anorexia, appetite increased, constipation, diarrhea, glossodynia, mouth ulceration, nausea, oral candidiasis, oral discomfort/pain, oral mucosal disorder, stomatitis, taste abnormal, tooth discoloration, vomiting, xerostomia

Genitourinary: Urinary retention

Hepatic: Hepatic function tests abnormal

Neuromuscular & skeletal: Dysarthria, fall, weakness

Ocular: Vision blurred

Renal: Hematuria

Respiratory: Throat irritation

Miscellaneous: Drunken feeling

Rare but important or life-threatening: Delusions, hypertension, illusion, urinary infection

Drug Interactions

Metabolism/Transport Effects Refer to individual components.

Avoid Concomitant Use There are no known interactions where it is recommended to avoid concomitant use.

Increased Effect/Toxicity

Tetrahydrocannabinol and Cannabidiol may increase the levels/effects of: Alcohol (Ethyl); CNS Depressants; Sympathomimetics

The levels/effects of Tetrahydrocannabinol and Cannabidiol may be increased by: Anticholinergic Agents; Cocaine; CYP2C9 Inhibitors (Moderate); CYP2C9 Inhibitors (Strong); CYP3A4 Inhibitors (Moderate); CYP3A4 Inhibitors (Strong); MAO Inhibitors

Decreased Effect

The levels/effects of Tetrahydrocannabinol and Cannabidiol may be decreased by: CYP3A4 Inducers (Strong); St Johns Wort

Storage/Stability Store unopened at 2°C to 8°C (36°F to 46°F); do not freeze. After opening, may be stored at room temperature of 15°C to 25°C (59°F to 77°F) for up to 28 days (5.5 mL vial) or 42 days (10 mL vial). Avoid heat and direct sunlight.

Mechanism of Action Stimulates cannabinoid receptors CB1 and CB2 in the CNS and dorsal root ganglia as well as other sites in the body. Cannabinoid receptors in the pain pathways of the brain and spinal cord mediate cannabinoid-induced analgesia. Peripheral CB2 receptors modulate immune function through cytokine release.

Pharmacodynamics/Kinetics

Absorption: Rapidly absorbed from the buccal mucosa

Distribution: Widely distributed, particularly to fatty tissues

Protein binding: Extensive

Metabolism: Hepatic, via CYP isoenzymes (2C9, 2C19, 2D6 and 3A4) to THC metabolite 11-hydroxy-tetrahydrocannabinol (11-OH-THC, psycho-active) and CBD metabolite 7-hydroxy-cannabidiol.

Half-life elimination: Biphasic: Initial: 1-2 hours; Terminal: 24-36 hours (or longer) secondary to redistribution from fatty tissue

Time to peak, plasma: 2-4 hours

Excretion: As metabolites, urine and feces

Dosage Buccal spray: Adults: Spasticity or neuropathic pain associated with multiple sclerosis (MS), cancer pain:

Initial: One spray in the morning and one spray in the afternoon or evening (maximum initial dose: 2 sprays on first day)

Titration and individualization: Dosage is self-titrated by the patient. After initiation of therapy, the dose may be increased each subsequent day by one spray as needed and tolerated. Usual dosage: 4-8 sprays daily. Most patients require ≤12 sprays daily. Experience is limited with dosage of >12 sprays daily, though some patients may require and tolerate higher dosing. Sprays should be evenly distributed over the course of the day during initial titration.

Elderly: Refer to adult dosing. Use with caution and monitor closely.

Dosage adjustment for toxicity: If adverse reactions, including intoxication-type symptoms, are noted the dosage should be suspended until resolution of the symptoms; a dosage reduction or extension of the interval between doses may be used to avoid a recurrence of symptoms. Retitration may be required in the event of adverse reactions and/or worsening of symptoms.

Dosage adjustment in renal impairment: No dosage adjustment provided in manufacturer's labeling (has not been studied). Use with caution.

Dosage adjustment in hepatic impairment: No dosage adjustment provided in manufacturer's labeling (has not been studied). Use with caution.

Administration Note: For buccal use only. Do not inhale, spray into nose, or apply spray to sore or inflamed mucosa.

Shake vial before use and remove protective cap; replace protective cap following use.

Priming: Vial should be held in an upright position and primed into a tissue prior to the initial use by depression of the actuator 2-3 times until a fine spray appears. Priming should not be required for subsequent uses. Do not spray near children, pets, or an open flame.

Normal use: Hold vial in upright position and spray into mouth; spray should be directed below the tongue or on the inside of the cheeks, avoiding direction to the pharynx. Initiate therapy by administering 1 spray in the morning and 1 spray in the afternoon or evening (between 4 pm and bedtime) on day 1. With subsequent titration, allow at least 15 minutes between sprays; however, during initial titration, sprays should be evenly spaced throughout the day. The application site should be varied.

Monitoring Parameters Mental status, response to pain; mucosal integrity and inflammation

Product Availability Not available in U.S.

Dosage Forms: Canada

Solution, buccal [spray]:

Sativex®: Delta-9 tetrahydrocannabinol 27 mg/mL and cannabidiol 25 mg/mL (5.5 mL, 10 mL)

◆ **Tetraiodothyronine and Triiodothyronine** *see* Thyroid, Desiccated *on page 2031*

◆ **2,2,2-tetramine** *see* Trientine *on page 2102*

Tetrastarch (TET ra starch)

Brand Names: U.S. Voluven

Brand Names: Canada Volulyte; Voluven

Index Terms Etherified Starch; HES; HES 130/0.4; Hydroxyethyl Starch

Pharmacologic Category Plasma Volume Expander, Colloid

Use Blood volume expander used in treatment and prevention of hypovolemia

Pregnancy Risk Factor C

Dosage IV infusion: Plasma volume expansion: **Note:** With severe dehydration, administer crystalloid first. Daily dose and rate of infusion dependent on amount of blood lost, on maintenance or restoration of hemodynamics, and on amount of hemodilution. Titrate to individual colloid needs, hemodynamics, and hydration status. Do not use in the critically ill including patients with sepsis, those with preexisting renal dysfunction or receiving dialysis, those with preexisting bleeding disorders or those with intracranial bleeding.

Children ≤12 years and Adolescents: May administer up to 50 mL/kg/day (or up to 3500 mL per day in a 70 kg patient); may administer repetitively over several days.

Mean daily dose ± SD in pediatric clinical trials:

Children <2 years: 16 ± 9 mL/kg

Children 2-12 years: 36 ± 11 mL/kg

Adults: May administer up to 50 mL/kg/day (or up to 3500 mL per day in a 70 kg patient); may administer repetitively over several days

Dosage adjustment in renal impairment: Avoid use in patients with preexisting renal dysfunction. Use is contraindicated in oliguric/anuric renal failure unrelated to hypovolemia or patients receiving dialysis. Discontinue use at the first sign of renal injury.

Dosage adjustment in hepatic impairment: No dosage adjustment provided in manufacturer's labeling; use is contraindicated in severe liver disease.

Additional Information Complete prescribing information should be consulted for additional detail.

Dosage Forms

Solution, Intravenous:

Voluven: 6% (500 mL)

Dosage Forms: Canada

Infusion, premixed in isotonic electrolyte solution:

Volulyte: 6% (250 mL, 500 mL)

◆ **TetraVisc** *see* Tetracaine (Ophthalmic) *on page 2017*

◆ **TetraVisc Forte** *see* Tetracaine (Ophthalmic) *on page 2017*

Tetrazepam [INT] (tet RA ze pam)

International Brand Names Megavix (FR); MTW-Tetrazepam (DE); Musapam (DE); Musaril (AT, DE); Muskelat (DE); Myolastan (AT, BE, CZ, ES, FR, LU); Myospasmal (DE); Panos (FR); Rilex (DE); Tepam-BASF (DE); Tethexal (DE); Tetra Flam (DE); Tetra-saar (DE); Tetramdura (DE); Tetrarelax (DE); Tetrazep 1A Pharma (DE); Tetrazep AbZ (DE); tetrazep von ct (DE); Tetrazepam AL (DE); Tetrazepam beta (DE); Tetrazepam Heumann (DE); Tetrazepam Stada (DE); Tetrazepam-neuraxpharm (DE); Tetrazepam-ratiopharm (DE); Tetrazepam-Teva (DE)

Pharmacologic Category Benzodiazepine

Reported Use Treatment of painful muscular contractions

Dosage Range Adults: Oral: 50 mg at bedtime; may be increased by 25 mg/day until the maximum dose of 150 mg is reached; may be taken 2-3 times/day with the larger dose given in the evening

Product Availability Product available in various countries; not currently available in the U.S.

Dosage Forms

Tablet: 50 mg

◆ **Teva-Acebutolol (Can)** *see* Acebutolol *on page 29*

◆ **Teva-Acyclovir (Can)** *see* Acyclovir (Systemic) *on page 47*

◆ **Teva-Alendronate (Can)** *see* Alendronate *on page 79*

◆ **Teva-Alfuzosin PR (Can)** *see* Alfuzosin *on page 84*

◆ **Teva-Alprazolam (Can)** *see* ALPRAZolam *on page 94*

◆ **Teva-Amiodarone (Can)** *see* Amiodarone *on page 114*

◆ **Teva-Amlodipine (Can)** *see* AmLODIPine *on page 123*

◆ **Teva-Anastrozole (Can)** *see* Anastrozole *on page 148*

◆ **Teva-Atenolol (Can)** *see* Atenolol *on page 189*

◆ **Teva-Atomoxetine (Can)** *see* AtoMOXetine *on page 191*

◆ **Teva-Azathioprine (Can)** *see* AzaTHIOprine *on page 210*

◆ **Teva-Betahistine (Can)** *see* Betahistine [CAN/INT] *on page 252*

◆ **Teva-Bisoprolol (Can)** *see* Bisoprolol *on page 266*

◆ **Teva-Bosentan (Can)** *see* Bosentan *on page 280*

◆ **Teva-Candesartan (Can)** *see* Candesartan *on page 335*

◆ **Teva-Candesartan/HCTZ (Can)** *see* Candesartan and Hydrochlorothiazide *on page 338*

◆ **Teva-Capecitabine (Can)** *see* Capecitabine *on page 339*

◆ **Teva-Carbamazepine (Can)** *see* CarBAMazepine *on page 346*

◆ **Teva-Cefadroxil (Can)** *see* Cefadroxil *on page 372*

◆ **Teva-Cephalexin (Can)** *see* Cephalexin *on page 405*

◆ **Teva-Chlorpromazine (Can)** *see* ChlorproMAZINE *on page 429*

◆ **Teva-Citalopram (Can)** *see* Citalopram *on page 451*

◆ **Teva-Clarithromycin (Can)** *see* Clarithromycin *on page 456*

◆ **Teva-Clindamycin (Can)** *see* Clindamycin (Systemic) *on page 460*

◆ **Teva-Clonazepam (Can)** *see* ClonazePAM *on page 478*

◆ **Teva-Clopidogrel (Can)** *see* Clopidogrel *on page 484*

◆ **Teva-Combo Sterinebs (Can)** *see* Ipratropium and Albuterol *on page 1109*

◆ **Teva-Diclofenac (Can)** *see* Diclofenac (Systemic) *on page 617*

◆ **Teva-Diclofenac EC (Can)** *see* Diclofenac (Systemic) *on page 617*

◆ **Teva-Diclofenac K (Can)** *see* Diclofenac (Systemic) *on page 617*

◆ **Teva-Diclofenac SR (Can)** *see* Diclofenac (Systemic) *on page 617*

◆ **Teva-Diltiazem (Can)** *see* Diltiazem *on page 634*

◆ **Teva-Diltiazem CD (Can)** *see* Diltiazem *on page 634*

◆ **Teva-Diltiazem HCL ER Capsules (Can)** *see* Diltiazem *on page 634*

◆ **Teva-Docusate Sodium [OTC] (Can)** *see* Docusate *on page 661*

◆ **Teva-Domperidone (Can)** *see* Domperidone [CAN/INT] *on page 666*

◆ **Teva-Donepezil (Can)** *see* Donepezil *on page 668*

◆ **Teva-Doxazosin (Can)** *see* Doxazosin *on page 674*

◆ **Teva-Doxycycline (Can)** *see* Doxycycline *on page 689*

◆ **Teva-Dutasteride (Can)** *see* Dutasteride *on page 702*

◆ **Teva-Efavirenz (Can)** *see* Efavirenz *on page 707*

◆ **Teva-Enalapril (Can)** *see* Enalapril *on page 722*

◆ **Teva-Entacapone (Can)** *see* Entacapone *on page 730*

◆ **Teva-Escitalopram (Can)** *see* Escitalopram *on page 765*

◆ **Teva-Ezetimibe (Can)** *see* Ezetimibe *on page 832*

◆ **Teva-Famotidine (Can)** *see* Famotidine *on page 845*

◆ **Teva-Fenofibrate S (Can)** *see* Fenofibrate and Derivatives *on page 852*

◆ **Teva-Fentanyl (Can)** *see* FentaNYL *on page 857*

◆ **Teva-Finasteride (Can)** *see* Finasteride *on page 878*

◆ **Teva-Fluoxetine (Can)** *see* FLUoxetine *on page 899*

◆ **Teva-Flutamide (Can)** *see* Flutamide *on page 907*

- ◆ **Teva-Fluvastatin (Can)** *see* Fluvastatin *on page 915*
- ◆ **Teva-Fosinopril (Can)** *see* Fosinopril *on page 932*
- ◆ **Teva-Furosemide (Can)** *see* Furosemide *on page 940*
- ◆ **Teva-Gabapentin (Can)** *see* Gabapentin *on page 943*
- ◆ **Teva-Galantamine ER (Can)** *see* Galantamine *on page 946*
- ◆ **Teva-Gliclazide (Can)** *see* Gliclazide [CAN/INT] *on page 964*
- ◆ **Teva-Glyburide (Can)** *see* GlyBURIDE *on page 972*
- ◆ **Tevagrastim** *see* Filgrastim *on page 875*
- ◆ **Teva-Hydrochlorothiazide (Can)** *see* Hydrochlorothiazide *on page 1009*
- ◆ **Teva-Hydromorphone (Can)** *see* HYDROmorphone *on page 1016*
- ◆ **Teva-Imatinib (Can)** *see* Imatinib *on page 1047*
- ◆ **Teva-Ipratropium Sterinebs (Can)** *see* Ipratropium (Systemic) *on page 1108*
- ◆ **Teva-Irbesartan (Can)** *see* Irbesartan *on page 1110*
- ◆ **Teva-Irbesartan HCTZ (Can)** *see* Irbesartan and Hydrochlorothiazide *on page 1112*
- ◆ **Teva-Ketoconazole (Can)** *see* Ketoconazole (Systemic) *on page 1144*
- ◆ **Teva-Lactulose (Can)** *see* Lactulose *on page 1156*
- ◆ **Teva-Lamivudine/Zidovudine (Can)** *see* Lamivudine and Zidovudine *on page 1160*
- ◆ **Teva-Lamotrigine (Can)** *see* LamoTRIgine *on page 1160*
- ◆ **Teva-Lansoprazole (Can)** *see* Lansoprazole *on page 1166*
- ◆ **Teva-Leflunomide (Can)** *see* Leflunomide *on page 1174*
- ◆ **Teva-Letrozole (Can)** *see* Letrozole *on page 1181*
- ◆ **Teva-Levocarbidopa (Can)** *see* Carbidopa and Levodopa *on page 351*
- ◆ **Teva-Lisinopril/Hctz (Type P) (Can)** *see* Lisinopril and Hydrochlorothiazide *on page 1229*
- ◆ **Teva-Lisinopril/Hctz (Type Z) (Can)** *see* Lisinopril and Hydrochlorothiazide *on page 1229*
- ◆ **Teva-Lisinopril (Type P) (Can)** *see* Lisinopril *on page 1226*
- ◆ **Teva-Lisinopril (Type Z) (Can)** *see* Lisinopril *on page 1226*
- ◆ **Teva-Lorazepam (Can)** *see* LORazepam *on page 1243*
- ◆ **Teva-Losartan (Can)** *see* Losartan *on page 1248*
- ◆ **Teva-Losartan/HCTZ (Can)** *see* Losartan and Hydrochlorothiazide *on page 1250*
- ◆ **Teva-Lovastatin (Can)** *see* Lovastatin *on page 1252*
- ◆ **Teva-Maprotiline (Can)** *see* Maprotiline *on page 1271*
- ◆ **Teva-Medroxyprogesterone (Can)** *see* MedroxyPROGESTERone *on page 1277*
- ◆ **Teva-Meloxicam (Can)** *see* Meloxicam *on page 1283*
- ◆ **Teva-Metformin (Can)** *see* MetFORMIN *on page 1307*
- ◆ **Teva-Methylphenidate ER-C (Can)** *see* Methylphenidate *on page 1336*
- ◆ **Teva-Metoprolol (Can)** *see* Metoprolol *on page 1350*
- ◆ **Teva-Mirtazapine (Can)** *see* Mirtazapine *on page 1376*
- ◆ **Teva-Mirtazapine OD (Can)** *see* Mirtazapine *on page 1376*
- ◆ **Teva-Moclobemide (Can)** *see* Moclobemide [CAN/INT] *on page 1384*
- ◆ **Teva-Modafinil (Can)** *see* Modafinil *on page 1386*
- ◆ **Teva-Montelukast (Can)** *see* Montelukast *on page 1392*
- ◆ **Teva-Morphine SR (Can)** *see* Morphine (Systemic) *on page 1394*
- ◆ **Teva-Nadolol (Can)** *see* Nadolol *on page 1411*
- ◆ **Teva-Naproxen (Can)** *see* Naproxen *on page 1427*
- ◆ **Teva-Naproxen EC (Can)** *see* Naproxen *on page 1427*
- ◆ **Teva-Naproxen Sodium (Can)** *see* Naproxen *on page 1427*
- ◆ **Teva-Naproxen Sodium DS (Can)** *see* Naproxen *on page 1427*
- ◆ **Teva-Naproxen SR (Can)** *see* Naproxen *on page 1427*
- ◆ **Teva-Naratriptan (Can)** *see* Naratriptan *on page 1430*
- ◆ **Teva-Nevirapine (Can)** *see* Nevirapine *on page 1440*
- ◆ **Teva-Nitrofurantoin (Can)** *see* Nitrofurantoin *on page 1463*
- ◆ **Teva-Nortriptyline (Can)** *see* Nortriptyline *on page 1476*
- ◆ **Teva-Olanzapine (Can)** *see* OLANZapine *on page 1491*
- ◆ **Teva-Olanzapine OD (Can)** *see* OLANZapine *on page 1491*
- ◆ **Teva-Omeprazole (Can)** *see* Omeprazole *on page 1508*
- ◆ **Teva-Ondansetron (Can)** *see* Ondansetron *on page 1513*
- ◆ **Teva-Pantoprazole (Can)** *see* Pantoprazole *on page 1570*
- ◆ **Teva-Paroxetine (Can)** *see* PARoxetine *on page 1579*
- ◆ **Teva-Pindolol (Can)** *see* Pindolol *on page 1652*
- ◆ **Teva-Pioglitazone (Can)** *see* Pioglitazone *on page 1654*
- ◆ **Teva-Pramipexole (Can)** *see* Pramipexole *on page 1695*
- ◆ **Teva-Pravastatin (Can)** *see* Pravastatin *on page 1700*
- ◆ **Teva-Prazosin (Can)** *see* Prazosin *on page 1703*
- ◆ **Teva-Pregabalin (Can)** *see* Pregabalin *on page 1710*
- ◆ **Teva-Propranolol (Can)** *see* Propranolol *on page 1731*
- ◆ **Teva-Quetiapine (Can)** *see* QUEtiapine *on page 1751*
- ◆ **Teva-Quetiapine XR (Can)** *see* QUEtiapine *on page 1751*
- ◆ **Teva-Rabeprazole EC (Can)** *see* RABEprazole *on page 1762*
- ◆ **Teva-Raloxifene (Can)** *see* Raloxifene *on page 1765*
- ◆ **Teva-Ramipril (Can)** *see* Ramipril *on page 1771*
- ◆ **Teva-Ranitidine (Can)** *see* Ranitidine *on page 1777*
- ◆ **Teva-Risedronate (Can)** *see* Risedronate *on page 1816*
- ◆ **Teva-Risperidone (Can)** *see* RisperiDONE *on page 1818*
- ◆ **Teva-Rosuvastatin (Can)** *see* Rosuvastatin *on page 1848*
- ◆ **Teva-Salbutamol (Can)** *see* Albuterol *on page 69*
- ◆ **Teva-Salbutamol Sterinebs P.F. (Can)** *see* Albuterol *on page 69*
- ◆ **Teva-Sertraline (Can)** *see* Sertraline *on page 1878*
- ◆ **Teva-Sildenafil (Can)** *see* Sildenafil *on page 1882*
- ◆ **Teva-Simvastatin (Can)** *see* Simvastatin *on page 1890*
- ◆ **Teva-Spironolactone (Can)** *see* Spironolactone *on page 1931*
- ◆ **Teva-Sucralfate (Can)** *see* Sucralfate *on page 1940*
- ◆ **Teva-Sulindac (Can)** *see* Sulindac *on page 1953*
- ◆ **Teva-Sumatriptan (Can)** *see* SUMAtriptan *on page 1953*
- ◆ **Teva-Sumatriptan DF (Can)** *see* SUMAtriptan *on page 1953*
- ◆ **Teva-Tamoxifen (Can)** *see* Tamoxifen *on page 1971*
- ◆ **Teva-Tamsulosin (Can)** *see* Tamsulosin *on page 1974*
- ◆ **Teva-Tamsulosin CR (Can)** *see* Tamsulosin *on page 1974*

- ◆ **Teva-Telmisartan (Can)** *see* Telmisartan *on page 1988*
- ◆ **Teva-Telmisartan HCTZ (Can)** *see* Telmisartan and Hydrochlorothiazide *on page 1990*
- ◆ **Teva-Terazosin (Can)** *see* Terazosin *on page 2001*
- ◆ **Teva-Terbinafine (Can)** *see* Terbinafine (Systemic) *on page 2002*
- ◆ **Teva-Theophylline SR (Can)** *see* Theophylline *on page 2026*
- ◆ **Teva-Tiaprofenic Acid (Can)** *see* Tiaprofenic Acid [CAN/INT] *on page 2034*
- ◆ **Teva-Ticlopidine (Can)** *see* Ticlopidine *on page 2040*
- ◆ **Teva-Timolol (Can)** *see* Timolol (Systemic) *on page 2042*
- ◆ **TEVA-Topiramate (Can)** *see* Topiramate *on page 2065*
- ◆ **TEVA-Tramadol/Acetaminophen (Can)** *see* Acetaminophen and Tramadol *on page 37*
- ◆ **Teva-Travoprost Z Ophthalmic Solution (Can)** *see* Travoprost *on page 2089*
- ◆ **Teva-Trazodone (Can)** *see* TraZODone *on page 2091*
- ◆ **Teva-Triamterene HCTZ (Can)** *see* Hydrochlorothiazide and Triamterene *on page 1012*
- ◆ **Teva-Trimel (Can)** *see* Sulfamethoxazole and Trimethoprim *on page 1946*
- ◆ **Teva-Trimel DS (Can)** *see* Sulfamethoxazole and Trimethoprim *on page 1946*
- ◆ **Teva-Valsartan (Can)** *see* Valsartan *on page 2127*
- ◆ **Teva-Valsartan HCTZ (Can)** *see* Valsartan and Hydrochlorothiazide *on page 2129*
- ◆ **Teva-Venlafaxine XR (Can)** *see* Venlafaxine *on page 2150*
- ◆ **Teva-Voriconazole (Can)** *see* Voriconazole *on page 2176*
- ◆ **Teva-Zolmitriptan (Can)** *see* ZOLMitriptan *on page 2210*
- ◆ **Teva-Zolmitriptan OD (Can)** *see* ZOLMitriptan *on page 2210*
- ◆ **Teveten** *see* Eprosartan *on page 748*
- ◆ **Teveten HCT** *see* Eprosartan and Hydrochlorothiazide *on page 750*
- ◆ **Teveten Plus (Can)** *see* Eprosartan and Hydrochlorothiazide *on page 750*
- ◆ **Tev-Tropin** *see* Somatropin *on page 1918*
- ◆ **Texacort** *see* Hydrocortisone (Topical) *on page 1014*
- ◆ **TG** *see* Thioguanine *on page 2029*
- ◆ **6-TG (error-prone abbreviation)** *see* Thioguanine *on page 2029*
- ◆ **TH9507** *see* Tesamorelin *on page 2010*

Thalidomide (tha LI doe mide)

Brand Names: U.S. Thalomid

Brand Names: Canada Thalomid

Pharmacologic Category Angiogenesis Inhibitor; Antineoplastic Agent; Immunomodulator, Systemic

Use

Erythema nodosum leprosum: Acute treatment of cutaneous manifestations of moderate to severe erythema nodosum leprosum; maintenance treatment for prevention and suppression of cutaneous manifestations of erythema nodosum leprosum recurrence

Multiple myeloma: Treatment of newly-diagnosed multiple myeloma (in combination with dexamethasone)

Pregnancy Risk Factor X

Pregnancy Considerations [U.S. Boxed Warning]: Thalidomide may cause severe birth defects or embryo-fetal death if taken during pregnancy. Thalidomide cannot be used in women who are pregnant or may become pregnant during therapy as even a single dose may cause severe birth defects. In order to decrease the risk of fetal exposure, thalidomide is available only through a special restricted distribution program (Thalomid REMS). Reproduction studies in animals and data from pregnant women have shown evidence of fetal abnormalities; use is contraindicated in women who are or may become pregnant. Anomalies observed in humans include amelia, phocomelia, bone defects, ear and eye abnormalities, facial palsy, congenital heart defects, urinary and genital tract malformations; mortality in ~40% of infants at or shortly after birth has also been reported.

Women of reproductive potential must avoid pregnancy 4 weeks prior to therapy, during therapy, during therapy interruptions, and for ≥4 weeks after therapy is discontinued. Two forms of effective contraception or total abstinence from heterosexual intercourse must be used by females who are not infertile or who have not had a hysterectomy. A negative pregnancy test (sensitivity of at least 50 mIU/mL) 10 to 14 days prior to therapy, within 24 hours prior to beginning therapy, weekly during the first 4 weeks, and every 4 weeks (every 2 weeks for women with irregular menstrual cycles) thereafter is required for women of childbearing potential. Thalidomide must be immediately discontinued for a missed period, abnormal pregnancy test or abnormal menstrual bleeding; refer patient to a reproductive toxicity specialist if pregnancy occurs during treatment.

Females of reproductive potential (including health care workers and caregivers) must also avoid contact with thalidomide capsules.

Thalidomide is also present in the semen of males. Males (even those vasectomized) must use a latex or synthetic condom during any sexual contact with women of childbearing potential and for up to 28 days following discontinuation of therapy. Males taking thalidomide must not donate sperm.

The parent or legal guardian for patients between 12 to 18 years of age must agree to ensure compliance with the required guidelines.

If pregnancy occurs during treatment, thalidomide must be immediately discontinued and the patient referred to a reproductive toxicity specialist. Any suspected fetal exposure to thalidomide must be reported to the FDA via the MedWatch program (1-800-FDA-1088) and to Celgene Corporation (1-888-423-5436). In Canada, thalidomide is available only through a restricted-distribution program called RevAid (1-888-738-2431).

Breast-Feeding Considerations It is not known if thalidomide is excreted in breast milk. Due to the potential for serious adverse reactions in the infant, a decision should be made to discontinue nursing or discontinue treatment with thalidomide, taking into account the importance of treatment to the mother. Use in breast-feeding women is contraindicated in the Canadian labeling.

Contraindications Hypersensitivity to thalidomide or any component of the formulation; pregnancy

Canadian labeling: Additional contraindications (not in U.S. labeling): Hypersensitivity to lenalidomide; breast-feeding

Warnings/Precautions Hazardous agent - use appropriate precautions for handling and disposal (NIOSH 2014 [group 2]).

Avoid exposure to non-intact capsules and body fluids of patients receiving thalidomide. If exposure occurs, wash area with soap and water. Wear gloves to prevent cutaneous exposure.

[U.S. Boxed Warning]: Thalidomide use for the treatment of multiple myeloma is associated with an increased risk for venous thromboembolism (VTE), including deep vein thrombosis (DVT) and pulmonary embolism (PE); the risk is increased when used in combination with standard chemotherapy agents, including dexamethasone. In one controlled study, the incidence of VTE was 22.5% in patients receiving thalidomide in combination with dexamethasone, compared to 4.9% for dexamethasone alone. Monitor for signs and symptoms of thromboembolism (shortness of breath, chest pain, or arm or leg swelling) and instruct patients to seek prompt medical attention with development of these symptoms. Consider thromboprophylaxis based on risk factors. Ischemic heart disease, including MI and stroke, also occurred at a higher rate (compared to placebo) in myeloma patients receiving thalidomide plus dexamethasone who had not received prior treatment. Assess individual risk factors for thromboembolism and consider thromboprophylaxis. The NCCN multiple myeloma guidelines (v.2.2014) recommend anticoagulant prophylaxis with thalidomide-based therapy. Anticoagulant prophylaxis should be individualized and selected based on the venous thromboembolism risk of the combination treatment regimen, using the safest and easiest to administer (Palumbo, 2008). The Canadian labeling recommends anticoagulant prophylaxis for at least the first 5 months of thalidomide-based therapy. Monitor for signs/symptoms of thromboembolism and advise patients to seek immediate care if symptoms (shortness of breath, chest pain, arm/leg swelling) develop. Other medications that are also associated with thromboembolism should be used with caution.

May cause leukopenia and neutropenia; avoid initiating therapy if ANC <750/mm^3; monitor blood counts. Persistent neutropenia may require treatment interruption. Anemia and thrombocytopenia have also been observed. May cause bradycardia; use with caution when administering concomitantly with medications that may also decrease heart rate. May require thalidomide dose reduction or discontinuation. Stevens-Johnson syndrome (SJS) and toxic epidermal necrolysis (TEN) have been reported (may be fatal); withhold therapy and evaluate if skin rash occurs; permanently discontinue if rash is exfoliative, purpuric, bullous or if SJS or TEN is suspected. Hypersensitivity, including erythematous macular rash, possibly associated with fever, tachycardia and hypotension has been reported. May require treatment interruption for severe reactions; discontinue if recurs with rechallenge.

Increased incidence of second primary malignancies (SPMs), including acute myeloid leukemia (AML) and myelodysplastic syndrome (MDS), has been observed in previously untreated multiple myeloma patients receiving thalidomide in combination with melphalan, and prednisone. In addition to AML and MDS, solid tumors have been reported with thalidomide maintenance treatment for multiple myeloma (Usmani, 2012). Carefully evaluate patients for SPMs prior to and during treatment and manage as clinically indicated.

Thalidomide is commonly associated with peripheral neuropathy; may be irreversible. Neuropathy generally occurs following chronic use (over months), but may occur with short-term use; onset may be delayed. Use caution with other medications that may also cause peripheral neuropathy. Monitor for signs/symptoms of neuropathy monthly for the first 3 months of therapy and regularly thereafter. Electrophysiological testing may be considered at baseline and every 6 months to detect asymptomatic neuropathy. To limit further damage, immediately discontinue (if clinically appropriate) in patients who develop neuropathy. Reinitiate therapy only if neuropathy returns to baseline; may require dosage reduction or permanent discontinuation. Seizures (including grand mal convulsions) have been reported in postmarketing data; monitor closely for clinical changes indicating potential seizure activity in patients with a history of seizures, concurrent therapy with drugs that alter seizure threshold, or conditions that predispose to seizures. May cause dizziness, drowsiness, and/or somnolence; caution patients about performing tasks that require mental alertness (eg, operating machinery or driving). Avoid ethanol and concomitant medications that may exacerbate these symptoms; dose reductions may be necessary for excessive drowsiness or somnolence. May cause orthostatic hypotension; use with caution in patients who would not tolerate transient hypotensive episodes. When arising from a recumbent position, advise patients to sit upright for a few minutes prior to standing. Constipation may commonly occur. May require treatment interruption or dosage reduction. Certain adverse reactions (constipation, fatigue, weakness, nausea, hypokalemia, hyperglycemia, DVT, pulmonary embolism, atrial fibrillation) are more likely in elderly patients. In studies conducted prior to the use of highly active antiretroviral therapy, thalidomide use was associated with increased viral loads in HIV infected patients. Monitor viral load after the 1st and 3rd months of therapy and every 3 months thereafter. Patients with a high tumor burden may be at risk for tumor lysis syndrome; monitor closely; institute appropriate management for hyperuricemia.

Potentially significant drug-drug interactions may exist, requiring dose or frequency adjustment, additional monitoring, and/or selection of alternative therapy. Patients should not donate blood during thalidomide treatment and for 1 month after therapy discontinuation

[U.S. Boxed Warning]: Thalidomide may cause severe birth defects or embryo-fetal death if taken during pregnancy. Thalidomide cannot be used in women who are pregnant or may become pregnant during therapy as even a single dose may cause severe birth defects. In order to decrease the risk of fetal exposure, thalidomide is available only through a special restricted distribution program (Thalomid REMS). Use is contraindicated in women who are or may become pregnant. Pregnancy must be excluded prior to therapy initiation with 2 negative pregnancy tests. Women of reproductive potential must avoid pregnancy 4 weeks prior to therapy, during therapy, during therapy interruptions, and for ≥4 weeks after therapy is discontinued; two reliable methods of birth control, or abstinence from heterosexual intercourse, must be used. Males taking thalidomide (even those vasectomized) must use a latex or synthetic condom during any sexual contact with women of childbearing potential and for up to 28 days following discontinuation of therapy. Males taking thalidomide must not donate sperm. Some forms of contraception may not be appropriate in certain patients. An intrauterine device (IUD) or implantable contraceptive may increase the risk of infection or bleeding; estrogen containing products may increase the risk of thromboembolism.

Due to the embryo-fetal risk, thalidomide is only available through a restricted program under the Thalomid REMS program. Prescribers and pharmacies must be certified with the program to prescribe or dispense thalidomide. Patients must sign an agreement and comply with the REMS program requirements.

Adverse Reactions

Cardiovascular: Edema, facial edema, hypotension, peripheral edema, thrombosis/embolism

Central nervous system: Agitation/anxiety, confusion, dizziness, fatigue, fever, headache, insomnia, malaise, motor neuropathy, nervousness, pain, sensory neuropathy, somnolence, vertigo

Dermatologic: Acne, dermatitis (fungal), desquamation, dry skin, maculopapular rash, nail disorder, pruritus, rash
Endocrine & metabolic: Hyperlipemia, hypocalcemia
Gastrointestinal: Anorexia, constipation, diarrhea, flatulence, nausea, oral moniliasis, tooth pain, weight gain/loss, xerostomia
Genitourinary: Impotence
Hematologic: Anemia, leukopenia, lymphadenopathy, neutropenia
Hepatic: AST increased, bilirubin increased, LFTs abnormal
Neuromuscular & skeletal: Arthralgia, back pain, muscle weakness, myalgia, neck pain/rigidity, neuropathy, paresthesia, tremor, weakness
Renal: Albuminuria, hematuria
Respiratory: Dyspnea, pharyngitis, rhinitis, sinusitis
Miscellaneous: Diaphoresis, infection
Rare but important or life-threatening: Acute renal failure, alkaline phosphatase increased, ALT increased, amenorrhea, angioedema, aphthous stomatitis, arrhythmia, atrial fibrillation, bile duct obstruction, bradycardia, BUN increased, carpal tunnel, cerebral vascular accident, CML, creatinine clearance decreased, creatinine increased, deafness, depression, diplopia, dysesthesia, ECG abnormalities, enuresis, eosinophilia, epistaxis, erythema multiforme, erythema nodosum, erythroleukemia, exfoliative dermatitis, febrile neutropenia, foot drop, galactorrhea, granulocytopenia, gynecomastia, hearing loss, hepatomegaly, Hodgkin's disease, hypercalcemia, hyper-/hypokalemia, hypersensitivity, hypertension, hyper-/hypothyroidism, hypersensitivity, hyperuricemia, hypomagnesemia, hyponatremia, hypoproteinemia, intestinal obstruction, intestinal perforation, interstitial pneumonitis, LDH increased, lethargy, leukocytosis, loss of consciousness, lymphedema, lymphopenia, mental status changes, metrorrhagia, MI, myxedema, nystagmus, oliguria, orthostatic hypotension, pancytopenia, paresthesia, petechiae, peripheral neuritis, photosensitivity, pleural effusion, prothrombin time changes, psychosis, pulmonary embolus, pulmonary hypertension, purpura, Raynaud's syndrome, renal failure, secondary malignancy (AML, MDS, solid tumors), seizure, sepsis, septic shock, sexual dysfunction, sick sinus syndrome, status epilepticus, Stevens-Johnson syndrome, stomach ulcer, stupor, suicide attempt, syncope, tachycardia, thrombocytopenia, toxic epidermal necrolysis, transient ischemic attack, tumor lysis syndrome, urticaria

Drug Interactions

Metabolism/Transport Effects None known.

Avoid Concomitant Use

Avoid concomitant use of Thalidomide with any of the following: Abatacept; Anakinra; Azelastine (Nasal); BCG; Canakinumab; Certolizumab Pegol; CloZAPine; CNS Depressants; Dipyrone; Natalizumab; Orphenadrine; Paraldehyde; Pimecrolimus; Rilonacept; Tacrolimus (Topical); Tocilizumab; Tofacitinib; Vaccines (Live); Vedolizumab

Increased Effect/Toxicity

Thalidomide may increase the levels/effects of: Abatacept; Alcohol (Ethyl); Anakinra; Azelastine (Nasal); Bisphosphonate Derivatives; Canakinumab; Certolizumab Pegol; CloZAPine; Leflunomide; Metyrosine; Natalizumab; Orphenadrine; Pamidronate; Paraldehyde; Pramipexole; Rilonacept; ROPINIRole; Rotigotine; Selective Serotonin Reuptake Inhibitors; Tofacitinib; Vaccines (Live); Vedolizumab; Zoledronic Acid

The levels/effects of Thalidomide may be increased by: Brimonidine (Topical); Cannabis; CNS Depressants; Contraceptives (Estrogens); Contraceptives (Progestins); Denosumab; Dexamethasone (Systemic); Dipyrone; Dronabinol; Erythropoiesis-Stimulating Agents; Estrogen Derivatives; Kava Kava; Magnesium Sulfate; Nabilone; Pimecrolimus; Roflumilast; Rufinamide; Tacrolimus (Topical); Tetrahydrocannabinol; Tocilizumab; Trastuzumab

Decreased Effect

Thalidomide may decrease the levels/effects of: BCG; Coccidioides immitis Skin Test; Sipuleucel-T; Vaccines (Inactivated); Vaccines (Live)

The levels/effects of Thalidomide may be decreased by: Echinacea

Storage/Stability Store at 20°C to 25°C (68°F to 77°F); excursions are permitted between 15°C and 30°C (59°F and 86°F). Protect from light. Keep in original package.

Mechanism of Action Immunomodulatory and antiangiogenic characteristics; immunologic effects may vary based on conditions; may suppress excessive tumor necrosis factor-alpha production in patients with ENL, yet may increase plasma tumor necrosis factor-alpha levels in HIV-positive patients. In multiple myeloma, thalidomide is associated with an increase in natural killer cells and increased levels of interleukin-2 and interferon gamma. Other proposed mechanisms of action include suppression of angiogenesis, prevention of free-radical-mediated DNA damage, increased cell mediated cytotoxic effects, and altered expression of cellular adhesion molecules.

Pharmacodynamics/Kinetics

Absorption: Slow, good
Protein binding: 55% to 66%
Metabolism: Minimal (unchanged drug is the predominant circulating component)
Half-life elimination: 5.5 to 7.3 hours
Time to peak, plasma: ~2 to 5 hours
Excretion: Urine (92%; <4% of the dose as unchanged drug); feces (<2%)

Dosage

Chronic graft-versus-host disease (refractory), treatment (off-label second-line use; limited data): Children ≥3 years: Oral: 3 mg/kg 4 times daily (dose adjusted to goal thalidomide concentration of ≥5 mcg/mL 2 hours post-dose) (Vogelsang, 1992) **or** Initial: 3 to 6 mg/kg/day in 2 to 4 divided doses; target dose 12 mg/kg/day; Maximum daily dose: 800 mg (Rovelli, 1998)

Erythema nodosum leprosum, acute cutaneous: Children ≥12 years and Adults: Oral: Initial: 100 to 300 mg once daily at bedtime, continue until signs/symptoms subside (usually ~2 weeks), then taper off in 50 mg decrements every 2 to 4 weeks. For severe cases with moderate-to-severe neuritis, corticosteroids may be initiated with thalidomide (taper off and discontinue corticosteroids when neuritis improves).

Patients weighing <50 kg: Initiate at lower end of the dosing range

Severe cutaneous reaction or patients previously requiring high doses: May be initiated at up to 400 mg once daily at bedtime or in divided doses

Erythema nodosum leprosum, maintenance (prevention/suppression, or with flares during tapering attempts): Children ≥12 years and Adults: Oral: Maintain on the minimum dosage necessary to control the reaction; efforts to taper should be repeated every 3 to 6 months, in decrements of 50 mg every 2 to 4 weeks.

Multiple myeloma: Adults: Oral: 200 mg once daily at bedtime (in combination with dexamethasone)

Multiple myeloma (off-label dosing):

In combination with bortezomib and dexamethasone (off-label combination): Induction therapy: 100 mg once daily for the first 14 days, then 200 mg once daily for 3 (21-day) cycles (Cavo, 2010) **or** 100 mg once daily for up to 8 (21-day) cycles (Kaufman, 2010)

In combination with melphalan and prednisone (off-label combination in U.S.): 200 to 400 mg once daily (Facon, 2007) **or** 100 mg once daily (Palumbo, 2008)

Canadian labeling: Adults ≥65 years: 200 mg once daily; maximum: 12 six-week cycles (in combination with melphalan and prednisone)

Multiple myeloma, maintenance (following autologous stem cell transplant; off-label use): 200 mg once daily starting 3 to 6 months after transplant; continue until disease progression or unacceptable toxicity (Brinker, 2006) or 100 mg once daily starting 42 to 60 days following transplant; increase to 200 mg once daily after 2 weeks if tolerated; continue for up to 12 months (in combination with prednisolone) (Spencer, 2009)

Multiple myeloma, salvage therapy: Initial: 200 mg once daily at bedtime; may increase daily dose by 200 mg every 2 weeks for 6 weeks (if tolerated) to a maximum of 800 mg once daily at bedtime (Singhal, 1999) **or** 100 mg once daily (in combination with dexamethasone) (Palumbo, 2001) **or** 200 mg once daily (in combination with bortezomib and dexamethasone) for 1 year (Garderet, 2012) **or** 400 mg once daily at bedtime (in combination with dexamethasone, cisplatin, doxorubicin, cyclophosphamide and etoposide) (Lee, 2003)

AIDS-related aphthous stomatitis (off-label use): Adults: Oral: 200 mg once daily at bedtime for up to 8 weeks, if no response, then 200 mg twice daily for 4 weeks (Jacobson, 1997)

Chronic graft-versus-host disease (refractory), treatment (off-label second-line use; optimum dose not determined): Adults: Oral: Initial: 100 mg once daily at bedtime, with dose escalation up to 400 mg daily in 3 to 4 divided doses (Wolff, 2010) **or** Initial: 50 to 100 mg 3 times daily; maximum dose: 600 to 1,200 mg daily (Kulkarni, 2003) **or** 200 mg 4 times daily (dose adjusted to goal thalidomide concentration of ≥5 mcg/mL 2 hours postdose) (Vogelsang, 1992) **or** 100 to 300 mg 4 times daily (Parker, 1995)

Systemic light chain amyloidosis (off-label use): Adults: Oral: 200 mg once daily (starting dose 50 to 100 mg once daily; titrate at 4-week intervals) in combination with cyclophosphamide and dexamethasone (Wechalekar, 2007)

Waldenström's macroglobulinemia (off-label use): Adults: Oral: ≤200 mg once daily for up to 52 weeks (in combination with rituximab) (Treon, 2008)

Dosing adjustment for toxicity:

ANC ≤750/mm^3: Withhold treatment if clinically appropriate

Multiple myeloma:

U.S. labeling: Constipation, oversedation, peripheral neuropathy: Temporarily withhold or continue with a reduced dose

Canadian labeling:

ANC <1500/mm^3: Withhold melphalan and prednisone for 1 week; resume melphalan and prednisone after 1 week if ANC >1500/mm^3 **or** if ANC 1000 to 1500/mm^3 reduce melphalan dose by 50% **or** if ANC <1000/mm^3 adjust chemotherapy dose based on clinical status of patient.

Constipation, oversedation: Temporarily withhold thalidomide treatment or continue with a reduced dose

Peripheral neuropathy, Grade 1 (paresthesia, weakness and/or loss of reflexes) without loss of function): Evaluate patient and consider dose reduction with worsening of symptoms; symptom improvement may not follow dose reduction, however.

Peripheral neuropathy, Grade 2 (interferes with function but not with daily activities), Grade 3 (interferes with daily activities), or Grade 4 (disabling neuropathy): Discontinue thalidomide treatment

Thromboembolic events: Withhold therapy and initiate standard anticoagulant treatment; may resume thalidomide therapy at original dose following stabilization of patient and resolution of thromboembolic event; maintain anticoagulant treatment for duration of thalidomide therapy

Off-label dosage adjustment (Richardson, 2012): Peripheral neuropathy:

Grade 1: Reduce dose by 50%

Grade 2: Temporarily interrupt therapy; once resolved to ≤ grade 1, resume therapy with a 50% dosage reduction (if clinically appropriate)

Grade 3 or higher: Discontinue therapy

Dosage adjustment in renal impairment: No dosage adjustment necessary for patients with renal impairment and on dialysis (per manufacturer). In a study of 6 patients with end-stage renal disease on dialysis, although clearance was increased by dialysis, a supplemental dose was not needed (Eriksson, 2003).

Multiple myeloma: An evaluation of 29 newly-diagnosed myeloma patients with renal failure (serum creatinine ≥2 mg/dL) treated with thalidomide and dexamethasone (some also received cyclophosphamide) found that toxicities and efficacy were similar to patients with normal renal function (Seol, 2010). A study evaluating induction therapy with thalidomide and dexamethasone in 31 newly-diagnosed myeloma patients with renal failure (CrCl <50 mL/minute), including 16 patients with severe renal impairment (CrCl <30 mL/minute) and 7 patients on chronic hemodialysis found that toxicities were similar to patients without renal impairment and that thalidomide and dexamethasone could be administered safely (Tosi, 2009).

Dosage adjustment in hepatic impairment: No dosage adjustment provided in manufacturer's labeling (has not been studied). However, thalidomide does not appear to undergo significant hepatic metabolism.

Administration Do not open or crush capsules. Avoid extensive handling of capsules; capsules should remain in blister pack until ingestion. If exposed to the powder content from broken capsules or body fluids from patients receiving thalidomide, the exposed area should be washed with soap and water.

U.S. labeling: Administer orally with water, preferably at bedtime once daily, at least 1 hour after the evening meal. Doses >400 mg/day may be given in divided doses at least 1 hour after meals. For missed doses, if <12 hours patient may receive dose; if >12 hours wait till next dose due.

Canadian labeling: Administer orally as a single dose at the same time each day; may be taken without regard to meals. May be administered at bedtime to decrease somnolence. Capsules should be swallowed whole, preferably with water.

Hazardous agent; use appropriate precautions for handling and disposal (NIOSH 2014 [group 2]). Wear gloves to prevent cutaneous exposure.

Monitoring Parameters CBC with differential, platelets; thyroid function tests (TSH at baseline then every 2 to 3 months during thalidomide treatment [Hamnvik, 2011]). In HIV-seropositive patients: viral load after 1 and 3 months, then every 3 months. Pregnancy testing (sensitivity of at least 50 mIU/mL) is required within 24 hours prior to initiation of therapy, weekly during the first 4 weeks, then every 4 weeks in women with regular menstrual cycles or every 2 weeks in women with irregular menstrual cycles. Signs of neuropathy monthly for the first 3 months, then periodically during treatment; consider monitoring of sensory nerve application potential amplitudes (at baseline and every 6 months) to detect asymptomatic neuropathy. Monitor for signs and symptoms of thromboembolism (shortness of breath, chest pain, arm/leg swelling), tumor lysis syndrome, bradycardia and syncope; monitor for clinical changes indicating potential seizure activity (in patients with a history of seizure).

Reference Range Graft-vs-host disease: Therapeutic plasma thalidomide levels are 5 to 8 mcg/mL, although it has been suggested that lower plasma levels (0.5 to 1.5 mcg/mL) may be therapeutic; peak serum thalidomide level after a 200 mg dose: 1.8 mcg/mL

Dosage Forms

Capsule, Oral:

Thalomid: 50 mg, 100 mg, 150 mg, 200 mg

Extemporaneous Preparations Hazardous agent; use appropriate precautions for handling and disposal (NIOSH 2014 [group 2]).

A 20 mg/mL oral suspension may be prepared with capsules and a 1:1 mixture of Ora-Sweet and Ora-Plus. Empty the contents of twelve 100 mg capsules into a glass mortar. Add small portions of the vehicle and mix to a uniform paste; mix while adding the vehicle in incremental proportions to almost 60 mL; transfer to an amber calibrated bottle, rinse mortar with vehicle, and add quantity of vehicle sufficient to make 60 mL. Label "shake well," "protect from light," and "refrigerate". Stable for 35 days refrigerated.

Kraft S, Johnson CE, and Tyler RP, "Stability of an Extemporaneously Prepared Thalidomide Suspension," *Am J Health Syst Pharm*, 2011, 69(1):56-8.

◆ **Thalomid** *see* Thalidomide *on page 2022*

◆ **Tham** *see* Tromethamine *on page 2107*

◆ **THC** *see* Dronabinol *on page 694*

◆ **THC and CBD** *see* Tetrahydrocannabinol and Cannabidiol [CAN/INT] *on page 2018*

◆ **The Magic Bullet [OTC]** *see* Bisacodyl *on page 265*

◆ **The Magic Bullett [OTC] (Can)** *see* Bisacodyl *on page 265*

◆ **Theo-24** *see* Theophylline *on page 2026*

◆ **Theochron** *see* Theophylline *on page 2026*

◆ **Theo ER (Can)** *see* Theophylline *on page 2026*

◆ **Theolair (Can)** *see* Theophylline *on page 2026*

Theophylline (thee OFF i lin)

Brand Names: U.S. Elixophyllin; Theo-24; Theochron

Brand Names: Canada Apo-Theo LA®; Novo-Theophyl SR; PMS-Theophylline; Pulmophylline; ratio-Theo-Bronc; Teva-Theophylline SR; Theo ER; Theolair; Uniphyl

Index Terms Theophylline Anhydrous

Pharmacologic Category Phosphodiesterase Enzyme Inhibitor, Nonselective

Use Treatment of symptoms and reversible airway obstruction due to chronic asthma, or other chronic lung diseases

Note: The Global Initiative for Asthma Guidelines (2009) and the National Heart, Lung and Blood Institute Guidelines (2007) do not recommend oral theophylline as a long-term control medication for asthma in children ≤5 years of age; use has been shown to be effective as an add-on (but not preferred) agent in older children and adults with severe asthma treated with inhaled or oral glucocorticoids. The guidelines do not recommend theophylline for the treatment of exacerbations of asthma.

The Global Initiative for Chronic Obstructive Lung Disease Guidelines (2013) suggest that while higher doses of slow release formulations of theophylline have been proven to be effective for use in COPD, it is not a preferred agent due to its potential for toxicity.

Pregnancy Risk Factor C

Pregnancy Considerations Teratogenic effects were observed in animal reproduction studies. Theophylline crosses the placenta; adverse effects may be seen in the newborn. Use is generally safe when used at the recommended doses (serum concentrations 5-12 mcg/mL) however maternal adverse events may be increased and efficacy may be decreased in pregnant women. Theophylline metabolism may change during pregnancy; the half-life is similar to that observed in otherwise healthy, nonsmoking adults with asthma during the first and second trimesters (~8.7 hours), but may increase to 13 hours (range: 8-18 hours) during the third trimester. The volume of distribution is also increased during the third trimester. Monitor serum levels. The recommendations for the use of theophylline in pregnant women with asthma are similar to those used in nonpregnant adults (National Heart, Lung, and Blood Institute Guidelines, 2004).

Breast-Feeding Considerations The concentration of theophylline in breast milk is similar to the maternal serum concentration. Irritability may be observed in the nursing infant. Serious adverse events in the infant are unlikely unless toxic serum levels are present in the mother.

Contraindications Hypersensitivity to theophylline or any component of the formulation; premixed injection may contain corn-derived dextrose and its use is contraindicated in patients with allergy to corn-related products

Warnings/Precautions If a patient develops signs and symptoms of theophylline toxicity (eg, persistent, repetitive vomiting), a serum theophylline level should be measured and subsequent doses held. Serum theophylline monitoring may be lessened as lower therapeutic ranges are established. More intense monitoring may be required during acute illness or when interacting drugs are introduced into the regimen. Use with caution in patients with peptic ulcer, hyperthyroidism, seizure disorders, and patients with tachyarrhythmias (eg, sinus tachycardia, atrial fibrillation); use may exacerbate these conditions. Theophylline-induced nonconvulsive status epilepticus has been reported (rarely) and should be considered in patients who develop CNS abnormalities. Theophylline clearance may be decreased in patients with acute pulmonary edema, congestive heart failure, cor-pulmonale, fever, hepatic disease, acute hepatitis, cirrhosis, hypothyroidism, sepsis with multiorgan failure, and shock; clearance may also be decreased in neonates, infants <3 months of age with decreased renal function, infants <1 year of age, the elderly >60 years, and patients following cessation of smoking.

Adverse Reactions Adverse events observed at therapeutic serum levels:

Cardiovascular: Flutter, tachycardia

Central nervous system: Headache, hyperactivity (children), insomnia, restlessness, seizures, status epilepticus (nonconvulsive)

Endocrine & metabolic: Hypercalcemia (with concomitant hyperthyroid disease)

Gastrointestinal: Nausea, reflux or ulcer aggravation, vomiting

Genitourinary: Difficulty urinating (elderly males with prostatism)

Neuromuscular & skeletal: Tremor

Renal: Diuresis (transient)

Drug Interactions

Metabolism/Transport Effects Substrate of CYP1A2 (major), CYP2C9 (minor), CYP2D6 (minor), CYP2E1 (major), CYP3A4 (major); **Note:** Assignment of Major/Minor substrate status based on clinically relevant drug interaction potential; **Inhibits** CYP1A2 (weak)

Avoid Concomitant Use

Avoid concomitant use of Theophylline with any of the following: Conivaptan; Deferasirox; Fusidic Acid (Systemic); Idelalisib; Iobenguane I 123; Riociguat; Stiripentol

Increased Effect/Toxicity

Theophylline may increase the levels/effects of: Formoterol; Indacaterol; Olodaterol; Pancuronium; Riociguat; Sympathomimetics

The levels/effects of Theophylline may be increased by: Abiraterone Acetate; Alcohol (Ethyl); Allopurinol; Antithyroid Agents; Aprepitant; AtoMOXetine; Cannabinoid-Containing Products; Ceritinib; Cimetidine; Conivaptan; CYP1A2 Inhibitors (Moderate); CYP1A2 Inhibitors (Strong); CYP3A4 Inhibitors (Moderate); CYP3A4 Inhibitors (Strong); Dasatinib; Deferasirox; Disulfiram; Estrogen Derivatives; Febuxostat; FluvoxaMINE; Fosaprepitant; Fusidic Acid (Systemic); Idelalisib; Interferons; Isoniazid; Ivacaftor; Linezolid; Luliconazole; Macrolide Antibiotics; Methotrexate; Metreleptin; Mexiletine; Mifepristone; Netupitant; Peginterferon Alfa-2b; Pentoxifylline; Propafenone; QuiNINE; Quinolone Antibiotics; Simeprevir; Stiripentol; Tedizolid; Thiabendazole; Ticlopidine; Vemurafenib; Zafirlukast; Zileuton

Decreased Effect

Theophylline may decrease the levels/effects of: Adenosine; Benzodiazepines; CarBAMazepine; Fosphenytoin; Iobenguane I 123; Lithium; Pancuronium; Phenytoin; Regadenoson; Zafirlukast

The levels/effects of Theophylline may be decreased by: Adalimumab; Aminoglutethimide; Barbiturates; Beta-Blockers (Beta1 Selective); Beta-Blockers (Nonselective); Bosentan; Cannabis; CarBAMazepine; CYP1A2 Inducers (Strong); CYP3A4 Inducers (Moderate); CYP3A4 Inducers (Strong); Cyproterone; Dabrafenib; Fosphenytoin; Isoproterenol; Metreleptin; Mitotane; Phenytoin; Protease Inhibitors; Siltuximab; St Johns Wort; Teriflunomide; Thyroid Products; Tocilizumab

Food Interactions

Ethanol: Ethanol may decrease theophylline clearance. Management: Avoid or limit ethanol.

Food: Food does not appreciably affect the absorption of liquid, fast-release products, and most sustained release products; however, food may induce a sudden release (dose-dumping) of once-daily sustained release products resulting in an increase in serum drug levels and potential toxicity. Changes in diet may affect the elimination of theophylline; charbroiled foods may increase elimination, reducing half-life by 50%. Management: Should be taken with water 1 hour before or 2 hours after meals. Avoid extremes of dietary protein and carbohydrate intake.

Storage/Stability Tablet, premixed infusion, solution: Store at controlled room temperature of 25°C (77°F).

Mechanism of Action Causes bronchodilatation, diuresis, CNS and cardiac stimulation, and gastric acid secretion by blocking phosphodiesterase which increases tissue concentrations of cyclic adenine monophosphate (cAMP) which in turn promotes catecholamine stimulation of lipolysis, glycogenolysis, and gluconeogenesis and induces release of epinephrine from adrenal medulla cells

Pharmacodynamics/Kinetics

Absorption: Oral: Dosage form dependent

Distribution: 0.45 L/kg (range: 0.3-0.7 L/kg) based on ideal body weight; distributes poorly into body fat; V_d may increase in premature neonates, patients with hepatic cirrhosis, acidemia (uncorrected), the elderly

Metabolism: Children >1 year and Adults: Hepatic; involves CYP1A2, 2E1 and 3A4; forms active metabolites (caffeine and 3-methylxanthine)

Protein binding: 40%, primarily to albumin

Half-life elimination: Highly variable and dependent upon age, liver function, cardiac function, lung disease, and smoking history

- Premature infants, postnatal age 3-15 days: 30 hours (range: 17-43 hours)
- Premature infants, postnatal age 25-57 days: 20 hours (range: 9.4-30.6 hours)
- Children 6-17 years: 3.7 hours (range: 1.5-5.9 hours)
- Adults 16-60 years with asthma, nonsmoking, otherwise healthy: 8.7 hours (range: 6.1-12.8 hours)

Time to peak, serum:
- Oral: Liquid: 1 hour
- IV: Within 30 minutes

Excretion: Urine
- Neonates: 50% as unchanged theophylline
- Children >3 months and Adults: ~10% as unchanged theophylline

Dosage Doses should be individualized based on steady-state serum concentrations and ideal body weight.

Acute symptoms: Loading dose: Children and Adults: Oral, IV:

Asthma exacerbations: While theophylline may be considered for relief of asthma symptoms, the role of treating exacerbations is not supported by current practice.

COPD treatment: Theophylline is currently considered second-line intravenous therapy in the emergency department or hospital setting when there is inadequate or insufficient response to short acting bronchodilators (Global Initiative for COPD Guidelines, 2013).

If no theophylline received within the previous 24 hours: 4.6 mg/kg loading dose (~5.8 mg/kg hydrous aminophylline) IV or 5 mg/kg orally. Loading dose intended to achieve a serum level of approximately 10 mcg/mL; loading doses should be given intravenously (preferred) or with a rapidly absorbed oral product (not an extended-release product). **Note:** On the average, for every 1 mg/kg theophylline given, blood levels will rise 2 mcg/mL.

If theophylline has been administered in the previous 24 hours: A loading dose is not recommended without obtaining a serum theophylline concentration. The loading dose should be calculated as follows:

Dose = (desired serum theophylline concentration - measured serum theophylline concentration) (V_d)

Acute symptoms: Maintenance dose: Children and Adults: IV: **Note:** To achieve a target concentration of 10 mcg/mL unless otherwise noted. Lower initial doses may be required in patients with reduced theophylline clearance. Dosage should be adjusted according to serum level measurements during the first 12- to 24-hour period.

- Infants 6-52 weeks: mg/kg/hour = (0.008) (age in weeks) + 0.21
- Children 1-9 years: 0.8 mg/kg/hour
- Children 9-12 years: 0.7 mg/kg/hour
- Adolescents 12-16 years (cigarette or marijuana smokers): 0.7 mg/kg/hour
- Adolescents 12-16 years (nonsmokers): 0.5 mg/kg/hour; maximum: 900 mg/day unless serum levels indicate need for larger dose
- Adults 16-60 years (otherwise healthy, nonsmokers): 0.4 mg/kg/hour; maximum: 900 mg/day unless serum levels indicate need for larger dose
- Adults >60 years: 0.3 mg/kg/hour; maximum: 400 mg/day unless serum levels indicate need for larger dose

Treatment of chronic conditions: With newer guidelines suggesting lower therapeutic theophylline ranges, it is unlikely that doses larger than >10 mg/kg/day will be required in children ≥1 year or adults.

Oral solution:

Infants <1 year: **Note:** Doses should be adjusted to maintain the peak steady state serum concentrations. The time to reach steady state will vary based on age and the presence of risk factors which may affect theophylline clearance.

Full-term Infants and Infants <26 weeks: Total daily dose (mg)= [(0.2 x age in weeks) +5] x (weight in kg); divide dose into 3 equal amounts and administer at 8-hour intervals

Full-term Infants and Infants ≥26 weeks and <52 weeks: Total daily dose (mg) = [(0.2 x age in weeks) +5] x (weight in kg); divide dose into 4 equal amounts and administer at 6-hour intervals

Children ≥1 year and <45 kg: Initial dose: 10-14 mg/kg/day (maximum: 300 mg/day) administered in divided doses every 4-6 hours; Maintenance: Up to 20 mg/kg/day (maximum: 600 mg/day)

Children >45 kg and Adults: Initial dose: 300 mg/day administered in divided doses every 6-8 hours; Maintenance: 400-600 mg/day (maximum: 600 mg/day)

Oral extended release formulations:

Children ≥1 year and <45 kg: Initial: 10-14 mg/kg once daily (maximum: 300 mg/day); Maintenance up to 20 mg/kg/day (maximum: 600 mg/day)

Children >45 kg and Adults: Initial dose: 300-400 mg once daily; Maintenance: 400-600 mg once daily (maximum: 600 mg/day)

Dosage adjustment in renal impairment: Oral, IV:

Infants 1-3 months: Consider dose reduction and frequent monitoring of serum theophylline concentrations.

Infants >3 months, Children, Adolescents, and Adults: No dosage adjustment necessary.

Dosage adjustment in hepatic impairment:

Oral: Infants, Children, Adolescents, and Adults: No dosage adjustment provided in manufacturer's labeling. However, dose reduction and frequent monitoring of serum theophylline concentration are required in patients with decreased hepatic function (eg, cirrhosis, acute hepatitis, cholestasis). Maximum dose: 400 mg daily

IV: Infants, Children, Adolescents, and Adults: Initial: 0.2 mg/kg/hour; maximum dose: 400 mg daily unless serum concentrations indicate need for larger dose. Use with caution and monitor serum theophylline concentrations frequently.

Dosing in obesity: Use ideal body weight for obese patients.

Dosage adjustment after serum theophylline measurement: Asthma: Within normal limits: Children: 5-10 mcg/mL; Adults: 5-15 mcg/mL: Maintain dosage if tolerated. Recheck serum theophylline concentration at 24-hour intervals (for acute IV dosing) or at 6- to 12-month intervals (for oral dosing). Finer adjustments in dosage may be needed for some patients. If levels ≥15 mcg/mL, consider 10% dose reduction to improve safety margin.

Note: Recheck serum theophylline levels after 3 days when using oral dosing, or after 12 hours (children) or 24 hours (adults) when dosing intravenously. Patients maintained with oral therapy may be reassessed at 6- to 12-month intervals.

Dietary Considerations Should be taken with water 1 hour before or 2 hours after meals. Premixed injection may contain corn-derived dextrose and its use is contraindicated in patients with allergy to corn-related products.

Administration

IV: Administer loading dose over 30 minutes; follow with a continuous infusion as appropriate

Oral: Long-acting preparations should be taken with a full glass of water, swallowed whole, or cut in half if scored. Do **not** crush. Extended release capsule forms may be opened and the contents sprinkled on soft foods; do **not** chew beads.

Monitoring Parameters Monitor heart rate, CNS effects (insomnia, irritability); respiratory rate (COPD patients often have resting controlled respiratory rates in low 20s); arterial or capillary blood gases (if applicable)

Theophylline levels: Serum theophylline levels should be monitored prior to making dose increases; in the presence of signs or symptoms of toxicity; or when a new illness, worsening of a present illness, or medication changes occur that may change theophylline clearance

IV loading dose: Measure serum concentrations 30 minutes after the end of an IV loading dose

IV infusion: Measure serum concentrations one half-life after starting a continuous infusion, then every 12-24 hours

Reference Range Therapeutic levels: Asthma:

Children: 5-10 mcg/mL

Adults: 5-15 mcg/mL

Dosage Forms

Capsule Extended Release 24 Hour, Oral:

Theo-24: 100 mg, 200 mg, 300 mg, 400 mg

Elixir, Oral:

Elixophyllin: 80 mg/15 mL (473 mL)

Solution, Intravenous:

Generic: 400 mg (250 mL, 500 mL); 800 mg (500 mL)

Solution, Oral:

Generic: 80 mg/15 mL (473 mL)

Tablet Extended Release 12 Hour, Oral:

Theochron: 100 mg, 200 mg, 300 mg

Generic: 100 mg, 200 mg, 300 mg, 450 mg

Tablet Extended Release 24 Hour, Oral:

Generic: 400 mg, 600 mg

Extemporaneous Preparations Note: An alcohol-containing commercial oral solution is available (80 mg/15mL).

A 5 mg/mL oral suspension may be made with tablets. Crush one 300 mg extended release tablet in a mortar and reduce to a fine powder. Add small portions of a 1:1 mixture of Ora-Sweet® and Ora-Plus® and mix to a uniform paste; mix while adding the vehicle in equal proportions to **almost** 60 mL; transfer to a calibrated bottle, rinse mortar with vehicle, and add sufficient quantity of vehicle to make 60 mL. Label "shake well". Stable for 90 days at room temperature.

Johnson CE, VanDeKoppel S, and Myers E, "Stability of Anhydrous Theophylline in Extemporaneously Prepared Alcohol-Free Oral Suspensions," *Am J Health-Syst Pharm*, 2005, 62(23):2518-20.

- **Theophylline and Ephedrine** *see* Ephedrine and Theophylline [INT] *on page 734*
- **Theophylline Anhydrous** *see* Theophylline *on page 2026*
- **TheraCIM hR3** *see* Nimotuzumab [INT] *on page 1457*
- **TheraCort [OTC]** *see* Hydrocortisone (Topical) *on page 1014*
- **TheraCys** *see* BCG *on page 229*
- **Thera-Ear [OTC]** *see* Carbamide Peroxide *on page 350*
- **Thera-Gesic [OTC]** *see* Methyl Salicylate and Menthol *on page 1344*
- **Thera-Gesic Plus [OTC]** *see* Methyl Salicylate and Menthol *on page 1344*
- **Theraloc** *see* Nimotuzumab [INT] *on page 1457*
- **Thermazene [DSC]** *see* Silver Sulfadiazine *on page 1887*
- **Thiacetazone and Isoniazid** *see* Isoniazid and Thiacetazone [INT] *on page 1124*
- **Thiamazole** *see* Methimazole *on page 1319*
- **Thiamin** *see* Thiamine *on page 2028*

Thiamine (THYE a min)

Brand Names: Canada Betaxin

Index Terms Aneurine Hydrochloride; Thiamin; Thiamine Hydrochloride; Thiaminium Chloride Hydrochloride; Vitamin B_1

Pharmacologic Category Vitamin, Water Soluble

Use Treatment of thiamine deficiency including beriberi, Wernicke's encephalopathy, Korsakoff's syndrome, neuritis associated with pregnancy, or in alcoholic patients; dietary supplement

Pregnancy Risk Factor A

Dosage

Adequate Intake:

0-6 months: 0.2 mg/day
7-12 months: 0.3 mg/day

Recommended daily intake:

1-3 years: 0.5 mg
4-8 years: 0.6 mg
9-13 years: 0.9 mg
14-18 years: Females: 1 mg; Males: 1.2 mg
≥19 years: Females: 1.1 mg; Males: 1.2 mg
Pregnancy, lactation: 1.4 mg

Parenteral nutrition supplementation:

Infants: 1.2 mg/day
Adults: 6 mg/day; may be increased to 25-50 mg/day with history of alcohol abuse

Thiamine deficiency (beriberi):

Children: 10-25 mg/dose IM or IV daily (if critically ill), or 10-50 mg/dose orally every day for 2 weeks, then 5-10 mg/dose orally daily for 1 month

Adults: 5-30 mg/dose IM or IV 3 times/day (if critically ill); then orally 5-30 mg/day in single or divided doses 3 times/day for 1 month

Alcohol withdrawal syndrome: Adults: 100 mg/day IM or IV for several days, followed by 50-100 mg/day orally

Wernicke's encephalopathy: Adults: Treatment (manufacturer labeling): Initial: 100 mg IV, then 50-100 mg/day IM or IV until consuming a regular, balanced diet. However, larger doses may be required based on failure of lower doses to produce clinical improvement in some patients.

Alternate dosage: The Royal College of Physicians (U.K.) has recommended the use of higher doses of thiamine (in combination with other B vitamins, ascorbic acid, potassium, phosphate, and magnesium) for the management of Wernicke's encephalopathy (Thomson, 2002):

Prophylaxis: 250 mg IV once daily for 3-5 days

Treatment: Initial: 500 mg IV 3 times/day for 3 days. If response to thiamine after 3 days, continue with 250 mg IM or IV once daily for an additional 5 days or until clinical improvement.

Dosage adjustment in renal impairment: No dosage adjustment provided in manufacturer's labeling.

Dosage adjustment in hepatic impairment: No dosage adjustment provided in manufacturer's labeling.

Additional Information Complete prescribing information should be consulted for additional detail.

Dosage Forms

Capsule, Oral:
Generic: 50 mg

Solution, Injection:
Generic: 100 mg/mL (2 mL)

Tablet, Oral:
Generic: 50 mg, 100 mg, 250 mg

Tablet, Oral [preservative free]:
Generic: 100 mg

◆ **Thiamine Hydrochloride** *see* Thiamine *on page 2028*

◆ **Thiaminium Chloride Hydrochloride** *see* Thiamine *on page 2028*

Thioguanine (thye oh GWAH neen)

Brand Names: U.S. Tabloid

Brand Names: Canada Lanvis®

Index Terms 2-Amino-6-Mercaptopurine; 6-TG (error-prone abbreviation); 6-Thioguanine (error-prone abbreviation); TG; Tioguanine

Pharmacologic Category Antineoplastic Agent, Antimetabolite; Antineoplastic Agent, Antimetabolite (Purine Analog)

Use Treatment of acute myelogenous (nonlymphocytic) leukemia (AML)

Pregnancy Risk Factor D

Dosage Oral: Children: Pediatric ALL (off-label use; combination therapy): Delayed intensification treatment phase: 60 mg/m^2/day for 14 days (Lange, 2002; Nachman, 1998)

Dosing comments in renal impairment: Children: No adjustment required (Aronoff, 2007).

Dosing comments in hepatic impairment: Deterioration in transaminases, alkaline phosphatase or bilirubin, toxic hepatitis, biliary stasis, clinical jaundice, evidence of hepatic sinusoidal obstruction syndrome (veno-occlusive disease), or evidence of portal hypertension: Discontinue treatment.

Additional Information Complete prescribing information should be consulted for additional detail.

Dosage Forms

Tablet, Oral:
Tabloid: 40 mg

◆ **6-Thioguanine (error-prone abbreviation)** *see* Thioguanine *on page 2029*

Thiopental [INT] (thye oh PEN tal)

International Brand Names Anesthal (IN); Bensulf (AR); Bitol Sodium (PK); Farmotal (IT); Intraval (AE, BB, BH, BM, BS, BZ, CY, EG, GB, GY, IQ, IR, JM, JO, KW, LB, LY, OM, PR, QA, SA, SR, SY, TT, YE); Intraval Sodium (IN); Nesdonal (HR, LU); Pantul (PE); Pensodital (MX); Pental (TR); Pentarim (MX); Pentazol (PH); Penthal (PH); Penthotal (CN); Pentocur (DK, FI, NO); Pentotal (KR); Pentotex (MY); Pentothal (AU, BB, BM, BS, BZ, CH, FR, GR, GY, ID, IT, JM, LU, MX, NL, NZ, PH, PT, PY, SE, SG, SR, TT, TW, UY); Pentothal Sodico (ES); Pentothal Sodium (ES, PL); Thiojex (PE); Thiopen (PK, TH); Thiopental (AE, BH, CY, EG, IQ, IR, JO, KW, LB, LY, OM, PL, QA, SA, SY, YE); Thiopental Biochemie (AT); Thiopentax (BR, PY); Tiobarbital (ES); Tiopental (CO, CR, GT, HN, HR, NI, PY, VE); Tiopental Sodico (AR); Tiopnetal (UY); Trapanal (DE, HU)

Index Terms Thiopental Sodium; Thiopentone

Pharmacologic Category Anticonvulsant, Barbiturate; Barbiturate; General Anesthetic

Reported Use Induction of anesthesia and adjunctive agent for anesthesia; treatment of convulsive states and of elevated intracranial pressure

Dosage Range Note: Dose ranges are not intended to guide prescribing; consult local prescribing information for additional information.

IV:

Induction anesthesia:
Children: 2-5 mg/kg
Adults: 3-6 mg/kg; maintenance: 25-100 mg as needed
Elderly: Refer to adult dosing; smaller doses are advisable

Seizures: Adults: 75-250 mg/dose

Increased intracranial pressure:
Children: 1-2 mg/kg/dose
Adults: 1.5-3 mg/kg/dose

Dosage adjustment in renal impairment: No dosage adjustment provided in manufacturer's labeling; however, use with caution as hypnotic effect may be prolonged or potentiated.

Dosage adjustment in hepatic impairment: No dosage adjustment provided in manufacturer's labeling; however, because thiopental is metabolized by the liver doses should be reduced in patients with hepatic impairment.

Product Availability Product available in various countries; not currently available in the U.S.

Dosage Forms

Injection, reconstituted, as sodium: 500 mg

- **Thiopental Sodium** *see* Thiopental [INT] *on page 2029*
- **Thiopentone** *see* Thiopental [INT] *on page 2029*
- **Thiophosphoramide** *see* Thiotepa *on page 2030*
- **Thioplex** *see* Thiotepa *on page 2030*

Thioridazine (thye oh RID a zeen)

Index Terms Mellaril; Thioridazine Hydrochloride

Pharmacologic Category First Generation (Typical) Antipsychotic

Additional Appendix Information

Beers Criteria – Potentially Inappropriate Medications for Geriatrics *on page 2271*

Use Management of schizophrenic patients who fail to respond adequately to treatment with other antipsychotic drugs, either because of insufficient effectiveness or the inability to achieve an effective dose due to intolerable adverse effects from those medications

Dosage Oral:

Children >2-12 years (off-label use): Range: 0.5-3 mg/kg/day in 2-3 divided doses; usual: 1 mg/kg/day; maximum: 3 mg/kg/day

Behavior problems (off-label use): Initial: 10 mg 2-3 times/day, increase gradually

Severe psychoses (off-label use): Initial: 25 mg 2-3 times/day, increase gradually

Children >12 years (off-label use) and Adults:

Schizophrenia/psychoses: Initial: 50-100 mg 3 times/day with gradual increments as needed and tolerated; maximum: 800 mg/day in 2-4 divided doses

Depressive disorders/dementia (off-label use): Initial: 25 mg 3 times/day; maintenance dose: 20-200 mg/day

Elderly: Behavioral symptoms associated with dementia (off-label use): Oral: Initial: 10-25 mg 1-2 times/day; increase at 4- to 7-day intervals by 10-25 mg/day; increase dose intervals (once daily, twice daily, etc) as necessary to control response or side effects. Maximum daily dose: 400 mg; gradual increases (titration) may prevent some side effects or decrease their severity.

Dosage adjustment in renal impairment: No dosage adjustment provided in manufacturer's labeling

Hemodialysis: Not dialyzable (0% to 5%)

Dosage adjustment in hepatic impairment: No dosage adjustment provided in manufacturer's labeling

Additional Information Complete prescribing information should be consulted for additional detail.

Dosage Forms

Tablet, Oral:

Generic: 10 mg, 25 mg, 50 mg, 100 mg

- **Thioridazine Hydrochloride** *see* Thioridazine *on page 2030*
- **Thiosulfuric Acid Disodium Salt** *see* Sodium Thiosulfate *on page 1915*

Thiotepa (thye oh TEP a)

Index Terms TESPA; Thiophosphoramide; Thioplex; Triethylenethiophosphoramide; TSPA

Pharmacologic Category Antineoplastic Agent, Alkylating Agent

Use Treatment of superficial papillary bladder cancer; palliative treatment of adenocarcinoma of breast or ovary; controlling intracavitary effusions caused by metastatic tumors

Pregnancy Risk Factor D

Dosage Note: In children, thiotepa is associated with a high emetic potential at doses ≥300 mg/m^2; antiemetics are recommended to prevent nausea and vomiting (Dupuis, 2011).

Children: HSCT for CNS malignancy (off-label use; combination chemotherapy): IV: 300 mg/m^2/day for 3 days beginning 8 days prior to transplant (Gilheeney, 2010) **or** 300 mg/m^2/day for 3 days beginning 5 days prior to transplant (Dunkel, 2010; Grodman, 2009)

Adults:

Bladder cancer: Intravesical: 60 mg in 30 to 60 mL NS retained for 2 hours once weekly for 4 weeks

Ovarian, breast cancer: IV: 0.3 to 0.4 mg/kg every 1 to 4 weeks

Effusions: Intracavitary: 0.6 to 0.8 mg/kg

Leptomeningeal metastases (off-label use/route): Intrathecal: 10 mg twice a week (on days 1 and 4 each week) for 8 weeks (Grossman, 1993)

Hematopoietic stem cell transplant (HSCT) for CNS malignancy (off-label use; combination chemotherapy): IV: 250 mg/m^2/day for 3 days beginning 9 days prior to transplant (Soussain, 2008) **or** 150 mg/m^2/dose every 12 hours for 6 doses, followed by stem cell reinfusion 96 hours after completion of thiotepa (Abrey, 2006)

Dosage adjustment for hematologic toxicity: IV:

WBC ≤3000/mm^3: Discontinue treatment.

Platelets ≤150,000/mm^3: Discontinue treatment.

Note: Use may be contraindicated with preexisting marrow damage and should be limited to cases where benefit outweighs risk.

Dosage adjustment in renal impairment: There are no dosage adjustments provided in the manufacturer's labeling. Use with caution; reduced dose may be warranted. Use may be contraindicated with existing renal impairment and should be limited to cases where benefit outweighs risk.

Dosage adjustment in hepatic impairment: There are no dosage adjustment provided in the manufacturer's labeling. Use with caution; reduced dose may be warranted. Use may be contraindicated with existing hepatic impairment and should be limited to cases where benefit outweighs risk.

Dosing in obesity:

*ASCO Guidelines for appropriate chemotherapy dosing in obese adults with cancer (**Note:** Excludes HSCT dosing):* Utilize patient's actual body weight (full weight) for calculation of body surface area- or weight-based dosing, particularly when the intent of therapy is curative; manage regimen-related toxicities in the same manner as for nonobese patients; if a dose reduction is utilized due to toxicity, consider resumption of full weight-based dosing with subsequent cycles, especially if cause of toxicity (eg, hepatic or renal impairment) is resolved (Griggs, 2012).

American Society for Blood and Marrow Transplantation (ASBMT) practice guideline committee position statement on chemotherapy dosing in obesity: Utilize actual body weight (full weight) for calculation of body surface area in thiotepa dosing for hematopoietic stem cell transplant conditioning regimens in adult patients weighing ≤120% of their ideal body weight (IBW). In patients weighing >120% IBW, utilize adjusted body weight 40% (ABW40) to calculate BSA (Bubalo, 2014).

ABW40: Adjusted wt (kg) = Ideal body weight (kg) + 0.4 [actual wt (kg) - ideal body weight (kg)]

Additional Information Complete prescribing information should be consulted for additional detail.

Thiothixene (thye oh THIKS een)

Brand Names: Canada Navane

Index Terms Navane; Tiotixene

Pharmacologic Category First Generation (Typical) Antipsychotic

Additional Appendix Information

Beers Criteria – Potentially Inappropriate Medications for Geriatrics *on page 2271*

Use Schizophrenia: For the management of schizophrenia

Dosage Schizophrenia: Children >12 years (off-label use), Adolescents (off-label use), and Adults: Oral: Initial: Mild-to-moderate symptoms: 2 mg 3 times daily; usual dose 15 mg daily; severe symptoms: 5 mg 2 times daily; usual dose 20-30 mg daily. Increase dose gradually. Maximum: 60 mg daily.

Dosage adjustment in renal impairment: No dosage adjustment provided in manufacturer's labeling.

Dosage adjustment in hepatic impairment: No dosage adjustment provided in manufacturer's labeling.

Additional Information Complete prescribing information should be consulted for additional detail.

Dosage Forms

Capsule, Oral:

Generic: 1 mg, 2 mg, 5 mg, 10 mg

- ◆ **Thonzonium, Neomycin, Colistin, and Hydrocortisone** *see* Neomycin, Colistin, Hydrocortisone, and Thonzonium *on page 1437*
- ◆ **Thorazine** *see* ChlorproMAZINE *on page 429*
- ◆ **Three-Factor PCC** *see* Factor IX Complex (Human) [(Factors II, IX, X)] *on page 838*
- ◆ **Thrive [OTC]** *see* Nicotine *on page 1449*
- ◆ **Thrombate III** *see* Antithrombin *on page 156*
- ◆ **Thrombate III® (Can)** *see* Antithrombin *on page 156*
- ◆ **Thymocyte Stimulating Factor** *see* Aldesleukin *on page 72*
- ◆ **Thymoglobulin** *see* Antithymocyte Globulin (Rabbit) *on page 158*
- ◆ **Thyrogen** *see* Thyrotropin Alfa *on page 2031*

Thyroid, Desiccated (THYE roid DES i kay tid)

Brand Names: U.S. Armour Thyroid; Nature-Throid; NP Thyroid; Westhroid; Westhroid-P [DSC]; WP Thyroid

Index Terms Desiccated Thyroid; Levothyroxine and Liothyronine; Tetraiodothyronine and Triiodothyronine; Thyroid Extract; Thyroid USP

Pharmacologic Category Thyroid Product

Additional Appendix Information

Beers Criteria – Potentially Inappropriate Medications for Geriatrics *on page 2271*

Use Replacement or supplemental therapy in hypothyroidism; pituitary TSH suppressants (thyroid nodules, thyroiditis, multinodular goiter, thyroid cancer)

Pregnancy Risk Factor A

Dosage Oral: **Note:** The American Association of Clinical Endocrinologists does not recommend the use of desiccated thyroid for thyroid replacement therapy for hypothyroidism (Baskin, 2002). Tablet strengths may vary by manufacturer in terms of grains or mg; dosing recommendations are based on general clinical equivalencies that 1 grain = 60 mg or 65 mg; 1/2 grain = 30 mg or 32.5 mg; and 1/4 grain = 15 mg or 16.25 mg.

Children: See table.

Recommended Pediatric Dosage for Congenital Hypothyroidism

Age	Daily Dose (mg)	Daily Dose/kg (mg)
0-6 mo	15-30	4.8-6
6-12 mo	30-45	3.6-4.8
1-5 y	45-60	3-3.6
6-12 y	60-90	2.4-3
>12 y	>90	1.2-1.8

Adults: Initial: 15-30 mg; increase with 15 mg increments every 2-3 weeks; use 15 mg in patients with cardiovascular disease or long-standing myxedema. Maintenance dose: Usually 60-120 mg/day; monitor TSH and clinical symptoms.

Dosage adjustment in renal impairment: No dosage adjustment provided in manufacturer's labeling.

Dosage adjustment in hepatic impairment: No dosage adjustment provided in manufacturer's labeling.

Additional Information Complete prescribing information should be consulted for additional detail.

Dosage Forms

Tablet, Oral:

Armour Thyroid: 15 mg, 30 mg, 60 mg, 90 mg, 120 mg, 180 mg, 240 mg, 300 mg

Nature-Throid: 16.25 mg, 32.5 mg, 48.75 mg, 65 mg, 81.25 mg, 97.5 mg, 113.75 mg, 130 mg, 146.25 mg, 162.5 mg, 195 mg, 260 mg, 325 mg

NP Thyroid: 30 mg, 60 mg, 90 mg

Westhroid: 16.25 mg, 32.5 mg, 48.75 mg, 65 mg, 81.25 mg, 97.5 mg, 113.75 mg, 130 mg, 146.25 mg, 162.5 mg, 195 mg, 260 mg, 325 mg

WP Thyroid: 16.25 mg, 32.5 mg, 48.75 mg, 65 mg, 81.25 mg, 97.5 mg, 113.75 mg, 130 mg

- ◆ **Thyroid Extract** *see* Thyroid, Desiccated *on page 2031*
- ◆ **Thyroid USP** *see* Thyroid, Desiccated *on page 2031*
- ◆ **Thyrolar®** *see* Liotrix *on page 1221*
- ◆ **ThyroShield [OTC]** *see* Potassium Iodide *on page 1690*

Thyrotropin Alfa (thye roe TROH pin AL fa)

Brand Names: U.S. Thyrogen

Brand Names: Canada Thyrogen

Index Terms Human Thyroid Stimulating Hormone; Recombinant Human Thyrotropin; Rh-TSH; Thyrotropin Alpha; TSH

Pharmacologic Category Diagnostic Agent

Use

Diagnostic imaging: Adjunctive diagnostic tool for serum thyroglobulin (Tg) testing (with or without radioiodine imaging) in follow up of patients with well-differentiated thyroid cancer who have previously undergone thyroidectomy.

Limitations of use: Thyrotropin alfa-stimulated Tg levels are generally lower than and do not correlate with Tg levels after thyroid hormone withdrawal; even when thyrotropin alfa-stimulated Tg testing is performed in combination with radioiodine imaging, there is a risk of missing a thyroid cancer diagnosis or of underestimating disease extent; anti-Tg antibodies may confound Tg assay and render Tg levels uninterpretable, in such cases, even with a negative or low-stage thyrotropin alfa radioiodine scan, consider further patient evaluation.

Thyroid tissue remnant ablation: Adjunctive treatment for radioiodine ablation of thyroid tissue remnants after total or near-total thyroidectomy in patients with well-differentiated thyroid cancer without evidence of metastatic disease

Limitations of use: The effect of thyrotropin alfa on long-term thyroid cancer outcomes has not been determined. Due to relatively small clinical experience, it is not possible to conclude if long-term thyroid cancer outcomes would be equivalent after thyrotropin alfa use or withholding thyroid hormone for TSH elevation prior to remnant ablation.

Pregnancy Risk Factor C

Dosage Note: Consider pretreatment with glucocorticoids for patients in whom local tumor expansion may compromise vital anatomic structures (such as trachea, CNS, or extensive macroscopic lung metastases).

Diagnostic imaging: Adults: IM: 0.9 mg, followed 24 hours later by a second 0.9 mg dose; obtain serum Tg sample 72 hours after the second thyrotropin alfa injection

Thyroid tissue remnant ablation: Adults: IM: 0.9 mg, followed 24 hours later by a second 0.9 mg dose

Radioiodine administration should be given 24 hours following the second thyrotropin alfa injection (for diagnostic scanning and remnant ablation). Perform diagnostic scanning 48 hours after radioiodine administration (72 hours after the second thyrotropin alfa injection). Post-therapy scanning may be delayed (additional days) to allow decline of background activity.

Dosage adjustment in renal impairment: There are no dosage adjustments provided in the manufacturer's labeling; however, elimination is significantly slower in dialysis-dependent end-stage renal impairment and TSH level elevation may be prolonged.

Dosage adjustment in hepatic impairment: There are no dosage adjustments provided in the manufacturer's labeling (has not been studied).

Additional Information Complete prescribing information should be consulted for additional detail.

Dosage Forms

Solution Reconstituted, Intramuscular:

Thyrogen: 1.1 mg (1 ea)

◆ **Thyrotropin Alpha** *see* Thyrotropin Alfa *on page 2031*

◆ **Tiacumicin B** *see* Fidaxomicin *on page 875*

TiaGABine (tye AG a been)

Brand Names: U.S. Gabitril

Index Terms Tiagabine Hydrochloride

Pharmacologic Category Anticonvulsant, Miscellaneous

Use Adjunctive therapy in adults and children ≥12 years of age in the treatment of partial seizures

Pregnancy Risk Factor C

Pregnancy Considerations Adverse events were observed in animal reproduction studies. Patients exposed to tiagabine during pregnancy are encouraged to enroll themselves into the AED Pregnancy Registry by calling 1-888-233-2334. Additional information is available at www.aedpregnancyregistry.org.

Breast-Feeding Considerations Levels of excretion of tiagabine and/or its metabolites in human milk have not been determined and effects on the nursing infant are unknown. According to the manufacturer, the decision to continue or discontinue breast-feeding during therapy should take into account the risk of exposure to the infant and the benefits of treatment to the mother.

Contraindications Hypersensitivity to tiagabine or any component of the formulation

Warnings/Precautions Antiepileptics are associated with an increased risk of suicidal behavior/thoughts with use (regardless of indication); patients should be monitored for signs/symptoms of depression, suicidal tendencies, and other unusual behavior changes during therapy and instructed to inform their healthcare provider immediately if symptoms occur. New-onset seizures and status epilepticus have been associated with tiagabine use when taken for off-label indications. Often these seizures have occurred shortly after the initiation of treatment or shortly after a dosage increase. Seizures have also occurred with very low doses or after several months of therapy. In most cases, patients were using concomitant medications (eg, antidepressants, antipsychotics, stimulants, opioids). In these instances, the discontinuation of tiagabine, followed by an evaluation for an underlying seizure disorder, is suggested. Use for unapproved indications, however, has not been proven to be safe or effective and is not recommended. When tiagabine is used as an adjunct in partial seizures (an FDA-approved indication), it should not be abruptly discontinued because of the possibility of increasing seizure frequency, unless safety concerns require a more rapid withdrawal. Rarely, nonconvulsive status epilepticus has been reported following abrupt discontinuation or dosage reduction.

Use with caution in patients with hepatic impairment. Experience in patients not receiving enzyme-inducing drugs has been limited; caution should be used in treating any patient who is not receiving one of these medications (decreased dose and slower titration may be required). Weakness, sedation, and confusion may occur with tiagabine use. Patients must be cautioned about performing tasks which require mental alertness (eg, operating machinery or driving). Effects with other sedative drugs or ethanol may be potentiated. May cause serious rash, including Stevens-Johnson syndrome.

Adverse Reactions

Cardiovascular: Chest pain, edema, hypertension, palpitation, peripheral edema, syncope, tachycardia, vasodilation

Central nervous system: Agitation, ataxia, chills, concentration decreased, confusion, confusion, depersonalization, depression, difficulty with memory, dizziness, euphoria, hallucination, hostility, insomnia, malaise, migraine, nervousness, paranoid reaction, personality disorder, somnolence, speech disorder

Dermatologic: Alopecia, bruising, dry skin, pruritus, rash

Gastrointestinal: Abdominal pain, diarrhea, gingivitis, increased appetite, mouth ulceration, nausea, stomatitis, vomiting, weight gain/loss

Neuromuscular & skeletal: Abnormal gait, arthralgia, dysarthria, hyper-/hypokinesia, hyper-/hypotonia, myasthenia, myalgia, myoclonus, neck pain, paresthesia, reflexes decreased, stupor, tremor, twitching, vertigo, weakness

Ocular: Abnormal vision, amblyopia, nystagmus

Otic: Ear pain, hearing impairment, otitis media, tinnitus

Respiratory: Bronchitis, cough, dyspnea, epistaxis, pneumonia

Miscellaneous: Allergic reaction, cyst, diaphoresis, flu-like syndrome, lymphadenopathy

Rare but important or life-threatening: Abortion, abscess, anemia, angina, apnea, asthma, blepharitis, blindness, cellulitis, cerebral ischemia, cholelithiasis, CNS neoplasm, coma, deafness, dehydration, dysphagia, dystonia, electrocardiogram abnormal, encephalopathy, hemorrhage, erythrocytes abnormal, fecal incontinence, herpes simplex/zoster, glossitis, goiter, hematuria, hemoptysis, hepatomegaly, hypercholesteremia, hyper-/hypoglycemia, hyperlipemia, hypokalemia, hyponatremia, hypotension, hypothyroidism, impotence, kidney failure, leukopenia, liver function tests abnormal, MI, neoplasm, peripheral vascular disorder, paralysis, photophobia, psychosis, petechia, photosensitivity, seizure (when used for unlabeled uses), sepsis, spasm, suicide attempt, thrombocytopenia, thrombophlebitis, urinary retention, urinary urgency, urticaria, visual field defect

Drug Interactions

Metabolism/Transport Effects Substrate of CYP3A4 (major); **Note:** Assignment of Major/Minor substrate status based on clinically relevant drug interaction potential

Avoid Concomitant Use

Avoid concomitant use of TiaGABine with any of the following: Azelastine (Nasal); Conivaptan; Fusidic Acid (Systemic); Idelalisib; Orphenadrine; Paraldehyde; Thalidomide

Increased Effect/Toxicity

TiaGABine may increase the levels/effects of: Alcohol (Ethyl); Azelastine (Nasal); Buprenorphine; CNS Depressants; Hydrocodone; Methotrimeprazine; Metyrosine; Mirtazapine; Orphenadrine; Paraldehyde; Pramipexole; ROPINIRole; Rotigotine; Selective Serotonin Reuptake Inhibitors; Suvorexant; Thalidomide; Zolpidem

The levels/effects of TiaGABine may be increased by: Aprepitant; Brimonidine (Topical); Cannabis; Ceritinib; Conivaptan; CYP3A4 Inhibitors (Moderate); CYP3A4 Inhibitors (Strong); Dasatinib; Doxylamine; Dronabinol; Droperidol; Fosaprepitant; Fusidic Acid (Systemic); HydrOXYzine; Idelalisib; Ivacaftor; Kava Kava; Luliconazole; Magnesium Sulfate; Methotrimeprazine; Mifepristone; Nabilone; Netupitant; Perampanel; Rufinamide; Simeprevir; Sodium Oxybate; Stiripentol; Tapentadol; Tetrahydrocannabinol

Decreased Effect

The levels/effects of TiaGABine may be decreased by: Bosentan; CYP3A4 Inducers (Moderate); CYP3A4 Inducers (Strong); Dabrafenib; Deferasirox; Mefloquine; Mianserin; Mitotane; Orlistat; Siltuximab; St Johns Wort; Tocilizumab

Food Interactions Food reduces the rate but not the extent of absorption. Management: Administer with food.

Storage/Stability Store at controlled room temperature of 20°C to 25°C (68°F to 77°F). Protect from moisture and light.

Mechanism of Action The exact mechanism by which tiagabine exerts antiseizure activity is not definitively known; however, *in vitro* experiments demonstrate that it enhances the activity of gamma aminobutyric acid (GABA), the major neuroinhibitory transmitter in the nervous system; it is thought that binding to the GABA uptake carrier inhibits the uptake of GABA into presynaptic neurons, allowing an increased amount of GABA to be available to postsynaptic neurons; based on *in vitro* studies, tiagabine does not inhibit the uptake of dopamine, norepinephrine, serotonin, glutamate, or choline

Pharmacodynamics/Kinetics

Absorption: Rapid (45 minutes); prolonged with food

Protein binding: 96%, primarily to albumin and α_1-acid glycoprotein

Metabolism: Hepatic via CYP (primarily 3A4)

Bioavailability: Oral: Absolute: 90%

Half-life elimination: 2-5 hours when administered with enzyme inducers; 7-9 hours when administered without enzyme inducers

Time to peak, plasma: 45 minutes

Excretion: Feces (63%); urine (25%); 2% as unchanged drug; primarily as metabolites

Dosage Oral (administer with food):

Patients receiving enzyme-inducing AED regimens:

Children 12-18 years: 4 mg once daily for 1 week; may increase to 8 mg daily in 2 divided doses for 1 week; then may increase by 4-8 mg weekly to response or up to 32 mg daily in 2-4 divided doses

Adults: 4 mg once daily for 1 week; may increase by 4-8 mg weekly to response or up to 56 mg daily in 2-4 divided doses; usual maintenance: 32-56 mg/day

Patients **not** receiving enzyme-inducing AED regimens: The estimated plasma concentrations of tiagabine in patients not taking enzyme-inducing medications is twice that of patients receiving enzyme-inducing AEDs. Lower doses are required; slower titration may be necessary.

Dosage adjustment in renal impairment: No dosage adjustment necessary.

Dosage adjustment in hepatic impairment: No specific dosage adjustment provided in manufacturer's labeling. However, dosage reduction may be necessary since clearance is reduced in the setting of hepatic impairment.

Dietary Considerations Take with food.

Monitoring Parameters A reduction in seizure frequency is indicative of therapeutic response to tiagabine in patients with partial seizures; complete blood counts, renal function tests, liver function tests, and routine blood chemistry should be monitored periodically during therapy; suicidality (eg, suicidal thoughts, depression, behavioral changes)

Reference Range Maximal plasma level after a 24 mg/dose: 552 ng/mL

Additional Information Animal studies suggest that tiagabine may bind to retina and uvea; however, no treatment-related ophthalmoscopic changes were seen long-term; periodic monitoring may be considered.

Dosage Forms

Tablet, Oral:

Gabitril: 2 mg, 4 mg, 12 mg, 16 mg

Generic: 2 mg, 4 mg

Extemporaneous Preparations A 1 mg/mL tiagabine hydrochloride oral suspension may be made with tablets and a 1:1 mixture of Ora-Sweet® and Ora-Plus®. Crush ten 12 mg tablets in a mortar and reduce to a fine powder. Add small portions of the vehicle and mix to a uniform paste; mix while adding the vehicle in incremental proportions to **almost** 120 mL; transfer to a graduated cylinder; rinse mortar with vehicle, and add quantity of vehicle sufficient to make 120 mL. Label "shake well" and "refrigerate". Store in amber plastic prescription bottles; stable for 70 days at room temperature or 91 days refrigerated (preferred).

A 1 mg/mL oral suspension may be made with tablets and a 6:1 mixture of simple syrup, NF and methylcellulose 1%. Crush ten 12 mg tablets in a mortar and reduce to a fine powder. Add 17 mL of methylcellulose 1% gel and mix to a uniform paste; mix while adding simple syrup, NF in incremental proportions to **almost** 120 mL; transfer to a graduated cylinder, rinse mortar with syrup, and add quantity of syrup sufficient to make 120 mL. Label "shake well" and "refrigerate". Store in amber plastic prescription bottles; stable for 42 days at room temperature or 91 days refrigerated (preferred).

Nahata MC, Pai VB, and Hipple TF, *Pediatric Drug Formulations*, 5th ed, Cincinnati, OH: Harvey Whitney Books Co, 2004.

◆ **Tiagabine Hydrochloride** *see* TiaGABine *on page 2032*

◆ **Tiamol® (Can)** *see* Fluocinonide *on page 894*

Tianeptine [INT] (tye ah NEP teen)

International Brand Names Antinepte (RO); Coaxil (BG, CZ, EE, HR, HU, PL, RO, RU, SI, SK); Lyxit (RO); Salymbra (EE); Stablon (AR, AT, BH, BR, EG, FR, ID, IN, KW, MX, MY, PK, PT, QA, SA, SG, TH, TR, VE, VN); Staborin (KR); Stiron (KR); Tatinol (CN); Tianeurax (DE); Tynept (IN)

Index Terms Tianeptine Sodium

Pharmacologic Category Antidepressant, Serotonin Reuptake Facilitator

Reported Use Major depressive episodes (mild, moderate, or severe)

Dosage Range
Children ≥15 years and Adults: 12.5 mg 3 times/day, before meals
Adults >70 years: Lower dose
Dosage adjustment for renal impairment: Lower dose
Product Availability Product available in various countries; not currently available in the U.S.
Dosage Forms
Tablet: 12.5 mg

◆ **Tianeptine Sodium** *see* Tianeptine [INT] *on page 2033*

Tiaprofenic Acid [CAN/INT]
(tye ah PRO fen ik AS id)

Brand Names: Canada Apo-Tiaprofenic; Dom-Tiaprofenic; PMS-Tiaprofenic; Teva-Tiaprofenic Acid
Pharmacologic Category Nonsteroidal Anti-inflammatory Drug (NSAID), Oral
Use Note: Not approved in U.S.
Relief of signs and symptoms of rheumatoid arthritis and osteoarthritis (degenerative joint disease)
Pregnancy Considerations Adverse effects were observed in animal reproduction studies. Tiaprofenic acid crosses the human placenta. Fetal exposure to NSAIDs late in pregnancy is associated with premature closure of ductus arteriosus. An increased number of stillbirths as well as delayed and prolonged labor were observed in animal studies. NSAID exposure during the first trimester is not strongly associated with congenital malformations; however, cardiovascular anomalies and cleft palate have been observed following NSAID exposure in some studies. The use of an NSAID close to conception may be associated with an increased risk of miscarriage. Nonteratogenic effects have been observed following NSAID administration during the third trimester including myocardial degenerative changes, prenatal constriction of the ductus arteriosus, fetal tricuspid regurgitation, failure of the ductus arteriosus to close postnatally; renal dysfunction or failure, oligohydramnios; gastrointestinal bleeding or perforation, increased risk of necrotizing enterocolitis; intracranial bleeding (including intraventricular hemorrhage), platelet dysfunction with resultant bleeding; pulmonary hypertension. Because they may cause premature closure of the ductus arteriosus, use of NSAIDs late in pregnancy should be avoided (use after 31 or 32 weeks gestation is not recommended by some clinicians). The chronic use of NSAIDs in women of reproductive age may be associated with infertility that is reversible upon discontinuation of the medication. Use of tiaprofenic acid is not recommended during pregnancy.
Breast-Feeding Considerations It is not known if tiaprofenic acid is excreted in breast milk. Breast-feeding is not recommended by the manufacturer.
Contraindications Hypersensitivity to tiaprofenic acid, any component of the formulation, aspirin, or other nonsteroidal anti-inflammatory drugs (NSAIDs); patients who experience acute asthma attacks, urticaria, rhinitis or other allergic manifestations with aspirin or NSAID therapy; peptic ulcer or active GI inflammatory disease
Warnings/Precautions Fatal asthmatic and anaphylactoid reactions have occurred in patients with "aspirin triad." Do not use in patients who experience bronchospasm, asthma, rhinitis, or urticaria with NSAID or aspirin therapy. NSAIDs are associated with an increased risk of adverse cardiovascular events, including MI, stroke, and new-onset or worsening of preexisting hypertension. Risk may be increased with duration of use or preexisting cardiovascular risk factors or disease. Carefully evaluate individual cardiovascular risk profiles prior to prescribing. Use caution with fluid retention and in heart failure. Use the lowest effective dose for the shortest duration of time, consistent with individual patient goals, to reduce risk of cardiovascular events; alternate therapies should be considered for patients at high risk. Use with caution in patients with decreased renal or hepatic function, history of GI disease (bleeding, ulcers, or previous GI symptoms with NSAID use), or those receiving anticoagulants and/or corticosteroids. Platelet adhesion and aggregation may be decreased; may prolong bleeding time; patients with coagulation disorders or who are receiving anticoagulants should be monitored closely. Anemia may occur; patients on long-term NSAID therapy should be monitored for anemia. Rarely, NSAID use has been associated with potentially severe blood dyscrasias (eg, agranulocytosis, thrombocytopenia, aplastic anemia). Gastrointestinal bleeding may occur without prior symptoms of gastrointestinal irritation. When used concomitantly with ≤325 mg of aspirin, a substantial increase in the risk of gastrointestinal complications (eg, ulcer) occurs; concomitant gastroprotective therapy (eg, proton pump inhibitors) is recommended (Bhatt, 2008).

NSAID use may compromise existing renal function; dose-dependent decreases in prostaglandin synthesis may result from NSAID use, reducing renal blood flow which may cause renal decompensation. NSAID use may increase the risk for hyperkalemia. Patients with impaired renal function, dehydration, heart failure, liver dysfunction, those taking diuretics, and ACE inhibitors, and the elderly are at greater risk of renal toxicity and hyperkalemia. Rehydrate patient before starting therapy; monitor renal function closely. Long-term NSAID use may result in renal papillary necrosis. The elderly are at increased risk for adverse effects (especially peptic ulceration, CNS effects, renal toxicity) from NSAIDs even at low doses. Withhold for at least 4-6 half-lives prior to surgical or dental procedures.

NSAIDS may cause drowsiness, dizziness, blurred vision, and other neurologic effects which may impair physical or mental abilities; patients must be cautioned about performing tasks which require mental alertness (eg, operating machinery or driving). Discontinue use with blurred or diminished vision and perform ophthalmologic exam. Monitor vision with long-term therapy.

Patients with autoimmune disorders may be at greater risk of developing aseptic meningitis, as rare adverse reaction associated with some NSAIDs. Avoid use in patients with prior history of urinary symptoms and discontinue at first sign of genitourinary problems. Severe cases of cystitis (bladder pain, dysuria, urinary frequency, hematuria) due to tiaprofenic acid have been reported.
Adverse Reactions
Cardiovascular: Edema, flushing
Central nervous system: Depression, dizziness, drowsiness, headache
Dermatologic: Erythema, pruritus, rash
Endocrine & metabolic: Hyperkalemia
Gastrointestinal: Abdominal pain, constipation, diarrhea, dyspepsia, epigastric distress, flatulence, heartburn, nausea, stomatitis, vomiting, xerostomia
Hematologic: Hemoglobin/hematocrit decreased
Renal: BUN increased
Respiratory: Epistaxis
Rare but important or life-threatening: Alkaline phosphatase increased, anaphylaxis, angina, angioedema, anorexia, anxiety, asthma, AST increased, bronchospasm, bruising, conjunctivitis, cramps, cystalgia, cystitis, diaphoresis, disorientation, duodenal ulcer, dyspnea, dysuria, enterocolitis, erythema multiforme, eye ulcer, fluid retention, gastric ulcer, gastrointestinal hemorrhage, GGT increased, hematuria, hepatotoxicity, hepatitis (fatal), hypertension, incontinence, insomnia, interstitial nephritis, intestinal perforation, jaundice, leukocytosis, leukopenia, melena, menstrual irregularities, oliguria, onycholysis, palpebral edema, palpitation, paresthesia,

photosensitivity, pollakiuria, polyuria, renal failure, serum creatinine increased, Stevens-Johnson syndrome, thrombocytopenia, tinnitus, toxic epidermal necrolysis, tremor, urticaria, vaginal bleeding, vertigo, vision blurred, weakness, weight gain. **Note:** Aseptic meningitis, neutropenia, and leukopenia have been associated rarely with NSAIDs.

Drug Interactions

Metabolism/Transport Effects None known.

Avoid Concomitant Use

Avoid concomitant use of Tiaprofenic Acid with any of the following: Dexketoprofen; Floctafenine; Ketorolac (Nasal); Ketorolac (Systemic); NSAID (COX-2 Inhibitor); Omacetaxine; Urokinase

Increased Effect/Toxicity

Tiaprofenic Acid may increase the levels/effects of: 5-ASA Derivatives; Agents with Antiplatelet Properties; Aliskiren; Aminoglycosides; Anticoagulants; Apixaban; Bisphosphonate Derivatives; Collagenase (Systemic); CycloSPORINE (Systemic); Dabigatran Etexilate; Deferasirox; Desmopressin; Digoxin; Eplerenone; Haloperidol; Ibritumomab; Lithium; Methotrexate; Nonsteroidal Anti-Inflammatory Agents; NSAID (COX-2 Inhibitor); Obinutuzumab; Omacetaxine; PEMEtrexed; Porfimer; Potassium-Sparing Diuretics; PRALAtrexate; Quinolone Antibiotics; Rivaroxaban; Salicylates; Tacrolimus (Systemic); Tenofovir; Thrombolytic Agents; Tositumomab and Iodine I 131 Tositumomab; Urokinase; Vancomycin; Verteporfin; Vitamin K Antagonists

The levels/effects of Tiaprofenic Acid may be increased by: ACE Inhibitors; Angiotensin II Receptor Blockers; Antidepressants (Tricyclic, Tertiary Amine); Corticosteroids (Systemic); CycloSPORINE (Systemic); Dasatinib; Dexketoprofen; Diclofenac (Systemic); Floctafenine; Glucosamine; Herbs (Anticoagulant/Antiplatelet Properties); Ibrutinib; Ketorolac (Nasal); Ketorolac (Systemic); Limaprost; Multivitamins/Fluoride (with ADE); Multivitamins/Minerals (with ADEK, Folate, Iron); Multivitamins/Minerals (with AE, No Iron); Omega-3 Fatty Acids; Pentosan Polysulfate Sodium; Pentoxifylline; Probenecid; Prostacyclin Analogues; Selective Serotonin Reuptake Inhibitors; Serotonin/Norepinephrine Reuptake Inhibitors; Sodium Phosphates; Tipranavir; Treprostinil; Vitamin E

Decreased Effect

Tiaprofenic Acid may decrease the levels/effects of: ACE Inhibitors; Aliskiren; Angiotensin II Receptor Blockers; Beta-Blockers; Eplerenone; HydrALAZINE; Loop Diuretics; Potassium-Sparing Diuretics; Prostaglandins (Ophthalmic); Salicylates; Selective Serotonin Reuptake Inhibitors; Thiazide Diuretics

The levels/effects of Tiaprofenic Acid may be decreased by: Bile Acid Sequestrants; Salicylates

Food Interactions Tiaprofenic acid peak serum levels may be decreased if taken with food. Management: Administer with food or milk.

Storage/Stability Store at 15°C to 30°C (59°F to 86°F).

Mechanism of Action Reversibly inhibits cyclooxygenase-1 and 2 (COX-1 and 2) enzymes, which results in decreased formation of prostaglandin precursors; has antipyretic, analgesic, and anti-inflammatory properties

Other proposed mechanisms not fully elucidated (and possibly contributing to the anti-inflammatory effect to varying degrees), include inhibiting chemotaxis, altering lymphocyte activity, inhibiting neutrophil aggregation/activation, and decreasing proinflammatory cytokine levels.

Pharmacodynamics/Kinetics

Absorption: Rapid

Protein binding: ~98%

Metabolism: Minimal (10%) to inactive metabolites

Half-life elimination: ~2 hours

Time to peak: 30-90 minutes

Excretion: Urine (50% as unchanged drug; <10% as metabolites)

Dosage Oral:

Adults:

Osteoarthritis: Usual initial and maintenance dose: 600 mg/day in 2-3 divided doses; rarely, patients may be maintained on 300 mg/day in divided doses; maximum daily dose: 600 mg

Rheumatoid arthritis: Usual initial and maintenance dose: 600 mg/day in 2-3 divided doses; maximum daily dose: 600 mg

Elderly: May consider lower initial dosing.

Dosage adjustment in renal impairment: No specific dosage adjustment provided in manufacturer's labeling. However, dosage adjustment is recommended since primarily renally eliminated.

Dosage adjustment in hepatic impairment: No dosage adjustment provided in manufacturer's labeling. Use with caution.

Dietary Considerations Should be taken with food or milk.

Administration Administer with food or milk.

Monitoring Parameters CBC; occult blood loss; periodic liver function tests; renal function (urine output, BUN, creatinine); electrolytes; monitor response (pain, range of motion, grip strength, mobility, ADL function), inflammation; observe for weight gain, edema; observe for bleeding, bruising; evaluate gastrointestinal effects (abdominal pain, bleeding, dyspepsia); mental confusion, disorientation; with long-term therapy, periodic ophthalmic exams

Product Availability Not available in U.S.

Dosage Forms: Canada

Tablet, oral: 200 mg, 300 mg

◆ **Tiazac** *see* Diltiazem *on page 634*

◆ **Tiazac XC (Can)** *see* Diltiazem *on page 634*

Tibolone [INT] (TYE boe lone)

International Brand Names Amena (PH); Boltin (ES); Cervictal (AR); Climabel (VN); Climafen (CL); Discretal (AR); Heria (BE); Klimater (BR); Libron (KR); Lirex (PY); Livial (AE, AU, BE, BG, BH, BR, CH, CL, CN, CO, CR, CY, CZ, DK, DO, EE, FI, FR, GB, GR, GT, HK, HN, HR, ID, IE, IL, IN, IS, IT, JO, KR, KW, LB, LT, MX, MY, NI, NL, NO, NZ, PA, PE, PH, PK, PL, PT, QA, RO, RU, SA, SE, SG, SI, SK, SV, TH, TR, TW, VE, VN); Liviel (AT); Liviella (DE); Livifem (ZA); Menotrix (EC); Tibofem (UY); Tibolux (EC); Tibona (UY); Tinox (CO, PE, PY, VE); Xyvion (AU)

Pharmacologic Category Estrogen and Progestin Combination

Reported Use Prevention of postmenopausal osteoporosis; symptomatic treatment of hot flushes and associated sweating resulting from menopause (surgical or natural); improvement of bone mineral density in patients with established postmenopausal osteoporosis and contraindications/intolerances to first-line therapy

Dosage Range Adults: Female: Oral: 2.5 mg once daily

Product Availability Product available in various countries; not currently available in the U.S.

Dosage Forms

Tablet: 2.5 mg

Ticagrelor (tye KA grel or)

Brand Names: U.S. Brilinta

Brand Names: Canada Brilinta

Index Terms AZD6140

Pharmacologic Category Antiplatelet Agent; Antiplatelet Agent, Cyclopentyltriazolopyrimidine

Additional Appendix Information

Oral Antiplatelet Comparison Chart *on page 2239*

Use Used in conjunction with aspirin for secondary prevention of thrombotic events in patients with unstable angina (UA), non-ST-elevation myocardial infarction (NSTEMI), or ST-elevation myocardial infarction (STEMI) managed medically or with percutaneous coronary intervention (PCI) and/or coronary artery bypass graft (CABG)

Pregnancy Risk Factor C

Pregnancy Considerations Fetal mortality and/or abnormalities were observed in animal studies at doses greater than maximum recommended human doses. There are no adequate and well-controlled studies in pregnant women. Use only if potential benefits outweigh potential risk to fetus. The Canadian labeling recommends women of childbearing potential use appropriate contraceptive measures.

Breast-Feeding Considerations Excretion into breast milk is unknown; use is not recommended.

Contraindications Hypersensitivity (eg, angioedema) to ticagrelor or any component of the formulation; active pathological bleeding (eg, peptic ulcer or intracranial hemorrhage); history of intracranial hemorrhage; severe hepatic impairment

Canadian labeling: Additional contraindications (not in U.S. labeling): Moderate hepatic impairment; concomitant use of strong CYP3A4 inhibitors (eg, ketoconazole, clarithromycin, ritonavir, atazanavir, nefazodone)

Warnings/Precautions [U.S. Boxed Warning]: Ticagrelor increases the risk of bleeding including significant and sometimes fatal bleeding. Use is contraindicated in patients with active pathological bleeding and presence or history of intracranial hemorrhage. Additional risk factors for bleeding include propensity to bleed (eg, recent trauma or surgery, recent or recurrent GI bleeding, active PUD, moderate-to-severe hepatic impairment), CABG or other surgical procedure, concomitant use of medications that increase risk of bleeding (eg, warfarin, NSAIDs), and advanced age. Bleeding should be suspected if patient becomes hypotensive after undergoing recent coronary angiography, PCI, CABG, or other surgical procedure even if overt signs of bleeding do not exist. **Where possible, manage bleeding without discontinuing ticagrelor as the risk of cardiovascular events is increased upon discontinuation.** If discontinuation of ticagrelor is necessary, resume as soon as possible after the bleeding source is identified and controlled. Hemostatic benefits of platelet transfusions are not known; may inhibit transfused platelets. Premature discontinuation of therapy may increase the risk of cardiac events (eg, stent thrombosis with subsequent fatal or nonfatal MI). Duration of therapy, in general, is determined by the type of stent placed (bare metal or drug eluting) and whether an ACS event was ongoing at the time of placement. Use with caution in patients who are at an increased risk of bradycardia (eg, second- or third-degree AV block, sick sinus syndrome) or taking other bradycardic-inducing agents (eg, beta blockers, nondihydropyridine calcium channel blockers). Ventricular pauses ≥3 seconds were noted more frequently with ticagrelor than with clopidogrel in a substudy of the Platelet Inhibition and Patient Outcomes (PLATO) trial. Dyspnea (often mild-to-moderate and transient) was observed more frequently in patients receiving ticagrelor than clopidogrel during clinical trials. Ticagrelor-related dyspnea does not require specific treatment nor does it warrant therapy interruption; however, therapy should be discontinued in patients unable to tolerate ticagrelor-related dyspnea.

[U.S. Boxed Warning]: Maintenance doses of aspirin greater than 100 mg/day reduce the efficacy of ticagrelor and should be avoided. Use of higher maintenance doses of aspirin (ie, >100 mg/day) was associated with relatively unfavorable outcomes for ticagrelor versus clopidogrel in the PLATO trial (Gaglia, 2011; Wallentin, 2009). Canadian labeling recommends a maximum maintenance aspirin dose of 150 mg/day.

[U.S. Boxed Warning]: Avoid initiation of ticagrelor when urgent CABG surgery is planned; when possible discontinue use at least 5 days before any surgery. Discontinue 5 days before elective surgery (except in patients with cardiac stents that have not completed their full course of dual antiplatelet therapy; patient-specific situations need to be discussed with cardiologist); restart ticagrelor as soon as possible after surgery (ACCF/AHA [Hillis, 2011]). The ACCF/AHA STEMI guidelines recommend discontinuation for at least 24 hours prior to on-pump CABG if possible; off-pump CABG may be performed within 24 hours of ticagrelor administration if the benefits of prompt revascularization outweigh the risks of bleeding (ACCF/AHA [O'Gara, 2013]).

Use is contraindicated in patients with severe hepatic impairment (Canadian labeling also contraindicates use in moderate-to-severe hepatic impairment). Use with caution in patients with renal impairment, a history of hyperuricemia or gouty arthritis. Canadian labeling does not recommend use in patients with uric acid nephropathy. Avoid concomitant use with strong CYP3A4 inhibitors (eg, ketoconazole, ritonavir, nefazodone) or strong CYP3A4 inducers (eg, rifampin, carbamazepine, dexamethasone, phenobarbital, phenytoin). Canadian labeling contraindicates use with strong CYP3A4 inhibitors.

Adverse Reactions Note: As with all drugs which may affect hemostasis, bleeding is associated with ticagrelor. Hemorrhage may occur at virtually any site. Risk is dependent on multiple variables, including the concurrent use of multiple agents which alter hemostasis and patient susceptibility.

Cardiovascular: Angina, atrial fibrillation, bradycardia, cardiac failure, hyper-/hypotension, palpitation, peripheral edema, syncope, ventricular extrasystoles, ventricular fibrillation, ventricular pauses, ventricular tachycardia

Central nervous system: Anxiety, depression, dizziness, fatigue, fever, headache, insomnia, vertigo

Dermatologic: Bruising, pruritus, rash, subcutaneous or dermal bleeding

Endocrine & metabolic: Diabetes mellitus, dyslipidemia, hypercholesterolemia, hypokalemia, uric acid increased

Gastrointestinal: Abdominal pain, constipation, diarrhea, dyspepsia, GI hemorrhage, nausea, vomiting

Genitourinary: Urinary tract bleeding, urinary tract infection

Hematologic: Anemia, hematoma, major bleeding (composite of major fatal/life threatening and other major bleeding events), minor bleeding, postprocedural hemorrhage

Local: Puncture site hematoma

Neuromuscular & skeletal: Arthralgia, back pain, noncardiac chest pain, extremity pain, musculoskeletal pain, myalgia, weakness

Renal: Creatinine increased (mechanism undetermined), hematuria, renal failure

Respiratory: Bronchitis, cough, dyspnea, epistaxis, nasopharyngitis, pneumonia

Rare but important or life-threatening: Angioedema, confusion, conjunctival hemorrhage, gastritis, gout, gynecomastia, hemarthrosis, hemoptysis, hypersensitivity, intracranial hemorrhage (including fatalities), intraocular hemorrhage, paresthesia, retinal hemorrhage, retroperitoneal hemorrhage

Drug Interactions

Metabolism/Transport Effects Substrate of CYP3A4 (major); **Note:** Assignment of Major/Minor substrate status based on clinically relevant drug interaction potential; **Inhibits** CYP2B6 (weak), CYP2C9 (moderate), CYP2D6 (weak)

Avoid Concomitant Use

Avoid concomitant use of Ticagrelor with any of the following: CYP3A4 Inducers (Strong); CYP3A4 Inhibitors (Strong); Dexamethasone (Systemic); Urokinase

Increased Effect/Toxicity

Ticagrelor may increase the levels/effects of: Agents with Antiplatelet Properties; Anticoagulants; Apixaban; ARIPiprazole; Bosentan; Cannabis; Carvedilol; Collagenase (Systemic); CYP2C9 Substrates; Dabigatran Etexilate; Digoxin; Dronabinol; Ibritumomab; Lovastatin; Obinutuzumab; Rivaroxaban; Salicylates; Simvastatin; Tetrahydrocannabinol; Thrombolytic Agents; Tositumomab and Iodine I 131 Tositumomab; Urokinase

The levels/effects of Ticagrelor may be increased by: Aspirin; CycloSPORINE (Systemic); CYP3A4 Inhibitors (Strong); Dasatinib; Glucosamine; Grapefruit Juice; Herbs (Anticoagulant/Antiplatelet Properties); Ibrutinib; Limaprost; Multivitamins/Fluoride (with ADE); Multivitamins/Minerals (with ADEK, Folate, Iron); Multivitamins/Minerals (with AE, No Iron); Omega-3 Fatty Acids; Pentosan Polysulfate Sodium; Pentoxifylline; Prostacyclin Analogues; Tipranavir; Vitamin E

Decreased Effect

The levels/effects of Ticagrelor may be decreased by: Aspirin; Bosentan; CYP3A4 Inducers (Moderate); CYP3A4 Inducers (Strong); CYP3A4 Inhibitors (Strong); Dabrafenib; Deferasirox; Dexamethasone (Systemic); Siltuximab; St Johns Wort; Tocilizumab

Storage/Stability Store at 25°C (77°F); excursions permitted to 15°C to 30°C (59°F to 86°F).

Mechanism of Action Reversibly and noncompetitively binds the adenosine diphosphate (ADP) $P2Y_{12}$ receptor on the platelet surface which prevents ADP-mediated activation of the GPIIb/IIIa receptor complex thereby reducing platelet aggregation. Due to the reversible antagonism of the $P2Y_{12}$ receptor, recovery of platelet function is likely to depend on serum concentrations of ticagrelor and its active metabolite.

Pharmacodynamics/Kinetics

Onset of inhibition of platelet aggregation (IPA): 180 mg loading dose: ~41% within 30 minutes (similar to clopidogrel 600 mg at 8 hours)

Peak effect: Time to maximal IPA: 180 mg loading dose: IPA ~88% at 2 hours post administration

Duration of IPA: 180 mg loading dose: 87% to 89% maintained from 2-8 hours; 24 hours after the last maintenance dose, IPA is 58% (similar to maintenance clopidogrel)

Time after discontinuation when IPA is 30%: ~56 hours; IPA 10%: ~110 hours (Gurbel, 2009). Mean IPA observed with ticagrelor at 3 days post-discontinuation was comparable to that observed with clopidogrel at 5 days post discontinuation.

Absorption: Rapid

Distribution: 88 L

Protein binding: >99% (parent drug and active metabolite)

Metabolism: Hepatic via CYP3A4/5 to active metabolite (AR-C124910XX)

Bioavailability: ~36% (range: 30% to 42%)

Half-life elimination: Parent drug: ~7 hours; active metabolite: ~9 hours

Time to peak: Parent drug: ~1.5 hours; active metabolite (AR-C124910XX): ~2.5 hours

Excretion: Feces (58%); urine (26%); actual amount of parent drug and active metabolite excreted in urine was <1% of total dose administered

Dosage Oral, NG: Adults:

Acute coronary syndrome: Unstable angina, non-ST-segment elevation myocardial infarction (NSTEMI), ST-segment elevation myocardial infarction (STEMI): Initial: 180 mg loading dose (with a loading dose of aspirin [eg, 325 mg] if not already receiving); Maintenance: 90 mg twice daily; initiated 12 hours after initial loading dose (with low-dose aspirin 75 to 100 mg/day or 81 mg/day in patients with UA/NSTEMI or STEMI as recommended by ACCF/AHA/SCAI). For UA/NSTEMI patients managed medically, continue ticagrelor for up to 12 months (ACCF/AHA [Anderson, 2013]). **Note**: Canadian labeling recommends a maintenance aspirin dose of 75-150 mg/day. Safety and efficacy of therapy beyond 12 months has not been established.

Duration of ticagrelor (in combination with aspirin) after stent placement: **Premature interruption of therapy may result in stent thrombosis with subsequent fatal and nonfatal MI.** According to the ACCF/AHA/SCAI PCI guidelines, those with ACS receiving either stent type (bare metal [BMS] or drug-eluting stent [DES]) or those receiving a DES for a non-ACS indication, ticagrelor for at least 12 months is recommended (ACCF/AHA/SCAI [Levine, 2011]). The ACCF/AHA guidelines for the management of UA/NSTEMI recommend up to 12 months of ticagrelor in patients with ACS who receive a BMS (ACCF/AHA [Anderson, 2013]). A duration >12 months may be considered in patients with DES placement. Recent data has demonstrated that continued dual antiplatelet therapy (ticagrelor not included in clinical trial) for a total of 30 months (compared to 12 months) significantly reduced the risk of stent thrombosis and major adverse cardiovascular/cerebrovascular events but was associated with a higher risk of bleeding (Mauri, 2014). Those receiving a BMS for a non-ACS indication should be given ticagrelor for at least 1 month and ideally up to 12 months; if patient is at increased risk of bleeding, give for a minimum of 2 weeks (ACCF/AHA/SCAI [Levine, 2011]).

Conversion from clopidogrel to ticagrelor: May initiate ticagrelor 90 mg twice daily beginning 24 hours after last clopidogrel dose (loading or maintenance). Patients who are in the acute phase of an acute coronary syndrome, especially if determined to be clopidogrel nonresponsive, may be considered for administration of ticagrelor 180 mg loading dose followed by 90 mg twice daily regardless of previous clopidogrel exposure, taking into consideration the administration of other antiplatelet agents (eg, GP IIb/IIIa inhibitors) (Gurbel, 2010; Wallentin, 2009). In one single blinded study, patients with ACS receiving ongoing clopidogrel treatment who were converted to ticagrelor *without* a loading dose did not experience a reduction in platelet inhibition compared to those who received a loading dose of ticagrelor (Caiazzo, 2014). **Note:** In general, conversion to ticagrelor results in an absolute inhibition of platelet aggregation (IPA) increase of 26.4%.

Dosage adjustment in renal impairment: No dosage adjustment necessary.

Hemodialysis: Use caution; drug is thought to be nondialyzable

Dosage adjustment in hepatic impairment:

Mild impairment: No dosage adjustment necessary.

Moderate impairment: There are no dosage adjustments provided in the manufacturer's labeling (has not been studied); however, undergoes hepatic metabolism; use caution. Use is contraindicated in the Canadian labeling.

Severe impairment: Use is contraindicated.

Dietary Considerations May be taken without regard to meals.

Administration May be administered without regard to meals. Missed doses should be taken at their next regularly scheduled time. For patients unable to swallow whole, tablets may be crushed to create a suspension for oral or NG use (Crean, 2013; Parodi, 2015).

Monitoring Parameters Signs of bleeding; hemoglobin and hematocrit periodically; renal function; uric acid levels (patients with gout or at risk of hyperuricemia); signs/symptoms of dyspnea; may consider platelet function testing to determine platelet inhibitory response if results of testing may alter management (ACCF/AHA [Anderson, 2013]).

Additional Information Unlike thienopyridines (eg, clopidogrel, prasugrel) which are prodrugs and require metabolic transformation to their active metabolites for their activity, ticagrelor and its active metabolite both exhibit antiplatelet activity by reversibly and noncompetitively binding to the adenosine diphosphate (ADP) $P2Y_{12}$ receptor on the platelet surface. Due to the reversible antagonism of the $P2Y_{12}$ receptor, recovery of platelet function is faster than with use of irreversible $P2Y_{12}$ receptor antagonists such as clopidogrel or prasugrel.

Dosage Forms

Tablet, Oral:

Brilinta: 90 mg

Dosage Forms: Canada

Tablet, oral:

Brilinta: 90 mg

Extemporaneous Preparations A suspension for oral administration may be prepared by crushing one or two 90 mg tablets in a mortar (for 60 seconds) and placing in a dosing cup. To ensure the full dose is received, rinse mortar with 100 mL purified water, transfer to dosing cup, and repeat rinse (Crean, 2013; Parodi, 2015).

A suspension for NG tube administration may be prepared by crushing one or two 90 mg tablets in a mortar (for 60 seconds); add 50 mL purified water to mortar and stir (for 60 seconds); transfer the suspension to a 50 mL oral enteral syringe and administer via NG tube. To ensure the full dose is received, add another 50 mL purified water to the mortar and stir for 60 seconds; using the same 50 mL oral enteral syringe, withdraw the suspension and administer entire amount via NG tube (Crean, 2013).

When stored in a PVC oral syringe for up to 2 hours, there was no degradation of the suspension detected (Crean, 2013).

Ticarcillin and Clavulanate Potassium [CAN/INT]

(tye kar SIL in & klav yoo LAN ate poe TASS ee um)

Brand Names: U.S. Timentin [DSC]

Brand Names: Canada Timentin

Index Terms Ticarcillin and Clavulanic Acid

Pharmacologic Category Antibiotic, Penicillin

Use

Bone and joint infections: Treatment of bone and joint infections caused by beta-lactamase-producing isolates of *Staphylococcus aureus*.

Endometritis: Treatment of endometritis caused by beta-lactamase-producing isolates of *Prevotella melaninogenicus*, *Enterobacter* species (including *E. cloacae*), *Klebsiella pneumoniae*, *Escherichia coli*, *S. aureus*, or *Staphylococcus epidermidis*.

Lower respiratory tract infections: Treatment of lower respiratory tract infections caused by beta-lactamase-producing isolates of *S. aureus*, *Haemophilus influenzae*, or *Klebsiella* species.

Peritonitis: Treatment of peritonitis caused by beta-lactamase-producing isolates of *E. coli*, *K. pneumonia*, or *Bacteroides fragilis* group.

Septicemia: Treatment of septicemia (including bacteremia) caused by beta-lactamase-producing isolates of *Klebsiella* species, *E. coli*, *S. aureus*, or *Pseudomonas aeruginosa* (or other *Pseudomonas* species).

Skin and skin structure infections: Treatment of skin and skin structure infections caused by beta-lactamase-producing isolates of *S. aureus*, *Klebsiella* species, or *E. coli*.

Urinary tract infections: Treatment of complicated and uncomplicated urinary tract infections caused by beta-lactamase-producing isolates of *E. coli*, *Klebsiella* species, *P. aeruginosa* (and other *Pseudomonas* species), *Citrobacter* species, *Enterobacter cloacae*, *Serratia marcescens*, or *S. aureus*.

Pregnancy Risk Factor B

Pregnancy Considerations Adverse events were not observed in animal reproduction studies. Ticarcillin and clavulanate cross the placenta (Maberry, 1992). Maternal use of penicillins has generally not resulted in an increased risk of adverse fetal effects (Crider, 2009; Santos, 2011). Ticarcillin/clavulanate is approved for the treatment of postpartum gynecologic infections, including endometritis, caused by susceptible organisms.

Breast-Feeding Considerations Small amounts of ticarcillin are found in breast milk (Matsuda, 1984; von Kobyletzki, 1983); however, it is not orally absorbed (Brogden, 1980). The manufacturer recommends that caution be exercised when administering ticarcillin/clavulanate to nursing women.

Contraindications Hypersensitivity (history of a serious reaction [eg, anaphylaxis, Stevens-Johnson syndrome]) to ticarcillin, clavulanate, or to other beta-lactams (eg, penicillins, cephalosporins)

Warnings/Precautions Serious and occasionally severe or fatal hypersensitivity (anaphylactic) reactions have been reported in patients on penicillin therapy (especially with a history of beta-lactam hypersensitivity and/or a history of sensitivity to multiple allergens); use with caution in patients with seizures and in patients with HF due to high sodium load. Hypokalemia has been reported; monitor serum potassium in patients with fluid and electrolyte imbalance and in patients receiving prolonged therapy. Use with caution and modify dosage in patients with renal impairment; Bleeding disorders have been observed (particularly in renal impairment); discontinue if thrombocytopenia or bleeding occurs. Prolonged use may result in fungal or bacterial superinfection, including *C. difficile*-associated diarrhea (CDAD) and pseudomembranous colitis; CDAD has been observed >2 months postantibiotic treatment.

Adverse Reactions

Cardiovascular: Local thrombophlebitis (with IV injection)

Central nervous system: Confusion, drowsiness, headache, seizure

Dermatologic: Skin rash

Endocrine & metabolic: Electrolyte disturbance, hypernatremia, hypokalemia

Gastrointestinal: *Clostridium difficile* diarrhea, diarrhea, nausea

Genitourinary: Proteinuria (false positive)

Hematologic & oncologic: Bleeding complication, eosinophilia, hemolytic anemia, positive direct Coombs' test (false positive)

Hepatic: Hepatotoxicity, increased serum ALT, increased serum AST, jaundice

Immunologic: Jarisch Herxheimer reaction

Infection: Superinfection (fungal or bacterial)

Renal: Interstitial nephritis (acute)

Miscellaneous: Anaphylaxis

Rare but important or life-threatening: Altered sense of smell, chest discomfort, chills, decreased hematocrit, decreased hemoglobin, decreased serum potassium, dizziness, dysgeusia, erythema multiforme, flatulence, headache, hemorrhagic cystitis, hypersensitivity reaction, hypouricemia, increased blood urea nitrogen, increased lactate dehydrogenase, increased serum alkaline phosphatase, increased serum creatinine, injection site reaction (burning, induration, pain, swelling), leukopenia, myalgia, myoclonus, neutropenia, prolonged prothrombin time, pruritus, pseudomembranous colitis (during or after antibacterial treatment), Stevens-Johnson syndrome, stomatitis, thrombocytopenia, toxic epidermal necrolysis, urticaria

Drug Interactions

Metabolism/Transport Effects None known.

Avoid Concomitant Use

Avoid concomitant use of Ticarcillin and Clavulanate Potassium with any of the following: BCG; Probenecid

Increased Effect/Toxicity

Ticarcillin and Clavulanate Potassium may increase the levels/effects of: Methotrexate; Vitamin K Antagonists

The levels/effects of Ticarcillin and Clavulanate Potassium may be increased by: Probenecid

Decreased Effect

Ticarcillin and Clavulanate Potassium may decrease the levels/effects of: Aminoglycosides; BCG; Mycophenolate; Sodium Picosulfate; Typhoid Vaccine

The levels/effects of Ticarcillin and Clavulanate Potassium may be decreased by: Tetracycline Derivatives

Preparation for Administration Reconstitute 3.1 g vials with 13 mL sterile water for injection or NS; shake well; resulting concentration is ticarcillin 200 mg/mL and clavulanic acid 6.7 mg/mL. Reconstitute 31 g bulk vials with 76 mL sterile water for injection or NS; shake well; resulting concentration is ticarcillin 300 mg/mL and clavulanic acid 10 mg/mL. Further dilute to a final concentration of 10-100 mg/mL in D_5W, LR, or NS.

Storage/Stability

Vials: Store intact vials at ≤24°C (≤75°F). Reconstituted solution is stable for 6 hours at room temperature and 72 hours when refrigerated. IV infusion in NS or LR is stable for 24 hours at room temperature (21°C to 24°C [70°F to 75°F]), 7 days when refrigerated (4°C [39°F]), or 30 days when frozen (-18°C [0°F]). IV infusion in D_5W solution is stable for 24 hours at room temperature (21°C to 24°C [70°F to 75°F]), 3 days when refrigerated (4°C [39°F]), or 7 days when frozen (-18°C [0°F]. After freezing, thawed solution is stable for 8 hours at room temperature. Do not refreeze. Darkening of drug indicates loss of potency of clavulanate potassium.

Premixed solution: Store frozen at ≤-20°C (-4°F). Thawed solution is stable for 24 hours at room temperature (22°C [72°F]) or 7 days under refrigeration at (4°C [39°F]); do not refreeze.

Mechanism of Action Inhibits bacterial cell wall synthesis by binding to one or more of the penicillin-binding proteins (PBPs), which in turn inhibits the final transpeptidation step of peptidoglycan synthesis in bacterial cell walls, thus inhibiting cell wall biosynthesis. Bacteria eventually lyse due to ongoing activity of cell wall autolytic enzymes (autolysins and murein hydrolases) while cell wall assembly is arrested.

Pharmacodynamics/Kinetics

Protein binding: Ticarcillin: ~45%; Clavulanic acid: ~25%

Half-life elimination: Ticarcillin: 1.1 hours; Clavulanic acid: 1.1 hours

Time to peak, plasma: Immediately following completion of 30-minute infusion

Excretion: Ticarcillin: Urine (60% to 70%); Clavulanic acid: Urine (35% to 45% as unchanged drug)

Dosage Note: Timentin (ticarcillin/clavulanate) is a combination product; each 3.1 g dosage form contains 3 g ticarcillin disodium and 0.1 g clavulanic acid.

Usual dosage range: Note: Dosage adjustment recommended in patients with renal impairment.

Infants ≥3 months, Children, Adolescents, and Adults: IV:

<60 kg: 200-300 mg ticarcillin/kg/day in divided doses every 4-6 hours (maximum: 18 g daily)

≥60 kg: 3.1 g every 4-6 hours

Indication-specific dosing:

Infants ≥3 months, Children, and Adolescents:

Mild to moderate infections: IV:

<60 kg: 200 mg ticarcillin/kg/day in divided doses every 6 hours (maximum: 12 g daily)

≥60 kg: 3.1 g every 6 hours

Severe infections: IV:

<60 kg: 300 mg ticarcillin/kg/day in divided doses every 4 hours. (maximum: 18 g daily)

≥60 kg: 3.1 g every 4 hours

Cystic fibrosis (off-label use): IV: 400 mg ticarcillin/kg/day in divided doses every 6 hours; higher doses have been used: 400-750 mg ticarcillin/kg/day in divided doses every 6 hours (maximum: 24-30 g ticarcillin daily) (Zobell, 2013)

Intra-abdominal infection, complicated (off-label use): IV: 200-300 mg ticarcillin/kg/day in divided every 4-6 hours (Solomkin, 2010)

Adults:

Gynecologic infections (eg, endometritis): IV:

Moderate infections: 200 mg ticarcillin/kg/day in divided doses every 6 hours (maximum: 12 g daily)

Severe infections: 300 mg ticarcillin/kg/day in divided doses every 4 hours (maximum: 18 g daily)

Systemic infections, urinary tract infections: IV:

<60 kg: 200-300 mg ticarcillin/kg/day in divided doses every 4-6 hours (maximum: 18 g daily)

≥60 kg: 3.1 g every 4-6 hours

Intra-abdominal infection, complicated, community-acquired, mild-to-moderate (off-label use): 3.1 g every 6 hours for 4-7 days (provided source controlled) (Solomkin, 2010)

Dosing adjustment in renal impairment: Loading dose: IV: 3.1 g one dose, followed by maintenance dose based on creatinine clearance:

CrCl 30-60 mL/minute: Administer 2 g of ticarcillin component every 4 hours

CrCl 10-30 mL/minute: Administer 2 g of ticarcillin component every 8 hours

CrCl <10 mL/minute: Administer 2 g of ticarcillin component every 12 hours

CrCl <10 mL/minute with concomitant hepatic dysfunction: 2 g of ticarcillin component every 24 hours

Intermittent hemodialysis (IHD) (administer after hemodialysis on dialysis days): Dialyzable (20% to 50%): 2 g of ticarcillin component every 12 hours; supplemented with 3.1 g (ticarcillin/clavulanate) after each dialysis session. Alternatively, administer 2 g every 8 hours without a supplemental dose for deep-seated infections (Heintz, 2009). **Note:** Dosing dependent on the assumption of 3 times/week, complete IHD sessions.

Peritoneal dialysis (PD): 3.1 g every 12 hours

Continuous renal replacement therapy (CRRT) (Heintz, 2009; Trotman, 2005): Drug clearance is highly dependent on the method of renal replacement, filter type, and flow rate. Appropriate dosing requires close monitoring of pharmacologic response, signs of adverse reactions due to drug accumulation, as well as drug concentrations in relation to target trough (if appropriate). The following are general recommendations only (based on dialysate flow/ultrafiltration rates of 1-2 L/hour and minimal residual renal function) and should not supersede clinical judgment:

CVVH: Loading dose of 3.1g followed by 2 g every 6-8 hours

CVVHD: Loading dose of 3.1 g followed by 3.1 g every 6-8 hours

CVVHDF: Loading dose of 3.1 g followed by 3.1 g every 6 hours

Note: Do not administer in intervals exceeding every 8 hours. Clavulanate component is hepatically eliminated; extending the dosing interval beyond 8 hours may result in loss of beta-lactamase inhibition.

Dosing adjustment in hepatic dysfunction: With concomitant renal dysfunction (CrCl <10 mL/minute): 2 g of ticarcillin component every 24 hours

Dietary Considerations Some products may contain potassium and/or sodium.

Administration Infuse over 30 minutes.

Some penicillins (eg, carbenicillin, ticarcillin, and piperacillin) have been shown to inactivate aminoglycosides *in vitro*. This has been observed to a greater extent with tobramycin and gentamicin, while amikacin has shown greater stability against inactivation. Concurrent use of these agents may pose a risk of reduced antibacterial efficacy *in vivo*, particularly in the setting of profound renal impairment. However, definitive clinical evidence is lacking. If combination penicillin/aminoglycoside therapy is desired in a patient with renal dysfunction, separation of doses (if feasible), and routine monitoring of aminoglycoside levels, CBC, and clinical response should be considered.

Monitoring Parameters Observe for signs and symptoms of anaphylaxis during first dose; serum electrolytes, bleeding time, and periodic tests of renal, hepatic, and hematologic function

Product Availability Not available in the U.S.

Dosage Forms: Canada

Injection, powder for reconstitution:

Timentin: Ticarcillin 3 g and clavulanic acid 0.1 g (3.1 g, 31 g) [contains sodium 4.5 mEq and potassium 0.15 mEq per g]

◆ **Ticarcillin and Clavulanic Acid** *see* Ticarcillin and Clavulanate Potassium [CAN/INT] *on page 2038*

◆ **Tice BCG** *see* BCG *on page 229*

Ticlopidine (tye KLOE pi deen)

Brand Names: Canada Apo-Ticlopidine; Dom-Ticlopidine; Gen-Ticlopidine; Mylan-Ticlopidine; Novo-Ticlopidine; Nu-Ticlopidine; PMS-Ticlopidine; Sandoz-Ticlopidine; Teva-Ticlopidine

Index Terms Ticlopidine Hydrochloride

Pharmacologic Category Antiplatelet Agent; Antiplatelet Agent, Thienopyridine

Additional Appendix Information

Beers Criteria – Potentially Inappropriate Medications for Geriatrics *on page 2271*

Oral Antiplatelet Comparison Chart *on page 2239*

Use Platelet aggregation inhibitor that reduces the risk of thrombotic stroke in patients who have had a stroke or stroke precursors (**Note:** Due to its association with life-threatening hematologic disorders, ticlopidine should be reserved for patients who are intolerant to aspirin, or who have failed aspirin therapy); adjunctive therapy (with aspirin) following successful coronary stent implantation to reduce the incidence of subacute stent thrombosis.

Pregnancy Risk Factor B

Dosage Oral: Adults:

Stroke prevention: 250 mg twice daily

Coronary artery stenting (initiate after successful implantation): 250 mg twice daily (in combination with antiplatelet doses of aspirin). If initiated prior to percutaneous coronary intervention, a loading dose of 500 mg may be administered (Berger, 1999). May continue treatment for up to 30 days per the manufacturer; however, in general, duration of therapy may extend up to 12 months in patients with drug-eluting stents or those with stent implantation (bare metal or drug eluting) for acute coronary syndrome (Levine, 2011).

Note: Overall, the use of ticlopidine has largely been replaced by newer $P2Y_{12}$ inhibitors (ie, clopidogrel, prasugrel, ticagrelor).

Dosage adjustment in renal impairment: No dosage adjustment provided in manufacturer's labeling. While there were no statistically significant differences in ADP-induced platelet aggregation, AUC increases and clearance decreases were seen in patients with mild to moderate renal impairment. However, bleeding time may be prolonged in patients with moderate renal impairment

Dosage adjustment in hepatic impairment: No dosage adjustment provided in manufacturer's labeling. Use with caution. Use is contraindicated in severe hepatic impairment.

Additional Information Complete prescribing information should be consulted for additional detail.

Dosage Forms

Tablet, Oral:

Generic: 250 mg

◆ **Ticlopidine Hydrochloride** *see* Ticlopidine *on page 2040*

◆ **TIG** *see* Tetanus Immune Globulin (Human) *on page 2015*

◆ **Tigan** *see* Trimethobenzamide *on page 2104*

Tigecycline (tye ge SYE kleen)

Brand Names: U.S. Tygacil

Brand Names: Canada Tygacil

Index Terms GAR-936

Pharmacologic Category Antibiotic, Glycylcycline

Use

Community-acquired bacterial pneumonia: Treatment of community-acquired pneumonia in patients 18 years and older caused by *Streptococcus pneumoniae* (penicillin-susceptible isolates), including cases with concurrent bacteremia, *Haemophilus influenzae* (beta-lactamase negative isolates), and *Legionella pneumophila*.

Complicated intra-abdominal infections: Treatment of complicated intra-abdominal infections in patients 18 years and older caused by *Citrobacter freundii*, *Enterobacter cloacae*, *Escherichia coli*, *Klebsiella oxytoca*, *Klebsiella pneumoniae*, *Enterococcus faecalis* (vancomycin-susceptible isolates), *Staphylococcus aureus* (methicillin-susceptible and methicillin-resistant isolates), *Streptococcus anginosus* group (includes *S. anginosus*, *Streptococcus intermedius*, and *Streptococcus constellatus*), *Bacteroides fragilis*, *Bacteroides thetaiotaomicron*, *Bacteroides uniformis*, *Bacteroides vulgatus*, *Clostridium perfringens*, and *Peptostreptococcus micros*.

Complicated skin and skin structure infections: Treatment of skin and skin structure infections in patients 18 years and older caused by *E. coli*, *E. faecalis* (vancomycin-susceptible isolates), *S. aureus* (methicillin-susceptible and methicillin-resistant isolates), *Streptococcus agalactiae*, *S. anginosus* group (includes *S. anginosus*, *S. intermedius*, and *S. constellatus*), *Streptococcus pyogenes*, *E. cloacae*, *K. pneumoniae*, and *B. fragilis*.

Pregnancy Risk Factor D

Pregnancy Considerations Because adverse effects were observed in animals and because of the potential for permanent tooth discoloration, tigecycline is classified pregnancy category D. Tigecycline frequently causes nausea and vomiting and, therefore, may not be ideal for use in a patient with pregnancy-related nausea.

Breast-Feeding Considerations It is not known if tigecycline is found in breast milk. The manufacturer recommends caution if giving tigecycline to a nursing woman. Nondose-related effects could include modification of bowel flora.

Contraindications

Hypersensitivity to tigecycline or any component of the formulation

Documentation of allergenic cross-reactivity for tetracyclines is limited. However, because of similarities in chemical structure and/or pharmacologic actions, the possibility of cross-sensitivity cannot be ruled out with certainty.

Canadian labeling: Additional contraindications (not in U.S. labeling): Hypersensitivity to tetracycline class of antibiotics

Warnings/Precautions [U.S. Boxed Warning]: In Phase 3 and 4 clinical trials, an increase in all-cause mortality was observed in patients treated with tigecycline compared to those treated with comparator antibiotics; cause has not been established. Use should be reserved for situations in which alternative treatments are not appropriate. In general, deaths were the result of worsening infection, complications of infection, or underlying comorbidity. May cause life-threatening anaphylaxis/anaphylactoid reactions. Due to structural similarity with tetracyclines, use caution in patients with prior hypersensitivity and/or severe adverse reactions associated with tetracycline use (Canadian labeling contraindicates use in patients with hypersensitivity to tetracyclines). Due to structural similarities with tetracyclines, may be associated with photosensitivity, pseudotumor cerebri, pancreatitis, and antianabolic effects (including increased BUN, azotemia, acidosis, and hyperphosphatemia) observed with this class. Acute pancreatitis (including fatalities) has been reported, including patients without known risk factors; discontinue use when suspected. May cause fetal harm if used during pregnancy; patients should be advised of potential risks associated with use. Permanent discoloration of the teeth may occur if used during tooth development (fetal stage through children up to 8 years of age).

Safety and efficacy in children <18 years of age have not been established due to increased mortality observed in trials of adult patients. Use only if no alternative antibiotics are available. Because of effects on tooth development (yellow-gray-brown discoloration), use in patients <8 years is not recommended.

Use caution in hepatic impairment; dosage adjustment recommended in severe hepatic impairment. Abnormal liver function tests (increased total bilirubin, prothrombin time, transaminases) have been reported. Isolated cases of significant hepatic dysfunction and hepatic failure have occurred. Closely monitor for worsening hepatic function in patients that develop abnormal liver function tests during therapy. Adverse hepatic effects may occur after drug discontinuation.

Prolonged use may result in fungal or bacterial superinfection, including *C. difficile*-associated diarrhea (CDAD) and pseudomembranous colitis; CDAD has been observed >2 months postantibiotic treatment. Use with caution if using as monotherapy for patients with intestinal perforation (in the small sample of available cases, septic shock occurred more frequently than patients treated with imipenem/cilastatin comparator). Do not use for diabetic foot infections; on-inferiority was not demonstrated in studies. Do not use for healthcare-acquired pneumonia (HAP) or ventilator-associated pneumonia (VAP); increased mortality and decreased efficacy have been reported in HAP and VAP trials.

Adverse Reactions

Cardiovascular: Localized phlebitis

Central nervous system: Dizziness, headache

Dermatologic: Skin rash

Endocrine & metabolic: Hyponatremia, increased amylase

Gastrointestinal: Abdominal pain, diarrhea, dyspepsia, nausea, vomiting

Hematologic & oncologic: Anemia, hypoproteinemia

Hepatic: Hyperbilirubinemia, increased serum ALT, increased serum AST, increased serum alkaline phosphatase

Infection: Abscess, infection

Neuromuscular & skeletal: Weakness

Renal: Increased blood urea nitrogen

Respiratory: Pneumonia

Miscellaneous: Abnormal healing

Rare but important or life-threatening: Acute pancreatitis, allergic skin reaction, anaphylactoid reaction, anaphylaxis, anorexia, *Clostridium difficile* associated diarrhea, dysgeusia, eosinophilia, hepatic insufficiency, hepatic failure, hypocalcemia, hypoglycemia, increased INR, increased serum creatinine, increased serum transaminases, increased INR, increased serum creatinine, increased serum transaminases, prolonged partial thromboplastin time, prolonged prothrombin time, pruritus, septic shock, Stevens-Johnson syndrome, swelling at injection site, thrombocytopenia, thrombophlebitis, vaginal moniliasis, vaginitis

Drug Interactions

Metabolism/Transport Effects None known.

Avoid Concomitant Use There are no known interactions where it is recommended to avoid concomitant use.

Increased Effect/Toxicity

Tigecycline may increase the levels/effects of: Warfarin

Decreased Effect There are no known significant interactions involving a decrease in effect.

Preparation for Administration Add 5.3 mL NS, D_5W, or LR to each 50 mg vial. Swirl gently to dissolve. Resulting solution is 10 mg/mL. Reconstituted solution must be further diluted to allow IV administration. Transfer to 100 mL IV bag for infusion (final concentration should not exceed 1 mg/mL). Reconstituted solution should be yellow-orange; discard if not this color.

Storage/Stability Prior to reconstitution, store at 20°C to 25°C (68°F to 77°F); excursions are permitted between 15°C and 30°C (59°F and 86°F). Reconstituted solution may be stored at room temperature (not to exceed 25°C [77°F]) for up to 6 hours in the vial or up to 24 hours if further diluted in a compatible IV solution. Alternatively, may be stored refrigerated at 2°C to 8°C (36°F to 46°F) for up to 48 hours following immediate transfer of the reconstituted solution into NS or D_5W.

Mechanism of Action A glycylcycline antibiotic that binds to the 30S ribosomal subunit of susceptible bacteria, thereby, inhibiting protein synthesis. Generally considered bacteriostatic; however, bactericidal activity has been demonstrated against isolates of *S. pneumoniae* and *L. pneumophila*. Tigecycline is a derivative of minocycline (9-t-butylglycylamido minocycline), and while not classified as a tetracycline, it may share some class-associated adverse effects. Tigecycline has demonstrated activity against a variety of gram-positive and -negative bacterial pathogens including methicillin-resistant staphylococci.

Pharmacodynamics/Kinetics

Distribution: V_d: 7-9 L/kg; extensive tissue distribution

Protein binding: 71% to 89%

Metabolism: Hepatic, via glucuronidation, N-acetylation, and epimerization to several metabolites, each <10% of the dose

Half-life elimination: Single dose: 27 hours; following multiple doses: 42 hours

Excretion: Feces (59%, primarily as unchanged drug); urine (33%, with 22% of the total dose as unchanged drug)

Dosage

Children ≥8 years and Adolescents: Limited data available: **Note:** Use should be reserved for situations when no effective alternative therapy is available

General dosing, susceptible infection: IV: Dosing based on data from pharmacokinetic trials.

Children 8-11 years: 1.2 mg/kg/dose every 12 hours; maximum dose: 50 mg

Children ≥12 years and Adolescents: 50 mg every 12 hours

Adults: **Note:** Duration of therapy dependent on severity/site of infection and clinical status and response to therapy.

Intra-abdominal infections, complicated (cIAI): IV: Initial: 100 mg as a single dose; Maintenance dose: 50 mg every 12 hours for 5-14 days; **Note:** 2010 IDSA guidelines recommend a treatment duration of 4-7 days (provided source controlled) for community-acquired, mild-to-moderate IAI

Pneumonia, community-acquired: IV: Initial: 100 mg as a single dose; Maintenance dose: 50 mg every 12 hours for 7-14 days

Skin/skin structure infections, complicated: IV: Initial: 100 mg as a single dose; Maintenance dose: 50 mg every 12 hours for 5-14 days

Dosage adjustment in renal impairment: No dosage adjustment necessary.

Poorly dialyzed; no supplemental dose or dosage adjustment necessary, including patients on intermittent hemodialysis, peritoneal dialysis, or continuous renal replacement therapy (eg, CVVHD).

Dosage adjustment in hepatic impairment:

Mild to moderate hepatic impairment (Child-Pugh class A or B): No dosage adjustment necessary.

Severe hepatic impairment (Child-Pugh class C): Initial: 100 mg single dose; Maintenance: 25 mg every 12 hours

Administration Infuse over 30-60 minutes through dedicated line or via Y-site

Dosage Forms

Solution Reconstituted, Intravenous:

Tygacil: 50 mg (1 ea)

◆ **Tikosyn** *see* Dofetilide *on page 662*

◆ **Tilia Fe** *see* Ethinyl Estradiol and Norethindrone *on page 808*

Tiludronate (tye LOO droe nate)

Brand Names: U.S. Skelid

Index Terms Tiludronate Disodium

Pharmacologic Category Bisphosphonate Derivative

Use Treatment of Paget's disease of the bone (osteitis deformans) in patients who have a level of serum alkaline phosphatase (SAP) at least twice the upper limit of normal, or who are symptomatic, or who are at risk for future complications of their disease

Pregnancy Risk Factor C

Dosage Oral: Adults: 400 mg (2 tablets of tiludronic acid) daily for a period of 3 months; allow an interval of 3 months to assess response

Dosage adjustment in renal impairment: No dosage adjustment provided in manufacturer's labeling. However, tiludronate is excreted renally. It is not recommended for use in patients with severe renal impairment (CrCl <30 mL/minute) and is not removed by dialysis.

Dosage adjustment in hepatic impairment: No dosage adjustment necessary.

Additional Information Complete prescribing information should be consulted for additional detail.

Dosage Forms

Tablet, Oral:

Skelid: 200 mg

◆ **Tiludronate Disodium** *see* Tiludronate *on page 2042*

◆ **Tim-AK (Can)** *see* Timolol (Ophthalmic) *on page 2043*

◆ **Timentin [DSC]** *see* Ticarcillin and Clavulanate Potassium [CAN/INT] *on page 2038*

◆ **Timentin (Can)** *see* Ticarcillin and Clavulanate Potassium [CAN/INT] *on page 2038*

Timolol (Systemic) (TIM oh lol)

Brand Names: Canada Apo-Timol®; Nu-Timolol; Teva-Timolol

Index Terms Timolol Maleate

Pharmacologic Category Antihypertensive; Beta-Blocker, Nonselective

Use Treatment of hypertension and angina; to reduce mortality following myocardial infarction; prophylaxis of migraine

The 2014 guideline for the management of high blood pressure in adults (JNC 8) recommends initiation of pharmacologic treatment to lower blood pressure for the following patients (JNC8 [James, 2013]):

- Patients ≥60 years of age, with systolic blood pressure (SBP) ≥150 mm Hg or diastolic blood pressure (DBP) ≥90 mm Hg. Goal of therapy is SBP <150 mm Hg and DBP <90 mm Hg.
- Patients <60 years of age, with SBP ≥140 mm Hg or DBP ≥90 mm Hg. Goal of therapy is SBP <140 mm Hg and DBP <90 mm Hg.
- Patients ≥18 years of age with diabetes, with SBP ≥140 mm Hg or DBP ≥90 mm Hg. Goal of therapy is SBP <140 mm Hg and DBP <90 mm Hg.
- Patients ≥18 years of age with chronic kidney disease (CKD), with SBP ≥140 mm Hg or DBP ≥90 mm Hg. Goal of therapy is SBP <140 mm Hg and DBP <90 mm Hg.

In patients with chronic kidney disease (CKD), regardless of race or diabetes status, the use of an ACE inhibitor (ACEI) or angiotensin receptor blocker (ARB) as initial therapy is recommended to improve kidney outcomes. In the general nonblack population (without CKD) including those with diabetes, initial antihypertensive treatment should consist of a thiazide-type diuretic, calcium channel blocker, ACEI, or ARB. In the general black population (without CKD) including those with diabetes, initial antihypertensive treatment should consist of a thiazide-type diuretic or a calcium channel blocker **instead of** an ACEI or ARB.

Pregnancy Risk Factor C

Dosage Oral: Adults:

Hypertension: Initial: 10 mg twice daily, increase gradually every 7 days, usual dosage: 20-40 mg/day in 2 divided doses; maximum: 60 mg/day

Prevention of myocardial infarction: 10 mg twice daily initiated within 1-4 weeks after infarction

Migraine headache: Initial: 10 mg twice daily, increase to maximum of 30 mg/day

Dosage adjustment in renal impairment: No specific dosage adjustment provided in manufacturer's labeling. However, timolol is primarily eliminated renally; dosage reduction may be necessary. Significant hypotension has been seen in patients with severe impairment and undergoing dialysis. Use with caution.

Dosage adjustment in hepatic impairment: No specific dosage adjustment provided in manufacturer's labeling. However, timolol is partially metabolized by the liver; dosage reduction may be necessary.

Additional Information Complete prescribing information should be consulted for additional detail.

Dosage Forms

Tablet, Oral:

Generic: 5 mg, 10 mg, 20 mg

Timolol (Ophthalmic) (TIM oh lol)

Brand Names: U.S. Betimol; Istalol; Timoptic; Timoptic Ocudose; Timoptic-XE

Brand Names: Canada Apo-Timop®; Dom-Timolol; Mylan-Timolol; Novo-Timol; PMS-Timolol; Sandoz-Timolol; Tim-AK; Timolol Maleate-EX; Timoptic-XE®; Timoptic®

Index Terms Timolol Hemihydrate; Timolol Maleate

Pharmacologic Category Beta-Blocker, Nonselective; Ophthalmic Agent, Antiglaucoma

Use Treatment of elevated intraocular pressure such as glaucoma or ocular hypertension

Pregnancy Risk Factor C

Dosage Ophthalmic:

Children and Adults:

Solution: Initial: Instill 1 drop (0.25% solution) into affected eye(s) twice daily; increase to 0.5% solution if response not adequate; decrease to 1 drop/day if controlled; do not exceed 1 drop twice daily of 0.5% solution

Gel-forming solution (Timolol GFS, Timoptic-XE®): Instill 1 drop (either 0.25% or 0.5% solution) once daily

Adults: Solution (Istalol®): Instill 1 drop (0.5% solution) once daily in the morning

Dosage adjustment in renal impairment: No dosage adjustment provided in manufacturer's labeling.

Dosage adjustment in hepatic impairment: No dosage adjustment provided in manufacturer's labeling.

Additional Information Complete prescribing information should be consulted for additional detail.

Dosage Forms

Gel Forming Solution, Ophthalmic:

Timoptic-XE: 0.25% (5 mL); 0.5% (5 mL)

Generic: 0.25% (5 mL); 0.5% (5 mL)

Solution, Ophthalmic:

Betimol: 0.25% (5 mL); 0.5% (5 mL, 10 mL, 15 mL)

Istalol: 0.5% (2.5 mL, 5 mL)

Timoptic: 0.25% (5 mL); 0.5% (5 mL, 10 mL)

Generic: 0.25% (5 mL, 10 mL, 15 mL); 0.5% (5 mL, 10 mL, 15 mL)

Solution, Ophthalmic [preservative free]:

Timoptic Ocudose: 0.25% (60 ea); 0.5% (60 ea)

- **Timolol and Bimatoprost** *see* Bimatoprost and Timolol [INT] *on page 264*
- **Timolol and Brimonidine** *see* Brimonidine and Timolol *on page 288*
- **Timolol and Dorzolamide** *see* Dorzolamide and Timolol *on page 673*
- **Timolol Hemihydrate** *see* Timolol (Ophthalmic) *on page 2043*
- **Timolol Maleate** *see* Timolol (Ophthalmic) *on page 2043*
- **Timolol Maleate** *see* Timolol (Systemic) *on page 2042*
- **Timolol Maleate and Brinzolamide** *see* Brinzolamide and Timolol [CAN/INT] *on page 289*
- **Timolol Maleate and Latanoprost** *see* Latanoprost and Timolol [CAN/INT] *on page 1172*
- **Timolol Maleate and Travoprost** *see* Travoprost and Timolol [CAN/INT] *on page 2090*
- **Timolol Maleate-EX (Can)** *see* Timolol (Ophthalmic) *on page 2043*
- **Timoptic** *see* Timolol (Ophthalmic) *on page 2043*
- **Timoptic® (Can)** *see* Timolol (Ophthalmic) *on page 2043*
- **Timoptic Ocudose** *see* Timolol (Ophthalmic) *on page 2043*
- **Timoptic-XE** *see* Timolol (Ophthalmic) *on page 2043*
- **Timoptic-XE® (Can)** *see* Timolol (Ophthalmic) *on page 2043*
- **Tinactin [OTC]** *see* Tolnaftate *on page 2063*
- **Tinactin Deodorant [OTC]** *see* Tolnaftate *on page 2063*
- **Tinactin Jock Itch [OTC]** *see* Tolnaftate *on page 2063*
- **Tinaspore [OTC]** *see* Tolnaftate *on page 2063*
- **Tincture of Opium** *see* Opium Tincture *on page 1518*

Tinzaparin (tin ZA pa rin)

Brand Names: Canada Innohep®

Index Terms Tinzaparin Sodium

Pharmacologic Category Anticoagulant; Anticoagulant, Low Molecular Weight Heparin

Use Treatment of deep vein thrombosis (DVT) and/or pulmonary embolism (PE) (except in patients with severe hemodynamic instability); prevention of venous thromboembolism (VTE) following orthopedic surgery or following general surgery in patients at high risk of VTE; prevention of clotting in indwelling intravenous lines and extracorporeal circuit during hemodialysis (in patients without high bleeding risk)

Pregnancy Considerations Teratogenic events were not observed in animal reproduction studies. Tinzaparin does not cross the human placenta. A pharmacokinetic study in pregnant women found no dose adjustment was needed during pregnancy. Vaginal bleeding was reported in ~10% of pregnant patients during tinzaparin therapy. LMWH is recommended over unfractionated heparin for the treatment of acute venous thromboembolism (VTE) in pregnant women. LMWH is also recommended over unfractionated heparin for VTE prophylaxis in pregnant women with certain risk factors. LMWH should be discontinued prior to induction of labor or a planned cesarean delivery. When choosing therapy, fetal outcomes (ie, pregnancy loss, malformations), maternal outcomes (ie, VTE, hemorrhage), burden of therapy, and maternal preference should be considered (Guyatt, 2012). Contains benzyl alcohol; use with caution in pregnant women due to association with gasping syndrome in premature infants.

Breast-Feeding Considerations Small amounts of LMWH have been detected in breast milk; however, because it has a low oral bioavailability, it is unlikely to cause adverse events in a nursing infant. Use of LMWH may be continued in breast-feeding women (Guyatt, 2012).

Contraindications Hypersensitivity to tinzaparin sodium, heparin or other low molecular weight heparins (LMWH), or any component of the formulation; active bleeding; history of confirmed or suspected immunologically mediated heparin-induced thrombocytopenia (HIT) or positive *in vitro* platelet-aggregation test in the presence of tinzaparin; acute or subacute endocarditis; generalized hemorrhage tendency and other conditions involving increased risks of hemorrhage (eg, severe hepatic insufficiency, imminent abortion); hemophilia or major blood clotting disorders; acute cerebral insult or hemorrhagic cerebrovascular accidents without systemic emboli; uncontrolled severe hypertension; diabetic or hemorrhagic retinopathy; injury or surgery involving the brain, spinal cord, eyes or ears; spinal/epidural anesthesia in patients requiring treatment dosages of tinzaparin; use of multidose vials containing benzyl alcohol in children <2 years of age, premature infants, and neonates

Note: Use of tinzaparin in patients with current HIT or HIT with thrombosis is **not** recommended and considered contraindicated due to high cross-reactivity to heparin-platelet factor-4 antibody (Guyatt [ACCP], 2012; Warkentin, 1999).

Warnings/Precautions Spinal or epidural hematomas, including subsequent paralysis, may occur with recent or anticipated neuraxial anesthesia (epidural or spinal) or spinal puncture in patients anticoagulated with low molecular weight heparin (LMWH) or heparinoids. Consider risk versus benefit prior to spinal procedures; risk is increased by the use of concomitant agents which may alter hemostasis, the use of indwelling epidural catheters for analgesia, a history of spinal deformity or spinal surgery, as well as traumatic or repeated epidural or spinal punctures. Avoid invasive spinal procedures for 12 hours following tinzaparin administration and withhold the next tinzaparin dose for at least 2 hours after the spinal procedure. Patient should be observed closely for signs and symptoms of neurological impairment. Not to be used interchangeably (unit for unit) with heparin or any other LMWHs.

Monitor patient closely for signs or symptoms of bleeding. Certain patients are at increased risk of bleeding. Risk factors include bacterial endocarditis; congenital or acquired bleeding disorders; active ulcerative or angiodysplastic GI diseases; severe uncontrolled hypertension; history of hemorrhagic stroke; use shortly after brain, spinal, or ophthalmologic surgery; those concomitantly treated with drugs that increase bleeding risk (eg, antiplatelet agents, anticoagulants); recent GI bleeding; thrombocytopenia or platelet defects; severe liver disease; hypertensive or diabetic retinopathy; or in patients undergoing invasive procedures. Withhold or discontinue for minor bleeding. Protamine infusion may be necessary for serious bleeding. Cases of thrombocytopenia including thrombocytopenia with thrombosis have occurred. Use with caution in patients with history of thrombocytopenia (drug-induced or congenital) or platelet defects; monitor platelet count closely. Use is contraindicated in patients with history of confirmed or suspected heparin-induced thrombocytopenia (HIT) or positive *in vitro* test for antiplatelet antibodies in the presence of tinzaparin. Discontinue therapy and consider alternative treatment if platelets are <100,000/mm^3 and/or thrombosis develops. Asymptomatic thrombocytosis has been observed with use, particularly in patients undergoing orthopedic surgery or with concurrent inflammatory process; discontinue use with increased platelet counts and evaluate the risks/necessity of further therapy. Prosthetic valve thrombosis has been reported in patients receiving thromboprophylaxis therapy with LMWHs. Pregnant women may be at increased risk.

Use with caution in hepatic impairment; associated with transient, dose-dependent increases in AST/ALT which typically resolve within 2 to 4 weeks of therapy discontinuation. Use with caution in patients with renal insufficiency. Reduced tinzaparin clearance has been observed in patients with moderate-to-severe renal impairment; Consider dosage reduction in patients with CrCl <30 mL/minute. Use with caution in the elderly (delayed elimination may occur). Use is not recommended in patients >70 years of age with renal impairment. An increase in all-cause mortality has been observed in patients ≥70 years (mean age: >82 years) with CrCl ≤60 mL/minute treated with tinzaparin compared to unfractionated heparin for acute DVT (Leizorovicz, 2011).

Heparin can cause hyperkalemia by suppressing aldosterone production; similar reactions could occur with LMWHs. Monitor for hyperkalemia which most commonly occurs in patients with risk factors for the development of hyperkalemia (eg, renal dysfunction, concomitant use of potassium-sparing diuretics or potassium supplements, hematoma in body tissues). For subcutaneous use only; do not administer intramuscularly or intravenously. Use with caution in patients <45 kg or >120 kg; limited experience in these patients. Individualized clinical and laboratory monitoring are recommended. Derived from porcine intestinal mucosa. Some dosage forms may contain sodium metabisulfite.

Benzyl alcohol and derivatives: Some dosage forms may contain benzyl alcohol and should not be used in pregnant women. In neonates, large amounts of benzyl alcohol (≥99 mg/kg/day) have been associated with a potentially fatal toxicity ("gasping syndrome"); the "gasping syndrome" consists of metabolic acidosis, respiratory distress, gasping respirations, CNS dysfunction (including convulsions, intracranial hemorrhage), hypotension, and cardiovascular collapse (AAP, 1997; CDC, 1982); some data suggests that benzoate displaces bilirubin from protein binding sites (Ahlfors, 2001); avoid or use dosage forms containing benzyl alcohol with caution in neonates. See manufacturer's labeling.

Adverse Reactions As with all anticoagulants, bleeding is the major adverse effect of tinzaparin. Hemorrhage may occur at virtually any site. Risk is dependent on multiple variables.

Cardiovascular: Angina pectoris, arrhythmia, chest pain, coronary thrombosis/MI, dependent edema, thromboembolism

Central nervous system: Fever, headache, pain

Dermatologic: Bullous eruption, erythematous rash, maculopapular rash, skin necrosis,

Gastrointestinal: Abdominal pain, constipation, diarrhea, nausea, vomiting

Genitourinary: Urinary tract infection

Hematologic: Bleeding events (major events including intracranial, retroperitoneal, or bleeding into a major prosthetic joint); hemorrhage site not specified; other bleeding events reported include anorectal bleeding, GI hemorrhage, hemarthrosis, hematemesis, hematuria, hemopericardium, injection site bleeding, melena, purpura, intra-abdominal bleeding, vaginal bleeding, wound hemorrhage); granulocytopenia, thrombocytopenia

Hepatic: ALT increased, AST increased

Local: Injection site cellulitis, injection site hematoma

Neuromuscular & skeletal: Back pain

Respiratory: Dyspnea, epistaxis

Miscellaneous: Allergic reaction, neoplasm

Rare but important or life-threatening: Agranulocytosis, angioedema, anaphylactoid reaction, GGT increased, hemoptysis, hypoaldosteronism, hyperkalemia, LDH increased, lipase increased, metabolic acidosis, ocular hemorrhage, osteopenia, osteoporosis, priapism, pruritus, rash, spinal epidural hematoma, Stevens-Johnson syndrome, thrombocytosis, toxic epidermal necrolysis, urticaria

Drug Interactions

Metabolism/Transport Effects None known.

Avoid Concomitant Use

Avoid concomitant use of Tinzaparin with any of the following: Apixaban; Dabigatran Etexilate; Edoxaban; Omacetaxine; Rivaroxaban; Urokinase; Vorapaxar

Increased Effect/Toxicity

Tinzaparin may increase the levels/effects of: ACE Inhibitors; Aliskiren; Angiotensin II Receptor Blockers; Anticoagulants; Canagliflozin; Collagenase (Systemic); Deferasirox; Eplerenone; Ibritumomab; Nintedanib; Obinutuzumab; Omacetaxine; Palifermin; Potassium Salts; Potassium-Sparing Diuretics; Rivaroxaban; Tositumomab and Iodine I 131 Tositumomab

The levels/effects of Tinzaparin may be increased by: 5-ASA Derivatives; Agents with Antiplatelet Properties; Apixaban; Dabigatran Etexilate; Dasatinib; Edoxaban; Herbs (Anticoagulant/Antiplatelet Properties); Ibrutinib; Limaprost; Nonsteroidal Anti-Inflammatory Agents; Omega-3 Fatty Acids; Pentosan Polysulfate Sodium; Pentoxifylline; Prostacyclin Analogues; Salicylates; Sugammadex; Thrombolytic Agents; Tibolone; Tipranavir; Urokinase; Vitamin E; Vorapaxar

Decreased Effect

The levels/effects of Tinzaparin may be decreased by: Estrogen Derivatives; Progestins

Storage/Stability Store at 15°C to 25°C (59°F to 77°F).

Mechanism of Action Tinzaparin is a low molecular weight heparin (average molecular weight ranges between 5500 and 7500 daltons, distributed as <2000 daltons [<10%], 2000-8000 daltons [60% to 72%], and >8000 daltons [22% to 36%]) that binds antithrombin III, enhancing the inhibition of several clotting factors, particularly factor Xa. Tinzaparin anti-Xa activity (70-120 units/mg) is greater than anti-IIa activity (~55 units/mg) and it has a higher ratio of antifactor Xa to antifactor IIa activity compared to unfractionated heparin. Low molecular weight heparins have a small effect on the activated partial thromboplastin time.

Pharmacodynamics/Kinetics Note: Values reflective of anti-Xa activity.

Onset of action: 2-3 hours

Duration: Detectable anti-Xa activity persists for 24 hours

Absorption: Slow; absorption half-life ~3 hours after subcutaneous administration

Distribution: 4 L

Metabolism: Does not undergo hepatic metabolism

Bioavailability: SubQ: ~90%

Half-life elimination: 82 minutes; prolonged in renal impairment

Time to peak: 4-6 hours

Excretion: Urine

Dosage Note: 1 mg of tinzaparin equals 70-120 units of anti-Xa activity

SubQ:

Infants, Children, and Adolescents: VTE treatment (off-label use; Monagle, 2012): **Note:** May initiate a vitamin K antagonist on day 1 of tinzaparin therapy; discontinue tinzaparin on day 6 or later if INR is not >2.

Birth to 2 months: 275 anti-Xa units/kg once daily

2-12 months: 250 anti-Xa units/kg once daily

1-5 years: 240 anti-Xa units/kg once daily

5-10 years: 200 anti-Xa units/kg once daily

10-16 years: 175 anti-Xa units/kg once daily

Adults:

DVT and/or PE treatment: 175 anti-Xa units/kg once daily (maximum: 18,000 anti-Xa units/day). The 2012 *Chest* guidelines recommend starting warfarin on the first or second treatment day and continuing tinzaparin until INR is ≥2 for at least 24 hours (usually 5-7 days) (Guyatt, 2012). Body weight dosing using prefilled syringes may also be considered. Refer to manufacturer labeling for detailed dosing recommendations.

DVT prophylaxis:

Hip replacement surgery: **Note:** The American College of Chest Physicians recommends initiation of LMWH ≥12 hours preoperatively **or** ≥12 hours postoperatively; extended duration up to 35 days suggested (Guyatt, 2012).

Preoperative regimen: 50 anti-Xa units/kg given 2 hours preoperatively followed by 50 anti-Xa units/kg once daily for 7-10 days

Postoperative regimen: 75 anti-Xa units/kg once daily, with initial dose given postoperatively and continued for 7-10 days

Knee replacement surgery: 75 anti-Xa units/kg once daily, with initial dose given postoperatively and continued for 7-10 days. **Note:** The American College of Chest Physicians recommends initiation of LMWH ≥12 hours preoperatively **or** ≥12 hours postoperatively; extended duration of up to 35 days suggested (Guyatt, 2012). Body weight dosing using prefilled syringes may also be considered. Refer to manufacturer labeling for detailed dosing recommendations.

General surgery: 3500 anti-Xa units once daily, with initial dose given 2 hours prior to surgery and then continued postoperatively for 7-10 days

IV: Adults: Anticoagulant in extracorporeal circuit during hemodialysis (recommendations apply to stable patients with chronic renal failure):

Dialysis session ≤4 hours (no hemorrhage risk): Initial bolus (via arterial side of circuit or IV): 4500 anti-Xa units at beginning of dialysis; typically achieves plasma concentrations of 0.5-1 anti-Xa units/mL; may give larger bolus for dialysis sessions >4 hours. For subsequent dialysis sessions, may adjust dose as necessary in increments of 500 anti-Xa units based on previous outcome.

Dialysis session ≤4 hours (hemorrhage risk): Initial bolus (IV only): 2250 anti-Xa units at beginning of dialysis (do not add to dialysis circuit). A smaller second IV dose may be administered during dialysis sessions >4 hours. For subsequent dialysis sessions, adjust dose as necessary to achieve plasma concentrations of 0.2-0.4 anti-Xa units/mL.

Elderly: No significant differences in safety or response were seen when used in patients ≥65 years of age. However, increased sensitivity to tinzaparin in elderly patients may be possible due to a decline in renal function. Use is not recommended in patients >70 years of age with renal impairment.

Dosage adjustment in renal impairment:

CrCl ≥30 mL/minute: No dosage adjustment provided in manufacturer's labeling; however, primarily undergoes renal elimination. Clearance is decreased in renal impairment; use with caution.

CrCl <30 mL/minute: Manufacturer's labeling suggests that a reduction in dose be considered but does not provide specific dose recommendations. Use with caution.

Dosage adjustment in hepatic impairment: No dosage adjustment provided in manufacturer's labeling. Does not undergo hepatic metabolism; however, has been associated with transient increases in transaminase levels; use with caution.

Dosing in obesity: A pharmacokinetic study confirmed that weight-based dosing (single doses of 75 or 175 units/kg) using actual body weight in heavy/obese patients between 100 and 165 kg led to achievement of similar anti-Xa activity levels compared to normal-weight patients (Hainer, 2002). However, there is limited clinical experience in patients with a BMI >40 kg/m^2.

Administration Patient should be lying down or sitting. Administer by deep SubQ injection into the lower abdomen, outer thigh, lower back, or upper arm. Injection site should be varied daily. To minimize bruising, do not rub the injection site. In hemodialysis patients, may be administered IV (patients with high or low hemorrhage risk) or added to the dialyzer circuit (patients with low hemorrhage risk).

Monitoring Parameters CBC (at baseline then twice weekly throughout therapy); renal function (use Cockcroft-Gault formula); hepatic function; potassium (baseline in patients at risk for hyperkalemia, monitor regularly if duration >7 days); stool for occult blood. Routine monitoring of anti-Xa levels is generally not recommended; however, anti-Xa levels may be beneficial in certain patients (eg, children, obese patients, patients with severe renal insufficiency receiving therapeutic doses, and possibly pregnant women receiving therapeutic doses) (Guyatt, 2012). Peak anti-Xa levels are measured 4-6 hours after administration. Monitoring of PT and/or aPTT is not of clinical benefit.

Reference Range Anti-Xa level (measured 4 hours after administration): Fixed-dose (3500 units): 0.15 anti-Xa units/mL; weight-based (75-175 units/kg): 0.34-0.70 anti-Xa units/mL; in treatment of venous thromboembolism, a target of 0.85 anti-Xa units/mL has been recommended (Garcia, 2012)

Children: Target anti-Xa level: 0.5-1 anti-Xa units/mL 4-6 hours after administration or 0.5-0.8 anti-Xa units/mL 2-6 hours after administration (Monagle, 2012)

Additional Information Neutralization of tinzaparin (in overdose) with protamine 1% solution: Manufacturer's recommendations: 1 mg protamine for each 100 anti-Xa units of tinzaparin; if PTT prolonged 2-4 hours after first dose (or if bleeding continues), consider additional dose of 0.5 mg for each 100 anti-Xa units of tinzaparin.

Dosage Forms: Canada

Injection, solution:

Innohep®: 10,000 anti-Xa units/mL (2 mL)

Innohep®: 20,000 anti-Xa units/mL (0.5 mL, 0.7 mL, 0.9 mL, 2 mL)

Injection, solution [preservative free]:

Innohep®: 10,000 anti-Xa units/mL (0.25 mL, 0.35 mL, 0.45 mL)

◆ **Tinzaparin Sodium** *see* Tinzaparin *on page 2043*

◆ **Tioguanine** *see* Thioguanine *on page 2029*

◆ **Tiotixene** *see* Thiothixene *on page 2031*

Tiotropium (ty oh TRO pee um)

Brand Names: U.S. Spiriva HandiHaler; Spiriva Respimat

Brand Names: Canada Spiriva

Index Terms Tiotropium Bromide Monohydrate

Pharmacologic Category Anticholinergic Agent; Anticholinergic Agent, Long-Acting

Use Chronic obstructive pulmonary disease: Maintenance treatment of bronchospasm associated with chronic obstructive pulmonary disease (COPD), including chronic bronchitis and emphysema; reduction of COPD exacerbations

Pregnancy Risk Factor C

Pregnancy Considerations Adverse events have been observed in animal reproduction studies.

Breast-Feeding Considerations It is not known if tiotropium is excreted in breast milk. The manufacturer recommends that caution be exercised when administering tiotropium to nursing women.

Contraindications Hypersensitivity to ipratropium, tiotropium, or any component of the formulation

Warnings/Precautions Paradoxical bronchospasm may occur with use of inhaled agents; discontinue use and consider other therapy if bronchospasm occurs. May cause dizziness and blurred vision; patients must be cautioned about performing tasks that require mental alertness (eg, operating machinery or driving).

Not indicated for the initial (rescue) treatment of acute episodes of bronchospasm. Use with caution in patients with narrow-angle glaucoma, prostatic hyperplasia, moderate-severe renal impairment, or bladder neck obstruction; avoid inadvertent instillation into the eyes. Immediate hypersensitivity reactions may occur; discontinue immediately if signs/symptoms occur. Use with caution in patients with a history of hypersensitivity to atropine.

The contents of Spiriva capsules are for inhalation only via the HandiHaler device. There have been reports of incorrect administration (swallowing of the capsules). Capsule for oral inhalation contains lactose; use with caution in patients with severe milk protein allergy. The contents of Spiriva inhalation spray are for inhalation only via the Respimat inhaler. Potentially significant interactions may exist, requiring dose or frequency adjustment, additional monitoring, and/or selection of alternative therapy.

Adverse Reactions

Cardiovascular: Angina pectoris (includes exacerbation of angina pectoris), chest pain, edema (dependent), palpitations (powder and solution)

Central nervous system: Depression,dizziness (powder and solution), headache, insomnia (powder and solution), paresthesia, voice disorder (powder and solution)

Dermatologic: Pruritus (powder and solution), skin rash (powder and solution)

Endocrine & metabolic: Hypercholesterolemia, hyperglycemia

Gastrointestinal: Abdominal pain, constipation (powder and solution), dyspepsia, gastroesophageal reflux disease (powder and solution), gastrointestinal disease (not otherwise specified), omitting, oropharyngeal candidiasis (powder and solution), stomatitis (includes ulcerative stomatitis; powder and solution), xerostomia (powder and solution)

Genitourinary: Urinary tract infection (powder and solution)

Hypersensitivity: Hypersensitivity reaction (powder and solution)

Infection: Candidiasis, herpes zoster, infection

Neuromuscular & skeletal: Arthralgia, arthritis, leg pain, myalgia, skeletal pain

Ophthalmic: Cataract

Respiratory: Cough, epistaxis (powder and solution), flu-like symptoms, laryngitis (powder and solution), pharyngitis (powder and solution), rhinitis, sinusitis, upper respiratory tract infection

Rare but important or life-threatening: Anaphylaxis, application site irritation (powder; includes glossitis, oral mucosa ulcer, pharyngolaryngeal pain), atrial fibrillation, blurred vision, dehydration, dermal ulcer, dysphagia, dysuria, gingivitis, glaucoma, glossitis, hoarseness, intestinal obstruction (includes paralytic ileus), joint swelling, paradoxical bronchospasm, skin infection, supraventricular tachycardia, tachycardia, urinary retention, xeroderma

Drug Interactions

Metabolism/Transport Effects Substrate of CYP2D6 (minor), CYP3A4 (minor); **Note:** Assignment of Major/Minor substrate status based on clinically relevant drug interaction potential

Avoid Concomitant Use

Avoid concomitant use of Tiotropium with any of the following: Aclidinium; Anticholinergic Agents; Glucagon; Ipratropium (Oral Inhalation); Potassium Chloride; Umeclidinium

Increased Effect/Toxicity

Tiotropium may increase the levels/effects of: AbobotulinumtoxinA; Analgesics (Opioid); Anticholinergic Agents; Cannabinoid-Containing Products; Glucagon; Mirabegron; OnabotulinumtoxinA; Potassium Chloride; RimabotulinumtoxinB; Thiazide Diuretics; Topiramate

The levels/effects of Tiotropium may be increased by: Aclidinium; Anticholinergic Agents; Ipratropium (Oral Inhalation); Mianserin; Pramlintide; Umeclidinium

Decreased Effect

Tiotropium may decrease the levels/effects of: Acetylcholinesterase Inhibitors; Itopride; Secretin

The levels/effects of Tiotropium may be decreased by: Acetylcholinesterase Inhibitors

Storage/Stability Spiriva HandiHaler: Store at 25°C (77°F); excursions are permitted between 15°C and 30°C (59°F and 86°F). Avoid excessive temperatures and moisture. Do not store capsules in HandiHaler device. Capsules should be stored in the blister pack and only removed immediately before use. Once protective foil is peeled back and/or removed, the capsule should be used immediately; if capsule is not used immediately it should be discarded.

Spiriva Respimat: Store at 25°C (77°F); excursions are permitted between 15°C and 30°C (59°F and 86°F). Avoid freezing.

Mechanism of Action Competitively and reversibly inhibits the action of acetylcholine at type 3 muscarinic (M_3) receptors in bronchial smooth muscle causing bronchodilation

Pharmacodynamics/Kinetics

Absorption: Poorly absorbed from GI tract, systemic absorption may occur from lung

Distribution: V_d: 32 L/kg

Protein binding: 72%

Metabolism: Hepatic (minimal), via CYP2D6 and CYP3A4

Bioavailability: Following inhalation, 19.5% (dry powder inhalation) or ~33% (inhalation solution); Oral solution: 2% to 3%

Half-life elimination: 5 to 6 days (dry powder inhalation)

Time to peak, plasma:

Spiriva HandiHaler: 5 minutes (following inhalation)

Spiriva Respimat: 5 to 7 minutes (following inhalation)

Excretion: Urine (14% of an inhaled dose [Spiriva HandiHaler]; 18.6% of an inhaled dose [Spiriva Respimat]); feces (primarily nonabsorbed drug)

Dosage

COPD: Adults: Oral inhalation:

Spiriva HandiHaler: Contents of 1 capsule (18 mcg) inhaled once daily using HandiHaler device. **Note:** To ensure drug delivery, the contents of each capsule should be inhaled twice.

Spiriva Respimat: Two inhalations (5 mcg) once daily (maximum: 2 inhalations per 24 hours).

Dosage adjustment in renal impairment: No dosage adjustment necessary; use caution in moderate to severe renal impairment; monitor closely.

Dosage adjustment in hepatic impairment: No dosage adjustment necessary.

Administration For oral inhalation only.

Spiriva Handihaler: Capsule should not be swallowed. Administer once daily at the same time each day. Remove capsule from foil blister immediately before use. Place capsule in the center chamber of the HandiHaler Inhaler. Must only use the HandiHaler Inhaler. Close mouthpiece firmly until a click is heard, leaving dustcap open. The capsule is pierced by pressing and releasing the green piercing button on the side of the HandiHaler device. Exhale fully. Close lips tightly around mouthpiece; do not exhale into inhaler. Tilt head slightly back and inhale (rapidly, steadily, and deeply); the capsule vibration (rattle) may be heard within the device. Hold breath for a few seconds then repeat procedure using the same tiotropium capsule. Throw away empty capsule by tipping into a trash can without touching it; do not leave in inhaler. Keep capsules and inhaler dry.

Spiriva Respimat: Prior to first use, insert cartridge into the inhaler and prime the unit by actuating the inhaler toward the ground until an aerosol cloud is visible; repeat three more times and then the unit is primed and ready for use. If not used for more than 3 days, actuate the inhaler once to prepare the inhaler for use. If not used for more than 21 days, actuate the inhaler until an aerosol cloud is visible and then repeat the process three more times to prepare the inhaler for use.

Monitoring Parameters FEV_1, peak flow (or other pulmonary function studies); anticholinergic adverse reactions (patients with CrCl ≤50 mL/min); signs and symptoms of narrow angle glaucoma and urinary retention

Dosage Forms

Aerosol Solution, Inhalation:

Spiriva Respimat: 2.5 mcg/actuation (4 g)

Capsule, Inhalation:

Spiriva HandiHaler: 18 mcg

Dosage Forms: Canada

Powder, for oral inhalation:

Spiriva: 18 mcg/capsule (10s)

◆ **Tiotropium Bromide Monohydrate** *see* Tiotropium *on page 2046*

Tipranavir (tip RA na veer)

Brand Names: U.S. Aptivus

Brand Names: Canada Aptivus

Index Terms PNU-140690E; TPV

Pharmacologic Category Antiretroviral, Protease Inhibitor (Anti-HIV)

Use Treatment of HIV-1 infections in combination with ritonavir and other antiretroviral agents; limited to highly treatment-experienced or multiprotease inhibitor-resistant patients.

Pregnancy Risk Factor C

Pregnancy Considerations Adverse events were observed in some animal reproduction studies. Tipranavir crosses the human placenta. The DHHS Perinatal HIV Guidelines note there are insufficient data to recommend use during pregnancy; however, if used, tipranavir must be given with low-dose ritonavir boosting. A small increased risk of preterm birth has been associated with maternal use of protease inhibitor-based combination antiretroviral (ARV) therapy during pregnancy; however, the benefits of use generally outweigh this risk and protease inhibitors (PIs) should not be withheld if otherwise recommended. Hyperglycemia, new onset of diabetes mellitus, or diabetic ketoacidosis have been reported with PIs; it is not clear if pregnancy increases this risk.

Regardless of CD4 count or HIV RNA copy number, all HIV-infected pregnant women should receive a combination ARV drug regimen. A combination of antepartum, intrapartum, and infant ARV prophylaxis is recommended. ARV therapy should be started as soon as possible in women with symptomatic infection. Although earlier initiation may be more effective in reducing the perinatal transmission of HIV, initiation may be delayed until after 12 weeks' gestation in women who do not require immediate treatment after careful consideration of maternal conditions (eg, nausea and vomiting) and the potential risks of first trimester fetal exposure for specific agents. A scheduled cesarean delivery at 38 weeks' gestation is recommended for all women with HIV RNA >1000 copies/mL or unknown concentrations near delivery in order to decrease transmission. If ARV therapy must be interrupted for <24 hours during the peripartum period, stop then restart all medications simultaneously in order to decrease the chance of developing resistance. Long-term follow-up is recommended for all infants exposed to ARV medications. In couples who want to conceive, the HIV-infected partner should attain maximum viral suppression prior to conception.

Health care providers are encouraged to enroll pregnant women exposed to antiretroviral medications in the Antiretroviral Pregnancy Registry (1-800-258-4263 or www.APRegistry.com). Health care providers caring for HIV-infected women and their infants may contact the National Perinatal HIV Hotline (888-448-8765) for clinical consultation (HHS [perinatal], 2014).

Women receiving estrogen (as hormonal contraception or replacement therapy) may have an increased incidence of rash.

Breast-Feeding Considerations It is not known if tipranavir is excreted into breast milk. Maternal or infant antiretroviral therapy does not completely eliminate the risk of postnatal HIV transmission. In addition, multiclass-resistant virus has been detected in breast-feeding infants despite maternal therapy. Therefore, in the United States, where formula is accessible, affordable, safe, and sustainable, and the risk of infant mortality due to diarrhea and respiratory infections is low, complete avoidance of breast-feeding by HIV-infected women is recommended to decrease potential transmission of HIV (HHS [perinatal], 2014).

Contraindications Concurrent therapy of tipranavir/ritonavir with alfuzosin, amiodarone, bepridil, cisapride, ergot derivatives (eg, dihydroergotamine, ergonovine, ergotamine, methylergonovine), flecainide, lovastatin, midazolam (oral), pimozide, propafenone, quinidine, rifampin, sildenafil (for pulmonary arterial hypertension [eg, Revatio®]), simvastatin, St John's wort, and triazolam; moderate-to-severe hepatic impairment (Child-Pugh class B or C)

Warnings/Precautions [U.S. Boxed Warning]: In combination with ritonavir, may cause hepatitis (including fatalities) and/or exacerbate preexisting hepatic dysfunction (causal relationship not established); patients with chronic hepatitis B or C are at increased risk. Monitor patients closely; discontinue use if signs or symptoms of toxicity occur or if asymptomatic AST/ALT elevations >10 times upper limit of normal or AST/ALT elevations >5-10 times upper limit of normal concurrently with total bilirubin >2.5 times the upper limit of normal occur. Use with caution in patients with mild hepatic impairment; contraindicated in moderate-to-severe impairment. May be associated with fat redistribution (buffalo hump, increased abdominal girth, breast engorgement, facial atrophy). Use caution in hemophilia. May increase cholesterol and/or triglycerides; hypertriglyceridemia may increase risk of pancreatitis. May cause hyperglycemia. Use with caution in patients with sulfonamide allergy. Protease inhibitors have been associated with a variety of hypersensitivity events (some severe), including rash, anaphylaxis (rare), angioedema, bronchospasm, erythema multiforme, and/or Stevens-Johnson syndrome (rare). It is generally recommended to discontinue treatment if severe rash or moderate symptoms accompanied by other systemic symptoms occur. Patients may develop immune reconstitution syndrome resulting in the occurrence of an inflammatory response to an indolent or residual opportunistic infection during initial HIV treatment or activation of autoimmune disorders (eg, Graves' disease, polymyositis, Guillain-Barré syndrome) later in therapy; further evaluation and treatment may be required.

[U.S. Boxed Warning]: Tipranavir in combination with ritonavir has been associated with rare reports of fatal and nonfatal intracranial hemorrhage; causal relationship not established. Events often occurred in patients with medical conditions (eg, CNS lesions, head trauma, recent neurosurgery, coagulopathy, alcohol abuse) or concurrent therapy which may have influenced these events. Tipranavir may inhibit platelet aggregation. Use with caution in patients who may be at risk for increased bleeding (trauma, surgery or other medical conditions) or in patients receiving concurrent medications which may increase the risk of bleeding, including antiplatelet agents and anticoagulants.

High potential for drug interactions; concomitant use of tipranavir with some drugs may require cautious use, may not be recommended, may require dosage adjustments, or may be contraindicated. Capsules contain dehydrated alcohol 7% w/w (0.1 g per capsule).

Adverse Reactions

Central nervous system: Fatigue, fever, headache
Dermatologic: Rash
Endocrine & metabolic: Dehydration, hypercholesterolemia, hypertriglyceridemia
Gastrointestinal: Abdominal pain, amylase increased, diarrhea, nausea, vomiting, weight loss
Hepatic: ALT increased, AST increased, GGT increased, transaminases increased
Hematologic: Anemia, bleeding, neutropenia, WBC decreased
Neuromuscular & skeletal: CPK increased, myalgia
Respiratory: Cough, dyspnea, epistaxis
Rare but important or life-threatening: Abdominal distension, anorexia, appetite decreased, diabetes mellitus, dizziness, dyspepsia, exanthem, facial wasting, flatulence, flu-like syndrome, gastroesophageal reflux, hepatic failure, hepatic steatosis, hepatitis, hyperbilirubinemia, hyperglycemia, hypersensitivity, immune reconstitution syndrome, insomnia, intracranial hemorrhage, lipase increased, lipoatrophy, lipodystrophy (acquired), lipohypertrophy, malaise, mitochondrial toxicity, muscle cramp, neuropathy (peripheral), pancreatitis, pruritus, renal insufficiency, sleep disorder, somnolence, thrombocytopenia

Drug Interactions

Metabolism/Transport Effects Substrate of CYP3A4 (major); **Note:** Assignment of Major/Minor substrate status based on clinically relevant drug interaction potential; **Inhibits** CYP2D6 (strong); **Induces** P-glycoprotein

Avoid Concomitant Use

Avoid concomitant use of Tipranavir with any of the following: Alfuzosin; Amiodarone; AtorvaSTATin; Bepridil [Off Market]; Boceprevir; Cisapride; Dabigatran Etexilate; Ergot Derivatives; Etravirine; Flecainide; Fluticasone (Nasal); Fluticasone (Oral Inhalation); Ledipasvir; Lomitapide; Lovastatin; Midazolam; Pimozide; Propafenone; Protease Inhibitors; QuiNIDine; Rifampin; Salmeterol; Simeprevir; Simvastatin; Sofosbuvir; St Johns Wort; Tadalafil; Tamoxifen; Telaprevir; Thioridazine; Triazolam; VinCRIStine (Liposomal)

Increased Effect/Toxicity

Tipranavir may increase the levels/effects of: Agents with Antiplatelet Properties; Alfuzosin; ALPRAZolam; Amiodarone; Anticoagulants; ARIPiprazole; AtoMOXetine; AtorvaSTATin; Bepridil [Off Market]; Bosentan; Calcium Channel Blockers (Dihydropyridine); Calcium Channel Blockers (Nondihydropyridine); CarBAMazepine; Cisapride; Clarithromycin; Colchicine; Contraceptives (Progestins); Cyclophosphamide; CycloSPORINE (Systemic); CYP2D6 Substrates; Digoxin; DOXOrubicin (Conventional); Eliglustat; Enfuvirtide; Ergot Derivatives; Fesoterodine; Flecainide; Fluticasone (Nasal); Fluticasone (Oral Inhalation); Iloperidone; Itraconazole; Ketoconazole

(Systemic); Lomitapide; Lovastatin; Meperidine; Metoprolol; Midazolam; Nebivolol; Nefazodone; Pimozide; Propafenone; Protease Inhibitors; QuiNIDine; Rifabutin; Riociguat; Rosuvastatin; Salmeterol; Sildenafil; Simeprevir; Simvastatin; Tacrolimus (Systemic); Tacrolimus (Topical); Tadalafil; Temsirolimus; Tetrabenazine; Thioridazine; TraZODone; Triazolam; Tricyclic Antidepressants; Vitamin E; Vortioxetine

The levels/effects of Tipranavir may be increased by: Clarithromycin; CycloSPORINE (Systemic); Delavirdine; Disulfiram; Enfuvirtide; Estrogen Derivatives; Fluconazole; MetroNIDAZOLE (Systemic); MetroNIDAZOLE (Topical); Simeprevir

Decreased Effect

Tipranavir may decrease the levels/effects of: Abacavir; Afatinib; Boceprevir; Brentuximab Vedotin; Clarithromycin; Codeine; Dabigatran Etexilate; Delavirdine; Didanosine; Dolutegravir; DOXOrubicin (Conventional); Estrogen Derivatives; Etravirine; Fosphenytoin; Iloperidone; Ledipasvir; Linagliptin; Meperidine; Methadone; P-glycoprotein/ABCB1 Substrates; PHENobarbital; Phenytoin; Protease Inhibitors; Proton Pump Inhibitors; Raltegravir; Sofosbuvir; Tamoxifen; Telaprevir; Tenofovir; Theophylline Derivatives; TraMADol; Valproic Acid and Derivatives; VinCRIStine (Liposomal); Zidovudine

The levels/effects of Tipranavir may be decreased by: Antacids; Boceprevir; Bosentan; CarBAMazepine; CYP3A4 Inducers (Moderate); CYP3A4 Inducers (Strong); Dabrafenib; Deferasirox; Fosphenytoin; Garlic; Mitotane; PHENobarbital; Phenytoin; Rifampin; Siltuximab; St Johns Wort; Tenofovir; Tocilizumab

Storage/Stability

Capsule: Prior to opening bottle, store under refrigeration at 2°C to 8°C (36°F to 46°F). After bottle is opened, may be stored at controlled room temperature of 25°C (77°F) for up to 60 days.

Oral solution: Store at 15°C to 30°C (59°F to 86°F). After bottle is open, use within 60 days. Do not refrigerate or freeze oral solution.

Mechanism of Action Binds to the site of HIV-1 protease activity and inhibits cleavage of viral Gag-Pol polyprotein precursors into individual functional proteins required for infectious HIV. This results in the formation of immature, noninfectious viral particles.

Pharmacodynamics/Kinetics

Absorption: Incomplete (percentage not established)

Distribution: V_d: 7.7-10 L

Protein binding: >99% (albumin, $alpha_1$-acid glycoprotein)

Metabolism: Hepatic, via CYP3A4 (minimal when coadministered with ritonavir)

Bioavailability: Not established

Half-life elimination: Children 2-<6 years of age: ~8 hours, 6-<12 years of age: ~7 hours, 12-18 years: ~5 hours; Adults: 6 hours

Time to peak, plasma: 3 hours

Excretion: Feces (82%); urine (4%); primarily as unchanged drug (when coadministered with ritonavir)

Dosage Oral:

Children ≥2 years: 14 mg/kg or 375 mg/m^2 (maximum: 500 mg/dose) twice daily. **Note:** Coadministration with ritonavir (6 mg/kg or 150 mg/m^2 [maximum: 200 mg/dose] twice daily) is required.

If intolerance or toxicity develops and virus is not resistant to multiple protease inhibitors: May decrease dose to 12 mg/kg or 290 mg/m^2 twice daily. **Note:** Coadministration with ritonavir (5 mg/kg or 115 mg/m^2 twice daily) is required.

Adults: 500 mg twice daily; **Note:** Coadministration with ritonavir (200 mg twice daily) is required.

Dosage adjustment in renal impairment: There are no dosage adjustments provided in the manufacturer's labeling (has not been studied). However, dosage adjustment not expected since renal clearance is negligible. Guidelines state that dosage adjustment is not required (HHS [adult], 2014).

Dosage adjustment in hepatic impairment:

Mild impairment (Child-Pugh class A): There are no dosage adjustments provided in the manufacturer's labeling; guidelines recommend to use with caution (HHS [adult], 2014).

Moderate-to-severe impairment (Child-Pugh class B or C): Concurrent use is contraindicated

Dietary Considerations Capsule contains dehydrated ethanol. Oral solution formulation contains vitamin E; additional vitamin E supplements should be avoided.

Administration Tipranavir must be coadministered with ritonavir. When using ritonavir tablets, administer with food (HHS [adult], 2014; (HHS [pediatric], 2014). When using ritonavir capsules or solution, administer with food for pediatric patients (HHS [pediatric], 2014); may be administered without regard to meals for adult patients (HHS [adult], 2014).

Monitoring Parameters Viral load, CD4, serum glucose, liver function tests, bilirubin

Dosage Forms

Capsule, Oral:

Aptivus: 250 mg

Solution, Oral:

Aptivus: 100 mg/mL (95 mL)

Tirofiban (tye roe FYE ban)

Brand Names: U.S. Aggrastat

Brand Names: Canada Aggrastat

Index Terms MK383; Tirofiban Hydrochloride

Pharmacologic Category Antiplatelet Agent, Glycoprotein IIb/IIIa Inhibitor

Use Unstable angina/non-ST-elevation myocardial infarction: To decrease the rate of thrombotic cardiovascular events (combined end point of death, MI, or refractory ischemia/repeat cardiac procedure) in patients with non-ST-elevation acute coronary syndrome (unstable angina/non-ST-elevation myocardial infarction [UA/NSTEMI]).

Pregnancy Risk Factor B

Pregnancy Considerations Adverse events have not been observed in animal reproduction studies. Information related to use in pregnancy is limited; successful use during pregnancy has been described in a case report (Boztosun, 2008).

Breast-Feeding Considerations It is not known if tirofiban is excreted in breast milk. Due to the potential for serious adverse reactions in the nursing infant, a decision should be made whether to discontinue nursing or to discontinue the drug, taking into account the importance of treatment to the mother.

Contraindications Severe hypersensitivity reaction (ie, anaphylactic reaction) to tirofiban or any component of the formulation; history of thrombocytopenia following prior exposure to tirofiban; active internal bleeding or a history of bleeding diathesis, major surgical procedure, or severe physical trauma within the previous month

Warnings/Precautions Bleeding is the most common complication encountered during this therapy; most major bleeding occurs at the arterial access site for cardiac catheterization. Caution in patients with platelets <150,000/mm^3; patients with hemorrhagic retinopathy; chronic dialysis patients; when used in combination with other drugs impacting on coagulation. Percutaneous coronary intervention (off-label use): Prior to pulling the sheath, ACT should be <180 seconds or aPTT <50 seconds (ACCF/AHA/SCAI [Levine, 2011]). Use standard compression techniques after sheath removal. Watch the site closely afterwards for further bleeding. Sheath hemostasis should be achieved at least 4 hours before hospital discharge. Other trauma and vascular punctures should be minimized. Avoid obtaining vascular access through a noncompressible site (eg, subclavian or jugular vein).

Profound thrombocytopenia has been reported with use of tirofiban. If during therapy platelet count decreases to <90,000/mm^3, monitor platelet counts to exclude pseudothrombocytopenia. If thrombocytopenia is confirmed, discontinue tirofiban and heparin if administered concurrently. Previous exposure to a glycoprotein IIb/IIIa inhibitor may increase the risk of thrombocytopenia. Use is contraindicated in patients with a history of thrombocytopenia following exposure to tirofiban.

Discontinue at least 2 to 4 hours prior to coronary artery bypass graft surgery (ACCF/AHA [Anderson, 2013]; ACCF/AHA [Hillis, 2011]). Dosage reduction of the maintenance infusion rate is necessary in patients with CrCl ≤60 mL/minute.

Adverse Reactions Bleeding is the major drug-related adverse effect. Patients received background treatment with aspirin and heparin. Adverse reactions reported are derived from both the high-dose bolus regimen **and** the dosing regimen used in studies that established the effectiveness of tirofiban.

Cardiovascular: Bradycardia, coronary artery dissection, edema, vasodepressor syncope
Central nervous system: Dizziness, headache
Dermatologic: Diaphoresis
Gastrointestinal: Nausea
Genitourinary: Pelvic pain
Hematologic & oncologic: Major hemorrhage (TIMI criteria major bleeding: Including hematoma [femoral] [Valgimigli, 2005], intracranial bleeding, GI bleeding, retroperitoneal bleeding [Aydin, 2003], GU bleeding, pulmonary alveolar hemorrhage [Guo, 2012], spinal-epidural hematoma), minor hemorrhage (TIMI criteria minor bleeding), thrombocytopenia
Neuromuscular & skeletal: Leg pain
Miscellaneous: Fever
Rare but important or life-threatening: Anaphylaxis, hemopericardium, hypersensitivity

Drug Interactions

Metabolism/Transport Effects None known.

Avoid Concomitant Use

Avoid concomitant use of Tirofiban with any of the following: Urokinase

Increased Effect/Toxicity

Tirofiban may increase the levels/effects of: Agents with Antiplatelet Properties; Anticoagulants; Apixaban; Collagenase (Systemic); Dabigatran Etexilate; Ibritumomab; Obinutuzumab; Rivaroxaban; Salicylates; Thrombolytic Agents; Tositumomab and Iodine I 131 Tositumomab; Urokinase

The levels/effects of Tirofiban may be increased by: Dasatinib; Glucosamine; Herbs (Anticoagulant/Antiplatelet Properties); Ibrutinib; Limaprost; Multivitamins/Fluoride (with ADE); Multivitamins/Minerals (with ADEK, Folate, Iron); Multivitamins/Minerals (with AE, No Iron); Omega-3 Fatty Acids; Pentosan Polysulfate Sodium; Pentoxifylline; Prostacyclin Analogues; Tipranavir; Vitamin E

Decreased Effect There are no known significant interactions involving a decrease in effect.

Storage/Stability Store at 25°C (77°F); excursions are permitted between 15°C and 30°C (59°F and 86°F); do not freeze. Protect from light during storage.

Mechanism of Action A reversible antagonist of fibrinogen binding to the glycoprotein (GP) IIb/IIIa receptor, the major platelet surface receptor involved in platelet aggregation. When administered intravenously, it inhibits *ex vivo* platelet aggregation in a dose- and concentration-dependent manner. When given according to the recommended regimen, >90% inhibition is attained within 10 minutes after initiation. Platelet aggregation inhibition is reversible following cessation of the infusion.

Pharmacodynamics/Kinetics

Onset: >90% inhibition of platelet aggregation (reversible after discontinuation) seen within 10 minutes
Distribution: V_{dss}: 22-42 L
Protein Binding: 65% (concentration dependent)
Metabolism: Negligible
Half-life elimination: 2 hours; **Note:** In ~90% of patients, *ex vivo* platelet aggregation returns to near baseline in 4-8 hours after discontinuation.
Excretion: Urine (65%) and feces (25%) primarily as unchanged drug

Dosage Adults: IV:

Unstable angina/non-ST-elevation myocardial infarction (UA/NSTEMI): Loading dose: 25 mcg/kg over 3 minutes; Maintenance infusion: 0.15 mcg/kg/minute continued for up to 18 hours.

Percutaneous coronary intervention (PCI): Loading dose: 25 mcg/kg over 3 minutes at the time of PCI; Maintenance infusion: 0.15 mcg/kg/minute continued for up to 18 hours (ACCF/AHA [Anderson, 2013]; ACCF/AHASCAI [Levine, 2011]; Valgimigli, 2004).

Stable ischemic heart disease (high-risk features) undergoing elective PCI (off-label use): Loading dose: 25 mcg/kg over 3 minutes at the time of PCI; Maintenance infusion: 0.15 mcg/kg/minute; was continued for up to 48 hours in the clinical trial (ACCF/AHA/SCAI [Levine, 2011]; Valgimigli, 2004). **Note**: Reserve for patients who were not pretreated with clopidogrel or who are undergoing elective PCI with stent implantation with adequate clopidogrel pretreatment (ACCF/AHA/SCAI [Levine, 2011]).

ST-elevation myocardial infarction (STEMI) undergoing primary PCI (off-label use): Loading dose: 25 mcg/kg over 3 minutes at the time of PCI; Maintenance infusion: 0.15 mcg/kg/minute in combination with heparin or bivalirudin in selected patients; was continued for 18 to 24 hours in clinical trials (ACCF/AHA [O'Gara, 2013]; ACCF/AHA/SCAI [Levine, 2011]; Valgimigli, 2008; Van't Hof, 2008).

Dosage adjustment in renal impairment:
CrCl >60 mL/minute: No dosage reduction necessary
CrCl ≤60 mL/minute: Loading dose: 25 mcg/kg over 3 minutes; Maintenance infusion: 0.075 mcg/kg/minute continued for up to 18 hours.

Administration IV: Infuse loading dose over 3 minutes, followed by continuous infusion. May be administered through the same catheter as heparin.

Monitoring Parameters Platelet count (baseline; 6 hours after initiation and daily thereafter during therapy). Monitor platelet counts more closely in patients who have had previous exposure to glycoprotein IIb/IIa antagonists. Persistent reductions of platelet counts <90,000/mm^3 may require interruption or discontinuation of infusion; hemoglobin and hematocrit; signs of bleeding.

Standard post-PCI assessment if patient undergoes PCI (eg, monitoring vascular access site, monitoring for chest pain and signs of bleeding)

Dosage Forms

Solution, Intravenous:

Aggrastat: 50 mcg/mL (100 mL, 250 mL)

◆ **Tirofiban Hydrochloride** *see* Tirofiban *on page 2049*

◆ **Tirosint** *see* Levothyroxine *on page 1205*

- **Titralac [OTC]** *see* Calcium Carbonate *on page 327*
- **Ti-U-Lac® H (Can)** *see* Urea and Hydrocortisone *on page 2115*
- **TIV (Trivalent Inactivated Influenza Vaccine)** *see* Influenza Virus Vaccine (Inactivated) *on page 1075*

TiZANidine (tye ZAN i deen)

Brand Names: U.S. Zanaflex

Brand Names: Canada Apo-Tizanidine; Gen-Tizanidine; Mylan-Tizanidine; Pal-Tizanidine; Zanaflex

Index Terms Sirdalud

Pharmacologic Category Alpha$_2$-Adrenergic Agonist

Additional Appendix Information

Beers Criteria - Potentially Inappropriate Medications for Geriatrics *on page 2271*

Use Muscle spasticity: Management of spasticity; reserve treatment with tizanidine for daily activities and times when relief of spasticity is most important.

Pregnancy Risk Factor C

Pregnancy Considerations Adverse events were observed in some animal reproduction studies.

Breast-Feeding Considerations Excretion in breast milk is unknown, but expected due to lipid solubility.

Contraindications Concomitant therapy with ciprofloxacin or fluvoxamine (potent CYP1A2 inhibitors)

Warnings/Precautions Significant hypotension, syncope, and sedation may occur; use caution in patients at risk for severe hypotensive effects (eg, patients taking concurrent medications which may predispose to hypotension) or sedative effects (patients must be cautioned about performing tasks which require mental alertness [eg, operating machinery or driving]). Effects with other sedative drugs or ethanol may be potentiated.Potentially significant drug-drug interactions may exist, requiring dose or frequency adjustment, additional monitoring, and/or selection of alternative therapy. Use caution in any patient with renal impairment. Clearance decreased significantly in patients with severe impairment (CrCl <25 mL/minute); dose reductions recommended. Use not recommended in patients with hepatic impairment; potential for hepatotoxicity likely due to extensive hepatic metabolism. Monitor aminotransferases prior to and during use or if hepatic injury is suspected.

May be inappropriate in older adults depending on comorbidities (eg, dementia, delirium) due to its potent anticholinergic effects (Beers Criteria). Use with caution; clearance decreased fourfold in the elderly; may increase risk of adverse effects and/or duration of effects. Elderly with severe renal impairment (CrCl <25 mL/minute) may have clearance reduced by >50% compared to healthy elderly subjects.

Use has been associated with visual hallucinations or delusions; use caution in patients with psychiatric disorders. Consider discontinuation of therapy if hallucinations occur. Withdrawal resulting in rebound hypertension, tachycardia, and hypertonia may occur upon discontinuation; doses should be decreased slowly, particularly in patients taking concomitant narcotics or receiving high doses (20 to 28 mg daily) for prolonged periods (≥9 weeks). Food alters absorption profile relative to administration under fasting conditions. In addition, bioequivalence between capsules and tablets is altered by food; capsules and tablets are bioequivalent under fasting conditions, but not under nonfasting conditions.

Adverse Reactions

Cardiovascular: Bradycardia, hypotension

Central nervous system: Anxiety, depression, dizziness, fever, nervousness, somnolence, speech disorder, visual hallucinations/delusions (generally occurring in first 6 weeks of therapy)

Dermatologic: Rash, skin ulcer

Gastrointestinal: Abdominal pain, constipation, diarrhea, dyspepsia, vomiting, xerostomia

Genitourinary: Urinary frequency, UTI

Hepatic: Liver enzymes increased

Neuromuscular & skeletal: Back pain, dyskinesia, myasthenia, paresthesia, weakness

Ocular: Blurred vision

Respiratory: Pharyngitis, rhinitis

Miscellaneous: Diaphoresis, flu-like syndrome, infection

Rare but important or life-threatening: Abnormal dreams, abnormal thinking, abscess, adrenal insufficiency, allergic reaction, anemia, angina pectoris, arrhythmia, carcinoma (including skin), cholelithiasis, deafness, dementia, depersonalization, dyslipidemia, gastrointestinal hemorrhage, glaucoma, heart failure, hepatomegaly, hemiplegia, hepatic failure, hepatitis, hepatoma, herpes infections, hypercholesterolemia, hyperglycemia, hypokalemia, hyponatremia, hypoproteinemia, hypothyroidism, intestinal obstruction, jaundice, leukopenia, leukocytosis, MI, migraine, neuralgia, optic neuritis, orthostatic hypotension, palpitation, paralysis, psychotic-like symptoms, pulmonary embolus, purpura, respiratory acidosis, retinal hemorrhage, seizure, sepsis, suicide attempt, syncope, thrombocythemia, thrombocytopenia, ventricular extrasystoles, ventricular tachycardia, vertigo

Drug Interactions

Metabolism/Transport Effects Substrate of CYP1A2 (major); **Note:** Assignment of Major/Minor substrate status based on clinically relevant drug interaction potential

Avoid Concomitant Use

Avoid concomitant use of TiZANidine with any of the following: Azelastine (Nasal); Ceritinib; Ciprofloxacin (Systemic); FluvoxaMINE; Iobenguane I 123; Orphenadrine; Paraldehyde; Thalidomide

Increased Effect/Toxicity

TiZANidine may increase the levels/effects of: ACE Inhibitors; Alcohol (Ethyl); Azelastine (Nasal); Beta-Blockers; Bradycardia-Causing Agents; Buprenorphine; Ceritinib; CNS Depressants; DULoxetine; Highest Risk QTc-Prolonging Agents; Hydrocodone; Hypotensive Agents; Lacosamide; Levodopa; Lisinopril; Methotrimeprazine; Metyrosine; Moderate Risk QTc-Prolonging Agents; Orphenadrine; Paraldehyde; Pramipexole; RisperiDONE; ROPINIRole; Rotigotine; Selective Serotonin Reuptake Inhibitors; Suvorexant; Thalidomide; Zolpidem

The levels/effects of TiZANidine may be increased by: Abiraterone Acetate; Barbiturates; Beta-Blockers; Bretylium; Brimonidine (Topical); Cannabis; Ciprofloxacin (Systemic); Contraceptives (Estrogens); CYP1A2 Inhibitors (Moderate); CYP1A2 Inhibitors (Strong); Deferasirox; Doxylamine; Dronabinol; Droperidol; FluvoxaMINE; HydrOXYzine; Kava Kava; Magnesium Sulfate; MAO Inhibitors; Methotrimeprazine; Mifepristone; Nabilone; Nicorandil; Peginterferon Alfa-2b; Perampanel; Rufinamide; Sodium Oxybate; Tapentadol; Tetrahydrocannabinol; Tofacitinib; Vemurafenib

Decreased Effect

TiZANidine may decrease the levels/effects of: Iobenguane I 123

The levels/effects of TiZANidine may be decreased by: Mirtazapine; Serotonin/Norepinephrine Reuptake Inhibitors; Tricyclic Antidepressants

Food Interactions The tablet and capsule dosage forms are not bioequivalent when administered with food. Food increases both the time to peak concentration and the extent of absorption for both the tablet and capsule. However, maximal concentrations of tizanidine achieved when administered with food were increased by 30% for the tablet, but decreased by 20% for the capsule. Under fed conditions, the capsule is approximately 80% bioavailable relative to the tablet. Management: Administer with or without food, but keep consistent.

Storage/Stability Store at 25°C (77°F); excursions are permitted between 15°C and 30°C (59°F and 86°F).

Mechanism of Action An alpha$_2$-adrenergic agonist agent which decreases spasticity by increasing presynaptic inhibition; effects are greatest on polysynaptic pathways; overall effect is to reduce facilitation of spinal motor neurons.

Pharmacodynamics/Kinetics

Onset: Single dose (8 mg): Peak effect: 1-2 hours

Duration: Single dose (8 mg): 3-6 hours

Absorption: Tablets and capsules are bioequivalent under fasting conditions, but not under nonfasting conditions.

Tablets administered with food: Peak plasma concentration is increased by ~30%; time to peak increased by 25 minutes; extent of absorption increased by ~30%.

Capsules administered with food: Peak plasma concentration decreased by 20%; time to peak increased by 2-3 hours; extent of absorption increased by ~10%.

Capsules opened and sprinkled on applesauce are not bioequivalent to administration of intact capsules under fasting conditions. Peak plasma concentration and AUC are increased by 15% to 20%; time to peak decreased by 15 minutes.

Distribution: IV: 2.4 L/kg

Protein binding: ~30%

Metabolism: Extensively hepatic via CYP1A2 to inactive metabolites

Bioavailability: ~40% (extensive first-pass metabolism)

Half-life elimination: ~2.5 hours

Time to peak, serum:

Fasting state: Capsule, tablet: 1 hour

Fed state: Capsule: 3-4 hours, Tablet: 1.5 hours

Excretion: Urine (60%); feces (20%)

Dosage Spasticity: Oral:

Adults: Initial: 2 mg up to 3 times daily (at 6- to 8-hour intervals) as needed; may titrate to optimal effect in 2-4 mg increments per dose (with a minimum of 1-4 days between dose increases); maximum: 36 mg daily. **Note:** Single doses >16 mg have not been studied.

Discontinuation of therapy: Gradually taper dose by 2-4 mg daily.

Elderly: Refer to adult dosing. Use with caution; clearance is decreased.

Dosage adjustment in renal impairment:

CrCl ≥25 mL/minute: No dosage adjustment provided in manufacturer's labeling; however, caution may be needed as creatinine clearance decreases.

CrCl <25 mL/minute: Use with caution; clearance reduced >50%. During initial dose titration, use reduced doses. If higher doses are necessary, increase dose instead of increasing dosing frequency.

Dosage adjustment in hepatic impairment: Avoid use in hepatic impairment; if used, reduce dose during initial dose titration. If higher doses are necessary, increase dose instead of increasing dosing frequency. Monitor aminotransferases.

Dietary Considerations Administration with food compared to administration in the fasting state results in clinically-significant differences in absorption and other pharmacokinetic parameters. Patients should be consistent and should not switch administration of the tablets or the capsules between the fasting and nonfasting state. In addition, switching between the capsules and the tablets in the fed state will also result in significant differences. Opening capsule contents to sprinkle on applesauce compared to swallowing intact capsules whole will also result in significant absorption differences. Patients should be consistent with regards to administration.

Administration Capsules may be opened and contents sprinkled on food; however, extent of absorption is increased up to 20% relative to administration of the capsule under fasted conditions.

Monitoring Parameters Monitor liver function (aminotransferases) at baseline and 1 month after maximum dose achieved or if hepatic injury suspected; blood pressure; renal function

Dosage Forms

Capsule, Oral:

Zanaflex: 2 mg, 4 mg, 6 mg

Generic: 2 mg, 4 mg, 6 mg

Tablet, Oral:

Zanaflex: 4 mg

Generic: 2 mg, 4 mg

- ◆ **TL Hydroquinone** *see* Hydroquinone *on page 1020*
- ◆ **TMC-114** *see* Darunavir *on page 569*
- ◆ **TMC125** *see* Etravirine *on page 821*
- ◆ **TMC207** *see* Bedaquiline *on page 233*
- ◆ **TMC278** *see* Rilpivirine *on page 1810*
- ◆ **TMC435** *see* Simeprevir *on page 1887*
- ◆ **TMP** *see* Trimethoprim *on page 2104*
- ◆ **TMP-SMX** *see* Sulfamethoxazole and Trimethoprim *on page 1946*
- ◆ **TMP-SMZ** *see* Sulfamethoxazole and Trimethoprim *on page 1946*
- ◆ **TMX-67** *see* Febuxostat *on page 848*
- ◆ **TMZ** *see* Temozolomide *on page 1991*
- ◆ **TNG** *see* Nitroglycerin *on page 1465*
- ◆ **TNKase** *see* Tenecteplase *on page 1996*
- ◆ **TNKase® (Can)** *see* Tenecteplase *on page 1996*
- ◆ **Tobi** *see* Tobramycin (Systemic, Oral Inhalation) *on page 2052*
- ◆ **TOBI (Can)** *see* Tobramycin (Systemic, Oral Inhalation) *on page 2052*
- ◆ **Tobi Podhaler** *see* Tobramycin (Systemic, Oral Inhalation) *on page 2052*
- ◆ **TOBI Podhaler (Can)** *see* Tobramycin (Systemic, Oral Inhalation) *on page 2052*
- ◆ **TobraDex®** *see* Tobramycin and Dexamethasone *on page 2056*
- ◆ **Tobradex® (Can)** *see* Tobramycin and Dexamethasone *on page 2056*
- ◆ **TobraDex® ST** *see* Tobramycin and Dexamethasone *on page 2056*

Tobramycin (Systemic, Oral Inhalation)

(toe bra MYE sin)

Brand Names: U.S. Bethkis; Kitabis Pak; Tobi; Tobi Podhaler

Brand Names: Canada Apo-Tobramycin; JAMP-Tobramycin; TOBI; TOBI Podhaler; Tobramycin Injection, USP

Index Terms Kitabis Pak; Tobramycin Sulfate

Pharmacologic Category Antibiotic, Aminoglycoside

Use Treatment of documented or suspected infections caused by susceptible gram-negative bacilli, including *Pseudomonas aeruginosa*. Tobramycin solution for inhalation and powder for inhalation are indicated for the management of cystic fibrosis patients with *Pseudomonas aeruginosa*.

Pregnancy Risk Factor D

Pregnancy Considerations **[U.S. Boxed Warning]: Aminoglycosides may cause fetal harm if administered to a pregnant woman.** There are several reports of total irreversible bilateral congenital deafness in children whose mothers received another aminoglycoside (streptomycin) during pregnancy; therefore, tobramycin is classified as pregnancy category D. Tobramycin crosses the placenta and produces detectable serum levels in the fetus. Although serious side effects to the fetus have not been reported following maternal use of tobramycin, a potential for harm exists.

Due to pregnancy-induced physiologic changes, some pharmacokinetic parameters of tobramycin may be altered. Pregnant women have an average-to-larger volume of distribution which may result in lower serum peak levels than for the same dose in nonpregnant women. Serum half-life is also shorter.

Breast-Feeding Considerations Tobramycin is excreted into breast milk and breast-feeding is not recommended by the manufacturer; however, tobramycin is not well absorbed when taken orally. This limited oral absorption may minimize exposure to the nursing infant. Nondose-related effects could include modification of bowel flora.

Contraindications Hypersensitivity to tobramycin, other aminoglycosides, or any component of the formulation

Warnings/Precautions **[U.S. Boxed Warning]: Aminoglycosides may cause neurotoxicity and/or nephrotoxicity;** usual risk factors include preexisting renal impairment, concomitant neuro-/nephrotoxic medications, advanced age, and dehydration. Ototoxicity may be directly proportional to the amount of drug given and the duration of treatment; tinnitus or vertigo are indications of vestibular injury and impending hearing loss; renal damage is usually reversible. Tinnitus and/or hearing loss have also been reported. May cause neuromuscular blockade, respiratory failure, and prolonged respiratory paralysis, especially when given soon after anesthesia or muscle relaxants. **[U.S. Boxed Warnings]: Aminoglycosides may cause fetal harm if administered to a pregnant woman.**

Not intended for long-term therapy due to toxic hazards associated with extended administration; use caution in preexisting renal insufficiency, vestibular or cochlear impairment, myasthenia gravis, Parkinson's disease, hypocalcemia, and conditions which depress neuromuscular transmission. Dosage modification required in patients with impaired renal function during systemic therapy. Prolonged use may result in fungal or bacterial superinfection, including *C. difficile*-associated diarrhea (CDAD) and pseudomembranous colitis; CDAD has been observed >2 months postantibiotic treatment. Solution may contain sodium metabisulfate; use caution in patients with sulfite allergy. Solution for injection may contain sodium metabisulfate; use caution in patients with sulfite allergy. Bronchospasm may occur with tobramycin solution for inhalation; bronchospasm or wheezing should be treated appropriately if either arise. Safety and efficacy of the solution for inhalation have not been demonstrated in patients with FEV_1 <40% or >80% predicted (Bethkis, TOBI), or FEV_1 <25% or >80% predicted (TOBI Podhaler) or FEV_1 <25% or >75% predicted (Kitabis Pak), in patients colonized with *Burkholderia cepacia*, or in patients <6 years of age. With powder for inhalation, consider baseline audiogram in patients at increased risk of auditory dysfunction. If any patient experiences tinnitus or hearing loss during treatment, audiological assessment should be performed. Serum tobramycin concentrations do not need to be monitored; one hour after powder inhalation, serum concentrations of 1-2 mcg/mL have been observed. If ototoxicity or nephrotoxicity occur, discontinue therapy until serum concentrations fall below 2 mcg/mL.

Potentially significant drug-drug interactions may exist, requiring dose or frequency adjustment, additional monitoring, and/or selection of alternative therapy.

Adverse Reactions

Injection: Frequency not defined:

Central nervous system: Confusion, disorientation, dizziness, headache, lethargy, vertigo

Dermatologic: Exfoliative dermatitis, pruritus, skin rash, urticaria

Endocrine & metabolic: Decreased serum calcium, decreased serum magnesium, decreased serum potassium and/or decreased serum sodium, increased lactate dehydrogenase

Gastrointestinal: Diarrhea, nausea, vomiting

Genitourinary: Casts in urine, oliguria, proteinuria

Hematologic & oncologic: Anemia, eosinophilia, granulocytopenia, leukocytosis, leukopenia, thrombocytopenia

Hepatic: Increased serum ALT, increased serum AST, increased serum bilirubin

Local: Pain at injection site

Miscellaneous: Fever

Otic: Auditory ototoxicity, hearing loss, tinnitus, vestibular ototoxicity

Renal: Increased blood urea nitrogen, increased serum creatinine

Inhalation

Cardiovascular: Chest discomfort

Central nervous system: Headache, malaise, voice disorder

Dermatologic: Skin rash

Endocrine: Increased serum glucose

Gastrointestinal: Diarrhea, dysgeusia, nausea, vomiting, xerostomia

Hematologic & oncologic: Eosinophilia, increased erythrocyte sedimentation rate, increased serum immunoglobulins

Miscellaneous: Fever

Neuromuscular & skeletal: Musculoskeletal chest pain, myalgia

Otic: Deafness (including unilateral deafness, reported as mild to moderate hearing loss or increased hearing loss), hypoacusis, tinnitus

Respiratory: Bronchitis, bronchospasm, cough, discoloration of sputum, dyspnea, epistaxis, hemoptysis, laryngitis, nasal congestion, oropharyngeal pain, pharyngolaryngeal pain, productive cough, pulmonary disease (includes pulmonary or cystic fibrosis exacerbations), rales, reduced forced expiratory volume, respiratory depression, rhinitis, throat irritation, tonsillitis, upper respiratory tract infection, wheezing

Rare but important or life-threatening: Abnormal breath sounds, decreased exercise tolerance, decrease in forced vital capacity, hypersensitivity reaction, increased bronchial secretions, lower respiratory tract infection, obstructive pulmonary disease, oral candidiasis, pneumonitis, pruritus, pulmonary congestion, urticaria

Drug Interactions

Metabolism/Transport Effects None known.

Avoid Concomitant Use

Avoid concomitant use of Tobramycin (Systemic, Oral Inhalation) with any of the following: BCG; Foscarnet; Mannitol

Increased Effect/Toxicity

Tobramycin (Systemic, Oral Inhalation) may increase the levels/effects of: AbobotulinumtoxinA; Bisphosphonate Derivatives; CARBOplatin; Colistimethate; CycloSPORINE (Systemic); Neuromuscular-Blocking Agents; OnabotulinumtoxinA; RimabotulinumtoxinB; Tenofovir

The levels/effects of Tobramycin (Systemic, Oral Inhalation) may be increased by: Amphotericin B; Capreomycin; Cephalosporins (2nd Generation); Cephalosporins (3rd Generation); Cephalosporins (4th Generation); CISplatin; Foscarnet; Loop Diuretics; Mannitol; Nonsteroidal Anti-Inflammatory Agents; Tenofovir; Vancomycin

Decreased Effect

Tobramycin (Systemic, Oral Inhalation) may decrease the levels/effects of: BCG; Sodium Picosulfate; Typhoid Vaccine

The levels/effects of Tobramycin (Systemic, Oral Inhalation) may be decreased by: Penicillins

Preparation for Administration Solution for injection: Dilute in 50-100 mL NS or D_5W for IV infusion.

Storage/Stability

Injection: Stable at room temperature both as the clear, colorless solution and as the dry powder. Reconstituted solutions remain stable for 24 hours at room temperature and 96 hours when refrigerated.

Powder, for inhalation (TOBI Podhaler): Store in original package at 25°C (77°F); excursions permitted to 15°C to 30°C (59°F to 86°F). Protect from moisture.

Solution, for inhalation (Bethkis, Kitabis Pak, TOBI): Store under refrigeration at 2°C to 8°C (36°F to 46°F). May be stored in foil pouch (opened or unopened) at room temperature of 25°C (77°F) for up to 28 days. Protect from light. The colorless to pale yellow solution may darken over time if not stored under refrigeration; however, the color change does not affect product quality. Do not use if solution has been stored at room temperature for >28 days.

Mechanism of Action Interferes with bacterial protein synthesis by binding to 30S and 50S ribosomal subunits, resulting in a defective bacterial cell membrane

Pharmacodynamics/Kinetics

Absorption:
- Oral: Poorly absorbed
- IM: Rapid and complete
- Inhalation: Peak serum concentrations:
  - Solution for inhalation: ~1 mcg/mL following a 300 mg dose
  - Powder for inhalation: ~1 mcg/mL (range: 0.49 to 1.55 mcg/mL) following a 112 mg dose

Distribution: V_d: 0.2 to 0.3 L/kg; Pediatrics: 0.2 to 0.7 L/kg; to extracellular fluid, including serum, abscesses, ascitic, pericardial, pleural, synovial, lymphatic, and peritoneal fluids; poor penetration into CSF, eye, bone, prostate
- Inhalation: Tobramycin remains concentrated primarily in the airways
  - Powder for inhalation: V_d (central compartment) for a typical cystic fibrosis patient: 85.1 L

Protein binding: <30%

Half-life elimination:
- Neonates: ≤1200 g: 11 hours; >1200 g: 2 to 9 hours
- Adults: IV: 2 to 3 hours; directly dependent upon glomerular filtration rate; Inhalation: ~4 hours
- Adults with impaired renal function: 5 to 70 hours
- Inhalation: Powder for inhalation: Serum clearance: 14.5 L/hour; Half-life: ~3 hours after 112 mg single dose

Time to peak, serum: IM: 30 to 60 minutes; IV: ~30 minutes

Excretion: Normal renal function: Urine (~90% to 95%) within 24 hours

Dosage Note: Dosage individualization is **critical** because of the low therapeutic index.

In underweight and nonobese patients, use of total body weight (TBW) instead of ideal body weight for determining the initial mg/kg/dose is widely accepted (Nicolau, 1995). Ideal body weight (IBW) also may be used to determine doses for patients who are neither underweight nor obese (Gilbert, 2009).

Initial and periodic plasma drug levels (eg, peak and trough with conventional dosing, post dose level at a prespecified time with extended-interval dosing) should be determined, particularly in critically-ill patients with serious infections or in disease states known to significantly alter aminoglycoside pharmacokinetics (eg, cystic fibrosis, burns, or major surgery).

Usual dosage range:

Infants and Children <5 years: IM, IV: 2.5 mg/kg/dose every 8 hours

Children ≥5 years: IM, IV: 2 to 2.5 mg/kg/dose every 8 hours

Note: Higher individual doses and/or more frequent intervals (eg, every 6 hours) may be required in selected clinical situations (cystic fibrosis) or serum levels document the need.

Children ≥6 years, Adolescents, and Adults: Inhalation:
- Bethkis, Kitabis Pak, TOBI: 300 mg every 12 hours (do not administer doses <6 hours apart); administer in repeated cycles of 28 days on drug followed by 28 days off drug.
- TOBI Podhaler: 112 mg (4 x 28 mg capsules) every 12 hours (do not administer doses <6 hours apart); administer in repeated cycles of 28 days on drug followed by 28 days off drug.

Adults: IM, IV:
- Conventional: 1 to 2.5 mg/kg/dose every 8 to 12 hours; to ensure adequate peak concentrations early in therapy, higher initial dosage may be considered in selected patients when extracellular water is increased (edema, septic shock, postsurgical, and/or trauma)
- Once-daily: 4 to 7 mg/kg/dose once daily; some clinicians recommend this approach for all patients with normal renal function; this dose is at least as efficacious with similar, if not less, toxicity than conventional dosing.

Indication-specific dosing:

Children:

CNS shunt infection: Intrathecal (off-label route): Refer to adult dosing

Cystic fibrosis:
- IM, IV: 2.5 to 3.3 mg/kg every 6 to 8 hours; **Note:** Some patients may require larger or more frequent doses if serum levels document the need (eg, cystic fibrosis or febrile granulocytopenic patients).
- Inhalation: Children ≥6 years and Adolescents: Refer to adult dosing.

Adults:

IM, IV:

Brucellosis: 240 mg (IM) daily or 5 mg/kg (IV) daily for 7 days; either regimen recommended in combination with doxycycline

Cholangitis: 4 to 6 mg/kg once daily with ampicillin

Diverticulitis, complicated: 1.5 to 2 mg/kg every 8 hours (with ampicillin and metronidazole)

Infective endocarditis (*Pseudomonas aeruginosa*) (off-label use): IM, IV: 8 mg/kg once daily (in combination with an extended-spectrum penicillin, or ceftazidime or cefepime) for a minimum of 6 weeks; adjust doses to maintain peak concentrations of 15 to 20 mcg/mL and trough concentrations ≤2 mcg/mL (AHA/IDSA [Baddour, 2005]; Rybak, 1986)

Meningitis *(Enterococcus or Pseudomonas aeruginosa)*: IV: Loading dose: 2 mg/kg, then 1.7 mg/kg/dose every 8 hours (administered with another bactericidal drug)

Pelvic inflammatory disease: Loading dose: 2 mg/kg, then 1.5 mg/kg every 8 hours **or** 4.5 mg/kg once daily

Plague *(Yersinia pestis)*: Treatment: 5 mg/kg/day, followed by postexposure prophylaxis with doxycycline

Pneumonia, hospital- or ventilator-associated: 7 mg/kg/day (with antipseudomonal beta-lactam or carbapenem)

Prophylaxis against endocarditis (dental, oral, upper respiratory procedures, GI/GU procedures): 1.5 mg/kg with ampicillin (50 mg/kg) 30 minutes prior to procedure. **Note:** AHA guidelines now recommend prophylaxis only in patients undergoing invasive procedures and in whom underlying cardiac conditions may predispose to a higher risk of adverse outcomes should infection occur. As of April 2007, routine prophylaxis no longer recommended by the AHA.

Tularemia: 5 mg/kg/day divided every 8 hours for 1 to 2 weeks

Urinary tract infection: 1.5 mg/kg/dose every 8 hours

Inhalation: **Cystic fibrosis:**

Bethkis, Kitabis Pak, TOBI: 300 mg every 12 hours (do not administer doses <6 hours apart); administer in repeated cycles of 28 days on drug followed by 28 days off drug.

TOBI Podhaler: 112 mg (4 x 28 mg capsules) every 12 hours (do not administer doses <6 hours apart); administer in repeated cycles of 28 days on drug followed by 28 days off drug.

Intrathecal (off-label route): **CNS shunt infection:** 5 to 20 mg/day (Tunkel, 2004)

Dosing in obesity: IM, IV: In moderate obesity (TBW/IBW ≥1.25) or greater, (eg, morbid obesity [TBW/IBW >2]), initial dosage requirement may be estimated using a dosing weight of IBW + 0.4 (TBW - IBW) (Traynor, 1995).

Dosage adjustment in renal impairment:

IM, IV

Conventional dosing:

CrCl ≥60 mL/minute: Administer every 8 hours
CrCl 40 to 60 mL/minute: Administer every 12 hours
CrCl 20 to 40 mL/minute: Administer every 24 hours
CrCl 10 to 20 mL/minute: Administer every 48 hours
CrCl <10 mL/minute: Administer every 72 hours

High-dose therapy: Interval may be extended (eg, every 48 hours) in patients with moderate renal impairment (CrCl 30 to 59 mL/minute) and/or adjusted based on serum level determinations.

Intermittent hemodialysis (IHD) (administer after hemodialysis on dialysis days) (Heintz, 2009): Dialyzable (25% to 70%; variable; dependent on filter, duration, and type of HD): IV:

Loading dose of 2 to 3 mg/kg, followed by:

Mild UTI or synergy: IV: 1 mg/kg every 48 to 72 hours; consider redosing for pre-HD or post-HD concentrations <1 mg/L

Moderate-to-severe UTI: IV 1 to 1.5 mg/kg every 48 to 72 hours; consider redosing for pre-HD concentrations <1.5 to 2 mg/L or post-HD concentrations <1 mg/L

Systemic gram-negative infection: IV: 1.5 to 2 mg/kg every 48 to 72 hours; consider redosing for pre-HD concentrations <3 to 5 mg/L or post-HD concentrations <2 mg/L

Note: Dosing dependent on the assumption of 3 times/week, complete IHD sessions.

Peritoneal dialysis (PD):

Administration via peritoneal dialysis (PD) fluid:

Gram-negative infection: 4 to 8 mg/L (4 to 8 mcg/mL) of PD fluid

Gram-positive infection (ie, synergy): 3 to 4 mg/L (3 to 4 mcg/mL) of PD fluid

Administration IVPB/IM: Dose as for CrCl <10 mL/minute and follow levels

Continuous renal replacement therapy (CRRT) (Heintz, 2009; Trotman, 2005): Drug clearance is highly dependent on the method of renal replacement, filter type, and flow rate. Appropriate dosing requires close monitoring of pharmacologic response, signs of adverse reactions due to drug accumulation, as well as drug concentrations in relation to target trough (if appropriate). The following are general recommendations only (based on dialysate flow/ultrafiltration rates of 1 to 2 L/hour and minimal residual renal function) and should not supersede clinical judgment:

CVVH/CVVHD/CVVHDF: IV: Loading dose of 2 to 3 mg/kg, followed by:

Mild UTI or synergy: IV 1 mg/kg every 24 to 36 hours (redose when concentration <1 mg/L)

Moderate-severe UTI: IV: 1 to 1.5 mg/kg every 24 to 36 hours (redose when concentration <1.5 to 2 mg/L)

Systemic gram-negative infection: IV: 1.5 to 2.5 mg/kg every 24 to 48 hours (redose when concentration <3 to 5 mg/L)

Inhalation: There are no dosage adjustments provided in the manufacturer's labeling (has not been studied).

Dosing adjustment in hepatic impairment: No dosage adjustment necessary; does not undergo hepatic metabolism.

Dietary Considerations May require supplementation of calcium, magnesium, potassium.

Administration

IV: Infuse over 30 to 60 minutes. Flush with saline before and after administration.

Inhalation:

Bethkis, Kitabis Pak, TOBI: To be inhaled over ~15 minutes using a handheld reusable nebulizer (PARI-LC PLUS) with a PARI Vios air compressor (Bethkis) or a DeVilbiss Pulmo-Aide air compressor (Kitabis Pak, TOBI). If multiple different nebulizer treatments are required, administer bronchodilator first, followed by chest physiotherapy, any other nebulized medications, and then tobramycin last. Do not mix with other nebulizer medications.

TOBI Podhaler: Capsules should be administered by oral inhalation via Podhaler device following manufacturer recommendations for use and handling. Capsules should be removed from the blister packaging immediately prior to use and should not be swallowed. Patients requiring bronchodilator therapy should administer the bronchodilator 15 to 90 minutes prior to TOBI Podhaler. The sequence of chest physiotherapy and additional inhaled therapies is at the discretion of the healthcare provider; however, TOBI Podhaler should always be administered last. The Canadian labeling recommends that patients requiring bronchodilator therapy should administer the bronchodilator 15 to 90 minutes prior to administering TOBI Podhaler.

Some penicillins (eg, carbenicillin, ticarcillin, and piperacillin) have been shown to inactivate aminoglycosides *in vitro*. This has been observed to a greater extent with tobramycin and gentamicin, while amikacin has shown greater stability against inactivation. Concurrent use of these agents may pose a risk of reduced antibacterial efficacy *in vivo*, particularly in the setting of profound renal impairment. However, definitive clinical evidence is lacking. If combination penicillin/aminoglycoside therapy is desired in a patient with renal dysfunction, separation of doses (if feasible), and routine monitoring of aminoglycoside levels, CBC, and clinical response should be considered.

Monitoring Parameters Urinalysis, urine output, BUN, serum creatinine, peak and trough plasma tobramycin levels. Levels are typically obtained after the third dose in conventional dosing. Be alert to ototoxicity; hearing should be tested before and during treatment

Some penicillin derivatives may accelerate the degradation of aminoglycosides *in vitro*. This may be clinically-significant for certain penicillin (ticarcillin, piperacillin, carbenicillin) and aminoglycoside (gentamicin, tobramycin) combination therapy in patients with significant renal impairment. Close monitoring of aminoglycoside levels is warranted.

Inhalation: The utility of monitoring serum concentrations in patients with renal impairment should be per health care provider discretion; serum concentrations achieved following inhalation are significantly less than those achieved following parenteral therapy in patients with normal renal function. Monitor serum tobramycin concentrations in patients with known or history of auditory dysfunction, renal dysfunction, and/or concomitant use of nephrotoxic drugs. One hour after inhalation, serum concentrations of 1 to 2 mcg/mL have been observed.

Reference Range

Timing of serum samples: Draw peak 30 minutes after 30-minute infusion has been completed or 1 hour following IM injection or beginning of infusion; draw trough immediately before next dose

Therapeutic levels:

Peak:

Serious infections: 6 to 8 mcg/mL (SI: 13 to 17 micromole/L)

Life-threatening infections: 8 to 10 mcg/mL (SI: 17 to 21 micromole/L)

Urinary tract infections: 4 to 6 mcg/mL (SI: 9 to 13 micromole/L)

Infective endocarditis (*Pseudomonas aeruginosa*): 15 to 20 mcg/mL (SI: 32 to 43 micromole/L)

Trough:

Serious infections: 0.5 to 1 mcg/mL

Life-threatening infections: 1 to 2 mcg/mL

The American Thoracic Society (ATS) recommends trough levels of <1 mcg/mL for patients with hospital-acquired pneumonia.

Monitor serum creatinine and urine output; obtain drug levels after the third dose unless otherwise directed

Inhalation: Serum levels are ~1 mcg/mL one hour following a 300 mg dose in patients with normal renal function.

Additional Information Once-daily dosing: Higher peak serum drug concentration to MIC ratios, demonstrated aminoglycoside postantibiotic effect, decreased renal cortex drug uptake, and improved cost-time efficiency are supportive reasons for the use of once daily dosing regimens for aminoglycosides. Current research indicates these regimens to be as effective for non-life-threatening infections, with no higher incidence of nephrotoxicity, than those requiring multiple daily doses. Doses are determined by calculating the entire day's dose via usual multiple dose calculation techniques and administering this quantity as a single dose. Doses are then adjusted to maintain mean serum concentrations above the MIC(s) of the causative organism(s). (Example: 2.5 to 5 mg/kg as a single dose; expected Cp_{max}: 10 to 20 mcg/mL and Cp_{min}: <1 mcg/mL). Further research is needed for universal recommendation in all patient populations and gram-negative disease; exceptions may include those with known high clearance (eg, children, patients with cystic fibrosis, or burns who may require shorter dosage intervals) and patients with renal function impairment for whom longer than conventional dosage intervals are usually required.

Product Availability Kitabis Pak: FDA approved December 2014. Kitabis Pak is a co-packaged kit containing a reusable nebulizer and tobramycin inhalation solution.

Dosage Forms

Capsule, Inhalation:

Tobi Podhaler: 28 mg

Nebulization Solution, Inhalation [preservative free]:

Bethkis: 300 mg/4 mL (4 mL)

Kitabis Pak: 300 mg/5 mL (5 mL)

Tobi: 300 mg/5 mL (5 mL)

Generic: 300 mg/5 mL (5 mL)

Solution, Injection:

Generic: 10 mg/mL (2 mL); 80 mg/2 mL (2 mL); 1.2 g/30 mL (30 mL); 2 g/50 mL (50 mL)

Solution, Intravenous:

Generic: 80 mg (100 mL)

Solution Reconstituted, Injection:

Generic: 1.2 g (1 ea)

Solution Reconstituted, Injection [preservative free]:

Generic: 1.2 g (1 ea)

Dosage Forms: Canada

Powder, for oral inhalation [capsule]:

TOBI Podhaler: 28 mg/capsule (224s)

Tobramycin (Ophthalmic) (toe bra MYE sin)

Brand Names: U.S. Tobrex

Brand Names: Canada PMS-Tobramycin; Sandoz-Tobramycin; Tobrex®

Index Terms Tobramycin Sulfate

Pharmacologic Category Antibiotic, Aminoglycoside; Antibiotic, Ophthalmic

Use Treatment of superficial ophthalmic infections caused by susceptible bacteria

Pregnancy Risk Factor B

Dosage Ophthalmic: Children ≥2 months and Adults:

Ointment: Instill 1/2" (1.25 cm) 2-3 times/day; for severe infections, apply every 3-4 hours

Solution: Instill 1-2 drops every 2-4 hours; for severe infections, instill up to 2 drops every hour until improved, then reduce to less frequent intervals

Additional Information Complete prescribing information should be consulted for additional detail.

Dosage Forms

Ointment, Ophthalmic:

Tobrex: 0.3% (3.5 g)

Solution, Ophthalmic:

Tobrex: 0.3% (5 mL)

Generic: 0.3% (5 mL)

Tobramycin and Dexamethasone

(toe bra MYE sin & deks a METH a sone)

Brand Names: U.S. TobraDex®; TobraDex® ST

Brand Names: Canada Tobradex®

Index Terms Dexamethasone and Tobramycin

Pharmacologic Category Antibiotic/Corticosteroid, Ophthalmic

Use Treatment of external ocular infection caused by susceptible gram-negative bacteria and steroid responsive inflammatory conditions of the palpebral and bulbar conjunctiva, cornea, and anterior segment of the globe

Pregnancy Risk Factor C

Dosage Ophthalmic: Children ≥2 years and Adults: Ocular infection/inflammation:

Ointment: Apply a small amount (~1/2-inch ribbon of ointment) up to 3-4 times/day

Suspension: Instill 1-2 drops every 4-6 hours; may be increased to 1-2 drops every 2 hours for the first 24-48 hours, then reduce to less frequent intervals

Additional Information Complete prescribing information should be consulted for additional detail.

Dosage Forms

Ointment, ophthalmic:

TobraDex®: Tobramycin 0.3% and dexamethasone 0.1% (3.5 g)

Suspension, ophthalmic: Tobramycin 0.3% and dexamethasone 0.1% (2.5 mL, 5 mL, 10 mL)

TobraDex®: Tobramycin 0.3% and dexamethasone 0.1% (2.5 mL, 5 mL, 10 mL)

TobraDex® ST: Tobramycin 0.3% and dexamethasone 0.05% (5 mL)

◆ **Tobramycin and Loteprednol Etabonate** *see* Loteprednol and Tobramycin *on page 1251*

◆ **Tobramycin Injection, USP (Can)** *see* Tobramycin (Systemic, Oral Inhalation) *on page 2052*

◆ **Tobramycin Sulfate** *see* Tobramycin (Ophthalmic) *on page 2056*

◆ **Tobramycin Sulfate** *see* Tobramycin (Systemic, Oral Inhalation) *on page 2052*

◆ **Tobrex** *see* Tobramycin (Ophthalmic) *on page 2056*

◆ **Tobrex® (Can)** *see* Tobramycin (Ophthalmic) *on page 2056*

Tocilizumab (toe si LIZ oo mab)

Brand Names: U.S. Actemra

Brand Names: Canada Actemra

Index Terms Atlizumab; MRA; R-1569; RoActemra

Pharmacologic Category Antirheumatic, Disease Modifying; Interleukin-6 Receptor Antagonist

Use

Polyarticular juvenile idiopathic arthritis: Treatment of active polyarticular juvenile idiopathic arthritis in patients 2 years and older.

Rheumatoid arthritis: Treatment of adults with moderately to severely active rheumatoid arthritis (RA) who have had an inadequate response to one or more disease-modifying antirheumatic drugs (DMARDs).

Systemic juvenile idiopathic arthritis: Treatment of active systemic juvenile idiopathic arthritis in patients 2 years and older.

Pregnancy Risk Factor C

Pregnancy Considerations Adverse events have been observed in some animal reproduction studies. Monoclonal antibodies cross the placenta, with the largest amount transferred during the third trimester. A pregnancy registry has been established to monitor outcomes of women exposed to tocilizumab during pregnancy (877-311-8972).

Breast-Feeding Considerations It is not known if tocilizumab is excreted in human milk. Because many immunoglobulins are excreted in human milk and the potential for serious adverse reactions exists, a decision should be made whether to discontinue nursing or to discontinue the drug, taking into account the importance of the drug to the mother.

Contraindications

Hypersensitivity to tocilizumab or any component of the formulation

Canadian labeling: Additional contraindications (not in U.S. labeling): Active infections

Warnings/Precautions [U.S. Boxed Warning]: Serious and potentially fatal infections (including active tuberculosis, invasive fungal, bacterial, viral, protozoal, and other opportunistic infections) have been reported in patients receiving tocilizumab; infection may lead to hospitalization or death. Most of the serious infections have occurred in patients on concomitant immunosuppressive therapy. Patients should be closely monitored for signs and symptoms of infection during and after treatment. If serious infection occurs during treatment, withhold tocilizumab until infection is controlled. Prior to treatment initiation, carefully consider risk versus benefit in patients with chronic or recurrent infections, tuberculosis exposure, history of or current opportunistic infection, underlying conditions predisposing to infection, or patients residing in or with travel to areas of endemic tuberculosis or endemic mycosis, The most common serious infections occurring have included pneumonia, UTI, cellulitis, herpes zoster, gastroenteritis, diverticulitis, sepsis, and bacterial arthritis. Do not administer tocilizumab to a patient with an active infection, including localized infection. Interrupt treatment for opportunistic infection or sepsis. **[U.S. Boxed Warning]: Tuberculosis (pulmonary or extrapulmonary) has been reported in patients receiving tocilizumab; both reactivation of latent infection and new infections have been reported. Patients should be tested for latent tuberculosis infection before and during therapy; consider treatment of latent tuberculosis prior to tocilizumab treatment. Some patients who test negative prior to therapy may develop active infection; monitor for signs and symptoms of tuberculosis during and after treatment in all patients.** Patients should be evaluated for tuberculosis risk factors with a tuberculin skin test prior to starting therapy. Consider antituberculosis treatment in patients with a history of latent or active tuberculosis if adequate treatment course cannot be confirmed, and for patients with risk factors for tuberculosis despite a negative test. Rare reactivation of herpes zoster has been reported. Patients should be brought up to date with all immunizations before initiating therapy. Live vaccines should not be given concurrently; there is no data available concerning secondary transmission of infection from live vaccines in patients receiving therapy.

Use of tocilizumab may affect defenses against malignancies; impact on the development and course of malignancies is not fully defined, however, malignancies were observed in clinical trials. Use with caution in patients with preexisting or recent onset CNS demyelinating disorders; rare cases of CNS demyelinating disorders (eg, multiple sclerosis) have occurred. All patients should be monitored for signs and symptoms of demyelinating disorders. May cause hypersensitivity or anaphylaxis; anaphylactic events including fatalities have been reported with IV administration; hypersensitivity reactions have occurred in patients who were premedicated, in patients with and without a prior history of hypersensitivity, and as early as the first infusion. Medications for the treatment of hypersensitivity reactions should be available for immediate use. Patients should seek medical attention if symptoms of hypersensitivity reaction occur with subcutaneous use. Stop infusion and permanently discontinue treatment in patients who develop a hypersensitivity reaction to tocilizumab. In clinical studies, reactions requiring treatment discontinuation included generalized erythema, rash, and urticaria. Use is not recommended in patients with active hepatic disease or hepatic impairment. Monitor ALT and AST. Do not initiate treatment if ALT or AST is >1.5 times ULN. Use with caution in patients at increased risk for gastrointestinal perforation; perforation has been reported, typically secondary to diverticulitis. Monitor for new-onset abdominal symptoms; promptly evaluate if new symptoms occur.

Use may cause increases in total cholesterol, triglycerides, LDL and HDL cholesterol; monitor ~4-8 weeks after initiation, then approximately every 6 months; hyperlipidemia should be managed according to current guidelines. Neutropenia and thrombocytopenia may occur; may require treatment interruption, dose or interval modification, or discontinuation. Monitor neutrophils and platelets. Do not initiate treatment in patients with an ANC <2000/mm^3 or platelet count <100,000/mm^3; discontinue treatment for ANC <500/mm^3 or platelet count <50,000/mm^3. Monitor transaminases; treatment should be discontinued in patients who develop elevated ALT or AST >5 x ULN. Patients receiving concomitant hepatotoxic drugs (eg, methotrexate) are at an increased risk of developing elevated transaminases; elevations are typically reversible and do not result in clinically evident hepatic injury.

Potentially significant drug/drug interactions may exist, requiring dose or frequency adjustment, additional monitoring, and/or selection of alternative therapy. Concomitant use with other biological DMARDs (eg, TNF blockers, IL-1 receptor blockers, anti-CD20 monoclonal antibodies, selective costimulation modulators) has not been studied and should should be avoided. Cautious use is recommended in elderly patients due to an increased incidence of serious infections. Subcutaneous administration is only indicated for adult patients with rheumatoid arthritis. Do not use subcutaneous injection for IV infusion. Product may contain polysorbate 80.

Adverse Reactions As reported for monotherapy, except where noted. Combination therapy refers to use in rheumatoid arthritis with nonbiological DMARDs or use in SJIA or PJIA in trials where most patients (~70% to 80%) were taking methotrexate at baseline.

Cardiovascular: Hypertension, peripheral edema

Central nervous system: Dizziness, headache

Dermatologic: Dermatological reaction (combination therapy; includes pruritus, urticaria), skin rash

Endocrine & metabolic: Hypothyroidism, increased LDL cholesterol (>1.5-2 x ULN; combination therapy; children and adolescents), increased serum cholesterol (>240 mg/dL; >1.5-2 x ULN; combination therapy; children and adolescents)

Gastrointestinal: Abdominal pain, diarrhea (children and adolescents), gastric ulcer, gastritis, oral mucosa ulcer, stomatitis, weight gain

Hematologic & oncologic: Leukopenia, neutropenia (combination therapy), thrombocytopenia (combination therapy)

Hepatic: Increased serum ALT, increased serum AST, increased serum bilirubin

Immunologic: Antibody development

Infection: Herpes simplex infection

Local: Injection site reaction (SubQ: Including erythema, pruritus, pain, and hematoma)

Ophthalmic: Conjunctivitis

Renal: Nephrolithiasis

Respiratory: Bronchitis, cough, dyspnea, nasopharyngitis, upper respiratory tract infection

Miscellaneous: Infusion-related reaction (combination therapy)

Rare but important or life-threatening: Anaphylaxis, anaphylactoid reaction, angioedema, aspergillosis, candidiasis, cellulitis, chronic inflammatory demyelinating polyneuropathy, cryptococcosis, diverticulitis, gastroenteritis, gastrointestinal perforation, herpes zoster, hypersensitivity, hypersensitivity pneumonitis, hypertriglyceridemia, hypotension, increased HDL cholesterol, malignant neoplasm (including breast and colon cancer), multiple sclerosis, otitis media, pneumonia, pneumocystosis, reactivation of latent Epstein-Barr virus, septic arthritis, sepsis, Stevens-Johnson syndrome, tuberculosis, urinary tract infection, varicella

Drug Interactions

Metabolism/Transport Effects None known.

Avoid Concomitant Use

Avoid concomitant use of Tocilizumab with any of the following: Abatacept; Anti-TNF Agents; BCG; Belimumab; Natalizumab; Pimecrolimus; Tacrolimus (Topical); Tofacitinib; Vaccines (Live)

Increased Effect/Toxicity

Tocilizumab may increase the levels/effects of: Abatacept; Anti-TNF Agents; Belimumab; Leflunomide; Natalizumab; Tofacitinib; Vaccines (Live)

The levels/effects of Tocilizumab may be increased by: Denosumab; Pimecrolimus; Roflumilast; Tacrolimus (Topical); Trastuzumab

Decreased Effect

Tocilizumab may decrease the levels/effects of: BCG; Coccidioides immitis Skin Test; CYP3A4 Substrates; Sipuleucel-T; Vaccines (Inactivated); Vaccines (Live)

The levels/effects of Tocilizumab may be decreased by: Echinacea

Preparation for Administration IV: Prior to administration, dilute to 50 mL (children <30 kg) or 100 mL (children ≥30 kg and adults) by slowly adding to 0.9% sodium chloride. Use vials for IV to prepare infusion solutions; do **not** use prefilled SubQ syringes to prepare IV solutions. Withdraw equal volume of 0.9% sodium chloride to the volume of tocilizumab required for dose; slowly add tocilizumab dose into infusion bag or bottle. Gently invert to mix (avoid foaming). Diluted solutions may be stored under refrigeration or at room temperature for up to 24 hours (protected from light) and are compatible with polypropylene, polyethylene (PE), polyvinyl chloride (PVC), and glass infusion containers. Allow diluted solution to reach room temperature prior to infusion.

Storage/Stability Store intact vials/syringes at 2°C to 8°C (36°F to 46°F). Do not freeze. Protect vials and syringes from light (store in the original package until time of use); keep syringes dry. Solutions diluted for IV infusion may be stored at 2°C to 8°C (36°F to 46°F) or room temperature for up to 24 hours and should be protected from light. Discard unused product remaining in the vials.

Mechanism of Action Antagonist of the interleukin-6 (IL-6) receptor. Endogenous IL-6 is induced by inflammatory stimuli and mediates a variety of immunological responses. Inhibition of IL-6 receptors by tocilizumab leads to a reduction in cytokine and acute phase reactant production.

Pharmacodynamics/Kinetics

Distribution: V_{dss}: Children: 2.54-4.08 L; Adults: 6.4 L

Bioavailability: SubQ: 80%

Half life elimination:

IV: Terminal, single dose: 6.3 days (concentration-dependent; may be increased up to 16-23 days [children] or 11-13 days [adults] at steady state)

SubQ: Concentration dependent: Adults: Up to 5 days (every other week dosing) or 13 days (every week dosing)

Dosage Note: Do not initiate if ANC is <2000/mm^3, platelets are <100,000/mm^3 or if ALT or AST are >1.5 times ULN.

Polyarticular juvenile idiopathic arthritis (PJIA): Children ≥2 years: IV: **Note:** Dose adjustment should not be made based solely on a single-visit body weight measurement due to fluctuations in body weight. May be used as monotherapy or in combination with methotrexate.

<30 kg: 10 mg/kg every 4 weeks

≥30 kg: 8 mg/kg every 4 weeks

Systemic juvenile idiopathic arthritis (SJIA): Children ≥2 years: IV: **Note:** Dose adjustment should not be made based solely on a single-visit body weight measurement due to fluctuations in body weight. May be used as monotherapy or in combination with methotrexate.

<30 kg: 12 mg/kg every 2 weeks

≥30 kg: 8 mg/kg every 2 weeks

Rheumatoid arthritis: Adults: **Note:** Methotrexate or other *nonbiologic* disease-modifying antirheumatic drugs (DMARDs) may be continued for the treatment of rheumatoid arthritis. Tocilizumab should not be used in combination with *biologic* DMARDs.

IV: Initial: 4 mg/kg every 4 weeks; increase to 8 mg/kg based on clinical response (maximum dose: 800 mg)

SubQ:

<100 kg: 162 mg every other week; increase to every week based on clinical response

≥100 kg: 162 mg every week

Transitioning from IV therapy to SubQ therapy: Administer the first SubQ dose instead of the next scheduled IV dose.

Dosage adjustment for toxicity:

Hypersensitivity (anaphylaxis or other clinically-significant hypersensitivity reaction): Stop immediately and discontinue permanently.

Infection (serious infection, opportunistic infection or sepsis): Interrupt treatment until the infection is controlled.

Polyarticular and systemic juvenile idiopathic arthritis: Dose reductions have not been studied; however, dose interruptions are recommended for liver enzyme abnormalities, low neutrophil counts, and low platelets similar to recommendations provided for rheumatoid arthritis. In addition, consider interrupting or discontinuing concomitant methotrexate and/or other medications and hold tocilizumab dosing until the clinical situation has been assessed.

Rheumatoid arthritis (RA):

Low absolute neutrophil counts (ANC):

ANC >1000 cells/mm^3: Maintain dose.

ANC 500-1000 cells/mm^3: Interrupt therapy; when ANC >1000 cells/mm^3, resume IV tocilizumab at 4 mg/kg (may increase to 8 mg/kg as clinically appropriate) or resume SubQ tocilizumab at every other week dosing (increase frequency to every week as clinically appropriate).

ANC <500 cells/mm^3: Discontinue.

Low platelet counts:

Platelets 50,000-100,000 cells/mm^3: Interrupt therapy; when platelet count is >100,000 cells/mm^3, resume IV tocilizumab at 4 mg/kg (may increase to 8 mg/kg as clinically appropriate) or resume SubQ tocilizumab at every other week dosing (increase frequency to every week as clinically appropriate).

Platelets <50,000 cells/mm^3: Discontinue.

Dosage adjustment for renal impairment:

Mild renal impairment: No dosage adjustment necessary.

Moderate-to-severe renal impairment: There are no dosage adjustments provided in the manufacturer's labeling (has not been studied).

Dosage adjustment for hepatic impairment: There are no dosage adjustments provided in the manufacturer's labeling (has not been studied). Not recommended for use in patients with active hepatic disease or hepatic impairment. Do not initiate therapy if ALT or AST are >1.5 times ULN.

Hepatotoxicity during treatment: Rheumatoid arthritis:

>1 to 3 x ULN: Adjust concomitant DMARDs as appropriate. For patients receiving IV therapy with persistent increases >1 to 3 x ULN, reduce dose to 4 mg/kg or interrupt until ALT/AST have normalized. For patients receiving SubQ therapy with persistent increases >1 to 3 x ULN, reduce injection frequency to every other week or interrupt until ALT/AST have normalized; increase frequency to every week as clinically appropriate.

>3 to 5 x ULN (confirmed with repeat testing): Interrupt until ALT/AST <3 x ULN and follow dosage adjustments recommended for liver enzyme abnormalities >1 to 3 x ULN. For persistent increases >3 x ULN, discontinue.

>5 x ULN: Discontinue.

Administration

IV: Allow diluted solution for infusion to reach room temperature prior to administration; infuse over 60 minutes using a dedicated IV line. Do not infuse other agents through same IV line. Do not administer IV push or IV bolus. Do not use if opaque particles or discoloration is visible.

SubQ: Rheumatoid arthritis: When transitioning from IV administration to SubQ administration, give the first SubQ dose instead of the next scheduled IV dose. Administer the full amount in the prefilled syringe. Allow to reach room temperature prior to use. Do not use if particulate matter or discoloration is visible; solution should be clear and colorless to pale yellow. Rotate injection sites; avoid injecting into moles, scars, or tender, bruised, red, or hard skin. Prefilled syringe is available for use by patients (self-administration).

Monitoring Parameters Latent TB screening prior to therapy initiation; neutrophils, platelets, ALT/AST (prior to therapy, 4-8 weeks after start of therapy, and every 3 months thereafter [RA]); neutrophils, platelets, ALT/AST (prior to therapy, at second infusion, and every 2-4 weeks [SJIA, U.S. labeling; SJIA and PJIA, Canadian labeling] or 4-8 weeks [PJIA, U.S. labeling] thereafter); additional liver function tests (eg, bilirubin) as clinically indicated; lipid panel (prior to, at 4-8 weeks following initiation, and every ~6 months during therapy); signs and symptoms of infection (prior to, during, and after therapy); signs and symptoms of CNS demyelinating disorders

Dosage Forms

Solution, Intravenous [preservative free]:

Actemra: 80 mg/4 mL (4 mL); 200 mg/10 mL (10 mL); 400 mg/20 mL (20 mL)

Solution Prefilled Syringe, Subcutaneous [preservative free]:

Actemra: 162 mg/0.9 mL (0.9 mL)

◆ **Toctino (Can)** *see* Alitretinoin (Systemic) [CAN/INT] *on page 88*

◆ **Today Sponge [OTC]** *see* Nonoxynol 9 *on page 1471*

Tofacitinib (toe fa SYE ti nib)

Brand Names: U.S. Xeljanz

Brand Names: Canada Xeljanz

Index Terms CP-690, 550; Tofacitinib Citrate

Pharmacologic Category Antirheumatic Miscellaneous; Antirheumatic, Disease Modifying; Janus Associated Kinase Inhibitor

Use Rheumatoid arthritis: Treatment of moderately- to severely-active rheumatoid arthritis (as monotherapy or in combination with methotrexate or other nonbiologic disease-modifying antirheumatic drugs [DMARDs]) in adults who have had an inadequate response to, or are intolerant of, methotrexate

Pregnancy Risk Factor C

Pregnancy Considerations Adverse events have been observed in animal reproduction studies. Healthcare providers are encouraged to enroll women exposed to tofacitinib during pregnancy in the Xeljanz Pregnancy Registry (877-311-8972); patients may also enroll themselves. Canadian labeling recommends avoiding use during pregnancy.

Breast-Feeding Considerations It is not known if tofacitinib is excreted in breast milk. Due to the potential for adverse reactions in a nursing infant, the decision to continue or discontinue breast-feeding during therapy should take into account the risk of exposure to the infant and the benefits of treatment to the mother.

Contraindications

There are no contraindications listed in the manufacturer's U.S. labeling.

Canadian labeling: Hypersensitivity to tofacitinib or any component of the formulation.

Warnings/Precautions [U.S. Boxed Warning]: Patients receiving tofacitinib are at increased risk for serious infections, which may result in hospitalization and/or fatality; infections often developed in patients receiving concomitant immunosuppressive agents (eg,

methotrexate or corticosteroids) and may present as disseminated disease. Active tuberculosis (disseminated or extrapulmonary), invasive fungal (including cryptococcosis and pneumocystosis) and bacterial, viral or other opportunistic infections (including esophageal candidiasis, multidermatomal herpes zoster, cytomegalovirus, and BK virus) have been reported in patients receiving tofacitinib. Reactivation of viral infections (eg, herpes zoster) was observed in clinical trials; the incidence of chronic viral hepatitis reactivation is unknown. Use with caution in patients that have been exposed to tuberculosis, with a history of serious or opportunistic infection, taking concomitant immunosuppressants, with comorbid conditions that predispose them to infections (eg, diabetes), or in patients who live in or travel to/from areas of endemic mycoses (ie, blastomycosis, coccidioidomycosis, histoplasmosis). Consider risks versus benefits prior to use in patients with a history of chronic or recurrent infection; do not initiate tofacitinib in patients with active infections, including localized infections. Monitor closely for signs/symptoms of infection during therapy; interrupt therapy if serious infections or sepsis develop. Use with caution in elderly patients; general incidence of infection is higher in elderly. Use with caution in Asian patients; an increased incidence of adverse reactions has been observed (Wollenhaupt, 2014; Xeljanz Canadian product monograph, 2014).

[U.S. Boxed Warning]: Tuberculosis (disseminated or extrapulmonary) has been reported in patients receiving tofacitinib. Patients should be evaluated for tuberculosis risk factors and active or latent infection (with a tuberculin skin test) before and during therapy. Treatment of latent tuberculosis should be initiated before use. Patients with initial negative tuberculin skin tests should receive continued monitoring for tuberculosis throughout treatment; active tuberculosis has developed in this population during treatment with tofacitinib. Use with caution in patients who have resided in regions where tuberculosis is endemic. Consider antituberculosis therapy if an adequate course of treatment cannot be confirmed in patients with a history of latent or active tuberculosis or for patients with risk factors despite negative skin test.

[U.S. Boxed Warning]: Lymphoma and other malignancies have been reported in patients receiving tofacitinib; Epstein Barr Virus-associated post-transplant lymphoproliferative disorder has been observed at an increased rate in renal transplant patients receiving tofacitinib and concomitant immunosuppressive medications. The most common types of malignancy observed were lung, breast, gastric, colorectal, renal cell, prostate, lymphoma, and malignant melanoma. Consider risks versus benefits prior to use in patients with a known malignancy (other than successfully treated nonmelanoma skin cancers [NMSCs]) or when continuing tofacitinib in patients who develop a new malignancy. NMSCs have been reported; patients at increased risk for skin cancer should have periodic skin examinations.

Lymphocytopenia (after an initial lymphocytosis), neutropenia (<2000 cells/mm^3), and anemia have been observed with tofacitinib therapy. Lymphocyte counts <500 cells/mm^3 were associated with increased incidence of treated and serious infections; avoid tofacitinib initiation in patients with lymphocytes <500 cells/mm^3 at baseline. Avoid use in patients with ANC <1000 cells/mm^3 at baseline; interrupt therapy if ANC is persistently between 500-1000 cells/mm^3 or if ANC <500 cells/mm^3 during treatment. Consider resuming tofacitinib when ANC ≥1000 cells/mm^3. Avoid use in patients with hemoglobin <9 g/dL; interrupt therapy if hemoglobin decreases >2 g/dL or if hemoglobin <8 g/dL. Monitor lymphocyte counts at baseline and every 3 months thereafter; ANC, platelet counts, and hemoglobin should be assessed at baseline, after 4-8 weeks of therapy, and every 3 months thereafter.

Use with caution in patients at increased risk for gastrointestinal perforation (eg, history of diverticulitis); perforations have been reported in clinical trials. Promptly evaluate new-onset abdominal symptoms in patients taking tofacitinib. Increases in lipid parameters (eg, total cholesterol, LDL, and HDL cholesterol) were observed in patients receiving tofacitinib; maximum lipid increases were typically seen within 6 weeks of initiation. Assess lipids 4-8 weeks after tofacitinib initiation and manage lipid abnormalities accordingly. Increased incidence of liver enzyme elevation was observed in patients taking tofacitinib compared to placebo. Routine liver function test monitoring is recommended; interrupt therapy if drug-induced liver injury is suspected.

A decrease in heart rate and prolonged PR interval have been reported with tofacitinib in clinical trials. Use caution in patients with baseline heart rate <60 bpm, conduction abnormalities, syncope or arrhythmia, ischemic heart disease, heart failure, or receiving concomitant therapy known to decrease heart rate or prolong the PR interval (Xeljanz Canadian product monograph, 2014). Interstitial lung disease (ILD) has been reported; patients developing ILD were receiving concomitant therapy associated with ILD (eg, methotrexate). Use with caution in patients with risk/history of ILD (Xeljanz Canadian product monograph, 2014).

Immunization status should be current before initiating therapy. Live vaccines should not be given concomitantly with tofacitinib; no data are available concerning vaccination response or secondary transmission of infection by live vaccines in patients receiving therapy.

Potentially significant drug-drug interactions may exist, requiring dose or frequency adjustment, additional monitoring, and/or selection of alternative therapy. Tofacitinib should not be administered in combination with strong immunosuppressive medications (eg, azathioprine, tacrolimus, cyclosporine) due to the risk of additive immunosuppression; such combinations have not been studied in rheumatoid arthritis. Tofacitinib should not be administered in combination with biologic DMARDs.

Use is not recommended in patients with severe hepatic impairment; dosage reduction required in patients with moderate hepatic impairment. Dosage reduction required in patients with moderate or severe renal impairment.

Adverse Reactions Frequencies may vary for specific doses; consult prescribing information.

Cardiovascular: Hypertension

Central nervous system: Headache

Gastrointestinal: Diarrhea

Genitourinary: Urinary tract infection

Hepatic: Increased serum ALT (>3 x upper limit of normal)

Infection: Infection (including serious infection)

Renal: Increased serum creatinine

Respiratory: Nasopharyngitis, upper respiratory tract infection

Rare but important or life-threatening: Abdominal pain, anemia, BK virus, cellulitis, cryptococcosis, cytomegalovirus disease, decreased heart rate, dehydration, dyspepsia, erythema, esophageal candidiasis, gastritis, hepatotoxicity, herpes zoster, increased creatine kinase, increased serum AST, interstitial pulmonary disease, liver steatosis, lymphocytopenia, malignant neoplasm, musculoskeletal pain, neutropenia, paresthesia, peripheral edema, pneumocystosis, pneumonia, prolongation P-R interval on ECG, pruritus, rhabdomyolysis, sinus congestion, skin carcinoma, skin rash, tendonitis, tuberculosis

Drug Interactions

Metabolism/Transport Effects Substrate of CYP2C19 (minor), CYP3A4 (major); **Note:** Assignment of Major/Minor substrate status based on clinically relevant drug interaction potential

Avoid Concomitant Use

Avoid concomitant use of Tofacitinib with any of the following: Abatacept; Anakinra; Anti-TNF Agents; BCG; CloZAPine; Conivaptan; CYP3A4 Inducers (Strong); Dipyrone; Fusidic Acid (Systemic); Idelalisib; Immunosuppressants; Natalizumab; Pimecrolimus; RiTUXimab; Tacrolimus (Topical); Tocilizumab; Vaccines (Live)

Increased Effect/Toxicity

Tofacitinib may increase the levels/effects of: Bradycardia-Causing Agents; CloZAPine; Natalizumab; Vaccines (Live)

The levels/effects of Tofacitinib may be increased by: Abatacept; Anakinra; Anti-TNF Agents; Aprepitant; Ceritinib; Conivaptan; CYP3A4 Inhibitors (Moderate); CYP3A4 Inhibitors (Strong); Denosumab; Dipyrone; Fluconazole; Fosaprepitant; Fusidic Acid (Systemic); Idelalisib; Immunosuppressants; Ivacaftor; Luliconazole; Methotrexate; Mifepristone; Netupitant; Pimecrolimus; RiTUXimab; Roflumilast; Simeprevir; Sitaxentan; Stiripentol; Tacrolimus (Topical); Tocilizumab; Trastuzumab

Decreased Effect

Tofacitinib may decrease the levels/effects of: BCG; Coccidioides immitis Skin Test; Sipuleucel-T; Vaccines (Inactivated); Vaccines (Live)

The levels/effects of Tofacitinib may be decreased by: Bosentan; CYP3A4 Inducers (Moderate); CYP3A4 Inducers (Strong); Dabrafenib; Deferasirox; Echinacea; St Johns Wort

Storage/Stability Store between 20°C and 25°C (68°F to 77°F).

Mechanism of Action Tofacitinib inhibits Janus kinase (JAK) enzymes, which are intracellular enzymes involved in stimulating hematopoiesis and immune cell function through a signaling pathway. In response to extracellular cytokine or growth factor signaling, JAKs activate signal transducers and activators of transcription (STATs), which regulate gene expression and intracellular activity. Inhibition of JAKs prevents cytokine- or growth factor-mediated gene expression and intracellular activity of immune cells, reduces circulating CD16/56+ natural killer cells, serum IgG, IgM, IgA, and C-reactive protein, and increases B cells.

Pharmacodynamics/Kinetics

Absorption: Oral: Rapid (74%); C_{max} is reduced by 32% when administered with high-fat meal, but AUC remains unchanged.

Distribution: V_d: 87 L

Protein binding: ~40% (predominantly to albumin)

Metabolism: Hepatic (70%): CYP3A4 and CYP2C19 to inactive metabolites

Half-life elimination: ~3 hours

Time to peak: 0.5-1 hour

Excretion: Primarily urine (30%) as unchanged drug

Dosage Rheumatoid arthritis (monotherapy or in combination with nonbiologic disease-modifying antirheumatic drugs (DMARDs): Adults: Oral: 5 mg twice daily

Note: Tofacitinib should not be used in combination with biologic DMARDs or with strong immunosuppressants, such as azathioprine, tacrolimus, or cyclosporine. Do not initiate therapy in patients with an absolute lymphocyte count <500 cells/mm^3, absolute neutrophil count <1000 cells/mm^3, or hemoglobin <9 g/dL.

Dosage adjustment for toxicity:

Lymphopenia (lymphocytes ≥500 cells/mm^3): Maintain dose.

Lymphopenia (lymphocytes <500 cells/mm^3): Discontinue therapy.

Neutropenia (ANC >1000 cells/mm^3): Maintain dose.

Neutropenia (ANC persistently between 500-1000 cells/mm^3): Interrupt therapy; resume when ANC >1000 cells/mm^3.

Neutropenia (ANC <500 cells/mm^3): Discontinue therapy.

Anemia (hemoglobin ≥9 g/dL **and** decrease ≤2 g/dL): Maintain dose.

Anemia (hemoglobin <8 g/dL **or** decrease >2 g/dL): Interrupt therapy until hemoglobin values have normalized.

Dosage adjustment for strong CYP3A4 inducers (eg, rifampin): Coadministration is not recommended

Dosage adjustment for strong CYP3A4 inhibitors (eg, ketoconazole): Reduce dose to 5 mg daily

Dosage adjustment for concomitant moderate CYP3A4 inhibitors and potent CYP2C19 inhibitors (eg, fluconazole): Reduce dose to 5 mg daily

Dosage adjustment in renal impairment:

Mild impairment: No dosage adjustment necessary.

Moderate-to-severe impairment: Reduce dose to 5 mg once daily. **Note:** Tofacitinib has not been studied in patients with baseline CrCl <40 mL/minute.

Dosage adjustment in hepatic impairment:

Mild impairment: No dosage adjustment necessary.

Moderate impairment: Reduce dose to 5 mg once daily.

Severe impairment: Use is not recommended (has not been studied in patients with severe hepatic impairment or in patients with hepatitis B or hepatitis C viruses).

Administration May be taken without regard to food.

Monitoring Parameters Lymphocyte count (baseline and every 3 months thereafter); neutrophil/platelet counts (baseline, after 4-8 weeks, and every 3 months thereafter); hemoglobin (baseline, after 4-8 weeks, and every 3 months thereafter); lipids (4-8 weeks after therapy initiation and periodically); LFTs; viral hepatitis (prior to initiating therapy in accordance with clinical guidelines); signs/symptoms of infections (including tuberculosis) during and after therapy; abdominal symptoms; skin examinations (periodically, in patients at increased risk for skin cancer); heart rate and blood pressure at baseline and periodically thereafter.

Dosage Forms

Tablet, Oral:

Xeljanz: 5 mg

◆ **Tofacitinib Citrate** *see* Tofacitinib *on page 2059*

Tofisopam [INT] (toe FIS oh pam)

International Brand Names Bydaxin (JP); Grandaxin (BG, CZ, HU, JP, KR, PK, RU, TH); Tifis (JP)

Pharmacologic Category Benzodiazepine

Reported Use Short-term treatment of anxiety; premedication for sleep induction

Dosage Range Adults: Oral: 50-300 mg/day

Product Availability Product available in various countries; not currently available in the U.S.

Dosage Forms

Tablet: 50 mg

◆ **Tofranil** *see* Imipramine *on page 1054*

◆ **Tofranil-PM** *see* Imipramine *on page 1054*

TOLAZamide (tole AZ a mide)

Pharmacologic Category Antidiabetic Agent, Sulfonylurea

Use Adjunct to diet for the management of mild-to-moderately severe, stable, type 2 diabetes mellitus (noninsulin dependent, NIDDM)

Pregnancy Risk Factor C

Dosage Oral: Adults: Doses >500 mg/day should be given in 2 divided doses:

Initial: 100-250 mg/day with breakfast or the first main meal of the day

Fasting blood sugar <200 mg/dL: 100 mg/day

Fasting blood sugar >200 mg/dL: 250 mg/day

Patient is malnourished, underweight, elderly, or not eating properly: 100 mg/day

Adjust dose in increments of 100-250 mg/day at weekly intervals to response; maximum daily dose: 1 g (doses >1 g/day are not likely to improve control)

Conversion from insulin to tolazamide:

<20 units day = 100 mg/day

21-<40 units/day = 250 mg/day

≥40 units/day = 250 mg/day and 50% of insulin dose

Dosing adjustment in renal impairment: No dosage adjustment provided in manufacturer's labeling. However, conservative initial and maintenance doses are recommended because tolazamide is metabolized to active metabolites, which are eliminated in the urine

Dosing comments in hepatic impairment: No dosage adjustment provided in manufacturer's labeling. However, conservative initial and maintenance doses and careful monitoring of blood glucose are recommended

Additional Information Complete prescribing information should be consulted for additional detail.

Dosage Forms

Tablet, Oral:

Generic: 250 mg, 500 mg

TOLBUTamide (tole BYOO ta mide)

Brand Names: Canada Apo-Tolbutamide®

Index Terms Orinase; Tolbutamide Sodium

Pharmacologic Category Antidiabetic Agent, Sulfonylurea

Use Adjunct to diet for the management of type 2 diabetes mellitus (noninsulin dependent, NIDDM)

Pregnancy Risk Factor C

Dosage Oral: **Note:** Divided doses may improve gastrointestinal tolerance.

Adults: Initial: 1-2 g/day as a single dose in the morning or in divided doses throughout the day. Maintenance dose: 0.25-3 g/day; however, a maintenance dose >2 g/day is seldom required.

Elderly: Initial: 250 mg 1-3 times/day; usual: 500-2000 mg; maximum: 3 g/day

Dosage adjustment in renal impairment: No dosage adjustment provided in manufacturer's labeling. However, conservative initial and maintenance doses are recommended.

Hemodialysis: Not dialyzable (0% to 5%)

Dosage adjustment in hepatic impairment: No dosage adjustment provided in manufacturer's labeling. However, conservative initial and maintenance doses and careful monitoring of blood glucose are recommended.

Additional Information Complete prescribing information should be consulted for additional detail.

Dosage Forms

Tablet, Oral:

Generic: 500 mg

◆ **Tolbutamide Sodium** *see* TOLBUTamide *on page 2062*

Tolcapone (TOLE ka pone)

Brand Names: U.S. Tasmar

Pharmacologic Category Anti-Parkinson's Agent, COMT Inhibitor

Use Adjunct to levodopa and carbidopa for the treatment of signs and symptoms of idiopathic Parkinson's disease in patients with motor fluctuations not responsive to other therapies

Pregnancy Risk Factor C

Dosage Note: Tolcapone is only appropriate in patients receiving concomitant carbidopa and levodopa. If clinical improvement is not observed after 3 weeks of therapy (regardless of dose), tolcapone treatment should be discontinued.

Parkinson's disease: Adults: Oral: Initial: 100 mg 3 times daily; may increase as tolerated to 200 mg 3 times daily only if clinical benefit is justified (dosage associated with an increased incidence of ALT elevations). **Note:** Levodopa dose may need to be decreased upon initiation of tolcapone (average reduction in clinical trials was 30%). As many as 70% of patients receiving levodopa doses >600 mg daily required levodopa dosage reduction in clinical trials. Patients with moderate-to-severe dyskinesia prior to initiation are also more likely to require dosage reduction.

Dosage adjustment in renal impairment:

Mild-to-moderate impairment (CrCl≥25 mL/minute): No dosage adjustment necessary.

Severe impairment (CrCl <25 mL/minute): No dosage adjustment provided in manufacturer's labeling (has not been studied). Use with caution.

Dosage adjustment in hepatic impairment: Use is contraindicated in patients with liver disease. Discontinue immediately if signs/symptoms of hepatic impairment develop.

Additional Information Complete prescribing information should be consulted for additional detail.

Dosage Forms

Tablet, Oral:

Tasmar: 100 mg

Tolciclate [INT] (tole SYE klate)

International Brand Names Fungifos (DE); Kilmicen (CH, MX); Tolmicen (CZ, IT, PT)

Pharmacologic Category Antifungal Agent, Topical

Reported Use Topical treatment of fungal infections

Dosage Range Adults: Topical: Apply to affected area 2-3 times/day

Product Availability Product available in various countries; not currently available in the U.S.

Dosage Forms

Cream: 1% (30 g)

Lotion: 1% (30 mL)

Powder: 0.5% (100 g)

◆ **Tolectin** *see* Tolmetin *on page 2062*

Tolmetin (TOLE met in)

Index Terms Tolectin; Tolmetin Sodium

Pharmacologic Category Nonsteroidal Anti-inflammatory Drug (NSAID), Oral

Additional Appendix Information

Beers Criteria - Potentially Inappropriate Medications for Geriatrics *on page 2271*

Use Treatment of rheumatoid arthritis and osteoarthritis, juvenile idiopathic arthritis (JIA)

Pregnancy Risk Factor C

Dosage Oral:

Children ≥2 years:

Juvenile idiopathic arthritis (JIA): Initial: 20 mg/kg/day in 3-4 divided doses, then 15-30 mg/kg/day in 3-4 divided doses (maximum dose: 30 mg/kg/day)

Analgesic (off-label use): 5-7 mg/kg/dose every 6-8 hours

Adults: RA, osteoarthritis: 400 mg 3 times/day; usual dose: 600 mg to 1.8 g/day; maximum: 1.8 g/day

Dosage adjustment in renal impairment: No dosage adjustment provided in manufacturer's labeling. However, use may precipitate or worsen renal injury. Use is not recommended in patients with advanced renal disease.

Dosage adjustment in hepatic impairment: No dosage adjustment provided in manufacturer's labeling.

Additional Information Complete prescribing information should be consulted for additional detail.

Dosage Forms

Capsule, Oral:

Generic: 400 mg

Tablet, Oral:

Generic: 200 mg, 600 mg

◆ **Tolmetin Sodium** *see* Tolmetin *on page 2062*

Tolnaftate (tole NAF tate)

Brand Names: U.S. Anti-Fungal [OTC]; Antifungal [OTC]; Athletes Foot Spray [OTC]; Dr Gs Clear Nail [OTC]; Fungi-Guard [OTC]; Fungoid-D [OTC]; Jock Itch Spray [OTC]; LamISIL AF Defense [OTC]; Medi-First Anti-Fungal [OTC]; Mycocide Clinical NS [OTC]; Podactin [OTC]; Tinactin Deodorant [OTC]; Tinactin Jock Itch [OTC]; Tinactin [OTC]; Tinaspore [OTC]; Tolnaftate Antifungal [OTC]

Brand Names: Canada Pitrex

Pharmacologic Category Antifungal Agent, Topical

Use Treatment of tinea pedis, tinea cruris, tinea corporis

Dosage Children ≥2 years and Adults: Topical: Wash and dry affected area; spray aerosol or apply 1-3 drops of solution or a small amount of cream, or powder and rub into the affected areas 2 times/day

Note: May use for up to 4 weeks for tinea pedis or tinea corporis, and up to 2 weeks for tinea cruris

Additional Information Complete prescribing information should be consulted for additional detail.

Dosage Forms

Aerosol, External:

Athletes Foot Spray [OTC]: 1% (150 g)
Tinactin [OTC]: 1% (150 g)

Aerosol Powder, External:

Jock Itch Spray [OTC]: 1% (130 g)
LamISIL AF Defense [OTC]: 1% (133 g)
Tinactin [OTC]: 1% (133 g)
Tinactin Deodorant [OTC]: 1% (133 g)

Cream, External:

Antifungal [OTC]: 1% (15 g)
Fungi-Guard [OTC]: 1% (15 g)
Fungoid-D [OTC]: 1% (113 g)
Medi-First Anti-Fungal [OTC]: 1% (1 ea)
Tinactin [OTC]: 1% (15 g, 30 g)
Tinactin Jock Itch [OTC]: 1% (15 g)
Tolnaftate Antifungal [OTC]: 1% (114 g)
Generic: 1% (15 g, 20 g, 28.3 g, 30 g)

Powder, External:

Anti-Fungal [OTC]: 1% (45 g)
LamISIL AF Defense [OTC]: 1% (113 g)
Podactin [OTC]: 1% (45 g)
Tinactin [OTC]: 1% (108 g)
Generic: 1% (45 g)

Solution, External:

Dr Gs Clear Nail [OTC]: 1% (18 mL)
Mycocide Clinical NS [OTC]: 1% (30 mL)
Tinaspore [OTC]: 1% (10 mL)
Generic: 1% (10 mL)

◆ **Tolnaftate Antifungal [OTC]** *see* Tolnaftate *on page 2063*

◆ **Toloxin (Can)** *see* Digoxin *on page 627*

Tolterodine (tole TER oh deen)

Brand Names: U.S. Detrol; Detrol LA

Brand Names: Canada Detrol®; Detrol® LA; Unidet®

Index Terms Tolterodine Tartrate

Pharmacologic Category Anticholinergic Agent

Additional Appendix Information

Beers Criteria - Potentially Inappropriate Medications for Geriatrics *on page 2271*

Use Treatment of patients with an overactive bladder with symptoms of urinary frequency, urgency, or urge incontinence

Pregnancy Risk Factor C

Pregnancy Considerations Teratogenic effects were observed in some animal reproduction studies.

Breast-Feeding Considerations It is not known if tolterodine is excreted in breast milk. Due to the potential for serious adverse reactions in the nursing infant, a decision should be made whether to discontinue nursing or to discontinue the drug, taking into account the importance of treatment to the mother.

Contraindications Hypersensitivity to tolterodine or fesoterodine (both are metabolized to 5-hydroxymethyl tolterodine) or any component of the formulation; urinary retention; gastric retention; uncontrolled narrow-angle glaucoma

Warnings/Precautions Cases of angioedema have been reported; some cases have occurred after a single dose. Discontinue immediately if angioedema and associated difficulty breathing, airway obstruction, or hypotension develop. May cause drowsiness, dizziness, and/or blurred vision, which may impair physical or mental abilities; patients must be cautioned about performing tasks which require mental alertness (eg, operating machinery or driving). Consider dose reduction or discontinuation if CNS effects occur. Use with caution in patients with bladder flow obstruction, may increase the risk of urinary retention. Use with caution in patients with gastrointestinal obstructive disorders (ie, pyloric stenosis), may increase the risk of gastric retention. Use with caution in patients with myasthenia gravis and controlled (treated) narrow-angle glaucoma; metabolized in the liver and excreted in the urine and feces, dosage adjustment is required for patients with renal or hepatic impairment. Tolterodine has been associated with QTc prolongation at high (supratherapeutic) doses. The manufacturer recommends caution in patients with congenital prolonged QT or in patients receiving concurrent therapy with QTc-prolonging drugs (class Ia or III antiarrhythmics). However, the mean change in QTc even at supratherapeutic dosages was less than 15 msec. Individuals who are CYP2D6 poor metabolizers or in the presence of inhibitors of CYP2D6 and CYP3A4 may be more likely to exhibit prolongation. Dosage adjustment is recommended in patients receiving CYP3A4 inhibitors (a lower dose of tolterodine is recommended). This medication is associated with potent anticholinergic properties which may be inappropriate in older adults depending on comorbidities (eg, dementia, delirium) (Beers Criteria).

Adverse Reactions

Cardiovascular: Chest pain

Central nervous system: Anxiety, dizziness, fatigue, headache, somnolence

Dermatologic: Dry skin

Gastrointestinal: Dry mouth

Gastrointestinal: Abdominal pain, constipation, diarrhea, dyspepsia, weight gain

Genitourinary: Dysuria

Neuromuscular & skeletal: Arthralgia

Ocular: Abnormal vision, dry eyes

Respiratory: Bronchitis, sinusitis

Miscellaneous: Flu-like syndrome, infection

Rare but important or life-threatening: Anaphylaxis, angioedema, confusion, dementia aggravated, disorientation, hallucinations, memory impairment, palpitation, peripheral edema, QTc prolongation, tachycardia

Drug Interactions

Metabolism/Transport Effects Substrate of CYP2C19 (minor), CYP2C9 (minor), CYP2D6 (major), CYP3A4 (major); **Note:** Assignment of Major/Minor substrate status based on clinically relevant drug interaction potential

Avoid Concomitant Use

Avoid concomitant use of Tolterodine with any of the following: Aclidinium; Conivaptan; Fusidic Acid (Systemic); Glucagon; Idelalisib; Ipratropium (Oral Inhalation); Potassium Chloride; Tiotropium; Umeclidinium

Increased Effect/Toxicity

Tolterodine may increase the levels/effects of: AbobotulinumtoxinA; Analgesics (Opioid); Anticholinergic Agents; Cannabinoid-Containing Products; Glucagon; Highest Risk QTc-Prolonging Agents; Mirabegron; Moderate Risk QTc-Prolonging Agents; OnabotulinumtoxinA; Potassium Chloride; RimabotulinumtoxinB; Thiazide Diuretics; Tiotropium; Topiramate; Warfarin

The levels/effects of Tolterodine may be increased by: Abiraterone Acetate; Aclidinium; Aprepitant; Ceritinib; Conivaptan; CYP2D6 Inhibitors (Moderate); CYP2D6 Inhibitors (Strong); CYP3A4 Inhibitors (Moderate); CYP3A4 Inhibitors (Strong); Dasatinib; Fosaprepitant; Fusidic Acid (Systemic); Idelalisib; Ipratropium (Oral Inhalation); Ivacaftor; Luliconazole; Mianserin; Mifepristone; Netupitant; Peginterferon Alfa-2b; Pramlintide; Simeprevir; Stiripentol; Umeclidinium; VinBLAStine

Decreased Effect

Tolterodine may decrease the levels/effects of: Acetylcholinesterase Inhibitors; Itopride; Secretin

The levels/effects of Tolterodine may be decreased by: Acetylcholinesterase Inhibitors; Bosentan; CYP3A4 Inducers (Moderate); CYP3A4 Inducers (Strong); Dabrafenib; Deferasirox; Mitotane; Peginterferon Alfa-2b; Siltuximab; St Johns Wort; Tocilizumab

Food Interactions Food increases bioavailability (~53% increase) of tolterodine tablets (dose adjustment not necessary); does not affect the pharmacokinetics of tolterodine extended release capsules. As a CYP3A4 inhibitor, grapefruit juice may increase the serum level and/or toxicity of tolterodine, but unlikely secondary to high oral bioavailability. Management: Monitor patients closely with concurrent grapefruit juice use.

Storage/Stability Store at 25°C (77°F); excursions permitted to 15°C to 30°C (59°F to 86°F). Protect from light.

Mechanism of Action Tolterodine is a competitive antagonist of muscarinic receptors. In animal models, tolterodine demonstrates selectivity for urinary bladder receptors over salivary receptors. Urinary bladder contraction is mediated by muscarinic receptors. Tolterodine increases residual urine volume and decreases detrusor muscle pressure.

Pharmacodynamics/Kinetics

Absorption: Immediate release tablet: Rapid; ≥77%

Distribution: IV: V_d: 113 ± 27 L

Protein binding: >96% (primarily to alpha$_1$-acid glycoprotein)

Metabolism: Extensively hepatic, primarily via CYP2D6 to 5-hydroxymethyltolterodine (active) and 3A4 usually (minor pathway). In patients with a genetic deficiency of CYP2D6, metabolism via 3A4 predominates.

Bioavailability: Immediate release tablet: Increased 53% with food

Half-life elimination:

Immediate release tablet: Extensive metabolizers: ~2 hours; Poor metabolizers: ~10 hours

Extended release capsule: Extensive metabolizers: ~7 hours; Poor metabolizers: ~18 hours

Time to peak: Immediate release tablet: 1-2 hours; Extended release capsule: 2-6 hours

Excretion: Urine (77%); feces (17%); primarily as metabolites (<1% unchanged drug) of which the active 5-hydroxymethyl metabolite accounts for 5% to 14% (<1% in poor metabolizers); as unchanged drug (<1%; <2.5% in poor metabolizers)

Dosage

Oral: Adults: Treatment of overactive bladder:

Immediate release tablet: 2 mg twice daily; the dose may be lowered to 1 mg twice daily based on individual response and tolerability

Dosing adjustment in patients concurrently taking strong CYP3A4 inhibitors (eg, ketoconazole, clarithromycin, ritonavir): 1 mg twice daily

Extended release capsule: 4 mg once daily; dose may be lowered to 2 mg once daily based on individual response and tolerability

Dosing adjustment in patients concurrently taking strong CYP3A4 inhibitors (eg, ketoconazole, clarithromycin, ritonavir): 2 mg once daily

Elderly: Safety and efficacy in patients >64 years was found to be similar to that in younger patients; no dosage adjustment is needed based on age

Dosing adjustment in renal impairment:

Immediate release tablet: Significantly reduced renal function (studies conducted in patients with CrCl 10-30 mL/minute): 1 mg twice daily; use with caution

Extended release capsule:

CrCl 10-30 mL/minute: 2 mg once daily

CrCl <10 mL/minute: Use is not recommended; has not been studied.

Dosing adjustment in hepatic impairment:

Immediate release tablet: Significantly reduced hepatic function: 1 mg twice daily; use with caution

Extended release capsule:

Mild-to-moderate impairment (Child-Pugh class A or B): 2 mg once daily

Severe impairment (Child-Pugh class C): Use is not recommended; has not been studied.

Administration Extended release capsule: Swallow whole; do not crush, chew, or open

Monitoring Parameters Renal function (BUN, creatinine); hepatic function

Dosage Forms

Capsule Extended Release 24 Hour, Oral:

Detrol LA: 2 mg, 4 mg

Generic: 2 mg, 4 mg

Tablet, Oral:

Detrol: 1 mg, 2 mg

Generic: 1 mg, 2 mg

◆ **Tolterodine Tartrate** *see* Tolterodine *on page 2063*

Tolvaptan (tol VAP tan)

Brand Names: U.S. Samsca

Brand Names: Canada Samsca™

Index Terms OPC-41061

Pharmacologic Category Vasopressin Antagonist

Use Treatment of clinically significant hypervolemic or euvolemic hyponatremia associated with heart failure or SIADH with either a serum sodium <125 mEq/L or less marked hyponatremia that is symptomatic and resistant to fluid restriction

Pregnancy Risk Factor C

Dosage Oral: Adults: Hyponatremia: Initial: 15 mg once daily; after at least 24 hours, may increase to 30 mg once daily to a maximum of 60 mg once daily titrating at 24-hour intervals to desired serum sodium concentration. Avoid fluid restriction during the first 24 hours of therapy. Do not use for more than 30 days due to the risk of hepatotoxicity.

Dosage adjustment in renal impairment:
CrCl ≥10 mL/minute: No dosage adjustment necessary
CrCl <10 mL/minute: Use not recommended (not studied); contraindicated in anuria (no benefit expected)

Dosage adjustment in hepatic impairment: Avoid use in patients with underlying liver disease, including cirrhosis.

Additional Information Complete prescribing information should be consulted for additional detail.

Dosage Forms

Tablet, Oral:
Samsca: 15 mg, 30 mg

Dosage Forms: Canada

Tablet, oral:
Samsca™: 15 mg, 30 mg, 60 mg

- ◆ **Tomoxetine** *see* AtoMOXetine *on page 191*
- ◆ **Tomudex (Can)** *see* Raltitrexed [CAN/INT] *on page 1769*
- ◆ **Topactin (Can)** *see* Fluocinonide *on page 894*
- ◆ **Topamax** *see* Topiramate *on page 2065*
- ◆ **Topamax Sprinkle** *see* Topiramate *on page 2065*
- ◆ **TopCare® Pain Relief PM [OTC]** *see* Acetaminophen and Diphenhydramine *on page 36*
- ◆ **Topex Topical Anesthetic** *see* Benzocaine *on page 246*
- ◆ **Topicaine [OTC]** *see* Lidocaine (Topical) *on page 1211*
- ◆ **Topicaine 5 [OTC]** *see* Lidocaine (Topical) *on page 1211*
- ◆ **Topicort** *see* Desoximetasone *on page 598*
- ◆ **Topicort® (Can)** *see* Desoximetasone *on page 598*
- ◆ **Topicort® Gel (Can)** *see* Desoximetasone *on page 598*
- ◆ **Topicort® Mild (Can)** *see* Desoximetasone *on page 598*
- ◆ **Topicort® Ointment (Can)** *see* Desoximetasone *on page 598*
- ◆ **Topicort Spray** *see* Desoximetasone *on page 598*
- ◆ **Topiragen** *see* Topiramate *on page 2065*

Topiramate (toe PYRE a mate)

Brand Names: U.S. Qudexy XR; Topamax; Topamax Sprinkle; Topiragen; Trokendi XR

Brand Names: Canada Abbott-Topiramate; ACT Topiramate; Apo-Topiramate; AURO-Topiramate; Dom-Topiramate; GD-Topiramate; Mint-Topiramate; Mylan-Topiramate; PHL-Topiramate; PMS-Topiramate; PRO-Topiramate; Q-Topiramate; RAN-Topiramate; Sandoz-Topiramate; TEVA-Topiramate; Topamax

Pharmacologic Category Anticonvulsant, Miscellaneous

Use

Epilepsy:
Monotherapy: As initial monotherapy in patients 2 years and older (immediate release) or 10 years and older (extended release [ER]) with partial-onset or primary generalized tonic-clonic seizures
Adjunctive therapy: As adjunctive therapy in patients 2 years and older (immediate release and Qudexy XR only) or 6 years and older (Trokendi XR only) with partial-onset seizures, primary generalized tonic-clonic seizures, or seizures associated with Lennox-Gastaut syndrome

Migraine (immediate release only): Prophylaxis of migraine headache in adults and adolescents 12 years and older.

Pregnancy Risk Factor D

Pregnancy Considerations Adverse events have been observed in animal reproduction studies. Based on limited data (n=5), topiramate was found to cross the placenta and could be detected in neonatal serum (Ohman, 2002). Topiramate may cause fetal harm if administered to a pregnant woman. An increased risk of oral clefts (cleft lip and/or palate) has been observed following first trimester exposure. Data from the North American Antiepileptic Drug (NAAED) Pregnancy Registry reported that the prevalence of oral clefts was 1.2% for infants exposed to topiramate during the first trimester of pregnancy, versus 0.39% to 0.46% for infants exposed to other antiepileptic drugs and 0.12% with no exposure. Although not evaluated during pregnancy, metabolic acidosis may be induced by topiramate. In general, metabolic acidosis during pregnancy may result in adverse effects and fetal death. Pregnant women and their newborns should be monitored for metabolic acidosis. Maternal serum concentrations may decrease during the second and third trimesters of pregnancy therefore therapeutic drug monitoring should be considered in pregnant women who require therapy (Ohman, 2009; Westin, 2009).

Use for migraine prophylaxis is contraindicated per the Canadian labeling in pregnant women or women of childbearing potential who are not using effective contraception.

Patients exposed to topiramate during pregnancy are encouraged to enroll themselves into the AED Pregnancy Registry by calling 1-888-233-2334. Additional information is available at www.aedpregnancyregistry.org.

Breast-Feeding Considerations Topiramate is excreted into breast milk. Based on information from five nursing infants, infant plasma concentrations of topiramate have been reported as 10% to 20% of the maternal plasma concentration. The manufacturer recommends that caution be used if administered to a nursing woman.

Contraindications

Extended release: Recent alcohol use (ie, within 6 hours prior to and 6 hours after administration) (Trokendi XR only); patients with metabolic acidosis who are taking concomitant metformin

Immediate release: There are no contraindications listed in the manufacturer's labeling.

Canadian labeling (not in U.S. labeling): Hypersensitivity to topiramate or any component of the formulation or container; pregnancy and women in childbearing years not using effective contraception (migraine prophylaxis only)

Warnings/Precautions Hazardous agent – use appropriate precautions for handling and disposal (NIOSH 2014 [group 3]).

Antiepileptics are associated with an increased risk of suicidal behavior/thoughts with use (regardless of indication); patients should be monitored for signs/symptoms of depression, suicidal tendencies, and other unusual behavior changes during therapy and instructed to inform their healthcare provider immediately if symptoms occur. Use with caution in patients with hepatic, respiratory, or renal impairment. Topiramate may decrease serum bicarbonate concentrations (up to 67% of epilepsy patients and 77% of migraine patients). Risk may be increased in patients with a predisposing condition (organ dysfunction, diarrhea, ketogenic diet, status epilepticus, or concurrent treatment with other drugs which may cause acidosis). Metabolic acidosis may occur at dosages as low as 50 mg/day.

Monitor serum bicarbonate as well as potential complications of chronic acidosis (nephrolithiasis, nephrocalcinosis, osteomalacia/osteoporosis, and reduced growth rates and/ or weight in children). Kidney stones have been reported in both children and adults; the risk of kidney stones is about 2-4 times that of the untreated population; consider avoiding use in patients on a ketogenic diet; the risk of kidney stones may be reduced by increasing fluid intake.

Cognitive dysfunction (confusion, psychomotor slowing, difficultly with concentration/attention, difficultly with memory, speech or language problems), psychiatric disturbances (depression or mood disorders), and sedation (somnolence or fatigue) may occur with topiramate use; incidence may be related to rapid titration and higher doses. Patients must be cautioned about performing tasks which require mental alertness (eg, operating machinery or driving). Effects with other sedative drugs or ethanol may be potentiated. Topiramate may also cause paresthesia, dizziness, and ataxia. Topiramate has been associated with acute myopia and secondary angle-closure glaucoma in adults and children, typically within 1 month of initiation; discontinue in patients with acute onset of decreased visual acuity and/or ocular pain. Visual field defects have also been reported independent of increased intraocular pressure; generally reversible upon discontinuation. Consider discontinuation if visual problems occur at any time during treatment. Hyperammonemia with or without encephalopathy may occur with or without concomitant valproate administration; valproic acid dose-dependency was observed in limited pediatric studies; use with caution in patients with inborn errors of metabolism or decreased hepatic mitochondrial activity. Hypothermia (core body temperature <35°C [95°F]) has been reported with concomitant use of topiramate and valproic acid; may occur with or without associated hyperammonemia and may develop after topiramate initiation or dosage increase; discontinuation of topiramate or valproic acid may be necessary. Topiramate may be associated with oligohydrosis and hyperthermia, most frequently in children; use caution and monitor closely during strenuous exercise, during exposure to high environmental temperature, or in patients receiving receiving other carbonic anhydrase inhibitors and drugs with anticholinergic activity. Use with caution in the elderly; dosage adjustment may be required.

Potentially significant drug-drug interactions may exist, requiring dose or frequency adjustment, additional monitoring, and/or selection of alternative therapy. Avoid abrupt withdrawal of topiramate therapy; it should be withdrawn/ tapered slowly to minimize the potential of increased seizure frequency. Doses were also gradually withdrawn in migraine prophylaxis studies.

Adverse Reactions Adverse events are reported for adult and pediatric patients for various indications and regimens. **Note:** A wide range of dosages were studied. Incidence of adverse events was frequently lower in the pediatric population studied.

Cardiovascular: Angina pectoris, atrioventricular block, bradycardia (adjunctive therapy for epilepsy in children 2 to 16 years, chest pain, deep vein thrombosis, edema, facial edema, flushing, hypertension, hypotension, orthostatic hypotension, phlebitis, pulmonary embolism, syncope, vasodilatation

Central nervous system: Abnormal electroencephalogram, abnormal gait, aggressive behavior, agitation, altered sense of smell, anxiety, apathy, aphasia, apraxia, ataxia, behavioral problems (adjunctive therapy for epilepsy in children 2 to 16 years), brain disease, cognitive dysfunction, confusion, delirium, delusions, depersonalization, depression, dizziness, drowsiness, dysarthria, dystonia, emotional lability, euphoria, exacerbation of depression, exacerbation of migraine headache, fatigue, hallucination, headache, hyperesthesia, hypertonia, hypoesthesia, hyporeflexia (adjunctive therapy for epilepsy in children 2 to 16 years), insomnia, irritability, lack of concentration, language problems, memory impairment, mood disorder, nervousness, neuropathy, pain, paranoia, paresthesia, psychomotor retardation, psychosis, psychoneurosis (adjunctive therapy for epilepsy in children 2 to 16 years), rigors, sensory disturbance, speech disturbance, stupor, tonic-clonic seizures (adjunctive therapy for epilepsy in children 2 to 16 years), vertigo, voice disorder, weight loss

Dermatologic: Abnormal hair texture, acne vulgaris, alopecia, body odor, dermatitis (adjunctive therapy for epilepsy in children 2 to 16 years), dermatological disease, diaphoresis, eczema (adjunctive therapy for epilepsy in children 2 to 16 years), erythematous rash, hypertrichosis (adjunctive therapy for epilepsy in children 2 to 16 years), pallor (adjunctive therapy for epilepsy in children 2 to 16 years), pruritus, seborrhea (adjunctive therapy for epilepsy in children 2 to 16 years), skin discoloration (adjunctive therapy for epilepsy in children 2 to 16 years), skin photosensitivity, skin rash, urticaria

Endocrine & metabolic: Albuminuria, amenorrhea, decreased libido, decreased serum bicarbonate, decreased serum phosphate, dehydration, diabetes mellitus, hot flash, hyperammonemia with/without encephalopathy with/without valproate (migraine therapy in adolescents 12 to 17 years), hyperglycemia, hyperlipidemia, hypermenorrhea, hyperthyroidism (migraine therapy in adolescents 12 to 17 years), hypocalcemia, hypoglycemia (adjunctive therapy for epilepsy in children 2 to 16 years), increased gamma-glutamyl transferase, increased thirst, intermenstrual bleeding, menstrual disease, weight gain (adjunctive therapy for epilepsy in children 2 to 16 years)

Gastrointestinal: Abdominal pain, ageusia, anorexia, constipation, decreased appetite, diarrhea, dysgeusia, dyspepsia, dysphagia (adjunctive therapy for epilepsy in children 2 to 16 years), enlargement of abdomen, esophagitis, fecal incontinence (adjunctive therapy for epilepsy in children 2 to 16 years), flatulence (adjunctive therapy for epilepsy in children 2 to 16 years), gastritis, gastroenteritis, gastroesophageal reflux disease, gastrointestinal disease, gingival hemorrhage, gingival hyperplasia (adjunctive therapy for epilepsy in children 2 to 16 years), gingivitis, glossitis (adjunctive therapy for epilepsy in children 2 to 16 years), hemorrhoids, increased appetite (adjunctive therapy for epilepsy in children 2 to 16 years), melena, nausea, sialorrhea (adjunctive therapy for epilepsy in children 2 to 16 years), stomatitis, vomiting, xerostomia

Genitourinary: Cystitis, dysuria, ejaculatory disorder, genital candidiasis, hematuria, impotence, leukorrhea (adjunctive therapy for epilepsy in children 2 to 16 years), mastalgia, nipple discharge, nocturia (adjunctive therapy for epilepsy in children 2 to 16 years), oliguria, premature ejaculation, prostatic disease, urinary frequency, urinary incontinence, urinary retention, urinary tract infection, urine abnormality, vaginal hemorrhage

Hematologic & oncologic: Anemia, eosinophilia, granulocytopenia, hematoma (adjunctive therapy for epilepsy in children 2 to 16 years), hemorrhage, leukopenia, lymphadenopathy, lymphocytopenia, neoplasm, prolonged prothrombin time (adjunctive therapy for epilepsy in children 2 to 16 years), purpura (adjunctive therapy for epilepsy in children 2 to 16 years), thrombocythemia, thrombocytopenia (adjunctive therapy for epilepsy in children 2 to 16 years)

Hepatic: Increased serum alkaline phosphatase, increased serum ALT, increased serum AST

Hypersensitivity: Hypersensitivity reaction

Infection: Candidiasis, infection, viral infection

Neuromuscular & skeletal: Arthralgia, arthropathy, back pain, dyskinesia, hyperkinesia (adjunctive therapy for epilepsy in children 2 to 16 years), leg cramps, leg pain, muscle spasm, myalgia, skeletal pain, tremor, weakness

Ophthalmic: Abnormal lacrimation (adjunctive therapy for epilepsy in children 2 to 16 years), accommodation disturbance, blepharoptosis, blurred vision, conjunctivitis, diplopia, eye disease, eye pain, myopia (adjunctive therapy for epilepsy in children 2 to 16 years), nystagmus, photophobia, scotoma, strabismus, visual disturbance, visual field defect, xerophthalmia

Otic: Hearing loss, otitis media, tinnitus

Renal: Increased serum creatinine, nephrolithiasis, polyuria, renal pain

Respiratory: Asthma, bronchitis, cough, dyspnea, epistaxis, flu-like symptoms, laryngitis (migraine therapy in adolescents 12 to 17 years), pharyngeal edema (migraine therapy in adolescents 12 to 17 years), pharyngitis, pneumonia, respiratory tract disease (adjunctive therapy for epilepsy in children 2 to 16 years), rhinitis, sinusitis, upper respiratory tract infection

Miscellaneous: Fever, trauma

Rare but important or life-threatening: Acute myopia with secondary angle-closure glaucoma, bone marrow depression (epilepsy), cerebellar syndrome (epilepsy), decreased serum phosphate (migraine therapy in adolescents 12 to 17 years), erythema multiforme, hepatic failure (including fatalities), hyperthermia, hypohidrosis, hypothermia (with valproate, with or without hyperammonemia), hypokalemia (adjunctive therapy in adults with partial-onset seizures), lymphocytosis (epilepsy), maculopathy, metabolic acidosis (hyperchloremia, nonanion gap), pancreatitis, pancytopenia (epilepsy), pemphigus, renal tubular acidosis, Stevens-Johnson syndrome, suicidal ideation, tongue edema (epilepsy), upper motor neuron lesion (epilepsy), vasospasm (epilepsy)

Drug Interactions

Metabolism/Transport Effects **Inhibits** CYP2C19 (weak); **Induces** CYP3A4 (weak)

Avoid Concomitant Use

Avoid concomitant use of Topiramate with any of the following: Alcohol (Ethyl); Azelastine (Nasal); Carbonic Anhydrase Inhibitors; Orphenadrine; Paraldehyde; Thalidomide; Ulipristal

Increased Effect/Toxicity

Topiramate may increase the levels/effects of: Alpha-/Beta-Agonists (Indirect-Acting); Amitriptyline; Amphetamines; Azelastine (Nasal); Buprenorphine; Carbonic Anhydrase Inhibitors; CNS Depressants; Flecainide; Fosphenytoin; Hydrocodone; Lithium; Memantine; MetFORMIN; Methotrimeprazine; Metyrosine; Mirtazapine; Orphenadrine; Paraldehyde; Phenytoin; Pramipexole; Primidone; QuiNIDine; ROPINIRole; Rotigotine; Selective Serotonin Reuptake Inhibitors; Suvorexant; Thalidomide; Valproic Acid and Derivatives; Zolpidem

The levels/effects of Topiramate may be increased by: Alcohol (Ethyl); Anticholinergic Agents; Brimonidine (Topical); Cannabis; Doxylamine; Dronabinol; Droperidol; HydrOXYzine; Kava Kava; Loop Diuretics; Magnesium Sulfate; Methotrimeprazine; Nabilone; Perampanel; Rufinamide; Salicylates; Sodium Oxybate; Tapentadol; Tetrahydrocannabinol; Thiazide Diuretics

Decreased Effect

Topiramate may decrease the levels/effects of: ARIPiprazole; Contraceptives (Estrogens); Contraceptives (Progestins); Methenamine; Primidone; Saxagliptin; Ulipristal

The levels/effects of Topiramate may be decreased by: CarBAMazepine; Fosphenytoin; Mefloquine; Mianserin; Orlistat; Phenytoin

Food Interactions Ketogenic diet may increase the possibility of acidosis and/or kidney stones. Management: Monitor for symptoms of acidosis or kidney stones.

Storage/Stability

Extended release capsules: Store at 15°C to 30°C (59°F to 86°F). Protect from moisture. Protect from light.

Sprinkle capsules: Store at or below 25°C (77°F). Protect from moisture.

Tablets: Store at 15°C to 30°C (59°F to 86°F). Protect from moisture.

Mechanism of Action Anticonvulsant activity may be due to a combination of potential mechanisms: Blocks neuronal voltage-dependent sodium channels, enhances GABA(A) activity, antagonizes AMPA/kainate glutamate receptors, and weakly inhibits carbonic anhydrase.

Pharmacodynamics/Kinetics

Absorption: Good, rapid; immediate release formulation is unaffected by food. A single Trokendi XR dose with a high-fat meal increased the C_{max} by 37% and shortened the T_{max} to approximately 8 hours; this effect is significantly reduced following repeat administrations. A single Qudexy XR dose with a high-fat meal delayed the T_{max} by 4 hours.

Protein binding: 15% to 41% (inversely related to plasma concentrations)

Metabolism: Minor amounts metabolized in liver via hydroxylation, hydrolysis, and glucuronidation; there is evidence of renal tubular reabsorption; percentage of dose metabolized in liver and clearance are increased in patients receiving enzyme inducers (eg, carbamazepine, phenytoin)

Bioavailability: ~80% (immediate release)

Half-life elimination: 21 hours (immediate release); ~31 hours (Trokendi XR); ~56 hours (Qudexy XR)

Time to peak, serum: ~1-4 hours (immediate release); ~24 hours (Trokendi XR); ~20 hours (Qudexy XR)

Excretion: Urine (~70% as unchanged drug)

Dosage Note: Do not abruptly discontinue therapy; taper dosage gradually to prevent rebound effects. (In clinical trials, adult doses were withdrawn by decreasing in weekly intervals of 50-100 mg daily gradually over 2-8 weeks for seizure treatment, and by decreasing in weekly intervals by 25-50 mg daily for migraine prophylaxis.) Bioequivalence has not been demonstrated between Trokendi XR and Qudexy XR.

Epilepsy, monotherapy: Partial-onset seizure and primary generalized tonic-clonic seizure:

Children 2-9 years: Oral:

Immediate release: Initial: 25 mg once daily (in evening); may increase to 25 mg twice daily in week 2; thereafter, may increase by 25-50 mg daily at weekly intervals over 5-7 weeks up to the following minimum recommended maintenance dose:

≤11 kg: 150 mg daily in 2 divided doses
12-22 kg: 200 mg daily in 2 divided doses
23-31 kg: 200 mg daily in 2 divided doses
32-38 kg: 250 mg daily in 2 divided doses
≥39 kg: 250 mg daily in 2 divided doses

Maximum maintenance dose: If additional seizure control is needed and therapy is tolerated, may further increase by 25-50 mg daily at weekly intervals up to the following maximum recommended maintenance dose:

≤11 kg: 250 mg daily in 2 divided doses
12-22 kg: 300 mg daily in 2 divided doses
23-31 kg: 350 mg daily in 2 divided doses
32-38 kg: 350 mg daily in 2 divided doses
≥39 kg: 400 mg daily in 2 divided doses

Children ≥10 years and Adults: Oral:

Immediate release: Initial: 25 mg twice daily; may increase weekly by 50 mg daily up to 100 mg twice daily (week 4 dose); thereafter, may further increase weekly by 100 mg daily up to the recommended dose of 200 mg twice daily.

Extended release: Initial: 50 mg daily for 1 week; may increase weekly by 50 mg daily up to 200 mg once daily (week 4 dose); thereafter, may further increase weekly by 100 mg daily up to the recommended dose of 400 mg once daily.

Canadian labeling: Children ≥6 years and Adults: Oral: Immediate release: Initial: 25 mg once daily (in evening); may increase to 25 mg twice daily in weeks 2 or 3, and up to 50 mg twice daily by weeks 3 or 4; may further increase weekly in increments of 50 mg daily up to recommended maximum of 200 mg twice daily.

Epilepsy, adjunctive therapy: Partial-onset seizure, primary generalized tonic-clonic seizure, or Lennox-Gastaut syndrome:

Children 2-6 years: Oral:

Immediate release: Initial: 25 mg (1-3 mg/kg/day) once daily (in evening) for 1 week; may increase every 1-2 weeks in increments of 1-3 mg/kg/day up to the recommended dose of 5-9 mg/kg/day in 2 divided doses.

Extended-release (Qudexy XR only): Initial: 25 mg (1-3 mg/kg/day) once daily (in evening) for 1 week; may increase every 1-2 weeks in increments of 1-3 mg/kg/day up to the recommended dose of 5-9 mg/kg once daily.

Children 6-16 years: Oral:

Immediate release: Initial: 25 mg (1-3 mg/kg/day) once daily (in evening) for 1 week; may increase every 1-2 weeks in increments of 1-3 mg/kg/day up to the recommended dose of 5-9 mg/kg/day in 2 divided doses.

Extended-release (Qudexy XR and Trokendi XR): Initial: 25 mg (1-3 mg/kg/day) once daily (in evening) for 1 week; may increase every 1-2 weeks in increments of 1-3 mg/kg/day up to the recommended dose of 5-9 mg/kg once daily.

Adolescents ≥17 years and Adults: Oral: **Note:** Doses >1600 mg have not been studied.

Immediate release: Initial: 25 mg once or twice daily for 1 week; may increase weekly by 25-50 mg daily until response; usual maintenance dose: 100-200 mg twice daily (partial-onset seizures) or 200 mg twice daily (primary generalized tonic-clonic seizures). Doses >400 mg daily have not shown additional benefit for treatment of partial-onset seizures.

Extended release: Initial: 25-50 mg once daily for 1 week; may increase weekly by 25-50 mg daily until response; usual maintenance dose: 200-400 mg once daily (partial-onset seizures, Lennox-Gastaut syndrome) or 400 mg once daily (primary generalized tonic-clonic seizures). Doses >400 mg daily have not shown additional benefit for treatment of partial-onset seizures.

Canadian labeling: Oral: Immediate release: Initial: 25 mg once or twice daily; may increase weekly by 50 mg daily up to the recommended dose of 100-200 mg twice daily (maximum recommended dose: 800 mg daily; doses >400 mg daily have shown no additional benefit).

Migraine prophylaxis: Adolescents ≥12 years and Adults: Oral: Immediate release: Initial: 25 mg once daily (in evening); may increase weekly by 25 mg daily up to the recommended dose of 100 mg daily given in 2 divided doses. Increased intervals between dose adjustments may be considered. Doses >100 mg daily have shown no additional benefit.

Cluster headache prophylaxis (off-label use): Adults: Initial: 25 mg daily, titrated at weekly intervals in 25 mg increments, up to 200 mg daily (Pascual, 2007)

Dosage adjustment in renal impairment: CrCl <70 mL/minute/1.73 m^2: Administer 50% dose and titrate more slowly

Hemodialysis: Supplemental dose may be needed during hemodialysis

Dosage adjustment in hepatic impairment: There are no dosage adjustments provided in the manufacturer's labeling. However, topiramate clearance in hepatic impairment may be reduced. Use with caution.

Administration Administer without regard to meals. Administer the immediate release formulation in divided doses. It is not recommended to crush, break, or chew immediate release tablets due to bitter taste. Swallow extended release (ER) and sprinkle capsules whole. Sprinkle capsules and Qudexy XR capsules may also be opened to sprinkle the entire contents on a small amount (~1 teaspoon) of soft food; swallow immediately and do not chew. Do not store drug/food mixture for future use. Do not sprinkle Trokendi XR capsules on food, chew, or crush. Avoid alcohol use with Trokendi XR capsules within 6 hours prior to and 6 hours after administration.

Hazardous agent; use appropriate precautions for handling and disposal (NIOSH 2014 [group 3]).

Monitoring Parameters Seizure frequency, hydration status; electrolytes (recommended monitoring includes serum bicarbonate at baseline and periodically during treatment), serum creatinine; monitor for symptoms of acute acidosis and complications of long-term acidosis (nephrolithiasis, nephrocalcinosis, osteomalacia/osteoporosis, and reduced growth rates and/or weight in children); ammonia level in patients with unexplained lethargy, vomiting, or mental status changes; intraocular pressure, symptoms of secondary angle closure glaucoma; suicidality (eg, suicidal thoughts, depression, behavioral changes)

Additional Information May be associated with weight loss in some patients

Dosage Forms

Capsule ER 24 Hour Sprinkle, Oral:

Qudexy XR: 25 mg (30 ea, 500 ea); 50 mg (30 ea, 500 ea); 100 mg (30 ea, 500 ea); 150 mg (30 ea, 500 ea); 200 mg (30 ea, 500 ea)

Generic: 25 mg (30 ea, 500 ea); 50 mg (30 ea, 500 ea); 100 mg (30 ea, 500 ea); 150 mg (30 ea, 500 ea); 200 mg (30 ea, 500 ea)

Capsule Extended Release 24 Hour, Oral:

Trokendi XR: 25 mg, 50 mg, 100 mg, 200 mg

Capsule Sprinkle, Oral:

Topamax Sprinkle: 15 mg, 25 mg

Generic: 15 mg, 25 mg

Tablet, Oral:

Topamax: 25 mg, 50 mg, 100 mg, 200 mg

Topiragen: 25 mg, 50 mg, 100 mg, 200 mg

Generic: 25 mg, 50 mg, 100 mg, 200 mg

Dosage Forms: Canada Refer to Dosage Forms. **Note:** Extended release capsules not available in Canada.

Extemporaneous Preparations Hazardous agent; use appropriate precautions for handling and disposal (NIOSH 2014 [group 3]).

A 6 mg/mL topiramate oral suspension may be made with tablets and one of two different vehicles (a 1:1 mixture of Ora-Sweet and Ora-Plus, or a mixture of Simple Syrup, NF and methylcellulose 1% with parabens). Crush six 100 mg tablets in a mortar and reduce to a fine powder. Add a small amount of methylcellulose gel and mix to a uniform paste (**Note:** Use a small amount of methylcellulose gel when using the 1:1 Ora-Sweet and Ora-Plus mixture as the vehicle; use 10 mL methylcellulose 1% with parabens when using Simple Syrup, NF as the vehicle); mix while adding the chosen vehicle in incremental proportions to **almost** 100 mL; transfer to a graduated cylinder; rinse mortar with vehicle, and add quantity of vehicle sufficient to make 100 mL. Store in plastic prescription bottles; label "shake well" and "refrigerate". Stable for 90 days refrigerated (preferred) or at room temperature.

Nahata MC, Pai VB, and Hipple TF, *Pediatric Drug Formulations*, 5th ed, Cincinnati, OH: Harvey Whitney Books Co, 2004.

◆ **Toposar** *see* Etoposide *on page 816*

Topotecan (toe poe TEE kan)

Brand Names: U.S. Hycamtin

Brand Names: Canada Hycamtin; Topotecan For Injection; Topotecan Hydrochloride For Injection

Index Terms Hycamptamine; SKF 104864; SKF 104864-A; Topotecan Hydrochloride

Pharmacologic Category Antineoplastic Agent, Camptothecin; Antineoplastic Agent, Topoisomerase I Inhibitor

Use

Cervical cancer: Treatment of recurrent or resistant (stage IVB) cervical cancer (in combination with cisplatin) which is not amenable to curative treatment with surgery and/or radiation therapy

Ovarian cancer: Treatment of metastatic ovarian cancer after failure of initial or subsequent chemotherapy

Small cell lung cancer: Treatment of relapsed or refractory small cell lung cancer (SCLC) in patients with a prior complete or partial response and who are at least 2 to 3 months from the end of first-line chemotherapy

Pregnancy Risk Factor D

Pregnancy Considerations Adverse effects were observed in animal reproduction studies. May cause fetal harm in pregnant women. Women of childbearing potential should use highly effective contraception to prevent pregnancy during treatment and for at least 1 month after therapy discontinuation.

Breast-Feeding Considerations It is not known if topotecan is excreted in breast milk. Due to the potential for serious adverse reactions in the nursing infant, the manufacturer recommends to discontinue breast-feeding in women who are receiving topotecan.

Contraindications

Hypersensitivity to topotecan or any component of the formulation; severe bone marrow depression (IV formulation)

Canadian labeling: Additional contraindications (not in U.S. labeling): Severe renal impairment (CrCl <20 mL/minute); pregnancy; breast-feeding

Warnings/Precautions Hazardous agent - use appropriate precautions for handling and disposal (NIOSH 2014 [group 1]). **[U.S. Boxed Warning]: May cause neutropenia, which may be severe or lead to infection or fatalities. Monitor blood counts frequently. Do NOT administer to patients with baseline neutrophils <1500/mm^3 and platelets <100,000/mm^3.** The dose-limiting toxicity is bone marrow suppression (primarily neutropenia); may also cause thrombocytopenia and anemia. Neutropenia is not cumulative overtime. Nadir neutrophil, platelet, and red blood cell counts occurred at a median of 12 days, 15 days, and 15 days, respectively. In a clinical study comparing IV to oral topotecan, G-CSF support was administered in a higher percentage of patients receiving oral topotecan (Eckardt, 2007). Bone marrow suppression may require dosage reduction and/or growth factor support. Topotecan-induced neutropenia may lead to neutropenic colitis (including fatalities); should be considered in patients presenting with neutropenia, fever and abdominal pain.

Diarrhea has been reported with oral topotecan; may be severe (requiring hospitalization); incidence may be higher in the elderly; educate patients on early recognition and proper management, including diet changes, increase in fluid intake, antidiarrheals, and antibiotics. The median time to onset of diarrhea (grade 2 or worse) was 9 days. The incidence of diarrhea may be higher in the elderly. Do not administer in patients with grade 3 or 4 diarrhea; reduce dose upon recovery to ≤ grade 1 toxicity. Interstitial lung disease (ILD) (with fatalities) has been reported; discontinue use in patients with confirmed ILD diagnosis; risk factors for ILD include a history of ILD, pulmonary fibrosis, lung cancer, thoracic radiation, and the use of colony-stimulating factors or medication with pulmonary toxicity; monitor pulmonary symptoms (cough, fever, dyspnea, and/or hypoxia). Use caution in renal impairment; may require dose adjustment (use in severe renal impairment is contraindicated in the Canadian labeling). Potentially significant drug-drug interactions may exist, requiring dose or frequency adjustment, additional monitoring, and/or selection of alternative therapy. Topotecan exposure is increased when oral topotecan is used concurrently with P-glycoprotein inhibitors; avoid concurrent use. Topotecan overdoses have been reported; potential causes include omission of the leading zero and missing the decimal point when prescribing, preparing, and administering. Recommended intravenous doses should generally not exceed 4 mg in adults; verify dose prior to administration.

Adverse Reactions

Central nervous system: Fatigue, fever, headache, pain

Dermatologic: Alopecia (reversible), rash

Gastrointestinal: Abdominal pain, anorexia, constipation, diarrhea, nausea, obstruction, stomatitis, vomiting

Hematologic: Anemia, leukopenia, neutropenia (nadir 8-11 days; recovery <21 days), neutropenic fever/sepsis, thrombocytopenia

Hepatic: BUN increased, liver enzymes increased (transient)

Neuromuscular & skeletal: Paresthesia, weakness

Respiratory: Cough, dyspnea, pneumonia

Miscellaneous: Infection, sepsis

Rare but important or life-threatening: Allergic reactions, anaphylactoid reactions, angioedema, bleeding (severe, associated with thrombocytopenia), dermatitis (severe), extravasation (inadvertent), interstitial lung disease (ILD), neutropenic colitis, pancytopenia, pruritus (severe)

Drug Interactions

Metabolism/Transport Effects Substrate of BCRP

Avoid Concomitant Use

Avoid concomitant use of Topotecan with any of the following: BCG; CloZAPine; Dipyrone; Natalizumab; P-glycoprotein/ABCB1 Inhibitors; Pimecrolimus; Tacrolimus (Topical); Tofacitinib; Vaccines (Live)

Increased Effect/Toxicity

Topotecan may increase the levels/effects of: CloZAPine; Leflunomide; Natalizumab; Tofacitinib; Vaccines (Live)

The levels/effects of Topotecan may be increased by: BCRP/ABCG2 Inhibitors; Denosumab; Dipyrone; Filgrastim; P-glycoprotein/ABCB1 Inhibitors; Pimecrolimus; Platinum Derivatives; Roflumilast; Tacrolimus (Topical); Trastuzumab

Decreased Effect

Topotecan may decrease the levels/effects of: BCG; Coccidioides immitis Skin Test; Sipuleucel-T; Vaccines (Inactivated); Vaccines (Live)

The levels/effects of Topotecan may be decreased by: Echinacea; Fosphenytoin-Phenytoin

Preparation for Administration Hazardous agent; use appropriate precautions for handling and disposal (NIOSH 2014 [group 1]). Reconstitute lyophilized powder with 4 mL SWFI. Reconstituted lyophilized powder and solution for injection should be further diluted in D_5W or NS for infusion.

Storage/Stability

IV:

Solution for injection: Store intact vials at 2°C to 8°C (36°F to 45°F). Protect from light. Single-use vials should be discarded after initial vial entry. Stability of solutions diluted for infusion is variable; refer to specific product information for details.

Lyophilized powder: Store intact vials at 20°C to 25°C (68°F to 77°F). Protect from light. Reconstituted solution is stable for up to 28 days at 20°C to 25°C (68°F to 77°F), although the manufacturer recommends use immediately after reconstitution. Solutions diluted in D_5W or NS are stable for 24 hours at room temperature (manufacturer recommendation) or up to 7 days under refrigeration (Craig, 1997). Reconstituted solution for injection (reconstituted with bacteriostatic SWFI to 1 mg/mL) for oral administration is stable for 14 days at 4°C in plastic syringes (Daw, 2004).

Oral: Store at 2°C to 8°C (36°F to 46°F). Protect from light.

Mechanism of Action Binds to topoisomerase I and stabilizes the cleavable complex so that religation of the cleaved DNA strand cannot occur. This results in the accumulation of cleavable complexes and single-strand DNA breaks. Topotecan acts in S phase of the cell cycle.

Pharmacodynamics/Kinetics

Absorption: Oral: Rapid

Distribution: V_d: 25 to 75 L/m^2 (Hartmann, 2006)

Protein binding: ~35%

Metabolism: Undergoes a rapid, pH-dependent hydrolysis of the lactone ring to yield a relatively inactive hydroxy acid in plasma; metabolized in the liver to N-demethylated metabolite

Bioavailability: Oral: ~40%

Half-life elimination: IV: 2 to 3 hours; renal impairment: ~5 hours; Oral: 3 to 6 hours

Time to peak, plasma: Oral: 1 to 2 hours; delayed with high-fat meal (3 to 4 hours)

Excretion:

IV: Urine (51%; 3% as N-desmethyl topotecan); feces (18%; 2% as N-desmethyl topotecan)

Oral: Urine (20%; 2% as N-desmethyl topotecan); feces (33%; <2% as N-desmethyl topotecan)

Dosage Note: Baseline neutrophil count should be ≥1500/mm^3 and platelets should be ≥100,000/mm^3 prior to treatment; for retreatment, neutrophil count should be >1000/mm^3; platelets >100,000/mm^3 and hemoglobin ≥9 g/dL. Intravenous doses should generally not exceed 4 mg; verify dose prior to administration.

Cervical cancer, recurrent or resistant: Adults: IV: 0.75 mg/m^2/day for 3 days (followed by cisplatin on day 1 only [with hydration]) every 21 days

Ovarian cancer, metastatic: Adults: IV: 1.5 mg/m^2/day for 5 consecutive days every 21 days, minimum of 4 cycles recommended in the absence of tumor progression **or** (off-label dosing) 1.25 mg/m^2/day for 5 days every 21 days until disease progression or unacceptable toxicity or a maximum of 12 months (Sehouli, 2011) **or** (weekly administration; off-label dosing) 4 mg/m^2 on days 1, 8, and 15 every 28 days until disease progression or unacceptable toxicity or a maximum of 12 months (Sehouli, 2011)

Small cell lung cancer (SCLC), relapsed or refractory: Adults:

IV: 1.5 mg/m^2/day for 5 consecutive days every 21 days, minimum of 4 cycles recommended in the absence of tumor progression

Oral: 2.3 mg/m^2/day for 5 consecutive days every 21 days (round dose to the nearest 0.25 mg); if patient vomits after dose is administered, do not give a replacement dose.

CNS malignancy, recurrent/refractory (off-label use; based on limited data): Children: Oral: 0.8 mg/m^2/day for 21 consecutive days every 4 weeks for ≥12 cycles (Minturn, 2011); additional data may be necessary to further define the role of topotecan in this condition

Ewing's sarcoma, relapsed/refractory or metastatic (off-label use): Children and Adults: IV: 0.75 mg/m^2/day for 5 consecutive days every 21 days (in combination with cyclophosphamide) (Hunold, 2006; Saylors, 2001)

Neuroblastoma, relapsed/refractory (off-label use): Children: IV: 0.75 mg/m^2/day for 5 days every 21 days (in combination with cyclophosphamide) (Ashraf, 2013; London, 2010) **or** 2 mg/m^2/day for 5 days every 21 days (monotherapy) (London, 2010)

Rhabdomyosarcoma, metastatic (off-label use): Children and Adults <21 years: IV: 0.75 mg/m^2/day for 5 consecutive days every 21 days for 2 cycles (window therapy; in combination with cyclophosphamide); if objective response occurred by week 6, follow with alternating cycles of vincristine, topotecan, and cyclophosphamide (VTC) with vincristine, dactinomycin, and cyclophosphamide (VAC) (Walterhouse, 2004)

Dosage adjustment for toxicity:

Cervical cancer (cisplatin may also require dosage adjustment): IV: Severe febrile neutropenia (<1000/mm^3 with temperature of 38°C) or platelet count <25,000/mm^3: Reduce topotecan to 0.6 mg/m^2/day for subsequent cycles (may consider G-CSF support [beginning on day 4] prior to instituting dose reduction for neutropenic fever).

For neutropenic fever despite G-CSF use, reduce dose to 0.45 mg/m^2/day for subsequent cycles.

Ovarian cancer: IV: Dosage adjustment for hematological effects: Severe neutropenia (<500/mm^3) or platelet count <25,000/mm^3: Reduce dose to 1.25 mg/m^2/day for subsequent cycles (may consider G-CSF support [beginning on day 6] prior to instituting dose reduction for severe neutropenia). **Note:** The Canadian labeling states that the dose may be further reduced to 1 mg/m^2/day if necessary.

Small cell lung cancer (SCLC):

IV: Dosage adjustment for hematological effects: Severe neutropenia (<500/mm^3) or platelet count <25,000/mm^3: Reduce dose to 1.25 mg/m^2/day for subsequent cycles (may consider G-CSF support [beginning on day 6] prior to instituting dose reduction for severe neutropenia). **Note:** The Canadian labeling states that the dose may be further reduced to 1 mg/m^2/day if necessary.

Oral:

Severe neutropenia (neutrophils <500/mm^3 associated with fever or infection or lasting ≥7 days) or prolonged neutropenia (neutrophils 500/mm^3 to 1000/mm^3 lasting beyond day 21) or platelets <25,000/mm^3: Reduce dose by 0.4 mg/m^2/day for subsequent cycles.

Diarrhea (grade 3 or 4): Do not administer to patients with grade 3 or 4 diarrhea. Upon recovery to ≤ grade 1 toxicity, reduce dose by 0.4 mg/m^2/day for subsequent cycles.

Dosage adjustment in renal impairment:

Manufacturer's recommendations:

IV:

CrCl ≥40 mL/minute: No dosage adjustment necessary.

CrCl 20 to 39 mL/minute: Reduce dose to 0.75 mg/m^2/dose

CrCl <20 mL/minute: There are no dosage adjustments provided in manufacturer's U.S. labeling (insufficient data available for dosing recommendation); use is contraindicated in the Canadian labeling.

Note: For topotecan in combination with cisplatin for cervical cancer, do not initiate treatment in patients with serum creatinine >1.5 mg/dL; consider discontinuing treatment in patients with serum creatinine >1.5 mg/dL in subsequent cycles.

Oral:

CrCl ≥50 mL/minute: No dosage adjustment necessary.

CrCl 30 to 49 mL/minute: Reduce dose to 1.5 mg/m^2/day; may increase after the 1st cycle by 0.4 mg/m^2/day if no severe hematologic or gastrointestinal toxicities occur.

CrCl <30 mL/minute: Reduce dose to 0.6 mg/m^2/day; may increase after the 1st cycle by 0.4 mg/m^2/day if no severe hematologic or gastrointestinal toxicities occur.

Alternate recommendations:

Aronoff, 2007: IV:

Children:

CrCl 30 to 50 mL/minute: Administer 75% of dose

CrCl 10 to 29 mL/minute: Administer 50% of dose

CrCl <10 mL/minute: Administer 25% of dose

Continuous renal replacement therapy (CRRT): Administer 50% of dose

Adults:

CrCl >50 mL/minute: Administer 75% of dose

CrCl 10 to 50 mL/minute: Administer 50% of dose

CrCl <10 mL/minute: Administer 25% of dose

Hemodialysis: Avoid use

Continuous ambulatory peritoneal dialysis (CAPD): Avoid use

Continuous renal replacement therapy (CRRT): 0.75 mg/m^2

Kintzel, 1995: IV:

CrCl 46 to 60 mL/minute: Administer 80% of dose

CrCl 31 to 45 mL/minute: Administer 75% of dose

CrCl ≤30 mL/minute: Administer 70% of dose

Dosage adjustment in hepatic impairment: *Manufacturer's labeling:*

IV: Bilirubin 1.7 to 15 mg/dL (U.S. labeling) or >1.5 to <10 mg/dL (Canadian labeling): No dosage adjustment necessary (the half-life is increased slightly; usual doses are generally tolerated).

Oral: There is no dosage adjustment provided in the manufacturer's labeling; however, dosage adjustment is likely not necessary as the pharmacokinetics of topotecan do not differ significantly based on serum bilirubin, ALT, or AST.

Dosing in obesity: *ASCO Guidelines for appropriate chemotherapy dosing in obese adults with cancer:* Utilize patient's actual body weight (full weight) for calculation of body surface area- or weight-based dosing, particularly when the intent of therapy is curative; manage regimen-related toxicities in the same manner as for nonobese patients; if a dose reduction is utilized due to toxicity, consider resumption of full weight-based dosing with subsequent cycles, especially if cause of toxicity (eg, hepatic or renal impairment) is resolved (Griggs, 2012).

Administration

IV: Administer IVPB over 30 minutes. For combination chemotherapy with cisplatin, administer pretreatment hydration.

Oral: Administer without regard to meals. Swallow whole; do not open, crush, chew, or divide capsule. If vomiting occurs after dose, do not take replacement dose. For patients unable to swallow capsules whole, reconstituted topotecan solution for injection (1 mg/mL concentration) may be mixed with up to 30 mL of acidic fruit juice (eg, apple, orange, grape) immediately prior to oral administration (Daw, 2004).

Hazardous agent; use appropriate precautions for handling and disposal (NIOSH 2014 [group 1]).

Monitoring Parameters CBC with differential and platelet count, renal function tests, bilirubin; monitor for symptoms of interstitial lung disease; diarrhea symptoms/hydration status

Dosage Forms

Capsule, Oral:

Hycamtin: 0.25 mg, 1 mg

Solution, Intravenous:

Generic: 4 mg/4 mL (4 mL)

Solution, Intravenous [preservative free]:

Generic: 4 mg/4 mL (4 mL)

Solution Reconstituted, Intravenous:

Hycamtin: 4 mg (1 ea)

Generic: 4 mg (1 ea)

Solution Reconstituted, Intravenous [preservative free]:

Generic: 4 mg (1 ea)

Extemporaneous Preparations

Hazardous agent; use appropriate precautions for handling and disposal (NIOSH 2014 [group 1]).

For patients unable to swallow capsules whole, reconstituted topotecan solution for injection (1 mg/mL concentration) may be mixed with up to 30 mL of acidic fruit juice (eg, apple, orange, grape) immediately prior to oral administration.

Daw NC, Santana VM, Iacono LC, et al. Phase I and pharmacokinetic study of topotecan administered orally once daily for 5 days for 2 consecutive weeks to pediatric patients with refractory solid tumors. *J Clin Oncol*. 2004;22(5):829-837.

◆ **Topotecan For Injection (Can)** *see* Topotecan *on page 2069*

◆ **Topotecan Hydrochloride** *see* Topotecan *on page 2069*

◆ **Topotecan Hydrochloride For Injection (Can)** *see* Topotecan *on page 2069*

◆ **Toprol XL** *see* Metoprolol *on page 1350*

◆ **Topsyn® (Can)** *see* Fluocinonide *on page 894*

◆ **Toradol** *see* Ketorolac (Systemic) *on page 1146*

◆ **Toradol® (Can)** *see* Ketorolac (Systemic) *on page 1146*

◆ **Toradol® IM (Can)** *see* Ketorolac (Systemic) *on page 1146*

◆ **Torasemide** *see* Torsemide *on page 2071*

Toremifene (tore EM i feen)

Brand Names: U.S. Fareston

Brand Names: Canada Fareston®

Index Terms FC1157a; Toremifene Citrate

Pharmacologic Category Antineoplastic Agent, Estrogen Receptor Antagonist; Selective Estrogen Receptor Modulator (SERM)

Use Treatment of metastatic breast cancer in postmenopausal women with estrogen receptor positive or estrogen receptor status unknown

Pregnancy Risk Factor D

Dosage Oral: Adults: Metastatic breast cancer (postmenopausal): 60 mg once daily, continue until disease progression

Dosage adjustment in renal impairment: No dosage adjustment necessary.

Dosage adjustment in hepatic impairment: No dosage adjustment provided in manufacturer's labeling. However, hepatic impairment increases systemic exposure to toremifene. Use with caution.

Additional Information Complete prescribing information should be consulted for additional detail.

Dosage Forms

Tablet, Oral:

Fareston: 60 mg

◆ **Toremifene Citrate** *see* Toremifene *on page 2071*

◆ **Torezolid** *see* Tedizolid *on page 1981*

◆ **Torisel** *see* Temsirolimus *on page 1994*

Torsemide (TORE se mide)

Brand Names: U.S. Demadex

Index Terms Torasemide

Pharmacologic Category Antihypertensive; Diuretic, Loop

Use

Management of edema associated with heart failure and hepatic or renal disease (including chronic renal failure); treatment of hypertension

Note: According to the Eighth Joint National Committee (JNC 8) guidelines, loop diuretics are not recommended for the initial treatment of hypertension (James, 2013). In patients with chronic kidney disease (ie, eGFR <30 mL/minute/1.73 m^2), the American Society of Hypertension/International Society of Hypertension (ASH/ISH) suggests that the use of a loop diuretic may be necessary (Weber, 2014).

Pregnancy Risk Factor B

Pregnancy Considerations A decrease in fetal weight, an increase in fetal resorption, and delayed fetal ossification has occurred in animal studies.

Breast-Feeding Considerations It is not known if torsemide is excreted in breast milk. The manufacturer recommends that caution be exercised when administering torsemide to nursing women.

Contraindications Hypersensitivity to torsemide, any component of the formulation, or any sulfonylurea; anuria

Warnings/Precautions Loop diuretics are potent diuretics; excess amounts can lead to profound diuresis with fluid and electrolyte loss; close medical supervision and dose evaluation are required. Potassium supplementation and/or use of potassium-sparing diuretics may be necessary to prevent hypokalemia. Use with caution in patients with cirrhosis; avoid sudden changes in fluid and electrolyte balance and acid/base status which may lead to hepatic encephalopathy. Administration with an aldosterone antagonist or potassium-sparing diuretic may provide additional diuretic efficacy and maintain normokalemia. Coadministration of antihypertensives may increase the risk of hypotension.

Monitor fluid status and renal function in an attempt to prevent oliguria, azotemia, and reversible increases in BUN and creatinine; close medical supervision of aggressive diuresis required. Ototoxicity has been demonstrated following oral administration of torsemide and following rapid IV administration of other loop diuretics. Other possible risk factors may include use in renal impairment, excessive doses, and concurrent use of other ototoxins (eg, aminoglycosides).

Chemical similarities are present among sulfonamides, sulfonylureas, carbonic anhydrase inhibitors, thiazides, and loop diuretics (except ethacrynic acid). Use in patients with sulfonylurea allergy is specifically contraindicated in product labeling; a risk of cross-reaction exists in patients with allergy to any of these compounds; avoid use when previous reaction has been severe. Discontinue if signs of hypersensitivity are noted.

Adverse Reactions

Cardiovascular: Chest pain, ECG abnormality

Central nervous system: Nervousness

Gastrointestinal: Constipation, diarrhea, dyspepsia, nausea, sore throat

Genitourinary: Excessive urination

Neuromuscular & skeletal: Arthralgia, myalgia, weakness

Respiratory: Cough, rhinitis

Rare but important or life-threatening: Angioedema, arthritis, atrial fibrillation, esophageal hemorrhage, GI hemorrhage, hyperglycemia, hyperuricemia, hypokalemia, hyponatremia, hypotension, hypovolemia, impotence, leukopenia, pancreatitis, rash, rectal bleeding, shunt thrombosis, Stevens-Johnson syndrome, syncope, thirst, thrombocytopenia, toxic epidermal necrolysis, ventricular tachycardia, vomiting

Drug Interactions

Metabolism/Transport Effects **Substrate** of CYP2C8 (minor), CYP2C9 (major), SLCO1B1; **Note:** Assignment of Major/Minor substrate status based on clinically relevant drug interaction potential

Avoid Concomitant Use There are no known interactions where it is recommended to avoid concomitant use.

Increased Effect/Toxicity

Torsemide may increase the levels/effects of: ACE Inhibitors; Allopurinol; Amifostine; Aminoglycosides; Antihypertensives; Cardiac Glycosides; CISplatin; Dofetilide; DULoxetine; Foscarnet; Hypotensive Agents; Ivabradine; Levodopa; Lithium; Methotrexate; Neuromuscular-Blocking Agents; Obinutuzumab; RisperiDONE; RiTUXimab; Salicylates; Sodium Phosphates; Topiramate; Warfarin

The levels/effects of Torsemide may be increased by: Alfuzosin; Analgesics (Opioid); Barbiturates; Beta2-Agonists; Brimonidine (Topical); Canagliflozin; Ceritinib; Corticosteroids (Orally Inhaled); Corticosteroids (Systemic); CycloSPORINE (Systemic); CYP2C9 Inhibitors (Moderate); CYP2C9 Inhibitors (Strong); Diazoxide; Eltrombopag; Herbs (Hypotensive Properties); Licorice; MAO Inhibitors; Methotrexate; Mifepristone; Nicorandil; Pentoxifylline; Phosphodiesterase 5 Inhibitors; Probenecid; Prostacyclin Analogues; Teriflunomide

Decreased Effect

Torsemide may decrease the levels/effects of: Hypoglycemic Agents; Lithium; Neuromuscular-Blocking Agents

The levels/effects of Torsemide may be decreased by: Bile Acid Sequestrants; CYP2C9 Inducers (Strong); Dabrafenib; Herbs (Hypertensive Properties); Methotrexate; Methylphenidate; Nonsteroidal Anti-Inflammatory Agents; Probenecid; Salicylates; Yohimbine

Storage/Stability

IV: Store at 15°C to 30°C (59°F to 86°F). If torsemide is to be administered via continuous infusion, stability has been demonstrated through 24 hours at room temperature in plastic containers for the following fluids and concentrations:

200 mg torsemide (10 mg/mL) added to 250 mL D_5W, 250 mL NS or 500 mL 0.45% sodium chloride

50 mg torsemide (10 mg/mL) added to 500 mL D_5W, 500 mL NS, or 500 mL 0.45% sodium chloride

Tablets: Store at 15°C to 30°C (59°F to 86°F).

Mechanism of Action Inhibits reabsorption of sodium and chloride in the ascending loop of Henle and distal renal tubule, interfering with the chloride-binding cotransport system, thus causing increased excretion of water, sodium, chloride, magnesium, and calcium; does not alter GFR, renal plasma flow, or acid-base balance

Pharmacodynamics/Kinetics

Onset of action: Diuresis: Oral: Within 1hour

Peak effect: Diuresis: Oral: 1-2 hours; Antihypertensive: Oral: 4-6 weeks (up to 12 weeks)

Duration: Diuresis: Oral: ~6-8 hours

Absorption: Oral: Rapid

Distribution: V_d: 12-15 L; Cirrhosis: Approximately doubled

Protein binding: >99%

Metabolism: Hepatic (~80%) via CYP

Bioavailability: ~80%

Half-life elimination: ~3.5 hours; Cirrhosis: 7-8 hours

Time to peak, plasma: Oral: 1 hour; delayed ~30 minutes when administered with food

Excretion: Urine (~20% as unchanged drug)

Dosage Adults: **Note:** IV and oral dosing are equivalent.

Edema:

Chronic renal failure: Oral, IV: Initial: 20 mg once daily; may increase gradually by doubling dose until the desired diuretic response is obtained (maximum recommended daily dose: 200 mg)

Heart failure:

Oral: Initial: 10 to 20 mg once daily; may increase gradually by doubling dose until the desired diuretic response is obtained. **Note:** ACCF/AHA 2013 guidelines for heart failure maximum recommended daily dose: 200 mg (Yancy, 2013).

IV: Initial: 10 to 20 mg; may repeat every 2 hours with double the dose as needed.

Continuous IV infusion (off-label dose): Initial: 20 mg IV load, then 5 to 20 mg/hour; repeat loading dose before increasing infusion rate. **Note:** With lower baseline creatinine clearance (eg, CrCl <25 mL/minute), the upper end of the initial infusion dosage range should be considered (ACCF/AHA [Yancy, 2013]; Brater, 1998).

Hepatic cirrhosis: Oral: Initial: 5 to 10 mg once daily; may increase gradually by doubling dose until the desired diuretic response is obtained (maximum recommended single dose: 40 mg). **Note:** Administer with an aldosterone antagonist or a potassium-sparing diuretic.

Hypertension: Oral: Initial: 5 mg once daily; may increase to 10 mg once daily after 4 to 6 weeks if adequate antihypertensive response is not apparent; if still not effective, an additional antihypertensive agent may be added. Usual dosage range (ASH/ISH [Weber, 2014]): 10 mg daily.

Dosage adjustment in renal impairment: No dosage adjustment necessary. However, higher doses may be required to achieve diuretic response.

Dosage adjustment in hepatic impairment: There are no dosage adjustments provided in manufacturer's labeling; use with caution.

Dietary Considerations May be taken without regard to meals; however, food slows the rate and reduces the extent of absorption and may reduce diuretic efficacy (Bard, 2004). May require increased intake of potassium-rich foods.

Administration

IV: Administer over ≥2 minutes; reserve IV administration for situations which require rapid onset of action

Oral: Administer without regard to meals; patients may be switched from the IV form to the oral (and vice-versa) with no change in dose

Monitoring Parameters Renal function, electrolytes, and fluid status (weight and I & O), blood pressure

Additional Information 10-20 mg torsemide is approximately equivalent to furosemide 40 mg or bumetanide 1 mg.

Dosage Forms

Solution, Intravenous:

Generic: 20 mg/2 mL (2 mL); 50 mg/5 mL (5 mL)

Tablet, Oral:

Demadex: 5 mg, 10 mg, 20 mg, 100 mg

Generic: 5 mg, 10 mg, 20 mg, 100 mg

◆ **Total Allergy [OTC]** *see* DiphenhydrAMINE (Systemic) *on page 641*

◆ **Total Allergy Medicine [OTC]** *see* DiphenhydrAMINE (Systemic) *on page 641*

Total Parenteral Nutrition

(TOE tal par EN ter al noo TRISH un)

Brand Names: U.S. Kabiven

Index Terms Hyperal; Hyperalimentation; Parenteral Nutrition; PN; TPN

Pharmacologic Category Caloric Agent; Intravenous Nutritional Therapy

Use Infusion of nutrient solutions into the bloodstream to support nutritional needs during a time when patient is unable to absorb nutrients via the gastrointestinal tract, cannot take adequate nutrition orally or enterally, or have had (or are expected to have) inadequate oral intake for 7-14 days.

Dosage PN is a highly-individualized therapy. The following general guidelines may be used in the estimation of needs. Electrolytes, vitamins, and trace minerals should be added to TPN mixtures based on patients individualized needs.

Children: IV: **Note:** Give within 5-7 days if unable to meet needs orally or with enteral nutrition:

Total calories:

<6 months: 85-105 kcal/kg/day

6-12 months: 80-100 kcal/kg/day

1-7 years: 75-90 kcal/kg/day

7-12 years: 50-75 kcal/kg/day

12-18 years: 30-50 kcal/kg/day

Fluid:

2-10 kg: 100 mL/kg

>10-20 kg: 1000 mL for 10 kg plus 50 mL/kg for each kg >10

>20 kg: 1500 mL for 10 kg plus 20 mL/kg for each kg >20

Carbohydrate (dextrose): 40% to 50% of caloric intake

<1 year: Initial: 6-8 mg/kg/minute; goal: 10-14 mg/kg/minute

1-10 years: Initial: 10% to 12.5%; daily increase: 5% increments (maximum: 15 mg/kg/minute)

>10 years: Initial: 10% to 15%; daily increase: 5% increments (maximum: 8.5 mg/kg/minute)

Protein (amino acids):

1-12 months: Initial: 2-3 g/kg/day; daily increase: 1 g/kg/day (maximum: 3 g/kg/day)

1-10 years: Initial: 1-2 g/kg/day; daily increase: 1 g/kg/day (maximum: 2-2.5 g/kg/day)

>10 years: Initial: 0.8-1.5 g/kg/day; daily increase: 1 g/kg/day (maximum: 1.5-2 g/kg/day)

Fat: Initial: 1 g/kg/day; daily increase: 1 g/kg/day (maximum: 3 g/kg/day); **Note:** Monitor triglycerides while receiving intralipids.

Adults: IV:

Total calories: Calculate using Harris-Benedict equation or based on stress level as indicated below:

Harris-Benedict Equation (BEE):

Females: 655.1 + [(9.56 x W) + (1.85 x H) - (4.68 x A)]

Males: 66.47 + [(13.75 x W) + (5 x H) - (6.76 x A)]

Then multiply BEE x (activity factor) x (stress factor)

W = weight in kg; H = height in cm; A = age in years

Activity factor = 1.2 sedentary, 1.3 normal activity, 1.4 active, 1.5 very active

Stress factor = 1.5 for trauma, stressed, or surgical patients and underweight (to promote weight gain); 2.0 for severe burn patients

Stress level:

Normal/mild stress level: 20-25 kcal/kg/day

Moderate stress level: 25-30 kcal/kg/day

Severe stress level: 30-40 kcal/kg/day

Pregnant women in second or third trimester: Add an additional 300 kcal/day

Fluid: mL/day = 30-40 mL/kg

Carbohydrate (dextrose):

5 g/kg/day or 3.5 mg/kg/minute (maximum rate: 4-7 mg/kg/minute)

Minimum recommended amount: 400 calories/day or 100 g/day

Protein (amino acids):

Maintenance: 0.8-1 g/kg/day

Normal/mild stress level: 1-1.2 g/kg/day

Moderate stress level: 1.2-1.5 g/kg/day

Severe stress level: 1.5-2 g/kg/day

Burn patients (severe): Increase protein until significant wound healing achieved

Solid organ transplant: Perioperative: 1.5-2 g/kg/day

Renal failure:
Acute (severely malnourished or hypercatabolic): 1.5-1.8 g/kg/day
Chronic, with dialysis: 1.2-1.3 g/kg/day
Chronic, without dialysis: 0.6-0.8 g/kg/day
Continuous hemofiltration: ≥1 g/kg/day
Hepatic failure:
Acute management when other treatments have failed:
With encephalopathy: 0.6-1 g/kg/day
Without encephalopathy: 1-1.5 g/kg/day
Chronic encephalopathy: Use branch chain amino acid enriched diets only if unresponsive to pharmacotherapy
Pregnant women in second or third trimester: Add an additional 10-14 g/day

Fat:
Initial: 20% to 40% of total calories (maximum: 60% of total calories or 2.5 g/kg/day); **Note:** Monitor triglycerides while receiving intralipids.
Safe for use in pregnancy
IV lipids are safe in adults with pancreatitis if triglyceride levels <400 mg/dL

Additional Information Complete prescribing information should be consulted for additional detail.

Dosage Forms

Emulsion, Intravenous:
Kabiven: (1026 mL, 1540 mL, 2053 mL, 2566 mL)
Perikabiven: (1440 mL,1920 mL, 2400 mL)

◆ **Totect** *see* Dexrazoxane *on page 606*
◆ **Toviaz** *see* Fesoterodine *on page 872*
◆ **tPA** *see* Alteplase *on page 99*
◆ **TPN** *see* Total Parenteral Nutrition *on page 2073*
◆ **TPV** *see* Tipranavir *on page 2047*
◆ **TR-700** *see* Tedizolid *on page 1981*
◆ **TR-701 FA** *see* Tedizolid *on page 1981*
◆ **tRA** *see* Tretinoin (Systemic) *on page 2096*
◆ **Tracleer** *see* Bosentan *on page 280*
◆ **Tradjenta** *see* Linagliptin *on page 1215*
◆ **Trajenta** *see* Linagliptin *on page 1215*
◆ **Tramacet (Can)** *see* Acetaminophen and Tramadol *on page 37*

TraMADol (TRA ma dole)

Brand Names: U.S. Active-Tramadol; ConZip; EnovaRX-Tramadol; Synapryn FusePaq; Ultram; Ultram ER

Brand Names: Canada Apo-Tramadol; Durela; Ralivia; Tridural; Ultram; Zytram XL

Index Terms Tramadol Hydrochloride

Pharmacologic Category Analgesic, Opioid

Use Relief of moderate to moderately-severe pain
Extended release formulations are indicated for patients requiring around-the-clock management of moderate to moderately-severe pain for an extended period of time

Pregnancy Risk Factor C

Pregnancy Considerations Adverse events were observed in animal reproduction studies. Tramadol has been shown to cross the human placenta when administered during labor. Postmarketing reports following tramadol use during pregnancy include neonatal seizures, withdrawal syndrome, fetal death, and stillbirth. Tramadol is not recommended for use during labor and delivery. Some Canadian products are contraindicated for use in pregnant women.

If chronic opioid exposure occurs in pregnancy, adverse events in the newborn (including withdrawal) may occur; monitoring of the neonate is recommended (Chou, 2009). Neonatal abstinence syndrome following opioid exposure may present with autonomic (eg, fever, temperature instability), gastrointestinal (eg, diarrhea, vomiting, poor feeding/weight gain), or neurologic (eg, high-pitched crying, increased muscle tone, irritability, seizure, tremor) symptoms (Dow, 2012; Hudak, 2012).

Breast-Feeding Considerations Tramadol is excreted into breast milk. Sixteen hours following a single 100 mg IV dose, the amount of tramadol found in breast milk was 0.1% of the maternal dose. Use is not recommended by the manufacturer for postdelivery analgesia in nursing mothers. Some Canadian products are contraindicated for use in nursing women. Nursing infants exposed to large doses of opioids should be monitored for apnea and sedation (Montgomery, 2012).

Contraindications Hypersensitivity to tramadol, opioids, or any component of the formulation
Additional contraindications for Ultram®, Rybix™ ODT, and Ultram® ER: Any situation where opioids are contraindicated, including acute intoxication with alcohol, hypnotics, centrally-acting analgesics, opioids, or psychotropic drugs
Additional contraindications for ConZip: Severe/acute bronchial asthma, hypercapnia, or significant respiratory depression in the absence of appropriately monitored setting and/or resuscitative equipment

Canadian product labeling:
Tramadol is contraindicated during or within 14 days following MAO inhibitor therapy
Extended release formulations: Additional contraindications:
Ralivia™, Tridural™: Severe (CrCl <30 mL/minute) renal dysfunction, severe (Child-Pugh class C) hepatic dysfunction
Durela™ and Zytram® XL: Severe (CrCl <30 mL/minute) renal dysfunction, severe (Child-Pugh class C) hepatic dysfunction; known or suspected mechanical GI obstruction or any disease/condition that affects bowel transit; mild, intermittent or short-duration pain that can be managed with other pain medication; management of peri-operative pain; obstructive airway, acute respiratory depression, cor pulmonale, delirium tremens, seizure disorder, severe CNS depression, increased cerebrospinal or intracranial pressure, head injury, breast-feeding, pregnancy; use during labor and delivery

Warnings/Precautions Rare but serious anaphylactoid reactions (including fatalities) often following initial dosing have been reported. Pruritus, hives, bronchospasm, angioedema, toxic epidermal necrolysis (TEN) and Stevens-Johnson syndrome also have been reported with use. Previous anaphylactoid reactions to opioids may increase risks for similar reactions to tramadol. Caution patients to swallow extended release tablets whole. Rapid release and absorption of tramadol from extended release tablets that are broken, crushed, or chewed may lead to a potentially lethal overdose. May cause CNS depression, which may impair physical or mental abilities; patients must be cautioned about performing tasks which require mental alertness (eg, operating machinery or driving). Effects with other sedative drugs or ethanol may be potentiated. May cause CNS depression and/or respiratory depression, particularly when combined with other CNS depressants. Use with caution and reduce dosage when administered to patients receiving other CNS depressants. An increased risk of seizures may occur in patients receiving serotonin reuptake inhibitors (SSRIs or anorectics), tricyclic antidepressants or other cyclic compounds (including cyclobenzaprine, promethazine), neuroleptics, drugs which may lower seizure threshold, or drugs which impair metabolism of tramadol (ie, CYP2D6 and 3A4 inhibitors). Patients with a history of seizures, or with a risk of seizures (head trauma, metabolic disorders, CNS infection, or malignancy, or during ethanol/drug withdrawal) are also at increased risk. Potentially significant drug interactions may exist, requiring dose or frequency adjustment, additional monitoring, and/or selection of alternative therapy.

Elderly (particularly >75 years of age), debilitated patients and patients with chronic respiratory disorders may be at greater risk of adverse events. Use with caution in patients with increased intracranial pressure or head injury. Avoid use in patients who are suicidal or addiction prone; use with caution in patients taking tranquilizers and/or antidepressants, or those with an emotional disturbance including depression. Healthcare provider should be alert to problems of abuse, misuse, and diversion. Use caution in heavy alcohol users. Use caution in treatment of acute abdominal conditions; may mask pain. Use tramadol with caution and reduce dosage in patients with liver disease or renal dysfunction. Avoid using extended release tablets in severe hepatic impairment. Tolerance or drug dependence may result from extended use (withdrawal symptoms have been reported); abrupt discontinuation should be avoided. Tapering of dose at the time of discontinuation limits the risk of withdrawal symptoms. Some products may contain phenylalanine.

After chronic maternal exposure to opioids, neonatal withdrawal syndrome may occur in the newborn; monitor neonate closely. Signs and symptoms include irritability, hyperactivity and abnormal sleep pattern, high pitched cry, tremor, vomiting, diarrhea and failure to gain weight. Onset, duration and severity depend on the drug used, duration of use, maternal dose, and rate of drug elimination by the newborn. Opioid withdrawal syndrome in the neonate, unlike in adults, may be life-threatening and should be treated according to protocols developed by neonatology experts.

Adverse Reactions

Cardiovascular: Chest pain, flushing, hypertension, orthostatic hypotension, peripheral edema, vasodilation

Central nervous system: Agitation, anxiety, apathy, ataxia, central nervous system stimulation, chills, confusion, depersonalization, depression, dizziness, drowsiness, euphoria, fatigue, headache, hypertonia, hypoesthesia, insomnia, lethargy, malaise, nervousness, pain, paresthesia, restlessness, rigors, sleep disorder, vertigo, withdrawal syndrome

Dermatologic: Dermatitis, diaphoresis, pruritus, skin rash

Endocrine & metabolic: Hot flash, hyperglycemia, weight loss

Gastrointestinal: Abdominal pain, anorexia, constipation, decreased appetite, diarrhea, dyspepsia, flatulence, nausea, sore throat, vomiting, xerostomia

Genitourinary: Menopausal symptoms, pelvic pain, prostatic disease, urine abnormality, urinary frequency, urinary retention, urinary tract infection

Neuromuscular & skeletal: Arthralgia, back pain, increased creatine phosphokinase, myalgia, neck pain, tremor, weakness

Ophthalmic: Blurred vision, miosis, visual disturbance

Respiratory: Bronchitis, cough, dyspnea, nasopharyngitis, pharyngitis, respiratory congestion, rhinitis, rhinorrhea, sinusitis, sneezing, upper respiratory tract infection

Miscellaneous: Accidental injury, fever, flu-like syndrome

Rare but important or life-threatening: Abnormal gait, anemia, appendicitis, bradycardia, cataract, cellulitis, cholecystitis, cholelithiasis, cognitive dysfunction, deafness, dysphagia, dysuria, ECG abnormality, edema, fecal impaction, gastroenteritis, gastrointestinal hemorrhage, gout, hematuria, hepatic failure, hypersensitivity reaction, hypoglycemia, increased blood urea nitrogen, increased gamma-glutamyl transferase, increased liver enzymes, increased serum creatinine, ischemic heart disease, menstrual disease, migraine, muscle spasm, mydriasis, night sweats, otitis, palpitations, pancreatitis, peripheral ischemia, pneumonia, proteinuria, pulmonary edema, pulmonary embolism, sedation, seizure, serotonin syndrome, skin vesicle, speech disturbance, Stevens-Johnson syndrome, stomatitis, suicidal tendencies, syncope, tachycardia, thrombocytopenia

Drug Interactions

Metabolism/Transport Effects Substrate of CYP2B6 (minor), CYP2D6 (major), CYP3A4 (major); **Note:** Assignment of Major/Minor substrate status based on clinically relevant drug interaction potential

Avoid Concomitant Use

Avoid concomitant use of TraMADol with any of the following: Azelastine (Nasal); CarBAMazepine; Conivaptan; Dapoxetine; Fusidic Acid (Systemic); Idelalisib; Orphenadrine; Paraldehyde; Thalidomide

Increased Effect/Toxicity

TraMADol may increase the levels/effects of: Alcohol (Ethyl); Alvimopan; Antipsychotic Agents; Azelastine (Nasal); Buprenorphine; CarBAMazepine; CNS Depressants; Desmopressin; Diuretics; Hydrocodone; MAO Inhibitors; Methotrimeprazine; Metoclopramide; Metyrosine; Orphenadrine; Paraldehyde; Pramipexole; ROPINIRole; Rotigotine; Selective Serotonin Reuptake Inhibitors; Serotonin Modulators; Suvorexant; Thalidomide; Tricyclic Antidepressants; Vitamin K Antagonists; Zolpidem

The levels/effects of TraMADol may be increased by: Amphetamines; Anticholinergic Agents; Antipsychotic Agents; Antipsychotic Agents (Phenothiazines); Aprepitant; Brimonidine (Topical); Cannabis; Ceritinib; Conivaptan; Cyclobenzaprine; CYP3A4 Inhibitors (Moderate); CYP3A4 Inhibitors (Strong); Dapoxetine; Dasatinib; Doxylamine; Dronabinol; Droperidol; Fosaprepitant; Fusidic Acid (Systemic); HydrOXYzine; Idelalisib; Ivacaftor; Kava Kava; Luliconazole; Magnesium Sulfate; Methotrimeprazine; Mifepristone; Nabilone; Netupitant; Perampanel; Rufinamide; Selective Serotonin Reuptake Inhibitors; Simeprevir; Sodium Oxybate; Stiripentol; Succinylcholine; Tapentadol; Tetrahydrocannabinol; Tricyclic Antidepressants

Decreased Effect

TraMADol may decrease the levels/effects of: CarBAMazepine; Pegvisomant

The levels/effects of TraMADol may be decreased by: Ammonium Chloride; Antiemetics (5HT3 Antagonists); Bosentan; CarBAMazepine; CYP2D6 Inhibitors (Moderate); CYP2D6 Inhibitors (Strong); CYP3A4 Inducers (Moderate); CYP3A4 Inducers (Strong); Dabrafenib; Deferasirox; Mitotane; Mixed Agonist / Antagonist Opioids; Naltrexone; Siltuximab; St Johns Wort; Tocilizumab

Food Interactions

Immediate release tablet: Rate and extent of absorption were not significantly affected by food. Management: Administer without regard to meals.

Extended release:

ConZip™: Rate and extent of absorption were unaffected by food. Management: Administer without regard to meals.

Ultram® ER: High-fat meal reduced C_{max} and AUC, and increased T_{max} by 3 hours. Management: Administer with or without food, but keep consistent.

Orally disintegrating tablet: Food delays the time to peak serum concentration by 30 minutes; extent of absorption was not significantly affected. Management: Administer without regard to meals.

Storage/Stability Store at 25°C (77°F); excursions permitted to 15°C to 30°C (59°F to 86°F).

Mechanism of Action Tramadol and its active metabolite (M1) binds to μ-opiate receptors in the CNS causing inhibition of ascending pain pathways, altering the perception of and response to pain; also inhibits the reuptake of norepinephrine and serotonin, which are neurotransmitters involved in the descending inhibitory pain pathway responsible for pain relief (Grond, 2004)

Pharmacodynamics/Kinetics

Onset of action: Immediate release: ~1 hour

Duration: 9 hours

Absorption: Immediate release formulation: Rapid and complete; Extended release formulation: Delayed

Distribution: V_d: 2.5-3 L/kg

Protein binding, plasma: ~20%

Metabolism: Extensively hepatic via demethylation (mediated by CYP3A4 and CYP2B6), glucuronidation, and sulfation; has pharmacologically active metabolite formed by CYP2D6 (M1; O-desmethyl tramadol)

Bioavailability: Immediate release: 75%; Extended release: Ultram® ER: 85% to 90% (as compared to immediate release), Zytram® XL, Tridural™: 70%

Half-life elimination: Tramadol: ~6-8 hours; Active metabolite: 7-9 hours; prolonged in elderly, hepatic or renal impairment; Zytram® XL: Apparent half-life: ~16 hours; Durela™, Ralivia™, Tridural™: ~5-9 hours

Time to peak: Immediate release: ~2 hours; Extended release: ConZip™: ~10-12 hours, Tridural™: ~4 hours; Durela™, Ultram® ER: ~12 hours

Excretion: Urine (30% as unchanged drug; 60% as metabolites)

Dosage Oral: Moderate-to-severe pain:

Children ≥17 years and Adults:

Immediate release: 50-100 mg every 4-6 hours (not to exceed 400 mg/day).For patients not requiring rapid onset of effect, tolerability may be improved by starting dose at 25 mg/day and titrating dose by 25 mg every 3 days, until reaching 25 mg 4 times/day. The total daily dose may then be increased by 50 mg every 3 days as tolerated, to reach dose of 50 mg 4 times/day. After titration, 50-100 mg may be given every 4-6 hours as needed up to a maximum 400 mg/day.

Orally-disintegrating tablet (Rybix™ ODT): 50-100 mg every 4-6 hours (not to exceed 400 mg/day); for patients not requiring rapid onset of effect, tolerability may be improved by starting dose at 50 mg/day and titrating dose by 50 mg every 3 days, until reaching 50 mg 4 times/day. After titration, 50-100 mg may be given every 4-6 hours as needed up to a maximum 400 mg/day.

Adults: Extended release:

U.S. labeling: ConZip™, Ultram® ER:

Patients not currently on immediate-release tramadol: 100 mg once daily; titrate every 5 days (ConZip™, Ultram® ER); maximum dose: 300 mg daily

Patients currently on immediate-release tramadol: Calculate 24-hour immediate release total dose and initiate total extended release daily dose (round dose to the next lowest 100 mg increment); titrate as tolerated to desired effect (maximum: 300 mg daily)

Canadian labeling: **Note:** Patients currently on immediate-release tramadol: When switching to extended release, initiate at the same or lowest nearest total daily tramadol dose. Not to exceed recommended maximum daily dosing.

Durela™, Ralivia™, Tridural™: Patients not currently on immediate-release tramadol or opioids: Initial: 100 mg once daily; titrate every 5 days (Durela™, Ralivia™) or every 2 days (Tridural™) as needed based on clinical response and severity of pain (maximum: 300 mg daily)

Zytram® XL: Patients not currently on immediate-release tramadol or opioids: 150 mg once daily; if pain relief is not achieved may titrate by increasing dosage incrementally, with sufficient time to evaluate effect of increased dosage; generally not more often than every 7 days (maximum: 400 mg daily)

Elderly >65 years: Use caution and initiate at the lower end of the dosing range

Elderly >75 years:

Immediate release: Do not exceed 300 mg/day; see Dosing adjustments for renal and hepatic impairment.

Extended release: Use with great caution. See adult, renal, and hepatic dosing.

Dosage adjustment in renal impairment:

Immediate release: CrCl <30 mL/minute: Administer 50-100 mg dose every 12 hours (maximum: 200 mg daily)

Extended release: Should not be used in patients with CrCl <30 mL/minute

Dosage adjustment in hepatic impairment:

Immediate release: Cirrhosis: Recommended dose: 50 mg every 12 hours

Extended release: Should not be used in patients with severe (Child-Pugh class C) hepatic dysfunction.

Dietary Considerations Some products may contain phenylalanine.

Administration

Immediate release: Administer without regard to meals.

Extended release: Swallow whole; do not crush, chew, or split. **Note:** Durela™, Ralivia™, and Tridural™: Canadian availability; products not available in U.S.:

ConZip™, Zytram® XL, Durela™: May administer without regard to meals.

Ultram® ER, Ralivia™, Tridural™: May administer without regard to meals, but administer in a consistent manner of either with or without meals.

Orally-disintegrating tablet: Remove from foil blister by peeling back (do not push tablet through the foil). Place tablet on tongue and allow to dissolve (may take ~1 minute); water is not needed, but may be administered with water. Do not chew, break, or split tablet.

Monitoring Parameters Pain relief, respiratory rate, blood pressure, and pulse; signs of tolerance, abuse, or suicidal ideation

Reference Range 100-300 ng/mL; however, serum level monitoring is not required

Dosage Forms Considerations

ConZip extended release capsules are formulated as a biphasic product, providing immediate and extended release components:

100 mg: 25 mg (immediate release) and 75 mg (extended release)

200 mg: 50 mg (immediate release) and 150 mg (extended release)

300 mg: 50 mg (immediate release) and 250 mg (extended release)

EnovaRX-Tramadol and Active-Tramadol are compounding kits. Refer to manufacturer's package insert for compounding instructions.

Synapryn FusePaq is a compounding kit for the preparation of an oral suspension. Refer to manufacturer's labeling for compounding instructions.

Dosage Forms

Capsule Extended Release 24 Hour, Oral:

ConZip: 100 mg, 200 mg, 300 mg

Generic: 150 mg

Cream, External:

Active-Tramadol: 8% (120 g)

EnovaRX-Tramadol: 5% (60 g, 120 g)

Suspension Reconstituted, Oral:

Synapryn FusePaq: 10 mg/mL (500 mL)

Tablet, Oral:
Ultram: 50 mg
Generic: 50 mg
Tablet Extended Release 24 Hour, Oral:
Ultram ER: 100 mg, 200 mg, 300 mg
Generic: 100 mg, 200 mg, 300 mg
Dosage Forms: Canada
Capsule Extended Release 24 Hour, Oral:
Durela: 100 mg, 200 mg, 300 mg
Tablet Extended Release 24 Hour, Oral:
Ralivia, Tridural: 100 mg, 200 mg, 300 mg
Zytram XL: 75 mg, 100 mg, 150 mg, 200 mg, 300 mg, 400 mg

Extemporaneous Preparations A 5 mg/mL oral suspension may be made with tablets and either Ora-Sweet® SF or a mixture of 30 mL Ora-Plus® and 30 mL strawberry syrup. Crush six 50 mg tramadol tablets in a mortar and reduce to a fine powder. Add small portions of the chosen vehicle and mix to a uniform paste; mix while adding vehicle in incremental proportions to **almost** 60 mL; transfer to a calibrated bottle, rinse mortar with vehicle, and add quantity of vehicle sufficient to make 60 mL. Label "shake well before use". Stable for 90 days refrigerated or at room temperature.

Wagner DS, Johnson CE, Cichon-Hensley BK, et al, "Stability of Oral Liquid Preparations of Tramadol in Strawberry Syrup and a Sugar-Free Vehicle," *Am J Health Syst Pharm*, 2003, 60(12):1268-70.

◆ **Tramadol Hydrochloride** *see* TraMADol *on page 2074*

◆ **Tramadol Hydrochloride and Acetaminophen** *see* Acetaminophen and Tramadol *on page 37*

◆ **Tramaphen-Odan (Can)** *see* Acetaminophen and Tramadol *on page 37*

Trametinib (tra ME ti nib)

Brand Names: U.S. Mekinist
Brand Names: Canada Mekinist
Index Terms GSK1120212
Pharmacologic Category Antineoplastic Agent, MEK Inhibitor
Use Melanoma: Treatment of unresectable or metastatic melanoma in patients with a BRAF V600E or BRAF V600K mutation (as detected by an approved test), either as a single-agent or in combination with dabrafenib. **Note:** Trametinib as a single-agent is not recommended in patients who have received prior BRAF-inhibitor therapy.
Pregnancy Risk Factor D
Pregnancy Considerations Adverse effects were observed in animal reproduction studies. Based on its mechanism of action, trametinib would be expected to cause fetal harm if administered to a pregnant woman. Females of reproductive potential should use a highly effective contraceptive during therapy and for 4 months after treatment is complete. When trametinib is used in combination with dabrafenib, a highly effective nonhormonal contraceptive method should be used (dabrafenib may diminish efficacy of hormonal contraceptives). Fertility may also be impaired in females. Due to a risk for impaired spermatogenesis, males who may want to father a child should seek fertility/family planning counseling prior to initiating combination therapy with dabrafenib.
Breast-Feeding Considerations It is not known if trametinib is excreted into breast milk. Due to the potential for serious adverse reactions in the nursing infant, the manufacturer recommends a decision be made whether to discontinue nursing or to discontinue the drug, taking into account the importance of treatment to the mother.
Contraindications There are no contraindications listed in the manufacturer's U.S. labeling.
Canadian labeling: Hypersensitivity to trametinib or any component of the formulation.

Warnings/Precautions Hazardous agent - use appropriate precautions for handling and disposal (meets NIOSH 2014 criteria). Cardiac events such as heart failure, left ventricular dysfunction, or decreased left ventricular ejection fraction (LVEF) were observed in clinical trials (for single-agent trametinib and when used in combination with dabrafenib); the median time to onset of cardiomyopathy for single-agent trametinib was ~2 months (range: 16-156 days) and ~3 months (range: 27-253 days) when used in combination with dabrafenib. Assess LVEF (by echocardiogram or MUGA scan) prior to therapy initiation, at one month, and then at 2- to 3-month intervals while on therapy. Cardiac dysfunction may require treatment interruption, dosage reduction, or discontinuation; such measures resulted in resolution of cardiomyopathy in some patients. May cause hypertension; monitor blood pressure. Venous thromboembolism events (some fatal) may occur when trametinib is used in combination with dabrafenib. DVT and PE occurred at an increased incidence with combination therapy. Patients should seek immediate medical attention with symptoms of DVT or PE (shortness of breath, chest pain, arm/leg swelling). Withhold trametinib for uncomplicated DVT or PE; permanently discontinue trametinib (and dabrafenib) for life-threatening PE. Interstitial lung disease and pneumonitis were observed in clinical trials; median time to initial presentation was 160 days (range: 60-172 days). Monitor for new or progressive pulmonary symptoms (eg, cough, dyspnea, hypoxia, pleural effusion, infiltrates); may require therapy interruption or permanent discontinuation.

Dermatologic toxicity (eg, rash, dermatitis, acneiform rash, palmar-plantar erythrodysesthesia syndrome, and erythema) was commonly observed in trametinib-treated patients (either as a single-agent or when used in combination with dabrafenib); some patients required hospitalization for severe toxicity or for secondary skin infections. The median time to onset and resolution of skin toxicity for single-agent trametinib was 15 days (range: 1-221 days) and 48 days (range: 1-282 days), respectively. The median time to onset and resolution of skin toxicity for combination therapy was 37 days (range: 1-225 days) and 33 days (range: 3-421 days), respectively. Monitor for dermatologic toxicity and signs/symptoms of secondary infections. Treatment interruption, dose reductions, and/or therapy discontinuation may be necessary. New primary cutaneous malignancies (which are associated with dabrafenib as single-agent therapy) may occur at a higher rate when trametinib is given in combination with dabrafenib. The incidence of basal cell carcinoma (BCC) is 9% for combination therapy versus 2% for single-agent dabrafenib. The time to BCC diagnosis ranged from 28 to 249 days for patients receiving combination therapy. Cutaneous squamous cell carcinomas (SCC), including keratoacanthoma, occurred at a lower rate for combination therapy compared to single-agent dabrafenib (7% vs 19%, respectively), with a time to diagnosis ranging from 136 to 197 days for combination therapy. Dermatologic exams should be performed prior to initiation of combination therapy, every 2 months while receiving combination treatment, and for up to 6 months following discontinuation.

Retinal pigment epithelial detachments (RPED) and retinal vein occlusion were seen in clinical trials (rare). Detachments were typically bilateral and multifocal and occurred in the macular area of the retina. RPED resolution occurred after a median of 11.5 days (range: 3-71 days) following therapy interruption, although some visual disturbances persisted beyond 1 month. Retinal vein occlusion may lead to macular edema, degeneration, decreased visual function, neovascularization, and glaucoma. Promptly refer patients for ophthalmological evaluations if loss of vision or other visual disturbances occur; trametinib therapy interruption and/or discontinuation may be ▶

required. In clinical trials, ophthalmic exams (including retinal evaluation) were performed prior to and regularly during treatment. Uveitis and iritis have been reported when trametinib is used in combination with dabrafenib and are managed symptomatically with ophthalmic steroid and mydriatic drops (does not require alteration in trametinib therapy).

Serious febrile reactions and fever (any severity) accompanied by hypotension, rigors/chills, dehydration, or renal failure may occur when trametinib is used in combination with dabrafenib. The incidence and severity were higher with combination therapy than with single-agent dabrafenib; the median time to onset of fever was 30 days and duration was 6 days for patients receiving combination therapy. Withhold trametinib for fever >104°F (if using in combination, withhold dabrafenib for fever ≥101.3°F) or for any fever with rigors/chills, hypotension, dehydration, or renal failure (evaluate for infection); may require prophylactic antipyretics upon therapy resumption. Hemorrhage, including symptomatic bleeding in a critical area/organ, may occur when trametinib is used in combination with dabrafenib. Major bleeding events (some fatal) included intracranial or gastrointestinal hemorrhage; may require treatment interruption and dosage reduction; permanently discontinue trametinib (and dabrafenib) for all grade 4 hemorrhagic events and any grade 3 event that does not improve with therapy interruption. While not reported with single-agent trametinib, hyperglycemia may occur while on combination therapy with dabrafenib; may require initiation of insulin or oral hypoglycemic agent therapy (or an increased dose if already taking); monitor serum glucose as clinically necessary, particularly in patients with preexisting diabetes or hyperglycemia. Instruct patients to report symptoms of severe hyperglycemia (eg, polydipsia, polyuria).

Prior to initiating therapy, confirm BRAF mutation status with an approved test; approved for use in patients with BRAF V600K and BRAF V600E mutations. Current data regarding use in patients with BRAF V600K mutation is limited; compared to BRAF V600E mutation, lower response rates have been observed with BRAF V600K mutation. Data regarding other less common BRAF V600 mutations is lacking. There are case reports of non-cutaneous malignancies, including pancreatic cancer (KRAS mutation-positive), colorectal cancer (recurrent NRAS mutation-positive), hand and neck cancer, and glioblastoma, with combination therapy; monitor for signs/symptoms of non-cutaneous malignancies. No trametinib dosage modification is necessary for new primary cutaneous and non-cutaneous malignancies; dabrafenib should be permanently discontinued if RAS mutation-positive non-cutaneous malignancies develop. Serious adverse reactions (tumor promotion, hemolytic anemia), which occur with single-agent dabrafenib, may also occur when trametinib is administered in combination with dabrafenib. Potentially significant drug-drug interactions may exist, requiring dose or frequency adjustment, additional monitoring, and/or selection of alternative therapy.

Adverse Reactions

Adverse reactions reported with monotherapy:

Cardiovascular: Bradycardia, cardiomyopathy (defined as cardiac failure, decreased left ventricular ejection fraction, or left ventricular dysfunction), decreased left ventricular ejection fraction (≥20% below baseline), hypertension

Central nervous system: Dizziness

Dermatologic: Acneiform eruption, cellulitis, folliculitis, paronychia, pruritus, pustular rash, skin rash, skin toxicity (most commonly skin rash, dermatitis acneiform rash, erythema, severe toxicity and secondary skin infection requiring hospitalization), xeroderma

Endocrine & metabolic: Hypoalbuminemia

Gastrointestinal: Abdominal pain, diarrhea, dysgeusia, stomatitis, xerostomia

Hematologic & oncologic: Anemia, hemorrhage (includes conjunctival hemorrhage, epistaxis, gingival bleeding, hematochezia, hematuria, hemorrhoidal hemorrhage, melena, rectal hemorrhage, vaginal hemorrhage), lymphedema (includes edema, peripheral edema)

Hepatic: Increased serum alkaline phosphatase, increased serum ALT, increased serum AST

Neuromuscular & skeletal: Rhabdomyolysis

Ophthalmic: Blurred vision, dry eye syndrome

Respiratory: Interstitial lung disease (or pneumonitis)

Rare but important or life-threatening: Palmar-plantar erythrodysesthesia, retinal detachment, retinal vein occlusion

Adverse reactions reported with dual therapy (trametinib plus dabrafenib):

Cardiovascular: Cardiomyopathy, hypertension, peripheral edema (includes edema and lymphedema), prolonged Q-T Interval on ECG

Central nervous system: Chills, dizziness, fatigue, headache, insomnia

Dermatologic: Acneiform eruption, cellulitis, erythema, folliculitis, hyperhidrosis, hyperkeratosis, night sweats, palmar-plantar erythrodysesthesia, paronychia, pruritus, pustular rash, skin rash (includes erythematous rash, generalized rash, macular rash, maculopapular rash, papular rash, pruritic rash, vesicular rash), skin toxicity, xeroderma

Endocrine & metabolic: Dehydration, hypercalcemia, hyperglycemia, hyperkalemia, hypoalbuminemia, hypocalcemia, hypokalemia, hypomagnesemia, hyponatremia, hypophosphatemia, increased gamma-glutamyl transferase

Gastrointestinal: Abdominal pain, constipation, decreased appetite, diarrhea, nausea, pancreatitis, stomatitis, vomiting, xerostomia

Genitourinary: Urinary tract infection

Hematologic & oncologic: Anemia, basal cell carcinoma, cutaneous papilloma, hemorrhage (includes brain stem hemorrhage, cerebral hemorrhage, epistaxis, eye hemorrhage, gastric hemorrhage, gingival hemorrhage, hematuria, intracranial hemorrhage, vaginal hemorrhage, vitreous hemorrhage), leukopenia, lymphocytopenia, major hemorrhage (gastric or intracranial hemorrhage), neutropenia, squamous cell carcinoma of skin (including keratoacanthoma), thrombocytopenia

Hepatic: Hyperbilirubinemia, increased serum alkaline phosphatase, increased serum ALT, increased serum AST

Infection: Actinic keratosis

Neuromuscular & skeletal: Arthralgia, back pain, limb pain, muscle spasm, myalgia, weakness

Ophthalmic: Blurred vision, transient blindness, uveitis

Renal: Increased serum creatinine, renal failure (includes acute renal failure)

Respiratory: Cough, oropharyngeal pain

Miscellaneous: Febrile reaction (can be complicated with chills/rigors, dehydration, renal failure, or syncope, or accompanied by hypotension, rigors or chills), fever

Rare but important or life-threatening: Deep vein thrombosis, pulmonary embolism

Drug combination trials:

Cardiovascular: Decreased left ventricular ejection fraction (≥20% below baseline)

Drug Interactions

Metabolism/Transport Effects Inhibits CYP2C8 (weak); **Induces** CYP3A4 (weak)

Avoid Concomitant Use There are no known interactions where it is recommended to avoid concomitant use.

Increased Effect/Toxicity

Trametinib may increase the levels/effects of: Dabrafenib

Decreased Effect

Trametinib may decrease the levels/effects of: ARIPiprazole; Hydrocodone; Saxagliptin

Food Interactions Administration with a high-fat, high-calorie meal decreased AUC by 24%, C_{max} by 70%, and delayed T_{max} by ~4 hours. Management: Administer 1 hour before or 2 hours after a meal.

Storage/Stability Store refrigerated at 2°C to 8°C (36°F to 46°F); do not freeze. Dispense in original bottle; do not remove desiccant. Protect from light and moisture. Do not transfer to pill boxes.

Mechanism of Action Reversibly and selectively inhibits mitogen-activated extracellular kinase (MEK) 1 and 2 activation and kinase activity. MEK is a downstream effector of the protein kinase B-raf (BRAF); BRAF V600 mutations result in constitutive activation of the BRAF pathway (including MEK1 and MEK2). Through inhibition of MEK 1 and 2 kinase activity, trametinib causes decreased cellular proliferation, cell cycle arrest, and increased apoptosis (Kim, 2013). The combination of trametinib and dabrafenib allows for greater inhibition of the MAPK pathway, resulting in BRAF V600 melanoma cell death (Flaherty, 2012).

Pharmacodynamics/Kinetics

Absorption: Rapid; decreased with a high-fat, high-calorie meal

Distribution: 214 L

Protein binding: ~97% to plasma proteins

Metabolism: Predominantly deacetylation (via hydrolytic enzymes) alone or with mono-oxygenation or in combination with glucuronidation

Bioavailability: 72%

Half-life elimination: 4-5 days

Time to peak: 1.5 hours; delayed with a high-fat, high-calorie meal

Excretion: Feces (>80%); urine (<20% with <0.1% as unchanged drug)

Dosage Melanoma, metastatic or unresectable (with BRAF V600E or BRAF V600K mutations): Adults: Oral: 2 mg once daily (either as a single-agent or in combination with dabrafenib), continue until disease progression or unacceptable toxicity

Missed doses: Do not take a missed dose within 12 hours of the next dose.

Dosage adjustment for toxicity:

Recommended trametinib dose reductions for toxicity:

First dose reduction: 1.5 mg once daily

Second dose reduction: 1 mg once daily

Subsequent modification (if unable to tolerate 1 mg once daily): Permanently discontinue

Note: If using combination therapy, refer to Dabrafenib monograph for recommended dabrafenib dose reductions.

Cardiac:

Asymptomatic, 10% or greater absolute decrease in LVEF from baseline and LVEF is below institutional lower limits of normal (LLN) from pretreatment value: Interrupt trametinib therapy for up to 4 weeks. If LVEF improves to normal within 4 weeks following therapy interruption, resume at a lower dose level. If LVEF does not improve to normal within 4 weeks following therapy interruption, permanently discontinue trametinib.

>20% absolute decrease in LVEF from baseline and LVEF is below institutional LLN: Permanently discontinue trametinib.

Symptomatic heart failure: Permanently discontinue trametinib.

Dermatologic:

Intolerable Grade 2 skin toxicity or Grade 3 or 4 skin toxicity: Interrupt trametinib therapy for up to 3 weeks. If toxicity improves within 3 weeks, resume at a lower dose level. If toxicity does not improve within 3 weeks following therapy interruption, permanently discontinue trametinib.

New primary cutaneous malignancies: No trametinib dosage modification is necessary.

Fever: Fever >40°C (104°F) or fever (any severity) complicated by rigors, hypotension, dehydration, or renal failure: Interrupt trametinib therapy until fever resolves, then resume at the same or a lower dose level. May require prophylactic antipyretics upon resumption.

Hemorrhage:

Grade 3 hemorrhage: Interrupt trametinib therapy for up to 3 weeks. If hemorrhage improves within 3 weeks, resume at a lower dose level. If hemorrhage does not improve within 3 weeks following therapy interruption, permanently discontinue trametinib.

Grade 4 hemorrhage: Permanently discontinue trametinib.

Ocular:

Uveitis and iritis: No trametinib dosage modification necessary.

Grade 2 or 3 retinal pigment epithelial detachments (RPED): Interrupt trametinib therapy for up to 3 weeks. If improves to ≤ grade 1 within 3 weeks following therapy interruption, resume at a lower dose level. If RPED does not improve within 3 weeks following therapy interruption, permanently discontinue trametinib.

Recurrence of RPED (any grade) after dose reduction/ therapy interruption: *Canadian labeling (not in U.S. labeling):* Permanently discontinue trametinib.

Retinal vein occlusion: Permanently discontinue trametinib.

Pulmonary: Interstitial lung disease or pneumonitis: Permanently discontinue trametinib.

Venous thromboembolism:

Uncomplicated DVT or PE: Interrupt trametinib therapy for up to 3 weeks. If improves to ≤ grade 1 within 3 weeks following therapy interruption, resume at a lower dose level. If toxicity does not improve within 3 weeks following therapy interruption, permanently discontinue trametinib.

Life-threatening PE: Permanently discontinue trametinib.

Other toxicity:

Intolerable Grade 2 adverse reaction or any Grade 3 adverse reaction: Interrupt trametinib therapy for up to 3 weeks. If toxicity improves to ≤ grade 1 within 3 weeks following therapy interruption, resume at a lower dose level. If toxicity does not improve within 3 weeks following therapy interruption, permanently discontinue trametinib.

Grade 4 adverse reaction, first occurrence: Interrupt trametinib therapy until improves to ≤ grade 1, then resume at a lower dose level **or** permanently discontinue trametinib.

Grade 4 adverse reaction, recurrent: Permanently discontinue trametinib.

New primary noncutaneous malignancy: No trametinib dosage modification is necessary.

Dosage adjustment for renal impairment:

Mild to moderate impairment (GFR ≥30 mL/minute/1.73 m^2): No dosage adjustment necessary.

Severe impairment (GFR <30 mL/minute/1.73 m^2): No dosage adjustment provided in manufacturer's labeling (has not been studied); however, renal excretion is low and is unlikely to affect drug exposure.

Dosage adjustment for hepatic impairment:

Mild impairment (total bilirubin ≤ ULN and AST > ULN **or** total bilirubin >1-1.5 times ULN with any AST): No dosage adjustment necessary.

Moderate to severe impairment: No dosage adjustment provided in manufacturer's labeling (has not been studied).

Dietary Considerations Take at least 1 hour before or 2 hours after a meal.

Administration Administer at least 1 hour before or 2 hours after a meal. Do not take a missed dose within 12 hours of the next dose. When administered in combination with dabrafenib, take the once daily trametinib dose at the same time each day with either the morning or evening dose of dabrafenib.

Hazardous agent; use appropriate precautions for handling and disposal (meets NIOSH 2014 criteria).

Monitoring Parameters CBC and liver function tests at baseline and periodically; assess LVEF (by echocardiogram or MUGA scan) at baseline, 1 month after therapy initiation, and then at 2- to 3-month intervals; ophthalmological evaluation as necessary (if reports of visual disturbance); monitor for signs/symptoms of pulmonary toxicity (eg, cough dyspnea, hypoxia, pleural effusion, or infiltrates); monitor for dermatologic toxicity and secondary skin infections; blood pressure; diarrhea.

For patients receiving combination therapy with dabrafenib: Dermatologic exams should be performed prior to treatment initiation, every 2 months while receiving combination treatment, and for up to 6 months following therapy discontinuation. Monitor for signs/symptoms of non-cutaneous malignancies.

Dosage Forms

Tablet, Oral:

Mekinist: 0.5 mg, 2 mg

◆ **Trandate** *see* Labetalol *on page 1151*

Trandolapril (tran DOE la pril)

Brand Names: U.S. Mavik

Brand Names: Canada Mavik

Pharmacologic Category Angiotensin-Converting Enzyme (ACE) Inhibitor; Antihypertensive

Use Treatment of hypertension alone or in combination with other antihypertensive agents; treatment of post-myocardial infarction (MI) heart failure (HF) or post-MI left ventricular (LV) dysfunction after myocardial infarction (MI)

The 2014 guideline for the management of high blood pressure in adults (Eighth Joint National Committee [JNC 8]) recommends initiation of pharmacologic treatment to lower blood pressure for the following patients:

- Patients ≥60 years of age with systolic blood pressure (SBP) ≥150 mm Hg or diastolic blood pressure (DBP) ≥90 mm Hg. Goal of therapy is SBP <150 mm Hg and DBP <90 mm Hg.
- Patients <60 years of age with SBP ≥140 mm Hg or DBP is ≥90 mm Hg. Goal of therapy is SBP <140 mm Hg and DBP <90 mm Hg.
- Patients ≥18 years of age with diabetes and SBP ≥140 mm Hg or DBP ≥90 mm Hg. Goal of therapy is SBP <140 mm Hg and DBP <90 mm Hg.
- Patients ≥18 years of age with chronic kidney disease (CKD) and SBP ≥140 mm Hg or DBP ≥90 mm Hg. Goal of therapy is SBP <140 mm Hg and DBP <90 mm Hg.

In patients with CKD, regardless of race or diabetes status, the use of an ACE inhibitor (ACEI) or angiotensin receptor blocker (ARB) as initial therapy is recommended to improve kidney outcomes. In the general nonblack population (without CKD) including those with diabetes, initial antihypertensive treatment should consist of a thiazide-type diuretic, calcium channel blocker, ACEI, or ARB. In the general black population (without CKD) including those with diabetes, initial antihypertensive treatment should consist of a thiazide-type diuretic or a calcium channel blocker **instead of** an ACEI or ARB.

Note: The American College of Cardiology Foundation/American Heart Association (ACCF/AHA) 2013 heart failure guidelines recommend the use of ACE inhibitors, along with other guideline directed medical therapies, to prevent heart failure in patients with a reduced ejection fraction who have a history of MI (Stage B HF), to prevent heart failure in any patient with a reduced ejection fraction (Stage B HF), or to treat those with heart failure and reduced ejection fraction (Stage C HFrEF) (ACCF/AHA [Yancy, 2013]).

The 2013 ACCF/AHA guidelines for the management of patients with ST-elevation myocardial infarction (STEMI) states that an ACE inhibitor should be initiated within the first 24 hours after STEMI in patients with anterior MI, heart failure, or left ventricular ejection fraction (LVEF) of 0.4 or less. It is also reasonable to initiate an ACE inhibitor in all patients with STEMI (O'Gara, 2013).

Pregnancy Risk Factor D

Dosage Adults: Oral:

Hypertension: Initial dose in patients not receiving a diuretic: 1 mg once daily (2 mg daily in black patients). Adjust dosage at intervals of ≥1 week according to blood pressure response; usual dosage (ASH/ISH [Weber, 2014]): 2 to 8 mg daily. There is little experience with doses >8 mg daily. Patients inadequately treated with once daily dosing at 4 mg may be treated with twice daily dosing. If blood pressure is not adequately controlled with trandolapril monotherapy, a diuretic may be added.

Post-MI heart failure or LV dysfunction: Initial: 1 mg once daily; titrate (as tolerated) towards target dose of 4 mg once daily. If 4 mg dose is not tolerated, patients may continue therapy with the greatest tolerated dose. The American College of Cardiology Foundation/American Heart Association guidelines recommend the use of a 0.5 mg test dose with titration up to 4 mg daily as tolerated (O'Gara, 2013).

Heart failure with reduced ejection fraction (HFrEF) (off-label use): Initial: 1 mg once daily; target dose: 4 mg once daily (ACCF/AHA [Yancy, 2013]).

Dosage adjustment in renal impairment: CrCl <30 mL/minute: Recommended starting dose: 0.5 mg once daily

Dosage adjustment in hepatic impairment: Cirrhosis: Recommended starting dose: 0.5 mg once daily

Additional Information Complete prescribing information should be consulted for additional detail.

Dosage Forms

Tablet, Oral:

Mavik: 1 mg, 2 mg, 4 mg

Generic: 1 mg, 2 mg, 4 mg

Dosage Forms: Canada

Capsule, Oral:

Mavik: 0.5 mg, 1 mg, 2 mg, 4 mg

Trandolapril and Verapamil

(tran DOE la pril & ver AP a mil)

Brand Names: U.S. Tarka®

Brand Names: Canada Tarka®

Index Terms Verapamil and Trandolapril

Pharmacologic Category Angiotensin-Converting Enzyme (ACE) Inhibitor; Antihypertensive; Calcium Channel Blocker

Use Treatment of hypertension; however, not indicated for initial treatment of hypertension

Pregnancy Risk Factor D

Dosage Dose is individualized

Dosage adjustment in renal impairment: Usual regimen need not be adjusted unless patient's creatinine clearance is <30 mL/minute. Titration of individual components must be done prior to switching to combination product

Dosage adjustment in hepatic impairment: No dosage adjustment provided in manufacturer's labeling (has not been studied). However, verapamil is hepatically metabolized; adjustment of dosage in hepatic impairment is recommended.

Additional Information Complete prescribing information should be consulted for additional detail.

Dosage Forms

Tablet, variable release: Trandolapril 2 mg [immediate release] and verapamil 180 mg [sustained release]; Trandolapril 2 mg [immediate release] and verapamil 240 mg [sustained release]; Trandolapril 4 mg [immediate release] and verapamil 240 mg [sustained release]

Tarka®:

1/240: Trandolapril 1 mg [immediate release] and verapamil 240 mg [sustained release]

2/180: Trandolapril 2 mg [immediate release] and verapamil 180 mg [sustained release]

2/240: Trandolapril 2 mg [immediate release] and verapamil 240 mg [sustained release]

4/240: Trandolapril 4 mg [immediate release] and verapamil 240 mg [sustained release]

Tranexamic Acid (tran eks AM ik AS id)

Brand Names: U.S. Cyklokapron; Lysteda

Brand Names: Canada Cyklokapron; Tranexamic Acid Injection BP

Pharmacologic Category Antifibrinolytic Agent; Antihemophilic Agent; Hemostatic Agent; Lysine Analog

Use

Tooth extraction in patients with hemophilia (injection): Short-term use (2 to 8 days) in hemophilia patients to reduce or prevent hemorrhage and reduce need for replacement therapy during and following tooth extraction

Cyclic heavy menstrual bleeding (oral): Treatment of cyclic heavy menstrual bleeding

Pregnancy Risk Factor B

Dosage

Oral:

Children ≥12 years, Adolescents, and Adults: Menorrhagia: 1300 mg 3 times daily (3900 mg daily) for up to 5 days during monthly menstruation

Children:

Hereditary angioedema (HAE) (off-label use):

Long-term prophylaxis: 20-40 mg/kg/day in 2-3 divided doses (maximum dose: 3000 mg daily) (Farkas, 2007) **or** 50 mg/kg/day (or 1000-2000 mg daily; depending on age and size of patient); may consider alternate-day regimen or twice-weekly regimen when frequency of attacks reduces; diarrhea may be a dose-limiting side effect (Gompels, 2005)

Short-term prophylaxis: 20-40 mg/kg/day in 2-3 divided doses (maximum dose: 3000 mg daily) (Farkas, 2007) **or** 500 mg 4 times daily (Gompels, 2005). **Note:** For short-term prophylaxis (eg, dental work), initiate 2-5 days before and continue for 2 days after the procedure (Bowen, 2004; Gompels, 2005).

Children and Adults: Traumatic hyphema (off-label use): 25 mg/kg administered 3 times daily for 5-7 days (Rahmani, 1999; Vangsted, 1983; Varnek, 1980). **Note:** This same regimen may also be used for secondary hemorrhage after an initial traumatic hyphema event.

Adults:

Hereditary angioedema (HAE) (off-label use):

Long-term prophylaxis: 1000-1500 mg 2-3 times daily; reduce to 500 mg/dose once or twice daily when frequency of attacks reduces (Gompels, 2005; Levy, 2010) **or** 25 mg/kg/dose administered 2-3 times daily (Bowen, 2004)

Short-term prophylaxis (eg, for dental work): 75 mg/kg/day divided 2-3 times daily for 5 days before and 2 days after the event (Bowen, 2004) **or** 1000 mg 4 times daily for 48 hours before and after procedure (Gompels, 2005)

Treatment of acute HAE attack: 25 mg/kg/dose (maximum single dose: 1000 mg) every 3-4 hours (maximum: 75 mg/kg/day) (Bowen, 2004) **or** 1000 mg 4 times daily for 48 hours (Gompels, 2005)

Prevention of dental procedure bleeding in patients on oral anticoagulant therapy (off-label use): Oral rinse: 4.8% solution: Hold 10 mL in mouth and rinse for 2 minutes then spit out. Repeat 4 times daily for 2 days after procedure. **Note:** Patient should not eat or drink for 1 hour after using oral rinse (Carter, 2003).

Transurethral prostatectomy, blood loss reduction (off-label use): 2000 mg 3 times daily on the operative and first postoperative day (Rannikko, 2004)

IV:

Children:

Prevention of perioperative bleeding associated with cardiac surgery (off-label use): 10 mg/kg given over 30 minutes prior to incision, 10 mg/kg while on cardiopulmonary bypass, and 10 mg/kg administered after protamine reversal (Chauhan, 2004; Chauhan, 2004)

or

Loading dose of 100 mg/kg over 15 minutes prior to incision, followed by 10 mg/kg/hour infusion (continued until ICU transport); add 100 mg/kg to pump reservoir when cardiopulmonary bypass initiated (Reid, 1997)

Prevention of perioperative bleeding associated with craniosynostosis surgery (off-label use): Loading dose of 50 mg/kg over 15 minutes prior to incision, followed by 5 mg/kg/hour (Goobie, 2011) **or** 15 mg/kg over 15 minutes prior to incision, followed by 10 mg/kg/hour until skin closure (Dadure, 2011)

Children and Adolescents:

Prevention of perioperative bleeding associated with spinal surgery (eg, spinal fusion) (off-label use): 10 mg/kg given over 15 minutes prior to incision followed by 1 mg/kg/hour for the remainder of the surgery; discontinue at time of wound closure (Neilipovitz, 2001; Verma, 2010)

or

100 mg/kg over 15 minutes prior to incision followed by 10 mg/kg/hour until skin closure (Sethna, 2005)

or

30 mg/kg over 20 minutes prior to incision followed by 1 mg/kg/hour during surgery and for 5 hours postoperatively (Elwatidy, 2008)

Children and Adults: Tooth extraction in patients with hemophilia (in combination with appropriate factor replacement therapy): 10 mg/kg immediately before surgery, then 10 mg/kg/dose 3-4 times daily; may be used for 2-8 days

Adults:

Elective cesarean section, blood loss reduction (off-label use): 1000 mg over 5 minutes at least 10 minutes prior to skin incision (Gungorduk, 2011)

Hereditary angioedema (HAE), treatment of acute attack (off-label use): 25 mg/kg/dose (maximum single dose: 1000 mg) every 3-4 hours (maximum: 75 mg/kg/day) (Bowen, 2004) **or** 1000 mg 4 times daily for 48 hours (Gompels, 2005)

Hip fracture surgery, blood conservation (off-label use): 15 mg/kg administered at the time of skin incision followed by a second dose (15 mg/kg) 3 hours later (Zufferey, 2010). Additional data may be necessary to further define the role of tranexamic acid in this setting.

Orthognathic surgery, blood loss reduction (off-label use): 20 mg/kg over 15 minutes prior to incision (Choi, 2009)

Prevention of perioperative bleeding associated with cardiac surgery (off-label use): Loading dose of 30 mg/kg over 30 minutes (total loading dose includes a test dose administered over the first 10 minutes followed by the remainder of dose) prior to incision, followed by 16 mg/kg/hour until sternal closure; add an additional 2 mg/kg to cardiopulmonary bypass circuit (Fergusson, 2008)

or

Loading dose of 10 mg/kg over 20 minutes prior to incision followed by 2 mg/kg/hour continued for 2 hours after transfer to ICU; add a prime dose of 50 mg for a 2.5 L cardiopulmonary bypass circuit; maintenance infusion adjusted for renal insufficiency (Nuttall, 2008)

or

Loading dose of 10-15 mg/kg over 10-15 minutes, followed by 1-1.5 mg/kg/hour. The authors suggest adding 2–2.5 mg/kg to cardiopulmonary bypass circuit; however, amounts have varied widely in clinical trials (Gravlee, 2008).

Prevention of perioperative bleeding associated with spinal surgery (eg, spinal fusion) (off-label use): 2000 mg over 20 minutes prior to incision followed by 100 mg/hour during surgery and for 5 hours postoperatively (Elwatidy, 2008) **or** 10 mg/kg prior to incision followed by 1 mg/kg/hour for the remainder of the surgery; discontinue at time of wound closure (Wong, 2008)

Total hip replacement surgery, blood conservation (off-label use): 10 to 15 mg/kg (or 1000 mg) administered over 5 to 10 minutes immediately before the operation or 15 minutes before skin incision; the preoperative dose may be followed by 10 mg/kg administered 3 to 12 hours after the operation. Postoperative doses ranged from a 10 mg/kg IV bolus (or 1000 mg) to a 1 mg/kg/hour infusion over 10 hours (Gandhi, 2013; Oremus, 2014).

Note: Multiple regimens have been evaluated in varying degrees of evidence quality. The regimen listed here reflects the more commonly used dosing based on a number of prospective randomized controlled trials (Johansson 2005; McConnell 2011; Niskanen, 2005; Oremus, 2014). Metaanalyses have also been conducted demonstrating significant reduction in blood loss perioperatively without an increased risk of thromboembolic events (Gandhi, 2013; Sukeik, 2011; Zhou, 2013). The use of *intra-articular* tranexamic acid (ie, 1000 mg/50 mL of NaCl 0.9% sprayed into the wound at the end of the procedure) has also been evaluated demonstrating effectiveness (Alshryda, 2014a; Alshryda, 2014b).

Total knee replacement surgery, blood conservation (off-label use):

Bilateral total knee replacement:

Simultaneous: 10 mg/kg over 10 minutes approximately 10 minutes before deflation of the first tourniquet with a second dose (10 mg/kg) 3 hours after the first dose (Dhillon, 2011)

Staged (3 days apart): For each total knee replacement, 1000 mg administered 15 minutes before skin incision and 1000 mg upon deflation of the tourniquet (Kelley, 2014)

Unilateral total knee replacement: 10 mg/kg administered either 10-30 minutes before inflation of tourniquet or 30 minutes before deflation of the tourniquet with a second dose (10 mg/kg) administered either 3 hours after the first dose or immediately after tourniquet release (Alvarez, 2008; Camarasa, 2006; Lozano, 2008). Instead of the second dose, may also administer an infusion of 1 mg/kg/hour beginning at the end of the operation and continuing for 6 hours postoperatively (Alvarez, 2008).

Trauma-associated hemorrhage (off-label use): Loading dose: 1000 mg over 10 minutes, followed by 1000 mg over the next 8 hours. **Note:** Clinical trial included patients with significant hemorrhage (SBP <90 mm Hg, heart rate >110 bpm, or both) or those at risk of significant hemorrhage. Treatment began within 8 hours of injury (CRASH-2 Trial Collaborators, 2010).

Dosing adjustment/interval in renal impairment:

IV formulation:

Tooth extraction in patients with hemophilia:

Serum creatinine 1.36-2.83 mg/dL: Maintenance dose of 10 mg/kg/dose twice daily

Serum creatinine 2.83-5.66 mg/dL: Maintenance dose of 10 mg/kg/dose once daily

Serum creatinine >5.66 mg/dL: Maintenance dose of 10 mg/kg/dose every 48 hours **or** 5 mg/kg/dose once daily

Cardiac surgery (the following dose adjustments have been recommended [Nuttall, 2008]):

Serum creatinine 1.6-3.3 mg/dL: Reduce maintenance infusion to 1.5 mg/kg/hour (based on a 25% reduction from 2 mg/kg/hour)

Serum creatinine 3.3-6.6 mg/dL: Reduce maintenance infusion to 1 mg/kg/hour (based on a 50% reduction from 2 mg/kg/hour)

Serum creatinine >6.6 mg/dL: Reduce maintenance infusion to 0.5 mg/kg/hour (based on a 75% reduction from 2 mg/kg/hour)

Oral formulation: *Cyclic heavy menstrual bleeding:*

Serum creatinine >1.4-2.8 mg/dL: 1300 mg twice daily (2600 mg daily) for up to 5 days

Serum creatinine 2.9-5.7 mg/dL: 1300 mg once daily for up to 5 days

Serum creatinine >5.7 mg/dL: 650 mg once daily for up to 5 days

Dosing adjustment in hepatic impairment: No dosage adjustment is necessary.

Additional Information Complete prescribing information should be consulted for additional detail.

Dosage Forms

Solution, Intravenous:

Cyklokapron: 100 mg/mL (10 mL)

Generic: 100 mg/mL (10 mL)

Solution, Intravenous [preservative free]:

Generic: 100 mg/mL (10 mL)

Tablet, Oral:

Lysteda: 650 mg

Generic: 650 mg

◆ **Tranexamic Acid Injection BP (Can)** *see* Tranexamic Acid *on page 2081*

◆ **Transamine Sulphate** *see* Tranylcypromine *on page 2083*

◆ **Transderm-V (Can)** *see* Scopolamine (Systemic) *on page 1870*

◆ **Transderm-Nitro (Can)** *see* Nitroglycerin *on page 1465*

- ◆ **Transderm-Scop** *see* Scopolamine (Systemic) *on page 1870*
- ◆ ***trans*-Retinoic Acid** *see* Tretinoin (Systemic) *on page 2096*
- ◆ ***trans*-Retinoic Acid** *see* Tretinoin (Topical) *on page 2099*
- ◆ ***trans* Vitamin A Acid** *see* Tretinoin (Systemic) *on page 2096*
- ◆ **Tranxene-T** *see* Clorazepate *on page 487*
- ◆ **Tranxene T-Tab** *see* Clorazepate *on page 487*

Tranylcypromine (tran il SIP roe meen)

Brand Names: U.S. Parnate

Brand Names: Canada Parnate®

Index Terms Transamine Sulphate; Tranylcypromine Sulfate

Pharmacologic Category Antidepressant, Monoamine Oxidase Inhibitor

Use Treatment of major depressive episode without melancholia

Pregnancy Considerations Adverse events were observed in animal reproduction studies.

Breast-Feeding Considerations Tranylcypromine is excreted in breast milk.

Contraindications

Cardiovascular disease (including hypertension); cerebrovascular defect; history of headache; history of hepatic disease or abnormal liver function tests; pheochromocytoma

Concurrent use of antihistamines, antihypertensives, antiparkinson drugs, bupropion, buspirone, caffeine (excessive use), CNS depressants (including ethanol and opioids), dextromethorphan, diuretics, elective surgery requiring general anesthesia (discontinue tranylcypromine ≥10 days prior to elective surgery), local vasoconstrictors, meperidine, MAO inhibitors or dibenzazepine derivatives (eg, amitriptyline, clomipramine, desipramine, imipramine, nortriptyline, protriptyline, doxepin, carbamazepine, cyclobenzaprine, amoxapine, maprotiline, trimipramine), SSRIs or SNRIs, spinal anesthesia (hypotension may be exaggerated), sympathomimetics (including amphetamines, cocaine, phenylephrine, pseudoephedrine) or related compounds (methyldopa, reserpine, levodopa, tryptophan), or foods high in tyramine content

Bupropion: At least 14 days should elapse between MAO inhibitor discontinuation and bupropion initiation.

Buspirone: At least 10 days should elapse between tranylcypromine discontinuation and buspirone initiation.

MAO inhibitors or dibenzazepine derivatives: At least 1-2 weeks should elapse between the use of another MAO inhibitor or dibenzazepine derivative and tranylcypromine use.

Meperidine: At least 2-3 weeks should elapse between MAO inhibitor discontinuation and meperidine use.

SSRIs or SNRIs: At least 2 weeks should elapse between the discontinuation of sertraline or paroxetine and the initiation of tranylcypromine. At least 5 weeks should elapse between the discontinuation of fluoxetine and the initiation of tranylcypromine. At least 1 week should elapse between discontinuation of a SNRI and the initiation of tranylcypromine. At least 2 weeks should elapse between the discontinuation of tranylcypromine and the initiation of SNRIs and SSRIs.

Warnings/Precautions **Risk of suicide: [U.S. Boxed Warning]: Antidepressants increase the risk of suicidal thinking and behavior in children, adolescents, and young adults (18-24 years of age) with major depressive disorder (MDD) and other psychiatric disorders;** consider risk prior to prescribing. Short-term studies did not show an increased risk in patients >24 years of age and showed a decreased risk inpatients >65 years. Closely monitor for clinical worsening, suicidality, or unusual changes in behavior such as anxiety, agitation, panic attacks, insomnia, irritability, hostility, impulsivity, akathisia, hypomania, and mania. The patient's family or caregiver should be instructed to closely observe the patient and communicate condition with healthcare provider. Such observation would generally include at least weekly face-to-face contact with patients or their family members or caregivers during the first 4 weeks of treatment, then every other week visits for the next 4 weeks, then at 12 weeks, and as clinically indicated beyond 12 weeks. Additional contact by telephone may be appropriate between face-to-face visits. A medication guide should be dispensed with each prescription. **Tranylcypromine is not FDA approved for treatment of children and adolescents.**

All patients treated with antidepressants should be observed similarly for clinical worsening and suicidality, especially during the initial few months of a course of drug therapy, or at times of dose changes, either increases or decreases. The possibility of a suicide attempt is inherent in major depression and may persist until remission occurs. Worsening depression and severe abrupt suicidality that are not part of the presenting symptoms may require discontinuation or modification of drug therapy. Use caution in high-risk patients during initiation of therapy. Prescriptions should be written for the smallest quantity consistent with good patient care.

Hypertensive crisis may occur with foods/supplements high in tyramine, tryptophan, phenylalanine, or tyrosine content; treatment with phentolamine is recommended for hypertensive crisis. Use with caution in patients who have glaucoma, hyperthyroidism, diabetes or hypotension. May cause orthostatic hypotension (especially at dosages >30 mg/day). Use with caution in patients at risk of seizures, or in patients receiving other drugs which may lower seizure threshold. Use with caution in patients with a history of drug abuse or acute alcoholism; potential for drug dependency exists especially in patients using excessive doses. Discontinue at least 48 hours prior to myelography. May increase the risks associated with electroconvulsive therapy. Use with caution in patients with renal impairment. Do not use with other MAO inhibitors or antidepressants. Avoid products containing sympathomimetic stimulants or dextromethorphan. Concurrent use with antihypertensive agents may lead to exaggeration of hypotensive effects. Effects may be potentiated when used with other sedative drugs or ethanol. Tranylcypromine is not generally considered a first-line agent for the treatment of depression; tranylcypromine is typically used in patients who have failed to respond to other treatments. May worsen psychosis in some patients or precipitate a shift to mania or hypomania in patients with bipolar disorder. **Tranylcypromine is not FDA approved for the treatment of bipolar depression.**

Abrupt discontinuation or interruption of antidepressant therapy has been associated with a discontinuation syndrome. Symptoms arising may vary with antidepressant however commonly include nausea, vomiting, diarrhea, headaches, lightheadedness, dizziness, diminished appetite, sweating, chills, tremors, paresthesias, fatigue, somnolence, and sleep disturbances (eg, vivid dreams, insomnia). Greater risks for developing a discontinuation syndrome have been associated with antidepressants with shorter half-lives, longer durations of treatment, and abrupt discontinuation. More severe symptoms have also been associated with MAO inhibitors. For antidepressants of short or intermediate half-lives, symptoms may emerge within 2-5 days after treatment discontinuation and last

7-14 days (APA, 2010; Fava, 2006; Haddad, 2001; Shelton, 2001; Warner, 2006).

Adverse Reactions

Cardiovascular: Edema, orthostatic hypotension, palpitation, tachycardia

Central nervous system: Agitation, anxiety, chills, dizziness, drowsiness, headache, insomnia, mania, restlessness

Dermatologic: Alopecia (rare), rash (rare), urticaria

Endocrine & metabolic: Sexual dysfunction (anorgasmia, ejaculatory disturbances, impotence); SIADH

Gastrointestinal: Abdominal pain, anorexia, constipation, diarrhea, nausea, xerostomia

Genitourinary: Urinary retention

Hematologic: Agranulocytosis, anemia, leukopenia, thrombocytopenia

Hepatic: Hepatitis (rare)

Neuromuscular & skeletal: Muscle spasm, myoclonus, numbness, paresthesia, tremor, weakness

Ocular: Blurred vision

Otic: Tinnitus

Miscellaneous: Diaphoresis

Postmarketing and/or case reports: Akinesia, ataxia, confusion, cystic acne, disorientation, memory loss, mouth fissures, polyuria, scleroderma (localized), urinary incontinence, urticaria, withdrawal symptoms

Drug Interactions

Metabolism/Transport Effects Inhibits CYP1A2 (moderate), CYP2A6 (strong), CYP2C19 (moderate), CYP2C8 (weak), CYP2C9 (weak), CYP2D6 (moderate), CYP2E1 (weak), CYP3A4 (weak), Monoamine Oxidase

Avoid Concomitant Use

Avoid concomitant use of Tranylcypromine with any of the following: Aclidinium; Alcohol (Ethyl); Alpha-/Beta-Agonists (Indirect-Acting); Alpha1-Agonists; Amphetamines; Anilidopiperidine Opioids; Antidepressants (Serotonin Reuptake Inhibitor/Antagonist); Apraclonidine; AtoMOXetine; Bezafibrate; Buprenorphine; BuPROPion; BusPIRone; CarBAMazepine; Cyclobenzaprine; Cyproheptadine; Dapoxetine; Dexmethylphenidate; Dextromethorphan; Diethylpropion; Glucagon; Hydrocodone; HYDROmorphone; Ipratropium (Oral Inhalation); Isometheptene; Levonordefrin; Linezolid; Maprotiline; Meperidine; Methyldopa; Methylene Blue; Methylphenidate; Mianserin; Mirtazapine; Morphine (Liposomal); Morphine (Systemic); Oxymorphone; Pholcodine; Pimozide; Pizotifen; Potassium Chloride; Selective Serotonin Reuptake Inhibitors; Serotonin 5-HT1D Receptor Agonists; Serotonin/Norepinephrine Reuptake Inhibitors; Tapentadol; Tegafur; Tetrabenazine; Tetrahydrozoline (Nasal); Thioridazine; Tiotropium; Tricyclic Antidepressants; Tryptophan; Umeclidinium

Increased Effect/Toxicity

Tranylcypromine may increase the levels/effects of: AbobotulinumtoxinA; Agomelatine; Alpha-/Beta-Agonists (Indirect-Acting); Alpha1-Agonists; Amphetamines; Analgesics (Opioid); Anticholinergic Agents; Antidepressants (Serotonin Reuptake Inhibitor/Antagonist); Antihypertensives; Antipsychotic Agents; Apraclonidine; ARIPiprazole; AtoMOXetine; Beta2-Agonists; Betahistine; Bezafibrate; Brimonidine (Ophthalmic); Brimonidine (Topical); BuPROPion; Cannabinoid-Containing Products; CYP1A2 Substrates; CYP2A6 Substrates; CYP2C19 Substrates; CYP2D6 Substrates; Cyproheptadine; Dexmethylphenidate; Dextromethorphan; Diethylpropion; Dofetilide; Domperidone; Doxapram; DOXOrubicin (Conventional); Doxylamine; Eliglustat; EPINEPHrine (Nasal); Epinephrine (Racemic); EPINEPHrine (Systemic, Oral Inhalation); Fesoterodine; Glucagon; Hydrocodone; HYDROmorphone; Hypoglycemic Agents; Isometheptene; Levonordefrin; Linezolid; Lithium; Lomitapide; Meperidine; Methadone; Methyldopa; Methylene Blue; Methylphenidate; Metoclopramide; Metoprolol; Mianserin; Mirabegron; Mirtazapine; Morphine (Liposomal); Morphine (Systemic); Nebivolol; Norepinephrine; OnabotulinumtoxinA; Orthostatic Hypotension Producing Agents; OxyCODONE; Pimozide; Pirfenidone; Pizotifen; Potassium Chloride; Reserpine; RimabotulinumtoxinB; Selective Serotonin Reuptake Inhibitors; Serotonin 5-HT1D Receptor Agonists; Serotonin Modulators; Serotonin/Norepinephrine Reuptake Inhibitors; Tetrahydrozoline (Nasal); Thiazide Diuretics; Thioridazine; Tiotropium; Topiramate; Tricyclic Antidepressants

The levels/effects of Tranylcypromine may be increased by: Aclidinium; Alcohol (Ethyl); Altretamine; Anilidopiperidine Opioids; Antiemetics (5HT3 Antagonists); Antipsychotic Agents; Buprenorphine; BusPIRone; CarBAMazepine; COMT Inhibitors; Cyclobenzaprine; Dapoxetine; Ipratropium (Oral Inhalation); Levodopa; MAO Inhibitors; Maprotiline; Oxymorphone; Pholcodine; Pramlintide; Propafenone; Tapentadol; Tedizolid; Tetrabenazine; TraMADol; Tryptophan; Umeclidinium

Decreased Effect

Tranylcypromine may decrease the levels/effects of: Acetylcholinesterase Inhibitors; Clopidogrel; Codeine; Domperidone; Itopride; Secretin; Tamoxifen; Tegafur

The levels/effects of Tranylcypromine may be decreased by: Acetylcholinesterase Inhibitors; Cyproheptadine; Domperidone

Food Interactions Concurrent ingestion of foods rich in tyramine, dopamine, tyrosine, phenylalanine, tryptophan, or caffeine may cause sudden and severe high blood pressure (hypertensive crisis or serotonin syndrome). Beverages containing tyramine (eg, hearty red wine and beer) may increase toxic effects. Management: Avoid tyramine-containing foods (aged or matured cheese, air-dried or cured meats including sausages and salamis; fava or broad bean pods, tap/draft beers, Marmite concentrate, sauerkraut, soy sauce, and other soybean condiments). Food's freshness is also an important concern; improperly stored or spoiled food can create an environment in which tyramine concentrations may increase. Avoid foods containing dopamine, tyrosine, phenylalanine, tryptophan, or caffeine. Avoid beverages containing tyramine.

Storage/Stability Store at room temperature of 15°C to 30°C (59°F to 86°F).

Mechanism of Action Tranylcypromine is a nonhydrazine monoamine oxidase inhibitor. It increases endogenous concentrations of epinephrine, norepinephrine, dopamine, and serotonin through inhibition of the enzyme (monoamine oxidase) responsible for the breakdown of these neurotransmitters.

Pharmacodynamics/Kinetics

Onset of action: Therapeutic: 2 days to 3 weeks continued dosing

Duration: MAO inhibition may persist for up to 10 days following discontinuation

Half-life elimination: 90-190 minutes

Time to peak, serum: ~2 hours

Excretion: Urine

Dosage Note: 20 mg of tranylcypromine = 45 mg phenelzine = 40 mg of isocarboxazid (Sheehan 1980)

Adults: Oral: Usual effective dose: 30 mg/day in divided doses; if symptoms don't improve after 2 weeks, increase by 10 mg increments at 1- to 3-week intervals; maximum: 60 mg/day

Discontinuation of therapy: Upon discontinuation of antidepressant therapy, gradually taper the dose to minimize the incidence of withdrawal symptoms and allow for the detection of re-emerging symptoms. Evidence supporting ideal taper rates is limited. APA and NICE guidelines suggest tapering therapy over at least several weeks with consideration to the half-life of the antidepressant; antidepressants with a shorter half-life and MAO inhibitors may need to be tapered more conservatively. In addition for long-term treated patients, WFSBP guidelines recommend tapering over 4-6 months. If intolerable withdrawal symptoms occur following a dose reduction, consider resuming the previously prescribed dose and/or decrease dose at a more gradual rate (APA, 2010; Bauer, 2002; Haddad, 2001; NCCMH, 2010; Schatzberg, 2006; Shelton, 2001; Warner, 2006).

MAO inhibitor recommendations:

Switching to or from an MAO inhibitor intended to treat psychiatric disorders:

Allow 14 days to elapse between discontinuing an alternative antidepressant without long half-life metabolites (eg, TCAs, paroxetine, fluvoxamine, venlafaxine) or MAO inhibitor intended to treat psychiatric disorders and initiation of tranylcypromine.

Allow 5 weeks to elapse between discontinuing fluoxetine (with long half-life metabolites) intended to treat psychiatric disorders and initiation of tranylcypromine.

Allow at least 7-14 days days to elapse between discontinuing tranylcypromine and initiation of an alternative antidepressant or MAO inhibitor intended to treat psychiatric disorders.

Use with other MAO inhibitors (such as linezolid or IV methylene blue):

Do not initiate tranylcypromine in patients receiving linezolid or IV methylene blue; consider other interventions for psychiatric condition.

If urgent treatment with linezolid or IV methylene blue is required in a patient already receiving tranylcypromine and potential benefits outweigh potential risks, discontinue tranylcypromine promptly and administer linezolid or IV methylene blue. Monitor for serotonin syndrome for 2 weeks or until 24 hours after the last dose of linezolid or IV methylene blue, whichever comes first. May resume tranylcypromine 24 hours after the last dose of linezolid or IV methylene blue.

Dosage adjustment in renal impairment: No dosage adjustment provided in manufacturer's labeling.

Dosage adjustment in hepatic impairment: No dosage adjustment provided in manufacturer's labeling. Use is contraindicated in patients with a history of liver disease or abnormal liver function tests.

Dietary Considerations Avoid tyramine-containing foods/beverages. Some examples include aged or matured cheese, air-dried or cured meats (including sausages and salamis), fava or broad bean pods, tap/draft beers, Marmite concentrate, sauerkraut, soy sauce and other soybean condiments. Food's freshness is also an important concern; improperly stored or spoiled food can create an environment where tyramine concentrations may increase.

Monitoring Parameters Blood glucose; blood pressure, mental status, suicide ideation (especially at the beginning of therapy or when doses are increased or decreased)

Additional Information Tranylcypromine has a more rapid onset of therapeutic effect than other MAO inhibitors, but causes more severe hypertensive reactions.

Dosage Forms

Tablet, Oral:

Parnate: 10 mg

Generic: 10 mg

◆ **Tranylcypromine Sulfate** *see* Tranylcypromine *on page 2083*

Trapidil [INT] (TRA pi dil)

International Brand Names Avantrin (IT); Rocornal (AT, DE, JP, KR); Travisco (BR, IT)

Pharmacologic Category Antiplatelet Agent; Growth Factor, Platelet-Derived; Vasodilator

Reported Use Management of ischemic heart disease

Dosage Range Adults: Oral: 400-600 mg/day in divided doses

Product Availability Product available in various countries; not currently available in the U.S.

Dosage Forms

Capsule: 200 mg

Tablet: 200 mg

Trastuzumab (tras TU zoo mab)

Brand Names: U.S. Herceptin

Brand Names: Canada Herceptin

Index Terms anti-c-erB-2; anti-ERB-2; Conventional Trastuzumab; MOAB HER2; rhuMAb HER2; Trastuzumab (Conventional)

Pharmacologic Category Antineoplastic Agent, Anti-HER2; Antineoplastic Agent, Monoclonal Antibody

Use

Breast cancer, adjuvant treatment: Treatment (adjuvant) of human epidermal growth receptor 2 (HER2)-overexpressing node positive or node negative (estrogen receptor/progesterone receptor negative or with 1 high risk feature) breast cancer as part of a treatment regimen consisting of doxorubicin, cyclophosphamide, and either paclitaxel or docetaxel; with docetaxel and carboplatin; or as a single agent following multimodality anthracycline-based therapy.

Breast cancer, metastatic: First-line treatment of HER2-overexpressing metastatic breast cancer (in combination with paclitaxel); single agent treatment of HER2-overexpressing breast cancer in patients who have received 1 or more chemotherapy regimens for metastatic disease.

Gastric cancer, metastatic: Treatment of HER2-overexpressing metastatic gastric or gastroesophageal junction adenocarcinoma (in combination with cisplatin and either capecitabine or 5-fluorouracil) in patients who have not received prior treatment for metastatic disease.

Pregnancy Risk Factor D

Pregnancy Considerations Adverse events were not observed in animal reproduction studies. However, trastuzumab inhibits HER2 protein, which has a role in embryonic development. **[U.S. Boxed Warning]: Trastuzumab exposure during pregnancy may result in oligohydramnios and oligohydramnios sequence (pulmonary hypoplasia, skeletal malformations and neonatal death).** Oligohydramnios (reversible in some cases) has been reported with trastuzumab use alone or with combination chemotherapy. If trastuzumab exposure occurs during pregnancy, monitor for oligohydramnios. Effective contraception is recommended during and for 6 months after treatment for women of childbearing potential. Women exposed to trastuzumab during pregnancy are encouraged to enroll in MotHER (the Herceptin Pregnancy Registry; 1-800-690-6720).

The National Comprehensive Cancer Network (NCCN) breast cancer guidelines (v.2.2014) advise against use during pregnancy and recommend (if indicated) administering trastuzumab in the postpartum period.

Breast-Feeding Considerations It is not known whether trastuzumab is secreted in human milk. Because many immunoglobulins are secreted in milk, and the potential for serious adverse reactions in the nursing infant exists, the decision to discontinue trastuzumab or discontinue breast-feeding during treatment should take in account the benefits of treatment to the mother. The extended half-life should also be considered for decisions regarding breast-feeding after therapy completion.

Contraindications

There are no contraindications listed in the manufacturer's labeling.

Canadian labeling: Hypersensitivity to trastuzumab, Chinese hamster ovary (CHO) cell proteins, or any component of the formulation

Warnings/Precautions Hazardous agent - use appropriate precautions for handling and disposal (meets NIOSH 2014 criteria). **[U.S. Boxed Warning]: Trastuzumab is associated with symptomatic and asymptomatic reductions in left ventricular ejection fraction (LVEF) and heart failure (HF); the incidence is highest in patients receiving trastuzumab with an anthracycline-containing chemotherapy regimen. Evaluate LVEF in all patients prior to and during treatment; discontinue for cardiomyopathy.** Extreme caution should be used in patients with preexisting cardiac disease or dysfunction. Prior or concurrent exposure to anthracyclines or radiation therapy significantly increases the risk of cardiomyopathy; other potential risk factors include advanced age, high or low body mass index, smoking, diabetes, hypertension, and hyper-/hypothyroidism. Discontinuation should be strongly considered in patients who develop a clinically significant reduction in LVEF during therapy; treatment with HF medications (eg, ACE inhibitors, beta-blockers) should be initiated. Withhold treatment for ≥16% decrease from pretreatment levels or LVEF below normal limits and ≥10% decrease from baseline (see Dosage adjustment for cardiotoxicity). Cardiomyopathy due to trastuzumab is generally reversible over a period of 1-3 months after discontinuation. Trastuzumab is also associated with arrhythmias, hypertension, mural thrombus formation, stroke, and even cardiac death.

[U.S. Boxed Warning]: Serious adverse events, including hypersensitivity reaction (anaphylaxis), infusion reactions (including fatalities), and pulmonary events (including acute respiratory distress syndrome [ARDS]) have been associated with trastuzumab. Discontinue for anaphylaxis, angioedema, ARDS or interstitial pneumonitis. Most of these events occur with the first infusion; pulmonary events may occur during or within 24 hours of the first infusion; delayed reactions have occurred. Interrupt infusion for dyspnea or significant hypotension; monitor until symptoms resolve. Infusion reactions may consist of fever and chills, and may also include nausea, vomiting, pain, headache, dizziness, dyspnea, hypotension, rash, and weakness. Retreatment of patients who experienced severe hypersensitivity reactions has been attempted (with premedication). Some patients tolerated retreatment, while others experienced a second severe reaction. When used in combination with myelosuppressive chemotherapy, trastuzumab may increase the incidence of neutropenia (moderate-to-severe) and febrile neutropenia; the incidence of anemia may be higher when trastuzumab is added to chemotherapy. Rare cases of nephrotic syndrome with evidence of glomerulopathy have been reported, with an onset of 4-18 months from trastuzumab initiation; complications may include volume overload and HF. The incidence of renal impairment was increased in metastatic gastric cancer patients when trastuzumab is added to chemotherapy.

May cause serious pulmonary toxicity (dyspnea, hypoxia, interstitial pneumonitis, pulmonary infiltrates, pleural effusion, noncardiogenic pulmonary edema, pulmonary insufficiency, acute respiratory distress syndrome, and/or pulmonary fibrosis); use caution in patients with preexisting pulmonary disease or patients with extensive pulmonary tumor involvement. Establish HER2 status prior to treatment; has only been studied in patients with evidence of HER2 protein overexpression, either by validated immunohistochemistry (IHC) assay or fluorescence *in situ* hybridization (FISH) assay. Tests appropriate for the specific tumor type (breast or gastric) should be used to assess HER2 status. **[U.S. Boxed Warning]: Trastuzumab exposure during pregnancy may result in oligohydramnios and oligohydramnios sequence (pulmonary hypoplasia, skeletal malformations and neonatal death).** Effective contraception is recommended during and for 6 months after treatment for women of childbearing potential. Conventional trastuzumab and ado-trastuzumab emtansine are **not** interchangeable; verify product label prior to reconstitution and administration to prevent medication errors. Dosing and treatment schedules between conventional trastuzumab (Herceptin) and ado-trastuzumab emtansine (Kadcyla) are different; confusion between the products may potentially cause harm to the patient. Potentially significant drug-drug interactions may exist, requiring dose or frequency adjustment, additional monitoring, and/or selection of alternative therapy.

Adverse Reactions

Cardiovascular: Arrhythmia, edema, cardiac failure, decreased left ventricular ejection fraction, hypertension, palpitations, peripheral edema, tachycardia

Central nervous system: Chills, depression, dizziness, headache, insomnia, neuropathy, pain, paresthesia, peripheral neuritis

Dermatologic: Acne vulgaris, nail disease, pruritus, skin rash

Gastrointestinal: Abdominal pain, anorexia, constipation, diarrhea, dyspepsia, nausea, vomiting

Genitourinary: Urinary tract infection

Hematologic: Anemia, leukopenia

Hypersensitivity: Hypersensitivity reaction

Infection: Herpes simplex infection, infection, influenza

Neuromuscular & skeletal: Arthralgia, muscle spasm, myalgia, ostealgia, weakness

Respiratory: Cough, dyspnea, epistaxis, flu-like syndrome, nasopharyngitis, pharyngolaryngeal pain, pharyngitis, rhinitis, sinusitis, upper respiratory tract infection

Miscellaneous: Accidental injury, fever, infusion related reaction (chills, fever most common)

Rare but important or life-threatening (as a single-agent or with combination chemotherapy): Adult respiratory distress syndrome, amblyopia, anaphylaxis, apnea, ascites, asthma, ataxia, blood coagulation disorder, bronchitis, cardiogenic shock, cardiomyopathy, cellulitis, cerebrovascular accident, colitis, coma, confusion, deafness, dermal ulcer, erysipelas, esophageal ulcer, febrile neutropenia, gastroenteritis, glomerulopathy, hematemesis, hemorrhage, hemorrhagic cystitis, hepatic failure, hepatitis, herpes zoster, hydrocephalus, hydronephrosis, hypercalcemia, hypotension, hypothyroidism, hypoxia, intestinal obstruction, interstitial pneumonitis, leukemia (acute), lymphangitis, madarosis, mania, meningitis, myopathy, neutropenia, neutropenic sepsis, oligohydramnios, onychoclasis, osteonecrosis, pancreatitis, pancytopenia, paresis, paroxysmal nocturnal dyspnea, pathological fracture, pericardial effusion, pleural effusion, pneumonitis, pneumothorax, pulmonary edema (noncardiogenic), pulmonary fibrosis, pulmonary hypertension, pyelonephritis, radiation injury, renal failure, respiratory failure, seizure, sepsis, syncope, stomatitis, thyroiditis (autoimmune), ventricular dysfunction

Drug Interactions

Metabolism/Transport Effects None known.

Avoid Concomitant Use

Avoid concomitant use of Trastuzumab with any of the following: Belimumab

Increased Effect/Toxicity

Trastuzumab may increase the levels/effects of: Antineoplastic Agents (Anthracycline, Systemic); Belimumab; Immunosuppressants

The levels/effects of Trastuzumab may be increased by: PACLitaxel

Decreased Effect

Trastuzumab may decrease the levels/effects of: PACLitaxel

Preparation for Administration Hazardous agent; use appropriate precautions for handling and disposal (meets NIOSH 2014 criteria). Check vial labels to assure appropriate product is being reconstituted (conventional trastuzumab and ado-trastuzumab emtansine are different products and are **NOT** interchangeable).

Reconstitute each vial with 20 mL of bacteriostatic sterile water for injection to a concentration of 21 mg/mL. Swirl gently; do not shake. Allow vial to rest for ~5 minutes. If the patient has a known hypersensitivity to benzyl alcohol, trastuzumab may be reconstituted with sterile water for injection without preservatives, which must be used immediately. Further dilute the appropriate volume for the trastuzumab dose in 250 mL NS prior to administration. Gently invert bag to mix.

Storage/Stability Prior to reconstitution, store intact vials under refrigeration at 2°C to 8°C (36°F to 46°F). Following reconstitution with bacteriostatic SWFI, the solution in the vial is stable refrigerated for 28 days from the date of reconstitution; do not freeze. Solutions reconstituted with sterile water for injection without preservatives must be used immediately. The solution diluted in 250 mL NS for infusion may be stored refrigerated for up to 24 hours prior to use; do not freeze.

Mechanism of Action Trastuzumab is a monoclonal antibody which binds to the extracellular domain of the human epidermal growth factor receptor 2 protein (HER-2); it mediates antibody-dependent cellular cytotoxicity by inhibiting proliferation of cells which overexpress HER-2 protein.

Pharmacodynamics/Kinetics

Distribution: V_d: 44 mL/kg; not likely to cross the (intact) blood-brain barrier (due to the large molecule size)

Half-life elimination: Weekly dosing: Mean: 6 days (range: 1-32 days); every 3 week regimen: Mean: 16 days (range: 11-23 days)

Dosage Note: Do **NOT** substitute conventional trastuzumab for or with ado-trastuzumab emtansine; products are different and are **NOT** interchangeable.

Breast cancer, adjuvant treatment, HER2+: Adults: IV:

Note: Extending adjuvant treatment beyond 1 year is not recommended

With concurrent paclitaxel or docetaxel:

Initial loading dose: 4 mg/kg infused over 90 minutes, followed by

Maintenance dose: 2 mg/kg infused over 30 minutes weekly for total of 12 weeks, followed 1 week later (when concurrent chemotherapy completed) by 6 mg/kg infused over 30-90 minutes every 3 weeks for total therapy duration of 52 weeks

With concurrent docetaxel/carboplatin:

Initial loading dose: 4 mg/kg infused over 90 minutes, followed by

Maintenance dose: 2 mg/kg infused over 30 minutes weekly for total of 18 weeks, followed 1 week later (when concurrent chemotherapy completed) by 6 mg/kg infused over 30-90 minutes every 3 weeks for total therapy duration of 52 weeks

Following completion of anthracycline-based chemotherapy:

Initial loading dose: 8 mg/kg infused over 90 minutes, followed by

Maintenance dose: 6 mg/kg infused over 30-90 minutes every 3 weeks for total therapy duration of 52 weeks

Breast cancer, metastatic, HER2+ (either as a single agent or in combination with paclitaxel): Adults: IV:

Initial loading dose: 4 mg/kg infused over 90 minutes, followed by

Maintenance dose: 2 mg/kg infused over 30 minutes weekly until disease progression

Gastric cancer, metastatic, HER2+ (in combination with cisplatin and either capecitabine or fluorouracil for 6 cycles followed by trastuzumab monotherapy; Bang, 2010): Adults: IV:

Initial loading dose: 8 mg/kg infused over 90 minutes, followed by

Maintenance dose: 6 mg/kg infused over 30-90 minutes every 3 weeks until disease progression

Missed doses *(Canadian labeling, 2013):* If a dose is missed by ≤1 week, the usual maintenance dose (based on patient's schedule) should be administered as soon as possible (do not wait until the next planned cycle); if a dose is missed by >1 week, then a loading dose (4 mg/kg if patient receives trastuzumab weekly; 8 mg/kg if on an every-3-week schedule) should be administered, followed by the usual maintenance dose and schedule.

Breast cancer (early stage, locally advanced, or inflammatory), neoadjuvant treatment, HER2+ (off-label use): Adults: IV: Trastuzumab, pertuzumab, and docetaxel (in patients with operable disease who have received no prior chemotherapy): Initial: 8 mg/kg (cycle 1) followed by 6 mg/kg every 3 weeks for a total of 4 neoadjuvant cycles; postoperatively, administer 3 cycles of adjuvant FEC [fluorouracil, epirubicin, and cyclophosphamide] chemotherapy and continue trastuzumab to complete 1 year of treatment (Gianni, 2012)

Breast cancer, metastatic, HER2+ (off-label combinations): Adults: IV:

Trastuzumab, pertuzumab, and docetaxel (in patients with no prior anti-HER2 therapy or chemotherapy to treat metastatic disease): Initial: 8 mg/kg followed by a maintenance dose of 6 mg/kg every 3 weeks until disease progression or unacceptable toxicity (Baselga, 2012)

Trastuzumab and lapatinib (in patients with progression on prior trastuzumab containing therapy): Initial: 4 mg/kg followed by a maintenance dose of 2 mg/kg every week (Blackwell, 2010; Blackwell, 2012)

Dosage adjustment for toxicity:

Cardiotoxicity: LVEF ≥16% decrease from baseline or LVEF below normal limits and ≥10% decrease from baseline: Withhold treatment for at least 4 weeks and repeat LVEF every 4 weeks. May resume trastuzumab treatment if LVEF returns to normal limits within 4-8 weeks and remains at ≤15% decrease from baseline value. Discontinue permanently for persistent (>8 weeks) LVEF decline or for >3 incidents of treatment interruptions for cardiomyopathy.

Infusion-related events:

Mild-moderate infusion reactions: Decrease infusion rate

Dyspnea, clinically significant hypotension: Interrupt infusion

Severe or life-threatening infusion reactions: Discontinue

Dosing adjustment in renal impairment: There are no dosage adjustments provided in the manufacturer's labeling, although data suggest that the disposition of trastuzumab is not altered based on serum creatinine (up to 2 mg/dL).

Dosing adjustment in hepatic impairment: There are no dosage adjustments provided in the manufacturer's labeling.

Administration Check label to ensure appropriate product is being administered (conventional trastuzumab and ado-trastuzumab emtansine are different products and are **NOT** interchangeable).

Administered by IV infusion; loading doses are infused over 90 minutes; maintenance doses may be infused over 30 minutes if tolerated. Do not administer with D_5W. **Do not administer IV push or by rapid bolus. Do not mix with any other medications.**

Observe patients closely during the infusion for fever, chills, or other infusion-related symptoms. Treatment with acetaminophen, diphenhydramine, and/or meperidine is usually effective for managing infusion-related events.

Hazardous agent; use appropriate precautions for handling and disposal (meets NIOSH 2014 criteria).

Monitoring Parameters Assessment for HER2 overexpression and HER2 gene amplification by validated immunohistochemistry (IHC) or fluorescence *in situ* hybridization (FISH) methodology (pretherapy); test should be specific for cancer type (breast vs gastric cancer). Pregnancy test (prior to treatment). Monitor vital signs during infusion; signs and symptoms of cardiac dysfunction; LVEF (baseline, every 3 months during treatment, upon therapy completion and if component of adjuvant therapy, every 6 months for at least 2 years; if treatment is withheld for significant LVEF dysfunction, monitor LVEF at 4-week intervals); signs and symptoms of infusion reaction or pulmonary toxicity; if pregnancy inadvertently occurs during treatment, monitor amniotic fluid volume

Dosage Forms

Solution Reconstituted, Intravenous:

Herceptin: 440 mg (1 ea)

- ◆ **Trastuzumab-MCC-DM1** *see* Ado-Trastuzumab Emtansine *on page 58*
- ◆ **Trastuzumab (Conventional)** *see* Trastuzumab *on page 2085*
- ◆ **Trastuzumab-DM1** *see* Ado-Trastuzumab Emtansine *on page 58*
- ◆ **Trastuzumab Emtansine** *see* Ado-Trastuzumab Emtansine *on page 58*
- ◆ **Trasylol [DSC]** *see* Aprotinin *on page 168*
- ◆ **Trasylol (Can)** *see* Aprotinin *on page 168*
- ◆ **Travatan Z** *see* Travoprost *on page 2089*

Travelers' Diarrhea and Cholera Vaccine [CAN/INT]

(TRAV uh lerz dahy uh REE uh & KOL er uh vak SEEN)

Brand Names: Canada Dukoral®

Index Terms *Vibrio cholera* and Enterotoxigenic *Escherichia coli Vaccine*; Cholera and Traveler's Diarrhea Vaccine; Cholera Vaccine; Enterotoxigenic *Escherichia coli* and *Vibrio cholera* Vaccine; Oral Cholera Vaccine; Traveller's Diarrhea Vaccine and Cholera; WC-rBS

Pharmacologic Category Vaccine

Additional Appendix Information

Immunization Administration Recommendations *on page 2250*

Immunization Recommendations *on page 2255*

Use Note: Not approved in U.S.

Protection against travelers' diarrhea and/or cholera in adults and children ≥2 years of age who will be visiting areas where there is a risk of contracting travelers' diarrhea caused by enterotoxigenic *E. coli* (ETEC) or cholera caused by *V. cholerae* O1 (classical and El Tor biotypes; Inaba and Ogawa serotypes)

Note: The Centers for Disease Control and Prevention (CDC) *Health Information for International Travel* ("The Yellow Book") categorizes the following areas of risk (CDC, 2012):

- Low-risk countries include the United States, Canada, Australia, New Zealand, Japan, and countries in Northern and Western Europe.
- Intermediate-risk countries include those in Eastern Europe, South Africa, and some of the Caribbean islands.
- High-risk areas include most of Asia, the Middle East, Africa, Mexico, and Central and South America.

Pregnancy Considerations Safety and efficacy in pregnant women have not been established; the vaccine is not recommended for use during pregnancy. However, since the vaccine is given orally in an inactivated form, acts locally in the gut, and does not replicate, it may not (in theory) cause a risk to the fetus. Use should only be considered if the potential benefit to the mother outweighs the potential risk to the fetus.

Breast-Feeding Considerations The manufacturer states that the vaccine may be given to lactating women.

Contraindications Hypersensitivity to any component of the formulation or packaging; acute illness (excluding minor illnesses such as a mild upper respiratory tract infection)

Warnings/Precautions Immediate treatment for anaphylactoid and/or hypersensitivity reactions should be available during vaccine administration. Vaccination may not result in effective immunity in all patients. Response depends upon multiple factors (eg, type of vaccine, age of patient) and may be improved by administering the vaccine at the recommended dose, route, and interval. Vaccines may not be effective if administered during periods of altered immune competence (CDC, 2011). Use with caution in severely immunocompromised patients (eg, patients receiving chemo/radiation therapy or other immunosuppressive therapy [including high-dose corticosteroids]); may have a reduced response to vaccination. In general, inactivated vaccines should be administered ≥2 weeks prior to planned immunosuppression when feasible (Rubin, 2014). Vaccine has not been shown to protect against cholera caused by *V. cholerae* serogroup O139 or other species of *Vibrio*. Vaccine may be administered to patients with HIV infection. No specific studies have been conducted in this patient population; however, a field study exhibited 84% immunity in a population with ~25% HIV prevalence.

The World Health Organization (WHO) recommends vaccination, in conjunction with other preventive and control strategies (eg, provision of safe water and sanitation efforts), in endemic areas (eg, south and southeast Asia and Africa) and in areas at risk for outbreaks. Vaccination should be targeted at high-risk populations (eg, children) when resources are limited. Reactive vaccination may be considered to control the spread of current outbreaks. In addition, the WHO recommends vaccination for travelers who are at an increased risk for the disease (eg, emergency relief and health workers in refugee situations) (WHO, 2010). The Public Health Agency of Canada currently includes cholera vaccination on its list of recommended vaccines for Canadian travelers. Currently, the U.S Center for Disease Control (CDC) does not recommend oral cholera vaccination for most U.S. travelers due to the low risk of cholera to travelers and the brief and incomplete immunity the vaccines confer (CDC, 2009). In order to maximize vaccination rates, the Canadian Immunization Guide recommends simultaneous administration of all age-appropriate vaccines (live or inactivated) for which a person is eligible at a single clinic visit, unless contraindications exist.

Some dosage forms may contain trace amounts of formaldehyde. Avoid oral administration of other medications (including oral vaccines) for 1 hour before and 1 hour after vaccine administration.

Adverse Reactions All serious adverse reactions related to the administration of the product should be reported to local provincial/territorial health agencies or to the Vaccine Safety Section at Public Health Agency of Canada (1-866-844-0018) and to the Senior Product Safety Officer, Pharmacovigilance Department, Aventis Pasteur Limited, 1755 Steeles Avenue West, Toronto, ON, M2R 3T4, Canada. 1-888-621-1146 (phone) or 416-667-2435 (fax).

Rare but important or life-threatening: Abdominal cramps/discomfort/pain, angioedema, appetite decreased, chills, cough, dehydration, diaphoresis, diarrhea, dizziness, drowsiness, dyspepsia, dyspnea, fainting, fatigue, fever, flatulence, flu-like syndrome, gastroenteritis, headache, hypertension, insomnia, joint pain, lymphadenitis, malaise, nausea, pain, paresthesia, pruritus, rash, rhinitis, shivering, sore throat, sputum increased, taste disturbance, urticaria, vomiting, weakness

Drug Interactions

Metabolism/Transport Effects None known.

Avoid Concomitant Use There are no known interactions where it is recommended to avoid concomitant use.

Increased Effect/Toxicity There are no known significant interactions involving an increase in effect.

Decreased Effect

The levels/effects of Travelers' Diarrhea and Cholera Vaccine may be decreased by: Belimumab; Immunosuppressants

Food Interactions May affect efficacy of vaccine. Management: Avoid food 1 hour before and 1 hour following vaccine administration.

Preparation for Administration To prepare the buffer solution, dissolve the effervescent granules contained in the sachet in 150 mL of cool water; do not use juice, milk, or other liquids or beverages. When preparing the vaccine for children 2-6 years of age, discard half the amount of the buffer solution before adding the vaccine. The vial containing the vaccine should be shaken and the entire contents should be added to the buffer solution and mixed.

Storage/Stability Dukoral® is supplied as a vial of oral vaccine and a sachet of sodium hydrogen carbonate effervescent granules.

Store unused vials at 2°C to 8°C (35°F to 46°F); do not freeze. Vials may be stored at room temperature (<27°C) for up to 2 weeks on one occasion only. The sachet may be stored separate from the vial at room temperature (<27°C). The vaccine-buffer solution mixture should be used immediately, but may be stored at room temperature (<27°C) for up to 2 hours after mixing.

Mechanism of Action Contains killed *V. cholerae* O1 bacteria and recombinant cholera toxin B subunit (CTB); the toxin of enterotoxigenic *E. coli* (ETEC) is structurally, functionally, and immunologically similar to CTB and is neutralized by antibodies against CTB. Vaccine administration induces immunity and an IgA antitoxic and antibacterial response locally within the gastrointestinal tract; immunity is specific to *V. cholerae* O1 (classical and El Tor biotypes; Inaba and Ogawa serotypes) and ETEC.

Pharmacodynamics/Kinetics

Onset of action: ETEC diarrhea and cholera immunity: ~1 week after primary immunization

Duration: ETEC immunity: 3 months after primary immunization; Cholera immunity: Children 2-6 years of age: 6 months after primary immunization; Children ≥6 years and Adults: 2 years after primary immunization

Dosage Oral:

Cholera:

Primary immunization:

Children 2-6 years: 3 doses given at intervals of ≥1 week and completed at least 1 week prior to trip to endemic/epidemic areas; restart treatment if interval between doses >6 weeks

Children >6 years and Adults: 2 doses given at intervals of ≥1 week and completed at least 1 week prior to trip to endemic/epidemic areas; restart treatment if interval between doses >6 weeks

Booster:

Children 2-6 years:

6 months to 5 years **since last dose**: 1 booster dose

>5 years **since last dose**: Repeat primary immunization schedule

Children >6 years and Adults:

2-5 years **since last dose**: 1 booster dose

>5 years **since last dose**: Repeat primary immunization schedule

ETEC:

Primary immunization: Children ≥2 years and Adults: 2 doses given at intervals of ≥1 week and completed at least 1 week prior to departure; restart treatment if interval between doses >6 weeks

Booster: Children ≥2 years and Adults:

3 months to 5 years **since last dose**: 1 booster dose

>5 years **since last dose**: Repeat primary immunization schedule

Dietary Considerations Food may affect efficacy of vaccine; avoid 1 hour before and 1 hour following vaccine administration.

Administration For oral use only; do not administer IM, IV, or SubQ. Oral administration of other medications, vaccines, and consumption of food or drink should be avoided 1 hour before and 1 hour following vaccine administration.

Administration with other vaccines (manufacturer recommendations): *Typhoid vaccine, oral:* Separate by at least 8 hours

Acetaminophen may be used when needed to provide comfort; however, routine prophylactic administration of acetaminophen to prevent fever due to vaccine use is not recommended. There is evidence of a decreased immune response to some vaccines associated with acetaminophen administration; the clinical significance of this reduction in immune response has not been established.

Product Availability Not available in U.S.

Dosage Forms: Canada

Suspension [vial]:

Dukoral®: 2.5 x 10^{10} of each of the following *Vibrio cholerae* O1 strains: Inaba classic (heat inactivated), Inaba El Tor (formalin inactivated), Ogawa classic (heat inactivated), Ogawa classic (formalin inactivated), and 1 mg recombinant cholera toxin B subunit (rCTB) (3 mL)

◆ **Traveller's Diarrhea Vaccine and Cholera** *see* Travelers' Diarrhea and Cholera Vaccine [CAN/INT] *on page 2088*

◆ **Travel Sickness [OTC]** *see* Meclizine *on page 1277*

◆ **Travel Tabs [OTC] (Can)** *see* DimenhyDRINATE *on page 637*

Travoprost (TRA voe prost)

Brand Names: U.S. Travatan Z

Brand Names: Canada Apo-Travoprost Z; Sandoz-Travoprost; Teva-Travoprost Z Ophthalmic Solution; Travatan Z

Index Terms Izba

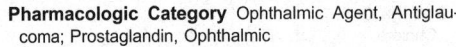

Pharmacologic Category Ophthalmic Agent, Antiglaucoma; Prostaglandin, Ophthalmic

Use Elevated intraocular pressure: Reduction of elevated intraocular pressure in patients with open-angle glaucoma or ocular hypertension

Pregnancy Risk Factor C

Dosage

Elevated intraocular pressure:

U.S. labeling: Adolescents ≥16 years and Adults: Ophthalmic: Instill 1 drop into affected eye(s) once daily in the evening; do not exceed once-daily dosing (may decrease IOP-lowering effect).

Canadian labeling: Adults: Ophthalmic: Instill 1 drop into affected eye(s) once daily in the evening; do not exceed once-daily dosing (may decrease IOP-lowering effect).

Dosage adjustment in renal impairment: There are no dosage adjustments provided in the manufacturer's labeling. However, dosage adjustments are unlikely due to low systemic absorption.

Dosage adjustment in hepatic impairment: There are no dosage adjustments provided in the manufacturer's labeling. However, dosage adjustments are unlikely due to low systemic absorption.

Additional Information Complete prescribing information should be consulted for additional detail.

Product Availability Izba (travoprost 0.003% ophthalmic solution): FDA approved May 2014; anticipated availability is currently unknown.

Dosage Forms

Solution, Ophthalmic:

Travatan Z: 0.004% (2.5 mL, 5 mL)

Generic: 0.004% (2.5 mL, 5 mL)

Travoprost and Timolol [CAN/INT]

(TRA voe prost & TIM oh lol)

Brand Names: Canada DuoTrav PQ

Index Terms Timolol Maleate and Travoprost

Pharmacologic Category Beta-Blocker, Nonselective; Ophthalmic Agent, Antiglaucoma; Prostaglandin, Ophthalmic

Use Note: Not approved in U.S.

Elevated intraocular pressure: For the reduction of intraocular pressure (IOP) in patients with open-angle glaucoma or ocular hypertension who inadequately respond to topical beta-blockers, prostaglandin analogues, or other IOP-reducing agents and in whom combination therapy is appropriate.. Not indicated for initial therapy.

Pregnancy Considerations Use of the combination product is contraindicated in women who are pregnant or attempting to become pregnant.

Breast-Feeding Considerations Timolol has been detected in human breast milk following ophthalmic administration. It is not known if travoprost is excreted in human milk. Per the manufacturer, the decision to discontinue nursing or discontinue the drug should take into account the importance of the drug to the mother. Also see individual agents.

Contraindications Hypersensitivity to travoprost, timolol, or any other component of the formulation; reactive airway diseases including bronchial asthma; history of bronchial asthma; severe chronic obstructive pulmonary disease (COPD); sick sinus syndrome or sino-atrial block; sinus bradycardia; second- or third-degree atrioventricular block; overt cardiac failure; cardiogenic shock; women who are pregnant or attempting to become pregnant. Also see individual agents.

Warnings/Precautions See individual agents.

Adverse Reactions Also see individual agents. Based on long-term studies:

Ocular: Blurred vision, dry eyes, eye irritant, eyelash growth, eye pain, eye pruritus, hyperemia, iris pigmentation changes, photophobia, punctuate keratitis

Rare but important or life-threatening: Allergic conjunctivitis, anterior chamber flare, arrhythmia, asthenopia, blepharitis, bradycardia, bronchospasm, chromaturia, conjunctival hemorrhage, contact dermatitis, cough, corneal staining, distichiasis, dizziness, dyspnea, extremity pain, eye allergy, eyelid dermatitis, eyelid edema, eyelid erythema, eyelid irritation, eyelid pain, eye swelling, headache, hyper-/hypotension, hypertrichosis, lacrimation increased, nervousness, ocular discomfort, periorbital disorder, postnasal drip, skin hyperpigmentation, thirst, throat irritation, urticaria, visual disturbance, xerophthalmia

Drug Interactions

Metabolism/Transport Effects Refer to individual components.

Avoid Concomitant Use

Avoid concomitant use of Travoprost and Timolol with any of the following: Beta2-Agonists; Ceritinib; Floctafenine; Methacholine

Increased Effect/Toxicity

Travoprost and Timolol may increase the levels/effects of: Alpha-/Beta-Agonists (Direct-Acting); Alpha1-Blockers; Alpha2-Agonists; Antipsychotic Agents (Phenothiazines); ARIPiprazole; Bradycardia-Causing Agents; Bupivacaine; Cardiac Glycosides; Ceritinib; Cholinergic Agonists; Disopyramide; DULoxetine; Ergot Derivatives; Fingolimod; Grass Pollen Allergen Extract (5 Grass Extract); Hypotensive Agents; Insulin; Lacosamide; Levodopa; Lidocaine (Systemic); Lidocaine (Topical); Mepivacaine; Methacholine; Midodrine; RisperiDONE; Sulfonylureas

The levels/effects of Travoprost and Timolol may be increased by: Abiraterone Acetate; Acetylcholinesterase Inhibitors; Alpha2-Agonists; Aminoquinolines (Antimalarial); Amiodarone; Anilidopiperidine Opioids; Antipsychotic Agents (Phenothiazines); Barbiturates; Bretylium; Calcium Channel Blockers (Dihydropyridine); Calcium Channel Blockers (Nondihydropyridine); Cobicistat; CYP2D6 Inhibitors (Moderate); CYP2D6 Inhibitors (Strong); Darunavir; Dipyridamole; Disopyramide; Dronedarone; Floctafenine; MAO Inhibitors; Nicorandil; Peginterferon Alfa-2b; Propafenone; Regorafenib; Reserpine; Selective Serotonin Reuptake Inhibitors; Tofacitinib

Decreased Effect

Travoprost and Timolol may decrease the levels/effects of: Beta2-Agonists; Theophylline Derivatives

The levels/effects of Travoprost and Timolol may be decreased by: Barbiturates; Nonsteroidal Anti-Inflammatory Agents; Peginterferon Alfa-2b; Rifamycin Derivatives

Storage/Stability Store between 2°C to 25°C (36°F to 77°F).

Mechanism of Action

Travoprost: Selective FP prostanoid receptor agonist which lowers intraocular pressure by increasing trabecular meshwork and outflow

Timolol: Blocks both $beta_1$- and $beta_2$-adrenergic receptors, reduces intraocular pressure by reducing aqueous humor production or possibly outflow; reduces blood pressure by blocking adrenergic receptors and decreasing sympathetic outflow, produces a negative chronotropic and inotropic activity through an unknown mechanism

Pharmacodynamics/Kinetics See individual agents.

Dosage Control of intraocular pressure: Adults: Ophthalmic: Instill 1 drop into affected eye(s) once daily in the morning or evening.

Administration Wash hands prior to use. Remove contact lenses prior to administration; wait 15 minutes before reinserting. Tilt head back, pull down lower eyelid and instill drop into pocket between eyelid and eye. Avoid touching bottle tip. Separate administration of other ophthalmic agents by 5 minutes.

Monitoring Parameters IOP, iris color changes, eyelash changes; systemic effects of beta blockade with ophthalmic administration

Product Availability Not available in U.S.

Dosage Forms: Canada

Solution, ophthalmic:

DuoTrav PQ: Travoprost 0.004% and timolol 0.5%: (2.5 mL, 5 mL)

TraZODone (TRAZ oh done)

Brand Names: U.S. Oleptro

Brand Names: Canada Apo-Trazodone; Apo-Trazodone D; Dom-Trazodone; Mylan-Trazodone; Novo-Trazodone; Nu-Trazodone; Nu-Trazodone D; Oleptro; PHL-Trazodone; PMS-Trazodone; ratio-Trazodone; Teva-Trazodone; Trazorel; ZYM-Trazodone

Index Terms Desyrel; Trazodone Hydrochloride

Pharmacologic Category Antidepressant, Serotonin Reuptake Inhibitor/Antagonist

Use Treatment of major depressive disorder

Pregnancy Risk Factor C

Pregnancy Considerations Adverse effects were observed in some animal reproduction studies. When trazodone is taken during pregnancy, an increased risk of major malformations has not been observed in the limited number of pregnancies studied (Einarson, 2003; Einarson, 2009). The long-term effects of *in utero* trazodone exposure on infant development and behavior are not known.

The ACOG recommends that therapy with antidepressants during pregnancy be individualized; treatment of depression during pregnancy should incorporate the clinical expertise of the mental health clinician, obstetrician, primary healthcare provider, and pediatrician. According to the American Psychiatric Association (APA), the risks of medication treatment should be weighed against other treatment options and untreated depression. Consideration should be given to using agents with safety data in pregnancy. For women who discontinue antidepressant medications during pregnancy and who may be at high risk for postpartum depression, the medications can be restarted following delivery. Treatment algorithms have been developed by the ACOG and the APA for the management of depression in women prior to conception and during pregnancy (ACOG, 2008; APA, 2010; Yonkers, 2009).

Breast-Feeding Considerations Trazodone is excreted into breast milk; breast milk concentrations peak ~2 hours following administration. It is not known if the trazodone metabolite is found in breast milk (Verbeeck, 1986). The long-term effects on neurobehavior have not been studied. The manufacturer recommends that caution be exercised when administering trazodone to nursing women.

Contraindications Hypersensitivity to trazodone or any component of the formulation; use of MAO inhibitors intended to treat psychiatric disorders (concurrently or within 14 days of discontinuing either trazodone or the MAO inhibitor); initiation of trazodone in a patient receiving linezolid or intravenous methylene blue

Warnings/Precautions [U.S. Boxed Warning]: Antidepressants increase the risk of suicidal thinking and behavior in children, adolescents, and young adults (18 to 24 years of age) with major depressive disorder (MDD) and other psychiatric disorders; consider risk prior to prescribing. Short-term studies did not show an increased risk in patients >24 years of age and showed a decreased risk in patients ≥65 years of age. Closely monitor for clinical worsening, suicidality, or unusual changes in behavior, particularly during the initial 1 to 2 months of therapy or during periods of dosage adjustments (increases or decreases); the patient's family or caregiver should be instructed to closely observe the patient and communicate condition with healthcare provider. A medication guide should be dispensed with each prescription. **Trazodone is not FDA approved for use in children.**

The possibility of a suicide attempt is inherent in major depression and may persist until remission occurs. Worsening depression and severe abrupt suicidality that are not part of the presenting symptoms may require discontinuation or modification of drug therapy. The patient's family or caregiver should be alerted to monitor patients for the emergence of suicidality and associated behaviors (such as agitation, irritability, hostility, impulsivity, and hypomania) and call healthcare provider.

May worsen psychosis in some patients or precipitate a shift to mania or hypomania in patients with bipolar disorder. Patients presenting with depressive symptoms should be screened for bipolar disorder. Monotherapy in patients with bipolar disorder should be avoided. **Trazodone is not FDA approved for the treatment of bipolar depression.**

Priapism, including cases resulting in permanent dysfunction, has occurred with the use of trazodone. Instruct patient to seek medical assistance for erection lasting >4 hours; use with caution in patients who have conditions which may predispose them to priapism (eg, sickle cell anemia, multiple myeloma, leukemia). Not recommended for use in a patient during the acute recovery phase of MI. The risks of sedation, postural hypotension, and/or syncope are high relative to other antidepressants. Trazodone frequently causes sedation, which may result in impaired performance of tasks requiring alertness (eg, operating machinery or driving).

Use with caution in patients with a history of cardiovascular disease (including previous MI, stroke, tachycardia, or conduction abnormalities). Although the risk of conduction abnormalities with this agent is low relative to other antidepressants, QT prolongation (with or without torsade de pointes), ventricular tachycardia, and other arrhythmias have been observed with the use of trazodone (reports limited to immediate-release formulation); use with caution in patients with preexisting cardiac disease. May impair platelet aggregation resulting in increased risk of bleeding events (eg, epistaxis, life threatening bleeding).

Potentially life-threatening serotonin syndrome (SS) has occurred with serotonergic agents (eg, SSRIs, SNRIs), particularly when used in combination with other serotonergic agents (eg, triptans, TCAs, fentanyl, lithium, tramadol, buspirone, St John's wort, tryptophan) or agents that impair metabolism of serotonin (eg, MAO inhibitors intended to treat psychiatric disorders, other MAO inhibitors [ie, linezolid and intravenous methylene blue]). Discontinue treatment (and any concomitant serotonergic agent) immediately if signs/symptoms arise.

Serotonin syndrome (SS)/neuroleptic malignant syndrome (NMS)-like reactions may occur with trazodone when used alone, particularly if used with other serotonergic agents (eg, serotonin/norepinephrine reuptake inhibitors [SNRIs], selective serotonin reuptake inhibitors [SSRIs], or triptans), drugs that impair serotonin metabolism (eg, MAO inhibitors), or antidopaminergic agents (eg, antipsychotics). If concurrent use is clinically warranted, carefully observe patient during treatment initiation and dose increases. Do not use concurrently with serotonin precursors (eg, tryptophan).

Use caution in patients with a previous seizure disorder or condition predisposing to seizures such as brain damage, or alcoholism. Bone fractures have been associated with antidepressant treatment. Consider the possibility of a fragility fracture if an antidepressant-treated patient presents with unexplained bone pain, point tenderness, swelling, or bruising (Rabenda, 2013; Rizzoli, 2012). Use with caution in patients with hepatic or renal dysfunction and in elderly patients. May cause SIADH and hyponatremia, predominantly in the elderly; volume depletion and/or concurrent use of diuretics likely increases risk. May cause mild pupillary dilation which in susceptible individuals can lead to an episode of narrow-angle glaucoma. Consider evaluating patients who have not had an iridectomy for narrow-angle glaucoma risk factors. Potentially significant drug-drug interactions may exist, requiring dose or frequency adjustment, additional monitoring, and/or selection of alternative therapy.

Abrupt discontinuation or interruption of antidepressant therapy has been associated with a discontinuation syndrome. Symptoms arising may vary with antidepressant however commonly include nausea, vomiting, diarrhea, headaches, lightheadedness, dizziness, diminished appetite, sweating, chills, tremors, paresthesias, fatigue, somnolence, and sleep disturbances (eg, vivid dreams, insomnia). Greater risks for developing a discontinuation syndrome have been associated with antidepressants with shorter half-lives, longer durations of treatment, and abrupt discontinuation. For antidepressants of short or intermediate half-lives, symptoms may emerge within 2 to 5 days after treatment discontinuation and last 7 to 14 days (APA, 2010; Fava, 2006; Haddad, 2001; Shelton, 2001; Warner, 2006).

Adverse Reactions

Cardiovascular: Edema

Central nervous system: Agitation, ataxia, confusion, disorientation, dizziness, fatigue, headache, memory impairment, migraine, sedation

Dermatologic: Night sweats

Endocrine & metabolic: Decreased libido

Gastrointestinal: Abdominal pain, constipation, dysgeusia, nausea, vomiting, xerostomia

Genitourinary: Ejaculatory disorder, urinary urgency

Neuromuscular & skeletal: Back pain, myalgia, tremor

Ophthalmic: Blurred vision, visual disturbance

Respiratory: Dyspnea

Rare but important and life-threatening: Abnormal dreams, abnormal orgasm, acne, akathisia, allergic reactions, alopecia, amylase increased, anemia, angle-closure glaucoma, anxiety, aphasia, apnea, appetite increased, arrhythmia, ataxia, atrial fibrillation, bladder pain, bradycardia, breast enlargement/engorgement, cardiac arrest, cardiospasm, cerebrovascular accident, chest pain, CHF, chills, cholestasis, clitorism, conduction block, diplopia, dry eyes, early menses, erectile dysfunction, extrapyramidal symptoms, eye pain, flushing, gait disturbance, hallucination, hearing loss (partial), hematuria, hemolytic anemia, hepatitis, hirsutism, hyperbilirubinemia, hyperhidrosis, hypersalivation, hypersensitivity, hypoesthesia, hypomania, impaired speech, impotence, insomnia, jaundice, lactation, leukocytosis, leukonychia, libido increased, liver enzyme alteration, methemoglobinemia, MI, muscle twitching, orthostatic hypotension, palpitation, paranoia, photophobia, photosensitivity reaction, priapism, pruritus, psoriasis, psychosis, QT prolongation, rash, reflux esophagitis, retrograde ejaculation, salivation increased, seizure, SIADH, speech impairment, stupor, tachycardia, tardive dyskinesia, tinnitus, torsade de pointes, urinary frequency increased, urinary incontinence, urinary retention, urticaria, vasodilation, ventricular ectopy, ventricular tachycardia, vertigo, weakness

Drug Interactions

Metabolism/Transport Effects Substrate of CYP2D6 (minor), CYP3A4 (major); **Note:** Assignment of Major/Minor substrate status based on clinically relevant drug interaction potential; **Inhibits** CYP3A4 (weak); **Induces** P-glycoprotein

Avoid Concomitant Use

Avoid concomitant use of TraZODone with any of the following: Conivaptan; Dapoxetine; Fusidic Acid (Systemic); Highest Risk QTc-Prolonging Agents; Idelalisib; Ivabradine; Linezolid; Lopinavir; MAO Inhibitors; Methylene Blue; Mifepristone; Pimozide; Saquinavir

Increased Effect/Toxicity

TraZODone may increase the levels/effects of: Antipsychotic Agents; Antipsychotic Agents (Phenothiazines); ARIPiprazole; Fosphenytoin; Highest Risk QTc-Prolonging Agents; Hydrocodone; Lomitapide; Methylene Blue; Metoclopramide; Moderate Risk QTc-Prolonging Agents; Phenytoin; Pimozide; Serotonin Modulators

The levels/effects of TraZODone may be increased by: Alcohol (Ethyl); Antiemetics (5HT3 Antagonists); Antipsychotic Agents; Antipsychotic Agents (Phenothiazines); Aprepitant; Atazanavir; Boceprevir; BusPIRone; Conivaptan; CYP3A4 Inhibitors (Moderate); CYP3A4 Inhibitors (Strong); Dapoxetine; Darunavir; Dasatinib; Fosamprenavir; Fosaprepitant; Fusidic Acid (Systemic); Idelalisib; Indinavir; Ivabradine; Ivacaftor; Linezolid; Lopinavir; Luliconazole; MAO Inhibitors; Mifepristone; Nelfinavir; Netupitant; QTc-Prolonging Agents (Indeterminate Risk and Risk Modifying); Ritonavir; Saquinavir; Selective Serotonin Reuptake Inhibitors; Simeprevir; Stiripentol; Tedizolid; Telaprevir; Tipranavir; Venlafaxine

Decreased Effect

TraZODone may decrease the levels/effects of: Warfarin

The levels/effects of TraZODone may be decreased by: Bosentan; CYP3A4 Inducers (Moderate); CYP3A4 Inducers (Strong); Dabrafenib; Deferasirox; Fosphenytoin; Mitotane; Phenytoin; Siltuximab; St Johns Wort; Tocilizumab

Food Interactions Time to peak serum levels may be increased if immediate release trazodone is taken with food. Management: Administer immediate release after meals to decrease lightheadedness and postural hypotension. Administer extended release on an empty stomach.

Storage/Stability

Immediate release tablet: Store at room temperature; avoid temperatures >40°C (>104°F). Protect from light.

Extended release tablet: Store at room temperature of 15°C to 30°C (59°F to 86°F). Protect from light.

Mechanism of Action Inhibits reuptake of serotonin, causes adrenoreceptor subsensitivity, and induces significant changes in 5-HT presynaptic receptor adrenoreceptors. Trazodone also significantly blocks histamine (H_1) and alpha$_1$-adrenergic receptors.

Pharmacodynamics/Kinetics

Onset of action: Therapeutic (antidepressant): Up to 6 weeks; sleep aid: 1 to 3 hours

Absorption: Well absorbed; Extended release: C_{max} increases ~86% when taken shortly after ingestion of a high-fat meal compared to fasting conditions

Protein binding: 85% to 95%

Metabolism: Hepatic via CYP3A4 (extensive) to an active metabolite (mCPP)

Half-life elimination: 7 to 10 hours

Time to peak, serum:

Immediate release: 30 to 100 minutes; delayed with food (up to 2.5 hours)

Extended release: 9 hours; not significantly affected by food

Excretion: Primarily urine (<1% excreted unchanged); secondarily feces

Dosage Oral: Therapeutic effects may take up to 6 weeks to occur; therapy is normally maintained for 6 to 12 months after optimum response is reached to prevent recurrence of depression. Use of once daily doses at bedtime may be considered for the treatment of depression to minimize adverse effects (Haria,1994; Rawls,1982).

Children 6 to 12 years: Depression (off-label use): Initial: 1.5 to 2 mg/kg/day in divided doses; increase gradually every 3 to 4 days as needed; maximum: 6 mg/kg/day in 3 divided doses

Adolescents: Depression (off-label use): Initial: 25 to 50 mg daily; increase to 100 to 150 mg daily in divided doses

Adults:

Depression: Initial: 150 mg daily in divided doses (may increase by 50 mg daily every 3 to 4 days); maximum dose: 600 mg daily

Extended release formulation: Initial: 150 mg once daily at bedtime (may increase by 75 mg daily every 3 days); maximum dose: 375 mg daily; once adequate response obtained, gradually reduce with adjustment based on therapeutic response

Note: Therapeutic effects may take up to 6 weeks. Therapy is normally maintained for 6 to 12 months after optimum response is reached to prevent recurrence of depression.

Insomnia (off-label use): Immediate release: 50 mg to 100 mg at bedtime (Haffmans, 1999; Mashiko, 1999; Saletu-Zyhlarz, 2002; Walsh, 1998)

Elderly: 25 to 50 mg at bedtime with 25 to 50 mg daily dose increase every 3 days for inpatients and weekly for outpatients, if tolerated; usual dose: 75 to 150 mg daily

Discontinuation of therapy: Upon discontinuation of antidepressant therapy, gradually taper the dose to minimize the incidence of withdrawal symptoms and allow for the detection of re-emerging symptoms. Evidence supporting ideal taper rates is limited. APA and NICE guidelines suggest tapering therapy over at least several weeks with consideration to the half-life of the antidepressant; antidepressants with a shorter half-life may need to be tapered more conservatively. In addition for long-term treated patients, WFSBP guidelines recommend tapering over 4 to 6 months. If intolerable withdrawal symptoms occur following a dose reduction, consider resuming the previously prescribed dose and/or decrease dose at a more gradual rate (APA, 2010; Bauer, 2002; Haddad, 2001; NCCMH, 2010; Schatzberg, 2006; Shelton, 2001; Warner, 2006).

MAO inhibitor recommendations:

Switching to or from an MAO inhibitor intended to treat psychiatric disorders:

Allow 14 days to elapse between discontinuing an MAO inhibitor intended to treat psychiatric disorders and initiation of trazodone.

Allow 14 days to elapse between discontinuing trazodone and initiation of an MAO inhibitor intended to treat psychiatric disorders.

Use with other MAO inhibitors (linezolid or IV methylene blue):

Do not initiate trazodone in patients receiving linezolid or IV methylene blue; consider other interventions for psychiatric condition.

If urgent treatment with linezolid or IV methylene blue is required in a patient already receiving trazodone and potential benefits outweigh potential risks, discontinue trazodone promptly and administer linezolid or IV methylene blue. Monitor for serotonin syndrome for 2 weeks or until 24 hours after the last dose of linezolid or IV methylene blue, whichever comes first. May resume trazodone 24 hours after the last dose of linezolid or IV methylene blue.

Dosage adjustment in renal impairment: There are no dosage adjustments provided in manufacturer's labeling (has not been studied). Use with caution.

Dosage adjustment in hepatic impairment: There are no dosage adjustments provided in manufacturer's labeling (has not been studied). Use with caution.

Administration

Immediate release tablet: Dosing after meals may decrease lightheadedness and postural hypotension

Extended release tablet: Take on an empty stomach; swallow whole or as a half tablet without food. Tablet may be broken along the score line, but do not crush or chew.

Monitoring Parameters Baseline liver function prior to and periodically during therapy; suicide ideation (especially at the beginning of therapy or when doses are increased or decreased); suicide ideation (especially at the beginning of therapy or when doses are increased or decreased); signs/symptoms of serotonin syndrome

Reference Range

Plasma levels do not always correlate with clinical effectiveness

Therapeutic: 0.5 to 2.5 mcg/mL

Potentially toxic: >2.5 mcg/mL

Toxic: >4 mcg/mL

Dosage Forms

Tablet, Oral:

Generic: 50 mg, 100 mg, 150 mg, 300 mg

Tablet Extended Release 24 Hour, Oral:

Oleptro: 150 mg, 300 mg

◆ **Trazodone Hydrochloride** *see* TraZODone *on page 2091*

◆ **Trazorel (Can)** *see* TraZODone *on page 2091*

◆ **Treanda** *see* Bendamustine *on page 241*

◆ **Trelstar (Can)** *see* Triptorelin *on page 2107*

◆ **Trelstar Depot** *see* Triptorelin *on page 2107*

◆ **Trelstar Depot Mixject** *see* Triptorelin *on page 2107*

◆ **Trelstar LA** *see* Triptorelin *on page 2107*

◆ **Trelstar LA Mixject** *see* Triptorelin *on page 2107*

◆ **Trelstar Mixject** *see* Triptorelin *on page 2107*

◆ **Tremytoine Inj (Can)** *see* Phenytoin *on page 1640*

◆ **TRENtal [DSC]** *see* Pentoxifylline *on page 1618*

Treprostinil (tre PROST in il)

Brand Names: U.S. Orenitram; Remodulin; Tyvaso; Tyvaso Refill; Tyvaso Starter

Brand Names: Canada Remodulin

Index Terms Treprostinil Sodium

Pharmacologic Category Prostacyclin; Prostaglandin; Vasodilator

Use Pulmonary arterial hypertension:

Injection: Treatment of pulmonary arterial hypertension (PAH) (WHO Group I) in patients with NYHA class II-IV symptoms to decrease exercise-associated symptoms; to diminish clinical deterioration when transitioning from epoprostenol (IV)

Inhalation: Treatment of pulmonary arterial hypertension (PAH) (WHO Group I) in patients with NYHA class III symptoms to improve exercise ability. **Note:** Nearly all controlled clinical trial experience has been with concomitant bosentan or sildenafil.

Oral: Treatment of pulmonary arterial hypertension (PAH) (WHO Group 1) in patients with WHO functional class II-III symptoms to improve exercise capacity.

Pregnancy Risk Factor B/C (product specific)

Pregnancy Considerations Adverse events were observed in some animal reproduction studies. Women with pulmonary arterial hypertension (PAH) are encouraged to avoid pregnancy (McLaughlin, 2009).

Breast-Feeding Considerations It is not known if treprostinil is excreted in breast milk. The manufacturers of the injection recommend that caution be exercised when administering treprostinil to nursing women. The manufacturer of the oral product recommends that a decision be made whether to discontinue nursing or to discontinue the drug.

Contraindications

Injection/inhalation: There are no contraindications listed in the manufacturer's labeling.

Oral: Severe hepatic impairment (Child-Pugh class C).

Documentation of allergenic cross-reactivity for prostaglandins is limited. However, because of similarities in chemical structure and/or pharmacologic actions, the possibility of cross-sensitivity cannot be ruled out with certainty.

Warnings/Precautions May produce symptomatic hypotension; use with caution in patients with low systemic arterial blood pressure. Abrupt withdrawal/large dosage reductions may worsen symptoms of pulmonary arterial hypertension (PAH). If a SubQ or IV infusion is restarted within a few hours of discontinuation, the same dose rate may be used. Interruptions for longer periods may require retitration. Regardless of administration route (inhalation, IV, oral, or SubQ), treatment interruptions should be avoided. Immediate access to medication, back-up inhalation device, or pump and infusion sets is essential to prevent treatment interruptions. Chronic continuous IV infusion of treprostinil via a chronic indwelling central venous catheter has been associated with serious blood stream infections. This method of administration should be reserved for patients who are intolerant of the SubQ route or in whom the benefit outweighs the potential risks. Treprostinil injection should only be used by clinicians experienced in the treatment of PAH. Prior to initiation, patients should be carefully evaluated for ability to administer treprostinil, either as an IV/SubQ infusion or inhalation, and care for the infusion system/inhalation device. Initiation of infusion must occur in a setting where adequate personnel and equipment necessary for hemodynamic monitoring and emergency treatment is available.

Use with caution in patients with hepatic impairment. IV/SubQ: Dose reduction is recommended for the initial dose in patients with mild to moderate hepatic insufficiency; titrate dose slowly in patients with hepatic insufficiency; has not been studied in severe hepatic impairment. Oral: Dose reduction is recommended for patients with mild hepatic impairment. Avoid use in patients with moderate impairment; use is contraindicated in patients with severe impairment.

Has not been studied in renal impairment (inhalation/IV/SubQ); use with caution in renal impairment; titrate dose slowly in patients with renal insufficiency. May inhibit platelet aggregation and increases the risk of bleeding. Inhalation: Safety and efficacy have not been established in patients with underlying pulmonary disease (eg, asthma, COPD). Patients with acute pulmonary infections should be monitored closely for exacerbation or reduced efficacy. Tablets can lodge in diverticulum; use with caution in patients with diverticulosis; should not be administered with ethanol since the release of treprostinil from the tablet may occur at a faster rate than intended. Potentially significant drug-drug interactions may exist, requiring dose or frequency adjustment, additional monitoring, and/or selection of alternative therapy.

Adverse Reactions

Cardiovascular: Edema, flushing, hypotension, syncope (Inhalation)

Central nervous system: Dizziness, headache

Dermatologic: Pruritus, skin rash

Endocrine & metabolic: Hypokalemia (Oral)

Gastrointestinal: Abdominal distress (Oral), diarrhea, nausea

Local: Infusion site reaction (SubQ), pain at injection site (SubQ; may improve after several months of therapy)

Neuromuscular & skeletal: Jaw pain, limb pain (Oral)

Respiratory: Cough (Inhalation), epistaxis (Inhalation), hemoptysis, pharyngolaryngeal pain (Inhalation), pneumonia, throat irritation (Inhalation), wheezing (Inhalation)

Rare but important or life-threatening: Angioedema, catheter infection (central venous), catheter sepsis (central venous), cellulitis, decreased platelet aggregation, hematoma, ostealgia, pain, paresthesia, swelling of extremities, thrombocytopenia, thrombophlebitis

Drug Interactions

Metabolism/Transport Effects Substrate of CYP2C8 (minor), CYP2C9 (minor); **Note:** Assignment of Major/Minor substrate status based on clinically relevant drug interaction potential

Avoid Concomitant Use There are no known interactions where it is recommended to avoid concomitant use.

Increased Effect/Toxicity

Treprostinil may increase the levels/effects of: Agents with Antiplatelet Properties; Anticoagulants; Antihypertensives; Highest Risk QTc-Prolonging Agents; Moderate Risk QTc-Prolonging Agents; Nonsteroidal Anti-Inflammatory Agents; Salicylates

The levels/effects of Treprostinil may be increased by: Alcohol (Ethyl); CYP2C8 Inhibitors (Strong); Mifepristone; Thrombolytic Agents

Decreased Effect

The levels/effects of Treprostinil may be decreased by: CYP2C8 Inducers (Strong)

Preparation for Administration Injection solution: For SubQ infusion, **product should not be diluted prior to use**. For IV infusion, dilute in SWFI, NS, Remodulin sterile diluent, or Flolan sterile diluent to a final volume of either 50 mL or 100 mL (dependent on system reservoir and calculated dose).

Storage/Stability

Injection solution: Store vials at 25°C (77°F); excursions are permitted between 15°C and 30°C (59°F and 86°F). Contents of a vial should not be used past 30 days after initial needle access into the vial. Stability for up to 14 days at 37°C has been shown for IV infusion concentrations as low as 4,000 ng/mL.

Solution for inhalation: Store ampuls in foil packs at 25°C (77°F); excursions are permitted between 15°C and 30°C (59°F and 86°F). Protect from light. Once foil pack is opened, ampules should be used within 7 days. Following transfer of solution to inhalation device, solution should remain in device for no more than 24 hours; discard unused portion.

Tablets: Store at 25°C (77°F); excursions are permitted between 15°C and 30°C (59°F and 86°F).

Mechanism of Action Treprostinil is a direct vasodilator of both pulmonary and systemic arterial vascular beds; also inhibits platelet aggregation.

Pharmacodynamics/Kinetics

Absorption: SubQ: Rapidly and completely

Distribution: 14 L/70 kg ideal body weight

Protein binding: 91% to 96%
Metabolism: Hepatic (primarily by CYP2C8); forms 5 inactive metabolites (HU1-HU5)
Bioavailability: Inhalation: 64% to 72% (dose-dependent); SubQ: 100%; Oral: ~17%
Half-life elimination: Terminal: ~4 hours
Time to peak: Oral: 4-6 hours
Excretion:
Urine (79%; 4% as unchanged drug, 64% as metabolites); feces (13%)
Oral: urine (0.19% as unchanged drug); feces (1.13% as unchanged drug)

Dosage Pulmonary arterial hypertension (PAH):
Children: SubQ; IV infusion: Limited experience in patients ≤16 years of age.
Adults:
Inhalation: **Note:** Prior to initiation, patients should be carefully evaluated for ability to administer treprostinil and care for the inhalation system and accessories required for administration. Immediate access to a back-up inhalation device, accessories, and medication is essential to prevent treatment interruptions.
Initial: 18 mcg (or 3 inhalations) every 4 hours 4 times/day; if 3 inhalations are not tolerated, reduce to 1 to 2 inhalations, then increase to 3 inhalations as tolerated
Maintenance: If tolerated, increase dose by an additional 3 inhalations at approximately 1- to 2-week intervals; target dose and maximum dose: 54 mcg (or 9 inhalations) 4 times/day
Oral: Initial: 0.25 mg every 12 hours or 0.125 mg every 8 hours; may increase dose in increments of 0.25 mg or 0.5 mg every 12 hours, or 0.125 mg every 8 hours every 3 to 4 days as tolerated to achieve optimal clinical response. If dose increments are not tolerated, consider slower titration. Maximum dose is determined by tolerability. If intolerable effects occur, decrease dose in increments of 0.25 mg; avoid abrupt discontinuation. Upon discontinuation, reduce the dose in increments of 0.5 mg to 1 mg daily.
Missed doses: If a dose is missed, take the missed dose as soon as possible. If ≥2 doses are missed, restart at a lower dose and retitrate.
Dosage adjustment for concurrent use in patients receiving strong CYP2C8 inhibitors (eg, gemfibrozil): Initiate a starting dose of 0.125 mg every 12 hours; increase in increments of 0.125 mg every 12 hours every 3 to 4 days.
Planned short-term treatment interruption: If patients are unable to continue oral treatment, a temporary infusion of subcutaneous or IV treprostinil may be considered. Divide the oral total daily dose by 5 to calculate the total daily dose (mg) of parenteral treprostinil.
SubQ (preferred) or IV infusion: **Note:** Prior to initiation, patients should be carefully evaluated for ability to administer treprostinil and care for the infusion system outside of inpatient setting. Immediate access to a back-up pump, infusion sets, and medication is essential to prevent treatment interruptions.
New to prostacyclin therapy: Initial: 1.25 ng/kg/minute; if dose cannot be tolerated due to systemic effects, reduce to 0.625 ng/kg/minute. Increase dose in increments of 1.25 ng/kg/minute per week for first 4 weeks, followed by increments of 2.5 ng/kg/minute per week for remainder of therapy. Limited experience with doses >40 ng/kg/minute. **Note:** Dose must be carefully and individually titrated (symptom improvement with minimal adverse effects). Avoid abrupt withdrawal. If infusion is restarted within a few hours of discontinuation, the same dose rate may be used. Interruptions for longer periods may require retitration.
Transitioning from epoprostenol (see table): **Note:** Transition should occur in a hospital setting to follow response (eg, walking distance, sign/symptoms of disease progression). May take 24 to 48 hours to transition. Transition is accomplished by initiating the infusion of treprostinil, and increasing it while simultaneously reducing the dose of intravenous epoprostenol. During transition, increases in PAH symptoms should be first treated with an increase in treprostinil dose. Occurrence of prostacyclin associated side effects should be treated by decreasing the dose of epoprostenol.

Transitioning From IV Epoprostenol to SubQ (Preferred) or IV Treprostinil

Step	Epoprostenol Dose	Treprostinil Dose
1	Maintain current dose	Initiate at 10% initial epoprostenol dose
2	Decrease to 80% initial dose	Increase to 30% initial epoprostenol dose
3	Decrease to 60% initial dose	Increase to 50% initial epoprostenol dose
4	Decrease to 40% initial dose	Increase to 70% initial epoprostenol dose
5	Decrease to 20% initial dose	Increase to 90% initial epoprostenol dose
6	Decrease to 5% initial dose	Increase to 110% initial epoprostenol dose
7	Discontinue epoprostenol	Maintain current dose plus additional 5% to 10% as needed

Elderly: Refer to adult dosing. Limited experience in patients ≥65 years; use caution.

Dosage adjustment in renal impairment:
Inhalation, SubQ infusion, IV infusion: There are no dosage adjustments provided in manufacturer's labeling (has not been studied). Use with caution and titrate slowly.
Oral: No dosage adjustment necessary.
Hemodialysis: Treprostinil is not removed by dialysis.

Dosage adjustment in hepatic impairment:
Inhalation: There are no dosage adjustments provided in manufacturer's labeling. However, hepatic impairment increases systemic exposure to treprostinil. Use with caution and titrate slowly.
SubQ infusion, IV infusion:
Mild to moderate impairment: Initial: 0.625 ng/kg/minute (ideal body weight). Use with caution and titrate slowly.
Severe impairment: There are no dosage adjustments provided in manufacturer's labeling (has not been studied). Use with caution and titrate slowly.
Oral:
Mild impairment (Child-Pugh class A): Initial: 0.125 mg every 12 hours; increase in increments of 0.125 mg every 12 hours every 3 to 4 days.
Moderate impairment (Child-Pugh class B): Avoid use.
Severe impairment (Child-Pugh class C): Use is contraindicated by the manufacturer.

Administration Avoid treatment interruptions or rapid large dosage reductions with use of inhalation, IV, or SubQ formulations. Immediate access to medication, a back-up inhalation device, or pump and infusion sets is essential to prevent treatment interruptions.
Inhalation: Do not mix with other medications. For inhalation only via the Tyvaso Inhalation System. Prior to the first treatment session of each day, transfer the entire contents of one ampule into the medicine chamber; one ampule contains sufficient volume of medication for all 4 treatment sessions in a single day. Between each session, the device should be capped and stored upright with the remaining medication inside. At the end of each day, the medicine chamber and any remaining medication

must be discarded. Avoid contact of solution with eyes or skin; wash hands after handling.

IV infusion: IV use is recommended when SubQ infusion is not tolerated or when the benefit outweighs the potential risks of an indwelling central venous catheter. Solution must be diluted in SWFI, NS, Remodulin sterile diluent, or Flolan sterile diluent prior to use and administered by continuous infusion using a central indwelling catheter and infusion pump. The ambulatory infusion pump should be small and lightweight; have occlusion/no delivery, low battery, programming error, and motor malfunction alarms; have ± 6% accuracy of the programmed rate; and be positive pressure driven. The reservoir should be made of polyvinyl chloride, polypropylene, or glass. Peripheral infusion may be used temporarily until central line is established. Infusion sets with an in-line 0.22 or 0.2 micron filter should be used for central and peripheral administration.

Oral: Administer with food. Swallow tablets whole; do not crush, split or chew; use only intact tablets.

SubQ infusion (preferred): Administer undiluted via continuous SubQ infusion using an appropriately designed infusion pump. The ambulatory infusion pump should be small and lightweight; be able to adjust infusion rates in ~0.002 mL/hour increments; have occlusion/no delivery, low battery, programming error, and motor malfunction alarms; have ± 6% accuracy of the programmed rate; and be positive pressure driven. The reservoir should be made of polyvinyl chloride, polypropylene, or glass. Infusion site reactions may be helped by moving the infusion site every 3 days, local application of topical hot and cold packs, topical or oral analgesics. Injection site pain and erythema may improve after several months of treprostinil therapy.

Monitoring Parameters BP, dyspnea, fatigue, activity tolerance, symptoms of excessive dose (eg, headache, nausea, vomiting)

Dosage Forms

Solution, Inhalation:

Tyvaso: 0.6 mg/mL (2.9 mL)

Tyvaso Refill: 0.6 mg/mL (2.9 mL)

Tyvaso Starter: 0.6 mg/mL (2.9 mL)

Solution, Injection:

Remodulin: 1 mg/mL (20 mL); 2.5 mg/mL (20 mL); 5 mg/mL (20 mL); 10 mg/mL (20 mL)

Tablet Extended Release, Oral:

Orenitram: 0.125 mg, 0.25 mg, 1 mg, 2.5 mg

◆ **Treprostinil Sodium** *see* Treprostinil *on page 2093*

◆ **Tretin-X** *see* Tretinoin (Topical) *on page 2099*

◆ **Tretinoin and Clindamycin** *see* Clindamycin and Tretinoin *on page 464*

◆ **Tretinoin, Fluocinolone Acetonide, and Hydroquinone** *see* Fluocinolone, Hydroquinone, and Tretinoin *on page 894*

Tretinoin (Systemic) (TRET i noyn)

Brand Names: Canada Vesanoid

Index Terms *trans* Vitamin A Acid; *trans*-Retinoic Acid; All-*trans* Retinoic Acid; All-*trans* Vitamin A Acid; ATRA; Ro 5488; tRA; Tretinoinum; Vesanoid

Pharmacologic Category Antineoplastic Agent, Retinoic Acid Derivative; Retinoic Acid Derivative

Use Induction of remission in patients with acute promyelocytic leukemia (APL), French American British (FAB) classification M3 (including the M3 variant) characterized by t(15;17) translocation and/or PML/RARα gene presence

Pregnancy Risk Factor D

Pregnancy Considerations Adverse events were observed in animal reproduction studies. **[U.S. Boxed Warning]: High risk of teratogenicity; if treatment with tretinoin is required in women of childbearing potential, two reliable forms of contraception should be used simultaneously during and for 1 month after treatment, unless abstinence is the chosen method. Within 1 week prior to starting therapy, serum or urine pregnancy test (sensitivity at least 50 mIU/mL) should be collected. If possible, delay therapy until results are available. Repeat pregnancy testing and contraception counseling monthly throughout the period of treatment.** Contraception must be used even when there is a history of infertility or menopause, unless a hysterectomy has been preformed. Tretinoin was detected in the serum of a neonate at birth following maternal use of standard doses during pregnancy (Takitani, 2005). Use in humans for the treatment of acute promyelocytic leukemia (APL) is limited and exposure occurred after the first trimester in most cases (Valappil, 2007). However, major fetal abnormalities and spontaneous abortions have been reported with other retinoids; some of these abnormalities were fatal. If the clinical condition of a patient presenting with APL during pregnancy warrants immediate treatment, tretinoin use should be avoided in the first trimester; treatment with tretinoin may be considered in the second and third trimester with careful fetal monitoring, including cardiac monitoring (Sanz, 2009).

Breast-Feeding Considerations It is not known if tretinoin is excreted in breast milk. Due to the potential for serious adverse reactions in the nursing infant, breast-feeding should be discontinued prior to treatment initiation.

Contraindications Hypersensitivity to tretinoin, other retinoids, parabens, or any component of the formulation

Warnings/Precautions Hazardous agent: Use appropriate precautions for handling and disposal (NIOSH 2014 [group 3]).

[U.S. Boxed Warning]: About 25% of patients with APL treated with tretinoin have experienced APL differentiation syndrome (DS) (formerly called retinoic-acid-APL [RA-APL] syndrome), which is characterized by fever, dyspnea, acute respiratory distress, weight gain, radiographic pulmonary infiltrates and pleural or pericardial effusions, edema, and hepatic, renal, and/or multiorgan failure. DS usually occurs during the first month of treatment, with some cases reported following the first dose. DS has been observed with or without concomitant leukocytosis and has occasionally been accompanied by impaired myocardial contractility and episodic hypotension; endotracheal intubation and mechanical ventilation have been required in some cases due to progressive hypoxemia, and several patients have expired with multiorgan failure. About one-half of DS cases are severe, which is associated with increased mortality. Management has not been defined, although high-dose steroids given at the first suspicion appear to reduce morbidity and mortality. Regardless of the leukocyte count, at the first signs suggestive of DS, immediately initiate steroid therapy with dexamethasone 10 mg IV every 12 hours for 3-5 days; taper off over 2 weeks. Most patients do not require termination of tretinoin therapy during treatment of DS.

[U.S. Boxed Warning]: During treatment, ~40% of patients will develop rapidly evolving leukocytosis. A high WBC at diagnosis increases the risk for further leukocytosis and may be associated with a higher risk of life-threatening complications. If signs and symptoms of the APL-DS syndrome are present together with leukocytosis, initiate treatment with high-dose steroids immediately. Consider adding full-dose chemotherapy (including an anthracycline, if not contraindicated) to the tretinoin therapy on day 1 or 2 for patients presenting with a WBC count of >5 x 10^9/L. Consider adding chemotherapy immediately in patients who presented with a WBC count of <5 x 10^9/L, yet the WBC count reaches ≥6 x 10^9/L by day 5, or ≥10 x 10^9/L by day 10, or ≥15 x 10^9/L by day 28.

[U.S. Boxed Warning]: High risk of teratogenicity; if treatment with tretinoin is required in women of childbearing potential, two reliable forms of contraception should be used during and for 1 month after treatment. Microdosed progesterone products ("minipill") may provide inadequate pregnancy protection. Repeat pregnancy testing and contraception counseling monthly throughout the period of treatment. If possible, initiation of treatment with tretinoin should be delayed until negative pregnancy test result is confirmed.

Retinoids have been associated with pseudotumor cerebri (benign intracranial hypertension), especially in children. Concurrent use of other drugs associated with this effect (eg, tetracyclines) may increase risk. Early signs and symptoms include papilledema, headache, nausea, vomiting, visual disturbances, intracranial noises, or pulsate tinnitus.

Up to 60% of patients experienced hypercholesterolemia or hypertriglyceridemia, which were reversible upon completion of treatment. Venous thrombosis and MI have been reported in patient without risk factors for thrombosis or MI; the risk for thrombosis (arterial and venous) is increased during the first month of treatment. Use with caution with antifibrinolytic agents; thrombotic complications have been reported (rarely) with concomitant use. Elevated liver function test results occur in 50% to 60% of patients during treatment. Carefully monitor liver function test results during treatment and give consideration to a temporary withdrawal of tretinoin if test results reach >5 times the upper limit of normal. Most liver function test abnormalities will resolve without interruption of treatment or after therapy completion. May cause headache, malaise, and/or dizziness; caution patients about performing tasks which require mental alertness (eg, operating machinery or driving). Effects may be potentiated when used with other sedative drugs or ethanol. Patients with APL are at high risk and can have severe adverse reactions to tretinoin. **[U.S. Boxed Warning]: Should be administered under the supervision of an experienced cancer chemotherapy physician.** Tretinoin treatment for APL should be initiated early, discontinue if pending cytogenetic analysis does not confirm APL by t(15;17) translocation or the presence of the PML/RARα fusion protein (caused by translocation of the promyelocytic [PML] gene on chromosome 15 and retinoic acid receptor [RAR] alpha gene on chromosome 17).

Tretinoin (which is also known as all-*trans* retinoic acid, or ATRA) and isotretinoin may be confused, while both products may be used in cancer treatment, they are **not** interchangeable; verify product prior to dispensing and administration to prevent medication errors.

Adverse Reactions Most patients will experience drug-related toxicity, especially headache, fever, weakness and fatigue. These are seldom permanent or irreversible and do not typically require therapy interruption.

Cardiovascular: Arrhythmias, cardiac arrest, cardiac failure, cardiomyopathy, chest discomfort, cerebral hemorrhage, edema, facial edema, flushing, heart enlarged, heart murmur, hyper-/hypotension, ischemia, MI, myocarditis, pallor, pericarditis, peripheral edema, secondary cardiomyopathy, stroke

Central nervous system: Agitation, anxiety, aphasia, cerebellar edema, CNS depression, coma, confusion, dementia, depression, dizziness, encephalopathy, facial paralysis, fever, forgetfulness, hallucination, headache, hypotaxia, hypothermia, insomnia, Intracranial hypertension, light reflex absent, malaise, pain, seizure, slow speech, somnolence, spinal cord disorder, unconsciousness

Dermatologic: Alopecia, cellulitis, pruritus, rash, skin changes, skin/mucous membrane dryness

Endocrine & metabolic: Acidosis, fluid imbalance, hypercholesterolemia and/or hypertriglyceridemia

Gastrointestinal: Abdominal distention, abdominal pain, anorexia, constipation, diarrhea, dyspepsia, GI hemorrhage, hepatitis, hepatosplenomegaly, liver function tests increased, mucositis, nausea/vomiting, ulcer, weight gain/loss

Genitourinary: Dysuria, micturition frequency, prostate enlarged

Hematologic: Disseminated intravascular coagulation, hemorrhage, leukocytosis

Hepatic: Ascites, hepatitis, liver function tests increased

Local: Phlebitis

Neuromuscular & skeletal: Abnormal gait, asterixis, bone inflammation, bone pain, dysarthria, flank pain, hemiplegia hyporeflexia leg weakness, myalgia, paresthesia, tremor

Ocular: Agnosia, ocular disorder, visual acuity change, visual disturbance, visual field deficit

Otic: Earache/ear fullness, hearing loss

Renal: Acute renal failure, renal insufficiency, renal tubular necrosis

Respiratory: Bronchial asthma, dyspnea, expiratory wheezing, larynx edema, lower respiratory tract disorders, pleural effusion, pneumonia, pulmonary hypertension, pulmonary infiltration, rales, respiratory insufficiency, upper respiratory tract disorders

Miscellaneous: Diaphoresis, infection, lymph disorder, shivering, retinoic acid-acute promyelocytic leukemia syndrome/differentiation syndrome

Rare but important or life-threatening: Arterial thrombosis, basophilia, erythema nodosum, genital ulceration, hypercalcemia, hyperhistaminemia, irreversible hearing loss, myositis, organomegaly, pancreatitis, pseudotumor cerebri, renal infarct, Sweet's syndrome, thrombocytosis, vasculitis (skin), venous thrombosis

Drug Interactions

Metabolism/Transport Effects Substrate of CYP2A6 (minor), CYP2B6 (minor), CYP2C8 (major), CYP2C9 (minor); **Note:** Assignment of Major/Minor substrate status based on clinically relevant drug interaction potential; **Inhibits** CYP2C9 (weak); **Induces** CYP2E1 (moderate)

Avoid Concomitant Use

Avoid concomitant use of Tretinoin (Systemic) with any of the following: BCG; Multivitamins/Fluoride (with ADE); Multivitamins/Minerals (with ADEK, Folate, Iron); Multivitamins/Minerals (with AE, No Iron); Natalizumab; Pimecrolimus; Tacrolimus (Topical); Tetracycline Derivatives; Tofacitinib; Vaccines (Live); Vitamin A

Increased Effect/Toxicity

Tretinoin (Systemic) may increase the levels/effects of: Antifibrinolytic Agents; Leflunomide; Natalizumab; Porfimer; Tofacitinib; Vaccines (Live); Verteporfin; Vitamin A

The levels/effects of Tretinoin (Systemic) may be increased by: CYP2C8 Inhibitors (Moderate); CYP2C8 Inhibitors (Strong); Deferasirox; Denosumab; Mifepristone; Multivitamins/Fluoride (with ADE); Multivitamins/Minerals (with ADEK, Folate, Iron); Multivitamins/Minerals (with AE, No Iron); Pimecrolimus; Roflumilast; Tacrolimus (Topical); Tetracycline Derivatives; Trastuzumab

Decreased Effect

Tretinoin (Systemic) may decrease the levels/effects of: BCG; Coccidioides immitis Skin Test; Contraceptives (Estrogens); Contraceptives (Progestins); Sipuleucel-T; Vaccines (Inactivated); Vaccines (Live)

The levels/effects of Tretinoin (Systemic) may be decreased by: CYP2C8 Inducers (Strong); Dabrafenib; Echinacea

Food Interactions Absorption of retinoids has been shown to be enhanced when taken with food. Management: Administer with a meal.

Storage/Stability Store capsule at 20°C to 25°C (68°F to 77°F). Protect from light.

Mechanism of Action Tretinoin appears to bind one or more nuclear receptors and decreases proliferation and induces differentiation of APL cells; initially produces maturation of primitive promyelocytes and repopulates the marrow and peripheral blood with normal hematopoietic cells to achieve complete remission

Pharmacodynamics/Kinetics

Absorption: Well absorbed

Protein binding: >95%, predominantly to albumin

Metabolism: Hepatic via CYP; primary metabolite: 4-oxo-all-*trans*-retinoic acid; displays autometabolism

Half-life elimination: Terminal: Parent drug: 0.5-2 hours

Time to peak, serum: 1-2 hours

Excretion: Urine (63%); feces (30%)

Dosage Details concerning dosing in combination regimens should also be consulted. **Note:** Induction treatment of APL with tretinoin should be initiated early; discontinue if pending cytogenetic analysis does not confirm t(15;17) translocation or the presence of the PML/RARα fusion protein.

Acute promyelocytic leukemia (APL): Oral:

Remission induction: Children and Adults: 45 mg/m^2/day in 2 equally divided doses until documentation of complete remission (CR); discontinue 30 days after CR or after 90 days of treatment, whichever occurs first

Remission induction (in combination with an anthracycline ± cytarabine; off-label use):

Children: 25 mg/m^2/day in 2 equally divided doses until complete remission or 90 days (Ortega, 2005)

Adults: 45 mg/m^2/day in 2 equally divided doses until complete remission or 90 days (Powell, 2010) or until complete hematologic remission (Ades, 2008; Sanz, 2008; Sanz, 2010)

Remission induction (in combination with arsenic trioxide; off-label use): Adults: 45 mg/m^2/day in 2 equally divided doses until <5% blasts in marrow and no abnormal promyelocytes or up to 85 days (Estey, 2006; Ravandi, 2009)

Consolidation therapy (off-label use):

Children: 25 mg/m^2/day in 2 equally divided doses for 15 days each month for 3 months (Ortega, 2005)

Adults: 45 mg/m^2/day in 2 equally divided doses for 15 days each month for 3 months (in combination with chemotherapy) (Lo-Coco, 2010; Sanz 2010) **or** 45 mg/m^2/day for 14 days every 4 weeks for 7 cycles (in combination with arsenic trioxide) (Ravandi, 2009)

Maintenance therapy, intermediate- and high-risk patients (off-label use):

Children: 25 mg/m^2/day in 2 equally divided doses for 15 days every 3 months for 2 years (Ortega, 2005)

Adults: 45 mg/m^2/day in 2 equally divided doses for 15 days every 3 months for 2 years (Sanz, 2004)

Dosage adjustment for toxicity:

APL differentiation syndrome: Initiate dexamethasone 10 mg IV every 12 hours for 3-5 days; consider interrupting tretinoin until resolution of hypoxia

Liver function tests >5 times the upper limit of normal: Consider temporarily withholding treatment.

Dosage adjustment in renal impairment: No dosage adjustment provided in the manufacturer's labeling (has not been studied).

Dosage adjustment in hepatic impairment: No dosage adjustment provided in the manufacturer's labeling (has not been studied).

Dosing in obesity: *ASCO Guidelines for appropriate chemotherapy dosing in obese adults with cancer:* Utilize patient's actual body weight (full weight) for calculation of body surface area- or weight-based dosing, particularly when the intent of therapy is curative; manage regimen-related toxicities in the same manner as for nonobese patients; if a dose reduction is utilized due to toxicity, consider resumption of full weight-based dosing with subsequent cycles, especially if cause of toxicity (eg, hepatic or renal impairment) is resolved (Griggs, 2012).

Dietary Considerations The absorption of retinoids (as a class) is enhanced when taken with food. Capsule contains soybean oil.

Administration Administer orally with a meal; do not crush capsules.

Although the manufacturer does not recommend the use of the capsule contents to extemporaneously prepare tretinoin suspension, there are limited case reports of use in patients who are unable to swallow the capsules whole. In a patient with a nasogastric (NG) tube, tretinoin capsules were cut open, with partial aspiration of the contents into a glass syringe, the residual capsule contents were mixed with soy bean oil and aspirated into the same syringe and administered (Shaw, 1995). Tretinoin capsules have also been mixed with sterile water (~20 mL) and heated in a water bath (37°C) to melt the capsules and create an oily suspension for NG tube administration (Bargetzi, 1996). Tretinoin has also been administered sublingually by squeezing the capsule contents beneath the tongue (Kueh, 1999). Low plasma concentrations have been reported when tretinoin has been administered through a feeding tube, although patient-specific impaired absorption or a lack of excipient (eg, soybean oil) may have been a contributing factor (Takitani, 2004).

Hazardous agent - use appropriate precautions for handling and disposal (NIOSH 2014 [group 3]).

Monitoring Parameters Bone marrow cytology to confirm t(15;17) translocation or the presence of the PML/RARα fusion protein (do not withhold treatment initiation for results); monitor CBC with differential, coagulation profile, liver function test results, and triglyceride and cholesterol levels frequently; monitor closely for signs of APL differentiation syndrome (eg, monitor volume status, pulmonary status, temperature, respiration)

Dosage Forms

Capsule, Oral:

Generic: 10 mg

Extemporaneous Preparations Hazardous agent: Use appropriate precautions for handling and disposal (NIOSH 2014 [group 3]).

Although the manufacturer does not recommend the use of the capsule contents to extemporaneously prepare a suspension of tretinoin (due to reports of low plasma levels) (Vesanoid® data on file), there are limited case reports of use in patients who are unable to swallow the capsules whole. In a patient with a nasogastric (NG) tube, tretinoin capsules were cut open, with partial aspiration of the contents aspirated into a glass syringe. The residual capsule contents were mixed with soybean oil, aspirated into the syringe, and administered (Shaw, 1995). Tretinoin capsules have also been mixed with sterile water (~20 mL) and heated in a water bath to melt the capsules and create an oily suspension for NG tube administration (Bargetzi, 1996). Tretinoin has also been administered sublingually by squeezing the capsule contents beneath the tongue (Kueh, 1999).

Bargetzi MJ, Tichelli A, Gratwohl A, et al, "Oral All-Transretinoic Acid Administration in Intubated Patients With Acute Promyelocytic Leukemia," *Schweiz Med Wochenschr*, 1996, 126(45):1944-5.

Kueh YK, Liew PP, Ho PC, et al, "Sublingual Administration of All-*Trans*-Retinoic Acid to a Comatose Patient With Acute Promyelocytic Leukemia," *Ann Pharmacother*, 1999, 33(4):503-5.

Shaw PJ, Atkins MC, Nath CE, et al, "ATRA Administration in the Critically Ill Patient," *Leukemia*, 1995, 9(7):1288.

Vesanoid® data on file, Roche Pharmaceuticals

Tretinoin (Topical) (TRET i noyn)

Brand Names: U.S. Atralin; Avita; Refissa; Renova; Renova Pump; Retin-A; Retin-A Micro; Retin-A Micro Pump; Tretin-X

Brand Names: Canada Rejuva-A; Renova; Retin-A; Retin-A Micro; Retinova; Stieva-A; Vitamin A Acid

Index Terms *trans*-Retinoic Acid; Retinoic Acid; Vitamin A Acid

Pharmacologic Category Acne Products; Retinoic Acid Derivative; Topical Skin Product, Acne

Use

Acne vulgaris: Atralin, Avita, Retin-A, Retin-A Micro, Tretin-X: Treatment of acne vulgaris.

Palliation of fine wrinkles: Renova: Adjunctive treatment for mitigation (palliation) of fine wrinkles in patients who use comprehensive skin care and sun avoidance programs.

Palliation of fine wrinkles, mottled hyperpigmentation, and facial skin roughness: Refissa: Adjunctive treatment for mitigation (palliation) of fine wrinkles, mottled hyperpigmentation, and tactile roughness of facial skin in patients who do not achieve such palliation using comprehensive skin care and sun avoidance programs alone.

Pregnancy Risk Factor C

Dosage Topical:

Acne vulgaris: Children ≥10 years (Atralin only) or Children ≥12 years, Adolescents, and Adults: Apply once daily to affected area before bedtime or in the evening.

Palliation of fine wrinkles (Refissa/Renova), mottled hyperpigmentation, and tactile roughness of facial skin (Refissa): Adults: Apply a pea-sized amount of cream to entire face once daily in the evening or before bedtime.

Elderly: Refer to adult dosing; safety/efficacy of Refissa has not been established in patients >50 years of age; safety/efficacy of Renova has not been established in patients >71 years of age.

Dosage adjustment in renal impairment: There are no dosage adjustments provided in the manufacturer's labeling.

Dosage adjustment in hepatic impairment: There are no dosage adjustments provided in the manufacturer's labeling.

Additional Information Complete prescribing information should be consulted for additional detail.

Dosage Forms

Cream, External:

Avita: 0.025% (20 g, 45 g)
Refissa: 0.05% (20 g, 40 g)
Renova: 0.02% (40 g, 60 g)
Renova Pump: 0.02% (44 g)
Retin-A: 0.025% (20 g, 45 g); 0.05% (20 g, 45 g); 0.1% (20 g, 45 g)
Tretin-X: 0.075% (35 g)
Generic: 0.025% (20 g, 45 g); 0.05% (20 g, 40 g, 45 g, 60 g); 0.1% (20 g, 45 g)

Gel, External:

Atralin: 0.05% (45 g)
Avita: 0.025% (20 g, 45 g)
Retin-A: 0.01% (15 g, 45 g); 0.025% (15 g, 45 g)
Retin-A Micro: 0.04% (20 g, 45 g); 0.1% (20 g, 45 g)
Retin-A Micro Pump: 0.04% (50 g); 0.08% (50 g); 0.1% (50 g)
Generic: 0.01% (15 g, 45 g); 0.025% (15 g, 45 g); 0.04% (20 g, 45 g, 50 g); 0.1% (20 g, 45 g, 50 g)

Kit, External:

Tretin-X: 0.025%, 0.05%, 0.1%

- ◆ **Tretinoinum** *see* Tretinoin (Systemic) *on page 2096*
- ◆ **Trexall** *see* Methotrexate *on page 1322*
- ◆ **Treximet** *see* Sumatriptan and Naproxen *on page 1957*
- ◆ **Triacetyluridine** *see* Uridine Triacetate *on page 2116*
- ◆ **Triaconazole** *see* Terconazole *on page 2006*
- ◆ **Triaderm (Can)** *see* Triamcinolone (Topical) *on page 2100*

Triamcinolone (Systemic) (trye am SIN oh lone)

Brand Names: U.S. Aristospan Intra-Articular; Aristospan Intralesional; Kenalog

Brand Names: Canada Aristospan

Index Terms Triamcinolone Acetonide, Parenteral; Triamcinolone Hexacetonide

Pharmacologic Category Corticosteroid, Systemic

Additional Appendix Information

Corticosteroids Systemic Equivalencies *on page 2228*

Use

Intra-articular (soft tissue): Acute gouty arthritis, acute/subacute bursitis, acute tenosynovitis, epicondylitis, rheumatoid arthritis, synovitis of osteoarthritis

Intralesional: Alopecia areata, discoid lupus erythematosus, keloids, granuloma annulare lesions (localized hypertrophic, infiltrated, or inflammatory), lichen planus plaques, lichen simplex chronicus plaques, psoriatic plaques, necrobiosis lipoidica diabeticorum, cystic tumors of aponeurosis or tendon (ganglia)

Systemic: Adrenocortical insufficiency, dermatologic diseases, endocrine disorders, gastrointestinal diseases, hematologic and neoplastic disorders, nervous system disorders, nephrotic syndrome, rheumatic disorders, allergic states, respiratory diseases, systemic lupus erythematosus (SLE), and other diseases requiring anti-inflammatory or immunosuppressive effects

Pregnancy Risk Factor C

Dosage The lowest possible dose should be used to control the condition; when dose reduction is possible, the dose should be reduced gradually.

Injection:

Acetonide:

Intra-articular, intrabursal, tendon sheaths: Adults: Initial: Smaller joints: 2.5 to 5 mg, larger joints: 5 to 15 mg; may require up to 10 mg for small joints and up to 40 mg for large joints; maximum dose/treatment (several joints at one time): 20 to 80 mg

Intradermal: Adults: Initial: 1 mg

IM: Range: 2.5 to 100 mg/day

Children: Initial: 0.11 to 1.6 mg/kg/day in 3 to 4 divided doses

Children 6 to 12 years: Initial: 40 mg

Children >12 years and Adults: Initial: 60 mg

Hay fever/pollen asthma: 40 to 100 mg as a single injection/season

Multiple sclerosis (acute exacerbation): 160 mg daily for 1 week, followed by 64 mg every other day for 1 month

Hexacetonide: Adults:

Intralesional, sublesional: Up to 0.5 mg/square inch of affected skin; range: 2 to 48 mg/day

Intra-articular: Average dose: 2 to 20 mg; smaller joints: 2 to 6 mg; larger joints: 10 to 20 mg. Frequency of injection into a single joint is every 3 to 4 weeks as necessary; to avoid possible joint destruction use as infrequently as possible.

Triamcinolone Dosing

	Acetonide	Hexacetonide
Intrasynovial	5-40 mg	
Intralesional	1-30 mg (usually 1 mg per injection site); 10 mg/mL suspension usually used	Up to 0.5 mg/sq inch affected area
Sublesional	1-30 mg	
Systemic IM	2.5-60 mg/dose (usual adult dose: 60 mg; may repeat with 20-100 mg dose when symptoms recur)	
Intra-articular	2.5-40 mg	2-20 mg average
large joints	5-15 mg	10-20 mg
small joints	2.5-5 mg	2-6 mg
Tendon sheaths	2.5-10 mg	
Intradermal	1 mg/site	

Dosage adjustment in renal impairment: No dosage adjustment provided in the manufacturer's labeling; use with caution.

Dosage adjustment in hepatic impairment: No dosage adjustment provided in the manufacturer's labeling.

Additional Information Complete prescribing information should be consulted for additional detail.

Dosage Forms

Suspension, Injection:

Aristospan Intra-Articular: 20 mg/mL (1 mL, 5 mL)

Aristospan Intralesional: 5 mg/mL (5 mL)

Kenalog: 10 mg/mL (5 mL); 40 mg/mL (1 mL, 5 mL, 10 mL)

Triamcinolone (Nasal) (trye am SIN oh lone)

Brand Names: U.S. Nasacort Allergy 24HR [OTC]; Nasacort AQ

Brand Names: Canada Nasacort AQ; Trinasal

Index Terms Triamcinolone Acetonide

Pharmacologic Category Corticosteroid, Nasal

Use Allergic rhinitis:

Rx: Management of seasonal and perennial allergic rhinitis in adults and children 2 years and older

OTC: For the relief of hay fever and other upper respiratory allergies (eg, nasal congestion, runny nose, sneezing, itchy nose) in adults and children 2 years and older

Pregnancy Risk Factor C

Dosage Allergic rhinitis: Intranasal:

Children 2 to <6 years: One spray (55 mcg) in each nostril once daily (maximum: 1 spray [55 mcg] in each nostril once daily)

Children 6 to <12 years: Initial: One spray (55 mcg) in each nostril once daily; may increase to 2 sprays (110 mcg) in each nostril once daily if response not adequate; once symptoms controlled may reduce to 1 spray (55 mcg) in each nostril once daily (maximum: 2 sprays [110 mcg] in each nostril once daily)

Children ≥12 years, Adolescents, and Adults: Two sprays (110 mcg) in each nostril once daily; once symptoms controlled reduce to 1 spray (55 mcg) in each nostril once daily (maximum: 2 sprays [110 mcg] in each nostril once daily)

Dosage adjustment in renal impairment: No dosage adjustment provided in the manufacturer's labeling (has not been studied).

Dosage adjustment in hepatic impairment: No dosage adjustment provided in the manufacturer's labeling (has not been studied).

Additional Information Complete prescribing information should be consulted for additional detail.

Dosage Forms Considerations

Nasacort AQ 16.5 g bottles contain 120 sprays.

Dosage Forms

Aerosol, Nasal:

Nasacort Allergy 24HR [OTC]: 55 mcg/actuation (10.8 mL, 16.9 mL)

Nasacort AQ: 55 mcg/actuation (16.5 g)

Generic: 55 mcg/actuation (16.5 g)

Triamcinolone (Ophthalmic)

(trye am SIN oh lone)

Brand Names: U.S. Triesence

Index Terms Triamcinolone acetonide

Pharmacologic Category Corticosteroid, Ophthalmic

Use

Intavitreal: Treatment of sympathetic ophthalmia, temporal arteritis, uveitis, ocular inflammatory conditions unresponsive to topical corticosteroids

Triesence™: Visualization during vitrectomy

Pregnancy Risk Factor D

Dosage Ophthalmic injection: Intravitreal: Children and Adults:

Ocular disease: Initial: 4 mg as a single dose; additional doses may be given as needed over the course of treatment

Visualization during vitrectomy (Triesence™): 1-4 mg

Dosage adjustment in renal impairment: No dosage adjustment provided in the manufacturer's labeling.

Dosage adjustment in hepatic impairment: No dosage adjustment provided in the manufacturer's labeling.

Additional Information Complete prescribing information should be consulted for additional detail.

Dosage Forms

Suspension, Intraocular:

Triesence: 40 mg/mL (1 mL)

Triamcinolone (Topical) (trye am SIN oh lone)

Brand Names: U.S. Dermasorb TA; Kenalog; Oralone; Pediaderm TA; Trianex; Triderm

Brand Names: Canada Kenalog®; Oracort; Triaderm

Pharmacologic Category Corticosteroid, Topical

Additional Appendix Information

Topical Corticosteroids *on page 2230*

Use

Oral topical: Adjunctive treatment and temporary relief of symptoms associated with oral inflammatory lesions and ulcerative lesions resulting from trauma

Topical: Inflammatory dermatoses responsive to steroids

Pregnancy Risk Factor C

Dosage

Oral topical: Oral inflammatory lesions/ulcers: Press a small dab (about 1/4 inch) to the lesion until a thin film develops. A larger quantity may be required for coverage of some lesions. For optimal results use only enough to coat the lesion with a thin film; do not rub in.

Topical:

Cream, Ointment:

0.025% or 0.05%: Apply thin film to affected areas 2-4 times/day

0.1% or 0.5%: Apply thin film to affected areas 2-3 times/day

Spray: Apply to affected area 3-4 times/day

Additional Information Complete prescribing information should be consulted for additional detail.

Dosage Forms

Aerosol Solution, External:

Kenalog: (63 g, 100 g)

Cream, External:

Triderm: 0.1% (28.4 g, 85.2 g)

Generic: 0.025% (15 g, 80 g, 454 g); 0.1% (15 g, 30 g, 80 g, 453.6 g, 454 g); 0.5% (15 g)

Kit, External:

Dermasorb TA: 0.1%

Pediaderm TA: 0.1%

Lotion, External:

Generic: 0.025% (60 mL); 0.1% (60 mL)

Ointment, External:

Trianex: 0.05% (17 g, 85 g)

Generic: 0.025% (15 g, 80 g, 454 g); 0.1% (15 g, 80 g, 453.6 g, 454 g); 0.5% (15 g)

Paste, Mouth/Throat:

Oralone: 0.1% (5 g)

Generic: 0.1% (5 g)

◆ **Triamcinolone Acetonide** *see* Triamcinolone (Nasal) *on page 2100*

◆ **Triamcinolone acetonide** *see* Triamcinolone (Ophthalmic) *on page 2100*

◆ **Triamcinolone Acetonide, Parenteral** *see* Triamcinolone (Systemic) *on page 2099*

◆ **Triamcinolone and Nystatin** *see* Nystatin and Triamcinolone *on page 1482*

◆ **Triamcinolone Hexacetonide** *see* Triamcinolone (Systemic) *on page 2099*

◆ **Triaminic Allerchews [OTC]** *see* Loratadine *on page 1241*

◆ **Triaminic® Children's Chest & Nasal Congestion [OTC]** *see* Guaifenesin and Phenylephrine *on page 988*

◆ **Triaminic® Children's Cold & Allergy [OTC]** *see* Chlorpheniramine and Phenylephrine *on page 426*

◆ **Triaminic Children's Fever Reducer Pain Reliever [OTC]** *see* Acetaminophen *on page 32*

◆ **Triaminic® Children's Night Time Cold & Cough [OTC]** *see* Diphenhydramine and Phenylephrine *on page 644*

◆ **Triaminic® Children's Softchews® Cough & Runny Nose [OTC]** *see* Dextromethorphan and Chlorpheniramine *on page 610*

◆ **Triaminic® Cold & Allergy (Can)** *see* Chlorpheniramine and Pseudoephedrine *on page 427*

◆ **Triaminic Cough/Runny Nose [OTC]** *see* DiphenhydrAMINE (Systemic) *on page 641*

◆ **Triaminic® Day Time Cold & Cough [OTC]** *see* Dextromethorphan and Phenylephrine *on page 611*

Triamterene (trye AM ter een)

Brand Names: U.S. Dyrenium

Pharmacologic Category Antihypertensive; Diuretic, Potassium-Sparing

Use Edema: For the treatment of edema associated with congestive heart failure, cirrhosis of the liver and the nephrotic syndrome; also in steroid-induced edema, idiopathic edema and edema due to secondary hyperaldosteronism.

Pregnancy Risk Factor C

Dosage

Edema: Adults: Oral: 100 to 300 mg daily in 1 to 2 divided doses; maximum dose: 300 mg daily

Hypertension (off-label use):

Children ≥1 year and Adolescents: Oral: Initial: 1 to 2 mg/kg/day in 2 divided doses; maximum: 3 to 4 mg/kg/day, up to 300 mg daily (NHLBI, 2004)

Prevention of antihypertensive diuretic-induced hypokalemia (off-label use):

Adults: Oral: Usual dose (ASH/ISH [Weber, 2014]): 100 mg daily

Elderly: Consider lower initial doses and titrate to response (Aronow, 2011)

Dosage adjustment in renal impairment:

Mild-to-moderate impairment: No dosage adjustment provided in manufacturer's labeling.

Severe impairment or progressive kidney disease: Use is contraindicated.

The following adjustments have also been recommended (Aronoff, 2007); **Note:** Renal function may be estimated using the Cockcroft-Gault formula for dosage adjustment purposes: Adults:

CrCl >50 mL/minute: No dosage adjustment necessary.

CrCl ≤50 mL/minute: Use not recommended.

Dosage adjustment in hepatic impairment:

Mild-to-moderate impairment: No dosage adjustment provided in manufacturer's labeling (has not been studied).

Severe hepatic disease: Use is contraindicated.

Additional Information Complete prescribing information should be consulted for additional detail.

Dosage Forms

Capsule, Oral:

Dyrenium: 50 mg, 100 mg

◆ **Triamterene and Hydrochlorothiazide** *see* Hydrochlorothiazide and Triamterene *on page 1012*

◆ **Trianex** *see* Triamcinolone (Topical) *on page 2100*

◆ **Triatec-8 (Can)** *see* Acetaminophen and Codeine *on page 36*

◆ **Triatec-8 Strong (Can)** *see* Acetaminophen and Codeine *on page 36*

◆ **Triatec-30 (Can)** *see* Acetaminophen and Codeine *on page 36*

Triazolam (trye AY zoe lam)

Brand Names: U.S. Halcion

Pharmacologic Category Benzodiazepine

Additional Appendix Information

Beers Criteria – Potentially Inappropriate Medications for Geriatrics *on page 2271*

Use Insomnia: Short-term (generally 7 to 10 days) treatment of insomnia

Pregnancy Risk Factor X

Dosage

Insomnia (short-term use): Oral:

Adults: Usual dose: 0.25 mg at bedtime; 0.125 mg at bedtime may be sufficient in some patients, such as those with low body weight; maximum dose: 0.5 mg daily

Elderly and/or debilitated patients: Initial: 0.125 mg at bedtime; maximum dose: 0.25 mg daily

Dental preprocedure oral sedation (off-label use): Adults: 0.25 mg 1 hour before procedure; 0.125 mg used for elderly patients or patients sensitive to sedative effects (Dionne, 2006)

Dosage adjustment in renal impairment: There are no dosage adjustments provided in the manufacturer's labeling; use with caution.

Dosage adjustment in hepatic impairment: There are no dosage adjustments provided in the manufacturer's labeling; use with caution.

Additional Information Complete prescribing information should be consulted for additional detail.

Dosage Forms

Tablet, Oral:

Halcion: 0.25 mg

Generic: 0.125 mg, 0.25 mg

◆ **Tri-B® [OTC]** *see* Folic Acid, Cyanocobalamin, and Pyridoxine *on page 921*

◆ **Tribavirin** *see* Ribavirin *on page 1797*

◆ **Tribenzor™** *see* Olmesartan, Amlodipine, and Hydrochlorothiazide *on page 1498*

◆ **Tri-Buffered Aspirin [OTC]** *see* Aspirin *on page 180*

◆ **Tricardio B** *see* Folic Acid, Cyanocobalamin, and Pyridoxine *on page 921*

◆ **Trichloroacetaldehyde Monohydrate** *see* Chloral Hydrate [CAN/INT] *on page 418*

Triclabendazole [INT] (try KLUH bend uh zole)

International Brand Names Clabenzole (KR); Egaten (FR, GR, VN)

Index Terms Egaten

Pharmacologic Category Anthelmintic

Reported Use *Fasciola hepatica* (sheep liver fluke) infection

Dosage Range Oral: 10 mg/kg as a single dose, may repeat in 12-24 hours for severe infection

Product Availability Product available in various countries; not currently available in the U.S.

◆ **Tricode® GF** *see* Guaifenesin, Pseudoephedrine, and Codeine *on page 989*

◆ **Tricor** *see* Fenofibrate and Derivatives *on page 852*

◆ **Tricosal** *see* Choline Magnesium Trisalicylate *on page 431*

◆ **Tri-Cyclen (Can)** *see* Ethinyl Estradiol and Norgestimate *on page 810*

◆ **Tri-Cyclen Lo (Can)** *see* Ethinyl Estradiol and Norgestimate *on page 810*

◆ **Triderm** *see* Triamcinolone (Topical) *on page 2100*

◆ **Tridesilon (Can)** *see* Desonide *on page 597*

◆ **Tridil** *see* Nitroglycerin *on page 1465*

◆ **Tridural (Can)** *see* TraMADol *on page 2074*

◆ **Trien** *see* Trientine *on page 2102*

Trientine (TRYE en teen)

Brand Names: U.S. Syprine

Brand Names: Canada Syprine®

Index Terms 2,2,2-tetramine; Trien; Trientine Hydrochloride; Triethylene Tetramine Dihydrochloride

Pharmacologic Category Chelating Agent

Use Treatment of Wilson's disease in patients intolerant to penicillamine

Pregnancy Risk Factor C

Dosage Oral:

Children <12 years: 500-750 mg/day in divided doses 2-4 times/day; maximum: 1.5 g/day. AASLD practice guidelines suggest 20 mg/kg/day rounded off to the nearest 250 mg, given in 2-3 divided doses (Roberts, 2008).

Children ≥12 years and Adults: 750-1250 mg/day in divided doses 2-4 times/day; maximum dose: 2 g/day. AASLD practice guidelines suggest typical doses of 750-1500 mg/day in 2-3 divided doses with maintenance therapy of 750-1000 mg/day (Roberts, 2008).

Dosage adjustment in renal impairment: No dosage adjustment provided in manufacturer's labeling.

Dosage adjustment in hepatic impairment: No dosage adjustment provided in manufacturer's labeling.

Additional Information Complete prescribing information should be consulted for additional detail.

Dosage Forms

Capsule, Oral:

Syprine: 250 mg

◆ **Trientine Hydrochloride** *see* Trientine *on page 2102*

◆ **Triesence** *see* Triamcinolone (Ophthalmic) *on page 2100*

◆ **Tri-Estarylla** *see* Ethinyl Estradiol and Norgestimate *on page 810*

◆ **Triethylene Tetramine Dihydrochloride** *see* Trientine *on page 2102*

◆ **Triethylenethiophosphoramide** *see* Thiotepa *on page 2030*

Trifluoperazine (trye floo oh PER a zeen)

Brand Names: Canada Apo-Trifluoperazine®; Novo-Trifluzine; PMS-Trifluoperazine; Terfluzine

Index Terms Stelazine; Trifluoperazine Hydrochloride

Pharmacologic Category First Generation (Typical) Antipsychotic

Additional Appendix Information

Beers Criteria – Potentially Inappropriate Medications for Geriatrics *on page 2271*

Use Treatment of schizophrenia; short-term treatment of generalized nonpsychotic anxiety

Dosage Oral:

Children 6-12 years: Schizophrenia/psychoses: Hospitalized or well-supervised patients: Initial: 1 mg 1-2 times/day, gradually increase until symptoms are controlled or adverse effects become troublesome; maximum: 15 mg/day

Adults:

Schizophrenia/psychoses:

Outpatients: 1-2 mg twice daily

Hospitalized or well-supervised patients: Initial: 2-5 mg twice daily with optimum response in the 15-20 mg/day range; do not exceed 40 mg/day

Nonpsychotic anxiety: 1-2 mg twice daily; maximum: 6 mg/day; therapy for anxiety should not exceed 12 weeks; do not exceed 6 mg/day for longer than 12 weeks when treating anxiety; agitation, jitteriness, or insomnia may be confused with original neurotic or psychotic symptoms

Elderly:

Schizophrenia/psychoses: Refer to adult dosing. Dose selection should start at the low end of the dosage range and titration must be gradual.

Behavioral symptoms associated with dementia behavior (off-label use): Initial: 0.5-1 mg 1-2 times/day; increase dose at 4- to 7-day intervals by 0.5-1 mg/day; increase dosing intervals (bid, tid, etc) as necessary to control response or side effects. Maximum daily dose: 40 mg. Gradual increases (titration) may prevent some side effects or decrease their severity.

Dosage adjustment in renal impairment: No dosage adjustment provided in manufacturer's labeling.

Hemodialysis: Not dialyzable (0% to 5%)

Dosage adjustment in hepatic impairment: Use is contraindicated in preexisting liver injury.

Additional Information Complete prescribing information should be consulted for additional detail.

Dosage Forms

Tablet, Oral:

Generic: 1 mg, 2 mg, 5 mg, 10 mg

Dosage Forms: Canada Note: Refer also to Dosage Forms.

Tablet, Oral: 20 mg

◆ **Trifluoperazine Hydrochloride** *see* Trifluoperazine *on page 2102*

◆ **Trifluorothymidine** *see* Trifluridine *on page 2103*

Trifluridine (trye FLURE i deen)

Brand Names: U.S. Viroptic
Brand Names: Canada Sandoz-Trifluridine; Viroptic®
Index Terms F_3T; Trifluorothymidine
Pharmacologic Category Antiviral Agent, Ophthalmic
Use Treatment of primary keratoconjunctivitis and recurrent epithelial keratitis caused by herpes simplex virus types I and II
Pregnancy Risk Factor C
Dosage Children ≥6 years, Adolescents, and Adults: Instill 1 drop into affected eye every 2 hours while awake, to a maximum of 9 drops daily, until re-epithelialization of corneal ulcer occurs; then use 1 drop every 4 hours while awake for another 7 days (minimum daily dosage of 5 drops is recommended); do **not** exceed 21 days of treatment; if improvement has not taken place in 7-14 days, consider another form of therapy

Dosage adjustment in renal impairment: No dosage adjustment provided in manufacturer's labeling.
Dosage adjustment in hepatic impairment: No dosage adjustment provided in manufacturer's labeling.

Additional Information Complete prescribing information should be consulted for additional detail.
Dosage Forms
Solution, Ophthalmic:
Viroptic: 1% (7.5 mL)
Generic: 1% (7.5 mL)

Triflusal [INT] (tri FLU sal)

International Brand Names Aflen (GR); Anpeval (ES); Disgren (AR, BR, ES, HU, KR, KW, LB, MX, PK, PY, UY, VE); Flurant (KR); Grendis (ID, MY, PH, TH); Paspirin (KR); Reoflen (GR); Risal (KR); Tecnosal (PT); Triflux (IT); TRIOFLEN (BG)
Pharmacologic Category Antiplatelet Agent
Reported Use Prophylaxis and treatment of thrombotic complications
Dosage Range Oral: 600-900 mg/day with meals
Product Availability Product available in various countries; not currently available in the U.S.
Dosage Forms
Capsule: 300 mg

◆ **Triglide** *see* Fenofibrate and Derivatives *on page 852*

◆ **Triglycyl Lysine Vasopressin** *see* Terlipressin [INT] *on page 2010*

◆ **Trigofen DM [OTC]** *see* Chlorpheniramine, Phenylephrine, and Dextromethorphan *on page 428*

Trihexyphenidyl (trye heks ee FEN i dil)

Brand Names: Canada PMS-Trihexyphenidyl; Trihexyphenidyl
Index Terms Artane; Benzhexol Hydrochloride; Trihexyphenidyl Hydrochloride
Pharmacologic Category Anti-Parkinson's Agent, Anticholinergic; Anticholinergic Agent
Additional Appendix Information
Beers Criteria – Potentially Inappropriate Medications for Geriatrics *on page 2271*
Use
Drug-induced extrapyramidal disorders: Control of extrapyramidal disorders caused by CNS drugs (eg, dibenzoxazepines, phenothiazines, thioxanthenes, butyrophenones)
Parkinsonism: Treatment of all forms of parkinsonism (postencephalitic, arteriosclerotic, and idiopathic) as adjunctive therapy
Pregnancy Risk Factor C
Dosage
Adults: Oral:
Drug-induced extrapyramidal disorders: Initial: 1 mg/day; increase as necessary to usual range: 5 to 15 mg/day in 3 to 4 divided doses
Parkinsonism: Initial: 1 mg/day, increase by 2 mg increments at intervals of 3 to 5 days; usual dose: 6 to 10 mg/day in 3 to 4 divided doses; doses of 12 to 15 mg/day may be required
Use in combination with levodopa: When trihexyphenidyl is used concomitantly with levodopa, the usual dose of each may need to be reduced. Usual range: 3 to 6 mg/day in divided doses
Elderly: Oral: Refer to adult dosing. **Note:** Conservative initial doses and gradual titration is especially important in patients >60 years of age.

Dosage adjustment in renal impairment: There are no dosage adjustments provided in the manufacturer's labeling; use with caution.
Dosage adjustment in hepatic impairment: There are no dosage adjustments provided in the manufacturer's labeling; use with caution.

Additional Information Complete prescribing information should be consulted for additional detail.
Dosage Forms
Elixir, Oral:
Generic: 0.4 mg/mL (473 mL)
Tablet, Oral:
Generic: 2 mg, 5 mg

◆ **Trihexyphenidyl Hydrochloride** *see* Trihexyphenidyl *on page 2103*

◆ **Trilafon** *see* Perphenazine *on page 1627*

◆ **Tri-Legest Fe** *see* Ethinyl Estradiol and Norethindrone *on page 808*

◆ **Trileptal** *see* OXcarbazepine *on page 1532*

◆ **Trilipix** *see* Fenofibrate and Derivatives *on page 852*

◆ **Trilisate** *see* Choline Magnesium Trisalicylate *on page 431*

◆ **Tri-Luma®** *see* Fluocinolone, Hydroquinone, and Tretinoin *on page 894*

◆ **TriLyte** *see* Polyethylene Glycol-Electrolyte Solution *on page 1674*

Trimebutine [CAN/INT] (trye me BYOO teen)

Brand Names: Canada Modulon
Index Terms Trimebutine Maleate
Pharmacologic Category 5-HT_3 Receptor Antagonist
Use Note: Not approved in U.S.
Treatment and relief of symptoms associated with irritable bowel syndrome (IBS) (spastic colon). In postoperative paralytic ileus in order to accelerate the resumption of the intestinal transit following abdominal surgery
Pregnancy Considerations Adverse events were not observed in animal reproduction studies. Use in pregnancy is not recommended per manufacturer.
Contraindications Hypersensitivity to trimebutine or any component of the formulation
Warnings/Precautions May cause drowsiness; use with caution in patients with CNS depression; may increase sedation from CNS depressants and/or ethanol. Advise patient to avoid operating machinery/driving until response is known.

Adverse Reactions
Central nervous system: Anxiety, dizziness, drowsiness, dizziness, fatigue, headache
Dermatologic: Rash
Endocrine & metabolic: Gynecomastia, mastalgia, menstrual disorder
Gastrointestinal: Constipation, diarrhea, dyspepsia, epigastric discomfort, nausea, taste disorder, xerostomia
Genitourinary: Urinary retention
Otic: Hearing impairment
Miscellaneous: Hot/cold sensations

Drug Interactions
Metabolism/Transport Effects None known.
Avoid Concomitant Use There are no known interactions where it is recommended to avoid concomitant use.
Increased Effect/Toxicity There are no known significant interactions involving an increase in effect.
Decreased Effect There are no known significant interactions involving a decrease in effect.

Storage/Stability Store at room temperature of 15°C to 30°C (59°F to 86°F).

Mechanism of Action Spasmolytic agent with antiserotonergic activity and moderate opiate receptor affinity. Reduces abnormal motility; does not alter normal GI motility.

Pharmacodynamics/Kinetics Half-life elimination: ~3 hours

Dosage Oral: Children ≥12 years and Adults:
Irritable bowel syndrome (IBS): 200 mg 3 times/day
Postoperative paralytic ileus: 200 mg 3 times/day

Dietary Considerations Should be taken before meals.

Administration Administer before meals.

Product Availability Not available in U.S.

Dosage Forms: Canada Tablet, oral: 100 mg, 200 mg

◆ **Trimebutine Maleate** *see* Trimebutine [CAN/INT] *on page 2103*

Trimetazidine [INT] (trye met AZ i deen)

International Brand Names Adexor (HN); Angintriz MR (ID); Angirel (PH); Angirel MR (PH); Anpect (EE); Apstar (RO); Cardimax (IN); Carvidon (IN, PH); Carvidon-MR (IN, PH); Dinemic (PK); Idaptan (ES); Invidon (IN); Invidon-XR (IN); Latrimet (GR); Matenol (HK, TH); Matenol MR (TH); Metagard (SG); Metazin (KR, SG); Miozidine (ID); Moduxin (EE); Neotri MR (BG); Portora (CZ); Predozone (BG); Preductal (HN, PL, RO); Preductal MR (EE, HR); Preduxl (HK); Tacirel LM (PT); Tagidine (KR); Trimez (PK); Trivedon (HK); Trizedon MR (ID); Trizidine (TH); Vascotasin (BG); Vasorel (CN); Vasorel MR (CN); Vassapro (PH); Vastarel (AE, AR, CY, DK, EG, FR, GR, IE, IT, JO, LB, NO, PK, PT, QA, SA, SG, TR, VN); Vastarel LM (PT); Vastarel LP (AR); Vastarel MR (AE, BH, BR, CL, CO, CY, EG, HK, KW, PE, PH, PY, QA, SA, SG, TH, UY, VE, VN); Vastinan (KR); Vastinan MR (KR); Vastinol (TH); Vazidin (HR); Zilutra (CZ)

Index Terms Trimetazidine Dichorhydrate; Trimetazidine Dihydrochloride; Trimetazidine Hydrochloride

Pharmacologic Category Cardiovascular Agent, Other

Reported Use Adjunctive therapy for symptomatic treatment of stable angina pectoris in patients intolerant of or unsuccessfully treated with first-line antianginal therapy

Dosage Range Oral: Angina:
Immediate release tablet: Initial and maximum dose: 20 mg 3 times daily
Modified release tablet: Initial and maximum dose: 35 mg twice daily

Dosage adjustment in renal impairment:
CrCl 30-60 mL/minute:
Immediate release tablet: Initial and maximum dose: [illegible] twice daily
Modified release tablet: Initial and maximum dose: 35 mg once daily (preferably in the morning)
CrCl <30 mL/minute: Use is contraindicated

Product Availability Product available in various countries; not currently available in the U.S.

Dosage Forms
Tablet, as dihydrochloride: 20 mg
Tablet, modified release, as dihydrochloride: 35 mg

◆ **Trimetazidine Dichorhydrate** *see* Trimetazidine [INT] *on page 2104*

◆ **Trimetazidine Dihydrochloride** *see* Trimetazidine [INT] *on page 2104*

◆ **Trimetazidine Hydrochloride** *see* Trimetazidine [INT] *on page 2104*

Trimethobenzamide (trye meth oh BEN za mide)

Brand Names: U.S. Tigan
Brand Names: Canada Tigan
Index Terms Trimethobenzamide HCl; Trimethobenzamide Hydrochloride
Pharmacologic Category Antiemetic
Additional Appendix Information
Beers Criteria – Potentially Inappropriate Medications for Geriatrics *on page 2271*

Use Nausea and vomiting: Treatment of postoperative nausea and vomiting; treatment of nausea associated with gastroenteritis

Dosage
Nausea/vomiting: Adults:
Oral: 300 mg 3 or 4 times daily
IM: 200 mg 3 or 4 times daily
Elderly: According to the manufacturer, consider dosage reduction or increasing the dosing interval in elderly patients with renal impairment, although use should be avoided in this age group due to the risk of EPS adverse effects combined with lower efficacy, as compared to other antiemetics (Beers Criteria).

Dosage adjustment in renal impairment: CrCl ≤70 mL/minute/1.73 m^2: Although no specific dosage adjustment provided in the manufacturer's labeling, dosage reduction or increasing the dosing interval is recommended.
Dosage adjustment in hepatic impairment: No dosage adjustment provided in the manufacturer's labeling.

Additional Information Complete prescribing information should be consulted for additional detail.

Dosage Forms
Capsule, Oral:
Tigan: 300 mg
Generic: 300 mg
Solution, Intramuscular:
Tigan: 100 mg/mL (2 mL, 20 mL)

◆ **Trimethobenzamide HCl** *see* Trimethobenzamide *on page 2104*

◆ **Trimethobenzamide Hydrochloride** *see* Trimethobenzamide *on page 2104*

Trimethoprim (trye METH oh prim)

Brand Names: U.S. Primsol
Brand Names: Canada Apo-Trimethoprim®
Index Terms TMP
Pharmacologic Category Antibiotic, Miscellaneous
Use Treatment of urinary tract infections due to susceptible strains of *E. coli*, *P. mirabilis*, *K. pneumoniae*, *Enterobacter* spp and coagulase-negative *Staphylococcus* including *S. saprophyticus*; acute otitis media due to susceptible strains of *S. pneumoniae* and *H. influenzae* in children
Pregnancy Risk Factor C

Dosage Oral:
Children:
Susceptible infections: Children ≥2 months: 4-6 mg/kg/day in divided doses every 12 hours (dosing for UTI in Schleiss, 2007); **Note:** AAP guidelines on treatment of UTI recommend 6-12 mg trimethoprim/kg/day (in combination with sulfamethoxazole) in 2 divided doses (AAP, 1999)
Acute otitis media: Children ≥6 months: 10 mg/kg/day in divided doses every 12 hours for 10 days
Adults:
***Pneumocystis jirovecii* pneumonia, mild-to-moderate (off-label use) (CDC, 2009):** 15 mg/kg/day in 3 divided doses in combination with dapsone
Susceptible infections: 100 mg every 12 hours or 200 mg every 24 hours for 10 days
Urinary tract infection, uncomplicated (off-label duration):
Treatment: 100 mg every 12 hours for 3 days (Gupta, 2011)
Prophylaxis: 100 mg once daily (Kodner, 2010)

Dosage adjustment in renal impairment:
CrCl 15-30 mL/minute: Administer 50 mg every 12 hours
CrCl <15 mL/minute: Not recommended
Hemodialysis: Moderately dialyzable (20% to 50%)
Dosage adjustment in hepatic impairment: No dosage adjustment provided in manufacturer's labeling; use with caution.
Additional Information Complete prescribing information should be consulted for additional detail.
Dosage Forms
Solution, Oral:
Primsol: 50 mg/5 mL (473 mL)
Tablet, Oral:
Generic: 100 mg

Trimethoprim and Polymyxin B
(trye METH oh prim & pol i MIKS in bee)

Brand Names: U.S. Polytrim®
Brand Names: Canada PMS-Polytrimethoprim; Polytrim™
Index Terms Polymyxin B and Trimethoprim
Pharmacologic Category Antibiotic, Ophthalmic
Use Treatment of surface ocular bacterial conjunctivitis and blepharoconjunctivitis
Pregnancy Risk Factor C
Dosage Ophthalmic:
Children ≥2 months and Adults: Instill 1 drop in affected eye(s) every 3 hours (maximum: 6 doses per day) for 7-10 days; has also been used 4 times daily for 5-7 days (Williams, 2013; *The Wills Eye Manual*, 2004)
Elderly: No overall differences observed between elderly and other adults

Dosage adjustment in renal impairment: No dosage adjustment provided in manufacturer's labeling.
Dosage adjustment in hepatic impairment: No dosage adjustment provided in manufacturer's labeling.
Additional Information Complete prescribing information should be consulted for additional detail.
Dosage Forms
Solution, ophthalmic: Trimethoprim 1 mg and polymyxin B 10,000 units per 1 mL (10 mL)
Polytrim®: Trimethoprim 1 mg and polymyxin B 10,000 units per 1 mL (10 mL)

◆ **Trimethoprim and Sulfamethoxazole** *see* Sulfamethoxazole and Trimethoprim *on page 1946*
◆ **Trinasal (Can)** *see* Triamcinolone (Nasal) *on page 2100*
◆ **TriNessa** *see* Ethinyl Estradiol and Norgestimate *on page 810*
◆ **Trinipatch (Can)** *see* Nitroglycerin *on page 1465*
◆ **Tri-Norinyl** *see* Ethinyl Estradiol and Norethindrone *on page 808*
◆ **Trintellix (Can)** *see* Vortioxetine *on page 2183*
◆ **Triostat** *see* Liothyronine *on page 1221*
◆ **Tripedia** *see* Diphtheria and Tetanus Toxoids, and Acellular Pertussis Vaccine *on page 649*
◆ **Triphasil (Can)** *see* Ethinyl Estradiol and Levonorgestrel *on page 803*
◆ **Triple Antibiotic** *see* Bacitracin, Neomycin, and Polymyxin B *on page 223*
◆ **Triple Paste AF [OTC]** *see* Miconazole (Topical) *on page 1360*
◆ **Tri-Previfem** *see* Ethinyl Estradiol and Norgestimate *on page 810*

Triprolidine and Pseudoephedrine
(trye PROE li deen & soo doe e FED rin)

Brand Names: U.S. Aprodine [OTC]; Ed A-Hist PSE [OTC]; Entre-Hist PSE; Pediatex TD [DSC]
Brand Names: Canada Actifed®
Index Terms Pseudoephedrine and Triprolidine
Pharmacologic Category Alkylamine Derivative; Alpha/Beta Agonist; Decongestant; Histamine H_1 Antagonist; Histamine H_1 Antagonist, First Generation
Use Temporary relief of nasal congestion, decongest sinus openings, running nose, sneezing, itching of nose or throat and itchy, watery eyes due to common cold, hay fever, or other upper respiratory allergies
Dosage Oral:
Liquid (Pediatex® TD):
Children 6-12 years: 1.33 mL every 6 hours (maximum: 4 doses/24 hours)
Children ≥12 years and Adults: 2.67 mL every 6 hours (maximum: 4 doses/24 hours)
Syrup (Aprodine):
Children 6-12 years: 5 mL every 4-6 hours; do not exceed 4 doses in 24 hours
Children >12 years and Adults: 10 mL every 4-6 hours; do not exceed 4 doses in 24 hours
Tablet (Aprodine):
Children 6-12 years: 1/2 tablet every 4-6 hours; do not exceed 4 doses in 24 hours
Children >12 years and Adults: One tablet every 4-6 hours; do not exceed 4 doses in 24 hours
Additional Information Complete prescribing information should be consulted for additional detail.
Dosage Forms
Liquid, oral:
Entre-Hist PSE: Triprolidine 0.938 mg and pseudoephedrine 10 mg per 1 mL
Syrup, oral:
Aprodine [OTC]: Triprolidine 1.25 mg and pseudoephedrine 30 mg per 5 mL
Tablet, oral:
Aprodine [OTC]: Triprolidine 2.5 mg and pseudoephedrine 60 mg
Ed A-Hist PSE [OTC]: Triprolidine 2.5 mg and pseudoephedrine 60 mg

◆ **Triprolidine, Codeine, and Pseudoephedrine** *see* Triprolidine, Pseudoephedrine, and Codeine [CAN/INT] *on page 2105*

Triprolidine, Pseudoephedrine, and Codeine [CAN/INT]
(trye PROE li deen, soo doe e FED rin, & KOE deen)

Brand Names: Canada CoActifed; Covan; ratio-Cotridin

Index Terms Codeine, Pseudoephedrine, and Triprolidine; Codeine, Triprolidine, and Pseudoephedrine; Cotridin; Pseudoephedrine, Codeine, and Triprolidine; Pseudoephedrine, Triprolidine, and Codeine; Triprolidine, Codeine, and Pseudoephedrine

Pharmacologic Category Alkylamine Derivative; Alpha/Beta Agonist; Analgesic, Opioid; Antitussive; Decongestant; Histamine H_1 Antagonist; Histamine H_1 Antagonist, First Generation

Use Note: Not approved in U.S.

Symptomatic relief of upper respiratory symptoms and cough

Pregnancy Considerations See individual agents.

Breast-Feeding Considerations See individual agents.

Contraindications Hypersensitivity to triprolidine, pseudoephedrine, opioids, or any component of the formulation (some formulations contain ethanol); acute respiratory depression; CNS depression or coma; increased intracranial pressure (ICP)/head trauma; convulsive disorder; acute abdomen/obstruction; use of MAO inhibitors within 14 days

Warnings/Precautions

Codeine: Use with caution in patients with hypersensitivity reactions to other phenanthrene derivative opioid agonists (morphine, hydrocodone, hydromorphone, levorphanol, oxycodone, oxymorphone); respiratory diseases (including asthma, emphysema, COPD), severe liver or renal insufficiency, biliary tract impairment, adrenal insufficiency, or pancreatitis. Tolerance or drug dependence may result from extended use. Not recommended for use for cough control in patients with a productive cough; not recommended as an antitussive for children <2 years of age; the elderly may be particularly susceptible to the CNS depressant and confusion as well as constipating effects of opioids. Use caution in patients with two or more copies of the variant CYP2D6*2 allele; may have extensive conversion from codeine to morphine and thus increased opioid-mediated effects. Avoid the use of codeine in these patients; consider alternative analgesics such as morphine or a nonopioid agent (Crews, 2012). The occurrence of this phenotype is seen in 0.5% to 1% of Chinese and Japanese, 0.5% to 1% of Hispanics, 1% to 10% of Caucasians, 3% of African-Americans, and 16% to 28% of North Africans, Ethiopians, and Arabs. Potentially significant drug interactions may exist, requiring dose or frequency adjustment, additional monitoring, and/or selection of alternative therapy. After chronic maternal exposure to opioids, neonatal withdrawal syndrome may occur in the newborn; monitor neonate closely. Signs and symptoms include irritability, hyperactivity and abnormal sleep pattern, high pitched cry, tremor, vomiting, diarrhea and failure to gain weight. Onset, duration and severity depend on the drug used, duration of use, maternal dose, and rate of drug elimination by the newborn. Opioid withdrawal syndrome in the neonate, unlike in adults, may be life-threatening and should be treated according to protocols developed by neonatology experts.

Pseudoephedrine: Use with caution in patients >60 years of age; administer with caution to patients with hypertension, hyperthyroidism, diabetes mellitus, cardiovascular disease, ischemic heart disease, increased intraocular pressure, or prostatic hyperplasia. Elderly patients are more likely to experience adverse reactions to sympathomimetics. Overdosage may cause hallucinations, seizures, CNS depression, and death. Avoid prolonged use; generally limited to not more than 5 days.

Triprolidine: Causes sedation; caution must be used in performing tasks which require alertness (eg, operating machinery or driving). Sedative effects of CNS depressants or ethanol are potentiated. Use with caution in patients with angle-closure glaucoma, pyloroduodenal obstruction (including stenotic peptic ulcer), urinary tract obstruction (including bladder neck obstruction and symptomatic prostatic hyperplasia), hyperthyroidism, increased intraocular pressure, and cardiovascular disease (including hypertension and tachycardia). In the elderly, avoid use of this potent anticholinergic agent due to increased risk of confusion, dry mouth, constipation, and other anticholinergic effects; clearance decreases in patients of advanced age (Beers Criteria). May cause paradoxical excitation in pediatric patients, and can result in hallucinations, coma, and death in overdose.

Adverse Reactions

Cardiovascular: Hypotension

Central nervous system: Agitation, dizziness, drowsiness, drug dependence (physical or psychological, with continued use), dysphoria, euphoria, hallucination, headache, increased intracranial pressure, paresthesia, sedation, seizure, withdrawal syndrome

Dermatologic: Diaphoresis, pruritus, skin rash

Gastrointestinal: Anorexia, biliary tract spasm, constipation, dysgeusia, nausea, vomiting, xerostomia

Genitourinary: Genitourinary tract spasm, urinary retention

Neuromuscular & skeletal: Muscle rigidity (rare), tremor

Ophthalmic: Blurred vision, nystagmus

Respiratory: Respiratory depression

Rare but important or life-threatening: Hypogonadism (Brennan, 2013; Debono, 2011)

Drug Interactions

Metabolism/Transport Effects Refer to individual components.

Avoid Concomitant Use

Avoid concomitant use of Triprolidine, Pseudoephedrine, and Codeine with any of the following: Aclidinium; Azelastine (Nasal); Ergot Derivatives; Glucagon; Iobenguane I 123; Ipratropium (Oral Inhalation); MAO Inhibitors; Orphenadrine; Paraldehyde; Potassium Chloride; Thalidomide; Tiotropium; Umeclidinium

Increased Effect/Toxicity

Triprolidine, Pseudoephedrine, and Codeine may increase the levels/effects of: AbobotulinumtoxinA; Alcohol (Ethyl); Alvimopan; Analgesics (Opioid); Anticholinergic Agents; ARIPiprazole; Azelastine (Nasal); Buprenorphine; CNS Depressants; Desmopressin; Diuretics; Glucagon; Hydrocodone; Methotrimeprazine; Metyrosine; Mirabegron; Mirtazapine; OnabotulinumtoxinA; Orphenadrine; Paraldehyde; Potassium Chloride; Pramipexole; RimabotulinumtoxinB; ROPINIRole; Rotigotine; Selective Serotonin Reuptake Inhibitors; Suvorexant; Sympathomimetics; Thalidomide; Thiazide Diuretics; Tiotropium; Topiramate; Zolpidem

The levels/effects of Triprolidine, Pseudoephedrine, and Codeine may be increased by: Aclidinium; Alkalinizing Agents; Amphetamines; Anticholinergic Agents; AtoMOXetine; Brimonidine (Topical); Cannabis; Carbonic Anhydrase Inhibitors; Doxylamine; Dronabinol; Droperidol; Ergot Derivatives; HydrOXYzine; Ipratropium (Oral Inhalation); Kava Kava; Linezolid; Magnesium Sulfate; MAO Inhibitors; Methotrimeprazine; Mianserin; Nabilone; Perampanel; Pramlintide; Rufinamide; Serotonin/Norepinephrine Reuptake Inhibitors; Sodium Oxybate; Somatostatin Analogs; Succinylcholine; Tapentadol; Tedizolid; Tetrahydrocannabinol; Umeclidinium

Decreased Effect

Triprolidine, Pseudoephedrine, and Codeine may decrease the levels/effects of: Acetylcholinesterase Inhibitors; Benzylpenicilloyl Polylysine; Betahistine; FentaNYL; Hyaluronidase; Iobenguane I 123; Itopride; Pegvisomant; Secretin

The levels/effects of Triprolidine, Pseudoephedrine, and Codeine may be decreased by: Acetylcholinesterase Inhibitors; Alpha1-Blockers; Ammonium Chloride; Amphetamines; CYP2D6 Inhibitors (Moderate); CYP2D6

Inhibitors (Strong); Mixed Agonist / Antagonist Opioids; Naltrexone; Spironolactone; Urinary Acidifying Agents

Pharmacodynamics/Kinetics See Pseudoephedrine and Codeine monographs.

Dosage Oral:

Children:

2-6 years: 2.5 mL 4 times/day

7-12 years: 5 mL 4 times/day **or** 1/2 tablet 4 times/day

Children >12 years and Adults: 10 mL 4 times/day **or** 1 tablet 4 times/day

Dosage adjustment in renal impairment: No dosage adjustment provided in manufacturer's labeling; use with caution.

Dosage adjustment in hepatic impairment: No dosage adjustment provided in manufacturer's labeling; use with caution.

Monitoring Parameters Signs or symptoms of hypogonadism or hypoadrenalism (Brennan, 2013)

Product Availability Not available in U.S.

Dosage Forms: Canada

Syrup, oral:

CoActifed, ratio-Cotridin: Triprolidine 2 mg, pseudoephedrine 30 mg, and codeine 10 mg per 5 mL

CoVan: Triprolidine 2 mg, pseudoephedrine 30 mg, and codeine 10 mg per 5 mL (500 mL)

Tablet, oral:

CoActifed: Triprolidine 4 mg, pseudoephedrine 60 mg, and codeine 20 mg (50s)

Triptorelin (trip toe REL in)

Brand Names: U.S. Trelstar Depot; Trelstar Depot Mixject; Trelstar LA; Trelstar LA Mixject; Trelstar Mixject

Brand Names: Canada Decapeptyl; Trelstar

Index Terms AY-25650; CL-118,532; D-Trp(6)-LHRH; Detryptoreline; Triptorelin Pamoate; Tryptoreline

Pharmacologic Category Gonadotropin Releasing Hormone Agonist

Use

Advanced prostate cancer: Palliative treatment of advanced prostate cancer

Assisted reproductive technologies: Decapeptyl [Canadian product]: Adjunctive therapy in women undergoing controlled ovarian hyperstimulation for assisted reproductive technologies (ART)

Pregnancy Risk Factor X

Dosage

Prostate cancer, advanced: Adults: IM:

3.75 mg once every 4 weeks **or**

11.25 mg once every 12 weeks **or**

22.5 mg once every 24 weeks

Controlled ovarian hyperstimulation for assisted reproductive technologies (ART) (adjunctive therapy): Decapeptyl [Canadian product]: Adults: Females: SubQ: Usual dose: 0.1 mg once daily initiated on day 2 or 3 or days 21 to 23 of menstrual cycle (or 5 to 7 days prior to expected onset of menses). Dose may be adjusted according to ovarian response as measured by ovarian ultrasound with or without serum estradiol levels. Treatment is continued until follicles achieve suitable size (typically 4 to 7 weeks).

Treatment of paraphilia/hypersexuality (off-label use; Guay, 2009; Thibaut, 1993): Adults: Males:

Note: May cause an initial increase in androgen concentrations which may be treated with an antiandrogen (eg, flutamide, cyproterone) for 1 to 2 months (Guay, 2009). Avoid use in patients with osteoporosis or active pituitary pathology.

SubQ: Test dose: 1 mg (observe for hypersensitivity)

IM: 3.75 mg monthly

Dosage adjustment in renal impairment: There are no dosage adjustments provided in the manufacturer's labeling. However, renal impairment increases systemic exposure to triptorelin.

Dosage adjustment in hepatic impairment: There are no dosage adjustments provided in the manufacturer's labeling. However, hepatic impairment increases systemic exposure to triptorelin.

Additional Information Complete prescribing information should be consulted for additional detail.

Dosage Forms

Suspension Reconstituted, Intramuscular:

Trelstar Depot: 3.75 mg (1 ea)

Trelstar Depot Mixject: 3.75 mg (1 ea)

Trelstar LA: 11.25 mg (1 ea)

Trelstar LA Mixject: 11.25 mg (1 ea)

Trelstar Mixject: 22.5 mg (1 ea)

Dosage Forms: Canada

Injection, solution [preservative free]:

Decapeptyl: 100 mcg/mL (equivalent to 95.6 mcg triptorelin free base) (1 mL) [prefilled syringe]

- ◆ **Triptorelin Pamoate** *see* Triptorelin *on page 2107*
- ◆ **Triquilar (Can)** *see* Ethinyl Estradiol and Levonorgestrel *on page 803*
- ◆ **Tris Buffer** *see* Tromethamine *on page 2107*
- ◆ **Trisenox** *see* Arsenic Trioxide *on page 177*
- ◆ **Tris(hydroxymethyl)aminomethane** *see* Tromethamine *on page 2107*
- ◆ **Tri-Sprintec** *see* Ethinyl Estradiol and Norgestimate *on page 810*
- ◆ **Trisulfa (Can)** *see* Sulfamethoxazole and Trimethoprim *on page 1946*
- ◆ **Trisulfa DS (Can)** *see* Sulfamethoxazole and Trimethoprim *on page 1946*
- ◆ **Trisulfa S (Can)** *see* Sulfamethoxazole and Trimethoprim *on page 1946*
- ◆ **Triumeq** *see* Abacavir, Dolutegravir, and Lamivudine *on page 22*
- ◆ **Trivagizole-3® (Can)** *see* Clotrimazole (Topical) *on page 488*
- ◆ **Trivora** *see* Ethinyl Estradiol and Levonorgestrel *on page 803*
- ◆ **Trizivir** *see* Abacavir, Lamivudine, and Zidovudine *on page 22*
- ◆ **Trocaine Throat [OTC]** *see* Benzocaine *on page 246*
- ◆ **Trokendi XR** *see* Topiramate *on page 2065*
- ◆ **Trombovar (Can)** *see* Sodium Tetradecyl Sulfate *on page 1914*

Tromethamine (troe METH a meen)

Brand Names: U.S. Tham

Index Terms Tris Buffer; Tris(hydroxymethyl)aminomethane

Pharmacologic Category Alkalinizing Agent, Parenteral

Use Correction of metabolic acidosis associated with cardiac bypass surgery or cardiac arrest; to correct excess acidity of stored blood that is preserved with acid citrate dextrose (ACD); indicated in infants needing alkalinization after receiving maximum sodium bicarbonate (8-10 mEq/kg/24 hours)

Pregnancy Risk Factor C

Dosage Dose depends on buffer base deficit; when deficit is known: tromethamine (mL of 0.3 M solution) = body weight (kg) x base deficit (mEq/L) x 1.1

Metabolic acidosis with cardiac arrest: Adults:
IV: 3.6-10.8 g (111-333 mL); additional amounts may be required to control acidosis after arrest reversed
Open chest: Intraventricular: 2-6 g (62-185 mL). **Note:** Do not inject into cardiac muscle
Acidosis associated with cardiac bypass surgery: Adults: IV: Average dose: 9 mL/kg (2.7 mEq/kg); 500 mL is adequate for most adults; maximum dose: 500 mg/kg over at least 1 hour
Excess acidity of acid citrate dextrose (ACD) blood in cardiac bypass surgery: Adults: 15-77 mL of 0.3 molar solution added to each 500 mL of ACD blood

Dosage adjustment in renal impairment: No dosage adjustment provided in manufacturer's labeling. Tromethamine is substantially excreted by the kidneys; use with caution; monitor ECG and potassium levels.
Dosage adjustment in hepatic impairment: No dosage adjustment provided in manufacturer's labeling.

Additional Information Complete prescribing information should be consulted for additional detail.

Dosage Forms
Solution, Intravenous:
Tham: 30 mEq/100 mL (500 mL)

Tropicamide (troe PIK a mide)

Brand Names: U.S. Mydral; Mydriacyl
Brand Names: Canada Diotrope®; Mydriacyl®
Index Terms Bistropamide
Pharmacologic Category Ophthalmic Agent, Mydriatic
Use Short-acting mydriatic used in diagnostic procedures; as well as preoperatively and postoperatively; treatment of some cases of acute iritis, iridocyclitis, and keratitis
Pregnancy Risk Factor C
Dosage Ophthalmic: Children and Adults (individuals with heavily pigmented eyes may require larger doses):
Cycloplegia: Instill 1-2 drops (1%); may repeat in 5 minutes
Exam must be performed within 30 minutes after the repeat dose; if the patient is not examined within 20-30 minutes, instill an additional drop
Mydriasis: Instill 1-2 drops (0.5%) 15-20 minutes before exam; may repeat every 30 minutes as needed

Dosage adjustment in renal impairment: No dosage adjustment provided in manufacturer's labeling.
Dosage adjustment in hepatic impairment: No dosage adjustment provided in manufacturer's labeling.

Additional Information Complete prescribing information should be consulted for additional detail.

Dosage Forms
Solution, Ophthalmic:
Mydral: 0.5% (15 mL); 1% (15 mL)
Mydriacyl: 1% (3 mL, 15 mL)
Generic: 0.5% (15 mL); 1% (2 mL, 3 mL, 15 mL)

Tropisetron [INT] (troh PI se tron)

International Brand Names Abatoarin (MX); Di Ou Ping (CN); Guang Di (CN); Hensetron (PH); Navoban (AT, AU, BG, BH, CH, CN, EE, EG, FI, GR, HK, HN, ID, IT, JO, KR, LB, MX, MY, NL, NO, NZ, PE, PH, PK, PT, QA, RU, SA, SE, SI, TR, TW, VE, VN, ZA); Novaban (BE); Setrovel (ID)
Index Terms Tropisetron Hydrochloride
Pharmacologic Category Serotonin Antagonist
Reported Use Prevention of nausea and vomiting induced by cytotoxic chemotherapy; treatment and prevention of postoperative nausea/vomiting
Dosage Range Adults:
IV:
Chemotherapy-induced nausea and vomiting: 5 mg before chemotherapy followed by 5 days of oral therapy
Postoperative nausea/vomiting: 2 mg shortly before induction of anesthesia
Oral: Chemotherapy-induced nausea and vomiting: 5 mg/day for 5 days following I.V. dose given on day 1; take in the morning at least 1 hour before meals
Product Availability Product available in various countries; not currently available in the U.S.
Dosage Forms
Capsule: 5 mg
Injection, solution: 1 mg/mL (2 mL, 5 mL)

◆ **Tropisetron Hydrochloride** *see* Tropisetron [INT] *on page 2108*

◆ **Trosec (Can)** *see* Trospium *on page 2108*

Trospium (TROSE pee um)

Brand Names: U.S. Sanctura XR [DSC]; Sanctura [DSC]
Brand Names: Canada Sanctura® XR; Trosec
Index Terms Trospium Chloride
Pharmacologic Category Anticholinergic Agent
Additional Appendix Information
Beers Criteria – Potentially Inappropriate Medications for Geriatrics *on page 2271*
Use Treatment of overactive bladder with symptoms of urgency, incontinence, and urinary frequency
Pregnancy Risk Factor C
Pregnancy Considerations Adverse events were observed in animal studies. There are no adequate or well-controlled studies in pregnant women; use only if clearly needed.
Breast-Feeding Considerations It is not known if trospium is excreted in breast milk. According to the manufacturer, the decision to continue or discontinue breast-feeding during therapy should take into account the risk of exposure to the infant and the benefits of treatment to the mother.
Contraindications Hypersensitivity to trospium or any component of the formulation; urinary retention; gastric retention; uncontrolled narrow-angle glaucoma
Warnings/Precautions Cases of angioedema involving the face, lips, tongue, and/or larynx have been reported. Immediately discontinue if tongue, hypopharynx, or larynx are involved. May cause drowsiness, confusion, dizziness, hallucinations, and/or blurred vision, which may impair physical or mental abilities; patients must be cautioned about performing tasks which require mental alertness (eg, operating machinery or driving). Effects with other sedative drugs or ethanol may be potentiated. May occur in the presence of increased environmental temperature; use caution in hot weather and/or exercise. Use with caution in patients with bladder flow obstruction, may increase the risk of urinary retention. Use with caution in patients with gastrointestinal obstructive disorders (eg, pyloric stenosis); may increase the risk of gastric retention. Use caution in patients with decreased GI motility (eg, myasthenia gravis, ulcerative colitis). Use immediate release formulation with caution in renal dysfunction; dosage adjustment is required. Use of the extended release formulation is contraindicated in patients with severe renal impairment (CrCl <30 mL/minute). Ethanol should not be ingested within 2 hours of the administration of the extended release formulation. Concurrent ethanol use may increase the incidence of drowsiness. Active tubular secretion (ATS) is a route of elimination; use caution with other medications that are eliminated by ATS (eg, procainamide, pancuronium, vancomycin, morphine, metformin, and tenofovir). Use with extreme caution in patients with controlled (treated) narrow-angle glaucoma. Use caution in patients with moderate or severe hepatic dysfunction. Use caution in Alzheimer's patients. Use caution in the elderly (≥65 years of age); increased anticholinergic side effects

are seen. This medication is associated with potent anticholinergic properties which may be inappropriate in older adults depending on comorbidities (eg, dementia, delirium) (Beers Criteria).

Adverse Reactions

Cardiovascular: Tachycardia

Central nervous system: Fatigue, headache

Dermatologic: Skin rash, xeroderma

Gastrointestinal: Abdominal distention, abdominal pain, constipation, dysgeusia, dyspepsia, flatulence, nausea, vomiting, xerostomia

Genitourinary: Urinary retention, urinary tract infection

Infection: Influenza

Ophthalmic: Blurred vision, dry eye syndrome

Respiratory: Dry nose, nasopharyngitis

Rare but important or life-threatening: Anaphylaxis, angioedema, confusion, delirium, drowsiness, fecal impaction, gastritis, hallucination, heat intolerance, hypertensive crisis, inversion T wave on ECG, palpitations, rhabdomyolysis, Stevens-Johnson syndrome, supraventricular tachycardia, syncope, visual disturbance

Drug Interactions

Metabolism/Transport Effects None known.

Avoid Concomitant Use

Avoid concomitant use of Trospium with any of the following: Aclidinium; Glucagon; Ipratropium (Oral Inhalation); Potassium Chloride; Tiotropium; Umeclidinium

Increased Effect/Toxicity

Trospium may increase the levels/effects of: AbobotulinumtoxinA; Analgesics (Opioid); Anticholinergic Agents; Cannabinoid-Containing Products; Glucagon; Mirabegron; OnabotulinumtoxinA; Potassium Chloride; RimabotulinumtoxinB; Thiazide Diuretics; Tiotropium; Topiramate

The levels/effects of Trospium may be increased by: Aclidinium; Alcohol (Ethyl); Ipratropium (Oral Inhalation); Mianserin; Pramlintide; Umeclidinium

Decreased Effect

Trospium may decrease the levels/effects of: Acetylcholinesterase Inhibitors; Itopride; Secretin

The levels/effects of Trospium may be decreased by: Acetylcholinesterase Inhibitors; MetFORMIN

Food Interactions

Ethanol: Ethanol may increase the peak (maximum) serum concentration of trospium when consumed within 2 hours of taking extended release trospium. Management: Avoid consuming any alcohol within 2 hours of taking a dose of extended release trospium.

Food: Administration with a fatty meal reduces the absorption and bioavailability of trospium. Management: Administer 1 hour prior to meals or an empty stomach. Administer extended release capsules in the morning with a full glass of water.

Storage/Stability Store at 20°C to 25°C (68°F to 77°F); excursions permitted between 15°C to 30°C (59°F to 86°F).

Mechanism of Action Trospium antagonizes the effects of acetylcholine on muscarinic receptors in cholinergically innervated organs. It reduces the smooth muscle tone of the bladder.

Pharmacodynamics/Kinetics

Absorption: <10%; decreased with a high-fat meal

Distribution: V_d: 395 - >600 L, primarily in plasma

Protein binding: 48% to 85% *in vitro*

Metabolism: Hypothesized to be via esterase hydrolysis and conjugation; forms metabolites

Bioavailability: Immediate release formulation: ~10% (range: 4% to 16%)

Half-life elimination: Immediate release formulation: 20 hours

Severe renal insufficiency (CrCl <30 mL/minute): ~33 hours; extended release formulation: ~35 hours

Time to peak, plasma: 5-6 hours

Excretion: Feces (85%); urine (~6%; mostly as unchanged drug) primarily via active tubular secretion

Dosage Oral:

Adults:

Immediate release: 20 mg twice daily

Extended release: 60 mg once daily

Elderly ≥75 years: Immediate release: Consider initial dose of 20 mg once daily (based on tolerability); Extended release: Refer to adult dosing.

Dosage adjustment in renal impairment:

CrCl ≥30 mL/minute: No dosage adjustment provided in manufacturer's labeling. However, renal impairment increases systemic exposure to trospium. Monitor for increased adverse effects.

CrCl <30 mL/minute:

Immediate release: 20 mg once daily at bedtime

Extended release: Use not recommended

Dosage adjustment in hepatic impairment:

Mild impairment: No dosage adjustment provided in manufacturer's labeling.

Moderate to severe impairment: No dosage adjustment provided in manufacturer's labeling; use with caution.

Dietary Considerations Take1 hour prior to meals or on an empty stomach.

Administration Administer 1 hour prior to meals or on an empty stomach. Administer extended release capsules in the morning with a full glass of water.

Dosage Forms

Capsule Extended Release 24 Hour, Oral:

Generic: 60 mg

Tablet, Oral:

Generic: 20 mg

- ◆ **Trospium Chloride** *see* Trospium *on page 2108*
- ◆ **Trulicity** *see* Dulaglutide *on page 697*
- ◆ **Trusopt** *see* Dorzolamide *on page 673*
- ◆ **Trusopt® (Can)** *see* Dorzolamide *on page 673*
- ◆ **Truvada** *see* Emtricitabine and Tenofovir *on page 721*

Trypsin, Balsam Peru, and Castor Oil

(TRIP sin, BAL sam pe RUE, & KAS tor oyl)

Brand Names: U.S. Granulex®; TBC; Vasolex™; Xenaderm®

Index Terms Balsam Peru, Castor Oil, and Trypsin; Castor Oil, Trypsin, and Balsam Peru

Pharmacologic Category Protectant, Topical

Use

Granulex®: Treatment of decubitus ulcers, varicose ulcers, debridement of eschar, dehiscent wounds and sunburn; promote wound healing; reduce odor from necrotic wounds

Vasolex™, Xenaderm ®: Treatment of decubitus ulcers, varicose ulcers, and dehiscent wounds; promote wound healing; reduce odor from necrotic wounds

Dosage Topical: Apply a minimum of twice daily or as often as necessary

Additional Information Complete prescribing information should be consulted for additional detail.

Dosage Forms

Aerosol, spray, topical:

Granulex®: Trypsin 0.12 mg, balsam Peru 87 mg, and castor oil 788 mg per gram (60 g, 120 g)

TBC: Trypsin 0.1 mg, balsam Peru 72.5 mg, and castor oil 650 mg per 0.82 mL (60 g, 120 g)

Ointment, topical:
Vasolex™: Trypsin 90 USP units, balsam Peru 87 mg, and castor oil 788 mg per gram (5 g, 30 g, 60 g)
Xenaderm®: Trypsin 90 USP units, balsam Peru 87 mg, and castor oil 788 mg per gram (30 g, 60 g)

- **Tryptoreline** *see* Triptorelin *on page 2107*
- **TSH** *see* Thyrotropin Alfa *on page 2031*
- **TSPA** *see* Thiotepa *on page 2030*
- **TST** *see* Tuberculin Tests *on page 2110*
- **TT** *see* Tetanus Toxoid (Adsorbed) *on page 2016*
- **Tuberculin Purified Protein Derivative** *see* Tuberculin Tests *on page 2110*
- **Tuberculin Skin Test** *see* Tuberculin Tests *on page 2110*

Tuberculin Tests (too BER kyoo lin tests)

Brand Names: U.S. Aplisol; Tubersol
Index Terms Mantoux; PPD; TB Skin Test; TST; Tuberculin Purified Protein Derivative; Tuberculin Skin Test
Pharmacologic Category Diagnostic Agent
Use Skin test in diagnosis of tuberculosis
Pregnancy Risk Factor C
Dosage Children and Adults: Intradermal: 0.1 mL

TST interpretation: Criteria for positive TST read at 48-72 hours (see Note below for healthcare workers):
Induration ≥5 mm: Persons with HIV infection (or risk factors for HIV infection, but unknown status), recent close contact to person with known active TB, persons with chest x-ray consistent with healed TB, persons who are immunosuppressed
Induration ≥10 mm: Persons with clinical conditions which increase risk of TB infection, recent immigrants, IV drug users, residents and employees of high-risk settings, children <4 years of age
Induration ≥15 mm: Persons who do not meet any of the above criteria (no risk factors for TB)
Note: A two-step test is recommended when testing will be performed at regular intervals (eg, for healthcare workers). If the first test is negative, a second TST should be administered 1-3 weeks after the first test was read.

TST interpretation (CDC guidelines) in a healthcare setting:
Baseline test: ≥10 mm is positive (either first or second step)
Serial testing without known exposure: Increase of ≥10 mm is positive
Known exposure:
≥5 mm is positive in patients with baseline of 0 mm
≥10 mm is positive in patients with negative baseline or previous screening result of ≥0 mm
Read test at 48-72 hours following placement. Test results with 0 mm induration or measured induration less than the defined cutoff point are considered to signify absence of infection with *M. tuberculosis*. Test results should be documented in millimeters even if classified as negative. Erythema and redness of skin are not indicative of a positive test result.

Additional Information Complete prescribing information should be consulted for additional detail.

Dosage Forms
Solution, Intradermal:
Aplisol: 5 units/0.1 mL (1 mL, 5 mL)
Tubersol: 5 units/0.1 mL (1 mL, 5 mL)

- **Tubersol** *see* Tuberculin Tests *on page 2110*
- **Tums [OTC]** *see* Calcium Carbonate *on page 327*
- **Tums Chews Extra Strength (Can)** *see* Calcium Carbonate *on page 327*
- **Tums E-X 750 [OTC]** *see* Calcium Carbonate *on page 327*
- **Tums Extra Strength (Can)** *see* Calcium Carbonate *on page 327*
- **Tums Freshers [OTC]** *see* Calcium Carbonate *on page 327*
- **Tums Kids [OTC]** *see* Calcium Carbonate *on page 327*
- **Tums Lasting Effects [OTC]** *see* Calcium Carbonate *on page 327*
- **Tums Regular Strength (Can)** *see* Calcium Carbonate *on page 327*
- **Tums Smoothies (Can)** *see* Calcium Carbonate *on page 327*
- **Tums Ultra 1000 [OTC]** *see* Calcium Carbonate *on page 327*
- **Tums Ultra Strength (Can)** *see* Calcium Carbonate *on page 327*
- **Tusnel [OTC]** *see* Guaifenesin, Pseudoephedrine, and Dextromethorphan *on page 989*
- **Tusnel-DM Pediatric [OTC]** *see* Guaifenesin, Pseudoephedrine, and Dextromethorphan *on page 989*
- **Tusnel Pediatric [OTC]** *see* Guaifenesin, Pseudoephedrine, and Dextromethorphan *on page 989*
- **Tusscough DHC [DSC]** *see* Dihydrocodeine, Chlorpheniramine, and Phenylephrine *on page 633*
- **TussiCaps** *see* Hydrocodone and Chlorpheniramine *on page 1012*
- **Tussigon** *see* Hydrocodone and Homatropine *on page 1013*
- **Tussin [OTC]** *see* GuaiFENesin *on page 986*
- **Tussionex** *see* Hydrocodone and Chlorpheniramine *on page 1012*
- **Tussionex Pennkinetic** *see* Hydrocodone and Chlorpheniramine *on page 1012*
- **TVP-1012** *see* Rasagiline *on page 1781*
- **Twinject (Can)** *see* EPINEPHrine (Systemic, Oral Inhalation) *on page 735*
- **Twinrix®** *see* Hepatitis A and Hepatitis B Recombinant Vaccine *on page 1000*
- **Twinrix® Junior (Can)** *see* Hepatitis A and Hepatitis B Recombinant Vaccine *on page 1000*
- **Twynsta** *see* Telmisartan and Amlodipine *on page 1989*
- **Ty21a Vaccine** *see* Typhoid Vaccine *on page 2112*
- **Tybost** *see* Cobicistat *on page 495*
- **Tygacil** *see* Tigecycline *on page 2040*
- **Tykerb** *see* Lapatinib *on page 1169*
- **Tylenol [OTC]** *see* Acetaminophen *on page 32*
- **Tylenol (Can)** *see* Acetaminophen *on page 32*
- **Tylenol #2** *see* Acetaminophen and Codeine *on page 36*
- **Tylenol #3** *see* Acetaminophen and Codeine *on page 36*
- **Tylenol 8 Hour [OTC]** *see* Acetaminophen *on page 32*
- **Tylenol Arthritis Pain [OTC]** *see* Acetaminophen *on page 32*
- **Tylenol Children's [OTC]** *see* Acetaminophen *on page 32*
- **Tylenol Children's Meltaways [OTC]** *see* Acetaminophen *on page 32*
- **Tylenol Codeine** *see* Acetaminophen and Codeine *on page 36*
- **Tylenol Elixir with Codeine (Can)** *see* Acetaminophen and Codeine *on page 36*
- **Tylenol Extra Strength [OTC]** *see* Acetaminophen *on page 32*

- ◆ **Tylenol Jr. Meltaways [OTC]** *see* Acetaminophen *on page 32*
- ◆ **Tylenol No. 1 (Can)** *see* Acetaminophen and Codeine *on page 36*
- ◆ **Tylenol No. 1 Forte (Can)** *see* Acetaminophen and Codeine *on page 36*
- ◆ **Tylenol No. 2 with Codeine (Can)** *see* Acetaminophen and Codeine *on page 36*
- ◆ **Tylenol No. 3 with Codeine (Can)** *see* Acetaminophen and Codeine *on page 36*
- ◆ **Tylenol No. 4 with Codeine (Can)** *see* Acetaminophen and Codeine *on page 36*
- ◆ **Tylenol® PM [OTC]** *see* Acetaminophen and Diphenhydramine *on page 36*
- ◆ **Tylenol® Severe Allergy [OTC]** *see* Acetaminophen and Diphenhydramine *on page 36*
- ◆ **Tylenol® with Codeine No. 3** *see* Acetaminophen and Codeine *on page 36*
- ◆ **Tylenol® with Codeine No. 4** *see* Acetaminophen and Codeine *on page 36*
- ◆ **Tylox** *see* Oxycodone and Acetaminophen *on page 1541*
- ◆ **Typh-1** *see* Typhoid and Hepatitis A Vaccine [CAN/INT] *on page 2111*
- ◆ **Typherix (Can)** *see* Typhoid Vaccine *on page 2112*
- ◆ **Typhim Vi** *see* Typhoid Vaccine *on page 2112*

Typhoid and Hepatitis A Vaccine [CAN/INT] (TYE foid & hep a TYE tis aye vak SEEN)

Brand Names: Canada ViVAXIM®

Index Terms HA; Hepatitis A and Typhoid Vaccine; Typh-1

Pharmacologic Category Vaccine, Inactivated (Bacterial); Vaccine, Inactivated (Viral)

Additional Appendix Information

Immunization Administration Recommendations *on page 2250*

Immunization Recommendations *on page 2255*

Use Note: Not approved in U.S.

Active immunization against typhoid fever caused by *Salmonella typhi* and against disease caused by hepatitis A virus (HAV)

National Advisory Committee on Immunizations (NACI) does not recommend use for routine vaccination but does recommend that immunization be considered in the following groups:

- Travelers to areas with a prolonged risk (>4 weeks) of exposure to *S. typhi* or travelers to areas with endemic hepatitis A
- Persons with intimate exposure to a *S. typhi* carrier or who are residing in communities with high endemic rates of hepatitis A virus or at risk of outbreaks
- Laboratory technicians with frequent exposure to *S. typhi* or individuals involved in hepatitis A research or production of hepatitis A vaccine
- Travelers with achlorhydria or hypochlorhydria
- Military personnel, relief workers, or others relocated to areas with high rates of hepatitis A infection
- Persons with lifestyle risks for hepatitis A infection (eg, drug abusers, homosexual men), chronic liver disease, receiving hepatotoxic medication or with disease(s) which may necessitate use of hepatotoxic medications
- Persons with hemophilia A or B treated with plasma-derived clotting factors
- Zookeepers, veterinarians, and researchers who handle nonhuman primates

Pregnancy Considerations Reproduction studies have not been conducted. The Canadian labeling does not recommend use in pregnant women. Although the safety of vaccination during pregnancy has not been determined, the theoretical risk to the infant is expected to be low. Inactivated vaccines have not been shown to cause increased risks to the fetus (Canadian NACI, 2006; CDC, 2011).

Breast-Feeding Considerations Inactivated vaccines do not affect the safety of breast-feeding for the mother or the infant. Breast-feeding infants should be vaccinated according to the recommended schedules (Canadian NACI, 2006; CDC, 2011).

Contraindications Hypersensitivity to typhoid vaccine, hepatitis A vaccine or any component of the formulation

Warnings/Precautions Immediate treatment (including epinephrine 1:1000) for anaphylactoid and/or hypersensitivity reactions should be available during vaccine use. Defer administration in patients with acute or febrile illness; may administer to patients with mild acute illness with low-grade fever. Use with caution in patients with a history of bleeding disorders (including thrombocytopenia) and/or patients on anticoagulant therapy; bleeding/hematoma may occur from IM administration. Syncope has been reported with use of injectable vaccines and may be accompanied by transient visual disturbances, weakness, or tonic-clonic movements. Procedures should be in place to avoid injuries from falling and to restore cerebral perfusion if syncope occurs.

Vaccination may not result in effective immunity in all patients. Response depends upon multiple factors (eg, type of vaccine, age of patient) and is improved by administering the vaccine at the recommended dose, route, and interval. Vaccines may not be effective if administered during periods of altered immune competence (CDC, 2011). Due to the long incubation period for hepatitis, unrecognized hepatitis A infection may be present at time of vaccination; immunization may not prevent infection in these patients. Patients with chronic liver disease may have decreased antibody response. Should not be used to treat typhoid fever. Not all recipients of typhoid vaccine will be fully protected against typhoid fever. Travelers should take all necessary precautions to avoid contact or ingestion of potentially contaminated food or water sources.

Simultaneous administration of other vaccines at different injection sites is not likely to affect immune response. Hepatitis A seroconversion rates are not lower with simultaneous administration of immune globulins (at separate sites) however hepatitis A antibody titers may be lower. The NACI recommends simultaneous administration of all age-appropriate vaccines for which a person is eligible at a single clinic visit, unless contraindications exist.

Use with caution in severely immunocompromised patients (eg, patients receiving chemo/radiation therapy or other immunosuppressive therapy (including high dose corticosteroids); may have a reduced response to vaccination. If appropriate, consider delaying administration until after completion of immunosuppressive therapy. In general, household and close contacts of persons with altered immunocompetence may receive all age appropriate vaccines; inactivated vaccines should be administered ≥2 weeks prior to planned immunosuppression when feasible (Rubin, 2014).

Some dosage forms may contain polysorbate 80 (also known as Tweens). Hypersensitivity reactions, usually a delayed reaction, have been reported following exposure to pharmaceutical products containing polysorbate 80 in certain individuals (Isaksson, 2002; Lucente 2000; Shelley, 1995). Thrombocytopenia, ascites, pulmonary deterioration, and renal and hepatic failure have been reported in ▶

premature neonates after receiving parenteral products containing polysorbate 80 (Alade, 1986; CDC, 1984). See manufacturer's labeling. Formulation may contain neomycin.

Adverse Reactions In Canada, adverse reactions may be reported to local provincial/territorial health agencies or to the Vaccine Safety Section at Public Health Agency of Canada (1-866-844-0018).

Central nervous system: Dizziness, fever, headache, malaise

Gastrointestinal: Diarrhea, nausea

Local: Injection site: Erythema, induration/edema, pain

Neuromuscular & skeletal: Myalgia, weakness

Rare but important or life-threatening (reported with ViVAXIM®): Arthralgia, pruritus, rash

Drug Interactions

Metabolism/Transport Effects None known.

Avoid Concomitant Use There are no known interactions where it is recommended to avoid concomitant use.

Increased Effect/Toxicity There are no known significant interactions involving an increase in effect.

Decreased Effect

The levels/effects of Typhoid and Hepatitis A Vaccine may be decreased by: Belimumab; Immunosuppressants

Storage/Stability Store between 2°C to 8°C (35°F to 46°F); do not freeze. Discard if frozen. Administer vaccine immediately after mixing.

Mechanism of Action Provides active immunization against typhoid fever through production of antibodies (predominantly IgG) and against hepatitis A infection through production of antihepatitis A virus antibodies.

Pharmacodynamics/Kinetics

Onset: Seroprotection rate at 14 days: Hepatitis A: ~96%, typhoid: ~89%; Seroprotection at 28 days: Hepatitis A: ~100%, typhoid: ~90%

Duration: Kinetic models suggest antihepatitis A antibodies may persist ≥20 years (NACI, 2006); Typhoid: 3 years

Dosage IM: Children ≥16 years, Adults, and Elderly:

Immunization: 1 mL single dose at least 2 weeks prior to expected exposure

Booster: May administer 1 mL booster dose 3 years after previous dose in individuals requiring a booster dose

Administration Mix vaccine components immediately before administration according to manufacturer labeling instructions. Shake well until white, cloudy suspension is achieved. **Do not administer intravascularly or intradermally.** Intramuscular administration into deltoid muscle is preferred. Do not administer to gluteal region. May consider subcutaneous administration in individuals at risk of hemorrhage (eg, thrombocytopenia, hemophilia). Subcutaneous administration may be associated with greater risk of injection site reactions. **Note:** For patients at risk of hemorrhage following intramuscular injection, the NACI recommends weighing the benefits and risks of intramuscular vaccination. If the patient receives antihemophilia or other similar therapy, intramuscular vaccination can be scheduled shortly after such therapy is administered. A fine needle can be used for the vaccination and firm pressure applied to the site (without rubbing) for at least 5 minutes. Patients on low-dose aspirin or long-term anticoagulant therapy (warfarin, heparin) are not considered to be at greater risk of complications and should receive scheduled vaccinations (NACI, 2006).

Simultaneous administration of vaccines helps ensure patients will be fully vaccinated by the appropriate age. Simultaneous administration of vaccines is defined as administering >1 vaccine on the same day at different anatomic sites. Antipyretics have not been shown to prevent febrile seizures. Antipyretics may be used to treat fever or discomfort following vaccination (CDC, 2011). One study reported that routine prophylactic administration of acetaminophen to prevent fever prior to vaccination decreased the immune response of some vaccines; the clinical significance of this reduction in immune response has not been established (Prymula, 2009).

Monitoring Parameters Monitor for syncope for 15 minutes following administration. If seizure-like activity associated with syncope occurs, maintain patient in supine or Trendelenburg position to reestablish adequate cerebral perfusion.

Additional Information Name of medication, date of administration, the vaccine manufacturer, lot number of vaccine, should be entered into the patient's permanent medical record.

Product Availability Not available in the U.S.

Dosage Forms: Canada

Injection, solution:

ViVAXIM®: Purified Vi capsular polysaccharide 25 mcg and hepatitis A virus 160 antigen units per 1 mL [contains polysorbate 80 and neomycin]

Typhoid Vaccine (TYE foid vak SEEN)

Brand Names: U.S. Typhim Vi; Vivotif

Brand Names: Canada Typherix; Typhim Vi; Vivotif

Index Terms Ty21a Vaccine; Typhoid Vaccine Live Oral Ty21a; Vi Vaccine; ViCPS

Pharmacologic Category Vaccine, Inactivated (Bacterial); Vaccine, Live (Bacterial)

Additional Appendix Information

Immunization Administration Recommendations *on page 2250*

Immunization Recommendations *on page 2255*

Use Active immunization against typhoid fever caused by *Salmonella typhi*:

Oral: Immunization of adults and children >6 years of age; complete the vaccine regimen at least 1 week before potential exposure to typhoid bacteria.

Canadian labeling: Approved for use in patients ≥5 years of age.

Parenteral: Immunization of adults and children ≥2 years of age; complete the vaccine regimen at least 2 weeks before potential exposure to typhoid bacteria.

Not for routine vaccination. In the United States and Canada, use should be limited to:

- Travelers to areas with a recognized risk of exposure to *S. typhi*
- Persons with intimate exposure to a household contact with *S. typhi* fever or a known carrier
- Laboratory technicians with frequent exposure to *S. typhi*

Additional Canadian recommendations: May consider administration to travelers with achlorhydria, hypochlorhydria, or receiving acid suppression therapy; anatomic or functional asplenia (Canadian Immunization Guide)

Pregnancy Risk Factor C

Dosage Immunization:

Oral: Children ≥6 years (U.S. labeling) or ≥5 years (Canadian labeling), Adolescents, and Adults:

Primary immunization: One capsule on alternate days (day 1, 3, 5, and 7) for a total of 4 doses; all doses should be complete at least 1 week prior to potential exposure

Reimmunization (with repeated or continued exposure to typhoid fever):

U.S. labeling: Repeat full course of primary immunization every 5 years

Canadian labeling: Repeat full course of primary immunization every 7 years

IM: Children ≥2 years, Adolescents, and Adults: 0.5 mL given at least 2 weeks prior to expected exposure

Reimmunization (with repeated or continued exposure to typhoid fever):

Typhim Vi: 0.5 mL every 2 years

Typherix (Canadian labeling; not available in U.S.): 0.5 mL every 3 years

Dosage adjustment in renal impairment: There are no dosage adjustments provided in manufacturer's labeling.

Dosage adjustment in hepatic impairment: There are no dosage adjustments provided in manufacturer's labeling.

Additional Information Complete prescribing information should be consulted for additional detail.

Dosage Forms

Capsule, enteric coated:

Vivotif: Viable *S. typhi* Ty21a 2-6.8 x 10^9 colony-forming units and nonviable *S. typhi* Ty21a 5-50 x 10^9 bacterial cells [contains lactose 100-180 mg/capsule and sucrose 26-130 mg/capsule]

Injection, solution:

Typhim Vi: Purified Vi capsular polysaccharide 25 mcg/0.5 mL (0.5 mL, 10 mL) [derived from *S. typhi* Ty2 strain]

Dosage Forms: Canada

Injection, solution:

Typherix: Vi capsular polysaccharide 25 mcg/0.5 mL (0.5 mL) [derived from *S. typhi* Ty2 strain]

- ◆ **Typhoid Vaccine Live Oral Ty21a** *see* Typhoid Vaccine *on page 2112*
- ◆ **Tysabri** *see* Natalizumab *on page 1432*
- ◆ **Tyvaso** *see* Treprostinil *on page 2093*
- ◆ **Tyvaso Refill** *see* Treprostinil *on page 2093*
- ◆ **Tyvaso Starter** *see* Treprostinil *on page 2093*
- ◆ **506U78** *see* Nelarabine *on page 1435*
- ◆ **U-90152S** *see* Delavirdine *on page 587*
- ◆ **UCB-P071** *see* Cetirizine *on page 411*
- ◆ **Uceris** *see* Budesonide (Systemic) *on page 293*
- ◆ **U-Cort** *see* Urea and Hydrocortisone *on page 2115*
- ◆ **UK-88,525** *see* Darifenacin *on page 568*
- ◆ **UK-427,857** *see* Maraviroc *on page 1272*
- ◆ **UK92480** *see* Sildenafil *on page 1882*
- ◆ **UK109496** *see* Voriconazole *on page 2176*
- ◆ **U-Kera E** *see* Urea *on page 2114*
- ◆ **Ulcidine (Can)** *see* Famotidine *on page 845*
- ◆ **Ulesfia** *see* Benzyl Alcohol *on page 250*

Ulipristal (ue li PRIS tal)

Brand Names: U.S. Ella

Brand Names: Canada Fibristal

Index Terms CDB-2914; Ulipristal Acetate

Pharmacologic Category Contraceptive; Progestin Receptor Modulator

Use

Emergency contraceptive (Ella): Prevention of pregnancy following unprotected intercourse or a known or suspected contraceptive failure. Ulipristal is not intended for routine use as a contraceptive.

Uterine fibroids (Fibristal [Canadian product]): Treatment of moderate-to-severe signs/symptoms of uterine fibroids in premenopausal adult women eligible for surgery. **Note:** Treatment is limited to 3 months.

Pregnancy Risk Factor X

Dosage

Emergency contraception (Ella): Oral:

Children and Adolescents (prepubertal): Not indicated for use prior to menarche

Adolescents (postpubertal) and Adults: 30 mg as soon as possible, but within 120 hours (5 days) of unprotected intercourse or contraceptive failure

Treatment of moderate to severe signs/symptoms of uterine fibroids (Fibristal [Canadian product]): Oral: Adults: Females (premenopausal): 5 mg daily for 3 consecutive months. **Note:** Treatment is limited to 3 months.

Note: Not indicated for use in postmenopausal women.

Dosage adjustment in renal impairment:

U.S. labeling (Ella): There are no dosage adjustments provided in the manufacturer's labeling (has not been studied).

Canadian labeling (Fibristal): Use is not recommended in moderate-to-severe renal impairment unless patient is monitored closely.

Dosage adjustment in hepatic impairment:

U.S. labeling (Ella): There are no dosage adjustments provided in the manufacturer's labeling (has not been studied).

Canadian labeling (Fibristal): Use is not recommended in hepatic impairment unless patient is monitored closely.

Additional Information Complete prescribing information should be consulted for additional detail.

Dosage Forms

Tablet, Oral:

Ella: 30 mg

Dosage Forms: Canada

Tablet, Oral:

Fibristal: 5 mg

- ◆ **Ulipristal Acetate** *see* Ulipristal *on page 2113*
- ◆ **Uloric** *see* Febuxostat *on page 848*
- ◆ **Ultibro Breezhaler (Can)** *see* Indacaterol and Glycopyrronium [CAN/INT] *on page 1063*
- ◆ **Ultiva** *see* Remifentanil *on page 1789*
- ◆ **Ultiva® (Can)** *see* Remifentanil *on page 1789*
- ◆ **Ultracet®** *see* Acetaminophen and Tramadol *on page 37*
- ◆ **Ultram** *see* TraMADol *on page 2074*
- ◆ **Ultram ER** *see* TraMADol *on page 2074*
- ◆ **Ultra Mide 25 [OTC]** *see* Urea *on page 2114*
- ◆ **Ultraquin™ (Can)** *see* Hydroquinone *on page 1020*
- ◆ **Ultrase (Can)** *see* Pancrelipase *on page 1566*
- ◆ **Ultrase MT (Can)** *see* Pancrelipase *on page 1566*
- ◆ **Ultravate** *see* Halobetasol *on page 993*
- ◆ **Ultravate® (Can)** *see* Halobetasol *on page 993*
- ◆ **Ultresa** *see* Pancrelipase *on page 1566*

Umeclidinium (ue me kli DIN ee um)

Brand Names: U.S. Incruse Ellipta

Index Terms Umeclidinium Bromide

Pharmacologic Category Anticholinergic Agent; Anticholinergic Agent, Long-Acting

Use Chronic obstructive pulmonary disease: Maintenance treatment of airflow obstruction in patients with chronic obstructive pulmonary disease (COPD), including chronic bronchitis and/or emphysema

Pregnancy Risk Factor C

Pregnancy Considerations Adverse events were not observed in animal reproduction studies. Systemic absorption following oral inhalation in negligible.

Breast-Feeding Considerations It is not known if umeclidinium is excreted into breast milk; however, systemic absorption following oral inhalation in negligible. The manufacturer recommends a decision be made whether to discontinue nursing or to discontinue the drug, taking into account the importance of treatment to the mother.

Contraindications Hypersensitivity to umeclidinium or any component of the formulation; severe hypersensitivity to milk proteins

Warnings/Precautions Do not use for acute episodes of chronic obstructive pulmonary disease (COPD). Do not initiate in patients with significantly worsening or acutely deteriorating COPD. Do not increase the daily dose beyond the recommended dose. Paradoxical bronchospasm may occur with the use of inhaled agents, which may be life threatening; discontinue use immediately and consider other therapy if bronchospasm occurs. May worsen the symptoms of narrow angle glaucoma, prostatic hyperplasia, and/or bladder neck obstruction; use with caution. Hypersensitivity reactions, including anaphylaxis, may occur. Powder for oral inhalation contains lactose; use is contraindicated in patients with severe milk protein allergy.

Adverse Reactions

Cardiovascular: Tachycardia

Gastrointestinal: Toothache, upper abdominal pain

Hematologic & oncologic: Bruise

Neuromuscular & skeletal: Arthralgia, myalgia

Respiratory: Cough, nasopharyngitis, pharyngitis, upper respiratory tract infection, viral upper respiratory tract infection

Rare but important or life-threatening: Atrial fibrillation

Drug Interactions

Metabolism/Transport Effects Substrate of CYP2D6 (minor), P-glycoprotein; **Note:** Assignment of Major/Minor substrate status based on clinically relevant drug interaction potential

Avoid Concomitant Use

Avoid concomitant use of Umeclidinium with any of the following: Aclidinium; Anticholinergic Agents; Glucagon; Ipratropium (Oral Inhalation); Potassium Chloride; Tiotropium

Increased Effect/Toxicity

Umeclidinium may increase the levels/effects of: AbobotulinumtoxinA; Analgesics (Opioid); Anticholinergic Agents; Cannabinoid-Containing Products; Glucagon; Mirabegron; OnabotulinumtoxinA; Potassium Chloride; RimabotulinumtoxinB; Thiazide Diuretics; Tiotropium; Topiramate

The levels/effects of Umeclidinium may be increased by: Aclidinium; Ipratropium (Oral Inhalation); Mianserin; Pramlintide

Decreased Effect

Umeclidinium may decrease the levels/effects of: Acetylcholinesterase Inhibitors; Itopride; Secretin

The levels/effects of Umeclidinium may be decreased by: Acetylcholinesterase Inhibitors

Storage/Stability Store between 68°F and 77°F (20°C and 25°C); excursions are permitted between 59°F and 86°F (15°C and 30°C). Protect from moisture, heat or sunlight. Remove inhaler from tray immediately prior to initial use. Discard inhaler 6 weeks after opening the foil tray or after the labeled number of inhalations have reached zero, whichever comes first.

Mechanism of Action Competitively and reversibly inhibits the action of acetylcholine at type 3 muscarinic (M_3) receptors in bronchial smooth muscle causing bronchodilation.

Pharmacodynamics/Kinetics

Absorption: Lung; minimum contribution from oral absorption

Distribution: V_d: 86 L (following IV administration)

Protein binding: ~89%

Metabolism: Hepatic via CYP2D6 and is a substrate for the P-glycoprotein (P-gp) transporter.

Half-life elimination: 11 hours

Time to peak: 5 to 15 minutes

Excretion: Urine <1%; feces 92% (following oral administration)

Dosage Oral inhalation: Chronic obstructive pulmonary disease (COPD): Adults: One inhalation (62.5 mcg) once daily; maximum dose: 1 inhalation (62.5 mcg) once daily

Dosage adjustment in renal impairment: No dosage adjustment necessary.

Dosage adjustment in hepatic impairment:

Mild to moderate hepatic impairment: No dosage adjustment necessary.

Severe hepatic impairment: There are no dosage adjustments provided in the manufacturer's labeling (has not been studied).

Administration Administer via oral inhalation once daily at the same time each day; do not use more than 1 inhalation every 24 hours. Do not shake inhaler. Remove from sealed pouch immediately prior to first use. Slide cover of mouthpiece down until a "click" is heard. Prior to inhaling the dose, exhale fully (do not exhale into the inhaler); close lips tightly around the inhaler mouthpiece and inhale (rapidly, steadily, and deeply); do not breathe through nose or block air vent with fingers. Remove inhaler and hold breath for a few seconds then breathe out slowly and gently. Only open inhaler cover when ready for administration; opening and closing the cover without inhaling the medicine will cause a dose to be lost (the lost dose will be securely held inside the inhaler, but it will no longer be available to be inhaled). Do not close inhaler cover until medication has been inhaled.

Monitoring Parameters FEV_1, peak flow, and/or other pulmonary function tests; signs and symptoms of narrow angle glaucoma and urinary retention

Dosage Forms

Aerosol Powder Breath Activated, Inhalation:

Incruse Ellipta: 62.5 mcg/inhalation (7 ea, 30 ea)

- **Umeclidinium Bromide** *see* Umeclidinium *on page 2113*
- **Umecta** *see* Urea *on page 2114*
- **Umecta Mousse** *see* Urea *on page 2114*
- **Umecta Nail Film** *see* Urea *on page 2114*
- **Umecta PD** *see* Urea *on page 2114*
- **Unasyn** *see* Ampicillin and Sulbactam *on page 145*
- **Unidet® (Can)** *see* Tolterodine *on page 2063*
- **Uniphyl (Can)** *see* Theophylline *on page 2026*
- **Uniretic®** *see* Moexipril and Hydrochlorothiazide *on page 1388*
- **Unithroid** *see* Levothyroxine *on page 1205*
- **Unithroid Direct** *see* Levothyroxine *on page 1205*
- **Univasc [DSC]** *see* Moexipril *on page 1388*
- **UniVert** *see* Meclizine *on page 1277*
- **Unna's Boot** *see* Zinc Gelatin *on page 2200*
- **Unna's Paste** *see* Zinc Gelatin *on page 2200*
- **Uramaxin** *see* Urea *on page 2114*
- **Uramaxin GT** *see* Urea *on page 2114*
- **Urasal® (Can)** *see* Methenamine *on page 1317*
- **Urate Oxidase** *see* Rasburicase *on page 1783*
- **Urate Oxidase, Pegylated** *see* Pegloticase *on page 1602*

Urea (yoor EE a)

Brand Names: U.S. Aluvea; Aquaphilic/Carbamide [OTC]; Atrac-Tain [OTC]; Beta Care Betamide [OTC]; Carb-O-Lac HP [OTC]; Carb-O-Lac5 [OTC]; Carb-O-Philic/20 [OTC]; Carb-O-Philic/40; Carmol 10 [OTC]; Carmol 20 [OTC]; Carmol [OTC]; CEM-Urea; Cerovel; Dermal Therapy Finger Care [OTC]; Dermasorb XM; DPM [OTC]; Gordons Urea; Gordons Urea [OTC]; Gormel 10 [OTC]; Gormel [OTC]; Hydro 35; Hydro 40; Kerafoam; Kerafoam 42;

Keralac; Lanaphilic/Urea [OTC]; Latrix XM; Mycocide CX Callus Exfoliator [OTC]; Nutraplus [OTC]; Rea Lo 39; Rea Lo 40; Rea-Lo [OTC]; Remeven; U-Kera E; Ultra Mide 25 [OTC]; Umecta; Umecta Mousse; Umecta Nail Film; Umecta PD; Uramaxin; Uramaxin GT; Urea Hydrating; Urea Nail; Urea-C40; Ureacin-10 [OTC]; Ureacin-20 [OTC]; Utopic; X-Viate

Index Terms Carbamide

Pharmacologic Category Keratolytic Agent; Topical Skin Product

Use Hyperkeratotic conditions: Debridement and promotion of normal healing of hyperkeratotic surface lesions, particularly where healing is retarded by local infection, necrotic tissue, fibrinous or purulent debris, or eschar; treatment of hyperkeratotic conditions, such as dry, rough skin; skin cracks and fissures; dermatitis; psoriasis; xerosis; ichthyosis; eczema; keratosis; keratoderma; corns and calluses; damaged, ingrown, and devitalized nails.

Pregnancy Risk Factor B/C (manufacturer specific)

Dosage Hyperkeratotic conditions: Adults: Topical: Apply 1-3 times daily

Additional Information Complete prescribing information should be consulted for additional detail.

Dosage Forms

Cream, External:

Aluvea: 39% (227 g)
Atrac-Tain [OTC]: 10% (2 g, 57 g, 142 g)
Carb-O-Lac5 [OTC]: Urea 20% and Ammonium Lactate 10% (236 g)
Carb-O-Lac HP [OTC]: Urea 20% and Ammonium Lactate 10% (277 g)
Carb-O-Philic/20 [OTC]: 20% (85 g)
Carb-O-Philic/40: 40% (85 g, 200 g)
Carmol 20 [OTC]: 20% (85 g)
DPM [OTC]: (170 g)
Gormel [OTC]: 20% (75 g, 120 g, 480 g, 2400 g)
Keralac: 47% (142 g)
Mycocide CX Callus Exfoliator [OTC]: 12% (100 mL)
Nutraplus [OTC]: 10% (85 g, 453 g)
Rea Lo 39: 39% (227 g)
Rea Lo 40: 40% (28.3 g, 85 g, 198.4 g)
Rea-Lo [OTC]: 30% (227 g, 59 mL)
Remeven: 50% (142 g, 255 g)
U-Kera E: 40% (28.35 g, 85.05 g, 198.45 g)
Uramaxin: 45% (255 g)
Ureacin-20 [OTC]: 20% (113.4 g)
Utopic: 41% (227 g)
X-Viate: 40% (28.3 g, 85 g, 199 g)
Generic: 10% (85 g); 20% (85 g); 39% (226.8 g, 227 g); 40% (28.35 g, 85 g, 85.05 g, 198.4 g, 198.6 g); 45% (255 g); 47% (142 g); 50% (142 g, 255 g); 39% (227 g)

Emulsion, External:

Latrix XM: 45% (240 mL)
Umecta: 40% (120 g, 227 g)
Umecta PD: 40% (198.5 g)
Generic: 50% (284 g, 300 g)

Foam, External:

Hydro 35: 35% (150 g)
Hydro 40: 40% (150 g)
Kerafoam: 30% (60 g, 100 g)
Kerafoam 42: 42% (60 g, 100 g)
Umecta Mousse: 40% (113.4 g)
Uramaxin: 20% (100 g)
Urea Hydrating: 35% (150 g)

Gel, External:

Carb-O-Philic/40: 40% (15 g)
Cerovel: 40% (25 mL)
Uramaxin: 45% (28 mL)
Uramaxin GT: 45% (20 mL)
Urea Nail: 45% (28 mL)
X-Viate: 40% (15 mL)
Generic: 40% (15 mL)

Kit, External:

Dermasorb XM: 39%
Uramaxin GT: 45%
Urea Nail: 40 & 0.2%

Lotion, External:

Atrac-Tain [OTC]: 5% (118 mL, 237 mL)
Beta Care Betamide [OTC]: 25% (120 mL, 480 mL)
Carmol 10 [OTC]: 10% (177 mL)
Cerovel: 40% (325 mL)
Dermal Therapy Finger Care [OTC]: 20% (18 mL)
Gormel 10 [OTC]: 10% (240 mL)
Nutraplus [OTC]: 10% (236 mL, 473 mL)
Rea Lo 40: 40% (236.6 mL)
Rea-Lo [OTC]: 15% (120 mL)
Ultra Mide 25 [OTC]: 25% (236 mL)
Uramaxin: 45% (480 g)
Urea-C40: 40% (236.6 mL)
Ureacin-10 [OTC]: 10% (236.56 mL)
X-Viate: 40% (237 mL)
Generic: 10% (180 mL, 240 mL, 480 mL); 40% (226.8 g, 236.6 mL); 45% (480 g)

Ointment, External:

Aquaphilic/Carbamide [OTC]: 10% (180 g, 454 g); 20% (454 g)
Gordons Urea [OTC]: 22% (30 g); 40% (30 g)
Lanaphilic/Urea [OTC]: 10% (454 g); 20% (454 g)

Shampoo, External:

Carmol [OTC]: 10% (240 mL)

Solution, External:

CEM-Urea: 45% (20 mL)

Stick, External:

Urea Nail: 50% (2.4 mL)

Suspension, External:

Umecta: 40% (283.4 g)
Umecta Nail Film: 40% (3 g, 18 mL)
Umecta PD: 40% (255.1 g)
Generic: 40% (283.4 g, 18 mL); 50% (284 g)

Urea and Hydrocortisone

(yoor EE a & hye droe KOR ti sone)

Brand Names: U.S. Carmol-HC® [DSC]; U-Cort

Brand Names: Canada Ti-U-Lac® H; Uremol® HC

Index Terms Hydrocortisone and Urea

Pharmacologic Category Corticosteroid, Topical

Use Inflammation of corticosteroid-responsive dermatoses

Pregnancy Risk Factor C

Dosage Topical: Children and Adults: Steroid-responsive dermatoses: Apply thin film and rub in well 2-4 times/day. Therapy should be discontinued when control is achieved; if no improvement is seen, reassessment of diagnosis may be necessary.

Additional Information Complete prescribing information should be consulted for additional detail.

Dosage Forms

Cream:

U-Cort: Urea 10% and hydrocortisone acetate 1% (28 g)

- ◆ **Urea-C40** *see* Urea *on page 2114*
- ◆ **Ureacin-10 [OTC]** *see* Urea *on page 2114*
- ◆ **Ureacin-20 [OTC]** *see* Urea *on page 2114*
- ◆ **Urea Hydrating** *see* Urea *on page 2114*
- ◆ **Urea Nail** *see* Urea *on page 2114*
- ◆ **Urea Peroxide** *see* Carbamide Peroxide *on page 350*
- ◆ **Urecholine** *see* Bethanechol *on page 257*
- ◆ **Urelle** *see* Methenamine, Sodium Phosphate Monobasic, Phenyl Salicylate, Methylene Blue, and Hyoscyamine *on page 1318*
- ◆ **Uremol® HC (Can)** *see* Urea and Hydrocortisone *on page 2115*

- **Urex** *see* Methenamine *on page 1317*
- **Uribel** *see* Methenamine, Sodium Phosphate Monobasic, Phenyl Salicylate, Methylene Blue, and Hyoscyamine *on page 1318*

Uridine Triacetate (URE i deen trye AS e tate)

Index Terms PN401; Triacetyluridine; Vistonuridine
Pharmacologic Category Antidote
Dosage Oral: Adults: Fluorouracil overdose (off-label use): 10 g every 6 hours for 20 doses beginning as soon as possible (8 hours to 4 days) after fluorouracil overdose (von Borstel, 2009)
Additional Information Complete prescribing information should be consulted for additional detail.

- **Urimar-T** *see* Methenamine, Sodium Phosphate Monobasic, Phenyl Salicylate, Methylene Blue, and Hyoscyamine *on page 1318*
- **Urinary Pain Relief [OTC]** *see* Phenazopyridine *on page 1629*
- **Urispas** *see* FlavoxATE *on page 881*
- **Urispas® (Can)** *see* FlavoxATE *on page 881*
- **Uro-L** *see* Methenamine, Sodium Phosphate Monobasic, Phenyl Salicylate, Methylene Blue, and Hyoscyamine *on page 1318*

Urofollitropin (yoor oh fol li TROE pin)

Brand Names: U.S. Bravelle
Brand Names: Canada Bravelle
Index Terms Follicle-Stimulating Hormone, Human; FSH; hFSH
Pharmacologic Category Gonadotropin; Ovulation Stimulator
Use
Multifollicular development during ART: Development of multiple follicles with assisted reproductive technologies (ART) in women who have previously received pituitary suppression.
Limitations of use: Prior to therapy, perform a complete gynecologic exam (including demonstration of tubal patency) and endocrinologic evaluation (cause of infertility should be diagnosed prior to ART); exclude the possibility of pregnancy; evaluate the fertility status of the male partner; exclude a diagnosis of primary ovarian failure.
Ovulation induction: Ovulation induction in women who previously received GnRH agonist or antagonist for pituitary suppression.
Pregnancy Risk Factor X
Dosage Note: Dose should be individualized. Use the lowest dose consistent with the expectation of good results. Over the course of treatment, doses may vary depending on individual patient response.

Assisted reproductive technologies (ART): Adults: Females: SubQ: Starting on day 2 or 3 of cycle, administer 225 units once daily for the first 5 days; urofollitropin may be administered together with menotropins and the total initial dose of both products combined should not exceed 225 units (menotropins 150 units and urofollitropin 75 units; or menotropins 75 units and urofollitropin 150 units). Adjust dose after 5 days based on ultrasound monitoring of ovarian response and measurement of serum estradiol levels. Do not make additional adjustments more frequently than once every 2 days or by >75-150 units. Maximum daily dose: 450 units (of urofollitropin, or menotropins plus urofollitropin); treatment >12 days is not recommended; once adequate follicular development is evident, hCG should be administered. Withhold the hCG dose if ovarian monitoring suggests an increased risk of OHSS.
Ovulation induction: Adults: Females: IM, SubQ: Initial: 150 units once daily for 5 days in the first cycle of treatment. After 5 days, dose adjustments up to 75-150 units can be made every ≥2 days based on ultrasound monitoring of ovarian response and/or measurement of serum estradiol levels; maximum daily dose: 450 units; treatment >12 days is not recommended. If response to follitropin is appropriate, administer hCG; withhold the hCG dose if ovarian monitoring suggests an increased risk of OHSS and advise the patient to refrain from intercourse. For subsequent cycles, the starting dose and dosage adjustments should be determined based on historical ovarian response.

Dosage adjustment in renal impairment: There are no dosage adjustments provided in manufacturer's labeling (has not been studied).
Dosage adjustment in hepatic impairment: There are no dosage adjustments provided in manufacturer's labeling (has not been studied).
Additional Information Complete prescribing information should be consulted for additional detail.
Dosage Forms
Solution Reconstituted, Injection:
Bravelle: 75 units (1 ea)

- **Uro-Mag [OTC]** *see* Magnesium Oxide *on page 1265*
- **Uromax (Can)** *see* Oxybutynin *on page 1536*
- **Uromitexan (Can)** *see* Mesna *on page 1305*
- **Uro-MP** *see* Methenamine, Sodium Phosphate Monobasic, Phenyl Salicylate, Methylene Blue, and Hyoscyamine *on page 1318*
- **Uroqid-Acid® No. 2** *see* Methenamine and Sodium Acid Phosphate *on page 1318*
- **Uroxatral** *see* Alfuzosin *on page 84*
- **Urozide (Can)** *see* Hydrochlorothiazide *on page 1009*
- **Urso (Can)** *see* Ursodiol *on page 2116*
- **Urso 250** *see* Ursodiol *on page 2116*
- **Ursodeoxycholic Acid** *see* Ursodiol *on page 2116*
- **Ursodesoxycholic Acid** *see* Ursodiol *on page 2116*

Ursodiol (ur soe DYE ol)

Brand Names: U.S. Actigall; Urso 250; Urso Forte
Brand Names: Canada Dom-Ursodiol C; PHL-Ursodiol C; PMS-Ursodiol C; Urso; Urso DS
Index Terms Ursodeoxycholic Acid; Ursodesoxycholic Acid
Pharmacologic Category Gallstone Dissolution Agent
Use
Actigall: Gallbladder stone dissolution; prevention of gallstones in obese patients experiencing rapid weight loss
Urso, Urso Forte: Primary biliary cirrhosis
Pregnancy Risk Factor B
Dosage Oral: Adults:
Gallstone dissolution (Actigall): 8-10 mg/kg/day in 2-3 divided doses; use beyond 24 months is not established
Gallstone prevention (Actigall): 300 mg twice daily
Primary biliary cirrhosis (Urso, Urso Forte): 13-15 mg/kg/day in 2-4 divided doses (with food)

Dosage adjustment in renal impairment: No dosage adjustment provided in manufacturer's labeling.
Dosage adjustment in hepatic impairment: No dosage adjustment provided in manufacturer's labeling.
Additional Information Complete prescribing information should be consulted for additional detail.

Dosage Forms

Capsule, Oral:

Actigall: 300 mg

Generic: 300 mg

Tablet, Oral:

Urso 250: 250 mg

Urso Forte: 500 mg

Generic: 250 mg, 500 mg

◆ **Urso DS (Can)** *see* Ursodiol *on page 2116*

◆ **Urso Forte** *see* Ursodiol *on page 2116*

Ustekinumab (yoo stek in YOO mab)

Brand Names: U.S. Stelara

Brand Names: Canada Stelara

Index Terms CNTO 1275

Pharmacologic Category Antipsoriatic Agent; Interleukin-12 Inhibitor; Interleukin-23 Inhibitor; Monoclonal Antibody

Use

Plaque psoriasis: Treatment of adults with moderate-to-severe plaque psoriasis who are candidates for phototherapy or systemic therapy

Psoriatic arthritis: Treatment of adults with active psoriatic arthritis (as monotherapy or in combination with methotrexate)

Pregnancy Risk Factor B

Pregnancy Considerations Adverse events were not observed in animal reproduction studies. There is limited information related to the use of ustekinumab in pregnancy (Andrulonis, 2012). In general, other agents are preferred for the treatment of plaque psoriasis in pregnant women (Hsu, 2012). Patients exposed to ustekinumab during pregnancy are encouraged to enroll in the pregnancy registry by calling 877-311-8972.

Breast-Feeding Considerations It is not known whether ustekinumab is secreted in human milk. Because many immunoglobulins are secreted in milk it is expected that ustekinumab will be present in breast milk. The U.S. labeling recommends caution be used in nursing women. The Canadian labeling recommends discontinuing nursing or discontinuing ustekinumab.

Contraindications

Clinically significant hypersensitivity to ustekinumab or any component of the formulation

Canadian labeling: Additional contraindications (not in U.S. labeling): Severe infections such as sepsis, tuberculosis, and opportunistic infections

Warnings/Precautions May increase the risk for malignancy although the impact on the development and course of malignancies is not fully defined. Rapidly appearing cutaneous squamous cell carcinomas (multiple) have been reported in patients receiving ustekinumab who were at risk for developing nonmelanoma skin cancer. Monitor all patients closely for the development of nonmelanoma skin cancer; closely follow patients >60 years of age, with a history of prolonged immunosuppression, and in patients with a history of PUVA treatment. Use with caution in patients with prior malignancy (use not studied in this population).

May increase the risk for infections or reactivation of latent infections. Serious bacterial, fungal, and viral infections have been observed with use. Avoid use in patients with clinically important active infection. Caution should be exercised when considering use in patients with a history of new/recurrent infections, with conditions that predispose them to infections (eg, diabetes or residence/travel from areas of endemic mycoses), or with chronic, latent, or localized infections, or who are genetically deficient in IL-12/IL-23 (IL-12/IL-23 genetic deficiency may predispose patients to disseminated infection). Patients who develop a new infection while undergoing treatment should be monitored closely. If a patient develops a serious infection, therapy should be discontinued or withheld until successful resolution of infection.

Do not use in patients with active tuberculosis (TB). Patients should be evaluated for latent tuberculosis infection with a tuberculin skin test prior to starting therapy. Treatment of latent TB should be initiated before ustekinumab therapy is used. Consider antituberculosis treatment in patients with a history of latent or active tuberculosis if an adequate prior treatment course cannot be confirmed. During and following treatment, monitor for signs/symptoms of active TB.

Antibody formation to ustekinumab has been observed with therapy and has been associated with decreased serum levels and therapeutic response in some patients. Hypersensitivity, including anaphylaxis and angioedema, has been reported. Discontinue immediately with signs/symptoms of hypersensitivity reaction and treat appropriately as indicated. Reversible posterior leukoencephalopathy syndrome (RPLS) has been observed (rare). RPLS symptoms include headache, seizures, confusion, and visual disturbances; may be fatal. Monitor; discontinue ustekinumab if symptoms occur and administer appropriate therapy. Use in combination with other immunosuppressive drugs or phototherapy has not been studied. Patients should be brought up to date with all immunizations before initiating therapy. **Live vaccines should not be given concurrently;** inactivated or nonlive vaccines may be given concurrently, but may not elicit a proper immune response. BCG vaccines should not be given 1 year prior to, during, or 1 year following treatment. Patients >100 kg may require higher dose to achieve adequate serum levels. Use in hepatic or renal impairment has not been studied.

The packaging may contain latex. Some dosage forms may contain polysorbate 80 (also known as Tweens). Hypersensitivity reactions, usually a delayed reaction, have been reported following exposure to pharmaceutical products containing polysorbate 80 in certain individuals (Isaksson, 2002; Lucente 2000; Shelley, 1995). Thrombocytopenia, ascites, pulmonary deterioration, and renal and hepatic failure have been reported in premature neonates after receiving parenteral products containing polysorbate 80 (Alade, 1986; CDC, 1984). See manufacturer's labeling. Potentially significant interactions may exist, requiring dose or frequency adjustment, additional monitoring, and/or selection of alternative therapy.

Adverse Reactions

Central nervous system: Depression, dizziness, fatigue, headache

Dermatologic: Pruritus

Gastrointestinal: Nausea

Immunologic: Antibody development

Infection: Infection (including severe infection)

Local: Erythema at injection site

Neuromuscular & skeletal: Arthralgia, back pain

Respiratory: Pharyngolaryngeal pain

Rare but important or life-threatening: Anaphylaxis, angina pectoris, angioedema, appendicitis, bacterial infection, bleeding at injection site, bruising at injection site, cellulitis, cerebrovascular accident, cholecystitis, dactylitis, diverticulitis, erythrodermic psoriasis, exfoliative dermatitis, fungal infection, gastroenteritis, herpes zoster, hypersensitivity reaction, hypertension, induration at injection site, irritation at injection site, itching at injection site, malignant melanoma (*in situ*), malignant neoplasm (breast, colon, head and neck, kidney, prostate, thyroid); myocardial infarction, nephrolithiasis, osteomyelitis, pain at injection site, pneumonia, pustular psoriasis, reversible posterior leukoencephalopathy syndrome, sepsis, squamous cell carcinoma of skin, swelling at injection site, urinary tract infection, viral infection

Drug Interactions

Metabolism/Transport Effects None known.

Avoid Concomitant Use

Avoid concomitant use of Ustekinumab with any of the following: BCG; Belimumab; InFLIXimab; Natalizumab; Pimecrolimus; Tacrolimus (Topical); Tofacitinib; Vaccines (Live)

Increased Effect/Toxicity

Ustekinumab may increase the levels/effects of: Belimumab; InFLIXimab; Leflunomide; Natalizumab; Tofacitinib; Vaccines (Live)

The levels/effects of Ustekinumab may be increased by: Denosumab; Pimecrolimus; Roflumilast; Tacrolimus (Topical); Trastuzumab

Decreased Effect

Ustekinumab may decrease the levels/effects of: BCG; Coccidioides immitis Skin Test; Sipuleucel-T; Vaccines (Inactivated); Vaccines (Live)

The levels/effects of Ustekinumab may be decreased by: Echinacea

Storage/Stability Refrigerate at 2°C to 8°C (36°F to 46°F); do not freeze. Store vials upright. Keep the product in the original carton to protect from light until the time of use. Do not shake. Discard any unused portion.

Mechanism of Action Ustekinumab is a human monoclonal antibody that binds to and interferes with the proinflammatory cytokines, interleukin (IL)-12 and IL-23. Biological effects of IL-12 and IL-23 include natural killer (NK) cell activation, CD4+ T-cell differentiation and activation. Ustekinumab also interferes with the expression of monocyte chemotactic protein-1 (MCP-1), tumor necrosis factor-alpha (TNF-α), interferon-inducible protein-10 (IP-10), and interleukin-8 (IL-8). Significant clinical improvement in psoriasis and psoriatic arthritis patients is seen in association with reduction of these proinflammatory signalers.

Pharmacodynamics/Kinetics

Distribution: V_d (terminal elimination phase): 45 mg: 0.161 ± 0.065 L/kg; 90 mg: 0.179 ± 0.085 L/kg

Bioavailability: Absolute bioavailability: SubQ: ~57%

Half-life elimination: 10-126 days

Time to peak, plasma: 45 mg: 13.5 days; 90 mg: 7 days

Dosage

Plaque psoriasis: Adults: SubQ:

Initial and maintenance: **Note:** Following an interruption in therapy, retreatment may be initiated at the initial dosing interval. Consider therapy discontinuation in any patient failing to demonstrate a response after 12 weeks of therapy.

≤100 kg: 45 mg at 0- and 4 weeks, and then every 12 weeks thereafter

>100 kg: 90 mg at 0- and 4 weeks, and then every 12 weeks thereafter. **Note:** Doses of 45 mg given to patients >100 kg were also efficacious; however, 90 mg is the recommended dose in these patients due to greater efficacy.

Note: The Canadian labeling suggests that if the response is inadequate on every-12-week therapy, may consider increasing frequency to every 8 weeks.

Psoriatic arthritis: Adults: SubQ: **Note:** When used for psoriatic arthritis, may be administered alone or in combination with methotrexate.

U.S. labeling:

Initial and maintenance: 45 mg at 0- and 4 weeks, and then every 12 weeks thereafter.

Coexistent psoriatic arthritis and moderate-to-severe plaque psoriasis in patients >100 kg: Initial and maintenance: 90 mg at 0- and 4 weeks, and then every 12 weeks thereafter.

Canadian labeling: Initial and maintenance:

≤100 kg: 45 mg at 0- and 4 weeks, and then every 12 weeks thereafter.

>100 kg: 90 mg at 0- and 4 weeks, and then every 12 weeks thereafter.

Dosage adjustment in renal impairment: There are no dosage adjustment provided in the manufacturer's labeling (has not been studied).

Dosage adjustment in hepatic impairment: There are no dosage adjustment provided in the manufacturer's labeling (has not been studied).

Administration Do not use if cloudy or discolored. Administer by subcutaneous injection into the top of the thigh, abdomen, upper arms, or buttocks. Rotate sites. Do not inject into tender, bruised, erythematous, or indurated skin. Avoid areas of skin where psoriasis is present. Discard any unused portion.

Monitoring Parameters Tuberculosis screening (prior to initiating and periodically during therapy); CBC; ustekinumab-antibody formation; monitor for signs/symptoms of infection, reversible posterior leukoencephalopathy syndrome (RPLS), and squamous cell skin carcinoma

Dosage Forms

Solution Prefilled Syringe, Subcutaneous [preservative free]:

Stelara: 45 mg/0.5 mL (0.5 mL); 90 mg/mL (1 mL)

◆ **Ustell** *see* Methenamine, Sodium Phosphate Monobasic, Phenyl Salicylate, Methylene Blue, and Hyoscyamine *on page 1318*

◆ **Utira-C** *see* Methenamine, Sodium Phosphate Monobasic, Phenyl Salicylate, Methylene Blue, and Hyoscyamine *on page 1318*

◆ **Utopic** *see* Urea *on page 2114*

◆ **Utradol (Can)** *see* Etodolac *on page 815*

◆ **Uvadex** *see* Methoxsalen (Systemic) *on page 1330*

Vaccinia Immune Globulin (Intravenous)

(vax IN ee a i MYUN GLOB yoo lin IN tra VEE nus)

Brand Names: U.S. CNJ-016

Index Terms IV-VIG; VIG; VIGIV

Pharmacologic Category Blood Product Derivative; Immune Globulin

Use Vaccinia conditions: Treatment and/or modification of the following conditions:

- Aberrant infections induced by vaccinia virus that include its accidental implantation in eyes (except in cases of isolated keratitis), mouth, or other areas where vaccinia infection would constitute a special hazard.
- Eczema vaccinatum
- Progressive vaccinia
- Severe generalized vaccinia
- Vaccinia infections in individuals who have skin conditions such as burns, impetigo, varicella-zoster, or poison ivy; or in individuals who have eczematous skin lesions because of either the activity or extensiveness of such lesions

The Advisory Committee on Immunization Practices (ACIP) recommends the following (CDC 2009; CDC [Rotz 2001]; CDC [Wharton 2003]):

Use is recommended for:

- Inadvertent inoculation (considering severity, toxicity of affected person, and pain)
- Eczema vaccinatum
- Generalized vaccinia (severe form or if underlying illness is present)
- Progressive vaccinia

Use may be considered for:

- Severe ocular complications except isolated keratitis

Use is not recommended for:

- Inadvertent inoculation that is not severe
- Mild or limited generalized vaccinia
- Nonspecific rashes, erythema multiforme, or Stevens-Johnson syndrome
- Postvaccinial encephalitis or encephalomyelitis

Pregnancy Risk Factor C

Dosage Vaccinia treatment/modification: Adolescents ≥16 years and Adults: IV: 6,000 units/kg; may repeat dose based on severity of symptoms and response to treatment (specific data are lacking); 9,000 units/kg may be considered if patient does not respond to initial dose. Single doses up to 24,000 unit/kg were tolerated in healthy volunteers.

Dosage adjustment in renal impairment: There are no dosage adjustments provided in the manufacturer's labeling. Use caution. In patients at risk of renal dysfunction, the rate of infusion and concentration of solution should be minimized; discontinue if renal function deteriorates.

Dosage adjustment in hepatic impairment: There are no dosage adjustments provided in manufacturer's labeling.

Additional Information Complete prescribing information should be consulted for additional detail.

Dosage Forms Injection, solution [preservative free; solvent-detergent treated]:

CNJ-016: ≥50,000 units/15 mL (15 mL)

- ◆ **Vaccinia Vaccine** *see* Smallpox Vaccine *on page 1900*
- ◆ **Vacuant Mini-Enema [OTC] [DSC]** *see* Docusate *on page 661*
- ◆ **Vagifem** *see* Estradiol (Topical) *on page 780*
- ◆ **Vagifem10 (Can)** *see* Estradiol (Topical) *on page 780*
- ◆ **Vagistat-3 [OTC]** *see* Miconazole (Topical) *on page 1360*
- ◆ **VAL-13081** *see* Bromopride [INT] *on page 292*

ValACYclovir (val ay SYE kloe veer)

Brand Names: U.S. Valtrex

Brand Names: Canada Apo-Valacyclovir; CO Valacyclovir; DOM-Valacyclovir; Mylan-Valacyclovir; PHL-Valacyclovir; PMS-Valacyclovir; PRO-Valacyclovir; Riva-Valacyclovir; Valtrex

Index Terms Valacyclovir Hydrochloride

Pharmacologic Category Antiviral Agent; Antiviral Agent, Oral

Use Treatment of herpes zoster (shingles) in immunocompetent patients; treatment of first-episode and recurrent genital herpes; suppression of recurrent genital herpes and reduction of transmission of genital herpes in immunocompetent patients; suppression of genital herpes in HIV-infected individuals; treatment of herpes labialis (cold sores); chickenpox in immunocompetent children

Pregnancy Risk Factor B

Pregnancy Considerations Adverse events were not observed in animal reproduction studies. Valacyclovir is metabolized to acyclovir. In a pharmacokinetic study, maternal acyclovir serum concentrations were higher in pregnant women receiving valacyclovir than those given acyclovir for the suppression of recurrent herpes simplex virus (HSV) infection late in pregnancy. Amniotic fluid concentrations were also higher; however, there was no evidence that fetal exposure differed between the groups (Kimberlin, 1998). Data from an acyclovir pregnancy registry has shown no increased rate of birth defects than that of the general population; however, the registry is small and the manufacturer notes that use during pregnancy is only warranted if the potential benefit to the mother justifies the risk of the fetus. Because more data is available for acyclovir, that agent is preferred for the treatment of genital herpes in pregnant women (ACOG, 2000; CDC, 2010); however, valacyclovir may be considered for use due to its simplified dosing schedule (DHHS, 2013). Pregnant women who have a history of genital herpes recurrence, suppressive therapy is recommended starting at 36 weeks gestation (ACOG, 2000; DHHS, 2013).

Breast-Feeding Considerations Valacyclovir is metabolized to acyclovir; acyclovir (but not unchanged valacyclovir) can be detected in breast milk. Peak concentrations in breast milk range from 0.5-2.3 times the corresponding maternal acyclovir serum concentration. This is expected to provide a nursing infant with a dose of acyclovir equivalent to ~0.6 mg/kg/day following ingestion of valacyclovir 500 mg twice daily by the mother. The manufacturer recommends that caution be used if administered to a nursing woman. Other sources note that women with HSV infection taking valacyclovir may breast-feed as long as there are not lesions on the breast, body lesions are covered, and strict hand hygiene is practiced (ACOG, 2000; Jaiyeoba, 2012). Women with HSV who also have HIV infection should not breast-feed; complete avoidance of breast-feeding by HIV-infected women is recommended to decrease potential transmission of HIV (DHHS [perinatal], 2012).

Contraindications Hypersensitivity to valacyclovir, acyclovir, or any component of the formulation

Warnings/Precautions Thrombotic thrombocytopenic purpura/hemolytic uremic syndrome has occurred in immunocompromised patients (at doses of 8 g/day). Safety and efficacy have not been established for treatment/suppression of recurrent genital herpes or disseminated herpes in patients with profound immunosuppression (eg, advanced HIV with CD4 <100 cells/mm^3). CNS adverse effects (including agitation, hallucinations, confusion, delirium, seizures, and encephalopathy) have been reported. Use caution in patients with renal impairment, the elderly, and/or those receiving nephrotoxic agents. Acute renal failure has been observed in patients with renal dysfunction; dose adjustment may be required. Precipitation in renal tubules may occur leading to urinary precipitation; adequately hydrate patient. For cold sores, treatment should begin at with earliest symptom (tingling, itching, burning). For genital herpes, treatment should begin as soon as possible after the first signs and symptoms (within 72 hours of onset of first diagnosis or within 24 hours of onset of recurrent episodes). For herpes zoster, treatment should begin within 72 hours of onset of rash. For chickenpox, treatment should begin with earliest sign or symptom. Use with caution in the elderly; CNS effects have been reported.

Adverse Reactions

Central nervous system: Depression, dizziness, fatigue, fever, headache

Dermatologic: Rash

Endocrine: Dehydration, dysmenorrhea

Gastrointestinal: Abdominal pain, diarrhea, nausea, vomiting

Hematologic: Mild leukopenia, thrombocytopenia

Hepatic: Alkaline phosphatase increased, ALT increased, AST increased

Neuromuscular & skeletal: Arthralgia

Respiratory: Nasopharyngitis, rhinorrhea

Miscellaneous: Herpes simplex

Rare but important or life-threatening: Acute hypersensitivity reactions (angioedema, anaphylaxis, dyspnea, pruritus, rash, urticaria); aggression, agitation, alopecia, anemia, aplastic anemia, ataxia, creatinine increased, coma, confusion, consciousness decreased, delirium, dysarthria, encephalopathy, erythema multiforme, facial edema, hallucinations (auditory and visual), hemolytic uremic syndrome (HUS), hepatitis, hypertension, leukocytoclastic vasculitis, mania, photosensitivity reaction, psychosis, renal failure, renal pain, seizure, tachycardia, thrombotic thrombocytopenic purpura (TTP), tremor, urinary precipitation, visual disturbances

Drug Interactions

Metabolism/Transport Effects None known.

Avoid Concomitant Use

Avoid concomitant use of ValACYclovir with any of the following: Foscarnet; Zoster Vaccine

Increased Effect/Toxicity

ValACYclovir may increase the levels/effects of: Mycophenolate; Tenofovir; Zidovudine

The levels/effects of ValACYclovir may be increased by: Foscarnet; Mycophenolate

Decreased Effect

ValACYclovir may decrease the levels/effects of: Zoster Vaccine

Storage/Stability Store at 15°C to 25°C (59°F to 77°F).

Mechanism of Action Valacyclovir is rapidly and nearly completely converted to acyclovir by intestinal and hepatic metabolism. Acyclovir is converted to acyclovir monophosphate by virus-specific thymidine kinase then further converted to acyclovir triphosphate by other cellular enzymes. Acyclovir triphosphate inhibits DNA synthesis and viral replication by competing with deoxyguanosine triphosphate for viral DNA polymerase and being incorporated into viral DNA.

Pharmacodynamics/Kinetics

Absorption: Rapid

Distribution: Acyclovir is widely distributed throughout the body including brain, kidney, lungs, liver, spleen, muscle, uterus, vagina, and CSF

Protein binding: ~14% to 18%

Metabolism: Hepatic; valacyclovir is rapidly and nearly completely converted to acyclovir and L-valine by first-pass effect; acyclovir is hepatically metabolized to a very small extent by aldehyde oxidase and by alcohol and aldehyde dehydrogenase (inactive metabolites)

Bioavailability: ~55% once converted to acyclovir

Half-life elimination: Normal renal function: Adults: Acyclovir: 2.5-3.3 hours, Valacyclovir: ~30 minutes; End-stage renal disease: Acyclovir: 14 to 20 hours; During hemodialysis: 4 hours

Excretion: Urine, primarily as acyclovir (89%); **Note:** Following oral administration of radiolabeled valacyclovir, 46% of the label is eliminated in the feces (corresponding to nonabsorbed drug), while 47% of the radiolabel is eliminated in the urine.

Dosage Oral:

Children 2 to <18 years: Chickenpox: 20 mg/kg/dose 3 times/day for 5 days (maximum: 1 g 3 times/day)

Children ≥12 and Adults: Herpes labialis (cold sores): 2 g twice daily for 1 day (separate doses by ~12 hours)

Adults:

CMV prophylaxis in allogeneic HSCT recipients (off-label use): 2 g 4 times/day

Herpes zoster (shingles): 1 g 3 times/day for 7 days

HSV, VZV in cancer patients (off-label use): Prophylaxis: 500 mg 2-3 times/day; Treatment: 1 g 3 times/day

Genital herpes:

Initial episode: 1 g twice daily for 10 days

Recurrent episode: 500 mg twice daily for 3 days

Reduction of transmission: 500 mg once daily (source partner)

Suppressive therapy:

Immunocompetent patients: 1 g once daily (500 mg once daily in patients with ≤9 recurrences per year)

HIV-infected patients (CD4 ≥100 cells/mm^3): 500 mg twice daily

Dosage adjustment in renal impairment:

Herpes zoster: Adults:

CrCl 30-49 mL/minute: 1 g every 12 hours

CrCl 10-29 mL/minute: 1 g every 24 hours

CrCl <10 mL/minute: 500 mg every 24 hours

Genital herpes: Adults:

U.S. labeling:

Initial episode:

CrCl 10-29 mL/minute: 1 g every 24 hours

CrCl <10 mL/minute: 500 mg every 24 hours

Recurrent episode: CrCl <29 mL/minute: 500 mg every 24 hours

Suppressive therapy: CrCl <29 mL/minute:

For usual dose of 1 g every 24 hours, decrease dose to 500 mg every 24 hours

For usual dose of 500 mg every 24 hours, decrease dose to 500 mg every 48 hours

HIV-infected patients: 500 mg every 24 hours

Canadian labeling:

Initial episode:

CrCl 10-29 mL/minute: 1 g every 24 hours

CrCl <10 mL/minute: 500 mg every 24 hours

Recurrent episode:

CrCl 10-29 mL/minute: 500 mg every 24 hours

CrCl <10 mL/minute: 500 mg every 24 hours

Suppressive therapy:

CrCl 10-29 mL/minute:

Immunocompetent or HIV-infected patients: 500 mg every 24 hours

Immunocompetent patients with ≤9 recurrences/year: 500 mg every 48 hours

CrCl <10 mL/minute:

Immunocompetent or HIV-infected patients: 500 mg every 24 hours

Immunocompetent patients with ≤9 recurrences/year: 500 mg every 48 hours

Herpes labialis: Adolescents and Adults *(U.S. labeling)* or Adults *(Canadian labeling)*:

CrCl 30-49 mL/minute: 1 g every 12 hours for 2 doses

CrCl 10-29 mL/minute: 500 mg every 12 hours for 2 doses

CrCl <10 mL/minute: 500 mg as a single dose

Hemodialysis: Dialyzable (~33% removed during 4-hour session); administer dose postdialysis

Chronic ambulatory peritoneal dialysis/continuous arteriovenous hemofiltration dialysis: Pharmacokinetic parameters are similar to those in patients with ESRD; supplemental dose not needed following dialysis

Dosage adjustment in hepatic impairment: No dosage adjustment necessary.

Dietary Considerations May be taken with or without food.

Administration If GI upset occurs, administer with meals.

Monitoring Parameters Urinalysis, BUN, serum creatinine, liver enzymes, and CBC

Dosage Forms

Tablet, Oral:

Valtrex: 500 mg, 1 g

Generic: 500 mg, 1 g

Extemporaneous Preparations A 50 mg/mL oral suspension may be made with caplets and either Ora-Sweet® or Ora-Sweet SF®. Crush eighteen 500 mg caplets in a mortar and reduce to a fine powder. Add 5 mL portions of chosen vehicle (40 mL total) and mix to a uniform paste; transfer to a 180 mL calibrated amber glass bottle, rinse mortar with 10 mL of vehicle 5 times, and add quantity of vehicle sufficient to make 180 mL. Label "shake well" and "refrigerate". Stable for 21 days refrigerated.

Fish DN, Vidaurri VA, and Deeter RG, "Stability of Valacyclovir Hydrochloride in Extemporaneously Prepared Oral Liquids," *Am J Health Syst Pharm*, 1999, 56(19):1957-60.

◆ **Valacyclovir Hydrochloride** *see* ValACYclovir *on page 2119*

◆ **Valchlor** *see* Mechlorethamine (Topical) *on page 1276*

◆ **Valcyte** *see* ValGANciclovir *on page 2121*

◆ **10-Valent Pneumococcal Nontypeable *Haemophilus influenzae* Protein D Conjugate Vaccine** *see* Pneumococcal Conjugate Vaccine (10-Valent) [CAN/INT] *on page 1668*

◆ **23-Valent Pneumococcal Polysaccharide Vaccine** *see* Pneumococcal Polysaccharide Vaccine (23-Valent) *on page 1671*

ValGANciclovir (val gan SYE kloh veer)

Brand Names: U.S. Valcyte

Brand Names: Canada Apo-Valganciclovir; Valcyte

Index Terms Valganciclovir Hydrochloride

Pharmacologic Category Antiviral Agent

Use Treatment of cytomegalovirus (CMV) retinitis in patients with acquired immunodeficiency syndrome (AIDS); prevention of CMV disease in high-risk patients (donor CMV positive/recipient CMV negative) undergoing kidney, heart, or kidney/pancreas transplantation

Pregnancy Risk Factor C

Pregnancy Considerations Valganciclovir is converted to ganciclovir and shares its reproductive toxicity. **[U.S. Boxed Warning]: Ganciclovir may be teratogenic and cause aspermatogenesis.** Based on animal data, temporary or permanent impairment of fertility may occur in males and females. Ganciclovir is also teratogenic in animals. Females should use effective contraception during treatment and for 30 days after; males should use barrier contraception during treatment and for 90 days after.

Breast-Feeding Considerations HIV-infected mothers are discouraged from breast-feeding to decrease the potential transmission of HIV.

Contraindications Hypersensitivity to valganciclovir, ganciclovir, or any component of the formulation

Warnings/Precautions Hazardous agent - use appropriate precautions for handling and disposal (NIOSH 2014 [group 2]).

[U.S. Boxed Warning]: May cause dose- or therapy-limiting granulocytopenia, anemia, and/or thrombocytopenia; do not use in patients with an absolute neutrophil count <500/mm^3, platelet count <25,000/mm^3, or hemoglobin <8 g/dL. Use with caution in patients with impaired renal function (dose adjustment required). Acute renal failure (ARF) may occur; ensure adequate hydration and use with caution in patients receiving concomitant nephrotoxic agents. Elderly patients with or without preexisting renal impairment may develop ARF; use with caution and adjust dose as needed. **[U.S. Boxed Warning]: Ganciclovir may be teratogenic, carcinogenic, and cause aspermatogenesis.** Due to its teratogenic potential, contraceptive precautions for female and male patients need to be followed during and for at least 90 days after therapy with the drug. Fertility may be temporarily or permanently impaired in males and females. Due to differences in bioavailability, valganciclovir tablets cannot be substituted for ganciclovir capsules on a one-to-one basis. The preferred dosage form for pediatric patients is the oral solution; however, valganciclovir tablets may used so long as the calculated dose is within 10% of the available tablet strength (450 mg). Not indicated for use in liver transplant patients (higher incidence of tissue-invasive CMV relative to oral ganciclovir was observed in trials). Use of valganciclovir for the treatment of congenital CMV disease has not been evaluated.

Benzyl alcohol and derivatives: Some dosage forms may contain sodium benzoate/benzoic acid; benzoic acid (benzoate) is a metabolite of benzyl alcohol; large amounts of benzyl alcohol (≥99 mg/kg/day) have been associated with a potentially fatal toxicity ("gasping syndrome") in neonates; the "gasping syndrome" consists of metabolic acidosis, respiratory distress, gasping respirations, CNS dysfunction (including convulsions, intracranial hemorrhage), hypotension, and cardiovascular collapse (AAP, 1997; CDC, 1982); some data suggests that benzoate displaces bilirubin from protein binding sites (Ahlfors, 2001); avoid or use dosage forms containing benzyl alcohol derivative with caution in neonates. See manufacturer's labeling.

Adverse Reactions Valganciclovir is expected to share similar idiosyncratic or low incidence toxicities associated with ganciclovir.

Cardiovascular: Edema, hyper-/hypotension, peripheral edema

Central nervous system: Agitation, confusion, depression, dizziness, fatigue, fever, hallucination, headache, insomnia, pain, paresthesia, peripheral neuropathy, psychosis, seizure

Dermatologic: Acne, dermatitis, pruritus

Endocrine & metabolic: Dehydration, hyperglycemia, hyper-/hypokalemia, hypocalcemia, hypomagnesemia, hypophosphatemia

Gastrointestinal: Abdominal distention/pain, appetite (decreased), constipation, diarrhea, dyspepsia, nausea, vomiting

Genitourinary: Urinary tract infection

Hematologic: Anemia, aplastic anemia, bleeding (potentially life-threatening due to thrombocytopenia), bone marrow depression, neutropenia, pancytopenia,

Hepatic: Ascites, hepatic insufficiency

Immunologic: Graft rejection, organ transplant rejection

Local: Catheter infection

Neuromuscular & skeletal: Arthralgia, back pain, limb pain, muscle cramps, tremor, weakness

Ocular: Retinal detachment

Renal: Creatinine clearance (decreased), dysuria, renal impairment, serum creatinine increased

Respiratory: Cough, dyspnea, nasopharyngitis, pharyngitis, pleural effusion, rhinorrhea, upper respiratory tract infection

Miscellaneous: Allergic reaction, local and systemic infection (including sepsis)

Rare but important or life-threatening: Bone marrow aplasia, postoperative complication, postoperative pain, postoperative wound complication (infection, increased drainage, dehiscence)

Drug Interactions

Metabolism/Transport Effects None known.

Avoid Concomitant Use

Avoid concomitant use of ValGANciclovir with any of the following: Imipenem

Increased Effect/Toxicity

ValGANciclovir may increase the levels/effects of: Imipenem; Mycophenolate; Reverse Transcriptase Inhibitors (Nucleoside); Tenofovir

The levels/effects of ValGANciclovir may be increased by: Mycophenolate; Probenecid; Tenofovir

Decreased Effect There are no known significant interactions involving a decrease in effect.

Food Interactions Coadministration with a high-fat meal increased AUC by 30%. Management: Valganciclovir should be taken with meals.

Preparation for Administration Hazardous agent; use appropriate precautions for handling and disposal (NIOSH 2014 [group 2]).

Oral solution: Prior to dispensing, prepare the oral solution by adding 91 mL of purified water to the bottle; shake well. Discard any unused medication after 49 days. A reconstituted 100 mL bottle will only provide 88 mL of solution for administration.

Storage/Stability

Oral solution: Store dry powder at 25°C (77°F); excursions permitted to 15°C to 30°C (59°F to 86°F). Store oral solution under refrigeration at 2°C to 8°C (36°F to 46°F); do not freeze. Discard any unused medication after 49 days.

Tablet: Store at 25°C (77°F); excursions permitted to 15°C to 30°C (59°F to 86°F).

Mechanism of Action Valganciclovir is rapidly converted to ganciclovir in the body. The bioavailability of ganciclovir from valganciclovir is increased 10-fold compared to oral ganciclovir. A dose of 900 mg achieved systemic exposure of ganciclovir comparable to that achieved with the recommended doses of intravenous ganciclovir of 5 mg/kg. Ganciclovir is phosphorylated to a substrate which competitively inhibits the binding of deoxyguanosine triphosphate to DNA polymerase resulting in inhibition of viral DNA synthesis.

Pharmacodynamics/Kinetics

Absorption: Well absorbed; high-fat meal increases AUC by 30%

Distribution: V_{dss}: Ganciclovir: 0.7 L/kg; widely to all tissue including CSF and ocular tissue

Protein binding: Ganciclovir: 1% to 2%

Metabolism: Converted to ganciclovir by intestinal mucosal cells and hepatocytes

Bioavailability: With food: 60%

Half-life elimination: Ganciclovir: 4.08 hours; prolonged with renal impairment; Severe renal impairment: Up to 68 hours

Time to peak: Ganciclovir: 1-3 hours

Excretion: Urine (primarily as ganciclovir)

Dosage Oral:

Infants, Children, and Adolescents 4 months to 16 years: Prevention of CMV disease following kidney or heart transplantation: Dose (mg) = 7 x body surface area x creatinine clearance* once daily beginning within 10 days of transplantation; continue therapy until 100 days post-transplantation. Doses should be rounded to the nearest 25 mg increment; maximum dose: 900 mg/day.

*CrCl (mL/minute/1.73 m^2) = [k x Height (cm)] divided by serum creatinine (mg/dL)

Note: If the calculated CrCl is >150 mL/minute/1.73 m^2, then a maximum value of 150 mL/minute/1.73 m^2 should be used to calculate the dose.

Note: Calculated using *modified* Schwartz formula where k is as follows:

Patients <2 years: k = 0.45

Girls 2-16 years: k = 0.55

Boys 2 to <13 years: k = 0.55

Boys 13-16 years: k = 0.7

Adolescents >16 years and Adults:

CMV retinitis:

Induction: 900 mg twice daily for 21 days

Maintenance: Following induction treatment, or for patients with inactive CMV retinitis who require maintenance therapy: 900 mg once daily

Prevention of CMV disease following transplantation: 900 mg once daily beginning within 10 days of transplantation; continue therapy until 100 days (heart or kidney-pancreas transplant) or 200 days (kidney transplant) post-transplantation

Dosage adjustment in renal impairment:

Infants, Children, and Adolescents 4 months to 16 years: No dosage adjustment necessary; calculation adjusts for renal function.

Adolescents >16 years and Adults:

Induction dose:

CrCl ≥60 mL/minute: No dosage adjustment necessary

CrCl 40 to 59 mL/minute: 450 mg twice daily

CrCl 25 to 39 mL/minute: 450 mg once daily

CrCl 10 to 24 mL/minute: 450 mg every 2 days

CrCl <10 mL/minute:

Manufacturer's labeling: Use not recommended; ganciclovir (with appropriately specified renal dosage adjustment) should be used instead of valganciclovir

Alternate recommendations: HIV infected persons: Consider valganciclovir solution 200 mg 3 times weekly (Lucas, 2014).

Hemodialysis:

Manufacturer's labeling: Use not recommended; ganciclovir (with appropriately specified renal dosage adjustment) should be used instead of valganciclovir.

Alternate recommendations: HIV infected persons: Consider valganciclovir solution 200 mg 3 times weekly (Lucas, 2014); valganciclovir is dialyzable and should be administered following dialysis.

Maintenance/prevention dose:

CrCl ≥60 mL/minute: No dosage adjustment necessary

CrCl 40 to 59 mL/minute: 450 mg once daily

CrCl 25 to 39 mL/minute: 450 mg every 2 days

CrCl 10 to 24 mL/minute: 450 mg twice weekly

CrCl <10 mL/minute:

Manufacturer's labeling: Use not recommended; ganciclovir (with appropriately specified renal dosage adjustment) should be used instead of valganciclovir

Alternate recommendations: HIV infected persons: Consider valganciclovir solution 100 mg 3 times weekly (Lucas, 2014).

Hemodialysis:

Manufacturer's labeling: Use not recommended; ganciclovir (with appropriately specified renal dosage adjustment) should be used instead of valganciclovir.

Alternate recommendations: HIV-infected persons: Consider valganciclovir solution 100 mg 3 times weekly (Lucas, 2014); valganciclovir is dialyzable and should be administered following dialysis.

Dosage adjustment in hepatic impairment: There are no dosage adjustments provided in manufacturer's labeling (has not been studied).

Dietary Considerations Should be taken with meals.

Administration Valganciclovir should be taken with meals. The preferred dosage form for pediatric patients is the oral solution; however, valganciclovir tablets may used so long as the calculated dose is within 10% of the available tablet strength (450 mg).

Due to the carcinogenic and mutagenic potential, avoid direct contact with broken or crushed tablets, powder for oral solution, and oral solution. Consideration should be given to handling and disposal according to guidelines issued for antineoplastic drugs. However, there is no consensus on the need for these precautions.

Hazardous agent; use appropriate precautions for handling and disposal (NIOSH 2014 [group 2]).

Monitoring Parameters Retinal exam (at least every 4-6 weeks), CBC, platelet counts, serum creatinine

Dosage Forms

Solution Reconstituted, Oral:

Valcyte: 50 mg/mL (88 mL)

Tablet, Oral:

Valcyte: 450 mg

Generic: 450 mg

Extemporaneous Preparations Hazardous agent; use appropriate precautions for handling and disposal (NIOSH 2014 [group 2]).

Note: Commercial preparation is available (50 mg/mL)

A 60 mg/mL oral suspension may be with tablets and a 1:1 mixture of Ora-Sweet® and Ora-Plus®. Crush sixteen 450 mg tablets and reduce to a fine powder. Add 1 mL portions of chosen vehicle (10 mL total) and mix to a uniform paste; mix while adding the vehicle in incremental proportions to **almost** 120 mL; transfer to a calibrated amber glass bottle, rinse mortar with vehicle, and add quantity of vehicle sufficient to make 120 mL. Label "shake well" and "refrigerate". Stable for 35 days refrigerated.

Henkin CC, Griener JC, and Ten Eick AP, "Stability of Valganciclovir in Extemporaneously Compounded Liquid Formulations," *Am J Health Syst Pharm*, 2003, 60(7):687-90.

- **Valganciclovir Hydrochloride** *see* ValGANciclovir *on page 2121*
- **Valisone Scalp Lotion (Can)** *see* Betamethasone (Topical) *on page 255*
- **Valium** *see* Diazepam *on page 613*
- **Valium® (Can)** *see* Diazepam *on page 613*
- **Valorin [OTC]** *see* Acetaminophen *on page 32*
- **Valorin Extra [OTC]** *see* Acetaminophen *on page 32*
- **Valproate Semisodium** *see* Valproic Acid and Derivatives *on page 2123*
- **Valproate Sodium** *see* Valproic Acid and Derivatives *on page 2123*
- **Valproic Acid** *see* Valproic Acid and Derivatives *on page 2123*
- **Valproic Acid Derivative** *see* Valproic Acid and Derivatives *on page 2123*

Valproic Acid and Derivatives

(val PROE ik AS id & dah RIV ah tives)

Brand Names: U.S. Depacon; Depakene; Depakote; Depakote ER; Depakote Sprinkles; Stavzor

Brand Names: Canada Apo-Divalproex; Apo-Valproic; Depakene; Dom-Divalproex; Dom-Valproic Acid; Dom-Valproic Acid E.C.; Epival; Epival ECT; Mylan-Divalproex; Mylan-Valproic; Novo-Divalproex; Novo-Valproic; PHL-Divalproex; PHL-Valproic Acid; PHL-Valproic Acid E.C.; PMS-Divalproex; PMS-Valproic Acid; PMS-Valproic Acid E.C.; ratio-Valproic; Sandoz-Valproic

Index Terms 2-Propylpentanoic Acid; 2-Propylvaleric Acid; Dipropylacetic Acid; Divalproex Sodium; DPA; Valproate Semisodium; Valproate Sodium; Valproic Acid; Valproic Acid Derivative

Pharmacologic Category Anticonvulsant, Miscellaneous; Antimanic Agent; Histone Deacetylase Inhibitor

Use

Oral, IV: Monotherapy and adjunctive therapy in the treatment of patients with complex partial seizures; monotherapy and adjunctive therapy of simple and complex absence seizures; adjunctive therapy in patients with multiple seizure types that include absence seizures

Additional indications: Depakote, Depakote ER, Stavzor: Mania associated with bipolar disorder; migraine prophylaxis

Limitation of use: Do not administer to a woman of childbearing potential unless essential for the management of her condition.

Pregnancy Risk Factor X (migraine prophylaxis)/D (all other indications)

Pregnancy Considerations Adverse events have been observed in animal reproduction studies and in human pregnancies. **[U.S. Boxed Warning]: May cause major congenital malformations such as neural tube defects (eg, spina bifida) and decreased IQ scores following in utero exposure. Use is contraindicated in pregnant women for the prevention of migraine. Use is not recommended in women of childbearing potential for any other condition unless valproate is essential to manage her condition and alternative therapies are not appropriate. Effective contraception should be used during therapy.**

Valproic acid crosses the placenta (Harden 2009b). Neural tube defects, craniofacial defects, cardiovascular malformations and defects of other body systems have been reported. Information from the North American Antiepileptic Drug Pregnancy Registry notes a fourfold increase in congenital malformations with exposure to valproic acid monotherapy during the 1st trimester of pregnancy when compared to monotherapy with other antiepileptic drugs (AED). The risk of spinal bifida is ~1% to 2% (general population risk estimated to be 0.06% to 0.07%).

Nonteratogenic adverse effects have also been reported. Decreased IQ scores have been noted in children exposed to valproate in utero when compared to children exposed to other antiepileptic medications or no antiepileptic medications; the risk of autism spectrum disorders may also be increased. Fatal hepatic failure in the infant, and afibrinogenemia leading to fatal hemorrhage in the newborn have been noted in case reports following in utero exposure to valproic acid.

Current guidelines recommend complete avoidance of valproic acid and derivatives for the treatment of epilepsy in pregnant women whenever possible (Harden 2009a), especially when used for conditions not associated with permanent injury or risk of death. Effective contraception should be used during treatment. When pregnancy is being planned, consider tapering off of therapy prior to conception if appropriate; abrupt discontinuation of therapy may cause status epilepticus and lead to maternal and fetal hypoxia. Folic acid decreases the risk of neural tube defects in the general population; supplementation with folic acid should be used prior to conception and during pregnancy in all women, including those taking valproate.

A pregnancy registry is available for women who have been exposed to valproic acid. Patients may enroll themselves in the North American Antiepileptic Drug (NAAED) Pregnancy Registry by calling (888) 233-2334. Additional information is available at www.aedpregnancyregistry.org.

Breast-Feeding Considerations Valproate is excreted into breast milk. Breast milk concentrations of valproic acid have been reported as 1% to 10% of maternal concentration. The weight-adjusted dose to the infant has been calculated to be ~4% (Hagg, 2000). The manufacturer recommends that caution be used if administered to nursing women.

Contraindications Hypersensitivity to valproic acid, divalproex, derivatives, or any component of the formulation; hepatic disease or significant impairment; urea cycle disorders; pregnant women for the prevention of migraine; known mitochondrial disorders caused by mutations in mitochondrial DNA polymerase gamma (POLG; eg, Alpers-Huttenlocher syndrome [AHS]) or children <2 years of age suspected of having a POLG-related disorder

Warnings/Precautions Hazardous agent - use appropriate precautions for handling and disposal (NIOSH 2014 [groups 2 and 3]).

[U.S. Boxed Warning]: Hepatic failure resulting in fatalities has occurred in patients, usually in the initial 6 months of therapy; children <2 years of age are at considerable risk. Risk is also increased in patients with hereditary neurometabolic syndromes caused by DNA mutations of the mitochondrial DNA polymerase gamma (POLG) gene (eg, Alpers-Huttenlocher syndrome [AHS]). Other risk factors include organic brain disease, mental retardation with severe seizure disorders, congenital metabolic disorders, and patients on multiple anticonvulsants. Monitor patients closely for appearance of malaise, weakness, facial edema, anorexia, jaundice, and vomiting; discontinue immediately with signs/symptom of significant or suspected impairment. Liver function tests should be performed at baseline and at regular intervals after initiation of therapy, especially within the first 6 months. Hepatic dysfunction may progress despite discontinuing treatment. Should only be used as monotherapy and with extreme caution in children <2 years of age and/or patients at high risk for hepatotoxicity. Contraindicated with significant hepatic impairment.

[U.S. Boxed Warning]: Risk of valproate-induced acute liver failure and death is increased in patients with hereditary neurometabolic syndromes caused by DNA mutations of the mitochondrial polymerase gamma (POLG) gene (eg, Alpers-Huttenlocher syndrome [AHS]). Use is contraindicated in patients with known mitochondrial disorders caused by POLG mutations and children <2 years of age suspected of having a POLG-related disorder. Use in children ≥2 years of age suspected of having a POLG-related disorder only after other anticonvulsants have failed and with close monitoring for the development of acute liver injury. POLG mutation testing should be performed in accordance with current clinical practice.

[U.S. Boxed Warning]: Cases of life-threatening pancreatitis, occurring at the start of therapy or following years of use, have been reported in adults and children. Some cases have been hemorrhagic with rapid progression of initial symptoms to death. Promptly evaluate symptoms of abdominal pain, nausea, vomiting, and/or anorexia; should generally be discontinued if pancreatitis is diagnosed.

[U.S. Boxed Warning]: May cause major congenital malformations such as neural tube defects (eg, spina bifida) and decreased IQ scores following in utero exposure. Use is contraindicated in pregnant women for the prevention of migraine. Use is not recommended in women of childbearing potential for any other condition unless valproate is essential to manage her condition and alternative therapies are not appropriate. Effective contraception should be used during therapy.

May cause severe thrombocytopenia, inhibition of platelet aggregation, and bleeding. Hypersensitivity reactions affecting multiple organs have been reported in association with valproate use; may include dermatologic and/or hematologic changes (eosinophilia, neutropenia, thrombocytopenia) or symptoms of organ dysfunction.

Hyperammonemia and/or encephalopathy, sometimes fatal, have been reported following the initiation of valproate therapy and may be present with normal transaminase levels. Ammonia levels should be measured in patients who develop unexplained lethargy and vomiting, changes in mental status, or in patients who present with hypothermia (unintentional drop in core body temperature to <35°C/95°F). Discontinue therapy if ammonia levels are increased and evaluate for possible urea cycle disorder (UCD); contraindicated in patients with UCD. Evaluation of UCD should be considered for the following patients prior to the start of therapy: History of unexplained encephalopathy or coma; encephalopathy associated with protein load; pregnancy or postpartum encephalopathy; unexplained mental retardation; history of elevated plasma ammonia or glutamine; history of cyclical vomiting and lethargy; episodic extreme irritability, ataxia; low BUN or protein avoidance; family history of UCD or unexplained infant deaths (particularly male); or signs or symptoms of UCD (hyperammonemia, encephalopathy, respiratory alkalosis). Hypothermia has been reported with valproate therapy; hypothermia may or may not be associated with hyperammonemia; may also occur with concomitant topiramate therapy following topiramate initiation or dosage increase.

In vitro studies have suggested valproate stimulates the replication of HIV and CMV viruses under experimental conditions. The clinical consequence of this is unknown, but should be considered when monitoring affected patients.

Antiepileptics are associated with an increased risk of suicidal behavior/thoughts with use (regardless of indication); patients should be monitored for signs/symptoms of depression, suicidal tendencies, and other unusual behavior changes during therapy and instructed to inform their healthcare provider immediately if symptoms occur.

Intravenous valproate is not recommended for post-traumatic seizure prophylaxis in patients with acute head trauma; study results for this indication suggested increased mortality with IV valproate use compared to IV phenytoin. Anticonvulsants should not be discontinued abruptly because of the possibility of increasing seizure frequency; valproate should be withdrawn gradually to minimize the potential of increased seizure frequency, unless safety concerns require a more rapid withdrawal. Patients treated for bipolar disorder should be monitored closely for clinical worsening or suicidality; prescriptions should be written for the smallest quantity consistent with good patient care.

Reversible and irreversible cerebral and cerebellar atrophy have been reported; motor and cognitive function should be routinely monitored to assess for signs and symptoms of brain atrophy. CNS depression may occur with valproate use. Patients must be cautioned about performing tasks which require mental alertness (operating machinery or driving). Effects with other sedative drugs or ethanol may be potentiated. Use with caution in the elderly as the elderly may be more sensitive to sedating effects and dehydration; in some elderly patients with somnolence, concomitant decreases in nutritional intake and weight loss were observed. Reduce initial dosages in elderly and closely monitor fluid status, nutritional intake, somnolence, and other adverse events. Potentially significant drug-drug interactions may exist, requiring dose or frequency adjustment, additional monitoring, and/or selection of alternative therapy.

Medication residue in stool has been reported (rarely) with oral Depakote (divalproex sodium) formulations; some reports have occurred in patients with shortened GI transit times (eg, diarrhea) or anatomic GI disorders (eg, ileostomy, colostomy). In patients reporting medication residue in stool, it is recommended to monitor valproate level and clinical condition.

Adverse Reactions

Cardiovascular: Chest pain, edema, facial edema, hypertension, hypotension, orthostatic hypotension, palpitations, peripheral edema, tachycardia, vasodilatation

Central nervous system: Abnormal dreams, abnormal gait, abnormality in thinking, agitation, amnesia, anxiety, ataxia, catatonia, chills, confusion, depression, dizziness, drowsiness, dyskinesia, emotional lability, hallucination, headache, hyper-reflexia, hypertonia, insomnia, malaise, myasthenia, nervousness, pain, paresthesia, personality disorder, sleep disorder, speech disturbance, tardive dyskinesia, twitching, vertigo

Dermatologic: Alopecia, diaphoresis, erythema nodosum, furunculosis, maculopapular rash, pruritus, seborrhea, skin rash, vesiculobullous dermatitis, xeroderma

Endocrine & metabolic: Amenorrhea, menstrual disease, weight gain, weight loss

Gastrointestinal: Abdominal pain, anorexia, constipation, diarrhea, dysgeusia, dyspepsia, dysphagia, eructation, fecal incontinence, flatulence, gastroenteritis, gingival hemorrhage, glossitis, hematemesis, hiccups, increased appetite, nausea, oral mucosa ulcer, pancreatitis, periodontal abscess, stomatitis, vomiting, xerostomia

Genitourinary: Cystitis, dysmenorrhea, dysuria, urinary frequency, urinary incontinence, vaginal hemorrhage, vaginitis

Hematologic & oncologic: Ecchymoses, hypoproteinemia, petechia, prolonged bleeding time, thrombocytopenia (dose related)

Hepatic: Increased serum ALT, increased serum AST

Infection: Fungal infection, infection, viral infection

Local: Injection site reaction, pain at injection site

Neuromuscular & skeletal: Arthralgia, back pain, discoid lupus erythematosus, dysarthria, hypokinesia, leg cramps, myalgia, neck pain, neck stiffness, osteoarthritis, tremor, weakness

Ophthalmic: Conjunctivitis, diplopia, dry eye syndrome, eye pain, nystagmus, photophobia, visual disturbance (amblyopia, blurred vision)

Otic: Deafness, otitis media, tinnitus

Respiratory: Bronchitis, cough, dyspnea, epistaxis, flu-like symptoms, pharyngitis, pneumonia, rhinitis, sinusitis

Miscellaneous: Accidental injury, fever

Rare but important or life-threatening: Abnormal thyroid function tests, acute porphyria, aggressive behavior, agranulocytosis, anemia, aplastic anemia, bradycardia, brain disease (rare), breast hypertrophy, cerebral atrophy (reversible or irreversible), coma (rare), decreased bone mineral density, decreased plasma carnitine concentrations, decreased platelet aggregation, dementia, eosinophilia, erythema multiforme, Fanconi-like syndrome (rare, in children), galactorrhea, hemorrhage, hepatic failure, hepatotoxicity, hostility, hyperactivity, hyperammonemia, hyperammonemic encephalopathy (in patients with UCD), hyperglycinemia, hypersensitivity angiitis, hypersensitivity reaction, hypofibrinogenemia, hyponatremia, hypothermia, leukopenia, lupus erythematosus, lymphocytosis, macrocytosis, ostealgia, osteopenia, pancytopenia, parotid gland enlargement, polycystic ovary syndrome (rare), psychosis, severe hypersensitivity (with multiorgan dysfunction), SIADH, skin photosensitivity, sleep disorder, Stevens-Johnson syndrome, suicidal ideation, suicidal tendencies, toxic epidermal necrolysis (rare), urinary incontinence, urinary tract infection

Drug Interactions

Metabolism/Transport Effects **Substrate** of CYP2A6 (minor), CYP2B6 (minor), CYP2C19 (minor), CYP2C9 (minor), CYP2E1 (minor); **Note:** Assignment of Major/ Minor substrate status based on clinically relevant drug interaction potential; **Inhibits** CYP2C9 (weak); **Induces** CYP2A6 (moderate)

Avoid Concomitant Use

Avoid concomitant use of Valproic Acid and Derivatives with any of the following: Cosyntropin

Increased Effect/Toxicity

Valproic Acid and Derivatives may increase the levels/ effects of: Barbiturates; CarBAMazepine; Ethosuximide; LamoTRIgine; LORazepam; Paliperidone; Primidone; RisperiDONE; Rufinamide; Sodium Oxybate; Temozolomide; Tricyclic Antidepressants; Vorinostat; Zidovudine

The levels/effects of Valproic Acid and Derivatives may be increased by: ChlorproMAZINE; Cosyntropin; Felbamate; GuanFACINE; Primidone; Salicylates; Topiramate

Decreased Effect

Valproic Acid and Derivatives may decrease the levels/ effects of: Fosphenytoin-Phenytoin; OLANZapine; OXcarbazepine; Urea Cycle Disorder Agents

The levels/effects of Valproic Acid and Derivatives may be decreased by: Barbiturates; CarBAMazepine; Carbapenems; Ethosuximide; Fosphenytoin-Phenytoin; Mefloquine; Methylfolate; Mianserin; Orlistat; Protease Inhibitors; Rifampin

Food Interactions Food may delay but does not affect the extent of absorption. Management: May administer with food if GI upset occurs.

Preparation for Administration Hazardous agent; use appropriate precautions for handling and disposal (NIOSH 2014 [groups 2 and 3]).

IV: Prior to administration of the injectable solution, dilute in 50 mL of a compatible diluent.

Storage/Stability

Oral: Store at controlled room temperature.

IV: Store at controlled room temperature. Stable in D_5W, NS, and LR for at least 24 hours when stored in glass or PVC.

Mechanism of Action Causes increased availability of gamma-aminobutyric acid (GABA), an inhibitory neurotransmitter, to brain neurons or may enhance the action of GABA or mimic its action at postsynaptic receptor sites

Pharmacodynamics/Kinetics

Distribution: Total valproate: 11 L/1.73 m^2; free valproate 92 L/1.73 m^2

Protein binding (concentration dependent): 80% to 90%; free fraction: ~10% at 40 mcg/mL and ~18.5% at 130 mcg/mL; protein binding decreased in the elderly and with hepatic or renal dysfunction

Metabolism: Extensively hepatic via glucuronide conjugation (30% to 50% of administered dose) and 40% via mitochondrial beta-oxidation; other oxidative metabolic pathways occur to a lesser extent. The relationship between dose and total valproate concentration is nonlinear; concentration does not increase proportionally with the dose, but increases to a lesser extent due to saturable plasma protein binding. The kinetics of unbound drug are linear.

Bioavailability: Depakote ER: ~90% relative to IV dose and ~89% relative to delayed release formulation

Half-life elimination (increased in neonates, elderly and those with liver disease): Children >2 months: 7-13 hours; Adults: 9-19 hours

Time to peak, serum:

Oral: Depakote tablet: ~4 hours; Depakote ER: 4-17 hours; Stavzor: 2 hours

Rectal (off-label route): 1-3 hours (Graves, 1987)

Excretion: Urine (30% to 50% as glucuronide conjugate, <3% as unchanged drug)

Dosage

Seizure disorders: **Note:** Administer doses >250 mg daily in divided doses.

Oral:

Simple and complex absence seizures: Children and Adults: Initial: 15 mg/kg/day; increase by 5-10 mg/kg/ day at weekly intervals until therapeutic levels are achieved; maximum: 60 mg/kg/day. Larger maintenance doses may be required in younger children.

Complex partial seizures: Children ≥10 years and Adults: Initial: 10-15 mg/kg/day; increase by 5-10 mg/kg/day at weekly intervals until therapeutic levels are achieved; maximum: 60 mg/kg/day. Larger maintenance doses may be required in younger children.

Note: Regular release and delayed release formulations are usually given in 2-4 divided doses per day; extended release formulation (Depakote ER) is usually given once daily. Depakote ER is not recommended for use in children <10 years of age. In patients previously maintained on regular release valproic acid therapy (Depakene) who convert to delayed release valproate tablets or capsules (Depakote, Stavzor), the same daily dose and frequency as the regular release should be used; once therapy is stabilized, the frequency of Depakote or Stavzor may be adjusted to 2-3 times daily.

Conversion to Depakote ER from a stable dose of Depakote: Children ≥10 years and Adults: May require an increase in the total daily dose between 8% and 20% to maintain similar serum concentrations.

Conversion to monotherapy from adjunctive therapy: The concomitant antiepileptic drug (AED) can be decreased by ~25% every 2 weeks; dosage reduction of the concomitant AED may begin when valproate therapy is initiated or 1-2 weeks following valproate initiation.

IV: Total daily IV dose should be equivalent to the total daily dose of the oral valproate product; administer dose as a 60-minute infusion (≤20 mg/minute) with the same frequency as oral products; switch patient to oral products as soon as possible. Alternatively, rapid infusions of 1.5-6 mg/kg/minute have been used in clinical trials to quickly achieve therapeutic concentrations, and were generally well tolerated (Ramsay, 2003; Venkataraman, 1999; Wheless, 2004). One study reported undiluted valproic acid administered at ≤10 mg/kg/minute (dose of ≤30 mg/kg) was well tolerated (Limdi, 2007).

Rectal (off-label route): Children: Dilute syrup 1:1 with water for use as a retention enema; acute and maintenance dose: 6-15 mg/kg/dose (Graves, 1987)

Status epilepticus, refractory (off-label use): Adults: IV: Loading dose: 15-20 mg/kg administered at 20 mg/minute; maintenance dose: IV infusion: 1-5 mg/kg/hour (Gaitanis, 2003). Alternatively, median loading doses of 25-30 mg/kg (maximum dose: 45 mg/kg) administered at ≤6 mg/kg/minute have also been reported (Limdi, 2005; Misra, 2006; Sinha, 2000).

Mania: Adults: Oral:

Depakote tablet, Stavzor: Initial: 750 mg/day in divided doses; dose should be adjusted as rapidly as possible to desired clinical effect; maximum recommended dosage: 60 mg/kg/day

Depakote ER: Initial: 25 mg/kg/day given once daily; dose should be adjusted as rapidly as possible to desired clinical effect; maximum recommended dose: 60 mg/kg/day.

Migraine prophylaxis: Oral:

Children ≥12 years (Stavzor): 250 mg twice daily; adjust dose based on patient response, up to 1000 mg/day

Children ≥16 years and Adults (Depakote tablet): 250 mg twice daily; adjust dose based on patient response, up to 1000 mg/day

Adults (Depakote ER): 500 mg once daily for 7 days, then increase to 1000 mg once daily; adjust dose based on patient response; usual dosage range 500-1000 mg/day

Diabetic neuropathy (off-label use): Adults: Oral: 500-1200 mg/day (Bril, 2011)

Elderly: Oral, IV: Lower initial doses are recommended due to decreased elimination and increased incidences of somnolence in the elderly; no specific dosage recommendations are provided by the manufacturer. Upward titration should be done slowly and with close monitoring for adverse events (eg, sedation, dehydration, decreased nutritional intake). Safety and efficacy for use in patients >65 years have not been studied for migraine prophylaxis.

Dosage adjustment in renal impairment: Mild-to-severe impairment: No dosage adjustment necessary; however, due to decreased protein binding in renal impairment, monitoring only total valproate concentrations may be misleading.

Dosage adjustment in hepatic impairment:

Mild-to-moderate impairment: Not recommended for use in hepatic disease; clearance is decreased with liver impairment. Hepatic disease is also associated with decreased albumin concentrations and 2- to 2.6-fold increase in the unbound fraction. Free concentrations of valproate may be elevated while total concentrations appear normal, therefore, monitoring only total valproate concentrations may be misleading.

Severe impairment: Use is contraindicated.

Administration

Oral: Oral valproate products may cause GI upset; taking with food or slowly increasing the dose may decrease GI upset should it occur.

Depakote ER: Swallow whole; do not crush or chew.

Depakote Sprinkle capsules may be swallowed whole or capsule opened and sprinkled on small amount (1 teaspoonful) of soft food (eg, pudding, applesauce) to be used immediately (do not store or chew).

Depakene capsule, Stavzor: Swallow whole; do not chew.

IV: Following dilution to final concentration, manufacturer's labeling recommends administering over 60 minutes at a rate ≤20 mg/minute. Alternatively, more rapid infusion rates of 1.5-6 mg/kg/minute have been used in clinical trials to quickly achieve therapeutic concentrations, and were generally well tolerated (Ramsay, 2003; Wheless, 2004). One study reported undiluted valproic acid administered at ≤10 mg/kg/minute (dose of ≤30 mg/kg) was well tolerated (Limdi, 2007).

Hazardous agent - use appropriate precautions for handling and disposal (NIOSH 2014 [groups 2 and 3]).

Monitoring Parameters Liver enzymes (at baseline and frequently during therapy especially during the first 6 months), CBC with platelets (baseline and periodic intervals), PT/PTT (especially prior to surgery), serum ammonia (with symptoms of lethargy, mental status change), serum valproate levels; suicidality (eg, suicidal thoughts, depression, behavioral changes); motor and cognitive function (for signs or symptoms of brain atrophy)

Reference Range Note: In general, trough concentrations should be used to assess adequacy of therapy; peak concentrations may also be drawn if clinically necessary (eg, concentration-related toxicity). Within 2-4 days of initiation or dose adjustment, trough concentrations should be drawn just before the next dose (extended-release preparations) or before the morning dose (for immediate-release preparations). Patients with epilepsy should not delay taking their dose for >2-3 hours. Additional patient-specific factors must be taken into consideration when interpreting drug levels, including indication, age, clinical response, pregnancy status, adherence, comorbidities, adverse effects, and concomitant medications (Patsalos, 2008; Reed, 2006).

Therapeutic:

Epilepsy: 50-100 mcg/mL (SI: 350-700 micromole/L); although seizure control may improve at levels >100 mcg/mL (SI: 700 micromole/L), toxicity may occur at levels of 100-150 mcg/mL (SI: 700-1040 micromole/L)

Mania: 50-125 mcg/mL (SI: 350-875 micromole/L)

Toxic: Some laboratories may report >200 mcg/mL (SI: >1390 micromole/L) as a toxic threshold, although clinical toxicity can occur at lower concentrations. Probability of thrombocytopenia increases with total valproate levels ≥110 mcg/mL in females or ≥135 mcg/mL in males.

Epilepsy: Although seizure control may improve at levels >100 mcg/mL (SI: 700 micromole/L), toxicity may occur at levels of 100-150 mcg/mL (SI: 700-1050 micromole/L)

Mania: Clinical response seen with trough levels between 50-125 mcg/mL (SI: 350-875 micromole/L); risk of toxicity increases at levels >125 mcg/mL (SI: 875 micromole/L)

Additional Information Divalproex sodium is a compound of sodium valproate and valproic acid; divalproex dissociates to valproate in the GI tract.

Extended release tablets have 10% to 20% less fluctuation in serum concentration than delayed release tablets.

Extended release tablets are not bioequivalent to delayed release tablets.

Dosage Forms Considerations Strengths of divalproex sodium and valproate sodium products are expressed in terms of valproic acid

Dosage Forms

Capsule, Oral:
Depakene: 250 mg
Generic: 250 mg

Capsule Delayed Release, Oral:
Stavzor: 125 mg, 250 mg, 500 mg

Capsule Sprinkle, Oral:
Depakote Sprinkles: 125 mg
Generic: 125 mg

Solution, Intravenous:
Depacon: 100 mg/mL (5 mL)

Solution, Intravenous [preservative free]:
Generic: 100 mg/mL (5 mL); 500 mg/5 mL (5 mL)

Solution, Oral:
Generic: 250 mg/5 mL (473 mL)

Syrup, Oral:
Depakene: 250 mg/5 mL (480 mL)
Generic: 250 mg/5 mL (5 mL, 10 mL, 473 mL)

Tablet Delayed Release, Oral:
Depakote: 125 mg, 250 mg, 500 mg
Generic: 125 mg, 250 mg, 500 mg

Tablet Extended Release 24 Hour, Oral:
Depakote ER: 250 mg, 500 mg
Generic: 250 mg, 500 mg

Valrubicin (val ROO bi sin)

Brand Names: U.S. Valstar

Brand Names: Canada Valtaxin®

Index Terms *N*-trifluoroacetyladriamycin-14-valerate; AD32

Pharmacologic Category Antineoplastic Agent, Anthracycline; Antineoplastic Agent, Topoisomerase II Inhibitor

Use Intravesical treatment of BCG-refractory bladder carcinoma *in situ*

Pregnancy Risk Factor C

Dosage Adults: Intravesical: Bladder cancer: 800 mg once weekly (retain for 2 hours) for 6 weeks

Dosage adjustment for toxicity: In clinical trials (Steinberg, 2000), treatment was delayed for 1 week for the following adverse events: Grade 3 dysuria (not controlled with phenazopyridine), frequency/urgency lasting >24 hours, grade 2 gross hematuria (without clots) lasting >48 hours, grade 3 hematuria (with clots) lasting >48 hours. For local toxicities < grade 4 (eg, dysuria [not controlled with phenazopyridine] or severe bladder spasm), anticholinergic therapy (systemic or topical) or topical anesthesia was administered prior to subsequent instillations.

Dosage adjustment in renal impairment: No dosage adjustment provided in manufacturer's labeling. However, dosage adjustment unlikely due to low systemic absorption.

Dosage adjustment in hepatic impairment: No dosage adjustment provided in manufacturer's labeling. However, dosage adjustment unlikely due to low systemic absorption.

Additional Information Complete prescribing information should be consulted for additional detail.

Dosage Forms

Solution, Intravesical [preservative free]:
Valstar: 40 mg/mL (5 mL)

Valsartan (val SAR tan)

Brand Names: U.S. Diovan

Brand Names: Canada ACT Valsartan; Apo-Valsartan; Auro-Valsartan; Ava-Valsartan; Diovan; Mylan-Valsartan; PMS-Valsartan; Ran-Valsartan; Sandoz-Valsartan; Teva-Valsartan

Pharmacologic Category Angiotensin II Receptor Blocker; Antihypertensive

Use

Alone or in combination with other antihypertensive agents in the treatment of primary hypertension; reduction of cardiovascular mortality in patients with left ventricular dysfunction postmyocardial infarction; treatment of heart failure (NYHA Class II-IV)

The 2014 guideline for the management of high blood pressure in adults (Eighth Joint National Committee [JNC 8; James, 2013]) recommends initiation of pharmacologic treatment to lower blood pressure for the following patients:

- Patients ≥60 years of age with systolic blood pressure (SBP) ≥150 mm Hg or diastolic blood pressure (DBP) ≥90 mm Hg. Goal of therapy is SBP <150 mm Hg and DBP <90 mm Hg.
- Patients <60 years of age with SBP ≥140 mm Hg or DBP ≥90 mm Hg. Goal of therapy is SBP <140 mm Hg and DBP <90 mm Hg.
- Patients ≥18 years of age with diabetes and SBP ≥140 mm Hg or DBP ≥90 mm Hg. Goal of therapy is SBP <140 mm Hg and DBP <90 mm Hg.
- Patients ≥18 years of age with chronic kidney disease (CKD) and SBP ≥140 mm Hg or DBP ≥90 mm Hg. Goal of therapy is SBP <140 mm Hg and DBP <90 mm Hg.

In patients with CKD, regardless of race or diabetes status, the use of an ACE inhibitor (ACEI) or angiotensin receptor blocker (ARB) as initial therapy is recommended to improve kidney outcomes. In the general nonblack population (without CKD), including those with diabetes, initial antihypertensive treatment should consist of a thiazide-type diuretic, calcium channel blocker, ACEI, or ARB. In the general black population (without CKD), including those with diabetes, initial antihypertensive treatment should consist of a thiazide-type diuretic or a calcium channel blocker instead of an ACEI or ARB.

The ACCF/AHA 2013 heart failure guidelines recommend the use of ARBs (ie, candesartan, losartan, and valsartan) in patients with HF with reduced ejection fraction who cannot tolerate ACE inhibitors (due to cough) to reduce morbidity and mortality. They also suggest that ARBs are reasonable first-line alternatives to ACE inhibitors in patients already maintained on an ARB for other indications (ACCF/AHA [Yancy, 2013]).

According to the ACCF/AHA guidelines for the management of ST-elevation myocardial infarction (STEMI) and guidelines for the management of unstable angina/non-ST-elevation myocardial infarction (UA/NSTEMI), an angiotensin receptor blocker should be given to patients who, after STEMI or UA/NSTEMI, have indications for (eg, clinical or radiologic signs of heart failure or LVEF ≤0.4) but are intolerant to ACE inhibitors. Valsartan is preferred in patients with STEMI (ACCF/AHA [Anderson, 2013]; ACCF/AHA [O'Gara, 2013]).

Pregnancy Risk Factor D

Pregnancy Considerations **[U.S. Boxed Warning]: Drugs that act on the renin-angiotensin system can cause injury and death to the developing fetus. Discontinue as soon as possible once pregnancy is detected.** The use of drugs which act on the renin-angiotensin system are associated with oligohydramnios. Oligohydramnios, due to decreased fetal renal function, may lead to fetal lung hypoplasia and skeletal malformations. Use is also associated with anuria, hypotension, renal failure, skull hypoplasia, and death in the fetus/neonate. in The exposed fetus should be monitored for fetal growth, amniotic fluid volume, and organ formation. Infants exposed *in utero* should be monitored for hyperkalemia, hypotension, and oliguria (exchange transfusions or dialysis may be needed). These adverse events are generally associated with maternal use in the second and third trimesters.

Untreated chronic maternal hypertension is also associated with adverse events in the fetus, infant, and mother. The use of angiotensin II receptor blockers is not recommended to treat chronic uncomplicated hypertension in pregnant women and should generally be avoided in women of reproductive potential (ACOG, 2013).

Breast-Feeding Considerations It is not known if valsartan is found in breast milk. Due to the potential for serious adverse reactions in the nursing infant, the manufacturer recommends a decision be made whether to discontinue nursing or to discontinue the drug, taking into account the importance of treatment to the mother. The Canadian labeling contraindicates use in nursing women.

Contraindications Hypersensitivity to valsartan or any component of the formulation; concomitant use with aliskiren in patients with diabetes mellitus

Canadian labeling: Additional contraindications (not in U.S. labeling): Concomitant use with aliskiren in patients with moderate-to-severe renal impairment (GFR <60 mL/minute/1.73 m^2); pregnancy; breast-feeding

Warnings/Precautions [U.S. Boxed Warning]: Drugs that act on the renin-angiotensin system can cause injury and death to the developing fetus. Discontinue as soon as possible once pregnancy is detected. May cause hyperkalemia; avoid potassium supplementation unless specifically required by healthcare provider. During the initiation of therapy, hypotension may occur, particularly in patients with heart failure or post-MI patients. Use extreme caution with concurrent administration of potassium-sparing diuretics or potassium supplements, in patients with mild-to-moderate hepatic dysfunction (adjust dose), in those who may be sodium/water depleted (eg, on high-dose diuretics), and in the elderly; correct depletion first.

Use caution with unstented unilateral/bilateral renal artery stenosis. When unstented bilateral renal artery stenosis is present, use is generally avoided due to the elevated risk of deterioration in renal function unless possible benefits outweigh risks. Use with caution with preexisting renal insufficiency; significant aortic/mitral stenosis. May be associated with deterioration of renal function and/or increases in serum creatinine, particularly in patients with low renal blood flow (eg, renal artery stenosis, heart failure) whose glomerular filtration rate (GFR) is dependent on efferent arteriolar vasoconstriction by angiotensin II. Use caution in patients with severe renal impairment or significant hepatic dysfunction. Monitor renal function closely in patients with severe heart failure; changes in renal function should be anticipated and dosage adjustments of valsartan or concomitant medications may be needed. Potentially significant drug-drug interactions may exist, requiring dose or frequency adjustment, additional monitoring, and/or selection of alternative therapy. In surgical patients on chronic angiotensin receptor blocker (ARB) therapy, intraoperative hypotension may occur with induction and maintenance of general anesthesia.

Angioedema has been reported rarely with some angiotensin II receptor antagonists (ARBs) and may occur at any time during treatment (especially following first dose). It may involve the head and neck (potentially compromising airway) or the intestine (presenting with abdominal pain). Patients with idiopathic or hereditary angioedema or previous angioedema associated with ACE-inhibitor therapy may be at an increased risk. Prolonged frequent monitoring may be required, especially if tongue, glottis, or larynx are involved, as they are associated with airway obstruction. Patients with a history of airway surgery may have a higher risk of airway obstruction. Discontinue therapy immediately if angioedema occurs. Aggressive early management is critical. Intramuscular (IM) administration of epinephrine may be necessary. Do not readminister to patients who have had angioedema with ARBs.

Adverse Reactions

Cardiovascular: Hypotension, orthostatic hypotension, syncope

Central nervous system: Dizziness, fatigue, headache, orthostatic dizziness, vertigo

Endocrine & metabolic: Serum potassium increased, hyperkalemia

Gastrointestinal: Abdominal pain (including upper), diarrhea, nausea

Hematologic & oncologic: Neutropenia

Infection: Viral infection

Neuromuscular & skeletal: Arthralgia, back pain

Ophthalmic: Blurred vision

Otic: Vertigo

Renal: Increased blood urea nitrogen, increased serum creatinine, renal insufficiency

Respiratory: Cough

All indications: Rare but important or life-threatening: Alopecia, anaphylaxis, anemia, angioedema, anorexia, bullous dermatitis, decreased hematocrit, decreased hemoglobin, dyspepsia, flatulence, hepatitis (rare), hypersensitivity reaction, impotence, insomnia, liver function tests increased, microcytic anemia, myalgia, palpitation, paresthesia, photosensitivity, pruritus, renal failure, rhabdomyolysis, skin rash, taste disorder, thrombocytopenia (very rare), vasculitis, xerostomia

Drug Interactions

Metabolism/Transport Effects Substrate of SLCO1B1; **Inhibits** CYP2C9 (weak)

Avoid Concomitant Use There are no known interactions where it is recommended to avoid concomitant use.

Increased Effect/Toxicity

Valsartan may increase the levels/effects of: ACE Inhibitors; Amifostine; Antihypertensives; CycloSPORINE (Systemic); DULoxetine; Hydrochlorothiazide; Hypotensive Agents; Levodopa; Lithium; Nonsteroidal Anti-Inflammatory Agents; Obinutuzumab; Potassium-Sparing Diuretics; RisperiDONE; RiTUXimab; Sodium Phosphates

The levels/effects of Valsartan may be increased by: Alfuzosin; Aliskiren; Barbiturates; Brimonidine (Topical); Canagliflozin; Dapoxetine; Diazoxide; Eltrombopag; Eplerenone; Heparin; Heparin (Low Molecular Weight); Herbs (Hypotensive Properties); Hydrochlorothiazide; MAO Inhibitors; Nicorandil; Pentoxifylline; Phosphodiesterase 5 Inhibitors; Potassium Salts; Prostacyclin Analogues; Teriflunomide; Tolvaptan; Trimethoprim

Decreased Effect

The levels/effects of Valsartan may be decreased by: Herbs (Hypertensive Properties); Methylphenidate; Nonsteroidal Anti-Inflammatory Agents; Yohimbine

Food Interactions Food decreases the peak plasma concentration and extent of absorption by 50% and 40%, respectively. Management: Administer consistently with regard to food.

Storage/Stability Store at 25°C (77°F); excursions permitted to 15°C to 30°C (59°F to 86°F). Protect from moisture.

Mechanism of Action Valsartan produces direct antagonism of the angiotensin II (AT2) receptors, unlike the ACE inhibitors. It displaces angiotensin II from the AT1 receptor and produces its blood pressure-lowering effects by antagonizing AT1-induced vasoconstriction, aldosterone release, catecholamine release, arginine vasopressin release, water intake, and hypertrophic responses. This action results in more efficient blockade of the cardiovascular effects of angiotensin II and fewer side effects than the ACE inhibitors.

Pharmacodynamics/Kinetics

Onset of action: ~2 hours

Duration: 24 hours

Distribution: V_d: 17 L (adults)

Protein binding: 95%, primarily albumin

Metabolism: To inactive metabolite

Bioavailability: Tablet: 25% (range: 10% to 35%); suspension: ~40% (~1.6 times more than tablet)

Half-life elimination: ~6 hours

Time to peak, serum: 2 to 4 hours

Excretion: Feces (83%) and urine (13%) as unchanged drug

Dosage Oral:

Hypertension:

Children 6 to 16 years: Initial: 1.3 mg/kg once daily (maximum: 40 mg/day); dose may be increased to achieve desired effect; doses >2.7 mg/kg (maximum: 160 mg) have not been studied. **Note:** Use in patients <18 years of age is not approved in the Canadian labeling.

Adults: Initial: 80 mg or 160 mg once daily (in patients who are not volume depleted); dose may be increased to achieve desired effect; usual dosage range (ASH/ISH [Weber, 2014]): 80 to 320 mg daily; target dose (JNC8 [James, 2013]): 160 to 320 mg daily; maximum recommended dose: 320 mg daily

Heart failure: Adults: Initial: 40 mg twice daily; titrate dose to 80 to 160 mg twice daily, as tolerated; maximum daily dose: 320 mg. The ACCF/AHA 2013 heart failure guidelines suggest initial dose of 20 to 40 mg twice daily and a target dose of 160 mg twice daily (Yancy, 2013).

Left ventricular dysfunction after MI: Adults: Initial: 20 mg twice daily; titrate dose to target of 160 mg twice daily as tolerated; may initiate ≥12 hours following MI

Dosage adjustment in renal impairment:

CrCl ≥30 mL/minute: No dosage adjustment necessary.

CrCl <30 mL/minute: There are no dosage adjustments provided in the manufacturer's labeling; safety and efficacy have not been established.

Dialysis: Not significantly removed

Dosage adjustment in hepatic impairment:

Mild-to-moderate impairment: No dosage adjustment necessary; use caution in patients with liver disease. Patients with mild-to-moderate chronic disease have twice the exposure as healthy volunteers.

Severe impairment: There are no dosage adjustments provided in the manufacturer's labeling; has not been studied

Dietary Considerations Avoid salt substitutes which contain potassium. May be taken with or without food.

Administration Administer with or without food.

Monitoring Parameters Baseline and periodic electrolyte panels, renal function, BP; in HF, serum potassium during dose escalation and periodically thereafter

2013 ACCF/AHA Heart Failure guideline recommendations: Within 1 to 2 weeks after initiation, reassess blood pressure (including postural blood pressure changes), renal function, and serum potassium; follow closely after dose changes. Patients with systolic blood pressure <80 mm Hg, low serum sodium, diabetes mellitus, and impaired renal function should be closely monitored (Yancy, 2013)

Additional Information Valsartan may have an advantage over losartan due to minimal metabolism requirements and consequent use in mild-to-moderate hepatic impairment.

Dosage Forms

Tablet, Oral:

Diovan: 40 mg, 80 mg, 160 mg, 320 mg

Generic: 40 mg, 80 mg, 160 mg, 320 mg

Extemporaneous Preparations A 4 mg/mL oral suspension may be made from tablets, Ora-Plus®, and Ora-Sweet® SF. Add 80 mL of Ora-Plus® to an 8-ounce amber glass bottle containing eight valsartan 80 mg tablets. Shake well for ≥2 minutes. Allow the suspension to stand for a minimum of 1 hour, then shake for ≥1 minute. Add 80 mL of Ora-Sweet SF® to the bottle and shake for ≥10 seconds. Store in amber glass prescription bottles; label "shake well". Stable for 30 days at room temperature or 75 days refrigerated.

Diovan® prescribing information, Novartis Pharmaceuticals Corp, East Hanover, NJ, 2012.

◆ **Valsartan and Amlodipine** *see* Amlodipine and Valsartan *on page 126*

Valsartan and Hydrochlorothiazide

(val SAR tan & hye droe klor oh THYE a zide)

Brand Names: U.S. Diovan HCT

Brand Names: Canada Apo-Valsartan/HCTZ; Ava-Valsartan/HCT; Diovan HCT; Mylan-Valsartan HCTZ; Sandoz Valsartan HCT; Teva-Valsartan HCTZ; Valsartan-HCT; Valsartan-HCTZ

Index Terms Hydrochlorothiazide and Valsartan

Pharmacologic Category Angiotensin II Receptor Blocker; Antihypertensive; Diuretic, Thiazide

Use

U.S. labeling: Treatment of hypertension (initial, add-on, or as substitute for titrated components)

Canadian labeling: Treatment of mild-to-moderate hypertension where combination therapy is appropriate. Not indicated for initial treatment.

Pregnancy Risk Factor D

Dosage

Hypertension: Adults: Oral:

U.S. labeling: Dose is individualized; combination product may be used as initial therapy or substituted for individual components in patients currently maintained on both agents separately or in patients not adequately controlled with monotherapy (using one of the agents or an agent within same antihypertensive class).

Initial therapy: Valsartan 160 mg and hydrochlorothiazide 12.5 mg once daily; dose may be titrated after 1-2 weeks of therapy. Maximum recommended daily doses: Valsartan 320 mg; hydrochlorothiazide 25 mg.

Add-on/replacement therapy: Valsartan 80-320 mg and hydrochlorothiazide 12.5-25 mg once daily; dose may be titrated after 3-4 weeks of therapy. Maximum recommended daily dose: Valsartan 320 mg; hydrochlorothiazide 25 mg.

Canadian labeling: Dose is individualized; combination product may be used as substitute for individual components following successful titration of each component. Maximum recommended daily dose: Valsartan 320 mg; hydrochlorothiazide 25 mg. Not approved for initial therapy.

Dosage adjustment in renal impairment:

CrCl ≥30 mL/minute: No dosage adjustment necessary.

CrCl <30 mL/minute: No dosage adjustment provided in manufacturer's labeling (has not been studied). Use is contraindicated in patients with anuria (U.S. and Canadian labeling) and not recommended in severe impairment (Canadian labeling).

Dosage adjustment in hepatic impairment:

Mild-to-moderate impairment: No dosage adjustment necessary; use with caution. Patients with mild-to-moderate chronic disease have twice the exposure of valsartan as healthy volunteers.

Severe impairment: No dosage adjustment provided in manufacturer's labeling (has not been studied). The Canadian labeling does not recommend use in severe impairment.

Additional Information Complete prescribing information should be consulted for additional detail.

Dosage Forms

Tablet, oral: 80 mg/12.5 mg: Valsartan 80 mg and hydrochlorothiazide 12.5 mg; 160 mg/12.5 mg: Valsartan 160 mg and hydrochlorothiazide 12.5 mg; 160 mg/25 mg: Valsartan 160 mg and hydrochlorothiazide 25 mg; 320 mg/12.5 mg: Valsartan 320 mg and hydrochlorothiazide 12.5 mg; 320 mg/25 mg: Valsartan 320 mg and hydrochlorothiazide 25 mg

Diovan HCT®: 80 mg/12.5 mg: Valsartan 80 mg and hydrochlorothiazide 12.5 mg; 160 mg/12.5 mg: Valsartan 160 mg and hydrochlorothiazide 12.5 mg; 160 mg/25 mg: Valsartan 160 mg and hydrochlorothiazide 25 mg; 320 mg/12.5 mg: Valsartan 320 mg and hydrochlorothiazide 12.5 mg; 320 mg/25 mg: Valsartan 320 mg and hydrochlorothiazide 25 mg

◆ **Valsartan-HCT (Can)** *see* Valsartan and Hydrochlorothiazide *on page 2129*

◆ **Valsartan-HCTZ (Can)** *see* Valsartan and Hydrochlorothiazide *on page 2129*

◆ **Valsartan, Hydrochlorothiazide, and Amlodipine** *see* Amlodipine, Valsartan, and Hydrochlorothiazide *on page 127*

◆ **Valstar** *see* Valrubicin *on page 2127*

◆ **Valtaxin® (Can)** *see* Valrubicin *on page 2127*

◆ **Valtrex** *see* ValACYclovir *on page 2119*

◆ **Val-Vancomycin (Can)** *see* Vancomycin *on page 2130*

◆ **Vanceril** *see* Beclomethasone (Systemic) *on page 230*

◆ **Vancocin (Can)** *see* Vancomycin *on page 2130*

◆ **Vancocin HCl** *see* Vancomycin *on page 2130*

Vancomycin (van koe MYE sin)

Brand Names: U.S. First-Vancomycin 25; First-Vancomycin 50; Vancocin HCl

Brand Names: Canada JAMP-Vancomycin; PMS-Vancomycin; Sterile Vancomycin Hydrochloride, USP; Val-Vancomycin; Vancocin; Vancomycin Hydrochloride for Injection; Vancomycin Hydrochloride for Injection, USP

Index Terms Vancomycin Hydrochloride

Pharmacologic Category Glycopeptide

Use

IV: Treatment of patients with infections caused by staphylococcal species and streptococcal species

Oral: Treatment of *C. difficile*-associated diarrhea and treatment of enterocolitis caused by *Staphylococcus aureus* (including methicillin-resistant strains)

Pregnancy Risk Factor B (oral); C (injection)

Pregnancy Considerations Adverse events have not been observed in animal reproduction studies. Vancomycin crosses the placenta and can be detected in fetal serum, amniotic fluid, and cord blood (Bourget, 1991; Reyes, 1989). Adverse fetal effects, including sensorineural hearing loss or nephrotoxicity, have not been reported following maternal use during the second or third trimesters of pregnancy.

The pharmacokinetics of vancomycin may be altered during pregnancy and pregnant patients may need a higher dose of vancomycin. Maternal half-life is unchanged, but the volume of distribution and the total plasma clearance may be increased (Bourget, 1991). Individualization of therapy through serum concentration monitoring may be warranted. Vancomycin is recommended for the treatment of mild, moderate, or severe *Clostridium difficile* infections in pregnant women (ACG [Surawicz, 2013]). Vancomycin is recommended as an alternative agent to prevent the transmission of group B streptococcal (GBS) disease from mothers to newborns (ACOG, 2011; CDC, 2010).

Breast-Feeding Considerations Vancomycin is excreted in human milk following IV administration. If given orally to the mother, the minimal systemic absorption of the dose would limit the amount available to pass into the milk. Vancomycin is recommended for the treatment of mild, moderate, or severe *Clostridium difficile* infections in breast-feeding women (ACG [Surawicz, 2013]). Due to the potential for serious adverse reactions in the nursing infant, the manufacturer recommends a decision be made whether to discontinue nursing or to discontinue the drug, taking into account the importance of treatment to the mother. Nondose-related effects could include modification of bowel flora.

Contraindications Hypersensitivity to vancomycin or any component of the formulation

Warnings/Precautions May cause nephrotoxicity although limited data suggest direct causal relationship; usual risk factors include preexisting renal impairment, concomitant nephrotoxic medications, advanced age, and dehydration (nephrotoxicity has also been reported following treatment with oral vancomycin, typically in patients >65 years of age). If multiple sequential (≥2) serum creatinine concentrations demonstrate an increase of 0.5 mg/dL or ≥50% increase from baseline (whichever is greater) in the absence of an alternative explanation, the patient should be identified as having vancomycin-induced nephrotoxicity (Rybak, 2009). Discontinue treatment if signs of nephrotoxicity occur; renal damage is usually reversible.

May cause neurotoxicity; usual risk factors include preexisting renal impairment, concomitant neuro-/nephrotoxic medications, advanced age, and dehydration. Ototoxicity, although rarely associated with monotherapy, is proportional to the amount of drug given and the duration of treatment. Tinnitus or vertigo may be indications of vestibular injury and impending bilateral irreversible damage. Discontinue treatment if signs of ototoxicity occur. Prolonged therapy (>1 week) or total doses exceeding 25 g may increase the risk of neutropenia; prompt reversal of neutropenia is expected after discontinuation of therapy. Prolonged use may result in fungal or bacterial superinfection, including *C. difficile*-associated diarrhea (CDAD) and pseudomembranous colitis; CDAD has been observed >2 months postantibiotic treatment. Use with caution in patients with renal impairment or those receiving other nephrotoxic or ototoxic drugs; dosage modification required in patients with impaired renal function (especially elderly). Accumulation may occur after multiple oral doses of vancomycin in patients with renal impairment; consider monitoring trough concentrations in this circumstance.

Rapid IV administration may result in hypotension, flushing, erythema, urticaria, and/or pruritus. Oral vancomycin is only indicated for the treatment of pseudomembranous colitis due to *C. difficile* and enterocolitis due to *S. aureus* and is not effective for systemic infections; parenteral vancomycin is not effective for the treatment of colitis due to *C. difficile* and enterocolitis due to *S. aureus*. Clinically significant serum concentrations have been reported in patients with inflammatory disorders of the intestinal mucosa who have taken oral vancomycin (multiple doses) for the treatment of *C. difficile*-associated diarrhea. Although use may be warranted, the risk for adverse reactions may be higher in this situation; consider monitoring serum trough concentrations, especially with renal insufficiency, severe colitis, concurrent rectal vancomycin administration, and/or concomitant IV aminoglycosides. The Society for Healthcare Epidemiology of America (SHEA) and the Infectious Diseases Society of America (IDSA) suggest that it is appropriate to obtain trough concentrations when a patient is receiving long courses of ≥2 g/day in adults (SHEA/IDSA [Cohen, 2010]). **Note:** The SHEA, the IDSA, and the American College of Gastroenterology (ACG) recommend the use of oral metronidazole for initial treatment of mild to moderate *C. difficile* infection and the use of oral vancomycin for initial treatment of severe *C. difficile* infection (SHEA/IDSA [Cohen, 2010]; ACG [Surawicz, 2013]).

Adverse Reactions

Injection:

Cardiovascular: Hypotension accompanied by flushing

Central nervous system: Chills, drug fever

Dermatologic: Erythematous rash on face and upper body (red neck or red man syndrome)

Hematologic: Eosinophilia, reversible neutropenia

Local: Phlebitis

Rare but important or life-threatening: Drug rash with eosinophilia and systemic symptoms (DRESS), ototoxicity (rare; use of other ototoxic agents may increase risk), renal failure (limited data suggesting direct relationship), Stevens-Johnson syndrome, thrombocytopenia, vasculitis

Oral:

Cardiovascular: Peripheral edema

Central nervous system: Fatigue, fever, headache

Gastrointestinal: Abdominal pain, bad taste (with oral solution), diarrhea, flatulence, nausea, vomiting

Genitourinary: Urinary tract infection

Neuromuscular & skeletal: Back pain

Rare but important or life-threatening: Creatinine increased, interstitial nephritis, ototoxicity, renal failure, renal impairment, thrombocytopenia, vasculitis

Drug Interactions

Metabolism/Transport Effects None known.

Avoid Concomitant Use

Avoid concomitant use of Vancomycin with any of the following: BCG

Increased Effect/Toxicity

Vancomycin may increase the levels/effects of: Aminoglycosides; Colistimethate; Neuromuscular-Blocking Agents

The levels/effects of Vancomycin may be increased by: Nonsteroidal Anti-Inflammatory Agents; Piperacillin

Decreased Effect

Vancomycin may decrease the levels/effects of: BCG; Sodium Picosulfate; Typhoid Vaccine

The levels/effects of Vancomycin may be decreased by: Bile Acid Sequestrants

Preparation for Administration Injection: Reconstitute vials with 20 mL of SWFI for each 1 g of vancomycin (10 mL/500 mg vial; 20 mL/1 g vial; 100 mL/5 g vial; 200 mL/10 g vial). The reconstituted solution must be further diluted with at least 100 mL of a compatible diluent per 500 mg of vancomycin prior to parenteral administration.

Intrathecal (off-label route): Vancomycin is available as a powder for injection and may be diluted to 1-5 mg/mL concentration in preservative free 0.9% sodium chloride for administration into the CSF.

Storage/Stability

Capsules: Store at controlled room temperature of 15°C to 30°C (59°F to 86°F).

Injection: Reconstituted 500 mg and 1 g vials are stable for at either room temperature or under refrigeration for 14 days. **Note:** Vials contain no bacteriostatic agent. Solutions diluted for administration in either D_5W or NS are stable under refrigeration for 14 days or at room temperature for 7 days.

Premixed solution (manufacturer premixed): Store at -20°C (-4°F); once thawed, solutions are stable for 72 hours at room temperature or for 30 days refrigerated. Do not refreeze.

Mechanism of Action Inhibits bacterial cell wall synthesis by blocking glycopeptide polymerization through binding tightly to D-alanyl-D-alanine portion of cell wall precursor

Pharmacodynamics/Kinetics

Absorption: Oral: Poor; may be enhanced with bowel inflammation; IM: Erratic; Intraperitoneal: ~38%

Distribution: V_d: 0.4-1 L/kg; Distributes widely in body tissue and fluids, except for CSF

Relative diffusion from blood into CSF: Good only with inflammation (exceeds usual MICs)

Uninflamed meninges: 0-4 mcg/mL; serum concentration dependent

Inflamed meninges: 6-11 mcg/mL; serum concentration dependent

CSF:blood level ratio: Normal meninges: Nil; Inflamed meninges: 20% to 30%

Protein binding: ~50%

Half-life elimination: Biphasic: Terminal:

Newborns: 6-10 hours

Infants and Children 3 months to 4 years: 4 hours

Children >3 years: 2.2-3 hours

Adults: 5-11 hours; significantly prolonged with renal impairment

End-stage renal disease: 200-250 hours

Time to peak, serum: IV: Immediately after completion of infusion

Excretion: IV: Urine (80% to 90% as unchanged drug); Oral: Primarily feces

Dosage

Usual dosage range: Note: Initial IV dosing should be based on actual body weight; subsequent dosing adjusted based on serum trough vancomycin concentrations.

Infants >1 month, Children, and Adolescents: IV:

Manufacturer's labeling: 10 mg/kg/dose every 6 hours

Alternate recommendations: 15 mg/kg/dose (maximum: 2,000 mg/dose) every 6 hours (IDSA [Liu, 2011])

Adults:

IV:

Manufacturer's labeling: Usual dose: 500 mg every 6 hours **or** 1,000 mg every 12 hours

Alternate recommendations: 15 to 20 mg/kg/dose every 8 to 12 hours (ASHP/IDSA/SIDP [Rybak, 2009]); **Note:** Dose requires adjustment in renal impairment

Complicated infections in seriously ill patients: A loading dose of 25 to 30 mg/kg (based on actual body weight) may be used to rapidly achieve target concentrations (ASHP/IDSA/SIDP [Rybak, 2009]).

Oral: 500 to 2,000 mg daily in divided doses every 6 hours. **Note:** Not appropriate for systemic infections due to low absorption.

Indication-specific dosing:

Bacteremia (*S. aureus* [methicillin-resistant]) (off-label use): IV:

Children and Adolescents: 15 mg/kg/dose every 6 hours for 2 to 6 weeks depending on severity (IDSA [Liu, 2011])

Adults: 15 to 20 mg/kg/dose (based on actual body weight) every 8 to 12 hours for 2 to 6 weeks depending on severity. A loading dose of 25 to 30 mg/kg (based on actual body weight) may be used to rapidly achieve target concentrations in seriously ill patients (ASHP/IDSA/SIDP [Rybak, 2009]; IDSA [Liu, 2011]).

Brain abscess, subdural empyema, spinal epidural abscess (*S. aureus* [methicillin-resistant]) (off-label use): IV:

Children and Adolescents: 15 mg/kg/dose every 6 hours for 4 to 6 weeks (with or without rifampin) (IDSA [Liu, 2011])

Adults: 15 to 20 mg/kg/dose (based on actual body weight) every 8 to 12 hours for 4 to 6 weeks (with or without rifampin). A loading dose of 25 to 30 mg/kg (based on actual body weight) may be used to rapidly achieve target concentrations in seriously ill patients (ASHP/IDSA/SIDP [Rybak, 2009]; IDSA [Liu, 2011]).

Catheter-related infections (off-label use): Adults: Antibiotic lock technique (Mermel, 2009): 2 mg/mL ± 10 units heparin/mL **or** 2.5 mg/mL ± 2,500 **or** 5,000 units heparin/mL **or** 5 mg/mL ± 5,000 units heparin/mL (preferred regimen); instill into catheter port with a volume sufficient to fill the catheter (2 to 5 mL). **Note:** May use SWFI/NS or D_5W as diluents. Do not mix with any other solutions. Dwell times generally should not exceed 48 hours before renewal of lock solution. Remove lock solution prior to catheter use, then replace.

***C. difficile*-associated diarrhea (CDAD):**

Infants >1 month, Children, and Adolescents: Oral: 40 mg/kg/day in 3 to 4 divided doses for 7 to 10 days (maximum: 2,000 mg daily)

Adults:

Oral:

Manufacturer's labeling: 125 mg 4 times daily for 10 days

Alternate recommendations:

Mild to moderate disease unresponsive to metronidazole: 125 mg 4 times daily for 10 days (ACG [Surawicz, 2013])

Severe disease (defined as serum albumin <3 g/dL and either WBC ≥15,000 or abdominal tenderness): 125 mg times daily for 10 days (ACG [Surawicz, 2013])

Severe, complicated infection: 500 mg every 6 hours for 10 to 14 days with or without concurrent IV metronidazole. May consider vancomycin retention enema (in patients with complete ileus) (SHEA/IDSA [Cohen, 2010])

Severe and complicated disease, without abdominal distention: 125 mg 4 times daily with IV metronidazole (ACG [Surawicz, 2013])

Severe and complicated disease with significant abdominal distention, ileus, and/or toxic colon: 500 mg 4 times daily plus rectal vancomycin in combination with IV metronidazole (ACG [Surawicz, 2013])

Recurrent, severe infection (if initial regimen did not include vancomycin): 125 mg 4 times daily for 10 days (ACG [Surawicz, 2013])

Rectal (off-label route): Retention enema:

Severe, complicated infection in patients with ileus: 500 mg every 6 hours (in 100 mL 0.9% sodium chloride) with oral vancomycin with or without concurrent IV metronidazole (SHEA/IDSA [Cohen, 2010])

Severe and complicated disease with abdominal distention, ileus, and/or toxic colon: 500 mg 4 times daily (in 500 mL NS) in combination with oral vancomycin and IV metronidazole (ACG [Surawicz, 2013])

Endocarditis:

Native valve (*Enterococcus*, vancomycin MIC ≤4 mg/L) (off-label use): IV: Adults: 15 to 20 mg/kg/dose (based on actual body weight) every 8 to 12 hours. A loading dose of 25 to 30 mg/kg (based on actual body weight) may be used to rapidly achieve target concentrations in seriously ill patients (ASHP/IDSA/SIDP [Rybak, 2009]) **or** 1,000 mg every 12 hours for 4 to 6 weeks (combine with gentamicin for 4 to 6 weeks) (BSAC [Gould, 2012])

Native valve (*S. aureus* [methicillin-resistant]) (off-label use): IV:

Children: 15 mg/kg/dose every 6 hours for 6 weeks (AHA [Baddour, 2005]; IDSA [Liu, 2011])

Adults: 15 to 20 mg/kg/dose (based on actual body weight) every 8 to 12 hours for 6 weeks. A loading dose of 25 to 30 mg/kg (based on actual body weight) may be used to rapidly achieve target concentrations in seriously ill patients (ASHP/IDSA/SIDP [Rybak, 2009]; IDSA [Liu, 2011]). **Note:** European guidelines support the entire duration of therapy to be 4 weeks and in combination with rifampin (BSAC [Gould, 2012]).

Native or prosthetic valve (streptococcal [penicillin MIC >0.5 mg/L or patient intolerant to penicillin] (off-label use): IV: Adults: 15 to 20 mg/kg/dose (based on actual body weight) every 8 to 12 hours for 6 weeks. A loading dose of 25 to 30 mg/kg (based on actual body weight) may be used to rapidly achieve target concentrations in seriously ill patients (AHA [Baddour, 2005]; ASHP/IDSA/SIDP [Rybak, 2009]) **or** 1,000 mg every 12 hours for 4 to 6 weeks (combine with gentamicin for at least the first 2 weeks). **Note:** The longer duration of treatment (ie, 6 weeks) should be used for patients with prosthetic valve endocarditis (BSAC [Gould, 2012]).

Prosthetic valve (*Enterococcus*, vancomycin MIC ≤4 mg/L) (off-label use): IV: Adults: 15 to 20 mg/kg/dose (based on actual body weight) every 8 to 12 hours for 6 weeks. A loading dose of 25 to 30 mg/kg (based on actual body weight) may be used to rapidly achieve target concentrations in seriously ill patients (AHA [Baddour, 2005]; ASHP/IDSA/SIDP [Rybak, 2009]) **or** 1,000 mg every 12 hours for 6 weeks (combine with gentamicin for 6 weeks) (BSAC [Gould, 2012]).

Prosthetic valve (*S. aureus* [methicillin-resistant]) (off-label use): IV:

Children: 15 mg/kg/dose every 6 hours for at least 2 to 6 weeks depending on source, presence of endovascular infection, and metastatic foci of infection (IDSA [Liu, 2011]).

Adults: 15 to 20 mg/kg/dose (based on actual body weight) every 8 to 12 hours for at least 6 weeks (combine with rifampin for the entire duration of therapy and gentamicin for the first 2 weeks). A loading dose of 25 to 30 mg/kg (based on actual body weight) may be used to rapidly achieve target concentrations in seriously ill patients (ASHP/IDSA/SIDP [Rybak, 2009]; IDSA [Liu, 2011]).

Endophthalmitis (off-label use): Adults: Intravitreal: Usual dose: 1 mg/0.1 mL NS instilled into vitreum; may repeat administration, if necessary, in 2 to 3 days, usually in combination with ceftazidime or an aminoglycoside (Kelsey, 1995). **Note:** Based on concerns for retinotoxicity, some clinicians have recommended using a lower dose of 0.2 mg/0.1mL; may repeat in 3 to 4 days, if necessary (Gan, 2001).

Enterocolitis *(S. aureus):*

Infants >1 months, Children, and Adolescents: Oral: 40 mg/kg/day in 3 to 4 divided doses for 7 to 10 days (maximum: 2,000 mg/day)

Adults: Oral: 500 to 2,000 mg/day in 3 to 4 divided doses for 7 to 10 days (usual dose: 125 to 500 mg every 6 hours)

Group B streptococcus (neonatal prophylaxis): Adults: IV: 1000 mg every 12 hours until delivery. **Note:** Reserved for penicillin allergic patients at high risk for anaphylaxis if organism is resistant to clindamycin or where no susceptibility data are available (CDC, 2010).

Meningitis:

Infants >1 month, Children, and Adolescents:

IV: 15 mg/kg/dose every 6 hours (for empiric therapy, use in combination with a third-generation cephalosporin); duration of therapy should be individualized based upon clinical response (in general, 10 to 21 days) (IDSA [Tunkel, 2004]). For methicillin-resistant *S. aureus*, treat for 2 weeks (with or without rifampin) (IDSA [Liu, 2011]).

Intrathecal, intraventricular (off-label route): 5 to 20 mg/day (IDSA [Tunkel, 2004])

Adults:

IV: 15 to 20 mg/kg/dose (based on actual body weight) every 8 to 12 hours (for empiric therapy, use in combination with a third-generation cephalosporin; for patients >50 years, include ampicillin); duration of therapy should be individualized based upon clinical response (in general, 10 to 21 days). A loading dose of 25 to 30 mg/kg (based on actual body weight) may be used to rapidly achieve target concentration in seriously ill patients (ASHP/IDSA/SIDP [Rybak, 2009]; IDSA [Tunkel, 2004]). **Note:** For PCN-resistant *Streptococcus pneumoniae* (MIC ≥2 mcg/mL), combine with a third-generation cephalosporin (IDSA [Tunkel, 2004]). For methicillin-resistant *S. aureus*, treat for 2 weeks (with or without rifampin) (IDSA [Liu, 2011]).

Intrathecal, intraventricular (off-label route): 5 to 20 mg/day (IDSA [Tunkel, 2004])

Osteomyelitis (S. aureus [methicillin-resistant]) (off-label use): IV:

Children and Adolescents: 15 mg/kg/dose every 6 hours for 4 to 6 weeks (IDSA [Liu, 2011])

Adults: 15 to 20 mg/kg/dose (based on actual body weight) every 8 to 12 hours for a minimum of 8 weeks (with or without rifampin). A loading dose of 25 to 30 mg/kg (based on actual body weight) may be used to rapidly achieve target concentrations in seriously ill patients (ASHP/IDSA/SIDP [Rybak, 2009]; IDSA [Liu, 2011]).

Pneumonia:

Community-acquired pneumonia (CAP):

Infants >3 months and Children (IDSA/PIDS, 2011): IV:

Note: In children ≥5 years, a macrolide antibiotic should be added if atypical pneumonia cannot be ruled out.

Group A *Streptococcus* (alternative to ampicillin or penicillin in beta-lactam allergic patients): 40 to 60 mg/kg/day divided every 6 to 8 hours

Presumed bacterial (in addition to recommended antibiotic therapy), *S. pneumoniae*, moderate-to-severe infection (MICs to penicillin ≤2.0 mcg/mL) (alternative to ampicillin or penicillin): 40 to 60 mg/kg/day divided every 6 to 8 hours

S. aureus (methicillin-susceptible) (alternative to cefazolin/oxacillin): 40 to 60 mg/kg/day divided every 6 to 8 hours

S. aureus, moderate-to-severe infection (methicillin-resistant +/- clindamycin susceptible) (preferred): 40 to 60 mg/kg/day divided every 6 to 8 hours **or** dosing to achieve AUC/MIC >400

Alternate regimen: 60 mg/kg/day divided every 6 hours for 7 to 21 days, depending on severity (Liu, 2011)

S. pneumoniae, moderate-to-severe infection (MICs to penicillin ≥4.0 mcg/mL) (alternative to ceftriaxone in beta-lactam allergic patients): 40 to 60 mg/kg/day divided every 6 to 8 hours

Adults: *S. aureus* (methicillin-resistant): IV: 15 to 20 mg/kg/dose (based on actual body weight) every 8 to 12 hours for 7 to 21 days depending on severity. A loading dose of 25 to 30 mg/kg (based on actual body weight) may be used to rapidly achieve target concentrations in seriously ill patients (ASHP/IDSA/SIDP [Rybak, 2009]; IDSA [Liu, 2011]).

Healthcare-associated pneumonia (HAP): *S. aureus* (methicillin-resistant): IV:

Infants and Children: 60 mg/kg/day divided every 6 hours for 7 to 21 days depending on severity (IDSA [Liu, 2011])

Adults: 15 to 20 mg/kg/dose (based on actual body weight) every 8 to 12 hours for 7 to 21 days depending on severity. A loading dose of 25 to 30 mg/kg (based on actual body weight) may be used to rapidly achieve target concentrations in seriously ill patients (ASHP/IDSA/SIDP [Rybak, 2009]; IDSA [Liu, 2011]).

Prophylaxis against infective endocarditis: IV:

Children:

Dental, oral, or upper respiratory tract surgery: 20 mg/kg/dose administered 1 hour prior to the procedure. **Note:** American Heart Association (AHA) guidelines recommend prophylaxis only in patients undergoing invasive procedures and in whom underlying cardiac conditions may predispose to a higher risk of adverse outcomes should infection occur.

GI/GU procedure: 20 mg/kg (plus gentamicin 1.5 mg/kg) administered 1 hour prior to surgery. **Note:** Routine prophylaxis no longer recommended by the AHA.

Adults:

Dental, oral, or upper respiratory tract surgery: 1,000 mg 1 hour before surgery. **Note:** AHA guidelines now recommend prophylaxis only in patients undergoing invasive procedures and in whom underlying cardiac conditions may predispose to a higher risk of adverse outcomes should infection occur.

GI/GU procedure: 1,000 mg plus 1.5 mg/kg gentamicin 1 hour prior to surgery. **Note:** As of April 2007, routine prophylaxis no longer recommended by the AHA.

Prosthetic joint infection (off-label use): IV: Adults:

Enterococcus spp (penicillin-susceptible or -resistant), *Propionibacterium acnes*, streptococci (beta-hemolytic): 15 mg/kg every 12 hours for 4 to 6 weeks, followed by an oral antibiotic suppressive regimen (IDSA [Osman, 2013]).

Note: For penicillin-susceptible or -resistant *Enterococcus* spp, consider addition of an aminoglycoside; in penicillin-susceptible *Enterococcus*, beta-hemolytic streptococcus or *Propionibacterium acnes* infections, only use vancomycin if patient has penicillin allergy (IDSA [Osman, 2013]).

Staphylococci (oxacillin-susceptible or -resistant):15 mg/kg every 12 hours for 2 to 6 weeks in combination with rifampin followed by oral antibiotic treatment and suppressive regimens (IDSA [Osman, 2013]).

Sepsis/Septic shock (empiric treatment or treatment for specific sensitive organism): IV: Adults: 15 to 20 mg/kg/dose (based on actual body weight) every 8 to 12 hours. A loading dose of 25 to 30 mg/kg (based on actual body weight) may be used to rapidly achieve target concentrations in seriously ill patients (ASHP/IDSA/SIDP [Rybak, 2009]). The Society of Critical Care Medicine recommends administration of empiric antibiotics within 1 hour of identifying severe sepsis (SCCM [Dellinger, 2013]).

Septic arthritis (*S. aureus* [methicillin-resistant]) (off-label use): IV:

Children: 15 mg/kg/dose every 6 hours for minimum of 3 to 4 weeks (IDSA [Liu, 2011]).

Adults: 15 to 20 mg/kg/dose (based on actual body weight) every 8 to 12 hours for 3 to 4 weeks. A loading dose of 25 to 30 mg/kg (based on actual body weight) may be used to rapidly achieve target concentrations in seriously ill patients (ASHP/IDSA/SIDP [Rybak, 2009]; IDSA [Liu, 2011]).

Septic thrombosis of cavernous or dural venous sinus (*S. aureus* [methicillin-resistant]) (off-label use): IV:

Children: 15 mg/kg/dose every 6 hours for 4 to 6 weeks (with or without rifampin) (IDSA [Liu, 2011])

Adults: 15 to 20 mg/kg/dose (based on actual body weight) every 8 to 12 hours for 4 to 6 weeks (with or without rifampin). A loading dose of 25 to 30 mg/kg (based on actual body weight) may be used to rapidly achieve target concentrations in seriously ill patients (ASHP/IDSA/SIDP [Rybak, 2009]; IDSA [Liu, 2011]).

Skin and skin structure infections, complicated (*S. aureus* [methicillin-resistant]) (off-label use): IV:

Children: 15 mg/kg/dose every 6 hours for 7 to 14 days (IDSA, [Liu, 2011])

Adults: 15 to 20 mg/kg/dose (based on actual body weight) every 8 to 12 hours for 7 to 14 days. A loading dose of 25 to 30 mg/kg (based on actual body weight) may be used to rapidly achieve target concentrations in seriously ill patients (ASHP/IDSA/SIDP [Rybak, 2009]; IDSA [Liu, 2011]).

Surgical (perioperative) prophylaxis (off-label use): IV:

Children: 15 mg/kg/dose within 120 minutes prior to surgical incision. May be administered in combination with other antibiotics depending upon the surgical procedure (ASHP/IDSA/SIS/SHEA [Bratzler, 2013]).

Adults: 15 mg/kg within 120 minutes prior to surgical incision. May be administered in combination with other antibiotics depending upon the surgical procedure (ASHP/IDSA/SIS/SHEA [Bratzler, 2013]).

Note: For patients known to be colonized with methicillin-resistant *S. aureus*, a single 15 mg/kg preoperative dose may be added to other recommended agents for the specific procedure (ASHP/IDSA/SIS/SHEA [Bratzler, 2013]).

The Society of Thoracic Surgeons recommends 1,000 to 1,500 mg or 15 mg/kg over 60 minutes with completion within 1 hour of skin incision. Although not well established, a second dose of 7.5 mg/kg may be considered during cardiopulmonary bypass (STS [Engelman, 2007]).

Dosage adjustment in renal impairment:

Oral: No dosage adjustment provided in manufacturer's labeling, However, dosage adjustment unlikely due to low systemic absorption.

IV: Vancomycin levels should be monitored in patients with any renal impairment:

CrCl >50 mL/minute: Start with 15 to 20 mg/kg/dose (usual: 750 to 1,500 mg) every 8 to 12 hours

CrCl 20 to 49 mL/minute: Start with 15 to 20 mg/kg/dose (usual: 750 to 1,500 mg) every 24 hours

CrCl <20 mL/minute: Will need longer intervals; determine by serum concentration monitoring

Note: In the critically-ill patient with renal insufficiency, the initial loading dose (25 to 30 mg/kg) should not be reduced. However, subsequent dosage adjustments should be made based on renal function and trough serum concentrations.

Poorly dialyzable by intermittent hemodialysis (0% to 5%); however, use of high-flux membranes and continuous renal replacement therapy (CRRT) increases vancomycin clearance, and generally requires replacement dosing.

Intermittent hemodialysis (IHD) (administer after hemodialysis on dialysis days): Following loading dose of 15 to 25 mg/kg, give either 500 to 1,000 mg **or** 5 to 10 mg/kg after each dialysis session (Heintz, 2009). **Note:** Dosing dependent on the assumption of 3 times/week, complete IHD sessions.

Redosing based on pre-HD concentrations:

<10 mg/L: Administer 1,000 mg after HD

10 to 25 mg/L: Administer 500 to 750 mg after HD

>25 mg/L: Hold vancomycin

Redosing based on post-HD concentrations: <10 to 15 mg/L: Administer 500 to 1,000 mg

Peritoneal dialysis (PD):

Administration via PD fluid: 15 to 30 mg/L (15 to 30 mcg/mL) of PD fluid

Systemic: Loading dose of 1,000 mg, followed by 500 to 1,000 mg every 48 to 72 hours with close monitoring of levels

Continuous renal replacement therapy (CRRT) (Heintz, 2009; Trotman, 2005): Drug clearance is highly dependent on the method of renal replacement, filter type, and flow rate. Appropriate dosing requires close monitoring of pharmacologic response, signs of adverse reactions due to drug accumulation, as well as drug concentrations in relation to target trough (if appropriate). The following are general recommendations only (based on dialysate flow/ultrafiltration rates of 1 to 2 L/hour and minimal residual renal function) and should not supersede clinical judgment:

CVVH: Loading dose of 15 to 25 mg/kg, followed by either 1,000 mg every 48 hours **or** 10 to 15 mg/kg every 24 to 48 hours

CVVHD: Loading dose of 15 to 25 mg/kg, followed by either 1,000 mg every 24 hours **or** 10 to 15 mg/kg every 24 hours

CVVHDF: Loading dose of 15 to 25 mg/kg, followed by either 1,000 mg every 24 hours **or** 7.5 to 10 mg/kg every 12 hours

Note: Consider redosing patients receiving CRRT for vancomycin concentrations <10 to 15 mg/L.

Dosage adjustment in hepatic impairment:

Oral: No dosage adjustment provided in the manufacturer's labeling. However, dosage adjustment unlikely due to low systemic absorption.

IV: No dosage adjustment provided in manufacturer's labeling. However, degrees of hepatic dysfunction do not affect the pharmacokinetics of vancomycin (Marti, 1996).

Dietary Considerations May be taken with food.

Administration

Intravenous: Administer vancomycin with a final concentration not to exceed 5 mg/mL by IV intermittent infusion over at least 60 minutes (recommended infusion period of ≥30 minutes for every 500 mg administered). Not for IM administration.

If a maculopapular rash appears on the face, neck, trunk, and/or upper extremities (red man syndrome), slow the infusion rate to over 1½ to 2 hours and increase the dilution volume. Hypotension, shock, and cardiac arrest (rare) have also been reported with too rapid of infusion. Reactions are often treated with antihistamines and steroids.

Intrathecal (off-label route): Vancomycin is available as a powder for injection and may be diluted to 1 to 5 mg/mL concentration in preservative free 0.9% sodium chloride for intrathecal administration.

Intravitreal: (off-label use): Administer vancomycin intravitreally with a final concentration of 1.0 mg/0.1 mL NS (Kelsey, 1995). **Note:** Due to retinotoxicity, some clinicians recommend using a lower dose of 0.2 mg/0.1 mL NS (Gan, 2001).

Oral: Vancomycin powder for injection may be reconstituted and used for oral administration (SHEA/IDSA [Cohen, 2010]). Reconstituted powder for injection (not premixed solution) may be administered orally by diluting the reconstituted solution in 30 mL of water; common flavoring syrups may be added to improve taste. The unflavored, diluted solution may also be administered via nasogastric tube. Also see Extemporaneous Preparations section.

Rectal (off-label route): May be administered as a retention enema per rectum (SHEA/IDSA [Cohen, 2010]); 500 mg in 100 to 500 mL of NS, volume may depend on length of segment being treated. If sodium chloride causes hyperchloremia could use solution with lower chloride concentration (eg, LR) (ACG [Surawicz, 2013]).

Extravasation treatment: Monitor IV site closely; extravasation will cause serious injury with possible necrosis and tissue sloughing. Rotate infusion site frequently.

Monitoring Parameters Intravenous: Periodic renal function tests, urinalysis, WBC; serum trough vancomycin concentrations in select patients (eg, aggressive dosing, unstable renal function, concurrent nephrotoxins, prolonged courses)

Suggested frequency of trough vancomycin concentration monitoring (Rybak, 2009):

Hemodynamically stable patients: Draw trough concentrations at least once-weekly.

Hemodynamically unstable patients: Draw trough concentrations more frequently or in some instances daily.

Prolonged courses (>3-5 days): Draw at least one steady-state trough concentration; repeat as clinically appropriate.

Note: Drawing >1 trough concentration prior to the fourth dose for short course (<3 days) or lower intensity dosing (target trough concentrations <15 mcg/mL) is not recommended.

Oral/rectal therapy: Serum sample monitoring is not typically required; consider monitoring serum trough concentrations, especially with renal insufficiency, severe colitis, concurrent rectal vancomycin administration, and/or concomitant IV aminoglycosides.

Reference Range

Timing of serum samples: Draw trough just before the administration of a dose at steady-state conditions. Steady state conditions generally occur approximately after the fourth dose. Drawing peak concentrations is no longer recommended.

Therapeutic levels: Trough: ≥10 mcg/mL. For pathogens with an MIC ≤1 mcg/mL, the minimum trough concentration should be 15 mcg/mL to meet target AUC/MIC of ≥400 (see **"Note"** below). For complicated infections (eg, bacteremia, endocarditis, osteomyelitis, meningitis, and hospital-acquired pneumonia caused by *S. aureus*), trough concentrations of 15-20 mcg/mL are recommended to improve penetration and improve clinical outcomes (Liu, 2011; Rybak, 2009). The American Thoracic Society (ATS) guidelines for hospital-acquired pneumonia and the Infectious Disease Society of America (IDSA) meningitis guidelines also recommend trough concentrations of 15-20 mcg/mL.

Note: Although AUC/MIC is the preferred pharmacokinetic-pharmacodynamic parameter used to determine clinical effectiveness, trough serum concentrations may be used as a surrogate marker for AUC and are recommended as the most accurate and practical method of vancomycin monitoring (Liu, 2011; Rybak, 2009).

Toxic: >80 mcg/mL (SI: >54 micromole/L)

Additional Information Because of its long half-life, vancomycin should be dosed on an every 8- to 12-hour basis. Monitoring of trough serum concentrations is advisable in certain situations. "Red man syndrome", characterized by skin rash and hypotension, is not an allergic reaction but rather is associated with too rapid infusion of the drug. To alleviate or prevent the reaction, infuse vancomycin at a rate of ≥30 minutes for each 500 mg of drug being administered (eg, 1 g over ≥60 minutes); 1.5 g over ≥90 minutes.

Dosage Forms

Capsule, Oral:

Vancocin HCl: 125 mg, 250 mg

Generic: 125 mg, 250 mg

Solution, Intravenous:

Generic: 500 mg/100 mL (100 mL); 750 mg/150 mL (150 mL); 1 g/200 mL (200 mL)

Solution, Oral:

First-Vancomycin 25: 25 mg/mL (150 mL, 300 mL)

First-Vancomycin 50: 50 mg/mL (150 mL, 210 mL, 300 mL)

Solution Reconstituted, Intravenous:

Generic: 500 mg (1 ea); 750 mg (1 ea); 1000 mg (1 ea); 5000 mg (1 ea); 10 g (1 ea)

Solution Reconstituted, Intravenous [preservative free]:

Generic: 1000 mg (1 ea); 5000 mg (1 ea); 10 g (1 ea)

Extemporaneous Preparations Note: A vancomycin (25 mg/mL or 50 mg/mL) suspension is commercially available as a compounding kit (First-Vancomycin).

Using a vial of vancomycin powder for injection (reconstituted to 50 mg/mL), add the appropriate volume for the dose to 30 mL of water and administer orally or via NG tube. For oral administration, common flavoring syrups may be added to improve taste.

Vancomycin Hydrochloride for Injection, USP (prescribing information), Schaumburg, Il, APP Pharmaceuticals, LLC, 2011.

A vancomycin 25 mg/mL solution in Ora-Sweet® and water (1:1) may be prepared by reconstituting vancomycin for injection with sterile water, then dilute with a 1:1 mixture of Ora-Sweet® and distilled water to a final concentration of 25 mg/mL; transfer to amber prescription bottle. Stable for 75 days refrigerated or for 26 days at room temperature.

Ensom MH, Decarie D, and Lakhani A, "Stability of Vancomycin 25 mg/mL in Ora-Sweet and Water in Unit-Dose Cups and Plastic Bottles at 4°C and 25°C," *Can J Hosp Pharm*, 2010, 63(5):366-72.

◆ **Vancomycin Hydrochloride** *see* Vancomycin *on page 2130*

◆ **Vancomycin Hydrochloride for Injection (Can)** *see* Vancomycin *on page 2130*

◆ **Vancomycin Hydrochloride for Injection, USP (Can)** *see* Vancomycin *on page 2130*

◆ **Vandazole** *see* MetroNIDAZOLE (Topical) *on page 1357*

Vandetanib (van DET a nib)

Brand Names: U.S. Caprelsa

Brand Names: Canada Caprelsa

Index Terms AZD6474; Zactima; ZD6474; Zictifa

Pharmacologic Category Antineoplastic Agent, Epidermal Growth Factor Receptor (EGFR) Inhibitor; Antineoplastic Agent, Tyrosine Kinase Inhibitor; Antineoplastic Agent, Vascular Endothelial Growth Factor (VEGF) Inhibitor

Use Thyroid cancer: Treatment of metastatic or unresectable locally-advanced medullary thyroid cancer (symptomatic or progressive)

Pregnancy Risk Factor D

Pregnancy Considerations Animal reproduction studies have demonstrated teratogenic effects and fetal loss. Because vandetanib inhibits angiogenesis, a critical component of fetal development, adverse effects on pregnancy would be expected. Women of childbearing potential should be advised to avoid pregnancy and use effective contraception during and for 4 months following treatment with vandetanib. Canadian labeling recommends that nonsterile males employ reliable contraceptive methods (barrier method in conjunction with spermicide) during and for 2 months after vandetanib treatment.

Breast-Feeding Considerations It is not known if vandetanib is excreted in human breast milk. Due to the potential for serious adverse reactions in the nursing infant, a decision should be made to discontinue vandetanib or to discontinue breast-feeding, taking into account the importance of treatment to the mother.

Contraindications Congenital long QT syndrome

Canadian labeling: Additional contraindications (not in U.S. labeling): Hypersensitivity to vandetanib or any component of the formulation; persistent Fridericia-corrected QT interval (QTcF) ≥500 ms; uncorrected hypokalemia, hypomagnesemia, or hypocalcemia; uncontrolled hypertension

Warnings/Precautions Hazardous agent - use appropriate precautions for handling and disposal (NIOSH 2014 [group 1]). **[U.S. Boxed Warning]: May prolong the QT interval; torsade de pointes and sudden death have been reported. Do not use in patients with hypocalcemia, hypokalemia, hypomagnesemia, or long QT syndrome. Correct electrolyte imbalance prior to initiating therapy. Monitor electrolytes and ECG (to monitor QT interval) at baseline, at 2-4 weeks, at 8-12 weeks, and every 3 months thereafter; monitoring (at the same frequency) is required following dose reductions for QT prolongation or with dose interruptions >2 weeks. Avoid the use of QT-prolonging agents; if concomitant use with QT prolonging agents cannot be avoided, monitor ECG more frequently. Vandetanib has a long half-life (19 days), therefore, adverse reactions (including QT prolongation) may resolve slowly; monitor appropriately.** Ventricular tachycardia has also been reported. The potential for QT prolongation is dose-dependent. Do not initiate treatment unless QT interval, Fridericia-corrected QT interval (QTcF) is <450 msec. During treatment, if QTcF >500 msec, withhold vandetanib and resume at a reduced dose when QTcF is <450 msec. Do not use in patients with a history of torsade de pointes, congenital long QT syndrome, bradyarrhythmias or uncompensated heart failure. Patients with ventricular arrhythmias or recent MI were excluded from clinical trials. To reduce the risk of QT prolongation, maintain serum calcium and magnesium within normal limits and maintain serum potassium ≥4 mEq/L. Heart failure (HF) has been reported; monitor for signs and symptoms of HF; may require discontinuation (HF may not be reversible upon discontinuation). Hypertension and hypertensive crisis have been observed with vandetanib; monitor blood pressure and initiate or adjust antihypertensive therapy as needed; may require vandetanib dosage adjustment or treatment interruption; discontinue vandetanib (permanently) if blood pressure cannot be adequately controlled. Canadian labeling contraindicates use in uncontrolled hypertension.

Diarrhea has been reported with use; may cause electrolyte imbalance (closely monitor electrolytes and ECGs to detect QT prolongation resulting from dehydration); routine antidiarrheals are recommended; withhold vandetanib treatment until resolution for severe diarrhea; dose reduction is recommended when treatment is resumed. Stevens-Johnson syndrome and other serious skin reactions (including fatal) have been reported. Mild-to-moderate skin reactions, including acne, dermatitis, dry skin, palmar-plantar erythrodysesthesia syndrome, pruritus, and rash have also been reported. Withhold treatment for dermatologic toxicity of grade 3 or higher; consider a reduced dose or permanent discontinuation upon improvement in symptoms. Consider discontinuation for severe dermatologic toxicity. Mild-to-moderate toxicity has responded to corticosteroids (systemic or topical), oral antihistamines, and antibiotics (topical or systemic). Increased risk of photosensitivity is associated with use; effective sunscreen and protective clothing are recommended during and for at least 4 months after treatment discontinuation.

Reversible posterior leukoencephalopathy syndrome (RPLS) been observed with vandetanib; symptoms of RPLS include altered mental function, confusion, headache, seizure, or visual disturbances; generally associated with hypertension; consider discontinuing treatment if RPLS occurs. Serious and sometimes fatal hemorrhagic events have been reported with use; discontinue in patients with severe hemorrhage; do not administer in patients with a recent history of hemoptysis with ≥2.5 mL of red blood. Ischemic cerebrovascular events (some fatal) have been observed with vandetanib; discontinue treatment in patients with severe ischemic events (the safety of resuming treatment after an ischemic event has not been studied). Interstitial lung disease (ILD) or pneumonitis (including fatalities) has been reported with vandetanib. Patients should be advised to report any new or worsening respiratory symptoms; ILD should be suspected with nonspecific respiratory symptoms such as hypoxia, pleural effusion, cough or dyspnea. Interrupt therapy for acute or worsening pulmonary symptoms; discontinue if ILD diagnosis is confirmed.

Increased doses of thyroid replacement therapy have been required in patients with prior thyroidectomy; obtain TSH at baseline, at 2-4 weeks, 8-12 weeks, and every 3 months after vandetanib initiation; if signs and symptoms of hypothyroidism occur during treatment, evaluate thyroid hormone levels and adjust replacement therapy if needed. Dosage reduction is recommended in patients with moderate-to-severe renal impairment. Exposure is increased in patients with impaired renal function; closely monitor QT interval; has not been studied in patients with end stage renal disease requiring dialysis. Not recommended for use in patients with moderate-to-severe hepatic impairment. Potentially significant drug-drug interactions may exist, requiring dose or frequency adjustment, additional monitoring, and/or selection of alternative therapy. Due to the risk for serious treatment-related adverse events, use in patients whose disease is not progressive or symptomatic should be only be undertaken after careful consideration. **[U.S. Boxed Warning]: Vandetanib is only available through a restricted access program; prescribers and pharmacies must be certified with the restricted distribution program to prescribe and dispense vandetanib.**

Adverse Reactions

Cardiovascular: Cardiac failure, cerebral ischemia, hypertension, prolonged Q-T interval on ECG

Central nervous system: Depression, fatigue, headache, insomnia

Dermatologic: Acne vulgaris, alopecia, nail disease (inflammation, tenderness, paronychia), pruritus, skin photosensitivity, skin rash, xeroderma

Endocrine & metabolic: Hypercalcemia, hyperglycemia, hyperkalemia, hypermagnesemia, hypocalcemia, hypoglycemia, hypokalemia, hypomagnesemia, hypothyroidism, weight loss

Gastrointestinal: Abdominal pain, decreased appetite, dysgeusia, dyspepsia, nausea, pseudomembranous colitis, vomiting, xerostomia

Hematologic & oncologic: Anemia, hemorrhage, leukopenia, neutropenia, thrombocytopenia

Infection: Sepsis

Hepatic: Increased serum ALT, increased serum bilirubin

Neuromuscular & skeletal: Muscle spasm, weakness

Ophthalmic: Blurred vision, corneal changes (corneal edema, corneal opacity, corneal dystrophy, iris hyperpigmentation, keratopathy, arcus lipoides, corneal deposits, acquired corneal dystrophy)

Renal: Increased serum creatinine

Respiratory: Aspiration pneumonia, cough, nasopharyngitis, respiratory arrest, respiratory failure, upper respiratory tract infection

Rare but important or life-threatening: Cardiorespiratory arrest, interstitial pulmonary disease, palmar-plantar erythrodysesthesia, pancreatitis, pneumonitis, reversible posterior leukoencephalopathy syndrome, Stevens-Johnson syndrome, torsades de pointes, ventricular tachycardia

Drug Interactions

Metabolism/Transport Effects Substrate of CYP3A4 (major); **Note:** Assignment of Major/Minor substrate status based on clinically relevant drug interaction potential; **Inhibits** BCRP, P-glycoprotein

Avoid Concomitant Use

Avoid concomitant use of Vandetanib with any of the following: Bosutinib; CYP3A4 Inducers (Strong); Highest Risk QTc-Prolonging Agents; Ivabradine; Mifepristone; Moderate Risk QTc-Prolonging Agents; PAZOPanib; Silodosin; St Johns Wort; Topotecan; VinCRIStine (Liposomal)

Increased Effect/Toxicity

Vandetanib may increase the levels/effects of: Afatinib; Bisphosphonate Derivatives; Bosutinib; Brentuximab Vedotin; Colchicine; Dabigatran Etexilate; Digoxin; DOXOrubicin (Conventional); Edoxaban; Everolimus; Highest Risk QTc-Prolonging Agents; Ledipasvir; MetFORMIN; Naloxegol; PAZOPanib; P-glycoprotein/ABCB1 Substrates; Prucalopride; Rifaximin; Rivaroxaban; Silodosin; Topotecan; VinCRIStine (Liposomal)

The levels/effects of Vandetanib may be increased by: Ivabradine; Mifepristone; Moderate Risk QTc-Prolonging Agents; QTc-Prolonging Agents (Indeterminate Risk and Risk Modifying)

Decreased Effect

The levels/effects of Vandetanib may be decreased by: Bosentan; CYP3A4 Inducers (Moderate); CYP3A4 Inducers (Strong); Dabrafenib; Deferasirox; Siltuximab; St Johns Wort; Tocilizumab

Storage/Stability Store at 25°C (77°F); excursions permitted to 15°C to 30°C (59°F to 86°F).

Mechanism of Action Multikinase inhibitor; inhibits tyrosine kinases including epidermal growth factor reception (EGFR), vascular endothelial growth factor (VEGF), rearranged during transfection (RET), protein tyrosine kinase 6 (BRK), TIE2, EPH kinase receptors and SRC kinase receptors, selectively blocking intracellular signaling, angiogenesis and cellular proliferation

Pharmacodynamics/Kinetics

Absorption: Slow

Protein binding: ~90%; to albumin and alpha 1-acid-glycoprotein

Distribution: V_d: ~7450 L

Metabolism: Hepatic, via CYP3A4 to N-desmethyl vandetanib and via flavin-containing monooxygenase enzymes to vandetanib-N-oxide

Bioavailability: Not affected by food

Half life, elimination: 19 days

Time to peak: 6 hours (range: 4-10 hours)

Excretion: Feces (~44%); urine (~25%)

Dosage Note: Do not initiate treatment unless QTcF <450 msec. Avoid concomitant use of QT-prolonging agents and strong CYP3A4 inducers. To reduce the risk of QT prolongation, maintain serum calcium and magnesium within normal limits and maintain serum potassium ≥4 mEq/L.

Medullary thyroid cancer, locally-advanced or metastatic: Adults: Oral: 300 mg once daily, continue treatment until no longer clinically benefiting or until unacceptable toxicity

Dosage adjustment for toxicity:

Toxicity ≥ grade 3: Interrupt dose until resolves or improves to grade 1, then resume at a reduced dose

Dosage reduction: Reduce from 300 mg once daily to 200 mg once daily, further reduce if needed to 100 mg once daily. For recurrent toxicities, reduce dose to 100 mg once daily after symptom improvement to ≤ grade 1 toxicity, if continued treatment is warranted.

Management of specific toxicities:

Cardiac: QTcF >500 msec: Withhold dose until QTcF returns to <450 msec, then resume at a reduced dose

Diarrhea (severe): Withhold treatment until resolution. Dose reduction is recommended when treatment is resumed. Routine antidiarrheals are recommended. Closely monitor electrolytes and ECGs to detect QT prolongation resulting from dehydration.

Heart failure: May require discontinuation.

Hemorrhage (severe): Discontinue.

Hypertension: Initiate or adjust antihypertensive therapy as needed; may require vandetanib dosage adjustment or treatment interruption; discontinue permanently if blood pressure cannot be adequately controlled.

Interstitial lung disease (ILD)/pneumonitis: Interrupt therapy for acute or worsening pulmonary symptoms. Discontinue if ILD diagnosis is confirmed.

Ischemic cerebrovascular events (severe): Discontinue treatment (safety of resuming treatment after an ischemic event has not been studied).

Reversible posterior leukoencephalopathy syndrome (RPLS): Discontinue treatment.

Skin reactions: Withhold treatment for dermatologic toxicity of grade 3 or higher. Consider a reduced dose or permanent discontinuation upon improvement in symptoms. Consider permanent discontinuation for severe dermatologic toxicity. Mild-to-moderate toxicity has responded to corticosteroids (systemic or topical), oral antihistamines, and antibiotics (topical or systemic).

Dosage adjustment in renal impairment:

CrCl ≥50 mL/minute: No dosage adjustment necessary

CrCl <50 mL/minute: Reduce initial dose to 200 mg once daily; closely monitor QT interval

Dosage adjustment in hepatic impairment:

Mild impairment (Child-Pugh class A): No dosage adjustment provided in manufacturer's labeling.

Moderate and severe impairment (Child-Pugh class B or C): Use is not recommended.

Dietary Considerations May be taken with or without food.

Administration May be administered with or without food. Missed doses should be omitted if within 12 hours of the next scheduled dose. Do not crush tablet. If unable to swallow tablet whole or if nasogastric or gastrostomy tube administration is necessary, disperse one tablet in 2 ounces of water (noncarbonated only) and stir for 10 minutes to disperse (will not dissolve completely) and administer immediately. Rinse residue in glass with additional 4 ounces of water (noncarbonated only) and administer.

Hazardous agent; use appropriate precautions for handling and disposal (NIOSH 2014 [group 1]).

Monitoring Parameters Monitor electrolytes (calcium, magnesium, potassium), TSH, and ECG (QT interval) at baseline, at 2-4 weeks, at 8-12 weeks, and every 3 months thereafter; also monitor QT interval at same frequency for dose reduction due to QT interval or treatment delays >2 weeks (monitor electrolytes and ECG more frequently if diarrhea). Monitor renal function, hepatic function, blood pressure; monitor for signs and symptoms of heart failure, reversible posterior leukoencephalopathy syndrome (RPLS), pulmonary and skin toxicities

Dosage Forms

Tablet, Oral:

Caprelsa: 100 mg, 300 mg

Extemporaneous Preparations Hazardous agent: Use appropriate precautions for handling and disposal (NIOSH 2014 [group 1]).

An oral solution may be prepared using the tablet. Disperse one tablet in 2 ounces of water (noncarbonated only) and stir for 10 minutes to disperse (will not dissolve completely) and administer immediately. Rinse residue in glass with additional 4 ounces of water (noncarbonated only) and administer.

◆ **Vaniqa** *see* Eflornithine *on page 710*

◆ **Vaniqa® (Can)** *see* Eflornithine *on page 710*

◆ **Vanos** *see* Fluocinonide *on page 894*

◆ **Vanoxide-HC®** *see* Benzoyl Peroxide and Hydrocortisone *on page 248*

◆ **Vanquish Extra Strength Pain Reliever [OTC]** *see* Acetaminophen, Aspirin, and Caffeine *on page 37*

◆ **Vantas** *see* Histrelin *on page 1005*

◆ **Vantin** *see* Cefpodoxime *on page 388*

◆ **Vaprisol** *see* Conivaptan *on page 507*

◆ **VAQTA** *see* Hepatitis A Vaccine *on page 1001*

◆ **VAR** *see* Varicella Virus Vaccine *on page 2141*

Vardenafil (var DEN a fil)

Brand Names: U.S. Levitra; Staxyn

Brand Names: Canada Levitra; Staxyn

Index Terms Vardenafil Hydrochloride

Pharmacologic Category Phosphodiesterase-5 Enzyme Inhibitor

Use Erectile dysfunction: Treatment of erectile dysfunction (ED)

Pregnancy Risk Factor B

Pregnancy Considerations Teratogenic effects were not observed in animal studies; however, vardenafil is not indicated for use in women. No effects on sperm motility or morphology were observed in healthy males.

Breast-Feeding Considerations It is not known if vardenafil is excreted in breast milk. Vardenafil is not indicated for use in women.

Contraindications Coadministration with nitrates (either regularly and/or intermittently) and nitric oxide donors; hypersensitivity to vardenafil or any component of the formulation.

Warnings/Precautions There is a degree of cardiac risk associated with sexual activity; therefore, physicians may wish to consider the patient's cardiovascular status prior to initiating any treatment for erectile dysfunction. Use caution in patients with anatomical deformation of the penis (angulation, cavernosal fibrosis, or Peyronie's disease) and in patients who have conditions which may predispose them to priapism (sickle cell anemia, multiple myeloma, leukemia). Priapism, painful erection >6 hours in duration has been reported (rarely). Instruct patients to seek immediate medical attention if erection persists >4 hours.

Use is not recommended in patients with hypotension (<90/50 mm Hg); uncontrolled hypertension (>170/100 mm Hg); unstable angina or angina during intercourse; life-threatening arrhythmias, stroke, or MI within the last 6 months; cardiac failure or coronary artery disease causing unstable angina. Safety and efficacy have not been studied in these patients. Use caution in patients with left ventricular outflow obstruction (eg, aortic stenosis, idiopathic hypertrophic subaortic stenosis). Use caution with the elderly or those with hepatic impairment (Child-Pugh class B); dosage adjustment is needed. Potentially significant drug-drug interactions may exist, requiring dose or frequency adjustment, additional monitoring, and/or selection of alternative therapy. Concomitant use with all forms of nitrates is contraindicated. If nitrate administration is medically necessary, it is not known when nitrates can be safely administered following the use of vardenafil; however, when a 20 mg (film-coated tablet) was administered 24 hours prior to a 0.4 mg sublingual dose of nitroglycerin, no changes in blood pressure or heart rate were detected.

Rare cases of nonarteritic ischemic optic neuropathy (NAION) have been reported; patients who have already experienced NAION are at an increased risk of recurrence. Other risk factors for NAION include heart disease, diabetes, hypertension, smoking, age >50 years, or history of certain eye problems. Use with caution in these patients only when the benefits outweigh the risks. Sudden decrease or loss of hearing has been reported rarely; hearing changes may be accompanied by tinnitus and dizziness.

Safety and efficacy have not been studied in patients with the following conditions, therefore, use in these patients is not recommended at this time: Congenital QT prolongation, patients taking medications known to prolong the QT interval (avoid use in patients taking Class Ia or III antiarrhythmics); severe hepatic impairment (Child-Pugh class C); end-stage renal disease requiring dialysis; retinitis pigmentosa or other degenerative retinal disorders. Potential underlying causes of erectile dysfunction should be evaluated prior to treatment. Some products may contain phylalanine. Some products may contain sorbitol; do not use in patients with fructose intolerance.

Adverse Reactions

Cardiovascular: Flushing

Central nervous system: Headache

Central nervous system: Dizziness

Gastrointestinal: Dyspepsia, nausea

Neuromuscular & skeletal: Back pain, CPK increased

Respiratory: Nasal congestion, rhinitis, sinusitis

Miscellaneous: Flu-like syndrome

Rare but important or life-threatening: Abnormal ejaculation, amnesia (transient global), anaphylactic reaction, angina, angioedema, arthralgia, dyspnea, hearing decreased, hearing loss, hyper-/hypotension, insomnia, liver function tests abnormal, MI, myalgia, nonarteritic ischemic optic neuropathy (NAION), orthostatic hypotension, pain, photophobia, photosensitivity, priapism, pruritus, rash, somnolence, syncope, tachycardia, tinnitus, ventricular tachyarrhythmia, vertigo, vision abnormal, visual acuity reduced, visual field defects, vision loss (temporary or permanent)

Drug Interactions

Metabolism/Transport Effects Substrate of CYP3A4 (major); **Note:** Assignment of Major/Minor substrate status based on clinically relevant drug interaction potential

Avoid Concomitant Use

Avoid concomitant use of Vardenafil with any of the following: Alprostadil; Amyl Nitrite; Cobicistat; Conivaptan; Dapoxetine; Fusidic Acid (Systemic); Idelalisib; Phosphodiesterase 5 Inhibitors; Riociguat; Vasodilators (Organic Nitrates)

Increased Effect/Toxicity

Vardenafil may increase the levels/effects of: Alpha1-Blockers; Alprostadil; Amyl Nitrite; Antihypertensives; Bosentan; Highest Risk QTc-Prolonging Agents; Moderate Risk QTc-Prolonging Agents; Phosphodiesterase 5 Inhibitors; Riociguat; Vasodilators (Organic Nitrates)

The levels/effects of Vardenafil may be increased by: Alcohol (Ethyl); Aprepitant; Boceprevir; Ceritinib; Clarithromycin; Cobicistat; Conivaptan; CYP3A4 Inhibitors (Moderate); CYP3A4 Inhibitors (Strong); Dapoxetine; Dasatinib; Erythromycin (Systemic); Fluconazole; Fosaprepitant; Fusidic Acid (Systemic); Idelalisib; Itraconazole; Ivacaftor; Ketoconazole (Systemic); Lorcaserin; Luliconazole; Mifepristone; Netupitant; Posaconazole; Sapropterin; Simeprevir; Stiripentol; Telaprevir; Voriconazole

Decreased Effect

The levels/effects of Vardenafil may be decreased by: Bosentan; Etravirine

Food Interactions High-fat meals decrease maximum serum concentration 18% to 50%. Serum concentrations/toxicity may be increased with grapefruit juice. Management: Do not take with a high-fat meal. Avoid grapefruit juice.

Storage/Stability Store at 25°C (77°F); excursions permitted to 15°C to 30°C (59°F to 86°F). Keep oral disintegrating tablets sealed in blisterpack until ready to use.

Mechanism of Action Does not directly cause penile erections, but affects the response to sexual stimulation. The physiologic mechanism of erection of the penis involves release of nitric oxide (NO) in the corpus cavernosum during sexual stimulation. NO then activates the enzyme guanylate cyclase, which results in increased levels of cyclic guanosine monophosphate (cGMP), producing smooth muscle relaxation and inflow of blood to the corpus cavernosum. Vardenafil enhances the effect of NO by inhibiting phosphodiesterase type 5 (PDE-5), which is responsible for degradation of cGMP in the corpus cavernosum; when sexual stimulation causes local release of NO, inhibition of PDE-5 by vardenafil causes increased levels of cGMP in the corpus cavernosum, resulting in smooth muscle relaxation and inflow of blood to the corpus cavernosum; at recommended doses, it has no effect in the absence of sexual stimulation.

Pharmacodynamics/Kinetics

Onset of action: ~60 minutes

Absorption: Rapid

Distribution: V_d: 208 L

Protein binding: ~95% (parent drug and metabolite)

Metabolism: Hepatic via CYP3A4 (major), CYP2C and 3A5 (minor); forms metabolite (active)

Bioavailability: ~15%

Film-coated tablet: Elderly (≥65 years): AUC increased by 52%; Hepatic impairment (moderate, Child-Pugh class B): AUC increased by 160%

Oral disintegrating tablet: Elderly (≥65 years): AUC increased by 21% more compared to film-coated tablet. When administered with water, AUC decreases by 29%.

Half-life elimination: Terminal: Vardenafil and metabolite: 4 to 6 hours

Time to peak, plasma: 0.5 to 2 hours

Excretion: Feces (~91% to 95% as metabolites); urine (~2% to 6%)

Dosage Note: Oral disintegrating tablets should not be used interchangeably with film-coated tablets; patients requiring a dose other than 10 mg should use the film-coated tablets.

Oral: Erectile dysfunction:

Adults:

Film-coated tablet (Levitra): 10 mg administered ~60 minutes prior to sexual activity; dosing range: 5 to 20 mg; taken as one single dose and not taken more than once daily; maximum 20 mg daily

Oral disintegrating tablet (Staxyn): 10 mg administered ~60 minutes prior to sexual activity; maximum: 10 mg daily

Elderly ≥65 years: Film-coated tablet (Levitra): Consider a starting dose of 5 mg administered ~60 minutes prior to sexual activity; taken as one single dose and not taken more than once daily

Dosing adjustment with concomitant medications:

Alpha-blocker (dose should be stable at time of vardenafil initiation):

Film-coated tablet (Levitra): Initial vardenafil dose: 5 mg per day; if an alpha-blocker is added to vardenafil therapy, it should be initiated at the smallest possible dose and titrated carefully.

Oral disintegrating tablet (Staxyn): Do not use to initiate therapy. Initial therapy should be with film-coated tablets at lower doses. Patients who have previously used film-coated tablets may be switched to oral disintegrating tablets as recommended by healthcare provider. With coadministration, consider a time interval between dosing (eg, 6-hour interval).

CYP3A4 inhibitors:

Film-coated tablet (Levitra): The dosage of vardenafil may require adjustment in patients receiving potent CYP3A4 inhibitors (eg, atazanavir, clarithromycin, erythromycin, indinavir, itraconazole, ketoconazole, ritonavir, saquinavir).

For ritonavir, a single dose of vardenafil 2.5 mg should not be exceeded in a 72-hour period.

For indinavir, saquinavir, atazanavir, ketoconazole 400 mg daily, itraconazole 400 mg daily, and clarithromycin, a single dose of vardenafil 2.5 mg should not be exceeded in a 24-hour period.

For ketoconazole 200 mg daily, itraconazole 200 mg daily, and erythromycin, a single dose of vardenafil 5 mg should not be exceeded in a 24-hour period.

Oral disintegrating tablet (Staxyn): Concurrent use not recommended with potent or moderate CYP3A4 inhibitors (atazanavir, clarithromycin, erythromycin, indinavir, itraconazole, ketoconazole, ritonavir, saquinavir)

Dosage adjustment in renal impairment:

Mild, moderate, or severe impairment: No dosage adjustment necessary.

Hemodialysis: Use not recommended.

Dosage adjustment in hepatic impairment:

Mild impairment (Child-Pugh class A): No dosage adjustment necessary.

Moderate impairment (Child-Pugh class B):

Film-coated tablet (Levitra): Initial: 5 mg administered ~60 minutes prior to sexual activity (maximum dose: 10 mg daily); taken as one single dose and not taken more than once daily

Oral disintegrating tablet (Staxyn): Use not recommended.

Severe impairment (Child-Pugh class C): Has not been studied; use is not recommended by the manufacturer.

Dietary Considerations Avoid grapefruit juice. Some products may contain phenylalanine. Some products may contain sorbitol; do not use in patients with fructose intolerance.

Administration May be administered with or without food, 60 minutes prior to sexual activity.

Oral disintegrating tablet should not be removed from blister pack until administered. Using dry hands, place immediately on tongue. Tablet will dissolve within seconds; do not take with liquid. Do not crush, split, or chew.

Monitoring Parameters Monitor for response, adverse reactions, blood pressure, and heart rate.

Dosage Forms

Tablet, Oral:

Levitra: 2.5 mg, 5 mg, 10 mg, 20 mg

Tablet Dispersible, Oral:

Staxyn: 10 mg

◆ **Vardenafil Hydrochloride** *see* Vardenafil *on page 2138*

Varenicline (var e NI kleen)

Brand Names: U.S. Chantix; Chantix Continuing Month Pak; Chantix Starting Month Pak

Brand Names: Canada Champix®

Index Terms Varenicline Tartrate

Pharmacologic Category Partial Nicotine Agonist; Smoking Cessation Aid

Use Smoking cessation: As an aid to smoking cessation treatment

Pregnancy Risk Factor C

Pregnancy Considerations Adverse events have been observed in animal reproduction studies.

Breast-Feeding Considerations It is not known if varenicline is excreted in breast milk. Due to the potential for serious adverse reactions in the nursing infant, the manufacturer recommends a decision be made whether to discontinue nursing or to discontinue the drug, taking into account the importance of treatment to the mother.

Contraindications Serious hypersensitivity reactions or skin reactions to varenicline or any component of the formulation

Warnings/Precautions [U.S. Boxed Warning]: Serious neuropsychiatric events (including depression, suicidal thoughts, and suicide) have been reported with ▶

use; some cases may have been complicated by symptoms of nicotine withdrawal following smoking cessation. Smoking cessation (with or without treatment) is associated with nicotine withdrawal symptoms and the exacerbation of underlying psychiatric illness; however, some of the behavioral disturbances were reported in treated patients who continued to smoke. Neuropsychiatric symptoms (eg, mood disturbances, psychosis, hostility) have occurred in patients with and without preexisting psychiatric disease; many cases resolved following therapy discontinuation although in some cases, symptoms persisted. Monitor all patients for behavioral changes and psychiatric symptoms (eg, agitation, depression, suicidal behavior, suicidal ideation); inform patients to discontinue treatment and contact their healthcare provider immediately if they experience any behavioral and/or mood changes. Patients with preexisting psychiatric illness (eg, bipolar disorder, major severe depression, schizophrenia) were not studied in premarketing clinical trials and limited safety data is available from postmarketing studies. Due to rare neuropsychiatric events, caution is warranted if treatment is initiated; worsening of psychiatric illness has been reported. **[U.S. Boxed Warning]: Before prescribing, the risks of serious neuropsychiatric events must be weighed against the immediate and long term benefits of smoking abstinence for each patient.**

Post-marketing reports of hypersensitivity reactions (including angioedema) and rare cases of serious skin reactions (including Stevens-Johnson syndrome and erythema multiforme) have been reported. Patients should be instructed to discontinue use and contact healthcare provider if signs/symptoms occur. Treatment may increase risk of cardiovascular events. A meta-analysis of 15 clinical trials, including a placebo-controlled trial in patients with stable cardiovascular disease, showed an increased incidence of major cardiovascular events (combined outcome of cardiovascular-related death, nonfatal MI, nonfatal stroke) in patients using varenicline compared with placebo. Cardiovascular events were uncommon in both the varenicline and placebo groups. These findings did not reach statistical significance, although data was consistent. Events occurred primarily in patients with known cardiovascular disease. The meta-analysis also showed a lower incidence of all-cause and cardiovascular mortality in varenicline-treated patients, although this was not statistically significant either. Seizures have been reported in patients with or without a history of seizures. Seizures generally occurred within the first month of therapy. Consider the risks against the benefits before initiating in patients with a history of seizures or other factors that can lower the seizure threshold; discontinue use if seizures occur during therapy. Dose-dependent nausea may occur; both transient and persistent nausea has been reported. Dosage reduction may be considered for intolerable nausea. May cause CNS depression, which may impair physical or mental abilities; patients must be cautioned about performing tasks which require mental alertness (eg, operating machinery or driving). There have been postmarketing reports of traffic accidents, near-miss incidents in traffic, or other accidental injuries in patients taking varenicline.

Use caution in renal dysfunction; dosage adjustment required with severe impairment. Potentially significant drug-drug interactions may exist, requiring dose or frequency adjustment, additional monitoring, and/or selection of alternative therapy. Consult drug interactions database for more detailed information.

Adverse Reactions

Cardiovascular: Angina pectoris, chest pain, myocardial infarction, peripheral edema

Central nervous system: Abnormal dreams, agitation, depression, drowsiness, headache, hostility, insomnia, irritability, lethargy, malaise, nightmares, sleep disorder, suicidal ideation, tension

Dermatologic: Skin rash

Gastrointestinal: Abdominal pain, anorexia, constipation, diarrhea, dysgeusia, dyspepsia, flatulence, gastroesophageal reflux disease, increased appetite, nausea, vomiting, xerostomia

Respiratory: Dyspnea, rhinorrhea, upper respiratory tract infection

Rare but important or life-threatening: Acute renal failure, amnesia, anemia, atrial fibrillation, Bell's palsy, cataract (subcapsular), cerebrovascular accident, conjunctivitis, cor pulmonale, coronary artery disease, decreased visual acuity, diabetes mellitus, dissociative disorder, dysarthria, dysphagia, ECG abnormality, eczema, enterocolitis, erectile dysfunction, erythema multiforme, gallbladder disease, gastrointestinal hemorrhage, homicidal ideation, hyperhidrosis, hyperlipidemia, hypersensitivity, hypoglycemia, hypokalemia, intestinal obstruction, leukocytosis, loss of consciousness, lymphadenopathy, mania, Meniere's disease, migraine, multiple sclerosis, myositis, nephrolithiasis, nocturnal amblyopia, nystagmus, ophthalmic vascular disease, oral mucosa ulcer, osteoporosis, pancreatitis, panic, photophobia, psychomotor agitation, psychomotor retardation, psychosis, pulmonary embolism, restless leg syndrome, seizure, skin photosensitivity, splenomegaly, Stevens-Johnson syndrome, syncope, tachycardia, thrombocytopenia, thrombosis, thyroid disease, transient blindness, transient ischemic attacks, urinary retention, ventricular premature contractions

Drug Interactions

Metabolism/Transport Effects **Substrate** of OCT2

Avoid Concomitant Use There are no known interactions where it is recommended to avoid concomitant use.

Increased Effect/Toxicity

Varenicline may increase the levels/effects of: Alcohol (Ethyl)

The levels/effects of Varenicline may be increased by: BuPROPion; H2-Antagonists; Quinolone Antibiotics; Trimethoprim

Decreased Effect There are no known significant interactions involving a decrease in effect.

Storage/Stability Store at 25°C (77°F); excursions permitted to 15°C to 30°C (59°F to 86°F).

Mechanism of Action Partial neuronal α_4 β_2 nicotinic receptor agonist; prevents nicotine stimulation of mesolimbic dopamine system associated with nicotine addiction. Also binds to 5-HT_3 receptor (significance not determined) with moderate affinity. Varenicline stimulates dopamine activity but to a much smaller degree than nicotine does, resulting in decreased craving and withdrawal symptoms.

Pharmacodynamics/Kinetics

Absorption: Well absorbed; unaffected by food

Protein binding: ≤20%

Metabolism: Minimal (<10% of clearance is through metabolism)

Bioavailability: ~90%

Half-life elimination: ~24 hours

Time to peak, plasma: ~3 to 4 hours

Excretion: Urine (92% as unchanged drug)

Dosage Smoking cessation: Adults: Oral:

Initial:

- Days 1 to 3: 0.5 mg once daily
- Days 4 to 7: 0.5 mg twice daily

Maintenance (≥ Day 8):

- U.S. labeling: 1 mg twice daily for 11 weeks
- Canadian labeling: 0.5 to 1 mg twice daily for 11 weeks

Note: Start 1 week before target quit date. Alternatively, patients may consider setting a quit date up to 35 days after initiation of varenicline and then quit smoking between 8 to 35 days of treatment (some data suggest that an extended pretreatment regimen may result in higher abstinence rates [Hajek, 2011]). If patient successfully quits smoking at the end of the 12 weeks, may continue for another 12 weeks to help maintain success. Patients who are motivated to quit and do not succeed in stopping smoking during prior therapy, or who relapse after treatment, should be encouraged to make another attempt with varenicline once factors contributing to the failed attempt have been identified and addressed.

Dosage adjustment for toxicity: Patients who cannot tolerate adverse events may require temporary (or permanent) reduction in dose.

Dosage adjustment in renal impairment:

CrCl ≥30 mL/minute: No dosage adjustment necessary.

CrCl <30 mL/minute: Initial: 0.5 mg once daily; maximum dose: 0.5 mg twice daily

End-stage renal disease (ESRD) (receiving hemodialysis): Maximum dose: 0.5 mg once daily

Dosage adjustment in hepatic impairment: No dosage adjustment necessary.

Dietary Considerations Take after eating and with a full glass of water to decrease gastric upset.

Administration Administer after eating and with a full glass of water.

Monitoring Parameters Monitor for behavioral changes and psychiatric symptoms (eg, agitation, depression, suicidal behavior, suicidal ideation).

Additional Information In all studies, patients received an educational booklet on smoking cessation and received up to 10 minutes of counseling at each weekly visit. Dosing started 1 week before target quit date. Successful cessation of smoking may alter pharmacokinetic properties of other medications (eg, theophylline, warfarin, insulin).

Dosage Forms

Tablet, Oral:

Chantix: 0.5 mg, 1 mg

Chantix Continuing Month Pak: 1 mg

Chantix Starting Month Pak: 0.5 mg x 11 & 1 mg x 42

◆ **Varenicline Tartrate** *see* Varenicline *on page 2139*

◆ **Varicella, Measles, Mumps, and Rubella Vaccine** *see* Measles, Mumps, Rubella, and Varicella Virus Vaccine *on page 1274*

Varicella Virus Vaccine

(var i SEL a VYE rus vak SEEN)

Brand Names: U.S. Varivax

Brand Names: Canada Varilrix; Varivax III

Index Terms Chickenpox Vaccine; VAR; Varicella-Zoster Virus (VZV) Vaccine (Varicella); VZV Vaccine (Varicella)

Pharmacologic Category Vaccine, Live (Viral)

Additional Appendix Information

Immunization Administration Recommendations *on page 2250*

Immunization Recommendations *on page 2255*

Use

Varicella prevention: For the prevention of varicella in persons 12 months and older

The Advisory Committee on Immunization Practices (ACIP) recommends vaccination for all children, adolescents, and adults who do not have evidence of immunity (CDC/ACIP [Marin, 2007]). Vaccination is especially important for:

- Healthcare personnel
- Household contacts of immunocompromised persons
- Persons living or working in environments where transmission is likely (teachers, child-care workers, residents and staff of institutional settings)
- Persons in environments where transmission has been reported
- Nonpregnant women of childbearing age
- Adolescents and adults in households with children
- International travelers

Dosage Varicella Immunization: Sub Q:

U.S. labeling:

Children ≥12 months: SubQ: 0.5 mL; a second dose may be administered ≥3 months later

Note: The ACIP recommends the routine childhood vaccination be 2 doses, with the first dose administered at 12 to 15 months of age. The second dose should be administered at 4 to 6 years of age before school entry, but it may be administered earlier provided ≥3 months have elapsed after the first dose. All children and adolescents who received only 1 dose of vaccine should receive a second dose (CDC/ACIP [Marin, 2007]). If the second dose was administered ≥4 weeks after the first dose, it may be considered as valid (CDC/ACIP [Akinsany-Beysolow, 2014]).

Adolescents ≥13 years and Adults: SubQ: Two doses of 0.5 mL separated by ≥4 weeks (4 to 8 weeks apart per ACIP). **Note:** The ACIP recommends that all children and adults without evidence of immunity receive 2 doses of the vaccine; those who received only 1 dose of vaccine receive a second dose (CDC/ACIP [Marin, 2007]).

Canadian labeling:

Children ≥12 months:

Varilrix: Two doses of 0.5 mL separated by ≥6 weeks

Varivax III: 0.5 mL as a single dose

Alternative recommendations (NACI, 2012): Two doses of 0.5 mL with first dose administered at 12 to 15 months of age. Separate doses by ≥3 months; however, if rapid protection is necessary, may administer second dose after ≥6 weeks.

Adolescents ≥13 years and Adults: Two single doses 0.5 mL separated by 4 to 8 weeks (Varivax III) or ≥6 weeks (Varilrix); **Note:** The NACI recommends that adolescents (≥13 years of age) and adults (<50 years of age) who received only 1 dose of vaccine receive a second dose (NACI, 2012).

Postexposure prophylaxis (healthy, previously unvaccinated individuals) (off-label use): Children ≥12 months, Adolescents, and Adults: SubQ: 0.5 mL administered ideally within 72 hours postexposure but may be used up to 120 hours (5 days) postexposure (CDC/ACIP [Marin, 2007]).

Dosage adjustment in renal impairment: There are no dosage adjustments provided in the manufacturer's labeling.

Dosage adjustment in hepatic impairment: There are no dosage adjustments provided in the manufacturer's labeling.

Additional Information Complete prescribing information should be consulted for additional detail.

Dosage Forms

Injectable, Subcutaneous [preservative free]:

Varivax: 1350 PFU/0.5 mL (1 ea)

Dosage Forms: Canada

Injection, powder for reconstitution [preservative free]:

Varivax III: 1350 plaque-forming units (PFU)

Injection, powder for reconstitution:

Valrilix: $10^{3.3}$ plaque-forming units (PFU)

◆ **Varicella Zoster** *see* Varicella-Zoster Immune Globulin (Human) *on page 2142*

Varicella-Zoster Immune Globulin (Human)

(var i SEL a- ZOS ter i MYUN GLOB yoo lin HYU man)

Brand Names: U.S. VariZIG
Brand Names: Canada VariZIG
Index Terms Varicella Zoster; VZIG
Pharmacologic Category Blood Product Derivative; Immune Globulin
Additional Appendix Information

Immunization Administration Recommendations *on page 2250*
Immunization Recommendations *on page 2255*

Use

U.S. labeling: Postexposure prophylaxis of varicella in high-risk individuals. High-risk groups include:
- Immunocompromised children and adults
- Newborns of mothers with varicella shortly before or after delivery
- Premature infants
- Neonates and infants <1 year of age
- Adults without evidence of immunity
- Pregnant women

Canadian labeling: In pregnant women, for the prevention or reduction in severity of maternal infection within 4 days of exposure to the varicella zoster virus.

The Advisory Committee on Immunization Practices (ACIP) recommends varicella-zoster immune globulin (VZIG) to patients who are at high risk for severe varicella infection and complications; and who were exposed to varicella or herpes zoster; and for whom varicella vaccine is contraindicated. The decision to use VZIG should take into consideration if the patient lacks evidence of immunity; if exposure is likely to result in an infection; and if the patient is at greater risk for varicella complications than the general population. The following are patient groups for whom VZIG is recommended (CDC, 2013):

- Immunocompromised patients without evidence of immunity (seronegative), including those with neoplastic disease (eg, leukemia or lymphoma); primary or acquired immunodeficiency; immunosuppressive therapy (including steroid therapy equivalent to prednisone ≥2 mg/kg or 20 mg/day)
- Newborn of mother who had onset of varicella (chickenpox) within 5 days before delivery or within 48 hours after delivery
- Hospitalized premature infants (≥28 weeks gestation) who were exposed during the neonatal period and whose mother has no evidence of immunity
- Hospitalized premature infants (<28 weeks gestation or ≤1000 g) regardless of maternal history and who were exposed during the neonatal period
- Pregnant women without evidence of immunity who have been exposed

Pregnancy Risk Factor C
Dosage

U.S. labeling: Postexposure prophylaxis: Children, Adolescents, and Adults: IM: Administer a single dose based on body weight. Dose may be repeated for high-risk patients with additional exposure >3 weeks after initial administration. The minimum dose is 62.5 units and the maximum dose is 625 units:
≤2 kg: 62.5 units
2.1 to 10 kg: 125 units
10.1 to 20 kg: 250 units
20.1 to 30 kg: 375 units
30.1 to 40 kg: 500 units
≥40.1 kg: 625 units

Note: Administration should begin as soon as possible and within 10 days after exposure (CDC, 2013). Administration should begin within 96 hours (ideally 48 hours) in hematopoietic cell transplant (HCT) recipients who are exposed to varicella or zoster or a varicella zoster vaccine vaccinee who develops a varicella-like rash (Tomblyn, 2009).

Canadian labeling: Prevention or reduction of maternal infection: Adults: IM, IV: 125 units/10 kg (minimum dose: 125 units; maximum dose: 625 units). Administer within 96 hours of exposure.

Additional Information Complete prescribing information should be consulted for additional detail.
Dosage Forms

Solution Reconstituted, Injection [preservative free]:
VariZIG: 125 units (1 ea)

◆ **Varicella-Zoster Virus (VZV) Vaccine (Varicella)** *see* Varicella Virus Vaccine *on page 2141*

◆ **Varilrix (Can)** *see* Varicella Virus Vaccine *on page 2141*

◆ **Varithena** *see* Polidocanol *on page 1672*

◆ **Varivax** *see* Varicella Virus Vaccine *on page 2141*

◆ **Varivax III (Can)** *see* Varicella Virus Vaccine *on page 2141*

◆ **VariZIG** *see* Varicella-Zoster Immune Globulin (Human) *on page 2142*

◆ **Vascepa** *see* Omega-3 Fatty Acids *on page 1507*

◆ **Vascular Endothelial Growth Factor Trap** *see* Ziv-Aflibercept (Systemic) *on page 2204*

◆ **Vaseretic** *see* Enalapril and Hydrochlorothiazide *on page 725*

◆ **VasoClear [OTC]** *see* Naphazoline (Ophthalmic) *on page 1426*

◆ **VasoClear-A [OTC]** *see* Naphazoline (Ophthalmic) *on page 1426*

◆ **Vasocon® (Can)** *see* Naphazoline (Ophthalmic) *on page 1426*

◆ **Vasolex™** *see* Trypsin, Balsam Peru, and Castor Oil *on page 2109*

Vasopressin (vay soe PRES in)

Brand Names: U.S. Pitressin Synthetic [DSC]; Vasostrict
Brand Names: Canada Pressyn; Pressyn AR
Index Terms 8-Arginine Vasopressin; ADH; Antidiuretic Hormone; AVP
Pharmacologic Category Antidiuretic Hormone Analog; Hormone, Posterior Pituitary
Use

Diabetes Insipidus (Pitressin Synthetic only): Treatment of central diabetes insipidus; differential diagnosis of diabetes insipidus

Vasodilatory shock (Vasostrict only): To increase blood pressure in adults patients with vasodilatory shock (eg, postcardiotomy or sepsis) who remain hypotensive despite fluids and catecholamines

Pregnancy Risk Factor C
Pregnancy Considerations Animal reproduction studies have not been conducted. Vasopressin may produce tonic uterine contractions; however, doses sufficient for diabetes insipidus are not likely to produce this effect.
Breast-Feeding Considerations It is not known if vasopressin is excreted in breast milk. Oral absorption by a nursing infant is unlikely because vasopressin is rapidly destroyed in the GI tract; however, consider pumping and discarding breast milk for 1.5 hours after receiving vasopressin (Vasostrict only) to minimize potential exposure to the breast-fed infant. The manufacturer recommends that

caution be exercised when administering vasopressin to nursing women.

Contraindications Hypersensitivity to vasopressin or any component of the formulation; hypersensitivity to chlorobutanol (Vasostrict only); uncorrected chronic nephritis with nitrogen retention (Pitressin Synthetic only)

Warnings/Precautions Use with caution in patients with seizure disorders, migraine, asthma, vascular disease, renal disease, cardiovascular disease, including arteriosclerosis; goiter with cardiac complications. IV administration (off-label route): Vesicant; ensure proper needle or catheter placement prior to and during infusion; extravasation may lead to severe vasoconstriction and localized tissue necrosis, gangrene of extremities, tongue, and ischemic colitis; avoid extravasation. May cause water intoxication; early signs include drowsiness, listlessness, and headache, these should be recognized to prevent coma and seizures. Elderly patients should be cautioned not to increase their fluid intake beyond that sufficient to satisfy their thirst in order to avoid water intoxication and hyponatremia; under experimental conditions, the elderly have shown to have a decreased responsiveness to vasopressin with respect to its effects on water homeostasis.

Adverse Reactions

Cardiovascular: Angina pectoris, atrial fibrillation, bradycardia, cardiac arrest, cardiac arrhythmia, ischemic heart disease, limb ischemia (distal), localized blanching, low cardiac output, myocardial infarction, right heart failure, shock, vasoconstriction (peripheral)

Central nervous system: Headache (pounding), vertigo

Dermatologic: Circumoral pallor, diaphoresis, gangrene of skin or other tissues, skin lesion (ischemic), urticaria

Endocrine & metabolic: Hyponatremia, hypovolemic shock, water intoxication

Gastrointestinal: Abdominal cramps, flatulence, mesenteric ischemia, nausea, vomiting

Hematologic & oncologic: Decreased platelet count, hemorrhage (intractable)

Hepatic: Increased serum bilirubin

Hypersensitivity: Anaphylaxis

Neuromuscular & skeletal: Tremor

Renal: Renal insufficiency

Respiratory: Bronchoconstriction

Drug Interactions

Metabolism/Transport Effects None known.

Avoid Concomitant Use There are no known interactions where it is recommended to avoid concomitant use.

Increased Effect/Toxicity There are no known significant interactions involving an increase in effect.

Decreased Effect There are no known significant interactions involving a decrease in effect.

Food Interactions Ethanol may decrease the antidiuretic effect. Management: Avoid ethanol.

Preparation for Administration Vasostrict: **Note:** Discard unused diluted solution after 18 hours at room temperature or 24 hours under refrigeration. Discard vial after 48 hours after first entry.

No fluid restriction: Final concentration vasopressin 0.1 units/mL: Reconstitute vasopressin 50 units (2.5 mL) with 500 mL NS or D_5W.

Fluid restriction: Final concentration 1 unit/mL: Reconstitute vasopressin 100 units (5 mL) with 100 mL NS or D_5W.

Storage/Stability Store between 2°C and 8°C (36°F and 46°F). Do not freeze.

Mechanism of Action Increases cyclic adenosine monophosphate (cAMP) which increases water permeability at the renal tubule resulting in decreased urine volume and increased osmolality; causes peristalsis by directly stimulating the smooth muscle in the GI tract; direct vasoconstrictor without inotropic or chronotropic effects. In vasodilatory shock, vasopressin increases systemic vascular resistance and mean arterial blood pressure and decreases heart rate and cardiac output.

Pharmacodynamics/Kinetics

Onset of action: Nasal: 1 hour; IV: ≤15 minutes

Duration: Nasal: 3 to 8 hours; IM, SubQ: 2 to 8 hours; IV: ≤20 minutes

Metabolism: Nasal/Parenteral: Hepatic, renal (inactive metabolites)

Half-life elimination: Nasal: 15 minutes; Parenteral: 10 to 20 minutes

Excretion: Nasal: Urine; SubQ: Urine (5% as unchanged drug) after 4 hours; IV: Urine (~6% as unchanged drug)

Dosage

Central diabetes insipidus: **Note:** Dosage is highly variable; titrate based on serum and urine sodium and osmolality in addition to fluid balance and urine output. Use of vasopressin is impractical for chronic therapy.

IM, SubQ:

Children: 2.5 to 10 units 2 to 4 times daily as needed

Adults: 5 to 10 units 2 to 4 times daily as needed

Continuous IV infusion (off-label route): **Note:** The optimum rate of infusion has not been well established; many protocols exist.

Children: Initial: 0.0005 units/kg/hour; increase dose by 0.0005 units/kg/hour increments every 5 to 10 minutes as needed to adequately reduce urine output (maximum dose: 0.01 unit/kg/hour) (Wise-Faberowski, 2004). **Note:** Although clinical trial titrated every 5 to 10 minutes, a reduced frequency of titration (eg, every 30 minutes) may be more appropriate given the half-life of vasopressin. To provide the infusion dose, the concentration used during the study was 20 units in 500 mL (0.04 units/mL) in D_5W.

Adults: Continuous infusion has not been formally evaluated in the post-neurosurgical adult. However, some convert IM/SubQ requirement to an hourly continuous IV infusion rate.

Vasodilatory shock: IV: Adults: **Note:** Dosage provided is empirical; titrate to lowest dose compatible with an acceptable response.

Post-cardiotomy shock: Initial: 0.03 units per minute. If the target blood pressure response is not achieved, titrate up by 0.005 units per minute at 10- to 15-minute intervals (maximum dose: 0.1 units per minute). After target blood pressure has been maintained for 8 hours without the use of catecholamines, taper by 0.005 units per minute every hour as tolerated to maintain target blood pressure.

Septic shock:

Surviving Sepsis Campaign recommendations: 0.03 units per minute added to norepinephrine to raise MAP to target or to decrease norepinephrine dose. Doses >0.03 units per minute may have more cardiovascular side effects and should only be reserved for salvage therapy (ie, failure to achieve MAP goal with other vasopressors) (SCCM [Dellinger, 2013]). To prevent subsequent hypotension after withdrawal of vasopressors, vasopressin should be slowly tapered (eg, titrated down by 0.01 units per minute every 30 minutes) **after** the catecholamine(s) are discontinued until no longer required (Bauer, 2010).

Manufacturer recommendations: Initial: 0.01 units per minute. If the target blood pressure response is not achieved, titrate up by 0.005 units per minute at 10- to 15-minute intervals (maximum dose: 0.07 units per minute). After target blood pressure has been maintained for 8 hours without the use of catecholamines, taper by 0.005 units per minute every hour as tolerated to maintain target blood pressure.

Central diabetes insipidus, post-traumatic (off-label use): Adults: IV: Initial: 2.5 units/hour; titrate to adequately reduce urine output (Levitt, 1984)

Donor management in brain-dead patients (hormone replacement therapy) (off-label use): Adults: IV: Initial: 1 unit bolus followed by 0.5 to 4 units/hour (Rosendale, 2003; UNOS Critical Pathway, 2002)

GI/variceal hemorrhage (off-label use): Continuous IV infusion: Dilute in NS or D_5W to 0.1 to 1 unit/mL. **Note:** Other therapies may be preferred.

GI hemorrhage (off-label use): Children: Initial IV bolus: 0.3 unit/kg (maximum: 20 units) may be given. Continuous IV infusion: 0.001 to 0.01 units/kg/minute; titrate dose as needed; maximum: 0.01 unit/kg/minute; if bleeding controlled for 12 to 24 hours, then taper off over 24 to 36 hours

Variceal hemorrhage (off-label use) [AASLD guidelines, 2007]: Adults: Initial: 0.2 to 0.4 units per minute, may titrate dose as needed to a maximum dose of 0.8 units per minute; maximum duration: 24 hours at highest effective dose continuously (to reduce incidence of adverse effects). Patient should also receive IV nitroglycerin concurrently to prevent myocardial ischemic complications; monitor closely for signs/symptoms of ischemia (myocardial, peripheral, bowel)

Pulseless arrest (off-label use) [ACLS, 2010]: Adults: IV, I.O.: 40 units; may give 1 dose to replace first or second dose of epinephrine. IV/I.O. drug administration is preferred, but if no access, may give endotracheally. ACLS guidelines do not recommend a specific endotracheal dose; however, may be given endotracheally using the same IV dose (ACLS, 2010; Wenzel, 1997).

Dosage adjustment in renal impairment: There are no dosage adjustments provided in the manufacturer's labeling.

Dosage adjustment in hepatic impairment: There are no dosage adjustments provided in the manufacturer's labeling.

Usual Infusion Concentrations: Adult IV infusion: 50 units in 500 mL (concentration: 0.1 unit/mL) **or** 100 units in 100 mL (concentration: 1 unit/mL) of D_5W or NS

Administration Pitressin Synthetic: For IM or SubQ administration (per manufacturer).

IV: May administer as IV bolus over seconds (ACLS, 2010) or as a continuous IV infusion (refer to indication-specific infusion rates in dosing for detailed recommendations); when administered as a continuous IV infusion for vasodilatory shock, the use of a central venous catheter is recommended. Use extreme caution to avoid extravasation because of risk of necrosis and gangrene. In treatment of varices, infusions are often supplemented with nitroglycerin infusions to minimize cardiac effects.

Vesicant; ensure proper needle or catheter placement prior to and during infusion; avoid extravasation.

Extravasation management: If extravasation occurs, stop infusion immediately and disconnect (leave cannula/needle in place); gently aspirate extravasated solution (do **NOT** flush the line); remove needle/cannula; elevate extremity. Initiate phentolamine (or alternative antidote).

Phentolamine: Dilute 5 to 10 mg in 10 to 15 mL NS and administer into extravasation site as soon as possible after extravasation (Peberdy, 2010).

Alternatives to phentolamine (due to shortage):

Nitroglycerin topical 2% ointment (based on limited case reports in neonates/infants): Apply 4 mm/kg as a thin ribbon to the affected areas; may repeat after 8 hours if needed (Wong, 1992) **or** apply a 1-inch strip on the affected site (Denkler, 1989).

Terbutaline (based on limited case reports): Infiltrate extravasation area using a solution of terbutaline 1 mg diluted to 10 mL in NS (large extravasation site; administration volume varied from 3 to 10 mL) **or** 1 mg diluted in 1 mL NS (small/distal extravasation site; administration volume varied from 0.5 to 1 mL) (Stier, 1999).

Intranasal (topical administration on nasal mucosa; off-label route): Administer injectable vasopressin on cotton plugs, as nasal spray, or by dropper. Should not be inhaled.

Endotracheal (off-label route): If no IV or intraosseous access, may give endotracheally. ACLS guidelines do not recommend a specific endotracheal dose; however, may be given endotracheally using the same IV dose (ACLS, 2010; Wenzel, 1997). Mix with 5 to 10 mL of water or normal saline, and administer down the endotracheal tube.

Monitoring Parameters Serum and urine sodium, urine specific gravity, urine and serum osmolality; urine output, fluid input and output, blood pressure, heart rate

Consult individual institutional policies and procedures.

Additional Information Vasopressin increases factor VIII levels and may be useful in hemophiliacs.

Dosage Forms

Solution, Injection:

Generic: 20 units/mL (0.5 mL, 1 mL, 10 mL)

Solution, Intravenous:

Vasostrict: 20 units/mL (1 mL)

◆ **Vasostrict** *see* Vasopressin *on page 2142*

◆ **Vasotec** *see* Enalapril *on page 722*

◆ **Vaxigrip (Can)** *see* Influenza Virus Vaccine (Inactivated) *on page 1075*

◆ **Vazculep** *see* Phenylephrine (Systemic) *on page 1638*

◆ **VCF Vaginal Contraceptive [OTC]** *see* Nonoxynol 9 *on page 1471*

◆ **VEC-162** *see* Tasimelteon *on page 1979*

◆ **Vectibix** *see* Panitumumab *on page 1568*

◆ **Vectical** *see* Calcitriol *on page 323*

Vecuronium (vek ue ROE nee um)

Brand Names: Canada Norcuron®

Index Terms Norcuron; ORG NC 45

Pharmacologic Category Neuromuscular Blocker Agent, Nondepolarizing

Use To facilitate endotracheal intubation and to relax skeletal muscles during surgery; to facilitate mechanical ventilation in ICU patients; does not relieve pain or produce sedation

Pregnancy Risk Factor C

Pregnancy Considerations Animal reproduction studies have not been conducted. The pharmacokinetics of vecuronium are altered during pregnancy. Use in cesarean section has been reported; umbilical venous concentrations were 11% of maternal values at delivery.

Breast-Feeding Considerations It is not known if vecuronium is excreted in breast milk. The manufacturer recommends that caution be exercised when administering vecuronium to nursing women.

Contraindications Hypersensitivity to vecuronium or any component of the formulation

Warnings/Precautions Ventilation must be supported during neuromuscular blockade. Vecuronium does not relieve pain or produce sedation; use should include appropriate anesthesia, pain control, and sedation. In patients requiring long-term administration, use of a peripheral nerve stimulator to monitor drug effects is strongly recommended. Additional doses of vecuronium or any other neuromuscular-blocking agent should be avoided unless nerve stimulation response suggests inadequate neuromuscular blockade. Certain clinical conditions may result in potentiation (dosage reduction may be necessary) or antagonism (dosage increase may be necessary) of neuromuscular blockade:

Antagonism: Alkalosis, hypercalcemia, demyelinating lesions, peripheral neuropathies, denervation, immobilization, infection, and muscle trauma

Potentiation: Electrolyte abnormalities, severe hyponatremia, severe hypocalcemia, severe hypokalemia, hypermagnesemia, cachexia, neuromuscular diseases, acidosis, Eaton-Lambert syndrome, and myasthenia gravis

Resistance may occur in burn patients (>30% of body) for period of 5-70 days postinjury. Hypothermia may prolong the duration of action. Use with caution in patients with hepatic impairment; clinical duration may be prolonged. Use with caution in patients who are anephric; clinical duration may be prolonged. Use with caution in patients who have underlying respiratory disease. Some patients may experience delayed recovery of neuromuscular function after administration (especially after prolonged use). Other factors associated with delayed recovery should be considered (eg, corticosteroid use, disease-related conditions). Cross-sensitivity with other neuromuscular-blocking agents may occur; use extreme caution in patients with previous anaphylactic reactions. Use caution in the elderly; dosage reduction may be considered. Children 1-10 years of age may require slightly higher initial doses and slightly more frequent supplementation. **[U.S. Boxed Warning]: Should be administered by adequately trained individuals familiar with its use.**

Benzyl alcohol and derivatives: Diluent may contain benzyl alcohol; large amounts of benzyl alcohol (≥99 mg/kg/day) have been associated with a potentially fatal toxicity ("gasping syndrome") in neonates; the "gasping syndrome" consists of metabolic acidosis, respiratory distress, gasping respirations, CNS dysfunction (including convulsions, intracranial hemorrhage), hypotension, and cardiovascular collapse (AAP, 1997; CDC, 1982); some data suggests that benzoate displaces bilirubin from protein binding sites (Ahlfors, 2001); avoid or use dosage forms containing benzyl alcohol with caution in neonates. See manufacturer's labeling.

Adverse Reactions Rare but important or life-threatening: Acute quadriplegic myopathy syndrome (prolonged use), Bradycardia, circulatory collapse, edema, flushing; hypersensitivity reaction (hypotension, tachycardia, erythema, rash, urticaria); itching, myositis ossificans (prolonged use), rash

Drug Interactions

Metabolism/Transport Effects None known.

Avoid Concomitant Use

Avoid concomitant use of Vecuronium with any of the following: QuiNINE

Increased Effect/Toxicity

Vecuronium may increase the levels/effects of: Cardiac Glycosides; Corticosteroids (Systemic); OnabotulinumtoxinA; RimabotulinumtoxinB

The levels/effects of Vecuronium may be increased by: AbobotulinumtoxinA; Aminoglycosides; Calcium Channel Blockers; Capreomycin; Clindamycin (Topical); Colistimethate; CycloSPORINE (Systemic); Dantrolene; Fosphenytoin-Phenytoin; Inhalational Anesthetics; Ketorolac (Nasal); Ketorolac (Systemic); Lincosamide Antibiotics; Lithium; Loop Diuretics; Magnesium Salts; Piperacillin; Polymyxin B; Procainamide; QuiNIDine; QuiNINE; Spironolactone; Tetracycline Derivatives; Vancomycin

Decreased Effect

The levels/effects of Vecuronium may be decreased by: Acetylcholinesterase Inhibitors; CarBAMazepine; Fosphenytoin-Phenytoin; Loop Diuretics

Preparation for Administration Reconstitute with compatible solution for injection to final concentration of 1 mg/mL. May further dilute reconstituted vial to 0.1-0.2 mg/mL in a compatible solution for IV infusion.

Storage/Stability Store intact vials of powder for injection at room temperature 20°C to 25°C (68°F to 77°F). Vials reconstituted with bacteriostatic water for injection (BWFI) may be stored for 5 days under refrigeration or at room temperature. Vials reconstituted with other compatible diluents (nonbacteriostatic) should be stored under refrigeration and used within 24 hours.

Mechanism of Action Blocks acetylcholine from binding to receptors on motor endplate inhibiting depolarization

Pharmacodynamics/Kinetics

Onset of action:

Good intubation conditions: Within 2.5-3 minutes

Maximum neuromuscular blockade: Within 3-5 minutes

Duration: Under balanced anesthesia (time to recovery to 25% of control): 25-40 minutes; recovery 95% complete ~45-65 minutes after injection of intubating dose

Distribution: V_d: 0.3-0.4 L/kg

Protein binding: 60% to 80%

Metabolism: Active metabolite: 3-desacetyl vecuronium (1/2 the activity of parent drug)

Half-life elimination: Healthy surgical patients and renal failure patients undergoing transplant surgery: 65-75 minutes; Late pregnancy: 35-40 minutes

Excretion: Primarily feces (40% to 75%); urine (30% as unchanged drug and metabolites)

Dosage Administer IV; dose to effect; doses will vary due to interpatient variability:

Children: ICU paralysis (eg, facilitate mechanical ventilation) in selected adequately sedated patients (off-label; Martin, 1999): Initial bolus dose: 0.1-0.15 mg/kg, then a continuous IV infusion of 1-2.5 **mcg**/kg/**minute** (0.06-0.15 **mg**/kg/**hour**); monitor depth of blockade using peripheral nerve stimulator every 2-3 hours initially until stable dose, then every 8-12 hours

Intermittent bolus dosing (Eldadah, 1989): 0.1 mg/kg every 1 hour as needed

Children ≥1 year and Adults: Surgical relaxation: **Note:** Children 1-10 years may require slightly higher initial doses and more frequent supplementation.

Tracheal intubation: IV: Initial: 0.08-0.1 mg/kg. **Note:** If intubation is performed using succinylcholine (not preferred agent in pediatric patients), the initial dose of vecuronium may be reduced to 0.04-0.06 mg/kg with inhalation anesthesia and 0.05-0.06 mg/kg with balanced anesthesia.

Obesity: For obese (≥130% of IBW) adult patients, may use ideal body weight (IBW) (Erstad, 2004; Schwartz, 1992; Weinstein, 1988); onset time may be slightly delayed using IBW.

Pretreatment/priming: Adults: 10% of intubating dose given 3-5 minutes before intubating dose

Maintenance for continued surgical relaxation (only after return of neuromuscular function): Intermittent dosing: 0.01-0.015 mg/kg **or** continuous infusion of 0.8-1.2 **mcg**/kg/**minute** (0.048-0.072 **mg**/kg/**hour**).

Note: Use lower end of the dosing range when anesthesia is maintained with an inhaled anesthetic agent, with the redosing interval guided by monitoring with a peripheral nerve stimulator.

Adults:

ICU paralysis (eg, facilitate mechanical ventilation) in selected adequately sedated patients (Darrah, 1989; Greenberg, 2013; Murray, 2002; Rudis, 1997): Initial bolus dose: 0.08-0.1 mg/kg, then a continuous IV infusion of 0.8-1.7 **mcg**/kg/**minute** (0.048-0.102 **mg**/kg/**hour**); monitor depth of blockade every 1-2 hours initially until stable dose, then every 8-12 hours. Usual maintenance infusion dose range: 0.8-1.2 **mcg**/kg/**minute** (0.048-0.072 **mg**/kg/**hour**).

Dosage adjustment (Rudis, 1996; Rudis, 1997): Adjust rate of administration in increments of 0.3 **mcg**/kg/**minute** (0.018 **mg**/kg/**hour**) or by 50% reductions of previous dose according to peripheral nerve stimulation response or desired clinical response. Discontinue infusion if neuromuscular function does not return.

Note: When possible, minimize depth and duration of paralysis. Stopping the infusion daily for some time until forced to restart based on patient condition is recommended to reduce post-paralytic complications (eg, acute quadriplegic myopathy syndrome [AQMS]) (Murray, 2002; Segredo, 1992).

Intermittent bolus dosing (Hunter, 1985): 0.1-0.2 mg/kg/dose; may be repeated when neuromuscular function returns

Control of refractory shivering in adequately sedated patients during therapeutic hypothermia after cardiac arrest (off-label use; Bernard, 2002; Nolan, 2003; Polderman, 2009): IV: 8-12 mg; redose as needed to control shivering. **Note:** Duration of action prolonged in hypothermic patients. May mask seizure activity.

Elderly: No specific guidelines available; refer to adult dosing. Dose selection should be cautious, at low end of dosage range, and titration should be slower to evaluate response.

Dosage adjustment in renal impairment: No dosage adjustment provided in manufacturer's labeling. However, patients with renal impairment do not experience clinically significant prolongation of neuromuscular blockade with vecuronium; however, in patients who are anephric, the clinical duration is prolonged.

Dosage adjustment in hepatic impairment: No dosage adjustment provided in manufacturer's labeling. However, dosage reduction may be necessary in patients with liver disease.

Usual Infusion Concentrations: Pediatric IV infusion: 0.1 mg/mL, 0.2 mg/mL, 1 mg/mL

Usual Infusion Concentrations: Adult IV infusion: 10 mg in 100 mL (concentration: 0.1 mg/mL), 20 mg in 100 mL (concentration: 0.2 mg/mL), **or** 50 mg in 50 mL (concentration: 1 mg/mL) of D_5W or NS

Administration Concentration of 1 mg/mL may be administered by rapid IV injection; may also be used for IV infusion in fluid-restricted patients.

Monitoring Parameters Blood pressure, heart rate; peripheral nerve stimulation (eg, train-of-four [TOF] count)

Additional Information Vecuronium is classified as an intermediate-duration neuromuscular-blocking agent. It produces minimal, if any, histamine release; does not relieve pain or produce sedation. It may produce cumulative effect on duration of blockade.

Dosage Forms

Solution Reconstituted, Intravenous:

Generic: 10 mg (1 ea); 20 mg (1 ea)

Solution Reconstituted, Intravenous [preservative free]:

Generic: 10 mg (1 ea); 20 mg (1 ea)

Vedolizumab (ve doe LIZ ue mab)

Brand Names: U.S. Entyvio

Pharmacologic Category Gastrointestinal Agent, Miscellaneous; Monoclonal Antibody; Monoclonal Antibody, Selective Adhesion-Molecule Inhibitor

Use

Crohn disease: Treatment of moderately to severely active Crohn disease in patients who have had an inadequate response with, lost response to, or were intolerant to inhibitors of tumor necrosis factor-alpha (TNF-alpha) blocker or immunomodulator; or had an inadequate response with, were intolerant to, or demonstrated dependence on corticosteroids.

Ulcerative colitis Treatment of moderately to severely active ulcerative colitis in patients who have had an inadequate response with, were intolerant to inhibitors of tumor necrosis factor-alpha (TNF-alpha) blocker or immunomodulator; or had an inadequate response with, were intolerant to, or demonstrated dependence on corticosteroids.

Pregnancy Risk Factor B

Pregnancy Considerations Adverse events have not been observed in animal reproduction studies. Monoclonal antibodies are transported across the placenta in a linear fashion as pregnancy progresses, with the largest amount transferred during the third trimester. Any adverse pregnancy effect would likely be greater during the second and third trimesters of pregnancy.

Health care providers are encouraged to enroll women exposed to vedolizumab during pregnancy in a pregnancy exposure registry. Information about the registry can be obtained by calling 1-877-825-3327.

Breast-Feeding Considerations It is not known if vedolizumab is excreted in breast milk. The manufacturer recommends that caution be exercised when administering vedolizumab to nursing women.

Contraindications Serious or severe hypersensitivity to vedolizumab or any component of the formulation

Warnings/Precautions Hypersensitivity reactions have been reported including anaphylaxis. Allergic reactions including dyspnea, bronchospasm, urticaria, flushing, rash, and increased blood pressure and heart rate have also been observed. Symptom onset may vary from during the infusion, immediately post-infusion, to several hours post-infusion. If serious reactions occur, discontinue administration immediately. Use may be associated with an increased risk for developing infections; most commonly reported infections included upper respiratory and nasal mucosa. Serious infections have also been reported in patients treated, including anal abscess, sepsis (some fatal), tuberculosis, salmonella sepsis, *Listeria* meningitis, giardiasis, and cytomegaloviral colitis. Therapy is not recommended in patients with uncontrolled, active, severe infections. If a patient develops a serious infection, consider discontinuing therapy. Use with caution in patients with a history of recurring severe infections. Screening for tuberculosis should be considered.

Integrin receptor antagonists have been associated with progressive multifocal leukoencephalopathy (PML), a rare and often fatal opportunistic infection of the central nervous system caused by the John Cunningham (JC) virus. Monitor patients for any new onset or worsening of neurological signs and symptoms including progressive weakness on one side of the body or clumsiness of limbs, disturbance of vision, and changes in thinking, memory, and orientation leading to confusion and personality changes. Symptoms may progress over days to weeks and can lead to death or severe disability in weeks to months. If PML is suspected withhold therapy and refer to a neurologist; if confirmed, discontinue therapy permanently. Elevations of transaminase and/or bilirubin have been reported in patients receiving vedolizumab. Discontinue therapy in patients with jaundice or other evidence of significant liver injury such as fatigue, anorexia, right upper abdominal discomfort, or dark urine. Patients should be brought up to date with all immunizations according to immunization guidelines before initiating therapy. Live vaccines should not be given concurrently unless the benefits outweigh the risks; there are no data on the secondary transmission of infection by live vaccines with vedolizumab. Non-live vaccines may be given concurrently.

Adverse Reactions

Central nervous system: Fatigue, headache

Dermatologic: Pruritus, skin rash

Gastrointestinal: Nausea

Hepatic: Increased serum ALT (≥3 x ULN), increased serum AST (≥3 x ULN)

Immunologic: Antibody development (may be neutralizing)

Infection: Influenza

Neuromuscular & skeletal: Arthralgia, back pain, limb pain

Respiratory: Bronchitis, cough, nasopharyngitis, oropharyngeal pain, sinusitis, upper respiratory tract infection

Miscellaneous: Fever, infusion related reaction

Rare but important or life-threatening: Hepatitis, hypersensitivity reaction, infection (including anal abscess, sepsis, tuberculosis, salmonella sepsis, listeria meningitis, giardiasis, cytomegaloviral colitis), malignant neoplasm (excluding dysplasia and basal cell carcinoma)

Drug Interactions

Metabolism/Transport Effects None known.

Avoid Concomitant Use

Avoid concomitant use of Vedolizumab with any of the following: Anti-TNF Agents; BCG; Belimumab; Natalizumab; Pimecrolimus; Tacrolimus (Topical); Tofacitinib; Vaccines (Live)

Increased Effect/Toxicity

Vedolizumab may increase the levels/effects of: Belimumab; Leflunomide; Natalizumab; Tofacitinib; Vaccines (Live)

The levels/effects of Vedolizumab may be increased by: Anti-TNF Agents; Denosumab; Pimecrolimus; Roflumilast; Tacrolimus (Topical); Trastuzumab

Decreased Effect

Vedolizumab may decrease the levels/effects of: BCG; Cholera Vaccine; Coccidioides immitis Skin Test; Sipuleucel-T; Vaccines (Inactivated); Vaccines (Live)

The levels/effects of Vedolizumab may be decreased by: Echinacea

Preparation for Administration Reconstitute at room temperature with 4.8 mL of sterile water for injection. Gently swirl vial for at least 15 seconds; do not vigorously shake or invert. Allow the solution to sit for up to 20 minutes at room temperature to allow for reconstitution and for any foam to settle; the vial can be swirled and inspected for dissolution during this time. If not fully dissolved after 20 minutes, allow another 10 minutes for dissolution. Do not use the vial if the drug product is not dissolved within 30 minutes. Solution should be clear or opalescent, colorless to light brownish yellow and free of visible particulates. Do not administer reconstituted solution showing uncharacteristic color or containing particulates.

Prior to withdrawing the reconstituted vedolizumab solution from the vial for dilution, gently invert vial 3 times. Add the 5 mL (300 mg) of reconstituted vedolizumab solution to 250 mL of sterile sodium chloride 0.9% and gently mix the infusion bag. Once reconstituted and diluted, use the infusion solution as soon as possible.

Storage/Stability Refrigerate unopened vials at 2°C to 8°C (36°F to 46°F). Retain in original package to protect from light. Following reconstitution and dilution, the infusion solution may be stored for up to 4 hours at 2°C to 8°C (36°F to 46°F). Do not freeze. Discard any unused portion.

Mechanism of Action Vedolizumab is a humanized monoclonal antibody that binds to the alpha4beta7 integrin and blocks the interaction of alpha4beta7 integrin with mucosal addressin cell adhesion molecule-1 (MAdCAM-1) and inhibits the migration of memory T-lymphocytes across the endothelium into inflamed gastrointestinal parenchymal tissue. The interaction of the alpha4beta7 integrin with MAdCAM-1 has been implicated as an important contributor to the chronic inflammation that is a hallmark of ulcerative colitis and Crohn disease.

Pharmacodynamics/Kinetics

Distribution: V_d: 5 L

Half-life elimination: 25 days (serum, at 300 mg dosage)

Dosage Note: Prior to initiating treatment, all patients should be brought up to date with all immunizations according to current immunization guidelines.

Crohn disease or ulcerative colitis: Adults: IV: 300 mg at 0, 2, and 6 weeks and then every 8 weeks thereafter. Discontinue therapy in patients who show no evidence of therapeutic benefit by week 14.

Elderly: Refer to adult dosing.

Dosage adjustment in renal impairment: There are no dosage adjustments provided in the manufacturer's labeling (has not been studied).

Dosage adjustment in hepatic impairment: There are no dosage adjustments provided in the manufacturer's labeling (has not been studied). Discontinue use with jaundice or signs/symptoms of hepatic injury.

Administration IV: Infuse over 30 minutes. Do not administer by IV push or bolus. Following infusion, flush with 30 mL of sterile 0.9% sodium chloride injection. Observe patients during infusion (until complete) and monitor for hypersensitivity reactions; discontinue if a reaction occurs.

Monitoring Parameters Observe patients during infusion (until complete) and monitor for hypersensitivity reactions; LFTs; tuberculosis screening according to local practice; signs/symptoms of infection; any new onset or worsening of neurological signs and symptoms

Dosage Forms

Solution Reconstituted, Intravenous [preservative free]: Entyvio: 300 mg (1 ea)

◆ **VEGF Trap** *see* Aflibercept (Ophthalmic) *on page 63*

◆ **VEGF Trap** *see* Ziv-Aflibercept (Systemic) *on page 2204*

◆ **VEGF Trap-Eye** *see* Aflibercept (Ophthalmic) *on page 63*

◆ **VEGF Trap R1R2** *see* Ziv-Aflibercept (Systemic) *on page 2204*

Velaglucerase Alfa (vel a GLOO ser ase AL fa)

Brand Names: U.S. Vpriv

Brand Names: Canada VPRIV

Index Terms Gene-Activated Human Acid-Beta-Glucosidase; GlcCerase

Pharmacologic Category Enzyme

Use Gaucher disease: For long-term enzyme replacement therapy for pediatric and adult patients with type 1 Gaucher disease.

Pregnancy Risk Factor B

Dosage Note: Pretreatment with antihistamines and/or corticosteroids can be considered for prevention of subsequent infusion reactions in patients with hypersensitivity reactions requiring symptomatic treatment; during clinical studies, patients were not routinely premedicated prior to infusion.

IV: Children ≥4 years, Adolescents, and Adults: Gaucher's disease (type 1): 60 units/kg every 2 weeks; adjust dose based upon disease activity (range: 15-60 units/kg evaluated in clinical trials)

Note: When switching from imiglucerase to velaglucerase alfa in stable patients, initiate treatment 2 weeks after the last imiglucerase dose and at the same dose.

Dosage adjustment in renal impairment: No dosage adjustment provided in manufacturer's labeling.

Dosage adjustment in hepatic impairment: No dosage adjustment provided in manufacturer's labeling.

Additional Information Complete prescribing information should be consulted for additional detail.

Dosage Forms

Solution Reconstituted, Intravenous [preservative free]:

Vpriv: 400 units (1 ea)

◆ **Velban** *see* VinBLAStine *on page 2160*

◆ **Velcade** *see* Bortezomib *on page 276*

◆ **Veletri** *see* Epoprostenol *on page 746*

◆ **Velivet** *see* Ethinyl Estradiol and Desogestrel *on page 799*

◆ **Velphoro** *see* Sucroferric Oxyhydroxide *on page 1941*

◆ **Veltin™** *see* Clindamycin and Tretinoin *on page 464*

Vemurafenib (vem ue RAF e nib)

Brand Names: U.S. Zelboraf

Brand Names: Canada Zelboraf

Index Terms BRAF(V600E) Kinase Inhibitor RO5185426; PLX4032; RG7204; RO5185426

Pharmacologic Category Antineoplastic Agent, BRAF Kinase Inhibitor

Use Melanoma:

U.S. labeling: Treatment of unresectable or metastatic melanoma in patients with a BRAFV600E mutation (as detected by an approved test).

Canadian labeling: Treatment of unresectable or metastatic melanoma in patients with a BRAFV600 mutation (as identified by a validated test).

Limitations of use: Vemurafenib is not indicated in patients with wild-type BRAF melanoma.

Pregnancy Risk Factor D

Pregnancy Considerations Adverse effects were not demonstrated in animal reproduction studies. Based on the mechanism of action, vemurafenib may cause fetal harm if administered during pregnancy or in patients who become pregnant during treatment. Women of childbearing potential and men of reproductive potential should use adequate contraception methods during and for at least 2 months after treatment (Canadian labeling recommends during and for at least 6 months after treatment).

Breast-Feeding Considerations It is not known if vemurafenib is excreted in breast milk. Due to the potential for serious adverse reactions in the nursing infant, the manufacturer recommends a decision be made whether to discontinue nursing or to discontinue the drug, taking into account the importance of treatment to the mother.

Contraindications There are no contraindications listed in the manufacturer's labeling.

Canadian labeling: Hypersensitivity to vemurafenib or any component of the formulation.

Warnings/Precautions Hazardous agent - use appropriate precautions for handling and disposal (NIOSH 2014 [group 1]). Only patients with a BRAFV600 mutation-positive melanoma (including BRAFV600E) will benefit from treatment; mutation must be detected and confirmed by an approved test prior to treatment. The cobas 4800 BRAF V600 Mutation Test was used in clinical trials and is FDA-approved to detect BRAFV600E mutation.

Cutaneous squamous cell carcinomas (cuSCC), keratoacanthomas, and melanoma have been reported (at a higher rate in patients receiving vemurafenib compared to control). Cutaneous SCC generally occurs early in the treatment course (median onset: 7 to 8 weeks) and is managed with excision (while continuing vemurafenib treatment). Approximately one-third of patients experienced >1 cuSCC occurrence and the median time between occurrences was 6 weeks. Potential risk factors for cuSCC include age ≥65 years, history of skin cancer, or chronic sun exposure. Monitor for skin lesions (with dermatology evaluation) at baseline and every 2 months during treatment; consider continued monitoring for 6 months after treatment. Noncutaneous squamous cell carcinomas (SCC) of the head and neck have also been observed; monitor closely for signs/symptoms. Vemurafenib may promote malignancies correlated with RAS activation; monitor for signs/symptoms of other malignancies.

Dermatologic reactions have been observed, including case reports of Stevens-Johnson syndrome and toxic epidermal necrolysis; discontinue (permanently) for severe dermatologic toxicity. Photosensitivity ranging from mild to severe has been reported. Advise patients to avoid sun exposure and wear protective clothing and use effective UVA/UVB sunscreen and lip balm (SPF ≥30) when outdoors. Dosage modifications are recommended for intolerable photosensitivity consisting of erythema ≥10% to 30% of body surface area. Uveitis (including iritis), blurred vision, and photophobia may occur; monitor for signs and symptoms. Uveitis may be managed with corticosteroid and mydriatic eye drops. Retinal vein occlusion has been reported in clinical trials.

QT prolongation (dose-dependent) has been observed; may lead to increased risk for ventricular arrhythmia, including torsade de pointes. Monitor electrolytes (calcium, magnesium and potassium) at baseline and with dosage adjustments. Monitor ECG at baseline, 15 days after initiation, then monthly for 3 months, then every 3 months thereafter (more frequently if clinically appropriate); also monitor with dosage adjustments. Do not initiate treatment if baseline QTc >500 msec. During treatment, if QTc >500 msec, temporarily interrupt treatment; correct electrolytes and control other risk factors for QT prolongation. May reinitiate with a dose reduction once QTc falls to <500 msec. Discontinue (permanently), if after correction of risk factors, both the QTc continues to increase >500 msec and there is >60 msec change above baseline. Do not initiate treatment in patients with electrolyte abnormalities which are not correctable, long QT syndrome, or taking concomitant medication known to prolong the QT interval.

Liver injury has been reported with use, and may cause functional impairment such as coagulopathy or other organ dysfunction. Monitor transaminases, alkaline phosphatase and bilirubin at baseline and monthly during therapy, or as clinically necessary. May require dosage reduction, therapy interruption, or discontinuation. Anaphylaxis and severe hypersensitivity may occur during treatment or upon reinitiation. Serious reactions have included generalized rash, erythema, hypotension, and drug rash with eosinophilia and systemic symptoms (DRESS syndrome). Discontinue (permanently) with severe hypersensitivity reaction. Pancreatitis has been reported (case reports), with onset generally occurring within 2 weeks of initiation (Muluneh, 2013; Zelboraf Canadian product monograph, 2015); exacerbation of pancreatitis has also occurred upon rechallenge. Patients with unexplained abdominal pain should be promptly evaluated for pancreatitis (eg, serum lipase and amylase; abdominal CT) as clinically indicated. Elderly patients may be at increased risk for adverse effects; in clinical trials, there was an increased incidence of cuSCC and keratoacanthoma, atrial fibrillation, peripheral edema, and nausea/decreased appetite in patients ≥65 years of age. Potentially significant drug-drug interactions may exist, requiring dose or frequency adjustment, additional monitoring, and/or selection of alternative therapy.

Adverse Reactions

Cardiovascular: Atrial fibrillation, hypotension, peripheral edema, prolonged Q-T interval on ECG, retinal vein occlusion, vasculitis

Central nervous system: Cranial nerve palsy (facial), dizziness, fatigue, headache, peripheral neuropathy

Dermatologic: alopecia, erythema, erythema nodosum, folliculitis, hyperkeratosis (actinic, seborrheic, pilaris), maculopapular rash, palmar-plantar erythrodysesthesia, papular rash, pruritus, skin photosensitivity, skin rash, Stevens-Johnson syndrome, sunburn, toxic epidermal necrolysis, xeroderma

Endocrine & metabolic: Weight loss

Gastrointestinal: Constipation, decreased appetite, diarrhea, dysgeusia, nausea, vomiting

Hematologic & oncologic: Basal cell carcinoma, cutaneous papilloma, malignant melanoma (new primary), squamous cell carcinoma of skin, squamous cell carcinoma (oropharyngeal)

Hepatic: Increased gamma-glutamyl transferase, Increased serum alkaline phosphatase, increased serum ALT, increased serum AST, increased serum bilirubin

Hypersensitivity: Anaphylaxis, hypersensitivity

Neuromuscular & skeletal: Arthralgia, arthritis, back pain, myalgia, limb pain, musculoskeletal pain, weakness

Ophthalmic: Blurred vision, iritis, photophobia, uveitis

Renal: Increased serum creatinine

Respiratory: Cough

Miscellaneous: Fever

Rare but important or life-threatening: Chronic myelomonocytic leukemia with NRAS mutation (progression of preexisting condition), drug reaction with eosinophilia and systemic symptoms (DRESS syndrome), febrile neutropenia, hepatic failure, neutropenia, panniculitis

Drug Interactions

Metabolism/Transport Effects **Substrate** of BCRP, CYP3A4 (major), P-glycoprotein; **Note:** Assignment of Major/Minor substrate status based on clinically relevant drug interaction potential; **Inhibits** BCRP, CYP1A2 (moderate), CYP2D6 (weak), P-glycoprotein; **Induces** CYP3A4 (weak)

Avoid Concomitant Use

Avoid concomitant use of Vemurafenib with any of the following: Bosutinib; Conivaptan; CYP3A4 Inducers (Strong); CYP3A4 Inhibitors (Strong); Fusidic Acid (Systemic); Highest Risk QTc-Prolonging Agents; Idelalisib; Ivabradine; Mifepristone; Moderate Risk QTc-Prolonging Agents; PAZOPanib; Silodosin; Topotecan; VinCRIStine (Liposomal)

Increased Effect/Toxicity

Vemurafenib may increase the levels/effects of: Afatinib; Bosutinib; Brentuximab Vedotin; Colchicine; CYP1A2 Substrates; Dabigatran Etexilate; DOXOrubicin (Conventional); Edoxaban; Everolimus; Highest Risk QTc-Prolonging Agents; Ledipasvir; Naloxegol; PAZOPanib; P-glycoprotein/ABCB1 Substrates; Pirfenidone; Porfimer; Prucalopride; Rifaximin; Rivaroxaban; Silodosin; Topotecan; Verteporfin; VinCRIStine (Liposomal); Warfarin

The levels/effects of Vemurafenib may be increased by: Aprepitant; Conivaptan; CYP3A4 Inhibitors (Moderate); CYP3A4 Inhibitors (Strong); Fosaprepitant; Fusidic Acid (Systemic); Idelalisib; Ipilimumab; Ivabradine; Ivacaftor; Luliconazole; Mifepristone; Moderate Risk QTc-Prolonging Agents; Netupitant; P-glycoprotein/ABCB1 Inhibitors; QTc-Prolonging Agents (Indeterminate Risk and Risk Modifying); Simeprevir

Decreased Effect

Vemurafenib may decrease the levels/effects of: ARIPiprazole; Hydrocodone; Saxagliptin

The levels/effects of Vemurafenib may be decreased by: Bosentan; CYP3A4 Inducers (Moderate); CYP3A4 Inducers (Strong); Dabrafenib; Deferasirox; P-glycoprotein/ABCB1 Inducers; Siltuximab; St Johns Wort; Tocilizumab

Storage/Stability Store at room temperature of 20°C to 25°C (68°F to 77°F); excursions permitted to 15°C and 30°C (59°F and 86°F). Store in the original container with the lid tightly closed.

Mechanism of Action BRAF kinase inhibitor (potent) which inhibits tumor growth in melanomas by inhibiting kinase activity of certain mutated forms of BRAF, including BRAF with V600E mutation, thereby blocking cellular proliferation in melanoma cells with the mutation. Does not have activity against cells with wild-type BRAF. BRAFV600E activating mutations are present in ~50% of melanomas; V600E mutation involves the substitution of glutamic acid for valine at amino acid 600. The cobas 4800 BRAF V600 mutation test is approved to detect BRAFV600E mutation.

Pharmacodynamics/Kinetics

Distribution: V_d: ~106 L

Protein binding: >99%, to albumin and α_1-acid glycoprotein

Half-life, elimination: 57 hours (range: 30 to 120 hours)

Time to peak: ~3 hours

Excretion: Feces (~94%); urine (~1%)

Dosage

U.S. labeling: Melanoma, metastatic or unresectable (with BRAFV600E mutation): 960 mg twice daily; continue until disease progression or unacceptable toxicity.

Canadian labeling: Melanoma, metastatic or unresectable (with BRAFV600 mutation): 960 mg twice daily; continue until disease progression or unacceptable toxicity.

Missed doses: A missed dose may be taken up to 4 hours prior to the next scheduled dose. If it is within 4 hours of the next scheduled dose, administer the next dose at the regular schedule. If vomiting occurs after a dose is taken, do not take an additional dose; continue with the next scheduled dose.

Dosing adjustment for toxicity: Note: Do not dose reduce below 480 mg twice daily. NCI Common Terminology Criteria for Adverse Events (CTC-AE) version 4.0 used for adverse event grades.

Grade 1 or grade 2 (tolerable) toxicity: No dosage adjustment recommended.

Grade 2 (intolerable) or grade 3 toxicity:

First incident: Interrupt treatment until toxicity returns to grade 0 or 1, then resume at 720 mg twice daily.

Second incident: Interrupt treatment until toxicity returns to grade 0 or 1, then resume at 480 mg twice daily.

Third incident: Discontinue permanently

Grade 4 toxicity:

First incident: Interrupt treatment until toxicity returns to grade 0 or 1, then resume at 480 mg twice daily **or** discontinue permanently.

Second incident: Discontinue permanently.

Specific toxicities:

Severe hypersensitivity or severe dermatologic toxicity: Discontinue permanently.

QTc interval changes:

U.S. labeling:

QTc >500 msec (grade ≥3): Temporarily withhold treatment, correct electrolytes and control risk factors for QT prolongation; may reinitiate with a dose reduction once QTc ≤500 msec.

QTc persistently >500 msec and >60 msec above baseline: Discontinue permanently.

Canadian labeling:

QTc >500 msec during treatment and ≤60 msec change from baseline:

First incident: Interrupt treatment until QTc <500 msec, then resume at 720 mg twice daily or 480 mg twice daily if dose previously reduced.

Second incident: Interrupt treatment until QTc <500 msec, then resume at 480 mg twice daily or discontinue permanently if dose previously reduced to 480 mg twice daily.

Third incident: Discontinue permanently.

QTc >500 msec during treatment and >60 msec above baseline: Discontinue permanently.

Dosage adjustment in renal impairment:

U.S. labeling:

Mild to moderate impairment (preexisting): No dosage adjustment necessary.

Severe impairment (preexisting): There are no dosage adjustments provided in the manufacturer's labeling (data are insufficient to determine if dosage adjustment is necessary); use with caution.

Canadian labeling: There are no dosage adjustments provided in the manufacturer's labeling.

Dosage adjustment in hepatic impairment:

Mild to moderate impairment (preexisting): No dosage adjustment necessary.

Severe impairment (preexisting): There are no dosage adjustments provided in the manufacturer's labeling (data are insufficient to determine if dosage adjustment is necessary); use with caution.

Hepatotoxicity/lab abnormalities during treatment: Refer to Dosage adjustment for toxicity and manage with dose reduction, treatment interruption, or discontinuation.

Administration Doses should be administered orally in the morning and evening, ~12 hours apart. Swallow whole with a glass of water; do not crush or chew. May be taken with or without a meal. If vomiting occurs after a dose is taken, do not take an additional dose; continue with the next scheduled dose.

Hazardous agent; use appropriate precautions for handling and disposal (NIOSH 2014 [group 1]).

Monitoring Parameters Liver transaminases, alkaline phosphatase and bilirubin at baseline and monthly during treatment (or as clinically appropriate). Electrolytes (calcium, magnesium and potassium) at baseline and after dosage modification. ECG at baseline, 15 days after initiation, then monthly for 3 months, then every 3 months thereafter (more frequently if clinically appropriate) and with dosage adjustments. Dermatology evaluation (for new skin lesions) at baseline and every 2 months during treatment; also consider continued monitoring for 6 months after completion of treatment. Signs/symptoms of hypersensitivity reactions, uveitis, and malignancies.

Dosage Forms

Tablet, Oral:

Zelboraf: 240 mg

Venlafaxine (ven la FAX een)

Brand Names: U.S. Effexor XR

Brand Names: Canada ACT Venlafaxine XR; Apo-Venlafaxine XR; Dom-Venlafaxine XR; Effexor XR; GD-Venlafaxine XR; Mylan-Venlafaxine XR; PMS-Venlafaxine XR; Ran-Venlafaxine XR; Riva-Venlafaxine XR; Sandoz-Venlafaxine XR; Teva-Venlafaxine XR; Venlafaxine XR

Pharmacologic Category Antidepressant, Serotonin/Norepinephrine Reuptake Inhibitor

Use

Generalized anxiety disorder (extended-release capsules only): Treatment of generalized anxiety disorder (GAD) as defined in the *Diagnostic and Statistical Manual of Mental Disorders (Fourth Edition) (DSM-IV)*.

Major depressive disorder (MDD): Treatment of MDD.

Panic disorder (extended-release capsules only): Treatment of panic disorder, with or without agoraphobia, as defined in *DSM-IV*.

Social anxiety disorder (extended-release capsules and tablets only): Treatment of social anxiety disorder, also known as social phobia, as defined in *DSM-IV*.

Pregnancy Risk Factor C

Pregnancy Considerations Adverse events have been observed in some animal reproduction studies. Venlafaxine and its active metabolite ODV cross the human placenta. An increased risk of teratogenic effects following venlafaxine exposure during pregnancy has not been observed, based on available data. The risk of spontaneous abortion may be increased. Neonatal seizures and neonatal abstinence syndrome have been noted in case reports following maternal use of venlafaxine during pregnancy. Nonteratogenic effects in the newborn following SSRI/SNRI exposure late in the third trimester include respiratory distress, cyanosis, apnea, seizures, temperature instability, feeding difficulty, vomiting, hypoglycemia, hyper- or hypotonia, hyper-reflexia, jitteriness, irritability, constant crying, and tremor. Symptoms may be due to the toxicity of the SNRI or a discontinuation syndrome and may be consistent with serotonin syndrome associated with treatment. The long-term effects of *in utero* SNRI/SSRI exposure on infant development and behavior are not known.

Due to pregnancy-induced physiologic changes, some pharmacokinetic parameters of venlafaxine may be altered. Women should be monitored for decreased efficacy. The ACOG recommends that therapy with SSRIs or SNRIs during pregnancy be individualized; treatment of depression during pregnancy should incorporate the clinical expertise of the mental health clinician, obstetrician, primary healthcare provider, and pediatrician. According to the American Psychiatric Association (APA), the risks of medication treatment should be weighed against other treatment options and untreated depression. For women who discontinue antidepressant medications during pregnancy and who may be at high risk for postpartum depression, the medications can be restarted following delivery. Treatment algorithms have been developed by the ACOG and the APA for the management of depression in women prior to conception and during pregnancy.

Breast-Feeding Considerations Venlafaxine and ODV are found in breast milk and the serum of nursing infants. Adverse events have not been observed; however, it is recommended to monitor the infant for adverse events if the decision to breast-feed has been made. The long-term effects on neurobehavior have not been studied, thus one should prescribe venlafaxine to a mother who is breast-feeding only when the benefits outweigh the potential risks. The manufacturer does not recommend breast-feeding during therapy.

Contraindications Hypersensitivity to venlafaxine or any component of the formulation; use of MAO inhibitors intended to treat psychiatric disorders (concurrently or within 14 days of discontinuing the MAO inhibitor); initiation of MAO inhibitor intended to treat psychiatric disorders within 7 days of discontinuing venlafaxine; initiation in patients receiving linezolid or intravenous methylene blue

Warnings/Precautions [U.S. Boxed Warning]: Antidepressants increase the risk of suicidal thinking and behavior in children, adolescents, and young adults (18-24 years of age) with major depressive disorder (MDD) and other psychiatric disorders; consider risk prior to prescribing. Short-term studies did not show an increased risk in patients >24 years of age and showed a decreased risk in patients ≥65 years. Closely monitor for clinical worsening, suicidality, or unusual changes in behavior, particularly during the first few months of therapy or during periods of dosage adjustments (increases or decreases); the patient's family or caregiver should be instructed to closely observe the patient and communicate condition with healthcare provider. Reduced growth rate has been observed with venlafaxine therapy in children. A medication guide should be dispensed with each prescription.

The possibility of a suicide attempt is inherent in major depression and may persist until remission occurs. Use caution in high-risk patients. Worsening depression and severe abrupt suicidality that are not part of the presenting symptoms may require discontinuation or modification of drug therapy. The patient's family or caregiver should be alerted to monitor patients for the emergence of suicidality and associated behaviors (such as agitation, irritability, hostility, impulsivity, and hypomania) and call healthcare provider.

May precipitate a shift to mania or hypomania in patients with bipolar disorder. Patients presenting with depressive symptoms should be screened for bipolar disorder, including details regarding family history of suicide, bipolar disorder, and depression. Monotherapy in patients with bipolar disorder should be avoided. **Venlafaxine is not FDA approved for the treatment of bipolar depression.**

Potentially life-threatening serotonin syndrome (SS) has occurred with serotonergic agents (eg, SSRIs, SNRIs), particularly when used in combination with other serotonergic agents (eg, triptans, TCAs, fentanyl, lithium, tramadol, buspirone, St John's wort, tryptophan) or agents that impair metabolism of serotonin (eg, MAO inhibitors intended to treat psychiatric disorders, other MAO inhibitors [ie, linezolid and intravenous methylene blue]). Discontinue treatment (and any concomitant serotonergic agent) immediately if signs/symptoms arise.

May cause sustained increase in blood pressure or tachycardia; dose related and increases are generally modest (12-15 mm Hg diastolic). Control preexisting hypertension prior to initiation of venlafaxine. Use caution in patients with recent history of MI, unstable heart disease, cerebrovascular conditions, or hyperthyroidism; may cause increase in anxiety, nervousness, insomnia; may cause weight loss (use with caution in patients where weight loss is undesirable); may cause increases in serum cholesterol and triglycerides; monitor during long-term treatment. Use caution with hepatic or renal impairment; dosage adjustments recommended. May cause hyponatremia/SIADH, age (the elderly), volume depletion and/or concurrent use of diuretics likely increases risk. Discontinue treatment in patients with symptomatic hyponatremia.

May impair platelet aggregation resulting in increased risk of bleeding events, particularly if used concomitantly with aspirin, or NSAIDs, warfarin, or other anticoagulants. Bleeding related to SSRI or SNRI use has been reported to range from relatively minor bruising and epistaxis to life-threatening hemorrhage. Interstitial lung disease and eosinophilic pneumonia have been rarely reported; may present as progressive dyspnea, cough, and/or chest pain. Prompt evaluation and possible discontinuation of therapy may be necessary. Venlafaxine may increase the risks associated with electroconvulsive therapy. Use cautiously in patients with previous seizure disorder. The risks of cognitive or motor impairment, as well as the potential for anticholinergic effects are very low. May cause or exacerbate sexual dysfunction. Bone fractures have been associated with antidepressant treatment. Consider the possibility of a fragility fracture if an antidepressant-treated patient presents with unexplained bone pain, point tenderness, swelling, or bruising (Rabenda, 2013; Rizzoli, 2012).

Use caution in elderly patients; may cause or exacerbate syndrome of inappropriate antidiuretic hormone secretion or hyponatremia; monitor sodium closely with initiation or dosage adjustments in older adults (Beers Criteria). Use caution in patients with increased intraocular pressure or at risk of acute narrow-angle glaucoma (angle-closure glaucoma). Potentially significant drug-drug interactions may exist, requiring dose or frequency adjustment, additional monitoring, and/or selection of alternative therapy.

Abrupt discontinuation or interruption of antidepressant therapy has been associated with a discontinuation syndrome. Symptoms arising may vary with antidepressant however commonly include nausea, vomiting, diarrhea, headaches, lightheadedness, dizziness, diminished appetite, sweating, chills, tremors, paresthesias, fatigue, somnolence, and sleep disturbances (eg, vivid dreams, insomnia). Greater risks for developing a discontinuation syndrome have been associated with antidepressants with shorter half-lives, longer durations of treatment, and abrupt discontinuation. For antidepressants of short or intermediate half-lives, symptoms may emerge within 2-5 days after treatment discontinuation and last 7-14 days (APA, 2010; Fava, 2006; Haddad, 2001; Shelton, 2001; Warner, 2006).

Adverse Reactions

Cardiovascular: Chest pain, edema, hypertension (dose related), palpitations, tachycardia, vasodilation

Central nervous system: Abnormal dreams, abnormality in thinking, agitation, amnesia, anorgasmia (female), anxiety, chills, confusion, depersonalization, depression, dizziness, drowsiness, headache, hypertonia, hypoesthesia, insomnia, migraine, nervousness, paresthesia, trismus, twitching, vertigo, yawning

Dermatologic: Diaphoresis, ecchymoses, pruritus

Endocrine & metabolic: Albuminuria, decreased libido, hypercholesterolemia, increased serum triglycerides, orgasm abnormal, weight gain, weight loss (more common in children & adolescents)

Gastrointestinal: Abdominal pain, anorexia, constipation, diarrhea, dysgeusia, dyspepsia, flatulence, increased appetite, nausea, vomiting, xerostomia

Genitourinary: Abnormal ejaculation, impotence, urinary disorder

Neuromuscular & skeletal: Neck pain, tremor, weakness

Ophthalmic: Accommodation disturbance, mydriasis, visual disturbance

Respiratory: Dyspnea, increased cough, pharyngitis

Miscellaneous: Accidental injury, fever

Rare but important or life-threatening: Abnormal behavior, abnormal gait, abnormal healing, abortion, acne vulgaris, adjustment disorder, ageusia, agranulocytosis, alcohol abuse, alcohol intolerance, alcohol intoxication, alopecia, altered sense of smell, amenorrhea, anaphylaxis, anemia, aneurysm, angina pectoris, angle-closure glaucoma, apathy, aphasia, appendicitis, arthritis, arthropathy, asthma, atelectasis, atrophic striae, attempted suicide, bacteremia, balanitis, basophilia, bigeminy, biliary colic, bladder pain, blepharitis, bone spur, bradycardia, bruxism, buccoglossal syndrome, bundle branch block, bursitis, candidiasis, carcinoma, cardiac arrhythmia (including atrial fibrillation, supraventricular tachycardia, ventricular extrasystoles, ventricular fibrillation, ventricular tachycardia, and torsades de pointes), cardiovascular disease (mitral valve and circulatory disturbance), cataract, cellulitis, central nervous system stimulation, cerebrovascular accident, cervicitis, changes in LDH, cheilitis, chest congestion, cholecystitis, cholelithiasis, chromatopsia, colitis, congenital anomalies, congestive heart failure, conjunctival edema, conjunctivitis, corneal lesion, coronary artery disease, crystalluria, cystitis, deafness, decreased pupillary reflex, deep vein thrombosis, dehydration, delirium, delusions, dementia, diabetes mellitus, diplopia, duodenitis, dysphagia, dysuria, eczema, electric shock-like sensation, emotional lability, endometriosis, eosinophilia, erythema multiforme, esophagitis, extrapyramidal reaction, eye pain, facial paralysis, first degree atrioventricular block, furunculosis, gastroenteritis, gastroesophageal reflux disease, gastrointestinal ulcer, gingivitis, glossitis, glycosuria, goiter, gout, granuloma, Guillain-Barré syndrome, hair discoloration, hematoma, hemochromatosis, hemorrhage (eye, GI, gum, mucocutaneous, rectal, retinal, subconjunctival, uterine, vaginal), hemorrhoids, hepatic effects (including GGT elevation; abnormalities of unspecified liver function tests; liver damage, necrosis, or failure; and fatty liver), hepatitis, homicidal ideation, hostility, hyperacidity, hyperacusis, hypercalciuria, hyperesthesia, hyperreflexia, hyperthyroidism, hyperuricemia, hyperventilation, hypoglycemia, hypohidrosis, hypokalemia, hypokinesia, hypomenorrhea, hyponatremia, hypophosphatemia, hyporeflexia, hypotension, hypothyroidism, hypotonia, hypoventilation, hysteria, ileitis, impulse control disorder, increased energy, increased libido, increased serum prolactin, interstitial pulmonary disease (including eosinophilic pneumonia), intestinal obstruction, keratitis, labyrinthitis, laryngismus, laryngitis, leukocytosis, leukoderma, leukopenia, leukorrhea, lichenoid dermatitis, loss of consciousness, lymphadenopathy, lymphocytosis, melena, menopause, miliaria, miosis, multiple myeloma, muscle spasm, myasthenia, nephrolithiasis, neuralgia, neuritis, neuropathy, neutropenia, night sweats, nystagmus, oliguria, onychia sicca, oral candidiasis, oral mucosa ulcer, oral paresthesia, orchitis, ostealgia, osteoporosis, osteosclerosis, otitis externa, otitis media, ovarian cyst, pancreatitis, pancytopenia, panic, papilledema, paranoia, paresis, parotitis, pathological fracture, pelvic pain, periodontitis, peripheral vascular disease, petechial rash, plantar fasciitis, pleurisy, pneumonia, polyuria, proctitis, prolonged bleeding time, prolonged erection, prostatic disease, pruritic rash, psoriasis, psychosis, psychotic depression, pulmonary embolism, purpura, pustular rash, pyelonephritis, pyuria, rectal disease, renal failure, renal function abnormality, renal pain, rhabdomyolysis, rheumatoid arthritis, rupture of tendon, salpingitis, scleritis, seborrhea, seizure, serotonin syndrome, SIADH, sialorrhea, sinus arrhythmia, skin atrophy, skin discoloration, skin hypertrophy, skin photosensitivity, sleep apnea, speech disturbance, Stevens-Johnson syndrome, stomatitis, stupor, suicidal ideation (reported at a frequency up to 2% in children/adolescents with major depressive disorder), tenosynovitis, thrombocythemia, thrombocytopenia, thyroiditis, thyroid nodule, tongue discoloration, uremia, urinary incontinence, urinary urgency, urolithiasis, urticaria, uterine spasm, uveitis, vaginal dryness, vaginitis, vesicobullous dermatitis, visual field defect, voice disorder, withdrawal syndrome, xeroderma, xerophthalmia

Drug Interactions

Metabolism/Transport Effects Substrate of CYP2C19 (minor), CYP2C9 (minor), CYP2D6 (major), CYP3A4 (major); **Note:** Assignment of Major/Minor substrate status based on clinically relevant drug interaction potential; **Inhibits** CYP2B6 (weak), CYP2D6 (weak), CYP3A4 (weak)

Avoid Concomitant Use

Avoid concomitant use of Venlafaxine with any of the following: Conivaptan; Dapoxetine; Fusidic Acid (Systemic); Idelalisib; Iobenguane I 123; Linezolid; MAO Inhibitors; Methylene Blue; Pimozide; Urokinase

Increased Effect/Toxicity

Venlafaxine may increase the levels/effects of: Agents with Antiplatelet Properties; Alpha-/Beta-Agonists; Anticoagulants; Antipsychotic Agents; Apixaban; ARIPiprazole; Aspirin; Collagenase (Systemic); Dabigatran Etexilate; Highest Risk QTc-Prolonging Agents; Hydrocodone; Ibritumomab; Lomitapide; Methylene Blue; Moderate Risk QTc-Prolonging Agents; NSAID (Nonselective); Obinutuzumab; Pimozide; Rivaroxaban; Salicylates; Serotonin Modulators; Thrombolytic Agents; Tositumomab and Iodine I 131 Tositumomab; TraZODone; Urokinase; Vitamin K Antagonists

The levels/effects of Venlafaxine may be increased by: Abiraterone Acetate; Alcohol (Ethyl); Antiemetics (5HT3 Antagonists); Antipsychotic Agents; Aprepitant; Ceritinib; Conivaptan; CYP2D6 Inhibitors (Moderate); CYP2D6 Inhibitors (Strong); CYP3A4 Inhibitors (Moderate); CYP3A4 Inhibitors (Strong); Dapoxetine; Dasatinib; Fosaprepitant; Fusidic Acid (Systemic); Glucosamine; Herbs (Anticoagulant/Antiplatelet Properties); Ibrutinib; Idelalisib; Ivacaftor; Limaprost; Linezolid; Luliconazole; MAO Inhibitors; Metoclopramide; Mifepristone; Multivitamins/Fluoride (with ADE); Multivitamins/Minerals (with ADEK, Folate, Iron); Multivitamins/Minerals (with AE, No Iron); Netupitant; Omega-3 Fatty Acids; Peginterferon Alfa-2b; Pentosan Polysulfate Sodium; Pentoxifylline; Propafenone; Prostacyclin Analogues; Simeprevir; Stiripentol; Tedizolid; Vitamin E; Voriconazole

Decreased Effect

Venlafaxine may decrease the levels/effects of: Alpha2-Agonists; Indinavir; Iobenguane I 123; Ioflupane I 123

The levels/effects of Venlafaxine may be decreased by: Bosentan; CYP3A4 Inducers (Moderate); CYP3A4 Inducers (Strong); Dabrafenib; Deferasirox; Mitotane; Peginterferon Alfa-2b; Siltuximab; St Johns Wort; Tocilizumab

Storage/Stability Store immediate-release tablets and extended-release capsules at 20°C to 25°C (68°F to 77°F). Store extended-release tablets at 25°C (77°F); excursions are permitted between 15°C and 30°C (59°F and 86°F).

Mechanism of Action Venlafaxine and its active metabolite, O-desmethylvenlafaxine (ODV), are potent inhibitors of neuronal serotonin and norepinephrine reuptake and weak inhibitors of dopamine reuptake. Venlafaxine and ODV have no significant activity for muscarinic cholinergic, H_1-histaminergic, or alpha$_2$-adrenergic receptors. Venlafaxine and ODV do not possess MAO-inhibitory activity. Venlafaxine functions like an SSRI in low doses (37.5 mg/day) and as a dual mechanism agent affecting serotonin and norepinephrine at doses above 225 mg/day (Harvey, 2000; Kelsey, 1996).

Pharmacodynamics/Kinetics

Absorption: Oral: ≥92%

Distribution: V_{dss}: Venlafaxine 7.5 ± 3.7 L/kg, ODV 5.7 ± 1.8 L/kg

Protein binding: Venlafaxine 27% ± 2%, ODV 30% ± 12%

Metabolism: Hepatic via CYP2D6 to active metabolite, O-desmethylvenlafaxine (ODV); other metabolites include N-desmethylvenlafaxine and N,O-didesmethylvenlafaxine

Bioavailability: Oral: ~45%

Half-life elimination: Venlafaxine: 5 ± 2 hours; ODV: 11 ± 2 hours; prolonged with cirrhosis (venlafaxine: ~30%, ODV: ~60%), renal impairment (venlafaxine: ~50%, ODV: ~40%), and during dialysis (venlafaxine: ~180%, ODV: ~142%)

Time to peak:

Immediate release: Venlafaxine: 2 hours, ODV: 3 hours

Extended release: Venlafaxine: 5.5 hours, ODV: 9 hours

Excretion: Urine (~87%; 5% of total dose as unchanged drug; 29% of total dose as unconjugated ODV; 26% of total dose as conjugated ODV; 27% of total dose as minor inactive metabolites)

Dosage Oral:

Children and Adolescents:

Attention-deficit/hyperactivity disorder (off-label use; Olvera, 1996): Initial: 12.5 mg/day

Children <40 kg: Increase by 12.5 mg/week to maximum of 50 mg/day in 2 divided doses

Children ≥40 kg: Increase by 25 mg/week to maximum of 75 mg/day in 3 divided doses.

Mean dose: 60 mg or 1.4 mg/kg administered in 2 to 3 divided doses

Adults:

Depression:

Immediate-release tablets: Initial: 37.5 to 75 mg/day, administered in 2 or 3 divided doses; may increase in ≤75 mg/day increments at intervals of ≥4 days as tolerated; usual dosage: 75 to 225 mg once daily (maximum daily dose: 375 mg) (APA, 2010)

Extended-release capsules or tablets: Initial: 37.5 to 75 mg once daily; in patients who are initiated at 37.5 mg once daily, may increase to 75 mg once daily after 4 to 7 days; dose may then be increased by ≤75 mg/day increments at intervals of ≥4 days as tolerated; usual dosage: 75 to 225 mg once daily (maximum daily dose: 225 mg)

Note: Patients treated with a therapeutic dose with venlafaxine immediate release may be switched to venlafaxine extended release (ER) at the nearest equivalent dose (mg/day). Following the formulation switch individual dosage adjustments may be necessary.

Generalized anxiety disorder: Extended-release capsules: Initial: 37.5 to 75 mg once daily; in patients who are initiated at 37.5 mg once daily, may increase to 75 mg once daily after 4 to 7 days; may then be increased by ≤75 mg/day increments at intervals of ≥4 days as tolerated; usual dosage: 75 to 225 mg once daily (maximum daily dose: 225 mg)

Panic disorder: Extended-release capsules: Initial: 37.5 mg once daily for 1 week; may increase to 75 mg once daily after 7 days, may then be increased by ≤75 mg/day increments at intervals of ≥7 days; usual dosage: 75 to 225 mg once daily (maximum daily dose: 225 mg).

Social anxiety disorder: Extended-release capsules or tablets: 75 mg once daily (maximum daily dose: 75 mg); no evidence that doses >75 mg/day offer any additional benefit

Obsessive-compulsive disorder (off-label use): Titrate to usual dosage range of 150 to 300 mg/day; however, doses up to 375 mg/day have been used; response may be seen in 4 weeks (Phelps, 2005)

Neuropathic pain (includes diabetic neuropathy) (off-label use): Immediate-release and extended release: Dosage range studied: 75 mg to 225 mg daily; therapy may be initiated with 37.5 mg once or twice daily to minimize adverse effects, and titrated by 75 mg per week to a maximum of 225 mg daily administered in a single daily dose or in divided doses (Bril, 2011; Chong, 2007; Dworkin, 2007; Grothe 2004)

Hot flashes (off-label use): Immediate-release and extended release: Dosage range studied: 37.5 to 150 mg daily; therapy usually initiated with 37.5 mg daily to minimize adverse effects; dose may remain at 37.5 mg daily or titrated by 37.5 mg per week to a dose of 75 mg or 150 mg daily administered in a single daily dose or in divided doses (AACE [Goodman, 2011]; Evans, 2005; Loibl, 2007; Loprinzi, 2000; Loprinzi, 2006)

Attention-deficit disorder (off-label use): Initial: Doses vary between 18.75 to 75 mg/day; may increase after 4 weeks to 150 mg/day; if tolerated, doses up to 225 mg/day have been used (Maidment, 2003)

Post-traumatic stress disorder (PTSD) (off-label use): Extended release formulation: 37.5 to 300 mg/day (Bandelow, 2008; Benedek, 2009)

Elderly: Refer to adult dosing. No specific recommendations for elderly; use with caution.

Discontinuation of therapy: Upon discontinuation of antidepressant therapy, gradually taper the dose to minimize the incidence of withdrawal symptoms and allow for the detection of re-emerging symptoms. Evidence supporting ideal taper rates is limited. APA and NICE guidelines suggest tapering therapy over at least several weeks with consideration to the half-life of the antidepressant; antidepressants with a shorter half-life may need to be tapered more conservatively. In addition for long-term treated patients, WFSBP guidelines recommend tapering over 4 to 6 months. If intolerable withdrawal symptoms occur following a dose reduction, consider resuming the previously prescribed dose and/or decrease dose at a more gradual rate (APA, 2010; Bauer, 2002; Haddad, 2001; NCCMH, 2010; Schatzberg, 2006; Shelton, 2001; Warner, 2006).

MAO inhibitor recommendations:

Switching to or from an MAO inhibitor intended to treat psychiatric disorders:

Allow 14 days to elapse between discontinuing an MAO inhibitor intended to treat psychiatric disorders and initiation of venlafaxine.

Allow 7 days to elapse between discontinuing venlafaxine and initiation of an MAO inhibitor intended to treat psychiatric disorders.

Use with other MAO inhibitors (linezolid or IV methylene blue):

Do not initiate venlafaxine in patients receiving linezolid or IV methylene blue; consider other interventions for psychiatric condition.

If urgent treatment with linezolid or IV methylene blue is required in a patient already receiving venlafaxine and potential benefits outweigh potential risks, discontinue venlafaxine promptly and administer linezolid or IV methylene blue. Monitor for SS for 7 days or until 24 hours after the last dose of linezolid or IV methylene blue, whichever comes first. May resume venlafaxine 24 hours after the last dose of linezolid or IV methylene blue.

Dosage adjustment in renal impairment:

Mild to moderate impairment (CrCl 30 to 89 mL/minute):

Extended release: Reduce total daily dose by 25% to 50%

Immediate release: Reduce total daily dose by 25%

Severe impairment: (CrCl <30 mL/minute): Reduce total daily dose by 50% or more

Hemodialysis: Reduce total daily dose by 50% or more

Dosage adjustment in hepatic impairment:

Mild to moderate impairment (Child-Pugh score 5 to 9): Reduce total daily dose by 50%

Severe impairment (Child-Pugh score 10 to 15) or cirrhosis: Reduce total daily dose by 50% or more

Dietary Considerations Administer with food.

Administration Administer with food.

Extended-release formulations: Swallow capsule or tablet whole with fluid; do not divide, crush, chew, or place in water. Contents of capsule may be sprinkled on a spoonful of applesauce and swallowed immediately without chewing; followed with a glass of water to ensure complete swallowing of the pellets.

Monitoring Parameters Blood pressure should be regularly monitored, especially in patients with a high baseline blood pressure; may cause mean increase in heart rate of 4-9 beats/minute; cholesterol; mental status for depression, suicide ideation (especially at the beginning of therapy or when doses are increased or decreased), anxiety, social functioning, mania, panic attacks; signs/symptoms of serotonin syndrome, hyponatremia, discontinuation symptoms; height and weight should be monitored in children; intraocular pressure and mydriasis (in patients with raised ocular pressure or at risk of acute narrow angle glaucoma) (APA, 2010)

Dosage Forms

Capsule Extended Release 24 Hour, Oral:
Effexor XR: 37.5 mg, 75 mg, 150 mg
Generic: 37.5 mg, 75 mg, 150 mg

Tablet, Oral:
Generic: 25 mg, 37.5 mg, 50 mg, 75 mg, 100 mg

Tablet Extended Release 24 Hour, Oral:
Generic: 37.5 mg, 75 mg, 150 mg, 225 mg

◆ **Venlafaxine XR (Can)** *see* Venlafaxine *on page 2150*

◆ **Venofer** *see* Iron Sucrose *on page 1118*

◆ **Ventavis** *see* Iloprost *on page 1046*

◆ **Ventolin Diskus (Can)** *see* Albuterol *on page 69*

◆ **Ventolin HFA** *see* Albuterol *on page 69*

◆ **Ventolin I.V. Infusion (Can)** *see* Albuterol *on page 69*

◆ **Ventolin Nebules P.F. (Can)** *see* Albuterol *on page 69*

◆ **VePesid** *see* Etoposide *on page 816*

◆ **Vepesid (Can)** *see* Etoposide *on page 816*

◆ **Veramyst** *see* Fluticasone (Nasal) *on page 910*

Verapamil (ver AP a mil)

Brand Names: U.S. Calan; Calan SR; Isoptin SR; Verelan; Verelan PM

Brand Names: Canada Apo-Verap; Apo-Verap SR; Covera; Covera-HS; Dom-Verapamil SR; Isoptin SR; Mylan-Verapamil; Mylan-Verapamil SR; Novo-Veramil; Novo-Veramil SR; Nu-Verap; Nu-Verap SR; PHL-Verapamil SR; PMS-Verapamil SR; PRO-Verapamil SR; Riva-Verapamil SR; Verapamil Hydrochloride Injection, USP; Verapamil SR; Verelan

Index Terms Iproveratril Hydrochloride; Verapamil Hydrochloride

Pharmacologic Category Antianginal Agent; Antiarrhythmic Agent, Class IV; Antihypertensive; Calcium Channel Blocker; Calcium Channel Blocker, Nondihydropyridine

Use

IV: Supraventricular tachyarrhythmia (PSVT, atrial fibrillation/flutter [rate control])

Oral: Treatment of hypertension; angina pectoris (vasospastic, chronic stable, unstable) (Calan, Covera-HS); supraventricular tachyarrhythmia (PSVT, atrial fibrillation/flutter [rate control])

The 2014 guideline for the management of high blood pressure in adults (JNC 8) recommends initiation of pharmacologic treatment to lower blood pressure for the following patients (JNC 8 [James, 2013]):

- Patients ≥60 years of age with systolic blood pressure (SBP) ≥150 mm Hg or diastolic blood pressure (DBP) ≥90 mm Hg. Goal of therapy is SBP <150 mm Hg and DBP <90 mm Hg.
- Patients <60 years of age with SBP ≥140 mm Hg or DBP ≥90 mm Hg. Goal of therapy is SBP <140 mm Hg and DBP <90 mm Hg.
- Patients ≥18 years of age with diabetes with SBP ≥140 mm Hg or DBP ≥90 mm Hg. Goal of therapy is SBP <140 mm Hg and DBP <90 mm Hg.
- Patients ≥18 years of age with chronic kidney disease (CKD) with SBP ≥140 mm Hg or DBP ≥90 mm Hg. Goal of therapy is SBP <140 mm Hg and DBP <90 mm Hg.

In patients with chronic kidney disease (CKD), regardless of race or diabetes status, the use of an ACE inhibitor (ACEI) or angiotensin receptor blocker (ARB) as initial therapy is recommended to improve kidney outcomes. In the general nonblack population (without CKD) including those with diabetes, initial antihypertensive treatment should consist of a thiazide-type diuretic, calcium channel blocker, ACEI, or ARB. In the general black population (without CKD) including those with diabetes, initial antihypertensive treatment should consist of a thiazide-type diuretic or a calcium channel blocker instead of an ACEI or ARB.

The ACCF/AHA guidelines for the management of unstable angina/non-ST-elevation myocardial infarction recommend verapamil to treat hypertension or ongoing ischemia if beta-blocker therapy is ineffective or contraindicated and in the absence of left ventricular dysfunction, pulmonary congestion, or AV block (ACCF/AHA [Anderson, 2013]).

Pregnancy Risk Factor C

Pregnancy Considerations Adverse events were observed in some animal reproduction studies in doses which also caused maternal toxicity. Verapamil crosses the placenta. Use during pregnancy may cause adverse fetal effects (bradycardia, heart block, hypotension) (Tan, 2001). Women with hypertrophic cardiomyopathy who are controlled with verapamil prior to pregnancy may continue therapy, but increased fetal monitoring is recommended (Gersh, 2011). Verapamil is not the preferred treatment for paroxysmal supraventricular tachycardia (PSVT) in pregnant women (Blomström-Lundqvist, 2003). Untreated chronic maternal hypertension is associated with adverse events in the fetus, infant, and mother. If treatment for hypertension during pregnancy is needed, other agents are preferred (ACOG, 2013).

Breast-Feeding Considerations Verapamil is excreted into breast milk; the estimated exposure to the nursing infant is <1% of the maternal dose. Breast-feeding is not recommended by some manufacturers.

Contraindications Hypersensitivity to verapamil or any component of the formulation; severe left ventricular dysfunction; hypotension (systolic pressure <90 mm Hg) or cardiogenic shock; sick sinus syndrome (except in patients with a functioning artificial ventricular pacemaker); second- or third-degree AV block (except in patients with a functioning artificial ventricular pacemaker); atrial flutter or fibrillation and an accessory bypass tract (Wolff-Parkinson-White [WPW] syndrome, Lown-Ganong-Levine syndrome)

IV: Additional contraindications include concurrent use of IV beta-blocking agents; ventricular tachycardia

Warnings/Precautions Avoid use in heart failure; can exacerbate condition; use is contraindicated in severe left ventricular dysfunction. Symptomatic hypotension with or without syncope can rarely occur; blood pressure must be lowered at a rate appropriate for the patient's clinical condition. Rare increases in hepatic enzymes can be observed. Can cause first-degree AV block or sinus bradycardia; use is contraindicated in patients with sick sinus syndrome, second- or third-degree AV block (except in patients with a functioning artificial pacemaker), or an accessory bypass tract (eg, WPW syndrome). Other conduction abnormalities are rare. Considered contraindicated in patients with wide complex tachycardias unless known to be supraventricular in origin; severe hypotension likely to occur upon administration (ACLS, 2010). Use caution when using verapamil together with a beta-blocker. Administration of IV verapamil and an IV beta-blocker within a few hours of each other may result in asystole and should be avoided; simultaneous administration is contraindicated. Use with other agents known to reduce SA node function and/or AV nodal conduction (eg, digoxin) or reduce sympathetic outflow (eg, clonidine) may increase the risk of serious bradycardia. Verapamil significantly increases digoxin serum concentrations; adjust digoxin dose. Use with caution in patients with HCM with outflow tract obstruction (especially those with high gradients, advanced heart failure, or sinus bradycardia); may be used in patients who cannot tolerate beta-blockade. Verapamil should not be used in those with systemic hypotension or severe dyspnea at rest (Gersh, 2011; Nishimura, 2004).

Decreased neuromuscular transmission has been reported with verapamil; use with caution in patients with attenuated neuromuscular transmission (Duchenne's muscular dystrophy, myasthenia gravis); dosage reduction may be required. Use with caution in renal impairment; monitor hemodynamics and possibly ECG if severe impairment, particularly if concomitant hepatic impairment. Use with caution in patients with hepatic impairment; dosage reduction may be required; monitor hemodynamics and possibly ECG if severe impairment. May prolong recovery from nondepolarizing neuromuscular-blocking agents. Use Covera-HS (extended-release delivery system) with caution in patients with severe GI narrowing. In patients with extremely short GI transit times (eg, <7 hours), dosage adjustment may be required; inadequate pharmacokinetic data. In neonates and young infants, avoid IV use for SVT due to severe apnea, bradycardia, hypotensive reactions, and cardiac arrest; in children, use IV with caution as myocardial depression and hypotension may occur.

Adverse Reactions

Cardiovascular: AV block, bradycardia, CHF/pulmonary edema, flushing, hypotension, peripheral edema

Central nervous system: Dizziness, fatigue, headache, lethargy, pain, sleep disturbance

Dermatologic: Rash

Gastrointestinal: Constipation, diarrhea, dyspnea, gingival hyperplasia, nausea

Hepatic: Liver enzymes increased

Neuromuscular & skeletal: Myalgia, paresthesia

Respiratory: Dyspnea

Miscellaneous: Flu-like syndrome

Rare but important or life-threatening:

Oral: Abdominal discomfort, alopecia, angina, arthralgia, atrioventricular dissociation, blurred vision, bruising, cerebrovascular accident, chest pain, claudication, confusion, diaphoresis, ECG abnormal, equilibrium disorders, erythema multiforme, exanthema, extrapyramidal symptoms, galactorrhea/hyperprolactinemia, gastrointestinal distress, gynecomastia, hyperkeratosis, impotence, insomnia, macules, MI, muscle cramps, palpitation, psychosis, purpura (vasculitis), shakiness, somnolence, spotty menstruation, Stevens-Johnson syndrome, syncope, tinnitus, urination increased, urticaria, weakness, xerostomia

IV: Bronchi/laryngeal spasm, depression, diaphoresis, itching, muscle fatigue, respiratory failure, rotary nystagmus, seizure, sleepiness, urticaria, vertigo

Postmarketing and/or case reports: Asystole, eosinophilia, EPS, exfoliative dermatitis, GI obstruction, hair color change, paralytic ileus, Parkinsonian syndrome, pulseless electrical activity, shock, ventricular fibrillation

Drug Interactions

Metabolism/Transport Effects **Substrate** of CYP1A2 (minor), CYP2B6 (minor), CYP2C9 (minor), CYP2E1 (minor), CYP3A4 (major), P-glycoprotein; **Note:** Assignment of Major/Minor substrate status based on clinically relevant drug interaction potential; **Inhibits** CYP1A2 (weak), CYP2C9 (weak), CYP2D6 (weak), CYP3A4 (moderate), P-glycoprotein

Avoid Concomitant Use

Avoid concomitant use of Verapamil with any of the following: Bosutinib; Ceritinib; Conivaptan; Dantrolene; Disopyramide; Dofetilide; Fusidic Acid (Systemic); Ibrutinib; Idelalisib; Ivabradine; Lomitapide; Naloxegol; Olaparib; PAZOPanib; Pimozide; Silodosin; Simeprevir; Tolvaptan; Topotecan; Trabectedin; Ulipristal; VinCRIStine (Liposomal)

Increased Effect/Toxicity

Verapamil may increase the levels/effects of: Afatinib; Alcohol (Ethyl); Aliskiren; Amifostine; Amiodarone; Antihypertensives; ARIPiprazole; AtorvaSTATin; Atosiban; Avanafil; Beta-Blockers; Bosentan; Bosutinib; Bradycardia-Causing Agents; Brentuximab Vedotin; Budesonide (Systemic, Oral Inhalation); BusPIRone; Calcium Channel Blockers (Dihydropyridine); Cannabis; CarBAMazepine; Cardiac Glycosides; Ceritinib; Colchicine; CycloSPORINE (Systemic); CYP3A4 Substrates; Dabigatran Etexilate; Dapoxetine; Disopyramide; Dofetilide; DOXOrubicin (Conventional); Dronabinol; Dronedarone; DULoxetine; Edoxaban; Eletriptan; Eliglustat; Eplerenone; Everolimus; FentaNYL; Fexofenadine; Fingolimod; Flecainide; Fosphenytoin; Halofantrine; Hydrocodone; Hypotensive Agents; Ibrutinib; Imatinib; Ivabradine; Ivacaftor; Lacosamide; Ledipasvir; Levodopa; Lithium; Lomitapide; Lovastatin; Lurasidone; Magnesium Salts; Midodrine; Naloxegol; Neuromuscular-Blocking Agents (Nondepolarizing); Nintedanib; Nitroprusside; Obinutuzumab; Olaparib; OxyCODONE; PAZOPanib; P-glycoprotein/ABCB1 Substrates; Phenytoin; Pimecrolimus; Pimozide; Propafenone; Prucalopride; QuiNIDine; Ranolazine; Red Yeast Rice; Rifaximin; RisperiDONE; RiTUXimab; Rivaroxaban; Salicylates; Salmeterol; Saxagliptin; Silodosin; Simeprevir; Simvastatin; Suvorexant; Tacrolimus (Systemic); Tacrolimus (Topical); Tetrahydrocannabinol; Tolvaptan; Topotecan; Trabectedin; Ulipristal; Vilazodone; VinCRIStine (Liposomal); Zopiclone; Zuclopenthixol

The levels/effects of Verapamil may be increased by: Alfuzosin; Alpha1-Blockers; Anilidopiperidine Opioids; Antifungal Agents (Azole Derivatives, Systemic); Aprepitant; AtorvaSTATin; Barbiturates; Bretylium; Brimonidine (Topical); Calcium Channel Blockers (Dihydropyridine); Cimetidine; CloNIDine; Conivaptan; CycloSPORINE (Systemic); CYP3A4 Inhibitors (Moderate); CYP3A4 Inhibitors (Strong); Dantrolene; Dasatinib; Diazoxide; Dronedarone; Fluconazole; Fosaprepitant; Fusidic Acid (Systemic); Grapefruit Juice; Herbs (Hypotensive Properties); Idelalisib; Ivabradine; Luliconazole; Macrolide Antibiotics; Magnesium Salts; MAO Inhibitors; Mifepristone; Netupitant; Nicorandil; Pentoxifylline; P-glycoprotein/ABCB1 Inhibitors; Phosphodiesterase 5 Inhibitors; Prostacyclin Analogues; Protease Inhibitors; QuiNIDine; Regorafenib; Stiripentol; Telithromycin; Tofacitinib

Decreased Effect

Verapamil may decrease the levels/effects of: Clopidogrel; Ifosfamide; MetFORMIN

The levels/effects of Verapamil may be decreased by: Barbiturates; Bosentan; Calcium Salts; CarBAMazepine; CYP3A4 Inducers (Moderate); CYP3A4 Inducers (Strong); Dabrafenib; Deferasirox; Efavirenz; Herbs (Hypertensive Properties); Methylphenidate; Mitotane; Nafcillin; P-glycoprotein/ABCB1 Inducers; Rifamycin Derivatives; Siltuximab; St Johns Wort; Tocilizumab; Yohimbine

Food Interactions

Ethanol: Verapamil may increase ethanol levels. Management: Monitor patients and caution about increased effects.

Food: Grapefruit juice may increase the serum concentration of verapamil. Management: Avoid grapefruit juice or use with caution and monitor for effects.

Storage/Stability Store at controlled room temperature of 15°C to 30°C (59°F to 86°F). Protect from light.

Mechanism of Action Inhibits calcium ion from entering the "slow channels" or select voltage-sensitive areas of vascular smooth muscle and myocardium during depolarization; produces relaxation of coronary vascular smooth muscle and coronary vasodilation; increases myocardial oxygen delivery in patients with vasospastic angina; slows automaticity and conduction of AV node.

Pharmacodynamics/Kinetics

Onset of action: Peak effect: Oral: Immediate release: 1-2 hours; IV: 1-5 minutes

Duration: Oral: Immediate release tablets: 6-8 hours; IV: 10-20 minutes

Absorption: Well absorbed

Distribution: V_d: 3.89 L/kg (Storstein, 1984)

Protein binding: ~90%

Metabolism: Hepatic (extensive first-pass effect) via multiple CYP isoenzymes; primary metabolite is norverapamil (20% pharmacologic activity of verapamil)

Bioavailability: Oral: 20% to 35%

Half-life elimination: Infants: 4.4-6.9 hours; Adults: Single dose: 3-7 hours, Multiple doses: 4.5-12 hours; severe hepatic impairment: 14-16 hours

Time to peak, serum: Oral:

Immediate release: 1-2 hours

Extended release (Covera-HS, Verelan PM): ~11 hours, drug release delayed ~4-5 hours

Sustained release: 5.21 hours (Calan SR, Isoptin SR); 7-9 hours (Verelan)

Excretion: Urine (70% as metabolites, 3% to 4% as unchanged drug); feces (16%)

Dosage

Children: **Note:** Verapamil is no longer included in the Pediatric Advanced Life Support (PALS) tachyarrhythmia algorithm.

Children: 1-15 years: SVT: IV: 0.1-0.3 mg/kg/dose over 2 minutes; maximum: 5 mg/dose, may repeat dose in 30 minutes if inadequate response; maximum for second dose: 10 mg

Adults:

Atrial fibrillation (rate control):

IV: 0.075 to 0.15 mg/kg (~5 to 10 mg for a 70-kg patient) administered as a bolus over 2 minutes; may give an additional 10 mg after 30 minutes if no response, then 0.005 mg/kg/minute as a continuous infusion (AHA/ACC/HRS [January, 2014])

Oral:

Extended release (off-label use): Usual maintenance dose range: 180 to 480 mg once daily (AHA/ACC/HRS [January, 2014])

Immediate release: 240 to 480 mg daily in 3 to 4 divided doses

SVT (ACLS, 2010): IV: 2.5 to 5 mg over 2 minutes; second dose of 5 to 10 mg (~0.15 mg/kg) may be given 15 to 30 minutes after the initial dose if patient tolerates, but does not respond to initial dose; maximum total dose: 20 to 30 mg

Angina: Oral: **Note:** When switching from immediate-release to extended/sustained release formulations, the total daily dose remains the same unless formulation strength does not allow for equal conversion.

Immediate release: Initial: 80 to 120 mg 3 times daily (elderly or small stature: 40 mg 3 times daily); Usual dose range (Gibbons, 2003): 80 to 160 mg 3 times daily

Extended release (Covera-HS): Initial: 180 mg once daily at bedtime; if inadequate response, may increase dose at weekly intervals to 240 mg once daily, then 360 mg once daily, then 480 mg once daily; maximum dose: 480 mg daily

PSVT prophylaxis: Oral: Immediate release: 240 to 480 mg/day in 3 to 4 divided doses

Hypertension: Oral: **Note:** When switching from immediate-release to extended/sustained release formulations, the total daily dose remains the same unless formulation strength does not allow for equal conversion.

Immediate release: Initial: 80 mg 3 times daily; usual dosage range (ASH/ISH [Weber, 2014]): 240 to 480 mg daily

Sustained release: Usual dosage range (ASH/ISH [Weber, 2014]): 240 to 480 mg daily; **Note:** There is no evidence of additional benefit with doses >360 mg/day.

Calan SR, Isoptin SR: Initial: 180 mg once daily in the morning (elderly or small stature: 120 mg daily); if inadequate response, may increase dose at weekly intervals to 240 mg once daily, then 180 mg twice daily (or 240 mg in the morning followed by 120 mg in the evening); maximum dose: 240 mg twice daily.

Verelan: Initial: 180 mg once daily in the morning (elderly or small stature: 120 mg daily); if inadequate response, may increase dose at weekly intervals to 240 mg once daily, then 360 mg once daily, then 480 mg once daily; maximum dose: 480 mg daily

Extended release: Usual dosage range (ASH/ISH [Weber, 2014]): 240 to 480 mg daily

Covera-HS: Initial: 180 mg once daily at bedtime; if inadequate response, may increase dose at weekly intervals to 240 mg once daily, then 360 mg once daily, then 480 mg once daily; maximum dose: 480 mg daily

Verelan PM: Initial: 200 mg once daily at bedtime (elderly or small stature: 100 mg daily); if inadequate response, may increase dose at weekly intervals to 300 mg once daily, then 400 mg once daily; maximum dose: 400 mg daily

Elderly: Hypertension: Oral: **Note:** When switching from immediate release to extended or sustained release formulations, the total daily dose remains the same unless formulation strength does not allow for equal conversion.

Manufacturer's recommendations:

Immediate release: Initial: 40 mg 3 times daily

Sustained release: Calan SR, Isoptin SR,Verelan: Initial: 120 mg once daily in the morning

Extended release:

Covera-HS: Initial: 180 mg once daily at bedtime

Verelan PM: Initial: 100 mg once daily at bedtime

ACCF/AHA Expert Consensus recommendations: Consider lower initial doses and titrating to response (Aronow, 2011)

Dosage adjustment in renal impairment: Manufacturer recommends caution and additional ECG monitoring in patients with renal insufficiency. The manufacturer of Verelan PM recommends an initial dose of 100 mg daily at bedtime. **Note:** A multiple dose study in adults suggests reduced renal clearance of verapamil and its metabolite (norverapamil) with advanced renal failure (Storstein, 1984). Additionally, several clinical papers report adverse effects of verapamil in patients with chronic renal failure receiving recommended doses of verapamil (Pritza, 1991; Váquez, 1996). In contrast, a number of single dose studies show no difference in verapamil (or norverapamil metabolite) disposition between chronic renal failure and control patients (Beyerlein, 1990; Hanyok, 1988; Mooy, 1985; Zachariah, 1991).

Dialysis: Not removed by hemodialysis (Mooy, 1985); supplemental dose is not necessary.

Dosage adjustment/comments in hepatic disease: In cirrhosis, reduce dose to 20% and 50% of normal for oral and intravenous administration, respectively, and monitor ECG (Somogyi, 1981). The manufacturer of Verelan PM recommends an initial adult dose of 100 mg/day at bedtime. The manufacturers of Calan, Calan SR, Covera-HS, Isoptin SR, and Verelan recommend giving 30% of the normal dose to patients with severe hepatic impairment.

Dietary Considerations Calan SR and Isoptin SR products may be taken with food or milk, other formulations may be administered without regard to meals; sprinkling contents of Verelan or Verelan PM capsule onto applesauce does not affect oral absorption.

Administration

Oral: Do not crush or chew sustained or extended release products.

Calan SR, Isoptin SR: Administer with food.

Verelan, Verelan PM: Capsules may be opened and the contents sprinkled on 1 tablespoonful of applesauce, then swallowed immediately without chewing. Do not subdivide contents of capsules.

IV: Rate of infusion: Over 2 minutes; over 3 minutes in older patients (ACLS, 2010)

Monitoring Parameters Monitor blood pressure and heart rate; periodic liver function tests; ECG, especially with renal and/or hepatic impairment

Consult individual institutional policies and procedures.

Dosage Forms

Capsule Extended Release 24 Hour, Oral:

Verelan: 120 mg, 180 mg, 240 mg, 360 mg

Verelan PM: 100 mg, 200 mg, 300 mg

Generic: 100 mg, 120 mg, 180 mg, 200 mg, 240 mg, 300 mg, 360 mg

Solution, Intravenous:

Generic: 2.5 mg/mL (2 mL, 4 mL)

Tablet, Oral:

Calan: 80 mg, 120 mg

Generic: 40 mg, 80 mg, 120 mg

Tablet Extended Release, Oral:

Calan SR: 120 mg, 180 mg, 240 mg

Isoptin SR: 120 mg, 180 mg, 240 mg

Generic: 120 mg, 180 mg, 240 mg

Extemporaneous Preparations A 50 mg/mL oral suspension may be made with immediate release tablets and either a 1:1 mixture of Ora-Sweet and Ora-Plus or a 1:1 mixture of Ora-Sweet SF and Ora-Plus or cherry syrup. When using cherry syrup, dilute cherry syrup concentrate 1:4 with simple syrup, NF. Crush seventy-five verapamil hydrochloride 80 mg tablets in a mortar and reduce to a fine powder. Add small portions of chosen vehicle (40 mL total) and mix to a uniform paste; mix while adding the vehicle in incremental proportions to **almost** 120 mL; transfer to a calibrated bottle, rinse mortar with vehicle, and add quantity of vehicle sufficient to make 120 mL. Label "shake well", "refrigerate", and "protect from light". Stable for 60 days refrigerated (preferred) or at room temperature (Allen, 1996).

A 50 mg/mL oral suspension may be made with immediate release tablets, a 1:1 preparation of methylcellulose 1% and simple syrup, and purified water. Crush twenty 80 mg verapamil tablets in a mortar and reduce to a fine powder. Add 3 mL purified water USP and mix to a uniform paste; mix while adding the vehicle incremental proportions to **almost** 32 mL; transfer to a calibrated bottle, rinse mortar with vehicle, and add quantity of vehicle sufficient to make 32 mL. Label "shake well" and "refrigerate". Stable for 91 days refrigerated (preferred) or at room temperature (Nahata, 1997).

Allen LV Jr and Erickson MA 3rd, "Stability of Labetalol Hydrochloride, Metoprolol Tartrate, Verapamil Hydrochloride, and Spironolactone With Hydrochlorothiazide in Extemporaneously Compounded Oral Liquids," *Am J Health Syst Pharm*, 1996, 53(19):304-9.

Nahata MC, "Stability of Verapamil in an Extemporaneous Liquid Dosage Form," *J Appl Ther Res*, 1997,1(3):271-3.

◆ **Verapamil and Trandolapril** *see* Trandolapril and Verapamil *on page 2080*

◆ **Verapamil Hydrochloride** *see* Verapamil *on page 2154*

◆ **Verapamil Hydrochloride Injection, USP (Can)** *see* Verapamil *on page 2154*

◆ **Verapamil SR (Can)** *see* Verapamil *on page 2154*

◆ **Verdeso** *see* Desonide *on page 597*

◆ **Verdrocet** *see* Hydrocodone and Acetaminophen *on page 1012*

◆ **Verelan** *see* Verapamil *on page 2154*

◆ **Verelan PM** *see* Verapamil *on page 2154*

◆ **Veripred 20** *see* PrednisoLONE (Systemic) *on page 1703*

◆ **Vermox** *see* Mebendazole [CAN/INT] *on page 1274*

Vernakalant [INT] (ver NAK a lant hye)

Index Terms Vernakalant HCL; Vernakalant Hydrochloride

Pharmacologic Category Antiarrhythmic Agent, Class I; Antiarrhythmic Agent, Class III

Reported Use Pharmacologic conversion of atrial fibrillation (AF) to normal sinus rhythm in post-cardiac surgery patients with AF ≤3 days duration and non-surgery patients with AF for ≤7 days duration

Dosage Range Note: Dose ranges are not intended to guide prescribing; consult local prescribing information for additional dosage and administration information

Atrial fibrillation (cardioversion): IV: Initial: 3 mg/kg over 10 minutes (maximum dose: 339 mg); may administer second dose of 2 mg/kg over 10 minutes (maximum dose: 226 mg) if conversion to normal sinus rhythm does not occur within 15 minutes after end of initial infusion; maximum cumulative dose: 5 mg/kg in 24 hours

Product Availability Product available in various countries; not currently available in the U.S.

Dosage Forms

Solution, Intravenous, as hydrochloride: 20 mg/mL

◆ **Vernakalant HCL** *see* Vernakalant [INT] *on page 2157*

◆ **Vernakalant Hydrochloride** *see* Vernakalant [INT] *on page 2157*

◆ **Versacloz** *see* CloZAPine *on page 490*

◆ **Versed** *see* Midazolam *on page 1361*

◆ **Versel® (Can)** *see* Selenium Sulfide *on page 1877*

◆ **Vertin-32 [OTC]** *see* Meclizine *on page 1277*

◆ **Verti-sulf** *see* Sulfur and Sulfacetamide *on page 1953*

◆ **Vesanoid** *see* Tretinoin (Systemic) *on page 2096*

◆ **VESIcare** *see* Solifenacin *on page 1917*

◆ **Vestura** *see* Ethinyl Estradiol and Drospirenone *on page 801*

◆ **Vexol** *see* Rimexolone *on page 1814*

◆ **Vexol® (Can)** *see* Rimexolone *on page 1814*

◆ **Vfend** *see* Voriconazole *on page 2176*

◆ **VFEND (Can)** *see* Voriconazole *on page 2176*

◆ **Vfend IV** *see* Voriconazole *on page 2176*

◆ **VFEND For Injection (Can)** *see* Voriconazole *on page 2176*

◆ **Viagra** *see* Sildenafil *on page 1882*

◆ **Vibativ** *see* Telavancin *on page 1986*

◆ **Vibramycin** *see* Doxycycline *on page 689*

◆ **Vibra-Tabs (Can)** *see* Doxycycline *on page 689*

◆ ***Vibrio cholera*** **and Enterotoxigenic** ***Escherichia coli Vaccine*** *see* Travelers' Diarrhea and Cholera Vaccine [CAN/INT] *on page 2088*

◆ **Vicks 44E [OTC]** *see* Guaifenesin and Dextromethorphan *on page 987*

◆ **Vicks DayQuil Mucus Control DM [OTC]** *see* Guaifenesin and Dextromethorphan *on page 987*

◆ **Vicks Nature Fusion Cough & Chest Congestion [OTC]** *see* Guaifenesin and Dextromethorphan *on page 987*

◆ **Vicks Pediatric Formula 44E [OTC]** *see* Guaifenesin and Dextromethorphan *on page 987*

◆ **Vicodin®** *see* Hydrocodone and Acetaminophen *on page 1012*

◆ **Vicodin ES** *see* Hydrocodone and Acetaminophen *on page 1012*

◆ **Vicodin HP** *see* Hydrocodone and Acetaminophen *on page 1012*

◆ **Vicoprofen** *see* Hydrocodone and Ibuprofen *on page 1013*

◆ **ViCPS** *see* Typhoid Vaccine *on page 2112*

◆ **Victoza** *see* Liraglutide *on page 1222*

◆ **Victrelis** *see* Boceprevir *on page 273*

◆ **Vidaza** *see* AzaCITIDine *on page 209*

◆ **Videx** *see* Didanosine *on page 622*

◆ **Videx EC** *see* Didanosine *on page 622*

◆ **Viekira Pak** *see* Ombitasvir, Paritaprevir, Ritonavir, and Dasabuvir *on page 1505*

◆ **VIG** *see* Vaccinia Immune Globulin (Intravenous) *on page 2118*

Vigabatrin (vye GA ba trin)

Brand Names: U.S. Sabril

Brand Names: Canada Sabril

Pharmacologic Category Anticonvulsant, Miscellaneous

Use

Infantile spasms: As monotherapy for pediatric patients 1 month to 2 years of age with infantile spasms for whom the potential benefits outweigh the potential risk of vision loss.

Refractory complex partial seizures: As adjunctive therapy for adults and pediatric patients 10 years and older with refractory complex partial seizures who have inadequately responded to several alternative treatments and for whom the potential benefits outweigh the risk of vision loss.

Canadian labeling: Additional uses (not in U.S. labeling): Active management of partial or secondary generalized seizures not controlled by usual treatments

Pregnancy Risk Factor C

Dosage

Infantile spasms: Oral: Infants and Children 1 month to 2 years: Initial dosing: 50 mg/kg/day divided twice daily; may titrate upwards by 25-50 mg/kg/day increments every 3 days to a maximum of 150 mg/kg/day divided twice daily

Note: To taper, decrease dose by 25-50 mg/kg/day increments every 3-4 days

Adjunctive treatment of seizures (Canadian labeling; not in U.S. labeling): Children: Oral: Initial: 40 mg/kg/day divided twice daily; maintenance dosages based on patient weight:

10-15 kg: 500-1000 mg daily divided twice daily
16-30 kg: 1000-1500 mg daily divided twice daily
31-50 kg: 1500-3000 mg daily divided twice daily
>50 kg: 2000-3000 mg daily divided twice daily

Refractory complex partial seizures: Oral:

Children and Adolescents 10 to <17 years and 25-60 kg: Initial: 250 mg twice daily; increase daily dose at weekly intervals based on response and tolerability. Recommended dose: 1000 mg twice daily

Note: To taper, decrease daily dose by one-third every week for 3 weeks.

Children ≥10 years and >60 kg, Adolescents ≥17 years, and Adults: Initial: 500 mg twice daily; increase daily dose by 500 mg increments at weekly intervals based on response and tolerability. Recommended dose: 1500 mg twice daily. (**Note:** Canadian labeling suggests that initial doses up to 2000 mg daily may be considered in patients with severe seizures.)

Note: To taper, decrease dose by 1000 mg daily on a weekly basis

Elderly: Initiate at low end of dosage range (refer to adult dosing); monitor closely for sedation and confusion

Dosage adjustment in renal impairment: Note: Renal function may be estimated using the Schwartz equation (children 10 to <12 years) and the Cockcroft-Gault formula (children ≥12 years, adolescents, and adults): Children ≥10 years, Adolescents, and Adults:

CrCl >50-80 mL/minute: Decrease dose by 25%
CrCl >30-50 mL/minute: Decrease dose by 50%
CrCl >10-30 mL/minute: Decrease dose by 75%

Dosage adjustment in hepatic impairment: No dosage adjustment provided in manufacturer's labeling; has not been studied. However, does not undergo appreciable hepatic metabolism.

Additional Information Complete prescribing information should be consulted for additional detail.

Dosage Forms

Packet, Oral:
Sabril: 500 mg (50 ea)

Tablet, Oral:
Sabril: 500 mg

Dosage Forms: Canada

Powder for suspension, oral [sachets]:
Sabril: 0.5 g

◆ **Vigamox** *see* Moxifloxacin (Ophthalmic) *on page 1403*

◆ **VIGIV** *see* Vaccinia Immune Globulin (Intravenous) *on page 2118*

◆ **Viibryd** *see* Vilazodone *on page 2158*

◆ **Vilanterol and Fluticasone** *see* Fluticasone and Vilanterol *on page 914*

◆ **Vilanterol and Fluticasone Furoate** *see* Fluticasone and Vilanterol *on page 914*

Vilazodone (vil AZ oh done)

Brand Names: U.S. Viibryd

Index Terms EMD 68843; SB659746-A; Vilazodone Hydrochloride

Pharmacologic Category Antidepressant, Selective Serotonin Reuptake Inhibitor/5-HT_{1A} Receptor Partial Agonist

Use Treatment of major depressive disorder

Pregnancy Risk Factor C

Pregnancy Considerations Adverse events have been observed in animal reproduction studies. An increased risk of teratogenic effects may be associated with maternal use of other SSRIs. However, available information is conflicting and information specific to the use of vilazodone has not been located. Nonteratogenic effects in the newborn following SSRI/SNRI exposure late in the third trimester include respiratory distress, cyanosis, apnea, seizures, temperature instability, feeding difficulty, vomiting, hypoglycemia, hypo- or hypertonia, hyper-reflexia, jitteriness, irritability, constant crying, and tremor. Symptoms may be due to the toxicity of the SSRIs/SNRIs or a discontinuation syndrome and may be consistent with serotonin syndrome associated with SSRI treatment. Persistent pulmonary hypertension of the newborn (PPHN) has also been reported with SSRI exposure. The long-term effects of *in utero* SSRI exposure on infant development and behavior are not known.

The ACOG recommends that therapy with SSRIs or SNRIs during pregnancy be individualized; treatment of depression during pregnancy should incorporate the clinical expertise of the mental health clinician, obstetrician, primary healthcare provider, and pediatrician. According to the American Psychiatric Association (APA), the risks of medication treatment should be weighed against other treatment options and untreated depression. For women who discontinue antidepressant medications during pregnancy and who may be at high risk for postpartum depression, the medications can be restarted following delivery. Treatment algorithms have been developed by the ACOG and the APA for the management of depression in women prior to conception and during pregnancy. Consideration should be given to using an agent with some safety information in pregnant women.

Breast-Feeding Considerations It is not known if vilazodone is excreted in breast milk. According to the manufacturer, the decision to continue or discontinue breastfeeding during therapy should take into account the risk of exposure to the infant and the benefits of treatment to the mother. Maternal use of an SSRI during pregnancy may cause delayed milk secretion. Long-term effects on development and behavior have not been studied.

Contraindications Use of MAO inhibitors intended to treat psychiatric disorders (concurrently or within 14 days of discontinuing either vilazodone or the MAO inhibitor); initiation of vilazodone in a patient receiving linezolid or intravenous methylene blue

Warnings/Precautions [U.S. Boxed Warning]: Antidepressants increase the risk of suicidal thinking and behavior in children, adolescents, and young adults (18-24 years of age) with major depressive disorder (MDD) and other psychiatric disorders; consider risk prior to prescribing. Short-term studies did not show an increased risk in patients >24 years of age and showed a decreased risk in patients ≥65 years. Closely monitor patients for clinical worsening, suicidality, or unusual changes in behavior, particularly during the initial 1-2 months of therapy or during periods of dosage adjustments (increases or decreases); the patient's family or caregiver should be instructed to closely observe the patient and communicate condition with healthcare provider. A medication guide concerning the use of antidepressants should be dispensed with each prescription. **Vilazodone is not FDA approved for use in children.**

The possibility of a suicide attempt is inherent in major depression and may persist until remission occurs. Use caution in high-risk patients. Worsening depression and severe abrupt suicidality that are not part of the presenting symptoms may require discontinuation or modification of drug therapy. The patient's family or caregiver should be alerted to monitor patients for the emergence of suicidality and associated behaviors (such as agitation, irritability, hostility, impulsivity, and hypomania) and call healthcare provider.

May worsen psychosis in some patients or precipitate a shift to mania or hypomania in patients with bipolar disorder. Patients presenting with depressive symptoms should be screened for bipolar disorder. Monotherapy in patients with bipolar disorder should be avoided. **Vilazodone is not FDA approved for the treatment of bipolar depression.**

Potentially life-threatening serotonin syndrome (SS) has occurred with serotonergic agents (eg, SSRIs, SNRIs), particularly when used in combination with other serotonergic agents (eg, triptans, TCAs, fentanyl, lithium, tramadol, buspirone, St John's wort, tryptophan) or agents that impair metabolism of serotonin (eg, MAO inhibitors intended to treat psychiatric disorders, other MAO inhibitors [ie, linezolid and intravenous methylene blue]). Discontinue treatment (and any concomitant serotonergic agent) immediately if signs/symptoms arise. May increase the risks associated with electroconvulsive therapy. Bone fractures have been associated with antidepressant treatment. Consider the possibility of a fragility fracture if an antidepressant-treated patient presents with unexplained bone pain, point tenderness, swelling, or bruising (Rabenda, 2013; Rizzoli, 2012). Has a low potential to impair cognitive or motor performance; caution operating hazardous machinery or driving. Potentially significant drug-drug interactions may exist, requiring dose or frequency adjustment, additional monitoring, and/or selection of alternative therapy.

Use with caution in patients with hepatic impairment or seizure disorders. Use caution in elderly patients; may be potentially inappropriate in patients with a history of falls or fractures, and may cause or exacerbate syndrome of inappropriate antidiuretic hormone secretion or hyponatremia; monitor sodium closely with initiation or dosage adjustments in older adults (Beers Criteria). May cause or exacerbate sexual dysfunction. May cause mild pupillary dilation which in susceptible individuals can lead to an episode of narrow-angle glaucoma. Consider evaluating patients who have not had an iridectomy for narrow-angle glaucoma risk factors.

Abrupt discontinuation or interruption of antidepressant therapy has been associated with a discontinuation syndrome. Symptoms arising may vary with antidepressant however commonly include nausea, vomiting, diarrhea, headaches, light-headedness, dizziness, diminished appetite, sweating, chills, tremors, paresthesias, fatigue, somnolence, and sleep disturbances (eg, vivid dreams, insomnia). Greater risks for developing a discontinuation syndrome have been associated with antidepressants with shorter half-lives, longer durations of treatment, and abrupt discontinuation. For antidepressants of short or intermediate half-lives, symptoms may emerge within 2-5 days after treatment discontinuation and last 7-14 days (APA, 2010; Fava, 2006; Haddad, 2001; Shelton, 2001; Warner, 2006).

Adverse Reactions

Cardiovascular: Palpitations

Central nervous system: Abnormal dreams, delayed ejaculation, dizziness, drowsiness, fatigue, insomnia, migraine, nervousness, paresthesia, restlessness, sedation

Dermatologic: Hyperhidrosis, night sweats

Endocrine & metabolic: Decreased libido

Gastrointestinal: Decreased appetite, diarrhea, dyspepsia, flatulence, gastroenteritis, increased appetite, nausea, vomiting, xerostomia

Genitourinary: Erectile dysfunction, orgasm disturbance, sexual disorder

Neuromuscular & skeletal: Arthralgia, tremor

Ophthalmic: Blurred vision, xerophthalmia

Rare but important or life-threatening: Angle-closure glaucoma, cataract, hallucination, hyponatremia, irritability, mania, panic attacks, pollakiuria, serotonin syndrome, suicidal tendencies, ventricular premature contractions

Drug Interactions

Metabolism/Transport Effects Substrate of CYP2C19 (minor), CYP2D6 (minor), CYP3A4 (major); **Note:** Assignment of Major/Minor substrate status based on clinically relevant drug interaction potential; **Inhibits** CYP2C8 (weak), CYP2D6 (weak); **Induces** CYP2C19 (moderate)

Avoid Concomitant Use

Avoid concomitant use of Vilazodone with any of the following: Dapoxetine; Dosulepin; Iobenguane I 123; Linezolid; MAO Inhibitors; Methylene Blue; Pimozide; Tryptophan; Urokinase

Increased Effect/Toxicity

Vilazodone may increase the levels/effects of: Agents with Antiplatelet Properties; Anticoagulants; Antidepressants (Serotonin Reuptake Inhibitor/Antagonist); Antipsychotic Agents; Apixaban; ARIPiprazole; Aspirin; Beta-Blockers; BusPIRone; CarBAMazepine; CloZAPine; Collagenase (Systemic); Dabigatran Etexilate; Desmopressin; Dextromethorphan; Dosulepin; Galantamine;

Hypoglycemic Agents; Ibritumomab; Methadone; Methylene Blue; Mexiletine; NSAID (COX-2 Inhibitor); NSAID (Nonselective); Obinutuzumab; Pimozide; RisperiDONE; Rivaroxaban; Salicylates; Serotonin Modulators; Thiazide Diuretics; Thrombolytic Agents; Tositumomab and Iodine I 131 Tositumomab; TraMADol; Urokinase; Vitamin K Antagonists

The levels/effects of Vilazodone may be increased by: Alcohol (Ethyl); Analgesics (Opioid); Antiemetics (5HT3 Antagonists); Antipsychotic Agents; BusPIRone; Cimetidine; CNS Depressants; CYP3A4 Inhibitors (Moderate); CYP3A4 Inhibitors (Strong); Dapoxetine; Dasatinib; Glucosamine; Herbs (Anticoagulant/Antiplatelet Properties); Ibrutinib; Limaprost; Linezolid; Lithium; MAO Inhibitors; Metoclopramide; Metyrosine; Multivitamins/Fluoride (with ADE); Multivitamins/Minerals (with ADEK, Folate, Iron); Multivitamins/Minerals (with AE, No Iron); Omega-3 Fatty Acids; Pentosan Polysulfate Sodium; Pentoxifylline; Prostacyclin Analogues; Tedizolid; Tipranavir; TraMADol; Tryptophan; Vitamin E

Decreased Effect

Vilazodone may decrease the levels/effects of: Iobenguane I 123; Ioflupane I 123; Thyroid Products

The levels/effects of Vilazodone may be decreased by: Bosentan; CarBAMazepine; CYP3A4 Inducers (Moderate); CYP3A4 Inducers (Strong); Cyproheptadine; Dabrafenib; Deferasirox; Mitotane; NSAID (COX-2 Inhibitor); NSAID (Nonselective); Siltuximab; St Johns Wort; Tocilizumab

Food Interactions Vilazodone concentrations in the fasted state can be decreased by ~50% compared to the fed state, and may result in a decreased effect in some patients. Management: Administer with food.

Storage/Stability Store at 25°C (77°F); excursions permitted to 15°C to 30°C (50°F to 86°F).

Mechanism of Action Vilazodone inhibits CNS neuron serotonin uptake; minimal or no effect on reuptake of norepinephrine or dopamine. It also binds selectively with high affinity to 5-HT_{1A} receptors and is a 5-HT_{1A} receptor partial agonist. 5-HT_{1A} receptor activity may be altered in depression and anxiety.

Pharmacodynamics/Kinetics

Protein binding: ~96% to 99%

Metabolism: Extensively hepatic, via CYP3A4 (major pathway) and 2C19 and 2D6 (minor pathways)

Bioavailability: 72% (with food); blood concentrations (AUC) may be decreased ~50% in the fasted state

Half-life elimination: Terminal: ~25 hours

Time to peak, serum: 4-5 hours

Excretion: Urine (1% as unchanged drug); feces (2% as unchanged drug)

Dosage Adults: Oral: Depression: Initial: 10 mg once daily for 7 days, then increase to 20 mg once daily for 7 days, then to recommended dose of 40 mg once daily

Discontinuation of therapy: Upon discontinuation of antidepressant therapy, gradually taper the dose to minimize the incidence of withdrawal symptoms and allow for the detection of re-emerging symptoms. Evidence supporting ideal taper rates is limited. APA and NICE guidelines suggest tapering therapy over at least several weeks with consideration to the half-life of the antidepressant; antidepressants with a shorter half-life may need to be tapered more conservatively. In addition for long-term treated patients, WFSBP guidelines recommend tapering over 4-6 months. If intolerable withdrawal symptoms occur following a dose reduction, consider resuming the previously prescribed dose and/or decrease dose at a more gradual rate (APA, 2010; Bauer, 2002; Haddad, 2001; NCCMH, 2010; Schatzberg, 2006; Shelton, 2001; Warner, 2006).

MAO inhibitor recommendations:

Switching to or from an MAO inhibitor intended to treat psychiatric disorders:

Allow 14 days to elapse between discontinuing an MAO inhibitor intended to treat psychiatric disorders and initiation of vilazodone.

Allow 14 days to elapse between discontinuing vilazodone and initiation of an MAO inhibitor intended to treat psychiatric disorders.

Use with other MAO inhibitors (linezolid or IV methylene blue):

Do not initiate vilazodone in patients receiving linezolid or IV methylene blue; consider other interventions for psychiatric condition.

If urgent treatment with linezolid or IV methylene blue is required in a patient already receiving vilazodone and potential benefits outweigh potential risks, discontinue vilazodone promptly and administer linezolid or IV methylene blue. Monitor for serotonin syndrome for 2 weeks or until 24 hours after the last dose of linezolid or IV methylene blue, whichever comes first. May resume vilazodone 24 hours after the last dose of linezolid or IV methylene blue.

Dosing adjustment for concomitant medications:

Strong CYP3A4 inhibitors (eg, ketoconazole): Reduce vilazodone dose to 20 mg once daily. Readjust vilazodone to original dose when CYP3A4 inhibitor is discontinued.

Moderate CYP3A4 inhibitors (eg, erythromycin): Reduce vilazodone dose to 20 mg once daily in patients with intolerable side effects. Readjust vilazodone to original dose when CYP3A4 inhibitor is discontinued.

Strong CYP3A4 inducers (eg, carbamazepine): Based on clinical response, consider increasing the dose 2-fold when used concomitantly for >14 days. Maximum daily dose: 80 mg. If CYP3A4 inducer is discontinued, reduce vilazodone dose to original level in 14 days.

Dosage adjustment in renal impairment: No dosage adjustment necessary.

Dosage adjustment in hepatic impairment: No dosage adjustment necessary.

Dietary Considerations Take with food.

Administration Administer with food.

Monitoring Parameters Monitor patient periodically for symptom resolution, mental status for depression, suicidal ideation (especially at the beginning of therapy or when doses are increased or decreased), anxiety, social functioning, mania, panic attacks, signs/symptoms of serotonin syndrome; akathisia

Dosage Forms

Kit, Oral:

Viibryd: 10 & 20 & 40 mg

Tablet, Oral:

Viibryd: 10 mg, 20 mg, 40 mg

◆ **Vilazodone Hydrochloride** *see* Vilazodone *on page 2158*

◆ **Vimizim** *see* Elosulfase Alfa *on page 714*

◆ **Vimpat** *see* Lacosamide *on page 1154*

VinBLAStine (vin BLAS teen)

Brand Names: Canada Vinblastine Sulphate Injection

Index Terms Velban; Vinblastine Sulfate; Vincaleukoblastine; VLB

Pharmacologic Category Antineoplastic Agent, Antimicrotubular; Antineoplastic Agent, Vinca Alkaloid

Use Treatment of Hodgkin lymphoma; lymphocytic lymphoma; histiocytic lymphoma; mycosis fungoides; testicular cancer; Kaposi sarcoma; histiocytosis X (Letterer-Siwe disease); has also been used for the treatment of refractory/resistant breast cancer and choriocarcinoma

Pregnancy Risk Factor D

Pregnancy Considerations Adverse effects were observed in animal reproduction studies. May cause fetal harm if administered during pregnancy. Women of childbearing potential should avoid becoming pregnant during vinblastine treatment. Aspermia has been reported in males who have received treatment with vinblastine.

Breast-Feeding Considerations It is not known if vinblastine is excreted in breast milk. Due to the potential for serious adverse reactions in the nursing infant, a decision should be made whether to discontinue vinblastine or to discontinue breast-feeding, taking into account the importance of treatment to the mother.

Contraindications Significant granulocytopenia (unless as a result of condition being treated); presence of bacterial infection

Warnings/Precautions Hazardous agent - use appropriate precautions for handling and disposal (NIOSH 2014 [group 1]). Avoid eye contamination (exposure may cause severe irritation). **[U.S. Boxed Warning]: For IV use only. Intrathecal administration may result in death.** To prevent administration errors, the Institute for Safe Medication Practices (ISMP) Targeted Medication Safety Best Practices for Hospitals initiative strongly recommends dispensing vinblastine diluted in a minibag (ISMP, 2014). **If not dispensed in a minibag, affix an auxiliary label stating "For intravenous use only - fatal if given by other routes" and also place in an overwrap labeled "Do not remove covering until moment of injection."** Vinblastine should **NOT** be prepared during the preparation of any intrathecal medications. After preparation, keep vinblastine in a location **away** from the separate storage location recommended for intrathecal medications. Vinblastine should **NOT** be delivered to the patient at the same time with any medications intended for central nervous system administration.

[U.S. Boxed Warning]: Vinblastine is a vesicant; ensure proper needle or catheter placement prior to and during infusion. Avoid extravasation. Extravasation may cause significant irritation. Individuals administering should be experienced in vinblastine administration. If extravasation occurs, discontinue immediately and initiate appropriate extravasation management, including local injection of hyaluronidase and moderate heat application to the affected area. Use a separate vein to complete administration.

Leukopenia commonly occurs; granulocytopenia may be severe with higher doses. The leukocyte nadir generally occurs 5 to 10 days after administration; recovery typically occurs 7 to 14 days later. Monitor for infections if WBC <2,000/mm^3. Leukopenia may be more pronounced in cachectic patients and patients with skin ulceration and may be less pronounced with lower doses used for maintenance therapy. Leukocytes and platelets may fall considerably with moderate doses when marrow is infiltrated with malignant cells (further use in this situation is not recommended). Thrombocytopenia and anemia may occur rarely.

May rarely cause disabling neurotoxicity; usually reversible. Seizures and severe and permanent CNS damage has occurred with higher then recommended doses and/or when administered more frequently than recommended. Acute shortness of breath and severe bronchospasm have been reported, most often in association with concurrent administration of mitomycin; may occur within minutes to several hours following vinblastine administration or up to 14 days following mitomycin administration; use caution in patients with preexisting pulmonary disease. Use with caution in patients with hepatic impairment; toxicity may be increased; may require dosage modification. Use with caution in patients with ischemic heart disease. Stomatitis may occur (rare); may be disabling, but is usually reversible.

Potentially significant drug-drug interactions may exist, requiring dose or frequency adjustment, additional monitoring, and/or selection of alternative therapy. **[U.S. Boxed Warning]: Should be administered under the supervision of an experienced cancer chemotherapy physician.**

Benzyl alcohol and derivatives: Some dosage forms may contain benzyl alcohol; large amounts of benzyl alcohol (≥99 mg/kg/day) have been associated with a potentially fatal toxicity ("gasping syndrome") in neonates; the "gasping syndrome" consists of metabolic acidosis, respiratory distress, gasping respirations, CNS dysfunction (including convulsions, intracranial hemorrhage), hypotension, and cardiovascular collapse (AAP, 1997; CDC, 1982); some data suggests that benzoate displaces bilirubin from protein binding sites (Ahlfors, 2001); avoid or use dosage forms containing benzyl alcohol with caution in neonates. See manufacturer's labeling.

Adverse Reactions

Common:

Cardiovascular: Hypertension
Central nervous system: Malaise
Dermatologic: Alopecia
Gastrointestinal: Constipation
Hematologic: Myelosuppression, leukopenia/granulocytopenia (nadir: 5-10 days; recovery: 7-14 days; dose-limiting toxicity)
Neuromuscular & skeletal: Bone pain, jaw pain, tumor pain

Less common:

Cardiovascular: Angina, cerebrovascular accident, coronary ischemia, ECG abnormalities, limb ischemia, MI, myocardial ischemia, Raynaud's phenomenon
Central nervous system: Depression, dizziness, headache, neurotoxicity (duration: >24 hours), seizure, vertigo
Dermatologic: Dermatitis, photosensitivity (rare), rash, skin blistering
Endocrine & metabolic: Aspermia, hyperuricemia, SIADH
Gastrointestinal: Abdominal pain, anorexia, diarrhea, gastrointestinal bleeding, hemorrhagic enterocolitis, ileus, metallic taste, nausea (mild), paralytic ileus, rectal bleeding, stomatitis, toxic megacolon, vomiting (mild)
Genitourinary: Urinary retention
Hematologic: Anemia, thrombocytopenia (recovery within a few days), thrombotic thrombocytopenic purpura
Local: Cellulitis (with extravasation), irritation, phlebitis (with extravasation), radiation recall
Neuromuscular & skeletal: Deep tendon reflex loss, myalgia, paresthesia, peripheral neuritis, weakness
Ocular: Nystagmus
Otic: Auditory damage, deafness, vestibular damage
Renal: Hemolytic uremic syndrome
Respiratory: Bronchospasm, dyspnea, pharyngitis

Drug Interactions

Metabolism/Transport Effects Substrate of CYP2D6 (minor), CYP3A4 (major), P-glycoprotein; **Note:** Assignment of Major/Minor substrate status based on clinically relevant drug interaction potential; **Inhibits** CYP2D6 (weak), CYP3A4 (weak); **Induces** P-glycoprotein

Avoid Concomitant Use

Avoid concomitant use of VinBLAStine with any of the following: BCG; CloZAPine; Conivaptan; Dabigatran Etexilate; Dipyrone; Fusidic Acid (Systemic); Idelalisib; Ledipasvir; Natalizumab; Pimecrolimus; Pimozide;

Sofosbuvir; Tacrolimus (Topical); Tofacitinib; Vaccines (Live); VinCRIStine (Liposomal)

Increased Effect/Toxicity

VinBLAStine may increase the levels/effects of: ARIPiprazole; CloZAPine; Dofetilide; Hydrocodone; Leflunomide; Lomitapide; MitoMYcin (Systemic); Natalizumab; Pimozide; Tofacitinib; Tolterodine; Vaccines (Live)

The levels/effects of VinBLAStine may be increased by: Aprepitant; Ceritinib; Conivaptan; CYP3A4 Inhibitors (Moderate); CYP3A4 Inhibitors (Strong); Dasatinib; Denosumab; Dipyrone; Fosaprepitant; Fusidic Acid (Systemic); Idelalisib; Itraconazole; Ivacaftor; Lopinavir; Luliconazole; Macrolide Antibiotics; MAO Inhibitors; Mifepristone; Netupitant; P-glycoprotein/ABCB1 Inhibitors; Pimecrolimus; Posaconazole; Ritonavir; Roflumilast; Simeprevir; Stiripentol; Tacrolimus (Topical); Trastuzumab; Voriconazole

Decreased Effect

VinBLAStine may decrease the levels/effects of: Afatinib; BCG; Brentuximab Vedotin; Coccidioides immitis Skin Test; Dabigatran Etexilate; DOXOrubicin (Conventional); Ledipasvir; Linagliptin; P-glycoprotein/ABCB1 Substrates; Sipuleucel-T; Sofosbuvir; Vaccines (Inactivated); Vaccines (Live); VinCRIStine (Liposomal)

The levels/effects of VinBLAStine may be decreased by: Bosentan; CYP3A4 Inducers (Moderate); CYP3A4 Inducers (Strong); Dabrafenib; Deferasirox; Echinacea; Mitotane; P-glycoprotein/ABCB1 Inducers; Siltuximab; St Johns Wort; Tocilizumab

Preparation for Administration Hazardous agent; use appropriate precautions for handling and disposal (NIOSH 2014 [group 1]). For infusion, may dilute in 25 to 50 mL NS or D_5W; dilution in larger volumes (≥100 mL) of IV fluids is not recommended. **Note:** In order to prevent inadvertent intrathecal administration, the Institute for Safe Medication Practices (ISMP) strongly recommends dispensing vinblastine in a minibag (**NOT** in a syringe).

Storage/Stability Note: Dispense in an overwrap which bears the statement "Do not remove covering until the moment of injection. Fatal if given intrathecally. For IV use only." If dispensing in a syringe (minibag is preferred) should be labeled: "Fatal if given intrathecally. For IV use only."

Store intact vials under refrigeration at 2°C to 8°C (36°F to 46°F). Protect from light.

Mechanism of Action Vinblastine binds to tubulin and inhibits microtubule formation, therefore, arresting the cell at metaphase by disrupting the formation of the mitotic spindle; it is specific for the M and S phases. Vinblastine may also interfere with nucleic acid and protein synthesis by blocking glutamic acid utilization.

Pharmacodynamics/Kinetics

Metabolism: Hepatic (via CYP3A) to active metabolite

Half-life elimination: Terminal: ~25 hours

Excretion: Feces (30% to 36%); urine (12% to 17%)

Dosage Note: Frequency and duration of therapy may vary by indication, concomitant combination chemotherapy and hematologic response. **For IV use only.** In order to prevent inadvertent intrathecal administration, the Institute for Safe Medication Practices (ISMP) strongly recommends dispensing vinblastine in a minibag (**NOT** a syringe).

Manufacturer's labeling:

Hodgkin lymphoma: Pediatric: IV: Initial dose: 6 mg/m²; do not administer more frequently than every 7 days

Letterer-Siwe disease: Pediatric: IV: Initial dose: 6.5 mg/m²; do not administer more frequently than every 7 days

Testicular cancer: Pediatric: IV: Initial dose: 3 mg/m²; do not administer more frequently than every 7 days

Hodgkin lymphoma, lymphocytic lymphoma, histiocytic lymphoma, mycosis fungoides, testicular cancer, Kaposi sarcoma, histiocytosis X (Letterer-Siwe disease): Adults: IV: Initial: 3.7 mg/m²; adjust dose every 7 days (based on white blood cell response) up to 5.5 mg/m² (second dose); 7.4 mg/m² (third dose); 9.25 mg/m² (fourth dose); and 11.1 mg/m² (fifth dose); do not administer more frequently than every 7 days. Usual dosage range: 5.5 to 7.4 mg/m² every 7 days; Maximum dose: 18.5 mg/m²; dosage adjustment goal is to reduce white blood cell count to ~3,000/mm³

Off-label and/or indication-specific dosing:

Hodgkin lymphoma (off-label dosing): IV:

ABVD regimen: Pediatric: 6 mg/m² days 1 and 15 of a 28-day cycle (in combination with doxorubicin, bleomycin, and dacarbazine) for 6 cycles (Hutchinson, 1998)

ABVD regimen: Adults: 6 mg/m² days 1 and 15 of a 28-day cycle (in combination with doxorubicin, bleomycin, and dacarbazine) for 2 cycles (early/favorable disease) or for 4 cycles (unfavorable disease) (Eich, 2010; Engert, 2007)

Stanford V regimen: Adults: 6 mg/m² weeks 1, 3, 5, 7, 9, and 11 (in combination with doxorubicin, mechlorethamine, vincristine, bleomycin, etoposide, and prednisone) (Bartlett, 1995; Horning, 2002)

Testicular cancer (off-label dosing): VeIP regimen: Adults: IV: 0.11 mg/kg daily for 2 days every 21 days (in combination with ifosfamide, cisplatin, and mesna) for 4 cycles (Loehrer, 1988; Loehrer, 1988 [correction]; Loehrer, 1998)

Bladder cancer (off-label use): Adults: IV:

Metastatic disease:

Dose-dense MVAC regimen: 3 mg/m² day 2 every 14 days (in combination with methotrexate, doxorubicin, and cisplatin) until disease progression or unacceptable toxicity (Sternberg, 2001; Sternberg, 2006)

MVAC regimen: 3 mg/m² days 2, 15, and 22 every 28 days (in combination with methotrexate, doxorubicin, and cisplatin) for up to 6 cycles (von der Maase, 2000) **or** 3 mg/m² days 2, 15, and 22 every 28 days (in combination with methotrexate, doxorubicin, and cisplatin) until disease progression or unacceptable toxicity (Sternberg, 2001; Sternberg, 2006) **or** 3 mg/m² days 1, 15, and 22 every 28 days (in combination with methotrexate, doxorubicin, and cisplatin) for up to 6 cycles (Bamias, 2004)

Neoadjuvant treatment:

MVAC regimen: 3 mg/m² days 2, 15, and 22 every 28 days (in combination with methotrexate, doxorubicin, and cisplatin) for 3 cycles (Grossman, 2003)

CMV regimen: 4 mg/m² days 1 and 8 every 21 days (in combination with methotrexate, cisplatin, and leucovorin) for 3 cycles (Griffiths, 2011)

Melanoma, metastatic (off-label use): Adults: IV:

CVD regimen: 2 mg/m² days 1 to 4 and 22 to 25 of a 6-week treatment cycle (in combination with cisplatin and dacarbazine); may repeat if tumor response (Eton, 2002)

CVD + immunotherapy regimen: 1.5 mg/m² days 1 to 4 and 22 to 25 of a 6-week treatment cycle (in combination with cisplatin, dacarbazine, aldesleukin, and interferon alfa-2b); may repeat if tumor response (Eton, 2002)

Non-small cell lung cancer (off-label use): Adults: IV:

Adjuvant treatment after complete resection: 4 mg/m² days 1, 8, 15, 22, and 29, then every 2 weeks (in combination with cisplatin) until last cisplatin dose (Arriagada, 2004)

Concurrent radiation: 5 mg/m² days 1, 8, 15, 22, and 29 (in combination with cisplatin and concurrent radiation therapy) (Curran, 2011)

Soft tissue sarcoma (desmoid tumors, aggressive fibromatosis), advanced (off-label use): Adults: IV: 6 mg/m^2 every 7 to 10 days (dose usually rounded to 10 mg) in combination with methotrexate for 1 year (Azzarelli, 2001)

Dosage adjustment in renal impairment: No dosage adjustment necessary.

Dosage adjustment in hepatic impairment:

The manufacturer's labeling recommends the following adjustment: Serum bilirubin >3 mg/dL: Administer 50% of dose

The following adjustments have also been recommended (Floyd, 2006; Superfin, 2007):

Serum bilirubin 1.5 to 3 mg/dL or transaminases 2 to 3 times ULN: Administer 50% of dose

Serum bilirubin >3 times ULN: Avoid use.

Dosing in obesity: *ASCO Guidelines for appropriate chemotherapy dosing in obese adults with cancer:* Utilize patient's actual body weight (full weight) for calculation of body surface area- or weight-based dosing, particularly when the intent of therapy is curative; manage regimen-related toxicities in the same manner as for nonobese patients; if a dose reduction is utilized due to toxicity, consider resumption of full weight-based dosing with subsequent cycles, especially if cause of toxicity (eg, hepatic or renal impairment) is resolved (Griggs, 2012).

Administration In order to prevent inadvertent intrathecal administration, the Institute for Safe Medication Practices (ISMP) strongly recommends dispensing vinblastine in a minibag (NOT in a syringe). For IV administration only. **Fatal if given intrathecally.** The preferred administration is as a short infusion in a 25 to 50 mL minibag. If administration via a minibag is not possible, may also be administered as an undiluted 1-minute infusion into a free flowing IV line to prevent venous irritation/extravasation. Prolonged administration times (≥30 to 60 minutes) and/or increased administration volumes may increase the risk of vein irritation and extravasation.

Vesicant; ensure proper needle or catheter placement prior to and during infusion. Avoid extravasation.

Extravasation management: If extravasation occurs, stop infusion immediately and disconnect (leave cannula/needle in place); gently aspirate extravasated solution (do **NOT** flush the line); initiate hyaluronidase antidote; remove needle/cannula; apply dry warm compresses for 20 minutes 4 times a day for 1-2 days; elevate extremity (Perez Fidalgo, 2012). Remaining portion of the vinblastine dose should be infused through a separate vein.

Hyaluronidase: If needle/cannula still in place, administer 1-6 mL hyaluronidase (150 units/mL) into the existing IV line; the usual dose is 1 mL hyaluronidase for each 1 mL of extravasated drug (Perez Fidalgo, 2012; Schulmeister, 2011). If needle/cannula was removed, inject 1-6 mL (150 units/mL) subcutaneously in a clockwise manner using 1 mL for each 1 mL of drug extravasated (Schulmeister, 2011) **or** administer 1 mL (150 units/mL) as 5 separate 0.2 mL injections (using a 25-gauge needle) subcutaneously into the extravasation site (Polovich, 2009).

Hazardous agent; use appropriate precautions for handling and disposal (NIOSH 2014 [group 1]).

Monitoring Parameters CBC with differential and platelet count, serum uric acid, hepatic function tests

Dosage Forms

Solution, Intravenous:

Generic: 1 mg/mL (10 mL)

Solution Reconstituted, Intravenous:

Generic: 10 mg (1 ea)

- ◆ **Vinblastine Sulfate** *see* VinBLAStine *on page 2160*
- ◆ **Vinblastine Sulphate Injection (Can)** *see* VinBLAStine *on page 2160*
- ◆ **Vincaleukoblastine** *see* VinBLAStine *on page 2160*
- ◆ **Vincasar PFS** *see* VinCRIStine *on page 2163*

VinCRIStine (vin KRIS teen)

Brand Names: U.S. Vincasar PFS

Brand Names: Canada Vincristine Sulfate Injection; Vincristine Sulfate Injection USP

Index Terms Conventional Vincristine; Leurocristine Sulfate; Oncovin; Vincristine (Conventional); Vincristine Sulfate

Pharmacologic Category Antineoplastic Agent, Antimicrotubular; Antineoplastic Agent, Vinca Alkaloid

Additional Appendix Information

Beers Criteria – Potentially Inappropriate Medications for Geriatrics *on page 2271*

Use Treatment of acute lymphocytic leukemia (ALL), Hodgkin lymphoma, non-Hodgkin lymphomas, Wilms' tumor, neuroblastoma, rhabdomyosarcoma

Pregnancy Risk Factor D

Pregnancy Considerations Animal reproduction studies have demonstrated teratogenicity and fetal loss. May cause fetal harm if administered during pregnancy. Women of childbearing potential should avoid becoming pregnant during treatment.

Breast-Feeding Considerations It is not known if vincristine is excreted in breast milk. Due to the potential for serious adverse reactions in the nursing infant, the decision to discontinue vincristine or to discontinue breast-feeding should take into account the benefits of treatment to the mother.

Contraindications Patients with the demyelinating form of Charcot-Marie-Tooth syndrome

Warnings/Precautions Hazardous agent - use appropriate precautions for handling and disposal (NIOSH 2014 [group 1]); avoid eye contamination.

[U.S. Boxed Warning]: For IV administration only; inadvertent intrathecal administration usually results in death. To prevent administration errors, the Institute for Safe Medication Practices (ISMP) Targeted Medication Safety Best Practices for Hospitals initiative and the World Health Organization strongly recommend dispensing vincristine diluted in a minibag (ISMP, 2014; WHO, 2007), **if not dispensed in a minibag, affix an auxiliary label stating "For intravenous use only - fatal if given by other routes" and also place in an overwrap labeled "Do not remove covering until moment of injection."** Vincristine should **NOT** be prepared during the preparation of any intrathecal medications. After preparation, keep vincristine in a location **away** from the separate storage location recommended for intrathecal medications. Vincristine should **NOT** be delivered to the patient at the same time with any medications intended for central nervous system administration.

[U.S. Boxed Warning]: Vincristine is a vesicant; ensure proper needle or catheter placement prior to and during infusion. Avoid extravasation. Individuals administering should be experienced in vincristine administration. Extravasation may cause significant irritation. If extravasation occurs, discontinue immediately and initiate appropriate extravasation management, including local injection of hyaluronidase and moderate heat application to the affected area. Use a separate vein to complete administration.

Neurotoxicity, including alterations in mental status such as depression, confusion, or insomnia may occur; neurologic effects are dose-limiting (may require dosage reduction) and may be additive with those of other neurotoxic agents and spinal cord irradiation. Use with caution in patients with preexisting neuromuscular disease and/or with concomitant neurotoxic agents. Constipation, paralytic ileus, intestinal necrosis and/or perforation may occur; constipation may present as upper colon impaction with an empty rectum (may require flat film of abdomen for diagnosis); generally responds to high enemas and laxatives. All patients should be on a prophylactic bowel management regimen.

Potentially significant drug-drug interactions may exist, requiring dose or frequency adjustment, additional monitoring, and/or selection of alternative therapy. Acute shortness of breath and severe bronchospasm have been reported with vinca alkaloids, usually when used in combination with mitomycin. Onset may be several minutes to hours after vincristine administration and up to 2 weeks after mitomycin. Progressive dyspnea may occur. Permanently discontinue vincristine if pulmonary dysfunction occurs.

Use with caution in patients with hepatic impairment; dosage modification required. May be associated with hepatic sinusoidal obstruction syndrome (SOS; formerly called veno-occlusive disease), increased risk in children <3 years of age; use with caution in hepatobiliary dysfunction. Monitor for signs or symptoms of hepatic SOS, including bilirubin >1.4 mg/dL, unexplained weight gain, ascites, hepatomegaly, or unexplained right upper quadrant pain (Arndt, 2004). Acute uric acid nephropathy has been reported with vincristine. Use with caution in the elderly; may cause or exacerbate syndrome of inappropriate antidiuretic hormone secretion or hyponatremia; monitor sodium closely with initiation or dosage adjustments in older adults (Beers Criteria).

Adverse Reactions

Cardiovascular: Edema, hyper-/hypotension, MI, myocardial ischemia

Central nervous system: Ataxia, coma, cranial nerve dysfunction (auditory damage, extraocular muscle impairment, laryngeal muscle impairment, paralysis, paresis, vestibular damage, vocal cord paralysis), dizziness, fever, headache, neurotoxicity (dose-related), neuropathic pain (common), seizure, vertigo

Dermatologic toxicity: Alopecia (common), rash

Endocrine & metabolic: Hyperuricemia, parotid pain, SIADH (rare)

Gastrointestinal: Abdominal cramps, abdominal pain, anorexia, constipation (common), diarrhea, intestinal necrosis, intestinal perforation, nausea, oral ulcers, paralytic ileus, vomiting, weight loss

Genitourinary: Bladder atony, dysuria, polyuria, urinary retention

Hematologic: Anemia (mild), leukopenia (mild), thrombocytopenia (mild), thrombotic thrombocytopenic purpura

Hepatic: Hepatic sinusoidal obstruction syndrome (SOS; veno-occlusive liver disease)

Local: Phlebitis, tissue irritation/necrosis (if infiltrated)

Neuromuscular & skeletal: Back pain, bone pain, deep tendon reflex loss, difficulty walking, foot drop, gait changes, jaw pain, limb pain, motor difficulties, muscle wasting, myalgia, paralysis, paresthesia, peripheral neuropathy (common), sensorimotor dysfunction, sensory loss

Ocular: Cortical blindness (transient), nystagmus, optic atrophy with blindness

Otic: Deafness

Renal: Acute uric acid nephropathy, hemolytic uremic syndrome

Respiratory: Bronchospasm, dyspnea, pharyngeal pain

Miscellaneous: Allergic reactions (rare), anaphylaxis (rare), hypersensitivity (rare)

Drug Interactions

Metabolism/Transport Effects Substrate of CYP3A4 (major), P-glycoprotein; **Note:** Assignment of Major/Minor substrate status based on clinically relevant drug interaction potential; **Inhibits** CYP3A4 (weak)

Avoid Concomitant Use

Avoid concomitant use of VinCRIStine with any of the following: BCG; Conivaptan; Fusidic Acid (Systemic); Idelalisib; Natalizumab; Pimecrolimus; Pimozide; Tacrolimus (Topical); Tofacitinib; Vaccines (Live)

Increased Effect/Toxicity

VinCRIStine may increase the levels/effects of: ARIPiprazole; Dofetilide; Hydrocodone; Leflunomide; Lomitapide; MitoMYcin (Systemic); Natalizumab; Pimozide; Tofacitinib; Vaccines (Live)

The levels/effects of VinCRIStine may be increased by: Aprepitant; Ceritinib; Conivaptan; CYP3A4 Inhibitors (Moderate); CYP3A4 Inhibitors (Strong); Dasatinib; Denosumab; Fosaprepitant; Fusidic Acid (Systemic); Idelalisib; Itraconazole; Ivacaftor; Lopinavir; Luliconazole; Macrolide Antibiotics; MAO Inhibitors; Mifepristone; Netupitant; NIFEdipine; P-glycoprotein/ABCB1 Inhibitors; Pimecrolimus; Posaconazole; Ritonavir; Roflumilast; Simeprevir; Stiripentol; Tacrolimus (Topical); Teniposide; Trastuzumab; Voriconazole

Decreased Effect

VinCRIStine may decrease the levels/effects of: BCG; Coccidioides immitis Skin Test; Fosphenytoin; Phenytoin; Sipuleucel-T; Vaccines (Inactivated); Vaccines (Live)

The levels/effects of VinCRIStine may be decreased by: Bosentan; CYP3A4 Inducers (Moderate); CYP3A4 Inducers (Strong); Dabrafenib; Deferasirox; Echinacea; Fosphenytoin; Mitotane; P-glycoprotein/ABCB1 Inducers; Phenytoin; Siltuximab; St Johns Wort; Tocilizumab

Preparation for Administration Hazardous agent; use appropriate precautions for handling and disposal (NIOSH 2014 [group 1]).

Solutions for IV infusion may be mixed in NS or D_5W. **Note:** In order to prevent inadvertent intrathecal administration the World Health Organization (WHO) and the Institute for Safe Medication Practices (ISMP) strongly recommend dispensing vincristine in a minibag (**NOT** in a syringe). Vincristine should **NOT** be prepared during the preparation of any intrathecal medications. If dispensing vincristine in a syringe, affix an auxiliary label stating **"For intravenous use only - fatal if given by other routes"** to the syringe, and the syringe must also be packaged in the manufacturer-provided overwrap which bears the statement **"Do not remove covering until the moment of injection. For intravenous use only. Fatal if given intrathecally."**

Storage/Stability Store intact vials refrigerated at 2°C to 8°C (36°F to 46°F). Protect from light.

IV solution: Diluted in 25 to 50 mL NS or D_5W, stable for 7 days under refrigeration, or 2 days at room temperature. In ambulatory pumps, solution is stable for 7 days at room temperature. After preparation, keep vincristine in a location away from the separate storage location recommended for intrathecal medications.

Mechanism of Action Binds to tubulin and inhibits microtubule formation, therefore, arresting the cell at metaphase by disrupting the formation of the mitotic spindle; it is specific for the M and S phases. Vincristine may also interfere with nucleic acid and protein synthesis by blocking glutamic acid utilization.

Pharmacodynamics/Kinetics

Distribution: Rapidly removed from bloodstream and tightly bound to tissues; penetrates blood-brain barrier poorly

Metabolism: Extensively hepatic, via CYP3A4

Half-life elimination: Terminal: 85 hours (range: 19-155 hours)

Excretion: Feces (~80%); urine (10% to 20%; <1% as unchanged drug)

Dosage Note: Doses may be capped at a maximum of 2 mg/dose. Dosing and frequency may vary by protocol and/or treatment phase; refer to specific protocol. In order to prevent inadvertent intrathecal administration, the World Health Organization (WHO) and the Institute for Safe Medication Practices (ISMP) strongly recommend dispensing vincristine in a minibag (**NOT** in a syringe).

Doses in the manufacturer's U.S. labeling: IV:

Children ≤10 kg: 0.05 mg/kg/dose once weekly

Children >10 kg: 1.5-2 mg/m²/dose; frequency may vary based on protocol

Adults: 1.4 mg/m²/dose; frequency may vary based on protocol

Additional dosing in combination therapy; indication-specific and/or off-label dosing:

Children:

ALL: IV: Induction phase: 1.5 mg/m²/dose days 0, 7, 14, and 21; Consolidation phase: 1.5 mg/m²/dose days 0, 28, and 56; Delayed intensification phase: 1.5 mg/m²/dose days 0, 7, and 14; Maintenance phase: 1.5 mg/m²/dose days 0, 28, and 56 (Bostrom, 2003) **or** Induction phase: 1.5 mg/m²/dose days 0, 7, 14, and 21; Consolidation phase: 1.5 mg/m²/dose days 0, 28, and 56; Interim maintenance phases: 1.5 mg/m²/dose days 0 and 28; Delayed intensification phase: 1.5 mg/m²/dose days 0, 7, and 14; Maintenance phase: 1.5 mg/m²/dose every 4 weeks (Avramis, 2002)

Burkitt lymphoma and B-cell ALL: IV: 1.5 mg/m² (maximum dose: 2 mg) on days 4 and 11 of initial phase cycle (initial phase is in combination with cyclophosphamide, doxorubicin, and CNS prophylaxis; alternates with secondary phase) for a total of 4 cycles of each phase (Bowman, 1996) **or** 1.5 mg/m² (maximum dose: 2 mg) on day 1 of cycle AA (in combination with dexamethasone, ifosfamide, methotrexate, cytarabine, etoposide and CNS prophylaxis) and on day 1 of cycle BB (in combination with dexamethasone, cyclophosphamide, methotrexate, doxorubicin, and CNS prophylaxis) (Reiter, 1999)

Ewing's sarcoma (off-label use): IV: 2 mg/m²/dose (maximum dose: 2 mg) on day 1 of a 21-day cycle, administer either every cycle or during odd-numbered cycles (Grier, 2003) **or** 0.67 mg/m²/day continuous infusion days 1, 2, and 3 (total 2 mg/m²/cycle; maximum dose/cycle: 2 mg) during cycles 1, 2, 3, and 6 (Kolb, 2003)

Hodgkin lymphoma: IV: BEACOPP regimen: 2 mg/m²/dose (maximum dose: 2 mg) on day 7 of a 21-day treatment cycle (Kelly, 2002)

Neuroblastoma: IV:

CE-CAdO regimen: 1.5 mg/m² (maximum dose: 2 mg) days 1 and 5 every 21 days for 2 cycles (Rubie, 1998) **or** 0.05 mg/kg days 1 and 5 for 2 cycles (Rubie, 2001)

CAV-P/VP regimen (off-label dosing): 0.033 mg/kg/day continuous infusion days 1, 2, and 3, then 1.5 mg/m² bolus day 9 of courses 1, 2, 4, and 6 (Kushner, 1994)

Retinoblastoma (off-label use): IV:

Children: 0.05 mg/kg on day 1 every 21 days (in combination with carboplatin) for 8 cycles (Rodriguez-Galindo, 2003)

or

Children ≤36 months: 0.05 mg/kg on day 0 every 28 days (in combination with carboplatin and etoposide) for 6 cycles (Freidman, 2000)

or

Children >36 months: 1.5 mg/m² (maximum dose: 2 mg) on day 0 every 28 days (in combination with carboplatin and etoposide) for 6 cycles (Friedman, 2000)

Rhabdomyosarcoma: IV:

VA regimen: 1.5 mg/m²/dose (maximum dose: 2 mg) weeks 1-8, weeks 13-20, and weeks 25-32 (Crist, 2001)

VAC regimen: 1.5 mg/m²/dose (maximum dose: 2 mg) weeks 0-12, week 16, weeks 20-25; Continuation therapy: Weeks 29-34, and weeks 38-43 (Crist, 2001)

Wilms' tumor: IV:

Children <1 year: 0.75 mg/m²/dose weekly for 10-11 weeks, then every 3 weeks for 15 additional weeks (total 25-26 weeks) (Pritchard, 1995)

Children ≥1 year: 1.5 mg/m²/dose weekly for 10-11 weeks, then every 3 weeks for 15 additional weeks (total 25-26 weeks) (Pritchard, 1995)

or

Children ≤30 kg: 0.05 mg/kg/dose (maximum dose: 2 mg) weeks 1, 2, 4, 5, 6, 7, 8, 10, and 11, followed by 0.067 mg/kg/dose (maximum dose: 2 mg) weeks 12, 13, 18, and 24 (Green, 2007)

Children >30 kg: 1.5 mg/m²/dose (maximum dose: 2 mg) weeks 1, 2, 4, 5, 6, 7, 8, 10, and 11, followed by 2 mg/m²/dose (maximum dose: 2 mg) weeks 12, 13, 18, and 24 (Green, 2007)

Adults:

ALL: IV:

Hyper-CVAD regimen: 2 mg/dose days 4 and 11 during odd-numbered cycles (cycles 1, 3, 5, 7) of an 8-cycle phase, followed by maintenance treatment (if needed) of 2 mg monthly for 2 years (Kantarjian, 2004)

CALBG 8811 regimen: Induction phase: 2 mg/dose days 1, 8, 15, and 22 (4-week treatment cycle); Early intensification phase: 2 mg/dose days 15, and 22 (4-week treatment cycle, repeat once); Late intensification phase: 2 mg/dose days 1, 8, 15 (8-week treatment cycle); Maintenance phase: 2 mg/dose day 1 every 4 weeks until 24 months from diagnosis (Larson, 1995)

Central nervous system tumors: PCV regimen: IV: 1.4 mg/m²/dose (maximum dose: 2 mg) on days 8 and 29 of a 6-week treatment cycle for a total of 6 cycles (van de Bent, 2006) **or** 1.4 mg/m²/dose (no maximum dose) on days 8 and 29 of a 6-week treatment cycle for up to 4 cycles (Cairncross, 2006)

Hodgkin lymphoma: IV:

BEACOPP regimen: 1.4 mg/m²/dose (maximum dose: 2 mg) on day 8 of a 21-day treatment cycle (Diehl, 2003)

Stanford-V regimen: 1.4 mg/m²/dose (maximum dose: 2 mg) in weeks 2, 4, 6, 8, 10, and 12 (Horning, 2000; Horning, 2002)

Non-Hodgkin lymphoma: IV:

Burkitt lymphoma:

CODOX-M/IVAC: Cycles 1 and 3 (CODOX-M): 1.5 mg/m² (no maximum dose) days 1 and 8 of cycle 1 and days 1, 8, and 15 of cycle 3 (Magrath, 1996) **or** 1.5 mg/m² (maximum dose: 2 mg) days 1 and 8 of cycles 1 and 3 (Mead 2002; Mead 2008); CODOX-M is in combination with cyclophosphamide, doxorubicin, methotrexate, and CNS prophylaxis and alternates with IVAC (etoposide, ifosfamide, mesna, cytarabine, and CNS prophylaxis) for a total of 4 cycles

Hyper-CVAD: 2 mg (flat dose) days 4 and 11 of courses 1, 3, 5, and 7 (in combination with cyclophosphamide, doxorubicin, and dexamethasone) and alternates with even courses 2, 4, 6, and 8 (methotrexate and cytarabine) (Thomas, 2006)

Follicular lymphoma: CVP regimen: 1.4 mg/m²/dose (maximum dose: 2 mg) on day 1 of a 21-day treatment cycle (in combination with cyclophosphamide and prednisone) for 8 cycles (Marcus, 2005)

Large B-cell lymphoma:

CHOP regimen: 1.4 mg/m²/dose (maximum dose: 2 mg) on day 1 of a 21-day treatment cycle for 8 cycles (Coiffier, 2002)

EPOCH regimen: 0.4 mg/m²/day continuous infusion for 4 days (over 96 hours) (total 1.6 mg/m²/cycle; dose not usually capped) of a 21-day treatment cycle (Wilson, 2002)

Ewing's sarcoma (off-label use): IV: VAC/IE regimen: VAC: 2 mg/m² (maximum dose: 2 mg) on day 1 of a 21-day treatment cycle (in combination with doxorubicin and cyclophosphamide), alternates with IE (ifosfamide and etoposide) for a total of 17 cycles (Grier, 2003)

Gestational trophoblastic tumors, high-risk (off-label use): IV: EMA/CO regimen: 1 mg/m² on day 8 of 2-week treatment cycle (in combination with etoposide methotrexate, dactinomycin, and cyclophosphamide), continue for at least 2 treatment cycles after a normal hCG level (Escobar, 2003)

Multiple myeloma (off-label use): IV:

DVD regimen: 1.4 mg/m²/dose (maximum dose: 2 mg) on day 1 of a 28-day treatment cycle (Rifkin, 2006)

VAD regimen: 0.4 mg/day continuous infusion for 4 days (over 96 hours) (total 1.6 mg/cycle) of a 28-day treatment cycle (Rifkin, 2006)

Ovarian cancer (off-label use): IV: VAC regimen: 1.5 mg/m²/dose (maximum dose: 2 mg) weekly for 8-12 weeks (Slayton, 1985)

Small cell lung cancer (off-label use): IV: CAV regimen: 1.4 mg/m²/dose day 1 of a 21-day treatment cycle (Hong, 1989) **or** 2 mg/dose on day 1 of a 21-day treatment cycle (von Pawel, 1999)

Thymoma, advanced (off-label use): IV: ADOC regimen: 0.6 mg/m² on day 3 every 3 weeks (in combination with cisplatin, doxorubicin, and cyclophosphamide) (Fornasiero, 1991)

Dosage adjustment in renal impairment: No dosage adjustment necessary (Kintzel, 1995).

Dosage adjustment in hepatic impairment:

The manufacturer's labeling recommends the following adjustment: Serum bilirubin >3 mg/dL: Administer 50% of normal dose.

The following adjustments have also been recommended:

Floyd, 2006: Serum bilirubin 1.5-3 mg/dL or transaminases 2-3 times ULN or alkaline phosphatase increased: Administer 50% of dose.

Superfin, 2007:

Serum bilirubin 1.5-3 mg/dL: Administer 50% of dose.

Serum bilirubin >3 mg/dL: Avoid use.

Dosing in obesity: *ASCO Guidelines for appropriate chemotherapy dosing in obese adults with cancer:* Adults: Dose should be capped at a maximum of 2 mg due to neurotoxicity concerns (Griggs, 2012).

Administration For IV administration only. FATAL IF GIVEN INTRATHECALLY.

In order to prevent inadvertent intrathecal administration, the World Health Organization (WHO) and the Institute for Safe Medication Practices (ISMP) strongly recommend dispensing vincristine in a minibag (NOT in a syringe). Vincristine should **NOT** be delivered to the patient at the same time with any medications intended for central nervous system administration.

IV: Preferred administration is as a short 5- to 10-minute infusion in a 25 to 50 mL minibag. If administration via minibag is not possible, may also be administered as a slow (1-minute) push. Some protocols utilize a 24-hour continuous infusion.

Vesicant; ensure proper needle or catheter placement prior to and during infusion. Avoid extravasation.

Extravasation management: If extravasation occurs, stop infusion immediately and disconnect (leave cannula/needle in place); gently aspirate extravasated solution (do **NOT** flush the line); initiate hyaluronidase antidote; remove needle/cannula; apply dry warm compresses for 20 minutes 4 times a day for 1 to 2 days; elevate (Perez Fidalgo, 2012). Remaining portion of the vincristine dose should be infused through a separate vein.

Hyaluronidase: If needle/cannula still in place, administer 1 to 6 mL hyaluronidase (150 units/mL) into the existing IV line; the usual dose is 1 mL hyaluronidase for each 1 mL of extravasated drug (Perez Fidalgo, 2012; Schulmeister, 2011). If needle/cannula was removed, inject 1 to 6 mL (150 units/mL) subcutaneously in a clockwise manner using 1 mL for each 1 mL of drug extravasated (Schulmeister, 2011) **or** administer 1 mL (150 units/mL) as 5 separate 0.2 mL injections (using a 25-gauge needle) subcutaneously into the extravasation site (Polovich, 2009).

Hazardous agent; use appropriate precautions for handling and disposal (NIOSH 2014 [group 1]).

Monitoring Parameters Serum electrolytes (sodium), hepatic function tests, CBC with differential, serum uric acid; monitor infusion site; neurologic examination, monitor for constipation/ileus and for signs/symptoms of peripheral neuropathy

Dosage Forms

Solution, Intravenous:

Vincasar PFS: 1 mg/mL (1 mL, 2 mL)

Solution, Intravenous [preservative free]:

Generic: 1 mg/mL (1 mL, 2 mL)

VinCRIStine (Liposomal)

(vin KRIS teen lye po SO mal)

Brand Names: U.S. Marqibo

Index Terms Liposomal Vincristine; Liposome Vincristine; Vincristine Liposome; Vincristine Sulfate Liposome; VSLI

Pharmacologic Category Antineoplastic Agent, Antimicrotubular; Antineoplastic Agent, Vinca Alkaloid

Use Treatment of relapsed Philadelphia chromosome-negative (Ph-) acute lymphoblastic leukemia (ALL) in adult patients whose disease has progressed after two or more antileukemic therapies

Pregnancy Risk Factor D

Pregnancy Considerations Adverse events (fetal malformations, decreased fetal weight, and fetal loss) were observed in animal reproduction studies at doses less than the recommended human dose. Given the mechanism of action, adverse fetal events would be expected to occur with use in pregnant women. Women of childbearing potential should avoid becoming pregnant during therapy.

Breast-Feeding Considerations Due to the potential for adverse reactions in the nursing infant, the decision to discontinue breast-feeding or to discontinue liposomal vincristine should take into account the benefits of treatment to the mother.

Contraindications Hypersensitivity to vincristine, liposomal vincristine, or any component of the formulation; patients with Charcot-Marie-Tooth syndrome or other demyelinating conditions; administration via the intrathecal route

Warnings/Precautions Hazardous agent - use appropriate precautions for handling and disposal (NIOSH 2014 [group 1]). **[U.S. Boxed Warning]: For IV administration only. Intrathecal administration is contraindicated; inadvertent intrathecal administration has resulted in death.** Liposomal vincristine should **NOT** be prepared during the preparation of any intrathecal medications. After preparation, keep liposomal vincristine in a location **away** from the separate storage location recommended for intrathecal medications. Liposomal vincristine should **NOT** be delivered to the patient at the same time with any medications intended for central nervous system administration.

[U.S. Boxed Warning]: Vincristine LIPOSOME and conventional vincristine are NOT interchangeable. Dosing differs between formulations; verify intended product and dose prior to preparation and administration to avoid overdoses. Avoid extravasation of liposomal vincristine (conventional vincristine is a vesicant). Only individuals experienced with vesicant administration should administer liposomal vincristine. Check for proper needle placement; if extravasation occurs, discontinue liposomal vincristine infusion immediately and institute appropriate extravasation management procedures.

Grade 3 and greater neutropenia, anemia, and thrombocytopenia were observed in clinical trials. Monitor blood counts closely and adjust dose or withhold therapy if necessary. Constipation, ileus, bowel obstruction, and colonic pseudo-obstruction have occurred with liposomal vincristine. Patients should be initiated on a prophylactic bowel regimen including a stool softener, dietary fiber, and hydration; laxative treatments may be considered. Severe fatigue was noted in clinical trials; treatment delay, dosage adjustment, or discontinuation may be necessary.

Neuropathies (sensory and motor) are common and cumulative. Neuropathy symptoms may include paresthesia, hyper-/hypoesthesia, hyporeflexia or areflexia, neuralgia, jaw pain, cranial neuropathy, ileus, arthralgia, myalgia, muscle spasm, and/or weakness. Evaluate neurologic status of patients closely prior to liposomal vincristine administration; neurologic toxicity risk is greater when given to patients with preexisting neuromuscular conditions or when used concomitantly with other neurotoxic agents. Treatment delay, dosage adjustment, and/or discontinuation may be necessary. Tumor lysis syndrome may occur as a consequence of therapy; monitor closely for signs and symptoms and manage accordingly.

Hepatotoxicity (including fatal cases) and increased AST have been reported. Monitor hepatic function tests; reduce dose or interrupt therapy if necessary. Use caution in patients with hepatic impairment; liposomal vincristine has not been studied in patients with severe hepatic impairment. In a study in a limited number of melanoma patients with moderate (Child-Pugh class B) hepatic impairment secondary to liver metastases, C_{max} and AUC were comparable to those in patients with normal hepatic function; patients with hepatic impairment received a dose of 1 mg/m^2 every 2 weeks versus 2 mg/m^2 in subjects with normal hepatic function (Bedikian, 2011). Avoid concomitant therapy with strong CYP3A4 or P-glycoprotein (P-gp) inducers or inhibitors. Use with caution in the elderly patient population; conventional vincristine may cause or exacerbate hyponatremia or syndrome of inappropriate antidiuretic hormone secretion; monitor sodium closely with therapy initiation or dosage adjustments (Beers Criteria).

Adverse Reactions

Cardiovascular: Cardiac arrest, hypotension

Central nervous system: Fatigue, fever, insomnia, mental status changes, pain

Gastrointestinal: Abdominal pain, appetite decreased, constipation, diarrhea, ileus, nausea

Hematologic: Anemia, neutropenia, neutropenic fever, thrombocytopenia

Hepatic: AST increased

Neuromuscular & skeletal: Muscle weakness, peripheral neuropathy, weakness

Respiratory: Pneumonia, respiratory distress, respiratory failure

Miscellaneous: Septic shock, staphylococcal infection

Drug Interactions

Metabolism/Transport Effects Substrate of CYP3A4 (major), P-glycoprotein; **Note:** Assignment of Major/Minor substrate status based on clinically relevant drug interaction potential; **Inhibits** CYP3A4 (weak)

Avoid Concomitant Use

Avoid concomitant use of VinCRIStine (Liposomal) with any of the following: BCG; CloZAPine; Conivaptan; CYP3A4 Inducers (Strong); CYP3A4 Inhibitors (Strong); Dexamethasone (Systemic); Dipyrone; Fusidic Acid (Systemic); Idelalisib; Natalizumab; P-glycoprotein/ABCB1 Inducers; P-glycoprotein/ABCB1 Inhibitors; Pimecrolimus; Pimozide; St Johns Wort; Tacrolimus (Topical); Tofacitinib; Vaccines (Live)

Increased Effect/Toxicity

VinCRIStine (Liposomal) may increase the levels/effects of: ARIPiprazole; CloZAPine; Dofetilide; Hydrocodone; Leflunomide; MitoMYcin (Systemic); Natalizumab; Pimozide; Tofacitinib; Vaccines (Live)

The levels/effects of VinCRIStine (Liposomal) may be increased by: Aprepitant; Ceritinib; Conivaptan; CYP3A4 Inhibitors (Moderate); CYP3A4 Inhibitors (Strong); Dasatinib; Denosumab; Dipyrone; Fosaprepitant; Fusidic Acid (Systemic); Idelalisib; Luliconazole; Macrolide Antibiotics; MAO Inhibitors; Mifepristone; Netupitant; NIFEdipine; P-glycoprotein/ABCB1 Inhibitors; Pimecrolimus; Roflumilast; Tacrolimus (Topical); Teniposide; Trastuzumab

Decreased Effect

VinCRIStine (Liposomal) may decrease the levels/effects of: BCG; Coccidioides immitis Skin Test; Sipuleucel-T; Vaccines (Inactivated); Vaccines (Live)

The levels/effects of VinCRIStine (Liposomal) may be decreased by: Bosentan; CYP3A4 Inducers (Moderate); CYP3A4 Inducers (Strong); Dabrafenib; Deferasirox; Dexamethasone (Systemic); Echinacea; P-glycoprotein/ABCB1 Inducers; Siltuximab; St Johns Wort; Tocilizumab

Preparation for Administration Hazardous agent; use appropriate precautions for handling and disposal (NIOSH 2014 [group 1]). Vincristine liposome preparation requires 60-90 minutes of dedicated time utilizing the manufacturer supplied kit. Do not reuse kit components with future doses.

1). Outside the sterile area, fill a water bath to a depth of at least 8 cm (3.2 inches); water should be heated to and maintained at **63°C to 67°C** (145.4°F to 152.6°F) for the entire procedure (use calibrated thermometer to monitor temperature). Maintain water depth of at least 8 cm (3.2 inches) throughout process. Water bath must remain outside the sterile area.

2). In a biological safety cabinet, vent the sodium phosphate vial with a sterile venting needle (with a 0.2 micron filter or other suitable venting device). Venting needle should always be kept above liquid level. Remove 1 mL of sphingomyelin/cholesterol liposome injection and inject into the sodium phosphate vial. Withdraw 5 mL of vincristine sulfate injection and inject into the sodium phosphate vial. Remove the venting needle and gently invert the sodium phosphate vial 5 times to mix (do **not** shake). Place flotation ring on the sodium phosphate vial.

3). Confirm the water bath is maintained between **63°C to 67°C** (145.4°F to 152.6°F). Outside the sterile area, place constituted sodium phosphate vial in the water bath for 10 minutes. Record constitution start and stop time, as well as starting and ending water temperature. After 10 minutes, remove the vial (with tongs), remove flotation ring, then dry the vial, affix vial overlabel, and gently invert 5 times to mix (do **not** shake). Allow the vial to equilibrate for at least 30 minutes at room temperature of 15°C to 30°C (59°F to 86°F), but for no longer than 12 hours. Once prepared, vincristine sulfate liposome concentration is 5 mg/31 mL (0.16 mg/mL).

4). Return vial to biologic safety cabinet. Calculate patient's vincristine liposome dose (based on actual BSA); remove corresponding volume from 100 mL NS or D_5W infusion bag. Inject vincristine liposome dose into the infusion bag (final volume of 100 mL). Do not use if a precipitate or other foreign matter is present in the vial or infusion bag. The amount contained in each vial may exceed the prescribed dose; use care with dosage and volume calculations. Discard unused portion of the vial. After preparation, keep liposomal vincristine in a location away from the separate storage location recommended for intrathecal medications.

Storage/Stability Store intact kit (containing vincristine vial, sphingomyelin/cholesterol liposome vial, and sodium phosphate vial) refrigerated at 2°C to 8°C (36°F to 46°F); do not freeze. Use appropriate precautions for handling and disposal. Once prepared, liposomal vincristine is stable for no more than 12 hours at room temperature. After preparation, keep liposomal vincristine in a location away from the separate storage location recommended for intrathecal medications.

Mechanism of Action Vincristine is a cell cycle specific agent which binds to tubulin, leading to microtubule depolymerization and cellular apoptosis. The liposomal formulation increases the half-life, allowing for enhanced cytotoxic activity in tumor cells.

Pharmacodynamics/Kinetics

Distribution: V_{dss}: 2.7 L (Bedikian, 2006)

Metabolism: Primarily hepatic

Half-life elimination: 45 hours (urinary half-life); dependent on rate of vincristine release from sphingosome (Bedikian, 2006)

Excretion: Feces (69%); urine (<8%)

Dosage Adults: **Note:** Vincristine liposomal and conventional vincristine are **NOT** interchangeable. Dosing differs between formulations; verify intended product and dose prior to preparation and administration. The liposomal vincristine dose is based on actual body surface area (BSA) and was not capped in studies (O'Brien, 2009; Rodriguez, 2009; Silverman, 2010).

Acute lymphoblastic leukemia (ALL; Philadelphia chromosome-negative), relapsed: IV: 2.25 mg/m^2 once every 7 days

Dosage adjustment for toxicity:

Fatigue, severe: Consider dose delay, reduction, or therapy discontinuation.

Hematologic toxicity: Grade 3 or 4 neutropenia, thrombocytopenia, or anemia: Consider dose reduction or modification.

Hepatic toxicity: Reduce dose or interrupt treatment.

Peripheral neuropathy:

Grade 3 or persistent grade 2 toxicity: Interrupt therapy until recovery to grade 1 or 2, then reduce dose to 2 mg/m^2. If grade 3 toxicity persists or if grade 4 toxicity occurs, discontinue liposomal vincristine.

Persistent grade 2 toxicity after first dose reduction to 2 mg/m^2: Interrupt therapy for up to 7 days until recovery to grade 1, then reduce dose to 1.825 mg/m^2. If neuropathy increases to grade 3 or 4, discontinue liposomal vincristine.

Persistent grade 2 toxicity after second dose reduction to 1.825 mg/m^2: Interrupt therapy for up to 7 days until recovery to grade 1, then reduce dose to 1.5 mg/m^2. If neuropathy increases to grade 3 or 4, discontinue liposomal vincristine.

Preexisting neuropathy, severe: Assess treatment benefit versus risk.

Dosage adjustment in renal impairment: No dosage adjustment provided in manufacturer's labeling (has not been studied); however, liposomal vincristine is minimally excreted by the kidney and like the conventional formulation, likely does not require dosage adjustment in renal impairment.

Dosage adjustment in hepatic impairment:

Moderate impairment (Child-Pugh class B): In a study in a limited number of melanoma patients with moderate (Child-Pugh class B) hepatic impairment secondary to liver metastases, C_{max} and AUC were comparable to those in patients with normal hepatic function; patients with hepatic impairment received a dose of 1 mg/m^2 every 2 weeks versus 2 mg/m^2 in subjects with normal hepatic function (Bedikian, 2011).

Severe impairment (Child-Pugh class C): No dosage adjustment provided in manufacturer's labeling (has not been studied).

Hepatotoxicity during treatment: Reduce dose or interrupt treatment.

Dosing in obesity: *ASCO Guidelines for appropriate chemotherapy dosing in obese adults with cancer:* Utilize patient's actual body weight (full weight) for calculation of body surface area- or weight-based dosing, particularly when the intent of therapy is curative; manage regimen-related toxicities in the same manner as for nonobese patients; if a dose reduction is utilized due to toxicity, consider resumption of full weight-based dosing with subsequent cycles, especially if cause of toxicity (eg, hepatic or renal impairment) is resolved (Griggs, 2012).

Administration Conventional vincristine is a vesicant. Limited information is available regarding liposomal vincristine extravasation, but may cause inflammation if extravasated; avoid extravasation. **For IV administration only. FATAL IF GIVEN INTRATHECALLY.** Liposomal vincristine should **NOT** be delivered to the patient at the same time as any medications intended for central nervous system administration.

IV: Infuse over 1 hour. Do not administer IV push or bolus; do not use with in-line filters. Infusion must be completed within 12 hours of preparation.

Hazardous agent; use appropriate precautions for handling and disposal (NIOSH 2014 [group 1]).

Monitoring Parameters CBC with differential and platelets; hepatic function; signs/symptoms of peripheral neuropathy or other neurologic toxicities; sodium (in elderly patients; conventional vincristine may cause or exacerbate hyponatremia or syndrome of inappropriate antidiuretic hormone secretion); signs/symptoms of tumor lysis syndrome; symptoms of constipation; monitor infusion site for extravasation

Additional Information The liposomal formulation of vincristine consists of vincristine encapsulated in sphingosomes, which are composed of sphingomyelin and cholesterol (Bedikian, 2006).

Dosage Forms

Suspension, Intravenous:

Marqibo: 5 mg/31 mL (1 ea)

- ◆ **Vincristine (Conventional)** *see* VinCRIStine *on page 2163*
- ◆ **Vincristine Liposome** *see* VinCRIStine (Liposomal) *on page 2166*
- ◆ **Vincristine Sulfate** *see* VinCRIStine *on page 2163*
- ◆ **Vincristine Sulfate Injection (Can)** *see* VinCRIStine *on page 2163*
- ◆ **Vincristine Sulfate Injection USP (Can)** *see* VinCRIStine *on page 2163*
- ◆ **Vincristine Sulfate Liposome** *see* VinCRIStine (Liposomal) *on page 2166*

Vinorelbine (vi NOR el been)

Brand Names: U.S. Navelbine

Brand Names: Canada Navelbine; Vinorelbine Injection, USP; Vinorelbine Tartrate for Injection

Index Terms Dihydroxydeoxynorvinkaleukoblastine; Vinorelbine Tartrate

Pharmacologic Category Antineoplastic Agent, Antimicrotubular; Antineoplastic Agent, Vinca Alkaloid

Use Treatment of non-small cell lung cancer (NSCLC)

Pregnancy Risk Factor D

Pregnancy Considerations Animal reproduction studies have demonstrated embryotoxicity, fetotoxicity, decreased fetal weight, and delayed ossification. May cause fetal harm if administered during pregnancy. Women of childbearing potential should avoid becoming pregnant during vinorelbine treatment.

Breast-Feeding Considerations It is not known if vinorelbine is excreted in breast milk. Due to the potential for serious adverse reactions in the nursing infant, breastfeeding should be discontinued during treatment.

Contraindications Pretreatment granulocyte counts $<1000/mm^3$

Warnings/Precautions Hazardous agent - use appropriate precautions for handling and disposal (NIOSH 2014 [group 1]). **[U.S. Boxed Warning]: For IV use only; intrathecal administration of other vinca alkaloids has resulted in death. If dispensed in a syringe, should be labeled "for intravenous use only - fatal if given intrathecally". [U.S. Boxed Warning]: Vesicant; ensure proper needle or catheter placement prior to and during infusion. Avoid extravasation. Extravasation may cause local tissue necrosis and/or thrombophlebitis. [U.S. Boxed Warning]: Severe granulocytopenia may occur with treatment (may lead to infection); granulocyte counts should be ≥1000 cells/mm^3 prior to treatment initiation; dosage adjustment may be required based on blood counts (monitor blood counts prior to each dose).** Granulocytopenia is a dose-limiting toxicity; nadir is generally 7-10 days after administration and recovery occurs within the following 7-14 days. Monitor closely for infections and/or fever in patients with severe granulocytopenia. Use with extreme caution in patients with compromised marrow reserve due to prior chemotherapy or radiation therapy.

Fatal cases of interstitial pulmonary changes and ARDS have been reported (with single-agent therapy (mean onset of symptoms: 1 week); promptly evaluate changes in baseline pulmonary symptoms or any new onset pulmonary symptoms (eg, dyspnea, cough, hypoxia). Acute shortness of breath and severe bronchospasm have been reported with vinca alkaloids; usually associated with the concurrent administration of mitomycin.

Vinorelbine should **NOT** be prepared during the preparation of any intrathecal medications. After preparation, keep vinorelbine in a location **away** from the separate storage location recommended for intrathecal medications. Elimination is predominantly hepatic; while there is no evidence that toxicity is enhanced in patients with elevated transaminases, use with caution in patients with severe hepatic injury or impairment; dosage modification required for elevated total bilirubin. May cause new onset or worsening of preexisting neuropathy; use with caution in patients with neuropathy; monitor for new or worsening sign/symptoms of neuropathy; dosage adjustment required. May cause severe constipation (grade 3-4), paralytic ileus, intestinal obstruction, necrosis, and/or perforation; some events were fatal. Oral vinorelbine (not available in the U.S.) is associated with a moderate antiemetic potential; antiemetics are recommended to prevent nausea/vomiting (Dupuis, 2011; Roila, 2010); IV vinorelbine has a minimal emetic potential (Dupuis, 2011; Roila, 2010). Potentially significant drug-drug interactions may exist, requiring dose or frequency adjustment, additional monitoring, and/or selection of alternative therapy. May have radiosensitizing effects with prior or concurrent radiation therapy; radiation recall reactions may occur in patients who have received prior radiation therapy. Avoid eye contamination (exposure may cause severe irritation). **[U.S. Boxed Warning]: Should be administered under the supervision of an experienced cancer chemotherapy physician.**

Adverse Reactions

Cardiovascular: Chest pain

Central nervous system: Fatigue

Dermatologic: Alopecia, rash

Gastrointestinal: Constipation, diarrhea, nausea, paralytic ileus, vomiting

Hematologic: Anemia, granulocytopenia (nadir: 7-10 days; recovery 14-21 days), leukopenia, neutropenia, neutropenic fever/sepsis, thrombocytopenia

Hepatic: AST increased, total bilirubin increased

Local: Injection site pain, injection site reaction (includes erythema and vein discoloration), phlebitis

Neuromuscular & skeletal: Arthralgia, jaw pain, myalgia, peripheral neuropathy, loss of deep tendon reflexes, weakness

Otic: Ototoxicity

Respiratory: Dyspnea

Rare but important or life-threatening: Abdominal pain, allergic reactions, anaphylaxis, angioedema, back pain, DVT, dysphagia, esophagitis, flushing, gait instability, headache, hemolytic uremic syndrome, hemorrhagic cystitis, hyper-/hypotension, hyponatremia, intestinal necrosis, intestinal obstruction, intestinal perforation, interstitial pulmonary changes, local rash, local urticaria, MI (rare), mucositis, muscle weakness, myocardial ischemia, pancreatitis, paralytic ileus, pneumonia, pruritus, pulmonary edema, pulmonary embolus, radiation recall (dermatitis, esophagitis), skin blistering, syndrome of inappropriate ADH secretion, tachycardia, thromboembolic events, thrombotic thrombocytopenic purpura, tumor pain, urticaria, vasodilation

Drug Interactions

Metabolism/Transport Effects Substrate of CYP2D6 (minor), CYP3A4 (major); **Note:** Assignment of Major/Minor substrate status based on clinically relevant drug interaction potential; **Inhibits** CYP2D6 (weak), CYP3A4 (weak)

Avoid Concomitant Use

Avoid concomitant use of Vinorelbine with any of the following: BCG; CloZAPine; Conivaptan; Dipyrone; Fusidic Acid (Systemic); Idelalisib; Natalizumab; Pimecrolimus; Pimozide; Tacrolimus (Topical); Tofacitinib; Vaccines (Live)

Increased Effect/Toxicity

Vinorelbine may increase the levels/effects of: ARIPiprazole; CloZAPine; Dofetilide; Hydrocodone; Leflunomide; Lomitapide; MitoMYcin (Systemic); Natalizumab; Pimozide; Tofacitinib; Vaccines (Live)

The levels/effects of Vinorelbine may be increased by: Aprepitant; Ceritinib; CISplatin; Conivaptan; CYP3A4 Inhibitors (Moderate); CYP3A4 Inhibitors (Strong); Dasatinib; Denosumab; Dipyrone; Fosaprepitant; Fusidic Acid (Systemic); Gefitinib; Idelalisib; Itraconazole; Ivacaftor; Luliconazole; Macrolide Antibiotics; Mifepristone; Netupitant; PACLitaxel; PACLitaxel (Protein Bound); Pimecrolimus; Posaconazole; Roflumilast; Simeprevir; Stiripentol; Tacrolimus (Topical); Trastuzumab; Voriconazole

Decreased Effect

Vinorelbine may decrease the levels/effects of: BCG; Coccidioides immitis Skin Test; Sipuleucel-T; Vaccines (Inactivated); Vaccines (Live)

The levels/effects of Vinorelbine may be decreased by: Bosentan; CYP3A4 Inducers (Moderate); CYP3A4 Inducers (Strong); Dabrafenib; Deferasirox; Echinacea; Mitotane; Siltuximab; St Johns Wort; Tocilizumab

Preparation for Administration Hazardous agent; use appropriate precautions for handling and disposal (NIOSH 2014 [group 1]). Dilute in D_5W or NS to a final concentration of 1.5-3 mg/mL (for syringe) or D_5W, NS, 1/2NS, $D_5$1/2NS, LR, or Ringer's to a final concentration of 0.5-2 mg/mL (for IV bag). Vinorelbine should **NOT** be prepared during the preparation of any intrathecal medications.

Storage/Stability Store intact vials refrigerated at 2°C to 8°C (36°F to 46°F); do not freeze. Protect from light. Intact vials are stable at room temperature of 25°C (77°F) for up to 72 hours. Solutions diluted for infusion in polypropylene syringes or polyvinyl chloride bags are stable for 24 hours at 5°C to 30°C (41°F to 86°F). After preparation, keep vinorelbine in a location **away** from the separate storage location recommended for intrathecal medications.

Mechanism of Action Semisynthetic vinca alkaloid which binds to tubulin and inhibits microtubule formation, therefore, arresting the cell at metaphase by disrupting the formation of the mitotic spindle; it is specific for the M and S phases. Vinorelbine may also interfere with nucleic acid and protein synthesis by blocking glutamic acid utilization.

Pharmacodynamics/Kinetics

Distribution: V_d: 25-40 L/kg; binds extensively to human platelets and lymphocytes (80% to 91%)

Protein binding: 80% to 91%

Metabolism: Extensively hepatic, via CYP3A4, to two metabolites, deacetylvinorelbine (active) and vinorelbine N-oxide

Half-life elimination: Triphasic: Terminal: 28-44 hours

Excretion: Feces (46%); urine (18%, 10% to 12% as unchanged drug)

Dosage

Non-small cell lung cancer (NSCLC): Adults: IV:

Single-agent therapy: 30 mg/m² every 7 days until disease progression or unacceptable toxicity

Combination therapy: 25-30 mg/m² every 7 days (in combination with cisplatin)

Off-label dosing: 25 mg/m² days 1 and 8 every 21 days (in combination with cisplatin and cetuximab) for up to 6 cycles (Pirker, 2009) **or** 25-30 mg/m² days 1, 8, and 15 every 28 days (in combination with gemcitabine) for 6 cycles **or** until disease progression or unacceptable toxicity (Herbst, 2002; Greco, 2007)

Breast cancer, metastatic (off-label use): Adults: IV: 25 mg/m² every 7 days (as a single agent) until disease progression or unacceptable toxicity (Zelek, 2001) **or** 30 mg/m² every 7 days (as a single agent); after 13 weeks, may administer every 14 days for patient convenience, continue until disease progression or unacceptable toxicity (Vogel, 1999) **or** 25 mg/m² every 7 days (in combination with trastuzumab) until disease progression or unacceptable toxicity (Burstein, 2001; Burstein, 2007) **or** 30 or 35 mg/m² days 1 and 8 every 21 days (in combination with trastuzumab) until disease progression or unacceptable toxicity (Andersson, 2011)

Cervical cancer (off-label use): Adults: IV: 30 mg/m² days 1 and 8 of a of a 21-day treatment cycle (Muggia, 2004; Muggia, 2005)

Hodgkin lymphoma, relapsed or refractory (off-label use): Adults: IV:

GVD regimen: 15 mg/m² (post-transplant patients) or 20 mg/m² (transplant-naïve patients) on days 1 and 8 of a 21-day cycle (in combination with gemcitabine and doxorubicin liposomal) for 2 to 6 cycles (Bartlett, 2007)

IGEV regimen: 20 mg/m² on day 1 of a 21-day cycle (in combination with ifosfamide, mesna, gemcitabine, and prednisolone) for 4 cycles (Santoro, 2007)

Malignant pleural mesothelioma (off-label use): Adults: IV: 30 mg/m² (maximum dose: 60 mg) every 7 days per 6-week treatment cycle, continue until disease progression (Stebbing, 2009) **or** 30 mg/m² (maximum dose: 60 mg) every 7 days for 6 weeks, off 2 weeks, then repeat cycle (Muers, 2008)

Ovarian cancer, relapsed (off-label use): Adults: IV: 25 mg/m² every 7 days (Bajetta, 1996) **or** 30 mg/m² days 1 and 8 of a 21-day treatment cycle (Rothenberg, 2004) until disease progression or unacceptable toxicity

Salivary gland cancer, recurrent (off-label use): Adults: IV: 25 mg/m² on days 1 and 8 of a 21-day cycle (in combination with cisplatin) for a minimum of 3 cycles and for up to 6 cycles (Airoldi, 2001) **or** 30 mg/m² every 7 days (monotherapy) for a minimum of 9 weeks and for up to 6 cycles (Airoldi, 2001)

Small cell lung cancer, refractory (off-label use): Adults: IV: 25 or 30 mg/m² every 7 days until disease progression or unacceptable toxicity (Furuse, 1996; Jessem, 1993)

Soft tissue sarcoma, advanced (off-label use): Adults: IV: 25 mg/m² days 1 and 8 of a 21-day treatment cycle (in combination with gemcitabine) until disease progression or unacceptable toxicity (Dileo, 2007)

Dosage adjustment in hematological toxicity: Granulocyte counts should be ≥1000 cells/mm³ prior to the administration of vinorelbine. Adjustments in the dosage of vinorelbine should be based on granulocyte counts obtained on the day of treatment as follows:

Granulocytes ≥1500 cells/mm³ on day of treatment: Administer 100% of starting dose

Granulocytes 1000-1499 cells/mm³ on day of treatment: Administer 50% of starting dose

Granulocytes <1000 cells/mm³ on day of treatment: Do not administer. Repeat granulocyte count in one week; if 3 consecutive doses are held because granulocyte count is <1000 cells/mm³, discontinue vinorelbine.

For patients who, during treatment, have experienced fever and/or sepsis while granulocytopenic or had 2 consecutive weekly doses held due to granulocytopenia, subsequent doses of vinorelbine should be:

75% of starting dose for granulocytes ≥1500 cells/mm³

37.5% of starting dose for granulocytes 1000-1499 cells/mm³

Dosage adjustment for neurotoxicity: Neurotoxicity ≥ grade 2: Discontinue treatment

Dosage adjustment for other adverse events: Severe adverse events: Reduce dose or discontinue treatment

Dosage adjustment in renal impairment:

Renal insufficiency: No dosage adjustment necessary.

Hemodialysis: Initial: IV: Reduce dose to 20 mg/m²/week; administer either after dialysis (on dialysis days) or on nondialysis days (Janus, 2010)

Dosing adjustment in hepatic impairment: Administer with caution in patients with hepatic insufficiency. In patients who develop hyperbilirubinemia during treatment with vinorelbine, the dose should be adjusted for total bilirubin as follows:

Serum bilirubin ≤2 mg/dL: Administer 100% of dose

Serum bilirubin 2.1-3 mg/dL: Administer 50% of dose (Ecklund, 2005; Floyd, 2006; Superfin, 2006)

Serum bilirubin >3 mg/dL: Administer 25% of dose (Ecklund, 2005; Floyd, 2006; Superfin, 2006)

Patients (breast cancer) with extensive liver metastases (>75% of liver volume): Administer 50% of dose (Ecklund, 2005; Superfin, 2006)

Dosing adjustment in patients with concurrent hematologic toxicity and hepatic impairment: Administer the lower of the doses determined from the adjustment recommendations.

Dosing in obesity: *ASCO Guidelines for appropriate chemotherapy dosing in obese adults with cancer:* Utilize patient's actual body weight (full weight) for calculation of body surface area- or weight-based dosing, particularly when the intent of therapy is curative; manage regimen-related toxicities in the same manner as for nonobese patients; if a dose reduction is utilized due to toxicity, consider resumption of full weight-based dosing with subsequent cycles, especially if cause of toxicity (eg, hepatic or renal impairment) is resolved (Griggs, 2012).

Administration For IV use only; FATAL IF GIVEN INTRATHECALLY. Administer as a direct intravenous push or rapid bolus, over 6-10 minutes (up to 30 minutes). Longer infusions may increase the risk of pain and phlebitis. Intravenous doses should be followed by at least 75-125 mL of saline or D_5W to reduce the incidence of phlebitis and inflammation.

Vesicant; ensure proper needle or catheter position prior to administration. Avoid extravasation.

Extravasation management: If extravasation occurs, stop infusion immediately and disconnect (leave cannula/needle in place); gently aspirate extravasated solution (do **NOT** flush the line); initiate hyaluronidase antidote; remove needle/cannula; apply dry warm compresses for 20 minutes 4 times a day for 1-2 days; elevate extremity (Perez Fidalgo, 2012). Remaining portion of the vinorelbine dose should be infused through a separate vein.

Hyaluronidase: If needle/cannula still in place, administer 1-6 mL hyaluronidase (150 units/mL) into the existing IV line; the usual dose is 1 mL hyaluronidase for each 1 mL of extravasated drug (Perez Fidalgo, 2012; Schulmeister, 2011). If needle/cannula was removed, inject 1-6 mL (150 units/mL) subcutaneously in a clockwise manner using 1mL for each 1 mL of drug extravasated (Schulmeister, 2011) **or** administer 1 mL (150 units/mL) as 5 separate 0.2 mL injections (using a 25-gauge needle) subcutaneously into the extravasation site (Polovich, 2009).

Hazardous agent; use appropriate precautions for handling and disposal (NIOSH 2014 [group 1]).

Monitoring Parameters CBC with differential and platelet count (prior to each dose, and after treatment), hepatic function tests; monitor for new-onset pulmonary symptoms (or worsening from baseline); monitor for neuropathy (new or worsening symptoms; monitor infusion site; monitor for signs symptoms of constipation/ileus

Dosage Forms

Solution, Intravenous:

Navelbine: 10 mg/mL (1 mL); 50 mg/5 mL (5 mL)

Generic: 10 mg/mL (1 mL); 50 mg/5 mL (5 mL)

Solution, Intravenous [preservative free]:

Generic: 10 mg/mL (1 mL); 50 mg/5 mL (5 mL)

- ◆ **Vinorelbine Injection, USP (Can)** *see* Vinorelbine *on page 2168*
- ◆ **Vinorelbine Tartrate** *see* Vinorelbine *on page 2168*
- ◆ **Vinorelbine Tartrate for Injection (Can)** *see* Vinorelbine *on page 2168*
- ◆ **Viokace** *see* Pancrelipase *on page 1566*
- ◆ **Viokase (Can)** *see* Pancrelipase *on page 1566*
- ◆ **Viorele** *see* Ethinyl Estradiol and Desogestrel *on page 799*
- ◆ **Viosterol** *see* Ergocalciferol *on page 753*
- ◆ **Viracept** *see* Nelfinavir *on page 1436*
- ◆ **Viramune** *see* Nevirapine *on page 1440*
- ◆ **Viramune XR** *see* Nevirapine *on page 1440*
- ◆ **Virazole** *see* Ribavirin *on page 1797*
- ◆ **Virdec [OTC]** *see* Chlorpheniramine and Phenylephrine *on page 426*
- ◆ **Virdec DM [OTC]** *see* Chlorpheniramine, Phenylephrine, and Dextromethorphan *on page 428*
- ◆ **Viread** *see* Tenofovir *on page 1998*
- ◆ **Viroptic** *see* Trifluridine *on page 2103*
- ◆ **Viroptic® (Can)** *see* Trifluridine *on page 2103*
- ◆ **Virt-Phos 250 Neutral** *see* Potassium Phosphate and Sodium Phosphate *on page 1692*
- ◆ **Virtrate-3** *see* Citric Acid, Sodium Citrate, and Potassium Citrate *on page 455*
- ◆ **Virtussin A/C** *see* Guaifenesin and Codeine *on page 987*
- ◆ **Virt-Vite** *see* Folic Acid, Cyanocobalamin, and Pyridoxine *on page 921*
- ◆ **Virt-Vite Forte** *see* Folic Acid, Cyanocobalamin, and Pyridoxine *on page 921*
- ◆ **Visanne® (Can)** *see* Dienogest [CAN/INT] *on page 623*
- ◆ **Viscoat®** *see* Sodium Chondroitin Sulfate and Sodium Hyaluronate *on page 1905*
- ◆ **Viscous Lidocaine** *see* Lidocaine (Topical) *on page 1211*
- ◆ **Visine-A [OTC]** *see* Naphazoline and Pheniramine *on page 1426*
- ◆ **Visine Advanced Allergy (Can)** *see* Naphazoline and Pheniramine *on page 1426*
- ◆ **Viskazide (Can)** *see* Pindolol and Hydrochlorothiazide [CAN/INT] *on page 1653*
- ◆ **Visken (Can)** *see* Pindolol *on page 1652*

Vismodegib (vis moe DEG ib)

Brand Names: U.S. Erivedge

Brand Names: Canada Erivedge

Index Terms GDC-0449; Hedgehog Antagonist GDC-0449

Pharmacologic Category Antineoplastic Agent, Hedgehog Pathway Inhibitor

Use Basal cell carcinoma: Treatment of metastatic basal cell carcinoma, or locally-advanced basal cell carcinoma that has recurred following surgery or in patients who are not candidates for surgery, and not candidates for radiation therapy

Pregnancy Risk Factor D

Pregnancy Considerations [U.S. Boxed Warning]: May result in severe birth defects or embryo-fetal death. Teratogenic effects (severe midline defects, missing digits, and other irreversible malformations), embryotoxic, and fetotoxic events were observed in animal reproduction studies when administered in doses less than the normal human dose. Based on its mechanism of action adverse effects on pregnancy would be expected. **[U.S. Boxed Warning]: Verify pregnancy status prior to initiating treatment and advise patients (female and male) of the risk of birth defects, the need for contraception and risk of exposure through semen.** In females of childbearing potential, obtain pregnancy test within 7 days prior to treatment initiation; after the negative pregnancy test, initiate highly effective contraception prior to the first vismodegib dose and continue during and for 7 months after treatment. During treatment (including treatment interruptions) and for 2 months after treatment, male patients should not donate sperm and should use condoms with spermicide (even after vasectomy) if their partner is of childbearing potential. Women exposed to vismodegib during pregnancy (directly or via seminal fluid) are encouraged to participate in the Erivedge Pregnancy Pharmacovigilance program by contacting the Genentech Adverse Event Line (1-888-835-2555). Pregnancies occurring during or within 7 months after treatment should be reported to the Genentech Adverse Event Line.

The Canadian labeling recommends that females of child-bearing potential use 2 simultaneous forms of effective contraception beginning at least 4 weeks prior to treatment initiation, during treatment (including treatment interruptions), and for 24 months after discontinuation. Pregnancy testing should be performed within 7 days prior to treatment initiation, monthly during treatment (including treatment interruptions) and for 24 months after discontinuation. For females of child bearing potential, a new prescription is required each month to allow for monthly pregnancy testing. Any suspected exposure (directly or via seminal fluid) during pregnancy should be immediately reported to the Erivedge Pregnancy Prevention Program (EPPP) at 1-888-748-8926.

Breast-Feeding Considerations It is not known if vismodegib is excreted in human milk. Due to the potential for serious adverse reactions in the nursing infant or child, the decision to discontinue breast-feeding or to discontinue vismodegib should take into account the benefits of treatment to the mother. The Canadian labeling contraindicates use in women who are nursing and recommends that women abstain from nursing for 24 months after discontinuation of therapy.

Contraindications

U.S. labeling: There are no contraindications listed within the manufacturer's labeling.

Canadian labeling: Hypersensitivity to vismodegib or any component of the formulation; pregnancy or females at risk of becoming pregnant; breast-feeding; male patients or female patients of childbearing potential who do not comply with the Erivedge Pregnancy Prevention Program; children and adolescents <18 years of age.

Warnings/Precautions Hazardous agent - use appropriate precautions for handling and disposal (meets NIOSH 2014 criteria). **[U.S. Boxed Warnings]: May result in severe birth defects or embryo-fetal death. Teratogenic effects (severe midline defects, missing digits, and other irreversible malformations), embryotoxic, and fetotoxic events were observed in animal reproduction studies. Verify pregnancy status prior to initiating treatment and advise patients (female and male) of the risk of birth defects, the need for contraception and risk of exposure through semen.** Amenorrhea was observed in women of reproductive potential; it is unknown if this is reversible.

Cardiac events (eg, cardiac failure, atrial fibrillation, left ventricular dysfunction, restrictive cardiomyopathy, myocardial infarction) have been observed during treatment. All events ≥ grade 3 occurred in patients with a history of significant cardiac disease. Cases of cutaneous squamous cell cancer (cuSCC) have been reported. Patients with advanced basal cell carcinoma are at risk for developing cuSCC; monitor during treatment. Vismodegib is associated with a moderate emetic potential; antiemetics may be needed to prevent nausea and vomiting. Diarrhea, constipation, abdominal pain, and decreased appetite may also occur.

Vismodegib metabolism is primarily hepatic; use with caution in patients with hepatic dysfunction. Elevated hepatic enzymes (mostly grades 1 and 2) have been observed with use; transient elevations ≥ grade 3 have been observed but did not require treatment interruption or discontinuation in most cases. Use with caution in patients with renal impairment (has not been studied). However, population pharmacokinetic analyses demonstrate that creatinine clearance (range: 30-80 mL/minute) does not have a clinically meaningful effect on systemic exposure; urinary excretion is <5%.

Advise patients not to donate blood or blood products during vismodegib treatment and for at least 7 months after the last vismodegib dose. The Canadian labeling recommends patients not donate blood or blood products during treatment (including treatment interruptions) and for 24 months after discontinuation.

Adverse Reactions

Central nervous system: Fatigue

Dermatologic: Alopecia

Endocrine & metabolic: Amenorrhea, hypokalemia, hyponatremia

Gastrointestinal: Abnormal taste, appetite decreased, constipation, diarrhea, loss of taste perception, nausea, vomiting, weight loss

Neuromuscular & skeletal: Arthralgia, muscle spasm

Renal: Azotemia

Rare but important or life-threatening: Abdominal pain, alkaline phosphatase increased, aspiration, atrial fibrillation, back pain, corneal abrasion, dehydration, dyspnea, hyperkalemia, hypocalcemia, keratitis, lymphopenia, pneumonia, urinary tract infection

Drug Interactions

Metabolism/Transport Effects Substrate of CYP2C9 (minor), CYP3A4 (minor), P-glycoprotein; **Note:** Assignment of Major/Minor substrate status based on clinically relevant drug interaction potential; **Inhibits** BCRP, CYP2C19 (weak), CYP2C8 (weak), CYP2C9 (weak)

Avoid Concomitant Use There are no known interactions where it is recommended to avoid concomitant use.

Increased Effect/Toxicity

The levels/effects of Vismodegib may be increased by: P-glycoprotein/ABCB1 Inhibitors

Decreased Effect

The levels/effects of Vismodegib may be decreased by: Antacids; H2-Antagonists; P-glycoprotein/ABCB1 Inducers; Proton Pump Inhibitors

Storage/Stability Store at 20°C to 25°C (68°F to 77°F); excursions permitted to 15°C to 30°C (59°F to 86°F).

Mechanism of Action Basal cell cancer is associated with mutations in Hedgehog pathway components. Hedgehog regulates cell growth and differentiation in embryogenesis; while generally not active in adult tissue, Hedgehog mutations associated with basal cell cancer can activate the pathway resulting in unrestricted proliferation of skin basal cells. Vismodegib is a selective Hedgehog pathway inhibitor which binds to and inhibits Smoothened homologue (SMO), the transmembrane protein involved in Hedgehog signal transduction.

Pharmacodynamics/Kinetics

Distribution: V_d: 16.4 to 26.6 L

Protein binding: >99%; primarily to serum albumin and $alpha_1$ acid glycoprotein (AAG)

Metabolism: Metabolized by oxidation, glucuronidation, and pyridine ring cleavage, although >98% of circulating components are as the parent drug

Bioavailability: ~32%

Half-life, elimination: Continuous daily dosing: ~4 days; Single dose: ~12 days

Time to peak: ~2.4 days (Graham, 2011)

Excretion: Feces (82%); urine (4%)

Dosage Note: Vismodegib is associated with a moderate emetic potential; antiemetics may be needed to prevent nausea and vomiting.

Basal cell cancer, metastatic or locally advanced: Adults: Oral: 150 mg once daily until disease progression or unacceptable toxicity. In clinical trials, treatment interruptions up to 4 weeks were allowed for toxicity recovery (Sekulik, 2012).

Missed doses: If a dose is missed, do not make up; resume dosing with the next scheduled dose.

Dosage adjustment in renal impairment: There are no dosage adjustments provided in manufacturer's labeling (has not been studied).

Dosage adjustment in hepatic impairment: There are no dosage adjustments provided in manufacturer's labeling (has not been studied).

Dietary Considerations May be taken without regard to food.

Administration Oral: May be taken with or without food. Swallow capsules whole; do not open or crush. Vismodegib is associated with a moderate emetic potential; antiemetics may be needed to prevent nausea and vomiting. Hazardous agent; use appropriate precautions for handling and disposal (meets NIOSH 2014 criteria).

Monitoring Parameters Pregnancy test within 1 week prior to treatment initiation.

Canadian labeling: Pregnancy testing (minimum sensitivity of 25 mIU/mL) within 1 week prior to treatment initiation, monthly during treatment (including during treatment interruptions), and for 24 months after discontinuation; CBC with differential and comprehensive metabolic panel at baseline and every 4 weeks thereafter; skin examination routinely during therapy.

Additional Information In a study of vismodegib in patients with basal cell nevus syndrome (not an approved use), with discontinuation of vismodegib treatment, taste alteration and muscle cramps abated within 1 month, and scalp and body hair began to regrow within 3 months (Tang, 2012).

Dosage Forms

Capsule, Oral:

Erivedge: 150 mg

◆ **Vistaril** *see* HydrOXYzine *on page 1024*

◆ **Vistide** *see* Cidofovir *on page 433*

◆ **Vistonuridine** *see* Uridine Triacetate *on page 2116*

◆ **VIT 45** *see* Ferric Carboxymaltose *on page 868*

◆ **Vita-C [OTC]** *see* Ascorbic Acid *on page 178*

◆ **Vitamin C** *see* Ascorbic Acid *on page 178*

◆ **Vitamin D_3 and Alendronate** *see* Alendronate and Cholecalciferol *on page 81*

◆ **Vitamin D and Calcium Carbonate** *see* Calcium and Vitamin D *on page 326*

Vitamin A (VYE ta min aye)

Brand Names: U.S. A-25 [OTC]; AFirm 1X [OTC]; AFirm 2X [OTC]; AFirm 3X [OTC]; Aquasol A; Gordons-Vite A [OTC]; Vitamin A Fish [OTC]

Index Terms Oleovitamin A

Pharmacologic Category Vitamin, Fat Soluble

Use Treatment and prevention of vitamin A deficiency; parenteral (IM) route is indicated when oral administration is not feasible or when absorption is insufficient (malabsorption syndrome); dietary supplement (OTC)

Pregnancy Risk Factor X

Dosage

Oral:

Dietary Reference Intake for vitamin A (presented as retinol activity equivalent [RAE]) (IOM, 2000):

Adequate intake (AI):

1-6 months: 400 mcg/day (1330 units/day)

7-12 months: 500 mcg/day (1670 units/day)

Recommended dietary allowance (RDA):

1-3 years: 300 mcg/day (1000 units/day)

4-8 years: 400 mcg/day (1330 units/day)

9-13 years: 600 mcg/day (2000 units/day)

Males >13 years: 900 mcg/day (3000 units/day)

Females >13 years: 700 mcg/day (2330 units/day)

Pregnant females:

14-18 years: 750 mcg/day (2500 units/day)

≥19 years: 770 mcg/day (2560 units/day)

Lactating females:

14-18 years: 1200 mcg/day (4000 units/day)

≥19 years: 1300 mcg/day (4330 units/day)

Treatment of measles (off-label use) (WHO, 2004; WHO, 2010): **Note:** Repeat with single dose in 2-4 weeks if severe malnutrition exists or ophthalmic evidence of a vitamin deficiency is present:

Infants <6 months: 50,000 units once daily for 2 days

Infants 6-11 months: 100,000 units once daily for 2 days

Children >11 months to 5 years: 200,000 units once daily for 2 days

Treatment of xerophthalmia (off-label use):

Infants <6 months: 50,000 units once daily for 2 days; repeat with single dose after 2 weeks (WHO, 2010)

Infants 6-12 months: 100,000 units once daily for 2 days; repeat with single dose after 2 weeks (WHO, 2010)

Children >1 year and Adults (except females of reproductive age): 200,000 units once daily for 2 days; repeat with single dose after 2 weeks (WHO, 2008)

Females of reproductive age (WHO, 1997; WHO, 2008):

With night blindness or Bitot's spots (less severe xerophthalmia): 5000-10,000 units daily (maximum 10,000 units/day) or ≤25,000 units once weekly for ≥4 weeks

Severe xerophthalmia: Refer to adult dosing.

High-dose supplementation in patients at high risk for deficiency (off-label dose) (eg, persons living in developing areas of the world where deficiency is a public health problem, especially persons with severe infectious disease or malnutrition):

Infants <6 months: Not recommended (WHO, 2011a)

Infants 6-12 months: 100,000 units/dose; repeat every 4-6 months, but do not readminister within 30 days of previous dose (WHO, 1997; WHO, 2010)

Children >1 year: 200,000 units/dose; repeat every 4-6 months, but do not readminister within 30 days of previous dose (WHO, 1997; WHO, 2010)

Adults: 200,000 units/dose every 6 months (WHO, 2008)

Pregnant females: Maximum: 10,000 units daily or 25,000 units once weekly. Administer for a minimum of 12 weeks during pregnancy or until delivery (WHO, 2008; WHO, 2011c)

Postpartum females: 200,000 units at delivery or within 8 weeks of delivery (WHO, 2008)

IM: **Deficiency (manufacturer recommendation): Note:** IM route is indicated when oral administration is not feasible or when absorption is insufficient (malabsorption syndrome):

Infants: 7500-15,000 units/day for 10 days

Children 1-8 years: 17,500-35,000 units/day for 10 days

Children >8 years and Adults: 100,000 units/day for 3 days, followed by 50,000 units/day for 2 weeks

Note: Follow-up therapy with an oral therapeutic multivitamin (containing additional vitamin A) is recommended: Oral:

Low Birth Weight Infants: Additional vitamin A is recommended; however, no dosage amount has been established.

Children ≤8 years: 5000-10,000 units/day for 2 months

Children >8 years and Adults: 10,000-20,000 units/day for 2 months

Additional Information Complete prescribing information should be consulted for additional detail.

Dosage Forms

Capsule, Oral:
A-25 [OTC]: 25,000 units
Vitamin A Fish [OTC]: 7500 units
Generic: 10,000 units

Capsule, Oral [preservative free]:
A-25 [OTC]: 25,000 units
Generic: 8000 units

Cream, External:
AFirm 1X [OTC]: 0.15% (30 g)
AFirm 2X [OTC]: 0.3% (30 g)
AFirm 3X [OTC]: 0.6% (30 g)
Gordons-Vite A [OTC]: 100,000 units/g (75 g, 120 g, 480 g, 2400 g)

Lotion, External:
Gordons-Vite A [OTC]: 100,000 units (120 mL, 4000 mL)

Solution, Intramuscular:
Aquasol A: 50,000 units/mL (2 mL)

Tablet, Oral:
Generic: 10,000 units, 15,000 units, Vitamin A 10000 units and beta carotene 1000 units

◆ **Vitamin A Acid** *see* Tretinoin (Topical) *on page* 2099

Vitamin A and Vitamin D (Systemic)

(VYE ta min aye & VYE ta min dee)

Brand Names: U.S. A&D Jr. [OTC]; D-Natural-5 [OTC]

Index Terms Cod Liver Oil

Pharmacologic Category Vitamin, Fat Soluble

Use Dietary supplement

Dosage Oral: Adults: Dietary supplement: One tablet or capsule once daily.

Additional Information Complete prescribing information should be consulted for additional detail.

Dosage Forms

Capsule, softgel, oral: Vitamin A 1250 units and vitamin D 130 units, Vitamin A 1250 units and vitamin D 135 units, Vitamin A 5,000 units and vitamin D 400 units, Vitamin A 10,000 units and vitamin D 400 units, Vitamin A 25,000 units and vitamin D 1000 units
A&D Jr. [OTC]: Vitamin A 10,000 units and vitamin D 400 units
D-Natural-5 [OTC]: Vitamin A 10,000 units and vitamin D 5000 units

Oil, oral: Vitamin A 5000 units and vitamin D 500 units per 5 mL (120 mL, 473 mL)

Tablet, oral: Vitamin A 10,000 units and vitamin D 400 units

Vitamin A and Vitamin D (Topical)

(VYE ta min aye & VYE ta min dee)

Brand Names: U.S. A+D® Original [OTC]; Baza® Clear [OTC]; Sween Cream® [OTC]

Index Terms Cod Liver Oil

Pharmacologic Category Topical Skin Product

Use Temporary relief of discomfort due to chapped skin or lips, cuts and scrapes, diaper rash, or minor burns

Dosage Topical: Children and Adults:
Diaper rash: Apply with each diaper change and any time prolonged exposure to wet diapers may occur (ie, at bedtime).
Skin protectant: Apply to affected areas as needed.

Additional Information Complete prescribing information should be consulted for additional detail.

Dosage Forms

Cream, topical:
Sween Cream® [OTC]: (2 g, 14 g, 57 g, 85 g, 142 g, 184 g, 339 g)

Ointment, topical: (0.9 g, 5 g, 60 g, 120 g, 454 g)
A+D® Original [OTC]: (42.5 g); (120 g); (454 g)
Baza® Clear [OTC]: (50 g, 142 g, 227 g)

◆ **Vitamin A Fish [OTC]** *see* Vitamin A *on page* 2173
◆ **Vitamin B_1** *see* Thiamine *on page* 2028
◆ **Vitamin B_2** *see* Riboflavin *on page* 1803
◆ **Vitamin B_3** *see* Niacin *on page* 1443
◆ **Vitamin B_3** *see* Niacinamide *on page* 1446
◆ **Vitamin B_6** *see* Pyridoxine *on page* 1747
◆ **Vitamin B_{12}** *see* Cyanocobalamin *on page* 515
◆ **Vitamin B_{12a}** *see* Hydroxocobalamin *on page* 1020
◆ **Vitamin D2** *see* Ergocalciferol *on page* 753

Vitamin E (VYE ta min ee)

Brand Names: U.S. Alph-E [OTC]; Alph-E-Mixed 1000 [OTC]; Alph-E-Mixed [OTC]; Aquasol E [OTC]; Aquavit-E [OTC]; Aqueous Vitamin E [OTC]; E-400 [OTC]; E-400-Clear [OTC]; E-400-Mixed [OTC]; E-Max-1000 [OTC]; E-Pherol [OTC]; Formula E 400 [OTC]; Gordons-Vite E [OTC]; Natural Vitamin E [OTC]; Nutr-E-Sol [OTC]; Vita-Plus E [OTC]; Vitamin E Beauty [OTC]; Vitec [OTC]; Xtra-Care [OTC]

Index Terms *d*-Alpha Tocopherol; *dl*-Alpha Tocopherol

Pharmacologic Category Vitamin, Fat Soluble

Use Dietary supplement

Note: According to the 2014 USPSTF recommendations for the primary prevention of cardiovascular disease and cancer, the use of vitamin E supplements are not recommended (Moyer, 2014).

Dosage Vitamin E may be expressed as alpha-tocopherol equivalents (ATE), which refer to the biologically-active (R) stereoisomer content.

Oral:

Adequate intake (AI) (IOM, 2000): Infants (RDA not established):
1-6 months: 4 mg
7-12 months: 5 mg

Recommended daily allowance (RDA) (IOM, 2000):
Children:
1-3 years: 6 mg; upper limit of intake should not exceed 200 mg/day
4-8 years: 7 mg; upper limit of intake should not exceed 300 mg/day
9-13 years: 11 mg; upper limit of intake should not exceed 600 mg/day
14-18 years: 15 mg; upper limit of intake should not exceed 800 mg/day
Adults: 15 mg; upper limit of intake should not exceed 1000 mg/day
Pregnant female:
≤18 years: 15 mg; upper level of intake should not exceed 800 mg/day
19-50 years: 15 mg; upper level of intake should not exceed 1000 mg/day
Lactating female:
≤18 years: 19 mg; upper level of intake should not exceed 800 mg/day
19-50 years: 19 mg; upper level of intake should not exceed 1000 mg/day

Vitamin E deficiency:
Children (with malabsorption syndrome): 1 unit/kg/day of water miscible vitamin E (to raise plasma tocopherol concentrations to the normal range within 2 months and to maintain normal plasma concentrations)
Adults: 60-75 units/day

Cystic fibrosis supplementation (Borowitz 2002): Infants and Children:
1-12 months: 40-50 units/day
1-3 years: 80-150 units/day
4-8 years: 100-200 units/day
>8 years: 200-400 units/day

Topical: Adults: Apply a thin layer over affected area

Additional Information Complete prescribing information should be consulted for additional detail.

Dosage Forms

Capsule, Oral:
Alph-E [OTC]: 400 units
Alph-E-Mixed [OTC]: 200 units, 400 units
Alph-E-Mixed 1000 [OTC]: 1000 units
Formula E 400 [OTC]: 400 units
Vita-Plus E [OTC]: 400 units
Generic: 100 units, 200 units, 400 units, 1000 units

Capsule, Oral [preservative free]:
E-400 [OTC]: 400 units
E-400-Clear [OTC]: 400 units
E-400-Mixed [OTC]: 400 units
E-Max-1000 [OTC]: 1000 units
Generic: 100 units, 400 units

Cream, External:
Gordons-Vite E [OTC]: 1500 units/30 g (15 g, 75 g, 480 g, 2400 g)
Generic: 1000 units (112 g)

Liquid, External:
Generic: 920 units/mL (28.5 mL, 57 mL, 114 mL)

Liquid, Oral:
Nutr-E-Sol [OTC]: 400 units/15 mL (473 mL)

Lotion, External:
Vitec [OTC]: (113 g)
Xtra-Care [OTC]: (2 mL, 59 mL, 118 mL, 237 mL, 621 mL, 1000 mL, 3840 mL)

Oil, External:
Vitamin E Beauty [OTC]: 24,000 units/52 mL (52 mL); 49,000 units/52 mL (52 mL)

Solution, Oral:
Aquasol E [OTC]: 15 units/0.3 mL (12 mL, 30 mL)
Aquavit-E [OTC]: 15 units/0.3 mL (30 mL)
Aqueous Vitamin E [OTC]: 15 units/0.3 mL (30 mL)
Generic: 15 units/0.3 mL (12 mL)

Tablet, Oral:
E-Pherol [OTC]: 400 units
Natural Vitamin E [OTC]: 200 units, 400 units
Generic: 100 units, 200 units, 400 units

- **Vitamin E Beauty [OTC]** *see* Vitamin E *on page 2174*
- **Vitamin G** *see* Riboflavin *on page 1803*
- **Vitamin K** *see* Phytonadione *on page 1647*
- **Vitamin K_1** *see* Phytonadione *on page 1647*
- **Vita-Plus E [OTC]** *see* Vitamin E *on page 2174*
- **Vita-Respa®** *see* Folic Acid, Cyanocobalamin, and Pyridoxine *on page 921*
- **Vitec [OTC]** *see* Vitamin E *on page 2174*
- **Vitekta** *see* Elvitegravir *on page 717*
- **Vitekta** *see* Elvitegravir *on page 717*
- **Vituz** *see* Hydrocodone and Chlorpheniramine *on page 1012*
- **Vi Vaccine** *see* Typhoid Vaccine *on page 2112*
- **Vivactil [DSC]** *see* Protriptyline *on page 1740*
- **Vivarin® [OTC]** *see* Caffeine *on page 319*
- **ViVAXIM® (Can)** *see* Typhoid and Hepatitis A Vaccine [CAN/INT] *on page 2111*
- **Vivelle-Dot** *see* Estradiol (Systemic) *on page 775*
- **Vivitrol** *see* Naltrexone *on page 1422*
- **Vivotif** *see* Typhoid Vaccine *on page 2112*
- **VLB** *see* VinBLAStine *on page 2160*
- **VM-26** *see* Teniposide *on page 1997*
- **Vogelxo** *see* Testosterone *on page 2010*
- **Vogelxo Pump** *see* Testosterone *on page 2010*
- **Volibris (Can)** *see* Ambrisentan *on page 107*
- **Voltaren** *see* Diclofenac (Systemic) *on page 617*
- **Voltaren Ophtha (Can)** *see* Diclofenac (Ophthalmic) *on page 621*
- **Voltaren Rapide (Can)** *see* Diclofenac (Systemic) *on page 617*
- **Voltaren SR (Can)** *see* Diclofenac (Systemic) *on page 617*
- **Voltaren-XR** *see* Diclofenac (Systemic) *on page 617*
- **Volulyte (Can)** *see* Tetrastarch *on page 2019*
- **Voluven** *see* Tetrastarch *on page 2019*
- **von Willebrand Factor/Factor VIII Complex** *see* Antihemophilic Factor/von Willebrand Factor Complex (Human) *on page 154*

Vorapaxar (vor a PAX ar)

Brand Names: U.S. Zontivity

Index Terms SCH530348; Vorapaxar Sulfate

Pharmacologic Category Antiplatelet Agent; Protease-Activated Receptor-1 (PAR-1) Antagonist

Use History of myocardial infarction or established peripheral arterial disease: To reduce thrombotic cardiovascular events (cardiovascular death, MI, stroke, urgent coronary revascularization) in patients with a history of myocardial infarction (MI) or with peripheral arterial disease (PAD)

Pregnancy Risk Factor B

Pregnancy Considerations Adverse events have not been observed in animal reproduction studies.

Breast-Feeding Considerations It is not known if vorapaxar is excreted in breast milk. Breast-feeding is not recommended by the manufacturer.

Contraindications History of stroke, transient ischemic attack (TIA), or intracranial hemorrhage (ICH); active pathological bleeding (eg, ICH, peptic ulcer bleeding)

Warnings/Precautions [U.S. Boxed Warning]: Use is contraindicated in patients with history of stroke, TIA, or ICH; or active pathological bleeding. Vorapaxar increases the risk of bleeding, including ICH and fatal bleeding. The risk of bleeding is proportional to the patient's underlying bleeding risk. General risk factors for bleeding include older age, low body weight, reduced renal or hepatic function, history of bleeding disorders, and concomitant use of medications known to increase the risk of bleeding (eg, anticoagulants, NSAIDS, selective serotonin reuptake inhibitors [SSRIs], serotonin norepinephrine reuptake inhibitors [SNRIs]); avoid use with warfarin or other anticoagulants. **Note:** No specific antidote exists for vorapaxar reversal. Significant inhibition of platelet aggregation remains 4 weeks after discontinuation.

Due to increased risk of bleeding, use is not recommended in patients with severe hepatic impairment; use with caution in patients with mild or moderate hepatic impairment and in patients with renal impairment. Potentially significant interactions may exist, requiring dose or frequency adjustment, additional monitoring, and/or selection of alternative therapy.

Adverse Reactions
Central nervous system: Depression
Dermatologic: Skin rash (includes cutaneous eruptions and exanthemas)
Endocrine & metabolic: Iron deficiency
Gastrointestinal: Gastrointestinal hemorrhage

Hematologic and oncologic: Anemia; hemorrhage; major hemorrhage (includes GUSTO [Global Utilization of Streptokinase and Tissue Plasminogen Activator for Occluded Arteries] bleeding categories "moderate or severe" and "severe"); major hemorrhage, life-threatening (clinically significant bleeding, including any bleeding requiring medical attention such as intracranial hemorrhage, or clinically significant overt signs of hemorrhage associated with a drop in hemoglobin of ≥3 g/dL [or when hemoglobin is unavailable, an absolute drop in hematocrit of ≥15% or a fall in hematocrit of 9% to <15%])

Ophthalmic: Retinopathy

Rare but important or life-threatening: Hemorrhagic death, intracranial hemorrhage

Drug Interactions

Metabolism/Transport Effects Substrate of CYP2J2 (minor), CYP3A4 (minor); **Note:** Assignment of Major/Minor substrate status based on clinically relevant drug interaction potential; **Inhibits** P-glycoprotein

Avoid Concomitant Use

Avoid concomitant use of Vorapaxar with any of the following: Anticoagulants; CYP3A4 Inducers (Strong); CYP3A4 Inhibitors (Strong); St Johns Wort; Urokinase

Increased Effect/Toxicity

Vorapaxar may increase the levels/effects of: Agents with Antiplatelet Properties; Anticoagulants; Collagenase (Systemic); Ibritumomab; Obinutuzumab; Salicylates; Thrombolytic Agents; Tositumomab and Iodine I 131 Tositumomab; Urokinase

The levels/effects of Vorapaxar may be increased by: CYP3A4 Inhibitors (Strong); Dasatinib; Glucosamine; Herbs (Anticoagulant/Antiplatelet Properties); Ibrutinib; Limaprost; Multivitamins/Fluoride (with ADE); Multivitamins/Minerals (with ADEK, Folate, Iron); Multivitamins/Minerals (with AE, No Iron); Omega-3 Fatty Acids; Pentosan Polysulfate Sodium; Pentoxifylline; Prostacyclin Analogues; Tipranavir; Vitamin E

Decreased Effect

The levels/effects of Vorapaxar may be decreased by: CYP3A4 Inducers (Strong); St Johns Wort

Storage/Stability Store at 20°C to 25°C (68°F to 77°F); excursions are permitted between 15°C and 30°C (59°F and 86°F). Store in the original package; protect from moisture. Keep the desiccant in the bottle.

Mechanism of Action Vorapaxar, a reversible antagonist of the protease-activated receptor-1 (PAR-1) expressed on platelets, inhibits thrombin-induced and thrombin receptor agonist peptide (TRAP)-induced platelet aggregation. Due to the very long half-life, vorapaxar is effectively irreversible.

Pharmacodynamics/Kinetics

Onset of action: ≥80% inhibition of TRAP-induced platelet aggregation within 1 week

Duration: Dose and concentration dependent; with the recommended dosing, inhibition of TRAP-induced platelet aggregation at a level of 50% can be expected 4 weeks after discontinuation

Absorption: Rapidly absorbed (Kosoglou, 2012)

Distribution: ~424 L

Protein binding: ≥99% to albumin

Metabolism: Hepatic via CYP3A4 and CYP2J2. Major active metabolite: M20 (accounts for ~20% of exposure to vorapaxar)

Bioavailability: ~100%

Half-life elimination: Effective half-life: 3 to 4 days; Terminal elimination half-life (vorapaxar and active metabolite): ~8 days (range: 5 to 13 days)

Time to peak: 1 to 2 hours

Excretion: Primarily in the form of metabolites through feces (58%); urine (25%)

Dosage History of myocardial infarction (MI) or established peripheral arterial disease (PAD): Adults: Oral: 2.08 mg once daily in combination with aspirin and/or clopidogrel. **Note:** No experience with use of vorapaxar as monotherapy or with antiplatelet agents other than aspirin and clopidogrel.

Dosage adjustment in renal impairment: No dosage adjustment necessary.

Dosage adjustment in hepatic impairment:

Mild to moderate impairment: No dosage adjustment necessary.

Severe impairment: Use is not recommended.

Administration Administer with or without food.

Monitoring Parameters Signs of bleeding; hemoglobin and hematocrit periodically

Dosage Forms

Tablet, Oral:

Zontivity: 2.08 mg

◆ **Vorapaxar Sulfate** *see* Vorapaxar *on page* 2175

◆ **Voraxaze** *see* Glucarpidase *on page* 971

Voriconazole (vor i KOE na zole)

Brand Names: U.S. Vfend; Vfend IV

Brand Names: Canada Apo-Voriconazole; Sandoz-Voriconazole; Teva-Voriconazole; VFEND; VFEND For Injection; Voriconazole For Injection

Index Terms UK109496

Pharmacologic Category Antifungal Agent, Oral; Antifungal Agent, Parenteral

Use Treatment of fungal infections: Treatment of invasive aspergillosis; treatment of esophageal candidiasis; treatment of candidemia (in non-neutropenic patients); treatment of disseminated *Candida* infections of the skin and abdomen, kidney, bladder wall and wounds; treatment of serious fungal infections caused by *Scedosporium apiospermum* and *Fusarium* spp (including *Fusarium solani*) in patients intolerant of, or refractory to, other therapy in children >12 years of age, adolescents and adults

Pregnancy Risk Factor D

Pregnancy Considerations Voriconazole can cause fetal harm when administered to a pregnant woman. Voriconazole was teratogenic and embryotoxic in animal studies, and lowered plasma estradiol in animal models. Women of childbearing potential should use effective contraception during treatment. Should be used in pregnant woman only if benefit to mother justifies potential risk to the fetus.

Breast-Feeding Considerations It is not known if voriconazole is excreted in breast milk. Due to the potential for serious adverse reactions in the nursing infant, the manufacturer recommends a decision be made whether to discontinue nursing or to discontinue the drug, taking into account the importance of treatment to the mother.

Contraindications Hypersensitivity to voriconazole or any component of the formulation; coadministration with astemizole, barbiturates (long acting), carbamazepine, cisapride, efavirenz (≥400 mg daily), ergot derivatives (ergotamine and dihydroergotamine), pimozide, quinidine, rifampin, rifabutin, ritonavir (≥800 mg daily), sirolimus, St John's wort, terfenadine

Documentation of allergenic cross-reactivity for imidazole antifungals is limited. However, because of similarities in chemical structure and/or pharmacologic actions, the possibility of cross-sensitivity cannot be ruled out with certainty.

Warnings/Precautions Hazardous agent - use appropriate precautions for handling and disposal (NIOSH 2014 [group 3]).

Visual changes, including blurred vision, changes in visual acuity, color perception, and photophobia, are commonly associated with treatment; postmarketing cases of optic neuritis and papilledema (lasting >1 month) have also been reported. Patients should be warned to avoid tasks which depend on vision, including operating machinery or driving. Changes are reversible on discontinuation following brief exposure/treatment regimens (≤28 days).

Serious (and rarely fatal) hepatic reactions (eg, hepatitis, cholestasis, fulminant failure) have been observed with voriconazole. In lung transplant recipients, median time to hepatic toxicity was 14 days with the majority occurring within 30 days of therapy initiation (Luong, 2012). Use with caution in patients with serious underlying medical conditions (eg, hematologic malignancy); hepatic reactions have occurred in patients with no identifiable underlying risk factors. Liver dysfunction is usually reversible upon therapy discontinuation. Monitor liver function and bilirubin at baseline and periodically during therapy. If elevations occur, evaluate further for severe hepatic injury; discontinuation may be warranted.

Voriconazole tablets contain lactose; avoid administration in hereditary galactose intolerance, Lapp lactase deficiency, or glucose-galactose malabsorption. Suspension contains sucrose; use caution with fructose intolerance, sucrase-isomaltase deficiency, or glucose-galactose malabsorption. Avoid/limit use of intravenous formulation in patients with moderate to severe renal impairment (CrCl <50 mL/minute); injection contains excipient cyclodextrin (sulfobutyl ether beta-cyclodextrin [SBECD]), which may accumulate, although the clinical significance of this finding is uncertain (Luke, 2010); consider using oral voriconazole in these patients unless benefit of injection outweighs the risk. If injection is used in patients CrCl <50 mL/minute, monitor serum creatinine closely; if increases occur, consider changing therapy to oral voriconazole.

Anaphylactoid-type reactions (eg, flushing, fever, sweating, tachycardia, chest tightness, dyspnea, nausea, pruritus, rash) may occur with IV infusion. Consider discontinuation of infusion should these reactions occur. Acute renal failure has been observed in severely ill patients; use with caution in patients receiving concomitant nephrotoxic medications. Evaluate renal function (particularly serum creatinine) at baseline and periodically during therapy.

Potentially significant drug-drug interactions may exist, requiring dose or frequency adjustment, additional monitoring, and/or selection of alternative therapy. QT interval prolongation has been associated with voriconazole use; rare cases of arrhythmia (including torsade de pointes), cardiac arrest, and sudden death have been reported, usually in seriously ill patients with comorbidities and/or risk factors (eg, prior cardiotoxic chemotherapy, cardiomyopathy, electrolyte imbalance, or concomitant QTc-prolonging drugs). Use with caution in these patient populations; correct electrolyte abnormalities (eg, hypokalemia, hypomagnesemia, hypocalcemia) prior to initiating therapy. Do not infuse concomitantly with blood products or short-term concentrated electrolyte solutions, even if the two infusions are running in separate intravenous lines (or cannulas).

Rare cases of malignancy (melanoma, squamous cell carcinoma [SCC]) have been reported in patients with prior onset of severe photosensitivity reactions or exposure to standard dose long-term voriconazole therapy (in lung transplant recipients, SCC increased by ~6% per 60 days with a 28% absolute risk increase at 5 years [Singer, 2012]). Other serious exfoliative cutaneous reactions, including Stevens-Johnson syndrome, have also been reported. Patient should avoid intense or prolonged exposure to direct sunlight; may cause photosensitivity, especially with long-term use. Discontinue use in patients who develop an exfoliative cutaneous reaction or a skin lesion consistent with squamous cell carcinoma or melanoma. Periodic total body skin examinations should be performed, particularly with prolonged use. Fluorosis and/or periostitis may occur during long-term therapy. If patient develops skeletal pain and radiologic findings of fluorosis or periostitis, discontinue therapy.

Voriconazole demonstrates nonlinear pharmacokinetics. Dose modifications may result in unpredictable changes in serum concentrations and contribute to toxicity. It is important to note that cutoff trough threshold values ranged widely among studies; however, an upper limit of <5.0 mg/L would be reasonable for most disease states (see CDC recommendations for *Exserohilum rostratum* in Reference Range section) (CDC, 2012). In patients >14 years of age or 12-14 years and weighing >50 kg, data suggest that pharmacokinetics are similar to adults (Friberg, 2012). In patients <12 years of age, the full pharmacokinetic profile for voriconazole is not completely defined, and for patients <2 years, the data are sparse. In children 2 to <12 years, current data suggests voriconazole undergoes a high degree of variability in exposure with linear elimination at lower doses and nonlinear elimination at higher doses; therefore, to achieve similar AUC as adults, increased dosage is necessary in children (Friberg, 2012; Karlsson, 2009; Walsh, 2010).

Correct electrolyte abnormalities (eg, hypokalemia, hypomagnesemia, hypocalcemia) prior to initiating therapy. Monitor pancreatic function in patients (children and adults) at risk for acute pancreatitis (eg, recent chemotherapy or hematopoietic stem cell transplantation). Pancreatitis has occurred in pediatric patients.

Benzyl alcohol and derivatives: Some dosage forms may contain sodium benzoate/benzoic acid; benzoic acid (benzoate) is a metabolite of benzyl alcohol; large amounts of benzyl alcohol (≥99 mg/kg/day) have been associated with a potentially fatal toxicity ("gasping syndrome") in neonates; the "gasping syndrome" consists of metabolic acidosis, respiratory distress, gasping respirations, CNS dysfunction (including convulsions, intracranial hemorrhage), hypotension, and cardiovascular collapse (AAP, 1997; CDC, 1982); some data suggests that benzoate displaces bilirubin from protein binding sites (Ahlfors, 2001); avoid or use dosage forms containing benzyl alcohol derivative with caution in neonates. See manufacturer's labeling.

Adverse Reactions

Cardiovascular: Tachycardia

Central nervous system: Chills, hallucinations, headache

Dermatologic: Skin rash

Endocrine & metabolic: Hypokalemia

Gastrointestinal: Nausea, vomiting

Hepatic: Cholestatic jaundice, increased serum alkaline phosphatase, increased serum ALT, increased serum AST

Ophthalmic: Photophobia, visual disturbance

Renal: Increased serum creatinine

Miscellaneous: Fever

Rare but important or life-threatening: Acute renal failure, adrenocortical insufficiency, agranulocytosis, alopecia, anaphylactoid reaction, anemia (aplastic, hemolytic, macrocytic, megaloblastic, or microcytic), angioedema, anorexia, anuria, arthritis, ascites, ataxia, atrial arrhythmia, atrial fibrillation, atrioventricular block, bacterial infection, bigeminy, blighted ovum, bone marrow depression, bradycardia, brain disease, bundle branch block, cardiac arrest, cardiac failure, cardiomegaly, cardiomyopathy, cellulitis, cerebral edema, cerebral hemorrhage, cerebral ischemia, cerebrovascular accident, chest pain, cholecystitis, cholelithiasis, cholestasis, chromatopsia, color blindness, coma, confusion, convulsions, corneal opacity, cyanosis, deafness, deep vein thrombophlebitis, deep vein thrombosis, delirium, dementia, dental fluorosis, depersonalization, depression, diabetes insipidus, diarrhea, discoid lupus erythematosus, disseminated intravascular coagulation, drowsiness, duodenal ulcer (active), duodenitis, dyspnea, eczema, edema, encephalitis, endocarditis, eosinophilia, erythema multiforme, esophageal ulcer, exfoliative dermatitis, extrapyramidal reaction, extrasystoles, fixed drug eruption, fungal infection, gastric ulcer, gastrointestinal hemorrhage, glucose tolerance decreased, graft versus host disease, Guillain-Barre syndrome, hematemesis, hemorrhagic cystitis, hepatic coma, hepatic failure, hepatitis, hepatomegaly, herpes simplex infection, hydronephrosis, hyperbilirubinemia, hypercholesterolemia, hyper-/hypocalcemia, hyper-/hypoglycemia, hyper-/hypomagnesemia, hyper-/hyponatremia, hyper-/hypotension, hyper-/hypothyroidism, hyperkalemia, hypersensitivity reaction, hyperuricemia, hypophosphatemia, hypoxia, impotence, increased blood urea nitrogen, increased gamma-glutamyl transferase, increased lactate dehydrogenase, increased susceptibility to infection, intestinal perforation, intracranial hypertension, jaundice, leukopenia, lymphadenopathy, lymphangitis, maculopapular rash, malignant melanoma, melanosis, multi-organ failure, myasthenia, myocardial infarction, myopathy, nephritis, nephrosis, neuropathy, nocturnal amblyopia, nodal arrhythmia, nodule, nystagmus, oculogyric crisis, optic atrophy, optic neuritis, orthostatic hypotension, osteomalacia, osteonecrosis, osteoporosis, otitis externa, palpitations, pancreatitis, pancytopenia, papilledema, paresthesia, perforated duodenal ulcer, periosteal disease, peripheral edema, peritonitis, petechia, pleural effusion, pneumonia, prolonged bleeding time, prolonged QT interval on ECG, pruritus, pseudomembranous colitis, pseudoporphyria, psoriasis, psychosis, pulmonary edema, pulmonary embolism, purpura, rectal hemorrhage, renal insufficiency, renal tubular necrosis, respiratory distress syndrome, respiratory tract infection, retinal hemorrhage, retinitis, seizure, sepsis, skin discoloration, skin photosensitivity, splenomegaly, squamous cell carcinoma, Stevens-Johnson syndrome, subconjunctival hemorrhage, substernal pain, suicidal ideation, supraventricular extrasystole, supraventricular tachycardia, syncope, thrombocytopenia, thrombophlebitis, thrombotic thrombocytopenic purpura, tongue edema, tonic-clonic seizures, torsades de pointes, toxic epidermal necrolysis, uremia, urinary incontinence, urinary retention, urinary tract infection, urticaria, uterine hemorrhage, uveitis, vaginal hemorrhage, vasodilation, ventricular arrhythmia, ventricular fibrillation, ventricular tachycardia, visual field defect

Drug Interactions

Metabolism/Transport Effects Substrate of CYP2C19 (major), CYP2C9 (major), CYP3A4 (minor); **Note:** Assignment of Major/Minor substrate status based on clinically relevant drug interaction potential; **Inhibits** CYP2C19 (moderate), CYP2C9 (moderate), CYP3A4 (strong)

Avoid Concomitant Use

Avoid concomitant use of Voriconazole with any of the following: Ado-Trastuzumab Emtansine; Alfuzosin; Apixaban; Astemizole; Atazanavir; Avanafil; Axitinib; Barbiturates; Bosutinib; Cabozantinib; CarBAMazepine; Ceritinib; Cisapride; Conivaptan; Crizotinib; Dapoxetine; Darunavir; Dihydroergotamine; Dofetilide; Dronedarone; Eletriptan; Eplerenone; Ergoloid Mesylates; Ergonovine; Ergotamine; Everolimus; Fluconazole; Halofantrine; Highest Risk QTc-Prolonging Agents; Ibrutinib; Irinotecan; Ivabradine; Lapatinib; Lercanidipine; Lomitapide; Lopinavir; Lovastatin; Lurasidone; Macitentan; Methylergonovine; Mifepristone; Naloxegol; Nilotinib; Nisoldipine; Olaparib; Pimozide; QuiNIDine; Ranolazine; Red Yeast Rice; Regorafenib; Rifamycin Derivatives; Ritonavir; Rivaroxaban; Saccharomyces boulardii; Salmeterol; Silodosin; Simeprevir; Simvastatin; Sirolimus; St Johns Wort; Suvorexant; Tamsulosin; Terfenadine; Ticagrelor; Tolvaptan; Toremifene; Trabectedin; Ulipristal; Vemurafenib; VinCRIStine (Liposomal); Vorapaxar

Increased Effect/Toxicity

Voriconazole may increase the levels/effects of: Ado-Trastuzumab Emtansine; Alfuzosin; Almotriptan; Alosetron; Antineoplastic Agents (Vinca Alkaloids); Apixaban; ARIPiprazole; Astemizole; AtorvaSTATin; Avanafil; Axitinib; Bedaquiline; Boceprevir; Bortezomib; Bosentan; Bosutinib; Brentuximab Vedotin; Brinzolamide; Budesonide (Nasal); Budesonide (Systemic, Oral Inhalation); BusPIRone; Busulfan; Cabazitaxel; Cabozantinib; Calcium Channel Blockers; Cannabis; Carvedilol; Ceritinib; Cilostazol; Cisapride; Cobicistat; Colchicine; Conivaptan; Contraceptives (Estrogens); Contraceptives (Progestins); Corticosteroids (Orally Inhaled); Corticosteroids (Systemic); Crizotinib; CycloSPORINE (Systemic); CYP2C19 Substrates; CYP2C9 Substrates; CYP3A4 Substrates; Dapoxetine; Dasatinib; Diclofenac (Systemic); Diclofenac (Topical); Dienogest; Dihydroergotamine; DOCEtaxel; Dofetilide; DOXOrubicin (Conventional); Dronabinol; Dronedarone; Dutasteride; Efavirenz; Eletriptan; Elvitegravir; Enzalutamide; Eplerenone; Ergoloid Mesylates; Ergonovine; Ergotamine; Erlotinib; Etizolam; Etravirine; Everolimus; FentaNYL; Fesoterodine; Fluticasone (Nasal); Fluticasone (Oral Inhalation); Fosamprenavir; Fosphenytoin; GuanFACINE; Halofantrine; Highest Risk QTc-Prolonging Agents; Hydrocodone; Ibrutinib; Ibuprofen; Idelalisib; Imatinib; Imidafenacin; Irinotecan; Ivabradine; Ivacaftor; Ixabepilone; Lacosamide; Lapatinib; Lercanidipine; Levobupivacaine; Levomilnacipran; Lomitapide; Losartan; Lovastatin; Lurasidone; Macitentan; Macrolide Antibiotics; Maraviroc; Meloxicam; Methadone; Methylergonovine; MethylPREDNISolone; Moderate Risk QTc-Prolonging Agents; Naloxegol; Nelfinavir; Nilotinib; Nisoldipine; Olaparib; Ospemifene; OxyCODONE; Paricalcitol; PAZOPanib; Phenytoin; Pimecrolimus; Pimozide; PONATinib; Porfimer; Pranlukast; PrednisoLONE (Systemic); PredniSONE; Proton Pump Inhibitors; QuiNIDine; Ranolazine; Red Yeast Rice; Regorafenib; Repaglinide; Retapamulin; Reverse Transcriptase Inhibitors (Non-Nucleoside); Rifamycin Derivatives; Rilpivirine; Rivaroxaban; Ruxolitinib; Salmeterol; Saxagliptin; Sildenafil; Silodosin; Simeprevir; Simvastatin; Sirolimus; Solifenacin; Sulfonylureas; SUNItinib; Suvorexant; Tacrolimus (Systemic); Tacrolimus (Topical); Tadalafil; Tamsulosin; Telaprevir; Terfenadine; Tetrahydrocannabinol; Ticagrelor; Tofacitinib; Tolterodine; Tolvaptan; Toremifene; Trabectedin; Ulipristal; Vardenafil; Vemurafenib; Venlafaxine; Verteporfin; Vilazodone; VinCRIStine (Liposomal); Vitamin K Antagonists; Vorapaxar; Zolpidem; Zopiclone

The levels/effects of Voriconazole may be increased by: Atazanavir; Boceprevir; Chloramphenicol; Cobicistat; Contraceptives (Estrogens); Contraceptives (Progestins); CYP2C19 Inhibitors (Moderate); CYP2C19 Inhibitors (Strong); CYP2C9 Inhibitors (Moderate); CYP2C9 Inhibitors (Strong); Etravirine; Fluconazole; Fosamprenavir; Ivabradine; Luliconazole; Macrolide Antibiotics; Mifepristone; Proton Pump Inhibitors; QTc-Prolonging Agents (Indeterminate Risk and Risk Modifying); Telaprevir

Decreased Effect

Voriconazole may decrease the levels/effects of: Amphotericin B; Atazanavir; Clopidogrel; Ifosfamide; Prasugrel; Saccharomyces boulardii; Ticagrelor

The levels/effects of Voriconazole may be decreased by: Atazanavir; Barbiturates; CarBAMazepine; CYP2C19 Inducers (Strong); CYP2C9 Inducers (Strong);

Dabrafenib; Darunavir; Didanosine; Efavirenz; Etravirine; Fosphenytoin; Lopinavir; Phenytoin; Reverse Transcriptase Inhibitors (Non-Nucleoside); Rifamycin Derivatives; Ritonavir; St Johns Wort; Sucralfate; Telaprevir

Food Interactions Food may decrease voriconazole absorption. Management: Oral voriconazole should be taken 1 hour before or 1 hour after a meal. Maintain adequate hydration unless instructed to restrict fluid intake.

Preparation for Administration

Powder for injection: Reconstitute 200 mg vial with 19 mL of sterile water for injection (use of automated syringe is not recommended). Resultant solution (20 mL) has a concentration of 10 mg/mL. Prior to infusion, must dilute to <5 mg/mL with NS, LR, D_5WLR, $D_5W^1/_2$NS, D_5W, D_5W with KCl 20 mEq, $^1/_2$NS, or D_5WNS. Do not dilute with 4.2% sodium bicarbonate infusion.

Powder for oral suspension: Add 46 mL of water to the bottle to make 40 mg/mL suspension. Shake vigorously for ~1 minute. Do not refrigerate or freeze.

Hazardous agent - use appropriate precautions for handling and disposal (NIOSH 2014 [group 3]).

Storage/Stability

Powder for injection: Store vials between 15°C to 30°C (59°F to 86°F). Reconstituted solutions are stable for up to 24 hours under refrigeration at 2°C to 8°C (36°F to 46°F).

Powder for oral suspension: Store at 2°C to 8°C (36°F to 46°F). Reconstituted oral suspension is stable for up to 14 days if stored at 15°C to 30°C (59°F to 86°F). Do not refrigerate or freeze.

Tablets: Store at 15°C to 30°C (59°F to 86°F).

Mechanism of Action Interferes with fungal cytochrome P450 activity (selectively inhibits 14-alpha-lanosterol demethylation), decreasing ergosterol synthesis (principal sterol in fungal cell membrane) and inhibiting fungal cell membrane formation.

Pharmacodynamics/Kinetics

Absorption: Well absorbed after oral administration; multiple doses administered with high-fat meals demonstrate decreased C_{max} and AUC

Distribution: V_d: 4.6 L/kg

Protein binding: 58%

Metabolism: Hepatic, via CYP2C19 (major pathway) and CYP2C9 and CYP3A4 (less significant); saturable (may demonstrate nonlinearity); the N-oxide major metabolite has minimal antifungal activity

Bioavailability: 96%

Half-life elimination: Variable, dose-dependent. **Note:** Steady-state trough concentrations are achieved within 1 day when an IV loading dose is administered and 5 days if no loading dose is used.

Time to peak: Oral: 1 to 2 hours

Excretion: Urine (<2% as unchanged drug)

Dosage Note: Actual body weight should be used for all weight-based dosing calculations.

Usual dosage ranges:

Children <12 years: Dosage not established

Children ≥12 years, Adolescents, and Adults:

Oral: 100 to 300 mg every 12 hours

IV: 6 mg/kg every 12 hours for 2 doses; followed by maintenance dose of 4 mg/kg every 12 hours

Indication-specific dosing:

Children >2 to <12 years (<40 kg):

Aspergillosis, invasive including disseminated and extrapulmonary infection treatment: (off-label use): Duration of therapy should be a minimum of 6 to 12 weeks or throughout period of immunosuppression (Walsh, 2008):

IV: **Note:** Data suggest higher doses (mg/kg) are required; consider using a loading dose: 9 mg/kg/dose every 12 hours for 2 doses on day 1, followed by a maintenance dose: 8 to 9 mg/kg/dose every 12 hours; maximum dose: 350 mg. Monitoring of concentrations may be warranted (Driscoll, 2011; *Red Book* [AAP], 2012).

Non-HIV-exposed/-positive (Walsh, 2008): 5 to 7 mg/kg/dose every 12 hours; see **Note** regarding higher dose recommendations

HIV-exposed/-positive (CDC, 2009): See **Note** regarding higher dose recommendations.

Initial: 6 to 8 mg/kg/dose (maximum: 400 mg/dose) every 12 hours for 2 doses on day 1

Maintenance: 7 mg/kg/dose (maximum: 200 mg/dose) every 12 hours; change to oral administration when able; duration of therapy (IV and oral combined): ≥12 weeks but should be individualized

Oral suspension: May consider oral therapy once the patient is stable

Non-HIV-exposed/-positive (Red Book [AAP], 2012): 9 mg/kg/dose every 12 hours

HIV-exposed/-positive (CDC, 2009): **Note:** Data suggest higher doses (mg/kg) are required (9 mg/kg every 12 hours) (*Red Book* [AAP], 2012)

Initial: 8 mg/kg/dose (maximum: 400 mg/dose) every 12 hours for 2 doses on day 1

Maintenance: 7 mg/kg/dose (maximum: 200 mg/dose) every 12 hours

Candidiasis or other serious fungal infection, treatment (off-label use; Driscoll, 2011; *Red Book* [AAP], 2012): IV:Loading dose: 9 mg/kg/dose every 12 hours for 2 doses on day 1, followed by a maintenance dose: 8 to 9 mg/kg/dose every 12 hours; maximum dose: 350 mg

Catheter-related bloodstream infections due to *Malassezia furfur* (off-label use; Mermel, 2009): IV: **Note:** Recent data suggest higher doses (mg/kg) than described in the guideline may be required (Driscoll, 2011):

Initial: 6 mg/kg every 12 hours for 2 doses.

Maintenance: 4 mg/kg every 12 hours.

Infection prophylaxis in graft-versus-host disease (GVHD) (off-label use; Tomblyn, 2009; Wingard, 2010): Note: The optimal duration of prophylaxis in GVHD has not been determined.

Oral:

Weight <20 kg: 50 mg every 12 hours

Weight ≥20 kg: 100 mg every 12 hours

IV: 4 mg/kg every 12 hours (maximum dose not to exceed weight-based oral dose)

Children ≥12 years and Adolescents (>40 kg):

Esophageal candidiasis (fluconazole-refractory, HIV-exposed/-positive patients) (off-label use; DHHS [pediatric] 2013): IV:

Initial: 6 mg/kg every 12 hours for 2 doses

Maintenance: 4 mg/kg every 12 hours. **Note:** Convert to oral therapy, when possible, at a dose of 200 mg every 12 hours

Children ≥12 years, Adolescents, and Adults:

Aspergillosis, invasive, including disseminated and extrapulmonary infection: Duration of therapy should be a minimum of 6 to 12 weeks or throughout period of immunosuppression (Walsh, 2008):

IV:

Initial: 6 mg/kg every 12 hours for 2 doses

Maintenance dose: 4 mg/kg every 12 hours

Oral: Maintenance dose:

Manufacturer's recommendations: **Note:** If patient has inadequate clinical response, titrate in 50 mg/dose increments for weight <40 kg and 100 mg/dose increments for weight ≥40 kg.

Weight <40 kg: 100 mg every 12 hours

Weight ≥40 kg: 200 mg every 12 hours

IDSA recommendations (Walsh, 2008): May consider oral therapy in place of IV with dosing of 4 mg/kg (rounded up to convenient tablet dosage form) every 12 hours; however, IV administration is preferred in serious infections since comparative efficacy with the oral formulation has not been established.

Candidemia in non-neutropenic patients and disseminated *Candida* infections in skin, and infections in abdomen, kidney, bladder wall and wounds: Treatment should continue for a minimum of 14 days following resolution of symptoms or following last positive culture, whichever is longer.

IV:

Initial: 6 mg/kg every 12 hours for 2 doses

Maintenance: 3 to 4 mg/kg every 12 hours

Oral:

Manufacturer's recommendations: Maintenance dose: **Note:** If patient has inadequate clinical response, titrate in 50 mg/dose increments for weight <40 kg and 100 mg/dose increments for weight ≥40 kg

Weight <40 kg: 100 mg every 12 hours

Weight ≥40 kg: 200 mg every 12 hours

Alternate recommendations (Pappas, 2009):

Initial: 400 mg every 12 hours for 2 doses

Maintenance: 200 mg every 12 hours

Esophageal candidiasis: Oral: Treatment should continue for a minimum of 14 days, and for at least 7 days following resolution of symptoms. **Note:** If patient has inadequate clinical response, titrate in 50 mg/dose increments for weight <40 kg and 100 mg/dose increments for weight ≥40 kg

Weight <40 kg: 100 mg every 12 hours; maximum: 300 mg daily

Weight ≥40 kg: 200 mg every 12 hours; maximum: 600 mg daily

Scedosporiosis, fusariosis:

IV:

Initial: 6 mg/kg every 12 hours for 2 doses

Maintenance dose: 4 mg/kg every 12 hours for >7 days

Oral: Maintenance dose: **Note:** If patient has inadequate clinical response, titrate in 50 mg/dose increments for weight <40 kg and 100 mg/dose increments for weight ≥40 kg.

Weight <40 kg: 100 mg every 12 hours

Weight ≥40 kg: 200 mg every 12 hours

Endophthalmitis, fungal (off-label use; Pappas, 2009): IV: 6 mg/kg every 12 hours for 2 doses, then 3 to 4 mg/kg every 12 hours.

Infection prophylaxis in graft-versus-host disease (GVHD) (high-risk patients; off-label use; Maertens, 2011; Tomblyn, 2009; Wingard, 2010): Note: The optimal duration of prophylaxis in GVHD has not been determined.

Oral: Weight >40 kg: 200 mg every 12 hours

IV: Weight >40 kg: 4 mg/kg every 12 hours

Meningitis (secondary to contaminated [eg, *Exserohilum rostratum*] steroid products) (off-label use) (CDC [parameningeal], 2012; Kauffman, 2013): Note: Consult an infectious disease specialist and current CDC guidelines for specific treatment recommendations. Therapy duration is ≥3 months; trough serum concentrations must be maintained between 2 to 5 mcg/mL.

IV: 6 mg/kg every 12 hours. If patient does not improve or has severe disease, consider adding amphotericin B (liposomal).

Oral (only in mild disease in adherent patients whose trough concentrations/response to therapy can be closely monitored): 6 mg/kg every 12 hours (CDC [parameningeal], 2012).

Osteoarticular infection involving the spine, discitis, epidural abscess or vertebral osteomyelitis (secondary to contaminated [eg, *Exserohilum rostratum*] steroid products) (off-label use) (CDC [osteoarticular], 2012; Kauffman, 2013): IV: 6 mg/kg every 12 hours for ≥3 months. **Note:** Consult an infectious disease specialist and current CDC guidelines for specific treatment recommendations. Trough serum concentrations must be maintained between 2 to 5 mcg/mL. If patient has severe disease, consider adding amphotericin B (liposomal). Patients may be switched to oral therapy if condition has improved or stabilized.

Osteoarticular infection not involving the spine (secondary to contaminated [eg, *Exserohilum rostratum*] steroid products) (off-label use) (CDC [osteoarticular], 2012; Kauffman, 2013): Note: Consult an infectious disease specialist and current CDC guidelines for specific treatment recommendations. Therapy duration is ≥3 months. Trough serum concentrations must be maintained between 2 to 5 mcg/mL.

IV: 6 mg/kg every 12 hours for 2 doses, then 4 mg/kg every 12 hours. If patient has severe disease, consider adding amphotericin B (liposomal)

Oral (only in mild disease in adherent patients whose trough concentrations/response to therapy can be closely monitored): 6 mg/kg every 12 hours for 2 doses, then 4 mg/kg every 12 hours

Adolescents and Adults (>40 kg):

Infection prophylaxis in standard- or high-risk patients with allogeneic hematopoietic stem cell transplant (HSCT) or certain autologous HSCT (off-label use; Castagna, 2012; Maertens, 2011; Tomblyn, 2009; Wingard, 2010): Note: Begin prophylaxis at the start of chemotherapy or the day of transplantation. The ASBMT recommends continuing prophylaxis until engraftment (ie, ~30 days) or for 7 days after the ANC reaches >1000 cells/mm^3 (Tomblyn, 2009). The IDSA recommends antimold prophylaxis in allograft HSCT patients "through the neutropenic period and beyond," based on a demonstrated survival advantage in patients receiving prophylaxis for ≥75 days post-HSCT, or until cessation of immunosuppressive therapy (Freifeld, 2011); some pediatric guidelines do not include voriconazole as an option for primary prophylaxis in cancer patients or HSCT recipients (Science, 2014).

Oral: Weight >40 kg: 200 mg every 12 hours

IV: Weight >40 kg: 4 mg/kg every 12 hours

Dosage adjustment in patients with inadequate response:

IV: Maintenance dose may be increased from 3 mg/kg every 12 hours to 4 mg/kg every 12 hours, depending upon condition.

Oral: Maintenance dose may be increased from 200 mg every 12 hours to 300 mg every 12 hours in patients weighing ≥40 kg (or to 150 mg every 12 hours in patients <40 kg), depending upon condition.

Dosage adjustment in patients unable to tolerate treatment:

IV: Maintenance dose may be reduced from 4 mg/kg every 12 hours to 3 mg/kg every 12 hours, depending upon condition.

Oral: Maintenance dose may be reduced in 50 mg decrements to a minimum dosage of 200 mg every 12 hours in patients weighing ≥40 kg (or to 100 mg every 12 hours in patients <40 kg), depending upon condition.

Dosage adjustment in patients receiving concomitant CYP450 enzyme inducers or substrates:

Efavirenz: Oral: Increase maintenance dose of voriconazole to 400 mg every 12 hours and reduce efavirenz dose to 300 mg once daily; upon discontinuation of voriconazole, return to the initial dose of efavirenz.

Phenytoin:
IV: Increase voriconazole maintenance dose to 5 mg/kg every 12 hours.
Oral: Increase voriconazole maintenance dose to 400 mg every 12 hours in patients ≥40 kg (200 mg every 12 hours in patients <40 kg).

Dosage adjustment in renal impairment:
IV:
CrCl ≥50 mL/minute: There are no dosage adjustments provided in the manufacturer's labeling.
CrCl <50 mL/minute: There are no specific dosage adjustments provided in the manufacturer's labeling. Due to accumulation of the intravenous vehicle (cyclodextrin), the manufacturer recommends the use of oral voriconazole in these patients unless an assessment of the benefit:risk justifies the use of IV voriconazole; if IV therapy is used, closely monitor serum creatinine and change to oral voriconazole when possible. IV therapy has been used in select patients with CrCl <50 mL/minute using varying doses (median duration of treatment 7 to 10 days) (Neofytos, 2012; Oude Lashof, 2012).
Oral:
Mild to severe impairment: No dosage adjustment necessary.
Dialysis: Poorly dialyzed; no supplemental dose or dosage adjustment necessary, including patients on intermittent hemodialysis (IHD) with thrice weekly sessions or peritoneal dialysis.
Continuous renal replacement therapy (CRRT) (Heintz, 2009): Drug clearance is highly dependent on the method of renal replacement, filter type, and flow rate. Appropriate dosing requires close monitoring of pharmacologic response, signs of adverse reactions due to drug accumulation, as well as drug concentrations in relation to target trough (if appropriate). The following are general recommendations only (based on dialysate flow/ultrafiltration rates of 1 to 2 L/hour and minimal residual renal function) and should not supersede clinical judgment:
CVVH, CVVHD, and CVVHDF: Loading dose of 400 mg every 12 hours for 2 doses, followed by 200 mg every 12 hours.

Dosage adjustment in hepatic impairment:
Mild to moderate impairment (Child-Pugh class A or B): Following standard loading dose, reduce maintenance dosage by 50%.
Severe impairment (Child-Pugh class C): There are no dosage adjustments provided in manufacturer's labeling (has not been studied). Should only be used if benefit outweighs risk; monitor closely for toxicity.

Administration
Oral: Administer 1 hour before or 1 hour after a meal. Shake oral suspension for approximately 10 seconds before each use. Enteral tube feedings may decrease oral absorption; may hold tube feedings for 1 hour before and 1 hour after a voriconazole dose (Williams, 2012).
IV: Infuse over 1 to 2 hours (rate not to exceed 3 mg/kg/hour). Do not administer as an IV bolus injection. Do not infuse **concomitantly** into same line or cannula with other drug infusions. Do not infuse **concomitantly** even in separate lines or cannulas with concentrated electrolyte solutions or blood products. May be infused simultaneously with nonconcentrated electrolytes or TPN through a separate IV line. If TPN is infused through a multiple lumen catheter, use a different port than used for voriconazole.

Hazardous agent - use appropriate precautions for handling and disposal (NIOSH 2014 [group 3]).

Monitoring Parameters Hepatic function at initiation and during course of treatment; renal function; serum electrolytes (particularly calcium, magnesium and potassium) prior to therapy initiation; visual function (visual acuity, visual field and color perception) if treatment course continues >28 days; monitor trough serum concentrations on day 5 of therapy and weekly thereafter for 4 to 6 weeks or when dosing adjustments are made; for infections other than meningitis or osteoarticular infections, may consider obtaining voriconazole trough level to assure therapeutics serum concentrations, in patients failing therapy or in those exhibiting signs of toxicity; pancreatic function (in patients at risk for acute pancreatitis); total body skin examination yearly (more frequently if lesions noted)

Trough recommendations in adult patients:
Meningitis or osteoarticular infections for *Exserohilum rostratum* (CDC, 2012): 2 to 5 mcg/mL
Other infections (Dolton, 2012; Hamada, 2012; Mitsani, 2012; Park, 2012):
Efficacy: >1.0 mcg/mL
Toxicity: <4.0 mcg/mL
Therapeutic range in adult patients (CDC, 2012; Dolton, 2012; Hamada, 2012; Mitsani, 2012; Park, 2012; Tomblyn, 2009): 1 to 5 mcg/mL

Refer to Additional Information for detailed discussion of these data and data in pediatric patients.

Reference Range Note: Refer to Additional Information for detailed discussion of these data and data in pediatric patients.

Trough recommendations in adult patients:
Meningitis or osteoarticular infections for *Exserohilum rostratum* (CDC, 2012): 2 to 5 mcg/mL
Other infections (Dolton, 2012; Hamada, 2012; Mitsani, 2012; Park, 2012):
Efficacy: >1.0 mcg/mL
Toxicity: <4.0 mcg/mL
Therapeutic range in adult patients (CDC, 2012; Dolton, 2012; Hamada, 2012; Mitsani, 2012; Park, 2012; Tomblyn, 2009): 1 to 5 mcg/mL

Additional Information The rationale supporting proposed therapeutic drug monitoring for voriconazole includes variable and unpredictable pharmacokinetics and drug toxicities. The metabolism of voriconazole is greatly influenced by hepatic enzyme saturation and genetic polymorphisms in the CYP2C19 isoenzyme system. These factors result in a nonlinear pharmacokinetic profile and wide inter-subject variability and poor dose-concentration relationship. Several studies have been published that have attempted to use therapeutic drug monitoring to decrease trough variability among patients receiving voriconazole. In one study, only 50% of patients achieved voriconazole trough concentrations within the target trough range without dose adjustments; the authors adjusted the dose of voriconazole to achieve a range of 1.0 to 5.5 mcg/mL (Park, 2012). Regarding the utility of therapeutic drug monitoring and treatment outcomes, several recent studies have reported a relationship between voriconazole trough concentrations and clinical success (Dolton, 2012; Hamada, 2012; Mitsani, 2012; Park, 2012; Soler-Palacin, 2012). Although there is variability among studies regarding the cutoff trough value associated with improved outcomes, it does appear that the probability of a positive outcome has been strongest when the voriconazole trough concentration is >1.0 mcg/mL. For toxicity, the strongest correlations have been made between voriconazole trough concentrations and neurological and dermatological adverse events (Dolton, 2012; Hamada, 2012; Mitsani, 2012; Park, 2012; Soler-Palacin, 2012). In these reports, the authors generally noted increased toxicity when trough concentrations exceeded threshold values. There are much less data supporting the existence between a cutoff threshold and hepatotoxicity. It is important to note that cutoff trough values ranged widely among studies; however, an upper limit <5.0 mcg/mL would be reasonable for most infections based on the available literature (see CDC recommendations for *Exserohilum rostratum* which follow).

Another controversy is determining in which patients drug levels should be obtained. Most clinical laboratories do not perform on-site drug analysis for voriconazole. Therefore, the utility of routine drug levels may be limited in the acute management of patients. Therapeutic drug monitoring of voriconazole troughs may be reasonable if a patient is not responding to therapy or if they are being placed on long-term prophylaxis or treatment. In response to the outbreak of infections secondary to contaminated (eg, *Exserohilum rostratum*) steroid products, the CDC has recommended that trough serum concentrations for treatment of *Exserohilum rostratum* must be maintained between 2 to 5 mcg/mL (CDC, 2012).

Trough recommendations in adult patients:

Meningitis or osteoarticular infections for *Exserohilum rostratum* (CDC, 2012): 2 to 5 mcg/mL

Other infections (Dolton, 2012; Hamada, 2012; Mitsani, 2012; Park, 2012):

Efficacy: >1.0 mcg/mL

Toxicity: <4.0 mcg/mL

Therapeutic range in adult patients (CDC, 2012; Dolton, 2012; Hamada, 2012; Mitsani, 2012; Park, 2012; Tomblyn, 2009): 1 to 5 mcg/mL

In children, plasma voriconazole levels vary widely; in older children, voriconazole pharmacokinetics trend toward nonlinear relationships. In one study, the median doses to achieve therapeutic levels for children <5 years of age and for children >5 years of age were 38 mg/kg/day and 15 mg/kg/day, respectively (Soler-Palacin, 2012). Trough concentration recommendations for children have not been determined.

Dosage Forms

Solution Reconstituted, Intravenous:

Generic: 200 mg (1 ea)

Solution Reconstituted, Intravenous [preservative free]:

Vfend IV: 200 mg (1 ea)

Suspension Reconstituted, Oral:

Vfend: 40 mg/mL (75 mL)

Generic: 40 mg/mL (75 mL)

Tablet, Oral:

Vfend: 50 mg, 200 mg

Generic: 50 mg, 200 mg

◆ **Voriconazole For Injection (Can)** *see* Voriconazole *on page 2176*

Vorinostat (vor IN oh stat)

Brand Names: U.S. Zolinza

Brand Names: Canada Zolinza

Index Terms SAHA; Suberoylanilide Hydroxamic Acid

Pharmacologic Category Antineoplastic Agent, Histone Deacetylase Inhibitor

Use Cutaneous T-cell lymphoma: Treatment of cutaneous manifestations of cutaneous T-cell lymphoma (CTCL) with progressive, persistent, or recurrent disease on or following 2 systemic treatments

Pregnancy Risk Factor D

Pregnancy Considerations Adverse events were observed in animal reproduction studies. Based on the mechanism of action, may cause fetal harm if administered during pregnancy. Inform patient of potential hazard if used during pregnancy or if pregnancy occurs during treatment.

Breast-Feeding Considerations It is not known if vorinostat is excreted in breast milk. Due to the potential for serious adverse reactions in the nursing infant, the decision to discontinue vorinostat or to discontinue breast-feeding should take into account the benefits of treatment to the mother.

Contraindications There are no contraindications in the manufacturer's U.S. labeling.

Canadian labeling: Hypersensitivity to vorinostat or any component of the formulation; severe hepatic impairment (total bilirubin ≥3 times ULN)

Warnings/Precautions Hazardous agent - use appropriate precautions for handling and disposal (NIOSH 2014 [group 1]). Pulmonary embolism and deep vein thrombosis (DVT) have been reported; monitor for signs/symptoms; use caution in patients with a history of thrombotic events. Dose-related thrombocytopenia and/or anemia may occur; may require dosage adjustments or discontinuation; monitor blood counts (every 2 weeks for 2 months, then monthly). Gastrointestinal bleeding due to severe thrombocytopenia has been reported in patients receiving vorinostat in combination with other histone deacetylase inhibitors (eg, valproic acid); monitor platelet counts more frequently in patients receiving concomitant histone deacetylase inhibitor therapy. QTc prolongation has been observed; baseline and periodic ECGs were done in clinical trials (Duvic, 2007; Olsen, 2007). Correct electrolyte abnormalities prior to treatment and monitor and correct potassium, calcium, and magnesium levels during therapy. Use caution in patients with a history of QTc prolongation or with medications known to prolong the QT interval. May cause hyperglycemia (may be severe); monitor serum glucose and use with caution in diabetics; may require diet and/or therapy modifications. Nausea, vomiting, and diarrhea may occur; antiemetics and antidiarrheals may be required; control preexisting nausea, vomiting, and diarrhea prior to treatment initiation; replace fluids and electrolytes to avoid dehydration. Adverse anastomotic healing events have occurred in patients recovering from bowel surgery; use with caution in the perioperative period in patients requiring bowel surgery. May cause dizziness or fatigue; caution patients about performing tasks which require mental alertness (eg, operating machinery or driving). Use with caution in patients with hepatic impairment; dose reductions are recommended (elimination is predominantly hepatic). The Canadian labeling does not recommend use in patients with moderate hepatic impairment (total bilirubin 1.5 to 3 times ULN) and contraindicates use in severe hepatic impairment (bilirubin ≥3 times ULN). Potentially significant drug-drug interactions may exist, requiring dose or frequency adjustment, additional monitoring, and/or selection of alternative therapy.

Adverse Reactions

Cardiovascular: Peripheral edema, QTc prolongation

Central nervous system: Chills, dizziness, fatigue, fever, headache

Dermatologic: Alopecia, pruritus, squamous cell carcinoma

Endocrine & metabolic: Dehydration, hyperglycemia

Gastrointestinal: Anorexia, appetite decreased, constipation, diarrhea, nausea, taste perversion, vomiting, weight loss, xerostomia

Hematologic: Anemia, thrombocytopenia

Neuromuscular & skeletal: Muscle spasm

Renal: Creatinine increased, proteinuria

Respiratory: Cough, dyspnea, pulmonary embolism, upper respiratory infection

Rare but important or life-threatening: Abdominal pain, angioneurotic edema, blurred vision, chest pain, cholecystitis, deafness, diverticulitis, dysphagia, DVT, enterococcal infection, exfoliative dermatitis, gastrointestinal bleeding, gastrointestinal hemorrhage, Guillain-Barré syndrome, hemoptysis, hypertension, hypokalemia, hyponatremia, infection, lethargy, leukopenia, MI, neutropenia, pneumonia, renal failure, sepsis, spinal cord injury, streptococcal bacteremia, stroke (ischemic), syncope, T-cell lymphoma, tumor hemorrhage, ureteric obstruction, ureteropelvic junction obstruction, urinary retention, vasculitis, weakness

Drug Interactions

Metabolism/Transport Effects None known.

Avoid Concomitant Use

Avoid concomitant use of Vorinostat with any of the following: CloZAPine; Dipyrone

Increased Effect/Toxicity

Vorinostat may increase the levels/effects of: CloZAPine; Highest Risk QTc-Prolonging Agents; Moderate Risk QTc-Prolonging Agents; Vitamin K Antagonists

The levels/effects of Vorinostat may be increased by: Dipyrone; Mifepristone; Valproic Acid and Derivatives

Decreased Effect There are no known significant interactions involving a decrease in effect.

Storage/Stability Store at 20°C to 25°C (68°F to 77°F); excursions permitted to 15°C to 30°C (59°F to 86°F).

Mechanism of Action Inhibits histone deacetylase enzymes, HDAC1, HDAC2, HDAC3, and HDAC6, which catalyze acetyl group removal from protein lysine residues (including histones and transcription factors). Histone deacetylase inhibition results in accumulation of acetyl groups, which alters chromatin structure and transcription factor activation; cell growth is terminated and apoptosis occurs.

Pharmacodynamics/Kinetics

Protein binding: ~71%

Metabolism: Glucuronidated and hydrolyzed (followed by beta-oxidation) to inactive metabolites

Bioavailability: Fasting: ~43%

Half-life elimination: ~2 hours

Time to peak, plasma: With high-fat meal: ~4 hours (range: 2 to 10 hours)

Excretion: Urine: 52% (~52% as inactive metabolites; <1% as unchanged drug)

Dosage Cutaneous T-cell lymphoma (CTCL): Adults: Oral: 400 mg once daily until disease progression or unacceptable toxicity

Dosage adjustment for toxicity:

U.S. labeling: Intolerance: Reduce dose to 300 mg once daily; if needed, may further reduce to 300 mg daily for 5 consecutive days per week

Canadian labeling: Grade 3 or 4 toxicity: Interrupt therapy until resolves to ≤ grade 1 (excluding grade 3 anemia and thrombocytopenia). Upon recovery, may reduce dose to 300 mg once daily. If necessary, may further reduce dose to 300 mg once daily for 5 consecutive days per week.

Additionally, in clinical trials, **dose reductions** were instituted for the following adverse events: Increased serum creatinine, decreased appetite, hypokalemia, leukopenia, nausea, neutropenia, thrombocytopenia, and vomiting. Vorinostat was **discontinued** for the following adverse events: Anemia, angioneurotic edema, weakness, chest pain, exfoliative dermatitis, DVT, ischemic stroke, lethargy, pulmonary embolism, and spinal cord injury.

Treatment was withheld in clinical trials for grade 4 anemia or thrombocytopenia or other grade 3 or 4 drug related toxicity, until resolved to ≤ grade 1. Treatment was reinitiated with dose reduction (Olsen, 2007).

Dosage adjustment in renal impairment: There are no dosage adjustments provided in the manufacturer's labeling (has not studied). However, based on the minimal renal elimination, adjustment not expected. Use with caution.

Dosage adjustment in hepatic impairment:

U.S. labeling: Initial:

Mild-to-moderate impairment (total bilirubin 1 to 3 times ULN **or** AST >ULN): 300 mg once daily

Severe impairment (total bilirubin >3 times ULN): There are no dosage adjustments provided in manufacturer's labeling (evidence is insufficient for a starting dose recommendation). Doses of 100 to 200 mg once daily were studied in a limited number of patients with severe impairment (Ramalingam, 2010); according to the manufacturer, the maximum dose used was 200 mg once daily.

Canadian labeling:

Mild impairment (total bilirubin >1 to 1.5 times ULN or total bilirubin ≤ULN and AST >ULN): 300 mg once daily

Moderate impairment (total bilirubin 1.5 to 3 times ULN): Use is not recommended

Severe impairment (total bilirubin ≥3 times ULN): Use is contraindicated

Administration Administer with food. Do not open, crush, break, or chew capsules. Maintain adequate hydration (≥2 L/day fluids) during treatment.

Hazardous agent; use appropriate precautions for handling and disposal (NIOSH 2014 [group 1]). Avoid direct skin or mucous membrane contact with crushed or broken capsules and/or capsule contents.

Monitoring Parameters CBC with differential and serum chemistries, including calcium, magnesium, potassium, glucose and creatinine (baseline, then every 2 weeks for 2 months, then monthly, or as clinically necessary), hepatic function, INR (if on concomitant warfarin therapy), fluid status, signs/symptoms of thromboembolism. Baseline and periodic ECGs were done in clinical trials (and are recommended in the Canadian labeling).

Dosage Forms

Capsule, Oral:

Zolinza: 100 mg

Extemporaneous Preparations Hazardous agent: Use appropriate precautions for handling and disposal (NIOSH 2014 [group 1]).

Although not recommended by the manufacturer, a 50 mg/mL oral suspension may be prepared with capsules. Add 20 mL Ora-Plus® into a glass bottle (≥4 oz). Add the contents of twenty 100 mg capsules and shake thoroughly to disperse (may take up to 3 minutes). Add 20 mL Ora-Sweet® and shake to disperse. Label "shake well". Stable for 14 days at room temperature.

Fouladi M, Park JR, Stewart CF, et al, "Pediatric Phase I Trial and Pharmacokinetic Study of Vorinostat: A Children's Oncology Group Phase I Consortium Report," *J Clin Oncol*, 2010, 28(22):3623-9.

Vortioxetine (vor tye OX e teen)

Brand Names: U.S. Brintellix

Brand Names: Canada Trintellix

Index Terms Lu AA21004; Vortioxetine Hydrobromide

Pharmacologic Category Antidepressant, Selective Serotonin Reuptake Inhibitor; Serotonin 5-HT_{1A} Receptor Agonist; Serotonin 5-HT_3 Receptor Antagonist

Use Major depressive disorder: Treatment of major depressive disorder (MDD)

Pregnancy Risk Factor C

Pregnancy Considerations Adverse events were observed in animal reproduction studies. Nonteratogenic effects in the newborn following SSRI/SNRI exposure late in the third trimester include respiratory distress, cyanosis, apnea, seizures, temperature instability, feeding difficulty, vomiting, hypoglycemia, hypo- or hypertonia, hyperreflexia, jitteriness, irritability, constant crying, and tremor. Symptoms may be due to the toxicity of the SSRIs/SNRIs or a discontinuation syndrome and may be consistent with serotonin syndrome associated with SSRI treatment. Persistent pulmonary hypertension of the newborn (PPHN) has also been reported with SSRI exposure.

The ACOG recommends that therapy with SSRIs or SNRIs during pregnancy be individualized; treatment of depression during pregnancy should incorporate the clinical expertise of the mental health clinician, obstetrician, primary healthcare provider, and pediatrician (ACOG, 2008). According to the American Psychiatric Association (APA), the risks of medication treatment should be weighed against other treatment options and untreated depression. For women who discontinue antidepressant medications during pregnancy and who may be at high risk for postpartum depression, the medications can be restarted following delivery (APA, 2010). Treatment algorithms have been developed by the ACOG and the APA for the management of depression in women prior to conception and during pregnancy (Yonkers, 2009).

Breast-Feeding Considerations It is not known if vortioxetine is excreted into breast milk. Due to the potential for serious adverse reactions in the nursing infant, the manufacturer recommends a decision be made whether to discontinue nursing or to discontinue the drug, taking into account the importance of treatment to the mother.

Contraindications Hypersensitivity to vortioxetine or any component of the formulation; use of MAO inhibitors intended to treat psychiatric disorders (concurrently or within 21 days of discontinuing vortioxetine or within 14 days of discontinuing the MAO inhibitor); initiation of vortioxetine in a patient receiving linezolid or intravenous methylene blue

Warnings/Precautions [U.S. Boxed Warning]: Antidepressants increase the risk of suicidal thinking and behavior in children, adolescents, and young adults (18 to 24 years of age) with major depressive disorder (MDD) and other psychiatric disorders; consider risk prior to prescribing. Short-term studies did not show an increased risk in patients >24 years of age and showed a decreased risk in patients ≥65 years. Closely monitor patients for clinical worsening, suicidality, or unusual changes in behavior, particularly during the initial 1 to 2 months of therapy or during periods of dosage adjustments (increases or decreases); the patient's family or caregiver should be instructed to closely observe the patient and communicate condition with healthcare provider. A medication guide concerning the use of antidepressants should be dispensed with each prescription. **Vortioxetine is not approved for use in children.**

The possibility of a suicide attempt is inherent in major depression and may persist until remission occurs. Use caution in high-risk patients. Worsening depression and severe abrupt suicidality that are not part of the presenting symptoms may require discontinuation or modification of drug therapy. The patient's family or caregiver should be alerted to monitor patients for the emergence of suicidality and associated behaviors (such as agitation, irritability, hostility, aggressiveness, impulsivity, and hypomania) and call healthcare provider.

May worsen psychosis in some patients or precipitate a mixed/manic episode in patients at risk for bipolar disorder. Use with caution in patients with a family history of bipolar disorder, mania, or hypomania. Patients presenting with depressive symptoms should be screened for bipolar disorder. **Vortioxetine is not FDA approved for the treatment of bipolar depression.**

Potentially life-threatening serotonin syndrome (SS) has occurred with serotonergic antidepressants (eg, SSRIs, SNRIs), particularly when used in combination with other serotonergic agents (eg, triptans, TCAs, fentanyl, lithium, tramadol, buspirone, St John's wort, tryptophan) or agents that impair metabolism of serotonin (eg, MAO inhibitors intended to treat psychiatric disorders, other MAO inhibitors [ie, linezolid and intravenous methylene blue]). Discontinue treatment (and any concomitant serotonergic agent) immediately if signs/symptoms arise.

May impair platelet aggregation resulting in increased risk of bleeding events, particularly if used concomitantly with aspirin, NSAIDs, warfarin or other anticoagulants. Bleeding related to antidepressant use has been reported to range from relatively minor bruising and epistaxis to life-threatening hemorrhage. May cause hyponatremia/SIADH (elderly at increased risk); volume depletion (diuretics may increase risk) may occur. Bone fractures have been associated with antidepressant treatment. Consider the possibility of a fragility fracture if an antidepressant-treated patient presents with unexplained bone pain, point tenderness, swelling, or bruising (Rabenda, 2013; Rizzoli, 2012). Use caution in elderly patients; may be potentially inappropriate in patients with a history of falls or fractures, and may cause or exacerbate syndrome of inappropriate antidiuretic hormone secretion or hyponatremia; monitor sodium closely with initiation or dosage adjustments in older adults (Beers Criteria). May cause mild pupillary dilation which in susceptible individuals can lead to an episode of narrow-angle glaucoma. Consider evaluating patients who have not had an iridectomy for narrow-angle glaucoma risk factors. May cause CNS depression, which may impair physical or mental abilities; patients must be cautioned about performing tasks that require mental alertness (eg, operating machinery or driving). Angioedema has been reported. Use with caution in patients with seizure disorders; seizures (rare) have been reported in patients without a prior history of seizures. Potentially significant drug-drug interactions may exist, requiring dose or frequency adjustment, additional monitoring, and/or selection of alternative therapy. Use is not recommended in severe hepatic impairment.

Abrupt discontinuation or interruption of antidepressant therapy has been associated with a discontinuation syndrome. Symptoms arising may vary with antidepressant however commonly include nausea, vomiting, diarrhea, headaches, lightheadedness, dizziness, diminished appetite, sweating, chills, tremors, paresthesias, fatigue, somnolence, and sleep disturbances (eg, vivid dreams, insomnia). Greater risks for developing a discontinuation syndrome have been associated with antidepressants with shorter half-lives, longer durations of treatment, and abrupt discontinuation. For antidepressants of short or intermediate half-lives, symptoms may emerge within 2 to 5 days after treatment discontinuation and last 7 to 14 days (APA, 2010; Fava, 2006; Haddad, 2001; Shelton, 2001; Warner, 2006).

Adverse Reactions

Central nervous system: Abnormal dreams, dizziness, female sexual disorder, male sexual disorder

Dermatologic: Pruritus

Gastrointestinal: Constipation, diarrhea, flatulence, nausea (dose-related, females >males; commonly occurs within the first week of treatment, then decreases in frequency but can persist in some patients), vomiting, xerostomia

Rare but important or life-threatening: Angle-closure glaucoma, hypomania, hyponatremia, mania, seizure, serotonin syndrome, withdrawal syndrome

Drug Interactions

Metabolism/Transport Effects Substrate of CYP2A6 (minor), CYP2B6 (minor), CYP2C19 (minor), CYP2C8 (minor), CYP2C9 (minor), CYP2D6 (major), CYP3A4 (major); **Note:** Assignment of Major/Minor substrate status based on clinically relevant drug interaction potential

Avoid Concomitant Use

Avoid concomitant use of Vortioxetine with any of the following: Dapoxetine; Dosulepin; Iobenguane I 123; Linezolid; MAO Inhibitors; Methylene Blue; Pimozide; Tryptophan; Urokinase

Increased Effect/Toxicity

Vortioxetine may increase the levels/effects of: Agents with Antiplatelet Properties; Anticoagulants; Antidepressants (Serotonin Reuptake Inhibitor/Antagonist); Antipsychotic Agents; Apixaban; Aspirin; Beta-Blockers; BusPIRone; CarBAMazepine; CloZAPine; Collagenase (Systemic); Dabigatran Etexilate; Desmopressin; Dextromethorphan; Dosulepin; Galantamine; Hypoglycemic Agents; Ibritumomab; Methadone; Methylene Blue; Mexiletine; NSAID (COX-2 Inhibitor); NSAID (Nonselective); Obinutuzumab; Pimozide; RisperiDONE; Rivaroxaban; Salicylates; Serotonin Modulators; Thiazide Diuretics; Thrombolytic Agents; Tositumomab and Iodine I 131 Tositumomab; TraMADol; Urokinase; Vitamin K Antagonists

The levels/effects of Vortioxetine may be increased by: Abiraterone Acetate; Alcohol (Ethyl); Analgesics (Opioid); Antiemetics (5HT3 Antagonists); Antipsychotic Agents; BuPROPion; BusPIRone; Cimetidine; CNS Depressants; Cobicistat; CYP2D6 Inhibitors (Moderate); CYP2D6 Inhibitors (Strong); Dapoxetine; Darunavir; Dasatinib; Glucosamine; Herbs (Anticoagulant/Antiplatelet Properties); Ibrutinib; Limaprost; Linezolid; Lithium; Macrolide Antibiotics; MAO Inhibitors; Metoclopramide; Metyrosine; Multivitamins/Fluoride (with ADE); Multivitamins/Minerals (with ADEK, Folate, Iron); Multivitamins/Minerals (with AE, No Iron); Omega-3 Fatty Acids; Peginterferon Alfa-2b; Pentosan Polysulfate Sodium; Pentoxifylline; Prostacyclin Analogues; Tedizolid; TraMADol; Tryptophan; Vitamin E

Decreased Effect

Vortioxetine may decrease the levels/effects of: Iobenguane I 123; Ioflupane I 123; Thyroid Products

The levels/effects of Vortioxetine may be decreased by: Bosentan; CarBAMazepine; CYP3A4 Inducers (Moderate); CYP3A4 Inducers (Strong); Cyproheptadine; Dabrafenib; Deferasirox; Mitotane; NSAID (COX-2 Inhibitor); NSAID (Nonselective); Peginterferon Alfa-2b; Siltuximab; St Johns Wort; Tocilizumab

Storage/Stability Store at 25°C (77°F); excursions are permitted between 15°C and 30°C (59°F and 86°F).

Mechanism of Action Inhibits reuptake of serotonin (5-HT); also has agonist activity at the 5-HT_{1A} receptor and antagonist activity at the 5-HT_3 receptor.

Pharmacodynamics/Kinetics

Absorption: Not affected by food

Distribution: V_d: 2600 L

Protein binding: 98%

Metabolism: Hepatic primarily through oxidation via CYP450 isoenzymes, primarily CYP2D6, and subsequent glucuronic acid conjugation to an inactive carboxylic acid metabolite

Bioavailability: 75%

Half-life elimination: ~66 hours

Time to peak: 7-11 hours

Excretion: Urine (59%); feces (26%)

Dosage

Major depressive disorder: Oral:

Adults: Initial: 10 mg once daily; increase to 20 mg once daily as tolerated; consider 5 mg once daily for patients who do not tolerate higher doses. Maintenance: 5-20 mg once daily.

Elderly:

U.S. labeling: No dosage adjustment necessary; refer to adult dosing.

Canadian labeling: Initial: 5 mg once daily; may increase to 10 mg once daily as tolerated. Use caution with doses >10 mg daily (maximum: 20 mg daily).

Dosage adjustment for CYP2D6 poor metabolizers: Maximum dose: 10 mg once daily.

Dosage adjustment for concomitant therapy with strong CYP2D6 inhibitors: Reduce total daily dose by one half when a strong CYP2D6 inhibitor (eg, bupropion, fluoxetine, paroxetine, or quinidine) is coadministered. Increase dose to original level when the CYP2D6 inhibitor is discontinued.

Dosage adjustment for concomitant strong CYP inducers: Consider increasing the dose when a strong CYP inducer (eg, rifampin, carbamazepine, phenytoin) is coadministered for >14 days. Maximum dose should not exceed three times the original dose. Reduce the dose to the original level within 14 days of discontinuing the CYP inducer.

Discontinuation of therapy: Upon discontinuation of antidepressant therapy, gradually taper the dose to minimize the incidence of withdrawal symptoms and allow for the detection of re-emerging symptoms. Evidence supporting ideal taper rates is limited. APA and NICE guidelines suggest tapering therapy over at least several weeks with consideration to the half-life of the antidepressant; antidepressants with a shorter half-life may need to be tapered more conservatively. In addition for long-term treated patients, WFSBP guidelines recommend tapering over 4-6 months. If intolerable withdrawal symptoms occur following a dose reduction, consider resuming the previously prescribed dose and/or decrease dose at a more gradual rate (APA, 2010; Bauer, 2002; Haddad, 2001; NCCMH, 2010; Schatzberg, 2006; Shelton, 2001; Warner, 2006).

Vortioxetine doses of 15 mg once daily or more are recommended by the manufacturer to be decreased to 10 mg once daily for one week before full discontinuation to prevent withdrawal symptoms.

MAO inhibitor recommendations:

Switching to or from an MAO inhibitor intended to treat psychiatric disorders:

Allow 14 days to elapse between discontinuing an MAO inhibitor intended to treat psychiatric disorders and initiation of vortioxetine.

Allow 21 days to elapse between discontinuing vortioxetine and initiation of an MAO inhibitor intended to treat psychiatric disorders.

Use with other MAO inhibitors (linezolid or IV methylene blue):

Do not initiate vortioxetine in patients receiving linezolid or IV methylene blue; consider other interventions for psychiatric condition.

If urgent treatment with linezolid or IV methylene blue is required in a patient already receiving vortioxetine and potential benefits outweigh potential risks, discontinue vortioxetine promptly and administer linezolid or IV methylene blue. Monitor for serotonin syndrome for 21 days or until 24 hours after the last dose of linezolid or IV methylene blue, whichever comes first. May resume vortioxetine 24 hours after the last dose of linezolid or IV methylene blue.

Dosage adjustment in renal impairment: No dosage adjustment necessary.

Dosage adjustment in hepatic impairment:

Mild-to-moderate impairment: No dosage adjustment necessary.

Severe impairment: Use not recommended (has not been studied).

Administration Administer without regard to meals.

Monitoring Parameters Mental status for depression, suicidal ideation (especially at the beginning of therapy or when doses are increased or decreased), anxiety, social functioning, mania, panic attacks; akathisia; signs/symptoms of serotonin syndrome and/or hyponatremia; hepatic function (baseline).

Dosage Forms

Tablet, Oral:

Brintellix: 5 mg, 10 mg, 20 mg

Dosage Forms: Canada

Tablet, Oral:

Trintellix: 5 mg, 10 mg, 20 mg

- ◆ **Vortioxetine Hydrobromide** *see* Vortioxetine *on page 2183*
- ◆ **VoSol® HC [DSC]** *see* Acetic Acid, Propylene Glycol Diacetate, and Hydrocortisone *on page 40*
- ◆ **VoSpire ER** *see* Albuterol *on page 69*
- ◆ **Votrient** *see* PAZOPanib *on page 1584*
- ◆ **VP-16** *see* Etoposide *on page 816*
- ◆ **VP-16-213** *see* Etoposide *on page 816*
- ◆ **VPI-Baclofen Intrathecal (Can)** *see* Baclofen *on page 223*
- ◆ **Vpriv** *see* Velaglucerase Alfa *on page 2147*
- ◆ **VPRIV (Can)** *see* Velaglucerase Alfa *on page 2147*
- ◆ **VRT111950** *see* Telaprevir *on page 1983*
- ◆ **VSLI** *see* VinCRIStine (Liposomal) *on page 2166*
- ◆ **Vumon® (Can)** *see* Teniposide *on page 1997*
- ◆ **VWF/FVIII Concentrate** *see* Antihemophilic Factor/von Willebrand Factor Complex (Human) *on page 154*
- ◆ **VWF:RCo** *see* Antihemophilic Factor/von Willebrand Factor Complex (Human) *on page 154*
- ◆ **vWF:RCof** *see* Antihemophilic Factor/von Willebrand Factor Complex (Human) *on page 154*
- ◆ **VX-770** *see* Ivacaftor *on page 1135*
- ◆ **VX-950** *see* Telaprevir *on page 1983*
- ◆ **Vyfemla** *see* Ethinyl Estradiol and Norethindrone *on page 808*
- ◆ **Vyloma (Can)** *see* Imiquimod *on page 1055*
- ◆ **Vytone** *see* Iodoquinol and Hydrocortisone *on page 1105*
- ◆ **Vytorin** *see* Ezetimibe and Simvastatin *on page 834*
- ◆ **Vyvanse** *see* Lisdexamfetamine *on page 1224*
- ◆ **VZIG** *see* Varicella-Zoster Immune Globulin (Human) *on page 2142*
- ◆ **VZV Vaccine (Varicella)** *see* Varicella Virus Vaccine *on page 2141*
- ◆ **VZV Vaccine (Zoster)** *see* Zoster Vaccine *on page 2218*

Warfarin (WAR far in)

Brand Names: U.S. Coumadin; Jantoven

Brand Names: Canada Apo-Warfarin; Coumadin; Mylan-Warfarin; Novo-Warfarin; Taro-Warfarin

Index Terms Warfarin Sodium

Pharmacologic Category Anticoagulant; Anticoagulant, Vitamin K Antagonist

Additional Appendix Information

Oral Anticoagulant Comparison Chart *on page 2233*

Reversal of Oral Anticoagulants *on page 2235*

Use

Prophylaxis and treatment of thromboembolic disorders (eg, venous, pulmonary) and embolic complications arising from atrial fibrillation or cardiac valve replacement: The 2014 American Heart Association/American College of Cardiology/Heart Rhythm Society guidelines for the management of AF recommend oral anticoagulation for patients with nonvalvular AF or atrial flutter with prior stroke, TIA, or a CHA_2DS_2-VASc score ≥2. In patients with AF or atrial flutter of ≥48 hours duration or when the duration is unknown, anticoagulation with warfarin is recommended for at least 3 weeks prior to and 4 weeks after cardioversion regardless of the CHA_2DS_2-VASc score and method used to restore sinus rhythm (January, 2014).

Adjunct to reduce risk of systemic embolism (eg, recurrent MI, stroke) after myocardial infarction: According to the American College of Cardiology/American Heart Association (ACCF/AHA) guidelines for the management of patients with ST-elevation myocardial infarction (STEMI), warfarin should be administered to patients with STEMI and AF and a $CHADS_2$ score of 2 or more, mechanical valve, venous thromboembolism, or hypercoagulable disorder. Use is reasonable in patients with STEMI and asymptomatic LV mural thrombi and may be considered in patients with STEMI and anterior apical akinesis or dyskinesis (O'Gara, 2013).

Pregnancy Risk Factor D (women with mechanical heart valves)/X (other indications)

Pregnancy Considerations Warfarin crosses the placenta; concentrations in the fetal plasma are similar to maternal values. Teratogenic effects have been reported following first trimester exposure and may include coumarin embryopathy (nasal hypoplasia and/or stippled epiphyses; limb hypoplasia may also be present). Adverse CNS events to the fetus have also been observed following exposure during any trimester and may include CNS abnormalities (including ventral midline dysplasia, dorsal midline dysplasia). Spontaneous abortion, fetal hemorrhage, and fetal death may also occur. Use is contraindicated during pregnancy (or in women of reproductive potential) except in women with mechanical heart valves who are at high risk for thromboembolism; use is also contraindicated in women with threatened abortion, eclampsia, or preeclampsia. Frequent pregnancy tests are recommended for women who are planning to become pregnant and adjusted-dose heparin or low molecular weight heparin (LMWH) should be substituted as soon as pregnancy is confirmed or adjusted-dose heparin or LMWH should be used instead of warfarin prior to conception.

In pregnant women with high-risk mechanical heart valves, the benefits of warfarin therapy should be discussed with the risks of available treatments (ACCP [Bates, 2012]; AHA/ACC [Nishimura, 2014]); when possible avoid warfarin use during the first trimester (ACCP [Bates, 2012]) and close to delivery (ACCP [Bates, 2012]; AHA/ACC [Nishimura, 2014]). Use of warfarin during the first trimester may be considered if the therapeutic INR can be achieved with a dose ≤5 mg/day (AHA/ACC [Nishimura, 2014]). Adjusted-dose LMWH or adjusted-dose heparin may be used throughout pregnancy or until week 13 of gestation when therapy can be changed to warfarin. LMWH or heparin should be resumed close to delivery. In women who are at a very high risk for thromboembolism (older generation mechanical prosthesis in mitral position or history of thromboembolism), warfarin can be used throughout pregnancy and replaced with LMWH or heparin near term; the use of low-dose aspirin is also recommended (ACCP [Bates, 2012] AHA/ACC [Nishimura, 2014]). Women who require long-term anticoagulation with warfarin and who are considering pregnancy, LMWH substitution should be done prior to conception when possible.

If anti-Xa monitoring cannot be done, do not use LMWH therapy in pregnant patients with a mechanical prosthetic valve (AHA/ACC [Nishimura, 2014]). When choosing therapy, fetal outcomes (ie, pregnancy loss, malformations), maternal outcomes (ie, VTE, hemorrhage), burden of therapy, and maternal preference should be considered (ACCP [Bates, 2012]).

Breast-Feeding Considerations Breast-feeding women may be treated with warfarin. Based on available data, warfarin does not pass into breast milk. Women who are breast-feeding should be carefully monitored to avoid excessive anticoagulation. According to the American College of Chest Physicians (ACCP), warfarin may be used in lactating women who wish to breast-feed their infants (Bates, 2012). Monitor nursing infants for bruising or bleeding (per manufacturer).

Contraindications Hypersensitivity to warfarin or any component of the formulation; hemorrhagic tendencies (eg, patients bleeding from the GI, respiratory, or GU tract; cerebral aneurysm; cerebrovascular hemorrhage; dissecting aortic aneurysm; spinal puncture and other diagnostic or therapeutic procedures with potential for significant bleeding; history of bleeding diathesis); recent or potential surgery of the eye or CNS; major regional lumbar block anesthesia or traumatic surgery resulting in large, open surfaces; blood dyscrasias; severe uncontrolled or malignant hypertension; pericarditis or pericardial effusion; bacterial endocarditis; unsupervised patients with conditions associated with a high potential for noncompliance; eclampsia/pre-eclampsia, threatened abortion, pregnancy (except in women with mechanical heart valves at high risk for thromboembolism)

Warnings/Precautions Hazardous agent; use appropriate precautions for handling and disposal (NIOSH 2014 [group 3]).

Use care in the selection of patients appropriate for this treatment. Ensure patient cooperation especially from the alcoholic, illicit drug user, demented, or psychotic patient; ability to comply with routine laboratory monitoring is essential. Use with caution in trauma, acute infection, moderate-severe renal insufficiency, prolonged dietary insufficiencies, moderate-severe hypertension, polycythemia vera, vasculitis, open wound, active TB, any disruption in normal GI flora, history of PUD, anaphylactic disorders, indwelling catheters, severe diabetes, and menstruating and postpartum women. Use with caution in patients with thyroid disease; warfarin responsiveness may increase (Ageno, 2012). Use with caution in protein C deficiency. Use with caution in patients with heparin-induced thrombocytopenia and DVT. Warfarin monotherapy is contraindicated in the initial treatment of active HIT. Reduced liver function, regardless of etiology, may impair synthesis of coagulation factors leading to increased warfarin sensitivity.

[U.S. Boxed Warning]: May cause major or fatal bleeding. Risk factors for bleeding include high intensity anticoagulation (INR >4), age (>65 years), variable INRs, history of GI bleeding, hypertension, cerebrovascular disease, serious heart disease, anemia, malignancy, trauma, renal insufficiency, drug-drug interactions, long duration of therapy, or known genetic deficiency in CYP2C9 activity. Patient must be instructed to report bleeding, accidents, or falls. Unrecognized bleeding sites (eg, colon cancer) may be uncovered by anticoagulation. Patient must also report any new or discontinued medications, herbal or alternative products used, or significant changes in smoking or dietary habits. Necrosis or gangrene of the skin and other tissue can occur, usually in conjunction with protein C or S deficiency. Consider alternative therapies if anticoagulation is necessary. Warfarin therapy may release atheromatous plaque emboli; symptoms depend on site of embolization, most commonly kidneys, pancreas, liver, and spleen. In some cases may lead to necrosis or death. "Purple toes syndrome," due to cholesterol microembolization, may rarely occur. The elderly may be more sensitive to anticoagulant therapy.

Presence of the CYP2C9*2 or *3 allele and/or polymorphism of the vitamin K oxidoreductase (VKORC1) gene may increase the risk of bleeding. Lower doses may be required in these patients; genetic testing may help determine appropriate dosing.

When temporary interruption is necessary before surgery, discontinue for approximately 5 days before surgery; when there is adequate hemostasis, may reinstitute warfarin therapy ~12-24 hours after surgery (evening of or next morning). Decision to safely continue warfarin therapy through the procedure and whether or not bridging of anticoagulation is necessary is dependent upon risk of perioperative bleeding and risk of thromboembolism, respectively. If risk of thromboembolism is elevated, consider bridging warfarin therapy with an alternative anticoagulant (eg, unfractionated heparin, LMWH) (Guyatt, 2012).

Adverse Reactions Bleeding is the major adverse effect of warfarin. Hemorrhage may occur at virtually any site. Risk is dependent on multiple variables, including the intensity of anticoagulation and patient susceptibility.

Cardiovascular: Vasculitis

Central nervous system: Signs/symptoms of bleeding (eg, dizziness, fatigue, fever, headache, lethargy, malaise, pain)

Dermatologic: Alopecia, bullous eruptions, dermatitis, rash, pruritus, urticaria

Gastrointestinal: Abdominal pain, diarrhea, flatulence, gastrointestinal bleeding, nausea, taste disturbance, vomiting

Genitourinary: Hematuria

Hematologic: Anemia, retroperitoneal hematoma, unrecognized bleeding sites (eg, colon cancer) may be uncovered by anticoagulation

Hepatic: Hepatitis (including cholestatic hepatitis), transaminases increased

Neuromuscular & skeletal: Osteoporosis (potential association with long-term use), paralysis, paresthesia, weakness

Respiratory: Respiratory tract bleeding, tracheobronchial calcification

Miscellaneous: Anaphylactic reaction, hypersensitivity/allergic reactions, skin necrosis, gangrene, "purple toes" syndrome

Drug Interactions

Metabolism/Transport Effects **Substrate** of CYP1A2 (minor), CYP2C19 (minor), CYP2C9 (major), CYP3A4 (minor); **Note:** Assignment of Major/Minor substrate status based on clinically relevant drug interaction potential; **Inhibits** CYP2C19 (weak), CYP2C9 (weak)

Avoid Concomitant Use

Avoid concomitant use of Warfarin with any of the following: Apixaban; Dabigatran Etexilate; Edoxaban; Enzalutamide; Omacetaxine; Rivaroxaban; Streptokinase; Tamoxifen; Urokinase; Vorapaxar

Increased Effect/Toxicity

Warfarin may increase the levels/effects of: Anticoagulants; Collagenase (Systemic); Deferasirox; Ethotoin; Fosphenytoin; Ibritumomab; Nintedanib; Obinutuzumab; Omacetaxine; Phenytoin; Regorafenib; Rivaroxaban; Sulfonylureas; Tositumomab and Iodine I 131 Tositumomab

The levels/effects of Warfarin may be increased by: Acetaminophen; Agents with Antiplatelet Properties; Allopurinol; Amiodarone; Androgens; Apixaban; Atazanavir; Bicalutamide; Boceprevir; Capecitabine; Cephalosporins; Ceritinib; Chloral Hydrate; Chloramphenicol; Cimetidine; Clopidogrel; Cloxacillin; Cobicistat; Corticosteroids (Systemic); Cranberry; CYP2C9 Inhibitors (Moderate); CYP2C9 Inhibitors (Strong); Dabigatran Etexilate; Dasatinib; Desvenlafaxine; Dexmethylphenidate; Disulfiram; Dronedarone; Econazole; Edoxaban; Efavirenz; Erlotinib; Erythromycin (Ophthalmic); Esomeprazole; Ethacrynic Acid; Ethotoin; Etoposide; Exenatide; Fenofibrate and Derivatives; Fenugreek; Fibric Acid Derivatives; Fluconazole; Fluorouracil (Systemic); Fluorouracil (Topical); Fosamprenavir; Fosphenytoin; Fusidic Acid (Systemic); Gefitinib; Gemcitabine; Ginkgo Biloba; Glucagon; Green Tea; Herbs (Anticoagulant/Antiplatelet Properties); HMG-CoA Reductase Inhibitors; Ibrutinib; Ifosfamide; Imatinib; Itraconazole; Ivermectin (Systemic); Ketoconazole (Systemic); Lansoprazole; Leflunomide; Levomilnacipran; Limaprost; Lomitapide; Macrolide Antibiotics; Methylphenidate; Metreleptin; MetroNIDAZOLE (Systemic); Miconazole (Oral); Miconazole (Topical); Mifepristone; Milnacipran; Mirtazapine; Multivitamins/Fluoride (with ADE); Multivitamins/Minerals (with ADEK, Folate, Iron); Multivitamins/Minerals (with AE, No Iron); Nelfinavir; Neomycin; Nonsteroidal Anti-Inflammatory Agents; NSAID (COX-2 Inhibitor); NSAID (Nonselective); Omega-3 Fatty Acids; Omeprazole; Oritavancin; Orlistat; Penicillins; Pentosan Polysulfate Sodium; Pentoxifylline; Phenytoin; Posaconazole; Proguanil; Propafenone; Prostacyclin Analogues; QuiNIDine; QuiNINE; Quinolone Antibiotics; Ranitidine; RomiDEPsin; Salicylates; Saquinavir; Selective Serotonin Reuptake Inhibitors; Sitaxentan; SORAfenib; Streptokinase; Sugammadex; Sulfinpyrazone [Off Market]; Sulfonamide Derivatives; Sulfonylureas; Tamoxifen; Tegafur; Telaprevir; Tetracycline Derivatives; Thrombolytic Agents; Thyroid Products; Tibolone; Tigecycline; Tipranavir; Tolterodine; Toremifene; Torsemide; TraMADol; Tricyclic Antidepressants; Urokinase; Vemurafenib; Venlafaxine; Vitamin E; Vorapaxar; Voriconazole; Vorinostat; Zafirlukast; Zileuton

Decreased Effect

The levels/effects of Warfarin may be decreased by: Adalimumab; Alcohol (Ethyl); Aminoglutethimide; Antithyroid Agents; Aprepitant; AzaTHIOprine; Barbiturates; Bile Acid Sequestrants; Boceprevir; Bosentan; CarBAMazepine; Cloxacillin; Coenzyme Q-10; Contraceptives (Estrogens); Contraceptives (Progestins); CYP2C9 Inducers (Strong); Dabrafenib; Darunavir; Dicloxacillin; Efavirenz; Elvitegravir; Enzalutamide; Eslicarbazepine; Estrogen Derivatives; Flucloxacillin; Fosaprepitant; Ginseng (American); Glutethimide; Green Tea; Griseofulvin; Lixisenatide; Lopinavir; Mercaptopurine; Metreleptin; Multivitamins/Minerals (with ADEK, Folate, Iron); Nafcillin; Nelfinavir; Phytonadione; Progestins; Rifamycin Derivatives; Ritonavir; St Johns Wort; Sucralfate; Telaprevir; Teriflunomide; TraZODone

Food Interactions

Ethanol: Acute ethanol ingestion (binge drinking) decreases the metabolism of oral anticoagulants and increases PT/INR. Chronic daily ethanol use increases the metabolism of oral anticoagulants and decreases PT/INR. Management: Avoid ethanol.

Food: The anticoagulant effects of warfarin may be decreased if taken with foods rich in vitamin K. Vitamin E may increase warfarin effect. Cranberry juice may increase warfarin effect. Management: Maintain a consistent diet; consult prescriber before making changes in diet. Take warfarin at the same time each day.

Preparation for Administration Reconstitute with 2.7 mL of sterile water (yields 2 mg/mL solution).

Hazardous agent; use appropriate precautions for handling and disposal (NIOSH 2014 [group 3]).

Storage/Stability

Injection: Prior to reconstitution, store at 15°C to 30°C (59°F to 86°F). Following reconstitution with 2.7 mL of sterile water (yields 2 mg/mL solution), stable for 4 hours at 15°C to 30°C (59°F to 86°F). Protect from light.

Tablet: Store at 15°C to 30°C (59°F to 86°F). Protect from light.

Mechanism of Action Hepatic synthesis of coagulation factors II, VII, IX, and X, as well as proteins C and S, requires the presence of vitamin K. These clotting factors are biologically activated by the addition of carboxyl groups to key glutamic acid residues within the proteins' structure. In the process, "active" vitamin K is oxidatively converted to an "inactive" form, which is then subsequently reactivated by vitamin K epoxide reductase complex 1 (VKORC1). Warfarin competitively inhibits the subunit 1 of the multi-unit VKOR complex, thus depleting functional vitamin K reserves and hence reduces synthesis of active clotting factors.

Pharmacodynamics/Kinetics

Onset of action: Anticoagulation: Oral: 24-72 hours

Peak effect: Full therapeutic effect: 5-7 days; INR may increase in 36-72 hours

Duration: 2-5 days

Absorption: Oral: Rapid, complete

Distribution: 0.14 L/kg

Protein binding: 99%

Metabolism: Hepatic, primarily via CYP2C9; minor pathways include CYP2C8, 2C18, 2C19, 1A2, and 3A4

Genomic variants: Approximately 37% reduced clearance of S-warfarin in patients heterozygous for 2C9 (*1/*2 or *1/*3), and ~70% reduced in patients homozygous for reduced function alleles (*2/*2, *2/*3, or *3/*3)

Half-life elimination: 20-60 hours; Mean: 40 hours; highly variable among individuals

Time to peak, plasma: Oral: ~4 hours

Excretion: Urine (92%, primarily as metabolites)

Dosage Note: Labeling identifies genetic factors which may increase patient sensitivity to warfarin. Specifically, genetic variations in the proteins CYP2C9 and VKORC1, responsible for warfarin's primary metabolism and pharmacodynamic activity, respectively, have been identified as predisposing factors associated with decreased dose requirement and increased bleeding risk. Genotyping tests are available, and may provide guidance on initiation of anticoagulant therapy. The American College of Chest Physicians recommends against the use of routine pharmacogenomic testing to guide dosing (Guyatt, 2012). For management of elevated INRs as a result of warfarin therapy, see Additional Information for guidance.

Oral:

Infants and Children (off-label use): Initial loading dose (if baseline INR is 1-1.3): 0.2 mg/kg (maximum: 10 mg/dose); adjust dose based on INR (reported ranges to maintain INR of 2-3: 0.09-0.33 mg/kg/day). Infants <12 months of age may require doses at or near the high end of this range; consistent anticoagulation may be difficult to maintain in children <5 years of age (Monagle, 2012).

Adults: Initial dosing must be individualized. Consider the patient (hepatic function, cardiac function, age, nutritional status, concurrent therapy, risk of bleeding) in addition to prior dose response (if available) and the clinical situation. Start 2-5 mg once daily for 2 days **or** for healthy individuals, 10 mg once daily for 2 days; lower doses (eg, 5 mg once daily) recommended for patients with confirmed HIT once platelet recovery has occurred (Guyatt, 2012). In patients with acute venous thromboembolism, initiation may begin on the first or second day of low molecular weight heparin or unfractionated heparin therapy (Guyatt, 2012). Adjust dose according to INR results; usual maintenance dose ranges from 2-10 mg daily (individual patients may require loading and maintenance doses outside these general guidelines).

Note: Lower starting doses may be required for patients with hepatic impairment, poor nutrition, CHF, elderly, high risk of bleeding, or patients who are debilitated, or those with reduced function genomic variants of the catabolic enzymes CYP2C9 (*2 or *3 alleles) or VKORC1 (-1639 polymorphism); see table. Higher initial doses may be reasonable in selected patients (ie, receiving enzyme-inducing agents and with low risk of bleeding).

Range[1] of Expected Therapeutic Maintenance Dose Based on CYP2C9[2] and VKORC1[3] Genotypes

VKORC1	CYP2C9					
	*1/*1	*1/*2	*1/*3	*2/*2	*2/*3	*3/*3
GG	5-7 mg	5-7 mg	3-4 mg	3-4 mg	3-4 mg	0.5-2 mg
AG	5-7 mg	3-4 mg	3-4 mg	3-4 mg	0.5-2 mg	0.5-2 mg
AA	3-4 mg	3-4 mg	0.5-2 mg	0.5-2 mg	0.5-2 mg	0.5-2 mg

Note: Must also take into account other patient related factors when determining initial dose (eg, age, body weight, concomitant medications, comorbidities). The American College of Chest Physicians recommends against the use of routine pharmacogenomic testing to guide dosing (Guyatt, 2012).

[1]Ranges derived from multiple published clinical studies.

[2]Patients with CYP2C9 *1/*3, *2/*2, *2/*3, and *3/*3 alleles may take up to 4 weeks to achieve maximum INR with a given dose regimen.

[3]VKORC1 -1639G>A (rs 9923231) variant is used in this table; other VKORC1 variants may also be important determinants of dose.

IV: Adults: 2-5 mg/day administered as a slow bolus injection

Dosage adjustment in renal disease: No dosage adjustment necessary. However, patients with renal failure have an increased risk of bleeding complications; monitor closely.

Dosage adjustment in hepatic disease: No dosage adjustment provided in manufacturer's labeling. However, the response to oral anticoagulants may be markedly enhanced in obstructive jaundice, hepatitis, and cirrhosis. INR should be closely monitored.

Dietary Considerations Foods high in vitamin K (eg, leafy green vegetables) inhibit anticoagulant effect. The list of usual foods with high vitamin K content is well known, however, some unique ones include green tea (*Camellia sinensis*), chewing tobacco, a variety of oils (canola, corn, olive, peanut, safflower, sesame seed, soybean, and sunflower) (Booth, 1999; Kuykendall, 2004; Nutescu, 2011). Snack foods containing Olestra have 80 mcg of vitamin K added to each ounce (Harrell, 1999). Some natural products may contain hidden sources of vitamin K (Nutescu, 2006). Avoid drastic changes in diet (eg, intake of large amounts of alfalfa, asparagus, broccoli, Brussels sprouts, cabbage, cauliflower, green teas, kale, lettuce, spinach, turnip greens, watercress) which decrease efficacy of warfarin. A balanced diet with a consistent intake of vitamin K is essential. The recommended dietary allowance for vitamin K in adults is 75 to 120 mcg/day (USDA Dietary Reference Intake).

Administration

Oral: Administer with or without food. Take at the same time each day.

IV: Administer as a slow bolus injection over 1-2 minutes; avoid all IM injections

Hazardous agent; use appropriate precautions for handling and disposal (NIOSH 2014 [group 3]).

Monitoring Parameters Prothrombin time, hematocrit; INR (frequency varies depending on INR stability); may consider genotyping of CYP2C9 and VKORC1 prior to initiation of therapy, if available

Reference Range

INR = patient prothrombin time/mean normal prothrombin time

ISI = international sensitivity index

INR should be increased by 2-3.5 times depending upon indication. An INR >4 does not generally add additional therapeutic benefit and is associated with increased risk of bleeding. **Note:** To prevent gastrointestinal bleeding events in patients receiving the combination of warfarin, aspirin, and clopidogrel, an INR of 2-2.5 is recommended unless condition requires a higher INR target (eg, certain mechanical heart valves) (Bhatt, 2008).

Adult Target INR Ranges Based Upon Indication

Indication	Targeted INR	Targeted INR Range
Cardiac		
Anterior myocardial infarction with LV thrombus or high risk for LV thrombus (EF<40%, anteroapical wall motion abnormality)[1,2,3]	2.5	2-3
Atrial fibrillation (nonvalvular)[4] or atrial flutter	2.5	2-3
LV systolic dysfunction (without established CAD) (eg, Takotsubo cardiomyopathy) with an LV thrombus	2.5	2-3
Valvular		
Carbomedics or St. Jude Medical bileaflet or Medtronic Hall tilting disk mechanical aortic valve in normal sinus rhythm and normal LA size[5]	2.5	2-3
Bileaflet or tilting disk mechanical mitral valve[5]	3	2.5-3.5
Caged ball or caged disk mechanical valve[5]	3	2.5-3.5
Mechanical aortic valve[6]	2.5	2-3
Mechanical mitral valve **or** mechanical valves in both the aortic and mitral positions[6]	3	2.5-3.5
Bioprosthetic mitral valve[7]	2.5	2-3
Rheumatic mitral valve disease (particularly mitral stenosis) and normal sinus rhythm (LA diameter >5.5 cm), AF, previous systemic embolism, or LA thrombus	2.5	2-3
Thromboembolism Treatment		
Venous thromboembolism[8]	2.5	2-3
Thromboprophylaxis		
Idiopathic pulmonary artery hypertension (IPAH)[9]	2	1.5-2.5
Antiphospholipid syndrome (no other risk factors)	2.5	2-3
Antiphospholipid syndrome and recurrent thromboembolism	2.5	2-3
Total hip or knee replacement or hip fracture surgery[10]	2.5	2-3

(continued)

Adult Target INR Ranges Based Upon Indication *(continued)*

Indication	Targeted INR	Targeted INR Range
Other Indications		
Ischemic stroke due to AF[11]	2.5	2-3
Cryptogenic stroke (recurrent) and either patent foramen ovale (PFO) or atrial septal aneurysm	2.5	2-3

Note: Unless otherwise noted, all recommendations derived from "Antithrombotic Therapy and Prevention of Thrombosis, 9th ed: American College of Chest Physicians Evidence-Based Clinical Practice Guidelines."

[1]If coronary stent placed, triple therapy (warfarin, low-dose aspirin, and clopidogrel) is recommended for 1 month (bare-metal stent) or 3-6 months (drug-eluting stent) followed by discontinuation of warfarin and use of dual antiplatelet therapy (eg, aspirin and clopidogrel) for up to 12 months.

[2]If coronary stent **not** placed, maintain anticoagulation (in combination with low-dose aspirin) for 3 months followed by discontinuation of warfarin and use of dual antiplatelet therapy (eg, aspirin and clopidogrel) for up to 12 months.

[3]The ACCF/AHA guidelines for the management of STEMI, suggest that a lower INR range of 2-2.5 might be considered in patients with STEMI receiving dual antiplatelet therapy (O'Gara, 2013).

[4]Recommended for those patients with nonvalvular AF or atrial flutter with prior stroke, TIA, or a CHA_2DS_2-VASc score ≥2 (AHA/ACC/HRS [January, 2014]).

[5]Recommendation from Stein, 2001.

[6]If at low risk of bleeding, combine with aspirin 81 mg/day.

[7]Maintain anticoagulation for 3 months after valve insertion then switch to aspirin 81 mg/day if no other indications for warfarin exist or clinically reassess need for warfarin in patients with prior history of systemic embolism.

[8]Treat for 3 months in patients with provoked VTE due to transient reversible risk factor. Treat for a minimum of 3 months in patients with unprovoked VTE and evaluate for extended anticoagulant therapy (ie, >3 months of therapy without a scheduled stop date). Other risk groups (eg, cancer) may require extended anticoagulant therapy.

[9]Recommendation from the ACCF/AHA 2009 Expert Consensus Document on Pulmonary Hypertension (McLaughlin, 2009)

[10]Continue for at least 10-14 days; up to 35 days after surgery is suggested.

[11]Instead of adjusted dose warfarin, the use of dabigatran has been suggested. In either case, oral anticoagulation should be initiated within 1-2 weeks after stroke onset or earlier in patients at low bleeding risk; bridging with aspirin may be required.

Warfarin levels are not used for monitoring degree of anticoagulation. They may be useful if a patient with unexplained coagulopathy is using the drug surreptitiously or if it is unclear whether clinical resistance is due to true drug resistance or lack of drug intake.

Normal prothrombin time (PT): 10.9-12.9 seconds. Healthy premature newborns have prolonged coagulation test screening results (eg, PT, aPTT, TT) which return to normal adult values at approximately 6 months of age. Healthy prematures, however, do not develop spontaneous hemorrhage or thrombotic complications because of a balance between procoagulants and inhibitors.

Additional Information

Pharmacogenomic Testing: The American College of Chest Physicians recommends against the use of routine pharmacogenomic testing to guide dosing (Guyatt, 2012). However, prospective genotyping is available, and may provide guidance on initiation of anticoagulant therapy. Commercial testing with PGxPredict™: WARFARIN is available from PGxHealth™ (Division of Clinical Data, Inc, New Haven, CT). The test genotypes patients for presence of the CYP2C9*2 or *3 alleles and the VKORC1 -1639G>A polymorphism. The results of the test allow patients to be phenotyped as extensive, intermediate, or poor metabolizers (CYP2C9) and as low, intermediate, or high warfarin sensitivity (VKORC1). Ordering information is available at 888-592-7327 or warfarininfo@pgxhealth.com.

Management of Elevated INR:

If INR above therapeutic range to <4.5 (no evidence of bleeding): Lower or hold next dose and monitor frequently; when INR approaches desired range, resume dosing with a lower dose (Patriquin, 2011).

If INR 4.5-10 (no evidence of bleeding): The 2012 ACCP guidelines recommend against routine vitamin K administration in this setting (Guyatt, 2012). Previously, the 2008 ACCP guidelines recommended if no risk factors for bleeding exist, to omit next 1 or 2 doses, monitor INR more frequently, and resume with an appropriately adjusted dose when INR in desired range; may consider administering vitamin K orally 1-2.5 mg if other risk factors for bleeding exist (Hirsh, 2008). Others have recommended consideration of vitamin K 1 mg orally or 0.5 mg IV (Patriquin, 2011).

If INR >10 (no evidence of bleeding): The 2012 ACCP guidelines recommend administration of oral vitamin K (dose not specified) in this setting (Guyatt, 2012). Previously, the 2008 ACCP guidelines recommended to hold warfarin, administer vitamin K orally 2.5-5 mg, expect INR to be reduced within 24-48 hours, monitor INR more frequently and give additional vitamin K at an appropriate dose if necessary; resume warfarin at an appropriately adjusted dose when INR is in desired range (Hirsh, 2008). Others have recommended consideration of vitamin K 2-2.5 mg orally or 0.5-1 mg IV (Patriquin, 2011).

If minor bleeding at any INR elevation: Hold warfarin, may administer vitamin K orally 2.5-5 mg, monitor INR more frequently, may repeat dose after 24 hours if INR correction incomplete; resume warfarin at an appropriately adjusted dose when INR is in desired range (Patriquin, 2011).

If major bleeding at any INR elevation: The 2012 ACCP guidelines recommend administration of four-factor prothrombin complex concentrate (PCC) and IV vitamin K 5-10 mg in this setting (Guyatt, 2012). Four-factor PCCs include Beriplex P/N, Cofact, Kcentra (available in U.S.), or Octaplex (available in Canada). Previously, the 2008 ACCP guidelines recommended to hold warfarin, administer vitamin K 10 mg by slow IV infusion and supplement with PCC depending on the urgency of the situation; IV vitamin K may be repeated every 12 hours (Hirsh, 2008).

Note: Use of high doses of vitamin K (eg, 10-15 mg) may cause warfarin resistance for ≥1 week. During this period of resistance, heparin or low-molecular-weight heparin (LMWH) may be given until INR responds.

Dosage Forms

Tablet, Oral:

Coumadin: 1 mg, 2 mg, 2.5 mg, 3 mg, 4 mg, 5 mg, 6 mg, 7.5 mg, 10 mg

Jantoven: 1 mg, 2 mg, 2.5 mg, 3 mg, 4 mg, 5 mg, 6 mg, 7.5 mg, 10 mg

Generic: 1 mg, 2 mg, 2.5 mg, 3 mg, 4 mg, 5 mg, 6 mg, 7.5 mg, 10 mg

◆ **Warfarin Sodium** *see* Warfarin *on page 2186*

◆ **4-Way Saline [OTC]** *see* Sodium Chloride *on page 1902*

◆ **WC-rBS** *see* Travelers' Diarrhea and Cholera Vaccine [CAN/INT] *on page 2088*

◆ **Welchol** *see* Colesevelam *on page 503*

◆ **Wellbutrin** *see* BuPROPion *on page 305*

◆ **Wellbutrin XL** *see* BuPROPion *on page 305*

◆ **Wellbutrin SR** *see* BuPROPion *on page 305*

◆ **Wera** *see* Ethinyl Estradiol and Norethindrone *on page 808*

◆ **Westcort** *see* Hydrocortisone (Topical) *on page 1014*

◆ **Westcort® (Can)** *see* Hydrocortisone (Topical) *on page 1014*

◆ **Westhroid** *see* Thyroid, Desiccated *on page 2031*

◆ **Westhroid-P [DSC]** *see* Thyroid, Desiccated *on page 2031*

Wheat Dextrin (weet DEKS trin)

Brand Names: U.S. Benefiber Drink Mix [OTC]; Benefiber For Children [OTC]; Benefiber Plus Calcium [OTC]; Benefiber [OTC]

Index Terms Dextrin; Resistant Dextrin; Resistant Maltodextrin

Pharmacologic Category Fiber Supplement; Laxative, Bulk-Producing

Use OTC labeling: Dietary fiber supplement

Dosage Oral: General dosing guidelines; consult specific product labeling.

Adequate intake for total fiber: **Note:** The definition of "fiber" varies; however, the soluble fiber in wheat dextrin is only one type of fiber which makes up the daily recommended intake of total fiber.

Children 1-3 years: 19 g/day
Children 4-8 years: 25 g/day
Children 9-13 years: Male: 31 g/day; Female: 26 g/day
Children 14-18 years: Male: 38 g/day; Female: 26 g/day
Adults 19-50 years: Male: 38 g/day; Female: 25 g/day
Adults ≥51 years: Male: 30 g/day; Female: 21 g/day
Pregnancy: 28 g/day
Lactation: 29 g/day

Additional Information Complete prescribing information should be consulted for additional detail.

Dosage Forms

Packet, Oral:
Benefiber Drink Mix [OTC]: (8 ea, 16 ea, 24 ea, 28 ea)

Powder, Oral:
Benefiber [OTC]: (80 g, 155 g, 245 g, 267 g, 350 g, 477 g, 529 g, 730 g)
Benefiber For Children [OTC]: (155 g)
Benefiber Plus Calcium [OTC]: (305 g, 423.8 g)

Tablet, Oral:
Benefiber [OTC]:

Tablet Chewable, Oral:
Benefiber [OTC]:
Benefiber Plus Calcium [OTC]:

- **Wilate** *see* Antihemophilic Factor/von Willebrand Factor Complex (Human) *on page 154*
- **Winpred (Can)** *see* PredniSONE *on page 1706*
- **WinRho SDF** *see* Rh_o(D) Immune Globulin *on page 1794*
- **Woman's Laxative [OTC] (Can)** *see* Bisacodyl *on page 265*
- **Womens Laxative [OTC]** *see* Bisacodyl *on page 265*
- **Wound Wash Saline [OTC]** *see* Sodium Chloride *on page 1902*
- **WP Thyroid** *see* Thyroid, Desiccated *on page 2031*
- **WR-2721** *see* Amifostine *on page 109*
- **WR-139007** *see* Dacarbazine *on page 549*
- **WR-139013** *see* Chlorambucil *on page 419*
- **WR-139021** *see* Carmustine *on page 364*
- **Wycillin** *see* Penicillin G Procaine *on page 1613*
- **Wycillin® (Can)** *see* Penicillin G Procaine *on page 1613*
- **Wymzya Fe** *see* Ethinyl Estradiol and Norethindrone *on page 808*
- **Xalacom (Can)** *see* Latanoprost and Timolol [CAN/INT] *on page 1172*
- **Xalatan** *see* Latanoprost *on page 1172*
- **Xalkori** *see* Crizotinib *on page 511*
- **Xanax** *see* ALPRAZolam *on page 94*
- **Xanax® (Can)** *see* ALPRAZolam *on page 94*
- **Xanax TS™ (Can)** *see* ALPRAZolam *on page 94*
- **Xanax XR** *see* ALPRAZolam *on page 94*
- **Xarelto** *see* Rivaroxaban *on page 1830*
- **Xarelto Starter Pack** *see* Rivaroxaban *on page 1830*
- **Xartemis XR** *see* Oxycodone and Acetaminophen *on page 1541*
- **Xatral (Can)** *see* Alfuzosin *on page 84*
- **Xeljanz** *see* Tofacitinib *on page 2059*
- **Xeloda** *see* Capecitabine *on page 339*
- **Xenaderm®** *see* Trypsin, Balsam Peru, and Castor Oil *on page 2109*
- **Xenazine** *see* Tetrabenazine *on page 2016*
- **Xenical** *see* Orlistat *on page 1520*
- **Xeomin** *see* IncobotulinumtoxinA *on page 1062*
- **Xeomin® (Can)** *see* IncobotulinumtoxinA *on page 1062*
- **Xeomin Cosmetic™ (Can)** *see* IncobotulinumtoxinA *on page 1062*
- **Xgeva** *see* Denosumab *on page 589*
- **Xiaflex** *see* Collagenase (Systemic) *on page 506*
- **Xifaxan** *see* Rifaximin *on page 1809*
- **Xigduo XR** *see* Dapagliflozin and Metformin *on page 561*
- **Xilep** *see* Rufinamide *on page 1854*
- **Ximino™** *see* Minocycline *on page 1371*

Xipamide [INT] (ZI pa mide)

International Brand Names Aquaphoril (AT, PY); Diurexan (GB, KR, PT); Xipamid (IN)

Pharmacologic Category Diuretic, Thiazide

Reported Use Treatment of edema; hypertension

Dosage Range Adults: Oral:

Edema: Initial: 40 mg in the morning; may increase to 80 mg in resistant cases; maintenance dose: 20 mg in the morning

Hypertension: 20 mg in the morning

Product Availability Product available in various countries; not currently available in the U.S.

Dosage Forms

Tablet: 20 mg

- **Xodol 5/300** *see* Hydrocodone and Acetaminophen *on page 1012*
- **Xodol 7.5/300** *see* Hydrocodone and Acetaminophen *on page 1012*
- **Xodol 10/300** *see* Hydrocodone and Acetaminophen *on page 1012*
- **Xolair** *see* Omalizumab *on page 1503*
- **Xolegel** *see* Ketoconazole (Topical) *on page 1145*
- **Xolido XP [OTC]** *see* Lidocaine (Topical) *on page 1211*
- **Xolox [DSC]** *see* Oxycodone and Acetaminophen *on page 1541*
- **Xopenex** *see* Levalbuterol *on page 1189*
- **Xopenex Concentrate** *see* Levalbuterol *on page 1189*
- **Xopenex HFA** *see* Levalbuterol *on page 1189*
- **XP13512** *see* Gabapentin Enacarbil *on page 946*
- **Xpect [OTC]** *see* GuaiFENesin *on page 986*
- **X-Pur Chlorhexidine (Can)** *see* Chlorhexidine Gluconate *on page 422*
- **XRP6258** *see* Cabazitaxel *on page 316*
- **Xtandi** *see* Enzalutamide *on page 733*
- **Xtra-Care [OTC]** *see* Vitamin E *on page 2174*
- **Xulane** *see* Ethinyl Estradiol and Norelgestromin *on page 807*
- **X-Viate** *see* Urea *on page 2114*
- **Xylac (Can)** *see* Loxapine *on page 1255*
- **Xylocaine** *see* Lidocaine (Systemic) *on page 1208*
- **Xylocaine** *see* Lidocaine (Topical) *on page 1211*
- **Xylocaine (Cardiac)** *see* Lidocaine (Systemic) *on page 1208*
- **Xylocaine-MPF** *see* Lidocaine (Systemic) *on page 1208*
- **Xylocaine® MPF With Epinephrine** *see* Lidocaine and Epinephrine *on page 1212*
- **Xylocaine Viscous** *see* Lidocaine (Topical) *on page 1211*

- ◆ **Xylocaine® With Epinephrine** *see* Lidocaine and Epinephrine *on page 1212*
- ◆ **Xylocard (Can)** *see* Lidocaine (Systemic) *on page 1208*
- ◆ **Xyntha** *see* Antihemophilic Factor (Recombinant) *on page 152*
- ◆ **Xyntha Solofuse** *see* Antihemophilic Factor (Recombinant) *on page 152*
- ◆ **Xyrem** *see* Sodium Oxybate *on page 1908*
- ◆ **Xyzal** *see* Levocetirizine *on page 1196*
- ◆ **Yasmin** *see* Ethinyl Estradiol and Drospirenone *on page 801*
- ◆ **Yaz** *see* Ethinyl Estradiol and Drospirenone *on page 801*
- ◆ **Yaz Plus (Can)** *see* Ethinyl Estradiol, Drospirenone, and Levomefolate *on page 812*

Yellow Fever Vaccine (YEL oh FEE ver vak SEEN)

Brand Names: U.S. YF-VAX
Brand Names: Canada YF-VAX
Pharmacologic Category Vaccine, Live (Viral)
Additional Appendix Information

Immunization Administration Recommendations *on page 2250*

Immunization Recommendations *on page 2255*

Use Induction of active immunity against yellow fever virus, primarily among persons traveling or living in areas where yellow fever infection exists and laboratory workers who may be exposed to the virus; vaccination may also be required for some international travelers

The Advisory Committee on Immunization Practices (ACIP) (CDC, 2010) recommends vaccination for:

- Persons traveling to or living in areas at risk for yellow fever transmission
- Persons traveling to countries which require vaccination for international travel
- Laboratory personnel who may be exposed to the yellow fever virus or concentrated preparations of the vaccine

Although the vaccine is approved for use in children ≥9 months of age, the CDC recommends use in children as young as 6 months under unusual circumstances (eg, travel to an area where exposure is unavoidable). Children <6 months of age should **never** receive the vaccine.

Pregnancy Risk Factor C

Dosage SubQ:

Children ≥6 months (off-label use): One dose (0.5 mL) ≥10 days before travel; Booster: Every 10 years for those at continued risk of exposure (CDC, 2010)

Children ≥9 months (per manufacturer), Adolescents, and Adults: One dose (0.5 mL) ≥10 days before travel; Booster: Every 10 years for those at continued risk of exposure

Note: Based on currently available data, the World Health Organization (WHO) has determined that vaccine failure is rare and booster doses are not needed. Future studies may determine if there are specific risk groups who could benefit from a booster dose (WHO, 2013).

Elderly: Monitor closely due to an increased incidence of serious adverse events in patients ≥60 years of age, particularly in patients receiving their first dose. The ACIP guidelines note that if travel is unavoidable, the decision to vaccinate travelers ≥60 years should be made after weighing the risks vs benefits (CDC, 2010).

Dosage adjustment in renal impairment: No dosage adjustment provided in manufacturer's labeling.

Dosage adjustment in hepatic impairment: No dosage adjustment provided in manufacturer's labeling.

Additional Information Complete prescribing information should be consulted for additional detail.

Dosage Forms

Injection, powder for reconstitution [17D-204 strain]:

YF-VAX®: ≥4.74 Log_{10} plaque-forming units (PFU) per 0.5 mL dose

- ◆ **Yervoy** *see* Ipilimumab *on page 1106*
- ◆ **Yervoy® (Can)** *see* Ipilimumab *on page 1106*
- ◆ **YF-VAX** *see* Yellow Fever Vaccine *on page 2192*
- ◆ **YM087** *see* Conivaptan *on page 507*
- ◆ **YM-178** *see* Mirabegron *on page 1375*
- ◆ **YM905** *see* Solifenacin *on page 1917*
- ◆ **YM-08310** *see* Amifostine *on page 109*
- ◆ **Yodoxin** *see* Iodoquinol *on page 1105*
- ◆ **Z4942** *see* Ifosfamide *on page 1040*
- ◆ **Zactima** *see* Vandetanib *on page 2135*
- ◆ **Zaditen® (Can)** *see* Ketotifen (Systemic) [CAN/INT] *on page 1149*
- ◆ **Zaditor [OTC]** *see* Ketotifen (Ophthalmic) *on page 1150*
- ◆ **Zaditor® (Can)** *see* Ketotifen (Ophthalmic) *on page 1150*

Zafirlukast (za FIR loo kast)

Brand Names: U.S. Accolate
Brand Names: Canada Accolate®
Index Terms ICI-204,219
Pharmacologic Category Leukotriene-Receptor Antagonist
Use Prophylaxis and chronic treatment of asthma
Pregnancy Risk Factor B
Pregnancy Considerations Adverse events were not observed in animal reproduction studies except with doses that were also maternally toxic. Based on limited data, an increased risk of teratogenic effects has not been observed with zafirlukast use in pregnancy (Bakhireva, 2007). Uncontrolled asthma is associated with adverse events on pregnancy (increased risk of perinatal mortality, pre-eclampsia, preterm birth, low birth weight infants). Zafirlukast may be considered for use in women who had a favorable response prior to becoming pregnant; however, initiating a leukotriene receptor antagonist during pregnancy is an alternative (but not preferred) treatment option for mild persistent asthma (NAEPP, 2005).

Breast-Feeding Considerations Zafirlukast is excreted into breast milk. In women receiving zafirlukast 40 mg twice daily, maternal serum concentrations were 225 ng/mL and breast milk concentrations were 50 ng/mL. Due to the potential for adverse reactions in the nursing infant, breast-feeding is not recommended by the manufacturer.

Contraindications Hypersensitivity to zafirlukast or any component of the formulation; hepatic impairment (including hepatic cirrhosis)

Canadian labeling: Additional contraindications (not in U.S. labeling): Patients in whom zafirlukast was discontinued due to treatment related hepatotoxicity

Warnings/Precautions Zafirlukast is not approved for use in the reversal of bronchospasm in acute asthma attacks, including status asthmaticus. Therapy with zafirlukast can be continued during acute exacerbations of asthma.

Hepatic adverse events (including hepatitis, hyperbilirubinemia, and hepatic failure) have been reported; female patients may be at greater risk. Periodic testing of liver function may be considered (early detection coupled with therapy discontinuation is generally believed to improve the likelihood of recovery). Advise patients to be alert for and to immediately report symptoms (eg, anorexia, right upper quadrant abdominal pain, nausea). If hepatic dysfunction is suspected (due to clinical signs/symptoms), discontinue use immediately and measure liver function tests (particularly ALT); resolution observed in most but not all cases upon discontinuation of therapy. Do not resume or restart if hepatic function studies indicate dysfunction. Use in patients with hepatic impairment (including hepatic cirrhosis) is contraindicated. Postmarketing reports of behavioral changes (ie, depression, insomnia) have been noted. Instruct patients to report neuropsychiatric symptoms/events during therapy.

Monitor INR closely with concomitant warfarin use. Rare cases of eosinophilic vasculitis (Churg-Strauss) have been reported in patients receiving zafirlukast (usually, but not always, associated with reduction in concurrent steroid dosage). No causal relationship established. Monitor for eosinophilic vasculitis, rash, pulmonary symptoms, cardiac symptoms, or neuropathy.

Clearance is decreased in elderly patients; C_{max} and AUC are increased approximately two- to threefold in adults ≥65 years compared to younger adults; however, no dosage adjustments are recommended in this age group. An increased proportion of zafirlukast patients >55 years of age reported infections as compared to placebo-treated patients. These infections were mostly mild or moderate in intensity and predominantly affected the respiratory tract. Infections occurred equally in both sexes, were dose-proportional to total milligrams of zafirlukast exposure, and were associated with coadministration of inhaled corticosteroids.

Adverse Reactions

Central nervous system: Dizziness, fever, headache, pain
Gastrointestinal: Abdominal pain, diarrhea, dyspepsia, nausea, vomiting
Hepatic: ALT increased
Neuromuscular & skeletal: Back pain, myalgia, weakness
Miscellaneous: Infection
Rare but important or life-threatening: Agranulocytosis, angioedema, arthralgia, bleeding, bruising, depression, edema, eosinophilia (systemic), eosinophilic pneumonia, hepatic failure, hepatitis, hyperbilirubinemia, hypersensitivity reactions, insomnia, malaise, pruritus, rash, urticaria, vasculitis with clinical features of Churg-Strauss syndrome (rare)

Drug Interactions

Metabolism/Transport Effects Substrate of CYP2C9 (major); **Note:** Assignment of Major/Minor substrate status based on clinically relevant drug interaction potential; **Inhibits** CYP1A2 (weak), CYP2C19 (weak), CYP2C8 (weak), CYP2C9 (moderate), CYP2D6 (weak), CYP3A4 (weak)

Avoid Concomitant Use

Avoid concomitant use of Zafirlukast with any of the following: Pimozide

Increased Effect/Toxicity

Zafirlukast may increase the levels/effects of: ARIPiprazole; Bosentan; Cannabis; Carvedilol; CYP2C9 Substrates; Dofetilide; Dronabinol; Hydrocodone; Lomitapide; Pimozide; Tetrahydrocannabinol; Theophylline Derivatives; Vitamin K Antagonists

The levels/effects of Zafirlukast may be increased by: Ceritinib; CYP2C9 Inhibitors (Moderate); CYP2C9 Inhibitors (Strong); Mifepristone

Decreased Effect

The levels/effects of Zafirlukast may be decreased by: CYP2C9 Inducers (Strong); Dabrafenib; Erythromycin (Systemic); Theophylline Derivatives

Food Interactions Food decreases bioavailability of zafirlukast by 40%. Management: Take on an empty stomach 1 hour before or 2 hours after meals.

Storage/Stability Store tablets at controlled room temperature of 20°C to 25°C (68°F to 77°F). Protect from light and moisture; dispense in original airtight container.

Mechanism of Action Zafirlukast is a selectively and competitive leukotriene-receptor antagonist (LTRA) of leukotriene D4 and E4 (LTD4 and LTE4), components of slow-reacting substance of anaphylaxis (SRSA). Cysteinyl leukotriene production and receptor occupation have been correlated with the pathophysiology of asthma, including airway edema, smooth muscle constriction, and altered cellular activity associated with the inflammatory process, which contribute to the signs and symptoms of asthma.

Pharmacodynamics/Kinetics

Distribution: V_{dss}: ~70 L
Protein binding: >99%, primarily to albumin
Metabolism: Extensively hepatic via CYP2C9
Bioavailability: Reduced 40% with food
Half-life elimination: ~10 hours
Time to peak, serum: 3 hours
Excretion: Feces (~90%); Urine (~10%)

Dosage Oral:

U.S. labeling:
Children 5-11 years: 10 mg twice daily
Children ≥12 years and Adults: 20 mg twice daily
Canadian labeling: Children ≥12 years and Adults: 20 mg twice daily
Elderly: Refer to adult dosing.

Dosage adjustment in renal impairment: No dosage adjustment necessary.

Dosage adjustment in hepatic impairment: Use is contraindicated.

Dietary Considerations Should be taken on an empty stomach (1 hour before or 2 hours after meals).

Administration Administer at least 1 hour before or 2 hours after a meal.

Monitoring Parameters Monitor for improvements in air flow; monitor closely for sign/symptoms of hepatic injury; periodic monitoring of LFTs may be considered (not proved to prevent serious injury, but early detection may enhance recovery)

Dosage Forms

Tablet, Oral:
Accolate: 10 mg, 20 mg
Generic: 10 mg, 20 mg

Zaleplon (ZAL e plon)

Brand Names: U.S. Sonata

Pharmacologic Category Hypnotic, Miscellaneous

Additional Appendix Information

Beers Criteria – Potentially Inappropriate Medications for Geriatrics *on page 2271*

Use Insomnia: Short-term treatment of insomnia.

Pregnancy Risk Factor C

Dosage Insomnia: Oral:

Adults: Usual dosage: 10 mg immediately before bedtime (range: 5 to 20 mg); 5 mg may be sufficient for certain low weight patients (maximum dose: 20 mg daily). Has been used for up to 5 weeks of treatment in controlled trial setting.
Debilitated patients: Usual dosage: 5 mg immediately before bedtime (maximum dose: 10 mg daily)
Elderly: Usual dosage: 5 mg immediately before bedtime (maximum dose: 10 mg daily)

Concomitant therapy: 5 mg initially should be given to patients concomitantly taking cimetidine.

Dosage adjustment in renal impairment:
Mild to moderate impairment: No dosage adjustment necessary.

Severe impairment: There are no dosage adjustments provided in the manufacturer's labeling (has not been studied).

Dosage adjustment in hepatic impairment:

Mild to moderate impairment: 5 mg immediately before bedtime

Severe impairment: Use is not recommended.

Additional Information Complete prescribing information should be consulted for additional detail.

Dosage Forms

Capsule, Oral:

Sonata: 5 mg, 10 mg

Generic: 5 mg, 10 mg

◆ **Zaltrap** *see* Ziv-Aflibercept (Systemic) *on page 2204*

◆ **Zamicet [DSC]** *see* Hydrocodone and Acetaminophen *on page 1012*

◆ **Zamine (Can)** *see* Ethinyl Estradiol and Drospirenone *on page 801*

◆ **Zanaflex** *see* TiZANidine *on page 2051*

Zanamivir (za NA mi veer)

Brand Names: U.S. Relenza Diskhaler

Brand Names: Canada Relenza®

Pharmacologic Category Antiviral Agent; Neuraminidase Inhibitor

Use Treatment of uncomplicated acute illness due to influenza virus A and B in patients who have been symptomatic for no more than 2 days; prophylaxis against influenza virus A and B

The Advisory Committee on Immunization Practices (ACIP) recommends that **treatment** be considered for the following:

- Persons with severe, complicated or progressive illness
- Hospitalized persons
- Persons at higher risk for influenza complications:
  - Children <2 years of age (highest risk in children <6 months of age)
  - Adults ≥65 years of age
  - Persons with chronic disorders of the pulmonary (including asthma) or cardiovascular systems (except hypertension)
  - Persons with chronic metabolic diseases (including diabetes mellitus), hepatic disease, renal dysfunction, hematologic disorders (including sickle cell disease), or immunosuppression (including immunosuppression caused by medications or HIV)
  - Persons with neurologic/neuromuscular conditions (including conditions such as spinal cord injuries, seizure disorders, cerebral palsy, stroke, mental retardation, moderate to severe developmental delay, or muscular dystrophy) which may compromise respiratory function, the handling of respiratory secretions, or that can increase the risk of aspiration
  - Pregnant or postpartum women (≤2 weeks after delivery)
  - Persons <19 years of age on long-term aspirin therapy
  - American Indians and Alaskan Natives
  - Persons who are morbidly obese (BMI ≥40)
  - Residents of nursing homes or other chronic care facilities
- Use may also be considered for previously healthy, nonhigh-risk outpatients with confirmed or suspected influenza based on clinical judgment when treatment can be started within 48 hours of illness onset.

The ACIP recommends that **prophylaxis** be considered for the following:

- Postexposure prophylaxis may be considered for family or close contacts of suspected or confirmed cases, who are at higher risk of influenza complications, and who have not been vaccinated against the circulating strain at the time of the exposure.
- Postexposure prophylaxis may be considered for unvaccinated healthcare workers who had occupational exposure without protective equipment.
- Pre-exposure prophylaxis should only be used for persons at very high risk of influenza complications who cannot be otherwise protected at times of high risk for exposure.
- Prophylaxis should also be administered to all eligible residents of institutions that house patients at high risk when needed to control outbreaks.

Pregnancy Risk Factor C

Pregnancy Considerations Adverse events were not observed in animal reproduction studies. An increased risk of adverse neonatal or maternal outcomes has not been observed following use of zanamivir during pregnancy. Untreated influenza infection is associated with an increased risk of adverse events to the fetus and an increased risk of complications or death to the mother. Neuraminidase inhibitors are currently recommended for the treatment or prophylaxis of influenza in pregnant women and women up to 2 weeks postpartum (CDC 60 [1], 2011; CDC March 13, 2014; January 2015).

Breast-Feeding Considerations It is not known if zanamivir is found in human milk and the manufacturer recommends that caution be exercised when administering zanamivir to nursing women. Influenza may cause serious illness in postpartum women and prompt evaluation for febrile respiratory illnesses is recommended (Louie, 2011).

Contraindications Hypersensitivity to zanamivir or any component of the formulation (contains milk proteins)

Warnings/Precautions Allergic-like reactions, including anaphylaxis, oropharyngeal edema, and serious skin rashes have been reported. Rare occurrences of neuropsychiatric events (including confusion, delirium, hallucinations, and/or self-injury) have been reported from postmarketing surveillance; direct causation is difficult to establish (influenza infection may also be associated with behavioral and neurologic changes). Patients must be instructed in the use of the delivery system. Antiviral treatment should begin within 48 hours of symptom onset. However, the CDC recommends that treatment may still be beneficial and should be started in hospitalized patients with severe, complicated or progressive illness if >48 hours. Treatment should not be delayed while awaiting results of laboratory tests for influenza. Nonhospitalized persons who are not at high risk for developing severe or complicated illness and who have a mild disease are not likely to benefit if treatment is started >48 hours after symptom onset. Nonhospitalized persons who are already beginning to recover do not need treatment. Effectiveness has not been established in patients with significant underlying medical conditions or for prophylaxis of influenza in nursing home patients (per manufacturer). The CDC recommends zanamivir to be used to control institutional outbreaks of influenza when circulating strains are suspected of being resistant to oseltamivir (refer to current guidelines). Not recommended for use in patients with underlying respiratory disease, such as asthma or COPD, due to lack of efficacy and risk of serious adverse effects. Bronchospasm, decreased lung function, and other serious adverse reactions, including those with fatal outcomes, have been reported in patients with and without airway disease; discontinue with bronchospasm or signs of decreased lung function. For a patient with an underlying airway disease where a medical decision has been made to use zanamivir, a fast-acting bronchodilator should be made available, and used prior to each dose. Not a substitute for annual flu vaccination; has not been shown to reduce risk of transmission of influenza to others. Consider primary or concomitant bacterial infections. Powder for oral inhalation contains lactose; use contraindicated in patients allergic to milk proteins. The inhalation powder should only be administered via inhalation using the provided Diskhaler® delivery device. The commercially available formulation is **not** intended to be solubilized or administered via any nebulizer/mechanical ventilator; inappropriate administration has resulted in death. Safety and efficacy of repeated courses or use with hepatic impairment or severe renal impairment have not been established. Indicated for children ≥5 years of age (for influenza prophylaxis) and children ≥7 years of age (for influenza treatment); children ages 5-6 years may have inadequate inhalation (via Diskhaler®) for the treatment of influenza.

Adverse Reactions

Central nervous system: Dizziness, fatigue, fever/chills, headache, malaise

Dermatologic: Urticaria

Gastrointestinal: Abdominal pain, anorexia, appetite decreased, diarrhea, nausea, throat/tonsil discomfort/pain, vomiting

Neuromuscular & skeletal: Arthralgia, articular rheumatism, muscle pain, musculoskeletal pain

Respiratory: Bronchitis, cough, infection, nasal inflammation, nasal signs and symptoms, sinusitis

Miscellaneous: Viral infection

Rare but important or life-threatening: Allergic or allergic-like reaction (including oropharyngeal edema), arrhythmia, bronchospasm, consciousness altered, delusions, dyspnea, hallucinations, neuropsychiatric events (self-injury, confusion, delirium), nightmares, rash (including serious cutaneous reactions [eg, erythema multiforme, Stevens-Johnson syndrome, toxic epidermal necrolysis]), seizure, syncope

Drug Interactions

Metabolism/Transport Effects None known.

Avoid Concomitant Use There are no known interactions where it is recommended to avoid concomitant use.

Increased Effect/Toxicity There are no known significant interactions involving an increase in effect.

Decreased Effect

Zanamivir may decrease the levels/effects of: Influenza Virus Vaccine (Live/Attenuated)

Storage/Stability Store at 25°C (77°F); excursions permitted to 15°C to 30°C (59°F to 86°F). Do not puncture blister until taking a dose using the Diskhaler®.

Mechanism of Action Zanamivir inhibits influenza virus neuraminidase enzymes, potentially altering virus particle aggregation and release.

Pharmacodynamics/Kinetics

Absorption: Inhalation: Systemic: ~4% to 17%

Protein binding, plasma: <10%

Metabolism: None

Half-life elimination, serum: 2.5-5.1 hours; Mild-to-moderate renal impairment: 4.7 hours; Severe renal impairment: 18.5 hours

Time to peak, plasma: 1-2 hours

Excretion: Urine (as unchanged drug); feces (unabsorbed drug)

Dosage Oral inhalation: Influenza virus A and B:

Manufacturer's recommendations:

Prophylaxis, household setting: Children ≥5 years and Adults: Two inhalations (10 mg) once daily for 10 days. Begin within 36 hours following onset of signs or symptoms of index case.

Prophylaxis, community outbreak: Adolescents and Adults: Two inhalations (10 mg) once daily for 28 days. Begin within 5 days of outbreak.

Treatment: Children ≥7 years and Adults: Two inhalations (10 mg total) twice daily for 5 days. Doses on first day should be separated by at least 2 hours; on subsequent days, doses should be spaced by ~12 hours. Begin within 2 days of signs or symptoms. Longer treatment may be considered for patients who remain severely ill after 5 days.

Alternate recommendations:

Prophylaxis (household exposure, CDC, 2012): Children ≥5 years and Adults: Two inhalations (10 mg) once daily for 7 days after last known exposure

Prophylaxis (institutional outbreak, CDC, 2012): Children ≥5 years and Adults: Two inhalations (10 mg) once daily; continue for ≥2 weeks and until ~7 days after identification of illness onset in the last patient. Zanamivir is to be used to control institutional outbreaks of influenza when circulating strains are suspected of being resistant to oseltamivir.

Prophylaxis (community outbreak, IDSA/PIDS, 2011): Children ≥5 years and Adults: Two inhalations (10 mg) once daily; continue until influenza activity in community subsides or immunity obtained from immunization; up to 28 days has been well tolerated (CDC, 2011)

Dosage adjustment for renal impairment: Adjustment not necessary following a 5-day course of treatment due to low systemic absorption; however the potential for drug accumulation should be considered.

Dosage adjustment in hepatic impairment: No dosage adjustment provided in manufacturer's labeling (has not been studied).

Administration Inhalation: Must be used with Diskhaler® delivery device. The foil blister disk containing zanamivir inhalation powder should not be manipulated, solubilized, or administered via a nebulizer. Patients who are scheduled to use an inhaled bronchodilator should use their bronchodilator prior to zanamivir. With the exception of the initial dose when used for treatment, administer at the same time each day.

Additional Information Majority of patients included in clinical trials were infected with influenza A, however, a number of patients with influenza B infections were also enrolled. Patients with lower temperature or less severe symptoms appeared to derive less benefit from therapy. No consistent treatment benefit was demonstrated in patients with chronic underlying medical conditions.

The absence of symptoms does not rule out viral influenza infection and clinical judgment should guide the decision for therapy. Treatment should not be delayed while waiting for the results of diagnostic tests. Treatment should be considered for high-risk patients with symptoms despite a negative rapid influenza test when the illness cannot be contributed to another cause. Use of zanamivir is not a substitute for vaccination (when available); susceptibility to influenza infection returns once therapy is discontinued.

Dosage Forms

Aerosol Powder Breath Activated, Inhalation:

Relenza Diskhaler: 5 mg/blister (20 ea)

- ◆ **Zantac** *see* Ranitidine *on page 1777*
- ◆ **Zantac 75 [OTC]** *see* Ranitidine *on page 1777*
- ◆ **Zantac 75 (Can)** *see* Ranitidine *on page 1777*
- ◆ **Zantac 150 Maximum Strength [OTC]** *see* Ranitidine *on page 1777*
- ◆ **Zantac Maximum Strength Non-Prescription (Can)** *see* Ranitidine *on page 1777*
- ◆ **Zarah** *see* Ethinyl Estradiol and Drospirenone *on page 801*
- ◆ **Zarontin** *see* Ethosuximide *on page 813*
- ◆ **Zarontin® (Can)** *see* Ethosuximide *on page 813*
- ◆ **Zaroxolyn [DSC]** *see* Metolazone *on page 1348*
- ◆ **Zaroxolyn (Can)** *see* Metolazone *on page 1348*

- ♦ **Zavesca** *see* Miglustat *on page 1367*
- ♦ **Zazole** *see* Terconazole *on page 2006*
- ♦ **Z-chlopenthixol** *see* Zuclopenthixol [CAN/INT] *on page 2219*
- ♦ **Z-Cof 1 [OTC] [DSC]** *see* Guaifenesin, Pseudoephedrine, and Dextromethorphan *on page 989*
- ♦ **Z-Cof 12 DM [OTC] [DSC]** *see* Guaifenesin, Pseudoephedrine, and Dextromethorphan *on page 989*
- ♦ **ZD1033** *see* Anastrozole *on page 148*
- ♦ **ZD1694** *see* Raltitrexed [CAN/INT] *on page 1769*
- ♦ **ZD1839** *see* Gefitinib [CAN/INT] *on page 950*
- ♦ **ZD6474** *see* Vandetanib *on page 2135*
- ♦ **ZD9238** *see* Fulvestrant *on page 939*
- ♦ **ZDV** *see* Zidovudine *on page 2196*
- ♦ **ZDV, Abacavir, and Lamivudine** *see* Abacavir, Lamivudine, and Zidovudine *on page 22*
- ♦ **ZDX** *see* Goserelin *on page 981*
- ♦ **Zeasorb-AF [OTC]** *see* Miconazole (Topical) *on page 1360*
- ♦ **Zebeta** *see* Bisoprolol *on page 266*
- ♦ **Zebutal** *see* Butalbital, Acetaminophen, and Caffeine *on page 313*
- ♦ **Zecuity** *see* SUMAtriptan *on page 1953*
- ♦ **Zegerid** *see* Omeprazole and Sodium Bicarbonate *on page 1511*
- ♦ **Zegerid OTC [OTC]** *see* Omeprazole and Sodium Bicarbonate *on page 1511*
- ♦ **Zelapar** *see* Selegiline *on page 1873*
- ♦ **Zelboraf** *see* Vemurafenib *on page 2148*
- ♦ **Zeldox** *see* Ziprasidone *on page 2201*
- ♦ **Zemplar** *see* Paricalcitol *on page 1577*
- ♦ **Zemuron** *see* Rocuronium *on page 1838*
- ♦ **Zemuron® (Can)** *see* Rocuronium *on page 1838*
- ♦ **Zenatane** *see* ISOtretinoin *on page 1127*
- ♦ **Zenchent** *see* Ethinyl Estradiol and Norethindrone *on page 808*
- ♦ **Zenchent Fe** *see* Ethinyl Estradiol and Norethindrone *on page 808*
- ♦ **Zencia** *see* Sulfur and Sulfacetamide *on page 1953*
- ♦ **Zenhale (Can)** *see* Mometasone and Formoterol *on page 1392*
- ♦ **Zenpep** *see* Pancrelipase *on page 1566*
- ♦ **Zenzedi** *see* Dextroamphetamine *on page 607*
- ♦ **Zephrex-D [OTC]** *see* Pseudoephedrine *on page 1742*
- ♦ **Zerbaxa** *see* Ceftolozane and Tazobactam *on page 394*
- ♦ **Zerit** *see* Stavudine *on page 1934*
- ♦ **Zestoretic** *see* Lisinopril and Hydrochlorothiazide *on page 1229*
- ♦ **Zestril** *see* Lisinopril *on page 1226*
- ♦ **Zetia** *see* Ezetimibe *on page 832*
- ♦ **Zetonna** *see* Ciclesonide (Nasal) *on page 432*
- ♦ **Zeven** *see* Dalbavancin *on page 551*
- ♦ **Ziac®** *see* Bisoprolol and Hydrochlorothiazide *on page 267*
- ♦ **Ziagen** *see* Abacavir *on page 20*
- ♦ **Ziagen® (Can)** *see* Abacavir *on page 20*
- ♦ **Ziana®** *see* Clindamycin and Tretinoin *on page 464*

Ziconotide (zi KOE no tide)

Brand Names: U.S. Prialt

Pharmacologic Category Analgesic, Nonopioid; Calcium Channel Blocker, N-Type

Use Management of severe chronic pain in patients requiring intrathecal therapy and who are intolerant or refractory to other therapies

Pregnancy Risk Factor C

Dosage Intrathecal:

Adults: Chronic pain: Initial dose: ≤2.4 mcg/day (0.1 mcg/hour)

Dose may be titrated by ≤2.4 mcg/day (0.1 mcg/hour) at intervals ≤2-3 times/week to a maximum dose of 19.2 mcg/day (0.8 mcg/hour) by day 21; average dose at day 21: 6.9 mcg/day (0.29 mcg/hour). A faster titration should be used only if the urgent need for analgesia outweighs the possible risk to patient safety.

Dosage adjustment for toxicity:

Cognitive impairment: Reduce dose or discontinue. Effects are generally reversible within 3-15 days of discontinuation.

Reduced level of consciousness: Discontinue until event resolves.

CK elevation with neuromuscular symptoms: Consider dose reduction or discontinuation.

Elderly: Refer to adult dosing; use with caution.

Dosage adjustment in renal impairment: No dosage adjustment provided in manufacturer's labeling (has not been studied).

Dosage adjustment in hepatic impairment: No dosage adjustment provided in manufacturer's labeling (has not been studied).

Additional Information Complete prescribing information should be consulted for additional detail.

Dosage Forms

Solution, Intrathecal [preservative free]:

Prialt: 500 mcg/20 mL (20 mL); 100 mcg/mL (1 mL); 500 mcg/5 mL (5 mL)

♦ **Zictifa** *see* Vandetanib *on page 2135*

Zidovudine (zye DOE vyoo deen)

Brand Names: U.S. Retrovir

Brand Names: Canada Apo-Zidovudine; AZT; Novo-AZT; Retrovir; Retrovir (AZT)

Index Terms Azidothymidine; AZT (error-prone abbreviation); Compound S; ZDV

Pharmacologic Category Antiretroviral, Reverse Transcriptase Inhibitor, Nucleoside (Anti-HIV)

Use Treatment of HIV infection in combination with at least two other antiretroviral agents; prevention of maternal/fetal HIV transmission

Pregnancy Risk Factor C

Pregnancy Considerations Adverse events have been observed in some animal reproduction studies. Zidovudine has a high level of transfer across the human placenta and the placenta also metabolizes zidovudine to the active metabolite. No increased risk of overall birth defects has been observed following first trimester exposure according to data collected by the antiretroviral pregnancy registry. The pharmacokinetics of zidovudine are not significantly altered in pregnancy and dosing adjustment is not needed. The HHS Perinatal HIV Guidelines consider zidovudine in combination with lamivudine to be a preferred NRTI backbone for use in antiretroviral-naïve pregnant women. Zidovudine should be administered IV near delivery regardless of antepartum regimen or mode of delivery in women with HIV RNA >1000 copies/mL or unknown HIV RNA status.

Cases of lactic acidosis/hepatic steatosis syndrome related to mitochondrial toxicity have been reported in pregnant women with prolonged use of nucleoside analogues. It is not known if pregnancy itself potentiates this known side effect; however, women may be at increased risk of lactic acidosis and liver damage. In addition, these adverse events are similar to other rare but life-threatening syndromes which occur during pregnancy (eg, HELLP syndrome). Hepatic enzymes and electrolytes should be monitored in women receiving nucleoside analogues and clinicians should watch for early signs of the syndrome. In addition, mitochondrial dysfunction may develop in infants following *in utero* exposure.

Regardless of CD4 count or HIV RNA copy number, all HIV-infected pregnant women should receive a combination antiretroviral (ARV) drug regimen. A combination of antepartum, intrapartum, and infant ARV prophylaxis is recommended. ARV therapy should be started as soon as possible in women with symptomatic infection. Although earlier initiation may be more effective in reducing the perinatal transmission of HIV, initiation may be delayed until after 12 weeks' gestation in women who do not require immediate treatment after careful consideration of maternal conditions (eg, nausea and vomiting) and the potential risks of first trimester fetal exposure for specific agents. A scheduled cesarean delivery at 38 weeks' gestation is recommended for all women with HIV RNA >1000 copies/mL or unknown concentrations near delivery in order to decrease transmission. If ARV therapy must be interrupted for <24 hours during the peripartum period, stop then restart all medications simultaneously in order to decrease the chance of developing resistance. Long-term follow-up is recommended for all infants exposed to ARV medications. In couples who want to conceive, the HIV-infected partner should attain maximum viral suppression prior to conception.

Health care providers are encouraged to enroll pregnant women exposed to antiretroviral medications in the Antiretroviral Pregnancy Registry (1-800-258-4263 or www.-APRegistry.com). Health care providers caring for HIV-infected women and their infants may contact the National Perinatal HIV Hotline (888-448-8765) for clinical consultation (HHS [perinatal], 2014).

Breast-Feeding Considerations Zidovudine is excreted into breast milk. Concentrations of zidovudine in breast milk are similar to those in the maternal serum. Maternal or infant antiretroviral therapy does not completely eliminate the risk of postnatal HIV transmission. In addition, multi-class-resistant virus has been detected in breast-feeding infants despite maternal therapy. Therefore, in the United States, where formula is accessible, affordable, safe, and sustainable, and the risk of infant mortality due to diarrhea and respiratory infections is low, complete avoidance of breast-feeding by HIV-infected women is recommended to decrease potential transmission of HIV (HHS [perinatal], 2014).

Contraindications Life-threatening hypersensitivity to zidovudine or any component of the formulation

Canadian labeling: Additional contraindications (not in U.S. labeling): Neutrophil count <750/mm^3 or hemoglobin <7.5 g/dL (4.65 mmol/L)

Warnings/Precautions Hazardous agent - use appropriate precautions for handling and disposal (NIOSH 2014 [group 2]).

[U.S. Boxed Warning]: Hematologic toxicity, including neutropenia and severe anemia have been reported with use. Toxicity may be related to duration of use and prior bone marrow reserve. Use with caution in patients with bone marrow compromise (granulocytes <1000 cells/mm^3 or hemoglobin <9.5 mg/dL); dose interruption may be required in patients who develop anemia or neutropenia. **[U.S. Boxed Warning]: Lactic acidosis and severe hepatomegaly with steatosis have been reported, including fatal cases.** Risks may be increased with liver disease, obesity, pregnancy, prolonged exposure, or in females. Suspend treatment with zidovudine in any patient who develops clinical or laboratory findings suggestive of lactic acidosis (transaminase elevation may/may not accompany hepatomegaly and steatosis). Use caution in combination with interferon alfa with or without ribavirin in HIV/HCV coinfected patients; monitor closely for hepatic decompensation, anemia, or neutropenia; dose reduction or discontinuation of interferon and/or ribavirin may be required if toxicity evident.

Zidovudine newborn prophylaxis may affect diagnostic virologic assays in HIV-exposed infants. If a virologic assay result is negative while the infant is receiving combination antiretroviral prophylaxis, repeat virologic testing should be considered 2 to 4 weeks after cessation of antiretroviral prophylaxis (HHS [pediatric], 2014).

[U.S. Boxed Warning]: Prolonged use has been associated with symptomatic myopathy and myositis. May cause redistribution of fat (eg, buffalo hump, peripheral wasting with increased abdominal girth, cushingoid appearance). Immune reconstitution syndrome may develop resulting in the occurrence of an inflammatory response to an indolent or residual opportunistic infection during initial HIV treatment or activation of autoimmune disorders (eg, Graves disease, polymyositis, Guillain-Barré syndrome) later in therapy; further evaluation and treatment may be required. Hematologic toxicity may be increased due to increased serum concentrations in patients with severe hepatic impairment. Use with caution in patients with severe renal impairment; dosage adjustment recommended. Reduce dose in patients with severe renal impairment. Do not administer with combination products that contain zidovudine as one of their components (eg, COMBIVIR [lamivudine and zidovudine] or TRIZIVIR [abacavir sulfate, lamivudine, and zidovudine]).

Benzyl alcohol and derivatives: Some dosage forms may contain sodium benzoate/benzoic acid; benzoic acid (benzoate) is a metabolite of benzyl alcohol; large amounts of benzyl alcohol (≥99 mg/kg/day) have been associated with a potentially fatal toxicity ("gasping syndrome") in neonates; the "gasping syndrome" consists of metabolic acidosis, respiratory distress, gasping respirations, CNS dysfunction (including convulsions, intracranial hemorrhage), hypotension, and cardiovascular collapse (AAP, 1997; CDC, 1982); some data suggests that benzoate displaces bilirubin from protein binding sites (Ahlfors, 2001); avoid or use dosage forms containing benzyl alcohol derivative with caution in neonates. See manufacturer's labeling.

Adverse Reactions

Cardiovascular: ECG abnormality (children), edema (children), heart failure (children), left ventricular dilation (children)

Central nervous system: Chills, fatigue, fever (children), headache, insomnia, irritability (children), malaise, nervousness (children)

Dermatologic: Rash (more common in children)

Gastrointestinal: Abdominal cramps, abdominal pain, anorexia, constipation (adults), diarrhea (children), dyspepsia, nausea (more common in adults), vomiting (more common in adults), weight loss (children)

Genitourinary: Hematuria (children)

Hematologic: Anemia (more common in neonates), granulocytopenia, macrocytosis (children), neutropenia (children), thrombocytopenia (children)

Hepatic: Hepatomegaly (children), transaminases increased

Neuromuscular & skeletal: Arthralgia, musculoskeletal pain, myalgia, neuropathy, weakness

Otic: Hearing loss

Respiratory: Cough (children)

Rare but important or life-threatening: Allergic reactions, amblyopia, anaphylaxis, angioedema, anxiety, aplastic anemia, back pain, body fat redistribution, cardiomyopathy, confusion, CPK increased, depression, diabetes, dizziness, dyslipidemias, dyspnea, gynecomastia, hearing loss, hemolytic anemia, hepatitis, hepatomegaly with steatosis, immune reconstitution syndrome, insulin resistance, jaundice, lactic acidosis, LDH increased, leukopenia, loss of mental acuity, lymphadenopathy, macular edema, mania, myopathy, myositis, oral mucosa pigmentation, pancreatitis, pancytopenia with marrow hypoplasia, paresthesia, photophobia, pruritus, pure red cell aplasia, rhabdomyolysis, seizure, skin/nail pigmentation changes (blue), Stevens-Johnson syndrome, syncope, taste perversion, toxic epidermal necrolysis, tremor, urticaria, vertigo

Drug Interactions

Metabolism/Transport Effects Substrate of CYP2A6 (minor), CYP2C19 (minor), CYP2C9 (minor), CYP3A4 (minor), OAT3; **Note:** Assignment of Major/Minor substrate status based on clinically relevant drug interaction potential

Avoid Concomitant Use

Avoid concomitant use of Zidovudine with any of the following: CloZAPine; Dipyrone; Stavudine

Increased Effect/Toxicity

Zidovudine may increase the levels/effects of: CloZAPine; Ribavirin

The levels/effects of Zidovudine may be increased by: Acyclovir-Valacyclovir; Clarithromycin; Dexketoprofen; Dipyrone; DOXOrubicin (Conventional); DOXOrubicin (Liposomal); Fluconazole; Ganciclovir-Valganciclovir; Interferons; Methadone; Probenecid; Raltegravir; Teriflunomide; Valproic Acid and Derivatives

Decreased Effect

Zidovudine may decrease the levels/effects of: Stavudine

The levels/effects of Zidovudine may be decreased by: Clarithromycin; DOXOrubicin (Conventional); DOXOrubicin (Liposomal); Protease Inhibitors; Rifamycin Derivatives

Preparation for Administration Hazardous agent; use appropriate precautions for handling and disposal (NIOSH 2014 [group 2]).

Solution for injection should be diluted with D_5W to a concentration ≤4 mg/mL.

Storage/Stability

IV: Store undiluted vials at 15°C to 25°C (59°F to 77°F). Protect from light. When diluted, solution is physically and chemically stable for 24 hours at room temperature and 48 hours if refrigerated. Attempt to administer diluted solution within 8 hours if stored at room temperature or 24 hours if refrigerated to minimize potential for microbial-contaminated solutions (vials are single-use and do not contain preservative).

Tablets, capsules, syrup: Store at 15°C to 25°C (59°F to 77°F). Protect capsules from moisture.

Mechanism of Action Zidovudine is a thymidine analog which interferes with the HIV viral RNA-dependent DNA polymerase resulting in inhibition of viral replication; nucleoside reverse transcriptase inhibitor

Pharmacodynamics/Kinetics

Distribution: Significant penetration into the CSF

V_d: 1-2.2 L/kg

Relative diffusion from blood into CSF: Adequate with or without inflammation (exceeds usual MICs)

CSF:blood level ratio: Normal meninges: ~60%

Protein binding: 25% to 38%

Metabolism: Hepatic via glucuronidation to inactive metabolites; extensive first-pass effect

Bioavailability: 54% to 74%

Half-life elimination: Terminal: 0.5-3 hours

Time to peak, serum: 30-90 minutes

Excretion:

Oral: Urine (72% to 74% as metabolites, 14% to 18% as unchanged drug)

IV: Urine (45% to 60% as metabolites, 18% to 29% as unchanged drug)

Dosage Note: Patients should receive IV therapy only until oral therapy can be administered.

Prevention of perinatal HIV transmission: **Note:** Start as soon as possible after birth, preferably within 6 to 12 hours of delivery. Continue dose from birth through 6 weeks of age (a 4-week course may be considered if the mother received ART therapy during pregnancy consistent with viral suppression and there are no concerns related to adherence with the regimen). Use zidovudine in combination with nevirapine in select situations (eg, infants born to mothers with only intrapartum therapy or no therapy) (HHS [perinatal], 2014).

Oral:

Manufacturer's labeling: Full-term infants: 2 mg/kg every 6 hours

AIDS*info* guidelines (HHS [perinatal], 2014):

Infants ≥35 weeks: 4 mg/kg/dose twice daily

Infants ≥30 weeks and <35 weeks gestation at birth: 2 mg/kg/dose every 12 hours; at 15 days of age, advance to 3 mg/kg/dose every 12 hours

Infants <30 weeks gestation at birth: 2 mg/kg/dose every 12 hours; at 4 weeks of age, advance to 3 mg/kg/dose every 12 hours

IV: Infants unable to receive oral dosing (start as soon as possible after birth, preferably within 6 to 12 hours of delivery; continue dose from birth through 6 weeks of age) (HHS [perinatal], 2014):

Infants ≥35 weeks: 3 mg/kg/dose every 12 hours

Infants ≥30 weeks and <35 weeks gestation at birth: 1.5 mg/kg/dose every 12 hours; at 15 days of age, advance to 2.3 mg/kg/dose every 12 hours

Infants <30 weeks gestation at birth: 1.5 mg/kg/dose every 12 hours; at 4 weeks of age, advance to 2.3 mg/kg/dose every 12 hours

Maternal: Oral: Dose adjustment not required in pregnant women. Begin oral therapy with usual recommended dose based on current treatment guidelines. Zidovudine should be administered by continuous IV infusion near delivery regardless of antepartum regimen or mode of delivery in women with HIV RNA >1000 copies/mL or unknown HIV RNA status. If oral zidovudine was part of the antepartum regimen, discontinue during intrapartum IV infusion. Other antiretroviral agents should be continued orally. Zidovudine IV is not required in women receiving combination antiretroviral therapy who have HIV RNA <1000 copies/mL near delivery and there are no concerns related to adherence with the regimen (HHS [perinatal], 2014).

During labor and delivery, administer zidovudine IV at 2 mg/kg as loading dose followed by a continuous IV infusion of 1 mg/kg/hour until delivery. For scheduled cesarean delivery, begin IV zidovudine 3 hours before surgery.

Treatment of HIV infection:

Children 4 weeks to <18 years (U.S. labeling) or 3 months to ≤12 years (Canadian labeling):

Oral: Dose should be calculated by body weight (in kg) or body surface area and should not exceed the recommended adult dose. **Note:** Doses calculated by body weight may not be the same as those calculated by body surface area.

Dosing based on body surface area: 240 mg/m² twice daily (maximum: 300 mg twice daily) **or** 160 mg/m²/dose 3 times daily (maximum: 200 mg 3 times daily)

Dosing based on weight (**Note:** 3 times daily dose is approved but rarely used in clinical practice):
4 to <9 kg: 12 mg/kg/dose twice daily **or** 8 mg/kg/dose 3 times/day
≥9 to <30 kg: 9 mg/kg/dose twice daily **or** 6 mg/kg/dose 3 times/day
≥30 kg: 300 mg twice daily **or** 200 mg 3 times/day
Children 3 months to ≤12 years (Canadian labeling): IV intermittent infusion: 120 mg/m²/dose every 6 hours (maximum: 160 mg/dose)
Children ≥12 years: IV intermittent infusion: 1 mg/kg/dose every 4 hours around-the-clock (5-6 doses/day)
Adults:
Oral: 300 mg twice daily or 200 mg 3 times/day
IV:
U.S. labeling: 1 mg/kg/dose administered every 4 hours around-the-clock (5 to 6 doses/day)
Canadian labeling: 1 to 2 mg/kg/dose administered every 4 hours around-the-clock (6 doses/day)

Postexposure prophylaxis (off-label use): Adults: Oral: 300 mg twice daily or 200 mg 3 times daily in combination with lamivudine or emtricitabine. A third agent may be added for high risk exposures. Therapy should be started within hours of exposure and continued for 4 weeks (CDC, 2005).

Dosage adjustment for hematologic toxicity: Consider dose interruption for significant anemia (hemoglobin <7.5 g/dL or >25% reduction from baseline) and/or neutropenia (granulocyte count <750 cells/mm³ or >50% reduction from baseline) until evidence of recovery. Anemia associated with chronic zidovudine may warrant dose reduction.

Dosage adjustment in renal impairment: CrCl <15 mL/minute including hemo-/peritoneal dialysis (administer dose after dialysis on dialysis days [HHS [adult], 2014]):
Oral: 100 mg every 6 to 8 hours (manufacturers labeling); 100 mg 3 times daily or 300 mg once daily (HHS [adult], 2014)
IV: 1 mg/kg every 6 to 8 hours
Continuous renal replacement therapy (CRRT): No adjustment needed (Aronoff, 2007)

Dosage adjustment in hepatic impairment: No specific dosage adjustment provided in manufacturer's labeling (has not been studied). However, adjustment may be necessary due to extensive hepatic metabolism.

Dietary Considerations May be taken without regard to meals.

Administration
Oral: Administer around-the-clock to promote less variation in peak and trough serum levels; may be administered without regard to meals
IV: Avoid rapid infusion or bolus injection. Do not administer IM
Neonates: Infuse over 30 minutes
Adults: Infuse over 1 hour; in pregnant women, infuse loading dose over 1 hour followed by continuous infusion

Hazardous agent; use appropriate precautions for handling and disposal (NIOSH 2014 [group 2]).

Monitoring Parameters
Monitor viral load (2 to 8 weeks after initiation/modification of therapy, and then every 3 to 6 months); CBC with differential (every 3 to 6 months); liver function tests (every 6 to 12 months); lipids, glucose (yearly if normal); observe for appearance of opportunistic infections [DHHS (adult), 2014])
Monitor CD4 count every 3 to 6 months; every 6 to 12 months once clinically stable. For patients who have been on ART for at least 2 years with consistent viral suppression, CD4 count frequency may be reduced to every 12 months for CD4 count 300 to 500 cells/mm³ and is considered optional for CD4 count >500 cells/mm³. Resume more frequent CD4 count monitoring in patients with viral rebound, new HIV-associated clinical symptoms, or when there are conditions or a new therapy that may reduce CD4 cell count (DHHS [adult], 2014]).

Additional Information Potential compliance problems, frequency of administration, and adverse effects should be discussed with patients before initiating therapy to help prevent the emergence of resistance.

Dosage Forms
Capsule, Oral:
Retrovir: 100 mg
Generic: 100 mg
Solution, Intravenous [preservative free]:
Retrovir: 10 mg/mL (20 mL)
Syrup, Oral:
Retrovir: 50 mg/5 mL (240 mL)
Generic: 50 mg/5 mL (240 mL)
Tablet, Oral:
Generic: 300 mg

- ◆ **Zidovudine, Abacavir, and Lamivudine** *see* Abacavir, Lamivudine, and Zidovudine *on page* 22
- ◆ **Zidovudine and Lamivudine** *see* Lamivudine and Zidovudine *on page* 1160
- ◆ **Zilactin [OTC]** *see* Benzyl Alcohol *on page* 250
- ◆ **Zilactin-B® (Can)** *see* Benzocaine *on page* 246
- ◆ **Zilactin Baby [OTC]** *see* Benzocaine *on page* 246
- ◆ **Zilactin Baby® (Can)** *see* Benzocaine *on page* 246

Zileuton (zye LOO ton)

Brand Names: U.S. Zyflo; Zyflo CR
Pharmacologic Category 5-Lipoxygenase Inhibitor
Use Prophylaxis and chronic treatment of asthma
Pregnancy Risk Factor C
Dosage Oral: Children ≥12 years and Adults:
Immediate release: 600 mg 4 times/day
Extended release: 1200 mg twice daily

Dosage adjustment in renal impairment: No dosage adjustment necessary.
Dosage adjustment in hepatic impairment: Contraindicated with hepatic impairment.

Additional Information Complete prescribing information should be consulted for additional detail.

Dosage Forms
Tablet, Oral:
Zyflo: 600 mg
Tablet Extended Release 12 Hour, Oral:
Zyflo CR: 600 mg

- ◆ **Zinacef** *see* Cefuroxime *on page* 399
- ◆ **Zinacef in Sterile Water** *see* Cefuroxime *on page* 399
- ◆ **Zinc 15 [OTC]** *see* Zinc Sulfate *on page* 2200
- ◆ **Zinc-220 [OTC]** *see* Zinc Sulfate *on page* 2200

Zinc Acetate (zink AS e tate)

Brand Names: U.S. Galzin
Pharmacologic Category Trace Element
Use Maintenance treatment of Wilson's disease following initial chelation therapy
Pregnancy Risk Factor A
Dosage Oral: Wilson's disease: **Note:** Dose expressed in mg elemental zinc:
Children ≥10 years: 75 mg/day in 3 divided doses; may increase to 150 mg/day in 3 divided doses if inadequate response to lower dose

American Association for the Study of Liver Diseases (AASLD) practice guideline recommendations (Roberts, 2008):

Children <50 kg and >5 years: 75 mg/day in 3 divided doses

Children >50 kg: 150 mg/day in 3 divided doses

Adults:

Males and nonpregnant females: 150 mg/day in 3 divided doses

Pregnant females: 75 mg/day in 3 divided doses; may increase to 150 mg/day in 3 divided doses if inadequate response to lower dose

Dosage adjustment in renal impairment: No dosage adjustment provided in manufacturer's labeling.

Dosage adjustment in hepatic impairment: No dosage adjustment provided in manufacturer's labeling.

Additional Information Complete prescribing information should be consulted for additional detail.

Dosage Forms Considerations

Strength of Galzin capsule is expressed as elemental zinc

Dosage Forms

Capsule, Oral:

Galzin: 25 mg, 50 mg

◆ **Zincate [DSC]** *see* Zinc Sulfate *on page 2200*

Zinc Chloride (zink KLOR ide)

Pharmacologic Category Trace Element

Use Cofactor for replacement therapy to different enzymes; helps maintain normal growth rates, normal skin hydration, and senses of taste and smell

Pregnancy Risk Factor C

Dosage Clinical response may not occur for up to 6-8 weeks

Supplemental to IV solutions:

Premature Infants <1500 g, up to 3 kg: 300 mcg/kg/day

Infants (full term) and Children ≤5 years: 100 mcg/kg/day

Adults:

Stable with fluid loss from small bowel: 12.2 mg zinc/L TPN or 17.1 mg zinc/kg (added to 1000 mL IV fluids) of stool or ileostomy output

Metabolically stable: 2.5-4 mg/day; add 2 mg/day for acute catabolic states

Dosage adjustment in renal impairment: No dosage adjustment provided in manufacturer's labeling. However, dosage adjustment may be necessary in severe impairment since zinc is primarily renally excreted. Additionally, aluminum accumulation may occur in the setting of renal impairment.

Dosage adjustment in hepatic impairment: No dosage adjustment provided in manufacturer's labeling.

Additional Information Complete prescribing information should be consulted for additional detail.

Dosage Forms Considerations

Strength of zinc chloride injection is expressed as elemental zinc

Dosage Forms

Solution, Intravenous:

Generic: 1 mg/mL (10 mL)

◆ **Zincfrin (Can)** *see* Phenylephrine and Zinc Sulfate [CAN/INT] *on page 1640*

Zinc Gelatin (zink JEL ah tin)

Brand Names: U.S. Gelucast®

Index Terms Dome Paste Bandage; Unna's Boot; Unna's Paste; Zinc Gelatin Boot

Pharmacologic Category Topical Skin Product

Use As a protectant and to support varicosities and similar lesions of the lower limbs

Dosage Topical: Apply externally as an occlusive boot

Additional Information Complete prescribing information should be consulted for additional detail.

Dosage Forms

Bandage: 3" x 10 yards; 4" x 10 yards

Gelucast®: 3" x 10 yards; 4" x 10 yards

◆ **Zinc Gelatin Boot** *see* Zinc Gelatin *on page 2200*

◆ **Zincofax® (Can)** *see* Zinc Oxide *on page 2200*

Zinc Oxide (zink OKS ide)

Brand Names: U.S. Ammens® Original Medicated [OTC]; Ammens® Shower Fresh [OTC]; Balmex® [OTC]; Boudreaux's® Butt Paste [OTC]; Critic-Aid Skin Care® [OTC]; Desitin® Creamy [OTC]; Desitin® [OTC]

Brand Names: Canada Zincofax®

Index Terms Base Ointment; Lassar's Zinc Paste

Pharmacologic Category Topical Skin Product

Use Protective coating for mild skin irritations and abrasions; soothing and protective ointment to promote healing of chapped skin, diaper rash

Dosage Infants, Children, and Adults: Topical: Apply as required for affected areas several times daily

Additional Information Complete prescribing information should be consulted for additional detail.

Dosage Forms

Cream, topical:

Balmex® [OTC]: 11.3% (60 g, 120 g, 480 g)

Cream, topical [stick]:

Balmex® [OTC]: 11.3% (56 g)

Ointment, topical: 20% (30 g, 60 g, 454 g); 40% (120 g)

Desitin® [OTC]: 40% (30 g, 60 g, 90 g, 120 g, 270 g, 480 g)

Desitin® Creamy [OTC]: 10% (60 g, 120 g)

Paste, topical:

Boudreaux's® Butt Paste [OTC]: 16% (30 g, 60 g, 120 g, 480 g)

Critic-Aid Skin Care® [OTC]: 20% (71 g, 170 g)

Powder, topical:

Ammens® Original Medicated [OTC], Ammens® Shower Fresh [OTC]: 9.1% (312 g)

Zinc Sulfate (zink SUL fate)

Brand Names: U.S. Eye-Sed [OTC]; Orazinc [OTC]; Zinc 15 [OTC]; Zinc-220 [OTC]; Zincate [DSC]

Brand Names: Canada Anuzinc; Rivasol

Index Terms $ZnSO_4$ (error-prone abbreviation)

Pharmacologic Category Trace Element

Use Zinc supplement (oral and parenteral); may improve wound healing in those who are deficient

Pregnancy Risk Factor C

Dosage

Oral (dose expressed as elemental zinc):

Adequate intake (AI): 1-6 months: 2.0 mg/day

Recommended daily allowance (RDA):

7-12 months: 3 mg/day

1-3 years: 3 mg/day

4-8 years: 5 mg/day

9-13 years: 8 mg/day

14-18 years:

Males: 11 mg/day

Females: 9 mg/day

Pregnancy: 12 mg/day

Lactation: 13 mg/day

≥19 years:
Males: 11 mg/day
Females: 8 mg/day
Pregnancy: 11 mg/day
Lactation: 12 mg/day
Parenteral TPN: IV:
Infants (premature, birth weight <1500 g up to 3 kg): 300 mcg/kg/day
Infants (full term) and Children ≤5 years: 100 mcg/kg/day
Adults:
Acute metabolic states: 4.5-6 mg/day
Metabolically stable: 2.5-4 mg/day
Replacement for small bowel fluid loss (metabolically stable): An additional 12.2 mg zinc/L of fluid lost, or an additional 17.1 mg zinc per kg of stool or ileostomy output

Additional Information Complete prescribing information should be consulted for additional detail.

Dosage Forms Considerations

Strength of zinc sulfate injection is expressed as elemental zinc

Oral zinc sulfate is approximately 23% elemental zinc

Dosage Forms

Capsule, Oral:
Orazinc [OTC]: 220 mg
Zinc-220 [OTC]: 220 mg
Generic: 220 mg

Solution, Intravenous:
Generic: 1 mg/mL (10 mL); 5 mg/mL (5 mL)

Solution, Ophthalmic:
Eye-Sed [OTC]: 0.217% (15 mL)

Tablet, Oral:
Orazinc [OTC]: 110 mg
Zinc 15 [OTC]: 66 mg
Generic: 220 mg

Tablet, Oral [preservative free]:
Generic: 220 mg

◆ **Zinc Sulfate and Phenylephrine** *see* Phenylephrine and Zinc Sulfate [CAN/INT] *on page 1640*

◆ **Zinda-Anastrozole (Can)** *see* Anastrozole *on page 148*

◆ **Zinda-Letrozole (Can)** *see* Letrozole *on page 1181*

◆ **Zinecard** *see* Dexrazoxane *on page 606*

◆ **Zingo** *see* Lidocaine (Topical) *on page 1211*

Ziprasidone (zi PRAS i done)

Brand Names: U.S. Geodon

Brand Names: Canada Zeldox

Index Terms Zeldox; Ziprasidone Hydrochloride; Ziprasidone Mesylate

Pharmacologic Category Second Generation (Atypical) Antipsychotic

Additional Appendix Information

Beers Criteria – Potentially Inappropriate Medications for Geriatrics *on page 2271*

Use Treatment of schizophrenia; treatment of acute manic or mixed episodes associated with bipolar disorder with or without psychosis; maintenance treatment of bipolar disorder as an adjunct to lithium or valproate; acute agitation in patients with schizophrenia

Pregnancy Risk Factor C

Pregnancy Considerations Adverse events were observed in animal reproduction studies. Antipsychotic use during the third trimester of pregnancy has a risk for abnormal muscle movements (extrapyramidal symptoms [EPS]) and/or withdrawal symptoms in newborns following delivery. Symptoms in the newborn may include agitation, feeding disorder, hypertonia, hypotonia, respiratory distress, somnolence, and tremor; these effects may be self-limiting or require hospitalization. Ziprasidone may cause hyperprolactinemia, which may decrease reproductive function in both males and females.

The ACOG recommends that therapy during pregnancy be individualized; treatment with psychiatric medications during pregnancy should incorporate the clinical expertise of the mental health clinician, obstetrician, primary healthcare provider, and pediatrician. Safety data related to atypical antipsychotics during pregnancy is limited and routine use is not recommended. However, if a woman is inadvertently exposed to an atypical antipsychotic while pregnant, continuing therapy may be preferable to switching to a typical antipsychotic that the fetus has not yet been exposed to; consider risk:benefit (ACOG, 2008).

Healthcare providers are encouraged to enroll women 18-45 years of age exposed to ziprasidone during pregnancy in the Atypical Antipsychotics Pregnancy Registry (1-866-961-2388 or http://www.womensmentalhealth.org/pregnancyregistry).

Breast-Feeding Considerations It is not known if ziprasidone is excreted into breast milk. Breast-feeding is not recommended by the manufacturer.

Contraindications Hypersensitivity to ziprasidone or any component of the formulation; history of (or current) prolonged QT; congenital long QT syndrome; recent myocardial infarction; uncompensated heart failure; concurrent use of other QTc-prolonging agents including arsenic trioxide, chlorpromazine, class Ia antiarrhythmics (eg, disopyramide, quinidine, procainamide), class III antiarrhythmics (eg, amiodarone, dofetilide, ibutilide, sotalol), dolasetron, droperidol, gatifloxacin, halofantrine, levomethadyl, mefloquine, mesoridazine, moxifloxacin, pentamidine, pimozide, probucol, sparfloxacin, tacrolimus, and thioridazine

Warnings/Precautions Hazardous agent - use appropriate precautions for handling and disposal (NIOSH 2014 [group 3]). **[U.S. Boxed Warning]: Elderly patients with dementia-related behavioral disorders treated with antipsychotics are at an increased risk of death compared to placebo.** Most deaths appeared to be either cardiovascular (eg, heart failure, sudden death) or infectious (eg, pneumonia) in nature. Ziprasidone is not approved for the treatment of dementia-related psychosis.

May result in QTc prolongation (dose related), which has been associated with the development of malignant ventricular arrhythmias (torsade de pointes) and sudden death. Note contraindications related to this effect. Observed prolongation was greater than with other atypical antipsychotic agents (risperidone, olanzapine, quetiapine), but less than with thioridazine. Correct electrolyte disturbances, especially hypokalemia or hypomagnesemia, prior to use and throughout therapy. Use caution in patients with bradycardia. Discontinue in patients found to have persistent QTc intervals >500 msec. Patients with symptoms of dizziness, palpitations, or syncope should receive further cardiac evaluation. May cause orthostatic hypotension. Use is contraindicated in patients with recent acute myocardial infarction (MI), QT prolongation, or uncompensated heart failure. Avoid use in patients with a history of cardiac arrhythmias; use with caution in patients with history of MI or unstable heart disease. Dyslipidemia has been reported with atypical antipsychotics; risk profile may differ between agents.

Leukopenia, neutropenia, and agranulocytosis (sometimes fatal) have been reported in clinical trials and postmarketing reports with antipsychotic use; presence of risk factors (eg, preexisting low WBC or history of drug-induced leuko-/neutropenia) should prompt periodic blood count assessment. Discontinue therapy at first signs of blood dyscrasias or if absolute neutrophil count <1000/mm^3. Potentially serious, sometimes fatal drug reaction with eosinophilia and systemic symptoms (DRESS), also known as multiorgan hypersensitivity reactions, have also been reported with ziprasidone. Monitor for signs and symptoms of possible disparate manifestations associated with lymphatic, hepatic, renal, cardiovascular, and/or hematologic organ systems; discontinuation and conversion to alternate therapy may be required.

May cause extrapyramidal symptoms (EPS). Risk of dystonia (and probably other EPS) may be greater with increased doses, use of conventional antipsychotics, males, and younger patients. Impaired core body temperature regulation may occur; caution with strenuous exercise, heat exposure, dehydration, and concomitant medication possessing anticholinergic effects; not reported in premarketing trials of ziprasidone. Antipsychotic use may also be associated with neuroleptic malignant syndrome (NMS). Use with caution in patients at risk of seizures.

Atypical antipsychotics have been associated with development of hyperglycemia. There is limited documentation with ziprasidone and specific risk associated with this agent is not known. Use caution in patients with diabetes or other disorders of glucose regulation; monitor for worsening of glucose control. May increase prolactin levels; clinical significance of hyperprolactinemia in patients with breast cancer or other prolactin-dependent tumors is unknown.

Use in elderly patients with dementia is associated with an increased risk of mortality and cerebrovascular accidents; avoid antipsychotic use for behavioral problems associated with dementia unless alternative nonpharmacologic therapies have failed and patient may harm self or others. In addition, use may cause or exacerbate syndrome of inappropriate antidiuretic hormone secretion or hyponatremia; monitor sodium closely with initiation or dosage adjustments in older adults (Beers Criteria).

Cognitive and/or motor impairment (sedation) is common with ziprasidone. CNS effects may be potentiated when used with other sedative drugs or ethanol. Use with caution in disorders where CNS depression is a feature. Use with caution in Parkinson's disease. Antipsychotic use has been associated with esophageal dysmotility and aspiration; use with caution in patients at risk of pneumonia (ie, Alzheimer's disease). Use caution in hepatic impairment. Ziprasidone has been associated with a fairly high incidence of rash (5%). Significant weight gain has been observed with antipsychotic therapy; incidence varies with product. Monitor waist circumference and BMI. Rare cases of priapism have been reported. Use the intramuscular formulation with caution in patients with renal impairment; formulation contains cyclodextrin, an excipient which may accumulate in renal insufficiency.

The possibility of a suicide attempt is inherent in psychotic illness or bipolar disorder; use caution in high-risk patients during initiation of therapy. Prescriptions should be written for the smallest quantity consistent with good patient care.

Adverse Reactions

Cardiovascular: Bradycardia, chest pain, facial edema, hypertension, orthostatic hypotension, tachycardia, vasodilatation

Central nervous system: Agitation, akathisia, akinesia, amnesia, anxiety, ataxia, chills, confusion, delirium, dizziness, drowsiness, dystonia, extrapyramidal symptoms, fever, headache, hostility, hypothermia, insomnia, oculogyric crisis, personality disorder, psychosis, speech disturbance, vertigo

Dermatologic: Fungal dermatitis, photosensitivity reaction, skin rash

Endocrine & metabolic: Dysmenorrhea

Gastrointestinal: Abdominal pain, anorexia, buccoglossal syndrome, constipation, diarrhea, dyspepsia, dysphagia, nausea, rectal hemorrhage, sialorrhea, tongue edema, vomiting, weight gain, xerostomia

Genitourinary: Priapism

Local: Pain at injection site

Neuromuscular & skeletal: Abnormal gait, back pain, choreoathetosis, cogwheel rigidity, dysarthria, dyskinesia, hyperkinesia, hypertonia, hypoesthesia, hypokinesia, hypotonia, myalgia, neuropathy, paresthesia, tremor, twitching, weakness

Ophthalmic: Diplopia, visual disturbance

Respiratory: Cough, dyspnea, infection, pharyngitis, rhinitis

Miscellaneous: Diaphoresis, flank pain, flu-like syndrome, furunculosis, withdrawal syndrome

Rare but important or life-threatening: Abnormal ejaculation, albuminuria, alkaline phosphatase increased, alopecia, amenorrhea, anemia, angina pectoris, angioedema, atrial fibrillation, basophilia, blepharitis, bruising, bundle branch block, cardiomegaly, cataract, cerebrovascular accident, cholestatic jaundice, circumoral paresthesia, conjunctivitis, contact dermatitis, creatinine (serum) increased, depression, DRESS syndrome, dry eyes, eczema, eosinophilia, epistaxis, exfoliative dermatitis, facial droop, fecal impaction, first degree atrioventricular, galactorrhea, gingival bleeding, gynecomastia, hematemesis, hematuria, hemoptysis, hepatitis, hepatomegaly, hyperchloremia, hypercholesterolemia, hyperglycemia, hyperkalemia, hypermenorrea, hyperreflexia, hypersensitivity reaction, hyperthyroidism, hyperuricemia, hypocalcemia, hypochloremia, hypocholesterolemia, hypoglycemia, hypokalemia, hypomagnesemia, hypomania, hyponatremia, hypoproteinemia, hypothyroidism, impotence, increased blood urea nitrogen, increased creatine phosphokinase, increased gamma-glutamyl transferase, increased monocytes, jaundice, keratitis, keratoconjunctivitis, ketosis, lactation (female), laryngismus, LDH increased, leukocytosis, leukopenia, leukoplakia (mouth), liver steatosis, lymphadenopathy, lymphedema, lymphocytosis, maculopapular rash, mania, melena, myocarditis, myoclonus, myopathy, neuroleptic malignant syndrome, nocturia, nystagmus, ocular hemorrhage, oliguria, paralysis, peripheral edema, phlebitis, photophobia, pneumonia, polycythemia, polyuria, prolonged Q-T interval on ECG (>500 msec), pulmonary embolism, respiratory alkalosis, seizure, serotonin syndrome, sexual dysfunction (male and female), syncope, tardive dyskinesia, tenosynovitis, thirst, thrombocythemia, thrombocytopenia, thrombophlebitis, thyroiditis, tinnitus, torsade de pointes, torticollis, transaminases increased, trismus, urinary incontinence, urinary retention, urticaria, uterine hemorrhage, vaginal hemorrhage, vesiculobullous dermatitis, visual field defect

Drug Interactions

Metabolism/Transport Effects Substrate of CYP1A2 (minor), CYP3A4 (minor); **Note:** Assignment of Major/Minor substrate status based on clinically relevant drug interaction potential; **Inhibits** CYP2D6 (weak), CYP3A4 (weak)

Avoid Concomitant Use

Avoid concomitant use of Ziprasidone with any of the following: Amisulpride; Azelastine (Nasal); FLUoxetine; Highest Risk QTc-Prolonging Agents; Ivabradine; Metoclopramide; Mifepristone; Moderate Risk QTc-Prolonging Agents; Orphenadrine; Paraldehyde; Pimozide; Sulpiride; Thalidomide

Increased Effect/Toxicity

Ziprasidone may increase the levels/effects of: Alcohol (Ethyl); Amisulpride; Azelastine (Nasal); Buprenorphine; CNS Depressants; FLUoxetine; Highest Risk QTc-Prolonging Agents; Hydrocodone; Lomitapide;

Methotrimeprazine; Methylphenidate; Metyrosine; Orphenadrine; Paraldehyde; Pimozide; Selective Serotonin Reuptake Inhibitors; Serotonin Modulators; Sulpiride; Suvorexant; Thalidomide; Zolpidem

The levels/effects of Ziprasidone may be increased by: Acetylcholinesterase Inhibitors (Central); Brimonidine (Topical); Cannabis; Doxylamine; Dronabinol; FLUoxetine; Ivabradine; Kava Kava; Magnesium Sulfate; Methotrimeprazine; Methylphenidate; Metoclopramide; Metyrosine; Mifepristone; Moderate Risk QTc-Prolonging Agents; Nabilone; Perampanel; QTc-Prolonging Agents (Indeterminate Risk and Risk Modifying); Rufinamide; Serotonin Modulators; Sodium Oxybate; Tapentadol; Tetrahydrocannabinol

Decreased Effect

Ziprasidone may decrease the levels/effects of: Amphetamines; Anti-Parkinson's Agents (Dopamine Agonist); Quinagolide

The levels/effects of Ziprasidone may be decreased by: CarBAMazepine

Food Interactions Administration with a meal containing at least 500 calories increases serum levels ~80%. Management: Administer with a meal containing at least 500 calories (Lincoln, 2010).

Preparation for Administration Hazardous agent; use appropriate precautions for handling and disposal (NIOSH 2014 [group 3]).

Each vial should be reconstituted with 1.2 mL SWFI. Shake vigorously; will form a pale, pink solution containing 20 mg/mL ziprasidone.

Storage/Stability

Capsule: Store at 25°C (77°F); excursion permitted to 15°C to 30°C (59°F to 86°F).

Vials for injection: Store at 25°C (77°F); excursion permitted to 15°C to 30°C (59°F to 86°F). Protect from light. Following reconstitution, injection may be stored at room temperature up to 24 hours or under refrigeration for up to 7 days. Protect from light.

Mechanism of Action Ziprasidone is a benzylisothiazolylpiperazine antipsychotic. The exact mechanism of action is unknown. However, *in vitro* radioligand studies show that ziprasidone has high affinity for D_2, D_3, 5-HT_{2A}, 5-HT_{1A}, 5-HT_{2C}, 5-HT_{1D}, and alpha$_1$-adrenergic; moderate affinity for histamine H_1 receptors; and no appreciable affinity for alpha$_2$-adrenergic receptors, beta-adrenergic, 5-HT_3, 5-HT_4, cholinergic, mu, sigma, or benzodiazepine receptors. Ziprasidone functions as an antagonist at the D_2, 5-HT_{2A}, and 5-HT_{1D} receptors and as an agonist at the 5-HT_{1A} receptor. Ziprasidone moderately inhibits the reuptake of serotonin and norepinephrine.

Pharmacodynamics/Kinetics

Absorption: Well absorbed; administration with 500-calorie meals increases serum levels ~80% (Lincoln, 2010).

Distribution: V_d: 1.5 L/kg

Protein binding: >99%, primarily to albumin and alpha$_1$-acid glycoprotein

Metabolism: Extensively hepatic, primarily chemical and enzymatic reductions via glutathione and aldehyde oxidase, respectively; less than 1/3 of total metabolism via CYP3A4 and CYP1A2 (minor)

Bioavailability: Oral (with food): 60%; IM: 100%

Half-life elimination: Oral: Mean terminal half-life: 7 hours; IM: Mean half-life: 2 to 5 hours

Time to peak: Oral: 6 to 8 hours; IM: ≤60 minutes

Excretion: Feces (~66%; <4% of total dose as unchanged drug); urine (~20%; <1% of total dose as unchanged drug)

Dosage

Bipolar disorder (acute and maintenance as adjunct to lithium or valproate): Adults: Oral: Initial: 40 mg twice daily; may increase to 60 mg or 80 mg twice daily on second day of treatment; subsequently adjust dose based on response and tolerability. Usual dosage: 40 to 80 mg twice daily.

Schizophrenia: Adults: Oral: Initial: 20 mg twice daily (U.S. labeling) or 20 to 40 mg twice daily (Canadian labeling). Increase dose based on response and tolerability no more frequently than every 2 days; ordinarily patients should be observed for improvement over several weeks before adjusting the dose. Usual dosage: 40 to 100 mg twice daily. Note: Dosages up to 320 mg per day appear safe; however, there is no data suggesting improved efficacy at higher doses (APA, 2004).

Acute agitation (schizophrenia): Adults: IM: 10 mg every 2 hours **or** 20 mg every 4 hours; maximum: 40 mg daily; oral therapy should replace IM administration as soon as possible

Elderly: No dosage adjustment is recommended; consider initiating at a low end of the dosage range, with slower titration

Dosage adjustment in renal impairment:

Oral: No dosage adjustment necessary

IM: Cyclodextrin, an excipient in the IM formulation, is cleared by renal filtration; use with caution.

Ziprasidone is not removed by hemodialysis.

Dosage adjustment in hepatic impairment:

U.S. labeling: There are no dosage adjustments provided in the manufacturer's labeling; however, drug undergoes extensive hepatic metabolism and systemic exposure may be increased. Use with caution.

Canadian labeling: Manufacturer labeling suggests that dose reductions should be considered but does not provide specific dosing recommendations.

Dietary Considerations Capsule: Take with food.

Administration

Oral: Administer with a meal containing at least 500 calories (Lincoln, 2010).

Injection: For IM administration only.

Hazardous agent; use appropriate precautions for handling and disposal (NIOSH 2014 [group 3]).

Monitoring Parameters Mental status; vital signs (as clinically indicated); blood pressure (baseline; repeat 3 months after antipsychotic initiation, then yearly); ECG (as clinically indicated); weight, height, BMI, waist circumference (baseline; repeat at 4, 8, and 12 weeks after initiating or changing therapy, then quarterly; consider switching to a different antipsychotic for a weight gain ≥5% of initial weight); CBC (as clinically indicated; monitor frequently during the first few months of therapy in patients with preexisting low WBC or history of drug-induced leukopenia/neutropenia); electrolytes (annually and as clinically indicated; perform baseline potassium and magnesium measurements in patients at risk for electrolyte disturbances and periodically monitor if diuretics are initiated during ziprasidone treatment); liver function (annually and as clinically indicated); personal and family history of obesity, diabetes, dyslipidemia, hypertension, or cardiovascular disease (baseline; repeat annually); fasting plasma glucose level/HbA_{1c} (baseline; repeat 3 months after starting antipsychotic, then yearly); fasting lipid panel (baseline; repeat 3 months after initiation of antipsychotic; if LDL level is normal repeat at 2-5 year intervals or more frequently if clinical indicated); changes in menstruation, libido, development of galactorrhea, erectile and ejaculatory function (at each visit for the first 12 weeks after the antipsychotic is initiated or until the dose is stable, then yearly); abnormal involuntary movements or parkinsonian signs (baseline; repeat weekly until dose stabilized for at least 2 weeks after introduction and for 2 weeks after any significant dose increase); tardive dyskinesia (every 12 months; high-risk patients every 6 months); ocular examination (yearly in patients >40 years; every 2 years in younger patients) (ADA, 2004; Lehman, 2004; Marder, 2004).

Additional Information The increased potential to prolong QTc, as compared to other available antipsychotic agents, should be considered in the evaluation of available alternatives.

Dosage Forms

Capsule, Oral:

Geodon: 20 mg, 40 mg, 60 mg, 80 mg

Generic: 20 mg, 40 mg, 60 mg, 80 mg

Solution Reconstituted, Intramuscular:

Geodon: 20 mg (1 ea)

Dosage Forms: Canada

Capsule, Oral:

Zeldox: 20 mg, 40 mg, 60 mg, 80 mg

Extemporaneous Preparations Hazardous agent: Use appropriate precautions for handling and disposal (NIOSH 2014 [group 3]).

A 2.5 mg/mL oral solution may be made with the injection. Use 8 vials of the 20 mg injectable powder. Add 1.2 mL of distilled water to each vial to make a 20 mg/mL solution. Once dissolved, transfer 7.5 mL to a calibrated bottle and add quantity of vehicle (Ora-Sweet®) sufficient to make 60 mL. Label "shake well" and "refrigerate". Stable for 14 days at room temperature or 42 days refrigerated (preferred).

Green K and Parish RC, "Stability of Ziprasidone Mesylate in an Extemporaneously Compounded Oral Solution," *J Pediatr Pharmacol Ther*, 2010, 15:138-41.

- **Ziprasidone Hydrochloride** *see* Ziprasidone *on page 2201*
- **Ziprasidone Mesylate** *see* Ziprasidone *on page 2201*
- **Zipsor** *see* Diclofenac (Systemic) *on page 617*
- **Zithranol** *see* Anthralin *on page 150*
- **Zithranol-RR** *see* Anthralin *on page 150*
- **Zithromax** *see* Azithromycin (Systemic) *on page 216*
- **Zithromax For Intravenous Injection (Can)** *see* Azithromycin (Systemic) *on page 216*
- **Zithromax TRI-PAK** *see* Azithromycin (Systemic) *on page 216*
- **Zithromax Tri-Pak** *see* Azithromycin (Systemic) *on page 216*
- **Zithromax Z-PAK** *see* Azithromycin (Systemic) *on page 216*
- **Zithromax Z-Pak** *see* Azithromycin (Systemic) *on page 216*

Ziv-Aflibercept (Systemic) (ziv a FLIB er sept)

Brand Names: U.S. Zaltrap

Index Terms Aflibercept I.V.; Vascular Endothelial Growth Factor Trap; VEGF Trap; VEGF Trap R1R2

Pharmacologic Category Antineoplastic Agent; Vascular Endothelial Growth Factor (VEGF) Inhibitor

Use Colorectal cancer, metastatic: Treatment of metastatic colorectal cancer (in combination with fluorouracil, leucovorin, and irinotecan [FOLFIRI]) in patients who are resistant to or have progressed on an oxaliplatin-based regimen

Pregnancy Risk Factor C

Pregnancy Considerations Adverse events were observed in animal reproduction studies with doses providing systemic exposure equivalent to ~30% of a human dose. The incidence of fetal malformations increased with increasing doses. Patients (male and female) should use effective contraception during therapy and for at least 3 months following treatment.

Breast-Feeding Considerations It is not known if ziv-aflibercept is excreted into breast milk. Due to the potential for serious adverse reactions in the nursing infant, the manufacturer recommends a decision to be made whether to discontinue nursing or to discontinue aflibercept, taking into account the importance of treatment to the mother.

Contraindications There are no contraindications listed in the manufacturer's labeling.

Warnings/Precautions The risk for hemorrhage is increased with ziv-aflibercept. **[U.S. Boxed Warning]: Severe and occasionally fatal hemorrhage, including gastrointestinal (GI) bleeding, has been reported with ziv-aflibercept/FOLFIRI. Monitor for signs and symptoms of GI and other severe bleeding events; do not administer to patients with severe hemorrhage;** discontinue if severe hemorrhage develops. Hemorrhagic events have also included hematuria, postprocedural hemorrhage, intracranial hemorrhage, and pulmonary hemorrhage/hemoptysis.

[U.S. Boxed Warning]: Severe or fatal GI perforation is a possibility; discontinue ziv-aflibercept if GI perforation occurs; monitor for signs/symptoms of GI perforation. The risk for GI and non-GI fistulas is increased with ziv-aflibercept; fistula sites have included anal, enterovesical, enterocutaneous, colovaginal and intestinal; discontinue in patients who develop fistula. Severe diarrhea and dehydration have been reported; the incidence of diarrhea is increased in patients ≥65 years of age; monitor elderly patients closely for diarrhea.

Proteinuria, nephrotic syndrome, and thrombotic microangiopathy (TMA) have been associated with ziv-aflibercept. Evaluate for proteinuria during treatment with urine dipstick and/or urinary protein creatinine ratio (UPCR); if dipstick ≥2+ for protein or UPCR >1, obtain 24-hour urine collection. Withhold ziv-aflibercept for proteinuria ≥2 g per 24 hours; for recurrent proteinuria, withhold treatment until <2 g per 24 hours and then resume with permanent dose reduction. Discontinue treatment for nephrotic syndrome or TMA.

The risk for grades 3/4 hypertension is increased; onset is generally within the first 2 treatment cycles. Monitor blood pressure every 2 weeks (more frequently if clinically indicated); treat with appropriate antihypertensive therapy (may require adjustment of existing antihypertensives); temporarily withhold treatment with uncontrolled hypertension; may reinitiate with permanent dose reduction when controlled. Discontinue for hypertensive crisis or encephalopathy. Patients with NYHA class III or IV heart failure were excluded from clinical trials.

[U.S. Boxed Warning]: Severely compromised wound healing may occur with ziv-aflibercept/FOLFIRI. Discontinue ziv-aflibercept with compromised wound healing. Withhold ziv-aflibercept at least 4 weeks prior to elective surgery. Do not resume ziv-aflibercept treatment until at least 4 weeks after major surgery AND until the surgical wound is completely healed. For minor surgeries (eg, central venous access port placement, biopsy, or tooth extraction), ziv-aflibercept may be resumed or initiated as soon as the surgical wound is fully healed.

A higher incidence of neutropenia and complications due to neutropenia (neutropenic fever and infection) occurred in patients receiving ziv-aflibercept; leukopenia and thrombocytopenia were also observed in clinical trials; monitor CBC with differential (baseline and prior to each cycle); delay treatment until ANC is ≥1,500/mm^3. Cases of reversible posterior leukoencephalopathy syndrome (RPLS) have been reported; confirm diagnosis with MRI; discontinue ziv-aflibercept if verified; symptoms generally resolve or improve within days, although persistent neurologic symptoms and death have been reported. Arterial thrombotic events (ATE), including transient ischemic attack, cerebrovascular accidents, and angina have occurred. Discontinue ziv-aflibercept in patients who experience

ATEs. Certain adverse events, such as diarrhea, dizziness, weakness, weight loss, and dehydration, occurred at a higher incidence in elderly compared to younger adults; monitor closely during treatment.

Adverse Reactions Note: Reactions reported in combination therapy with fluorouracil, leucovorin, and irinotecan (FOLFIRI).

Cardiovascular: Arterial thromboembolic events, hypertension, venous thromboembolic events

Central nervous system: Dysphonia, fatigue, headache, reversible posterior encephalopathy syndrome (RPLS)

Dermatologic: Hyperpigmentation, palmar-plantar erythrodysesthesia

Endocrine & metabolic: Dehydration

Gastrointestinal: Abdominal pain, appetite decreased, diarrhea, gastrointestinal perforation, hemorrhoids, proctalgia, rectal hemorrhage, stomatitis, upper abdominal pain, weight loss

Genitourinary: Urinary tract infection

Hematologic: Bleeding, leukopenia, neutropenia, neutropenic fever, neutropenic infection/sepsis, thrombocytopenia

Hepatic: AST increased, ALT increased

Neuromuscular & skeletal: Weakness

Renal: Creatinine increased, nephrotic syndrome, proteinuria

Respiratory: Dyspnea, epistaxis, oropharyngeal pain, pulmonary embolism, rhinorrhea

Miscellaneous: Antibody formation, fistula formation, infection

Rare but important or life-threatening: Hypersensitivity reactions, thrombotic microangiopathy, wound healing impaired

Drug Interactions

Metabolism/Transport Effects None known.

Avoid Concomitant Use

Avoid concomitant use of Ziv-Aflibercept (Systemic) with any of the following: CloZAPine; Dipyrone

Increased Effect/Toxicity

Ziv-Aflibercept (Systemic) may increase the levels/effects of: Bisphosphonate Derivatives; CloZAPine

The levels/effects of Ziv-Aflibercept (Systemic) may be increased by: Dipyrone

Decreased Effect There are no known significant interactions involving a decrease in effect.

Preparation for Administration Prior to infusion, dilute in D_5W or NS to a final concentration of 0.6-8 mg/mL. Use polyvinyl chloride (PVC) infusion bags containing DEHP or polyolefin bags. After initial vial puncture, do not re-enter; discard any unused portion of the vial. Do not mix with other medications.

Storage/Stability Store intact vials refrigerated at 2°C to 8°C (36°F to 46°F). Protect from light (store in original outer carton).

Solutions diluted for infusion may be stored in refrigerator for up to 24 hours, or at 20°C to 25°C (68°F to 77°F) for up to 8 hours.

Mechanism of Action Also known as VEGF-trap, ziv-aflibercept is a recombinant fusion protein which is comprised of portions of binding domains for vascular endothelial growth factor (VEGF) receptors 1 and 2, attached to the Fc portion of human IgG1. Ziv-aflibercept acts as a decoy receptor for VEGF-A, VEGF-B, and placental growth factor (PlGF) which prevent VEGF receptor binding/activation to their receptors (an action critical to angiogenesis), thus leading to antiangiogenesis and tumor regression.

Pharmacodynamics/Kinetics Half-life elimination: ~6 days (range: 4 to 7 days)

Dosage Colorectal cancer, metastatic: Adults: IV: 4 mg/kg every 2 weeks (in combination with fluorouracil, leucovorin, and irinotecan [FOLFIRI]), continue until disease progression or unacceptable toxicity

Dosage adjustment for toxicity:

Arterial thrombotic events: Discontinue treatment.

Fistula formation: Discontinue treatment.

Gastrointestinal perforation: Discontinue treatment.

Hemorrhage, severe: Discontinue treatment.

Hypertension:

Recurrent or severe hypertension: Temporarily withhold treatment until controlled, and then resume with a permanent dose reduction to 2 mg/kg every 2 weeks.

Hypertensive crisis or hypertensive encephalopathy: Discontinue treatment.

Neutropenia: Temporarily withhold treatment until ANC is ≥1500/mm^3.

Renal effects:

Proteinuria (≥2 g/24 hours): Temporarily withhold treatment until proteinuria <2 g/24 hours and then resume at previous dose.

Recurrent proteinuria: Temporarily withhold treatment until proteinuria <2 g/24 hours, and then resume with a permanent dose reduction to 2 mg/kg every 2 weeks.

Nephrotic syndrome or thrombotic microangiopathy: Discontinue treatment.

Reversible posterior leukoencephalopathy syndrome (RPLS): Discontinue treatment.

Surgery/wound healing impairment:

Elective surgery: Temporarily withhold treatment for at least 4 weeks prior to elective surgery; do not resume until at least 4 weeks after major surgery AND until wound is fully healed; for minor surgery (eg, biopsy, central venous port placement, tooth extraction), may be resumed after wound is fully healed.

Wound healing impaired: Discontinue treatment.

Note: For toxicities related to FOLFIRI, refer to individual Fluorouracil (Systemic) or Irinotecan monographs.

Dosage adjustment in renal impairment: There are no dosage adjustments provided in the manufacturer's labeling; however, need for adjustment is not likely because exposure in patients with mild, moderate, and severe impairment was similar to that of patients with normal renal function.

Dosage adjustment in hepatic impairment:

Mild (total bilirubin >1-1.5 times ULN) to moderate (total bilirubin >1.5-3 times ULN) impairment: There are no dosage adjustments provided in the manufacturer's labeling; however, need for adjustment is not likely because exposure was similar to that of patients with normal hepatic function.

Severe impairment (total bilirubin >3 times ULN): There are no dosage adjustments provided in the manufacturer's labeling (no data available).

Administration IV: Infuse over 1 hour. Do not administer as an IV push or bolus. Administer prior to any FOLFIRI component. Do not administer other medications through the same intravenous line.

Infuse via a 0.2 micron polyethersulfone filter; do not use filters made of polyvinylidene fluoride (PVDF) or nylon. Administer with one of the following types of infusion sets: Polyvinyl chloride (PVC) containing DEHP, DEHP-free PVC containing trioctyl-trimellitate (TOTM), polypropylene, polyethylene lined PVC, or polyurethane.

Monitoring Parameters CBC with differential (baseline and prior to each cycle); urine protein (dipstick analysis and/or urinary protein creatinine ratio [UPCR], obtain 24-hour urine collection if dipstick ≥2+ for protein or UPCR >1); blood pressure (every 2 weeks; more frequently if clinically indicated); monitor for signs/symptoms of hemorrhage or GI perforation; monitor elderly patients closely for diarrhea and/or dehydration. Monitor wounds for healing impairment.

Dosage Forms

Solution, Intravenous [preservative free]:
Zaltrap: 100 mg/4 mL (4 mL); 200 mg/8 mL (8 mL)

- **Zmax** *see* Azithromycin (Systemic) *on page 216*
- **Zmax SR (Can)** *see* Azithromycin (Systemic) *on page 216*
- **$ZnSO_4$ (error-prone abbreviation)** *see* Zinc Sulfate *on page 2200*
- **Zocor** *see* Simvastatin *on page 1890*

Zofenopril [INT] (zoe FEN oh pril)

International Brand Names Bifracard (MX); Bifril (AT, DE, DK, FI, GB, IE, IS, IT, LB, NO, SE, SG); Presiam (AR); Teoula (FR); Zocardis (RU); Zofecard (HR); Zofen (BG); Zofenil (AT, BE, DE, DK, ES, FI, FR, GB, IE, IS, KR, LU, NO, PT, SE); Zofepril (GR, IT); Zofil (NL); Zofistar (EE, LT); Zomen (RO); Zopranol (BE, ES, GR, IT, LU, NL, PT)

Pharmacologic Category Angiotensin-Converting Enzyme (ACE) Inhibitor

Reported Use Management of hypertension; treatment of acute anterior wall myocardial infarction

Dosage Range Oral: Adults:

Acute anterior wall myocardial infarction: Begin 24 hours after onset of symptoms and continue dose for 6 weeks; initial: 7.5 mg every 12 hours for 2 days, then 15 mg every 12 hours for 2 days, then 30 mg every 12 hours; target dose: 30 mg every 12 hours

Hypertension: Initial: 15 mg once daily, may increase dose at 4-week intervals; usual effective dose: 30 mg once daily; maximum daily dose: 60 mg/day, administer once daily or in two divided doses

Note: Diuretics should be discontinued 2-3 days prior to initiating zofenopril, if possible. Restart diuretic after blood pressure is stable, if needed. If diuretic can be discontinued prior to therapy, begin with 15 mg/day with close supervision until stable blood pressure. Start dose at 7.5 mg/day if these measures cannot be taken.

Dosage adjustment in renal impairment: Hypertension:
CrCl ≤45 mL/minute: Decrease daily dosage by 50%
CrCl >45 mL/minute: No adjustment required

Dialysis: Initial and maintenance dose: Decrease dose by 75%

Dosage adjustment in hepatic impairment: Hypertension:
Mild-to-moderate impairment: Decrease daily dosage by 50%
Severe impairment: Use is contraindicated

Product Availability Product available in various countries; not currently available in the U.S.

Dosage Forms

Tablet: 7.5 mg, 30 mg, 60 mg

- **Zofran** *see* Ondansetron *on page 1513*
- **Zofran ODT** *see* Ondansetron *on page 1513*
- **Zol 446** *see* Zoledronic Acid *on page 2206*
- **Zoladex** *see* Goserelin *on page 981*
- **Zoladex LA (Can)** *see* Goserelin *on page 981*
- **Zoledronate** *see* Zoledronic Acid *on page 2206*

Zoledronic Acid (zoe le DRON ik AS id)

Brand Names: U.S. Reclast; Zometa

Brand Names: Canada Aclasta; Taro-Zoledronic Acid; Taro-Zoledronic Acid Concentrate; Zoledronic Acid Injection; Zoledronic Acid for Injection; Zoledronic Acid Z; Zometa Concentrate

Index Terms CGP-42446; Zol 446; Zoledronate

Pharmacologic Category Bisphosphonate Derivative

Use

Glucocorticoid-induced osteoporosis (Reclast): Treatment and prevention of glucocorticoid-induced osteoporosis in men and women who are initiating or continuing systemic glucocorticoids in a daily dose equivalent to 7.5 mg or more of prednisone and who are expected to remain on glucocorticoids for at least 12 months.

Hypercalcemia of malignancy (Zometa): Treatment of hypercalcemia (albumin-corrected serum calcium ≥12 mg/dL) of malignancy.

Multiple myeloma and bone metastases from solid tumors (Zometa): Treatment of patients with multiple myeloma and patients with documented bone metastases from solid tumors, in conjunction with standard antineoplastic therapy.

Osteoporosis in men (Reclast): To increase bone mass in men with osteoporosis.

Paget disease of bone (Reclast): Treatment of Paget disease of bone in men and women.

Postmenopausal osteoporosis (Reclast): Treatment and prevention of osteoporosis in postmenopausal women.

Pregnancy Risk Factor D

Pregnancy Considerations Adverse events were observed in animal reproduction studies. It is not known if bisphosphonates cross the placenta, but fetal exposure is expected (Djokanovic, 2008; Stathopoulos, 2011). Bisphosphonates are incorporated into the bone matrix and gradually released over time. The amount available in the systemic circulation varies by dose and duration of therapy. Theoretically, there may be a risk of fetal harm when pregnancy follows the completion of therapy; however, available data have not shown that exposure to bisphosphonates during pregnancy significantly increases the risk of adverse fetal events (Djokanovic, 2008; Levy, 2009; Stathopoulos, 2011). Until additional data is available, most sources recommend discontinuing bisphosphonate therapy in women of reproductive potential as early as possible prior to a planned pregnancy; use in premenopausal women should be reserved for special circumstances when rapid bone loss is occurring (Bhalla, 2010; Pereira, 2012; Stathopoulos, 2011). Because hypocalcemia has been described following *in utero* bisphosphonate exposure, exposed infants should be monitored for hypocalcemia after birth (Djokanovic, 2008; Stathopoulos, 2011). Use in pregnant women is contraindicated per the Canadian labeling.

Breast-Feeding Considerations It is not known if zoledronic acid is excreted into breast milk. Due to the potential for serious adverse reactions in the nursing infant, the U.S. manufacturer recommends a decision be made whether to discontinue nursing or to discontinue the drug, taking into account the importance of treatment to the mother. Use in nursing women is contraindicated per the Canadian labeling.

Contraindications

U.S. labeling:

Hypersensitivity to zoledronic acid or any component of the product; hypocalcemia (Reclast only); CrCl <35 mL/minute and in those with evidence of acute renal impairment (Reclast only).

Documentation of allergenic cross-reactivity for bisphosphonates is limited. However, because of similarities in chemical structure and/or pharmacologic actions, the possibility of cross-sensitivity cannot be ruled out with certainty.

Canadian labeling:

All indications: Hypersensitivity to zoledronic acid or other bisphosphonates, or any component of the formulation; uncorrected hypocalcemia at the time of infusion; pregnancy, breast-feeding

Nononcology uses: Additional contraindications: Use in patients with CrCl <35 mL/minute and use in patients with evidence of acute renal impairment due to an increased risk of renal failure

Warnings/Precautions Hazardous agent - use appropriate precautions for handling and disposal (NIOSH 2014 [group 3]).

Osteonecrosis of the jaw (ONJ) has been reported in patients receiving bisphosphonates. Risk factors include invasive dental procedures (eg, tooth extraction, dental implants, boney surgery); a diagnosis of cancer, with concomitant chemotherapy, radiotherapy, or corticosteroids; poor oral hygiene, ill-fitting dentures; and comorbid disorders (anemia, coagulopathy, infection, preexisting dental disease). Most reported cases occurred after IV bisphosphonate therapy; however, cases have been reported following oral therapy. A dental exam and preventive dentistry should be performed prior to placing patients with risk factors on chronic bisphosphonate therapy. The manufacturer's labeling states that there are no data to suggest whether discontinuing bisphosphonates in patients requiring invasive dental procedures reduces the risk of ONJ. However, other experts suggest that there is no evidence that discontinuing therapy reduces the risk of developing ONJ (Assael, 2009). The benefit/risk must be assessed by the treating physician and/or dentist/surgeon prior to any invasive dental procedure. Patients developing ONJ while on bisphosphonates should receive care by an oral surgeon.

Atypical, low-energy, or low-trauma femur fractures have been reported in patients receiving bisphosphonates. The fractures include subtrochanteric femur (bone just below the hip joint) and diaphyseal femur (long segment of the thigh bone). Some patients experience prodromal pain weeks or months before the fracture occurs. It is unclear if bisphosphonate therapy is the cause for these fractures; atypical femur fractures have also been reported in patients not taking bisphosphonates, and in patients receiving glucocorticoids. Patients receiving long-term (>3-5 years) bisphosphonate therapy may be at an increased risk. Patients presenting with thigh or groin pain with a history of receiving bisphosphonates should be evaluated for femur fracture. Consider interrupting bisphosphonate therapy in patients who develop a femoral shaft fracture; assess for fracture in the contralateral limb.

Infrequently, severe (and occasionally debilitating) musculoskeletal (bone, joint, and/or muscle) pain have been reported during bisphosphonate treatment. The onset of pain ranged from a single day to several months. Consider discontinuing therapy in patients who experience severe symptoms; symptoms usually resolve upon discontinuation. Some patients experienced recurrence when rechallenged with same drug or another bisphosphonate; avoid use in patients with a history of these symptoms in association with bisphosphonate therapy.

May cause a significant risk of hypocalcemia in patients with Paget's disease, in whom the pretreatment rate of bone turnover may be greatly elevated. Hypocalcemia, including severe and life-threatening hypocalcemia, has also been reported with oncology-related uses. Hypocalcemia must be corrected before initiation of therapy in patients with Paget's disease, osteoporosis, or oncology indications. Ensure adequate calcium and vitamin D intake during therapy. Use caution in patients with disturbances of calcium and mineral metabolism (eg, hypoparathyroidism, thyroid/parathyroid, surgery, malabsorption syndromes, excision of small intestine).

Nononcology indications: Use is contraindicated in patients with CrCl <35 mL/minute and in patients with evidence of acute renal impairment due to an increased risk of renal failure. Obtain serum creatinine and calculate creatinine clearance (using actual body weight) with the Cockcroft-Gault formula prior to each administration. In the management of osteoporosis, re-evaluate the need for continued therapy periodically; the optimal duration of treatment has not yet been determined. Consider discontinuing after 3-5 years of use in patients at low risk for fracture; following discontinuation, re-evaluate fracture risk periodically.

Oncology indications: Use caution in mild-to-moderate renal dysfunction; dosage adjustment required. In cancer patients, renal toxicity has been reported with doses >4 mg or infusions administered over 15 minutes. Risk factors for renal deterioration include preexisting renal insufficiency and repeated doses of zoledronic acid and other bisphosphonates. Dehydration and the use of other nephrotoxic drugs which may contribute to renal deterioration should be identified and managed. Use is not recommended in patients with severe renal impairment (serum creatinine >3 mg/dL or CrCl <30 mL/minute) and bone metastases (limited data); use in patients with hypercalcemia of malignancy and severe renal impairment (serum creatinine >4.5 mg/dL for hypercalcemia of malignancy) should only be done if the benefits outweigh the risks. Diuretics should not be used before correcting hypovolemia. Renal deterioration, resulting in renal failure and dialysis has occurred in patients treated with zoledronic acid after single and multiple infusions at recommended doses of 4 mg over 15 minutes. Assess renal function prior to treatment and withhold for renal deterioration [increase in serum creatinine of 0.5 mg/dL (if baseline level normal) or increase of 1 mg/dL (if baseline level abnormal)]; treatment should be withheld until renal function returns to within 10% of baseline.

According to the American Society of Clinical Oncology (ASCO) guidelines for bisphosphonates in multiple myeloma, treatment with zoledronic acid is not recommended for asymptomatic (smoldering) or indolent myeloma or with solitary plasmacytoma (Kyle, 2007). The National Comprehensive Cancer Network (NCCN) multiple myeloma guidelines (v.2.2013) recommend bisphosphonates for all patients receiving treatment for symptomatic disease; the use of bisphosphonates in stage 1 or smoldering disease may be considered, although preferably as part of a clinical trial.

Adequate hydration is required during treatment (urine output ~2 L/day); avoid overhydration, especially in patients with heart failure. Preexisting renal compromise, severe dehydration, and concurrent use with diuretics or other nephrotoxic drugs may increase the risk for renal impairment. Single and multiple infusions in patients with both normal and impaired renal function have been associated with renal deterioration, resulting in renal failure and dialysis or death (rare). Patients with underlying moderate-to-severe renal impairment, increased age, concurrent use of nephrotoxic or diuretic medications, or severe dehydration prior to or after zoledronic acid administration may have an increased risk of acute renal impairment or renal failure. Others with increased risk include patients with renal impairment or dehydration secondary to fever, sepsis, gastrointestinal losses, or diuretic use. If history or physical exam suggests dehydration, treatment should not be given until the patient is normovolemic. Transient increases in serum creatinine may be more pronounced in patients with impaired renal function; consider monitoring creatinine clearance in at-risk patients taking other renally-eliminated drugs.

Conjunctivitis, uveitis, episcleritis, iritis, scleritis, and orbital inflammation have been reported (infrequently) with use; further ophthalmic evaluation (and possibly therapy discontinuation) may be necessary in patients with complicated infection. Use caution in patients with aspirin-sensitive asthma (may cause bronchoconstriction) and the elderly (because decreased renal function occurs more commonly in elderly patients). Rare cases of urticaria and angioedema and very rare cases of anaphylactic reactions/shock have been reported. Do not administer Zometa and Reclast (Aclasta [Canadian brand]) to the same patient for different indications.

Adverse Reactions Note: An acute reaction (eg, arthralgia, fever, flu-like symptoms, myalgia) may occur within the first 3 days following infusion in up to 44% of patients; usually resolves within 3-4 days of onset, although may take up to 14 days to resolve. The incidence may be decreased with acetaminophen (prior to infusion and for 72 hours postinfusion).

Oncology indications:

Cardiovascular: Chest pain, hypotension, lower extremity edema

Central nervous system: Agitation, anxiety, confusion, depression, dizziness, fatigue, headache, hypoesthesia, insomnia, rigors

Dermatologic: Alopecia, dermatitis

Endocrine & metabolic: Dehydration, hyper-/hypomagnesemia, hypocalcemia, hypokalemia, hypophosphatemia

Gastrointestinal: Abdominal pain, anorexia, constipation, decreased appetite, diarrhea, dyspepsia, dysphagia, mucositis, nausea, sore throat, stomatitis, vomiting, weight loss

Genitourinary: Urinary tract infection

Hematologic & oncologic: Anemia, granulocytopenia, neutropenia, pancytopenia, progression of cancer, thrombocytopenia

Infection: Candidiasis, infection (nonspecific)

Neuromuscular & skeletal: Arthralgia, back pain, limb pain, myalgia, ostealgia, paresthesia, skeletal pain, weakness

Renal: Increased serum creatinine, renal insufficiency

Respiratory: Cough, dyspnea, upper respiratory tract infection

Miscellaneous: Fever

Nononcology indications:

Cardiovascular: Atrial fibrillation, chest pain, palpitations, peripheral edema, hypertension

Central nervous system: Chills, dizziness, fatigue, fever, headache, hyperthermia, hypoesthesia, lethargy, malaise, pain, paresthesia, rigors, vertigo

Dermatologic: Hyperhidrosis, skin rash

Endocrine & metabolic: Hypocalcemia

Gastrointestinal: Abdominal discomfort, abdominal pain, anorexia, constipation, diarrhea, dyspepsia, nausea, vomiting

Hematologic & oncologic: Change in serum protein (C-reactive protein increased)

Immunologic: Infusion related reaction

Neuromuscular & skeletal: Arthralgia, arthritis, back pain, jaw pain, joint swelling, limb pain, muscle spasm, musculoskeletal pain, myalgia, neck pain, ostealgia, shoulder pain, stiffness, weakness

Ophthalmic: Eye pain

Renal: Increased serum creatinine

Respiratory: Dyspnea, flu-like symptoms

All indications: Rare but important or life-threatening: Acute renal failure (requiring hospitalization/dialysis), arthralgia (sometimes severe and/or incapacitating), bradycardia, femur fracture (diaphyseal or subtrochanteric), hematuria, hyperesthesia, hyperparathyroidism, hypersensitivity, injection site reaction (eg, itching, pain, redness), interstitial lung disease, iritis, myalgia (sometimes severe and/or incapacitating), osteonecrosis (primarily of the jaws), periorbital swelling, scleritis, Stevens-Johnson syndrome, toxic epidermal necrolysis

Drug Interactions

Metabolism/Transport Effects None known.

Avoid Concomitant Use There are no known interactions where it is recommended to avoid concomitant use.

Increased Effect/Toxicity

Zoledronic Acid may increase the levels/effects of: Deferasirox; Phosphate Supplements

The levels/effects of Zoledronic Acid may be increased by: Aminoglycosides; Calcitonin; Nonsteroidal Anti-Inflammatory Agents; Systemic Angiogenesis Inhibitors; Thalidomide

Decreased Effect

The levels/effects of Zoledronic Acid may be decreased by: Proton Pump Inhibitors

Preparation for Administration Hazardous agent; use appropriate precautions for handling and disposal (NIOSH 2014 [group 3]).

Solution for injection:

Reclast, Aclasta (Canadian brand): No further preparation is necessary.

Zometa concentrate vials: Further dilute in 100 mL NS or D_5W prior to administration.

Zometa ready-to-use bottles: No further preparation is necessary. If reduced doses are required for patients with renal impairment, withdraw the appropriate volume of solution and replace with an equal amount of NS or D_5W.

Storage/Stability Solution for injection:

Aclasta (Canadian brand): Store at room temperature of 15°C to 30°C (59°F to 86°F). Keep sealed in original package until administration.

Reclast: Store at room temperature of 25°C (77°F); excursions permitted to 15°C to 30°C (59°F to 86°F). After opening, stable for 24 hours at 2°C to 8°C (36°F to 46°F). If refrigerated, allow the refrigerated solution to reach room temperature before administration.

Zometa: Store concentrate vials and ready-to-use bottles at 25°C (77°F); excursions permitted to 15°C to 30°C (59°F to 86°F). Diluted solutions for infusion which are not used immediately after preparation should be refrigerated at 2°C to 8°C (36°F to 46°F). Infusion of solution must be completed within 24 hours of preparation. The ready-to-use bottles are for single use only; if any preparation is necessary (preparing reduced dosage for patients with renal impairment), the prepared, diluted solution may be refrigerated at 2°C to 8°C (36°F to 46°F) if not used immediately. Infusion of solution must be completed within 24 hours of preparation. The previously withdrawn volume from the ready-to-use solution should be discarded; do not store or reuse.

Mechanism of Action A bisphosphonate which inhibits bone resorption via actions on osteoclasts or on osteoclast precursors; inhibits osteoclastic activity and skeletal calcium release induced by tumors. Decreases serum calcium and phosphorus, and increases their elimination. In osteoporosis, zoledronic acid inhibits osteoclast-mediated resorption, therefore reducing bone turnover.

Pharmacodynamics/Kinetics

Distribution: Binds to bone

Protein binding: 23% to 53%

Metabolism: Primarily eliminated intact via the kidney; metabolism not likely

Half-life elimination: Triphasic; Terminal: 146 hours

Excretion: Urine (39% ± 16% as unchanged drug) within 24 hours; feces (<3%)

Dosage Note: Acetaminophen administration after the infusion may reduce symptoms of acute-phase reactions. Patients treated for multiple myeloma and Paget's disease should receive a daily calcium and vitamin D supplement, and patients with osteoporosis should receive calcium and vitamin D supplementation if dietary intake is inadequate.

Hypercalcemia of malignancy (albumin-corrected serum calcium ≥12 mg/dL) (Zometa): Adults: IV: 4 mg (maximum) given as a single dose. Wait at least 7 days before considering retreatment.

Multiple myeloma or metastatic bone lesions from solid tumors (Zometa): Adults: IV: 4 mg once every 3-4 weeks

Osteoporosis, glucocorticoid-induced, treatment and prevention (Reclast, Aclasta [Canadian brand]): Adults: IV: 5 mg once a year

Osteoporosis, prevention: Adults: IV:

Reclast: 5 mg once every 2 years

Aclasta (Canadian brand): 5 mg as a single (one-time) dose

Osteoporosis, treatment (Reclast, Aclasta [Canadian brand]): Adults: IV: 5 mg once a year; consider discontinuing after 3-5 years of use in patients at low risk for fracture

Paget's disease: Adults: IV:

Reclast: 5 mg as a single dose. **Note:** Data concerning retreatment is not available; retreatment may be considered for relapse (increase in alkaline phosphatase) if appropriate, for inadequate response, or in patients who are symptomatic.

Aclasta (Canadian brand): 5 mg as a single dose. Data concerning retreatment is limited; retreatment with 5 mg (single dose) may be considered for relapse after an interval of at least 1 year from initial treatment.

Prevention of aromatase inhibitor-induced bone loss in breast cancer (off-label use): Adults: IV: 4 mg once every 6 months for 5 years (Brufsky, 2012)

Prevention of androgen deprivation-induced bone loss in nonmetastatic prostate cancer (off-label use): Adults: IV: 4 mg once every 3 months for 1 year (Smith, 2003) or 4 mg once every 12 months (Michaelson, 2007)

Dosage adjustment in renal impairment (at treatment initiation): Note: Prior to each dose, obtain serum creatinine and calculate the creatinine clearance using the Cockcroft-Gault formula.

***Nononcology uses:* Note:** Use actual body weight in the Cockcroft-Gault formula when calculating clearance for nononcology uses.

CrCl ≥35 mL/minute: No dosage adjustment required.

CrCl <35 mL/minute: Use is contraindicated.

Oncology uses:

Multiple myeloma and bone metastases:

CrCl >60 mL/minute: 4 mg (no dosage adjustment necessary)

CrCl 50-60 mL/minute: Reduce dose to 3.5 mg

CrCl 40-49 mL/minute: Reduce dose to 3.3 mg

CrCl 30-39 mL/minute: Reduce dose to 3 mg

CrCl <30 mL/minute: Use is not recommended.

Hypercalcemia of malignancy:

Mild-to-moderate impairment: No dosage adjustment necessary.

Severe impairment (serum creatinine >4.5 mg/dL):

U.S. labeling: Evaluate risk versus benefit

Canadian labeling: Use is not recommended.

Dosage adjustment for renal toxicity (during treatment):

Hypercalcemia of malignancy: Evidence of renal deterioration: Evaluate risk versus benefit.

Multiple myeloma and bone metastases: Evidence of renal deterioration: Withhold dose until renal function returns to within 10% of baseline; renal deterioration defined as follows:

Normal baseline creatinine: Increase of 0.5 mg/dL

Abnormal baseline creatinine: Increase of 1 mg/dL

Reinitiate therapy at the same dose administered prior to treatment interruption.

Multiple myeloma: Albuminuria >500 mg/24 hours (unexplained): Withhold dose until return to baseline, then reevaluate every 3-4 weeks; consider reinitiating with a longer infusion time of at least 30 minutes (Kyle, 2007).

Dosage adjustment in hepatic impairment: No dosage adjustment provided in the manufacturer's labeling (has not been studied); however, zoledronic acid is not metabolized hepatically.

Dietary Considerations

Multiple myeloma or metastatic bone lesions from solid tumors: Take daily calcium supplement (500 mg) and daily multivitamin (with 400 units vitamin D).

Osteoporosis: Ensure adequate calcium and vitamin D intake; if dietary intake is inadequate, dietary supplementation is recommended. Women and men should consume:

Calcium: 1000 mg/day (men: 50-70 years) **or** 1200 mg/day (women ≥51 years and men ≥71 years) (IOM, 2011; NOF, 2013)

Vitamin D: 800-1000 IU/day (men and women ≥50 years) (NOF, 2013). Recommended Dietary Allowance (RDA): 600 IU/day (men and women ≤70 years) **or** 800 IU/day (men and women ≥71 years) (IOM, 2011).

Paget's disease: Take elemental calcium 1500 mg/day (750 mg twice daily or 500 mg 3 times/day) and vitamin D 800 units/day, particularly during the first 2 weeks after administration.

Administration If refrigerated, allow solution to reach room temperature before administration. Infuse over at least 15 minutes. Flush IV line with 10 mL NS flush following infusion. Infuse in a line separate from other medications. Patients must be appropriately hydrated prior to treatment. Acetaminophen after administration may reduce the incidence of acute reaction (eg, arthralgia, fever, flu-like symptoms, myalgia).

Hazardous agent; use appropriate precautions for handling and disposal (NIOSH 2014 [group 3]).

Monitoring Parameters Prior to initiation of therapy, dental exam and preventive dentistry for patients at risk for osteonecrosis, including all cancer patients

Nononcology uses: Serum creatinine prior to each dose, especially in patients with risk factors, calculate creatinine clearance before each treatment (consider interim monitoring in patients at risk for acute renal failure), evaluate fluid status and adequately hydrate patients prior to and following administration.

Osteoporosis: Bone mineral density (BMD) should be reevaluated every 2 years (or more frequently) after initiating therapy (NOF, 2013); in patients with combined zoledronic acid and glucocorticoid treatment, BMD should be made at initiation of therapy and repeated after 6-12 months; serum calcium and 25(OH)D; annual measurements of height and weight, assessment of chronic back pain; serum calcium and 25(OH)D; phosphorus and magnesium; may consider monitoring biochemical markers of bone turnover

Paget's disease: Alkaline phosphatase; pain; serum calcium and 25(OH)D; phosphorus and magnesium; symptoms of hypocalcemia

Oncology uses: Serum creatinine prior to each dose; serum electrolytes, phosphate, magnesium, and hemoglobin/hematocrit should be evaluated regularly. Monitor serum calcium to assess response and avoid overtreatment. In patients with multiple myeloma, monitor urine every 3-6 months for albuminuria.

Reference Range

Calcium (total): Adults: 9.0-11.0 mg/dL (2.05-2.54 mmol/L), may slightly decrease with aging

Phosphorus: 2.5-4.5 mg/dL (0.81-1.45 mmol/L)

Vitamin D: There is no clear consensus on a reference range for total serum 25(OH)D concentrations or the validity of this level as it relates clinically to bone health. In addition, there is significant variability in the reporting of serum 25(OH)D levels as a result of different assay types in use; however, the following ranges have been suggested:

Adults (IOM, 2011): Sufficient levels in practically all persons: ≥20 ng/mL (50 nmol/L); concern for risk of toxicity: >50 ng/mL (125 nmol/L)

Osteoporosis patients (NOF, 2013): Recommended level to reach and maintain: ~30 ng/mL (75 nmol/L)

Additional Information Oncology Comment:

Metastatic breast cancer: The American Society of Clinical Oncology (ASCO) guidelines on the role of bone-modifying agents (BMAs) in the prevention and treatment of skeletal-related events for metastatic breast cancer patients were updated (Van Poznak, 2011). The guidelines recommend initiating a BMA (denosumab, pamidronate, zoledronic acid) in patients with a diagnosis of metastatic breast cancer to the bone. There is currently no literature indicating the superiority of one particular BMA over another. The optimal duration has yet to be defined; however, the guidelines recommend continuing therapy until substantial decline in patient's performance status. In patients with normal creatinine clearance (>60 mL/minute), no dosage/interval/infusion rate changes for pamidronate or zoledronic acid are necessary. For patients with CrCl <30 mL/minute, pamidronate and zoledronic acid are not recommended. While no renal dose adjustments are recommended for denosumab, close monitoring is advised for risk of hypocalcemia in patients with CrCl <30 mL/minute or on dialysis. The ASCO guidelines are in alignment with package insert guidelines for dosing, renal dose adjustments, infusion times, prevention and management of osteonecrosis of the jaw, and monitoring of laboratory parameter recommendations. BMAs are not the first-line therapy for pain. BMAs are to be used as adjunctive therapy for cancer-related bone pain associated with bone metastasis, demonstrating a modest pain control benefit. BMAs should be used in conjunction with agents such as NSAIDS, opioid and nonopioid analgesics, corticosteroids, radiation/surgery, interventional procedures.

Multiple myeloma: The American Society of Clinical Oncology (ASCO) also has guidelines published on the use of bisphosphonates for prevention and treatment of bone disease in multiple myeloma (Kyle, 2007). Pamidronate or zoledronic acid use is recommended in multiple myeloma patients with lytic bone destruction or compression spine fracture from osteopenia. Clodronate (not available in the U.S.; available in Canada), administered orally or IV, is an alternative treatment. The use of the bisphosphonates pamidronate and zoledronic acid may be considered in patients with pain secondary to osteolytic disease, adjunct therapy to stabilize fractures or impending fractures, and IV bisphosphonates for multiple myeloma patients with osteopenia but no radiographic evidence of lytic bone disease. Bisphosphonates are not recommended in patients with solitary plasmacytoma, smoldering (asymptomatic) or indolent myeloma, or monoclonal gammopathy of undetermined significance. The guidelines recommend monthly treatment for a period of 2 years. At that time, physicians need to consider discontinuing in responsive and stable patients, and reinitiate if new-onset skeletal-related event occurs. The ASCO guidelines are in alignment with package insert guidelines for dosing, renal dose adjustments, infusion times, prevention and management of osteonecrosis of the jaw, and monitoring of laboratory parameter recommendations. The guidelines also state in patients with a serum creatinine >3 mg/dL or CrCl <30 mL/minute or extensive bone disease, pamidronate at a dose of 90 mg over 4-6 hours is recommended (unless preexisting renal disease at which a reduced dose should be considered). The ASCO committee also recommends monitoring for the presence of albuminuria every 3-6 months. In patients with albuminuria >500 mg/24 hours, withhold the dose until level returns to baseline, then recheck every 3-4 weeks. Pamidronate may be reinitiated at a dose not to exceed 90 mg every 4 weeks with a longer infusion time of at least 4 hours. The committee also recommends considering increasing the infusion time of zoledronic acid to at least 30 minutes. However, one study has demonstrated that extending the infusion to 30 minutes did not change the safety profile (Berenson, 2011).

Dosage Forms

Concentrate, Intravenous:

Zometa: 4 mg/5 mL (5 mL)

Generic: 4 mg/5 mL (5 mL)

Concentrate, Intravenous [preservative free]:

Generic: 4 mg/5 mL (5 mL)

Solution, Intravenous:

Reclast: 5 mg/100 mL (100 mL)

Zometa: 4 mg/100 mL (100 mL)

Generic: 5 mg/100 mL (100 mL)

Solution, Intravenous [preservative free]:

Generic: 4 mg/100 mL (100 mL); 5 mg/100 mL (100 mL)

Solution Reconstituted, Intravenous:

Generic: 4 mg (1 ea)

Dosage Forms: Canada

Concentrate, Intravenous:

Zometa: 4 mg/5 mL (5 mL)

Infusion, Solution [premixed]:

Aclasta: 5 mg/100 mL

◆ **Zoledronic Acid for Injection (Can)** *see* Zoledronic Acid *on page 2206*

◆ **Zoledronic Acid Injection (Can)** *see* Zoledronic Acid *on page 2206*

◆ **Zoledronic Acid Z (Can)** *see* Zoledronic Acid *on page 2206*

◆ **Zolinza** *see* Vorinostat *on page 2182*

ZOLMitriptan (zohl mi TRIP tan)

Brand Names: U.S. Zomig; Zomig ZMT

Brand Names: Canada Dom-Zolmitriptan; JAMP-Zolmitriptan; Mylan-Zolmitriptan; Mylan-Zolmitriptan ODT; PMS-Zolmitriptan; PMS-Zolmitriptan ODT; Riva-Zolmitriptan; Sandoz-Zolmitriptan; Sandoz-Zolmitriptan ODT; Teva-Zolmitriptan; Teva-Zolmitriptan OD; Zolmitriptan ODT; Zomig; Zomig Nasal Spray; Zomig Rapimelt

Index Terms 311C90

Pharmacologic Category Antimigraine Agent; Serotonin 5-$HT_{1B,\ 1D}$ Receptor Agonist

Use Migraines: Acute treatment of migraine with or without aura in adults

Pregnancy Risk Factor C

Pregnancy Considerations Adverse events were observed in animal reproduction studies. Information related to zolmitriptan use in pregnancy is limited (Källén, 2011; Nezvalová-Henriksen, 2010; Nezvalová-Henriksen, 2012). Until additional information is available, other agents are preferred for the initial treatment of migraine in pregnancy (Da Silva, 2012; MacGregor, 2012; Williams, 2012).

Breast-Feeding Considerations It is not known if zolmitriptan is excreted in breast milk. Due to the potential for serious adverse reactions in the nursing infant, the decision to continue or discontinue breast-feeding during therapy should take into account the risk of exposure to the infant and the benefits of treatment to the mother.

Contraindications

Ischemic coronary artery disease (angina pectoris, history of myocardial infarction [MI], or documented silent ischemia); coronary artery vasospasm, including Prinzmetal variant angina, or other significant underlying cardiovascular disease; Wolff-Parkinson-White syndrome or arrhythmias associated with other cardiac accessory conduction pathway disorders; peripheral vascular disease; ischemic bowel disease; uncontrolled hypertension; recent use (within 24 hours) of treatment with another 5-HT_1 agonist, or an ergotamine-containing or ergot-type medication like dihydroergotamine or methysergide; history of stroke, transient ischemic attack, or history of hemiplegic or basilar migraine; coadministration of monoamine oxidase A (MAO A) inhibitors or use of zolmitriptan within 2 weeks of discontinuation of MAO A inhibitor therapy; hypersensitivity to zolmitriptan or any component of the formulation.

Documentation of allergenic cross-reactivity for triptans is limited. However, because of similarities in chemical structure and/or pharmacologic actions, the possibility of cross-sensitivity cannot be ruled out with certainty.

Warnings/Precautions Zolmitriptan is indicated only in patient populations with a clear diagnosis of migraine. If a patient does not respond to the first dose, the diagnosis of migraine should be reconsidered; rule out underlying neurologic disease in patients with atypical headache and in patients with no prior history of migraine. Not indicated for migraine prophylaxis (may be used off-label for menstrual migraine prophylaxis) or for the treatment of cluster headache. Acute migraine agents (eg, triptans, opioids, ergotamine, or a combination of the agents) used for 10 or more days per month may lead to worsening of headaches (medication overuse headache); withdrawal treatment may be necessary in the setting of overuse. Not for prophylactic treatment of migraine headaches. Cardiac events (coronary artery vasospasm, transient ischemia, myocardial infarction, ventricular tachycardia/fibrillation, cardiac arrest, and death) have been reported within a few hours of 5-HT_1 agonist administration; use in contraindicated in patients with ischemic or vasospastic coronary artery disease. Patients who experience sensations of chest pain/pressure/tightness or symptoms suggestive of angina following dosing should be evaluated for coronary artery disease or Prinzmetal's angina before receiving additional doses; if dosing is resumed and similar symptoms recur, monitor with ECG. Patients with Prinzmetal's variant angina, Wolff-Parkinson-White Syndrome or arrhythmias associated with other cardiac accessory conduction pathway disorders should not receive zolmitriptan. Should not be given to patients who have risk factors for CAD (eg, hypertension, hypercholesterolemia, smoker, obesity, diabetes, strong family history of CAD, menopause, male >40 years of age) without adequate cardiac evaluation. Patients with suspected CAD should have cardiovascular evaluation to rule out CAD before considering zolmitriptan's use; if cardiovascular evaluation negative, first dose would be safest if given in the healthcare provider's office (consider ECG monitoring). Periodic evaluation of those without cardiovascular disease, but with continued risk factors, should be done. Significant elevation in blood pressure, including hypertensive crisis, has been reported in patients with and without a history of hypertension. Use is contraindicated in patients with uncontrolled hypertension. Peripheral vascular ischemia, gastrointestinal vascular ischemia, and infarction (presenting with abdominal pain and bloody diarrhea, splenic infarction, and Raynaud's syndrome have been reported with 5-HT_1 agonists. In patients who experience signs or symptoms suggestive of a vasospastic reaction following use of a 5-HT_1 agonist, rule out a vasospastic reaction before receiving additional doses. Cerebral/subarachnoid hemorrhage and stroke have been reported with 5-HT_1 agonist administration and some have resulted in fatalities. Do not administer to patients with a history of stroke or TIA; discontinue use if a cerebrovascular event occurs. Rarely, partial vision loss and blindness (transient and permanent) have been reported with 5-HT_1 agonists. Use with caution in patients with hepatic impairment. Zomig-ZMT tablets contain phenylalanine. Symptoms of agitation, confusion, hallucinations, labile blood pressure, hyper-reflexia, incoordination, myoclonus, shivering, and tachycardia (serotonin syndrome) may occur with concomitant proserotonergic drugs (eg, SSRIs, SNRIs, TCAs, MAO inhibitors, or triptans) or agents which reduce zolmitriptan's metabolism. Elderly patients are more likely to have underlying cardiovascular disease and hepatic or renal impairment; use with caution. Cardiovascular evaluation is recommended for elderly patients with other cardiovascular risk factors prior to initiation of therapy. Zomig-ZMT tablets contain phenylalanine.

Adverse Reactions

Cardiovascular: Chest pain, facial edema, palpitations

Central nervous system: Chills, depersonalization, dizziness, drowsiness, flushing sensation, headache, hyperesthesia, hypoesthesia, insomnia, local alterations in temperature sensations, myasthenia, pain, paresthesia, sensation of pressure, vertigo

Dermatologic: Application site irritation (nasal spray), diaphoresis

Gastrointestinal: Abdominal pain, dyspepsia, dysphagia, nausea, unpleasant taste, vomiting, xerostomia

Hypersensitivity: Hypersensitivity reaction

Local: Local pain (neck/throat/jaw)

Neuromuscular & skeletal: Arthralgia, myalgia, weakness

Respiratory: Constriction of the pharynx, nasal discomfort (nasal spray), pressure on pharynx

Rare but important or life-threatening: Amblyopia, anaphylactoid reaction, anaphylaxis, angina pectoris, apnea, arthritis, ataxia, atrial fibrillation, bradycardia, breast carcinoma, breast neoplasm, cardiac arrhythmia, cerebral ischemia, confusion, coronary artery vasospasm, cyanosis, eosinophilia, erythema multiforme, esophagitis, fibrocystic breast disease, gastrointestinal carcinoma, gastrointestinal infarction, gastrointestinal necrosis, genitourinary neoplasm, hallucination, hematemesis, hepatic neoplasm, hypertension, hypertensive crisis, hyperthyroidism, infection, intestinal obstruction, ischemic colitis, ischemic heart disease, mania, melena, myocardial infarction, neoplasm, pancreatitis, pneumonia, prolonged Q-T interval on ECG, psychosis, pyelonephritis, seizure, serotonin syndrome, sialadenitis, skin neoplasm, skin photosensitivity, splenic infarction, syncope, tardive dyskinesia, tetany, thrombocytopenia, ulcer, urinary tract infection, uterine fibroid enlargement, vaginitis, vasodilatation, visual field defects

Drug Interactions

Metabolism/Transport Effects **Substrate** of CYP1A2 (minor); **Note:** Assignment of Major/Minor substrate status based on clinically relevant drug interaction potential

Avoid Concomitant Use

Avoid concomitant use of ZOLMitriptan with any of the following: Dapoxetine; Ergot Derivatives; MAO Inhibitors

Increased Effect/Toxicity

ZOLMitriptan may increase the levels/effects of: Antipsychotic Agents; Droxidopa; Ergot Derivatives; Metoclopramide; Serotonin Modulators

The levels/effects of ZOLMitriptan may be increased by: Antiemetics (5HT3 Antagonists); Antipsychotic Agents; Cimetidine; Dapoxetine; Ergot Derivatives; MAO Inhibitors; Propranolol

Decreased Effect There are no known significant interactions involving a decrease in effect.

Storage/Stability Store at 20°C to 25°C (68°F to 77°F). Protect tablets from light and moisture.

Mechanism of Action Selective agonist for serotonin ($5\text{-}HT_{1B}$ and $5\text{-}HT_{1D}$ receptors) in cranial arteries and sensory nerves of the trigeminal system; causes vasoconstriction and reduces inflammation associated with antidromic neuronal transmission correlating with relief of migraine

Pharmacodynamics/Kinetics

Absorption: Well absorbed

Distribution: V_d: Oral: 7 L/kg; Nasal spray: 8.4 L/kg

Protein binding: 25%

Metabolism: Converted to an active N-desmethyl metabolite (2-6 times more potent than zolmitriptan at $5\text{-}HT_{1B}$ and $5\text{-}HT_{1D}$ receptors)

Bioavailability: 40% (not impacted by food); mean bioavailability of nasal spray compared with oral tablet: 102%

Half-life elimination: 3 hours

Time to peak, serum: Tablet: 1.5 hours; Orally-disintegrating tablet and nasal spray: 3 hours

Excretion: Urine (~60% to 65% total dose; 8% of total dose as unchanged drug; 4% of total dose as N-desmethyl metabolite); feces (30%)

Dosage Adults:

Migraine:

Initial dose: **Note:** Administer at the onset of migraine headache.

Nasal inhalation: 2.5 mg (maximum 5 mg)

Oral:

Tablet: 1.25-2.5 mg (maximum: 5 mg)

Orally-disintegrating tablet: 2.5 mg (maximum: 5 mg)

Second dose (either nasal inhalation or oral): May repeat in 2 hours if the migraine headache has not resolved or returns after transient improvement (maximum daily dose: 10 mg)

Menstrual migraine, prophylaxis (off-label use): Oral: 2.5 mg 2-3 times daily starting 2 days prior to the expected onset of menses and continued through to 5 days after the onset of menses (7 days total) (Tuchman, 2008)

Elderly: Initiate therapy at the low end of the dosing range.

Dosage adjustment for concomitant therapy with cimetidine: Maximum single dose: 2.5 mg (maximum daily dose: 5 mg)

Dosage adjustment in renal impairment: No dosage adjustment provided in manufacturer's labeling; however, zolmitriptan clearance is reduced in patients with severe renal impairment (CrCl 5-25 mL/minute).

Dosage adjustment in hepatic impairment:

Tablet: Moderate to severe impairment: Initial: 1.25 mg (maximum daily dose: 5 mg)

Orally disintegrating tablet: Not recommended in patients with moderate or severe hepatic impairment; oral disintegrating tablets should not be broken in half.

Nasal inhalation: Not recommended in patients with moderate or severe hepatic impairment

Dietary Considerations Some products may contain phenylalanine.

Administration Administer as soon as migraine headache starts.

Tablet: May be broken in half to achieve a smaller initial dose.

Orally-disintegrating tablet: Must be taken whole; do not break, crush, or chew. Place on tongue and allow to dissolve. Administration with liquid is not required.

Nasal spray: Blow nose gently prior to use. After removing protective cap, instill device into nostril. Block opposite nostril; breathe in gently through nose while pressing plunger of spray device. Breathe gently through mouth for 5-10 seconds.

Monitoring Parameters Headache severity, signs/symptoms suggestive of angina; blood pressure; ECG with first dose in patients with likelihood of unrecognized coronary disease, such as patients with significant hypertension, hypercholesterolemia, obese patients, patients with diabetes, smokers with other risk factors or strong family history of coronary artery disease

Dosage Forms

Solution, Nasal:

Zomig: 2.5 mg (6 ea); 5 mg (6 ea)

Tablet, Oral:

Zomig: 2.5 mg, 5 mg

Generic: 2.5 mg, 5 mg

Tablet Dispersible, Oral:

Zomig ZMT: 2.5 mg, 5 mg

Generic: 2.5 mg, 5 mg

◆ **Zolmitriptan ODT (Can)** *see* ZOLMitriptan *on page* 2210

◆ **Zoloft** *see* Sertraline *on page* 1878

Zolpidem (zole PI dem)

Brand Names: U.S. Ambien; Ambien CR; Edluar; Intermezzo; Zolpimist

Brand Names: Canada Sublinox

Index Terms Zolpidem Tartrate

Pharmacologic Category Hypnotic, Miscellaneous

Additional Appendix Information

Beers Criteria – Potentially Inappropriate Medications for Geriatrics *on page* 2271

Use Insomnia:

Ambien, Edluar, Zolpimist: Short-term treatment of insomnia with difficulty of sleep onset

Ambien CR: Treatment of insomnia with difficulty of sleep onset and/or sleep maintenance

Intermezzo: "As needed" treatment of insomnia when middle-of-the-night awakening is followed by difficulty returning to sleep and the patient has ≥4 hours of sleep time remaining

Sublinox [Canadian product]: Short-term treatment of insomnia (with difficulty of sleep onset, frequent awakenings, and/or early awakenings)

Pregnancy Risk Factor C

Pregnancy Considerations Adverse events were observed in some animal reproduction studies. Zolpidem crosses the placenta (Juric, 2009). Severe neonatal respiratory depression has been reported when zolpidem was used at the end of pregnancy, especially when used concurrently with other CNS depressants. Children born of mothers taking sedative/hypnotics may be at risk for withdrawal; neonatal flaccidity has been reported in infants following maternal use of sedative/hypnotics during pregnancy. Additional adverse effects to the fetus/newborn have been noted in some studies (Wang, 2010; Wikner, 2011).

Breast-Feeding Considerations Zolpidem is excreted in breast milk. The manufacturer recommends that caution be exercised when administering zolpidem to nursing women.

Contraindications Hypersensitivity to zolpidem or any component of the formulation

Canadian labeling: Additional contraindications (not in U.S. labeling): Significant obstructive sleep apnea syndrome and acute and/or severe impairment of respiratory function; myasthenia gravis; severe hepatic impairment; personal or family history of sleepwalking

Warnings/Precautions Should be used only after evaluation of potential causes of sleep disturbance. Failure of sleep disturbance to resolve after 7-10 days may indicate the need for psychiatric and/or medical illness reevaluation. Hypnotics/sedatives have been associated with abnormal thinking and behavior changes including decreased inhibition, aggression, bizarre behavior, agitation, visual and auditory hallucinations, and depersonalization. These changes may occur unpredictably and may indicate previously unrecognized psychiatric disorders; evaluate appropriately. Sedative/hypnotics may produce withdrawal symptoms following abrupt discontinuation. Use with caution in patients with depression; worsening of depression, including suicide or suicidal ideation has been reported with the use of hypnotics. Intentional overdose may be an issue in this population. The minimum dose that will effectively treat the individual patient should be used. Prescriptions should be written for the smallest quantity consistent with good patient care. May cause CNS depression impairing physical and mental capabilities; patients must be cautioned about performing tasks which require mental alertness (operating machinery or driving). Drowsiness and a decreased level of consciousness may lead to falls and severe injuries; hip fractures and intracranial hemorrhage have been reported. Zolpidem should only be administered when the patient is able to stay in bed a full night (7 to 8 hours) before being active again. Intermezzo should be taken in bed if patient awakes in the middle of the night (ie, if ≥4 hours left before waking) and there is difficulty in returning to sleep.

Potentially significant drug-drug interactions may exist, requiring dose or frequency adjustment, additional monitoring, and/or selection of alternative therapy.

Use caution in patients with myasthenia gravis (contraindicated in the Canadian labeling). Avoid use in patients with sleep apnea or a history of sedative-hypnotic abuse. Postmarketing studies have indicated that the use of hypnotic/sedative agents (including zolpidem) for sleep has been associated with hypersensitivity reactions including anaphylaxis as well as angioedema. Do not rechallenge patient if such reactions occur. An increased risk for hazardous sleep-related activities such as sleep-driving; cooking and eating food, making phone calls or having sex while asleep have also been noted; amnesia, anxiety, and other neuropsychiatric symptoms may also occur. Discontinue treatment in patients who report any sleep-related episodes. Canadian labeling recommends avoiding use in patients with disorders (eg, restless legs syndrome, periodic limb movement disorder, sleep apnea) that may disrupt sleep and cause frequent awakenings, potentially increasing the risk of complex sleep-related behaviors. Use with caution in patients with a history of drug dependence. Risk of abuse is increased in patients with a history or family history of alcohol or drug abuse or mental illness.

Use caution with respiratory disease (Canadian labeling contraindicates use with acute and/or severe impairment of respiratory function). Use caution with hepatic impairment (Canadian labeling contraindicates use in severe impairment); dose adjustment required. Because of the rapid onset of action, administer immediately prior to bedtime, after the patient has gone to bed and is having difficulty falling asleep, or during the middle of the night when at least 4 hours are left before waking (Intermezzo).

Use caution in the elderly; dose adjustment recommended. Closely monitor elderly or debilitated patients for impaired cognitive and/or motor performance, confusion, and potential for falling. Avoid chronic use (>90 days) in older adults; adverse events, including delirium, falls, fractures, have been observed with nonbenzodiazepine hypnotic use in the elderly similar to events observed with benzodiazepines. Data suggests improvements in sleep duration and latency are minimal (Beers Criteria).

Dosage adjustment is recommended for females; pharmacokinetic studies involving zolpidem showed a significant increase in maximum concentration and exposure in females compared to males at the same dose. When studied for the unapproved use of insomnia associated with ADHD in children, a higher incidence (~7%) of hallucinations was reported. In addition, sleep latency did not decrease compared to placebo.

Some dosage forms may contain polysorbate 80 (also known as Tweens). Hypersensitivity reactions, usually a delayed reaction, have been reported following exposure to pharmaceutical products containing polysorbate 80 in certain individuals (Isaksson, 2002; Lucente 2000; Shelley, 1995). Thrombocytopenia, ascites, pulmonary deterioration, and renal and hepatic failure have been reported in premature neonates after receiving parenteral products containing polysorbate 80 (Alade, 1986; CDC, 1984). See manufacturer's labeling.

Adverse Reactions

Cardiovascular: Chest discomfort, increased blood pressure, palpitations

Central nervous system: Abnormal dreams, amnesia, anxiety, apathy, ataxia, burning sensation, confusion, depersonalization, depression, disinhibition, disorientation, dizziness, drowsiness, drugged feeling, eating disorder (binge eating), emotional lability, equilibrium disturbance, euphoria, fatigue, hallucination, headache, hypoesthesia, increased body temperature, insomnia, lack of concentration, lethargy, memory impairment, paresthesia, psychomotor retardation, sleep disorder, stress, vertigo

Dermatologic: Skin rash, urticaria, wrinkling of skin

Endocrine & metabolic: Hypermenorrhea

Gastrointestinal: Abdominal distress, abdominal tenderness, change in appetite, constipation, diarrhea, dyspepsia, flatulence, frequent bowel movements, gastroenteritis, gastroesophageal reflux disease, hiccups, nausea, vomiting, xerostomia

Genitourinary: Dysuria, urinary tract infection, vaginal dryness

Hypersensitivity: Hypersensitivity reaction

Neuromuscular & skeletal: Arthralgia, back pain, muscle cramps, muscle spasm, myalgia, neck pain, tremor, weakness

Ophthalmic: Accommodation disturbance, asthenopia, blurred vision, diplopia, eye redness, visual disturbance (including altered depth perception)

Otic: Labyrinthitis, tinnitus

Respiratory: Dry throat, flu-like symptoms, lower respiratory tract infection, pharyngitis, sinusitis, throat irritation, upper respiratory tract infection

Miscellaneous: Fever

Rare but important or life-threatening: Abnormal hepatic function tests, acute renal failure, aggressive behavior, anaphylaxis, anemia, angina pectoris, angioedema, anorexia, arteritis, arthritis, breast fibroadenosis, breast neoplasm, bronchitis, cardiac arrhythmia, cerebrovascular disease, circulatory shock, cognitive dysfunction, corneal ulcer, delusions, dementia, dermatitis, drug tolerance, dysarthria, dysphagia, edema, extrasystoles, glaucoma, hepatic insufficiency, hyperbilirubinemia, hyperglycemia, hyperlipidemia, hypertension, hypotension, hysteria, illusion, impotence, leukopenia, lymphadenopathy, migraine, myocardial infarction, neuralgia, neuritis, neuropathy, orthostatic hypotension, panic disorder, personality disorder, psychoneurosis, pulmonary edema, pulmonary embolism, pyelonephritis, respiratory depression, restless leg syndrome, rhinitis, scleritis, somnambulism, syncope, tachycardia, tenesmus, tetany, thrombosis, urinary incontinence, vaginitis, ventricular tachycardia

Drug Interactions

Metabolism/Transport Effects **Substrate** of CYP1A2 (minor), CYP2C19 (minor), CYP2C9 (minor), CYP2D6 (minor), CYP3A4 (major); **Note:** Assignment of Major/Minor substrate status based on clinically relevant drug interaction potential

Avoid Concomitant Use

Avoid concomitant use of Zolpidem with any of the following: Azelastine (Nasal); Conivaptan; Fusidic Acid (Systemic); Idelalisib; Orphenadrine; Paraldehyde; Sodium Oxybate; Thalidomide

Increased Effect/Toxicity

Zolpidem may increase the levels/effects of: Alcohol (Ethyl); Azelastine (Nasal); Buprenorphine; CarBAMazepine; Hydrocodone; Methotrimeprazine; Metyrosine; Orphenadrine; Paraldehyde; Pramipexole; ROPINIRole; Rotigotine; Selective Serotonin Reuptake Inhibitors; Sodium Oxybate; Suvorexant; Thalidomide

The levels/effects of Zolpidem may be increased by: Antifungal Agents (Azole Derivatives, Systemic); Aprepitant; Brimonidine (Topical); Cannabis; Ceritinib; CNS Depressants; Conivaptan; CYP3A4 Inhibitors (Moderate); CYP3A4 Inhibitors (Strong); Dasatinib; Dronabinol; Droperidol; FluvoxaMINE; Fosaprepitant; Fusidic Acid (Systemic); Idelalisib; Ivacaftor; Kava Kava; Luliconazole; Magnesium Sulfate; Methotrimeprazine; Mifepristone; Nabilone; Netupitant; Perampanel; Rufinamide; Simeprevir; Stiripentol; Tapentadol; Tetrahydrocannabinol

Decreased Effect

The levels/effects of Zolpidem may be decreased by: Bosentan; CarBAMazepine; CYP3A4 Inducers (Moderate); CYP3A4 Inducers (Strong); Dabrafenib; Deferasirox; Flumazenil; Mitotane; Rifamycin Derivatives; Siltuximab; St Johns Wort; Telaprevir; Tocilizumab

Food Interactions Maximum plasma concentration and bioavailability are decreased with food; time to peak plasma concentration is increased; half-life remains unchanged. Grapefruit juice may decrease the metabolism of zolpidem. Management: Do not administer with (or immediately after) a meal. Avoid grapefruit juice.

Storage/Stability

Ambien, Edluar, Intermezzo: Store at 20°C to 25°C (68°F to 77°F). Protect sublingual tablets from light and moisture.

Ambien CR: Store at 15°C to 25°C (59°F to 77°F); limited excursions permitted up to 30°C (86°F).

Zolpimist: Store upright at 25°C (77°F); excursions are permitted to 15°C to 30 °C (59°F to 86 °F). Do not freeze. Avoid prolonged exposure to temperatures >30°C (86°F).

Sublinox [Canadian product]: Store at 15°C to 30°C (59°F to 86°F); protect from light and moisture.

Mechanism of Action Zolpidem, an imidazopyridine hypnotic that is structurally dissimilar to benzodiazepines, enhances the activity of the inhibitory neurotransmitter, γ-aminobutyric acid (GABA), via selective agonism at the benzodiazepine-1 (BZ_1) receptor; the result is increased chloride conductance, neuronal hyperpolarization, inhibition of the action potential, and a decrease in neuronal excitability leading to sedative and hypnotic effects. Because of its selectivity for the BZ_1 receptor site over the BZ_2 receptor site, zolpidem exhibits minimal anxiolytic, myorelaxant, and anticonvulsant properties (effects largely attributed to agonism at the BZ_2 receptor site).

Pharmacodynamics/Kinetics

Onset of action: Immediate release: 30 minutes

Duration: Immediate release: 6-8 hours

Absorption: Rapid; C_{max} and AUC is increased by ~45% in females compared to male subjects

Distribution: V_d: 0.54 L/kg after an IV dose (Holm, 2000)

Protein binding: ~93%

Metabolism: Hepatic methylation and hydroxylation via CYP3A4 (~60%), CYP2C9 (~22%), CYP1A2 (~14%), CYP2D6 (~3%), and CYP2C19 (~3%) to 3 inactive metabolites (Holm, 2000)

Bioavailability: Immediate-release tablet: 70% (Holm, 2000)

Half-life elimination:

Immediate release, Extended release: ~2.5 hours (range: 1.4-4.5 hours); Cirrhosis: Up to 9.9 hours; Elderly: Prolonged up to 32%

Spray: ~3 hours (range: 1.7-8.4)

Sublingual tablet (Edluar, Intermezzo): ~3 hours (range: 1.4-6.7 hours)

Time to peak, plasma:

Immediate release: 1.6 hours; 2.2 hours with food

Extended release: 1.5 hours; 4 hours with food

Spray: ~0.9 hours

Sublingual tablet: Edluar: ~1.4 hours, ~1.8 hours with food; Intermezzo: 0.6-1.3 hours, ~3 hours with food

Excretion: Urine (48% to 67%, primarily as metabolites); feces (29% to 42%, primarily as metabolites)

Dosage Oral:

Adults: **Note:** The lowest effective dose should be used; higher doses may be more likely to impair next morning activities.

Immediate release tablet, spray: 5 mg (females) or 5 to 10 mg (males) immediately before bedtime; maximum dose: 10 mg daily

Extended release tablet: 6.25 mg (females) or 6.25 to 12.5 mg (males) immediately before bedtime; maximum dose: 12.5 mg

Sublingual tablet:

Edluar, Sublinox [Canadian product]: 5 mg (females) or 5 to 10 mg (males) immediately before bedtime; if 5 mg dose is ineffective may increase to 10 mg (maximum dose: 10 mg daily)

Intermezzo: **Note:** Take in bed only if ≥4 hours left before waking and there is difficulty in returning to sleep.

Females: 1.75 mg once per night as needed (maximum: 1.75 mg/night)

Males: 3.5 mg once per night as needed (maximum: 3.5 mg/night)

Dosage adjustment with concomitant CNS depressants: Females and males: 1.75 mg once per night as needed; dose adjustment of concomitant CNS depressant(s) may be necessary.

Debilitated:

Immediate release tablet, spray: 5 mg immediately before bedtime

Sublingual tablet:

Edluar, Sublinox [Canadian product]: 5 mg immediately before bedtime

Extended release tablet: 6.25 mg immediately before bedtime

Elderly:

Immediate release tablet, spray: 5 mg immediately before bedtime

Sublingual tablet:

Edluar, Sublinox [Canadian product]: 5 mg immediately before bedtime

Intermezzo: Females and males: 1.75 mg once per night as needed (maximum: 1.75 mg/night). **Note:** Take only if ≥4 hours left before waking and there is difficulty in returning to sleep.

Extended release tablet: 6.25 mg immediately before bedtime

Dosage adjustment in renal impairment: No dosage adjustment necessary. Use with caution and monitor patients with renal impairment closely. Not dialyzable.

Hemodialysis: Not dialyzable

Dosage adjustment in hepatic impairment:

U.S. labeling:

Immediate release tablet, spray: 5 mg immediately before bedtime

Extended release tablet: 6.25 mg immediately before bedtime

Sublingual tablet:

Edluar: 5 mg immediately before bedtime

Intermezzo: Females and males: 1.75 mg once per night as needed. **Note:** Take only if ≥4 hours left before waking and there is difficulty in returning to sleep.

Canadian labeling: Sublingual tablet: Sublinox:

Mild-to-moderate impairment: 5 mg immediately before bedtime

Severe impairment: Use is contraindicated.

Dietary Considerations For faster sleep onset, do not administer with (or immediately after) a meal.

Administration Ingest immediately before bedtime due to rapid onset of action. Regardless of dosage form, do not administer with or immediately after a meal. Intermezzo should be taken in bed if patient awakes in the middle of the night (ie, if ≥4 hours left before waking) and there is difficulty in returning to sleep.

Ambien CR tablets should be swallowed whole; do not divide, crush, or chew.

Edluar, Intermezzo, or Sublinox [Canadian product] sublingual tablets should be placed under the tongue and allowed to disintegrate; do not swallow or administer Edluar or Sublinox with water.

Zolpimist oral spray should be sprayed directly into the mouth over the tongue. Prior to initial use, pump should be primed by spraying 5 times. If pump is not used for at least 14 days, reprime pump with 1 spray.

Monitoring Parameters Daytime alertness; fall risk, respiratory rate; behavior profile; tolerance, abuse, and dependence; reevaluate if insomnia persists after 7 to 10 days of use.

Additional Information Causes fewer disturbances in sleep stages as compared to benzodiazepines. Time spent in sleep stages 3 and 4 are maintained; zolpidem decreases sleep latency; should not be prescribed in quantities exceeding a 1-month supply.

Dosage Forms

Solution, Oral:

Zolpimist: 5 mg/actuation (7.7 mL)

Tablet, Oral:

Ambien: 5 mg, 10 mg

Generic: 5 mg, 10 mg

Tablet Extended Release, Oral:

Ambien CR: 6.25 mg, 12.5 mg

Generic: 6.25 mg, 12.5 mg

Tablet Sublingual, Sublingual:

Edluar: 5 mg, 10 mg

Intermezzo: 1.75 mg, 3.5 mg

Dosage Forms: Canada

Tablet, sublingual:

Sublinox: 5 mg, 10 mg

◆ **Zolpidem Tartrate** *see* Zolpidem *on page 2212*

◆ **Zolpimist** *see* Zolpidem *on page 2212*

◆ **Zolvit [DSC]** *see* Hydrocodone and Acetaminophen *on page 1012*

◆ **Zometa** *see* Zoledronic Acid *on page 2206*

◆ **Zometa Concentrate (Can)** *see* Zoledronic Acid *on page 2206*

◆ **Zomig** *see* ZOLMitriptan *on page 2210*

◆ **Zomig Nasal Spray (Can)** *see* ZOLMitriptan *on page 2210*

◆ **Zomig Rapimelt (Can)** *see* ZOLMitriptan *on page 2210*

◆ **Zomig ZMT** *see* ZOLMitriptan *on page 2210*

◆ **Zonalon** *see* Doxepin (Topical) *on page 678*

◆ **Zonalon (Can)** *see* Doxepin (Systemic) *on page 676*

◆ **Zonalon® (Can)** *see* Doxepin (Topical) *on page 678*

◆ **Zonatuss** *see* Benzonatate *on page 247*

◆ **Zonegran** *see* Zonisamide *on page 2215*

Zonisamide (zoe NIS a mide)

Brand Names: U.S. Zonegran

Pharmacologic Category Anticonvulsant, Miscellaneous

Use Adjunct treatment of partial seizures in children >16 years of age and adults with epilepsy

Pregnancy Risk Factor C

Pregnancy Considerations Teratogenic effects were observed in animal reproduction studies; therefore, zonisamide is classified as pregnancy category C. Zonisamide crosses the placenta and can be detected in the newborn following delivery. Although adverse fetal events have been reported, the risk of teratogenic effects following maternal use of zonisamide in not clearly defined. Other agents may be preferred until additional data is available. Newborns should be monitored for transient metabolic acidosis after birth. Zonisamide clearance may increase in the second trimester of pregnancy, requiring dosage adjustment. Women of childbearing potential are advised to use effective contraception during therapy.

Patients exposed to zonisamide during pregnancy are encouraged to enroll themselves into the AED Pregnancy Registry by calling 1-888-233-2334. Additional information is available at http://www.aedpregnancyregistry.org.

Breast-Feeding Considerations Zonisamide is excreted into breast milk in concentrations similar to those in the maternal plasma and has been detected in the plasma of a nursing infant. According to the manufacturer, the decision to continue or discontinue breast-feeding during therapy should take into account the risk of exposure to the infant and the benefits of treatment to the mother.

Contraindications Hypersensitivity to zonisamide, sulfonamides, or any component of the formulation

Warnings/Precautions Hazardous agent - use appropriate precautions for handling and disposal (NIOSH 2014 [group 3]).

Rare, but potentially fatal sulfonamide reactions have occurred following the use of zonisamide. These reactions include Stevens-Johnson syndrome, fulminant hepatic necrosis, agranulocytosis, aplastic anemia, and toxic epidermal necrolysis, usually appearing within 2-16 weeks of drug initiation. Discontinue zonisamide if rash develops. Chemical similarities are present among sulfonamides, sulfonylureas, carbonic anhydrase inhibitors, thiazides, and loop diuretics (except ethacrynic acid). Use in patients with sulfonamide allergy is specifically contraindicated in product labeling, however, a risk of cross-reaction exists in patients with allergy to any of these compounds; avoid use when previous reaction has been severe. Use may be associated with the development of metabolic acidosis (generally dose-dependent) in certain patients; predisposing conditions/therapies include renal disease, severe respiratory disease, diarrhea, surgery, ketogenic diet, and other medications. Pediatric patients may also be at an increased risk for and may have more severe metabolic acidosis. Serum bicarbonate should be monitored in all patients prior to and during use; if metabolic acidosis occurs, consider decreasing the dose or tapering the dose to discontinue. If use continued despite acidosis, alkali treatment should be considered. Untreated metabolic acidosis may increase the risk of developing nephrolithiasis, nephrocalcinosis, osteomalacia (or rickets in children), or osteoporosis; pediatric patients may also have decreased growth rates.

Pooled analysis of trials involving various antiepileptics (regardless of indication) showed an increased risk of suicidal thoughts/behavior (incidence rate: 0.43% treated patients compared to 0.24% of patients receiving placebo); risk observed as early as 1 week after initiation and continued through duration of trials (most trials ≤24 weeks). Monitor all patients for notable changes in behavior that might indicate suicidal thoughts or depression; notify healthcare provider immediately if symptoms occur.

Discontinue zonisamide in patients who develop acute renal failure or a significant sustained increase in creatinine/BUN concentration. Kidney stones have been reported. Do not use in patients with renal impairment (GFR <50 mL/minute); use with caution in patients with hepatic impairment.

Significant CNS effects include psychiatric symptoms, psychomotor slowing, and fatigue or somnolence. Fatigue and somnolence occur within the first month of treatment, most commonly at doses of 300 to 500 mg/day in adults. Effects with other sedative drugs or ethanol may be potentiated. May cause sedation, which may impair physical or mental abilities; patients must be cautioned about performing tasks which require mental alertness (eg, operating machinery or driving). Abrupt withdrawal may precipitate seizures; discontinue or reduce doses gradually.

Decreased sweating (oligohydrosis) and hyperthermia requiring hospitalization have been reported in children. Pediatric patients may also be at an increased risk and may have more severe metabolic acidosis.

Adverse Reactions

Central nervous system: Agitation/irritability, anxiety, ataxia, concentration decreased, confusion, depression, difficulty in verbal expression, dizziness fatigue, headache, hyperesthesia, incoordination, insomnia, memory impairment, mental slowing, nervousness, schizophrenic/schizophreniform behavior, seizure, somnolence, speech disorders, status epilepticus, tiredness, tremor

Dermatologic: Bruising, pruritus, rash

Gastrointestinal: Abdominal pain, anorexia, constipation, diarrhea, dyspepsia, diarrhea, dyspepsia, nausea, taste perversion, vomiting, weight loss, xerostomia

Neuromuscular & skeletal: Abnormal gait, paresthesia, weakness

Ocular: Amblyopia, diplopia, nystagmus

Otic: Tinnitus

Renal: Kidney stones

Respiratory: Cough increased, pharyngitis, rhinitis

Rare (but important or life threatening symptoms): Agranulocytosis, allergic reaction, alopecia, amenorrhea, aplastic anemia, apnea, arthritis, atrial fibrillation, bladder calculus, bradycardia, cerebrovascular accident, cholangitis, cholecystitis, cholestatic jaundice, colitis, deafness, duodenitis, encephalopathy, fecal incontinence, gingivitis, GI ulcer, glaucoma, heart failure, hematuria, hemoptysis, hirsutism, hyper-/hypotension, hyperthermia, hypoglycemia, hyponatremia, immunodeficiency, impotence, iritis, leukopenia, lupus erythematosus, lymphadenopathy, mastitis, menorrhagia, metabolic acidosis, neuropathy, oculogyric crisis, oligohidrosis (children), pancreatitis, photophobia, pulmonary embolus, rectal hemorrhage, Stevens-Johnson syndrome, stroke, suicidal behavior/ideation, syncope, thrombocytopenia, thrombophlebitis, toxic epidermal necrolysis, urinary incontinence, ventricular extrasystoles

Drug Interactions

Metabolism/Transport Effects Substrate of CYP2C19 (minor), CYP3A4 (major); **Note:** Assignment of Major/Minor substrate status based on clinically relevant drug interaction potential

Avoid Concomitant Use

Avoid concomitant use of Zonisamide with any of the following: Azelastine (Nasal); Carbonic Anhydrase Inhibitors; Conivaptan; Fusidic Acid (Systemic); Idelalisib; Orphenadrine; Paraldehyde; Thalidomide

Increased Effect/Toxicity

Zonisamide may increase the levels/effects of: Alcohol (Ethyl); Alpha-/Beta-Agonists (Indirect-Acting); Amphetamines; Azelastine (Nasal); Buprenorphine; Carbonic Anhydrase Inhibitors; CNS Depressants; Flecainide; Hydrocodone; Memantine; MetFORMIN; Methotrimeprazine; Metyrosine; Mirtazapine; Orphenadrine; Paraldehyde; Pramipexole; QuiNIDine; ROPINIRole; Rotigotine; Selective Serotonin Reuptake Inhibitors; Suvorexant; Thalidomide; Zolpidem

The levels/effects of Zonisamide may be increased by: Aprepitant; Brimonidine (Topical); Cannabis; Ceritinib; Conivaptan; CYP3A4 Inhibitors (Moderate); CYP3A4 Inhibitors (Strong); Dasatinib; Doxylamine; Dronabinol; Droperidol; Fosaprepitant; Fusidic Acid (Systemic); HydrOXYzine; Idelalisib; Ivacaftor; Kava Kava; Luliconazole; Magnesium Sulfate; Methotrimeprazine; Mifepristone; Nabilone; Netupitant; Perampanel; Rufinamide; Salicylates; Simeprevir; Sodium Oxybate; Stiripentol; Tapentadol; Tetrahydrocannabinol

Decreased Effect

Zonisamide may decrease the levels/effects of: Lithium; Methenamine

The levels/effects of Zonisamide may be decreased by: Bosentan; CYP3A4 Inducers (Moderate); CYP3A4 Inducers (Strong); Dabrafenib; Deferasirox; Fosphenytoin; Mefloquine; Mianserin; Mitotane; Orlistat; PHENobarbital; Phenytoin; Siltuximab; St Johns Wort; Tocilizumab

Food Interactions Food delays time to maximum concentration, but does not affect bioavailability. Management: Administer without regard to meals.

Storage/Stability Store at controlled room temperature 25°C (77°F). Protect from moisture and light.

Mechanism of Action The exact mechanism of action is not known. May stabilize neuronal membranes and suppress neuronal hypersynchronization through action at sodium and calcium channels. Does not affect GABA activity.

Pharmacodynamics/Kinetics

Distribution: V_d: 1.45 L/kg

Protein binding: 40%

Metabolism: Hepatic via CYP3A4; forms N-acetyl zonisamide and 2-sulfamoylacetyl phenol (SMAP)

Half-life elimination: Plasma: ~63 hours

Time to peak: 2-6 hours

Excretion: Urine (62%, 35% as unchanged drug, 65% as metabolites); feces (3%)

Dosage Oral:

Children >16 years and Adults:

Adjunctive treatment of partial seizures: Initial: 100 mg/day; dose may be increased to 200 mg/day after 2 weeks. Further dosage increases to 300 mg/day and 400 mg/day can then be made with a minimum of 2 weeks between adjustments, in order to reach steady state at each dosage level. Doses of up to 600 mg/day have been studied, however, there is no evidence of increased response with doses above 400 mg/day.

Mania (off-label use): Initial: 100-200 mg/day; maximum: 600 mg/day (Kanba, 1994)

Elderly: Data from clinical trials is insufficient for patients >65 years; begin dosing at the low end of the dosing range.

Dosage adjustment in renal impairment:

GFR ≥50 mL/minute: No dosage adjustment provided in manufacturer's labeling. However, slower titration and frequent monitoring are indicated in patients with renal disease; use with caution.

GFR <50 mL/minute: Use is not recommended. Marked renal impairment (CrCl <20 mL/minute) was associated with a 35% increase in AUC.

Dosage adjustment in hepatic impairment: No dosage adjustment provided in manufacturer's labeling (has not been studied). However, slower titration and frequent monitoring are indicated in patients with hepatic impairment; use with caution.

Dietary Considerations May be taken without regard to meals.

Administration Capsules should be swallowed whole. Dose may be administered once or twice daily. Doses of 300 mg/day and higher are associated with increased side effects. Steady-state levels are reached in 14 days.

Hazardous agent; use appropriate precautions for handling and disposal (NIOSH 2014 [group 3]).

Monitoring Parameters Metabolic profile, specifically BUN, serum creatinine; serum bicarbonate (prior to initiation and periodically during therapy); suicidality (eg, suicidal thoughts, depression, behavioral changes)

Dosage Forms

Capsule, Oral:

Zonegran: 25 mg, 100 mg

Generic: 25 mg, 50 mg, 100 mg

Extemporaneous Preparations Hazardous agent; use appropriate precautions during preparation and disposal (NIOSH 2014 [group 3]).

A 10 mg/mL suspension may be made using capsules and either simple syrup or methylcellulose 0.5%. Empty contents of ten 100 mg capsules into glass mortar. Reduce to a fine powder and add a small amount of Simple Syrup, NF and mix to a uniform paste; mix while adding the chosen vehicle in incremental proportions to **almost** 100 mL; transfer to an amber calibrated plastic bottle, rinse mortar with vehicle, and add quantity of vehicle sufficient to make 100 mL. Label "shake well" and "refrigerate". When using simple syrup vehicle, stable 28 days at room temperature or refrigerated (preferred). When using methylcellulose vehicle, stable 7 days at room temperature or 28 days refrigerated. **Note:** Although no visual evidence of microbial growth was observed, storage under refrigeration would be recommended to minimize microbial contamination.

Abobo CV, Wei B, and Liang D, "Stability of Zonisamide in Extemporaneously Compounded Oral Suspensions," *Am J Health Syst Pharm*, 2009, 66(12):1105-9.

◆ **Zontivity** *see* Vorapaxar *on page 2175*

Zopiclone [CAN/INT] (ZOE pi clone)

Brand Names: Canada ACT Zopiclone; Apo-Zopiclone; Dom-Zopiclone; Imovane; JAMP-Zopiclone; Mar-Zopiclone; Mint-Zopiclone; Mylan-Zopiclone; Novo-Zopiclone; PHL-Zopiclone; PMS-Zopiclone; PRO-Zopiclone; Q-Zopiclone; RAN-Zopiclone; ratio-Zopiclone; Rhovane; Riva-Zopiclone; Sandoz-Zopiclone; Septa-Zopiclone

Pharmacologic Category Hypnotic, Miscellaneous

Use Note: Not approved in U.S.

Insomnia: Short-term and symptomatic relief of insomnia (typically treatment should not exceed 7 to 10 consecutive days).

Pregnancy Considerations There is insufficient data on safety in pregnancy; however, benzodiazepines may cause congenital malformations during the 1st trimester and neonatal CNS depression during the last few weeks of pregnancy; it is expected zopiclone may do the same. Use is not recommended during pregnancy.

Breast-Feeding Considerations Zopiclone is excreted in human milk and its concentration may reach 50% of plasma levels; therefore, it is not recommended to use while breast-feeding.

Contraindications Hypersensitivity to zopiclone or any component of the formulation; severe respiratory impairment (eg, significant sleep apnea syndrome); myasthenia gravis; severe hepatic insufficiency

Warnings/Precautions CNS depression impairing physical and mental capabilities may occur and in some cases may persist into the following day (driving performance may be impaired up to 11 hours following administration [Leufkens, 2014]). Risk of persistent effects is increased if taken without a full night's sleep, with higher dosages, and/or concomitant use of other CNS depressants or drugs that increase zopiclone. Some patients may experience persistent effects at recommended dosages. Use with caution in patients who previously manifested paradoxical reactions to ethanol or other sedatives. Symptomatic treatment of insomnia should be initiated only after careful evaluation of potential causes of sleep disturbance. Failure of sleep disturbance to resolve after 7 to 10 days may indicate psychiatric and/or medical illness; should not be administered for more than 7 to 10 days consecutively. Use with caution in patients with mild-moderate hepatic impairment; dosage adjustment recommended. Use is contraindicated in severe hepatic insufficiency. Use with caution in patients with chronic respiratory disease. Use is contraindicated in patients with severe respiratory insufficiency. Accumulation of zopiclone or its metabolites is not anticipated in renal impairment; the manufacturer labeling however recommends a dose reduction. Use with caution in the elderly (more susceptible to adverse reactions), debilitated patients, and in patients with depression.

Amnesia can occur; do not take unless a full night's sleep is possible. An increased risk for hazardous sleep-related activities such as sleep-driving; cooking and eating food, and making phone calls while asleep have also been noted; patients with a personal or family history of sleepwalking or disorders that affect sleep (eg, restless leg syndrome, sleep apnea, periodic limb movement) may be at increased risk. Hypnotics/sedatives have been associated with abnormal thinking and behavior changes including decreased inhibition, aggression, bizarre behavior, agitation, hallucinations, and depersonalization. These changes may occur unpredictably and may indicate previously unrecognized psychiatric disorders; evaluate appropriately. May cause dependence; withdrawal symptoms can occur with abrupt discontinuation; the risk of dependence is increased in patients with a history of alcoholism and drug abuse. Use caution when reducing dose or withdrawing therapy; decrease slowly and monitor for withdrawal symptoms. Flumazenil may cause acute withdrawal in patients receiving long-term benzodiazepine therapy.

Potentially significant drug-drug interactions may exist, requiring dose or frequency adjustment, additional monitoring, and/or selection of alternative therapy. Because of the rapid onset of action, administer immediately prior to bedtime or after the patient has gone to bed and is having difficulty falling asleep. Angioedema and signs of anaphylaxis have been reported (rarely) with administration, including after the initial dose. Patients developing angioedema should discontinue therapy and should not be rechallenged.

Adverse Reactions

Cardiovascular: Palpitations

Central nervous system: Aggressiveness behavior, anterograde amnesia (rare; dose-related; elderly are at particular risk), anxiety, ataxia, bitter taste, confusion, depression, dizziness, drowsiness, euphoria, hypotonia, impaired morning arousal, intoxicated feeling, memory impairment, nervousness, speech disturbance

Dermatological: Diaphoresis

Gastrointestinal: Anorexia, constipation, coated tongue, halitosis, increased appetite, sialorrhea, xerostomia

Neuromuscular & skeletal: Tremor, weakness

Rare but important or life-threatening: Abnormal behavior (possibly associated with amnesia), anaphylactoid reaction, anaphylaxis, angioedema (rare; includes angioedema of the tongue, oropharyngeal edema, laryngeal edema), constriction of the pharynx (has occurred with angioedema; suggests anaphylaxis), delusions, diplopia, disinhibition, disturbance in attention, drug dependence, dyspepsia, dyspnea (has occurred with angioedema; suggests anaphylaxis), hostility, increased serum alkaline phosphatase (mild to moderate; very rare), increased serum transaminases (mild to moderate; very rare), lack of concentration, myasthenia, nausea (has occurred with angioedema; suggests anaphylaxis), paresthesia (not associated with withdrawal), psychotic symptoms (includes agitation, depersonalization, hallucination, irritability, nightmares), rebound insomnia (upon withdrawal), respiratory depression, restlessness, sleep disorder (complex sleep-related behaviors, usually without recall of the event; includes sleep driving, sleep eating, preparing food, and making telephone calls while not fully awake), somnambulism, vomiting (has occurred with angioedema; suggests anaphylaxis), withdrawal syndrome

Drug Interactions

Metabolism/Transport Effects **Substrate** of CYP2C8 (minor), CYP3A4 (major); **Note:** Assignment of Major/Minor substrate status based on clinically relevant drug interaction potential

Avoid Concomitant Use

Avoid concomitant use of Zopiclone with any of the following: Alcohol (Ethyl); Azelastine (Nasal); Conivaptan; Fusidic Acid (Systemic); Idelalisib; Orphenadrine; Paraldehyde; Sodium Oxybate; Thalidomide

Increased Effect/Toxicity

Zopiclone may increase the levels/effects of: Azelastine (Nasal); Buprenorphine; CNS Depressants; Hydrocodone; Methotrimeprazine; Metyrosine; Mirtazapine; Orphenadrine; Paraldehyde; Pramipexole; Prilocaine; ROPINIRole; Rotigotine; Selective Serotonin Reuptake Inhibitors; Sodium Nitrite; Sodium Oxybate; Suvorexant; Thalidomide; Zolpidem

The levels/effects of Zopiclone may be increased by: Alcohol (Ethyl); Brimonidine (Topical); Cannabis; Conivaptan; CYP3A4 Inhibitors (Moderate); CYP3A4 Inhibitors (Strong); Dasatinib; Doxylamine; Dronabinol; Droperidol; Fusidic Acid (Systemic); HydrOXYzine; Idelalisib; Ivacaftor; Kava Kava; Luliconazole; Magnesium Sulfate; Methotrimeprazine; Mifepristone; Nabilone; Nitric Oxide; Perampanel; Rufinamide; Simeprevir; Stiripentol; Tapentadol; Tetrahydrocannabinol

Decreased Effect

The levels/effects of Zopiclone may be decreased by: Bosentan; CYP3A4 Inducers (Moderate); CYP3A4 Inducers (Strong); Dabrafenib; Deferasirox; Flumazenil; Mitotane; Siltuximab; St Johns Wort; Tocilizumab

Food Interactions Effect/toxicity may be increased by grapefruit juice. Management: Avoid concurrent use.

Storage/Stability Store at room temperature of 15°C to 30°C (59°F to 86°F). Protect from light and moisture.

Mechanism of Action Zopiclone is a cyclopyrrolone derivative and has a pharmacological profile similar to benzodiazepines. Zopiclone reduces sleep latency, increases duration of sleep, and decreases the number of nocturnal awakenings.

Pharmacodynamics/Kinetics

Distribution: V_d: ~92 to 105 L; occurs rapidly from vascular compartment

Protein binding: ~45%

Metabolism: Extensively hepatic via CYP3A4 and CYP2C8 (Becquemont, 1999); metabolites have minimal or no activity

Bioavailability: 77%

Half-life elimination: ~5 hours; Elderly: ~7 hours; Hepatic impairment: ~12 hours

Time to peak, serum: <2 hours; Hepatic impairment: 3.5 hours

Excretion: Urine (75%; ~4% to 5% as unchanged drug); feces (16%)

Dosage Note: Treatment should generally not exceed 7 to 10 consecutive days.

Insomnia: Oral:

Adults: Initial: 3.75 mg once daily at bedtime; may increase to 5 mg and then to 7.5 mg once daily if necessary (maximum: 7.5 mg once daily)

Patients with chronic respiratory insufficiency: Initial: 3.75 mg once daily at bedtime; may increase as tolerated up to 7.5 mg once daily with caution if clinically indicated. Use is contraindicated in patients with severe respiratory function insufficiency.

Elderly/debilitated: Initial: 3.75 mg once daily at bedtime; may increase up to 5 mg once daily if necessary (maximum: 5 mg once daily)

Dosage adjustment for concomitant therapy: Potent CYP3A4 inhibitors: Initial zopiclone dose: 3.75 mg once daily at bedtime; may increase to 5 mg once daily with caution if clinically indicated.

Dosage adjustment in renal impairment: Initial: 3.75 mg once daily at bedtime; may increase up to 5 mg once daily with caution if clinically indicated.

Dosage adjustment in hepatic impairment:

Mild-to-moderate hepatic impairment: Initial: 3.75 mg once daily at bedtime; may increase up to 5 mg once daily with caution if clinically indicated.

Severe hepatic impairment: Use is contraindicated.

Administration Administer just before bedtime.

Monitoring Parameters Monitor for confusion, excessive drowsiness (especially in elderly), and/or respiratory depression. Monitor patients with hepatic insufficiency or with chronic respiratory insufficiency closely.

Product Availability Not available in U.S.

Dosage Forms: Canada

Tablet, oral: 5 mg, 7.5 mg

◆ **Zorbtive** *see* Somatropin *on page 1918*

◆ **Zortress** *see* Everolimus *on page 822*

◆ **Zorvolex** *see* Diclofenac (Systemic) *on page 617*

◆ **Zostavax** *see* Zoster Vaccine *on page 2218*

Zoster Vaccine (ZOS ter vak SEEN)

Brand Names: U.S. Zostavax

Brand Names: Canada Zostavax

Index Terms Herpes Zoster Vaccine; HZV; Shingles Vaccine; VZV Vaccine (Zoster)

Pharmacologic Category Vaccine, Live (Viral)

Additional Appendix Information

Immunization Administration Recommendations *on page 2250*

Immunization Recommendations *on page 2255*

Use

Herpes zoster prevention: Prevention of herpes zoster (shingles) in patients ≥50 years of age

The Advisory Committee on Immunization Practices (ACIP) recommends:

Routine vaccination of **all patients ≥60 years of age, including** patients who report a previous episode of zoster; patients with chronic medical conditions (eg, chronic renal failure, diabetes mellitus, rheumatoid arthritis, chronic pulmonary disease) unless those conditions are contraindications; and residents of nursing homes and other long-term care facilities ≥60 years of age without contraindications (CDC/ACIP [Harpaz, 2008]).

Limitations of use: Not indicated for treatment of zoster or postherpetic neuralgia (PHN); not indicated for prophylaxis of primary varicella infection (chickenpox).

Dosage SubQ: Adults ≥50 years: 0.65 mL administered as a single dose; there are no data to support readministration of the vaccine (CDC/ACIP [Harpaz, 2008])

Dosage adjustment in renal impairment: There are no dosage adjustments provided in the manufacturer's labeling.

Dosage adjustment in hepatic impairment: There are no dosage adjustments provided in the manufacturer's labeling.

Additional Information Complete prescribing information should be consulted for additional detail.

Dosage Forms

Solution Reconstituted, Subcutaneous [preservative free]:

Zostavax: 19,400 units/0.65 mL (1 ea)

- **Zosyn** *see* Piperacillin and Tazobactam *on page 1657*
- **Zovia®** *see* Ethinyl Estradiol and Ethynodiol Diacetate *on page 801*
- **Zovirax** *see* Acyclovir (Systemic) *on page 47*
- **Zovirax** *see* Acyclovir (Topical) *on page 51*
- **Z-Pak** *see* Azithromycin (Systemic) *on page 216*
- **Zubsolv** *see* Buprenorphine and Naloxone *on page 304*

Zuclopenthixol [CAN/INT] (zoo kloe pen THIX ol)

Brand Names: Canada Clopixol; Clopixol Depot; Clopixol-Acuphase

Index Terms Z-chlopenthixol; Zuclopenthixol Acetate; Zuclopenthixol Decanoate; Zuclopenthixol Dihydrochloride; Zuclopenthixol Hydrochloride; Zuclopentixol Acetate; Zuclopentixol Decanoate; Zuclopentixol Hydrochloride

Pharmacologic Category First Generation (Typical) Antipsychotic

Use Note: Not approved in U.S.

Schizophrenia: Management of schizophrenia; acetate injection is intended for short-term acute treatment; decanoate injection is for long-term management; tablets may be used in either the initial or maintenance phase

Pregnancy Considerations Adverse events were observed in animal reproduction studies. Antipsychotic use during the third trimester of pregnancy has a risk for abnormal muscle movements (extrapyramidal symptoms [EPS]) and withdrawal symptoms in newborns following delivery. Symptoms in the newborn may include agitation, feeding disorder, hypertonia, hypotonia, respiratory distress, somnolence, and tremor; these effects may be self-limiting or require hospitalization.

Contraindications Hypersensitivity to zuclopenthixol, thioxanthenes, or any component of the formulation; acute intoxication (ethanol, barbiturate, or opioid); CNS depression; coma; suspected or established subcortical brain damage; circulatory collapse

Warnings/Precautions [Canadian Boxed Warning]: Neuroleptic malignant syndrome (NMS) has been associated with use of antipsychotic agents, including zuclopenthixol; monitor for mental status changes, fever, muscle rigidity, and/or autonomic instability (risk may be increased in patients with Parkinson disease or Lewy body dementia). Discontinue treatment immediately with onset of NMS; recurrence has been reported in patients rechallenged with antipsychotic therapy.

Elderly patients with dementia-related psychosis treated with antipsychotics are at an increased risk of death compared to placebo. Most deaths appeared to be either cardiovascular (eg, heart failure, sudden death) or infectious (eg, pneumonia) in nature. An increased incidence of cerebrovascular adverse events (including fatalities) has been reported in elderly patients with dementia-related psychosis. Zuclopenthixol is not approved for use in elderly patients with dementia or dementia-related psychosis.

May alter cardiac conduction; life-threatening arrhythmias have occurred with therapeutic doses of antipsychotics. Avoid use in patients with underlying QT prolongation, in those taking medicines that prolong the QT interval, or cause polymorphic ventricular tachycardia; monitor ECG closely for dose-related QT effects. Adverse effects of decanoate may be prolonged. May cause orthostatic hypotension; use with caution in patients at risk of this effect or in those who would not tolerate transient hypotensive episodes (cerebrovascular disease, cardiovascular disease, hypovolemia, or concurrent medication use which may predispose to hypotension/bradycardia). Venous thromboembolism (VTE) has been reported with antipsychotics; evaluate VTE risk prior to and during therapy. Use of antipsychotic agents may cause or exacerbate syndrome of inappropriate antidiuretic hormone secretion or hyponatremia; monitor sodium closely with initiation or dosage adjustments in older adults (Beers Criteria). First generation antipsychotics may also be inappropriate in older adults depending on comorbidities (eg, dementia, delirium) due to potent anticholinergic effects (Beers Criteria).

Antipsychotic use has been associated with esophageal dysmotility and aspiration; use with caution in patients at risk of pneumonia (ie, Alzheimer disease). May cause extrapyramidal symptoms, including pseudoparkinsonism, acute dystonic reactions, akathisia, and tardive dyskinesia. Risk of dystonia (and possibly other EPS) may be greater with increased doses, use of conventional antipsychotics, males, and younger patients. Risk of tardive dyskinesia and potential for irreversibility may be increased in elderly patients (particularly women), prolonged therapy, and higher total cumulative dose.

Use with caution in patients with cardiovascular disease, hepatic impairment, Parkinson disease, renal impairment, or seizure disorder. May cause anticholinergic effects (constipation, xerostomia, blurred vision, urinary retention); use with caution in patients with decreased gastrointestinal motility, paralytic ileus, urinary retention, BPH, xerostomia, or visual problems. Advise patients to report onset or worsening of anticholinergic effects. Use is not recommended in narrow-angle glaucoma. Similar drugs have been associated with pigmentary retinopathy, corneal deposits, and photosensitivity. Relative to other neuroleptics, zuclopenthixol has a low potency of cholinergic blockade. Use has been associated with increased prolactin levels; dosage adjustment or therapy discontinuation may be necessary with clinically significant hyperprolactinemia. Use with caution in patients with breast cancer, other prolactin-dependent tumors, and pituitary gland tumors. Prolonged hyperprolactinemia in association with hypogonadism may result in decreased bone mineral density in females and males. Cases of diabetic ketoacidosis have occurred in patients with no reported history of hyperglycemia. Obtain blood glucose level and body weight prior to initiation and then periodically thereafter.

Myelosuppression (eg, leukopenia, granulocytopenia, agranulocytosis) has been observed with antipsychotic use. Obtain blood counts prior to initiation and then periodically thereafter. Impaired core body temperature regulation may occur; caution with strenuous exercise, heat exposure, dehydration, and concomitant medication possessing anticholinergic effects. May be sedating, use with caution in disorders where CNS depression is a feature; patients must be cautioned about performing tasks which require mental alertness (eg, operating machinery or driving). Potentially significant drug interactions may exist, requiring dose or frequency adjustment, additional monitoring, and/or selection of alternative therapy. Use caution when withdrawing therapy; decrease slowly and monitor for withdrawal symptoms (eg, nausea, vomiting, or insomnia). Symptoms usually observed within 4 days of withdrawal and subside within 1 to 2 weeks. Decreased libido, menstrual disorders, erectile dysfunction (including priapism rarely) and ejaculation failure have been reported; significant dysfunction may require dosage adjustment or discontinuation of therapy. Effects are reversible upon discontinuation.

Adverse Reactions

Cardiovascular: Hypotension, orthostatic hypotension, palpitations, syncope, tachycardia

Central nervous system: Abnormal dreams, abnormal gait, agitation, akathisia, amnesia, anorgasmia (females), anxiety, apathy, confusion, depression, dizziness, drowsiness, dystonia, extrapyramidal reaction, hallucination, headache, hypertonia, insomnia, lack of concentration, malaise, pain, paresthesia, tardive dyskinesia, vertigo

Dermatologic: Diaphoresis, pallor, pruritus, seborrhea

Endocrine & metabolic: Decreased libido, increased thirst, menstrual disease, weight gain, weight loss

Gastrointestinal: Anorexia, constipation, diarrhea, dyspepsia, increased appetite, nausea, sialorrhea, vomiting, xerostomia

Genitourinary: Ejaculatory disorder, urination disorder

Neuromuscular & skeletal: Hypokinesia, myalgia, tremor, weakness

Ophthalmic: Accommodation disturbance, visual disturbance

Rare but important or life-threatening: Agranulocytosis, apnea, arthritis, cataract, cholestatic hepatitis, convulsions, drug dependence, drug-induced Parkinson's disease, dyschromia, dysphagia, gastric ulcer, glossitis, hepatic insufficiency, hyperacusis, hyperglycemia, hyperlipidemia, hyperprolactinemia, hyperreflexia, hypersensitivity reaction, hypothermia, hypotonia, leukopenia, mydriasis, neuroleptic malignant syndrome, oculogyric crisis, peripheral edema, pharyngitis, prolonged Q-T interval on ECG, skin photosensitivity, skin rash (including erythematous and psoriasiform rash), thrombocytopenia, torsades de pointes, torticollis, trismus, ventricular fibrillation, ventricular tachycardia

Drug Interactions

Metabolism/Transport Effects **Substrate** of CYP2D6 (major), CYP3A4 (minor); **Note:** Assignment of Major/Minor substrate status based on clinically relevant drug interaction potential

Avoid Concomitant Use

Avoid concomitant use of Zuclopenthixol with any of the following: Aclidinium; Amisulpride; Azelastine (Nasal); Glucagon; Highest Risk QTc-Prolonging Agents; Ipratropium (Oral Inhalation); Ivabradine; Metoclopramide; Mifepristone; Moderate Risk QTc-Prolonging Agents; Orphenadrine; Paraldehyde; Potassium Chloride; Sulpiride; Thalidomide; Tiotropium; Umeclidinium

Increased Effect/Toxicity

Zuclopenthixol may increase the levels/effects of: AbobotulinumtoxinA; Alcohol (Ethyl); Amisulpride; Analgesics (Opioid); Anticholinergic Agents; Azelastine (Nasal); Buprenorphine; CNS Depressants; Glucagon; Highest Risk QTc-Prolonging Agents; Hydrocodone; Methotrimeprazine; Methylphenidate; Metyrosine; OnabotulinumtoxinA; Orphenadrine; Paraldehyde; Potassium Chloride; RimabotulinumtoxinB; Selective Serotonin Reuptake Inhibitors; Serotonin Modulators; Sulpiride; Suvorexant; Thalidomide; Thiazide Diuretics; Tiotropium; Topiramate; Zolpidem

The levels/effects of Zuclopenthixol may be increased by: Abiraterone Acetate; Acetylcholinesterase Inhibitors (Central); Aclidinium; Brimonidine (Topical); Cannabis; CYP2D6 Inhibitors (Moderate); CYP2D6 Inhibitors (Strong); CYP3A4 Inhibitors (Moderate); CYP3A4 Inhibitors (Strong); Doxylamine; Dronabinol; Ipratropium (Oral Inhalation); Ivabradine; Kava Kava; Magnesium Sulfate; Methotrimeprazine; Methylphenidate; Metoclopramide; Metyrosine; Mifepristone; Moderate Risk QTc-Prolonging Agents; Nabilone; Peginterferon Alfa-2b; Perampanel; Pramlintide; QTc-Prolonging Agents (Indeterminate Risk and Risk Modifying); Rufinamide; Serotonin Modulators; Sodium Oxybate; Tapentadol; Tetrahydrocannabinol; Umeclidinium

Decreased Effect

Zuclopenthixol may decrease the levels/effects of: Acetylcholinesterase Inhibitors; Amphetamines; Anti-Parkinson's Agents (Dopamine Agonist); Itopride; Quinagolide; Secretin

The levels/effects of Zuclopenthixol may be decreased by: Acetylcholinesterase Inhibitors; Anti-Parkinson's Agents (Dopamine Agonist); CYP3A4 Inducers (Strong); Peginterferon Alfa-2b

Storage/Stability

Ampuls/vials: Store at 15°C to 25°C (59°F to 77°F). Protect from light. Acuphase® and depot injections may be mixed together in the same syringe.

Tablets: Store at 15°C to 25°C (59°F to 77°F).

Mechanism of Action Zuclopenthixol is a thioxanthene antipsychotic with a piperazine side chain; related to fluphenazine, the cis(z)-clopenthixol is the active isomer of this neuroleptic; blocks postsynaptic dopaminergic (D_1 and D_2) brain receptors. Also has high affinity for 5-HT_2 and alpha-1 adrenergic receptors, and a weaker affinity for $histamine_1$-receptors.

Pharmacodynamics/Kinetics

Onset of action: Acetate injection: Sedation within 2 hours

Duration: Acetate injection: 2-3 days; Decanoate injection: 2 weeks

Distribution: V_d: 20 L/kg

Protein binding: ~98%

Metabolism: Hepatic via sulfoxidation, and N-dealkylation; (*in vitro* data suggests that metabolism may occur via CYP2D6 and CYP3A4 [Davies, 2010]); also undergoes glucuronidation. Metabolites are inactive.

Half-life elimination: Terminal: Oral: ~20 hours; Depot: 19 days

Time to peak: Tablet: ~4 hours; Acetate injection: 24-48 hours; Decanoate injection: 3-7 days

Excretion: Mostly feces; urine (~10%; minimal amount as unchanged drug)

Dosage Adults: Schizophrenia/psychosis:

Oral:

Acute psychosis: Initial: 10 to 50 mg daily in 2 to 3 divided doses; may titrate dose upward by 10 to 20 mg every 2 to 3 days; usual dosage range: 20 to 60 mg daily; maximum dose: 100 mg daily

Maintenance therapy: Maintain lowest effective dose; usual maintenance dose: 20 to 40 mg daily; may be given as a single dose

IM:

Acute psychosis: Zuclopenthixol acetate: Usual dose: 50 to 150 mg; may be repeated in 2 to 3 days (some patients may require an additional dose 1 to 2 days after the initial dose and then repeat every 2 to 3 days as necessary); no more than 400 mg or 4 injections should be given in the course of treatment

Transfer of patients from IM acetate to oral tablets: **Note:** Allow 2 to 3 days after final injection before initiating oral therapy:

50 mg of acetate injection every 2 to 3 days = 20 mg daily of oral tablets

100 mg of acetate injection every 2 to 3 days = 40 mg daily of oral tablets

150 mg of acetate injection every 2 to 3 days = 60 mg daily of oral tablets

Long-term management of psychosis: Zuclopenthixol decanoate: Maintenance therapy: Usual maintenance dose: 150 to 300 mg every 2 to 4 weeks; dose increase or reduction and/or more frequent administration may be required in some patients. Maintain lowest effective dose.

Transfer of patients from oral tablets to IM decanoate: **Note:** Supplemental oral dosing, with subsequent tapering, may be required during the transition period.

≤20 mg daily of oral tablets = 100 mg of decanoate injection every 2 weeks

25 to 40 mg daily of oral tablets = 200 mg of decanoate injection every 2 weeks

50 to 75 mg daily of oral tablets = 300 mg of decanoate injection every 2 weeks

>75 mg/day of oral tablets = 400 mg of decanoate injection every 2 weeks

Transfer of patients from IM acetate to IM decanoate: **Note:** When initiating maintenance therapy with decanoate, may administer initial dose concomitantly with final acetate injection:

50 mg of acetate injection every 2 to 3 days = 100 mg of decanoate injection every 2 weeks

100 mg of acetate injection every 2 to 3 days = 200 mg of decanoate injection every 2 weeks

150 mg of acetate injection every 2 to 3 days = 300 mg of decanoate injection every 2 weeks

Dosage adjustment in renal impairment: There are no dosage adjustments provided in manufacturer's labeling (has not been studied). Renal impairment is not likely to influence systemic exposure as the drug undergoes extensive hepatic metabolism and is primarily excreted in the feces. Use with caution.

Dosage adjustment in hepatic impairment: There are no dosage adjustments provided in manufacturer's labeling (has not been studied). Use with caution; zuclopenthixol undergoes extensive hepatic metabolism.

Administration

IM: Acetate or decanoate: Administer by deep injection into the gluteal region. Injection volumes exceeding 2 mL should be distributed between 2 injection sites. When administration of the acetate **and** decanoate formulations is necessary (eg, exacerbation of chronic psychosis), may mix the acetate and decanoate formulations in the same syringe and administer as a single injection.

Oral: Tablets should be administered in 2 or 3 divided doses with initial dosing; may switch to once-daily administration at bedtime during maintenance treatment. May be administered without regards to meals.

Monitoring Parameters Vital signs; hepatic function, lipid profile, blood glucose (baseline and periodically thereafter); HbA_{1c}; BMI; CBC (baseline and periodically thereafter); mental status, abnormal involuntary movement scale (AIMS), extrapyramidal symptoms (EPS)

Product Availability Not available in U.S.

Dosage Forms: Canada

Injection:

Clopixol Acuphase: 50 mg/mL [zuclopenthixol 42.5 mg/mL] (1 mL, 2 mL)

Clopixol Depot: 200 mg/mL [zuclopenthixol 144.4 mg/mL] (10 mL)

Tablet, oral:

Clopixol: 10 mg, 25 mg

- ◆ **Zuclopenthixol Acetate** *see* Zuclopenthixol [CAN/INT] *on page 2219*
- ◆ **Zuclopenthixol Decanoate** *see* Zuclopenthixol [CAN/INT] *on page 2219*
- ◆ **Zuclopenthixol Dihydrochloride** *see* Zuclopenthixol [CAN/INT] *on page 2219*
- ◆ **Zuclopenthixol Hydrochloride** *see* Zuclopenthixol [CAN/INT] *on page 2219*
- ◆ **Zuclopentixol Acetate** *see* Zuclopenthixol [CAN/INT] *on page 2219*
- ◆ **Zuclopentixol Decanoate** *see* Zuclopenthixol [CAN/INT] *on page 2219*
- ◆ **Zuclopentixol Hydrochloride** *see* Zuclopenthixol [CAN/INT] *on page 2219*
- ◆ **Zuplenz** *see* Ondansetron *on page 1513*
- ◆ **Zyban** *see* BuPROPion *on page 305*
- ◆ **Zyclara** *see* Imiquimod *on page 1055*
- ◆ **Zyclara Pump** *see* Imiquimod *on page 1055*
- ◆ **Zydelig** *see* Idelalisib *on page 1038*
- ◆ **Zydone [DSC]** *see* Hydrocodone and Acetaminophen *on page 1012*
- ◆ **Zyflo** *see* Zileuton *on page 2199*
- ◆ **Zyflo CR** *see* Zileuton *on page 2199*
- ◆ **Zykadia** *see* Ceritinib *on page 407*
- ◆ **Zylet®** *see* Loteprednol and Tobramycin *on page 1251*
- ◆ **Zyloprim** *see* Allopurinol *on page 90*
- ◆ **Zymar (Can)** *see* Gatifloxacin *on page 949*
- ◆ **Zymaxid** *see* Gatifloxacin *on page 949*
- ◆ **ZYM-Cholestyramine-Light (Can)** *see* Cholestyramine Resin *on page 431*
- ◆ **ZYM-Cholestyramine-Regular (Can)** *see* Cholestyramine Resin *on page 431*
- ◆ **ZYM-Clonazepam (Can)** *see* ClonazePAM *on page 478*
- ◆ **ZYM-Cyclobenzaprine (Can)** *see* Cyclobenzaprine *on page 516*
- ◆ **ZYM-Fluoxetine (Can)** *see* FLUoxetine *on page 899*
- ◆ **ZYM-Mirtazapine (Can)** *see* Mirtazapine *on page 1376*
- ◆ **ZYM-Sotalol (Can)** *see* Sotalol *on page 1927*
- ◆ **ZYM-Trazodone (Can)** *see* TraZODone *on page 2091*
- ◆ **Zyncof [OTC]** *see* Guaifenesin and Dextromethorphan *on page 987*
- ◆ **Zypram™** *see* Pramoxine and Hydrocortisone *on page 1698*
- ◆ **ZyPREXA** *see* OLANZapine *on page 1491*
- ◆ **Zyprexa (Can)** *see* OLANZapine *on page 1491*
- ◆ **Zyprexa Intramuscular (Can)** *see* OLANZapine *on page 1491*
- ◆ **ZyPREXA Relprevv** *see* OLANZapine *on page 1491*
- ◆ **Zyprexa Zydis** *see* OLANZapine *on page 1491*

◆ **ZyPREXA Zydis** *see* OLANZapine *on page 1491*

◆ **ZyrTEC Allergy [OTC]** *see* Cetirizine *on page 411*

◆ **ZyrTEC Allergy Childrens [OTC]** *see* Cetirizine *on page 411*

◆ **ZyrTEC Childrens Allergy [OTC]** *see* Cetirizine *on page 411*

◆ **ZyrTEC Childrens Hives Relief [OTC]** *see* Cetirizine *on page 411*

◆ **ZyrTEC Hives Relief [OTC]** *see* Cetirizine *on page 411*

◆ **ZyrTEC Itchy Eye [OTC]** *see* Ketotifen (Ophthalmic) *on page 1150*

◆ **Zytiga** *see* Abiraterone Acetate *on page 26*

◆ **Zytram XL (Can)** *see* TraMADol *on page 2074*

◆ **Zyvox** *see* Linezolid *on page 1217*

◆ **Zyvoxam (Can)** *see* Linezolid *on page 1217*

◆ **ZzzQuil [OTC]** *see* DiphenhydrAMINE (Systemic) *on page 641*

APPENDIX TABLE OF CONTENTS

Assessment of Liver Function
- Assessment of Liver Function.......... 2224

Assessment of Renal Function
- Renal Function Estimation in Adult Patients.......... 2225

Comparative Drug Charts
- Corticosteroids Systemic Equivalencies.......... 2228
- Inhaled Corticosteroids.......... 2229
- Topical Corticosteroids.......... 2230
- Opioid Conversion Table.......... 2232
- Oral Anticoagulant Comparison Chart.......... 2233
- Reversal of Oral Anticoagulants.......... 2235
- Oral Antiplatelet Comparison Chart.......... 2239

Cytochrome P450 and Drug Interactions
- Cytochrome P450 Enzymes: Substrates, Inhibitors, and Inducers.......... 2241

Immunizations and Vaccinations
- Immunization Administration Recommendations.......... 2250
- Immunization Recommendations.......... 2255

Therapy Recommendations
- Beers Criteria – Potentially Inappropriate Medications for Geriatrics.......... 2271

Miscellaneous
- Oral Dosages That Should Not Be Crushed.......... 2276

ASSESSMENT OF LIVER FUNCTION

Child-Pugh Score

Component	Score Given for Observed Findings		
	1	2	3
Encephalopathy grade[1]	None	1 to 2	3 to 4
Ascites	None	Mild or controlled by diuretics	Moderate or refractory despite diuretics
Albumin (g/dL)	>3.5	2.8 to 3.5	<2.8
Total bilirubin (mg/dL)	<2 (<34 micromoles/L)	2 to 3 (34 to 50 micromoles/L)	>3 (>50 micromoles/L)
or			
Modified total bilirubin[2]	<4	4 to 7	>7
Prothrombin time (seconds prolonged)	<4	4 to 6	>6
or			
INR	<1.7	1.7 to 2.3	>2.3

[1]**Encephalopathy Grades**

Grade 0: Normal consciousness, personality, neurological examination, electroencephalogram
Grade 1: Restless, sleep disturbed, irritable/agitated, tremor, impaired handwriting, 5 cps waves
Grade 2: Lethargic, time-disoriented, inappropriate, asterixis, ataxia, slow triphasic waves
Grade 3: Somnolent, stuporous, place-disoriented, hyperactive reflexes, rigidity, slower waves
Grade 4: Unrousable coma, no personality/behavior, decerebrate, slow 2 to 3 cps delta activity

Alternative Encephalopathy Grades

Grade 1: Mild confusion, anxiety, restlessness, fine tremor, slowed coordination
Grade 2: Drowsiness, disorientation, asterixis
Grade 3: Somnolent but rousable, marked confusion, incomprehensible speech, incontinent, hyperventilation
Grade 4: Coma, decerebrate posturing, flaccidity

[2]Modified total bilirubin used to score patients who have Gilbert syndrome or who are taking indinavir.

CHILD-PUGH CLASSIFICATION

Class A (mild hepatic impairment): Score 5 to 6
Class B (moderate hepatic impairment): Score 7 to 9
Class C (severe hepatic impairment): Score 10 to 15

REFERENCES

Centers for Disease Control and Prevention (CDC). Report of the NIH panel to define principles of therapy of HIV infection and guidelines for the use of antiretroviral agents in HIV-infected adults and adolescents. March 2004. Available at http://www.aidsinfo.nih.gov

U.S. Department of Health and Human Services Food and Drug Administration. Guidance for industry, pharmacokinetics in patients with impaired hepatic function: study design, data analysis, and impact on dosing and labeling. May 2003. Available at http://www.fda.gov/OHRMS/DOCKETS/98fr/99D-5047-GDL00002.pdf

RENAL FUNCTION ESTIMATION IN ADULT PATIENTS

Evaluation of a patient's renal function often includes the use of equations to estimate glomerular filtration rate (GFR) (eg, estimated GFR [eGFR] creatinine clearance [CrCl]) using an endogenous filtration marker (eg, serum creatinine) and other patient variables. For example, the Cockcroft-Gault equation estimates renal function by calculating CrCl and is typically used to steer medication dosing. Equations which calculate eGFR are primarily used to categorize chronic kidney disease (CKD) staging and monitor progression. The rate of creatinine clearance does not always accurately represent GFR; creatinine may be cleared by other renal mechanisms in addition to glomerular filtration and serum creatinine concentrations may be affected by nonrenal factors (eg, age, gender, race, body habitus, illness, diet). In addition, these equations were developed based on studies in limited populations and may either over- or underestimate the renal function of a specific patient.

Nevertheless, most clinicians estimate renal function using CrCl as an indicator of actual renal function for the purpose of adjusting medication doses. For medications that require dose adjustment for renal impairment, utilization of eGFR (ie, Modification of Diet in Renal Disease [MDRD]) may overestimate renal function by up to 40% which may result in supra-therapeutic medication doses (Hermsen 2009). These equations should only be used in the clinical context of patient-specific factors noted during the physical exam/work-up. The 2012 National Kidney Foundation (NKF)-Kidney Disease Improving Global Outcomes (KDIGO) CKD guidelines state that drug dosing should be based on an e-GFR which is **not** adjusted for body surface area (BSA) (ie, reported in units of mL/minute/1.73 m^2) since the effect of eGFR adjusted for BSA compared to eGFR without adjustments for BSA has not been extensively studied. **Decisions regarding drug therapy and doses must be based on clinical judgment.**

RENAL FUNCTION ESTIMATION EQUATIONS

Commonly used equations to estimate renal function utilizing the endogenous filtration marker serum creatinine include the Cockcroft-Gault, Jelliffe, four-variable Modification of Diet in Renal Disease (MDRD), six-variable MDRD (aka, MDRD extended), and Chronic Kidney Disease Epidemiology Collaboration (CKD-EPI). All of these equations, except for the CKD-EPI, were originally developed using a serum creatinine assay measured by the alkaline picrate-based (Jaffe) method. Many substances, including proteins, can interfere with the accuracy of this assay and overestimate serum creatinine concentration. The NKF and The National Kidney Disease Education Program (NDKEP) advocated for a universal creatinine assay, in order to ensure an accurate estimate of renal function in patients. As a result, a more specific enzymatic assay with an isotope dilution mass spectrometry (IDMS)-traceable international standard was developed. Compared to the older methods, IDMS-traceable assays may report lower serum creatinine values and may, therefore, overestimate renal function when used in the original equations not re-expressed for use with a standardized serum creatinine assay (eg, Cockcroft-Gault, Jelliffe, original MDRD). Updated four-variable MDRD and six-variable MDRD equations based on serum creatinine measured by the IDMS-traceable method has been proposed for adults (Levey 2006); the Cockcroft-Gault and Jelliffe equations have not been re-expressed and may overestimate renal function when used with a serum creatinine measured by the IDMS-traceable method. However, at this point, all laboratories should be using creatinine methods calibrated to be IDMS traceable.

The CKD-EPI creatinine equation, published in 2009, uses the same four variables as the four-variable MDRD (serum creatinine, age, sex, and race), but allows for more precision when estimating higher GFR values (eg, eGFR >60 mL/minute/1.73 m^2) as compared to the MDRD equation. The NKDEP has not made a recommendation on the general implementation of the CKD-EPI equation but does suggest that laboratories which report numeric values for eGFR >60 mL/minute/1.73 m^2 should consider the use of CKD-EPI. The NKD-KDIGO 2012 CKD guidelines recommend that clinicians use a creatinine-derived equation for the evaluation and management of CKD and specifically recommend that clinical laboratories use the 2009 CKD-EPI equation when reporting eGFR in adults.

The following factors may contribute to an inaccurate estimation of renal function (Stevens 2006):

- Increased creatinine generation (may underestimate renal function):
  - Black or African American patients
  - Muscular body habitus
  - Ingestion of cooked meats
- Decreased creatinine generation (may overestimate renal function):
  - Increased age
  - Female patients
  - Hispanic patients
  - Asian patients
  - Amputees
  - Malnutrition, inflammation, or deconditioning (eg, cancer, severe cardiovascular disease, hospitalized patients)
  - Neuromuscular disease
  - Vegetarian diet
- Rapidly changing serum creatinine (either up or down): In patients with rapidly rising serum creatinines (ie, increasing by >0.5 to 0.7 mg/dL/day), it is best to assume that the patient's renal function is severely impaired

RENAL FUNCTION ESTIMATION IN ADULT PATIENTS

Use extreme caution when estimating renal function in the following patient populations:

- Low body weight (actual body weight < ideal body weight)
- Liver transplant
- Elderly (>90 years of age)
- Dehydration
- Recent kidney transplantation (serum creatinine values may decrease rapidly and can lead to renal function underestimation; conversely, delayed graft function may be present)

Note: In most situations, the use of the patient's ideal body weight (IBW) is recommended for estimating renal function, except when the patient's actual body weight (ABW) is less than ideal. Use of actual body weight (ABW) in obese patients (and possibly patients with ascites) may significantly overestimate renal function. Some clinicians prefer to use an adjusted body weight in such cases [eg, IBW + 0.4 (ABW - IBW)]; the adjustment factor may vary based on practitioner and/or institutional preference.

IDMS-traceable methods

Method 1: MDRD equation[1]:

eGFR = 175 X $(\text{Creatinine})^{-1.154}$ X $(\text{Age})^{-0.203}$ X (Gender) X (Race)
where:
eGFR = estimated GFR; calculated in mL/minute/1.73 m^2
Creatinine is input in mg/dL
Age is input in years
Gender: Females: Gender = 0.742; Males: Gender = 1
Race: Black: Race = 1.212; White or other: Race = 1

Method 2: MDRD Extended equation:

eGFR = 161.5 X $(\text{Creatinine})^{-0.999}$ X $(\text{Age})^{-0.176}$ X $(\text{SUN})^{-0.170}$ X $(\text{Albumin})^{0.318}$ X (Gender) X (Race)
where:
eGFR = estimated GFR; calculated in mL/minute/1.73 m^2
Creatinine is input in mg/dL
Age is input in years
SUN = Serum Urea Nitrogen; input in mg/dL
Albumin = Serum Albumin; input in g/dL
Gender: Females: Gender = 0.762; Males: Gender = 1
Race: Black: Race = 1.18; White or other: Race = 1

Method 3: CKD-EPI equation[2]:

eGFR = 141 X $(\text{Creatinine/k})^{\text{Exp}}$ X $(0.993)^{\text{Age}}$ X (Gender) X (Race)
where:
eGFR = estimated GFR; calculated in mL/minute/1.73 m^2
(Creatinine/k):
Creatinine is input in mg/dL
k: Females: k = 0.7; Males: k = 0.9
Exp:
When (Creatinine/k) is ≤1: Females: Exp = -0.329; Males: Exp = -0.411
When (Creatinine/k) is >1: Exp = -1.209
Age is input in years
Gender: Females: Gender = 1.018; Males: Gender = 1
Race: Black: Race = 1.159; White or other: Race = 1

Alkaline picrate-based (Jaffe) methods

Note: These equations have not been updated for use with serum creatinine methods traceable to IDMS. Use with IDMS-traceable serum creatinine methods may overestimate renal function; use with caution.

Method 1: MDRD equation:

eGFR = 186 X $(\text{Creatinine})^{-1.154}$ X $(\text{Age})^{-0.203}$ X (Gender) X (Race)
where:
eGFR = estimated GFR; calculated in mL/minute/1.73 m^2
Creatinine is input in mg/dL
Age is input in years
Gender: Females: Gender = 0.742; Males: Gender = 1
Race: Black: Race = 1.212; White or other: Race = 1

Method 2: MDRD Extended equation:

eGFR = 170 X $(\text{Creatinine})^{-0.999}$ X $(\text{Age})^{-0.176}$ X $(\text{SUN})^{-0.170}$ X $(\text{Albumin})^{0.318}$ X (Gender) X (Race)
where:
eGFR = estimated GFR; calculated in mL/minute/1.73 m^2
Creatinine is input in mg/dL
Age is input in years
SUN = Serum Urea Nitrogen; input in mg/dL
Albumin = Serum Albumin; input in g/dL
Gender: Females: Gender = 0.762; Males: Gender = 1
Race: Black: Race = 1.18; White or other: Race = 1

Method 3: Cockroft-Gault equation[3]

Males: CrCl = [(140 - Age) X Weight] / (72 X Creatinine)
Females: CrCl = {[(140 - Age) X Weight] / (72 X Creatinine)} X 0.85
where:
CrCl = creatinine clearance; calculated in mL/minute
Age is input in years
Weight is input in kg
Creatinine is input in mg/dL

Method 4: Jelliffe equation

Males: CrCl = {98 - [0.8 X (Age - 20)]} / (Creatinine)
Females: CrCl = Use above equation, then multiply result by 0.9
where:
CrCl = creatinine clearance; calculated in mL/minute/1.73 m^2
Age is input in years
Creatinine is input in mg/dL

FOOTNOTES

[1]Preferred equation for CKD staging National Kidney Disease Education Program
[2]Recommended equation for the reporting of eGFR by the NKD-KDIGO guidelines
[3]Equation typically used for adjusting medication doses

REFERENCES

Cockcroft DW, Gault MH. Prediction of creatinine clearance from serum creatinine. *Nephron.* 1976;16(1):31-41.

Dowling TC, Matzke GR, Murphy JE, Burckart GJ. Evaluation of renal drug dosing: prescribing information and clinical pharmacist approaches. *Pharmacotherapy.* 2010;30(8):776-786.

Hermsen ED, Maiefski M, Florescu MC, Qiu F, Rupp ME. Comparison of the modification of diet in renal disease and Cockcroft-Gault equations for dosing antimicrobials. *Pharmacotherapy.* 2009;29(6):649-655.

Jelliffe RW. Letter: creatinine clearance: bedside estimate. *Ann Intern Med.* 1973;79(4):604-605.

Kidney disease: improving global outcomes (KDIGO) CKD work group. KDIGO 2012 clinical practice guidelines for the evaluation and management of chronic kidney disease. *Kidney Inter.* 2013;3:1-150. http://www.kdigo.org/clinical_practice_guidelines/pdf/CKD/KDIGO_2012_CKD_GL.pdf

Levey AS, Bosch JP, Lewis JB, Greene T, Rogers N, Roth D. A more accurate method to estimate glomerular filtration rate from serum creatinine: a new prediction equation. Modification of diet in renal disease study group. *Ann Intern Med.* 1999;16;130(6):461–470.

Levey AS, Coresh J, Greene T, et al. Using standardized serum creatinine values in the modification of diet in renal disease study equation for estimating glomerular filtration rate. *Ann Intern Med.* 2006;145(4):247-254.

Levey AS, Stevens LA, Schmid CH, et al. A new equation to estimate glomerular filtration rate. *Ann Intern Med.* 2009;150(9):604-612.

National Kidney Disease Education Program. GFR calculators. http://www.nkdep.nih.gov/professionals/gfr_calculators. Accessed April 24, 2013.

Stevens LA, Coresh J, Greene T, Levey AS. Assessing kidney function – measured and estimated glomerular filtration rate. *N Engl J Med.* 2006;354 (23):2473-2483.

CORTICOSTEROIDS SYSTEMIC EQUIVALENCIES

Glucocorticoid	Approximate Equivalent Dose (mg)	Routes of Administration	Relative Anti-inflammatory Potency	Relative Mineralocorticoid Potency	Protein Binding (%)	Half-life Plasma (min)
		Short-Acting				
Cortisone	25	PO, IM	0.8	0.8	90	30
Hydrocortisone	20	IM, IV	1	1	90	90
		Intermediate-Acting				
MethylPREDNISolone[1]	4	PO, IM, IV	5	0	—	180
PrednisoLONE	5	PO, IM, IV, intra-articular, intradermal, soft tissue injection	4	0.8	90 to 95	200
PredniSONE	5	PO	4	0.8	70	60
Triamcinolone[1]	4	IM, intra-articular, intradermal, intrasynovial, soft tissue injection	5	0	—	300
		Long-Acting				
Betamethasone	0.75	PO, IM, intra-articular, intradermal, intrasynovial, soft tissue injection	25	0	64	100 to 300
Dexamethasone	0.75	PO, IM, IV, intra-articular, intradermal, soft tissue injection	25 to 30	0	—	100 to 300
		Mineralocorticoids				
Fludrocortisone	—	PO	10	125	42	200

[1]May contain propylene glycol as an excipient in injectable forms

Asare K. Diagnosis and treatment of adrenal insufficiency in the critically ill patient. *Pharmacotherapy*. 2007;27(11):1512-1528.

INHALED CORTICOSTEROIDS

Estimated Comparative Daily Dosage

Children ≥12 Years of Age and Adults

Drug	Low Daily Dose	Medium Daily Dose	High Daily Dose
Beclomethasone aerosol solution inhalation	80 to 240 mcg	>240 to 480 mcg	>480 mcg
Budesonide aerosol powder breath-activated inhalation	180 to 600 mcg	>600 to 1,200 mcg	>1,200 mcg
Ciclesonide HFA	160 to 320 mcg	>320 to 640 mcg	>640 mcg
Flunisolide aerosol solution inhalation	320 mcg	>320 to 640 mcg	>640 mcg
Fluticasone HFA	88 to 264 mcg	>264 to 440 mcg	>440 mcg
Fluticasone aerosol powder breath-activated inhalation	100 to 300 mcg	>300 to 500 mcg	>500 mcg
Mometasone aerosol powder breath-activated inhalation	200 mcg	400 mcg	>400 mcg

HFA = hydrofluoroalkane

Children <12 Years of Age

Drug	Low Daily Dose	Medium Daily Dose	High Daily Dose
Beclomethasone inhalation	0 to 4 years: NA 5 to 11 years: 80 to 160 mcg	0 to 4 years: NA 5 to 11 years: >160 to 320 mcg	0 to 4 years: NA 5 to 11 years: >320 mcg
Budesonide aerosol powder breath-activated inhalation	0 to 4 years: NA 5 to 11 years: 180 to 400 mcg	0 to 4 years: NA 5 to 11 years: >400 to 800 mcg	0 to 4 years: NA 5 to 11 years: >800 mcg
Budesonide nebulized	0 to 4 years: 0.25 to 0.5 mg 5 to 11 years: 0.5 mg	0 to 4 years: >0.5 to 1 mg 5 to 11 years: 1 mg	0 to 4 years: >1 mg 5 to 11 years: 2 mg
Ciclesonide HFA	0 to 4 years: NA 5 to 11 years: 80 to 160 mcg	0 to 4 years: NA 5 to 11 years: >160 to 320 mcg	0 to 4 years: NA 5 to 11 years: >320 mcg
Flunisolide aerosol solution inhalation	0 to 4 years: NA 5 to 11 years: 160 mcg	0 to 4 years: NA 5 to 11 years: 320 mcg	0 to 4 years: NA 5 to 11 years: ≥640 mcg
Fluticasone HFA	0 to 4 years: 176 mcg 5 to 11 years: 88 to 176 mcg	0 to 11 years: >176 to 352 mcg	0 to 11 years: >352 mcg
Fluticasone aerosol powder breath-activated inhalation	0 to 4 years: NA 5 to 11 years: 100 to 200 mcg	0 to 4 years: NA 5 to 11 years: >200 to 400 mcg	0 to 4 years: NA 5 to 11 years: >400 mcg
Mometasone aerosol powder breath-activated inhalation	NA	NA	NA

HFA = hydrofluoroalkane, NA = not approved for use in this age group or no data available

REFERENCE

Expert Panel Report 3. Guidelines for the diagnosis and management of asthma. *Clinical Practice Guidelines*, National Institutes of Health, National Heart, Lung, and Blood Institute, NIH Publication No. 08-4051. Available at http://www.nhlbi.nih.gov/guidelines/asthma/asthgdln.htm

TOPICAL CORTICOSTEROIDS

GUIDELINES FOR SELECTION AND USE OF TOPICAL CORTICOSTEROIDS

The quantity prescribed and the frequency of refills should be monitored to reduce the risk of adrenal suppression. In general, short courses of high-potency agents are preferable to prolonged use of low potency. After control is achieved, control should be maintained with a low potency preparation.

1. Low-to-medium potency agents are usually effective for treating thin, acute, inflammatory skin lesions; whereas, high or super-potent agents are often required for treating chronic, hyperkeratotic, or lichenified lesions.
2. Since the stratum corneum is thin on the face and intertriginous areas, low-potency agents are preferred but a higher potency agent may be used for 2 weeks.
3. Because the palms and soles have a thick stratum corneum, high or super-potent agents are frequently required.
4. Low potency agents are preferred for infants and the elderly. Infants have a high body surface area to weight ratio; elderly patients have thin, fragile skin.
5. The vehicle in which the topical corticosteroid is formulated influences the absorption and potency of the drug. Ointment bases are preferred for thick, lichenified lesions; they enhance penetration of the drug. Creams are preferred for acute and subacute dermatoses; they may be used on moist skin areas or intertriginous areas. Solutions, gels, and sprays are preferred for the scalp or for areas where a nonoil-based vehicle is needed.
6. In general, super-potent agents should not be used for longer than 2 to 3 weeks unless the lesion is limited to a small body area. Medium- to high-potency agents usually cause only rare adverse effects when treatment is limited to 3 months or less, and use on the face and intertriginous areas are avoided. If long-term treatment is needed, intermittent vs continued treatment is recommended.
7. Most preparations are applied once or twice daily. More frequent application may be necessary for the palms or soles because the preparation is easily removed by normal activity and penetration is poor due to a thick stratum corneum. Every-other-day or weekend-only application may be effective for treating some chronic conditions.

Relative Potency of Selected Topical Corticosteroids

	Steroid	Dosage Form
	Very High Potency	
0.05%	Betamethasone dipropionate, augmented	Cream, gel, lotion, ointment
0.05%	Clobetasol propionate	Cream, foam, gel, lotion, ointment, shampoo, spray
0.05%	Diflorasone diacetate	Ointment
0.05%	Halobetasol propionate	Cream, ointment
	High Potency	
0.1%	Amcinonide	Cream, ointment, lotion
0.05%	Betamethasone dipropionate, augmented	Cream
0.05%	Betamethasone dipropionate	Cream, ointment
0.1%	Betamethasone valerate	Ointment
0.05%	Desoximetasone	Gel
0.25%	Desoximetasone	Cream, ointment
0.05%	Diflorasone diacetate	Cream, ointment
0.05%	Fluocinonide	Cream, ointment, gel
0.1%	Halcinonide	Cream, ointment
0.5%	Triamcinolone acetonide	Cream, spray
	Intermediate Potency	
0.05%	Betamethasone dipropionate	Lotion
0.1%	Betamethasone valerate	Cream
0.1%	Clocortolone pivalate	Cream
0.05%	Desoximetasone	Cream
0.1%	Diflucortolone	Cream, oily cream, ointment
0.02%	Flumethasone pivalate	Cream
0.025%	Fluocinolone acetonide	Cream, ointment
0.05%	Flurandrenolide	Cream, ointment, lotion, tape
0.005%	Fluticasone propionate	Ointment
0.05%	Fluticasone propionate	Cream, lotion
0.1%	Hydrocortisone butyrate[1]	Ointment, solution
0.2%	Hydrocortisone valerate[1]	Cream, ointment
0.1%	Mometasone furoate[1]	Cream, ointment, lotion
0.1%	Prednicarbate	Cream, ointment
0.025%	Triamcinolone acetonide	Cream, ointment, lotion
0.1%	Triamcinolone acetonide	Cream, ointment, lotion

Relative Potency of Selected Topical Corticosteroids *(continued)*

	Steroid	Dosage Form
	Low Potency	
0.05%	Alclometasone dipropionate[1]	Cream, ointment
0.05%	Desonide	Cream, ointment
0.01%	Fluocinolone acetonide	Cream, solution
0.5%	Hydrocortisone[1]	Cream, ointment, lotion
0.5%	Hydrocortisone acetate[1]	Cream, ointment
1%	Hydrocortisone acetate[1]	Cream, ointment
1%	Hydrocortisone[1]	Cream, ointment, lotion, solution
2.5%	Hydrocortisone[1]	Cream, ointment, lotion

[1]Not fluorinated

OPIOID CONVERSION TABLE

This table serves as a general guide to opioid conversion. Utilization of a direct conversion without a detailed patients and medication assessment is not recommended and may result in over- or underdosing. Chronic administration may alter pharmacokinetics and change parenteral:oral ratio.

Opioid Analgesics – Initial Oral Dosing Commonly Used for Severe Pain

Drug	Equianalgesic Dose (mg)		Initial Oral Dose	
	Oral[1]	Parenteral[2]	Children[3] (mg/kg)	Adults (mg)
Buprenorphine	—	0.4	—	—
Butorphanol	—	2	—	—
FentaNYL	—	0.1	—	—
HYDROmorphone	7.5	1.5	0.06	4 to 8
Levorphanol	Acute: 4 Chronic: 1	Acute: 2 Chronic: 1	0.04	2 to 4
Meperidine[4]	300	75	Not recommended	
Methadone[5]	See Guidelines for Conversion to Oral Methadone in Adults	Variable	0.2	5 to 10
Morphine	30	10	0.3	15 to 30
Nalbuphine	—	10	—	—
OxyCODONE	20	—	0.2	10 to 20
Oxymorphone	10	1	—	5 to 10
Pentazocine	50	30	—	—

Guidelines for Conversion to Oral Methadone in Adults[5]

Oral Morphine Dose or Equivalent (mg/day)	Oral Morphine:Oral Methadone (Conversion Ratio)
<90	4:1
90 to 300	8:1
>300	12:1

[1]Elderly: Starting dose should be lower for this population group.

[2]Standard parenteral doses (IM) for acute pain in adults; can be used to convert doses for IV infusions and repeated small IV boluses. For single IV boluses, use half the IM dose.

[3]The pharmacokinetics of opioids in children and infants >6 months old are similar to adults, but infants <6 months old, especially premature or physically compromised ones, are at risk of apnea.

[4]Not recommended for routine use

[5]Conversion of higher doses may be guided by the following (consult a pain or palliative care specialist if unfamiliar with methadone prescribing): As the total daily chronic dose of morphine increases, the equianalgesic dose ratio (morphine:methadone) changes (American Pain Society 2008). Total daily dose should be divided by 3; delivered every 8 hours. Methadone is significantly more potent with repetitive dosing (due to its active metabolite). Begin methadone at lower doses and gradually titrate. Applicability to pediatric patients is unknown.

REFERENCES

National Cancer Institute. Pain (PDQ). Last modified May 7, 2009. Available at http://www.cancer.gov/cancertopics/pdq/supportivecare/pain/HealthProfessional/page1

National Comprehensive Cancer Network (NCCN). Clinical practice guidelines in oncology: adult cancer pain. Version 1, 2009. Available at http://www.nccn.org/professionals/physician_gls/PDF/pain.pdf

Patanwala AE, Duby J, Waters D, Erstad BL. Opioid conversions in acute care. *Ann Pharmacother.* 2007;41(2):255-266.

Principles of Analgesic Use in the Treatment of Acute Pain and Cancer Pain. 6th ed. Glenview, IL: American Pain Society; 2008.

ORAL ANTICOAGULANT COMPARISON CHART

Medication	Mechanism of Action	Metabolism	Monitoring Parameters	Pharmacotherapy Pearls	Reversal Strategies[1]	Preoperative/Preprocedure Management (General Guide)
Warfarin	• Inhibits formation of vitamin K-dependent clotting factors II, VII, IX, X, and proteins C and S	• CYP2C9 • CYP1A2 • CYP3A4 • CYP2C19	• PT/INR (individualized; depends on INR stability)	• CYP1A2, 3A4, 2C9, and 2C19 drug interactions and vitamin K-containing food interactions • Full therapeutic effect usually seen within 5 to 7 days • Half-life is ~40 hours	• Vitamin K (route and dose will depend on clinical situation and INR) • For major bleeding (at any INR): Consider PCC with vitamin K ± FFP	• Hold at least 5 days before surgery; depending on urgency of surgery/procedure, may administer low-dose IV or oral vitamin K • Minor dental and minor dermatological procedures or cataract surgery: Continue warfarin (with hemostatic agent [dental] or local hemostasis [dermatological]); may also discontinue use 2 to 3 days prior to dental procedures. Patients with prior stroke undergoing dental procedures should routinely continue warfarin.
Dabigatran (Pradaxa)	• Directly inhibits thrombin	• Hepatic glucuronidation • P-gp substrate	• Routine lab monitoring not required; aPTT, ECT (if available), TT (most sensitive) may be used to detect presence of dabigatran • Renal function	• Compliance issues (BID dosing) • Specific conversions to/from warfarin, parenteral anticoagulants • Renal dosing adjustment required; per ACCP, contraindicated with CrCl ≤30 mL/minute • Use with caution in patients ≥80 years of age • Dose reduction or avoidance required if used with dronedarone, ketoconazole, P-gp inhibitors • P-gp drug interactions • Half-life is 12 to 17 hours; considerably prolonged with severe renal impairment	• No specific antidote; for major bleeding, may consider activated PCC (ie, FEIBA NF), recombinant factor VIIa[2], or concentrates of factors II, IX, or X[3] • Use of a 4-factor PCC was shown **not** to be effective • Dabigatran is ~60% dialyzable • Activated charcoal may be used if ingestion occurred <2 hours prior to presentation	• CrCl ≥50 mL/minute: Hold 1 to 2 days before surgery • CrCl <50 mL/minute: Hold 3 to 5 days before surgery • May consider holding for >5 days in patients undergoing major surgery, spinal puncture, or insertion of a spinal or epidural catheter or port

Medication	Mechanism of Action	Metabolism	Monitoring Parameters	Pharmacotherapy Pearls	Reversal Strategies[1]	Preoperative/Preprocedure Management (General Guide)
Rivaroxaban (Xarelto)	• Directly inhibits factor Xa	• CYP3A4 • CYP3A5 • CYP2J2 • P-gp substrate	• Routine lab monitoring not required; may use PT to detect presence of rivaroxaban • Renal and hepatic function	• Administer doses ≥15 mg/day with food • Dosing frequency depends on indication • Specific conversions to/from warfarin, parenteral anticoagulants • Renal dosing adjustment required • Avoid in moderate or severe hepatic impairment • CYP3A4 and P-gp drug interactions • Half-life is 5 to 9 hours; slightly prolonged with renal impairment	• No specific antidote; for major bleeding, may consider PCC, activated PCC (ie, FEIBA NF), or recombinant factor VIIa[3] • Rivaroxaban is **not** dialyzable	• Hold at least 24 hours before surgery; longer duration of treatment cessation may be necessary based on individual patient situation and physician clinical judgment
Apixaban (Eliquis)	• Directly inhibits factor Xa	• CYP3A4 • P-gp substrate	• Routine lab monitoring not required; PT, INR, and aPTT may be used to detect presence of apixaban	• Compliance issues (BID dosing) • Specific conversions to/from warfarin, parenteral anticoagulants • Renal dosing adjustment required (NVAF); the AHA/ASA recommends to avoid use with CrCl <25 mL/minute • Not recommended in patients with severe liver impairment • CYP3A4 and P-gp drug interactions • Half-life is ~8 to 15 hours; slightly prolonged with renal impairment	• No specific antidote; for major bleeding, may consider PCC, activated PCC (ie, FEIBA NF), or recombinant factor VIIa • Apixaban is **not** dialyzable • Activated charcoal may be used if ingestion occurred within 2 to 6 hours of presentation	• Hold at least 24 to 48 hours, depending on risk or location of bleeding, before elective surgery or invasive procedures.

Abbreviations: ACCP = American College of Chest Physicians, AHA/ASA = American Heart Association/American Stroke Association, aPTT = activated partial thromboplastin time, BID = twice daily, ECT = ecarin clotting time, FFP = fresh frozen plasma, INR = international normalized ratio, NVAF = nonvalvular atrial fibrillation, PCC = prothrombin complex concentrate, P-gp = P-glycoprotein, PT = prothrombin time, TT = thrombin time

Note: Recommendations listed reflect only the U.S. labeling or U.S. clinical practice guidelines.

[1]Management of anticoagulant-associated bleeding requires careful consideration of the indication for anticoagulant therapy and bleeding extent (eg, epistaxis vs intracranial hemorrhage); minor bleeding may only require local hemostasis.

[2]The use of rFVIIa in healthy subjects treated with another direct thrombin inhibitor, melagatran (not FDA-approved), did not reverse the anticoagulant effects of melagatran.

[3]The evidence in support of these reversal strategies is limited; an exception to this may be the use of a 4-factor PCC for rivaroxaban reversal. The only available 4-factor PCC currently in the U.S. is Kcentra. Other 4-factor PCCs **not** available in the U.S. include Beriplex P/N, Cofact, and Octaplex. Bebulin VH and Profilnine SD **do not** contain adequate levels of factor VII and are considered 3-factor PCCs.

Armstrong MJ, Gronseth G, Anderson DC, et al. Summary of evidence-based guideline: periprocedural management of antithrombotic medications in patients with ischemic cerebrovascular disease: report of the Guideline Development Subcommittee of the American Academy of Neurology. *Neurology*. 2013;80(22):2065-2069.

Furie KL, Goldstein LB, Albers GW, et al. Oral antithrombotic agents for the prevention of stroke in nonvalvular atrial fibrillation: a science advisory for health care professionals from the American Heart Association/American Stroke Association. *Stroke*. 2012;43(12):3442-3453.

Guyatt GH, Akl EA, Crowther M, et al. Executive summary: antithrombotic therapy and prevention of thrombosis, 9th ed: American College of Chest Physicians evidence-based clinical practice guidelines. *Chest*. 2012;141(2 Suppl):7S-47S.

Kaatz S, Kouides PA, Garcia DA, et al. Guidance on the emergent reversal of oral thrombin and factor Xa inhibitors. *Am J Hematol*. 2012;87(Suppl 1):S141-S145.

Levi M, Eerenberg E, Kamphuisen PW. Bleeding risk and reversal strategies for old and new anticoagulants and antiplatelet agents. *J Thromb Haemost*. 2011;9(9):1705-1712.

Poulsen BK, Grove EL, Husted SE. New oral anticoagulants: a review of the literature with particular emphasis on patients with impaired renal function. *Drugs*. 2012;72(13):1739-1753.

Wolzt M, Levi M, Sarich TC, et al. Effect of recombinant factor VIIa on melagatran-induced inhibition of thrombin generation and platelet activation in healthy volunteers. *Thromb Haemost*. 2004;91(6):1090-1096.

REVERSAL OF ORAL ANTICOAGULANTS

Both oral and parenteral anticoagulants have established use in the prevention and treatment of a variety of thrombotic conditions (eg, acute coronary syndrome, venous thromboembolism, stroke). Although much has been done to prevent bleeding events associated with these agents, hemorrhagic events still continue to occur. Therefore, a thorough understanding of how best to reverse these agents when bleeding does occur is imperative. Information in this area is surfacing rapidly and recommendations may be changing. Refer to the most recent literature or guidelines for more detail and guidance. Reversal of parenteral anticoagulants, such as heparin and low molecular weight heparin (LMWH), and management of bleeding associated with these agents is established and beyond the focus of this piece.

For many years, vitamin K antagonists (eg, warfarin, acenocoumarol) were the only effective oral anticoagulants available. Recently, newer oral anticoagulants have been developed and are now marketed for prevention of stroke in patients with nonvalvular atrial fibrillation and prevention and treatment of venous thromboembolism. These include dabigatran, apixaban, and rivaroxaban. Dabigatran is an oral direct thrombin inhibitor. Apixaban and rivaroxaban are both oral factor Xa inhibitors.

VITAMIN K ANTAGONIST-INDUCED BLEEDING

Warfarin is the most common vitamin K antagonist (VKA) used in North America. The management of bleeding and reversal of other VKAs is the same. Therefore, the term VKA will be used here. VKAs interfere with the cyclic interconversion of vitamin K and vitamin K epoxide, ultimately resulting in lowered production of effective factors II, VII, IX, and X. VKAs also inhibit the production of proteins C, S, and Z which may result in procoagulation. The half-life of racemic warfarin ranges from 36 to 42 hours. Other VKAs, such as acenocoumarol, have significantly shorter half-lives. Warfarin, due to metabolism via the cytochrome P450 enzyme system (specifically CYP2C9, CYP3A4, CYP1A2, and CYP2C19), is subject to a number of drug-drug interactions which may occur by inhibiting these isoenzymes, leading to reduced metabolism and elevated warfarin concentrations. Intensity of anticoagulation with VKAs can predict the incidence of bleeding events. When the INR is greater than 5, the incidence of bleeding increases dramatically; patient factors also play a major role in risk of bleeding (eg, prior history of bleeding, advanced age, renal insufficiency) (Ageno 2012).

Patients with elevated INR may not need reversal unless undergoing an invasive procedure. If the invasive procedure is elective, the procedure should be delayed until INR is acceptable for the procedure. In general, for patients with an INR of 6 to 10, up to ~2.5 days may elapse before the INR reduces to <4 (Patel 2000). Some patients may require bridging with a parenteral anticoagulant during this time to prevent thrombosis.

Patients who are bleeding may require reversal with vitamin K (or phytonadione). Rapid reversal is necessary if the bleeding is life-threatening. In this case, the use of intravenous vitamin K and either fresh frozen plasma (FFP), prothrombin complex concentrates (PCC), or recombinant factor VIIa (rFVIIa) becomes imperative. Currently, the American College of Chest Physicians recommends an intravenous vitamin K dose of 5 to 10 mg administered slowly. Due to the occurrence of anaphylactoid reaction with rapid intravenous administration with vitamin K, intravenous vitamin K should always be diluted in a minimum of 50 mL of a compatible solution and infused over at least 20 minutes (Ageno 2012). Reduction of INR with intravenous administration usually begins within 2 hours of administration. Subcutaneous administration of vitamin K is not recommended due to slower resolution of elevated INR.

The choice as to which coagulation factor (FFP, PCC, or rFVIIa) to use in addition to intravenous vitamin K for the patient who has life-threatening bleeding has not been established. Advantages and disadvantages exist with all the coagulation factors. Regardless of which one is chosen, the target INR for the patient with a life-threatening bleed is typically <1.5. FFP contains all of the factors inhibited by warfarin (factors II, VII, IX, and X) and would be an ideal agent to use for reversal. However, high volumes of FFP may be problematic in patients who are sensitive to rapid fluid shifts (eg, heart failure). FFP also has the disadvantages of possible allergic reaction, transfusion-related lung injury (TRALI), transmission of infection, and prolonged preparation time due to frozen storage. A new plasma substitute (OctaplaseLG) is now available. OctaplaseLG, labeled for the rapid reversal of VKA-induced anticoagulation, is solvent-detergent treated and has been shown to not cause TRALI and other side effects seen with FFP. PCCs, although more costly compared to FFP, are advantageous in that they have a lower infusion volume, lower transmission rate of infection, can be administered rapidly with rapid reversal of VKA-associated coagulopathy, do not require cross-matching, and are associated with less complications. Currently, the American College of Chest Physicians recommends the use of four-factor PCCs over FFP and rFVIIa. The only available four-factor PCC in the U.S. is Kcentra (known as Beriplex P/N outside the U.S.). Other four-factor PCCs not available in the U.S. include Cofact, Kanokad, and Octaplex. Bebulin VH and Profilnine SD do not contain adequate levels of factor VII and are considered three-factor PCCs (see Table next page).

Composition of Prothrombin Complex Concentrates

Prothrombin Complex Concentrate	Factor II	Factor VII	Factor IX	Factor X	Heparin	Human Antithrombin III	Protein C	Protein S	Protein Z
"Three-Factor (minimal factor VII component) PCCs"									
Bebulin VH	24 to 38 IU/mL	<5 IU/mL	24 to 38 IU/mL	24 to 38 IU/mL	<0.15 IU/IU FIX	–	–	–	–
Profilnine SD	NMT 150 units per 100 FIX units	NMT 35 units per 100 FIX units	100 units	NMT 100 units per 100 FIX units	–	–	–	–	–
"Four-Factor PCCs"									
Cofact[a]	14 to 35 IU/mL	7 to 20 IU/mL	25 IU/mL	14 to 35 IU/mL	–	<0.6 IU/mL	11 to 39 IU/mL	1 to 8 IU/mL	–
Kanokad[a]	14 to 35 IU/mL	7 to 20 IU/mL	25 IU/mL	14 to 35 IU/mL	–	–	–	–	–
Kcentra (known as Beriplex P/N outside the U.S.)	19 to 40 IU/mL	10 to 25 IU/mL	20 to 31 IU/mL	25 to 51 IU/mL	0.4 to 2 IU/mL	0.2 to 1.5 IU/mL	21 to 41 IU/mL	12 to 34 IU/mL	–
Octaplex[a]	14 to 38 IU/mL	9 to 24 IU/mL	25 IU/mL	18 to 30 IU/mL	5 to 12.5 IU/mL	–	13 to 31 IU/mL	12 to 32 IU/mL	–
"Activated PCC"									
FEIBA NF	1.3 IU/IU[b]	0.9 IU/IU	1.4 IU/IU[b]	1.1 IU/IU[b]	–	–	1.1 IU/IU	–	–

FIX = Factor IX, NMT = not more than

[a]Not available in the U.S.

[b]Mainly nonactivated form

The use of rFVIIa gained some interest; however, it has not been shown to be superior to PCC or FFP and is the most expensive agent of the three. The combination of rFVIIa and three-factor PCC (along with intravenous vitamin K) has been used with some success (Sarode 2012); however, the combination cannot be recommended at this time.

DABIGATRAN-INDUCED BLEEDING

Dabigatran is a new oral direct thrombin inhibitor with an elimination half-life of 12 to 17 hours. Dabigatran is 80% excreted in the urine as unchanged drug and therefore elimination half-life is prolonged in patients with renal impairment (up to 28 hours with severe impairment). Dabigatran is hepatically metabolized via glucuronidation to active acylglucuronide isomers. Although not a substrate for CYP450, dabigatran is a substrate of P-glycoprotein (gp). Therefore, P-gp inhibitors may increase dabigatran concentrations, resulting in a higher risk of bleeding events.

Similar to its parenteral counterparts (eg, argatroban), dabigatran does not have a specific reversal agent. Although the INR may be elevated with dabigatran use, vitamin K is not effective for dabigatran-induced bleeding. In addition, the aPTT rises as dabigatran concentrations increase; however, the use of protamine will not reverse these effects on the aPTT. Based on limited evidence for reversal strategies, several different recommendations have been put forth. Activated charcoal should be administered if oral intake was recent (ie, within a couple of hours of presentation). Hemodialysis, although this may be impractical, has been shown to remove 62% to 68% over 2 to 4 hours (Stangier 2010). The use of a four-factor PCC (Cofact; not available in the U.S.) has been shown to be ineffective for dabigatran reversal (Eerenberg 2011). In addition, other coagulation factors (eg, FFP, rFVIIa) have not adequately demonstrated benefit in humans and therefore cannot be formally recommended.

ORAL FACTOR XA INHIBITOR-INDUCED BLEEDING

Apixaban and rivaroxaban are oral factor Xa inhibitors. Apixaban has an elimination half-life of 8 to 15 hours and is metabolized to a minor degree via the cytochrome P450 system (specifically CYP2C19, CYP2C8, CYP2C9, and CYP3A4) and is a P-gp substrate. Apixaban is also partially excreted (~27%) as unchanged drug in the urine. Rivaroxaban has an elimination half-life of 5 to 9 hours and is excreted (~36%) as unchanged drug in the urine. Rivaroxaban is hepatically metabolized via CYP3A4/5 and CYP2J2 and is a substrate of P-gp as well.

The use of rFVIIa has been shown to decrease the bleeding time in animal models; however, it does not reverse the anticoagulant effect of rivaroxaban. The use of rFVIIa has not been formally evaluated in humans treated with rivaroxaban or apixaban. The use of a four-factor PCC (Cofact; not available in the U.S.) has been shown to reverse the anticoagulant effect of rivaroxaban in humans (Eerenberg 2011). Therefore, because of the lack of data in humans, the use of PCC or rFVIIa cannot be formally recommended for rapid reversal in patients receiving apixaban or rivaroxaban.

CONCLUSION

The approach to the bleeding patient receiving oral anticoagulation is challenging. Unfortunately, data supporting specific reversal agents is lacking beyond the known antidotes used for specific therapies (eg, warfarin). Research in this area is expanding the knowledge; however, much research is still needed to further define specific approaches to patients receiving newer oral anticoagulants. Reversal agents for some of these new oral anticoagulants are being developed, such as the recombinant antidote PRT064445, and future oral anticoagulants will likely be released with a reversal agent (eg, betrixaban and its specific antidote PRT4445).

REFERENCES

Ageno W, Gallus AS, Wittkowsky A, et al. Oral anticoagulant therapy: antithrombotic therapy and prevention of thrombosis, 9th ed: American College of Chest Physicians evidence-based clinical practice guidelines. *Chest.* 2012;141(2 Suppl):e44S-e88S.

Bauer KA. Reversal of antithrombotic agents. *Am J Hematol.* 2012;87(Suppl 1):S119-S126.

Bechtel BF, Nunez TC, Lyon JA, Cotton BA, Barrett TW. Treatments for reversing warfarin anticoagulation in patients with acute intracranial hemorrhage: a structured literature review. *Int J Emerg Med.* 2011;4(1):40.

Dager WE. Developing a management plan for oral anticoagulant reversal. *Am J Health Syst Pharm.* 2013;70(10 Suppl 1):S21-S31.

Dager WE, Gosselin RC, Kitchen S, Dwyre D. Dabigatran effects on the international normalized ratio, activated partial thromboplastin time, thrombin time, and fibrinogen: a multicenter, *in vitro* study. *Ann Pharmacother.* 2012;46(12):1627-1636.

Dumkow LE, Voss JR, Peters M, Jennings DL. Reversal of dabigatran-induced bleeding with a prothrombin complex concentrate and fresh frozen plasma. *Am J Health Syst Pharm.* 2012;69(19):1646-1650.

Eerenberg ES, Kamphuisen PW, Sijpkens MK, Meijers JC, Buller HR, Levi M. Reversal of rivaroxaban and dabigatran by prothrombin complex concentrate: a randomized, placebo-controlled, crossover study in healthy subjects. *Circulation.* 2011;124(14):1573-1579.

Holbrook A, Schulman S, Witt DM, et al. Evidence-based management of anticoagulant therapy: antithrombotic therapy and prevention of thrombosis, 9th ed: American College of Chest Physicians evidence-based clinical practice guidelines. *Chest.* 2012;141(2 Suppl):e152S-e184S.

Kaatz S, Kouides PA, Garcia DA, et al. Guidance on the emergent reversal of oral thrombin and factor Xa inhibitors. *Am J Hematol.* 2012;87(Suppl 1): S141-S145.

Marlu R, Hodaj E, Paris A, Albaladejo P, Cracowski JL, Pernod G. Effect of non-specific reversal agents on anticoagulant activity of dabigatran and rivaroxaban: a randomised crossover *ex vivo* study in healthy volunteers. *Thromb Haemost.* 2012;108(2):217-224.

Miesbach W, Seifried E. New direct oral anticoagulants – current therapeutic options and treatment recommendations for bleeding complications. *Thromb Haemost.* 2012;108(4):625-632.

Miyares MA, Davis K. Newer oral anticoagulants: a review of laboratory monitoring options and reversal agents in the hemorrhagic patient. *Am J Health Syst Pharm.* 2012;69(17):1473-1484.

Ortel TL. Perioperative management of patients on chronic antithrombotic therapy. *Hematology Am Soc Hematol Educ Program.* 2012;2012:529-535.

Patel RJ, Witt DM, Saseen JJ, Tillman DJ, Wilkinson DS. Randomized, placebo-controlled trial of oral phytonadione for excessive anticoagulation. *Pharmacotherapy.* 2000;20(10):1159-1166.

Patriquin C, Crowther M. Treatment of warfarin-associated coagulopathy with vitamin K. *Expert Rev Hematol.* 2011;4(6):657-665.

Sarode R, Matevosyan K, Bhagat R, Rutherford C, Madden C, Beshay JE. Rapid warfarin reversal: a 3-factor prothrombin complex concentrate and recombinant factor VIIa cocktail for intracerebral hemorrhage. *J Neurosurg*. 2012;116(3):491-497.

Sarode R, Milling TJ Jr, Refaai MA, et al. Efficacy and safety of a four-factor prothrombin complex concentrate (4F-PCC) in patients on vitamin K antagonists presenting with major bleeding: a randomized, plasma-controlled, phase IIIb study. *Circulation*. 2013.

Siegal DM, Crowther MA. Acute management of bleeding in patients on novel oral anticoagulants. *Eur Heart J*. 2013;34(7):489-498b.

Stangier J, Rathgen K, Stähle H, Mazur D. Influence of renal impairment on the pharmacokinetics and pharmacodynamics of oral dabigatran etexilate: an open-label, parallel-group, single-centre study. *Clin Pharmacokinet*. 2010;49(4):259-268.

van Ryn J, Stangier J, Haertter S, et al. Dabigatran etexilate – a novel, reversible, oral direct thrombin inhibitor: interpretation of coagulation assays and reversal of anticoagulant activity. *Thromb Haemost*. 2010;103(6):1116-1127.

Wanek MR, Horn ET, Elapavaluru S, Baroody SC, Sokos G. Safe use of hemodialysis for dabigatran removal before cardiac surgery. *Ann Pharmacother*. 2012;46(9):e21.

Weitz JI, Eikelboom JW, Samama MM; American College of Chest Physicians. New antithrombotic drugs: antithrombotic therapy and prevention of thrombosis, 9th ed: American College of Chest Physicians evidence-based clinical practice guidelines. *Chest*. 2012;141(2 Suppl):e120S-e151S.

ORAL ANTIPLATELET COMPARISON CHART

Medication	Mechanism of Action	Reversible Platelet Inhibition	Prodrug	Metabolism	Pharmacotherapy Pearls	Reversal Strategies[1]	Preoperative/Preprocedure Management (General Guide)
Aspirin	Inhibits cyclooxygenase-1 and 2	No	No	• CYP2C9	• Chronic NSAID use can compromise antiplatelet effects • Monitor for GI ulceration	• No specific antidote • Consider platelet transfusion ± DDAVP • Normal platelet function returns within 7 to 10 days after discontinuation	• Hold 7 to 10 days before surgery • May be continued through surgery for CABG or noncardiac surgery in patients with moderate to high cardiac risk • Minor dental or dermatological procedures or cataract surgery: Continue through procedure. AAN recommends continuation when undergoing any dental procedure for patients taking aspirin for ischemic stroke prevention.
Cilostazol (Pletal)	Inhibits platelet phosphodiesterase III	Yes	No	• CYP3A4 • CYP2C19 • CYP1A2 • CYP2D6	• Administer before or 2 hours after meals • Contraindicated in patients with heart failure of any severity • CYP3A4 and 2C19 drug interactions	• No specific antidote • Normal platelet function returns within 4 days after discontinuation	• Hold 2 to 3 days before surgery
Clopidogrel (Plavix)	Inhibits $P2Y_{12}$ component of ADP receptors	No	Yes	• CYP2C19 • CYP3A4	• CYP2C19 inhibitors may reduce concentrations of active metabolite • CYP2C19 polymorphisms may affect clopidogrel efficacy	• No specific antidote • Consider platelet transfusion ± DDAVP • Normal platelet function returns within 7 to 10 days after discontinuation	• Hold 5 to 10 days before surgery[2]
Prasugrel (Effient)	Inhibits $P2Y_{12}$ component of ADP receptors	No	Yes	• CYP3A4 • CYP2B6	• Reduce maintenance dose to 5 mg in patients <60 kg • Contraindicated in patients with history of stroke, TIA • Not recommended in patients ≥75 years of age	• No specific antidote • Consider platelet transfusion ± DDAVP • Normal platelet function returns within 5 to 9 days after discontinuation	• Hold 5 to 7 days before surgery[2]

Medication	Mechanism of Action	Reversible Platelet Inhibition	Prodrug	Metabolism	Pharmacotherapy Pearls	Reversal Strategies[1]	Preoperative/Preprocedure Management (General Guide)
Ticagrelor (Brilinta)	Inhibits $P2Y_{12}$ component of ADP receptors	Yes	No	• CYP3A4 • CYP3A5	• Used in combination with aspirin; daily maintenance aspirin dose should not exceed 81 mg • CYP3A4 drug interactions • BID dosing • Monitor closely for dyspnea, bradyarrhythmia (including ventricular pauses)	• No specific antidote • Consider aminocaproic acid, tranexamic acid, recombinant factor VIIa • Normal platelet function returns within 3 to 5 days after discontinuation	• Hold at least 5 days before surgery[2]
Ticlopidine	Inhibits $P2Y_{12}$ component of ADP receptors	No	Yes	• CYP3A4	• Black Box warning on hematologic toxicities (aplastic anemia, TTP) • Frequent CBC monitoring required • BID dosing	• No specific antidote • Consider platelet transfusion ± DDAVP • Normal platelet function returns within 5 to 10 days after discontinuation	• Hold 10 to 14 days before surgery

[1]Management of antiplatelet-associated bleeding requires careful consideration of the indication for antiplatelet therapy and bleeding extent (eg, epistaxis vs intracranial hemorrhage); minor bleeding may only require local hemostasis.

[2]When urgent CABG is necessary, the ACCF/AHA CABG guidelines recommend discontinuation for at least 24 hours prior to surgery (Hillis 2011).

Armstrong MJ, Gronseth G, Anderson DC, et al. Summary of evidence-based guideline: periprocedural management of antithrombotic medications in patients with ischemic cerebrovascular disease: report of the Guideline Development Subcommittee of the American Academy of Neurology. *Neurology*. 2013;80(22):2065-2069.

Hillis LD, Smith PK, Anderson JL, et al. 2011 ACCF/AHA guideline for coronary artery bypass graft surgery: executive summary: a report of the American College of Cardiology Foundation/American Heart Association task force on practice guidelines. *Circulation*. 2011;124(23):2610-2642.

Levi M, Eerenberg E, Kamphuisen PW. Bleeding risk and reversal strategies for old and new anticoagulants and antiplatelet agents. *J Thromb Haemost*. 2011;9(9):1705-1712.

Patrono C, Andreotti F, Arnesen H, et al. Antiplatelet agents for the treatment and prevention of atherothrombosis. *Eur Heart J*. 2011;32(23):2922-2932.

CYTOCHROME P450 ENZYMES: SUBSTRATES, INHIBITORS, AND INDUCERS

INTRODUCTION

Most drugs are eliminated from the body, at least in part, by being chemically altered to less lipid-soluble products (ie, metabolized), and thus are more likely to be excreted via the kidneys or the bile. Phase I metabolism includes drug hydrolysis, oxidation, and reduction, and results in drugs that are more polar in their chemical structure, while Phase II metabolism involves the attachment of an additional molecule onto the drug (or partially metabolized drug) in order to create an inactive and/or more water soluble compound. Phase II processes include (primarily) glucuronidation, sulfation, glutathione conjugation, acetylation, and methylation.

Virtually any of the Phase I and II enzymes can be inhibited by some xenobiotic or drug. Some of the Phase I and II enzymes can be induced. Inhibition of the activity of metabolic enzymes will result in increased concentrations of the substrate (drug), whereas induction of the activity of metabolic enzymes will result in decreased concentrations of the substrate. For example, the well-documented enzyme-inducing effects of phenobarbital may include a combination of Phase I and II enzymes. Phase II glucuronidation may be increased via induced UDP-glucuronosyltransferase (UGT) activity, whereas Phase I oxidation may be increased via induced cytochrome P450 (CYP) activity. However, for most drugs, the primary route of metabolism (and the primary focus of drug-drug interaction) is Phase I oxidation.

CYP enzymes may be responsible for the metabolism (at least partial metabolism) of ~75% of all drugs, with the CYP3A subfamily responsible for nearly half of this activity. Found throughout plant, animal, and bacterial species, CYP enzymes represent a superfamily of xenobiotic metabolizing proteins. There have been several hundred CYP enzymes identified in nature, each of which has been assigned to a family (1, 2, 3, etc), subfamily (A, B, C, etc), and given a specific enzyme number (1, 2, 3, etc) according to the similarity in amino acid sequence that it shares with other enzymes. Of these many enzymes, only a few are found in humans, and even fewer appear to be involved in the metabolism of xenobiotics (eg, drugs). The key human enzyme subfamilies include CYP1A, CYP2A, CYP2B, CYP2C, CYP2D, CYP2E, and CYP3A. However, the number of distinct isozymes (eg, CYP2C9) found to be functionally active in humans, as well as, the number of genetically variant forms of these isozymes (eg, CYP2C9*2) in individuals continues to expand.

CYP enzymes are found in the endoplasmic reticulum of cells in a variety of human tissues (eg, skin, kidneys, brain, lungs), but their predominant sites of concentration and activity are the liver and intestine. Though the abundance of CYP enzymes throughout the body is relatively equally distributed among the various subfamilies, the relative contribution to drug metabolism is (in decreasing order of magnitude) CYP3A4 (nearly 50%), CYP2D6 (nearly 25%), CYP2C8/9 (nearly 15%), then CYP1A2, CYP2C19, CYP2A6, and CYP2E1. Owing to their potential for numerous drug-drug interactions, those drugs that are identified in preclinical studies as substrates of CYP3A enzymes are often given a lower priority for continued research and development in favor of drugs that appear to be less affected by (or less likely to affect) this enzyme subfamily.

Each enzyme subfamily possesses unique selectivity toward potential substrates. For example, CYP1A2 preferentially binds medium-sized, planar, lipophilic molecules, while CYP2D6 preferentially binds molecules that possess a basic nitrogen atom. Some CYP subfamilies exhibit polymorphism (ie, genetic variation that results in a modified enzyme with small changes in amino acid sequences that may manifest differing catalytic properties). The best described polymorphisms involve CYP2C9, CYP2C19, and CYP2D6. Individuals possessing "wild type" genes exhibit normal functioning CYP capacity. Others, however, possess genetic variants that leave the person with a subnormal level of catalytic potential (so called "poor metabolizers"). Poor metabolizers would be more likely to experience toxicity from drugs metabolized by the affected enzymes (or less effects if the enzyme is responsible for converting a prodrug to it's active form as in the case of codeine). The percentage of people classified as poor metabolizers varies by enzyme and population group. As an example, ~7% of Caucasians and only about 1% of Asians appear to be CYP2D6 poor metabolizers.

CYP enzymes can be both inhibited and induced by other drugs, leading to increased or decreased serum concentrations (along with the associated effects), respectively. Induction occurs when a drug causes an increase in the amount of smooth endoplasmic reticulum, secondary to increasing the amount of the affected CYP enzymes in the tissues. This "revving up" of the CYP enzyme system may take several days to reach peak activity, and likewise, may take several days, even months, to return to normal following discontinuation of the inducing agent.

CYP inhibition occurs via several potential mechanisms. Most commonly, a CYP inhibitor competitively (and reversibly) binds to the active site on the enzyme, thus preventing the substrate from binding to the same site, and preventing the substrate from being metabolized. The affinity of an inhibitor for an enzyme may be expressed by an inhibition constant (Ki) or IC50 (defined as the concentration of the inhibitor required to cause 50% inhibition under a given set of conditions). In addition to reversible competition for an enzyme site, drugs may inhibit enzyme activity by binding to sites on the enzyme other than that to which the substrate would bind, and thereby cause a change in the functionality or physical structure of the enzyme. A drug may also bind to the enzyme in an irreversible (ie, "suicide") fashion. In such a case, it is not the concentration of drug at the enzyme site that is important (constantly binding and releasing), but the number of molecules available for binding (once bound, always bound).

Although an inhibitor or inducer may be known to affect a variety of CYP subfamilies, it may only inhibit one or two in a clinically important fashion. Likewise, although a substrate is known to be at least partially metabolized by a variety of CYP enzymes, only one or two enzymes may contribute significantly enough to its overall metabolism to warrant concern when used with potential inducers or inhibitors. Therefore, when attempting to predict the level of risk of using two drugs that may affect each other via altered CYP function, it is important to identify the relative effectiveness of the inhibiting/inducing drug on the CYP subfamilies that significantly contribute to the metabolism of the substrate. The contribution of a specific CYP pathway to substrate metabolism should be considered not only in light of other known CYP pathways, but also other nonoxidative pathways for substrate metabolism (eg, glucuronidation) and transporter proteins (eg, P-glycoprotein) that may affect the presentation of a substrate to a metabolic pathway.

HOW TO USE THIS TABLE

The following table provides a clinically relevant perspective on drugs that are affected by, or affect, cytochrome P450 (CYP) enzymes. Not all human, drug-metabolizing CYP enzymes are specifically (or separately) included in the table. Some enzymes have been excluded because they do not appear to significantly contribute to the metabolism of marketed drugs (eg, CYP2C18). In the case of CYP3A4, the industry routinely uses this single enzyme designation to represent all enzymes in the CYP3A subfamily. CYP3A7 is present in fetal livers. It is effectively absent from adult livers. CYP3A4 (adult) and CYP3A7 (fetal) appear to share similar properties in their respective hosts. The impact of CYP3A7 in fetal and neonatal drug interactions has not been investigated.

An enzyme that appears to play a clinically significant (major) role in a drug's metabolism is indicated by "S". A clinically significant designation is the result of a two-phase review. The first phase considered the contribution of each CYP enzyme to the overall metabolism of the drug. The enzyme pathway was considered potentially clinically relevant if it was responsible for at least 30% of the metabolism of the drug. If so, the drug was subjected to a second phase. The second phase considered the clinical relevance of a substrate's concentration being increased twofold, or decreased by one-half (such as might be observed if combined with an effective CYP inhibitor or inducer, respectively). If either of these changes was considered to present a clinically significant concern, the CYP pathway for the drug was designated "major." If neither change would appear to present a clinically significant concern, or if the CYP enzyme was responsible for a smaller portion of the overall metabolism (ie, <30%), then no association between the enzyme and the drug will appear in the table.

Enzymes that are strongly or moderately inhibited by a drug are indicated by "↓". Enzymes that are weakly inhibited are not identified in the table. The designations are the result of a review of published clinical reports, available Ki data, and assessments published by other experts in the field. As it pertains to Ki values set in a ratio with achievable serum drug concentrations ([I]) under normal dosing conditions, the following parameters were employed: [I]/Ki ≥1 = strong; [I]/Ki 0.1 to 1 = moderate; [I]/Ki <0.1 = weak.

Enzymes that appear to be effectively induced by a drug are indicated by "↑". This designation is the result of a review of published clinical reports and assessments published by experts in the field.

In general, clinically significant interactions are more likely to occur between substrates ("S") and either inhibitors or inducers of the same enzyme(s), which have been indicated by "↓" and "↑", respectively. However, these assessments possess a degree of subjectivity, at times based on limited indications regarding the significance of CYP effects of particular agents. An attempt has been made to balance a conservative, clinically-sensitive presentation of the data with a desire to avoid the numbing effect of a "beware of everything" approach. It is important to note that information related to CYP metabolism of drugs is expanding at a rapid pace, and thus, the contents of this table should only be considered to represent a "snapshot" of the information available at the time of publication.

SELECTED READINGS

Bjornsson TD, Callaghan JT, Einolf HJ, et al. The conduct of *in vitro* and *in vivo* drug-drug interaction studies: a PhRMA perspective. *J Clin Pharmacol.* 2003;43(5):443-469.

Drug-Drug Interactions. Rodrigues AD, ed. New York, NY: Marcel Dekker, Inc; 2002.

Metabolic Drug Interactions. Levy RH, Thummel KE, Trager WF, et al, eds. Philadelphia, PA: Lippincott Williams & Wilkins; 2000.

Michalets EL. Update: clinically significant cytochrome P-450 drug interactions. *Pharmacotherapy.* 1998;18(1):84-112.

Thummel KE, Wilkinson GR. *In vitro* and *in vivo* drug interactions involving human CYP3A. *Annu Rev Pharmacol Toxicol.* 1998;38:389-430.

Zhang Y, Benet LZ. The gut as a barrier to drug absorption: combined role of cytochrome P450 3A and P-Glycoprotein. *Clin Pharmacokinet.* 2001;40 (3):159-168.

SELECTED WEBSITES

http://www.imm.ki.se/CYPalleles

http://medicine.iupui.edu/flockhart

http://www.fda.gov/Drugs/DevelopmentApprovalProcess/DevelopmentResources/DrugInteractionsLabeling/ucm080499.htm

CYP: Substrates, Inhibitors, Inducers

S = substrate; ↓ = inhibitor; ↑ = inducer

Drug	1A2	2A6	2B6	2C8	2C9	2C19	2D6	2E1	3A4
Acenocoumarol	S				S				
Alfentanil									S
Alfuzosin									S
Alosetron	S								
ALPRAZolam									S
Ambrisentan						S			S
Aminophylline	S								
Amiodarone		↓		S	↓		↓		S, ↓
Amitriptyline							S		
AmLODIPine	↓								S
Amobarbital		↑							
Amoxapine							S		
Aprepitant									S, ↓
ARIPiprazole							S		S
Armodafinil						↓			S, ↑
Atazanavir									S, ↓
Atomoxetine							S		
Atorvastatin									S
Benzphetamine									S
Betaxolol	S						S		
Bisoprolol									S
Bortezomib						S, ↓			S
Bosentan					S, ↑				S, ↑
Bromazepam									S
Bromocriptine									S
Budesonide									S
Buprenorphine									S
BuPROPion			S						
BusPIRone									S
Busulfan									S
Caffeine	S								↓
Captopril							S		
CarBAMazepine	↑		↑	↑	↑	↑			S, ↑
Carisoprodol						S			
Carvedilol					S		S		
Celecoxib				↓	S				
ChlordiazePOXIDE									S
Chloroquine							S, ↓		S
Chlorpheniramine									S
ChlorproMAZINE							S, ↓		
Chlorzoxazone								S	
Ciclesonide									S
Cilostazol									S
Cimetidine	↓					↓	↓		↓
Cinacalcet							↓		
Ciprofloxacin	↓								
Cisapride									S
Citalopram						S			S

CYP: Substrates, Inhibitors, Inducers *(continued)*

Drug	1A2	2A6	2B6	2C8	2C9	2C19	2D6	2E1	3A4
Clarithromycin									S, ↓
Clobazam						S			S
ClomiPRAMINE	S					S	S, ↓		
ClonazePAM									S
Clorazepate									S
Clotrimazole									↓
CloZAPine	S						↓		
Cobicistat									S, ↓
Cocaine							↓		S
Codeine[1]							S		
Colchicine									S
Conivaptan									S, ↓
Cyclobenzaprine	S								
Cyclophosphamide[2]			S						S
CycloSPORINE									S, ↓
Dacarbazine	S							S	
Dantrolene									S
Dapsone					S				S
Darifenacin							↓		S
Darunavir									S
Dasatinib									S
Delavirdine					↓	↓	↓		S, ↓
Desipramine		↓	↓				S, ↓		↓
Desogestrel						S			
Dexamethasone									S, ↑
Dexlansoprazole						S, ↓			S
Dexmedetomidine		S					↓		
Dextromethorphan							S		
Diazepam						S			S
Diclofenac	↓								
Dihydroergotamine									S
Diltiazem									S, ↓
DiphenhydrAMINE							↓		
Disopyramide									S
Disulfiram								↓	
DOCEtaxel									S
Doxepin							S		
DOXOrubicin			↓				S		S
Doxycycline									↓
DULoxetine	S						S, ↓		
Efavirenz[3]			S		↓	↓			S, ↓, ↑
Eletriptan									S
Enflurane								S	
Eplerenone									S
Ergoloid mesylates									S
Ergonovine									S
Ergotamine									S
Erlotinib									S
Erythromycin									S, ↓
Escitalopram						S			S
Esomeprazole						S, ↓			S
Estradiol	S								S

CYP: Substrates, Inhibitors, Inducers *(continued)*

Drug	1A2	2A6	2B6	2C8	2C9	2C19	2D6	2E1	3A4
Estrogens, conjugated A/synthetic	S								S
Estrogens, conjugated equine	S								S
Estrogens, esterified	S								S
Estropipate	S								S
Eszopiclone									S
Ethinyl estradiol									S
Ethosuximide									S
Etoposide									S
Exemestane									S
Felbamate									S
Felodipine				↓					S
FentaNYL									S
Flecainide							S		
Fluconazole					↓	↓			↓
Flunisolide									S
FLUoxetine	↓				S	↓	S, ↓		
FluPHENAZine							S		
Flurazepam									S
Flurbiprofen					↓				
Flutamide	S								S
Fluticasone									S
Fluvastatin					S, ↓				
FluvoxaMINE	S, ↓					↓	S		
Fosamprenavir (as amprenavir)									S, ↓
Fosaprepitant									S, ↓
Fosphenytoin (as phenytoin)			↑	↑	S, ↑	S, ↑			↑
Fospropofol	↓		S		S	↓			↓
Gefitinib									S
Gemfibrozil	↓			↓	↓	↓			
Glimepiride					S				
GlipiZIDE					S				
Guanabenz	S								
Haloperidol							S, ↓		S, ↓
Halothane								S	
Ibuprofen					↓				
Ifosfamide[4]		S				S			S
Imatinib							↓		S, ↓
Imipramine						S	S, ↓		
Indinavir									S, ↓
Indomethacin					↓				
Irbesartan				↓	↓				
Irinotecan			S						S
Isoflurane								S	
Isoniazid		↓				↓	↓	S, ↓	
Isosorbide dinitrate									S
Isosorbide mononitrate									S
Isradipine									S
Itraconazole									S, ↓
Ixabepilone									S
Ketamine			S		S				S
Ketoconazole	↓	↓			↓	↓	↓		S, ↓
Lansoprazole						S, ↓			S

CYP: Substrates, Inhibitors, Inducers *(continued)*

Drug	1A2	2A6	2B6	2C8	2C9	2C19	2D6	2E1	3A4
Lapatinib									S
Letrozole		↓							
Levonorgestrel									S
Lidocaine							S, ↓		S, ↓
Lomustine							S		
Lopinavir									S
Loratadine						↓			
Losartan				↓	S, ↓				S
Lovastatin									S
Maprotiline							S		
Maraviroc									S
MedroxyPROGESTERone									S
Mefenamic acid					↓				
Mefloquine									S
Mephobarbital						S			
Mestranol[5]					S				S
Methadone							↓		S
Methamphetamine							S		
Methoxsalen	↓	↓							
Methsuximide						S			
Methylergonovine									S
MethylPREDNISolone									S
Metoprolol							S		
MetroNIDAZOLE									↓
Mexiletine	S, ↓						S		
Miconazole	↓	↓			↓	↓	↓	↓	S, ↓
Midazolam									S
Mirtazapine	S						S		S
Moclobemide						S	S		
Modafinil						↓			S
Montelukast					S				S
Nafcillin									↑
Nateglinide					S				S
Nebivolol							S		
Nefazodone							S		S, ↓
Nelfinavir						S			S, ↓
Nevirapine			↑						S, ↑
NiCARdipine					↓	↓	↓		S, ↓
NIFEdipine	↓								S
Nilotinib									S
Nilutamide						S			
NiMODipine									S
Nisoldipine									S
Norethindrone									S
Norfloxacin	↓								↓
Norgestrel									S
Nortriptyline							S		
Ofloxacin	↓								
OLANZapine	S								
Omeprazole					↓	S, ↓			S
Ondansetron									S
OXcarbazepine									↑

CYP: Substrates, Inhibitors, Inducers *(continued)*

Drug	1A2	2A6	2B6	2C8	2C9	2C19	2D6	2E1	3A4
PACLitaxel				S	S				S
Pantoprazole						S, ↓			
Paricalcitol									S
PARoxetine			↓				S, ↓		
PAZOPanib									S
Pentamidine						S			
PENTobarbital		↑							↑
Perphenazine							S		
PHENobarbital	↑	↑	↑	↑	↑	S			↑
Phenytoin			↑	↑	S, ↑	S, ↑			↑
Pimozide	S								S
Pindolol							S		
Pioglitazone				S, ↓					
Piroxicam					↓				
Posaconazole									↓
Primaquine	↓								S
Primidone	↑		↑	↑	↑				↑
Procainamide							S		
Progesterone						S			S
Promethazine			S				S		
Propafenone							S		
Propofol	↓		S		S	↓			↓
Propranolol	S						S		
Protriptyline							S		
Pyrimethamine					↓				
Quazepam						S			S
QUEtiapine									S
QuiNIDine							↓		S, ↓
QuiNINE				↓	↓		↓		S
RABEprazole				↓		S, ↓			S
Ramelteon	S								
Ranolazine							↓		S
Rasagiline	S								
Repaglinide				S					S
Rifabutin									S, ↑
Rifampin	↑	↑	↑	↑	↑	↑			↑
Rifapentine				↑	↑				↑
Riluzole	S								
RisperiDONE							S		
Ritonavir				↓			S, ↓		S, ↓
ROPINIRole	S								
Ropivacaine	S								
Rosiglitazone				S, ↓					
Salmeterol									S
Saquinavir									S, ↓
Secobarbital		↑		↑	↑				
Selegiline			S						
Sertraline			↓			S, ↓	S, ↓		↓
Sevoflurane								S	
Sibutramine									S
Sildenafil									S
Simvastatin									S

CYP: Substrates, Inhibitors, Inducers *(continued)*

Drug	1A2	2A6	2B6	2C8	2C9	2C19	2D6	2E1	3A4
Sirolimus									S
Sitaxsentan					↓	↓			↓
Solifenacin									S
SORAfenib			↓	↓	↓				
Spiramycin									S
SUFentanil									S
SulfADIAZINE					S, ↓				
Sulfamethoxazole					S, ↓				
SUNItinib									S
Tacrine	S								
Tacrolimus									S
Tadalafil									S
Tamoxifen				↓	S		S		S
Tamsulosin							S		S
Telithromycin									S, ↓
Temsirolimus									S
Teniposide									S
Terbinafine							↓		
Tetracycline									S, ↓
Theophylline	S							S	S
Thiabendazole	↓								
Thioridazine							S, ↓		
Thiotepa			↓						
Thiothixene	S								
TiaGABine									S
Ticlopidine						↓	↓		S
Timolol							S		
Tinidazole									S
Tipranavir									S
TiZANidine	S								
TOLBUTamide					S, ↓				
Tolterodine							S		S
Toremifene									S
Torsemide					S				
TraMADol[1]							S		S
Tranylcypromine	↓	↓				↓	↓		
TraZODone									S
Tretinoin				S					
Triazolam									S
Trifluoperazine	S								
Trimethoprim				↓	S, ↓				S
Trimipramine						S	S		S
Vardenafil									S
Venlafaxine							S		S
Verapamil									S, ↓
VinBLAStine									S
VinCRIStine									S
Vinorelbine									S
Voriconazole					S	S			↓
Warfarin					S, ↓				

CYP: Substrates, Inhibitors, Inducers *(continued)*

Drug	1A2	2A6	2B6	2C8	2C9	2C19	2D6	2E1	3A4
Zafirlukast					S, ↓				
Zileuton	↓								
Zolpidem									S
Zonisamide									S
Zopiclone					S				S
Zuclopenthixol							S		

[1]This opioid analgesic is bioactivated *in vivo* via CYP2D6. Inhibiting this enzyme would decrease the effects of the analgesic. The active metabolite might also affect, or be affected by, CYP enzymes.

[2]Cyclophosphamide is bioactivated *in vivo* to acrolein via CYP2B6 and 3A4. Inhibiting these enzymes would decrease the effects of cyclophosphamide.

[3]Data have shown both induction (*in vivo*) and inhibition (*in vitro*) of CYP3A4.

[4]Ifosfamide is bioactivated *in vivo* to acrolein via CYP3A4. Inhibiting this enzyme would decrease the effects of ifosfamide.

[5]Mestranol is bioactivated *in vivo* to ethinyl estradiol via CYP2C8/9. See Ethinyl Estradiol for additional CYP information.

IMMUNIZATION ADMINISTRATION RECOMMENDATIONS

The following tables are taken from the General Recommendations on Immunization 2011:

- Guidelines for Spacing of Live and Inactivated Antigens
- Guidelines for Administering Antibody-Containing Products and Vaccines
- Recommended Intervals Between Administration of Antibody-Containing Products and Measles- or Varicella-Containing Vaccine, by Product and Indication for Vaccination
- Vaccination of persons with Primary and Secondary Immunodeficiencies
- Needle length and Injection Site of IM injections

Guidelines for Spacing of Live and Inactivated Antigens

Antigen Combination	Recommended Minimum Interval Between Doses
Two or more inactivated[1]	May be administered simultaneously or at any interval between doses
Inactivated and live	May be administered simultaneously or at any interval between doses
Two or more live injectable[2]	28 days minimum interval, if not administered simultaneously

[1]Certain experts suggest a 28-day interval between tetanus toxoid, reduced diphtheria toxoid, and reduced acellular pertussis (Tdap) vaccine and tetravalent meningococcal conjugate vaccine if they are not administered simultaneously.

[2]Live oral vaccines (eg, Ty21a typhoid vaccine and rotavirus vaccine) may be administered simultaneously or at any interval before or after inactivated or live injectable vaccines.

Adapted from American Academy of Pediatrics. Pertussis. Pickering LK, Baker CJ, Kimberlin DW, et al, eds. *Red Book*: 2009 Report of the Committee on Infectious Diseases. 28th ed. Elk Grove Village, IL: American Academy of Pediatrics; 2009;22.

Guidelines for Administering Antibody-Containing Products[1] and Vaccines

Simultaneous Administration (during the same office visit)

Products Administered	Recommended Minimum Interval Between Doses
Antibody-containing products and inactivated antigen	Can be administered simultaneously at different anatomic sites or at any time interval between doses.
Antibody-containing products and live antigen	Should **not** be administered simultaneously.[2] If simultaneous administration of measles-containing vaccine or varicella vaccine is unavoidable, administer at different sites and revaccinate or test for seroconversion after the recommended interval.

Nonsimultaneous Administration

Products Administered		Recommended Minimum Interval Between Doses
Administered first	**Administered second**	
Antibody-containing products	Inactivated antigen	No interval necessary
Inactivated antigen	Antibody-containing products	No interval necessary
Antibody-containing products	Live antigen	Dose-related[2,3]
Live antigen	Antibody-containing products	2 weeks[2]

[1]Blood products containing substantial amounts of immune globulin include intramuscular and intravenous immune globulin, specific hyperimmune globulin (eg, hepatitis B immune globulin, tetanus immune globulin, varicella zoster immune globulin, and rabies immune globulin), whole blood, packed red blood cells, plasma, and platelet products.

[2]Yellow fever vaccine, rotavirus vaccine, oral Ty21a typhoid vaccine, live-attenuated influenza vaccine, and zoster vaccine are exceptions to these recommendations. These live-attenuated vaccines can be administered at any time before, after, or simultaneously with an antibody-containing product.

[3]The duration of interference of antibody-containing products with the immune response to the measles component of measles-containing vaccine, and possibly varicella vaccine, is dose-related.

Recommended Intervals Between Administration of Antibody-Containing Products and Measles- or Varicella-Containing Vaccine, by Product and Indication for Vaccination

Product/Indication	Dose (mg IgG/kg) and Route[1]	Recommended Interval Before Measles- or Varicella-Containing Vaccine[2] Administration (mo)
Tetanus IG	IM: 250 units (10 mg IgG/kg)	3
Hepatitis A IG		
Contact prophylaxis	IM: 0.02 mL/kg (3.3 mg IgG/kg)	3
International travel	IM: 0.06 mL/kg (10 mg IgG/kg)	3
Hepatitis B IG	IM: 0.06 mL/kg (10 mg IgG/kg)	3
Rabies IG	IM: 20 int. units/kg (22 mg IgG/kg)	4
Varicella IG	IM: 125 units/10 kg (60 to 200 mg IgG/kg) (maximum: 625 units)	5
Measles prophylaxis IG		
Standard (ie, nonimmunocompromised) contact	IM: 0.25 mL/kg (40 mg IgG/kg)	5
Immunocompromised contact	IM: 0.50 mL/kg (80 mg IgG/kg)	6
Blood transfusion		
Red blood cells (RBCs), washed	IV: 10 mL/kg (negligible IgG/kg)	None
RBCs, adenine-saline added	IV: 10 mL/kg (10 mg IgG/kg)	3
Packed RBCs (hematocrit 65%)[3]	IV: 10 mL/kg (60 mg IgG/kg)	6
Whole blood cells (hematocrit 35% to 50%)[3]	IV: 10 mL/kg (80 to 100 mg IgG/kg)	6
Plasma/platelet products	IV: 10 mL/kg (160 mg IgG/kg)	7
Cytomegalovirus intravenous immune globulin (IGIV)	150 mg/kg maximum	6
IGIV		
Replacement therapy for immune deficiencies[4]	IV: 300 to 400 mg/kg[4]	8
Immune thrombocytopenic purpura treatment	IV: 400 mg/kg	8
Postexposure varicella prophylaxis[5]	IV: 400 mg/kg	8
Immune thrombocytopenic purpura treatment	IV: 1000 mg/kg	10
Kawasaki disease	IV: 2 g/kg	11
Monoclonal antibody to respiratory syncytial virus F protein (Synagis [Medimmune])[6]	IM: 15 mg/kg	None

HIV = human immunodeficiency virus, IG = immune globulin, IgG = immune globulin G, IGIV = intravenous immune globulin, mg IgG/kg = milligrams of immune globulin G per kilogram of body weight, IM = intramuscular, IV = intravenous, RBCs = red blood cells

[1]This table is not intended for determining the correct indications and dosages for using antibody-containing products. Unvaccinated persons might not be fully protected against measles during the entire recommended interval, and additional doses of IG or measles vaccine might be indicated after measles exposure. Concentrations of measles antibody in an IG preparation can vary by manufacturer's lot. Rates of antibody clearance after receipt of an IG preparation also might vary. Recommended intervals are extrapolated from an estimated half-life of 30 days for passively acquired antibody and an observed interference with the immune response to measles vaccine for 5 months after a dose of 80 mg IgG/kg.

[2]Does not include zoster vaccine. Zoster vaccine may be given with antibody-containing blood products.

[3]Assumes a serum IgG concentration of 16 mg/mL

[4]Measles and varicella vaccinations are recommended for children with asymptomatic or mildly symptomatic HIV infection but are contraindicated for persons with severe immunosuppression from HIV or any other immunosuppressive disorder.

[5]The investigational product VariZIG, similar to licensed varicella-zoster IG (VZIG), is a purified human IG preparation made from plasma containing high levels of anti-varicella antibodies (IgG). The interval between VariZIG and varicella vaccine (Var or MMRV) is 5 months.

[6]Contains antibody only to respiratory syncytial virus

Vaccination of Persons With Primary and Secondary Immunodeficiencies

Category	Specific Immunodeficiency	Contraindicated Vaccines[1]	Risk-Specific Recommended Vaccines[1]	Effectiveness and Comments
Primary				
B-lymphocyte (humoral)	Severe antibody deficiencies (eg, X-linked agammaglobulinemia and common variable immunodeficiency)	Oral poliovirus (OPV)[2] Smallpox Live-attenuated influenza vaccine (LAIV) BCG Ty21a (live oral typhoid) Yellow fever	Pneumococcal Consider measles and varicella vaccination	The effectiveness of any vaccine is uncertain if it depends only on the humoral response (eg, PPSV or MPSV4) IGIV interferes with the immune response to measles vaccine and possibly varicella vaccine
	Less severe antibody deficiencies (eg, selective IgA deficiency and IgG subclass deficiency)	OPV[2] BCG Yellow Fever Other live-vaccines appear to be safe	Pneumococcal	All vaccines likely effective; immune response may be attenuated
T-lymphocyte (cell-mediated and humoral)	Complete defects (eg, severe combined immunodeficiency [SCID] disease, complete DiGeorge syndrome)	All live vaccines[3,4,5]	Pneumococcal	Vaccines might be ineffective
	Partial defects (eg, most patients with DiGeorge syndrome, Wiskott-Aldrich syndrome, ataxia- telangiectasia)	All live vaccines[3,4,5]	Pneumococcal Meningococcal Hib (if not administered in infancy)	Effectiveness of any vaccine depends on degree of immune suppression
Complement	Persistent complement, properdin, or factor B deficiency	None	Pneumococcal Meningococcal	All routine vaccines likely effective
Phagocytic function	Chronic granulomatous disease, leukocyte adhesion defect, and myeloperoxidase deficiency	Live bacterial vaccines[3]	Pneumococcal[6]	All inactivated vaccines safe and likely effective; live viral vaccines likely safe and effective

Vaccination of Persons With Primary and Secondary Immunodeficiencies *continued*

Category	Specific Immunodeficiency	Contraindicated Vaccines[1]	Risk-Specific Recommended Vaccines[1]	Effectiveness and Comments
Secondary				
	HIV/AIDS	OPV[2] Smallpox BCG LAIV Withhold MMR and varicella in severely immunocompromised persons Yellow fever vaccine might have a contraindication or a precaution depending on clinical parameters of immune function[9]	Pneumococcal Consider Hib (if not administered in infancy) and meningococcal vaccination.	MMR, varicella, rotavirus, and all inactivated vaccines, including inactivated influenza, might be effective.[7]
	Malignant neoplasm, transplantation, immunosuppressive or radiation therapy	Live viral and bacterial, depending on immune status[3,4]	Pneumococcal	Effectiveness of any vaccine depends on degree of immune suppression
	Asplenia	None	Pneumococcal Meningococcal Hib (if not administered in infancy)	All routine vaccines likely effective
	Chronic renal disease	LAIV	Pneumococcal Hepatitis B[8]	All routine vaccines likely effective

AIDS = acquired immunodeficiency syndrome; BCG = bacille Calmette-Guerin; Hib = *Haemophilus influenzae* type b; HIV = human immunodeficiency virus; IG = immunoglobulin; IGIV = immune globulin intravenous; LAIV = live, attenuated influenza vaccine; MMR = measles, mumps, and rubella; MPSV4 = quadrivalent meningococcal polysaccharide vaccine; OPV = oral poliovirus vaccine (live); PPSV = pneumococcal polysaccharide vaccine; TIV = trivalent inactivated influenza vaccine

[1]Other vaccines that are universally or routinely recommended should be administered if not contraindicated.

[2]OPV is no longer available in the United States.

[3]Live bacterial vaccines: BCG and oral Ty21a *Salmonella typhi* vaccine

[4]Live viral vaccines: MMR, MMRV, OPV, LAIV, yellow fever, zoster, rotavirus, varicella, and vaccinia (smallpox). Smallpox vaccine is not recommended for children or the general public.

[5]Regarding T-lymphocyte immunodeficiency as a contraindication for rotavirus vaccine, data exist only for severe combined immunodeficiency.

[6]Pneumococcal vaccine is not indicated for children with chronic granulomatous disease beyond age-based universal recommendations for PCV. Children with chronic granulomatous disease are not at increased risk for pneumococcal disease.

[7]HIV-infected children should receive IG after exposure to measles and may receive varicella and measles vaccine if $CD4^+$ lymphocyte count is ≥15%.

[8]Indicated based on the risk from dialysis-based bloodborne transmission

[9]Symptomatic HIV infection or $CD4^+$ T-lymphocyte count of <200/mm^3 or <15% of total lymphocytes for children aged <6 years is a containdication to yellow fever vaccine administration. Asymptomatic HIV infection with $CD4^+$ T-lymphocyte count of 200 to 499/mm^3 for persons aged ≥6 years or 15% to 24% of total lymphocytes for children aged <6 years is a precaution for yellow fever vaccine administration. Details of yellow fever vaccine recommendations are available from the CDC. (CDC. Yellow fever vaccine: recommendations of the Advisory Committee on Immunization Practices [ACIP]. *MMWR Recomm Rep*. 2010;59[No. RR-7].)

Adapted from American Academy of Pediatrics. Passive immunization. Pickering LK, Baker CJ, Kimberline DW, et al, eds. *Red Book*: 2009 Report of the Committee on Infectious Diseases. 28th ed. Elk Grove Village, IL: American Academy of Pediatrics; 2009;74-75.

Needle Length and Injection Site of IM for Children Aged ≤18 years (by age) and Adults Aged ≥19 years (by sex and weight)

Age Group	Needle Length	Injection Site
Children (birth to 18 y)		
Neonates[1]	5/8" (16 mm)[2]	Anterolateral thigh
Infant 1 to 12 mo	1" (25 mm)	Anterolateral thigh
Toddler 1 to 2 y	1 to 1 1/4" (25 to 32 mm)	Anterolateral thigh[3]
	5/8[2] to 1" (16 to 25 mm)	Deltoid muscle of the arm
Children 3 to 18 y	5/8[2] to 1" (16 to 25 mm)	Deltoid muscle of the arm[3]
	1 to 1 1/4" (25 to 32 mm)	Anterolateral thigh
Adults ≥19 y		
Men and women <60 kg (130 lb)	1" (25 mm)[4]	Deltoid muscle of the arm
Men and women 60 to 70 kg (130 to 152 lb)	1" (25 mm)	
Men 70 to 118 kg (152 to 260 lb)	1 to 1 1/2" (25 to 38 mm)	
Women 70 to 90 kg (152 to 200 lb)		
Men >118 kg (260 lb)	1 1/2" (38 mm)	
Women >90 kg (200 lb)		

IM = intramuscular

[1]First 28 days of life

[2]If skin is stretched tightly and subcutaneous tissues are not bunched

[3]Preferred site

[4]Some experts recommend a 5/8" needle for men and women who weigh <60 kg.

Adapted from Poland GA, Borrud A, Jacobsen RM, et al. Determination of deltoid fat pad thickness: implications for needle length in adult immunization. *JAMA*. 1997;277:1709-1711.

RECOMMENDATIONS FOR TRAVELERS

The Centers for Disease Control and Prevention (CDC) also provides guidance to assist travelers and their health care providers in deciding the vaccines, medications, and other measures necessary to prevent illness and injury during international travel. Available at http://wwwnc.cdc.gov/travel

REFERENCE

Centers for Disease Control and Prevention (CDC). Recommendations of the Advisory Committee on Immunization Practices (ACIP): general recommendations on immunization. *MMWR Recomm Rep*. 2011;60(2):1-61.

IMMUNIZATION RECOMMENDATIONS

Recommended Immunization Schedule for Persons 0 to 18 Years of Age — United States, 2014[a]

Vaccine	Birth	1 mo	2 mos	4 mos	6 mos	9 mos	12 mos	15 mos	18 mos	19–23 mos	2–3 yrs	4–6 yrs	7–10 yrs	11–12 yrs	13–15 yrs	16–18 yrs
Hepatitis B[1] (HepB)	1st dose	2nd dose					3rd dose									
Rotavirus[2] (RV) RV-1 (2-dose series); RV-5 (3-dose series)			1st dose	2nd dose	see foot-note 2											
Diphtheria, tetanus & acellular pertussis[3] (DTaP: <7 yrs)			1st dose	2nd dose	3rd dose			4th dose				5th dose				
Tetanus & diphtheria & acellular pertussis[4] (Tdap: ≥ 7 yrs)														(Tdap)		
Haemophilus influenzae type b[5] (Hib)			1st dose	2nd dose	see foot-note 5		3rd or 4th dose, see footnote 5									
Pneumococcal conjugate[6] (PCV13)			1st dose	2nd dose	3rd dose		4th dose									
Pneumococcal polysaccharide[6] (PPSV23)																
Inactivated poliovirus[7] (IPV) (<18 years)			1st dose	2nd dose			3rd dose					4th dose				
Influenza[8] (IIV;LAIV) 2 doses for some: see footnote 8					Annual vaccination (IIV only)						Annual vaccination (IIV or LAIV)					
Measles, mumps, rubella[9] (MMR)							1st dose					2nd dose				
Varicella[10] (VAR)							1st dose					2nd dose				
Hepatitis A[11] (Hep A)							2 dose series see footnote 11									
Human papillomavirus[12] (HPV2: females only; HPV4: males and females)														(3 dose series)		
Meningococcal[13] (Hib-MenCY ≥ 6 wks; MenACWY-D ≥ 9 mos; MenACWY-CRM ≥ 2 mos.)			see footnote 13											1st dose		booster

Key	
Range of recommended ages for all children.	Range of recommended ages for catch-up immunization.
Range of recommended ages for certain high-risk groups.	Range of recommended ages during which catch-up is encouraged and for certain high-risk groups.
Not routinely recommended.	

NOTE: The recommendations in the tables must be read along with the following footnotes.

[a] This schedule includes recommendations in effect as of January 1, 2014. Any dose not administered at the recommended age should be administered at a subsequent visit, when indicated and feasible. The use of a combination vaccine generally is preferred over separate injections of its equivalent component vaccines. Vaccination providers should consult the relevant Advisory Committee on Immunization Practices (ACIP) statement for detailed recommendations, available online at http://www.cdc.gov/vaccines/hcp/acip-recs/index.html. Clinically significant adverse events that follow vaccination should be reported to the Vaccine Adverse Event Reporting System (VAERS) online (http://www.vaers.hhs.gov) or by telephone (800-822-7967).Suspected cases of vaccine-preventable diseases should be reported to the state or local health department. Additional information, including precautions and contraindications for vaccination, is available from CDC online (http://www.cdc.gov/vaccines/recs/vac-admin/contraindications.htm) or by telephone (800-CDC-INFO [800-232-4636]). This schedule is approved by the Advisory Committee on Immunization Practices (http//www.cdc.gov/vaccines/acip), the American Academy of Pediatrics (http://www.aap.org), the American Academy of Family Physicians (http://www.aafp.org), and the American College of Obstetricians and Gynecologists (http://www.acog.org).

This schedule includes recommendations in effect as of January 1, 2014. Any dose not administered at the recommended age should be administered at a subsequent visit, when indicated and feasible. The use of a combination vaccine generally is preferred over separate injections of its equivalent component vaccines. Vaccination providers should consult the relevant Advisory Committee on Immunization Practices (ACIP) statement for detailed recommendations, available at **http://www.cdc.gov/vaccines/hcp/acip-recs/index.html**. Clinically significant adverse events that follow vaccination should be reported to the Vaccine Adverse Event Reporting System (VAERS), available at http://vaers.hhs.gov/index or by telephone at **(800) 822-7967**. Also see the footnotes after the following "Catch-up Immunization Schedule" for more specific information about the vaccines.

Catch-up Immunization Schedule for Persons 4 Months to 18 Years of Age Who Start Late or Who Are >1 Month Behind – United States, 2014

This table provides catch-up schedules and minimum intervals between doses for children whose vaccinations have been delayed. A vaccine series does not need to be restarted, regardless of the time that has elapsed between doses. Use the section appropriate for the child's age. Always use this table in conjunction with the previous "Recommended immunization schedule for persons aged 0 through 18 years" and the footnotes that follow.

Vaccine	Minimum Age for Dose 1	Minimum Interval Between Doses			
		Dose 1 to Dose 2	Dose 2 to Dose 3	Dose 3 to Dose 4	Dose 4 to Dose 5
Catch-up Schedule for Persons 4 Months to 6 Years of Age					
Hepatitis B[1]	Birth	**4 weeks**	**8 weeks** and ≥16 weeks after first dose; minimum age for final dose is 24 weeks		
Rotavirus[2]	6 weeks	**4 weeks**	**4 weeks**[2]		
Diphtheria, tetanus, and acellular pertussis[3]	6 weeks	**4 weeks**	**4 weeks**	**6 months**	**6 months**[3]
Haemophilus influenzae type b[5]	6 weeks	**4 weeks** if first dose administered at <12 months of age **8 weeks** (as final dose) if first dose administered at 12 to 14 months of age **No further doses needed** if first dose administered at ≥15 months of age	**4 weeks**[5] if currently <12 months of age and first dose administered at <7 months of age **8 weeks** and 12 to 59 months of age (as final dose)[5] if currently <12 months of age and first dose administered between 7 to 11 months of age (regardless of Hib vaccine [PRP-T or PRP-OMP] used for first dose); **or** if currently 12 to 59 months of age and first dose administered at <12 months of age; **or** first 2 doses were PRP-OMP and administered at <12 months of age **No further doses needed** if previous dose administered at ≥15 months of age	**8 weeks** (as final dose) This dose only necessary for children 12 to 59 months of age who received 3 (PRP-T) doses before 12 months of age and started primary series before 7 months of age	
Pneumococcal[6]	6 weeks	**4 weeks** if first dose administered at <12 months of age **8 weeks** (as final dose for healthy children) if first dose administered at ≥12 months of age **No further doses needed** for healthy children if first dose administered at ≥24 months of age	**4 weeks** if currently <12 months of age **8 weeks** (as final dose for healthy children) if currently ≥12 months of age **No further doses needed** for healthy children if previous dose administered at ≥24 months of age	**8 weeks** (as final dose) This dose only necessary for children 12 to 59 months of age who received 3 doses before 12 months of age or for children at high risk who received 3 doses at any age	
Inactivated poliovirus[7]	6 weeks	**4 weeks**[7]	**4 weeks**[7]	**6 months**[7] minimum 4 years of age for final dose	
Meningococcal[13]	6 weeks	**8 weeks**[13]	See footnote 13	See footnote 13	
Measles, mumps, rubella[9]	12 months	**4 weeks**			
Varicella[10]	12 months	**3 months**			
Hepatitits A[11]	12 months	**6 months**			

Vaccine	Minimum Age for Dose 1	Minimum Interval Between Doses			
		Dose 1 to Dose 2	**Dose 2 to Dose 3**	**Dose 3 to Dose 4**	**Dose 4 to Dose 5**
Catch-up Schedule for Persons 7 to 18 Years of Age					
Tetanus, diphtheria; tetanus, diphtheria, and acellular pertussis[4]	7 years[4]	**4 weeks**	**4 weeks** if first dose of DTaP/DT administered at <12 months of age **6 months** if first dose of DTaP/DT administered at ≥12 months of age and then no further doses needed for catch-up	**6 months** if first dose of DTaP/DT administered at <12 months of age	
Human papillomavirus[12]	9 years	Routine dosing intervals are recommended[12]			
Hepatitis A[11]	12 months	**6 months**			
Hepatitis B[1]	Birth	**4 weeks**	**8 weeks** (and ≥16 weeks after first dose)		
Inactivated poliovirus[7]	6 weeks	**4 weeks**	**4 weeks**[7]	**6 months**[7]	
Meningococcal[13]	6 weeks	**8 weeks**[13]			
Measles, mumps, rubella[9]	12 months	**4 weeks**			
Varicella[10]	12 months	**3 months** if person is <13 years of age **4 weeks** if person is ≥13 years of age			

Footnotes to Recommended Immunization Schedule for Persons 0 to 18 Years of Age and the Catch-up Immunization Schedule

Note: For further guidance on the use of the vaccines mentioned below, see http://www.cdc.gov/vaccines/hcp/acip-recs/index.html. For vaccine recommendations for persons ≥19 years of age, see the adult immunization schedule.

[1]**Hepatitis B vaccine (HepB)** *(Minimum age: Birth)*

Routine vaccination:

At birth:

- Administer monovalent HepB vaccine to all newborns before hospital discharge.
- For infants born to hepatitis B surface antigen (HBsAg)-positive mothers, administer HepB vaccine and 0.5 mL of hepatitis B immune globulin (HBIG) within 12 hours of birth. These infants should be tested for HBsAg and antibody to HBsAg (anti-HBs) 1 to 2 months after completion of the HepB series at 9 to 18 months of age (preferably at the next well-child visit).
- If the mother's HBsAg status is unknown, within 12 hours of birth, administer HepB vaccine to all infants regardless of birth weight. For infants weighing <2,000 grams, administer HBIG in addition to HepB vaccine within 12 hours of birth. Determine the mother's HBsAg status as soon as possible and, if she is HBsAg-positive, also administer HBIG for infants weighing ≥2,000 grams as soon as possible but no later than 7 days of age.

Doses following the birth dose:

- The second dose should be administered at 1 or 2 months of age. Monovalent HepB vaccine should be used for doses administered before 6 weeks of age.
- Infants who did not receive a birth dose should receive 3 doses of a HepB-containing vaccine on a schedule of 0, 1 to 2 months, and 6 months of age starting as soon as feasible. See the previous "Catch-up Immunization Schedule".
- Administer the second dose 1 to 2 months after the first dose (minimum interval of 4 weeks); administer the third dose at least 8 weeks after the second dose **and** at least 16 weeks after the **first** dose. The final (third of fourth) dose in the HepB vaccine series should be administered **no earlier than 24 weeks of age**.
- Administration of a total of 4 doses of HepB vaccine is permitted when a combination vaccine containing HepB is administered after the birth dose.

Catch-up vaccination:

- Unvaccinated persons should complete a 3-dose series.
- A 2-dose series (doses separated by at least 4 months) of adult formulation Recombivax HB is licensed for use in children 11 to 15 years of age.
- For other catch-up guidance, see the previous "Catch-up Immunization Schedule".

[2]**Rotavirus vaccine (RV)** *(Minimum age: 6 weeks for both RV-1 [Rotarix] and RV-5 [RotaTeq])*

Routine vaccination:

- Administer a series of RV vaccine to all infants as follows:
  - If Rotarix is used, administer a 2-dose series at 2 and 4 months of age.
  - If RotaTeq is used, administer a 3-dose series at ages 2, 4, and 6 months of age.
  - If any dose in the series was RotaTeq or vaccine product is unknown for any dose in the series, a total of 3 doses of RV vaccine should be administered.

Catch-up vaccination:

- The maximum age for the first dose in the series is 14 weeks, 6 days; vaccination should not be initiated for infants ≥15 weeks, 0 days of age.
- The maximum age for the final dose in the series is 8 months, 0 days.
- For other catch-up guidance, see the previous "Catch-up Immunization Schedule".

[3]**Diphtheria and tetanus toxoids and acellular pertussis vaccine (DTaP)** *(Minimum age: 6 weeks; exception: DTaP-IPV [Kinrix]: 4 years)*

Routine vaccination:

- Administer a 5-dose series of DTaP vaccine at 2, 4, 6, and 15 to 18 months of age, and at 4 to 6 years of age. The fourth dose may be administered as early as 12 months of age, provided at least 6 months have elapsed since the third dose.

Catch-up vaccination:

- The fifth dose of DTaP vaccine is not necessary if the fourth dose was administered at ≥4 years of age.
- For other catch-up guidance, see the previous "Catch-up Immunization Schedule".

[4]**Tetanus and diphtheria toxoids and acellular pertussis vaccine (Tdap)** *(Minimum age: 10 years for Adacel and Boostrix)*

Routine vaccination:

- Administer 1 dose of Tdap vaccine to all adolescents 11 to 12 years of age.
- Tdap can be administered regardless of the interval since the last tetanus and diphtheria toxoid-containing vaccine.
- Administer 1 dose of Tdap vaccine to pregnant adolescents during each pregnancy (preferred during 27 to 36 weeks gestation), regardless of time since prior Td or Tdap vaccination.

Catch-up vaccination:

- Persons ≥7 years of age who are not fully immunized with DTaP vaccine series should receive Tdap vaccine as 1 (preferably the first) dose in the catch-up series; if additional doses are needed, use Td vaccine. For children 7 to 10 years of age who receive a dose of Tdap as part of the catch-up series, an adolescent Tdap vaccine dose at 11 to 12 years of age should **not** be administered. Td should be administered instead 10 years after the Tdap dose.
- Persons 11 to 18 years of age who have not received Tdap vaccine should receive a dose, followed by tetanus and diphtheria toxoids (Td) booster doses every 10 years thereafter.
- Inadvertent doses of DTaP vaccine:
  - If administered inadvertently to a child 7 to 10 years of age, may count as part of the catch-up series. This dose can count as the adolescent Tdap dose or the child can later receive a Tdap booster dose at 11 to 12 years of age.
  - If administered inadvertently to an adolescent 11 to 18 years of age, the dose should be counted as the adolescent Tdap booster.
- For other catch-up guidance, see the previous "Catch-up Immunization Schedule".

[5]***Haemophilus influenzae* type b conjugate vaccine (Hib)** *(Minimum age: 6 weeks for PRP-T [ActHIB, DTaP-IPV/Hib (Pentacel), and Hib-MenCY (MenHibrix)], PRP-OMP [PedvaxHIB or COMVAX], 12 months for PRP-T [Hiberix])*

Routine vaccination:

- Administer a 2- or 3-dose Hib vaccine primary series and a booster dose (dose 3 or 4 depending on vaccine used in primary series) at 12 to 15 months of age to complete a full Hib vaccine series.
- The primary series with ActHIB, MenHibrix, or Pentacel consists of 3 doses and should be administered at 2, 4, and 6 months of age. The primary series with PedvaxHib or COMVAX consists of 2 doses and should be administered at 2 and 4 months of age; a dose at 6 months of age is not indicated.
- One booster dose (dose 3 or 4 depending on vaccine used in primary series) of any Hib vaccine should be administered at 12 to 15 months of age. An exception is Hiberix vaccine. Hiberix should only be used for the booster (final) dose in children 12 months to 4 years of age who have received at least 1 prior dose of Hib-containing vaccine.
- For recommendations on the use of MenHibrix in patients at increased risk for meningococcal disease, please refer to the meningococcal vaccine footnotes and also to *MMWR*. 2013;62(RR02);1-22. Available at http://www.cdc.gov/mmwr/pdf/rr/rr6202.pdf.

Catch-up vaccination:

- If dose 1 was administered at 12 to 14 months of age, administer a second (final) dose at least 8 weeks after dose 1, regardless of Hib vaccine used in the primary series.
- If the first 2 doses were PRP-OMP (PedvaxHIB or COMVAX) and were administered at ≤11 months of age, the third (and final) dose should be administered at 12 to 15 months of age and at least 8 weeks after the second dose.
- If the first dose was administered at 7 to 11 months of age, administer the second dose at least 4 weeks later and a third (and final) dose at 12 to 15 months of age or 8 weeks after the second dose, whichever is later, regardless of Hib vaccine used for the first dose.
- If the first dose is administered at <12 months of age and the second dose is given between 12 to 14 months of age, a third (and final) dose should be given 8 weeks later.
- For unvaccinated children ≥15 months of age, administer only 1 dose.
- For other catch-up guidance, see the previous "Catch-up Immunization Schedule". For catch-up guidance related to MenHibrix, please see the meningococcal vaccine footnotes and also *MMWR*. 2013;62(RR02);1-22. Available at http://www.cdc.gov/mmwr/pdf/rr/rr6202.pdf.

Vaccination of persons with high-risk conditions:

- Children 12 to 59 months of age who are at increased risk for Hib disease, including chemotherapy recipients and whose with anatomic or functional asplenia (including sickle cell disease), human immunodeficiency virus (HIV) infection, immunoglobulin deficiency, or early component complement deficiency, who have received either no doses or only 1 dose of Hib vaccine before 12 months of age, should receive 2 additional doses of Hib vaccine 8 weeks apart; children who received ≥2 doses of Hib vaccine before 12 months of age should receive 1 additional dose.
- For patients <5 years of age undergoing chemotherapy or radiation treatment who received a Hib vaccine dose(s) within 14 days of starting therapy or during therapy, repeat the dose(s) at least 3 months following therapy completion.
- Recipients of hematopoietic stem cell transplant (HSCT) should be revaccinated with a 3-dose regimen of Hib vaccine starting 6 to 12 months after successful transplant, regardless of vaccination history; doses should be administered at elast 4 weeks apart.
- A single dose of any Hib-containing vaccine should be administered to unimmunized* children and adolescents ≥15 months of age undergoing an elective splenectomy; if possible, vaccine should be administered at least 14 days before the procedure.
- Hib vaccine is not routinely recommended for patients ≥5 years of age. However, 1 dose of Hib vaccine should be administered to unimmunized* persons ≥5 years of age who have anatomic or functional asplenia (including sickle cell disease) and unvaccinated persons 5 to 18 years of age with human immunodeficiency virus (HIV) infection.

*Patients who have not received a primary series and booster dose or at least 1 dose of Hib vaccine after 14 months of age are considered unimmunized.

[6]**Pneumococcal vaccines** *(Minimum age: 6 weeks for PCV13, 2 years for PPSV23)*

Routine vaccination with PCV13:

- Administer a 4-dose series of PCV13 vaccine at 2, 4, 6, and 12 to 15 months of age.
- For children 14 to 59 months of age who have received an age-appropriate series of 7-valent PCV (PCV7), administer a single supplemental dose of 13-valent PCV (PCV13).

Catch-up vaccination with PCV13:

- Administer 1 dose of PCV13 to all healthy children 24 to 59 months of age who are not completely vaccinated for their age.
- For other catch-up guidance, see the previous "Catch-up Immunization Schedule".

Vaccination of persons with high-risk conditions with PCV13 and PPSV23:

- All recommended PCV13 doses should be administered prior to PPSV23 vaccination if possible.
- For children 2 to 5 years of age with any of the following conditions: Chronic heart disease (particularly cyanotic congenital heart disease and cardiac failure); chronic lung disease (including asthma if treated with high-dose oral corticosteroid therapy); diabetes mellitus; cerebrospinal fluid leak; cochlear implant; sickle cell disease and other hemoglobuinopathies; anatomic or functional asplenia; HIV infection; chronic renal failure; nephrotic syndrome; diseases associated with treatment with immunosuppressive drugs or radiation therapy, including malignant neoplasms, leukemias, lymphomas, and Hodgkin disease; solid organ transplantation; or congenital immunodeficiency:
    1. Administer 1 dose of PCV13 if 3 doses of PCV (PCV7 and/or PCV13) were received previously.
    2. Administer 2 doses of PCV13 at least 8 weeks apart if fewer than 3 doses of PCV (PCV7 and/or PCV13) were received previously.
    3. Administer 1 supplemental dose of PCV13 if 4 doses of PCV7 or other age-appropriate complete PCV7 series was received previously.
    4. The minimum interval between doses of PCV (PCV7 or PCV13) is 8 weeks.
    5. For children with no history of PPSV23 vaccination, administer PPSV23 at least 8 weeks after the most recent dose of PCV13.
- For children 6 to 18 years of age who have cerebrospinal fluid leak; cochlear implant; sickle cell disease and other hemoglobinopathies; anatomic or functional asplenia; congenital or acquired immunodeficiencies; HIV infection; chronic renal failure; nephrotic syndrome; diseases associated with treatment with immunosuppressive drugs or radiation therapy, including malignant neoplasms, leukemias, lymphomas, and Hodgkin disease; generalized malignancy; solid organ transplantation; or multiple myeloma:
    1. If neither PCV13 nor PPSV23 has been received previously, administer 1 dose of PCV13 now and 1 dose of PPSV23 at least 8 weeks later.
    2. If PCV13 has been received previously but PPSV23 has not, administer 1 dose of PPSV23 at least 8 weeks after the most recent dose of PCV13.
    3. If PPSV23 has been received but PCV13 has not, administer 1 dose of PCV13 at least 8 weeks after the most recent dose of PPSV23.
- For children 6 to 18 years of age with chronic heart disease (particularly cyanotic congenital heart disease and cardiac failure), chronic lung disease (including asthma if treated with high-dose oral corticosteroid therapy), diabetes mellitus, alcoholism, or chronic liver disease, who have not received PPSV23, administer 1 dose of PPSV23. If PCV13 has been received previously, then PPSV23 should be administered at least 8 weeks after any prior PCV13 dose.
- A single revaccination with PPSV23 should be administered 5 years after the first dose to children with sickle cell disease or other hemoglobinopathies; anatomic or functional asplenia; congenital or acquired immunodeficiencies; HIV infection; chronic renal failure; nephrotic syndrome; diseases associated with treatment with immunosuppressive drugs or radiation therapy, including malignant neoplasms, leukemias, lymphomas, and Hodgkin disease; generalized malignancy; solid organ transplantation; or multiple myeloma.

[7]**Inactivated poliovirus vaccine (IPV)** *(Minimum age: 6 weeks)*

Routine vaccination:

- Administer a 4-dose series of IPV at 2, 4, and 6 to 18 months of age and at 4 to 6 years of age. The final dose in the series should be administered on or after the fourth birthday and at least 6 months after the previous dose.

Catch-up vaccination:

- In the first 6 months of life, minimum age and minimum intervals are only recommended if the person is at risk for imminent exposure to circulating poliovirus (ie, travel to a polio-endemic region or during an outbreak).
- If ≥4 doses are administered before 4 years of age, an additional dose should be administered at 4 to 6 years of age and at least 6 months after the previous dose.
- A fourth dose is not necessary if the third dose was administered at ≥4 years of age and at least 6 months after the previous dose.
- If both OPV and IPV were administered as part of a series, a total of 4 doses should be administered, regardless of the child's current age. IPV is not routinely recommended for U.S. residents ≥18 years of age.
- For other catch-up guidance, see the previous "Catch-up Immunization Schedule".

[8]**Influenza vaccines** *(Minimum age: 6 months for inactivated influenza vaccine [IIV]; 2 years for live, attenuated influenza vaccine [LAIV])*

Routine vaccination:

- Administer influenza vaccine annually to all children beginning at 6 months of age. For most healthy, nonpregnant persons 2 to 49 years of age, either LAIV or IIV may be used. However, LAIV should **not** be administered to some persons, including 1) those with asthma, 2) children 2 to 4 years of age who had wheezing in the past 12 months, or 3) those who have any other underlying medical conditions that predispose them to influenza complications. For all other contraindications to use of LAIV, see *MMWR*. 2013;62(No. RR-7);1-43. Available at http://www.cdc.gov/mmwr/pdf/rr/rr6207.pdf.

For children 6 months to 8 years of age:

- For the 2013 to 2014 season, administer 2 doses (separated by at least 4 weeks) to children who are receiving influenza vaccine for the first time. Some children in this age group who have been vaccinated previously will also need 2 doses. For additional guidance, follow dosing guidelines in the 2013 to 2014 ACIP influenza vaccine recommendations. See *MMWR*. 2013;62(No. RR-7);1-43. Available at http://www.cdc.gov/mmwr/pdf/rr/rr6207.pdf.
- For the 2014 to 2015 season, follow dosing guidelines in the 2014 ACIP influenza vaccine recommendations.

For persons ≥9 years of age:

- Administer 1 dose.

[9]**Measles, mumps, and rubella vaccine (MMR)** *(Minimum age: 12 months for routine vaccination)*

Routine vaccination:

- Administer a 2-dose series of MMR vaccine at 12 to 15 months of age and 4 to 6 years of age. The second dose may be administered before 4 years of age, provided at least 4 weeks have elapsed since the first dose.
- Administer 1 dose of MMR vaccine to infants 6 to 11 months of age before departure from the United States for international travel. These children should be revaccinated with 2 doses of MMR vaccine, the first at 12 to 15 months of age (12 months if the child remains in an area where disease risk is high) and the second dose at least 4 weeks later.
- Administer 2 doses of MMR vaccine to children ≥12 months of age before departure from the United States for international travel. The first dose should be administered at ≥12 months of age and the second dose at least 4 weeks later.

Catch-up vaccination:

- Ensure that all school-aged children and adolescents have had 2 doses of MMR vaccine; the minimum interval between the 2 doses is 4 weeks.
- For other catch-up guidance, see the previous "Catch-up Immunization Schedule".

[10]**Varicella vaccine (VAR)** *(Minimum age: 12 months)*

Routine vaccination:

- Administer a 2-dose series of VAR vaccine at 12 to 15 months of age and 4 to 6 years of age. The second dose may be administered before 4 years of age, provided at least 3 months have elapsed since the first dose. If the second dose was administered at least 4 weeks after the first dose, it can be accepted as valid.

Catch-up vaccination:

- Ensure that all persons 7 to 18 years of age without evidence of immunity (see *MMWR*. 2007;56[No. RR-4]. Available at http://www.cdc.gov/mmwr/pdf/rr/rr5604.pdf) have 2 doses of varicella vaccine. For children 7 to 12 years of age, the recommended minimum interval between doses is 3 months (if the second dose was administered at least 4 weeks after the first dose, it can be accepted as valid); for persons ≥13 years of age, the minimum interval between doses is 4 weeks.
- For other catch-up guidance, see the previous "Catch-up Immunization Schedule".

[11]**Hepatitis A vaccine (HepA)** *(Minimum age: 12 months)*

Routine vaccination:

- Initiate the 2-dose HepA vaccine series at 12 to 23 months of age; separate the 2 doses by 6 to 18 months.
- Children who have received 1 dose of HepA vaccine before 24 months of age should receive a second dose 6 to 18 months after the first dose.
- For any person ≥2 years of age who has not already received the HepA vaccine series, 2 doses of HepA vaccine separated by 6 to 18 months may be administered if immunity against hepatitis A virus infection is desired.

Catch-up vaccination:

- The minimum interval between the 2 doses is 6 months.
- For other catch-up guidance, see the previous "Catch-up Immunization Schedule".

Special populations:

- Administer 2 doses of HepA vaccine at least 6 months apart to previously unvaccinated persons who live in areas where vaccination programs target older children or who are at increased risk for infection. This includes persons traveling to or working in countries that have high or intermediate endemicity of infection; men having sex with men; users of injection and noninjection illicit drugs; persons who work with HAV-infected primates or with HAV in a research laboratory; persons with clotting-factor disorders; persons with chronic liver disease; and persons who anticipate close, personal contact (eg, household or regular babysitting) with an international adoptee during the first 60 days after arrival in the United States from a country with high or intermediate endemicity. The first dose should be administered as soon as the adoption is planned, ideally ≥2 weeks before the arrival of the adoptee.

[12]**Human papillomavirus vaccines (HPV)** *(Minimum age: 9 years for HPV2 [Cervarix] and HPV4 [Gardasil])*

Routine vaccination:

- Administer a 3-dose series of HPV vaccine on a schedule of 0, 1 to 2, and 6 months to all adolescents 11 to 12 years of age. Either HPV4 or HPV2 may be used for females and only HPV4 may be used for males.
- The vaccine series can be started beginning at 9 years of age.
- Administer the second dose 1 to 2 months after the first dose (minimum interval of 4 weeks) and administer the third dose 24 weeks after the first dose and 16 weeks after the second dose (minimum interval of 12 weeks).

Catch-up vaccination:

- Administer the vaccine series to females (either HPV2 or HPV4) and males (HPV4) at 13 to 18 years of age if not previously vaccinated.
- Use recommended routine dosing intervals (see above) for vaccine series catch-up.
- For other catch-up guidance, see the previous "Catch-up Immunization Schedule".

[13]**Meningococcal conjugate vaccines (MCV)** *(Minimum age: 6 weeks for Hib-MenCY [MenHibrix], 9 months for MenACWY-D [Menactra], 2 months for MenACWY-CRM [Menveo])*

Routine vaccination:

- Administer a single dose of Menactra or Menveo vaccine at 11 to 12 years of age with a booster dose at 16 years of age.
- Adolescents 11 to 18 years of age with human immunodeficiency virus (HIV) infection should receive a 2-dose primary series of Menactra or Menveo with at least 8 weeks between doses.
- For children 2 months to 18 years of age with high-risk conditions, see below.

Catch-up vaccination:

- Administer Menactra or Menveo vaccine at 13 to 18 years of age if not previously vaccinated.
- If the first dose is administered at 13 to 15 years of age, a booster dose should be administered at 16 to 18 years of age with a minimum interval of at least 8 weeks between doses.
- If the first dose is administered at ≥16 years of age, a booster dose is not needed.
- For other catch-up guidance, see the previous "Catch-up Immunization Schedule".

Vaccination of persons with high-risk conditions and other persons at increased risk of disease:

- Children with anatomic or functional asplenia (including sickle cell disease):
  1. For children <19 months of age, administer a 4-dose infant series of MenHibrix or Menveo at 2, 4, 6, and 12 to 15 months of age.
  2. For children 19 to 23 months of age who have not completed a series of MenHibrix or Menveo, administer 2 primary doses of Menveo at least 3 months apart.
  3. For children ≥24 months of age who have not received a complete series of MenHibrix, Menveo, or Menactra, administer 2 primary doses of either Menactra or Menveo at least 2 months apart. If Menactra is administered to a child with asplenia (including sickle cell disease), do not administer Menactra until 2 years of age and at least 4 weeks after the completion of all PCV13 doses.
- Children with persistent complement component deficiency:
  1. For children <19 months of age, administer a 4-dose infant series of either MenHibrix or Menveo at 2, 4, 6, and 12 to 15 months of age.
  2. For children 7 to 23 months of age who have not initiated vaccination, two options exist depending on age and vaccine brand:
     a. For children who initiate vaccination with Menveo at 7 to 23 months of age, a 2-dose series should be administered with the second dose after 12 months of age and at least 3 months after the first dose.
     b. For children who initiate vaccination with Menactra at 9 to 23 months of age, a 2-dose series of Menactra should be administered at least 3 months apart.
     c. For children ≥24 months of age who have not received a complete series of MenHibrix, Menveo, or Menactra, administer 2 primary doses of either Menactra or Menveo at least 2 months apart.
- For children who travel to or reside in countries in which meningoccoal disease is hyperendemic or epidemic, including countries in the African meningitis belt or the Hajj, administer an age-appropriate formulation and series of Menactra or Menveo for protection against serogroups A and W meningococcal disease. Prior receipt of MenHibrix is not sufficient for children traveling to the meningitis belt or the Hajj because it does not contain serogroups A or W.
- For children at risk during a community outbreak attributable to a vaccine serogroup, administer or complete an age- and formulation-appropriate series of MenHibrix, Menactra, or Menveo.
- For booster doses among persons with high-risk conditions, refer to: *MMWR*. 2013;62(RR02);1-22. Available at http://www.cdc.gov/mmwr/preview/mmwrhtml/rr6202a1.htm.

Catch-up recommendations for persons with high-risk conditions:

1. If MenHibrix is administered to achieve protection against meningococcal disease, a complete age-appropriate series of MenHibrix should be administered.
2. If the first dose of MenHibrix is given at or after 12 months of age, a total of 2 doses should be given at least 8 weeks apart to ensure protection against serogroups C and Y meningococcal disease.
3. For children who initiate vaccination with Menveo at 7 to 9 months of age, a 2-dose series should be administered with the second dose after 12 months of age and at least 3 months after the first dose.
4. For other catch-up recommendations for these persons, refer to: *MMWR*. 2013;62(RR02);1-22. Available at http://www.cdc.gov/mmwr/preview/mmwrhtml/rr6202a1.htm.

For complete information on the use of meningococcal vaccines, including guidance related to vaccination of persons at increased risk of infection, see: *MMWR*. 2013;62(RR02);1-22. Available at http://www.cdc.gov/mmwr/preview/mmwrhtml/rr6202a1.htm

This schedule is approved by the Advisory Committee on Immunization Practices (**http://www.cdc.gov/vaccines/acip/index.html**), the American Academy of Pediatrics (**http://www.aap.org**), the American Academy of Family Physicians (**http://www.aafp.org**), and the American College of Obstetricians and Gynecologists (**http://www.acog.org**).

REFERENCE

Centers for Disease Control and Prevention (CDC). Advisory Committee on Immunization Practices (ACIP) recommended immunization schedules for persons aged 0 through 18 years and adults aged 19 years and older – United States, 2014. Available at http://www.cdc.gov/vaccines/schedules/hcp/child-adolescent.html

Recommended Adult Immunization Schedule by Vaccine and Age Group[1] — United States, 2014

Vaccine	Age group: 19 to 21 years	22 to 26 years	27 to 49 years	50 to 59 years	60 to 64 years	≥ 65 years
Influenza[2,*]	1 dose annually					
Tetanus, diphtheria, pertussis (Td/Tdap)[3,*]	Substitute 1-time dose of Tdap for Td booster; then boost with Td every 10 y					
Varicella[4,*]	2 doses					
Human papillomavirus (HPV) female[5,*]	3 doses					
Human papillomavirus (HPV) male[5,*]	3 doses	3 doses				
Zoster[6]					1 dose	
Measles, mumps, rubella (MMR)[7,*]	1 or 2 doses					
Pneumococcal 13-valent conjugate (PCV13)[8,*]	1 dose					
Pneumococcal polysaccharide (PPSV23)[9,10]	1 or 2 doses					1 dose
Meningococcal[11,*]	1 or more doses					
Hepatitis A[12,*]	2 doses					
Hepatitis B[13,*]	3 doses					
Haemophilus influenzae type b (Hib)[14,*]	1 or 3 doses					

*Covered by the Vaccine Injury Compensation Program.

For all persons in this category who meet the age requirements and who lack documentation of vaccination or have no evidence of previous infection; zoster vaccine reccommended regardless of prior episode of zoster.

Recommended if some other risk factor is present (eg, on the basis of medical, occupational, lifestyle, or other indication).

No recommendation.

NOTE: The recommendations in the tables must be read along with the following footnotes.

Vaccines That Might Be Indicated for Adults Based on Medical and Other Indications[1]

Vaccine	Pregnancy	Immunocompromising conditions (excluding human immunodeficiency virus [HIV])[4,6,7,8,15]	HIV infection CD4+ T lymphocyte count[4,6,7,8,15]: < 200 cells/μL	HIV infection CD4+ T lymphocyte count: ≥ 200 cells/μL	Men who have sex with men (MSM)	Kidney failure, end-stage renal disease, receipt of hemodialysis	Heart disease, chronic lung disease, chronic alcoholism	Asplenia (including elective splenectomy and persistent complement component deficiencies)[8,14]	Chronic liver disease	Diabetes	Healthcare personnel
Influenza[2,*]	1 dose IIV annually				1 dose IIV or LAIV annually	1 dose IIV annually					1 dose IIV or LAIV annually
Tetanus, diphtheria, pertussis (Td/Tdap)[3,*]	1 dose Tdap each pregnancy	Substitute 1-time dose of Tdap for Td booster; then boost with Td every 10 years									
Varicella[4,*]	Contraindicated			2 doses							
Human papillomavirus (HPV) female[5,*]		3 doses through age 26 yrs				3 doses through age 26 yrs					
Human papillomavirus (HPV) male[5,*]		3 doses through age 26 yrs				3 doses through age 21 yrs					
Zoster[6]	Contraindicated				1 dose						
Measles, mumps, rubella (MMR)[7,*]	Contraindicated			1 or 2 doses							
Pneumococcal 13-valent conjugate (PCV13)[8]						1 dose	1 dose				
Pneumococcal polysaccharide (PPSV23)[9,10]						1 or 2 doses					
Meningococcal[11,*]	1 or more doses										
Hepatitis A[12,*]	2 doses										
Hepatitis B[13,*]	3 doses										
Haemophilus influenzae type b (Hib)[14,*]		post-HSCT recipients only	1 or 3 doses								

*Covered by the Vaccine Injury Compensation Program.

For all persons in this category who meet the age requirements and who lack documentation of vaccination or have no evidence of previous infection; zoster vaccine reccommended regardless of prior episode of zoster.

Recommended if some other risk factor is present (eg, on the basis of medical, occupational, lifestyle, or other indication).

No recommendation.

NOTE: The recommendations in the tables must be read along with the following footnotes.

Footnotes to Recommended Adult Immunization Schedule

[1]Additional information

- Additional guidance for the use of the vaccines described in this supplement is available at http://www.cdc.gov/vaccines/hcp/acip-recs/.
- Information on vaccination recommendations when vaccination status is unknown and other general immunization information can be found in the General Recommendations on Immunization at http://www.cdc.gov/mmwr/preview/mmwrhtml/rr6002a1.htm.
- Information on travel vaccine requirements and recommendations (eg, for hepatitis A and B, meningococcal, other vaccines) is available at http://wwwnc.cdc.gov/travel/destinations/list.
- Additional information and resources regarding vaccination of pregnant women can be found at http://www.cdc.gov/vaccines/adults/rec-vac/pregnant.html.

[2]Influenza vaccine

- Annual vaccination against influenza is recommended for all persons ≥6 months of age.
- Persons ≥6 months of age, including pregnant women and persons with hives-only allergy to eggs, can receive the inactivated influenza vaccine (IIV). An age-appropriate IIV formulation should be used.
- Adults 18 to 49 years of age can receive the recombinant influenza vaccine (RIV) (FluBlok). RIV does not contain any egg protein.
- Healthy, nonpregnant persons 2 to 49 years of age without high-risk medical conditions can receive either intranasally administered live, attenuated influenza vaccine (LAIV) (FluMist) or IIV. Health care personnel who care for severely immunocompromised persons (ie, those who require care in a protected environment) should receive IIV or RIV, rather than LAIV.
- The intramuscularly or intradermally administered IIV are options for adults 18 to 64 years of age.
- Adults ≥65 years of age can receive the standard-dose IIV or the high-dose IIV (Fluzone High-Dose).

[3]Tetanus, diphtheria, and acellular pertussis vaccine (Td/Tdap)

- Administer 1 dose of Tdap vaccine to pregnant women during each pregnancy (preferred during 27 to 36 weeks' gestation), regardless of interval since prior Td or Tdap vaccination.
- Persons ≥11 years of age who have not received Tdap vaccine or for whom vaccine status is unknown should receive a dose of Tdap, followed by tetanus and diphtheria toxoids (Td) booster doses every 10 years thereafter. Tdap can be administered regardless of interval since the most recent tetanus or diphtheria-toxoid-containing vaccine.
- Adults with an unknown or incomplete history of completing a 3-dose primary vaccination series with Td-containing vaccines should begin or complete a primary vaccination series, including a Tdap dose.
- For unvaccinated adults, administer the first 2 doses at least 4 weeks apart and the third dose 6 to 12 months after the second.
- For incompletely vaccinated adults (ie, <3 doses), administer remaining doses.
- Refer to the ACIP statement for recommendations for administering Td/Tdap as prophylaxis in wound management (see footnote 1).

[4]Varicella vaccine

- All adults without evidence of immunity to varicella (as defined below) should receive 2 doses of single-antigen varicella vaccine or a second dose if they have received only 1 dose.
- Vaccination should be emphasized for those who have close contact with persons at high risk for severe disease (eg, health care personnel and family contacts of persons with immunocompromising conditions) or who are at high risk for exposure or transmission (eg, teachers; child care employees; residents and staff members of institutional settings, including correctional institutions; college students; military personnel; adolescents and adults living in households with children; nonpregnant women of childbearing age; international travelers).
- Pregnant women should be assessed for evidence of varicella immunity. Women who do not have evidence of immunity should receive the first dose of varicella vaccine upon completion or termination of pregnancy and before discharge from the health care facility. The second dose should be administered 4 to 8 weeks after the first dose.
- Evidence of immunity to varicella in adults includes any of the following:
  - Documentation of 2 doses of varicella vaccine at least 4 weeks apart
  - U.S.-born before 1980, except health care personnel and pregnant women
  - History of varicella based on diagnosis or verification of varicella disease by a health care provider
  - History of herpes zoster based on diagnosis or verification of herpes zoster disease by a health care provider, or
  - Laboratory evidence of immunity or laboratory confirmation of disease

[5]Human papillomavirus vaccine (HPV)

- Two vaccines are licensed for use in females, bivalent HPV vaccine (HPV2) and quadrivalent HPV vaccine (HPV4), and one HPV vaccine for use in males, HPV4.
- For females, either HPV4 or HPV2 is recommended in a 3-dose series for routine vaccination at 11 or 12 years of age, and for those 13 to 26 years of age, if not previously vaccinated.
- For males, HPV4 is recommended in a 3-dose series for routine vaccination at 11 or 12 years of age, and for those 13 to 21 years of age, if not previously vaccinated. Males 22 to 26 years of age may be vaccinated.
- HPV4 is recommended for men who have sex with men through 26 years of age for those who did not get any or all doses when they were younger.
- Vaccination is recommended for immunocompromised persons (including those with HIV infection) through 26 years of age for those who did not get any or all doses when they were younger.
- A complete series for either HPV4 or HPV2 consists of 3 doses. The second dose should be administered 4 to 8 weeks (minimum interval of 4 weeks) after the first dose; the third dose should be administered 24 weeks after the first dose and 16 weeks after the second dose (minimum interval of at least 12 weeks).
- HPV vaccines are not recommended for use in pregnant women. However, pregnancy testing is not needed before vaccination. If a woman is found to be pregnant after initiating the vaccination series, no intervention is needed; the remainder of the 3-dose series should be delayed until completion of pregnancy.

[6]Zoster vaccine

- A single dose of zoster vaccine is recommended for adults ≥60 years of age, regardless of whether they report a prior episode of herpes zoster. Although the vaccine is licensed by the U.S. Food and Drug Administration for use among and can be administered to persons ≥50 years of age, ACIP recommendes that vaccination begin at 60 years of age.
- Persons ≥60 years of age with chronic medical conditions may be vaccinated, unless their condition constitutes a contraindication, such as pregnancy or severe immunodeficiency.

[7]Measles, mumps, rubella vaccine (MMR)

- Adults born before 1957 generally are considered immune to measles and mumps. All adults born in 1957 or later should have documentation of ≥1 dose of MMR vaccine, unless they have a medical contraindication to the vaccine or laboratory evidence of immunity to each of the three diseases. Documentation of provider-diagnosed disease is not considered acceptable evidence of immunity for measles, mumps, or rubella.
- **Measles component:**
  - A routine second dose of MMR vaccine, administered a minimum of 28 days after the first dose, is recommended for adults who:
    - Are students in postsecondary educational institutions
    - Work in a health care facility, or
    - Plan to travel internationally
  - Persons who received inactivated (killed) measles vaccine or measles vaccine of unknown type during 1963–1967 should be revaccinated with 2 doses of MMR vaccine.
- **Mumps component:**
  - A routine second dose of MMR vaccine, administered a minimum of 28 days after the first dose, is recommended for adults who:
    - Are students in a postsecondary educational institution
    - Work in a health care facility, or
    - Plan to travel internationally
  - Persons vaccinated before 1979 with either killed mumps vaccine or mumps vaccine of unknown type who are at high risk for mumps infection (eg, persons who are working in a health care facility) should be considered for revaccination with 2 doses of MMR vaccine.
- **Rubella component:** For women of childbearing age, regardless of birth year, rubella immunity should be determined. If there is no evidence of immunity, women who are not pregnant should be vaccinated. Pregnant women who do not have evidence of immunity should receive MMR vaccine upon completion or termination of pregnancy and before discharge from the health care facility.
- **Health care personnel born before 1957:** For unvaccinated health care personnel born before 1957 who lack laboratory evidence of measles, mumps, and/or rubella immunity or laboratory confirmation of disease, health care facilities should consider vaccinating personnel with 2 doses of MMR vaccine at the appropriate interval for measles and mumps or 1 dose of MMR vaccine for rubella.

[8]Pneumococcal conjugate vaccine (PCV13)

- Adults ≥19 years of age with immunocompromising conditions (including chronic renal failure and nephrotic syndrome), functional or anatomic asplenia, cerebrospinal fluid leaks, or cochlear implants who have not previously received PCV13 or PPSV23 should receive a single dose of PCV13, followed by a dose of PPSV23 at least 8 weeks later.
- Adults ≥19 years of age with the aforementioned conditions who have previously received ≥1 dose of PPSV23 should receive a dose of PCV13 ≥1 year after the last PPSV23 dose was received. For adults who require additional doses of PPSV23, the first such dose should be given no sooner than 8 weeks after PCV13 and at least 5 years after the most recent dose of PPSV23.
- When indicated, PCV13 should be administered to patients who are uncertain of their vaccination status history and have no record of previous vaccination.
- Although PCV13 is licensed by the U.S. Food and Drug Administration for use among and can be administered to persons ≥50 years of age, ACIP recommends PCV13 for adults ≥19 years of age with the specific medical conditions noted above.

[9]Pneumococcal polysaccharide vaccine (PPSV23)

- When PCV13 is also indicated, PCV13 should be given first (see footnote 8).
- Vaccinate all persons with the following indications:
  - All adults ≥65 years of age
  - Adults <65 years of age with chronic lung disease (including chronic obstructive pulmonary disease, emphysema, and asthma), chronic cardiovascular diseases, diabetes mellitus, chronic renal failure, nephrotic syndrome, chronic liver disease (including cirrhosis), alcoholism, cochlear implants, cerebrospinal fluid leaks, immunocompromising conditions, and functional or anatomic asplenia (eg, sickle cell disease and other hemoglobinopathies, congenital or acquired asplenia, splenic dysfunction, or splenectomy [if elective splenectomy is planned, vaccinate ≥2 weeks before surgery])
  - Residents of nursing homes or long-term care facilities, and
  - Adults who smoke cigarettes
- Persons with immunocompromising conditions and other selected conditions are recommended to receive PCV13 and PPSV23 vaccines. See footnote 8 for information on timing of PCV13 and PPSV23 vaccinations.
- Persons with asymptomatic or symptomatic HIV infection should be vaccinated as soon as possible after their diagnosis.
- When cancer chemotherapy or other immunosuppressive therapy is being considered, the interval between vaccination and initiation of immunosuppresive therapy should be ≥2 weeks. Vaccination during chemotherapy or radiation therapy should be avoided.
- Routine use of PPSV23 is not recommended for American Indians/Alaska Natives or other persons <65 years of age, unless they have underlying medical conditions that are PPSV23 indications. However, public health authorities may consider recommending PPSV23 for American Indians/Alaska Natives who are living in areas where the risk for invasive pneumococcal disease is increased.
- When indicated, PPSV23 vaccine should be administered to patients who are uncertain of their vaccination status and have no record of vaccination.

[10]Revaccination with PPSV23

- One-time revaccination 5 years after the first dose of PPSV23 is recommended for persons 19 to 64 years of age with chronic renal failure or nephrotic syndrome, functional or anatomic asplenia (eg, sickle cell disease, splenectomy), or immunocompromising conditions.
- Persons who received 1 or 2 doses of PPSV23 before 65 years of age for any indication should receive another dose of the vaccine at ≥65 years of age if at least 5 years have passed since their previous dose.
- No further doses are needed for persons vaccinated with PPSV23 at ≥65 years of age.

[11]Meningococcal vaccine

- Administer 2 doses of quadrivalent meningococcal conjugate vaccine (MenACWY-D [Menactra]) at least 2 months apart to adults with functional asplenia or persistent complement component deficiencies. HIV infection is not an indication for routine vaccination with MenACWY-D. If an HIV-infected person of any age is vaccinated, 2 doses of MenACWY-D should be administered at least 2 months apart.
- Administer a single dose of meningococcal vaccine to microbiologists routinely exposed to isolates of *Neisseria meningitidis*, military recruits, persons at risk during an outbreak attributable to a vaccine serogroup, and persons who travel to or live in countries in which meningococcal disease is hyperendemic or epidemic.
- First-year college students ≤21 years of age who are living in residence halls should be vaccinated if they have not received a dose on or after their 16th birthday.
- MenACWY-D is preferred for adults with any of the preceding indications who are ≤55 years of age, as well as for adults ≥56 years of age: a) who were vaccinated previously with MenACWY-D and are recommended for revaccination or b) for whom multiple doses are anticipated. Meningococcal polysaccharide vaccine (MenACWY-CRM [Menveo]) is preferred for adults ≥56 years of age who have not received MenACWY-D previously and who require a single dose only (eg, travelers).

- Revaccination with MenACWY-D every 5 years is recommended for adults previously vaccinated with MenACWY-D or MenACWY-CRM who remain at increased risk for infection (eg, adults with anatomic or functional asplenia, persistent complement component deficiencies, or microbiologists).

[12]**Hepatitis A vaccine**

- Vaccinate any person seeking protection from hepatitis A virus (HAV) infection and persons with any of the following indications:
  - Men who have sex with men and persons who use injection or noninjection illicit drugs
  - Persons working with HAV-infected primates or with HAV in a research laboratory setting
  - Persons with chronic liver disease and persons who receive clotting factor concentrates
  - Persons traveling to or working in countries that have high or intermediate endemicity of hepatitis A, and
  - Unvaccinated persons who anticipate close personal contatct (eg, household, regular babysitting) with an international adoptee during the first 60 days after arrival in the United States from a country with high or intermediate endemicity (see footnote 1 for more information on travel recommendations). The first dose of the 2-dose hepatitis A vaccine series should be administered as soon as adoption is planned, ideally ≥2 weeks before the arrival of the adoptee.
- Single-antigen vaccine formulations should be administered in a 2-dose schedule at either 0 and 6 to 12 months (Havrix) or 0 and 6 to 18 months (Vaqta). If the combined hepatitis A and hepatitis B vaccine (Twinrix) is used, administer 3 doses at 0, 1, and 6 months; alternatively, a 4-dose schedule may be used, administered on days 0, 7, and 21 to 30, followed by a booster dose at month 12.

[13]**Hepatitis B vaccine**

- Vaccinate persons with any of the following indications and any person seeking protection from hepatitis B virus (HBV) infection:
  - Sexually active persons who are not in a long-term, mutually monogamous relationship (eg, persons with more than one sex partner during the previous 6 months), persons seeking evaluation or treatment for a sexually transmitted disease (STD), current or recent injection drug users, and men who have sex with men
  - Health care personnel and public safety workers who are potentially exposed to blood or other infectious body fluids
  - Persons with diabetes who are <60 years of age as soon as feasible after diagnosis and persons with diabetes who are ≥60 years of age at the discretion of the treating clinician, based on the likelihood of acquiring HBV infection, including the risk posed by an increased need for assisted blood glucose monitoring in long-term care facilities, the likelihood of experiencing chronic sequelae if infected with HBV, and the likelihood of immune response to vaccination.
  - Persons with end-stage renal disease, including patients receiving hemodialysis, persons with HIV infection, and persons with chronic liver disease
  - Household contacts and sex partners of hepatitis B surface antigen-positive persons, clients and staff members of institutions for persons with developmental disabilities, and international travelers to countries with high or intermediate prevalence of chronic HBV infection, and
  - All adults in the following settings: STD treatment facilities, HIV testing and treatment facilities, facilities providing drug-abuse treatment and prevention services, health care settings targeting services to injection drug users or men who have sex with men, correctional facilities, end-stage renal disease programs and facilities for chronic hemodialysis patients, and institutions and nonresidential day-care facilities for persons with developmental disabilities
- Administer missing doses to complete a 3-dose series of hepatitis B vaccine to those persons not vaccinated or not completely vaccinated. The second dose should be administered 1 month after the first dose; the third dose should be given at least 2 months after the second dose (and at least 4 months after the first dose). If the combined hepatitis A and hepatitis B vaccine (Twinrix) is used, give 3 doses at 0, 1, and 6 months; alternatively, a 4-dose Twinrix schedule, administered on days 0, 7, and 21 to 30, followed by a booster dose at month 12, may be used.
- Adult patients receiving hemodialysis or with other immunocompromising conditions should receive 1 dose of 40 mcg/mL (Recombivax HB) administered on a 3-dose schedule at 0, 1, and 6 months, or 2 doses of 20 mcg/mL (Engerix-B) administered simultaneously on a 4-dose schedule at 0, 1, 2, and 6 months.

[14]***Haemophilus influenzae* type b vaccine (Hib)**

- One dose of Hib vaccine should be administered to persons who have functional or anatomic asplenia or sickle cell disease or to those who are undergoing elective splenectomy if they have not previously received Hib vaccine. Hib vaccination ≥14 days before splenectomy is suggested.
- Receipients of a hematopoietic stem cell transplant should be vaccinated with a 3-dose regimen 6 to 12 months after a successful transplant, regardless of vaccination history; at least 4 weeks should separate doses.
- Hib vaccine is not recommended for adults with HIV infection since their risk for Hib infection is low.

[15]Immunocompromising conditions

- Inactivated vaccines generally are acceptable (eg, pneumococcal, meningococcal, inactivated influenza vaccine) and live vaccines generally are avoided in persons with immune deficiencies or immunocompromising conditions. Information on specific conditions is available at http://www.cdc.gov/vaccines/hcp/acip-recs/index.html.

REFERENCE

Centers for Disease Control and Prevention (CDC). Advisory Committee on Immunization Practices (ACIP) recommended immunization schedules for persons aged 0 through 18 years and adults aged 19 years and older – United States, 2014. Available at http://www.cdc.gov/vaccines/schedules/hcp/adult.html

VACCINE INJURY TABLE

The Vaccine Injury Table makes it easier for some people to get compensation. The table lists and explains injuries/conditions that are presumed to be caused by vaccines. It also lists time periods in which the first symptom of these injuries/conditions must occur after receiving the vaccine. If the first symptom of these injuries/conditions occurs within the listed time period, it is presumed that the vaccine was the cause of the injury or condition, unless another cause is found. For example, if the patient received the tetanus vaccines and had a severe allergic reaction (anaphylaxis) within 4 hours after receiving the vaccine, then it is presumed that the tetanus vaccine caused the injury if no other cause is found.

If the injury/condition is not on the table or if the injury/condition did not occur within the time period on the table, it must be proven that the vaccine caused the injury/condition. Such proof must be based on medical records or opinion, which may include expert witness testimony.

Vaccine Injury Table[1]

Vaccine		Illness, Disability, Injury, or Condition Covered	Time Period for First Symptom or Manifestation of Onset or of Significant Aggravation After Vaccine Administration
Vaccines containing tetanus toxoid (eg, DTaP, DTP, DT, Td, TT)	A.	Anaphylaxis or anaphylactic shock	4 hours
	B.	Brachial neuritis	2 to 28 days
	C.	Any acute complication or sequela (including death) of an illness, disability, injury, or condition referred to above which illness, disability, injury, or condition arose within the time period prescribed	Not applicable
Vaccines containing whole cell pertussis bacteria, extracted or partial cell pertussis bacteria, or specific pertussis antigen(s) (eg, DTP, DTaP, P, DTP-Hib)	A.	Anaphylaxis or anaphylactic shock	4 hours
	B.	Encephalopathy (or encephalitis)	72 hours
	C.	Any acute complication or sequela (including death) of an illness, disability, injury, or condition referred to above which illness, disability, injury, or condition arose within the time period prescribed	Not applicable
Measles, mumps, and rubella vaccine or any of its components (eg, MMR, MR, M, R)	A.	Anaphylaxis or anaphylactic shock	4 hours
	B.	Encephalopathy (or encephalitis)	5 to 15 days
	C.	Any acute complication or sequela (including death) of an illness, disability, injury, or condition referred to above which illness, disability, injury, or condition arose within the time period prescribed	Not applicable
Vaccines containing rubella virus (eg, MMR, MR, R)	A.	Chronic arthritis	7 to 42 days
	B.	Any acute complication or sequela (including death) of an illness, disability, injury, or condition referred to above which illness, disability, injury, or condition arose within the time period prescribed	Not applicable
Vaccines containing measles virus (eg, MMR, MR, M)	A.	Thrombocytopenic purpura	7 to 30 days
	B.	Vaccine-strain measles viral infection in an immunodeficient recipient	6 months
	C.	Any acute complication or sequela (including death) of an illness, disability, injury, or condition referred to above which illness, disability, injury, or condition arose within the time period prescribed	Not applicable
Vaccines containing polio live virus (OPV)	A.	Paralytic polio	
		• In a nonimmunodeficient recipient	30 days
		• In an immunodeficient recipient	6 months
		• In a vaccine-associated community case	Not applicable
	B.	Vaccine-strain polio viral infection	
		• In a nonimmunodeficient recipient	30 days
		• In an immunodeficient recipient	6 months
		• In a vaccine-associated community case	Not applicable
	C.	Any acute complication or sequela (including death) of an illness, disability, injury, or condition referred to above which illness, disability, injury, or condition arose within the time period prescribed	Not applicable
Vaccines containing polio inactivated (eg, IPV)	A.	Anaphylaxis or anaphylactic shock	4 hours
	B.	Any acute complication or sequela (including death) of an illness, disability, injury, or condition referred to above which illness, disability, injury, or condition arose within the time period prescribed	Not applicable

Vaccine Injury Table[1] *(continued)*

Vaccine		Illness, Disability, Injury, or Condition Covered	Time Period for First Symptom or Manifestation of Onset or of Significant Aggravation After Vaccine Administration
Hepatitis B vaccines	A.	Anaphylaxis or anaphylactic shock	4 hours
	B.	Any acute complication or sequela (including death) of an illness, disability, injury, or condition referred to above which illness, disability, injury, or condition arose within the time period prescribed	Not applicable
Hemophilus influenzae type b polysaccharide conjugate vaccines		No condition specified	Not applicable
Varicella vaccine		No condition specified	Not applicable
Rotavirus vaccine		No condition specified	Not applicable
Pneumococcal conjugate vaccines		No condition specified	Not applicable
Hepatitis A vaccines		No condition specified	Not applicable
Trivalent influenza vaccines		No condition specified	Not applicable
Meningococcal vaccines		No condition specified	Not applicable
Human papillomavirus (HPV) vaccines		No condition specified	Not applicable
Any new vaccine recommended by the Centers for Disease Control and Prevention for routine administration to children, after publication by the secretary of a notice of coverage*		No condition specified	Not applicable

*Now includes all vaccines against seasonal influenza (except trivalent influenza vaccines, which are already covered), effective November 12, 2013

[1]Effective date: July 22, 2011. Available at http://www.hrsa.gov/vaccinecompensation/vaccinetable.html

BEERS CRITERIA – POTENTIALLY INAPPROPRIATE MEDICATIONS FOR GERIATRICS

Criteria for Medications That Should Be Avoided or Used With Caution in Older Adults

Independent of Diagnoses or Conditions

Applicable Medications	Summary of Prescribing Concerns	Recommendation	Quality of Evidence	Strength of Recommendation
Alpha-1-blockers: Doxazosin, prazosin, terazosin	High risk of orthostatic hypotension; alternative agents preferred due to a more favorable risk:benefit profile	Avoid use as an antihypertensive	Moderate	Strong
Alpha-2 agonists: CloNIDine, guanabenz, guanFACINE, methyldopa Central monoamine-depleting agent: Reserpine (>0.1 mg/day)	High risk of CNS adverse effects; may also cause orthostatic hypotension and bradycardia; not recommended for routine use as an antihypertensive	Avoid clonidine as a first-line antihypertensive. Avoid others as listed.	Low	Strong
Antiarrhythmic drugs (Class Ia, Ic, III): Amiodarone, dofetilide, dronedarone, flecainide, ibutilide, procainamide, propafenone, quinidine, sotalol	In older adults, data suggest rate control may provide more benefits than risks compared to rhythm control for most patients. Amiodarone is associated with numerous toxicities (eg, thyroid disease, QT prolongation, pulmonary disorders).	Avoid antiarrhythmic drugs as first-line treatment of atrial fibrillation	High	Strong
Antihistamines, first generation (alone or in combination products): Brompheniramine, carbinoxamine, chlorpheniramine, clemastine, cyproheptadine, dexchlorpheniramine, diphenhydrAMINE (oral), doxylamine, hydrOXYzine, promethazine, triprolidine	First generation antihistamines have potent anticholinergic properties; older adults are at increased risk for anticholinergic effects and toxicity. Diphenhydramine use may be appropriate in certain situations such as the acute treatment of severe allergic reactions.	Avoid	High (hydroxyzine, promethazine) Moderate (all others)	Strong
Antiparkinson agents: Benztropine (oral), trihexyphenidyl	Alternative, more-efficacious agents preferred for treatment of Parkinson's disease. Not recommended for prevention of extrapyramidal symptoms associated with antipsychotics.	Avoid	Moderate	Strong
Antipsychotics, first generation **and** second generation: ARIPiprazole, asenapine, chlorproMAZINE, cloZAPine, fluPHENAZine, haloperidol, iloperidone, loxapine, lurasidone, olanzapine, paliperidone, perphenazine, pimozide, QUEtiapine, risperiDONE, thioridazine, thiothixene, trifluoperazine, ziprasidone, zuclopenthixol [Canadian product]	Increased risk of stroke and mortality in patients with dementia. In addition, use may cause or exacerbate syndrome of inappropriate antidiuretic hormone secretion or hyponatremia; monitor sodium closely with initiation or dosage adjustments in older adults.	Avoid use for behavioral problems of dementia unless nonpharmacological options have failed and patient is threat to self or others; SIADH risk: Use with caution	Moderate	Strong
Antispasmodic drugs: Belladonna alkaloids, clidinium and chlordiazepoxide, dicyclomine, hyoscyamine, propantheline, scopolamine	Potent anticholinergic properties and uncertain efficacy	Avoid except in short-term palliative care to decrease oral secretions	Moderate	Strong
Barbiturates: Amobarbital, butabarbital, butalbital, mephobarbital, PENTobarbital, PHENobarbital, secobarbital	Risk of overdose with low dosages, tolerance to sleep effects, and increased risk of physical dependence	Avoid	High	Strong
Benzodiazepines, long-acting: Amitriptyline and chlordiazepoxide, chlorazepate, chlordiazePOXIDE, clidinium and chlordiazepoxide, clonazePAM, diazepam, flurazepam, quazepam	In older adults, benzodiazepines increase the risk of impaired cognition, delirium, falls, fractures, and motor vehicle accidents. Increased sensitivity to benzodiazepines in this age group and slower metabolism of long-acting agents.	Avoid benzodiazepines (any type) for treatment of insomnia, agitation, or delirium	High	Strong
Benzodiazepines, short-acting: ALPRAZolam, estazolam, LORazepam, oxazepam, temazepam, triazolam	In older adults, benzodiazepines increase the risk of impaired cognition, delirium, falls, fractures, and motor vehicle accidents. Increased sensitivity in this age group to benzodiazepines.	Avoid benzodiazepines (any type) for treatment of insomnia, agitation, or delirium	High	Strong
CarBAMazepine	Use may cause or exacerbate syndrome of inappropriate antidiuretic hormone secretion or hyponatremia; monitor sodium closely with initiation or dosage adjustments in older adults.	Use with caution	Moderate	Strong

Criteria for Medications That Should Be Avoided or Used With Caution in Older Adults *continued*

Applicable Medications	Summary of Prescribing Concerns	Recommendation	Quality of Evidence	Strength of Recommendation
CARBOplatin	Use may cause or exacerbate syndrome of inappropriate antidiuretic hormone secretion or hyponatremia; monitor sodium closely with initiation or dosage adjustments in older adults.	Use with caution	Moderate	Strong
ChlorproPAMIDE	Prolonged half-life in elderly patients which could cause prolonged hypoglycemia. Additionally, causes SIADH.	Avoid	High	Strong
CISplatin	Use may cause or exacerbate syndrome of inappropriate antidiuretic hormone secretion or hyponatremia; monitor sodium closely with initiation or dosage adjustments in older adults.	Use with caution	Moderate	Strong
Dabigatran	Greater risk of bleeding in older adults aged ≥75 years (exceeds warfarin bleeding risk); lack of safety and efficacy in patients with CrCl <30 mL/minute	Use with caution in adults aged ≥75 years of if CrCl <30mL/minute	Moderate	Weak
Desiccated thyroid	Concerns about cardiac effects; safer alternatives available	Avoid	Low	Strong
Digoxin >0.125 mg/day	Decreased renal clearance may lead to increased risk of toxic effects. Higher doses are associated with no additional benefit in heart failure patients, and may increase the risk of toxicity.	Avoid	Moderate	Strong
Dipyridamole, oral (short-acting)	May cause orthostatic hypotension; more-efficacious alternative agents available	Avoid	Moderate	Strong
Disopyramide	Potent negative inotrope and therefore may induce heart failure in elderly patients. It is also strongly anticholinergic. Other antiarrhythmic drugs should be used.	Avoid	Low	Strong
Dronedarone	In patient with permanent atrial fibrillation or heart failure, worse outcomes have been reported with use. In general, rate control is preferred over rhythm control for atrial fibrillation.	Avoid in patients with permanent atrial fibrillation or heart failure	Moderate	Strong
Ergot mesylates	Have not been shown to be effective	Avoid	High	Strong
Estrogens (with or without progestins)	Evidence of the carcinogenic (breast and endometrial cancer) potential of these agents and lack of cardioprotective effect in older women Evidence for vaginal estrogens for treatment of vaginal dryness to be safe and effective in women with breast cancer, particularly at estradiol doses <25 mcg twice weekly	Avoid oral and topical patch. Topical vaginal cream: Acceptable to use low-dose intravaginal estrogen for the management of dyspareunia, lower urinary tract infections, and other vaginal symptoms	High (oral and patch formulations) Moderate (topical formulations)	Strong (oral and patch formulations) Weak (topical formulations)
Glyburide	Increased risk of severe, prolonged hypoglycemia in older adults	Avoid	High	Strong
Indomethacin	Of all available NSAIDs, this drug produces the most adverse effects. Non-COX-selective oral NSAID use associated with an increased risk of GI bleeding and peptic ulcer disease in older adults in high-risk category (eg, >75 years or age or receiving concomitant oral/parenteral corticosteroids, anticoagulants, or antiplatelet agents). Proton pump inhibitors or misoprostol use reduces risk, but does not eliminate it. Longer duration of NSAID use correlates with a trend towards increasing incidence GI ulcers, bleeding, or perforation.	Avoid	Moderate	Strong
Insulin, sliding scale	Regardless of care setting, an increased risk of hypoglycemia without improvement in management of hyperglycemia	Avoid	Moderate	Strong

Criteria for Medications That Should Be Avoided or Used With Caution in Older Adults *continued*

Applicable Medications	Summary of Prescribing Concerns	Recommendation	Quality of Evidence	Strength of Recommendation
Isoxsuprine	Lack of efficacy	Avoid	High	Strong
Ketorolac (includes parenteral)	Associated with an increased risk of GI bleeding and peptic ulcer disease in older adults in high-risk category (eg, >75 years or age or receiving concomitant oral/parenteral corticosteroids, anticoagulants, or antiplatelet agents). Proton pump inhibitors or misoprostol use reduces risk, but does not eliminate it. Longer duration of NSAID use correlates with a trend towards increasing incidence GI ulcers, bleeding, or perforation.	Avoid	High	Strong
Megestrol	Increased risk of thrombotic events and possibly death; effect on weight is minimal	Avoid	Moderate	Strong
Meperidine	Not an effective oral analgesic in doses commonly used. Safer alternative agents preferred due to potential for neurotoxicity.	Avoid	High	Strong
Meprobamate	Highly sedating anxiolytic with a high rate of physical dependence	Avoid	Moderate	Strong
MethylTESTOSTERone	Potential for cardiac problems; contraindicated in men with prostate cancer	Avoid unless indicated for moderate to severe hypogonadism	Moderate	Weak
Metoclopramide	May cause extrapyramidal effects (including tardive dyskinesia), particularly in frail older adults	Avoid, unless for gastroparesis	Moderate	Strong
Mineral oil	Potential for aspiration and adverse effects; safer alternatives available	Avoid	Moderate	Strong
Mirtazapine	Use may cause or exacerbate syndrome of inappropriate antidiuretic hormone secretion or hyponatremia; monitor sodium closely with initiation or dosage adjustments in older adults.	Use with caution	Moderate	Strong
NIFEdipine, short-acting	Potential for hypotension; risk of precipitating myocardial ischemia	Avoid	High	Strong
Nitrofurantoin	Potential for pulmonary toxicity; safer alternatives available; renal impairment (CrCl <60 mL/minute) results in inadequate drug concentration in urine and lack of efficacy	Avoid for long-term suppression; avoid in patients with CrCl <60 mL/minute	Moderate	Strong
Nonbenzodiazepine hypnotics: Eszopiclone, zolpidem, zaleplon	Similar adverse events (eg, delirium, falls, fractures) in older adults to events seen with benzodiazepine use; minimal improvement seen with sleep latency and duration	Avoid chronic use (>90 days)	Moderate	Strong
Non-COX-selective NSAIDS (oral): Aspirin (>325 mg/day), diclofenac, diflunisal, etodolac, fenoprofen, ibuprofen, ketoprofen, meclofenamate, mefenamic acid, meloxicam, nabumetone, naproxen, oxaprozin, piroxicam, sulindac, tolmetin	Use associated with an increased risk of GI bleeding and peptic ulcer disease in older adults in high risk category (eg, >75 years or age or receiving concomitant oral/parenteral corticosteroids, anticoagulants, or antiplatelet agents). Proton pump inhibitors or misoprostol use reduce risk, but do not eliminate it. Longer duration of NSAID use correlates with a trend towards increasing incidence GI ulcers, bleeding, or perforation.	Avoid chronic use unless other alternatives are not effective and patient can take gastroprotective agent (proton pump inhibitor or misoprostol)	Moderate	Strong
Pentazocine	Opioid analgesic that causes more CNS adverse effects, including confusion and hallucinations, more commonly than other opioid drugs. Additionally, it is a mixed agonist and antagonist; safer alternative agents are available.	Avoid	Low	Strong
Prasugrel	Risk of bleeding is increased in older adults; risk may be offset by benefit in older adults at highest risk (eg, prior MI or diabetes)	Use with caution in adults aged ≥75 years	Moderate	Weak
Serotonin-norepinephrine reuptake inhibitors and selective serotonin reuptake inhibitors	Use may cause or exacerbate syndrome of inappropriate antidiuretic hormone secretion or hyponatremia; monitor sodium closely with initiation or dosage adjustments in older adults.	Use with caution	Moderate	Strong

Criteria for Medications That Should Be Avoided or Used With Caution in Older Adults *continued*

Applicable Medications	Summary of Prescribing Concerns	Recommendation	Quality of Evidence	Strength of Recommendation
Skeletal muscle relaxants: Carisoprodol, chlorzoxazone, cyclobenzaprine, metaxalone, methocarbamol, orphenadrine	Most muscle relaxants are poorly tolerated by elderly patients, since these cause anticholinergic adverse effects, sedation, and risk of fracture. Additionally, efficacy is questionable at dosages tolerated by elderly patients.	Avoid	Moderate	Strong
Somatropin (growth hormone)	Body composition effects are minimal and use associated with edema, arthralgia, carpal tunnel syndrome, gynecomastia, and impaired fasting glucose.	Avoid, except as hormone replacement after pituitary gland removal	High	Strong
Spironolactone (>25 mg/day)	Risk of hyperkalemia is increased for heart failure patients receiving >25 mg/day, particularly if taking concomitant medications such as NSAIDS, ACE inhibitors, angiotensin receptor blockers, or potassium supplements.	Avoid in patients with heart failure or with a CrCl <30 mL/minute	Moderate	Strong
Testosterone	Potential for cardiac problems; contraindicated in men with prostate cancer	Avoid unless indicated for moderate to severe hypogonadism	Moderate	Weak
Thioridazine	Potent anticholinergic properties; risk of QT-interval prolongation	Avoid	Moderate	Strong
Ticlopidine	Safer, more effective alternatives exist.	Avoid	Moderate	Strong
Tricyclic antidepressants	Use may cause or exacerbate syndrome of inappropriate antidiuretic hormone secretion or hyponatremia; monitor sodium closely with initiation or dosage adjustments in older adults.	Use with caution	High	Strong
Tricyclic antidepressants, tertiary (alone or in combination): Amitriptyline, amitriptyline and chlordiazepoxide, clomiPRAMINE, doxepin >6 mg/day, imipramine, perphenazine and amitriptyline, trimipramine	Potent anticholinergic properties, sedating, and potential for orthostatic hypotension; doxepin at doses ≤6 mg/day has safety profile comparable to placebo	Avoid	High	Strong
Trimethobenzamide	One of the least effective antiemetic drugs and may cause extrapyramidal adverse effects	Avoid	Moderate	Strong
VinCRIStine	Use may cause or exacerbate syndrome of inappropriate antidiuretic hormone secretion or hyponatremia; monitor sodium closely with initiation or dosage adjustments in older adults.	Use with caution	Moderate	Strong

Drugs with Potent Anticholinergic Properties

Class of Drug	Individual Agents
Antihistamines	Brompheniramine, carbinoxamine, chlorpheniramine, clemastine, cyproheptadine, dimenhydrinate, diphenhydrAMINE, hydrOXYzine, loratadine, meclizine
Antidepressants	Amitriptyline, amoxapine, clomiPRAMINE, desipramine, doxepin, imipramine, nortriptyline, PARoxetine, protriptyline, trimipramine
Antimuscarinics (urinary incontinence)	Darifenacin, fesoterodine, flavoxATE, oxybutynin, solifenacin, tolterodine, trospium
Antiparkinson agents	Benztropine, trihexyphenidyl
Antipsychotics	ChlorproMAZINE, cloZAPine, fluPHENAZine, loxapine, OLANZapine, perphenazine, pimozide, prochlorperazine, promethazine, thioridazine, thiothixene, trifluoperazine
Antispasmodics	Atropine products, belladonna alkaloids, dicyclomine, homatropine, hyoscyamine products, propantheline, scopolamine
Skeletal muscle relaxants	Carisoprodol, cyclobenzaprine, orphenadrine, tiZANidine

REFERENCE

American Geriatrics Society 2012 Beers Criteria Update Expert Panel. American Geriatrics Society updated beers criteria for potentially inappropriate medication use in older adults. *J Am Geriatr Soc*. 2012;60(4):616-631.

ORAL DOSAGES THAT SHOULD NOT BE CRUSHED

There are a variety of reasons for crushing tablets or capsule contents prior to administering to the patient. Patients may have nasogastric tubes which do not permit the administration of tablets or capsules, an oral solution for a particular medication may not be available from the manufacturer or readily prepared by pharmacy, patients may have difficulty swallowing capsules or tablets, or mixing of powdered medication with food or drink may make the drug more palatable.

Generally, medications which should not be crushed fall into one of the following categories:

- **Extended Release Products:** The formulation of some tablets is specialized as to allow the medication within it to be slowly released into the body. This may be accomplished by centering the drug within the core of the tablet, with a subsequent shedding of multiple layers around the core. Wax melts in the GI tract, releasing drug contained within the wax matrix (eg, OxyCONTIN). Capsules may contain beads which have multiple layers which are slowly dissolved with time.

  Common Abbreviations for Extended Release Products

CD	Controlled dose
CR	Controlled release
CRT	Controlled release tablet
LA	Long-acting
SR	Sustained release
TR	Timed release
TD	Time delay
SA	Sustained action
XL	Extended release
XR	Extended release

- **Medications Which Are Irritating to the Stomach:** Tablets which are irritating to the stomach may be enteric-coated which delays release of the drug until the time when it reaches the small intestine. Enteric-coated aspirin is an example of this.
- **Foul-Tasting Medication:** Some drugs are quite unpleasant to taste so the manufacturer coats the tablet in a sugar coating to increase its palatability. By crushing the tablet, this sugar coating is lost and the patient tastes the unpleasant tasting medication.
- **Sublingual Medication:** Medication intended for use under the tongue should not be crushed. While it appears to be obvious, it is not always easy to determine if a medication is to be used sublingually. Sublingual medications should indicate on the package that they are intended for sublingual use.
- **Effervescent Tablets:** These are tablets which, when dropped into a liquid, quickly dissolve to yield a solution. Many effervescent tablets, when crushed, lose their ability to quickly dissolve.
- **Potentially Hazardous Substances:** Certain drugs, including antineoplastic agents, hormonal agents, some antivirals, some bioengineered agents, and other miscellaneous drugs, are considered potentially hazardous when used in humans based on their characteristics. Examples of these characteristics include carcinogenicity, teratogenicity, reproductive toxicity, organ toxicity at low doses, genotoxicity, or new drugs with structural and toxicity profiles similar to existing hazardous drugs. Exposure to these substances can result in adverse effects and should be avoided. Crushing or breaking a tablet or opening a capsule of a potentially hazardous substance may increase the risk of exposure to the substance through skin contact, inhalation, or accidental ingestion. The extent of exposure, potency, and toxicity of the hazardous substance determines the health risk. Institutions have policies and procedures to follow when handling any potentially hazardous substance. **Note:** All potentially hazardous substances may not be represented in this table. Refer to institution-specific guidelines for precautions to observe when handling hazardous substances.

RECOMMENDATIONS

1. It is not advisable to crush certain medications.
2. Consult individual monographs prior to crushing capsule or tablet.
3. If crushing a tablet or capsule is contraindicated, consult with your pharmacist to determine whether an oral solution exists or can be compounded.

Drug Product	Dosage Form	Dosage Reasons/Comments
Accutane	Capsule	Mucous membrane irritant; teratogenic potential
Aciphex	Tablet	Extended release
Aciphex Sprinkle	Capsule	Slow release. Capsule may be opened and contents sprinkled on soft food (eg, applesauce, fruit- or vegetable-based baby food, yogurt) or emptied into a small amount of liquid (eg, infant formula, apple juice, pediatric electrolyte solution). Granules should not be chewed or crushed.
Actiq	Lozenge	Slow release. This lollipop delivery system requires the patient to dissolve it slowly.
Actoplus Met XR	Tablet	Variable release
Actonel	Tablet	Irritant. Chewed, crushed, or sucked tablets may cause oropharyngeal irritation.
Adalat CC	Tablet	Extended release
Adderall XR	Capsule	Extended release[1]
Adenovirus (Types 4, 7) Vaccine	Tablet	Teratogenic potential; enteric-coated; do not disrupt tablet to avoid releasing live adenovirus in upper respiratory tract
Advicor	Tablet	Variable release
Afeditab CR	Tablet	Extended release
Afinitor	Tablet	Mucous membrane irritant; teratogenic potential; hazardous substance[11]
Aggrenox	Capsule	Extended release. Capsule may be opened; contents include an aspirin tablet that may be chewed and dipyridamole pellets that may be sprinkled on applesauce.
Alavert Allergy and Sinus D-12	Tablet	Extended release
Allegra-D	Tablet	Extended release
ALPRAZolam ER	Tablet	Extended release
Altoprev	Tablet	Extended release
Ambien CR	Tablet	Extended release
Amitiza	Capsule	Manufacturer recommendation
Amnesteem	Capsule	Mucous membrane irritant; teratogenic potential
Ampyra	Tablet	Extended release
Amrix	Capsule	Extended release
Aplenzin	Tablet	Extended release
Apriso	Capsule	Extended release[1]; maintain pH at ≤6
Aptivus	Capsule	Taste. Oil emulsion within spheres
Aricept 23 mg	Tablet	Film-coated; chewing or crushing may increase rate of absorption
Arava	Tablet	Teratogenic potential; hazardous substance[11]
Arthrotec	Tablet	Delayed release; enteric-coated
Asacol	Tablet	Slow release
Aspirin enteric-coated	Capsule, tablet	Delayed release; enteric-coated
Astagraf XL	Capsule	Extended release
Atelvia	Tablet	Extended release; tablet coating is an important part of the delayed release
Augmentin XR	Tablet	Extended release[2,8]
AVINza	Capsule	Slow release[1] (not pudding)
Avodart	Capsule	Capsule should not be handled by pregnant women due to teratogenic potential[10]; hazardous substance[11]
Azulfidine EN-tabs	Tablet	Delayed release
Bayer Aspirin EC	Caplet	Enteric-coated
Bayer Aspirin, Low Adult 81 mg	Tablet	Enteric-coated
Bayer Aspirin, Regular Strength 325 mg	Caplet	Enteric-coated
Biaxin XL	Tablet	Extended release
Biltricide	Tablet	Taste[8]
Bisac-Evac	Tablet	Enteric-coated[3]
Bisacodyl	Tablet	Enteric-coated[3]

ORAL DOSAGES THAT SHOULD NOT BE CRUSHED

Drug Product	Dosage Form	Dosage Reasons/Comments
Boniva	Tablet	Irritant. Chewed, crushed, or sucked tablets may cause oropharyngeal irritation.
Bosulif	Tablet	Hazardous substance[11]
Budeprion SR	Tablet	Extended release
Buproban	Tablet	Extended release
BuPROPion SR	Tablet	Extended release
Calan SR	Tablet	Extended release[8]
Campral	Tablet	Delayed release; enteric-coated
Caprelsa	Tablet	Teratogenic potential; hazardous substance[11]
Carbatrol	Capsule	Extended release[1]
Cardene SR	Capsule	Extended release
Cardizem	Tablet	Not described as slow release but releases drug over 3 hours.
Cardizem CD	Capsule	Extended release
Cardizem LA	Tablet	Extended release
Cardura XL	Tablet	Extended release
Cartia XT	Capsule	Extended release
Casodex	Tablet	Teratogenic potential; hazardous substance[11]
CeeNU	Capsule	Teratogenic potential; hazardous substance[11]
Cefaclor extended release	Tablet	Extended release
Ceftin	Tablet	Taste[2]. Use suspension for children.
Cefuroxime	Tablet	Taste[2]. Use suspension for children.
CellCept	Capsule, tablet	Teratogenic potential; hazardous substance[9,11]
Charcoal Plus DS	Tablet	Enteric-coated
Chlor-Trimeton 12-Hour	Tablet	Extended release[2]
Cipro XR	Tablet	Extended release[2]
Claravis	Capsule	Mucous membrane irritant; teratogenic potential
Claritin-D 12-Hour	Tablet	Extended release[2]
Claritin-D 24-Hour	Tablet	Extended release[2]
Colace	Capsule	Taste[5]
Colestid	Tablet	Slow release
Cometriq	Capsule	Teratogenic potential; hazardous substance[11]
Commit	Lozenge	Integrity compromised by chewing or crushing
Concerta	Tablet	Extended release
Contrave	Tablet	Extended release
ConZip	Capsule	Variable release; tablet disruption may cause overdose
Coreg CR	Capsule	Extended release[1]; may add contents to chilled applesauce
Cotazym-S	Capsule	Enteric-coated[1]
Covera-HS	Tablet	Extended release
Creon	Capsule	Extended release[1]; enteric-coated contents
Crixivan	Capsule	Taste. Capsule may be opened and mixed with fruit puree (eg, banana).
Cyclophosphamide	Capsule, tablet	Hazardous substance[11]; manufacturer recommendation
Cymbalta	Capsule	Enteric-coated[1]; may add contents to apple juice or applesauce but not chocolate
Depakene	Capsule	Slow release; mucous membrane irritant[2]; hazardous substance[11]
Depakote	Tablet	Delayed release; hazardous substance[11]
Depakote ER	Tablet	Extended release; hazardous substance[11]
Depakote Sprinkles	Capsule	Extended release[1]
Detrol LA	Capsule	Extended release
Dexedrine	Capsule	Extended release
Dexilant	Capsule	Delayed release[1]
Diacomit	Capsule	Manufacturer recommendation[12]
Diamox Sequels	Capsule	Extended release
Dibenzyline	Capsule	Hazardous substance[11]

Drug Product	Dosage Form	Dosage Reasons/Comments
Diclegis	Tablet	Delayed release; manufacturer recommendation
Dilacor XR	Capsule	Extended release
Dilantin	Capsule	Extended release; manufacturer recommendation[12]
Dilatrate-SR	Capsule	Extended release
Dilt-CD	Capsule	Extended release
Dilt-XR	Capsule	Extended release
Diltia XT	Capsule	Extended release
Ditropan XL	Tablet	Extended release
Divalproex ER	Tablet	Extended release
Donnatal Extentab	Tablet	Extended release[2]
Doxidan	Tablet	Enteric-coated[3]
Drisdol	Capsule	Liquid filled[4]
Droxia	Capsule	May be opened; wear gloves to handle; hazardous substance[11]
Duavee	Tablet	Manufacturer recommendation; hazardous substance[11]
Dulcolax	Capsule	Liquid-filled
Dulcolax	Tablet	Enteric-coated[3]
EC-Naprosyn	Tablet	Delayed release; enteric-coated
Ecotrin Adult Low Strength	Tablet	Enteric-coated
Ecotrin Maximum Strength	Tablet	Enteric-coated
Ecotrin Regular Strength	Tablet	Enteric-coated
E.E.S.	Tablet	Enteric-coated[2]
Effer-K	Tablet	Effervescent tablet[6]
Effervescent Potassium	Tablet	Effervescent tablet[6]
Effexor XR	Capsule	Extended release
Embeda	Capsule	Extended release[1]; do not give via NG tube
E-Mycin	Tablet	Enteric-coated
Enablex	Tablet	Slow release
Entocort EC	Capsule	Extended release; enteric-coated[1]
Epanova	Capsule	Manufacturer recommendation
Equetro	Capsule	Extended release[1]
Ergomar	Tablet	Sublingual form[7]
Erivedge	Capsule	Teratogenic potential[11]
Eryc	Capsule	Enteric-coated
Ery-Tab	Tablet	Delayed release; enteric-coated
Erythromycin Stearate	Tablet	Enteric-coated
Erythromycin Base	Tablet	Enteric-coated
Erythromycin Delayed-Release	Capsule	Enteric-coated pellets[1]
Etoposide	Capsule	Hazardous substance[11]
Evista	Tablet	Taste; teratogenic potential[10]; hazardous substance[11]
Exalgo	Tablet	Extended release; breaking, chewing, crushing, or dissolving before ingestion or injecting increases the risk of overdose
Exjade	Tablet	Do not chew or swallow whole; do not give as tablets meant to be given as a liquid
Fareston	Tablet	Teratogenic potential; hazardous substance[11]
Feldene	Capsule	Mucous membrane irritant
Fentanyl	Lozenge	Slow release; lollipop delivery system requires the patient to slowly dissolve in mouth
Fentora	Tablet	Buccal tablet; swallowing whole or crushing may reduce effectiveness
Feosol	Tablet	Enteric-coated[2]
Fergon	Tablet	Enteric-coated
Ferro-Sequels	Tablet	Slow release
Fetzima	Capsule	Extended release
Flagyl ER	Tablet	Extended release

ORAL DOSAGES THAT SHOULD NOT BE CRUSHED

Drug Product	Dosage Form	Dosage Reasons/Comments
Fleet Laxative	Tablet	Enteric-coated[3]
Flomax	Capsule	Slow release
Focalin XR	Capsule	Extended release[1]
Forfivo XL	Capsule	Extended release
Fortamet	Tablet	Extended release
Fosamax	Tablet	Mucous membrane irritant
Fosamax Plus D	Tablet	Mucous membrane irritant
Fulyzaq	Tablet	Delayed release
Galzin	Capsule	Manufacturer recommendation[12]; possible gastric irritation
Gengraf	Capsule	Teratogenic potential; hazardous substance[11]
Geodon	Capsule	Hazardous substance[11]
Gleevec	Tablet	Taste[8]. May be dissolved in water or apple juice; hazardous substance[11]
GlipiZIDE XL	Tablet	Extended release
Glucophage XR	Tablet	Extended release
Glucotrol XL	Tablet	Extended release
Glumetza	Tablet	Extended release
Gralise	Tablet	Extended release
Halfprin	Tablet	Enteric-coated
Hetlioz	Capsule	Manufacturer recommendation
Hexalen	Capsule	Teratogenic potential; hazardous substance[11]
Horizant	Tablet	Extended release
Hycamtin	Capsule	Teratogenic potential; hazardous substance[11]
Hydrea	Capsule	Can be opened and mixed with water; wear gloves to handle; hazardous substance[11]
Iclusig	Tablet	Teratogenic potential; hazardous substance[11]
Imbruvica	Capsule	Teratogenic potential; hazardous substance[11]
Imdur	Tablet	Extended release[8]
Inderal LA	Capsule	Extended release
Indomethacin SR	Capsule	Slow release[1,2]
Inlyta	Tablet	Teratogenic potential; hazardous substance[11]
InnoPran XL	Capsule	Extended release
Intelence	Tablet	Tablet should be swallowed whole and not crushed; tablet may be dispersed in water
Intermezzo	Tablet	Sublingual form[7]
Intuniv	Tablet	Extended release
Invega	Tablet	Extended release
IsoDitrate	Tablet	Extended release
Isoptin SR	Tablet	Extended release[8]
Isosorbide Dinitrate Sublingual	Tablet	Sublingual form[7]
ISOtretinoin	Capsule	Mucous membrane irritant
Jalyn	Capsule	Capsule should not be handled by pregnant women due to teratogenic potential[10]; hazardous substance[9,11]
Janumet XR	Tablet	Extended release
Juxtapid	Capsule	Manufacturer recommendation
Kadian	Capsule	Extended release[1]. Do not give via NG tubes; may add contents to applesauce without crushing.
Kaletra	Tablet	Film-coated; pregnant women or women who may become pregnant should not handle crushed or broken tablets; active ingredients surrounded by wax matrix to prevent health care exposure
Kapidex	Capsule	Delayed release[1]
Kapvay	Tablet	Extended release
Kazano	Tablet	Not scored; manufacturer recommendation[12]
K-Dur	Tablet	Slow release
Keppra	Tablet	Taste[2]
Keppra XR	Tablet	Extended release[2]

Drug Product	Dosage Form	Dosage Reasons/Comments
Ketek	Tablet	Slow release
Khedezia	Tablet	Extended release
Klor-Con	Tablet	Extended release[2]
Klor-Con M	Tablet	Slow release[2]; some strengths are scored; to make liquid, place tablet in 120 mL of water; disperse 2 minutes; stir
K-Lyte/Cl	Tablet	Effervescent tablet[6]
Kombiglyze XR	Tablet	Extended release; tablet matrix may remain in stool
K-Tab	Tablet	Extended release[2]
LaMICtal XR	Tablet	Extended release
Lescol XL	Tablet	Extended release
Letairis	Tablet	Film-coated; slow release; hazardous substance[11]
Leukeran	Tablet	Teratogenic potential; hazardous substance[11]
Levbid	Tablet	Extended release[8]
Lialda	Tablet	Delayed release, enteric-coated
Lipitor	Tablet	Manufacturer recommendation
Lithium carbonate XR	Tablet	Extended release
Lithobid	Tablet	Extended release
Lovaza	Capsule	Contents of capsule may erode walls of styrofoam or plastic materials
Luvox CR	Capsule	Extended release
Lysodren	Tablet	Hazardous substance[11]
Mag-Tab SR	Tablet	Extended release
Matulane	Capsule	Teratogenic potential; hazardous substance[11]
Maxiphen DM	Tablet	Slow release[8]
Mestinon ER	Tablet	Extended release[2]
Metadate CD	Capsule	Extended release[1]
Metadate ER	Tablet	Extended release
Metoprolol ER	Tablet	Extended release
MicroK Extencaps	Capsule	Extended release[1,2]
Minocin	Capsule	Slow release
Mirapex ER	Tablet	Extended release
Morphine sulfate extended-release	Tablet	Extended release
Motrin	Tablet	Taste[5]
Moxatag	Tablet	Extended release
MS Contin	Tablet	Extended release[2]
Mucinex	Tablet	Slow release
Mucinex DM	Tablet	Slow release[2]
Multaq	Tablet	Hazardous substance[11]
Myfortic	Tablet	Delayed release; teratogenic potential; hazardous substance[11]
Myrbetriq	Tablet	Extended release
Namenda XR	Capsule	Extended release[1]
Naprelan	Tablet	Extended release
Neoral	Capsule	Teratogenic potential; hazardous substance[11]
NexIUM	Capsule	Delayed release[1]
Niaspan	Tablet	Extended release
Nicotinic Acid	Capsule, Tablet	Slow release[8]
Nifediac CC	Tablet	Extended release
Nifedical XL	Tablet	Extended release
NIFEdipine ER	Tablet	Extended release
Nitrostat	Tablet	Sublingual route[7]
Norpace CR	Capsule	Extended release; form within a special capsule
Norvir	Tablet	Crushing tablets has resulted in decreased bioavailability of drug[2]
Noxafil	Tablet	Delayed release

Drug Product	Dosage Form	Dosage Reasons/Comments
Nucynta ER	Tablet	Extended release; tablet disruption may cause a potentially fatal overdose
Ofev	Capsule	Taste; hazardous substance[11]
Oleptro	Tablet	Extended release[8]
Omtryg	Capsule	Manufacturer recommendation
Onglyza	Tablet	Film-coated
Opana ER	Tablet	Extended release; tablet disruption may cause a potentially fatal overdose
Opsumit	Tablet	Teratogenic potential; hazardous substance[11]
Oracea	Capsule	Delayed release
Oramorph SR	Tablet	Extended release[2]
Oravig	Tablet	Buccal tablet
Orphenadrine citrate ER	Tablet	Extended release
Oseni	Tablet	Manufacturer recommendation[12]
Otezla	Tablet	Manufacturer recommendation
Oxtellar XR	Tablet	Extended release
OxyCONTIN	Tablet	Extended release; surrounded by wax matrix; tablet disruption may cause a potentially fatal overdose
Oxymorphone ER	Tablet	Extended release
Pancrease MT	Capsule	Enteric-coated[1]
Pancreaze	Capsule	Slow-release[1]; enteric-coated contents
Pancrelipase	Capsule	Slow-release[1]; enteric-coated contents
Paxil CR	Tablet	Extended release
Pentasa	Capsule	Slow release[1]
Pertzye	Capsule	Slow-release[1]; enteric-coated contents
Pexeva	Tablet	Film-coated
Phenytek	Capsule	Extended release; manufacturer recommendation[12]
Plendil	Tablet	Extended release
Pomalyst	Capsule	Teratogenic potential; hazardous substance[11]; health care workers should avoid contact with capsule contents/body fluids
Pradaxa	Capsule	Bioavailability increases by 75% when the pellets are taken without the capsule shell
Prevacid	Capsule	Delayed release[1]
Prevacid	Suspension	Slow release. Contains enteric-coated granules. Not for use in NG tubes; mix with water only
Prevacid SoluTab	Tablet	Orally disintegrating. Do not swallow; dissolve in water only and dispense via dosing syringe or NG tube.
Prezcobix	Tablet	Film-coated
PriLOSEC	Capsule	Delayed release
PriLOSEC OTC	Tablet	Delayed release
Pristiq	Tablet	Extended release
Procardia XL	Tablet	Extended release
Procysbi	Capsule	Delayed release[1]
Prolopa	Capsule	Manufacturer recommendation
Propecia	Tablet	Women who are, or may become, pregnant should not handle crushed or broken tablets due to teratogenic potential[10]; hazardous substance[11]
Proscar	Tablet	Women who are, or may become, pregnant should not handle crushed or broken tablets due to teratogenic potential[10]; hazardous substance[11]
Protonix	Tablet	Slow release
PROzac Weekly	Capsule	Enteric-coated
Purinethol	Tablet	Teratogenic potential[10]; hazardous substance[11]
Pytest	Capsule	Hazardous substance[11]
Qudexy XR	Capsule	Extended release
QuiNIDine ER	Tablet	Extended release[8]; enteric-coated
Ranexa	Tablet	Slow release

Drug Product	Dosage Form	Dosage Reasons/Comments
Rapamune	Tablet	Hazardous substance[11]; pharmacokinetic NanoCrystal technology may be affected[2]
Rayos	Tablet	Delayed release; release is dependent upon intact coating
Razadyne ER	Capsule	Extended release
Renagel	Tablet	Expands in liquid if broken/crushed.
Renvela	Tablet	Enteric-coated[2]; expands in liquid if broken or crushed
Requip XL	Tablet	Extended release
Rescriptor	Tablet	If unable to swallow, may dissolve 100 mg tablets in water and drink; 200 mg tablets must be swallowed whole
Revlimid	Capsule	Teratogenic potential; hazardous substance[11]; health care workers should avoid contact with capsule contents/body fluids
RisperDAL M-Tab	Tablet	Orally disintegrating. Do not chew or break tablet; after dissolving under tongue, tablet may be swallowed
Ritalin LA	Capsule	Extended release[1]
Ritalin-SR	Tablet	Extended release
Rythmol SR	Capsule	Extended release
Ryzolt	Tablet	Extended release; tablet disruption may cause overdose
SandIMMUNE	Capsule	Teratogenic potential; hazardous substance[11]
Saphris	Tablet	Sublingual form[7]
Sensipar	Tablet	Tablets are not scored and cutting may cause inaccurate dosage
SEROquel XR	Tablet	Extended release
Sinemet CR	Tablet	Extended release[8]
Sitavig	Tablet	Buccal tablet; swallowing whole or crushing eliminates or reduces effectiveness
Slo-Niacin	Tablet	Slow release[8]
Slow-Mag	Tablet	Delayed release
Solodyn	Tablet	Extended release
Somnote	Capsule	Liquid filled
Soriatane	Capsule	Teratogenic potential; hazardous substance[11]
Sprycel	Tablet	Film-coated. Active ingredients are surrounded by a wax matrix to prevent health care exposure. Women who are, or may become pregnant, should not handle crushed or broken tablets; teratogenic potential; hazardous substance[11]
Stavzor	Capsule	Delayed release; hazardous substance[11]
Stivarga	Tablet	Manufacturer recommendation; teratogenic potential; hazardous substance[11]
Strattera	Capsule	Capsule contents can cause ocular irritation.
Sudafed 12-Hour	Capsule	Extended release[2]
Sudafed 24-Hour	Capsule	Extended release[2]
Sulfazine EC	Tablet	Delayed release, enteric-coated
Sular	Tablet	Extended release
Sustiva	Tablet	Tablets should not be broken (capsules should be used if dosage adjustment needed)
Symax Duotab	Tablet	Controlled release
Symax SR	Tablet	Extended release
Syprine	Capsule	Potential risk of contact dermatitis
Tabloid	Tablet	Teratogenic potential; hazardous substance[11]
Tafinlar	Capsule	Teratogenic potential; hazardous substance[11]
Tamoxifen	Tablet	Teratogenic potential; hazardous substance[11]
Targretin	Capsule	Manufacturer recommendation; teratogenic potential; hazardous substance[11]
Tasigna	Capsule	Hazardous substance[11]; altering capsule may lead to high blood levels, increasing the risk of toxicity
Taztia XT	Capsule	Extended release[1]
Tecfidera	Capsule	Manufacturer recommendation; delayed release; irritant
TEGretol-XR	Tablet	Extended release[2]
Temodar	Capsule	Teratogenic potential; hazardous substance[11]. **Note:** If capsules are accidentally opened or damaged, rigorous precautions should be taken to avoid inhalation or contact of contents with the skin or mucous membranes.

Drug Product	Dosage Form	Dosage Reasons/Comments
Tessalon Perles	Capsule	Swallow whole; pharmacologic action may cause choking if chewed or opened and swallowed.
Tetracycline	Capsule	Hazardous substance[11]
Thalomid	Capsule	Teratogenic potential; hazardous substance[11]
Theo-24	Capsule	Extended release[1]; contains beads that dissolve through GI tract
Theochron	Tablet	Extended release
Theophylline ER	Tablet	Extended release
Tiazac	Capsule	Extended release[1]
Topamax	Capsule	Taste[1]
Topamax	Tablet	Taste
Toprol XL	Tablet	Extended release[8]
Toviaz	Tablet	Extended release
Tracleer	Tablet	Teratogenic potential; hazardous substance[10,11]; women who are or may be pregnant should not handle crushed or broken tablets
TRENtal	Tablet	Extended release
Treximet	Tablet	Unique formulation enhances rapid drug absorption
TriLipix	Capsule	Extended release
Trokendi XR	Capsule	Extended release
Tylenol Arthritis Pain	Caplet	Controlled release
Tylenol 8 Hour	Caplet	Extended release
Uceris	Tablet	Extended release; coating on tablet designed to break down at pH of ≥7
Ultram ER	Tablet	Extended release. Tablet disruption my cause a potentially fatal overdose.
Ultresa	Capsule	Delayed release; enteric-coated contents
Ultrase	Capsule	Enteric-coated[1]
Ultrase MT	Capsule	Enteric-coated[1]
Uniphyl	Tablet	Slow release
Urocit-K	Tablet	Wax-coated; prevents upper GI release
Uroxatral	Tablet	Extended release
Valcyte	Tablet	Irritant potential[2]; teratogenic potential; hazardous substance[11]
Vascepa	Capsule	Manufacturer recommendation
Venlafaxine ER	Tablet	Extended release
Verapamil SR	Tablet	Extended release[8]
Verelan	Capsule	Sustained release[1]
Verelan PM	Capsule	Extended release[1]
Vesanoid	Capsule	Teratogenic potential; hazardous substance[11]
VESIcare	Tablet	Enteric-coated
Videx EC	Capsule	Delayed release
Vimovo	Tablet	Delayed release
Viokace	Tablet	Mucous membrane irritant
Viramune XR	Tablet	Extended release[2]
Voltaren-XR	Tablet	Extended release
VoSpire ER	Tablet	Extended release
Votrient	Tablet	Crushing significantly increases AUC and T_{max}; hazardous substance[11]; crushed or broken tablets may cause dangerous skin problems
Wellbutrin	Tablet	Film-coated
Wellbutrin SR	Tablet	Extended release
Wellbutrin XL	Tablet	Extended release
Xalkori	Capsule	Teratogenic potential; hazardous substance[11]
Xanax XR	Tablet	Extended release
Xeloda	Tablet	Teratogenic potential; hazardous substance[11].
Xigduo XR	Tablet	Extended release
Xtandi	Capsule	Teratogenic potential; hazardous substance[11]

Drug Product	Dosage Form	Dosage Reasons/Comments
Zegerid OTC	Capsule	Delayed release[2]
Zelboraf	Tablet	Teratogenic potential; hazardous substance[11]
Zenpep	Capsule	Delayed release[1]; enteric-coated contents
Zohydro ER	Capsule	Extended release; capsule disruption may cause a potentially fatal overdose
Zolinza	Capsule	Irritant; avoid contact with skin or mucous membranes; use gloves to handle; teratogenic potential; hazardous substance[11]
Zomig-ZMT	Tablet	Oral-disintegrating form[7]
Zortress	Tablet	Mucous membrane irritant; teratogenic potential; hazardous substance[11]
Zyban	Tablet	Slow release
Zydelig	Tablet	Manufacturer recommendation
Zyflo CR	Tablet	Extended release
ZyrTEC-D Allergy & Congestion	Tablet	Extended release
Zytiga	Tablet	Teratogenic potential; hazardous substance[11]; women who are or may be pregnant should wear gloves if handling tablets

[1]Capsule may be opened and the contents taken without crushing or chewing; soft food, such as applesauce or pudding, may facilitate administration; contents may generally be administered via nasogastric tube using an appropriate fluid, provided entire contents are washed down the tube.

[2]Liquid dosage forms of the product are available; however, dose, frequency of administration, and manufacturers may differ from that of the solid dosage form.

[3]Antacids and/or milk may prematurely dissolve the coating of the tablet.

[4]Capsule may be opened and the liquid contents removed for administration.

[5]The taste of this product in a liquid form would likely be unacceptable to the patient; administration via nasogastric tube should be acceptable.

[6]Effervescent tablets must be dissolved in the amount of diluent recommended by the manufacturer.

[7]Tablets are made to disintegrate under (or on) the tongue.

[8]Tablet is scored and may be broken in half without affecting release characteristics.

[9]Skin contact may enhance tumor production; avoid direct contact.

[10]Prescribing information recommends that women who are, or may become, pregnant should not handle medication, especially if crushed or broken; avoid direct contact.

[11]Potentially hazardous or hazardous substance; refer to institution-specific guidelines for precautions to observe when handling this substance.

[12]Altering (eg, chewing, crushing, splitting, opening) the dosage form has not been studied, according to the manufacturer.

REFERENCES

Mitchell JF. Oral dosage forms that should not be crushed. Available at http://www.ismp.org/tools/DoNotCrush.pdf. Accessed November 11, 2011.

National Institute for Occupational Safety and Health (NIOSH). NIOSH list of antineoplastic and other hazardous drugs in healthcare settings 2012. Available at http://www.cdc.gov/niosh/docs/2012-150/pdfs/2012-150.pdf. Accessed July 11, 2012.

PHARMACOLOGIC CATEGORY INDEX

Abortifacient
Carboprost Tromethamine ... 360
Dinoprostone ... 640
Mifepristone ... 1366

Acetylcholinesterase Inhibitor
Echothiophate Iodide ... 703
Edrophonium ... 706
Edrophonium and Atropine ... 706
Neostigmine ... 1438
Physostigmine ... 1647
Pyridostigmine ... 1746

Acetylcholinesterase Inhibitor (Central)
Donepezil ... 668
Galantamine ... 946
Rivastigmine ... 1833

Acne Products
Adapalene ... 54
Adapalene and Benzoyl Peroxide ... 54
Benzoyl Peroxide and Hydrocortisone ... 248
Clindamycin and Tretinoin ... 464
Cyproterone and Ethinyl Estradiol [CAN/INT] ... 532
Erythromycin and Benzoyl Peroxide ... 765
Erythromycin (Topical) ... 765
ISOtretinoin ... 1127
Sulfacetamide (Topical) ... 1943
Sulfur and Sulfacetamide ... 1953
Tazarotene ... 1980
Tretinoin (Topical) ... 2099

Activated Prothrombin Complex Concentrate (aPCC)
Anti-inhibitor Coagulant Complex (Human) ... 155

Adhesiolytic
Icodextrin ... 1037

Adrenergic Agonist Agent
DOBUTamine ... 654
DOPamine ... 669
Phenylephrine and Zinc Sulfate [CAN/INT] ... 1640

Aldehyde Dehydrogenase Inhibitor
Disulfiram ... 654

Alkalinizing Agent
Citric Acid, Sodium Citrate, and Potassium Citrate ... 455
Electrolyte Solution, Renal Replacement ... 710
Sodium Bicarbonate ... 1901

Alkalinizing Agent, Oral
Potassium Citrate and Citric Acid ... 1689
Sodium Citrate and Citric Acid ... 1905

Alkalinizing Agent, Parenteral
Tromethamine ... 2107

Alkylamine Derivative
Acrivastine and Pseudoephedrine ... 46
Brompheniramine ... 292
Chlorpheniramine and Acetaminophen ... 426
Chlorpheniramine and Phenylephrine ... 426
Chlorpheniramine and Pseudoephedrine ... 427
Chlorpheniramine, Phenylephrine, and Dextromethorphan ... 428
Chlorpheniramine, Pseudoephedrine, and Dextromethorphan ... 428
Dexchlorpheniramine ... 603
Dextromethorphan and Chlorpheniramine ... 610
Dihydrocodeine, Chlorpheniramine, and Phenylephrine ... 633
Hydrocodone and Chlorpheniramine ... 1012
Naphazoline and Pheniramine ... 1426
Triprolidine and Pseudoephedrine ... 2105
Triprolidine, Pseudoephedrine, and Codeine [CAN/INT] ... 2105

Allergen-Specific Immunotherapy
Grass Pollen Allergen Extract (Timothy Grass) ... 985

Alpha$_1$ Agonist
Midodrine ... 1365
Naphazoline and Pheniramine ... 1426
Naphazoline (Nasal) ... 1426
Naphazoline (Ophthalmic) ... 1426

Alpha$_1$ Blocker
Alfuzosin ... 84
Doxazosin ... 674
Dutasteride and Tamsulosin ... 702
Phenoxybenzamine ... 1635
Phentolamine ... 1636
Prazosin ... 1703
Silodosin ... 1885
Tamsulosin ... 1974
Terazosin ... 2001

Alpha$_2$-Adrenergic Agonist
Brimonidine (Topical) ... 288
CloNIDine ... 480
Dexmedetomidine ... 604
GuanFACINE ... 990
Lofexidine [INT] ... 1232
Methyldopa ... 1332
TiZANidine ... 2051

Alpha$_2$ Agonist, Ophthalmic
Apraclonidine ... 165
Brimonidine and Timolol ... 288
Brimonidine (Ophthalmic) ... 288

Alpha-Adrenergic Agonist
Chlorpheniramine and Phenylephrine ... 426
Chlorpheniramine, Phenylephrine, and Dextromethorphan ... 428
Dihydrocodeine, Chlorpheniramine, and Phenylephrine ... 633
Diphenhydramine and Phenylephrine ... 644
Phenylephrine (Systemic) ... 1638

Alpha-Adrenergic Blocking Agent, Oral
Indoramin [INT] ... 1070

Alpha/Beta Agonist
Acrivastine and Pseudoephedrine ... 46
Chlorpheniramine and Pseudoephedrine ... 427
Chlorpheniramine, Pseudoephedrine, and Dextromethorphan ... 428
Desloratadine and Pseudoephedrine ... 594
Dipivefrin ... 651
EPHEDrine (Systemic) ... 734
EPINEPHrine (Systemic, Oral Inhalation) ... 735
Etilefrine [INT] ... 815
Fexofenadine and Pseudoephedrine ... 874
Guaifenesin and Pseudoephedrine ... 989
Loratadine and Pseudoephedrine ... 1242
Norepinephrine ... 1472
Pseudoephedrine ... 1742
Triprolidine and Pseudoephedrine ... 2105
Triprolidine, Pseudoephedrine, and Codeine [CAN/INT] ... 2105

5 Alpha-Reductase Inhibitor
Dutasteride ... 702
Dutasteride and Tamsulosin ... 702
Finasteride ... 878

Amebicide
Iodoquinol ... 1105

MetroNIDAZOLE (Systemic) ... 1353
Paromomycin ... 1579

Amino Acid
Glutamine ... 971

Aminoquinoline (Antimalarial)
Chloroquine ... 424
Hydroxychloroquine ... 1021
Primaquine ... 1713

5-Aminosalicylic Acid Derivative
Balsalazide ... 226
Mesalamine ... 1301
Olsalazine ... 1500
SulfaSALAzine ... 1950

Ammonium Detoxicant
Lactulose ... 1156
Neomycin ... 1436

AMPA Glutamate Receptor Antagonist
Perampanel ... 1620

Amylinomimetic
Pramlintide ... 1697

Anabolic Steroid
Oxymetholone ... 1546

Analgesic Combination (Opioid)
Acetaminophen and Codeine ... 36
Acetaminophen and Tramadol ... 37
Belladonna and Opium ... 238
Hydrocodone and Acetaminophen ... 1012
Hydrocodone and Ibuprofen ... 1013
Oxycodone and Acetaminophen ... 1541
Oxycodone and Aspirin ... 1542
Oxycodone and Ibuprofen ... 1542

Analgesic, Miscellaneous
Acetaminophen ... 32
Acetaminophen and Diphenhydramine ... 36
Acetaminophen and Tramadol ... 37
Acetaminophen, Aspirin, and Caffeine ... 37
Acetaminophen, Codeine, and Doxylamine [CAN/INT] ... 37
Aspirin and Diphenhydramine ... 185
Butalbital and Acetaminophen ... 314
Chlorpheniramine and Acetaminophen ... 426
Pregabalin ... 1710
Tetrahydrocannabinol and Cannabidiol [CAN/INT] ... 2018

Analgesic, Nonopioid
Bupivacaine (Liposomal) ... 299
Methotrimeprazine [CAN/INT] ... 1329
Ziconotide ... 2196

Analgesic, Nonsteroidal Anti-inflammatory Drug
Aceclofenac [INT] ... 30
Azapropazone [INT] ... 210
Dexketoprofen [INT] ... 603
Dipyrone [INT] ... 653
Etoricoxib [INT] ... 821
Fenbufen [INT] ... 852
Niflumic Acid [INT] ... 1454
Nimesulide [INT] ... 1456
Parecoxib [INT] ... 1576
Tenoxicam [INT] ... 2001

Analgesic, Opioid
Acetaminophen and Codeine ... 36
Acetaminophen, Codeine, and Doxylamine [CAN/INT] ... 37
Alfentanil ... 83
Belladonna and Opium ... 238
Buprenorphine ... 300
Buprenorphine and Naloxone ... 304
Butorphanol ... 314
Codeine ... 497
Dihydrocodeine, Aspirin, and Caffeine ... 632
Dihydrocodeine, Chlorpheniramine, and Phenylephrine ... 633
FentaNYL ... 857
Hydrocodone and Acetaminophen ... 1012
Hydrocodone and Chlorpheniramine ... 1012
HYDROmorphone ... 1016
Levorphanol ... 1204
Meperidine ... 1293
Methadone ... 1311
Morphine (Liposomal) ... 1400
Morphine (Systemic) ... 1394
Nalbuphine ... 1416
Opium Tincture ... 1518
OxyCODONE ... 1538
Oxycodone and Acetaminophen ... 1541
Oxycodone and Aspirin ... 1542
Oxycodone and Ibuprofen ... 1542
Oxycodone and Naloxone ... 1542
Oxymorphone ... 1546
Paregoric ... 1577
Pentazocine ... 1616
Promethazine and Codeine ... 1725
Remifentanil ... 1789
SUFentanil ... 1941
Tapentadol ... 1975
TraMADol ... 2074
Triprolidine, Pseudoephedrine, and Codeine [CAN/INT] ... 2105

Analgesic, Opioid Partial Agonist
Buprenorphine ... 300
Buprenorphine and Naloxone ... 304
Butorphanol ... 314
Nalbuphine ... 1416
Pentazocine ... 1616

Analgesic, Topical
Benzyl Alcohol ... 250
Diethylamine Salicylate [INT] ... 624
Lidocaine and Tetracaine ... 1214
Lidocaine (Topical) ... 1211
Methyl Salicylate and Menthol ... 1344

Analgesic, Urinary
Pentosan Polysulfate Sodium ... 1617
Phenazopyridine ... 1629

Androgen
Danazol ... 558
Fluoxymesterone ... 903
Mesterolone [INT] ... 1307
MethylTESTOSTERone ... 1345
Oxandrolone ... 1531
Testosterone ... 2010

Anesthetic/Corticosteroid
Pramoxine and Hydrocortisone ... 1698

Anesthetic, Topical
Fluorescein and Benoxinate ... 895

Angiogenesis Inhibitor
Lenalidomide ... 1177
Pomalidomide ... 1677
Ranibizumab ... 1776
Thalidomide ... 2022

Angiotensin II Receptor Blocker
Amlodipine and Olmesartan ... 126
Amlodipine and Valsartan ... 126
Amlodipine, Valsartan, and Hydrochlorothiazide ... 127

Azilsartan 214
Azilsartan and Chlorthalidone 215
Candesartan 335
Candesartan and Hydrochlorothiazide 338
Eprosartan 748
Eprosartan and Hydrochlorothiazide 750
Irbesartan 1110
Irbesartan and Hydrochlorothiazide 1112
Losartan 1248
Losartan and Hydrochlorothiazide 1250
Olmesartan 1496
Olmesartan, Amlodipine, and Hydrochlorothiazide 1498
Olmesartan and Hydrochlorothiazide 1498
Telmisartan 1988
Telmisartan and Amlodipine 1989
Telmisartan and Hydrochlorothiazide 1990
Valsartan 2127
Valsartan and Hydrochlorothiazide 2129

Angiotensin-Converting Enzyme (ACE) Inhibitor

Amlodipine and Benazepril 125
Benazepril 238
Benazepril and Hydrochlorothiazide 240
Captopril 342
Captopril and Hydrochlorothiazide 345
Cilazapril [CAN/INT] 434
Cilazapril and Hydrochlorothiazide [CAN/INT] 436
Delapril [INT] 587
Enalapril 722
Enalapril and Hydrochlorothiazide 725
Fosinopril 932
Imidapril [INT] 1051
Lisinopril 1226
Lisinopril and Hydrochlorothiazide 1229
Moexipril 1388
Moexipril and Hydrochlorothiazide 1388
Perindopril 1623
Perindopril and Indapamide [CAN/INT] 1626
Quinapril 1756
Ramipril 1771
Ramipril and Hydrochlorothiazide [CAN/INT] 1773
Spirapril [INT] 1931
Temocapril [INT] 1991
Trandolapril 2080
Trandolapril and Verapamil 2080
Zofenopril [INT] 2206

Anilidopiperidine Opioid

Alfentanil 83
FentaNYL 857
Remifentanil 1789
SUFentanil 1941

Anorexiant

Diethylpropion 624
Lorcaserin 1246
Methamphetamine 1315
Naltrexone and Bupropion 1423
Phentermine 1635

Antacid

Aluminum Hydroxide 103
Aluminum Hydroxide and Magnesium Carbonate 103
Aluminum Hydroxide and Magnesium Hydroxide 103
Aluminum Hydroxide and Magnesium Trisilicate 103
Aluminum Hydroxide, Magnesium Hydroxide, and Simethicone 104
Calcium Carbonate 327
Calcium Carbonate and Magnesium Hydroxide 328
Magaldrate and Simethicone 1261
Magnesium Hydroxide 1263
Sodium Bicarbonate 1901

Anthelmintic

Albendazole 65
Ivermectin (Systemic) 1136
Mebendazole [CAN/INT] 1274
Praziquantel 1702
Pyrantel Pamoate 1744
Triclabendazole [INT] 2102

Anthraquinone

Diacerein [INT] 613

Antiandrogen

Abiraterone Acetate 26
Cyproterone [CAN/INT] 530
Dienogest [CAN/INT] 623

Antianginal Agent

Aliskiren, Amlodipine, and Hydrochlorothiazide 87
AmLODIPine 123
Amlodipine and Atorvastatin 124
Amlodipine and Benazepril 125
Amlodipine and Olmesartan 126
Amlodipine and Valsartan 126
Amlodipine, Valsartan, and Hydrochlorothiazide 127
Amyl Nitrite 147
Atenolol 189
Diltiazem 634
Isosorbide Dinitrate 1124
Isosorbide Mononitrate 1126
Metoprolol 1350
Nadolol 1411
NiCARdipine 1446
NIFEdipine 1451
Nitroglycerin 1465
Olmesartan, Amlodipine, and Hydrochlorothiazide 1498
Perhexiline [INT] 1621
Propranolol 1731
Ranolazine 1779
Telmisartan and Amlodipine 1989
Verapamil 2154

Antianxiety Agent

Carpipramine [INT] 367

Antianxiety Agent, Miscellaneous

BusPIRone 311
Meprobamate 1296

Antiarrhythmic Agent, Class I

Vernakalant [INT] 2157

Antiarrhythmic Agent, Class Ia

Disopyramide 653
Procainamide 1716
QuiNIDine 1759

Antiarrhythmic Agent, Class Ib

Lidocaine (Systemic) 1208
Mexiletine 1359

Antiarrhythmic Agent, Class Ic

Flecainide 882
Propafenone 1725

Antiarrhythmic Agent, Class II

Acebutolol 29
Esmolol 769
Propranolol 1731
Sotalol 1927

Antiarrhythmic Agent, Class III

Amiodarone 114
Dofetilide 662
Dronedarone 695
Ibutilide 1036

Sotalol ... 1927
Vernakalant [INT] ... 2157

Antiarrhythmic Agent, Class IV
Digitoxin [INT] ... 627
Diltiazem ... 634
Verapamil ... 2154

Antiarrhythmic Agent, Miscellaneous
Adenosine ... 55
Digoxin ... 627

Antiasthmatic
Bamifylline [INT] ... 227

Antibiotic, Aminoglycoside
Amikacin ... 111
Dibekacin [INT] ... 616
Gentamicin (Ophthalmic) ... 962
Gentamicin (Systemic) ... 959
Isepamicin [INT] ... 1120
Kanamycin ... 1142
Neomycin ... 1436
Streptomycin ... 1937
Tobramycin (Ophthalmic) ... 2056
Tobramycin (Systemic, Oral Inhalation) ... 2052

Antibiotic, Carbapenem
Doripenem ... 671
Ertapenem ... 760
Imipenem and Cilastatin ... 1051
Meropenem ... 1299

Antibiotic, Cephalosporin
Cefoperazone and Sulbactam [INT] ... 382

Antibiotic, Cephalosporin (First Generation)
Cefadroxil ... 372
CeFAZolin ... 373
Cephalexin ... 405

Antibiotic, Cephalosporin (Second Generation)
Cefaclor ... 372
CefoTEtan ... 385
CefOXitin ... 386
Cefprozil ... 389
Cefuroxime ... 399

Antibiotic, Cephalosporin (Third Generation)
Cefdinir ... 376
Cefditoren ... 378
Cefixime ... 380
Cefotaxime ... 382
Cefpodoxime ... 388
Cefsulodin [INT] ... 391
CefTAZidime ... 392
Ceftibuten ... 394
CefTRIAXone ... 396

Antibiotic, Cephalosporin (Fourth Generation)
Cefepime ... 378
Cefpirome [INT] ... 388

Antibiotic, Cephalosporin (Fifth Generation)
Ceftaroline Fosamil ... 391
Ceftolozane and Tazobactam ... 394

Antibiotic/Corticosteroid, Ophthalmic
Loteprednol and Tobramycin ... 1251
Neomycin, Polymyxin B, and Dexamethasone ... 1437
Neomycin, Polymyxin B, and Hydrocortisone ... 1438
Prednisolone and Gentamicin ... 1706
Sulfacetamide and Prednisolone ... 1944
Tobramycin and Dexamethasone ... 2056

Antibiotic/Corticosteroid, Otic
Ciprofloxacin and Dexamethasone ... 446
Ciprofloxacin and Hydrocortisone ... 446
Neomycin, Colistin, Hydrocortisone, and Thonzonium ... 1437
Neomycin, Polymyxin B, and Hydrocortisone ... 1438

Antibiotic/Corticosteroid, Topical
Neomycin, Polymyxin B, and Hydrocortisone ... 1438

Antibiotic, Cyclic Lipopeptide
DAPTOmycin ... 563

Antibiotic, Fluoroquinolone
Besifloxacin ... 251
Ciprofloxacin (Ophthalmic) ... 446
Ciprofloxacin (Otic) ... 446
Ciprofloxacin (Systemic) ... 441
Gatifloxacin ... 949
Gemifloxacin ... 957
Levofloxacin (Ophthalmic) ... 1200
Levofloxacin (Systemic) ... 1197
Moxifloxacin (Ophthalmic) ... 1403
Moxifloxacin (Systemic) ... 1401
Norfloxacin ... 1475
Ofloxacin (Ophthalmic) ... 1491
Ofloxacin (Otic) ... 1491
Ofloxacin (Systemic) ... 1490

Antibiotic, Glycylcycline
Tigecycline ... 2040

Antibiotic, Irrigation
Polymyxin B ... 1676

Antibiotic, Ketolide
Telithromycin ... 1987

Antibiotic, Lincosamide
Clindamycin (Systemic) ... 460
Clindamycin (Topical) ... 464

Antibiotic, Macrolide
Azithromycin (Ophthalmic) ... 219
Azithromycin (Systemic) ... 216
Clarithromycin ... 456
Erythromycin and Sulfisoxazole ... 765
Erythromycin (Ophthalmic) ... 764
Erythromycin (Systemic) ... 762
Erythromycin (Topical) ... 765
Fidaxomicin ... 875
Josamycin [INT] ... 1141
Midecamycin [INT] ... 1365
Roxithromycin [INT] ... 1853
Spiramycin [CAN/INT] ... 1931

Antibiotic, Macrolide Combination
Erythromycin and Sulfisoxazole ... 765
Lansoprazole, Amoxicillin, and Clarithromycin ... 1169
Omeprazole, Clarithromycin, and Amoxicillin ... 1511

Antibiotic, Miscellaneous
Aztreonam ... 220
Bacitracin (Systemic) ... 222
Chloramphenicol ... 421
Clofazimine [INT] ... 473
Colistimethate ... 504
Dapsone (Systemic) ... 561
Fosfomycin ... 932
Fusidic Acid (Ophthalmic) [CAN/INT] ... 942
Fusidic Acid (Systemic) [INT] ... 942
Fusidic Acid (Topical) [CAN/INT] ... 943
Methenamine ... 1317
Methenamine and Sodium Acid Phosphate ... 1318
Methenamine, Phenyl Salicylate, Methylene Blue, Benzoic Acid, and Hyoscyamine ... 1318

Methenamine, Sodium Phosphate Monobasic, Phenyl Salicylate, Methylene Blue, and Hyoscyamine ... 1318
MetroNIDAZOLE (Systemic) ... 1353
Nitrofurantoin ... 1463
Nitroxoline [INT] ... 1469
Polymyxin B ... 1676
Rifabutin ... 1803
Rifampin ... 1804
Rifaximin ... 1809
Secnidazole [INT] ... 1872
Sulfamethoxazole and Trimethoprim ... 1946
Teicoplanin [INT] ... 1983
Trimethoprim ... 2104

Antibiotic, Ophthalmic

Azithromycin (Ophthalmic) ... 219
Bacitracin and Polymyxin B ... 222
Bacitracin, Neomycin, and Polymyxin B ... 223
Bacitracin, Neomycin, Polymyxin B, and Hydrocortisone ... 223
Bacitracin (Ophthalmic) ... 222
Besifloxacin ... 251
Ciprofloxacin (Ophthalmic) ... 446
Erythromycin (Ophthalmic) ... 764
Framycetin [INT] ... 937
Fusidic Acid (Ophthalmic) [CAN/INT] ... 942
Gatifloxacin ... 949
Gentamicin (Ophthalmic) ... 962
Levofloxacin (Ophthalmic) ... 1200
Moxifloxacin (Ophthalmic) ... 1403
Neomycin, Polymyxin B, and Gramicidin ... 1437
Neomycin, Polymyxin B, and Hydrocortisone ... 1438
Ofloxacin (Ophthalmic) ... 1491
Sulfacetamide (Ophthalmic) ... 1943
Tobramycin (Ophthalmic) ... 2056
Trimethoprim and Polymyxin B ... 2105

Antibiotic, Oral Rinse

Chlorhexidine Gluconate ... 422

Antibiotic, Otic

Ciprofloxacin and Dexamethasone ... 446
Ciprofloxacin and Hydrocortisone ... 446
Ciprofloxacin (Otic) ... 446
Framycetin [INT] ... 937
Neomycin, Colistin, Hydrocortisone, and Thonzonium ... 1437
Neomycin, Polymyxin B, and Hydrocortisone ... 1438
Ofloxacin (Otic) ... 1491

Antibiotic, Oxazolidinone

Linezolid ... 1217
Tedizolid ... 1981

Antibiotic, Penicillin

Amoxicillin ... 130
Amoxicillin and Clavulanate ... 133
Amoxicillin and Cloxacillin [INT] ... 136
Ampicillin ... 141
Ampicillin and Cloxacillin [INT] ... 144
Ampicillin and Sulbactam ... 145
Cloxacillin [CAN/INT] ... 488
Dicloxacillin ... 621
Flucloxacillin [INT] ... 885
Lansoprazole, Amoxicillin, and Clarithromycin ... 1169
Nafcillin ... 1414
Omeprazole, Clarithromycin, and Amoxicillin ... 1511
Oxacillin ... 1528
Penicillin V Potassium ... 1614
Penicillin G Benzathine ... 1609
Penicillin G Benzathine and Penicillin G Procaine ... 1611
Penicillin G (Parenteral/Aqueous) ... 1611
Penicillin G Procaine ... 1613
Piperacillin [CAN/INT] ... 1656
Piperacillin and Tazobactam ... 1657
Pivmecillinam [INT] ... 1663
Ticarcillin and Clavulanate Potassium [CAN/INT] ... 2038

Antibiotic, Pleuromutilin

Retapamulin ... 1793

Antibiotic, Quinolone

Lomefloxacin [INT] ... 1233
Nadifloxacin [INT] ... 1411
Nalidixic Acid [INT] ... 1418
Pefloxacin [INT] ... 1588
Prulifloxacin [INT] ... 1742
Rufloxacin [INT] ... 1855
Sparfloxacin [INT] ... 1930

Antibiotic, Respiratory Fluoroquinolone

Gemifloxacin ... 957
Levofloxacin (Systemic) ... 1197
Moxifloxacin (Systemic) ... 1401

Antibiotic, Streptogramin

Quinupristin and Dalfopristin ... 1762

Antibiotic, Sulfonamide Derivative

Erythromycin and Sulfisoxazole ... 765
Sulfacetamide (Topical) ... 1943
SulfADIAZINE ... 1944
Sulfamethoxazole and Trimethoprim ... 1946
Sulfur and Sulfacetamide ... 1953

Antibiotic, Tetracycline Derivative

Demeclocycline ... 589
Doxycycline ... 689
Minocycline ... 1371
Tetracycline ... 2017

Antibiotic, Topical

Bacitracin and Polymyxin B ... 222
Bacitracin, Neomycin, and Polymyxin B ... 223
Bacitracin, Neomycin, Polymyxin B, and Hydrocortisone ... 223
Bacitracin (Topical) ... 222
Chlorhexidine Gluconate ... 422
Clioquinol and Flumethasone [CAN/INT] ... 465
Erythromycin (Topical) ... 765
Fusidic Acid (Topical) [CAN/INT] ... 943
Gentian Violet ... 962
Mafenide ... 1261
MetroNIDAZOLE (Topical) ... 1357
Mupirocin ... 1404
Neomycin ... 1436
Neomycin and Polymyxin B ... 1437
Neomycin, Polymyxin B, and Hydrocortisone ... 1438
Retapamulin ... 1793
Silver Nitrate ... 1886
Silver Sulfadiazine ... 1887

Anticholinergic Agent

Atropine ... 200
Atropine and Pralidoxime ... 203
Benztropine ... 248
Darifenacin ... 568
Dicyclomine ... 622
Edrophonium and Atropine ... 706
Fesoterodine ... 872
Glycopyrrolate ... 975
Hyoscyamine ... 1026
Hyoscyamine, Atropine, Scopolamine, and Phenobarbital ... 1027
Indacaterol and Glycopyrronium [CAN/INT] ... 1063
Ipratropium and Albuterol ... 1109
Ipratropium and Fenoterol [CAN/INT] ... 1109
Ipratropium (Nasal) ... 1109

Ipratropium (Systemic) ... 1108
Oxitropium [INT] ... 1536
Pirenzepine [INT] ... 1662
Prifinium [INT] ... 1712
Procyclidine [CAN/INT] ... 1721
Propantheline ... 1727
Propiverine [INT] ... 1728
Scopolamine (Systemic) ... 1870
Solifenacin ... 1917
Tiotropium ... 2046
Tolterodine ... 2063
Trihexyphenidyl ... 2103
Trospium ... 2108
Umeclidinium ... 2113

Anticholinergic Agent, Long-Acting
Tiotropium ... 2046
Umeclidinium ... 2113

Anticholinergic Agent, Ophthalmic
Atropine ... 200
Cyclopentolate ... 517
Homatropine ... 1005

Anticoagulant
Acenocoumarol [CAN/INT] ... 30
Antithrombin ... 156
Apixaban ... 158
Argatroban ... 168
Bivalirudin ... 268
Dabigatran Etexilate ... 542
Dalteparin ... 553
Danaparoid [CAN/INT] ... 556
Desirudin ... 593
Enoxaparin ... 726
Fondaparinux ... 924
Heparin ... 997
Nadroparin [CAN/INT] ... 1412
Rivaroxaban ... 1830
Tinzaparin ... 2043
Warfarin ... 2186

Anticoagulant, Coumarin Derivative
Phenprocoumon [INT] ... 1635

Anticoagulant, Direct Thrombin Inhibitor
Argatroban ... 168
Bivalirudin ... 268
Dabigatran Etexilate ... 542
Desirudin ... 593

Anticoagulant, Factor Xa Inhibitor
Apixaban ... 158
Fondaparinux ... 924
Rivaroxaban ... 1830

Anticoagulant, Heparin
Heparin ... 997

Anticoagulant, Heparinoid
Danaparoid [CAN/INT] ... 556

Anticoagulant, Indanedione
Fluindione [INT] ... 892

Anticoagulant, Low Molecular Weight Heparin
Dalteparin ... 553
Enoxaparin ... 726
Nadroparin [CAN/INT] ... 1412
Tinzaparin ... 2043

Anticoagulant, Vitamin K Antagonist
Acenocoumarol [CAN/INT] ... 30
Warfarin ... 2186

Anticonvulsant, Barbiturate
PENTobarbital ... 1617
PHENobarbital ... 1632
Thiopental [INT] ... 2029

Anticonvulsant, Hydantoin
Fosphenytoin ... 934
Phenytoin ... 1640

Anticonvulsant, Miscellaneous
AcetaZOLAMIDE ... 39
Barbexaclone [INT] ... 227
CarBAMazepine ... 346
Felbamate ... 850
Gabapentin ... 943
Gabapentin Enacarbil ... 946
Lacosamide ... 1154
LamoTRIgine ... 1160
LevETIRAcetam ... 1191
Magnesium Sulfate ... 1265
OXcarbazepine ... 1532
Paraldehyde [CAN/INT] ... 1575
Perampanel ... 1620
Pregabalin ... 1710
Primidone ... 1714
Stiripentol [CAN/INT] ... 1935
TiaGABine ... 2032
Topiramate ... 2065
Valproic Acid and Derivatives ... 2123
Vigabatrin ... 2158
Zonisamide ... 2215

Anticonvulsant, Neuronal Potassium Channel Opener
Ezogabine ... 835

Anticonvulsant, Succinimide
Ethosuximide ... 813
Methsuximide ... 1331

Anticonvulsant, Triazole Derivative
Rufinamide ... 1854

Anticystine Agent
Cysteamine (Ophthalmic) ... 535
Cysteamine (Systemic) ... 534

Antidepressant, Alpha-2 Antagonist
Mirtazapine ... 1376

Antidepressant, Dopamine/Norepinephrine-Reuptake Inhibitor
BuPROPion ... 305
Naltrexone and Bupropion ... 1423

Antidepressant, Monoamine Oxidase Inhibitor
Phenelzine ... 1630
Selegiline ... 1873
Tranylcypromine ... 2083

Antidepressant, Monoamine Oxidase Inhibitor, Reversible
Moclobemide [CAN/INT] ... 1384

Antidepressant, Selective Serotonin Reuptake Inhibitor
Citalopram ... 451
Escitalopram ... 765
FLUoxetine ... 899
FluvoxaMINE ... 916
PARoxetine ... 1579
Sertraline ... 1878
Vortioxetine ... 2183

Antidepressant, Selective Serotonin Reuptake Inhibitor/5-HT_{1A} Receptor Partial Agonist
Vilazodone ... 2158

Antidepressant, Serotonin/Norepinephrine Reuptake Inhibitor
Desvenlafaxine 598
DULoxetine 698
Milnacipran 1368
Venlafaxine 2150

Antidepressant, Serotonin Reuptake Facilitator
Tianeptine [INT] 2033

Antidepressant, Serotonin Reuptake Inhibitor/Antagonist
Nefazodone 1435
TraZODone 2091

Antidepressant, Tetracyclic
Maprotiline 1271

Antidepressant, Tricyclic
Dosulepin [INT] 673
Melitracen [INT] 1283

Antidepressant, Tricyclic (Secondary Amine)
Amoxapine 128
Desipramine 593
Nortriptyline 1476
Protriptyline 1740

Antidepressant, Tricyclic (Tertiary Amine)
Amitriptyline 119
Amitriptyline and Chlordiazepoxide 122
Amitriptyline and Perphenazine 122
ClomiPRAMINE 475
Doxepin (Systemic) 676
Imipramine 1054
Lofepramine [INT] 1232

Antidiabetic Agent
Pramlintide 1697

Antidiabetic Agent, Alpha-Glucosidase Inhibitor
Acarbose 29
Miglitol 1367

Antidiabetic Agent, Biguanide
Dapagliflozin and Metformin 561
Glipizide and Metformin 969
Glyburide and Metformin 974
Linagliptin and Metformin 1217
MetFORMIN 1307
Pioglitazone and Metformin 1655
Repaglinide and Metformin 1792
Rosiglitazone and Metformin 1847
Saxagliptin and Metformin 1869
Sitagliptin and Metformin 1898

Antidiabetic Agent, Dipeptidyl Peptidase IV (DPP-IV) Inhibitor
Linagliptin 1215
Linagliptin and Metformin 1217
Saxagliptin 1867
Saxagliptin and Metformin 1869
SitaGLIPtin 1897
Sitagliptin and Metformin 1898
Sitagliptin and Simvastatin 1899

Antidiabetic Agent, Dopamine Agonist
Bromocriptine 291

Antidiabetic Agent, Glucagon-Like Peptide-1 (GLP-1) Receptor Agonist
Albiglutide 66
Dulaglutide 697
Exenatide 830
Liraglutide 1222

Antidiabetic Agent, Meglitinide Analog
Nateglinide 1432
Repaglinide 1791
Repaglinide and Metformin 1792

Antidiabetic Agent, Sodium-Glucose Cotransporter 2 (SGLT2) Inhibitor
Dapagliflozin and Metformin 561
Empagliflozin 718

Antidiabetic Agent, Sulfonylurea
ChlorproPAMIDE 429
Gliclazide [CAN/INT] 964
Glimepiride 966
GlipiZIDE 967
Glipizide and Metformin 969
Gliquidone [INT] 970
GlyBURIDE 972
Glyburide and Metformin 974
Pioglitazone and Glimepiride 1654
Rosiglitazone and Glimepiride 1847
TOLAZamide 2062
TOLBUTamide 2062

Antidiabetic Agent, Thiazolidinedione
Pioglitazone 1654
Pioglitazone and Glimepiride 1654
Pioglitazone and Metformin 1655
Rosiglitazone 1847
Rosiglitazone and Glimepiride 1847
Rosiglitazone and Metformin 1847

Antidiarrheal
Attapulgite [CAN/INT] 204
Bismuth 265
Crofelemer 514
Diphenoxylate and Atropine 644
Loperamide 1236
Loperamide and Simethicone 1237
Nifuroxazide [INT] 1454
Octreotide 1485
Opium Tincture 1518
Paregoric 1577
Psyllium 1744

Antidiuretic Hormone Analog
Vasopressin 2142

Antidote
Acetylcysteine 40
Aluminum Hydroxide 103
Amifostine 109
Amyl Nitrite 147
Atropine 200
Atropine and Pralidoxime 203
Calcitonin 322
Calcium Acetate 326
Calcium Carbonate 327
Calcium Polystyrene Sulfonate [CAN/INT] 333
Carglumic Acid 362
Charcoal, Activated 416
Deferoxamine 586
Dexrazoxane 606
Digoxin Immune Fab 630
Dimercaprol 638
Edrophonium 706
Edrophonium and Atropine 706
Ferric Hexacyanoferrate 870
Flumazenil 892
Fomepizole 922
Glucagon 970
Glucarpidase 971
Hydroxocobalamin 1020
Leucovorin Calcium 1183
LEVOleucovorin 1200

Mesna ... 1305
Methylene Blue ... 1333
Naloxone ... 1419
Naltrexone ... 1422
Octreotide ... 1485
Phenoxybenzamine ... 1635
Physostigmine ... 1647
Potassium Iodide ... 1690
Pralidoxime ... 1694
Protamine ... 1737
Raxibacumab ... 1786
Sodium Nitrite ... 1907
Sodium Nitrite and Sodium Thiosulfate ... 1907
Sodium Phenylacetate and Sodium Benzoate ... 1908
Sodium Polystyrene Sulfonate ... 1912
Sodium Thiosulfate ... 1915
Succimer ... 1939
Sugammadex [INT] ... 1942
Uridine Triacetate ... 2116

Antidote, Extravasation

Dexrazoxane ... 606
Nitroglycerin ... 1465
Phentolamine ... 1636
Sodium Thiosulfate ... 1915
Terbutaline ... 2004

Antidote, Hypoglycemia

Diazoxide ... 616
Glucagon ... 970

Antiemetic

Aprepitant ... 166
Bromopride [INT] ... 292
Cinnarizine [INT] ... 440
Dexamethasone (Systemic) ... 599
Dolasetron ... 663
Dronabinol ... 694
Droperidol ... 695
Fosaprepitant ... 929
Granisetron ... 983
HydrOXYzine ... 1024
Meclizine ... 1277
Metoclopramide ... 1345
Netupitant and Palonosetron ... 1440
Ondansetron ... 1513
Palonosetron ... 1561
Perphenazine ... 1627
Prochlorperazine ... 1718
Promethazine ... 1723
Trimethobenzamide ... 2104

Antifibrinolytic Agent

Aminocaproic Acid ... 113
Tranexamic Acid ... 2081

Antiflatulent

Aluminum Hydroxide, Magnesium Hydroxide, and Simethicone ... 104
Loperamide and Simethicone ... 1237
Magaldrate and Simethicone ... 1261

Antifungal Agent

Fenticonazole [INT] ... 868
Pentamidine ... 1616

Antifungal Agent, Azole Derivative

Terconazole ... 2006

Antifungal Agent, Imidazole Derivative

Butoconazole ... 314
Clotrimazole (Oral) ... 488
Clotrimazole (Topical) ... 488
Econazole ... 703
Ketoconazole (Systemic) ... 1144
Ketoconazole (Topical) ... 1145
Miconazole (Topical) ... 1360
Omoconazole [INT] ... 1512
Oxiconazole ... 1536
Sertaconazole ... 1877
Sulconazole ... 1943

Antifungal Agent, Ophthalmic

Natamycin ... 1432

Antifungal Agent, Oral

Fluconazole ... 885
Flucytosine ... 889
Griseofulvin ... 985
Itraconazole ... 1130
Ketoconazole (Systemic) ... 1144
Posaconazole ... 1683
Terbinafine (Systemic) ... 2002
Voriconazole ... 2176

Antifungal Agent, Oral Nonabsorbed

Clotrimazole (Oral) ... 488
Nystatin (Oral) ... 1481

Antifungal Agent, Parenteral

Amphotericin B Cholesteryl Sulfate Complex ... 136
Amphotericin B (Conventional) ... 136
Amphotericin B (Lipid Complex) ... 138
Amphotericin B (Liposomal) ... 139
Anidulafungin ... 150
Caspofungin ... 370
Fluconazole ... 885
Micafungin ... 1359
Voriconazole ... 2176

Antifungal Agent, Topical

Amorolfine [INT] ... 128
Betamethasone and Clotrimazole ... 256
Bifonazole [INT] ... 264
Butenafine ... 314
Ciclopirox ... 433
Clioquinol and Flumethasone [CAN/INT] ... 465
Clotrimazole (Topical) ... 488
Econazole ... 703
Efinaconazole ... 710
Gentian Violet ... 962
Iodoquinol and Hydrocortisone ... 1105
Isoconazole [INT] ... 1120
Ketoconazole (Topical) ... 1145
Luliconazole ... 1256
Miconazole (Topical) ... 1360
Naftifine ... 1416
Nystatin and Triamcinolone ... 1482
Nystatin (Topical) ... 1482
Oxiconazole ... 1536
Sertaconazole ... 1877
Sulconazole ... 1943
Tavaborole ... 1980
Terbinafine (Topical) ... 2004
Tolciclate [INT] ... 2062
Tolnaftate ... 2063

Antifungal Agent, Vaginal

Butoconazole ... 314
Clotrimazole (Topical) ... 488
Metronidazole and Nystatin [CAN/INT] ... 1358
Miconazole (Topical) ... 1360
Sulfanilamide ... 1950
Terconazole ... 2006

Antigonadotropic Agent

Gestrinone [INT] ... 962

Antigout Agent

Allopurinol ... 90
Colchicine ... 500

Colchicine and Probenecid 503
Febuxostat 848

Antihemophilic Agent

Aminocaproic Acid 113
Antihemophilic Factor (Human) 152
Antihemophilic Factor (Recombinant [Porcine Sequence]) 153
Antihemophilic Factor/von Willebrand Factor Complex (Human) 154
Anti-inhibitor Coagulant Complex (Human) 155
Desmopressin 594
Factor IX Complex (Human) [(Factors II, IX, X)] 838
Factor IX (Human) 840
Factor IX (Recombinant) 841
Factor XIII Concentrate (Human) 843
Factor VIIa (Recombinant) 836
Tranexamic Acid 2081

Antihemorrhoidal Agent

Benzocaine 246
Hydrocortisone (Topical) 1014

Antihepaciviral, NS5A Inhibitor

Ledipasvir and Sofosbuvir 1173
Ombitasvir, Paritaprevir, Ritonavir, and Dasabuvir 1505

Antihepaciviral, Nucleoside (Anti-HCV)

Peginterferon Alfa-2a and Ribavirin [CAN/INT] 1592
Peginterferon Alfa-2b and Ribavirin [CAN/INT] 1598
Ribavirin 1797

Antihepaciviral, Polymerase Inhibitor (Anti-HCV)

Ledipasvir and Sofosbuvir 1173
Ombitasvir, Paritaprevir, Ritonavir, and Dasabuvir 1505
Sofosbuvir 1915

Antihepaciviral, Protease Inhibitor (Anti-HCV)

Boceprevir 273
Ombitasvir, Paritaprevir, Ritonavir, and Dasabuvir 1505
Simeprevir 1887
Telaprevir 1983

Antihepadnaviral, Reverse Transcriptase Inhibitor, Nucleoside (Anti-HBV)

Entecavir 731
LamiVUDine 1157

Antihepadnaviral, Reverse Transcriptase Inhibitor, Nucleotide (Anti-HBV)

Adefovir 54
Tenofovir 1998

Antihistamine

Dimethindene [INT] 638
Mebhydrolin [INT] 1276
Oxatomide [INT] 1532
Rupatadine [INT] 1855

Antihistamine, Low-Sedating

Mizolastine [INT] 1384

Antihistamine, Nonsedating

Ebastine [INT] 702

Antihyperlipidemic Agent, Apolipoprotein B Antisense Oligonucleotide

Mipomersen 1375

Antihypertensive

Acebutolol 29
Aliskiren, Amlodipine, and Hydrochlorothiazide 87
Aliskiren and Hydrochlorothiazide 87
AMILoride 113
AmLODIPine 123
Amlodipine and Atorvastatin 124
Amlodipine and Benazepril 125
Amlodipine and Olmesartan 126
Amlodipine and Valsartan 126
Amlodipine, Valsartan, and Hydrochlorothiazide 127
Atenolol 189
Azilsartan 214
Azilsartan and Chlorthalidone 215
Benazepril 238
Benazepril and Hydrochlorothiazide 240
Betaxolol (Systemic) 256
Bisoprolol 266
Bisoprolol and Hydrochlorothiazide 267
Bumetanide 297
Candesartan 335
Candesartan and Hydrochlorothiazide 338
Captopril 342
Captopril and Hydrochlorothiazide 345
Carvedilol 367
Chlorothiazide 426
Chlorthalidone 430
Cilazapril [CAN/INT] 434
Clevidipine 460
CloNIDine 480
Diltiazem 634
Doxazosin 674
Enalapril 722
Enalapril and Hydrochlorothiazide 725
Eplerenone 740
Eprosartan 748
Eprosartan and Hydrochlorothiazide 750
Esmolol 769
Felodipine 850
Fenoldopam 856
Fosinopril 932
Furosemide 940
GuanFACINE 990
HydrALAZINE 1007
Hydrochlorothiazide 1009
Hydrochlorothiazide and Triamterene 1012
Indapamide 1065
Irbesartan 1110
Irbesartan and Hydrochlorothiazide 1112
Isosorbide Dinitrate and Hydralazine 1126
Isradipine 1130
Labetalol 1151
Lisinopril 1226
Lisinopril and Hydrochlorothiazide 1229
Losartan 1248
Losartan and Hydrochlorothiazide 1250
Methyclothiazide 1331
Methyldopa 1332
Metoprolol 1350
Minoxidil (Systemic) 1374
Moexipril 1388
Moexipril and Hydrochlorothiazide 1388
Nadolol 1411
Nebivolol 1434
NiCARdipine 1446
NIFEdipine 1451
Nisoldipine 1459
Nitroprusside 1467
Olmesartan 1496
Olmesartan, Amlodipine, and Hydrochlorothiazide 1498
Perindopril 1623
Perindopril and Indapamide [CAN/INT] 1626
Phentolamine 1636
Pindolol 1652
Pindolol and Hydrochlorothiazide [CAN/INT] 1653
Prazosin 1703
Propranolol 1731

Quinapril 1756
Ramipril 1771
Ramipril and Hydrochlorothiazide [CAN/INT] 1773
Spironolactone 1931
Telmisartan 1988
Telmisartan and Amlodipine 1989
Telmisartan and Hydrochlorothiazide 1990
Terazosin 2001
Timolol (Systemic) 2042
Torsemide 2071
Trandolapril 2080
Trandolapril and Verapamil 2080
Triamterene 2101
Valsartan 2127
Valsartan and Hydrochlorothiazide 2129
Verapamil 2154

Anti-inflammatory Agent
Alitretinoin (Systemic) [CAN/INT] 88
Balsalazide 226
Colchicine and Probenecid 503
Dexamethasone (Systemic) 599
Etofenamate [INT] 815
Felbinac [INT] 850

Anti-inflammatory Agent, Ophthalmic
Dexamethasone (Ophthalmic) 602

Anti-inflammatory, Locally Applied
Carbamide Peroxide 350

Antilipemic Agent, 2-Azetidinone
Ezetimibe 832
Ezetimibe and Atorvastatin 833
Ezetimibe and Simvastatin 834

Antilipemic Agent, Bile Acid Sequestrant
Cholestyramine Resin 431
Colesevelam 503
Colestipol 504

Antilipemic Agent, Fibric Acid
Bezafibrate [CAN/INT] 261
Ciprofibrate [INT] 441
Fenofibrate and Derivatives 852
Gemfibrozil 956

Antilipemic Agent, HMG-CoA Reductase Inhibitor
Amlodipine and Atorvastatin 124
AtorvaSTATin 194
Ezetimibe and Atorvastatin 833
Ezetimibe and Simvastatin 834
Fluvastatin 915
Lovastatin 1252
Niacin and Lovastatin 1446
Pitavastatin 1663
Pravastatin 1700
Rosuvastatin 1848
Simvastatin 1890
Sitagliptin and Simvastatin 1899

Antilipemic Agent, Microsomal Triglyceride Transfer Protein (MTP) Inhibitor
Lomitapide 1233

Antilipemic Agent, Miscellaneous
Acipimox [INT] 43
Niacin 1443
Niacin and Lovastatin 1446

Antilipemic Agent, Omega-3 Fatty Acids
Omega-3 Fatty Acids 1507

Antimalarial Agent
Artemether and Lumefantrine 177
Artesunate 178
Atovaquone and Proguanil 198
Halofantrine [INT] 993
Mefloquine 1280
Pyrimethamine 1749
QuiNIDine 1759
QuiNINE 1761
Sulfadoxine and Pyrimethamine [INT] 1946

Antimanic Agent
Asenapine 179
ChlorproMAZINE 429
Lithium 1230
Methotrimeprazine [CAN/INT] 1329
OLANZapine 1491
RisperiDONE 1818
Valproic Acid and Derivatives 2123

Antimicrobial Agent
Pipemidic Acid [INT] 1655

Antimigraine Agent
Almotriptan 92
Dihydroergotamine 633
Eletriptan 711
Ergotamine 754
Frovatriptan 938
Naratriptan 1430
Rizatriptan 1836
SUMAtriptan 1953
Sumatriptan and Naproxen 1957
ZOLMitriptan 2210

Antimyoclonic, Miscellaneous
Piracetam [INT] 1661

Antineoplastic Agent
Bortezomib 276
Carfilzomib 361
Fotemustine [INT] 937
Ibrutinib 1030
Lenalidomide 1177
Pomalidomide 1677
Thalidomide 2022
Ziv-Aflibercept (Systemic) 2204

Antineoplastic Agent, Alkylating Agent
Bendamustine 241
Busulfan 312
CARBOplatin 357
Carmustine 364
Chlorambucil 419
CISplatin 448
Cyclophosphamide 517
Eptaplatin [INT] 751
Estramustine 782
Ifosfamide 1040
Lomustine 1235
Mechlorethamine (Systemic) 1276
Mechlorethamine (Topical) 1276
Melphalan 1283
Oxaliplatin 1528
Procarbazine 1717
Thiotepa 2030

Antineoplastic Agent, Alkylating Agent (Nitrogen Mustard)
Bendamustine 241
Chlorambucil 419
Cyclophosphamide 517
Ifosfamide 1040
Mechlorethamine (Systemic) 1276
Mechlorethamine (Topical) 1276
Melphalan 1283

Antineoplastic Agent, Alkylating Agent (Nitrosourea)
Carmustine ... 364
Fotemustine [INT] ... 937
Lomustine ... 1235
Nimustine [INT] ... 1457

Antineoplastic Agent, Alkylating Agent (Triazene)
Dacarbazine ... 549
Temozolomide ... 1991

Antineoplastic Agent, Anaplastic Lymphoma Kinase Inhibitor
Ceritinib ... 407
Crizotinib ... 511

Antineoplastic Agent, Anthracenedione
MitoXANtrone ... 1382

Antineoplastic Agent, Anthracycline
DAUNOrubicin (Conventional) ... 577
DAUNOrubicin (Liposomal) ... 580
DOXOrubicin (Conventional) ... 679
DOXOrubicin (Liposomal) ... 684
Epirubicin ... 739
IDArubicin ... 1037
Valrubicin ... 2127

Antineoplastic Agent, Antiandrogen
Abiraterone Acetate ... 26
Bicalutamide ... 262
Cyproterone [CAN/INT] ... 530
Enzalutamide ... 733
Flutamide ... 907
Nilutamide ... 1455

Antineoplastic Agent, Antibiotic
Bleomycin ... 270
DACTINomycin ... 551
MitoMYcin (Ophthalmic) ... 1382
MitoMYcin (Systemic) ... 1380

Antineoplastic Agent, Antibody Drug Conjugate
Ado-Trastuzumab Emtansine ... 58
Brentuximab Vedotin ... 286
Gemtuzumab Ozogamicin ... 957

Antineoplastic Agent, Anti-CD19/CD3
Blinatumomab ... 271

Antineoplastic Agent, Anti-CD20
Obinutuzumab ... 1482
Ofatumumab ... 1488
RiTUXimab ... 1825

Antineoplastic Agent, Anti-CD30
Brentuximab Vedotin ... 286

Antineoplastic Agent, Anti-CD33
Gemtuzumab Ozogamicin ... 957

Antineoplastic Agent, Anti-CD52
Alemtuzumab ... 75

Antineoplastic Agent, Anti-HER2
Ado-Trastuzumab Emtansine ... 58
Lapatinib ... 1169
Pertuzumab ... 1627
Trastuzumab ... 2085

Antineoplastic Agent, Antimetabolite
AzaCITIDine ... 209
Capecitabine ... 339
Cladribine ... 455
Clofarabine ... 470
Cytarabine (Conventional) ... 535
Cytarabine (Liposomal) ... 540
Decitabine ... 581
Fludarabine ... 890
Fluorouracil (Systemic) ... 896
Fluorouracil (Topical) ... 899
Gemcitabine ... 952
Mercaptopurine ... 1296
Nelarabine ... 1435
PEMEtrexed ... 1606
Pentostatin ... 1618
PRALAtrexate ... 1693
Raltitrexed [CAN/INT] ... 1769
Thioguanine ... 2029

Antineoplastic Agent, Antimetabolite (Antifolate)
Methotrexate ... 1322
PEMEtrexed ... 1606
PRALAtrexate ... 1693
Raltitrexed [CAN/INT] ... 1769

Antineoplastic Agent, Antimetabolite (Purine Analog)
Cladribine ... 455
Clofarabine ... 470
Fludarabine ... 890
Mercaptopurine ... 1296
Nelarabine ... 1435
Pentostatin ... 1618
Thioguanine ... 2029

Antineoplastic Agent, Antimetabolite (Pyrimidine Analog)
Capecitabine ... 339
Cytarabine (Conventional) ... 535
Cytarabine (Liposomal) ... 540
Fluorouracil (Systemic) ... 896
Fluorouracil (Topical) ... 899
Gemcitabine ... 952

Antineoplastic Agent, Antimicrotubular
Ado-Trastuzumab Emtansine ... 58
Cabazitaxel ... 316
DOCEtaxel ... 656
Eribulin ... 755
Estramustine ... 782
Ixabepilone ... 1138
PACLitaxel (Conventional) ... 1550
PACLitaxel (Protein Bound) ... 1554
VinBLAStine ... 2160
VinCRIStine ... 2163
VinCRIStine (Liposomal) ... 2166
Vinorelbine ... 2168

Antineoplastic Agent, Anti-PD-1 Monoclonal Antibody
Nivolumab ... 1469
Pembrolizumab ... 1604

Antineoplastic Agent, Aromatase Inhibitor
Anastrozole ... 148
Exemestane ... 828
Letrozole ... 1181

Antineoplastic Agent, BCR-ABL Tyrosine Kinase Inhibitor
Bosutinib ... 282
Dasatinib ... 574
Imatinib ... 1047
Nilotinib ... 1454
PONATinib ... 1680

Antineoplastic Agent, Biological Response Modulator
Aldesleukin ... 72
BCG ... 229

Interferon Alfa-2b 1096
Peginterferon Alfa-2b 1596

Antineoplastic Agent, BRAF Kinase Inhibitor
Dabrafenib 546
Vemurafenib 2148

Antineoplastic Agent, Bruton Tyrosine Kinase Inhibitor
Ibrutinib 1030

Antineoplastic Agent, Camptothecin
Irinotecan 1112
Topotecan 2069

Antineoplastic Agent, Cephalotaxine
Omacetaxine 1501

Antineoplastic Agent, DNA Methylation Inhibitor
AzaCITIDine 209
Decitabine 581

Antineoplastic Agent, Enzyme
Asparaginase (E. coli) 179
Asparaginase (Erwinia) 180
Pegaspargase 1588

Antineoplastic Agent, Epidermal Growth Factor Receptor (EGFR) Inhibitor
Afatinib 61
Cetuximab 413
Erlotinib 756
Gefitinib [CAN/INT] 950
Lapatinib 1169
Panitumumab 1568
Vandetanib 2135

Antineoplastic Agent, Epothilone B Analog
Ixabepilone 1138

Antineoplastic Agent, Estrogen Receptor Antagonist
Fulvestrant 939
Tamoxifen 1971
Toremifene 2071

Antineoplastic Agent, Gonadotropin-Releasing Hormone Agonist
Goserelin 981
Histrelin 1005
Leuprolide 1186

Antineoplastic Agent, Gonadotropin-Releasing Hormone Antagonist
Degarelix 587

Antineoplastic Agent, Hedgehog Pathway Inhibitor
Vismodegib 2171

Antineoplastic Agent, Histone Deacetylase Inhibitor
Belinostat 236
RomiDEPsin 1841
Vorinostat 2182

Antineoplastic Agent, Hormone
Megestrol 1281

Antineoplastic Agent, Hormone Antagonist
Mifepristone 1366

Antineoplastic Agent, Hormone (Estrogen/Nitrogen Mustard)
Estramustine 782

Antineoplastic Agent, Janus Associated Kinase Inhibitor
Ruxolitinib 1856

Antineoplastic Agent, MEK Inhibitor
Trametinib 2077

Antineoplastic Agent, Miscellaneous
Aldesleukin 72
Arsenic Trioxide 177
Asparaginase (E. coli) 179
Asparaginase (Erwinia) 180
Hydroxyurea 1021
Mitotane 1382
Pegaspargase 1588
Polyestradiol [INT] 1673
Porfimer 1682

Antineoplastic Agent, Monoclonal Antibody
Ado-Trastuzumab Emtansine 58
Alemtuzumab 75
Bevacizumab 257
Blinatumomab 271
Brentuximab Vedotin 286
Cetuximab 413
Gemtuzumab Ozogamicin 957
Ipilimumab 1106
Nimotuzumab [INT] 1457
Nivolumab 1469
Obinutuzumab 1482
Ofatumumab 1488
Panitumumab 1568
Pembrolizumab 1604
Pertuzumab 1627
Ramucirumab 1775
RiTUXimab 1825
Siltuximab 1885
Trastuzumab 2085

Antineoplastic Agent, mTOR Kinase Inhibitor
Everolimus 822
Temsirolimus 1994

Antineoplastic Agent, Phosphatidylinositol 3-Kinase Inhibitor
Idelalisib 1038

Antineoplastic Agent, Platinum Analog
CARBOplatin 357
CISplatin 448
Oxaliplatin 1528

Antineoplastic Agent, Podophyllotoxin Derivative
Etoposide 816
Etoposide Phosphate 820
Teniposide 1997

Antineoplastic Agent, Protein Synthesis Inhibitor
Omacetaxine 1501

Antineoplastic Agent, Retinoic Acid Derivative
Bexarotene (Systemic) 261
Bexarotene (Topical) 261
ISOtretinoin 1127
Tretinoin (Systemic) 2096

Antineoplastic Agent, Taxane Derivative
Cabazitaxel 316
DOCEtaxel 656
PACLitaxel (Conventional) 1550
PACLitaxel (Protein Bound) 1554

Antineoplastic Agent, Topoisomerase I Inhibitor
Irinotecan 1112
Topotecan 2069

Antineoplastic Agent, Topoisomerase II Inhibitor
DAUNOrubicin (Conventional) 577
DAUNOrubicin (Liposomal) 580
DOXOrubicin (Conventional) 679

DOXOrubicin (Liposomal) 684
Epirubicin 739
Etoposide 816
Etoposide Phosphate 820
IDArubicin 1037
MitoXANtrone 1382
Teniposide 1997
Valrubicin 2127

Antineoplastic Agent, Tyrosine Kinase Inhibitor
Afatinib 61
Axitinib 207
Bosutinib 282
Ceritinib 407
Crizotinib 511
Dasatinib 574
Erlotinib 756
Gefitinib [CAN/INT] 950
Ibrutinib 1030
Imatinib 1047
Lapatinib 1169
Nilotinib 1454
PAZOPanib 1584
PONATinib 1680
Regorafenib 1787
Ruxolitinib 1856
SORAfenib 1923
SUNItinib 1957
Vandetanib 2135

Antineoplastic Agent, Vascular Endothelial Growth Factor Receptor 2 (VEGFR2) Inhibitor
Ramucirumab 1775

Antineoplastic Agent, Vascular Endothelial Growth Factor (VEGF) Inhibitor
Axitinib 207
Bevacizumab 257
PAZOPanib 1584
Ramucirumab 1775
Regorafenib 1787
SORAfenib 1923
SUNItinib 1957
Vandetanib 2135

Antineoplastic Agent, Vinca Alkaloid
VinBLAStine 2160
VinCRIStine 2163
VinCRIStine (Liposomal) 2166
Vinorelbine 2168

Antiparasitic Agent, Topical
Benzyl Alcohol 250
Ivermectin (Topical) 1137
Lindane 1217
Malathion 1268
Permethrin 1627
Pyrethrins and Piperonyl Butoxide 1746
Spinosad 1930

Anti-Parkinson's Agent, Anticholinergic
Benztropine 248
Procyclidine [CAN/INT] 1721
Trihexyphenidyl 2103

Anti-Parkinson's Agent, COMT Inhibitor
Entacapone 730
Levodopa, Carbidopa, and Entacapone 1196
Tolcapone 2062

Anti-Parkinson's Agent, Decarboxylase Inhibitor
Carbidopa 351
Carbidopa and Levodopa 351
Levodopa, Carbidopa, and Entacapone 1196

Anti-Parkinson's Agent, Dopamine Agonist
Amantadine 105
Benserazide and Levodopa [CAN/INT] 244
Bromocriptine 291
Piribedil [INT] 1662
Pramipexole 1695
ROPINIRole 1844
Rotigotine 1851

Anti-Parkinson's Agent, Dopamine Precursor
Carbidopa and Levodopa 351
Levodopa, Carbidopa, and Entacapone 1196

Anti-Parkinson's Agent, MAO Type B Inhibitor
Rasagiline 1781
Selegiline 1873

Antiplatelet Agent
Anagrelide 147
Aspirin 180
Aspirin and Dipyridamole 185
Cilostazol 437
Clopidogrel 484
Dipyridamole 652
Indobufen [INT] 1067
Prasugrel 1699
Ticagrelor 2035
Ticlopidine 2040
Trapidil [INT] 2085
Triflusal [INT] 2103
Vorapaxar 2175

Antiplatelet Agent, Cyclopentyltriazolopyrimidine
Ticagrelor 2035

Antiplatelet Agent, Glycoprotein IIb/IIIa Inhibitor
Abciximab 24
Eptifibatide 751
Tirofiban 2049

Antiplatelet Agent, Thienopyridine
Clopidogrel 484
Prasugrel 1699
Ticlopidine 2040

Antiprogestin
Mifepristone 1366

Antiprotozoal
Atovaquone 197
Eflornithine 710
Furazolidone [INT] 940
Meglumine Antimoniate [INT] 1283
Nitazoxanide 1461
Ornidazole [INT] 1522
Pentamidine 1616
Secnidazole [INT] 1872
Sodium Stibogluconate [INT] 1913

Antiprotozoal, Nitroimidazole
Metronidazole and Nystatin [CAN/INT] 1358
MetroNIDAZOLE (Systemic) 1353

Antipsoriatic Agent
Anthralin 150
Golimumab 977
Ustekinumab 2117

Antipsychotic Agent, Atypical
Sertindole [INT] 1878

Antipsychotic Agent, Butyrophenone
Pipamperone [INT] 1655

Antipsychotic Agent, Typical, Phenothiazine
Benperidol [INT] 244
Bromperidol [INT] 292

Antipyretic
Dipyrone [INT] ... 653

Antiretroviral, CCR5 Antagonist (Anti-HIV)
Maraviroc ... 1272

Antiretroviral, Fusion Protein Inhibitor (Anti-HIV)
Enfuvirtide ... 726

Antiretroviral, Integrase Inhibitor (Anti-HIV)
Abacavir, Dolutegravir, and Lamivudine ... 22
Elvitegravir ... 717
Elvitegravir, Cobicistat, Emtricitabine, and Tenofovir ... 718
Raltegravir ... 1767

Antiretroviral, Protease Inhibitor (Anti-HIV)
Atazanavir ... 185
Darunavir ... 569
Darunavir and Cobicistat ... 572
Fosamprenavir ... 928
Indinavir ... 1066
Lopinavir and Ritonavir ... 1237
Nelfinavir ... 1436
Ritonavir ... 1822
Saquinavir ... 1865
Tipranavir ... 2047

Antiretroviral, Reverse Transcriptase Inhibitor, Non-nucleoside (Anti-HIV)
Delavirdine ... 587
Efavirenz ... 707
Efavirenz, Emtricitabine, and Tenofovir ... 709
Emtricitabine, Rilpivirine, and Tenofovir ... 722
Etravirine ... 821
Nevirapine ... 1440
Rilpivirine ... 1810

Antiretroviral, Reverse Transcriptase Inhibitor, Nucleoside (Anti-HIV)
Abacavir ... 20
Abacavir and Lamivudine ... 22
Abacavir, Dolutegravir, and Lamivudine ... 22
Abacavir, Lamivudine, and Zidovudine ... 22
Didanosine ... 622
Efavirenz, Emtricitabine, and Tenofovir ... 709
Elvitegravir, Cobicistat, Emtricitabine, and Tenofovir ... 718
Emtricitabine ... 720
Emtricitabine and Tenofovir ... 721
Emtricitabine, Rilpivirine, and Tenofovir ... 722
LamiVUDine ... 1157
Lamivudine and Zidovudine ... 1160
Stavudine ... 1934
Zidovudine ... 2196

Antiretroviral, Reverse Transcriptase Inhibitor, Nucleotide (Anti-HIV)
Efavirenz, Emtricitabine, and Tenofovir ... 709
Elvitegravir, Cobicistat, Emtricitabine, and Tenofovir ... 718
Emtricitabine and Tenofovir ... 721
Emtricitabine, Rilpivirine, and Tenofovir ... 722
Tenofovir ... 1998

Antirheumatic, Disease Modifying
Abatacept ... 23
Adalimumab ... 51
Anakinra ... 148
Certolizumab Pegol ... 409
Etanercept ... 795
Golimumab ... 977
InFLIXimab ... 1070
Leflunomide ... 1174
Methotrexate ... 1322
Tocilizumab ... 2057
Tofacitinib ... 2059

Antirheumatic Miscellaneous
Cyclophosphamide ... 517
Hyaluronate and Derivatives ... 1006
RiTUXimab ... 1825
Tofacitinib ... 2059

Antiseborrheic Agent, Topical
Sulfur and Sulfacetamide ... 1953

Antiseptic, Topical
Potassium Iodide and Iodine ... 1690

Antispasmodic Agent, Gastrointestinal
Alverine [INT] ... 104
Atropine ... 200
Clidinium and Chlordiazepoxide ... 460
Fenoverine [INT] ... 857
Hyoscyamine, Atropine, Scopolamine, and Phenobarbital ... 1027
Mebeverine [INT] ... 1275
Prifinium [INT] ... 1712

Antispasmodic Agent, Urinary
Belladonna and Opium ... 238
FlavoxATE ... 881
Oxybutynin ... 1536

Antithyroid Agent
Benzylthiouracil [INT] ... 250
Carbimazole [INT] ... 356
Methimazole ... 1319
Potassium Iodide ... 1690
Potassium Iodide and Iodine ... 1690
Propylthiouracil ... 1735

Antitubercular Agent
Bedaquiline ... 233
Ethambutol ... 798
Isoniazid ... 1120
Isoniazid and Thiacetazone [INT] ... 1124
Pyrazinamide ... 1745
Rifabutin ... 1803
Rifampin ... 1804
Rifapentine ... 1807
Streptomycin ... 1937

Antitussive
Acetaminophen, Codeine, and Doxylamine [CAN/INT] ... 37
Benzonatate ... 247
Chlorpheniramine, Phenylephrine, and Dextromethorphan ... 428
Chlorpheniramine, Pseudoephedrine, and Dextromethorphan ... 428
Clobutinol [INT] ... 468
Codeine ... 497
Dextromethorphan and Chlorpheniramine ... 610
Dextromethorphan and Phenylephrine ... 611
Dihydrocodeine, Chlorpheniramine, and Phenylephrine ... 633
Dimemorfan [INT] ... 637
Guaifenesin and Codeine ... 987
Guaifenesin and Dextromethorphan ... 987
Hydrocodone and Chlorpheniramine ... 1012
Hydrocodone and Homatropine ... 1013
Pholcodine [INT] ... 1646
Promethazine and Codeine ... 1725
Promethazine and Dextromethorphan ... 1725
Triprolidine, Pseudoephedrine, and Codeine [CAN/INT] ... 2105

Antitussive/Decongestant
Pseudoephedrine and Dextromethorphan ... 1743

Antitussive/Decongestant/Expectorant
Guaifenesin, Pseudoephedrine, and Codeine ... 989
Guaifenesin, Pseudoephedrine, and Dextromethorphan ... 989

Antivenin
Centruroides Immune $F(ab')_2$ (Equine) ... 405

Antiviral Agent
Aciclovir (Ophthalmic) [INT] ... 43
Acyclovir (Systemic) ... 47
Amantadine ... 105
Brivudine [INT] ... 289
Cidofovir ... 433
Famciclovir ... 843
Foscarnet ... 931
Ganciclovir (Systemic) ... 948
Oseltamivir ... 1523
Penciclovir ... 1608
Peramivir ... 1619
Rimantadine ... 1813
ValACYclovir ... 2119
ValGANciclovir ... 2121
Zanamivir ... 2194

Antiviral Agent, Adamantane
Amantadine ... 105
Rimantadine ... 1813

Antiviral Agent, Ophthalmic
Trifluridine ... 2103

Antiviral Agent, Oral
ValACYclovir ... 2119

Antiviral Agent, Topical
Acyclovir (Topical) ... 51
Docosanol ... 661

Anxiolytics, Sedatives, and Hypnotics, Miscellaneous
Paraldehyde [CAN/INT] ... 1575

Appetite Stimulant
Dronabinol ... 694
Megestrol ... 1281

Aromatase Inhibitor
Formestane [INT] ... 926

Artemisinin Derivative
Artesunate ... 178

Barbiturate
Amobarbital ... 128
Butabarbital ... 313
Butalbital, Acetaminophen, and Caffeine ... 313
Butalbital and Acetaminophen ... 314
Butalbital, Aspirin, and Caffeine ... 314
Methohexital ... 1321
PENTobarbital ... 1617
PHENobarbital ... 1632
Primidone ... 1714
Secobarbital ... 1872
Thiopental [INT] ... 2029

Benzodiazepine
ALPRAZolam ... 94
Amitriptyline and Chlordiazepoxide ... 122
Bromazepam [CAN/INT] ... 290
Brotizolam [INT] ... 293
ChlordiazePOXIDE ... 422
Clidinium and Chlordiazepoxide ... 460
CloBAZam ... 465
ClonazePAM ... 478
Clorazepate ... 487
Diazepam ... 613
Estazolam ... 775
Ketazolam [INT] ... 1144
Loprazolam [INT] ... 1241
LORazepam ... 1243
Lormetazepam [INT] ... 1247
Medazepam [INT] ... 1277
Midazolam ... 1361
Nitrazepam [CAN/INT] ... 1461
Oxazepam ... 1532
Pinazepam [INT] ... 1652
Prazepam [INT] ... 1702
Quazepam ... 1751
Temazepam ... 1990
Tetrazepam [INT] ... 2020
Tofisopam [INT] ... 2061
Triazolam ... 2101

$Beta_1$- & $Beta_2$-Adrenergic Agonist Agent
Isoproterenol ... 1124

$Beta_2$-Adrenergic Agonist
Arformoterol ... 168
Bambuterol [INT] ... 227
Clenbuterol [INT] ... 460
Ipratropium and Albuterol ... 1109
Ipratropium and Fenoterol [CAN/INT] ... 1109

$Beta_2$-Adrenergic Agonist, Long-Acting
Arformoterol ... 168
Budesonide and Formoterol ... 297
Fluticasone and Salmeterol ... 912
Fluticasone and Vilanterol ... 914
Formoterol ... 926
Indacaterol ... 1063
Indacaterol and Glycopyrronium [CAN/INT] ... 1063
Mometasone and Formoterol ... 1392
Olodaterol ... 1498
Salmeterol ... 1860

$Beta_2$ Agonist
Albuterol ... 69
Budesonide and Formoterol ... 297
Fluticasone and Salmeterol ... 912
Fluticasone and Vilanterol ... 914
Formoterol ... 926
Indacaterol ... 1063
Indacaterol and Glycopyrronium [CAN/INT] ... 1063
Levalbuterol ... 1189
Metaproterenol ... 1307
Olodaterol ... 1498
Pirbuterol ... 1662
Salmeterol ... 1860
Terbutaline ... 2004

$Beta_2$ Agonist, Long-Acting
Mometasone and Formoterol ... 1392

$Beta_3$ Agonist
Mirabegron ... 1375

Beta-Adrenergic Blocker, Nonselective
Bupranolol [INT] ... 300
Dorzolamide and Timolol ... 673
Levobunolol ... 1194
Propranolol ... 1731
Sotalol ... 1927

Beta-Adrenergic Blocker, Ophthalmic
Bupranolol [INT] ... 300

Beta-Blocker, Beta-1 Selective
Atenolol ... 189
Betaxolol (Systemic) ... 256
Bisoprolol ... 266
Bisoprolol and Hydrochlorothiazide ... 267
Esmolol ... 769

Metoprolol ... 1350
Nebivolol ... 1434

Beta Blocker, Intrinsic Sympathomimetic Activity (ISA)
Befunolol [INT] ... 233

Beta-Blocker, Nonselective
Brimonidine and Timolol ... 288
Brinzolamide and Timolol [CAN/INT] ... 289
Latanoprost and Timolol [CAN/INT] ... 1172
Metipranolol ... 1345
Nadolol ... 1411
Timolol (Ophthalmic) ... 2043
Timolol (Systemic) ... 2042
Travoprost and Timolol [CAN/INT] ... 2090

Beta-Blocker With Alpha-Blocking Activity
Carvedilol ... 367
Labetalol ... 1151

Beta-Blocker With Intrinsic Sympathomimetic Activity
Acebutolol ... 29
Pindolol ... 1652
Pindolol and Hydrochlorothiazide [CAN/INT] ... 1653

Bile Acid
Chenodiol ... 417

Biological, Miscellaneous
Glatiramer Acetate ... 963

Biological Response Modulator
Interferon Alfa-2b ... 1096
Oprelvekin ... 1519
Peginterferon Alfa-2b ... 1596
Peginterferon Beta-1a ... 1602

Bisphosphonate Derivative
Alendronate ... 79
Alendronate and Cholecalciferol ... 81
Clodronate [CAN/INT] ... 469
Etidronate ... 813
Etidronate and Calcium Carbonate [CAN/INT] ... 814
Ibandronate ... 1028
Ibandronic Acid [INT] ... 1030
Pamidronate ... 1563
Risedronate ... 1816
Tiludronate ... 2042
Zoledronic Acid ... 2206

Blood Product Derivative
Albumin ... 67
Antihemophilic Factor (Human) ... 152
Antihemophilic Factor/von Willebrand Factor Complex (Human) ... 154
Anti-inhibitor Coagulant Complex (Human) ... 155
Antithrombin ... 156
Aprotinin ... 168
Botulism Immune Globulin (Intravenous-Human) ... 284
C1 Inhibitor (Human) ... 315
Cytomegalovirus Immune Globulin (Intravenous-Human) ... 541
Factor IX Complex (Human) [(Factors II, IX, X)] ... 838
Factor IX (Human) ... 840
Factor XIII Concentrate (Human) ... 843
Fibrinogen Concentrate (Human) ... 874
Hepatitis B Immune Globulin (Human) ... 1002
Immune Globulin ... 1056
Protein C Concentrate (Human) ... 1738
Prothrombin Complex Concentrate (Human) [(Factors II, VII, IX, X), Protein C, and Protein S] ... 1738
Rabies Immune Globulin (Human) ... 1764
$Rh_o(D)$ Immune Globulin ... 1794
Tetanus Immune Globulin (Human) ... 2015
Vaccinia Immune Globulin (Intravenous) ... 2118
Varicella-Zoster Immune Globulin (Human) ... 2142

Blood Viscosity Reducer Agent
Pentoxifylline ... 1618

Bone-Modifying Agent
Denosumab ... 589

Bronchodilator
Doxofylline [INT] ... 679

C1 Esterase Inhibitor
C1 Inhibitor (Human) ... 315
C1 Inhibitor (Recombinant) ... 316

Calcimimetic
Cinacalcet ... 439

Calcineurin Inhibitor
CycloSPORINE (Ophthalmic) ... 529
CycloSPORINE (Systemic) ... 522
Pimecrolimus ... 1650
Tacrolimus (Systemic) ... 1962
Tacrolimus (Topical) ... 1968

Calcium Channel Antagonist, Gastrointestinal
Pinaverium [CAN/INT] ... 1651

Calcium Channel Blocker
Aliskiren, Amlodipine, and Hydrochlorothiazide ... 87
AmLODIPine ... 123
Amlodipine and Atorvastatin ... 124
Amlodipine and Benazepril ... 125
Amlodipine and Olmesartan ... 126
Amlodipine and Valsartan ... 126
Amlodipine, Valsartan, and Hydrochlorothiazide ... 127
Azelnidipine [INT] ... 214
Clevidipine ... 460
Diltiazem ... 634
Felodipine ... 850
Flunarizine [CAN/INT] ... 892
Isradipine ... 1130
Lacidipin [INT] ... 1154
Lercanidipine [INT] ... 1181
Manidipine [INT] ... 1269
NiCARdipine ... 1446
NIFEdipine ... 1451
Nilvadipine [INT] ... 1456
NiMODipine ... 1456
Nisoldipine ... 1459
Nitrendipine [INT] ... 1463
Olmesartan, Amlodipine, and Hydrochlorothiazide ... 1498
Telmisartan and Amlodipine ... 1989
Trandolapril and Verapamil ... 2080
Verapamil ... 2154

Calcium Channel Blocker, Dihydropyridine
Aliskiren, Amlodipine, and Hydrochlorothiazide ... 87
AmLODIPine ... 123
Amlodipine and Atorvastatin ... 124
Amlodipine and Benazepril ... 125
Amlodipine and Olmesartan ... 126
Amlodipine and Valsartan ... 126
Amlodipine, Valsartan, and Hydrochlorothiazide ... 127
Barnidipine [INT] ... 227
Clevidipine ... 460
Felodipine ... 850
Isradipine ... 1130
NiCARdipine ... 1446
NIFEdipine ... 1451
NiMODipine ... 1456
Nisoldipine ... 1459

Olmesartan, Amlodipine, and Hydrochlorothiazide 1498
Telmisartan and Amlodipine 1989

Calcium Channel Blocker, Nondihydropyridine
Diltiazem 634
Verapamil 2154

Calcium Channel Blocker, N-Type
Ziconotide 2196

Calcium Salt
Calcium Acetate 326
Calcium and Vitamin D 326
Calcium Carbonate 327
Calcium Chloride 328
Calcium Citrate 330
Calcium Glubionate 330
Calcium Gluconate 330
Etidronate and Calcium Carbonate [CAN/INT] 814

Caloric Agent
Fat Emulsion (Fish Oil Based) [CAN/INT] 847
Fat Emulsion (Plant Based) 848
Total Parenteral Nutrition 2073

Carbonic Anhydrase Inhibitor
AcetaZOLAMIDE 39
Methazolamide 1317

Carbonic Anhydrase Inhibitor (Ophthalmic)
Brinzolamide 288
Brinzolamide and Timolol [CAN/INT] 289
Dorzolamide 673
Dorzolamide and Timolol 673

Cardiac Glycoside
Digoxin 627

Cardiovascular Agent, Miscellaneous
Ranolazine 1779

Cardiovascular Agent, Other
Ivabradine [INT] 1134
Trimetazidine [INT] 2104

Cathartic
Sodium Phosphates 1909

Cauterizing Agent, Topical
Silver Nitrate 1886

Cellular Immunotherapy, Autologous
Sipuleucel-T 1893

Central Monoamine-Depleting Agent
Reserpine 1793
Tetrabenazine 2016

Central Nervous System Depressant
Sodium Oxybate 1908

Central Nervous System Stimulant
Armodafinil 175
Caffeine 319
Dexmethylphenidate 605
Dextroamphetamine 607
Dextroamphetamine and Amphetamine 609
Diethylpropion 624
Lisdexamfetamine 1224
Methamphetamine 1315
Methylphenidate 1336
Modafinil 1386
Phentermine 1635

Chelating Agent
Deferasirox 582
Deferiprone 585
Deferoxamine 586
Edetate CALCIUM Disodium 705
PenicillAMINE 1608
Trientine 2102

Chemoprotective Agent
Amifostine 109
Dexrazoxane 606
Mesna 1305
Palifermin 1555

Chemotherapy Modulating Agent
Leucovorin Calcium 1183
LEVOleucovorin 1200

Chloride Channel Activator
Lubiprostone 1255

Cholinergic Agonist
Acetylcholine 40
Bethanechol 257
Carbachol 346
Cevimeline 415
Pilocarpine (Systemic) 1649

Colony Stimulating Factor
Darbepoetin Alfa 565
Eltrombopag 714
Epoetin Alfa 742
Filgrastim 875
Lenograstim [INT] 1181
Molgramostim [INT] 1388
Pegfilgrastim 1589
RomiPLOStim 1842
Sargramostim 1865

Contraceptive
Estradiol and Dienogest 780
Ethinyl Estradiol and Desogestrel 799
Ethinyl Estradiol and Drospirenone 801
Ethinyl Estradiol and Ethynodiol Diacetate 801
Ethinyl Estradiol and Etonogestrel 802
Ethinyl Estradiol and Levonorgestrel 803
Ethinyl Estradiol and Norelgestromin 807
Ethinyl Estradiol and Norethindrone 808
Ethinyl Estradiol and Norgestimate 810
Ethinyl Estradiol and Norgestrel 812
Ethinyl Estradiol, Drospirenone, and Levomefolate 812
Levonorgestrel 1201
MedroxyPROGESTERone 1277
Nonoxynol 9 1471
Norethindrone 1473
Norethindrone and Mestranol 1475
Ulipristal 2113

Contraceptive, Oral (Progestin)
Desogestrel [INT] 597

Corticosteroid, Inhalant (Oral)
Beclomethasone (Systemic) 230
Budesonide and Formoterol 297
Budesonide (Systemic) 293
Ciclesonide (Systemic) 432
Fluticasone and Salmeterol 912
Fluticasone and Vilanterol 914
Fluticasone (Oral Inhalation) 907
Mometasone and Formoterol 1392
Mometasone (Oral Inhalation) 1389

Corticosteroid, Nasal
Azelastine and Fluticasone 214
Beclomethasone (Nasal) 232
Budesonide (Nasal) 296
Ciclesonide (Nasal) 432
Flunisolide (Nasal) 893

Fluticasone (Nasal) ... 910
Mometasone (Nasal) ... 1391
Triamcinolone (Nasal) ... 2100

Corticosteroid, Ophthalmic
Bacitracin, Neomycin, Polymyxin B, and Hydrocortisone ... 223
Dexamethasone (Ophthalmic) ... 602
Difluprednate ... 626
Fluorometholone ... 896
Loteprednol ... 1251
Neomycin, Polymyxin B, and Hydrocortisone ... 1438
PrednisoLONE (Ophthalmic) ... 1706
Rimexolone ... 1814
Triamcinolone (Ophthalmic) ... 2100

Corticosteroid, Otic
Ciprofloxacin and Dexamethasone ... 446
Ciprofloxacin and Hydrocortisone ... 446
Dexamethasone (Ophthalmic) ... 602
Neomycin, Colistin, Hydrocortisone, and Thonzonium ... 1437
Neomycin, Polymyxin B, and Hydrocortisone ... 1438

Corticosteroid, Rectal
Hydrocortisone (Topical) ... 1014

Corticosteroid, Systemic
Betamethasone (Systemic) ... 253
Budesonide (Systemic) ... 293
Cortisone ... 510
Cosyntropin ... 510
Deflazacort [INT] ... 587
Dexamethasone (Systemic) ... 599
Fludrocortisone ... 891
Hydrocortisone (Systemic) ... 1013
MethylPREDNISolone ... 1340
PrednisoLONE (Systemic) ... 1703
PredniSONE ... 1706
Triamcinolone (Systemic) ... 2099

Corticosteroid, Topical
Alclometasone ... 72
Bacitracin, Neomycin, Polymyxin B, and Hydrocortisone ... 223
Betamethasone and Clotrimazole ... 256
Betamethasone (Topical) ... 255
Calcipotriene and Betamethasone ... 321
Clioquinol and Flumethasone [CAN/INT] ... 465
Clobetasol ... 468
Clocortolone ... 469
Desonide ... 597
Desoximetasone ... 598
Diflorasone ... 625
Diflucortolone [CAN/INT] ... 625
Difluprednate (Topical) [INT] ... 627
Fluocinolone, Hydroquinone, and Tretinoin ... 894
Fluocinolone (Topical) ... 893
Fluocinonide ... 894
Flurandrenolide ... 906
Fluticasone (Topical) ... 911
Halcinonide ... 992
Halobetasol ... 993
Halometasone [INT] ... 993
Hydrocortisone (Topical) ... 1014
Iodoquinol and Hydrocortisone ... 1105
Mometasone (Topical) ... 1391
Neomycin, Polymyxin B, and Hydrocortisone ... 1438
Nystatin and Triamcinolone ... 1482
Prednicarbate ... 1703
Triamcinolone (Topical) ... 2100
Urea and Hydrocortisone ... 2115

Cortisol Receptor Blocker
Mifepristone ... 1366

Cosmetic Agent, Implant
Poly-L-Lactic Acid ... 1676

Cough Preparation
Guaifenesin and Codeine ... 987
Guaifenesin and Dextromethorphan ... 987

Cystic Fibrosis Transmembrane Conductance Regulator Potentiator
Ivacaftor ... 1135

Cytochrome P-450 Inhibitor
Cobicistat ... 495
Darunavir and Cobicistat ... 572
Elvitegravir, Cobicistat, Emtricitabine, and Tenofovir ... 718
Ombitasvir, Paritaprevir, Ritonavir, and Dasabuvir ... 1505

Cytoprotective Agent
Rebamipide [INT] ... 1786

Decongestant
Acrivastine and Pseudoephedrine ... 46
Chlorpheniramine and Phenylephrine ... 426
Chlorpheniramine and Pseudoephedrine ... 427
Chlorpheniramine, Phenylephrine, and Dextromethorphan ... 428
Chlorpheniramine, Pseudoephedrine, and Dextromethorphan ... 428
Desloratadine and Pseudoephedrine ... 594
Dextromethorphan and Phenylephrine ... 611
Dihydrocodeine, Chlorpheniramine, and Phenylephrine ... 633
Diphenhydramine and Phenylephrine ... 644
Fexofenadine and Pseudoephedrine ... 874
Guaifenesin and Phenylephrine ... 988
Loratadine and Pseudoephedrine ... 1242
Pseudoephedrine ... 1742
Triprolidine and Pseudoephedrine ... 2105
Triprolidine, Pseudoephedrine, and Codeine [CAN/INT] ... 2105

Decongestant/Analgesic
Pseudoephedrine and Ibuprofen ... 1743

Depigmenting Agent
Fluocinolone, Hydroquinone, and Tretinoin ... 894
Hydroquinone ... 1020

Diagnostic Agent
Adenosine ... 55
Arginine ... 171
Corticorelin ... 509
Cosyntropin ... 510
Edrophonium ... 706
Fluorescein ... 894
Fluorescein and Benoxinate ... 895
Glucagon ... 970
Mannitol ... 1269
Methacholine ... 1310
Proparacaine and Fluorescein ... 1728
Thyrotropin Alfa ... 2031
Tuberculin Tests ... 2110

Dietary Supplement
Manganese ... 1268
Methylfolate, Methylcobalamin, and Acetylcysteine ... 1334

Disinfectant, Antibacterial (Topical)
Sodium Hypochlorite Solution ... 1906

Diuretic
Pamabrom ... 1563

Diuretic, Carbonic Anhydrase Inhibitor
AcetaZOLAMIDE ... 39
Methazolamide ... 1317

Diuretic, Loop
Azosemide [INT] ... 220
Bumetanide ... 297
Ethacrynic Acid ... 797
Furosemide ... 940
Torsemide ... 2071

Diuretic, Miscellaneous
Mefruside [INT] ... 1281

Diuretic, Osmotic
Mannitol ... 1269

Diuretic, Potassium-Sparing
AMILoride ... 113
Eplerenone ... 740
Hydrochlorothiazide and Triamterene ... 1012
Spironolactone ... 1931
Triamterene ... 2101

Diuretic, Thiazide
Aliskiren, Amlodipine, and Hydrochlorothiazide ... 87
Aliskiren and Hydrochlorothiazide ... 87
Amlodipine, Valsartan, and Hydrochlorothiazide ... 127
Azilsartan and Chlorthalidone ... 215
Benazepril and Hydrochlorothiazide ... 240
Bisoprolol and Hydrochlorothiazide ... 267
Candesartan and Hydrochlorothiazide ... 338
Captopril and Hydrochlorothiazide ... 345
Chlorothiazide ... 426
Chlorthalidone ... 430
Cilazapril and Hydrochlorothiazide [CAN/INT] ... 436
Enalapril and Hydrochlorothiazide ... 725
Eprosartan and Hydrochlorothiazide ... 750
Hydrochlorothiazide ... 1009
Hydrochlorothiazide and Triamterene ... 1012
Irbesartan and Hydrochlorothiazide ... 1112
Lisinopril and Hydrochlorothiazide ... 1229
Losartan and Hydrochlorothiazide ... 1250
Methyclothiazide ... 1331
Moexipril and Hydrochlorothiazide ... 1388
Olmesartan, Amlodipine, and Hydrochlorothiazide ... 1498
Olmesartan and Hydrochlorothiazide ... 1498
Pindolol and Hydrochlorothiazide [CAN/INT] ... 1653
Ramipril and Hydrochlorothiazide [CAN/INT] ... 1773
Telmisartan and Hydrochlorothiazide ... 1990
Valsartan and Hydrochlorothiazide ... 2129
Xipamide [INT] ... 2191

Diuretic, Thiazide-Related
Indapamide ... 1065
Metolazone ... 1348
Perindopril and Indapamide [CAN/INT] ... 1626

Dopamine Agonist
Fenoldopam ... 856

Dopamine Antagonist
Domperidone [CAN/INT] ... 666

Echinocandin
Anidulafungin ... 150
Caspofungin ... 370
Micafungin ... 1359

Electrolyte Supplement
Electrolyte Solution, Renal Replacement ... 710
Magnesium L-lactate ... 1264

Electrolyte Supplement, Oral
Calcium and Vitamin D ... 326
Calcium Carbonate ... 327
Calcium Gluconate ... 330
Magnesium L-aspartate Hydrochloride ... 1264
Magnesium Chloride ... 1261
Magnesium Gluconate ... 1263
Magnesium Oxide ... 1265
Potassium Bicarbonate and Potassium Chloride ... 1687
Potassium Bicarbonate and Potassium Citrate ... 1687
Potassium Chloride ... 1687
Potassium Gluconate ... 1690
Potassium Phosphate and Sodium Phosphate ... 1692
Sodium Bicarbonate ... 1901

Electrolyte Supplement, Parenteral
Ammonium Chloride ... 127
Calcium Chloride ... 328
Calcium Gluconate ... 330
Magnesium Chloride ... 1261
Magnesium Sulfate ... 1265
Potassium Acetate ... 1686
Potassium Chloride ... 1687
Potassium Phosphate ... 1691
Sodium Acetate ... 1900
Sodium Bicarbonate ... 1901
Sodium Chloride ... 1902
Sodium Glycerophosphate Pentahydrate ... 1906
Sodium Phosphates ... 1909

Endocannabinoid CB1 Receptor Antagonist
Rimonabant [INT] ... 1814

Endothelin Receptor Antagonist
Ambrisentan ... 107
Bosentan ... 280

Enkephalinase Inhibitor
Racecadotril [INT] ... 1765

Enzyme
Agalsidase Alfa [CAN/INT] ... 63
Agalsidase Beta ... 64
Alglucosidase Alfa ... 85
Alpha-Galactosidase ... 94
Collagenase (Systemic) ... 506
Dornase Alfa ... 672
Elosulfase Alfa ... 714
Glucarpidase ... 971
Idursulfase ... 1040
Imiglucerase ... 1051
Laronidase ... 1172
Pancrelipase ... 1566
Pegademase Bovine ... 1588
Pegloticase ... 1602
Protein C Concentrate (Human) ... 1738
Rasburicase ... 1783
Taliglucerase Alfa ... 1971
Velaglucerase Alfa ... 2147

Enzyme Cofactor
Sapropterin ... 1864

Enzyme, Gastrointestinal
Sacrosidase ... 1860

Enzyme Inhibitor
Eliglustat ... 712
Miglustat ... 1367

Enzyme, Topical Debridement
Collagenase (Topical) ... 507

Enzyme, Urate-Oxidase (Recombinant)
Pegloticase ... 1602
Rasburicase ... 1783

Epidermal Growth Factor Receptor (EGFR) Inhibitor
Nimotuzumab [INT] 1457

Ergot Derivative
Bromocriptine 291
Cabergoline 319
Dihydroergotamine 633
Ergonovine [CAN/INT] 754
Ergotamine 754
Methylergonovine 1333
Oxytocin and Ergometrine Maleate [INT] 1550

Erythropoiesis-Stimulating Agent (ESA)
Darbepoetin Alfa 565
Epoetin Alfa 742

Estrogen and Progestin Combination
Cyproterone and Ethinyl Estradiol [CAN/INT] 532
Estradiol and Dienogest 780
Estradiol and Levonorgestrel 781
Estradiol and Norethindrone 781
Ethinyl Estradiol and Desogestrel 799
Ethinyl Estradiol and Drospirenone 801
Ethinyl Estradiol and Ethynodiol Diacetate 801
Ethinyl Estradiol and Etonogestrel 802
Ethinyl Estradiol and Levonorgestrel 803
Ethinyl Estradiol and Norelgestromin 807
Ethinyl Estradiol and Norethindrone 808
Ethinyl Estradiol and Norgestimate 810
Ethinyl Estradiol and Norgestrel 812
Ethinyl Estradiol, Drospirenone, and Levomefolate 812
Norethindrone and Mestranol 1475
Tibolone [INT] 2035

Estrogen Derivative
Estradiol (Systemic) 775
Estradiol (Topical) 780
Estrogens (Conjugated A/Synthetic) 782
Estrogens (Conjugated B/Synthetic) 785
Estrogens (Conjugated/Equine) and Bazedoxifene 782
Estrogens (Conjugated/Equine, Systemic) 787
Estrogens (Conjugated/Equine, Topical) 790
Estrogens (Esterified) 790
Estropipate 793
Polyestradiol [INT] 1673

Ethanolamine Derivative
Acetaminophen, Codeine, and Doxylamine [CAN/INT] 37
Carbinoxamine 356
Clemastine 459
DimenhyDRINATE 637
Diphenhydramine and Phenylephrine 644
DiphenhydrAMINE (Systemic) 641
Doxylamine and Pyridoxine 693

Expectorant
GuaiFENesin 986
Guaifenesin and Codeine 987
Guaifenesin and Dextromethorphan 987
Guaifenesin and Phenylephrine 988
Guaifenesin and Pseudoephedrine 989
Potassium Iodide 1690

Fiber Supplement
Psyllium 1744
Wheat Dextrin 2190

First Generation (Typical) Antipsychotic
Amitriptyline and Perphenazine 122
ChlorproMAZINE 429
Droperidol 695
Flupentixol [CAN/INT] 903
FluPHENAZine 905
Haloperidol 993
Loxapine 1255
Methotrimeprazine [CAN/INT] 1329
Periciazine [CAN/INT] 1621
Perphenazine 1627
Pimozide 1651
Pipotiazine [CAN/INT] 1660
Prochlorperazine 1718
Thioridazine 2030
Thiothixene 2031
Trifluoperazine 2102
Zuclopenthixol [CAN/INT] 2219

Fumaric Acid Derivative
Dimethyl Fumarate 639

GABA Agonist/Glutamate Antagonist
Acamprosate 28

GABA Analog
Gabapentin 943

Gallstone Dissolution Agent
Ursodiol 2116

Gastrointestinal Agent, Miscellaneous
Adalimumab 51
Alvimopan 104
Carbenoxolone [INT] 350
Certolizumab Pegol 409
Glutamine 971
InFLIXimab 1070
Lansoprazole, Amoxicillin, and Clarithromycin 1169
Linaclotide 1215
Lubiprostone 1255
Methylnaltrexone 1334
Naloxegol 1418
Natalizumab 1432
Omeprazole, Clarithromycin, and Amoxicillin 1511
Sucralfate 1940
Vedolizumab 2146

Gastrointestinal Agent, Prokinetic
Bromopride [INT] 292
Domperidone [CAN/INT] 666
Itopride [INT] 1130
Metoclopramide 1345
Mosapride [INT] 1401

Gastrointestinal Agent, Stimulant
Dexpanthenol 606

General Anesthetic
Etomidate 816
FentaNYL 857
Ketamine 1143
Methohexital 1321
Propofol 1728
SUFentanil 1941
Thiopental [INT] 2029

Genitourinary Irrigant
Mannitol 1269
Neomycin and Polymyxin B 1437
Sodium Chloride 1902
Sorbitol 1927

Glucagon-Like Peptide-2 (GLP-2) Analog
Teduglutide 1982

Glucocorticoid
Deflazacort [INT] 587

Glucosylceramide Synthase Inhibitor
Eliglustat ... 712
Miglustat ... 1367

Glutamate Inhibitor
Riluzole ... 1812

Glycopeptide
Dalbavancin ... 551
Oritavancin ... 1519
Telavancin ... 1986
Vancomycin ... 2130

Gold Compound
Auranofin ... 204

Gonadotropin
Chorionic Gonadotropin (Human) ... 431
Chorionic Gonadotropin (Recombinant) ... 432
Follitropin Alfa ... 921
Follitropin Beta ... 921
Gonadorelin [CAN/INT] ... 980
Lutropin Alfa [CAN/INT] ... 1259
Menotropins ... 1292
Urofollitropin ... 2116

Gonadotropin Releasing Hormone Agonist
Buserelin [CAN/INT] ... 309
Goserelin ... 981
Histrelin ... 1005
Leuprolide ... 1186
Leuprolide and Norethindrone ... 1189
Nafarelin ... 1414
Triptorelin ... 2107

Gonadotropin Releasing Hormone Antagonist
Cetrorelix ... 413
Degarelix ... 587
Ganirelix ... 949

Growth Factor, Platelet-Derived
Becaplermin ... 230
Trapidil [INT] ... 2085

Growth Hormone
Somatropin ... 1918

Growth Hormone Receptor Antagonist
Pegvisomant ... 1604

Growth Hormone Releasing Factor
Tesamorelin ... 2010

Hematopoietic Agent
Darbepoetin Alfa ... 565
Eltrombopag ... 714
Epoetin Alfa ... 742
Filgrastim ... 875
Pegfilgrastim ... 1589
Plerixafor ... 1665
RomiPLOStim ... 1842
Sargramostim ... 1865

Hematopoietic Stem Cell Mobilizer
Plerixafor ... 1665

Hemostatic Agent
Aminocaproic Acid ... 113
Aprotinin ... 168
Desmopressin ... 594
Etamsylate [INT] ... 795
Prothrombin Complex Concentrate (Human) [(Factors II, VII, IX, X), Protein C, and Protein S] ... 1738
Tranexamic Acid ... 2081

Histamine H_1 Agonist
Betahistine [CAN/INT] ... 252

Histamine H_1 Antagonist
Acetaminophen, Codeine, and Doxylamine [CAN/INT] ... 37
Acrivastine and Pseudoephedrine ... 46
Azelastine (Nasal) ... 213
Azelastine (Ophthalmic) ... 213
Bepotastine ... 250
Brompheniramine ... 292
Carbinoxamine ... 356
Cetirizine ... 411
Chlorpheniramine and Acetaminophen ... 426
Chlorpheniramine and Phenylephrine ... 426
Chlorpheniramine and Pseudoephedrine ... 427
Chlorpheniramine, Phenylephrine, and Dextromethorphan ... 428
Chlorpheniramine, Pseudoephedrine, and Dextromethorphan ... 428
Clemastine ... 459
Cyproheptadine ... 529
Desloratadine ... 594
Desloratadine and Pseudoephedrine ... 594
Dexchlorpheniramine ... 603
Dextromethorphan and Chlorpheniramine ... 610
Dihydrocodeine, Chlorpheniramine, and Phenylephrine ... 633
DimenhyDRINATE ... 637
Diphenhydramine and Phenylephrine ... 644
DiphenhydrAMINE (Systemic) ... 641
Doxylamine and Pyridoxine ... 693
Fexofenadine ... 873
Fexofenadine and Pseudoephedrine ... 874
Hydrocodone and Chlorpheniramine ... 1012
HydrOXYzine ... 1024
Ketotifen (Ophthalmic) ... 1150
Ketotifen (Systemic) [CAN/INT] ... 1149
Levocabastine (Nasal) [CAN/INT] ... 1194
Levocabastine (Ophthalmic) [CAN/INT] ... 1195
Levocetirizine ... 1196
Loratadine ... 1241
Loratadine and Pseudoephedrine ... 1242
Meclizine ... 1277
Naphazoline and Pheniramine ... 1426
Olopatadine (Nasal) ... 1500
Olopatadine (Ophthalmic) ... 1500
Promethazine ... 1723
Promethazine and Codeine ... 1725
Promethazine and Dextromethorphan ... 1725
Triprolidine and Pseudoephedrine ... 2105
Triprolidine, Pseudoephedrine, and Codeine [CAN/INT] ... 2105

Histamine H_1 Antagonist, First Generation
Acetaminophen, Codeine, and Doxylamine [CAN/INT] ... 37
Brompheniramine ... 292
Carbinoxamine ... 356
Chlorpheniramine and Acetaminophen ... 426
Chlorpheniramine and Phenylephrine ... 426
Chlorpheniramine and Pseudoephedrine ... 427
Chlorpheniramine, Phenylephrine, and Dextromethorphan ... 428
Chlorpheniramine, Pseudoephedrine, and Dextromethorphan ... 428
Clemastine ... 459
Cyproheptadine ... 529
Dexchlorpheniramine ... 603
Dextromethorphan and Chlorpheniramine ... 610
Dihydrocodeine, Chlorpheniramine, and Phenylephrine ... 633
DimenhyDRINATE ... 637
Diphenhydramine and Phenylephrine ... 644
DiphenhydrAMINE (Systemic) ... 641
Doxylamine and Pyridoxine ... 693

Hydrocodone and Chlorpheniramine 1012
HydrOXYzine 1024
Meclizine 1277
Naphazoline and Pheniramine 1426
Promethazine 1723
Promethazine and Codeine 1725
Promethazine and Dextromethorphan 1725
Triprolidine and Pseudoephedrine 2105
Triprolidine, Pseudoephedrine, and Codeine [CAN/INT] 2105

Histamine H_1 Antagonist, Second Generation

Acrivastine and Pseudoephedrine 46
Azelastine and Fluticasone 214
Azelastine (Nasal) 213
Azelastine (Ophthalmic) 213
Bepotastine 250
Cetirizine 411
Desloratadine 594
Desloratadine and Pseudoephedrine 594
Fexofenadine 873
Fexofenadine and Pseudoephedrine 874
Ketotifen (Ophthalmic) 1150
Ketotifen (Systemic) [CAN/INT] 1149
Levocabastine (Nasal) [CAN/INT] 1194
Levocabastine (Ophthalmic) [CAN/INT] 1195
Levocetirizine 1196
Loratadine 1241
Loratadine and Pseudoephedrine 1242
Olopatadine (Nasal) 1500
Olopatadine (Ophthalmic) 1500

Histamine H_2 Antagonist

Cimetidine 438
Famotidine 845
Lafutidine [INT] 1157
Nizatidine 1471
Ranitidine 1777

Histamine H_3 Antagonist

Betahistine [CAN/INT] 252

Histone Deacetylase Inhibitor

Valproic Acid and Derivatives 2123

Homocystinuria, Treatment Agent

Betaine 252

Hormone

Calcitonin 322

Hormone, Posterior Pituitary

Desmopressin 594
Terlipressin [INT] 2010
Vasopressin 2142

5-HT_3 Receptor Antagonist

Ramosetron [INT] 1774
Trimebutine [CAN/INT] 2103

Human Growth Factor

Oprelvekin 1519

4-Hydroxyphenylpyruvate Dioxygenase Inhibitor

Nitisinone 1461

Hyperprolactinemia Agent, Dopamine (D_2) Agonist

Quinagolide [CAN/INT] 1755

Hypnotic, Benzodiazepine

Flurazepam 906

Hypnotic, Miscellaneous

Chloral Hydrate [CAN/INT] 418
Eszopiclone 793
Ramelteon 1770
Suvorexant 1961
Tasimelteon 1979
Zaleplon 2193
Zolpidem 2212
Zopiclone [CAN/INT] 2217

Imidazoline Derivative

Naphazoline and Pheniramine 1426
Naphazoline (Nasal) 1426
Naphazoline (Ophthalmic) 1426

Immune Globulin

Antithymocyte Globulin (Equine) 157
Antithymocyte Globulin (Rabbit) 158
Botulism Immune Globulin (Intravenous-Human) 284
Cytomegalovirus Immune Globulin (Intravenous-Human) 541
Hepatitis B Immune Globulin (Human) 1002
Immune Globulin 1056
Rabies Immune Globulin (Human) 1764
Rh_o(D) Immune Globulin 1794
Tetanus Immune Globulin (Human) 2015
Vaccinia Immune Globulin (Intravenous) 2118
Varicella-Zoster Immune Globulin (Human) 2142

Immunomodulator, Systemic

Alitretinoin (Systemic) [CAN/INT] 88
Dimethyl Fumarate 639
Interferon Alfa-2b 1096
Lenalidomide 1177
Peginterferon Alfa-2b 1596
Peginterferon Beta-1a 1602
Pomalidomide 1677
Thalidomide 2022

Immunosuppressant Agent

Antithymocyte Globulin (Equine) 157
Antithymocyte Globulin (Rabbit) 158
AzaTHIOprine 210
Basiliximab 228
Cyclophosphamide 517
CycloSPORINE (Ophthalmic) 529
CycloSPORINE (Systemic) 522
Everolimus 822
InFLIXimab 1070
Mercaptopurine 1296
Methotrexate 1322
Mycophenolate 1405
Pimecrolimus 1650
RiTUXimab 1825
Sirolimus 1893
Tacrolimus (Systemic) 1962
Tacrolimus (Topical) 1968

Inotrope

DOBUTamine 654
DOPamine 669
Milrinone 1370

Insulin, Combination

Insulin Aspart Protamine and Insulin Aspart 1084
Insulin Lispro Protamine and Insulin Lispro 1088
Insulin NPH and Insulin Regular 1090

Insulin, Intermediate-Acting

Insulin NPH 1089

Insulin, Intermediate- to Long-Acting

Insulin Detemir 1085

Insulin, Long-Acting

Insulin Glargine 1086

Insulin, Rapid-Acting

Insulin Aspart 1083
Insulin Glulisine 1086
Insulin Lispro 1087

Insulin, Short-Acting
Insulin Regular 1091

Interferon
Interferon Alfa-2b 1096
Interferon Alfacon-1 1100
Interferon Alfa-n3 1100
Interferon Alpha, Multi-Subtype [INT] 1100
Interferon Beta-1a 1100
Interferon Beta-1b 1103
Interferon Gamma-1b 1104
Peginterferon Alfa-2a 1590
Peginterferon Alfa-2a and Ribavirin [CAN/INT] 1592
Peginterferon Alfa-2b 1596
Peginterferon Alfa-2b and Ribavirin [CAN/INT] 1598
Peginterferon Beta-1a 1602

Interleukin-1 Beta Inhibitor
Canakinumab 335

Interleukin-1 Inhibitor
Canakinumab 335
Rilonacept 1810

Interleukin-1 Receptor Antagonist
Anakinra 148

Interleukin-6 Receptor Antagonist
Siltuximab 1885
Tocilizumab 2057

Interleukin-12 Inhibitor
Ustekinumab 2117

Interleukin-23 Inhibitor
Ustekinumab 2117

Intravenous Nutritional Therapy
Total Parenteral Nutrition 2073

Iron Salt
Ferric Carboxymaltose 868
Ferric Gluconate 869
Ferrous Fumarate 870
Ferrous Gluconate 870
Ferrous Sulfate 871
Ferumoxytol 871
Iron Dextran Complex 1117
Iron Sucrose 1118
Polysaccharide-Iron Complex 1677

Irrigant
Sodium Chloride 1902

Janus Associated Kinase Inhibitor
Ruxolitinib 1856
Tofacitinib 2059

Kallikrein Inhibitor
Ecallantide 703

Keratinocyte Growth Factor
Palifermin 1555

Keratolytic Agent
Anthralin 150
Cantharidin [CAN/INT] 338
Podophyllum Resin 1672
Tazarotene 1980
Urea 2114

Laxative
Magnesium Hydroxide 1263
Magnesium Hydroxide and Mineral Oil 1264

Laxative, Bowel Evacuant
Sodium Phosphates 1909

Laxative, Bulk-Producing
Psyllium 1744
Wheat Dextrin 2190

Laxative, Osmotic
Lactulose 1156
Polyethylene Glycol 3350 1674
Polyethylene Glycol-Electrolyte Solution 1674
Sodium Picosulfate, Magnesium Oxide, and Citric Acid 1911
Sodium Sulfate, Potassium Sulfate, and Magnesium Sulfate 1914
Sodium Sulfate, Potassium Sulfate, Magnesium Sulfate, and Polyethylene Glycol-Electrolyte Solution 1914
Sorbitol 1927

Laxative, Saline
Magnesium Citrate 1262

Laxative, Stimulant
Bisacodyl 265
Docusate and Senna 662
Sodium Picosulfate, Magnesium Oxide, and Citric Acid 1911

Leptin Analog
Metreleptin 1353

Leukotriene-Receptor Antagonist
Montelukast 1392
Zafirlukast 2192

Lipase Inhibitor
Orlistat 1520

5-Lipoxygenase Inhibitor
Zileuton 2199

Local Anesthetic
Benzocaine 246
Benzocaine, Butamben, and Tetracaine 247
Bupivacaine 299
Cetylpyridinium and Benzocaine [CAN/INT] 415
Chloroprocaine 423
Cocaine 497
Levobupivacaine [INT] 1194
Lidocaine and Epinephrine 1212
Lidocaine and Prilocaine 1213
Lidocaine and Tetracaine 1214
Lidocaine (Systemic) 1208
Lidocaine (Topical) 1211
Mepivacaine 1295
Proparacaine and Fluorescein 1728
Ropivacaine 1846
Tetracaine (Ophthalmic) 2017
Tetracaine (Systemic) 2017
Tetracaine (Topical) 2017

Local Anesthetic, Ophthalmic
Proparacaine 1728

Local Anesthetic, Oral
Benzydamine [CAN/INT] 249
Dyclonine 702

Lubricant, Ocular
Sodium Chloride 1902

Lung Surfactant
Beractant 250
Bovine Lipid Extract Surfactant [CAN/INT] 285
Calfactant 334
Lucinactant 1256

Lysine Analog
Aminocaproic Acid ... 113
Tranexamic Acid ... 2081

Magnesium Salt
Magnesium L-aspartate Hydrochloride ... 1264
Magnesium L-lactate ... 1264
Magnesium Chloride ... 1261
Magnesium Citrate ... 1262
Magnesium Glucoheptonate [CAN/INT] ... 1262
Magnesium Gluconate ... 1263
Magnesium Hydroxide ... 1263
Magnesium Oxide ... 1265
Magnesium Sulfate ... 1265

Mast Cell Stabilizer
Bepotastine ... 250
Cromolyn (Nasal) ... 514
Cromolyn (Ophthalmic) ... 514
Ketotifen (Ophthalmic) ... 1150
Ketotifen (Systemic) [CAN/INT] ... 1149
Lodoxamide ... 1232
Nedocromil ... 1435

Melatonin Receptor Agonist
Ramelteon ... 1770
Tasimelteon ... 1979

Metabolic Alkalosis Agent
Carglumic Acid ... 362

Monoclonal Antibody
Adalimumab ... 51
Alemtuzumab ... 75
Basiliximab ... 228
Belimumab ... 235
Canakinumab ... 335
Denosumab ... 589
Eculizumab ... 703
Golimumab ... 977
InFLIXimab ... 1070
Palivizumab ... 1560
Ranibizumab ... 1776
Raxibacumab ... 1786
RiTUXimab ... 1825
Ustekinumab ... 2117
Vedolizumab ... 2146

Monoclonal Antibody, Anti-Asthmatic
Omalizumab ... 1503

Monoclonal Antibody, Complement Inhibitor
Eculizumab ... 703

Monoclonal Antibody, Selective Adhesion-Molecule Inhibitor
Natalizumab ... 1432
Vedolizumab ... 2146

mTOR Kinase Inhibitor
Everolimus ... 822
Sirolimus ... 1893

Mucolytic Agent
Acetylcysteine ... 40
Ambroxol [INT] ... 109
Bromhexine [INT] ... 291
Carbocisteine [INT] ... 357
Dornase Alfa ... 672
Erdosteine [INT] ... 753
Mecysteine [INT] ... 1277

Natriuretic Peptide, B-Type, Human
Nesiritide ... 1439

Neuraminidase Inhibitor
Oseltamivir ... 1523
Peramivir ... 1619
Zanamivir ... 2194

Neuromuscular Blocker Agent, Depolarizing
Succinylcholine ... 1939

Neuromuscular Blocker Agent, Nondepolarizing
Atracurium ... 198
Cisatracurium ... 447
Pancuronium ... 1567
Rocuronium ... 1838
Vecuronium ... 2144

Neuromuscular Blocker Agent, Toxin
AbobotulinumtoxinA ... 28
IncobotulinumtoxinA ... 1062
OnabotulinumtoxinA ... 1512
RimabotulinumtoxinB ... 1813

N-Methyl-D-Aspartate Receptor Antagonist
Dextromethorphan and Quinidine ... 611
Memantine ... 1286

Nonsteroidal Anti-inflammatory Drug (NSAID)
Diclofenac (Ophthalmic) ... 621
Diclofenac (Systemic) ... 617

Nonsteroidal Anti-inflammatory Drug (NSAID), COX-2 Selective
Celecoxib ... 402
Etoricoxib [INT] ... 821
Parecoxib [INT] ... 1576

Nonsteroidal Anti-inflammatory Drug (NSAID), Nasal
Ketorolac (Nasal) ... 1149

Nonsteroidal Anti-inflammatory Drug (NSAID), Ophthalmic
Bromfenac ... 291
Diclofenac (Ophthalmic) ... 621
Flurbiprofen (Ophthalmic) ... 906
Ketorolac (Ophthalmic) ... 1149
Nepafenac ... 1439

Nonsteroidal Anti-inflammatory Drug (NSAID), Oral
Acemetacin [INT] ... 30
Diclofenac and Misoprostol ... 621
Diclofenac (Systemic) ... 617
Diflunisal ... 626
Dipyrone [INT] ... 653
Etodolac ... 815
Fenoprofen ... 857
Floctafenine [CAN/INT] ... 883
Flurbiprofen (Systemic) ... 906
Hydrocodone and Ibuprofen ... 1013
Ibuprofen ... 1032
Indomethacin ... 1067
Ketoprofen ... 1145
Ketorolac (Systemic) ... 1146
Lornoxicam [INT] ... 1248
Loxoprofen [INT] ... 1255
Mefenamic Acid ... 1280
Meloxicam ... 1283
Nabumetone ... 1411
Naproxen ... 1427
Niflumic Acid [INT] ... 1454
Nimesulide [INT] ... 1456
Oxaprozin ... 1532
Oxycodone and Ibuprofen ... 1542
Piroxicam ... 1662
Sulindac ... 1953
Sumatriptan and Naproxen ... 1957
Tenoxicam [INT] ... 2001
Tiaprofenic Acid [CAN/INT] ... 2034
Tolmetin ... 2062

Nonsteroidal Anti-inflammatory Drug (NSAID), Parenteral
Dipyrone [INT] ... 653
Ibuprofen ... 1032
Indomethacin ... 1067
Ketorolac (Systemic) ... 1146
Lornoxicam [INT] ... 1248

Nonsteroidal Anti-inflammatory Drug (NSAID), Suppository
Dipyrone [INT] ... 653

Nootropic
Aniracetam [INT] ... 150
Piracetam [INT] ... 1661

Norepinephrine Reuptake Inhibitor, Selective
AtoMOXetine ... 191
Reboxetine [INT] ... 1786

Nutritional Supplement
Fluoride ... 895

Ophthalmic Agent
Aflibercept (Ophthalmic) ... 63
Cysteamine (Ophthalmic) ... 535
Fluorescein and Benoxinate ... 895
Ocriplasmin ... 1484
Pegaptanib ... 1588
Ranibizumab ... 1776

Ophthalmic Agent, Antiglaucoma
AcetaZOLAMIDE ... 39
Betaxolol (Ophthalmic) ... 257
Bimatoprost ... 264
Bimatoprost and Timolol [INT] ... 264
Brimonidine and Timolol ... 288
Brimonidine (Ophthalmic) ... 288
Brinzolamide ... 288
Brinzolamide and Timolol [CAN/INT] ... 289
Carbachol ... 346
Dipivefrin ... 651
Dorzolamide ... 673
Dorzolamide and Timolol ... 673
Echothiophate Iodide ... 703
Latanoprost ... 1172
Latanoprost and Timolol [CAN/INT] ... 1172
Levobunolol ... 1194
Methazolamide ... 1317
Metipranolol ... 1345
Pilocarpine (Ophthalmic) ... 1649
Timolol (Ophthalmic) ... 2043
Travoprost ... 2089
Travoprost and Timolol [CAN/INT] ... 2090

Ophthalmic Agent, Miotic
Acetylcholine ... 40
Carbachol ... 346
Echothiophate Iodide ... 703
Pilocarpine (Ophthalmic) ... 1649

Ophthalmic Agent, Miscellaneous
MitoMYcin (Ophthalmic) ... 1382

Ophthalmic Agent, Mydriatic
Atropine ... 200
Cyclopentolate and Phenylephrine ... 517
Homatropine ... 1005
Tropicamide ... 2108

Ophthalmic Agent, Toxin
IncobotulinumtoxinA ... 1062
OnabotulinumtoxinA ... 1512

Ophthalmic Agent, Vasoconstrictor
Dipivefrin ... 651
Naphazoline and Pheniramine ... 1426
Naphazoline (Ophthalmic) ... 1426

Ophthalmic Agent, Viscoelastic
Hyaluronate and Derivatives ... 1006
Sodium Chondroitin Sulfate and Sodium Hyaluronate ... 1905

Opioid Antagonist
Naloxone ... 1419
Naltrexone ... 1422
Naltrexone and Bupropion ... 1423
Oxycodone and Naloxone ... 1542

Opioid Antagonist, Peripherally-Acting
Alvimopan ... 104
Methylnaltrexone ... 1334
Naloxegol ... 1418

Orexin Receptor Antagonist
Suvorexant ... 1961

Otic Agent, Analgesic
Antipyrine and Benzocaine ... 156

Otic Agent, Anti-infective
Acetic Acid ... 39
Acetic Acid, Propylene Glycol Diacetate, and Hydrocortisone ... 40

Otic Agent, Cerumenolytic
Antipyrine and Benzocaine ... 156
Carbamide Peroxide ... 350

Ovulation Stimulator
Chorionic Gonadotropin (Human) ... 431
Chorionic Gonadotropin (Recombinant) ... 432
ClomiPHENE ... 473
Follitropin Alfa ... 921
Follitropin Beta ... 921
Lutropin Alfa [CAN/INT] ... 1259
Menotropins ... 1292
Urofollitropin ... 2116

Oxytocic Agent
Carbetocin [CAN/INT] ... 350
Oxytocin ... 1549
Oxytocin and Ergometrine Maleate [INT] ... 1550

Parathyroid Hormone Analog
Teriparatide ... 2008

Partial Nicotine Agonist
Varenicline ... 2139

Pediculocide
Benzyl Alcohol ... 250
Ivermectin (Topical) ... 1137
Lindane ... 1217
Malathion ... 1268
Permethrin ... 1627
Pyrethrins and Piperonyl Butoxide ... 1746
Spinosad ... 1930

Peritoneal Dialysate, Osmotic
Icodextrin ... 1037

Phenothiazine Derivative
Promethazine ... 1723
Promethazine and Codeine ... 1725
Promethazine and Dextromethorphan ... 1725

Phosphate Binder
Calcium Acetate ... 326
Ferric Citrate ... 869
Lanthanum ... 1169
Sevelamer ... 1881
Sucroferric Oxyhydroxide ... 1941

Phosphodiesterase-3 Enzyme Inhibitor
Anagrelide ... 147
Cilostazol ... 437
Milrinone ... 1370

Phosphodiesterase-4 Enzyme Inhibitor
Apremilast ... 165
Roflumilast ... 1840

Phosphodiesterase-5 Enzyme Inhibitor
Avanafil ... 205
Sildenafil ... 1882
Tadalafil ... 1968
Vardenafil ... 2138

Phosphodiesterase Enzyme Inhibitor
Enoximone [INT] ... 730

Phosphodiesterase Enzyme Inhibitor, Nonselective
Caffeine ... 319
Theophylline ... 2026

Photosensitizing Agent, Topical
Aminolevulinic Acid ... 114
Methyl Aminolevulinate ... 1332

Piperazine Derivative
Cetirizine ... 411
HydrOXYzine ... 1024
Levocetirizine ... 1196
Meclizine ... 1277

Piperidine Derivative
Cyproheptadine ... 529
Desloratadine ... 594
Desloratadine and Pseudoephedrine ... 594
Fexofenadine ... 873
Fexofenadine and Pseudoephedrine ... 874
Ketotifen (Ophthalmic) ... 1150
Ketotifen (Systemic) [CAN/INT] ... 1149
Levocabastine (Nasal) [CAN/INT] ... 1194
Levocabastine (Ophthalmic) [CAN/INT] ... 1195
Loratadine ... 1241
Loratadine and Pseudoephedrine ... 1242
Olopatadine (Nasal) ... 1500
Olopatadine (Ophthalmic) ... 1500

Plasma Volume Expander, Colloid
Albumin ... 67
Dextran ... 607
Hetastarch ... 1004
Tetrastarch ... 2019

Polyclonal Antibody
Antithymocyte Globulin (Equine) ... 157
Antithymocyte Globulin (Rabbit) ... 158

Potassium Channel Blocker
Dalfampridine ... 552

Progestin
Dydrogesterone [INT] ... 702
Hydroxyprogesterone Caproate ... 1021
Leuprolide and Norethindrone ... 1189
Levonorgestrel ... 1201
Lynestrenol [INT] ... 1261
MedroxyPROGESTERone ... 1277
Megestrol ... 1281
Norethindrone ... 1473
Progesterone ... 1722

Progestin Receptor Modulator
Ulipristal ... 2113

Prostacyclin
Epoprostenol ... 746
Iloprost ... 1046
Treprostinil ... 2093

Prostaglandin
Alprostadil ... 96
Beraprost [INT] ... 251
Carboprost Tromethamine ... 360
Diclofenac and Misoprostol ... 621
Dinoprostone ... 640
Epoprostenol ... 746
Iloprost ... 1046
Misoprostol ... 1379
Treprostinil ... 2093

Prostaglandin, Ophthalmic
Bimatoprost ... 264
Bimatoprost and Timolol [INT] ... 264
Latanoprost ... 1172
Latanoprost and Timolol [CAN/INT] ... 1172
Travoprost ... 2089
Travoprost and Timolol [CAN/INT] ... 2090

Protease-Activated Receptor-1 (PAR-1) Antagonist
Vorapaxar ... 2175

Proteasome Inhibitor
Bortezomib ... 276
Carfilzomib ... 361

Protectant, Topical
Aluminum Hydroxide ... 103
Trypsin, Balsam Peru, and Castor Oil ... 2109

Protein C
Protein C Concentrate (Human) ... 1738

Prothrombin Complex Concentrate (PCC)
Factor IX Complex (Human) [(Factors II, IX, X)] ... 838
Prothrombin Complex Concentrate (Human) [(Factors II, VII, IX, X), Protein C, and Protein S] ... 1738

Proton Pump Inhibitor
Dexlansoprazole ... 603
Esomeprazole ... 771
Lansoprazole ... 1166
Lansoprazole, Amoxicillin, and Clarithromycin ... 1169
Omeprazole ... 1508
Omeprazole and Sodium Bicarbonate ... 1511
Omeprazole, Clarithromycin, and Amoxicillin ... 1511
Pantoprazole ... 1570
RABEprazole ... 1762

Psoralen
Methoxsalen (Systemic) ... 1330
Methoxsalen (Topical) ... 1331

Pyrimidine Synthesis Inhibitor
Teriflunomide ... 2006

Rauwolfia Alkaloid
Reserpine ... 1793

Renin Inhibitor
Aliskiren ... 85
Aliskiren, Amlodipine, and Hydrochlorothiazide ... 87
Aliskiren and Hydrochlorothiazide ... 87

Rescue Agent (Chemotherapy)
Leucovorin Calcium ... 1183
LEVOleucovorin ... 1200

Respiratory Stimulant
Almitrine [INT] ... 92
Doxapram ... 673

Retinoic Acid Derivative
Alitretinoin (Systemic) [CAN/INT] ... 88
Clindamycin and Tretinoin ... 464

Fluocinolone, Hydroquinone, and Tretinoin 894
ISOtretinoin 1127
Tretinoin (Systemic) 2096
Tretinoin (Topical) 2099

Retinoid-Like Compound
Acitretin 43

Salicylate
Aspirin 180
Choline Magnesium Trisalicylate 431
Magnesium Salicylate 1265
Methyl Salicylate and Menthol 1344
Salsalate 1862

Scabicidal Agent
Crotamiton 514
Lindane 1217
Malathion 1268
Permethrin 1627

Sclerosing Agent
Ethanolamine Oleate 799
Morrhuate Sodium 1401
Polidocanol 1672
Sodium Tetradecyl Sulfate 1914
Talc (Sterile) 1971

Second Generation (Atypical) Antipsychotic
ARIPiprazole 171
Asenapine 179
CloZAPine 490
Iloperidone 1044
Lurasidone 1256
OLANZapine 1491
Paliperidone 1556
QUEtiapine 1751
RisperiDONE 1818
Ziprasidone 2201

Sedative
Dexmedetomidine 604

Selective 5-HT$_3$ Receptor Antagonist
Dolasetron 663
Granisetron 983
Netupitant and Palonosetron 1440
Ondansetron 1513
Palonosetron 1561

Selective Aldosterone Blocker
Eplerenone 740
Spironolactone 1931

Selective Bradykinin B2 Receptor Antagonist
Icatibant 1037

Selective Estrogen Receptor Modulator (SERM)
ClomiPHENE 473
Estrogens (Conjugated/Equine) and Bazedoxifene 782
Ospemifene 1527
Raloxifene 1765
Tamoxifen 1971
Toremifene 2071

Selective Serotonin Reuptake Inhibitor (SSRI)
Dapoxetine [INT] 561

Selective T-Cell Costimulation Blocker
Abatacept 23
Belatacept 233

Serotonin 5-HT$_{1B, 1D}$ Receptor Agonist
Almotriptan 92
Eletriptan 711
Frovatriptan 938
Naratriptan 1430
Rizatriptan 1836
SUMAtriptan 1953
Sumatriptan and Naproxen 1957
ZOLMitriptan 2210

Serotonin 5-HT$_4$ Receptor Agonist
Prucalopride [CAN/INT] 1741

Serotonin 5-HT$_{2C}$ Receptor Agonist
Lorcaserin 1246

Serotonin 5-HT$_3$ Receptor Antagonist
Vortioxetine 2183

Serotonin and Histamine Antagonist
Pizotifen [CAN/INT] 1664

Serotonin Antagonist
Ketanserin [INT] 1144
Tropisetron [INT] 2108

Shampoo, Pediculocide
Pyrethrins and Piperonyl Butoxide 1746

Skeletal Muscle Relaxant
Baclofen 223
Carisoprodol 363
Carisoprodol and Aspirin 364
Carisoprodol, Aspirin, and Codeine 364
Chlorzoxazone 430
Cyclobenzaprine 516
Dantrolene 559
Gallamine Triethiodide [INT] 948
Idrocilamide [INT] 1040
Metaxalone 1307
Methocarbamol 1320
Orphenadrine 1522
Orphenadrine, Aspirin, and Caffeine 1522

Skin and Mucous Membrane Agent
Imiquimod 1055

Skin and Mucous Membrane Agent, Miscellaneous
Hyaluronate and Derivatives 1006

Smoking Cessation Aid
BuPROPion 305
Nicotine 1449
Varenicline 2139

Sodium-Glucose Cotransporter 2 (SGLT2) Inhibitor
Dapagliflozin and Metformin 561
Empagliflozin 718

Sodium Salt
Sodium Chloride 1902

Soluble Guanylate Cyclase (sGC) Stimulator
Riociguat 1814

Somatostatin Analog
Lanreotide 1165
Octreotide 1485
Pasireotide 1583

Spermicide
Nonoxynol 9 1471

Sphingosine 1-Phosphate (S1P) Receptor Modulator
Fingolimod 879

Stem Cell Factor, Human
Ancestim [INT] 150

Stool Softener
Docusate 661
Docusate and Senna 662

Strontium Salt
Strontium Ranelate [INT] ... 1938

Substance P/Neurokinin 1 Receptor Antagonist
Aprepitant ... 166
Fosaprepitant ... 929
Netupitant and Palonosetron ... 1440

Substituted Benzimidazole
Dexlansoprazole ... 603
Esomeprazole ... 771
Lansoprazole ... 1166
Lansoprazole, Amoxicillin, and Clarithromycin ... 1169
Omeprazole ... 1508
Omeprazole and Sodium Bicarbonate ... 1511
Omeprazole, Clarithromycin, and Amoxicillin ... 1511
Pantoprazole ... 1570
RABEprazole ... 1762

Sympathomimetic
Diethylpropion ... 624
Dopexamine [INT] ... 671
Methamphetamine ... 1315
Phentermine ... 1635

Theophylline Derivative
Doxofylline [INT] ... 679
Ephedrine and Theophylline [INT] ... 734

Thioamide
Methimazole ... 1319
Propylthiouracil ... 1735

Thrombolytic Agent
Alteplase ... 99
Reteplase ... 1794
Tenecteplase ... 1996

Thrombopoietic Agent
Eltrombopag ... 714
RomiPLOStim ... 1842

Thyroid Product
Levothyroxine ... 1205
Liothyronine ... 1221
Liotrix ... 1221
Thyroid, Desiccated ... 2031

Tissue-Selective Estrogen Complex (TSEC)
Estrogens (Conjugated/Equine) and Bazedoxifene ... 782

Tocolytic Agent
Atosiban [INT] ... 197

Topical Skin Product
Acetic Acid ... 39
Adapalene and Benzoyl Peroxide ... 54
Aminolevulinic Acid ... 114
Becaplermin ... 230
Bentoquatam ... 246
Benzoyl Peroxide and Hydrocortisone ... 248
Benzyl Alcohol ... 250
Calamine ... 321
Calcipotriene ... 321
Clindamycin and Tretinoin ... 464
Dexpanthenol ... 606
Doxepin (Topical) ... 678
Eflornithine ... 710
Erythromycin (Topical) ... 765
Fluorouracil (Topical) ... 899
Imiquimod ... 1055
Ingenol Mebutate ... 1083
Methyl Aminolevulinate ... 1332
Methyl Salicylate and Menthol ... 1344
Minoxidil (Topical) ... 1374
Pimecrolimus ... 1650
Selenium Sulfide ... 1877
Tacrolimus (Topical) ... 1968
Urea ... 2114
Vitamin A and Vitamin D (Topical) ... 2174
Zinc Gelatin ... 2200
Zinc Oxide ... 2200

Topical Skin Product, Acne
Adapalene ... 54
Adapalene and Benzoyl Peroxide ... 54
Azelaic Acid ... 213
Benzoyl Peroxide and Hydrocortisone ... 248
Clindamycin and Tretinoin ... 464
Clindamycin (Topical) ... 464
Erythromycin and Benzoyl Peroxide ... 765
Erythromycin (Topical) ... 765
Sulfacetamide (Topical) ... 1943
Sulfur and Sulfacetamide ... 1953
Tazarotene ... 1980
Tretinoin (Topical) ... 2099

Topical Skin Product, Antibacterial
Silver Nitrate ... 1886

Trace Element
Zinc Acetate ... 2199
Zinc Chloride ... 2200
Zinc Sulfate ... 2200

Trace Element, Parenteral
Copper ... 509
Manganese ... 1268
Selenium ... 1876

Tumor Necrosis Factor (TNF) Blocking Agent
Adalimumab ... 51
Certolizumab Pegol ... 409
Etanercept ... 795
Golimumab ... 977
InFLIXimab ... 1070

Tyrosine Hydroxylase Inhibitor
Metyrosine ... 1359

Tyrosine Kinase Inhibitor
Nintedanib ... 1458

Urea Cycle Disorder (UCD) Treatment Agent
Carglumic Acid ... 362
Sodium Phenylacetate and Sodium Benzoate ... 1908
Sodium Phenylbutyrate ... 1908

Uricosuric Agent
Colchicine and Probenecid ... 503
Probenecid ... 1716

Urinary Acidifying Agent
Potassium Acid Phosphate ... 1687

Urinary Tract Product
Cysteamine (Systemic) ... 534

Vaccine
Meningococcal Group C-CRM197 Conjugate Vaccine [CAN/INT] ... 1288
Travelers' Diarrhea and Cholera Vaccine [CAN/INT] ... 2088

Vaccine, Inactivated (Bacterial)
Anthrax Vaccine Adsorbed ... 151
Diphtheria and Tetanus Toxoid ... 645
Diphtheria and Tetanus Toxoids, Acellular Pertussis, and Poliovirus Vaccine ... 646
Diphtheria and Tetanus Toxoids, Acellular Pertussis, Poliovirus and Haemophilus b Conjugate Vaccine ... 648

Diphtheria and Tetanus Toxoids, and Acellular Pertussis Vaccine 649
Diphtheria, Tetanus Toxoids, Acellular Pertussis, Hepatitis B (Recombinant), and Poliovirus (Inactivated) Vaccine 651
Haemophilus b Conjugate and Hepatitis B Vaccine 991
Haemophilus b Conjugate Vaccine 991
Meningococcal (Groups A / C / Y and W-135) Diphtheria Conjugate Vaccine 1289
Meningococcal Polysaccharide (Groups C and Y) and Haemophilus b Tetanus Toxoid Conjugate Vaccine 1291
Meningococcal Polysaccharide (Groups A / C / Y and W-135) Tetanus Toxoid Conjugate Vaccine [CAN/INT] 1290
Meningococcal Polysaccharide Vaccine (Groups A / C / Y and W-135) 1292
Pneumococcal Conjugate Vaccine (10-Valent) [CAN/INT] 1668
Pneumococcal Conjugate Vaccine (13-Valent) 1670
Pneumococcal Polysaccharide Vaccine (23-Valent) 1671
Tetanus Toxoid (Adsorbed) 2016
Typhoid and Hepatitis A Vaccine [CAN/INT] 2111
Typhoid Vaccine 2112

Vaccine, Inactivated (Bacterial, Viral)

Diphtheria and Tetanus Toxoids, Acellular Pertussis, Hepatitis B (Recombinant), Poliovirus (Inactivated), and Haemophilus influenzae B Conjugate (Adsorbed) Vaccine [CAN/INT] 647

Vaccine, Inactivated (Viral)

Diphtheria and Tetanus Toxoids, Acellular Pertussis, and Poliovirus Vaccine 646
Diphtheria and Tetanus Toxoids, Acellular Pertussis, Poliovirus and Haemophilus b Conjugate Vaccine 648
Diphtheria, Tetanus Toxoids, Acellular Pertussis, Hepatitis B (Recombinant), and Poliovirus (Inactivated) Vaccine 651
Haemophilus b Conjugate and Hepatitis B Vaccine 991
Hepatitis A and Hepatitis B Recombinant Vaccine 1000
Hepatitis A Vaccine 1001
Hepatitis B Vaccine (Recombinant) 1002
Influenza A Virus Vaccine (H5N1) 1074
Influenza Virus Vaccine (Inactivated) 1075
Japanese Encephalitis Virus Vaccine (Inactivated) 1141
Papillomavirus (Types 6, 11, 16, 18) Vaccine (Human, Recombinant) 1574
Papillomavirus (Types 16, 18) Vaccine (Human, Recombinant) 1574
Poliovirus Vaccine (Inactivated) 1673
Rabies Vaccine 1764
Typhoid and Hepatitis A Vaccine [CAN/INT] 2111

Vaccine, Live (Bacterial)

BCG 229
Typhoid Vaccine 2112

Vaccine, Live (Viral)

Influenza Virus Vaccine (Live/Attenuated) 1080
Measles, Mumps, and Rubella Virus Vaccine 1273
Measles, Mumps, Rubella, and Varicella Virus Vaccine 1274
Rotavirus Vaccine 1851
Smallpox Vaccine 1900
Varicella Virus Vaccine 2141
Yellow Fever Vaccine 2192
Zoster Vaccine 2218

Vascular Endothelial Growth Factor (VEGF) Inhibitor

Aflibercept (Ophthalmic) 63
Bevacizumab 257
Pegaptanib 1588
Ranibizumab 1776
SUNItinib 1957
Ziv-Aflibercept (Systemic) 2204

Vasoconstrictor

Ornipressin [INT] 1522

Vasodilator

Alprostadil 96
Ambrisentan 107
Amyl Nitrite 147
Bencyclane [INT] 241
Bosentan 280
Dipyridamole 652
Epoprostenol 746
HydrALAZINE 1007
Iloprost 1046
Isosorbide Dinitrate 1124
Isosorbide Dinitrate and Hydralazine 1126
Isosorbide Mononitrate 1126
Levosimendan [INT] 1205
Naftidrofuryl [INT] 1416
Nicorandil [INT] 1449
Nitroglycerin 1465
Nitroprusside 1467
Papaverine 1573
Trapidil [INT] 2085
Treprostinil 2093

Vasodilator, Direct-Acting

Diazoxide 616
Minoxidil (Systemic) 1374

Vasopressin Analog, Synthetic

Desmopressin 594

Vasopressin Antagonist

Conivaptan 507
Tolvaptan 2064

Vitamin

Folic Acid, Cyanocobalamin, and Pyridoxine 921

Vitamin D Analog

Alendronate and Cholecalciferol 81
Alfacalcidol [CAN/INT] 82
Calcipotriene 321
Calcipotriene and Betamethasone 321
Calcitriol 323
Doxercalciferol 679
Ergocalciferol 753
Paricalcitol 1577

Vitamin, Fat Soluble

Beta-Carotene 251
Calcium and Vitamin D 326
Phytonadione 1647
Vitamin A 2173
Vitamin A and Vitamin D (Systemic) 2174
Vitamin E 2174

Vitamin K Antagonist

Phenprocoumon [INT] 1635

Vitamin, Water Soluble

Ascorbic Acid 178
Cyanocobalamin 515
Doxylamine and Pyridoxine 693
Folic Acid 919
Hydroxocobalamin 1020
Leucovorin Calcium 1183

Niacin 1443
Niacinamide 1446
Pyridoxine 1747
Riboflavin 1803
Thiamine 2028

Vitreolytic

Ocriplasmin 1484

Xanthine Oxidase Inhibitor

Allopurinol 90
Febuxostat 848

INTERNATIONAL TRADE NAMES INDEX

The following countries are included in this index and are abbreviated as follows:

Argentina (AR)
Australia (AU)
Austria (AT)
Bahamas (BS)
Bahrain (BH)
Bangladesh (BD)
Barbados (BB)
Belgium (BE)
Belize (BZ)
Benin (BJ)
Bermuda (BM)
Bolivia (BO)
Brazil (BR)
Bulgaria (BG)
Burkina Faso (BF)
Chile (CL)
China (CN)
Colombia (CO)
Costa Rica (CR)
Côte D' Ivoire (CI)
Croatia (HR)
Cuba (CU)
Cyprus (CY)
Czech Republic (CZ)
Denmark (DK)
Dominican Republic (DO)
Ecuador (EC)
Egypt (EG)
El Salvador (SV)
Estonia (EE)
Ethiopia (ET)
Finland (FI)
France (FR)
Gambia (GM)
Germany (DE)
Ghana (GH)
Great Britain [UK] (GB)
Greece (GR)
Guatemala (GT)
Guinea (GN)
Guyana (GY)
Honduras (HN)
Hong Kong (HK)
Hungary (HU)
Iceland (IS)
India (IN)
Indonesia (ID)
Iran (IR)
Iraq (IQ)
Ireland (IE)
Israel (IL)
Italy (IT)
Jamaica (JM)
Japan (JP)
Jordan (JO)
Kenya (KE)
Korea, Republic of (KR)
Kuwait (KW)
Latvia (LV)
Lebanon (LB)
Liberia (LR)
Libya (LY)
Lithuania (LT)
Luxembourg (LU)
Malawi (MW)
Malaysia (MY)
Mali (ML)
Malta (MT)
Mauritania (MR)
Mauritius (MU)
Mexico (MX)
Morocco (MA)
Netherlands (NL)
New Zealand (NZ)
Nicaragua (NI)
Niger (NE)
Nigeria (NG)
Norway (NO)
Oman (OM)
Pakistan (PK)
Panama (PA)
Paraguay (PY)
Peru (PE)
Philippines (PH)
Poland (PL)
Portugal (PT)
Puerto Rico (PR)
Qatar (QA)
Romania (RO)
Russian Federation (RU)
Saudi Arabia (SA)
Senegal (SN)
Seychelles (SC)
Sierra Leone (SL)
Singapore (SG)
Slovakia (SK)
Slovenia (SI)
South Africa (ZA)
Spain (ES)
Sudan (SD)
Surinam (SR)
Sweden (SE)
Switzerland (CH)
Syrian Arab Republic (SY)
Taiwan, Province of China (TW)
Tanzania (TZ)
Thailand (TH)
Trinidad and Tobago (TT)
Tunisia (TN)
Turkey (TR)
Uganda (UG)
United Arab Emirates (AE)
Uruguay (UY)
Venezuela (VE)
Vietnam (VN)
Yemen (YE)
Zambia (ZM)
Zimbabwe (ZW)

A313 (FR) *see* Vitamin A 2173
AAA Spray (GB) *see* Benzocaine 246
Aacidexam (BE) *see* Dexamethasone (Systemic) 599
A-Acido (AR) *see* Tretinoin (Topical) 2099
AAFact (ID) *see* Antihemophilic Factor (Human) 152
AAS (AR, BR, ES) *see* Aspirin 180
Abacin (IT) *see* Sulfamethoxazole and Trimethoprim 1946
Abaktal (BG, CZ, HN, PL, RU, SI, SK) *see* Pefloxacin [INT] 1588
Abamune (IN, LB, UY) *see* Abacavir 20
Abapril (HR) *see* Cilazapril [CAN/INT] 434
Abaprim (IT) *see* Trimethoprim 2104
A-Basedock (JP) *see* Furosemide 940
Abatoarin (MX) *see* Tropisetron [INT] 2108
Abatrio (VN) *see* Abacavir, Lamivudine, and Zidovudine 22
Abavan (CO, PE) *see* Abacavir 20
Abbocillin VK (AU) *see* Penicillin V Potassium 1614
Abbosynagis (IL) *see* Palivizumab 1560
Abbotic XL (ID) *see* Clarithromycin 456
Abbotic Granule (ID) *see* Clarithromycin 456
Abbotic (ID) *see* Clarithromycin 456
Abboticin (DK) *see* Erythromycin (Systemic) 762
Abbottselsun (ES) *see* Selenium Sulfide 1877
Abdal (IN) *see* Aceclofenac [INT] 30
Abec (IN) *see* Abacavir 20
Abefen (MX) *see* Chloramphenicol 421
Abelcet (AR, AT, AU, BE, BR, CY, CZ, DK, FI, FR, GB, GR, HN, HR, HU, IE, IT, LB, NL, NO, NZ, SE, SG, SK, TR) *see* Amphotericin B (Lipid Complex) 138
Abel (IN) *see* Bambuterol [INT] 227
Abemide (JP, TW) *see* ChlorproPAMIDE 429
Aberela (NO, SE) *see* Tretinoin (Topical) 2099
Abernil (TR, VN) *see* Naltrexone 1422
Abery (JP) *see* Thiamine 2028
Abhayrab (TH) *see* Rabies Vaccine 1764
Abilify (AE, AT, AU, BE, BG, BH, BR, CH, CL, CN, CO, CY, CZ, DE, DK, EE, ES, FI, FR, GB, GR, HK, HN, HR, HU, ID, IE, IL, IS, IT, JP, KR, KW, LB, LT, MT, MX, MY, NL, NO, PH, PL, PT, PY, QA, RO, RU, SA, SE, SG, SI, SK, TH, TR, TW, VE, VN, ZA) *see* ARIPiprazole 171
Abilify Discmelt (PH) *see* ARIPiprazole 171
Abilify ODT (NZ) *see* ARIPiprazole 171
Abine (AR) *see* Gemcitabine 952
Abinol (CL) *see* LORazepam 1243
Abiplatin (IL, NZ, TW) *see* CISplatin 448
Abirom (ID) *see* Cefpirome [INT] 388
A-Bite (MY) *see* Crotamiton 514
Abitren (IL) *see* Diclofenac (Systemic) 617
Abitrexate (IL, SG, TH, TW) *see* Methotrexate 1322
Abixa (PH) *see* Memantine 1286
Ablok (BR) *see* Atenolol 189
Abomacetin (JP) *see* Erythromycin (Systemic) 762
Aboprost (IN) *see* Misoprostol 1379
Aboren (AR) *see* Midecamycin [INT] 1365
Abortom (IN) *see* Mifepristone 1366
Abran (KR) *see* Loprazolam [INT] 1241
Abraxane (AE, AR, AU, CN, CY, CZ, DE, DK, EE, FR, GB, GR, HK, HR, HU, IE, IN, JP, KR, LT, NL, NO, NZ, PL, PT, RO, SE, SG, SI, SK, TR) *see* PACLitaxel (Protein Bound) 1554
Abrax (IL) *see* Docosanol 661
Abraxil (CL) *see* Doxycycline 689
Abretia (CL, PE, UY) *see* AtoMOXetine 191
Abrolen (GR, LB) *see* Ambroxol [INT] 109
Abseamed (TR) *see* Epoetin Alfa 742
Absenor (SE) *see* Valproic Acid and Derivatives 2123
Abstral (BM, GB, HR, TR) *see* FentaNYL 857
Abutol (TW) *see* Acebutolol 29
A-B Vask (ID) *see* AmLODIPine 123
ABZ (IN) *see* Albendazole 65
Acabel (AR, ES, PT, VE) *see* Lornoxicam [INT] 1248
Acalix (AR, PY, VE) *see* Diltiazem 634
Acamed (TH) *see* Trihexyphenidyl 2103
Acamol (CL, IL) *see* Acetaminophen 32
Acamoli Baby (IL) *see* Acetaminophen 32
Acamoli Forte suppositories for Kids (IL) *see* Acetaminophen 32
Acamol Night (IL) *see* Acetaminophen and Diphenhydramine 36
Acamol To-Go (IL) *see* Acetaminophen 32
Acampral (KR) *see* Acamprosate 28
Acamprol (IN) *see* Acamprosate 28
ACA (MY) *see* Trihexyphenidyl 2103
Acantex (AR, CL) *see* CefTRIAXone 396
Acarbixin (MX) *see* Amoxicillin and Clavulanate 133
Acard (PL) *see* Aspirin 180
Acarol Dry Syrup (KR) *see* Formoterol 926
ACB (IN) *see* Aceclofenac [INT] 30
ACB (NZ) *see* Acebutolol 29
ACC 200 (AE, BH, EE, KW, QA) *see* Acetylcysteine 40
Accarb (NZ) *see* Acarbose 29
ACC (AR, HU, LB, LU, MX, RU, SA, ZA) *see* Acetylcysteine 40
Accelio (JP) *see* Acetaminophen 32
Accent (JP) *see* Furosemide 940
Accolate (AE, AR, AU, BB, BE, BF, BH, BJ, BM, BS, BZ, CH, CI, CL, CN, CZ, ES, ET, FI, GB, GH, GM, GN, GY, HK, HN, HU, ID, IE, IL, JM, JO, KE, KR, LR, MA, ML, MR, MU, MW, MX, NE, NG, NL, NO, NZ, PE, PH, PK, PL, PR, PT, QA, RU, SA, SC, SD, SG, SI, SK, SL, SN, SR, TN, TR, TT, TW, TZ, UG, UY, VE, ZA, ZM, ZW) *see* Zafirlukast 2192
Accoleit (IT) *see* Zafirlukast 2192
Accord (PY) *see* Losartan 1248
Accotin (DK) *see* ISOtretinoin 1127
Accupril (AR, AU, BE, BO, BZ, CL, CO, CR, DO, EC, GT, HK, HN, ID, KR, LU, MX, NI, NZ, PA, PE, PH, PK, PR, PY, SV, TH, TW, TZ, UG, UY, VE, VN, ZA, ZM, ZW) *see* Quinapril 1756
Accuprin (IT) *see* Quinapril 1756
Accupro (AT, BG, CH, CZ, DE, DK, EE, FI, GB, HR, HU, IE, LT, PL, RO, RU, SE, SK) *see* Quinapril 1756
Accupron (GR) *see* Quinapril 1756
Ac-De (MX) *see* DACTINomycin 551
Acderma (JP) *see* Fluocinonide 894
Acea Gel (GB, IE) *see* MetroNIDAZOLE (Topical) 1357
AC Ear Drops (IN) *see* Ciprofloxacin (Otic) 446
AC Ear Drops (IN) *see* Ciprofloxacin (Systemic) 441
Acebitor (PH) *see* Enalapril 722
Ace-Bloc (TW) *see* Captopril 342
Acebumin (PE) *see* Albumin 67
Aceclofar (AE) *see* Aceclofenac [INT] 30
Aceclonac (CY) *see* Aceclofenac [INT] 30
Acecol (JP, KR) *see* Temocapril [INT] 1991
Acecor (CZ) *see* Acebutolol 29
Acecpar (VN) *see* Aceclofenac [INT] 30
Acediur (IT) *see* Captopril and Hydrochlorothiazide 345
Acedrin (PY) *see* Cefepime 378
Aceler (MX) *see* Fusidic Acid (Topical) [CAN/INT] 943
Acemetacin Heumann (DE) *see* Acemetacin [INT] 30
Acemetacin intermuti (DE) *see* Acemetacin [INT] 30
Acemetacin Stada (DE) *see* Acemetacin [INT] 30
acemetacin von ct (DE) *see* Acemetacin [INT] 30
Acemet (MY, PE) *see* Acemetacin [INT] 30
Acemin (AT) *see* Lisinopril 1226
Acemix (IT) *see* Acemetacin [INT] 30
Acemol (VN) *see* Acetaminophen 32
Acemuk (AR) *see* Acetylcysteine 40
Acemycin (TW) *see* Amikacin 111
Acenac (PK) *see* Aceclofenac [INT] 30
Acenal (IN) *see* Aceclofenac [INT] 30
Acenor-M (ID) *see* Fosinopril 932
Acenox (CL) *see* Acenocoumarol [CAN/INT] 30

Aceo (TH) *see* Acemetacin [INT] ... 30
Acephlogont (DE) *see* Acemetacin [INT] ... 30
Acepin (TW) *see* Acebutolol ... 29
Aceplus (IT, NL) *see* Captopril and Hydrochlorothiazide ... 345
Acepramin (HN, HU) *see* Aminocaproic Acid ... 113
Aceprax (PY, UY) *see* ALPRAZolam ... 94
Acepress (ID, IT) *see* Captopril ... 342
Acepril (GB) *see* Captopril ... 342
Acepril (MY) *see* Lisinopril ... 1226
Aceprin (HK, MY) *see* Aspirin ... 180
Acequin (IT) *see* Quinapril ... 1756
Acerbon (DE) *see* Lisinopril ... 1226
Acercomp (DE) *see* Lisinopril and Hydrochlorothiazide ... 1229
Acerdil (CL, PE, PY) *see* Lisinopril ... 1226
Acerdil D (CL, PY) *see* Lisinopril and Hydrochlorothiazide ... 1229
Aceren (KR) *see* Diacerein [INT] ... 613
Aceril (IL) *see* Captopril ... 342
Acernix (PH) *see* Pantoprazole ... 1570
Acerpril (KR) *see* Perindopril ... 1623
Acertil AR (HK) *see* Perindopril ... 1623
Acertil (CN, KR, TW) *see* Perindopril ... 1623
Acertil Plus Arginine (KR) *see* Perindopril and Indapamide [CAN/INT] ... 1626
Acertil Plus (HK, KR, TW) *see* Perindopril and Indapamide [CAN/INT] ... 1626
Acer (VN) *see* Aceclofenac [INT] ... 30
Acesistem (IT) *see* Enalapril and Hydrochlorothiazide ... 725
Acetab (AE) *see* Captopril ... 342
Acetab (VN) *see* Acetaminophen ... 32
Acetadiazol (MX) *see* AcetaZOLAMIDE ... 39
Acetadote (AU, NZ) *see* Acetylcysteine ... 40
Acetak (PE) *see* AcetaZOLAMIDE ... 39
Acetalgin (CH) *see* Acetaminophen ... 32
Acetal (PY) *see* Amiodarone ... 114
Acetamol (IT) *see* Acetaminophen ... 32
Acetan HCT (MY) *see* Losartan and Hydrochlorothiazide ... 1250
Acetanol (JP) *see* Acebutolol ... 29
Acetard (FI) *see* Aspirin ... 180
Acetar (PT) *see* Piracetam [INT] ... 1661
Acetec (IN) *see* Acitretin ... 43
Acetec (MY) *see* Enalapril ... 722
Acetec (TW) *see* Perindopril ... 1623
Aceten (IN) *see* Captopril ... 342
Acetensa (ID) *see* Losartan ... 1248
Acetensil (ES) *see* Enalapril ... 722
Aceterin (EE) *see* Cetirizine ... 411
Aceticil (BR) *see* Aspirin ... 180
Acetilcolina Colirio (AR) *see* Acetylcholine ... 40
Acetilcolina Cusi (ES) *see* Acetylcholine ... 40
Acetin (ID, MY) *see* Acetylcysteine ... 40
Acetopt (NZ) *see* Sulfacetamide (Ophthalmic) ... 1943
Acetram (ID) *see* Acetaminophen and Tramadol ... 37
Acetram-Semi (KR) *see* Acetaminophen and Tramadol ... 37
Acetretin (AE) *see* Tretinoin (Topical) ... 2099
ACET suppositories (SG) *see* Acetaminophen ... 32
Acet (TW) *see* Acetylcysteine ... 40
Acetylcystein NM Pharma (SE) *see* Acetylcysteine ... 40
Acetylcystein Tika (SE) *see* Acetylcysteine ... 40
Acetylspiramycin (JP) *see* Spiramycin [CAN/INT] ... 1931
Acetysal (BG) *see* Aspirin ... 180
Acezide (GB) *see* Captopril and Hydrochlorothiazide ... 345
Acfen-A (MX) *see* Tretinoin (Topical) ... 2099
Acfol (ES, PT) *see* Folic Acid ... 919
Achromycin V (AE, BH, CY, EG, IQ, IR, JO, JP, KW, LB, LY, OM, QA, SA, SY, YE) *see* Tetracycline ... 2017
Achromycin (AE, AT, BH, CY, EG, IN, IQ, IR, JO, JP, KW, LB, LY, OM, PK, QA, SA, SY, YE, ZA) *see* Tetracycline ... 2017
Achromycin Ear/Eye Oint (NZ) *see* Tetracycline ... 2017
Acibiogel (CO) *see* Aluminum Hydroxide, Magnesium Hydroxide, and Simethicone ... 104
Acic (AE, BH, EE, KW, QA) *see* Acyclovir (Systemic) ... 47
Acic (AE, CY, EE, KW, QA) *see* Acyclovir (Topical) ... 51
Acicard (TW) *see* Ranitidine ... 1777
Acic Creme (DE) *see* Acyclovir (Topical) ... 51
Aciclidan (DK) *see* Acyclovir (Topical) ... 51
Aciclodan (DK) *see* Acyclovir (Systemic) ... 47
Aciclomed (BE) *see* Acyclovir (Topical) ... 51
Aciclor (VE) *see* Aciclovir (Ophthalmic) [INT] ... 43
Aciclor (VE) *see* Acyclovir (Systemic) ... 47
Aciclor (VE) *see* Acyclovir (Topical) ... 51
Aciclosina (PT) *see* Acyclovir (Systemic) ... 47
Aciclosina (PT) *see* Acyclovir (Topical) ... 51
Acicone-S (QA) *see* Magaldrate and Simethicone ... 1261
Acic-Ophtal (DE) *see* Aciclovir (Ophthalmic) [INT] ... 43
Acicur-P (PY) *see* Acetaminophen ... 32
Acicvir (NZ) *see* Acyclovir (Systemic) ... 47
Acid A Vit (NL) *see* Tretinoin (Topical) ... 2099
Acide Folique CCD (FR) *see* Folic Acid ... 919
Acidex (AR) *see* Ranitidine ... 1777
Acid Mantle (MX) *see* Calcium Acetate ... 326
Acidnor (AE, BH, CY, EG, IQ, IR, JO, KW, LB, LY, OM, QA, SA, SY, YE) *see* Cimetidine ... 438
Ácido ascórbico (MX) *see* Ascorbic Acid ... 178
Acido Folico (AR, CO, EC, PE) *see* Folic Acid ... 919
Acido Folico Fada (AR) *see* Folic Acid ... 919
Acido Folinico/Leucovorina (CL) *see* Leucovorin Calcium ... 1183
Acido Nalidixico Prodes (ES) *see* Nalidixic Acid [INT] ... 1418
Acido Nicotinico (CO) *see* Niacin ... 1443
Acidum e-aminocapronicum (PL) *see* Aminocaproic Acid ... 113
Acidum nicotinicum (HU) *see* Niacin ... 1443
Acifam (JO) *see* Famotidine ... 845
Acifar (ID) *see* Acyclovir (Topical) ... 51
Aciflux (CL) *see* Ranitidine ... 1777
Acifol (AR) *see* Folic Acid ... 919
Acifox (PH) *see* CefOXitin ... 386
Aciherpin (PH) *see* Acyclovir (Systemic) ... 47
Aciherpin (PH) *see* Acyclovir (Topical) ... 51
Acihexal (AU) *see* Acyclovir (Systemic) ... 47
Acilax Cream (HK) *see* Acyclovir (Topical) ... 51
Acilina (PY) *see* Amoxicillin ... 130
Aciloc (BF, BJ, CI, CZ, ET, GH, GM, GN, IN, KE, LR, MA, ML, MR, MU, MW, NE, NG, SC, SD, SL, SN, TN, TW, TZ, UG, VN, ZM, ZW) *see* Ranitidine ... 1777
Aciloc (DK, FI) *see* Cimetidine ... 438
Acimax (AU) *see* Omeprazole ... 1508
Aci-Med (ZA) *see* Cimetidine ... 438
Acimox (MX) *see* Amoxicillin ... 130
Acinil (DK, SE) *see* Cimetidine ... 438
Acinon (JP) *see* Nizatidine ... 1471
Acipan (HR, SI) *see* Pantoprazole ... 1570
Aciphen (HU) *see* Diethylamine Salicylate [INT] ... 624
Aciprazol (AE, BH, CY, EG, IQ, IR, JO, KW, LB, LY, OM, QA, SA, SY, YE) *see* RABEprazole ... 1762
Acipredex (PH) *see* Ciprofloxacin and Dexamethasone ... 446
Acipro (PH) *see* Ciprofloxacin (Systemic) ... 441
Acirax (VN) *see* Acyclovir (Systemic) ... 47
Acirax (VN) *see* Acyclovir (Topical) ... 51
Aciren (KR) *see* Ciprofloxacin (Systemic) ... 441
Acitidine (KR) *see* Nizatidine ... 1471
Acitidin (KR) *see* Nizatidine ... 1471
Acitral (ID) *see* Aluminum Hydroxide, Magnesium Hydroxide, and Simethicone ... 104
Acitrexol (PE) *see* Acitretin ... 43
Acitrom (IN) *see* Acenocoumarol [CAN/INT] ... 30
Acivir (CH, IL, IN, QA) *see* Acyclovir (Topical) ... 51
Acivir Cold Sore Cream (AU) *see* Acyclovir (Topical) ... 51

Acivirex (GT, HN, NI, SV) *see* Acyclovir (Systemic) 47
Acivirex (GT, HN, NI, SV) *see* Acyclovir (Topical) 51
Acivir Eye (IN) *see* Aciclovir (Ophthalmic) [INT] 43
Acivir Eye (IN) *see* Acyclovir (Systemic) 47
Aclam (ID) *see* Amoxicillin and Clavulanate 133
Aclasta (AE, AR, AT, AU, BE, BG, BH, BR, CH, CL, CN, CO, CR, CZ, DE, DK, DO, EC, EE, ES, FI, FR, GB, GR, GT, HK, HN, HR, HU, ID, IE, IL, IS, IT, KR, KW, LB, LT, MT, MY, NI, NL, NO, NZ, PA, PE, PH, PL, PT, QA, RO, RU, SA, SE, SG, SI, SK, SV, TH, TR, TW, UY, VN, ZA) *see* Zoledronic Acid 2206
Aclear (HK) *see* Adapalene 54
Aclene (KR) *see* Adapalene 54
Acler (AR) *see* Fluorouracil (Topical) 899
Aclexa (EE, HR) *see* Celecoxib 402
Aclin (AU, HK, NZ) *see* Sulindac 1953
Aclipak (SG) *see* PACLitaxel (Conventional) 1550
Aclixel (MX) *see* PACLitaxel (Conventional) 1550
Acloderm (CZ, RU) *see* Alclometasone 72
Aclon (VN) *see* Aceclofenac [INT] 30
Acloral (MX) *see* Ranitidine 1777
Aclor (AU) *see* Cefaclor 372
Aclosone (NL) *see* Alclometasone 72
Aclotine (FR) *see* Antithrombin 156
Aclovir (FI, TH, TW) *see* Acyclovir (Systemic) 47
Acnal SC (KR) *see* ISOtretinoin 1127
Acnatac (DE) *see* Tretinoin (Topical) 2099
Acnatac (DK, FI, RO) *see* Clindamycin and Tretinoin 464
Acnean (TW) *see* Azelaic Acid 213
Acneclin (AR) *see* Minocycline 1371
Acnecur (PY) *see* ISOtretinoin 1127
Acnederm (AE, SA) *see* Azelaic Acid 213
Acnederm (BG) *see* Tretinoin (Topical) 2099
Acnederm Ery Gel (DE) *see* Erythromycin (Topical) 765
Acnederm (IN) *see* Erythromycin (Topical) 765
Acnederm Medicated Lotion (SG) *see* Azelaic Acid 213
Acne Foundation (ID) *see* Azelaic Acid 213
Acnefug-EL (CZ, EE) *see* Erythromycin (Topical) 765
Acne Hermal (GR) *see* Erythromycin (Topical) 765
Acnelene (PK) *see* Adapalene 54
Acnemin (ES) *see* ISOtretinoin 1127
Acneryne (BE) *see* Erythromycin (Topical) 765
Acnetrex (PH) *see* ISOtretinoin 1127
Acnetrim (IL, TW) *see* Erythromycin (Topical) 765
Acnin (KR) *see* Clindamycin (Topical) 464
Acnocin (TH) *see* Clindamycin (Systemic) 460
Acnotin (EC, HK, SG, TH) *see* ISOtretinoin 1127
Acnu (CH, DE, NL) *see* Nimustine [INT] 1457
Acocard (MX) *see* Dacarbazine 549
Acomexol (MX) *see* Crotamiton 514
Acomplia (AE, BH, IS, LU, MX, SE) *see* Rimonabant [INT] 1814
Acondro (GB) *see* Ethinyl Estradiol and Drospirenone 801
Acortiz (MX) *see* Hydrochlorothiazide 1009
Acostin (IN) *see* Colistimethate 504
Acotril (PH) *see* Glimepiride 966
Acovil (ES) *see* Ramipril 1771
Acoxxel (RU) *see* Etoricoxib [INT] 821
Acpan (AR) *see* Glycopyrrolate 975
Acpio (AU) *see* Pioglitazone 1654
Acquin (AU) *see* Quinapril 1756
Acran (ID) *see* Ranitidine 1777
Acref (JP) *see* FentaNYL 857
Acrios (ID) *see* Acarbose 29
Acrium (KR) *see* Atracurium 198
Acrocef (EC) *see* CefTRIAXone 396
Acromax (AT) *see* Cromolyn (Ophthalmic) 514
Acromicina (MX) *see* Tetracycline 2017
Acronitol (GR) *see* Potassium Chloride 1687
Acrose (IL) *see* Acarbose 29
Acrovastin (EC) *see* AtorvaSTATin 194
Acrovir (EC) *see* ValACYclovir 2119
ACS (KR) *see* Acyclovir (Systemic) 47
Acsolve-C (IN) *see* Clindamycin and Tretinoin 464
Acstin (KR) *see* Pioglitazone 1654
Actabone (ID) *see* Clodronate [CAN/INT] 469
Actaclo (PH) *see* Clopidogrel 484
Actacode (AU) *see* Codeine 497
Actalipid (ID) *see* AtorvaSTATin 194
Actamin (JP) *see* Thiamine 2028
Actan (CL, PY) *see* FLUoxetine 899
Actanac (CZ) *see* Clindamycin and Tretinoin 464
Actapin (HK, ID, SG) *see* AmLODIPine 123
Actapril (SK) *see* Trandolapril 2080
Actapulgite (BE, CH, FR, VN) *see* Attapulgite [CAN/INT] 204
Actazolam (ID) *see* ALPRAZolam 94
Actemra (AE, AR, AU, BR, CL, CN, CO, EC, HK, ID, IL, IN, JP, KR, LB, MY, NZ, PE, PH, QA, SG, TH, TW, VN) *see* Tocilizumab 2057
Actensil Plus (ES) *see* Enalapril and Hydrochlorothiazide 725
Act-HIB (BE, BG, BR, CL, CN, DK, EE, FR, GR, IL, KR, PE, PK, PY, SE, UY) *see* Haemophilus b Conjugate Vaccine 991
Acthiol (BR) *see* Mecysteine [INT] 1277
Actibile (PH) *see* Ursodiol 2116
Acticarb (AE, EG) *see* Charcoal, Activated 416
Actiderm (AR) *see* Desoximetasone 598
Actifed (AE, AU, BB, BE, BF, BH, BJ, BM, BS, BZ, CI, CY, EE, EG, ET, GH, GM, GN, GY, ID, IQ, IR, JM, JO, KE, KR, KW, LB, LR, LY, MA, ML, MR, MU, MW, MX, MY, NE, NG, NL, OM, PE, PY, QA, SA, SC, SD, SG, SL, SN, SR, SY, TN, TT, TZ, UG, VE, YE, ZA, ZM, ZW) *see* Triprolidine and Pseudoephedrine 2105
Actifed Antitusivo (PE) *see* Triprolidine, Pseudoephedrine, and Codeine [CAN/INT] 2105
Actifed Compound Linctus (AE, BF, BH, BJ, CI, CY, EG, ET, GH, GM, GN, HK, IQ, IR, JO, KE, KW, LB, LR, LY, MA, ML, MR, MU, MW, NE, NG, OM, QA, SA, SC, SD, SL, SN, SY, TZ, UG, YE, ZA, ZM, ZW) *see* Triprolidine, Pseudoephedrine, and Codeine [CAN/INT] 2105
Actifed Compound (TH) *see* Triprolidine, Pseudoephedrine, and Codeine [CAN/INT] 2105
Actifedrin (AR, BR, CL) *see* Triprolidine and Pseudoephedrine 2105
Actifen CR (PH) *see* Diclofenac (Systemic) 617
Actigall (NZ) *see* Ursodiol 2116
Actilax (AU) *see* Lactulose 1156
Actilyse (AE, AR, AT, AU, BD, BE, BF, BG, BH, BJ, BR, CH, CI, CL, CN, CO, CY, CZ, DE, DK, EC, EE, EG, ES, ET, FI, FR, GB, GH, GM, GN, GR, HK, HN, HR, HU, ID, IE, IL, IN, IQ, IR, IS, IT, JO, KE, KR, KW, LB, LR, LT, LU, LY, MA, ML, MR, MU, MW, MX, MY, NE, NG, NL, NO, NZ, OM, PE, PH, PK, PL, PT, PY, QA, RO, RU, SA, SC, SD, SE, SG, SI, SK, SL, SN, SY, TH, TN, TR, TW, TZ, UG, UY, VE, VN, YE, ZA, ZM, ZW) *see* Alteplase 99
Actimibe Plus (PY) *see* Ezetimibe and Simvastatin 834
Actimin (MY) *see* Triprolidine and Pseudoephedrine 2105
Actinerval (AR, PY) *see* CarBAMazepine 346
Actinium (CR, DO, GT, HN, MX, NI, PA, SV) *see* OXcarbazepine 1532
Actiol (IT) *see* Mecysteine [INT] 1277
Actiq (AU, CH, DE, DK, ES, FI, FR, GB, IE, IL, KR, NO, PT, SE) *see* FentaNYL 857
Actium (PY) *see* BusPIRone 311
Activacin (JP) *see* Alteplase 99
Activelle (AE, AR, CH, DK, FI, FR, HK, HR, IL, IS, KR, KW, LT, NL, QA, SE, SG, SI, SK, TW, UY, VN) *see* Estradiol and Norethindrone 781
Activelle (AR, FI, HK, IL, KR, MY, SE, SG, TH, TW, UY) *see* Ethinyl Estradiol and Norethindrone 808
Activigil (UY) *see* Modafinil 1386
Activir (FR) *see* Acyclovir (Systemic) 47

Activir (FR) *see* Acyclovir (Topical) ... 51
Activon (CH) *see* Etofenamate [INT] ... 815
Actixim (VN) *see* Cefuroxime ... 399
Actol (AT, DE, ES) *see* Niflumic Acid [INT] ... 1454
Actonace (PH) *see* Triamcinolone (Nasal) ... 2100
Actonaze (PH) *see* Triamcinolone (Systemic) ... 2099
Actonel (AE, AR, AT, AU, BB, BE, BG, BH, BM, BO, BR, BS, BZ, CH, CL, CO, CR, CY, CZ, DE, DO, EC, EE, EG, ES, FR, GB, GR, GT, GY, HK, HN, HR, ID, IE, IL, IT, JM, JO, JP, KR, KW, LB, MX, MY, NI, NL, PA, PE, PL, PR, PT, PY, QA, RO, SG, SI, SR, SV, TH, TR, TT, TW, UY, VE, VN) *see* Risedronate ... 1816
Actonel Once A Month (ID, IL) *see* Risedronate ... 1816
Actonel Once A Week (BH, IL, KW, LB, VN, ZA) *see* Risedronate ... 1816
Actonel once A Week (CY) *see* Risedronate ... 1816
Actoplatin (ID) *see* CARBOplatin ... 357
Actoril (AR) *see* Pioglitazone and Glimepiride ... 1654
Actoril (KR) *see* Risedronate ... 1816
Actos M (AR) *see* Pioglitazone and Metformin ... 1655
Actos (AE, AR, AT, AU, BB, BE, BG, BH, BM, BO, BR, BS, BZ, CH, CL, CN, CO, CR, CZ, DE, DK, DO, EC, EE, ES, FI, FR, GB, GR, GT, GY, HK, HN, HR, ID, IE, IT, JM, JO, JP, KR, KW, LB, LT, MT, MY, NI, NL, NO, NZ, PA, PE, PH, PL, PR, PT, QA, RO, RU, SA, SE, SG, SI, SK, SR, SV, TH, TR, TT, TW, VE) *see* Pioglitazone ... 1654
Actos Met (CL, EC, PE) *see* Pioglitazone and Metformin ... 1655
Actosmet (HK, ID, KR, PH, TH, TW) *see* Pioglitazone and Metformin ... 1655
Actosryl (KR) *see* Pioglitazone and Glimepiride ... 1654
Actozon (KR) *see* Pioglitazone ... 1654
Actraphane 30 (CZ) *see* Insulin NPH and Insulin Regular ... 1090
Actrapid (DK, ES, SG) *see* Insulin Regular ... 1091
Actron (PY, UY) *see* Ibuprofen ... 1032
Actuss (AU) *see* Pholcodine [INT] ... 1646
Acuatim (ID, JP) *see* Nadifloxacin [INT] ... 1411
Acuco (ZA) *see* Sulfamethoxazole and Trimethoprim ... 1946
Acudor (PT) *see* Etodolac ... 815
Acuflam (PH) *see* Diclofenac (Systemic) ... 617
Acugen (PH) *see* ISOtretinoin ... 1127
Acugrain (MY) *see* Pizotifen [CAN/INT] ... 1664
Acuitel (AE, BH, CY, EG, FR, IL, IQ, IR, JO, KW, LB, LY, MU, OM, QA, SA, SY, TR, YE) *see* Quinapril ... 1756
Acular (AE, AR, AT, BM, BR, CH, CL, CN, CR, DE, DK, DO, EG, FI, FR, GB, GT, HN, IE, IN, IT, JO, KR, KW, LB, MY, NI, NL, PA, PE, PH, SA, SG, SV, TH, TR, TW, VN, ZA) *see* Ketorolac (Ophthalmic) ... 1149
Aculare (BE) *see* Ketorolac (Ophthalmic) ... 1149
Acular LS (AE, AR, CO, HK, KW, LB, SA) *see* Ketorolac (Ophthalmic) ... 1149
Aculex (KR) *see* Atracurium ... 198
Acunaso (ZA) *see* Pseudoephedrine ... 1742
Acuphlem (ZA) *see* Carbocisteine [INT] ... 357
Acupil (IN) *see* Quinapril ... 1756
Acupressin (IN) *see* Terlipressin [INT] ... 2010
Acupril (MX, NL, PT) *see* Quinapril ... 1756
Acure (PK) *see* Albendazole ... 65
Acure (TW) *see* Adapalene ... 54
Acusprain (ZA) *see* Naproxen ... 1427
A.C.V. (TH) *see* Acyclovir (Topical) ... 51
ACWY Vax (GB) *see* Meningococcal (Groups A / C / Y and W-135) Diphtheria Conjugate Vaccine ... 1289
Acyclo-V (AU, BH) *see* Acyclovir (Systemic) ... 47
Acyclovenir (IL) *see* Acyclovir (Systemic) ... 47
Acylene (MY) *see* Acyclovir (Systemic) ... 47
Acypront (HK) *see* Acetylcysteine ... 40
Acyrax (FI) *see* Acyclovir (Systemic) ... 47
Acyvir (EC) *see* Acyclovir (Topical) ... 51
Acyvir (EC, IT, VN) *see* Acyclovir (Systemic) ... 47
Aczebri (PH) *see* Cefaclor ... 372
Adacai (DO) *see* Ezetimibe and Simvastatin ... 834
Adacel (AU, HR, PH, RO, SG) *see* Diphtheria and Tetanus Toxoids, and Acellular Pertussis Vaccine ... 649
Adaferin (CR, DO, GR, GT, HN, IN, MX, NI, PA, SV, TR) *see* Adapalene ... 54
Adaferin Gel (IL) *see* Adapalene ... 54
Adagen (CA) *see* Pegademase Bovine ... 1588
Adalat 10 (AU) *see* NIFEdipine ... 1451
Adalat 20 (AU) *see* NIFEdipine ... 1451
Adalat L (JP) *see* NIFEdipine ... 1451
Adalat (AE, AR, AT, BE, BF, BH, BJ, BR, CH, CI, CL, CR, CZ, DE, DK, EE, EG, ES, ET, FI, GB, GH, GM, GN, GR, GT, HK, HN, HR, HU, ID, IE, IT, JO, JP, KE, KR, KW, LR, LU, MA, ML, MR, MU, MW, MX, MY, NE, NG, NI, NO, PA, PE, PH, PK, PL, PT, QA, RU, SA, SC, SD, SE, SL, SN, SV, TN, TR, TZ, UG, UY, VE, VN, ZA, ZM, ZW) *see* NIFEdipine ... 1451
Adalat CR (BG, CH, CY, GR, JP, RO, TH) *see* NIFEdipine ... 1451
Adalat Crono (IT) *see* NIFEdipine ... 1451
Adalate (FR) *see* NIFEdipine ... 1451
Adalat GITS 30 (PH) *see* NIFEdipine ... 1451
Adalat GITS (CN, HK) *see* NIFEdipine ... 1451
Adalat LA (BH, GB, KW, LB, MY, SG) *see* NIFEdipine ... 1451
Adalat LP (FR) *see* NIFEdipine ... 1451
Adalat Oros (AU, BB, BM, BR, BS, BZ, CL, CO, DK, DO, EC, EE, ES, FI, GY, ID, IS, JM, KR, NL, NO, NZ, PE, PR, PY, SE, SI, SR, TT, TW, UY, VE) *see* NIFEdipine ... 1451
Adalat Retard (AE, AT, BF, BH, BJ, CI, CL, CR, CZ, DE, EG, ES, ET, GB, GH, GM, GN, GR, GT, HK, HN, ID, IQ, IR, JO, KE, KW, LR, LY, MA, ML, MR, MU, MW, MY, NE, NG, NI, OM, PA, PE, PH, PL, PY, QA, SA, SC, SD, SL, SN, SV, SY, TN, TZ, UG, YE, ZM, ZW) *see* NIFEdipine ... 1451
Adalken (MX) *see* PenicillAMINE ... 1608
Adamon (AR, CR, DO, GT, HN, NI, PA, PY, SV) *see* TraMADol ... 2074
Adancor (FR) *see* Nicorandil [INT] ... 1449
Adant Dispo (ID) *see* Hyaluronate and Derivatives ... 1006
Adaphen XL (ZA) *see* Methylphenidate ... 1336
Adaphen (ZA) *see* Methylphenidate ... 1336
Adartrel (CH, FR, GB, IE, NO, SE) *see* ROPINIRole ... 1844
Adasuve (CZ, DE, EE, ES, LT, NL, SE, SI, SK) *see* Loxapine ... 1255
Adax (EC) *see* ALPRAZolam ... 94
Adax Retard (EC) *see* ALPRAZolam ... 94
Adazol (EC) *see* Albendazole ... 65
Adbiotin (CO) *see* Amoxicillin ... 130
Adcapone (IN) *see* Entacapone ... 730
Adcef (IN) *see* Cefdinir ... 376
Adcetris (AU, BE, CH, CZ, DE, DK, EE, FR, GB, HR, IE, JP, KR, LT, NL, NO, RO, SE, SG, SI, SK) *see* Brentuximab Vedotin ... 286
Adcirca (AT, AU, BE, BR, CZ, DK, EE, FR, GB, HR, IE, IS, JP, LT, MX, NL, NO, PT, RO, SE, SI, SK) *see* Tadalafil ... 1968
Adco-Sulindac (ZA) *see* Sulindac ... 1953
Addcef (VN) *see* Cefdinir ... 376
Addcomp (DE) *see* Captopril and Hydrochlorothiazide ... 345
Addex (PH) *see* Amoxicillin and Clavulanate ... 133
Addex-Tham (SE) *see* Tromethamine ... 2107
Addictex (TR) *see* Buprenorphine ... 300
Addi-K (BF, BJ, CI, ET, GH, GM, GN, KE, LR, MA, ML, MR, MU, MW, MY, NE, NG, SC, SD, SL, SN, TH, TN, TZ, UG, ZA, ZM, ZW) *see* Potassium Chloride ... 1687
Additiva Calcium (PL) *see* Calcium Carbonate ... 327
Additiva Ferrum (PL) *see* Ferrous Gluconate ... 870
Addos XR (AU) *see* NIFEdipine ... 1451

Adecard (VN) *see* Adenosine 55
Adecco (ID) *see* MetFORMIN 1307
Adec (TW) *see* Mebendazole [CAN/INT] 1274
Adecur (CL, MX, PY) *see* Terazosin 2001
Adecut (JP) *see* Delapril [INT] 587
Adefin XL (AU) *see* NIFEdipine 1451
Adefin (AU) *see* NIFEdipine 1451
Adeflo (PH) *see* Fluticasone and Salmeterol 912
Adekin (GR) *see* Cyproheptadine 529
Adekon (MX) *see* Ergocalciferol 753
Adel (MX) *see* Clarithromycin 456
Adelone (GR) *see* PrednisoLONE (Ophthalmic) 1706
Ademan (TW) *see* HydrALAZINE 1007
Adempas (AU, CH, CZ, DE, DK, EE, ES, GB, HR, JP, KR, LT, NL, NO, RO, SE, SG, SI, SK) *see* Riociguat 1814
Adenex (PE) *see* Terazosin 2001
Adenocard (BR) *see* Adenosine 55
Adenock (JP) *see* Allopurinol 90
Adenocor (AU, BE, BG, CY, CZ, DK, EE, EG, ES, FI, GB, GR, HN, HU, IE, IL, JO, KR, LU, MY, NL, NO, NZ, PE, PL, PT, SA, SE, SG, SI, SK, TH, TR, TW, UY, VE, ZA) *see* Adenosine 55
Adenoject (IN) *see* Adenosine 55
Adenophos (QA) *see* Adenosine 55
Adenoscan (AU, ES, HK, JP) *see* Adenosine 55
Adenosina Biol (AR) *see* Adenosine 55
Adenozer (TW) *see* Adenosine 55
Adenuric (BE, CY, CZ, DE, DK, EE, FR, GB, GR, HR, IE, IT, LT, NL, NZ, PT, RO, SE, SI, SK, TR) *see* Febuxostat 848
Adepact (KR) *see* Adefovir 54
Adepam (KR) *see* Adefovir 54
Adepend (BG, GB, HR, LT, SI, SK) *see* Naltrexone 1422
Adepril (IT) *see* Amitriptyline 119
Adepssir (PH) *see* FLUoxetine 899
Adeptin (KR) *see* Adefovir 54
Adermina (CL) *see* Fluocinolone (Topical) 893
Aderowest (MX) *see* Ergocalciferol 753
Adesera (IN) *see* Adefovir 54
Adesil (KR) *see* Adefovir 54
Adex 200 (IL) *see* Ibuprofen 1032
A-Dex (KR) *see* Anastrozole 148
Adex Liqui-Gels (IL) *see* Ibuprofen 1032
Adexor (HN) *see* Trimetazidine [INT] 2104
Adezan (GR) *see* Dipyridamole 652
Adezio (HK, SG) *see* Cetirizine 411
Adiaben (HR) *see* ChlorproPAMIDE 429
Adiamil (PY) *see* Adapalene 54
Adiazine (FR) *see* SulfADIAZINE 1944
Adiazin (FI) *see* SulfADIAZINE 1944
Adifen SR (MY) *see* NIFEdipine 1451
Adiflox (IN) *see* Ciprofloxacin (Otic) 446
Adiflox (IN) *see* Ciprofloxacin (Systemic) 441
Adimicin (HR) *see* Vancomycin 2130
Adin (AU, NZ) *see* Desmopressin 594
Adine (CL) *see* Norepinephrine 1472
Adin Melt (AU) *see* Desmopressin 594
Adinol (MX) *see* Acetaminophen 32
Adinos (BR) *see* Desonide 597
Adin Spray (IL) *see* Desmopressin 594
Adipam (KR) *see* HydrOXYzine 1024
Adipex (CH, KR) *see* Phentermine 1635
Adipex Retard (AT, CZ, MY) *see* Phentermine 1635
Adipine XL (GB) *see* NIFEdipine 1451
Adipin (VN) *see* AmLODIPine 123
Adiprin EC (JO) *see* Aspirin 180
Adiro (MX, VE) *see* Aspirin 180
Adisen (KR) *see* Amoxapine 128
Aditor (JO, LB) *see* AtorvaSTATin 194
Adiuretin-SD (CZ, HN, PL) *see* Desmopressin 594
Adiuretin SD (HU) *see* Desmopressin 594
Adizem-XL (IE) *see* Diltiazem 634
Adizem XL (LB, TR) *see* Diltiazem 634
Adizem-CD (IL) *see* Diltiazem 634
Adizem (IE, LU) *see* Diltiazem 634
Adlox (IN) *see* Levofloxacin (Systemic) 1197
Admed (KR) *see* Memantine 1286
Admenta (IN) *see* Memantine 1286
Admon (ES) *see* NiMODipine 1456
A.D. Mycin (JO) *see* DOXOrubicin (Conventional) 679
AD Mycin (KR) *see* DOXOrubicin (Conventional) 679
A.D.Mycin (TH) *see* DOXOrubicin (Conventional) 679
Adobe (KR) *see* Amlodipine and Atorvastatin 124
Adocor (DE) *see* Captopril 342
Adofen (ES) *see* FLUoxetine 899
Adolan (IL) *see* Methadone 1311
Adol (EG, JO, KW, LB, QA) *see* Acetaminophen 32
Adolonta (ES) *see* TraMADol 2074
Adomed (AT) *see* Bupranolol [INT] 300
Adomir (JP) *see* Fluticasone and Salmeterol 912
Adonix (PH) *see* Sildenafil 1882
Adopal (FI) *see* Methyldopa 1332
Adoport (GB) *see* Tacrolimus (Systemic) 1962
Adorem (CO) *see* Acetaminophen 32
Adormix (CL) *see* Zolpidem 2212
Adorucin (VN) *see* DOXOrubicin (Conventional) 679
Adovi (ID) *see* Zidovudine 2196
Adracon (PE) *see* SUMAtriptan 1953
Adreject (CL) *see* EPINEPHrine (Systemic, Oral Inhalation) 735
Adreject Jr (CL) *see* EPINEPHrine (Systemic, Oral Inhalation) 735
Adrekar (AT, DE) *see* Adenosine 55
Adrelan (PH) *see* MethylPREDNISolone 1340
Adrenalina (IT) *see* EPINEPHrine (Systemic, Oral Inhalation) 735
Adrenalin (BG, FI, NO) *see* EPINEPHrine (Systemic, Oral Inhalation) 735
Adrenam (DE) *see* Etilefrine [INT] 815
Adrenor (ES, IN) *see* Norepinephrine 1472
Adreson (BE, HN, HU, LU, NL, PL) *see* Cortisone 510
Adriablastina (BG) *see* DOXOrubicin (Conventional) 679
Adriablastina RD (HR) *see* DOXOrubicin (Conventional) 679
Adriacin (JP) *see* DOXOrubicin (Conventional) 679
Adriamycin (AU, CN, DK, GB, IS, NO, NZ, SE) *see* DOXOrubicin (Conventional) 679
Adriamycin CS (SG) *see* DOXOrubicin (Conventional) 679
Adriamycin PFS (KR) *see* DOXOrubicin (Conventional) 679
Adriamycin RDF (KR) *see* DOXOrubicin (Conventional) 679
Adriblastina (AE, AR, BE, BH, CY, CZ, EG, HU, IT, JO, LB, LU, MX, NL, PK, PL, QA, RO, SA, SK, TR, VE) *see* DOXOrubicin (Conventional) 679
Adriblastina CS (CO) *see* DOXOrubicin (Conventional) 679
Adriblastina PFS (EE) *see* DOXOrubicin (Conventional) 679
Adriblastina RTU (CL) *see* DOXOrubicin (Conventional) 679
Adriblastina Soluzione Pronta (IT) *see* DOXOrubicin (Conventional) 679
Adriblastin (AT, CH, IL) *see* DOXOrubicin (Conventional) 679
Adriblastine (FR) *see* DOXOrubicin (Conventional) 679
AdriCept (DE) *see* DOXOrubicin (Conventional) 679
Adricin (ID) *see* DOXOrubicin (Conventional) 679
Adride P (IN) *see* Pioglitazone and Glimepiride 1654
Adrimedac (DE) *see* DOXOrubicin (Conventional) 679
Adrim (IN, JO, VN) *see* DOXOrubicin (Conventional) 679
Adronat (AU) *see* Alendronate 79
Adrosal (PH) *see* DOXOrubicin (Conventional) 679
Adroten (MY) *see* Bisoprolol 266

Adrovance (FR) *see* Alendronate and Cholecalciferol 81
Adroxef (CL) *see* Cefadroxil 372
Adroyd (IN) *see* Oxymetholone 1546
Adsorbed DT COQ (HK, TW) *see* Diphtheria and Tetanus Toxoids, and Acellular Pertussis Vaccine 649
ADT Booster (AU) *see* Diphtheria and Tetanus Toxoid 645
Adumbran (AT, DE, GR) *see* Oxazepam 1532
A Duo Ting (CN) *see* Erdosteine [INT] 753
Adursal (FI) *see* Ursodiol 2116
Advacan (IN) *see* Everolimus 822
Advagraf (BE, CN, CZ, DE, DK, EE, FR, GB, HK, HR, IE, IS, LT, PH, RO, SE, SK, TH, TW, VN) *see* Tacrolimus (Systemic) 1962
Advair (BM) *see* Fluticasone and Salmeterol 912
Advantan (MX) *see* MethylPREDNISolone 1340
Advaquenil (JO) *see* Hydroxychloroquine 1021
Advarone (JO) *see* Amiodarone 114
Advate (AR, AT, AU, BE, CH, CY, CZ, DE, DK, EE, FR, GB, GR, HK, HR, HU, IE, IT, JP, KR, MY, NL, NO, NZ, QA, RO, SE, SG) *see* Antihemophilic Factor (Recombinant) 152
Advecit (TR) *see* Temozolomide 1991
Advicor (CA) *see* Niacin and Lovastatin 1446
Advil (AU, BR, CO, CR, DO, EE, ES, FR, GT, HK, HN, IL, LB, MX, NI, PA, PH, PL, RO, SA, SV, VE, VN, ZA) *see* Ibuprofen 1032
Advil Cold and Sinus (SA) *see* Pseudoephedrine and Ibuprofen 1743
Advil Cold & Sinus (AE, BH, IL, KW, LB) *see* Pseudoephedrine and Ibuprofen 1743
Advil Cold-Sinus (EC) *see* Pseudoephedrine and Ibuprofen 1743
Aedon (IN) *see* CloBAZam 465
Aequamen (DE) *see* Betahistine [CAN/INT] 252
Aerinaze (BE, CR, CZ, GR, IE, LT, NL, PT, RO, SK, TR) *see* Desloratadine and Pseudoephedrine 594
Aerius D-12 (ID) *see* Desloratadine and Pseudoephedrine 594
Aerius D (CL) *see* Desloratadine and Pseudoephedrine 594
Aerius (AE, AR, AT, BE, BG, BH, CH, CL, CN, CO, CR, CY, CZ, DE, DK, DO, EE, ES, FI, FR, GB, GR, GT, HK, HN, HR, HU, ID, IE, IL, IS, IT, KR, KW, LB, LT, MT, MY, NI, NL, NO, NZ, PA, PH, PL, PT, QA, RO, RU, SA, SE, SG, SK, SV, TH, TR, TW, VE, VN) *see* Desloratadine 594
Aerius D12 (PE, SG) *see* Desloratadine and Pseudoephedrine 594
AeroBec (DK, NO, SE) *see* Beclomethasone (Nasal) 232
AeroBec (DK, NO, SE) *see* Beclomethasone (Systemic) 230
Aerobin (DE) *see* Theophylline 2026
Aerobroncol (UY) *see* Ambroxol [INT] 109
Aerocef (AT) *see* Cefixime 380
Aerocort (MY) *see* Beclomethasone (Nasal) 232
Aerocort (MY) *see* Beclomethasone (Systemic) 230
Aerodiol (AT, BE) *see* Estradiol (Systemic) 775
Aerodual (TH) *see* Ipratropium and Fenoterol [CAN/INT] 1109
Aerolin (BR, CN, GR) *see* Albuterol 69
Aeromax (DE) *see* Salmeterol 1860
Aeromol (TH) *see* Albuterol 69
Aeron (AU) *see* Ipratropium (Systemic) 1108
Aeronide (TH) *see* Budesonide (Systemic) 293
Aeronid (PE) *see* Fluticasone and Salmeterol 912
Aerosolv (AT) *see* Acetylcysteine 40
Aerosporin (IN) *see* Polymyxin B 1676
Aerotina (AR) *see* Loratadine 1241
Aerotrop (AR) *see* Ipratropium (Nasal) 1109
Aerotrop (AR, PY) *see* Ipratropium (Systemic) 1108
Aerovent (EG, IL, IQ, IR, LY, OM, YE) *see* Ipratropium (Systemic) 1108
Aerovent (IN) *see* Beclomethasone (Nasal) 232
Aerovent (IN) *see* Beclomethasone (Systemic) 230
Aero-Vent (PH) *see* Albuterol 69
Aeroxina (AR) *see* Clarithromycin 456
AET (AR) *see* Polidocanol 1672
Aethoxyscerol (BE, CZ) *see* Polidocanol 1672
Aethoxysklerol (AT, AU, CH, DK, FI, NL, NO, PY, SE, SK, TH) *see* Polidocanol 1672
Aethoxysklreol (EG, SI) *see* Polidocanol 1672
Aethylcarbonis Chinin (ID) *see* QuiNINE 1761
Aetoxisclerol (FR) *see* Polidocanol 1672
Afalpi Syrup (IL) *see* Pseudoephedrine 1742
Afazol Z (MX) *see* Zinc Sulfate 2200
Afebril (EC, PY) *see* Ibuprofen 1032
Afebrin (HK) *see* Acetaminophen 32
Afebryl (LU) *see* Acetaminophen 32
Afeme (AR) *see* Dexchlorpheniramine 603
Affusine (NL) *see* Fusidic Acid (Topical) [CAN/INT] 943
Afiancen (AR) *see* Fenbufen [INT] 852
AFI-B6 (NO) *see* Pyridoxine 1747
AFI-B (NO) *see* Thiamine 2028
AFI-D2 forte (NO) *see* Ergocalciferol 753
Afidil (VN) *see* Triprolidine and Pseudoephedrine 2105
AFI-Fluor (NO) *see* Fluoride 895
Afifon (IL) *see* Beclomethasone (Nasal) 232
Afinitor (AE, AR, AU, BE, BR, CH, CL, CN, CO, CY, CZ, DE, DK, EE, ES, FR, GB, HK, HR, ID, IL, IS, JP, KR, KW, LB, LT, MY, NO, NZ, PH, QA, RO, SA, SE, SG, SI, SK, TH, TR, TW, VN) *see* Everolimus 822
Afipran (NO) *see* Metoclopramide 1345
Aflacin (SG) *see* Ofloxacin (Ophthalmic) 1491
Aflamax (PE) *see* Naproxen 1427
Aflamid (MX) *see* Meloxicam 1283
Aflamil (BG, SK) *see* Aceclofenac [INT] 30
Aflarex (CL, CO, PE, VE) *see* Fluorometholone 896
Aflem (PH) *see* Carbocisteine [INT] 357
Aflen (GR) *see* Triflusal [INT] 2103
Afloc (KR) *see* Levofloxacin (Ophthalmic) 1200
Afloderm (HR, SK) *see* Alclometasone 72
Afloxx (PE) *see* Meloxicam 1283
Afloyan (ES) *see* Mirtazapine 1376
Afluon (GR, TR) *see* Azelastine (Nasal) 213
Aflusan (AR) *see* Itopride [INT] 1130
Afluteston (AT) *see* Fluoxymesterone 903
Aflux (CO) *see* Acetylcysteine 40
Afoliva (KR) *see* Adefovir 54
Afongan (AR, GR) *see* Omoconazole [INT] 1512
Aforbes (PH) *see* AmLODIPine 123
Aforglim (PH) *see* Glimepiride 966
Afrolate (ES) *see* Etofenamate [INT] 815
Aftab (DE) *see* Triamcinolone (Systemic) 2099
Aftab (DE) *see* Triamcinolone (Topical) 2100
Aftate (AE) *see* Tolnaftate 2063
Afucid (ID) *see* Fusidic Acid (Topical) [CAN/INT] 943
Afungil (MX) *see* Fluconazole 885
A.F. Valdecasas (MX) *see* Folic Acid 919
Agalin (PL) *see* Lindane 1217
Agapurin (HU, PK, VN) *see* Pentoxifylline 1618
Agarol (CH) *see* Sorbitol 1927
Agasten (BR) *see* Clemastine 459
Agatiflox (PH) *see* Gatifloxacin 949
Agelmin (GR, SG) *see* Cetirizine 411
Agemo (PK) *see* Omega-3 Fatty Acids 1507
Agen (EE) *see* AmLODIPine 123
Agentam (PH) *see* Gentamicin (Systemic) 959
Agglad Ofteno (CL, CO, PE, VE) *see* Brimonidine (Ophthalmic) 288
Agglutek (TW) *see* Heparin 997
Aggrastat (AE, AT, AU, BB, BE, BG, BM, BS, BZ, CH, CN, CY, CZ, DE, DK, EE, EG, FI, GB, GR, GY, HK, HU, IE, IL, IN, IT, JM, JO, LB, LT, MY, NL, NO, NZ, PH, PK, PL, PR, PT, QA, SA, SE, SG, SI, SR, TR, TT, TW) *see* Tirofiban 2049
Aggravan (ID, PH) *see* Cilostazol 437

Aggrenox (AE, BE, BH, CO, CZ, DE, GR, HK, ID, IL, IT, KW, PH, PT, QA, RO, RU, SK, TH, TW, VN) *see* Aspirin and Dipyridamole 185
Agilam (VE) *see* Domperidone [CAN/INT] 666
Agilex (AR) *see* Indomethacin 1067
Agiserc (IL) *see* Betahistine [CAN/INT] 252
Agisten (IL) *see* Clotrimazole (Topical) 488
Aglicem (ES) *see* TOLBUTamide 2062
Aglycid (IT) *see* TOLBUTamide 2062
Agnicin (MX) *see* Amikacin 111
Agolene (BE) *see* DimenhyDRINATE 637
AGON SR (NZ) *see* Felodipine 850
Agopton (AT, CH, DE) *see* Lansoprazole 1166
Agrastat (AR, BR, CL, CO, CR, EC, ES, FR, GT, HN, KR, MX, NI, PA, PE, SV, UY, VE) *see* Tirofiban 2049
Agrelid (AR) *see* Anagrelide 147
Agremol (TH) *see* Dipyridamole 652
A Grin (MX) *see* Vitamin A 2173
Agrylin (AU, HK, ID, IL, KR, PH, SG, TH, TW) *see* Anagrelide 147
AGT Ray (IN) *see* Ambroxol [INT] 109
Aguder (CL) *see* Tazarotene 1980
Agudol (PY) *see* Nimesulide [INT] 1456
Agyrax (BE, FR) *see* Meclizine 1277
Ahbina (KR) *see* Triamcinolone (Systemic) 2099
Ai Ben (CN) *see* Ibandronate 1028
Ai Bo Ding (CN) *see* Cladribine 455
Aifude (CN) *see* Prulifloxacin [INT] 1742
Ai Ge (CN) *see* Furosemide 940
Ai Jia Xing (CN) *see* Erythromycin (Systemic) 762
Ai Luo (CN) *see* Esmolol 769
Aimafix (TH) *see* Factor IX (Human) 840
Ainedix (CO) *see* Nilutamide 1455
Ainex (CO) *see* Nimesulide [INT] 1456
Aipexin (KR) *see* Diclofenac (Ophthalmic) 621
Airest (IT) *see* Bamifylline [INT] 227
Airet (CO) *see* Loratadine and Pseudoephedrine 1242
Airex (PH) *see* Cephalexin 405
Airlukast (PE) *see* Montelukast 1392
Airmax (CO) *see* Albuterol 69
Airol (AE, BH, CH, DE, GR, IT, KW, MY, PH, PK, PL, QA, TW) *see* Tretinoin (Topical) 2099
Airomir (AU, BE, CR, DK, ES, FI, FR, GB, GT, HN, LU, NI, NO, NZ, PA, SE, SV, TW, UY) *see* Albuterol 69
Air-Tal (BE) *see* Aceclofenac [INT] 30
Airtal (DO, IE, IT, PY, RU, TR) *see* Aceclofenac [INT] 30
Airum (CL) *see* Clenbuterol [INT] 460
Airuohua (CN) *see* Leflunomide 1174
Aisike (CN) *see* Acyclovir (Systemic) 47
Aisile (CN) *see* Acyclovir (Systemic) 47
Aizea (GB) *see* Desogestrel [INT] 597
Ajuloxon (KR) *see* Loxoprofen [INT] 1255
Ajustin (KR) *see* Azithromycin (Systemic) 216
Akabar (MX) *see* Nifuroxazide [INT] 1454
Akacin (MX, TH) *see* Amikacin 111
Aka-Fluor (PE) *see* Fluorescein 894
Akamigis (VN) *see* Amikacin 111
Akamin (AU) *see* Minocycline 1371
Akamon (JO, MY, TR, TW) *see* Bromazepam [CAN/INT] 290
Akatinol (CO, DO, GT, HN, PA, PY, SV, UY) *see* Memantine 1286
Akdara (KW) *see* Imiquimod 1055
AK-Dilate (PE) *see* Phenylephrine (Systemic) 1638
A-Keftal (IN) *see* Artesunate 178
Akenex (AR) *see* Moclobemide [CAN/INT] 1384
AK-Espore (PE) *see* Neomycin, Polymyxin B, and Gramicidin 1437
Akfen (IE) *see* GuanFACINE 990
Akicin (TH) *see* Amikacin 111
Akilen (ID, SG) *see* Ofloxacin (Systemic) 1490
Akim (EC) *see* Amikacin 111
Akinol (KR) *see* ISOtretinoin 1127
Aklis (UY) *see* Lisinopril 1226
Aklonil (TR) *see* ClonazePAM 478
Akne-Mycin (AE, HK, IL, JO, KW, MY, NL, PT, QA, SG, SI) *see* Erythromycin (Topical) 765
Aknemycin (BE, CZ, DE) *see* Erythromycin (Topical) 765
Aknenormin (DE) *see* ISOtretinoin 1127
Aknilox (CH, TR) *see* Erythromycin (Topical) 765
Akoset (MY) *see* Furosemide 940
Akrotiazina (PY) *see* Pipotiazine [CAN/INT] 1660
Aktiferrin (HU) *see* Ferrous Sulfate 871
AK-Trol (PE) *see* Neomycin, Polymyxin B, and Dexamethasone 1437
Alabel (JP) *see* Aminolevulinic Acid 114
Alacir (UY) *see* DULoxetine 698
ALA (CN) *see* Aminolevulinic Acid 114
Alaglio (JP) *see* Aminolevulinic Acid 114
Alagyl (JP) *see* Clemastine 459
Alanase (NZ, TW) *see* Beclomethasone (Nasal) 232
Alapren (ZA) *see* Enalapril 722
Alapril (IT) *see* Lisinopril 1226
Alastina (ES) *see* Ebastine [INT] 702
Alatrol (MY) *see* Cetirizine 411
Alaxa (IT) *see* Bisacodyl 265
Alba (IN) *see* Albumin 67
Albalon (AE, BH, CH, CY, EG, HK, IQ, IR, JO, KW, LB, LY, NL, OM, QA, SA, SY, TH, YE) *see* Naphazoline (Ophthalmic) 1426
Albalon Liquifilm (AU, NZ) *see* Naphazoline (Ophthalmic) 1426
Albalon Relief (AU, NZ) *see* Phenylephrine (Systemic) 1638
Albapure (ID, TW) *see* Albumin 67
Albasol (CO) *see* Naphazoline (Ophthalmic) 1426
Albatel (TH) *see* Albendazole 65
Albatrina (MX) *see* Loratadine 1241
Alben (BR) *see* Albendazole 65
Albenda (AE, BH, KW, LB, QA, SA) *see* Albendazole 65
Albentel (PE) *see* Albendazole 65
Alben-VC (TH) *see* Albendazole 65
Albenzol (EC) *see* Albendazole 65
Albetol (FI) *see* Labetalol 1151
Albex (AE, BH, CY, EG, IQ, IR, JO, KW, LB, LY, OM, QA, SA, SY, VN, YE) *see* Albendazole 65
Albezole (IN) *see* Albendazole 65
Albicort (BE) *see* Triamcinolone (Systemic) 2099
Albigone (TR) *see* Lisinopril 1226
Albiomin (TH) *see* Albumin 67
Albiotin (ID) *see* Clindamycin (Systemic) 460
Albistat (LU) *see* Miconazole (Topical) 1360
Albix (KR) *see* Memantine 1286
Alborina (ES) *see* Roxithromycin [INT] 1853
Albotein (IT) *see* Albumin 67
Albox (JP) *see* AcetaZOLAMIDE 39
Albucid (AE, BF, BH, BJ, CI, CY, EG, ET, GH, GM, GN, ID, IN, IQ, IR, JO, KE, KW, LB, LR, LY, MA, ML, MR, MU, MW, NE, NG, OM, QA, SA, SC, SD, SL, SN, SY, TN, TZ, UG, YE, ZM, ZW) *see* Sulfacetamide (Ophthalmic) 1943
Albuman 20% (ID) *see* Albumin 67
Albuman (IS) *see* Albumin 67
Albumer (BF, BJ, CI, ET, GH, GM, GN, KE, LR, MA, ML, MR, MU, MW, NE, NG, SC, SD, SL, SN, TN, TZ, UG, ZM, ZW) *see* Albumin 67
Albumex 20 (HK) *see* Albumin 67
Albumex (AU, NZ) *see* Albumin 67
Albumin 5% (CH) *see* Albumin 67
Albumin 5% Human (DE) *see* Albumin 67
Albumina Humana (BR) *see* Albumin 67
Albuminar (BR, ID, IL, VN) *see* Albumin 67
Albuminativ (AT, NO, SE) *see* Albumin 67
Albuminative (SA) *see* Albumin 67
Albumin Human Salzarm 25% (DE) *see* Albumin 67
Albunorm (BG, HR, RO, SI) *see* Albumin 67

Alburel (PH) *see* Albumin 67
Alburex (CO, CY) *see* Albumin 67
Alburx (CN) *see* Albumin 67
Albusol (ZA) *see* Albumin 67
Albutein 25% (BR, CN, HK) *see* Albumin 67
Albutein (AE, BH, HR, LB, PH, SA, VN) *see* Albumin 67
Albyl-E (NO) *see* Aspirin 180
Alcaine (AE, AU, BE, BF, BH, BJ, CH, CI, CN, CY, EG, ET, GH, GM, GN, GR, HK, IL, IQ, IR, IS, JO, KE, KR, KW, LB, LR, LT, LY, MA, ML, MR, MU, MW, MY, NE, NG, NO, OM, PH, PK, PL, QA, RU, SC, SD, SI, SL, SN, SY, TN, TR, TW, TZ, UG, YE, ZA, ZM, ZW) *see* Proparacaine 1728
Alcain (SA) *see* Proparacaine 1728
Alcavixin (PH) *see* VinCRIStine 2163
Alcelam (TH) *see* ALPRAZolam 94
Alcetam (IN) *see* Piracetam [INT] 1661
Alcidol (TH) *see* Alfacalcidol [CAN/INT] 82
Alcloxidine (IL) *see* Chlorhexidine Gluconate 422
Alcobon (AE, BH, CY, EG, IL, IQ, IR, JO, KW, LB, LY, NZ, OM, QA, SA, SY, YE) *see* Flucytosine 889
Alcobuse (TH) *see* Disulfiram 654
Alcocin (IN) *see* Acetaminophen 32
Alcohol Stop (KR) *see* Disulfiram 654
Alcolbing (KR) *see* Disulfiram 654
Alcomicin (AE, BF, BH, BJ, CI, CY, EG, ET, GH, GM, GN, IQ, IR, JO, KE, KW, LB, LR, LY, MA, ML, MR, MU, MW, NE, NG, OM, QA, SA, SC, SD, SL, SN, SY, TN, TZ, UG, YE, ZM, ZW) *see* Gentamicin (Systemic) 959
Alcon Cilox (CO, ID) *see* Ciprofloxacin (Ophthalmic) 446
Alcon Cilox (CO, ID) *see* Ciprofloxacin (Systemic) 441
Alconmide (PH) *see* Lodoxamide 1232
Alcon-Mydril (AR, PY, UY) *see* Tropicamide 2108
Alcorim-F (IN) *see* Sulfamethoxazole and Trimethoprim 1946
Alcosept (IL) *see* Chlorhexidine Gluconate 422
Alcover (HN, HU) *see* Sodium Oxybate 1908
Alcrovan (KR) *see* Alclometasone 72
Aldactin (TW) *see* Spironolactone 1931
Aldactone A (AR, BB, BM, BS, BZ, EC, ES, GY, JM, SR, TT, UY) *see* Spironolactone 1931
Aldactone (AE, AT, AU, BE, BF, BH, BJ, BR, CH, CI, CO, CR, CY, DE, EC, EE, EG, ES, ET, FI, FR, GB, GH, GM, GN, GR, HK, HR, HU, IE, IN, IQ, IR, IS, IT, JO, KE, KR, KW, LB, LR, LU, LY, MA, ML, MR, MT, MU, MW, MX, NE, NG, NL, NO, OM, PA, PE, PH, PK, PL, PT, QA, RU, SA, SC, SD, SE, SG, SI, SK, SL, SN, SY, TH, TN, TW, TZ, UG, VE, VN, YE, ZA, ZM, ZW) *see* Spironolactone 1931
Aldacton (TR) *see* Spironolactone 1931
Aldapres (ID) *see* Indapamide 1065
Aldara (AE, AT, AU, BE, BG, BH, CH, CL, CN, CR, CY, CZ, DE, DK, EE, ES, FI, FR, GB, GR, GT, HK, HN, HR, IE, IL, IS, IT, KR, LB, LT, MT, MX, MY, NL, NO, NZ, PA, PH, PL, PT, QA, RO, RU, SA, SE, SI, SK, SV, TH, TR, TW, VN) *see* Imiquimod 1055
Aldarin (BF, BJ, CI, ET, GH, GM, GN, KE, LR, MA, ML, MR, MU, MW, NE, NG, SC, SD, SL, SN, TN, TZ, UG, ZM, ZW) *see* Amiodarone 114
Aldarone (TH) *see* Amiodarone 114
Aldar (UY) *see* Trimebutine [CAN/INT] 2103
Aldazine (AU, NZ) *see* Thioridazine 2030
Aldazol (PH) *see* Albendazole 65
Aldecin (BG) *see* Beclomethasone (Nasal) 232
Aldinam (CL) *see* Lacosamide 1154
Aldin (IN) *see* Ranitidine 1777
Aldin (TW) *see* Methyldopa 1332
Aldisa-SR (ID) *see* Loratadine and Pseudoephedrine 1242
Aldizem (HR, SI) *see* Diltiazem 634
Aldocumar (ES) *see* Warfarin 2186
Aldolan (TR) *see* Meperidine 1293
Aldomer (ID) *see* Donepezil 668
Aldomet (AE, AR, AU, BE, BF, BH, BJ, BR, CH, CI, CR, CY, DK, EG, ES, ET, FR, GB, GH, GM, GN, GR, GT, HN, IE, IL, IQ, IR, IT, JO, KE, KW, LB, LR, LU, LY, MA, ML, MR, MU, MW, MX, NE, NG, NI, NL, NO, OM, PA, PE, PH, PK, PT, PY, QA, SA, SC, SD, SE, SG, SL, SN, SV, SY, TN, TZ, UG, UY, VE, VN, YE, ZM, ZW) *see* Methyldopa 1332
Aldomet-Forte (HK) *see* Methyldopa 1332
Aldometil (AT) *see* Methyldopa 1332
Aldopam (IN) *see* Pralidoxime 1694
Aldopa (PY) *see* Methyldopa 1332
Aldoquin (CO) *see* Hydroquinone 1020
Aldoron (AR) *see* Nimesulide [INT] 1456
Aldo-Silvederma (HK) *see* Silver Sulfadiazine 1887
Aldosomnil (ES) *see* Lormetazepam [INT] 1247
Aldospirone (IL) *see* Spironolactone 1931
Aldoxol (PY) *see* Spironolactone 1931
Aldren 70 (PH, TH) *see* Alendronate 79
Aldron (HR) *see* Alendronate 79
Aldrox (CL) *see* Alendronate 79
Aldrox (BE) *see* Aluminum Hydroxide 103
Aldurazyme (AT, AU, BE, BG, BR, CH, CL, CY, CZ, DE, DK, EE, ES, FI, FR, GB, GR, HK, HN, HR, IE, IL, IT, JP, KR, LT, MT, MY, NL, NO, NZ, PL, PT, RO, RU, SE, SG, SI, SK, TH, TR, TW) *see* Laronidase 1172
Ale (CN) *see* AtorvaSTATin 194
Aledo Gel (TW) *see* Clindamycin (Systemic) 460
Aledo Gel (TW) *see* Clindamycin (Topical) 464
Alenato (AR) *see* Alendronate 79
Alend (KR) *see* Alendronate 79
Alendomax (JO) *see* Alendronate 79
Alendovenir (IL) *see* Alendronate 79
Alendra (PH) *see* Alendronate 79
Alendrate (NZ) *see* Alendronate 79
Alendrex (NZ) *see* Alendronate 79
Alendro (AU, SA) *see* Alendronate 79
Alendrobell (AU) *see* Alendronate 79
Alendronate (TH) *see* Alendronate 79
Alendro Once Weekly (KW) *see* Alendronate 79
Alendros (KR) *see* Alendronate 79
Alendroxl (PH) *see* Alendronate 79
Alenfos (KR) *see* Alendronate 79
Alenvona (GB) *see* Ethinyl Estradiol and Desogestrel 799
Alenys (AR) *see* Fluticasone (Nasal) 910
Alepam (AU, TW) *see* Oxazepam 1532
Aleprozil (MX) *see* Omeprazole 1508
Alepsal (MX) *see* PHENobarbital 1632
Aleptiz (PH) *see* Valproic Acid and Derivatives 2123
Alercet (EC, GT, PA, PE, SV) *see* Cetirizine 411
Alerest (TH) *see* Cetirizine 411
Alerfast (PE) *see* Loratadine 1241
Alerfedine D (AR) *see* Fexofenadine and Pseudoephedrine 874
Alerfedine (AR) *see* Fexofenadine 873
Alergical SF (PE) *see* Chlorpheniramine and Pseudoephedrine 427
Alergicol LP (PE) *see* Loratadine and Pseudoephedrine 1242
Alergiol (PY) *see* Olopatadine (Ophthalmic) 1500
Alergit (EC) *see* Loratadine 1241
Alergocit (PK) *see* Levocetirizine 1196
Alergoliber (ES) *see* Rupatadine [INT] 1855
Alergone (PH) *see* Cetirizine 411
Alergorom (RO) *see* Cromolyn (Nasal) 514
Alergorom (RO) *see* Cromolyn (Ophthalmic) 514
Alergot (VE) *see* Azelastine (Ophthalmic) 213
Alerid (AE, BH, CY, EG, IQ, IR, JO, KW, LB, LY, OM, QA, SA, SY, YE) *see* Cetirizine 411
Alermax (PY) *see* Levocetirizine 1196
Alernitis (ID) *see* Loratadine 1241
Aleros (ID) *see* Desloratadine 594
Alertasa (ES) *see* Pyridoxine 1747

Alertex (CL, EC) *see* Modafinil 1386
Alertop (CL, PY) *see* Cetirizine 411
Alerviden (CO) *see* Cetirizine 411
Aletor (PH) *see* Cetirizine 411
Aleudrina (ES) *see* Isoproterenol 1124
Aleval (MX) *see* Sertraline 1878
Aleva (PH) *see* Ebastine [INT] 702
Aleve (EE, PL, PY, SG, UY) *see* Naproxen 1427
Aleviate (AU, HK) *see* Antihemophilic Factor/von Willebrand Factor Complex (Human) 154
Aleviatin (JP, TW) *see* Phenytoin 1640
Alexan (AE, AT, BG, CH, CL, CZ, DK, EC, GB, HK, HN, HR, HU, ID, IE, IT, JO, LB, PL, PT, RO, RU, SA, SE, SI, SK, TH, TR, VN, ZA) *see* Cytarabine (Conventional) 535
Alexia-D (PY) *see* Fexofenadine and Pseudoephedrine 874
Alexia (PY) *see* Fexofenadine 873
{alexia SR (SI) *see* Tapentadol 1975
Alexin (IN) *see* Cephalexin 405
Alfacan (CN) *see* Alfacalcidol [CAN/INT] 82
Alfa Caps (IN) *see* Alfacalcidol [CAN/INT] 82
Alfacid (DE) *see* Rifabutin 1803
Alfa Cloromicol (EC) *see* Chloramphenicol 421
Alfacort (AE, AR, BH, JO, KW, QA, SA) *see* Hydrocortisone (Topical) 1014
Alfacort (UY) *see* PredniSONE 1706
Alfadil XL (PH) *see* Doxazosin 674
Alfadil (SE) *see* Doxazosin 674
Alfadina (ES) *see* Brimonidine (Ophthalmic) 288
Alfadiol (PL) *see* Alfacalcidol [CAN/INT] 82
Alfadrops (IN) *see* Apraclonidine 165
Alfaken (MX) *see* Lisinopril 1226
Alfamedin (DE) *see* Doxazosin 674
Alfamet (TR) *see* Methyldopa 1332
Alfamox (IT) *see* Amoxicillin 130
Alfarol (JP, TW) *see* Alfacalcidol [CAN/INT] 82
Alfason (DE) *see* Hydrocortisone (Topical) 1014
Alfast (BR) *see* Alfentanil 83
Alfatil (FR) *see* Cefaclor 372
Alfatil LP (FR) *see* Cefaclor 372
Alfazole (VN) *see* CeFAZolin 373
Alfenil (KR) *see* Alfentanil 83
Alferon N (CA) *see* Interferon Alfa-n3 1100
Alficetin (AR) *see* Colistimethate 504
Alfinor (HK, MY) *see* Betahistine [CAN/INT] 252
Alfron XL (KR) *see* Alfuzosin 84
Alfsin XL (KR) *see* Alfuzosin 84
Alfuca (TH) *see* Albendazole 65
Alfu-Kal XL (IL) *see* Alfuzosin 84
Alfumax (PH) *see* Alfuzosin 84
Alfurix XL (KR) *see* Alfuzosin 84
Alfusin (IN) *see* Alfuzosin 84
Alfuzin (PH) *see* Alfuzosin 84
Alfuzo XL (TW) *see* Alfuzosin 84
Alfuzon XL (KR) *see* Alfuzosin 84
Alfuzostad (CZ) *see* Alfuzosin 84
Alganex (SE) *see* Tenoxicam [INT] 2001
Algeldraat (NL) *see* Aluminum Hydroxide 103
Algesal[+Myrtecaine] (AT, CH, CZ, DE, ES, FI, GB, HU, NL, SE) *see* Diethylamine Salicylate [INT] 624
Algesal (BE, IT, NO) *see* Diethylamine Salicylate [INT] 624
Algesalona E (DE) *see* Etofenamate [INT] 815
Algex (CL) *see* Mefenamic Acid 1280
Algiderma (PT) *see* Diethylamine Salicylate [INT] 624
Algifort (PH) *see* Mefenamic Acid 1280
Algimabo (ES) *see* Dipyrone [INT] 653
Algimesil (IT) *see* Nimesulide [INT] 1456
Algimide (CO) *see* Acetaminophen and Codeine 36
Algimide F (CO) *see* Acetaminophen and Codeine 36
Algina (PY) *see* Aspirin 180
Alginox (EC) *see* Acetaminophen 32
Algirona (BR) *see* Dipyrone [INT] 653
Algocetil (IT) *see* Sulindac 1953
Algoderm (ES) *see* Diethylamine Salicylate [INT] 624
Algofen (IT) *see* Ibuprofen 1032
Algoflex (IT) *see* Diethylamine Salicylate [INT] 624
Algolider (IT) *see* Nimesulide [INT] 1456
Algopyrin (HU) *see* Dipyrone [INT] 653
Algor (PY) *see* Rosiglitazone 1847
Algoxib (BG) *see* Celecoxib 402
Aliaron D 10 (JP) *see* Thiamine 2028
A-Lices 1% (MY, NZ, PH, SG, TH) *see* Malathion 1268
A-Lices (VN) *see* Malathion 1268
Alimax (TR) *see* Telmisartan 1988
Alimta (AE, AR, AT, AU, BE, BG, BH, BR, CH, CL, CN, CO, CY, CZ, DE, DK, EE, ES, FI, FR, GB, GR, HK, HN, HR, HU, ID, IE, IL, IS, IT, JO, JP, KR, LB, LT, MT, MX, MY, NL, NO, NZ, PE, PL, PT, PY, QA, RO, RU, SA, SE, SG, SI, SK, TH, TR, TW, VN) *see* PEMEtrexed 1606
Alin (CR, DO, GT, NI, PA, SV) *see* Dexamethasone (Systemic) 599
Alinol (TH) *see* Allopurinol 90
Alipase (FR) *see* Pancrelipase 1566
Alipid (VN) *see* AtorvaSTATin 194
Alipza (IE) *see* Pitavastatin 1663
Alisade (EE) *see* Fluticasone (Nasal) 910
Aliserin (IT) *see* DiphenhydrAMINE (Systemic) 641
Aliseum (IT) *see* Diazepam 613
Alista (ID) *see* Cilostazol 437
Alisyd (MX) *see* Prednicarbate 1703
Alitoc (KR) *see* Alitretinoin (Systemic) [CAN/INT] 88
Ali Veg (ES) *see* Cimetidine 438
Aliviofta1 (CO) *see* Naphazoline (Ophthalmic) 1426
Alizar (CL) *see* Spironolactone 1931
Alkerana (AR) *see* Melphalan 1283
Alkeran (AE, AT, AU, BE, BF, BH, BJ, BR, CH, CI, CL, CN, CY, CZ, DE, DK, EE, EG, ET, FI, FR, GB, GH, GM, GN, GR, HK, HN, HR, HU, ID, IE, IL, IN, IQ, IR, IS, IT, JO, KE, KR, KW, LB, LR, LT, LU, LY, MA, ML, MR, MT, MU, MW, MX, MY, NE, NG, NL, NO, NZ, OM, PH, PL, PT, QA, RU, SA, SC, SD, SE, SG, SI, SK, SL, SN, SY, TH, TN, TR, TW, TZ, UG, UY, VN, YE, ZA, ZM, ZW) *see* Melphalan 1283
Alkil (ID) *see* Cefadroxil 372
Alkonatrem Gel (FR) *see* Demeclocycline 589
Alkyloxan (KR, SG) *see* Cyclophosphamide 517
Alkyroxan (KR) *see* Cyclophosphamide 517
Allard (IN) *see* Cefpirome [INT] 388
Allase (PH) *see* GlyBURIDE 972
Allbacom (KR) *see* Albendazole 65
All Clear (HK) *see* Naphazoline (Ophthalmic) 1426
AllDone (BG) *see* Nimesulide [INT] 1456
Alledine (AU) *see* Loratadine 1241
Allegra 180 (CL) *see* Fexofenadine 873
Allegra D (CL) *see* Fexofenadine and Pseudoephedrine 874
Allegra-D (BB, BM, BR, BS, BZ, CO, CR, DO, EC, GT, GY, HN, JM, KR, MX, NI, NL, PA, PE, PR, PY, SR, SV, TT, UY, VE) *see* Fexofenadine and Pseudoephedrine 874
Allegra (BB, BM, BR, BS, BZ, CO, CR, DO, EC, GT, GY, HN, IN, JM, JP, KR, MX, NI, NL, PA, PE, PR, PY, SR, SV, TT, TW, UY, VE) *see* Fexofenadine 873
Allegro (DE) *see* Frovatriptan 938
Allegro (IL) *see* Fluticasone (Nasal) 910
Allegro (IL) *see* Fluticasone (Oral Inhalation) 907
Allegron (AU, GB, IE) *see* Nortriptyline 1476
Allemax (PE) *see* Fexofenadine 873
Allentop (HK) *see* Alendronate 79
Allepatadine (KR) *see* Olopatadine (Ophthalmic) 1500
Allercort (TW) *see* Budesonide (Nasal) 296
Allercrom (IN) *see* Cromolyn (Ophthalmic) 514
Allereze (AU) *see* Loratadine 1241
Allerfen (IT) *see* Promethazine 1723

Allerfen (KR) *see* Ketotifen (Systemic) [CAN/INT] 1149
Allergefon (FR, VN) *see* Carbinoxamine 356
Allergetin (AE, BH, KW, QA, SA) *see* Chlorpheniramine and Pseudoephedrine 427
Allerglobuline (BF, BJ, CI, ET, GH, GM, GN, KE, LR, MA, ML, MR, MU, MW, NE, NG, SC, SD, SL, SN, TN, TZ, UG, ZM, ZW) *see* Immune Globulin 1056
Allergocrom (MY, SG, TW) *see* Cromolyn (Ophthalmic) 514
Allergodil (AE, AT, BE, BG, CH, CZ, DE, DK, EE, FR, HN, IT, LB, LT, NL, PL, PT, RO, RU, SA, SI, SK, TR, VE) *see* Azelastine (Nasal) 213
Allergodil (AT, BE, CH, CZ, DE, DK, EE, FR, HR, IT, LT, NL, PT, RO, RU, SK) *see* Azelastine (Ophthalmic) 213
Allergy-Care (IL) *see* Cetirizine 411
Allergyx (IL) *see* Loratadine 1241
Allerkid (PH) *see* Cetirizine 411
Allermin (JP) *see* DiphenhydrAMINE (Systemic) 641
Allermist (JP) *see* Fluticasone (Nasal) 910
Allerpid (MY) *see* Loratadine and Pseudoephedrine 1242
Allersoothe (AU, NZ) *see* Promethazine 1723
Allerta (PH) *see* Loratadine 1241
Allertec (SG) *see* Cetirizine 411
Allertyn (HK, SG) *see* Loratadine 1241
Allerzet (PH) *see* Levocetirizine 1196
Allerzine (MY) *see* Cetirizine 411
Allevisone (TW) *see* Fluticasone (Oral Inhalation) 907
Allevisone (TW) *see* Fluticasone (Topical) 911
Alli (HK, NZ, TW) *see* Orlistat 1520
Allo (CO) *see* Allopurinol 90
Allogut (TR) *see* Allopurinol 90
Allohexal (NZ) *see* Allopurinol 90
Allohex (ID) *see* Loratadine 1241
Allopin (TH) *see* Allopurinol 90
Alloprim (PH) *see* Allopurinol 90
Allopur (CH, NO) *see* Allopurinol 90
Allo-Puren (DE) *see* Allopurinol 90
Allopurinol-ratiopharm (LU) *see* Allopurinol 90
Allor (HK) *see* Loratadine 1241
Alloric (TH) *see* Allopurinol 90
Alloril (IL) *see* Allopurinol 90
Allorin (AU) *see* Allopurinol 90
Alloris (SG) *see* Loratadine 1241
Allosig (AU) *see* Allopurinol 90
Allozym (JP) *see* Allopurinol 90
Allpargin (LU) *see* Allopurinol 90
Allurase (PH) *see* Allopurinol 90
Allurit (IT) *see* Allopurinol 90
Allvoran (DE) *see* Diclofenac (Systemic) 617
Almacin (HR) *see* Amoxicillin 130
Almarytm (IT) *see* Flecainide 882
Almax (CO) *see* Phenazopyridine 1629
Almedon (PK) *see* Domperidone [CAN/INT] 666
Almeta (JP) *see* Alclometasone 72
Almetec (MX) *see* Olmesartan 1496
Almex (MY) *see* Albendazole 65
Almide (FR) *see* Lodoxamide 1232
Alminth (IN) *see* Albendazole 65
Almiral (AE, BF, BH, BJ, CI, CY, EG, ET, GH, GM, GN, IQ, IR, JO, KE, KW, LB, LR, LY, MA, ML, MR, MU, MW, NE, NG, OM, QA, SA, SC, SD, SL, SN, SY, TN, TW, TZ, UG, YE, ZM, ZW) *see* Diclofenac (Systemic) 617
Almodan (GB) *see* Amoxicillin 130
Almogran (AT, BE, CH, DE, DK, ES, FI, FR, GB, IE, IS, IT, JP, KR, NL, NO, PT, SE) *see* Almotriptan 92
Almorsan (AR) *see* Amoxicillin 130
Almycetin (PY) *see* Chloramphenicol 421
Alna (AT, DE) *see* Tamsulosin 1974
Alnacort (IN) *see* Deflazacort [INT] 587
Alnagon (RO) *see* OxyCODONE 1538
Alnax (TH) *see* ALPRAZolam 94
Alnex (MX) *see* Dipyrone [INT] 653
Alodan "Gerot" (AT) *see* Meperidine 1293
Alodorm (AU, HK) *see* Nitrazepam [CAN/INT] 1461
Alofecid (KR) *see* Finasteride 878
Aloginan (JP) *see* Clemastine 459
Aloid (MX) *see* Miconazole (Topical) 1360
Alomax (HR) *see* Minoxidil (Topical) 1374
Alomide (AE, AT, BE, BF, BG, BH, BJ, CH, CI, CN, CO, CZ, DE, DK, EG, ES, ET, FI, GB, GH, GM, GN, GR, HK, HN, HR, HU, ID, IE, IL, IT, JO, KE, KR, KW, LB, LR, LU, MA, ML, MR, MU, MW, MX, MY, NE, NG, NO, PE, PK, PL, PT, PY, QA, RU, SC, SD, SG, SI, SL, SN, TH, TN, TR, TW, TZ, UG, VE, VN, ZA, ZM, ZW) *see* Lodoxamide 1232
Alonet (HK) *see* Atenolol 189
Alonix-S (TW) *see* NIFEdipine 1451
Alopam (DK, NO) *see* Oxazepam 1532
Aloperidin (GR) *see* Haloperidol 993
Alopexy (AE, BE, IL, KW, LB, RO, VN) *see* Minoxidil (Topical) 1374
Alopexyl (FR) *see* Minoxidil (Topical) 1374
Alopine (TW) *see* AmLODIPine 123
Alopron (BB, BM, BS, GY, JM, SR, TR, TT) *see* Allopurinol 90
Alopurinol (HR) *see* Allopurinol 90
Aloret (PK) *see* Desloratadine 594
Alositol (JP) *see* Allopurinol 90
Alosol (MX) *see* Neomycin and Polymyxin B 1437
Alosol (MX) *see* Polymyxin B 1676
Alosot (UY) *see* Sotalol 1927
Alostil (FR) *see* Minoxidil (Topical) 1374
Alostil (ID) *see* Amikacin 111
Alostin (KR) *see* Alprostadil 96
Alovell (ID, PH, VN) *see* Alendronate 79
Alovent (VE) *see* Ipratropium (Systemic) 1108
Aloxi (AT, AU, BE, BG, CH, CY, CZ, DE, DK, EE, ES, FI, FR, GB, GR, HR, HU, IE, IS, IT, JP, KR, LT, MT, MY, NL, NO, NZ, PH, PL, PT, RO, RU, SE, SG, SI, SK, TH, TR, TW, VN) *see* Palonosetron 1561
Aloxid (ID) *see* Minoxidil (Topical) 1374
Aloxidil (BR) *see* Minoxidil (Topical) 1374
Aloxtra (ID) *see* Donepezil 668
Alozex (BR) *see* Anastrozole 148
Alpax (AE, BH, CY, EG, IQ, IR, JO, KW, LB, LY, OM, QA, SA, SY, YE) *see* Pancuronium 1567
Alpaz (PE) *see* ALPRAZolam 94
Alpentin (ID) *see* Gabapentin 943
AL (PH) *see* Allopurinol 90
Alpha-Baclofen (NZ) *see* Baclofen 223
Alphabrin (BR) *see* Brimonidine (Ophthalmic) 288
Alphabrin P (BR) *see* Brimonidine (Ophthalmic) 288
Alphacal (GR) *see* Alfacalcidol [CAN/INT] 82
Alphacin (NZ) *see* Ampicillin 141
Alpha D3 (AR, CZ, EE, GR, HR, IL, IT, PH, PY, RO, RU, SG, SK, TH, TR, VE, VN) *see* Alfacalcidol [CAN/INT] 82
Alphaderm (GB) *see* Urea and Hydrocortisone 2115
Alphadopa (IN) *see* Methyldopa 1332
Alphadrate (NL) *see* Urea 2114
Alphagan (AR, AT, AU, BE, BR, CH, CL, CN, CZ, DE, DK, EC, EG, ES, FI, FR, GB, GR, HR, IN, IS, IT, JO, JP, KW, LB, MX, NL, NO, NZ, PL, PT, SE, TR, TW, VN, ZA) *see* Brimonidine (Ophthalmic) 288
Alphagan P (AE, AR, AU, BR, CL, CN, CO, HK, IL, KR, KW, LB, MY, NZ, PH, SA, SG, TH, TW, VE) *see* Brimonidine (Ophthalmic) 288
Alphagram (PH) *see* Chloramphenicol 421
1 Alpha Leo (BE) *see* Alfacalcidol [CAN/INT] 82
Alphamin (JP) *see* Clemastine 459
Alphamox (AU) *see* Amoxicillin 130
Alphanate (CL, HK, MY, PH, SG, TH) *see* Antihemophilic Factor/von Willebrand Factor Complex (Human) 154
Alphanine SD (AE, HK, SG, TH, TW) *see* Factor IX (Human) 840
Alphapen (MX) *see* Ampicillin 141

Alphapres (PH) *see* CloNIDine 480
Alphapress (AU) *see* HydrALAZINE 1007
Alplax (AR) *see* ALPRAZolam 94
Alplucine[vet.] (FR) *see* Josamycin [INT] 1141
Alporin (KR) *see* Cefuroxime 399
Alpralid (IL) *see* ALPRAZolam 94
Alpraline (MY) *see* ALPRAZolam 94
Alpranax (KR, MY) *see* ALPRAZolam 94
Alprax (AU, HK, IN, TH) *see* ALPRAZolam 94
Alpraz (LU) *see* ALPRAZolam 94
Alprida (AR) *see* Mosapride [INT] 1401
Alprim (AU, SG) *see* Trimethoprim 2104
Alprocontin (IN) *see* ALPRAZolam 94
Alprostan (RU) *see* Alprostadil 96
Alprostapint (BG, HU) *see* Alprostadil 96
Alprox (HU, IL, LB, TW) *see* ALPRAZolam 94
Alpurase (PH) *see* Allopurinol 90
Alpuric (LU) *see* Allopurinol 90
Alpurin (PH) *see* Allopurinol 90
Alrex (BR, HK, TH) *see* Loteprednol 1251
Alsoben (KR, VN) *see* Misoprostol 1379
Alspiron (RO) *see* Spironolactone 1931
Alsucral (EC, FI, MY) *see* Sucralfate 1940
Alsylax (CL) *see* Bisacodyl 265
Altacef (PH) *see* Cefuroxime 399
Altace Plus (VE) *see* Ramipril and Hydrochlorothiazide [CAN/INT] 1773
Altace (VE) *see* Ramipril 1771
Altapres (PH) *see* NIFEdipine 1451
Altargo (AR, AT, AU, BE, BR, CL, CO, CR, CY, CZ, DE, DK, DO, EE, GB, GR, GT, HN, HR, IE, IN, IS, IT, KR, LT, MX, MY, NI, NL, NO, PA, PE, PH, PL, PT, RO, SA, SE, SG, SI, SK, SV, TR) *see* Retapamulin 1793
Altazolin (HR, SI) *see* CeFAZolin 373
Altec (IN) *see* Ambroxol [INT] 109
Alteisduo (FR) *see* Olmesartan and Hydrochlorothiazide 1498
Alteis (FR) *see* Olmesartan 1496
Alten (MY) *see* Tretinoin (Topical) 2099
Altesona (ES) *see* Cortisone 510
Althea (PH) *see* Cyproterone and Ethinyl Estradiol [CAN/INT] 532
Altiazem (BG, HK, IT) *see* Diltiazem 634
Altiazem Retard (IT) *see* Diltiazem 634
Altiazem RR (EE, RU) *see* Diltiazem 634
Altilev (UY) *see* Nortriptyline 1476
Altinate (IN) *see* Artesunate 178
Altirin (KR) *see* Cetirizine 411
Altodor (DE) *see* Etamsylate [INT] 795
Altol (IN) *see* Atenolol 189
Altone (TH) *see* Spironolactone 1931
Altramet (HR, PL) *see* Cimetidine 438
Altraz (IN) *see* Anastrozole 148
Altren (BE) *see* Acemetacin [INT] 30
Altriabak (BE) *see* Ketotifen (Ophthalmic) 1150
Altrol (MX) *see* Calcitriol 323
Altrom (EC) *see* Ketorolac (Systemic) 1146
Altrox (PH) *see* ALPRAZolam 94
Altruline (CR, DO, GT, HN, MX, NI, PA, SV) *see* Sertraline 1878
Altven (AU) *see* Venlafaxine 2150
Alu-Cap (AE, BF, BH, BJ, CI, CY, EG, ET, GH, GM, GN, IL, IQ, IR, JO, KE, KW, LB, LR, LY, MA, ML, MR, MU, MW, NE, NG, OM, QA, SA, SC, SD, SL, SN, SY, TN, TZ, UG, YE, ZM, ZW) *see* Aluminum Hydroxide 103
Alucol (IT) *see* Aluminum Hydroxide 103
Aludrox (DE) *see* Aluminum Hydroxide 103
Alugel (DE) *see* Aluminum Hydroxide 103
Alumbra (CL) *see* Misoprostol 1379
Alumigel (JP) *see* Aluminum Hydroxide 103
Alunlan (TW) *see* Allopurinol 90
Alupent (AE, AT, BH, CY, EG, GB, GR, ID, IE, IL, IN, IQ, IR, IT, JO, KR, KW, LB, LY, NL, OM, PE, QA, RU, SY, YE) *see* Metaproterenol 1307
Aluprex (MX) *see* Sertraline 1878
Aluric (LB) *see* Allopurinol 90
Alurin (BZ, GT) *see* Allopurinol 90
Aluron (VE) *see* Allopurinol 90
Alusac (UY) *see* Sucralfate 1940
Alusulin (HU) *see* Sucralfate 1940
Alu-Tab (AU, HK, PH, SG) *see* Aluminum Hydroxide 103
Alutab (MY) *see* Aluminum Hydroxide 103
Aluvia (CN, EC, ID, PE, TH) *see* Lopinavir and Ritonavir 1237
Alvedon (SE) *see* Acetaminophen 32
Alvelol (KR) *see* Carvedilol 367
Alventa (HR, RO) *see* Venlafaxine 2150
Alveoxina (AR) *see* Colistimethate 504
Alverix (CY, TR) *see* AMILoride 113
Alverix (KR) *see* Alverine [INT] 104
Alvesco (AE, AR, AU, BE, BR, CH, CO, CY, CZ, DE, EE, FI, GB, GR, HK, HN, HR, IE, IL, JP, KR, LT, MY, NL, NO, NZ, PL, PT, RO, SA, SE, SG, SK, TR, TW, VE) *see* Ciclesonide (Systemic) 432
Alvigo (LB) *see* Betahistine [CAN/INT] 252
Alviz (ID) *see* ALPRAZolam 94
Alvo (JP) *see* Oxaprozin 1532
Alvonamid (HR) *see* Indapamide 1065
Alzaimax (AR) *see* Donepezil 668
Alzam (MX, ZA) *see* ALPRAZolam 94
Alzax (KR) *see* ALPRAZolam 94
Alzedon (HK) *see* Donepezil 668
Alzene (AU) *see* Cetirizine 411
Alzene (CO) *see* PACLitaxel (Conventional) 1550
Alzental (AE, BH, CY, EG, IQ, IR, JO, KW, LB, LY, OM, QA, SA, SG, SY, YE) *see* Albendazole 65
Alzepil (LB) *see* Donepezil 668
Alzim (ID) *see* Donepezil 668
Alzinox (PH) *see* Aluminum Hydroxide 103
Alzit (PA) *see* Donepezil 668
Alzolam (IN, SG) *see* ALPRAZolam 94
Alzol (TH) *see* Albendazole 65
Alzone-S (IN) *see* Cefoperazone and Sulbactam [INT] 382
Alzor CCB (PH) *see* Amlodipine and Olmesartan 126
Alzor HCT (PH) *see* Olmesartan and Hydrochlorothiazide 1498
Alzor (PH) *see* Olmesartan 1496
Alzytec (SG) *see* Cetirizine 411
Amaday (PH) *see* AmLODIPine 123
Amadiab (ID) *see* Glimepiride 966
Amadol (AU) *see* Acetaminophen 32
Amagesen Solutab (DE) *see* Amoxicillin 130
Amalar (VN) *see* Sulfadoxine and Pyrimethamine [INT] 1946
Amanda (TH) *see* TraMADol 2074
Amanda (TW) *see* Amantadine 105
Amandine (UY) *see* Amantadine 105
Amandin (TW) *see* Amantadine 105
Amantadina Juventus (ES) *see* Amantadine 105
Amantadina Llorente (ES) *see* Amantadine 105
Amantadin (EE) *see* Amantadine 105
Amanta (KR) *see* Amantadine 105
Amantan (BE, LU) *see* Amantadine 105
Amantix (CO, PL) *see* Amantadine 105
Amantrel (IN) *see* Amantadine 105
Amarax (TH) *see* Glimepiride 966
Amarel (FR) *see* Glimepiride 966
Amarine (TW) *see* Glimepiride 966
Amaryl (AE, AR, AT, AU, BB, BF, BG, BH, BJ, BM, BO, BR, BS, BZ, CH, CI, CL, CN, CO, CR, CY, CZ, DE, DK, DO, EE, EG, ES, ET, FI, GB, GH, GM, GN, GT, GY, HK, HN, HR, ID, IE, IL, IN, IS, IT, JM, JO, KE, KR, KW, LB, LR, LT, MA, ML, MR, MU, MW, MX, MY, NE, NG, NI, NL,

NO, PA, PE, PK, PL, PR, PT, PY, QA, RO, RU, SA, SC, SD, SE, SI, SK, SL, SN, SR, SV, TH, TN, TR, TT, TW, TZ, UG, UY, VE, VN, ZA, ZM, ZW) *see* Glimepiride ... 966
Amarylle (BE) *see* Glimepiride ... 966
Amat (IN) *see* Amlodipine and Atorvastatin ... 124
Amazolon (JP) *see* Amantadine ... 105
Ambacillin (TW) *see* Ampicillin and Sulbactam ... 145
Ambacitam (TH) *see* Ampicillin and Sulbactam ... 145
Ambamida (AR) *see* Erythromycin (Systemic) ... 762
Ambe 12 (LU) *see* Cyanocobalamin ... 515
Amben (TR) *see* Cefadroxil ... 372
Ambese (VE) *see* Secnidazole [INT] ... 1872
Ambesyl (PH) *see* AmLODIPine ... 123
Ambien (BB, BM, BS, BZ, GY, JM, PR, SR, TT) *see* Zolpidem ... 2212
Ambien CR (AR, IL) *see* Zolpidem ... 2212
Ambigram (CO, DO, GT, HN, PA, SV) *see* Norfloxacin ... 1475
Ambilan (CL) *see* Amoxicillin and Clavulanate ... 133
Ambiopi (ID) *see* Ampicillin ... 141
Ambirix (AT, BE, BG, CH, CZ, DE, DK, EE, ES, FI, FR, GB, GR, IE, IT, MT, NL, NO, PL, PT, RU, SE, SK, TR) *see* Hepatitis A and Hepatitis B Recombinant Vaccine ... 1000
AmBisome (AE, AR, AT, AU, BE, CH, CY, DE, DK, ES, FI, FR, GB, GR, HK, HN, IE, IL, IT, JP, KR, KW, LB, NL, NO, PL, PY, RU, SE, SG, TH, TR, TW) *see* Amphotericin B (Liposomal) ... 139
Ambisome (BR, HU, IS, SI) *see* Amphotericin B (Liposomal) ... 139
Ambistryn-S (IN) *see* Streptomycin ... 1937
Ambix (UY) *see* Amlodipine and Benazepril ... 125
Amblum (PK) *see* Artemether and Lumefantrine ... 177
Ambotetra (MX) *see* Tetracycline ... 2017
Ambramicina (CO, IT) *see* Tetracycline ... 2017
Ambrex (BG) *see* Ambroxol [INT] ... 109
Ambril (AR, VE, VN) *see* Ambroxol [INT] ... 109
Ambrobene (AT, CZ, HU) *see* Ambroxol [INT] ... 109
Ambrocol (KR) *see* Ambroxol [INT] ... 109
Ambrolan (EE) *see* Ambroxol [INT] ... 109
Ambrolar (SA) *see* Ambroxol [INT] ... 109
Ambrol (BR) *see* Ambroxol [INT] ... 109
Ambrolex (AU, PH, TH) *see* Ambroxol [INT] ... 109
Ambron (HK) *see* Ambroxol [INT] ... 109
Ambronox (TH) *see* Ambroxol [INT] ... 109
Ambrosan (CZ, PL) *see* Ambroxol [INT] ... 109
Ambrosia (SA) *see* Ambroxol [INT] ... 109
Ambroten (BR) *see* Ambroxol [INT] ... 109
Ambrotos (PY) *see* Ambroxol [INT] ... 109
!Ambroxol Basics (DE) *see* Ambroxol [INT] ... 109
Ambulax-2 (IN) *see* Zolpidem ... 2212
Ambutol (MY) *see* Ethambutol ... 798
Amcal Dry Cough Forte (AU) *see* Pholcodine [INT] ... 1646
Amcal (PH) *see* AmLODIPine ... 123
Amcardia (TH) *see* AmLODIPine ... 123
Amcard (IN) *see* AmLODIPine ... 123
Amcef (MX) *see* CefTRIAXone ... 396
Amchafibrin (ES) *see* Tranexamic Acid ... 2081
Amcillin (KR) *see* Ampicillin ... 141
Amclo (IN) *see* Amoxicillin and Cloxacillin [INT] ... 136
Amcopen (PK) *see* Ampicillin ... 141
Amdepin (BF, BJ, CI, ET, GH, GM, GN, KE, LR, MA, ML, MR, MU, MW, NE, NG, SC, SD, SL, SN, TN, TZ, UG, ZM, ZW) *see* AmLODIPine ... 123
Amdhapine (SG) *see* AmLODIPine ... 123
Amdipin (CO, PE) *see* AmLODIPine ... 123
Amdixal (ID) *see* AmLODIPine ... 123
Amedin (HK) *see* AmLODIPine ... 123
A Mei (TW) *see* Naftifine ... 1416
Ameloz (EE) *see* Aminolevulinic Acid ... 114
AmeLuz (DK) *see* Aminolevulinic Acid ... 114
Ameluz (GB, HR, NL, NO) *see* Aminolevulinic Acid ... 114
Amena (PH) *see* Tibolone [INT] ... 2035
Ameparomo (JP) *see* Paromomycin ... 1579
Amepirise (TW) *see* Glimepiride ... 966
Amerge (JP) *see* Naratriptan ... 1430
Amermycin (HK, TH) *see* Doxycycline ... 689
Amethocaine (BH, JO) *see* Tetracaine (Ophthalmic) ... 2017
Ametic (ZA) *see* Metoclopramide ... 1345
Ametik (IT) *see* Trimethobenzamide ... 2104
Ametop (GB, IE, NZ) *see* Tetracaine (Topical) ... 2017
Ametrex (CO) *see* Acetaminophen ... 32
Ametycine (FR) *see* MitoMYcin (Systemic) ... 1380
Amevan (EC) *see* MetroNIDAZOLE (Systemic) ... 1353
Am-Fam 400 (IN) *see* Ibuprofen ... 1032
Amfazol (VN) *see* Ketoconazole (Topical) ... 1145
Amfipen (AE, BH, CY, EG, GB, IE, IQ, IR, JO, KW, LB, LY, OM, QA, SA, SY, YE) *see* Ampicillin ... 141
Amfucin (PH) *see* Amphotericin B (Conventional) ... 136
Amfulan (TW) *see* Fluocinonide ... 894
Amias (GB, IE) *see* Candesartan ... 335
Amican (HK) *see* Candesartan ... 335
Amicar (AE, AU, BH, CY, EG, IL, IQ, IR, JO, KW, LB, LY, OM, QA, SA, SY, YE, ZA) *see* Aminocaproic Acid ... 113
Amicare (PH) *see* Amikacin ... 111
Amicasil (IT) *see* Amikacin ... 111
Amicil (MX) *see* Amoxicillin ... 130
Amicilon (BR) *see* Amikacin ... 111
Amicin (IN) *see* Amikacin ... 111
Amiclaran (CZ) *see* AMILoride ... 113
Amicor H (HR) *see* Lisinopril and Hydrochlorothiazide ... 1229
Amicor (RO) *see* AtorvaSTATin ... 194
Amicrobin (ES) *see* Norfloxacin ... 1475
Amidona (CN) *see* Methadone ... 1311
Amidrone (JO) *see* Amiodarone ... 114
Amiduret Trom (DE) *see* AMILoride ... 113
Amifos (PK) *see* Amifostine ... 109
A-Migdobis (MX) *see* Bismuth ... 265
Amignul (GR) *see* Almotriptan ... 92
Amikabiot (PE) *see* Amikacin ... 111
Amikacina (CL) *see* Amikacin ... 111
Amikacina Medical (ES) *see* Amikacin ... 111
Amikacina Normon (ES, PT) *see* Amikacin ... 111
Amikacin Fresenius (DE) *see* Amikacin ... 111
Amikafur (MX) *see* Amikacin ... 111
Amikagram (PE) *see* Amikacin ... 111
Amikal (DK) *see* AMILoride ... 113
Amikan (IT) *see* Amikacin ... 111
Amikaxing (CN) *see* Amikacin ... 111
Amikayect (MX) *see* Amikacin ... 111
Amikin. (MX) *see* Amikacin ... 111
Amikin (BF, BG, BJ, CH, CI, CO, CZ, EC, EE, EG, ET, GB, GH, GM, GN, HK, HU, IE, JO, KE, KR, KW, LR, MA, ML, MR, MU, MW, NE, NG, NZ, PE, PK, PL, QA, SA, SC, SD, SL, SN, TN, TZ, UG, ZA, ZM, ZW) *see* Amikacin ... 111
Amiklin (FR) *see* Amikacin ... 111
Amikozit (AE, BH, CY, EG, IL, IQ, IR, JO, KW, LB, LY, OM, QA, RO, RU, SA, SY, TR, YE) *see* Amikacin ... 111
Amiktam (KR) *see* Amikacin ... 111
Amilamont (GB) *see* AMILoride ... 113
Amilit (IT) *see* Amitriptyline ... 119
Amiloberag (DE) *see* AMILoride ... 113
Amilo (KR) *see* AMILoride ... 113
Amilorid NM Pharma (SE) *see* AMILoride ... 113
Amilo (TW) *see* AmLODIPine ... 123
Amilozid (HN) *see* AMILoride ... 113
Amimox (SE) *see* Amoxicillin ... 130
Aminazin (RU) *see* ChlorproMAZINE ... 429
Amineurin (DE) *see* Amitriptyline ... 119
Aminomux (AR, PY, UY, VE) *see* Pamidronate ... 1563

Aminor (AE, BH, CY, EG, IL, IQ, IR, JO, KW, LB, LY, OM, QA, SA, SY, YE) *see* Norethindrone 1473
Aminosidine (JP) *see* Paromomycin 1579
Amiocar (AR) *see* Amiodarone 114
Amiodacore (IL) *see* Amiodarone 114
Amiodarex (DE) *see* Amiodarone 114
Amiodarona (CL) *see* Amiodarone 114
Amiohexal (DE) *see* Amiodarone 114
Amio (PH) *see* Amiodarone 114
Amiorel (AR) *see* Bromhexine [INT] 291
Amiorit (CO) *see* Amiodarone 114
Amiosin (ID) *see* Amikacin 111
Amipenix (JP) *see* Ampicillin 141
Amiphos (IN) *see* Amifostine 109
Amipril (PH) *see* Ramipril 1771
Amiprin (JP) *see* Amitriptyline 119
Amira (AU) *see* Moclobemide [CAN/INT] 1384
Amiram (JO) *see* Amitriptyline 119
Amiride (IL) *see* AMILoride 113
Amirone (AE) *see* Amiodarone 114
Amiron (KR) *see* Amiodarone 114
Amitab (IN) *see* Secnidazole [INT] 1872
Amital (KR) *see* Amobarbital 128
Amitax (PH) *see* Amikacin 111
Amitiza (CH, JP) *see* Lubiprostone 1255
Amitone (HK, MY, SG) *see* Ketotifen (Systemic) [CAN/INT] 1149
Amitrip (NZ) *see* Amitriptyline 119
Amitriptylinum (PL) *see* Amitriptyline 119
Ami (TW) *see* Azelaic Acid 213
Amivalex (HU) *see* Lactulose 1156
Amizil (PH) *see* Terbinafine (Systemic) 2002
Amizil (PH) *see* Terbinafine (Topical) 2004
AMK (HK, TH) *see* Amoxicillin and Clavulanate 133
Amlate (ZA) *see* AmLODIPine 123
Amlibon B (VE) *see* Amlodipine and Benazepril 125
Amlibon (MY) *see* AmLODIPine 123
Amlo-M (KR) *see* AmLODIPine 123
Amloc (AR, CL) *see* AmLODIPine 123
Amlocar (PE) *see* AmLODIPine 123
Amlodac (MY, TW) *see* AmLODIPine 123
Amlodar (AE, KW, LB) *see* AmLODIPine 123
Amlod (HK, TH) *see* AmLODIPine 123
Amlodigamma (HK) *see* AmLODIPine 123
Amlodine (PH, TW) *see* AmLODIPine 123
Amlodin (JP) *see* AmLODIPine 123
Amlodipin Plus (CH) *see* Amlodipine and Atorvastatin 124
Amlogrix (ID) *see* AmLODIPine 123
Amlong (HK, MY, SG) *see* AmLODIPine 123
Amlopine (TH) *see* AmLODIPine 123
Amlopin (HR, KR, PL) *see* AmLODIPine 123
Amlopres (HK) *see* AmLODIPine 123
Amlopress (SA) *see* AmLODIPine 123
Amlor (BE, FR, IL, LU, SA) *see* AmLODIPine 123
Amlostar (KR) *see* AmLODIPine 123
Amlosyn (CO) *see* AmLODIPine 123
Amlotens (SG) *see* AmLODIPine 123
Amlotrene (PH) *see* AmLODIPine 123
Amlovasc (CH) *see* AmLODIPine 123
Amlovas (CR, DO, GT, HN, NI, PA, SV, VN) *see* AmLODIPine 123
Amlozen (HK) *see* AmLODIPine 123
Ammimox (TH) *see* Amoxicillin 130
Ammonaps (AT, CZ, DE, DK, ES, FR, GB, HR, IT, LT, NL, PL, PT, RO, SE, SI, SK) *see* Sodium Phenylbutyrate 1908
Amoban (JP) *see* Zopiclone [CAN/INT] 2217
Amobay (MX) *see* Amoxicillin 130
Amobay Cl (MX) *see* Amoxicillin and Clavulanate 133
Amocla (KR) *see* Amoxicillin and Clavulanate 133
Amoclan (AE, BH, CY, EG, IQ, IR, JO, KW, LB, LY, OM, QA, SA, SY, TW, YE) *see* Amoxicillin and Clavulanate 133
Amoclan (QA) *see* Amoxicillin 130
Amoclav (DE) *see* Amoxicillin and Clavulanate 133
Amoclave (ES) *see* Amoxicillin 130
Amoclen (CZ) *see* Amoxicillin 130
Amocoat (TW) *see* Amorolfine [INT] 128
Amocure (TW) *see* NiMODipine 1456
Amodex (FR) *see* Amoxicillin 130
Amodin (KR) *see* AmLODIPine 123
Amodipin (KR) *see* AmLODIPine 123
Amoflux (BR) *see* Amoxicillin 130
Amoksiclav (TH) *see* Amoxicillin and Clavulanate 133
Amol (AE, BH, CY, EG, IQ, IR, JO, KW, LB, LY, OM, QA, SA, SY, YE) *see* Acetaminophen 32
Amolin (IE) *see* Atenolol 189
Amolin (TW) *see* Amoxicillin 130
A-Mol (TH) *see* Acetaminophen 32
Amorin (KR) *see* Glimepiride 966
Amoron (HR) *see* Indapamide 1065
Amosyt (SE) *see* DimenhyDRINATE 637
Amotaks (PL) *see* Amoxicillin 130
Amotril (AE, BH, CY, EG, IQ, IR, JO, KW, LB, LY, OM, QA, SA, SY, YE) *see* ClonazePAM 478
Amoval (PE) *see* Amoxicillin 130
Amox (AE, BH, CY, EG, IQ, IR, IT, JO, KW, LB, LY, OM, QA, SA, SY, YE) *see* Amoxicillin 130
Amoxal (VE) *see* Amoxicillin 130
Amoxapen (CY, TR) *see* Amoxicillin 130
Amoxcillin (TH) *see* Amoxicillin 130
Amoxcin (TW) *see* Amoxicillin 130
Amoxi-basan (DE) *see* Amoxicillin 130
Amoxicap (HK, PK) *see* Amoxicillin 130
Amoxic Comp (IS) *see* Amoxicillin and Clavulanate 133
Amoxicilina (CO, EC) *see* Amoxicillin 130
Amoxiclav (MX) *see* Amoxicillin and Clavulanate 133
Amoxiclav-BID (MX) *see* Amoxicillin and Clavulanate 133
Amoxiclav-Teva (IL) *see* Amoxicillin and Clavulanate 133
Amoxicle (KR) *see* Amoxicillin and Clavulanate 133
Amoxiclin (PE) *see* Amoxicillin 130
Amoxico (PH) *see* Amoxicillin 130
Amoxidal (AR, UY) *see* Amoxicillin 130
Amoxidin 7 (PE) *see* Amoxicillin 130
Amoxidin (AE, BF, BH, BJ, CI, CY, EG, ET, GH, GM, GN, IQ, IR, JO, KE, KW, LB, LR, LY, MA, ML, MR, MU, MW, NE, NG, OM, QA, SA, SC, SD, SL, SN, SY, TN, TZ, UG, YE, ZM, ZW) *see* Amoxicillin 130
Amoxiflox (PH) *see* Moxifloxacin (Ophthalmic) 1403
Amoxifur (MX) *see* Amoxicillin 130
Amoxiga (CO) *see* Amoxicillin 130
Amoxigran (HK) *see* Amoxicillin 130
Amoxihexal (DE) *see* Amoxicillin 130
Amoxi (IL) *see* Amoxicillin 130
Amoxil (AE, AU, BF, BH, BJ, BR, CI, CY, EC, EG, ET, GB, GH, GM, GN, GR, ID, IE, IQ, IR, JO, KE, KW, LB, LR, LY, MA, ML, MR, MU, MW, MX, NE, NG, NZ, OM, PE, QA, SA, SC, SD, SL, SN, SY, TN, TR, TZ, UG, YE, ZA, ZM, ZW) *see* Amoxicillin 130
Amoxillin (IL, IT) *see* Amoxicillin 130
Amoxin (FI, IS) *see* Amoxicillin 130
Amoxinova (MX) *see* Amoxicillin 130
Amoxipen (AE, JO, SA, VN) *see* Amoxicillin 130
Amoxipenil (CL) *see* Amoxicillin 130
Amoxi Plus (PY) *see* Amoxicillin and Clavulanate 133
Amoxisol (MX) *see* Amoxicillin 130
Amoxitab (HK) *see* Amoxicillin 130
Amoxi TO (TH) *see* Amoxicillin 130
Amoxivan (IN) *see* Amoxicillin 130
Amoxivet (MX) *see* Amoxicillin 130
Amoxsan Forte (ID) *see* Amoxicillin 130
Amoxsan (ID) *see* Amoxicillin 130

Amoxxlin (KR) *see* Amoxicillin and Clavulanate 133
Amoxyclav (IL) *see* Amoxicillin and Clavulanate 133
Amoxy (CN) *see* Amoxicillin 130
Amoxydar (AE, SA) *see* Amoxicillin 130
Amoxy-diolan (DE) *see* Amoxicillin 130
Amoxypen (DE, PE) *see* Amoxicillin 130
Ampamet (IT) *see* Aniracetam [INT] 150
Ampavit (TH) *see* Cyanocobalamin 515
Ampecu (EC) *see* Ampicillin 141
Ampen (VE) *see* Ampicillin 141
Amphocil (MX) *see* Amphotericin B (Conventional) 136
Amphocil (AT, AU, CZ, DK, FI, GB, GR, HK, HN, HR, HU, IL, IT, MX, MY, NL, PL, SE, SI, TH, TW) *see* Amphotericin B Cholesteryl Sulfate Complex 136
Amphogel (KR) *see* Aluminum Hydroxide 103
Amphojel (ZA) *see* Aluminum Hydroxide 103
Ampholin (TH) *see* Amphotericin B (Conventional) 136
Ampholip (IN, VN) *see* Amphotericin B (Lipid Complex) 138
Ampho-Moronal (CH) *see* Amphotericin B (Conventional) 136
Amphotec (CN) *see* Amphotericin B (Liposomal) 139
Amphotret (TH) *see* Amphotericin B (Conventional) 136
Ampi-1 (PH) *see* Ampicillin 141
Ampibex (EC) *see* Ampicillin 141
Ampiblan (CO) *see* Ampicillin 141
Ampicil (BR) *see* Ampicillin 141
Ampicilina (EC) *see* Ampicillin 141
Ampicillin (PL) *see* Ampicillin 141
Ampicin (PH) *see* Ampicillin 141
Ampiclin (PH) *see* Ampicillin 141
Ampiclox (AE, EG, PK) *see* Ampicillin and Cloxacillin [INT] 144
Ampiclox (NL) *see* Cloxacillin [CAN/INT] 488
Ampiclox (SG) *see* Ampicillin 141
Ampicyn (AU, QA) *see* Ampicillin 141
Ampidar (AE, BH, CY, EG, IL, IQ, IR, JO, KW, LB, LY, OM, QA, SA, SY, YE) *see* Ampicillin 141
Ampigen SB (AR) *see* Ampicillin and Sulbactam 145
Ampiger (BR) *see* Ampicillin 141
Ampilag (BF, BJ, CI, ET, GH, GM, GN, KE, LR, MA, ML, MR, MU, MW, NE, NG, SC, SD, SL, SN, TN, TZ, UG, ZM, ZW) *see* Ampicillin 141
Ampilin (IN) *see* Ampicillin 141
Ampillin (MY) *see* Ampicillin 141
Ampimax (PH) *see* Ampicillin and Sulbactam 145
Ampimedin (PY) *see* Ampicillin 141
Ampipen (IN, ZA) *see* Ampicillin 141
Ampipharm (JO) *see* Ampicillin 141
Ampi-quim (MX) *see* Abacavir 20
Ampisulciillin (BG) *see* Ampicillin and Sulbactam 145
Ampisulcillin (EE) *see* Ampicillin and Sulbactam 145
Ampitenk (AR) *see* Ampicillin 141
Ampitrex (PH) *see* Ampicillin 141
Ampivral (CO) *see* Ampicillin 141
Ampliactil (AR) *see* ChlorproMAZINE 429
Ampliar Duo (AR) *see* Ezetimibe and Atorvastatin 833
Ampliblan (CO) *see* Ampicillin 141
Amplictil (BR) *see* ChlorproMAZINE 429
Ampliron Plus (PY) *see* Amlodipine and Benazepril 125
Ampliron (PY) *see* AmLODIPine 123
Amplisul (EC) *see* Ampicillin and Sulbactam 145
Amplium (IT) *see* Ampicillin and Cloxacillin [INT] 144
Ampolin (TW) *see* Ampicillin 141
Amprace (AU, NZ) *see* Enalapril 722
Ampres (GB) *see* Chloroprocaine 423
Ampril HL (EE) *see* Ramipril and Hydrochlorothiazide [CAN/INT] 1773
Ampril (HR) *see* Ramipril 1771
Ampty (IN) *see* Itopride [INT] 1130
Amsapen (MX) *see* Ampicillin 141
Amsubac (TH) *see* Ampicillin and Sulbactam 145
Amtas (SG) *see* AmLODIPine 123
a.m.t. (DE) *see* Amantadine 105
Amtrel (TH) *see* Amlodipine and Benazepril 125
Amtuss (MY) *see* Ambroxol [INT] 109
Amukin (BE, LU, NL) *see* Amikacin 111
Amuno Retard (DE) *see* Indomethacin 1067
Amuprux (AR) *see* Bivalirudin 268
Amval (CO, GT) *see* Amlodipine and Valsartan 126
Amvasc (AE, QA) *see* AmLODIPine 123
Amvax B (PH) *see* Hepatitis B Vaccine (Recombinant) 1002
Amvisc (NL, PL) *see* Hyaluronate and Derivatives 1006
Amxol (HK, SG, TH) *see* Ambroxol [INT] 109
Amybital (TW) *see* Amobarbital 128
Amycal (NO) *see* Amobarbital 128
Amycor (FR) *see* Bifonazole [INT] 264
Amydramine-II (AE, LB) *see* DiphenhydrAMINE (Systemic) 641
Amydramkine-II (SA) *see* DiphenhydrAMINE (Systemic) 641
Amygra (PK) *see* Pyridostigmine 1746
Amyl Nitrite (NZ) *see* Amyl Nitrite 147
Amytal Sodium (AU) *see* Amobarbital 128
Amytal (TH) *see* Amobarbital 128
Amytril (BR) *see* Amitriptyline 119
Amyzol (HR) *see* Amitriptyline 119
Amze (AR, PY) *see* AmLODIPine 123
Anabet (PT) *see* Nadolol 1411
Anabon (KR) *see* Ibandronate 1028
Anaccord (NZ) *see* Anastrozole 148
Anaclosil (ES) *see* Cloxacillin [CAN/INT] 488
Anadip (KR) *see* Lercanidipine [INT] 1181
Anaerobex (AT) *see* MetroNIDAZOLE (Systemic) 1353
Anaestherit (AT) *see* Benzocaine 246
Anaesthesin (DE) *see* Benzocaine 246
Anafen (ID) *see* Ibuprofen 1032
Anafranil 25 (ID) *see* ClomiPRAMINE 475
Anafranil (AE, AR, AT, AU, BB, BE, BF, BG, BH, BJ, BM, BR, BS, BZ, CH, CI, CL, CN, CO, CY, CZ, DE, DK, EC, EE, EG, ES, ET, FI, FR, GB, GH, GM, GN, GR, GY, HK, HN, HR, HU, IE, IL, IN, IQ, IR, IS, IT, JM, JO, KE, KW, LB, LR, LT, LU, LY, MA, ML, MR, MT, MU, MW, MX, NE, NG, NL, NO, NZ, OM, PH, PK, PL, PT, PY, QA, RO, RU, SA, SC, SD, SE, SI, SK, SL, SN, SR, SY, TH, TN, TR, TT, TZ, UG, UY, VE, VN, YE, ZA, ZM, ZW) *see* ClomiPRAMINE 475
Anafranil Retard (AT, DK, FI, NL, SE) *see* ClomiPRAMINE 475
Anafranil SR 75 (IL) *see* ClomiPRAMINE 475
Anafranil SR (LB, MY, NZ, SG) *see* ClomiPRAMINE 475
Anagastra (ES) *see* Pantoprazole 1570
Anagregal (IT) *see* Ticlopidine 2040
Ana-Guard (ZA) *see* EPINEPHrine (Systemic, Oral Inhalation) 735
Analab (MY, TH) *see* TraMADol 2074
Analac (TW, VN) *see* Ketorolac (Systemic) 1146
Analept (GR) *see* Enalapril 722
Analeric (GR) *see* Diflunisal 626
Analgan Tram (EC) *see* Acetaminophen and Tramadol 37
Analgel (AR) *see* Acemetacin [INT] 30
Analgina (AR, PY) *see* Dipyrone [INT] 653
Analgin (BG, CZ, DE, EG, RU) *see* Dipyrone [INT] 653
Analgine (BE) *see* Dipyrone [INT] 653
Analgiser (AE, BH, CY, EG, IQ, IR, JO, KW, LB, LY, OM, QA, SA, SY, YE) *see* Acetaminophen 32
Analin (PH) *see* Nalbuphine 1416
Analphen (MX) *see* Acetaminophen 32
Analspec (ID) *see* Mefenamic Acid 1280
Analtram (ID) *see* Acetaminophen and Tramadol 37
Anamorph (AU) *see* Morphine (Systemic) 1394
Anandron (AR, AU, CH, CZ, FI, FR, GR, HN, HR, HU, MX, NL, NO, PL, PT, SE, VN) *see* Nilutamide 1455
Anan (JP) *see* Bisacodyl 265

Anapen (AU, BG, CH, CZ, DE, FR, GR, HU, PL, PT, SE, TR) *see* EPINEPHrine (Systemic, Oral Inhalation) 735
Anapenil (MX) *see* Penicillin V Potassium 1614
Anapolon (PL, QA) *see* Oxymetholone 1546
Anaprilan (RU) *see* Propranolol 1731
Anapril (SG, TH) *see* Enalapril 722
Anapril S Minitab (TH) *see* Enalapril 722
Anapsique (MX) *see* Amitriptyline 119
Anargil (MY, SK, TH, TR, VN) *see* Danazol 558
Anaromat (RO) *see* Anastrozole 148
Anaropin (VN) *see* Ropivacaine 1846
Anasteronal (ES) *see* Oxymetholone 1546
Anastil (VE) *see* Oxazepam 1532
Anastrol (AU, IL) *see* Anastrozole 148
Anatac (ES) *see* Carbocisteine [INT] 357
Anatan (KR) *see* Candesartan 335
Anatensol (BE, HK, IN, NL) *see* FluPHENAZine 905
Anatensol Decanoate (PE) *see* FluPHENAZine 905
Anatoxal Di Te Per Berna (PE) *see* Diphtheria and Tetanus Toxoids, and Acellular Pertussis Vaccine 649
Anatrole (NZ) *see* Anastrozole 148
Anausin (FR) *see* Metoclopramide 1345
Anautin (DK, EC) *see* DimenhyDRINATE 637
Anazol (AE) *see* MetroNIDAZOLE (Systemic) 1353
Anazole (PH) *see* Anastrozole 148
Anazo (TH) *see* Phenazopyridine 1629
Anazo (TW, VN) *see* Anastrozole 148
Anbacim (ID) *see* Cefuroxime 399
Anbin (ES) *see* Antithrombin 156
Anbinex (AR, IL, PY, SG) *see* Antithrombin 156
An Bu (CN) *see* Bromhexine [INT] 291
Ancaron (JP) *see* Amiodarone 114
Ancea (PH) *see* Cyproterone and Ethinyl Estradiol [CAN/INT] 532
Ancefa (ID) *see* Cefadroxil 372
Ancillin (TW) *see* Ampicillin 141
Ancobon (HK) *see* Flucytosine 889
Anco (DE) *see* Ibuprofen 1032
Ancotil (AE, AT, AU, BG, BH, BR, CH, CY, CZ, DE, DK, EG, FR, GB, GR, HR, IE, IL, IQ, IR, IT, JO, KW, LB, LY, NL, NO, OM, PL, QA, SA, SE, SG, SY, YE) *see* Flucytosine 889
Ancotyl (RU) *see* Flucytosine 889
Andante (RU) *see* Zaleplon 2193
Andapsin (SE) *see* Sucralfate 1940
Andaxin (HN, HU) *see* Meprobamate 1296
Andazol (TR) *see* Albendazole 65
Andepra (AU) *see* DULoxetine 698
Andiar (EC) *see* Montelukast 1392
Andocit (TH) *see* Indomethacin 1067
Andolex (NO, SE) *see* Benzydamine [CAN/INT] 249
Andol (HR) *see* Aspirin 180
Andosept (ZA) *see* Benzydamine [CAN/INT] 249
Andral (PH) *see* PHENobarbital 1632
Andrews TUMS Antacid (AU) *see* Calcium Carbonate 327
Andrin (PY) *see* Terazosin 2001
Androcur (AE, AR, AT, AU, BE, BG, BH, BR, CH, CN, CO, CY, CZ, DE, DK, DO, EC, EE, EG, ES, FI, FR, GB, GR, HK, HN, HR, HU, ID, IE, IL, IT, JO, JP, KR, KW, LB, MX, MY, NL, PE, PK, PL, PT, QA, RO, SA, SE, SG, SI, SK, TH, TR, TW, UY, VE, VN, ZA) *see* Cyproterone [CAN/INT] 530
Androcur Dep (QA) *see* Cyproterone [CAN/INT] 530
Androderm (AU, NZ) *see* Testosterone 2010
AndroForte (AU) *see* Testosterone 2010
Androgel (AE, BE, BH, CZ, EE, FR, HK, HN, HU, IE, IT, KW, MY, NL, QA, RU, SA, SG, TH, TW, VN) *see* Testosterone 2010
Androlic (TH) *see* Oxymetholone 1546
Andropatch (GR) *see* Testosterone 2010
Andros (PH) *see* Sildenafil 1882
Androstat (EC, PY) *see* Cyproterone [CAN/INT] 530
Androtin (MX) *see* Famotidine 845
Androxyl (MY, SG) *see* Cefadroxil 372
An Du Fen (CN) *see* Acetaminophen and Codeine 36
Anectine (AE, BB, BH, BM, BS, BZ, CY, EG, ES, GB, GY, IE, IQ, IR, JM, JO, KW, LB, LY, MX, OM, QA, SA, SR, SY, TT, YE) *see* Succinylcholine 1939
Aneiromox (ES) *see* Bumetanide 297
Anekain (HR) *see* Bupivacaine 299
Anekcin (PH) *see* Succinylcholine 1939
Anektil (PH) *see* Succinylcholine 1939
Anelmin (AE, BH, CY, EG, IQ, IR, JO, KW, LB, LY, OM, QA, SA, SY, YE) *see* Mebendazole [CAN/INT] 1274
Anelmin (PY) *see* Nitazoxanide 1461
Anemet (DE, HN) *see* Dolasetron 663
Anemolat (ID) *see* Folic Acid 919
Anepol (KR, TH) *see* Propofol 1728
Anerex (MX) *see* Thiamine 2028
Anerobizol (PH) *see* MetroNIDAZOLE (Systemic) 1353
Anerrum (TH) *see* Iron Sucrose 1118
Anesject (ID) *see* Ketamine 1143
Anespar (ID) *see* Midazolam 1361
Anespin (PH) *see* Atropine 200
Anestalcon (AR, BR, CL, PY) *see* Proparacaine 1728
Anestecin crema (CO) *see* Lidocaine and Prilocaine 1213
Anesthal (IN) *see* Thiopental [INT] 2029
Anestil (EC) *see* Lidocaine and Prilocaine 1213
Anesvan (TH) *see* Propofol 1728
Anetamin (JP) *see* Sodium Oxybate 1908
Aneurin-AS (DE) *see* Thiamine 2028
Anexate (AE, AT, AU, BE, BF, BG, BH, BJ, CH, CI, CN, CY, CZ, DE, EE, EG, ES, ET, FR, GH, GM, GN, GR, HK, HN, HR, HU, ID, IE, IL, IQ, IR, IT, JO, JP, KE, KR, KW, LB, LR, LU, LY, MA, ML, MR, MU, MW, MY, NE, NG, NL, NO, NZ, OM, PK, PL, PT, QA, RO, SA, SC, SD, SI, SK, SL, SN, SY, TH, TN, TR, TW, TZ, UG, VN, YE, ZA, ZM, ZW) *see* Flumazenil 892
Anexia (ID) *see* Ramipril 1771
Anexin (ID) *see* Sertraline 1878
Anexin (PY) *see* ClomiPHENE 473
Anexopen (GR) *see* Naproxen 1427
Anfertil (BR) *see* Ethinyl Estradiol and Norgestrel 812
Anfix (ID) *see* Cefixime 380
Anflupin (TW) *see* Flurbiprofen (Systemic) 906
Anfotericina B (DO, GT, PA) *see* Amphotericin B (Conventional) 136
Anfuramide (JP) *see* Furosemide 940
Ange 28 (JP) *see* Levonorgestrel 1201
Angela (TH) *see* Acetaminophen 32
Angeliq (AU, BB, BM, BS, BZ, CN, CO, CR, CY, DO, EC, EE, FR, GB, GT, GY, HK, HN, ID, IE, IL, JM, KR, KW, MY, NI, NL, PA, PH, PR, SA, SR, SV, TH, TT) *see* Ethinyl Estradiol and Drospirenone 801
Angibid SR (KR) *see* Isosorbide Dinitrate 1124
Angicor (DK) *see* Nicorandil [INT] 1449
Angiderm Patch (KR) *see* Nitroglycerin 1465
Angilol (IE) *see* Propranolol 1731
Angimet (PH) *see* Metoprolol 1350
Anginal (JP) *see* Dipyridamole 652
Anginine (AU) *see* Nitroglycerin 1465
Angintriz MR (ID) *see* Trimetazidine [INT] 2104
Angiodarona (BR) *see* Amiodarone 114
Angiolat (UY) *see* Nisoldipine 1459
Angiomax (AR, AU, CL, IL, IN, NZ) *see* Bivalirudin 268
Angiopril (IN) *see* Captopril 342
Angiopurin (HU) *see* Pentoxifylline 1618
Angioretic (EC) *see* Losartan and Hydrochlorothiazide 1250
Angiotec (JO) *see* Enalapril 722
Angioten (ID) *see* Losartan 1248
Angiotrofen (CR, DO, GT, HN, NI, PA, SV) *see* Diltiazem 634
Angiotrofin (MX) *see* Diltiazem 634

Angiotrofin Retard (MX) *see* Diltiazem 634
Angiovan (CO) *see* Cilostazol 437
Angiox (AT, BE, BG, CH, CZ, DE, DK, EE, ES, FI, FR, GB, GR, HN, HR, IE, IS, IT, LT, MT, NL, NO, PL, PT, RO, RU, SE, SI, SK, TR) *see* Bivalirudin 268
Angiozem (PH) *see* Diltiazem 634
Angiozide (AE, BH, CY, EG, IQ, IR, JO, KW, LB, LY, OM, QA, SA, SY, YE) *see* Enalapril and Hydrochlorothiazide 725
Angirel MR (PH) *see* Trimetazidine [INT] 2104
Angirel (PH) *see* Trimetazidine [INT] 2104
Angised (HR, SG) *see* Nitroglycerin 1465
Angistad (PH) *see* Isosorbide Mononitrate 1126
Angitrate (ZA) *see* Isosorbide Mononitrate 1126
Angitrit (SG) *see* Isosorbide Dinitrate 1124
Angizaar (SG) *see* Losartan 1248
Angizem (IT) *see* Diltiazem 634
Angonic (VN) *see* Enalapril 722
Angoron (GR) *see* Amiodarone 114
Angsobide (MY) *see* Isosorbide Dinitrate 1124
AnHe (CN) *see* Glyburide and Metformin 974
Anhigot (MX) *see* Dorzolamide and Timolol 673
Anhistan (JP) *see* Clemastine 459
Anicef (KR) *see* Cefdinir 376
Animex (UY) *see* Moclobemide [CAN/INT] 1384
Animin (TW) *see* Perphenazine 1627
Anin (IN) *see* Hydroxyprogesterone Caproate 1021
Anipen (PH) *see* Imipenem and Cilastatin 1051
Anistal (DO, GT, HN, NI, SV) *see* Ranitidine 1777
Anitdoxe (TW) *see* Doxepin (Topical) 678
Anitrim (MX) *see* Sulfamethoxazole and Trimethoprim 1946
Anjal (TW) *see* Hydrochlorothiazide and Triamterene 1012
Ankorme (TW) *see* Butenafine 314
Anli (CN) *see* Ofloxacin (Otic) 1491
Anlin (TW) *see* Diazepam 613
Anmatic (TH) *see* Piroxicam 1662
An Mei LIn (CN) *see* Cloxacillin [CAN/INT] 488
Annita (BR) *see* Nitazoxanide 1461
Anodyne (TW) *see* Indomethacin 1067
Anoion (PH) *see* Amiodarone 114
Anoldin (MY) *see* AmLODIPine 123
Anol (TW) *see* Mannitol 1269
Anoprolin (JP) *see* Allopurinol 90
Anorex (FR) *see* Diethylpropion 624
Anorex (KR) *see* Dantrolene 559
Anorsia (TH) *see* Pizotifen [CAN/INT] 1664
Anosin (KR) *see* Adenosine 55
Anpec (AU, TW) *see* Verapamil 2154
Anpechlor (PH) *see* Chloramphenicol 421
Anpect (EE) *see* Trimetazidine [INT] 2104
Anpeval (ES) *see* Triflusal [INT] 2103
An Pu Luo (CN) *see* Loxoprofen [INT] 1255
An Qi (CN) *see* Amoxicillin and Clavulanate 133
Anquil (GB, IE) *see* Benperidol [INT] 244
Anquin (IL) *see* Norfloxacin 1475
Ansaid (CL, CN, EC, PK) *see* Flurbiprofen (Systemic) 906
Ansal (NZ) *see* Diflunisal 626
Ansatipine (FR) *see* Rifabutin 1803
Ansatipin (ES, FI, SE) *see* Rifabutin 1803
Ansederm (FR) *see* Lidocaine and Prilocaine 1213
Anselol (AU) *see* Atenolol 189
Anseren (IT) *see* Ketazolam [INT] 1144
Ansial (AR) *see* BusPIRone 311
Ansieten (AR) *see* Ketazolam [INT] 1144
Ansietil (CL) *see* Ketazolam [INT] 1144
Ansifix SR (EC) *see* Venlafaxine 2150
Ansi (ID) *see* FLUoxetine 899
Ansilan (CO) *see* FLUoxetine 899
Ansilan (CZ) *see* Medazepam [INT] 1277
Ansilor (PT) *see* LORazepam 1243
Ansimar (IT, PH) *see* Doxofylline [INT] 679
Ansin (TW) *see* Aspirin 180
Ansiodex (PY) *see* Citalopram 451
Ansiolin (IT) *see* Diazepam 613
Ansiolit (EC) *see* ALPRAZolam 94
Ansiopax (UY) *see* Clorazepate 487
Ansiospaz (PE) *see* Clorazepate 487
Ansiowas (ES) *see* Meprobamate 1296
Ansitec (BR) *see* BusPIRone 311
Ansrin (KR) *see* Anthralin 150
Ansures (MY, PH) *see* MetFORMIN 1307
Ansutam (TW) *see* Ampicillin and Sulbactam 145
Ansuzole (MY) *see* Anastrozole 148
Antabenz (MY) *see* Flumazenil 892
Antabus (AT, CH, CL, CZ, DE, DK, EC, ES, FI, HR, IS, NL, NO, SE, SI, TR) *see* Disulfiram 654
Antabuse (AU, BE, GB, IE, IT, LU, MX, NZ, SG, ZA) *see* Disulfiram 654
Antacsal-E (MX) *see* Aspirin 180
Antadys (LB) *see* Flurbiprofen (Systemic) 906
Antaethyl (HN, HU) *see* Disulfiram 654
Antagonil (DE) *see* NiCARdipine 1446
Antagonin (BF, BJ, CI, ET, GH, GM, GN, KE, LR, MA, ML, MR, MU, MW, NE, NG, SC, SD, SL, SN, TN, TZ, UG, ZM, ZW) *see* Ranitidine 1777
Antagosan (DE, HR) *see* Aprotinin 168
Antak (BR) *see* Ranitidine 1777
Antalcol (RO) *see* Disulfiram 654
Antalgin (MX) *see* Indomethacin 1067
Antalgina (PE) *see* Dipyrone [INT] 653
Antalgin (ES) *see* Naproxen 1427
Antalgin (ID) *see* Dipyrone [INT] 653
Antalgo (IT) *see* Nimesulide [INT] 1456
Antalin (CL) *see* Amitriptyline 119
Antalip (CY) *see* Gemfibrozil 956
Antallpen (LB) *see* Ampicillin 141
Antamol (JO) *see* Acetaminophen 32
Antangping (CN) *see* Nateglinide 1432
Antarene (FR) *see* Ibuprofen 1032
Antaspan (VN) *see* ClonazePAM 478
Antasten (AR) *see* Captopril 342
Antasthmin (AT) *see* Isoproterenol 1124
Anta (TH) *see* LORazepam 1243
Antaxone (ES, IT, RU) *see* Naltrexone 1422
Antebor (BE) *see* Sulfacetamide (Ophthalmic) 1943
Antelepsin (HU) *see* ClonazePAM 478
Antemin (CH) *see* DimenhyDRINATE 637
Antenex (AU) *see* Diazepam 613
Anten (NZ) *see* Doxepin (Systemic) 676
Antens (KR) *see* Enalapril 722
Antepsin (AR, DK, FI, GB, IE, IS, IT, NO, TR) *see* Sucralfate 1940
Anterin (TW) *see* Diclofenac (Systemic) 617
Antex (PY) *see* Simvastatin 1890
Anthel (AU, TW) *see* Pyrantel Pamoate 1744
Anthelmin (PK) *see* Pyrantel Pamoate 1744
Anthramed (ID) *see* Anthralin 150
Anthranol (AE, BH, CY, EG, ES, FR, IQ, IR, JO, KW, LB, LY, OM, PH, QA, SA, SY, YE, ZA) *see* Anthralin 150
Anthrin (KR) *see* Anthralin 150
Anthrobin P (JP) *see* Antithrombin 156
Anthrom (PH) *see* Aspirin 180
Anti-D (SG) *see* ChlorproPAMIDE 429
Antiallersin (BG) *see* Promethazine 1723
Antiax (PY) *see* Magaldrate and Simethicone 1261
Anticholium (AT, DE) *see* Physostigmine 1647
Anticlot (VN) *see* Heparin 997
Anticol (PL) *see* Disulfiram 654
Anticude (ES) *see* Edrophonium 706
Antidep (IN) *see* Imipramine 1054
Antidiab (HR, PL) *see* GlipiZIDE 967
Antidoxe (TW) *see* Doxepin (Systemic) 676
Antietanol (BR) *see* Disulfiram 654

Antifan (CZ, EE) *see* Terbinafine (Topical) 2004
Antifin (CN, PK) *see* Terbinafine (Systemic) 2002
Antiflam (UY) *see* Famotidine 845
Antiflogil (BR) *see* Nimesulide [INT] 1456
Antiflog (IT) *see* Piroxicam 1662
Antifloxil (ES) *see* Nimesulide [INT] 1456
Antiflu (IN) *see* Oseltamivir 1523
Antif (PE) *see* Letrozole 1181
Antigeron (BR) *see* Cinnarizine [INT] 440
Antigone (FR) *see* Desogestrel [INT] 597
Antigreg (MY, SG) *see* Ticlopidine 2040
Antigrilin (IN) *see* Eptifibatide 751
Antihydral (CH, LU) *see* Methenamine 1317
Antikrein (JP) *see* Aprotinin 168
Antikun (ID) *see* Piracetam [INT] 1661
Antilon (TW) *see* Pyridostigmine 1746
Antimal (AE) *see* Chloroquine 424
Antimet (ZA) *see* Cinnarizine [INT] 440
Antimic (TH) *see* Isoniazid 1120
Antimigraine (TW) *see* Ergotamine 754
Antimigrin (AT) *see* Naratriptan 1430
Antimycolin (TW) *see* Oxiconazole 1536
Antinal (BE, CH) *see* Nifuroxazide [INT] 1454
Antinaus (NZ) *see* Prochlorperazine 1718
Antinepte (RO) *see* Tianeptine [INT] 2033
Antiox (PH) *see* Mebendazole [CAN/INT] 1274
Antiparkin (LU) *see* Selegiline 1873
Antiplar (PH) *see* Clopidogrel 484
Anti-Plate 75 (BF, BJ, CI, ET, GH, GM, GN, KE, LR, MA, ML, MR, MU, MW, NE, NG, SC, SD, SL, SN, TN, TZ, UG, ZM, ZW) *see* Dipyridamole 652
Antipois (VN) *see* Charcoal, Activated 416
Antipres (ID) *see* Sertraline 1878
Antipressan (GB, IE) *see* Atenolol 189
Antiprestin (ID) *see* FLUoxetine 899
Antiprotin (AE) *see* Bromocriptine 291
Antiroid (KR) *see* Propylthiouracil 1735
Antisacer (PT) *see* Phenytoin 1640
Anti (SE) *see* Acyclovir (Topical) 51
Antisek (EC) *see* Chlorhexidine Gluconate 422
Antisemin (TW) *see* Cyproheptadine 529
Antiss (CO) *see* Levocetirizine 1196
Antithrombin III (HK) *see* Antithrombin 156
Antithrombin III Immuno (HR, HU) *see* Antithrombin 156
Anti-Thyrox (IN) *see* Carbimazole [INT] 356
Antitussivum Burger (DE) *see* Codeine 497
Antivir (TH) *see* Zidovudine 2196
Antivom (HK) *see* Betahistine [CAN/INT] 252
Antivomit (FI) *see* DimenhyDRINATE 637
Antix (NO) *see* Acyclovir (Systemic) 47
Antix (NO) *see* Acyclovir (Topical) 51
Antizoal (PH) *see* MetroNIDAZOLE (Systemic) 1353
Antizol (GB, IE) *see* Fomepizole 922
Antodine (AE, BH, CY, EG, IQ, IR, JO, KW, LB, LY, OM, QA, SA, SY, YE) *see* Famotidine 845
Antol (TW) *see* Atropine 200
Anton (TW) *see* Diflunisal 626
Antox (CR, GT, HN, NI, PA, SV) *see* Ciprofloxacin (Systemic) 441
Antra (IT) *see* Omeprazole 1508
Antranol (BR) *see* Anthralin 150
Antrex (FI, PL, TW) *see* Leucovorin Calcium 1183
Antribid (PT) *see* Sulindac 1953
Antroquoril (AU) *see* Betamethasone (Topical) 255
Anuar (AR) *see* Roxithromycin [INT] 1853
Anulax (EC) *see* Bisacodyl 265
Anulette (CL, PE) *see* Ethinyl Estradiol and Levonorgestrel 803
Anulit (PY) *see* Ethinyl Estradiol and Levonorgestrel 803
Anuva (ID) *see* Diclofenac (Systemic) 617
Anwu (MY, TW) *see* FluvoxaMINE 916
Anxel (EE) *see* Pantoprazole 1570
Anxiar (RO) *see* LORazepam 1243
Anxidin (FI) *see* Clorazepate 487
Anxilet (TW) *see* RisperiDONE 1818
Anxiolan (TH) *see* BusPIRone 311
Anxiolit (AT, CH) *see* Oxazepam 1532
Anxiolit Retard (CH) *see* Oxazepam 1532
Anxira (TH) *see* LORazepam 1243
Anxirloc (ID) *see* CloBAZam 465
Anxiron (AE, BH, CY, EG, HN, HU, IQ, IR, JO, KW, LB, LY, OM, QA, SA, SY, YE) *see* BusPIRone 311
Anxokast (TW) *see* Montelukast 1392
Anxolipo (TW) *see* AtorvaSTATin 194
Anxopone (TW) *see* Entacapone 730
Anxotos (TW) *see* Pioglitazone 1654
Anxut (DE) *see* BusPIRone 311
Anxyl (LB) *see* Bromazepam [CAN/INT] 290
Anxyrex (FR) *see* Bromazepam [CAN/INT] 290
Anycef (KR) *see* Cefdinir 376
Anydipine (KR) *see* AmLODIPine 123
Anzapine (MY) *see* CloZAPine 490
Anzaplus (PH) *see* Losartan and Hydrochlorothiazide 1250
Anzatax (AE, AU, CN, EG, HK, KR, LB, MY, NZ, PH, SA, SG, TH, TW) *see* PACLitaxel (Conventional) 1550
Anzatax (PE) *see* ClonazePAM 478
Anzela (VN) *see* Azelaic Acid 213
Anzemet (AR, AT, AU, BG, CH, FR, GB, GR, IT, KR, MX, NL, PL, SE, VE) *see* Dolasetron 663
Anzepam (TW) *see* LORazepam 1243
Anzief (JP) *see* Allopurinol 90
Anzol (PH) *see* Anastrozole 148
Ao Bo Lin (CN) *see* Ornidazole [INT] 1522
Ao Er Fei (CN) *see* Oseltamivir 1523
Aofolin (CN) *see* Flucloxacillin [INT] 885
3-A Ofteno (CR, DO, GT, HN, NI, PA, SV, VE) *see* Diclofenac (Ophthalmic) 621
Aofuqing (CN) *see* Calcipotriene 321
Ao Gu Li (CN) *see* Ambroxol [INT] 109
Ao Ke An (CN) *see* MetroNIDAZOLE (Systemic) 1353
Ao Ning (CN) *see* Oxybutynin 1536
Ao Nuo Xian (CN) *see* Dexrazoxane 606
Ao Rui Xin (CN) *see* Balsalazide 226
Ao Sai Juo Xing (CN) *see* Oxytocin 1549
Ao Shu Xin (CN) *see* Erythromycin (Systemic) 762
Aotal (FR) *see* Acamprosate 28
Ao Wei Xian (CN) *see* Itopride [INT] 1130
Apacef (BE, FR, LU) *see* CefoTEtan 385
Apagrel (IN) *see* Prasugrel 1699
Apalin (MY) *see* Amikacin 111
Apamid (SE) *see* GlipiZIDE 967
Apano (TW) *see* Mifepristone 1366
Aparkan (HU) *see* Trihexyphenidyl 2103
Aparsonin (DE) *see* Bromhexine [INT] 291
Apatef (AU, DE, IT, PT) *see* CefoTEtan 385
Apaurin (HR, SI, SK) *see* Diazepam 613
Apecitab (AR) *see* Capecitabine 339
Apeton 4 (ID) *see* Cyproheptadine 529
Apetrol (KR) *see* Megestrol 1281
Aphenylbarbit (CH) *see* PHENobarbital 1632
Aphrodil (AE, BH, CY, EG, IQ, IR, JO, KW, LB, LY, OM, QA, SA, SY, YE) *see* Sildenafil 1882
Aphtiria (FR) *see* Lindane 1217
Apicarpine (JO) *see* Pilocarpine (Ophthalmic) 1649
Apiclof (JO) *see* Diclofenac (Ophthalmic) 621
Apicort (AE, BH, JO, QA, SA) *see* PrednisoLONE (Ophthalmic) 1706
Apicort Forte (AE, JO, QA, SA) *see* PrednisoLONE (Ophthalmic) 1706
Apicrom (JO) *see* Cromolyn (Ophthalmic) 514
Apidra (AE, AR, AT, AU, BB, BE, BG, BH, BR, BS, CH, CL, CN, CO, CR, CY, CZ, DE, DK, DO, EC, EE, ES, FI, FR, GB, GR, GT, HK, HN, HR, HU, ID, IE, IL, IN, IS, IT, JM, JP, KR, KW, LB, LT, MT, MX, MY, NI, NL, NO, NZ, PA, PE, PH, PL, PT, PY, QA, RO, RU, SA, SE, SG, SI,

SK, SV, TH, TR, TT, TW, UY, VN) *see* Insulin Glulisine 1086
Apiflox (AE, KW) *see* Norfloxacin 1475
Apifrin-Z (AE, SA) *see* Phenylephrine and Zinc Sulfate [CAN/INT] 1640
Apigen (AE, BH, JO, QA, SA) *see* Gentamicin (Ophthalmic) 962
Apigent (AE, BH, CY, EG, IQ, IR, JO, KW, LB, LY, OM, QA, SA, SY, YE) *see* Gentamicin (Systemic) 959
Apigrane (JO) *see* SUMAtriptan 1953
Apildon (HK) *see* Domperidone [CAN/INT] 666
Apilepsin (HR) *see* Valproic Acid and Derivatives 2123
Apimol (AE, JO) *see* Timolol (Ophthalmic) 2043
Apine (TW) *see* Atropine 200
Apisate (IE) *see* Diethylpropion 624
Apisopt (JO) *see* Dorzolamide 673
Apisulfa (BH, QA, SA) *see* Sulfacetamide (Ophthalmic) 1943
Apisulpha-20 (AE) *see* Sulfacetamide (Ophthalmic) 1943
Apitropin (AE, BH, JO, KW) *see* Atropine 200
Apixol (JO) *see* Betaxolol (Ophthalmic) 257
Apizolin (JO) *see* Naphazoline (Ophthalmic) 1426
Aplacasse (AR) *see* LORazepam 1243
Aplactan (JP) *see* Cinnarizine [INT] 440
Aplaket (HK, MY, SG, TH) *see* Ticlopidine 2040
Aplexal (JP) *see* Cinnarizine [INT] 440
Aplosyn (PH) *see* Fluocinolone (Topical) 893
Apo-Acetazolamide (MY) *see* AcetaZOLAMIDE 39
Apo-Alpraz (SG) *see* ALPRAZolam 94
Apo-Amoxi (MY) *see* Amoxicillin 130
Apo-Atenol (HK) *see* Atenolol 189
Apo-Bromocriptine (NZ) *see* Bromocriptine 291
Apo-Cal (HK, MY) *see* Calcium Carbonate 327
Apocanda (DE) *see* Clotrimazole (Topical) 488
Apo-Carbamazepine (MY) *see* CarBAMazepine 346
Apocard (ES, PT) *see* Flecainide 882
Apo-Chlorax (SG) *see* Clidinium and Chlordiazepoxide 460
Apo-Cimetidine (NZ) *see* Cimetidine 438
Apo-Cloxi (SG) *see* Cloxacillin [CAN/INT] 488
Apoclox (PK) *see* Ampicillin and Cloxacillin [INT] 144
Apocyclin (FI) *see* Tetracycline 2017
Apo-diazepam (CZ) *see* Diazepam 613
Apo-diltiazem CD (NZ) *see* Diltiazem 634
Apodorm (NO, SE) *see* Nitrazepam [CAN/INT] 1461
Apodruff (IN) *see* Ketoconazole (Topical) 1145
Apo-Folic (NZ) *see* Folic Acid 919
Apo-Gain (MY) *see* Minoxidil (Topical) 1374
Apogar (MX) *see* Pioglitazone 1654
Apo-Glibenclamide (NZ) *see* GlyBURIDE 972
Apo-Hydro (MY) *see* Hydrochlorothiazide 1009
Apo-ISMN (HK) *see* Isosorbide Mononitrate 1126
Apokalin (NO) *see* Neomycin 1436
Apo-K (JO, MY) *see* Potassium Chloride 1687
Apolar (FI, ID, NO, SE) *see* Desonide 597
Apolets (TH) *see* Clopidogrel 484
Apo-Levotard (MY) *see* Carbidopa and Levodopa 351
Apolide (MX) *see* Nimesulide [INT] 1456
Apomiterl (JP) *see* Cinnarizine [INT] 440
Apo-Nadolol (NZ) *see* Nadolol 1411
Apo-Nicotinic Acid (NZ) *see* Niacin 1443
Aponil (TR) *see* Nimesulide [INT] 1456
APO-Perphenazine (MY) *see* Perphenazine 1627
Apo-Pindolol (NZ) *see* Pindolol 1652
Apo-Prednisone (NZ) *see* PredniSONE 1706
Apo-Primidone (NZ) *see* Primidone 1714
Apo-Ranitidine (NZ) *see* Ranitidine 1777
Apo-Selegiline (NZ) *see* Selegiline 1873
Apo-Timop (NZ) *see* Timolol (Ophthalmic) 2043
Apotomin (JP) *see* Cinnarizine [INT] 440
Apo-triazide (HK) *see* Hydrochlorothiazide and Triamterene 1012
Apo-Trifluoperazine (PL) *see* Trifluoperazine 2102
Apo-Trihex (MY) *see* Trihexyphenidyl 2103
Apovent (IL) *see* Ipratropium (Systemic) 1108
Apozepam (DK) *see* Diazepam 613
Appese (AU) *see* ROPINIRole 1844
Appeton Activ-C (MY) *see* Ascorbic Acid 178
Approvel (DE) *see* Irbesartan 1110
Apranax (CR, DO, FR, GT, HN, NI, PA, RU, SV, VE, VN) *see* Naproxen 1427
Apraz (BR) *see* ALPRAZolam 94
Aprazo (TW) *see* ALPRAZolam 94
Aprednislon (AT) *see* PrednisoLONE (Systemic) 1703
Aprelax (PH) *see* Naproxen 1427
Aprelazine (TW) *see* HydrALAZINE 1007
Apresol (IN) *see* HydrALAZINE 1007
Apresolina (MX, PT, UY, VE) *see* HydrALAZINE 1007
Apresoline (AU, BB, BF, BH, BJ, BM, BS, BZ, CI, CY, EG, ET, GB, GH, GM, GN, GY, IE, JM, KE, LR, MA, ML, MR, MU, MW, NE, NG, NL, NZ, PH, QA, SA, SC, SD, SG, SL, SN, SR, TH, TN, TR, TT, TW, TZ, UG, ZM, ZW) *see* HydrALAZINE 1007
Apresolin (NO, SE) *see* HydrALAZINE 1007
Aprezin (TW) *see* HydrALAZINE 1007
Aprical (DE, LU) *see* NIFEdipine 1451
Apridal (PY) *see* Enalapril 722
Aprinol (JP) *see* Allopurinol 90
Aprion (ID) *see* Pregabalin 1710
Aprior (PH) *see* Nicorandil [INT] 1449
Aprix (CO) *see* Acetaminophen and Codeine 36
Aprix F (CO) *see* Acetaminophen and Codeine 36
Aprocin (HK) *see* Ciprofloxacin (Ophthalmic) 446
Aprocin (HK) *see* Ciprofloxacin (Systemic) 441
Aprodil (EC) *see* Finasteride 878
Aprokam (GB) *see* Cefuroxime 399
Apronal (TH) *see* Allopurinol 90
Apronax (EC) *see* Naproxen 1427
Aprotimbin (HR, KR) *see* Aprotinin 168
Aprovel (AE, AR, AT, BB, BE, BH, BO, BR, BS, CH, CL, CN, CO, CR, CZ, DE, DK, DO, EC, EE, ES, FI, FR, GB, GR, GT, HK, HN, HR, HU, ID, IE, IT, JM, JO, KR, KW, LB, LT, MT, MX, MY, NI, NL, NO, PA, PE, PH, PK, PL, PR, PT, PY, QA, RO, RU, SA, SE, SG, SI, SK, SV, TH, TR, TT, TW, UY, VE, VN) *see* Irbesartan 1110
Aproven (AU) *see* Ipratropium (Systemic) 1108
Aprozide (BR) *see* Irbesartan and Hydrochlorothiazide 1112
Aprtan (KR) *see* Irbesartan 1110
Aprurol (UY) *see* Lindane 1217
Apsatan (JP) *see* Cinnarizine [INT] 440
Apstar (RO) *see* Trimetazidine [INT] 2104
Aptamol (IN) *see* Acetaminophen 32
Aptivus (AR, AT, AU, BE, BG, CH, CZ, DE, DK, EE, ES, FI, FR, GB, GR, HN, HR, HU, IE, IS, IT, LT, MT, MX, NL, NO, NZ, PL, PT, RO, RU, SE, SI, SK, TR, TW) *see* Tipranavir 2047
Apton (PT) *see* Pantoprazole 1570
Aptor (ID) *see* Aspirin 180
Apulon (TW) *see* HydrALAZINE 1007
Apurin (FI, GR, NL) *see* Allopurinol 90
Apuzin (MY) *see* Captopril 342
Aquacaine (AU) *see* Penicillin G Procaine 1613
Aquacare HP (AU, NZ) *see* Urea 2114
Aquacort (DE) *see* Budesonide (Systemic) 293
Aquadon (IL) *see* Chlorthalidone 430
Aquadrate (GB, IE) *see* Urea 2114
Aquaear (AU) *see* Acetic Acid 39
Aquafol (KR) *see* Propofol 1728
Aquanase (MY) *see* Beclomethasone (Nasal) 232
Aquaphoril (AT, PY) *see* Xipamide [INT] 2191
Aquarid (ZA) *see* Furosemide 940
Aquarius (GR) *see* Ketoconazole (Topical) 1145
Aquasec (IN) *see* Racecadotril [INT] 1765
Aquasol AD (MX) *see* Ergocalciferol 753

Aquasol E (CO) *see* Vitamin E 2174
Aquaviron (IN) *see* Testosterone 2010
Aquavit-E (DO, HN, PA, SV) *see* Vitamin E 2174
Aquazone (ES) *see* Bumetanide 297
Aqucilina (ES) *see* Penicillin G Procaine 1613
Aqudol (EC) *see* Acetaminophen, Aspirin, and Caffeine 37
Aquimod Cream (IL) *see* Imiquimod 1055
Aquin (PK) *see* Gatifloxacin 949
Aquo-Cytobion (DE) *see* Hydroxocobalamin 1020
Aqurea (SG) *see* Urea 2114
Ara-C (AR) *see* Cytarabine (Conventional) 535
Arabine (DK, FI, FR) *see* Cytarabine (Conventional) 535
Arabitin (JP) *see* Cytarabine (Conventional) 535
Arabloc (AU, NZ) *see* Leflunomide 1174
Araclof (ID) *see* Diclofenac (Systemic) 617
Aracytin (CO, GR, IT, UY) *see* Cytarabine (Conventional) 535
Aracytine (FR) *see* Cytarabine (Conventional) 535
Aradix Retard (CL, PE, PY) *see* Methylphenidate 1336
Arados (EC) *see* Losartan 1248
Aragam (GB) *see* Immune Globulin 1056
Aragan (KR) *see* Hyaluronate and Derivatives 1006
Aragan Plus (MY) *see* Hyaluronate and Derivatives 1006
Aralen (MX) *see* Chloroquine 424
Aralen Phosphate (AE, BF, BH, BJ, CI, CY, EC, EG, ET, GH, GM, GN, IL, IQ, IR, JO, KE, KW, LB, LR, LY, MA, ML, MR, MU, MW, NE, NG, OM, PE, QA, SA, SC, SD, SL, SN, SY, TN, TZ, UG, YE, ZA, ZM, ZW) *see* Chloroquine 424
Arandin (KR) *see* Atenolol 189
Aranesp (AE, AT, AU, BE, BG, BH, CH, CY, CZ, DE, DK, EE, FI, FR, GB, GR, HK, HN, HR, IE, IL, IS, IT, JO, KW, LT, MX, NL, NO, NZ, PL, QA, RO, SA, SE, SI, SK, TR, TW) *see* Darbepoetin Alfa 565
Arasemide (JP) *see* Furosemide 940
Arastad (VN) *see* Leflunomide 1174
Aratac (AU, NZ, SG, TH, TW) *see* Amiodarone 114
Arava (AE, AR, AT, AU, BB, BD, BE, BG, BH, BO, BR, BS, CH, CL, CO, CR, CY, CZ, DE, DK, DO, EC, EE, FI, FR, GB, GR, GT, HK, HN, HR, HU, ID, IE, IL, IN, IS, IT, JM, JO, JP, KR, KW, LB, LT, MT, MX, MY, NI, NL, NO, NZ, PA, PE, PH, PK, PL, PR, PT, PY, QA, RO, RU, SA, SE, SG, SI, SK, SV, TH, TR, TT, TW, VE, VN) *see* Leflunomide 1174
Aravida (PE) *see* Leflunomide 1174
Arax (TW) *see* HydrOXYzine 1024
Arbeela Breezhaler (AU) *see* Indacaterol 1063
Arbistin (MX) *see* Carbocisteine [INT] 357
ARB (KR) *see* Losartan 1248
Arb-S (KR) *see* Olmesartan 1496
Arbutol (ID) *see* Ethambutol 798
Arcadipin (AT) *see* Nilvadipine [INT] 1456
Arcalyst (SE) *see* Rilonacept 1810
Arcanafenac (ZA) *see* Diclofenac (Systemic) 617
Arcavit-B!1 (AT) *see* Thiamine 2028
Arcavit-B!2 (AT) *see* Riboflavin 1803
Arcdone (TW) *see* Donepezil 668
Archhifen eye (TH) *see* Chloramphenicol 421
Archifar (HR, SG) *see* Meropenem 1299
Arcolane (CO) *see* Ketoconazole (Topical) 1145
Arcored (ID) *see* Cyanocobalamin 515
Arcosal (DK) *see* TOLBUTamide 2062
Arcoxia (AE, AR, AT, AU, BE, BG, BH, BR, CH, CL, CN, CO, CY, CZ, DE, DK, EC, EE, FI, FR, GB, GR, HK, HN, HR, ID, IE, IL, IS, IT, KW, LB, LT, MY, NL, NO, NZ, PE, PH, PT, QA, RO, RU, SA, SE, SG, SI, SK, TH, TR, TW, UY, VE, VN, ZA) *see* Etoricoxib [INT] 821
Arcoxib (PH) *see* Etoricoxib [INT] 821
Ardeanutrisol SO (CZ) *see* Sorbitol 1927
Ardeaosmosol MA (CZ) *see* Mannitol 1269
Ardin (SG) *see* Loratadine 1241
Arechin (PL) *see* Chloroquine 424
Aredia (AE, AT, AU, BB, BE, BF, BG, BH, BJ, BM, BS, BZ, CH, CI, CL, CN, CO, CY, CZ, DE, DK, EE, EG, ET, FI, FR, GB, GH, GM, GN, GR, GY, HK, HN, HR, HU, ID, IE, IL, IN, IQ, IR, IT, JM, JO, JP, KE, KW, LB, LR, LU, LY, MA, ML, MR, MT, MU, MW, NE, NG, NL, NO, OM, PE, PH, PK, PL, PT, QA, RO, RU, SA, SC, SD, SE, SG, SI, SK, SL, SN, SR, SY, TH, TN, TR, TT, TW, TZ, UG, VN, YE, ZA, ZM, ZW) *see* Pamidronate 1563
Aremed 1 (SG) *see* Anastrozole 148
Aremed (TH, TW) *see* Anastrozole 148
Aremis (ES) *see* Sertraline 1878
Arem (ZA) *see* Nitrazepam [CAN/INT] 1461
Arendal (PE) *see* Alendronate 79
Ares (HR) *see* RABEprazole 1762
Arespin (ID) *see* Norepinephrine 1472
Arestal (KR) *see* Loperamide 1236
Arestin (IL) *see* Minocycline 1371
Areta (BG) *see* Lercanidipine [INT] 1181
Arfen (BF, BJ, CI, ET, GH, GM, GN, KE, LR, MA, ML, MR, MU, MW, MY, NE, NG, SC, SD, SL, SN, TN, TZ, UG, ZM, ZW) *see* Acetaminophen 32
Arfen (ID) *see* Ibuprofen 1032
Arficin (HR) *see* Rifampin 1804
Arflex Retard (BR) *see* Nimesulide [INT] 1456
Arflur (IN) *see* Flurbiprofen (Systemic) 906
Argamate (KR) *see* Calcium Polystyrene Sulfonate [CAN/INT] 333
Arganova (NL) *see* Argatroban 168
Argata (AT) *see* Argatroban 168
Argatra (DE) *see* Argatroban 168
Argentafil (CR, NI, PA, SV) *see* Silver Sulfadiazine 1887
Argentamicina (PE) *see* Silver Sulfadiazine 1887
Argenzil (UY) *see* Silver Sulfadiazine 1887
Argilex (AR) *see* Indomethacin 1067
Arginina (PL) *see* Arginine 171
Argocytromag (PL) *see* Magnesium Citrate 1262
Arheuma (TW) *see* Leflunomide 1174
Ariane (PH) *see* Cyproterone and Ethinyl Estradiol [CAN/INT] 532
Arianna (AU) *see* Anastrozole 148
Aricept D (JP) *see* Donepezil 668
Aricept-D (NZ) *see* Donepezil 668
Aricept (AE, AT, AU, BD, BE, BF, BG, BH, BJ, CH, CI, CN, CY, CZ, DE, DK, EE, EG, ES, ET, FI, FR, GB, GH, GM, GN, GR, HK, HN, HR, HU, ID, IE, IL, IQ, IR, IS, IT, JO, JP, KE, KR, KW, LB, LR, LY, MA, ML, MR, MU, MW, MY, NE, NG, NO, NZ, OM, PH, PK, PL, PT, QA, RO, RU, SA, SC, SD, SE, SG, SI, SK, SL, SN, SY, TN, TR, TW, TZ, UG, VN, YE, ZA, ZM, ZW) *see* Donepezil 668
Aricept Evess (HK, ID, MY, PH, SG, TH, VN) *see* Donepezil 668
Aricept Evis (KR) *see* Donepezil 668
Ariclaim (AT, BE, BG, CH, CZ, DE, DK, EE, ES, FI, FR, GB, GR, HN, IE, IT, MT, NL, NO, PL, PT, RO, RU, SE, SK, TR) *see* DULoxetine 698
Aridol (AU, CH, FI, FR, GR, NO, PT, SE, SG) *see* Mannitol 1269
Ariel TDDS (HK) *see* Scopolamine (Systemic) 1870
Arifenicol (BR) *see* Chloramphenicol 421
Arika (TW) *see* ARIPiprazole 171
Arilex (CL) *see* ARIPiprazole 171
Arilin (DE) *see* MetroNIDAZOLE (Systemic) 1353
Arilvax (NL, ZA) *see* Yellow Fever Vaccine 2192
Arimidex (AE, AR, AT, AU, BB, BD, BE, BF, BG, BH, BJ, BM, BO, BR, BS, BZ, CH, CI, CL, CN, CO, CR, CY, CZ, DE, DK, DO, EC, EE, ES, ET, FI, FR, GB, GH, GM, GN, GR, GT, GY, HK, HN, HR, HU, ID, IE, IL, IS, IT, JM, JO, JP, KE, KR, LB, LR, LT, LU, MA, ML, MR, MU, MW, MX, MY, NE, NG, NI, NL, NO, NZ, PA, PE, PH, PK, PL, PR, PT, QA, RO, RU, SA, SC, SD, SE, SG, SI, SL, SN, SR, SV, TH, TN, TR, TT, TW, TZ, UG, UY, VE, VN, ZA, ZM, ZW) *see* Anastrozole 148

Arinac (IN) *see* Pseudoephedrine and Ibuprofen 1743
Aripax (GR) *see* LORazepam 1243
Aripe (KR) *see* Donepezil 668
Ariple (TW) *see* ARIPiprazole 171
Ariprazol (GT, PA) *see* ARIPiprazole 171
Ariski (ID) *see* ARIPiprazole 171
Aristab (BR) *see* ARIPiprazole 171
Aristen (HK) *see* Clotrimazole (Topical) 488
Aristocor (AT) *see* Flecainide 882
Aristocort A (MY, TH) *see* Triamcinolone (Systemic) 2099
Aristocort A (MY, TH) *see* Triamcinolone (Topical) 2100
Aristophen (HK) *see* Chloramphenicol 421
Ariva (HR) *see* Amorolfine [INT] 128
Arive (IN) *see* ARIPiprazole 171
Arixind (AR) *see* ARIPiprazole 171
Arixtra (AE, AR, AT, AU, BB, BE, BG, BH, BM, BR, BS, BZ, CH, CL, CN, CO, CR, CY, CZ, DE, DK, DO, EC, EE, FI, FR, GB, GR, GT, GY, HN, HR, HU, ID, IE, IL, IN, IS, IT, JM, JP, KR, KW, LB, LT, MT, MX, MY, NI, NL, NO, PA, PE, PH, PL, PR, PT, QA, RO, RU, SA, SE, SG, SI, SK, SR, SV, TH, TR, TT, TW, UY, VN) *see* Fondaparinux 924
Arizil (PH) *see* Donepezil 668
Arizole (TW) *see* ARIPiprazole 171
Arizol (UY) *see* ARIPiprazole 171
Arkamin (IN) *see* CloNIDine 480
Arket (CN) *see* Ketoprofen 1145
Arketis (RO) *see* PARoxetine 1579
Arkine (ID) *see* Trihexyphenidyl 2103
Arlemide (AR) *see* ARIPiprazole 171
Arlette (CL, CO, PE, PY, VE) *see* Desogestrel [INT] 597
Arluy (MX) *see* Mebeverine [INT] 1275
Armisetin (TR) *see* Chloramphenicol 421
Armocur (IL) *see* Cyproterone [CAN/INT] 530
Armod (IN) *see* Armodafinil 175
Armol (DO, GT, HN, NI, PA, SV) *see* Alendronate 79
Arnetin (MY) *see* Ranitidine 1777
Arodoc C (JP) *see* ChlorproPAMIDE 429
Aroflo-50 (PH) *see* Fluticasone and Salmeterol 912
Aroflo-125 (PH) *see* Fluticasone and Salmeterol 912
Aroflo-250 (PH) *see* Fluticasone and Salmeterol 912
Aroglycem (JP) *see* Diazoxide 616
Aromacin (JO) *see* Exemestane 828
Aromasil (ES) *see* Exemestane 828
Aromasin (AE, AR, AT, AU, BE, BG, BH, BR, CH, CL, CN, CO, CR, CY, CZ, DE, DK, DO, EC, EE, EG, FI, GB, GR, GT, HK, HN, HR, ID, IE, IL, IQ, IR, IS, IT, KR, KW, LB, LT, LY, MY, NI, NL, NO, NZ, OM, PA, PE, PH, PL, PT, QA, RO, RU, SA, SE, SG, SI, SK, SV, SY, TH, TR, TW, UY, VE, VN, YE, ZA) *see* Exemestane 828
Aromasine (FR) *see* Exemestane 828
Aropax 20 (AR, AU, BE, BR, NZ, PY, UY, ZA) *see* PARoxetine 1579
Aropax (LU, MX) *see* PARoxetine 1579
Arovit (AE, BE, BH, BR, CO, CY, EC, EG, IL, IQ, IR, IT, JO, KW, LB, LY, OM, PE, QA, SA, SE, SY, YE) *see* Vitamin A 2173
Aroxat (CL) *see* PARoxetine 1579
Aroxin (SG) *see* Amoxicillin 130
Arpimune (PH) *see* CycloSPORINE (Systemic) 522
Arpolax (HK) *see* Citalopram 451
Arranon G (JP) *see* Nelarabine 1435
Arrest (JP) *see* Clemastine 459
Arring (TW) *see* Triazolam 2101
Arrop (MX) *see* Naltrexone 1422
Arrox (HK, MY) *see* Meloxicam 1283
Arslide (PK) *see* Nimesulide [INT] 1456
Artagen (IN) *see* Naproxen 1427
Artal (FI) *see* Pentoxifylline 1618
Artamin (AE, AT, CY, JO, KR, MY, PL, QA, SA) *see* PenicillAMINE 1608
Artamine (EG) *see* PenicillAMINE 1608
Artane (AE, AR, AT, AU, BE, BH, BR, CH, CL, CY, DE, EG, ES, FI, FR, GR, HR, IE, IL, IQ, IR, IT, JO, KW, LB, LU, LY, NL, OM, PE, PT, QA, SA, SI, SY, YE, ZA) *see* Trihexyphenidyl 2103
Artan (VN) *see* Trihexyphenidyl 2103
Artate (JP) *see* Cinnarizine [INT] 440
Artazide (PH) *see* Losartan and Hydrochlorothiazide 1250
Artedil (ES) *see* Manidipine [INT] 1269
Artelife (MX) *see* Pentoxifylline 1618
Artemether-Plus (VN) *see* Artemether and Lumefantrine 177
Artepid (ID) *see* Clopidogrel 484
Arterenol (DE) *see* Norepinephrine 1472
Artesol (CL) *see* Cilostazol 437
Art (FR, IL) *see* Diacerein [INT] 613
Artheogrel (PH) *see* Clopidogrel 484
Arthirinal (CY) *see* Tenoxicam [INT] 2001
Arthrexin (AU, ZA) *see* Indomethacin 1067
Arthrifen (PH) *see* Diclofenac (Systemic) 617
Arthrocine (FR) *see* Sulindac 1953
Arthrofar (GR) *see* Diacerein [INT] 613
Arthrofluor (HU) *see* Fluoride 895
Arthrotec 50 (AU) *see* Diclofenac and Misoprostol 621
Arthrotec (AE, BF, BG, BH, BJ, CI, CN, CY, CZ, DK, EE, EG, ET, FI, GB, GH, GM, GN, GR, HK, HN, IE, IL, IQ, IR, IS, JO, KE, KW, LB, LR, LY, MA, ML, MR, MU, MW, NE, NG, NL, NO, OM, QA, RO, SA, SC, SD, SE, SL, SN, SY, TN, TZ, UG, VE, YE, ZA, ZM, ZW) *see* Diclofenac and Misoprostol 621
ArthrotecForte (SK) *see* Diclofenac and Misoprostol 621
Articel (HR) *see* Perindopril 1623
Articlox (GR) *see* Hydroxocobalamin 1020
Artifar (GR) *see* Carisoprodol 363
Artiflam (BE, LU) *see* Tiaprofenic Acid [CAN/INT] 2034
Artilog (ES) *see* Celecoxib 402
Artison (AE, BH, CY, EG, IQ, IR, JO, KW, LB, LY, OM, QA, SA, SY, YE) *see* TOLBUTamide 2062
Artizona (CL) *see* Diacerein [INT] 613
Artlex (KR) *see* AtoMOXetine 191
Artocoron (DE) *see* Naftidrofuryl [INT] 1416
Artoflam (ID) *see* Diacerein [INT] 613
Artok (AT) *see* Lornoxicam [INT] 1248
Artonil (SE) *see* Ranitidine 1777
Artose (VN) *see* Celecoxib 402
Artosin (DE, JP, MX, NL) *see* TOLBUTamide 2062
Artotec (FR, RU) *see* Diclofenac and Misoprostol 621
Artrait (AR, PE) *see* Methotrexate 1322
Artrichine (EC) *see* Colchicine 500
Artriclox (CO) *see* Meloxicam 1283
Artrilab (CL) *see* Leflunomide 1174
Artrilona S (UY) *see* Indomethacin 1067
Artrinovo (ES) *see* Indomethacin 1067
Artrites (CO) *see* Diclofenac (Systemic) 617
Artriunic (ES) *see* Tenoxicam [INT] 2001
Artrizan (ES) *see* Diacerein [INT] 613
Artrocam (CZ, HR) *see* Tenoxicam [INT] 2001
Artrocaptin (ES) *see* Tolmetin 2062
Artroda (KR) *see* Diacerein [INT] 613
Artrodar (AR, BR, CN, CO, CZ, HK, ID, IN, MY, SK, TH, VN) *see* Diacerein [INT] 613
Artroglobina (PE, UY) *see* Diacerein [INT] 613
Artrogota (ES) *see* Diethylamine Salicylate [INT] 624
Artrolyt (AT, PT) *see* Diacerein [INT] 613
Artrotec (ES, IT, MX, PE) *see* Diclofenac and Misoprostol 621
Artroxen (IT) *see* Naproxen 1427
Artz (CN) *see* Hyaluronate and Derivatives 1006
Aruclonin (HU) *see* CloNIDine 480
Arvekap (GR) *see* Triptorelin 2107
Arvind (HR) *see* LamoTRIgine 1160
Arvolac (PH) *see* Ketorolac (Systemic) 1146
Arxeda (RO) *see* Capecitabine 339

Arya (PH) *see* Glimepiride 966
Arythmol (GB, IE) *see* Propafenone 1725
Arzerra (AT, AU, CH, CZ, DE, DK, EE, FR, GB, HR, IE, IS, JP, LT, NL, NO, PL, PT, RO, SE, SI) *see* Ofatumumab 1488
Arzimol (ES) *see* Cefprozil 389
Arzobema (MX) *see* Imipenem and Cilastatin 1051
5-ASA 400 (AR, PY) *see* Mesalamine 1301
Asacol (AE, BE, BH, CH, CY, DK, EG, FI, GB, GR, HR, IL, IT, JO, JP, KW, LB, LU, MX, NL, NO, NZ, PK, PT, QA, SA, SE, SG, TW) *see* Mesalamine 1301
Asacolon (CO, IE) *see* Mesalamine 1301
Asacor (TW) *see* Lovastatin 1252
Asadin (MY, TW) *see* Arsenic Trioxide 177
Asalit (BR) *see* Mesalamine 1301
Asamid (HR) *see* Ethosuximide 813
Asapor (FI) *see* Aspirin 180
Asasantine LP (FR) *see* Aspirin and Dipyridamole 185
Asasantin (HN, NL) *see* Aspirin and Dipyridamole 185
Asasantin Retard (CH, DK, FI, GB, IE, NO, NZ, SE) *see* Aspirin and Dipyridamole 185
Asasantin SR (AU) *see* Aspirin and Dipyridamole 185
Asawin (CO) *see* Aspirin 180
A-Scabs (HK, MY, VN) *see* Permethrin 1627
A Scabs (ID) *see* Permethrin 1627
Ascapil (IN) *see* Ivermectin (Systemic) 1136
Ascardia (ID) *see* Aspirin 180
Ascarol (EC) *see* Albendazole 65
Ascochrom (GR) *see* Halcinonide 992
Ascofer (LU) *see* Ascorbic Acid 178
Ascofer (PL) *see* Ferrous Gluconate 870
Asconvita (PH) *see* Ascorbic Acid 178
Ascorbin (PH) *see* Ascorbic Acid 178
Ascorbovit (QA) *see* Ascorbic Acid 178
Ascormin (TW) *see* Ascorbic Acid 178
Ascorvit (DE) *see* Ascorbic Acid 178
Ascotop (DE) *see* ZOLMitriptan 2210
Asec (KR) *see* Aceclofenac [INT] 30
Asenapt (IN) *see* Asenapine 179
Asendin (ID) *see* Amoxapine 128
Asenta (IL) *see* Donepezil 668
Asenza Plus (PH) *see* Pioglitazone and Glimepiride 1654
Aseptone (MY) *see* Methadone 1311
Aseranox (GR) *see* Ketanserin [INT] 1144
Asiadexa (VN) *see* Dexamethasone (Systemic) 599
Asiazole (TH) *see* MetroNIDAZOLE (Systemic) 1353
A Si Ke Ding (CN) *see* DOPamine 669
Asima (KR) *see* Doxofylline [INT] 679
Asisten (UY) *see* Captopril 342
Asklerol (IN) *see* Polidocanol 1672
Askorbin (ID) *see* Ascorbic Acid 178
Askorbinsyre "Dak" (DK) *see* Ascorbic Acid 178
Aslene (MY) *see* Orlistat 1520
Asmaact (HK) *see* Montelukast 1392
Asmabec Clickhaler (FR, IE) *see* Beclomethasone (Systemic) 230
Asmabec (IE) *see* Beclomethasone (Nasal) 232
Asmacaire (PH) *see* Albuterol 69
Asmadex (ID) *see* Ephedrine and Theophylline [INT] 734
Asmadil (BF, BJ, CI, ET, GH, GM, GN, JO, KE, LR, MA, ML, MR, MU, MW, NE, NG, SA, SC, SD, SL, SN, TN, TZ, UG, ZM, ZW) *see* Albuterol 69
Asmadren (NO) *see* Isoproterenol 1124
Asmalat (LB) *see* Albuterol 69
Asmalin Pulmoneb (PH) *see* Albuterol 69
Asmalin (SG) *see* Terbutaline 2004
Asmanex (JP, RO) *see* Mometasone (Oral Inhalation) 1389
Asmanex Twisthaler (AE, BH, KW, VN) *see* Mometasone (Oral Inhalation) 1389
Asmano (ID) *see* Ephedrine and Theophylline [INT] 734
Asmasolon (ID) *see* Ephedrine and Theophylline [INT] 734
Asmaten (MY) *see* Ketotifen (Systemic) [CAN/INT] 1149
Asmatol (AR) *see* Albuterol 69
Asmelor Novolizer (FR) *see* Formoterol 926
Asmidon (JP) *see* Albuterol 69
Asmol CFC-Free (AU) *see* Albuterol 69
Asmol (SG) *see* Albuterol 69
Asodoc (MX) *see* DOCEtaxel 656
Asolan (MY) *see* ALPRAZolam 94
Asolfena (BG) *see* Solifenacin 1917
Asotax (AR, MX) *see* PACLitaxel (Conventional) 1550
Asovorin (AR) *see* Leucovorin Calcium 1183
Asparaginase medac (PL) *see* Asparaginase (E. coli) 179
Aspa (TW) *see* Aspirin 180
Aspax (VN) *see* Sparfloxacin [INT] 1930
Aspec (NZ) *see* Aspirin 180
Aspen Bromocriptine (ZA) *see* Bromocriptine 291
Aspendos (RO) *see* Modafinil 1386
Aspen (PH) *see* Aspirin 180
Aspent (TH) *see* Aspirin 180
Aspersinal (AR) *see* ChlorproMAZINE 429
Aspex (IL) *see* Aspirin 180
ASP (HK) *see* Aspirin 180
Aspicard (SA) *see* Aspirin 180
Aspicot (LB) *see* Aspirin 180
Aspidon (PH) *see* RisperiDONE 1818
Aspilets EC (PH) *see* Aspirin 180
Aspilets (ID, PH, VN) *see* Aspirin 180
Aspimed (AE) *see* Aspirin 180
Aspinal (EG, QA) *see* Aspirin 180
Aspirax (RO) *see* Aspirin 180
Aspirem (BB, BM, BS, BZ, CY, GY, JM, PR, SR, TT) *see* Aspirin 180
Aspire (TW) *see* Aspirin 180
Aspirina (CL, CO, EC) *see* Aspirin 180
Aspirin (AE, BF, BH, BJ, CI, CY, EG, ET, GH, GM, GN, HK, IL, IQ, IR, JO, KE, KW, LB, LR, LY, MA, ML, MR, MU, MW, NE, NG, OM, QA, SA, SC, SD, SL, SN, SY, TN, TZ, UG, YE, ZM, ZW) *see* Aspirin 180
Aspirina efervescente (MX) *see* Aspirin 180
Aspirina Junior (MX) *see* Aspirin 180
Aspirin Bayer (HK) *see* Aspirin 180
Aspirin Cardio (IL, SG) *see* Aspirin 180
Aspitor (PH) *see* Aspirin 180
Aspro (AT, CH, CZ, FR, GB, IT, NL, NZ, SA) *see* Aspirin 180
Aspro Junior (QA) *see* Aspirin 180
Asprovit (EE) *see* Aspirin 180
Asrina (TH) *see* Aspirin 180
Assal (MX) *see* Albuterol 69
ASS (DE) *see* Aspirin 180
Assival (IL) *see* Diazepam 613
Assoral (IT) *see* Roxithromycin [INT] 1853
Assure (TW) *see* Bismuth 265
Assy (AR) *see* Permethrin 1627
Astair (TH) *see* Montelukast 1392
Astator (SI) *see* AtorvaSTATin 194
Astaz-P (TH) *see* Piperacillin and Tazobactam 1657
Astelin (PK) *see* Azelastine (Nasal) 213
Asthafen (IN) *see* Ketotifen (Systemic) [CAN/INT] 1149
Asthalin HFA (HK) *see* Albuterol 69
Asthalin (IN, LB) *see* Albuterol 69
Asthamxine (SG) *see* Bromhexine [INT] 291
Asthan (TW) *see* Ketotifen (Systemic) [CAN/INT] 1149
Asthator (RO) *see* Montelukast 1392
Asthavent (AE, ZA) *see* Albuterol 69
Asthenopin (PH) *see* Pilocarpine (Ophthalmic) 1649
Asthma (MY) *see* Ephedrine and Theophylline [INT] 734
Asthmasian (TH) *see* Terbutaline 2004

Asthma Soho (ID) *see* Ephedrine and Theophylline [INT] ... 734
Asthmatin (HK) *see* Montelukast ... 1392
Asthromed (PH) *see* Aspirin ... 180
Asthterol (KR) *see* Bambuterol [INT] ... 227
Astin (MX) *see* Pravastatin ... 1700
Astinon (PH) *see* Pyridostigmine ... 1746
Astmopent (PL) *see* Metaproterenol ... 1307
Asto (JP) *see* TOLBUTamide ... 2062
Astomin (JP) *see* Dimemorfan [INT] ... 637
Astonin (ES) *see* Fludrocortisone ... 891
Astonin H (AT, CO, CZ, DE, HN, RO) *see* Fludrocortisone ... 891
Astonin-H (HR, HU, LU) *see* Fludrocortisone ... 891
Astrix (PH) *see* Aspirin ... 180
Astromide (AU, NZ) *see* Temozolomide ... 1991
Astrozol (PH) *see* Anastrozole ... 148
Astudal (ES) *see* AmLODIPine ... 123
Asumalife (MY, SG, VN) *see* Ketotifen (Systemic) [CAN/INT] ... 1149
Asvimol (PH) *see* Albuterol ... 69
Atacand D (AR) *see* Candesartan and Hydrochlorothiazide ... 338
Atacand (AE, AR, AT, AU, BB, BE, BF, BG, BH, BJ, BM, BR, BS, BZ, CH, CI, CL, CO, CR, CY, CZ, DE, DK, DO, EE, EG, ES, ET, FI, FR, GH, GM, GN, GR, GT, HN, HR, HU, IE, IL, IS, JM, JO, KE, KR, KW, LB, LR, LT, MA, ML, MR, MU, MW, MX, MY, NE, NG, NI, NL, NO, NZ, PA, PE, PL, PR, PT, QA, RO, RU, SA, SC, SD, SE, SG, SI, SK, SL, SN, SV, TN, TR, TT, TZ, UG, UY, ZA, ZM, ZW) *see* Candesartan ... 335
Atacand HCT (BR) *see* Candesartan and Hydrochlorothiazide ... 338
Atacand Plus (AE, AU, BB, BE, BF, BJ, BM, BS, BZ, CH, CI, CO, CR, CY, CZ, DK, DO, EE, ES, ET, FI, GH, GM, GN, GR, GT, GY, HN, HR, HU, IE, IL, IS, JM, JO, KE, KR, KW, LB, LR, MA, ML, MR, MU, MW, MX, MY, NE, NG, NI, NL, NO, PA, PE, PR, QA, RO, SA, SC, SD, SE, SG, SI, SK, SL, SN, SR, SV, TN, TR, TT, TZ, UG, VE, ZA, ZM, ZW) *see* Candesartan and Hydrochlorothiazide ... 338
Atacor (HK) *see* AtorvaSTATin ... 194
Atacure (JO, LB) *see* Atracurium ... 198
Atadin (TW) *see* Amantadine ... 105
Ataline (MY) *see* Terbutaline ... 2004
Atamel (PE) *see* Acetaminophen ... 32
Atamir (DK) *see* PenicillAMINE ... 1608
Atanaal Softcap (TW) *see* NIFEdipine ... 1451
Atarax (AE, AT, AU, BB, BE, BG, BH, BM, BS, BZ, CH, CY, CZ, DE, DK, DO, EC, EE, EG, ES, FI, FR, GB, GR, GT, GY, HK, HN, HU, IN, IS, IT, JM, JO, KW, LB, LU, MT, MX, MY, NI, NL, NO, PE, PL, PT, QA, RU, SA, SE, SI, SK, SR, SV, TH, TR, TT, TW, VN) *see* HydrOXYzine ... 1024
Ataraxone (AR, UY) *see* HydrOXYzine ... 1024
Atarax Uce (PK) *see* HydrOXYzine ... 1024
Atarin (CL, FI) *see* Amantadine ... 105
Atarox (PY) *see* Atenolol ... 189
Atarva (AR) *see* AtorvaSTATin ... 194
Atasart-H (VN) *see* Candesartan and Hydrochlorothiazide ... 338
Atasart (PH, VN) *see* Candesartan ... 335
Atazor (IN) *see* Atazanavir ... 185
Atcord (MX) *see* Atenolol ... 189
Ateben (AR) *see* Nortriptyline ... 1476
Atecard (IN) *see* Atenolol ... 189
AteHexal (DE, NZ) *see* Atenolol ... 189
Atehexal (LU) *see* Atenolol ... 189
Atelol (BF, BJ, CI, ET, GH, GM, GN, JO, KE, LR, MA, ML, MR, MU, MW, NE, NG, SC, SD, SL, SN, TN, TZ, UG, ZM, ZW) *see* Atenolol ... 189
Atem (AE, BH, CY, EG, IQ, IR, IT, JO, KW, LB, LY, OM, PK, QA, SA, SY, YE) *see* Ipratropium (Systemic) ... 1108
Atemur Mite (DE) *see* Fluticasone (Oral Inhalation) ... 907
Atenal (KR) *see* Atenolol ... 189
Atenativ 500 (AT, CH, HN) *see* Antithrombin ... 156
Atenativ (CZ, DE, DK, ES, FI, GR, HR, HU, IT, NL, NO, SE, SK) *see* Antithrombin ... 156
Atend (MX) *see* Antithrombin ... 156
Atendol (DE) *see* Atenolol ... 189
Atenet (DK) *see* Atenolol ... 189
Ateni (IL) *see* Atenolol ... 189
Atenil (CH) *see* Atenolol ... 189
Ateno (AE, BH, CY, EG, IQ, IR, JO, KW, LB, LY, OM, QA, SA, SY, YE) *see* Atenolol ... 189
Atenobene (HU) *see* Atenolol ... 189
Atenocor (RO) *see* Atenolol ... 189
Atenogamma (DE) *see* Atenolol ... 189
Atenolin (KR) *see* Atenolol ... 189
Atenol (IT) *see* Atenolol ... 189
Atenolol-B (HU) *see* Atenolol ... 189
Atenolol Pharmavit (HU) *see* Atenolol ... 189
Atenolol von ct (LU) *see* Atenolol ... 189
Atensina (BR) *see* CloNIDine ... 480
Atensin (BF, BJ, CI, ET, GH, GM, GN, JO, KE, LR, MA, ML, MR, MU, MW, NE, NG, SC, SD, SL, SN, TN, TZ, UG, ZM, ZW) *see* Propranolol ... 1731
Atenual (PE) *see* Ketazolam [INT] ... 1144
Atenurix (PH) *see* Febuxostat ... 848
Ateplax (EC, PE) *see* Clopidogrel ... 484
Atepros (PH) *see* Finasteride ... 878
Aterax (ZA) *see* HydrOXYzine ... 1024
Aterkey (LB) *see* Lovastatin ... 1252
Ateroclar Duo (AR) *see* Ezetimibe and Atorvastatin ... 833
A-Terol (KR) *see* Bambuterol [INT] ... 227
Atestad (PH) *see* Atenolol ... 189
Atgam (AU, BG, IN, KR, MX, MY, NZ, SG, SI) *see* Antithymocyte Globulin (Equine) ... 157
ATG-Fresenius (CY) *see* Antithymocyte Globulin (Rabbit) ... 158
ATG-Fresinius (EE, SE) *see* Antithymocyte Globulin (Rabbit) ... 158
Athlete's Foot (AR, HU) *see* Tolnaftate ... 2063
Athletes Foot Powder (IL) *see* Tolnaftate ... 2063
Athyrazol (HR) *see* Methimazole ... 1319
Atidem (PE) *see* Piroxicam ... 1662
Atifan (CZ, EE) *see* Terbinafine (Systemic) ... 2002
Atimos (BG, RO) *see* Formoterol ... 926
Atimos Modulite (GB) *see* Formoterol ... 926
Atinol (TW) *see* Atenolol ... 189
Atisenap (AR) *see* Asenapine ... 179
Atisuril (MX) *see* Allopurinol ... 90
Ativan (AE, AU, BF, BH, BJ, CI, CO, CR, DO, EC, EG, ET, GB, GH, GM, GN, GT, HN, IE, IN, JO, KE, KR, KW, LR, MA, ML, MR, MU, MW, MX, NE, NG, NI, NZ, PA, PE, PH, PK, QA, SA, SC, SD, SG, SL, SN, SV, TN, TW, TZ, UG, UY, VE, VN, ZA, ZM, ZW) *see* LORazepam ... 1243
Atizor (CL) *see* Azithromycin (Systemic) ... 216
Atlacne (AR) *see* ISOtretinoin ... 1127
Atlansil (AR, BR, CL, PE, UY) *see* Amiodarone ... 114
Atmose (PH) *see* Mefenamic Acid ... 1280
Atock (JP, KR, TW) *see* Formoterol ... 926
Atodel (MY, PH, TR) *see* Prazosin ... 1703
Atofar (ID) *see* AtorvaSTATin ... 194
Atoken (MX) *see* Atenolol ... 189
Atokken (RO) *see* Irbesartan ... 1110
Atolow (KR) *see* AtorvaSTATin ... 194
Atomase (NZ) *see* Beclomethasone (Nasal) ... 232
Atonium (LB) *see* Atenolol ... 189
Atopitar (PH) *see* AtorvaSTATin ... 194
Ator (AE, BH, CY, EG, IQ, IR, JO, KW, LB, LY, OM, PH, QA, SA, SY, YE) *see* AtorvaSTATin ... 194

Atorcal (TW) *see* AtorvaSTATin 194
Atorin (TW) *see* AtorvaSTATin 194
Atoris (BE, HU, LT, RU, SG) *see* AtorvaSTATin 194
Atorlip (CO, HK, LB, PE) *see* AtorvaSTATin 194
Atormin (AE, BH, KW, QA, SA) *see* Atenolol 189
Atorphil (PH) *see* AtorvaSTATin 194
Atorsan (ID, TH) *see* AtorvaSTATin 194
Atorvachol (AU) *see* AtorvaSTATin 194
Atorva (KR, SA) *see* AtorvaSTATin 194
Atorvaright (HK) *see* AtorvaSTATin 194
Atorwin (ID, PH) *see* AtorvaSTATin 194
Atosil (DE) *see* Promethazine 1723
Atossisclerol (IT) *see* Polidocanol 1672
Atoty (TW) *see* AtorvaSTATin 194
Atoxan (PK) *see* Oxatomide [INT] 1532
Atozet (AU, HR) *see* Ezetimibe and Atorvastatin 833
Atracor (PH) *see* Atracurium 198
Atractil (LU) *see* Diethylpropion 624
Atra (KR, TH) *see* Atracurium 198
Atralex (MY) *see* Atracurium 198
Atravell (PH) *see* Atracurium 198
Atrexel (MX) *see* Methotrexate 1322
Atriance (AT, BE, CH, CZ, DE, DK, EE, FR, GB, GR, HR, IE, IL, IT, LT, NL, NO, PL, PT, RO, RU, SE, SI, SK) *see* Nelarabine 1435
Atri (KR) *see* Hyaluronate and Derivatives 1006
Atripla (AR, AT, AU, BE, CH, CL, CY, CZ, DE, DK, EE, FR, GB, GR, HK, HR, IE, IL, IS, IT, LT, MX, NL, NO, NZ, PL, PT, RO, SE, SI, SK, TH, TR) *see* Efavirenz, Emtricitabine, and Tenofovir 709
Atroact-10 (PH) *see* AtorvaSTATin 194
Atrocox (ID) *see* Meloxicam 1283
Atrodar (TR, VE) *see* Diacerein [INT] 613
Atrodual (FI) *see* Ipratropium and Albuterol 1109
Atrofen (DO) *see* PHENobarbital 1632
Atrolin (TW) *see* Ipratropium and Albuterol 1109
Atrombin (FI) *see* Dipyridamole 652
Atronase (DK) *see* Ipratropium (Nasal) 1109
Atropan (PH) *see* Atropine 200
Atropina Braun (ES) *see* Atropine 200
Atropina (IT) *see* Atropine 200
Atropina Llorens (ES) *see* Atropine 200
Atropina Sulfato Serra (ES) *see* Atropine 200
Atropin "Dak" (DK) *see* Atropine 200
Atropin (DE, FI, HR) *see* Atropine 200
Atropin Dispersa (LU) *see* Atropine 200
Atropine (GR) *see* Atropine 200
Atropine Martinet (FR) *see* Atropine 200
Atropine Sulfate (IL) *see* Atropine 200
Atropine Sulfate Tablets (GB) *see* Atropine 200
Atropini sulfas (HR) *see* Atropine 200
Atropin Minims (NO) *see* Atropine 200
Atropinsulfat Braun (LU) *see* Atropine 200
Atropinsulfat Lannacher (AT) *see* Atropine 200
Atropinsulfatloesung Fresenius (LU) *see* Atropine 200
Atropinum Sulfuricum (HU, PL) *see* Atropine 200
Atropinum Sulfuricum Nycomed (AT) *see* Atropine 200
Atropocil (PT) *see* Atropine 200
Atrop (SG) *see* Atropine 200
Atroptal (PH) *see* Atropine 200
Atropt (AU, NZ) *see* Atropine 200
Atrosol (TR) *see* Atropine 200
Atrovent (AE, AR, AT, AU, BD, BE, BG, BH, BR, CH, CL, CN, CO, CR, CY, CZ, DK, DO, EC, EE, EG, FI, FR, GB, GR, GT, HK, HN, HR, ID, IE, IS, JO, JP, KW, LB, MT, MY, NI, NL, NO, NZ, PA, PE, PH, PK, PL, PT, PY, QA, RU, SA, SE, SG, SK, SV, SY, TR, TW, UY) *see* Ipratropium (Systemic) 1108
Atrovent (AE, AU, CL, CR, CZ, DK, DO, EE, FI, FR, GT, HN, IS, LT, NI, PA, SE, SI, SK, SV, VN) *see* Ipratropium (Nasal) 1109
Atrovent Aerosol (NZ) *see* Ipratropium (Systemic) 1108
Atrovent Comp (FI) *see* Ipratropium and Fenoterol [CAN/INT] 1109
Atrovent Nasal (NZ) *see* Ipratropium (Systemic) 1108
Atrovent N (SG) *see* Ipratropium (Systemic) 1108
Atrovent UDV (KR) *see* Ipratropium (Systemic) 1108
Atryn (CZ, GR, HR, LT, NL, RO, SK) *see* Antithrombin 156
ATryn (GB, PL, PT) *see* Antithrombin 156
Atswift (SG) *see* AtorvaSTATin 194
Attenta (AU) *see* Methylphenidate 1336
Attentho (CO) *see* AtoMOXetine 191
Attentrol (IN) *see* AtoMOXetine 191
Atural (PE) *see* Ranitidine 1777
Atus (IT) *see* Ambroxol [INT] 109
Atzirut X (IL) *see* Bisacodyl 265
Aubagio (AU, CH, CZ, DE, DK, EE, GB, HR, IL, IS, KR, LT, NL, NO, NZ, RO, SE, SI, SK) *see* Teriflunomide 2006
Aubrex (PH) *see* Celecoxib 402
Audiwax (PH) *see* Docusate 661
Audmonal Forte (GB) *see* Alverine [INT] 104
Audmonal (GB) *see* Alverine [INT] 104
Augamox (AE, BH, CY, EG, IQ, IR, JO, KW, LB, LY, OM, QA, SA, SY, YE) *see* Amoxicillin and Clavulanate 133
AugMaxcil (ZA) *see* Amoxicillin and Clavulanate 133
Augmentan (DE) *see* Amoxicillin and Clavulanate 133
Augmentin (AE, AT, AU, BB, BE, BF, BG, BH, BJ, BM, BS, BZ, CH, CI, CR, CY, CZ, DO, EC, EE, EG, ES, ET, FI, FR, GB, GH, GM, GN, GR, GT, GY, HK, HN, HR, HU, IE, IL, IN, IQ, IR, IS, IT, JM, JO, JP, KE, KR, KW, LB, LR, LY, MA, ML, MR, MT, MU, MW, MX, MY, NE, NG, NI, NL, NO, NZ, OM, PA, PE, PK, PL, PT, QA, RO, RU, SA, SC, SD, SI, SK, SL, SN, SR, SV, SY, TH, TN, TR, TT, TZ, UG, UY, VE, VN, YE, ZA, ZM, ZW) *see* Amoxicillin and Clavulanate 133
Augmentine (ES) *see* Amoxicillin and Clavulanate 133
Augmentin ES (IL) *see* Amoxicillin and Clavulanate 133
Augmentin SR (TH) *see* Amoxicillin and Clavulanate 133
Augmex (VN) *see* Amoxicillin and Clavulanate 133
Aulin (AR, BG, CH, CZ, GR, HR, IE, IT, PL, PT, RO, VE) *see* Nimesulide [INT] 1456
Aulzadin (HK) *see* Famotidine 845
Aumax (VN) *see* CefTRIAXone 396
Aunativ (AE, BH, CY, EG, IQ, IR, JO, KW, LB, LY, OM, QA, SA, SY, YE) *see* Immune Globulin 1056
Auradol (IT) *see* Frovatriptan 938
Auralgan (AE, BH, CY, EG, IL, IQ, IR, JO, KW, LB, LY, NZ, OM, QA, SA, SY, YE) *see* Antipyrine and Benzocaine 156
Auralgan (non-prescription) (AU) *see* Antipyrine and Benzocaine 156
Auralyt (MX) *see* Benzocaine 246
Auralyt (CO) *see* Antipyrine and Benzocaine 156
Aurinol (PH) *see* Allopurinol 90
Aurium (PY) *see* Methylphenidate 1336
Aurnida (IN) *see* Ornidazole [INT] 1522
Aurofox (MX) *see* CefTRIAXone 396
Auronim (IN, RU) *see* Nimesulide [INT] 1456
Auropan (HN, HR, HU, RU) *see* Auranofin 204
Auropennz (CL) *see* Ampicillin and Sulbactam 145
Aurorex (EC, MX, PE) *see* Moclobemide [CAN/INT] 1384
Aurorix (AE, AR, AT, AU, BE, BG, BH, BR, CH, CL, CZ, DK, EE, EG, FI, GR, HK, HN, HR, HU, ID, IS, IT, KR, KW, LU, NL, NO, PH, PK, PL, PT, QA, SA, SE, SI, SK, TH, TR, UY) *see* Moclobemide [CAN/INT] 1384
Aurotaz (QA) *see* Piperacillin and Tazobactam 1657
Aurozapine (VN) *see* Mirtazapine 1376
Auscap (AU) *see* FLUoxetine 899
Ausfam (AU) *see* Famotidine 845
Ausgem (AU) *see* Gemfibrozil 956
Auspilic (ID) *see* Amoxicillin and Clavulanate 133
Auspril (AU) *see* Enalapril 722

Ausran (AU) *see* Ranitidine 1777
Austrapen (AU) *see* Ampicillin 141
Austyn (KR) *see* Theophylline 2026
Aut (AR) *see* Pyrantel Pamoate 1744
Autoplex (JP) *see* Anti-inhibitor Coagulant Complex (Human) 155
Autoplex-T (IL) *see* Anti-inhibitor Coagulant Complex (Human) 155
Auxxil (CL, PY) *see* Levofloxacin (Systemic) 1197
Avadol (MY) *see* Acetaminophen 32
Avagal (UY) *see* Colistimethate 504
Avage (NZ, SG) *see* Tazarotene 1980
Avaglim (AT, BE, BG, CH, CZ, DE, DK, ES, FI, FR, GB, GR, HN, IE, IT, NL, NO, PT, RU, SE, TR) *see* Rosiglitazone and Glimepiride 1847
Avalide (BZ, SR) *see* Irbesartan and Hydrochlorothiazide 1112
Avalox (AE, BH, BR, CH, CY, DE, EG, IQ, IR, IT, JO, KW, LB, LY, OM, QA, SA, SY, YE) *see* Moxifloxacin (Systemic) 1401
Avamax (PH) *see* AtorvaSTATin 194
Avamigran (PH) *see* Ergotamine 754
Avamys (AE, AU, BE, BH, BR, CH, CL, CO, CR, CY, CZ, DE, DK, DO, EC, EE, FR, GB, GR, GT, HK, HN, HR, ID, IE, IL, IS, IT, KR, KW, LB, LT, MY, NI, NL, NO, NZ, PA, PE, PH, PL, PT, QA, RO, SA, SE, SG, SI, SK, SV, TH, TR, TW, UY, VN) *see* Fluticasone (Nasal) 910
Avandamet (AE, AR, AT, AU, BB, BE, BG, BH, BM, BR, BS, BZ, CH, CL, CO, CR, CZ, DE, DK, DO, EC, FI, FR, GB, GR, GT, GY, HK, HN, ID, IE, IL, IT, JM, KR, KW, MT, MY, NI, NL, NO, NZ, PA, PE, PH, PL, PR, PT, QA, RO, RU, SA, SE, SG, SI, SK, SR, SV, TH, TR, TT, TW, UY, VE, VN) *see* Rosiglitazone and Metformin 1847
Avandaryl (AR, BH, EC, ID, KR, KW, MX, PH, SA) *see* Rosiglitazone and Glimepiride 1847
Avandia (AE, AR, AT, AU, BB, BE, BG, BH, BM, BO, BR, BS, BZ, CH, CL, CR, CZ, DE, DK, DO, EC, EG, ES, FI, FR, GB, GR, GT, GY, HK, HN, ID, IE, IL, IT, JM, JO, KR, KW, MX, MY, NI, NL, NO, NZ, PA, PH, PK, PL, PR, PT, QA, RU, SA, SE, SG, SR, SV, TH, TR, TT, UY, VE, VN) *see* Rosiglitazone 1847
Avanep (IN) *see* Nepafenac 1439
Avantrin (IT) *see* Trapidil [INT] 2085
Avanza (AU, NZ) *see* Mirtazapine 1376
Avanza Soltab (AU) *see* Mirtazapine 1376
Avapro (AR, AU, BM, BZ, GY, JP, MX, SR) *see* Irbesartan 1110
Avapro HCT (AR, AU) *see* Irbesartan and Hydrochlorothiazide 1112
Avastin (AE, AR, AT, AU, BE, BG, BH, BR, CH, CL, CN, CO, CY, CZ, DE, DK, EC, EE, ES, FI, FR, GB, GR, HK, HN, HR, HU, ID, IE, IL, IS, IT, JO, JP, KR, KW, LB, LT, MT, MX, MY, NL, NO, NZ, PE, PH, PL, PT, PY, QA, RO, RU, SE, SG, SI, SK, TH, TR, TW, UY, VN) *see* Bevacizumab 257
Avastinee (HK) *see* Simvastatin 1890
Avaxim (AE, AR, AU, BG, CO, CY, EC, GB, HK, ID, IE, IL, KR, KW, LB, SA, SG, TH, VN) *see* Hepatitis A Vaccine 1001
Avazinc (IL) *see* Zinc Sulfate 2200
Avedox-FC (MX) *see* Albuterol 69
Avegesic (MY) *see* Meloxicam 1283
Avelon (ZA) *see* Moxifloxacin (Systemic) 1401
Avelox (AR, AU, BB, BE, BF, BG, BJ, BM, BS, BZ, CI, CL, CN, CO, CR, CZ, DK, DO, EC, EE, ET, FI, GB, GH, GM, GN, GT, GY, HK, HN, HR, ID, IE, JM, JP, KE, KR, LR, LT, MA, ML, MR, MU, MW, MY, NE, NG, NI, NL, NZ, PA, PE, PH, PK, PL, PR, PY, RO, RU, SC, SD, SE, SG, SK, SL, SN, SR, SV, TH, TN, TR, TT, TZ, UG, UY, VE, VN, ZM, ZW) *see* Moxifloxacin (Systemic) 1401
Aventyl (MY) *see* Nortriptyline 1476
Averinal (VN) *see* Alverine [INT] 104
Avernol (TR) *see* Carvedilol 367
Avessa (LU) *see* Ondansetron 1513
Avestra (SE) *see* Risedronate 1816
Aveten (MY) *see* Atenolol 189
Avevasc (MY, SG) *see* AmLODIPine 123
Avexus (MY) *see* Clarithromycin 456
Avezol (MY) *see* Fluconazole 885
Av F Aza Acne Foundation (ID) *see* Azelaic Acid 213
Aviant (MX) *see* Desloratadine 594
Avibon (FR) *see* Vitamin A 2173
Avidart (ES) *see* Dutasteride 702
Avigilen (DE) *see* Piracetam [INT] 1661
Aviomarin (HR, PL) *see* DimenhyDRINATE 637
Aviral (CO) *see* Zidovudine 2196
Aviran (MX) *see* Indinavir 1066
Avir (VE) *see* Acyclovir (Systemic) 47
Avir (VE) *see* Acyclovir (Topical) 51
Avirzid (ID) *see* Zidovudine 2196
Avistar (MX) *see* AmLODIPine 123
Avitan (GR) *see* Vitamin A 2173
Avitcid (FI) *see* Tretinoin (Topical) 2099
Avitina (IT) *see* Vitamin A 2173
Avitol (AT) *see* Vitamin A 2173
Avlocardyl (FR, VN) *see* Propranolol 1731
Avloclor (BF, BJ, CI, ET, GB, GH, GM, GN, IE, KE, LR, MA, ML, MR, MU, MW, NE, NG, SC, SD, SL, SN, TN, TZ, UG, ZA, ZM, ZW) *see* Chloroquine 424
Avocel (ID) *see* Levocetirizine 1196
Avocin (ES) *see* Piperacillin [CAN/INT] 1656
Avodart (AE, AR, AT, AU, BB, BE, BG, BH, BM, BR, BS, BZ, CH, CL, CN, CO, CR, CY, CZ, DE, DK, DO, EC, EE, FI, FR, GB, GR, GT, GY, HK, HN, HR, ID, IE, IL, IS, IT, JM, KR, LB, LT, MX, MY, NI, NL, NO, NZ, PA, PE, PH, PL, PR, PT, QA, RO, RU, SA, SE, SG, SI, SK, SR, SV, TH, TR, TT, TW, VN) *see* Dutasteride 702
Avolve (JP) *see* Dutasteride 702
Avomine (TR) *see* Promethazine 1723
Avomit (HR) *see* Letrozole 1181
Avonex (AE, AR, AT, AU, BE, BG, BH, BR, CH, CL, CO, CY, CZ, DE, DK, EE, ES, FI, FR, GB, GR, HK, HR, HU, IE, IL, IS, IT, JO, JP, KR, KW, LB, LT, MT, NL, NO, NZ, PE, PL, PT, PY, QA, RO, RU, SA, SE, SI, SK, TR, UY, VE) *see* Interferon Beta-1a 1100
Avorax (HK) *see* Acyclovir (Systemic) 47
Avorax (SG) *see* Acyclovir (Topical) 51
Avotyne (MY) *see* Loratadine 1241
Avoxin (HR) *see* FluvoxaMINE 916
Avoxin (JO) *see* Levofloxacin (Systemic) 1197
Avural (PY) *see* Indinavir 1066
Axacef (HK) *see* Cefuroxime 399
Axadine (KR) *see* Nizatidine 1471
Axal (PH) *see* ALPRAZolam 94
Axasol (CL) *see* Clotrimazole (Topical) 488
A-Xat CR (KR) *see* PARoxetine 1579
Axcel (MY) *see* Acetaminophen 32
Axed (MX) *see* Ergocalciferol 753
Axel Bromhexine (SG) *see* Bromhexine [INT] 291
Axeler (FR) *see* Amlodipine and Olmesartan 126
Axella (PH) *see* Cetirizine 411
Axepim (FR) *see* Cefepime 378
Axepta (IN) *see* AtoMOXetine 191
Axeptyl (GT) *see* Amitriptyline 119
Axera (PH) *see* Cefepime 378
Axetef (PH) *see* Cefixime 380
Axetine (CN, NZ, PH, SG) *see* Cefuroxime 399
Axet (PH) *see* Cefuroxime 399
Axibin (PH) *see* DOXOrubicin (Conventional) 679
Axid (AE, BH, CN, CY, CZ, HR, HU, LB, MX, QA, SA, VN) *see* Nizatidine 1471
Axid Pulvules (BF, BG, BJ, CI, ET, GB, GH, GM, GN, GR, ID, IE, KE, KR, LR, MA, ML, MR, MU, MW, MY, NE, NG, PK, PL, SC, SD, SE, SG, SL, SN, TN, TR, TZ, UG, VE, ZA, ZM, ZW) *see* Nizatidine 1471

Axilin (MX) *see* Flunarizine [CAN/INT] 892
Axilium (IT) *see* Lormetazepam [INT] 1247
Axim (HK) *see* Cefuroxime 399
Axira (HR) *see* Cyproterone and Ethinyl Estradiol [CAN/INT] 532
Axiron (AU) *see* Testosterone 2010
Axit (AU) *see* Mirtazapine 1376
A Xi Ya (CN) *see* Furosemide 940
Axo (DO, GT, HN, NI, PA, SV) *see* AtorvaSTATin 194
Axofin (MX) *see* Doxofylline [INT] 679
Axoflon (PH) *see* Levofloxacin (Systemic) 1197
Axol (MX, MY, SG) *see* Ambroxol [INT] 109
Axone (AE, BH, CY, EG, IQ, IR, JO, KW, LB, LY, OM, QA, SA, SY, YE) *see* CefTRIAXone 396
Axonyl (FR) *see* Piracetam [INT] 1661
Axoptic (MY) *see* Betaxolol (Ophthalmic) 257
Axotide (CH) *see* Fluticasone (Oral Inhalation) 907
Axtar (MX) *see* CefTRIAXone 396
Axual (AR) *see* Pregabalin 1710
Axura (AT, BE, BG, CH, CZ, DE, DK, EE, ES, FI, FR, GB, GR, IE, IT, MT, NL, NO, PL, PT, RO, RU, SE, SK, TR) *see* Memantine 1286
Axurocef (TW) *see* Cefuroxime 399
Aylehning (TW) *see* Chenodiol 417
Aylide (AU) *see* Glimepiride 966
Aza-250 (HK) *see* Azithromycin (Systemic) 216
Aza-500 (HK) *see* Azithromycin (Systemic) 216
Azacortid (AR, CL, PY, UY) *see* Deflazacort [INT] 587
Azactam (AT, AU, BB, BE, BF, BG, BH, BJ, BM, BS, BZ, CH, CI, CN, CO, DE, DK, EE, EG, ES, ET, FI, FR, GB, GH, GM, GN, GR, GY, HN, IE, IT, JM, JO, JP, KE, LB, LR, MA, ML, MR, MT, MU, MW, NE, NG, NO, NZ, PK, PL, PT, QA, RU, SC, SD, SE, SG, SK, SL, SN, SR, TN, TR, TT, TW, TZ, UG, VE, ZA, ZM, ZW) *see* Aztreonam 220
Azadose (FR) *see* Azithromycin (Systemic) 216
Azadus (TH) *see* AzaTHIOprine 210
Azafalk (DE) *see* AzaTHIOprine 210
Azalea (KR) *see* Azelaic Acid 213
Azalia (BG, CZ, ES, HU, PL) *see* Desogestrel [INT] 597
Azamun (AE, AU, MY, NZ, SA, TW) *see* AzaTHIOprine 210
Azamune (GB) *see* AzaTHIOprine 210
Azanem (BR) *see* Aztreonam 220
Azanin (JP) *see* AzaTHIOprine 210
Azantac (FR, MX) *see* Ranitidine 1777
Azapin (AU) *see* AzaTHIOprine 210
Azapress (ZA) *see* AzaTHIOprine 210
Azaprin (AE, KW, SA) *see* AzaTHIOprine 210
Azaprine (KR) *see* AzaTHIOprine 210
Aza-Q (DE) *see* AzaTHIOprine 210
Azarekhexal (EE) *see* AzaTHIOprine 210
Azarex (DE) *see* AzaTHIOprine 210
Azarga (AR, AU, BE, CH, CL, CO, CY, CZ, DE, DK, EC, EE, FR, GB, GR, HK, HR, HU, IE, IL, IS, IT, KW, LT, MY, NL, NZ, PE, PH, PL, PT, QA, RO, SA, SE, SG, SI, SK, TH, TR, TW) *see* Brinzolamide and Timolol [CAN/INT] 289
Azaron (BE) *see* DiphenhydrAMINE (Systemic) 641
Azas (KR) *see* Azithromycin (Systemic) 216
Azathiodura (DE) *see* AzaTHIOprine 210
Azatioprina (PE) *see* AzaTHIOprine 210
Azatioprina Wellcome (IT) *see* AzaTHIOprine 210
Azatol (RO) *see* Pantoprazole 1570
Azatril (EE) *see* Azithromycin (Systemic) 216
Azatrilem (MX) *see* AzaTHIOprine 210
Aze-Air (VN) *see* Azelastine (Nasal) 213
Azeat (DE) *see* Acemetacin [INT] 30
Azeclear (HK) *see* Azelaic Acid 213
Azee (HK) *see* Azithromycin (Systemic) 216
Azeemycin (PH) *see* Azithromycin (Systemic) 216
Azeflo (IN) *see* Azelastine and Fluticasone 214
Azelan (BR) *see* Azelaic Acid 213
Azelan (KR) *see* Azelastine (Nasal) 213
Azelan (KR) *see* Azelastine (Ophthalmic) 213
Azela (PH, TW) *see* Azelastine (Nasal) 213
Azel (CO) *see* Azelastine (Ophthalmic) 213
Azelin (VN) *see* Azelaic Acid 213
Azel (TW) *see* Azelaic Acid 213
Azelvin (NO, SE) *see* Azelastine (Nasal) 213
Azenam (IN) *see* Aztreonam 220
Azenil (IL) *see* Azithromycin (Systemic) 216
Azepal (HU) *see* CarBAMazepine 346
Azepan (AE, BH, CY, EG, IQ, IR, JO, KW, LB, LY, OM, QA, SA, SY, YE) *see* Diazepam 613
Azep (CN, IN, NZ, SG) *see* Azelastine (Nasal) 213
Azep Eye Drops (HK) *see* Azelastine (Ophthalmic) 213
Azep Nasal Spray (AU, HK, NZ) *see* Azelastine (Nasal) 213
Azeptil (TR) *see* Tranexamic Acid 2081
Azeptin Nasal (KR) *see* Azelastine (Nasal) 213
Azerra (SK) *see* Ofatumumab 1488
Azerty (FR) *see* Nalbuphine 1416
Azetin (TW) *see* Azelastine (Nasal) 213
Azi-500 (PH) *see* Azithromycin (Systemic) 216
Azibact (DE) *see* Azithromycin (Systemic) 216
Azibiot (RO) *see* Azithromycin (Systemic) 216
Azicine (HK) *see* Azithromycin (Systemic) 216
Azide (AU) *see* Chlorothiazide 426
Azide (PK) *see* Gliclazide [CAN/INT] 964
Aziderm (IN) *see* Azelaic Acid 213
Azidex (AT) *see* Pantoprazole 1570
Azidomine (KR) *see* Zidovudine 2196
Azilect (AT, AU, BE, BG, CH, CY, CZ, DE, DK, EE, ES, FI, FR, GB, GR, HN, HR, IE, IL, IS, IT, KR, LT, MT, NL, NO, PH, PL, PT, RO, RU, SE, SI, SK, TH, TR, TW) *see* Rasagiline 1781
Azillin (CH) *see* Amoxicillin 130
Azilva (JP) *see* Azilsartan 214
Azimac (SA) *see* Azithromycin (Systemic) 216
Azimax (MY) *see* Azithromycin (Systemic) 216
Azimed (HR) *see* Azithromycin (Systemic) 216
Azimet (PH) *see* Ketotifen (Systemic) [CAN/INT] 1149
Azinobin (CO) *see* Azithromycin (Systemic) 216
Azin (PH) *see* Azithromycin (Systemic) 216
Azinza (PE) *see* Vorinostat 2182
Azirocin (KR) *see* Azithromycin (Systemic) 216
Azith (AU, TH) *see* Azithromycin (Systemic) 216
Azithral (IN) *see* Azithromycin (Systemic) 216
Azithrom (TW) *see* Azithromycin (Systemic) 216
Azithro (MY) *see* Azithromycin (Systemic) 216
Azitops (KR) *see* Azithromycin (Systemic) 216
Azitrex (EC) *see* Azithromycin (Systemic) 216
Azitrix (PT) *see* Azithromycin (Systemic) 216
Azitrocin (IT) *see* Azithromycin (Systemic) 216
Azitromax (NO, SE) *see* Azithromycin (Systemic) 216
Azitrox (SK) *see* Azithromycin (Systemic) 216
Aziwok (BF, BJ, CI, ET, GH, GM, GN, IN, KE, LR, MA, ML, MR, MU, MW, NE, NG, SC, SD, SL, SN, TN, TZ, UG, ZM, ZW) *see* Azithromycin (Systemic) 216
Azmacon (ID) *see* Albuterol 69
Azmacort (NZ, PK) *see* Triamcinolone (Systemic) 2099
Azo Cefasabal (PE) *see* Phenazopyridine 1629
Azoel (PY) *see* Mebendazole [CAN/INT] 1274
Az Ofteno (CL, CR, DO, GT, HN, NI, PA, SV, VE) *see* Azelastine (Ophthalmic) 213
Azol (AU, ID, TW) *see* Danazol 558
Azolin (IN) *see* CeFAZolin 373
Azolmen (IT) *see* Bifonazole [INT] 264
Azol NCP (TW) *see* AcetaZOLAMIDE 39
Azomax (BH, KW) *see* Azithromycin (Systemic) 216
Azomycin (AE, KW, QA, SA) *see* Azithromycin (Systemic) 216
Azomyne (JO, LB, QA) *see* Azithromycin (Systemic) 216

Azomyr (AR, AT, CH, CZ, DE, DK, EE, ES, FI, FR, GB, GR, IE, IT, LT, MT, MX, NL, NO, PL, PT, RU, SE, SK, TR) *see* Desloratadine ... 594
Azona (IN) *see* Ziprasidone ... 2201
Azonet (HR) *see* Anastrozole ... 148
Azonit (JO, LB) *see* Isoconazole [INT] ... 1120
Azonz (FI) *see* TraZODone ... 2091
Azopi (IL) *see* AzaTHIOprine ... 210
Azopt (AE, AR, AT, AU, BE, BG, BH, BR, CH, CL, CN, CO, CR, CY, CZ, DE, DK, EC, EE, EG, ES, FI, FR, GB, GR, GT, HK, HN, HR, HU, ID, IE, IL, IS, IT, JO, KR, KW, LB, LT, MT, MX, MY, NI, NL, NO, NZ, PA, PE, PH, PL, PT, PY, QA, RO, RU, SA, SE, SG, SI, SK, SV, TH, TR, TW, UY, VE, VN) *see* Brinzolamide ... 288
Azoptic (ZA) *see* Brinzolamide ... 288
Azoran (MX) *see* Omeprazole ... 1508
Azoran (ID) *see* Amiodarone ... 114
Azoran (IN) *see* AzaTHIOprine ... 210
Azoren (HK, MY, SG) *see* Amlodipine and Olmesartan ... 126
Azorga (BR, JP) *see* Brinzolamide and Timolol [CAN/INT] ... 289
Azor (ZA) *see* ALPRAZolam ... 94
Azosin SR (TW) *see* Alfuzosin ... 84
Azox (JO) *see* Azithromycin (Systemic) ... 216
Azro (AE, BH, CY, EG, IQ, IR, JO, KW, LB, LY, OM, QA, SA, SY, YE) *see* Azithromycin (Systemic) ... 216
Aztor EZ (PE) *see* Ezetimibe and Atorvastatin ... 833
Aztram (PH) *see* Aztreonam ... 220
Aztrin (ID) *see* Azithromycin (Systemic) ... 216
Azudoxat (DE) *see* Doxycycline ... 689
Azukon (IN) *see* Gliclazide [CAN/INT] ... 964
Azukon MR (BR, IN, PH) *see* Gliclazide [CAN/INT] ... 964
Azulfidina (MX) *see* SulfaSALAzine ... 1950
Azulfidine (CL, DE, VE) *see* SulfaSALAzine ... 1950
Azulfidine-EN (CL) *see* SulfaSALAzine ... 1950
Azulfidine EN-tabs (AR) *see* SulfaSALAzine ... 1950
Azulfin (BR) *see* SulfaSALAzine ... 1950
Azulix (BR, PH) *see* Glimepiride ... 966
Azunaftil (DE) *see* Naftidrofuryl [INT] ... 1416
Azupel (PY) *see* Gentamicin (Systemic) ... 959
Azurex (TH) *see* Cetirizine ... 411
Azymol (PE, PY) *see* ARIPiprazole ... 171
Azyter (DE, FR, GB, HK, HR, ID, IE, PT, RO, TH) *see* Azithromycin (Ophthalmic) ... 219
Azyth (PH) *see* Azithromycin (Systemic) ... 216
B!1!2-Depot-Vicotrat (DE) *see* Hydroxocobalamin ... 1020
B1-ASmedic (DE) *see* Thiamine ... 2028
B!1-Vicotrat (DE) *see* Thiamine ... 2028
B2-ASmedic (DE) *see* Riboflavin ... 1803
B(6)-Vicotrat (DE) *see* Pyridoxine ... 1747
B12 Ankermann (PL) *see* Cyanocobalamin ... 515
B12-Depot-Hevert (DE) *see* Hydroxocobalamin ... 1020
B12 Depot-Rotexmedica (DE) *see* Hydroxocobalamin ... 1020
B12-Depot-Vicotrat (DE) *see* Hydroxocobalamin ... 1020
B12 Latino (ES) *see* Cyanocobalamin ... 515
Babette (DE) *see* Desogestrel [INT] ... 597
Baburol (TW) *see* Bambuterol [INT] ... 227
Baby Agisten (IL) *see* Clotrimazole (Topical) ... 488
Babydent (CZ) *see* Benzocaine ... 246
Baby Orajel (PL) *see* Benzocaine ... 246
Babypasmil (AR) *see* Dicyclomine ... 622
Bacbutol (ID) *see* Ethambutol ... 798
Baccidal (JP, KR, TW) *see* Norfloxacin ... 1475
Baccillin (KR) *see* Ampicillin and Sulbactam ... 145
Bacda-B (TH) *see* Betamethasone and Clotrimazole ... 256
Bacdan (TW) *see* Sulfamethoxazole and Trimethoprim ... 1946
Bacflocin (TW) *see* Levofloxacin (Systemic) ... 1197
Bacidal (TH) *see* Mupirocin ... 1404
Baciderm (VE) *see* Bacitracin (Topical) ... 222
Bacifurane (BE, LU) *see* Nifuroxazide [INT] ... 1454
Bacihexal (PH) *see* Amoxicillin ... 130
Bacin (MY, SG, TH) *see* Sulfamethoxazole and Trimethoprim ... 1946
Bacitran (KR) *see* Bacitracin (Topical) ... 222
Baclan (KR) *see* Baclofen ... 223
Baclecin (HK) *see* Clarithromycin ... 456
Baclofene (FR) *see* Baclofen ... 223
Baclofen-ratiopharm (LU) *see* Baclofen ... 223
Baclon (FI, TW) *see* Baclofen ... 223
Baclopar (IE) *see* Baclofen ... 223
Baclosal (IL) *see* Baclofen ... 223
Baclosan (RU) *see* Baclofen ... 223
Baclosol (VN) *see* Baclofen ... 223
Bacofen (KR) *see* Baclofen ... 223
Bacort (PY) *see* Betamethasone (Topical) ... 255
Bacperazone (RU) *see* Cefoperazone and Sulbactam [INT] ... 382
Bacquinor (ID) *see* Ciprofloxacin (Systemic) ... 441
Bacqure (TH) *see* Imipenem and Cilastatin ... 1051
Bacron (KR) *see* Baclofen ... 223
Bactacin (KR) *see* Ampicillin and Sulbactam ... 145
Bactamox (VE) *see* Amoxicillin ... 130
Bactazon (ID) *see* Cefoperazone and Sulbactam [INT] ... 382
Bactelan (MX) *see* Sulfamethoxazole and Trimethoprim ... 1946
Bacterfin (EC) *see* Clarithromycin ... 456
Bacteric (MX) *see* Sulfamethoxazole and Trimethoprim ... 1946
Bactermin (TW) *see* Mupirocin ... 1404
Bacterol (CL) *see* Sulfamethoxazole and Trimethoprim ... 1946
Bacterol (CO) *see* Moxifloxacin (Systemic) ... 1401
Bacterol Forte (CL) *see* Sulfamethoxazole and Trimethoprim ... 1946
Bactesyn (ID) *see* Ampicillin and Sulbactam ... 145
Bactevo (VN) *see* Levofloxacin (Systemic) ... 1197
Bactex (TH) *see* Mupirocin ... 1404
Bacticef (IN) *see* Cefuroxime ... 399
Bacticel (AR, DO, GT, HN, NI, PA, SV) *see* Sulfamethoxazole and Trimethoprim ... 1946
Bacticep (TH) *see* Cefoperazone and Sulbactam [INT] ... 382
Bactidox (PH) *see* Doxycycline ... 689
Bactiflox (BF, BJ, CI, ET, GH, GM, GN, KE, LR, MA, ML, MR, MU, MW, NE, NG, SC, SD, SG, SL, SN, TN, TZ, UG, ZM, ZW) *see* Ciprofloxacin (Systemic) ... 441
Bactifree (PH) *see* Mupirocin ... 1404
Bactigen (VN) *see* Gentamicin (Ophthalmic) ... 962
Bactil (ES) *see* Ebastine [INT] ... 702
Bactiver (MX) *see* Sulfamethoxazole and Trimethoprim ... 1946
Bactiv (PH) *see* Amoxicillin and Clavulanate ... 133
Bactocin (BR, PH) *see* Mupirocin ... 1404
Bactoclav (PH) *see* Amoxicillin and Clavulanate ... 133
Bactoderm (ID, IL) *see* Mupirocin ... 1404
Bactokil (TH) *see* Mupirocin ... 1404
Bactoprim (TH) *see* Sulfamethoxazole and Trimethoprim ... 1946
Bactox (EE) *see* Amoxicillin ... 130
Bactox Ge (FR) *see* Amoxicillin ... 130
Bactramin (JP) *see* Sulfamethoxazole and Trimethoprim ... 1946
Bactrim (AE, AR, AT, AU, BE, BH, BR, CH, CY, CZ, DE, DK, EC, EE, EG, ES, FR, ID, IN, IQ, IR, IT, JO, KW, LB, LY, MT, MX, NO, OM, PK, PT, QA, SA, SE, SK, SY, TH, TR, VN, YE) *see* Sulfamethoxazole and Trimethoprim ... 1946
Bactrim DS (AU) *see* Sulfamethoxazole and Trimethoprim ... 1946
Bactrimel (GR, VE) *see* Sulfamethoxazole and Trimethoprim ... 1946

Bactrim F (CO) *see* Sulfamethoxazole and Trimethoprim ... 1946
Bactrim Forte (AT, FI, FR, PT, SE) *see* Sulfamethoxazole and Trimethoprim ... 1946
Bactrobaan (DE) *see* Mupirocin ... 1404
Bactroban (AE, AR, AT, AU, BB, BD, BE, BF, BG, BH, BJ, BM, BR, BS, BZ, CH, CI, CL, CN, CR, CY, CZ, DK, DO, EG, ES, ET, FI, FR, GB, GH, GM, GN, GR, GT, GY, HK, HN, HU, ID, IE, IL, IN, IQ, IR, IS, IT, JM, JO, JP, KE, KR, KW, LB, LR, LU, LY, MA, ML, MR, MU, MW, MX, MY, NE, NG, NI, NL, NO, NZ, OM, PA, PH, PK, PL, PR, PT, PY, QA, RU, SA, SC, SD, SE, SG, SI, SK, SL, SN, SR, SV, SY, TH, TN, TR, TT, TW, TZ, UG, UY, VE, YE, ZA, ZM, ZW) *see* Mupirocin ... 1404
Bactroban Nasal Ointment (AU) *see* Mupirocin ... 1404
Bactromax (CO) *see* Rifampin ... 1804
Bactropin (MX) *see* Sulfamethoxazole and Trimethoprim ... 1946
Baduson (TW) *see* FlavoxATE ... 881
Baflox (CO) *see* Ciprofloxacin (Systemic) ... 441
Bagobiotic (EC) *see* Mupirocin ... 1404
Bagomicina (CL, EC) *see* Minocycline ... 1371
Bagotanilo (MX) *see* CARBOplatin ... 357
Bai Er Luo (CN) *see* Propranolol ... 1731
Baietta (MX) *see* Exenatide ... 830
Bai Kang (CN) *see* Glyburide and Metformin ... 974
Bain (TW) *see* Nalbuphine ... 1416
Bai Yue (CN) *see* Carbocisteine [INT] ... 357
Bajapres (CO) *see* Albuterol ... 69
Bajaten (CL) *see* Enalapril ... 722
Baknyl (EC) *see* Erythromycin (Systemic) ... 762
Balad (AE) *see* Fusidic Acid (Topical) [CAN/INT] ... 943
Balcor (BR) *see* Diltiazem ... 634
B.A.L. (DE, FR, IN, IT) *see* Dimercaprol ... 638
Balidon (CL) *see* Triazolam ... 2101
Balidon (CO) *see* CARBOplatin ... 357
BAL (IE) *see* Dimercaprol ... 638
BAL In Oil (GR, MY) *see* Dimercaprol ... 638
Balisa (DE) *see* Urea ... 2114
Balkaprofen (BF, BJ, CI, ET, GH, GM, GN, KE, LR, MA, ML, MR, MU, MW, NE, NG, SC, SD, SL, SN, TN, TZ, UG, ZM, ZW) *see* Ibuprofen ... 1032
Balminil DM D (CA) *see* Pseudoephedrine and Dextromethorphan ... 1743
Balminil DM + Decongestant + Expectorant (CA) *see* Guaifenesin, Pseudoephedrine, and Dextromethorphan ... 989
Balminil (ES) *see* Nitrendipine [INT] ... 1463
Balmox (PT) *see* Nabumetone ... 1411
Balon (TW) *see* Metoclopramide ... 1345
Balticin (ID) *see* Gentamicin (Systemic) ... 959
Balurol (BR) *see* Pipemidic Acid [INT] ... 1655
Balzide (IT) *see* Balsalazide ... 226
Bambec (AT, BH, BR, CN, DE, DK, EG, GB, KR, NO, PH, PK, QA, SE, SG, TH, TW, VN) *see* Bambuterol [INT] ... 227
Bambudil (IN) *see* Bambuterol [INT] ... 227
Bamgetol (ID) *see* CarBAMazepine ... 346
Bamifen (VN) *see* Baclofen ... 223
Bamifix (BR, IT) *see* Bamifylline [INT] ... 227
Bami-med (BE, CH) *see* Bamifylline [INT] ... 227
Bamiphil (KR) *see* Bamifylline [INT] ... 227
Bamyl (SE) *see* Aspirin ... 180
Bamyxin (IL) *see* Bacitracin, Neomycin, and Polymyxin B ... 223
Banadoz (ID) *see* Cefpodoxime ... 388
Banan (CN, HK, JP, KR, TH) *see* Cefpodoxime ... 388
Banan Dry Syrup (KR) *see* Cefpodoxime ... 388
Banbact (TH) *see* Mupirocin ... 1404
Bandotan (AR) *see* Didanosine ... 622
Bandrobon (AR) *see* Ibandronate ... 1028
BangNi (CN) *see* Nimesulide [INT] ... 1456
Bang Yi (CN) *see* Rifaximin ... 1809
Banjil (KR) *see* Urea ... 2114
Banlice Mousse (AU) *see* Pyrethrins and Piperonyl Butoxide ... 1746
Ban Su (CN) *see* Ticlopidine ... 2040
Bantix (CN, PY) *see* Mupirocin ... 1404
Baogin (TW) *see* Diazepam ... 613
Baojen (TW) *see* Fluoxymesterone ... 903
Bapex (MX) *see* Gabapentin ... 943
Baphil (KR) *see* Bamifylline [INT] ... 227
Bapter (IN) *see* Tolterodine ... 2063
Baquinor (ID) *see* Ciprofloxacin (Ophthalmic) ... 446
Baquinor (ID) *see* Ciprofloxacin (Systemic) ... 441
Baraclude (AE, AR, AT, AU, BE, BG, BH, BR, CH, CL, CN, CO, CR, CY, CZ, DE, DK, DO, EE, ES, FI, FR, GB, GR, GT, HK, HN, HR, HU, ID, IE, IL, IS, IT, JO, JP, KR, KW, LB, LT, MT, MY, NI, NL, NO, NZ, PA, PE, PH, PK, PL, PT, QA, RO, RU, SA, SE, SG, SI, SK, SV, TH, TR, TW, UY, VN) *see* Entecavir ... 731
Barapa (KR) *see* Baclofen ... 223
Baratol (GB, IE, ZA) *see* Indoramin [INT] ... 1070
Barbamyl (IL) *see* Amobarbital ... 128
Barbilettae (FI) *see* PHENobarbital ... 1632
Barbiphenyl (FI) *see* PHENobarbital ... 1632
Barbloc (AU, TW) *see* Pindolol ... 1652
Barcan (DK, FI, SE) *see* Aceclofenac [INT] ... 30
Barizin (HR) *see* NiCARdipine ... 1446
Barlolin (TW) *see* Bromocriptine ... 291
Barnix (ES) *see* Barnidipine [INT] ... 227
Barole (PH) *see* RABEprazole ... 1762
Barolyn (FI) *see* Metolazone ... 1348
Barontin (KR) *see* Gabapentin ... 943
Bartolium (ID) *see* Flunarizine [CAN/INT] ... 892
Barzepin (ID) *see* OXcarbazepine ... 1532
Basal-H-Insulin (DE) *see* Insulin NPH ... 1089
Basalin (TH) *see* Insulin Glargine ... 1086
Basazyde (TW) *see* Balsalazide ... 226
Basdene (FR) *see* Benzylthiouracil [INT] ... 250
Based (TW) *see* Methimazole ... 1319
Basiflux (PT) *see* Bromhexine [INT] ... 291
Basocef (DE) *see* CeFAZolin ... 373
Basodexan (DE) *see* Urea ... 2114
Basofortina (AR, PY) *see* Methylergonovine ... 1333
Basolest (NL) *see* Carbimazole [INT] ... 356
B-Aspirin (TH) *see* Aspirin ... 180
Bassado (IT) *see* Doxycycline ... 689
Baten (CR, DO, EC, GT, HN, NI, PA, SV) *see* Fluconazole ... 885
Batmen (ES) *see* Prednicarbate ... 1703
Batrafan (IN) *see* Ciclopirox ... 433
Batrafen (AE, AT, BB, BD, BG, BH, BM, BS, BZ, CH, CL, CY, CZ, DE, EC, EE, EG, GY, HK, HN, HR, HU, ID, IQ, IR, IT, JM, JO, JP, KW, LB, LY, NL, NZ, OM, PE, PK, PL, PR, PY, QA, RU, SA, SG, SK, SR, SY, TR, TT, UY, VE, YE) *see* Ciclopirox ... 433
Batrafen Gel (DE) *see* Ciclopirox ... 433
Batrafen Nail Lacquer (IL) *see* Ciclopirox ... 433
Baxan (GB) *see* Cefadroxil ... 372
Baxidyme (PH) *see* CefTAZidime ... 392
Baxmicin (BR) *see* MitoMYcin (Systemic) ... 1380
Baxo (JP) *see* Piroxicam ... 1662
Baxol (KR) *see* Rimexolone ... 1814
Bayaspirina (AR) *see* Aspirin ... 180
Bayaspirin Protect 100 (CN) *see* Aspirin ... 180
Baycaron (DE, GB, IE, NL, NO) *see* Mefruside [INT] ... 1281
Baycip (CL) *see* Ciprofloxacin (Systemic) ... 441
Baydol (CO) *see* Acemetacin [INT] ... 30
Baydol LP (CO) *see* Acemetacin [INT] ... 30
Bayer Aspirin Cardio (ZA) *see* Aspirin ... 180
Bayer Bayrab Rabies Immune Globulin (PH) *see* Rabies Immune Globulin (Human) ... 1764
Bayhep (PK) *see* Hepatitis B Immune Globulin (Human) ... 1002

Baylotensin (JP) *see* Nitrendipine [INT] 1463
Baymycard (BG, DE, HN, HU, JP) *see* Nisoldipine 1459
Bayotensin (DE) *see* Nitrendipine [INT] 1463
Baypresol (ES) *see* Nitrendipine [INT] 1463
Baypress (AR, AT, BE, CH, CZ, DK, FR, HU, IT, LU, NL, PL) *see* Nitrendipine [INT] 1463
Bayprin EC (PH) *see* Aspirin 180
Bayrab (PK) *see* Rabies Immune Globulin (Human) 1764
BayRHo-D (ID) *see* $Rh_o(D)$ Immune Globulin 1794
Bay Rho-D (IL) *see* $Rh_o(D)$ Immune Globulin 1794
Bayrogel (AR, BR) *see* Etofenamate [INT] 815
Bayro (IT, MX) *see* Etofenamate [INT] 815
BayTet (MX, PK) *see* Tetanus Immune Globulin (Human) 2015
Bazetham (HR) *see* Tamsulosin 1974
B-Beta (ID) *see* Bisoprolol 266
BB (TW) *see* Clindamycin (Systemic) 460
BCG-Medac (TH) *see* BCG 229
Bcnu (BG, HN) *see* Carmustine 364
B-Cor (JO, LB) *see* Bisoprolol 266
B Cort (CO) *see* Budesonide (Systemic) 293
Beacon K SR (MY) *see* Potassium Chloride 1687
Beafemic (MY, SG) *see* Mefenamic Acid 1280
Beahexol (SG) *see* Trihexyphenidyl 2103
Beamodium (MY) *see* Loperamide 1236
Beamotil (MY, SG) *see* Diphenoxylate and Atropine 644
Beamoxy (MY) *see* Amoxicillin 130
Beanamine (SG) *see* DiphenhydrAMINE (Systemic) 641
Beapen VK (MY) *see* Penicillin V Potassium 1614
Beaphenicol (SG) *see* Chloramphenicol 421
Beaptin SR (SG) *see* Verapamil 2154
Bearantel (SG) *see* Pyrantel Pamoate 1744
Bearax (SG) *see* Acyclovir (Systemic) 47
Bearclor (VN) *see* Cefaclor 372
Bearfina (KR) *see* Finasteride 878
Beartec (KR) *see* Enalapril 722
Beartra (KR) *see* Acetaminophen and Tramadol 37
Bearverin (VN) *see* Propiverine [INT] 1728
Beatacycline (SG) *see* Tetracycline 2017
Beatafed (MY) *see* Triprolidine and Pseudoephedrine 2105
Beatizem (SG) *see* Diltiazem 634
Beautipex (KR) *see* Betahistine [CAN/INT] 252
Beautyface (TW) *see* Adapalene 54
Beavate (MY) *see* Betamethasone (Topical) 255
Bebulin Team 4 (RU) *see* Factor IX (Human) 840
Bebulin TIM 4 (HN) *see* Factor IX (Human) 840
Bebyzal (KR) *see* Ibuprofen 1032
Becanden (TW) *see* Triprolidine and Pseudoephedrine 2105
Becantex (ID) *see* Rebamipide [INT] 1786
Becaplex (LB) *see* Becaplermin 230
Becaps (BR) *see* Thiamine 2028
Becarin (MY) *see* Miconazole (Topical) 1360
Becenun (BR, FI, NO) *see* Carmustine 364
Becilan (FR) *see* Pyridoxine 1747
Beclate (HK, IN, MY, ZA) *see* Beclomethasone (Nasal) 232
Beclate (ZA) *see* Beclomethasone (Systemic) 230
Beclazide MR (TH) *see* Gliclazide [CAN/INT] 964
Beclazone (BH, CY, HK, KW, LB, NZ, SA, TR, VN) *see* Beclomethasone (Systemic) 230
Beclazone (HK, NZ) *see* Beclomethasone (Nasal) 232
Beclo-Asma CFC Free (SG) *see* Beclomethasone (Nasal) 232
Becloforte (AE, BH, CY, EG, IQ, IR, JO, KW, LB, LY, OM, QA, SA, SY, YE) *see* Beclomethasone (Nasal) 232
Becloforte (AE, BH, JO, QA, SA) *see* Beclomethasone (Systemic) 230
Beclomet (CH, DK, FI, MY, NO, SE, SG, TW) *see* Beclomethasone (Nasal) 232
Beclomet (DK, FI, NO, SE, SG, TH) *see* Beclomethasone (Systemic) 230
Beclomet Easyhaler (TH) *see* Beclomethasone (Nasal) 232
Beclomin (PK) *see* Beclomethasone (Nasal) 232
Beclomin (PK) *see* Beclomethasone (Systemic) 230
Beclonasal (EE, FI) *see* Beclomethasone (Nasal) 232
Beclone (FR) *see* Beclomethasone (Nasal) 232
Beclone (FR) *see* Beclomethasone (Systemic) 230
Beclophar (GB) *see* Beclomethasone (Nasal) 232
Beclophar (GB, IE) *see* Beclomethasone (Systemic) 230
Beclo-Rhino (FR) *see* Beclomethasone (Nasal) 232
Beclosol Aquoso (BR) *see* Beclomethasone (Nasal) 232
Beclovent Inhalador (CO) *see* Beclomethasone (Nasal) 232
Beclovent Inhalador (CO) *see* Beclomethasone (Systemic) 230
Beconase (AE, AT, BB, BF, BH, BJ, BM, BS, CH, CI, CO, CR, CY, DO, EE, EG, ET, FI, FR, GB, GH, GM, GN, GT, GY, HN, IQ, IR, JM, JO, KE, KW, LB, LR, LY, MA, ML, MR, MU, MW, MY, NE, NG, NI, NL, NZ, OM, PA, PE, PK, PR, PT, QA, SA, SC, SD, SL, SN, SV, SY, TH, TN, TT, TZ, UG, VE, YE, ZA, ZM, ZW) *see* Beclomethasone (Nasal) 232
Beconase Allergy & Hayfever 12 Hour (AU) *see* Beclomethasone (Nasal) 232
Beconase (VE) *see* Beclomethasone (Systemic) 230
Becotide (AE, AT, BE, BF, BG, BH, BJ, CI, CR, CY, CZ, DO, EE, ET, FR, GB, GH, GM, GN, GT, HK, HN, IE, IL, IQ, IR, IT, JO, KE, KW, LB, LR, LY, MA, ML, MR, MT, MU, MW, NE, NG, NI, NO, OM, PA, PT, QA, RU, SA, SC, SD, SG, SK, SL, SN, SV, SY, TN, TW, TZ, UG, YE, ZA, ZM, ZW) *see* Beclomethasone (Nasal) 232
Becotide (AE, BH, CH, CN, CR, CZ, DO, EG, GT, HN, IE, JO, NI, PA, QA, SA, SV) *see* Beclomethasone (Systemic) 230
Becta (KR) *see* Almitrine [INT] 92
Bedoc (GR) *see* Cyanocobalamin 515
Bedodeka (IL) *see* Cyanocobalamin 515
Bedol (GB, IE) *see* Estradiol (Systemic) 775
Bedoral (ZA) *see* Ketorolac (Systemic) 1146
Bedoxine (BE, LU) *see* Pyridoxine 1747
Bedoyecta (MX) *see* Pyridoxine 1747
Bedoyecta Pediátrica (MX) *see* Folic Acid, Cyanocobalamin, and Pyridoxine 921
Bedozane (LU) *see* Flutamide 907
Bedoze (PT) *see* Cyanocobalamin 515
Bedozil (BR) *see* Cyanocobalamin 515
Bedoz (KR) *see* Beraprost [INT] 251
Bedranol (AE, BB, BF, BJ, BM, BS, BZ, CI, ET, GH, GM, GN, GY, JM, KE, LB, LR, MA, ML, MR, MU, MW, NE, NG, SC, SD, SL, SN, SR, TN, TT, TZ, UG, ZM, ZW) *see* Propranolol 1731
Bedriol (UY) *see* Flunarizine [CAN/INT] 892
Beesix (ZA) *see* Pyridoxine 1747
Befarin (TH) *see* Warfarin 2186
Befibrat (DE) *see* Bezafibrate [CAN/INT] 261
Befizal (FR) *see* Bezafibrate [CAN/INT] 261
Beflavine (FR) *see* Riboflavin 1803
Beforal (CZ, PL) *see* Butorphanol 314
Befrin (KR) *see* Trifluoperazine 2102
Befurine (TW) *see* Clobetasol 468
Beglunina (ES) *see* Pyridoxine 1747
Behepan (SE) *see* Cyanocobalamin 515
Behepan (SE) *see* Hydroxocobalamin 1020
Behistin (TH) *see* Betahistine [CAN/INT] 252
Beibeisha (CN) *see* Josamycin [INT] 1141
Bei Ka Ming (CN) *see* Ketotifen (Ophthalmic) 1150
BeiKe (CN) *see* Tolterodine 2063
Bei Li (CN) *see* Naproxen 1427
Bei Luo (CN) *see* Loxoprofen [INT] 1255
Beinuoke (CN) *see* Cefaclor 372
Beiqi (CN) *see* Azelnidipine [INT] 214

Bei Shi Li (CN) *see* Betamethasone (Systemic) 253
Beisong (CN) *see* Betamethasone (Topical) 255
Bekanta (JP) *see* Methyldopa 1332
Bekarbon (ID) *see* Charcoal, Activated 416
Bekunis B (LU) *see* Bisacodyl 265
Belarmin (TR) *see* DiphenhydrAMINE (Systemic) 641
Belax (MY) *see* Beclomethasone (Nasal) 232
Belestar (AR) *see* Estrogens (Conjugated/Equine, Systemic) 787
Belifax (VN) *see* Omeprazole 1508
Bellacina (PY) *see* ChlorproMAZINE 429
Bellaface (EC, GT) *see* Estradiol and Dienogest 780
Bellafit N (CH) *see* Atropine 200
Bellapan (PL) *see* Atropine 200
Bellasthman Medihaler (DE) *see* Isoproterenol 1124
Belloid (IN) *see* Scopolamine (Systemic) 1870
Bellpino-Artin (IN) *see* Atropine 200
Bellune (HR) *see* Cyproterone and Ethinyl Estradiol [CAN/INT] 532
Belnarl (JP) *see* Beraprost [INT] 251
Beloc (CL) *see* Acebutolol 29
Beloc (AR, AT, CO, DE) *see* Metoprolol 1350
Beloc Duriles (AT) *see* Metoprolol 1350
Beloc Zok (CH) *see* Metoprolol 1350
Beloderm (HR, SK) *see* Betamethasone (Topical) 255
Beloken (IE) *see* Metoprolol 1350
Belomet (HR) *see* Cimetidine 438
Belotaxel (KR) *see* DOCEtaxel 656
Belustine (ES, FR, HN, IT, RU, TR) *see* Lomustine 1235
Bemase (TH) *see* Beclomethasone (Nasal) 232
Bemedrex Easyhaler (FR) *see* Beclomethasone (Nasal) 232
Bemedrex (FR) *see* Beclomethasone (Systemic) 230
Bemefor (PH) *see* Glyburide and Metformin 974
Bemfola (GB) *see* Follitropin Alfa 921
Bemin (EC) *see* Albuterol 69
Bemon (DE) *see* Betamethasone (Topical) 255
Benace (IN) *see* Benazepril 238
Benacid (TH) *see* Probenecid 1716
Benadon (AR, AT, CH, ES, GB, IE, IT, PT, SE) *see* Pyridoxine 1747
Benadryl Allergy Liquid Release (GB) *see* Cetirizine 411
Benadryl Allergy (PE) *see* DiphenhydrAMINE (Systemic) 641
Benadryl (AR, CO, EC, GR, IN, MY, PH, PK, TH, VE, VN) *see* DiphenhydrAMINE (Systemic) 641
Benadryl A (UY) *see* DiphenhydrAMINE (Systemic) 641
Benadryl for the Family Original (AU) *see* DiphenhydrAMINE (Systemic) 641
Benadryl One (PH) *see* Cetirizine 411
Benadryl Plus (GB) *see* Acrivastine and Pseudoephedrine 46
Bena (HK) *see* DiphenhydrAMINE (Systemic) 641
Benalipril (DE) *see* Enalapril 722
Benamine (KR) *see* Benzydamine [CAN/INT] 249
Benamine (TW) *see* DiphenhydrAMINE (Systemic) 641
Benanzyl (JP) *see* Clemastine 459
Benaprost (AR) *see* Terazosin 2001
Benaxima (MX) *see* Cefotaxime 382
Benaxona (MX) *see* CefTRIAXone 396
Bencavir (LU) *see* Famciclovir 843
Bencid (IN, TH) *see* Probenecid 1716
Bencipen (PE) *see* Aztreonam 220
Benclamet (IN) *see* Glyburide and Metformin 974
Bendam (AR) *see* Bendamustine 241
Bendamina (PE) *see* Benzydamine [CAN/INT] 249
Benda (TH) *see* Mebendazole [CAN/INT] 1274
Bendazole (JO) *see* Mebendazole [CAN/INT] 1274
Bendex-400 (ZA) *see* Albendazole 65
Bendinfus (BG) *see* Bendamustine 241
Bendit (IN) *see* Bendamustine 241
Bendol (HK) *see* DiphenhydrAMINE (Systemic) 641
Benecid Valdecasas (MX) *see* Probenecid 1716
Benedorm (AR) *see* Bromazepam [CAN/INT] 290
Benefix (AR, AT, AU, BE, BG, CN, CO, CY, CZ, DE, DK, EE, ES, FR, GB, GR, HK, HN, HR, IE, IL, IS, IT, JP, KR, LT, MT, NL, NO, PL, RO, RU, SA, SE, SI, SK, TR) *see* Factor IX (Recombinant) 841
Beneflur (ES, MX) *see* Fludarabine 890
Benemicin (RU, SK) *see* Rifampin 1804
Benemide (FR) *see* Probenecid 1716
Benemid (GB, GR, IE, NL, QA) *see* Probenecid 1716
Benerva (AE, AR, BB, BE, BH, BM, BR, BS, BZ, CH, CY, EG, ES, FR, GB, GH, GR, GY, IL, IQ, IR, IT, JM, JO, KE, KW, LB, LU, LY, NL, OM, PE, QA, SA, SE, SR, SY, TT, TZ, UG, YE, ZM) *see* Thiamine 2028
Benestan OD (PT) *see* Alfuzosin 84
Benestan (PT) *see* Alfuzosin 84
Benet (JP) *see* Risedronate 1816
Benetor (IE) *see* Olmesartan 1496
Beneuran (AT) *see* Thiamine 2028
Beneurol (LU) *see* Thiamine 2028
Beneuron (IN) *see* Thiamine 2028
Benflux (PT) *see* Ambroxol [INT] 109
Benhex Cream (NZ) *see* Lindane 1217
Benicar HCT (CR, GT, HN, NI, PA, SV) *see* Olmesartan and Hydrochlorothiazide 1498
Benil (HR) *see* Naphazoline (Nasal) 1426
Benil (SG) *see* GlyBURIDE 972
Benlysta (AU, BE, BR, CH, CY, CZ, DE, DK, EE, FR, GB, HK, HR, IL, IS, KR, LT, NL, NO, PH, RO, SA, SE, SG, SI, SK, TR) *see* Belimumab 235
Bennaston (MY) *see* Methadone 1311
Benocten (AE, CH) *see* DiphenhydrAMINE (Systemic) 641
Benofomin (ID) *see* MetFORMIN 1307
Benomet (ID) *see* Cimetidine 438
Benoquin (AR) *see* Balsalazide 226
Benosone (MY) *see* Betamethasone (Topical) 255
Benoxuric (ID) *see* Allopurinol 90
Benpen (AU, NZ) *see* Penicillin G (Parenteral/ Aqueous) 1611
Benperidol-neuraxpharm (DE) *see* Benperidol [INT] 244
Benpine (MY, SG, TH) *see* ChlordiazePOXIDE 422
Benstat (TH) *see* Finasteride 878
Bensulf (AR) *see* Thiopental [INT] 2029
Bentapen (PH) *see* Penicillin G (Parenteral/ Aqueous) 1611
Bentic (PY) *see* MetFORMIN 1307
Bentos (FR, JP, KR) *see* Befunolol [INT] 233
Bentril (KR) *see* Bromopride [INT] 292
Bentrop (AU, NZ) *see* Benztropine 248
Bentyl (BR, MX, TW) *see* Dicyclomine 622
Ben-U-Ron (CH, PT) *see* Acetaminophen 32
ben-u-ron (HU) *see* Acetaminophen 32
Benuron (JP) *see* Acetaminophen 32
Benuryl (IL) *see* Probenecid 1716
Benylan (DK) *see* DiphenhydrAMINE (Systemic) 641
Benylin 3.3 mg-D-E (CA) *see* Guaifenesin, Pseudoephedrine, and Codeine 989
Benylin DM-D (CA) *see* Pseudoephedrine and Dextromethorphan 1743
Benylin DM-D-E (CA) *see* Guaifenesin, Pseudoephedrine, and Dextromethorphan 989
Benzac Eritromicina (BR) *see* Erythromycin and Benzoyl Peroxide 765
Benzac Kombi (CO) *see* Erythromycin and Benzoyl Peroxide 765
Benzac Plus (CR, DO, GT, HN, NI, PA, PE, SV) *see* Erythromycin and Benzoyl Peroxide 765
Benzamin (KR) *see* Cyclobenzaprine 516
Benzamycin (CN, CY, KR, MX, MY, PH, SG, TR) *see* Erythromycin and Benzoyl Peroxide 765
Benzapen (PH) *see* Penicillin G Benzathine 1609
Benzetacil (MX) *see* Penicillin G Procaine 1613

Benzetacil (BR, EC, ES, MX) *see* Penicillin G Benzathine ... 1609
Benzetacil L.A. (AR, CO, PE, PY, UY, VE) *see* Penicillin G Benzathine ... 1609
Benzhexol (CN, LB, TH, TW, ZA) *see* Trihexyphenidyl ... 2103
Benzirin (CO) *see* Benzydamine [CAN/INT] ... 249
Benzol (PH) *see* Albendazole ... 65
Benzopain (JO) *see* OLANZapine ... 1491
Benzopin (ZA) *see* Diazepam ... 613
Benzoral (AR) *see* Hydroxocobalamin ... 1020
Benzycol Verde (CO) *see* Benzydamine [CAN/INT] ... 249
Beofenac (DE) *see* Aceclofenac [INT] ... 30
Beof (PY, UY) *see* Betaxolol (Systemic) ... 256
Bepanten (IT) *see* Dexpanthenol ... 606
Bepanthen (AE, AU, BE, CH, DE, EE, FI, HN, ID, KR, KW, LB, LT, LU, NZ, QA, RU, SA, SG, TH) *see* Dexpanthenol ... 606
Bepanthene (ES, PT, TR, UY) *see* Dexpanthenol ... 606
Bepanthol (EC) *see* Dexpanthenol ... 606
Bepantol (BR, ZA) *see* Dexpanthenol ... 606
Bepella (CZ) *see* Niacinamide ... 1446
Bephen (HK, LU) *see* Trifluridine ... 2103
Beporin (KR) *see* Bepotastine ... 250
Beprogel (HK, SG, TH) *see* Betamethasone (Topical) ... 255
Beprol (AU) *see* Bisoprolol ... 266
Bepronate (TH) *see* Betamethasone (Topical) ... 255
Beprosone (HK, ID, PH, SG, TH) *see* Betamethasone (Topical) ... 255
Bepsar (PH) *see* Losartan ... 1248
Beracle (KR) *see* Beraprost [INT] ... 251
Berasil (KR) *see* Beraprost [INT] ... 251
Berast (KR) *see* Beraprost [INT] ... 251
Berasus (JP) *see* Beraprost [INT] ... 251
Berea (ID) *see* Ambroxol [INT] ... 109
Bergoline (AU) *see* Cabergoline ... 319
Berifen (CR, GT, HN, NI, PA, SV) *see* Diclofenac (Systemic) ... 617
Beriglobina (BR) *see* Immune Globulin ... 1056
Beriglobin (AE, AT, BH, CH, CY, DE, EG, IQ, IR, JO, KW, LB, LY, OM, QA, SA, SE, SY, YE) *see* Immune Globulin ... 1056
Beriglobina P (CL) *see* Immune Globulin ... 1056
Beriglobin P (AR, TW) *see* Immune Globulin ... 1056
Berinert (AT, AU, BE, CH, CY, CZ, DK, ES, FI, FR, GB, HU, IL, KR, NL, NO, PT, RO, SE, SI, SK, TR) *see* C1 Inhibitor (Human) ... 315
Berinert P (AR) *see* C1 Inhibitor (Human) ... 315
Berinin P (CO) *see* Factor IX (Human) ... 840
Beriplex (IL) *see* Prothrombin Complex Concentrate (Human) [(Factors II, VII, IX, X), Protein C, and Protein S] ... 1738
Beriplex P/N (AR, AU, BR, DE, ES, GB, NL, SI) *see* Prothrombin Complex Concentrate (Human) [(Factors II, VII, IX, X), Protein C, and Protein S] ... 1738
Berivine (LU) *see* Riboflavin ... 1803
Berkamil (IE) *see* AMILoride ... 113
Berkolol (HK) *see* Propranolol ... 1731
Berlinsulin H 30 70 (DE) *see* Insulin NPH and Insulin Regular ... 1090
Berlipril (BG, HR) *see* Enalapril ... 722
Berlthyrox (DE) *see* Levothyroxine ... 1205
Bermin B (JP) *see* Thiamine ... 2028
Bernoflox (ID) *see* Ciprofloxacin (Systemic) ... 441
Berodan (KR) *see* Halcinonide ... 992
Berodual (AE, AR, AT, CL, CO, CZ, DE, DK, GR, HN, ID, KR, MY, NL, PH, PL, PT, PY, QA, RU, SI, TH, TW, UY, VE, VN) *see* Ipratropium and Fenoterol [CAN/INT] ... 1109
Berodual HFA (EC, PE) *see* Ipratropium and Fenoterol [CAN/INT] ... 1109
Berodualin (AT) *see* Ipratropium and Fenoterol [CAN/INT] ... 1109
Berodual N (CH, DE, EE, LT, MY, RO, SG, SI, SK) *see* Ipratropium and Fenoterol [CAN/INT] ... 1109
Berodual Solution (SG) *see* Ipratropium and Fenoterol [CAN/INT] ... 1109
Berotec (AE, AR, AT, AU, BE, BH, BR, CH, CZ, DE, DK, EC, EG, ES, FI, FR, GB, HR, HU, IE, KW, LU, NL, NO, NZ, PL, PT, QA, SA, SE, SI, VN) *see* Fenoterol [INT] ... 857
Berotec N (LT, PL, RO, SK) *see* Fenoterol [INT] ... 857
Berovent (GR) *see* Ipratropium and Albuterol ... 1109
Berrab P (HK) *see* Rabies Vaccine ... 1764
Bertocil (PT) *see* Betaxolol (Ophthalmic) ... 257
Bertocil (PT) *see* Betaxolol (Systemic) ... 256
Berubi-long (DE) *see* Hydroxocobalamin ... 1020
Besanta (TH) *see* Irbesartan ... 1110
Besartin (SG) *see* Irbesartan ... 1110
Besavar (GB) *see* Alfuzosin ... 84
Bescamin (PE) *see* Thalidomide ... 2022
Beselna (JP) *see* Imiquimod ... 1055
Besivance (AR, AU, HK, KR, MY, SG, TH) *see* Besifloxacin ... 251
Besmate (TW) *see* Ipratropium and Albuterol ... 1109
Besone (MY, TH) *see* Betamethasone (Topical) ... 255
Besonin Aqua (MY, TH) *see* Budesonide (Nasal) ... 296
Bespar (DE, GR) *see* BusPIRone ... 311
Besser (MX) *see* Dorzolamide and Timolol ... 673
Bestafen (MX) *see* Ibuprofen ... 1032
Bestalin (ID) *see* HydrOXYzine ... 1024
Bestatin (PH) *see* AtorvaSTATin ... 194
Bestatin (TH) *see* Simvastatin ... 1890
Bestidine (KR) *see* Famotidine ... 845
Besutin (TW) *see* Betahistine [CAN/INT] ... 252
Beta-2 (KR) *see* Terbutaline ... 2004
Betabactyl (DE) *see* Ticarcillin and Clavulanate Potassium [CAN/INT] ... 2038
Betabion (DE, ES) *see* Thiamine ... 2028
Betablok (ID) *see* Atenolol ... 189
Betacaine (IL) *see* Lidocaine (Topical) ... 1211
Betacar-15 (TH) *see* Beta-Carotene ... 251
Betacar (CL) *see* Atenolol ... 189
Betacard (IN, RU) *see* Atenolol ... 189
Beta-Cardone (GB, IE) *see* Sotalol ... 1927
Betacard (PH) *see* Carvedilol ... 367
Betac (BG, JO, KR, MY, PH, RO, SG, TR, TW) *see* Betaxolol (Systemic) ... 256
Betaclar (IT) *see* Befunolol [INT] ... 233
Betacor (AE, BH, CY, EG, IL, IQ, IR, JO, KW, LB, LY, OM, QA, SA, SY, YE) *see* Sotalol ... 1927
Betacorten (IL) *see* Betamethasone (Topical) ... 255
Betacortone (CH) *see* Halcinonide ... 992
Betacorton Solution (CZ, EE) *see* Halcinonide ... 992
Betacort (PK) *see* Betamethasone (Topical) ... 255
Betacor (TW) *see* Bisoprolol ... 266
Betaday (TH) *see* Atenolol ... 189
Betaderm (RO, VE) *see* Betamethasone (Topical) ... 255
Betades (IT) *see* Sotalol ... 1927
Betadran (FR) *see* Bupranolol [INT] ... 300
betadrenol (DE, IT) *see* Bupranolol [INT] ... 300
Betadrenol (SG) *see* Bupranolol [INT] ... 300
Betafact (IL, LB) *see* Factor IX (Human) ... 840
Betaferon (AE, AR, AT, AU, BE, BG, BH, BR, CH, CL, CN, CO, CR, CY, CZ, DE, DK, DO, EC, EE, ES, FI, FR, GB, GR, GT, HK, HN, HR, HU, ID, IE, IL, IS, IT, JO, KR, KW, LB, LT, MT, MX, MY, NI, NL, NO, NZ, PA, PE, PH, PL, PT, QA, RO, RU, SA, SE, SG, SI, SK, SV, TH, TR, TW, UY, ZA) *see* Interferon Beta-1b ... 1103
Betagalen (DE) *see* Betamethasone (Topical) ... 255
Betagan (AE, AR, AU, BE, BH, BR, CN, CY, DK, EG, ES, FR, GB, HK, IE, IL, IN, IQ, IR, JO, KR, KW, LB, LU, LY,

MX, MY, NL, NZ, OM, PT, QA, SA, SG, SY, TR, UY, YE, ZA) *see* Levobunolol 1194
Betagen (CL) *see* Levobunolol 1194
Betagen (AE) *see* Betahistine [CAN/INT] 252
Betaglid (HR) *see* Glimepiride 966
Betahistine-Eurogenerics (LU) *see* Betahistine [CAN/INT] 252
Betalans (ID) *see* Lansoprazole 1166
Betalitik (ID) *see* Ambroxol [INT] 109
Betalmic (SK) *see* Betaxolol (Ophthalmic) 257
Betaloc (AU, CN, CO, GB, HK, HN, HU, IN, KR, LT, MY, PH, PL, RO, RU, SI, SK, VN) *see* Metoprolol 1350
Betaloc CR (NZ) *see* Metoprolol 1350
Betaloc Zoc (BF, BJ, CI, ET, GH, GM, GN, KE, LR, MA, ML, MR, MU, MW, NE, NG, SC, SD, SL, SN, TN, TZ, UG, ZM, ZW) *see* Metoprolol 1350
Betaloc Zok (BH, CO, CY, EC, EE, HK, HR, HU, JO, KW, LT, PE, PK, PL, RO, SK, TR, TW) *see* Metoprolol 1350
Betaloc ZOK (VN) *see* Metoprolol 1350
Betaloc Zox (CN) *see* Metoprolol 1350
Betalol (TH) *see* Propranolol 1731
Betamana (PL) *see* Metipranolol 1345
Betamann (DE, LU) *see* Metipranolol 1345
Betamazole (TW) *see* Betamethasone and Clotrimazole 256
Betamed (AE) *see* Betamethasone (Topical) 255
Betamin (AU) *see* Thiamine 2028
Betamine (LU) *see* Thiamine 2028
Betam-Ophtal (ID) *see* Dexamethasone (Ophthalmic) 602
Betamox (MY) *see* Amoxicillin 130
Betamycin (TW) *see* Piperacillin and Tazobactam 1657
Betanase (AE, BH, CY, EG, IQ, IR, JO, KW, LB, LY, OM, QA, SA, SY, YE) *see* GlyBURIDE 972
Betanese 5 (BF, BJ, CI, ET, GH, GM, GN, KE, LR, MA, ML, MR, MU, MW, NE, NG, SC, SD, SL, SN, TN, TZ, UG, ZM, ZW) *see* GlyBURIDE 972
Betanis (JP) *see* Mirabegron 1375
Betanoid (ZA) *see* Betamethasone (Systemic) 253
Betanol (FR) *see* Metipranolol 1345
Beta (NZ) *see* Betamethasone (Topical) 255
Beta-One (ID, KR) *see* Bisoprolol 266
Beta Ophtiole (AT, BE, NL, PH, PT, SG, TW) *see* Metipranolol 1345
Betaperamide (ZA) *see* Loperamide 1236
Betaplex (CL) *see* Carvedilol 367
Betaren (IL) *see* Diclofenac (Systemic) 617
Betarretin (PE) *see* Tretinoin (Topical) 2099
Betarun (TW) *see* Betaxolol (Systemic) 256
Betasaerc (JO) *see* Betahistine [CAN/INT] 252
Betascan (TW) *see* Propranolol 1731
Betasel (AR) *see* Betaxolol (Ophthalmic) 257
Betasel (AR) *see* Betaxolol (Systemic) 256
Betasel S (AR) *see* Betaxolol (Ophthalmic) 257
Betasel S (AR) *see* Betaxolol (Systemic) 256
Betaserc (AE, AT, BE, BG, BH, BR, CH, CY, CZ, DK, EC, EE, EG, FI, GR, HK, HN, HR, HU, ID, KW, LT, LU, MY, NL, NO, PE, PH, PL, PT, QA, RO, RU, SA, SG, SI, TR, TW, VN) *see* Betahistine [CAN/INT] 252
Beta-Sol (AU) *see* Thiamine 2028
Betasone (AE) *see* Betamethasone (Systemic) 253
Betasone (HK, LB, SA) *see* Betamethasone (Topical) 255
Betastin (JO) *see* Betahistine [CAN/INT] 252
Beta-Tabs (AU) *see* Thiamine 2028
Beta-Timelets (AE, BH, CY, EG, IL, IQ, IR, JO, KW, LB, LY, OM, QA, SA, SY, YE) *see* Propranolol 1731
Betatop Ge (FR) *see* Atenolol 189
Betaval (BH, JO) *see* Betamethasone (Topical) 255
Betavate (KR) *see* Clobetasol 468
Betavert (PH) *see* Betahistine [CAN/INT] 252
Betavin (CO) *see* Beta-Carotene 251
Betawin (MY) *see* Metoprolol 1350
Betaxa (BG) *see* Betaxolol (Ophthalmic) 257
Betaxen (PK) *see* Betaxolol (Ophthalmic) 257
Betaxen (PK) *see* Betaxolol (Systemic) 256
Betaxol (VE) *see* Betaxolol (Ophthalmic) 257
Betaxol (VE) *see* Betaxolol (Systemic) 256
Betazok (PH) *see* Metoprolol 1350
Betazon (BG) *see* Betamethasone (Topical) 255
Beten (MY) *see* Atenolol 189
Betenol (KR) *see* Atenolol 189
Betesil (GB) *see* Betamethasone (Topical) 255
Betetrim (TW) *see* BuPROPion 305
Bethacil (IT) *see* Ampicillin and Sulbactam 145
Betiral (GR) *see* Ornidazole [INT] 1522
Betistin (UY) *see* Betahistine [CAN/INT] 252
Betmiga (AU, BE, CH, CY, CZ, DE, DK, EE, ES, FR, GB, HK, HR, IS, KR, LT, NL, NO, RO, SE, SI, SK, TR) *see* Mirabegron 1375
Betnelan (IN, PK) *see* Betamethasone (Systemic) 253
Betnelan (QA) *see* Betamethasone (Topical) 255
Betnesol (BE, CH, FR, IL, IN, PK) *see* Betamethasone (Systemic) 253
Betneval (FR) *see* Betamethasone (Topical) 255
Betnoderm (SE) *see* Betamethasone (Topical) 255
Betnovat (DK, IS, LT, NO, SE) *see* Betamethasone (Topical) 255
Betnovate (AE, AT, AU, BG, BH, BR, CH, CL, CY, CZ, EE, ES, GB, GR, HK, IL, IN, JO, KW, LB, MX, NZ, PH, PT, QA, SA, SG, TH, TR, UY, VE, VN) *see* Betamethasone (Topical) 255
Betolvex (CH, DK, FI, NO, SE) *see* Cyanocobalamin 515
Betolvex[inj.] (SE) *see* Cyanocobalamin 515
Betoptic (AE, AT, AU, BE, BF, BH, BJ, BR, CI, CL, CO, CY, CZ, DK, EG, ET, FR, GB, GH, GM, GN, GR, HN, HR, IE, IQ, IR, IT, JO, KE, KR, KW, LB, LR, LY, MA, ML, MR, MT, MU, MW, MY, NE, NG, NL, NO, NZ, OM, PK, PT, PY, QA, RO, RU, SA, SC, SD, SE, SK, SL, SN, SY, TN, TR, TW, TZ, UG, UY, YE, ZA, ZM, ZW) *see* Betaxolol (Ophthalmic) 257
Betoptic S (AU, BG, BR, CH, CL, CN, CO, CR, CZ, EE, FI, GT, HK, HU, IL, KR, MY, NI, NO, NZ, PA, PH, PL, PY, RO, SE, SG, SV, TH, TR, TW, UY, VE, VN, ZA) *see* Betaxolol (Ophthalmic) 257
Betoptima (DE, ID) *see* Betaxolol (Ophthalmic) 257
Betoptima (DE, ID) *see* Betaxolol (Systemic) 256
Betoquin (AU) *see* Betaxolol (Ophthalmic) 257
Betoquin (AU) *see* Betaxolol (Systemic) 256
Betram (PH) *see* TraMADol 2074
Betrion (HR) *see* Mupirocin 1404
Betris (TH) *see* Betahistine [CAN/INT] 252
Betsol "Z" (MX) *see* Sodium Bicarbonate 1901
Bettamousse (IL) *see* Betamethasone (Topical) 255
Bevacol (JO, LB, SA) *see* Mebeverine [INT] 1275
Bevidam (VE) *see* Benzydamine [CAN/INT] 249
Bevispas (ZA) *see* Mebeverine [INT] 1275
Bevitine (FR) *see* Thiamine 2028
Bevitol (AT) *see* Thiamine 2028
Bevoren (LU) *see* GlyBURIDE 972
Bewel 300 (TH) *see* Irbesartan 1110
Bexedan (UY) *see* Bromhexine [INT] 291
Bexidermil (ES) *see* Magnesium Salicylate 1265
Bexil (PH) *see* DiphenhydrAMINE (Systemic) 641
Bexinor (SG) *see* Norfloxacin 1475
Bexivit (GR) *see* Pyridoxine 1747
Bexolo (TW) *see* Betaxolol (Systemic) 256
Bextra (BR) *see* Parecoxib [INT] 1576
Bexxam (PH) *see* Meloxicam 1283
Bezacur (LU) *see* Bezafibrate [CAN/INT] 261
Bezafibrat (DE, DK) *see* Bezafibrate [CAN/INT] 261
Bezalip (AE, AR, AT, BH, CY, CZ, EG, FI, GB, GR, HK, HN, HU, IE, IN, IT, JO, JP, KW, MX, NL, NO, NZ, PK, PT, QA, SA, SE, TH, TW, VE, ZA) *see* Bezafibrate [CAN/INT] 261

Bezalip PR (TR) *see* Bezafibrate [CAN/INT] 261
Bezalip Retard (BH, EC, HK, IN, KR, KW, MX, NZ, PE, PT, QA, SA, TW, UY) *see* Bezafibrate [CAN/INT] 261
Bezalip Rwetard (AE) *see* Bezafibrate [CAN/INT] 261
Bezalon (TW) *see* Benzydamine [CAN/INT] 249
Bezamidin (CZ, HR, HU, PL) *see* Bezafibrate [CAN/INT] 261
Bezamil (TH) *see* Bezafibrate [CAN/INT] 261
Bezam (PH) *see* AmLODIPine 123
Bezart (PH) *see* Irbesartan 1110
Bezastad (PH) *see* Bezafibrate [CAN/INT] 261
Bezatol SR (JP) *see* Bezafibrate [CAN/INT] 261
Bglau (PT) *see* Brimonidine (Ophthalmic) 288
Bialminal (PT) *see* PHENobarbital 1632
Bianos (EC, PE) *see* Secnidazole [INT] 1872
Biascor (AR, PY) *see* Labetalol 1151
Biatron (ID) *see* MetroNIDAZOLE (Systemic) 1353
Biaxin HP (DE) *see* Clarithromycin 456
Biaxsig (AU) *see* Roxithromycin [INT] 1853
Bica (AR) *see* Calcium Carbonate 327
Bicadex (HR, PH) *see* Bicalutamide 262
Bicalan (EE) *see* Bicalutamide 262
Bicalox (NZ) *see* Bicalutamide 262
Bicalude (KR) *see* Bicalutamide 262
Bicalu (KR) *see* Bicalutamide 262
Bicamide (IL, LB) *see* Bicalutamide 262
Bicapros (PH) *see* Bicalutamide 262
Bicard (AU) *see* Bisoprolol 266
Bicebid (VN) *see* Cefixime 380
Bicillin L-A (AU, NZ) *see* Penicillin G Benzathine 1609
Bicillin LA 1.2 (ZA) *see* Penicillin G Benzathine 1609
Bicillin LA 2.4 (ZA) *see* Penicillin G Benzathine 1609
Biclar (BE, LU) *see* Clarithromycin 456
Biclin (ES, MX, PT) *see* Amikacin 111
Bicloc (EC) *see* Bicalutamide 262
Bicnu (CL, HU) *see* Carmustine 364
BiCNU (AR, CO, CZ, FR, GB, IE, KR, MX, NZ, PH, PT, TW, UY, ZA) *see* Carmustine 364
BICNU (EC, VN) *see* Carmustine 364
Bicolax (ID) *see* Bisacodyl 265
Bicol (TR) *see* Carvedilol 367
Biconcilina BZ (EC) *see* Penicillin G Benzathine 1609
Biconcor (BR, MX) *see* Bisoprolol and Hydrochlorothiazide 267
Bicor (AU) *see* Bisoprolol 266
Bicosa (KR) *see* Losartan 1248
Bicrolid (ID, SG) *see* Clarithromycin 456
Bidicef (ID) *see* Cefadroxil 372
Bidimalaquin (VN) *see* Chloroquine 424
Bidopar (TW) *see* Carbidopa and Levodopa 351
Bidrostat (AR, PY) *see* Bicalutamide 262
Bi-Euglucon M "5" (MX) *see* Glyburide and Metformin 974
Bi-Euglucon M (EC, PE, UY) *see* Glyburide and Metformin 974
Bi-Euglucon (CO, IT, VE) *see* Glyburide and Metformin 974
Bifantrel (CO) *see* Pyrantel Pamoate 1744
Bifazol (IT) *see* Bifonazole [INT] 264
Bifen Cataplasma (KR) *see* Flurbiprofen (Systemic) 906
Bifene (PT) *see* Fenbufen [INT] 852
Bifen (HK, SG) *see* Ibuprofen 1032
Biferce (ID, SG) *see* Ascorbic Acid 178
Bifiteral (BE, DE, LU) *see* Lactulose 1156
Bifix (FR) *see* Nifuroxazide [INT] 1454
Bifokey (ES) *see* Bifonazole [INT] 264
Bifomyk (DE) *see* Bifonazole [INT] 264
Bifonal (AR) *see* Bifonazole [INT] 264
Bifonazol R.O. (AR) *see* Bifonazole [INT] 264
Bifon (DE) *see* Bifonazole [INT] 264
Biforge (KR) *see* Amlodipine and Valsartan 126
Bifosa (IN) *see* Alendronate 79
Bifracard (MX) *see* Zofenopril [INT] 2206
Bifril (AT, DE, DK, FI, GB, IE, IS, IT, LB, NO, SE, SG) *see* Zofenopril [INT] 2206
Big-Ben (TH) *see* Mebendazole [CAN/INT] 1274
Bigemax (VN) *see* Gemcitabine 952
Biguax (CO) *see* MetFORMIN 1307
Bikalen (TR) *see* Bicalutamide 262
Biklin (AR, AT, DE, FI, SE, VE) *see* Amikacin 111
Bilaten (CL) *see* Candesartan 335
Bileco (AR) *see* Bleomycin 270
Bilem (TH) *see* Tamoxifen 1971
Bileni (EE, LT) *see* Azelastine and Fluticasone 214
Bilenzima (BR) *see* Bromopride [INT] 292
Bilgrel (VN) *see* Clopidogrel 484
Bi Li (CN) *see* Bromhexine [INT] 291
Bilina (ES) *see* Levocabastine (Ophthalmic) [CAN/INT] 1195
Bi-Love-G (JP) *see* Riboflavin 1803
Biloxcin (VN) *see* Ofloxacin (Systemic) 1490
Biltricide (AE, AU, BF, BH, BJ, CI, CY, DE, EG, ET, FR, GH, GM, GN, GR, HK, IL, IQ, IR, JO, KE, KW, LB, LR, LY, MA, ML, MR, MU, MW, NE, NG, NL, OM, QA, SA, SC, SD, SL, SN, SY, TN, TZ, UG, YE, ZA, ZM, ZW) *see* Praziquantel 1702
Bimat-T (VN) *see* Bimatoprost and Timolol [INT] 264
Bimat (VN) *see* Bimatoprost 264
Bimaz (VN) *see* Carbimazole [INT] 356
Bimicot (AR) *see* Bifonazole [INT] 264
Bimxan (MX) *see* Amoxicillin 130
Binaldan (CH) *see* Loperamide 1236
Binarin (MX) *see* Epirubicin 739
Binelax ER (KR) *see* Cyclobenzaprine 516
Bingsaiyou (CN) *see* Propylthiouracil 1735
Binicapin (KR) *see* NiCARdipine 1446
Binoclar (CR, DO, GT, NI, PA, SV, VN) *see* Clarithromycin 456
Binocrit (CH, GB, HR, MY, RO, TR) *see* Epoetin Alfa 742
Binotal (AT, BR, CO, MX, UY) *see* Ampicillin 141
Binozyt (ID, KR, SG, TH, VN) *see* Azithromycin (Systemic) 216
Biocaf (AE, BH, CY, EG, IL, IQ, IR, JO, KW, LB, LY, OM, QA, SA, SY, YE) *see* Chloramphenicol 421
Biocalyptol (FR) *see* Pholcodine [INT] 1646
Biocarbon (MY) *see* Charcoal, Activated 416
Biocardin (BG) *see* Dipyridamole 652
Biocatines D2 (ES) *see* Ergocalciferol 753
Biocef (AT) *see* Cefpodoxime 388
Biocef (ES) *see* Ceftibuten 394
Biocilin (MX) *see* Filgrastim 875
Biocil (MY) *see* Ampicillin 141
Bioclavid (AE, BH, CY, DE, DK, EG, IQ, IR, JO, KW, LB, LY, OM, PH, QA, SA, SE, SY, YE) *see* Amoxicillin and Clavulanate 133
Bioclavid Forte (PH) *see* Amoxicillin and Clavulanate 133
Bioclox (IN) *see* Cloxacillin [CAN/INT] 488
Biocort (PH) *see* Hydrocortisone (Systemic) 1013
Biocort (ZA) *see* Hydrocortisone (Topical) 1014
Biocoryl (ES) *see* Procainamide 1716
Biocristin (IN) *see* VinCRIStine 2163
Biocronil (CO) *see* Enalapril 722
Biocronil (CO) *see* Enalapril and Hydrochlorothiazide 725
Biodacyna (LT) *see* Amikacin 111
Biodalgic (FR) *see* TraMADol 2074
Biodexan Ofteno (MX) *see* Neomycin, Polymyxin B, and Dexamethasone 1437
Biodexan Ofteno (MX) *see* Polymyxin B 1676
Biodiabes (UY) *see* ChlorproPAMIDE 429
Biodone Extra Forte (NZ) *see* Methadone 1311
Biodone Forte (AU, NZ) *see* Methadone 1311
Biodone (NZ) *see* Methadone 1311
Biodoxi (IN) *see* Doxycycline 689
Biodramina (ES) *see* DimenhyDRINATE 637

Biodribin (PL) *see* Cladribine 455
Biodrop (AR) *see* Dorzolamide 673
Biodroxil (AE, BG, BH, CY, EG, IL, IQ, IR, JO, KW, LB, LY, OM, PE, QA, SA, SY, VN, YE) *see* Cefadroxil 372
Biodroxyl (VE) *see* Cefadroxil 372
Bioepicyna (PL) *see* Epirubicin 739
Biofanal (DE) *see* Nystatin (Topical) 1482
Biofazolin (PL) *see* CeFAZolin 373
Biofenac (BE, CZ, GR, NL, PT) *see* Aceclofenac [INT] 30
Bioferon (PY, TH, UY) *see* Interferon Alfa-2b 1096
Biofigran (CO) *see* Filgrastim 875
Biofilen (MX) *see* Atenolol 189
Biofilgran (MX) *see* Filgrastim 875
Biofloxin (IN) *see* Norfloxacin 1475
Bioflutin-N (DE) *see* Etilefrine [INT] 815
Bio-Folic (BE) *see* Folic Acid 919
Biofradin (ES) *see* Neomycin 1436
Biogam Ca (BE) *see* Calcium Gluconate 330
Biogam F (BE) *see* Fluoride 895
Biogam Fe (BE) *see* Ferrous Gluconate 870
Biogam Mg (BE, CH) *see* Magnesium Gluconate 1263
Biogaracin (IN) *see* Gentamicin (Systemic) 959
Biogen (JP) *see* Thiamine 2028
Biogen (PE) *see* ClomiPHENE 473
Biogenta Oftalmica (CO) *see* Gentamicin (Ophthalmic) 962
Biogenta Oftalmica (CO) *see* Gentamicin (Systemic) 959
Biogesic (SG) *see* Acetaminophen 32
Biogesic Suspension (HK) *see* Acetaminophen 32
Bioglumin (ES) *see* ChlorproPAMIDE 429
Biogrisin (PL) *see* Griseofulvin 985
Bio-Hep-B (IL) *see* Hepatitis B Vaccine (Recombinant) 1002
Biohulin NPH (KR) *see* Insulin NPH 1089
Biojoint (IN) *see* Diacerein [INT] 613
Biokacin (MX, PY) *see* Amikacin 111
Biolac (PH) *see* Lactulose 1156
Biol (CH) *see* Bisoprolol 266
Biol Comp (CH) *see* Bisoprolol and Hydrochlorothiazide 267
Biolectra (AT) *see* Calcium Carbonate 327
Biolon (IL, KR) *see* Hyaluronate and Derivatives 1006
Biolytan (MX) *see* Disopyramide 653
Biomab EGFR (IN) *see* Nimotuzumab [INT] 1457
Biomag (IT) *see* Cimetidine 438
Biomixin (MX) *see* Doxycycline 689
Biopain (PH) *see* Acetaminophen 32
Bioplatino (PE) *see* CISplatin 448
Bioprexum (ID) *see* Perindopril 1623
Bioprexum Plus (ID) *see* Perindopril and Indapamide [CAN/INT] 1626
Biopulmin (CL) *see* Erdosteine [INT] 753
Bioquin (CL) *see* Erythromycin and Sulfisoxazole 765
Bioreucam (PT) *see* Tenoxicam [INT] 2001
Biorgan (AR) *see* Trimebutine [CAN/INT] 2103
Biorix (TW) *see* Moclobemide [CAN/INT] 1384
Biorphen (GB) *see* Orphenadrine 1522
Biorrub (BR) *see* DOXOrubicin (Conventional) 679
Biosal (IT) *see* Nimesulide [INT] 1456
Bioselenium (CR, DO, GT, HN, NI, PA, SV) *see* Selenium Sulfide 1877
Biosim (IN) *see* Simvastatin 1890
Biosint (MX) *see* Cefotaxime 382
Biosoviran (IT) *see* Pipemidic Acid [INT] 1655
Biosporin (EC) *see* CycloSPORINE (Systemic) 522
Biostate (AU, HK, NZ, SG) *see* Antihemophilic Factor/von Willebrand Factor Complex (Human) 154
Biosupressin (HU) *see* Hydroxyurea 1021
Biotamoxal (AR) *see* Amoxicillin 130
Biotam (VN) *see* Oxacillin 1528
Biotax (IL) *see* PACLitaxel (Conventional) 1550
Biotax (IN) *see* Cefotaxime 382
Biotine (SG) *see* Tetracycline 2017
Biotonus (PE) *see* Mosapride [INT] 1401
Biotrexate (IN) *see* Methotrexate 1322
Biotriax (ID) *see* CefTRIAXone 396
Biotum (PL) *see* CefTAZidime 392
Biovinate (PH) *see* CARBOplatin 357
Biovir (BR) *see* Lamivudine and Zidovudine 1160
Biovital Vitamin C (HU) *see* Ascorbic Acid 178
Bioyl (TW) *see* Bisacodyl 265
Biozac (BG) *see* FLUoxetine 899
Biozole (MY) *see* Fluconazole 885
Bipax (LB) *see* Clidinium and Chlordiazepoxide 460
Biphasil (ZA) *see* Ethinyl Estradiol and Levonorgestrel 803
Biplatinex (VE) *see* CARBOplatin 357
Biprel (CN) *see* Perindopril and Indapamide [CAN/INT] 1626
BiPreterax (AR, BB, BM, BS, BZ, CO, CR, DE, DO, FR, GT, GY, HN, IE, JM, NI, NL, PA, PE, PH, PK, PR, SR, SV, TT, VE) *see* Perindopril and Indapamide [CAN/INT] 1626
Bipreterax Arginine (AE, KW, LB, SA) *see* Perindopril and Indapamide [CAN/INT] 1626
Bipreterax (BH, QA) *see* Perindopril and Indapamide [CAN/INT] 1626
Biprin (CO) *see* Pyridoxine 1747
Bi-Profenid (BB, BS, FR, JM, NL) *see* Ketoprofen 1145
Bipro (ID) *see* Bisoprolol 266
Biprosta (IN) *see* Bicalutamide 262
Biraxin (PH) *see* Acyclovir (Systemic) 47
Birobin (AT) *see* Metolazone 1348
Bi-Rofenid (BE) *see* Ketoprofen 1145
Bisacod (TH) *see* Bisacodyl 265
Bisakodils (EE) *see* Bisacodyl 265
Bisalax (AU, BG) *see* Bisacodyl 265
Bisanorin (JP) *see* Riboflavin 1803
Bisbacter (CO) *see* Bismuth 265
Bisbon (KR) *see* Alendronate 79
Bisco (PH) *see* Bisacodyl 265
Biscor (ID, JO, SA, TW) *see* Bisoprolol 266
Biscosal (JP) *see* Fluocinonide 894
Biseko (PL) *see* Albumin 67
Biseptol (BG) *see* Sulfamethoxazole and Trimethoprim 1946
Bi Si Ling (CN) *see* Aniracetam [INT] 150
Bislan (MY, SG) *see* Bromhexine [INT] 291
Bisloc (TH) *see* Bisoprolol 266
Bismucar (PE) *see* Bismuth 265
Bismultin (GR) *see* Econazole 703
Bismuthum subgallicum (PL) *see* Bismuth 265
Bismutol (EC, PE) *see* Bismuth 265
Bismutsubsalicylat-Steigerwald (DE) *see* Bismuth 265
Biso 5 (TW) *see* Bisoprolol 266
Bisocor (LB) *see* Bisoprolol 266
Bisofan (HK) *see* Bromhexine [INT] 291
Bisohexal (SG) *see* Bisoprolol 266
Bisolangin (NL) *see* Ambroxol [INT] 109
Bisolex (HR) *see* Bromhexine [INT] 291
Bisol (MY) *see* Bisoprolol 266
Bisolol (IL) *see* Bisoprolol 266
Bisolvex (PH) *see* Bromhexine [INT] 291
Bisolvon (AE, AR, AT, AU, BE, BH, BR, CH, CL, CO, CY, CZ, DE, DK, EG, ES, FI, FR, GR, HN, HR, ID, IE, IN, IT, JO, KR, KW, LB, LU, MX, NL, NO, NZ, PE, PH, PK, PT, PY, QA, SA, SE, SI, TH, UY, VE, VN) *see* Bromhexine [INT] 291
Bisolvon[vet.] (CH) *see* Bromhexine [INT] 291
Bisolvon Chesty (AU) *see* Bromhexine [INT] 291
Bisomerck (DE) *see* Bisoprolol 266
Bisono Tape (JP) *see* Bisoprolol 266
Bisosten (PH) *see* Bisoprolol 266
Bisoten (JO) *see* Bisoprolol 266
Bisovell (ID) *see* Bisoprolol 266
Bispec (IN) *see* Solifenacin 1917

Bispro (AU) *see* Bisoprolol ... 266
Bi Su Fu (CN) *see* Diclofenac (Systemic) ... 617
Bisulase (JP) *see* Riboflavin ... 1803
Bisuran (BR) *see* Bromhexine [INT] ... 291
Bitammon (CZ) *see* Ampicillin and Sulbactam ... 145
Biteven (TW) *see* Bisoprolol ... 266
Bi-Tildiem (FR) *see* Diltiazem ... 634
Bitol Sodium (PK) *see* Thiopental [INT] ... 2029
Bittle (HK) *see* Clindamycin (Topical) ... 464
Bituvitan (JP) *see* Riboflavin ... 1803
Bivaflo (IN) *see* Bivalirudin ... 268
Bivasave (IN) *see* Bivalirudin ... 268
Bivit (IT) *see* Pyridoxine ... 1747
Bladderon (JP) *see* FlavoxATE ... 881
Bladuril (AR, CO, DO, EC, PE, PY) *see* FlavoxATE ... 881
Blastocarb (CL) *see* CARBOplatin ... 357
Blastocarb RU (MX) *see* CARBOplatin ... 357
Blastolem (CL, CO) *see* CISplatin ... 448
Blastolem RU (MX) *see* CISplatin ... 448
Blastomat (HR, RO) *see* Temozolomide ... 1991
Blastovin PF (IL) *see* VinBLAStine ... 2160
Blastovin (PY) *see* VinBLAStine ... 2160
Blaztere (IN) *see* Zoledronic Acid ... 2206
Bledstop (ID) *see* Methylergonovine ... 1333
Blef-10 (CO, PE) *see* Sulfacetamide (Ophthalmic) ... 1943
Blefamide (CO) *see* Sulfacetamide and Prednisolone ... 1944
Blefamide SF (EC, MX) *see* Sulfacetamide and Prednisolone ... 1944
Blefamide SOP (CO, MX) *see* Sulfacetamide and Prednisolone ... 1944
Bleminal (DE) *see* Allopurinol ... 90
Blenamax (AU, RU, SG, TW) *see* Bleomycin ... 270
Blend-A-Med (DE) *see* Chlorhexidine Gluconate ... 422
Blenoxane (BR, EC, EG, ZA) *see* Bleomycin ... 270
Bleocin (AE, BG, CZ, EE, EG, GR, HK, HN, HU, ID, IN, JO, JP, KR, LB, MY, PE, PL, PT, QA, SA, SG, TH, TR, TW, VN) *see* Bleomycin ... 270
Bleocina (UY) *see* Bleomycin ... 270
Bleocin-S (MY) *see* Bleomycin ... 270
Bleocip (LB) *see* Bleomycin ... 270
Bleocris (PY) *see* Bleomycin ... 270
Bleo (HK) *see* Bleomycin ... 270
Bleolem (CO, MX, TH) *see* Bleomycin ... 270
Bleomax (MX) *see* Bleomycin ... 270
Bleomicina (ES, IT) *see* Bleomycin ... 270
Bleomycin (AT, CH, DK, FI, GB, NO, SE) *see* Bleomycin ... 270
Bleomycine (BE, FR, LU, NL) *see* Bleomycin ... 270
Bleomycin PFI (IL) *see* Bleomycin ... 270
Bleomycinum (DE) *see* Bleomycin ... 270
Bleph-10 (AE, AU, BH, CY, EG, IQ, IR, JO, KW, LB, LY, NZ, OM, QA, SA, SY, YE) *see* Sulfacetamide (Ophthalmic) ... 1943
Bleph-30 (AE, BH, CY, EG, IQ, IR, JO, KW, LB, LY, OM, QA, SA, SY, YE) *see* Sulfacetamide (Ophthalmic) ... 1943
Blephamide (AT, AU, BG, BH, CH, DE, EG, KW, LB, QA, SA, TW) *see* Sulfacetamide and Prednisolone ... 1944
Blesifen (ID) *see* ClomiPHENE ... 473
Blexit (CL) *see* Bleomycin ... 270
Blisscolic (PK) *see* Dicyclomine ... 622
Blistra (ID) *see* NiCARdipine ... 1446
Blocadren (AT, IT, LB, QA) *see* Timolol (Systemic) ... 2042
Blocalcin (HU, SK) *see* Diltiazem ... 634
Blocamine (AR) *see* Labetalol ... 1151
Blocanol (FI) *see* Timolol (Ophthalmic) ... 2043
Bloc-Med (PH) *see* Captopril ... 342
Bloflex (PH) *see* Cephalexin ... 405
Bloicin-S (PH) *see* Bleomycin ... 270
Bloket (PY) *see* Atenolol ... 189
Blokium (AE, BF, BH, BJ, CI, CY, EG, ET, GH, GM, GN, GR, HU, IQ, IR, JO, KE, KW, LB, LR, LY, MA, ML, MR, MU, MW, NE, NG, OM, PY, QA, SA, SC, SD, SL, SN, SY, TN, TZ, UG, VE, YE, ZA, ZM, ZW) *see* Atenolol ... 189
Blopresid (IT) *see* Candesartan and Hydrochlorothiazide ... 338
Blopress-D (CL) *see* Candesartan and Hydrochlorothiazide ... 338
Blopress (AE, AT, BB, BH, BM, BR, BS, BZ, CH, CN, CR, CY, DE, DO, EC, EG, GT, GY, HK, HN, ID, IQ, IR, IT, JM, JO, JP, KW, LB, LY, MX, MY, NI, NL, OM, PA, PE, PH, PK, PR, QA, SA, SG, SR, SV, SY, TH, TT, TW, VE, YE) *see* Candesartan ... 335
Blopress Comp (SE) *see* Candesartan and Hydrochlorothiazide ... 338
Blopress Plus (AE, BH, CH, CR, EC, GT, HK, HN, ID, JO, KW, LB, NI, PA, PE, PH, QA, SA, SV, TH, TW, UY) *see* Candesartan and Hydrochlorothiazide ... 338
Blorec (ID) *see* Carvedilol ... 367
Blossom (CN) *see* Venlafaxine ... 2150
Blotex (MX) *see* Atenolol ... 189
Blow (CO) *see* Montelukast ... 1392
Blox 8 (PY) *see* Candesartan ... 335
Blox (CL) *see* Candesartan ... 335
Blox-D (CL, EC, PY) *see* Candesartan and Hydrochlorothiazide ... 338
Bloxan (HR, RO) *see* Metoprolol ... 1350
Bloxiverz (BM) *see* Neostigmine ... 1438
Bluetec (VN) *see* Cetirizine ... 411
Blugat (MX) *see* Gabapentin ... 943
Blunid (PK) *see* Nimesulide [INT] ... 1456
Bluxantron (EC) *see* MitoXANtrone ... 1382
Bo Bang Lin (CN) *see* Aniracetam [INT] ... 150
Bobei (CN) *see* CARBOplatin ... 357
Bobrusie (PL) *see* Fluoride ... 895
Bocartin (VN) *see* CARBOplatin ... 357
Bocatriol (DE) *see* Calcitriol ... 323
Bocycline (TW) *see* Tetracycline ... 2017
Bocytin (TH) *see* Carbocisteine [INT] ... 357
Boda (CN) *see* Doxapram ... 673
Bodrexin Pilek Alergi (ID) *see* Chlorpheniramine and Pseudoephedrine ... 427
Boidan (JP) *see* Amantadine ... 105
Bokey (SG, TW) *see* Aspirin ... 180
Bolano (TW) *see* Dorzolamide ... 673
Bolaxin (TW) *see* Methocarbamol ... 1320
Bolenic (TW) *see* Zoledronic Acid ... 2206
Boltin (ES) *see* Tibolone [INT] ... 2035
Bomecon (TW) *see* SulfaSALAzine ... 1950
Bomex (MY, SG) *see* Brompheniramine ... 292
Bomine (TH) *see* Brompheniramine ... 292
Bonabon B!2 (JP) *see* Riboflavin ... 1803
Bonacal (SG) *see* Calcium Carbonate ... 327
Bonac Gel (PE) *see* Erythromycin (Topical) ... 765
Bonadoxina (CR, GT, HN, MX, NI, PA, SV) *see* Meclizine ... 1277
Bonaid (KR) *see* Alendronate ... 79
Bonalerg - D (GT) *see* Loratadine and Pseudoephedrine ... 1242
Bonalerg (GT) *see* Loratadine ... 1241
Bonaling-A (KR) *see* DimenhyDRINATE ... 637
Bonalon (JP) *see* Alendronate ... 79
Bonamina (CN) *see* Meclizine ... 1277
Bonamine (PH) *see* Meclizine ... 1277
Bonapex (EG) *see* Alendronate ... 79
Bonat (IL) *see* Ibandronate ... 1028
Bonatranquan (DE) *see* LORazepam ... 1243
Boncordin (AR) *see* Benazepril ... 238
Bondi (ID) *see* Diacerein [INT] ... 613
Bondiol (DE) *see* Alfacalcidol [CAN/INT] ... 82
Bondormin (IL) *see* Brotizolam [INT] ... 293
Bondronat IV (PH) *see* Ibandronate ... 1028
Bondronat (AE, AT, AU, BE, BH, CH, CL, CN, CO, CZ, DE, DK, EC, EE, FR, GR, HK, HR, HU, ID, IE, IS, IT,

KW, LB, MX, NL, NO, NZ, PE, PL, QA, RO, RU, SA, SE, SI, SK, TH, TW) *see* Ibandronate 1028
Bondronat (AT, CH, DE, DK, ES, FR, SE) *see* Ibandronic Acid [INT] 1030
Bo-Ne-Ca (TH) *see* Calcium Carbonate 327
Bonefos (AT, BE, BG, BH, BR, CH, CN, CO, CZ, DK, EE, ES, FI, GB, GR, HK, HN, HR, ID, IE, IL, KW, MX, MY, NL, NO, PE, PH, PK, PL, QA, RO, RU, SA, SE, SG, SI, SK, TH, TR, TW, VN) *see* Clodronate [CAN/INT] 469
Bone-One (VN) *see* Alfacalcidol [CAN/INT] 82
Bonglixan (MX) *see* Insulin Glargine 1086
Boni-M (KR) *see* Ibandronate 1028
Bonil (UY) *see* Imipramine 1054
Bonky (HK, KR) *see* Calcitriol 323
Bonmax (IN) *see* Raloxifene 1765
Bonmax (JO) *see* Alendronate 79
BonMax (TH) *see* Alendronate 79
Bon-One (CN, HK, ID, MY, TH) *see* Alfacalcidol [CAN/INT] 82
Bonoq (DE) *see* Gatifloxacin 949
Bonoq-Uro (DE) *see* Gatifloxacin 949
Bontoss (BR) *see* Bromhexine [INT] 291
Bonumin (FI) *see* Diethylpropion 624
Bonviva (AE, AT, BE, BG, BH, BR, CH, CL, CO, CY, CZ, DE, DK, EC, EE, ES, FI, FR, GB, GR, HK, HR, HU, ID, IE, IS, IT, JP, KR, KW, LB, LT, MT, MX, MY, NL, NO, NZ, PE, PH, PL, PT, PY, QA, RO, RU, SA, SE, SG, SI, SK, TH, TR, TW, UY, VN) *see* Ibandronate 1028
Bonviva (AT, SE) *see* Ibandronic Acid [INT] 1030
Bonyl (DK) *see* Naproxen 1427
Bookey (IN) *see* Doxylamine and Pyridoxine 693
Boostrix (AE, AT, AU, CO, CY, CZ, DE, FI, HK, IL, MX, NZ, PH, SG) *see* Diphtheria and Tetanus Toxoids, and Acellular Pertussis Vaccine 649
Bopacatin (SK) *see* CARBOplatin 357
Bo Ping (CN) *see* Nisoldipine 1459
Boravid (IE) *see* Ofloxacin (Systemic) 1490
Boro-Scopal (DE) *see* Scopolamine (Systemic) 1870
Bo Rui Te (CN) *see* Cinnarizine [INT] 440
Borymycin (MY, SG, TW) *see* Minocycline 1371
Bosentas (IN) *see* Bosentan 280
Bosmin (KR, TW) *see* EPINEPHrine (Systemic, Oral Inhalation) 735
Bosnum (HK, TH) *see* Fexofenadine 873
Bosporon (ES, PT) *see* Lornoxicam [INT] 1248
Bosulif (AU, BE, CH, CZ, DE, DK, FR, GB, HR, IS, LT, NL, NO, RO, SE, SI, SK, TR) *see* Bosutinib 282
Bosvate (NZ) *see* Bisoprolol 266
Botox (AE, AR, AU, BH, CH, CZ, DE, DK, ES, FI, FR, GB, HR, HU, IE, IS, IT, JO, KW, LB, LU, NL, NO, PL, QA, SA, SE, SI, SK, VN) *see* OnabotulinumtoxinA 1512
B-Platin (BR) *see* CARBOplatin 357
BPNorm (PH) *see* Fosinopril 932
BPros (KR) *see* ChlorproPAMIDE 429
BPzide (IN) *see* Hydrochlorothiazide 1009
BQL (BF, BJ, CI, ET, GH, GM, GN, IN, KE, LR, MA, ML, MR, MU, MW, NE, NG, SC, SD, SL, SN, TN, TZ, UG, ZM, ZW) *see* Enalapril 722
Bradirubra (IT) *see* Hydroxocobalamin 1020
Brainal (ES) *see* NiMODipine 1456
Braintop (BE, LU) *see* Piracetam [INT] 1661
Brakhor (MX) *see* Pravastatin 1700
Bralifex (ID) *see* Tobramycin (Ophthalmic) 2056
Bralifex Plus (ID) *see* Tobramycin and Dexamethasone 2056
Bralix (AE, BB, BH, BM, BS, BZ, CY, GY, IL, JM, JO, LB, LY, NL, OM, PR, QA, SA, SR, SY, TR, TT, YE) *see* Clidinium and Chlordiazepoxide 460
Brameston (BB, BM, BS, BZ, EC, GY, JM, PR, SG, SR, TT) *see* Bromocriptine 291
Bramitob (CO, CZ) *see* Tobramycin (Systemic, Oral Inhalation) 2052
Branzol (AR) *see* Ambroxol [INT] 109
Branzol (UY) *see* Pantoprazole 1570
Bratofil (VE) *see* Fluocinolone (Topical) 893
Bravelle (AE, AT, BH, BR, CY, DE, ES, GB, GR, HK, HR, ID, IE, IL, KW, LB, LT, MY, NO, PH, QA, RO, SA, SE, SG, SI, SK, TR, VN) *see* Urofollitropin 2116
Brawmicin (VN) *see* Cinnarizine [INT] 440
Braxan (MX) *see* Amiodarone 114
Braxidin (ID) *see* Clidinium and Chlordiazepoxide 460
Brazaves (JP) *see* Miglustat 1367
Brazepam (ZA) *see* Bromazepam [CAN/INT] 290
Bre-A-Col (MX) *see* Guaifenesin and Dextromethorphan 987
Breakyl (GB) *see* FentaNYL 857
Brecare (PH) *see* Montelukast 1392
Brecio (KR) *see* Almitrine [INT] 92
Breinox (EC, VE) *see* Piracetam [INT] 1661
Breminal (AR) *see* Tolterodine 2063
Brenfed (IN) *see* Pseudoephedrine and Ibuprofen 1743
Brentan (DK) *see* Miconazole (Topical) 1360
Breo Ellipta (AU, BM) *see* Fluticasone and Vilanterol 914
Bretra (KR) *see* Letrozole 1181
Brevafen (AR) *see* Alfentanil 83
Breva (IT) *see* Ipratropium and Albuterol 1109
Brevibloc (AE, AR, AT, AU, BE, BR, CH, CZ, DK, ES, FI, FR, GB, GR, HK, HN, HR, HU, IE, IT, KR, MX, NL, NO, NZ, PL, SE, SI, TH, TR, TW, UY, VN) *see* Esmolol 769
Breviblo (PK) *see* Esmolol 769
Brevicilina (ES) *see* Penicillin G Benzathine 1609
Brevimytal Natrium (DE) *see* Methohexital 1321
Brevinarcon (PL) *see* Butabarbital 313
Brevinaze (ZA) *see* Ketamine 1143
Brevinor (AU, BF, BJ, CI, ET, GH, GM, GN, KE, LR, MA, ML, MR, MU, MW, NE, NG, NZ, SC, SD, SL, SN, TN, TZ, UG, ZM, ZW) *see* Ethinyl Estradiol and Norethindrone 808
Brevital (BF, BJ, CI, ET, GH, GM, GN, KE, LR, MA, ML, MR, MU, MW, NE, NG, SC, SD, SL, SN, TN, TZ, UG, ZA, ZM, ZW) *see* Methohexital 1321
Brexel (ID) *see* DOCEtaxel 656
Brexen (PH) *see* Celecoxib 402
Brexic (IN) *see* Piroxicam 1662
Brexin (AE, BH, CY, EG, IL, IQ, IR, JO, KW, LB, LY, OM, QA, SA, SY, TW, VN, YE) *see* Piroxicam 1662
Bricalin (IL) *see* Terbutaline 2004
Bricanil (VE) *see* Terbutaline 2004
Bricanyl (AE, AR, AT, AU, BB, BE, BF, BH, BJ, BM, BR, BS, BZ, CH, CI, CN, CY, CZ, DK, EG, ET, FI, FR, GB, GH, GM, GN, GY, HK, HN, HU, IE, IL, IN, IQ, IR, IS, IT, JM, JO, KE, KR, KW, LB, LR, LU, LY, MA, ML, MR, MU, MW, MY, NE, NG, NL, NO, NZ, OM, PE, PH, PK, PT, QA, SA, SC, SD, SE, SG, SL, SN, SR, SY, TN, TR, TT, TW, TZ, UG, VN, YE, ZA, ZM, ZW) *see* Terbutaline 2004
Bricanyl retard (NL) *see* Terbutaline 2004
Bricanyl Turbuhaler (HU, PL) *see* Terbutaline 2004
Bricasma (ID) *see* Terbutaline 2004
Briclin (UY) *see* Amikacin 111
Bridic (PT) *see* Brivudine [INT] 289
Bridin-T (KR) *see* Brimonidine (Ophthalmic) 288
Bridion (AR, AT, AU, BE, BR, CH, CL, CO, CY, CZ, DK, EE, ES, FR, GB, GR, HR, HU, IL, IS, JP, KR, LB, LT, MX, MY, NL, NO, NZ, PE, PH, PL, PT, RO, RU, SE, SG, SI, SK, TH, TR) *see* Sugammadex [INT] 1942
Bridopen (PH) *see* Ampicillin 141
Brietal (DK, FI, GB, HN, HU, NO, PL, SE, TW) *see* Methohexital 1321
Brietal sodique (FR, LU) *see* Methohexital 1321
Brietal Sodium (AT, BF, BJ, CH, CI, ET, GB, GH, GM, GN, KE, LR, MA, ML, MR, MU, MW, NE, NG, NL, RU, SC, SD, SL, SN, TN, TZ, UG, ZA, ZM, ZW) *see* Methohexital 1321
Brietal-Sodium (AU, CZ, HU) *see* Methohexital 1321
Briglau (NL) *see* Brimonidine (Ophthalmic) 288

Briklin (GR) *see* Amikacin ... 111
Brilinta (AR, AU, BR, CL, CN, CO, HK, ID, IL, KR, MY, NZ, PE, PH, QA, SA, SG, TH, VN) *see* Ticagrelor ... 2035
Brilique (BE, CH, CY, CZ, DE, DK, EE, FR, GB, HR, IE, IS, LT, NL, NO, PL, PT, RO, SE, SI, SK, TR) *see* Ticagrelor ... 2035
Brilizid (PH) *see* GlipiZIDE ... 967
Brimexate (IT) *see* Methotrexate ... 1322
Brimicon (CN) *see* Brimonidine (Ophthalmic) ... 288
Brimo (AE, TW) *see* Brimonidine (Ophthalmic) ... 288
Brimocom (IN) *see* Brimonidine (Ophthalmic) ... 288
Brimodin (PE) *see* Acetylcysteine ... 40
Brimonal (RO) *see* Brimonidine (Ophthalmic) ... 288
Brimontal (TR) *see* Brimonidine (Ophthalmic) ... 288
Brimo Ophtal (DE) *see* Brimonidine (Ophthalmic) ... 288
Brimopress (AR, CL, PY, UY) *see* Brimonidine (Ophthalmic) ... 288
Brimorand (SE) *see* Brimonidine (Ophthalmic) ... 288
Brimoratio (NO) *see* Brimonidine (Ophthalmic) ... 288
Brimot (HR) *see* Brimonidine (Ophthalmic) ... 288
Brinex (KR) *see* Bumetanide ... 297
Brintellix (AU, CZ, EE, ES, HR, IS, LT, NL, RO, SE, SI, SK) *see* Vortioxetine ... 2183
Brintenal (AR) *see* Selegiline ... 1873
BrinzoQuin (AU) *see* Brinzolamide ... 288
Briofil (IT) *see* Bamifylline [INT] ... 227
Brionil (ES) *see* Nedocromil ... 1435
Briop (CO, MX) *see* Brimonidine (Ophthalmic) ... 288
Brisofer (PH) *see* Ferrous Sulfate ... 871
Brisoral (ES) *see* Cefprozil ... 389
Brispen (MX) *see* Dicloxacillin ... 621
Bristaciclina (ES) *see* Tetracycline ... 2017
Bristacol (ES) *see* Pravastatin ... 1700
Bristaflam (CR, GT, HN, NI, PA, SV, VE) *see* Aceclofenac [INT] ... 30
Bristamox (FR) *see* Amoxicillin ... 130
Bristaxol (MX) *see* PACLitaxel (Conventional) ... 1550
Bristol-Videx EC (CO) *see* Didanosine ... 622
Bristopen (FR) *see* Oxacillin ... 1528
Britaline (MY) *see* Terbutaline ... 2004
Britaxol (CL) *see* PACLitaxel (Conventional) ... 1550
BritLofex (GB) *see* Lofexidine [INT] ... 1232
Brival (RO) *see* Brivudine [INT] ... 289
Brivex (CH) *see* Brivudine [INT] ... 289
Brivirac (IT) *see* Brivudine [INT] ... 289
Brivir (BG, GR) *see* Brivudine [INT] ... 289
Brivox (CR, DO, GT, HN, NI, PA, SV) *see* Brivudine [INT] ... 289
Brivozost (HR) *see* Brivudine [INT] ... 289
Brivumen (EE) *see* Brivudine [INT] ... 289
Brixia (AR, CL, PY, UY) *see* Azelastine (Ophthalmic) ... 213
Broadced (ID) *see* CefTRIAXone ... 396
Brochlor (GB) *see* Chloramphenicol ... 421
Brocid (TW) *see* Probenecid ... 1716
Brodilan (VE) *see* Clenbuterol [INT] ... 460
Broflex (GB) *see* Trihexyphenidyl ... 2103
Brogamax (MX) *see* Sulfamethoxazole and Trimethoprim ... 1946
Bromax (PT) *see* Ambroxol [INT] ... 109
Bromazanil (LU) *see* Bromazepam [CAN/INT] ... 290
Bromazepam-Eurogenerics (LU) *see* Bromazepam [CAN/INT] ... 290
Bromaze (ZA) *see* Bromazepam [CAN/INT] ... 290
Bromazin (TW) *see* Bromazepam [CAN/INT] ... 290
Bromergon (HR, TH) *see* Bromocriptine ... 291
Bromex (BE, IN, LU, TH) *see* Bromhexine [INT] ... 291
Bromexidryl (AR) *see* Bromhexine [INT] ... 291
Bromexina-ratiopharm (PT) *see* Bromhexine [INT] ... 291
Bromexin (PY) *see* Bromhexine [INT] ... 291
Bromfluex (RO) *see* Bromhexine [INT] ... 291
Bromhexina Austral (AR) *see* Bromhexine [INT] ... 291
Bromhexin ACO (SE) *see* Bromhexine [INT] ... 291
Bromhexina Lafedar (AR) *see* Bromhexine [INT] ... 291
Bromhexina Sintesina (AR) *see* Bromhexine [INT] ... 291
Bromhexina Vannier (AR) *see* Bromhexine [INT] ... 291
Bromhexin BC (DE) *see* Bromhexine [INT] ... 291
Bromhexin Berlin-Chemie (DE) *see* Bromhexine [INT] ... 291
Bromhexin (DE, DK) *see* Bromhexine [INT] ... 291
Bromhexine EG (BE) *see* Bromhexine [INT] ... 291
Bromhexine-Eurogenerics (LU) *see* Bromhexine [INT] ... 291
Bromhexine-ratiopharm (BE) *see* Bromhexine [INT] ... 291
Bromhexin Eu Rho (DE) *see* Bromhexine [INT] ... 291
Bromhexin Funcke (DE) *see* Bromhexine [INT] ... 291
Bromhexin Losung Funcke (DE) *see* Bromhexine [INT] ... 291
Bromhexin-ratiopharm (DE) *see* Bromhexine [INT] ... 291
bromhexin von ct (DE, LU) *see* Bromhexine [INT] ... 291
Bromhexin "Dak" (DK) *see* Bromhexine [INT] ... 291
Bromhex (SE) *see* Bromhexine [INT] ... 291
Brom (HK) *see* Bromhexine [INT] ... 291
Bromhydrate d'homatropine-Chauvin (LU) *see* Homatropine ... 1005
Bromicof (MX) *see* Bromhexine [INT] ... 291
Bromidem (LU) *see* Bromazepam [CAN/INT] ... 290
Bromidol Depot (DK) *see* Bromperidol [INT] ... 292
Bromidol (DK) *see* Bromperidol [INT] ... 292
Bromika (ID) *see* Bromhexine [INT] ... 291
Bromine (TW) *see* Brompheniramine ... 292
Brom (KR) *see* Bromperidol [INT] ... 292
Bromocorn (PL) *see* Bromocriptine ... 291
Bromocriptina (CO) *see* Bromocriptine ... 291
Bromocriptin-Richter (HU) *see* Bromocriptine ... 291
Bromodol (AR, GR) *see* Bromperidol [INT] ... 292
Bromodol Decanoato (AR) *see* Bromperidol [INT] ... 292
Bromo-Kin (FR) *see* Bromocriptine ... 291
Bromopan (BR) *see* Bromopride [INT] ... 292
Bromox (VE) *see* Bromhexine [INT] ... 291
Bromselon (ES) *see* Ebastine [INT] ... 702
Bromuc (BR) *see* Acetylcysteine ... 40
Bromurex (CO) *see* Pancuronium ... 1567
Bromxine (GR, HN, SG) *see* Bromhexine [INT] ... 291
Bronac (KR) *see* Bromfenac ... 291
Bronair (EC) *see* Bromhexine [INT] ... 291
Bronchathiol (FR) *see* Carbocisteine [INT] ... 357
Bronchicum (DE) *see* Codeine ... 497
Bronchitol (AU, GB, HR) *see* Mannitol ... 1269
Broncho D (IL) *see* DiphenhydrAMINE (Systemic) ... 641
Bronchodam (PH) *see* Terbutaline ... 2004
Bronchodine (BE) *see* Codeine ... 497
Bronchodual (FR) *see* Ipratropium and Fenoterol [CAN/INT] ... 1109
Broncholit (ID) *see* Carbocisteine [INT] ... 357
Bronchoretard (DE) *see* Theophylline ... 2026
Bronchosan (SK) *see* Bromhexine [INT] ... 291
Bronchosol (TH) *see* Albuterol ... 69
Bronco Asmo (TH) *see* Terbutaline ... 2004
Broncobiot (PE) *see* Penicillin G (Parenteral/ Aqueous) ... 1611
Broncocalmine (AR) *see* Bromhexine [INT] ... 291
Broncocor (IT) *see* Pirbuterol ... 1662
Broncodil (IT) *see* Clenbuterol [INT] ... 460
Broncofenil (BR) *see* GuaiFENesin ... 986
Broncoflem (PH) *see* Acetylcysteine ... 40
Broncokin (IT) *see* Bromhexine [INT] ... 291
Broncolin (MY, PH) *see* Albuterol ... 69
Broncolit (PY) *see* Clenbuterol [INT] ... 460
Bronconox (CO) *see* Beclomethasone (Nasal) ... 232
Bronconox (CO) *see* Beclomethasone (Systemic) ... 230
Bronconox Forte (CO) *see* Beclomethasone (Nasal) ... 232
Bronconox Forte (CO) *see* Beclomethasone (Systemic) ... 230
Bronconyl (TH) *see* Terbutaline ... 2004
Broncoral (ES) *see* Formoterol ... 926
Broncot (CL) *see* Ambroxol [INT] ... 109

Broncoterol (PT) *see* Clenbuterol [INT] ... 460
Brondisal (ID) *see* Albuterol ... 69
Bronex (PH) *see* Budesonide (Systemic) ... 293
Bronilide (FR) *see* Flunisolide (Nasal) ... 893
Bronkese (ZA) *see* Bromhexine [INT] ... 291
Bronket (VN) *see* Ketotifen (Systemic) [CAN/INT] ... 1149
Bronq-C (AR) *see* Clenbuterol [INT] ... 460
Bronquisedan Elixir (AR) *see* Bromhexine [INT] ... 291
Bronsolvan (ID) *see* Theophylline ... 2026
Brontel (PY) *see* Clenbuterol [INT] ... 460
Brontex (EE) *see* Ambroxol [INT] ... 109
Brontol (CO) *see* Bromhexine [INT] ... 291
Bronuck (JP) *see* Bromfenac ... 291
Bronxol (MX, PT) *see* Ambroxol [INT] ... 109
Bropasmo (PY) *see* Domperidone [CAN/INT] ... 666
Bropavol (CL) *see* Bromhexine [INT] ... 291
Bropil (CL) *see* Albuterol ... 69
Broquial-PM (PE) *see* Carbocisteine [INT] ... 357
Broramin (TW) *see* Brompheniramine ... 292
Brospec (ID) *see* CefTRIAXone ... 396
Brospina (MX) *see* Buprenorphine ... 300
Brostagin (PL) *see* Pyridostigmine ... 1746
Brosur (IN) *see* Bromfenac ... 291
Brothine (TW) *see* Terbutaline ... 2004
Brotussol (DE) *see* Bromhexine [INT] ... 291
Brozil (MY, SG) *see* Gemfibrozil ... 956
Brucam (MX) *see* Piroxicam ... 1662
Brucarcer (MX) *see* CarBAMazepine ... 346
Brucen (MX) *see* GlyBURIDE ... 972
Brufen 400 (IL) *see* Ibuprofen ... 1032
Brufen (AE, AT, AU, BD, BE, BH, CH, CY, CZ, DE, DK, EE, EG, ES, FI, FR, GB, GR, HK, HR, ID, IE, IQ, IR, IT, JO, JP, KR, KW, LB, LT, LY, MT, MY, NL, NO, NZ, OM, PH, PK, PT, QA, RO, RU, SA, SE, SG, SI, SK, SY, TR, TW, VN, YE, ZA) *see* Ibuprofen ... 1032
Brufen Forte (ID) *see* Ibuprofen ... 1032
Brufen Retard (SG) *see* Ibuprofen ... 1032
Brufen Syrup for Children (KR) *see* Ibuprofen ... 1032
Brufincol (MX) *see* Pravastatin ... 1700
Brufort (IT) *see* Ibuprofen ... 1032
Brulamycin (HN, PL) *see* Tobramycin (Systemic, Oral Inhalation) ... 2052
Brumetidina (IT, VN) *see* Cimetidine ... 438
Brumixol (IT, TW) *see* Ciclopirox ... 433
Brumox-500 (PH) *see* Amoxicillin ... 130
Brupen (MX) *see* Ampicillin ... 141
Brurem (MX) *see* Sulindac ... 1953
Bruzol (MX) *see* Albendazole ... 65
Brytolin (PH) *see* Albuterol ... 69
B-Tablock (BR) *see* Levobunolol ... 1194
B-Tene (AU) *see* Beta-Carotene ... 251
Bucain (DE, HU, ID) *see* Bupivacaine ... 299
Bucaine (AE, BH, CY, EG, IQ, IR, JO, KW, LB, LY, OM, QA, SA, SY, YE) *see* Bupivacaine ... 299
Bucanil (MY) *see* Terbutaline ... 2004
Bucaril (TH) *see* Terbutaline ... 2004
Buccastem 3 (AE, BH, CY, EG, IQ, IR, JO, KW, LB, LY, OM, QA, SA, SY, YE) *see* Prochlorperazine ... 1718
Buccastem (NZ) *see* Prochlorperazine ... 1718
Buccolam (GB) *see* Midazolam ... 1361
Bucco Tantum (CH) *see* Benzydamine [CAN/INT] ... 249
Buclen (VE) *see* Clenbuterol [INT] ... 460
Bucodrin (PE) *see* Benzydamine [CAN/INT] ... 249
Bucogel (AR) *see* Chlorhexidine Gluconate ... 422
Bucoglobin (UY) *see* Chlorhexidine Gluconate ... 422
Bucoxidina (PE) *see* Chlorhexidine Gluconate ... 422
Budair (MY) *see* Budesonide (Systemic) ... 293
Budamax (AU) *see* Budesonide (Nasal) ... 296
Budecort DP (MY) *see* Budesonide (Systemic) ... 293
Budecort Nasal (PH) *see* Budesonide (Nasal) ... 296
Budeflam (ZA) *see* Budesonide (Nasal) ... 296
Budema (TW) *see* Bumetanide ... 297
Budena (HK) *see* Budesonide (Nasal) ... 296
Budenase AQ (HK) *see* Budesonide (Nasal) ... 296
Budenofalk (AU, DE, HK, KR, PH, RO, SG) *see* Budesonide (Systemic) ... 293
Budeson Aqua (AR) *see* Budesonide (Systemic) ... 293
Budeson Aqua (TW) *see* Budesonide (Nasal) ... 296
Budeson (AR) *see* Budesonide (Systemic) ... 293
BudeSpray (TH) *see* Budesonide (Systemic) ... 293
Budiair (KR) *see* Budesonide (Systemic) ... 293
Budicort Respules (IL) *see* Budesonide (Systemic) ... 293
Buenox (EC) *see* Magaldrate and Simethicone ... 1261
Bufabron (ID) *see* Theophylline ... 2026
Bufamoxy (ID) *see* Amoxicillin ... 130
Bufect Forte (ID) *see* Ibuprofen ... 1032
Bufect (ID) *see* Ibuprofen ... 1032
Bufencon (MY) *see* Betamethasone (Systemic) ... 253
Bufferin Advance (TW) *see* Acetaminophen, Aspirin, and Caffeine ... 37
Bufferin (JO, UY) *see* Aspirin ... 180
Bufigen (MX) *see* Nalbuphine ... 1416
Buflin (MX) *see* Flunarizine [CAN/INT] ... 892
Build (TW) *see* MethylTESTOSTERone ... 1345
Bultis Film (KR) *see* Sildenafil ... 1882
Bu Luo Na Tai (CN) *see* Nesiritide ... 1439
Bumaflex N (PY) *see* Naproxen ... 1427
Bumelex (VE) *see* Bumetanide ... 297
Bumetanid (CY) *see* Bumetanide ... 297
Bumet (DO, GT, HN, IN, PA, SV) *see* Bumetanide ... 297
Bumetin (CO) *see* Trimebutine [CAN/INT] ... 2103
Bumetone (KR, TH) *see* Nabumetone ... 1411
Buminate 25% (HK, PH) *see* Albumin ... 67
Bunafine (TW) *see* Butenafine ... 314
Bunascan Spinal (ID) *see* Bupivacaine ... 299
Bunase (TH) *see* Budesonide (Systemic) ... 293
Bunolgan (TW) *see* Levobunolol ... 1194
Bunol (KR) *see* Butorphanol ... 314
Bupasmol (UY) *see* Scopolamine (Systemic) ... 1870
Bupensan (LT) *see* Buprenorphine ... 300
Bupep SR (IN) *see* BuPROPion ... 305
Buphenyl (JP, KR, TW) *see* Sodium Phenylbutyrate ... 1908
Bupicaina (AR) *see* Bupivacaine ... 299
Bupine (PK) *see* Bupivacaine ... 299
Bupinest S.P. (PE) *see* Bupivacaine ... 299
Bupinex (PY, UY) *see* Bupivacaine ... 299
Bupivacaine Aguettant (FR) *see* Bupivacaine ... 299
Bupivacaine B. Braun (FR) *see* Bupivacaine ... 299
Bupivacain Jenapharm (DE) *see* Bupivacaine ... 299
Bupivacain-RPR CO!2 (DE) *see* Bupivacaine ... 299
Bupivacain-RPR (DE) *see* Bupivacaine ... 299
Bupralex (AU) *see* Buprenorphine ... 300
Bupren (AR) *see* Buprenorphine ... 300
Buprex (EC) *see* Ibuprofen ... 1032
Buprine (TH) *see* Buprenorphine ... 300
Buprotrin (TW) *see* BuPROPion ... 305
Buradol (KR) *see* Carisoprodol ... 363
Burana (FI) *see* Ibuprofen ... 1032
Burgerstein Vitamin B!6 (CH) *see* Pyridoxine ... 1747
Burinax (BR) *see* Bumetanide ... 297
Burinex (AE, AT, AU, BB, BE, BF, BJ, BM, BS, BZ, CH, CI, CR, DE, DK, EG, ET, FI, FR, GB, GH, GM, GN, GR, GY, HK, IE, JM, JO, KE, LB, LR, LU, MA, ML, MR, MU, MW, MY, NE, NG, NL, NO, NZ, PH, PK, PR, QA, SA, SC, SD, SE, SG, SI, SL, SN, SR, TH, TN, TT, TZ, UG, ZA, ZM, ZW) *see* Bumetanide ... 297
Burnax (EC) *see* Fluconazole ... 885
Burnazin (ID) *see* Silver Sulfadiazine ... 1887
Burn-Gel (ES) *see* Neomycin ... 1436
Burnsil (PH) *see* Silver Sulfadiazine ... 1887
Buscapina (AR, CO, CR, GT, HN, NI, PA, PE, PY, SV, UY, VE) *see* Scopolamine (Systemic) ... 1870
Buscolax (PH) *see* Bisacodyl ... 265
Buscopan (AT, AU, BE, BH, BR, CH, CN, CY, CZ, DK, EG, FI, GB, GR, HK, HR, IE, IN, IS, IT, KR, KW, LT,

MY, NZ, PH, PK, PL, PT, QA, RO, RU, SA, SE, SG, SI, SK, TH, TR, TW) *see* Scopolamine (Systemic) 1870
Buscopina (CL) *see* Scopolamine (Systemic) 1870
Buscotica (ID) *see* Scopolamine (Systemic) 1870
Busetal (PE) *see* Disulfiram 654
Busidril (ES) *see* Ebastine [INT] 702
Busilvex (AT, BE, BG, CH, CZ, DE, DK, EE, FI, FR, GB, GR, HN, HR, IE, IT, MT, MX, NL, NO, PL, PT, RO, RU, SE, SK, TR) *see* Busulfan 312
Busiral (AE, BH, CY, EG, IQ, IR, JO, KW, LB, LY, OM, QA, SA, SY, YE) *see* BusPIRone 311
Buspar (AT, BE, BH, CH, CZ, DK, EC, EE, EG, ES, FI, FR, GB, HK, IE, IT, KR, KW, LU, MT, MX, NL, NO, NZ, PK, PT, QA, RU, SA, SE, SK, TR, ZA) *see* BusPIRone 311
Busparium (UY) *see* BusPIRone 311
Busphen (KR) *see* Butorphanol 314
Buspin (IN) *see* BusPIRone 311
Buspon (TR) *see* BusPIRone 311
Busp (TW) *see* BusPIRone 311
Busulfex (AU, CN, HK, IL, JP, KR, MY, SG, TH, TW) *see* Busulfan 312
Busulf (PK) *see* Busulfan 312
Busulif (EE) *see* Bosutinib 282
Busvir (BR) *see* Ritonavir 1822
Butacort (NZ) *see* Budesonide (Nasal) 296
Butaline (MY) *see* Terbutaline 2004
Butalin (JO, LB, SA) *see* Albuterol 69
Butamide (JP) *see* TOLBUTamide 2062
Butamine (IL) *see* DOBUTamine 654
Butamol (AR, AU, PY) *see* Albuterol 69
Butaro (TW) *see* Butorphanol 314
Butavate (GR) *see* Clobetasol 468
Butavent (MY) *see* Albuterol 69
Butefin (TW) *see* Butenafine 314
Butinat (AR) *see* Bumetanide 297
Butin (TW) *see* Bromocriptine 291
Butipalen (KR) *see* Adapalene 54
Butirid (JP) *see* Riboflavin 1803
Butix (FR) *see* DiphenhydrAMINE (Systemic) 641
Buto-Air (ES) *see* Albuterol 69
Buto-Asma (BG, HK, PK, TH) *see* Albuterol 69
Butobloc (ZA) *see* Acebutolol 29
Butop (IN) *see* Butenafine 314
Butotal (CN) *see* Albuterol 69
Butrans (GB, IE, IL) *see* Buprenorphine 300
Butrum (IN) *see* Butorphanol 314
Butyl (TH) *see* Scopolamine (Systemic) 1870
Butyn (PK) *see* Oxybutynin 1536
Buvacaina (EC) *see* Bupivacaine 299
Buvacainas (CO) *see* Bupivacaine 299
Buvanest Spinal (ID) *see* Bupivacaine 299
Buventol (AE, AT, CZ, EE, NO, SG, TW) *see* Albuterol 69
Buventol Easyhaler (FR, TH) *see* Albuterol 69
Buwecon (TW) *see* Hyoscyamine 1026
Buxon (CL) *see* BuPROPion 305
B-Vasc (ZA) *see* Atenolol 189
Byanodine (HU) *see* PenicillAMINE 1608
Bydaxin (JP) *see* Tofisopam [INT] 2061
Bydureon (AU, CH, CZ, DE, DK, GB, IL, JP, KR, LT, NL, NO, SE, SI, SK) *see* Exenatide 830
Byetta (AE, AR, AT, AU, BE, BG, BR, CH, CL, CN, CO, CY, DE, DK, EC, EE, ES, FI, FR, GB, GR, HK, HN, HR, HU, IE, IL, IS, IT, JP, KR, KW, LB, LT, MT, MY, NL, NO, NZ, PH, PK, PL, PT, QA, RO, RU, SA, SE, SG, SI, SK, TH, TR, TW) *see* Exenatide 830
Bykomycin (AT, CZ, DE) *see* Neomycin 1436
Bypro (TH, TW) *see* Bicalutamide 262
Bysclas (PH) *see* Clarithromycin 456
Cabal (AR) *see* Cetirizine 411
Cabaser (AR, AU, CH, DK, FI, GB, IE, IL, IT, SE) *see* Cabergoline 319
Cabergoline-Pharmacia (LU) *see* Cabergoline 319
Caberlin (IN) *see* Cabergoline 319
Cabexa (HR) *see* Cabergoline 319
Cabotin (TW) *see* Carbocisteine [INT] 357
Cabotrim (IL) *see* Cabergoline 319
Cacare (TH) *see* Calcitriol 323
Cacepin (KR) *see* QUEtiapine 1751
Cadatin (AU) *see* Amlodipine and Atorvastatin 124
Cadauet (JP) *see* Amlodipine and Atorvastatin 124
Cadef Elixir Pediatric (KR) *see* Digoxin 627
Cadens (FR) *see* Calcitonin 322
Caderma (KR) *see* Prednicarbate 1703
Cadex (IL) *see* Doxazosin 674
Cadicon (TH) *see* Gliclazide [CAN/INT] 964
Cadicycline (BF, BJ, CI, ET, GH, GM, GN, KE, LR, MA, ML, MR, MU, MW, NE, NG, SC, SD, SL, SN, TN, TZ, UG, ZM, ZW) *see* Tetracycline 2017
Cadil (HR) *see* Carvedilol 367
Cadil (KR) *see* Doxazosin 674
Cadimycetin (BF, BJ, CI, ET, GH, GM, GN, KE, LR, MA, ML, MR, MU, MW, NE, NG, SC, SD, SL, SN, TN, TZ, UG, ZM, ZW) *see* Chloramphenicol 421
Cadiquin (BF, BJ, CI, ET, GH, GM, GN, KE, LR, MA, ML, MR, MU, MW, NE, NG, SC, SD, SL, SN, TN, TZ, UG, ZA, ZM, ZW) *see* Chloroquine 424
Caditar (PE) *see* Celecoxib 402
Cadlin (KR) *see* Doxazosin 674
Cadotin (TH) *see* Calcitonin 322
Cadotril (PE) *see* Racecadotril [INT] 1765
Caduet (AE, AT, AU, BG, BH, CH, CL, CN, CR, CZ, DO, ES, FR, GT, HK, HN, HR, HU, ID, IL, KR, KW, LB, LT, MX, MY, NI, PA, PT, QA, RO, RU, SA, SG, SI, SK, SV, TH, TR, TW, VE) *see* Amlodipine and Atorvastatin 124
Caedax (AT, GR, PT) *see* Ceftibuten 394
Caelyx (AE, AR, AT, AU, BE, BH, BR, CH, CL, CN, CO, CY, CZ, DE, DK, EC, EE, ES, FI, FR, GB, GR, HR, HU, ID, IE, IL, IN, IS, IT, JO, KR, LB, LT, MT, MX, MY, NL, NO, NZ, PE, PH, PL, PT, QA, RO, RU, SE, SG, SI, SK, TH, TR, TW, UY, VE, VN) *see* DOXOrubicin (Liposomal) 684
Cafalogen (PE) *see* CefTRIAXone 396
Cafcit (GR, VN) *see* Caffeine 319
Cafergot (MX, SE) *see* Ergotamine 754
Cafeton (TW) *see* Ergotamine 754
Cafnea (AU) *see* Caffeine 319
Cafonate (PH) *see* Leucovorin Calcium 1183
Cafona (TW) *see* Leucovorin Calcium 1183
Caftar (MX) *see* Ergotamine 754
Calabren (CZ) *see* GlyBURIDE 972
Calapol (ID) *see* Acetaminophen 32
Calaptin (IN) *see* Verapamil 2154
Calbivas (ID) *see* AmLODIPine 123
Calblock (JP) *see* Azelnidipine [INT] 214
Calbloc (PH) *see* AmLODIPine 123
Calbone (PH) *see* Calcium Carbonate 327
Calbo (TW) *see* Calcium Citrate 330
Calcanate (TH) *see* Calcium Carbonate 327
Calcedon (DE) *see* Calcium Gluconate 330
Calcefor (CL, PE) *see* Calcium Carbonate 327
Calchek (IN) *see* AmLODIPine 123
Calchicine Houde (PY) *see* Colchicine 500
Calci-10 (TH) *see* Calcitonin 322
Calci Aid (PH) *see* Calcium Carbonate 327
Calcibloc OD (PH) *see* NIFEdipine 1451
Calcibloc (PH) *see* NIFEdipine 1451
Calcibon (CO) *see* Calcium Citrate 330
Calcicard (GB) *see* Diltiazem 634
Calcichew (FI, GB, IE, LU) *see* Calcium Carbonate 327
Calcifar (PL) *see* Calcium Carbonate 327
Calciferol BD (TH) *see* Ergocalciferol 753
Calciferol (CZ) *see* Ergocalciferol 753
Calcigamma (DE) *see* Calcium Carbonate 327
Calcigard (IN, SG, TH) *see* NIFEdipine 1451
Calcigran Sine (EE) *see* Calcium Carbonate 327

Calcii Gluconas (FI) *see* Calcium Gluconate 330
Calcijex (AE, AU, CN, GB, HU, LU, MY, SA, TW) *see* Calcitriol 323
Calcilos (DE) *see* Calcium Carbonate 327
Calcimate (PH) *see* Calcium Carbonate 327
Calcimusc (HU) *see* Calcium Gluconate 330
Calcinate (PH) *see* Calcium Gluconate 330
Calcinin (TW) *see* Calcitonin 322
Calcio 600 + D (CO) *see* Calcium and Vitamin D 326
Calcio Gluconato (AR, IT) *see* Calcium Gluconate 330
Calcioral (PT) *see* Calcium Carbonate 327
Calcit (BE, FR, IT, NL) *see* Calcium Carbonate 327
Calcite (KR) *see* Calcium Citrate 330
Calcit (ID) *see* Calcitriol 323
Calcitoran (JP) *see* Calcitonin 322
Calcitriol (CO) *see* Calcitriol 323
Calcit SG (TH) *see* Calcitriol 323
Calcium 20 Madariaga (ES) *see* Calcium Carbonate 327
Calcium (BE, NO) *see* Calcium Glubionate 330
Calcium (BG, PL) *see* Calcium Carbonate 327
Calcium Braun (DE) *see* Calcium Gluconate 330
Calciumcarbonat-Dial (AT) *see* Calcium Carbonate 327
Calcium Carbonate (FR) *see* Calcium Carbonate 327
Calciumcarbonat Fresenius (CH) *see* Calcium Carbonate 327
Calcium-Carbonat Salmon Pharma (CH) *see* Calcium Carbonate 327
Calcium chloratum (PL) *see* Calcium Chloride 328
Calcium Dago (DE) *see* Calcium Carbonate 327
Calcium Disodium Versenate (AU) *see* Edetate CALCIUM Disodium 705
Calcium Edetate de Sodium (FR) *see* Edetate CALCIUM Disodium 705
Calcium effervescens (PL) *see* Calcium Carbonate 327
Calciumfolinat-Ebewe (PL, TW) *see* Leucovorin Calcium 1183
Calcium Folinate (NZ) *see* Leucovorin Calcium 1183
Calciumfolinat Faulding (SE) *see* Leucovorin Calcium 1183
Calciumfolinat Pharmalink (SE) *see* Leucovorin Calcium 1183
Calciumfolinat "Faulding" (DK) *see* Leucovorin Calcium 1183
Calcium Genericon (AT) *see* Calcium Carbonate 327
Calcium Gluconate (AU) *see* Calcium Gluconate 330
Calcium Gluconicum (BG, PL) *see* Calcium Gluconate 330
Calcium Gluconicum Granulatum (PL) *see* Calcium Gluconate 330
Calcium Klopfer (AT) *see* Calcium Carbonate 327
Calcium-Phosphatbinder Bichsel (CH) *see* Calcium Carbonate 327
Calcium Pliva (PL) *see* Calcium Glubionate 330
Calcium Pliva (PL) *see* Calcium Gluconate 330
Calcium Polfa (PL) *see* Calcium Glubionate 330
Calcium Polfa (PL) *see* Calcium Gluconate 330
Calcium Resonium (AU, HK, IE, IN, KW, SA) *see* Calcium Polystyrene Sulfonate [CAN/INT] 333
Calcium Sandoz (AT, ES, FI, HR, NL) *see* Calcium Glubionate 330
Calcium-Sandoz (CH, DK, FR, IN, SE, ZA) *see* Calcium Glubionate 330
Calcium-Sandoz Forte (BG) *see* Calcium Carbonate 327
Calcival D (MX) *see* Calcium Citrate 330
Calco [salmon] (HU) *see* Calcitonin 322
Calcorrt (EC) *see* Deflazacort [INT] 587
Calcort (BB, BR, BS, CH, DE, GB, JM, KR, LU, MX, PE, TT, VE) *see* Deflazacort [INT] 587
Calco (TH) *see* Calcitonin 322
Calcuim Resonium (CN) *see* Calcium Polystyrene Sulfonate [CAN/INT] 333
Calcuren (FI) *see* Calcium Carbonate 327
Caldine (FR) *see* Lacidipin [INT] 1154
Caldine (PH) *see* Manidipine [INT] 1269
Caleobrol (PY) *see* Calcitriol 323
Calfate (PT) *see* Sucralfate 1940
Calfonat (DK) *see* Leucovorin Calcium 1183
Calibral (PT) *see* Tenoxicam [INT] 2001
Calidron (JO) *see* Alendronate 79
Calith (TW) *see* Lithium 1230
Calixta (HR) *see* Mirtazapine 1376
Callexe (AR) *see* LevETIRAcetam 1191
Callexe XR (AR) *see* LevETIRAcetam 1191
Calmaben (BG) *see* DiphenhydrAMINE (Systemic) 641
Calmador (AR) *see* TraMADol 2074
Calmaxid (CH) *see* Nizatidine 1471
Calmdown (TW) *see* Venlafaxine 2150
Calmex (PY) *see* Acetaminophen and Tramadol 37
Calm-EZ (TW) *see* QUEtiapine 1751
Calmofilase (CO) *see* HydrOXYzine 1024
Calmol (UY) *see* TraMADol 2074
Calmpent (PH) *see* Gabapentin 943
Calmpose (BF, BJ, CI, ET, GH, GM, GN, IN, KE, LR, MA, ML, MR, MU, MW, NE, NG, SC, SD, SL, SN, TN, TZ, UG, ZA, ZM, ZW) *see* Diazepam 613
Calm U (NZ) *see* DiphenhydrAMINE (Systemic) 641
Calmurid (CL) *see* Hydrocortisone (Topical) 1014
Calmurid (BE, DE, LU, NL, PT) *see* Urea 2114
Calmuril (FI, SE) *see* Urea 2114
Calmylin with Codeine (CA) *see* Guaifenesin, Pseudoephedrine, and Codeine 989
Calnat (ID) *see* Calcium Carbonate 327
Calner (CL) *see* Clorazepate 487
Calnit (ES) *see* NiMODipine 1456
Calnurs (JP) *see* Diltiazem 634
Calos (ID) *see* Calcium Carbonate 327
Calperos (CH, PL) *see* Calcium Carbonate 327
Calperos D3 (HK) *see* Calcium and Vitamin D 326
Calpol (AE, BF, BH, BJ, CI, CY, EG, ET, GH, GM, GN, IE, IQ, IR, JO, JP, KE, KW, LB, LR, LY, MA, ML, MR, MU, MW, NE, NG, OM, PR, QA, SA, SC, SD, SI, SL, SN, SY, TN, TZ, UG, YE, ZM, ZW) *see* Acetaminophen 32
Calporosis D (ID) *see* Calcium and Vitamin D 326
Calsan (CH, MX, PH) *see* Calcium Carbonate 327
Calsical (ID) *see* Calcium and Vitamin D 326
Calskin (TW) *see* Calcipotriene 321
Calslot (JP) *see* Manidipine [INT] 1269
Calsuba (ZA) *see* Calcium Carbonate 327
Calsum Forte (TH) *see* Calcium Carbonate 327
Calsum (TH) *see* Calcium Carbonate 327
Cal-Sup (AU) *see* Calcium Carbonate 327
Calsynar (BR, TW) *see* Calcitonin 322
Calsynar [salmon] (HU, LU) *see* Calcitonin 322
Caltab (TH) *see* Calcium Carbonate 327
Calteo (KR) *see* Calcium Citrate 330
Caltess (PL) *see* Calcium Carbonate 327
Caltrate + D 300 (HK) *see* Calcium and Vitamin D 326
Caltrate 600 (CO, CR, DO, GT, HN, NI, PA, PE, SV, VE) *see* Calcium Carbonate 327
Caltrate (AE, AU, BB, BH, BM, BS, BZ, CO, CY, EG, GY, IL, IQ, IR, JM, JO, KW, LB, LY, MX, MY, OM, PL, PR, QA, SA, SR, SY, TT, VN, YE) *see* Calcium Carbonate 327
Caltrón (MX) *see* Calcium Carbonate 327
Caltum (ID) *see* CefTAZidime 392
Calumide (PH) *see* Bicalutamide 262
Calumid (MY, TH, VN) *see* Bicalutamide 262
Calumin (PH) *see* Bicalutamide 262
Calutex (AU) *see* Bicalutamide 262
Calutide-50 (IN) *see* Bicalutamide 262
Calutol (EC) *see* Bicalutamide 262
Calvase (NZ) *see* AmLODIPine 123
Calypsol (AE, BB, BG, BH, BM, BS, BZ, CY, CZ, EG, GY, HN, HU, IQ, IR, JM, JO, KW, LB, LY, OM, PK, PL, PR, QA, RO, RU, SA, SR, SY, TH, TT, VN, YE) *see* Ketamine 1143

Calzepin (VN) *see* CarBAMazepine 346
Camapine (TW) *see* CarBAMazepine 346
Camazol (MY, SG) *see* Carbimazole [INT] 356
Cambic-15 (TH) *see* Meloxicam 1283
Camcolit (BE, BH, CY, EG, IE, IQ, IR, KW, LB, LU, LY, OM, PK, QA, SA, SG, SY, TW, YE) *see* Lithium 1230
Camcolite (AE, JO) *see* Lithium 1230
Camelia (AR) *see* Desogestrel [INT] 597
Camen (KR) *see* Carbimazole [INT] 356
Camezol (BF, BJ, CI, ET, GH, GM, GN, KE, LR, MA, ML, MR, MU, MW, NE, NG, SC, SD, SL, SN, TN, TZ, UG, ZM, ZW) *see* MetroNIDAZOLE (Systemic) 1353
Camicil (BF, BJ, CI, ET, GH, GM, GN, KE, LR, MA, ML, MR, MU, MW, NE, NG, SC, SD, SL, SN, TN, TZ, UG, ZM, ZW) *see* Ampicillin 141
Camidexon (ID) *see* Dexamethasone (Systemic) 599
Camisan (MY) *see* Terbinafine (Systemic) 2002
Camnovate (SG) *see* Betamethasone (Topical) 255
Campain (ID) *see* Piroxicam 1662
Campanex (GR) *see* Cimetidine 438
Campath (PE, UY) *see* Alemtuzumab 75
Campos (DO, GT, HN, NI, SV) *see* Desloratadine 594
Campral (AR, AT, AU, BE, BG, BR, CH, CN, CZ, DE, DK, EE, ES, FI, GB, GR, HN, IE, IT, MT, MX, NL, NO, PL, PT, RU, SE, SG, SK, TR) *see* Acamprosate 28
Campto (AE, AT, BE, BF, BG, BH, BJ, CH, CI, CN, CY, CZ, DE, DK, EE, ES, ET, FI, FR, GB, GH, GM, GN, GR, HK, HN, HR, ID, IE, IL, IT, JO, JP, KE, KR, LR, MA, ML, MR, MT, MU, MW, MY, NE, NG, NL, NO, PH, PK, PL, PT, QA, RO, RU, SA, SC, SD, SE, SG, SI, SK, SL, SN, TH, TN, TR, TW, TZ, UG, VN, ZA, ZM, ZW) *see* Irinotecan 1112
Camptosar (AR, AU, BO, BR, CL, CO, CR, DO, GT, MX, NI, NZ, PA, PE, PR, SV, UY, VE) *see* Irinotecan 1112
Camri (IN) *see* Lornoxicam [INT] 1248
Camrox (KR) *see* Meloxicam 1283
Camsilon (GB) *see* Edrophonium 706
Camtecan (KR) *see* Irinotecan 1112
Canadiol (ES) *see* Itraconazole 1130
Canasa (CO) *see* Mesalamine 1301
Canasone C.B. (TH) *see* Betamethasone and Clotrimazole 256
Canazol (TH) *see* Clotrimazole (Topical) 488
Canceren (KR) *see* Methotrexate 1322
Cancetil (KR) *see* Candesartan 335
Cancetil Plus (KR) *see* Candesartan and Hydrochlorothiazide 338
Cancidas (AE, AR, AT, AU, BE, BG, BR, CH, CL, CN, CO, CR, CY, CZ, DE, DK, DO, EC, EE, ES, FI, FR, GB, GR, GT, HK, HN, HR, HU, IE, IL, IN, IS, IT, JO, JP, KR, KW, LT, MT, MX, MY, NI, NL, NO, NZ, PA, PE, PH, PL, PT, QA, RO, RU, SA, SE, SG, SI, SK, SV, TH, TR, TW, UY, VE) *see* Caspofungin 370
Cancyt (PH) *see* Cytarabine (Conventional) 535
Candazole (HK, ID, MY, SG, TH) *see* Clotrimazole (Topical) 488
Candecard H (BG) *see* Candesartan and Hydrochlorothiazide 338
Candelotan (KR) *see* Candesartan 335
Candepress (TR) *see* Candesartan 335
Canderin (ID) *see* Candesartan 335
Candesa Plus (KR) *see* Candesartan and Hydrochlorothiazide 338
Candesar-H (IN) *see* Candesartan and Hydrochlorothiazide 338
Candesar (IN, KR) *see* Candesartan 335
Candexin (PH) *see* Clotrimazole (Topical) 488
Candez (PH) *see* Candesartan 335
Candez Plus (PH) *see* Candesartan and Hydrochlorothiazide 338
Candibene (CZ) *see* Clotrimazole (Topical) 488
Candid (BF, BJ, CI, ET, GH, GM, GN, KE, LR, MA, ML, MR, MU, MW, NE, NG, SC, SD, SL, SN, TN, TZ, UG, VE, ZM, ZW) *see* Clotrimazole (Topical) 488
Candid-B (MY) *see* Betamethasone and Clotrimazole 256
Candio-Hermal (DE) *see* Nystatin (Topical) 1482
Candiplas (SG, TR) *see* Miconazole (Topical) 1360
Candistat (IN) *see* Itraconazole 1130
Canditral (PE, PH, SG, VN) *see* Itraconazole 1130
Candiva (PH) *see* Clotrimazole (Topical) 488
Candizol (AE, BH, CY, EG, IQ, IR, JO, KW, LB, LY, OM, QA, SA, SY, YE) *see* Miconazole (Topical) 1360
Candizole (BE) *see* Fluconazole 885
Candizole (ZA) *see* Clotrimazole (Topical) 488
Candizol oral (AE, BH, CY, EG, IQ, IR, JO, KW, LB, LY, OM, QA, SA, SY, YE) *see* Miconazole (Topical) 1360
Candyl-D (NZ) *see* Piroxicam 1662
Canesoral (AU) *see* Fluconazole 885
Canesten 1 (KR) *see* Clotrimazole (Topical) 488
Canesten (AE, AT, AU, BF, BG, BH, BJ, BO, BR, CH, CI, CL, CO, CY, CZ, DK, EC, EE, EG, ET, FI, GB, GH, GM, GN, GR, HK, HR, ID, IE, IN, IQ, IR, IS, IT, JO, KE, KR, KW, LB, LR, LY, MA, ML, MR, MT, MU, MW, MY, NE, NG, NL, NO, NZ, OM, PE, PH, PK, PL, PT, QA, RO, RU, SA, SC, SD, SE, SG, SI, SK, SL, SN, SY, TH, TN, TR, TW, TZ, UG, UY, VE, VN, YE, ZA, ZM, ZW) *see* Clotrimazole (Topical) 488
Canesten (AU, DE) *see* Bifonazole [INT] 264
Canestene (BE) *see* Clotrimazole (Topical) 488
Canesten Extra Bifonazol (DE) *see* Bifonazole [INT] 264
Canesten (IS) *see* Clotrimazole (Oral) 488
Canflame (TW) *see* Silver Sulfadiazine 1887
Canifug (DE) *see* Clotrimazole (Topical) 488
Canison (PH) *see* Clotrimazole (Topical) 488
Canlin (TW) *see* Ursodiol 2116
Canolen (TR) *see* Ciclopirox 433
Cansartan (KR) *see* Candesartan 335
Cansartan Plus (KR) *see* Candesartan and Hydrochlorothiazide 338
Cantacid (KR) *see* Calcium Carbonate 327
Cantar (IN, VN) *see* Candesartan 335
Cantex (TR) *see* Voriconazole 2176
Canthacur (CA) *see* Cantharidin [CAN/INT] 338
Cantharone (CA) *see* Cantharidin [CAN/INT] 338
Canzeal (VN) *see* Glimepiride 966
Caosina (ES) *see* Calcium Carbonate 327
Capace (ZA) *see* Captopril 342
Capebina (VN) *see* Capecitabine 339
Capecitabina (PE) *see* Capecitabine 339
Capetero (PH) *see* Capecitabine 339
Capexion (GB) *see* Tacrolimus (Systemic) 1962
Capibine (IN) *see* Capecitabine 339
Capicet (IN) *see* Cinacalcet 439
Capillus (KR) *see* Minoxidil (Topical) 1374
Capimune (GB) *see* CycloSPORINE (Systemic) 522
Caplenal (GB) *see* Allopurinol 90
Capmerin (PH) *see* Mercaptopurine 1296
Capocard (JO, KW, QA, SA) *see* Captopril 342
Capomed (PH) *see* Captopril 342
Capool (TW) *see* Calcium Carbonate 327
Capotec (PH) *see* Captopril 342
Capotena (MX) *see* Captopril 342
Capoten (AE, AU, BB, BE, BH, BM, BR, BS, BZ, CL, CN, CO, CY, CZ, DK, EC, EG, ES, ET, FI, GB, GR, GY, HK, IE, IT, JM, JO, KE, KW, LB, LU, NG, NL, NO, NZ, PH, PK, PL, PT, QA, SA, SE, SR, TR, TT, TZ, UG, VE, ZA, ZM) *see* Captopril 342
Capotril (AE, BH, CY, EG, IQ, IR, JO, KW, LB, LY, OM, QA, SA, SY, YE) *see* Captopril 342
Capozid (DK) *see* Captopril and Hydrochlorothiazide 345
Capozide (BB, BH, BM, BS, BZ, CH, CY, EG, GY, ID, IE, JM, KW, MX, NL, NZ, PE, PH, PK, QA, RU, SA, SR, TT, VE, ZA) *see* Captopril and Hydrochlorothiazide 345

Capozide Forte (AT) *see* Captopril and Hydrochlorothiazide 345
Capozit (KR) *see* Captopril and Hydrochlorothiazide 345
Caprelsa (AR, AU, BE, BR, CH, CZ, DE, DK, EE, ES, FR, GB, HK, HR, IL, IS, KR, LT, MX, NL, NO, RO, SE, SI, SK) *see* Vandetanib 2135
Caprifim (ID) *see* Cefepime 378
Capril (KR, SA, TH) *see* Captopril 342
Caprilon (FI) *see* Tranexamic Acid 2081
Caprin (GB) *see* Aspirin 180
Caprin (IN) *see* Heparin 997
Caprizide (BH, CY, EG, IQ, IR, JO, KW, LB, LY, OM, QA, SA, SY, YE) *see* Captopril and Hydrochlorothiazide 345
Caproamin (ES, VE) *see* Aminocaproic Acid 113
Caproamin Fides (ES) *see* Aminocaproic Acid 113
Caprolest (NL) *see* Aminocaproic Acid 113
Caprol (ID) *see* Pantoprazole 1570
Caprolisin (IT) *see* Aminocaproic Acid 113
Capsinat (ID) *see* Amoxicillin and Clavulanate 133
Captace (AE, PH) *see* Captopril 342
Captarsan (VN) *see* Captopril 342
Captaton (AR) *see* FLUoxetine 899
Captea (FR) *see* Captopril and Hydrochlorothiazide 345
Captensin (ID) *see* Captopril 342
Captodoc (DE) *see* Captopril 342
Captoflux (DE) *see* Captopril 342
Captohexal (EE, LU, NZ) *see* Captopril 342
Captolane (FR) *see* Captopril 342
Captomed (QA) *see* Captopril 342
Captopren (AE, BH, CY, EG, IL, IQ, IR, JO, KW, LB, LY, OM, QA, SA, SY, YE) *see* Captopril 342
Captopress (GR) *see* Captopril and Hydrochlorothiazide 345
Captoprilan-D (DO) *see* Captopril and Hydrochlorothiazide 345
Captopril (DO) *see* Captopril 342
Captopril-H (IN) *see* Captopril and Hydrochlorothiazide 345
Captopril Pharmavit (HU) *see* Captopril 342
Captotec (BR) *see* Captopril 342
Captral (MX) *see* Captopril 342
Caraben (KR) *see* Calcitriol 323
Carace 20 (GB) *see* Lisinopril and Hydrochlorothiazide 1229
Carace Plus (GB, IE) *see* Lisinopril and Hydrochlorothiazide 1229
Caradine (TH) *see* Loratadine 1241
Carafate (AU, NZ) *see* Sucralfate 1940
Caraten (TH) *see* Carvedilol 367
Carazepin (AE, BH, CY, EG, IQ, IR, JO, KW, LB, LY, OM, QA, SA, SY, YE) *see* CarBAMazepine 346
Carbachol (PL) *see* Carbachol 346
Carbadac (BF, BJ, CI, ET, GH, GM, GN, KE, LR, MA, ML, MR, MU, MW, NE, NG, SC, SD, SL, SN, TN, TZ, UG, ZM, ZW) *see* CarBAMazepine 346
Carbaderme (PT) *see* Urea 2114
Carbaderm (NO) *see* Urea 2114
Carbaflex (HN, NI, SV) *see* Methocarbamol 1320
Carbagen (GB) *see* CarBAMazepine 346
Carbaglu (AT, BE, CZ, DE, DK, EE, FR, GB, HR, IL, IT, LT, NL, PL, PT, RO, SE, SI, SK) *see* Carglumic Acid 362
Carbalex (EE) *see* CarBAMazepine 346
Carbal (TW) *see* Carbachol 346
Carbamazepin-B (HU) *see* CarBAMazepine 346
Carbam (EC) *see* CarBAMazepine 346
Carbamid (LU) *see* Urea 2114
Carbamid Widmer (DE) *see* Urea 2114
Carbamol (KR) *see* Methocarbamol 1320
Carbapin (PE) *see* CarBAMazepine 346
Carbatin (TW) *see* Gabapentin 943
Carbatol (AE, BH, IN, JO, TW) *see* CarBAMazepine 346
Carbatol CR (SG) *see* CarBAMazepine 346
Carbazene (TH) *see* CarBAMazepine 346
Carbazina (MX) *see* CarBAMazepine 346
Carbidol (BR) *see* Carbidopa and Levodopa 351
Carbilev (ZA) *see* Carbidopa and Levodopa 351
Carbimazol Aliud (AT) *see* Carbimazole [INT] 356
Carbimazol Henning (DE) *see* Carbimazole [INT] 356
Carbinib (PT) *see* AcetaZOLAMIDE 39
Carbizole (PK) *see* Carbimazole [INT] 356
Carbloxal (ID) *see* Carvedilol 367
Carbocaina (IT) *see* Mepivacaine 1295
Carbocain Dental (NO) *see* Mepivacaine 1295
Carbocain (DK, SE) *see* Mepivacaine 1295
Carbocaine Dental (PL, ZA) *see* Mepivacaine 1295
Carbocaine HCl (FR) *see* Mepivacaine 1295
Carbocal (ES) *see* Calcium Carbonate 327
Carbocin (BR) *see* Carbocisteine [INT] 357
Carboflem (PH) *see* Carbocisteine [INT] 357
Carbolim (BR) *see* Lithium 1230
Carbolit (CL, CO, MX) *see* Lithium 1230
Carbolithium (IT) *see* Lithium 1230
Carbo Medicinalis (PL) *see* Charcoal, Activated 416
Carbomint (VN) *see* Charcoal, Activated 416
Carbomix (FR, SE, TR, TW) *see* Charcoal, Activated 416
Carbon Natural (UY) *see* Charcoal, Activated 416
Ca-R-Bon (TH) *see* Charcoal, Activated 416
Carboplat (AR, DE, MX) *see* CARBOplatin 357
Carboplatin Abic (TH) *see* CARBOplatin 357
Carboplatin (AE, AU, CY, DK, IL, JO, KW, LB, NO, NZ, SA) *see* CARBOplatin 357
Carboplatin a (PT) *see* CARBOplatin 357
Carboplatin-David Bull (LU) *see* CARBOplatin 357
Carboplatin DBL (MY) *see* CARBOplatin 357
Carboplatin dbl (PT) *see* CARBOplatin 357
Carboplatin-Medac (LU) *see* CARBOplatin 357
Carboplatin-Teva (HU) *see* CARBOplatin 357
Carboplatinum Cytosafe-Delta West (LU) *see* CARBOplatin 357
Carboplatin "Delta West" (HR) *see* CARBOplatin 357
Carbosin (BE, GR, ID, KR, NO, PH) *see* CARBOplatin 357
Carbosin Lundbeck (FI) *see* CARBOplatin 357
Carbosorb X (AU, NZ) *see* Charcoal, Activated 416
Carbosorb (NZ) *see* Charcoal, Activated 416
Carbosorb XS (AU, NZ) *see* Charcoal, Activated 416
Carbostesin (AT, CH, DE) *see* Bupivacaine 299
Carbotec (MX) *see* CARBOplatin 357
Carbotinol (PH) *see* CARBOplatin 357
Carbotos (CL) *see* Carbocisteine [INT] 357
Carbotox (SK) *see* Charcoal, Activated 416
Carbotural (MX) *see* Charcoal, Activated 416
Carbox (PH) *see* OXcarbazepine 1532
Cardace-H (IN) *see* Ramipril and Hydrochlorothiazide [CAN/INT] 1773
Cardace (ID, IN) *see* Ramipril 1771
Cardanat (DE) *see* Etilefrine [INT] 815
Cardcor (BR) *see* Digoxin 627
Cardease (PH) *see* DOBUTamine 654
Cardeloc (TH) *see* Metoprolol 1350
Cardem (ES) *see* Celiprolol [INT] 404
Cardenalin (JP) *see* Doxazosin 674
Cardene (IE, NL) *see* NiCARdipine 1446
Cardene SR (GB, NL) *see* NiCARdipine 1446
Cardensiel (FR) *see* Bisoprolol 266
Cardepine (MY) *see* NiCARdipine 1446
Cardepine SR (MY) *see* NiCARdipine 1446
Cardiacin (TW) *see* Digoxin 627
Cardiagen (DE) *see* Captopril 342
Cardialgine (DE) *see* Etilefrine [INT] 815
Cardiamed (MY) *see* Norepinephrine 1472
Cardiazem (KR) *see* Diltiazem 634
Cardibloc SR (SG) *see* NiCARdipine 1446
Cardiblok (ZA) *see* Propranolol 1731
Cardibrain (TW) *see* NiCARdipine 1446

Cardicor (DK, IE) *see* Bisoprolol 266
Cardifen (ZA) *see* NIFEdipine 1451
Cardiiopine (AE) *see* NIFEdipine 1451
Cardiject (ID, IN, TH, ZA) *see* DOBUTamine 654
Cardil (AE, BG, BH, DK, IS, LT, MY, QA, RU) *see* Diltiazem 634
Cardiloc (IL) *see* Bisoprolol 266
Cardilol (AE) *see* Propranolol 1731
Cardilol (JO, LB, PH) *see* Carvedilol 367
Cardilor (MY, TH) *see* Amiodarone 114
Cardil (PY) *see* Isosorbide Dinitrate 1124
Cardil Retard (GR) *see* Diltiazem 634
Cardimax (IN) *see* Trimetazidine [INT] 2104
Cardimax (PE) *see* Adenosine 55
Cardin (KR) *see* QuiNIDine 1759
Cardinol LA (NZ) *see* Propranolol 1731
Cardinol (NZ) *see* Propranolol 1731
Cardinorm (AU) *see* Amiodarone 114
Cardioaspirina (CO, PE) *see* Aspirin 180
Cardiogoxin (AR) *see* Digoxin 627
Cardiolen (CL) *see* Verapamil 2154
Cardiol (FI, MY) *see* Carvedilol 367
Cardioplus (CL) *see* Olmesartan 1496
Cardioplus AM (CL) *see* Amlodipine and Olmesartan 126
Cardiopril (CH) *see* Spirapril [INT] 1931
Cardioprin 100 (IL) *see* Aspirin 180
Cardioprin (HR, TW) *see* Aspirin 180
Cardioquina (UY) *see* QuiNIDine 1759
Cardioquinol (EC) *see* QuiNIDine 1759
Cardiorona (CR, DO, GT, HN, NI, PA, SV) *see* Amiodarone 114
Cardiorytmin (FI) *see* Procainamide 1716
Cardiosel-OD (PH) *see* Metoprolol 1350
Cardiosel (PH) *see* Metoprolol 1350
Cardiostat (PH) *see* Metoprolol 1350
Cardiotab (PH) *see* Metoprolol 1350
Cardioten (PH) *see* Atenolol 189
Cardiotensin (PL) *see* Moexipril 1388
Cardiotone (ID) *see* DOBUTamine 654
Cardioton (PE) *see* Aspirin 180
Cardiovasc (EC) *see* Losartan and Hydrochlorothiazide 1250
Cardiovasc (IT) *see* Lercanidipine [INT] 1181
Cardioxane (AR, AT, BR, CL, CO, CZ, DK, EC, EG, ES, FI, FR, GB, GT, HN, HU, IL, IT, KR, MX, NI, NL, PE, PL, PY, SI, SV, UY, VE) *see* Dexrazoxane 606
Cardioxin (PH) *see* Digoxin 627
Cardipair (KR) *see* Amlodipine and Atorvastatin 124
Cardipene (TH) *see* NiCARdipine 1446
Cardipres (PH) *see* Carvedilol 367
Cardipril (PT, TR) *see* Imidapril [INT] 1051
Cardiprin (HK) *see* Aspirin 180
Cardismo (ID) *see* Isosorbide Mononitrate 1126
Cardisorb (HU) *see* Isosorbide Mononitrate 1126
Cardispare (ZA) *see* Propranolol 1731
Cardispray (AE) *see* Nitroglycerin 1465
Carditoxin (HU) *see* Digitoxin [INT] 627
Cardium (SG) *see* Diltiazem 634
Cardivas (IN, VN) *see* Carvedilol 367
Cardiwell (IN) *see* Dipyridamole 652
Cardizem CD (AU, BR, NZ) *see* Diltiazem 634
Cardizem (AU, BR, DK, FI, NO, NZ, SE) *see* Diltiazem 634
Cardizem Retard (DK, FI, SE, TW) *see* Diltiazem 634
Cardizem SR (BR) *see* Diltiazem 634
Cardizem Unotard (TW) *see* Diltiazem 634
Cardnit (PK) *see* Nitroglycerin 1465
Cardol (AU, TW) *see* Sotalol 1927
Cardolol (TW) *see* Propranolol 1731
Cardol (PH) *see* AmLODIPine 123
Cardomel (ES) *see* Enoximone [INT] 730
Cardomin (PH) *see* DOBUTamine 654
Cardonit (HU) *see* Isosorbide Dinitrate 1124
Cardopar (SG) *see* Carbidopa and Levodopa 351
Cardopax (DK) *see* Isosorbide Dinitrate 1124
Cardoxin Forte (IL) *see* Dipyridamole 652
Cardoxin (IL) *see* Digoxin 627
Cardoxin (IL) *see* Dipyridamole 652
Cardoxone (TR) *see* Metoprolol 1350
Cardoxx (HR) *see* Isosorbide Mononitrate 1126
Cardular (DE, LB) *see* Doxazosin 674
Cardular PP (DE) *see* Doxazosin 674
Cardular Uro (DE) *see* Doxazosin 674
Cardura XL (CL, CN, CO, CR, DO, EC, EE, GT, HK, HN, LT, MY, NI, PA, PE, PL, RO, SI, SK, SV, TH) *see* Doxazosin 674
Cardura-XL S.R. (KR) *see* Doxazosin 674
Cardura (AE, AR, BG, BH, CL, CO, CR, CY, CZ, DO, EG, GB, GR, GT, HK, HN, HU, ID, IE, IQ, IR, JO, KW, LT, LY, MX, MY, NI, NL, OM, PA, PK, PT, QA, RU, SA, SG, SV, SY, TH, TR, UY, VE, YE, ZA, ZM) *see* Doxazosin 674
Cardura CR (CH) *see* Doxazosin 674
Carduran XL (BR) *see* Doxazosin 674
Carduran (AU, ES, NO, VN) *see* Doxazosin 674
Carduran Neo (ES) *see* Doxazosin 674
Carduran Retard (DK, IS) *see* Doxazosin 674
Cardyl (ES) *see* AtorvaSTATin 194
Carecin (JP) *see* Cinnarizine [INT] 440
Carencil (PE) *see* Donepezil 668
Cargen (KR) *see* Carvedilol 367
Carident (NO) *see* Fluoride 895
Carim (EC, UY) *see* Modafinil 1386
Carimycin (TW) *see* Clarithromycin 456
Carin (MY) *see* Loratadine 1241
Carinose (TH) *see* Loratadine 1241
Carinox (MY) *see* Loratadine and Pseudoephedrine 1242
Carisoma (GB, IN, VN) *see* Carisoprodol 363
Carlevod (AR) *see* Carbidopa and Levodopa 351
Carlipin (HK) *see* Acarbose 29
Carlit (PY) *see* Lithium 1230
Carlmycin (TW) *see* Kanamycin 1142
Carloc (ZA) *see* Carvedilol 367
Carlov (PK) *see* Carvedilol 367
Carmapine (TH) *see* CarBAMazepine 346
Carmaz (IN) *see* CarBAMazepine 346
Carmed (ID) *see* Urea 2114
Carmen (DE) *see* Lercanidipine [INT] 1181
Carmian (CL) *see* CarBAMazepine 346
Carmin (AR, UY) *see* Desogestrel [INT] 597
Carmine (KR) *see* CarBAMazepine 346
Carmubris (AT, DE) *see* Carmustine 364
Carnet (CN) *see* Foscarnet 931
Carnotprim (MX) *see* Metoclopramide 1345
Carnyl (DK) *see* Aspirin 180
Carodiet (KR) *see* Amlodipine and Atorvastatin 124
Carol (KR) *see* Ibuprofen 1032
Caronem (ID) *see* Meropenem 1299
Caropraml (IN) *see* Doxapram 673
Carotaben (AT, CH, CZ, DE, NO) *see* Beta-Carotene 251
Carotan (PE) *see* CefTRIAXone 396
Carpin (MX) *see* CarBAMazepine 346
Carplan (KR) *see* CARBOplatin 357
Carrier (PY) *see* Memantine 1286
Carsemex (TH) *see* Carbocisteine [INT] 357
Carsive (ID) *see* NiCARdipine 1446
Carsodil (KR) *see* Isosorbide Dinitrate 1124
Cartia (PT) *see* Aspirin 180
Cartigen (MX) *see* Diacerein [INT] 613
Cartivix (PT) *see* Diacerein [INT] 613
Cartrex (FR) *see* Aceclofenac [INT] 30
Cartrilet (ID) *see* Ticlopidine 2040
Caruderma (HK) *see* Urea 2114
Carvasin (IT) *see* Isosorbide Dinitrate 1124
Carvastin (PH) *see* AtorvaSTATin 194
Carvedexxon (IL) *see* Carvedilol 367

Carvedil (EC) *see* Carvedilol ... 367
Carvedlol (KR) *see* Carvedilol ... 367
Carvelol (KR, NZ) *see* Carvedilol ... 367
Carvenal (KR) *see* Carvedilol ... 367
Carvepen (SG) *see* Carvedilol ... 367
Carveta (KR) *see* Carvedilol ... 367
Carvidex (TR) *see* Carvedilol ... 367
Carvidil (RU) *see* Carvedilol ... 367
Carvidol (CN, JO) *see* Carvedilol ... 367
Carvidon (IN, PH) *see* Trimetazidine [INT] ... 2104
Carvidon-MR (IN, PH) *see* Trimetazidine [INT] ... 2104
Carvid (PH) *see* Carvedilol ... 367
Carvilar (DO) *see* Carvedilol ... 367
Carvisken (JP) *see* Pindolol ... 1652
Carvo (TW) *see* Carvedilol ... 367
Caryolysine (FR, GR) *see* Mechlorethamine (Systemic) ... 1276
Carzepin (HK, MY) *see* CarBAMazepine ... 346
Casartan (PH) *see* Candesartan ... 335
Cascor XL (TH) *see* Diltiazem ... 634
Casobit (KR) *see* Bicalutamide ... 262
Casodex (AE, AR, AT, BB, BD, BE, BF, BG, BH, BJ, BM, BR, BS, BZ, CH, CI, CL, CN, CO, CR, CY, CZ, DE, DK, DO, EE, ES, ET, FI, FR, GB, GH, GM, GN, GR, GT, GY, HK, HN, HR, HU, ID, IE, IL, IT, JM, JO, JP, KE, KR, KW, LB, LR, LT, LU, MA, ML, MR, MT, MU, MW, MX, MY, NE, NG, NI, NL, NO, PA, PE, PH, PK, PL, PR, PT, QA, RO, RU, SC, SD, SE, SG, SI, SK, SL, SN, SR, SV, TH, TN, TR, TT, TW, TZ, UG, UY, VE, VN, ZA, ZM, ZW) *see* Bicalutamide ... 262
Caspirin (MY) *see* Aspirin ... 180
Cassadan (DE) *see* ALPRAZolam ... 94
Castilium (PT) *see* CloBAZam ... 465
Catabon (JP) *see* DOPamine ... 669
Catacrom (GB) *see* Cromolyn (Ophthalmic) ... 514
Catafast (SA) *see* Diclofenac (Systemic) ... 617
Cataflam D (ID) *see* Diclofenac (Systemic) ... 617
Cataflam (AE, BE, BH, CL, CY, EC, EE, EG, HK, ID, IE, IL, IQ, IR, JO, KW, LB, LT, LY, NL, NO, OM, PE, PT, QA, SA, SY, TR, TW, UY, VE, YE) *see* Diclofenac (Systemic) ... 617
Cataflam (BH, CY, SG) *see* Diclofenac (Ophthalmic) ... 621
Cataflam Drops (MY) *see* Diclofenac (Systemic) ... 617
Catanac (TH) *see* Diclofenac (Systemic) ... 617
Catapin (PH) *see* CloNIDine ... 480
Catapresan (AR, AT, CH, CL, CO, CR, DE, DK, DO, EC, ES, FI, GR, GT, HN, HR, IS, IT, NI, NL, NO, PA, PE, PT, SE, SI, SV, VE) *see* CloNIDine ... 480
Catapresan Depot (CZ, DE) *see* CloNIDine ... 480
Catapresan TTS (IT) *see* CloNIDine ... 480
Catapres (AU, BB, BD, BF, BH, BJ, BM, BS, BZ, CI, CY, ET, GB, GH, GM, GN, GY, HK, ID, IE, IL, IN, IQ, IR, JM, JO, JP, KE, KR, KW, LR, MA, ML, MR, MU, MW, MY, NE, NG, NZ, OM, PH, PK, PR, QA, SA, SC, SD, SG, SL, SN, SR, TN, TT, TW, TZ, UG, ZM, ZW) *see* CloNIDine ... 480
Catapress (AE, EG) *see* CloNIDine ... 480
Catapressan (BE, FR, LU, VN) *see* CloNIDine ... 480
Catarrosine (AR) *see* Bromhexine [INT] ... 291
Catas (KR) *see* Diclofenac (Systemic) ... 617
Catenol (BF, BJ, CI, ET, GH, GM, GN, KE, LR, MA, ML, MR, MU, MW, NE, NG, SC, SD, SL, SN, TH, TN, TZ, UG, ZM, ZW) *see* Atenolol ... 189
Catepsin (PY) *see* QUEtiapine ... 1751
Catin (TW) *see* Trimethoprim ... 2104
Catlep (JP) *see* Indomethacin ... 1067
Cato-Bell (IN) *see* Potassium Iodide ... 1690
Catoplin (SG) *see* Captopril ... 342
Causalon (AR) *see* Acetaminophen ... 32
Causalon (UY) *see* Dipyrone [INT] ... 653
Cavel (MY) *see* Carvedilol ... 367
Caveril (AE, BB, BH, BM, BS, BZ, CY, ET, GH, GY, IL, JM, JO, KE, LB, MU, OM, PR, QA, SR, SY, TT, TZ, YE) *see* Verapamil ... 2154
Caverject (AE, AR, AT, BB, BH, BM, BO, BR, BS, BZ, CL, CO, CR, CY, CZ, DE, DO, EC, EE, EG, FR, GB, GT, GY, HU, IE, IQ, IR, IS, JM, JO, KR, KW, LB, LU, LY, MX, MY, NI, NL, NO, NZ, OM, PA, PE, PR, PT, PY, QA, SA, SE, SG, SI, SR, SV, SY, TR, TT, TW, UY, VE, VN, YE, ZA) *see* Alprostadil ... 96
Caverject Dual Chamber (FR, HK) *see* Alprostadil ... 96
Caverject Impulse (AU) *see* Alprostadil ... 96
Caverjet (IL) *see* Alprostadil ... 96
Cavumox (MY, TH) *see* Amoxicillin and Clavulanate ... 133
Caxin (PH) *see* Cloxacillin [CAN/INT] ... 488
Caxlem (PH) *see* Meloxicam ... 1283
Cayston (NL) *see* Aztreonam ... 220
Cazosin (TH) *see* Doxazosin ... 674
CB-400 (TH) *see* Albendazole ... 65
C-Clarin (KR) *see* Clarithromycin ... 456
CC-Nefro 500 (DE) *see* Calcium Carbonate ... 327
CCNU (AE, BH, CY, EG, GB, IL, IQ, IR, JO, KW, LB, LY, OM, PK, QA, SA, SY, TR, YE) *see* Lomustine ... 1235
C.C.N.U. (ES) *see* Lomustine ... 1235
Ccombigan (HU) *see* Brimonidine and Timolol ... 288
CD Jevax (KR, TH) *see* Japanese Encephalitis Virus Vaccine (Inactivated) ... 1141
C-Dose (BE) *see* Ascorbic Acid ... 178
CDR Fortos (ID) *see* Calcium and Vitamin D ... 326
CDT Vaccine (NZ) *see* Diphtheria and Tetanus Toxoid ... 645
Ceact (IN) *see* Piracetam [INT] ... 1661
Cealb (AE) *see* Albumin ... 67
Cebactam (CO) *see* Cefoperazone and Sulbactam [INT] ... 382
Cebenicol (FR) *see* Chloramphenicol ... 421
Cebion (AE, AT, BH, CL, CY, EG, ES, GR, IL, IQ, IR, IT, JO, KW, LB, LY, OM, PE, PL, PT, QA, SA, SY, YE) *see* Ascorbic Acid ... 178
Cebralat C (BR) *see* Cilostazol ... 437
Cebridin (UY) *see* Cinnarizine [INT] ... 440
Cebrium (TH) *see* Flunarizine [CAN/INT] ... 892
Cebrotonin (DE, EC, MY, SG) *see* Piracetam [INT] ... 1661
Cebutid (FR) *see* Flurbiprofen (Systemic) ... 906
CEC 500 (DE) *see* Cefaclor ... 372
Cec (MX) *see* Cefaclor ... 372
Cecai (TW) *see* Ascorbic Acid ... 178
Cecan (PY) *see* Cephalexin ... 405
Cecap (HK) *see* Ascorbic Acid ... 178
CEC (AT, BG, DO, ZA) *see* Cefaclor ... 372
CeCe (KR) *see* Ascorbic Acid ... 178
Cecenu (BE, DE, GR, NL, PL) *see* Lomustine ... 1235
Ceclobid (PH) *see* Cefaclor ... 372
Ceclodyne (RO) *see* Cefaclor ... 372
Ceclor CD (AU) *see* Cefaclor ... 372
Ceclor (AE, AT, AU, BB, BF, BH, BJ, BM, BR, BS, BZ, CH, CI, CN, CO, EC, EG, ES, ET, GH, GM, GN, GR, GY, HK, HN, HU, JM, KE, KR, LB, LR, MA, ML, MR, MU, MW, MX, NE, NG, NL, PE, PH, PK, PL, PT, QA, RO, RU, SA, SC, SD, SL, SN, SR, TN, TR, TT, TZ, UG, VE, ZM, ZW) *see* Cefaclor ... 372
Ceclor AF (PE) *see* Cefaclor ... 372
Ceclor DS (PH) *see* Cefaclor ... 372
Ceclor MR (BF, BH, BJ, CI, CY, ET, GH, GM, GN, HK, KE, KW, LB, LR, MA, ML, MR, MU, MW, NE, NG, SA, SC, SD, SL, SN, TN, TZ, UG, ZM, ZW) *see* Cefaclor ... 372
Ceclor PDR (CY) *see* Cefaclor ... 372
Ceclor Retard (CH, ES) *see* Cefaclor ... 372
Ceclor SR (NZ) *see* Cefaclor ... 372
Cecon (BB, BM, BS, BZ, GY, JM, PH, PR, SR, TT) *see* Ascorbic Acid ... 178
Cecon Drops (AU) *see* Ascorbic Acid ... 178
Cecrun (KR) *see* Cefaclor ... 372
Cedantron (ID) *see* Ondansetron ... 1513

Cedar (CO) *see* HydrOXYzine ... 1024
Cedax (AE, AR, BB, BG, BH, BM, BS, BZ, CH, CR, CZ, DO, EC, FI, GB, GT, GY, HK, HN, HR, HU, ID, IE, IT, JM, MX, MY, NI, NL, PA, PH, PL, QA, RO, RU, SE, SG, SI, SK, SR, SV, TH, TT, VE, VN) *see* Ceftibuten ... 394
Cedocard (AE, AT, BE, CY, GB, ID, IE, LU, NL, QA, TR) *see* Isosorbide Dinitrate ... 1124
Cedocard Retard (AT, ID, NL) *see* Isosorbide Dinitrate ... 1124
Cedrox (AE, BH, CY, EG, IQ, IR, JO, KW, LB, LY, OM, QA, SA, SK, SY, YE) *see* Cefadroxil ... 372
Cedroxil (BR) *see* Cefadroxil ... 372
Cedur (BE, BR, DE, LU) *see* Bezafibrate [CAN/INT] ... 261
Cedur Retard (CH) *see* Bezafibrate [CAN/INT] ... 261
Ceelin (SG) *see* Ascorbic Acid ... 178
CEENU (AR, CN, MX, SG, UY) *see* Lomustine ... 1235
CeeNU (AU, BF, BJ, CI, CL, ET, GH, GM, GN, HK, KE, KR, LR, MA, ML, MR, MU, MW, NE, NG, NZ, PH, SC, SD, SL, SN, TN, TZ, UG, ZA, ZM, ZW) *see* Lomustine ... 1235
Ceenu (CZ) *see* Lomustine ... 1235
Ceetrotide (BH) *see* Cetrorelix ... 413
Cefabac (AE, BH, CY, EG, IL, IQ, IR, JO, KW, LB, LY, OM, QA, SA, SY, YE) *see* Cefaclor ... 372
Cefabiot (MX) *see* Cefuroxime ... 399
Cefabiotic (ID) *see* Cephalexin ... 405
Cefacar (AR) *see* Cefadroxil ... 372
Cefacell (KR) *see* Cefadroxil ... 372
Cefacet (FR) *see* Cephalexin ... 405
Cefacidal (EC, LU, PE, VE, ZA) *see* CeFAZolin ... 373
Cefacin-M (HK) *see* Cephalexin ... 405
Cefacle (KR) *see* Cefaclor ... 372
Cefacolin (AR) *see* Cefotaxime ... 382
Cefacrol (PE) *see* CefTRIAXone ... 396
Cefactam (PY, UY) *see* Cefoperazone and Sulbactam [INT] ... 382
Cefadal (BF, BJ, CI, ET, GH, GM, GN, KE, LR, MA, ML, MR, MU, MW, NE, NG, SC, SD, SL, SN, TN, TZ, UG, ZA, ZM, ZW) *see* Cephalexin ... 405
Cefadime (TW) *see* CefTAZidime ... 392
Cefadin (EC) *see* Cephalexin ... 405
Cefadox (PH) *see* Cefpodoxime ... 388
Cefadril (IT, LB, QA, SA) *see* Cefadroxil ... 372
Cefadrol (IN) *see* Cefadroxil ... 372
Cefadrox (AE, KW, PH, PY, SA) *see* Cefadroxil ... 372
Cefadur (MY) *see* Cefadroxil ... 372
Cefadyl (BF, BJ, CI, ET, GH, GM, GN, KE, LR, MA, ML, MR, MU, MW, NE, NG, SC, SD, SL, SN, TN, TZ, UG, ZM, ZW) *see* Cephalexin ... 405
Cefalekol (HU) *see* Cefotaxime ... 382
Cefalin (ID, PH) *see* Cephalexin ... 405
Cefaloc (PH) *see* Cefaclor ... 372
Cefalom (GR) *see* Cefadroxil ... 372
Cefalver (MX) *see* Cephalexin ... 405
Cefamax (TH) *see* Cefepime ... 378
Cefamezin (AE, EG, HR, JP, KR, QA, RU, SA, TH, TR) *see* CeFAZolin ... 373
Cefamox (SE) *see* Cefadroxil ... 372
Cefanozix (PY) *see* Cefoperazone and Sulbactam [INT] ... 382
Cefarad (AE, BF, BH, BJ, CI, CY, EG, ET, GH, GM, GN, IQ, IR, JO, KE, KW, LB, LR, LY, MA, ML, MR, MU, MW, NE, NG, OM, QA, SA, SC, SD, SL, SN, SY, TN, TZ, UG, YE, ZM, ZW) *see* CeFAZolin ... 373
Cefarox (ID) *see* Cefixime ... 380
Cefastad (HK) *see* Cephalexin ... 405
Cefasun (IN) *see* Cefuroxime ... 399
Cefat (ID) *see* Cefadroxil ... 372
Cefatum (MY) *see* CefTAZidime ... 392
Cefa (TW) *see* CeFAZolin ... 373
Cefaxicina (ES) *see* CefOXitin ... 386
Cefaxin (KR) *see* Ciprofloxacin (Systemic) ... 441
Cefaxona (MX) *see* CefTRIAXone ... 396
Cefaxone (KR, MY, SG) *see* CefTRIAXone ... 396
Cefaz (HR) *see* CefTAZidime ... 392
Cefazime (SG) *see* CefTAZidime ... 392
Cefazin (TW) *see* CeFAZolin ... 373
Cefazol (ID, TH) *see* CeFAZolin ... 373
Cefazolina (LB) *see* CeFAZolin ... 373
Cefazoline Panpharma (FR) *see* CeFAZolin ... 373
Cefazovit (PH) *see* CeFAZolin ... 373
Cefclor (TH) *see* Cefaclor ... 372
Cefdiar (KR) *see* Cefdinir ... 376
Cefdoxime (KR) *see* Cefpodoxime ... 388
Cefemax (TW) *see* Cefepime ... 378
Cefen (TH) *see* Ibuprofen ... 1032
Cefepima (CO) *see* Cefepime ... 378
Ceferom (TW) *see* Cefpirome [INT] ... 388
Cefexin (HR) *see* Cefixime ... 380
Cef-H (MY) *see* CefTAZidime ... 392
Ceficad (IN) *see* Cefepime ... 378
Cefinov (ID) *see* Cefepime ... 378
Cefin (SG) *see* CefTRIAXone ... 396
Cefipex (LB) *see* Cefepime ... 378
Cefirad (KR) *see* Cefotaxime ... 382
Cefirax (EC, PE, PY) *see* Cefpodoxime ... 388
Cefirax (KR) *see* Cefixime ... 380
Cefire (VN) *see* Cefpirome [INT] ... 388
Cefix (AE, BH, CY, EG, IQ, IR, JO, KR, KW, LB, LY, MY, OM, QA, SA, SY, YE) *see* Cefixime ... 380
Cefixmycin (PH, TW) *see* Cefixime ... 380
Cefizol (TR) *see* CeFAZolin ... 373
Cefkizon (KR) *see* CefTRIAXone ... 396
Cefkor (AU) *see* Cefaclor ... 372
Ceflacid (MX) *see* Cefaclor ... 372
Ceflour (MY) *see* Cefuroxime ... 399
Ceflox (IN) *see* Ciprofloxacin (Ophthalmic) ... 446
Ceflox (IN) *see* Ciprofloxacin (Otic) ... 446
Ceflox (IN) *see* Ciprofloxacin (Systemic) ... 441
Cefmate (IN) *see* Cefoperazone and Sulbactam [INT] ... 382
Cefmed (PH) *see* Cefaclor ... 372
Cefmono (PH) *see* Cefuroxime ... 399
Cefmore (TW) *see* CefOXitin ... 386
Cefnaxl (PH) *see* Cefdinir ... 376
Cefnir (PK) *see* Cefdinir ... 376
Cefobacatam (PH) *see* Cefoperazone and Sulbactam [INT] ... 382
Cefobactam DI (ID) *see* Cefoperazone and Sulbactam [INT] ... 382
Cefobeta (IN) *see* Cefoperazone and Sulbactam [INT] ... 382
Cefocam (PY) *see* Cefotaxime ... 382
Cefodox (AE, BH, CY, EG, IE, IL, IQ, IR, IT, JO, KW, LB, LU, LY, OM, QA, SA, SY, YE) *see* Cefpodoxime ... 388
Cefolatam (KR) *see* Cefoperazone and Sulbactam [INT] ... 382
Ceforal (IL) *see* Cephalexin ... 405
Ceforal (PT) *see* Cefadroxil ... 372
Ceforan (RO) *see* Cefadroxil ... 372
Cefortam (PT) *see* CefTAZidime ... 392
Cefort (RO) *see* CefTRIAXone ... 396
Cefotaksim (HR) *see* Cefotaxime ... 382
Cefotax (AE, BH, CY, EG, IQ, IR, JO, JP, KW, LB, LY, OM, QA, RO, SA, SY, YE) *see* Cefotaxime ... 382
Cefotaxim (DE, NO) *see* Cefotaxime ... 382
Cefot (DO) *see* Cefotaxime ... 382
Cefotrial (PE) *see* Cefotaxime ... 382
Cefovit (IL) *see* Cephalexin ... 405
Cefoxim (KR) *see* Cefotaxime ... 382
Cefoxitin Sodium (AU) *see* CefOXitin ... 386
Cefoxivit (PH) *see* CefOXitin ... 386
Cefox (PH) *see* Cefotaxime ... 382
Cefpar SB (TH) *see* Cefoperazone and Sulbactam [INT] ... 382

Cefper (MY, TH) *see* Cefoperazone and Sulbactam [INT] ... 382
Cefpiran (KR) *see* Cefotaxime ... 382
Cefpiran (PE) *see* CefTAZidime ... 392
Cefproz (AE, LB, SA) *see* Cefprozil ... 389
Cefraden (MX) *see* CefTRIAXone ... 396
Cefralin (PE) *see* Cefdinir ... 376
Cefratam (ID) *see* Cefoperazone and Sulbactam [INT] ... 382
Cefrax (TR) *see* Cephalexin ... 405
Cefriex (ID) *see* CefTRIAXone ... 396
Cefrin (PH) *see* Cefpirome [INT] ... 388
Cefrom (AT, CN, FR, GR, ID, IN, KW, PK, SA, TW, ZA) *see* Cefpirome [INT] ... 388
Cefrozil (KR) *see* Cefprozil ... 389
Cefspan (CN, ID, JP, PK, TH, TW, VN) *see* Cefixime ... 380
Cef-S (PH) *see* CefTRIAXone ... 396
Ceftamil (RO) *see* CefTAZidime ... 392
Ceftax (AE, BH, JO, QA, SA) *see* Cefotaxime ... 382
Ceftem (KR) *see* Ceftibuten ... 394
Ceftenon (AT) *see* CefoTEtan ... 385
Ceftidin (IN) *see* CefTAZidime ... 392
Ceftil (KR) *see* Cefuroxime ... 399
Ceftim (IT, PT) *see* CefTAZidime ... 392
Ceftoral (GR) *see* Cefixime ... 380
Ceftrex (MX, TH) *see* CefTRIAXone ... 396
Ceftrian (EC) *see* CefTRIAXone ... 396
Ceftrianol (MX) *see* CefTRIAXone ... 396
Ceftriax-1 (PH) *see* CefTRIAXone ... 396
Ceftrilem (MX) *see* CefTRIAXone ... 396
Ceftum (ID, JO) *see* CefTAZidime ... 392
Cefudura (DE) *see* Cefuroxime ... 399
Cefuhexal (DE) *see* Cefuroxime ... 399
Cefumax (LB, PH) *see* Cefuroxime ... 399
Cefuracet (MX) *see* Cefuroxime ... 399
Cefurax (DE) *see* Cefuroxime ... 399
Cefuro-Puren (DE) *see* Cefuroxime ... 399
Cefurox (TH) *see* Cefuroxime ... 399
Cefurox-wolff (DE) *see* Cefuroxime ... 399
Cefutil (AE, BH, CY, EG, IQ, IR, JO, KW, LB, LY, OM, QA, SA, SY, YE) *see* Cefuroxime ... 399
Cefutin (KR) *see* Cefuroxime ... 399
Cefuxime (HK, KR) *see* Cefuroxime ... 399
Cefxin (SG) *see* Cefuroxime ... 399
Cefxitin (TH) *see* CefOXitin ... 386
Cefxon (ID) *see* CefTRIAXone ... 396
Cefzalin (AE) *see* CeFAZolin ... 373
Cefzil (AE, BB, BG, BH, BM, BS, BZ, CN, CZ, EE, EG, GB, GR, GY, HN, JM, KR, KW, LB, LT, NL, PL, QA, SA, SI, SK, SR, TT) *see* Cefprozil ... 389
Cefzime (PH) *see* Cefuroxime ... 399
Cefzon (CN, JP) *see* Cefdinir ... 376
Cef-Zone (TH) *see* CefTRIAXone ... 396
Ceglution 300 (EC) *see* Lithium ... 1230
Ceglution (AR) *see* Lithium ... 1230
Ceksentri (SI) *see* Maraviroc ... 1272
Cektin (KR) *see* Cefaclor ... 372
Celamine (TH) *see* Imipramine ... 1054
Celapram (AU, NZ) *see* Citalopram ... 451
Celbexx (PK) *see* Celecoxib ... 402
Celcox (IL) *see* Celecoxib ... 402
Celcoxx (PH, VN) *see* Celecoxib ... 402
Celea (BE) *see* Desogestrel [INT] ... 597
Celebra (BR, CL, CR, DK, DO, FI, GT, HN, IL, IS, NI, NO, PA, SE, SV, UY) *see* Celecoxib ... 402
Celebral (GR) *see* Piracetam [INT] ... 1661
Celebrex (AE, AR, AT, AU, BD, BE, BF, BG, BH, BJ, CH, CI, CN, CO, CY, CZ, DE, DK, EC, EE, EG, ES, FR, GB, GH, GM, GN, GR, HK, HR, ID, IQ, IR, IT, JO, JP, KE, KR, KW, LB, LR, LT, LY, MA, ML, MR, MU, MW, MX, MY, NE, NG, NL, NZ, OM, PE, PH, PK, PL, PT, QA, RO, RU, SA, SC, SD, SG, SK, SL, SN, SY, TH, TN, TR, TW, TZ, UG, VE, VN, YE, ZM, ZW) *see* Celecoxib ... 402
Celecox (AE, BH, CY, EG, IQ, IR, JO, JP, KW, LB, LY, OM, QA, SA, SY, YE) *see* Celecoxib ... 402
Celectan (CO, VE) *see* Nitazoxanide ... 1461
Celectol (CZ, FR, GB, PL, VN) *see* Celiprolol [INT] ... 404
Celenid (MY, SG) *see* Cinnarizine [INT] ... 440
Celestan Depot (DE) *see* Betamethasone (Systemic) ... 253
Celestene Chronodose (FR) *see* Betamethasone (Systemic) ... 253
Celestoderm (FR) *see* Betamethasone (Topical) ... 255
Celeston Chronodose (FI, NO, TR) *see* Betamethasone (Systemic) ... 253
Celestone (AE, AR, BE, BH, CO, DE, EG, KR, LB, MX, PE, PL, PT, QA, SA, UY) *see* Betamethasone (Systemic) ... 253
Celestone Chronodose (AE, AU, CH, ES, GR, IL, LB, NZ) *see* Betamethasone (Systemic) ... 253
Celestone Cronodose (PE, PY, UY) *see* Betamethasone (Systemic) ... 253
Celestone Soluspan (MX) *see* Betamethasone (Systemic) ... 253
Celeston (SE) *see* Betamethasone (Systemic) ... 253
Celeuk (JP) *see* Aldesleukin ... 72
Celexib (PH) *see* Celecoxib ... 402
Celexil (AU) *see* Celecoxib ... 402
Celexin (HK) *see* Cephalexin ... 405
Celib (IN) *see* Celecoxib ... 402
Celica (AU) *see* Citalopram ... 451
Celin (IN) *see* Ascorbic Acid ... 178
Celipres (PL) *see* Celiprolol [INT] ... 404
Celipro-Lich (DE) *see* Celiprolol [INT] ... 404
Celiprol (RU) *see* Celiprolol [INT] ... 404
Celium (TH) *see* Medazepam [INT] ... 1277
Cellcept (AE, BH, CL, CN, CY, HR, HU, IS, JO, KW, LB, LT, QA, RO, SA, VN) *see* Mycophenolate ... 1405
CellCept (BB, BF, BJ, BM, BS, BZ, CI, ET, GH, GM, GN, GY, HK, JM, KE, LR, MA, ML, MR, MT, MU, MW, NE, NG, NZ, PY, SC, SD, SI, SK, SL, SN, SR, TN, TR, TT, TZ, UG, ZA, ZM, ZW) *see* Mycophenolate ... 1405
Cellidrin (DE) *see* Allopurinol ... 90
Cellmune (IN) *see* Mycophenolate ... 1405
Cell (PY) *see* Gemfibrozil ... 956
Celltop (FR) *see* Etoposide ... 816
Celltriaxon (MY) *see* CefTRIAXone ... 396
Celmetin (NO) *see* CeFAZolin ... 373
Celocid (ID) *see* Cefuroxime ... 399
Celocurine (BE, FR) *see* Succinylcholine ... 1939
Celocurin (SE) *see* Succinylcholine ... 1939
Celodim (ID) *see* CefTAZidime ... 392
Celon (BE) *see* Ascorbic Acid ... 178
Celoxin (EC) *see* Ethinyl Estradiol and Desogestrel ... 799
Celsentri (AR, AU, BE, BR, CH, CL, CN, CO, CY, CZ, DE, DK, EC, EE, FR, GB, GR, HK, HR, IE, IL, IS, IT, JP, LT, NL, NO, NZ, PE, PL, PT, RO, SA, SE, SG, SK, TH, TR, TW) *see* Maraviroc ... 1272
Celtax (JO) *see* PACLitaxel (Conventional) ... 1550
Celtect (JP) *see* Oxatomide [INT] ... 1532
Celtium (EC) *see* Escitalopram ... 765
Celupan (ES) *see* Naltrexone ... 1422
Celvista (TH) *see* Raloxifene ... 1765
Cemedin 400 (IL) *see* Cimetidine ... 438
Cemediz (VN) *see* Cetirizine ... 411
Cementin (SG) *see* Cimetidine ... 438
Cemidon (ES) *see* Isoniazid ... 1120
Cemol (TH) *see* Acetaminophen ... 32
Cenacert (AR) *see* Oxatomide [INT] ... 1532
Cencamat (TH) *see* Cimetidine ... 438
Cencenac (TH) *see* Diclofenac (Systemic) ... 617
Cendo Fluorescein (ID) *see* Fluorescein ... 894
Cenestin (CA) *see* Estrogens (Conjugated A/Synthetic) ... 782
Cenilene (PT) *see* FluPHENAZine ... 905
Cenlidac (TH) *see* Sulindac ... 1953

Cenol (LU) *see* Ascorbic Acid 178
Cenomycin (JP) *see* CefOXitin 386
Cenparkin (TW) *see* Benserazide and Levodopa [CAN/INT] 244
Cenpidine (TH) *see* Ticlopidine 2040
Cental (TW) *see* Pentoxifylline 1618
Centex (PY) *see* Ezetimibe 832
Centilax (KR) *see* HydrOXYzine 1024
Centocort (TH) *see* Triamcinolone (Systemic) 2099
Centocort (TH) *see* Triamcinolone (Topical) 2100
Centrac (GR) *see* Prazepam [INT] 1702
Centrax (IE) *see* Prazepam [INT] 1702
Centryl (TW) *see* Meprobamate 1296
Cepacaina (BR, MX) *see* Cetylpyridinium and Benzocaine [CAN/INT] 415
Cepacaine (AU, ZA) *see* Cetylpyridinium and Benzocaine [CAN/INT] 415
Cepacilina (ES) *see* Penicillin G Benzathine 1609
Cepezet (ID) *see* ChlorproMAZINE 429
Cephalen (SG) *see* Cephalexin 405
Cephalex (DE) *see* Cephalexin 405
Cephalexyl (TH) *see* Cephalexin 405
Cephanmycin (MY, SG) *see* Cephalexin 405
Cephlor (AE, BH, CY, EG, IL, IQ, IR, JO, KW, LB, LY, OM, QA, SA, SY, YE) *see* Cefaclor ... 372
Cephoral (CH, DE, PL) *see* Cefixime 380
Cepiram (PH) *see* Cefepime 378
Cepodem (IN, LB, ZA) *see* Cefpodoxime 388
Ceporex (AU, BB, BH, BM, BS, BZ, CY, EG, GB, GY, IQ, IR, IT, JM, JO, KW, LB, LY, MX, NZ, OM, PH, PT, QA, SA, SR, SY, TT, VN, YE, ZA) *see* Cephalexin ... 405
Ceporex Forte (PT) *see* Cephalexin 405
Ceporexin (AR) *see* Cephalexin 405
Ceprax (CO) *see* Cephalexin 405
Ceprazol (CL) *see* Albendazole 65
Ceprosim (KR) *see* Cefuroxime 399
Ceprotin (AT, AU, BE, BG, CH, CZ, DE, DK, EE, ES, FI, FR, GB, GR, HN, HR, IE, IS, IT, LT, MT, NL, NO, PL, PT, RO, RU, SE, SI, SK, TR) *see* Protein C Concentrate (Human) ... 1738
Ceptaxone (KR) *see* CefTRIAXone 396
Ceptolate (AU) *see* Mycophenolate 1405
Ceracal (IN) *see* Cinacalcet 439
Ceracl (KR) *see* Cefaclor 372
Cerafix (ID) *see* Cefixime 380
Ceralin (HR) *see* Cephalexin 405
Ceranade (KR) *see* Clopidogrel 484
Ceratex (HK) *see* Cetirizine 411
Cerator (MY, TH) *see* Pentoxifylline 1618
Cerazet (ES, IT) *see* Desogestrel [INT] 597
Cerazette (AE, AR, AT, BE, BH, BR, CH, CL, CO, CR, CZ, DE, DK, DO, EC, EE, FI, FR, GB, GR, GT, HK, HN, HR, HU, ID, IE, IL, IN, IS, IT, JO, KW, LB, LT, MY, NI, NL, NO, NZ, PA, PE, PH, PL, PT, QA, RO, RU, SA, SE, SG, SI, SK, SV, TH, UY, VE) *see* Desogestrel [INT] ... 597
Cercine (JP) *see* Diazepam 613
Cerebolan (JP) *see* Cinnarizine [INT] 440
Cerebrex (KR) *see* Celecoxib 402
Cerebrin (PK) *see* Cinnarizine [INT] 440
Cerebroforte (DE) *see* Piracetam [INT] 1661
Cerebrol (EC) *see* Piracetam [INT] 1661
Cerebropan (IT) *see* Piracetam [INT] 1661
Cerebrosteril (DE) *see* Piracetam [INT] 1661
Cerebryl (AT, HU) *see* Piracetam [INT] 1661
Cerebyx (KR) *see* Fosphenytoin 934
Ceregulart (JP) *see* Diazepam 613
Cerekinon (CN, HK, JP, MY, SG, TH) *see* Trimebutine [CAN/INT] 2103
Cerelle (GB) *see* Desogestrel [INT] 597
Cereluc (AR) *see* Pioglitazone 1654
Cereluc Met (AR) *see* Pioglitazone and Metformin 1655
Ceremin (PK) *see* Piracetam [INT] 1661
Cereneu (TH) *see* Fosphenytoin 934
Cerenicol (VN) *see* Chloramphenicol 421
Cerepar (CH, HN, SA) *see* Cinnarizine [INT] 440
Cerepar N (DE) *see* Piracetam [INT] 1661
Ceretal (TW) *see* Pentoxifylline 1618
Cerexin (ZA) *see* Cephalexin 405
Cerezyme (AT, AU, BE, BG, BR, CH, CL, CN, CY, CZ, DE, DK, EE, ES, FI, FR, GB, GR, HK, HN, HR, IE, IL, IT, KR, LB, LT, MT, MY, NL, NO, NZ, PL, PT, RO, RU, SE, SG, SK, TH, TR, TW) *see* Imiglucerase ... 1051
Cerezyzme (SI) *see* Imiglucerase 1051
Cerhein (KR) *see* Diacerein [INT] 613
Cerini (ID) *see* Cetirizine 411
Ceris (FR, VN) *see* Trospium 2108
Ceritec (MY, SG) *see* Cetirizine 411
Cerixon (KR) *see* CefTRIAXone 396
Cermox (AR) *see* CycloSPORINE (Systemic) 522
Cerofazil (KR) *see* Cefprozil 389
Cerosel (PL) *see* Selenium 1876
Cero (TW) *see* Cefaclor 372
Ceroxim (IL, ZA) *see* Cefuroxime 399
Cerson (HR) *see* Nitrazepam [CAN/INT] 1461
Certican (AE, AR, AT, AU, BE, BG, BH, BR, CH, CL, CN, CO, CY, CZ, DE, DK, EC, EE, ES, FI, FR, GR, HK, HN, HR, ID, IL, IN, IS, IT, JP, KR, KW, LB, LT, MY, NL, NO, NZ, PE, PH, PK, PL, PT, PY, QA, RO, SA, SE, SG, SI, SK, TH, TR, TW, UY, VE, VN) *see* Everolimus ... 822
Cerubidin (AE, BH, CY, DK, EG, FI, GB, HK, HN, IE, IQ, KW, LB, LY, MY, NO, OM, QA, SA, SE, SY, YE) *see* DAUNOrubicin (Conventional) ... 577
Cerubidine (BE, CH, CL, CZ, FR, IL, LU, NL, NZ, PL, RU, TR, UY) *see* DAUNOrubicin (Conventional) ... 577
Cerucal (DE, EE, HU) *see* Metoclopramide 1345
Ceruvin (TH) *see* Clopidogrel 484
Cervarix (AE, AR, AT, AU, BE, BH, CH, CL, CO, CR, CY, CZ, DE, DK, DO, EC, EE, ES, FR, GB, GR, GT, HK, HN, HR, HU, IL, IS, IT, JP, KR, KW, LB, LT, MX, MY, NI, NL, NO, NZ, PA, PE, PH, PL, PT, QA, RO, RU, SA, SE, SG, SI, SK, SV, TH, TR, TW, UY, VN) *see* Papillomavirus (Types 16, 18) Vaccine (Human, Recombinant) ... 1574
Cervasal (BG) *see* Dihydroergotamine 633
Cervictal (AR) *see* Tibolone [INT] 2035
Cervidil (AU, NZ) *see* Dinoprostone 640
Cerviprime (IN, VN) *see* Dinoprostone 640
Cerviprost (AT, RU) *see* Dinoprostone 640
Cerylana (VE) *see* DiphenhydrAMINE (Systemic) 641
Cesbron (PT) *see* Clenbuterol [INT] 460
Cesilpro (KR) *see* Cefprozil 389
Ceso (IN) *see* Esomeprazole 771
Cesol (DE, MX, PL) *see* Praziquantel 1702
Cesoline-W (TH) *see* HydrALAZINE 1007
Cesoline Y (TH) *see* HydrALAZINE 1007
Cesplon (ES) *see* Captopril 342
Cestazid (PH) *see* CefTAZidime 392
Cetabrium (ID) *see* ChlordiazePOXIDE 422
Cetacin (KR) *see* Acemetacin [INT] 30
Cetadol (PH) *see* Acetaminophen and Tramadol 37
Cetadop (ID) *see* DOPamine 669
Cetalerg (DE) *see* Cetirizine 411
Cetamadole (KR) *see* Acetaminophen and Tramadol 37
Cetamid (PH) *see* AcetaZOLAMIDE 39
Cetamine (BE, LU) *see* Ascorbic Acid 178
Cetam (IT, SG) *see* Piracetam [INT] 1661
Cetapain (ID) *see* Acetaminophen 32
Cetatrex (ID) *see* SUMAtriptan 1953
Cetavlex (FR) *see* Chlorhexidine Gluconate 422
Cetavlon (FR) *see* Chlorhexidine Gluconate 422
Cetaxin (PE) *see* Ciprofibrate [INT] 441
Cetax (TW) *see* Cefotaxime 382
Cetazine (TW) *see* CefTAZidime 392
Cetazum (ID) *see* CefTAZidime 392
Cetebe (BG, HU) *see* Ascorbic Acid 178
Cethis (HK, TH) *see* Cetirizine 411

Cethixim (ID) *see* Cefuroxime ... 399
Cetihis (MY) *see* Cetirizine ... 411
Cetilan (PH) *see* Acetylcysteine ... 40
Cetil (IN, PE) *see* Cefuroxime ... 399
Cetimer (GT, HN, NI, SV) *see* Levocetirizine ... 1196
Cetimil (ES) *see* Nedocromil ... 1435
Cetirax (CO) *see* Cetirizine ... 411
Cetirin (HK) *see* Cetirizine ... 411
Cetitev (MX) *see* Cetirizine ... 411
Cetizal (RO) *see* Levocetirizine ... 1196
Cetodol (PH) *see* Acetaminophen and Tramadol ... 37
Cetoxil (MX) *see* Cefuroxime ... 399
Cetra (PH) *see* Acetaminophen and Tramadol ... 37
Cetraxal (CR, DO, GT, HN, NI, PA, SV) *see* Ciprofloxacin (Systemic) ... 441
Cetriaf (DO) *see* CefTRIAXone ... 396
Cetriler (PE) *see* Levocetirizine ... 1196
Cetrimed (TH) *see* Cetirizine ... 411
Cetrine (CN, CO, EC) *see* Cetirizine ... 411
Cetrinets (MY) *see* Ascorbic Acid ... 178
Cetrizin (TH) *see* Cetirizine ... 411
Cetron (AR) *see* Ondansetron ... 1513
Cetro (QA) *see* Cetirizine ... 411
Cetrotide (AE, AR, AT, AU, BE, BG, BR, CH, CN, CO, CY, CZ, DE, DK, EC, EE, ES, FI, FR, GB, GR, HK, HN, HR, ID, IE, IL, IN, IT, JP, KR, KW, LB, LT, MT, MX, MY, NL, NO, NZ, PE, PH, PL, PT, RO, RU, SA, SE, SG, SI, SK, TR, TW, VE, VN) *see* Cetrorelix ... 413
Cetta (TH) *see* Acetaminophen ... 32
Cety (TW) *see* Cetirizine ... 411
Ceumid (EC, UY) *see* LevETIRAcetam ... 1191
Cevacl (KR) *see* Cefaclor ... 372
Cevadil (ID) *see* Flunarizine [CAN/INT] ... 892
Cevalin (MX) *see* Ascorbic Acid ... 178
Cevidrops (BE) *see* Ascorbic Acid ... 178
Cevi Drops (LU) *see* Ascorbic Acid ... 178
Ce-Vi-Sol (CR, DO, GT, HN, NI, PA, PH, SV) *see* Ascorbic Acid ... 178
Cevitil (QA) *see* Ascorbic Acid ... 178
Cewin (BR) *see* Ascorbic Acid ... 178
Cexil (KR) *see* Cefuroxime ... 399
Cexima (PY) *see* Cefixime ... 380
Cexim (HU) *see* Cefuroxime ... 399
Cexim (TW) *see* Cefixime ... 380
Cexyl (RO) *see* Cefadroxil ... 372
C-Flox (AU, UY) *see* Ciprofloxacin (Systemic) ... 441
Chalocaine Jelly (TH) *see* Lidocaine (Topical) ... 1211
Chalocaine (TH) *see* Lidocaine (Systemic) ... 1208
Chalocaine with Adrenaline (TH) *see* Lidocaine and Epinephrine ... 1212
Chamberlain`s Cough Remedy (ZA) *see* GuaiFENesin ... 986
Champix (AE, AR, AT, AU, BE, BG, BH, BR, BZ, CH, CL, CN, CO, CR, CY, CZ, DE, DK, EC, EE, ES, FI, FR, GB, GR, GT, HK, HN, HR, ID, IE, IL, IS, IT, JP, KR, KW, LT, MT, MX, MY, NI, NL, NO, NZ, PA, PE, PH, PL, PT, QA, RO, RU, SA, SE, SG, SI, SK, SV, TH, TR, TW, UY, VE, VN) *see* Varenicline ... 2139
Champ Syrup (KR) *see* Acetaminophen ... 32
Chang Mei (CN) *see* Olsalazine ... 1500
Charcodote (GB, HK, KR, SG) *see* Charcoal, Activated ... 416
Charcotrace (AU) *see* Charcoal, Activated ... 416
Chebil (PT) *see* Chenodiol ... 417
Chef (TW) *see* CefTRIAXone ... 396
Chemacin (IT) *see* Amikacin ... 111
Chemet (AT, BM) *see* Succimer ... 1939
Chemicetina (IT) *see* Chloramphenicol ... 421
Chemiofurin (ES) *see* Nitrofurantoin ... 1463
Chemists' Own Cold Sore Cream (AU) *see* Acyclovir (Topical) ... 51
Chemist's Own Dolased Day/Night Pain Relief (AU) *see* Acetaminophen, Codeine, and Doxylamine [CAN/INT] ... 37
Chemists' Own Sinus Relief (AU) *see* Pseudoephedrine ... 1742
Chemochin (HR) *see* Chloroquine ... 424
Chenday (TW) *see* Labetalol ... 1151
Chendol (GB, MY, PT) *see* Chenodiol ... 417
Chen Jing (CN) *see* Diclofenac (Ophthalmic) ... 621
Chenofalk (AT, BE, CH, CZ, DE, GB, HK, HN, ID, IT, MY, NL, PH) *see* Chenodiol ... 417
Chenossil (IT) *see* Chenodiol ... 417
Cheno (TW) *see* Chenodiol ... 417
Cheracol D (MX) *see* Guaifenesin and Dextromethorphan ... 987
Chewette C (HK) *see* Ascorbic Acid ... 178
Chibro-Proscar (FR) *see* Finasteride ... 878
Chibroxin (AE, BR, CN, CY, EG, ES, HR, IQ, IR, JO, LB, LY, OM, PE, QA, SA, SY, VE, YE) *see* Norfloxacin ... 1475
Chibroxine (BH, FR, KW, UY) *see* Norfloxacin ... 1475
Chibroxol (LU) *see* Norfloxacin ... 1475
Chiclida (CO) *see* Meclizine ... 1277
Children's Bufferin (CN) *see* Acetaminophen ... 32
Children's S Tylenol (KR) *see* Acetaminophen ... 32
Chinacin-T (TH) *see* Clindamycin (Systemic) ... 460
Chinacin-T (TH) *see* Clindamycin (Topical) ... 464
Chingazol (TH) *see* Clotrimazole (Topical) ... 488
Chinidin (BG) *see* QuiNIDine ... 1759
Chinidin Retard (HN) *see* QuiNIDine ... 1759
Chinidinum prolongatum (PL) *see* QuiNIDine ... 1759
Chinidinum sulfuricum (PL) *see* QuiNIDine ... 1759
Chinofungin (HU, PL) *see* Tolnaftate ... 2063
Chinoplus (PL) *see* Prulifloxacin [INT] ... 1742
Chinotal (HU) *see* Pentoxifylline ... 1618
Chirocaina (CL, VE) *see* Levobupivacaine [INT] ... 1194
Chirocaina (VE) *see* Bupivacaine ... 299
Chirocaine (AT, AU, BE, BH, CH, CN, CZ, FI, FR, GB, GR, HK, HN, HR, ID, IE, IT, JP, KR, KW, MY, NL, NO, PE, PH, PL, QA, SE, SG, SI, SK, TH, TR, TW, VN) *see* Levobupivacaine [INT] ... 1194
Chistait (JP) *see* Mecysteine [INT] ... 1277
Chizocin (TW) *see* Naftifine ... 1416
Chlobax (SG) *see* Clidinium and Chlordiazepoxide ... 460
Chloguin (TW) *see* Hydroxychloroquine ... 1021
Chlomazin (KR) *see* ChlorproMAZINE ... 429
Chlophazolin (BG) *see* CloNIDine ... 480
Chloradorm (AU) *see* Chloral Hydrate [CAN/INT] ... 418
Chlorafast (NZ) *see* Chloramphenicol ... 421
Chloraldurat (DE, NL) *see* Chloral Hydrate [CAN/INT] ... 418
Chloralhydrat 500 (ID) *see* Chloral Hydrate [CAN/INT] ... 418
Chloramex (ZA) *see* Chloramphenicol ... 421
Chloraminophene (FR) *see* Chlorambucil ... 419
Chloramphenicol (BE) *see* Chloramphenicol ... 421
Chloramphenicol Faure, Ophthadoses (CH) *see* Chloramphenicol ... 421
Chloram-P (TH) *see* Chloramphenicol ... 421
Chloraprep (GB) *see* Chlorhexidine Gluconate ... 422
Chlorazin (BG, CH) *see* ChlorproMAZINE ... 429
Chlorcol (ZA) *see* Chloramphenicol ... 421
Chlordiazepoxid L.F.M. (HU) *see* ChlordiazePOXIDE ... 422
Chlordiazepoxidum (NL) *see* ChlordiazePOXIDE ... 422
Chlorek Sodowy 24Na (PL) *see* Sodium Chloride ... 1902
Chlorhexamed (AT, CH) *see* Chlorhexidine Gluconate ... 422
Chlorhexidine Obstetric Lotion (AU) *see* Chlorhexidine Gluconate ... 422
Chlorhex (TH) *see* Chlorhexidine Gluconate ... 422
Chlorhydrate de Bupivacaine Dakota (FR) *see* Bupivacaine ... 299

Chlorhydrate de cyclopentolate (LU) *see* Cyclopentolate ... 517
Chlormide (JP) *see* ChlorproPAMIDE ... 429
Chlornicol (ZA) *see* Chloramphenicol ... 421
Chlornitromycin (BG) *see* Chloramphenicol ... 421
Chlorochin (CH, HR) *see* Chloroquine ... 424
Chlorofoz (PH) *see* Chloroquine ... 424
Chlorohex (SG) *see* Chlorhexidine Gluconate ... 422
Chloromax (PH) *see* Chloroquine ... 424
Chloromycetin (AR, AU, CR, DO, ES, FI, HN, IE, IS, IT, MX, NI, PA, PH, QA, SE, TW, ZA) *see* Chloramphenicol ... 421
Chloromycetin Eye Preparations (AU, NZ) *see* Chloramphenicol ... 421
Chloropernazinum (PL) *see* Prochlorperazine ... 1718
Chloropotassuril (BE) *see* Potassium Chloride ... 1687
Chloroptic (AE, BH, CY, EG, GR, IE, IQ, IR, JO, KW, LB, LY, OM, PH, PK, QA, SA, SY, YE, ZA) *see* Chloramphenicol ... 421
Chloroquini Diphosphas (NL) *see* Chloroquine ... 424
Chlorosal (IL) *see* Chlorothiazide ... 426
Chlorosan (AE, BH, CY, EG, IQ, IR, JO, KW, LB, LY, OM, QA, SA, SY, YE) *see* Chloramphenicol ... 421
Chlorpromed (TH) *see* ChlorproMAZINE ... 429
Chlorpropamid (PL) *see* ChlorproPAMIDE ... 429
Chlorquin (AU, NZ) *see* Chloroquine ... 424
Chlorsig Eye Preparations (AU) *see* Chloramphenicol ... 421
Chlorsig (HK, NZ) *see* Chloramphenicol ... 421
Chlorsuccillin (PL) *see* Succinylcholine ... 1939
Chlorumagene (FR) *see* Magnesium Hydroxide ... 1263
Chlorvescent (NZ) *see* Potassium Chloride ... 1687
Chlothia (JP) *see* Hydrochlorothiazide ... 1009
Chlotride (AU, NL) *see* Chlorothiazide ... 426
Chlovas (TH) *see* AtorvaSTATin ... 194
Chme (TW) *see* Itraconazole ... 1130
Cholal modificado (MX) *see* Magnesium Sulfate ... 1265
Cholchicin "Agepha" (AT) *see* Colchicine ... 500
Cholespar (ID) *see* Pravastatin ... 1700
Cholestabyl (DE) *see* Colestipol ... 504
Cholestagel (CZ, DK, EE, GB, HR, NO, RO, SE, TR) *see* Colesevelam ... 503
Cholestat (ID) *see* Simvastatin ... 1890
Choles (TW) *see* Cholestyramine Resin ... 431
Cholstat (AU) *see* Pravastatin ... 1700
Cholstatin (VN) *see* Lovastatin ... 1252
Cholvastin (ID) *see* Lovastatin ... 1252
Chooz Antacid Gum 500 (AE, BH, CY, EG, IQ, IR, JO, KW, LB, LY, OM, QA, SA, SY, YE) *see* Calcium Carbonate ... 327
Choreazine (JP) *see* Tetrabenazine ... 2016
Christamol (HK) *see* Acetaminophen ... 32
Chromalux (ID) *see* Misoprostol ... 1379
Chronadalate LP (FR) *see* NIFEdipine ... 1451
Chrono-Indocid (FR) *see* Indomethacin ... 1067
Chronol (TH) *see* Disulfiram ... 654
Chrytemin (JP) *see* Imipramine ... 1054
Ciaflam (VN) *see* Aceclofenac [INT] ... 30
Cialis (AE, AR, AT, AU, BB, BE, BF, BG, BH, BJ, BR, BS, CH, CI, CL, CN, CO, CR, CY, CZ, DE, DK, DO, EE, ES, ET, FI, FR, GB, GH, GM, GN, GR, HK, HN, HR, ID, IE, IL, IS, IT, JM, JP, KE, KR, KW, LB, LR, LT, MA, ML, MR, MT, MU, MW, MX, MY, NE, NG, NI, NL, NO, NZ, PA, PE, PH, PL, PT, QA, RO, RU, SA, SC, SD, SE, SG, SI, SK, SL, SN, SV, TH, TN, TR, TT, TW, TZ, UG, VE, VN, ZA, ZM, ZW) *see* Tadalafil ... 1968
Cianocobalamina B12 Davi (PT) *see* Cyanocobalamin ... 515
Ciatyl-Z Acuphase (DE) *see* Zuclopenthixol [CAN/INT] ... 2219
Ciatyl-Z (DE) *see* Zuclopenthixol [CAN/INT] ... 2219
Ciatyl-Z Depot (DE) *see* Zuclopenthixol [CAN/INT] ... 2219
Ciazil (AU) *see* Citalopram ... 451
Ciazil (VN) *see* Epirubicin ... 739
Cibacalcin (AE, BH, CY, EG, GR, IL, IQ, IR, JO, KW, LB, LY, OM, QA, SA, SY, YE) *see* Calcitonin ... 322
Cibacalcine [human] (LU) *see* Calcitonin ... 322
Cibacen (AE, AT, BB, BE, BF, BH, BJ, BM, BS, BZ, CH, CI, CY, DE, EG, ES, ET, GH, GM, GN, GR, GY, ID, IE, IL, IQ, IR, IT, JM, JO, KE, KR, KW, LB, LR, LU, LY, MA, ML, MR, MU, MW, NE, NG, NL, NZ, OM, PH, PT, QA, SA, SC, SD, SE, SL, SN, SR, SY, TN, TR, TT, TW, TZ, UG, VN, YE, ZA, ZM, ZW) *see* Benazepril ... 238
Cibacene (FR) *see* Benazepril ... 238
Cibacen HCT (PT) *see* Benazepril and Hydrochlorothiazide ... 240
Cibadrex (AE, AT, BB, BF, BG, BH, BJ, BM, BS, BZ, CH, CI, CY, DE, EG, ET, FR, GH, GM, GN, GR, GY, IL, IQ, IR, IT, JM, JO, KE, KW, LB, LR, LY, MA, ML, MR, MU, MW, NE, NG, NL, NZ, OM, PR, QA, SA, SC, SD, SL, SN, SR, SY, TN, TR, TT, TZ, UG, VN, YE, ZA, ZM, ZW) *see* Benazepril and Hydrochlorothiazide ... 240
Ciblex (CL, PY) *see* Mirtazapine ... 1376
Cibradex (CN) *see* Benazepril and Hydrochlorothiazide ... 240
Cibrato (BR) *see* Ciprofibrate [INT] ... 441
Cicamin (PY) *see* Loperamide ... 1236
Ciclamil (CL) *see* Cyclobenzaprine ... 516
Cicleno (CL) *see* DULoxetine ... 698
Cicletex (AR) *see* Ciclesonide (Systemic) ... 432
Ciclidon (CL, PE) *see* Ethinyl Estradiol and Desogestrel ... 799
Ciclo 21 (BR) *see* Ethinyl Estradiol and Levonorgestrel ... 803
Ciclobiotico (PT) *see* Tetracycline ... 2017
Ciclochem (ES) *see* Ciclopirox ... 433
Ciclodin (PH) *see* Ciprofloxacin (Systemic) ... 441
Ciclofalina (ES) *see* Piracetam [INT] ... 1661
Cicloferon (CR, DO, GT, MX, NI, PA, SV) *see* Acyclovir (Systemic) ... 47
Cicloferon (CR, DO, GT, PA, SV) *see* Acyclovir (Topical) ... 51
Ciclohale (LB) *see* Ciclesonide (Systemic) ... 432
Ciclohexal (ZA) *see* CycloSPORINE (Systemic) ... 522
Ciclokapron (VE) *see* Tranexamic Acid ... 2081
Ciclolato (BR) *see* Cyclopentolate ... 517
Ciclolux (IT) *see* Cyclopentolate ... 517
Ciclonal (MX) *see* Doxycycline ... 689
Ciclopar (CO) *see* Albendazole ... 65
Ciclopejico (ES) *see* Cyclopentolate ... 517
Ciclopenal (AR, PY) *see* Cyclopentolate ... 517
Ciclople (ES) *see* Cyclopentolate ... 517
Cicloplegic (ES) *see* Cyclopentolate ... 517
Cicloplejico Llorens (ES) *see* Cyclopentolate ... 517
Cicloral (AU, DE) *see* CycloSPORINE (Systemic) ... 522
Ciclotetryl (AR) *see* Tetracycline ... 2017
Cicloviral (CO) *see* Aciclovir (Ophthalmic) [INT] ... 43
Cicloviral (CO) *see* Acyclovir (Systemic) ... 47
Cicloviral (CO) *see* Acyclovir (Topical) ... 51
Cicloxal (ES) *see* Cyclophosphamide ... 517
Ciclox (PH) *see* Acyclovir (Systemic) ... 47
Cicough (TH) *see* Carbocisteine [INT] ... 357
Cidanchin (ES) *see* Chloroquine ... 424
Cidan-Cilina 900 (ES) *see* Penicillin G Procaine ... 1613
Cidine (TH) *see* Cimetidine ... 438
Cidomycin (AE, BH, CY, EG, GB, IQ, IR, JO, KW, LB, LY, OM, QA, SA, SY, YE, ZA) *see* Gentamicin (Systemic) ... 959
Cidoten (CL) *see* Betamethasone (Systemic) ... 253
Cifacure (PH) *see* Cefixime ... 380
Cifespasma (AR) *see* Scopolamine (Systemic) ... 1870
Cifex (PH) *see* Ciprofloxacin (Systemic) ... 441
Cifex (TR) *see* Cefixime ... 380
Cifloc (ZA) *see* Ciprofloxacin (Systemic) ... 441
Ciflodal (PH) *see* Ciprofloxacin (Systemic) ... 441
Cifloptic (PE) *see* Ciprofloxacin (Ophthalmic) ... 446

Cifloptic (PE) *see* Ciprofloxacin (Systemic) 441
Ciflox (AE, FR, HR, KW, QA, VE) *see* Ciprofloxacin (Systemic) 441
Ciflox (DK) *see* Ciprofloxacin and Hydrocortisone 446
Cifloxin (HK, PH) *see* Ciprofloxacin (Systemic) 441
Cifran (AU, BF, BJ, CI, CN, ET, GH, GM, GN, IN, KE, LR, MA, ML, MR, MU, MW, NE, NG, RO, SC, SD, SL, SN, TN, TZ, UG, VN, ZM, ZW) *see* Ciprofloxacin (Systemic) 441
Cifran DPS (IN) *see* Ciprofloxacin (Ophthalmic) 446
Cigamet (TH) *see* Cimetidine 438
Ciganclor (PY, UY) *see* Ganciclovir (Systemic) 948
Cikedrix (PH) *see* CefTRIAXone 396
Cilamin (IN) *see* PenicillAMINE 1608
Cilamox (AU) *see* Amoxicillin 130
Cilapenem (KR, TH) *see* Imipenem and Cilastatin 1051
Cilaril (IL) *see* Cilazapril [CAN/INT] 434
Cilazil (HR) *see* Cilazapril [CAN/INT] 434
Cilest (AE, AR, BE, BG, BH, CH, CO, CR, CY, CZ, DE, DK, DO, EE, FI, FR, GB, GT, HN, HR, IE, IT, KW, LT, MX, NI, NL, PA, PE, PL, PY, QA, RO, RU, SA, SE, SI, SK, SV, TH, TR, UY) *see* Ethinyl Estradiol and Norgestimate 810
Cileste (AT) *see* Ethinyl Estradiol and Norgestimate 810
Ciletin (PH) *see* Cilostazol 437
Cilex (AU) *see* Cephalexin 405
Cilicaine Syringe (AU) *see* Penicillin G Procaine 1613
Cilicaine VK (AU, NZ) *see* Penicillin V Potassium 1614
Cilisod (TW) *see* Ampicillin 141
Cilo V (KR) *see* Cilostazol 437
Cilobact (CO) *see* Ciprofloxacin (Ophthalmic) 446
Cilobact (CO) *see* Ciprofloxacin (Systemic) 441
Cilodes (KR) *see* Ciprofloxacin and Dexamethasone 446
Cilodex (BR, CL, CO, DE, DK, IL, KR, MX, NZ, PE, PY, SG, UY, ZA) *see* Ciprofloxacin and Dexamethasone 446
Cilopen VK (AU) *see* Penicillin V Potassium 1614
CiloQuin (AU) *see* Ciprofloxacin (Ophthalmic) 446
Cilosol (KR, TH) *see* Cilostazol 437
Cilostal (CR, DO, EC, GT, HN, NI, PA, PE, SV) *see* Cilostazol 437
Cilost (VN) *see* Cilostazol 437
Ciloxadex (AR) *see* Ciprofloxacin and Dexamethasone 446
Ciloxan (AE, AR, AT, AU, BE, BG, BH, BR, CH, CL, CY, CZ, DE, DK, EE, EG, FR, GB, GR, HK, HR, HU, IE, IL, JO, KW, LB, LT, MY, NL, NZ, PH, PK, PL, PY, QA, SA, SE, SK, TH, TR, TW, UY, VE, VN, ZA) *see* Ciprofloxacin (Ophthalmic) 446
Ciloxan (AU) *see* Ciprofloxacin (Otic) 446
Cilox (NO) *see* Ciprofloxacin (Ophthalmic) 446
Cilox (NO) *see* Ciprofloxacin (Systemic) 441
Cilroton (GR) *see* Domperidone [CAN/INT] 666
CIMAher (AR, BR, CO) *see* Nimotuzumab [INT] 1457
Cimal (CO) *see* DULoxetine 698
Cimascal (ES) *see* Calcium Carbonate 327
Cimbene (BB, BM, BS, BZ, GY, JM, SR, TT) *see* Cimetidine 438
Cimedine (AE, BH, CY, EG, IQ, IR, JO, KW, LB, LY, OM, QA, SA, SY, YE) *see* Cimetidine 438
Cimehexal (HU, LU) *see* Cimetidine 438
Cimeldine (HU) *see* Cimetidine 438
Cimetag (AE, AT, BH, KW, QA) *see* Cimetidine 438
Cimetase (MX) *see* Cimetidine 438
Cimetidina (CL, PY) *see* Cimetidine 438
Cimetidina Inexfa (ES) *see* Cimetidine 438
Cimetidin AL (HU) *see* Cimetidine 438
Cimetidina Merck (ES) *see* Cimetidine 438
Cimetidin (BG, CH, DE, NO) *see* Cimetidine 438
Cimetidine (CZ) *see* Cimetidine 438
Cimetin (CZ, EC, IN) *see* Cimetidine 438
Cimet (TH) *see* Cimetidine 438
Cimewell (TW) *see* Cimetidine 438
Cimex (FI) *see* Cimetidine 438
Cimexol (ID) *see* Cimetidine 438
Cimizt (GB) *see* Ethinyl Estradiol and Desogestrel 799
CimLich (LU) *see* Cimetidine 438
Cimoxin (PE) *see* Ciprofloxacin (Systemic) 441
Cimulcer (MY, PH) *see* Cimetidine 438
Cimzia (AR, AT, AU, BE, BR, CH, CO, CY, CZ, DE, DK, EE, FR, GB, HR, HU, JP, LT, MX, MY, NL, NO, NZ, PL, PT, RO, SE, SI, SK, TR) *see* Certolizumab Pegol 409
Cinabioquim (AR) *see* Cinnarizine [INT] 440
Cinact (IN) *see* Cinnarizine [INT] 440
Cinadil (PE, PY) *see* Cinnarizine [INT] 440
Cinadine (ZA) *see* Cimetidine 438
Cinaflox (PE) *see* Ciprofloxacin (Systemic) 441
Cinageron (BR) *see* Cinnarizine [INT] 440
Cinam (ID) *see* Ampicillin and Sulbactam 145
Cinaren (VE) *see* Cinnarizine [INT] 440
Cinarin (LB, PH) *see* Cinnarizine [INT] 440
Cinarizina (AR, BR, ES) *see* Cinnarizine [INT] 440
Cinarizina Ratiopharm (ES, PT) *see* Cinnarizine [INT] 440
Cinarizin (HR) *see* Cinnarizine [INT] 440
Cinar (JO) *see* Cinnarizine [INT] 440
Cinaziere (GB) *see* Cinnarizine [INT] 440
Cinazin (CH) *see* Cinnarizine [INT] 440
Cinazyn (IT) *see* Cinnarizine [INT] 440
Cincomil Bedoce (ES) *see* Cyanocobalamin 515
Cincopal (ES) *see* Fenbufen [INT] 852
Cincordil (BR) *see* Isosorbide Mononitrate 1126
Cinedil (HR) *see* Cinnarizine [INT] 440
Cinergil (CL) *see* Cinnarizine [INT] 440
Cinfamar (ES) *see* DimenhyDRINATE 637
Cinmik (PH) *see* Amikacin 111
Cinnabene (AT, CZ) *see* Cinnarizine [INT] 440
Cinnabloc (PH) *see* Cinnarizine [INT] 440
Cinna (DE, MY, SG, TH) *see* Cinnarizine [INT] 440
Cinnaforte (DE) *see* Cinnarizine [INT] 440
Cinnageron (CH) *see* Cinnarizine [INT] 440
Cinnamed (CH) *see* Cinnarizine [INT] 440
Cinnamin (JP) *see* Azapropazone [INT] 210
Cinnarizin AL (DE) *see* Cinnarizine [INT] 440
Cinnarizin R.A.N. (DE) *see* Cinnarizine [INT] 440
Cinnarizin-ratiopharm (DE) *see* Cinnarizine [INT] 440
Cinnarizin Siegfried (DE) *see* Cinnarizine [INT] 440
cinnarizin von ct (DE) *see* Cinnarizine [INT] 440
Cinnaron (CY, SG) *see* Cinnarizine [INT] 440
Cinnar (SG) *see* Cinnarizine [INT] 440
Cinnipirine (NL) *see* Cinnarizine [INT] 440
Cinolon (ID) *see* Fluocinolone (Topical) 893
Cinon Forte (PT) *see* Cinnarizine [INT] 440
Cinopal (DK) *see* Fenbufen [INT] 852
Cinryze (CZ, DK, EE, GB, LT, SE, SK) *see* C1 Inhibitor (Human) 315
Cintag (BR) *see* Cimetidine 438
Cintigo (ID) *see* Cinnarizine [INT] 440
Cintilan (BR) *see* Piracetam [INT] 1661
Cinulcus (ES) *see* Cimetidine 438
Cipatin (TR) *see* Capecitabine 339
Cipcal (IN) *see* Calcium Carbonate 327
Cipcin (TW) *see* Ciprofloxacin (Ophthalmic) 446
Cipen (KR) *see* Levocetirizine 1196
Cipflox (NZ) *see* Ciprofloxacin (Systemic) 441
Cipide (BR) *see* Ciprofibrate [INT] 441
Cipla-Actin (ZA) *see* Cyproheptadine 529
Ciplactin (IN, VN) *see* Cyproheptadine 529
Cipladanogen (CO) *see* Danazol 558
Cipladinex (CO) *see* Didanosine 622
Cipladuovir (CO) *see* Lamivudine and Zidovudine 1160
Ciplametazon Inhalador Nasal (CO) *see* Beclomethasone (Nasal) 232
Ciplanevimune (CO) *see* Nevirapine 1440
Ciplar (IN) *see* Propranolol 1731
Ciploc (PK) *see* Ciprofloxacin (Systemic) 441

Ciplox (BF, BJ, CI, ET, GH, GM, GN, HK, KE, LR, MA, ML, MR, MU, MW, NE, NG, SC, SD, SK, SL, SN, TN, TZ, UG, ZA, ZM, ZW) *see* Ciprofloxacin (Systemic) 441
Ciplus (KR) *see* Ciprofloxacin (Ophthalmic) 446
Ciplus (KR) *see* Ciprofloxacin (Systemic) 441
Cipocal (TR) *see* Calcipotriene 321
Cipol (KR) *see* CycloSPORINE (Systemic) 522
Cipol-N (KR) *see* CycloSPORINE (Systemic) 522
Cipotriol (HK) *see* Calcipotriene 321
Cipralex (AE, AT, BG, BH, CH, CY, CZ, DE, DK, EE, EG, ES, FI, GB, GR, HR, HU, ID, IE, IL, IN, IQ, IR, IS, IT, JO, KW, LB, LT, LY, NO, OM, PK, PL, PT, QA, RO, RU, SA, SE, SI, SK, SY, TR, YE) *see* Escitalopram 765
Cipram (AE, BF, BH, BJ, CI, CY, EG, ET, GH, GM, GN, GR, HK, ID, IQ, IR, JO, KE, KR, KW, LB, LR, LY, MA, ML, MR, MU, MW, MY, NE, NG, OM, PK, QA, SA, SC, SD, SG, SL, SN, SY, TH, TN, TR, TW, TZ, UG, YE, ZM, ZW) *see* Citalopram 451
Cipramil (AU, BE, BR, CL, CN, DE, DK, EE, FI, GB, IE, IL, LU, NL, NO, NZ, PE, PL, RU, SE, VN, ZA) *see* Citalopram 451
Ciprane (BR) *see* Cyproterone and Ethinyl Estradiol [CAN/INT] 532
Ciprecu (EC) *see* Ciprofloxacin (Systemic) 441
Cipridanol (PY) *see* MethylPREDNISolone 1340
Ciprid (EC) *see* Sucralfate 1940
Cipril - H (IN) *see* Lisinopril and Hydrochlorothiazide 1229
Cipril (HK, IN) *see* Lisinopril 1226
Ciprinol (BG, EE, RO) *see* Ciprofloxacin (Systemic) 441
Cipro (AR, BR, CO, JO, PY) *see* Ciprofloxacin (Systemic) 441
Ciprobay (AE, BG, BH, CY, CZ, EG, IQ, IR, JO, KR, KW, LB, LY, MY, OM, PH, PL, QA, SA, SY, TH, VN, YE, ZA) *see* Ciprofloxacin (Systemic) 441
Ciprobay Ear Drop (VN) *see* Ciprofloxacin and Hydrocortisone 446
Ciprobay HC (EE, KR, SG, ZA) *see* Ciprofloxacin and Hydrocortisone 446
Ciprobay HC Otic (AE, KW, QA) *see* Ciprofloxacin and Hydrocortisone 446
Ciprobay Uro (DE) *see* Ciprofloxacin (Systemic) 441
Ciprobay (VN) *see* Ciprofloxacin (Otic) 446
Ciprobeta (DE) *see* Ciprofloxacin (Systemic) 441
Ciprobid (AE, BF, BH, BJ, CI, CY, EG, ET, GH, GM, GN, IQ, IR, JO, KE, KW, LB, LR, LY, MA, ML, MR, MU, MW, NE, NG, OM, QA, SA, SC, SD, SL, SN, SY, TH, TN, TZ, UG, YE, ZM, ZW) *see* Ciprofloxacin (Systemic) 441
Ciprobiotic (GT, HN, ID, NI) *see* Ciprofloxacin (Systemic) 441
Ciprocan (KR) *see* Ciprofloxacin (Systemic) 441
Ciprocep (TH) *see* Ciprofloxacin (Systemic) 441
Ciprocin (AE, BH, CY, EG, IQ, IR, JO, KW, LB, LY, OM, QA, SA, SY, YE) *see* Ciprofloxacin (Systemic) 441
Ciprocin (EG) *see* Ciprofloxacin (Ophthalmic) 446
Ciprodar (AE, BH, CY, EG, HK, IQ, IR, JO, KW, LB, LY, OM, QA, SA, SY, YE) *see* Ciprofloxacin (Systemic) 441
Ciprodar (HK) *see* Ciprofloxacin (Otic) 446
Ciprodar (HK, JO, SA) *see* Ciprofloxacin (Ophthalmic) 446
Ciprodex (EC, PE, PY, UY) *see* Ciprofloxacin and Dexamethasone 446
Ciprodex (IL) *see* Ciprofloxacin (Systemic) 441
Ciproflox (CY, PE, SA) *see* Ciprofloxacin (Systemic) 441
Ciprogal (UY) *see* Cyproheptadine 529
Ciprogis (IL) *see* Ciprofloxacin (Systemic) 441
Ciproglen (MY) *see* Ciprofloxacin (Systemic) 441
Cipro HC (BR) *see* Ciprofloxacin and Hydrocortisone 446
Cipro HC Otic (HK) *see* Ciprofloxacin and Hydrocortisone 446
Ciprolak (PE) *see* Ciprofloxacin (Ophthalmic) 446
Ciprolak (PE) *see* Ciprofloxacin (Systemic) 441
Ciprol (AU) *see* Ciprofloxacin (Systemic) 441
Ciprolet (SG) *see* Ciprofloxacin (Systemic) 441
Ciprolin (PE) *see* Ciprofloxacin (Systemic) 441
Ciprolip (BR) *see* Ciprofibrate [INT] 441
Ciprolon (AE, BH, CY, EG, IQ, IR, JO, KW, LB, LY, OM, QA, SA, SY, YE) *see* Ciprofloxacin (Systemic) 441
Cipromed (PE) *see* Ciprofloxacin (Systemic) 441
Cipromycin (GR) *see* Ciprofloxacin (Systemic) 441
Cipropharm (AE, BH, CY, EG, IQ, IR, JO, KW, LB, LY, OM, QA, SA, SY, YE) *see* Ciprofloxacin (Systemic) 441
Ciprophil (PH) *see* Ciprofloxacin (Systemic) 441
Ciproplex (PY) *see* Cyproterone [CAN/INT] 530
Ciproral (DE) *see* Cyproheptadine 529
Ciprotal (PH) *see* Ciprofloxacin (Ophthalmic) 446
Ciprotal (PH) *see* Ciprofloxacin (Systemic) 441
Ciproterona (CL) *see* Cyproterone [CAN/INT] 530
Ciproton (MX) *see* Pantoprazole 1570
Ciprouro SR (KR) *see* Ciprofloxacin (Systemic) 441
Ciproval (CL) *see* Ciprofloxacin (Systemic) 441
Ciprovit-A (PE) *see* Cyproheptadine 529
Ciprox (AE, BH, CY, EG, IQ, IR, JO, KW, LB, LY, MY, OM, QA, SA, SY, YE) *see* Ciprofloxacin (Systemic) 441
Ciproxan (JP) *see* Ciprofloxacin (Systemic) 441
Ciproxina (BB, BM, BS, BZ, CR, DO, EC, GT, HN, JM, NI, NL, PA, PR, PT, SR, SV, TT) *see* Ciprofloxacin (Systemic) 441
Ciproxina (ES) *see* Ciprofloxacin and Hydrocortisone 446
Ciproxin (AT, AU, CH, DK, FI, GB, GR, HK, ID, IE, IT, KR, NO, NZ, SE, TR, TW) *see* Ciprofloxacin (Systemic) 441
Ciproxine (BE) *see* Ciprofloxacin (Systemic) 441
Ciproxin HC (CH) *see* Ciprofloxacin and Hydrocortisone 446
Ciproxin HC ear drops (AU) *see* Ciprofloxacin and Hydrocortisone 446
Ciproxin HC Otic Drops (NZ) *see* Ciprofloxacin and Hydrocortisone 446
Ciproxin-Hydrocortisone (IS) *see* Ciprofloxacin and Hydrocortisone 446
Cipro XR (BM) *see* Ciprofloxacin (Systemic) 441
Ciproxxak (PE) *see* Ciprofloxacin and Dexamethasone 446
Ciproxyl (HK, TH) *see* Ciprofloxacin (Systemic) 441
Ciram (SG) *see* Citalopram 451
Circlevein (KR) *see* Aspirin 180
Circonyl (AR) *see* QuiNINE 1761
Circulaid (JO) *see* Pentoxifylline 1618
Circupon (AT, CH, DE) *see* Etilefrine [INT] 815
Circuvit (AR) *see* Warfarin 2186
Circuvit E (DE) *see* Etilefrine [INT] 815
Ciriax Otic (AR, PE) *see* Ciprofloxacin and Hydrocortisone 446
Ciriax (PE) *see* Ciprofloxacin (Systemic) 441
Cirok (PH, SG) *see* Ciprofloxacin (Systemic) 441
Ciroxin (TW) *see* Ciprofloxacin (Ophthalmic) 446
Ciroxin (TW) *see* Ciprofloxacin (Systemic) 441
Cirpobay (CN) *see* Ciprofloxacin (Systemic) 441
Cisaken[tabs] (MX) *see* Cinnarizine [INT] 440
Cisly (LU) *see* CISplatin 448
Cismetin (KR) *see* Cimetidine 438
Cisordinol Acutard (CL, EE, FI, PE, PT, SE) *see* Zuclopenthixol [CAN/INT] 2219
Cisordinol-Acutard[inj.] (HU) *see* Zuclopenthixol [CAN/INT] 2219
Cisordinol-Acutard (NO) *see* Zuclopenthixol [CAN/INT] 2219
Cisordinol (AT, CL, CZ, DK, EE, FI, HN, HU, NO, PE, PT, SE) *see* Zuclopenthixol [CAN/INT] 2219
Cisordinol Depot (AT, CL, DK, EE, FI, HN, HU, NO, PE, PT, SE) *see* Zuclopenthixol [CAN/INT] 2219
Cispatin (KR) *see* CISplatin 448

Cisplan (KR) *see* CISplatin ... 448
Cisplatin (AU, ID, IN, NZ) *see* CISplatin ... 448
Cisplatin Ebewe (HU) *see* CISplatin ... 448
Cisplatin-Ebewe (MY) *see* CISplatin ... 448
Cisplatine-Lilly (LU) *see* CISplatin ... 448
Cisplatin medac (LU) *see* CISplatin ... 448
Cisplatino (CO, EC, ES, PE) *see* CISplatin ... 448
Cisplatin Teva (HU) *see* CISplatin ... 448
Cisplatinum Cytosafe-Delta West (LU) *see* CISplatin ... 448
Cisplatyl (FR) *see* CISplatin ... 448
Cistalgina (AR) *see* Phenazopyridine ... 1629
Cistamine (TH) *see* Cetirizine ... 411
Cistazol (TW) *see* Cilostazol ... 437
Cisteen (PH) *see* CISplatin ... 448
Cisticid (BR, CL, MX, PE, VE) *see* Praziquantel ... 1702
Cistomid (IT) *see* Pipemidic Acid [INT] ... 1655
Citaalogen (JO) *see* Citalopram ... 451
Citafam (AR) *see* Cytarabine (Conventional) ... 535
Citakey (VN) *see* Cilostazol ... 437
Cital (MY) *see* Citalopram ... 451
Citalogen (AE, BH, KW, QA, SA) *see* Citalopram ... 451
Citalo (KR) *see* Escitalopram ... 765
Citalon (HR) *see* Citalopram ... 451
Citalor (BR) *see* AtorvaSTATin ... 194
Citao (TW) *see* Citalopram ... 451
Citao (TW) *see* Escitalopram ... 765
Citaplex (KR) *see* Escitalopram ... 765
Citarabina (ES) *see* Cytarabine (Conventional) ... 535
Citaz (ID) *see* Cilostazol ... 437
Citazol (TH, TW) *see* Cilostazol ... 437
Citazone (CO) *see* Citalopram ... 451
Citidine (HK) *see* Cimetidine ... 438
Citilat (IT) *see* NIFEdipine ... 1451
Citius (AE, BH, CY, EG, ES, IQ, IR, JO, KW, LB, LY, OM, QA, SA, SY, YE) *see* Cimetidine ... 438
Citodon (SE) *see* Acetaminophen and Codeine ... 36
Citodox (AR) *see* Etoposide ... 816
Citofen (HR) *see* Tamoxifen ... 1971
Citol Brim (PY) *see* Brimonidine (Ophthalmic) ... 288
Citol Clor (PY) *see* Chloramphenicol ... 421
Citol Dorzo (PY) *see* Dorzolamide ... 673
Citol Dorzotim (PY) *see* Dorzolamide and Timolol ... 673
Citol Gentamicina (PY) *see* Gentamicin (Ophthalmic) ... 962
Citomid RU (MX, TH) *see* VinCRIStine ... 2163
Citonina (AR) *see* Calcitonin ... 322
Citopam (IN) *see* Citalopram ... 451
Citopcin (KR) *see* Ciprofloxacin (Systemic) ... 441
Citoplatino (IT) *see* CISplatin ... 448
Citoplax (BR) *see* CISplatin ... 448
Citox (MX) *see* Citalopram ... 451
CitraFleet (DE, DK, FI, FR, IE, IS, NO, PT, SE, SK) *see* Sodium Picosulfate, Magnesium Oxide, and Citric Acid ... 1911
Citramag (GB) *see* Magnesium Citrate ... 1262
Citravite (IN, NZ) *see* Ascorbic Acid ... 178
Citrokalcium (HN) *see* Calcium Citrate ... 330
Civar (LB) *see* Acyclovir (Topical) ... 51
Civeran (ES) *see* Loratadine ... 1241
Cixa (TW) *see* Ciprofloxacin (Systemic) ... 441
Cizo (PH) *see* CeFAZolin ... 373
Clabenzole (KR) *see* Triclabendazole [INT] ... 2102
Clabet (PH) *see* Clarithromycin ... 456
Clacef (ID) *see* Cefotaxime ... 382
Clacillin Duo Dry Syrup (KR) *see* Amoxicillin and Clavulanate ... 133
Clacina (TH) *see* Clarithromycin ... 456
Cladex (PH) *see* Cefotaxime ... 382
Cladrim (IN) *see* Cladribine ... 455
Claforan (AE, AT, AU, BB, BE, BF, BG, BH, BJ, BM, BR, BS, BZ, CH, CI, CR, CY, DK, EC, EE, EG, ES, ET, FI, FR, GB, GH, GM, GN, GR, GT, GY, HK, HN, HR, HU, ID, IE, IL, IN, IQ, IR, IT, JM, JO, KE, KR, KW, LB, LR, LU, LY, MA, ML, MR, MT, MU, MW, MY, NE, NG, NI, NL, NZ, OM, PA, PH, PK, PY, QA, RU, SA, SC, SD, SE, SG, SI, SK, SL, SN, SR, SV, SY, TH, TN, TR, TT, TW, TZ, UG, VE, YE, ZA, ZM, ZW) *see* Cefotaxime ... 382
Clafotax (BH, JO, KW, QA, SA) *see* Cefotaxime ... 382
Clairette (KR) *see* Cyproterone and Ethinyl Estradiol [CAN/INT] ... 532
Clalodine (TH) *see* Loratadine ... 1241
Clamentin (ZA) *see* Amoxicillin and Clavulanate ... 133
Clamiben (BR) *see* GlyBURIDE ... 972
Clamide (HK) *see* GlyBURIDE ... 972
Clamisin (KR) *see* Clarithromycin ... 456
Clamist (IN) *see* Clemastine ... 459
Clamovid (HK, MY, SG) *see* Amoxicillin and Clavulanate ... 133
Clamoxin (MX) *see* Amoxicillin and Clavulanate ... 133
Clamoxyl (AT, AU, BB, BE, BM, BS, BZ, CH, FR, GY, JM, NL, NZ, PE, PR, PT, SR, TT) *see* Amoxicillin ... 130
Clamoxyl (AU) *see* Amoxicillin and Clavulanate ... 133
Clamoxyl Duo 400 (AU) *see* Amoxicillin and Clavulanate ... 133
Clamycin (AE, BH, KW, LB, PH, QA, SA) *see* Clarithromycin ... 456
Clanza CR (PH) *see* Aceclofenac [INT] ... 30
Clanza (PH) *see* Aceclofenac [INT] ... 30
Clarac (AU, NZ) *see* Clarithromycin ... 456
Claradol Codeine (FR) *see* Acetaminophen and Codeine ... 36
Claradol (MA) *see* Acetaminophen ... 32
Claral (ES) *see* Diflucortolone [CAN/INT] ... 625
Claramax (NZ) *see* Desloratadine ... 594
Claramida (AR) *see* Roxithromycin [INT] ... 1853
Claramid (BE, FR, LU) *see* Roxithromycin [INT] ... 1853
Claranta (PH) *see* Clarithromycin ... 456
Clara (QA, SA) *see* Loratadine ... 1241
Claratyne (AU, CY, NZ) *see* Loratadine ... 1241
Claravis (BM) *see* ISOtretinoin ... 1127
Claraxim (TH) *see* Cefotaxime ... 382
Clarazole (AE, KW, QA) *see* Ketoconazole (Systemic) ... 1144
Clareal (FR) *see* Desogestrel [INT] ... 597
Clarelux Foam (GB, IE) *see* Clobetasol ... 468
Clarelux (HR) *see* Clobetasol ... 468
Clarexid (HR) *see* Clarithromycin ... 456
Claribax (PH) *see* Clarithromycin ... 456
Claribid (IN) *see* Clarithromycin ... 456
Claricin-P (TH) *see* Clarithromycin ... 456
Claridar (AE, BH, CY, EG, IQ, IR, JO, KW, LB, LY, OM, QA, SA, SY, YE) *see* Clarithromycin ... 456
Clarid (TH) *see* Loratadine ... 1241
Clariflu (MX) *see* Loratadine and Pseudoephedrine ... 1242
Clarifriol (MX) *see* Loratadine and Pseudoephedrine ... 1242
Clarihexal (AU) *see* Clarithromycin ... 456
Clarihist (PH) *see* Loratadine ... 1241
Clari (KR, SG) *see* Clarithromycin ... 456
Clarimac (IN) *see* Clarithromycin ... 456
Clarimax (CL) *see* Clarithromycin ... 456
Clarimed (PE) *see* Clarithromycin ... 456
Clarin (AE, BH, CY, EG, IQ, IR, JO, KW, LB, LY, OM, QA, SA, SY, YE) *see* Loratadine ... 1241
Clarinase 24 Hour Extended Release (MY, SG) *see* Loratadine and Pseudoephedrine ... 1242
Clarinase 24 Hour Relief (AU) *see* Loratadine and Pseudoephedrine ... 1242
Clarinase (AE, BH, CY, EG, HK, HR, ID, IL, IQ, IR, IS, JO, KR, KW, LB, LY, MY, OM, PH, QA, SA, SI, SK, SY, TH, TW, VE, VN, YE) *see* Loratadine and Pseudoephedrine ... 1242
Clarinase Repetabs (CN, NZ) *see* Loratadine and Pseudoephedrine ... 1242
Clarinese (ZA) *see* Loratadine ... 1241

Claripel (AR) *see* Hydroquinone 1020
Claripen (SG) *see* Clarithromycin 456
Clariston (EC) *see* Clarithromycin 456
Clarith (JP, TH) *see* Clarithromycin 456
Clarithro (AU) *see* Clarithromycin 456
Claritin (BR, ID, PH) *see* Loratadine 1241
Claritine-D (RO) *see* Loratadine and Pseudoephedrine 1242
Claritine (AE, BB, BE, BF, BG, BH, BJ, BM, BS, BZ, CH, CI, CY, CZ, EE, EG, ET, GH, GM, GN, GY, HR, HU, IQ, IR, JM, JO, KE, KW, LB, LR, LT, LU, LY, MA, ML, MR, MU, MW, NE, NG, NL, OM, PK, PL, PT, QA, RO, RU, SA, SC, SD, SI, SK, SL, SN, SR, SY, TN, TR, TT, TZ, UG, YE, ZM, ZW) *see* Loratadine 1241
Clarityn (AT, DK, FI, GB, IE, IS, IT, NO, SE) *see* Loratadine 1241
Clarityne-D (CR, DO, GR, GT, HN, NI, PA, PY, SV, TR, UY) *see* Loratadine and Pseudoephedrine 1242
Clarityne D Repetabs (CO, PE) *see* Loratadine and Pseudoephedrine 1242
Clarityne (MX) *see* Loratadine and Pseudoephedrine 1242
Clarityne (AR, CL, CN, CO, CR, DO, ES, FR, GR, GT, HK, HN, KR, MX, MY, PA, PE, PY, SV, TH, TW, UY, VE, VN) *see* Loratadine 1241
Clarium (DE) *see* Piribedil [INT] 1662
Clariwin (SG) *see* Clarithromycin 456
Clarix (AE, BH, CY, EG, IQ, IR, JO, KW, LB, LY, OM, QA, SA, SY, YE) *see* Clarithromycin 456
Clarmyl (ES) *see* CloBAZam 465
Claroftal (AR, PY) *see* Cromolyn (Ophthalmic) 514
Claroft (BR) *see* Naphazoline (Ophthalmic) 1426
Claroma (KR) *see* Clarithromycin 456
Claron (TH) *see* Clarithromycin 456
Clarosin (KR) *see* Clarithromycin 456
Clarzole (BH) *see* Ketoconazole (Systemic) 1144
Clasifel (PY, UY) *see* Hydroquinone 1020
Clasine (PE) *see* Clarithromycin 456
Clasteon (IT, TR) *see* Clodronate [CAN/INT] 469
Clatax (ID) *see* Cefotaxime 382
Claudemor (PT) *see* Benzocaine 246
Claudia (BE) *see* Cyproterone and Ethinyl Estradiol [CAN/INT] 532
Claudine (SK) *see* Cilostazol 437
Clavamox (CH, DE, ID, IN) *see* Amoxicillin and Clavulanate 133
Clavant (MX) *see* Amoxicillin and Clavulanate 133
Clavar (AE, BH, CY, EG, IQ, IR, JO, KW, LB, LY, OM, QA, SA, SY, YE) *see* Amoxicillin and Clavulanate 133
Claventin (FR) *see* Ticarcillin and Clavulanate Potassium [CAN/INT] 2038
Claventin (IL) *see* Amoxicillin and Clavulanate 133
Claversal (AT, BE, DE, ES, IT, LU, PT) *see* Mesalamine 1301
Clavicin (MY) *see* Amoxicillin and Clavulanate 133
Clavigrenin akut (DE) *see* Ergotamine 754
Clavinex (CL, EC) *see* Amoxicillin and Clavulanate 133
Clavipen (MX) *see* Amoxicillin and Clavulanate 133
Clavmex (PH) *see* Amoxicillin and Clavulanate 133
Clavodar (AE, BH, CY, EG, IQ, IR, JO, KW, LB, LY, OM, QA, SA, SY, YE) *see* Amoxicillin and Clavulanate 133
Clavoxil (BR) *see* Amoxicillin and Clavulanate 133
Clavox (TW) *see* Cefotaxime 382
Clavucyd (MX) *see* Amoxicillin and Clavulanate 133
Clavulin (BF, BJ, CI, CO, ET, GH, GM, GN, KE, LR, MA, ML, MR, MU, MW, MX, NE, NG, SC, SD, SL, SN, TN, TZ, UG, ZM, ZW) *see* Amoxicillin and Clavulanate 133
Clavulox Duo (AR, PY) *see* Amoxicillin and Clavulanate 133
Clavumox (DE, PE, ZA) *see* Amoxicillin and Clavulanate 133
Clavuser (MX) *see* Amoxicillin and Clavulanate 133
Claxin (KR) *see* Clarithromycin 456
Clazic SR (VN) *see* Gliclazide [CAN/INT] 964
Clazol (PH) *see* Cilostazol 437
Cleancef (SG, VN) *see* Cefaclor 372
Cleanxate (MY, SG) *see* FlavoxATE 881
Cleardent (IL) *see* Chlorhexidine Gluconate 422
Clear Eyes (NZ) *see* Naphazoline (Ophthalmic) 1426
Clearine (IN) *see* Naphazoline (Ophthalmic) 1426
Clearol (TW) *see* Gemfibrozil 956
Cleating (CN) *see* Diflunisal 626
Clebudan (CL) *see* Budesonide (Systemic) 293
Clefan (MY) *see* Fluticasone (Nasal) 910
Clemanil (JP) *see* Clemastine 459
Clemastinum (PL) *see* Clemastine 459
Clem (PY) *see* Pentoxifylline 1618
Clenasma (IT) *see* Clenbuterol [INT] 460
Clenbunal (VE) *see* Clenbuterol [INT] 460
Clenil (AE, AR, BH, BR, CY, EG, IL, IQ, IR, IT, JO, KW, LB, LY, OM, QA, SA, SG, SY, TW, YE) *see* Beclomethasone (Nasal) 232
Clenil (AE, BR, CN, IT, SG, TW) *see* Beclomethasone (Systemic) 230
Clenil Forte (CY) *see* Beclomethasone (Systemic) 230
Clenil Forte (ID) *see* Beclomethasone (Nasal) 232
Clenil Modulite (GB) *see* Beclomethasone (Nasal) 232
Clenox (CO, PE) *see* Enoxaparin 726
Clensan (TW) *see* Betahistine [CAN/INT] 252
Clentel (EC) *see* Clopidogrel 484
Cleocin HCl (AU, PK, TW) *see* Clindamycin (Systemic) 460
Cleocin T (KR, TR, TW) *see* Clindamycin (Topical) 464
Cleocin T (TR, TW) *see* Clindamycin (Systemic) 460
Cleosensa (GB) *see* Ethinyl Estradiol and Drospirenone 801
Cleo (TW) *see* Tobramycin (Ophthalmic) 2056
Cleridium (FR, PH) *see* Dipyridamole 652
Clerinax (PY) *see* Naproxen 1427
Clerin LR (PY) *see* Phenytoin 1640
Clerin (PY) *see* Phenytoin 1640
Cleron (SG, TR) *see* Clarithromycin 456
Clesin (KR) *see* Cromolyn (Nasal) 514
Clesin (KR) *see* Cromolyn (Ophthalmic) 514
Cleveral (IT) *see* Piracetam [INT] 1661
Clever (IT) *see* Ebastine [INT] 702
Cleviprex (AU, CH, DE, ES, NL, NZ, SE) *see* Clevidipine 460
Clexane (AE, AR, AU, BB, BE, BF, BG, BH, BJ, BM, BS, CH, CI, CL, CN, CO, CR, CY, CZ, DE, DO, EC, EE, EG, ES, ET, GB, GH, GM, GN, GR, GT, GY, HK, HN, HR, HU, IE, IL, IN, IT, JM, JO, JP, KE, KR, KW, LR, LT, LU, MA, ML, MR, MU, MW, MX, MY, NE, NG, NI, NL, NZ, PA, PE, PH, PK, PL, PR, PY, QA, RO, RU, SA, SC, SD, SG, SI, SK, SL, SN, SV, TH, TN, TR, TT, TW, TZ, UG, UY, VE, VN, ZM, ZW) *see* Enoxaparin 726
Clexane Forte (AU, IL, SG) *see* Enoxaparin 726
Clex (KR) *see* Cefaclor 372
Cliad (ID) *see* Clidinium and Chlordiazepoxide 460
Clibon (DO, GT, HN, NI) *see* Estradiol and Norethindrone 781
Clicin (VN) *see* Clindamycin (Systemic) 460
Clidets (VE) *see* Clindamycin (Systemic) 460
Clid (KR) *see* Ticlopidine 2040
Clidol (KR) *see* Sulindac 1953
Clidorel (ID) *see* Clopidogrel 484
Climabel (VN) *see* Tibolone [INT] 2035
Climadan (ID, SG) *see* Clindamycin (Systemic) 460
Climaderm (BR, VE) *see* Estradiol (Systemic) 775
Climafen (CL) *see* Tibolone [INT] 2035
Climanor (GB, IE, TR) *see* MedroxyPROGESTERone 1277
Climara (AT, AU, BE, BG, CH, CZ, EE, FI, FR, IE, KR, NZ, PH, PL, RU, TH, ZA) *see* Estradiol (Systemic) 775
Climara (RO) *see* Estradiol (Topical) 780

Climarest (DE) *see* Estrogens (Conjugated/Equine, Systemic) ... 787
Climatrol (CO) *see* Estrogens (Conjugated/Equine, Systemic) ... 787
Climatrol E (CL, PY, VE) *see* Estrogens (Conjugated/ Equine, Systemic) ... 787
Climene (DO) *see* Cyproterone and Ethinyl Estradiol [CAN/INT] ... 532
Climodien (AT, BE, NO, PT, SE) *see* Estradiol and Dienogest ... 780
Climodiene (FR) *see* Estradiol and Dienogest ... 780
Clinacin (AE, BH, CY, EG, IQ, IR, JO, KW, LB, LY, OM, QA, SA, SY, YE) *see* Clindamycin (Systemic) ... 460
Clinadol Forte (AR, UY) *see* Flurbiprofen (Systemic) ... 906
Clinbercin (ID) *see* Clindamycin (Systemic) ... 460
Clincin (TW) *see* Clindamycin (Systemic) ... 460
Clincor (VE) *see* Tetracycline ... 2017
Clindac-A (IN) *see* Clindamycin (Systemic) ... 460
Clindac-A (IN) *see* Clindamycin (Topical) ... 464
Clindacid (PY) *see* Clindamycin (Systemic) ... 460
Clindacin (AE, BH, CY, EG, IQ, IR, JO, KW, LB, LY, OM, PE, QA, SA, SY, YE) *see* Clindamycin (Systemic) ... 460
Clindacin T (KW, SA) *see* Clindamycin (Topical) ... 464
Clinda (DE) *see* Clindamycin (Systemic) ... 460
Clindagel (SG) *see* Clindamycin (Topical) ... 464
Clindala (ID) *see* Clindamycin (Systemic) ... 460
Clindal AZ (BR, HK) *see* Azithromycin (Systemic) ... 216
Clindalin (TH) *see* Clindamycin (Systemic) ... 460
Clindal (PH) *see* Clindamycin (Systemic) ... 460
Clinda-P (TH) *see* Clindamycin (Systemic) ... 460
ClindaTech (AU, NZ, PH) *see* Clindamycin (Topical) ... 464
Clindatec (PH) *see* Clindamycin (Systemic) ... 460
Clindavid (TH) *see* Clindamycin (Systemic) ... 460
Clinderm (PH) *see* Clindamycin (Topical) ... 464
Clindox (JO) *see* Clindamycin (Systemic) ... 460
Clindox (PE) *see* Clindamycin (Topical) ... 464
Clinfar (BR) *see* Simvastatin ... 1890
Clinika (ID) *see* Clindamycin (Topical) ... 464
Clinivate (TH) *see* Betamethasone (Topical) ... 255
Clinmax (HK) *see* Clindamycin (Topical) ... 464
Clinofem (DE) *see* MedroxyPROGESTERone ... 1277
Clinoina (AR) *see* Clindamycin and Tretinoin ... 464
Clinorette (GB, IE) *see* Estradiol and Norethindrone ... 781
Clinoril (AE, AT, BE, BF, BH, BJ, CH, CI, CY, EG, ET, GB, GH, GM, GN, HN, IE, IL, IQ, IR, IT, JO, KE, KW, LB, LR, LY, MA, ML, MR, MU, MW, MX, NE, NG, NL, NO, OM, PL, QA, SA, SC, SD, SE, SL, SN, SY, TH, TN, TZ, UG, VE, YE, ZM, ZW) *see* Sulindac ... 1953
Clinott (TH) *see* Clindamycin (Systemic) ... 460
Clinovir (ID, TH) *see* Acyclovir (Systemic) ... 47
Clinovir (ID, TH) *see* Acyclovir (Topical) ... 51
Clint (BF, BJ, CI, ET, GH, GM, GN, KE, LR, MA, ML, MR, MU, MW, NE, NG, SC, SD, SL, SN, TN, TW, TZ, UG, ZM, ZW) *see* Allopurinol ... 90
Cliovelle (KR) *see* Estradiol and Norethindrone ... 781
Clipper (BE, GB) *see* Beclomethasone (Nasal) ... 232
Clison (MX) *see* Sulindac ... 1953
Clistin (IN) *see* Carbinoxamine ... 356
Clitaxel (VE) *see* PACLitaxel (Conventional) ... 1550
Clizid (PH) *see* Gliclazide [CAN/INT] ... 964
Clizine (TW) *see* Meclizine ... 1277
Cliz (PH) *see* Clindamycin (Systemic) ... 460
Clo V (KR) *see* Clopidogrel ... 484
Cloart (KR) *see* Clopidogrel ... 484
Clobamax (PE) *see* CloBAZam ... 465
Clobam (PK) *see* CloBAZam ... 465
Clobasone (TH) *see* Clobetasol ... 468
Clobator (IN) *see* CloBAZam ... 465
Clobax (CO) *see* Deflazacort [INT] ... 587
Clobazam (PE) *see* CloBAZam ... 465
Clobemix (AU) *see* Moclobemide [CAN/INT] ... 1384
Clobenate (PE) *see* Clobetasol ... 468
Clobesan (ID) *see* Clobetasol ... 468
Clobesol (AR, BR, HK, IT, MX) *see* Clobetasol ... 468
Clobet (TH) *see* Clobetasol ... 468
Clobex (HK, ID, NZ, PH, SG, TW) *see* Clobetasol ... 468
Clobexpro (MX) *see* Clobetasol ... 468
Clobezan (CO, EC) *see* Clobetasol ... 468
Clobutol (PT) *see* Ethambutol ... 798
Cloderm (AE, BH, CY, EG, HK, IQ, IR, JO, KR, KW, LB, LY, OM, QA, SA, SG, SY, TH, VN, YE) *see* Clobetasol ... 468
Cloderm (DE) *see* Clotrimazole (Topical) ... 488
Cloderm (ID) *see* Alclometasone ... 72
Clodine (IL) *see* Chlorhexidine Gluconate ... 422
Clodor (LB) *see* Clopidogrel ... 484
Clodron (DE) *see* Clodronate [CAN/INT] ... 469
Clofazic (AR, CL, PE) *see* Clofarabine ... 470
Clofec (TH) *see* Diclofenac (Systemic) ... 617
Clofen (AE, JO, KW, LB, QA, SA) *see* Diclofenac (Systemic) ... 617
Clofen (AU) *see* Baclofen ... 223
Clofenex-50 (HK) *see* Diclofenac (Systemic) ... 617
Clofen Retard (AE, KW) *see* Diclofenac (Systemic) ... 617
Clofibral (PY) *see* Bezafibrate [CAN/INT] ... 261
Clofix (TW) *see* Clopidogrel ... 484
Clofoam (LB) *see* Clobetasol ... 468
Clofozine (IN) *see* Clofazimine [INT] ... 473
Clofranil (IN, PH) *see* ClomiPRAMINE ... 475
Clofritis (ID) *see* CloBAZam ... 465
Cloftal (VE) *see* Chloramphenicol ... 421
Clogin (ID) *see* Clopidogrel ... 484
Clojac (KR) *see* ClomiPRAMINE ... 475
Clo-Kit Junior (IN) *see* Chloroquine ... 424
Clolar (MX) *see* Clofarabine ... 470
Clomazol (EC, NZ) *see* Clotrimazole (Topical) ... 488
Clomene (PH) *see* ClomiPHENE ... 473
Clomentin (TR) *see* Escitalopram ... 765
Clomhexal (AU) *see* ClomiPHENE ... 473
Clomid (AE, AR, AU, BE, BH, CH, CY, EG, FR, GB, IE, IQ, IR, IT, JO, KW, LB, LY, MY, NL, OM, PH, PK, QA, SA, SG, SY, TH, TW, YE) *see* ClomiPHENE ... 473
Clomidep (VN) *see* ClomiPRAMINE ... 475
Clomifen (FI) *see* ClomiPHENE ... 473
Clomihexal (ZA) *see* ClomiPHENE ... 473
Clomipen (KR) *see* ClomiPHENE ... 473
Clomitene (PH) *see* Metoclopramide ... 1345
Clomoval (AE, BH, CY, EG, IQ, IR, JO, KW, LB, LY, OM, QA, SA, SY, YE) *see* ClomiPHENE ... 473
Clonac (AU) *see* Diclofenac (Systemic) ... 617
Clonapilep (MX) *see* ClonazePAM ... 478
Clonaril (TH) *see* ClonazePAM ... 478
Clonate (MY, PH) *see* Clobetasol ... 468
Clonatril (JO) *see* ClonazePAM ... 478
Clonatryl (CO) *see* ClonazePAM ... 478
Clonazepamum (HU) *see* ClonazePAM ... 478
Clonazine (IE) *see* ChlorproMAZINE ... 429
Clonea (AU) *see* Clotrimazole (Topical) ... 488
Clonex (IL) *see* ClonazePAM ... 478
Clonidina Larjan (AR) *see* CloNIDine ... 480
Clonidural (AR) *see* CloNIDine ... 480
Clonigen (PH) *see* CloNIDine ... 480
Clonilou (ES) *see* CloNIDine ... 480
Clonin (TW) *see* ClomiPHENE ... 473
Clonipresan (PY) *see* CloNIDine ... 480
Clonipress (PH) *see* CloNIDine ... 480
Clonopam (TW) *see* ClonazePAM ... 478
Clonotril (CY, PH, SG, TR) *see* ClonazePAM ... 478
Clonovate (SG) *see* Clobetasol ... 468
Clont (DE) *see* MetroNIDAZOLE (Systemic) ... 1353
Clood (IL) *see* Clopidogrel ... 484
Clopamon (ZA) *see* Metoclopramide ... 1345
Clopax (ES) *see* CloBAZam ... 465
Clopedin (ID) *see* Meperidine ... 1293
Clopes (ID) *see* Acyclovir (Systemic) ... 47
Clopidexcel (IL) *see* Clopidogrel ... 484

Clopidrol (PH) *see* Clopidogrel 484
Clopilet (IN) *see* Clopidogrel 484
Clopimet (PH) *see* Clopidogrel 484
Clopin (CH) *see* CloZAPine 490
Clopine (AU, ID, MY, NZ, TW) *see* CloZAPine 490
Clopiright (HK) *see* Clopidogrel 484
Clopistad (HK) *see* Clopidogrel 484
Clopivas (HK) *see* Clopidogrel 484
Clopivaz (PH) *see* Clopidogrel 484
Clopivid (HK, MY) *see* Clopidogrel 484
Clopixol Acuphase (AE, AU, BH, BR, CN, EG, HK, HR, IL, IN, IT, LB, MX, MY, PK, RO, SA, SI, ZA) *see* Zuclopenthixol [CAN/INT] 2219
Clopixol Acutard (CH) *see* Zuclopenthixol [CAN/INT] 2219
Clopixol (AE, AR, AU, BE, BG, BH, BR, CH, CN, CY, ES, FR, GB, GR, HK, HR, IE, IL, IT, JO, KR, KW, LB, LU, MX, MY, NL, PK, PL, RO, RU, SA, SG, TH, TR, TW, VN, ZA) *see* Zuclopenthixol [CAN/INT] 2219
Clopixol Depot (AE, AU, BH, BR, CH, CY, EG, HK, HR, IL, IN, IT, LB, LU, MX, MY, NL, PK, QA, RO, SA, SG, SI, TH, TW, ZA) *see* Zuclopenthixol [CAN/INT] 2219
Clopram (BF, BJ, CI, ET, GH, GM, GN, JO, KE, LR, MA, ML, MR, MU, MW, NE, NG, SC, SD, SL, SN, TN, TZ, UG, ZM, ZW) *see* Metoclopramide 1345
Clopran (TW) *see* ClomiPRAMINE 475
Clopsine (MX) *see* CloZAPine 490
Cloracef (ID) *see* Cefaclor 372
Cloracef MR (AE, BH, CY, EG, IL, IQ, IR, JO, KW, LB, LY, OM, QA, SA, SY, YE) *see* Cefaclor 372
Cloramfeni Ofteno (GT, MX, SV) *see* Chloramphenicol 421
Cloramidina Ophth Oint (ID) *see* Chloramphenicol 421
Cloran (MX) *see* Chloramphenicol 421
Clorana (BR) *see* Hydrochlorothiazide 1009
Cloranfenicol (VE) *see* Chloramphenicol 421
Cloranxen (PL) *see* Clorazepate 487
Cloraxin (VN) *see* Chloramphenicol 421
Clorcef (PH) *see* Cefaclor 372
Clordil (MX) *see* Chloramphenicol 421
Clordox (BR) *see* Doxycycline 689
Cloril (TH) *see* CloZAPine 490
Clorimax (PY) *see* ClomiPRAMINE 475
Clorix (ZA) *see* Moclobemide [CAN/INT] 1384
Clormicin (CO) *see* Clarithromycin 456
Clorochina Bayer (IT) *see* Chloroquine 424
Clorochina Bifosfato (IT) *see* Chloroquine 424
Cloromisan (PE) *see* Chloramphenicol 421
Cloroptic (CO) *see* Chloramphenicol 421
Cloroquina Llorente (ES) *see* Chloroquine 424
Clorotir (NZ) *see* Cefaclor 372
Clorpromaz (BR) *see* ChlorproMAZINE 429
Clortalil (BR) *see* Chlorthalidone 430
Closderm (PH) *see* Clobetasol 468
Clostilbegyt (AE, BB, BG, BH, BM, BS, BZ, CY, EG, GY, HN, IQ, IR, JM, JO, KW, LB, LY, OM, PL, PR, QA, RU, SA, SR, SY, TT, VN, YE) *see* ClomiPHENE 473
Clostil (PH) *see* ClomiPHENE 473
Clothree (IL) *see* Clotrimazole (Topical) 488
Clotinab (KR, PY, TH) *see* Abciximab 24
Clotinil (TW) *see* Clopidogrel 484
Clotiz (PH) *see* Clopidogrel 484
Clotrasone (CN) *see* Clotrimazole (Topical) 488
Clotrasone (CN, ES, PH) *see* Betamethasone and Clotrimazole 256
Clotrex (DO) *see* Clotrimazole (Topical) 488
Clotrimaderm (IL, NZ) *see* Clotrimazole (Topical) 488
Clotrisone (IL) *see* Betamethasone and Clotrimazole 256
Clovate (ES) *see* Clobetasol 468
Clovertil (ID) *see* ClomiPHENE 473
Clovex (JO) *see* Clopidogrel 484
Clovika (ID) *see* Acyclovir (Systemic) 47
Clovillin (PH) *see* Ampicillin 141
Clovir (KR, PH, PY) *see* Acyclovir (Systemic) 47
Clovir (TW) *see* Acyclovir (Topical) 51
Clovisone (PH) *see* Hydrocortisone (Systemic) 1013
Clovix (MY) *see* Clopidogrel 484
Clovixx (TW) *see* Clopidogrel 484
Clovizole (PH) *see* MetroNIDAZOLE (Systemic) 1353
Cloviz (PH) *see* CeFAZolin 373
Cloxacap (HK, SG) *see* Cloxacillin [CAN/INT] 488
Cloxacap (SG) *see* Oxacillin 1528
Cloxam (TH) *see* Cloxacillin [CAN/INT] 488
Cloxapene (IN) *see* Ampicillin and Cloxacillin [INT] 144
Cloxcin (SG) *see* Oxacillin 1528
Cloxgen (TH) *see* Cloxacillin [CAN/INT] 488
Cloxidil (VN) *see* Cloxacillin [CAN/INT] 488
Cloxipen (AE) *see* Ampicillin and Cloxacillin [INT] 144
Cloxomed (TW) *see* Cloxacillin [CAN/INT] 488
Clox (PH) *see* Cloxacillin [CAN/INT] 488
Clozamed (TH) *see* CloZAPine 490
Clozarem (MY) *see* CloZAPine 490
Clozaril (AU, GB, HK, ID, IE, JP, KR, MY, NZ, PK, SG, TH, TW) *see* CloZAPine 490
Clozene (TW) *see* Clorazepate 487
Clozer (MX) *see* ClonazePAM 478
Clozine (IN) *see* ChlorproMAZINE 429
Cluyer (AR) *see* Meperidine 1293
CMaxid (HK) *see* Cefuroxime 399
CoActifed (CA) *see* Triprolidine, Pseudoephedrine, and Codeine [CAN/INT] 2105
Coalbi (KR) *see* Levocetirizine 1196
Coamox (TH) *see* Amoxicillin 130
Coaparin (PL) *see* Heparin 997
CoApprovel (DE) *see* Irbesartan and Hydrochlorothiazide 1112
CoAprovel (MX, VN) *see* Irbesartan and Hydrochlorothiazide 1112
Coaprovel (AE, AR, AT, BB, BE, BG, BH, BM, BS, CH, CL, CN, CO, CR, CZ, DE, DK, DO, EC, EE, ES, FI, FR, GB, GR, GT, GY, HK, HN, HR, HU, ID, IE, IT, JM, JO, KR, KW, LB, LT, MT, MY, NI, NL, NO, PA, PE, PH, PR, PT, PY, QA, RO, RU, SA, SE, SG, SI, SK, SV, TH, TT, TW, UY, VE) *see* Irbesartan and Hydrochlorothiazide 1112
Co-Aprovel (HK, TH) *see* Irbesartan and Hydrochlorothiazide 1112
Coartem (ID, PE, PH, QA, VN) *see* Artemether and Lumefantrine 177
Coaxil (BG, CZ, EE, HR, HU, PL, RO, RU, SI, SK) *see* Tianeptine [INT] 2033
Cobalin (AE, BH, CY, EG, IQ, IR, JO, KW, LB, LY, OM, QA, SA, SY, YE) *see* Cyanocobalamin 515
Cobalin-H (AE, GB, QA) *see* Hydroxocobalamin 1020
Cobalmin (PE) *see* CARBOplatin 357
Cobalparen (DE) *see* Hydroxocobalamin 1020
Cobalvit (IT) *see* Hydroxocobalamin 1020
Cobamin Ophth Soln (HK) *see* Cyanocobalamin 515
Cobasol (AU) *see* Cabergoline 319
Cobay-500 (PH) *see* Ciprofloxacin (Systemic) 441
Cobay (TH) *see* Ciprofloxacin (Systemic) 441
Cobiona (ES) *see* Oxatomide [INT] 1532
Cobisk (KR) *see* AmLODIPine 123
Cobis (KR) *see* Bisoprolol and Hydrochlorothiazide 267
Cobitussin (TW) *see* Codeine 497
Cobizal (KR) *see* Mometasone (Nasal) 1391
Cocine (TW) *see* Colchicine 500
Co-Codamol (HK) *see* Acetaminophen and Codeine 36
Cocol (JP) *see* Flucytosine 889
Codabrol (IL) *see* Acetaminophen and Codeine 36
Cod-Acamol 10/500 (IL) *see* Acetaminophen and Codeine 36
Cod-Acamol 15/325 (IL) *see* Acetaminophen and Codeine 36
Codalgin (AU, NZ) *see* Acetaminophen and Codeine 36
Codant (IE) *see* Codeine 497

Codapane (AU) *see* Acetaminophen and Codeine 36
Codapane Forte (AU) *see* Acetaminophen and Codeine 36
Codedrill sans sucre (FR) *see* Codeine 497
Codein (AR, KR, PY) *see* Codeine 497
Codeine Linctus (GB) *see* Codeine 497
Codeine Phosphate (CY, CZ, NZ) *see* Codeine 497
Codeini phosphatis (HR) *see* Codeine 497
Codeinsaft von ct (DE) *see* Codeine 497
Codeintropfen Ribbeck (DE) *see* Codeine 497
Codeintropfen von ct (DE) *see* Codeine 497
Codeinum Phosphorcum (PL) *see* Codeine 497
Codeinum phosphoricum Berlin-Chemie (DE) *see* Codeine 497
Codeinum phosphoricum Compretten (DE) *see* Codeine 497
Codeisan (PT) *see* Codeine 497
Codelpar (CL) *see* Acetaminophen and Codeine 36
Codenfan (FR) *see* Codeine 497
Coderit (MX) *see* Codeine 497
Coderpina (GT, HN, SV) *see* Codeine 497
Codicaps (DE) *see* Codeine 497
Codicet (TH) *see* Acetaminophen and Codeine 36
Codicompren (DE) *see* Codeine 497
Codicontin (BE, CH, LU) *see* Dihydrocodeine, Aspirin, and Caffeine 632
Codidol (AT) *see* Dihydrocodeine, Aspirin, and Caffeine 632
Codiforton (DE) *see* Codeine 497
Codilprane Enfant (FR) *see* Acetaminophen and Codeine 36
Codimal (PH) *see* GuaiFENesin 986
Codin Linctus (IN) *see* Codeine 497
Co-Dio (JP) *see* Valsartan and Hydrochlorothiazide 2129
Co-Diopass (KR) *see* Valsartan and Hydrochlorothiazide 2129
codi OPT (DE) *see* Codeine 497
Codiortan (KR) *see* Valsartan and Hydrochlorothiazide 2129
Co-Diovan (AE, AT, AU, BG, BH, CH, CY, CZ, EE, GR, HK, HR, ID, IL, JO, KW, LB, LT, MY, NL, NZ, PH, PK, PL, PT, RU, SA, SG, SI, SK, TH, TR, TW, VN) *see* Valsartan and Hydrochlorothiazide 2129
CoDiovan (DE, GB, IE, KR, MX) *see* Valsartan and Hydrochlorothiazide 2129
Co-Diovane (BE) *see* Valsartan and Hydrochlorothiazide 2129
Codipar (GB, IE) *see* Acetaminophen and Codeine 36
Codipertussin (DE) *see* Codeine 497
Codipront mono (DE, LU) *see* Codeine 497
Codipront N (PH) *see* Codeine 497
Codiqvan (KR) *see* Valsartan and Hydrochlorothiazide 2129
Codisol (DK) *see* Pholcodine [INT] 1646
Coditam (ID) *see* Acetaminophen and Codeine 36
Codoliprane Enfant (FR) *see* Acetaminophen and Codeine 36
Codoliprane (FR) *see* Acetaminophen and Codeine 36
Codotussyl (SG) *see* Acetylcysteine 40
Codotussyl toux seche (FR) *see* Pholcodine [INT] 1646
Codral Dry Cough Liquid (AU) *see* Pholcodine [INT] 1646
Coedarone (MX) *see* Amiodarone 114
Cofact (BE, NL) *see* Prothrombin Complex Concentrate (Human) [(Factors II, VII, IX, X), Protein C, and Protein S] 1738
Cofarin (TW) *see* Warfarin 2186
Cofen (SG) *see* GuaiFENesin 986
Cofexor XL ER (KR) *see* Venlafaxine 2150
Coffeinum Natrium Benzoicum (PL) *see* Caffeine 319
Co-Flem (ZA) *see* Carbocisteine [INT] 357
Cogentin (AT, AU, EG, GB, HK, IE, KW, MY, NZ, PT, SA, SE, SG, TH) *see* Benztropine 248
Cogetine (TH) *see* Chloramphenicol 421
Cognil (PY) *see* Methylphenidate 1336
Cognitive (VN) *see* Selegiline 1873
Cognitiv (RU) *see* Selegiline 1873
Cohemin Depot (FI) *see* Hydroxocobalamin 1020
Co-Hypace (PH) *see* Enalapril and Hydrochlorothiazide 725
Co-Irvebal (ID) *see* Irbesartan and Hydrochlorothiazide 1112
Co-Ivyzar (PH) *see* Irbesartan and Hydrochlorothiazide 1112
Cokenzen (FR) *see* Candesartan and Hydrochlorothiazide 338
Coklav (TH) *see* Amoxicillin and Clavulanate 133
Col-Alphar (MX) *see* Pravastatin 1700
Colaspase (JO) *see* Asparaginase (E. coli) 179
Colazal (KR) *see* Balsalazide 226
Colazide (AT, AU, GB, NZ) *see* Balsalazide 226
Colazid (NO, SE) *see* Balsalazide 226
Colchicin Agepha (AT) *see* Colchicine 500
Colchicina Lirca (IT) *see* Colchicine 500
Colchicina Phoenix (AR) *see* Colchicine 500
Colchicine capsules (NL) *see* Colchicine 500
Colchicine Houde (AR, BE, ES, FR, LU, PT) *see* Colchicine 500
Colchicine (IL) *see* Colchicine 500
Colchicum-Dispert (BG, DE, HU, PL, TR) *see* Colchicine 500
Colchifar (VN) *see* Colchicine 500
Colchily (TH) *see* Colchicine 500
Colchimedio (CO, CR, DO, GT, HN, NI, PA, SV) *see* Colchicine 500
Colchin (KR) *see* Colchicine 500
Colchiquim (MX) *see* Colchicine 500
Colchis (BR) *see* Colchicine 500
Colchisol (PE) *see* Colchicine 500
Colchysat Burger (DE) *see* Colchicine 500
Colcine (TH) *see* Colchicine 500
Colcitex (SG) *see* Colchicine 500
Coldacrom (AT) *see* Cromolyn (Ophthalmic) 514
Coldin (CL) *see* Carbocisteine [INT] 357
Coldrex Broncho (PL) *see* GuaiFENesin 986
Colese (AU) *see* Mebeverine [INT] 1275
Colese (TW) *see* Maprotiline 1271
Colesken (MX) *see* Simvastatin 1890
Colestid (AT, AU, BB, BE, BG, BH, BM, BS, BZ, CH, CZ, ES, GB, GY, HN, HR, HU, IE, IL, IT, JM, LU, NL, NZ, PL, PT, SA, SR, TT) *see* Colestipol 504
Colestiramina (CL, CO, PY) *see* Cholestyramine Resin 431
Colestrol (IT) *see* Cholestyramine Resin 431
Colfarit (CZ, HN) *see* Aspirin 180
Colfed (BF, BJ, CI, ET, GH, GM, GN, KE, LR, MA, ML, MR, MU, MW, NE, NG, SC, SD, SL, SN, TN, TZ, UG, ZA, ZM, ZW) *see* Triprolidine and Pseudoephedrine 2105
Colfinair (ES) *see* Colistimethate 504
Colgout (AU, HK, NZ) *see* Colchicine 500
Colhidrol (AR) *see* DOXOrubicin (Conventional) 679
Colidac (IN) *see* Cilostazol 437
Colidimin (AT) *see* Rifaximin 1809
Colidium (ID) *see* Loperamide 1236
Colifilm (AR) *see* Loperamide 1236
Colifin (CH, DE) *see* Colistimethate 504
Colifoam (AE, AT) *see* Hydrocortisone (Systemic) 1013
Colifoam (AU, GR) *see* Hydrocortisone (Topical) 1014
Coligon (IN) *see* Dicyclomine 622
Coliman (TW) *see* ChlorproMAZINE 429
Colimicina IM (IT) *see* Colistimethate 504
Colimycin (CL) *see* Colistimethate 504
Colimycine (FR, SK) *see* Colistimethate 504

Colinsan (DE) *see* AzaTHIOprine 210
Coliper (CL) *see* Loperamide 1236
Coliracin (IL) *see* Colistimethate 504
Colircusi Atropina (ES) *see* Atropine 200
Colircusi Cicloplejico (ES) *see* Cyclopentolate 517
Colircusi Cloramfenicol (ES) *see* Chloramphenicol 421
Colircusi Fluoresceina (ES) *see* Fluorescein 894
Colircusi Tropicamida (ES) *see* Tropicamide 2108
Coliriocilina Neomicina (ES) *see* Neomycin 1436
Colirio Collado Cortioftal (ES) *see* Cortisone 510
Colirio Ocul Atropina (ES) *see* Atropine 200
Colirio Ocul Cicloplejic (ES) *see* Cyclopentolate 517
Colirio Ocul Fluorescein (ES) *see* Fluorescein 894
Colis (KR) *see* Colistimethate 504
Colistate (TH) *see* Colistimethate 504
Colistimixin (AU) *see* Colistimethate 504
Colistin (CH, NL) *see* Colistimethate 504
Colistineb (BE) *see* Colistimethate 504
Colistin Link (AU, NZ) *see* Colistimethate 504
Colitofalk (BE, LU) *see* Mesalamine 1301
Colixin (PT) *see* Colistimethate 504
Colizole DS (IN) *see* Sulfamethoxazole and Trimethoprim 1946
Colizole (IN) *see* Sulfamethoxazole and Trimethoprim 1946
Colliprol (MX) *see* Propranolol 1731
Colmibe (EC) *see* Ezetimibe and Simvastatin 834
Colmibe (EC, PE, PY, UY) *see* Ezetimibe and Atorvastatin 833
Colmifen (SG) *see* Baclofen 223
Colobreathe (BE, CZ, EE, GB, NL, SE) *see* Colistimethate 504
Colobutine (BG, CZ) *see* Trimebutine [CAN/INT] 2103
Colodium (HK) *see* Loperamide 1236
Colofac (AT, AU, GB, IE, PK, TH, ZA) *see* Mebeverine [INT] 1275
Colofiber (BE) *see* Psyllium 1744
Colomycin (CZ, GB, GR, HK, HN, IE, SG, SI) *see* Colistimethate 504
Coloncure (TW) *see* Mesalamine 1301
Colo-Pleon (DE) *see* SulfaSALAzine 1950
Colopriv (FR) *see* Mebeverine [INT] 1275
Colorex (IN) *see* Balsalazide 226
Colospa (ID, IN) *see* Mebeverine [INT] 1275
Colospan (HK) *see* Scopolamine (Systemic) 1870
Colospa Retard (HR) *see* Mebeverine [INT] 1275
Colospasmin (AE, BH, EG, KW, QA, RO) *see* Mebeverine [INT] 1275
Colotal (IL) *see* Mebeverine [INT] 1275
Coloximina (AR) *see* Rifaximin 1809
Coloxyl (AU, NZ) *see* Docusate 661
Colpradin (MX) *see* Pravastatin 1700
Colsancetine (ID) *see* Chloramphenicol 421
Colufase (EC, PE) *see* Nitazoxanide 1461
Coluquim (PE) *see* Nitazoxanide 1461
Co-Lutem (VN) *see* Artemether and Lumefantrine 177
Colypan (EC) *see* Trimebutine [CAN/INT] 2103
Coly (TH) *see* Mefenamic Acid 1280
Comadex (EC) *see* Tamsulosin 1974
Combantril (CH) *see* Pyrantel Pamoate 1744
Combantrin-1 (NZ) *see* Mebendazole [CAN/INT] 1274
Combantrin-1 with mebendazole (AU) *see* Mebendazole [CAN/INT] 1274
Combantrin (AT, BG, BH, CL, CO, EC, EG, FR, GB, GR, IT, KR, NZ, PE, PH, PT, QA, SA, VE, VN, ZA) *see* Pyrantel Pamoate 1744
Combetzar (PH) *see* Losartan and Hydrochlorothiazide 1250
Combigan (AE, AR, AT, AU, BE, BR, CH, CL, CO, CZ, DE, DK, EC, FI, FR, GB, GR, HK, HN, HR, IE, IL, IN, IT, KR, KW, LB, LT, MY, NL, NO, NZ, PE, PH, PL, PT, SA, SE, SG, SI, SK, TH, TW, VN, ZA) *see* Brimonidine and Timolol 288
Combiginor (UY) *see* Norethindrone and Mestranol 1475
Combipul (PH) *see* Ipratropium and Albuterol 1109
Combivent (AE, AR, AT, BB, BE, BF, BH, BJ, BM, BR, BS, BZ, CI, CL, CN, CO, CR, CY, DK, DO, EC, EE, EG, ES, ET, FR, GH, GM, GN, GT, GY, HK, HN, ID, IE, IL, IQ, IR, JM, JO, KE, KR, KW, LB, LR, LY, MA, ML, MR, MU, MW, MX, NE, NG, NI, NL, OM, PA, PE, PH, PY, QA, SA, SC, SD, SE, SG, SL, SN, SR, SV, SY, TH, TN, TR, TT, TW, TZ, UG, UY, VE, VN, YE, ZA, ZM, ZW) *see* Ipratropium and Albuterol 1109
Combivent Aerosol (AU, NZ) *see* Ipratropium and Albuterol 1109
Combivent UDV (GB, IE) *see* Ipratropium and Albuterol 1109
Combivir (AE, AT, AU, BE, BF, BG, BH, BJ, CH, CI, CL, CN, CO, CR, CY, CZ, DE, DK, DO, EE, EG, ET, FI, FR, GB, GH, GM, GN, GR, GT, HK, HN, HR, HU, IE, IL, IN, IQ, IR, IS, IT, JO, KE, KR, KW, LB, LR, LT, LY, MA, ML, MR, MT, MU, MW, MX, MY, NE, NG, NI, NL, NO, NZ, OM, PA, PE, PH, PL, PT, QA, RO, RU, SA, SC, SD, SE, SG, SI, SK, SL, SN, SV, SY, TN, TR, TW, TZ, UG, UY, VE, VN, YE, ZA, ZM, ZW) *see* Lamivudine and Zidovudine 1160
Combiwave SF (PH) *see* Fluticasone and Salmeterol 912
Combodart (BE, BR, DK, EE, FR, GB, IE, LT, NL, PT, SI) *see* Dutasteride and Tamsulosin 702
Comboglyze (TR) *see* Saxagliptin and Metformin 1869
Combutol (IN) *see* Ethambutol 798
Comcerta (VE) *see* Methylphenidate 1336
Comdipin (ID) *see* AmLODIPine 123
Comenazol (VN) *see* Pantoprazole 1570
Comenter (EC) *see* Selegiline 1873
Comfora (IN) *see* Pentosan Polysulfate Sodium 1617
Cominar (AR) *see* Diacerein [INT] 613
Comizial (IT) *see* PHENobarbital 1632
Comoprin (TH) *see* Aspirin 180
Compaz (BR) *see* Diazepam 613
Competact (AT, CH, CZ, DE, EE, FR, GB, HN, HR, HU, IE, IT, LT, MT, NL, NO, PL, PT, RO, RU, SE, SK, TR) *see* Pioglitazone and Metformin 1655
Complamin (EC) *see* Cyproheptadine 529
Compleciclin (ES) *see* Demeclocycline 589
Comploment Continus (AE, BH, CH, CY, EG, IE, IL, IQ, IR, JO, KW, LB, LY, OM, QA, SA, SY, YE) *see* Pyridoxine 1747
Compretten (DE) *see* Codeine 497
Comtade (CO) *see* Entacapone 730
Comtan (AE, AR, AT, AU, BE, BG, BH, BR, CH, CL, CN, CY, CZ, DE, DK, EC, EE, EG, ES, FI, FR, GB, GR, HK, HN, HR, HU, ID, IE, IL, IT, JO, JP, KR, KW, LT, MT, MX, MY, NL, NO, NZ, PE, PH, PL, PT, QA, RO, RU, SA, SE, SK, TH, TR, TW, UY, VE) *see* Entacapone 730
Comtess (AT, BE, BG, CH, CZ, DE, DK, EE, ES, FR, GB, GR, HN, IE, IS, IT, LT, MT, NL, NO, PL, PT, RU, SE, SK, TR) *see* Entacapone 730
Comvax (MX) *see* Haemophilus b Conjugate and Hepatitis B Vaccine 991
Comycin (TW) *see* Kanamycin 1142
Conacid (AR) *see* Folic Acid 919
Conamic (TH) *see* Mefenamic Acid 1280
Conazole (JO) *see* Itraconazole 1130
Concatag (AR) *see* Neomycin 1436
Concerta XL (GB) *see* Methylphenidate 1336
Concerta (AE, AR, AT, AU, BB, BE, BG, BH, BM, BR, BS, BZ, CH, CL, CN, CO, CR, CY, DE, DK, DO, EC, EE, ES, FI, GR, GT, GY, HK, HR, ID, IL, IS, JM, JP, KW, LB, LT, MX, MY, NI, NL, NO, NZ, PA, PE, PH, PL, PR, PT, QA, RO, SA, SE, SG, SI, SK, SR, SV, TH, TR, TT, TW, UY, VN) *see* Methylphenidate 1336
Concerta LP (FR) *see* Methylphenidate 1336
Concerta Oros (KR) *see* Methylphenidate 1336

Concilium (AR) *see* Benperidol [INT] ... 244
Concor 5 Plus (AE, SA) *see* Bisoprolol and Hydrochlorothiazide ... 267
Concor (AE, AR, AT, BB, BG, BH, BR, BS, CH, CL, CN, CO, CR, CY, CZ, DE, EC, EE, EG, GT, HK, HN, HR, HU, ID, IN, IT, JM, JO, KR, KW, LB, LU, MX, MY, NI, NL, PA, PE, PK, PL, PT, QA, RO, RU, SA, SI, SK, SV, TH, TR, TT, TW, VE, VN, ZA) *see* Bisoprolol ... 266
Concor COR (DE, HR, VN) *see* Bisoprolol ... 266
Concorda (NZ) *see* Donepezil ... 668
Concordin (DK, GB, IE) *see* Protriptyline ... 1740
Concore (PH) *see* Bisoprolol ... 266
Concor Plus (AT, CH, HN, PT) *see* Bisoprolol and Hydrochlorothiazide ... 267
Condencia (KR) *see* ClomiPRAMINE ... 475
Condep (MY) *see* MedroxyPROGESTERone ... 1277
Condition (JP) *see* Diazepam ... 613
Condiver (CO) *see* Podophyllum Resin ... 1672
Conductasa (ES) *see* Pyridoxine ... 1747
Conexine (EC) *see* Sertraline ... 1878
Conferon (HU) *see* Ferrous Sulfate ... 871
Confidex (BE, FR) *see* Prothrombin Complex Concentrate (Human) [(Factors II, VII, IX, X), Protein C, and Protein S] ... 1738
Confidol (DE) *see* Etilefrine [INT] ... 815
Confortid (AE, BH, CY, DK, EG, FI, IQ, IR, IS, JO, KW, LB, LY, NO, OM, QA, SA, SE, SY, YE) *see* Indomethacin ... 1067
Confumin (TW) *see* Halcinonide ... 992
Congen (PH) *see* Crotamiton ... 514
Conicine (TW) *see* Colchicine ... 500
Conlax-10 (HK) *see* Bisacodyl ... 265
Conmel (CO, VE) *see* Dipyrone [INT] ... 653
Conmycin (ID) *see* Tetracycline ... 2017
Conmy (MY, PH, TW) *see* Terazosin ... 2001
Co-Normoten (PH) *see* Losartan and Hydrochlorothiazide ... 1250
Conpac (TW) *see* Dalteparin ... 553
Conpanzole (MY) *see* Pantoprazole ... 1570
Conpin (DE) *see* Isosorbide Mononitrate ... 1126
Conquer (TW) *see* Mebendazole [CAN/INT] ... 1274
Consac (PH) *see* Tobramycin (Ophthalmic) ... 2056
Consec (IN) *see* Ranitidine ... 1777
Conserve (PK) *see* AMILoride ... 113
Constan (JP) *see* ALPRAZolam ... 94
Constantia (ID) *see* Nystatin (Oral) ... 1481
Constella (CH, CZ, DE, DK, EE, ES, GB, HR, IS, LT, NL, NO, SE, SK) *see* Linaclotide ... 1215
Constipen (ID) *see* Lactulose ... 1156
Consudine (TH) *see* Triprolidine and Pseudoephedrine ... 2105
Consupren (AE, BH, CY, EG, IQ, IR, JO, KW, LB, LY, OM, QA, SA, SY, YE) *see* CycloSPORINE (Systemic) ... 522
Contalax (FR, LB) *see* Bisacodyl ... 265
Contalgin (DK, IS) *see* Morphine (Systemic) ... 1394
Contemnol (CZ) *see* Lithium ... 1230
Contem (PY) *see* Loperamide ... 1236
Contimit (DE) *see* Terbutaline ... 2004
Contracid (PH) *see* Ranitidine ... 1777
Contracne (FR) *see* ISOtretinoin ... 1127
Contramal (BE, FR, HU, IN, IT, TR) *see* TraMADol ... 2074
Contramal LP (FR) *see* TraMADol ... 2074
Contramareo (ES) *see* DimenhyDRINATE ... 637
Contrapect (DE) *see* Codeine ... 497
Contrasmina (IT) *see* Clenbuterol [INT] ... 460
Contraspasmin (CZ, DE) *see* Clenbuterol [INT] ... 460
Contrathion (AR, BR, FR, GR, IT, TR) *see* Pralidoxime ... 1694
Control (IT) *see* LORazepam ... 1243
Controloc (BG, CZ, EE, EG, HR, HU, IL, IR, JO, LT, MY, PK, PL, RO, RU, SE, SG, SI, SK, TH, ZA) *see* Pantoprazole ... 1570
Contrycal (EE) *see* Aprotinin ... 168
Contrykal (DE) *see* Aprotinin ... 168
Contugesic (ES) *see* Dihydrocodeine, Aspirin, and Caffeine ... 632
Converium (TR) *see* Irbesartan ... 1110
Convertal D (UY) *see* Losartan and Hydrochlorothiazide ... 1250
Convertal (PE) *see* NiCARdipine ... 1446
Convertal (PY, UY) *see* Losartan ... 1248
Converten (IN) *see* Enalapril ... 722
Convertin (IL) *see* Enalapril ... 722
Convolsil (TH) *see* ClonazePAM ... 478
Convulax (AE, KW) *see* CarBAMazepine ... 346
Convulex (AT, BE, BG, CH, CZ, DE, EE, GB, HN, HU, IE, LU, PL, RU, SG, TR, TW) *see* Valproic Acid and Derivatives ... 2123
Conyx (KR) *see* Zolpidem ... 2212
Coochil (TW) *see* Dicyclomine ... 622
CoOLMETEC (FR) *see* Olmesartan and Hydrochlorothiazide ... 1498
Copalex (HK) *see* Clopidogrel ... 484
Copalia (EE, HR, PT, SE) *see* Amlodipine and Valsartan ... 126
Copamide (IN) *see* ChlorproPAMIDE ... 429
Copan (KR) *see* Clenbuterol [INT] ... 460
Copan (MY) *see* Scopolamine (Systemic) ... 1870
Copaxone (AR, AT, AU, BE, BG, BR, CH, CO, CY, CZ, DE, DK, EE, ES, FI, FR, GB, GR, HN, HR, HU, IE, IL, IS, IT, KR, LT, NL, NO, NZ, PE, PL, PY, RO, RU, SE, SI, SK, TR, TW, UY) *see* Glatiramer Acetate ... 963
Copegrel (VN) *see* Clopidogrel ... 484
Copegus (AE, AR, AT, AU, BE, BG, BH, CH, CO, CY, CZ, DE, DK, EC, EE, FI, FR, GB, GR, HK, IE, IL, IS, IT, JO, JP, KW, LB, LT, MX, NL, NO, PL, PT, QA, SA, SE, SI, SK, TH, UY) *see* Ribavirin ... 1797
Co-Prenessa (RO) *see* Perindopril and Indapamide [CAN/INT] ... 1626
Coquan (CO) *see* ClonazePAM ... 478
Coracten (AE, BH, CY, DE, EG, GB, IQ, IR, JO, KW, LB, LY, OM, QA, SA, SY, YE) *see* NIFEdipine ... 1451
Coralan (AU, HK, ID, IL, IN, MY, PH, SG, TH) *see* Ivabradine [INT] ... 1134
Coral (IT) *see* NIFEdipine ... 1451
Co-ramipril (BE) *see* Ramipril and Hydrochlorothiazide [CAN/INT] ... 1773
Corangin (CH, NZ) *see* Isosorbide Mononitrate ... 1126
Corangin SR (TW) *see* Isosorbide Mononitrate ... 1126
Coras (AU) *see* Diltiazem ... 634
Co-Rasilez (RU, TW) *see* Aliskiren and Hydrochlorothiazide ... 87
Corasol (CL) *see* Nisoldipine ... 1459
Corathiem (HN, JP) *see* Cinnarizine [INT] ... 440
Coraxan (RU) *see* Ivabradine [INT] ... 1134
Corbeta (IN) *see* Propranolol ... 1731
Corbionax (FR) *see* Amiodarone ... 114
Corbis (AR) *see* Bisoprolol ... 266
Corcanfol (AR) *see* Etilefrine [INT] ... 815
Cordaflex (BG, HU, VN) *see* NIFEdipine ... 1451
Cordarene (BR) *see* AmLODIPine ... 123
Cordarex (DE) *see* Amiodarone ... 114
Cordarone X (AU, GB, IE, IN, NZ, ZA) *see* Amiodarone ... 114
Cordarone (AE, BB, BE, BF, BG, BH, BJ, BM, BS, BZ, CH, CI, CN, CO, CR, CY, CZ, DO, EC, EE, EG, ET, FI, FR, GH, GM, GN, GT, GY, HK, HN, HR, HU, ID, IQ, IR, IS, IT, JM, JO, KE, KR, KW, LB, LR, LY, MA, ML, MR, MU, MW, MY, NE, NG, NI, NL, NO, OM, PA, PE, PH, PK, PL, PR, PT, PY, QA, RO, RU, SA, SC, SD, SE, SG, SI, SK, SL, SN, SR, SV, SY, TH, TN, TR, TT, TW, TZ, UG, VN, YE, ZM, ZW) *see* Amiodarone ... 114
Cordes VAS (DE) *see* Tretinoin (Topical) ... 2099
Cordiax (IT) *see* Celiprolol [INT] ... 404
Cordila SR (ID) *see* Diltiazem ... 634

Cordilat (MX) *see* NIFEdipine ... 1451
Cordilat (BR) *see* Verapamil ... 2154
Cordilox SR (AU) *see* Verapamil ... 2154
Cordipen Retard (SG) *see* NIFEdipine ... 1451
Cordipen (SG) *see* NIFEdipine ... 1451
Cordipin XL (HR) *see* NIFEdipine ... 1451
Cordipin (HK, HR) *see* NIFEdipine ... 1451
Cordipin Retard (HR) *see* NIFEdipine ... 1451
Cordizem (MY) *see* Diltiazem ... 634
Cordodopa Forte (PT) *see* DOPamine ... 669
Cordralan (PE) *see* Diclofenac (Systemic) ... 617
Cordure (CO) *see* Memantine ... 1286
Coreg (BB, BM, BR, BS, BZ, GY, JM, SR, TT) *see* Carvedilol ... 367
Co-Renitec (AE, AT, BE, BF, BG, BH, BJ, BR, CI, CY, CZ, EG, ET, FR, GH, GM, GN, GR, HK, IQ, IR, JO, KE, KW, LB, LR, LY, MA, ML, MR, MU, MW, MX, NE, NG, NZ, OM, PE, PH, PK, QA, RU, SA, SC, SD, SG, SL, SN, SY, TN, TZ, UG, VE, YE, ZA, ZM, ZW) *see* Enalapril and Hydrochlorothiazide ... 725
Corenitec (AR, NL) *see* Enalapril and Hydrochlorothiazide ... 725
Co-Reniten (CH) *see* Enalapril and Hydrochlorothiazide ... 725
Corentel D (PY, UY) *see* Bisoprolol and Hydrochlorothiazide ... 267
Corentel (PE, PY, UY) *see* Bisoprolol ... 266
Corflo (IN) *see* Nicorandil [INT] ... 1449
Corgard (AR, BB, BE, BM, BR, BS, BZ, CH, CO, CZ, EG, ES, FR, GB, GY, IE, IT, JM, JO, KE, KW, LU, MX, MY, NG, NL, PE, PH, PK, PL, QA, RU, SR, TR, TT, TW, TZ, UG, UY, VE, ZA, ZM) *see* Nadolol ... 1411
Coric (DE) *see* Lisinopril ... 1226
Coric Plus (DE) *see* Lisinopril and Hydrochlorothiazide ... 1229
Corifam (ID) *see* Rifampin ... 1804
Corifeo (DE) *see* Lercanidipine [INT] ... 1181
Coriminic (IN) *see* Chlorpheniramine and Pseudoephedrine ... 427
Corinfar (HU) *see* NIFEdipine ... 1451
Coriodal (CL) *see* Propranolol ... 1731
Corion (IN) *see* Chorionic Gonadotropin (Human) ... 431
Coripen (UY) *see* Hydrocortisone (Systemic) ... 1013
Coritensil (AR) *see* Carvedilol ... 367
Coritrope (ID) *see* Milrinone ... 1370
Corlentor (EE, HR, NL, RO) *see* Ivabradine [INT] ... 1134
Corlopam (CA) *see* Fenoldopam ... 856
Cornalgin (ID) *see* Dipyrone [INT] ... 653
Corneregel (GR, HK, HU, LU, PH, SK, TW) *see* Dexpanthenol ... 606
Cornutamin (CZ) *see* Ergotamine ... 754
Corocyd (ID) *see* Famotidine ... 845
Corodex (UY) *see* Dexamethasone (Systemic) ... 599
Corodil (DK) *see* Enalapril ... 722
Corodin-D (CL, PY) *see* Losartan and Hydrochlorothiazide ... 1250
Coronair (BE) *see* Dipyridamole ... 652
Coronex (NZ) *see* Isosorbide Dinitrate ... 1124
Coronovo (AR) *see* Amiodarone ... 114
Corotenol (AE, BH, CY, EG, IQ, IR, JO, KW, LB, LY, OM, QA, SA, SY, YE) *see* Atenolol ... 189
Corotrend (DE) *see* NIFEdipine ... 1451
Corotrop (AT, CH, CZ, ES, SE) *see* Milrinone ... 1370
Corotrope (AR, BE, CL, CO, ES, FR, GR, HN, LU, NL, PE, PL, SI, SK, UY, VE) *see* Milrinone ... 1370
Corpotasin CL (MX) *see* Potassium Bicarbonate and Potassium Chloride ... 1687
Corpotasin (MX) *see* Potassium Chloride ... 1687
Corpril (TH) *see* Ramipril ... 1771
Corsodyl (AE, BE, BH, DE, HK, IE, IL, IS, IT, KW, NL, NO, PL, PT, QA, SA, SE, SI, SK, ZA) *see* Chlorhexidine Gluconate ... 422
Corsodyl Mint (BG, CZ, EE, LT) *see* Chlorhexidine Gluconate ... 422
Corstat (HK) *see* Simvastatin ... 1890
Cortaid Cream (AU) *see* Hydrocortisone (Topical) ... 1014
Cortal (PH) *see* Aspirin ... 180
Cortal (SE) *see* Cortisone ... 510
Cortancyl (FR, LB) *see* PredniSONE ... 1706
Cortate (AU, HK, MY) *see* Cortisone ... 510
Cort Dome (CO, EC) *see* Hydrocortisone (Topical) ... 1014
Cortef (HR) *see* Hydrocortisone (Systemic) ... 1013
Corteroid (AR) *see* Betamethasone (Systemic) ... 253
Cortic-DS (AU) *see* Hydrocortisone (Topical) ... 1014
Cortiderm (BH, KW, QA, SA) *see* Hydrocortisone (Topical) ... 1014
Cortiderm (IN) *see* Betamethasone (Topical) ... 255
Cortiflam-D (IN) *see* Dexchlorpheniramine ... 603
Cortiflex (PE) *see* Triamcinolone (Systemic) ... 2099
Cortiflex (PE) *see* Triamcinolone (Topical) ... 2100
Cortifoam (IL) *see* Hydrocortisone (Systemic) ... 1013
Cortilate (IN) *see* Halcinonide ... 992
Cortineff (BG, PL, RU) *see* Fludrocortisone ... 891
Cortin (PH) *see* Hydrocortisone (Systemic) ... 1013
Cortioftal (ES) *see* Cortisone ... 510
Cortiol (PT) *see* PredniSONE ... 1706
Cortiprex (CL, PE, PY) *see* PredniSONE ... 1706
Cortis-100 (PH) *see* Hydrocortisone (Systemic) ... 1013
Cortisate (DK) *see* Cortisone ... 510
Cortisol L.C.H. (CL) *see* Hydrocortisone (Systemic) ... 1013
Cortison Augensalbe Dr. Winzer (DE) *see* Cortisone ... 510
Cortison Ciba (CH, DE) *see* Cortisone ... 510
Cortisone Acetate (CY, IL) *see* Cortisone ... 510
Cortisone (FR, NZ, PL) *see* Cortisone ... 510
Cortison (NL) *see* Cortisone ... 510
Cortison Nycomed (NO) *see* Cortisone ... 510
Cortisporin Cream (BB, BM, BS, BZ, GY, JM, NL, PK, SR, TT) *see* Neomycin, Polymyxin B, and Hydrocortisone ... 1438
Cortisporin Ear (BB, BM, BS, BZ, GY, JM, NL, PH, SR, TT) *see* Neomycin, Polymyxin B, and Hydrocortisone ... 1438
Cortisporin Ophthalmic Suspension (BB, BM, BS, BZ, GY, JM, NL, SR, TT) *see* Neomycin, Polymyxin B, and Hydrocortisone ... 1438
Cortisporin Otico (MX) *see* Polymyxin B ... 1676
Cortistab (GB) *see* Cortisone ... 510
Cortisyl (GB, IE) *see* Cortisone ... 510
Cortival (AU) *see* Betamethasone (Topical) ... 255
Cortixyl Depot (PE) *see* Betamethasone (Systemic) ... 253
Cortoderm (ZA) *see* Fluocinolone (Topical) ... 893
Cortone-Azetat (AT) *see* Cortisone ... 510
Cortone (IT) *see* Cortisone ... 510
Cortope (JO) *see* PrednisoLONE (Systemic) ... 1703
Cortrosinta Depot (PT) *see* Cosyntropin ... 510
Cortrosyn (BE, HU) *see* Cosyntropin ... 510
Cortrosyn Depot (AE, BE, BF, BG, BH, BJ, CI, CY, CZ, EG, ET, FR, GH, GM, GN, HK, HN, HU, IQ, IR, IT, JO, KE, KW, LB, LR, LY, MA, ML, MR, MU, MW, NE, NG, NL, OM, QA, SA, SC, SD, SL, SN, SY, TH, TN, TW, TZ, UG, YE, ZA, ZM, ZW) *see* Cosyntropin ... 510
Cort-S (IN) *see* Hydrocortisone (Systemic) ... 1013
Cortum (PH) *see* Cefuroxime ... 399
Cortyk (CL) *see* Dexamethasone (Systemic) ... 599
Corubin (EC) *see* Carvedilol ... 367
Corus-H (BR) *see* Losartan and Hydrochlorothiazide ... 1250
Corvert (AT, CH, FI, FR, GR, IT, NL, NO, SE) *see* Ibutilide ... 1036
Corvo (CR, PA) *see* Enalapril ... 722
Corvox (ID) *see* Levofloxacin (Systemic) ... 1197
Corycardon (TR) *see* Irbesartan and Hydrochlorothiazide ... 1112
Coryol (CO, CR, GT, NI, PA, RO, SV) *see* Carvedilol ... 367

Corzem (JO) *see* Diltiazem ... 634
Corzepin (ES) *see* Perhexiline [INT] ... 1621
Cosaar (AT, CH) *see* Losartan ... 1248
Cosaar Plus (AT, CH) *see* Losartan and Hydrochlorothiazide ... 1250
Cosac (HK) *see* Pseudoephedrine ... 1742
Cosadin (PH) *see* Bisacodyl ... 265
Cosal (KR) *see* Losartan ... 1248
Cosamide (AU) *see* Bicalutamide ... 262
Cosca (KR) *see* Losartan ... 1248
Cosca Plus-F (KR) *see* Losartan and Hydrochlorothiazide ... 1250
Cosca Plus (KR) *see* Losartan and Hydrochlorothiazide ... 1250
Cosflox (IN) *see* Ciprofloxacin (Systemic) ... 441
Cosmegen (AR, AT, AU, BE, BG, BM, BR, CH, DE, EE, EG, ES, FI, FR, GB, GR, HN, IE, IT, KR, MT, NL, NO, NZ, PH, PK, PT, PY, RU, SE, SI, SK, TR, TW) *see* DACTINomycin ... 551
Cosmegen, Lyovac (GB, HK) *see* DACTINomycin ... 551
Cosmin (PK) *see* ISOtretinoin ... 1127
Cosmofer (AE, AT, CN, DE, DK, FI, GB, GR, ID, IE, JO, KR, LT, NL, NO, PH, PT, SA, SE, TH, VE) *see* Iron Dextran Complex ... 1117
Cosopt (AE, AR, AT, AU, BB, BE, BH, BM, BR, BS, BZ, CH, CL, CO, CY, CZ, DE, DK, EC, ES, FI, FR, GR, GY, HK, HR, HU, IL, IS, IT, JM, JO, JP, KR, KW, LB, LT, MX, MY, NL, NZ, PE, PH, PK, PL, PR, PT, QA, RO, RU, SA, SE, SG, SI, SR, TH, TR, TT, TW, UY, VE) *see* Dorzolamide and Timolol ... 673
Cost (AR, BR) *see* Ketamine ... 1143
Costil (ID) *see* Domperidone [CAN/INT] ... 666
Costim (TW) *see* Colistimethate ... 504
Costi (TW) *see* Domperidone [CAN/INT] ... 666
Cosudex (AU, NZ) *see* Bicalutamide ... 262
Cosue (KR) *see* Pseudoephedrine ... 1742
Cotareg (FR, IT, KR, TW) *see* Valsartan and Hydrochlorothiazide ... 2129
Co-Tareg (PH) *see* Valsartan and Hydrochlorothiazide ... 2129
Co-Tazo (TW) *see* Piperacillin and Tazobactam ... 1657
Cotazym-S (AU) *see* Pancrelipase ... 1566
Cotazym-S Forte (AU) *see* Pancrelipase ... 1566
Cotemp (TH) *see* Acetaminophen ... 32
Co Teveten (FR) *see* Eprosartan and Hydrochlorothiazide ... 750
Cotol (TW) *see* Clopidogrel ... 484
Cotran (TW) *see* Albuterol ... 69
Cotren (TH) *see* Clotrimazole (Topical) ... 488
Cotriatec (FR) *see* Ramipril and Hydrochlorothiazide [CAN/INT] ... 1773
Cotrim (BF, BJ, CI, ET, GH, GM, GN, KE, KR, LR, MA, ML, MR, MU, MW, MY, NE, NG, SC, SD, SL, SN, TN, TZ, UG, ZM, ZW) *see* Sulfamethoxazole and Trimethoprim ... 1946
Cotrim DS (MY) *see* Sulfamethoxazole and Trimethoprim ... 1946
Cotrimel (HK) *see* Sulfamethoxazole and Trimethoprim ... 1946
Co-Tritace (AE, KW, QA) *see* Ramipril and Hydrochlorothiazide [CAN/INT] ... 1773
Cotrix (AE, BH, CY, EG, IQ, IR, JO, KW, LB, LY, OM, QA, SA, SY, YE) *see* Sulfamethoxazole and Trimethoprim ... 1946
Cotrizol (TW) *see* Sulfamethoxazole and Trimethoprim ... 1946
Coumadan (AR) *see* Warfarin ... 2186
Coumadin (AE, AU, BF, BH, BJ, CI, CL, CY, DE, EC, EG, ET, GH, GM, GN, IL, IQ, IR, IT, JO, KE, KR, KW, LB, LR, LY, MA, ML, MR, MU, MW, MX, NE, NG, NZ, OM, PH, PK, QA, SA, SC, SD, SL, SN, SY, TN, TR, TZ, UG, VE, YE, ZM, ZW) *see* Warfarin ... 2186
Coumadine (FR, VN) *see* Warfarin ... 2186
Covan (CA) *see* Triprolidine, Pseudoephedrine, and Codeine [CAN/INT] ... 2105
Covapril (MY) *see* Perindopril ... 1623
Covaratan (KR) *see* Valsartan and Hydrochlorothiazide ... 2129
Covasc (MY) *see* AmLODIPine ... 123
Covastin (HK, MY, SG) *see* Simvastatin ... 1890
Covelay (PH) *see* Acyclovir (Systemic) ... 47
Covelay (PH) *see* Acyclovir (Topical) ... 51
Coverene (AR) *see* Perindopril ... 1623
Coverex (BG, CZ, HN, HU, PL, SE) *see* Perindopril ... 1623
Covergim (VN) *see* Perindopril ... 1623
Coversum (AT, CH, DE) *see* Perindopril ... 1623
Coversum Combi (DE) *see* Perindopril and Indapamide [CAN/INT] ... 1626
Coversyl (AE, BB, BE, BH, BM, BR, BS, BZ, CL, CO, CR, CY, DK, DO, EG, ES, FI, FR, GB, GR, GT, GY, IE, IN, IS, IT, JM, JO, JP, KW, LB, LU, MT, MX, MY, NI, NL, NZ, PA, PE, PH, PK, PR, PT, PY, QA, SA, SG, SI, SR, SV, TH, TR, TT, UY, VE, VN, ZA) *see* Perindopril ... 1623
Coversyl Comp (DK, FI, SE) *see* Perindopril and Indapamide [CAN/INT] ... 1626
Coversyl Plus (AU, BE, BR, GB, IN, MY, PH, SG, TH, UY, VN) *see* Perindopril and Indapamide [CAN/INT] ... 1626
Coversyl Plus LD (AU) *see* Perindopril and Indapamide [CAN/INT] ... 1626
Covinace (MY) *see* Perindopril ... 1623
Covina (TW) *see* Estradiol and Norethindrone ... 781
Covina (TW) *see* Ethinyl Estradiol and Norethindrone ... 808
Covir Cream (TH) *see* Acyclovir (Topical) ... 51
Co Vitam B12 (ES) *see* Cyanocobalamin ... 515
Covospor (ZA) *see* Clotrimazole (Topical) ... 488
Covrix (TH) *see* Perindopril ... 1623
Cox-2 (PH) *see* Celecoxib ... 402
Coxco (TW) *see* Losartan ... 1248
Coxicam (EC) *see* Meloxicam ... 1283
Cox (IN) *see* Etoricoxib [INT] ... 821
Coxine SR (TW) *see* Isosorbide Mononitrate ... 1126
Coxine (TW) *see* Isosorbide Mononitrate ... 1126
Coxoral (PH) *see* Celecoxib ... 402
Coxtral (PL, RU) *see* Nimesulide [INT] ... 1456
Coxylate (IN) *see* Doxofylline [INT] ... 679
Coxzan (PH) *see* Celecoxib ... 402
Coyarin (ID) *see* Amoxicillin and Clavulanate ... 133
Cozaar (AE, AU, BB, BE, BH, BM, BR, BS, BZ, CL, CN, CR, CY, CZ, DK, EC, EE, EG, ES, FI, FR, GB, GR, GT, GY, HK, HN, HR, HU, ID, IE, IS, JM, JO, KR, KW, LB, LT, LU, MT, MX, MY, NI, NL, NO, NZ, PA, PE, PH, PK, PL, PT, QA, RO, RU, SA, SE, SG, SI, SK, SR, SV, TH, TR, TT, TW, VE, VN) *see* Losartan ... 1248
Cozaar-Comp (FI, GB, IE, NO) *see* Losartan and Hydrochlorothiazide ... 1250
Cozaar Comp (IS) *see* Losartan and Hydrochlorothiazide ... 1250
Cozaarex D (AR) *see* Losartan and Hydrochlorothiazide ... 1250
Cozaarex (AR) *see* Losartan ... 1248
Cozaar Plus (DK, ES, KR, PT) *see* Losartan and Hydrochlorothiazide ... 1250
Cozavan (AU) *see* Losartan ... 1248
Cozep (TH) *see* ChlordiazePOXIDE ... 422
CPG (ID) *see* Clopidogrel ... 484
C-Phenicol (PH) *see* Chloramphenicol ... 421
CPLoradine (HK) *see* Loratadine ... 1241
CP-Lovac (HK) *see* AmLODIPine ... 123
CP-Pyridine (HK) *see* Phenazopyridine ... 1629
Crabcan (KR) *see* Irinotecan ... 1112
Cramon Duo (KR) *see* Amoxicillin and Clavulanate ... 133
Cramotin (KR) *see* Amoxicillin and Clavulanate ... 133

Cranoc (DE) *see* Fluvastatin 915
Crasigen Duo (KR) *see* Amoxicillin and Clavulanate 133
Crasnitin (AT, CH, HN, PT) *see* Asparaginase (E. coli) 179
Cravit (CN, HK, ID, JP, MY, PK, SG, TH, TW, VN) *see* Levofloxacin (Systemic) 1197
Cravit (CN, JP, KR, SG, TH, TW, VN) *see* Levofloxacin (Ophthalmic) 1200
Cravit Ophthalmic (HK, ID, MY) *see* Levofloxacin (Ophthalmic) 1200
Cravox (ID) *see* Levofloxacin (Systemic) 1197
Creliverol-12 (PE) *see* Cyanocobalamin 515
Crema Blanca Bustillos (MX) *see* Hydroquinone 1020
Cremirit (CL) *see* Betamethasone (Topical) 255
Cremoquinona (CO, EC) *see* Hydroquinone 1020
Crenble (KR) *see* Clenbuterol [INT] 460
Creobic (VN) *see* Tolnaftate 2063
Cresart (PH) *see* Olmesartan 1496
Crestor (AE, AR, AT, AU, BB, BE, BF, BG, BH, BJ, BM, BR, BS, BZ, CH, CI, CL, CN, CO, CR, CY, CZ, DK, DO, EC, EE, ET, FI, FR, GB, GH, GM, GN, GR, GT, GY, HK, HN, HR, ID, IE, IL, IS, IT, JM, JP, KE, KR, KW, LB, LR, LT, MA, ML, MR, MU, MW, MX, NE, NG, NI, NL, NO, NZ, PA, PE, PH, PR, PT, PY, QA, RO, RU, SA, SC, SD, SE, SG, SI, SK, SL, SN, SR, SV, TH, TN, TR, TT, TW, TZ, UG, UY, VE, VN, ZA, ZM, ZW) *see* Rosuvastatin 1848
CRH (AT, DE, NL) *see* Corticorelin 509
CRH-Ferring (KR) *see* Corticorelin 509
Crinone (AR, AU, BE, BH, CH, CN, CY, DE, DK, ES, FI, GB, GR, HK, HR, ID, IE, IL, IT, KR, KW, LB, MY, NO, NZ, PH, RU, SE, SG, TR, TW, UY, VE, VN) *see* Progesterone 1722
Cripsa (ID) *see* Bromocriptine 291
Crisafeno (PY) *see* Tamoxifen 1971
Crisapla (UY) *see* Oxaliplatin 1528
Crismel (HU) *see* Omeprazole 1508
Crispin (JP) *see* TraMADol 2074
Cristalmina Film Gel (ES) *see* Chlorhexidine Gluconate 422
Cristalomicina (AR) *see* Kanamycin 1142
Cristovin (IL) *see* VinCRIStine 2163
Criten (CL) *see* Bromocriptine 291
Crixan OD (PH) *see* Clarithromycin 456
Crixivan (AE, AT, AU, BB, BE, BG, BH, BM, BO, BS, BZ, CH, CN, CR, CY, CZ, DE, DK, DO, EC, EE, ES, FI, FR, GB, GR, GT, HK, HN, HR, HU, IE, IL, IS, IT, JM, KR, LB, LT, LU, MT, MX, MY, NI, NL, NO, NZ, PA, PE, PH, PL, PR, PT, QA, RO, RU, SE, SG, SI, SK, SV, TR, TT, TW, UY, VE, VN) *see* Indinavir 1066
Crobate (KR) *see* Clobetasol 468
Crocan (KR) *see* Chloroquine 424
Croix Blanche (LU) *see* Acetaminophen 32
Cromabak (BE, IT, PH, PT) *see* Cromolyn (Ophthalmic) 514
Cromadoses (FR) *see* Cromolyn (Ophthalmic) 514
Cromal AQ (IN, MY) *see* Cromolyn (Nasal) 514
Cromal (TH, VN) *see* Cromolyn (Ophthalmic) 514
Croma (QA) *see* Cromolyn (Ophthalmic) 514
Cromatonbic B12 (ES) *see* Cyanocobalamin 515
Cromatonferro (IT) *see* Ferrous Gluconate 870
Cromisol (VE) *see* Cromolyn (Ophthalmic) 514
Cromoftal (VE) *see* Cromolyn (Ophthalmic) 514
Cromohexal (CZ, HN, PL, TW, ZA) *see* Cromolyn (Nasal) 514
Cromohexal (CZ, PL, TR, ZA) *see* Cromolyn (Ophthalmic) 514
Cromolerg (BR) *see* Cromolyn (Ophthalmic) 514
Cromolux (AU, NZ) *see* Cromolyn (Ophthalmic) 514
Cromonal (QA) *see* Cromolyn (Nasal) 514
Crom-Ophtal (ID) *see* Cromolyn (Ophthalmic) 514
Cromoptic (FR, IL) *see* Cromolyn (Ophthalmic) 514
Cromorhinol (FR) *see* Cromolyn (Nasal) 514
Cromorom (BG) *see* Cromolyn (Ophthalmic) 514
Cromus (CO, DO, HN, PA) *see* Tacrolimus (Topical) 1968
Cronase (ID) *see* Loratadine and Pseudoephedrine 1242
Cronase (IL) *see* Cromolyn (Nasal) 514
Cronitin (ID) *see* Loratadine 1241
Cronizat (IT) *see* Nizatidine 1471
Cronocef (IT) *see* Cefprozil 389
Cronogeron (BR) *see* Cinnarizine [INT] 440
Cronopen (AR) *see* Azithromycin (Systemic) 216
Cronovera (MX) *see* Verapamil 2154
Crotamitex (DE) *see* Crotamiton 514
Crotamiton (PL) *see* Crotamiton 514
Crotanol (VE) *see* Crotamiton 514
Crotan (PK) *see* Crotamiton 514
Crotorax (IN) *see* Crotamiton 514
Croydoxin-FM (IN) *see* Sulfadoxine and Pyrimethamine [INT] 1946
Cryofaxol (MX) *see* Cyclophosphamide 517
Cryosid (MX) *see* Etoposide 816
Cryosolona (MX) *see* MethylPREDNISolone 1340
Cryostatin (MX) *see* Octreotide 1485
Cryoxet (MX) *see* PACLitaxel (Conventional) 1550
Cryptal (ID) *see* Fluconazole 885
Cryptocur (GR, NL) *see* Gonadorelin [CAN/INT] 980
Crysanal (AU) *see* Naproxen 1427
Crytion (UY) *see* Auranofin 204
C-Tri T (TH) *see* Cefuroxime 399
Cuantil (AR, PY) *see* Ifosfamide 1040
Cubicin (AR, AT, AU, BE, BG, BR, CH, CL, CN, CO, CY, CZ, DE, DK, EE, ES, FI, FR, GB, GR, HK, HN, HR, IE, IL, IN, IS, IT, JP, KR, KW, LT, MT, MY, NL, NO, NZ, PH, PL, PT, QA, RO, RU, SE, SG, SI, SK, TH, TR, TW, VN) *see* DAPTOmycin 563
Cubraxis (MX) *see* Montelukast 1392
Cumatil (CO) *see* Phenytoin 1640
Cupid (VN) *see* Sildenafil 1882
Cuprenil (BG, HN, PL) *see* PenicillAMINE 1608
Cuprimine (MY, NL, NO, TH, TW) *see* PenicillAMINE 1608
Cuprimune (AR, BR) *see* PenicillAMINE 1608
Cupripen (AR, ES) *see* PenicillAMINE 1608
Cuprofen (TH) *see* Ibuprofen 1032
Curacil (ID) *see* Fluorouracil (Systemic) 896
Curacit (NO) *see* Succinylcholine 1939
Curacne (AE, JO, KW) *see* ISOtretinoin 1127
Curacne Ge (FR) *see* ISOtretinoin 1127
Curacne (KW) *see* Tretinoin (Topical) 2099
Curafen (PH) *see* Diclofenac (Systemic) 617
Curakne (CH) *see* ISOtretinoin 1127
Curalest (NL) *see* Succinylcholine 1939
Curam (AE, AU, BH, CO, HK, JO, KW, LB, MY, PE, SA, SG, TH, TW) *see* Amoxicillin and Clavulanate 133
Curanail (FR) *see* Amorolfine [INT] 128
Curanel (CH) *see* Amorolfine [INT] 128
Curash (AU, NZ, PH) *see* Zinc Oxide 2200
Curatane (IL) *see* ISOtretinoin 1127
Curazid Forte (PH) *see* Isoniazid 1120
Curestat (JO) *see* Flutamide 907
Curionialis (MX) *see* Rocuronium 1838
Curiosin (HU) *see* Hyaluronate and Derivatives 1006
Curisafe (AE, BH, CY, EG, IQ, IR, JO, KW, LB, LY, OM, QA, SA, SY, YE) *see* Cefadroxil 372
Curocef (AT, CL) *see* Cefuroxime 399
Curofen (KR) *see* Baclofen 223
Curon-B (ZA) *see* Pancuronium 1567
Curovix (KR) *see* Clopidogrel 484
Curoxime (PT) *see* Cefuroxime 399
Curpol (LU) *see* Acetaminophen 32
Currun (TH) *see* Triamcinolone (Systemic) 2099
Curyken (MX) *see* Loratadine 1241
Cusate (TH) *see* Docusate 661

Cusicrom (BH, EG, LB, SA) *see* Cromolyn (Nasal) 514
Cusicrom (BH, JO, KW, SA, TW) *see* Cromolyn (Ophthalmic) 514
Cusigel (AE) *see* Fluocinonide 894
Cusimolol (AE, BH, EG, JO, KW, LB, MY, QA, SA) *see* Timolol (Ophthalmic) 2043
Cusiviral (HK, MY, SG) *see* Aciclovir (Ophthalmic) [INT] 43
Cusiviral (MY, SG) *see* Acyclovir (Systemic) 47
Cuspa (IN) *see* Mebeverine [INT] 1275
Custodiol (ID) *see* Bisacodyl 265
Cutacelan (AR, CO, EC, PE, VE) *see* Azelaic Acid 213
Cutaclin (CR, DO, GT, HN, NI, PA, SV) *see* Clindamycin (Topical) 464
Cutason (DE) *see* PredniSONE 1706
Cutinolone (AE) *see* Triamcinolone (Topical) 2100
Cutivat (DK, IS) *see* Fluticasone (Topical) 911
Cutivate (AE, AR, AT, BB, BE, BG, BH, BM, BS, CH, CN, CR, CY, CZ, DO, EC, EE, EG, GB, GT, GY, HK, HN, JM, KR, KW, LB, LT, MY, NL, PA, PE, PH, PK, PL, PR, PT, PY, QA, RO, RU, SA, SG, SI, SV, TR, TT, TW, UY, VE, VN) *see* Fluticasone (Topical) 911
Cuvarlix (MY) *see* Orlistat 1520
Cuxabrain (DE) *see* Piracetam [INT] 1661
C-Vimin (FI, NO, SE) *see* Ascorbic Acid 178
C-Vital (LB, SA) *see* Ascorbic Acid 178
C Vitamin Pharmavit (HU) *see* Ascorbic Acid 178
C-Will (BE, LU, TH) *see* Ascorbic Acid 178
Cyanokit (FR, HR) *see* Hydroxocobalamin 1020
Cyano Kit (JP) *see* Hydroxocobalamin 1020
Cybelle (PH) *see* Cyproterone and Ethinyl Estradiol [CAN/INT] 532
Cybens (KR) *see* Cyclobenzaprine 516
Cybutol (ID) *see* Albuterol 69
Cycin (KR, SG) *see* Ciprofloxacin (Systemic) 441
Cyclabid (ZA) *see* Tetracycline 2017
Cyclidox (ZA) *see* Doxycycline 689
Cyclimycin (ZA) *see* Minocycline 1371
Cyclindox (VN) *see* Doxycycline 689
Cyclivex (ZA) *see* Acyclovir (Systemic) 47
Cycloblastin (AU, NZ) *see* Cyclophosphamide 517
Cycloblastine (LU) *see* Cyclophosphamide 517
Cyclocide (TW) *see* Cytarabine (Conventional) 535
Cycloflex (IL) *see* Cyclobenzaprine 516
Cyclogest (AE, BH, CY, EG, IQ, IR, JO, KW, LB, LY, MY, OM, PK, QA, SA, SG, SY, VN, YE, ZA) *see* Progesterone 1722
Cyclogyl (AE, AU, BE, BF, BG, BH, BJ, CH, CI, CL, CO, CY, DK, EG, ET, GH, GM, GN, GR, IL, IN, IQ, IR, IS, JO, KE, KR, KW, LB, LR, LY, MA, ML, MR, MU, MW, NE, NG, NL, NZ, OM, PK, QA, SA, SC, SD, SE, SG, SL, SN, SY, TH, TN, TR, TW, TZ, UG, UY, VE, YE, ZA, ZM, ZW) *see* Cyclopentolate 517
Cyclogynon (ID) *see* Ethinyl Estradiol and Levonorgestrel 803
Cycloherp (HK) *see* Acyclovir (Systemic) 47
Cycloherp (HK, JO) *see* Acyclovir (Topical) 51
Cyclokapron (IS) *see* Tranexamic Acid 2081
Cyclolady (TW) *see* Danazol 558
Cyclomed (IL) *see* Acyclovir (Topical) 51
Cyclominol (IN) *see* Dicyclomine 622
Cyclomune (IN) *see* CycloSPORINE (Ophthalmic) 529
Cyclomycin-K (GR) *see* Cefadroxil 372
Cyclopent (HU) *see* Cyclopentolate 517
Cyclopentolat (AT, NO) *see* Cyclopentolate 517
Cyclopentolate (CZ) *see* Cyclopentolate 517
Cyclopentolate Eye Drops (PH) *see* Cyclopentolate 517
Cyclopentol (LU) *see* Cyclopentolate 517
Cyclopen (TW) *see* Cyclopentolate 517
Cycloplatin (CZ, HU, PL) *see* CARBOplatin 357
Cyclorine (JO) *see* CycloSPORINE (Systemic) 522
Cyclostad (PH) *see* Acyclovir (Systemic) 47
Cyclostad (PH) *see* Acyclovir (Topical) 51
Cyclostin (DE) *see* Cyclophosphamide 517
Cyclostin N (DE) *see* Cyclophosphamide 517
Cyclothil (AE) *see* Cyclopentolate 517
Cyclovax (HK, TR) *see* Acyclovir (Topical) 51
Cyclovax (TR) *see* Acyclovir (Systemic) 47
Cyclovex (LB) *see* Acyclovir (Systemic) 47
Cyclovir (BF, BJ, CI, ET, GH, GM, GN, KE, LR, MA, ML, MR, MU, MW, NE, NG, SC, SD, SL, SN, TN, TZ, UG, ZM, ZW) *see* Acyclovir (Systemic) 47
Cyclovir (IN) *see* Aciclovir (Ophthalmic) [INT] 43
Cyclovir (IN) *see* Acyclovir (Topical) 51
Cycogyl (CN, HK) *see* Cyclopentolate 517
Cycortide (HK) *see* Budesonide (Systemic) 293
Cycram (VN) *see* Cyclophosphamide 517
Cycrin (AR, NZ) *see* MedroxyPROGESTERone 1277
Cydipin (ID) *see* AmLODIPine 123
Cygest (ID) *see* Progesterone 1722
Cyheptine (TH) *see* Cyproheptadine 529
Cyklokapron (AE, AT, AU, BH, CH, CY, DE, DK, EE, EG, FI, GB, IE, IQ, IR, JO, KW, LB, LY, NL, NO, NZ, OM, QA, SA, SE, SG, SY, YE, ZA) *see* Tranexamic Acid 2081
Cyllanvir (PH) *see* Acyclovir (Systemic) 47
Cylocide (JP) *see* Cytarabine (Conventional) 535
Cymalium (ID) *see* Flunarizine [CAN/INT] 892
Cymbalta (AE, AR, AT, AU, BE, BG, BH, BR, CH, CL, CN, CO, CR, CY, CZ, DE, DK, DO, EC, EE, ES, FI, FR, GB, GT, HK, HN, HR, HU, ID, IE, IL, IT, JP, KR, KW, LB, LT, MT, MX, MY, NI, NL, NO, NZ, PA, PE, PH, PL, QA, RO, RU, SA, SE, SG, SK, TH, TR, TW) *see* DULoxetine 698
Cymevan (FR) *see* Ganciclovir (Systemic) 948
Cymeven (CY) *see* Ganciclovir (Systemic) 948
Cymevene (AE, AR, AT, AU, BE, BF, BG, BH, BJ, BR, CH, CI, CL, CN, CO, CZ, DK, EC, EE, EG, ET, FI, GB, GH, GM, GN, GR, HK, HN, HR, ID, IL, IN, IQ, IR, IS, IT, JO, KE, KR, KW, LB, LR, LT, LY, MA, ML, MR, MT, MU, MW, MY, NE, NG, NL, NO, NZ, OM, PE, PH, PL, PY, QA, RO, SA, SC, SD, SE, SI, SK, SL, SN, SY, TH, TN, TR, TW, TZ, UG, VE, VN, YE, ZM, ZW) *see* Ganciclovir (Systemic) 948
Cynocuatro (MX) *see* Levothyroxine 1205
Cynomel (BF, BJ, CI, ET, FR, GH, GM, GN, KE, LR, MA, ML, MR, MU, MW, MX, NE, NG, PE, SC, SD, SL, SN, TN, TZ, UG, ZA, ZM, ZW) *see* Liothyronine 1221
Cynomycin (IN) *see* Minocycline 1371
Cypestra-35 (CH) *see* Cyproterone and Ethinyl Estradiol [CAN/INT] 532
Cyplegin (JP) *see* Cyclopentolate 517
Cyplox (HK) *see* Ciprofloxacin (Systemic) 441
Cypral (VE) *see* Ciprofloxacin (Systemic) 441
Cypress (MY, TH) *see* Cyproterone and Ethinyl Estradiol [CAN/INT] 532
Cypress (NL) *see* Barnidipine [INT] 227
Cyprodin (TW) *see* Cyproheptadine 529
Cyprogin (HK, TH) *see* Cyproheptadine 529
Cyprohexal (AU) *see* Cyproterone [CAN/INT] 530
Cypro (KR) *see* Ciprofloxacin (Systemic) 441
Cypromin (JP, TW) *see* Cyproheptadine 529
Cypron 50 (IL, MY) *see* Cyproterone [CAN/INT] 530
Cyprone (AU) *see* Cyproterone [CAN/INT] 530
Cyprono (TH) *see* Cyproheptadine 529
Cyproplex (BE, TW) *see* Cyproterone [CAN/INT] 530
Cyprosian (TH) *see* Cyproheptadine 529
Cyprostat (AU, GB) *see* Cyproterone [CAN/INT] 530
Cyprostol (AT) *see* Misoprostol 1379
Cyprotin (SG) *see* Cyproheptadine 529
Cyprotol (BG) *see* Cyproheptadine 529
Cyral (AT) *see* Primidone 1714
Cyrdanex (RO) *see* Dexrazoxane 606
Cyrin (PH) *see* CycloSPORINE (Systemic) 522
Cyrona (TW) *see* Cyproterone [CAN/INT] 530
Cysplack (PH) *see* CISplatin 448
Cystadan (AU, IL) *see* Betaine 252

Cystadane (CZ, DK, EE, IS, JP, KR, LT, SE, SI, SK) *see* Betaine ... 252
Cystagon (AT, AU, BE, BG, CH, CZ, DE, DK, EE, FI, FR, GB, GR, HN, HR, IE, IS, IT, MT, NL, NO, PL, PT, RO, RU, SE, SI, SK, TR, TW) *see* Cysteamine (Systemic) ... 534
Cystaline (TH) *see* Acetylcysteine ... 40
Cystazole (JO) *see* Albendazole ... 65
Cysten (JP) *see* Cinnarizine [INT] ... 440
Cysticide (IN) *see* Praziquantel ... 1702
Cysto-Myacyne N (DE) *see* Neomycin ... 1436
Cysto-Saar (DE) *see* Nitroxoline [INT] ... 1469
Cystosol (SE) *see* Sorbitol ... 1927
Cystrin (GB) *see* Oxybutynin ... 1536
Cytadine (TW) *see* Cyproheptadine ... 529
Cytamen (AU, GB, IE) *see* Cyanocobalamin ... 515
Cytarabin (DE, NO) *see* Cytarabine (Conventional) ... 535
Cytarabine (AU) *see* Cytarabine (Conventional) ... 535
Cytarabine Injection (AU, GB, NZ) *see* Cytarabine (Conventional) ... 535
Cytarabinum-Delta West (LU) *see* Cytarabine (Conventional) ... 535
Cytarine (IN, SG, TH, VN) *see* Cytarabine (Conventional) ... 535
Cytil (CO) *see* Misoprostol ... 1379
Cytine (NZ) *see* Cimetidine ... 438
Cytoblastin (BG, IN, VN) *see* VinBLAStine ... 2160
Cytocarb (LB) *see* CARBOplatin ... 357
Cytocristin (BG, IN, VN) *see* VinCRIStine ... 2163
Cytodrox (JO) *see* Hydroxyurea ... 1021
Cytofine (PE) *see* Misoprostol ... 1379
Cytogem (ID) *see* Gemcitabine ... 952
Cytolog (IN) *see* Misoprostol ... 1379
Cytomel 25 (IL) *see* Liothyronine ... 1221
Cytomel (BE, LU, NL) *see* Liothyronine ... 1221
Cytomid-250 (IN) *see* Flutamide ... 907
Cytonal (RU, TR) *see* Cytarabine (Conventional) ... 535
Cytosar (AE, AT, BE, BG, BH, CH, CY, CZ, EE, EG, FI, GB, GH, HK, HN, HR, HU, IL, IQ, IR, JO, KE, KW, LB, LY, NL, OM, PE, PK, PT, QA, RO, SA, SY, TH, TZ, UG, VN, YE, ZM) *see* Cytarabine (Conventional) ... 535
Cytosar-U (ID, KR, MY, VE) *see* Cytarabine (Conventional) ... 535
Cytosat (CN) *see* Cytarabine (Conventional) ... 535
Cytosa U (KR) *see* Cytarabine (Conventional) ... 535
Cytotec (AE, AU, BE, BF, BG, BH, BJ, CH, CI, CN, CO, CR, CY, CZ, DE, DK, EC, EE, EG, ES, ET, FI, FR, GB, GH, GM, GN, GR, HK, HN, HU, ID, IE, IL, IQ, IR, IS, IT, JO, JP, KE, KR, KW, LB, LR, LU, LY, MA, ML, MR, MT, MU, MW, MX, MY, NE, NG, NI, NL, NO, NZ, OM, PA, PE, PL, PT, QA, RU, SA, SC, SD, SE, SG, SI, SK, SL, SN, SV, SY, TH, TN, TR, TW, TZ, UG, VE, YE, ZA, ZM, ZW) *see* Misoprostol ... 1379
Cytotect (PL) *see* Cytomegalovirus Immune Globulin (Intravenous-Human) ... 541
Cytoxan (CO, HU, ID) *see* Cyclophosphamide ... 517
Cytox (PH) *see* Cytarabine (Conventional) ... 535
Cytragen (PH) *see* Doxycycline ... 689
Cytribin (PL) *see* Bismuth ... 265
Cytropil (ID) *see* Piracetam [INT] ... 1661
Dabaz (IN, PE) *see* Dacarbazine ... 549
Da Bei (CN) *see* Argatroban ... 168
Daberol (KR) *see* Betaxolol (Systemic) ... 256
Dabex (MX) *see* MetFORMIN ... 1307
Dabinese (VE) *see* ChlorproPAMIDE ... 429
Dabroston (HR) *see* Dydrogesterone [INT] ... 702
Dacam (FI) *see* Piroxicam ... 1662
Dacam RL (CL) *see* Betamethasone (Systemic) ... 253
Dacarbazina (ES) *see* Dacarbazine ... 549
Dacarbazin (BG, CZ, HN, HU) *see* Dacarbazine ... 549
Dacarbazine DBL (MY) *see* Dacarbazine ... 549
Dacarbazine Dome (DK) *see* Dacarbazine ... 549
Dacarbazine For Injection (AU) *see* Dacarbazine ... 549
Dacarbazine (NZ) *see* Dacarbazine ... 549
Dacarb (BR) *see* Dacarbazine ... 549
Dacarel (PY, UY) *see* NiCARdipine ... 1446
Dacarzin (PY) *see* Dacarbazine ... 549
Dacatic (FI) *see* Dacarbazine ... 549
Dacef (ZA) *see* Cefadroxil ... 372
Dacin (CH) *see* Dacarbazine ... 549
Dacin (SG) *see* Clindamycin (Systemic) ... 460
DAC (KR, SG) *see* Dacarbazine ... 549
Dacmozen (IN) *see* DACTINomycin ... 551
Dacogen (AR, BE, BR, CH, CL, CN, CO, CY, CZ, DE, DK, EE, GB, HR, IE, IL, IN, KR, LT, MY, NL, NO, PE, PH, RO, RU, SE, SG, SI, SK, TH, TR) *see* Decitabine ... 581
Dacortin (CH, ES) *see* PredniSONE ... 1706
Dacotin (IN) *see* Oxaliplatin ... 1528
Dacplat (AR) *see* Oxaliplatin ... 1528
Dacta Oral Gel (AE, BH, CY, EG, IQ, IR, JO, KW, LB, LY, OM, QA, SA, SY, YE) *see* Miconazole (Topical) ... 1360
Dacta Topical Gel (AE, BH, CY, EG, IQ, IR, JO, KW, LB, LY, OM, QA, SA, SY, YE) *see* Miconazole (Topical) ... 1360
Dacten D (PY) *see* Candesartan and Hydrochlorothiazide ... 338
Dacten (PY) *see* Candesartan ... 335
Dacticin (VN) *see* DACTINomycin ... 551
Dactilon (PE) *see* DACTINomycin ... 551
Dactinomicina Ac-De (PE) *see* DACTINomycin ... 551
Dactin (VN) *see* DACTINomycin ... 551
Dadcrome (HK) *see* Cromolyn (Nasal) ... 514
Dadcrome (HK) *see* Cromolyn (Ophthalmic) ... 514
Daedalon (HU) *see* DimenhyDRINATE ... 637
Daedox (VN) *see* Cefpodoxime ... 388
Dafalgan (BE, LU) *see* Acetaminophen ... 32
Dafalgan Codeine (FR) *see* Acetaminophen and Codeine ... 36
Dafalgan odis (LU) *see* Acetaminophen ... 32
Da Fei Xin (CN) *see* Minoxidil (Topical) ... 1374
Dafil (AR) *see* NiCARdipine ... 1446
Dafne 35 (TH) *see* Cyproterone and Ethinyl Estradiol [CAN/INT] ... 532
Daforin (BR) *see* FLUoxetine ... 899
Dafrin (TW) *see* Miconazole (Topical) ... 1360
Dagla (DO, GT, MX) *see* Itopride [INT] ... 1130
Dagonal (UY) *see* Warfarin ... 2186
Dagramycine (LU) *see* Doxycycline ... 689
Dagravit B!1 (ES) *see* Thiamine ... 2028
Dagravit B1 (PT) *see* Thiamine ... 2028
Dagrilan (GR) *see* FLUoxetine ... 899
Dailix (KR) *see* Furosemide ... 940
Daily Ge (FR) *see* Ethinyl Estradiol and Levonorgestrel ... 803
DAILYvasc (PH) *see* AmLODIPine ... 123
Dainipron (HK) *see* MetFORMIN ... 1307
Dainol (KR) *see* Etidronate ... 813
Daisy (TH) *see* Ethinyl Estradiol and Desogestrel ... 799
Daiteren F (JP) *see* Furosemide ... 940
Daivobet (AU, BG, BH, BR, CH, CL, CN, CO, CR, CZ, DE, DK, DO, EC, EE, ES, FI, FR, GT, HK, HN, HU, ID, IL, IS, KR, KW, LB, LT, MX, MY, NO, NZ, PA, PH, PK, PL, PT, QA, RO, SA, SE, SG, SI, SK, SV, TH, TW, VN) *see* Calcipotriene and Betamethasone ... 321
Daivonex (AE, AR, AU, BB, BE, BG, BH, BM, BR, BS, BZ, CH, CL, CN, CO, CR, CZ, DE, DK, DO, EC, EE, FI, FR, GT, GY, HK, HN, ID, IL, IN, IT, JM, JO, KR, KW, MX, MY, NL, NO, NZ, PA, PH, PK, PL, PR, PT, QA, RU, SA, SE, SI, SK, SR, SV, TH, TT, TW, UY, VE, VN) *see* Calcipotriene ... 321
Dakar (LU) *see* Lansoprazole ... 1166
Daklin (PH) *see* Clindamycin (Systemic) ... 460
Daksol (CO, VE) *see* Secnidazole [INT] ... 1872
DaktaGOLD (AU, NZ) *see* Ketoconazole (Topical) ... 1145
Daktarin (AR, AT, AU, BB, BD, BE, BF, BG, BJ, BM, BR, BS, BZ, CH, CI, CL, CN, CO, CZ, EC, EE, EG, ES, ET,

FI, FR, GB, GH, GM, GN, GR, GY, HK, HR, ID, IE, IL, IT, JM, JP, KE, KR, LR, LT, LU, MA, ML, MR, MU, MW, MX, NE, NG, NL, NZ, PE, PH, PK, PL, PT, PY, RU, SC, SD, SG, SI, SL, SN, SR, TH, TN, TR, TT, TZ, UG, UY, VE, VN, ZA, ZM, ZW) *see* Miconazole (Topical) ... 1360
Daktar (LU, NO, SE) *see* Miconazole (Topical) ... 1360
Dalacin C (AT, AU, BE, BF, BG, BH, BJ, BR, CH, CI, CL, CN, CO, CY, CZ, DK, EC, EE, EG, ET, GB, GH, GM, GN, GR, HK, HR, ID, IE, IL, IN, IQ, IR, IT, KE, KW, LB, LR, LT, LY, MA, ML, MR, MU, MW, MY, NE, NG, NL, NZ, OM, PE, PH, PL, PT, RO, SA, SC, SD, SG, SI, SK, SL, SN, SY, TH, TN, TR, TZ, UG, UY, VN, YE, ZA, ZM, ZW) *see* Clindamycin (Systemic) ... 460
Dalacin (AE, CR, DO, GT, HN, HU, IS, JO, NI, PA, QA, SV, TH) *see* Clindamycin (Systemic) ... 460
Dalacin (DK, FI, IE, SE) *see* Clindamycin (Topical) ... 464
Dalacine (FR) *see* Clindamycin (Systemic) ... 460
Dalacine (FR) *see* Clindamycin (Topical) ... 464
Dalacine T (FR) *see* Clindamycin (Topical) ... 464
Dalacin T (AE, AR, AU, BG, BH, BR, CH, CL, CN, CO, EE, EG, HK, IE, IT, JO, KW, MY, NL, PE, PK, PL, QA, SA, SI, SK, TH, VE, VN, ZA) *see* Clindamycin (Topical) ... 464
Dalaclin (PH) *see* Clindamycin (Systemic) ... 460
Dalagis T (IL) *see* Clindamycin (Topical) ... 464
Dalam (AR, JO, PY) *see* Midazolam ... 1361
Dalamed (PH) *see* Clindamycin (Systemic) ... 460
Dalben (HR) *see* Albendazole ... 65
Dalcap (IN) *see* Clindamycin (Systemic) ... 460
Dalcipran (AR, PT) *see* Milnacipran ... 1368
Daleron (HR, SI) *see* Acetaminophen ... 32
Dalfaz (AR, ES, PL, RU) *see* Alfuzosin ... 84
Dalgen (CO) *see* Doxazosin ... 674
Daliding (CN) *see* CefOXitin ... 386
Dalidome (MX) *see* Zinc Sulfate ... 2200
Dalipaitan (CN) *see* Cefoperazone and Sulbactam [INT] ... 382
Daliresp (CZ, EE, HR, TR) *see* Roflumilast ... 1840
Dalisol (MX) *see* Leucovorin Calcium ... 1183
Dalivit (BR) *see* Riboflavin ... 1803
Dalmadorm (BR, CH, GH, GR, GT, HK, ID, IT, KE, KR, NL, NO, PT, SG, TH, TW, TZ, UG, ZM) *see* Flurazepam ... 906
Dalmam AQ (HK) *see* Fluticasone (Nasal) ... 910
Dalman AQ (HK) *see* Fluticasone (Oral Inhalation) ... 907
Dalmane (GH, IE, KE, NO, TZ, UG, ZM) *see* Flurazepam ... 906
Dalpam (TW) *see* Flurazepam ... 906
Dalpas (VE) *see* BusPIRone ... 311
Dalpic Forte (CL) *see* Trimebutine [CAN/INT] ... 2103
Dal (PY) *see* Ethinyl Estradiol and Desogestrel ... 799
Da Lu (CN) *see* Lornoxicam [INT] ... 1248
Dalys (PE, PY, UY) *see* PACLitaxel (Conventional) ... 1550
Dalzad (HN) *see* Valsartan ... 2127
Damacir (CO) *see* Dicloxacillin ... 621
Dama-Lax (ES) *see* Docusate ... 661
Damicine (CO) *see* Clindamycin (Systemic) ... 460
Damiclin V (CO) *see* Clindamycin (Systemic) ... 460
Damide (IT) *see* Indapamide ... 1065
Damin (TW) *see* Prazosin ... 1703
Damopecia (KR) *see* Finasteride ... 878
Dampurine (TW) *see* Bethanechol ... 257
Danac (MX) *see* Ondansetron ... 1513
Danafusin (DK, SE) *see* Alfuzosin ... 84
Danalax (VN) *see* Bisacodyl ... 265
Danantizol (AR, PY) *see* Methimazole ... 1319
Danarem (VN) *see* Danazol ... 558
Danasin (TR) *see* Danazol ... 558
Danatrol (BE, CH, ES, FR, GR, IT, LU, NL, PT) *see* Danazol ... 558
Danazol Jean Marie (HK) *see* Danazol ... 558
Danazol (KR, PL) *see* Danazol ... 558
Danazol-ratiopharm (DE) *see* Danazol ... 558
Dancin (PH) *see* Ampicillin ... 141
Dancor (AT, CH, NL) *see* Nicorandil [INT] ... 1449
Danilax (HK) *see* Lactulose ... 1156
Danitin (PH) *see* Ranitidine ... 1777
Danizax (VN) *see* Triamcinolone (Systemic) ... 2099
Danlixin (CN) *see* Isosorbide Mononitrate ... 1126
Danocil (KR) *see* Danazol ... 558
Danoclav (ID) *see* Amoxicillin and Clavulanate ... 133
Danocrine (BB, BM, BS, BZ, DK, FI, GY, HK, ID, JM, NO, PK, SE, SR, TT) *see* Danazol ... 558
Danodiol (AE, BB, BH, BM, BS, BZ, CY, EC, EG, GH, GY, IL, JM, JO, KE, LB, LY, MU, OM, PR, QA, SA, SR, SY, TT, TZ, YE) *see* Danazol ... 558
Danoflox (ID) *see* Ofloxacin (Systemic) ... 1490
Danogar (CL) *see* Danazol ... 558
Danogen (HN, IN) *see* Danazol ... 558
Danokrin (AT) *see* Danazol ... 558
Danol (AE, BH, CY, EE, EG, GB, HN, IE, IL, IQ, IR, JO, KW, LB, LY, OM, QA, SA, SY, YE) *see* Danazol ... 558
Danoprox (DE) *see* Oxatomide [INT] ... 1532
Danoval (BG, CZ, HN, HR, HU, PL, RU) *see* Danazol ... 558
Danovir (ID) *see* Acyclovir (Topical) ... 51
Danoxilin (ID) *see* Amoxicillin ... 130
Danssan (MY) *see* Enalapril ... 722
Dantamacrin (BG, CH, DE) *see* Dantrolene ... 559
Dantrium (AU, BE, DK, FR, GB, GR, IE, IL, IT, JP, LU, NL, NZ, PT, QA, SI, TR, VN, ZA) *see* Dantrolene ... 559
Dantrolen (AR, AT, BG, BR, CZ, PL, RU) *see* Dantrolene ... 559
Dantron (MY, TH, ZA) *see* Ondansetron ... 1513
Dantum (HK) *see* Benzydamine [CAN/INT] ... 249
Danzamin (KR) *see* DiphenhydrAMINE (Systemic) ... 641
Daonil (AE, AR, AU, BD, BE, BF, BH, BJ, BO, BR, CH, CI, CL, CR, CY, DK, DO, EG, ET, FR, GH, GM, GN, GR, GT, HK, HN, HR, ID, IE, IN, IQ, IR, IT, JO, JP, KE, KR, KW, LB, LR, LU, LY, MA, ML, MR, MU, MW, MY, NE, NG, NI, NO, NZ, OM, PA, PH, PT, PY, QA, RU, SA, SC, SD, SG, SL, SN, SV, SY, TH, TN, TR, TW, TZ, UG, UY, VE, VN, YE, ZA, ZM, ZW) *see* GlyBURIDE ... 972
Daonil + Metformin (MY) *see* Glyburide and Metformin ... 974
Dapalix (MY) *see* Indapamide ... 1065
Dapamax (TZ, UG, ZA, ZM, ZW) *see* Indapamide ... 1065
Dapa (MY) *see* Indapamide ... 1065
Dapa-tabs (AU) *see* Indapamide ... 1065
Dapaz (ES) *see* Meprobamate ... 1296
Daphne (BE) *see* Cyproterone and Ethinyl Estradiol [CAN/INT] ... 532
Dapotum D (CH, HN) *see* FluPHENAZine ... 905
Dapotum (AT) *see* FluPHENAZine ... 905
Dapotum d (HN) *see* FluPHENAZine ... 905
Dapril (AE, BF, BJ, CI, ET, GH, GM, GN, KE, LR, LT, MA, ML, MR, MU, MW, MY, NE, NG, RU, SC, SD, SG, SK, SL, SN, TN, TR, TZ, UG, ZM, ZW) *see* Lisinopril ... 1226
Dapriton (HK) *see* Dexchlorpheniramine ... 603
Daprolin (ID) *see* Leuprolide ... 1186
Daprox (DK) *see* Naproxen ... 1427
Daps (AR) *see* Dapsone (Systemic) ... 561
Dapsona (CO) *see* Dapsone (Systemic) ... 561
Dapson (DK, EG, KR, NL, NO) *see* Dapsone (Systemic) ... 561
Dapsone (AU) *see* Dapsone (Systemic) ... 561
Dapson-Fatol (DE) *see* Dapsone (Systemic) ... 561
Dapuaa (KR) *see* Lansoprazole ... 1166
Daraprim (AE, AR, AT, AU, BB, BE, BF, BG, BH, BJ, BM, BS, BZ, CH, CI, CL, CY, CZ, DE, EG, ES, ET, GB, GH, GM, GN, GR, GY, HK, IE, IL, IN, IQ, IR, JM, JO, KE, KR, KW, LB, LR, LU, LY, MA, ML, MR, MU, MW, MX, NE, NG, NL, NO, OM, PE, PL, QA, SA, SC, SD, SI,

SL, SN, SR, SY, TN, TT, TW, TZ, UG, UY, YE, ZA, ZM, ZW) *see* Pyrimethamine ... 1749
Daraprin (BR) *see* Pyrimethamine ... 1749
Darbin (BR, PY) *see* Cytarabine (Conventional) ... 535
Dardex (ES) *see* Isoniazid ... 1120
Darfin (MX) *see* Amiodarone ... 114
Darflox (TH) *see* Prulifloxacin [INT] ... 1742
Daribur (MX) *see* Zinc Sulfate ... 2200
Daric (PY) *see* Finasteride ... 878
Dariten OD (IN) *see* Darifenacin ... 568
Darlibose (VN) *see* Miglitol ... 1367
Darob (AT, BG, HR, RO) *see* Sotalol ... 1927
Darolan (NL) *see* Bromhexine [INT] ... 291
Daronal (CO) *see* Amiodarone ... 114
Daroxime (LB) *see* Cefuroxime ... 399
Dartelin (HR) *see* Pentoxifylline ... 1618
Darvilen (DE) *see* CefoTEtan ... 385
Darvine (TW) *see* Clemastine ... 459
Daryant-Tulle (ID) *see* Framycetin [INT] ... 937
Daryazinc (ID) *see* Zinc Sulfate ... 2200
Darzitil Plus (AR) *see* Amoxicillin and Clavulanate ... 133
Dasav (MX) *see* Diltiazem ... 634
Dasten (AR) *see* Oxatomide [INT] ... 1532
Dastosin (ES) *see* Dimemorfan [INT] ... 637
Dasuen (ES) *see* Temazepam ... 1990
Dasutra (IN) *see* Dapoxetine [INT] ... 561
Datan Forte (ID) *see* Mefenamic Acid ... 1280
Datisan (AR) *see* MitoMYcin (Systemic) ... 1380
Datolan (ES) *see* Zopiclone [CAN/INT] ... 2217
Daunobin (IN) *see* DAUNOrubicin (Conventional) ... 577
Daunoblastina (AE, AR, BH, BR, CN, CY, CZ, EG, ES, GR, HR, HU, IQ, IR, IT, JO, KR, KW, LB, LY, OM, PT, QA, SA, SY, TW, VE, VN, YE) *see* DAUNOrubicin (Conventional) ... 577
Daunoblastin (AT, DE, ZA) *see* DAUNOrubicin (Conventional) ... 577
Daunocin (BR, ID, KR, SG, VN) *see* DAUNOrubicin (Conventional) ... 577
Daunorrubicina (EC, PY) *see* DAUNOrubicin (Conventional) ... 577
Daunorubicin Injection (AU) *see* DAUNOrubicin (Conventional) ... 577
DaunoXome (AT, DK, FI, FR, GB, IT, NO, SE) *see* DAUNOrubicin (Liposomal) ... 580
DaunoXome (ES, FI, LU) *see* DAUNOrubicin (Conventional) ... 577
Davesol (EC) *see* Lindane ... 1217
Davinefrina (PT) *see* Phenylephrine (Systemic) ... 1638
Davitamon A (AE, BH, CY, EG, IL, IQ, IR, JO, KW, LB, LY, OM, QA, SA, SY, YE) *see* Vitamin A ... 2173
Daxar (BE) *see* Lansoprazole ... 1166
Daxas (AR, BR, CH, CO, CZ, DE, DK, EE, FR, GB, HK, HR, ID, IE, IS, KR, LB, LT, MY, NL, NO, PH, PL, PT, RO, SA, SE, SI, SK, TH) *see* Roflumilast ... 1840
Daxim (CL, VE) *see* Levosimendan [INT] ... 1205
Daxol Plus (PY) *see* Albendazole ... 65
Daxol (PY) *see* Mebendazole [CAN/INT] ... 1274
Daxon (MX) *see* Nitazoxanide ... 1461
Daxotel (PH, TH, VE) *see* DOCEtaxel ... 656
Daxxas (MX) *see* Roflumilast ... 1840
Dayflu N (PE) *see* Pseudoephedrine and Ibuprofen ... 1743
Daypro (PK) *see* Oxaprozin ... 1532
Dayrun (BG, CZ, EE) *see* Oxaprozin ... 1532
Dayvital (NL) *see* Ascorbic Acid ... 178
Dazil (AE, BH, CY, EG, IQ, IR, JO, KW, LB, LY, OM, QA, SA, SY, YE) *see* Diltiazem ... 634
Dazolin (AR, UY) *see* Naphazoline (Nasal) ... 1426
Dazolin (CO) *see* Donepezil ... 668
DB-10 (PH) *see* MedroxyPROGESTERone ... 1277
DBL (TW) *see* Gemcitabine ... 952
D-CAL (CN) *see* Calcium and Vitamin D ... 326
DDAVP (BR, CL, IT) *see* Desmopressin ... 594
DDAVP Desmopressin (PT) *see* Desmopressin ... 594
Deadict (IN) *see* Disulfiram ... 654
Deallergy (TW) *see* Cetirizine ... 411
Deaten (CL) *see* AtoMOXetine ... 191
Debax (AT) *see* Captopril ... 342
Debecylina (PL) *see* Penicillin G Benzathine ... 1609
Debekacyl (JP, LU) *see* Dibekacin [INT] ... 616
Debelex (AR) *see* Azapropazone [INT] ... 210
Debequin C (MX) *see* Guaifenesin and Dextromethorphan ... 987
Deblaston (AT, DE, ZA) *see* Pipemidic Acid [INT] ... 1655
Debretin (PL) *see* Trimebutine [CAN/INT] ... 2103
Debridat AF (CL) *see* Trimebutine [CAN/INT] ... 2103
Debridat (AR, AT, CH, EG, FR, HU, IT, LB, MX, PL, PT, RO, SA, VE, VN) *see* Trimebutine [CAN/INT] ... 2103
Decabicin (ES) *see* Dibekacin [INT] ... 616
Deca (CN, MY, TH) *see* FluPHENAZine ... 905
Decadol (PL) *see* Haloperidol ... 993
Decadron (AE, BH, CO, CY, EC, IT, JO, KW, LB, PY, QA, SA) *see* Dexamethasone (Systemic) ... 599
Decadron (CO, EC) *see* Dexamethasone (Ophthalmic) ... 602
Decalogiflox (FR) *see* Lomefloxacin [INT] ... 1233
Decan (PH, SG, TW) *see* Dexamethasone (Systemic) ... 599
Decantin (PH) *see* Azithromycin (Systemic) ... 216
Decaparil (ID) *see* Ramipril ... 1771
Decapeptyl (AE, AR, BE, BG, BH, CL, CN, CO, CY, CZ, DE, EC, EG, ES, FR, GB, HK, HN, HR, HU, IE, IL, IQ, IR, IT, JO, KW, LB, LU, LY, MY, NL, OM, PL, PT, PY, QA, RU, SA, SK, SY, TR, UY, VE, YE) *see* Triptorelin ... 2107
Decapeptyl CR (AE, BH, CY, EG, HR, IL, IQ, IR, JO, KR, KW, LB, LY, MY, NZ, OM, PH, QA, SA, SG, SY, TH, YE) *see* Triptorelin ... 2107
Decapeptyl Depot (AT, CZ, DE, DK, EE, FI, IS, KR, LT, MY, SE, SK) *see* Triptorelin ... 2107
Decapeptyl LP (FR) *see* Triptorelin ... 2107
Decapeptyl Retard (CH) *see* Triptorelin ... 2107
Decapeptyl SR (PK) *see* Triptorelin ... 2107
Decarbay (TW) *see* Acarbose ... 29
Decasone (ZA) *see* Dexamethasone (Systemic) ... 599
Decasurik (ID) *see* Allopurinol ... 90
Decatocin (ID) *see* Oxytocin ... 1549
Decatona (ID) *see* Phenytoin ... 1640
Decdan (IN) *see* Dexamethasone (Systemic) ... 599
Decentan (AT, DE, ES) *see* Perphenazine ... 1627
Decilone Forte (PH) *see* Desoximetasone ... 598
Decilone (PH) *see* Desoximetasone ... 598
Decipar (ES) *see* Enoxaparin ... 726
Declage (KR) *see* Somatropin ... 1918
Decloban (ES) *see* Clobetasol ... 468
Declophen (AE, BH, CY, EG, IQ, IR, JO, KW, LB, LY, OM, QA, SA, SY, YE) *see* Diclofenac (Systemic) ... 617
Declot (TW) *see* Ticlopidine ... 2040
Declovir (HK) *see* Acyclovir (Topical) ... 51
Decoin (KR) *see* Codeine ... 497
De-Cold (SG) *see* Loratadine and Pseudoephedrine ... 1242
Decomit (SG) *see* Beclomethasone (Nasal) ... 232
Decortin (DE, HR) *see* PredniSONE ... 1706
Decortin H (BG) *see* PrednisoLONE (Systemic) ... 1703
Decortisyl (IE) *see* PredniSONE ... 1706
Decostriol (DE, TH) *see* Calcitriol ... 323
Decrelip (PY) *see* Simvastatin ... 1890
Decreten (ID) *see* Pindolol ... 1652
Decrilip (ID) *see* Bezafibrate [CAN/INT] ... 261
Dectancyl (VN) *see* Dexamethasone (Systemic) ... 599
Deculin (ID) *see* Pioglitazone ... 1654
Dedralen (IT) *see* Doxazosin ... 674
Defam (MX) *see* Nimesulide [INT] ... 1456
Defanyl (FR) *see* Amoxapine ... 128
Defas (AR) *see* Deflazacort [INT] ... 587

Defense (TW) *see* Cimetidine 438
Defetol (HK) *see* Chlorpheniramine, Pseudoephedrine, and Dextromethorphan 428
Defiltran (FR) *see* AcetaZOLAMIDE 39
Defin (MX) *see* Dipyrone [INT] 653
Defirin (GR) *see* Desmopressin 594
Deflamon (IT) *see* MetroNIDAZOLE (Systemic) 1353
Deflam (ZA) *see* Oxaprozin 1532
Deflan (GR, IT) *see* Deflazacort [INT] 587
Deflenol (MX) *see* GuaiFENesin 986
Deflogen (BR) *see* Nimesulide [INT] 1456
Deflox (ES) *see* Terazosin 2001
Deftan (ES) *see* Lofepramine [INT] 1232
Defur (PL) *see* Tolterodine 2063
Degison (TW) *see* Dantrolene 559
Degiton (TW) *see* Ibuprofen 1032
Deglu (TW) *see* Acarbose 29
Degraler (CL, EC, PE) *see* Levocetirizine 1196
Degranol (ZA) *see* CarBAMazepine 346
Deherp (TH, TW) *see* Acyclovir (Systemic) 47
Deherp (TW) *see* Acyclovir (Topical) 51
Dehidrobenzoperidol (PT) *see* Droperidol 695
Dehidrobenzperidol (ES) *see* Droperidol 695
Dehydrobenzperidol (AE, AT, BE, BH, CY, CZ, DE, DK, EG, FI, IL, IQ, IR, JO, KW, LB, LU, LY, NL, OM, QA, SA, SY, TH, TR, YE) *see* Droperidol 695
Dehydrocortison (BG) *see* PredniSONE 1706
Deiron (ES) *see* Etofenamate [INT] 815
Deiten (IT) *see* Nitrendipine [INT] 1463
Dekatravel (BE) *see* DimenhyDRINATE 637
Dekstran 40000 (PL) *see* Dextran 607
Dekstran 70000 (PL) *see* Dextran 607
Delagil (BB, BM, BS, BZ, GY, HN, HU, JM, PR, RU, SR, TT) *see* Chloroquine 424
Delaien (CN) *see* Celiprolol [INT] 404
Delaket (IT) *see* Delapril [INT] 587
Delamin (TW) *see* Dexchlorpheniramine 603
Delanin (TH) *see* Hydroquinone 1020
Delaxin (PY) *see* Fexofenadine 873
Delcortin (DK) *see* PredniSONE 1706
Delepsine (DK) *see* Valproic Acid and Derivatives 2123
Delfen II (ZA) *see* Nonoxynol 9 1471
Delfen Foam (AE) *see* Nonoxynol 9 1471
Delfen (IL, IN, PT) *see* Nonoxynol 9 1471
Delfos (IT) *see* Nimesulide [INT] 1456
Delgamer (ES) *see* Diethylpropion 624
Delice (TW) *see* Lindane 1217
Delifon (CO) *see* Oxybutynin 1536
Delinar (AR) *see* Mesna 1305
Deline (LB) *see* Desloratadine 594
Delipo (JP) *see* Fluocinonide 894
De Li Shu (CN) *see* Aspirin and Dipyridamole 185
Delitex (DE) *see* Lindane 1217
Delix (DE, TR) *see* Ramipril 1771
Dellegra (JP) *see* Fexofenadine and Pseudoephedrine 874
Delmofulvina (IT) *see* Griseofulvin 985
Delnil (CL) *see* Minocycline 1371
Delok (IN) *see* DULoxetine 698
Delonal (DE) *see* Alclometasone 72
Delopa (PH) *see* Desloratadine 594
Delor (AE, BH, CY, EG, IQ, IR, JO, KW, LB, LY, OM, QA, SA, SY, YE) *see* Clobetasol 468
Delorat (UY) *see* Desloratadine 594
Delos (AR) *see* Roxithromycin [INT] 1853
Delphicort (AT, DE) *see* Triamcinolone (Systemic) 2099
Delphicort (AT, DE) *see* Triamcinolone (Topical) 2100
Delphi Creme (BE, NL) *see* Triamcinolone (Topical) 2100
Delsoralen (ID) *see* Methoxsalen (Systemic) 1330
Delster (HK) *see* Hydrocortisone (Topical) 1014
Deltacarbon (TH) *see* Charcoal, Activated 416
Deltacef (TR) *see* Cefepime 378
Deltacortene (IT) *see* PredniSONE 1706
Deltacortril (EG, PK) *see* PrednisoLONE (Systemic) 1703
Deltamid Ofteno (GT, HN, NI, PA) *see* Sulfacetamide and Prednisolone 1944
Deltasolone (VN) *see* PrednisoLONE (Systemic) 1703
Deltasone (HK) *see* PredniSONE 1706
Delta West Carboplatin (ID, PH) *see* CARBOplatin 357
Deltazen (FR) *see* Diltiazem 634
Deltison (SE) *see* PredniSONE 1706
Deltrox (AR) *see* Cefuroxime 399
Delucon (AU) *see* QUEtiapine 1751
Demanitol (PE) *see* Mannitol 1269
Demare (TW) *see* Zaleplon 2193
Demar (VE) *see* Lindane 1217
Demazin 6 Hour Relief (AU) *see* Chlorpheniramine and Pseudoephedrine 427
Demecline (TW) *see* Demeclocycline 589
Deme (PH) *see* Meperidine 1293
Demergin (GR) *see* Methylergonovine 1333
Demerol HCl (MX, PH) *see* Meperidine 1293
Demero (VE) *see* Meperidine 1293
Demetrin (AT, CH, CZ, DE, ES, HR, PT, QA) *see* Prazepam [INT] 1702
Demiderm (VE) *see* Alclometasone 72
Demil (TW) *see* Bromocriptine 291
Demofenac (IL) *see* Diclofenac (Systemic) 617
Demolox (AE, DK, IN) *see* Amoxapine 128
Demoquin (GR) *see* Chloroquine 424
Demser (CA) *see* Metyrosine 1359
Denamol (TH) *see* Acetaminophen 32
Denapol (JP) *see* Cinnarizine [INT] 440
Denapranil (MY) *see* ClomiPRAMINE 475
Denason (BR) *see* Phenylephrine (Systemic) 1638
Dencorub (AU) *see* Magnesium Salicylate 1265
Denecort (PH) *see* Budesonide (Systemic) 293
Denerel (MY, SG, TW) *see* Ketotifen (Systemic) [CAN/INT] 1149
Denex (MY, SG, TR) *see* Metoprolol 1350
Denim (TH) *see* DimenhyDRINATE 637
Denirin (KR) *see* Desmopressin 594
De-nol (PL) *see* Bismuth 265
Denosin 5 (TW) *see* Desloratadine 594
Denosin (KR, VN) *see* Adenosine 55
Denpax (AU) *see* FentaNYL 857
Denpru (AR) *see* Protamine 1737
Densate (AU) *see* Alendronate 79
Densical (ES) *see* Calcium Carbonate 327
Dentacline (KR) *see* Doxycycline 689
Dentalfluoro (IT) *see* Fluoride 895
Dentan (SE) *see* Fluoride 895
Dentispray (ES, PL) *see* Benzocaine 246
Dentistar (KR) *see* Doxycycline 689
Dentocar (HU) *see* Fluoride 895
Dentodex (PE) *see* Chlorhexidine Gluconate 422
Dentodrin (PE) *see* Benzydamine [CAN/INT] 249
Denufam (ID) *see* Famotidine 845
Denvar (CR, DO, ES, GT, HN, MX, NI, PA, SV) *see* Cefixime 380
Denvercort (AR) *see* Betamethasone (Topical) 255
Denzapine (GB, IE) *see* CloZAPine 490
Deopens (ZA) *see* Magnesium Hydroxide 1263
Deoxon Gel (KR) *see* Desoximetasone 598
Deoxon Lotion (KR) *see* Desoximetasone 598
Deoxymykoin (CZ) *see* Doxycycline 689
Depacon (KP, PH) *see* Valproic Acid and Derivatives 2123
Depain (KR) *see* Diclofenac (Systemic) 617
Depain Plaster (KR) *see* Diclofenac (Systemic) 617
Depakene (AR, CN, CO, ID, JP, PE, PH, PY, UY) *see* Valproic Acid and Derivatives 2123
Depakine (AE, AT, BE, BG, BH, CH, CY, EE, EG, ES, FR, GR, HN, HU, IQ, IR, JO, KW, LB, LU, LY, OM, PL, PT,

QA, RU, SA, SY, TH, VE, YE) *see* Valproic Acid and Derivatives ... 2123
Depakine Chrono (KP, LU, TH, TW) *see* Valproic Acid and Derivatives ... 2123
Depakin (IT, PK, RU, TR) *see* Valproic Acid and Derivatives ... 2123
Depakote (BZ, SR) *see* Valproic Acid and Derivatives ... 2123
Depermide (TW) *see* Indapamide ... 1065
D'epifrin (PL) *see* Dipivefrin ... 651
Depin-E Retard (TH) *see* NIFEdipine ... 1451
Depin (IN) *see* NIFEdipine ... 1451
Depix (JP) *see* Furosemide ... 940
Depixol (GB) *see* Flupentixol [CAN/INT] ... 903
Deplatt (SG) *see* Clopidogrel ... 484
Deplat (TW) *see* Clopidogrel ... 484
Depo-M (TH) *see* MedroxyPROGESTERone ... 1277
Depocyte (AT, BE, BG, CH, CZ, DE, DK, EE, FI, FR, GB, GR, HN, HR, IE, IS, IT, MT, NL, NO, PL, PT, RO, RU, SE, SI, SK, TR) *see* Cytarabine (Liposomal) ... 540
DepoCyte (KR) *see* Cytarabine (Liposomal) ... 540
Depofemme (PH) *see* MedroxyPROGESTERone ... 1277
Depofin (MX) *see* Iodoquinol ... 1105
Depolan (FI) *see* Morphine (Systemic) ... 1394
Depo Medrol (AE, BH, KW, LB, QA, SA) *see* MethylPREDNISolone ... 1340
Depo-Medrol (EG, IS, LU, MX, SI, SK, VN) *see* MethylPREDNISolone ... 1340
Deponeo (ID) *see* MedroxyPROGESTERone ... 1277
Deponit (CN, DE, HU, LU, MY, PE, PH) *see* Nitroglycerin ... 1465
Deponit NT (IL) *see* Nitroglycerin ... 1465
Depon (TR) *see* Acetaminophen ... 32
Depo-Prodasone (FR) *see* MedroxyPROGESTERone ... 1277
Depo Progestin (ID) *see* MedroxyPROGESTERone ... 1277
Depo-Provera (AE, AU, BH, CN, CY, EG, IL, IQ, IR, JO, KW, LB, LY, OM, PH, QA, SA, SG, SY, VN, YE) *see* MedroxyPROGESTERone ... 1277
Depo-Ralovera (AU) *see* MedroxyPROGESTERone ... 1277
Deporeva (PH) *see* MedroxyPROGESTERone ... 1277
Depo-Testosterone (ZA) *see* Testosterone ... 2010
Depo-Test (TH) *see* Testosterone ... 2010
Depotrust (PH) *see* MedroxyPROGESTERone ... 1277
Depovit-B12 (AE, QA) *see* Hydroxocobalamin ... 1020
Depovit-B 12 (EG) *see* Hydroxocobalamin ... 1020
Deppreo (VN) *see* BuPROPion ... 305
Deprakine (DK, FI, NO) *see* Valproic Acid and Derivatives ... 2123
Depramina (BR) *see* Imipramine ... 1054
Depranil (SG) *see* ClomiPRAMINE ... 475
Deprax (CL, PY) *see* Sertraline ... 1878
Deprax (ES) *see* TraZODone ... 2091
Deprazolin (CZ) *see* Prazosin ... 1703
Deprectal (MX) *see* OXcarbazepine ... 1532
Deprefax (AR) *see* Nefazodone ... 1435
Deprel (PK) *see* TraZODone ... 2091
Deprenyl (FR) *see* Selegiline ... 1873
Depresil (PH) *see* TraZODone ... 2091
Deprexan (IL) *see* Desipramine ... 593
Deprexin (BB, BM, BS, BZ, GY, HU, JM, SR, TT) *see* FLUoxetine ... 899
Depridat (PK) *see* Trimebutine [CAN/INT] ... 2103
Depridol (HN, HU) *see* Methadone ... 1311
Deprimil (PT) *see* Lofepramine [INT] ... 1232
Deprine (LB) *see* Sertraline ... 1878
Deprizac (PH) *see* FLUoxetine ... 899
Deprolac (TW) *see* Bromocriptine ... 291
Depropin (MY) *see* Dosulepin [INT] ... 673
Deproxin (TH) *see* FLUoxetine ... 899
Deproz (ID) *see* FLUoxetine ... 899
Deprozol (BR) *see* Secnidazole [INT] ... 1872
Depsol (IN) *see* Imipramine ... 1054
Depsonil (IN) *see* Imipramine ... 1054
Deptral (ID) *see* Sertraline ... 1878
Deptran (AU) *see* Doxepin (Systemic) ... 676
DePURA (BR) *see* Ergocalciferol ... 753
Dequaspray (GB) *see* Lidocaine (Systemic) ... 1208
Dequazol Oral (PE) *see* MetroNIDAZOLE (Systemic) ... 1353
Dequin (MX) *see* Guaifenesin and Dextromethorphan ... 987
Deralin (AU, IL) *see* Propranolol ... 1731
Derbac-M (IE, NZ) *see* Malathion ... 1268
Derbisol (KR) *see* Clobetasol ... 468
Dercason (ID) *see* Desoximetasone ... 598
Dergelasen (CO) *see* BusPIRone ... 311
Dergott (JP) *see* Dihydroergotamine ... 633
Derilate (ES) *see* Tiaprofenic Acid [CAN/INT] ... 2034
Derimine (JP) *see* Oxiconazole ... 1536
Deriva MS (MY) *see* Adapalene ... 54
Dermacaine (TH) *see* Lidocaine and Prilocaine ... 1213
Dermacom (CL) *see* Butenafine ... 314
Dermacorte (TH) *see* Desoximetasone ... 598
Dermacort (HK, MY) *see* Triamcinolone (Topical) ... 2100
Dermacortine (PE) *see* Mometasone (Topical) ... 1391
Dermacort (MY) *see* Triamcinolone (Systemic) ... 2099
Derma-Coryl (CY, EG, IQ, IR, JO, LY, OM, QA, SY, YE) *see* Econazole ... 703
Dermacrin HC Lotion (KR) *see* Hydrocortisone (Topical) ... 1014
Dermadex (PH) *see* Fluocinonide ... 894
Dermadrate Dry Skin Treatment Cream (SG) *see* Urea ... 2114
Dermafin (MY) *see* Terbinafine (Systemic) ... 2002
Dermafin (MY) *see* Terbinafine (Topical) ... 2004
Derm-Aid (AE, CY) *see* Hydrocortisone (Topical) ... 1014
Dermalar (IL) *see* Fluocinolone (Topical) ... 893
Derma-Lomexin (SA) *see* Fenticonazole [INT] ... 868
Dermanide (ID) *see* Desonide ... 597
Derm A (PH) *see* Tretinoin (Topical) ... 2099
Dermasafe (TW) *see* Mupirocin ... 1404
Dermaseb (AR) *see* Sulfacetamide (Ophthalmic) ... 1943
Dermaser (PY) *see* Sulfacetamide (Ophthalmic) ... 1943
Dermasil (IL) *see* Terbinafine (Systemic) ... 2002
Dermasil (IL) *see* Terbinafine (Topical) ... 2004
Dermasolon Gel (ID) *see* Fluocinolone (Topical) ... 893
Dermasone (SG) *see* Betamethasone (Topical) ... 255
Dermatane (AU) *see* ISOtretinoin ... 1127
Dermatech Bantix (CO) *see* Mupirocin ... 1404
Dermatin (AE, BH, CY, EG, IQ, IR, JO, KW, LB, LY, OM, QA, SA, SY, YE) *see* Clotrimazole (Topical) ... 488
Dermatin (DE) *see* Terbinafine (Systemic) ... 2002
Dermatol (DE, PL) *see* Bismuth ... 265
Dermatop (BG, BR, CZ, DE, HR, ID, IT, KR, TH, TR) *see* Prednicarbate ... 1703
Dermatovate (MX) *see* Clobetasol ... 468
Dermax (ZA) *see* Terbinafine (Systemic) ... 2002
Dermazin (HK, PL, RU, SI, SK, TH) *see* Silver Sulfadiazine ... 1887
Dermestril (BE, CZ, DE, FI, IT, PT) *see* Estradiol (Systemic) ... 775
Dermestril Septem (FR) *see* Estradiol (Systemic) ... 775
Dermin Cream (KR) *see* Prednicarbate ... 1703
Dermizole (TH) *see* Clotrimazole (Topical) ... 488
Dermo 6 (FR) *see* Pyridoxine ... 1747
Dermocare (KR) *see* Hydrocortisone (Topical) ... 1014
Dermocare (TW) *see* Clobetasol ... 468
Dermo Chabre B6 (ES) *see* Pyridoxine ... 1747
Dermocort (BG) *see* Betamethasone (Topical) ... 255
Dermofix (BE, EG, ES, ID, KR, KW, LB, PT, QA, SA) *see* Sertaconazole ... 1877
Dermolar (AE, BH, QA, SA) *see* Fluocinolone (Topical) ... 893

Dermol (NZ) *see* Clobetasol 468
Dermomax (BR) *see* Lidocaine (Topical) 1211
Dermome (TW) *see* Mometasone (Topical) 1391
Dermon (HK, MY) *see* Miconazole (Topical) 1360
Dermonide (KR) *see* Desonide 597
Dermonistat (AE, BH, CY, EG, IQ, IR, JO, KW, LB, LY, OM, QA, SA, SY, YE) *see* Miconazole (Topical) 1360
Dermopur (PL) *see* Benzocaine 246
Dermorelle (FR) *see* Vitamin E 2174
Dermosol (KR) *see* Clobetasol 468
Dermosupril (EC, PE) *see* Desonide 597
Dermotasone (KR) *see* Mometasone (Topical) 1391
Dermotop (HR, QA) *see* Prednicarbate 1703
Dermoval (FR) *see* Clobetasol 468
Dermovat (DK, FI, IS, NO, SE) *see* Clobetasol 468
Dermovate (AE, AT, BB, BD, BE, BF, BG, BH, BJ, BM, BS, BZ, CH, CI, CL, CO, CY, CZ, EC, EE, EG, ET, GB, GH, GM, GN, GT, GY, HK, HN, HU, IE, IL, IQ, IR, JM, JO, JP, KE, KR, KW, LB, LR, LT, LY, MA, ML, MR, MU, MW, MY, NE, NG, NL, OM, PA, PE, PH, PK, PL, PR, PT, PY, QA, RO, RU, SA, SC, SD, SG, SL, SN, SR, SV, SY, TH, TN, TR, TT, TW, TZ, UG, UY, VE, VN, YE, ZM, ZW) *see* Clobetasol 468
Dermovel (ID) *see* Mometasone (Topical) 1391
Dermoxin (DE) *see* Clobetasol 468
Deronga (DE) *see* Natamycin 1432
Derox-5 (PH) *see* AmLODIPine 123
Deroxat (CH, FR) *see* PARoxetine 1579
Derozin (GR) *see* Cinnarizine [INT] 440
Derzid-C (HK, TH) *see* Betamethasone and Clotrimazole 256
Derzid (HK, SG) *see* Betamethasone (Topical) 255
Desagit 5 (PY) *see* Trihexyphenidyl 2103
Desalark (IT) *see* Dexamethasone (Systemic) 599
Desalex (BR, CO) *see* Desloratadine 594
Desal (PL) *see* Furosemide 940
Desaltan (KR) *see* Candesartan 335
Desaltan Plus (KR) *see* Candesartan and Hydrochlorothiazide 338
Desbly (FR) *see* GuaiFENesin 986
Deschu (TW) *see* Desloratadine 594
Desconex (ES) *see* Loxapine 1255
Desec (TH) *see* Omeprazole 1508
Desentol (SE) *see* DiphenhydrAMINE (Systemic) 641
Desferal (AE, AR, AT, AU, BB, BE, BF, BG, BH, BJ, BM, BR, BS, BZ, CH, CI, CL, CN, CY, CZ, DE, DK, EE, EG, ES, ET, FI, FR, GB, GH, GM, GN, GR, GY, HK, HN, HU, ID, IE, IL, IN, IQ, IR, IS, IT, JM, JO, KE, KR, KW, LB, LR, LU, LY, MA, ML, MR, MT, MU, MW, MX, MY, NE, NG, NL, NO, OM, PH, PK, PL, PT, QA, RO, RU, SA, SC, SD, SE, SG, SI, SK, SL, SN, SR, SY, TH, TN, TR, TT, TW, TZ, UG, UY, VE, VN, YE, ZA, ZM, ZW) *see* Deferoxamine 586
Desick (VN) *see* DimenhyDRINATE 637
Desiken (MX) *see* Ribavirin 1797
Desintan (FI, GB) *see* Lindane 1217
Desirel (TH) *see* TraZODone 2091
Desirett (EE) *see* Desogestrel [INT] 597
Desitic (DE) *see* Ticlopidine 2040
Desitin (MX) *see* Zinc Oxide 2200
Desitrend (GB) *see* LevETIRAcetam 1191
Desketo (CL) *see* Dexketoprofen [INT] 603
Desketo (IT) *see* Clobutinol [INT] 468
Deslafax (AR) *see* Desvenlafaxine 598
Deslodine (PH) *see* Desloratadine 594
Deslogen (PH) *see* Desloratadine 594
Deslora (HK) *see* Desloratadine 594
Desloran (EC) *see* Desloratadine 594
Deslorastal (PH) *see* Desloratadine 594
Deslor (IN) *see* Desloratadine 594
Desman (TW) *see* Iron Dextran Complex 1117
Desmin (DE) *see* Ethinyl Estradiol and Desogestrel 799
Desmin (KR) *see* Desmopressin 594
Desmogalen (DE) *see* Desmopressin 594
Desmomelt (GB, IE) *see* Desmopressin 594
Desmop ODIFS Powder (KR) *see* Desmopressin 594
Desmopresin DDAVP (AR) *see* Desmopressin 594
Desmospray (GB, IE, PT) *see* Desmopressin 594
Desmotab (GB, IE) *see* Desmopressin 594
Desmotabs (DE) *see* Desmopressin 594
Desoclin (KR) *see* Desonide 597
Desolett 28 (SE) *see* Ethinyl Estradiol and Desogestrel 799
Desolett (TR) *see* Ethinyl Estradiol and Desogestrel 799
Desolex (ID) *see* Desonide 597
Desomono (GB) *see* Desogestrel [INT] 597
Desone (TW) *see* Desoximetasone 598
Deson (HK, TH) *see* MetFORMIN 1307
Desonia (KR) *see* Desonide 597
Desorate (TH) *see* Valproic Acid and Derivatives 2123
Desora (TW) *see* Desloratadine 594
Desoren (CH) *see* Ethinyl Estradiol and Desogestrel 799
Desorox (GB) *see* Desogestrel [INT] 597
Desowen (AR, AU, CL, CR, DO, GT, HK, HN, IN, MX, NI, PH, SG, UY, VE) *see* Desonide 597
Desowon Lotion (KR) *see* Desonide 597
Desoxyn (BM) *see* Methamphetamine 1315
Despej (PE) *see* Desloratadine 594
Desproxyl (MX) *see* Rocuronium 1838
Destap (CL) *see* Beclomethasone (Nasal) 232
Destap FS (CL) *see* Beclomethasone (Systemic) 230
Destina (PK) *see* Desloratadine 594
Destolit (PE) *see* Permethrin 1627
Destramin (BG) *see* Dexchlorpheniramine 603
Destrim (CO) *see* Trimethoprim and Polymyxin B 2105
Desumide (TW) *see* TOLAZamide 2062
Desyrel (JP) *see* TraZODone 2091
Detebencil (AR) *see* Ivermectin (Systemic) 1136
Detemes Retard (AT) *see* Dihydroergotamine 633
Detenler (AR) *see* Methotrimeprazine [CAN/INT] 1329
Detensiel (FR) *see* Bisoprolol 266
Detension (KR) *see* Valsartan and Hydrochlorothiazide 2129
Deten (TH) *see* AmLODIPine 123
Deterodine SR (IE) *see* Tolterodine 2063
Dethasone (KR) *see* Desoximetasone 598
Deticene (AR, CL, CZ, EG, FR, GR, HN, HR, IL, IT, KR, NL, PL, PT, RU, SA, TR, UY, VN) *see* Dacarbazine 549
Deticine (HU) *see* Dacarbazine 549
Detilem (MX) *see* Dacarbazine 549
Detimedac (DE) *see* Dacarbazine 549
Detms (LU) *see* Dihydroergotamine 633
Detreomycyna (PL) *see* Chloramphenicol 421
Detrichol (ID) *see* Gemfibrozil 956
Detrodin SR (KR) *see* Tolterodine 2063
Detrunorm XL (GB) *see* Propiverine [INT] 1728
Detrunorm (GB, HR, ZA) *see* Propiverine [INT] 1728
Detrunorm XR (HR) *see* Propiverine [INT] 1728
Detrusitol XL (GB, IE) *see* Tolterodine 2063
Detrusitol (AE, AR, AT, AU, BE, BG, BH, BR, BZ, CL, CN, CO, CR, CY, CZ, DE, DO, EC, EE, EG, ES, FI, FR, GB, GR, GT, HK, HN, HU, ID, IE, IL, IN, IQ, IR, IS, IT, JO, JP, KW, LB, LT, LY, MX, MY, NI, NL, NO, NZ, OM, PA, PE, PH, PK, PL, QA, RU, SA, SE, SG, SI, SK, SV, SY, TR, TW, VE, YE) *see* Tolterodine 2063
Detrusitol Retard (BR, DK, KW, PT, SA) *see* Tolterodine 2063
Detrusitol SR (BG, CH, CL, CO, CZ, HR, IL, KR, LT, MY, NO, PE, RO, SE, SG, SK, TH, VE) *see* Tolterodine 2063
Deursil (IT) *see* Ursodiol 2116
Deustin (KR) *see* Amlodipine and Atorvastatin 124
Devastin (VN) *see* Rosuvastatin 1848
Devidon (HR) *see* TraZODone 2091
Devincil (LU) *see* Verapamil 2154

Deviplat (MX) *see* Clopidogrel 484
Devirus (TW) *see* Acyclovir (Ophthalmic) [INT] 43
Devitol (AT, FI) *see* Ergocalciferol 753
Devom (PK) *see* DimenhyDRINATE 637
Devoxim (CO) *see* Cefixime 380
Dexabion (MX) *see* Thiamine 2028
Dexacap (ID, SG, VN) *see* Captopril 342
Dexacort Forte (IL) *see* Dexamethasone (Systemic) 599
Dexaflam (DE) *see* Dexamethasone (Systemic) 599
Dexaflox (ID) *see* Pefloxacin [INT] 1588
Dexafree (CH, FR, GB, PL, PT) *see* Dexamethasone (Ophthalmic) 602
Dexafree (CH, FR, PL, PT) *see* Dexamethasone (Systemic) 599
Dexagel (TH) *see* Dexamethasone (Ophthalmic) 602
Dexak (PL) *see* Dexketoprofen [INT] 603
Dexambutol (FR) *see* Ethambutol 798
Dexamed (CZ, JO, RO, SG, TR) *see* Dexamethasone (Systemic) 599
Dexamol PM (IL) *see* Acetaminophen and Diphenhydramine 36
Dexamphetamine (AU) *see* Dextroamphetamine 607
Dexamphetamini Sulfas (CH) *see* Dextroamphetamine 607
Dexan (CL) *see* Pseudoephedrine 1742
Dexanorm (ID) *see* Repaglinide 1791
Dexanta (ID) *see* Aluminum Hydroxide, Magnesium Hydroxide, and Simethicone 104
Dex Antihist (HK) *see* Dexchlorpheniramine 603
Dexarazoxane Martian (AR) *see* Dexrazoxane 606
Dexaron Plus (AE, BH, CY, EG, IQ, IR, JO, KW, LB, LY, OM, QA, SA, SY, YE) *see* Neomycin, Polymyxin B, and Dexamethasone 1437
Dexa-Sine (BE) *see* Dexamethasone (Ophthalmic) 602
Dexa-Sine (BE) *see* Dexamethasone (Systemic) 599
Dexa-Sine SE (NO) *see* Dexamethasone (Ophthalmic) 602
Dexa-Sine SE (NO) *see* Dexamethasone (Systemic) 599
Dexatamin (MY, SG) *see* Dexchlorpheniramine 603
Dexazol (ID) *see* Ketoconazole (Systemic) 1144
Dexdor (HR, RO, TR) *see* Dexmedetomidine 604
Dexedrine (GB, NO) *see* Dextroamphetamine 607
Dexferin (TW) *see* Dexchlorpheniramine 603
Dexidex (MX) *see* Nitazoxanide 1461
Dexigen (ID) *see* Desoximetasone 598
Dexilant DR (KR) *see* Dexlansoprazole 603
Dexilant (HK, LT, MY, PH, SE, SG, TH) *see* Dexlansoprazole 603
Deximune (GB, IL, SG) *see* CycloSPORINE (Systemic) 522
Dexmethsone (AU, NZ) *see* Dexamethasone (Systemic) 599
Dexocort (ID) *see* Desoximetasone 598
Dexofen (BG) *see* Dexketoprofen [INT] 603
Dexoket (CZ) *see* Dexketoprofen [INT] 603
Dexolut (ID) *see* Bromhexine [INT] 291
Dexomen (HR) *see* Dexketoprofen [INT] 603
Dexometorfano-Guaifenesina (MX) *see* Guaifenesin and Dextromethorphan 987
Dexona (IN) *see* Dexamethasone (Systemic) 599
Dexopral (AR) *see* Dexlansoprazole 603
Dexo (PY) *see* Ursodiol 2116
Dexosyn Plus (IN) *see* Neomycin, Polymyxin B, and Dexamethasone 1437
Dexotel (IN) *see* DOCEtaxel 656
Dexrazoxane Chiron (AR) *see* Dexrazoxane 606
Dexsul (MX) *see* Neomycin, Polymyxin B, and Dexamethasone 1437
Dexsul (MX) *see* Polymyxin B 1676
Dextamina B1 (ES) *see* Thiamine 2028
Dextamina B6 (ES) *see* Pyridoxine 1747
Dextran-1 B. Braun (CH) *see* Dextran 607
Dextran 40 Injection (AU) *see* Dextran 607
Dextran 40 Vifor (CH) *see* Dextran 607
Dextran 70 Injection (AU) *see* Dextran 607
Dextran 70 Vifor (CH) *see* Dextran 607
Dextran Spofa (CZ) *see* Dextran 607
Dextricyl (PH) *see* GuaiFENesin 986
Dextril 70 (FI) *see* Dextran 607
DextroPlus (HK) *see* Guaifenesin, Pseudoephedrine, and Dextromethorphan 989
Dezacor (ES) *see* Deflazacort [INT] 587
Dezartal (CL, CO) *see* Deflazacort [INT] 587
Dezor Cream (MY, SG, TH) *see* Ketoconazole (Topical) 1145
Dezor (ID) *see* Ketoconazole (Topical) 1145
Dezor Kem (VN) *see* Ketoconazole (Topical) 1145
Dezor Shampoo (MY, PH) *see* Ketoconazole (Topical) 1145
DF 118 Forte (GB) *see* Dihydrocodeine, Aspirin, and Caffeine 632
DF 118 (IE) *see* Dihydrocodeine, Aspirin, and Caffeine 632
D-Fiam (TH) *see* Diclofenac (Systemic) 617
D-forte (FI) *see* Ergocalciferol 753
DFZ (IN) *see* Deflazacort [INT] 587
Dhabesol (HK, KR, MY) *see* Clobetasol 468
Dhacillin (HK, MY) *see* Ampicillin 141
Dhacocin (MY, SG) *see* Vancomycin 2130
Dhacopan (HK) *see* Scopolamine (Systemic) 1870
DHAcort (HK, MY) *see* Hydrocortisone (Topical) 1014
Dhactulose (HK, MY, SG) *see* Lactulose 1156
Dhamotil (HK, MY) *see* Diphenoxylate and Atropine 644
Dhaperazine (HK, MY) *see* Prochlorperazine 1718
Dhartisone-100 (ID, MY) *see* Hydrocortisone (Systemic) 1013
Dhatifen (HK, MY) *see* Ketotifen (Systemic) [CAN/INT] 1149
Dhatracin (SG) *see* Tetracycline 2017
Dhatrim (MY) *see* Sulfamethoxazole and Trimethoprim 1946
DHC Continus (GB, HU, IE, PL) *see* Dihydrocodeine, Aspirin, and Caffeine 632
DHC Mundipharma (DE) *see* Dihydrocodeine, Aspirin, and Caffeine 632
DH-Ergotamin (PL) *see* Dihydroergotamine 633
DHT (AR) *see* Dihydroergotamine 633
Diabacil (ES) *see* Rifampin 1804
Diaban (TW) *see* Miglitol 1367
DiabeDerm (TH) *see* Urea 2114
Diabemet (MY) *see* MetFORMIN 1307
Diabemide (BF, BJ, CI, ET, GH, GM, GN, IT, KE, LR, MA, ML, MR, MU, MW, NE, NG, SC, SD, SL, SN, TN, TZ, UG, ZM, ZW) *see* ChlorproPAMIDE 429
Diaben (AE, BH, CY, EG, IQ, IR, JO, KW, LB, LY, OM, QA, SA, SY, YE) *see* GlyBURIDE 972
Diabenese (AE, BB, BF, BH, BJ, BM, BS, BZ, CI, CO, CR, CY, DO, EG, ET, GB, GH, GM, GN, GR, GT, GY, HN, IL, IQ, IR, IT, JM, JO, KE, KW, LB, LR, LY, MA, ML, MR, MU, MW, MX, NE, NG, NI, NL, OM, PA, PR, PT, QA, SC, SD, SL, SN, SR, SV, SY, TN, TT, TZ, UG, YE, ZA, ZM, ZW) *see* ChlorproPAMIDE 429
Diaben (JP) *see* TOLBUTamide 2062
Diabenol (TH) *see* GlyBURIDE 972
Diabeside (TH) *see* Gliclazide [CAN/INT] 964
Diabes (TW) *see* GlipiZIDE 967
Diabesulf (EC) *see* GlyBURIDE 972
Diabetase (DE) *see* MetFORMIN 1307
Diabet (ES) *see* ChlorproPAMIDE 429
Diabetin (TW) *see* GlyBURIDE 972
Diabetmin (HK, MY) *see* MetFORMIN 1307
Diabetmin Retard (HK) *see* MetFORMIN 1307
Diabetol (PL) *see* TOLBUTamide 2062
Diabetol (PY) *see* MetFORMIN 1307
Diabetone (PH) *see* Pioglitazone 1654
Diabeton Metilato (IT) *see* TOLBUTamide 2062

Diabeton (RU) *see* Gliclazide [CAN/INT] 964
Diabetose (JP) *see* TOLBUTamide 2062
Diabewas (IT) *see* TOLAZamide 2062
Diabex (AU) *see* MetFORMIN 1307
Diabex XR (AU) *see* MetFORMIN 1307
Diabezin (TW) *see* ChlorproPAMIDE 429
Diabinese (AR, AU, BE, BR, CH, CL, EC, ES, HK, HR, IE, KR, LU, NO, PE, PH, PK, PL, SA, TH, TR, UY) *see* ChlorproPAMIDE 429
Diabines (SE) *see* ChlorproPAMIDE 429
Diabitex (BB, BM, BS, BZ, GY, JM, NL, SR, TT, ZA) *see* ChlorproPAMIDE 429
Diacarb (RU) *see* AcetaZOLAMIDE 39
Dia-Colon (IT) *see* Lactulose 1156
Diacomit (AT, BE, CY, CZ, DE, DK, EE, ES, FI, FR, GB, GR, HR, HU, IE, IS, IT, JP, KR, LT, LU, NL, NO, PL, PT, RO, SE, SI, SK) *see* Stiripentol [CAN/INT] 1935
Diacor (CL) *see* Mebendazole [CAN/INT] 1274
Diacordin (SK) *see* Diltiazem 634
Diacor LP (FR) *see* Diltiazem 634
Di-Actane (FR) *see* Naftidrofuryl [INT] 1416
Diacyclan (GR) *see* Bencyclane [INT] 241
Diadium (ID) *see* Loperamide 1236
Diafat (PH) *see* MetFORMIN 1307
Diafen (PY, UY) *see* Baclofen 223
Diaformina LP (UY) *see* MetFORMIN 1307
Diaformina (UY) *see* MetFORMIN 1307
Diaformin (BR, HK, TW) *see* MetFORMIN 1307
Diaformin XR (AU) *see* MetFORMIN 1307
Diafusor (LU) *see* Nitroglycerin 1465
Diaglime (ID) *see* Glimepiride 966
Diaglinex (PE) *see* Rosiglitazone 1847
Diaglip (TH) *see* Glimepiride 966
Diakarmon (AE, BF, BH, BJ, CI, CY, EG, ET, GH, GM, GN, IQ, IR, JO, KE, KW, LB, LR, LY, MA, ML, MR, MU, MW, NE, NG, OM, QA, SA, SC, SD, SL, SN, SY, TN, TZ, UG, YE, ZM, ZW) *see* Gentamicin (Systemic) 959
Dialag (BF, BJ, CI, ET, GH, GM, GN, KE, LR, MA, ML, MR, MU, MW, NE, NG, SC, SD, SL, SN, TN, TZ, UG, ZM, ZW) *see* Diazepam 613
Dialens (CH) *see* Dextran 607
Dialgin (BG) *see* Dipyrone [INT] 653
Dialifer (ID) *see* Iron Sucrose 1118
Dialon (AE, BH, KW, LB, QA, SA) *see* MetFORMIN 1307
Dialon (ID) *see* Diflunisal 626
Dialosa (GR, SG) *see* Glimepiride 966
Diamet (JO) *see* MetFORMIN 1307
Diamicron (AE, AR, AT, BE, BH, BR, CH, CL, CO, DE, DK, EC, EG, ES, FR, GB, GR, IE, IN, IT, KR, LB, LU, MX, MY, NZ, PE, PH, PK, PT, SA, TH, TW, UY, VE, VN, ZA) *see* Gliclazide [CAN/INT] 964
Diamicron MR (AR, BB, BH, BM, BR, BS, BZ, CH, CL, CN, CO, CR, CY, DO, EG, GB, GT, GY, HK, ID, JM, JO, KR, KW, LB, MY, NI, NL, NZ, PA, PE, PH, PR, PY, QA, SA, SR, SV, TH, TR, TT, TW, UY, VE, VN) *see* Gliclazide [CAN/INT] 964
Diamicron Uno (IS) *see* Gliclazide [CAN/INT] 964
Diamide (MY) *see* Glyburide and Metformin 974
Diamide (NZ) *see* Loperamide 1236
Diamid (JO) *see* Gliclazide [CAN/INT] 964
Diamig (IN, IT) *see* Miglitol 1367
Diamilla (DK, EE) *see* Desogestrel [INT] 597
Diamine (TW) *see* DiphenhydrAMINE (Systemic) 641
Diaminocillina (IT) *see* Penicillin G Benzathine 1609
Diamox (AE, AR, AT, AU, BD, BE, BG, BH, BR, CH, CO, CY, DK, EE, EG, ES, FR, GB, GR, HK, HR, IE, IN, IQ, IR, IS, IT, JO, JP, KR, KW, LB, LU, LY, MT, MY, NL, NO, NZ, OM, QA, RU, SA, SE, SG, SI, SK, SY, TH, VE, VN, YE, ZA) *see* AcetaZOLAMIDE 39
Diamox Sustets (CO) *see* AcetaZOLAMIDE 39
Diamsalina (MX) *see* Dicloxacillin 621
Dianben (ES) *see* MetFORMIN 1307
Diane-35 (AE, BB, BH, BM, BS, BZ, CO, DO, GY, JM, JO, KW, LB, NL, PR, QA, SA, SR, TT, UY, VE, ZA) *see* Cyproterone and Ethinyl Estradiol [CAN/INT] 532
Diane 35 (AR, BG, BR, CH, CL, CR, CZ, DK, DO, EC, EE, EG, FR, GT, HK, HN, HR, ID, IL, KR, MY, NI, PA, PE, PH, PK, PY, RO, SG, SI, SK, SV, TH, TW) *see* Cyproterone and Ethinyl Estradiol [CAN/INT] 532
Diane 35 Diario (ES) *see* Cyproterone and Ethinyl Estradiol [CAN/INT] 532
Diane-35 ED (AU, NZ) *see* Cyproterone and Ethinyl Estradiol [CAN/INT] 532
Diane (AT, BE, EE, FI, IN, MX, NO, RU, SE, TR, VN) *see* Cyproterone and Ethinyl Estradiol [CAN/INT] 532
Diane Mite (IS) *see* Cyproterone and Ethinyl Estradiol [CAN/INT] 532
Dianette (IE) *see* Cyproterone and Ethinyl Estradiol [CAN/INT] 532
Dianicotyl (GR) *see* Isoniazid 1120
Dianid (MY) *see* Gliclazide [CAN/INT] 964
Dianorm (PH) *see* Gliclazide [CAN/INT] 964
Dian Shu (CN) *see* Dexamethasone (Ophthalmic) 602
Di An Song (CN) *see* Betamethasone (Topical) 255
Diapam (FI, TR) *see* Diazepam 613
Diapectolin (PH) *see* Furazolidone [INT] 940
Diaperol (MX) *see* Loperamide 1236
Diaphyllin (VN) *see* Theophylline 2026
Diapine (MY, SG, TH, TW) *see* Diazepam 613
Diapo (MY) *see* Diazepam 613
Diaprel (BG, CZ, EE, HN, HR, HU, PL, SI) *see* Gliclazide [CAN/INT] 964
Diaprel MR (BG, CZ, HR, LT, RO) *see* Gliclazide [CAN/INT] 964
Diapride (AU, HK, JO, KW, LB, MY, SG) *see* Glimepiride 966
Diarase (MY) *see* Diphenoxylate and Atropine 644
Diareze (AU) *see* Loperamide 1236
Diarlop (IN) *see* Loperamide 1236
Diarodil (TH) *see* Loperamide 1236
Diarona (UY) *see* Amiodarone 114
Diarret (IT) *see* Nifuroxazide [INT] 1454
Diarsed (AE, FR, VN) *see* Diphenoxylate and Atropine 644
Diasectral (FI) *see* Acebutolol 29
Diasef (SG) *see* GlipiZIDE 967
Diaseptyl (FR) *see* Chlorhexidine Gluconate 422
Diaslim (TH) *see* MetFORMIN 1307
Diastabol (AT, CH, CZ, DE, FI, FR, GR, HN, IE, MX, NL, PL, PT, SE, SI) *see* Miglitol 1367
Diastop (NZ) *see* Diphenoxylate and Atropine 644
Diatabs (PH) *see* Loperamide 1236
Diat (JP) *see* Azosemide [INT] 220
Diatol (NZ) *see* TOLBUTamide 2062
Diatracin (ES) *see* Vancomycin 2130
Diatrim (IL) *see* Diacerein [INT] 613
Diatrol (SG) *see* Loperamide 1236
Diavista-M (IN) *see* Pioglitazone and Metformin 1655
Diaxine (SA) *see* Diphenoxylate and Atropine 644
Diazem (TR) *see* Diazepam 613
Diazemuls (GB, IT) *see* Diazepam 613
Diazepam Desitin (HU) *see* Diazepam 613
Diazepam-Eurogenerics (LU) *see* Diazepam 613
Diazepam (HK) *see* Diazepam 613
Diazepam-ratiopharm (LU) *see* Diazepam 613
Diazepan (AE, BF, BH, BJ, CI, CY, EG, ES, ET, GH, GM, GN, IQ, IR, JO, KE, KW, LB, LR, LY, MA, ML, MR, MU, MW, NE, NG, OM, QA, SA, SC, SD, SL, SN, SY, TN, TZ, UG, YE, ZM, ZW) *see* Diazepam 613
Diazid (JP) *see* Isoniazid 1120
Diazomid (TR) *see* AcetaZOLAMIDE 39
Diazon (SG, TH) *see* Ketoconazole (Systemic) 1144
Dibacilina (MX) *see* Ampicillin 141
Dibactil (PY) *see* Ciprofloxacin (Systemic) 441

Dibaprim (MX) *see* Sulfamethoxazole and Trimethoprim 1946
Dibecon (TH) *see* ChlorproPAMIDE 429
Dibelet (MY) *see* GlyBURIDE 972
DiBendryl (TH) *see* DiphenhydrAMINE (Systemic) 641
Dibenyline (AE, AU, BE, BF, BH, BJ, CI, CY, EG, ET, GB, GH, GM, GN, GR, HK, IL, IQ, IR, JO, KE, KW, LB, LR, LU, LY, MA, ML, MR, MU, MW, NE, NG, NL, OM, QA, SA, SC, SD, SL, SN, SY, TN, TZ, UG, YE, ZA, ZM, ZW) *see* Phenoxybenzamine 1635
Dibenzyran (AT, DE) *see* Phenoxybenzamine 1635
Dibertil (BE, LU) *see* Metoclopramide 1345
Dibizide (MY) *see* GlipiZIDE 967
Diblocin (DE) *see* Doxazosin 674
Diblocin PP (DE) *see* Doxazosin 674
Diblocin Uro (DE) *see* Doxazosin 674
Dibose (MY) *see* Acarbose 29
Dibrondrin (AT) *see* DiphenhydrAMINE (Systemic) 641
Dicaptol (HU) *see* Dimercaprol 638
Dicarz (AU) *see* Carvedilol 367
Dicetel (AE, AR, AT, BE, BG, BH, BR, CH, CN, CO, CY, CZ, FR, GR, HN, HR, HU, IT, KR, KW, LU, MY, NL, PE, PT, QA, SA, SK, TH, TR, TW, UY, VE) *see* Pinaverium [CAN/INT] 1651
Dichinalex (IT) *see* Chloroquine 424
Dichlorzid (KR) *see* Hydrochlorothiazide 1009
Dichlotride (BE, DK, HK, LU, NL, PT, TH) *see* Hydrochlorothiazide 1009
Dicil (EC) *see* Terbinafine (Systemic) 2002
Dicinone (BR, CH, ES) *see* Etamsylate [INT] 795
Diclac (CN) *see* Diclofenac (Systemic) 617
Dicladox (AR) *see* DOXOrubicin (Conventional) 679
Diclax SR (NZ) *see* Diclofenac (Systemic) 617
Diclex (TH) *see* Dicloxacillin 621
Dicloabak (BE) *see* Diclofenac (Ophthalmic) 621
Diclobene (AT) *see* Diclofenac (Systemic) 617
Dicloced (FR) *see* Diclofenac (Ophthalmic) 621
Diclocil (DK, EC, FI, GR, NO, PT, SE, VE) *see* Dicloxacillin 621
Diclofenac (CO) *see* Diclofenac (Systemic) 617
Diclofen (AE, BH, CY, EG, IQ, IR, JO, KW, LB, LY, OM, QA, SA, SY, TW, YE) *see* Diclofenac (Systemic) 617
Diclofen Cremogel (AE, BH, CY, EG, IQ, IR, JO, KW, LB, LY, OM, QA, SA, SY, YE) *see* Diclofenac (Systemic) 617
Dicloflam (ZA) *see* Diclofenac (Systemic) 617
Dicloftil (IL) *see* Diclofenac (Ophthalmic) 621
Diclo (IT) *see* Dicloxacillin 621
Diclomax (IN) *see* Diclofenac (Systemic) 617
Diclomine (TH) *see* Dicyclomine 622
Diclon (DK) *see* Diclofenac (Systemic) 617
Diclonox (TH) *see* Dicloxacillin 621
Dicloran Gel (BF, BJ, CI, ET, GH, GM, GN, KE, LR, MA, ML, MR, MU, MW, NE, NG, SC, SD, SL, SN, TN, TZ, UG, ZM, ZW) *see* Diclofenac (Systemic) 617
Diclosan SR (AE, BH, CY, EG, IQ, IR, JO, KW, LB, LY, OM, QA, SA, SY, YE) *see* Diclofenac (Systemic) 617
Diclosian (TH) *see* Diclofenac (Systemic) 617
Diclowal (CR, DO, GT, HN, NI, PA, SV) *see* Diclofenac (Systemic) 617
Dicloxane-F (TH) *see* Dicloxacillin 621
Dicloxane (TH) *see* Dicloxacillin 621
Dicloxno (TH) *see* Dicloxacillin 621
Dicloxsig (AU) *see* Dicloxacillin 621
Dicodin (FR) *see* Dihydrocodeine, Aspirin, and Caffeine 632
Diconpin (DE) *see* Isosorbide Dinitrate 1124
Dicorantil-F (BR) *see* Disopyramide 653
Dicorvin (ES) *see* Spiramycin [CAN/INT] 1931
Dicorynan (ES) *see* Disopyramide 653
Dicron (KR) *see* Diflorasone 625
Dicton (DE, LU) *see* Codeine 497
Dicyclin Forte (IN) *see* Tetracycline 2017
Dicymine (HK, TH) *see* Dicyclomine 622
Dicynene (CH, GB, IE) *see* Etamsylate [INT] 795
Dicynone (BE, CH, FR, HR, HU, IT, LU) *see* Etamsylate [INT] 795
Didasten (MX) *see* Didanosine 622
Dideral (TR) *see* Propranolol 1731
Didralin (SG, TR) *see* Hydrochlorothiazide 1009
Didronate/Calcium (DK) *see* Etidronate and Calcium Carbonate [CAN/INT] 814
Didronate + Calcium (FI, NO, SE) *see* Etidronate and Calcium Carbonate [CAN/INT] 814
Didronate (DK, FI, NO, SE) *see* Etidronate 813
Didronat (TR) *see* Etidronate 813
Didronel (AT, CH, DE, FR, GR, HK, IE, JP, LU, NL, PT) *see* Etidronate 813
Didronel PMO (GB, IE) *see* Etidronate and Calcium Carbonate [CAN/INT] 814
Die Li (CN) *see* Gabapentin 943
Diemon (AR) *see* Tamoxifen 1971
Dienille (BG) *see* Estradiol and Dienogest 780
Diergospray (FR) *see* Dihydroergotamine 633
Di-Ertride (SG) *see* Hydrochlorothiazide 1009
Dietil Retard (BE) *see* Diethylpropion 624
Dietil-retard (LU) *see* Diethylpropion 624
Di-Eudrin (VE) *see* Hydrochlorothiazide 1009
Difena (TW) *see* Diclofenac (Systemic) 617
Difene (IE) *see* Diclofenac (Systemic) 617
Difengesic Gel (TH) *see* Diclofenac (Systemic) 617
Difenidrin (BR) *see* DiphenhydrAMINE (Systemic) 641
Difetoin (HR) *see* Phenytoin 1640
Differin (AE, AR, AU, BR, CL, CN, CO, EE, FI, HK, HU, IS, JO, KR, KW, LT, MY, NL, NO, NZ, PE, PH, PL, PT, PY, RU, SA, SG, SI, TH, TR, TW, UY, VE, VN, ZA) *see* Adapalene 54
Differine (CZ, ES, FR, LB, SK) *see* Adapalene 54
Differin Gel (AT, BE, CH, DE, GB, IE, IL, IT, SE) *see* Adapalene 54
Difflam (AU, BH, CY, GB, HK, IE, KW, MY, PH, QA, SG, TH, TW) *see* Benzydamine [CAN/INT] 249
Difflam Forte (TH) *see* Benzydamine [CAN/INT] 249
Diffu-K (FR) *see* Potassium Chloride 1687
Diffutab SR 600 (KR) *see* Ibuprofen 1032
Dificid (AU, NZ) *see* Fidaxomicin 875
Dificlir (CY, CZ, DE, DK, EE, ES, FR, GB, HR, IS, LT, NL, NO, RO, SE, SI, SK, TR) *see* Fidaxomicin 875
Difiram (TH) *see* Disulfiram 654
Diflazon (VN) *see* Fluconazole 885
Diflonid (NO) *see* Diflunisal 626
Diflorate (IN) *see* Diflorasone 625
Diflosid (PH) *see* Diclofenac (Systemic) 617
Diflucan (AE, AT, AU, BB, BE, BF, BG, BH, BJ, BM, BS, BZ, CH, CI, CL, CN, CR, CZ, DE, DK, DO, EE, ES, ET, FI, GB, GH, GM, GN, GT, GY, HK, HN, HR, HU, ID, IE, IS, IT, JM, JO, JP, KE, KR, KW, LB, LR, LT, LU, MA, ML, MR, MT, MU, MW, MX, MY, NE, NG, NI, NL, NO, NZ, PA, PE, PH, PL, PT, QA, RO, RU, SA, SC, SD, SE, SI, SK, SL, SN, SR, SV, TH, TN, TR, TT, TW, TZ, UG, VN, ZA, ZM, ZW) *see* Fluconazole 885
DiflucanOne (AU) *see* Fluconazole 885
Diflucor (IN) *see* Diflucortolone [CAN/INT] 625
Difluvid (MY) *see* Fluconazole 885
Difluzole (KR) *see* Fluconazole 885
Difnazol (KR) *see* Fluconazole 885
Diformin (FI) *see* MetFORMIN 1307
Diformin Retard (FI) *see* MetFORMIN 1307
Difosfen (AR, CO, MY, SG, TH, UY) *see* Etidronate 813
Dif per tet all (MY, PH, PK) *see* Diphtheria and Tetanus Toxoids, and Acellular Pertussis Vaccine 649
Dif tet all (IT, PK) *see* Diphtheria and Tetanus Toxoid 645
Diftet (HK) *see* Diphtheria and Tetanus Toxoid 645
Difuco (KR) *see* Diflucortolone [CAN/INT] 625
Difusin (TH) *see* Fusidic Acid (Topical) [CAN/INT] 943
Digalo (TW) *see* Dihydroergotamine 633

Digaol (FR) *see* Timolol (Ophthalmic) 2043
Digaril (ES) *see* Fluvastatin 915
Digedrat (BR) *see* Trimebutine [CAN/INT] 2103
Digerent (IT) *see* Trimebutine [CAN/INT] 2103
Digerex (BR) *see* Bromopride [INT] 292
Digeril (EC) *see* Magaldrate and Simethicone 1261
Digesan (BR) *see* Bromopride [INT] 292
Digesprid (BR) *see* Bromopride [INT] 292
Digest (ID) *see* Lansoprazole 1166
Digestil (BR) *see* Bromopride [INT] 292
Digestina (BR) *see* Bromopride [INT] 292
Digezanol (MX) *see* Albendazole 65
Digibind (GB, NO) *see* Digoxin Immune Fab 630
Digifab (SG) *see* Digoxin Immune Fab 630
DigiFab (TW) *see* Digoxin Immune Fab 630
Digimed (DE) *see* Digitoxin [INT] 627
Digimerck (AT, DE, HN, HU, TR) *see* Digitoxin [INT] 627
Digitalina Nativelle (IT) *see* Digitoxin [INT] 627
Digitaline (GR, PT) *see* Digitoxin [INT] 627
Digitaline Nativelle (BE, BR, CH, FR, LU) *see* Digitoxin [INT] 627
Digitossina (IT) *see* Digitoxin [INT] 627
Digitoxin Nyco (NO) *see* Digitoxin [INT] 627
Digitoxin Streuli (CH) *see* Digitoxin [INT] 627
Digitrin (NO, SE) *see* Digitoxin [INT] 627
Diglucron (TH) *see* Gliclazide [CAN/INT] 964
Dignokonstant (DE) *see* NIFEdipine 1451
Digosin (JP, KR) *see* Digoxin 627
Digoxil (PY) *see* Digoxin 627
Digoxina Boehringer (ES) *see* Digoxin 627
Digoxina (CO, ES, GT, HN, NI, PE) *see* Digoxin 627
Digoxin-Actavis (HK) *see* Digoxin 627
Digoxine Nativelle (LU) *see* Digoxin 627
Digoxine Navtivelle (FR) *see* Digoxin 627
Digoxin Immune FAB (Ovine) Digibind (AU) *see* Digoxin Immune Fab 630
Digoxin NI (ID) *see* Digoxin 627
Digoxin (PL) *see* Digoxin 627
Digoxin-Sandoz (BF, BJ, CH, CI, ET, GH, GM, GN, ID, JP, KE, LR, MA, ML, MR, MU, MW, NE, NG, SC, SD, SL, SN, TN, TZ, UG, ZM, ZW) *see* Digoxin 627
Digoxin-Zori (IL) *see* Digoxin 627
Digoxin "Dak" (DK) *see* Digoxin 627
Digram (PY) *see* Tadalafil 1968
Digrasil (CO, PE) *see* Orlistat 1520
Digrin (KR) *see* GlipiZIDE 967
Dihalar (HR) *see* Ketotifen (Ophthalmic) 1150
Di-Hydan (FR, LU, VN) *see* Phenytoin 1640
Dihydergot (AU, BE, BF, BJ, BR, CH, CI, CZ, ES, ET, GH, GM, GN, GR, ID, IL, KE, LR, LU, MA, ML, MR, MU, MW, NE, NG, NL, NO, PE, SC, SD, SL, SN, TN, TR, TZ, UG, VE, ZA, ZM, ZW) *see* Dihydroergotamine 633
Dihydergot Sandoz (AT) *see* Dihydroergotamine 633
Dihydrocodeine (CY, GB) *see* Dihydrocodeine, Aspirin, and Caffeine 632
Dihydroergotaminum Methansulfonicum (PL) *see* Dihydroergotamine 633
Dihydroergotaminum Tartaricum (PL) *see* Dihydroergotamine 633
Dihydroergotamin "Dak" (DK) *see* Dihydroergotamine 633
Dikacine (BE, LU) *see* Dibekacin [INT] 616
Dilacoran (BR, MX) *see* Verapamil 2154
Dilacor (AR) *see* Barnidipine [INT] 227
Dilacor (BG) *see* Digoxin 627
Diladel (IT) *see* Diltiazem 634
Dilahex (PH) *see* Felodipine 850
Dilamet (AR) *see* Lormetazepam [INT] 1247
Dilanacin (CY, EG, IQ, JO, SD) *see* Digoxin 627
Dilanorm (NL) *see* Celiprolol [INT] 404
Dilantin (AU, FR, HK, ID, IN, MY, NZ, PH, PK, SG, TH, VE, VN) *see* Phenytoin 1640
Dilasig (AU) *see* Carvedilol 367
Dilatam 120 SR (IL) *see* Diltiazem 634
Dilatam 240 CD (IL) *see* Diltiazem 634
Dilatame (AT) *see* Diltiazem 634
Dilatam (ZA) *see* Diltiazem 634
Dilatrate-SR (BM) *see* Isosorbide Dinitrate 1124
Dilatrend (AE, AR, AT, AU, BF, BG, BH, BJ, CH, CI, CL, CN, CY, CZ, DE, EC, EE, EG, ET, GH, GM, GN, GR, HK, HR, HU, IT, JO, KE, KR, KW, LB, LR, MA, ML, MR, MU, MW, MX, NE, NG, NO, NZ, PE, PH, PL, PY, QA, RO, SA, SC, SD, SG, SL, SN, TH, TN, TR, TW, TZ, UG, UY, VE, VN, ZM, ZW) *see* Carvedilol 367
Dilaudid (AT, AU) *see* HYDROmorphone 1016
Dilbloc (PT) *see* Carvedilol 367
Dilbres (ID) *see* Diltiazem 634
Dilcardia (BF, BJ, CI, ET, GB, GH, GM, GN, IN, KE, LR, MA, ML, MR, MU, MW, NE, NG, SC, SD, SL, SN, TH, TN, TZ, UG, ZA, ZM, ZW) *see* Diltiazem 634
Dilcor (DK) *see* Diltiazem 634
Dilem SR (TH) *see* Diltiazem 634
Dilfar (PT) *see* Diltiazem 634
Dilid (KR) *see* HYDROmorphone 1016
Dilitair (PH) *see* Doxofylline [INT] 679
Dilofen ER (PH) *see* Felodipine 850
Dilopin (KR) *see* Felodipine 850
Dilox (CL) *see* Ketorolac (Systemic) 1146
Diloxin (TH) *see* Dicloxacillin 621
Dilrene (CZ, FR, HU) *see* Diltiazem 634
Diltahexal CD (AU) *see* Diltiazem 634
Diltahexal (DE, LU) *see* Diltiazem 634
Dilta-Hexal (LU) *see* Diltiazem 634
Diltam (IE) *see* Diltiazem 634
Diltan (BB, BM, BS, BZ, GY, HU, JM, SR, TT) *see* Diltiazem 634
Diltan SR (AE, BH, CY, EG, IQ, IR, JO, KW, LB, LY, OM, QA, SA, SY, YE) *see* Diltiazem 634
Diltelan Depot (IE) *see* Diltiazem 634
Diltelan (KR, TW) *see* Diltiazem 634
Dilteran SR (KR) *see* Diltiazem 634
Diltiazem-B (HU) *see* Diltiazem 634
Diltiazem-Ethypharm (LU) *see* Diltiazem 634
Diltiazem-XI (LU) *see* Diltiazem 634
Diltiazyn (CO) *see* Diltiazem 634
Diltime (BF, BJ, CI, ET, GH, GM, GN, KE, LR, MA, ML, MR, MU, MW, NE, NG, SC, SD, SL, SN, TN, TZ, UG, ZM, ZW) *see* Diltiazem 634
Dilucid (MX) *see* Lovastatin 1252
Dilucort (ZA) *see* Hydrocortisone (Topical) 1014
Diluran (CZ) *see* AcetaZOLAMIDE 39
Dilutol (EC, VN) *see* Enoxaparin 726
Dilzanton (DE) *see* Diltiazem 634
Dilzem CD (AU) *see* Diltiazem 634
Dilzem (AE, AT, AU, BH, CH, CY, CZ, DE, EG, FI, HR, HU, IE, IN, IQ, IR, JO, KW, LB, LY, NZ, OM, PK, PL, QA, RO, SA, SY, TH, YE) *see* Diltiazem 634
Dilzem LA (NZ) *see* Diltiazem 634
Dilzem Retard (AE, AT, BH, CY, CZ, DE, EG, IQ, IR, JO, KW, LB, LY, OM, QA, SA, SY, YE) *see* Diltiazem 634
Dilzem RR (CH) *see* Diltiazem 634
Dilzem SR (CY, GB, NZ, VN) *see* Diltiazem 634
Dilzene (IT) *see* Diltiazem 634
Dilzereal 90 Retard (DE) *see* Diltiazem 634
Dilzicardin (DE) *see* Diltiazem 634
Dimacol (MX) *see* Guaifenesin and Dextromethorphan 987
Dimard (CO, EC) *see* Hydroxychloroquine 1021
Dimcef (KR) *see* CefTAZidime 392
Dimecaina (CL) *see* Lidocaine (Topical) 1211
Dimefor (CO, MX, PE) *see* MetFORMIN 1307
Dimegan D (MX) *see* Loratadine and Pseudoephedrine 1242
Dimegan (MX) *see* Loratadine 1241
Dimegan (FR) *see* Brompheniramine 292
Dimenate (HK, MY) *see* DimenhyDRINATE 637

Dimenhidrinato (MX) *see* DimenhyDRINATE 637
Dimenidrinato (IT) *see* DimenhyDRINATE 637
Dimetane (AE, GR, QA, TW) *see* Brompheniramine 292
Dimetriose (AU, IE, PT) *see* Gestrinone [INT] 962
Dimetrose (BE, BR, IT, LU) *see* Gestrinone [INT] 962
Dimetus (TH) *see* Gliclazide [CAN/INT] 964
Dimicaps (MX) *see* DimenhyDRINATE 637
Dimipra (PH) *see* Cefepime 378
Dimirel (AU) *see* Glimepiride 966
Dimitone (DK) *see* Carvedilol 367
Dimodan (MX) *see* Disopyramide 653
Dimopen (MX) *see* Amoxicillin 130
Dimorf (BR) *see* Morphine (Systemic) 1394
Dimorf SP (PY) *see* Morphine (Systemic) 1394
Dimotil (HK) *see* Diphenoxylate and Atropine 644
Dimycon (HR) *see* Fluconazole 885
Dimzef (PH) *see* CefTAZidime 392
Dinadom (AR) *see* Desmopressin 594
Dinagen (MX) *see* Piracetam [INT] 1661
Dinagest (JP) *see* Dienogest [CAN/INT] 623
Dinegal (CO) *see* Flunarizine [CAN/INT] 892
Dinemic (PK) *see* Trimetazidine [INT] 2104
Dineurin (CL) *see* Gabapentin 943
Dineurol (PY) *see* Gabapentin 943
Dinex EC (PE) *see* Didanosine 622
Dinex (IN) *see* Didanosine 622
Dinisor (ES) *see* Diltiazem 634
Dinisor Retard (ES) *see* Diltiazem 634
Dinobroxol (ES) *see* Ambroxol [INT] 109
Dinoldin (ES) *see* Rifampin 1804
Dinol (KR) *see* Etidronate 813
Dinpen (PH) *see* Ampicillin 141
Dintaxin (PH) *see* CefOXitin 386
Dintoina (IT) *see* Phenytoin 1640
Dioctyl (GB) *see* Docusate 661
Diondel (AR, CL, UY) *see* Flecainide 882
Diondel (ES) *see* Metolazone 1348
Diopass (KR) *see* Valsartan 2127
Diopine-C (MX) *see* Dipivefrin 651
Diopine (ES, GR) *see* Dipivefrin 651
Diosfen (VN) *see* Etidronate 813
Dioten (KR) *see* Valsartan 2127
Di Ou Ping (CN) *see* Tropisetron [INT] 2108
Diovan D (AR, PY, UY) *see* Valsartan and Hydrochlorothiazide 2129
Diovan (AE, AR, AT, AU, BB, BD, BG, BH, BM, BO, BR, BS, BZ, CH, CN, CO, CR, CY, CZ, DE, DK, DO, EC, EE, EG, ES, FI, GB, GR, GT, GY, HK, HR, ID, IE, IL, IN, IQ, IR, IS, JM, JO, JP, KR, KW, LB, LT, LY, MX, MY, NI, NL, NO, NZ, OM, PA, PE, PH, PK, PL, PR, PT, PY, QA, RO, RU, SA, SE, SG, SI, SK, SR, SV, SY, TH, TR, TT, TW, UY, VE, VN, YE) *see* Valsartan 2127
Diovan/Amlibon (VE) *see* Amlodipine and Valsartan 126
Diovan Comp (DK, IS, NO, SE) *see* Valsartan and Hydrochlorothiazide 2129
Diovane (BG) *see* Valsartan 2127
Diovan HCT (BR, CO, EC, HN, PE, VE) *see* Valsartan and Hydrochlorothiazide 2129
Dioxaflex (DO, GT, HN, NI, PA, SV) *see* Diclofenac (Systemic) 617
Dipam (HR) *see* Indapamide 1065
Dipazide (TH) *see* GlipiZIDE 967
Dip (CO, EC) *see* Sucralfate 1940
Dipentum (AE, AR, AT, AU, BH, CH, CY, DE, DK, EG, FI, FR, GB, GR, HK, HN, HU, IE, IL, IQ, IR, IS, IT, JO, KR, KW, LB, LY, NL, NO, NZ, OM, PT, QA, SA, SE, SY, TR, YE, ZA) *see* Olsalazine 1500
Diperpen (IT) *see* Pipemidic Acid [INT] 1655
Dipezona (AR) *see* Diazepam 613
Diphedan (HU) *see* Phenytoin 1640
Diphenoxylate A (MY) *see* Diphenoxylate and Atropine 644
Diphereline (AU, RO, VN) *see* Triptorelin 2107
Diphereline PR (HK, KR, TW) *see* Triptorelin 2107
Diphergan (PL) *see* Promethazine 1723
Diphos (DE) *see* Etidronate 813
Dipinkor (ID) *see* NIFEdipine 1451
Dipion (KR) *see* Diethylpropion 624
Dipiperon (BE, CH, DE, DK, FR, GR, LU, NL) *see* Pipamperone [INT] 1655
Dipoquin (NZ) *see* Dipivefrin 651
Diporax (TW) *see* Clidinium and Chlordiazepoxide 460
Dipot (TH) *see* Clorazepate 487
Dipoxido (TW) *see* ChlordiazePOXIDE 422
Dipresan (HR) *see* GuanFACINE 990
Diprin (BR) *see* Dipyrone [INT] 653
Diprine (TW) *see* Dipivefrin 651
Diprivan (AE, AR, AT, AU, BB, BE, BF, BG, BH, BJ, BM, BR, BS, BZ, CI, CL, CN, CO, CR, CY, CZ, DE, DK, DO, EE, EG, ES, ET, FI, FR, GB, GH, GM, GN, GR, GT, GY, HK, HN, HR, HU, ID, IE, IL, IN, IQ, IR, IT, JM, JO, KE, KW, LB, LR, LU, LY, MA, ML, MR, MT, MU, MW, MX, MY, NE, NG, NI, NL, NO, NZ, OM, PA, PE, PH, PK, PL, PR, PT, QA, RU, SA, SC, SD, SE, SI, SK, SL, SN, SR, SV, SY, TN, TR, TT, TW, TZ, UG, UY, VE, VN, YE, ZA, ZM, ZW) *see* Propofol 1728
Diprocel (HK, MY) *see* Betamethasone (Topical) 255
Diproderm (AT, DK, ES, FI, IS, NO, SE) *see* Betamethasone (Topical) 255
Diprofen (TW) *see* Propofol 1728
Diprofol (IL) *see* Propofol 1728
Diprofos Depot (DK, PT) *see* Betamethasone (Systemic) 253
Diprolen (CH, DK, FI) *see* Betamethasone (Topical) 255
Diprolene (AE, BE, BH, FR, KW, NL, PH, PK, PL, QA, SA, TR) *see* Betamethasone (Topical) 255
Di-Promal (AT) *see* Ipratropium and Albuterol 1109
Diprophos (BG, CH, HU, SK) *see* Betamethasone (Systemic) 253
Diprosone (AU, BE, BG, BH, BR, CO, CZ, DE, EG, FR, GB, HK, IT, KW, LB, MY, NL, NZ, PE, PH, PT, PY, QA, SA, SI, TH, VN) *see* Betamethasone (Topical) 255
Diprosone Depot (DE) *see* Betamethasone (Systemic) 253
Diprospan (CN, DK, HK, IS, SG, TH, VN) *see* Betamethasone (Systemic) 253
Diprotop (TH) *see* Betamethasone (Topical) 255
Dipyrol (ZA) *see* Dipyridamole 652
Diqvan (KR) *see* Valsartan 2127
Diralox (ID) *see* Furazolidone [INT] 940
Dirastan (CZ) *see* TOLBUTamide 2062
Dirine (MY) *see* Furosemide 940
Diroquine (TH) *see* Chloroquine 424
Diroton (EE, SK) *see* Lisinopril 1226
Dirox (AR) *see* Acetaminophen 32
Dirpasid (MX) *see* Metoclopramide 1345
Dirytmin (LU, NL, SE) *see* Disopyramide 653
Disalazin (PE) *see* SulfaSALAzine 1950
Disalcid (BB, BM, BS, BZ, GY, JM, NL, SR, TT) *see* Salsalate 1862
Disal (KR, TW) *see* Salsalate 1862
Disalunil (BG, PL) *see* Hydrochlorothiazide 1009
Disalunil (PL) *see* Chlorothiazide 426
Disartan (TW) *see* Valsartan 2127
Disbronc (CL) *see* Ciclesonide (Systemic) 432
Discral (MX) *see* Sucralfate 1940
Discretal (AR) *see* Tibolone [INT] 2035
Disemide (TW) *see* Furosemide 940
Diseptyl (IL) *see* Sulfamethoxazole and Trimethoprim 1946
Disflam (EC) *see* Diclofenac (Systemic) 617
Disgren (AR, BR, ES, HU, KR, KW, LB, MX, PK, PY, UY, VE) *see* Triflusal [INT] 2103
Di Shuang (CN) *see* Dipyrone [INT] 653
Disipal (CH, CZ, IE, IT, LU, NO, SE) *see* Orphenadrine 1522

Dislipen (PY) *see* Ciprofibrate [INT] 441
Dismam L (PE) *see* Lactulose 1156
Dismaren (AR) *see* Cinnarizine [INT] 440
Dismifen (MX) *see* Acetaminophen 32
Disocor (PL) *see* Disopyramide 653
Disofrol (SE) *see* Pseudoephedrine 1742
Disol (HK) *see* Bromhexine [INT] 291
Disomet (FI) *see* Disopyramide 653
Disonate (IN) *see* Etidronate 813
Disoprivan (CH, HR) *see* Propofol 1728
Disorat (AE) *see* Metipranolol 1345
Disothiazide (IL) *see* Hydrochlorothiazide 1009
Dispamet (AE, BH, CY, EG, IQ, IR, JO, KW, LB, LY, OM, QA, SA, SY, YE) *see* Cimetidine 438
Dispatim (DE) *see* Timolol (Ophthalmic) 2043
Dispel (PH) *see* Domperidone [CAN/INT] 666
Dispercort (UY) *see* Deflazacort [INT] 587
Dispon (IT) *see* Liothyronine 1221
Dispril (AE, BE, BH, CY, EG, IQ, IR, JO, KW, LB, LY, NO, OM, QA, SA, SY, TR, YE) *see* Aspirin 180
Disprin (BB, BF, BJ, BM, BS, BZ, CI, ET, GB, GH, GM, GN, GY, HK, IE, IN, JM, KE, LR, MA, ML, MR, MU, MW, NE, NG, NZ, PK, PR, SC, SD, SG, SL, SN, SR, TN, TT, TZ, UG, ZM, ZW) *see* Aspirin 180
Disron-P (JP) *see* HydrOXYzine 1024
Dissenten (IT) *see* Loperamide 1236
Dissilax (AE, BH, CY, EG, IQ, IR, JO, KW, LB, LY, OM, QA, SA, SY, YE) *see* Bisacodyl 265
Distaclor (CO, GB, IE, MY, SG, TH) *see* Cefaclor 372
Distamine (GB, IE, NL) *see* PenicillAMINE 1608
Distaph (AU) *see* Dicloxacillin 621
Distaxid (ES) *see* Nizatidine 1471
Distensil (PE) *see* Succinylcholine 1939
Distex (CL, CN) *see* Flurbiprofen (Systemic) 906
Distinon (IN) *see* Pyridostigmine 1746
Distocide (AE, BH, CY, EG, IL, IN, IQ, IR, JO, KR, KW, LB, LY, OM, QA, SA, SG, SY, VN, YE) *see* Praziquantel 1702
Distrin (KR) *see* Diacerein [INT] 613
Disudrin (ID) *see* Pseudoephedrine 1742
Disuf (HK) *see* Fusidic Acid (Topical) [CAN/INT] 943
Disulfix (AR) *see* Disulfiram 654
Disulone (FR) *see* Dapsone (Systemic) 561
Ditamin (HR, PL) *see* Dihydroergotamine 633
DiTe Anatoxal Berna Adults (NZ) *see* Diphtheria and Tetanus Toxoid 645
DiTe Anatoxal Berna Children (NZ) *see* Diphtheria and Tetanus Toxoid 645
DITE Anatoxal Berna (PH, TH) *see* Diphtheria and Tetanus Toxoid 645
diTe Booster (DK) *see* Diphtheria and Tetanus Toxoid 645
Ditenaten (DE) *see* Theophylline 2026
DiTePer Anatoxal Berna Vaccine (HK, MY, PH) *see* Diphtheria and Tetanus Toxoids, and Acellular Pertussis Vaccine 649
Dithiazide (AU) *see* Hydrochlorothiazide 1009
Dithrasis (FR) *see* Anthralin 150
Dithrocream (GB, IE, IL) *see* Anthralin 150
Ditoin (HK, MY, TH) *see* Phenytoin 1640
Ditranol FNA (NL) *see* Anthralin 150
Ditropan (AE, AR, AT, AU, BE, CH, CY, CZ, FI, FR, GB, GR, HN, HU, IT, JO, KR, KW, LB, LU, PL, PT, SE, TW) *see* Oxybutynin 1536
Ditterolina (MX) *see* Dicloxacillin 621
Diubiz (PH) *see* Hydrochlorothiazide 1009
Diulactone (PH) *see* Spironolactone 1931
Diulo (AU, PT) *see* Metolazone 1348
Diupill (PH) *see* Furosemide 940
Diurace (PE) *see* Hydrochlorothiazide 1009
Diuracet-K (PE) *see* Hydrochlorothiazide and Triamterene 1012
Diural (DK, NO, SE) *see* Furosemide 940
Diural (UY) *see* AcetaZOLAMIDE 39
Diuramid (PL) *see* AcetaZOLAMIDE 39
Diurecide (PE) *see* Mannitol 1269
Diuremid CR (RO) *see* Indapamide 1065
Diuremid SR (RO) *see* Indapamide 1065
Diuresal (AE, BF, BH, BJ, CI, CY, EG, ET, GH, GM, GN, IQ, IR, JO, KE, KW, LB, LR, LY, MA, ML, MR, MU, MW, NE, NG, OM, QA, SA, SC, SD, SL, SN, SY, TN, TZ, UG, YE, ZM, ZW) *see* Furosemide 940
Diures (PH) *see* Hydrochlorothiazide 1009
Diuret-P (TH) *see* Hydrochlorothiazide 1009
Diurexan (GB, KR, PT) *see* Xipamide [INT] 2191
Diurex (AR, PY) *see* Hydrochlorothiazide 1009
Diurilix (FR) *see* Chlorothiazide 426
Diurin (NZ) *see* Furosemide 940
Diurix (BR) *see* Hydrochlorothiazide 1009
Diurone (AU) *see* Chlorothiazide 426
Diuron (HR) *see* Eplerenone 740
Diurosulfona (ES) *see* Chlorothiazide 426
Diursan (PY) *see* Hydrochlorothiazide 1009
Diusemide (BF, BJ, CI, ET, GH, GM, GN, KE, LR, MA, ML, MR, MU, MW, NE, NG, SC, SD, SL, SN, TN, TZ, UG, ZM, ZW) *see* Furosemide 940
Diutropan (TH) *see* Oxybutynin 1536
Diuvar (ID) *see* Furosemide 940
Diuver (CZ, PL, RU) *see* Torsemide 2071
Diuzid (PH) *see* Hydrochlorothiazide 1009
Diva-35 (ZA) *see* Cyproterone and Ethinyl Estradiol [CAN/INT] 532
Divaltan (KR) *see* Valsartan 2127
Divarius (FR) *see* PARoxetine 1579
Divigel (CH, DK, EE, IN, MY, SE, SG, TH, TW) *see* Estradiol (Systemic) 775
Divir (PY) *see* Didanosine 622
Divoltar (ID) *see* Diclofenac (Systemic) 617
Divonal (PE) *see* DimenhyDRINATE 637
Dixamid (GR) *see* Indapamide 1065
Dixarit (LU, NZ) *see* CloNIDine 480
Dixeran (AT, BE, CH) *see* Melitracen [INT] 1283
Dixi-35 (CL, PE, PY) *see* Cyproterone and Ethinyl Estradiol [CAN/INT] 532
Dixin (CO) *see* ALPRAZolam 94
Dizine (ID) *see* Flunarizine [CAN/INT] 892
Dizinil (AE, BH, KW, QA, SA) *see* DimenhyDRINATE 637
Dizitab (PH) *see* Meclizine 1277
Dizoflox (PH) *see* Ofloxacin (Otic) 1491
Dizole One (AU) *see* Fluconazole 885
Dizzigo (IN) *see* Cinnarizine [INT] 440
Dizzinon (PH) *see* Cinnarizine [INT] 440
DKB-GT (JP) *see* Dibekacin [INT] 616
D-Mannitol (KR) *see* Mannitol 1269
DMPS-Heyl (NO) *see* Dimercaprol 638
DMZone (KR) *see* Pioglitazone 1654
Doang (TW) *see* DimenhyDRINATE 637
Dobamin (KR) *see* DOBUTamine 654
Dobesin (DK) *see* Diethylpropion 624
Dobetin (IT, VE) *see* Cyanocobalamin 515
Dobtan (BR) *see* DOBUTamine 654
Dobucard (MY, PH) *see* DOBUTamine 654
Dobucor (ES) *see* DOBUTamine 654
Dobu-Hameln (PE) *see* DOBUTamine 654
Dobuject (AE, BH, CZ, DK, FI, ID, IL, JO, KR, MX, NZ, PH, PK, PL, RU, SA, SE, SG, TW) *see* DOBUTamine 654
Dobunex (PH) *see* DOBUTamine 654
Dobupal (ES) *see* Venlafaxine 2150
Doburan (ID, KR, PH, VE) *see* DOBUTamine 654
Dobusafe (CO, VN) *see* DOBUTamine 654
Dobutamina Abbott (ES) *see* DOBUTamine 654
Dobutamina (EC) *see* DOBUTamine 654
Dobutamina Inibsa (ES) *see* DOBUTamine 654
Dobutamina Rovi (ES) *see* DOBUTamine 654
Dobutamine Aguettant (FR) *see* DOBUTamine 654
Dobutamine Hydrochloride (GB) *see* DOBUTamine 654

Dobutamine Panpharma (FR) *see* DOBUTamine 654
Dobutamin Hexal (DE, HU) *see* DOBUTamine 654
Dobutamin-Ratiopharm (DE) *see* DOBUTamine 654
Dobutel (PH, TH) *see* DOBUTamine 654
Dobutrex (AU, BE, BF, BG, BH, BJ, CH, CI, CZ, DK, EG, ES, ET, FR, GB, GH, GM, GN, HN, HR, HU, IE, IN, IT, JO, KE, KR, LR, MA, ML, MR, MU, MW, MX, MY, NE, NG, NL, NO, PY, QA, RU, SA, SC, SD, SE, SI, SL, SN, TN, TR, TZ, UG, VN, ZM, ZW) *see* DOBUTamine 654
Docaciclo (BE) *see* Acyclovir (Systemic) 47
Docatone (ES) *see* Doxapram 673
Doccefaclo (BE) *see* Cefaclor 372
Docetax (PH) *see* DOCEtaxel 656
Docetere (ID) *see* DOCEtaxel 656
Docilen (PE, PY, UY) *see* Zopiclone [CAN/INT] 2217
Docin (TH) *see* Indomethacin 1067
Dociton (DE) *see* Propranolol 1731
Docpirace (BE) *see* Piracetam [INT] 1661
Docusaat FNA (NL) *see* Docusate 661
Docusoft (IL) *see* Docusate 661
Docusol (GB) *see* Docusate 661
Docyl (TH) *see* Doxycycline 689
Dodecavit (FR) *see* Hydroxocobalamin 1020
Dodec (TR) *see* Cyanocobalamin 515
Dodemina (MX) *see* Pyridoxine 1747
Doflex (IN) *see* Diclofenac (Systemic) 617
Dofu (TW) *see* Doxepin (Systemic) 676
Dofu (TW) *see* Doxepin (Topical) 678
Doinmycin (TW) *see* Doxycycline 689
Doka (HR) *see* Doxazosin 674
Dokard (PH) *see* DOPamine 669
Dokat (TR) *see* Doxycycline 689
Doketrol (AR) *see* Nitroprusside 1467
Doksiciklin (HR) *see* Doxycycline 689
Doksin (TR) *see* Doxycycline 689
Doktacillin (SE) *see* Ampicillin 141
Dolac (BF, BJ, CI, ET, GH, GM, GN, ID, KE, LR, MA, ML, MR, MU, MW, NE, NG, RU, SC, SD, SL, SN, TN, TZ, UG, ZM, ZW) *see* Ketorolac (Systemic) 1146
Dolafen (PH) *see* Ibuprofen 1032
Dolaforte (AU) *see* Acetaminophen and Codeine 36
Dolanaest (DE) *see* Bupivacaine 299
Dolanet (PY) *see* Dipyrone [INT] 653
Dolan FP (PH) *see* Ibuprofen 1032
Dolan Infantil (GT, HN, NI, SV) *see* Acetaminophen 32
Dolantag (EC, PE) *see* Acetaminophen and Tramadol 37
Dolantina (BR) *see* Meperidine 1293
Dolantin (DE) *see* Meperidine 1293
Dolantine (BE) *see* Meperidine 1293
Dolapent (FI, PL) *see* Pentazocine 1616
Dolapril (AU, VN) *see* Trandolapril 2080
Dolargan (HN, PL) *see* Meperidine 1293
Dolcet (PH) *see* Acetaminophen and Tramadol 37
Dolchis (VN) *see* Etodolac 815
Dolcol (JP) *see* Pipemidic Acid [INT] 1655
Dolcontin Depottab (NO) *see* Morphine (Systemic) 1394
Dolcontin (FI, SE) *see* Morphine (Systemic) 1394
Dolcontin (GR) *see* Dihydrocodeine, Aspirin, and Caffeine 632
Dolemicin (ES) *see* Dipyrone [INT] 653
Dolestine (IL) *see* Meperidine 1293
Doletran (PY) *see* DOCEtaxel 656
Doleven (JP) *see* Hydroxocobalamin 1020
Dolex (UY) *see* Acetaminophen 32
Dolezine (VN) *see* Olmesartan 1496
Dolforin (BG) *see* FentaNYL 857
Dolgan (MX) *see* Dipyrone [INT] 653
Dolgesic (ES) *see* Acetaminophen 32
Dolgit (AE, BH, CY, DE, EG, IQ, IR, JO, KW, LB, LY, OM, QA, SA, SY, YE) *see* Ibuprofen 1032
Dolinac (IT) *see* Felbinac [INT] 850
Dolipol (FR) *see* TOLBUTamide 2062
Doliprane (FR, IN, LB, MA) *see* Acetaminophen 32
Dolisec (GR) *see* Sucralfate 1940
Dolitabs (FR) *see* Acetaminophen 32
Dolmal (PH) *see* TraMADol 2074
Dolmed (FI) *see* Methadone 1311
Dolmen (EE) *see* Dexketoprofen [INT] 603
Dolmen (IT) *see* Tenoxicam [INT] 2001
Dolobid (AE, BF, BH, BJ, CI, CZ, ET, GH, GM, GN, KE, KW, LR, MA, ML, MR, MU, MW, MX, NE, NG, PT, QA, RU, SA, SC, SD, SL, SN, TH, TN, TZ, UG, ZA, ZM, ZW) *see* Diflunisal 626
Doloc (CL) *see* Nimesulide [INT] 1456
Dolocaine (PH) *see* Lidocaine (Systemic) 1208
Dolocalma (PT) *see* Dipyrone [INT] 653
Dolocid (NL) *see* Diflunisal 626
Doloctaprin (AR) *see* Nimesulide [INT] 1456
Dolocyl (CH) *see* Ibuprofen 1032
Dolodent (DK) *see* Benzocaine 246
Dolodol (ES) *see* TraMADol 2074
Dolofar (CL) *see* Ketoprofen 1145
Dolofast (EC) *see* Ketoprofen 1145
Doloflam (PH) *see* Diclofenac (Systemic) 617
Dologesic (PH) *see* Acetaminophen and Tramadol 37
Dolomax (CO) *see* Ketoprofen 1145
Dolomax (PE) *see* Ibuprofen 1032
Dolomol (AE, BH, CY, EG, IQ, IR, JO, KW, LB, LY, OM, QA, SA, SY, YE) *see* Acetaminophen 32
Dolonac (VN) *see* Clidinium and Chlordiazepoxide 460
Dolones (ID) *see* Lidocaine and Prilocaine 1213
Dolonex (IN) *see* Piroxicam 1662
Dolonime (CO) *see* Nimesulide [INT] 1456
Dolonovag (AR) *see* HYDROmorphone 1016
Doloral (PE) *see* Ibuprofen 1032
Dolorex Gel (PE) *see* Ketorolac (Systemic) 1146
Dolorex (PE) *see* Ketorolac (Systemic) 1146
Dolormin (DE) *see* Ibuprofen 1032
Dolorol Forte (ZA) *see* Acetaminophen and Codeine 36
Dolorol (ZA) *see* Acetaminophen 32
Dolosal (BR) *see* Meperidine 1293
Dolostan (LB) *see* Mefenamic Acid 1280
Dolo Target (CH) *see* Felbinac [INT] 850
Dolotral (PH) *see* TraMADol 2074
Dolotren (DO, GT, HN, NI, PA, SV) *see* Diclofenac (Systemic) 617
Doloverina (PY) *see* Mebeverine [INT] 1275
Dolpaz (PH) *see* TraMADol 2074
Dolprone (LU) *see* Acetaminophen 32
Dol-Proxyvon (IN) *see* Tapentadol 1975
Dolquine (ES) *see* Hydroxychloroquine 1021
Dolquine (SG) *see* Chloroquine 424
Dolsin (CZ) *see* Meperidine 1293
Dol-Stop (LU) *see* Acetaminophen 32
Doltard (DK, EE) *see* Morphine (Systemic) 1394
Dolten (AR, PY) *see* Ketorolac (Systemic) 1146
Doltramcet (KR) *see* Acetaminophen and Tramadol 37
Doluvital (MX) *see* Acetaminophen 32
Dolvifen (MX) *see* Pyridoxine 1747
Dolviran (MX) *see* Acetaminophen 32
Dolzam (LU) *see* TraMADol 2074
Domar (HK, IT, SG, TH) *see* Pinazepam [INT] 1652
Domecin (JP) *see* Methyldopa 1332
Dome (ID) *see* Domperidone [CAN/INT] 666
Domer (MX) *see* Omeprazole 1508
Domeran (ID) *see* Domperidone [CAN/INT] 666
Domerdon (TH) *see* Domperidone [CAN/INT] 666
Domes (IT) *see* Nimesulide [INT] 1456
Domical (GB) *see* Amitriptyline 119
Domide (MY) *see* Thalidomide 2022
Domiken (MX) *see* Doxycycline 689
Domilium (TW) *see* Trifluoperazine 2102
Domi (MY) *see* Midazolam 1361
Domina (HK, VN) *see* Hydroquinone 1020
Dominal (ID) *see* Domperidone [CAN/INT] 666

Dominic (ID) *see* DOBUTamine ... 654
Dominium (EC) *see* FLUoxetine ... 899
Dominum (CO) *see* Sertraline ... 1878
Domitrone (PH) *see* MitoXANtrone ... 1382
Domnamid (DK, NO) *see* Estazolam ... 775
Domp-M (TH) *see* Domperidone [CAN/INT] ... 666
Domperid (CN) *see* Domperidone [CAN/INT] ... 666
Domperine (KR) *see* Domperidone [CAN/INT] ... 666
Domper (PH, TW) *see* Domperidone [CAN/INT] ... 666
Dompe (TW) *see* Domperidone [CAN/INT] ... 666
Dompil (VN) *see* Domperidone [CAN/INT] ... 666
Domp (TH) *see* Domperidone [CAN/INT] ... 666
Dompy (AE, QA) *see* Domperidone [CAN/INT] ... 666
Domstal (IN) *see* Domperidone [CAN/INT] ... 666
Donafan (PE) *see* Loperamide ... 1236
Donalgin (HU) *see* Niflumic Acid [INT] ... 1454
Donamed F (PE) *see* Loperamide ... 1236
Don-A (PH) *see* Domperidone [CAN/INT] ... 666
Donaren (BR) *see* TraZODone ... 2091
Donaren Retard (BR) *see* TraZODone ... 2091
Donataxel (EC) *see* DOCEtaxel ... 656
Donaz (IN) *see* Donepezil ... 668
Done-5 (PH) *see* Donepezil ... 668
Donecept (HK, TR) *see* Donepezil ... 668
Donecil (PE) *see* Donepezil ... 668
Donept (TH) *see* Donepezil ... 668
Doneurin (DE) *see* Doxepin (Systemic) ... 676
Donezel (PH) *see* Donepezil ... 668
Donezil (KR, MY) *see* Donepezil ... 668
Dong Kang Ming (CN) *see* Ofloxacin (Ophthalmic) ... 1491
Dong Koo Dermo Lotion (KR) *see* Desonide ... 597
Donnatal Ekixir (TH) *see* Hyoscyamine, Atropine, Scopolamine, and Phenobarbital ... 1027
Donnatal (ZA) *see* Hyoscyamine, Atropine, Scopolamine, and Phenobarbital ... 1027
Donobid (NO, SE) *see* Diflunisal ... 626
Donobin (PK) *see* DAUNOrubicin (Conventional) ... 577
Donulide (PT) *see* Nimesulide [INT] ... 1456
Dopacard (CH, DE, DK, FR, GB, IE, NL, SE) *see* Dopexamine [INT] ... 671
Dopacris (BR) *see* DOPamine ... 669
Dopadura (DE) *see* Carbidopa and Levodopa ... 351
Dopagyt (IN) *see* Methyldopa ... 1332
Dopamax (PH) *see* DOPamine ... 669
Dopamet (HK, ID, NO, PH, TR) *see* Methyldopa ... 1332
Dopamex (TH) *see* DOPamine ... 669
Dopamina (ES) *see* DOPamine ... 669
Dopamin AWD (HN) *see* DOPamine ... 669
Dopamin (BG, CH, NO) *see* DOPamine ... 669
Dopamine (FR, NL) *see* DOPamine ... 669
Dopamine Injection (AU) *see* DOPamine ... 669
Dopamine Pierre Fabre (LU) *see* DOPamine ... 669
Dopamin Giulini (HU, LU) *see* DOPamine ... 669
Dopamin Guilini (AT, DE, ID) *see* DOPamine ... 669
Dopamin Natterman (BG) *see* DOPamine ... 669
Dopaminum (PL) *see* DOPamine ... 669
Dopamix (KR) *see* DOPamine ... 669
Dopanore (AE, JO, SA) *see* Methyldopa ... 1332
Dopapro (KR) *see* ROPINIRole ... 1844
Dopareel (HK) *see* Zopiclone [CAN/INT] ... 2217
Doparine (PH) *see* Methyldopa ... 1332
Dopar (TW) *see* DOPamine ... 669
Dopatab M (HK) *see* Methyldopa ... 1332
Dopavate (TW) *see* DOPamine ... 669
Dopegyt (AE, BB, BG, BH, BM, BS, BZ, CY, CZ, EG, GY, HU, IL, IQ, IR, JM, JO, KW, LB, LY, MY, OM, PL, PR, QA, RO, RU, SA, SR, SY, TT, YE) *see* Methyldopa ... 1332
Dopezil (PH) *see* Donepezil ... 668
Dophilin (TW) *see* Doxazosin ... 674
Dopicar (IL) *see* Carbidopa and Levodopa ... 351
Dopil (HR) *see* Donepezil ... 668
Dopina (PE) *see* DOPamine ... 669
Dopinga (IN) *see* DOPamine ... 669
Dopin (TH) *see* Dosulepin [INT] ... 673
Dopmin (CZ, DK, EE, FI, MY, TR, TW) *see* DOPamine ... 669
Dopmin E (RU) *see* DOPamine ... 669
Dopram (AT, AU, BE, CH, DE, DK, EG, FI, FR, GR, IE, NL, SA, ZA) *see* Doxapram ... 673
Dopress (KR) *see* Methyldopa ... 1332
Dopress (NZ) *see* Dosulepin [INT] ... 673
Doprosone (AE) *see* Betamethasone (Topical) ... 255
Dopsan (TH) *see* Dapsone (Systemic) ... 561
Doralese (GB, IE) *see* Indoramin [INT] ... 1070
Doranit (ID) *see* Ranitidine ... 1777
Dorbantil (PY) *see* Doxazosin ... 674
Doremi (KR) *see* Alclometasone ... 72
Dorfene (PK) *see* Buprenorphine ... 300
Doribax (AR, AT, CO, CY, CZ, DE, EE, FR, GR, HK, HN, HR, HU, ID, IE, IL, LB, MY, NL, NO, PH, PL, QA, SA, SE, SG, SI, TH, TR, VN) *see* Doripenem ... 671
Doricox (IN) *see* Etoricoxib [INT] ... 821
Doricum (VE) *see* Midazolam ... 1361
Doriglen (IN) *see* Doripenem ... 671
Dorink (TW) *see* Danazol ... 558
Doriprex (RU) *see* Doripenem ... 671
Dorken (ES) *see* Clorazepate ... 487
Dorlotin (HU) *see* Amobarbital ... 128
Dorlotyn (HU) *see* Amobarbital ... 128
Dormatylan (AT) *see* Secobarbital ... 1872
Dormeben (CO) *see* Zolpidem ... 2212
Dormelox (BR) *see* Meloxicam ... 1283
Dormex (CL) *see* Brotizolam [INT] ... 293
Dormex (PE) *see* Zopiclone [CAN/INT] ... 2217
Dorme (ZA) *see* Quazepam ... 1751
Dormicum (AE, AR, AT, BB, BD, BE, BF, BG, BH, BJ, BM, BS, BZ, CH, CI, CN, CO, CY, CZ, DE, DK, EC, EE, EG, ES, ET, FI, GH, GM, GN, GR, GY, HK, HR, HU, ID, IQ, IR, IS, JM, JO, JP, KE, KR, KW, LB, LR, LT, LU, LY, MA, ML, MR, MT, MU, MW, MX, NE, NG, NL, NO, OM, PH, PK, PL, PT, PY, QA, RO, RU, SA, SC, SD, SE, SG, SI, SK, SL, SN, SR, SY, TH, TN, TR, TT, TW, TZ, UG, UY, VN, YE, ZA, ZM, ZW) *see* Midazolam ... 1361
Dormicum[inj.] (HR) *see* Midazolam ... 1361
Dormi (ID) *see* Scopolamine (Systemic) ... 1870
Dormirex (GT) *see* HydrOXYzine ... 1024
Dormital (PY) *see* PHENobarbital ... 1632
Dormital (UY) *see* PENTobarbital ... 1617
Dormizol (AU) *see* Zolpidem ... 2212
Dormizol (PH) *see* Midazolam ... 1361
Dormodor (ES, ZA) *see* Flurazepam ... 906
Dormonid (BR, CL, PE) *see* Midazolam ... 1361
Dormonoct (AR, BE, GB, IE, NL, PT, ZA) *see* Loprazolam [INT] ... 1241
Dormutil (DE) *see* DiphenhydrAMINE (Systemic) ... 641
Dormutil N (NO) *see* DiphenhydrAMINE (Systemic) ... 641
Dormyl (GR) *see* Quazepam ... 1751
Dorner (CN, ID, JP, PH, TH) *see* Beraprost [INT] ... 251
Dornot (BR) *see* Meperidine ... 1293
Dorocor (VN) *see* Cefaclor ... 372
Dortisop (KR) *see* Dorzolamide and Timolol ... 673
Doryl (FI) *see* Carbachol ... 346
Doryx (AU, NZ) *see* Doxycycline ... 689
Dorzolam (CO) *see* Dorzolamide ... 673
Dorzolol (CO) *see* Dorzolamide and Timolol ... 673
Dorzopt (CO) *see* Dorzolamide and Timolol ... 673
Dorzox (IN) *see* Dorzolamide ... 673
Dosabin (TW) *see* Doxazosin ... 674
Dosan (NZ) *see* Doxazosin ... 674
Dosberotec (DE, IT) *see* Fenoterol [INT] ... 857
Dosier (DO, EC, GT, HN, MX, NI, SV) *see* Mosapride [INT] ... 1401
Dosin (CL) *see* Domperidone [CAN/INT] ... 666
Dosiseptine (FR) *see* Chlorhexidine Gluconate ... 422

Dosixbe (AR) *see* Hydroxocobalamin 1020
Doslax (IN) *see* Docusate 661
Dosmin (KR) *see* Pyridostigmine 1746
Dospir (CH) *see* Ipratropium and Albuterol 1109
Dostan (AU) *see* Cabergoline 319
Dosteril (MX) *see* Lisinopril 1226
Dostinex (AE, AT, AU, BE, BG, BH, BR, CH, CL, CO, CR, CY, CZ, DE, DK, DO, EC, EE, EG, ES, FI, FR, GB, GR, GT, HK, HN, IE, IL, IQ, IR, IS, IT, JO, KR, KW, LB, LT, LU, LY, MT, MX, MY, NI, NL, NO, NZ, OM, PA, PE, PL, PT, QA, RO, RU, SA, SE, SG, SI, SK, SV, SY, TR, TW, UY, VE, YE, ZA) *see* Cabergoline 319
Dostin (PK) *see* Erdosteine [INT] 753
Dostol (EC) *see* Erdosteine [INT] 753
Dotaxel (KR) *see* DOCEtaxel 656
Dothapax (GB) *see* Dosulepin [INT] 673
Dothcin (IN) *see* Dosulepin [INT] 673
Dothep (AU, IE, MY) *see* Dosulepin [INT] 673
Dothip (IN) *see* Dosulepin [INT] 673
Dothrocyn (ID) *see* Erythromycin (Systemic) 762
Dotramol (ID) *see* Acetaminophen and Tramadol 37
Dotur (UY) *see* Doxycycline 689
Doulishu (TW) *see* Adapalene 54
Douzabin Retard Forte (LB) *see* Hydroxocobalamin 1020
Doval (ZA) *see* Diazepam 613
Dovate (ZA) *see* Clobetasol 468
Dovir (CO) *see* Hydrocodone and Ibuprofen 1013
Dovobet (BE, GB, GR, IE, IT, NL) *see* Calcipotriene and Betamethasone 321
Dovonex (EG, GB, GR, IE, JP, ZA) *see* Calcipotriene 321
Doxaben XL (TW) *see* Doxazosin 674
Doxaben (TW) *see* Doxazosin 674
Doxacard (IN) *see* Doxazosin 674
Doxacor (PE) *see* Doxazosin 674
Doxagamma (DE) *see* Doxazosin 674
Doxal (FI) *see* Doxepin (Systemic) 676
Doxan (TW) *see* Doxazosin 674
Doxapril (AR) *see* Lisinopril 1226
Doxa (PY) *see* DOBUTamine 654
Doxar (PH) *see* Losartan 1248
Doxat (BH, CY, EG, IQ, IR, JO, KW, LB, LY, OM, QA, SA, SY, VN, YE) *see* Doxycycline 689
Doxatensa (ES) *see* Doxazosin 674
Doxazone XL SR (KR) *see* Doxazosin 674
Doxazosina Alter (ES) *see* Doxazosin 674
Doxazosina Cinfa (ES) *see* Doxazosin 674
Doxazosina Combino Pharm (ES) *see* Doxazosin 674
Doxazosina Geminis (ES) *see* Doxazosin 674
Doxazosina Normon (ES) *see* Doxazosin 674
Doxazosina Pharmagenus (ES) *see* Doxazosin 674
Doxazosina Ratiopharm (ES) *see* Doxazosin 674
Doxazosina Ur (ES) *see* Doxazosin 674
Doxecal (PH) *see* DOCEtaxel 656
Doxecan (KR) *see* Doxepin (Systemic) 676
Doxepia (DE) *see* Doxepin (Systemic) 676
Doxetal (JO) *see* DOCEtaxel 656
Doxetar (IN) *see* Doxepin (Systemic) 676
Doxetasan (ID) *see* DOCEtaxel 656
Doxet (PE) *see* DULoxetine 698
Doxfree (IN) *see* Doxofylline [INT] 679
Doxican (PT) *see* Tenoxicam [INT] 2001
Doxiclat (ES) *see* Doxycycline 689
Doxil (IL) *see* DOXOrubicin (Liposomal) 684
Doximed (FI) *see* Doxycycline 689
Doxime (PY) *see* Sertraline 1878
Doximycin (FI) *see* Doxycycline 689
Doxine (NZ) *see* Doxycycline 689
Doxin (IN) *see* Doxepin (Systemic) 676
Doxin (PH, TH) *see* Doxycycline 689
Doxiplus (PE) *see* Doxycycline 689
DOXO-cell (DE) *see* DOXOrubicin (Conventional) 679
Doxocris (AR) *see* DOXOrubicin (Conventional) 679
Doxolbran (AR) *see* Doxazosin 674
Doxolem RU (MX) *see* DOXOrubicin (Conventional) 679
Doxopeg (AR, BR, CL, CR, DO, GT, HN, MX, PE, SV) *see* DOXOrubicin (Liposomal) 684
Doxopeg (CO) *see* DOXOrubicin (Conventional) 679
Doxorbin (AR) *see* DOXOrubicin (Conventional) 679
Doxorubicina (ES) *see* DOXOrubicin (Conventional) 679
Doxorubicin Azupharma (DE) *see* DOXOrubicin (Conventional) 679
Doxorubicin Bigmar (CH) *see* DOXOrubicin (Conventional) 679
Doxorubicin Bristol (CH) *see* DOXOrubicin (Conventional) 679
Doxorubicine Asta (FR) *see* DOXOrubicin (Conventional) 679
Doxorubicin Ebewe (CH) *see* DOXOrubicin (Conventional) 679
Doxorubicine Dakota (FR) *see* DOXOrubicin (Conventional) 679
Doxorubicin Hexal (DE) *see* DOXOrubicin (Conventional) 679
Doxorubicin (IN) *see* DOXOrubicin (Conventional) 679
Doxorubicin NC (DE) *see* DOXOrubicin (Conventional) 679
Doxorubicin R.P. (DE) *see* DOXOrubicin (Conventional) 679
Doxorubicin "Paranova" (DK) *see* DOXOrubicin (Conventional) 679
Doxorubin (CH, DK, GB, IN, MY, NL, TH) *see* DOXOrubicin (Conventional) 679
Doxosol (FI) *see* DOXOrubicin (Conventional) 679
Doxsig (AU) *see* Doxycycline 689
Doxtie (AR, EC) *see* DOXOrubicin (Conventional) 679
Doxure (IN) *see* Doxepin (Topical) 678
Doxy-1 (IN) *see* Doxycycline 689
Doxy-100 (DE, NZ) *see* Doxycycline 689
Doxy 200 (LU) *see* Doxycycline 689
Doxy M (EE) *see* Doxycycline 689
Doxybene (CZ) *see* Doxycycline 689
Doxycap (HK, SG) *see* Doxycycline 689
Doxycin (SA) *see* Doxycycline 689
Doxycline (LU, TH) *see* Doxycycline 689
Doxycyclin AL (HU) *see* Doxycycline 689
Doxycycline (BE) *see* Doxycycline 689
Doxycycline-Ethypharm (LU) *see* Doxycycline 689
Doxycycline-Eurogenerics (LU) *see* Doxycycline 689
Doxydar (JO, SA) *see* Doxycycline 689
Doxyhexal (CZ, HU, LU) *see* Doxycycline 689
Doxy Komb (LU) *see* Doxycycline 689
Doxylag (BB, BF, BH, BJ, BM, BS, BZ, CI, CY, EG, ET, GH, GM, GN, GY, IQ, IR, JM, JO, KE, KW, LB, LR, LY, MA, ML, MR, MU, MW, NE, NG, OM, QA, SA, SC, SD, SL, SN, SR, SY, TN, TT, TZ, UG, YE, ZM, ZW) *see* Doxycycline 689
Doxy (LB) *see* Doxycycline 689
Doxylcap (TH) *see* Doxycycline 689
Doxylets (LU) *see* Doxycycline 689
Doxylin (AU, IL, NO, NZ) *see* Doxycycline 689
Doxyline (SG) *see* Doxycycline 689
Doxylis (FR) *see* Doxycycline 689
Doxymycine (LU) *see* Doxycycline 689
Doxymycin (TW, ZA) *see* Doxycycline 689
Doxypharm (HU) *see* Doxycycline 689
Doxy SMB (LU) *see* Doxycycline 689
Dozic (CO, PY) *see* OLANZapine 1491
Dozil (ID) *see* Donepezil 668
Dozola (TW) *see* Dorzolamide and Timolol 673
Dozozin (TH) *see* Doxazosin 674
D-Pam (NZ) *see* Diazepam 613
D-Penamine (AU, NZ) *see* PenicillAMINE 1608
D-Penil (PE) *see* PenicillAMINE 1608
DPT (TW) *see* Diphtheria and Tetanus Toxoids, and Acellular Pertussis Vaccine 649

Draconyl (GR) *see* Terbutaline 2004
Draganon (IT, JP) *see* Aniracetam [INT] 150
Dralitem (CR, EC, GT, HN, NI, PY, SV) *see* Temozolomide 1991
Dramamine (AE, AR, AU, BB, BD, BE, BF, BH, BJ, BM, BS, BZ, CI, CO, EG, ET, GB, GH, GM, GN, GY, ID, IE, IN, JM, JP, KE, KR, KW, LR, LU, MA, ML, MR, MU, MW, MX, NE, NG, NL, NZ, PR, QA, SC, SD, SG, SL, SN, SR, TN, TT, TW, TZ, UG, VE, ZA, ZM, ZW) *see* DimenhyDRINATE 637
Dramavir (ES) *see* DimenhyDRINATE 637
Dramavol (GT, HN, NI, PA, SV) *see* DimenhyDRINATE 637
Dramina (HR) *see* DimenhyDRINATE 637
Dramin (BR) *see* DimenhyDRINATE 637
Dranolis (GR) *see* Pindolol 1652
Dravyr (MY) *see* Aciclovir (Ophthalmic) [INT] 43
Dravyr (MY, SG) *see* Acyclovir (Systemic) 47
Dravyr (SG) *see* Acyclovir (Topical) 51
Dreisacarb (AT) *see* Calcium Carbonate 327
Drenaflen (EC) *see* Acetylcysteine 40
Drenison (BR) *see* Flurandrenolide 906
Drenural (MX) *see* Bumetanide 297
Drexel (VE) *see* Nimesulide [INT] 1456
Dridase (DE, NL) *see* Oxybutynin 1536
Dridol (NO, SE) *see* Droperidol 695
Driken (MX) *see* Iron Dextran Complex 1117
Drill (HU) *see* Carbocisteine [INT] 357
Driminate Supp (MY) *see* DimenhyDRINATE 637
Drinexin (PE) *see* Orphenadrine 1522
Drin (GR) *see* Ibuprofen 1032
Driptane (EE, HR, LB, PH, RU, VN) *see* Oxybutynin 1536
Dristan Sinus (CO) *see* Pseudoephedrine and Ibuprofen 1743
Drocef (KR) *see* Cefadroxil 372
Drofen (VN) *see* Ibandronate 1028
Drogenil (GB, IE) *see* Flutamide 907
Droleptan (AU, FR, GB, IE, VN) *see* Droperidol 695
Dromadol (GB) *see* TraMADol 2074
Dromyl (NO) *see* DimenhyDRINATE 637
Dronalen Plus (AU) *see* Alendronate and Cholecalciferol 81
Droncit Vet (NO) *see* Praziquantel 1702
Dronol (PY) *see* Permethrin 1627
Dropedol (TW) *see* Droperidol 695
Dropel (TW) *see* Droperidol 695
Droperdal (BR) *see* Droperidol 695
Droperidol (PL) *see* Droperidol 695
Droperol (IN) *see* Droperidol 695
Droriate (PK) *see* Risedronate 1816
Drosyn (IN) *see* Phenylephrine (Systemic) 1638
Drovax (ID) *see* Cefadroxil 372
Drowsy (TW) *see* Triazolam 2101
Droxamida (PE) *see* Hydroxyurea 1021
Droxicef (AE, BH, CY, EG, IQ, IR, JO, KW, LB, LY, OM, QA, SA, SY, VN, YE) *see* Cefadroxil 372
Droxil (AE, BH, CY, EG, IQ, IR, JO, KW, LB, LY, OM, QA, SA, SY, YE) *see* Cefadroxil 372
Droxine (AU, NZ) *see* Levothyroxine 1205
Droxol (AR) *see* Pirenzepine [INT] 1662
Droxyl (IN) *see* Cefadroxil 372
Drozid (PH) *see* Cefadroxil 372
Druisel (AR) *see* Ibuprofen 1032
Drynalken (MX) *see* DOPamine 669
Dryptal (IE) *see* Furosemide 940
D-Stop-ratiopharm (LU) *see* Loperamide 1236
D.T. COQ (MY) *see* Diphtheria and Tetanus Toxoids, and Acellular Pertussis Vaccine 649
DTIC (AT, ZA) *see* Dacarbazine 549
D.T.I.C. (DE) *see* Dacarbazine 549
D.T.I.C.-Dome (AT, SE, ZA) *see* Dacarbazine 549
DTIC-Dome (BE, GB, KR) *see* Dacarbazine 549
DTI (HK, KR) *see* Dacarbazine 549
DTM (IN) *see* Diltiazem 634
D.T. Vax Vaccine (AE) *see* Diphtheria and Tetanus Toxoid 645
Duacillin (MY) *see* Ampicillin 141
Duact (DK, FI, KR) *see* Acrivastine and Pseudoephedrine 46
Duactin 5 (AE, BH, CY, EG, IQ, IR, JO, KW, LB, LY, OM, QA, SA, SY, YE) *see* AmLODIPine 123
Dual Antigen (IN) *see* Diphtheria and Tetanus Toxoid 645
Dual Down (KR) *see* Amlodipine and Valsartan 126
Duasma (TW) *see* Budesonide (Systemic) 293
Duavent (PH) *see* Ipratropium and Albuterol 1109
Duavive (CZ, EE, HR, KR, LT, NL, PT, SE) *see* Estrogens (Conjugated/Equine) and Bazedoxifene 782
Dublina (CL) *see* Ciprofibrate [INT] 441
Duboisine (FR) *see* Hyoscyamine 1026
Ducodine (MY) *see* Pholcodine [INT] 1646
Dudencer (HK) *see* Omeprazole 1508
Duellin [+ Levodopa] (PL) *see* Carbidopa 351
Dufaston (IT) *see* Dydrogesterone [INT] 702
Dufine (PT) *see* ClomiPHENE 473
Duinum (BF, BJ, CI, ET, GH, GM, GN, KE, LR, MA, ML, MR, MU, MW, MY, NE, NG, SC, SD, SG, SL, SN, TH, TN, TZ, UG, VN, ZM, ZW) *see* ClomiPHENE 473
Dukoral® (CA) *see* Travelers' Diarrhea and Cholera Vaccine [CAN/INT] 2088
Dulcolan (VE) *see* Bisacodyl 265
Dulcolax (AE, AR, AT, AU, BB, BE, BF, BG, BH, BJ, BM, BR, BS, BZ, CH, CI, CN, CO, CR, CY, CZ, DE, DK, DO, EG, ET, FR, GB, GH, GM, GN, GR, GT, GY, HK, HN, HR, IN, IQ, IR, IS, IT, JM, JO, KE, KR, KW, LB, LR, LU, LY, MA, ML, MR, MU, MW, MX, MY, NE, NG, NI, NL, NO, NZ, OM, PA, PE, PH, PK, PT, QA, RO, RU, SA, SC, SD, SE, SI, SK, SL, SN, SR, SV, SY, TH, TN, TR, TT, TW, TZ, UG, UY, VN, YE, ZM, ZW) *see* Bisacodyl 265
Dulco Laxo (ES) *see* Bisacodyl 265
Dulco-lax perles (GB) *see* Bisacodyl 265
Duloxa (KR) *see* DULoxetine 698
Dulox (CO) *see* Cilostazol 437
Duloxeteg (SV) *see* DULoxetine 698
Dultavax (IL) *see* Diphtheria and Tetanus Toxoid 645
Dumirox (DK, ES, KR, UY) *see* FluvoxaMINE 916
Dumolid (ID) *see* Nitrazepam [CAN/INT] 1461
Dumoxin (BH, CY, EG, ID, IQ, IR, JO, KW, LB, LY, NO, OM, QA, SA, SY, YE) *see* Doxycycline 689
Dumozol (AE, BH, CY, JO, KW, SA) *see* MetroNIDAZOLE (Systemic) 1353
Dumyrox (GR, PT) *see* FluvoxaMINE 916
Duna (ES) *see* Pinazepam [INT] 1652
Duobloc (PH) *see* Carvedilol 367
Duocaine (MY) *see* Lidocaine and Prilocaine 1213
Duocetz (TH) *see* Acetaminophen and Tramadol 37
Duocide (TW) *see* Sulfamethoxazole and Trimethoprim 1946
Duoclin (KR) *see* Clindamycin (Topical) 464
Duocom (PH) *see* Tobramycin and Dexamethasone 2056
Duodart (AR, AU, CH, CL, CY, CZ, DE, FI, HK, HR, ID, IL, IS, MY, NO, PH, PL, RO, SG, SK, TR, TW) *see* Dutasteride and Tamsulosin 702
Duo Di (CN) *see* Doxycycline 689
Duodopa (AU, HR, IL, RO, TH) *see* Carbidopa and Levodopa 351
DuoDopa (BE, GB, IE) *see* Carbidopa and Levodopa 351
Duodyne (KR) *see* Acetaminophen and Tramadol 37
duofem (DE) *see* Levonorgestrel 1201
Duogas (TH) *see* Omeprazole 1508
Duogastril (ES) *see* Cimetidine 438
Duoglyze (CH) *see* Saxagliptin and Metformin 1869
Duolin (IN, NZ) *see* Ipratropium and Albuterol 1109
Duolip (CO) *see* Ezetimibe and Simvastatin 834

Duoluton-L (IN) *see* Ethinyl Estradiol and Norgestrel 812
Duoluton (AR, IN, JP, TW) *see* Ethinyl Estradiol and Norgestrel 812
Duomox (BG, HN) *see* Amoxicillin 130
Duonase (IN) *see* Azelastine and Fluticasone 214
Duopidogrel (MY) *see* Clopidogrel 484
DuoResp Spiromax (GB) *see* Budesonide and Formoterol 297
Duosc (KR) *see* Amlodipine and Atorvastatin 124
Duotan (KR) *see* Valsartan and Hydrochlorothiazide 2129
Duotifen (VN) *see* Pizotifen [CAN/INT] 1664
Duotram XR (AU) *see* TraMADol 2074
DuoTrav (AE, AR, AT, AU, BE, BG, BH, CH, CL, CO, CR, CY, CZ, DE, DK, EE, FI, FR, GB, GR, GT, HK, HN, HR, HU, IE, IL, IS, IT, JP, KR, KW, LB, LT, MT, MY, NI, NL, NO, NZ, PE, PH, PL, PT, QA, RO, RU, SA, SE, SG, SI, SK, SV, TH, TR, TW, UY, VN) *see* Travoprost and Timolol [CAN/INT] 2090
Duo-Travatan (BR) *see* Travoprost and Timolol [CAN/INT] 2090
Duovan (KR) *see* Valsartan and Hydrochlorothiazide 2129
Duovent (BE, BR, DK, IT, MY, NO, NZ, VE, ZA) *see* Ipratropium and Fenoterol [CAN/INT] 1109
Duovent N (BR) *see* Ipratropium and Fenoterol [CAN/INT] 1109
Duovent UDVS (SG) *see* Ipratropium and Fenoterol [CAN/INT] 1109
Duovir-D (LB) *see* Lamivudine and Zidovudine 1160
Duovir (IN) *see* Lamivudine and Zidovudine 1160
Duphalac (AE, AT, AU, BE, BG, BH, CL, CN, CY, CZ, EC, EE, EG, ES, FI, FR, GB, GR, HK, HN, HR, HU, ID, IE, IQ, IR, IT, JO, KR, KW, LB, LT, LU, LY, MY, NL, NO, NZ, OM, PE, PH, PK, PL, PT, PY, QA, RO, RU, SA, SE, SG, SK, SY, TH, TR, TW, VN, YE, ZA) *see* Lactulose 1156
Duphaston (AE, AT, AU, BE, BH, BR, CH, CL, CO, CY, CZ, DE, EC, EE, EG, ES, FR, GB, GR, HK, HN, HR, HU, ID, IE, IL, IN, JO, KR, KW, LB, LT, LU, MY, NL, PH, PK, PL, PT, PY, QA, RO, RU, SA, SE, SG, SK, TH, TR, TW, VE, VN, ZA) *see* Dydrogesterone [INT] 702
Dupin (TW) *see* Diazepam 613
Duplamin (IT) *see* Promethazine 1723
Duplat (MX) *see* Pentoxifylline 1618
Duprost (IN) *see* Dutasteride 702
Du.Q (TW) *see* AmLODIPine 123
Durabeta (PH) *see* Atenolol 189
Duracaine (CL) *see* Bupivacaine 299
Duracef (AT, BE, BF, BG, BJ, CI, CZ, EC, EE, ES, ET, GH, GM, GN, HN, HU, KE, LR, MA, ML, MR, MU, MW, MX, NE, NG, PE, PL, SC, SD, SL, SN, TN, TZ, UG, ZA, ZM, ZW) *see* Cefadroxil 372
Duradox (AE, KW, QA) *see* Doxycycline 689
Duralis (LB) *see* Tadalafil 1968
Duralyn-CR (TH) *see* Theophylline 2026
duranifin (DE) *see* Mefruside [INT] 1281
Duranifin (DE) *see* NIFEdipine 1451
Duranol (PH) *see* Propranolol 1731
Duraphat (AT, DE, DK, FI, NO, PL, SE) *see* Fluoride 895
Duraprox (BE, CL, CO, GR, KR, TR) *see* Oxaprozin 1532
Durater (CR, DO, GT, HN, MX, NI, PA, SV) *see* Famotidine 845
Duratocin (AR, AU, BH, CL, CN, CZ, EC, HK, IT, KR, MY, NZ, PE, PH, SG, TH, UY, VN) *see* Carbetocin [CAN/INT] 350
Duratrimet (DE) *see* Sulfamethoxazole and Trimethoprim 1946
Durazanil (DE) *see* Bromazepam [CAN/INT] 290
Durbis[inj.] (DK) *see* Disopyramide 653
Durbis (DK, SE) *see* Disopyramide 653
Durbis Retard (NO, SE) *see* Disopyramide 653
Durekal (FI) *see* Potassium Chloride 1687
Dur-Elix (AU) *see* Bromhexine [INT] 291
Duricef (AE, BH, EG, KR, KW, LB, PK, QA, TR) *see* Cefadroxil 372
Duride (AU, NZ, TW) *see* Isosorbide Mononitrate 1126
Duroceptol (KR) *see* DULoxetine 698
Duroc (KR) *see* Hydroxychloroquine 1021
Durodor Retard (MX) *see* TraMADol 2074
Duroferon (FI, NO, SE) *see* Ferrous Sulfate 871
Durogesic D-Trans (BR) *see* FentaNYL 857
Durogesic D Trans (HK, KR, PE, TW) *see* FentaNYL 857
Durogesic (AE, AU, BH, CN, CO, CY, ID, IN, JO, LB, MX, NZ, PH, PK, PY, QA, SA, SG, TH, VN) *see* FentaNYL 857
Duro-K 600 (AU) *see* Potassium Chloride 1687
Durolane (ID) *see* Hyaluronate and Derivatives 1006
Duromine (AU, BB, BF, BJ, BM, BS, BZ, CI, CR, CY, DO, ET, GB, GH, GM, GN, GT, GY, HN, IE, JM, KE, KW, LB, LR, MA, ML, MR, MU, MW, NE, NG, NI, NL, NZ, PA, PR, SC, SD, SL, SN, SR, SV, TN, TT, TZ, UG, ZA, ZM, ZW) *see* Phentermine 1635
Durotep MT (JP) *see* FentaNYL 857
Duro-Tuss (AU, HK, MY, SG) *see* Pholcodine [INT] 1646
Duskare (IN) *see* Diacerein [INT] 613
Dusodril (AT, CZ, DE, HR) *see* Naftidrofuryl [INT] 1416
Duspamen (SA) *see* Mebeverine [INT] 1275
Duspatal (CL, DE, IT, NL, PT) *see* Mebeverine [INT] 1275
Duspatalin (AE, AR, BE, BH, BR, CH, CN, CY, CZ, DK, ES, FR, HK, HN, HU, ID, JO, KR, KW, LT, LU, MX, MY, PE, PH, PY, QA, RO, SA, SK, TW, UY, VN) *see* Mebeverine [INT] 1275
Duspatalin Retard (CO, EC, LB) *see* Mebeverine [INT] 1275
Duspatin (TH) *see* Mebeverine [INT] 1275
Duticin (PH, PK) *see* Dacarbazine 549
Dutonin (AT, ES, GB, IE) *see* Nefazodone 1435
Duvaline (PY) *see* BusPIRone 311
Duvig (AR) *see* DOBUTamine 654
Duvimex (AE, BH, CY, EG, IQ, IR, JO, KW, LB, LY, OM, QA, SA, SY, YE) *see* Acyclovir (Systemic) 47
Duxetin (AR, UY) *see* DULoxetine 698
Duxetine (TW) *see* DULoxetine 698
D-Veniz (IN) *see* Desvenlafaxine 598
D-VOID (IN) *see* Desmopressin 594
D-Worm (ZA) *see* Mebendazole [CAN/INT] 1274
Dyazide (AE, BB, BF, BH, BJ, BM, BS, BZ, CH, CI, CY, EG, ET, GB, GH, GM, GN, GY, IE, IL, IQ, IR, JM, JO, JP, KE, KW, LB, LR, LY, MA, ML, MR, MU, MW, MX, MY, NE, NG, OM, PH, PK, PT, QA, SA, SC, SD, SL, SN, SR, SY, TH, TN, TT, TW, TZ, UG, YE, ZA, ZM, ZW) *see* Hydrochlorothiazide and Triamterene 1012
Dyberzide (GR) *see* Hydrochlorothiazide and Triamterene 1012
Dycerin (KR) *see* Diacerein [INT] 613
Dyclobiot (PE) *see* Dicloxacillin 621
Dylastine (AU) *see* Azelastine and Fluticasone 214
Dymadon (AU) *see* Acetaminophen 32
Dymaten (MX) *see* Loratadine 1241
Dymista (AU, CH, DE, DK, EE, FI, GB, HR, IE, LT, RO, SE, SI, SK) *see* Azelastine and Fluticasone 214
Dymistalan (CZ, HR, SI) *see* Azelastine and Fluticasone 214
Dymistin (CZ) *see* Azelastine and Fluticasone 214
Dymoxin (TH) *see* Amoxicillin 130
Dynacil (DE) *see* Fosinopril 932
DynaCirc (AR) *see* Isradipine 1130
Dynacirc (BB, BM, BS, BZ, CO, GY, HK, JM, MX, MY, PH, PK, SR, TH, TR, TT, TW, VE) *see* Isradipine 1130
Dynacirc SR (KR) *see* Isradipine 1130
Dynacirc SRO (CO, MX, MY, NZ, SG, TH) *see* Isradipine 1130

Dynastat (AE, AT, AU, BE, BH, CN, CY, CZ, DE, DK, EE, FI, FR, GB, GR, HK, HR, ID, IE, IS, IT, KW, LT, MY, NL, NO, NZ, PE, PH, PL, PT, QA, RO, RU, SE, SG, SI, SK, TH, TR, TW) *see* Parecoxib [INT] ... 1576
Dynatra (BE, LU) *see* DOPamine ... 669
Dyneric (DE) *see* ClomiPHENE ... 473
Dynexan (CH, FR) *see* Lidocaine (Topical) ... 1211
Dynorm (DE) *see* Cilazapril [CAN/INT] ... 434
Dynos (ZA) *see* DOPamine ... 669
Dyren (KR) *see* Triamterene ... 2101
Dysmenalgit (DE) *see* Naproxen ... 1427
Dyspagon (LU) *see* Loperamide ... 1236
Dyspnoesan (NL) *see* Isoproterenol ... 1124
Dysport (AE, AR, AT, AU, BE, BG, BR, CH, CO, CY, CZ, DE, DK, EE, ES, FI, FR, GR, HK, HU, IL, IT, JO, KR, LB, MX, MY, NL, NO, NZ, PL, PT, RO, RU, SE, SG, SI, SK, TH, TR, VN, ZA) *see* AbobotulinumtoxinA ... 28
Dystonal (BE) *see* Dihydroergotamine ... 633
Dytenzide (BE, NL) *see* Hydrochlorothiazide and Triamterene ... 1012
Dytide H (AT, DE) *see* Hydrochlorothiazide and Triamterene ... 1012
Dytor (IN) *see* Torsemide ... 2071
Dyvistalin (SE) *see* Azelastine and Fluticasone ... 214
Dyvistanil (EE) *see* Azelastine and Fluticasone ... 214
Dyzolor (PH) *see* Fluconazole ... 885
D-Zol (NZ) *see* Danazol ... 558
DZP (MY) *see* Diazepam ... 613
EAC (DE) *see* Aminocaproic Acid ... 113
Earcalm (GB, IE) *see* Acetic Acid ... 39
Ear Clear for Swimmers Ear (AU) *see* Acetic Acid ... 39
Earclear (NZ) *see* Carbamide Peroxide ... 350
Earflo Otic (TW) *see* Ofloxacin (Otic) ... 1491
Early Bird (AU) *see* Pyrantel Pamoate ... 1744
Easy Acne (TW) *see* Adapalene ... 54
Easy Antiseptic (TW) *see* Chlorhexidine Gluconate ... 422
Easydobu (TW) *see* DOBUTamine ... 654
Easyfor SR (TW) *see* Venlafaxine ... 2150
Easyhaler Beclomethasone (GB, IE) *see* Beclomethasone (Nasal) ... 232
Easyhaler Salbutamol (GB, IE) *see* Albuterol ... 69
Easyn (MY) *see* Ampicillin and Sulbactam ... 145
Ebasitin (VN) *see* Ebastine [INT] ... 702
Ebastel (AE, AR, BR, CL, CY, DE, EC, ES, JP, KR, KW, LB, SA, TR, TW, VE) *see* Ebastine [INT] ... 702
Ebast (IN, PK) *see* Ebastine [INT] ... 702
Ebastin (TW) *see* Ebastine [INT] ... 702
Ebatis (KR) *see* Ebastine [INT] ... 702
Ebeposide (SG) *see* Etoposide ... 816
Eberubi (SG) *see* Epirubicin ... 739
Ebetaxel (AE, HK, ID, IL, LB, SA, SG) *see* PACLitaxel (Conventional) ... 1550
Ebetrexat (BG, HR, LB) *see* Methotrexate ... 1322
Ebexantron (SG) *see* MitoXANtrone ... 1382
Ebixa (AE, AR, AT, AU, BE, BG, BH, CH, CL, CN, CY, CZ, DE, DK, EE, ES, FI, FR, GB, GR, HK, HR, HU, IE, IL, IS, IT, KR, KW, LB, LT, MT, MX, MY, NL, NO, NZ, PK, PL, PT, QA, RO, RU, SA, SE, SG, SI, SK, TH, TR, TW) *see* Memantine ... 1286
Ebix (BR) *see* Memantine ... 1286
Ebost (VN) *see* Ebastine [INT] ... 702
E-Butol (SG) *see* Ethambutol ... 798
Ebutol (SG, TW) *see* Ethambutol ... 798
Ecalin (HR, RU) *see* Econazole ... 703
ECALTA (AR, BE, BR, CH, CL, CO, CY, CZ, DE, DK, EC, EE, FR, GR, HN, HR, HU, ID, IE, IT, LB, LT, NL, NO, PL, PT, QA, RO, SA, SE, SI, SK, TR) *see* Anidulafungin ... 150
Ecanol (IN) *see* Econazole ... 703
Ecaprinil-D (CR, DO, GT, HN, NI, PA, SV) *see* Enalapril and Hydrochlorothiazide ... 725
Ecaprinil (CR, PA) *see* Enalapril ... 722
ECARD (JP) *see* Candesartan and Hydrochlorothiazide ... 338
Ecasil (BR) *see* Aspirin ... 180
Ecaten (MX) *see* Captopril ... 342
Ecatrol (ID) *see* Calcitriol ... 323
Ecax (CL) *see* Meloxicam ... 1283
Ecazide (CL, FR) *see* Captopril and Hydrochlorothiazide ... 345
Ecclepia (RO) *see* Epirubicin ... 739
Eccoxolac (GB) *see* Etodolac ... 815
ECEEZ (IN) *see* Levonorgestrel ... 1201
Eclid (ID) *see* Acarbose ... 29
Eclosynt (CO) *see* Beclomethasone (Nasal) ... 232
Eclosynt (CO) *see* Beclomethasone (Systemic) ... 230
Ecobec (BG, EE, FR, PT) *see* Beclomethasone (Nasal) ... 232
Ecobec (BG, EE, PT) *see* Beclomethasone (Systemic) ... 230
Ecocain (AE, QA) *see* Lidocaine (Systemic) ... 1208
Ecocain w/Adrenaline (AE, KW) *see* Lidocaine and Epinephrine ... 1212
Ecodermac (UY) *see* Econazole ... 703
Ecoderm (ZA) *see* Econazole ... 703
Ecodipin (CH) *see* NIFEdipine ... 1451
Ecofenac (CH) *see* Diclofenac (Systemic) ... 617
Ecomi (HK, VN) *see* Econazole ... 703
Ecomucyl (CH) *see* Acetylcysteine ... 40
Econaderm (BB, BM, BS, BZ, GY, JM, SR, TT) *see* Econazole ... 703
Econopred (MY) *see* PrednisoLONE (Ophthalmic) ... 1706
Econopred Plus (AE, BF, BH, BJ, CI, CY, EG, ET, GH, GM, GN, HK, IQ, IR, JO, KE, KW, LB, LR, LY, MA, ML, MR, MU, MW, NE, NG, OM, QA, SA, SC, SD, SG, SL, SN, SY, TN, TZ, UG, YE, ZM, ZW) *see* PrednisoLONE (Ophthalmic) ... 1706
Econ (TH) *see* Econazole ... 703
Ecopan (CH) *see* Mefenamic Acid ... 1280
Ecosal (BG) *see* Albuterol ... 69
Ecostatin (GB, IE, NZ) *see* Econazole ... 703
Ecotrin (AR, CL, MX, NZ, TW) *see* Aspirin ... 180
Ecotrixon (ID) *see* CefTRIAXone ... 396
Ecovitamine B12 (FR) *see* Cyanocobalamin ... 515
Ecox (CO) *see* Ethambutol ... 798
Ecozar (PH) *see* Losartan ... 1248
Ecozar Plus (PH) *see* Losartan and Hydrochlorothiazide ... 1250
Ecozol-VT (HK) *see* Econazole ... 703
Ecron (ID) *see* Vecuronium ... 2144
Ectalin (UY) *see* Norfloxacin ... 1475
Ectaprim (MX) *see* Sulfamethoxazole and Trimethoprim ... 1946
Ectin (IN) *see* Ivermectin (Systemic) ... 1136
Ectopal (TH) *see* Danazol ... 558
Ectren (ES) *see* Quinapril ... 1756
Ectrin (PH) *see* Erdosteine [INT] ... 753
Ecuanil (UY) *see* Meprobamate ... 1296
Ecural (DE) *see* Mometasone (Topical) ... 1391
Ecutamol (EC) *see* Albuterol ... 69
Ecuvas (EC) *see* Simvastatin ... 1890
Ecuvir (EC) *see* Acyclovir (Systemic) ... 47
Ecuvir (EC) *see* Acyclovir (Topical) ... 51
Eczacort (PH) *see* Hydrocortisone (Topical) ... 1014
Edamox (HK) *see* Amoxicillin ... 130
Edarbi (CH, CZ, DE, EE, GB, HK, HR, IE, LT, NL, PH, RO, SE, SK, TH) *see* Azilsartan ... 214
Edarbi CLD (MX) *see* Azilsartan and Chlorthalidone ... 215
Edarbyclor (HK) *see* Azilsartan and Chlorthalidone ... 215
Edecam (MX) *see* Piroxicam ... 1662
Edecril (NL) *see* Ethacrynic Acid ... 797
Edecrina (SE) *see* Ethacrynic Acid ... 797
Edecrin (AT, AU, CZ, GB, IE, NL) *see* Ethacrynic Acid ... 797
Edee (KR) *see* Calcium Carbonate ... 327

Edegra (IN) *see* Sildenafil 1882
Edelsin (ES) *see* Ethinyl Estradiol and Norgestimate 810
Edemid (HR) *see* Furosemide 940
Edepin (TW) *see* AMILoride 113
Edetal-CA (DO) *see* Edetate CALCIUM Disodium 705
Edex (FR) *see* Alprostadil 96
Edhanol (BR) *see* PHENobarbital 1632
Edicin (BG, EE, HR, RO, TH) *see* Vancomycin 2130
Edifen (KR) *see* Ketotifen (Ophthalmic) 1150
Edifen (KR) *see* Ketotifen (Systemic) [CAN/INT] 1149
Edixim (HR) *see* Cefixime 380
Ednapron (MX) *see* PredniSONE 1706
Ednyt (BB, BM, BS, BZ, GY, HU, JM, SR, TT) *see* Enalapril 722
Edolfene (PT) *see* Flurbiprofen (Ophthalmic) 906
Edopect (ID) *see* Erdosteine [INT] 753
Edpa (KR) *see* Escitalopram 765
Edronax (AE, AT, AU, BE, BG, BH, CH, DE, DK, EE, EG, FI, GB, HN, HR, IE, IL, IS, IT, NO, NZ, PL, PT, QA, SA, SE, SI, TH, TR) *see* Reboxetine [INT] 1786
Edurant (AU, BE, CH, CY, CZ, DE, DK, EE, ES, FR, GB, HK, HR, IL, IS, JP, KR, LT, MY, NL, NO, NZ, RO, SE, SG, SI, SK, TH, TR) *see* Rilpivirine 1810
EES (AU) *see* Erythromycin (Systemic) 762
Efaclor (MY) *see* Cefaclor 372
Efatracina (UY) *see* Bacitracin (Ophthalmic) 222
Efatracina (UY) *see* Bacitracin (Topical) 222
Efavir (IN, LB, PE, PY) *see* Efavirenz 707
Efcortelan (BF, BJ, CI, ET, GH, GM, GN, KE, LR, MA, ML, MR, MU, MW, NE, NG, SC, SD, SL, SN, TN, TZ, UG, ZM, ZW) *see* Hydrocortisone (Topical) 1014
Efcortelan Soluble (AE, BH, CY, EG, IQ, IR, JO, KW, LB, LY, OM, QA, SA, SY, YE) *see* Hydrocortisone (Systemic) 1013
Efecient (IN) *see* Ferric Gluconate 869
Efectin (AT, CZ, HU, PL) *see* Venlafaxine 2150
Efectine (MX) *see* Loratadine 1241
Efectin EP (RO) *see* Venlafaxine 2150
Efectin ER (BG) *see* Venlafaxine 2150
Efectus (DO) *see* Cefepime 378
Efedrin (BR, DK, IS, NO, SE) *see* EPHEDrine (Systemic) 734
Efedrin NAF (NO) *see* EPHEDrine (Systemic) 734
Efermol (PY) *see* Acetaminophen 32
Efexiva (HR, SI) *see* Venlafaxine 2150
Efexor XL (ID) *see* Venlafaxine 2150
Efexor (AE, AR, BE, BH, BR, CH, CO, CR, DK, DO, EE, EG, FI, GB, GR, GT, HN, IE, IT, JO, LU, NI, NL, NO, PA, PE, PK, QA, SA, SE, SV, TR, ZA) *see* Venlafaxine 2150
Efexor Depot (FI, IS, NO, SE) *see* Venlafaxine 2150
Efexor ER (CH) *see* Venlafaxine 2150
Efexor XR (AE, AR, AU, BH, BR, CL, CN, CO, CR, CY, EC, EE, GT, HK, HN, IL, KR, KW, LB, LT, MX, MY, NI, NZ, PA, PE, PH, PT, QA, SA, SG, SV, TH, VE, VN) *see* Venlafaxine 2150
Effac (TW) *see* Tacrolimus (Topical) 1968
Effederm (FR) *see* Tretinoin (Topical) 2099
Effentora (EE, GB) *see* FentaNYL 857
Efferalgan 500 (CR, DO, EE, GT, HN, NI, PA, SV) *see* Acetaminophen 32
Efferalgan (HR, HU, LT, LU) *see* Acetaminophen 32
Efferalganodis (FR) *see* Acetaminophen 32
Effexor (FR) *see* Venlafaxine 2150
Effezel (MX) *see* Adapalene and Benzoyl Peroxide 54
Efficib (EE, HR, RO) *see* Sitagliptin and Metformin 1898
Effient (AR, AU, BR, CO, HK, IL, IN, KR, LB, MY, NZ, SG, TH) *see* Prasugrel 1699
Efflumidex (BG, CZ, DE, HN, HR, HU) *see* Fluorometholone 896
Effortil (AR, AT, BE, CH, CY, DE, FI, FR, HR, IT, LU, NO, PT, SE) *see* Etilefrine [INT] 815
Effortil[Vet.] (AT) *see* Etilefrine [INT] 815
Effortil[vet.] (CH, FR) *see* Etilefrine [INT] 815
Effortil PL (BE, LU) *see* Etilefrine [INT] 815
Effosomyl XL (GB) *see* Tolterodine 2063
Effox (PL) *see* Isosorbide Mononitrate 1126
Eficef (RO) *see* Cefixime 380
Efient (AT, BE, CH, CY, CZ, DE, DK, EE, FR, GB, HR, IE, IS, JP, LT, NL, NO, PL, PT, RO, SE, SI, SK, TR) *see* Prasugrel 1699
Efipres (IN) *see* EPHEDrine (Systemic) 734
Efixano (PY) *see* Irinotecan 1112
Efloran (CZ) *see* MetroNIDAZOLE (Systemic) 1353
Efortil (BR, ES) *see* Etilefrine [INT] 815
Efosin (TW) *see* Dipyridamole 652
Efotax (ID) *see* Cefotaxime 382
Efotin (PH) *see* Epoetin Alfa 742
Efox (HR) *see* Cefuroxime 399
Efracea (GB, IE) *see* Doxycycline 689
Efridol (IT) *see* Nimesulide [INT] 1456
Efrin-10 (IL) *see* Phenylephrine (Systemic) 1638
Efrinalin (BR) *see* Norepinephrine 1472
Eftipine (VN) *see* NiMODipine 1456
Efudix (AE, AR, AU, BE, BG, BH, CH, CL, CR, CY, DO, EG, FR, GB, GH, GT, HN, IE, IQ, IR, IT, JO, KE, KW, LB, LY, NI, NL, NO, NZ, OM, PA, PE, PL, PY, QA, RO, SA, SI, SK, SV, SY, TW, TZ, UG, UY, YE, ZM) *see* Fluorouracil (Topical) 899
Efurix (BR) *see* Fluorouracil (Topical) 899
Efurox (MY) *see* Cefuroxime 399
Egacene (NL) *see* Hyoscyamine 1026
Egaten (FR, GR, VN) *see* Triclabendazole [INT] 2102
Egazil Duretter (DK, FI, NO, SE) *see* Hyoscyamine 1026
E-Gen-C (ZA) *see* Ethinyl Estradiol and Levonorgestrel 803
Egery (FR) *see* Erythromycin (Topical) 765
Egifilin (HU) *see* Theophylline 2026
Egitinid (RO) *see* Imatinib 1047
Egitromb (BG) *see* Clopidogrel 484
Eglandin (KR) *see* Alprostadil 96
Eglen (JP) *see* Cinnarizine [INT] 440
Eglidon (AR) *see* Terazosin 2001
Egocort (AE) *see* Hydrocortisone (Topical) 1014
E (GR) *see* Diclofenac (Systemic) 617
EinsAlpha (DE) *see* Alfacalcidol [CAN/INT] 82
Ejertol (CO) *see* Sildenafil 1882
Ekmetacin (PT) *see* Indomethacin 1067
Ekvacillin (NO, SE) *see* Cloxacillin [CAN/INT] 488
Elacutan (DE, PL) *see* Urea 2114
Elafax (PY, UY) *see* Venlafaxine 2150
Elafax XR (PY, UY) *see* Venlafaxine 2150
Elan (IT) *see* Isosorbide Mononitrate 1126
Elantan (AE, AT, CR, CZ, DE, DO, EC, GT, HK, HN, ID, IE, JO, KR, LU, MX, MY, NI, PA, PE, PH, PK, SG, SV, VE) *see* Isosorbide Mononitrate 1126
Elantan LA (MY) *see* Isosorbide Mononitrate 1126
Elantan Long (CZ, DE, HK, LT, MY, PH, SG) *see* Isosorbide Mononitrate 1126
Elantan SR (KW) *see* Isosorbide Mononitrate 1126
Elaprase (AT, AU, BE, BG, BR, CH, CZ, DE, DK, EE, ES, FI, FR, GB, GR, HK, HN, HR, IE, IL, IT, JP, KR, LT, MT, MY, NL, NO, NZ, PL, PT, RU, SE, SG, SI, SK, TH, TR, TW) *see* Idursulfase 1040
elaprase (RO) *see* Idursulfase 1040
Elatrolet (IL) *see* Amitriptyline 119
Elatrol (IL) *see* Amitriptyline 119
Elavil (FR) *see* Amitriptyline 119
Elazop (KR) *see* Brinzolamide and Timolol [CAN/INT] 289
Elbrus (AR) *see* Rasagiline 1781
Elcion CR (IN) *see* Diazepam 613
Elcoman (AR) *see* Loperamide 1236
Elcrit (DE) *see* CloZAPine 490

Eldepryl (AU, BE, CN, DK, FI, GB, IE, NL, NO, NZ, SE, TW) *see* Selegiline 1873
Eldicet (CL, ES, IN, PH, PY) *see* Pinaverium [CAN/INT] 1651
Eldopaque (AE, BH, CY, EG, GR, IQ, IR, JO, KW, LB, LY, OM, PE, PH, QA, SA, SY, YE) *see* Hydroquinone 1020
Eldopaque Forte (AE, BH, CY, EG, IQ, IR, JO, KW, LB, LY, OM, PH, QA, SA, SY, YE) *see* Hydroquinone 1020
Eldoper Plus (IN) *see* Loperamide and Simethicone 1237
Eldoquin (AE, BH, CR, CY, EG, GT, HK, HN, IQ, IR, JO, KW, LB, LY, MX, NI, OM, PA, PE, PH, PK, PT, QA, SA, SV, SY, YE) *see* Hydroquinone 1020
Eldoquin Cream (NZ) *see* Hydroquinone 1020
Eldoquin Forte (AE, BH, CY, EG, HK, IQ, IR, JO, KW, LB, LY, OM, PH, QA, SA, SY, YE) *see* Hydroquinone 1020
Eldostam (KR) *see* Erdosteine [INT] 753
Eleadol (UY) *see* Ketorolac (Systemic) 1146
Elecor (ES) *see* Eplerenone 740
Elelyso (AU) *see* Taliglucerase Alfa 1971
Elenium (HN, HU, PK, PL, RU) *see* ChlordiazePOXIDE 422
Elentol (FR) *see* Lindane 1217
Elequine (BB, BM, BS, EC, JM, NL, PR, SR, TT) *see* Levofloxacin (Systemic) 1197
Eleuphrat (AU) *see* Betamethasone (Topical) 255
Eleva (AU) *see* Sertraline 1878
Elevat (ZA) *see* Dronabinol 694
Elevex (PH) *see* Timolol (Ophthalmic) 2043
Elevin (GB) *see* Ethinyl Estradiol and Levonorgestrel 803
Elfivir (PE) *see* Nelfinavir 1436
Elfonal (KR) *see* Enalapril 722
Elica (AE, BH, JO, KW, PH, QA, SA) *see* Mometasone (Topical) 1391
Elicca (LB) *see* Mometasone (Topical) 1391
Elicort (PH) *see* Mometasone (Topical) 1391
Elidel (AE, AR, AT, AU, BE, BG, BH, BR, CH, CL, CN, CO, CY, CZ, DE, DK, EC, EE, EG, ES, FI, GB, HK, HN, HR, ID, IL, IN, IS, IT, JO, KR, KW, LB, LT, MX, MY, NL, NO, NZ, PH, PL, PT, QA, RO, RU, SA, SE, SG, SI, SK, TH, TR, TW, UY, VE) *see* Pimecrolimus 1650
Eliflam (PY) *see* Celecoxib 402
Eligard (AU, BG, DE, EE, FR, HK, HR, IS, LT, NZ, RO, SI, SK, TH, TR, VN) *see* Leuprolide 1186
Elimicina Dermica (PY) *see* Erythromycin (Topical) 765
Elinap (TR) *see* Nimesulide [INT] 1456
Eliquis (AR, AU, BE, BR, CH, CN, CO, CY, CZ, DE, DK, EE, FR, GB, HK, HR, ID, IE, IL, IS, JP, KR, LT, MY, NL, NO, PH, PL, QA, RO, SE, SG, SI, SK, TH, TR) *see* Apixaban 158
Elisca (HK) *see* Chloramphenicol 421
Elisone (HK) *see* Mometasone (Topical) 1391
Elisor (FR) *see* Pravastatin 1700
Elitan (TR, VN) *see* Metoclopramide 1345
Elixine (CL) *see* Theophylline 2026
Elixir Ferrous Gluconate (ZA) *see* Ferrous Gluconate 870
Elizac (ID) *see* FLUoxetine 899
ella (HK) *see* Ulipristal 2113
Ella (IL, MY, SG) *see* Ulipristal 2113
Ellanco (HK, MY) *see* Lovastatin 1252
ellaOne (AT, BE, CH, CY, CZ, DE, DK, EE, FR, GB, HN, HR, KR, LT, NL, NO, PL, PT, RO, SE, SI, SK, TR) *see* Ulipristal 2113
Elle (PH) *see* Danazol 558
Elle (PK) *see* Eletriptan 711
Ellia (HK) *see* Adapalene 54
Elmego Spray (TH) *see* Indomethacin 1067
Elmetacin (AE, AU, BH, EC, EE, HU, KW, PK, PL, QA, SA, SK, VE) *see* Indomethacin 1067
Elmiron (AR, AU, HK, KR, PE, TW) *see* Pentosan Polysulfate Sodium 1617
Elmogan (HK, HR) *see* Gemfibrozil 956
Eloamin (CZ) *see* Acetylcysteine 40
Elobact (DE) *see* Cefuroxime 399
Elocom (AE, BE, BF, BG, BH, BJ, BR, CH, CI, CL, CO, CR, CZ, DO, EG, ET, GH, GM, GN, GT, HN, HR, IL, IQ, IR, JO, KE, KR, KW, LB, LR, LY, MA, ML, MR, MU, MW, NE, NG, NI, OM, PA, PE, PK, PL, PT, QA, RO, RU, SA, SC, SD, SI, SK, SL, SN, SV, SY, TN, TZ, UG, YE, ZM, ZW) *see* Mometasone (Topical) 1391
Elocon (AR, AT, CY, DK, EE, FI, GB, GR, ID, IE, IN, IS, IT, LT, NL, NO, PH, PY, SE, TR, UY, VE) *see* Mometasone (Topical) 1391
Elocon Cream (AU, NZ) *see* Mometasone (Topical) 1391
Elocon Ointment (AU, NZ) *see* Mometasone (Topical) 1391
Elodius (BR) *see* Tipranavir 2047
Elofuran (BR) *see* Pipemidic Acid [INT] 1655
Elohaes (HR, NL) *see* Hetastarch 1004
Elohaest (AT) *see* Hetastarch 1004
Elo Hes (ES) *see* Hetastarch 1004
Elomet (HK, MY, SG, TH, TW, VN) *see* Mometasone (Topical) 1391
Elonton SR (KR) *see* Isosorbide Mononitrate 1126
Elontril (EE, LT, RO, SK) *see* BuPROPion 305
Elonza (TH) *see* Sildenafil 1882
Eloquine (TR) *see* Mefloquine 1280
Elorgan (ES) *see* Pentoxifylline 1618
Eloson (CN) *see* Mometasone (Topical) 1391
Elosone (HK, SG) *see* Mometasone (Topical) 1391
Eloxatin (AE, AU, BE, BG, BH, BR, CH, CL, CN, CO, CR, CY, CZ, DE, DK, DO, EE, ES, FI, GB, GT, HK, HN, HR, ID, IE, IL, IT, JO, KR, KW, MX, MY, NI, NL, NO, NZ, PA, PE, PH, PL, QA, RO, SA, SE, SG, SI, SV, TH, TR, TW, VN) *see* Oxaliplatin 1528
Eloxatine (FR, LB, RU, VE) *see* Oxaliplatin 1528
Elozora (RO) *see* Letrozole 1181
Elpenor (DE) *see* CarBAMazepine 346
Elpicef (ID) *see* CefTRIAXone 396
Elpilip (AR) *see* Bezafibrate [CAN/INT] 261
Elplat (JP) *see* Oxaliplatin 1528
Elsep (FR) *see* MitoXANtrone 1382
Elspar (BR, MX) *see* Asparaginase (E. coli) 179
Elstatin (SG) *see* Lovastatin 1252
Eltair (MY) *see* Budesonide (Systemic) 293
Eltair (NZ, SG) *see* Budesonide (Nasal) 296
Elthon (CN, VN) *see* Itopride [INT] 1130
Elthyrone (BE) *see* Levothyroxine 1205
Elthyro (TH) *see* Levothyroxine 1205
Eltidine (KR) *see* Ranitidine 1777
Eltoven (CL, PY) *see* Tolterodine 2063
Eltroxin (AE, BD, BF, BH, BJ, BM, BZ, CH, CI, CY, CZ, DK, EG, ET, GB, GH, GM, GN, GY, HK, IL, IQ, IR, JO, JP, KE, KW, LB, LR, LY, MA, ML, MR, MU, MW, NE, NG, OM, PH, PK, QA, SA, SC, SD, SL, SN, SR, SY, TH, TN, TW, TZ, UG, YE, ZA, ZM, ZW) *see* Levothyroxine 1205
Elvanse (DK, GB, SE) *see* Lisdexamfetamine 1224
Elvecis (AR) *see* CISplatin 448
Elvefocal (AR) *see* Folic Acid 919
Elvenavir (AR) *see* Indinavir 1066
Elvorine (BE) *see* LEVOleucovorin 1200
Elyzol (FI) *see* MetroNIDAZOLE (Systemic) 1353
Elzar (ID) *see* Irbesartan 1110
Emadrin (PK) *see* Procyclidine [CAN/INT] 1721
Emanthal (IN) *see* Albendazole 65
Emaxen (CR, DO, EC, GT, HN, NI, PA, SV) *see* Interferon Beta-1a 1100
EMB (DE) *see* Ethambutol 798
Embevio (VN) *see* Desogestrel [INT] 597
EMB-Fatol (HK) *see* Ethambutol 798

Embol (TH) *see* Piracetam [INT] 1661
Emconcor (BE, DK, ES, FI, NO, SE) *see* Bisoprolol 266
Emcyt (MX) *see* Estramustine 782
Emdalen (ZA) *see* Lofepramine [INT] 1232
Emderm (IN) *see* Fluocinolone (Topical) 893
Emdon (TH) *see* Nimesulide [INT] 1456
Emdopa (IN) *see* Methyldopa 1332
Emef (IN) *see* Moxifloxacin (Ophthalmic) 1403
Emef (IN) *see* Moxifloxacin (Systemic) 1401
Emeliv (SG) *see* Metoclopramide 1345
Emend IV (AU, HK, IL, KR, NZ, SG) *see* Fosaprepitant 929
Emend (AR, AT, AU, BE, BG, BR, CH, CL, CN, CO, CR, CY, CZ, DE, DK, DO, EE, ES, FI, FR, GB, GR, GT, HN, HR, HU, IE, IL, IS, IT, JP, KR, KW, LT, MT, MX, MY, NI, NL, NO, NZ, PA, PE, PH, PT, PY, QA, RO, RU, SE, SG, SI, SK, SV, TH, TR, TW, VE) *see* Aprepitant 166
Emend Tri-Pack (HK) *see* Aprepitant 166
Emep (PH) *see* Esomeprazole 771
Emerade (GB) *see* EPINEPHrine (Systemic, Oral Inhalation) 735
Emergen (PE) *see* Sertraline 1878
Emeset (IN) *see* Ondansetron 1513
Emeside (GB, IE, TR) *see* Ethosuximide 813
Emestane (PH) *see* Exemestane 828
Emetiral (RO) *see* Prochlorperazine 1718
Emetron (HU) *see* Ondansetron 1513
Emflex (GB) *see* Acemetacin [INT] 30
Emforal (TR) *see* Propranolol 1731
Emgesan (FI, SE) *see* Magnesium Hydroxide 1263
Eminens (HR) *see* ROPINIRole 1844
Emipastin (MX) *see* Pravastatin 1700
Emistop (PH) *see* Ondansetron 1513
Emla (AE, AR, AT, AU, BB, BE, BF, BG, BH, BJ, BM, BS, BZ, CH, CI, CN, CY, CZ, DE, DK, EG, ET, FI, FR, GB, GH, GM, GN, GR, GY, HK, ID, IE, IL, IQ, IR, IS, IT, JM, JO, JP, KE, KW, LB, LR, LY, MA, ML, MR, MU, MW, MX, MY, NE, NG, NL, NO, NZ, OM, PE, PH, PL, PY, QA, RU, SA, SC, SD, SE, SI, SL, SN, SR, SY, TH, TN, TR, TT, TW, TZ, UG, VN, YE, ZA, ZM, ZW) *see* Lidocaine and Prilocaine 1213
Emla Cream (NZ) *see* Lidocaine and Prilocaine 1213
Emlansa (HK) *see* Lansoprazole 1166
Emla Patch (NZ) *see* Lidocaine and Prilocaine 1213
Emlocaine (PH) *see* Lidocaine and Prilocaine 1213
Emnorm (NZ) *see* MetFORMIN 1307
Emodan (PH) *see* Ondansetron 1513
Emodopan (PE) *see* DOPamine 669
Emoferrina (IT) *see* Ferrous Gluconate 870
Emotival (AR) *see* LORazepam 1243
E-Moxclav (AE, BH, CY, EG, IQ, IR, JO, KW, LB, LY, OM, QA, SA, SY, YE) *see* Amoxicillin and Clavulanate 133
Emozul (GB) *see* Esomeprazole 771
Emparis (VN) *see* Esomeprazole 771
Empecid (AR, PY) *see* Clotrimazole (Topical) 488
Emperal (DK) *see* Metoclopramide 1345
Emposil (ID) *see* Sildenafil 1882
Empurine (PH, TH) *see* Mercaptopurine 1296
Emquin (IN) *see* Chloroquine 424
Emselex (AT, BE, BG, CH, CZ, DE, DK, EE, ES, FI, FR, GB, GR, HN, HR, HU, IE, IS, IT, LT, MT, NL, NO, PE, PL, PT, RO, RU, SE, SI, SK, TR) *see* Darifenacin 568
Emthexate (AT, BE, GR, ID, JO, KW, NL, NO, PH, PK, PT, TH, TR, TW) *see* Methotrexate 1322
Emthexate PF (KR) *see* Methotrexate 1322
Emthexat (SE) *see* Methotrexate 1322
Emthrxate (SI) *see* Methotrexate 1322
Emtix (FI) *see* Docusate 661
Emtriva (AR, AT, AU, BE, BG, CH, CZ, DE, DK, EE, ES, FI, FR, GB, GR, HN, HR, HU, IE, IL, IS, IT, JP, LT, MT, MX, NL, NO, NZ, PL, PT, RO, RU, SE, SK, TR) *see* Emtricitabine 720
Emu-V E (BF, BJ, CI, ET, GH, GM, GN, KE, LR, MA, ML, MR, MU, MW, NE, NG, SC, SD, SL, SN, TN, TZ, UG, ZM, ZW) *see* Erythromycin (Systemic) 762
E-Mycin (AU, PK) *see* Erythromycin (Systemic) 762
Emzolam-100 (PH) *see* Temozolomide 1991
Enablex (AU, EC, NZ, PH, SA, ZA) *see* Darifenacin 568
Enablex/Emselex (CO) *see* Darifenacin 568
Enace-D (IN) *see* Enalapril and Hydrochlorothiazide 725
Enace (TH) *see* Enalapril 722
Enadiol (CL, PY) *see* Estradiol (Systemic) 775
Enaf-150 (TH) *see* MedroxyPROGESTERone 1277
Enafon (KR) *see* Amitriptyline 119
Enahexal (NZ) *see* Enalapril 722
Enakur (ID) *see* Metoclopramide 1345
Enalagamma (DE) *see* Enalapril 722
Enalapril (ES) *see* Enalapril 722
Enaloc (FI) *see* Enalapril 722
Enalten-D (EC) *see* Enalapril and Hydrochlorothiazide 725
Enanton Depot (DK, FI, NO, SE) *see* Leuprolide 1186
Enantone (AT, DE, FR) *see* Leuprolide 1186
Enantone Depot (IT) *see* Leuprolide 1186
Enantone LP (TH) *see* Leuprolide 1186
Enantone SR (CN, HK) *see* Leuprolide 1186
Enantyum (AR, AT, BE, CR, DO, GT, HN, NI, NL, PA, SE, SV) *see* Dexketoprofen [INT] 603
Enantyum (ES, IT) *see* Clobutinol [INT] 468
Enap (HK, HR, HU, RO, SG, SI, SK) *see* Enalapril 722
Enap HL (HR, RO, SG) *see* Enalapril and Hydrochlorothiazide 725
Enap H (PL, SI, SK) *see* Enalapril and Hydrochlorothiazide 725
Enap [inj.] (HU) *see* Enalapril 722
Enap i.v. (HR) *see* Enalapril 722
Enapren (IT) *see* Enalapril 722
Enaprin (KR) *see* Enalapril 722
Enaril (KR, TH) *see* Enalapril 722
Enatec (BB, BM, BS, BZ, GY, JM, SR, TT) *see* Enalapril 722
Enazil (PL) *see* Enalapril 722
Enbid-20 (PH) *see* Enalapril 722
Enbrel (AE, AR, AT, AU, BE, BG, BH, BR, CH, CL, CN, CO, CR, CY, CZ, DE, DK, EC, EE, ES, FI, FR, GB, GR, GT, HK, HN, HR, HU, ID, IE, IL, IN, IS, IT, JO, JP, KR, KW, LB, LT, MT, MX, MY, NI, NL, NO, NZ, PA, PE, PH, PL, PT, QA, RO, RU, SA, SE, SG, SI, SK, SV, TH, TR, TW, VE, VN) *see* Etanercept 795
Encavar (PH) *see* Amlodipine and Atorvastatin 124
Encefalux (ES) *see* Piracetam [INT] 1661
Encetrop (CH, DE) *see* Piracetam [INT] 1661
Encine EM (TW) *see* Aspirin 180
Enclor (MY, SG) *see* Chloramphenicol 421
Encloxil (PH) *see* Cloxacillin [CAN/INT] 488
Encore (TW) *see* Acetylcysteine 40
Encorton (PL) *see* PredniSONE 1706
Endace (IN) *see* Megestrol 1281
Endazole (PH) *see* MetroNIDAZOLE (Systemic) 1353
Endep (AU) *see* Amitriptyline 119
Endial (AR) *see* Glimepiride 966
Endo-D (IT) *see* Ergocalciferol 753
Endobulin (CZ, FI) *see* Immune Globulin 1056
Endofolin (BR) *see* Folic Acid 919
Endometrin (HK, IL) *see* Progesterone 1722
Endomixin (IT) *see* Neomycin 1436
Endone (AU) *see* OxyCODONE 1538
Endopryl (CY) *see* Selegiline 1873
Endosone (PH) *see* PredniSONE 1706
Endoxana (GB) *see* Cyclophosphamide 517
Endoxan-Asta (AE, AR, BH, CH, CY, FR, HK, ID, IN, IQ, IR, JO, KW, LB, LY, MY, OM, PH, QA, SA, SY, TH, TW, YE) *see* Cyclophosphamide 517
Endoxan (AT, AU, BE, BG, CL, CZ, DE, EC, EE, EG, GR, HN, HR, HU, IL, IT, KR, LU, NL, NZ, PK, PL, PT, RO,

RU, SG, SI, SK, TR, UY, VN, ZA) *see* Cyclophosphamide 517
Endoxon-Asta (AU) *see* Cyclophosphamide 517
Endrolin (ID, PH) *see* Leuprolide 1186
Endronax (BR) *see* Alendronate 79
Enduferon (PH) *see* Interferon Alfa-2b 1096
Endufil (PH) *see* Filgrastim 875
Enduron (AU, GB) *see* Methyclothiazide 1331
Endurpin (PH) *see* Nalbuphine 1416
Enduxan (BR) *see* Cyclophosphamide 517
Enelfa (LU) *see* Acetaminophen 32
Enem (TH) *see* Meropenem 1299
Enetege (UY) *see* Nitroglycerin 1465
Enetil (CO) *see* Enalapril 722
Enetra (BG) *see* Nimesulide [INT] 1456
Engaba (PK) *see* Gabapentin 943
Engerix-B (AE, AR, AT, AU, BB, BE, BG, BH, BM, BR, BS, BZ, CH, CL, CR, CY, CZ, DE, DK, DO, EC, EE, EG, FI, FR, GB, GR, GT, GY, HK, HN, HU, IE, IN, IS, IT, JM, KW, LB, LT, MT, MX, MY, NI, NL, NO, NZ, PA, PE, PK, PL, PT, PY, QA, RO, RU, SA, SE, SG, SI, SK, SR, SV, TH, TR, TT, TW, UY, VE, ZA) *see* Hepatitis B Vaccine (Recombinant) 1002
Engerix B (VN) *see* Hepatitis B Vaccine (Recombinant) 1002
Engtel (PK) *see* Telithromycin 1987
Enhancin (PH) *see* Amoxicillin and Clavulanate 133
Enhansid (PH) *see* Folic Acid 919
Eni (CR, DO, GT, HN, NI) *see* Ciprofloxacin (Systemic) 441
Enidin (AU) *see* Brimonidine (Ophthalmic) 288
Enidin P (AU) *see* Brimonidine (Ophthalmic) 288
Enidrel (AR) *see* Oxazepam 1532
Enipaxol (IN) *see* Loxapine 1255
Enkacetyn (ID) *see* Chloramphenicol 421
Enlafax-XR (AU) *see* Venlafaxine 2150
Ennafine (KR) *see* Butenafine 314
Ennamax (ID) *see* Cyproheptadine 529
Enoclex (PH) *see* Enoxaparin 726
Enolol (TH) *see* Atenolol 189
Enoxin (SG, TH) *see* Ciprofloxacin (Systemic) 441
Enpalevo (TW) *see* Carbidopa and Levodopa 351
Enpott (TH) *see* Potassium Chloride 1687
Enpril (KR) *see* Enalapril 722
Enselin-2G (IN) *see* Rosiglitazone and Glimepiride 1847
Enselin 2M (IN) *see* Rosiglitazone and Metformin 1847
Enset (PH) *see* Ondansetron 1513
Enteclud (VN) *see* Entecavir 731
Entegard (PH) *see* Entecavir 731
Enteromicina (PT) *see* Neomycin 1436
Entia (TH) *see* Oxaliplatin 1528
Entikav (HK) *see* Entecavir 731
Entir (SG, TH) *see* Acyclovir (Systemic) 47
Entir (TH) *see* Acyclovir (Topical) 51
Entizol (CZ) *see* MetroNIDAZOLE (Systemic) 1353
Entobar (KR) *see* PENTobarbital 1617
Entocort (AE, AR, AT, BE, BH, BR, CH, CZ, DK, FI, FR, GB, HK, HU, IE, IL, IS, IT, JO, KR, KW, NL, NO, PL, PT, SA, SE, SK, TR) *see* Budesonide (Systemic) 293
Entolon (JP) *see* Nalidixic Acid [INT] 1418
Entrydil (IE) *see* Diltiazem 634
Enturion (SG) *see* AtorvaSTATin 194
Entyvio (AU, CZ, DE, DK, EE, GB, HR, LT, NL, RO, SE, SI, SK) *see* Vedolizumab 2146
Envas (BF, BJ, CI, ET, GH, GM, GN, IN, KE, LR, MA, ML, MR, MU, MW, NE, NG, SC, SD, SL, SN, TN, TZ, UG, ZM, ZW) *see* Enalapril 722
Enviage (EE) *see* Aliskiren 85
Enxak (BR) *see* Ergotamine 754
Enzastar (VN) *see* PEMEtrexed 1606
Enzil (TW) *see* Amantadine 105
Enzimar (CO) *see* Metoclopramide 1345
Eoxy (TW) *see* Etoricoxib [INT] 821
Epalon (TR) *see* Maprotiline 1271
Epalon (TW) *see* Donepezil 668
Epamin (AR, BO, BR, CL, CO, CR, DO, EC, GT, HN, MX, NI, PA, PE, PR, SV, VE) *see* Phenytoin 1640
Epanutin (AE, AT, BE, BF, BH, BJ, CI, CY, CZ, DE, EG, ES, ET, FI, GB, GH, GM, GN, GR, HU, IE, IL, IQ, IR, JO, KE, KW, LB, LR, LU, LY, MA, ML, MR, MU, MW, NE, NG, NL, OM, PL, QA, SA, SC, SD, SE, SL, SN, SY, TN, TR, TZ, UG, UY, YE, ZA, ZM, ZW) *see* Phenytoin 1640
Epaxal (AE, BH, CO, GB, IE, IL) *see* Hepatitis A Vaccine 1001
Epax (EC) *see* Omega-3 Fatty Acids 1507
Epazin (PH) *see* CarBAMazepine 346
Epecoal (JP) *see* Mecysteine [INT] 1277
Epelon (TW) *see* Isoconazole [INT] 1120
Eperzan (CZ, EE, HR, NL, SE, SK) *see* Albiglutide 66
Epexol (ID) *see* Ambroxol [INT] 109
Ephedrine Hydrochloride (NZ) *see* EPHEDrine (Systemic) 734
Ephedrine Sulfate Inj (AU, NZ) *see* EPHEDrine (Systemic) 734
Ephynal (AT, BE, CH, ES, GR, IT, PT) *see* Vitamin E 2174
EPIAO (TH) *see* Epoetin Alfa 742
Epicin (TW) *see* Epirubicin 739
Epicort (CO) *see* Clotrimazole (Topical) 488
Epictal (IN) *see* LevETIRAcetam 1191
Epictal (JO) *see* LamoTRIgine 1160
Epidac (AR) *see* Doxylamine and Pyridoxine 693
Epidoxo (PY) *see* Epirubicin 739
Epiduo (AR, AU, BE, BR, CH, CL, CO, DE, DK, EC, FI, FR, GB, GR, HK, IE, IN, IS, IT, KR, KW, MY, NO, NZ, PH, PL, PT, SA, SE, SG, TH) *see* Adapalene and Benzoyl Peroxide 54
Epifenac (AE, BH, CY, EG, IQ, IR, JO, KW, LB, LY, OM, QA, SA, SY, YE) *see* Diclofenac (Systemic) 617
Epifil (AR) *see* Epirubicin 739
Epifoam (AE, BH, CY, EG, IL, IQ, IR, JO, KW, LB, LY, OM, QA, SA, SY, YE) *see* Pramoxine and Hydrocortisone 1698
Epigent (AE, BH, CY, EG, IQ, IR, JO, KW, LB, LY, OM, QA, SA, SY, YE) *see* Gentamicin (Systemic) 959
Epilan-D (AT, BG, CZ) *see* Phenytoin 1640
Epilem (MX, TH) *see* Epirubicin 739
Epilen (TW) *see* LevETIRAcetam 1191
Epileptol CR (KR) *see* CarBAMazepine 346
Epileptol (KR) *see* CarBAMazepine 346
Epiletam (RO) *see* LevETIRAcetam 1191
Epilev (HR) *see* LevETIRAcetam 1191
Epilim (AU, BF, BJ, CI, ET, GB, GH, GM, GN, HK, IE, KE, KP, LR, MA, ML, MR, MU, MW, MY, NE, NG, NZ, SC, SD, SL, SN, TN, TZ, UG, ZA, ZM, ZW) *see* Valproic Acid and Derivatives 2123
Epilim Chrono 500 (BB, BM, BS, GY, HK, JM, MY, NL, PR, TT) *see* Valproic Acid and Derivatives 2123
Epilramate (TW) *see* Topiramate 2065
Epimag (AE, EG) *see* Magnesium Citrate 1262
Epimate (PH) *see* Topiramate 2065
Epinat (NO) *see* Phenytoin 1640
Epinefrina (CL, EC) *see* EPINEPHrine (Systemic, Oral Inhalation) 735
Epinitril (FR) *see* Nitroglycerin 1465
Epipen (AR, AU, BE, CH, CZ, DK, FI, HK, IL, IS, JP, LT, NL, NO, NZ, PL, SE, SG, SI, SK, TH, TW) *see* EPINEPHrine (Systemic, Oral Inhalation) 735
Epipen Jr (AU, FI, HK, IL, NO, SE, SG, SK, TH, TW) *see* EPINEPHrine (Systemic, Oral Inhalation) 735
Epi-Pevaryl (DE) *see* Econazole 703
Epiphenicol (AE, BH, CY, EG, IQ, IR, JO, KW, LB, LY, OM, QA, SA, SY, YE) *see* Chloramphenicol 421

Epirax (AE, BH, CY, EG, IL, IQ, IR, JO, KW, LB, LY, OM, QA, SA, SY, YE) *see* Clidinium and Chlordiazepoxide 460
Epirazole (AE, BH, CY, EG, IQ, IR, JO, KW, LB, LY, OM, QA, SA, SY, YE) *see* Omeprazole 1508
Episan (ID) *see* Sucralfate 1940
Episenta (GB) *see* Valproic Acid and Derivatives 2123
Episindan (HK, HR, SG) *see* Epirubicin 739
Epitomax (FI, FR) *see* Topiramate 2065
Epitopic (AE, FR) *see* Difluprednate 626
Epitopic (AE, FR) *see* Difluprednate (Topical) [INT] 627
Epitop (PH) *see* Topiramate 2065
Epitrim (AE, BH, CY, EG, IQ, IR, JO, KW, LB, LY, OM, QA, RO, SA, SY, YE) *see* Sulfamethoxazole and Trimethoprim 1946
Epival (AE, BH, CR, CY, DO, EG, GT, IQ, IR, JO, KW, LB, LY, MX, NI, OM, PA, PH, QA, SA, SV, SY, YE) *see* Valproic Acid and Derivatives 2123
Epiven (ID; PH) *see* Gabapentin 943
Epivid (PH) *see* Epirubicin 739
Epivir 3TC (CL) *see* LamiVUDine 1157
Epivir (AE, AT, BE, BH, BR, CY, CZ, DE, DK, EE, EG, ES, FI, FR, GB, GR, HN, HR, HU, IE, IL, IQ, IR, IS, IT, JO, KW, LB, LT, LU, LY, MT, NL, NO, OM, PE, PL, PT, PY, QA, RO, RU, SA, SE, SG, SI, SK, SY, TH, TR, VE, VN, YE) *see* LamiVUDine 1157
Epleptin (ZA) *see* Gabapentin 943
Eplerona (AR) *see* Eplerenone 740
Eplerone (PY) *see* Eplerenone 740
E.P.Mycin (PH) *see* Epirubicin 739
Epogen (PH) *see* Epoetin Alfa 742
Epokine (PH) *see* Epoetin Alfa 742
Eporon (TH) *see* Epoetin Alfa 742
Eposal Retard (CO) *see* CarBAMazepine 346
Eposal (VE) *see* ChlordiazePOXIDE 422
Eposin (CO, MY, TH, TW) *see* Etoposide 816
Eposino (PH) *see* Epoetin Alfa 742
Eposis (KR, PH, TH) *see* Epoetin Alfa 742
Epotin (AE, KW, LB, QA) *see* Epoetin Alfa 742
Epovax (PH) *see* Epoetin Alfa 742
Epram (TW, UY) *see* Escitalopram 765
Eprex (AE, AR, AU, BB, BD, BE, BG, BH, BM, BR, BS, BZ, CH, CR, CY, CZ, DK, DO, EE, EG, ES, FI, FR, GB, GR, GT, GY, HK, HN, HR, HU, ID, IL, IN, IQ, IR, IT, JM, JO, KW, LB, LY, MX, MY, NI, NL, NO, NZ, OM, PA, PE, PH, PK, PL, PY, QA, RO, RU, SA, SE, SG, SR, SV, SY, TH, TR, TT, TW, UY, VE, VN, YE) *see* Epoetin Alfa 742
Eprocin (KR) *see* Ciprofloxacin (Systemic) 441
Epsamon (CH) *see* Aminocaproic Acid 113
Epsicaprom (PT) *see* Aminocaproic Acid 113
Epsidox (CL) *see* Etoposide 816
Epsilon (FI) *see* Aminocaproic Acid 113
Eptadone (GB, IT) *see* Methadone 1311
Eptoin (IN) *see* Phenytoin 1640
Eptus (IN) *see* Eplerenone 740
Epzicom (JP) *see* Abacavir and Lamivudine 22
Equaltha (MX) *see* Anidulafungin 150
Equanil (AU, FR, GB, IE, ZA) *see* Meprobamate 1296
Equasym XL (GB, IE) *see* Methylphenidate 1336
Equasym Depot (DK, NO, SE) *see* Methylphenidate 1336
Equasym Retard (DE) *see* Methylphenidate 1336
Equilibrium (IN) *see* ChlordiazePOXIDE 422
Equin (HK) *see* Estrogens (Conjugated/Equine, Systemic) 787
Equinorm (BF, BJ, CI, ET, GH, GM, GN, KE, LR, MA, ML, MR, MU, MW, NE, NG, SC, SD, SL, SN, TN, TZ, UG, ZA, ZM, ZW) *see* ClomiPRAMINE 475
Equipaz (AR) *see* Prazepam [INT] 1702
Equiplen (PE) *see* Omega-3 Fatty Acids 1507
Equirex (IN) *see* Clidinium and Chlordiazepoxide 460
Equoral (AE, EE, HR, RO, TH) *see* CycloSPORINE (Systemic) 522
Eraclox (PH) *see* Cloxacillin [CAN/INT] 488
Eradix (ID) *see* Meropenem 1299
ERA (NZ) *see* Erythromycin (Systemic) 762
Eranz (AR, BR, CL, CO, CR, EC, GT, MX, NI, SV, VE) *see* Donepezil 668
Erase (IN) *see* Erythromycin (Systemic) 762
Eraxis (AU, HK, IL, KR, MY, PH, SG, TH, TW) *see* Anidulafungin 150
ERAZABAN (CZ, EE, FR, IE, NL, PL, PT) *see* Docosanol 661
Erazaban (SK, TR) *see* Docosanol 661
Erazon (HR, RU) *see* Piroxicam 1662
Erbitux (AE, AR, AT, AU, BE, BG, BR, CH, CL, CN, CO, CR, CY, CZ, DE, DK, DO, EC, EE, ES, FI, FR, GB, GR, GT, HK, HN, HR, HU, ID, IE, IL, IS, IT, JP, KR, KW, LB, LT, MT, MY, NI, NL, NO, NZ, PA, PE, PH, PL, PT, QA, RO, RU, SE, SG, SI, SK, SV, TH, TR, TW, VE, VN, ZA) *see* Cetuximab 413
Ercefuryl (BE, ES, FR, IT, LU) *see* Nifuroxazide [INT] 1454
Erceryl (FR) *see* Nifuroxazide [INT] 1454
Ercofer (SE) *see* Ferrous Fumarate 870
Ercoquin (DK, NO) *see* Hydroxychloroquine 1021
Ercoril (DK) *see* Propantheline 1727
Ercotina (SE) *see* Propantheline 1727
Erdine (KR) *see* Erdosteine [INT] 753
Erdobat (ID) *see* Erdosteine [INT] 753
Erdoce (KR) *see* Erdosteine [INT] 753
Erdomac (IN) *see* Erdosteine [INT] 753
Erdomed (AT, BG, CZ, HN, PL, RO, SK) *see* Erdosteine [INT] 753
Erdopect (FI) *see* Erdosteine [INT] 753
Erdos (KR, TH) *see* Erdosteine [INT] 753
Erdotin (DK, GB, IE, IL, IT, PT) *see* Erdosteine [INT] 753
Erdozets (IN) *see* Erdosteine [INT] 753
Ereccil (PY) *see* Sildenafil 1882
Erectol (AR) *see* Sildenafil 1882
Eremfat (DE) *see* Rifampin 1804
Ergam (HU) *see* Ergotamine 754
Ergenyl (SE) *see* Valproic Acid and Derivatives 2123
Ergocaf (MX) *see* Ergotamine 754
Ergocalm (DE) *see* Lormetazepam [INT] 1247
Ergodryl Mono (AU) *see* Ergotamine 754
Ergojen (PH) *see* Methylergonovine 1333
Ergokapton (AT) *see* Ergotamine 754
Ergo-Kranit (DE) *see* Ergotamine 754
Ergolan (CN) *see* Diltiazem 634
Ergomet (PH) *see* Methylergonovine 1333
Ergometrina maleato (CL) *see* Ergonovine [CAN/INT] 754
Ergometrine (CN) *see* Ergonovine [CAN/INT] 754
ergo sanol (DE) *see* Ergotamine 754
Ergosanol (DE, LU) *see* Ergotamine 754
Ergosanol SL (CH) *see* Ergotamine 754
Ergosanol Spezial N (LU) *see* Ergotamine 754
Ergosia (TH) *see* Ergotamine 754
Ergosterina Irradiata (IT) *see* Ergocalciferol 753
Ergotab (IN) *see* Ergonovine [CAN/INT] 754
Ergotamina (PY) *see* Dihydroergotamine 633
Ergotamina tartrato (IT) *see* Ergotamine 754
Ergotamin (DE) *see* Ergotamine 754
Ergotamin Medihaler (DK) *see* Ergotamine 754
Ergotaminum Tartaricum (PL) *see* Ergotamine 754
Ergotamin "Dak" (DK) *see* Ergotamine 754
Ergotan (IT) *see* Ergotamine 754
Ergotartrat (AT) *see* Ergotamine 754
Ergoto (KR) *see* Ergonovine [CAN/INT] 754
Ergotrate (BR, MX, PE, PH) *see* Ergonovine [CAN/INT] 754
Ergovasan (AT) *see* Dihydroergotamine 633
Ergovin (TW) *see* Ergonovine [CAN/INT] 754
Eribell (PY) *see* Ferrous Sulfate 871
Eribiotic (BR) *see* Erythromycin (Systemic) 762

Ericina (CO) *see* Epirubicin 739
Erifor (MX) *see* Tetracycline 2017
Erifostine (AR) *see* Amifostine 109
Erigran (PY) *see* Erythromycin (Systemic) 762
Erilax (KR) *see* Orphenadrine 1522
Erilin (CO) *see* Sildenafil 1882
Erimicin (AR, PY, UY) *see* Erythromycin and Benzoyl Peroxide 765
Erinmet (IN) *see* Ergonovine [CAN/INT] 754
Erios (CH) *see* Erythromycin (Systemic) 762
Eriotib (AR) *see* Bendamustine 241
Erisul (CO) *see* Erythromycin and Sulfisoxazole 765
Eritrex (BR) *see* Erythromycin (Systemic) 762
Eritrocina (PT) *see* Erythromycin (Systemic) 762
Eritrogen (TH) *see* Epoetin Alfa 742
Eritrolag (AE, BF, BH, BJ, CI, CY, EG, ET, GH, GM, GN, IQ, IR, JO, KE, KW, LB, LR, LY, MA, ML, MR, MU, MW, NE, NG, OM, QA, SA, SC, SD, SL, SN, SY, TN, TZ, UG, YE, ZM, ZW) *see* Erythromycin (Systemic) 762
Eritromicina (CL) *see* Erythromycin (Systemic) 762
Eritromicin (HR) *see* Erythromycin (Systemic) 762
Erivedge (AU, CH, CY, CZ, DE, DK, EE, GB, HR, IL, IS, KR, LT, MX, NL, NO, NZ, RO, SE, SG, SI, SK, TR) *see* Vismodegib 2171
Erlibelle (GB) *see* Ethinyl Estradiol and Levonorgestrel 803
Erlvirax (SG) *see* Acyclovir (Systemic) 47
Ermycin (CY, SG, TR) *see* Erythromycin (Systemic) 762
Ernafil (HK, SG) *see* Sildenafil 1882
Ernex (AR, UY) *see* Benzydamine [CAN/INT] 249
Erocetin (PY, UY) *see* Cephalexin 405
Erocin (JO) *see* Erythromycin (Ophthalmic) 764
Erodium (AR) *see* Bromperidol [INT] 292
Erolin (BB, BM, BS, BZ, GY, JM, SR, TT) *see* Loratadine 1241
Eromel (ZA) *see* Erythromycin (Systemic) 762
Erostin (IN) *see* Ebastine [INT] 702
Erotab (SG) *see* Erythromycin (Systemic) 762
Erotadil (VN) *see* Tadalafil 1968
Eroton (BG) *see* Sildenafil 1882
Eroxet (PH) *see* CefTRIAXone 396
Eroxim (CO) *see* Sildenafil 1882
Eroxmit (PH) *see* Cefuroxime 399
Erphacef (ID) *see* CefTRIAXone 396
Erphadrox (ID) *see* Cefadroxil 372
Erradic (BR) *see* Omeprazole, Clarithromycin, and Amoxicillin 1511
Errkes (TR) *see* Ketorolac (Ophthalmic) 1149
Errolon (AR) *see* Furosemide 940
ERruvin (KR) *see* Methylergonovine 1333
Ertensi (ID) *see* AmLODIPine 123
Ertusin (ID) *see* Erdosteine [INT] 753
Erwinase (AR, AT, GR, IE, KR, LB, NL, NZ, PT, SE, SG, TH, VN) *see* Asparaginase (Erwinia) 180
Ery-V (PH) *see* Erythromycin (Ophthalmic) 764
Eryacne (AR, AU, CO, FR, GR, IT, KR, NZ, PY, SG, TH, VE) *see* Erythromycin (Topical) 765
Eryacnen (BR, CL, CR, DO, GT, HN, NI, PA, PE, SV) *see* Erythromycin (Topical) 765
Eryaknen (CH) *see* Erythromycin (Topical) 765
Erycin (MY, TH, TW) *see* Erythromycin (Systemic) 762
Eryc (KR, SA) *see* Erythromycin (Systemic) 762
Ery (DE) *see* Erythromycin (Systemic) 762
Eryderm (AE, NL, QA, SA) *see* Erythromycin (Topical) 765
Erydermec (DE) *see* Erythromycin (Topical) 765
Erydin (DK) *see* Isoproterenol 1124
Ery-Diolan (QA) *see* Erythromycin (Systemic) 762
Eryfluid (CZ, FR, LB, RO) *see* Erythromycin (Topical) 765
Erylik (HK) *see* Erythromycin (Topical) 765
Ery Max (IS) *see* Erythromycin (Systemic) 762
Erymed (ID) *see* Erythromycin (Topical) 765
Erymycin AF (ZA) *see* Erythromycin (Systemic) 762
Erypo (AT, DE) *see* Epoetin Alfa 742
Ery-Tab (BB, BM, BS, BZ, GY, JM, PR, SR, TT) *see* Erythromycin (Systemic) 762
Erytab-S (MY) *see* Erythromycin (Systemic) 762
Eryth-Mycin (TH) *see* Erythromycin (Systemic) 762
Erythran (TR) *see* Erythromycin (Systemic) 762
Erythrocin (AE, AT, BH, CY, EG, GB, GR, IE, IQ, IR, JO, KR, KW, LB, LY, OM, QA, SA, SY, TW, YE) *see* Erythromycin (Systemic) 762
Erythrocine (NL) *see* Erythromycin (Systemic) 762
Erythrodar (AE, BH, JO, QA, SA) *see* Erythromycin (Systemic) 762
Erythro (KR) *see* Erythromycin (Systemic) 762
Erythromil (AT, BE, BF, BG, BJ, CH, CI, CZ, DE, DK, EE, ET, FI, FR, GB, GH, GM, GN, GR, HN, IE, IT, KE, LR, MA, ML, MR, MT, MU, MW, NE, NG, NL, NO, PL, PT, RU, SC, SD, SE, SK, SL, SN, TN, TR, TZ, UG, ZM, ZW) *see* Erythromycin (Systemic) 762
Erythromycin (DE) *see* Erythromycin (Systemic) 762
Erythromycinum (NL) *see* Erythromycin (Systemic) 762
Erythropen (GR) *see* Erythromycin (Systemic) 762
Erythro-Teva (IL) *see* Erythromycin (Systemic) 762
Esacinone (AE, BH, CY, EG, IQ, IR, JO, KW, LB, LY, OM, QA, SA, SY, YE) *see* Fluocinolone (Topical) 893
Escapelle (HR, RO) *see* Levonorgestrel 1201
Escapin (PE) *see* Scopolamine (Systemic) 1870
Escital (KR) *see* Escitalopram 765
Escivex (PH) *see* Escitalopram 765
Escodaron (CH) *see* Amiodarone 114
Escoflex (CH) *see* Chlorzoxazone 430
Escoprim (CH) *see* Sulfamethoxazole and Trimethoprim 1946
Escor (AT, DE, DK, FI, LU) *see* Nilvadipine [INT] 1456
Escord (IN) *see* Esmolol 769
Escre (JP) *see* Chloral Hydrate [CAN/INT] 418
Esdedril (IT) *see* Naftidrofuryl [INT] 1416
Esdian (TW) *see* Cyproterone and Ethinyl Estradiol [CAN/INT] 532
Eselin (IT) *see* Etamsylate [INT] 795
Esfalon-D (CL) *see* Enalapril and Hydrochlorothiazide 725
Esgen (KR) *see* Estropipate 793
Esidep (TH) *see* Escitalopram 765
Esidrex (AE, AT, BB, BE, BF, BH, BJ, BM, BS, BZ, CH, CI, CY, EG, ET, FR, GH, GM, GN, GR, GY, IN, IQ, IR, IT, JM, JO, KE, KW, LB, LR, LU, LY, MA, ML, MR, MU, MW, NE, NG, NL, NO, OM, QA, SA, SC, SD, SE, SL, SN, SR, SY, TN, TT, TZ, UG, UY, YE, ZA, ZM, ZW) *see* Hydrochlorothiazide 1009
Esidrix (DE) *see* Hydrochlorothiazide 1009
Esilgan (ID, IT, JP, KR, PK) *see* Estazolam 775
ES (IN) *see* Lisinopril 1226
Esipram (AU) *see* Escitalopram 765
Esitalo (AU, HK) *see* Escitalopram 765
Eskaflam (MX) *see* Nimesulide [INT] 1456
Eskalith (BB, BM, BS, BZ, GY, JM, SR, TT) *see* Lithium 1230
Eskapar (MX) *see* Nifuroxazide [INT] 1454
Eskasole (MX) *see* Albendazole 65
Eskazine (ES) *see* Trifluoperazine 2102
Eskazole (AT, AU, DE, ES, GB, IL, JP, NL, NZ) *see* Albendazole 65
Eskotrin (VE) *see* Aspirin 180
Eslam (TW) *see* Estazolam 775
Eslax (JP) *see* Rocuronium 1838
Eslite (IN) *see* Hydroquinone 1020
Eslopran (CO) *see* Escitalopram 765
Esmara (KR) *see* Letrozole 1181
Esmeron (AE, AT, AU, BE, BG, BH, BR, CH, CL, CN, CR, CY, CZ, DE, DK, DO, EE, EG, ES, FI, FR, GB, GR, GT, HK, HN, HR, HU, IE, IL, IQ, IR, IS, IT, JO, KR, KW, LB, LT, LY, MT, MY, NI, NL, NO, NZ, OM, PA, PE, PH, PK,

PL, PT, QA, RO, RU, SA, SE, SG, SI, SK, SV, SY, TH, TR, TW, VE, VN, YE) *see* Rocuronium 1838
Esmind (JP) *see* ChlorproMAZINE 429
Esmirtal (PE) *see* Memantine 1286
Esmya (CH, DE, GB, SG) *see* Ulipristal 2113
Esoderm (AE) *see* Lindane 1217
Esofag (IN) *see* Esomeprazole 771
Esoflux (PH) *see* Esomeprazole 771
Esomed (IL) *see* Hydroquinone 1020
Esomep (PH) *see* Esomeprazole 771
Esonide (QA, SG) *see* Budesonide (Nasal) 296
Esoplex (LB) *see* Escitalopram 765
Esorest (IN) *see* Esomeprazole 771
Esoxium (VN) *see* Esomeprazole 771
Espadox (DE) *see* Doxepin (Systemic) 676
Espa-lepsin (DE) *see* CarBAMazepine 346
Espasmotab (EC) *see* Scopolamine (Systemic) 1870
Espast (PE) *see* Baclofen 223
Espazine (IN) *see* Trifluoperazine 2102
Espectrin (BR) *see* Sulfamethoxazole and Trimethoprim 1946
Esperal (BG, FR, IN, RU) *see* Disulfiram 654
Espercil (CL) *see* Tranexamic Acid 2081
Esperson (BD, BG, BR, CL, HK, ID, IN, JP, KR, MY, PH, PK, PT, SG, TH, TW) *see* Desoximetasone 598
Espin (SG) *see* Dosulepin [INT] 673
Espledol (ES) *see* Acemetacin [INT] 30
Espo (CN, JP) *see* Epoetin Alfa 742
Espogen (TH) *see* Epoetin Alfa 742
Esracain (IL) *see* Lidocaine (Systemic) 1208
Esracain Jelly (IL) *see* Lidocaine (Topical) 1211
Esram (HR) *see* Escitalopram 765
Esroban (KR) *see* Mupirocin 1404
Estalin (ID) *see* Estazolam 775
Estalis continuous (AU) *see* Estradiol and Norethindrone 781
Estalis Sequi (AU) *see* Estradiol and Norethindrone 781
Estaprol (AR, CL, UY) *see* Ciprofibrate [INT] 441
Estazolam (PL) *see* Estazolam 775
Estazor (ID) *see* Ursodiol 2116
Estel (KR) *see* Ebastine [INT] 702
Estelle-35 (AE) *see* Cyproterone and Ethinyl Estradiol [CAN/INT] 532
Estelle-35 ED (AU, ID, NZ) *see* Cyproterone and Ethinyl Estradiol [CAN/INT] 532
Estelle -35 (IL, MY, SG, TW) *see* Cyproterone and Ethinyl Estradiol [CAN/INT] 532
Estermax (CO) *see* Estrogens (Conjugated/Equine, Systemic) 787
Estima Ge (FR) *see* Progesterone 1722
Estimex (PY) *see* Escitalopram 765
Estimin (TW) *see* Ebastine [INT] 702
Estin (ID) *see* Cetirizine 411
Estinor (SG) *see* Levonorgestrel 1201
Estiva-600 (TH) *see* Efavirenz 707
Estival (GR) *see* Carbocisteine [INT] 357
Estivan (BE) *see* Ebastine [INT] 702
Esto (IL) *see* Escitalopram 765
Estomil (ES) *see* Lansoprazole 1166
Estracomb (AE, BH, CY, EG, IQ, IR, JO, KW, LB, LY, OM, QA, SA, SY, YE) *see* Estradiol and Norethindrone 781
Estracomb (IL) *see* Ethinyl Estradiol and Norethindrone 808
Estracomb TTS (SA) *see* Estradiol and Norethindrone 781
Estracyt (AE, AR, AT, BE, BG, BH, CH, CL, CN, CO, CY, CZ, DE, DK, EE, EG, ES, FI, FR, GB, GR, HK, HN, HR, IE, IL, IQ, IR, IS, IT, JO, JP, KR, KW, LB, LY, MT, MY, NL, NO, OM, PL, PT, QA, RO, RU, SA, SE, SG, SI, SK, SY, TR, TW, VE, VN, YE, ZA) *see* Estramustine 782
Estraderm MX (AU, IN, PT, SA, SG) *see* Estradiol (Systemic) 775
Estraderm (AU, CO, DK, SE, VN) *see* Estradiol (Systemic) 775
Estraderm TTS (AE, AT, BF, BH, BJ, CI, CO, CY, CZ, DE, EG, ET, FR, GB, GH, GM, GN, GR, IL, IQ, IR, IT, JO, KE, KR, KW, LB, LR, LY, MA, ML, MR, MU, MW, NE, NG, NZ, OM, PL, PY, QA, SC, SD, SL, SN, SY, TN, TR, TZ, UG, YE, ZA, ZM, ZW) *see* Estradiol (Systemic) 775
Estrade (TW) *see* Estradiol (Systemic) 775
Estradot (AU, BR, CZ, DE, FI, GB, GR, IE, NO, PT, SE, UY) *see* Estradiol (Systemic) 775
Estradot (HR) *see* Estradiol (Topical) 780
Estradurin (CH, DE, DK, ES, FI, NL, NO, SE) *see* Polyestradiol [INT] 1673
Estra Gel (TW) *see* Estradiol (Systemic) 775
Estragest TTS (AE, BH, CY, DE, EG, IQ, IR, JO, KW, LB, LY, OM, QA, SA, SY, YE) *see* Estradiol and Norethindrone 781
Estragest TTS (IL) *see* Ethinyl Estradiol and Norethindrone 808
Estranova (PE) *see* Estrogens (Conjugated/Equine, Systemic) 787
Estrapatch (FR) *see* Estradiol (Systemic) 775
Estrarona (UY) *see* Estrogens (Conjugated/Equine, Systemic) 787
Estratab (CA) *see* Estrogens (Esterified) 790
Estreptomicina (AR) *see* Streptomycin 1937
Estrepto-Monaxin (MX) *see* Streptomycin 1937
Estreva (DE, HK, PE, PT, TR, VN) *see* Estradiol (Systemic) 775
Estreva Gel (PE) *see* Estradiol (Systemic) 775
Estrifam (DE) *see* Estradiol (Systemic) 775
Estring (AT, CH, DE, DK, FI, NL, NO, SG, ZA) *see* Estradiol (Topical) 780
Estrinolon (BR) *see* Estrogens (Conjugated/Equine, Systemic) 787
Estrofem (AR, AT, AU, BE, BH, BR, CH, CN, CZ, DK, EE, FI, FR, HK, HU, IL, IN, IS, KR, KW, LB, LT, NZ, PH, RU, SA, SG, SI, TH, UY) *see* Estradiol (Systemic) 775
Estrofem Forte (BF, BJ, CI, ET, GH, GM, GN, KE, LR, MA, ML, MR, MU, MW, NE, NG, SC, SD, SL, SN, TN, TZ, UG, ZM, ZW) *see* Estradiol (Systemic) 775
Estrogel (VE) *see* Estradiol (Systemic) 775
Estromon FC (TH) *see* Estrogens (Conjugated/Equine, Systemic) 787
Estronorm (NO) *see* Estradiol (Systemic) 775
Estro-Pause (ZA) *see* Estradiol (Systemic) 775
Estroquin (PE) *see* Leucovorin Calcium 1183
Estulic (BE, BF, BJ, CH, CI, CZ, DE, ET, FR, GH, GM, GN, HN, HU, ID, JP, KE, LR, MA, ML, MR, MU, MW, NE, NG, NL, PH, PL, RU, SC, SD, SL, SN, TN, TZ, UG, ZA, ZM, ZW) *see* GuanFACINE 990
Esulin (TW) *see* TOLAZamide 2062
Esvat (ID) *see* Simvastatin 1890
Eszo 2 (TW) *see* Estazolam 775
Eszop (CL) *see* Eszopiclone 793
Etaconil (CL, PE) *see* Flutamide 907
Etalpha (AT, CL, CN, DK, FI, IS, NL, NO, PT, RU, SE) *see* Alfacalcidol [CAN/INT] 82
Etambutol (BG, HR) *see* Ethambutol 798
Etambutol Northia (AR) *see* Ethambutol 798
Etambutol Richet (AR) *see* Ethambutol 798
Etambutol Richmond (AR) *see* Ethambutol 798
Etamine (PH) *see* Ketamine 1143
Etanorden (BG) *see* Ibandronate 1028
Etapiam (IT) *see* Ethambutol 798
Etec 1000 (EC) *see* Vitamin E 2174
Eteophyl (KR) *see* Theophylline 2026
Eternal (MX) *see* Vitamin E 2174
Ethambin-PIN (PH) *see* Ethambutol 798
Ethambutol (PL) *see* Ethambutol 798
Ethamsyl (IN) *see* Etamsylate [INT] 795
Etham (TH) *see* Ethambutol 798

Ethbutol (TH) *see* Ethambutol 798
ETH Ciba 400 (ID) *see* Ethambutol 798
Ethicef (ID) *see* Cefadroxil 372
Ethicholine (MY, SG) *see* Succinylcholine 1939
Ethicol (ID) *see* Simvastatin 1890
Ethifrin (PK) *see* Phenylephrine (Systemic) 1638
Ethigent (ID) *see* Gentamicin (Systemic) 959
Ethimox (ID) *see* Amoxicillin 130
Ethipramine (ZA) *see* Imipramine 1054
Ethrimax DS (ID) *see* Azithromycin (Systemic) 216
Ethyfron (JP) *see* Etilefrine [INT] 815
Ethymal (NL) *see* Ethosuximide 813
Ethyol (AE, AR, AT, AU, BE, BG, BH, BR, CH, CL, CO, CR, CY, CZ, DE, DK, DO, EC, ES, FI, FR, GB, GR, GT, HK, HN, IE, IL, IT, KR, LU, MX, NI, NL, NZ, PA, PE, PH, PL, PT, QA, SE, SV, TR, TW, UY, VE) *see* Amifostine 109
Etibi (AT, ID, IT) *see* Ethambutol 798
Etibon (TW) *see* Etidronate 813
Etidoxina (CO) *see* Doxycycline 689
Etidronat Jenapharm (DE) *see* Etidronate 813
Etidron (IT) *see* Etidronate 813
Etifibrat (SV) *see* Bezafibrate [CAN/INT] 261
Etilefrina (AR) *see* Etilefrine [INT] 815
Etilefrina Denver Farma (AR) *see* Etilefrine [INT] 815
Etilefrina Fabra (AR) *see* Etilefrine [INT] 815
Etilefrina Larjan (AR) *see* Etilefrine [INT] 815
Etilefrin AL (DE) *see* Etilefrine [INT] 815
Etilefrin (DE) *see* Etilefrine [INT] 815
Etilefrin-Neosan (DE) *see* Etilefrine [INT] 815
Etilefrin-ratiopharm (DE) *see* Etilefrine [INT] 815
etil von ct (DE) *see* Etilefrine [INT] 815
Etindrax (MX) *see* Allopurinol 90
Etinoline (CN) *see* Albuterol 69
Etipramid (CN) *see* Theophylline 2026
Eti-Puren (DE) *see* Etilefrine [INT] 815
Etisec (IN) *see* Secnidazole [INT] 1872
Etisona 3 (PY) *see* PrednisoLONE (Systemic) 1703
ETL (TW) *see* Etodolac 815
Etnoderm (CL) *see* Hydroquinone 1020
Etocin (BF, BJ, CI, ET, GH, GM, GN, KE, LR, MA, ML, MR, MU, MW, NE, NG, SC, SD, SL, SN, TN, TZ, UG, ZM, ZW) *see* Erythromycin (Systemic) 762
Etocris (PY) *see* Etoposide 816
Etodagim (VN) *see* Etodolac 815
Etodine (LB) *see* Etodolac 815
Etodin Fort (BG) *see* Etodolac 815
Etofen (CH) *see* Etofenamate [INT] 815
Etoflam (PH) *see* Etodolac 815
Etogel (CZ) *see* Etofenamate [INT] 815
Etomal (FI) *see* Ethosuximide 813
Etomidat-Lipuro (CH, LU) *see* Etomidate 816
Etomidato-Lipuro (AR) *see* Etomidate 816
Etonalin F (JP) *see* Fluocinonide 894
Etonco (MX) *see* Etoposide 816
Etoniri (MX) *see* Irinotecan 1112
Etonox (TH) *see* Etodolac 815
Etopan XL (GB, IL) *see* Etodolac 815
Etopan (IL) *see* Etodolac 815
Etopofos (AT, DK, FI, NO, SE) *see* Etoposide Phosphate 820
Etopophos (AU, CH, FR, GB, IE, NL, NZ, ZA) *see* Etoposide Phosphate 820
Etopos (MX) *see* Etoposide 816
Etopos (MX) *see* Etoposide Phosphate 820
Etoposid (AE, CY, IL, JO, KW) *see* Etoposide 816
Etoposide (AU, IL, NZ) *see* Etoposide 816
Etoposide Pierre Fabre (LU) *see* Etoposide 816
Etoposide Teva (HU) *see* Etoposide 816
Etoposido (PE) *see* Etoposide 816
Etopul (ID, PH) *see* Etoposide 816
Etosid (IN, VE) *see* Etoposide 816
Etosuximida (ES) *see* Ethosuximide 813
Etova (IN) *see* Etodolac 815
Etoxin (BR) *see* Ethosuximide 813
Etoxisclerol (VE) *see* Polidocanol 1672
Etrivex (GB) *see* Clobetasol 468
Etron nistatina (EC) *see* Metronidazole and Nystatin [CAN/INT] 1358
Etrotab (MY) *see* Erythromycin (Systemic) 762
Etylu Aminobenzoesan (PL) *see* Benzocaine 246
EU2000 (TH) *see* Terbinafine (Systemic) 2002
Eubotol (VN) *see* Ethambutol 798
Eucardic (GB, IE, NL) *see* Carvedilol 367
Eucerin (DE) *see* Urea 2114
Euchlor (VN) *see* Chloramphenicol 421
Euclamin (PL) *see* GlyBURIDE 972
Eucor (EC) *see* Lisinopril 1226
Eucor (TH) *see* Simvastatin 1890
Eucycline (GR) *see* Ketotifen (Systemic) [CAN/INT] 1149
Eudemine (GB) *see* Diazoxide 616
Euderm (HK, MY, SG) *see* Urea 2114
Eudextran (IT) *see* Dextran 607
Eudigox (IT) *see* Digoxin 627
Eudyna (MY) *see* Tretinoin (Topical) 2099
Eufindol (CL) *see* TraMADol 2074
Euform Retard (PH) *see* MetFORMIN 1307
Eugenix (ID) *see* Benserazide and Levodopa [CAN/INT] 244
Eugen (TW) *see* Triprolidine and Pseudoephedrine 2105
Eugerial (AR, CO, PE) *see* NiMODipine 1456
Euglim (IN) *see* Glimepiride 966
Euglo Plus (PH) *see* Glyburide and Metformin 974
Euglotab (PH) *see* GlyBURIDE 972
Euglucan (FR) *see* GlyBURIDE 972
Euglucon (AE, AR, AT, AU, BD, BE, BF, BH, BJ, BO, CH, CI, CO, CY, CZ, DE, EC, EG, ES, ET, FI, GH, GM, GN, GR, HK, HR, IN, IQ, IR, IT, JO, JP, KE, KR, KW, LB, LR, LU, LY, MA, ML, MR, MU, MW, MX, MY, NE, NG, NZ, OM, PH, PK, PT, PY, QA, RU, SA, SC, SD, SE, SG, SL, SN, SY, TH, TN, TW, TZ, UG, YE, ZA, ZM, ZW) *see* GlyBURIDE 972
Eugynon 28 (DE) *see* Ethinyl Estradiol and Norgestrel 812
Eugynon 30 (IE) *see* Ethinyl Estradiol and Norgestrel 812
Euhypnos (BE, IE, LU, NZ) *see* Temazepam 1990
Euipnos (IT) *see* Temazepam 1990
Eukacin (TW) *see* Amikacin 111
Eulexin (AE, AR, AU, BE, BH, BR, CR, CY, DO, EG, FI, GT, HN, IR, IT, JO, KE, KR, KW, LB, LU, LY, MX, NI, NL, NO, NZ, OM, PA, PK, PT, QA, SA, SE, SV, SY, TR, VE) *see* Flutamide 907
Eulexine (FR) *see* Flutamide 907
Eulip (TW) *see* Bezafibrate [CAN/INT] 261
Eulitop (BE, ES) *see* Bezafibrate [CAN/INT] 261
Eumac (IN) *see* Pantoprazole 1570
Eumide (MY) *see* Flutamide 907
Eumitan (AT) *see* Frovatriptan 938
Eumotil (UY) *see* Trimebutine [CAN/INT] 2103
Eunice-35 (MX) *see* Cyproterone and Ethinyl Estradiol [CAN/INT] 532
Eunoctal (FR) *see* Amobarbital 128
Eunoctin (HN) *see* Nitrazepam [CAN/INT] 1461
Eupantol (FR) *see* Pantoprazole 1570
Eupept (BR) *see* Omeprazole 1508
Euphorin (JP) *see* Diazepam 613
Euphyllin (PL) *see* Theophylline 2026
Euphyllin Retard (ID) *see* Theophylline 2026
Euphyllin Retard Mite (ID) *see* Theophylline 2026
Euphylong (AE, BH, CY, EG, HK, HU, IQ, IR, JO, KW, LB, LY, OM, QA, SA, SY, YE) *see* Theophylline 2026
Euphylong Retardkaps (DE) *see* Theophylline 2026
Eupramin (HR) *see* Imipramine 1054
Euradal (ES) *see* Bisoprolol 266

Eurax (AE, AT, AU, BB, BE, BF, BH, BJ, BM, BS, BZ, CH, CI, CL, CO, CY, EG, ET, FR, GB, GH, GM, GN, GR, GY, HK, HR, IE, IL, IN, IQ, IR, IT, JM, JO, KE, KW, LB, LR, LU, LY, MA, ML, MR, MU, MW, MX, MY, NE, NG, NL, NO, NZ, OM, PE, PL, PT, QA, SA, SC, SD, SG, SI, SL, SN, SR, SY, TN, TT, TZ, UG, VN, YE, ZA, ZM, ZW) *see* Crotamiton ... 514
Euraxil (ES) *see* Crotamiton ... 514
Eurax-Lotio (AT) *see* Crotamiton ... 514
Eurepa (VN) *see* Repaglinide ... 1791
Eurobetsol (HK) *see* Clobetasol ... 468
Eurocin (PH) *see* Ampicillin ... 141
Euroclin V (CO, EC) *see* Clindamycin (Topical) ... 464
Euroclin (EC) *see* Clindamycin (Systemic) ... 460
Euroclovir (HK) *see* Acyclovir (Systemic) ... 47
Eurodal (PH) *see* Dalteparin ... 553
Eurodin (JP, TW) *see* Estazolam ... 775
Eurofenac (HK) *see* Diclofenac (Systemic) ... 617
Euroflox (AE, BH, CY, EG, IL, IQ, IR, JO, KW, LB, LY, OM, QA, SA, SY, YE) *see* Norfloxacin ... 1475
Eurolac (PH) *see* Ketorolac (Systemic) ... 1146
Eurolev (PH) *see* Levothyroxine ... 1205
Euromucil (PE) *see* Psyllium ... 1744
Europain (HK) *see* Acetaminophen ... 32
Eurovan (HK) *see* Zopiclone [CAN/INT] ... 2217
Eurovir (PY) *see* Acyclovir (Systemic) ... 47
Eurovir (PY) *see* Acyclovir (Topical) ... 51
Eurythmic (IN) *see* Amiodarone ... 114
Eusaprim (AT, BE, FI, IS, IT, NO, SE) *see* Sulfamethoxazole and Trimethoprim ... 1946
Euspiran (CZ) *see* Isoproterenol ... 1124
Eutac (TW) *see* Moclobemide [CAN/INT] ... 1384
Eutebrol (CR, EC, GT, HN, NI, PA, PE, SV) *see* Memantine ... 1286
Euthyral (VN) *see* Liotrix ... 1221
Euthyrox (AE, AR, AT, BE, BG, BH, BR, CH, CN, CY, CZ, DE, EE, HR, HU, ID, IS, JO, KW, LB, MY, PH, PL, QA, RO, RU, SA, SE, SG, SI, SK, TH, TR, VE) *see* Levothyroxine ... 1205
Eutirox (BB, BS, CL, CR, DO, ES, GT, HN, IT, JM, MX, NI, NL, PA, PE, SV, TT) *see* Levothyroxine ... 1205
Eutizon (HR) *see* Isoniazid ... 1120
Eutropin (BR, IN, KR, TH) *see* Somatropin ... 1918
Eutroxsig (AU, NZ) *see* Levothyroxine ... 1205
Euvax-B (KR) *see* Hepatitis B Immune Globulin (Human) ... 1002
Evaflox (MY) *see* Ofloxacin (Systemic) ... 1490
Evalen (ID) *see* Adapalene ... 54
Evalin (ID) *see* CeFAZolin ... 373
Evamox (PK) *see* AcetaZOLAMIDE ... 39
Evaprost (PH) *see* Carboprost Tromethamine ... 360
Evasc (KR) *see* AmLODIPine ... 123
Evastel (MX) *see* Ebastine [INT] ... 702
Evastel Z (MX) *see* Ebastine [INT] ... 702
Evatocin (PH) *see* Oxytocin ... 1549
Eveclin Half (KR) *see* Estradiol and Norethindrone ... 781
Eveclin Half (KR) *see* Ethinyl Estradiol and Norethindrone ... 808
Evelea MD (AR) *see* Ethinyl Estradiol and Levonorgestrel ... 803
Evepar (FR) *see* Cyproterone and Ethinyl Estradiol [CAN/INT] ... 532
Eveprem (KR) *see* Ethinyl Estradiol and Norethindrone ... 808
Everhepa (KR) *see* Adefovir ... 54
Everiden (HU) *see* Valproic Acid and Derivatives ... 2123
Everose (GB) *see* Calcium Acetate ... 326
Eviana (IL) *see* Estradiol and Norethindrone ... 781
Eviclin (KR) *see* Estradiol and Norethindrone ... 781
Eviclin (KR) *see* Ethinyl Estradiol and Norethindrone ... 808
Evicta (TH) *see* Bezafibrate [CAN/INT] ... 261
Evifyne (AU) *see* Raloxifene ... 1765
Eviline (HK) *see* Aluminum Hydroxide, Magnesium Hydroxide, and Simethicone ... 104
Evina (AR) *see* Ergonovine [CAN/INT] ... 754
Evion (IN) *see* Vitamin E ... 2174
Eviplera (AU, BE, CH, CY, CZ, DE, DK, EE, ES, FR, GB, IE, IL, IS, LT, NL, NO, NZ, SE, SI, SK) *see* Emtricitabine, Rilpivirine, and Tenofovir ... 722
Evista (AE, AR, AT, AU, BE, BF, BG, BH, BJ, BR, CH, CI, CL, CN, CO, CY, CZ, DE, DK, EE, ES, ET, FI, FR, GB, GH, GM, GN, GR, HK, HN, HR, HU, ID, IE, IL, IT, KE, KR, KW, LR, LT, MA, ML, MR, MT, MU, MW, MX, MY, NE, NG, NL, NO, NZ, PE, PH, PK, PL, PT, QA, RO, RU, SA, SC, SD, SE, SG, SI, SK, SL, SN, TN, TR, TW, TZ, UG, UY, VE, VN, ZA, ZM, ZW) *see* Raloxifene ... 1765
Evolox (RO) *see* Levofloxacin (Systemic) ... 1197
Evoltra (AT, AU, BE, CY, CZ, DE, DK, EE, FR, GB, GR, HK, HR, IE, IT, JP, KR, LT, MY, NL, NO, NZ, PL, PT, RO, SE, SG, SI, SK, TH, TR) *see* Clofarabine ... 470
Evomixan (BR) *see* MitoXANtrone ... 1382
Evoquin (AR, UY) *see* Hydroxychloroquine ... 1021
Evorel (AR, BB, BM, BS, DK, GY, IE, IL, JM, NL, NO, PR, SE, SR, TT, UY, ZA) *see* Estradiol (Systemic) ... 775
Evorelconti (MX) *see* Ethinyl Estradiol and Norethindrone ... 808
Evorel Conti (AR) *see* Estradiol and Norethindrone ... 781
Evorel Conti (AR) *see* Ethinyl Estradiol and Norethindrone ... 808
Evorel Conti (BB, BM, BS, GY, JM, NL, PR, SR, TT) *see* Estradiol (Systemic) ... 775
Evorel Cont (IL) *see* Estradiol and Norethindrone ... 781
Evorel Cont (IL) *see* Ethinyl Estradiol and Norethindrone ... 808
Evorel Sequi (IL) *see* Estradiol and Norethindrone ... 781
Evorel Sequi (IL) *see* Ethinyl Estradiol and Norethindrone ... 808
Evorel (TR) *see* Estradiol (Topical) ... 780
Evoxac (JP, TW) *see* Cevimeline ... 415
Evozar (BR) *see* Gentamicin (Systemic) ... 959
Evra (AE, AR, BB, BE, BH, BM, BR, BS, BZ, CH, CL, CO, CR, CZ, DE, DK, DO, EC, EE, FI, FR, GB, GR, GT, GY, HK, HN, HR, IE, IL, IS, IT, JM, KR, KW, LT, MT, MY, NI, NL, NO, PA, PE, PH, PL, PR, PT, PY, QA, RO, RU, SA, SE, SG, SI, SK, SR, SV, TH, TT, TW, UY, VE, VN) *see* Ethinyl Estradiol and Norelgestromin ... 807
Evy (TW) *see* Memantine ... 1286
Ewofex (RO) *see* Fexofenadine ... 873
Exaccord (AU) *see* Exemestane ... 828
Exacin (JP) *see* Isepamicin [INT] ... 1120
Exacol (MX) *see* Chloramphenicol ... 421
Exacyl (AE, BE, CZ, FR, HN, LB, LU, PL) *see* Tranexamic Acid ... 2081
Exafal (PK) *see* Artemether and Lumefantrine ... 177
Exastrin (MX) *see* Phenylephrine and Zinc Sulfate [CAN/INT] ... 1640
Exastrin (MX) *see* Zinc Sulfate ... 2200
Excaugh (HK) *see* GuaiFENesin ... 986
Excedrin (AE, CO, IL, KR, QA) *see* Acetaminophen, Aspirin, and Caffeine ... 37
Excegran (JP, KR) *see* Zonisamide ... 2215
Excillin (PH) *see* Ampicillin ... 141
Exel (MX) *see* Meloxicam ... 1283
Exelderm (GB, IE, IT, KR, TW) *see* Sulconazole ... 1943
Exelon (AE, AR, AT, AU, BE, BG, BH, BO, BR, CH, CL, CN, CO, CR, CY, CZ, DE, DK, DO, EC, EE, EG, FI, FR, GB, GR, GT, HK, HN, HU, ID, IE, IL, IS, IT, JO, JP, KR, KW, LB, LT, MT, MX, NI, NL, NO, NZ, PA, PE, PH, PK, PL, PR, PT, PY, QA, RO, RU, SA, SE, SG, SI, SK, SV, TH, TR, TW, UY, VE, VN, ZA) *see* Rivastigmine ... 1833
Exelon Parche (CL) *see* Rivastigmine ... 1833
Exelon Parches (AR, CO, EC) *see* Rivastigmine ... 1833

Exelon Patch (AE, AU, BR, CY, HK, HR, HU, IL, IS, KR, KW, LB, LT, MY, NZ, PE, PH, QA, RO, SG, SI, SK, TH) *see* Rivastigmine ... 1833
Exembol (GB) *see* Argatroban ... 168
Exempla (AR) *see* CefTRIAXone ... 396
Exepime (ID) *see* Cefepime ... 378
Exflem (PH) *see* Acetylcysteine ... 40
Exforge D (AR, CL) *see* Amlodipine, Valsartan, and Hydrochlorothiazide ... 127
Exforge (AE, AR, AU, BE, CH, CL, CN, CO, CY, CZ, DE, DK, EC, EE, ES, FR, GB, GR, HK, HR, HU, ID, IE, IL, IS, JP, KR, KW, LB, LT, MY, NL, NO, NZ, PE, PH, PT, QA, SA, SE, SG, SI, SK, TH, TW, VN) *see* Amlodipine and Valsartan ... 126
Exforge HCT (AT, AU, BE, BR, CH, CO, CY, CZ, DE, DK, EC, EE, FR, HK, HR, IE, KW, LB, LT, MY, NL, NO, PE, PH, PL, PT, QA, SA, SE, SG, SI, SK, TH, TR, TW, VN) *see* Amlodipine, Valsartan, and Hydrochlorothiazide ... 127
Exiadol (MX) *see* Guaifenesin and Dextromethorphan ... 987
Exidol (IL) *see* Acetaminophen, Aspirin, and Caffeine ... 37
Exigo (PH) *see* Betahistine [CAN/INT] ... 252
Exinef (DE) *see* Etoricoxib [INT] ... 821
Exinol (VE) *see* Sucralfate ... 1940
Exipan (IL) *see* Piroxicam ... 1662
Exirel (AT, GB) *see* Pirbuterol ... 1662
Exjade (AE, AR, AT, AU, BE, BG, BH, BR, CH, CL, CN, CO, CY, CZ, DE, DK, EC, EE, ES, FI, FR, GB, GR, HK, HN, HR, HU, ID, IE, IL, IS, IT, JP, KR, KW, LB, LT, MT, MX, MY, NL, NO, NZ, PE, PH, PL, PT, PY, QA, RO, RU, SA, SE, SG, SI, SK, TH, TR, TW, UY, VN) *see* Deferasirox ... 582
Exlip ER (KR) *see* Niacin ... 1443
Exlutena (SE) *see* Lynestrenol [INT] ... 1261
Exlutona (CH, DE, NO) *see* Lynestrenol [INT] ... 1261
Exluton (AR, BE, CZ, FI, FR, LU, MX, NL, PT, ZA) *see* Lynestrenol [INT] ... 1261
Exocin (DK, FI, GB, GR, IE, IT, NO, PK, PT, TR, ZA) *see* Ofloxacin (Ophthalmic) ... 1491
Exocine (FR) *see* Ofloxacin (Ophthalmic) ... 1491
Exoderil (AE, AT, BG, BH, CR, CY, CZ, DE, EE, EG, GR, GT, HK, HN, HR, ID, IL, IQ, IR, JO, KR, KW, LB, LT, LY, MY, NI, OM, PA, PK, PL, QA, RO, RU, SA, SI, SV, SY, TR, TW, YE) *see* Naftifine ... 1416
Exofen (JO) *see* Fexofenadine ... 873
Exomax (HK) *see* Fluconazole ... 885
Exomuc (FR, LU) *see* Acetylcysteine ... 40
Exoseptoplix (FR) *see* Chlorhexidine Gluconate ... 422
Expafusin (ES) *see* Hetastarch ... 1004
Expan (CO) *see* Doxepin (Systemic) ... 676
Expanfen (FR) *see* Ibuprofen ... 1032
Expelin (MX) *see* Carbocisteine [INT] ... 357
Expetan (HK) *see* Carbocisteine [INT] ... 357
Expetan Kids (HK) *see* Carbocisteine [INT] ... 357
Expit (UY) *see* Acyclovir (Systemic) ... 47
Expit (UY) *see* Acyclovir (Topical) ... 51
Expogin (TH) *see* Methylergonovine ... 1333
Exputex (IE) *see* Carbocisteine [INT] ... 357
Extavia (AU, BE, CZ, DK, EE, FR, GB, GR, HR, HU, IE, IT, LT, NL, NO, PL, PT, RO, SE, SI, TR) *see* Interferon Beta-1b ... 1103
Extencilline (FR, HR) *see* Penicillin G Benzathine ... 1609
Extensil (AR) *see* Dapoxetine [INT] ... 561
Extimon (ID) *see* CefTAZidime ... 392
Extine (AU) *see* PARoxetine ... 1579
Extovon (TH) *see* Bromhexine [INT] ... 291
Extracta (AR) *see* Darifenacin ... 568
Extraneal Dialysis Solution (AR, AU, BE, CH, CZ, DK, EE, FI, FR, HN, IE, IL, IT, NL, NO, NZ, SE, SG, TH, TW) *see* Icodextrin ... 1037
Extraneal (HR, KR, KW, LB, LT, QA, RO, SA, SI, SK, VN) *see* Icodextrin ... 1037
Extrapan Gel (HK) *see* Ibuprofen ... 1032
Extrapen (AE, BF, BH, BJ, CI, CY, EG, ET, GH, GM, GN, IQ, IR, JO, KE, KW, LB, LR, LY, MA, ML, MR, MU, MW, NE, NG, OM, QA, SA, SC, SD, SL, SN, SY, TN, TZ, UG, YE, ZM, ZW) *see* Ampicillin ... 141
Extreme (KR) *see* Pantoprazole ... 1570
Extur (ES) *see* Indapamide ... 1065
Exvan (KR) *see* Valsartan ... 2127
Exxiv (PT, RU) *see* Etoricoxib [INT] ... 821
Exzapine (PH) *see* OLANZapine ... 1491
Eyebrex (PH) *see* Tobramycin (Ophthalmic) ... 2056
Eyecon (IL) *see* Hyaluronate and Derivatives ... 1006
Eyefen (IN) *see* Flurbiprofen (Systemic) ... 906
Eyekas (JP) *see* Riboflavin ... 1803
Eyezep (AU, KR) *see* Azelastine (Ophthalmic) ... 213
Eylea (AU, BE, CH, CY, CZ, DE, DK, EE, FI, GB, HK, HR, IS, JP, KR, LT, MY, NO, NZ, PH, PL, RO, SE, SG, SI, SK) *see* Aflibercept (Ophthalmic) ... 63
Eyle (TR) *see* Aflibercept (Ophthalmic) ... 63
Eyosin (PH) *see* Hyoscyamine ... 1026
Eyzu (TW) *see* Estrogens (Conjugated/Equine, Systemic) ... 787
Ezator (CO, PE) *see* Ezetimibe and Atorvastatin ... 833
Ezede (SG) *see* Loratadine ... 1241
Ezenide (MY) *see* Desonide ... 597
E-Zentius (PE) *see* Escitalopram ... 765
Ezetib (IN) *see* Ezetimibe ... 832
Ezetrol (AE, AR, AT, AU, BE, BG, BH, CH, CL, CN, CO, CY, CZ, DE, DK, EC, EE, ES, FI, FR, GB, GR, HK, HN, HR, ID, IE, IL, IS, JO, KR, KW, LB, LT, MX, MY, NL, NO, NZ, PE, PH, PT, QA, RO, RU, SA, SE, SG, SI, SK, TH, TW, VE, VN) *see* Ezetimibe ... 832
Ezilax (BH, JO, KW) *see* Lactulose ... 1156
Ezipect (SA) *see* Bromhexine [INT] ... 291
Ezitoget (VN) *see* Ezetimibe ... 832
Ezolvin (SA) *see* Bromhexine [INT] ... 291
Ezon-T (JP) *see* Tolnaftate ... 2063
Ezopen Creme (BR) *see* Acyclovir (Topical) ... 51
Ezopta (GR) *see* Ranitidine ... 1777
Ezovir (AU) *see* Famciclovir ... 843
F-525 (GR) *see* Etofenamate [INT] ... 815
Fabahistin (GB, ZA) *see* Mebhydrolin [INT] ... 1276
Fabracin (AR) *see* Cinnarizine [INT] ... 440
Fabrazyme (AT, AU, BE, BG, CH, CL, CY, CZ, DE, DK, EE, ES, FI, FR, GB, GR, HK, HN, HR, HU, IE, IL, IS, IT, KR, LT, MT, MY, NL, NO, NZ, PL, PT, RO, RU, SE, SG, SI, SK, TH, TR, TW) *see* Agalsidase Beta ... 64
Fabrol (AT, GR) *see* Acetylcysteine ... 40
Fabuzest (IN) *see* Febuxostat ... 848
Facetik (CO) *see* Cyproterone and Ethinyl Estradiol [CAN/INT] ... 532
Facicam (MX) *see* Piroxicam ... 1662
Facidex (MX) *see* Famotidine ... 845
Facid (ID, IN) *see* Famotidine ... 845
Facidmol (MX) *see* Bismuth ... 265
Facnyne (KR) *see* Factor IX (Human) ... 840
Facort (TH) *see* Triamcinolone (Systemic) ... 2099
Facort (TH) *see* Triamcinolone (Topical) ... 2100
Factive (AE, CN, KR, KW, LB, QA, SA, TW, ZA) *see* Gemifloxacin ... 957
Factodin (GR) *see* Clotrimazole (Topical) ... 488
Fadaflumaz (AR) *see* Flumazenil ... 892
Fadalefrina (AR, UY) *see* Phenylephrine (Systemic) ... 1638
Fadastigmina (AR) *see* Neostigmine ... 1438
Fadine (AE, BH, CY, EG, IQ, IR, JO, KW, LB, LY, OM, QA, SA, SY, YE) *see* Famotidine ... 845
Fadin (TW, VN) *see* Famotidine ... 845
Fadrox (CO) *see* Cefadroxil ... 372
Fadul (DE) *see* Famotidine ... 845
Fagusan N Losung (DE) *see* GuaiFENesin ... 986
Falazine (EC) *see* SulfaSALAzine ... 1950
Falciat (IN) *see* Artesunate ... 178

Falcistat (TR) *see* Sulfadoxine and Pyrimethamine [INT] 1946
Falergi (ID) *see* Cetirizine 411
Falexin (KR) *see* Cephalexin 405
Falithrom (DE) *see* Phenprocoumon [INT] 1635
Falmmazine (VN) *see* Silver Sulfadiazine 1887
Falocef (ID) *see* Cefepime 378
Falvin (IT) *see* Fenticonazole [INT] 868
Famagen (KR) *see* Famotidine 845
Famcino (VN) *see* Famciclovir 843
Famcir (KR) *see* Famciclovir 843
Famcler (KR) *see* Famciclovir 843
Famcro (KR) *see* Famciclovir 843
Famel Broomhexine (NL) *see* Bromhexine [INT] 291
Famicle (KR) *see* Famciclovir 843
Family Care Baciracin (KR) *see* Bacitracin (Topical) 222
Famocid (AE, BF, BJ, CI, ET, GH, GM, GN, IN, KE, KW, LR, MA, ML, MR, MU, MW, NE, NG, QA, SA, SC, SD, SL, SN, TN, TZ, UG, ZM, ZW) *see* Famotidine 845
Famoc (SG) *see* Famotidine 845
Famodar (AE, BH, CY, EG, IQ, IR, JO, KW, LB, LY, OM, QA, SA, SY, YE) *see* Famotidine 845
Famodil (IT) *see* Famotidine 845
Famodine (AE, BH, CY, EG, IL, IQ, IR, JO, KW, LB, LY, MY, OM, PK, QA, SA, SY, YE) *see* Famotidine 845
Famodin (RO) *see* Famotidine 845
Famogal (CO) *see* Famotidine 845
Famogard (RU) *see* Famotidine 845
Famohexal (AU) *see* Famotidine 845
Famo (IL) *see* Famotidine 845
Famonerton (DE) *see* Famotidine 845
Famopsin (TR) *see* Famotidine 845
Famosan (CZ, EE, HR) *see* Famotidine 845
Famosia (TH) *see* Famotidine 845
Famotec (AE, QA) *see* Famotidine 845
Famotid (BR) *see* Famotidine 845
Famotin (SG) *see* Famotidine 845
Famowal (IN) *see* Famotidine 845
Famox (BR, NZ, TW) *see* Famotidine 845
Fampyra (AU, CZ, DE, DK, EE, ES, FR, GB, IE, IL, NO, NZ, SE) *see* Dalfampridine 552
Fampyra SR (KR) *see* Dalfampridine 552
Famtrex (IN) *see* Famciclovir 843
Famvir (AE, AT, AU, BB, BE, BF, BG, BH, BJ, BM, BS, BZ, CH, CI, CY, CZ, DE, DK, EE, EG, ES, ET, FI, GB, GH, GM, GN, GR, GY, HK, HN, HR, HU, ID, IE, IL, IS, IT, JM, JP, KE, KR, KW, LB, LR, LU, MA, ML, MR, MT, MU, MW, NE, NG, NL, NO, NZ, PK, PL, PT, QA, RU, SA, SC, SD, SE, SK, SL, SN, SR, TH, TN, TR, TT, TW, TZ, UG, ZA, ZM, ZW) *see* Famciclovir 843
Famvir[extern.] (CH) *see* Penciclovir 1608
Fanapt (IL) *see* Iloperidone 1044
Fanaxal (ES) *see* Alfentanil 83
Fandhi (IL) *see* Antihemophilic Factor (Human) 152
Fang Di (CL) *see* Naftifine 1416
Fangtan (CN) *see* CISplatin 448
Fanle (CN) *see* Famciclovir 843
Fanlin (CN) *see* Cefoperazone and Sulbactam [INT] 382
Fansidar (AE, AT, AU, BH, BR, CH, CY, EG, FR, GB, GH, GR, ID, IE, IL, IQ, IR, JO, KW, LB, LY, OM, PE, PH, PK, PL, QA, SA, SY, TZ, UG, VN, YE, ZM) *see* Sulfadoxine and Pyrimethamine [INT] 1946
Fansidol (IT) *see* Nimesulide [INT] 1456
Fansitab (AE, BH, CY, EG, IL, IQ, IR, JO, KW, LB, LY, OM, QA, SA, SY, YE) *see* Sulfadoxine and Pyrimethamine [INT] 1946
Fantamax (SG) *see* FentaNYL 857
Fanta (TW) *see* Aluminum Hydroxide and Magnesium Hydroxide 103
Fantil (UY) *see* PrednisoLONE (Systemic) 1703
Fapresor (ID) *see* Metoprolol 1350
Fapris (AR) *see* Desvenlafaxine 598
Farbivent (ID) *see* Ipratropium and Albuterol 1109
Farcolin (AE, BH, CY, EG, IQ, IR, JO, KW, LB, LY, OM, QA, SA, SY, YE) *see* Albuterol 69
Farconcil (AE, BH, CY, EG, IQ, IR, JO, KW, LB, LY, OM, QA, SA, SY, YE) *see* Amoxicillin 130
Farcopril (AE, BH, CY, EG, IQ, IR, JO, KW, LB, LY, OM, QA, SA, SY, YE) *see* Captopril 342
Farelax (ID) *see* Atracurium 198
Faremid (IT) *see* Pipemidic Acid [INT] 1655
Fareston (AE, AR, AT, AU, BE, BH, BM, BR, CH, CN, CZ, DE, EE, ES, FI, FR, GB, GR, HN, HR, HU, IE, IT, JP, KR, LT, LU, MT, MX, NL, NZ, PE, PL, PT, QA, RO, RU, SE, SI, SK, TH, TR, TW, UY) *see* Toremifene 2071
Farganesse (IT) *see* Promethazine 1723
Fargan (IT) *see* Promethazine 1723
Fargoxin (ID) *see* Digoxin 627
Farlac (BR) *see* Lactulose 1156
Farlutal (AE, BE, BR, CN, CY, EG, FR, IQ, IR, IT, JO, KR, KW, LB, LY, NL, OM, QA, SA, SY, TR, YE) *see* MedroxyPROGESTERone 1277
Farlutal (AE, EG, SA) *see* Progesterone 1722
Farlutal Depot (BH, EG, QA) *see* MedroxyPROGESTERone 1277
Farlutal Depot (BH, QA) *see* Progesterone 1722
Farmacef (TH) *see* Cefuroxime 399
Farmadiuril (ES) *see* Bumetanide 297
Farmadral (ID) *see* Propranolol 1731
Farmaflebon (CR, GT, HN, PA, SV) *see* Polidocanol 1672
Farmagard (ID) *see* Nadolol 1411
Farmalex (TH) *see* Cephalexin 405
Farmamide (DE) *see* Ifosfamide 1040
Farmapram (MX) *see* ALPRAZolam 94
Farmaproina (ES) *see* Penicillin G Procaine 1613
Farmiblastina (ES) *see* DOXOrubicin (Conventional) 679
Farmicetina (AR) *see* Chloramphenicol 421
Farmicina (UY) *see* Erythromycin (Systemic) 762
Farmistin CS (DE) *see* VinCRIStine 2163
Farmobion B6 (IT) *see* Pyridoxine 1747
Farmobion D2 (IT) *see* Ergocalciferol 753
Farmobion Pp (IT) *see* Niacinamide 1446
Farmorrubicina RTU (CL) *see* Epirubicin 739
Farmorubicina CS (BR, CO, EC) *see* Epirubicin 739
Farmorubicin (AE, AT, BH, CH, CY, CZ, DE, DK, EG, FI, GR, HN, HR, HU, IL, IN, IQ, IR, JO, JP, KW, LB, LU, LY, MX, NO, OM, PK, PL, QA, RU, SA, SE, SI, SK, SY, TR, VE, YE, ZA) *see* Epirubicin 739
Farmorubicina (ES, IT, PE, PT, VN) *see* Epirubicin 739
Farmorubicina R.D. (BR) *see* Epirubicin 739
Farmorubicin CSU (ZA) *see* Epirubicin 739
Farmorubicine (BE, FR, NL) *see* Epirubicin 739
Farmorubicin PFS (BG, EE) *see* Epirubicin 739
Farmorubicin RD (BG, EE, ID, MX, ZA) *see* Epirubicin 739
Farmotal (IT) *see* Thiopental [INT] 2029
Farmoten (ID) *see* Captopril 342
Farnat (ID) *see* MetroNIDAZOLE (Systemic) 1353
Farnitran (PT) *see* Nitrendipine [INT] 1463
Farotin (KR) *see* Famotidine 845
Farpain (ID) *see* Ketorolac (Systemic) 1146
Fascar (TH) *see* Clarithromycin 456
Fase (IT) *see* Aprotinin 168
Faslodex (AR, AT, AU, BE, BG, BR, CH, CL, CN, CO, CR, CY, CZ, DE, DK, DO, EE, ES, FI, FR, GB, GR, GT, HK, HN, HR, HU, IE, IL, IN, IS, IT, JP, KR, LT, MT, MX, MY, NI, NL, NO, NZ, PA, PE, PH, PL, PT, RO, RU, SE, SG, SI, SK, SV, TH, TR, TW, UY, VE) *see* Fulvestrant 939
Fasolan (MX) *see* Flunarizine [CAN/INT] 892
Fastfen (BR) *see* SUFentanil 1941
Fastfen (CO) *see* Acetaminophen and Tramadol 37
Fastic (JP, KR) *see* Nateglinide 1432
Fastum (AE, BH, CH, CR, CY, DO, EC, EG, GT, HN, HR, IT, KW, MY, NI, PA, PH, QA, RO, RU, SA, SV, VN) *see* Ketoprofen 1145

Fasturtec (AE, AT, AU, BE, BG, BR, CH, CY, CZ, DE, DK, EE, ES, FI, FR, GB, GR, HK, HN, HR, HU, IE, IN, IT, KR, LB, LT, MT, NL, NO, NZ, PL, PT, RO, RU, SE, SG, SI, SK, TR, TW, VE) *see* Rasburicase 1783
Fasulide (BR) *see* Nimesulide [INT] 1456
Fatral (ID) *see* Sertraline 1878
Fauldoso (PT) *see* DOXOrubicin (Conventional) 679
Faverin (AE, AU, BH, CY, EG, GB, HK, IE, IQ, IR, JO, KW, LB, LY, OM, PK, QA, SA, SG, SY, TH, TR, YE) *see* FluvoxaMINE 916
Favic (AU) *see* Famciclovir 843
Favint (NZ) *see* Tiotropium 2046
Favistan (AT, CZ, DE, HR, HU, PY) *see* Methimazole 1319
Favolip (IN) *see* Lovastatin 1252
Favoxil (IL) *see* FluvoxaMINE 916
Faxine (TW) *see* Venlafaxine 2150
Faxinorm (DK) *see* Rifaximin 1809
Fazol (FR) *see* Isoconazole [INT] 1120
Fazolin (TH) *see* CeFAZolin 373
Fazolon (BR) *see* CeFAZolin 373
FCZ Infusion (ID) *see* Fluconazole 885
Febin (TW) *see* Ketoprofen 1145
Febratic (MX) *see* Ibuprofen 1032
Febridol (AU) *see* Acetaminophen 32
Febrile Free (PH) *see* Acetaminophen 32
Feburic (HK, JP, KR, TW) *see* Febuxostat 848
Febuxtat (AR) *see* Febuxostat 848
Fecipil (TW) *see* Lacidipin [INT] 1154
Fectin (ID) *see* Chlorhexidine Gluconate 422
Fectrim (GB) *see* Sulfamethoxazole and Trimethoprim 1946
Fedac Compound (HK, MY) *see* Triprolidine, Pseudoephedrine, and Codeine [CAN/INT] 2105
Fedac (HK, MY) *see* Triprolidine and Pseudoephedrine 2105
Fedil SR (TH) *see* Felodipine 850
Fedil (TW) *see* Felodipine 850
Fedox (PY) *see* HydrOXYzine 1024
Feiba Tim 4 (KR, TW) *see* Anti-inhibitor Coagulant Complex (Human) 155
FeiLin (CN) *see* Fenoprofen 857
Feinalmin (JP) *see* Imipramine 1054
Feinardon (AR) *see* Tetrabenazine 2016
Felalgyl[vet.] (FR) *see* Niflumic Acid [INT] 1454
Felantin (PE) *see* Phenytoin 1640
Felbamyl (AR) *see* Felbamate 850
Felcam (TW) *see* Piroxicam 1662
Felden (AT, CH, DK, FI, NO) *see* Piroxicam 1662
Feldene (AE, AR, BB, BE, BF, BG, BH, BJ, BM, BS, BZ, CI, CL, CO, CY, EC, EE, EG, ET, FR, GB, GH, GM, GN, GR, GY, HK, ID, IE, IL, IQ, IR, IT, JM, JO, JP, KE, KR, KW, LB, LR, LY, MA, ML, MR, MU, MW, MX, MY, NE, NG, NL, OM, PE, PH, PK, PL, PT, QA, RO, SA, SC, SD, SG, SL, SN, SR, SY, TH, TN, TR, TT, TZ, UG, VE, VN, YE, ZM, ZW) *see* Piroxicam 1662
Feldene Gel (AU, BF, BJ, CI, ET, GH, GM, GN, KE, LR, MA, ML, MR, MU, MW, NE, NG, SC, SD, SL, SN, TH, TN, TZ, UG, ZM, ZW) *see* Piroxicam 1662
Felden Gel (IS) *see* Piroxicam 1662
Feldoral (QA) *see* Piroxicam 1662
Felexin (MY, TR) *see* Cephalexin 405
Feliz (PH) *see* Citalopram 451
Feliz S (PH) *see* Escitalopram 765
Feloact (PH) *see* Racecadotril [INT] 1765
Felo-Bits (AR) *see* Atenolol 189
Felocor (DE) *see* Felodipine 850
Felocor Retardtab (DE) *see* Felodipine 850
Felodil ER (VN) *see* Felodipine 850
Felodil XR (AU) *see* Felodipine 850
Felodur ER (AU) *see* Felodipine 850
Felo ER (NZ, TW) *see* Felodipine 850
Felogamma Retard (DE) *see* Felodipine 850
Felogard (IN) *see* Felodipine 850
Felopine 5 (TH) *see* Felodipine 850
Felopine-SR (TW) *see* Felodipine 850
Felostad 5 Retard (HK) *see* Felodipine 850
Feloten (TH) *see* Felodipine 850
Felox (ID) *see* Pefloxacin [INT] 1588
Felpin E.R. (PH) *see* Felodipine 850
Felpin (TW) *see* Felodipine 850
Femanest (SE) *see* Estradiol (Systemic) 775
Femara (AE, AR, AT, AU, BD, BE, BG, BH, BO, BR, CH, CL, CN, CO, CR, CY, CZ, DE, DK, DO, EC, EE, EG, ES, FI, FR, GB, GR, GT, HK, HN, HR, HU, ID, IE, IL, IQ, IR, IT, JO, JP, KR, KW, LB, LT, LY, MX, MY, NI, NL, NZ, OM, PA, PE, PH, PK, PL, PR, PT, PY, QA, RO, RU, SA, SE, SG, SI, SK, SV, SY, TH, TR, TW, UY, VE, VN, YE) *see* Letrozole 1181
Femarate (TH) *see* Ferrous Fumarate 870
Femar (IS, NO) *see* Letrozole 1181
Femas (JP) *see* Ferrous Sulfate 871
Fematrix (GB, IE) *see* Estradiol (Systemic) 775
Femavit (DE) *see* Estrogens (Conjugated/Equine, Systemic) 787
Fem (CN) *see* Estradiol (Systemic) 775
Femex (NL) *see* Naproxen 1427
Femgard (CO) *see* Letrozole 1181
Femide 500 (TH) *see* Furosemide 940
Femina-35 (EE) *see* Cyproterone and Ethinyl Estradiol [CAN/INT] 532
Feminac 35 (CH) *see* Cyproterone and Ethinyl Estradiol [CAN/INT] 532
Feminil (NO) *see* Cyproterone and Ethinyl Estradiol [CAN/INT] 532
Feminova (BE) *see* Estradiol (Systemic) 775
Fe Min (TW) *see* Fexofenadine 873
Femipres (IT) *see* Moexipril 1388
Femiprim (MX) *see* Ascorbic Acid 178
Femitranol (PY) *see* Methylergonovine 1333
Femizet (PH, TH) *see* Anastrozole 148
Femolet (AU) *see* Letrozole 1181
Femorum (TH) *see* Iron Sucrose 1118
Fempress (AT, CH, DE) *see* Moexipril 1388
Fempress Plus (DE) *see* Moexipril and Hydrochlorothiazide 1388
Femsept (FR) *see* Estradiol (Systemic) 775
Femseven (GB, IE) *see* Estradiol (Systemic) 775
Femstat One (CA) *see* Butoconazole 314
Femtran (AU, NZ) *see* Estradiol (Systemic) 775
Fenac (AR) *see* Bromfenac 291
Fenac (AU) *see* Diclofenac (Systemic) 617
Fenactil (PL) *see* ChlorproMAZINE 429
Fenadex (LB, SA) *see* Fexofenadine 873
Fenafex (TH) *see* Fexofenadine 873
Fenagesic (SG) *see* Mefenamic Acid 1280
Fenahex (PH) *see* Tamoxifen 1971
Fenam (AE) *see* Mefenamic Acid 1280
Fenamic (AE, BH, CY, EG, IL, IQ, IR, JO, KW, LB, LY, OM, QA, SA, SY, YE) *see* Mefenamic Acid 1280
Fenamin (ZA) *see* Mefenamic Acid 1280
Fenamol (AE, BH, CY, EG, IL, IQ, IR, JO, KW, LB, LY, OM, QA, SA, SY, YE) *see* Mefenamic Acid 1280
Fenamon (AE, BF, BH, BJ, CI, CY, EG, ET, GH, GM, GN, IQ, IR, JO, KE, KW, LB, LR, LY, MA, ML, MR, MU, MW, MY, NE, NG, OM, QA, SA, SC, SD, SL, SN, SY, TN, TZ, UG, YE, ZM, ZW) *see* NIFEdipine 1451
Fenampicin (ES) *see* Rifampin 1804
Fenatic (ID) *see* Ibuprofen 1032
Fenatoin NM (SE) *see* Phenytoin 1640
Fenatrop (AR) *see* Trimebutine [CAN/INT] 2103
Fenatussin (KR) *see* GuaiFENesin 986
Fenax (CH) *see* Etofenamate [INT] 815
Fenazil (IT) *see* Promethazine 1723
Fenazine (AE, BH, CY, EG, IQ, IR, JO, KW, LB, LY, OM, QA, SA, SY, YE) *see* Promethazine 1723

Fenbid (AE, BF, BH, BJ, CI, CY, EG, ET, GB, GH, GM, GN, IQ, IR, JO, KE, KW, LB, LR, LY, MA, ML, MR, MU, MW, NE, NG, OM, QA, SA, SC, SD, SL, SN, SY, TN, TZ, UG, YE, ZM, ZW) *see* Ibuprofen ... 1032
Fenbid Cream (CN) *see* Ibuprofen ... 1032
Fencino (GB) *see* FentaNYL ... 857
Fendex (ID) *see* Dexketoprofen [INT] ... 603
Fendrix (BE, BG, CZ, EE, FR, GB, GR, HR, IE, IT, MT, NL, NO, PT, RO, SE, SK, TR) *see* Hepatitis B Vaccine (Recombinant) ... 1002
Fenemal (DK, IS, NO) *see* PHENobarbital ... 1632
Fenemal NM Pharma (SE) *see* PHENobarbital ... 1632
Fenergan (AR, ES, PE, PT, PY, UY, VE) *see* Promethazine ... 1723
Fenevit (PH) *see* Phenytoin ... 1640
Fenfedrin (HK, SG) *see* Chlorpheniramine and Pseudoephedrine ... 427
Fengam (TH) *see* Tiaprofenic Acid [CAN/INT] ... 2034
Feng Du (CN) *see* Naloxone ... 1419
Feng Hai Lu (CN) *see* Mannitol ... 1269
Fengkesong (CN) *see* Amphotericin B (Liposomal) ... 139
Fenicol (ID) *see* Chloramphenicol ... 421
Fenidantoin S (MX) *see* Phenytoin ... 1640
Fenilefrina (BR) *see* Phenylephrine (Systemic) ... 1638
Fenitin (PH) *see* Phenytoin ... 1640
Fenitoina (ES) *see* Phenytoin ... 1640
Fenitoina Rubio (ES) *see* Phenytoin ... 1640
Fenitron (MX) *see* Phenytoin ... 1640
Fenivir (BG, TR) *see* Penciclovir ... 1608
Fenizolan (DE) *see* Fenticonazole [INT] ... 868
Fen Le (CN) *see* Hydroxychloroquine ... 1021
Fen Li (CN) *see* Dexketoprofen [INT] ... 603
Fenlips (IL) *see* Penciclovir ... 1608
Fenobarbital (EC, GT, NI, PE, SV) *see* PHENobarbital ... 1632
Fenobarbitale (IT) *see* PHENobarbital ... 1632
Fenobarbitale Sodico (IT) *see* PHENobarbital ... 1632
Fenobarbital FNA (NL) *see* PHENobarbital ... 1632
Fenocin (ID) *see* Penicillin V Potassium ... 1614
Fenogel (PT) *see* Etofenamate [INT] ... 815
Fenolax (CZ) *see* Bisacodyl ... 265
Fenolip (PT) *see* Cromolyn (Nasal) ... 514
Fenopron (GB, HK, IE, KR) *see* Fenoprofen ... 857
Fenorin (CZ) *see* Carbocisteine [INT] ... 357
Fenostad (AT) *see* Fenoterol [INT] ... 857
Fenotal (PY) *see* PHENobarbital ... 1632
Fenoterol (PL) *see* Fenoterol [INT] ... 857
Fenoxene (IN) *see* Phenoxybenzamine ... 1635
Fenpaed (NZ) *see* Ibuprofen ... 1032
Fensedyl (AR) *see* Oxatomide [INT] ... 1532
Fensel (ES) *see* Felodipine ... 850
Fensol (ZA) *see* Fenoterol [INT] ... 857
Fentadur Patch (KR) *see* FentaNYL ... 857
Fentafienil (IT) *see* SUFentanil ... 1941
Fenta (IL) *see* FentaNYL ... 857
Fentalim (IT) *see* Alfentanil ... 83
Fentalis (GB, IE) *see* FentaNYL ... 857
Fentamax Mat Patch (KR) *see* FentaNYL ... 857
Fentanest (BR, IT, MX, PY, UY) *see* FentaNYL ... 857
Fentanila (CL) *see* FentaNYL ... 857
Fentanilo (VE) *see* FentaNYL ... 857
Fentanor (IN) *see* Phentolamine ... 1636
Fentanyl Citrate (EC) *see* FentaNYL ... 857
Fentanyl (CR, DO, GT, NI, PA, SV) *see* FentaNYL ... 857
Fentax (PY) *see* FentaNYL ... 857
Fentazin (GB, IE) *see* Perphenazine ... 1627
Fentiazol (PY) *see* MetroNIDAZOLE (Systemic) ... 1353
Fentiderm (IT) *see* Fenticonazole [INT] ... 868
Fentigyn (IT) *see* Fenticonazole [INT] ... 868
Fentizol (BR) *see* Fenticonazole [INT] ... 868
Fenton (PK) *see* PHENobarbital ... 1632
Fentos Tape (JP) *see* FentaNYL ... 857
Fenuril (FI) *see* Urea ... 2114
Fenylefrinhydroklorid (NO) *see* Phenylephrine (Systemic) ... 1638
Fenytoin (DE, DK) *see* Phenytoin ... 1640
Fenzol (PK) *see* Fenticonazole [INT] ... 868
Feosol (PH) *see* Ferrous Sulfate ... 871
Feospan (AE, BF, BH, BJ, CI, CY, EG, ET, GH, GM, GN, HK, IQ, IR, JO, KE, KW, LB, LR, LY, MA, ML, MR, MU, MW, NE, NG, OM, QA, SA, SC, SD, SL, SN, SY, TN, TZ, UG, YE, ZA, ZM, ZW) *see* Ferrous Sulfate ... 871
Feospan Z (AE, QA) *see* Ferrous Sulfate ... 871
Feprapax (GB) *see* Lofepramine [INT] ... 1232
Feprax (ID) *see* ALPRAZolam ... 94
Fepron (TW) *see* Fenoprofen ... 857
Fera (AU) *see* Letrozole ... 1181
Feraken (MX) *see* Moclobemide [CAN/INT] ... 1384
Ferbon (KR) *see* Leucovorin Calcium ... 1183
Ferfacef (ID) *see* CefTRIAXone ... 396
Ferglobin (PH) *see* Ferrous Sulfate ... 871
Fergon (AE, AU, GB, IE) *see* Ferrous Gluconate ... 870
Ferinject (AR, AT, AU, BR, CH, CY, CZ, DE, DK, ES, FI, FR, GB, GR, HR, IL, IS, KR, LB, LT, NL, NO, NZ, PE, PT, RO, SE, SG, SK) *see* Ferric Carboxymaltose ... 868
Fer-In-Sol (AR, BR, CL, CZ, GR, HK, KW, PE, SA, VE) *see* Ferrous Sulfate ... 871
Feri (PH) *see* Folic Acid ... 919
Ferium (CL) *see* Ferric Carboxymaltose ... 868
Ferlea (AR) *see* Ferrous Sulfate ... 871
Fermig (MX) *see* SUMAtriptan ... 1953
Fermil (AU) *see* ClomiPHENE ... 473
Fernore (BE) *see* Ferrous Gluconate ... 870
Feroba (KR) *see* Ferrous Sulfate ... 871
Fero-Gradumet (BE, ES, LU, NL, PL) *see* Ferrous Sulfate ... 871
Ferome (TH) *see* Cefpirome [INT] ... 388
Feromin Oral Drops (SA) *see* Ferrous Sulfate ... 871
Feromin (QA) *see* Ferrous Sulfate ... 871
Ferotine (KR) *see* Famotidine ... 845
Ferrate (LB) *see* Ferrous Fumarate ... 870
Ferraton (EC) *see* Ferrous Fumarate ... 870
Ferrematos (IT) *see* Ferrous Gluconate ... 870
Ferriprox (AE, AR, AT, AU, BE, BH, BR, CH, CN, CY, CZ, DE, DK, EE, FI, FR, GB, GR, HK, HR, ID, IE, IL, IT, KR, KW, LT, NL, NO, NZ, PH, PT, QA, RO, SA, SE, SG, SI, SK, TH, TR, VN) *see* Deferiprone ... 585
Ferritin Oti (PT) *see* Ferric Gluconate ... 869
Ferrlecit (CZ, DE, HN, IL) *see* Ferric Gluconate ... 869
Ferrlecit (DE, HU) *see* Ferrous Gluconate ... 870
Ferro-Agepha (AT) *see* Ferrous Gluconate ... 870
Ferrobet (AT) *see* Ferrous Fumarate ... 870
Ferro Duretter (DK) *see* Ferrous Sulfate ... 871
Ferrofer (TH) *see* Iron Sucrose ... 1118
Ferrogamma (DE) *see* Ferrous Sulfate ... 871
Ferrogard (JO) *see* Ferrous Sulfate ... 871
Ferrogluconaat FNA (NL) *see* Ferrous Gluconate ... 870
Ferrograd (GB, IE) *see* Ferrous Sulfate ... 871
Ferro-grad (IT) *see* Ferrous Sulfate ... 871
Ferro-Gradumet (AE, AT, AU, BG, BH, CH, CY, EG, HU, ID, IL, IQ, IR, JO, KW, LB, LY, OM, PT, QA, SA, SY, YE) *see* Ferrous Sulfate ... 871
Ferro-Gradumet (BG) *see* Ferrous Gluconate ... 870
Ferrokapsul (DE) *see* Ferrous Fumarate ... 870
Ferroklinge (BR) *see* Ferrous Fumarate ... 870
Ferrolent (CR, DO, GT, HN, NI, PA, SV) *see* Ferrous Sulfate ... 871
Ferro-Liquid (AU) *see* Ferrous Sulfate ... 871
ferrominerase (DE) *see* Ferrous Gluconate ... 870
Ferronal (IL) *see* Ferrous Gluconate ... 870
Ferronat (BG, CZ) *see* Ferrous Fumarate ... 870
Ferronat (LB) *see* Ferrous Gluconate ... 870
Ferrophor (DE) *see* Ferrous Sulfate ... 871
Ferroplex "Era" (DK) *see* Ferrous Sulfate ... 871
Ferrostatin (JP) *see* Ferrous Sulfate ... 871
Ferrosterol (UY) *see* Ferrous Sulfate ... 871

Ferro-Tab (AU) *see* Ferrous Fumarate 870
FerroTab (NZ) *see* Ferrous Fumarate 870
Ferrovin (KR) *see* Iron Sucrose 1118
Ferrum Hausmann (BE, CH, DE, LU) *see* Ferrous Fumarate 870
Ferrum Verla (DE) *see* Ferrous Gluconate 870
Fersaday (GB, IE) *see* Ferrous Fumarate 870
Fersivag (MX) *see* Lisinopril 1226
Fertab (AE, KW) *see* ClomiPHENE 473
Fertec (CO) *see* ClomiPHENE 473
Ferticlo (PH) *see* ClomiPHENE 473
Fertilan (HK) *see* ClomiPHENE 473
Fertiline (JO, QA) *see* ClomiPHENE 473
Fertilin (TR) *see* ClomiPHENE 473
Fertilphen (ID) *see* ClomiPHENE 473
Fertinic (AE) *see* Ferrous Gluconate 870
Fertin (ID) *see* ClomiPHENE 473
Fertomid (IN) *see* ClomiPHENE 473
Ferumat (BE, LU, NL) *see* Ferrous Fumarate 870
Ferval (MX) *see* Ferrous Fumarate 870
Fervex (BR) *see* Acetaminophen 32
Fesema (CO) *see* Formoterol 926
Fetik (ID) *see* Ketoprofen 1145
Fetimin (HR) *see* Naftifine 1416
Fetinor (ID) *see* Gemfibrozil 956
Fevalax (PY) *see* FluvoxaMINE 916
Fevarin (BG, CZ, DK, EE, FI, HN, HR, HU, IT, NL, NO, PL, RO, RU, SE) *see* FluvoxaMINE 916
Fever-Free (PH) *see* Ibuprofen 1032
Fexibron (PE) *see* Iron Dextran Complex 1117
Fexin (PH) *see* Ciprofloxacin (Systemic) 441
Fexin (ZA) *see* Cephalexin 405
Fexiron (AR, PE, PY) *see* Iron Dextran Complex 1117
Fexodex (JO) *see* Fexofenadine 873
Fexodine (AE, BH, HK, KW, QA, SA) *see* Fexofenadine 873
Fexofast (TH) *see* Fexofenadine 873
Fexofed (ID) *see* Fexofenadine and Pseudoephedrine 874
Fexofin (MY) *see* Fexofenadine 873
Fexon (KR) *see* Fexofenadine 873
Fexoral (PH) *see* Fexofenadine 873
Fexotabs (AU) *see* Fexofenadine 873
Fexotene (TH) *see* Fexofenadine 873
Fexovid (MY) *see* Fexofenadine 873
Fexurix (CL) *see* Febuxostat 848
Fialgin (PY) *see* Thioridazine 2030
Fiberad (PK) *see* Psyllium 1744
Fibermate (PH, VN) *see* Psyllium 1744
Fibonel (CL) *see* Famotidine 845
Fibral (CO) *see* Psyllium 1744
Fibralgin (HR) *see* Acetaminophen 32
Fibrase (IT) *see* Pentosan Polysulfate Sodium 1617
Fibrezym (DE) *see* Pentosan Polysulfate Sodium 1617
Fibrocard (LU) *see* Verapamil 2154
Fibrocide (PT) *see* Pentosan Polysulfate Sodium 1617
Fibrocid (ES) *see* Pentosan Polysulfate Sodium 1617
Fibrocol (PK) *see* Psyllium 1744
Fibrogammin (AT, BE, DE, FR, GR) *see* Factor XIII Concentrate (Human) 843
Fibrogammin P (AR, AU, BR, CH, GB, IL) *see* Factor XIII Concentrate (Human) 843
Fibrolax (IT) *see* Psyllium 1744
Fibrolip (CO, UY) *see* Ciprofibrate [INT] 441
Fibro-Vein (AE, AR, AU, GB, HN, IE, IT, KW, NZ, SK, TW) *see* Sodium Tetradecyl Sulfate 1914
Fibro Vein (PL) *see* Sodium Tetradecyl Sulfate 1914
Fibrozol (ID) *see* Cilostazol 437
Fibsol (AU) *see* Lisinopril 1226
Fidium (ES) *see* Betahistine [CAN/INT] 252
Filabac (AR) *see* Abacavir 20
Filanc (MX) *see* Acetaminophen 32
Filatil (CR, DO, GT, HN, MX, NI, PA, SV) *see* Filgrastim 875
Filcrin (UY) *see* Vinorelbine 2168
Filgen (EC, TH) *see* Filgrastim 875
Filginase (AR) *see* Efavirenz 707
Filicine (GR) *see* Folic Acid 919
Filorose (GR) *see* Anthralin 150
Filosir (AU) *see* Fingolimod 879
Filpril (AU) *see* Quinapril 1756
Filtaten (MX) *see* FentaNYL 857
Filtroquinona (DO, EC, GT, HN, PA, SV) *see* Hydroquinone 1020
Fimazid (ES) *see* Isoniazid 1120
Fimizina (ES) *see* Rifampin 1804
Fimoplas (PH) *see* Tranexamic Acid 2081
Finaber (PY) *see* Ondansetron 1513
Finacea (AU, BG, FR, GB, IE, MX, SE) *see* Azelaic Acid 213
Finail (DK, SE) *see* Amorolfine [INT] 128
Finallerg (AE, BH, CY, EG, IQ, IR, JO, KW, LB, LY, OM, QA, SA, SY, YE) *see* Cetirizine 411
Finapros (PH) *see* Finasteride 878
Finarid (PH) *see* Finasteride 878
Finascar (JO) *see* Finasteride 878
Finaspros (CO) *see* Finasteride 878
Finaspro (TW) *see* Finasteride 878
Finas (SG) *see* Finasteride 878
Finasta (AU) *see* Finasteride 878
Finastar (KR) *see* Finasteride 878
Finastid (HR) *see* Finasteride 878
Finast (VN) *see* Finasteride 878
Finatra (CN) *see* Finasteride 878
Finatux (PT) *see* Carbocisteine [INT] 357
Fincar (HK, IN, KR) *see* Finasteride 878
Fines (KR) *see* Piroxicam 1662
Finex (PY) *see* Terbinafine (Systemic) 2002
Finex (PY) *see* Terbinafine (Topical) 2004
Finibax (JP, KR, TW) *see* Doripenem 671
Finide (PH) *see* Finasteride 878
Finiscar (QA) *see* Finasteride 878
Finlepsin (BG, HU, RO) *see* CarBAMazepine 346
Finnacar (AU) *see* Finasteride 878
Finoxal (CO) *see* Pyrantel Pamoate 1744
Finpro (ID, ZA) *see* Finasteride 878
Finska (TW) *see* Loratadine 1241
Fintel (PE) *see* Albendazole 65
Fintop (VN) *see* Butenafine 314
Finuret (AR) *see* Pipemidic Acid [INT] 1655
Fionat (ID) *see* Folic Acid 919
Fiorinal (AU) *see* Acetaminophen, Codeine, and Doxylamine [CAN/INT] 37
Fiorinal (CA) *see* Butalbital, Aspirin, and Caffeine 314
Fioritina (AR) *see* Norepinephrine 1472
Firazyr (AT, AU, BE, BR, CH, CZ, DE, DK, EE, FR, GB, GR, HR, IE, IL, LT, NL, NO, PL, PT, RO, RU, SE, SI, SK) *see* Icatibant 1037
Firide (TH) *see* Finasteride 878
Firmagon (AR, AT, AU, BE, BR, CH, CY, CZ, DE, DK, EE, FR, GB, HK, HR, IE, IL, IS, KR, LB, LT, MY, NL, NO, PE, PL, PT, QA, RO, SA, SE, SG, SI, SK, TH, TR) *see* Degarelix 587
Fisamox (AU) *see* Amoxicillin 130
Fisiodar (IT) *see* Diacerein [INT] 613
Fisostigmina Salicilato (IT) *see* Physostigmine 1647
Fisostin (IT) *see* Physostigmine 1647
Fistrin (CO) *see* Finasteride 878
Fit-C (ID) *see* Ascorbic Acid 178
Fitonal (AR) *see* Ketoconazole (Topical) 1145
Fivoflu (IN, JO, PH, VE) *see* Fluorouracil (Systemic) 896
Fivtum (PH) *see* CefTAZidime 392
Fixamicin HC (CO) *see* Ciprofloxacin and Hydrocortisone 446
Fix-A (PH) *see* Cefixime 380

Fixateur phospho-calcique Bichsel (CH) *see* Calcium Carbonate ... 327
Fixcef (PH) *see* Cefixime ... 380
Fixef (ID) *see* Cefixime ... 380
Fixeril (AR, UY) *see* Ciprofibrate [INT] ... 441
Fixical (FR) *see* Calcium Carbonate ... 327
Fixime (ZA) *see* Cefixime ... 380
Fixim (LB, NL) *see* Cefixime ... 380
Fixiphar (ID) *see* Cefixime ... 380
Fixit (AE, QA, SA) *see* Nizatidine ... 1471
Fixoten (MX) *see* Pentoxifylline ... 1618
Fixx (IN) *see* Cefixime ... 380
Flacort (PE) *see* Deflazacort [INT] ... 587
Fladex (ID) *see* MetroNIDAZOLE (Systemic) ... 1353
Fladystin (ID) *see* Metronidazole and Nystatin [CAN/INT] ... 1358
Flagentyl (KR, PH, PT, TR, VN) *see* Secnidazole [INT] ... 1872
Flagesol (UY) *see* MetroNIDAZOLE (Systemic) ... 1353
Flagizole (AE, BH, CY, EG, IQ, IR, JO, KW, LB, LY, OM, QA, SA, SY, YE) *see* MetroNIDAZOLE (Systemic) ... 1353
Flagyl (AR, AU, BE, BG, BH, BR, CH, CL, CO, CY, EC, EG, FR, GB, GR, HK, ID, IE, IL, IN, IS, JO, KR, KW, LB, NL, NO, NZ, PE, PH, PK, PT, QA, RO, RU, SA, SG, SI, TH, TR, TW, VE, VN) *see* MetroNIDAZOLE (Systemic) ... 1353
Flagyl Comp (FI) *see* Metronidazole and Nystatin [CAN/INT] ... 1358
Flagyl Nistatina (BR, CO) *see* Metronidazole and Nystatin [CAN/INT] ... 1358
Flagystatin V (CR, HN, MX, NI) *see* Metronidazole and Nystatin [CAN/INT] ... 1358
Flagystatin (AR, ID, PH, PY, SG, UY) *see* Metronidazole and Nystatin [CAN/INT] ... 1358
Flagystatine (PE) *see* Metronidazole and Nystatin [CAN/INT] ... 1358
Flake (TW) *see* Doxepin (Systemic) ... 676
Flake (TW) *see* Doxepin (Topical) ... 678
Flamaret (ZA) *see* Indomethacin ... 1067
Flamar Eye Drops (ID) *see* Diclofenac (Ophthalmic) ... 621
Flamarion (AR) *see* Acemetacin [INT] ... 30
Flamar (PH) *see* Celecoxib ... 402
Flamazine (AE, AU, BH, CY, DK, EG, FI, GB, IQ, IR, IS, JO, KW, LB, LY, NO, NZ, OM, PK, QA, SA, SY, TH, TW, YE, ZA) *see* Silver Sulfadiazine ... 1887
Flamergi (ID) *see* Naphazoline and Pheniramine ... 1426
Flamexin (RO) *see* Piroxicam ... 1662
Flamex (JO) *see* Celecoxib ... 402
Flamic Gel (TH) *see* Piroxicam ... 1662
Flamicina (MX) *see* Ampicillin ... 141
Flamicort (ID) *see* Triamcinolone (Systemic) ... 2099
Flamide (MX) *see* Nimesulide [INT] ... 1456
Flamirex (AR) *see* Deflazacort [INT] ... 587
Flammazine (AT, BE, BG, CH, DE, ES, FR, GR, NL, PH, PT) *see* Silver Sulfadiazine ... 1887
Flamon (BB, BM, BS, BZ, CH, GY, JM, MY, PR, SR, TT) *see* Verapamil ... 2154
Flamoxi (ID) *see* Meloxicam ... 1283
Flamquit (TW) *see* Diclofenac (Systemic) ... 617
Flanax (BR, EC) *see* Naproxen ... 1427
Flancox (BR) *see* Etodolac ... 815
Flantadin (GR, IT) *see* Deflazacort [INT] ... 587
Flarex (AE, AR, AT, AU, BF, BG, BH, BJ, CI, CN, CY, CZ, EG, ET, GH, GM, GN, HK, HN, IL, IQ, IR, IT, JO, KE, KR, KW, LB, LR, LY, MA, ML, MR, MU, MW, MY, NE, NG, NL, OM, PH, PL, PY, QA, RU, SA, SC, SD, SL, SN, SY, TH, TN, TW, TZ, UG, VN, YE, ZM, ZW) *see* Fluorometholone ... 896
Flaryzil (PY) *see* Flunarizine [CAN/INT] ... 892
Flasinyl (KR) *see* MetroNIDAZOLE (Systemic) ... 1353
Flason (ID) *see* MethylPREDNISolone ... 1340
Flavamed (BG, DK, EE, FI, HR, LT, PL, RU, TR) *see* Ambroxol [INT] ... 109
Flavate (IN) *see* FlavoxATE ... 881
Flavettes (SG) *see* Ascorbic Acid ... 178
Flavicina (AR) *see* DOXOrubicin (Conventional) ... 679
Flavis (IT) *see* Piracetam [INT] ... 1661
Flavitol (AT) *see* Riboflavin ... 1803
Flavorin (TH) *see* FlavoxATE ... 881
Flaxedil (AR, AU, GB, HR, NL) *see* Gallamine Triethiodide [INT] ... 948
Flaxedyl (HU) *see* Gallamine Triethiodide [INT] ... 948
Flaxel (PE) *see* Celecoxib ... 402
Flazal (BR) *see* Deflazacort [INT] ... 587
Flazinil (EC) *see* Zolpidem ... 2212
Flazol (AE, BH, CY, EG, IQ, IR, JO, KW, LB, LY, OM, QA, SA, SY, YE) *see* MetroNIDAZOLE (Systemic) ... 1353
Flebogamma (HK, IL, MY, SG, TH) *see* Immune Globulin ... 1056
Flebutol (VE) *see* Acebutolol ... 29
Flecadura (DE) *see* Flecainide ... 882
Flecaine (FR, VN) *see* Flecainide ... 882
Flecaine LP (FR) *see* Flecainide ... 882
Flecatab (AU, TW) *see* Flecainide ... 882
Flecoxin (CY) *see* Bromhexine [INT] ... 291
Flector (FR, LB) *see* Diclofenac (Systemic) ... 617
Flegamina (CZ, PL) *see* Bromhexine [INT] ... 291
Flekainid (SK) *see* Flecainide ... 882
Flemex-AC OD (TH) *see* Acetylcysteine ... 40
Flemex AC (TH) *see* Acetylcysteine ... 40
Flemex (VN) *see* Carbocisteine [INT] ... 357
Fleming (HK, TH, VN) *see* Amoxicillin and Clavulanate ... 133
Flemonex (PH) *see* GuaiFENesin ... 986
Flemoxin (AE, BH, CY, EG, IQ, IR, JO, KW, LB, LY, OM, QA, SA, SY, YE) *see* Amoxicillin ... 130
Fleur (CZ) *see* Desogestrel [INT] ... 597
Flexagen (ZA) *see* Diclofenac (Systemic) ... 617
Flexbumin (CZ, SK) *see* Albumin ... 67
Flexen (LB) *see* Ketoprofen ... 1145
Flexer (PE, TW) *see* Cyclobenzaprine ... 516
Flexfree (BE, LU) *see* Felbinac [INT] ... 850
Flexiban (AE, AR, IT, PT, QA) *see* Cyclobenzaprine ... 516
Flexicam (AE) *see* Meloxicam ... 1283
Flexid (HR) *see* Levofloxacin (Systemic) ... 1197
Flexilor (VN) *see* Lornoxicam [INT] ... 1248
Flexirox (FR) *see* Piroxicam ... 1662
Flexital CR (TH) *see* Pentoxifylline ... 1618
Flexium (BE) *see* Etofenamate [INT] ... 815
Flezacor (CR, GT, HN, PA, SV) *see* Deflazacort [INT] ... 587
Flindix (PT) *see* Isosorbide Dinitrate ... 1124
Fliven (TR) *see* Eplerenone ... 740
Flixonase (AR, AT, AU, BE, BG, BH, BR, CL, CN, CY, CZ, DK, DO, EC, EE, FI, FR, GB, HK, HN, HR, IE, IL, IS, IT, JM, JO, KR, KW, LB, LT, NL, NZ, PA, PE, PH, PL, PY, QA, RO, RU, SA, SG, SI, SK, SV, TH, TR, TT, TW, UY, VE, VN) *see* Fluticasone (Nasal) ... 910
Flixonase (AR, AT, AU, BE, BR, CZ, DK, DO, EC, EE, FI, FR, GB, HK, HN, ID, IE, IL, IT, KR, MY, NL, PA, PE, PL, PY, RU, SG, SV, TH, TW, UY, VE) *see* Fluticasone (Oral Inhalation) ... 907
Flixonase Nasule (IL) *see* Fluticasone (Nasal) ... 910
Flixonas (PK) *see* Fluticasone (Nasal) ... 910
Flixonas (PK) *see* Fluticasone (Oral Inhalation) ... 907
Flixotaide (PT) *see* Fluticasone (Oral Inhalation) ... 907
Flixotide (AE, AR, AT, BE, BG, BH, BR, CL, CN, CR, CY, CZ, DK, EC, EE, EG, FI, FR, GB, GR, GT, HK, HN, HR, ID, IE, IL, IQ, IR, IS, IT, JM, JO, KR, KW, LB, LT, LY, MY, NI, NL, NZ, OM, PA, PE, PH, PY, QA, RO, RU, SA, SE, SG, SI, SK, SV, SY, TH, TR, TT, TW, UY, VE, VN, YE) *see* Fluticasone (Oral Inhalation) ... 907
Flixotide Inhaler (AU) *see* Fluticasone (Oral Inhalation) ... 907

Flixotide Nebules (AU) *see* Fluticasone (Oral Inhalation) ... 907
Flixovate (FR) *see* Fluticasone (Oral Inhalation) ... 907
Flixovate (FR) *see* Fluticasone (Topical) ... 911
Floam (PL) *see* Fluoride ... 895
Flobacin (IT) *see* Ofloxacin (Systemic) ... 1490
Flocan (KR) *see* Fluconazole ... 885
Floctil (HK, MY, TH) *see* Azithromycin (Systemic) ... 216
Flodil LP (FR) *see* Felodipine ... 850
Flodin (PE) *see* Meloxicam ... 1283
Floginax (IT) *see* Naproxen ... 1427
Flogirax (BR) *see* Ofloxacin (Systemic) ... 1490
Flogocort (EC) *see* Mometasone (Topical) ... 1391
Flogol (AR) *see* Etofenamate [INT] ... 815
Flogoprofen (ES) *see* Etofenamate [INT] ... 815
Flogovital (AR) *see* Niflumic Acid [INT] ... 1454
Flogovital N.F. (AR) *see* Nimesulide [INT] ... 1456
Flogozan (CR, DO, GT, HN, NI, PA, SV) *see* Diclofenac (Systemic) ... 617
Flohale (AE) *see* Fluticasone (Oral Inhalation) ... 907
Flohale (ID) *see* Terbutaline ... 2004
Flolan (AT, AU, BE, CH, CZ, DK, EE, ES, FR, GB, GR, IE, IL, IT, NL, NO, PL, SG, TW) *see* Epoprostenol ... 746
Flolid (IT) *see* Nimesulide [INT] ... 1456
Flomax (NZ, TR) *see* Tamsulosin ... 1974
Flomaxtra XL (GB) *see* Tamsulosin ... 1974
Flomaxtra (AU, NZ) *see* Tamsulosin ... 1974
Flomist (MY) *see* Fluticasone (Nasal) ... 910
Flomist (MY) *see* Fluticasone (Oral Inhalation) ... 907
Flonida (IN) *see* Fluorouracil (Systemic) ... 896
Flonorm (CO, MX) *see* Rifaximin ... 1809
Flopen (AU) *see* Flucloxacillin [INT] ... 885
Floquin DPS (IN) *see* Levofloxacin (Ophthalmic) ... 1200
Floran (AU) *see* Fluoride ... 895
Floraquin (TW) *see* Iodoquinol ... 1105
Florate (BR) *see* Fluorometholone ... 896
Floricot (IN) *see* Fludrocortisone ... 891
Florinef (AU, CH, CL, DK, FI, GB, GR, HK, IE, IS, KR, MY, NL, NO, NZ, SE, SG, SI, TH, TW, VN, ZA) *see* Fludrocortisone ... 891
Florinefe (BR, UY, VE) *see* Fludrocortisone ... 891
Florizel (GB) *see* Gestrinone [INT] ... 962
Florocycline (FR) *see* Tetracycline ... 2017
Florom (PK) *see* Fluorometholone ... 896
Florone (DE, GR) *see* Diflorasone ... 625
Floroxin (AE, BH, CY, EG, IQ, IR, JO, KW, LB, LY, OM, QA, SA, SY, YE) *see* Ciprofloxacin (Systemic) ... 441
Flosef (IN) *see* Fluorometholone ... 896
Flosetron (BG) *see* Betamethasone (Systemic) ... 253
Flotavid (ID) *see* Ofloxacin (Systemic) ... 1490
Flotiran (PT) *see* Betamethasone and Clotrimazole ... 256
Flotral (LB, PE, VN) *see* Alfuzosin ... 84
Flotrin (DE) *see* Terazosin ... 2001
Flovas (IN) *see* Pitavastatin ... 1663
Flovid (HK, PH, SG) *see* Ofloxacin (Systemic) ... 1490
Floxacap (ID) *see* Levofloxacin (Systemic) ... 1197
Floxacin (MX) *see* Norfloxacin ... 1475
Floxal (AT, BG, CH, CZ, DE, HN, PL, RO, RU) *see* Ofloxacin (Ophthalmic) ... 1491
Floxapen (AE, AT, AU, BE, CH, GB, GR, KW, MX, NL, PT, SA, VE, ZA) *see* Flucloxacillin [INT] ... 885
Floxel (PH) *see* Levofloxacin (Systemic) ... 1197
Floxet (HK, HU, UY) *see* FLUoxetine ... 899
Floxil (AR) *see* Ofloxacin (Systemic) ... 1490
Floxin (KR) *see* Flucloxacillin [INT] ... 885
Floxin (VN) *see* Pefloxacin [INT] ... 1588
Floxsid (ID) *see* Ciprofloxacin (Systemic) ... 441
Floxstat (BB, BM, BS, CO, EC, GY, JM, NL, PR, SR, TT, VE) *see* Ofloxacin (Systemic) ... 1490
Floxyfral (AT, BE, CH, FR, LU) *see* FluvoxaMINE ... 916
Flu-21 (IT) *see* Fluocinonide ... 894
FLU-D (TW) *see* Fluconazole ... 885
Fluamar (CO) *see* Fluticasone and Salmeterol ... 912
Fluanxol (AE, AT, AU, BE, BG, BH, CH, CL, CN, CZ, DE, DK, EE, FI, GB, HK, IL, IN, JO, KW, LT, NL, NO, NZ, PE, PK, PL, PT, RU, SA, SE, SG, SI, TH, TR, TW, VN) *see* Flupentixol [CAN/INT] ... 903
Fluanxol Depot (AE, AT, BG, BH, CH, CN, CZ, DE, DK, EE, FI, HK, HN, IL, IN, IS, KW, LB, LT, MY, NO, PE, PH, QA, RO, SA, SE, SG, SI, SK, TH, TW, VN, ZA) *see* Flupentixol [CAN/INT] ... 903
Fluanxol Mite (IS) *see* Flupentixol [CAN/INT] ... 903
Fluaton (IT) *see* Fluorometholone ... 896
Flu-Base (JP) *see* Fluorometholone ... 896
Flubason (ES, IT) *see* Desoximetasone ... 598
Flubiol (JP) *see* Fluocinonide ... 894
Flubiotic (ES) *see* Amoxicillin ... 130
Flubron[vet.] (FR) *see* Bromhexine [INT] ... 291
Flucand (AE, BH, CY, EG, IQ, IR, JO, KW, LB, LY, OM, QA, SA, SY, YE) *see* Fluconazole ... 885
Flucanol (IL) *see* Fluconazole ... 885
Flucazol (AE, BH, BR, CY, EG, IQ, IR, JO, KW, LB, LY, OM, QA, SA, SY, YE) *see* Fluconazole ... 885
Flucazole (NZ) *see* Fluconazole ... 885
Fluccil (BR) *see* Metoclopramide ... 1345
Fluciderm (ID, MY, SG) *see* Fluocinolone (Topical) ... 893
Flucilium (TW) *see* Flunarizine [CAN/INT] ... 892
Flucil (NZ) *see* Flucloxacillin [INT] ... 885
Flucil (TH) *see* Acetylcysteine ... 40
Flucinar (BG, CZ, DE, HN, PL, VN) *see* Fluocinolone (Topical) ... 893
Flucinom (CH, CZ, GR) *see* Flutamide ... 907
Flucinome (HR) *see* Flutamide ... 907
Fluclox (DE, PH) *see* Flucloxacillin [INT] ... 885
Flucloxil (MY) *see* Flucloxacillin [INT] ... 885
Flucloxin (NZ) *see* Flucloxacillin [INT] ... 885
Flucogus (TW) *see* Fluconazole ... 885
Flucona (KR) *see* Fluconazole ... 885
Flucon (AU, BE, CH, CZ, FR, GR, HK, HN, HU, LU, NZ, PT, TR, TW) *see* Fluorometholone ... 896
Flucon (KR) *see* Fluconazole ... 885
Flucoral (ID) *see* Fluconazole ... 885
Flucoran (NZ) *see* Fluconazole ... 885
Flucort (IN, TW, VN) *see* Fluocinolone (Topical) ... 893
Flucortone (TW) *see* Fluocinolone (Topical) ... 893
Flucoxan (MX) *see* Fluconazole ... 885
Flucozal (BR, PK) *see* Fluconazole ... 885
Flucozol (EC) *see* Fludarabine ... 890
Fluctin (DE) *see* FLUoxetine ... 899
Fluctine (AT, CH) *see* FLUoxetine ... 899
Fludac (BF, BJ, CI, ET, GH, GM, GN, IN, KE, LR, MA, ML, MR, MU, MW, NE, NG, SC, SD, SL, SN, TN, TZ, UG, ZM, ZW) *see* FLUoxetine ... 899
Fludacel (PE) *see* Fludarabine ... 890
Fludalym (VN) *see* Fludarabine ... 890
Fludan (HK, MY) *see* Flunarizine [CAN/INT] ... 892
Fludara (AT, AU, BE, BG, BH, CH, CL, CN, CO, CY, CZ, DE, DK, DO, EE, FI, FR, GB, GR, HK, HN, HR, HU, ID, IE, IL, IN, IS, IT, JO, JP, KR, KW, LB, LT, LU, MY, NL, NO, NZ, PH, PL, PY, QA, RO, RU, SA, SE, SG, SI, SK, TH, TR, TW, UY, VE, VN, ZA) *see* Fludarabine ... 890
Fludecasine (JP) *see* FluPHENAZine ... 905
Fludecate (CL, IL) *see* FluPHENAZine ... 905
Fludecate Multidose (ZA) *see* FluPHENAZine ... 905
Fludent (FI, NO, SE) *see* Fluoride ... 895
Fludex (AT, BE, CH, DK, FR, GR, LB, LU, PT, TR, VN) *see* Indapamide ... 1065
Fludex SR (KR) *see* Indapamide ... 1065
Fludicon (HK) *see* Fluconazole ... 885
Fludilat (BR, DE, GR, ID, PT, TH, VE) *see* Bencyclane [INT] ... 241
Fludil (VE) *see* Flunarizine [CAN/INT] ... 892
Fluditec (EE) *see* Carbocisteine [INT] ... 357
Fludizol (TH) *see* Fluconazole ... 885
Flufenan (BR) *see* FluPHENAZine ... 905
Flugalin (PL) *see* Flurbiprofen (Systemic) ... 906

Flugen (TW) *see* Silver Sulfadiazine ... 1887
Flugerel (PL, TW) *see* Flutamide ... 907
Fluibron (BR, LB, PK) *see* Ambroxol [INT] ... 109
Fluidasa (AR) *see* Erdosteine [INT] ... 753
Fluidex (CZ) *see* Dextran ... 607
Fluidin (BR) *see* Ambroxol [INT] ... 109
Fluidin (ES) *see* GuaiFENesin ... 986
Fluifort (HK) *see* Carbocisteine [INT] ... 357
Fluimicil (CH, DE) *see* Acetylcysteine ... 40
Fluimiquil (LU) *see* Acetylcysteine ... 40
Fluimucil A (MY, PK) *see* Acetylcysteine ... 40
Fluimucil (AR, BG, BR, CL, CO, CZ, EC, HK, HU, ID, IT, MA, NL, PE, PL, RU, SG, TH, TW) *see* Acetylcysteine ... 40
Fluimukan (HR) *see* Acetylcysteine ... 40
Fluir (BR) *see* Formoterol ... 926
Fluken (MX) *see* Flutamide ... 907
Fluketin (SG) *see* FLUoxetine ... 899
Flulem (CO, MX, TH) *see* Flutamide ... 907
Flulium (TH) *see* Clorazepate ... 487
Flulone (AR) *see* Fluocinolone (Topical) ... 893
Flulon (PH) *see* Fluorometholone ... 896
Flumach (FR) *see* Spironolactone ... 1931
Flumage (AR) *see* Flumazenil ... 892
Flumax (KR) *see* Fluconazole ... 885
Flumazen (AU) *see* Flumazenil ... 892
Flumed (CL) *see* Bromhexine [INT] ... 291
Flumed (AE, KW, QA, SA) *see* Chlorpheniramine and Pseudoephedrine ... 427
Flumedil (MX) *see* GlipiZIDE ... 967
Flumelon (KR) *see* Fluorometholone ... 896
Flumetholone (KR) *see* Fluorometholone ... 896
Flumetholon (HK, JP, KR, TW) *see* Fluorometholone ... 896
Flumethyl (ID) *see* MethylPREDNISolone ... 1340
Flumetol NF (DO, GT, NI, PA, SV) *see* Fluorometholone ... 896
Flumetol NF Ofteno (MX) *see* Fluorometholone ... 896
Flumetol (QA, RO) *see* Fluorometholone ... 896
Flumex (BR, CO, EC) *see* Fluorometholone ... 896
Flumex (PH) *see* Acetylcysteine ... 40
Flumid (SG, VN) *see* Flutamide ... 907
Flumig (PH) *see* Flunarizine [CAN/INT] ... 892
Flumil (ES) *see* Acetylcysteine ... 40
Flumil (PY, UY) *see* Flumazenil ... 892
Flumixol (CO) *see* Acetylcysteine ... 40
Flunariz (PH) *see* Flunarizine [CAN/INT] ... 892
Flunatop (BE) *see* Flunarizine [CAN/INT] ... 892
Flunavert (DE) *see* Flunarizine [CAN/INT] ... 892
Flunazol (CY) *see* Fluconazole ... 885
Flunazole (TW) *see* Fluconazole ... 885
Flunco (TH) *see* Fluconazole ... 885
Flunexil (BR) *see* Flumazenil ... 892
Flunide (TW, VN) *see* Fluocinonide ... 894
Flunidor (PT) *see* Diflunisal ... 626
Flunil (IN) *see* FLUoxetine ... 899
Flunil (KR) *see* Flumazenil ... 892
Flunir (FR) *see* Niflumic Acid [INT] ... 1454
Flunolone-V (SG, TH) *see* Fluocinolone (Topical) ... 893
Flunolone (TW) *see* Fluocinolone (Topical) ... 893
Flunox (IT) *see* Flurazepam ... 906
Fluo-A (TW) *see* Fluocinolone (Topical) ... 893
Fluociclerc (PY) *see* Fluocinolone (Topical) ... 893
Fluocinolona (PY) *see* Fluocinolone (Topical) ... 893
Fluocyne (FR) *see* Fluorescein ... 894
Fluodel (BR) *see* Fluoride ... 895
Fluoderm (ZA) *see* Fluocinolone (Topical) ... 893
Fluodont (AT) *see* Fluoride ... 895
Fluodontyl (BE, ES, FR, LU) *see* Fluoride ... 895
Fluodrazin (BR) *see* Isoniazid ... 1120
Fluoen (IL) *see* Fluoride ... 895
Fluoftal (AT) *see* Fluorescein ... 894
Fluoftal (CO) *see* Fluorometholone ... 896
Fluogum (FR, PL) *see* Fluoride ... 895
Fluohexal (AU) *see* FLUoxetine ... 899
Fluonatril (HR) *see* Fluoride ... 895
Fluonco (PH) *see* Fluorouracil (Systemic) ... 896
Fluonid (MY) *see* Fluocinolone (Topical) ... 893
Fluoplexe (FR) *see* Fluoride ... 895
Fluor-I-Strip (NL) *see* Fluorescein ... 894
Fluor-A-Day (GB, IE) *see* Fluoride ... 895
Fluoralfa (IT) *see* Fluorescein ... 894
Fluor (BE) *see* Fluoride ... 895
Fluor Crinex (FR) *see* Fluoride ... 895
Fluorecite (NO) *see* Fluorescein ... 894
Fluoresceina (BR) *see* Fluorescein ... 894
Fluoresceina Oculos (ES) *see* Fluorescein ... 894
Fluorescein (DE, HR) *see* Fluorescein ... 894
Fluoresceine (IL, LU) *see* Fluorescein ... 894
Fluoresceine Ophtadose (BE) *see* Fluorescein ... 894
Fluoresceine SDU Faure (CH) *see* Fluorescein ... 894
Fluoresceinnatrium (SE) *see* Fluorescein ... 894
Fluorescite (AE, AR, AU, BF, BH, BJ, CI, CN, CY, CZ, EC, EE, EG, ET, GH, GM, GN, HK, HN, IL, IQ, IR, JO, KE, KR, KW, LB, LR, LY, MA, ML, MR, MU, MW, NE, NG, NZ, OM, PL, QA, SA, SC, SD, SG, SL, SN, SY, TH, TN, TR, TW, TZ, UG, YE, ZA, ZM, ZW) *see* Fluorescein ... 894
Fluore Stain Strips (IN) *see* Fluorescein ... 894
Fluoretas (UY) *see* Fluoride ... 895
Fluorets (AE, GB, HK, IE, MY, SA) *see* Fluorescein ... 894
Fluorette (DK, FI, NO, SE) *see* Fluoride ... 895
Fluoretten (DE) *see* Fluoride ... 895
Fluorex (FR) *see* Fluoride ... 895
Fluorid Gel DENTSPLY DeTrey (DE) *see* Fluoride ... 895
Fluorilette (FI) *see* Fluoride ... 895
Fluor Kin (ES) *see* Fluoride ... 895
Fluor Lacer (ES) *see* Fluoride ... 895
Fluor Microsol (FR) *see* Fluoride ... 895
Fluor Oligosol (FR) *see* Fluoride ... 895
Fluoropos (KR) *see* Fluorometholone ... 896
Fluoros (DE) *see* Fluoride ... 895
Fluor-Retard (NO) *see* Fluoride ... 895
Fluorscit (QA) *see* Fluorescein ... 894
Fluor-S.M.B. (BE) *see* Fluoride ... 895
Fluortabletjes (NL) *see* Fluoride ... 895
Fluor Unicophar (BE) *see* Fluoride ... 895
Fluorvitin (IT) *see* Fluoride ... 895
Fluossen (CZ, PL) *see* Fluoride ... 895
Fluotrat (BR) *see* Fluoride ... 895
Fluovex (MY) *see* FLUoxetine ... 899
Fluoxem (CL) *see* Flumazenil ... 892
Fluoxeren (IT) *see* FLUoxetine ... 899
Fluox (NZ) *see* FLUoxetine ... 899
Fluoxone (SG) *see* FLUoxetine ... 899
Fluox-Puren (DE) *see* FLUoxetine ... 899
Fluozoid (MX) *see* Ethosuximide ... 813
Flupazine (MX) *see* Trifluoperazine ... 2102
Flura (AU) *see* Fluoride ... 895
Flurablastin (DK, FI, NO, SE) *see* Fluorouracil (Systemic) ... 896
Fluracedyl (BE, MY, NL, PH) *see* Fluorouracil (Systemic) ... 896
Fluralema (VE) *see* Flurazepam ... 906
Flurant (KR) *see* Triflusal [INT] ... 2103
Fluraz (IN) *see* Flurazepam ... 906
Flurazin (TW) *see* Trifluoperazine ... 2102
Flurbic (AR) *see* Flurbiprofen (Systemic) ... 906
Flur Di Fen (TW) *see* Flurbiprofen (Ophthalmic) ... 906
Fluroblastine (BE) *see* Fluorouracil (Systemic) ... 896
Fluroblastin (VE) *see* Fluorouracil (Systemic) ... 896
Flurofen (GR) *see* Flurbiprofen (Systemic) ... 906
Flurofen Retard (DK) *see* Flurbiprofen (Systemic) ... 906
Flurolon (DK, NO) *see* Fluorometholone ... 896
Fluronin (TW) *see* FLUoxetine ... 899
Flurozin (TH) *see* Flurbiprofen (Systemic) ... 906
Fluseminal (GR) *see* Norfloxacin ... 1475
Fluserin (UY) *see* Tolterodine ... 2063

Flusine (TW) *see* Flucytosine 889
Flutacan (LU) *see* Flutamide 907
Fluta-Cell (ID) *see* Flutamide 907
Flutafin (TW) *see* Acetylcysteine 40
Flutaide (PT) *see* Fluticasone (Nasal) 910
Flutaide (PT) *see* Fluticasone (Oral Inhalation) 907
Flutamex (DE) *see* Flutamide 907
Flutam (HU) *see* Flutamide 907
Flutamid Abbott (HU) *see* Flutamide 907
Flutamid (RU) *see* Flutamide 907
Flutamin (AU, NZ) *see* Flutamide 907
Flutan (CY, JO, RO, SG, TH) *see* Flutamide 907
Flutanon (PH) *see* Flutamide 907
Flutaplex (CO, ID) *see* Flutamide 907
Flutasin (BG, HR, HU, RO) *see* Flutamide 907
Flutax (AR) *see* Flutamide 907
Flutexine (LB) *see* Flutamide 907
Flutica (DE) *see* Fluticasone (Nasal) 910
Flutica (DE) *see* Fluticasone (Oral Inhalation) 907
Flutide (DE, NO, SE) *see* Fluticasone (Oral Inhalation) 907
Flutide (NO, SE) *see* Fluticasone (Nasal) 910
Flutimar HFA (CO) *see* Fluticasone (Oral Inhalation) 907
Flutin (AE, CO, KW, MY, QA, SA) *see* FLUoxetine 899
Flutinasal (GR) *see* Fluticasone (Nasal) 910
Flutinasal (GR) *see* Fluticasone (Oral Inhalation) 907
Flutinase (CH) *see* Fluticasone (Nasal) 910
Flutinase (CH) *see* Fluticasone (Oral Inhalation) 907
Flutine (TH) *see* FLUoxetine 899
Flutinide (MY) *see* Fluticasone (Nasal) 910
Flutitrim (SG) *see* Fluticasone (Nasal) 910
Flutitrim (SG) *see* Fluticasone (Oral Inhalation) 907
Flutivate (BR, CL, DE, NO) *see* Fluticasone (Topical) 911
Flutivate (BR, DE, NO) *see* Fluticasone (Oral Inhalation) 907
Flutonin (VN) *see* FLUoxetine 899
Flutrax (EC, PY) *see* Flutamide 907
Fluval (HR) *see* FLUoxetine 899
Fluvir (IN) *see* Oseltamivir 1523
Fluvohexal (DE) *see* FluvoxaMINE 916
Fluvoxim (PE) *see* FluvoxaMINE 916
Fluvoxin (IN, TH) *see* FluvoxaMINE 916
Fluxar (ID) *see* Fluconazole 885
Flux (BR) *see* Indapamide 1065
Fluxen (TW) *see* FLUoxetine 899
Fluxet (DE) *see* FLUoxetine 899
Fluxetin (HK) *see* FLUoxetine 899
Fluxide (PH) *see* Praziquantel 1702
Fluxil (AE, BH, CY, EG, IQ, IR, JO, KW, LB, LY, OM, QA, SA, SG, SY, TR, YE) *see* FLUoxetine 899
Flux (NO) *see* Fluoride 895
Fluxus (EC, PY) *see* Flutamide 907
Fluzepam (HR) *see* Flurazepam 906
Fluzina (CR, DO, EC, GT, HN, NI, PA, SV) *see* Flunarizine [CAN/INT] 892
Fluzin (KR) *see* Fluconazole 885
Fluzole (AU) *see* Fluconazole 885
Fluzone (BF, BJ, CI, ET, GH, GM, GN, KE, LR, MA, ML, MR, MU, MW, NE, NG, SC, SD, SL, SN, TN, TZ, UG, ZM, ZW) *see* Fluconazole 885
Fluzone (GT) *see* Fluticasone (Nasal) 910
Fluzone (GT) *see* Fluticasone (Oral Inhalation) 907
Fluzoral (TH) *see* Fluconazole 885
FML (AE, AR, BE, BH, CN, CR, CY, EG, ES, GB, GR, HK, IE, IL, IQ, IR, JO, KW, LB, LY, MY, OM, PE, PH, QA, SA, SG, SY, TH, TW, VN, YE, ZA) *see* Fluorometholone 896
FML Damla (TR) *see* Fluorometholone 896
FML Liquifilm (AU, CH, FI, LU, NL, NZ) *see* Fluorometholone 896
F.M.L. (UY) *see* Fluorometholone 896
FNI 2B (MX) *see* Interferon Alfa-2b 1096
Foban (HK, ID, SG) *see* Fusidic Acid (Topical) [CAN/INT] 943
Focusan (AT, CH, CZ, NL) *see* Tolnaftate 2063
Focus (IT) *see* Ibuprofen 1032
Focus (TW) *see* Piroxicam 1662
Fogyl (MY) *see* MetroNIDAZOLE (Systemic) 1353
Fokusin (RO) *see* Tamsulosin 1974
Folacid (PL) *see* Folic Acid 919
Folacin (BR, HR, NO, RU, SE, TW) *see* Folic Acid 919
Folart (PH) *see* Folic Acid 919
Folavit (BE) *see* Folic Acid 919
Folbiol (TR) *see* Folic Acid 919
Folcasin (ID) *see* Leucovorin Calcium 1183
Folcodal (AR) *see* Cinnarizine [INT] 440
Foli 5 (IL) *see* Folic Acid 919
Foliage (PH) *see* Folic Acid 919
Foliamin (HK, JP, TH) *see* Folic Acid 919
Folic Acid DHA (MY) *see* Folic Acid 919
Folic Acid Pharm Ecologist (AR) *see* Folic Acid 919
Folical (CO) *see* Leucovorin Calcium 1183
Folicare (BH) *see* Folic Acid 919
Folicid (KR) *see* Folic Acid 919
Folicil (CY, PT) *see* Folic Acid 919
Folicum (AE, BH, KW, QA, SA) *see* Folic Acid 919
Foligan (DE) *see* Allopurinol 90
Foligem (IN) *see* Urofollitropin 2116
Folimax (PH) *see* Folic Acid 919
Folimet (DK) *see* Folic Acid 919
Folina 15 (TW) *see* Leucovorin Calcium 1183
Folina (IT) *see* Folic Acid 919
Folinato de Calcio Dakota Farma (PT) *see* Leucovorin Calcium 1183
Folin (BR) *see* Folic Acid 919
Folinsyre "Dak" (DK) *see* Folic Acid 919
Foliphar (BE) *see* Folic Acid 919
Foliront (JP) *see* Furosemide 940
Folivital (GT, HN, MX, NI, SV) *see* Folic Acid 919
Folivita (SA) *see* Folic Acid 919
Folivit (TH) *see* Folic Acid 919
Follegon (TW) *see* Urofollitropin 2116
Follimon (KR, TH) *see* Urofollitropin 2116
Follistim (JP) *see* Follitropin Beta 921
Follitrin (AR, CL, PY, UY) *see* Urofollitropin 2116
Foloicare (AE) *see* Folic Acid 919
Folotyn (KR) *see* PRALAtrexate 1693
Folsan (AT, HR) *see* Folic Acid 919
Folsmycin (TW) *see* Fosfomycin 932
Folsyre (NO) *see* Folic Acid 919
Folverlan (DE) *see* Folic Acid 919
Folvite (AE, BB, BH, BM, BS, BZ, CH, CY, EG, FI, GY, IL, IQ, IR, JM, JO, KW, LB, LY, NL, OM, QA, SA, SR, SY, TT, YE) *see* Folic Acid 919
FomepizoleAP-HP (FR) *see* Fomepizole 922
Fomicyt (GB) *see* Fosfomycin 932
Fomiken (MX) *see* Phenytoin 1640
Fonat (AU) *see* Alendronate 79
Fongamil (FR, GR, PT) *see* Omoconazole [INT] 1512
Fonosil (TW) *see* Fosinopril 932
Fontego (IT) *see* Bumetanide 297
Fontex (DK, FI, IS, NO, SE) *see* FLUoxetine 899
Fonurit (HU) *see* AcetaZOLAMIDE 39
Fonvicol (PH) *see* CeFAZolin 373
Fopo (TW) *see* Pimozide 1651
Foracort (MY) *see* Budesonide and Formoterol 297
Foradil Aerolizer (AE, BH, CO, CY, EG, IQ, IR, JO, KW, LB, LY, NZ, OM, QA, SA, SY, YE) *see* Formoterol 926
Foradil (AT, BE, BF, BJ, BR, CH, CI, CZ, DK, EE, ET, FI, FR, GH, GM, GN, GR, HK, IE, IL, IT, KE, LR, LT, MA, ML, MR, MU, MW, MX, NE, NG, NO, NZ, PE, PH, PL, PT, RU, SC, SD, SE, SG, SK, SL, SN, TN, TR, TZ, UG, UY, VE, ZA, ZM, ZW) *see* Formoterol 926
Foradile (AU) *see* Formoterol 926
Foradil P (DE) *see* Formoterol 926

Foragin (ID) *see* Dipyrone [INT] ... 653
Forair (PH) *see* Fluticasone and Salmeterol ... 912
Forasma (TW) *see* Formoterol ... 926
Forasm (KR) *see* EPHEDrine (Systemic) ... 734
Foratec (IN) *see* Formoterol ... 926
Forbatec (AE, BH, CY, EG, IL, IQ, IR, JO, KW, LB, LY, OM, QA, SA, SY, YE) *see* Cefaclor ... 372
For-BPH (PH) *see* Finasteride ... 878
Forcad (PH) *see* Simvastatin ... 1890
Forcaltonin (AT, BE, BG, CH, CZ, DE, DK, EE, ES, FI, FR, GB, GR, HN, IE, IL, IT, MT, NL, NO, PL, PT, RU, SE, SK, TR) *see* Calcitonin ... 322
Forcan (IN, VN) *see* Fluconazole ... 885
Forcilin (AR) *see* Modafinil ... 1386
Fordenta (ID) *see* Chlorhexidine Gluconate ... 422
Forderm (ID) *see* Clobetasol ... 468
Fordesia (ID) *see* Donepezil ... 668
Fordiuran (ES) *see* Bumetanide ... 297
Fordrim (AR) *see* Flurazepam ... 906
Forexo (RO, SK) *see* Cefpodoxime ... 388
Forgram (PH) *see* CefTRIAXone ... 396
Forifek (ID) *see* Cefaclor ... 372
Forilin (DK) *see* Roxithromycin [INT] ... 1853
Forimycin (DK) *see* Roxithromycin [INT] ... 1853
Forken (MX) *see* Amiodarone ... 114
Forknow (MY, SG) *see* Flunarizine [CAN/INT] ... 892
Formet (AU, JO, MY) *see* MetFORMIN ... 1307
Formin (IN) *see* MetFORMIN ... 1307
Formit (AE, BH, KW, QA, SA) *see* MetFORMIN ... 1307
Formoair (FR) *see* Formoterol ... 926
Formorol (TW) *see* Formoterol ... 926
For MR. (KR) *see* Sildenafil ... 1882
Formulaexpec (ES) *see* GuaiFENesin ... 986
Formyco (ID, SG) *see* Ketoconazole (Topical) ... 1145
Formyco (SG) *see* Ketoconazole (Systemic) ... 1144
Fornac (IN) *see* Aceclofenac [INT] ... 30
Fornax (PE) *see* Cefuroxime ... 399
Fornidd (PH) *see* MetFORMIN ... 1307
Forosa (PH) *see* Alendronate ... 79
Forsine (TW) *see* Fosinopril ... 932
Forsteo (AT, BE, BG, CH, CN, CY, CZ, DE, DK, EE, ES, FI, FR, GB, GR, HN, HU, IE, IS, IT, KR, LT, MT, NL, NO, PL, PT, RO, RU, SE, SI, SK, TR) *see* Teriparatide ... 2008
Forta B 5.000 (BE) *see* Hydroxocobalamin ... 1020
Forta B12 (BE, LU) *see* Hydroxocobalamin ... 1020
Fortal (BE, LU) *see* Pentazocine ... 1616
Fortalgesic[inj.] (CH) *see* Pentazocine ... 1616
Fortam (CH, ES, UY) *see* CefTAZidime ... 392
Fortanest (ID) *see* Midazolam ... 1361
Fortasec (ES) *see* Loperamide ... 1236
Fortaz (BR) *see* CefTAZidime ... 392
Fortecortin (AT, BG, CH, DE) *see* Dexamethasone (Systemic) ... 599
Forteo (AE, AR, AU, BH, BR, CL, CO, CR, DO, GT, HK, HR, JP, KW, LB, MX, MY, NZ, PA, PE, PY, QA, SA, SG, SV, TH, TW, VE) *see* Teriparatide ... 2008
Fortera Orally Soluble Film (KR) *see* Sildenafil ... 1882
Fortfen SR (ZA) *see* Diclofenac (Systemic) ... 617
Fortical (ES) *see* Calcium Carbonate ... 327
Fortical (IL) *see* Calcitonin ... 322
Fortius (IN) *see* Rosuvastatin ... 1848
Fortolin (HK) *see* Acetaminophen ... 32
Fortovase (AE, AR, BG, BH, IN, KW, MX, PE, QA, VE, VN) *see* Saquinavir ... 1865
Fortral (AT, AU, BG, CZ, DE, DK, GB, HR, IE, NZ, PL) *see* Pentazocine ... 1616
Fortralin (FI, NO) *see* Pentazocine ... 1616
Fortralin[inj./rect.] (NO) *see* Pentazocine ... 1616
Fortulin (HR) *see* Formoterol ... 926
Fortum (AE, AR, AT, AU, BB, BF, BG, BH, BJ, BM, BS, BZ, CI, CL, CN, CO, CR, CY, CZ, DE, DK, DO, EC, EE, EG, ET, FR, GB, GH, GM, GN, GT, GY, HK, HN, HU, ID, IE, IL, IN, IQ, IR, IS, JM, JO, KE, KR, KW, LB, LR, LT, LY, MA, ML, MR, MU, MW, MX, MY, NE, NG, NI, NL, NO, NZ, OM, PA, PE, PH, PR, PY, QA, RO, RU, SA, SC, SD, SE, SI, SK, SL, SN, SR, SV, SY, TH, TN, TR, TT, TW, TZ, UG, VE, VN, YE, ZA, ZM, ZW) *see* CefTAZidime ... 392
Fortum Pro (HN) *see* CefTAZidime ... 392
Fortumset (FR) *see* CefTAZidime ... 392
Fortwin (BF, BJ, CI, ET, GH, GM, GN, IN, KE, LR, MA, ML, MR, MU, MW, NE, NG, SC, SD, SL, SN, TN, TZ, UG, ZM, ZW) *see* Pentazocine ... 1616
Fortzaar (AE, BH, CY, EG, FR, HR, IT, KW, MY, PT, QA, RO, SA, SE, TH) *see* Losartan and Hydrochlorothiazide ... 1250
Forvey (ES) *see* Frovatriptan ... 938
For-You (TW) *see* ClomiPRAMINE ... 475
Forzaten (BE) *see* Amlodipine and Olmesartan ... 126
Forzest (IN) *see* Tadalafil ... 1968
Forzid (PH) *see* CefTAZidime ... 392
Forzyn Beta (PY) *see* Cefepime ... 378
Fosalan (IL) *see* Alendronate ... 79
Fosamax (AE, AR, AT, AU, BB, BE, BG, BH, BM, BR, BS, BZ, CH, CL, CN, CY, CZ, DE, DK, EC, EE, EG, ES, FI, FR, GB, GR, GY, HK, HR, IE, IT, JM, JO, KR, KW, LB, MX, NL, NO, NZ, PE, PK, PL, PR, PT, QA, RO, RU, SA, SE, SG, SI, SK, SR, TH, TR, TT, TW, VE, VN) *see* Alendronate ... 79
Fosamax Once Weekly (AE, BH, LB, SA) *see* Alendronate ... 79
Fosamax Plus (AR, CL, CN, CR, GT, HK, ID, KR, MX, MY, NI, NZ, PA, SG, SV, TH, TW, VN) *see* Alendronate and Cholecalciferol ... 81
Fosamax Plus Once Weekly (AU) *see* Alendronate and Cholecalciferol ... 81
Fosavance (AE, AT, BE, BG, BH, CH, CY, CZ, DE, DK, EE, ES, FI, FR, GB, GR, HN, HR, HU, IE, IL, IT, KW, LB, MT, NL, NO, PH, PT, QA, RO, RU, SE, SK, TR) *see* Alendronate and Cholecalciferol ... 81
Fosavis (SE) *see* Fosinopril ... 932
Foscarnet Elea (AR) *see* Foscarnet ... 931
Foscarnet Filaxis (AR) *see* Foscarnet ... 931
Foscarnet Richmond (AR) *see* Foscarnet ... 931
Foscavir (AR, AT, AU, BE, CH, CZ, DE, ES, FI, FR, GB, GR, HN, HU, IL, IT, JP, LU, NL, NO, NZ, PT, SE, SG) *see* Foscarnet ... 931
Fosfitone (AR, UY) *see* Succinylcholine ... 1939
Fosfocil (DO, GT, HN, PA, SV) *see* Fosfomycin ... 932
Fosfocina (EC, ES) *see* Fosfomycin ... 932
Fosfocine (FR, VN) *see* Fosfomycin ... 932
Fosfomin (TH) *see* Fosfomycin ... 932
Fosfurol (PY, UY) *see* Fosfomycin ... 932
Fosinil (BE, ES, LU) *see* Fosinopril ... 932
Fosinorm (DE) *see* Fosinopril ... 932
Fosipres (IT) *see* Fosinopril ... 932
Fosipril (AU) *see* Fosinopril ... 932
Fositen (CH, PT) *see* Fosinopril ... 932
Fositens (AT, CY, EG, ES, IL, IQ, IR, LY, OM, SY, YE) *see* Fosinopril ... 932
Foskina (PH) *see* Mupirocin ... 1404
Fosmicin-S (JP) *see* Fosfomycin ... 932
Fosmidex (ID) *see* Fosfomycin ... 932
Fosmin (EC, PE) *see* Alendronate ... 79
Fosolin (IN) *see* Fosphenytoin ... 934
Fosrenol (AT, AU, BE, BG, CH, CY, CZ, DE, DK, EE, FI, FR, GB, GR, HK, HN, ID, IL, IS, JP, KR, LT, MY, NL, NO, PH, PT, RO, SE, SG, SI, SK, TH, TR, TW) *see* Lanthanum ... 1169
Fostimon (AE, AT, BE, BG, BH, CH, CY, CZ, DK, FI, FR, GB, HN, IL, IT, KW, LB, MX, NL, PL, PT, QA, TR) *see* Urofollitropin ... 2116
Fostimon HP (SA) *see* Urofollitropin ... 2116
Fostipur (ES) *see* Urofollitropin ... 2116
Fostoin (JP) *see* Fosphenytoin ... 934

Fosval (PY) *see* Alendronate 79
Fot-Amsa (MX) *see* Cefotaxime 382
Fotexina (CO, EC, MX) *see* Cefotaxime 382
Fouch (GR) *see* Clindamycin (Topical) 464
Fovas (IN) *see* Fosinopril 932
Fovepta (VN) *see* Hepatitis B Immune Globulin (Human) 1002
Foxate (TW) *see* FlavoxATE 881
Foxitin (AE, JO, SA) *see* CefOXitin 386
Foxolin (KR) *see* Amoxicillin 130
Fozal (PH) *see* Alfuzosin 84
Fozitec (FR) *see* Fosinopril 932
Foznol (IE, IT) *see* Lanthanum 1169
Fozole (IN) *see* Pantoprazole 1570
Fracitin (SG) *see* Framycetin [INT] 937
Fractal (FR) *see* Fluvastatin 915
Fractal LP (FR) *see* Fluvastatin 915
Frade (IN) *see* Framycetin [INT] 937
Fradicilina (ES) *see* Penicillin G Procaine 1613
Fradyl (BE, LU) *see* Neomycin 1436
Fragmin (AE, AT, AU, BE, BG, BH, BR, CH, CL, CN, CO, CY, CZ, DE, DK, EC, EE, EG, ES, FI, GB, GR, HK, HN, HR, HU, IE, IL, IN, IQ, IR, IS, IT, JO, KR, KW, LB, LT, LY, MT, NL, NO, NZ, OM, PE, PK, PL, PT, QA, RO, RU, SA, SE, SG, SI, SK, SY, TR, TW, YE, ZA) *see* Dalteparin 553
Fragmine (FR) *see* Dalteparin 553
Fragmin P Forte (DE) *see* Dalteparin 553
Framycin (PK) *see* Framycetin [INT] 937
Franol (BR) *see* Ephedrine and Theophylline [INT] 734
Franol (TH) *see* Theophylline 2026
Frantel (VN) *see* Albendazole 65
Fraxiparina (BR, ES, IT, PT, VE) *see* Nadroparin [CAN/INT] 1412
Fraxiparin (AT, DE, DO, GT, HN, KW, NI, PA, SV) *see* Nadroparin [CAN/INT] 1412
Fraxiparine (AE, AR, AU, BE, BG, BH, CH, CL, CN, CY, CZ, EC, EE, EG, FI, FR, GR, HK, HR, HU, ID, IL, IN, KR, LB, LT, LU, MX, MY, NL, NO, NZ, PH, PK, PL, PY, QA, RO, RU, SE, SG, SI, SK, TH, TR, TW, UY, VN) *see* Nadroparin [CAN/INT] 1412
Fraxiparine Forte (PH, SG, TH) *see* Nadroparin [CAN/INT] 1412
Fraxiparine TX (CO, CR, MX, PE, UY) *see* Nadroparin [CAN/INT] 1412
Fraxodi (BE, GR) *see* Nadroparin [CAN/INT] 1412
Frazon (ID) *see* Ondansetron 1513
Freeya (KR) *see* Sildenafil 1882
Freez-Eze Throat Anesthetic Gel (SG) *see* Benzocaine 246
Frego (ID) *see* Flunarizine [CAN/INT] 892
Fremet (ES) *see* Cimetidine 438
Frenactil (BE, LU, NL) *see* Benperidol [INT] 244
Frenaler (CL) *see* Loratadine 1241
Frenolyn (TR) *see* Budesonide (Systemic) 293
Frenurin (BR) *see* Oxybutynin 1536
Fresofol (AU, KR, MY, NZ, PH, TW) *see* Propofol 1728
Fresofol MCT/LCT (HK, ID, TH) *see* Propofol 1728
Fretic (PH) *see* Furosemide 940
Frezitron (PH) *see* Granisetron 983
Fridalit (AR) *see* Hydrocortisone (Systemic) 1013
Fridep (ID) *see* Sertraline 1878
Frimania (ID) *see* Lithium 1230
Frina (GR) *see* Propranolol 1731
Frinova (ES) *see* Promethazine 1723
Frisium (AT, AU, BE, BR, CR, CY, CZ, DE, DK, DO, EG, FI, GB, GR, GT, HK, HN, HU, ID, IE, IL, IN, IT, LU, MY, NI, NL, NO, NZ, PA, PK, PL, QA, SG, SI, SK, SV, TH, TR, TW, UY, VE) *see* CloBAZam 465
Frisolona Forte (PT) *see* PrednisoLONE (Ophthalmic) 1706
Frisolona (PT) *see* PrednisoLONE (Ophthalmic) 1706
Fristamin (IT) *see* Loratadine 1241
Fritens (ID) *see* Irbesartan 1110
Frixopel (PY) *see* Propranolol 1731
Froben (AE, AT, BE, BH, CH, IN, KR, KW, NL, PK, PT, QA, SA, SG, ZA) *see* Flurbiprofen (Systemic) 906
Froben SR (AE, BH, QA, ZA) *see* Flurbiprofen (Systemic) 906
Fromena (RO) *see* Frovatriptan 938
Fromen (CZ) *see* Frovatriptan 938
Fromilid (HR, HU, RO, TR) *see* Clarithromycin 456
Fromirex (NL) *see* Frovatriptan 938
Fronil (TW) *see* Imipramine 1054
Frontal (BR) *see* ALPRAZolam 94
Frontin (HU, RO) *see* ALPRAZolam 94
Fropine (KR) *see* FLUoxetine 899
Frosit (ID) *see* Aspirin 180
Frotin (HK, MY, TW) *see* MetroNIDAZOLE (Systemic) 1353
Frovex (IE) *see* Frovatriptan 938
Froxime (AE, BH, CY, EG, IQ, IR, JO, KW, LB, LY, OM, QA, SA, SY, YE) *see* Cefuroxime 399
Froxtil (KR) *see* Cefpodoxime 388
FructiCal (PL) *see* Calcium Carbonate 327
Frumeron (SG, TH) *see* Indapamide 1065
Frusedan (BF, BJ, CI, ET, GH, GM, GN, KE, LR, MA, ML, MR, MU, MW, NE, NG, SC, SD, SL, SN, TN, TZ, UG, ZA, ZM, ZW) *see* Furosemide 940
Frusid (AU, HK, NZ) *see* Furosemide 940
FSME-Immun (DE) *see* Meningococcal (Groups A / C / Y and W-135) Diphtheria Conjugate Vaccine 1289
Ftazidime (GR) *see* CefTAZidime 392
Ftoracort (EE) *see* Triamcinolone (Topical) 2100
Ftorocort (VN) *see* Triamcinolone (Topical) 2100
Fucidin IV (ZA) *see* Fusidic Acid (Systemic) [INT] 942
Fucidin (AE, AR, AT, BB, BE, BH, CH, CL, CN, CO, CZ, DE, DK, EC, EE, FI, FR, GB, GR, HK, HU, ID, IE, IL, IS, IT, JO, KR, KW, LB, LT, MX, NL, NO, PE, PH, PK, PL, PY, QA, RU, SA, SE, SI, SK, TH, TR, TW, UY, VN, ZA) *see* Fusidic Acid (Topical) [CAN/INT] 943
Fucidin (AE, AU, CH, EG, FI, HK, IL, KR, KW, MY, NZ, PH, RO, SA, SG, SI, TH, UY) *see* Fusidic Acid (Systemic) [INT] 942
Fucidine (DK, ES, FR, PT, SE) *see* Fusidic Acid (Systemic) [INT] 942
Fucidine (ES) *see* Fusidic Acid (Ophthalmic) [CAN/INT] 942
Fucidine (ES) *see* Fusidic Acid (Topical) [CAN/INT] 943
Fucidin (IT) *see* Fusidic Acid (Ophthalmic) [CAN/INT] 942
Fucidin Topical (AU, NZ) *see* Fusidic Acid (Topical) [CAN/INT] 943
Fucid (PH) *see* Fusidic Acid (Topical) [CAN/INT] 943
Fucimycin (TW) *see* Fusidic Acid (Topical) [CAN/INT] 943
Fucinex (PH) *see* Fusidic Acid (Topical) [CAN/INT] 943
Fucithalmic (AT, BB, BE, BH, CH, CL, CO, DE, DK, EC, EE, EG, FI, HK, IE, IL, JO, KW, LB, MY, NL, NO, NZ, PH, PK, PT, RO, RU, SA, SE, TH, TR, ZA) *see* Fusidic Acid (Ophthalmic) [CAN/INT] 942
Fucithalmmic (CZ) *see* Fusidic Acid (Ophthalmic) [CAN/INT] 942
Fucotin (TW) *see* FlavoxATE 881
5-FU (DE, JP, KR) *see* Fluorouracil (Systemic) 896
Fudixing (CN) *see* Gatifloxacin 949
Fudone (BF, BJ, CI, ET, GH, GM, GN, KE, LR, MA, ML, MR, MU, MW, NE, NG, SC, SD, SL, SN, TN, TZ, UG, ZM, ZW) *see* Famotidine 845
Fugacar (TH, VN) *see* Mebendazole [CAN/INT] 1274
Fuganol (GR) *see* Sertaconazole 1877
Fugerel (AT, AU, CN, HU, PH, TH, VN) *see* Flutamide 907
Fuhe (CN) *see* Rifampin 1804
Fu-Iron (TW) *see* Ferric Gluconate 869
Fu Ke (CN) *see* Fluorouracil (Systemic) 896

Fukole (MY, PH) *see* Fluconazole 885
Fukricin (ID) *see* Natamycin 1432
Fulaidi (CN) *see* Repaglinide 1791
Fulaihe (CN) *see* Repaglinide and Metformin 1792
Fulcard (KR) *see* Flecainide 882
Fulcin (BR, EC, ES, FI, IT, NO, PT) *see* Griseofulvin 985
Fulcin Forte (MX) *see* Griseofulvin 985
Fulcin S (DE) *see* Griseofulvin 985
Fulcol (EC) *see* Sulconazole 1943
Fulgram (CL) *see* Norfloxacin 1475
Fullcilina (AR) *see* Amoxicillin 130
Ful Lee (TW) *see* Tazarotene 1980
Fullgram (KR) *see* Clindamycin (Systemic) 460
Fullicilina Plus (AR) *see* Amoxicillin and Clavulanate 133
Fulnite (IN) *see* Eszopiclone 793
Fuloan (TW) *see* Fluoxymesterone 903
Fulopin (ID) *see* AmLODIPine 123
Fuloren (KR) *see* FLUoxetine 899
Fulosin (TW) *see* Fusidic Acid (Topical) [CAN/INT] 943
Fulpen A (JP) *see* Bromhexine [INT] 291
Fulsadem (AR) *see* Zolpidem 2212
Fulsed (CN, IN, VN) *see* Midazolam 1361
Fulsix (JP) *see* Furosemide 940
Fulsovin (GB) *see* Griseofulvin 985
Fuluminol (JP) *see* Clemastine 459
Fuluson (KR) *see* Fluorometholone 896
Fuluvamide (JP) *see* Furosemide 940
Fulvicina (ES) *see* Griseofulvin 985
Fumafer (AE, FR, PT, SA, VE) *see* Ferrous Fumarate 870
Fumaresutin (JP) *see* Clemastine 459
Fumay (TW) *see* Fluconazole 885
Fumiron (DE) *see* Ferrous Fumarate 870
Funa (TH) *see* Fluconazole 885
Funazine-S (TW) *see* FluPHENAZine 905
Funazine (TW) *see* FluPHENAZine 905
Funazol (KR) *see* Fluconazole 885
Funcid (PH) *see* Butenafine 314
Funcional (EC) *see* Sildenafil 1882
Fundan (SE) *see* Ketoconazole (Topical) 1145
Funet (ID) *see* Ketoconazole (Systemic) 1144
Funex (CO) *see* Fluconazole 885
Fungata (AT, DE) *see* Fluconazole 885
Fungaway (TW) *see* Ketoconazole (Topical) 1145
Fungazol (PK) *see* Econazole 703
Fungazol (TH) *see* Ketoconazole (Systemic) 1144
Fungicare (IL) *see* Clotrimazole (Topical) 488
Fungicide (IN) *see* Ketoconazole (Systemic) 1144
Fungicide (TW) *see* Clotrimazole (Topical) 488
Fungicidin (CZ, SK) *see* Nystatin (Topical) 1482
Fungiderm (AT) *see* Bifonazole [INT] 264
Fungiderma (TW) *see* Nystatin and Triamcinolone 1482
Fungiderm-K (TH) *see* Ketoconazole (Topical) 1145
Fungifos (DE) *see* Tolciclate [INT] 2062
Fungilac (HR) *see* Amorolfine [INT] 128
Fungilin Lozenges (AU, NZ) *see* Amphotericin B (Conventional) 136
Fungilin (QA) *see* Amphotericin B (Conventional) 136
Funginix (DK) *see* Terbinafine (Systemic) 2002
Funginix (DK) *see* Terbinafine (Topical) 2004
Funginox (LB) *see* Itraconazole 1130
Funginox (TH) *see* Ketoconazole (Systemic) 1144
Fungistat 3 (BB, BM, BS, BZ, GY, JM, PR, SR, TT) *see* Terconazole 2006
Fungistat (CO, MX, VE) *see* Terconazole 2006
Fungistop (ID) *see* Griseofulvin 985
Fungitech (TW) *see* Terbinafine (Systemic) 2002
Fungitericin (PH) *see* Amphotericin B (Conventional) 136
Fungitrazol (ID) *see* Itraconazole 1130
Fungium (CL, PY) *see* Ketoconazole (Systemic) 1144
Fungium (CL, PY) *see* Ketoconazole (Topical) 1145
Fungivin (NO, PK) *see* Griseofulvin 985
Fungizid (DE) *see* Terbinafine (Systemic) 2002
Fungizid (DE) *see* Terbinafine (Topical) 2004
Fungizol (PH) *see* Ketoconazole (Systemic) 1144
Fungizon (CN, HN) *see* Amphotericin B (Conventional) 136
Fungizone (CH, CL, CO, DE, FI, FR, GR, IE, IN, IT, JO, KE, KR, NG, NL, NO, NZ, PE, PL, QA, SE, SI, TR, TW, TZ, UY, VE, ZA) *see* Amphotericin B (Conventional) 136
Fungoral (GR, NO, SE) *see* Ketoconazole (Systemic) 1144
Fungoral (IS, NO) *see* Ketoconazole (Topical) 1145
Fungostatin (GR) *see* Fluconazole 885
Fungoz (ID) *see* Fluconazole 885
Fungster (BE) *see* Terbinafine (Systemic) 2002
Fungster (BE) *see* Terbinafine (Topical) 2004
Fungtopic (PH) *see* Miconazole (Topical) 1360
Funguard (JP) *see* Micafungin 1359
Funjapin (TW) *see* Cefepime 378
Funnix (TW) *see* BuPROPion 305
Funxion (PH) *see* Pregabalin 1710
Funzal (CO) *see* Terbinafine (Systemic) 2002
Funzela (PH) *see* Fluconazole 885
Funzol (AE, HR, JO, LB, QA, SA) *see* Fluconazole 885
Fuprostatel (TW) *see* Flutamide 907
Furacam (EC) *see* Cefuroxime 399
Furadantina (AR, CL, MX) *see* Nitrofurantoin 1463
Furadantin (AT, IN, IS, NO, SE, SI) *see* Nitrofurantoin 1463
Furadantine MC (BE) *see* Nitrofurantoin 1463
Furadantine-MC (NL, PT) *see* Nitrofurantoin 1463
Furadantine (FR, LU) *see* Nitrofurantoin 1463
Furadantin Retard (CH) *see* Nitrofurantoin 1463
Furadina (VE) *see* Nitrofurantoin 1463
Furadin (PK) *see* Nitrofurantoin 1463
Furadonins (LT) *see* Nitrofurantoin 1463
Furanpur (UY) *see* Nitrofurantoin 1463
Furanthril (CZ) *see* Furosemide 940
Furantoina (ES) *see* Nitrofurantoin 1463
Furanturil (BG) *see* Furosemide 940
Furetic (TH) *see* Furosemide 940
Furic (PH) *see* Febuxostat 848
Furide (TW) *see* Furosemide 940
Furidona (AR) *see* Furazolidone [INT] 940
Furimin (KR) *see* Phentermine 1635
Furix (NO, SE) *see* Furosemide 940
Furobactina (ES) *see* Nitrofurantoin 1463
Furobioxin (MX) *see* Cefuroxime 399
Furolin (GR) *see* Nitrofurantoin 1463
Furolink (PH) *see* Furosemide 940
Furomen (FI) *see* Furosemide 940
Furomex (CZ) *see* Furosemide 940
Furomin (FI) *see* Furosemide 940
Furon (HU) *see* Furosemide 940
Furopine (VN) *see* Furazolidone [INT] 940
Furo-Puren (DE) *see* Furosemide 940
Furorese (DE, LU) *see* Furosemide 940
Furosedon (JP) *see* Furosemide 940
Furosemide-Eurogenerics (LU) *see* Furosemide 940
Furosemid (HR, HU) *see* Furosemide 940
Furosemid Pharmavit (HU) *see* Furosemide 940
Furosemid-ratiopharm (LU) *see* Furosemide 940
Furosemix (LU) *see* Furosemide 940
Furosetic (LB) *see* Furosemide 940
Furosix (BR) *see* Furosemide 940
Furovenir (IL) *see* Furosemide 940
Furoxime (TH) *see* Cefuroxime 399
Furoxim (PH) *see* Cefuroxime 399
Furoxona (CL, CO, MX, PE, VE) *see* Furazolidone [INT] 940
Furoxone (IN, PH, PK) *see* Furazolidone [INT] 940
Fursemid (HR) *see* Furosemide 940
Furudin (KR) *see* Bencyclane [INT] 241
Furuitong (CN) *see* Pioglitazone and Metformin 1655

Furusemide (JP) *see* Furosemide 940
Fusacid (HR, PL) *see* Fusidic Acid (Topical) [CAN/INT] 943
Fuseride (TH) *see* Furosemide 940
Fu Shi Ling (CN) *see* Foscarnet 931
Fu Shu Da (CN) *see* MetroNIDAZOLE (Systemic) 1353
Fusicutan (CH, DE) *see* Fusidic Acid (Topical) [CAN/INT] 943
Fusid (DE, IL) *see* Furosemide 940
Fusiderm (BH) *see* Fusidic Acid (Topical) [CAN/INT] 943
Fusid (TH) *see* Fusidic Acid (Topical) [CAN/INT] 943
Fusigra (ID) *see* Fusidic Acid (Topical) [CAN/INT] 943
Fusimex (PH) *see* Furosemide 940
Fusitop (EC) *see* Fusidic Acid (Topical) [CAN/INT] 943
Fuson (ID, PH) *see* Fusidic Acid (Topical) [CAN/INT] 943
Fusovin (TH) *see* Griseofulvin 985
Futeshu (CN) *see* Terbinafine (Topical) 2004
Futisone (TW) *see* Fluticasone (Oral Inhalation) 907
Futisone (TW) *see* Fluticasone (Topical) 911
Futuran (ES) *see* Eprosartan 748
Futuran Plus (ES) *see* Eprosartan and Hydrochlorothiazide 750
Fuweidin (TW) *see* Famotidine 845
Fuxetine (KR) *see* FLUoxetine 899
Fuxol (MX) *see* Furazolidone [INT] 940
Fuyunhon (HK) *see* Urea 2114
Fuzeon (AR, AT, AU, BE, BG, BR, CH, CL, CN, CO, CY, CZ, DE, DK, EC, EE, ES, FI, FR, GB, GR, HN, HR, HU, IE, IL, IT, LT, MT, MX, NL, NO, NZ, PE, PL, PT, RO, RU, SE, SG, SI, SK, TH, TR, TW, UY) *see* Enfuvirtide 726
Fuzine (TW) *see* Trifluoperazine 2102
Fuzocim (AE) *see* Alfuzosin 84
Fuzolan (ID) *see* Fluconazole 885
Fybogel (GB, IE, MY, NZ, SG, TH) *see* Psyllium 1744
Fycompa (AU, CH, CZ, DE, DK, EE, ES, FR, GB, HK, HR, IL, IS, LT, NO, SE, SI, SK) *see* Perampanel 1620
Fylin (TW) *see* Pentoxifylline 1618
Fynadin (TW) *see* Fexofenadine 873
Fynasid (TW) *see* Finasteride 878
Fynefta (AU) *see* Fingolimod 879
Fytosid (IN, PH, SG, TH, TW) *see* Etoposide Phosphate 820
Fytosid (VN) *see* Etoposide 816
GA-Amclav (AU) *see* Amoxicillin and Clavulanate 133
Gaap Ofteno (CR, DO, GT, HN, NI, PA, SV) *see* Latanoprost 1172
Gabacet (FR) *see* Piracetam [INT] 1661
Gabadin (PY) *see* Gabapentin 943
Gabalept (RO) *see* Gabapentin 943
Gabalon (JP) *see* Baclofen 223
Gabanet (JO, LB) *see* Gabapentin 943
Gabantin (MX) *see* Gabapentin 943
Gabapenin (KR) *see* Gabapentin 943
Gabapen (JP) *see* Gabapentin 943
Gabaran (AU) *see* Gabapentin 943
Gabaron (PH) *see* Gabapentin 943
Gabasant (ID) *see* Gabapentin 943
Gabatin (CH, KR) *see* Gabapentin 943
Gabatine (AU) *see* Gabapentin 943
Gabatopa (KR) *see* Topiramate 2065
Gabaz (MX) *see* GlipiZIDE 967
Gabbroral (BE, IT, LU) *see* Paromomycin 1579
Gabbryl (ID) *see* Paromomycin 1579
Gabenil (HK) *see* Gabapentin 943
Gabexol (ID) *see* Gabapentin 943
Gabica (PK) *see* Pregabalin 1710
GAB (IN) *see* Lindane 1217
Gabirol (CR, DO, GT, MX, NI, SV) *see* Rimantadine 1813
Gabitril (AT, AU, BE, BG, CH, CZ, DE, DK, ES, FI, FR, GB, GR, HN, IE, IT, LT, NO, PL, PT, SI) *see* TiaGABine 2032
Gabix (PH) *see* Gabapentin 943
Gabrilen (DE) *see* Ketoprofen 1145
Gabrilen Retard (DE) *see* Ketoprofen 1145
Gabrosidina (DO, GT, HN, NI, SV) *see* Paromomycin 1579
Gabutin (TH) *see* Gabapentin 943
Gadol (VE) *see* Cimetidine 438
Gadoserin (JP) *see* Diltiazem 634
Galaflax (AR) *see* Gallamine Triethiodide [INT] 948
Galamer (IN) *see* Galantamine 946
Galantyl (AU) *see* Galantamine 946
Galaxdar (ES) *see* Diacerein [INT] 613
Galcodine (GB) *see* Codeine 497
Galenphol (GB) *see* Pholcodine [INT] 1646
Galidrin (MX) *see* Ranitidine 1777
Galium (ID) *see* Flunarizine [CAN/INT] 892
Gallasin (KR) *see* Gallamine Triethiodide [INT] 948
Gallisal (FI) *see* Diethylamine Salicylate [INT] 624
Galonin (KR) *see* Gallamine Triethiodide [INT] 948
Galopran (AR) *see* Mosapride [INT] 1401
Galsya (RO) *see* Galantamine 946
Galusan (ES) *see* Pipemidic Acid [INT] 1655
Galzin (AR) *see* Zinc Acetate 2199
Gama Acaderm (CL) *see* Lindane 1217
Gamabenceno Plus (CO, GT, HN, SV) *see* Permethrin 1627
Gama (CN) *see* Interferon Gamma-1b 1104
Gamanil (GB, IE) *see* Lofepramine [INT] 1232
Gamastan Immune Globulin (IL) *see* Immune Globulin 1056
Gambex (ZA) *see* Lindane 1217
Gamicin (TW) *see* Gentamicin (Systemic) 959
Gamikal (MX) *see* Amikacin 111
Gamimune (KW, QA) *see* Immune Globulin 1056
Gamine XR (AU) *see* Galantamine 946
Gamma 16 (IL) *see* Immune Globulin 1056
Gammadyn F (BE) *see* Fluoride 895
Gammadyn Mg (BE) *see* Magnesium Gluconate 1263
Gammagard (BG, DK, FR, GB, HN, IT, NL, SE) *see* Immune Globulin 1056
Gammagard S/D (HK, IL, SA) *see* Immune Globulin 1056
Gamma I.V. (IN) *see* Immune Globulin 1056
Gammanorm (AE, FR, GB) *see* Immune Globulin 1056
Gammaplex (GB) *see* Immune Globulin 1056
Gammaraas (ID) *see* Immune Globulin 1056
Gammonativ (AE, BH, CY, DE, DK, EG, IQ, IR, JO, KW, LB, LY, NO, OM, QA, SA, SE, SY, YE) *see* Immune Globulin 1056
Gamocid (KR) *see* Mosapride [INT] 1401
Gamonil (CH, DE) *see* Lofepramine [INT] 1232
Gamunex-C (MY) *see* Immune Globulin 1056
Gamunex (AE, CY, ID, IL) *see* Immune Globulin 1056
Ganaton (IN, JP, KW, LB, PH, PK, RU, TH) *see* Itopride [INT] 1130
Ganfort (AE, AR, AT, AU, BE, BR, CH, CL, CN, CO, CY, CZ, DE, DK, EC, EE, ES, FI, FR, GB, GR, HK, HR, HU, IE, IL, IN, IS, IT, KR, KW, LB, LT, LU, MT, MY, NL, NO, NZ, PE, PH, PL, PT, RO, SA, SE, SG, SI, SK, TH, VN) *see* Bimatoprost and Timolol [INT] 264
Ganforti (MX) *see* Bimatoprost and Timolol [INT] 264
Ganguard (IN) *see* Ganciclovir (Systemic) 948
Ganin (ID) *see* Gabapentin 943
Ganirest (JP) *see* Ganirelix 949
Gantalyn (CL) *see* Gentamicin (Systemic) 959
Gantaprim (IT) *see* Sulfamethoxazole and Trimethoprim 1946
Gantin (AU) *see* Gabapentin 943
Gantrim (IT) *see* Sulfamethoxazole and Trimethoprim 1946
Ganvirel Duo (AR) *see* Lamivudine and Zidovudine 1160
Gaofen (CN) *see* Cloxacillin [CAN/INT] 488

Gapatin (TW) *see* Gabapentin ... 943
Gapraton (KR) *see* Itopride [INT] ... 1130
Gapride (KR) *see* Itopride [INT] ... 1130
Gapridol (MX) *see* Gabapentin ... 943
Garalone (PT) *see* Gentamicin (Systemic) ... 959
Garamicina (BR, CO, CR, DO, GT, HN, NI, PA, SV) *see* Gentamicin (Systemic) ... 959
Garamicina Oftalmica (CO, CR, DO, GT, HN, NI, PA, SV) *see* Gentamicin (Ophthalmic) ... 962
Garamicina Oftalmica (CO, CR, DO, GT, HN, NI, PA, SV) *see* Gentamicin (Systemic) ... 959
Garamicin (TH) *see* Gentamicin (Systemic) ... 959
Garamycin (AE, BH, CH, CY, CZ, EG, HK, HR, ID, IN, IQ, IR, JO, KW, LB, LY, NL, NO, OM, PL, QA, RU, SA, SE, SG, SY, TH, TR, TW, YE) *see* Gentamicin (Systemic) ... 959
Garamycin (BH, CH, EG, HK, ID, KW, MY, NO, PH, QA, SA, SG, TW) *see* Gentamicin (Ophthalmic) ... 962
Garapepsin (GR) *see* Trimebutine [CAN/INT] ... 2103
Garasent (MY, SG) *see* Gentamicin (Systemic) ... 959
Garasone (CZ) *see* Gentamicin (Ophthalmic) ... 962
Garasone (CZ) *see* Gentamicin (Systemic) ... 959
Garbose (MY) *see* Acarbose ... 29
Garcol (HK) *see* DimenhyDRINATE ... 637
Garcon (KR) *see* Glucagon ... 970
Gardan (BB, BM, BS, BZ, GY, JM, NL, SR, TT) *see* Mefenamic Acid ... 1280
Gardasil (AE, AR, AT, AU, BE, BG, BH, CH, CL, CO, CR, CZ, DE, DK, EC, EE, ES, FI, FR, GB, GR, GT, HK, HN, HR, ID, IE, IL, IS, IT, JP, KR, KW, LB, LT, MT, MY, NI, NL, NO, NZ, PA, PE, PH, PL, PT, QA, RO, RU, SA, SE, SG, SK, SV, TH, TR, TW, UY, VN) *see* Papillomavirus (Types 6, 11, 16, 18) Vaccine (Human, Recombinant) ... 1574
Gardenal (BE, BR, CZ, ES, FR, GR, IN, LB, LU, QA, TH, UY, VE, ZA) *see* PHENobarbital ... 1632
Gardenale (ES, IT) *see* PHENobarbital ... 1632
Gardenale[inj.] (IT) *see* PHENobarbital ... 1632
Gardenal Sodium (GB) *see* PHENobarbital ... 1632
Garexin (ID) *see* Gentamicin (Ophthalmic) ... 962
Garian (UY) *see* Balsalazide ... 226
Gartricin (ES) *see* Benzocaine ... 246
Gasafe (TW) *see* Famotidine ... 845
Gascop (MX) *see* Albendazole ... 65
Gascosin (PH) *see* Scopolamine (Systemic) ... 1870
Gasdol (CL) *see* Domperidone [CAN/INT] ... 666
Gasec (BB, BM, BS, BZ, GY, HK, JM, MY, SR, TT) *see* Omeprazole ... 1508
Gasec Gastrocaps (BF, BJ, CI, ET, GH, GM, GN, KE, LR, MA, ML, MR, MU, MW, NE, NG, SC, SD, SL, SN, TN, TZ, UG, ZM, ZW) *see* Omeprazole ... 1508
Gasidone (PH) *see* Domperidone [CAN/INT] ... 666
Gasmezol (VN) *see* Sucralfate ... 1940
Gasmodin (VN) *see* Famotidine ... 845
Gasmotin (CN, JP, PH, TH, VN) *see* Mosapride [INT] ... 1401
Gasprid (UY) *see* Mosapride [INT] ... 1401
Gasrobid (ID) *see* Isosorbide Dinitrate ... 1124
Gastec (AR) *see* Omeprazole ... 1508
Gastenz (AU) *see* Pantoprazole ... 1570
Gaster (CN, JP, KR, TW) *see* Famotidine ... 845
Gastevin (VN) *see* Lansoprazole ... 1166
Gastop (PE) *see* Omeprazole ... 1508
Gastracid (DE) *see* Omeprazole ... 1508
Gastracol (CH) *see* Aluminum Hydroxide ... 103
Gastrax (DE) *see* Nizatidine ... 1471
Gastren (PY) *see* Famotidine ... 845
Gastrial (AR) *see* Ranitidine ... 1777
Gastride (CO) *see* Mosapride [INT] ... 1401
Gastride (PH) *see* Scopolamine (Systemic) ... 1870
Gastridin (ID) *see* Ranitidine ... 1777
Gastridin (IT) *see* Famotidine ... 845
Gastril (MY) *see* Ranitidine ... 1777
Gastrium (PY) *see* Famotidine ... 845
Gastrix (PH) *see* Rebamipide [INT] ... 1786
Gastro-Bismol (TH) *see* Bismuth ... 265
Gastrobi S.R. (KR) *see* Metoclopramide ... 1345
Gastrocid (PH) *see* Calcium Carbonate ... 327
Gastrodine (CL) *see* RABEprazole ... 1762
Gastrodin (TW) *see* Cimetidine ... 438
Gastrodog[vet.] (FR) *see* Alverine [INT] ... 104
Gastrodomina (BF, BJ, CI, ET, GH, GM, GN, HU, KE, LR, MA, ML, MR, MU, MW, NE, NG, SC, SD, SL, SN, TN, TZ, UG, ZM, ZW) *see* Famotidine ... 845
Gastrofer (ID) *see* Omeprazole ... 1508
Gastroflux (GT) *see* Domperidone [CAN/INT] ... 666
Gastro H2 (ES) *see* Cimetidine ... 438
Gastro (IL) *see* Famotidine ... 845
Gastrokin (AR) *see* Mosapride [INT] ... 1401
Gastroloc (TW) *see* Pantoprazole ... 1570
Gastromax (AR) *see* Pantoprazole ... 1570
Gastrone (PH) *see* Ranitidine ... 1777
Gastronerton (DE, LU) *see* Metoclopramide ... 1345
Gastron (ZA) *see* Loperamide ... 1236
Gastropax (EC) *see* Clidinium and Chlordiazepoxide ... 460
Gastropiron (IT) *see* Pirenzepine [INT] ... 1662
Gastropyrin (FI) *see* SulfaSALAzine ... 1950
Gastrosedol (AR) *see* Ranitidine ... 1777
Gastrosil (CH, DE, LU, PH) *see* Metoclopramide ... 1345
Gastro-Stop (AU) *see* Loperamide ... 1236
Gastro-Timelets (LU) *see* Metoclopramide ... 1345
Gastrovex (MY) *see* Lansoprazole ... 1166
Gastrozepina (PT) *see* Pirenzepine [INT] ... 1662
Gastrozepin (AT, AU, CZ, DE, GR, JP, NL, RU, SI) *see* Pirenzepine [INT] ... 1662
Gastrul (ID) *see* Misoprostol ... 1379
Gastrum (CO) *see* Famotidine ... 845
Gatamine (TW) *see* Galantamine ... 946
Gatif (CL) *see* Gatifloxacin ... 949
Gatif Forte (AR) *see* Gatifloxacin ... 949
Gatiflo (JP, KR) *see* Gatifloxacin ... 949
Gatilox (PY) *see* Gatifloxacin ... 949
Gatof (KR) *see* Itopride [INT] ... 1130
Gatox (HR) *see* Lindane ... 1217
Gaty (TW) *see* Gabapentin ... 943
Gaverject (PK) *see* Alprostadil ... 96
Gavin (AR) *see* Pregabalin ... 1710
Gawei (TW) *see* Cimetidine ... 438
Gazyva (AU, NL) *see* Obinutuzumab ... 1482
Gazyvaro (HR, LT, SI, SK) *see* Obinutuzumab ... 1482
Geadol (NO) *see* TraMADol ... 2074
Geangin (NL) *see* Verapamil ... 2154
Geavir (DK, SE) *see* Acyclovir (Systemic) ... 47
Geavir (SE) *see* Aciclovir (Ophthalmic) [INT] ... 43
Gedare (GB) *see* Ethinyl Estradiol and Desogestrel ... 799
Gedum (AR) *see* Gemfibrozil ... 956
Geftilon (IN) *see* Gefitinib [CAN/INT] ... 950
Gelargin (CZ) *see* Fluocinolone (Topical) ... 893
Gelocatil (ES) *see* Acetaminophen ... 32
Geloderm (CL) *see* MetroNIDAZOLE (Topical) ... 1357
Geltim LP (FR) *see* Timolol (Ophthalmic) ... 2043
Geltim (RO) *see* Timolol (Ophthalmic) ... 2043
Geluprane 500 (FR) *see* Acetaminophen ... 32
Gelusil Plus (TW) *see* Aluminum Hydroxide, Magnesium Hydroxide, and Simethicone ... 104
Gelusil-S (ZA) *see* Aluminum Hydroxide, Magnesium Hydroxide, and Simethicone ... 104
Gembine (KR) *see* Gemcitabine ... 952
Gembio (PH) *see* Gemcitabine ... 952
Gemcibine (KR) *see* Gemcitabine ... 952
Gemcikal (ID, PH) *see* Gemcitabine ... 952
Gemcit (BR, PE, PH) *see* Gemcitabine ... 952
Gemcite (IN) *see* Gemcitabine ... 952
Gemd (SG, TW) *see* Gemfibrozil ... 956
Gemezar (JO) *see* Gemcitabine ... 952
Gemfibril (TH) *see* Gemfibrozil ... 956

Gemfi (DE) *see* Gemfibrozil 956
Gemflor (TW) *see* Gemcitabine 952
Gemicort (KR) *see* Triamcinolone (Systemic) 2099
Gemicort (KR) *see* Triamcinolone (Topical) 2100
Gemita (PH, TH, TW) *see* Gemcitabine 952
Gemitin (CL) *see* Chloramphenicol 421
Gemitin Oftalmico (CL) *see* Chloramphenicol 421
Gemivil (JO) *see* Imatinib 1047
Gemmis (TW) *see* Gemcitabine 952
Gemnpid (TW) *see* Gemfibrozil 956
Gemone (IN) *see* Gemifloxacin 957
Gemot (TR) *see* Irbesartan 1110
Gem-S (TW) *see* Gemfibrozil 956
Gemtan (KR) *see* Gemcitabine 952
Gemtavis (ID) *see* Gemcitabine 952
Gemtra (KR) *see* Gemcitabine 952
Gemtro (AR) *see* Gemcitabine 952
Gemxit (MX) *see* Gemcitabine 952
Gemycin (JO) *see* Gentamicin (Systemic) 959
Gemzar (AE, AT, AU, BE, BF, BG, BH, BJ, BO, BR, CH, CI, CL, CN, CO, CY, CZ, DE, DK, DO, EE, EG, ES, ET, FI, FR, GB, GH, GM, GN, GR, HK, HR, HU, ID, IE, IL, IS, IT, KE, KR, LB, LR, LT, LU, MA, ML, MR, MT, MU, MW, MX, MY, NE, NG, NL, NO, NZ, PA, PE, PH, PK, PL, PR, PT, PY, QA, RO, RU, SA, SC, SD, SE, SG, SI, SK, SL, SN, TH, TN, TR, TW, TZ, UG, UY, VE, VN, ZA, ZM, ZW) *see* Gemcitabine 952
Gemzil (TH) *see* Captopril 342
Genacin (PK) *see* Gentamicin (Systemic) 959
Genadine (TW) *see* Loratadine 1241
Genaflox (VN) *see* Flucloxacillin [INT] 885
Genaxol (TW) *see* PACLitaxel (Conventional) 1550
Genbexil (EC) *see* Gentamicin (Systemic) 959
Gencari (TW) *see* Carisoprodol 363
Gencet (AE) *see* Cetirizine 411
Genclav (PH) *see* Amoxicillin and Clavulanate 133
Genclone (TW) *see* Zopiclone [CAN/INT] 2217
Gencolax (TH) *see* Bisacodyl 265
Gendarin (SE) *see* Alendronate 79
Gendobu (TW) *see* DOBUTamine 654
Generlog (TH) *see* Triamcinolone (Systemic) 2099
Generlog (TH) *see* Triamcinolone (Topical) 2100
Genetaxyl (TH) *see* PACLitaxel (Conventional) 1550
Genfuxen (TW) *see* Sulconazole 1943
Gengigel (MY) *see* Hyaluronate and Derivatives 1006
Gengivarium (IT) *see* Benzocaine 246
Gengraf (AE, HK, MY, QA, SA, VN) *see* CycloSPORINE (Systemic) 522
Gengxian (CN) *see* Lovastatin 1252
Genheal (PH, TH) *see* Somatropin 1918
Genin (TH) *see* QuiNINE 1761
Geniol Flex (AR) *see* Magnesium Salicylate 1265
Geniquin (TW) *see* Hydroxychloroquine 1021
Genlac (AU) *see* Lactulose 1156
Genmisil (VN) *see* Gentamicin (Systemic) 959
Genmycin (IN) *see* Gentamicin (Ophthalmic) 962
Genobiotic-Doxi (MX) *see* Doxycycline 689
Genocin (TH) *see* Chloroquine 424
Genoclam (ID) *see* ClomiPHENE 473
Genocolan (AR) *see* Lactulose 1156
Genoestatina (MX) *see* Pravastatin 1700
Genogris (ES) *see* Piracetam [INT] 1661
Genoldene (MX) *see* Piroxicam 1662
Genopril (TW) *see* Lisinopril 1226
Genoptic (AE, AU, BH, CY, EG, IQ, IR, JO, KW, LB, LY, NZ, OM, QA, SA, SG, SY, YE) *see* Gentamicin (Systemic) 959
Genoptic (AU, NZ, SG) *see* Gentamicin (Ophthalmic) 962
Genoral (AU) *see* Estropipate 793
Genorin (VN) *see* FlavoxATE 881
Genotonorm (BE, FR) *see* Somatropin 1918
Genotonorm Miniquick (FR) *see* Somatropin 1918
Genotropin (AE, AR, AT, AU, BG, BH, BR, CH, CL, CN, CO, CR, CY, CZ, DE, DK, DO, EE, EG, FI, GB, GR, GT, HN, HR, HU, ID, IL, IN, IQ, IR, IS, IT, JO, KR, KW, LB, LT, LY, MX, NI, NL, NO, NZ, OM, PA, PE, PK, PL, PT, QA, RO, RU, SA, SE, SI, SK, SV, SY, TH, TR, UY, VE, YE) *see* Somatropin 1918
Genoxal (BR) *see* Cyclophosphamide 517
Genox (AU, NZ) *see* Tamoxifen 1971
Genozyl (MX) *see* Allopurinol 90
Genozym (PY) *see* ClomiPHENE 473
Gensia (ID) *see* AmLODIPine 123
Genso (TW) *see* Atracurium 198
Gensulin M30 (TH) *see* Insulin NPH and Insulin Regular 1090
Gensulin N (TH) *see* Insulin NPH 1089
Gensumycin (FI, NO, SE) *see* Gentamicin (Systemic) 959
Genta-590 (PE) *see* Gentamicin (Ophthalmic) 962
Genta-590 (PE) *see* Gentamicin (Systemic) 959
Gentabiotic (PE) *see* Gentamicin (Systemic) 959
Gentabrand (EC) *see* Gentamicin (Ophthalmic) 962
Gentabrand (EC) *see* Gentamicin (Systemic) 959
Gentacare (PH) *see* Gentamicin (Systemic) 959
Gentac (TW) *see* Gentamicin (Systemic) 959
Gentadar (AE, BH, JO, QA) *see* Gentamicin (Ophthalmic) 962
Gentaderm (AR) *see* Gentamicin (Systemic) 959
Gentagram (BR, PE) *see* Gentamicin (Ophthalmic) 962
Gentagram (BR, PE) *see* Gentamicin (Systemic) 959
Gentalline (FR) *see* Gentamicin (Ophthalmic) 962
Gentalline (FR) *see* Gentamicin (Systemic) 959
Gental (PY, TH) *see* Gentamicin (Ophthalmic) 962
Gental (PY, TH) *see* Gentamicin (Systemic) 959
Gentalyn (CL, VE) *see* Gentamicin (Ophthalmic) 962
Gentalyn (IT, PE, VE) *see* Gentamicin (Systemic) 959
Gentalyn Oftalmico-Otico (PE) *see* Gentamicin (Systemic) 959
Gentamax (EC) *see* Gentamicin (Systemic) 959
Gentamed (CY, JO) *see* Gentamicin (Systemic) 959
Gentamen (AE, BH, CY, EG, IQ, IR, JO, KW, LB, LY, OM, QA, SA, SY, YE) *see* Gentamicin (Systemic) 959
Gentamina (AR, PY) *see* Gentamicin (Systemic) 959
Gentam (SA) *see* Gentamicin (Systemic) 959
Gentamytrex (NL) *see* Gentamicin (Ophthalmic) 962
Gentamytrex (NL) *see* Gentamicin (Systemic) 959
Gentanal (ID) *see* Gentamicin (Ophthalmic) 962
Genta-Oph (TH) *see* Gentamicin (Ophthalmic) 962
Genta-Oph (TH) *see* Gentamicin (Systemic) 959
Gentapro (SG) *see* Gentamicin (Ophthalmic) 962
Gentapro (SG) *see* Gentamicin (Systemic) 959
Gentarad (AE, BH, CY, EG, IQ, IR, JO, KW, LB, LY, OM, QA, SA, SY, YE) *see* Gentamicin (Systemic) 959
Gentasil (PE) *see* Gentamicin (Systemic) 959
Gentasporin (IN) *see* Gentamicin (Systemic) 959
Gentatrim (IL) *see* Gentamicin (Systemic) 959
Gentawin (TH) *see* Gentamicin (Systemic) 959
Genticin (AE, BF, BH, BJ, CI, CY, EG, ET, GB, GH, GM, GN, IE, IQ, IR, JO, KE, KW, LB, LR, LY, MA, ML, MR, MU, MW, NE, NG, OM, QA, SA, SC, SD, SL, SN, SY, TN, TR, TZ, UG, YE, ZM, ZW) *see* Gentamicin (Systemic) 959
Genticin (CY, DK, GB, TR) *see* Gentamicin (Ophthalmic) 962
Genticyn (IN) *see* Gentamicin (Ophthalmic) 962
Genticyn (IN) *see* Gentamicin (Systemic) 959
Gentiderm (ID) *see* Gentamicin (Systemic) 959
Gentleclean (TW) *see* Hydroquinone 1020
Gentocil (PT) *see* Gentamicin (Ophthalmic) 962
Gentocil (PT) *see* Gentamicin (Systemic) 959
Gentolol (TW) *see* Acebutolol 29
Gent-Ophtal (DE) *see* Gentamicin (Ophthalmic) 962
Gent-Ophtal (DE) *see* Gentamicin (Systemic) 959
Gentran 40 (LU, NL) *see* Dextran 607

Gentran 70 (LU, NL) *see* Dextran 607
Gentus (IT) *see* Dimemorfan [INT] 637
Genurin (IT, SG, TW) *see* FlavoxATE 881
Genurin S (BR) *see* FlavoxATE 881
Genzamycin (LB) *see* Erythromycin and Benzoyl Peroxide 765
Genzosin (TW) *see* Doxazosin 674
Geocoxib (PH) *see* Celecoxib 402
Geodon (BR, BZ, CO, CR, DO, ES, GR, GT, HN, IE, IL, MX, NI, PA, SV, TR, TW, VE, ZA) *see* Ziprasidone 2201
Geozif (VN) *see* Azithromycin (Systemic) 216
Geozit (PH) *see* Azithromycin (Systemic) 216
Gepeprostin (BR) *see* Bicalutamide 262
Gepromi (MX) *see* Progesterone 1722
Gerafen (PH) *see* Chloramphenicol 421
Geramet (IE) *see* Cimetidine 438
Geram (FR) *see* Piracetam [INT] 1661
Geratam (BE, CZ, LU, SE) *see* Piracetam [INT] 1661
Gericarb SR (IE) *see* CarBAMazepine 346
Gericin (ES) *see* Nitrendipine [INT] 1463
Geriflox (IE) *see* Flucloxacillin [INT] 885
Geroam (KR) *see* Gemcitabine 952
Geroxalen (NL) *see* Methoxsalen (Topical) 1331
Gerucim (HR) *see* Cimetidine 438
Gervaken (MX) *see* Clarithromycin 456
Geser (CL) *see* Cinacalcet 439
Gesicain Jelly (IN) *see* Lidocaine (Topical) 1211
Gesicain Ointment (IN) *see* Lidocaine (Topical) 1211
Gesicain Viscous (IN) *see* Lidocaine (Topical) 1211
Gesica (TH) *see* Ibuprofen 1032
Geslutin (CO, DO, GT, HN, MX, NI) *see* Progesterone 1722
Geslutin PNM (EC, PE) *see* Progesterone 1722
GestaPolar (DE) *see* MedroxyPROGESTERone 1277
Gestapuran (FI, SE) *see* MedroxyPROGESTERone 1277
Ge Tai (CN) *see* Lomefloxacin [INT] 1233
Getanosan (ID) *see* Gemcitabine 952
Getcet (PH) *see* Levocetirizine 1196
Getidin (PH) *see* Cimetidine 438
Getran (TW) *see* Terbutaline 2004
Getryl (PH) *see* Glimepiride 966
Getzpraz (VN) *see* ALPRAZolam 94
Gevatran (FR) *see* Naftidrofuryl [INT] 1416
Gevilon (AT, BG, CH, CZ, DE, HR, HU, IS, PL) *see* Gemfibrozil 956
Gewacalm (AT) *see* Diazepam 613
Gexcil (PH) *see* Amoxicillin 130
Gezt (PY) *see* Gemcitabine 952
G.F.B.-600 (TH) *see* Gemfibrozil 956
Giabri (CL, CO) *see* Ciprofibrate [INT] 441
Giardil (AR) *see* Furazolidone [INT] 940
Giarlam (BR) *see* Furazolidone [INT] 940
Giasion (IT) *see* Cefditoren 378
Gibixen (IT) *see* Naproxen 1427
Gichtex (AT) *see* Allopurinol 90
GI Kit (IN) *see* Omeprazole, Clarithromycin, and Amoxicillin 1511
Gilemal (AT, HU) *see* GlyBURIDE 972
Gilenya (AR, AU, BE, BR, CH, CL, CO, CY, CZ, DE, DK, EE, FR, GB, GR, HK, HR, IE, IL, IS, JP, KR, LB, LT, MX, MY, NL, NO, NZ, PE, QA, RO, SA, SE, SG, SI, SK, TH, TR) *see* Fingolimod 879
Gilex (IL) *see* Doxepin (Systemic) 676
Gilucor (HR, HU) *see* Sotalol 1927
Giludop (DK, SE) *see* DOPamine 669
Gimaclav (MX) *see* Amoxicillin and Clavulanate 133
Gima (ID) *see* Procainamide 1716
Gimalxina (MX) *see* Amoxicillin 130
Ginarsan Forte (PE) *see* Tamoxifen 1971
Ginarsan (PE) *see* Tamoxifen 1971
Gine-Dermofix (LB) *see* Sertaconazole 1877
Ginet-63 (NZ) *see* Cyproterone and Ethinyl Estradiol [CAN/INT] 532
Ginet-84 (NZ) *see* Cyproterone and Ethinyl Estradiol [CAN/INT] 532
Ginet (PE) *see* Clotrimazole (Topical) 488
Ginoderm Gel (PY) *see* Estradiol (Systemic) 775
Ginomi (KR) *see* Hydroquinone 1020
GI Norm (PH) *see* Domperidone [CAN/INT] 666
Gino-Travogen (PT) *see* Isoconazole [INT] 1120
Giona Easyhaler (MY, SG, TH) *see* Budesonide (Systemic) 293
Giotrif (AU, BE, CH, CZ, DE, DK, EE, FR, GB, HR, JP, KR, LT, MY, NL, NO, RO, SE, SG, SI, SK) *see* Afatinib 61
Giprim (TW) *see* Trimethoprim 2104
Gipzide (TH) *see* GlipiZIDE 967
Gitazone (TH) *see* Pioglitazone 1654
Gitrabin (HK, HR, PH, RO, SG) *see* Gemcitabine 952
Gityl (DE) *see* Bromazepam [CAN/INT] 290
Givincef (ID) *see* Cefpirome [INT] 388
Givotan (PY) *see* Nitazoxanide 1461
Glactiv (JP) *see* SitaGLIPtin 1897
Gladem (AT, DE) *see* Sertraline 1878
Glafemak (GR) *see* Timolol (Ophthalmic) 2043
Glafornil (CL) *see* MetFORMIN 1307
Glamide (TH) *see* GlyBURIDE 972
Glamigan (BR) *see* Bimatoprost 264
Glanducorpin (HU) *see* Progesterone 1722
Glanique (EC, MX) *see* Levonorgestrel 1201
Glanyl (KR) *see* Cinnarizine [INT] 440
Glaritus (VN) *see* Insulin Glargine 1086
Glash Vista (JP) *see* Bimatoprost 264
Glaucomed (CO) *see* AcetaZOLAMIDE 39
Glauconex (AT, BE, DE, LU, NL) *see* Befunolol [INT] 233
Glauco Oph (HK, TH) *see* Timolol (Ophthalmic) 2043
Glaucosan (ZA) *see* Timolol (Ophthalmic) 2043
Glauco (TH) *see* Timolol (Ophthalmic) 2043
Glaucothil (AT) *see* Dipivefrin 651
Glaudin (DK, SE) *see* Brimonidine (Ophthalmic) 288
Glaudrops (ES) *see* Dipivefrin 651
Glauline (GB) *see* Metipranolol 1345
Glaumetax (AR) *see* Methazolamide 1317
Glaumox (AU, NZ) *see* AcetaZOLAMIDE 39
Glaupax (CH, DE, HR, JP, TH) *see* AcetaZOLAMIDE 39
Glauseta (ID) *see* AcetaZOLAMIDE 39
Glautan (IL) *see* Latanoprost 1172
Glautimol (BR) *see* Timolol (Ophthalmic) 2043
Glavis (KR) *see* MetFORMIN 1307
Glazer (TH) *see* Glimepiride 966
Glazidim (BE, FI, IT, LU) *see* CefTAZidime 392
Glemaz (EC) *see* Glimepiride 966
Glemont-CT (PH) *see* Montelukast 1392
Glemont-IR (PH) *see* Montelukast 1392
Glemont (MY) *see* Montelukast 1392
Glencet (MY, PH) *see* Levocetirizine 1196
Glentaz (VN) *see* Tazarotene 1980
Glevate (MY, PH) *see* Clobetasol 468
Glevo IV (PH) *see* Levofloxacin (Systemic) 1197
Glexil (VN) *see* Cephalexin 405
Glezone (KR) *see* Pioglitazone 1654
Gliabetes (ID) *see* Pioglitazone 1654
Gliadel (GR, IL, IT, JP, MY, NL, SG, TH, TW) *see* Carmustine 364
Gliadel Implant (AU, ES) *see* Carmustine 364
Glianimon (DE, GR) *see* Benperidol [INT] 244
Gliban (AE, BH, CY, EG, IQ, IR, JO, KW, LB, LY, OM, QA, SA, SY, YE) *see* GlyBURIDE 972
Glibedal (HR) *see* GlyBURIDE 972
Glibenclamid (HR) *see* GlyBURIDE 972
Glibenclamid Pharmavit (HU) *see* GlyBURIDE 972
Glibenclamid-ratiopharm (LU) *see* GlyBURIDE 972
Gliben-CP (HK) *see* GlyBURIDE 972
Glibenese (AE, AT, BE, BF, BH, BJ, CH, CI, CY, DE, DK, EG, ET, FI, FR, GH, GM, GN, GR, IL, IQ, IR, JO, KE,

KW, LB, LR, LU, LY, MA, ML, MR, MU, MW, NE, NG, NL, OM, PL, QA, RU, SA, SC, SD, SE, SL, SN, SY, TN, TZ, UG, YE, ZA, ZM, ZW) *see* GlipiZIDE 967
Glibenese GITS (PL) *see* GlipiZIDE 967
Glibenhexal (LU) *see* GlyBURIDE 972
Gliben (IT) *see* GlyBURIDE 972
Glibesyn (MY, SG, TH) *see* GlyBURIDE 972
Glibetic (IL) *see* GlyBURIDE 972
Glibet (IN) *see* GlyBURIDE 972
Glibetin (TW) *see* GlipiZIDE 967
Glibil-5 (SA) *see* GlyBURIDE 972
Glibil (AE, BH, CY, EG, IQ, IR, JO, KW, LB, LY, OM, QA, SA, SY, YE) *see* GlyBURIDE 972
Glibomet (AE, BG, CR, DO, GT, HN, IT, LB, NI, PA, SV) *see* Glyburide and Metformin 974
Gliboral (BF, BJ, CI, ET, GH, GM, GN, KE, LB, LR, MA, ML, MR, MU, MW, NE, NG, SC, SD, SL, SN, TN, TZ, UG, ZM, ZW) *see* GlyBURIDE 972
Glibos (TW) *see* Acarbose 29
Glibudon (TW) *see* MetFORMIN 1307
Glicada SR (HK) *see* Gliclazide [CAN/INT] 964
Glicalin (TW) *see* Gliclazide [CAN/INT] 964
Glican (SV) *see* GlipiZIDE 967
Glicenex (EC) *see* MetFORMIN 1307
Glicobase (IT) *see* Acarbose 29
Glicophage (RO) *see* MetFORMIN 1307
Glicorp (BR) *see* ChlorproPAMIDE 429
Glicron (TW) *see* Gliclazide [CAN/INT] 964
Glidiabet (PE) *see* GlyBURIDE 972
Glidiab (TW) *see* GlipiZIDE 967
Glidipion (RO) *see* Pioglitazone 1654
Glifage (BR) *see* MetFORMIN 1307
Gliformin (CO) *see* MetFORMIN 1307
Glihexal (VN) *see* GlyBURIDE 972
Glikamel (ID) *see* Gliclazide [CAN/INT] 964
Glimaccord (NZ) *see* Glimepiride 966
Glimaryl (HK, MY, TW) *see* Glimepiride 966
Glimatib (VN) *see* Imatinib 1047
Glimbax (GR) *see* Prulifloxacin [INT] 1742
Glimel (AU, HK) *see* GlyBURIDE 972
Glimepid (KR) *see* Glimepiride 966
Glimep (KR) *see* Glimepiride 966
Glimeryl (HK, JO) *see* Glimepiride 966
Glimicron (HK, JP, MY) *see* Gliclazide [CAN/INT] 964
Glimide (PE) *see* Glimepiride 966
Glimulin (VN) *see* Glimepiride 966
Glimxl (HK) *see* Glimepiride 966
Glinade (KR) *see* Nateglinide 1432
Glinate (IN) *see* Nateglinide 1432
Glinib (KR) *see* Imatinib 1047
Glin (TW) *see* Terbutaline 2004
Glinux 70/30 (MX) *see* Insulin NPH and Insulin Regular 1090
Glinux-R (MX) *see* Insulin Regular 1091
Gliolan (BE, CZ, DE, DK, EE, ES, FR, GR, HR, KR, NL, NO, PL, PT, RO, SE) *see* Aminolevulinic Acid 114
Glioten (BR, EC, PE, PY, SG) *see* Enalapril 722
Gliotenzide (EC, SG) *see* Enalapril and Hydrochlorothiazide 725
Gliozac (MX) *see* Pioglitazone 1654
Gliparil (TH) *see* Glimepiride 966
Glipid (NZ) *see* GlipiZIDE 967
Glipimed (TH) *see* GlipiZIDE 967
Glipizide BP (PL) *see* GlipiZIDE 967
Glipizide (PL) *see* GlipiZIDE 967
Glipom (AE, BH, SA) *see* GlipiZIDE 967
Glipressina (IT) *see* Terlipressin [INT] 2010
Glisulin (KR) *see* GlyBURIDE 972
Glisulin XR (CR, DO, GT, HN, NI, PA, SV) *see* MetFORMIN 1307
Glita (IN) *see* Pioglitazone 1654
Glitaz (PH) *see* Pioglitazone 1654
Glitisol (TR) *see* GlyBURIDE 972
Glitis (TW) *see* Pioglitazone 1654
Glitol (KR) *see* Miglitol 1367
Glito (VN) *see* Pioglitazone 1654
Glitter (PH) *see* Pioglitazone 1654
Glivec (AE, AR, AT, AU, BE, BG, BH, BR, CH, CL, CN, CO, CY, CZ, DE, DK, EC, EE, ES, FI, FR, GB, GR, HK, HN, HR, HU, ID, IE, IL, IS, IT, JO, JP, KR, KW, LB, LT, MT, MX, MY, NL, NO, PE, PH, PK, PL, PT, PY, QA, RO, RU, SA, SE, SG, SI, SK, TH, TR, TW, UY, VE, VN) *see* Imatinib 1047
Glivic (NZ) *see* Imatinib 1047
Glix (MY) *see* GlipiZIDE 967
Glizide (SG) *see* Gliclazide [CAN/INT] 964
Glizide (TH) *see* GlipiZIDE 967
Glizolan (ES) *see* Diacerein [INT] 613
Glizone (KR) *see* Pioglitazone 1654
Globazine (PH) *see* ChlorproMAZINE 429
Globenicol (NL) *see* Chloramphenicol 421
Globentyl (DK) *see* Aspirin 180
Globuman Berna (PH) *see* Immune Globulin 1056
Glocar (ID) *see* Aspirin 180
Glocef (ID) *see* Cefotaxime 382
Glocyp (ID) *see* Cyproheptadine 529
Glojaya (ID) *see* Ciprofloxacin (Systemic) 441
Glomin (ID) *see* DOPamine 669
Glomox (LB, SA) *see* Amoxicillin 130
Glopir (GR) *see* NIFEdipine 1451
Glopixin (VN) *see* Cephalexin 405
Gloryfen (LB) *see* Cefotaxime 382
Glosix (ID) *see* Furosemide 940
Glotrizine (AE, QA) *see* Cetirizine 411
Glotron (ID) *see* Ondansetron 1513
Glottyl (LU) *see* Codeine 497
Glu-A (KR) *see* MetFORMIN 1307
Glubacida (MX) *see* Bacitracin and Polymyxin B 222
Glubacida (MX) *see* Neomycin 1436
Glubacida (MX) *see* Polymyxin B 1676
Gluben (IL) *see* GlyBURIDE 972
Glubitor-OD (PH) *see* Gliclazide [CAN/INT] 964
Glubosil (TH) *see* Pioglitazone 1654
Glucagen (AE, AR, AU, BE, BH, BR, CH, CL, CO, CY, DE, DK, EC, FR, GR, HK, IE, IN, IT, JO, MY, NZ, PL, PY, SA, TH, UY, ZA) *see* Glucagon 970
GlucaGen (AT, FI, GB, HR, HU, IE, IL, IS, LT, LU, NL, PT, QA, SG, SI, SK, TR, VN) *see* Glucagon 970
Glucagen G (JP) *see* Glucagon 970
Glucagen Novo (HK) *see* Glucagon 970
Glucagon Novo Nordisk (SE) *see* Glucagon 970
Glucal (ZA) *see* Calcium Gluconate 330
Glucantime (BR, ES, FR) *see* Meglumine Antimoniate [INT] 1283
Glucantim (IT) *see* Meglumine Antimoniate [INT] 1283
Glucar (MY) *see* Acarbose 29
Glucemin (CO) *see* Pioglitazone 1654
Gluciophage XR (VN) *see* MetFORMIN 1307
Gluclean (KR) *see* Glyburide and Metformin 974
Glucobay (AE, AR, AT, AU, BB, BD, BE, BF, BG, BH, BJ, BM, BR, BS, BZ, CH, CI, CL, CN, CO, CR, CY, CZ, DE, DK, DO, EC, EG, ES, ET, FI, GB, GH, GM, GN, GT, GY, HK, HN, HR, HU, ID, IE, IN, IQ, IR, IS, IT, JM, JO, JP, KE, KR, KW, LB, LR, LU, LY, MA, ML, MR, MU, MW, MX, MY, NE, NG, NI, NL, NO, NZ, OM, PA, PE, PH, PK, PL, PR, PT, PY, QA, RO, RU, SA, SC, SD, SE, SG, SL, SN, SR, SV, SY, TH, TN, TR, TT, TW, TZ, UG, UY, VE, VN, YE, ZA, ZM, ZW) *see* Acarbose 29
Glucobene (HU) *see* GlyBURIDE 972
Glucodiab (TH) *see* GlipiZIDE 967
Glucodown (KR) *see* MetFORMIN 1307
Glucofage (EC, VE) *see* MetFORMIN 1307
Glucofer (JO) *see* Ferrous Gluconate 870
Glucoferro (IT) *see* Ferrous Gluconate 870
Glucofine (VN) *see* MetFORMIN 1307
Glucofor (ID) *see* MetFORMIN 1307

Glucoform (PH) *see* MetFORMIN ... 1307
Glucoles (TH) *see* MetFORMIN ... 1307
Glucolip (IN, PH) *see* GlipiZIDE ... 967
Glucomet (AU, SG) *see* MetFORMIN ... 1307
Glucomid (BF, BJ, CI, ET, GH, GM, GN, KE, LR, MA, ML, MR, MU, MW, NE, NG, SC, SD, SL, SN, TN, TZ, UG, ZM, ZW) *see* GlyBURIDE ... 972
Glucomine (TW) *see* MetFORMIN ... 1307
Glucomin (IL) *see* MetFORMIN ... 1307
Glucomol (IN) *see* Timolol (Ophthalmic) ... 2043
Gluconate de Calcium Lavoisier (FR) *see* Calcium Gluconate ... 330
Gluconato Calc Fresenius (ES) *see* Calcium Gluconate ... 330
Gluconato Calcico (ES) *see* Calcium Gluconate ... 330
Gluconic (ID) *see* GlyBURIDE ... 972
Gluconil (PH) *see* GlipiZIDE ... 967
Glucon (MY) *see* MetFORMIN ... 1307
Gluconon (KR) *see* Pioglitazone ... 1654
Glucophage (AE, AR, AT, AU, BB, BE, BF, BH, BJ, BM, BS, BZ, CH, CI, CN, CY, CZ, DK, EE, EG, ET, FI, FR, GB, GH, GM, GN, GR, GY, HK, HR, ID, IE, IL, IN, IQ, IR, IS, IT, JM, JO, KE, KW, LB, LR, LU, LY, MA, ML, MR, MU, MW, MX, MY, NE, NG, NO, OM, PE, PH, PK, PT, QA, RU, SA, SC, SD, SE, SI, SK, SL, SN, SR, SY, TN, TR, TT, TW, TZ, UG, VN, YE, ZA, ZM, ZW) *see* MetFORMIN ... 1307
Glucophage Forte (CZ, NL, PH) *see* MetFORMIN ... 1307
Glucophage-Mite (DE) *see* MetFORMIN ... 1307
Glucophage Retard (EG, IL, QA) *see* MetFORMIN ... 1307
Glucophage SR (GB, IE) *see* MetFORMIN ... 1307
Glucophage XR (AE, HK, KW, LB, MY) *see* MetFORMIN ... 1307
Glucored (ID) *see* Gliclazide [CAN/INT] ... 964
Glucor (FR) *see* Acarbose ... 29
Glucorid (MY) *see* Acarbose ... 29
Gluco-Rite (IL) *see* GlipiZIDE ... 967
Gluco (TH) *see* MetFORMIN ... 1307
Glucotika (ID) *see* MetFORMIN ... 1307
Glucotin (PH) *see* MetFORMIN ... 1307
Glucotrol XL (BB, BM, BS, BZ, CN, GY, HK, ID, JM, RO, SR, TT) *see* GlipiZIDE ... 967
Glucovance (AE, AU, BB, BE, BG, BH, BR, BS, CH, CL, CO, CY, CZ, EC, FR, HK, ID, JM, KR, KW, LB, MY, NL, PE, PH, PK, PT, QA, RO, RU, SA, SG, SI, SK, TH, TT, TW, VN) *see* Glyburide and Metformin ... 974
Glucoven (MX) *see* GlyBURIDE ... 972
Glucozen (PH) *see* Glimepiride ... 966
Glucozide (TW) *see* GlipiZIDE ... 967
Gluctam (EE, HU) *see* Gliclazide [CAN/INT] ... 964
Gludepatic (ID) *see* MetFORMIN ... 1307
Gludine (KR) *see* Glimepiride ... 966
Glufor (ID, IL) *see* MetFORMIN ... 1307
Glukamin (EC) *see* Amikacin ... 111
Glumet DC (MY) *see* MetFORMIN ... 1307
Glumet Forte (HK) *see* MetFORMIN ... 1307
Glumet (MY, PH) *see* MetFORMIN ... 1307
Glumet XR (PH) *see* MetFORMIN ... 1307
Glumida (ES) *see* Acarbose ... 29
Glumin (ID) *see* MetFORMIN ... 1307
Glumin XR (ID) *see* MetFORMIN ... 1307
Glunat (TW) *see* Nateglinide ... 1432
Glunor (PE) *see* MetFORMIN ... 1307
Glupa (KR) *see* MetFORMIN ... 1307
Glupizide (TW) *see* GlipiZIDE ... 967
Glurenor (DE, IT) *see* Gliquidone [INT] ... 970
Glurenorm (AT, BE, CZ, DE, HR, HU) *see* Gliquidone [INT] ... 970
Glustin (AE, AT, BE, BF, BG, BH, BJ, CH, CI, CY, CZ, DE, DK, EE, EG, ES, ET, FI, FR, GB, GH, GM, GN, GR, HN, IE, IL, IQ, IR, IT, KE, KW, LB, LR, LT, LY, MA, ML, MR, MT, MU, MW, NE, NG, NL, NO, OM, PT, QA, RU, SA, SC, SD, SE, SK, SL, SN, SY, TN, TZ, UG, YE, ZA, ZM, ZW) *see* Pioglitazone ... 1654
Glustress (TH) *see* MetFORMIN ... 1307
Glutarase (IT) *see* Pyridoxine ... 1747
Gluvas (ID) *see* Glimepiride ... 966
Gluzo (TH) *see* GlyBURIDE ... 972
Glyade (AU, HK, TW) *see* Gliclazide [CAN/INT] ... 964
Glybotic (ID) *see* Amikacin ... 111
Glycare (HK) *see* Glimepiride ... 966
Glyciphage (IN) *see* MetFORMIN ... 1307
Glycobase (JP) *see* Fluocinonide ... 894
Glycomet (SG) *see* MetFORMIN ... 1307
Glycomin (KR) *see* MetFORMIN ... 1307
Glycomin (ZA) *see* GlyBURIDE ... 972
Glycon MR (TH) *see* Gliclazide [CAN/INT] ... 964
Glycon (TH) *see* Gliclazide [CAN/INT] ... 964
Glycophos (CH, CN, DK, ES, FI, GB, GR, HK, LT, NL, NZ, PL, PT, RO, SE, SI, TH) *see* Sodium Glycerophosphate Pentahydrate ... 1906
Glycophose (TR) *see* Sodium Glycerophosphate Pentahydrate ... 1906
Glyco-P (IN) *see* Glycopyrrolate ... 975
Glycopyrodyn (TW) *see* Glycopyrrolate ... 975
Glycopyrrola (KR) *see* Glycopyrrolate ... 975
Glycovate (PH) *see* Acarbose ... 29
Glycylpressin (AT, DE) *see* Terlipressin [INT] ... 2010
Glyformin (TW) *see* MetFORMIN ... 1307
Glygen (TH) *see* GlipiZIDE ... 967
Glymet (AE, BH, CY, EG, IQ, IR, JO, KW, LB, LY, OM, QA, SA, SY, YE) *see* MetFORMIN ... 1307
Glymet (MY) *see* Glyburide and Metformin ... 974
Glynase (AE, QA) *see* GlyBURIDE ... 972
Glynase (IN, SG, VN) *see* GlipiZIDE ... 967
Glypressin (AR, AU, BE, CH, CN, CY, CZ, DK, EC, EE, EG, ES, FI, GB, GR, HK, HR, HU, IE, IL, IS, JO, KR, LT, LU, MY, NL, NO, NZ, PE, PH, PL, QA, RO, SA, SE, SG, SI, SK, TH, TR, TW, UY, VN) *see* Terlipressin [INT] ... 2010
Glypressine (FR, PT) *see* Terlipressin [INT] ... 2010
Glypride (AE) *see* Glimepiride ... 966
Glytan (PK) *see* Nateglinide ... 1432
Glyteol (BR) *see* GuaiFENesin ... 986
Glytop (AR) *see* Triamcinolone (Topical) ... 2100
Glytrin Spray (NZ, SG) *see* Nitroglycerin ... 1465
Glyverase (MX) *see* Terlipressin [INT] ... 2010
Glyzide (AE, BH, LB) *see* Gliclazide [CAN/INT] ... 964
Glyzip (IN) *see* GlipiZIDE ... 967
Gobbidona (AR) *see* Methadone ... 1311
Gobbifol (AR, PY) *see* Propofol ... 1728
Godabion B6 (ES) *see* Pyridoxine ... 1747
Godamed (IL) *see* Aspirin ... 180
Gofen (PH) *see* Ibuprofen ... 1032
Goflex (AE, BH, CY, EG, ID, IL, IQ, IR, JO, KW, LB, LY, OM, QA, SA, SY, YE) *see* Nabumetone ... 1411
Goldar (IN) *see* Auranofin ... 204
Gomcef (KR) *see* Cefuroxime ... 399
Gomcephin (KR) *see* CefTRIAXone ... 396
Gompron (VN) *see* Fenoprofen ... 857
Gomsetron (VN) *see* Granisetron ... 983
Gomsid (KR) *see* Mefruside [INT] ... 1281
Gonablok (IN) *see* Danazol ... 558
Gonacor (PE, PY) *see* Chorionic Gonadotropin (Human) ... 431
Gonalef (JP, VE) *see* Follitropin Alfa ... 921
Gonal-F (AE, AR, AT, AU, BE, BG, BH, BR, CH, CL, CN, CO, CR, CY, CZ, DE, DK, DO, EC, EE, EG, ES, FI, FR, GB, GR, GT, HK, HN, HR, HU, ID, IE, IL, IN, IS, IT, KR, KW, LB, LT, MT, MY, NI, NL, NO, NZ, PA, PE, PH, PK, PL, PT, QA, RO, RU, SA, SE, SG, SI, SK, SV, TR, TW, VN) *see* Follitropin Alfa ... 921
Gonapeptyl (AE, FR, GB, IE, JO, LB, PY, RO, VN) *see* Triptorelin ... 2107
Gonapeptyl CR (BH, QA) *see* Triptorelin ... 2107

Gonapeptyl,CR (LB) *see* Triptorelin 2107
GonapeptylCR (SA) *see* Triptorelin 2107
Gonapeptyl Daily (BR) *see* Triptorelin 2107
Gonax (JP) *see* Degarelix 587
Gondonar (PY) *see* Anastrozole 148
Gonnaz (PH) *see* Gabapentin 943
Gonocilin (BR) *see* Probenecid 1716
Gonorcin (TH) *see* Norfloxacin 1475
Go-On (PH) *see* Hyaluronate and Derivatives 1006
Gopten (AU, BE, BG, BR, CH, CO, CZ, EE, ES, HK, HN, HR, HU, ID, IE, IT, LB, LT, LU, MT, MX, NL, NO, NZ, PK, PL, PT, RO, RU, SE, SI, SK, TR, UY) *see* Trandolapril 2080
Gordox (HU, VN) *see* Aprotinin 168
Gotabiotic (AR) *see* Tobramycin (Ophthalmic) 2056
Gotik (PY) *see* Ticlopidine 2040
Gotinal (VE) *see* Naphazoline (Nasal) 1426
Gotland Bisoprex (CO) *see* Bisoprolol and Hydrochlorothiazide 267
Goutex (CO) *see* Febuxostat 848
Goutichine (TH) *see* Colchicine 500
Goutilex (TW) *see* Allopurinol 90
Goutix (VN) *see* Etoricoxib [INT] 821
Goutnil (IN, PH) *see* Colchicine 500
Goval (EC) *see* RisperiDONE 1818
Gozid (TH) *see* Gemfibrozil 956
GPO-A-Flu (TH) *see* Oseltamivir 1523
Graceptor (JP) *see* Tacrolimus (Systemic) 1962
Gracial 28 (AE, BH, CY, EG, IQ, IR, JO, KW, LB, LY, OM, PH, QA, SA, SY, YE) *see* Ethinyl Estradiol and Desogestrel 799
Gradiab (ID) *see* MetFORMIN 1307
Gradient (IT) *see* Flunarizine [CAN/INT] 892
Gradual (UY) *see* Oxybutynin 1536
Grafacetin (ID) *see* Chloramphenicol 421
Grafalin (ID) *see* Albuterol 69
Gralddep (MX) *see* Loratadine and Pseudoephedrine 1242
Gr-Alfa (IN) *see* Alfacalcidol [CAN/INT] 82
Gramagen (TH) *see* Gemcitabine 952
Gramal (MX) *see* Molgramostim [INT] 1388
Gramazine (TW) *see* Nalidixic Acid [INT] 1418
Grambiot (PY) *see* Meropenem 1299
Gramcil (PH) *see* Ampicillin 141
Gramet (ID) *see* Granisetron 983
Gramoneg (IN, TH) *see* Nalidixic Acid [INT] 1418
Gran (CN, JP, MY, SG, TH, VN) *see* Filgrastim 875
Grandaxin (BG, CZ, HU, JP, KR, PK, RU, TH) *see* Tofisopam [INT] 2061
Grandoxy (AE, QA) *see* Doxycycline 689
Graneodin-B (MX) *see* Benzocaine 246
Granicip (IN) *see* Granisetron 983
Granocyte (AR, AT, BE, BG, BR, CH, CL, CN, CY, DE, DK, EE, FI, FR, GB, GR, HN, HR, ID, IE, IL, IN, IT, KW, LT, MY, NL, NO, PH, PK, PL, QA, RU, SE, SG, SI, TH, TR, TW, VE) *see* Lenograstim [INT] 1181
Granon (ID) *see* Granisetron 983
Granored (HR) *see* Granisetron 983
Grantron (TW) *see* Granisetron 983
Granudoxy (FR, LU) *see* Doxycycline 689
Granulokine (BR) *see* Filgrastim 875
Grasin (KR) *see* Filgrastim 875
Gratril OD (KR) *see* Granisetron 983
Gratusminal (ES) *see* PHENobarbital 1632
Gravamin (PE) *see* DimenhyDRINATE 637
Gravask (ID) *see* AmLODIPine 123
Gravida (BE) *see* Folic Acid 919
Gravi-Fol (DE) *see* Folic Acid 919
Gravol (CR, DO, GT, HK, HN, IN, NI, PA, PE, PH, SV) *see* DimenhyDRINATE 637
Gravx (PK) *see* Nimesulide [INT] 1456
Green Eight (KR) *see* Antihemophilic Factor (Recombinant) 152
Green Nose (KR) *see* Triprolidine and Pseudoephedrine 2105
Grendis (ID, MY, PH, TH) *see* Triflusal [INT] 2103
Greosin (ES) *see* Griseofulvin 985
Grexa Plus (PE) *see* Rosiglitazone and Glimepiride 1847
Grexin (TH) *see* Digoxin 627
Gricin (CZ, DE, HU, PL) *see* Griseofulvin 985
Gridokline (HK) *see* Clopidogrel 484
Griflux (PT) *see* Carbocisteine [INT] 357
Grifobutol (CL) *see* Acebutolol 29
Grifoclobam (CL) *see* CloBAZam 465
Grifonimod (PE) *see* NiMODipine 1456
Grifoparkin (CL, PE) *see* Carbidopa and Levodopa 351
Grifopil (CL) *see* Enalapril 722
Grifotaxima (CL) *see* Cefotaxime 382
Grifulin Forte (IL) *see* Griseofulvin 985
Grifulvin (TH) *see* Griseofulvin 985
Grimatin (JP) *see* Filgrastim 875
Grinsul (AR) *see* Amoxicillin 130
Grisefuline (FR) *see* Griseofulvin 985
Grisenova (GR) *see* Griseofulvin 985
Grisen (TW) *see* Griseofulvin 985
Griseofulvina (IT) *see* Griseofulvin 985
Griseofulvin (HN, IE, PL) *see* Griseofulvin 985
Griseofulvin Leo (LU) *see* Griseofulvin 985
Griseofulvin Prafa (ID) *see* Griseofulvin 985
Griseomed (AT) *see* Griseofulvin 985
Griseovin (EG) *see* Griseofulvin 985
Griseovine (VN) *see* Griseofulvin 985
griseo von ct (DE) *see* Griseofulvin 985
Grisflavin (TH) *see* Griseofulvin 985
Grisfulvin V (PH) *see* Griseofulvin 985
Grisol (CH) *see* Griseofulvin 985
Grisomicon (PT) *see* Griseofulvin 985
Grisoral (IN) *see* Griseofulvin 985
Grisovin (AE, AT, AU, BH, CO, CY, CZ, EG, IQ, IR, JO, KW, LB, LY, MX, OM, PE, PT, QA, SA, SY, VE, YE) *see* Griseofulvin 985
Grisovina FP (IT) *see* Griseofulvin 985
Grisovin-FP (AR, PH, UY) *see* Griseofulvin 985
Grisuven (HK) *see* Griseofulvin 985
Grisuvin (MY) *see* Griseofulvin 985
Grivin Forte (ID) *see* Griseofulvin 985
Grivin (MY, TH) *see* Griseofulvin 985
Gromin (KR) *see* ClomiPRAMINE 475
Growell (SG) *see* Minoxidil (Topical) 1374
Growgen-GM (AR) *see* Molgramostim [INT] 1388
Growject BC (JP) *see* Somatropin 1918
Growtropin-II (KR) *see* Somatropin 1918
Growtropin II (VN) *see* Somatropin 1918
Growtropin-Aq (CO) *see* Somatropin 1918
Grunamox (EC) *see* Amoxicillin 130
Gruncef (DE) *see* Cefadroxil 372
Guafedrin (AE, QA, SA) *see* Guaifenesin and Pseudoephedrine 989
Guaiatussin (PL) *see* GuaiFENesin 986
Guajacuran (CZ) *see* GuaiFENesin 986
Guajazyl (PL) *see* GuaiFENesin 986
Guamet (HK) *see* MetFORMIN 1307
Guang Di (CN) *see* Tropisetron [INT] 2108
Guan Shuang (CN) *see* Pitavastatin 1663
Guaphan (SA) *see* GuaiFENesin 986
Guaxan (ES) *see* Nimesulide [INT] 1456
Guayaten (VE) *see* Minoxidil (Systemic) 1374
Gubamine (AR) *see* Cyproheptadine 529
Gubang (CN) *see* Alendronate 79
Gupisone (AE, BH, KW, QA, SA) *see* PrednisoLONE (Systemic) 1703
Gusong (CN) *see* Risedronate 1816
Gutron (AE, AR, AT, BG, CH, CL, CN, CZ, DE, EG, FR, GR, HK, HN, HU, IL, IT, LT, NL, NZ, PL, PT, QA, RO, RU, SA, SG, SI, SK, UY) *see* Midodrine 1365

Gwajafen (PL) *see* GuaiFENesin 986
Gymiso (AU, FR) *see* Misoprostol 1379
Gynalgia (AR) *see* Acemetacin [INT] 30
Gynatam (PH) *see* Tamoxifen 1971
Gynatrol (DK) *see* Ethinyl Estradiol and Levonorgestrel 803
Gynazole-1 (CA) *see* Butoconazole 314
Gyneamsa (MX) *see* Calcitriol 323
Gynergen (IT) *see* Ergotamine 754
Gyno Canesten (CN) *see* Clotrimazole (Topical) 488
Gyno-Coryl (CY, EG, IQ, IR, JO, LY, OM, QA, SY, YE) *see* Econazole 703
Gyno-Daktarin (AE, BD, BG, BH, CY, CZ, EE, EG, FI, HR, IQ, IR, JO, JP, KR, KW, LB, LU, LY, MX, OM, QA, RU, SA, SY, YE) *see* Miconazole (Topical) 1360
Gyno (EE) *see* Econazole 703
Gynofen 35 (GR) *see* Cyproterone and Ethinyl Estradiol [CAN/INT] 532
Gyno-Fungix (BR) *see* Terconazole 2006
Gynokadin (DE) *see* Estradiol (Systemic) 775
Gyno-Lomexin (SA) *see* Fenticonazole [INT] 868
Gynol-Plus (SE) *see* Nonoxynol 9 1471
Gyno-neuralgin (DE) *see* Ibuprofen 1032
Gynonys (IN) *see* Hydroxyprogesterone Caproate 1021
Gyno-Pevaryl (AE, BH, HU, IL, KW, LB, LU, SA) *see* Econazole 703
Gynoplix (HK) *see* MetroNIDAZOLE (Systemic) 1353
Gynosterone (IL) *see* MethylTESTOSTERone 1345
Gyno-Terazol (BE, CZ, LU, NL, PL) *see* Terconazole 2006
Gyno-Travogen (AE, AT, BH, CH) *see* Isoconazole [INT] 1120
Gynoxin (BE, GB, HU, NL, PL) *see* Fenticonazole [INT] 868
Gyno-Zalain (PE) *see* Sertaconazole 1877
GynPolar (DE) *see* Estradiol (Systemic) 775
Gynprogest (PY) *see* Progesterone 1722
Gyrablock (AE, BH, CY, EG, IQ, IR, JO, KW, LB, LY, OM, QA, SA, SG, SY, YE) *see* Norfloxacin 1475
Gyraxen (PH) *see* Tamoxifen 1971
H2 Blocker-ratiopharm (LU) *see* Cimetidine 438
H2 Bloc (PH) *see* Famotidine 845
H-2 (KR) *see* Cimetidine 438
Habitrol Gum (NZ) *see* Nicotine 1449
Hadarax (TH) *see* HydrOXYzine 1024
Haelan (GB) *see* Flurandrenolide 906
Haemate (DK, SE) *see* Antihemophilic Factor/von Willebrand Factor Complex (Human) 154
Haemate P (AR, CH, CO, CY, DE, HR, HU, IL, RO, SI, SK) *see* Antihemophilic Factor/von Willebrand Factor Complex (Human) 154
Haemiton (DE, IL) *see* CloNIDine 480
Haemocomplettan (AT, CH, CZ, DE, FR, GR, HN, NL, PT, RO, TR) *see* Fibrinogen Concentrate (Human) 874
Haemocomplettan P (TW) *see* Fibrinogen Concentrate (Human) 874
Haemoctin (GB) *see* Antihemophilic Factor (Human) 152
Haemoctin SDH (IL) *see* Antihemophilic Factor (Human) 152
Haemokion (AE, BH, CY, EG, IL, IQ, IR, JO, KW, LB, LY, OM, QA, SA, SY, YE) *see* Phytonadione 1647
Haemonine (GB) *see* Factor IX (Human) 840
Haemopressin (AT, CH, DE, FR, NL) *see* Terlipressin [INT] 2010
Haemoprotect (DE) *see* Ferrous Sulfate 871
Haemoprot (IN) *see* Aprotinin 168
Haemosolvate Factor VIII (ZA) *see* Antihemophilic Factor/von Willebrand Factor Complex (Human) 154
Haemosolvex (ZA) *see* Factor IX (Human) 840
Haes Esteril (ES) *see* Hetastarch 1004
HAES-steril (BE, HR, LU, NL, PL) *see* Hetastarch 1004
Haes-Steril (BG, BH, CH, CN, CZ, DE, GB, GR, HN, ID, IL, IN, PH, RU, SA, SG, TH) *see* Hetastarch 1004
Haes Steril (EG) *see* Hetastarch 1004
Hagen (TW) *see* Diltiazem 634
Haicin (PH) *see* Minocycline 1371
Hailon (CN) *see* Levofloxacin (Systemic) 1197
Haiprex (DK, IS) *see* Methenamine 1317
Hairex (IN) *see* Minoxidil (Topical) 1374
Hairgrow (AE, BH, HK, KW, LB, QA, RO, SA) *see* Minoxidil (Topical) 1374
Hair Max (PK) *see* Minoxidil (Topical) 1374
Hair-Treat Forte (IL) *see* Minoxidil (Topical) 1374
Hair-Treat (IL) *see* Minoxidil (Topical) 1374
Hakelon (JP) *see* Fluocinonide 894
Halamid (DE) *see* Nedocromil 1435
Halaven (AU, BE, CH, CZ, DE, DK, EE, ES, FR, GB, HK, HR, IL, IS, JP, KR, LT, MY, NL, NO, PH, RO, SE, SG, SI, SK, TH, TR) *see* Eribulin 755
Halciderm (AU, CH, GB, IE, IT, NL) *see* Halcinonide 992
Halciderm Crema Al (CR, DO, GT, HN, NI, PA, SV) *see* Halcinonide 992
Halciderme (PE) *see* Halcinonide 992
Halciion (QA) *see* Triazolam 2101
Halcion (AT, AU, BB, BE, BF, BG, BJ, BM, BR, BS, BZ, CH, CI, CR, CZ, DE, DK, EE, ES, ET, FI, FR, GB, GH, GM, GN, GR, GT, GY, HK, HN, HR, IE, IL, IS, IT, JM, KE, KR, LR, LT, LU, MA, ML, MR, MT, MU, MW, MX, NE, NG, NI, NL, NO, PA, PK, PT, RU, SC, SD, SE, SI, SK, SL, SN, SR, SV, TH, TN, TR, TT, TW, TZ, UG, ZA, ZM, ZW) *see* Triazolam 2101
Haldin (AE, BF, BH, BJ, CI, CY, EG, ET, GH, GM, GN, IQ, IR, JO, KE, KW, LB, LR, LY, MA, ML, MR, MU, MW, NE, NG, OM, QA, SA, SC, SD, SL, SN, SY, TN, TZ, UG, YE, ZM, ZW) *see* Cimetidine 438
Haldol (AT, BE, BH, BZ, CL, CY, DE, EG, GB, HR, IE, IS, JO, KW, LB, LU, MX, NI, NO, NZ, PA, PE, PK, PT, RO, SA, SE, SI, TR, VE) *see* Haloperidol 993
Haldol Decanoas (AE, BB, BF, BG, BH, BJ, BM, BS, CH, CI, CR, CY, CZ, DO, EC, EG, ET, FR, GH, GM, GN, GT, GY, HK, HN, ID, IL, IQ, IR, IT, JM, JO, KE, KR, KW, LB, LR, LY, MA, ML, MR, MU, MW, NE, NG, NL, OM, PR, PY, QA, SA, SC, SD, SL, SN, SR, SV, SY, TN, TT, TW, TZ, UG, UY, YE, ZM, ZW) *see* Haloperidol 993
Haldol decanoas (LU) *see* Haloperidol 993
Haldol Decanoate (AU) *see* Haloperidol 993
Haldol Decanoato (BR, CL) *see* Haloperidol 993
Haldol depo (HR) *see* Haloperidol 993
Ha Le Te (CN) *see* Halcinonide 992
Halfan (AE, AT, BE, BF, BH, BJ, CI, CO, CY, DE, EG, ES, ET, FR, GB, GH, GM, GN, IL, IQ, IR, JO, KE, KW, LB, LR, LU, LY, MA, ML, MR, MU, MW, NE, NG, NL, OM, PK, PT, QA, SA, SC, SD, SL, SN, SY, TN, TZ, UG, YE, ZA, ZM, ZW) *see* Halofantrine [INT] 993
Halidor (HU, PL, RU, TR) *see* Bencyclane [INT] 241
Halodin (TH) *see* Loratadine 1241
Halog (AT, BR, DE, DK, ES, FR, ID, KR, NO, VE) *see* Halcinonide 992
Halomycetin Augensalbe (AT) *see* Chloramphenicol 421
Haloper (DE, RU) *see* Haloperidol 993
Haloperidol Decanoat (HU) *see* Haloperidol 993
Haloperidol Esteve (ES) *see* Haloperidol 993
Haloperidol Prodes (ES) *see* Haloperidol 993
Haloperidol-ratiopharm (LU) *see* Haloperidol 993
Haloperil (MX) *see* Haloperidol 993
Halopidol decanoato (AR, CO) *see* Haloperidol 993
Halotestin (AU, BH, CI, CY, ET, FR, GH, GM, GN, GR, HU, IT, KE, LR, LY, ML, MR, MU, MW, NE, NG, NL, NO, SC, SD, SL, SN, TN, TZ, UG, ZA, ZM, ZW) *see* Fluoxymesterone 903
Halotri (ES) *see* Liothyronine 1221
Haloxen (SG) *see* Haloperidol 993
Haloxin (SG) *see* Chloroquine 424
Haloxin (SG) *see* Hydroxychloroquine 1021
Halubone (KR) *see* Hyaluronate and Derivatives 1006
Hamarin (GB) *see* Allopurinol 90

Hamidon (KR) *see* Domperidone [CAN/INT] 666
Hamostat (IN) *see* Aminocaproic Acid 113
Hanacef (KR) *see* Cefadroxil 372
Hancerom (KR) *see* Cefpirome [INT] 388
Hanlexin (CN) *see* Triazolam 2101
Hanmaryl (KR) *see* Glimepiride 966
Hansepran (IN) *see* Clofazimine [INT] 473
Hantracet (KR) *see* Acetaminophen and Tramadol 37
Hantrazol (KR) *see* Itraconazole 1130
Happigra Gran (KR) *see* Sildenafil 1882
Hapsen (ID) *see* Bisoprolol 266
Haridol-D (CN) *see* Haloperidol 993
Haridol Decanoate (TH) *see* Haloperidol 993
Harifin (TH) *see* Finasteride 878
Harmetone (CO) *see* Domperidone [CAN/INT] 666
Harmogen (CH, GB, IE) *see* Estropipate 793
Harmonise (AU) *see* Loperamide 1236
Harnal D (ID) *see* Tamsulosin 1974
Harnal (CN, HK, JP, PH) *see* Tamsulosin 1974
Harnalidge D (TW) *see* Tamsulosin 1974
Harnal OCAS (ID, MY, PH, SG, TH, VN) *see* Tamsulosin 1974
Harnin (JP) *see* FlavoxATE 881
Harond (KR) *see* Hydrocortisone (Systemic) 1013
Hartil (RU) *see* Ramipril 1771
Hart (PY) *see* Diltiazem 634
Hartsorb (TH) *see* Isosorbide Dinitrate 1124
Hartylox (PH) *see* Captopril 342
Harusin SR (KR) *see* Tamsulosin 1974
Harvoni (CZ, DE, DK, EE, GB, NZ, SE) *see* Ledipasvir and Sofosbuvir 1173
Havlane (FR) *see* Loprazolam [INT] 1241
HAVpur (DE) *see* Hepatitis A Vaccine 1001
Havrix 1440 (AU, BB, BM, BS, BZ, GY, HK, IN, JM, MX, PR, SR, TT) *see* Hepatitis A Vaccine 1001
Havrix (AT, BE, CH, CL, CN, CR, CZ, DK, DO, EC, EE, FI, FR, GB, GR, GT, HN, IE, IL, IS, IT, KR, LT, MY, NI, NL, NO, NZ, PA, PE, PH, PK, PL, PT, PY, RO, RU, SE, SG, SI, SK, SV, TR, TW, UY, VE, VN) *see* Hepatitis A Vaccine 1001
Havrix Junior (BB, BM, BS, BZ, GY, HK, IN, JM, MX, PR, SR, TT) *see* Hepatitis A Vaccine 1001
Havrix Monodose (AE, BH, CY, EG, IQ, IR, JO, KW, LB, LY, OM, QA, SA, SY, YE) *see* Hepatitis A Vaccine 1001
Haxifal (FR) *see* Cefaclor 372
Haxim (PH) *see* Cefotaxime 382
Hayospan (PH) *see* Scopolamine (Systemic) 1870
Hazidol (VN) *see* Haloperidol 993
H-B-Vax II (AT, AU, BE, BG, CH, CZ, DE, DK, EE, FI, FR, GR, IT, MT, NL, NO, PL, PT, RU, SE, SK, TR, TW) *see* Hepatitis B Vaccine (Recombinant) 1002
HB-Vax (AE, QA) *see* Hepatitis B Vaccine (Recombinant) 1002
HBvaxPRO (AT, BE, BG, CH, CZ, DE, DK, EE, FI, FR, GB, GR, IE, IT, MT, NL, NO, NZ, PL, PT, RU, SE, SK, TR) *see* Hepatitis B Vaccine (Recombinant) 1002
HCQS (PE, TH) *see* Hydroxychloroquine 1021
HCT (EC) *see* Hydrochlorothiazide 1009
H.C.T. (ID) *see* Hydrochlorothiazide 1009
HCTZ 25 (TH) *see* Hydrochlorothiazide 1009
Headache (KR) *see* Flunarizine [CAN/INT] 892
Healip (DK, FI, GR, SE) *see* Docosanol 661
Healon (CO, EC, HU, IN, LU, PK, TW, ZA) *see* Hyaluronate and Derivatives 1006
Healon GV (ZA) *see* Hyaluronate and Derivatives 1006
Healonid (AT, FR) *see* Hyaluronate and Derivatives 1006
Heana (TW) *see* Estradiol and Norethindrone 781
Heartoace (TW) *see* Disopyramide 653
Heartprilprotect (KR) *see* Ramipril 1771
Hebagam IM (ZA) *see* Hepatitis B Immune Globulin (Human) 1002
Heberon Alfa R (CO) *see* Interferon Alfa-2b 1096
Hecobac (ID) *see* Clarithromycin 456
Hectorol (CA) *see* Doxercalciferol 679
Hedex (IE) *see* Acetaminophen 32
Heferol (HR) *see* Ferrous Fumarate 870
Hegon (AR) *see* Zaleplon 2193
Heimdall Diurex (CO) *see* Indapamide 1065
Heiwin (PH) *see* Norfloxacin 1475
He Ke DiSi (CN) *see* Lafutidine [INT] 1157
Heksavit (FI) *see* Pyridoxine 1747
Helenil (AR, BR) *see* Ketoprofen 1145
Helen (TH) *see* Cyproterone and Ethinyl Estradiol [CAN/INT] 532
Helex (HR) *see* ALPRAZolam 94
Heliclam (EC) *see* Omeprazole, Clarithromycin, and Amoxicillin 1511
Heliclar (LU) *see* Clarithromycin 456
Heliclo (KR) *see* Clarithromycin 456
Helicobacter Test Infai (IT) *see* Urea 2114
Heliopar (FI) *see* Chloroquine 424
Heliton (AR) *see* Nitazoxanide 1461
Helixate (AT, GR, HU, IT, NL, PL) *see* Antihemophilic Factor (Recombinant) 152
Helixate Nexgen (AU, BE, CZ, DE, DK, EE, FR, NO, SE) *see* Antihemophilic Factor (Recombinant) 152
Helixate NexGen (GB, IE) *see* Antihemophilic Factor (Recombinant) 152
Helix SR (HU) *see* ALPRAZolam 94
Helizol (EC) *see* Omeprazole 1508
Helmex (DE) *see* Pyrantel Pamoate 1744
Helmiben (UY) *see* Albendazole 65
Helmidazole (AE, BH, CY, EG, IL, IQ, IR, JO, KW, LB, LY, OM, QA, SA, SY, YE) *see* Albendazole 65
Helminar (PE) *see* Granisetron 983
Helmintox (FR, RU) *see* Pyrantel Pamoate 1744
Helmizol (BR) *see* MetroNIDAZOLE (Systemic) 1353
Helocetin (KR) *see* Chloramphenicol 421
Heloc (NO) *see* Docosanol 661
Helpin (CZ, DE) *see* Brivudine [INT] 289
Helsibon (JP) *see* Diltiazem 634
Helvevir (CH) *see* Acyclovir (Systemic) 47
Hemabate (CN, GB, MY, SG, TW) *see* Carboprost Tromethamine 360
Hemaflow (PH) *see* Clopidogrel 484
Hema F (TW) *see* Ferrous Fumarate 870
Hema-K (PH) *see* Phytonadione 1647
Hemapo (ID, TH, VN) *see* Epoetin Alfa 742
Hemasol (SG) *see* Homatropine 1005
Hemastat (PH) *see* Heparin 997
Hemax (TH) *see* Epoetin Alfa 742
Hemi-Daonil (AR, FR, MA) *see* GlyBURIDE 972
Hemidol (TW) *see* Indapamide 1065
Hemo 141 (ES) *see* Etamsylate [INT] 795
Hemobion (MX) *see* Ferrous Sulfate 871
Hemocaprol (ES) *see* Aminocaproic Acid 113
Hemoced[vet.] (FR) *see* Etamsylate [INT] 795
Hemoclar (AE, BH, EG, FR, SA) *see* Pentosan Polysulfate Sodium 1617
Hemoclot (PH) *see* Tranexamic Acid 2081
Hemofil M (DE, FR, IT, TH, TW) *see* Antihemophilic Factor (Human) 152
Hemogenin (BR) *see* Oxymetholone 1546
Hemohes (AR, CL, LU, NL) *see* Hetastarch 1004
Hemonor (PE) *see* Heparin 997
Hemopressin (PK) *see* Vasopressin 2142
Hemostan (PH) *see* Tranexamic Acid 2081
Hemototal (PT) *see* Ferrous Gluconate 870
Hemotrex (PH) *see* Tranexamic Acid 2081
Hemovas (ES) *see* Pentoxifylline 1618
Heng En (CN) *see* MitoXANtrone 1382
Heng Li An (CN) *see* ZOLMitriptan 2210
Heng Yi (CN) *see* Aspirin and Dipyridamole 185
Henplatin (PH) *see* Oxaliplatin 1528

Hensetron (PH) *see* Tropisetron [INT] 2108
Hentaxel (PH) *see* DOCEtaxel 656
Hentrozole (PH) *see* Letrozole 1181
HepaBig (EG) *see* Hepatitis B Immune Globulin (Human) 1002
Hepabig (IN, KR, MY, PH) *see* Hepatitis B Immune Globulin (Human) 1002
Hepacaf (BE) *see* Hepatitis B Immune Globulin (Human) 1002
Hepaflex (FI, NO) *see* Heparin 997
Hepagam B (IL) *see* Hepatitis B Immune Globulin (Human) 1002
Hepalac (TH) *see* Lactulose 1156
Heparin (AT, BF, BG, BJ, CH, CI, CZ, DE, ET, FI, GB, GH, GM, GN, GR, HN, IL, KE, LR, MA, ML, MR, MU, MW, NE, NG, NO, SC, SD, SE, SL, SN, TN, TZ, UG, ZA, ZM, ZW) *see* Heparin 997
Heparine (BE, NL) *see* Heparin 997
Heparine Choay (FR) *see* Heparin 997
Heparine Novo (BE, NL) *see* Heparin 997
Heparin Injection B.P. (AU) *see* Heparin 997
Heparin Leo (DK, HK, ID, MY, PH, TW) *see* Heparin 997
Heparin Novo (TW) *see* Heparin 997
Heparin Sodium B Braun (ID, MY) *see* Heparin 997
Hepatect (AT, CH, CO, DE, EE, HN, IE, PL, PT, TR, TW) *see* Hepatitis B Immune Globulin (Human) 1002
Hepatect CP (VN) *see* Hepatitis B Immune Globulin (Human) 1002
Hepatitis B Immunoglobulin-VF (AU) *see* Hepatitis B Immune Globulin (Human) 1002
Hepatoum (FR) *see* Alverine [INT] 104
Hepatyrix (AT, DE, GB, IE, NZ) *see* Typhoid and Hepatitis A Vaccine [CAN/INT] 2111
Hepavax Gene (CO) *see* Hepatitis B Vaccine (Recombinant) 1002
Hepaviral (ID) *see* Ribavirin 1797
Hepavit (AT) *see* Hydroxocobalamin 1020
Hep-B Gammagee (AE) *see* Hepatitis B Immune Globulin (Human) 1002
HepBQuin (IN, NL) *see* Hepatitis B Immune Globulin (Human) 1002
Hepcure (KR) *see* Adefovir 54
Heplav (ID) *see* LamiVUDine 1157
Hepovir (PK) *see* Adefovir 54
Heprin (PH) *see* Heparin 997
Hepsal (SG) *see* Heparin 997
Hepsera (AE, AR, AT, AU, BE, BG, BR, CH, CL, CN, CO, CR, CY, CZ, DE, DK, DO, EC, EE, ES, FI, FR, GB, GR, GT, HK, HN, HR, HU, ID, IE, IL, IS, IT, JO, KR, KW, LT, MT, MY, NI, NL, NO, NZ, PA, PE, PH, PK, PL, PT, QA, RO, RU, SA, SE, SG, SI, SK, SV, TH, TR, TW, VE, VN) *see* Adefovir 54
Hepssel (KR) *see* Adefovir 54
Heptadon (AT) *see* Methadone 1311
Heptanon (HR) *see* Methadone 1311
Heptasan (ID) *see* Cyproheptadine 529
Heptin (PH) *see* Heparin 997
Heptodin (CN) *see* LamiVUDine 1157
Hepuman Berna (PE) *see* Hepatitis B Immune Globulin (Human) 1002
Heracillin (DK, SE) *see* Flucloxacillin [INT] 885
Herax (ID) *see* Acyclovir (Systemic) 47
Herben (KR) *see* Diltiazem 634
Herbesser 60 (MY, TH) *see* Diltiazem 634
Herbesser 90 SR (HK, MY, SG, TH) *see* Diltiazem 634
Herbesser 180 SR (HK) *see* Diltiazem 634
Herbesser (JP, MY, TH, TW) *see* Diltiazem 634
Herbesser R100 (HK, JP) *see* Diltiazem 634
Herbesser R200 (HK, JP) *see* Diltiazem 634
Herbessor 30 (MY) *see* Diltiazem 634
Herbessor (SG, VN) *see* Diltiazem 634
Herceptin (AE, AR, AT, AU, BB, BE, BF, BG, BH, BJ, BM, BR, BS, BZ, CH, CI, CL, CN, CO, CY, CZ, DE, DK, EC, EE, ES, ET, FI, FR, GB, GH, GM, GN, GR, GY, HK, HN, HR, HU, ID, IE, IL, IS, IT, JM, JO, KE, KR, LB, LR, LT, MA, ML, MR, MT, MU, MW, MX, MY, NE, NG, NL, NO, NZ, PE, PH, PL, PT, PY, QA, RO, RU, SA, SC, SD, SE, SG, SI, SK, SL, SN, SR, TH, TN, TR, TT, TW, TZ, UG, UY, VE, VN, ZA, ZM, ZW) *see* Trastuzumab 2085
Herclov (ID) *see* ValACYclovir 2119
Herem (AR) *see* Roxithromycin [INT] 1853
Herfam (KR) *see* Famciclovir 843
Heria (BE) *see* Tibolone [INT] 2035
Herklin (MX) *see* Lindane 1217
Hermolepsin (SE) *see* CarBAMazepine 346
Herocan (TW) *see* Irinotecan 1112
Herpavir (JO) *see* Acyclovir (Topical) 51
Herpecid (KR) *see* Acyclovir (Topical) 51
Herpesin (CZ) *see* Acyclovir (Topical) 51
Herpesin (CZ, SK) *see* Acyclovir (Systemic) 47
Herpetad (CR, DO, GT, HN, NI, PA, SV) *see* Acyclovir (Systemic) 47
Herpevex (MY) *see* Acyclovir (Systemic) 47
Herpevir (FR) *see* Acyclovir (Systemic) 47
Herpevir (FR) *see* Acyclovir (Topical) 51
Herpex (BH, IN, PH) *see* Acyclovir (Systemic) 47
Herpex (IN) *see* Acyclovir (Topical) 51
Herpizyg (TH) *see* Acyclovir (Systemic) 47
Herwont (IN) *see* Misoprostol 1379
Herzer (JP) *see* Nitroglycerin 1465
Hesor (TW) *see* Diltiazem 634
Hespander (JP) *see* Hetastarch 1004
Hestar-200 (CO, ID) *see* Hetastarch 1004
Hesteril (ES) *see* Hetastarch 1004
Hetailin (CN) *see* Aprotinin 168
Heviran (PL) *see* Acyclovir (Systemic) 47
Hexabiotin (DK) *see* Erythromycin (Systemic) 762
Hexacycline (FR) *see* Tetracycline 2017
Hexa-Defital (AR) *see* Lindane 1217
Hexadilat (DK) *see* NIFEdipine 1451
Hexakapron (IL) *see* Tranexamic Acid 2081
Hexalense (FR) *see* Aminocaproic Acid 113
Hexaler Plus (AR) *see* Desloratadine and Pseudoephedrine 594
Hexalgin (BG) *see* Dipyrone [INT] 653
Hexal Ranitic (AU) *see* Ranitidine 1777
Hexamandin (PL) *see* Methenamine 1317
Hexamet (ZA) *see* Cimetidine 438
Hexamycin (DK) *see* Gentamicin (Systemic) 959
Hexan (PY) *see* Glimepiride 966
Hexanurat (DK) *see* Allopurinol 90
Hexapindol (DK) *see* Pindolol 1652
Hexarone (ZA) *see* Amiodarone 114
Hexasoptin (DK, FI) *see* Verapamil 2154
Hexer (ID) *see* Ranitidine 1777
Hexidine (MY) *see* Chlorhexidine Gluconate 422
Hexiquin (ID) *see* Ciprofloxacin (Systemic) 441
Hexisept (BG) *see* Chlorhexidine Gluconate 422
Hexobion 100 (DE) *see* Pyridoxine 1747
Hexoderm (PY) *see* Betamethasone (Topical) 255
Hexvix (AT, BE, CH, CY, CZ, DE, DK, EE, ES, FI, FR, GR, IT, NL, NO, PT, SE) *see* Aminolevulinic Acid 114
Hexymer-2 (ID) *see* Trihexyphenidyl 2103
Hiace (JP) *see* Thiamine 2028
Hi-Alarzin (JP) *see* Tolnaftate 2063
Hialid (ID, PH) *see* Hyaluronate and Derivatives 1006
Hibechin (JP) *see* Promethazine 1723
Hiberix (AU, SI) *see* Haemophilus b Conjugate Vaccine 991
Hiberna (JP) *see* Promethazine 1723
Hibernal (HU, SE) *see* ChlorproMAZINE 429
HIBest (FR, IN) *see* Haemophilus b Conjugate Vaccine 991
Hibicet (AE) *see* Chlorhexidine Gluconate 422
Hibident (AT) *see* Chlorhexidine Gluconate 422

Hibiotic (AE, BH, CY, EG, IQ, IR, JO, KW, LB, LY, OM, QA, SA, SY, YE) *see* Amoxicillin and Clavulanate 133
Hibiscott (AR) *see* Chlorhexidine Gluconate 422
Hibiscrub (CH, FR, GB, HK, NL, PK, SG, TH) *see* Chlorhexidine Gluconate 422
Hibisol (AE, BF, BH, BJ, CI, CY, EG, ET, GH, GM, GN, HK, IQ, IR, JO, KE, KW, LB, LR, LY, MA, ML, MR, MU, MW, NE, NG, OM, QA, SA, SC, SD, SL, SN, SY, TN, TZ, UG, YE, ZM, ZW) *see* Chlorhexidine Gluconate 422
Hibitane (AE, BE, BH, CY, DK, EG, FR, HK, IQ, IR, IS, JO, KW, LB, LY, OM, QA, SA, SE, SY, YE) *see* Chlorhexidine Gluconate 422
Hibitane Antiseptic (AU) *see* Chlorhexidine Gluconate 422
Hibitane Concentrate (TH) *see* Chlorhexidine Gluconate 422
Hibitane Cream (GR) *see* Chlorhexidine Gluconate 422
Hibitane Solution (GR) *see* Chlorhexidine Gluconate 422
Hibitan (KR) *see* Chlorhexidine Gluconate 422
Hiblok (ID) *see* Atenolol 189
Hibon (JP) *see* Riboflavin 1803
HibTITER (AE, AT, BH, CY, DE, EG, FI, GB, HN, IL, IQ, IR, IT, JO, KW, LB, LY, NZ, OM, QA, SA, SY, YE) *see* Haemophilus b Conjugate Vaccine 991
Hicee (JP) *see* Ascorbic Acid 178
Hiconcil (BE, FR, JO, KW, VN) *see* Amoxicillin 130
Hidanil (CO) *see* Phenytoin 1640
Hidantoína (MX) *see* Phenytoin 1640
Hiderax (CO) *see* HydrOXYzine 1024
Hidil (SG, TH) *see* Gemfibrozil 956
Hidine (TH) *see* Chlorhexidine Gluconate 422
Hidipine (KR) *see* Felodipine 850
Hidonac (ID, MY, PH, TH, TW) *see* Acetylcysteine 40
Hidrafasa (ES) *see* Isoniazid 1120
Hidral (AR, UY) *see* HydrALAZINE 1007
Hidramox (MX) *see* Amoxicillin 130
Hidranison (ES) *see* Isoniazid 1120
Hidrasec (CL, CN, CO, CR, CZ, DO, EC, EE, FI, GB, GR, GT, HK, HN, HR, MX, MY, NI, PA, PH, PY, RO, SE, SG, TH, VE, VN) *see* Racecadotril [INT] 1765
Hidrasolco (ES) *see* Isoniazid 1120
Hidratan (PY) *see* Racecadotril [INT] 1765
Hidrazida (ES, PT) *see* Isoniazid 1120
Hidrociclina (MX) *see* Penicillin G Procaine 1613
Hidrocortif (EC) *see* Hydrocortisone (Systemic) 1013
Hidrocort (VE) *see* Hydrocortisone (Systemic) 1013
Hidrolid (AR) *see* Hydroxyurea 1021
Hidronol T (CL) *see* Hydrochlorothiazide and Triamterene 1012
Hidroronol (CL) *see* Hydrochlorothiazide 1009
Hidrosaluretil (ES) *see* Hydrochlorothiazide 1009
Hidrotisona (AR) *see* Hydrocortisone (Topical) 1014
Hidroxicarbamida (CL) *see* Hydroxyurea 1021
Hidroxina (EC) *see* HydrOXYzine 1024
Hidroxuber (ES) *see* Hydroxocobalamin 1020
Hierro (AR) *see* Ferrous Fumarate 870
Hifen (VN) *see* Terbinafine (Topical) 2004
Higan (TH) *see* Scopolamine (Systemic) 1870
Highduet (KR) *see* Amlodipine and Atorvastatin 124
Higrotona (ES) *see* Chlorthalidone 430
Higroton (BR, EC, MX, VE) *see* Chlorthalidone 430
Hilactan (JP) *see* Cinnarizine [INT] 440
Hiloca (TW) *see* QUEtiapine 1751
Himentin (SG) *see* Cimetidine 438
Hinecol (KR) *see* Bethanechol 257
Hinicol (TW) *see* Chloramphenicol 421
Hipecor (CL) *see* Sotalol 1927
Hipeksal (FI) *see* Methenamine 1317
Hipen (BF, BJ, CI, ET, GH, GM, GN, KE, LR, MA, ML, MR, MU, MW, NE, NG, SC, SD, SL, SN, TN, TZ, UG, ZM, ZW) *see* Amoxicillin 130
Hiperdipina (PT) *see* Nitrendipine [INT] 1463
Hiperil (PT) *see* Captopril 342
Hiperlex (ES) *see* Fosinopril 932
Hiperlipen (CO, EC, PE, PY, VE) *see* Ciprofibrate [INT] 441
Hipertensal (AR) *see* GuanFACINE 990
Hipertensal Combi (AR) *see* Amlodipine and Atorvastatin 124
Hiperton (MX) *see* Sodium Chloride 1902
Hipexal (CL) *see* GlyBURIDE 972
Hipnax (PT) *see* Nitrazepam [CAN/INT] 1461
Hipnoz (ID) *see* Midazolam 1361
Hipo Femme (MX) *see* Miconazole (Topical) 1360
Hipoge (CL) *see* Hydrocortisone (Topical) 1014
Hipokinon (MX) *see* Trihexyphenidyl 2103
Hipolixan (CL) *see* AtorvaSTATin 194
Hipolixan (PY) *see* Gemfibrozil 956
Hiposterol (CL) *see* Lovastatin 1252
Hipovastin (AR) *see* Lovastatin 1252
Hipover (PE) *see* Repaglinide 1791
Hippigra (HK) *see* Sildenafil 1882
Hippro Forte (TH) *see* Ciprofloxacin (Systemic) 441
Hippro (TH) *see* Ciprofloxacin (Systemic) 441
Hipranol (MY) *see* Propranolol 1731
Hiprex (AE, AT, AU, BB, BF, BJ, BM, BS, BZ, CI, CR, DO, ET, FI, GB, GH, GM, GN, GT, GY, HN, JM, KE, LR, MA, ML, MR, MU, MW, MX, MY, NE, NG, NO, NZ, OM, PA, PH, SC, SD, SE, SL, SN, SR, SV, TN, TT, TZ, UG, ZA, ZM, ZW) *see* Methenamine 1317
Hiprogin (MY) *see* Hydroxyprogesterone Caproate 1021
Hiprogress (IN) *see* Hydroxyprogesterone Caproate 1021
Hiramicin (HR) *see* Doxycycline 689
Hiranin (TW) *see* Carisoprodol 363
Hirapine (MY) *see* Nevirapine 1440
Hirdsyn (JP) *see* Cinnarizine [INT] 440
Hirnamin (TW) *see* Methotrimeprazine [CAN/INT] 1329
Hirobriz Breezhaler (CZ, DE, DK, EE, ES, HR, LT, PL, PT, SE, SI, SK) *see* Indacaterol 1063
Hisart (TW) *see* Losartan and Hydrochlorothiazide 1250
Hiscifed (TH) *see* Triprolidine and Pseudoephedrine 2105
Hishiherin-S (JP) *see* Etilefrine [INT] 815
Hismazine (MY) *see* Cetirizine 411
Hispen (PH) *see* Mefenamic Acid 1280
Hista-Bloc (PH) *see* Famotidine 845
Histac (BF, BH, BJ, CI, ET, GH, GM, GN, HU, IN, JO, KE, KW, LR, MA, ML, MR, MU, MW, NE, NG, SC, SD, SL, SN, TH, TN, TZ, UG, ZM, ZW) *see* Ranitidine 1777
Histafed (IL) *see* Triprolidine and Pseudoephedrine 2105
Histagone (PH) *see* Ebastine [INT] 702
Histaklor (ID) *see* Dexchlorpheniramine 603
Histak (ZA) *see* Ranitidine 1777
Histaloc (AE, BH, KW, SA) *see* Promethazine 1723
Histamine-Care (IL) *see* Triprolidine and Pseudoephedrine 2105
Histan (TH) *see* HydrOXYzine 1024
Histaplen (BR, UY) *see* Levocetirizine 1196
Histatec (CH) *see* Cetirizine 411
Histaverin (ES) *see* Codeine 497
Histazan (JO) *see* Promethazine 1723
Histazin (AE, BH, CY, EG, IQ, IR, JO, KW, LB, LY, OM, QA, SA, SY, YE) *see* Promethazine 1723
Histazine (IL, PH) *see* Cetirizine 411
Histergan (BF, BH, BJ, CI, CY, EG, ET, GH, GM, GN, IQ, IR, JO, KE, KW, LR, LY, MA, ML, MR, MU, MW, NE, NG, OM, QA, SC, SD, SL, SN, SY, TN, TZ, UG, YE, ZM, ZW) *see* DiphenhydrAMINE (Systemic) 641
Histigo (ID) *see* Betahistine [CAN/INT] 252
Histimet (AR, PL) *see* Levocabastine (Ophthalmic) [CAN/INT] 1195
Histin (TH) *see* Carbinoxamine 356

Histodil (HN, HU, RU, VN) *see* Cimetidine 438
Histodil[inj.] (HU) *see* Cimetidine 438
Histrine (ID) *see* Cetirizine 411
Hithia (JP) *see* Thiamine 2028
Hitolin (TW) *see* Mebendazole [CAN/INT] 1274
Hitrazole (KR) *see* Itraconazole 1130
Hitrin (CR, GT, HN, NI, PA, SV) *see* Terazosin 2001
Hitrol (ID) *see* Calcitriol 323
Hivent DS (PH) *see* Albuterol 69
Hizentra (GB) *see* Immune Globulin 1056
Hizin (SG, TH) *see* HydrOXYzine 1024
HMG (KR) *see* Menotropins 1292
HMG Lepori (ES) *see* Menotropins 1292
HMG Massone[inj.] (AR) *see* Menotropins 1292
H.M.G. Organon (ES) *see* Menotropins 1292
Hocular (TW) *see* Loperamide 1236
Hoemal (MY, SG) *see* Acetaminophen 32
Hofcomant (AT, FI) *see* Amantadine 105
Hogel (CO) *see* Clopidogrel 484
Holetar (EE) *see* Lovastatin 1252
Holgyeme (FR) *see* Cyproterone and Ethinyl Estradiol [CAN/INT] 532
Holoxan (AE, AT, AU, BD, BE, BG, BH, CH, CL, CN, CY, CZ, DE, DK, EC, EE, EG, ES, FI, FR, GR, HK, HN, HR, HU, ID, IE, IL, IQ, IR, IS, IT, JO, KR, KW, LB, LT, LU, LY, MT, MY, NL, NO, NZ, OM, PH, PK, PL, PT, QA, RO, RU, SA, SE, SG, SI, SK, SY, TH, TR, TW, UY, VN, YE) *see* Ifosfamide 1040
Holoxane (BR) *see* Ifosfamide 1040
Homarin Forte (IN) *see* Homatropine 1005
Homatropine (AU, BE, NL) *see* Homatropine 1005
Homatropine Faure (FR) *see* Homatropine 1005
Homatropin (HR, NO, PY) *see* Homatropine 1005
Homatropin-POS (DE) *see* Homatropine 1005
Homedin (VN) *see* Iloprost 1046
Homocodeina (ES) *see* Pholcodine [INT] 1646
Homonal (JP) *see* Mafenide 1261
H-One (PH) *see* Cetirizine 411
36 Horas (PY) *see* Tadalafil 1968
Horizon (JP) *see* Diazepam 613
Hosolvon (SG) *see* Bromhexine [INT] 291
Hostacortin (ID) *see* PredniSONE 1706
Hostacyclin (AT, GR) *see* Tetracycline 2017
Hostacycline (IN, PH, ZA) *see* Tetracycline 2017
Hostacycline-P (ZA) *see* Tetracycline 2017
Hostlos (DK) *see* Bromhexine [INT] 291
Hotemin (CZ, MY) *see* Piroxicam 1662
Hovasc (HK, MY) *see* AmLODIPine 123
Hovicor (PH) *see* Hydrocortisone (Topical) 1014
HRF (BE, GB, IE, LU) *see* Gonadorelin [CAN/INT] 980
Huacose (TW) *see* TOLAZamide 2062
Huanli (CN) *see* Ciclopirox 433
Huberdasen (ES) *see* Piracetam [INT] 1661
Hui Er Ding (CN) *see* Emtricitabine 720
Huining (CN) *see* Rebamipide [INT] 1786
Huiyuan (CL) *see* Bumetanide 297
Huma-Captopril (HU) *see* Captopril 342
Huma-Col-Asa (HU) *see* Mesalamine 1301
Huma-Fluoxetin (HU) *see* FLUoxetine 899
Huma-Folacid (HU) *see* Folic Acid 919
Humagel (FR) *see* Paromomycin 1579
Humalog 25 (CN) *see* Insulin Lispro Protamine and Insulin Lispro 1088
Humalog (AE, AT, AU, BB, BE, BF, BG, BH, BJ, BM, BR, BS, BZ, CH, CI, CL, CN, CO, CY, CZ, DE, DK, ET, FI, FR, GB, GH, GM, GN, GR, GY, HN, HR, HU, ID, IE, IN, IS, IT, JM, KE, KW, LB, LR, LT, MA, ML, MR, MU, MW, MX, NE, NG, NL, NO, PK, PT, PY, QA, RO, RU, SA, SC, SD, SE, SI, SK, SL, SN, SR, TH, TN, TR, TT, TW, TZ, UG, UY, VE, ZA, ZM, ZW) *see* Insulin Lispro 1087
Humalog Lispro (CR, GT, HN, IL, KR, NI, PA, PE, SV) *see* Insulin Lispro 1087
Humalog Mix 25 (AE, AU, BB, BH, BM, BR, BS, BZ, CL, CO, CR, CY, DO, GT, GY, HK, HN, ID, IL, JM, KR, KW, LB, MX, MY, NI, NL, NZ, PA, PE, PH, PR, QA, SA, SG, SR, SV, TH, TT, VE) *see* Insulin Lispro Protamine and Insulin Lispro 1088
Humalog Mix 50 (AE, AU, BH, CY, IL, KW, LB, MY, QA, SA) *see* Insulin Lispro Protamine and Insulin Lispro 1088
Humalog Mix (AT, BE, CH, DE, DK, EE, ES, FR, GB, GR, HR, HU, IL, IS, LT, NO, PT, RO, RU, SE, SI, SK, TR, TW) *see* Insulin Lispro Protamine and Insulin Lispro 1088
Humalog Mix NPL (AT, BE, BG, CH, CZ, DE, DK, FI, FR, GB, GR, HN, IE, IT, NL, NO, PT, RU, SE, TR) *see* Insulin Lispro 1087
Humalog NPL (AE, BH, IL, KW) *see* Insulin Lispro Protamine and Insulin Lispro 1088
Huma-Metoprol (HU) *see* Metoprolol 1350
Human Albumin 5% (DE) *see* Albumin 67
Human Albumin 25% (DE) *see* Albumin 67
Huma-Nifedin (HU) *see* NIFEdipine 1451
Human Insulatard (IN) *see* Insulin NPH 1089
Human Protaphane (GB, IE) *see* Insulin NPH 1089
Human PTH (JP) *see* Teriparatide 2008
Huma-Pindol (HU) *see* Pindolol 1652
Huma-Purol (HU) *see* Allopurinol 90
Huma-Ranidine (HU) *see* Ranitidine 1777
Huma-Salmol (HU) *see* Albuterol 69
Huma-Sorbide (HU) *see* Isosorbide Dinitrate 1124
Huma-Spiroton (HU) *see* Spironolactone 1931
Humatin (AT, CH, DE, ES, IT) *see* Paromomycin 1579
Humatrope (AR, AU, BF, BJ, BR, CI, CL, ET, GB, GH, GM, GN, KE, LR, MA, ML, MR, MU, MW, MX, MY, NE, NG, PE, SC, SD, SL, SN, TN, TW, TZ, UG, ZA, ZM, ZW) *see* Somatropin 1918
Huma-Zolamide (HN, HU) *see* AcetaZOLAMIDE 39
Humegon (AR, BF, BJ, CI, DE, ET, GH, GM, GN, GR, HN, IN, IT, KE, KR, LR, LU, MA, ML, MR, MU, MW, NE, NG, SC, SD, SL, SN, TN, TZ, UG, ZA, ZM, ZW) *see* Menotropins 1292
Humexcough (BG) *see* Carbocisteine [INT] 357
Humex Fournier (FR) *see* Pholcodine [INT] 1646
Humex Nosni (CZ) *see* Phenylephrine (Systemic) 1638
Huminsulin 30/70 (IN) *see* Insulin NPH and Insulin Regular 1090
Huminsulin 50-50 (IN) *see* Insulin NPH and Insulin Regular 1090
Huminsulin Basal (CH) *see* Insulin Regular 1091
Huminsulin Basal (NPH) (CH, DE) *see* Insulin NPH 1089
Huminsulin "Lilly" Basal (NPH) (AT) *see* Insulin NPH 1089
Huminsulin Normal (AT) *see* Insulin Regular 1091
Humira (AE, AR, AT, AU, BE, BG, BH, BR, CH, CL, CN, CO, CY, CZ, DE, DK, EC, EE, EG, FI, FR, GB, GR, HK, HN, HR, HU, IE, IL, IQ, IR, IS, IT, JO, JP, KR, KW, LB, LT, LY, MT, MX, MY, NL, NO, NZ, OM, PE, PL, PT, PY, QA, RO, RU, SA, SE, SG, SI, SK, SY, TR, TW, UY, VE, VN, YE, ZA) *see* Adalimumab 51
Humoglob (PH) *see* Immune Globulin 1056
Humorap (PY) *see* Citalopram 451
Humoxal (FR) *see* Phenylephrine (Systemic) 1638
Humulin I (IT) *see* Insulin NPH 1089
Humulin 30 70 (AE, AU, CR, DO, GT, HN, MY, NI, PA, SV) *see* Insulin NPH and Insulin Regular 1090
Humulin 30/70 (CY, ID, IT, NZ, PE, SE) *see* Insulin NPH and Insulin Regular 1090
Humulin 60/40 (KR) *see* Insulin NPH and Insulin Regular 1090
Humulin 70/30 (BB, BS, BZ, CL, CN, CO, GY, HK, IL, JM, JO, KR, LB, MX, PH, SR, TH, TT, VE, VN) *see* Insulin NPH and Insulin Regular 1090

Humulin 70 30 (KW, PK, SA) *see* Insulin NPH and Insulin Regular 1090
Humulin 80/20 (KR) *see* Insulin NPH and Insulin Regular 1090
Humulin 90/10 (KR) *see* Insulin NPH and Insulin Regular 1090
Humulin M 70/30 (TR) *see* Insulin NPH and Insulin Regular 1090
Humulin M 80/20 (TR) *see* Insulin NPH and Insulin Regular 1090
Humulina 30:70 (ES) *see* Insulin NPH and Insulin Regular 1090
Humulina (ES) *see* Insulin NPH 1089
Humulina Regular (ES) *see* Insulin Regular 1091
Humuline 30 70 (BE) *see* Insulin NPH and Insulin Regular 1090
Humuline 30/70 (NL) *see* Insulin NPH and Insulin Regular 1090
Humuline NPH (BE) *see* Insulin NPH 1089
Humuline R (BE) *see* Insulin Regular 1091
Humulin M3 (LT, SI, SK) *see* Insulin NPH and Insulin Regular 1090
Humulin M3 (Mixture 3) (GB) *see* Insulin NPH and Insulin Regular 1090
Humulin N (AE, AU, BB, BF, BG, BH, BJ, BM, BR, BS, BZ, CI, CO, CR, CY, DO, EE, EG, ET, GH, GM, GN, GT, GY, HK, HN, HR, IL, IQ, IR, JM, JO, KE, KR, KW, LB, LR, LT, LY, MA, ML, MR, MU, MW, MX, MY, NE, NG, NI, NL, OM, PA, PE, PK, PY, QA, RO, SA, SC, SD, SI, SK, SL, SN, SR, SV, SY, TH, TN, TT, TZ, UG, UY, VE, VN, YE, ZA, ZM, ZW) *see* Insulin NPH 1089
Humulin NPH (DK, GR, PH, SE, TW) *see* Insulin NPH 1089
Humulin R (AE, AU, BG, BH, BM, BZ, CL, CN, CO, CR, CY, CZ, DO, EE, GT, GY, HK, HR, HU, ID, IL, IT, JO, KR, KW, LB, MX, MY, NI, NZ, PA, PE, PK, PY, QA, RO, SA, SE, SI, SK, SR, SV, TH, TR, VN) *see* Insulin Regular 1091
Humulin Regular (DK, FI, GR, PT, RU) *see* Insulin Regular 1091
Humulin S (GB) *see* Insulin Regular 1091
Humullin NPH (IS) *see* Insulin NPH 1089
Hurricaine (ES, LU) *see* Benzocaine 246
Hurricaine Gel (IL) *see* Benzocaine 246
Hurricane Spray (SG) *see* Benzocaine 246
Husimba (KR) *see* Simvastatin 1890
Hustentabs-ratiopharm (DE, LU) *see* Bromhexine [INT] 291
Hustosol (CH) *see* Bromhexine [INT] 291
Hu Tai (CN) *see* Naphazoline (Nasal) 1426
Hyalein (JP) *see* Hyaluronate and Derivatives 1006
Hyal Forte (KR) *see* Hyaluronate and Derivatives 1006
Hyalgan (AT, BE, BG, BH, CY, CZ, DK, ES, FI, FR, HR, HU, IS, IT, LB, LT, RO, SA, SI, SK) *see* Hyaluronate and Derivatives 1006
HYalgan (TR) *see* Hyaluronate and Derivatives 1006
Hyal (MY) *see* Hyaluronate and Derivatives 1006
Hyaludrop (KR) *see* Hyaluronate and Derivatives 1006
Hyanit (DE) *see* Urea 2114
Hyan (TH) *see* Levonorgestrel 1201
Hybloc (NZ) *see* Labetalol 1151
Hycamtin (AE, AR, AT, AU, BE, BG, BH, BR, CH, CL, CN, CY, CZ, DE, DK, EE, ES, FI, FR, GB, GR, HK, HN, HR, HU, IE, IL, IS, IT, JO, KR, KW, LB, LT, MT, MY, NL, NO, NZ, PH, PK, PL, PT, QA, RO, RU, SA, SE, SG, SI, SK, TH, TR, TW, UY, VE, VN) *see* Topotecan 2069
Hycephen (HK) *see* Acetaminophen and Tramadol 37
Hychlozide (TH) *see* Hydrochlorothiazide 1009
Hycodone (KR) *see* Hydrocodone and Acetaminophen 1012
Hycomin (KR) *see* Hydroxocobalamin 1020
Hycortil (PH) *see* Hydrocortisone (Systemic) 1013
Hycort (MY, PH) *see* Hydrocortisone (Systemic) 1013
Hydab (PH) *see* Hydroxyurea 1021
Hydac (FI, SE) *see* Felodipine 850
Hydal (AT) *see* HYDROmorphone 1016
Hydantin (FI) *see* Phenytoin 1640
Hydantoin (KR) *see* Phenytoin 1640
Hydantol (JP) *see* Phenytoin 1640
Hydarax (VN) *see* HydrOXYzine 1024
Hydcort (KR) *see* Hydrocortisone (Topical) 1014
Hyde (KR) *see* Hydrocortisone (Topical) 1014
Hydiphen (DE) *see* ClomiPRAMINE 475
Hydol (IE) *see* Dihydrocodeine, Aspirin, and Caffeine 632
Hydopa (AU) *see* Methyldopa 1332
Hydracort (LB, VN) *see* Hydrocortisone (Topical) 1014
Hydramine (TW) *see* DiphenhydrAMINE (Systemic) 641
Hydrapres (AR, ES) *see* HydrALAZINE 1007
Hydrazin (TW) *see* Isoniazid 1120
Hydrea (AU, BE, BG, BR, CL, CO, DK, EE, EG, ES, FI, GB, GR, HK, ID, IE, JP, KR, LU, MX, NL, NZ, PK, RU, SE, TH, TW, UY, VN, ZA) *see* Hydroxyurea 1021
Hydrene (AU, NZ) *see* Hydrochlorothiazide and Triamterene 1012
Hydrex (FI, JO) *see* Hydrochlorothiazide 1009
Hydrex (HK) *see* Chlorhexidine Gluconate 422
Hydrinate (MY) *see* DimenhyDRINATE 637
Hydrine (SG) *see* Hydroxyurea 1021
Hydro-Adreson Aquosum (BF, BJ, CI, ET, GH, GM, GN, KE, LR, MA, ML, MR, MU, MW, NE, NG, SC, SD, SL, SN, TN, TZ, UG, ZM, ZW) *see* Hydrocortisone (Systemic) 1013
Hydrochlorothiazidum (PL) *see* Chlorothiazide 426
Hydrochlorothiazidum (PL) *see* Hydrochlorothiazide 1009
Hydrochlorzide (MY) *see* Hydrochlorothiazide 1009
Hydrocobamine (NL) *see* Hydroxocobalamin 1020
Hydrocodin (HU) *see* Dihydrocodeine, Aspirin, and Caffeine 632
Hydrocortancyl (FR) *see* PrednisoLONE (Systemic) 1703
Hydrocort (IL) *see* Hydrocortisone (Systemic) 1013
Hydrocortison (DE) *see* Hydrocortisone (Systemic) 1013
Hydrocortisone Upjohn (FR) *see* Hydrocortisone (Systemic) 1013
Hydrocort (JO, KW, SG) *see* Hydrocortisone (Topical) 1014
Hydrocortone (AT, PT) *see* Hydrocortisone (Systemic) 1013
Hydroderm (SG) *see* Hydrocortisone (Topical) 1014
Hydrokortison (EE) *see* Hydrocortisone (Topical) 1014
Hydroksyetyloskrobia (PL) *see* Hetastarch 1004
Hydromedin (DE) *see* Ethacrynic Acid 797
Hydromedin i.v.[inj.] (DE) *see* Ethacrynic Acid 797
Hydromet (MX) *see* Hydrocodone and Homatropine 1013
Hydromol Intensive (GB) *see* Urea 2114
Hydromycin (TH) *see* Tetracycline 2017
Hydroquine (TW) *see* Hydroxychloroquine 1021
Hydroquin (TH) *see* Hydroxychloroquine 1021
Hydro-Saluric (GB, IE) *see* Hydrochlorothiazide 1009
Hydrosil (HK) *see* Aluminum Hydroxide, Magnesium Hydroxide, and Simethicone 104
Hydrotopic (PH) *see* Hydrocortisone (Systemic) 1013
Hydrotopic (PH) *see* Hydrocortisone (Topical) 1014
Hydroxo 5.000 (FR, LU) *see* Hydroxocobalamin 1020
Hydroxo-B 12 (AU) *see* Hydroxocobalamin 1020
Hydroxycarbamid (PL) *see* Hydroxyurea 1021
Hydroxyurea medac (PL, SE) *see* Hydroxyurea 1021
Hydrozide (HK, TH) *see* Hydrochlorothiazide 1009
Hydrozole (AU) *see* Clotrimazole (Topical) 488
Hyemex (PH) *see* Albendazole 65
Hyflex (PY) *see* Meloxicam 1283
Hyflox (TH) *see* Ofloxacin (Systemic) 1490

Hygroton (AE, AR, AT, AU, BB, BE, BF, BH, BJ, BM, BS, BZ, CH, CI, CY, CZ, DE, DK, EE, EG, ES, ET, FI, FR, GB, GH, GM, GN, GR, GY, HN, HU, ID, IE, IQ, IR, JM, JO, KE, KR, KW, LB, LR, LY, MA, ML, MR, MT, MU, MW, MY, NE, NG, NL, NO, NZ, OM, PL, PT, PY, QA, RU, SA, SC, SD, SE, SI, SK, SL, SN, SR, SY, TN, TR, TT, TZ, UG, YE, ZA, ZM, ZW) *see* Chlorthalidone 430
Hykor (PH) *see* Terazosin 2001
Hyles (TH) *see* Spironolactone 1931
Hylo-Comod (DE) *see* Hyaluronate and Derivatives 1006
Hymox (BH, JO, KW) *see* Amoxicillin 130
Hynorex Retard (DE) *see* Lithium 1230
Hyomide (PH) *see* Scopolamine (Systemic) 1870
Hyospasmol (ZA) *see* Scopolamine (Systemic) 1870
Hypace (PH) *see* Enalapril 722
Hypam (NZ) *see* Triazolam 2101
Hypen (JP) *see* Etodolac 815
Hyperab (QA) *see* Rabies Immune Globulin (Human) 1764
Hypercor (TH) *see* Bisoprolol 266
Hypercrit (BR, CL) *see* Epoetin Alfa 742
Hypergo (PH) *see* Perindopril 1623
Hyper HAES (DK, EE, FI, NO, SE) *see* Hetastarch 1004
HyperHEP B (HK, IL, NZ, TW) *see* Hepatitis B Immune Globulin (Human) 1002
Hyperhep (QA) *see* Hepatitis B Immune Globulin (Human) 1002
Hyperhes (AT, FR) *see* Hetastarch 1004
Hyperil (ID) *see* Ramipril 1771
Hyperil (KR) *see* Enalapril 722
Hyperlipen (BE, CH) *see* Ciprofibrate [INT] 441
Hypernol (SG) *see* Atenolol 189
Hyperphen (ZA) *see* HydrALAZINE 1007
Hyperrab S D (IL) *see* Rabies Immune Globulin (Human) 1764
Hyperrho-D (TW) *see* $Rh_o(D)$ Immune Globulin 1794
Hypersil (SG) *see* Lisinopril 1226
Hyperstat (BE, CZ, ES, HR, HU, LU, SE) *see* Diazoxide 616
Hyper-Tet (HK, KR) *see* Tetanus Immune Globulin (Human) 2015
Hypertet (IL, TW) *see* Tetanus Immune Globulin (Human) 2015
Hypertonalum (DE) *see* Diazoxide 616
Hyperzine (PH) *see* HydrALAZINE 1007
Hypetor (PH) *see* Metoprolol 1350
Hyphen (PH) *see* DiphenhydrAMINE (Systemic) 641
Hypher (CN) *see* Amoxicillin 130
Hypnofast (HK) *see* Midazolam 1361
Hypnogen (EE) *see* Zolpidem 2212
Hypnomidate (AT, BE, BG, BR, CH, CZ, DE, ES, FR, GB, GR, HR, IE, LU, MX, NL, PL, PT, PY, RU, SI, TR, TW, ZA) *see* Etomidate 816
Hypnotex (IN) *see* Nitrazepam [CAN/INT] 1461
Hypnovel (AU, BE, CO, CR, DO, FR, GB, GT, HN, IE, NI, NZ, PA, SV) *see* Midazolam 1361
Hypoca (CN, JP, TW) *see* Barnidipine [INT] 227
Hypodine (TH) *see* CloNIDine 480
Hypodol (AR) *see* Lornoxicam [INT] 1248
Hypolag (BB, BF, BJ, BM, BS, BZ, CI, ET, GH, GM, GN, GY, JM, KE, LR, MA, ML, MR, MU, MW, NE, NG, PR, SC, SD, SL, SN, SR, TN, TT, TZ, UG, ZM, ZW) *see* Methyldopa 1332
Hypoloc (DK, SE) *see* Nebivolol 1434
Hypomide (ZA) *see* ChlorproPAMIDE 429
Hypophos (IN) *see* Calcium Acetate 326
Hypopress (AE, BH, CY, EG, IQ, IR, JO, KW, LB, LY, OM, QA, SA, SY, YE) *see* Captopril 342
Hyposec (AE, BH, CY, EG, IQ, IR, JO, KW, LB, LY, OM, QA, SA, SY, YE) *see* Omeprazole 1508
Hypoten (AE, BH, CY, EG, IQ, IR, JO, KW, LB, LY, OM, QA, SA, SY, YE) *see* Atenolol 189
Hypotens (IL) *see* Prazosin 1703
Hypotensor (GR) *see* Captopril 342
Hypothiazid (HN, HU, RU) *see* Hydrochlorothiazide 1009
Hy-po-tone (ZA) *see* Methyldopa 1332
Hypovase (GB, IE) *see* Prazosin 1703
Hypozam (PH) *see* Midazolam 1361
Hypren (AT) *see* Ramipril 1771
Hypril (PH) *see* Enalapril 722
Hyprosin (NZ, TW) *see* Prazosin 1703
Hyron (HU) *see* Terazosin 2001
Hyruan (KR) *see* Hyaluronate and Derivatives 1006
Hysix (JP) *see* Pyridoxine 1747
Hyskon (DE) *see* Dextran 607
Hysone (KR) *see* Hydrocortisone (Systemic) 1013
Hysone (PK) *see* Hydrocortisone (Topical) 1014
Hyson (TW) *see* Hydrocortisone (Systemic) 1013
Hytacand (FR, PT) *see* Candesartan and Hydrochlorothiazide 338
Hytas (BR) *see* Methotrexate 1322
Hytaz (PH) *see* Hydrochlorothiazide 1009
Hythalton (IN) *see* Chlorthalidone 430
Hytinon (VN) *see* Hydroxyurea 1021
Hytisone (TH) *see* Hydrocortisone (Topical) 1014
Hytone Lotion (KR) *see* Hydrocortisone (Topical) 1014
Hytracin (JP) *see* Terazosin 2001
Hytrin (AU, BB, BE, BM, BS, BZ, CL, CN, CO, CY, CZ, EC, GB, GR, GY, HK, HU, ID, IE, IL, IN, JM, KR, LU, MX, MY, NL, NZ, PE, PH, PK, PL, PR, PT, RU, SR, TH, TR, TT, TW, UY, VE, VN) *see* Terazosin 2001
Hytrin BPH (CH) *see* Terazosin 2001
Hytrine (FR) *see* Terazosin 2001
Hytrinex (SE) *see* Terazosin 2001
Hytrol (IN) *see* Enalapril 722
Hytroz (ID) *see* Terazosin 2001
Hyzaar (AE, AU, BB, BH, BM, BS, BZ, CL, CN, CR, CY, CZ, EC, EG, FR, GR, GY, HK, HR, ID, JM, JO, KW, LB, MX, MY, NL, NZ, PA, PE, PH, PK, PL, QA, RO, SA, SG, SI, SK, SR, TH, TR, TT, TW, VE, VN) *see* Losartan and Hydrochlorothiazide 1250
Hyzaar DS (PH) *see* Losartan and Hydrochlorothiazide 1250
Hyzaar Forte (HK, SG, TW) *see* Losartan and Hydrochlorothiazide 1250
Hyzaar Plus (HK, SG) *see* Losartan and Hydrochlorothiazide 1250
Hyzan (HK) *see* Ranitidine 1777
Hyzin (PH) *see* Terazosin 2001
IAL (ID, MY) *see* Hyaluronate and Derivatives 1006
Ibabon (KR) *see* Ibandronate 1028
Ibaril (BG, DK, FI, NL, NO) *see* Desoximetasone 598
Ibef (KR) *see* Irbesartan and Hydrochlorothiazide 1112
Ibefro (KR) *see* Irbesartan 1110
Ibekacin (AR) *see* Dibekacin [INT] 616
Ibera (KR) *see* Irbesartan 1110
Ibesaa (TW) *see* Irbesartan 1110
Ibetan (KR) *see* Irbesartan 1110
Ibet (PY) *see* Ezetimibe 832
Ibiamox (AE, BH, CY, EG, IQ, IR, JO, KW, LB, LY, OM, QA, SA, SY, TH, YE) *see* Amoxicillin 130
Ibicar (PH) *see* Beclomethasone (Systemic) 230
Ibicyn (TW) *see* Tetracycline 2017
Ibilex (AU, NZ, TH) *see* Cephalexin 405
Ibimycin (AU) *see* Ampicillin 141
Ibrac (EC) *see* Ibandronate 1028
Ibufac (MY) *see* Ibuprofen 1032
Ibufen (IL, KR) *see* Ibuprofen 1032
Ibuflam (MX) *see* Ibuprofen 1032
Ibufug (DE) *see* Ibuprofen 1032
Ibugesic (IN, LB) *see* Ibuprofen 1032

Ibulgan (AE, BB, BF, BH, BJ, BM, BS, BZ, CI, CY, EG, ET, GH, GM, GN, GY, IL, IQ, IR, JM, JO, KE, KW, LB, LR, LY, MA, ML, MR, MU, MW, NE, NG, OM, QA, SA, SC, SD, SL, SN, SR, SY, TN, TT, TZ, UG, YE, ZM, ZW) *see* Ibuprofen 1032
Ibumetin (DK, FI, NL, NO, SE) *see* Ibuprofen 1032
Ibupirac (AR, CL) *see* Ibuprofen 1032
Ibuprofen (HK) *see* Ibuprofen 1032
Ibuprox (ES) *see* Ibuprofen 1032
Ibusal (FI) *see* Ibuprofen 1032
Ibustrin (AT, CZ, HR, IT, MX, PT) *see* Indobufen [INT]....1067
Ibustrin[inj.] (IT) *see* Indobufen [INT] 1067
Ibutin (GR) *see* Trimebutine [CAN/INT] 2103
Icacine (FR) *see* Dibekacin [INT] 616
Icaden (BR, CO, CR, DO, EC, GT, HN, NI, PA, PE, PY, SV, UY, VE) *see* Isoconazole [INT] 1120
Icaz LP (FR) *see* Isradipine 1130
Icaz SRO (PH) *see* Isradipine 1130
Iclofar (ID) *see* ValACYclovir 2119
I-Clom (PH) *see* ClomiPHENE 473
Iclusig (CH, CZ, DE, DK, EE, FR, GB, HR, LT, NL, NO, SE, SI, SK) *see* PONATinib 1680
Icomein (TW) *see* Itraconazole 1130
Icoplax (AR) *see* Vancomycin 2130
Icox (PH) *see* Celecoxib 402
Ictus (BR) *see* Carvedilol 367
Icubron (UY) *see* Bromhexine [INT] 291
Icupen (IN) *see* Doripenem 671
Icystein (TW) *see* Acetylcysteine 40
Idalon (JP) *see* Floctafenine [CAN/INT] 883
Idaman (ID) *see* Tretinoin (Topical) 2099
Idamycin (MX) *see* IDArubicin 1037
Idaptan (ES) *see* Trimetazidine [INT] 2104
Idarac (FR, PK, QA, TH, VN) *see* Floctafenine [CAN/INT] 883
Idaralem (MX, TH) *see* IDArubicin 1037
IDC (TH) *see* Indomethacin 1067
Idena (CR, DO, EC, GT, HN, NI, SV) *see* Ibandronate 1028
Idicin (IN) *see* Indomethacin 1067
Idom (DE) *see* Dosulepin [INT] 673
Idomethine (JP) *see* Indomethacin 1067
Idon (PE, PY) *see* Domperidone [CAN/INT] 666
Idotrim (SE) *see* Trimethoprim 2104
Idotyl (DK) *see* Aspirin 180
Idroxocobalamina (IT) *see* Hydroxocobalamin 1020
I (IE) *see* Trimethoprim 2104
Ifadex (MX) *see* Ifosfamide 1040
Ifa Fonal (MX) *see* Diazepam 613
Ifaxim (CO) *see* Rifaximin 1809
Ifiral (IN) *see* Cromolyn (Nasal) 514
Ifirmasta (HR) *see* Irbesartan 1110
Ifistatin (SG) *see* Simvastatin 1890
Ifloxin (PH) *see* Ciprofloxacin (Ophthalmic) 446
Ifloxin (PH) *see* Ciprofloxacin (Systemic) 441
Ifolem (MX, TH) *see* Ifosfamide 1040
Ifomida (MX) *see* Ifosfamide 1040
Ifomide (JP) *see* Ifosfamide 1040
Ifos (LB, PE, PY) *see* Ifosfamide 1040
Igantet (AR, CL, MY, SG) *see* Tetanus Immune Globulin (Human) 2015
Igantibe (ID) *see* Hepatitis B Immune Globulin (Human) 1002
IG Gamma (IL) *see* Immune Globulin 1056
Iglodep (ID) *see* Sertraline 1878
Ignis (IN) *see* Esomeprazole 771
IGRHO (IL) *see* Rh_o(D) Immune Globulin 1794
Igroton (IT) *see* Chlorthalidone 430
Ig Vena NIV (ID) *see* Immune Globulin 1056
Ihope (PH) *see* CloZAPine 490
Ikaclomin (IL) *see* ClomiPHENE 473
Ikacor (IL) *see* Verapamil 2154
Ikagen (ID) *see* Gentamicin (Systemic) 959
Ikamicetin (ID) *see* Chloramphenicol 421
Ikamoxil (ID) *see* Amoxicillin 130
Ikaphen (ID) *see* Phenytoin 1640
Ikapress (IL) *see* Verapamil 2154
Ikaprim (ID) *see* Sulfamethoxazole and Trimethoprim 1946
Ikaran (FR, LU, VN) *see* Dihydroergotamine 633
Ikaran LP (FR) *see* Dihydroergotamine 633
Ikium (AR) *see* Desvenlafaxine 598
Ikonaz (HR) *see* Itraconazole 1130
Ikorel (AU, DK, FR, GR, IE, NL, NZ, TR) *see* Nicorandil [INT] 1449
Iktorivil (SE) *see* ClonazePAM 478
Ilacen (TW) *see* Diflunisal 626
Ilaris (AR, AT, AU, BE, BR, CH, CY, CZ, DE, DK, EE, FR, GB, HK, HR, IL, JP, LT, NL, NO, NZ, PH, PL, PT, QA, SA, SE, SG, SI, SK, TR) *see* Canakinumab 335
Ildor (ES) *see* Nedocromil 1435
Ilefrin (ID) *see* Phenylephrine and Zinc Sulfate [CAN/INT] 1640
Iletin-R (IN) *see* Insulin Regular 1091
Ileveran (MX) *see* Enalapril 722
Ilevox (PH) *see* Levofloxacin (Ophthalmic) 1200
Ilgaper (BG) *see* Repaglinide 1791
Ilimit (EC, PE, PY, UY) *see* ARIPiprazole 171
Ilocet (PH) *see* PrednisoLONE (Ophthalmic) 1706
Ilocet (PH) *see* PrednisoLONE (Systemic) 1703
Ilomedin (CH, CY, GR, HR, HU, IL, NZ, PL, RO, SE, SI, TH, TR, TW, VN) *see* Iloprost 1046
Ilosone (BR, KR, MX, PH, VE) *see* Erythromycin (Systemic) 762
Iloticina (AR, CO) *see* Erythromycin (Topical) 765
Ilotycin T.S. (ZA) *see* Erythromycin (Topical) 765
Ilozef (PH) *see* CeFAZolin 373
Iltux HCT (EC) *see* Olmesartan and Hydrochlorothiazide 1498
IM-75 (AR) *see* Indomethacin 1067
Imacillin (DK, NO, SE) *see* Amoxicillin 130
Imadrax (DK) *see* Amoxicillin 130
Imarem (TR) *see* Imatinib 1047
Imavir (AE) *see* Acyclovir (Topical) 51
Imaxetil (PY) *see* Leflunomide 1174
I-Max (PH) *see* MetFORMIN 1307
Imazol (DE, EE, VE) *see* Clotrimazole (Topical) 488
Imbaron (KR) *see* Sulindac 1953
Imdex CR (MY, SG) *see* Isosorbide Mononitrate 1126
Imdex (HK, TH) *see* Isosorbide Mononitrate 1126
Imdur 60 (MX, TW) *see* Isosorbide Mononitrate 1126
Imdur (AE, BF, BH, BJ, CI, CY, DK, EE, ET, GB, GH, GM, GN, HK, ID, IE, KE, KW, LR, LU, MA, ML, MR, MU, MW, NE, NG, PH, PT, SA, SC, SD, SE, SG, SL, SN, TN, TR, TZ, UG, VN, ZM, ZW) *see* Isosorbide Mononitrate 1126
Imdur Durules (AU, KR) *see* Isosorbide Mononitrate 1126
Imediat N (UY) *see* Levonorgestrel 1201
Imefu (TW) *see* Isoconazole [INT] 1120
Imenam (TW) *see* Imipenem and Cilastatin 1051
Imepen (TH) *see* Imipenem and Cilastatin 1051
Imeson (DE) *see* Nitrazepam [CAN/INT] 1461
Imet (BF, BJ, CI, ET, GH, GM, GN, KE, LR, MA, ML, MR, MU, MW, NE, NG, SC, SD, SL, SN, TN, TZ, UG, ZM, ZW) *see* Indomethacin 1067
Imexa (MY) *see* Azithromycin (Systemic) 216
Imex (BG, DE, EE, KR, LT, TR, TW) *see* Tetracycline 2017
Imferon (AE, BH, CY, EG, IL, IQ, IR, JO, KW, LB, LY, OM, QA, SA, SY, TR, YE) *see* Iron Dextran Complex 1117
Imflac (AU) *see* Diclofenac (Systemic) 617
Imiclast (ID) *see* Imipenem and Cilastatin 1051
Imidakin (TW) *see* Ornidazole [INT] 1522
Imidex (MX) *see* Lansoprazole 1166
Imidol (JP) *see* Imipramine 1054

Imiggran (IS) *see* SUMAtriptan 1953
Imigran (AE, AT, AU, BB, BG, BH, BM, BR, BS, BZ, CH, CL, CY, CZ, DE, DK, EC, EE, EG, ES, FI, GB, GR, GY, HK, HN, HR, HU, IE, IT, JM, JO, KR, KW, LB, LT, MX, MY, NL, NO, NZ, PE, PH, PK, PL, PT, QA, RO, RU, SA, SE, SI, SK, SR, TH, TR, TT, TW, UY, VE, VN) *see* SUMAtriptan 1953
Imigrane (FR) *see* SUMAtriptan 1953
Imigran Nasal Spray (SA) *see* SUMAtriptan 1953
Imigran Radis (GB, IE) *see* SUMAtriptan 1953
Imiject (FR) *see* SUMAtriptan 1953
Imilanyle (JP) *see* Imipramine 1054
Imimine (TW) *see* Imipramine 1054
Imimore (PE) *see* Imiquimod 1055
Iminam (PH) *see* Imipenem and Cilastatin 1051
Iminen (MX) *see* Imipenem and Cilastatin 1051
Imine (TW) *see* Imipramine 1054
Imipen (PH) *see* Imipenem and Cilastatin 1051
Imiquad (VN) *see* Imiquimod 1055
Imitrex (BE, IL, LU) *see* SUMAtriptan 1953
Immucyst (AR, AT, AU, BE, BG, CH, CN, CO, CZ, DE, EC, EE, FR, GB, GR, HK, HN, HR, HU, IL, IT, KR, MY, NZ, PT, PY, RO, SG, SI, SK, TH, TR, TW, VN) *see* BCG 229
Immukine (BE, NL) *see* Interferon Gamma-1b 1104
Immukin (HK) *see* Interferon Gamma-1b 1104
Immunate (TH) *see* Antihemophilic Factor/von Willebrand Factor Complex (Human) 154
Immunine (DE, EE, SE, TH) *see* Factor IX (Human) 840
IMMUNOHBs (TH) *see* Hepatitis B Immune Globulin (Human) 1002
Immunorel (PH) *see* Immune Globulin 1056
Immuthera (KR) *see* AzaTHIOprine 210
Imnovid (BE, CH, CY, DE, DK, EE, ES, FI, FR, GB, HR, IE, IL, LT, NL, NO, SE, SI, SK, TR) *see* Pomalidomide 1677
Imocam (VN) *see* Irinotecan 1112
Imodiuduo (FR) *see* Loperamide and Simethicone 1237
Imodium Advanced (AU, NZ) *see* Loperamide and Simethicone 1237
Imodium (AE, AT, AU, BB, BE, BF, BG, BH, BJ, BM, BS, CH, CI, CN, CO, CY, CZ, DE, DK, EC, EE, EG, ET, FI, FR, GB, GH, GM, GN, GR, GY, HK, HR, HU, ID, IE, IL, IN, IQ, IR, IS, IT, JM, JO, KE, KW, LB, LR, LT, LU, LY, MA, ML, MR, MU, MW, MX, MY, NE, NG, NL, NO, NZ, OM, PE, PH, PK, PL, PR, PT, PY, QA, RO, RU, SA, SC, SD, SE, SG, SK, SL, SN, SR, SY, TH, TN, TR, TT, TW, TZ, UG, UY, VE, VN, YE, ZA, ZM, ZW) *see* Loperamide 1236
Imodium Comp (NO) *see* Loperamide and Simethicone 1237
Imodium Duo (NL) *see* Loperamide and Simethicone 1237
Imodium med simethicon (DK) *see* Loperamide and Simethicone 1237
Imodium Plus (AT, BE, CH, CZ, DE, FI, GB, GR, HK, IE, IL, PL, PT, RU, SE, TH, ZA) *see* Loperamide and Simethicone 1237
Imodonil (HK) *see* Loperamide 1236
Imogam (AU) *see* Rabies Immune Globulin (Human) 1764
Imogam Rabia (AR, PY) *see* Rabies Immune Globulin (Human) 1764
Imogam Rabies (BF, BG, BJ, CI, EE, ET, GH, GM, GN, KE, LR, MA, ML, MR, MU, MW, NE, NG, PH, SC, SD, SL, SN, TN, TZ, UG, ZA, ZM, ZW) *see* Rabies Immune Globulin (Human) 1764
Imojev (HK, PH, SG, TH) *see* Japanese Encephalitis Virus Vaccine (Inactivated) 1141
Imonox (TH) *see* Loperamide 1236
Imosec (BR) *see* Loperamide 1236
Imosen (TW) *see* Loperamide 1236
Imossel (FR) *see* Loperamide 1236
Imot Ofteno al (CR, DO, GT, HN, NI, PA, SV) *see* Timolol (Ophthalmic) 2043
Imovane (AR, AU, BB, BE, BM, BR, BS, BZ, CH, CL, CN, CO, CZ, DK, EE, EG, FI, FR, GR, GY, HK, HN, HU, IL, IS, IT, JM, KR, LT, LU, MX, MY, NL, NO, NZ, PL, RO, RU, SE, SG, SR, TR, TT, TW, UY, VE, VN) *see* Zopiclone [CAN/INT] 2217
Imovax d.T. Adult (EE) *see* Diphtheria and Tetanus Toxoid 645
Imovax DT (CY, IL) *see* Diphtheria and Tetanus Toxoid 645
Imovax Polio (AR, BE, BG, CN, CZ, EE, FI, HK, HN, HR, IL, IS, IT, KR, LT, NO, PE, PK, PY, RO, SK, TW, UY, VN) *see* Poliovirus Vaccine (Inactivated) 1673
Imovax Rabbia (IT) *see* Rabies Vaccine 1764
Imovax Rabia (UY) *see* Rabies Vaccine 1764
Imovax Rabies (PL) *see* Rabies Vaccine 1764
Imoxy (BR) *see* Imiquimod 1055
Impedil (AR) *see* Etamsylate [INT] 795
Imperan (AE, BH, CY, EG, IQ, IR, JO, KW, LB, LY, OM, PY, QA, SA, SY, TW, YE) *see* Metoclopramide 1345
Imperon (ES) *see* Ferrous Gluconate 870
Implanta (KR) *see* CycloSPORINE (Systemic) 522
Imprida (CZ, EE, HR, PT, SE) *see* Amlodipine and Valsartan 126
Impromen (BE, DE, IT, LU, NL) *see* Bromperidol [INT] 292
Impromen decanoas (BE, LU, NL) *see* Bromperidol [INT] 292
Impromen Tropfen (DE) *see* Bromperidol [INT] 292
Improntal (ES) *see* Piroxicam 1662
Impugan (DK, ID, SE) *see* Furosemide 940
Imrest (AU) *see* Zopiclone [CAN/INT] 2217
Imtack (IE) *see* Isosorbide Dinitrate 1124
Imtrate (NZ) *see* Isosorbide Mononitrate 1126
Imtrate SR (AU) *see* Isosorbide Mononitrate 1126
Imufor (AR, AT) *see* Interferon Gamma-1b 1104
Imukin (AE, AT, AU, BH, CH, CO, CY, CZ, DE, DK, EG, ES, FI, FR, GB, GR, IL, IQ, IR, IT, JO, KW, LB, LY, NO, OM, PL, QA, SA, SE, SG, SY, TW, YE) *see* Interferon Gamma-1b 1104
Imukin Inj. (NZ) *see* Interferon Gamma-1b 1104
Imulate (AU, NZ) *see* Mycophenolate 1405
Imunen (BR) *see* AzaTHIOprine 210
Imuprin (AE, BB, BF, BH, BJ, BM, BS, BZ, CI, CY, EG, ET, FI, GH, GM, GN, GY, HK, IQ, IR, JM, JO, KE, KW, LB, LR, LY, MA, ML, MR, MU, MW, NE, NG, OM, PR, QA, SA, SC, SD, SL, SN, SR, SY, TH, TN, TT, TW, TZ, UG, YE, ZM, ZW) *see* AzaTHIOprine 210
Imuprine (NZ) *see* AzaTHIOprine 210
Imuran (AE, AR, AU, BB, BD, BE, BF, BG, BH, BJ, BM, BS, BZ, CI, CL, CN, CO, CY, CZ, EC, EE, EG, ET, GB, GH, GM, GN, GR, GY, HK, HN, HR, HU, ID, IE, IL, IN, IQ, IR, JM, JO, JP, KE, KR, KW, LB, LR, LT, LU, LY, MA, ML, MR, MU, MW, MX, MY, NE, NG, NL, NZ, OM, PH, PK, PL, PT, PY, QA, RU, SA, SC, SD, SG, SI, SK, SL, SN, SR, SY, TH, TN, TR, TT, TW, TZ, UG, UY, VN, YE, ZM, ZW) *see* AzaTHIOprine 210
Imurek (AT, CH, DE) *see* AzaTHIOprine 210
Imurel (DK, ES, FI, FR, IS, NO, SE, VN) *see* AzaTHIOprine 210
Imusera (JP) *see* Fingolimod 879
Imusporin (CO, IN) *see* CycloSPORINE (Systemic) 522
Inacid (ES) *see* Indomethacin 1067
Inac (SG) *see* Diclofenac (Systemic) 617
Inac TR (SG) *see* Diclofenac (Systemic) 617
Inamid (ID) *see* Loperamide 1236
Inapsin (ZA) *see* Droperidol 695
Inavir (TH) *see* Indinavir 1066
Inbestan (JP) *see* Clemastine 459
Inbumed (MX) *see* Albuterol 69
Incardel (MX) *see* Acarbose 29
Incel (BR, PY) *see* CISplatin 448

Incidal (NL) *see* Mebhydrolin [INT] 1276
Incidal-OD (ID) *see* Cetirizine 411
Incivo (AR, AU, BE, BR, CH, CL, CO, CY, CZ, DE, DK, EE, FR, GB, HR, IE, IL, IS, LT, NL, NO, NZ, QA, RO, SA, SE, SI, SK, TR) *see* Telaprevir 1983
Inclovir (ID) *see* ValACYclovir 2119
Incoril (EC) *see* Diltiazem 634
Inco (TW) *see* Ketorolac (Systemic) 1146
Incremin con hierro (MX) *see* Pyridoxine 1747
Incremin con Hierro (MX) *see* Thiamine 2028
Incruse Ellipta (AU, CZ, EE, FI, GB, HR, IE, LT, NL, PT, SE, SI, SK) *see* Umeclidinium 2113
Indacin (PK) *see* Indomethacin 1067
Indaflex (MX) *see* Indomethacin 1067
Indalgin (TW) *see* Indomethacin 1067
Indalix (HK, MY, ZA) *see* Indapamide 1065
Indanet (MX) *see* Indomethacin 1067
Indanorm (AE, BH, KW, QA) *see* Indapamide 1065
Indapamide-Eurogenerics (LU) *see* Indapamide 1065
Indapamide-Generics (LU) *see* Indapamide 1065
Indapress (CL) *see* Indapamide 1065
Indap (RU) *see* Indapamide 1065
Ind Clav (TH) *see* Amoxicillin and Clavulanate 133
Indecin (TW) *see* Indomethacin 1067
Indenol (KR) *see* Propranolol 1731
Inderal (AE, AR, AT, AU, BB, BE, BF, BG, BH, BJ, BM, BR, BS, BZ, CH, CI, CO, CY, DK, EC, EG, ET, GH, GM, GN, GR, GY, HN, IE, IQ, IR, IT, JM, JO, KE, KR, KW, LB, LR, LU, LY, MA, ML, MR, MU, MW, MY, NE, NG, NL, NO, OM, PE, PH, PK, PT, PY, QA, SA, SC, SD, SE, SG, SI, SL, SN, SR, SY, TN, TT, TW, TZ, UG, UY, VE, VN, YE, ZM, ZW) *see* Propranolol 1731
Inderalici (MX) *see* Propranolol 1731
Inderal LA (AE, BB, BF, BH, BJ, BM, BS, BZ, CI, CY, EG, ET, GH, GM, GN, GY, IE, IQ, IR, JM, JO, KE, KW, LB, LR, LY, MA, ML, MR, MU, MW, NE, NG, OM, PE, PT, QA, SA, SC, SD, SL, SN, SR, SY, TN, TT, TZ, UG, YE, ZM, ZW) *see* Propranolol 1731
Inderm Gel (BE, DE) *see* Erythromycin (Topical) 765
Indesol (KR) *see* Propranolol 1731
Indevus Spinal Heavy (ID) *see* Bupivacaine 299
Indicarb (IN) *see* Procarbazine 1717
Indicardin (BF, BJ, CI, ET, GH, GM, GN, KE, LR, MA, ML, MR, MU, MW, NE, NG, SC, SD, SL, SN, TN, TZ, UG, ZM, ZW) *see* Propranolol 1731
Indicontin Continus (HK) *see* Indapamide 1065
Indilan (MX) *see* Indinavir 1066
Indiurex (PH) *see* Furosemide 940
Indivan (PY) *see* Indinavir 1066
Indivir (IN) *see* Indinavir 1066
Indobact (PY) *see* Amikacin 111
Indobene (CZ, HU, SK) *see* Indomethacin 1067
Indocap (IN, PK) *see* Indomethacin 1067
Indocap S.R. (IN) *see* Indomethacin 1067
Indocid (AE, AT, AU, BB, BF, BH, BJ, BR, BS, BZ, CH, CI, CY, EG, ET, FR, GH, GM, GN, GR, IQ, IR, JM, JO, KE, KW, LB, LR, LY, MA, ML, MR, MU, MW, MX, NE, NG, NO, OM, PE, PH, PT, QA, SA, SC, SD, SL, SN, SY, TN, TT, TZ, UG, VE, YE, ZM, ZW) *see* Indomethacin 1067
Indocid PDA (AU) *see* Indomethacin 1067
Indocid-R (NZ) *see* Indomethacin 1067
Indocin (BM) *see* Indomethacin 1067
Indocin I.V. (IL, KR) *see* Indomethacin 1067
Indocolir (DE, TR) *see* Indomethacin 1067
Indocollirio (IT) *see* Indomethacin 1067
Indocollyre (AT, BE, CZ, FR, HK, HU, IL, JO, KR, LB, NL, PL, PT, RU) *see* Indomethacin 1067
Indoflam Eye (IN) *see* Indomethacin 1067
Indofol (MX) *see* Propofol 1728
Indogesic (AE, BH, CY, EG, IQ, IR, JO, KW, LB, LY, OM, QA, SA, SY, YE) *see* Indomethacin 1067
Indolag (AE, BF, BH, BJ, BM, CI, CY, EG, ET, GH, GM, GN, GY, IQ, IR, JO, KE, KW, LB, LR, LY, MA, ML, MR, MU, MW, NE, NG, OM, PR, QA, SA, SC, SD, SL, SN, SR, SY, TN, TZ, UG, YE, ZM, ZW) *see* Indomethacin 1067
Indolgina (CR, DO, GT, HN, NI, PA, SV) *see* Indomethacin 1067
Indomecin (CO) *see* Indomethacin 1067
Indomed F (TH) *see* Indomethacin 1067
Indomee (SE) *see* Indomethacin 1067
Indomelan (AT) *see* Indomethacin 1067
Indomen (MY, SG) *see* Indomethacin 1067
Indomet (AR, EE) *see* Indomethacin 1067
Indometin (FI) *see* Indomethacin 1067
Indomin (AE, BH, CY, EG, IQ, IR, JO, KW, LB, LY, OM, QA, RU, SA, SY, YE) *see* Indomethacin 1067
Indono (TH) *see* Indomethacin 1067
Indoplant (ID) *see* Levonorgestrel 1201
Indopril (AU) *see* Perindopril 1623
Indopril (VN) *see* Imidapril [INT] 1051
Indoprin M (PY) *see* Glyburide and Metformin 974
Indorem (BM, GY, PR, SR) *see* Indomethacin 1067
Indorene (IT) *see* Indoramin [INT] 1070
Indosan (AE, BH, CY, EG, IQ, IR, JO, KW, LB, LY, OM, QA, SA, SY, YE) *see* Indomethacin 1067
Indo (SG) *see* Indomethacin 1067
Indosima (PY) *see* Indomethacin 1067
Indosyl Mono (AU) *see* Perindopril 1623
Indotecan (KR) *see* Irinotecan 1112
Indovis (IL) *see* Indomethacin 1067
Indoxen (HK) *see* Indomethacin 1067
Indoy (TW) *see* Indomethacin 1067
Indozu (TW) *see* Indomethacin 1067
Inductal (AR, LB) *see* Eszopiclone 793
Indurit (PY) *see* Spironolactone 1931
Induxin (ID) *see* Oxytocin 1549
Indylon (BF, BJ, CI, ET, GH, GM, GN, KE, LR, MA, ML, MR, MU, MW, NE, NG, SC, SD, SL, SN, TN, TZ, UG, ZM, ZW) *see* Indomethacin 1067
Inedol (PE) *see* Azithromycin (Systemic) 216
Inegy (AE, AT, BE, BH, CH, CY, CZ, DE, DK, EE, ES, FI, FR, GB, GR, HR, IE, IL, IT, LB, NL, NO, PT, QA, RU, SA, SE, TR) *see* Ezetimibe and Simvastatin 834
Inem (PY) *see* Imipenem and Cilastatin 1051
Inerson (ID) *see* Desoximetasone 598
Inexium (FR) *see* Esomeprazole 771
Infacalm (HK) *see* Ibuprofen 1032
Infadin (CZ) *see* Ergocalciferol 753
Infanrix (AE, AT, BB, BE, BG, BM, BS, BZ, GY, HR, IT, JM, MX, NL, RO, SE, SR, TT, TW) *see* Diphtheria and Tetanus Toxoids, and Acellular Pertussis Vaccine 649
Infanrix Hexa (AE, AR, AT, AU, BE, CH, CL, CY, CZ, DE, ES, GR, HK, HR, ID, IE, IL, IT, LB, MX, MY, NL, NZ, PE, PH, PL, PT, QA, RO, SA, SE, TH, TR, VE, ZA) *see* Diphtheria and Tetanus Toxoids, Acellular Pertussis, Hepatitis B (Recombinant), Poliovirus (Inactivated), and Haemophilus influenzae B Conjugate (Adsorbed) Vaccine [CAN/INT] 647
Infanrix IPV Hib (CY, LB, SA) *see* Diphtheria and Tetanus Toxoids, Acellular Pertussis, Poliovirus and Haemophilus b Conjugate Vaccine 648
Infanrix IPV + Hib (DE, MY, PH) *see* Diphtheria and Tetanus Toxoids, Acellular Pertussis, Poliovirus and Haemophilus b Conjugate Vaccine 648
Infanrix-IPV+Hib (HR, SG) *see* Diphtheria and Tetanus Toxoids, Acellular Pertussis, Poliovirus and Haemophilus b Conjugate Vaccine 648
Infanrix IPV-Hib (NZ) *see* Diphtheria and Tetanus Toxoids, Acellular Pertussis, Poliovirus and Haemophilus b Conjugate Vaccine 648
Infanrix IPV + HIB (PE) *see* Diphtheria and Tetanus Toxoids, Acellular Pertussis, Poliovirus and Haemophilus b Conjugate Vaccine 648

Infanrix-IPV/Hib (TH) *see* Diphtheria and Tetanus Toxoids, Acellular Pertussis, Poliovirus and Haemophilus b Conjugate Vaccine 648
Infanrix-IPV+HIB (VE) *see* Diphtheria and Tetanus Toxoids, Acellular Pertussis, Poliovirus and Haemophilus b Conjugate Vaccine 648
Infanrix Penta (AU, CY, GR, NL, NZ, SE) *see* Diphtheria, Tetanus Toxoids, Acellular Pertussis, Hepatitis B (Recombinant), and Poliovirus (Inactivated) Vaccine 651
Infasurf (IL, KR, SG) *see* Calfactant 334
Infectofos (DE) *see* Fosfomycin 932
Infectopedicul (DE) *see* Permethrin 1627
Infectoroxit (DE) *see* Roxithromycin [INT] 1853
Infectoscab (CZ) *see* Permethrin 1627
Infectotrimet (DE) *see* Trimethoprim 2104
Infectrim (PE) *see* Sulfamethoxazole and Trimethoprim 1946
Infeld (ID) *see* Piroxicam 1662
Infen (IN) *see* Dexketoprofen [INT] 603
Infergen (AT, BE, BG, CH, CZ, DE, DK, ES, FI, FR, GB, GR, HN, IE, IT, NL, NO, PL, PT, RU, SE, TR) *see* Interferon Alfacon-1 1100
Inflacor (CO) *see* Betamethasone (Systemic) 253
Inflalid (BR) *see* Nimesulide [INT] 1456
Inflamac (CH) *see* Diclofenac (Systemic) 617
Inflamene (BR, ID) *see* Piroxicam 1662
Inflammide (PE) *see* Budesonide (Systemic) 293
Inflanac (HK, MY, TH) *see* Diclofenac (Systemic) 617
Inflanefran (DE) *see* PrednisoLONE (Ophthalmic) 1706
Inflasic (PH) *see* Mefenamic Acid 1280
Inflaxen (CO) *see* Leflunomide 1174
Inflectra (RO) *see* InFLIXimab 1070
Influ-A (IL) *see* Amantadine 105
Influ (TW) *see* Amantadine 105
Infukoll M 40 (DE) *see* Dextran 607
Infukoll HES (PL) *see* Hetastarch 1004
Infusan M20 (ID) *see* Mannitol 1269
Ingafol (IN) *see* Folic Acid 919
Ingagen-M (IN) *see* Methylergonovine 1333
Ingelan (AT, DE) *see* Isoproterenol 1124
INH Agepha (AT) *see* Isoniazid 1120
Inhavir (CO) *see* LamiVUDine 1157
Inhibace (AE, AR, AT, AU, BE, BG, BH, CH, CL, CN, CO, CZ, EE, ES, FI, GR, HK, HN, HU, IT, JP, KR, KW, LB, NL, NZ, PE, PK, PL, PT, QA, SA, SE, SG, TR, TW, UY, VE, ZA) *see* Cilazapril [CAN/INT] 434
Inhibitron (MX) *see* Omeprazole 1508
Inhipraz (ID) *see* Lansoprazole 1166
Inhipump (ID) *see* Omeprazole 1508
Inhitril (ID) *see* Lisinopril 1226
INH Lannacher (AT) *see* Isoniazid 1120
INH Waldheim (AT) *see* Isoniazid 1120
Inibace (LU) *see* Cilazapril [CAN/INT] 434
Inigrin (MX) *see* Loratadine 1241
Inipomp (FR) *see* Pantoprazole 1570
Iniprol (BE, FR, IT, LU) *see* Aprotinin 168
Inisia (KR) *see* Ulipristal 2113
Injectafer (BE) *see* Ferric Carboxymaltose 868
Inj. Magnesii Sulfurici (PL) *see* Magnesium Sulfate 1265
Inj. natrii chlorati isotonica (PL) *see* Sodium Chloride 1902
Inkotan (HR, RO) *see* Trospium 2108
Inltya (IS) *see* Axitinib 207
Inlyta (AR, AU, BE, CH, CY, CZ, DE, DK, EE, ES, GB, HK, HR, JP, KR, LT, MY, NL, NO, NZ, RO, SE, SG, SI, SK, TR) *see* Axitinib 207
Inmatrol (ID) *see* Neomycin, Polymyxin B, and Dexamethasone 1437
Inmox (CO) *see* DULoxetine 698
Inmuderm (CO) *see* Imiquimod 1055
Inmunef (MX) *see* Filgrastim 875
Inmunobron (PY) *see* Montelukast 1392
Inmunoprin (CL, CO, EC, PE, UY) *see* Thalidomide 2022
Innocan (TW) *see* Irinotecan 1112
Innogem (HU) *see* Gemfibrozil 956
Innohep (AE, AR, BE, BG, BH, CO, DE, DK, EG, ES, FI, FR, GB, GR, HK, IE, IT, JO, KW, LB, LU, MY, NL, NO, NZ, PH, PK, PT, QA, RO, SA, SE, SG, SI, TH, TR, TW) *see* Tinzaparin 2043
innohep (CH) *see* Tinzaparin 2043
Innosfen (BR, PY) *see* Alfacalcidol [CAN/INT] 82
Innovace (GB, IE) *see* Enalapril 722
Innoxalon (JP) *see* Nalidixic Acid [INT] 1418
Innozide (GB, IE) *see* Enalapril and Hydrochlorothiazide 725
Inocar (ES) *see* Cilazapril [CAN/INT] 434
Inoderm (ID) *see* Fluocinolone (Topical) 893
Inoflox (PH) *see* Ofloxacin (Ophthalmic) 1491
Inoflox (PH) *see* Ofloxacin (Otic) 1491
Inomet (TR) *see* Indomethacin 1067
Inopan (VN) *see* DOPamine 669
Inopin (TH) *see* DOPamine 669
Inopril (AE, BH, CY, EG, IQ, IR, JO, KW, LB, LY, OM, QA, SA, SY, YE) *see* Lisinopril 1226
Inotop (AT) *see* DOBUTamine 654
Inotrex (GR, PT) *see* DOBUTamine 654
Inotrop (ID) *see* DOBUTamine 654
Inotropin (AR) *see* DOPamine 669
Inovad (ID) *see* Milrinone 1370
Inovan (JP) *see* DOPamine 669
Inovelon (AT, CH, CY, CZ, DE, DK, EE, FR, GB, GR, HN, HR, IE, IL, IS, IT, JP, KR, LT, NL, NO, PL, PT, RO, SE, SI, SK, TR) *see* Rufinamide 1854
Inox (HK, MY, PH) *see* Itraconazole 1130
Inpamide (TH) *see* Indapamide 1065
Inpanol (HK) *see* Propranolol 1731
Inpepsa (ID) *see* Sucralfate 1940
Inphalex (ID) *see* Cephalexin 405
Inprax (MX) *see* Oxybutynin 1536
Inpront (CL) *see* Moclobemide [CAN/INT] 1384
Inpura (KR) *see* Mometasone (Topical) 1391
Insaar (ID) *see* Losartan 1248
Inselon (TW) *see* Aminocaproic Acid 113
Inshel (TW) *see* Ferrous Sulfate 871
Insig (AU) *see* Indapamide 1065
Insigrel (ID) *see* Clopidogrel 484
Insogen (MX) *see* ChlorproPAMIDE 429
Insomed (PH) *see* Acetaminophen and Diphenhydramine 36
Insomin (FI) *see* Nitrazepam [CAN/INT] 1461
Insopin (MY) *see* Zopiclone [CAN/INT] 2217
Inspra (AE, AT, AU, BE, BG, CH, CO, CY, CZ, DE, DK, EE, FI, FR, GB, GR, HK, HN, HR, IE, IL, IS, KW, LT, MY, NL, NO, NZ, PL, PT, QA, RO, SE, SG, SI, SK, TR, TW) *see* Eplerenone 740
Inspra IC (MX) *see* Eplerenone 740
Instanyl (AT, BE, CZ, DE, DK, EE, FR, HR, IS, LT, NL, SE, SI, SK) *see* FentaNYL 857
Instanyl Nasal (GB, NO) *see* FentaNYL 857
Insugen R (TH) *see* Insulin Regular 1091
Insuget R (PH) *see* Insulin Regular 1091
Insulact Forte (PH) *see* Pioglitazone 1654
Insulact (PH) *see* Pioglitazone 1654
Insulatard (DK) *see* Insulin NPH 1089
Insulatard HM (AE, BE, BF, BH, BJ, CI, CY, EG, ET, GH, GM, GN, IL, IQ, IR, JO, KE, KW, LB, LR, LY, MA, ML, MR, MU, MW, NE, NG, OM, QA, SA, SC, SD, SL, SN, SY, TN, TW, TZ, UG, YE, ZA, ZM, ZW) *see* Insulin NPH 1089
Insulatard Innolet (FR) *see* Insulin NPH 1089
Insulina Humulin 70/30 (AR) *see* Insulin NPH and Insulin Regular 1090
Insulina Humulin (AR, CL) *see* Insulin NPH 1089

Insulina Humulin R (AR) *see* Insulin Regular 1091
Insulina Levemir (AR) *see* Insulin Detemir 1085
Insulina Novorapid (AR, UY) *see* Insulin Aspart 1083
Insuline Humuline NPH (NL) *see* Insulin NPH 1089
Insuline Insulatard (NL) *see* Insulin NPH 1089
Insuline Isuhuman Basal (NL) *see* Insulin NPH 1089
Insuline Lispro Humalog (FR) *see* Insulin Lispro 1087
Insulin Humalog (PL) *see* Insulin Lispro 1087
Insulin Insulatard HM (CH) *see* Insulin Regular 1091
Insulin Insulatard Human (DE, TH) *see* Insulin NPH 1089
Insulin Mixtard 30 HM (IL) *see* Insulin NPH and Insulin Regular 1090
Insulin "Novo Nordisk" Insulatard HM (AT) *see* Insulin NPH 1089
Insulin Protaphane HM (DE) *see* Insulin NPH 1089
Insuman 25 (IE) *see* Insulin NPH and Insulin Regular 1090
Insuman 50 (IE) *see* Insulin NPH and Insulin Regular 1090
Insuman Basal (DE, TH) *see* Insulin NPH 1089
Insuman Basal (IE) *see* Insulin Regular 1091
Insuman Comb 25 (CH, DE) *see* Insulin NPH and Insulin Regular 1090
Insuman Comb 30 (TH) *see* Insulin NPH and Insulin Regular 1090
Insuman Comb (CZ, EE, GB) *see* Insulin NPH and Insulin Regular 1090
Insuman (EC) *see* Insulin NPH 1089
Insuman (NO) *see* Insulin Regular 1091
Insuman R (CL) *see* Insulin Regular 1091
Insuman Rapid (TH) *see* Insulin Regular 1091
Insumed (PH) *see* MetFORMIN 1307
Insumin (JP) *see* Flurazepam 906
Intacape (TH) *see* Capecitabine 339
Intal (BR) *see* Cromolyn (Nasal) 514
Intapan (MY) *see* Nalbuphine 1416
Intard (AE, BH, KW, QA) *see* Diphenoxylate and Atropine 644
Intaxel (IN, JO, TH, TW, VN) *see* PACLitaxel (Conventional) 1550
Intazide (IN) *see* Balsalazide 226
Integrex (CO) *see* Reboxetine [INT] 1786
Integrilin (AE, AR, AT, AU, BE, BG, BH, CH, CN, CO, CY, CZ, DE, DK, EE, ES, FI, FR, GB, GR, HK, HN, HR, HU, ID, IE, IL, IS, IT, KW, LT, MT, MY, NL, NO, PH, PK, PL, PT, QA, RO, RU, SE, SG, SI, SK, TH, TR, TW) *see* Eptifibatide 751
Integrillin (VN) *see* Eptifibatide 751
Intelence (AR, AT, AU, BE, BR, CH, CL, CN, CO, CY, CZ, DE, DK, EC, EE, FR, GB, GR, HK, HN, HR, IE, IL, IS, IT, JP, KR, LT, MY, NL, NO, NZ, PE, PL, PT, QA, RO, RU, SA, SE, SG, SI, SK, TH, TR, TW) *see* Etravirine 821
Inteluz (PY, UY) *see* Piracetam [INT] 1661
Intensit (AR) *see* Modafinil 1386
Interac (PY) *see* Rosiglitazone and Metformin 1847
Interberin (AT) *see* Sargramostim 1865
Interbi (HK, ID) *see* Terbinafine (Systemic) 2002
Interbi (HK, ID) *see* Terbinafine (Topical) 2004
Interbutol (PH) *see* Ethambutol 798
Intercon (ID) *see* Mometasone (Topical) 1391
Interdoxin (ID) *see* Doxycycline 689
Interfam (HK) *see* Famotidine 845
Interflox (ID) *see* Ciprofloxacin (Ophthalmic) 446
Interflox (ID) *see* Ciprofloxacin (Systemic) 441
Interleukina II (CL) *see* Aldesleukin 72
Interleukina 2 (PY) *see* Aldesleukin 72
Intermax gamma (KR) *see* Interferon Gamma-1b 1104
Internol (MX) *see* Atenolol 189
Internolol (ID) *see* Atenolol 189
Interprim (ID) *see* Cefepime 378
Intesul (AR) *see* Mosapride [INT] 1401
Intocel (AR) *see* Cladribine 455
Intrafat (TW) *see* Fat Emulsion (Plant Based) 848
Intrafer (AR) *see* Iron Dextran Complex 1117
Intragam P (AU, HK, ID) *see* Immune Globulin 1056
Intraglobin (CH, DE, IT, TW) *see* Immune Globulin 1056
Intraglobin F (IL) *see* Immune Globulin 1056
Intralipid (AE, AU, BG, BH, CH, CY, CZ, DK, EE, EG, FI, HK, ID, IL, IN, IQ, IR, IS, JO, KW, LB, LT, LY, MY, NL, NO, NZ, OM, PH, QA, RU, SA, SE, SI, SK, SY, TH, TR, YE) *see* Fat Emulsion (Plant Based) 848
Intralipos (HK, KR, MY, TH, TW) *see* Fat Emulsion (Plant Based) 848
Intramed (ZA) *see* Ampicillin 141
Intrasept (CH) *see* Penicillin G Procaine 1613
Intrastigmina (IL, PT) *see* Neostigmine 1438
Intratect (GB, HK) *see* Immune Globulin 1056
Intraval (AE, BB, BH, BM, BS, BZ, CY, EG, GB, GY, IQ, IR, JM, JO, KW, LB, LY, OM, PR, QA, SA, SR, SY, TT, YE) *see* Thiopental [INT] 2029
Intraval Sodium (IN) *see* Thiopental [INT] 2029
Intrenon (CZ) *see* Naloxone 1419
Intril SR (TH) *see* Indapamide 1065
Intrinsa Patch (FR, IE) *see* Testosterone 2010
Introcin (CL) *see* Sulfamethoxazole and Trimethoprim 1946
Intron A (AE, AR, AT, AU, BE, BH, CH, CL, CN, CO, CR, CY, CZ, DE, DK, DO, EE, EG, ES, FI, FR, GB, GR, GT, HK, HN, HR, HU, IE, IL, IS, IT, JO, JP, KE, LT, MT, NI, NL, NO, NZ, PA, PE, PH, PK, PL, PT, QA, RO, RU, SA, SE, SI, SK, SV, TR, TW, VE, VN) *see* Interferon Alfa-2b 1096
Introna (AT, DK, FI, FR, NO, SE) *see* Interferon Alfa-2b 1096
Intron-A (GR, ID, MY, SG) *see* Interferon Alfa-2b 1096
Intropin IV (MY) *see* DOPamine 669
Intropin (GB, IE, UY, ZA) *see* DOPamine 669
Invanz (AE, AR, AT, AU, BE, BG, BH, BO, BR, CH, CL, CN, CO, CR, CY, CZ, DE, DK, DO, EC, EE, ES, FI, FR, GB, GR, GT, HK, HN, HR, HU, ID, IE, IL, IN, IS, IT, KR, LB, LT, MT, MX, MY, NI, NL, NO, NZ, PA, PE, PH, PL, PR, PT, PY, QA, RO, RU, SA, SE, SG, SI, SK, SV, TH, TR, TW, UY, VE, VN) *see* Ertapenem 760
Inveda (MX) *see* Paliperidone 1556
Inveda Sustenna (MX) *see* Paliperidone 1556
Invega (AE, AR, AT, AU, BE, BH, BR, CH, CN, CO, CY, CZ, DE, DK, EE, GB, GR, HK, HN, HR, ID, IE, IL, IS, IT, JP, KR, KW, LB, LT, MY, NL, NZ, PH, PL, PT, QA, RO, RU, SA, SE, SG, SI, SK, TH, TR, TW, VN) *see* Paliperidone 1556
Invega SR (KR) *see* Paliperidone 1556
Invega Sustenna (AU, BR, CN, HK, IL, MY, NZ, PH, SG, TH, TW) *see* Paliperidone 1556
Invert Plaster (KR) *see* Triamcinolone (Systemic) 2099
Invert Plaster (KR) *see* Triamcinolone (Topical) 2100
Inviclot (ID) *see* Heparin 997
Invidon (IN) *see* Trimetazidine [INT] 2104
Invidon-XR (IN) *see* Trimetazidine [INT] 2104
Invigan (EC) *see* Ornidazole [INT] 1522
Invirase (AE, AT, AU, BB, BE, BF, BH, BJ, BM, BS, BZ, CH, CI, CL, CN, CO, CY, CZ, DE, DK, EC, EE, ES, ET, FI, FR, GB, GH, GM, GN, GR, GY, HK, HN, HR, HU, IE, IL, IS, IT, JM, JP, KE, KW, LR, LT, LU, MA, ML, MR, MT, MU, MW, MY, NE, NG, NL, NO, PH, PL, PT, PY, QA, RO, RU, SC, SD, SE, SG, SI, SK, SL, SN, SR, TH, TN, TR, TT, TW, TZ, UG, UY, VN, ZA, ZM, ZW) *see* Saquinavir 1865
Invitec (ID) *see* Misoprostol 1379
Invomit (ID) *see* Ondansetron 1513
Invoril (AE, BF, BJ, CI, ET, GH, GM, GN, IN, KE, LR, MA, ML, MR, MU, MW, NE, NG, SC, SD, SG, SL, SN, TH, TN, TZ, UG, ZM, ZW) *see* Enalapril 722
Invozide (IN) *see* Enalapril and Hydrochlorothiazide 725
Inza (AU, HK) *see* Naproxen 1427
Inzolam (MY) *see* Triazolam 2101

Iobolin (BR) *see* Liothyronine 1221
Iobrim (IN) *see* Brimonidine (Ophthalmic) 288
Iodid (BE) *see* Potassium Iodide 1690
Iodure de Potassium (FR) *see* Potassium Iodide 1690
Ioduro Potasico Rovi (ES) *see* Potassium Iodide 1690
Iolvisc (LU) *see* Hyaluronate and Derivatives 1006
Ionamin (BE, IE, LU) *see* Phentermine 1635
Ionamine (CH) *see* Phentermine 1635
Ion-K (CO) *see* Potassium Gluconate 1690
Ionsys (AT, BE, BG, CH, CZ, DE, DK, EE, ES, FI, FR, GB, GR, HN, IE, IT, MT, NL, NO, PL, PT, RU, SE, SK, TR) *see* FentaNYL 857
Iopidine (AR, AT, AU, BE, BF, BG, BJ, BR, CH, DE, DK, ET, FI, FR, GB, GH, GM, GN, GR, HK, HN, IE, IL, IT, KE, KR, LR, LU, MA, ML, MR, MU, MW, MY, NE, NG, NL, NO, NZ, PE, PL, PT, PY, SA, SC, SD, SE, SG, SL, SN, TH, TN, TR, TZ, UG, VE, ZA, ZM, ZW) *see* Apraclonidine 165
Iopimax (ES) *see* Apraclonidine 165
Iosalide (IT) *see* Josamycin [INT] 1141
Ipamide (IN) *see* Ifosfamide 1040
Ipamix (IT) *see* Indapamide 1065
Ipaton (HU, RO) *see* Ticlopidine 2040
I-Patrimol (PE) *see* Ipratropium (Systemic) 1108
Ipentol (TW, VN) *see* Pentoxifylline 1618
Iperol Forte (TH) *see* Ipratropium and Fenoterol [CAN/INT] 1109
Iperol (TH) *see* Ipratropium and Fenoterol [CAN/INT] 1109
Iperten (FR, HU, IT) *see* Manidipine [INT] 1269
Iphox (PH) *see* Ifosfamide 1040
Ipnovel (IT) *see* Midazolam 1361
Ipolab (IT) *see* Labetalol 1151
Ipolipid (AE, BF, BH, BJ, CI, CY, EG, ET, GH, GM, GN, IL, IQ, IR, JO, KE, KW, LB, LR, LY, MA, ML, MR, MU, MW, MY, NE, NG, OM, QA, RU, SA, SC, SD, SG, SL, SN, SY, TN, TR, TZ, UG, YE, ZM, ZW) *see* Gemfibrozil 956
Ipol (NZ) *see* Poliovirus Vaccine (Inactivated) 1673
Iporel (PL) *see* CloNIDine 480
Ipradual (AR) *see* Ipratropium and Fenoterol [CAN/INT] 1109
Ipramol (MY) *see* Ipratropium and Albuterol 1109
Ipran (CL, CO) *see* Escitalopram 765
Ipranase AQ (IN) *see* Ipratropium (Nasal) 1109
Ipratec (PK) *see* Ipratropium (Systemic) 1108
Ipravent (IN) *see* Ipratropium (Systemic) 1108
Ipraxa (NO) *see* Ipratropium (Systemic) 1108
Ipren (DK, RU, SE) *see* Ibuprofen 1032
Iprestan (SG) *see* Irbesartan 1110
Ipreziv (EE, NL) *see* Azilsartan 214
Iprofen (PY) *see* Ketoprofen 1145
Iprolan (PH) *see* Ciprofloxacin (Systemic) 441
Ipron (TW) *see* Aminocaproic Acid 113
Iprovent (SG) *see* Ipratropium (Systemic) 1108
Iprox (ID) *see* Ibuprofen 1032
Iprubac (PH) *see* Ciprofloxacin (Systemic) 441
Ipsilon (AR, BR, JP, PY, UY) *see* Aminocaproic Acid 113
Ipstyl (DK, IT, NO) *see* Lanreotide 1165
Ipufen (TW) *see* Ibuprofen 1032
Iqfadina (MX) *see* Ranitidine 1777
Irahex (MY, PH) *see* Piracetam [INT] 1661
Iraxen (PE) *see* Naproxen 1427
Irazem (AR) *see* ARIPiprazole 171
Irazol (PH) *see* Naphazoline and Pheniramine 1426
Irbec (BG) *see* Irbesartan 1110
Irbenox (TH) *see* Irbesartan 1110
Irbeprex H (CO) *see* Irbesartan and Hydrochlorothiazide 1112
Irbesan (HR) *see* Irbesartan 1110
Irbesel (PE) *see* Irbesartan 1110
Irbetan (JP, TW) *see* Irbesartan 1110
Irbett (EC) *see* Irbesartan 1110
Irbezyd-H (PH) *see* Irbesartan and Hydrochlorothiazide 1112
Irbezyd (PH) *see* Irbesartan 1110
Irbosyd (ID) *see* Mebeverine [INT] 1275
Ircodon (KR) *see* OxyCODONE 1538
Ircos (PH) *see* Neomycin, Polymyxin B, and Hydrocortisone 1438
Ircovas (VN) *see* Irbesartan 1110
Irebeprex (CO) *see* Irbesartan 1110
Iremofar (GR) *see* HydrOXYzine 1024
Irenax (TW) *see* Irinotecan 1112
Iressa (AE, AR, AU, BE, BH, BR, CH, CL, CN, CO, CR, CY, CZ, DE, DK, DO, EE, FR, GB, GR, GT, HK, HN, HR, ID, IE, IL, IS, KR, KW, LB, LT, MY, NI, NL, NO, NZ, PA, PE, PH, PL, QA, RO, RU, SE, SG, SI, SK, SV, TH, TR, TW, VE, VN) *see* Gefitinib [CAN/INT] 950
Iretensa (ID) *see* Irbesartan 1110
Iretien (PY) *see* Fusidic Acid (Topical) [CAN/INT] 943
Irfen (AE, BH, CH, CY, EG, IQ, IR, JO, KW, LB, LY, OM, QA, SA, SY, YE) *see* Ibuprofen 1032
Irican (PH) *see* Irinotecan 1112
Iridus (AR) *see* Naftidrofuryl [INT] 1416
Iridux (BR) *see* Naftidrofuryl [INT] 1416
Iridux F200 (BR) *see* Naftidrofuryl [INT] 1416
Irifone (GR) *see* Etofenamate [INT] 815
Irifrin (RU) *see* Phenylephrine (Systemic) 1638
Irinocyt (CO) *see* Irinotecan 1112
Irinogen (EC, PY) *see* Irinotecan 1112
Irinoll (TH) *see* Irinotecan 1112
Irinotel (IN, JO, TH, TW) *see* Irinotecan 1112
Irinotesin (HK, PH, SG, TH) *see* Irinotecan 1112
Irino (TH) *see* Irinotecan 1112
Iritecan (KR) *see* Irinotecan 1112
Irizz. (MX) *see* ALPRAZolam 94
Irnocam (MY) *see* Irinotecan 1112
Ironax (IT) *see* Ferrous Gluconate 870
Iroplex (AR) *see* Cinnarizine [INT] 440
Irovel-H (IN) *see* Irbesartan and Hydrochlorothiazide 1112
Irovel (IN) *see* Irbesartan 1110
Iroviton Calcium (AT) *see* Calcium Carbonate 327
Irprestan (HK) *see* Irbesartan 1110
Irribow (JP, KR, TH) *see* Ramosetron [INT] 1774
Irrigor (CL) *see* Flunarizine [CAN/INT] 892
Irrigor (PE) *see* NiMODipine 1456
Irta (KR) *see* Itraconazole 1130
Irtan (DE, MX) *see* Nedocromil 1435
Irtan (ID) *see* Irbesartan 1110
Irtan Plus (ID) *see* Irbesartan and Hydrochlorothiazide 1112
Irumed (HR) *see* Lisinopril 1226
Iruxol Mono (BE, BR, CH, CZ, FI, GR, ZA) *see* Collagenase (Topical) 507
Iruxol (PY, VE) *see* Collagenase (Topical) 507
Iruxol Simplex (CO, EC, PE) *see* Collagenase (Topical) 507
Irvebal (ID) *see* Irbesartan 1110
Irvell (ID) *see* Irbesartan 1110
Irwax (PH) *see* Docusate 661
Isabelle (AU) *see* Ethinyl Estradiol and Drospirenone 801
Iscotin (TW) *see* Isoniazid 1120
Iscover (AR, AT, AU, BE, BG, BR, CH, CZ, DE, DK, EE, ES, FR, GB, GR, HR, IE, IT, LT, MT, NO, PL, PT, RO, RU, SE, SK, TR) *see* Clopidogrel 484
ISDN AL (HU) *see* Isosorbide Dinitrate 1124
ISDN (DE) *see* Isosorbide Dinitrate 1124
ISDN-Q (HU) *see* Isosorbide Dinitrate 1124
ISDN-ratiopharm (LU) *see* Isosorbide Dinitrate 1124
Iselpin (PH) *see* Sucralfate 1940
Isentress (AE, AR, AU, BE, BR, CH, CL, CN, CO, CY, CZ, DE, DK, EC, EE, FR, GB, GR, HK, HN, HR, IE, IL, IS, IT, JP, KR, KW, LT, MY, NL, NO, NZ, PE, PL, PT, QA,

RO, SE, SG, SI, SK, TH, TR, TW, UY) *see* Raltegravir ... 1767
Isepacin (AT, IT, JP, MX, PT) *see* Isepamicin [INT] ... 1120
Isepacine (BE) *see* Isepamicin [INT] ... 1120
Isepalline (FR) *see* Isepamicin [INT] ... 1120
Isipen (HR, PL) *see* Piperacillin [CAN/INT] ... 1656
Iski (IN) *see* Diltiazem ... 634
Islotin (AR) *see* MetFORMIN ... 1307
Ismexin (FI) *see* Isosorbide Mononitrate ... 1126
ISMN AL (HU) *see* Isosorbide Mononitrate ... 1126
ISMN (AT, DE) *see* Isosorbide Mononitrate ... 1126
ISMN Genericon (HR) *see* Isosorbide Mononitrate ... 1126
ISMN Pharmavit (HU) *see* Isosorbide Mononitrate ... 1126
Ismo 20 (BB, BM, BS, BZ, GY, IN, JM, MY, NZ, PR, SR, TH, TT, TW, ZA) *see* Isosorbide Mononitrate ... 1126
Ismo-20 (BF, BJ, CI, ET, GH, GM, GN, KE, LR, MA, ML, MR, MU, MW, NE, NG, SC, SD, SL, SN, TN, TZ, UG, ZM, ZW) *see* Isosorbide Mononitrate ... 1126
ISMO (CL, DK, EG, GB, IE, IS, IT, NL, SE) *see* Isosorbide Mononitrate ... 1126
Ismo (AE, BH, LU, QA, SA) *see* Isosorbide Mononitrate ... 1126
Ismox (FI) *see* Isosorbide Mononitrate ... 1126
Isoamitil Sedante (ES) *see* Amobarbital ... 128
Isobide (TW) *see* Isosorbide Dinitrate ... 1124
Isobid (KR) *see* Isosorbide Mononitrate ... 1126
Isobinate (TH) *see* Isosorbide Dinitrate ... 1124
Isocaine 3% (IL) *see* Mepivacaine ... 1295
Isocaine (QA) *see* Mepivacaine ... 1295
Isocard (HR) *see* Isosorbide Mononitrate ... 1126
Isocard (LU) *see* Isosorbide Dinitrate ... 1124
Isocard Retard (AE, BH, CY, EG, IQ, IR, JO, KW, LB, LY, OM, QA, SA, SY, YE) *see* Isosorbide Dinitrate ... 1124
Isocon (PK) *see* Isoconazole [INT] ... 1120
Isocord (CO) *see* Isosorbide Dinitrate ... 1124
Isoday 40 (AE, BH, CY, EG, IQ, IR, JO, KW, LB, LY, OM, QA, SA, SY, YE) *see* Isosorbide Dinitrate ... 1124
Iso-Dexter (ES) *see* Isoniazid ... 1120
Isodinit (LU, RO) *see* Isosorbide Dinitrate ... 1124
Isodol (IT) *see* Nimesulide [INT] ... 1456
Isoface (DO, EC, GT, MX, PA, PE, PY, SV) *see* ISOtretinoin ... 1127
Isofem (EC) *see* Calcium Carbonate ... 327
Isofra (RU) *see* Framycetin [INT] ... 937
Isogen (IL) *see* Isoconazole [INT] ... 1120
Isoglaucon (ES, HU) *see* CloNIDine ... 480
Isoket (AE, AR, BG, CH, CN, CY, CZ, DE, EE, HK, HU, ID, IE, IL, JO, KW, LU, MY, PH, PL, PY, RU, SA, SG, TR, UY, VE, VN) *see* Isosorbide Dinitrate ... 1124
Isoket Retard (AE, CH, CZ, DE, EG, GB, HK, IN, KR, KW) *see* Isosorbide Dinitrate ... 1124
Isoket Spray (KR) *see* Isosorbide Dinitrate ... 1124
Isokin (IN) *see* Isoniazid ... 1120
Isoklon (CO) *see* Eszopiclone ... 793
Iso-Lacer (ES) *see* Isosorbide Dinitrate ... 1124
Isolan (AR) *see* Isosorbide Mononitrate ... 1126
Isolin (IN) *see* Isoproterenol ... 1124
Isolone (KR) *see* Diflucortolone [CAN/INT] ... 625
Isomack (AT, HU, LU, VN) *see* Isosorbide Dinitrate ... 1124
Iso Mack (CH, HU) *see* Isosorbide Dinitrate ... 1124
Iso Mack Retard (AE, BH, CY, EG, IQ, IR, JO, KW, LB, LY, OM, QA, SA, SY, YE) *see* Isosorbide Dinitrate ... 1124
Isomack Spray (KR) *see* Isosorbide Dinitrate ... 1124
Isomel (IE) *see* Isoproterenol ... 1124
Isomenyl (JP) *see* Isoproterenol ... 1124
Isomerine (AR) *see* Dexchlorpheniramine ... 603
Isomonat (AT, CZ) *see* Isosorbide Mononitrate ... 1126
Isomon (GR) *see* Isosorbide Mononitrate ... 1126
Isomonit (AU, DE, LU, PL) *see* Isosorbide Mononitrate ... 1126
Isomonit Retard (VN) *see* Isosorbide Mononitrate ... 1126
Isomytal (JP) *see* Amobarbital ... 128
Isonate (PH) *see* Isosorbide Mononitrate ... 1126
Isonazol (KR) *see* Isoconazole [INT] ... 1120
Isonefrine (PK) *see* Phenylephrine (Systemic) ... 1638
Isonep H (PH) *see* Neomycin, Polymyxin B, and Hydrocortisone ... 1438
Isonex (ID, IN) *see* Isoniazid ... 1120
Isoniac (AR) *see* Isoniazid ... 1120
Isoniazid Atlantic (HK) *see* Isoniazid ... 1120
Isoniazid (AU, NZ) *see* Isoniazid ... 1120
Isoniazide Drank FNA (NL) *see* Isoniazid ... 1120
Isoniazidum (PL) *see* Isoniazid ... 1120
Isoniazid "Dak" (DK) *see* Isoniazid ... 1120
Isoniazid "Oba" (DK) *see* Isoniazid ... 1120
Isonicid (HN) *see* Isoniazid ... 1120
Isopen-20 (TH) *see* Isosorbide Mononitrate ... 1126
Isoprenalina Cloridrato (IT) *see* Isoproterenol ... 1124
Isoprenalinhydrochlorid-Braun (LU) *see* Isoproterenol ... 1124
Isoprenalin (NO, SE) *see* Isoproterenol ... 1124
Isoptin (AE, AT, AU, BG, BH, CH, CO, CY, CZ, DE, DK, EC, EE, EG, FI, GR, HK, HR, HU, IE, IT, JO, KR, KW, LB, LU, MY, NL, NO, NZ, PE, PH, PK, PL, PT, QA, RO, RU, SA, SE, SG, SI, SK, TR, TW, VN, ZA) *see* Verapamil ... 2154
Isoptine (BE, FR) *see* Verapamil ... 2154
Isoptino (AR, PY, UY) *see* Verapamil ... 2154
Isoptin Retard (AT, CH, CR, DE, DO, EE, FI, GR, GT, HN, IS, IT, LT, NI, PA, PL, PT, SE, SV) *see* Verapamil ... 2154
Isoptin RR (HR, RO, SI) *see* Verapamil ... 2154
Isoptin SR (AE, AU, BG, BH, CN, CY, CZ, EG, HK, ID, JO, KR, KW, LB, NL, NZ, QA, SA, SG, SK, TW, ZA) *see* Verapamil ... 2154
Isopto Atropina (AR, CO, EC, PE, PY) *see* Atropine ... 200
Isopto Atropine (AE, BE, BF, BH, BJ, CI, CY, EG, ET, GH, GM, GN, IE, IQ, IR, JO, KE, KR, KW, LB, LR, LY, MA, ML, MR, MU, MW, MY, NE, NG, OM, PH, PK, QA, SA, SC, SD, SL, SN, SY, TH, TN, TZ, UG, YE, ZA, ZM, ZW) *see* Atropine ... 200
Isopto Atropin (SE) *see* Atropine ... 200
Isopto B12 (ES) *see* Cyanocobalamin ... 515
Isopto-Biotic (SE) *see* Polymyxin B ... 1676
Isopto Carbachol (AE, AU, BF, BH, BJ, CI, CY, DE, EG, ET, GB, GH, GM, GN, HR, IQ, IR, JO, KE, KW, LB, LR, LU, LY, MA, ML, MR, MU, MW, NE, NG, OM, QA, SA, SC, SD, SL, SN, SY, TN, TZ, UG, YE, ZA, ZM, ZW) *see* Carbachol ... 346
Isopto-Carbachol (FI, IE) *see* Carbachol ... 346
Isopto Carpina (AR, CO, PE, PY, UY, VE) *see* Pilocarpine (Ophthalmic) ... 1649
Isopto Carpine (AE, AU, BE, BF, BH, BJ, CI, CY, EE, EG, ET, FI, GH, GM, GN, GR, HK, HN, IE, IQ, IR, IS, JO, KE, KW, LB, LR, LY, MA, ML, MR, MU, MW, NE, NG, NL, NO, OM, PH, PL, QA, SA, SC, SD, SG, SL, SN, SY, TH, TN, TW, TZ, UG, YE, ZM, ZW) *see* Pilocarpine (Ophthalmic) ... 1649
Isopto-Carpine (VN) *see* Pilocarpine (Ophthalmic) ... 1649
Isopto Cetamide (AE, BE, BH, CY, EG, IQ, IR, JO, KW, LB, LY, OM, QA, SA, SY, YE) *see* Sulfacetamide (Ophthalmic) ... 1943
Isopto-Dex (DE) *see* Dexamethasone (Ophthalmic) ... 602
Isopto Fenicol (AE, AR, BH, CY, EG, IQ, IR, JO, KW, LB, LY, OM, PY, QA, SA, SY, YE) *see* Chloramphenicol ... 421
Isopto Flucon (ES) *see* Fluorometholone ... 896
Isopto Frin (AU, EC) *see* Phenylephrine (Systemic) ... 1638
Isopto (GB) *see* Atropine ... 200
Isopto Homatropine (AE, AU, BF, BH, BJ, CI, CY, EG, ET, FR, GH, GM, GN, IL, IQ, IR, JO, KE, KW, LB, LR, LY, MA, ML, MR, MU, MW, MY, NE, NG, NZ, OM, QA, SA, SC, SD, SL, SN, SY, TN, TZ, UG, YE, ZA, ZM, ZW) *see* Homatropine ... 1005

Isopto-Homatropine (BF, BJ, CI, ET, GH, GM, GN, KE, LR, MA, ML, MR, MU, MW, NE, NG, SC, SD, SL, SN, TN, TZ, UG, ZA, ZM, ZW) *see* Homatropine 1005
Isopto Karbakolin (SE) *see* Carbachol 346
Isopto-Maxidex (AR, CO, NO, PY) *see* Dexamethasone (Ophthalmic) 602
Isopto Maxitrol (GR) *see* Neomycin, Polymyxin B, and Dexamethasone 1437
Isopto Pilocarpina (CL) *see* Pilocarpine (Ophthalmic) 1649
Isopto Pilocarpine (FR) *see* Pilocarpine (Ophthalmic) 1649
Iso-Puren (DE) *see* Isosorbide Dinitrate 1124
Isorat (TR) *see* Isosorbide Mononitrate 1126
Isorbid (MX) *see* Isosorbide Dinitrate 1124
Isorbide (PE) *see* Isosorbide Dinitrate 1124
Isordil (AE, AR, AU, BH, BR, CY, EG, HN, ID, IE, IL, IN, IQ, IR, JO, KW, LB, LU, LY, NL, OM, PH, PK, PY, QA, SA, SY, TR, YE, ZA) *see* Isosorbide Dinitrate 1124
Isorem (TR) *see* Isosorbide Dinitrate 1124
Isore (PH) *see* Neomycin, Polymyxin B, and Dexamethasone 1437
Isoric (ID) *see* Allopurinol 90
Isosorbide (CY, HR) *see* Isosorbide Mononitrate 1126
Isospan SR (HU) *see* Isosorbide Mononitrate 1126
Isotane (TH) *see* ISOtretinoin 1127
Isoten (BE) *see* Bisoprolol 266
Isotera (TW) *see* DOCEtaxel 656
Isotic Adretor (ID) *see* Timolol (Ophthalmic) 2043
Isotic Tobryne (ID) *see* Tobramycin (Ophthalmic) 2056
Isotina (KR) *see* ISOtretinoin 1127
Isotinon (KR) *see* ISOtretinoin 1127
Isotol (IT) *see* Mannitol 1269
Isotonax (LU) *see* Isosorbide Dinitrate 1124
Isotren (KR) *see* ISOtretinoin 1127
Isotret-Hexal (DE) *see* ISOtretinoin 1127
Isotrex (AE, AU, BH, BR, CL, CR, CY, DK, GB, ID, IE, LU, MX, NI, PK, QA, SA, SG, TW) *see* ISOtretinoin 1127
Isotrex Gel (CO, DE, FR, HK, IL, IT, MY, NZ, PH, PL, TH) *see* ISOtretinoin 1127
Isotril ER (KR) *see* Isosorbide Mononitrate 1126
Isotrim (IT) *see* Sulfamethoxazole and Trimethoprim 1946
Isotroin (IN) *see* ISOtretinoin 1127
Isovorin (AT, CH, DK, FI, GB, GR, IS, NL, NO, PT, SE, ZA) *see* LEVOleucovorin 1200
Isox (DO, GT, HN, MX, PA, SV) *see* Itraconazole 1130
Isozid (DE) *see* Isoniazid 1120
Isozide (VN) *see* Isoniazid 1120
Ispidon (PE) *see* RisperiDONE 1818
Israel (IL) *see* Axitinib 207
Istalol (BM) *see* Timolol (Ophthalmic) 2043
Istam-Far (GR) *see* Cyproheptadine 529
Istin (GB, IE) *see* AmLODIPine 123
Istodax (AU, KR) *see* RomiDEPsin 1841
Istonil (PY) *see* Carbidopa and Levodopa 351
Istopril (TR) *see* Enalapril 722
Isuprel (EG, HU, LU) *see* Isoproterenol 1124
Isuprel HCl (BE, FR, HK, KR, TH) *see* Isoproterenol 1124
Isuprel Inj (AU, NZ) *see* Isoproterenol 1124
Isupril (JO) *see* Isoproterenol 1124
Italcefal (EC) *see* Cephalexin 405
Italconazol (EC) *see* Econazole 703
Itan (CL) *see* Metoclopramide 1345
Itapleno (MX) *see* Azelastine (Ophthalmic) 213
Itcozol (NZ) *see* Itraconazole 1130
Iterax (ID, PH) *see* HydrOXYzine 1024
Itiflox (PH) *see* Gatifloxacin 949
Itoprid (AR, IN) *see* Itopride [INT] 1130
Itrac (HR) *see* Itraconazole 1130
Itracon (HK, KR, SG, TH) *see* Itraconazole 1130
Itrafung (EC) *see* Itraconazole 1130
Itragen (CO) *see* Itraconazole 1130
Itranax (MX) *see* Itraconazole 1130
Itranol (IL) *see* Itraconazole 1130
Itrasix (TH) *see* Itraconazole 1130
Itraspor (TR) *see* Itraconazole 1130
Itra (TH) *see* Itraconazole 1130
Itrazole (NZ) *see* Itraconazole 1130
Itrin (AE, BH, EG, IT, JO, KW, LB, QA, SA) *see* Terazosin 2001
Itrizole (JP) *see* Itraconazole 1130
Itzodial (KR) *see* Itopride [INT] 1130
Itzol (ID) *see* Itraconazole 1130
Ivadal (AT) *see* Zolpidem 2212
Ivanes (ID) *see* Ketamine 1143
Ivemend (BE, CH, CZ, DE, DK, EE, FR, GB, GR, HR, IE, LT, NL, NO, PT, RO, SE, SI, SK, TR) *see* Fosaprepitant 929
Ivermectol (IN) *see* Ivermectin (Systemic) 1136
Ivermin (EC) *see* Ivermectin (Systemic) 1136
Ivertal (AR) *see* Ivermectin (Systemic) 1136
Iverx (CL) *see* Ivermectin (Systemic) 1136
Ivetra (PH) *see* LevETIRAcetam 1191
Ivexterm (CR, DO, GT, HN, MX, NI, PA, SV) *see* Ivermectin (Systemic) 1136
IV Globulin-S (KR) *see* Immune Globulin 1056
I.V.-Globulin SN (PH) *see* Immune Globulin 1056
IVheBex (FR, GR) *see* Hepatitis B Immune Globulin (Human) 1002
Ivomec (CH) *see* Ivermectin (Systemic) 1136
Ivracain (CH) *see* Chloroprocaine 423
Iwacillin (JP) *see* Ampicillin 141
Ixel (AE, AT, BG, BH, CO, CZ, EE, FI, FR, IL, KW, LB, PL, PT, QA, RU, TR, VN) *see* Milnacipran 1368
Ixempra (AR, CH, CL, CO, FR, IL, IN, KR, NZ, SG, TH, TW) *see* Ixabepilone 1138
Ixemprya (PE) *see* Ixabepilone 1138
Ixiaro (DE, DK, EE, FR, GB, HK, HR, LT, NL, NO, PT, SE, SG, SK) *see* Japanese Encephalitis Virus Vaccine (Inactivated) 1141
Ixime (AE, MY) *see* Cefixime 380
Ixopolet (MX) *see* Vitamin E 2174
Ixprim (FR) *see* Acetaminophen and Tramadol 37
Izacef (ZA) *see* CeFAZolin 373
Izadima (EC) *see* CefTAZidime 392
Izatan (KR) *see* Irbesartan 1110
Izilox (FR) *see* Moxifloxacin (Systemic) 1401
Izofran (CL, UY) *see* Ondansetron 1513
Izoltil (AE, BF, BH, BJ, CI, CY, EG, ET, GH, GM, GN, IQ, IR, JO, KE, KW, LB, LR, LY, MA, ML, MR, MU, MW, NE, NG, OM, QA, SA, SC, SD, SL, SN, SY, TN, TZ, UG, YE, ZM, ZW) *see* Amoxicillin 130
Jabasulide (PT) *see* Nimesulide [INT] 1456
Jacutin (AT, CH, CZ, DE, HN, LU, PL, SG) *see* Lindane 1217
Jadelle (EC, TH) *see* Levonorgestrel 1201
Jadin (KR) *see* Nizatidine 1471
Jaizzy (IN) *see* Diacerein [INT] 613
Jakavi (AR, AU, BE, CH, CL, CY, CZ, DE, DK, EE, FR, GB, HK, HR, IL, IS, KR, LT, NL, NO, RO, SE, SG, SI, SK, TR) *see* Ruxolitinib 1856
Jamylene (FR) *see* Docusate 661
Janacin (HK, MY, TH) *see* Norfloxacin 1475
Januet (IL) *see* Sitagliptin and Metformin 1898
Janumet (AE, AR, AT, AU, BE, BH, BR, CH, CL, CN, CO, CR, CY, CZ, DE, DK, EE, FR, GB, GR, GT, HK, HN, HR, ID, IE, IN, IS, IT, KR, KW, LB, LT, MY, NI, NL, NO, NZ, PE, PH, PL, PT, QA, RO, SA, SE, SG, SI, SK, SV, TH, TR, TW, VN) *see* Sitagliptin and Metformin 1898
Janumet XR (SG) *see* Sitagliptin and Metformin 1898
Januvia (AE, AR, AT, AU, BB, BE, BH, BM, BR, BS, BZ, CH, CL, CN, CO, CR, CY, CZ, DE, DK, EC, EE, FR, GB, GR, GT, GY, HK, HN, HR, ID, IE, IL, IN, IS, IT, JM, JP, KR, KW, LB, LT, MX, MY, NI, NL, NO, NZ, PE, PH,

PL, PR, PT, QA, RO, RU, SA, SE, SG, SI, SK, SR, SV, TH, TR, TT, TW, UY, VN) *see* SitaGLIPtin 1897
Japrolox (VN) *see* Loxoprofen [INT] 1255
Jardiance (AU, CH, CZ, DE, DK, EE, GB, HR, KR, LT, NL, NO, PT, RO, SE, SI, SK) *see* Empagliflozin 718
Jarontin (KR) *see* Ethosuximide 813
Jasmine (FR) *see* Ethinyl Estradiol and Drospirenone 801
Jasminelle (FR) *see* Ethinyl Estradiol and Drospirenone 801
Jatroneural (DE) *see* Trifluoperazine 2102
Jatroneural Retard (AT) *see* Trifluoperazine 2102
Jatrosom (DE) *see* Tranylcypromine 2083
Jatrox (DE) *see* Bismuth 265
Jayacin (ID) *see* Ciprofloxacin (Systemic) 441
Jaydess (CZ, GB) *see* Levonorgestrel 1201
Jeanine (BG, CZ, PL, RU) *see* Estradiol and Dienogest 780
Jectocef (PH) *see* Cefuroxime 399
Jeita (TW) *see* Piperacillin and Tazobactam 1657
Jeitin (KR) *see* CefOXitin 386
Jekovit (FI) *see* Ergocalciferol 753
Jellin (DE) *see* Fluocinolone (Topical) 893
Jenacillin O (DE) *see* Penicillin G Procaine 1613
Jenac (TW) *see* Etodolac 815
Jenasteron (KR) *see* Testosterone 2010
Jencevac (IN) *see* Japanese Encephalitis Virus Vaccine (Inactivated) 1141
Jenloga (BM) *see* CloNIDine 480
Jennifer 35 (DE) *see* Cyproterone and Ethinyl Estradiol [CAN/INT] 532
Jentadueto (BE, CH, CZ, DK, EE, ES, GB, HR, IE, LT, NL, RO, SE, SI, SK) *see* Linagliptin and Metformin 1217
Jespect (AU) *see* Japanese Encephalitis Virus Vaccine (Inactivated) 1141
Jetisopt (KR) *see* Dorzolamide and Timolol 673
Jetrea (BE, CZ, DE, DK, EE, FR, GB, HR, IE, LT, NL, NO, RO, SE, SI, SK) *see* Ocriplasmin 1484
Jevtana (AR, AU, BE, BR, CH, CL, CR, CY, CZ, DE, DK, DO, EE, FR, GB, GT, HK, HN, HR, ID, IE, IL, IS, KR, LB, LT, MX, MY, NI, NL, NO, PA, PE, PH, PL, QA, RO, SE, SG, SI, SK, SV, TH, TR) *see* Cabazitaxel 316
Jexit (TW) *see* Flupentixol [CAN/INT] 903
Jext (GB) *see* EPINEPHrine (Systemic, Oral Inhalation) 735
Jezil (AU) *see* Gemfibrozil 956
Jia-Cal (TW) *see* Calcium Citrate 330
Jia Met (TW) *see* Naftifine 1416
Jicsron (JP) *see* Nalidixic Acid [INT] 1418
Jie Baili (CN) *see* PEMEtrexed 1606
Jie Li Tai (CN) *see* Gentamicin (Systemic) 959
Jielite (CN) *see* Ampicillin and Cloxacillin [INT] 144
Jiesilin (CN) *see* Piracetam [INT] 1661
Jiexin (CN) *see* Filgrastim 875
Jijufen (CN) *see* Oprelvekin 1519
Jin Di Na (CN) *see* Rimantadine 1813
Jin Er Lun (CN) *see* Naloxone 1419
Jin Si Ping (CN) *see* Selegiline 1873
Jintum (TW) *see* Carbocisteine [INT] 357
Jiu Bao Ke (CN) *see* Enalapril and Hydrochlorothiazide 725
JL Bragg's Medicinal Charcoal (HK) *see* Charcoal, Activated 416
Jodam (PL) *see* Potassium Iodide 1690
Jodetten Henning (DE) *see* Potassium Iodide 1690
Jodgamma (DE) *see* Potassium Iodide 1690
Jodid (DE, HU, LU, PL) *see* Potassium Iodide 1690
Jodid Merck (AT) *see* Potassium Iodide 1690
Jodid-ratiopharm (DE) *see* Potassium Iodide 1690
Jodid Verla (DE) *see* Potassium Iodide 1690
Jodix (FI) *see* Potassium Iodide 1690
Jodostin (PL) *see* Potassium Iodide 1690
Jodox (PL) *see* Potassium Iodide 1690
Johnlax (TW) *see* Bisacodyl 265
Johnstal (TW) *see* Mefenamic Acid 1280
Jolindac (TW) *see* Sulindac 1953
Jomybel (BE) *see* Josamycin [INT] 1141
Jonamin (AU) *see* Phentermine 1635
Jonfa (VN) *see* Zolpidem 2212
Josacin (DE) *see* Josamycin [INT] 1141
Josacine (FR) *see* Josamycin [INT] 1141
Josalid (AT) *see* Josamycin [INT] 1141
Josamina (ES) *see* Josamycin [INT] 1141
Josaxin (ES, IT, JP) *see* Josamycin [INT] 1141
Josir (FR) *see* Tamsulosin 1974
Jovia (PH) *see* Escitalopram 765
J-Tadine (KR) *see* Loratadine 1241
Jufurix (DE) *see* Furosemide 940
Julab (TH) *see* Selegiline 1873
Juliet-35 ED (AU) *see* Cyproterone and Ethinyl Estradiol [CAN/INT] 532
Juliet (BR) *see* Desogestrel [INT] 597
Juliette (DE) *see* Cyproterone and Ethinyl Estradiol [CAN/INT] 532
Julitam (PH) *see* LevETIRAcetam 1191
Julphasole (MY) *see* Lansoprazole 1166
Jumexal (CH) *see* Selegiline 1873
Jumex (AR, AT, BG, CR, CY, CZ, DO, HN, HR, HU, IL, IT, KR, MY, NI, PH, PL, PT, PY, SI, SK, TH, UY, VE) *see* Selegiline 1873
Jumtab (PY) *see* Interferon Beta-1a 1100
Junate (IN) *see* Artesunate 178
Junizac (DE) *see* Ranitidine 1777
Jun Neng (CN) *see* Finasteride 878
Jurnista (AT, AU, CZ, DE, DK, EE, ES, HN, HU, ID, IT, MX, NZ, PH, PT, SG, SI) *see* HYDROmorphone 1016
Jurnista IR (KR) *see* HYDROmorphone 1016
Jurnista SR (KR) *see* HYDROmorphone 1016
Justin (ID) *see* Lovastatin 1252
Justor (FR) *see* Cilazapril [CAN/INT] 434
Justum (PY) *see* Cefadroxil 372
Jutabis (DE) *see* Bisoprolol 266
Jutabloc (DE) *see* Metoprolol 1350
Jutaclin (DE) *see* Clindamycin (Systemic) 460
Jutacor Comp (DE, EG, IL, IQ, IR, JO, LB, LY, OM, SY, YE) *see* Captopril and Hydrochlorothiazide 345
Jutadilat (DE) *see* NIFEdipine 1451
Jutalar (DE) *see* Doxazosin 674
Jutalex (DE) *see* Sotalol 1927
Jutamox (DE) *see* Amoxicillin 130
Jutapress (DE) *see* Nitrendipine [INT] 1463
Kaban (DE) *see* Clocortolone 469
Kabol (DO) *see* Cefepime 378
Kaboping (CN) *see* Acarbose 29
Kacinth-A (ZA) *see* Amikacin 111
Kadian (BM) *see* Morphine (Systemic) 1394
Kadiflam (ID) *see* Diclofenac (Systemic) 617
Kai Bao Wei Yuan (CN) *see* Pioglitazone 1654
Kai Er Ding (CN) *see* Lofexidine [INT] 1232
Kaifa (CN) *see* Ampicillin and Cloxacillin [INT] 144
Kaifa (CN) *see* Cloxacillin [CAN/INT] 488
Kaifu (CN) *see* Interferon Alfa-2b 1096
Kaiji (CN) *see* Pantoprazole 1570
KaiLaiTong (CN) *see* TiZANidine 2051
Kai Nai Yin (CN) *see* Aminocaproic Acid 113
Kainever (PT) *see* Estazolam 775
Kai Yin (CN) *see* Carbocisteine [INT] 357
Kaizem CD (IN) *see* Diltiazem 634
Kaizole (TW) *see* Mebendazole [CAN/INT] 1274
Kala Folic (AR) *see* Ethinyl Estradiol, Drospirenone, and Levomefolate 812
Kalbeten (IL) *see* Bismuth 265
Kalcide (TW) *see* Praziquantel 1702
Kalcidon (SE) *see* Calcium Carbonate 327
Kalcijev karbonat (HR) *see* Calcium Carbonate 327

Kalcij-folinat (HR) *see* Leucovorin Calcium 1183
Kalcij-karbonat (HR) *see* Calcium Carbonate 327
Kalcitena (SE) *see* Calcium Carbonate 327
Kaldrene (DO) *see* Hydrochlorothiazide and Triamterene 1012
Kaldyum (VN) *see* Potassium Chloride 1687
Kaleorid (DK, FR, IS, NO, SE, VN) *see* Potassium Chloride 1687
Kaletra (MX) *see* Ritonavir 1822
Kaletra (AE, AR, AT, AU, BB, BE, BG, BH, BM, BO, BR, BS, BZ, CH, CN, CO, CR, CY, CZ, DE, DK, DO, EC, EE, EG, ES, FI, FR, GB, GR, GT, GY, HK, HN, HR, HU, IE, IL, IQ, IR, IT, JM, JO, JP, KR, KW, LB, LT, LY, MT, MX, MY, NI, NL, NO, NZ, OM, PA, PE, PK, PL, PR, PT, PY, QA, RO, RU, SA, SE, SG, SI, SK, SR, SV, SY, TH, TR, TT, TW, UY, VE, VN, YE) *see* Lopinavir and Ritonavir 1237
Kalfoxim (ID) *see* Cefotaxime 382
Kaliale (FR) *see* Cyproterone [CAN/INT] 530
Kalicor (CZ) *see* Piracetam [INT] 1661
Kalimate (JP, MY, PH, TH, TW) *see* Calcium Polystyrene Sulfonate [CAN/INT] 333
Kalinorm (FI) *see* Potassium Chloride 1687
Kalinor-Retard P (DE) *see* Potassium Chloride 1687
Kalipoz (PL) *see* Potassium Chloride 1687
Kalitake (ID) *see* Calcium Polystyrene Sulfonate [CAN/INT] 333
Kalitaker (KR) *see* Calcium Polystyrene Sulfonate [CAN/INT] 333
Kalium (BF, BJ, CI, ET, GH, GM, GN, KE, LR, MA, ML, MR, MU, MW, NE, NG, NL, PH, SC, SD, SL, SN, TN, TZ, UG, ZA, ZM, ZW) *see* Potassium Chloride 1687
Kalium-Durettes (NL) *see* Potassium Chloride 1687
Kalium gluconicum (PL) *see* Potassium Gluconate 1690
Kaliumiodid BC (DE) *see* Potassium Iodide 1690
Kaliumiodid (CH) *see* Potassium Iodide 1690
Kalium jodatum (DE) *see* Potassium Iodide 1690
Kaliumjodid Lannacher (AT) *see* Potassium Iodide 1690
Kaliumjodid Recip (SE) *see* Potassium Iodide 1690
Kaliumjodid "Dak" (DK) *see* Potassium Iodide 1690
Kalium-R (CH, HN) *see* Potassium Chloride 1687
Kalixocin (AU) *see* Clarithromycin 456
Kallmiren (AE, BH, CY, EG, IQ, IR, JO, KW, LB, LY, OM, QA, SA, SY, YE) *see* BusPIRone 311
Kalma (AU) *see* ALPRAZolam 94
Kalmicetine (IN) *see* Chloramphenicol 421
Kalnex (ID) *see* Tranexamic Acid 2081
Kalquest (ID) *see* Calcium Polystyrene Sulfonate [CAN/INT] 333
Kaltrofen (ID) *see* Ketoprofen 1145
Kaluril (AU, TW) *see* AMILoride 113
Kalydeco (AU, CH, CZ, DE, DK, EE, FR, GB, HR, LT, NL, NO, NZ, SE, SK) *see* Ivacaftor 1135
Kalymin (BG, DE, EE, RU, TR) *see* Pyridostigmine 1746
Kalytes (PH) *see* Potassium Chloride 1687
Kal-Zarevet (IL) *see* Calcium Carbonate 327
Kalzonorm (AT) *see* Calcium Carbonate 327
Kamacaine (IL) *see* Bupivacaine 299
Kamez (VN) *see* Torsemide 2071
Kamicin (HK) *see* Clotrimazole (Topical) 488
Kamina (PT) *see* Amikacin 111
Kamin (PH) *see* Amikacin 111
Kamiren (HR, RO) *see* Doxazosin 674
Kamrab (KR) *see* Rabies Immune Globulin (Human) 1764
KamRho-D IV (IL) *see* $Rh_o(D)$ Immune Globulin 1794
KamRho-D IM (IL) *see* $Rh_o(D)$ Immune Globulin 1794
Kamycine (FR) *see* Kanamycin 1142
Kan-1000 (VN) *see* Kanamycin 1142
Kanacet (IT) *see* Kanamycin 1142
Kanacin (KR) *see* Kanamycin 1142
Kanacolirio (ES) *see* Kanamycin 1142
Kanacyn (BE, LU, PK) *see* Kanamycin 1142
Kanafil (IT) *see* Kanamycin 1142
Kanafluid (ES) *see* Kanamycin 1142
Kanahidro (ES) *see* Kanamycin 1142
Kanakion (PT) *see* Phytonadione 1647
Kanamac (IN) *see* Kanamycin 1142
Kanamicina Firma (IT) *see* Kanamycin 1142
Kanamicin (HR) *see* Kanamycin 1142
Kanamycin Capsules Meiji (TH) *see* Kanamycin 1142
Kanamycin Meiji (HK, PH, TW) *see* Kanamycin 1142
Kanamycin-POS (DE) *see* Kanamycin 1142
Kanamycin Sanbe (ID) *see* Kanamycin 1142
Kanamytrex (DE) *see* Kanamycin 1142
Kananeo (VN) *see* Kanamycin 1142
Kananovo (ES) *see* Kanamycin 1142
Kanapiam Orale (IT) *see* Kanamycin 1142
Kanaplus (ES) *see* Kanamycin 1142
Kanaqua (ES) *see* Kanamycin 1142
Kanarco (ID) *see* Kanamycin 1142
Kanasig (AU) *see* Kanamycin 1142
Kana-Stulln (DE) *see* Kanamycin 1142
Kanatrol (IT) *see* Kanamycin 1142
Kanavit (CZ) *see* Phytonadione 1647
Kanbine (ES) *see* Amikacin 111
Kancin-L (SG) *see* Kanamycin 1142
Kancin (IN, MY, PH, TH) *see* Kanamycin 1142
Kandepres (HR) *see* Candesartan 335
Kanescin (ES) *see* Kanamycin 1142
Kang Ling (CN) *see* Piracetam [INT] 1661
Kang Zan (CN) *see* Rufloxacin [INT] 1855
Kannasyn (GB, IE) *see* Kanamycin 1142
Kano (IT) *see* Kanamycin 1142
Kanolone (MY) *see* Triamcinolone (Systemic) 2099
Kanolone (MY) *see* Triamcinolone (Topical) 2100
Kan-Ophtal (DE) *see* Kanamycin 1142
Kanox (MY) *see* Ketamine 1143
Kantonel (KR) *see* Risedronate 1816
Kantrex (BF, BJ, CI, ES, ET, GH, GM, GN, KE, LR, MA, ML, MR, MU, MW, MX, NE, NG, PE, SC, SD, SL, SN, TN, TZ, UG, ZA, ZM, ZW) *see* Kanamycin 1142
Kaodene (GB) *see* Codeine 497
Kaonol (CL, PE) *see* Ivermectin (Systemic) 1136
Kaopectate (PL) *see* Attapulgite [CAN/INT] 204
Kapanol (AU) *see* Morphine (Systemic) 1394
Kapidin (BG, CZ) *see* Lercanidipine [INT] 1181
Kaportan (VN) *see* Olmesartan 1496
Kapril (TR) *see* Captopril 342
Kaprofen (TH) *see* Ketoprofen 1145
Kaptin II (AE, KW) *see* Attapulgite [CAN/INT] 204
Kapvay (BM) *see* CloNIDine 480
Kapvay ER (KR) *see* CloNIDine 480
Karbakolin Isopto (DK) *see* Carbachol 346
Karbamazepin (DK, NO) *see* CarBAMazepine 346
Kardak (HK) *see* Simvastatin 1890
Karden (AT) *see* NiCARdipine 1446
Karidine (CN) *see* Phenazopyridine 1629
Karidium (AR) *see* CloBAZam 465
Karil (LU) *see* Calcitonin 322
Karison Creme (DE) *see* Clobetasol 468
Karison Salbe (DE) *see* Clobetasol 468
Karlit (AR) *see* Lithium 1230
Karlor CD (AU) *see* Cefaclor 372
Karlor (AU) *see* Cefaclor 372
Karmikin (MX) *see* Amikacin 111
Karozaar (KR) *see* Losartan 1248
Karter (KR) *see* Carvedilol 367
Karvea (AT, AU, CY, ES, TR) *see* Irbesartan 1110
Karvezide (AT, AU, BG, CH, CZ, DE, DK, EE, ES, FI, FR, GB, GR, HR, IE, IT, LT, MT, NO, PT, RO, RU, SE, SK, TR) *see* Irbesartan and Hydrochlorothiazide 1112
Karvil (PH) *see* Carvedilol 367
Kasporin (TH) *see* CycloSPORINE (Systemic) 522

Kastair EZ (PH) *see* Montelukast ... 1392
Kastair (PH) *see* Montelukast ... 1392
Katalar (QA) *see* Ketamine ... 1143
Katimin-1 (TW) *see* Phytonadione ... 1647
Katlex (JP) *see* Furosemide ... 940
Katoseran (JP) *see* Cinnarizine [INT] ... 440
Katrina (EC) *see* Permethrin ... 1627
Kattwilon N (DE) *see* Isoproterenol ... 1124
Kay-Cee-L (GB, IE) *see* Potassium Chloride ... 1687
Kayexalate (BB, BE, BM, BS, BZ, FR, GY, IL, IT, JM, SR, TH, TT, VN) *see* Sodium Polystyrene Sulfonate ... 1912
Kaypen (IN) *see* Penicillin V Potassium ... 1614
KC-F (JP) *see* Fluocinonide ... 894
K-Chlor (PH) *see* Potassium Chloride ... 1687
KCL Retard (AE, AT, BH, CY, CZ, EG, GR, HN, IQ, IR, IT, JO, KW, LB, LY, OM, QA, SA, SY, YE) *see* Potassium Chloride ... 1687
K-Contin (BF, BJ, CI, ET, GH, GM, GN, KE, KR, LR, MA, ML, MR, MU, MW, NE, NG, SC, SD, SL, SN, TN, TZ, UG, ZA, ZM, ZW) *see* Potassium Chloride ... 1687
K-Contin Continus (AE) *see* Potassium Chloride ... 1687
K-Cor (IN) *see* Nicorandil [INT] ... 1449
K-Dur (MX) *see* Potassium Chloride ... 1687
Keal (FR, LU) *see* Sucralfate ... 1940
Keamotin (HK) *see* Famotidine ... 845
Kebanon (KR) *see* Ketoprofen ... 1145
Kebir (PY) *see* Oxaliplatin ... 1528
Ke Di (CN) *see* Nisoldipine ... 1459
Kedrialb (PH) *see* Albumin ... 67
Kedu (CN) *see* Zidovudine ... 2196
Kefacin (BH, CY, EG, IQ, IR, JO, KR, KW, LB, LY, OM, QA, SA, SY, YE) *see* Cephalexin ... 405
Kefaclor (TZ) *see* Cefaclor ... 372
Kefadim (BF, BJ, CI, ET, GH, GM, GN, KE, LR, LU, MA, ML, MR, MU, MW, NE, NG, PK, SC, SD, SL, SN, TN, TW, TZ, UG, VN, ZA, ZM, ZW) *see* CefTAZidime ... 392
Kefalex (FI) *see* Cephalexin ... 405
Kefalospes (GR) *see* Cephalexin ... 405
Kefarin (GR) *see* CeFAZolin ... 373
Kefaxin (GR, IE) *see* Cephalexin ... 405
Kefazim (AT) *see* CefTAZidime ... 392
Kefazin (IL) *see* CeFAZolin ... 373
Kefezy (PH) *see* Cefuroxime ... 399
Keflex (AE, AT, BB, BF, BH, BJ, BM, BR, BS, BZ, CI, CO, CY, DK, EE, ET, GB, GH, GM, GN, GR, GY, JM, JO, KE, KW, LB, LR, MA, ML, MR, MU, MW, MX, NE, NG, NO, PE, PH, PK, PL, PT, QA, RO, SA, SC, SD, SE, SL, SN, SR, TH, TN, TT, TZ, UG, ZM, ZW) *see* Cephalexin ... 405
Keflor CD (AU) *see* Cefaclor ... 372
Keflor (AU, IN) *see* Cefaclor ... 372
Kefloridina (ES) *see* Cephalexin ... 405
Kefnir (MY) *see* Cefdinir ... 376
Kefolor (FI) *see* Cefaclor ... 372
Keforal (AR, BE, FR, IT, NL, VE) *see* Cephalexin ... 405
Kefstar (PH) *see* Cefuroxime ... 399
Keftid (GB) *see* Cefaclor ... 372
Keftriaxone (IL) *see* CefTRIAXone ... 396
Kefurox (LU, QA) *see* Cefuroxime ... 399
Kefzim (CL) *see* CefTAZidime ... 392
Kefzol (AT, BE, BF, BJ, CH, CI, ET, GB, GH, GM, GN, HN, HR, HU, IE, IS, KE, LR, LU, MA, ML, MR, MU, MW, NE, NG, NL, PK, SC, SD, SL, SN, TN, TZ, UG, VN, ZM, ZW) *see* CeFAZolin ... 373
Keimax (DE) *see* Ceftibuten ... 394
Keimicina (IT) *see* Kanamycin ... 1142
Keiran (VE) *see* Ketamine ... 1143
Ke Jie (CN) *see* Piracetam [INT] ... 1661
Kelac (IN) *see* Ketorolac (Systemic) ... 1146
Kelafox (CO) *see* Calcium Acetate ... 326
Kelatin (BE, LU, NL) *see* PenicillAMINE ... 1608
Kelatine (PT) *see* PenicillAMINE ... 1608
Kelefusin (MX) *see* Potassium Chloride ... 1687
Kelfen (VE) *see* Ketoprofen ... 1145
Kelfer (AE, GR, IN, MY, SG, TH, TW, VN) *see* Deferiprone ... 585
Ke Li (CN) *see* Digoxin ... 627
Kelin (TW) *see* CeFAZolin ... 373
Keliping (CN) *see* Felodipine ... 850
Kelly (BR) *see* Desogestrel [INT] ... 597
Kemadrin (AE, AT, AU, BB, BE, BG, BH, BM, BS, BZ, CH, CY, CZ, DK, EE, EG, ES, FI, FR, GB, GR, GY, HN, HU, IE, IL, IN, IQ, IR, IT, JM, JO, KW, LB, LU, LY, MT, NL, NO, NZ, OM, PT, QA, RU, SA, SE, SI, SK, SR, SY, TR, TT, UY, YE) *see* Procyclidine [CAN/INT] ... 1721
Kemicetine (AE, BH, CY, EG, GR, HK, IQ, IR, JO, KW, LB, LY, OM, QA, SA, SY, YE) *see* Chloramphenicol ... 421
Kemocarb (JO, PH, SG, TH, TW, VN) *see* CARBOplatin ... 357
Kemocarb (VN) *see* CISplatin ... 448
Kemocin (KR) *see* Cefaclor ... 372
Kemoplat (IN, PH, SG, TW) *see* CISplatin ... 448
Kemzid (HK) *see* Triamcinolone (Systemic) ... 2099
Kenacin A (JO) *see* Triamcinolone (Topical) ... 2100
Kenacin (PY) *see* Minoxidil (Topical) ... 1374
Kenacort A (AE, AR, BE, CH, CL, PH) *see* Triamcinolone (Systemic) ... 2099
Kenacort-A (AU, BH, CN, EG, ID, KE, NZ, PE, TW, TZ, UG, UY) *see* Triamcinolone (Systemic) ... 2099
Kenacort-A (BH, EG, ID, KE, QA, TW, TZ, UG) *see* Triamcinolone (Topical) ... 2100
Kenacort A IA ID (BH, JO) *see* Triamcinolone (Systemic) ... 2099
Kenacort A I.M. (BH, IQ, JO, KW, LB, LY, OM, QA, SA, SY, YE) *see* Triamcinolone (Systemic) ... 2099
Kenacort A in Orabase (CH) *see* Triamcinolone (Systemic) ... 2099
Kenacort A in Orabase (CH) *see* Triamcinolone (Topical) ... 2100
Kenacort-A in Orabase (NL) *see* Triamcinolone (Topical) ... 2100
Kenacort A (NL) *see* Triamcinolone (Topical) ... 2100
Kenacort E (PE) *see* Triamcinolone (Systemic) ... 2099
Kenacort E (PE) *see* Triamcinolone (Topical) ... 2100
Kenacort (IN, VE, VN) *see* Triamcinolone (Systemic) ... 2099
Kenacort (PH, VE) *see* Triamcinolone (Topical) ... 2100
Kenacort Retard (FR) *see* Triamcinolone (Systemic) ... 2099
Kenacort T (FI, NO, SE) *see* Triamcinolone (Systemic) ... 2099
Kenacort T (FI, SE) *see* Triamcinolone (Topical) ... 2100
Kenacort T Munnsalve (NO) *see* Triamcinolone (Systemic) ... 2099
Kenadion (IN) *see* Phytonadione ... 1647
Kenalgesic (CO) *see* Ketorolac (Ophthalmic) ... 1149
Kenalgesic (CO) *see* Ketorolac (Systemic) ... 1146
Kena-Lite (TH) *see* Triamcinolone (Systemic) ... 2099
Kena-Lite (TH) *see* Triamcinolone (Topical) ... 2100
Kenalog (CN, DK, JO, PK) *see* Triamcinolone (Topical) ... 2100
Kenalog (DK, EE, GB, HR, HU, PK) *see* Triamcinolone (Systemic) ... 2099
Kenalog in Orabase (AU, BF, BJ, CI, ET, GH, GM, GN, ID, KE, LR, MA, ML, MR, MU, MW, NE, NG, NZ, SC, SD, SL, SN, TN, TZ, UG, ZA, ZM, ZW) *see* Triamcinolone (Systemic) ... 2099
Kenalog in Orabase (BH, ID, KW, SA, ZA) *see* Triamcinolone (Topical) ... 2100
Kenalon (TW) *see* Nystatin (Topical) ... 1482
Kenazole (AE, BH, CY, EG, IQ, IR, JO, KW, LB, LY, OM, QA, SA, SY, TW, YE) *see* Ketoconazole (Topical) ... 1145
Kenazol (TH) *see* Ketoconazole (Systemic) ... 1144
Kenco (TW) *see* Bisoprolol ... 266
Kendaron (ID) *see* Amiodarone ... 114

Kenergon (CH) *see* Lidocaine (Topical) ... 1211
Kenesil (ES) *see* NiMODipine ... 1456
Kenhancer (MY, SG) *see* Ketoprofen ... 1145
Ke Ni (CL) *see* Secnidazole [INT] ... 1872
Kenofen (MY) *see* Ketoprofen ... 1145
Kenoket (MX) *see* ClonazePAM ... 478
Keno (SG) *see* Triamcinolone (Systemic) ... 2099
Keno (SG) *see* Triamcinolone (Topical) ... 2100
Kenstatin (MX) *see* Pravastatin ... 1700
Kentadin (MX) *see* Pentoxifylline ... 1618
Kentera (AT, BE, BG, CH, CZ, DE, DK, EE, ES, FI, FR, GB, GR, HN, HR, IE, IT, MT, NL, NO, PL, PT, RO, RU, SE, SK, TR) *see* Oxybutynin ... 1536
Kentera Patch (GB, IE) *see* Oxybutynin ... 1536
Kenzar Plus (PH) *see* Losartan and Hydrochlorothiazide ... 1250
Kenzen (FR) *see* Candesartan ... 335
Kenzolol (MX) *see* NiMODipine ... 1456
Keon EC (PH) *see* Ketoprofen ... 1145
Keotsan (PE) *see* Ketoprofen ... 1145
Kepcet (AU, DE) *see* LevETIRAcetam ... 1191
Kepinol (DE) *see* Sulfamethoxazole and Trimethoprim ... 1946
Kepivance (AT, AU, BE, BG, CH, CZ, DE, DK, EE, ES, FI, FR, GB, GR, HN, HR, IE, IL, IS, IT, KR, LT, MT, NL, NO, PL, PT, RO, RU, SE, SI, SK, TR) *see* Palifermin ... 1555
Keplioon (JP) *see* Paliperidone ... 1556
Keppra (AE, AR, AT, AU, BB, BE, BG, BH, BM, BS, CH, CL, CN, CO, CR, CY, CZ, DE, DK, DO, EC, EE, ES, FI, FR, GB, GR, GT, HK, HN, HR, HU, ID, IE, IL, IN, IS, IT, JM, JO, JP, KR, KW, LB, LT, MT, MX, MY, NI, NL, NO, NZ, PA, PE, PH, PL, PR, PT, QA, RO, RU, SA, SE, SG, SI, SK, SV, TH, TR, TT, TW, VN) *see* LevETIRAcetam ... 1191
Keppra I.V. (AU) *see* LevETIRAcetam ... 1191
Keproline (TW) *see* Maprotiline ... 1271
Keptrix (PH) *see* CefTRIAXone ... 396
Keqi (CL) *see* Lomefloxacin [INT] ... 1233
Keracaine (FR, LU) *see* Proparacaine ... 1728
Keraflox (IT, PT) *see* Prulifloxacin [INT] ... 1742
Keral (GB, IE, KR) *see* Dexketoprofen [INT] ... 603
Keratinamin (JP) *see* Urea ... 2114
Kerdica (TH) *see* Manidipine [INT] ... 1269
Kerfenmycin (TW) *see* Cefaclor ... 372
Keritmon (MX) *see* Amiodarone ... 114
Kerlone (AT, BE, CN, DE, FR, GR, KR, KW, LB, MY, PY, QA, SA, TW, VN) *see* Betaxolol (Systemic) ... 256
Kerlon (FI, IT, JO, NL) *see* Betaxolol (Systemic) ... 256
Keromin (KR) *see* Ketorolac (Systemic) ... 1146
Keromycin (TW) *see* Chloramphenicol ... 421
Kerron (AU) *see* LevETIRAcetam ... 1191
Kertasin (AR) *see* Etilefrine [INT] ... 815
Kertonbose (TW) *see* Acarbose ... 29
Kesaquil (HK) *see* QUEtiapine ... 1751
Kessar (CL, FR, GR, IT, ZA) *see* Tamoxifen ... 1971
Kestine (AT, DK, EE, FI, GR, HK, IE, IS, IT, LT, NL, NO, PK, PT, RU, SE, SG, TR, ZA) *see* Ebastine [INT] ... 702
Kestin (FR) *see* Ebastine [INT] ... 702
Kestinlyo (FR) *see* Ebastine [INT] ... 702
Ketadom (HK) *see* Ketoprofen ... 1145
Ketalar (AE, AU, BB, BE, BH, BM, BS, BZ, CH, CY, DK, EE, EG, ES, FI, FR, GB, GR, GY, HK, ID, IE, IL, IN, IQ, IR, IT, JM, JO, KW, LB, LU, LY, MT, MY, NO, NZ, OM, PE, PT, QA, SA, SE, SK, SR, SY, TR, TT, TW, UY, YE) *see* Ketamine ... 1143
Ketalgin (CH) *see* Methadone ... 1311
Ketalin (MX) *see* Ketamine ... 1143
Ketamax (PH) *see* Ketamine ... 1143
Ketamin-S (+) (PY) *see* Ketamine ... 1143
Ketanest (AT, HR, NL, PL) *see* Ketamine ... 1143
Ketanine (SG) *see* Captopril ... 342
Ketanov (IN, PH, RO) *see* Ketorolac (Systemic) ... 1146
Ketanrift (JP) *see* Allopurinol ... 90
Ketashort (CO) *see* Ketamine ... 1143
Ketasma (IN) *see* Ketotifen (Systemic) [CAN/INT] ... 1149
Ketava (MY) *see* Ketamine ... 1143
Ketazol (AE, BH, CY, EG, IQ, IR, JO, KW, LB, LY, OM, QA, SA, SY, YE) *see* Ketoconazole (Topical) ... 1145
Ketazol (PH) *see* Ketamine ... 1143
Ketazol (ZA) *see* Ketoconazole (Systemic) ... 1144
Ketazon (AR) *see* Piroxicam ... 1662
Ketek (AE, AT, BE, BG, BH, CH, CN, CR, CY, CZ, DE, DK, DO, EC, EE, EG, ES, FI, FR, GB, GR, GT, HN, HR, IE, IL, IT, KR, KW, LT, MT, MX, NI, NL, NO, NZ, PA, PL, PT, RO, SA, SE, SG, SI, SK, SV, TH, TR, TW, VE) *see* Telithromycin ... 1987
Ketensin (NL) *see* Ketanserin [INT] ... 1144
Ketesse (AT, BE, CH, CO, CZ, DK, EC, EE, FI, FR, HK, ID, IT, KW, LB, LT, MY, PE, PH, PT, SA, SE, SG, SI, SK, TR) *see* Dexketoprofen [INT] ... 603
Ketesse (CH, ES, IT, LU) *see* Clobutinol [INT] ... 468
Ketfren (AR, BR) *see* Ketoprofen ... 1145
Ketifen (HK) *see* Ketotifen (Systemic) [CAN/INT] ... 1149
Ketilept (PH) *see* QUEtiapine ... 1751
Ketin (TW) *see* Ketoprofen ... 1145
Ketipinor (MY, SG) *see* QUEtiapine ... 1751
Ketmin (IN) *see* Ketamine ... 1143
Ketobet (PH) *see* Ketorolac (Systemic) ... 1146
Ketobun-A (JP) *see* Allopurinol ... 90
Ketocef (HR) *see* Cefuroxime ... 399
Ketoconazol (CR, DO, GT, HN, NI, PA, SV) *see* Ketoconazole (Systemic) ... 1144
Ketoconazol (CR, DO, GT, HN, NI, PA, SV) *see* Ketoconazole (Topical) ... 1145
Ketoco (TW) *see* Ketoconazole (Topical) ... 1145
Ketodar (JO) *see* Ketoconazole (Systemic) ... 1144
Ketoderm (FR) *see* Ketoconazole (Topical) ... 1145
Ketofain (KR) *see* Ketoprofen ... 1145
Ketofen (HK, IN, MY, PH, TW) *see* Ketoprofen ... 1145
Ketoflam (ZA) *see* Ketoprofen ... 1145
Ketof (LU) *see* Ketotifen (Ophthalmic) ... 1150
Ketogesic (VN) *see* Ketorolac (Systemic) ... 1146
Ketohexal (ZA) *see* Ketotifen (Ophthalmic) ... 1150
Ketohexal (ZA) *see* Ketotifen (Systemic) [CAN/INT] ... 1149
Keto (HK, ID, MY, PH, SG) *see* Ketorolac (Systemic) ... 1146
Ketokid (AR) *see* Ketotifen (Systemic) [CAN/INT] ... 1149
Ketolac (TH) *see* Ketorolac (Systemic) ... 1146
Ketolar (ES) *see* Ketamine ... 1143
Ketolgin (AE, BH, CY, EG, IQ, IR, JO, KW, LB, LY, OM, QA, SA, SY, YE) *see* Ketoprofen ... 1145
Ketolgin Gel (AE, BH, CY, EG, IQ, IR, JO, KW, LB, LY, OM, QA, SA, SY, YE) *see* Ketoprofen ... 1145
Ketolgin SR (AE, BH, CY, EG, IQ, IR, JO, KW, LB, LY, OM, QA, SA, SY, YE) *see* Ketoprofen ... 1145
Ketomed (PH) *see* Ketorolac (Systemic) ... 1146
Ketomex (FI) *see* Ketoprofen ... 1145
Ketomin (KR) *see* Ketamine ... 1143
Ketomin (TW) *see* Ketotifen (Systemic) [CAN/INT] ... 1149
Ketonal Forte (SK) *see* Ketoprofen ... 1145
Ketonal (HR, RO, SI, SK) *see* Ketoprofen ... 1145
Ketona (TW) *see* Ketoconazole (Systemic) ... 1144
Ketona (TW) *see* Ketoconazole (Topical) ... 1145
Ketopine (NZ) *see* Ketoconazole (Topical) ... 1145
Ketop (RO) *see* Ketotifen (Systemic) [CAN/INT] ... 1149
Ketoptic (VE) *see* Ketotifen (Ophthalmic) ... 1150
Ketoracin (KR) *see* Ketorolac (Systemic) ... 1146
Ketoral (AU) *see* Ketorolac (Systemic) ... 1146
Ketorin (FI) *see* Ketoprofen ... 1145
Ketorol (RO) *see* Ketorolac (Systemic) ... 1146
Ketoro (TW) *see* Ketorolac (Systemic) ... 1146
Ketor (TW) *see* Ketoprofen ... 1145
Ketosma (TW) *see* Ketotifen (Systemic) [CAN/INT] ... 1149

Ketospray (IL) *see* Ketoprofen ... 1145
Ketostix (AU) *see* Nitroprusside ... 1467
Keto (TH) *see* Ketotifen (Systemic) [CAN/INT] ... 1149
Ketotifeno MK (DO, GT, NI, PA, SV) *see* Ketotifen (Ophthalmic) ... 1150
Ketotifen-ratiopharm (LU) *see* Ketotifen (Ophthalmic) ... 1150
Ketotisin (CL) *see* Ketotifen (Systemic) [CAN/INT] ... 1149
Ketovent (IN) *see* Ketotifen (Systemic) [CAN/INT] ... 1149
Ketovid (PH) *see* Ketoconazole (Systemic) ... 1144
Ketozol (PH) *see* Ketoconazole (Topical) ... 1145
Ketozol Shampoo (IL) *see* Ketoconazole (Topical) ... 1145
Ketrel (HK) *see* Tretinoin (Topical) ... 2099
Ketricin (ID) *see* Triamcinolone (Systemic) ... 2099
Ketricin (ID) *see* Triamcinolone (Topical) ... 2100
Ketron (CO) *see* Ketorolac (Systemic) ... 1146
Ketros (ID) *see* Ketoprofen ... 1145
Ketum (CO) *see* Ketoprofen ... 1145
Kevatril (DE) *see* Granisetron ... 983
Kevtam (AU) *see* LevETIRAcetam ... 1191
Kexelate (ZA) *see* Sodium Polystyrene Sulfonate ... 1912
Keydipin ER (KR) *see* Felodipine ... 850
Keylyte (IN) *see* Potassium Chloride ... 1687
Keyou (CN) *see* Penciclovir ... 1608
Ke Ze Pu (CN) *see* Lidocaine (Systemic) ... 1208
Kezon (TH) *see* Ketoconazole (Topical) ... 1145
Kicesol (JO) *see* Pyrethrins and Piperonyl Butoxide ... 1746
Kicindal (KR) *see* Pefloxacin [INT] ... 1588
Kicker (KR) *see* Oxandrolone ... 1531
Kiddi Pharmaton (MX) *see* Cyanocobalamin ... 515
Kiddi Pharmaton (MX) *see* Folic Acid, Cyanocobalamin, and Pyridoxine ... 921
Kiddi Pharmaton (MX) *see* Magnesium Sulfate ... 1265
Kidiprin (JO) *see* Aspirin ... 180
Kidiron (TH) *see* Ferrous Sulfate ... 871
Kiditard (NL) *see* QuiNIDine ... 1759
Kidolex (TW) *see* Cephalexin ... 405
Kidonax (MX) *see* Nitazoxanide ... 1461
Kidrolase (AE, AR, BG, CO, EG, FR, IL, LB, PE, PL, UY) *see* Asparaginase (E. coli) ... 179
Kilmicen (CH, MX) *see* Tolciclate [INT] ... 2062
Kilonum (TR) *see* Lithium ... 1230
Kilox (EC, GT, HN, NI, PA) *see* Ivermectin (Systemic) ... 1136
Kimapan (MY) *see* Captopril ... 342
Kimite Pad (CN) *see* Scopolamine (Systemic) ... 1870
Kimite Patch (KR) *see* Scopolamine (Systemic) ... 1870
Kimite (VN) *see* Scopolamine (Systemic) ... 1870
Kimodin (TW) *see* Famotidine ... 845
Kimpron (VN) *see* Fenoprofen ... 857
Kinaplase (AR) *see* Zonisamide ... 2215
Kinax (TW) *see* ALPRAZolam ... 94
Kine (PE) *see* Ketorolac (Systemic) ... 1146
Kineret (AT, AU, CY, CZ, DE, DK, EE, FI, FR, GB, GR, HR, IE, IL, IS, IT, LT, NL, NO, PT, RO, SE, SG, SI, SK, TR) *see* Anakinra ... 148
Kinetix (IN) *see* Mosapride [INT] ... 1401
Kinetos (UY) *see* Leflunomide ... 1174
Kinflocin (TW) *see* Ofloxacin (Systemic) ... 1490
Kinidin (AE, BH, CY, CZ, EG, FI, GR, IE, IQ, IR, JO, KW, LB, LY, NO, OM, PH, SA, SE, SY, YE) *see* QuiNIDine ... 1759
Kinidin Durules (AU, QA) *see* QuiNIDine ... 1759
Kinidin durules (PL) *see* QuiNIDine ... 1759
Kinidine (NL) *see* QuiNIDine ... 1759
Kinilentin (PL) *see* QuiNIDine ... 1759
Kinin (DK, SE) *see* QuiNINE ... 1761
Kinitard (PL) *see* QuiNIDine ... 1759
Kinotomin (JP) *see* Clemastine ... 459
Kinoxacin (KR) *see* Ofloxacin (Systemic) ... 1490
Kinsol (AE, BH, CY, EG, IL, IQ, IR, JO, KW, LB, LY, OM, QA, SA, SY, YE) *see* Trihexyphenidyl ... 2103
Kinson (AU) *see* Carbidopa and Levodopa ... 351
Kinxaben (TW) *see* Doxazosin ... 674
Kinzalcomb (AT, BE, BG, CH, CZ, DE, DK, EE, ES, FI, FR, GB, HR, IE, IT, MT, NL, NO, PL, PT, RO, RU, SE, SK, TR) *see* Telmisartan and Hydrochlorothiazide ... 1990
Kinzalmono (AT, BE, CH, CZ, DE, DK, EE, FI, FR, GB, IE, IT, MT, NL, NO, PL, PT, RU, SE, SK, TR) *see* Telmisartan ... 1988
Kinzolam (TW) *see* Estazolam ... 775
Kinzosin (TW) *see* Terazosin ... 2001
Kiovig (AT, AU, BE, BG, CH, CZ, DE, DK, EE, FI, FR, GB, GR, HK, HN, IE, IL, IT, MT, NL, NO, PL, PT, RU, SE, SK, TR) *see* Immune Globulin ... 1056
Kipres (JP) *see* Montelukast ... 1392
Kirin B!1 (JP) *see* Thiamine ... 2028
Kitak (RO) *see* Cladribine ... 455
Kitapram (TW) *see* Citalopram ... 451
Kivexa (AR, AT, AU, BE, BG, BR, CH, CL, CO, CY, CZ, DE, DK, EC, EE, ES, FI, FR, GB, GR, HK, HN, HR, HU, IE, IL, IS, IT, KR, LT, MT, MX, MY, NL, NO, NZ, PL, PT, RO, RU, SE, SG, SI, SK, TH, TR, TW, UY) *see* Abacavir and Lamivudine ... 22
Klacid XL (AE, BH, CY, EG, IQ, IR, JO, KW, LB, LY, OM, QA, SA, SY, YE) *see* Clarithromycin ... 456
Klacid (AE, AT, AU, BG, BH, CH, CN, CR, CY, CZ, DE, DK, EE, EG, ES, FI, GT, HK, HN, HU, IE, IL, IQ, IR, IS, IT, JO, KR, KW, LB, LT, LY, MY, NI, NO, NZ, OM, PA, PL, PT, QA, RO, RU, SA, SE, SG, SI, SK, SV, SY, TH, TR, VN, YE) *see* Clarithromycin ... 456
Klacid HP7 (AU) *see* Omeprazole, Clarithromycin, and Amoxicillin ... 1511
Klacid MR (MY, VN) *see* Clarithromycin ... 456
Klamonex (KR) *see* Amoxicillin and Clavulanate ... 133
Klaribac (AE, BH, CY, EG, IQ, IR, JO, KW, LB, LY, OM, QA, SA, SY, YE) *see* Clarithromycin ... 456
Klaricid XL (KR) *see* Clarithromycin ... 456
Klaricid (AR, BB, BM, BR, BS, BZ, CL, CO, EC, GB, GR, GY, JM, KR, MX, NL, PE, PH, PK, PR, PY, SR, TT, TW, UY, VE) *see* Clarithromycin ... 456
Klaricid Pediatric (PH) *see* Clarithromycin ... 456
Klaricina (ES) *see* Penicillin G Procaine ... 1613
Klariderm (ES) *see* Fluocinonide ... 894
Klaridex (IL) *see* Clarithromycin ... 456
Klarid (PH) *see* Clarithromycin ... 456
Klarihist (AE, BH, CY, EG, IQ, IR, JO, KW, LB, LY, OM, QA, SA, SY, YE) *see* Loratadine ... 1241
Klarin (IL) *see* Clarithromycin ... 456
Klaris (KR) *see* Clarithromycin ... 456
Klarithan (ZA) *see* Clarithromycin ... 456
Klarith (TW) *see* Clarithromycin ... 456
Klarmyn (MX, PH) *see* Clarithromycin ... 456
Klarquine (PK) *see* Chloroquine ... 424
Klavic (PH) *see* Amoxicillin and Clavulanate ... 133
Klenzit-MS (PH) *see* Adapalene ... 54
Klenzit (PH) *see* Adapalene ... 54
Kleotrat (GR) *see* Cefadroxil ... 372
Klerimed (AE, BH, CY, EG, IQ, IR, JO, KW, LB, LY, MY, OM, QA, SA, SG, SY, YE) *see* Clarithromycin ... 456
Klerimid (AE, BH, CY, EG, IQ, IR, JO, KW, LB, LY, OM, QA, SA, SY, YE) *see* Clarithromycin ... 456
Klexane (DK, FI, IS, NO, SE) *see* Enoxaparin ... 726
Klidibrax (ID) *see* Clidinium and Chlordiazepoxide ... 460
Kliiogest (JO) *see* Estradiol and Norethindrone ... 781
Klimater (BR) *see* Tibolone [INT] ... 2035
Klimicin (CZ) *see* Clindamycin (Systemic) ... 460
Klimonorm (HK) *see* Ethinyl Estradiol and Levonorgestrel ... 803
Klincyn (PH) *see* Clindamycin (Systemic) ... 460
Klindamycin (TH) *see* Clindamycin (Systemic) ... 460
Klinda RX (TH) *see* Clindamycin (Systemic) ... 460
Klinidox (CO) *see* Fusidic Acid (Topical) [CAN/INT] ... 943
Klinits (CL) *see* Permethrin ... 1627

Klinomycin (LU) *see* Minocycline 1371
Klinset (ID) *see* Loratadine 1241
Kliogest (BF, BH, BJ, CI, ET, GH, GM, GN, KE, KW, LR, MA, ML, MR, MU, MW, NE, NG, PK, SC, SD, SL, SN, TN, TZ, UG, ZM, ZW) *see* Estradiol and Norethindrone 781
Kliogest (KR, PK, SG) *see* Ethinyl Estradiol and Norethindrone 808
Kliovance (AU) *see* Estradiol (Systemic) 775
Kliovance (AU, NZ) *see* Estradiol and Norethindrone 781
Klobamicina (ES) *see* Dibekacin [INT] 616
Kloderma (ID) *see* Clobetasol 468
Klomicina (AR) *see* Roxithromycin [INT] 1853
Klonalcrom (AR) *see* Cromolyn (Ophthalmic) 514
Klonastin (AR) *see* Simvastatin 1890
Klopoxid (DK) *see* ChlordiazePOXIDE 422
Kloral (DK) *see* Chloral Hydrate [CAN/INT] 418
Kloramfenicol (DK, NO, SE) *see* Chloramphenicol 421
Kloramfenikol (SE) *see* Chloramphenicol 421
Kloramphenicol (NO) *see* Chloramphenicol 421
Klorhexidin (NO) *see* Chlorhexidine Gluconate 422
Klorhexol (FI) *see* Chlorhexidine Gluconate 422
Klorokinfosfat (NO, SE) *see* Chloroquine 424
Klorpo (PH, SG) *see* ChlordiazePOXIDE 422
Klorproman (FI) *see* ChlorproMAZINE 429
Klorzoxazon (DK) *see* Chlorzoxazone 430
Klotrimasool (EE) *see* Clotrimazole (Topical) 488
Klovig (TH) *see* Immune Globulin 1056
Klox (IN) *see* Cloxacillin [CAN/INT] 488
klysma Sorbit (DE) *see* Sorbitol 1927
Klyx (FI, NL, NO, SE) *see* Docusate 661
Kmoxilin (KR) *see* Amoxicillin and Clavulanate 133
Koate-DVI (AR, CL, CO, CR, DO, GT, HK, HR, ID, IL, MX, PA, PH, SV, UY) *see* Antihemophilic Factor (Human) 152
Kodein (NO) *see* Codeine 497
Kodein Recip (SE) *see* Codeine 497
Kodein "Dak" (DK) *see* Codeine 497
Kodone (GT) *see* Hydrocodone and Acetaminophen 1012
Kofatol (TW) *see* CeFAZolin 373
Kofex (PL) *see* Caffeine 319
Koffex DM-D (CA) *see* Pseudoephedrine and Dextromethorphan 1743
Koffex DM + Decongestant + Expectorant (CA) *see* Guaifenesin, Pseudoephedrine, and Dextromethorphan 989
Kofixir (HK) *see* Fexofenadine 873
Kogenate (AT, BE, CH, CL, CY, CZ, DE, DK, EE, FR, GB, GR, HR, HU, IE, IT, JO, NL, NO, NZ, PL, SE, TW) *see* Antihemophilic Factor (Recombinant) 152
Kogenate FS (AR, AU, CN, CO, CR, EC, GT, HK, HN, ID, IL, LB, MY, PA, SA, SG, SV, TH, ZA) *see* Antihemophilic Factor (Recombinant) 152
Kogrel (MY) *see* Clopidogrel 484
Koinsar (ID) *see* Losartan 1248
Kokain (DK) *see* Cocaine 497
Kolestran (TR) *see* Cholestyramine Resin 431
Koligin (TW) *see* Meprobamate 1296
Kolincin (HK) *see* Clindamycin (Topical) 464
Kolkatriol F (ID) *see* Calcipotriene 321
Kolkatriol (ID) *see* Calcipotriene 321
Kolkatriol (ID) *see* Calcitriol 323
Kolkisin (NO) *see* Colchicine 500
Kollagenase (BR) *see* Collagenase (Topical) 507
Kolomycin (SK) *see* Colistimethate 504
Koloskol (ID) *see* Pravastatin 1700
Kombiglyze (AU, IN, VN) *see* Saxagliptin and Metformin 1869
Kombiglyze XR (AR, AU, BR, CL, HK, ID, IL, KR, MX, MY, PH, SA, SG, TH) *see* Saxagliptin and Metformin 1869
Komboglyze (BE, CY, CZ, DE, DK, EE, FR, GB, HR, HU, LT, NL, PL, RO, SE, SI, SK) *see* Saxagliptin and Metformin 1869
Komboglyze XR (CH) *see* Saxagliptin and Metformin 1869
Konakion (10 mg) (AE, AU, BG, BH, CY, DE, EC, EG, GB, GH, IE, IL, IQ, IR, IT, JO, KE, KW, LB, LY, NL, OM, QA, SA, SE, SY, TZ, UG, YE, ZM) *see* Phytonadione 1647
Konakion 10 mg (AT, FI, HN) *see* Phytonadione 1647
Konakion MM (BH, CL, HR, KW, LB, MX) *see* Phytonadione 1647
Konakion MM Paediatric (BB, BM, BS, BZ, GY, JM, SR, TT) *see* Phytonadione 1647
Konakion MM Pediatric (AR, AU, BR, CH, CO, NZ, PE, PK, PY, UY, VN) *see* Phytonadione 1647
Konakion (BE, DK, ES, HU, IS, LU, NO, SI, TR) *see* Phytonadione 1647
Konitra (KR) *see* Itraconazole 1130
Konshien (TW) *see* Piroxicam 1662
Konsyl (IL, TW) *see* Psyllium 1744
Kontil (TR) *see* Pyrantel Pamoate 1744
Kontram XL SR (KR) *see* TraMADol 2074
Konverge (IE) *see* Amlodipine and Olmesartan 126
Konveril Plus (TR) *see* Enalapril and Hydrochlorothiazide 725
Konzert (MY) *see* Sertaconazole 1877
Kop Gel (MY) *see* Ketoprofen 1145
Kopodex (CL, CO, PE, PY) *see* LevETIRAcetam 1191
Kopseu (KR) *see* Pseudoephedrine 1742
Koptin (CR, DO, GT, HN, NI, PA, SV) *see* Azithromycin (Systemic) 216
Korandil (TR) *see* Enalapril 722
Koreberon (CZ, DE, HU) *see* Fluoride 895
Korec (FR) *see* Quinapril 1756
Koridol (HK) *see* TraMADol 2074
Kormakin (PH) *see* Amikacin 111
Kortezor (PH) *see* Ketorolac (Systemic) 1146
Kosteo (AU) *see* Calcitriol 323
Kovan (TW) *see* Valsartan 2127
Kovent SF (PH) *see* Fluticasone and Salmeterol 912
Kovilen (IT) *see* Nedocromil 1435
Kovinal (IT) *see* Nedocromil 1435
Kovix (KR) *see* Clopidogrel 484
Kozosin (HK) *see* Terazosin 2001
Krabinex (PH) *see* Hydroxyurea 1021
Kratium (BB, BF, BJ, BM, BS, BZ, CI, ET, GH, GM, GN, GY, JM, KE, LR, MA, ML, MR, MU, MW, NE, NG, NL, PR, SC, SD, SL, SN, SR, TN, TR, TT, TZ, UG, ZM, ZW) *see* Diazepam 613
Kratol (IN) *see* Mannitol 1269
Kredex (AU, BE, ES, FR, LU, NO, SE) *see* Carvedilol 367
Kreislauf Katovit (DE) *see* Etilefrine [INT] 815
Krema-Rosa (AE, BH, CY, EG, IQ, IR, JO, KW, LB, LY, OM, QA, SA, SY, YE) *see* Clotrimazole (Topical) 488
Kremezin (TW) *see* Charcoal, Activated 416
Krem Ochronny z Tiosiarczanem Sodu A (PL) *see* Sodium Thiosulfate 1915
Krenosine (CH) *see* Adenosine 55
Krenosin (FR, IT, LU, MX) *see* Adenosine 55
Kriadex (MX) *see* ClonazePAM 478
Kridan Simple (ES) *see* Isoniazid 1120
Kripton (AU) *see* Bromocriptine 291
Krisovin (MY, SG) *see* Griseofulvin 985
Krobicin (MX) *see* Clarithromycin 456
Kromicin (CO) *see* Azithromycin (Systemic) 216
Kryobulin TIM 3 (CZ, HN) *see* Antihemophilic Factor (Recombinant) 152
Kryptocur (BE, CH, CZ, DE, HN, HR, IT, LU) *see* Gonadorelin [CAN/INT] 980
Krystexxa (CZ, EE, LT, NL, SE, SK) *see* Pegloticase 1602

KSR (HK, ID) *see* Potassium Chloride 1687
K-Tab (PK) *see* Potassium Chloride 1687
Kuanium (TW) *see* Clidinium and Chlordiazepoxide 460
Kudeq (AU) *see* Celecoxib 402
Kui La Lan (CN) *see* Dexketoprofen [INT] 603
Kulinet (GR) *see* Cyproheptadine 529
Kun Te (CN) *see* Flucloxacillin [INT] 885
Kunyrin (VN) *see* Leucovorin Calcium 1183
Kupbloicin (VN) *see* Bleomycin 270
Kupdina (VN) *see* Danazol 558
Kuppam (MX) *see* Pantoprazole 1570
Kuptamete (VN) *see* CefoTEtan 385
Kurtigo (ID) *see* Betahistine [CAN/INT] 252
Kusnarin (JP) *see* Nalidixic Acid [INT] 1418
Kutoin (ID) *see* Phenytoin 1640
Kutrix (JP) *see* Furosemide 940
Kutub (IN) *see* Dapoxetine [INT] 561
Kuvan (AR, AU, BE, CH, CN, CZ, DE, DK, EE, FR, GB, HN, HR, IE, IL, IS, KR, LT, NL, NO, NZ, PT, RO, SE, SI, SK, TW) *see* Sapropterin 1864
Kuzem (TW) *see* Sodium Polystyrene Sulfonate 1912
Kwellada (GR) *see* Lindane 1217
Kwell (AE, SA) *see* Lindane 1217
Kwell-P (TR) *see* Pyrethrins and Piperonyl Butoxide 1746
Kwells (IE) *see* Scopolamine (Systemic) 1870
Kybernin (ES, HR, HU) *see* Antithrombin 156
Kybernin P (BR, ES, ID) *see* Antithrombin 156
Kymoxin (KR) *see* Amoxicillin 130
Kynteles (AU) *see* Vedolizumab 2146
Kyocristine (JP) *see* VinCRIStine 2163
Kyotil (TW) *see* Granisetron 983
Kyprolis (IL) *see* Carfilzomib 361
Kyrin (TH) *see* Fluconazole 885
Kytril (AE, AR, AT, AU, BE, BF, BG, BH, BJ, BR, CH, CI, CL, CO, CY, CZ, DK, EC, EE, EG, ES, ET, FI, FR, GB, GH, GM, GN, GR, HK, HN, HR, HU, ID, IE, IL, IQ, IR, IT, JO, JP, KE, KR, KW, LB, LR, LU, LY, MA, ML, MR, MT, MU, MW, MX, NE, NG, NL, NO, OM, PE, PH, PK, PL, PT, QA, RO, RU, SA, SC, SD, SE, SG, SI, SK, SL, SN, SY, TH, TN, TR, TW, TZ, UG, UY, VE, YE, ZA, ZM, ZW) *see* Granisetron 983
Laaglyda MR (GB) *see* Gliclazide [CAN/INT] 964
Labdiazina (PT) *see* SulfADIAZINE 1944
Labedin (TW) *see* Labetalol 1151
Labenda (TH) *see* Albendazole 65
Labesin (KR) *see* Labetalol 1151
Labicitin (KR) *see* LamoTRIgine 1160
Labinpina (CO) *see* Scopolamine (Systemic) 1870
Labrea (BR) *see* Donepezil 668
Labuton (TW) *see* Nabumetone 1411
Lacasa (IN) *see* Lacosamide 1154
Lac-Dol (AU) *see* Lactulose 1156
Lacedim (ID) *see* CefTAZidime 392
Laceran (DE, PT) *see* Urea 2114
Lacflavin (JP) *see* Riboflavin 1803
Lacibloc (PH) *see* Lacidipin [INT] 1154
Lacin (TH) *see* Clindamycin (Systemic) 460
Lacipil (BG, BR, CL, CO, CZ, EE, EG, HN, HR, IT, LT, MY, NZ, PH, PL, PT, RO, RU, SG, SI, SK, TR, TW, VE, VN) *see* Lacidipin [INT] 1154
Lacivas FC (IN) *see* Lacidipin [INT] 1154
Lacoly (TW) *see* Lactulose 1156
Lacons (ID) *see* Lactulose 1156
Lacopen (CO) *see* Lansoprazole 1166
Lacosam (IN) *see* Lacosamide 1154
Lacoset (IN) *see* Lacosamide 1154
Lacotem (AR) *see* Lacosamide 1154
Lacoxa (TW) *see* Etodolac 815
Lacretin (JP) *see* Clemastine 459
Lacrima Plus (MX) *see* Dextran 607
Lacroemol (PH) *see* Chloramphenicol 421
Lacromid (CY, TR) *see* Bezafibrate [CAN/INT] 261
Lacromycin (IL) *see* Gentamicin (Ophthalmic) 962
Lacromycin (IL) *see* Gentamicin (Systemic) 959
Lacson (ZA) *see* Lactulose 1156
Lactafem (PE) *see* Desogestrel [INT] 597
Lacticare HC (PH) *see* Hydrocortisone (Topical) 1014
Lacticare-HC (VN) *see* Hydrocortisone (Topical) 1014
Lactinese (PE) *see* Cabergoline 319
Lactocol (ES) *see* GuaiFENesin 986
Lactocur (AU, LU) *see* Lactulose 1156
Lactrin (ID) *see* Erdosteine [INT] 753
Lactulax (EC, ID, MX, UY) *see* Lactulose 1156
Lactulen (CO) *see* Lactulose 1156
Lactul (MY, TW) *see* Lactulose 1156
Lactulon (PY) *see* Lactulose 1156
Lactulosa (EC) *see* Lactulose 1156
Lactulose-ratiopharm (LU) *see* Lactulose 1156
Lactumed (MY) *see* Lactulose 1156
Lactus (SG) *see* Lactulose 1156
Lactuverlan (DE) *see* Lactulose 1156
Lacure (KR) *see* Hyaluronate and Derivatives 1006
Ladazol (ZA) *see* Danazol 558
Ladevina (AR, VN) *see* Lenalidomide 1177
Ladiomil (HR) *see* Maprotiline 1271
Ladiwin (BF, BJ, CI, ET, GH, GM, GN, KE, LR, MA, ML, MR, MU, MW, NE, NG, SC, SD, SL, SN, TN, TZ, UG, ZA, ZM, ZW) *see* LamiVUDine 1157
Ladogal (AR, BR, MX, MY, PE, PH, TH, TW, UY, VE) *see* Danazol 558
L-Adrenalin (AT) *see* EPINEPHrine (Systemic, Oral Inhalation) 735
Lady-E35 (TH) *see* Cyproterone and Ethinyl Estradiol [CAN/INT] 532
Ladyline (KR) *see* Ferric Gluconate 869
Lady (PH) *see* Ethinyl Estradiol and Levonorgestrel 803
Lady-Ten 35 (CL) *see* Cyproterone and Ethinyl Estradiol [CAN/INT] 532
Laevolac (AT, CN, HK, HN, IL, IT, NZ, PT, TH, VN) *see* Lactulose 1156
Lafaxid (IN) *see* Lafutidine [INT] 1157
Lafigin (PY) *see* LamoTRIgine 1160
Lafuca (KR) *see* Lafutidine [INT] 1157
La-Fu (CZ) *see* Fluorouracil (Systemic) 896
Lafumac (IN) *see* Lafutidine [INT] 1157
Lafunomyl (FI, SE) *see* Alfuzosin 84
Lafuzo (TW) *see* Alfuzosin 84
Lagaquin (BB, BF, BJ, BM, BS, BZ, CI, ET, GH, GM, GN, GY, JM, KE, LR, MA, ML, MR, MU, MW, NE, NG, PR, SC, SD, SL, SN, SR, TN, TT, TZ, UG, ZA, ZM, ZW) *see* Chloroquine 424
Lagas (ID) *see* Lansoprazole 1166
Lagatrim (AE, BF, BH, BJ, CI, CY, EG, ET, GH, GM, GN, IQ, IR, JO, KE, KW, LB, LR, LY, MA, ML, MR, MU, MW, NE, NG, OM, QA, SA, SC, SD, SL, SN, SY, TN, TZ, UG, YE, ZM, ZW) *see* Sulfamethoxazole and Trimethoprim 1946
Lagatrim Forte (BB, BF, BJ, BM, BS, BZ, CI, ET, GH, GM, GN, GY, JM, KE, LB, LR, MA, ML, MR, MU, MW, NE, NG, NL, PR, SC, SD, SL, SN, SR, TN, TT, TZ, UG, ZM, ZW) *see* Sulfamethoxazole and Trimethoprim 1946
Lagavit B12 (AE, BB, BH, BM, BS, BZ, CY, EG, GY, IQ, IR, JM, JO, KW, LB, LY, NL, OM, PR, QA, SA, SR, SY, TT, YE) *see* Cyanocobalamin 515
Lagose (AR) *see* Dapoxetine [INT] 561
Lagricel Ofteno (CR, DO, GT, HN, NI, PA, SV) *see* Hyaluronate and Derivatives 1006
Laidec (TW) *see* Riluzole 1812
Laidor (IT) *see* Nimesulide [INT] 1456
Laila-35 ED (AU) *see* Cyproterone and Ethinyl Estradiol [CAN/INT] 532
Laining (TW) *see* Propranolol 1731
Laiping (CN) *see* Miglitol 1367
Lai Yi (CN) *see* Flumazenil 892

Lakshmi (KR) *see* Orlistat 1520
Lalaca (KR) *see* Pregabalin 1710
Lama (IN) *see* AmLODIPine 123
Lambanol (IT) *see* Docusate 661
Lambutol (TH) *see* Ethambutol 798
Lamcoin (TH) *see* Clofazimine [INT] 473
Lamda (ID) *see* Amiodarone 114
Lamdra SBK (MX) *see* LamoTRIgine 1160
Lamepil (IN) *see* LamoTRIgine 1160
Lametec (CO) *see* LamoTRIgine 1160
Lamictal (AE, AR, AT, AU, BB, BD, BE, BG, BH, BM, BO, BR, BS, BZ, CH, CL, CN, CO, CR, CY, CZ, DE, DK, DO, EC, EE, EG, ES, FI, FR, GB, GR, GT, GY, HK, HN, HR, HU, ID, IE, IL, IQ, IR, IS, IT, JM, JO, JP, KR, KW, LB, LT, LU, LY, MT, MX, MY, NI, NL, NO, NZ, OM, PA, PE, PH, PK, PL, PR, PT, PY, QA, RO, RU, SA, SE, SG, SI, SK, SR, SV, SY, TH, TR, TT, TW, UY, VE, VN, YE) *see* LamoTRIgine 1160
Lamidac (IN) *see* LamiVUDine 1157
Lamidine (TW) *see* LamiVUDine 1157
Lamidus (AU, TW) *see* LamoTRIgine 1160
Lamifen (AE, JO, PH, QA, SA) *see* Terbinafine (Systemic) 2002
Lamifen (PH) *see* Terbinafine (Topical) 2004
Lamiffix (KR) *see* LamiVUDine 1157
Lamiros (ID) *see* LamoTRIgine 1160
Lamisil (AE, AR, AT, AU, BE, BF, BG, BH, BJ, BR, CH, CI, CL, CN, CO, CY, CZ, DK, EC, EE, EG, ET, FI, FR, GB, GH, GM, GN, GR, HK, HN, HR, ID, IE, IL, IQ, IR, IS, IT, JO, JP, KE, KR, KW, LB, LR, LT, LY, MA, ML, MR, MT, MU, MW, MY, NE, NG, NL, NO, NZ, OM, PE, PH, PK, PL, PT, PY, QA, RO, RU, SA, SC, SD, SE, SG, SI, SK, SL, SN, SY, TH, TN, TR, TW, TZ, UG, UY, VE, VN, YE, ZM, ZW) *see* Terbinafine (Systemic) 2002
Lamisil (AE, AR, AT, AU, BE, BG, BR, CH, CL, CO, CZ, DK, EE, EG, FI, FR, GB, GR, HK, HN, HR, ID, IL, IS, IT, KR, LT, MY, NL, NO, PE, PH, PK, PL, PT, PY, RO, RU, SE, SG, SI, SK, TH, TR, TW, UY) *see* Terbinafine (Topical) 2004
Lamisilate (FR) *see* Terbinafine (Systemic) 2002
Lamisilate (FR) *see* Terbinafine (Topical) 2004
Lamisil AT (ID) *see* Terbinafine (Systemic) 2002
Lamisil AT (ID) *see* Terbinafine (Topical) 2004
Lamisil Dermgel (FR, IL) *see* Terbinafine (Systemic) 2002
Lamisil Once (AE, AU, HK, KR, KW, LB, PH, QA, SA, TH, VN) *see* Terbinafine (Systemic) 2002
Lamisil Once (AU, HK, PH, TH) *see* Terbinafine (Topical) 2004
Lamitol (HR) *see* Labetalol 1151
Lamitor (AE, PH) *see* LamoTRIgine 1160
Lamivir (LB, PE, TH) *see* LamiVUDine 1157
Lammifen (KW) *see* Terbinafine (Systemic) 2002
Lamodex (IL) *see* LamoTRIgine 1160
Lamogin (CO, TW) *see* LamoTRIgine 1160
Lamogine (AU, IL) *see* LamoTRIgine 1160
Lamor (JO) *see* LamoTRIgine 1160
La Morph (NZ) *see* Morphine (Systemic) 1394
Lamosyn (PH) *see* LamoTRIgine 1160
Lamotrin (HK) *see* LamoTRIgine 1160
Lamotrix (MY, PH, SG, TW, VN) *see* LamoTRIgine 1160
Lamox (HR) *see* LamoTRIgine 1160
Lamoxy (IN) *see* Amoxicillin 130
Lampicin Fort (HK) *see* Ampicillin and Cloxacillin [INT] 144
Lamprene (AU, CH, CZ, EG, FR, GR, HK, IR, MY, NZ, SA) *see* Clofazimine [INT] 473
Lampren (ES, JP, NL) *see* Clofazimine [INT] 473
Lamuna (DE) *see* Ethinyl Estradiol and Desogestrel 799
Lamuzid (BF, BJ, CI, ET, GH, GM, GN, KE, LR, MA, ML, MR, MU, MW, NE, NG, SC, SD, SL, SN, TN, TZ, UG, ZA, ZM, ZW) *see* Lamivudine and Zidovudine 1160
Lanacane (ES) *see* Benzocaine 246
Lanacin (AE, BH, CY, EG, IQ, IR, JO, KW, LB, LY, OM, QA, SA, SY, YE) *see* Clindamycin (Systemic) 460
Lanacordin (ES) *see* Digoxin 627
Lancef (ID) *see* Cefotaxime 382
Lancid (KR) *see* Lansoprazole 1166
Lanclic (KR) *see* FLUoxetine 899
Landacort (CO) *see* Deflazacort [INT] 587
Landip (IN) *see* Lercanidipine [INT] 1181
Lando (ID) *see* Clindamycin (Systemic) 460
Landstav (MX) *see* Stavudine 1934
Landuet (TW) *see* Enalapril and Hydrochlorothiazide 725
Lanexat (BB, BM, BR, BS, BZ, CL, CO, DK, EC, FI, GY, JM, MX, PE, PY, SE, SR, TT, UY, VE) *see* Flumazenil 892
Lanfast (AE, BH, KW, QA, SA) *see* Lansoprazole 1166
Lanfix (ID) *see* Cefixime 380
Langaton (KR) *see* Lansoprazole 1166
Langjing (CN) *see* Clemastine 459
Langoran (FR) *see* Isosorbide Dinitrate 1124
Langoran LP (FR) *see* Isosorbide Dinitrate 1124
Langtian (CN) *see* Moclobemide [CAN/INT] 1384
Lanicor (AE, AR, AT, BB, BF, BH, BJ, BM, BS, BZ, CI, CY, CZ, DE, EC, EG, ET, GH, GM, GN, GR, GY, HR, IQ, IR, JM, JO, KE, KW, LB, LR, LU, LY, MA, ML, MR, MU, MW, NE, NG, OM, QA, SA, SC, SD, SL, SN, SR, SY, TN, TT, TZ, UG, VE, YE, ZM, ZW) *see* Digoxin 627
Lanidem (KR) *see* Lacidipin [INT] 1154
Lanikor (RU) *see* Digoxin 627
Lanioxin (IS) *see* Digoxin 627
Lan Meishu (CN) *see* Terbinafine (Topical) 2004
Lanmer (ID) *see* Meropenem 1299
Lanobin (KR) *see* Hydroxocobalamin 1020
Lanodizol (MX) *see* Lansoprazole 1166
Lanomycin (GR) *see* Amikacin 111
Lanoprost (TW) *see* Latanoprost 1172
Lanotan (KR) *see* Latanoprost 1172
Lanoxin (AE, AR, AU, BB, BE, BF, BH, BJ, BM, BS, BZ, CI, CY, EG, ET, GB, GH, GM, GN, GR, GY, HK, IE, IL, IN, IQ, IR, IT, JM, JO, JP, KE, KR, KW, LB, LR, LU, LY, MA, ML, MR, MU, MW, MX, MY, NE, NG, NL, NO, NZ, OM, PH, PK, PT, PY, QA, RU, SA, SC, SD, SE, SG, SL, SN, SR, SY, TH, TN, TR, TT, TW, TZ, UG, UY, YE, ZM, ZW) *see* Digoxin 627
Lanoxin PG (NZ) *see* Digoxin 627
Lanox (PH) *see* Digoxin 627
Lanpraz (CO) *see* Lansoprazole 1166
Lanprol (AE, BH, CY, EG, IQ, IR, JO, KR, KW, LB, LY, OM, QA, SA, SY, YE) *see* Lansoprazole 1166
Lanpro (MY) *see* Lansoprazole 1166
Lanproton (CO) *see* Lansoprazole 1166
Lansal (FI) *see* Lansoprazole 1166
Lan Sha (CN) *see* Azilsartan 214
Lansiclav (ID) *see* Amoxicillin and Clavulanate 133
Lans-OD (MY) *see* Lansoprazole 1166
Lans OD (PH) *see* Lansoprazole 1166
Lanso (GR, IL, MY) *see* Lansoprazole 1166
Lansomid (QA) *see* Lansoprazole 1166
Lansone (HU) *see* Lansoprazole 1166
Lansopep (CO) *see* Lansoprazole 1166
Lansor (TR) *see* Lansoprazole 1166
Lansozole (KR) *see* Lansoprazole 1166
Lanspro-30 (PH) *see* Lansoprazole 1166
Lanster (KR) *see* Lansoprazole 1166
Lanston (KR) *see* Lansoprazole 1166
Lantadin (AT) *see* Deflazacort [INT] 587
Lantarel (DE) *see* Methotrexate 1322
Lanthonate (IN) *see* Lanthanum 1169
Lantidin (PH) *see* Phenytoin 1640
Lantiflam (ID) *see* Ketoprofen 1145
Lanton (IL) *see* Lansoprazole 1166
Lantron (JP) *see* Amitriptyline 119
Lantus (AE, AR, AT, AU, BB, BE, BG, BH, BM, BR, BS, BZ, CH, CL, CN, CO, CR, CY, CZ, DE, DK, DO, EC,

EE, FI, FR, GB, GR, GT, GY, HK, HN, HR, HU, ID, IE, IL, IN, IS, IT, JM, JO, KR, KW, LB, LT, MT, MX, MY, NI, NL, NO, NZ, PA, PE, PH, PK, PL, PR, PT, PY, QA, RO, RU, SA, SE, SG, SI, SK, SR, SV, TH, TR, TT, TW, UY, VE, VN) *see* Insulin Glargine 1086
Lanvell (PH) *see* Lansoprazole 1166
Lanvis (AE, AR, AU, BB, BE, BF, BH, BJ, BM, BR, BS, BZ, CH, CI, CL, CO, CY, CZ, EE, EG, ET, FR, GB, GH, GM, GN, GR, GY, HK, HN, HR, HU, IE, IL, IQ, IR, JM, JO, KE, KR, KW, LB, LR, LT, LY, MA, ML, MR, MU, MW, MY, NE, NG, NL, OM, PL, QA, SA, SC, SD, SE, SI, SK, SL, SN, SR, SY, TH, TN, TT, TW, TZ, UG, VN, YE, ZA, ZM, ZW) *see* Thioguanine 2029
Lanximed (CO) *see* Lansoprazole 1166
Lanzap (RO, RU) *see* Lansoprazole 1166
Lanzep (PH) *see* Lansoprazole 1166
Lanzo (DK, IS, SE) *see* Lansoprazole 1166
Lanzol-30 (IN) *see* Lansoprazole 1166
Lanzo Melt (NO) *see* Lansoprazole 1166
Lanzopral (AR, PE, PY, UY, VE) *see* Lansoprazole 1166
Lanzopral Heli-Pak (PE) *see* Lansoprazole, Amoxicillin, and Clarithromycin 1169
Lanzopran (AU) *see* Lansoprazole 1166
Lanzor (AE, BH, DE, EG, FR, JO, KW, LB, QA, SA) *see* Lansoprazole 1166
Lanzostad (LT) *see* Lansoprazole 1166
Lanzul (CZ, EE, HR, LT, PL, RO, SI, SK) *see* Lansoprazole 1166
Lapenax (AR) *see* CloZAPine 490
Laper (CO) *see* Dipyrone [INT] 653
Lapicef (ID) *see* Cefadroxil 372
Lapiderm (KR) *see* Terbinafine (Systemic) 2002
Lapifed (ID) *see* Triprolidine and Pseudoephedrine 2105
Lapimuc (ID) *see* Ambroxol [INT] 109
Lapixime (ID) *see* Cefotaxime 382
Lapraz (ID) *see* Lansoprazole 1166
Lapren (KR) *see* Clofazimine [INT] 473
Lapren SL (KR) *see* Clofazimine [INT] 473
Lapricef (GT, NI, PA, SV) *see* Cefadroxil 372
Lapril (JO, TH) *see* Enalapril 722
Laproton (ID) *see* Lansoprazole 1166
Laquifun (AR) *see* Amorolfine [INT] 128
Laracit (CO, MX) *see* Cytarabine (Conventional) 535
Laractyl (PH) *see* ChlorproMAZINE 429
Laredine (AE, BH, CY, EG, IQ, IR, JO, KW, LB, LY, OM, QA, SA, SY, YE) *see* Loratadine 1241
Largactil (AT, AU, BB, BE, BF, BH, BJ, BM, BS, BZ, CI, CL, CR, CY, DO, EG, ES, ET, FR, GB, GH, GM, GN, GR, GT, GY, HN, IE, IQ, IR, IT, JM, JO, KE, KW, LB, LR, LU, LY, MA, ML, MR, MU, MW, MX, NE, NG, NI, NL, NO, NZ, OM, PA, PK, PR, PT, QA, SA, SC, SD, SL, SN, SR, SV, SY, TN, TR, TT, TZ, UG, VE, YE, ZA, ZM, ZW) *see* ChlorproMAZINE 429
Largo (SG) *see* ChlorproMAZINE 429
Lariam (AE, AT, AU, BE, BF, BG, BH, BJ, CH, CI, CL, CY, CZ, DE, DK, EG, ES, ET, FI, FR, GB, GH, GM, GN, GR, HK, HN, IE, IL, IQ, IR, IT, JO, KE, KR, KW, LB, LR, LU, LY, MA, ML, MR, MU, MW, NE, NG, NL, NO, OM, PE, PH, PL, PT, QA, RU, SA, SC, SD, SE, SI, SK, SL, SN, SY, TN, TR, TZ, UG, UY, VN, YE, ZA, ZM, ZW) *see* Mefloquine 1280
Laricam (JP) *see* Mefloquine 1280
Laridox (IN) *see* Sulfadoxine and Pyrimethamine [INT] 1946
Larimef (IN) *see* Mefloquine 1280
Larineo (HR) *see* Trandolapril 2080
Laritol (MX) *see* Loratadine 1241
Larixin (JP) *see* Cephalexin 405
Larotin D (EC) *see* Loratadine and Pseudoephedrine 1242
Larotin (EC) *see* Loratadine 1241
Laroxyl (BF, BJ, CI, ET, FR, GH, GM, GN, IT, KE, LR, MA, ML, MR, MU, MW, NE, NG, SC, SD, SL, SN, TN, TZ, UG, VN, ZM, ZW) *see* Amitriptyline 119
Larpose (IN) *see* LORazepam 1243
Larry (TH) *see* Ketoconazole (Topical) 1145
Lartron (MX) *see* Ondansetron 1513
Lasa (TW) *see* Losartan 1248
Lascacilin (PY) *see* Penicillin G (Parenteral/ Aqueous) 1611
Laser (IT) *see* Naproxen 1427
Laservis (DE, MY) *see* Hyaluronate and Derivatives 1006
Lasgan (ID) *see* Lansoprazole 1166
Lasilix (FR, MA) *see* Furosemide 940
Lasix (AE, AT, AU, BB, BE, BF, BH, BJ, BM, BR, BS, BZ, CH, CI, CL, CO, CR, CY, CZ, DE, DK, DO, EC, EG, ET, FI, GB, GH, GM, GN, GR, GT, GY, HK, HN, HR, ID, IE, IN, IQ, IR, IT, JM, JO, KE, KR, KW, LB, LR, LU, LY, MA, ML, MR, MU, MW, MX, MY, NE, NG, NI, NL, NO, NZ, OM, PA, PE, PH, PK, PR, PT, PY, QA, RU, SA, SC, SD, SE, SG, SI, SL, SN, SR, SV, SY, TH, TN, TR, TT, TW, TZ, UG, UY, VE, VN, YE, ZM, ZW) *see* Furosemide 940
Lasix[inj.] (HR) *see* Furosemide 940
Lasix Retard (DK, EE, IS, LT, NO, PT, SE) *see* Furosemide 940
Lasma (AE, BH, CY, EG, GB, IQ, IR, JO, KW, LB, LY, OM, QA, SA, SY, YE) *see* Theophylline 2026
Lasoprol (SG) *see* Lansoprazole 1166
Laspar (ZA) *see* Asparaginase (E. coli) 179
Lastet (AE, BG, CL, HK, HU, IN, JO, JP, KR, MY, PE, SA, SG, TH, TW, VN) *see* Etoposide 816
Lastet-S (KR) *see* Etoposide 816
Lastin (FI, NO, SE) *see* Azelastine (Nasal) 213
Lastin (FI, SE) *see* Azelastine (Ophthalmic) 213
Lasyn (TW) *see* Lacidipin [INT] 1154
Latanocom (AU) *see* Latanoprost and Timolol [CAN/INT] 1172
Latanox (CO) *see* Latanoprost 1172
Latapres (HR) *see* Latanoprost 1172
Lataro (KR) *see* Latanoprost 1172
Laticort (BG, HN, PL) *see* Hydrocortisone (Topical) 1014
Latipress (ID, PH) *see* Latanoprost 1172
Latisse (AR, BR, CL, HK, KR, KW, NZ, SG) *see* Bimatoprost 264
Latof (PY) *see* Latanoprost 1172
Latof-T (EC, PY, UY) *see* Latanoprost and Timolol [CAN/INT] 1172
Latrigine (TW) *see* LamoTRIgine 1160
Latrimet (GR) *see* Trimetazidine [INT] 2104
Latuda (AU, CH, CZ, EE, GB, HR, LT, NL, NO, SE, SI, SK) *see* Lurasidone 1256
Latus AZT (PY) *see* Zidovudine 2196
Latycin (AE, BH, CY, EG, IQ, IR, JO, KW, LB, LY, OM, QA, SA, SY, YE) *see* Tetracycline 2017
Latys (GR) *see* Piracetam [INT] 1661
Laubeel (DE) *see* LORazepam 1243
Lauracalm (LU) *see* LORazepam 1243
Laura (ZA) *see* Loratadine 1241
Laurimic (ES) *see* Fenticonazole [INT] 868
Lavelia Lotion (KR) *see* Mometasone (Topical) 1391
Laveric (ID) *see* Furosemide 940
Laver (TH) *see* Triamcinolone (Systemic) 2099
Laver (TH) *see* Triamcinolone (Topical) 2100
Lavex (KR) *see* Nabumetone 1411
Laviquin (KR) *see* Hydroquinone 1020
Lawarin (CZ) *see* Warfarin 2186
Laxacod (ID) *see* Bisacodyl 265
Laxadilac (ID) *see* Lactulose 1156
Laxadine (ID) *see* Docusate 661
Laxadin (IL) *see* Bisacodyl 265

Laxadyl (AE, BF, BH, BJ, CI, CY, EG, ET, GH, GM, GN, IQ, IR, JO, KE, KW, LB, LR, LY, MA, ML, MR, MU, MW, NE, NG, OM, QA, SA, SC, SD, SL, SN, SY, TN, TZ, UG, YE, ZM, ZW) *see* Bisacodyl ... 265
Laxalan (PE) *see* Lactulose ... 1156
Laxal (PE) *see* Lactulose ... 1156
Laxamucil (FI) *see* Psyllium ... 1744
Laxana (ID) *see* Bisacodyl ... 265
Laxans-ratiopharm (LU) *see* Bisacodyl ... 265
Laxasium (ID) *see* Magnesium Hydroxide ... 1263
Laxatin (TW) *see* Bisacodyl ... 265
Laxcodyl (TH) *see* Bisacodyl ... 265
Laxette (ZA) *see* Lactulose ... 1156
Laxocodyl (AE, BH, JO, KW, QA, SA) *see* Bisacodyl ... 265
Laxol (PL) *see* Docusate ... 661
Laxomag (AE) *see* Magnesium Hydroxide ... 1263
Lax-Tab (AU, NZ) *see* Bisacodyl ... 265
Lazafin (ID) *see* SulfaSALAzine ... 1950
Laz (ID) *see* Lansoprazole ... 1166
Lazol (HR) *see* Lansoprazole ... 1166
L-Cimexyl (SG) *see* Acetylcysteine ... 40
LC-Lexin (PH) *see* Cephalexin ... 405
Leal (UY) *see* Piroxicam ... 1662
Lebocar (AR) *see* Carbidopa and Levodopa ... 351
Lecadin (KR) *see* Lercanidipine [INT] ... 1181
Lecasol (JP, KR) *see* Clemastine ... 459
Leche De Magnesia (CO, EC, PE) *see* Magnesium Hydroxide ... 1263
Lecital (LB, SA) *see* Citalopram ... 451
Lecrav (ID) *see* Levofloxacin (Systemic) ... 1197
Lecrolyn (EE, NO, RU) *see* Cromolyn (Ophthalmic) ... 514
Lectacin (VN) *see* Levofloxacin (Ophthalmic) ... 1200
Lectacin (VN) *see* Levofloxacin (Systemic) ... 1197
Lectil (FR) *see* Betahistine [CAN/INT] ... 252
Lectopam (KR) *see* Bromazepam [CAN/INT] ... 290
Ledamox (JP) *see* AcetaZOLAMIDE ... 39
Leder C (TW) *see* Ascorbic Acid ... 178
Ledercort (AE, AR, BH, CY, EG, IN, IQ, IR, JO, KW, LB, LY, OM, QA, SA, SY, YE) *see* Triamcinolone (Systemic) ... 2099
Ledercort (AR, IN, PK) *see* Triamcinolone (Topical) ... 2100
Lederderm (DE) *see* Minocycline ... 1371
Lederfen (AT, GB, LU) *see* Fenbufen [INT] ... 852
Lederfoline (FR, PT) *see* Leucovorin Calcium ... 1183
Lederfolin (ES, IE, IT) *see* Leucovorin Calcium ... 1183
Ledermicina (IT) *see* Demeclocycline ... 589
Ledermix (NO) *see* Triamcinolone (Topical) ... 2100
Ledermycin (AT, AU, BE, GB, GR, IE, IN, LU, NL, NZ, PK) *see* Demeclocycline ... 589
Lederplatin (DK) *see* CISplatin ... 448
Lederscan (HK) *see* Aluminum Hydroxide and Magnesium Hydroxide ... 103
Lederspan (AE) *see* Triamcinolone (Systemic) ... 2099
Ledertepa (BE, LU, NL) *see* Thiotepa ... 2030
Ledertrexate (BE, FR, LU, MX, NZ, PT) *see* Methotrexate ... 1322
Ledervorin Calcium (BE, LU, NL) *see* Leucovorin Calcium ... 1183
Ledocar (PH) *see* Carbidopa and Levodopa ... 351
Ledoren (IT) *see* Nimesulide [INT] ... 1456
Ledoxan (PH) *see* Cyclophosphamide ... 517
Ledoxina (MX) *see* Cyanocobalamin ... 515
Ledoxina (MX) *see* Cyclophosphamide ... 517
Leeyo (TW) *see* Escitalopram ... 765
Lefenine (TW) *see* Flurbiprofen (Systemic) ... 906
Leflodal (TW) *see* Levofloxacin (Systemic) ... 1197
Lefloxin (TH) *see* Levofloxacin (Systemic) ... 1197
Lefluar (AR) *see* Leflunomide ... 1174
Lefocin (KR) *see* Levofloxacin (Ophthalmic) ... 1200
Lefocin (KR) *see* Levofloxacin (Systemic) ... 1197
Lefos (ES) *see* Isoniazid ... 1120
Lefotil (KR) *see* Mexiletine ... 1359
Lefrina (ID) *see* Phenylephrine and Zinc Sulfate [CAN/INT] ... 1640
Legederm (IT) *see* Alclometasone ... 72
Legendal (CH) *see* Lactulose ... 1156
Legil (BR) *see* Tenoxicam [INT] ... 2001
Legir (UY) *see* Metoclopramide ... 1345
Lehydan (SE) *see* Phenytoin ... 1640
Lekadol (HR) *see* Acetaminophen ... 32
Lekap (TR) *see* Sildenafil ... 1882
Le Ke Ning (CN) *see* Doxepin (Topical) ... 678
Lekoptin (HR) *see* Verapamil ... 2154
Lekotam (HR, SI) *see* Bromazepam [CAN/INT] ... 290
Lemat (HR) *see* Imatinib ... 1047
Lematite (PK) *see* Pizotifen [CAN/INT] ... 1664
Lemblastine (CL, MX) *see* VinBLAStine ... 2160
Lembrol (AR) *see* Diazepam ... 613
Lemed (HK) *see* Levofloxacin (Systemic) ... 1197
Lemgrip (BE, LU) *see* Acetaminophen ... 32
Leminter (MX) *see* Pantoprazole ... 1570
Lemitens (HR) *see* Telmisartan ... 1988
Lemoxol (NZ) *see* CefTAZidime ... 392
Lemtrada (AU, CZ, DE, DK, EE, GB, HR, LT, NL, RO, SE, SI) *see* Alemtuzumab ... 75
Lemttrada (NO) *see* Alemtuzumab ... 75
Lemytriol (MX) *see* Calcitriol ... 323
Lenadex (JP) *see* Dexamethasone (Systemic) ... 599
Lenamet OTC (ZA) *see* Cimetidine ... 438
Lenamet (ZA) *see* Cimetidine ... 438
Lenangio (IN) *see* Lenalidomide ... 1177
Lenara (KR) *see* Letrozole ... 1181
Lenasone (ZA) *see* Betamethasone (Systemic) ... 253
Lencid (BE, LU) *see* Lindane ... 1217
Lendacin (HR, HU) *see* CefTRIAXone ... 396
Lendianon (BR) *see* Lindane ... 1217
Lenditro (ZA) *see* Oxybutynin ... 1536
Lendomax (AE) *see* Alendronate ... 79
Lendorm (AT, DE, DK) *see* Brotizolam [INT] ... 293
Lendormin (BE, CH, CN, DE, GR, HU, IE, IT, JP, KR, LU, NL, PT, VE) *see* Brotizolam [INT] ... 293
Lengout (AU) *see* Colchicine ... 500
Leniartil (IT) *see* Naproxen ... 1427
Lenide-T (ZA) *see* Loperamide ... 1236
Lenipril (KR) *see* Enalapril ... 722
Lenison (UY) *see* ChlorproMAZINE ... 429
Lenitin (IL) *see* Bromazepam [CAN/INT] ... 290
Lennon-Colchicine (ZA) *see* Colchicine ... 500
Lennon-Dapsone (ZA) *see* Dapsone (Systemic) ... 561
Lennon-Warfarin (ZA) *see* Warfarin ... 2186
Lenocef (ZA) *see* Cephalexin ... 405
Lenocin (TH) *see* Tetracycline ... 2017
Lenor (IN) *see* Lornoxicam [INT] ... 1248
Lenovate (ZA) *see* Betamethasone (Topical) ... 255
Lenoxin (DE) *see* Digoxin ... 627
Lensor (LU) *see* Omeprazole ... 1508
Lentaron (AR, AT, BE, CH, DE, DK, ES, HU, IT, LU, NL, PT) *see* Formestane [INT] ... 926
Lentocaine (MX) *see* Mepivacaine ... 1295
Lentocilin-S (PT) *see* Penicillin G Benzathine ... 1609
Lento-Kalium (IT) *see* Potassium Chloride ... 1687
Len V.K. (ZA) *see* Penicillin V Potassium ... 1614
Leomypen (DK) *see* Penicillin G Benzathine ... 1609
Leostesin Jelly (AE, BH, CY, EG, IQ, IR, JO, KW, LB, LY, OM, QA, SA, SY, YE) *see* Lidocaine (Topical) ... 1211
Leostesin Ointment (AE, BF, BH, BJ, CI, CY, EG, ET, GH, GM, GN, IQ, IR, JO, KE, KW, LB, LR, LY, MA, ML, MR, MU, MW, NE, NG, OM, QA, SA, SC, SD, SL, SN, SY, TN, TZ, UG, YE, ZM, ZW) *see* Lidocaine (Topical) ... 1211
Lepavent (TW) *see* Valproic Acid and Derivatives ... 2123
Lepax (TW) *see* Escitalopram ... 765
Lepigine (LB) *see* LamoTRIgine ... 1160
Leponex (AE, AT, BE, BG, BH, BR, CH, CL, CO, CY, CZ, DE, DK, EC, EE, EG, ES, FI, FR, GR, HN, HR, IL, IQ,

IR, IS, IT, JO, KW, LB, LT, LY, MX, NL, NO, OM, PE, PH, PL, PT, QA, RO, SA, SE, SI, SK, SY, TR, UY, VE, VN, YE) *see* CloZAPine ... 490
Leprofen (PY) *see* Anastrozole ... 148
Lepsitol (ID) *see* CarBAMazepine ... 346
Leptanal (NO, SE) *see* FentaNYL ... 857
Leptazine (VE) *see* Trifluoperazine ... 2102
Leptilan (BF, BJ, CI, ET, GH, GM, GN, KE, LR, MA, ML, MR, MU, MW, NE, NG, SC, SD, SL, SN, TN, TW, TZ, UG, ZA, ZM, ZW) *see* Valproic Acid and Derivatives ... 2123
Leptopsique (MX) *see* Perphenazine ... 1627
Leptosuccin (HR) *see* Succinylcholine ... 1939
Lercadip (AE, BH, ES, GR, IT, KW, LB, QA, SA, SE, TH) *see* Lercanidipine [INT] ... 1181
Lercal (SK) *see* Lercanidipine [INT] ... 1181
Lercamen (RU) *see* Lercanidipine [INT] ... 1181
Lercan (AU, FR) *see* Lercanidipine [INT] ... 1181
Lercapin (EE, KR, LT) *see* Lercanidipine [INT] ... 1181
Lercaton (HU) *see* Lercanidipine [INT] ... 1181
Lerdip (NL) *see* Lercanidipine [INT] ... 1181
Lergigan (SE) *see* Promethazine ... 1723
Lergium (PE) *see* Cetirizine ... 411
Lermex (TH) *see* Acyclovir (Systemic) ... 47
Lerogin (CN) *see* Clidinium and Chlordiazepoxide ... 460
Leroxacin (KR) *see* Levofloxacin (Systemic) ... 1197
Lertamine D (MX) *see* Loratadine and Pseudoephedrine ... 1242
Lertamine (MX) *see* Loratadine ... 1241
Lertamine Repetabs (CL) *see* Loratadine and Pseudoephedrine ... 1242
Lertazin (VN) *see* Levocetirizine ... 1196
Lertus CD (MX) *see* Codeine ... 497
Lervasc (IN) *see* Lercanidipine [INT] ... 1181
Lerzam (ES) *see* Lercanidipine [INT] ... 1181
Lesacin (KR) *see* Levofloxacin (Systemic) ... 1197
Lescol XL (AE, AR, AU, BG, BH, CO, CY, EC, GB, HR, ID, JO, KR, KW, LB, LT, MX, MY, PE, PH, QA, RO, SA, SG, SI, SK, TH, TW, VN) *see* Fluvastatin ... 915
Lescol (AE, AT, AU, BB, BE, BH, BM, BR, BS, BZ, CH, CN, CY, CZ, DK, EE, EG, FI, FR, GB, GR, GY, HK, HN, HR, HU, IE, IL, IQ, IR, IT, JM, JO, KR, KW, LB, LY, MX, MY, NL, NO, NZ, OM, PE, PH, PL, PT, QA, RO, RU, SA, SE, SG, SI, SK, SR, SY, TH, TR, TT, TW, VE, YE) *see* Fluvastatin ... 915
Lescol LP (FR) *see* Fluvastatin ... 915
Lesefer (CO) *see* Sertraline ... 1878
Lesflam (MY, SG) *see* Diclofenac (Systemic) ... 617
Lesofat (PH) *see* Orlistat ... 1520
Lesporina (CO) *see* Cefadroxil ... 372
Less-K (TH) *see* Calcium Polystyrene Sulfonate [CAN/INT] ... 333
Lestid (DK, FI, GR, NO, SE) *see* Colestipol ... 504
Lestramyl (GB) *see* Ethinyl Estradiol and Desogestrel ... 799
L'estrogel (JP) *see* Estradiol (Topical) ... 780
Lesvatin (ID) *see* Simvastatin ... 1890
Letara (AU, NZ) *see* Letrozole ... 1181
Letex (PY) *see* Meloxicam ... 1283
Lethira (ID) *see* LevETIRAcetam ... 1191
Lethyl (ZA) *see* PHENobarbital ... 1632
Letizen (HR) *see* Cetirizine ... 411
Letizia (PE) *see* Desloratadine ... 594
Letoripe (PH) *see* Letrozole ... 1181
Letram (PH) *see* LevETIRAcetam ... 1191
Letraz (ID) *see* Letrozole ... 1181
Letrizine (PH) *see* Levocetirizine ... 1196
Letroz (PY) *see* Letrozole ... 1181
Letzol (IN) *see* Letrozole ... 1181
Leubex (AR) *see* DOXOrubicin (Conventional) ... 679
Leucocalcin (PY) *see* Leucovorin Calcium ... 1183
Leucogen (ID) *see* Filgrastim ... 875
Leucomax (AR, AT, BE, BR, CH, CZ, DE, DK, ES, FI, FR, GB, HR, HU, IE, IT, LU, MX, NL, NO, PT, SE) *see* Molgramostim [INT] ... 1388
Leuconolver (VE) *see* Leucovorin Calcium ... 1183
Leuco-Plus (TH) *see* Filgrastim ... 875
Leucostim (JO, KR) *see* Filgrastim ... 875
Leucovorin (AE, AT, BG, CH, DE, EG, GR, IE, IL, JO, KW, LB, PL, SA, TH, UY) *see* Leucovorin Calcium ... 1183
Leucovorin Calcium (AU, CZ, HK, HN, ID, IN, MY, NZ, TH) *see* Leucovorin Calcium ... 1183
Leucovorin Ca (PL) *see* Leucovorin Calcium ... 1183
Leucovorine Abic (NL) *see* Leucovorin Calcium ... 1183
Leukase N (DE) *see* Framycetin [INT] ... 937
Leukast (PH) *see* Montelukast ... 1392
Leukeran (AE, AR, AT, AU, BB, BD, BE, BF, BG, BH, BJ, BM, BR, BS, BZ, CH, CI, CL, CN, CY, CZ, DE, DK, EE, EG, ES, ET, FI, FR, GB, GH, GM, GN, GR, GY, HK, HN, HR, HU, ID, IE, IL, IN, IQ, IR, IS, IT, JM, JO, JP, KE, KR, KW, LB, LR, LT, LU, LY, MA, ML, MR, MT, MU, MW, MX, MY, NE, NG, NL, NO, NZ, OM, PE, PH, PK, PL, PT, QA, RU, SA, SC, SD, SE, SG, SI, SK, SL, SN, SR, SY, TH, TN, TR, TT, TW, TZ, UG, UY, YE, ZA, ZM, ZW) *see* Chlorambucil ... 419
Leuko Fungex (NZ) *see* Miconazole (Topical) ... 1360
Leukokine (ID) *see* Filgrastim ... 875
Leunase (AU, BD, CN, HK, ID, IN, JP, KR, MY, NZ, PH, PK, SG, TH, TW, VN) *see* Asparaginase (E. coli) ... 179
Leuplin Depot (TW) *see* Leuprolide ... 1186
Leuplin (KR) *see* Leuprolide ... 1186
Leustat (AR, GB, IE) *see* Cladribine ... 455
Leustatin (AT, AU, BE, BG, BR, CH, CR, DO, ES, FI, GR, GT, HK, HN, IT, KR, LU, NI, NL, NO, NZ, PA, PH, PT, SE, SG, SV, TW, UY, VE) *see* Cladribine ... 455
Leustatine (FR) *see* Cladribine ... 455
Leuzotev (TH) *see* Zoledronic Acid ... 2206
Levact (BE, CZ, DK, FI, FR, GB, GR, IE, IS, IT, NL, NO, SI, SK, TR) *see* Bendamustine ... 241
Levaler (DO, GT, PA, SV) *see* Levocetirizine ... 1196
Levanxol (AT, BE, LU) *see* Temazepam ... 1990
Levaquin (AR, BR, CO, PE) *see* Levofloxacin (Systemic) ... 1197
Levaxin (SE) *see* Levothyroxine ... 1205
Levazide (ID) *see* Benserazide and Levodopa [CAN/INT] ... 244
Lev Desitin (CH) *see* LevETIRAcetam ... 1191
Levemir (AE, AT, AU, BE, BG, BH, BR, CH, CL, CN, CY, CZ, DE, DK, FI, FR, GB, GR, HN, HR, HU, ID, IE, IL, IS, IT, JO, JP, KR, KW, LB, LT, MX, MY, NL, NO, PE, PH, PT, QA, RO, RU, SA, SE, SG, SI, SK, TH, TR, TW, UY, VN) *see* Insulin Detemir ... 1085
Levensa SR (KR) *see* Venlafaxine ... 2150
Leverctin (BR) *see* Ivermectin (Systemic) ... 1136
Levest (GB) *see* Ethinyl Estradiol and Levonorgestrel ... 803
Levetam (UY) *see* LevETIRAcetam ... 1191
Levetrim (IL) *see* LevETIRAcetam ... 1191
Levhexal (MX) *see* Levothyroxine ... 1205
Levim (TW) *see* LevETIRAcetam ... 1191
Levit (PH) *see* LevETIRAcetam ... 1191
Levitra (AE, AR, AT, AU, BB, BE, BG, BH, BM, BR, BS, BZ, CH, CL, CN, CO, CR, CZ, DE, DK, DO, EC, EE, ES, FI, FR, GB, GR, GT, GY, HK, HN, HR, ID, IE, IL, IT, JM, JP, KR, KW, LB, LT, MT, MX, MY, NI, NL, NO, NZ, PA, PE, PH, PL, PR, PT, QA, RO, RU, SA, SE, SG, SI, SK, SR, SV, TH, TR, TT, TW, VE, VN) *see* Vardenafil ... 2138
Levitra ODT (EC, HK, KR) *see* Vardenafil ... 2138
Levitra Orodispersible (CY, IL) *see* Vardenafil ... 2138
Levium (DE) *see* Methotrimeprazine [CAN/INT] ... 1329
Levlen ED (AU, NZ) *see* Ethinyl Estradiol and Levonorgestrel ... 803
Levobact (PH) *see* Levofloxacin (Systemic) ... 1197

Levoben (ID) *see* Benserazide and Levodopa [CAN/INT] ... 244
Levocar (JO) *see* Carbidopa and Levodopa ... 351
Levocen (KR) *see* Levocetirizine ... 1196
Levocet (BR, EC, IN) *see* Levocetirizine ... 1196
Levocezal (KR) *see* Levocetirizine ... 1196
Levocin (ID, PH, TH) *see* Levofloxacin (Systemic) ... 1197
Levo (IL) *see* Levofloxacin (Systemic) ... 1197
Levokacin (KR) *see* Levofloxacin (Ophthalmic) ... 1200
Levokacin (KR) *see* Levofloxacin (Systemic) ... 1197
Levolac (FI, NO) *see* Lactulose ... 1156
Levomax (CO) *see* Levofloxacin (Ophthalmic) ... 1200
Levomed (MY) *see* Carbidopa and Levodopa ... 351
Levomet (HK, SG, TH) *see* Carbidopa and Levodopa ... 351
Levomicin (KR) *see* Levofloxacin (Systemic) ... 1197
Levomine (AR) *see* Levocetirizine ... 1196
Levonelle-2 (AU) *see* Levonorgestrel ... 1201
Levonelle (GB, IE, NZ) *see* Levonorgestrel ... 1201
Levonor (PL, PY, UY, VN) *see* Norepinephrine ... 1472
Levonova (SE) *see* Levonorgestrel ... 1201
Levopar (DE, ID) *see* Benserazide and Levodopa [CAN/INT] ... 244
Levopar Plus (IL) *see* Benserazide and Levodopa [CAN/INT] ... 244
Levophed Bitartrate (AE, AU, BE, BH, CY, EG, GR, IL, IQ, IR, JO, KR, KW, LB, LY, MY, NZ, OM, PH, QA, SA, SG, SY, TH, TW, YE) *see* Norepinephrine ... 1472
Levophed (GB, IE, LU) *see* Norepinephrine ... 1472
Levophta (FR, LB) *see* Levocabastine (Ophthalmic) [CAN/INT] ... 1195
Levoquin (HK, PH) *see* Levofloxacin (Systemic) ... 1197
Levores (ID) *see* Levofloxacin (Systemic) ... 1197
Levosan (PK) *see* Levobunolol ... 1194
Levospa (PH) *see* Levofloxacin (Ophthalmic) ... 1200
Levosta (KR) *see* Levofloxacin (Ophthalmic) ... 1200
Levostar-R (IN) *see* Rupatadine [INT] ... 1855
Levostrel (TW) *see* Levonorgestrel ... 1201
Levothyrox (FR) *see* Levothyroxine ... 1205
Levotiroxina (EC) *see* Levothyroxine ... 1205
Levotirox (IT) *see* Levothyroxine ... 1205
Levotra (KR) *see* Levofloxacin (Ophthalmic) ... 1200
Levoxacin (IT) *see* Levofloxacin (Systemic) ... 1197
Levoxacin (KR) *see* Levofloxacin (Ophthalmic) ... 1200
Levoxin (HK) *see* Levofloxacin (Systemic) ... 1197
Levox (JO, PH) *see* Levofloxacin (Systemic) ... 1197
Levoxl (HK) *see* Levofloxacin (Systemic) ... 1197
Levozine (SG, TW) *see* Levocetirizine ... 1196
Levozin (FI) *see* Methotrimeprazine [CAN/INT] ... 1329
Levrix (NZ) *see* Levocetirizine ... 1196
Levron (AR) *see* LevETIRAcetam ... 1191
Levsin SL (HK) *see* Hyoscyamine ... 1026
Levulan Kerastick (TH) *see* Aminolevulinic Acid ... 114
Levunid (PE) *see* Levofloxacin (Ophthalmic) ... 1200
Levunid (PE) *see* Levofloxacin (Systemic) ... 1197
Levunolol (AR) *see* Levobunolol ... 1194
Levviax (AT, BE, BG, CZ, DE, DK, EE, ES, FI, FR, GB, HN, IE, IT, MT, NL, NO, PL, PT, RU, SE, SK, TR) *see* Telithromycin ... 1987
Le Wei (CN) *see* Tazarotene ... 1980
Lexacort (ID) *see* PredniSONE ... 1706
Lexacorton (ID) *see* Hydrocortisone (Topical) ... 1014
Lexacure (KR) *see* Escitalopram ... 765
Lexam (AU) *see* Escitalopram ... 765
Lexapam (KR) *see* Escitalopram ... 765
Lexapro (AR, AU, BB, BM, BR, BS, BZ, CN, CR, DO, EC, GT, GY, HK, HN, IE, JM, JP, KR, MY, NI, NL, NZ, PA, PE, PH, PR, SG, SR, SV, TH, TT, TW, VE) *see* Escitalopram ... 765
Lexatin (ES) *see* Bromazepam [CAN/INT] ... 290
Lexatin (KR) *see* Escitalopram ... 765
Lexaurin (CZ, HR) *see* Bromazepam [CAN/INT] ... 290
Lexavrin (SK) *see* Bromazepam [CAN/INT] ... 290
Lexcitam (KR) *see* Escitalopram ... 765
Lexcomet (ID),*see* MethylPREDNISolone ... 1340
Lexfin (CO) *see* Celecoxib ... 402
Lexigo (ID) *see* Betahistine [CAN/INT] ... 252
Lexilium (CY, HR) *see* Bromazepam [CAN/INT] ... 290
Lexin (AE, JO, PE) *see* Cephalexin ... 405
Lexinor (BD, CL, ID, IN, JP, PK, SE, SG, TW) *see* Norfloxacin ... 1475
Lexipron (ID) *see* Cephalexin ... 405
Lexiva (IL, JP) *see* Fosamprenavir ... 928
Lexoma (KR) *see* Formoterol ... 926
Lexomil (FR, VN) *see* Bromazepam [CAN/INT] ... 290
Lexopam (JO) *see* Bromazepam [CAN/INT] ... 290
Lexostad (DE) *see* Bromazepam [CAN/INT] ... 290
Lexotan (AU, BE, BG, BR, DK, EC, HK, ID, IE, IS, IT, LU, MX, PE, PH, PL, PT, PY, RO, SG, TH, TW, UY, VN) *see* Bromazepam [CAN/INT] ... 290
Lexotanil (AE, AR, AT, BH, CH, CL, CY, DE, EG, GR, JO, KW, LB, LT, NL, NO, PK, QA, SA, TR, VE) *see* Bromazepam [CAN/INT] ... 290
Lexotanol (EE) *see* Bromazepam [CAN/INT] ... 290
Lexpec (GB, IE) *see* Folic Acid ... 919
Lexzepam (ID) *see* Bromazepam [CAN/INT] ... 290
Le Zai (CN) *see* Tolterodine ... 2063
Lezat (CO) *see* Levocetirizine ... 1196
Lezol (PH) *see* Letrozole ... 1181
Lezra (ID) *see* Letrozole ... 1181
Leztrol (PH) *see* AtorvaSTATin ... 194
Lghyal (IN) *see* Hyaluronate and Derivatives ... 1006
LH-RH Tanabe (TW) *see* Gonadorelin [CAN/INT] ... 980
Libbera (PE) *see* Levocetirizine ... 1196
Liberal (TH) *see* Flunarizine [CAN/INT] ... 892
Liberaxim (MX) *see* HYDROmorphone ... 1016
Libertek (CZ) *see* Roflumilast ... 1840
Libertrim (MX) *see* Trimebutine [CAN/INT] ... 2103
Liberty (KR) *see* ChlordiazePOXIDE ... 422
Li Bi Fu (CN) *see* Dolasetron ... 663
Libotasin (GR) *see* Cinnarizine [INT] ... 440
Libractam (PY, UY) *see* Ampicillin and Sulbactam ... 145
Libradin (ES, IT, NL) *see* Barnidipine [INT] ... 227
Librapamil (EC) *see* Verapamil ... 2154
Librax (AE, AR, BB, BE, BF, BH, BJ, BM, BS, BZ, CH, CI, CR, CY, DO, EG, ET, FI, FR, GH, GM, GN, GR, GT, GY, HK, HN, ID, IL, IQ, IR, IS, IT, JM, JO, KE, KR, KW, LB, LR, LY, MA, ML, MR, MU, MW, NE, NG, NI, NL, OM, PA, PE, PK, PT, QA, SA, SC, SD, SG, SL, SN, SR, SV, SY, TH, TN, TR, TT, TW, TZ, UG, VE, VN, YE, ZA, ZM, ZW) *see* Clidinium and Chlordiazepoxide ... 460
Libraxin (CN) *see* Clidinium and Chlordiazepoxide ... 460
Libretin (PH) *see* Albuterol ... 69
Librium (AE, BH, CY, EG, FR, GH, HK, HN, HU, ID, IE, IN, IQ, IR, IT, JO, KE, KW, LB, LY, OM, QA, SA, SG, SY, TZ, UG, YE, ZA, ZM) *see* ChlordiazePOXIDE ... 422
Librocol (CH) *see* Clidinium and Chlordiazepoxide ... 460
Librodan (ID) *see* Clindamycin (Systemic) ... 460
Libron (KR) *see* Tibolone [INT] ... 2035
Licab (IN) *see* Lithium ... 1230
Licarb (HK, TH) *see* Lithium ... 1230
Licarbium (IL) *see* Lithium ... 1230
Lice Care (SG) *see* Malathion ... 1268
Lice-Enz (GR) *see* Pyrethrins and Piperonyl Butoxide ... 1746
Lice-omite (PK) *see* Permethrin ... 1627
Lice Rid (AU) *see* Malathion ... 1268
Licesol (BH) *see* Pyrethrins and Piperonyl Butoxide ... 1746
Licodin (TW) *see* Ticlopidine ... 2040
Licorax (KR) *see* Naproxen ... 1427
Licovir (ID) *see* Acyclovir (Systemic) ... 47
Lidaltrin (ES) *see* Quinapril ... 1756
Lidaprim (AE, SA) *see* Sulfamethoxazole and Trimethoprim ... 1946

Lidaprim Forte (AE, SA) *see* Sulfamethoxazole and Trimethoprim 1946
Liderman (AT) *see* Oxiconazole 1536
Lidex (BE, BM, GR, KR, LU, PH) *see* Fluocinonide 894
Lidiprine (HK) *see* Lidocaine and Prilocaine 1213
Lidocadren Teva (IL) *see* Lidocaine and Epinephrine 1212
Lidocain Gel (FI) *see* Lidocaine (Topical) 1211
Lidocain Spray (BG) *see* Lidocaine (Topical) 1211
Lidocard (DK) *see* Lidocaine (Systemic) 1208
Lidoderm (GR, NO) *see* Lidocaine (Topical) 1211
Lidong (CN) *see* Lactulose 1156
Lidotop Cataplasma (KR) *see* Lidocaine (Topical) 1211
Lidoxin (SG) *see* Cloxacillin [CAN/INT] 488
Lifacor (PH) *see* Leucovorin Calcium 1183
Lifaton B1 (ES) *see* Thiamine 2028
Lifaton B12 (ES) *see* Cyanocobalamin 515
Lifezar (PH) *see* Losartan 1248
Lifibron (ID) *see* Gemfibrozil 956
Li Fu (CN) *see* MetroNIDAZOLE (Topical) 1357
Lignocaine Gel (AU) *see* Lidocaine (Topical) 1211
Lignopad (HK, MY) *see* Lidocaine (Topical) 1211
Ligofragmin (AR) *see* Dalteparin 553
Likacin (AE, BH, CY, EG, HU, IL, IQ, IR, JO, KW, LB, LY, OM, QA, SA, SG, SY, VN, YE) *see* Amikacin 111
Likelin (CN) *see* Leucovorin Calcium 1183
Li Ke Ning (CN) *see* Doxepin (Systemic) 676
Likodin (TW) *see* Cefadroxil 372
Likuden (DE) *see* Griseofulvin 985
Lilac (PH) *see* Lactulose 1156
Li Ling (CN) *see* Tretinoin (Topical) 2099
Liman (AT, DE) *see* Tenoxicam [INT] 2001
Limas (JP) *see* Lithium 1230
Limbatril (DE) *see* Amitriptyline and Chlordiazepoxide 122
Limbatrilin (CL) *see* Amitriptyline and Chlordiazepoxide 122
Limbial (IT) *see* Oxazepam 1532
Limbitrol (AE, AT, BE, BH, BR, CY, EG, FI, FR, GH, GR, ID, IL, IQ, IR, JO, KE, KW, LB, LY, NL, OM, QA, SA, SY, TW, TZ, UG, YE, ZM) *see* Amitriptyline and Chlordiazepoxide 122
Limbitryl (IT) *see* Amitriptyline and Chlordiazepoxide 122
Limcee (IN) *see* Ascorbic Acid 178
Limdopa (VN) *see* DOPamine 669
Limember (PE) *see* Memantine 1286
Limus (TW) *see* QUEtiapine 1751
Linatecan (PE) *see* Irinotecan 1112
Lincil (HN) *see* NiCARdipine 1446
Lincox (PH) *see* Celecoxib 402
Linctus Tussinol (AU) *see* Pholcodine [INT] 1646
Lindacin (TW) *see* Clindamycin (Systemic) 460
Lindan (ID) *see* Lindane 1217
Lindano (AR) *see* Lindane 1217
Lindano-GBHG (PY) *see* Lindane 1217
Lindella CD (CO) *see* Ethinyl Estradiol and Levonorgestrel 803
Lindella (CO) *see* Ethinyl Estradiol and Levonorgestrel 803
Lindell (PH) *see* Permethrin 1627
Linden Lotion (KR) *see* Lindane 1217
Lindex (EC) *see* Memantine 1286
Lindisc (AR, CO, CR, EC, GT, HN, NI, PA, SV) *see* Estradiol (Systemic) 775
Lindormin (MX) *see* Brotizolam [INT] 293
Lindoxyl (DE) *see* Ambroxol [INT] 109
Linea (GR, IT) *see* Diethylpropion 624
Linespan (LB) *see* Linezolid 1217
Linface (EC) *see* Cyproterone and Ethinyl Estradiol [CAN/INT] 532
Linfonex (CL, PY) *see* Mycophenolate 1405
Linglanxin (CN) *see* Cefoperazone and Sulbactam [INT] 382
Lingraine (GB, IE) *see* Ergotamine 754
Linisan (RO) *see* Citalopram 451
Linodiab (ID) *see* Gliclazide [CAN/INT] 964
Linoladiol N (EE) *see* Estradiol (Systemic) 775
Linola Urea (DE) *see* Urea 2114
Linopril (AE, BH, CY, EG, IQ, IR, JO, KW, LB, LY, OM, QA, SA, SY, YE) *see* Lisinopril 1226
Linox (IN) *see* Linezolid 1217
Lintos (IT) *see* Ambroxol [INT] 109
Li Nuo Ke (CN) *see* Nimesulide [INT] 1456
Linvas (IN) *see* Lisinopril 1226
Liobac (TH) *see* Baclofen 223
Liocarpina (IT) *see* Pilocarpine (Ophthalmic) 1649
Lioram (BR) *see* Zolpidem 2212
Lioresal (AE, AR, AT, AU, BB, BD, BE, BF, BG, BH, BJ, BM, BR, BS, BZ, CH, CI, CN, CO, CY, CZ, DE, DK, EE, EG, ES, ET, FI, FR, GB, GH, GM, GN, GR, GY, HK, HN, HR, HU, ID, IE, IL, IN, IQ, IR, IS, IT, JM, JO, JP, KE, KW, LB, LR, LU, LY, MA, ML, MR, MT, MU, MW, MY, NE, NG, NL, NO, NZ, OM, PH, PK, PL, PT, PY, QA, RO, RU, SA, SC, SD, SE, SG, SI, SL, SN, SR, SY, TH, TN, TR, TT, TZ, UG, VE, YE, ZA, ZM, ZW) *see* Baclofen 223
Lioresyl (CL) *see* Baclofen 223
Liothyronin (NO, PL, SE) *see* Liothyronine 1221
Lioton (RU) *see* Heparin 997
Lipaco (MY) *see* Simvastatin 1890
Lipacreon (JP) *see* Pancrelipase 1566
Lipanor (CZ, EE, FR, HN, IL, KR, PL, PT, RU) *see* Ciprofibrate [INT] 441
Lipazil (AU, NZ) *see* Gemfibrozil 956
Lipebin (AE, BH, CY, EG, IL, IQ, IR, JO, KW, LB, LY, OM, PE, QA, SA, SY, YE) *see* Lactulose 1156
Lipecor (KR) *see* Simvastatin 1890
Lipemol (ES) *see* Pravastatin 1700
Liperol (MX) *see* Lovastatin 1252
Liperox (AR) *see* Riboflavin 1803
Lipex (AU, HR, NZ) *see* Simvastatin 1890
Lipibec Duo (AR) *see* Ezetimibe and Atorvastatin 833
Lipicap (TH) *see* Gemfibrozil 956
Lipichek (PH) *see* Rosuvastatin 1848
Lipidoff (TW) *see* Simvastatin 1890
Lipidown (KR) *see* Orlistat 1520
Lipiduce (HK, MY) *see* AtorvaSTATin 194
Lipigem (PH) *see* Gemfibrozil 956
Lipigo (PH) *see* AtorvaSTATin 194
Lipikhan (HK, PH) *see* AtorvaSTATin 194
Lipilou (KR) *see* AtorvaSTATin 194
Lipinon (KR) *see* AtorvaSTATin 194
Lipinorm (ID) *see* Simvastatin 1890
Lipison (HK, SG) *see* Gemfibrozil 956
Lipistad (HK) *see* AtorvaSTATin 194
Lipista (VN) *see* Pravastatin 1700
Lipistorol (HK) *see* Gemfibrozil 956
Lipiterol (KR) *see* AtorvaSTATin 194
Lipitin (HR) *see* AtorvaSTATin 194
Lipitor (AE, AR, AU, BD, BE, BF, BH, BJ, BO, BR, CI, CL, CN, CO, CR, CY, DO, EC, EE, EG, ET, FI, GB, GH, GM, GN, GR, GT, HK, HN, ID, IE, IL, IQ, IR, JO, JP, KE, KR, KW, LB, LR, LY, MA, ML, MR, MU, MW, MX, MY, NE, NG, NI, NL, NO, NZ, OM, PA, PE, PH, PK, PR, PY, QA, SA, SC, SD, SE, SG, SL, SN, SV, SY, TH, TN, TR, TW, TZ, UG, UY, VE, VN, YE, ZA, ZM, ZW) *see* AtorvaSTATin 194
Lipitrop (ID) *see* Gemfibrozil 956
Lipivent (PH) *see* AtorvaSTATin 194
Lipiwon (KR) *see* AtorvaSTATin 194
Lipizile (PH) *see* Gemfibrozil 956
Liplat (ES) *see* Pravastatin 1700
Liplatin (KR) *see* Oxaliplatin 1528
Liple (JP) *see* Alprostadil 96
Lipless (BR) *see* Ciprofibrate [INT] 441

Lipneo (BR) *see* Ciprofibrate [INT] 441
Lipoactin (KR) *see* AtorvaSTATin 194
Lipobrand (EC) *see* Ciprofibrate [INT] 441
Lipocin (MX) *see* Bezafibrate [CAN/INT] 261
Lipoclin (BR) *see* Lovastatin 1252
Lipocol-Merz (DE) *see* Cholestyramine Resin 431
Lipocor (PK) *see* Bezafibrate [CAN/INT] 261
Lipocura (PY) *see* Rimonabant [INT] 1814
Lipodar (AE, BH, CY, EG, IQ, IR, JO, KW, LB, LY, OM, QA, SA, SY, YE) *see* AtorvaSTATin 194
Lipo-Dox (TH, TW) *see* DOXOrubicin (Liposomal) 684
Lipofol (TW) *see* Propofol 1728
Lipofor (JO, SG) *see* Gemfibrozil 956
Lipofundin-S (MY, TW) *see* Fat Emulsion (Plant Based) 848
Lipolo (TH) *see* Gemfibrozil 956
Lipomax 10 Plus (PY) *see* Ezetimibe and Atorvastatin 833
Lipomax 20 Plus (PY) *see* Ezetimibe and Atorvastatin 833
Lipomax (PY, QA, SA) *see* AtorvaSTATin 194
Lipomet (KR) *see* AtorvaSTATin 194
Lipomin (ES) *see* Diethylpropion 624
Liponorm (EC) *see* AtorvaSTATin 194
Liponorm (IT) *see* Simvastatin 1890
Lipostat (AE, AU, BG, BH, CZ, EE, EG, GB, HN, HU, IE, JO, KW, LB, PL, QA, SA) *see* Pravastatin 1700
Liposyn II (MX, PE) *see* Fat Emulsion (Plant Based) 848
Lipovas (JP) *see* Simvastatin 1890
Lipovenos (CL, PH) *see* Fat Emulsion (Plant Based) 848
Liprace (AU) *see* Lisinopril 1226
Lipres (ID) *see* Gemfibrozil 956
Liprevil (DE) *see* Pravastatin 1700
Liprido (TW) *see* Lidocaine and Prilocaine 1213
Liprikaine (TH) *see* Lidocaine and Prilocaine 1213
Lipril Cream (KR) *see* Lidocaine and Prilocaine 1213
Lipril (IN) *see* Lisinopril 1226
Liprolog (AT, BE, BG, CH, CZ, DE, DK, FI, FR, GB, GR, HN, IE, IT, NL, NO, PT, RU, SE, TR) *see* Insulin Lispro 1087
Lipro (MY) *see* Lidocaine and Prilocaine 1213
Liptan (AE, BH, CY, EG, IL, IQ, IR, JO, JP, KW, LB, LY, OM, QA, SA, SY, YE) *see* Ibuprofen 1032
Liptruzet (BM) *see* Ezetimibe and Atorvastatin 833
Lipur (FR) *see* Gemfibrozil 956
Lipuro (PH) *see* Propofol 1728
Liquemin (DE, IT) *see* Heparin 997
Liquemine (BE, TR) *see* Heparin 997
Liquifer (NL) *see* Ferrous Sulfate 871
Liramin (VE) *see* Dexchlorpheniramine 603
Lirex (PY) *see* Tibolone [INT] 2035
Lisdene (MY, SG) *see* Lisinopril 1226
Lishenbao (CN) *see* Urofollitropin 2116
Lisibeta (DE) *see* Lisinopril 1226
Lisidigal (VN) *see* Lisinopril 1226
Lisigamma (DE) *see* Lisinopril 1226
Lisihexal (DE) *see* Lisinopril 1226
Lisiletic (VE) *see* Lisinopril and Hydrochlorothiazide 1229
Lisim (MY, SG) *see* Terbinafine (Systemic) 2002
Lisim (SG) *see* Terbinafine (Topical) 2004
Lisino (DE) *see* Loratadine 1241
Lisipril (CO) *see* Lisinopril and Hydrochlorothiazide 1229
Lisipril (CO, DO) *see* Lisinopril 1226
Lisir (TH) *see* Lisinopril 1226
Liskantin (BG, CZ, DE, EE, LU) *see* Primidone 1714
Liskonum (AE, BH, CY, EG, IQ, IR, JO, KW, LB, LY, OM, QA, SA, SY, YE) *see* Lithium 1230
Lisobac (MX) *see* Amikacin 111
Lisodren (BR) *see* Mitotane 1382
Lisomucin (PT) *see* Bromhexine [INT] 291
Lisoneurin (AR) *see* Hydroxocobalamin 1020
Lisopress (BB, BM, BS, BZ, GY, HU, JM, NZ, SR, TT) *see* Lisinopril 1226
Lisopril (HK) *see* Lisinopril 1226
Lisoril (IN, SG) *see* Lisinopril 1226
Lisovyr (AR, CL) *see* Acyclovir (Systemic) 47
Lisovyr Cream (AR) *see* Acyclovir (Topical) 51
Lisovyr Crema (CL) *see* Acyclovir (Topical) 51
Lispecip (RO) *see* Pioglitazone 1654
Lispril (TH) *see* Lisinopril 1226
Listaflex (AR) *see* Carisoprodol 363
Listril (IN) *see* Lisinopril 1226
Litaduet (KR) *see* Amlodipine and Atorvastatin 124
Litak (AT, AU, BE, BG, CH, CZ, DE, DK, EE, ES, FI, FR, GB, GR, HN, HR, IE, IL, IT, LT, MT, NL, NO, PL, PT, RU, SE, SI, SK, TR, TW) *see* Cladribine 455
Litalir (AT, CH, CZ, HN, HR, HU) *see* Hydroxyurea 1021
Litamol (VN) *see* Ethambutol 798
Litangen (TW) *see* ChlorproPAMIDE 429
Litanin (ES) *see* Ursodiol 2116
Litarex (DK, NO) *see* Lithium 1230
L:ithan (KR) *see* Lithium 1230
Litheum 300 (MX) *see* Lithium 1230
Lithicarb (AU, MY) *see* Lithium 1230
Lithicarb FC (NZ) *see* Lithium 1230
Lithionit (NO, SE) *see* Lithium 1230
Lithium Carbonicum (PL) *see* Lithium 1230
Lithiumkarbonat "Oba" (DK) *see* Lithium 1230
Lithocap (IN) *see* Lithium 1230
Litiasin (PE) *see* Potassium Citrate and Citric Acid 1689
Liticarb (HN, HU) *see* Lithium 1230
Litij-karbonat (HR) *see* Lithium 1230
Litil (DO) *see* Lithium 1230
Litinol (VE) *see* Allopurinol 90
Lition (TW) *see* Phenoxybenzamine 1635
Litiumkarbonat "Dak" (DK) *see* Lithium 1230
Litocarb (PE) *see* Lithium 1230
Litocin (TW) *see* Oxytocin 1549
Lito (FI) *see* Lithium 1230
Litorcom (ID) *see* AtorvaSTATin 194
Litorva (IL) *see* AtorvaSTATin 194
Litrecan (AR) *see* Linezolid 1217
Litrol (ID) *see* Neomycin, Polymyxin B, and Dexamethasone 1437
Livalo (AU, CN, KR, TH, TW) *see* Pitavastatin 1663
Livazo (CH, DE, IE, LB, NL, SE) *see* Pitavastatin 1663
Livial (AE, AU, BE, BG, BH, BR, CH, CL, CN, CO, CR, CY, CZ, DK, DO, EE, FI, FR, GB, GR, GT, HK, HN, HR, ID, IE, IL, IN, IS, IT, JO, KR, KW, LB, LT, MX, MY, NI, NL, NO, NZ, PA, PE, PH, PK, PL, PT, QA, RO, RU, SA, SE, SG, SI, SK, SV, TH, TR, TW, VE, VN) *see* Tibolone [INT] 2035
Liviel (AT) *see* Tibolone [INT] 2035
Liviella (DE) *see* Tibolone [INT] 2035
Livifem (ZA) *see* Tibolone [INT] 2035
Livingpherol (KR) *see* Vitamin E 2174
Livocab (DE, ES, NL) *see* Levocabastine (Ophthalmic) [CAN/INT] 1195
Livocab (DE, NL) *see* Levocabastine (Nasal) [CAN/INT] 1194
Livo Luk (IN) *see* Lactulose 1156
Livomedrox (PY) *see* MedroxyPROGESTERone 1277
Livostin (AE, AT, AU, BE, BG, BH, CH, CL, CN, CO, CY, CZ, DK, EE, EG, FI, GB, GR, HN, HR, HU, IL, IQ, IR, IS, IT, JO, KR, KW, LB, LU, LY, MX, NO, NZ, OM, PT, PY, QA, SA, SE, SI, SY, UY, VE, YE, ZA) *see* Levocabastine (Ophthalmic) [CAN/INT] 1195
Livostin (AE, AT, AU, BE, CH, CN, CZ, DK, EG, FI, GR, IL, IS, JP, NO, NZ, PT, QA, SE, SI, VE, ZA) *see* Levocabastine (Nasal) [CAN/INT] 1194
Liza (MY, PH) *see* Ethinyl Estradiol and Drospirenone 801
Lizelle (MY, PH) *see* Ethinyl Estradiol and Drospirenone 801

Lizhu Yindefu (CN) *see* Interferon Gamma-1b 1104
Lizinna (GB) *see* Ethinyl Estradiol and Norgestimate 810
Liz (MY) *see* Ethinyl Estradiol and Drospirenone 801
Lizolid (VN) *see* Linezolid 1217
Lizor (ID) *see* Cefprozil 389
Llanol (PH, VN) *see* Allopurinol 90
LM Dextran L (ID) *see* Dextran 607
LM Dextran (ID) *see* Dextran 607
Lobate (IN) *see* Clobetasol 468
Lobesol (MY) *see* Clobetasol 468
Lobeta (DE) *see* Loratadine 1241
Lobevat (CR, DO, GT, HN, MX, NI, PA, SV) *see* Clobetasol 468
Lobione (LU) *see* Betahistine [CAN/INT] 252
Lobivon (GR, IT, NL, TR) *see* Nebivolol 1434
Locacid (IL, PT, SK) *see* Tretinoin (Topical) 2099
Locacorten Vioform (BH, EG, KW, LB, QA, SA) *see* Clioquinol and Flumethasone [CAN/INT] 465
Locacorten-Vioform (DE, DK, FI, NL, NO, SE) *see* Clioquinol and Flumethasone [CAN/INT] 465
Locacorten-Vioform Ear Drops (AU) *see* Clioquinol and Flumethasone [CAN/INT] 465
Localyn (IT) *see* Fluocinolone (Topical) 893
Locana (TH) *see* Lidocaine (Systemic) 1208
Locapred (CH, VN) *see* Desonide 597
Locarp (IN) *see* Pilocarpine (Ophthalmic) 1649
Locatop (CH, CZ, PL, VN) *see* Desonide 597
Locef (NZ) *see* Cefaclor 372
Locemine (TW) *see* Levocetirizine 1196
Locemix (AR) *see* Minoxidil (Topical) 1374
Loceride (PH) *see* Gemfibrozil 956
Loceryl (AE, AR, AT, BE, BH, BR, CH, CL, CN, CO, CR, CY, CZ, DE, DK, DO, EC, EE, FI, FR, GB, GR, GT, HK, HN, HU, IE, IL, IN, IS, KR, KW, LB, LT, MY, NI, NO, NZ, PA, PE, PL, QA, RU, SA, SE, SG, SI, SK, SV, TH, TR, TW, UY, VE, ZA) *see* Amorolfine [INT] 128
Loceryl Nail Lacquer (AU) *see* Amorolfine [INT] 128
Locetar (ES, IT, PH, PT) *see* Amorolfine [INT] 128
Lochol (JP) *see* Fluvastatin 915
Lochol (TH) *see* Simvastatin 1890
Locid (KR) *see* Ranitidine 1777
Lock 2 (BF, BJ, CI, ET, GH, GM, GN, IN, KE, LR, MA, ML, MR, MU, MW, NE, NG, SC, SD, SL, SN, TN, TZ, UG, ZM, ZW) *see* Cimetidine 438
Locoid (AE, BE, BH, BR, CH, CL, CN, CY, CZ, DK, EG, FI, FR, GB, HN, HU, IE, IQ, IR, IS, JO, KW, LB, LY, NL, NO, NZ, OM, PE, PT, QA, RO, RU, SA, SE, SK, SY, TR, TW, VN, YE) *see* Hydrocortisone (Topical) 1014
Locoid Lipo (IN) *see* Hydrocortisone (Topical) 1014
Locoidon (AT, IT, PE, SI) *see* Hydrocortisone (Topical) 1014
Locol (DE) *see* Fluvastatin 915
Locorten-Vioform (CY) *see* Clioquinol and Flumethasone [CAN/INT] 465
Locorten Vioform (NZ) *see* Clioquinol and Flumethasone [CAN/INT] 465
Locorten Vioformo (VE) *see* Clioquinol and Flumethasone [CAN/INT] 465
Locula (IN) *see* Sulfacetamide (Ophthalmic) 1943
Lodales (FR) *see* Simvastatin 1890
Lodexa-5 (TH) *see* Dexamethasone (Systemic) 599
Lodexa (TH) *see* Dexamethasone (Systemic) 599
Lodia (ID) *see* Loperamide 1236
Lodial (RO) *see* Losartan 1248
Lodibes (PH) *see* AmLODIPine 123
Lodil (KR) *see* Felodipine 850
Lodine XL (CN) *see* Etodolac 815
Lodine (AE, AT, BH, CH, FI, FR, IT, KR, KW, MX, PK, QA, SA, TR, VE) *see* Etodolac 815
Lodine Retard (MX) *see* Etodolac 815
Lodine SR (GB) *see* Etodolac 815
Lodin (PH) *see* AmLODIPine 123
Lodipin ER (KR) *see* Felodipine 850
Lodistad MR (PH) *see* Felodipine 850
Lodoc (AR) *see* Benzocaine 246
Lodotra (AU, GB, IL, KR, RO, SG, SK, TR) *see* PredniSONE 1706
Lodoz (AE, BE, BG, BH, CZ, EE, FI, HK, ID, IN, IT, KW, MY, NO, QA, SA, SG, TH, VN) *see* Bisoprolol and Hydrochlorothiazide 267
Lodulce (PH) *see* GlyBURIDE 972
Loette 21 (SG) *see* Ethinyl Estradiol and Levonorgestrel 803
Loette (HK, IN, MY, NZ, SG) *see* Ethinyl Estradiol and Levonorgestrel 803
Lofarbil (GR) *see* Metoprolol 1350
Lofatin (TW) *see* CefOXitin 386
Lofenoxal (AU) *see* Diphenoxylate and Atropine 644
Loflam (AE) *see* Aceclofenac [INT] 30
Lofral (HK, JO, MY) *see* AmLODIPine 123
Lofucin (KR) *see* Ciprofloxacin (Systemic) 441
Logastric (BE) *see* Omeprazole 1508
Logenate (RO) *see* Antihemophilic Factor (Recombinant) 152
Logicin Sinus (HK) *see* Pseudoephedrine 1742
Logiflox (FR) *see* Lomefloxacin [INT] 1233
Logiparin (AT, CZ, IN) *see* Tinzaparin 2043
Logoderm (NZ) *see* Alclometasone 72
Logomed Kreislauf-Tabletten (DE) *see* Etilefrine [INT] 815
Logos (ZA) *see* Famotidine 845
Logynon (AE, BF, BH, BJ, CI, CY, EG, ET, GH, GM, GN, IQ, IR, JO, KE, KW, LB, LR, LY, MA, ML, MR, MU, MW, NE, NG, OM, PH, QA, SA, SC, SD, SL, SN, SY, TN, TZ, UG, YE, ZM, ZW) *see* Ethinyl Estradiol and Levonorgestrel 803
Logynon ED (AU, ZA) *see* Ethinyl Estradiol and Levonorgestrel 803
Lohist (BH, JO, KW, SA) *see* Loratadine 1241
Lojuxta (CZ, DE, EE, GB, HR, LT, NL, RO, SE, SK) *see* Lomitapide 1233
Lokev (ID) *see* Omeprazole 1508
Lokilan (NO) *see* Flunisolide (Nasal) 893
Lokren (HN, PL, SK) *see* Betaxolol (Systemic) 256
Loksin (ID) *see* Mometasone (Topical) 1391
Lolita (TH) *see* Ketoprofen 1145
Lolomit (CO) *see* Timolol (Ophthalmic) 2043
Lomac (IN) *see* Omeprazole 1508
Lomaday (MY) *see* Lomefloxacin [INT] 1233
Lomakline (HK) *see* AmLODIPine 123
Lomarin (IT) *see* DimenhyDRINATE 637
Lomaxacin (KR) *see* Lomefloxacin [INT] 1233
Lomax (AE, BH, KW, SA) *see* Lomefloxacin [INT] 1233
L-Ombrix (MX) *see* Mebendazole [CAN/INT] 1274
Lomeane (PH) *see* Mometasone (Topical) 1391
Lomebact (TW) *see* Lomefloxacin [INT] 1233
Lomed D (PY) *see* Desloratadine and Pseudoephedrine 594
Lomedium (VN) *see* Loperamide 1236
Lomeflon (JP) *see* Lomefloxacin [INT] 1233
Lomeflox (DO, HK) *see* Lomefloxacin [INT] 1233
Lomesone (GR) *see* Alclometasone 72
Lomexin (AE, AR, AT, BG, BH, BR, CO, CY, CZ, DE, ES, FR, GR, IT, KR, KW, LB, LT, MX, PK, PT, QA, RO, RU, SG, SK, TR, TW, ZA) *see* Fenticonazole [INT] 868
Lomexin T (AE, BH, KW, LB) *see* Fenticonazole [INT] 868
Lomex (PY) *see* Omeprazole 1508
Lomflox (IN, SG) *see* Lomefloxacin [INT] 1233
Lomide (AU, NZ) *see* Lodoxamide 1232
Lomid (PY) *see* Desloratadine 594
Lomid SR (EG) *see* Isradipine 1130
Lomir (AE, AT, BE, BF, BH, BJ, BR, CH, CI, CY, CZ, DE, EG, ES, ET, FI, GH, GM, GN, GR, HN, HU, IE, IL, IQ, IR, JO, KE, KW, LB, LR, LU, LY, MA, ML, MR, MU, MW, NE, NG, NL, NO, OM, PL, PT, QA, RU, SA, SC,

SD, SE, SK, SL, SN, SY, TN, TR, TZ, UG, YE, ZA, ZM, ZW) *see* Isradipine 1130
Lomir Retard (DK, IS) *see* Isradipine 1130
Lomir SRO (AE, AT, BH, CH, CY, CZ, FI, HN, IT, KW, NL, NO, PL, PT, QA, SA, SE) *see* Isradipine 1130
Lomisat (DE, ES) *see* Clobutinol [INT] 468
Lomoh-40 (PH) *see* Enoxaparin 726
Lomoh-60 (PH) *see* Enoxaparin 726
Lomont (GB) *see* Lofepramine [INT] 1232
Lomotil (MX) *see* Loperamide 1236
Lomotil (AE, AU, BB, BF, BH, BJ, CI, CO, CY, EG, ET, GB, GH, GM, GN, HK, IN, JM, KE, KW, LR, MA, ML, MR, MU, MW, NE, NG, NL, PE, PT, QA, SA, SC, SD, SL, SN, TH, TN, TR, TT, TZ, UG, ZA, ZM, ZW) *see* Diphenoxylate and Atropine 644
Lomotine (AE, BH, CY, EG, IL, IQ, IR, JO, KW, LB, LY, OM, QA, SA, SY, YE) *see* Diphenoxylate and Atropine 644
Lomper (ES) *see* Mebendazole [CAN/INT] 1274
Lomsin (MX) *see* Albendazole 65
Lomudal (DK, FI, GR, IS, IT, NO, SE) *see* Cromolyn (Ophthalmic) 514
Lomudal (DK, FI, GR, NO, SE) *see* Cromolyn (Nasal) 514
Lomusol (AT) *see* Cromolyn (Ophthalmic) 514
Lomusol (AT, BE, FR, NL) *see* Cromolyn (Nasal) 514
Lomustine (IN, SE) *see* Lomustine 1235
Lomustine "Medac" (DK) *see* Lomustine 1235
Lomustinum (PL) *see* Lomustine 1235
Lonarid mono (LU) *see* Acetaminophen 32
Lonazep (IN) *see* ClonazePAM 478
Lonazet (CO) *see* OXcarbazepine 1532
Lonene (ID) *see* Etodolac 815
Longacef (AE, BH, CY, EG, IQ, IR, JO, KW, LB, LY, OM, QA, SA, SY, YE) *see* CefTRIAXone 396
Longacef (VE) *see* Cefixime 380
Longasteril 40° (DE, LU) *see* Dextran 607
Longcardio (TW) *see* Carvedilol 367
Longes (JP) *see* Lisinopril 1226
Longshutong (CN) *see* Bisacodyl 265
Longum 4 (NL) *see* Pipotiazine [CAN/INT] 1660
Lonikan (AR) *see* Fludrocortisone 891
Lonine (GR, TW) *see* Etodolac 815
Loniper (PH) *see* Loperamide 1236
Loniten (AT, AU, BR, CH, GB, GR, IE, IT, KR, NO, TH, TW) *see* Minoxidil (Systemic) 1374
Lonnoten (NL) *see* Minoxidil (Systemic) 1374
Lonocam (KR) *see* Lornoxicam [INT] 1248
Lonolox (DE) *see* Minoxidil (Systemic) 1374
Lonoten (FR) *see* Minoxidil (Systemic) 1374
Lonpra (CO) *see* Hydrochlorothiazide 1009
Lonseren (ES) *see* Pipotiazine [CAN/INT] 1660
Lontencin (PH) *see* Terazosin 2001
Lonza (TH) *see* LORazepam 1243
Lopac (TW) *see* Loxapine 1255
Lopamide (IN) *see* Loperamide 1236
Lopamol (LT) *see* AtorvaSTATin 194
Lopam (TW) *see* LORazepam 1243
Lopedin (TW) *see* Loperamide 1236
Lopedium (HU, LU) *see* Loperamide 1236
Lopemid (IT) *see* Loperamide 1236
Lopen (KR) *see* Loxoprofen [INT] 1255
Lopentac (KR) *see* Loxoprofen [INT] 1255
Loperamide-Eurogenerics (LU) *see* Loperamide 1236
Loperamide-Generics (LU) *see* Loperamide 1236
Loperamid-ratiopharm (LU) *see* Loperamide 1236
Loperamil (HK, SG) *see* Loperamide 1236
Loper (HK) *see* Loperamide 1236
Loperhoe (DE) *see* Loperamide 1236
Loperium (BB, BM, BS, BZ, GY, JM, NL, SR, TT) *see* Loperamide 1236
Lopermide (HK) *see* Loperamide 1236
Lopermid (TR) *see* Loperamide 1236
Lophakomp-B1 (DE) *see* Thiamine 2028
Lophakomp-B 12 Depot (DE) *see* Hydroxocobalamin 1020
Lopicare (IL) *see* Loperamide 1236
Lopid (AE, AR, AU, BE, BH, BR, CL, CO, CR, CY, DK, DO, EC, EG, FI, GB, GR, GT, HK, HN, ID, IE, IL, IQ, IR, IT, JO, KR, KW, LB, LU, LY, MX, NI, NL, NO, OM, PA, PE, PH, PK, PT, QA, SA, SE, SV, SY, TH, TR, TW, UY, VE, VN, YE, ZA) *see* Gemfibrozil 956
Lopid OD (PH) *see* Gemfibrozil 956
Lopirel (HK) *see* Clopidogrel 484
Lopiretic (PT) *see* Captopril and Hydrochlorothiazide 345
Lopirin (AT, CH, DE) *see* Captopril 342
Lopirin (TW) *see* Aspirin 180
Lopmin (KR) *see* Loperamide 1236
Lopram (AE, KW, QA) *see* Citalopram 451
Lopresor (AE, AR, AT, AU, BB, BE, BF, BH, BJ, BM, BS, BZ, CI, CL, CY, CZ, EG, ES, ET, GB, GH, GM, GN, GR, GY, IE, IQ, IR, IT, JM, JO, KE, KW, LR, LU, LY, MA, ML, MR, MU, MW, MX, NE, NG, NL, NZ, OM, PT, PY, QA, SA, SC, SD, SL, SN, SR, SY, TN, TT, TZ, UG, UY, VE, YE, ZA, ZM, ZW) *see* Metoprolol 1350
Lopresor Divitab (IL) *see* Metoprolol 1350
Lopresor OROS (LU) *see* Metoprolol 1350
Lopresor Retard (AE, AT, BH, CH, GR, IT, PT) *see* Metoprolol 1350
Lopresor SR (GB) *see* Metoprolol 1350
Lopressor (BR, FR, LB) *see* Metoprolol 1350
Lopress (TH) *see* Prazosin 1703
Loprex (IL) *see* Loperamide 1236
Loprid (RO) *see* Loperamide 1236
Lopril-D (BR) *see* Captopril and Hydrochlorothiazide 345
Lopril (FI, FR) *see* Captopril 342
Loprolol (ID) *see* Metoprolol 1350
Loprox (AR, BR, CR, DO, EC, GT, MX, NI, PA, SV, TH) *see* Ciclopirox 433
Loprox Laca (MX) *see* Ciclopirox 433
Loprox Nail Lacquer (ID) *see* Ciclopirox 433
Loprox Naillacquer (KR) *see* Ciclopirox 433
Lorabasics (DE) *see* Loratadine 1241
Lorabenz (DK) *see* LORazepam 1243
Loraclar (DE) *see* Loratadine 1241
Loraclear Hayfever Relief (NZ) *see* Loratadine 1241
Lora (CN) *see* LORazepam 1243
Loradad (LB) *see* Loratadine 1241
Loraderm (DE) *see* Loratadine 1241
Loradin (HK) *see* Loratadine 1241
Lorafen (PL) *see* LORazepam 1243
Lorahist (PH) *see* Loratadine 1241
Lorakine (QA) *see* Loratadine 1241
Loralergan (PE) *see* Desloratadine 594
Loralerg (DE) *see* Loratadine 1241
Lora-Lich (DE) *see* Loratadine 1241
Loramet (BE, CH, ES, GR, HK, NL, SG, TH, ZA) *see* Lormetazepam [INT] 1247
Loram (HR) *see* LORazepam 1243
Loramide (SG) *see* Loperamide 1236
Loranka (BE) *see* Lormetazepam [INT] 1247
Lorano (AU, DE, PH, ZA) *see* Loratadine 1241
Lorans (AE, BH, CY, EG, IQ, IR, IT, JO, KW, LB, LY, MY, OM, QA, SA, SY, YE) *see* LORazepam 1243
Loranta (TH) *see* Losartan 1248
Lorastine (IL) *see* Loratadine 1241
Lorastyne (AU) *see* Loratadine 1241
Lora-Tabs (NZ) *see* Loratadine 1241
Loratadura (DE) *see* Loratadine 1241
Loratan (AE, BH, CY, EG, IQ, IR, JO, KW, LB, LY, OM, QA, SA, SY, YE) *see* Loratadine 1241
Loratin (AE, QA) *see* Loratadine 1241
Loraton (HK) *see* Loratadine 1241
Loratrim (IL) *see* Loratadine 1241
Lora (TW) *see* Loratadine 1241
Loratyne (PH) *see* Loratadine 1241
Loravan (KR) *see* LORazepam 1243

Lorax (BR) *see* LORazepam 1243
Lorazepam-Efeka (LU) *see* LORazepam 1243
Lorazepam-Eurogenerics (LU) *see* LORazepam 1243
Lorazep (TH) *see* LORazepam 1243
Lorazin (TW) *see* LORazepam 1243
Lorbi (AR) *see* Bromhexine [INT] 291
Lorcam (JP) *see* Lornoxicam [INT] 1248
Lorcef (PH) *see* Cefaclor 372
Lordiar (HR) *see* Loperamide 1236
Lorelin (MX, PK) *see* Leuprolide 1186
Lorenin (PT) *see* LORazepam 1243
Loretam (DE) *see* Lormetazepam [INT] 1247
Loretsin (MX) *see* Pravastatin 1700
Lorfast-D (IN) *see* Loratadine and Pseudoephedrine 1242
Lorfast (BF, BJ, CI, ET, GH, GM, GN, IN, KE, LR, MA, ML, MR, MU, MW, NE, NG, SC, SD, SL, SN, TN, TZ, UG, ZM, ZW) *see* Loratadine 1241
Loric-100 (PH) *see* Allopurinol 90
Loric-300 (PH) *see* Allopurinol 90
Loridem (BE, LU) *see* LORazepam 1243
Loridin (BF, BJ, CI, ET, GH, GM, GN, KE, LR, MA, ML, MR, MU, MW, NE, NG, SC, SD, SG, SL, SN, TN, TZ, UG, ZM, ZW) *see* Loratadine 1241
Lorien (ZA) *see* FLUoxetine 899
Lorihis (ID) *see* Loratadine 1241
Lorimox (MX) *see* Loratadine 1241
Lorimox (MX) *see* Loratadine and Pseudoephedrine 1242
Lorinase (QA) *see* Loratadine and Pseudoephedrine 1242
Lorine (BH, JO, KW) *see* Loratadine 1241
Lorin (IN) *see* Loratadine 1241
Lorita (TH) *see* Loratadine 1241
Lorivan (IL, TR) *see* LORazepam 1243
Lormyx (GR) *see* Rifaximin 1809
Lornica (IN) *see* Lornoxicam [INT] 1248
Lornicam (CO) *see* Lornoxicam [INT] 1248
Lornox (AT) *see* Lornoxicam [INT] 1248
Lorsilan (HR) *see* LORazepam 1243
Lorstat (AU) *see* AtorvaSTATin 194
Lortaan (IT) *see* Losartan 1248
Lorvas (IN) *see* Indapamide 1065
Lorzaar (DE) *see* Losartan 1248
Lorzaar Plus (DE) *see* Losartan and Hydrochlorothiazide 1250
Losacar (IN, MY) *see* Losartan 1248
Losacor D (AR, PE) *see* Losartan and Hydrochlorothiazide 1250
Losacor (AR, HK, PE) *see* Losartan 1248
Losacor HCT (HK) *see* Losartan and Hydrochlorothiazide 1250
Losa K (KR) *see* Losartan 1248
Losalac (TH) *see* Lactulose 1156
Losaltan (KR) *see* Losartan 1248
Losanet (QA) *see* Losartan and Hydrochlorothiazide 1250
Losardex (IL) *see* Losartan 1248
Losardex PLus (IL) *see* Losartan and Hydrochlorothiazide 1250
Losargard (PH) *see* Losartan 1248
Losargard Plus (PH) *see* Losartan and Hydrochlorothiazide 1250
Losarmax (KR) *see* Losartan 1248
Losartan Plus (IL) *see* Losartan and Hydrochlorothiazide 1250
Losartas (SG) *see* Losartan 1248
Losart-H (PH) *see* Losartan and Hydrochlorothiazide 1250
Losartin (KR) *see* Losartan 1248
Losec (AE, AR, AT, AU, BB, BE, BF, BH, BJ, BM, BR, BS, BZ, CI, CN, CY, CZ, DK, EE, EG, ES, ET, FI, GB, GH, GM, GN, GR, GY, HK, HU, IE, IL, IQ, IR, IS, IT, JM, JO, KE, KW, LB, LR, LU, LY, MA, ML, MR, MU, MW, MX, MY, NE, NG, NL, NO, NZ, OM, PH, PK, PL, PT, PY, QA, RO, RU, SA, SC, SD, SE, SL, SN, SR, SY, TN, TR, TW, TZ, UG, UY, VE, VN, YE, ZM, ZW) *see* Omeprazole 1508
Losec MUPS (CO, MY, PH) *see* Omeprazole 1508
Losemin (TW) *see* Tropicamide 2108
Loseprazol (SI) *see* Omeprazole 1508
Losferon (FR) *see* Ferrous Gluconate 870
Losferron (DE, IT, LU, NL) *see* Ferrous Gluconate 870
Lo Solvan (CN) *see* Ambroxol [INT] 109
Lostacef (ID) *see* Cefadroxil 372
Lostad HCT (HK, MY) *see* Losartan and Hydrochlorothiazide 1250
Lostam (EC) *see* Tamsulosin 1974
Lostapres (AR) *see* Ramipril 1771
Lostatin (PE, SG) *see* Lovastatin 1252
Lostin (PE) *see* Lovastatin 1252
Losu-3 (TH) *see* Glimepiride 966
Lotan (MX) *see* Loratadine 1241
Lotan (HR) *see* Losartan 1248
Lotan Plus (IL) *see* Losartan and Hydrochlorothiazide 1250
Lotarin (TW) *see* Loratadine 1241
Lotasbat (ID) *see* Clobetasol 468
Lotemax (AE, AR, CN, CY, DE, GB, GR, HK, IE, IL, IT, JO, KR, KW, LB, LT, MY, PH, PL, SI, SK, TH, TR, UY, VN) *see* Loteprednol 1251
Lotemp (TH) *see* Acetaminophen 32
Lotenac (ID) *see* Atenolol 189
Lotenal (KR) *see* Atenolol 189
Lotense (LB, MY) *see* AmLODIPine 123
Lotensin (BR, CN, HN, HU, MX, PE, PL, RU) *see* Benazepril 238
Lotensin H (BR) *see* Benazepril and Hydrochlorothiazide 240
Lotensin HCT (HN, PL) *see* Benazepril and Hydrochlorothiazide 240
Lotepred (IN) *see* Loteprednol 1251
Loterex (MX) *see* Loteprednol 1251
Lotesoft (PY, VE) *see* Loteprednol 1251
Lote (TW) *see* FluvoxaMINE 916
Lothisil (VN) *see* Propylthiouracil 1735
Lotim (HR) *see* Losartan 1248
Lotramina (PE) *see* Clotrimazole (Topical) 488
Lotremin (MY) *see* Clotrimazole (Topical) 488
Lotrial D (AR, PY, UY) *see* Enalapril and Hydrochlorothiazide 725
Lotrial (AR, PE, UY) *see* Enalapril 722
Lotricomb (AR, DE, NZ, VE) *see* Betamethasone and Clotrimazole 256
Lotriderm (BE, BH, CH, CL, CO, CR, CY, DO, EG, GB, GT, HN, ID, JO, KW, LB, NI, PA, QA, SA, SV, ZA) *see* Betamethasone and Clotrimazole 256
Lotrimin AF (MX) *see* Miconazole (Topical) 1360
Louten (AR, CL, PY, UY) *see* Latanoprost 1172
Lovacel (KR) *see* Lovastatin 1252
Lovachol (ZA) *see* Lovastatin 1252
Lovacol (CL, FI) *see* Lovastatin 1252
Lovalord (KR) *see* Lovastatin 1252
Lovan (AU) *see* FLUoxetine 899
Lovastad (DK) *see* Lovastatin 1252
Lovasterol (CO) *see* Lovastatin 1252
Lovas (TH) *see* AmLODIPine 123
Lovastin (EC, KR, SG) *see* Lovastatin 1252
Lovaton (BR) *see* Lovastatin 1252
Lovenox (AT, FR, ID, LB, PT) *see* Enoxaparin 726
Lovequin (ID) *see* Levofloxacin (Systemic) 1197
Lovina (DE) *see* Ethinyl Estradiol and Desogestrel 799
Lovir (AE, AU, KW, NZ, PH, QA) *see* Acyclovir (Systemic) 47
Lovire (ZA) *see* Acyclovir (Systemic) 47
Lovire (ZA) *see* Acyclovir (Topical) 51

Lovispes (EE) *see* Nebivolol 1434
Lovorin (PH) *see* Leucovorin Calcium 1183
Lovrak (KW, QA) *see* Acyclovir (Topical) 51
Lowchol (JO) *see* Pravastatin 1700
Lowdep (VN) *see* Citalopram 451
Lowdipine (KR) *see* AmLODIPine 123
Lowiop (KR) *see* Dorzolamide and Timolol 673
Low-Lip (AE, BH, CY, EG, IL, IQ, IR, JO, KW, LB, LY, OM, QA, SA, SY, YE) *see* Gemfibrozil 956
Lowlipen (CO) *see* AtorvaSTATin 194
Lowpston (JP) *see* Furosemide 940
Lowsta (VN) *see* Lovastatin 1252
Lowtan (TW) *see* Losartan 1248
Lowtiyel (MX) *see* Testosterone 2010
Loxalate (AU) *see* Escitalopram 765
Loxamine (NZ) *see* PARoxetine 1579
Loxan (CO) *see* Ciprofloxacin (Systemic) 441
Loxapac (BE, DK, ES, FR, GB, GR, IE, IN, KR, LU, NL, TW) *see* Loxapine 1255
Loxaris (IN) *see* Loxapine 1255
Loxar (UY) *see* Raloxifene 1765
Loxazol (CH, NL) *see* Permethrin 1627
Loxen (FR, VN) *see* NiCARdipine 1446
Loxen LP (VN) *see* NiCARdipine 1446
Loxfen (VN) *see* Loxoprofen [INT] 1255
Loxfin (KR) *see* Loxoprofen [INT] 1255
Loxibest (MX) *see* Meloxicam 1283
Loxicam (JO) *see* Meloxicam 1283
Loxil (ID) *see* Meloxicam 1283
Loxinter (ID) *see* Ofloxacin (Systemic) 1490
Loxof (LB) *see* Levofloxacin (Systemic) 1197
Loxol (JO) *see* LamoTRIgine 1160
Loxonin (BR, CN, JP, MX, PE, TH, VE) *see* Loxoprofen [INT] 1255
Loxwin (VN) *see* Ofloxacin (Systemic) 1490
Lozap (BG) *see* Losartan 1248
Lozap H (BG, EE) *see* Losartan and Hydrochlorothiazide 1250
Lozapine (IL) *see* CloZAPine 490
Lozapin (IN) *see* CloZAPine 490
Lozaris (TH) *see* Losartan 1248
Lozarsin (KR) *see* Losartan and Hydrochlorothiazide 1250
Lozato (KR) *see* Losartan 1248
Lozence (KR) *see* Cilostazol 437
Lozetin Plus (KR) *see* Losartan and Hydrochlorothiazide 1250
Lozicum (HK) *see* LORazepam 1243
Lozil (BR) *see* Gemfibrozil 956
LPG (AU) *see* Penicillin G Benzathine 1609
L.P.V. (AU) *see* Penicillin V Potassium 1614
Lritecin (KR) *see* Irinotecan 1112
Luarprofeno (AR) *see* Flurbiprofen (Systemic) 906
Lubor (HR) *see* Piroxicam 1662
Lubowel (IN) *see* Lubiprostone 1255
Lubrirhin (DE) *see* Bromhexine [INT] 291
Lubrisec (AR) *see* Acetylcysteine 40
Lucassin (AU) *see* Terlipressin [INT] 2010
Lucentis (AE, AR, AT, AU, BE, BH, BR, CH, CL, CO, CY, CZ, DE, DK, EC, EE, ES, FR, GB, GR, HK, HR, HU, ID, IE, IL, IN, IT, JO, JP, KR, KW, LB, LT, MY, NO, NZ, PE, PH, PL, PT, QA, RO, RU, SA, SE, SG, SI, SK, TH, TR, TW, VN, ZA) *see* Ranibizumab 1776
Lucetam (BG, HU, PL, RO, RU) *see* Piracetam [INT] 1661
Lucette (GB) *see* Ethinyl Estradiol and Drospirenone 801
Luci (IN) *see* Fluocinolone (Topical) 893
Lucium (PY, UY) *see* CloBAZam 465
Lucon (HK) *see* Fluconazole 885
Lucostin (AT) *see* Lomustine 1235
Lucostine (FI) *see* Lomustine 1235
Lucrin (AU, MY, NZ, RU, SG, TR, VN) *see* Leuprolide 1186
Lucrin Depot (AU, BE, CH, CR, CZ, GT, HN, IL, KR, MX, NI, NZ, PA, PL, RO, SG, SV, TR) *see* Leuprolide 1186
Lucrin PDS (MY) *see* Leuprolide 1186
Luctor (DE) *see* Naftidrofuryl [INT] 1416
Ludeal Ge (FR) *see* Ethinyl Estradiol and Levonorgestrel 803
Ludex (MX) *see* Famotidine 845
Ludilat (AT) *see* Bencyclane [INT] 241
Ludiomil (AE, AR, AT, BB, BD, BE, BF, BG, BH, BJ, BM, BR, BS, BZ, CH, CI, CN, CO, CY, CZ, DE, DK, EE, EG, ES, ET, FI, FR, GB, GH, GM, GN, GR, GY, HK, HN, HU, ID, IE, IN, IQ, IR, IS, IT, JM, JO, JP, KE, KR, KW, LB, LR, LU, LY, MA, ML, MR, MT, MU, MW, MX, NE, NG, NL, NO, NZ, OM, PE, PH, PK, PL, PT, QA, RO, RU, SA, SC, SD, SE, SK, SL, SN, SR, SY, TH, TN, TR, TT, TW, TZ, UG, UY, VE, YE, ZA, ZM, ZW) *see* Maprotiline 1271
Ludiomil[inj.] (HU, LU) *see* Maprotiline 1271
Ludios (ID) *see* Maprotiline 1271
Luditec (MX) *see* GlipiZIDE 967
Lueva (BE, ES) *see* Desogestrel [INT] 597
Luforan (BE, ES) *see* Gonadorelin [CAN/INT] 980
Luften (ID) *see* CloZAPine 490
Lukadin (IT) *see* Amikacin 111
Lukair (KR) *see* Montelukast 1392
Lukakline (SG) *see* Montelukast 1392
Lukast (CO, JO) *see* Montelukast 1392
Lukodermine (PK) *see* Methoxsalen (Systemic) 1330
Lukodermine (PK) *see* Methoxsalen (Topical) 1331
Lulicon (JP) *see* Luliconazole 1256
Lulifin (IN) *see* Luliconazole 1256
Lumcalcio (ES) *see* PHENobarbital 1632
Lumelin 2 (TW) *see* Estradiol (Systemic) 775
Lumeran (HK) *see* Ranitidine 1777
Lumidol (HR) *see* TraMADol 2074
Lumifurex (FR) *see* Nifuroxazide [INT] 1454
Lumigan (AE, AR, AT, AU, BE, BG, BR, CH, CL, CN, CO, CR, CZ, DE, DK, EC, EE, ES, FI, FR, GB, GR, GT, HK, HN, HR, HU, IE, IL, IN, IS, IT, JO, JP, KR, KW, LB, LT, MT, MX, MY, NL, NO, NZ, PA, PE, PH, PK, PL, PT, RO, RU, SA, SE, SG, SI, SK, SV, TH, TR, TW, VE, VN, ZA) *see* Bimatoprost 264
Luminal (AR, CH, DE, ES, KR, PH, SK) *see* PHENobarbital 1632
Luminale (IT) *see* PHENobarbital 1632
Luminaletas (AR, ES) *see* PHENobarbital 1632
Luminalette (IT) *see* PHENobarbital 1632
Luminaletten (DE) *see* PHENobarbital 1632
Luminalum (PL) *see* PHENobarbital 1632
Lumirelax (FR) *see* Methocarbamol 1320
Lunabell (JP) *see* Ethinyl Estradiol and Norethindrone 808
Lunaline (SG) *see* Maprotiline 1271
Lunan Likang (CN) *see* Milrinone 1370
Lunar (PK) *see* Flunarizine [CAN/INT] 892
Lunelax (SE) *see* Psyllium 1744
Lunesta (JP) *see* Eszopiclone 793
Lunetoron (JP) *see* Bumetanide 297
Lunex (ID) *see* Tranexamic Acid 2081
Lungtec (TW, VN) *see* Bambuterol [INT] 227
Lunox 2 (UY) *see* Eszopiclone 793
Luobang (CN) *see* Cefpirome [INT] 388
Luobaomai (CN) *see* Loperamide 1236
Luodan (CN) *see* Omeprazole 1508
Luoqi (CN) *see* Simvastatin 1890
Luoqing (CN) *see* Clindamycin (Systemic) 460
Luo Te Wei (CN) *see* Rotavirus Vaccine 1851
Luoxu (CN) *see* Pantoprazole 1570
Luoyu (CN) *see* Nateglinide 1432
Luphere Depot (PH, VN) *see* Leuprolide 1186
Lupible (PH) *see* Ursodiol 2116
Lupibose (IN) *see* Bosentan 280

Lupin (ID) *see* AmLODIPine ... 123
Lupocet (HR) *see* Acetaminophen ... 32
Lupotus (HR) *see* Bromhexine [INT] ... 291
Luprac (JP) *see* Torsemide ... 2071
Lupride Depot (IN) *see* Leuprolide ... 1186
Lupride (IN) *see* Leuprolide ... 1186
Luprolex Depot (PH) *see* Leuprolide ... 1186
Luprolex (PH) *see* Leuprolide ... 1186
Lupron (AR, BB, BH, BM, BR, BS, CL, CO, EC, GY, JM, JO, NL, PR, PY, QA, SR, TT, UY, VE) *see* Leuprolide ... 1186
Lupron Depot (AE, AR, BH, BR, CL, EC, KW, PE, PY, SA, UY, VE) *see* Leuprolide ... 1186
Lupron SC (CO, PE) *see* Leuprolide ... 1186
Lupro (TW) *see* Leuprolide ... 1186
Lu Qi (CN) *see* Indomethacin ... 1067
Lura XL (KR) *see* Alfuzosin ... 84
Lurdex (MX) *see* Albendazole ... 65
Luret (DE) *see* Azosemide [INT] ... 220
Lusadeina Fuerte (PE) *see* Acetaminophen and Codeine ... 36
Luseck (JP) *see* Furosemide ... 940
Lusopress (IT) *see* Nitrendipine [INT] ... 1463
Lustral (BH, GB, IE, IL, QA, SA, TR) *see* Sertraline ... 1878
Lustraline (TW) *see* Sertraline ... 1878
Lutamidal (CL, PE, PY) *see* Bicalutamide ... 262
Lutamin (JP) *see* Gonadorelin [CAN/INT] ... 980
Luteina (PL) *see* Progesterone ... 1722
Lutisone (HK) *see* Fluticasone (Nasal) ... 910
Lutisone (HK) *see* Fluticasone (Oral Inhalation) ... 907
Lutrelef (BE, CH, FR, HU, PL, SE, SG) *see* Gonadorelin [CAN/INT] ... 980
Lutsnal (KR) *see* Tamsulosin ... 1974
Luvenil (PY) *see* RisperiDONE ... 1818
Luver-I.S. (MX) *see* Lutropin Alfa [CAN/INT] ... 1259
Luveris (AE, AR, AT, AU, BE, BR, CH, CL, CN, CY, CZ, DE, DK, EE, ES, FI, FR, GB, GR, HK, HN, HR, ID, IE, IL, IN, IT, KR, KW, LB, LT, MY, NL, NO, NZ, PH, PL, PT, RO, RU, SA, SE, SG, SI, SK, TR, TW, UY, VE, VN) *see* Lutropin Alfa [CAN/INT] ... 1259
Luvinsta (VN) *see* Fluvastatin ... 915
Luvmox (PH) *see* Amoxicillin and Clavulanate ... 133
Luvox (AR, AU, BR, CL, CN, EC, ID, MX, MY, NZ, PE, TW, VE, VN, ZA) *see* FluvoxaMINE ... 916
Luxfen (BG, CZ, LT) *see* Brimonidine (Ophthalmic) ... 288
Luzul (IT) *see* Lormetazepam [INT] ... 1247
L-Xapam (KR) *see* Escitalopram ... 765
Lyceft (IN) *see* CefTRIAXone ... 396
Lycinate (AU) *see* Nitroglycerin ... 1465
Lyclear (AU, GB, IE, TR) *see* Permethrin ... 1627
Lyclear Creme Rinse (AE, BH, CY, EG, IQ, IR, JO, KW, LB, LY, OM, QA, SA, SY, YE) *see* Permethrin ... 1627
Lyclear Dermal Cream (IL) *see* Permethrin ... 1627
Lyderm (NZ) *see* Permethrin ... 1627
Lydin (IN) *see* Ranitidine ... 1777
Lydocan (MY) *see* Lidocaine (Systemic) ... 1208
Lydol (BG) *see* Meperidine ... 1293
Lydroxil (IN) *see* Cefadroxil ... 372
Lyflex (GB, IE) *see* Baclofen ... 223
Lyforan (IN) *see* Cefotaxime ... 382
Lykavir (VN) *see* Artesunate ... 178
Lymetel (ES) *see* Fluvastatin ... 915
Lymphoglobuline (TW) *see* Antithymocyte Globulin (Equine) ... 157
Lyndavel (PH) *see* MedroxyPROGESTERone ... 1277
Lynlor (GB) *see* OxyCODONE ... 1538
Lyogen (DE) *see* FluPHENAZine ... 905
Lyogen Depot (DE) *see* FluPHENAZine ... 905
Lyophilisate (ID) *see* Cyclophosphamide ... 517
Lyoxatin (VN) *see* Oxaliplatin ... 1528
Lyphocin (NZ) *see* Vancomycin ... 2130
Lyramycin (IN) *see* Gentamicin (Systemic) ... 959
Lyrica (AE, AR, AT, AU, BE, BG, BH, BR, CH, CL, CN, CO, CR, CY, CZ, DE, DK, DO, EC, EE, ES, FI, FR, GB, GR, GT, HK, HN, HR, HU, ID, IE, IL, IN, IS, IT, JP, KR, KW, LB, LT, MT, MX, MY, NI, NL, NO, NZ, PA, PE, PH, PL, PT, QA, RO, RU, SA, SE, SG, SI, SK, SV, TH, TR, TW, UY, VE, VN) *see* Pregabalin ... 1710
Lyrimpin (VN) *see* Rifampin ... 1804
Lyrinel XL (GB) *see* Oxybutynin ... 1536
Lyrinel (IL, MX, TH) *see* Oxybutynin ... 1536
Lyrinel Oros SR (KR) *see* Oxybutynin ... 1536
Lysagor (ID) *see* Pizotifen [CAN/INT] ... 1664
Lysalgo (IT) *see* Mefenamic Acid ... 1280
Lysantin (DK) *see* Orphenadrine ... 1522
Lysanxia (BE, FR, LU) *see* Prazepam [INT] ... 1702
Lysodren (AT, BE, BG, CH, CZ, DE, DK, EE, ES, FI, FR, GB, GR, HN, HR, IE, IT, KR, LT, MT, NL, NO, PL, PT, RO, RU, SE, SI, SK, TR, TW) *see* Mitotane ... 1382
Lysomucil (LU) *see* Acetylcysteine ... 40
Lysopadol (IE) *see* Ambroxol [INT] ... 109
Lysopain (CH) *see* Ambroxol [INT] ... 109
Lysox (LU) *see* Acetylcysteine ... 40
Lyssavac N Berna (HK, MY, PH) *see* Rabies Vaccine ... 1764
Lysthenon (AE, AT, BG, CH, EE, RO, RU, SA, TR) *see* Succinylcholine ... 1939
Lystin (HK) *see* Nystatin (Topical) ... 1482
Lytelsen (JP) *see* Diltiazem ... 634
Lytenur (DE) *see* Piracetam [INT] ... 1661
Lyxit (RO) *see* Tianeptine [INT] ... 2033
L-Zet (PH) *see* Levocetirizine ... 1196
L-Zinc (ID) *see* Zinc Sulfate ... 2200
M-M-R II (AU, CZ, ID, MY, NZ, TH) *see* Measles, Mumps, and Rubella Virus Vaccine ... 1273
M-M-R Vax (AT, DE) *see* Measles, Mumps, and Rubella Virus Vaccine ... 1273
M-M-R Vaxpro (IS, LT, SI, SK) *see* Measles, Mumps, and Rubella Virus Vaccine ... 1273
Maalox (AT, BB, BS, CZ, DE, FR, GB, GR, HN, IE, IL, IT, JM, NL, PE, PH, PY, TH, TT, UY, VN) *see* Aluminum Hydroxide and Magnesium Hydroxide ... 103
Maalox Plus (CL, GR, MY) *see* Aluminum Hydroxide, Magnesium Hydroxide, and Simethicone ... 104
Maalox Plus (PE) *see* Aluminum Hydroxide and Magnesium Hydroxide ... 103
Maalox (TH) *see* Aluminum Hydroxide and Magnesium Trisilicate ... 103
Mabapenem (KR) *see* Meropenem ... 1299
MabCampath (AU, CY, FR, GB, HN, ID, IL, KR, MT, MY, NO, RU, SE, SG, SK, TH, TR, ZA) *see* Alemtuzumab ... 75
Mabcampath (JO) *see* Alemtuzumab ... 75
Mabertin (AR) *see* Temazepam ... 1990
Mabron (AE, BH, CY, EG, IQ, IR, JO, KW, LB, LY, MY, OM, QA, SA, SG, SY, YE) *see* TraMADol ... 2074
Mabthera (AE, AR, AT, AU, BB, BE, BF, BG, BH, BJ, BM, BR, BS, BZ, CH, CI, CL, CN, CO, CY, CZ, DE, DK, EC, EE, EG, ET, FI, FR, GB, GH, GM, GN, GR, GY, HK, HN, HR, HU, ID, IE, IL, IS, IT, JM, JO, KE, KR, LB, LR, LT, MA, ML, MR, MT, MU, MW, MX, MY, NE, NG, NL, NO, NZ, PE, PH, PK, PL, PT, PY, QA, RO, RU, SA, SC, SD, SE, SG, SI, SK, SL, SN, SR, TH, TN, TR, TT, TW, TZ, UG, UY, VE, VN, ZA, ZM, ZW) *see* RiTUXimab ... 1825
Macaine (ZA) *see* Bupivacaine ... 299
Macbutin (IN) *see* Rifabutin ... 1803
Maccabimol (IL) *see* Acetaminophen ... 32
Macdin (VN) *see* Linezolid ... 1217
Macef (ID) *see* Cefepime ... 378
Macepim (TW) *see* Cefepime ... 378
Macladin (IT) *see* Clarithromycin ... 456
Maclar (LU) *see* Clarithromycin ... 456
Macolme (VN) *see* Olmesartan ... 1496
Macolol (TW) *see* Calcitriol ... 323
Macperan (KR) *see* Metoclopramide ... 1345

Macrobid (GB, IE) *see* Nitrofurantoin 1463
Macrodantina (BR, CL, CO, CR, DO, GT, HN, MX, NI, PA, PE, SV) *see* Nitrofurantoin 1463
Macrodantin (AU, CY, EG, IL, IT, PH, QA, TR, ZA) *see* Nitrofurantoin 1463
Macrodex 6% (GB) *see* Dextran 607
Macrodex (DE, NL) *see* Dextran 607
Macrodin (CY) *see* Nitrofurantoin 1463
Macrodin (PH) *see* Clarithromycin 456
Macrofuran (ID) *see* Nitrofurantoin 1463
Macroleuco (PH) *see* Filgrastim 875
Macromax (PH) *see* Azithromycin (Systemic) 216
Macropen (BG, HR, JP, RU) *see* Midecamycin [INT] 1365
Macroral (IT) *see* Midecamycin [INT] 1365
Macrosil (ES) *see* Roxithromycin [INT] 1853
Macroxam (PH) *see* Piroxicam 1662
Macrozide (CO) *see* Pyrazinamide 1745
Macrozit (CO, PE) *see* Azithromycin (Systemic) 216
Mactex (PY) *see* Ethinyl Estradiol and Norgestimate 810
Macugen (AT, BE, BG, CH, CY, CZ, DE, DK, EE, FI, FR, GB, GR, HN, HR, IE, IT, JP, LT, MT, NL, NO, PE, PH, PL, PT, RO, RU, SE, SI, SK, TH, TR) *see* Pegaptanib 1588
Madame Pearl's Mucolytic (HK) *see* Acetylcysteine 40
Madipine (KR) *see* Manidipine [INT] 1269
Madiplot (TH) *see* Manidipine [INT] 1269
Madiprazole (TH) *see* Omeprazole 1508
Madlexin (ID) *see* Cephalexin 405
Madomed (TH) *see* MethylPREDNISolone 1340
Madomine (MY) *see* Sulfadoxine and Pyrimethamine [INT] 1946
Madonna (MY) *see* Levonorgestrel 1201
Madopar (AE, AR, AT, AU, BH, CH, CN, CO, CZ, DE, DK, EE, EG, ES, FI, GB, GR, HK, HN, HR, ID, IE, IS, IT, KR, LB, LT, MX, MY, NL, NO, NZ, PE, PH, PK, PL, PT, QA, RO, RU, SA, SG, SI, SK, TH, TR, TW, VE, VN) *see* Benserazide and Levodopa [CAN/INT] 244
Madopar-F (IN) *see* Benserazide and Levodopa [CAN/INT] 244
Madopark (SE) *see* Benserazide and Levodopa [CAN/INT] 244
Madoxy (TH) *see* Doxycycline 689
Maexeni (GB) *see* Ethinyl Estradiol and Levonorgestrel 803
Mafarin (TW) *see* Warfarin 2186
Mafatate (JP) *see* Mafenide 1261
Mafel (AR, PY) *see* Progesterone 1722
Mafidol (PE) *see* Acetaminophen 32
Maforan (TH) *see* Warfarin 2186
Maformin (TH) *see* MetFORMIN 1307
Magicul (AU) *see* Cimetidine 438
Magmil (KR) *see* Magnesium Hydroxide 1263
Magnacef (AE, BH, JO, LB, QA, SA) *see* Cefixime 380
Magnapen (PE) *see* Ampicillin 141
Magnaspor (TH) *see* Cefuroxime 399
Magnecyl (SE) *see* Aspirin 180
Magnelium (CA) *see* Magnesium Glucoheptonate [CAN/INT] 1262
Magnerot[inj.] (DE) *see* Magnesium Gluconate 1263
Magnesia san Pelligrino (IT) *see* Magnesium Hydroxide 1263
Magnesii Sulfas (PL) *see* Magnesium Sulfate 1265
Magnesii Sulfas Siccatus (PL) *see* Magnesium Sulfate 1265
Magnesio (AR) *see* Magnesium Gluconate 1263
Magnesium Gluconicum (AT) *see* Magnesium Gluconate 1263
Magnesium Oligosol (FR) *see* Magnesium Gluconate 1263
Magnesium Sulfuricum (PL) *see* Magnesium Sulfate 1265
Magnesol (PL) *see* Magnesium Citrate 1262
Magnez (PL) *see* Magnesium Oxide 1265
Magnimox (PE) *see* Amoxicillin 130
Magniton-R (GR) *see* Indapamide 1065
Magnolex (CA) *see* Magnesium Glucoheptonate [CAN/INT] 1262
Magnopyrol (BR) *see* Dipyrone [INT] 653
Magnorol Sirop (CA) *see* Magnesium Glucoheptonate [CAN/INT] 1262
Magnurol (ES) *see* Terazosin 2001
MAGO (KR) *see* Magnesium Oxide 1265
Magunesin (KR) *see* Magnesium Sulfate 1265
Magurol (JO, MY) *see* Doxazosin 674
Maikeding (CN) *see* Ivermectin (Systemic) 1136
Maikohis (JP) *see* Clemastine 459
Mailen (EC) *see* Desloratadine 594
Maintate (JP) *see* Bisoprolol 266
Majezik (TR) *see* Flurbiprofen (Systemic) 906
Majsolin (HR) *see* Primidone 1714
Makrocef (HR) *see* Cefotaxime 382
Malachlo (KR) *see* Chloroquine 424
Malafon (MY) *see* Sulfadoxine and Pyrimethamine [INT] 1946
Malafree (KR) *see* Primaquine 1713
Malanil (TH) *see* Atovaquone and Proguanil 198
Malaquin (AE, BH, CY, EG, IL, IQ, IR, JO, KW, LB, LY, OM, QA, SA, SY, YE) *see* Chloroquine 424
Malarex (AE, BH, CY, EG, ID, IL, IQ, IR, JO, KW, LB, LY, MY, OM, PH, QA, SA, SY, YE) *see* Chloroquine 424
Malarivon (BB, BM, BS, BZ, GY, JM, PR, SR, TT) *see* Chloroquine 424
Malarone (AT, AU, BE, BH, CH, CZ, DE, DK, EE, ES, FI, FR, GB, GR, HK, HN, IE, IL, IS, IT, JP, KR, KW, LT, MY, NL, NO, NZ, PE, PL, PT, QA, SA, SE, SG, SI, SK) *see* Atovaquone and Proguanil 198
Malation (EE, NO) *see* Malathion 1268
Malaviron (BF, BJ, CI, ET, GH, GM, GN, KE, LR, MA, ML, MR, MU, MW, NE, NG, SC, SD, SL, SN, TN, TZ, UG, ZA, ZM, ZW) *see* Chloroquine 424
Malend (KR) *see* Alendronate 79
Malergo (DO) *see* Ergonovine [CAN/INT] 754
Malerim (AE, BH, CY, EG, IL, IQ, IR, JO, KW, LB, LY, OM, QA, SA, SY, YE) *see* Sulfadoxine and Pyrimethamine [INT] 1946
Maliasin (AT, CH, DE, IT, PY, TR) *see* Barbexaclone [INT] 227
Malirid (IN) *see* Primaquine 1713
Malival (MX) *see* Indomethacin 1067
Mallermin-F (JP) *see* Clemastine 459
Malocide (FR) *see* Pyrimethamine 1749
Malocide (IN) *see* Sulfadoxine and Pyrimethamine [INT] 1946
Malon (MY) *see* Metoclopramide 1345
Malthionex (LU) *see* Malathion 1268
Mamofen (IN) *see* Tamoxifen 1971
Mamograf (AR) *see* Charcoal, Activated 416
Manace (MY) *see* Haloperidol 993
Manaslu (KR) *see* Nimesulide [INT] 1456
Mandehexan (PL) *see* Methenamine 1317
Mandelamine (PL) *see* Methenamine 1317
Mandolgin (DK) *see* TraMADol 2074
Mandroton (DE) *see* Etilefrine [INT] 815
Manerix (ES, GB, IE) *see* Moclobemide [CAN/INT] 1384
Manic (TH) *see* Mefenamic Acid 1280
Manidon (ES, VE) *see* Verapamil 2154
Manidon Retard (ES) *see* Verapamil 2154
Maninil (BG, EE) *see* GlyBURIDE 972
Maniprex (BE, LU) *see* Lithium 1230
Maniton (TW) *see* Mannitol 1269
Manivasc (BR) *see* Manidipine [INT] 1269
Manlsum (TW) *see* Flurazepam 906
Manmox (TH) *see* Amoxicillin 130
Mannisol B (PL) *see* Mannitol 1269

Mannisol (HN) *see* Mannitol 1269
Mannit-Losung (DE) *see* Mannitol 1269
Mannitol (KR, PL) *see* Mannitol 1269
Mannits (EE) *see* Mannitol 1269
Manobaxine (TH) *see* Methocarbamol 1320
Manobrozil (TH) *see* Gemfibrozil 956
Manodepo (TH) *see* MedroxyPROGESTERone 1277
Manodiol (TH) *see* Ethinyl Estradiol and Norgestrel 812
Manoflox (TH) *see* Norfloxacin 1475
Manoglucon (TH) *see* GlyBURIDE 972
Manolone (TH) *see* Triamcinolone (Systemic) 2099
Manolone (TH) *see* Triamcinolone (Topical) 2100
Manomet (TH) *see* Cimetidine 438
Manomic (TH) *see* Mefenamic Acid 1280
Manorifcin (TH) *see* Rifampin 1804
Manotin (TW) *see* Memantine 1286
Mano-Trim Forte (TH) *see* Sulfamethoxazole and Trimethoprim 1946
Mano-Trim (TH) *see* Sulfamethoxazole and Trimethoprim 1946
Manoxidil (TH) *see* Minoxidil (Systemic) 1374
Mansal (ES) *see* Cimetidine 438
Mantadan (IT) *see* Amantadine 105
Mantadix (FR, LU) *see* Amantadine 105
Mantidan (BR) *see* Amantadine 105
Manyper (DE, GR) *see* Manidipine [INT] 1269
Manzida (MX) *see* Ethambutol 798
Mao-B (KR) *see* Selegiline 1873
Maoblock (KR) *see* Pancuronium 1567
Maoread (JP) *see* Furosemide 940
MAOtil (DE) *see* Selegiline 1873
Mapenem (TH) *see* Meropenem 1299
Mapin (HK, MY) *see* Naloxone 1419
Mapluxin (MX) *see* Digoxin 627
Mapress (MY) *see* Haloperidol 993
Maprolu (HU, LU) *see* Maprotiline 1271
Mapryl (ID) *see* Glimepiride 966
MaQaid (JP) *see* Triamcinolone (Ophthalmic) 2100
Maquine (AE, BH, CY, EG, IL, IQ, IR, JO, KW, LB, LY, OM, QA, SA, SY, YE) *see* Chloroquine 424
Maradex (VE) *see* Dexamethasone (Ophthalmic) 602
Maradex (VE) *see* Dexamethasone (Systemic) 599
Marcaina (BR, GT, SV) *see* Bupivacaine 299
Marcain (AU, DK, FI, GB, HN, HU, ID, IE, IS, IT, JP, MY, NO, NZ, PT, RU, SE, SG, VN) *see* Bupivacaine 299
Marcaine (AE, BE, BG, BH, CY, CZ, EE, EG, FR, GR, HK, IL, IQ, IR, JO, KR, KW, LB, LT, LU, LY, NL, OM, PH, PL, QA, SA, SI, SK, SY, TH, TR, TW, YE) *see* Bupivacaine 299
Marcaine Heavy (KR) *see* Bupivacaine 299
Marcaine Plain (BF, BJ, CI, ET, GH, GM, GN, KE, LR, MA, ML, MR, MU, MW, NE, NG, SC, SD, SL, SN, TN, TZ, UG, ZM, ZW) *see* Bupivacaine 299
Marcaine Spinal Heavy (VN) *see* Bupivacaine 299
Marcain Spinal (BG, DK, EG, IS, LT, PL, SI, SK) *see* Bupivacaine 299
Marcen (ES) *see* Ketazolam [INT] 1144
Marcoumar (AT, BE, BR, DK, DE, NL, CH) *see* Phenprocoumon [INT] 1635
Marcumar (DE) *see* Phenprocoumon [INT] 1635
Marcuphen (DE) *see* Phenprocoumon [INT] 1635
Mareamin (CL) *see* DimenhyDRINATE 637
Mareosan (ES) *see* DimenhyDRINATE 637
Marevan (AE, AU, BE, BR, CN, DK, EE, FI, GB, IE, LU, NO, NZ, SG) *see* Warfarin 2186
Marfarin (HN) *see* Warfarin 2186
Margrilan (AE, BH, CY, EG, IQ, IR, JO, KW, LB, LY, OM, PH, QA, SA, SG, SY, YE) *see* FLUoxetine 899
Margyl (IT) *see* Phenelzine 1630
Maril (HK, SG, TH) *see* Metoclopramide 1345
Marinol (DE) *see* Dronabinol 694
Mariosea XL (GB) *see* Tolterodine 2063
Marivarin (HR) *see* Warfarin 2186
Marogel (KR) *see* Magnesium Hydroxide 1263
Marolin (ES) *see* DimenhyDRINATE 637
Maronil (IL) *see* ClomiPRAMINE 475
Marovilina (MX) *see* Ampicillin 141
Marsthine (JP, PH, TW) *see* Clemastine 459
Martapan (GB) *see* Dexamethasone (Systemic) 599
Martefarin (HR) *see* Warfarin 2186
Martesia (EC) *see* Pregabalin 1710
Martimil (ES) *see* Nortriptyline 1476
Marvelon 21 (NZ, TH, TW) *see* Ethinyl Estradiol and Desogestrel 799
Marvelon 28 (AU, DK, ID, NZ, PH, TH) *see* Ethinyl Estradiol and Desogestrel 799
Marvelon (AR, AT, BE, BF, BG, BH, BJ, CH, CI, CL, CN, CO, CY, CZ, DE, DK, EC, EE, EG, ET, FI, GB, GH, GM, GN, GR, HK, HN, IQ, IR, IS, JO, KE, KW, LB, LR, LT, LY, MA, ML, MR, MU, MW, MX, MY, NE, NG, NL, NO, OM, PE, PK, PL, PT, QA, RU, SA, SC, SD, SI, SK, SL, SN, SY, TN, TZ, UG, UY, VE, VN, YE, ZA, ZM, ZW) *see* Ethinyl Estradiol and Desogestrel 799
Marvical (UY) *see* Alendronate and Cholecalciferol 81
Marvil (LB, PE, UY) *see* Alendronate 79
Marviol (IE) *see* Ethinyl Estradiol and Desogestrel 799
Marvir (TH) *see* Acyclovir (Systemic) 47
Marvir (TH) *see* Acyclovir (Topical) 51
Marzolam (TH) *see* ALPRAZolam 94
Masaton (JP) *see* Allopurinol 90
Maschitt (JP) *see* Hydrochlorothiazide 1009
Masdil (ES) *see* Diltiazem 634
Masletine (JP) *see* Clemastine 459
Maspara w/Codeine (TH) *see* Acetaminophen and Codeine 36
Mastabloc (PY) *see* Olopatadine (Ophthalmic) 1500
Mastical (ES) *see* Calcium Carbonate 327
Mastodanatrol (PT) *see* Danazol 558
Matador (LB) *see* Levofloxacin (Systemic) 1197
Matalmin (TW) *see* Chlorzoxazone 430
Matcine (MY, SG, TH) *see* ChlorproMAZINE 429
Matenol (HK, TH) *see* Trimetazidine [INT] 2104
Matenol MR (TH) *see* Trimetazidine [INT] 2104
Matever (EE, SE) *see* LevETIRAcetam 1191
Matilina (PY) *see* Maprotiline 1271
Matoride XL (GB) *see* Methylphenidate 1336
Matosin (ID) *see* Oxytocin 1549
Matrifen (BE, DK, EE, GB) *see* FentaNYL 857
Matulane (KR, PH) *see* Procarbazine 1717
Mavid (DE) *see* Clarithromycin 456
Mavilex (MY) *see* Clenbuterol [INT] 460
Maxadol (ZA) *see* Acetaminophen and Codeine 36
Maxair Autohaler (FR) *see* Pirbuterol 1662
Maxair (CH) *see* Pirbuterol 1662
maxalt (AE) *see* Rizatriptan 1836
Maxalt (AR, AT, AU, BE, BG, BR, CH, CR, DE, DK, EE, ES, FI, FR, GB, GR, GT, HN, HR, HU, IS, IT, KR, LB, LT, MX, NL, NO, NZ, PA, PE, PL, PT, QA, RO, SA, SE, SI, SK, SV) *see* Rizatriptan 1836
Maxaltlyo (FR) *see* Rizatriptan 1836
Maxalt RPD (CL, PE, VE) *see* Rizatriptan 1836
Maxamox (AU) *see* Amoxicillin 130
Maxaquin (AU, CZ, EC, HK, IT, KR, MX, PK, PT, VE, ZA) *see* Lomefloxacin [INT] 1233
Maxcef (AR, BR, UY) *see* Cefepime 378
Maxcef (ID) *see* Cefadroxil 372
Maxcil (ZA) *see* Amoxicillin 130
Maxdio (KR) *see* Valsartan 2127
Maxdioplus (KR) *see* Valsartan and Hydrochlorothiazide 2129
Maxef (MX) *see* Cefepime 378
Maxeron (IN) *see* Metoclopramide 1345
Maxetibe Plus (PY) *see* Ezetimibe and Atorvastatin 833
Maxetibe (PY) *see* Ezetimibe 832
Maxfrom (AR) *see* Cefepime 378
Maxgrel (KR) *see* Clopidogrel 484

Max (HK, SG) *see* Ambroxol [INT] ... 109
MaxiBone 70 (IL) *see* Alendronate ... 79
MaxiBone (IL) *see* Alendronate ... 79
Maxi-calc (CH) *see* Calcium Carbonate ... 327
Maxicef (ID) *see* Cefepime ... 378
Maxicef (PE) *see* Cefixime ... 380
Maxidauno (AR) *see* DAUNOrubicin (Conventional) ... 577
Maxidene (TH) *see* Piroxicam ... 1662
Maxiderm (EC) *see* Desonide ... 597
Maxidex (AE, AU, BE, BF, BH, BJ, BR, CH, CI, CL, CY, CZ, DK, EC, EE, EG, ET, FR, GB, GH, GM, GN, GR, HN, HR, HU, IE, IL, IQ, IR, IS, JO, KE, KR, KW, LB, LR, LT, LY, MA, ML, MR, MU, MW, MY, NE, NG, NZ, OM, PE, PH, PK, QA, RO, RU, SA, SC, SD, SE, SG, SI, SL, SN, SY, TN, TR, TW, TZ, UG, VN, YE, ZA, ZM, ZW) *see* Dexamethasone (Ophthalmic) ... 602
Maxifer (PH) *see* Iron Sucrose ... 1118
Maxigen (PH) *see* Gentamicin (Systemic) ... 959
Maxi-Kalz (CZ) *see* Calcium Carbonate ... 327
Maxilan (ID) *see* Cefepime ... 378
Maxil (JO) *see* Cefuroxime ... 399
Maximus (PE) *see* Alendronate and Cholecalciferol ... 81
Maxipen (CO) *see* Ampicillin ... 141
Maxipime (AE, AT, BE, BG, BH, CH, CL, CN, CZ, DE, DK, EC, EE, EG, ES, FI, GR, HK, HN, HR, HU, IT, JO, JP, KR, KW, LB, LU, MX, MY, NL, PE, PK, PL, PT, QA, RU, SA, SE, SG, SI, SK, TR, TW, VE, VN, ZA) *see* Cefepime ... 378
Maxitrol (MX) *see* Neomycin and Polymyxin B ... 1437
Maxitrol (MX) *see* Polymyxin B ... 1676
Maxitrol (AE, BB, BE, BF, BG, BH, BJ, BM, BR, BS, BZ, CH, CI, CL, CO, CZ, EC, EE, EG, ET, FI, GB, GH, GM, GN, GY, HK, HR, IE, IL, IS, JM, KE, KR, KW, LR, LT, MA, ML, MR, MU, MW, MY, NE, NG, NL, NO, NZ, PE, PH, PK, PL, QA, RO, SA, SC, SD, SI, SL, SN, SR, TH, TN, TT, TW, TZ, UG, VE, VN, ZA, ZM, ZW) *see* Neomycin, Polymyxin B, and Dexamethasone ... 1437
Maxmor (ID) *see* Azithromycin (Systemic) ... 216
Maxolon (AE, AU, BB, BF, BH, BJ, BM, BS, BZ, CI, CY, EG, ET, GB, GH, GM, GN, GY, IE, IQ, IR, JM, JO, KE, KW, LB, LR, LY, MA, ML, MR, MU, MW, NE, NG, NZ, OM, QA, SA, SC, SD, SL, SN, SR, SY, TN, TT, TZ, UG, YE, ZA, ZM, ZW) *see* Metoclopramide ... 1345
Maxor (AU) *see* Omeprazole ... 1508
Maxpro (ID) *see* Cefixime ... 380
Maxpro (PH) *see* Ciprofloxacin (Systemic) ... 441
Maxtrex (GB) *see* Methotrexate ... 1322
Maxzide (BM) *see* Hydrochlorothiazide and Triamterene ... 1012
Maxzide (TW) *see* Triamterene ... 2101
Maycor (DE) *see* Isosorbide Dinitrate ... 1124
Maycor Retard (ES) *see* Isosorbide Dinitrate ... 1124
Maygace (ES) *see* Megestrol ... 1281
MBC (IN) *see* Mebeverine [INT] ... 1275
MB-Combi (SA) *see* Clofazimine [INT] ... 473
MCP-Beta Tropfen (DE) *see* Metoclopramide ... 1345
MCP-ratiopharm (LU) *see* Metoclopramide ... 1345
MCR (IL) *see* Morphine (Systemic) ... 1394
Meapron (KR) *see* MethylPREDNISolone ... 1340
Meaverin (DE) *see* Mepivacaine ... 1295
Mebagen (SA) *see* Mebeverine [INT] ... 1275
Mebedal (MX) *see* Mebendazole [CAN/INT] ... 1274
Mebemerck (DE) *see* Mebeverine [INT] ... 1275
Mebemint (CO) *see* Mebeverine [INT] ... 1275
Mebendazol (MX) *see* Mebendazole [CAN/INT] ... 1274
Mebenix (BR) *see* Albendazole ... 65
Mebensole (MX) *see* Mebendazole [CAN/INT] ... 1274
Mebetin (HK, MY, SG) *see* Mebeverine [INT] ... 1275
Mebeverine EG (BE) *see* Mebeverine [INT] ... 1275
Mebeverine Hydrochloride (GB) *see* Mebeverine [INT] ... 1275
Mebex (IN) *see* Mebendazole [CAN/INT] ... 1274
Mebezol (TW) *see* Mebendazole [CAN/INT] ... 1274
Mebrin (IN) *see* Mebeverine [INT] ... 1275
Mebumal (DK) *see* PENTobarbital ... 1617
Mebutan (NL) *see* Nabumetone ... 1411
Mebzol (AE, BH, KW, QA) *see* Mebendazole [CAN/INT] ... 1274
Mecapem (KR) *see* Meropenem ... 1299
Mecaron (KR) *see* Meloxicam ... 1283
Mecasel (VN) *see* Meloxicam ... 1283
Mechol (TW) *see* Pravastatin ... 1700
Mecid A (PH) *see* Mefenamic Acid ... 1280
Mecir LP (FR) *see* Tamsulosin ... 1974
Meclitab (PH) *see* Meclizine ... 1277
Meclomid (MX) *see* Metoclopramide ... 1345
Meclopstad (VN) *see* Metoclopramide ... 1345
Mecon (TW) *see* Meloxicam ... 1283
Mecox (ID) *see* Meloxicam ... 1283
Mectizan (BF, BJ, CI, ET, GH, GM, GN, KE, LR, MA, ML, MR, MU, MW, NE, NG, SC, SD, SL, SN, TN, TZ, UG, VN, ZA, ZM, ZW) *see* Ivermectin (Systemic) ... 1136
Medacef (AE, BH, KW, QA, SA) *see* Cefaclor ... 372
Medaject[inj.] (DE) *see* Procainamide ... 1716
Medazine (TH) *see* Medazepam [INT] ... 1277
Medazol (HR) *see* MetroNIDAZOLE (Systemic) ... 1353
Medcoflox (ID) *see* Ciprofloxacin (Systemic) ... 441
Medemycin (HK, JP) *see* Midecamycin [INT] ... 1365
Medene (TH) *see* AcetaZOLAMIDE ... 39
Mederantil[vet.] (CH, DE, FR) *see* Brotizolam [INT] ... 293
Medesup (ES) *see* Bisacodyl ... 265
Medevac (AU) *see* Sorbitol ... 1927
Medex (AR) *see* Bromhexine [INT] ... 291
Medfort (PE) *see* MetFORMIN ... 1307
Medibronc (FR) *see* Carbocisteine [INT] ... 357
Medicarpine (PK) *see* Pilocarpine (Ophthalmic) ... 1649
Medicefa (KR, VN) *see* Cefadroxil ... 372
Medicef (GT, NI) *see* Cephalexin ... 405
Medicol Advance (PH) *see* Ibuprofen ... 1032
Medicol (PH) *see* Ibuprofen ... 1032
Medicort (ID) *see* Fluticasone (Oral Inhalation) ... 907
Medicort (ID) *see* Fluticasone (Topical) ... 911
Medicort (PE) *see* Dexamethasone (Systemic) ... 599
Medifolin (PT) *see* Leucovorin Calcium ... 1183
Medihaler-Ergotamine (GB) *see* Ergotamine ... 754
Medihaler Ergotamine (NZ) *see* Ergotamine ... 754
Medihaler-Iso (GB, LU, NL, PT) *see* Isoproterenol ... 1124
Medikinet XL (EE) *see* Methylphenidate ... 1336
Medikinet (CH, DE, DK, EE, NO, PL, SE) *see* Methylphenidate ... 1336
Medikinet CR (DE) *see* Methylphenidate ... 1336
Medikinet Retard (KR) *see* Methylphenidate ... 1336
Mediklin (ID) *see* Clindamycin (Topical) ... 464
Medi-Klin TR (ID) *see* Clindamycin and Tretinoin ... 464
Medilax (DK, IS) *see* Lactulose ... 1156
Mediloxan (MX) *see* Lornoxicam [INT] ... 1248
Medinox Mono (DE) *see* PENTobarbital ... 1617
Medipekt (FI) *see* Bromhexine [INT] ... 291
Medipyrin (SK) *see* Acetaminophen ... 32
Mediruka (KR) *see* Montelukast ... 1392
Medisorbin (GT, HN, NI, SV) *see* Lovastatin ... 1252
Medistan (LB) *see* Nystatin (Oral) ... 1481
Meditabine (IL) *see* Gemcitabine ... 952
Meditaxel (PE) *see* PACLitaxel (Conventional) ... 1550
Meditrol (TH) *see* Calcitriol ... 323
Medixin (IT) *see* Sulfamethoxazole and Trimethoprim ... 1946
Medixon (ID, PH) *see* MethylPREDNISolone ... 1340
Medizol V (GT, SV) *see* Metronidazole and Nystatin [CAN/INT] ... 1358
Mednin (TW) *see* MethylPREDNISolone ... 1340
Medobeta (SG, TR) *see* Betamethasone (Topical) ... 255
Medoclor (BG, TR) *see* Cefaclor ... 372
Medocriptine (BG) *see* Bromocriptine ... 291
Medocycline (HK) *see* Tetracycline ... 2017
Medodarone (PH) *see* Amiodarone ... 114

Medodermone (SG, VN) *see* Clobetasol 468
Medofloxine (MY) *see* Ofloxacin (Systemic) 1490
Medoflucon (CN, SG) *see* Fluconazole 885
Medoflucon (SK) *see* Fluorometholone 896
Medolexin (MY) *see* Cephalexin 405
Medolin (SG) *see* Albuterol 69
Medomycin (BF, BJ, CI, ET, GH, GM, GN, KE, LR, MA, ML, MR, MU, MW, MY, NE, NG, SC, SD, SG, SL, SN, TH, TN, TW, TZ, UG, ZM, ZW) *see* Doxycycline 689
Medopa (JP, TH) *see* Methyldopa 1332
Medopam (ZA) *see* Oxazepam 1532
Medopa (PT) *see* DOPamine 669
Medopexol (TR) *see* Pramipexole 1695
Medophenicol (JO, TR) *see* Chloramphenicol 421
Medoprazole (BF, BJ, CI, ET, GH, GM, GN, KE, LR, MA, ML, MR, MU, MW, MY, NE, NG, SC, SD, SL, SN, TN, TZ, UG, ZM, ZW) *see* Omeprazole 1508
Medopred (TR) *see* PrednisoLONE (Systemic) 1703
Medoptic (PH) *see* Chloramphenicol 421
Medoram (JO) *see* Methyldopa 1332
Medostatin (AE, BG, BH, CY, EG, IL, IQ, IR, JO, KW, LB, LY, MY, OM, QA, SA, SG, SY, YE) *see* Lovastatin 1252
Medovir (AE, BF, BG, BH, BJ, CI, CY, EG, ET, GH, GM, GN, IQ, IR, JO, KE, KW, LB, LR, LY, MA, ML, MR, MU, MW, MY, NE, NG, OM, QA, SA, SC, SD, SG, SL, SN, SY, TN, TW, TZ, UG, YE, ZM, ZW) *see* Acyclovir (Systemic) 47
Medovir (MY) *see* Acyclovir (Topical) 51
Medoxicam (AE) *see* Meloxicam 1283
Medox (PH) *see* Doxycycline 689
Medrate (DE) *see* MethylPREDNISolone 1340
Medrexim (JP) *see* Fluocinonide 894
Medrocil (AR) *see* Hydrocortisone (Topical) 1014
Medrol (AE, BB, BE, BH, BM, BS, BZ, CH, CL, CN, CO, CR, CY, CZ, DE, DK, EC, EE, EG, ES, FI, FR, GB, GR, GT, GY, HN, HR, ID, IE, IL, IN, IQ, IR, IT, JM, JO, KR, KW, LB, LT, LU, LY, MT, NI, NL, NO, NZ, OM, PA, PE, PH, PL, PT, QA, RO, RU, SA, SE, SI, SK, SR, SV, SY, TR, TT, VE, VN, YE, ZA) *see* MethylPREDNISolone 1340
Medrone (GB) *see* MethylPREDNISolone 1340
Medrone (TW) *see* MedroxyPROGESTERone 1277
Medroxine (UY) *see* MedroxyPROGESTERone 1277
Medroxol (SA) *see* Ambroxol [INT] 109
Medsara (MX) *see* Cytarabine (Conventional) 535
Medsatrexate (MX) *see* Methotrexate 1322
Medsavorina (MX) *see* Leucovorin Calcium 1183
Medtax (PH) *see* Tamoxifen 1971
Medtol (VN) *see* Cefpirome [INT] 388
Medusit (PT) *see* Fluoride 895
Medxime (PH) *see* Cefuroxime 399
Medzart (PH) *see* Losartan 1248
Mefacit (PL) *see* Mefenamic Acid 1280
Mefac (PE) *see* Mefenamic Acid 1280
Mefeamina (ES) *see* Orphenadrine 1522
Mefede (KR) *see* Mafenide 1261
Mefen (HK) *see* Mefenamic Acid 1280
Mefenix (AR) *see* Tenoxicam [INT] 2001
Mefliam (ZA) *see* Mefloquine 1280
Meflupin (TW) *see* Meropenem 1299
Mefoxa (ID) *see* Ofloxacin (Systemic) 1490
Mefoxil (GR) *see* CefOXitin 386
Mefoxin (AE, AU, BB, BE, BF, BG, BH, BJ, BM, BS, BZ, CI, CY, CZ, EG, ET, FI, FR, GB, GH, GM, GN, GY, HN, HU, IE, IL, IQ, IR, IT, JM, JO, KE, KW, LB, LR, LU, LY, MA, ML, MR, MU, MW, NE, NG, NL, NZ, OM, PT, QA, SA, SC, SD, SL, SN, SR, SY, TN, TT, TW, TZ, UG, YE, ZA, ZM, ZW) *see* CefOXitin 386
Mefoxitin (AT, CH, DE, DK, ES, NO, SE) *see* CefOXitin 386
Mefpa (TH) *see* Methyldopa 1332
Mefurosan (ID) *see* Mometasone (Topical) 1391
Megace (AR, AT, AU, BD, BE, BG, CL, CN, CO, CZ, EE, EG, FR, GB, GR, HK, HN, HR, IE, IT, JO, JP, KR, KW, LB, LT, MY, NL, NO, NZ, PK, PL, PT, QA, RU, SA, SG, SI, TH, TR, TW, UY, VN) *see* Megestrol 1281
Megacef (PH) *see* CefTAZidime 392
Megacilina Oral (PE) *see* Penicillin V Potassium 1614
Megafol (AU) *see* Folic Acid 919
Megal (MX) *see* Guaifenesin and Dextromethorphan 987
Megalotect (IL, KR, TH) *see* Cytomegalovirus Immune Globulin (Intravenous-Human) 541
Megamilbedoce (ES) *see* Hydroxocobalamin 1020
Megamox (IN) *see* Amoxicillin and Cloxacillin [INT] 136
Megapen (IN) *see* Ampicillin and Cloxacillin [INT] 144
Megapime (MY, TH) *see* Cefepime 378
Megaplatin (LB) *see* CARBOplatin 357
Megaplex (ID, PH, RU) *see* Megestrol 1281
Megase (VE) *see* Megestrol 1281
Megastrol (PY) *see* Megestrol 1281
Megatil (IN) *see* ChlorproMAZINE 429
Megatus (TW) *see* Megestrol 1281
Megavix (FR) *see* Tetrazepam [INT] 2020
Megaxin (IL) *see* Moxifloxacin (Systemic) 1401
Megejohn (TW) *see* Megestrol 1281
Megesia (KR) *see* Megestrol 1281
Megesin (HK, RO) *see* Megestrol 1281
Megestat (BR, DE) *see* Megestrol 1281
Megestron (MX) *see* MedroxyPROGESTERone 1277
Megex-I (PE) *see* Megestrol 1281
Megion (AE, BH, CR, GT, HN, JO, KW, LB, MX, NI, PA, PH, QA, SA, SV) *see* CefTRIAXone 396
Meglucon (DE) *see* MetFORMIN 1307
Megostat (AU, HR) *see* Megestrol 1281
Meiact (AE, BH, CN, ES, JP, KR, KW, LB, QA, SA, TH, VN) *see* Cefditoren 378
Meibida (CN) *see* GlipiZIDE 967
Mei-Cal (TW) *see* Calcium Citrate 330
Mei Jia Xin (CN) *see* Midecamycin [INT] 1365
Meikam (ID) *see* Cloxacillin [CAN/INT] 488
Meilital (CN) *see* Midecamycin [INT] 1365
Mei Ou Ka (CN) *see* Midecamycin [INT] 1365
Meipril (ID) *see* Enalapril 722
Meisusheng (CN) *see* Methotrexate 1322
Meithromax (TH) *see* Azithromycin (Systemic) 216
Meixil (TH) *see* Amoxicillin 130
Mejoralito Junior (MX) *see* Acetaminophen 32
Mejoralito Pediátrico (MX) *see* Acetaminophen 32
Mekinist (AU, BM, CZ, HR, LT, NL, SE, SI, SK) *see* Trametinib 2077
Me-Korti (FI) *see* PredniSONE 1706
Melabon (DE) *see* Aspirin 180
Meladinina (CR, DO, GT, NI, PA, PY, SV) *see* Methoxsalen (Systemic) 1330
Meladinina (CR, DO, GT, NI, PA, SV) *see* Methoxsalen (Topical) 1331
Meladinine (AE, CN, FR, VN) *see* Methoxsalen (Topical) 1331
Meladinine (CN, FR, TH, VN) *see* Methoxsalen (Systemic) 1330
Melanocyl (IN) *see* Methoxsalen (Systemic) 1330
Melanocyl (IN) *see* Methoxsalen (Topical) 1331
Melanosa (KR) *see* Hydroquinone 1020
Melanox (ID) *see* Hydroquinone 1020
Melaoline (GR) *see* Methoxsalen (Topical) 1331
Melart (PH) *see* Meloxicam 1283
Melashine (MY) *see* Hydroquinone 1020
Melbin (HK, JP) *see* MetFORMIN 1307
Melcam (HK, TH) *see* Meloxicam 1283
Melcox (KR) *see* Meloxicam 1283
Meldian (HR) *see* ChlorproPAMIDE 429
Meleril (AR, CO, PY, UY, VE) *see* Thioridazine 2030
Meletin (MY, TW) *see* Mexiletine 1359
Melfalan (ES) *see* Melphalan 1283
Melflam (HK) *see* Meloxicam 1283

Meliam (HR) *see* Meloxicam 1283
Melicam (TW) *see* Meloxicam 1283
Melicin (TW) *see* Minocycline 1371
Melipramin (CZ, HN, HU, PL, SK) *see* Imipramine 1054
Melital (AE) *see* Glimepiride 966
Melix (AE, BB, BF, BH, BJ, BM, BS, BZ, CI, CY, EG, ET, GH, GM, GN, GY, IL, IQ, IR, JM, JO, KE, KW, LB, LR, LY, MA, ML, MR, MU, MW, NE, NG, NL, OM, PR, QA, SA, SC, SD, SL, SN, SR, SY, TN, TT, TZ, UG, YE, ZA, ZM, ZW) *see* GlyBURIDE 972
Melizide (AU, SG) *see* GlipiZIDE 967
Melizid (FI) *see* GlipiZIDE 967
Mellerette (IT) *see* Thioridazine 2030
Melleril (AE, AT, BE, BF, BG, BH, BJ, BR, CH, CI, CY, CZ, DE, DK, EE, EG, ES, ET, FR, GB, GH, GM, GN, GR, HN, ID, IE, IQ, IR, IT, JO, KE, KR, KW, LB, LR, LY, MA, ML, MR, MT, MU, MW, MX, NE, NG, NL, NO, OM, PE, PK, PT, QA, RU, SA, SC, SD, SE, SK, SL, SN, SY, TN, TR, TZ, UG, VN, YE, ZA, ZM, ZW) *see* Thioridazine 2030
Mellerzin (TW) *see* Thioridazine 2030
Mellistin (TH) *see* Colistimethate 504
Mellitos C (JP) *see* ChlorproPAMIDE 429
Mellitos D (JP) *see* TOLBUTamide 2062
Melloderm-HQ (TH) *see* Hydroquinone 1020
Melocam (AE, BH, CO, CY, EG, IL, IQ, IR, JO, KW, LB, LY, MY, OM, QA, SA, SY, YE) *see* Meloxicam 1283
Melocon (ID) *see* Mometasone (Topical) 1391
Melocox (KR, PH) *see* Meloxicam 1283
Melode (KR) *see* Diazepam 613
Melodia (TH) *see* Ethinyl Estradiol and Drospirenone 801
Melodil (IL) *see* Maprotiline 1271
Mel-OD (IN, MY, TH) *see* Meloxicam 1283
Melodyn (AT) *see* Meloxicam 1283
Meloflam (PH) *see* Meloxicam 1283
Melomet (MY) *see* Mometasone (Topical) 1391
Melone 16 (TW) *see* MethylPREDNISolone 1340
Melopen (TW) *see* Meropenem 1299
Melophar (AE) *see* Mefloquine 1280
Melosteral (MX) *see* Meloxicam 1283
Melox (AE, BH, CY, EG, IL, IQ, IR, JO, KR, KW, LB, LY, MY, OM, QA, RO, SA, SG, SY, TH, TW, YE) *see* Meloxicam 1283
Meloxibell (AU) *see* Meloxicam 1283
Meloxin (ID) *see* Meloxicam 1283
Melpha (PK) *see* Melphalan 1283
Melquine (TW) *see* Hydroquinone 1020
Melquin HP (KR) *see* Hydroquinone 1020
Melsone (IN) *see* MethylPREDNISolone 1340
Melzin (PH) *see* CloNIDine 480
Melzin (TW) *see* Thioridazine 2030
Memantin (GT, HN, NI) *see* Memantine 1286
Memanto (KR) *see* Memantine 1286
Memanxa (AU) *see* Memantine 1286
Memary (JP) *see* Memantine 1286
Memento (AR) *see* Pipemidic Acid [INT] 1655
Memoril (NZ) *see* Memantine 1286
Memoril (PY) *see* Piracetam [INT] 1661
Memorit (IL) *see* Donepezil 668
Memosprint (IT) *see* Pyridoxine 1747
Memotal (JO, RO) *see* Piracetam [INT] 1661
Memotropil (PL) *see* Piracetam [INT] 1661
Memovic (KR) *see* Meloxicam 1283
Memox (IL) *see* Memantine 1286
Memozet (MY) *see* Piracetam [INT] 1661
Mem (PH) *see* Methylergonovine 1333
Mempil (TH) *see* Piracetam [INT] 1661
Memry (PH) *see* Memantine 1286
Memxa (TH) *see* Memantine 1286
Menactra (HK, MY, PH, SG) *see* Meningococcal (Groups A / C / Y and W-135) Diphtheria Conjugate Vaccine 1289
Menamig (CH) *see* Frovatriptan 938
Menatriptan (CR, DO, GT, HN, NI, PA, SV) *see* Frovatriptan 938
Menaxol (CR, DO, GT, HN, NI, PA, SV) *see* Acetylcysteine 40
Menaxol Forte (CR, DO, GT, HN, NI, PA, SV) *see* Acetylcysteine 40
Mencetam (TH) *see* Piracetam [INT] 1661
Mencevax A/C/W/Y-135 (TH) *see* Meningococcal (Groups A / C / Y and W-135) Diphtheria Conjugate Vaccine 1289
Mencevax ACWY (AE, AT, AU, CH, DE, FI, HK, IL, IT, KW, MY, NO, NZ, PH, SA, SG) *see* Meningococcal (Groups A / C / Y and W-135) Diphtheria Conjugate Vaccine 1289
Mencevax (BE) *see* Meningococcal (Groups A / C / Y and W-135) Diphtheria Conjugate Vaccine 1289
Mendon (JP) *see* Clorazepate 487
Menegradil (AR) *see* Etilefrine [INT] 815
Menelat (PH) *see* Mirtazapine 1376
Menem IV (PH) *see* Meropenem 1299
Menest (AR, CA) *see* Estrogens (Esterified) 790
Menfazona (ES) *see* Nefazodone 1435
Meniace (JP, KR) *see* Betahistine [CAN/INT] 252
Menisone (TW) *see* MethylPREDNISolone 1340
Menistin (PE) *see* Betahistine [CAN/INT] 252
Menito (TW) *see* DimenhyDRINATE 637
Menjugate (AR, AU, BE, CH, CZ, DE, FI, GB, IE, SI) *see* Meningococcal Group C-CRM197 Conjugate Vaccine [CAN/INT] 1288
Menna (TW) *see* DiphenhydrAMINE (Systemic) 641
Menoaid Combipatch (JP) *see* Estradiol and Norethindrone 781
Menocal (KR) *see* Calcitonin 322
Menodin-Retard (CO) *see* Estradiol (Systemic) 775
Menogon 75 (AE, BH, CY, EG, HK, IL, IQ, IR, JO, KW, LB, LY, OM, QA, SA, SY, YE) *see* Menotropins 1292
Menogon (FR, HK, PH, PK, SG, TH) *see* Menotropins 1292
Menograine (ZA) *see* CloNIDine 480
Menomune (AU, PH) *see* Meningococcal (Groups A / C / Y and W-135) Diphtheria Conjugate Vaccine 1289
Menopur (AE, AT, AU, BE, BH, CH, CN, CY, CZ, DK, EG, FI, GB, HK, HR, HU, ID, IE, IL, IQ, IR, IS, JO, KR, KW, LB, LY, MY, NO, OM, PH, PL, PT, QA, RO, SA, SE, SI, SK, SY, TH, TR, TW, VN, YE) *see* Menotropins 1292
Menorest (AU, DE, IT) *see* Estradiol (Systemic) 775
Menosor (TH) *see* Mebeverine [INT] 1275
Menostat (VE) *see* Estrogens (Conjugated/Equine, Systemic) 787
Menotrix (EC) *see* Tibolone [INT] 2035
Mensil (PY) *see* Allopurinol 90
Mensoton (DE) *see* Ibuprofen 1032
Mentax (EE, IL, JP, KR, TW) *see* Butenafine 314
Mentix (CL) *see* Modafinil 1386
mentopin Hustenstiller (DE) *see* Clobutinol [INT] 468
Mentumir (PH) *see* Escitalopram 765
Menuix (CL) *see* Rasagiline 1781
Menveo (AU, HK, ID, KR, PH) *see* Meningococcal (Groups A / C / Y and W-135) Diphtheria Conjugate Vaccine 1289
Mepem (CN, TW) *see* Meropenem 1299
Meperdol (PY) *see* Meperidine 1293
Meperidol (UY) *see* Meperidine 1293
Mepha Gasec (CR, GT, HN, NI, PA, SV) *see* Omeprazole 1508
Mephanol (AE, BF, BH, BJ, CH, CI, CY, EG, ET, GH, GM, GN, IQ, IR, JO, KE, KW, LB, LR, LY, MA, ML, MR, MU, MW, MY, NE, NG, OM, QA, SA, SC, SD, SL, SN, SY, TN, TZ, UG, YE, ZM, ZW) *see* Allopurinol 90
Mephaquin (BB, BM, BS, BZ, CH, CR, EC, GT, GY, HK, HN, IL, JM, NI, PE, PT, SG, SR, SV, TT, VN) *see* Mefloquine 1280

Mephathiol (CH) *see* Carbocisteine [INT] 357
Mephenon (BE, LU) *see* Methadone 1311
Mephicetine (LB) *see* Chloramphenicol 421
Mephicycline (LB) *see* Tetracycline 2017
Mephipen (LB) *see* Ampicillin 141
Mepicaton 3% (TH) *see* Mepivacaine 1295
Mepicaton (SA) *see* Mepivacaine 1295
Mepidont (PL) *see* Mepivacaine 1295
Mepigobbi (AR) *see* Mepivacaine 1295
Mepigryl (KR) *see* Glimepiride 966
Mepivastesin (CZ, HK, IL, PL, SG) *see* Mepivacaine 1295
Mepracid (PH) *see* Omeprazole 1508
Meprate (GB) *see* Meprobamate 1296
Meprate (IN) *see* MedroxyPROGESTERone 1277
Meprazol (AU) *see* Omeprazole 1508
Meprednisona All Pro (AR) *see* MethylPREDNISolone 1340
Mepresone (PH) *see* MethylPREDNISolone 1340
Meprobamat (DE, GB, HR) *see* Meprobamate 1296
Mepro (BE) *see* Meprobamate 1296
Meprodat (FI) *see* Carisoprodol 363
Meprodil (CH) *see* Meprobamate 1296
Mepron (BB, BM, BS, BZ, GY, JM, PL, SR, TT) *see* Atovaquone 197
Meprosetil (ID) *see* ChlorproMAZINE 429
Meprospan (ES) *see* Meprobamate 1296
Mequin (TH) *see* Mefloquine 1280
Meraparon (MY) *see* Meropenem 1299
Merapiran (AR) *see* Meloxicam 1283
Merapiran (AR) *see* Piracetam [INT] 1661
Merapur (MX) *see* Menotropins 1292
Merbentyl (AE, EG) *see* Dicyclomine 622
Mercaptopurina Wellcome (ES) *see* Mercaptopurine 1296
Mercaptyl (CH) *see* PenicillAMINE 1608
Mercilon (CH, EC, FR, IS, KR, LT, PH, SG, SK, TW, VN) *see* Ethinyl Estradiol and Desogestrel 799
Merckformin (HU) *see* MetFORMIN 1307
Merflam (ID) *see* Diclofenac (Systemic) 617
Mergium (PH) *see* RABEprazole 1762
Mergon (TW) *see* Ergonovine [CAN/INT] 754
Mergot (PH) *see* Methylergonovine 1333
Mergotrex (PH) *see* Methylergonovine 1333
Mericle (KR) *see* Glimepiride 966
Meridian AP (UY) *see* Theophylline 2026
Merimono (DE) *see* Estradiol (Systemic) 775
Merional (GB) *see* Menotropins 1292
Meripramin (JP) *see* Imipramine 1054
Merislon (CN, CR, DO, GT, HK, ID, JP, MY, PH, SG, SV, TH, TW, VN) *see* Betahistine [CAN/INT] 252
Meristin (ID) *see* Betahistine [CAN/INT] 252
Merkaptopurin (TW) *see* Mercaptopurine 1296
Merlit (AT, RU) *see* LORazepam 1243
Merlopam (ID) *see* LORazepam 1243
Merobac I.V. (CO) *see* Meropenem 1299
Merofen (ID) *see* Meropenem 1299
Meromax (PH) *see* Meropenem 1299
Meronem (AE, BB, BE, BF, BG, BH, BJ, BM, BR, BS, BZ, CH, CI, CL, CO, CR, CY, CZ, DE, DK, DO, EC, EE, EG, ES, ET, FI, GB, GH, GM, GN, GR, GT, GY, HK, HN, HR, HU, ID, IE, IL, IN, IS, JM, JO, KE, LB, LR, LT, LU, MA, ML, MR, MU, MW, MY, NE, NG, NI, NL, NO, PA, PE, PH, PK, PL, PR, PT, QA, RO, RU, SA, SC, SD, SE, SG, SI, SK, SL, SN, SR, SV, TH, TN, TR, TT, TZ, UG, UY, VE, VN, ZA, ZM, ZW) *see* Meropenem 1299
Meropemed (PE) *see* Meropenem 1299
Meropen (JP, KR, PH) *see* Meropenem 1299
Merop (PH) *see* Meropenem 1299
Merosan (ID) *see* Meropenem 1299
Merosin (KR) *see* Meropenem 1299
Mero (TH) *see* Meropenem 1299
Meroxi (ID) *see* Meropenem 1299
Merozan (PH) *see* Meropenem 1299
Merozen (PY) *see* Meropenem 1299
Merpurin (PH) *see* Mercaptopurine 1296
Merrem (AU, IT, MX, NZ) *see* Meropenem 1299
Mersa (PH) *see* Vancomycin 2130
Mersikol (ID) *see* Gemfibrozil 956
Mersivas (ID) *see* Simvastatin 1890
Mertigo (ID, TH) *see* Betahistine [CAN/INT] 252
Mertus (ID) *see* Mupirocin 1404
Merval (PY) *see* Risedronate 1816
Merverin (UY) *see* Mebeverine [INT] 1275
Merxin (JP) *see* CefOXitin 386
Mesacol (BF, BJ, CI, ET, GH, GM, GN, IN, KE, LR, MA, ML, MR, MU, MW, NE, NG, SC, SD, SL, SN, TN, TZ, UG, ZM, ZW) *see* Mesalamine 1301
Mesacol (TW) *see* Bethanechol 257
Mesalin (KR) *see* Mesalamine 1301
Mesasal (AU, DK, NO, ZA) *see* Mesalamine 1301
Mescorit (DE) *see* MetFORMIN 1307
Mescryo (MX) *see* Mesna 1305
Mesid (IT) *see* Nimesulide [INT] 1456
Meslatin (PH) *see* Oxaliplatin 1528
M-Eslon (CL, CO, EC, PE) *see* Morphine (Systemic) 1394
Meslon (TW) *see* Betahistine [CAN/INT] 252
Mesnil (MX, PE, PY) *see* Mesna 1305
Mesodal (MX) *see* Mesna 1305
Mesofam (KR) *see* Aztreonam 220
Mesolone (KR) *see* MethylPREDNISolone 1340
Mesporin IV (BB, BM, BS, BZ, GY, HK, JM, PR, SR) *see* CefTRIAXone 396
Mesporin (AE, BF, BH, BJ, CI, CY, EE, EG, ET, GH, GM, GN, IQ, IR, JO, KE, KW, LB, LR, LY, MA, ML, MR, MU, MW, MY, NE, NG, OM, QA, SA, SC, SD, SL, SN, SY, TN, TT, TZ, UG, YE, ZM, ZW) *see* CefTRIAXone 396
Mesporin IM (BB, BM, BS, BZ, GY, HK, JM, PR, SR) *see* CefTRIAXone 396
Mestacine (FR) *see* Minocycline 1371
Mesteron (PL) *see* MethylTESTOSTERone 1345
Mestinon (AE, AR, AT, AU, BB, BE, BH, BM, BR, BS, BZ, CH, CL, CO, CR, CY, CZ, DK, DO, EG, ES, FI, FR, GB, GH, GR, GT, GY, HK, HN, HR, HU, ID, IE, IL, IQ, IR, IT, JM, JO, KR, KW, LB, LU, LY, MX, MY, NI, NO, OM, PA, PE, PH, PL, PT, PY, QA, SA, SE, SG, SI, SK, SR, SV, SY, TH, TR, TT, TW, TZ, UG, UY, VE, YE, ZM) *see* Pyridostigmine 1746
Mestinon Retard (NL) *see* Pyridostigmine 1746
Mestoranum (DE, DK, NO) *see* Mesterolone [INT] 1307
Mestrel (MX, TH) *see* Megestrol 1281
Mestrol (TW) *see* Megestrol 1281
Mesulid (BE, CZ, GR, HK, HU, IL, IN, IT, KR, LU, MX, PY) *see* Nimesulide [INT] 1456
Mesyrel (TW) *see* TraZODone 2091
Metabolin (JP) *see* Thiamine 2028
Metacain DS (PH) *see* Lidocaine and Prilocaine 1213
Metacalmans (AR) *see* Methadone 1311
Metacen (IT) *see* Indomethacin 1067
Metacort (PH) *see* Dexamethasone (Systemic) 599
Metact (JP) *see* Pioglitazone and Metformin 1655
Metadate CD SR (KR) *see* Methylphenidate 1336
Metadol (PE) *see* Methadone 1311
Metadon (DK, EE, IS, LT, NO, SE) *see* Methadone 1311
Metaflex (AR) *see* Nimesulide [INT] 1456
Metagard (SG) *see* Trimetazidine [INT] 2104
Metagesic (EC) *see* Acetaminophen and Tramadol 37
Metagesic (PH) *see* Acetaminophen 32
Metalcaptase[inj.] (CZ, HR) *see* PenicillAMINE 1608
Metalcaptase (DE, HR, JP, LU, TW) *see* PenicillAMINE 1608
Metalyse (AE, AT, AU, BE, BF, BG, BH, BJ, CH, CI, CL, CO, CY, CZ, DE, DK, EE, EG, ES, ET, FI, FR, GB, GH, GM, GN, GR, HK, HN, HR, HU, ID, IE, IL, IQ, IR, IS, IT,

JO, KE, KR, KW, LB, LR, LT, LY, MA, ML, MR, MT, MU, MW, MX, MY, NE, NG, NL, NO, NZ, OM, PE, PL, PT, QA, RO, RU, SA, SC, SD, SE, SG, SI, SK, SL, SN, SY, TH, TN, TR, TW, TZ, UG, VN, YE, ZA, ZM, ZW) *see* Tenecteplase ... 1996
Metamar (AR) *see* Betamethasone (Systemic) ... 253
Metamide (NZ) *see* Metoclopramide ... 1345
Metamizol (CL) *see* Dipyrone [INT] ... 653
Metamucil (AR, CL, HK, NL, NZ) *see* Psyllium ... 1744
Metaoxedrin (DK, NO) *see* Phenylephrine (Systemic) ... 1638
Metasedin (ES) *see* Methadone ... 1311
Metasolvens (CH) *see* Bromhexine [INT] ... 291
Metaspray (IN) *see* Mometasone (Nasal) ... 1391
Metastigmin[inj.] (FI) *see* Neostigmine ... 1438
Meta (TH) *see* Promethazine ... 1723
Metazem (IE) *see* Diltiazem ... 634
Metazin (KR, SG) *see* Trimetazidine [INT] ... 2104
Metazol (ZA) *see* MetroNIDAZOLE (Systemic) ... 1353
Metchek (NZ) *see* MetFORMIN ... 1307
Metcor (ID) *see* MethylPREDNISolone ... 1340
Metenix 5 (GB, GR, IE, SG) *see* Metolazone ... 1348
Metermine (AU) *see* Phentermine ... 1635
Meterone (TW) *see* MedroxyPROGESTERone ... 1277
Metex XR (AU) *see* MetFORMIN ... 1307
Metfogamma (DE) *see* MetFORMIN ... 1307
Metfor (AE, BH, QA) *see* MetFORMIN ... 1307
Metforal (CR, DO, EC, GT, HN, IT, LT, NI, PA, SG, SV) *see* MetFORMIN ... 1307
Metgluco (JP) *see* MetFORMIN ... 1307
Methacin (HK) *see* Indomethacin ... 1067
Methaddict (DE) *see* Methadone ... 1311
Methadone chlorhydrate (FR) *see* Methadone ... 1311
Methadone Hydrochloride (PL) *see* Methadone ... 1311
Methadose (CO) *see* Methadone ... 1311
Methapain (JP) *see* Methadone ... 1311
Methergin (AE, AT, BD, BE, BF, BG, BH, BJ, BR, CH, CI, CL, CO, CZ, DE, DK, EE, EG, ES, ET, FI, FR, GB, GH, GM, GN, HK, HN, ID, IE, IL, IS, IT, JO, JP, KE, KR, KW, LR, MA, ML, MR, MT, MU, MW, MX, MY, NE, NG, NL, NO, PE, PH, PK, PT, QA, RU, SC, SD, SE, SG, SI, SK, SL, SN, TN, TW, TZ, UG, UY, VE, VN, ZA, ZM, ZW) *see* Methylergonovine ... 1333
Methergine (CY, LB, SA, TR) *see* Methylergonovine ... 1333
Methimazol (PL) *see* Methimazole ... 1319
Methizol (DE) *see* Methimazole ... 1319
Methoblastin (AU, NZ) *see* Methotrexate ... 1322
Methocarbamol (PL) *see* Methocarbamol ... 1320
Metholen (KR) *see* Methoxsalen (Topical) ... 1331
Methoplain (JP) *see* Methyldopa ... 1332
Methotrexat Bigmar (CH) *see* Methotrexate ... 1322
Methotrexate (AU, HK, ID, IL, MY, PH, TH, TW) *see* Methotrexate ... 1322
Methotrexat Ebewe (CH) *see* Methotrexate ... 1322
Methotrexat-Ebewe (HU) *see* Methotrexate ... 1322
Methotrexate Faulding (SE) *see* Methotrexate ... 1322
Methotrexate[inj.] (HR, IT) *see* Methotrexate ... 1322
Methotrexate Pharmacia (SE) *see* Methotrexate ... 1322
Methotrexate Wyeth Lederle (SE) *see* Methotrexate ... 1322
Methotrexate "Lederle" (HU) *see* Methotrexate ... 1322
Methotrexat Farmos (CH) *see* Methotrexate ... 1322
Methotrexat (HR) *see* Methotrexate ... 1322
Methotrexat Lachema (HU) *see* Methotrexate ... 1322
Methotrexat Lederle (CH) *see* Methotrexate ... 1322
Methotrexato (AR, EC) *see* Methotrexate ... 1322
Methotrexat Teva (CH) *see* Methotrexate ... 1322
Methotrexat-Teva (HU) *see* Methotrexate ... 1322
Methozane (IL) *see* Methotrimeprazine [CAN/INT] ... 1329
Methylin (AR) *see* Methylphenidate ... 1336
Methylon (KR) *see* MethylPREDNISolone ... 1340
Methylpred (AU) *see* MethylPREDNISolone ... 1340
Methylprednisolone David Bull (LU) *see* MethylPREDNISolone ... 1340
Methysol (KR) *see* MethylPREDNISolone ... 1340
Metibasol (PT) *see* Methimazole ... 1319
Meticorten (AR, BR, CL, CO, CR, DO, GT, HN, MX, NI, PA, PE, PT, SV, VE) *see* PredniSONE ... 1706
Metildopa (CL, HR) *see* Methyldopa ... 1332
Metilpres (AR) *see* PredniSONE ... 1706
Metimyd (MX) *see* Sulfacetamide and Prednisolone ... 1944
Metindol (PL) *see* Indomethacin ... 1067
Metixane (MX) *see* Sucralfate ... 1940
Metizol (PL) *see* Methimazole ... 1319
Metlazel (AE, BH, CY, EG, IQ, IR, JO, KW, LB, LY, OM, QA, SA, SY, YE) *see* Metoclopramide ... 1345
Metligine (JP) *see* Midodrine ... 1365
Metocamol (KR) *see* Methocarbamol ... 1320
Metoclamid (LU) *see* Metoclopramide ... 1345
Metoclopramide-Eurogenerics (LU) *see* Metoclopramide ... 1345
Metoclox (EC) *see* Metoclopramide ... 1345
Metodik (AR) *see* Methotrexate ... 1322
Meto-Hennig (DE) *see* Metoprolol ... 1350
Metohexal (AU, HU, LU) *see* Metoprolol ... 1350
MetoHEXAL (VN) *see* Metoprolol ... 1350
Metoject (CZ, DK, ES, FR, HR, RO, SK) *see* Methotrexate ... 1322
Metolaz (IN) *see* Metolazone ... 1348
Metolol-CP (HK) *see* Metoprolol ... 1350
Metop (IE) *see* Metoprolol ... 1350
Metopram (FI) *see* Metoclopramide ... 1345
Metopril (ID) *see* Captopril ... 342
Metoprim (PH) *see* Metoprolol ... 1350
Metoprogamma (DE) *see* Metoprolol ... 1350
Metoprolol-B (HU) *see* Metoprolol ... 1350
Metoprolol-rpm (LU) *see* Metoprolol ... 1350
Metoprolol Stada (HU) *see* Metoprolol ... 1350
Metoral (MY, TH) *see* Triamcinolone (Systemic) ... 2099
Metoral (TH) *see* Triamcinolone (Topical) ... 2100
Metos (KR) *see* Metolazone ... 1348
Metostad (PH) *see* Metoprolol ... 1350
Metosyn (BB, BF, BJ, BS, BZ, CI, CZ, DK, ET, GB, GH, GM, GN, GY, IE, JM, KE, LR, MA, ML, MR, MU, MW, NE, NG, NO, PR, SC, SD, SL, SN, SR, TN, TT, TZ, UG, ZA, ZM, ZW) *see* Fluocinonide ... 894
Metothyrin (HU) *see* Methimazole ... 1319
Metotreksat (HR) *see* Methotrexate ... 1322
Metotressato Teva (IT) *see* Methotrexate ... 1322
Metotrexato (CL) *see* Methotrexate ... 1322
Metotrexato DBL (IT) *see* Methotrexate ... 1322
Metoxaleno (UY) *see* Methoxsalen (Systemic) ... 1330
Metoxiprim (MX) *see* Sulfamethoxazole and Trimethoprim ... 1946
Metoz (PH) *see* Metolazone ... 1348
Metpata (TH) *see* Methyldopa ... 1332
Metrergina (AR, PY) *see* Ergonovine [CAN/INT] ... 754
Metrex (PY) *see* Methotrexate ... 1322
Metrim (TH) *see* Sulfamethoxazole and Trimethoprim ... 1946
Metrix (ID) *see* Glimepiride ... 966
Metrocaps (DO, PA) *see* Metronidazole and Nystatin [CAN/INT] ... 1358
Metrocycline (PH) *see* Tetracycline ... 2017
Metroderme (PT) *see* MetroNIDAZOLE (Topical) ... 1357
Metrodin (HK) *see* Urofollitropin ... 2116
Metrodin HP (NZ) *see* Urofollitropin ... 2116
Metrogel (CR, DE, DO, GB, GT, HN, NI, PA, SV, TW) *see* MetroNIDAZOLE (Topical) ... 1357
Metrogyl (AU) *see* MetroNIDAZOLE (Systemic) ... 1353
Metrogyl Gel (TH, VN) *see* MetroNIDAZOLE (Topical) ... 1357
Metrolag (AE, BF, BH, BJ, CH, CI, CY, EG, ET, GH, GM, GN, IQ, IR, JO, KE, KW, LB, LR, LY, MA, ML, MR, MU,

MW, NE, NG, OM, QA, SA, SC, SD, SL, SN, SY, TN, TW, TZ, UG, YE, ZM, ZW) *see* MetroNIDAZOLE (Systemic) ... 1353
Metrol (AU) *see* Metoprolol ... 1350
Metrolex (TH) *see* MetroNIDAZOLE (Systemic) ... 1353
Metronidazole IV (AU, NZ) *see* MetroNIDAZOLE (Systemic) ... 1353
Metronide (AU) *see* MetroNIDAZOLE (Systemic) ... 1353
Metrosa (EE, HR) *see* MetroNIDAZOLE (Topical) ... 1357
Metrozin (CO) *see* MetroNIDAZOLE (Systemic) ... 1353
Metrozin Nistatina (CO) *see* Metronidazole and Nystatin [CAN/INT] ... 1358
Metsal AR (AU) *see* Magnesium Salicylate ... 1265
Metsil (PH) *see* Metoclopramide ... 1345
Metvell (ID) *see* Methylergonovine ... 1333
Metvix (AR, AT, AU, BE, BR, CH, CL, CZ, DE, DK, ES, FI, GB, GR, IE, IS, IT, KR, NL, NO, NZ, PT, SE, SG, SI, SK) *see* Methyl Aminolevulinate ... 1332
Metvixia (FR) *see* Methyl Aminolevulinate ... 1332
Mevac-A (PH) *see* Hepatitis A Vaccine ... 1001
Mevacor (AE, AT, BB, BH, BM, BS, BZ, CZ, DK, FI, GR, GY, HK, JM, KW, MX, NL, PK, PL, PR, QA, SR, TT) *see* Lovastatin ... 1252
Mevalotin (CN, DE, ID, JP, KR) *see* Pravastatin ... 1700
Mevalotin Protect (TH) *see* Pravastatin ... 1700
Mevamox (BR) *see* Meloxicam ... 1283
Mevan (KR) *see* Mepivacaine ... 1295
Meva (SA) *see* Mebeverine [INT] ... 1275
Meverina (PY) *see* Mebeverine [INT] ... 1275
Meverstin (KR) *see* Lovastatin ... 1252
Mevinacor (DE) *see* Lovastatin ... 1252
Mevir (AT) *see* Brivudine [INT] ... 289
Mex 24 (AR) *see* Pseudoephedrine ... 1742
Mexalen (AT, CZ, HU) *see* Acetaminophen ... 32
Mexat (CO) *see* Methotrexate ... 1322
Mexicord (PL) *see* Mexiletine ... 1359
Mexitec (ID) *see* Mexiletine ... 1359
Mexitil (AE, AT, AU, BB, BE, BG, BH, BM, BS, BZ, CH, CY, CZ, DE, DK, EE, EG, ES, FI, FR, GB, GR, GY, HN, HR, HU, IE, IL, IN, IQ, IR, IT, JM, JO, JP, KW, LB, LU, LY, MT, NL, NO, NZ, OM, PT, QA, RU, SA, SE, SK, SR, SY, TR, TT, TW, VN, YE) *see* Mexiletine ... 1359
Mexitilen (AR) *see* Mexiletine ... 1359
Mexpharm (ID) *see* Meloxicam ... 1283
Mexx (PH) *see* Meloxicam ... 1283
Mexylin (ID) *see* Amoxicillin ... 130
Mezacar (PH) *see* CarBAMazepine ... 346
Mezacar SR (PH) *see* CarBAMazepine ... 346
Mezacol (AE) *see* Mesalamine ... 1301
Mezactam (KR) *see* Aztreonam ... 220
Mezatrin (ID) *see* Azithromycin (Systemic) ... 216
Mezavant XL (GB) *see* Mesalamine ... 1301
Mezelol (MX) *see* Metoprolol ... 1350
Mezide (TW) *see* Gliclazide [CAN/INT] ... 964
Mezolar Matrix (GB) *see* FentaNYL ... 857
Mezomine (KR) *see* Methazolamide ... 1317
Mezo (PH) *see* Mometasone (Topical) ... 1391
Mezym Forte (BG) *see* Pancrelipase ... 1566
MF/110 (IT) *see* Nimesulide [INT] ... 1456
M-Flox (TH) *see* Norfloxacin ... 1475
MGR (IN) *see* Flunarizine [CAN/INT] ... 892
Miacalcic (AE, AU, BE, BG, BH, BR, CH, CL, CN, CO, CY, CZ, DE, DK, EC, EE, EG, ES, FI, FR, GR, HK, HN, ID, IE, IQ, IR, IS, JO, KW, LB, LY, MT, MX, MY, NO, NZ, OM, PE, PH, PL, PT, QA, RU, SA, SE, SG, SI, SK, SY, TH, TR, TW, VN, YE) *see* Calcitonin ... 322
Miacalcic [salmon] (HR, HU) *see* Calcitonin ... 322
Miacin (AE, BH, CY, EG, IL, IQ, IR, JO, KW, LB, LY, OM, QA, SA, SY, YE) *see* Amikacin ... 111
Miaryl (KR, MY) *see* Glimepiride ... 966
Mibetel (VN) *see* Telmisartan ... 1988
Mical (IL) *see* Carbocisteine [INT] ... 357
Micamin (RU) *see* Micafungin ... 1359
Micamlo (JP) *see* Telmisartan and Amlodipine ... 1989
Micanol (AT, AU, BE, DE, DK, IL, NO, NZ, PT, SE) *see* Anthralin ... 150
Micardis (AE, AR, AT, AU, BE, BF, BH, BJ, BR, CH, CI, CL, CN, CO, CR, CY, CZ, DE, DK, DO, EC, EE, EG, ET, FI, FR, GB, GH, GM, GN, GR, GT, HK, HN, HR, HU, ID, IE, IL, IQ, IR, IS, IT, JO, KE, KR, KW, LB, LR, LT, LY, MA, ML, MR, MT, MU, MW, MX, MY, NE, NG, NI, NL, NO, OM, PA, PH, PL, PT, PY, QA, RO, RU, SA, SC, SD, SE, SG, SI, SK, SL, SN, SV, SY, TH, TN, TR, TW, TZ, UG, UY, VN, YE, ZA, ZM, ZW) *see* Telmisartan ... 1988
Micardis Amlo (AR, CH, CL, CO, PE) *see* Telmisartan and Amlodipine ... 1989
Micardis Anlo (BR) *see* Telmisartan and Amlodipine ... 1989
Micardis HCT (BR) *see* Telmisartan and Hydrochlorothiazide ... 1990
Micardis Plus (AE, AR, AT, AU, BE, BG, BH, CH, CL, CN, CO, CR, CY, CZ, DE, DK, DO, EC, EE, ES, FI, FR, GB, GT, HK, HN, HR, HU, ID, IE, IS, IT, KR, KW, LB, LT, MT, MY, NI, NL, NO, NZ, PA, PE, PH, PL, PT, PY, QA, RO, RU, SA, SE, SG, SI, SK, SV, TH, TR, TW, UY, VE, VN) *see* Telmisartan and Hydrochlorothiazide ... 1990
Miccil (DO, GT, HN, MX, PA, PE, SV) *see* Bumetanide ... 297
MIC (IN) *see* Mosapride [INT] ... 1401
Miclast (IT) *see* Ciclopirox ... 433
Miclor (KR) *see* Cefaclor ... 372
Micobutina (AR) *see* Amorolfine [INT] ... 128
Micocept (HK) *see* Mycophenolate ... 1405
Micoderm (PE) *see* Isoconazole [INT] ... 1120
Micofulvin (ES) *see* Fenticonazole [INT] ... 868
Micofun (CO) *see* Bifonazole [INT] ... 264
Micogal (RO) *see* Itraconazole ... 1130
Micolis (AR, CL, EC, PE, PY, UY) *see* Econazole ... 703
Micombi (JP) *see* Telmisartan and Hydrochlorothiazide ... 1990
Micomedil (KR) *see* Miconazole (Topical) ... 1360
Miconacina (MX) *see* Natamycin ... 1432
Miconax (VE) *see* Econazole ... 703
Miconazol (MX) *see* Miconazole (Topical) ... 1360
Miconol (AR) *see* Miconazole (Topical) ... 1360
Micopirox (AR) *see* Ciclopirox ... 433
Micoral (AR, BR) *see* Ketoconazole (Systemic) ... 1144
Micoral (AR, BR) *see* Ketoconazole (Topical) ... 1145
Micoral (PE) *see* Itraconazole ... 1130
Micoset (CL) *see* Terbinafine (Systemic) ... 2002
Micoset (CL) *see* Terbinafine (Topical) ... 2004
Micosin (EC) *see* Ketoconazole (Topical) ... 1145
Micos (IT) *see* Econazole ... 703
Micosona (ES) *see* Naftifine ... 1416
Micostatin (CL) *see* Nystatin (Oral) ... 1481
Micostatin (MX, VE) *see* Nystatin (Topical) ... 1482
Micostyl (BR) *see* Econazole ... 703
Micotex (AR) *see* Econazole ... 703
Micoxolamina (IT) *see* Ciclopirox ... 433
Micozone (EC) *see* Terbinafine (Systemic) ... 2002
Micozone (EC) *see* Terbinafine (Topical) ... 2004
Micranil (AR) *see* SUMAtriptan ... 1953
Micreme (NZ) *see* Miconazole (Topical) ... 1360
Micril PP (PT) *see* Niacinamide ... 1446
Microcidal (ZA) *see* Griseofulvin ... 985
Microcilin (PH) *see* Ampicillin ... 141
Microdiol (BR, IL) *see* Ethinyl Estradiol and Desogestrel ... 799
Microdiol (ID) *see* Ethinyl Estradiol and Norgestrel ... 812
Microfemin CD (CO) *see* Ethinyl Estradiol and Levonorgestrel ... 803
Microfemin (CO) *see* Ethinyl Estradiol and Levonorgestrel ... 803
Microfer (GR) *see* Ferrous Sulfate ... 871

Microgyn (DK) *see* Ethinyl Estradiol and Levonorgestrel 803
Microgynon 20 ED (AU, NZ) *see* Ethinyl Estradiol and Levonorgestrel 803
Microgynon 21 (DE, PL) *see* Ethinyl Estradiol and Levonorgestrel 803
Microgynon 28 (DE) *see* Ethinyl Estradiol and Levonorgestrel 803
Microgynon 30 (AE, AT, BE, BF, BH, BJ, CH, CI, CY, DO, EG, ET, GB, GH, GM, GN, HK, IE, IQ, IR, JO, KE, KW, LB, LR, LY, MA, ML, MR, MU, MW, MY, NE, NG, NL, NZ, OM, QA, SA, SC, SD, SL, SN, SY, TN, TZ, UG, YE, ZM, ZW) *see* Ethinyl Estradiol and Levonorgestrel 803
Microgynon 30 ED (AU, BB, BM, BS, BZ, GY, HK, JM, NZ, PR, SR, TH, TT) *see* Ethinyl Estradiol and Levonorgestrel 803
Microgynon CD (CO, DO, EC, MX) *see* Ethinyl Estradiol and Levonorgestrel 803
Microgynon (CO, CR, CZ, DK, DO, EC, FI, GR, GT, HN, ID, IL, IS, IT, MX, NI, NO, PA, PE, PH, RU, SI, SK, SV, UY) *see* Ethinyl Estradiol and Levonorgestrel 803
Micro-Kalium Retard (AT) *see* Potassium Chloride 1687
Microlenyn 30 ED (TH) *see* Ethinyl Estradiol and Levonorgestrel 803
Microlut (CO, LU) *see* Levonorgestrel 1201
Micromycin (MX) *see* Minocycline 1371
Micronor (AE, AU, BF, BH, BJ, BR, CI, CY, EG, ET, GB, GH, GM, GN, IE, IL, IQ, IR, JO, KE, KW, LB, LR, LY, MA, ML, MR, MU, MW, NE, NG, OM, QA, SA, SC, SD, SL, SN, SY, TN, TZ, UG, YE, ZM, ZW) *see* Norethindrone 1473
Micro-Novom (ZA) *see* Norethindrone 1473
Micronovum (AT, CH, DE, ZA) *see* Norethindrone 1473
Microparin (DO, GT, SV) *see* Enoxaparin 726
Micropil (PH) *see* Ethinyl Estradiol and Norethindrone 808
Microser (AR, CL, EC, IT, PE, PK, VE) *see* Betahistine [CAN/INT] 252
Microshield (AU, IN, KR) *see* Chlorhexidine Gluconate 422
Microtrim (DE) *see* Sulfamethoxazole and Trimethoprim 1946
Microval (LU) *see* Levonorgestrel 1201
Microxin (MX) *see* Norfloxacin 1475
Microzide (JO) *see* Gliclazide [CAN/INT] 964
Mictonetten (DE) *see* Propiverine [INT] 1728
Mictonorm (AE, BE, CZ, DE, GR, HK, ID, PH, PT, SG, SI, SK, TR) *see* Propiverine [INT] 1728
Mictral (GB) *see* Nalidixic Acid [INT] 1418
Micturol Simple (ES) *see* Nitrofurantoin 1463
Midacum (ZA) *see* Midazolam 1361
Midamor (AT, CH, FI, GB, IE, NL, NO, NZ, SE) *see* AMILoride 113
Midarine (IN, JO, KW) *see* Succinylcholine 1939
Midax (PY) *see* OLANZapine 1491
Midazol (IL) *see* Midazolam 1361
Midazo (TW) *see* Midazolam 1361
MIDDLEEAST (IL) *see* Propranolol 1731
Midecin (IT) *see* Midecamycin [INT] 1365
Mide (TW) *see* Pyrazinamide 1745
Midfrin (KR) *see* Phenylephrine (Systemic) 1638
Midodrine Hydrochloride (ID) *see* Midodrine 1365
Midolam (IL) *see* Midazolam 1361
Midon (IE) *see* Midodrine 1365
Midopril (KW) *see* Captopril 342
Midorine (TW) *see* Midodrine 1365
Midotens (BR) *see* Lacidipin [INT] 1154
Midozor (MX) *see* Midazolam 1361
Midrat (MX) *see* Captopril 342
Midriafen (CO) *see* Phenylephrine (Systemic) 1638
Midric (ID) *see* Tropicamide 2108
Midriodavi (PT) *see* Cyclopentolate 517
Midron (KR) *see* Midodrine 1365
Midu (CN) *see* Methotrexate 1322
Mielogen (IT) *see* Molgramostim [INT] 1388
Mielucin (ES) *see* Busulfan 312
Mi Er Ning (CN) *see* Mirtazapine 1376
Mifegyne (AT, BE, CH, DE, DK, EE, FI, FR, GB, GR, IL, NL, NO, NZ, PT, RO, SE, SI, SK, ZA) *see* Mifepristone 1366
Mifegyn (RU) *see* Mifepristone 1366
Mifestad (VN) *see* Mifepristone 1366
Miflonid (CZ) *see* Budesonide (Systemic) 293
Miflonide (BE, DE, IL, IT, NZ, PT, TR) *see* Budesonide (Systemic) 293
Mifolian (CN) *see* Mifepristone 1366
Miformin (TH) *see* MetFORMIN 1307
Migard (DK, EE, FI, GB, GR, NO, SE) *see* Frovatriptan 938
Migbose (TW) *see* Miglitol 1367
Miglucan (FR) *see* GlyBURIDE 972
Migoff (TW) *see* Rizatriptan 1836
Migon (IN) *see* Flunarizine [CAN/INT] 892
Migragesin (CO) *see* SUMAtriptan 1953
Migranal (GB) *see* Dihydroergotamine 633
Migranil (IN) *see* Dihydroergotamine 633
Migranil (PK) *see* Ergotamine 754
Migrastat (IE) *see* SUMAtriptan 1953
Migraval (VE) *see* SUMAtriptan 1953
Migretamine (JP) *see* Ergotamine 754
Migrexa (DE, HR) *see* Ergotamine 754
Migson (IN) *see* Rizatriptan 1836
Miguard (KR) *see* Frovatriptan 938
Mikaciland (PY) *see* Amikacin 111
Mikacin (AE, BH, QA, SA) *see* Amikacin 111
Mikaject (ID) *see* Amikacin 111
Mikasin (ID) *see* Amikacin 111
Miketorin (JP) *see* Amitriptyline 119
Mikin (KR) *see* Amikacin 111
Mikogal (HU, RU) *see* Omoconazole [INT] 1512
Mikostat (AE) *see* Nystatin (Oral) 1481
Mikroplex Magnesium (DE) *see* Magnesium Gluconate 1263
Milamox-BIG (TH) *see* Amoxicillin 130
Milatus (PE) *see* Imatinib 1047
Milcopen (FI) *see* Penicillin V Potassium 1614
Milenium (CR, GT, PA, SV) *see* Esomeprazole 771
Milice (IT) *see* Pyrethrins and Piperonyl Butoxide 1746
Milicor (IN) *see* Milrinone 1370
Milinor (HR) *see* Lindane 1217
Milithin (GR) *see* Lithium 1230
Milk of Magnesia (IL, PL) *see* Magnesium Hydroxide 1263
Millibar (CN, TW) *see* Indapamide 1065
Millisrol (JP) *see* Nitroglycerin 1465
Milmag (PL) *see* Magnesium Hydroxide 1263
Miloderme (PT) *see* Alclometasone 72
Miloxam (AE, BH, CY, EG, IL, IQ, IR, JO, KW, LB, LY, OM, QA, SA, SY, YE) *see* Meloxicam 1283
Miloz (ID) *see* Midazolam 1361
Miltaun (AT) *see* Meprobamate 1296
Miltown (ES) *see* Meprobamate 1296
Milurit (BG, CZ, HN, HU, SK) *see* Allopurinol 90
Mimpara (AE, AT, BE, BG, BH, CH, CL, CY, CZ, DE, DK, EE, ES, FI, FR, GB, GR, HN, HR, HU, IE, IL, IS, IT, KW, LT, MT, MX, NL, NO, PL, PT, QA, RO, RU, SA, SE, SI, SK, TR) *see* Cinacalcet 439
Min-I-Jet Isoprenaline (GB) *see* Isoproterenol 1124
Min-I-Jet Naloxone (GB) *see* Naloxone 1419
Minalgin (CH) *see* Dipyrone [INT] 653
Minart (CR, DO, GT, HN, NI, PA, SV) *see* Candesartan 335
Minax (AU, HK, TW) *see* Metoprolol 1350
Minaxen (TR) *see* Minocycline 1371
Minazol (CO) *see* MitoMYcin (Systemic) 1380

Mindchange (VN) *see* Levonorgestrel 1201
Mindiab (DK, EE, FI, NO, PK, RU, SE) *see* GlipiZIDE 967
Minecin (KR) *see* Prazosin 1703
Minedrox (PE) *see* Hydroxocobalamin 1020
Minerva-35 (ZA) *see* Cyproterone and Ethinyl Estradiol [CAN/INT] 532
Minias (IT) *see* Lormetazepam [INT] 1247
Miniaspi 80 (ID) *see* Aspirin 180
Minidiab (AE, AT, AU, BE, BF, BG, BH, BJ, BR, CI, CL, CY, CZ, EG, ET, FR, GH, GM, GN, HN, HU, IL, IQ, IR, IS, IT, JO, KE, KW, LB, LR, LU, LY, MA, ML, MR, MU, MW, MY, NE, NG, OM, PH, PL, PT, QA, SA, SC, SD, SI, SK, SL, SN, SY, TH, TN, TR, TW, TZ, UG, VE, VN, YE, ZA, ZM, ZW) *see* GlipiZIDE 967
Minidril (FR) *see* Ethinyl Estradiol and Levonorgestrel 803
Minihep (AE, QA) *see* Heparin 997
Minilip (HU) *see* Gemfibrozil 956
Minims Atropine (AT) *see* Atropine 200
Minims-Atropine (IE) *see* Atropine 200
Minims Atropine Sulfaat (NL) *see* Atropine 200
Minims Atropine Sulfate (AE, BH, CY, EG, GB, HK, IQ, IR, JO, KW, LB, LY, OM, QA, SA, SY, YE) *see* Atropine 200
Minims Atropine Sulphate (FI) *see* Atropine 200
Minims-Atropinsulfat (AT) *see* Atropine 200
Minims Chloramphenicol (AE, BH, CY, EG, IQ, IR, JO, KW, LB, LY, OM, QA, SA, SY, YE) *see* Chloramphenicol 421
Minims Cyclopentolate Hydrocloride (AE, AU, BH, CY, EG, IL, IQ, IR, JO, KW, LB, LY, NZ, OM, QA, SA, SY, YE) *see* Cyclopentolate 517
Minims-Cyclopentolate (IE) *see* Cyclopentolate 517
Minims Fluoresceine (BE) *see* Fluorescein 894
Minims Fluorescein Sodium (FI, GB) *see* Fluorescein 894
Minims Homatropine (AE, BH, CY, EG, IL, IQ, IR, JO, KW, LB, LY, OM, QA, SA, SY, YE) *see* Homatropine 1005
Minims Homatropine HBr (HK) *see* Homatropine 1005
Minims Homatropine Hydrobromide (GB, IE) *see* Homatropine 1005
Minims-Homatropinhydrobromid (AT) *see* Homatropine 1005
Minims Metipranolol (GB) *see* Metipranolol 1345
Minims Neomycin (BE, NL) *see* Neomycin 1436
Minims Phenylephrine HCL 10% (ZA) *see* Phenylephrine (Systemic) 1638
Minims Phenylephrine Hydrochloride (GB, IE) *see* Phenylephrine (Systemic) 1638
Minims Proxymetacaine Hydrochloride (GB) *see* Proparacaine 1728
Minims Tropicamide (GB, IE) *see* Tropicamide 2108
Mini-PE (DK) *see* Norethindrone 1473
Minipil (PH) *see* Ethinyl Estradiol and Levonorgestrel 803
Miniplanor (JP) *see* Allopurinol 90
Minipres (BZ, CR, EC, ES, GT, MX, NI, PA, SV, VE) *see* Prazosin 1703
Minipres Retard (AR) *see* Prazosin 1703
Minipress XL (IN) *see* Prazosin 1703
Minipress (AE, AT, AU, BB, BE, BF, BG, BH, BJ, BM, BS, BZ, CI, CY, EG, ET, FR, GH, GM, GN, GR, GY, HN, ID, IL, IQ, IR, JM, JO, KE, KW, LB, LR, LY, MA, ML, MR, MU, MW, MY, NE, NG, NL, OM, PK, PL, QA, RO, SA, SC, SD, SG, SL, SN, SR, SY, TH, TN, TR, TT, TW, TZ, UG, YE, ZM, ZW) *see* Prazosin 1703
Minipres SR (CO) *see* Prazosin 1703
Minipress SR (BR) *see* Prazosin 1703
Minirin (AT, AU, BG, CH, CN, CO, DE, DK, EC, EE, FI, FR, HR, HU, IL, IS, LT, LU, MY, NO, NZ, PE, PH, PK, PT, PY, RU, SE, SG, SI, TR, TW) *see* Desmopressin 594
Minirin DDAVP (AE, BH, CY, GR, HK, IQ, IR, IT, JO, KW, LB, LY, OM, QA, SA, SY, TH, YE) *see* Desmopressin 594
Minirin Melt (AE, AU, CY, EG, IL, KW, LB, PH, QA, SA, TH) *see* Desmopressin 594
Minirinmelt (FR) *see* Desmopressin 594
Minirinmelt OD (JP) *see* Desmopressin 594
Minirin Nasal Spray (AU, NZ) *see* Desmopressin 594
Minisiston (TW) *see* Ethinyl Estradiol and Levonorgestrel 803
Minison (MY, TW) *see* Prazosin 1703
Minitent (AE, BH, CY, EG, IQ, IR, JO, KW, LB, LY, OM, QA, SA, SY, YE) *see* Captopril 342
Minitran (AU, BE, CR, DO, GR, GT, HN, LU, PA, SV, UY) *see* Nitroglycerin 1465
Minivlar (KR) *see* Ethinyl Estradiol and Levonorgestrel 803
Minixime (MY) *see* Cefixime 380
Minlife-P (TW) *see* Loratadine and Pseudoephedrine 1242
Minny 28 (TH) *see* Ethinyl Estradiol and Desogestrel 799
Minny (TH) *see* Ethinyl Estradiol and Desogestrel 799
Mino-50 (LU) *see* Minocycline 1371
Minocin (AE, BE, BH, BO, BR, CH, CN, CR, DO, EC, EG, ES, GB, GR, GT, HK, HN, ID, IT, KR, KW, LU, MX, NI, NL, PA, PE, PH, PK, PR, PT, PY, QA, SA, SV, UY, VE, VN) *see* Minocycline 1371
Minocin Akne (SI) *see* Minocycline 1371
Minocin SA (IE) *see* Minocycline 1371
Minoclin (IL) *see* Minocycline 1371
Minocyclin 50 Stada (DE) *see* Minocycline 1371
Minocyclin (CZ) *see* Minocycline 1371
Minodiab (AR, CR, ES, GB, GR, GT, IE, MX, NI, PA) *see* GlipiZIDE 967
Minodil (TH) *see* Minoxidil (Topical) 1374
Minogran (CO) *see* Minocycline 1371
Minoline (TW) *see* Minocycline 1371
Minolox (VN) *see* Minocycline 1371
Minomycin (AU, NZ) *see* Minocycline 1371
Minopan (KR) *see* Acetaminophen 32
Minoprin (BR) *see* Estrogens (Conjugated/Equine, Systemic) 787
Minostad (AT) *see* Minocycline 1371
Minotab 50 (BE, NZ, ZA) *see* Minocycline 1371
Minotab (LU) *see* Minocycline 1371
Minot (AR) *see* Sulconazole 1943
Minot (CO, EC, PE) *see* Minocycline 1371
Minoxi-5 (SG) *see* Minoxidil (Topical) 1374
Minoxidil Isac (PH) *see* Minoxidil (Topical) 1374
Minoximen (IT) *see* Minoxidil (Topical) 1374
Minoxiten (DO) *see* Minoxidil (Topical) 1374
Minoxyl (KR) *see* Minoxidil (Topical) 1374
Minoz MR (RO) *see* Minocycline 1371
Minprog (AT) *see* Alprostadil 96
Minprostin E(2) (DE, DK) *see* Dinoprostone 640
Minprostin (NO, SE) *see* Dinoprostone 640
Min Qi (CN) *see* Azelastine (Nasal) 213
Minrin (BE, LU, NL) *see* Desmopressin 594
Minurin (ES) *see* Desmopressin 594
Minzil (PH) *see* Oxacillin 1528
Miocacin (GR, PT) *see* Midecamycin [INT] 1365
Miocamen (CY, EG, GR, IT, LU) *see* Midecamycin [INT] 1365
Miocamycin (JP) *see* Midecamycin [INT] 1365
Miochol-E (AU, BE, CH, DE, DK, FI, GB, GR, HK, ID, IE, IL, IT, KR, LB, NL, NO, NZ, RO, SE, SG, SI, TR, ZA) *see* Acetylcholine 40
Miochole (FR) *see* Acetylcholine 40
Miochol (FI, LU, NL, PT) *see* Acetylcholine 40
Miodar (CO) *see* Celecoxib 402
Mioflex (ES) *see* Succinylcholine 1939
Miokar (ID) *see* Pilocarpine (Ophthalmic) 1649
Miomax (PK) *see* Midecamycin [INT] 1365

Mio-Relax (CO) *see* TiZANidine 2051
Mio Relax (ES) *see* Carisoprodol 363
Miosan (BR) *see* Cyclobenzaprine 516
Miosen (ES) *see* Dipyridamole 652
Miostat (AR, AU, BE, BR, CH, CZ, FR, HN, HU, IL, KR, LB, LU, MY, NL, NZ, PH, PK, PL, PY, SG, TH, TR, TW, VN) *see* Carbachol 346
Miostin (RO) *see* Neostigmine 1438
Mioticol (IT) *see* Carbachol 346
Miotin (TH, VN) *see* Midecamycin [INT] 1365
Miotonoachol (AR) *see* Bethanechol 257
Miovalis (AU) *see* Meloxicam 1283
Miowas (ES, IT) *see* Methocarbamol 1320
Miowas G (ES) *see* Gallamine Triethiodide [INT] 948
Miozidine (ID) *see* Trimetazidine [INT] 2104
Miquimod (EC) *see* Imiquimod 1055
Mirabril (PY) *see* RisperiDONE 1818
Miracet (KR) *see* Donepezil 668
Miracid (TH) *see* Omeprazole 1508
Miraclin (IT) *see* Doxycycline 689
Miragenta (CO) *see* Gentamicin (Ophthalmic) 962
Miragenta (CO) *see* Gentamicin (Systemic) 959
Miramycin (HK, SG, TH) *see* Gentamicin (Systemic) 959
Mirapex (AR, KR, TW, VE) *see* Pramipexole 1695
Mirapex ER (HK) *see* Pramipexole 1695
Mirapexin (AT, BE, BG, CH, CZ, DE, DK, FI, FR, GB, GR, HN, HR, HU, IE, IT, NL, NO, PL, PT, RO, RU, SE, TR) *see* Pramipexole 1695
Mirapex-LA (JP) *see* Pramipexole 1695
Mirapront (IT) *see* Phentermine 1635
Mirasan (AR) *see* Naphazoline (Ophthalmic) 1426
Mirastad (HK) *see* Mirtazapine 1376
Miratracina (CO) *see* Bacitracin and Polymyxin B 222
Miravelle Suave (CO) *see* Ethinyl Estradiol and Desogestrel 799
Miraxil (CO) *see* Proparacaine 1728
Mirazep (IN, PH) *see* Mirtazapine 1376
Mircol (PY) *see* Econazole 703
Mirena (AE, AR, AT, AU, BB, BE, BG, BH, BM, BS, BZ, CH, CO, CR, CY, CZ, DE, DO, EC, ES, GB, GT, GY, HK, HN, HR, HU, ID, IE, IL, IS, IT, JM, JP, KR, KW, LB, LT, LU, MY, NI, NL, NZ, PA, PE, PH, PR, PY, RO, RU, SA, SI, SR, SV, TR, TT, UY, VN, ZA) *see* Levonorgestrel 1201
Mirenil (PL) *see* FluPHENAZine 905
Mirgy (VN) *see* Gabapentin 943
M.I.R. (IL) *see* Morphine (Systemic) 1394
Mirocef (HR) *see* CefTAZidime 392
Mirosin (TW) *see* Minocycline 1371
Mirtapax (CO, EC) *see* Mirtazapine 1376
Mirtazon (AU) *see* Mirtazapine 1376
Mirubal (VE) *see* Phentermine 1635
Mirvaso (CZ, DE, DK, EE, FR, GB, HR, LT, NL, NO, RO, SE, SK) *see* Brimonidine (Topical) 288
Misar (HR) *see* ALPRAZolam 94
Misel (KR, SG) *see* Misoprostol 1379
Misodel (RO) *see* Misoprostol 1379
MisoOne (BG) *see* Misoprostol 1379
Misostol (PY, VE) *see* MitoXANtrone 1382
Misotrol (CL) *see* Misoprostol 1379
Mistabron (KR, LU, PH, VN) *see* Mesna 1305
Mistaline (FR) *see* Mizolastine [INT] 1384
Mistamine (BE, CH, GB) *see* Mizolastine [INT] 1384
Misulvan (CL) *see* Milnacipran 1368
Misyo (RO) *see* Methadone 1311
MISYO (SK) *see* Methadone 1311
Mitatonin (HK) *see* Norfloxacin 1475
Mite-X (IL) *see* Permethrin 1627
Mitexan (BR) *see* Mesna 1305
Mithra Folic (BE) *see* Folic Acid 919
Mitocyna (PY) *see* MitoMYcin (Systemic) 1380
Mitomicina-C (PT) *see* MitoMYcin (Systemic) 1380
Mitomicina (CL) *see* MitoMYcin (Systemic) 1380
Mitomycin-C (AT, BG, CH, CN, GR, HN, ID, IT, KR, NL, PH, RU, TH, TR, TW) *see* MitoMYcin (Systemic) 1380
Mitomycin C (ES, HK, IL, IN, PL) *see* MitoMYcin (Systemic) 1380
Mitomycin-C Kyowa (AU, CZ, GB, HU, LU, NZ) *see* MitoMYcin (Systemic) 1380
Mitomycin (DE, DK, MY, SE) *see* MitoMYcin (Systemic) 1380
Mitomycine (BE) *see* MitoMYcin (Systemic) 1380
Mitostat (FI) *see* MitoMYcin (Systemic) 1380
Mitotie (EC, MX) *see* MitoMYcin (Systemic) 1380
Mitoxana (GB) *see* Ifosfamide 1040
Mitoxgen (AR, MX) *see* MitoXANtrone 1382
Mitrotan (BG) *see* Methylergonovine 1333
Mitrotan (GR) *see* Ergonovine [CAN/INT] 754
Mitroxone (MX) *see* MitoXANtrone 1382
Mittoval (IT) *see* Alfuzosin 84
Mittrone (KR) *see* MitoXANtrone 1382
Miwana (PL) *see* Sodium Chloride 1902
Mixato (CO) *see* Pipemidic Acid [INT] 1655
Mi Xi Ning (CN) *see* MitoXANtrone 1382
MIXRE (TW) *see* AtoMOXetine 191
Mixtard 10 (GR) *see* Insulin NPH and Insulin Regular 1090
Mixtard 20 (GR) *see* Insulin NPH and Insulin Regular 1090
Mixtard 30 (AT, CZ, DK, GR, LB, MY, NZ, RO, SA, SG) *see* Insulin NPH and Insulin Regular 1090
Mixtard 30 HM (AE, BH, CI, EG, ET, GH, GM, GN, HK, IQ, IR, JO, KE, KW, LR, LY, MW, QA, RU, TW) *see* Insulin NPH and Insulin Regular 1090
Mixtard 40 (GR) *see* Insulin NPH and Insulin Regular 1090
Mixtard 50 (AT, GR, RO) *see* Insulin NPH and Insulin Regular 1090
Mixtard 50 HM (KW) *see* Insulin NPH and Insulin Regular 1090
Mixtura Alba (CZ) *see* Zinc Oxide 2200
Mizodin (PL) *see* Primidone 1714
Mizolam (MY) *see* Midazolam 1361
Mizollen (BE, CH, DE, DK, FR, GB, IT, NL, SE) *see* Mizolastine [INT] 1384
Mizosin (MY) *see* Prazosin 1703
MMR II (AE, AR, BH, CH, CN, GB, HK, NO, PH, QA, SA, SE, TW, VN) *see* Measles, Mumps, and Rubella Virus Vaccine 1273
MMR (EG) *see* Measles, Mumps, and Rubella Virus Vaccine 1273
M.M.R. Vaccine (KR) *see* Measles, Mumps, and Rubella Virus Vaccine 1273
MNI (PY) *see* Isosorbide Mononitrate 1126
Mobec (DE) *see* Meloxicam 1283
Mobemide (IL, SG) *see* Moclobemide [CAN/INT] 1384
Mobenac (PH) *see* Aceclofenac [INT] 30
Mobex (KR) *see* Meloxicam 1283
Mobic (AE, AR, AU, BB, BE, BF, BH, BJ, BM, BS, BZ, CI, CN, CO, CY, DK, EC, EG, ET, FI, FR, GB, GH, GM, GN, GY, HK, IE, IL, IQ, IR, IT, JM, JO, KE, KR, KW, LB, LR, LY, MA, ML, MR, MU, MW, MY, NE, NG, NO, NZ, OM, PE, PH, PY, QA, SA, SC, SD, SE, SG, SL, SN, SR, SY, TH, TN, TR, TT, TW, TZ, UG, UY, VE, VN, YE, ZA, ZM, ZW) *see* Meloxicam 1283
Mobicox (CH, CR, DO, GT, HN, MX, NI, PA, SV) *see* Meloxicam 1283
Mobiflex (GB, IE) *see* Tenoxicam [INT] 2001
Mobiflex (ID) *see* Meloxicam 1283
Mobilat (DE) *see* Indomethacin 1067
Mobilis (AU) *see* Piroxicam 1662
Mobilus D (AU) *see* Piroxicam 1662
Mobinul (KR) *see* Glycopyrrolate 975
Mobix (PK) *see* Meloxicam 1283
Mocetasin (VN) *see* Acemetacin [INT] 30

Moclamine (FR) *see* Moclobemide [CAN/INT] 1384
Moclod (TW) *see* Moclobemide [CAN/INT] 1384
Moclodura (DE) *see* Moclobemide [CAN/INT] 1384
Mocydone M (TH) *see* Domperidone [CAN/INT] 666
Modalert (IN) *see* Modafinil 1386
Modalim (CN, CY, ID, KW, MY, NL, PH, SA, SG, TR, VN) *see* Ciprofibrate [INT] 441
Modalina (IT) *see* Trifluoperazine 2102
Modamide (FR) *see* AMILoride 113
Modanil (KR) *see* Modafinil 1386
Modasomil (AT, CH) *see* Modafinil 1386
Modavigil (AU, NZ) *see* Modafinil 1386
Modecate (AU, BB, BH, BM, BS, BZ, ES, GB, GY, IE, JM, JO, NZ, PK, PR, QA, SG, SR, TT, UY, VN) *see* FluPHENAZine 905
Moderan (VE) *see* Lactulose 1156
Moderatan (FR) *see* Diethylpropion 624
Moderex (PY) *see* ALPRAZolam 94
Moderlax (PT) *see* Bisacodyl 265
Modezine (PH) *see* FluPHENAZine 905
Modfil (IN) *see* Modafinil 1386
Modifical (CO) *see* Ondansetron 1513
Modigraf (GB) *see* Tacrolimus (Systemic) 1962
Modik (BR) *see* Imiquimod 1055
Modin (PH) *see* Famotidine 845
Modiodal (DK, ES, FR, GR, IS, JP, MX, NL, NO, PT, SE, TR) *see* Modafinil 1386
Modip (CR, DO, GT, HN, NI, PA, SV) *see* NiMODipine 1456
Modip (DE) *see* Felodipine 850
Moditen (AE, BF, BH, BJ, CI, CZ, ET, FR, GH, GM, GN, HR, IQ, KE, KW, LR, MA, ML, MR, MU, MW, NE, NG, NL, OM, QA, SA, SC, SD, SL, SN, TN, TZ, UG, VE, YE, ZM, ZW) *see* FluPHENAZine 905
Moditen Depot (BG, HN) *see* FluPHENAZine 905
Modiur (CO) *see* Trifluoperazine 2102
Modiur (UY) *see* Hydrochlorothiazide 1009
Mododom (AE) *see* Domperidone [CAN/INT] 666
Modomed (TH) *see* Domperidone [CAN/INT] 666
Modopar (FR) *see* Benserazide and Levodopa [CAN/INT] 244
Modraderm (BE) *see* Alclometasone 72
Modrasone (GB, IE) *see* Alclometasone 72
Modulex (CO) *see* Lubiprostone 1255
Modul (PE) *see* Scopolamine (Systemic) 1870
Modup (TW) *see* Amitriptyline 119
Moduretic (Combinado con hidroclorotiazida) (MX) *see* AMILoride 113
Modus (ES) *see* NiMODipine 1456
Modusik-A Ofteno (CN, CR, DO, GT, HN, NI, PA, PE, SV) *see* CycloSPORINE (Ophthalmic) 529
Moduxin (EE) *see* Trimetazidine [INT] 2104
Moex (BG, CZ, DK, FR, HK, RU) *see* Moexipril 1388
Moex Plus (BG) *see* Moexipril and Hydrochlorothiazide 1388
Mofen (ID) *see* Ibuprofen 1032
Moflodal (TW) *see* Moxifloxacin (Systemic) 1401
Mofulex (ID) *see* Mometasone (Topical) 1391
Mofuroate (TW) *see* Mometasone (Topical) 1391
Mogadon (AE, AT, AU, BE, BH, CH, DK, EG, FR, IS, IT, MY, NL, NO, PK, SA, SE, SG, SI, TH) *see* Nitrazepam [CAN/INT] 1461
Mogasinte (PT) *see* Domperidone [CAN/INT] 666
Mogine (NZ) *see* LamoTRIgine 1160
Mohrus Patch (JP) *see* Ketoprofen 1145
Moisten (CN) *see* Chloramphenicol 421
Mokast (TW) *see* Montelukast 1392
Mokcell (PE) *see* Cytarabine (Conventional) 535
Moksacin (HR) *see* Moxifloxacin (Ophthalmic) 1403
Moladerm (ID) *see* Miconazole (Topical) 1360
Molason (ID) *see* Betamethasone (Topical) 255
Molavir (ID) *see* Acyclovir (Systemic) 47
Molazol (ID) *see* MetroNIDAZOLE (Systemic) 1353
Molcer (GB) *see* Docusate 661
Molden (KR) *see* Nimesulide [INT] 1456
Moldina (ES) *see* Bifonazole [INT] 264
Molelant (GR) *see* Cefotaxime 382
Molipaxin (GB, IE) *see* TraZODone 2091
Mol-Iron (CO) *see* Ferrous Sulfate 871
Moltanine (JP) *see* Mecysteine [INT] 1277
Moltoben (DO, GT, HN, PA, SV) *see* FLUoxetine 899
Momate (PH) *see* Mometasone (Topical) 1391
Momecort (PH) *see* Mometasone (Topical) 1391
Momegen (PH) *see* Mometasone (Topical) 1391
Momentum (LU) *see* Acetaminophen 32
Momet (ID) *see* Mometasone (Topical) 1391
Momicine (ES) *see* Midecamycin [INT] 1365
Monace (AU) *see* Fosinopril 932
Monasan (MY) *see* FluPHENAZine 905
Monaspor (AT, CZ, NL) *see* Cefsulodin [INT] 391
Monastar (KR) *see* Finasteride 878
Monazol (FR) *see* Sertaconazole 1877
Monem (MY, TH) *see* Meropenem 1299
Monest (HR) *see* Montelukast 1392
Moniarix (BF, BJ, CI, ET, GH, GM, GN, KE, LR, MA, ML, MR, MU, MW, NE, NG, SC, SD, SL, SN, TN, TZ, UG, ZA, ZM, ZW) *see* Pneumococcal Polysaccharide Vaccine (23-Valent) 1671
Monicor (FR) *see* Isosorbide Mononitrate 1126
Mo Ni Ka (CN) *see* Racecadotril [INT] 1765
Monilac (JP) *see* Lactulose 1156
Monis (CO) *see* Isosorbide Mononitrate 1126
Monis-XR (PH) *see* Isosorbide Mononitrate 1126
Monit 20 (IN) *see* Isosorbide Mononitrate 1126
Monitazon (KR) *see* Mometasone (Nasal) 1391
Monoalgic LP (FR) *see* TraMADol 2074
Monobeltin (ES) *see* Bupranolol [INT] 300
Monobide (EC) *see* Isosorbide Mononitrate 1126
Monocef (IN) *see* CefTRIAXone 396
Monocin (KR) *see* Doxycycline 689
Monoclair (DE) *see* Isosorbide Mononitrate 1126
Monoclarium (SG) *see* Clarithromycin 456
Monoclate-P (AT, DK, FR, GR, KR, SE, TW) *see* Antihemophilic Factor (Human) 152
Monoclate P (GB, IE) *see* Antihemophilic Factor (Human) 152
monoclox (BH) *see* Cloxacillin [CAN/INT] 488
Monoclox (CY, JO, MY, TR, VN) *see* Cloxacillin [CAN/INT] 488
Mono Corax (DE) *see* Isosorbide Mononitrate 1126
Mono Corax Retard (DE) *see* Isosorbide Mononitrate 1126
Monocord 40 (IL) *see* Isosorbide Mononitrate 1126
Monocord 50 SR (IL) *see* Isosorbide Mononitrate 1126
Monocor (TW) *see* Bisoprolol 266
Monocycline (PH) *see* Tetracycline 2017
Mono Demetrin (DE) *see* Prazepam [INT] 1702
Monodox (CO) *see* Doxycycline 689
Monodur Durules (AU) *see* Isosorbide Mononitrate 1126
Monofeme (NZ) *see* Ethinyl Estradiol and Levonorgestrel 803
MonoFIX-VF (AU, NZ) *see* Factor IX (Human) 840
Monoflam (CZ, DE) *see* Diclofenac (Systemic) 617
Mono-Getic (TW) *see* Salsalate 1862
Mono-Jod (DE) *see* Potassium Iodide 1690
Monoket (IT, NO, PY, SE, UY) *see* Isosorbide Mononitrate 1126
Monoket OD (NO, SE) *see* Isosorbide Mononitrate 1126
Monoket Retard (AT, IT) *see* Isosorbide Mononitrate 1126
Monolair (KR) *see* Montelukast 1392
Monolax (TH) *see* Bisacodyl 265
Monolitum (CR, DO, ES, GT, HN, NI, PA, SV) *see* Lansoprazole 1166
Monolong 40 (IL) *see* Isosorbide Mononitrate 1126

Monolong 60 (IL) *see* Isosorbide Mononitrate 1126
Monolong (DE) *see* Isosorbide Mononitrate 1126
Mono Mack (CY, HU, LU, MX) *see* Isosorbide Mononitrate 1126
Mono-Mack (CZ) *see* Isosorbide Mononitrate 1126
Mononaxy (FR) *see* Clarithromycin 456
Mononine (CZ, DE, FR, GB, GR, IE, NL, SE, SI, SK) *see* Factor IX (Human) 840
Mononit 20 (IL) *see* Isosorbide Mononitrate 1126
Mononit (PE, PL) *see* Isosorbide Mononitrate 1126
Monopost (GB, IE) *see* Latanoprost 1172
Monopress (ES) *see* Nitrendipine [INT] 1463
Monopril (AU, BB, BG, BM, BS, BZ, CN, CO, CZ, DK, EE, EG, GR, GY, HK, HN, HR, HU, JM, KR, MX, MY, NO, PE, PK, PL, RO, RU, SE, SR, TH, TR, TT, TW, VE, ZA) *see* Fosinopril 932
Monopront (FI) *see* Isosorbide Mononitrate 1126
Monorem (TR) *see* Isosorbide Mononitrate 1126
Monores (IT) *see* Clenbuterol [INT] 460
Mono-Sanorania (DE) *see* Isosorbide Mononitrate 1126
Monosan (RU) *see* Isosorbide Mononitrate 1126
Monos (IT) *see* Rufloxacin [INT] 1855
Monosorbitrate (IN) *see* Isosorbide Mononitrate 1126
Monosorb (TH) *see* Isosorbide Mononitrate 1126
Monosordil (GR) *see* Isosorbide Mononitrate 1126
Monostop (ES) *see* Bifonazole [INT] 264
Monotab (SK) *see* Isosorbide Mononitrate 1126
Monotaxel (KR) *see* DOCEtaxel 656
Monotildiem (BF, BJ, CI, ET, GH, GM, GN, KE, LR, MA, ML, MR, MU, MW, NE, NG, SC, SD, SL, SN, TN, TZ, UG, ZM, ZW) *see* Diltiazem 634
Mono-Tildiem (LU) *see* Diltiazem 634
Mono-Tildiem SR (SG) *see* Diltiazem 634
Monotramal LP (FR) *see* TraMADol 2074
Monotrate (IN) *see* Isosorbide Mononitrate 1126
Monotrim (AE, BF, BJ, CH, CI, ET, GH, GM, GN, IE, KE, LR, MA, ML, MR, MU, MW, NE, NG, NL, SC, SD, SL, SN, TN, TZ, UG, ZA, ZM, ZW) *see* Trimethoprim 2104
Monovel (AE, BH, CO, CY, EG, IL, IQ, IR, JO, KW, LB, LY, OM, QA, SA, SY, YE) *see* Mometasone (Topical) 1391
Mono Vitamine B12 (FR) *see* Cyanocobalamin 515
Monowel (PH) *see* CefOXitin 386
Monozide (AE, EG, JO) *see* Hydrochlorothiazide 1009
Montair (IN, PH) *see* Montelukast 1392
Montecad (PH) *see* Montelukast 1392
Montek-10 (TH) *see* Montelukast 1392
Montekast (PH) *see* Montelukast 1392
Monteka (TW) *see* Montelukast 1392
Montelair (HK, MY) *see* Montelukast 1392
Montelu V (KR) *see* Montelukast 1392
Montelukan (KR) *see* Montelukast 1392
Montelukan QDT (KR) *see* Montelukast 1392
Montemax (PH) *see* Montelukast 1392
Montena (KR) *see* Montelukast 1392
Montepect (KR) *see* Montelukast 1392
Montexin (TW) *see* Montelukast 1392
Montiget (PH) *see* Montelukast 1392
Montra (PH) *see* Isosorbide Mononitrate 1126
Monural (BG, HU, PL, RO, RU, SK) *see* Fosfomycin 932
Monuril (BR, CH, CO, DE, FR, ID, IE, LU, PT) *see* Fosfomycin 932
Monurol (AR, AT, BE, CL, CN, ES, FI, GR, HK, IL, IT, KR, LB, MX, MY, NL, PE, PH, PK, SA, SE, SG, TH, TR, TW, VN) *see* Fosfomycin 932
Mopen (IT) *see* Amoxicillin 130
Mopik (TW) *see* Meloxicam 1283
Mopral (FR, MX) *see* Omeprazole 1508
Mopram (KR) *see* Doxapram 673
Mopride (TW) *see* Mosapride [INT] 1401
Mopsalem (CO) *see* Methoxsalen (Systemic) 1330
Mopsalem (CO) *see* Methoxsalen (Topical) 1331
Mopsoralen (BE) *see* Methoxsalen (Systemic) 1330
Moradol (PL) *see* Butorphanol 314
Morbifurb (CN) *see* Sulfamethoxazole and Trimethoprim 1946
Morefine (TW) *see* ChlorproMAZINE 429
Morex (IN) *see* Moclobemide [CAN/INT] 1384
Morfarin (TH) *see* Warfarin 2186
Morficontin (GR) *see* Morphine (Systemic) 1394
Moricort (KR) *see* Mometasone (Topical) 1391
Moris Forte (ID) *see* Ibuprofen 1032
Moris (ID) *see* Ibuprofen 1032
Moronal (DE) *see* Nystatin (Topical) 1482
Morphanton (DE) *see* Morphine (Systemic) 1394
Morphgesic SR (GB) *see* Morphine (Systemic) 1394
Morphgesic (TR) *see* Morphine (Systemic) 1394
Mortin (VN) *see* Sulfamethoxazole and Trimethoprim 1946
Morupar (MX, PH) *see* Measles, Mumps, and Rubella Virus Vaccine 1273
Mor-Vita (PH) *see* Pizotifen [CAN/INT] 1664
Mosadil (KR) *see* Mosapride [INT] 1401
Mosamet (EC) *see* Mosapride [INT] 1401
Mosap (IN) *see* Mosapride [INT] 1401
Mosar (AR, KR, LB, UY) *see* Mosapride [INT] 1401
Mosardal (ID) *see* Levofloxacin (Systemic) 1197
Mosaro (KR) *see* Mosapride [INT] 1401
Mosasone (KR) *see* Mosapride [INT] 1401
Moscontin (FR) *see* Morphine (Systemic) 1394
Mosedin (AE, BH, CY, EG, IQ, IR, JO, KW, LB, LY, OM, QA, SA, SY, YE) *see* Loratadine 1241
Mosegor (AE, BH, CH, DE, EG, ES, GR, LU, PH, PK, PT, QA, SA) *see* Pizotifen [CAN/INT] 1664
Mosil (FR) *see* Midecamycin [INT] 1365
Mosone (PH) *see* Mometasone (Topical) 1391
Mostanol (DE) *see* Acemetacin [INT] 30
Motaderm (ID) *see* Mometasone (Topical) 1391
Mo Tai (CN) *see* Nisoldipine 1459
Motens (BE, CH, DK, GB, GR, NL) *see* Lacidipin [INT] 1154
Motiax (IT) *see* Famotidine 845
Moticlod (VN) *see* Clodronate [CAN/INT] 469
Motide (PE, PY) *see* Mosapride [INT] 1401
Motidine (HK) *see* Famotidine 845
Motidone (MY) *see* Domperidone [CAN/INT] 666
Motigut (MY) *see* Domperidone [CAN/INT] 666
Motilat (JO, LB) *see* Domperidone [CAN/INT] 666
Motilex (ID) *see* Loperamide 1236
Motilium (AE, AR, AT, AU, BB, BE, BG, BH, BM, BR, BS, BZ, CH, CN, CY, CZ, DE, DK, EC, EE, EG, FR, GB, GY, HK, HN, HU, ID, IE, IL, IT, JM, JO, KR, KW, LB, LT, LU, MX, MY, NL, NZ, PE, PH, PK, PR, PT, PY, QA, RO, RU, SG, SR, TR, TT, TW, UY, VN, ZA) *see* Domperidone [CAN/INT] 666
Motilium [tabs.] (PL) *see* Domperidone [CAN/INT] 666
Motinorm (IN, PH) *see* Domperidone [CAN/INT] 666
Motiron (DK) *see* Methylphenidate 1336
Motivan (SG) *see* Haloperidol 993
Motivan (TH) *see* DimenhyDRINATE 637
Motivest (PH) *see* FLUoxetine 899
Motozina (IT) *see* DimenhyDRINATE 637
Motrigine (PH) *see* LamoTRIgine 1160
Motrim (AT) *see* Trimethoprim 2104
Motrin (AE, BH, CO, CR, CY, EG, GT, HN, IQ, IR, JO, KW, LB, LY, MX, NI, OM, PA, PE, QA, SA, SV, SY, YE) *see* Ibuprofen 1032
Movalis (BG, CZ, EE, ES, HR, IS, PL, PT, RO, RU, SI, SK) *see* Meloxicam 1283
Mova Nitrat Pipette (PL) *see* Silver Nitrate 1886
Movectro (AU) *see* Cladribine 455
Movelax (PH) *see* Lactulose 1156
Movergan (DE, HR) *see* Selegiline 1873
Movex (IL) *see* Bromhexine [INT] 291
Movi-Cox (ID) *see* Meloxicam 1283

Movicox (NL) *see* Meloxicam 1283
Movigil (CL) *see* Modafinil 1386
Movistal (LU) *see* Metoclopramide 1345
Movon-20 (IN) *see* Piroxicam 1662
Movon Gel (IN) *see* Piroxicam 1662
Movox (AU) *see* FluvoxaMINE 916
Moxacef (GR) *see* Cefadroxil 372
Moxafen (AE, BH, CY, EG, IL, IQ, IR, JO, KR, KW, LB, LY, OM, QA, SA, SY, YE) *see* Tamoxifen 1971
Moxalid (GR) *see* Meloxicam 1283
Moxar (CO) *see* Mosapride [INT] 1401
Moxarin (AE, BH, CY, EG, IQ, IR, JO, KW, LB, LY, OM, QA, SA, SY, YE) *see* Amoxicillin 130
Moxaval (EC) *see* Moxifloxacin (Systemic) 1401
Moxicam (AU, KR) *see* Meloxicam 1283
Moxiclav (AE, BF, BH, BJ, CI, CY, EG, ET, GH, GM, GN, IQ, IR, JO, KE, KW, LB, LR, LY, MA, ML, MR, MU, MW, NE, NG, OM, QA, SA, SC, SD, SG, SL, SN, SY, TN, TZ, UG, YE, ZM, ZW) *see* Amoxicillin and Clavulanate 133
Moxicle (TH) *see* Amoxicillin and Clavulanate 133
Moxiclox (IN) *see* Amoxicillin and Cloxacillin [INT] 136
Moxidil (KR) *see* Minoxidil (Topical) 1374
Moxif (IN) *see* Moxifloxacin (Systemic) 1401
Moxiflo (KR) *see* Moxifloxacin (Ophthalmic) 1403
Moxiflo (KR) *see* Moxifloxacin (Systemic) 1401
Moxiflox (PH) *see* Moxifloxacin (Systemic) 1401
Moxiforce (KR) *see* Moxifloxacin (Ophthalmic) 1403
Moxilen (BF, BJ, CI, ET, GH, GM, GN, KE, LB, LR, MA, ML, MR, MU, MW, MY, NE, NG, SC, SD, SG, SL, SN, TN, TZ, UG, ZM, ZW) *see* Amoxicillin 130
Mox (IN) *see* Amoxicillin 130
Moxista (KR) *see* Moxifloxacin (Ophthalmic) 1403
Moxlin (MX) *see* Amoxicillin and Clavulanate 133
Moxylin (EC) *see* Amoxicillin 130
M-Oxy (PE) *see* OxyCODONE 1538
Moxypen (IL, ZA) *see* Amoxicillin 130
Moxyvit (IL) *see* Amoxicillin 130
Mozal (TW) *see* Albuterol 69
Moz-Bite (MY, SG, VN) *see* Crotamiton 514
Mozepam (PH) *see* Nitrazepam [CAN/INT] 1461
Mozep (IN) *see* Pimozide 1651
Mozobil (AT, AU, BE, BR, CY, CZ, DE, DK, EE, FR, GB, HK, HR, IE, IL, IS, KR, LT, MX, MY, NL, NO, PL, PT, RO, SE, SG, SI, SK, TH, TR) *see* Plerixafor 1665
MPA Gyn 5 (DE) *see* MedroxyPROGESTERone 1277
MPL Bica (PH) *see* Bicalutamide 262
MPL Coverin (PH) *see* Leucovorin Calcium 1183
MPL CYTA (PH) *see* Cytarabine (Conventional) 535
MPL Hi-Oxy (PH) *see* Hydroxyurea 1021
MPL Toposid (PH) *see* Etoposide 816
M-Prednihexal (DE) *see* MethylPREDNISolone 1340
MS Contin (AU, BE, CN, IT, NL, VE) *see* Morphine (Systemic) 1394
MS Contin CR (KR) *see* Morphine (Systemic) 1394
MS Mono (AU) *see* Morphine (Systemic) 1394
MSP (IL) *see* Morphine (Systemic) 1394
MST Continus (AE, AR, BF, BG, BH, BJ, CI, CY, CZ, EE, EG, ET, GB, GH, GM, GN, HK, HN, HR, ID, IE, IQ, IR, JO, KE, KW, LB, LR, LY, MA, ML, MR, MU, MW, MY, NE, NG, OM, PH, PK, PL, QA, RO, SA, SC, SD, SG, SK, SL, SN, SY, TH, TN, TR, TW, TZ, UG, YE, ZA, ZM, ZW) *see* Morphine (Systemic) 1394
MST Continus Retard (CH) *see* Morphine (Systemic) 1394
MST (PT) *see* Morphine (Systemic) 1394
MTW-Roxithromycin (DE) *see* Roxithromycin [INT] 1853
MTW-Tetrazepam (DE) *see* Tetrazepam [INT] 2020
MTX Hexal (LU) *see* Methotrexate 1322
Mubonet (MX) *see* Calcium Carbonate 327
Mucarin (PY) *see* Trimebutine [CAN/INT] 2103
Muchan (AR) *see* EPHEDrine (Systemic) 734
Mucibron (BR) *see* Ambroxol [INT] 109
Muciclar (AE, QA) *see* Carbocisteine [INT] 357
Mucinex (MY) *see* GuaiFENesin 986
Muclear (TH) *see* Acetylcysteine 40
Mucoangin (BE, CH, DE, DK, HU, SE) *see* Ambroxol [INT] 109
Mucocar (PE) *see* Acetylcysteine 40
Mucochem (CO) *see* Acetylcysteine 40
Mucocis (IT) *see* Carbocisteine [INT] 357
Mucoclear (SG) *see* Ambroxol [INT] 109
Mucodin (SG) *see* Carbocisteine [INT] 357
Mucodox (BE) *see* Erdosteine [INT] 753
Mucodrenol (PT) *see* Ambroxol [INT] 109
Mucodyne (GB, IN, JP) *see* Carbocisteine [INT] 357
Mucofalk (ID, MY, PH, SG) *see* Psyllium 1744
Mucofalk Orange (BG, EE) *see* Psyllium 1744
Mucofar (VE) *see* Carbocisteine [INT] 357
Mucofillin (JP) *see* Acetylcysteine 40
Mucofluid (ES) *see* Mesna 1305
Mucoflux (BR) *see* Carbocisteine [INT] 357
Mucofor (CH) *see* Erdosteine [INT] 753
Mucofree (SA) *see* Bromhexine [INT] 291
Mucolair (LU) *see* Acetylcysteine 40
Mucolan (AE) *see* Bromhexine [INT] 291
Mucolase (AE) *see* Carbocisteine [INT] 357
Mucolator (LU, MY) *see* Acetylcysteine 40
Mucoless (IL) *see* Bromhexine [INT] 291
Mucolex (MY) *see* Bromhexine [INT] 291
Mucolin (BR) *see* Ambroxol [INT] 109
Mucolitic (AR) *see* Carbocisteine [INT] 357
Mucolitico (CN) *see* Acetylcysteine 40
Mucolit (IL, UY) *see* Carbocisteine [INT] 357
Mucolix (HN, SG) *see* Bromhexine [INT] 291
Mucolyte (SA) *see* Bromhexine [INT] 291
Mucomiste (PT) *see* Acetylcysteine 40
Mucomyst (AT, BE, DK, FI, FR, KR, LU, NL, NO, SE) *see* Acetylcysteine 40
Mucomystendo (FR) *see* Acetylcysteine 40
Muconil (MY) *see* Ambroxol [INT] 109
Mucopect (KR) *see* Ambroxol [INT] 109
Mucopide (IN) *see* Rebamipide [INT] 1786
Mucopront (BH, EG, PY, QA, VE) *see* Carbocisteine [INT] 357
Mucopro (PH) *see* Rebamipide [INT] 1786
Mucoprotec (PH) *see* Rebamipide [INT] 1786
Mucoram (QA) *see* Ambroxol [INT] 109
Muco Rhinathiol (BE) *see* Carbocisteine [INT] 357
Mucosan (AT, ES) *see* Ambroxol [INT] 109
Mucoserin (KR) *see* Acetylcysteine 40
Mucosof (CL) *see* Acetylcysteine 40
Muco-Sol (KR) *see* Bromhexine [INT] 291
Mucosol (SG) *see* Bromhexine [INT] 291
Mucosolvan (AE, AR, AT, BG, BH, BR, CL, CN, CO, CY, CZ, DE, EG, GR, HK, HR, IT, KW, LB, MX, MY, PH, PL, PT, PY, QA, RO, RU, SA, SG, SK, TH, TR, UY, VE, VN) *see* Ambroxol [INT] 109
Mucosolvin (IN) *see* Ambroxol [INT] 109
Mucosolvon (PK) *see* Ambroxol [INT] 109
Mucosta (CN, ID, JP, KR, MY, PH, TH, VN) *see* Rebamipide [INT] 1786
Mucosten (KR) *see* Acetylcysteine 40
Mucosys (IN) *see* Acetylcysteine 40
Mucotablets (QA) *see* Carbocisteine [INT] 357
Mucotal (LB) *see* Carbocisteine [INT] 357
Mucotec (QA) *see* Erdosteine [INT] 753
Muco-Treat (IL) *see* Carbocisteine [INT] 357
Mucotrop (CO) *see* Bromhexine [INT] 291
Mucovin (FI) *see* Bromhexine [INT] 291
Mucoxolan (BR) *see* Ambroxol [INT] 109
Mucoza (TH) *see* Acetylcysteine 40
Mucum (AE, BH, SA) *see* Ambroxol [INT] 109
Mucylin (ID) *see* Acetylcysteine 40
Mudapenil (AR) *see* Penicillin G Procaine 1613

Mujonal (CN) *see* Terbinafine (Topical) 2004
Mukolit (ID) *see* Acetylcysteine 40
Mulax (ID) *see* Psyllium 1744
Mulax (TW) *see* Baclofen 223
Multaq (AT, AU, CH, CN, CO, CY, CZ, DE, DK, EE, FR, GB, HK, HN, HR, IE, IL, IN, IS, KR, KW, LT, MY, NL, NO, PE, PH, PL, PT, SE, SG, SI, SK, TH, TR, TW) *see* Dronedarone 695
Multiferon (BG, IN, MX, SE, ZA) *see* Interferon Alpha, Multi-Subtype [INT] 1100
Multigesic (IN) *see* Diethylamine Salicylate [INT] 624
Multimix (IN) *see* Ephedrine and Theophylline [INT] 734
Multiparin (NZ, PK) *see* Heparin 997
Multiscleran (DE) *see* Riboflavin 1803
Multivent (PH) *see* Ipratropium and Albuterol 1109
Multosin (DE) *see* Estramustine 782
Mumeru Vax (PH) *see* Measles, Mumps, and Rubella Virus Vaccine 1273
Mundidol Retard (AT) *see* Morphine (Systemic) 1394
Munobal (DE, KR, MX, VE) *see* Felodipine 850
Munobal Retard (AT, DE) *see* Felodipine 850
Munorm (IN) *see* Ambroxol [INT] 109
Mupaten (AR) *see* Isoconazole [INT] 1120
Muphoran (AT, AU, BE, BR, CN, FR, GR, IL, IT, PT, SI, TR) *see* Fotemustine [INT] 937
Mupicin (PH) *see* Mupirocin 1404
Mupiderm (FR) *see* Mupirocin 1404
Mupider (NZ, SG) *see* Mupirocin 1404
Mupiral (EC) *see* Mupirocin 1404
Mupiroban (KR) *see* Mupirocin 1404
Mupirox (AR, PE) *see* Mupirocin 1404
Mupirox Nasal (AR) *see* Mupirocin 1404
Muporin (TH) *see* Mupirocin 1404
Muprin (HK, ID, MY, PH) *see* Mupirocin 1404
Murazol (KR) *see* Terbinafine (Topical) 2004
Murelax (AU) *see* Oxazepam 1532
Murine Clear Eyes (AU) *see* Naphazoline (Ophthalmic) 1426
Murukos F (JP) *see* Fluocinonide 894
Murupe Patch 48 (KR) *see* Piroxicam 1662
Musant (BG) *see* TiZANidine 2051
Musapam (DE) *see* Tetrazepam [INT] 2020
Musaril (AT, DE) *see* Tetrazepam [INT] 2020
Muscaran (BE, LU) *see* Bethanechol 257
Muscol (TW) *see* Chlorzoxazone 430
Muse (AE, BH, CY, EG, GB, IE, IQ, IR, JO, KW, LB, LT, LY, OM, QA, SA, SY, YE, ZA) *see* Alprostadil 96
Musgud (TW) *see* Cyclobenzaprine 516
Muskelat (DE) *see* Tetrazepam [INT] 2020
Mustargen (IL) *see* Mechlorethamine (Systemic) 1276
Mustin (IN) *see* Bendamustine 241
Mustoforan (ES) *see* Fotemustine [INT] 937
Mustophoran (BG, CZ, HU, PL, RO, RU, SK) *see* Fotemustine [INT] 937
Mustopic Oint (IN) *see* Tacrolimus (Topical) 1968
Musxan (TH) *see* Methocarbamol 1320
Mutabon D (AE, AR, BH, CY, EG, ID, IL, IQ, IR, JO, KW, LB, LY, OM, PY, QA, SA, SY, YE) *see* Amitriptyline and Perphenazine 122
Mutabon-D (BB, BM, BS, BZ, GY, JM, NL, PR, SR, TT) *see* Amitriptyline and Perphenazine 122
Mutabon M (AE, BH, CY, EG, ID, IL, IQ, IR, JO, KW, LB, LY, OM, QA, SA, SY, YE) *see* Amitriptyline and Perphenazine 122
Mutabon-M (BB, BM, BS, BZ, GY, JM, NL, PR, SR, TT) *see* Amitriptyline and Perphenazine 122
Mutabon A (AE, BH, CY, EG, IL, IQ, IR, JO, KW, LB, LY, OM, QA, SA, SY, YE) *see* Amitriptyline and Perphenazine 122
Mutabon-A (BB, BM, BS, BZ, GY, JM, NL, PR, SR, TT) *see* Amitriptyline and Perphenazine 122
Mutabon F (AE, BH, CY, EG, IL, IQ, IR, JO, KW, LB, LY, OM, QA, SA, SY, YE) *see* Amitriptyline and Perphenazine 122
Mutabon-F (BB, BM, BS, BZ, GY, JM, NL, PR, SR, TT) *see* Amitriptyline and Perphenazine 122
Mutabon (IT) *see* Amitriptyline and Perphenazine 122
Mutacil (KR) *see* Psyllium 1744
Mutamycin (DK, EE, EG, FI, HR, JO, NO, PT, UY) *see* MitoMYcin (Systemic) 1380
Muterin (KR) *see* Acetylcysteine 40
Mutigan (VE) *see* Primidone 1714
Mutilium (SA) *see* Domperidone [CAN/INT] 666
Mutrim (PH) *see* Ibuprofen 1032
Mutsutamin (JP) *see* Thiamine 2028
Mutum (AR, PE, VE) *see* Fluconazole 885
Mutum CR (EC) *see* Oxybutynin 1536
Mutum (EC) *see* Oxybutynin 1536
Muvera (IN) *see* Meloxicam 1283
Muvett (DO, EC, GT, PA, SV) *see* Trimebutine [CAN/INT] 2103
Muxan (DE) *see* Docosanol 661
Muxatil (PY) *see* Acetylcysteine 40
Muxol (FR, LB, VN) *see* Ambroxol [INT] 109
Muzona (HK) *see* Terbinafine (Systemic) 2002
Muzoral (ID) *see* Ketoconazole (Systemic) 1144
M. V. I. 12 (MX) *see* Pyridoxine 1747
MXL (TW) *see* Morphine (Systemic) 1394
Myacyne (DE) *see* Neomycin 1436
Myambutol (AE, AT, AU, BE, BF, BJ, CH, CI, DE, DK, ES, ET, FR, GB, GH, GM, GN, GR, IE, IN, KE, KR, LR, LU, MA, ML, MR, MU, MW, MY, NE, NG, NL, NZ, PK, PT, SA, SC, SD, SE, SI, SL, SN, TH, TN, TZ, UG, ZM, ZW) *see* Ethambutol 798
My-B (TH) *see* Bacitracin, Neomycin, and Polymyxin B 223
Mycalcin (TH) *see* Calcitonin 322
Mycamiine (SK) *see* Micafungin 1359
Mycamine (AT, AU, BR, CH, CN, CY, CZ, DE, DK, EE, FR, GB, GR, HK, HN, HR, ID, IE, IN, IS, IT, KR, LB, LT, MY, NL, NO, PH, PL, PT, RO, SA, SE, SG, SI, TH, TR, TW) *see* Micafungin 1359
Mycefix (PH) *see* Cefixime 380
Mycelvan (DO, GT, PA, SV) *see* Terbinafine (Systemic) 2002
Mycelvan (DO, GT, PA, SV) *see* Terbinafine (Topical) 2004
Mycetin (IT) *see* Chloramphenicol 421
Mycil Healthy Feet (AU) *see* Tolnaftate 2063
Mycin (KR) *see* Penicillin G Benzathine 1609
Mycin (PH) *see* Gentamicin (Systemic) 959
Mycobutin (AT, AU, BE, BG, CH, CZ, DE, GB, GR, HK, HN, HU, IE, IL, IT, JP, KR, LU, NL, NZ, QA, RU, SI, TR, TW) *see* Rifabutin 1803
Mycobutol (BF, BJ, CI, ET, GH, GM, GN, KE, LR, MA, ML, MR, MU, MW, NE, NG, SC, SD, SL, SN, TN, TZ, UG, ZM, ZW) *see* Ethambutol 798
Mycocid (IN) *see* Clotrimazole (Topical) 488
Mycocyst (BB, BM, BS, BZ, GY, JM, SR, TT) *see* Fluconazole 885
Mycodermil (CH) *see* Fenticonazole [INT] 868
Mycofebrin (GR) *see* Ketoconazole (Topical) 1145
Mycofen (DK) *see* Ciclopirox 433
Mycofentin (VE) *see* Fenticonazole [INT] 868
Mycoheal Cream (AE, BH, CY, EG, IQ, IR, JO, KW, LB, LY, OM, QA, SA, SY, YE) *see* Miconazole (Topical) 1360
Mycoheal Oral Gel (AE, BH, CY, EG, IQ, IR, JO, KW, LB, LY, OM, QA, SA, SY, YE) *see* Miconazole (Topical) 1360
Mycohermal (AE) *see* Clotrimazole (Topical) 488
Myco-Hermal (IL) *see* Clotrimazole (Topical) 488
Mycol CR (NZ) *see* Metoprolol 1350
Myconail (IL) *see* Ciclopirox 433

Mycopen (PH) *see* Mycophenolate 1405
Mycophil (QA) *see* Nystatin (Oral) 1481
Mycorest (SG) *see* Fluconazole 885
Mycoril (SG, TW) *see* Clotrimazole (Topical) 488
Mycosporan (SE) *see* Bifonazole [INT] 264
Mycospor (AR, AU, BE, CZ, DE, ES, GR, HR, LU, MX, NL, NO, PT, ZA) *see* Bifonazole [INT] 264
Mycosporin (AT) *see* Bifonazole [INT] 264
Mycostatin (AR, AU, EG, ID, NZ, ZA) *see* Nystatin (Topical) 1482
Mycostatin EVT (CN) *see* Nystatin (Oral) 1481
Mycostatin (IS, JO, KW, QA, SA) *see* Nystatin (Oral) 1481
Mycostat (KW, QA, SA) *see* Nystatin (Oral) 1481
Mycoster (AE, FR, HR, IL, KW, LB, LU, PT, VN) *see* Ciclopirox 433
Mycosyst (HU) *see* Fluconazole 885
Mycotrazol (HK) *see* Itraconazole 1130
Mycozole (TH) *see* Clotrimazole (Topical) 488
Mycros (TW) *see* Metolazone 1348
Myden (RO) *see* Perindopril 1623
Mydfrin (AE, BG, BH, CN, CY, EG, HK, IQ, IR, JO, KW, LB, LY, MY, OM, PH, PY, QA, SA, SG, SY, UY, YE) *see* Phenylephrine (Systemic) 1638
Mydiatab (HK) *see* Glyburide and Metformin 974
Mydramide (IL) *see* Tropicamide 2108
Mydriacyl (AE, AU, BF, BH, BJ, BR, CI, CL, CO, CY, DK, EE, EG, ET, GB, GH, GM, GN, HK, HU, IE, IQ, IR, IS, JO, KE, KR, KW, LB, LR, LT, LY, MA, ML, MR, MU, MW, MY, NE, NG, NZ, OM, PE, PH, PK, PL, QA, RO, RU, SA, SC, SD, SE, SG, SI, SL, SN, SY, TH, TN, TW, TZ, UG, VE, VN, YE, ZA, ZM, ZW) *see* Tropicamide 2108
Mydriaticum (AT, CH, DE, FR, LU, NL) *see* Tropicamide 2108
Mydrilate (GB, IE) *see* Cyclopentolate 517
Mydrin-M (JP) *see* Tropicamide 2108
Mydrum (CZ, HN, HU) *see* Tropicamide 2108
Myfloxin (TH) *see* Norfloxacin 1475
Myfortic (AE, AR, AT, AU, BE, BG, BH, BR, CH, CL, CN, CO, CY, CZ, DE, DK, EC, EE, ES, FI, FR, GB, GR, HN, HR, ID, IE, IL, IS, IT, JO, KR, KW, LB, LT, MX, MY, NL, NO, PE, PH, PK, PL, PT, PY, QA, RO, RU, SA, SE, SG, SI, SK, TH, TR, TW, UY, VE, VN) *see* Mycophenolate 1405
Myfungar (CZ, DE, MX, RU) *see* Oxiconazole 1536
Myk 1 (BE, LU, NL) *see* Sulconazole 1943
Myk (FR) *see* Sulconazole 1943
Mykoderm (DE) *see* Miconazole (Topical) 1360
Mykyo (TW) *see* Metolazone 1348
Mylanta 2go Rolltabs (NZ) *see* Calcium Carbonate and Magnesium Hydroxide 328
Mylanta II (VN) *see* Aluminum Hydroxide, Magnesium Hydroxide, and Simethicone 104
Mylanta (AU, NZ, SG) *see* Aluminum Hydroxide, Magnesium Hydroxide, and Simethicone 104
Mylanta Rolltab (CO) *see* Calcium Carbonate and Magnesium Hydroxide 328
Mylepsinum (DE) *see* Primidone 1714
Myleran (AE, AR, AT, AU, BB, BE, BF, BG, BH, BJ, BM, BR, BS, BZ, CH, CI, CL, CY, CZ, DE, EC, EE, EG, ET, FR, GB, GH, GM, GN, GR, GY, HK, HN, HR, IE, IL, IN, IQ, IR, IS, IT, JM, JO, KE, KW, LB, LR, LT, LU, LY, MA, ML, MR, MT, MU, MW, MX, MY, NE, NG, NL, NZ, OM, PE, PL, PT, QA, RU, SA, SC, SD, SE, SG, SI, SK, SL, SN, SR, SY, TH, TN, TR, TT, TW, TZ, UG, UY, VN, YE, ZA, ZM, ZW) *see* Busulfan 312
Myleugyn LP (FR) *see* Econazole 703
Mylocort (ZA) *see* Hydrocortisone (Topical) 1014
Mylotarg (AR, BR, CO, GR, JP, KR) *see* Gemtuzumab Ozogamicin 957
Mynocine (FR) *see* Minocycline 1371
Myobloc (GR) *see* Diacerein [INT] 613
Myobloc (KR) *see* RimabotulinumtoxinB 1813
Myocard-DX (PH) *see* DOPamine 669
Myocard (PH) *see* DOPamine 669
Myocet (AT, BE, BG, CH, CY, CZ, DE, DK, EE, ES, FI, FR, GB, GR, HR, HU, IE, IL, IT, LT, MT, NL, NO, PL, PT, RO, SK, TR) *see* DOXOrubicin (Liposomal) 684
Myocholine-Glenwood (AT, DE, IT) *see* Bethanechol 257
Myocholine Glenwood (CH) *see* Bethanechol 257
Myocord (AR) *see* Atenolol 189
Myodial (PH) *see* Amiodarone 114
Myofast (CO) *see* DOBUTamine 654
Myofast (CO) *see* DOPamine 669
Myoflex (HR) *see* Chlorzoxazone 430
Myoflexin (HN, HU) *see* Chlorzoxazone 430
Myogard (AE, BH, CY, EG, IN, IQ, IR, JO, KW, LB, LY, OM, QA, SA, SY, YE) *see* NIFEdipine 1451
Myo Hermes (ES) *see* Bethanechol 257
Myolastan (AT, BE, CZ, ES, FR, LU) *see* Tetrazepam [INT] 2020
Myomethol (HK, VN) *see* Methocarbamol 1320
Myonil (DK) *see* Diltiazem 634
Myonil Retard (DK) *see* Diltiazem 634
Myoplegine (LU) *see* Succinylcholine 1939
Myores (ID) *see* TiZANidine 2051
Myorexin Inj (KR) *see* Methocarbamol 1320
Myos-Nor (CO) *see* TiZANidine 2051
Myospasmal (DE) *see* Tetrazepam [INT] 2020
Myotec (PH) *see* Mycophenolate 1405
Myotenlis (IT) *see* Succinylcholine 1939
Myotil (HK) *see* DOPamine 669
Myotonic (ID) *see* Methylergonovine 1333
Myotonine Chloride (GB, UY) *see* Bethanechol 257
Myotonin (KR) *see* Bethanechol 257
Myovin (IN) *see* Nitroglycerin 1465
Myoxam (ES) *see* Midecamycin [INT] 1365
Myozyme (AT, AU, BE, BG, CH, CY, CZ, DE, DK, EE, ES, FI, FR, GB, GR, HK, HN, HR, IE, IL, IT, JP, KR, LT, MT, MX, MY, NL, NO, NZ, PL, PT, RO, RU, SE, SG, SI, SK, TH, TR, TW) *see* Alglucosidase Alfa 85
Mypara (TH) *see* Acetaminophen 32
Myran (SG) *see* Busulfan 312
Myron (TW) *see* Meropenem 1299
Myser (JP) *see* Difluprednate (Topical) [INT] 627
Myslee (JP) *see* ZOLMitriptan 2210
Mysodelle (GB) *see* Misoprostol 1379
Mysoline (AE, AR, AT, AU, BE, BF, BG, BH, BJ, CH, CI, CL, CY, DK, EE, EG, ES, ET, FI, FR, GH, GM, GN, GR, HK, IE, IN, IQ, IR, IT, JO, KE, KW, LB, LR, LU, LY, MA, ML, MR, MT, MU, MW, MY, NE, NG, NL, NO, OM, PT, QA, RU, SA, SC, SD, SE, SG, SK, SL, SN, SY, TN, TR, TW, TZ, UG, UY, YE, ZA, ZM, ZW) *see* Primidone 1714
Mysoven (TH) *see* Acetylcysteine 40
Mytadon Cristalia (UY) *see* Methadone 1311
Mytedom (BR) *see* Methadone 1311
Mytodex (PH) *see* Tobramycin and Dexamethasone 2056
Mytomycin C (JP) *see* MitoMYcin (Systemic) 1380
Mytoxid (PH) *see* MitoMYcin (Systemic) 1380
Nabila (PE) *see* Nebivolol 1434
Nabone (TH) *see* Nabumetone 1411
Nabratin (CR, DO, GT, HN, NI, SV) *see* Clopidogrel 484
Nabuco (IL) *see* Nabumetone 1411
Nabucox (FR) *see* Nabumetone 1411
Nabuflam (IN) *see* Nabumetone 1411
Nabugesic (JO) *see* Nabumetone 1411
Naburen (CO, DO, GT, PA, SV) *see* Nabumetone 1411
Nabuser (IT) *see* Nabumetone 1411
N-Acc (ID) *see* Acetylcysteine 40
Nacetyl (PH) *see* Acetylcysteine 40
Na Chuan (CN) *see* SUMAtriptan 1953
Nacid (KR) *see* Nizatidine 1471
Naclex (ID) *see* Furosemide 940

Naclof (JO) *see* Diclofenac (Ophthalmic) 621
Nacomic (MX) *see* Miconazole (Topical) 1360
NAC-ratiopharm (LU) *see* Acetylcysteine 40
Nacrez (DK, GB) *see* Desogestrel [INT] 597
NAC (TR) *see* Acetylcysteine 40
Nadibact (IN) *see* Nadifloxacin [INT] 1411
Nadine (AE, BH, CY, EG, IQ, IR, JO, KW, LB, LY, OM, QA, SA, SY, YE) *see* Ranitidine 1777
Nadis (TW) *see* Furosemide 940
Nadixa (BG, CO, CR, DE, DO, EC, ES, GR, GT, HN, IT, KR, LB, MX, NI, PA, PE, PT, PY, SV, TR) *see* Nadifloxacin [INT] 1411
Nadoxin (LB, PH) *see* Nadifloxacin [INT] 1411
Nafacil-S (MX) *see* Cephalexin 405
Nafarin (ID) *see* Chlorpheniramine and Pseudoephedrine 427
Nafartol (MX) *see* Calcitriol 323
Nafasol (ZA) *see* Naproxen 1427
NAF (HR) *see* Fluoride 895
Nafiset (MX) *see* Desmopressin 594
Naflax (PH) *see* Naproxen 1427
Naflox (LB) *see* Norfloxacin 1475
Nafluor (AR) *see* Fluoride 895
NaFril (DE) *see* Fluoride 895
Nafrolen (CY) *see* Naftidrofuryl [INT] 1416
Naftazolina (IT) *see* Naphazoline (Ophthalmic) 1426
Naftilong (DE, HU, LU) *see* Naftidrofuryl [INT] 1416
Naftilux (FR) *see* Naftidrofuryl [INT] 1416
Nafti-Puren (DE) *see* Naftidrofuryl [INT] 1416
Nafti-ratiopharm (DE) *see* Naftidrofuryl [INT] 1416
Naftisol (AT) *see* Naftidrofuryl [INT] 1416
nafti von ct (DE) *see* Naftidrofuryl [INT] 1416
Naftodril (AT) *see* Naftidrofuryl [INT] 1416
Nagun (AR) *see* DOXOrubicin (Conventional) 679
Nail Batrafen (NZ) *see* Ciclopirox 433
Nailderm (IE) *see* Terbinafine (Systemic) 2002
Naillacquer (KR) *see* Ciclopirox 433
Nairet (VN) *see* Terbutaline 2004
Nakom (EE, HR, RO, RU, SI, SK) *see* Carbidopa and Levodopa 351
Nakom [+ Levodopa] (PL) *see* Carbidopa 351
Nal-Acid (GR) *see* Nalidixic Acid [INT] 1418
Nalbufina (UY) *see* Nalbuphine 1416
Nalbuphin OrPha (CH) *see* Nalbuphine 1416
Nalcryn SP (MX) *see* Nalbuphine 1416
Naldix (AE, BH, CY, EG, IL, IQ, IR, JO, KW, LB, LY, OM, QA, SA, SY, YE) *see* Nalidixic Acid [INT] 1418
Naldorex (RO) *see* Naproxen 1427
Nalerona (PE, PY) *see* Naltrexone 1422
Nalfon (AT, BB, BM, BS, BZ, GY, JM, MX, NL, RU, SR, TT) *see* Fenoprofen 857
Nalgesic (FR) *see* Fenoprofen 857
Nalgesik (ID) *see* Acetaminophen 32
Nalgesin (BG, HR) *see* Naproxen 1427
Nali 500 (UY) *see* Nalidixic Acid [INT] 1418
Nalidix (AE, BH, CY, EG, IL, IQ, IR, JO, KW, LB, LY, OM, QA, SA, SY, YE) *see* Nalidixic Acid [INT] 1418
Nalidixic (VN) *see* Nalidixic Acid [INT] 1418
Nalidixin (CZ) *see* Nalidixic Acid [INT] 1418
Nalidixol (ES) *see* Nalidixic Acid [INT] 1418
Nalion (TR) *see* ALPRAZolam 94
Nalitucsan (JP) *see* Nalidixic Acid [INT] 1418
Nalixan (FI) *see* Nalidixic Acid [INT] 1418
Nalixone (MX) *see* Nalidixic Acid [INT] 1418
Nalone (FR) *see* Naloxone 1419
Nalorex (BE, FR, GB, IE, NL, PT) *see* Naltrexone 1422
Nalox (AR) *see* MetroNIDAZOLE (Systemic) 1353
Naloxon (BG, CH, DE, IS) *see* Naloxone 1419
Naloxone Abello (ES) *see* Naloxone 1419
Naloxone Hydrochlorid (GB) *see* Naloxone 1419
Naloxonum Hydrochloricum (PL) *see* Naloxone 1419
Naloxonum Prolongatum (PL) *see* Naloxone 1419
Nalpain (DK, FI, PT, SE, SI) *see* Nalbuphine 1416
Naltrexin (KR) *see* Naltrexone 1422
Nametone (TH) *see* Nabumetone 1411
Namic (MY) *see* Mefenamic Acid 1280
Namir (AR) *see* Bromhexine [INT] 291
Nani Pre Dental (ES) *see* Benzocaine 246
Naniprus (PL) *see* Nitroprusside 1467
Nansius (DO) *see* Clorazepate 487
Napafen (EC) *see* Acetaminophen 32
Napageln (JP) *see* Felbinac [INT] 850
Napamide (MY, NZ, SG, TH) *see* Indapamide 1065
Napamol (ZA) *see* Acetaminophen 32
Napan (HK, MY) *see* Mefenamic Acid 1280
Napaton (TW) *see* Acetaminophen 32
Napha-Nasal (BG) *see* Naphazoline (Nasal) 1426
Naphcon-A (AE, AU, BE, BH, CL, CN, EC, EG, HK, ID, KR, KW, LB, MY, NZ, PE, PH, PK, QA, SA, SG, TH, VN) *see* Naphazoline and Pheniramine 1426
Naphcon (AE, BE, BF, BH, BJ, CI, CY, EG, ET, GH, GM, GN, GR, IQ, IR, JO, KE, KW, LB, LR, LY, MA, ML, MR, MU, MW, NE, NG, OM, QA, SA, SC, SD, SL, SN, SY, TN, TZ, UG, VE, YE, ZM, ZW) *see* Naphazoline (Ophthalmic) 1426
Naphcon-F (CO) *see* Naphazoline (Ophthalmic) 1426
Naphcon Forte (AE, AU, BF, BH, BJ, CI, CY, EG, ET, GH, GM, GN, IL, IQ, IR, JO, KE, KW, LB, LR, LY, MA, ML, MR, MU, MW, NE, NG, NZ, OM, QA, SA, SC, SD, SL, SN, SY, TN, TZ, UG, YE, ZM, ZW) *see* Naphazoline (Ophthalmic) 1426
Naphtears (CL, PE, PK, PY) *see* Naphazoline (Ophthalmic) 1426
Napizide (TW) *see* GlipiZIDE 967
Naposin (TW) *see* Naproxen 1427
Napoxen (PH) *see* Naproxen 1427
Napran (PH) *see* Acetaminophen 32
Naprex (ID) *see* Acetaminophen 32
Naprex (PK) *see* Naproxen 1427
Naprilate (PH) *see* Enalapril 722
Naprilene (IT) *see* Enalapril 722
Naprium (AE, BF, BH, BJ, CI, CY, EG, ET, GH, GM, GN, IQ, IR, JO, KE, KW, LB, LR, LY, MA, ML, MR, MU, MW, NE, NG, OM, QA, SA, SC, SD, SL, SN, SY, TN, TZ, UG, YE, ZM, ZW) *see* Naproxen 1427
Naprius (IT) *see* Naproxen 1427
Naprix (BR) *see* Ramipril 1771
Naprizide (IL) *see* Enalapril and Hydrochlorothiazide 725
Naprocap (PH) *see* Capecitabine 339
Naprodil (MX) *see* Naproxen 1427
Naproflex (TH) *see* Naproxen 1427
Naprontag (AR) *see* Naproxen 1427
Naproplat (PH) *see* CARBOplatin 357
Naprorex (AE, BH, CY, EG, IQ, IR, JO, KW, LB, LY, OM, QA, SA, SY, TR, YE) *see* Naproxen 1427
Naprosyn (AE, AU, BB, BF, BH, BJ, BM, BS, BZ, CI, CY, CZ, DK, EC, EG, ES, ET, FI, GB, GH, GM, GN, GR, GY, IE, IN, IQ, IR, IT, JM, JO, KE, KW, LB, LR, LY, MA, ML, MR, MU, MW, NE, NG, NO, OM, PE, PT, PY, QA, RU, SA, SC, SD, SE, SL, SN, SR, SY, TN, TT, TZ, UG, YE, ZM, ZW) *see* Naproxen 1427
Naprosyne (BE, FR, NL) *see* Naproxen 1427
Naprosyn LE (TH) *see* Naproxen 1427
Naprosyn LLE Forte (PH) *see* Naproxen 1427
Naprosyn LLE (PH) *see* Naproxen 1427
Naprosyn SR (AU) *see* Naproxen 1427
Naproxi 250 (IL) *see* Naproxen 1427
Naproxi 500 (IL) *see* Naproxen 1427
Naprux (AR) *see* Naproxen 1427
Naragran (DK) *see* Naratriptan 1430
Naramig (AE, AR, AU, BE, BG, BH, BR, CH, CL, CO, CY, CZ, DE, EC, EE, EG, FI, FR, GB, GR, HU, IL, IQ, IR, JO, KR, KW, LB, LT, LY, MX, NL, NO, NZ, OM, PE, PT, QA, RU, SA, SE, SG, SI, SY, TH, TR, UY, YE) *see* Naratriptan 1430
Narapril (AE, KR) *see* Enalapril 722

Naratrex (IN) *see* Naratriptan 1430
Narcan (AE, AU, BE, BF, BH, BJ, BR, CI, CY, EG, ET, FR, GB, GH, GM, GN, GR, IL, IQ, IR, IT, JO, KE, KR, KW, LB, LR, LU, LY, MA, ML, MR, MU, MW, NE, NG, NZ, OM, PK, PL, QA, SA, SC, SD, SG, SL, SN, SY, TN, TW, TZ, UG, VE, YE, ZM, ZW) *see* Naloxone 1419
Narcanti (AT, DK, HN, HU, MX, NO, PL, UY) *see* Naloxone 1419
Narcotan (IN) *see* Naloxone 1419
Nardelzine (BE, ES, LU) *see* Phenelzine 1630
Nardil (AE, AU, GB, IE, NZ) *see* Phenelzine 1630
Nardyl (DE) *see* DiphenhydrAMINE (Systemic) 641
Narebox (IN) *see* Reboxetine [INT] 1786
Narfoz (ID) *see* Ondansetron 1513
Narigix (JP) *see* Nalidixic Acid [INT] 1418
Narinex (KR) *see* Mometasone (Nasal) 1391
Nariplus (KR) *see* Enalapril and Hydrochlorothiazide 725
Narkamon (DE, PL) *see* Ketamine 1143
Narlox (PH) *see* Naloxone 1419
Narobic (ZA) *see* MetroNIDAZOLE (Systemic) 1353
Naropeine (FR, GR, PT, VN) *see* Ropivacaine 1846
Narop (IL, SE) *see* Ropivacaine 1846
Naropin (AE, AR, AT, AU, BB, BE, BH, BM, BS, BZ, CH, CN, CO, CY, CZ, DE, DK, EG, ES, FI, GB, GY, HK, HN, ID, IE, IQ, IR, IS, JM, JO, KR, KW, LB, LU, LY, MX, MY, NL, NO, NZ, OM, PH, PL, QA, RO, RU, SA, SG, SI, SR, SY, TH, TR, TT, VE, YE) *see* Ropivacaine 1846
Naropina (IT) *see* Ropivacaine 1846
Narpan (MY, SG) *see* Naltrexone 1422
Narsis (PK) *see* Medazepam [INT] 1277
Narval (UY) *see* Levothyroxine 1205
Narvin (TH) *see* AmLODIPine 123
Narxona (AR) *see* Naloxone 1419
Nasa-12 (LU) *see* Pseudoephedrine 1742
Nasacort AQ (AR, BG, CL, CO, CY, CZ, HK, KW, LB, MX, MY, PE, PY, UY, VE, VN) *see* Triamcinolone (Nasal) 2100
Nasacort (AT, BR, CH, DK, ES, FI, GB, GR, HR, ID, IT, KR, NL, NO, PK, PT, SE, SG, TH, TR, TW) *see* Triamcinolone (Nasal) 2100
Nasafed (ID) *see* Triprolidine and Pseudoephedrine 2105
Nasaflex (KR) *see* Mometasone (Nasal) 1391
Nasaga (TW) *see* Fexofenadine 873
Nasair (VE) *see* Beclomethasone (Nasal) 232
Nasalate Nose Cream (AU) *see* Phenylephrine (Systemic) 1638
Nasaler (PE) *see* Loratadine 1241
Nasaler Plus CL (PE) *see* Chlorpheniramine and Pseudoephedrine 427
Nasalide (FR, KR) *see* Flunisolide (Nasal) 893
Nasanyl (JP) *see* Nafarelin 1414
Nasarel (IN) *see* Nafarelin 1414
Nasative (KR) *see* Mometasone (Nasal) 1391
Nasa w/codeine (TH) *see* Acetaminophen and Codeine 36
Nasea (ID, JP, KR, PH, TH) *see* Ramosetron [INT] 1774
Nasenspray (CH) *see* Phenylephrine (Systemic) 1638
Naseron OD (PH) *see* Ramosetron [INT] 1774
Nasobec Aqueous (GR, HK, KR, PL) *see* Beclomethasone (Nasal) 232
Nasocobi (KR) *see* Mometasone (Nasal) 1391
Nasofan (HK) *see* Fluticasone (Nasal) 910
Nasofan (HK) *see* Fluticasone (Oral Inhalation) 907
Nasoflo (PH) *see* Fluticasone (Nasal) 910
Nasoflo (PH) *see* Fluticasone (Oral Inhalation) 907
Nasomet (PT) *see* Mometasone (Nasal) 1391
Nasonex (AE, AR, AT, AU, BE, BG, BH, BR, CH, CL, CN, CO, CR, CY, CZ, DE, DK, DO, FI, FR, GB, GR, GT, HK, HN, HR, HU, ID, IL, IS, IT, JP, KW, LB, LT, NI, NL, NO, PA, PE, PH, PL, QA, RO, RU, SA, SE, SI, SK, SV, TH, TR, TW, UY, VE, VN) *see* Mometasone (Nasal) 1391
Nasonex Nasal Spray (AU, DE, EE, GB, HK, ID, IE, KR, MY, PH, SG) *see* Mometasone (Nasal) 1391
Nasonide (MY) *see* Triamcinolone (Nasal) 2100
Nasoride (PH) *see* Budesonide (Nasal) 296
Naspro (ID) *see* Aspirin 180
Nastizol (EC) *see* Chlorpheniramine and Pseudoephedrine 427
Nastizol EX (MX) *see* Permethrin 1627
Nastizol Hidrospray (PY) *see* Budesonide (Nasal) 296
Natacyn (AR, CN, CO, KR, MY, PL, SG, TH, TW) *see* Natamycin 1432
Natadrops (IN) *see* Natamycin 1432
Natafucin (GB, IT) *see* Natamycin 1432
Natamycyna (PL) *see* Natamycin 1432
Natax (AR) *see* Bromfenac 291
Natead (FR) *see* Rh_o(D) Immune Globulin 1794
Natecal (ES) *see* Calcium Carbonate 327
Natele (MX) *see* Pyridoxine 1747
Natezhen (CN) *see* Natamycin 1432
Naticardina (IT) *see* QuiNIDine 1759
Natil-N (DE) *see* Flunarizine [CAN/INT] 892
Natispray (LU) *see* Nitroglycerin 1465
Natralgin (GR) *see* Dipyrone [INT] 653
Natravox (PH) *see* Amoxicillin and Clavulanate 133
Natrecor (BB, BM, BS, BZ, GY, ID, JM, NL, PR, QA, SG, SR, TT, VE) *see* Nesiritide 1439
Natrii chloridum 0,9% solutio pro irrigatione (PL) *see* Sodium Chloride 1902
Natrilix AP (VE) *see* Indapamide 1065
Natrilix (AR, AU, BF, BJ, BR, CI, CY, DE, EC, ET, FI, GB, GH, GM, GN, HK, ID, IN, IQ, IR, IT, KE, LB, LR, LY, MA, ML, MR, MU, MW, NE, NG, NZ, OM, PK, SC, SD, SL, SN, SY, TN, TZ, UG, UY, VE, YE, ZA, ZM, ZW) *see* Indapamide 1065
Natrilix Retard (IS, SE) *see* Indapamide 1065
Natrilix SR (AE, AU, BB, BH, BM, BS, BZ, CL, CR, DE, DO, EG, GT, GY, HN, IE, IN, JM, JO, KW, MY, NI, NL, PA, PE, PH, PR, PY, QA, SA, SG, SR, SV, TT, TW, UY, VN) *see* Indapamide 1065
Natrium bicarbonicum (PL) *see* Sodium Bicarbonate 1901
Natrium chloratum (PL) *see* Sodium Chloride 1902
Natrium Fluoratum (PL) *see* Fluoride 895
Natriumfluorid Baer (AT, DE, LU) *see* Fluoride 895
Natrix (KR) *see* Indapamide 1065
Natrix SR (KR) *see* Indapamide 1065
Natropas (AR) *see* Cinnarizine [INT] 440
Natulan (AE, AR, AT, AU, BE, BG, BH, CH, CY, CZ, DE, DK, EG, ES, FI, FR, GB, GH, GR, HN, HR, HU, IE, IL, IQ, IR, IT, JO, KW, LB, LU, LY, MY, NL, NO, OM, PK, PL, PT, QA, RU, SA, SE, SY, TR, TZ, UG, YE, ZM) *see* Procarbazine 1717
Natulanar (BR) *see* Procarbazine 1717
Natural Betacarotene (AU) *see* Beta-Carotene 251
Naturogest (IN) *see* Progesterone 1722
Nausedron (BR) *see* Ondansetron 1513
Nausetil (AU) *see* Prochlorperazine 1718
Nausicalm (FR) *see* DimenhyDRINATE 637
Nausil (TH) *see* Metoclopramide 1345
Nautisol (BF, BJ, CI, ET, GH, GM, GN, KE, LR, MA, ML, MR, MU, MW, MY, NE, NG, SC, SD, SL, SN, TN, TR, TZ, UG, VN, ZA, ZM, ZW) *see* Prochlorperazine 1718
Nauzelin (ES, JP) *see* Domperidone [CAN/INT] 666
Navamin (TH) *see* DimenhyDRINATE 637
Navane (AU, BR, NL) *see* Thiothixene 2031
Navelbine (AE, AR, AT, AU, BB, BG, BH, BM, BR, BS, BZ, CH, CL, CN, CY, CZ, DE, DK, EE, EG, ES, FI, FR, GB, GR, GY, ID, IE, IL, IQ, IR, IS, IT, JM, JO, KR, KW, LB, LT, LU, LY, MX, MY, NL, NO, NZ, OM, PK, PL, QA,

RO, RU, SA, SE, SI, SK, SR, SY, TH, TR, TT, TW, VN, YE) *see* Vinorelbine ... 2168
Navelbin (HN) *see* Vinorelbine ... 2168
Navicalm (PT) *see* Meclizine ... 1277
Navoban (AT, AU, BG, BH, CH, CN, EE, EG, FI, GR, HK, HN, ID, IT, JO, KR, LB, MX, MY, NL, NO, NZ, PE, PH, PK, PT, QA, RU, SA, SE, SI, TR, TW, VE, VN, ZA) *see* Tropisetron [INT] ... 2108
Naxen (MX, NZ) *see* Naproxen ... 1427
Naxen-F CR (KR) *see* Naproxen ... 1427
Naxen F (KR) *see* Naproxen ... 1427
Naxidine (NL) *see* Nizatidine ... 1471
Naxidin (HN, HU) *see* Nizatidine ... 1471
Naxone (AE, BH, CY, EG, IL, IQ, IR, JO, KW, LB, LY, OM, QA, SA, SY, YE) *see* Naloxone ... 1419
Naxopren (FI) *see* Naproxen ... 1427
Naxproglycem (KR) *see* Diazoxide ... 616
Naxy (FR) *see* Clarithromycin ... 456
Naxyn 250 (IL) *see* Naproxen ... 1427
Naxyn 500 (IL) *see* Naproxen ... 1427
Nazine (TH) *see* Cinnarizine [INT] ... 440
Nazin (SG) *see* Cinnarizine [INT] ... 440
Nazole (KR) *see* Ketoconazole (Topical) ... 1145
Nazol (HR) *see* Naphazoline (Nasal) ... 1426
Nazolin (AE) *see* Naphazoline (Nasal) ... 1426
Nazol (MY, SG) *see* Danazol ... 558
Nazotral (CO) *see* Cromolyn (Nasal) ... 514
Nazotral (CO) *see* Cromolyn (Ophthalmic) ... 514
Nazovell (ID) *see* Ketoprofen ... 1145
Neagel (AR) *see* Ganciclovir (Systemic) ... 948
Nebacetina (MX) *see* Bacitracin and Polymyxin B ... 222
Nebacetin N Spruhverband (DE) *see* Neomycin ... 1436
Nebapol B (AR) *see* Neomycin ... 1436
Nebapul (CL) *see* Methylphenidate ... 1336
Nebcin (AE, BF, BG, BH, BJ, CI, ET, GH, GM, GN, GR, KE, LR, MA, ML, MR, MU, MW, NE, NG, PK, SA, SC, SD, SL, SN, TN, TZ, UG, VN, ZM, ZW) *see* Tobramycin (Systemic, Oral Inhalation) ... 2052
Nebcina (NO, SE) *see* Tobramycin (Systemic, Oral Inhalation) ... 2052
Nebcine (FR) *see* Tobramycin (Systemic, Oral Inhalation) ... 2052
Nebibeta (KR) *see* Nebivolol ... 1434
Nebican (KR) *see* Nebivolol ... 1434
Nebicard (IN, PH) *see* Nebivolol ... 1434
Nebicar (PH) *see* Nebivolol ... 1434
Nebicina (IT) *see* Tobramycin (Systemic, Oral Inhalation) ... 2052
Nebilet (AE, AR, AU, BG, BR, CH, CL, CO, CR, CZ, DE, DO, EE, FI, GB, GT, HK, HN, HR, IE, JO, KR, KW, LB, LT, MY, NI, PA, PE, PH, PL, PT, RO, RU, SA, SE, SG, SI, SK, SV, TH, VE, VN, ZA) *see* Nebivolol ... 1434
Nebilox (FR) *see* Nebivolol ... 1434
Nebil (PH) *see* Nebivolol ... 1434
Nebinorm (RO) *see* Nebivolol ... 1434
Nebistar (IN) *see* Nebivolol ... 1434
Nebistol (KR) *see* Nebivolol ... 1434
Nebitlol (KR) *see* Nebivolol ... 1434
Neblock (BR) *see* Nebivolol ... 1434
NEBS (JP) *see* Acetaminophen ... 32
Nebyol (HR) *see* Nebivolol ... 1434
Necaxime (TH) *see* Cefotaxime ... 382
Neciblok (ID) *see* Sucralfate ... 1940
Neconase (CN) *see* Beclomethasone (Nasal) ... 232
Necopen (ES) *see* Cefixime ... 380
Nedax (BR) *see* Lindane ... 1217
Nedax Plus (BR) *see* Permethrin ... 1627
Nedipin (TW) *see* NIFEdipine ... 1451
Neditol XL (GB) *see* Tolterodine ... 2063
Nedocromil-Natrium "Schoeller Pharma" (AT) *see* Nedocromil ... 1435
Nedox (CO, PE) *see* Esomeprazole ... 771
Nefadar (CH, DE, DK, NO, SE) *see* Nefazodone ... 1435
Nefagrel (AR) *see* Prasugrel ... 1699
Nefalox (GR) *see* Cefadroxil ... 372
Nefaril (UY) *see* Nefazodone ... 1435
Nefazodone "BMS" (AT) *see* Nefazodone ... 1435
Nefoben (AR) *see* Theophylline ... 2026
Nefrecil (PL) *see* Phenazopyridine ... 1629
Nefrofer (ID) *see* Iron Sucrose ... 1118
Nefrofil (PY) *see* Chlorthalidone ... 430
Nefrotal Plus (DO) *see* Losartan and Hydrochlorothiazide ... 1250
Nefryl (MX) *see* Oxybutynin ... 1536
Negacef (AE, BH, KW, LB, QA, SA) *see* CefTAZidime ... 392
Negadix (IN) *see* Nalidixic Acid [INT] ... 1418
Negaflox (BG) *see* Norfloxacin ... 1475
Neg-Gram (IT) *see* Nalidixic Acid [INT] ... 1418
Negram (AE, AU, BH, CY, DE, EG, FR, GB, IE, IL, IQ, IR, JO, KW, LB, LY, NL, NO, OM, PK, QA, RU, SA, SY, TR, YE) *see* Nalidixic Acid [INT] ... 1418
Neksium (IN) *see* Esomeprazole ... 771
Neladix (BG) *see* Nalidixic Acid [INT] ... 1418
Nelapine (PH) *see* NIFEdipine ... 1451
Nelgen (PH) *see* Gentamicin (Systemic) ... 959
Nelvir (CO, IN, PY, VE) *see* Nelfinavir ... 1436
Nemacina (AR) *see* Nelfinavir ... 1436
Nemasole (AR) *see* Mebendazole [CAN/INT] ... 1274
Nembutal (AT) *see* PENTobarbital ... 1617
Nemcis (VN) *see* Imipenem and Cilastatin ... 1051
Nemestran (AR, CH, CZ, ES, MX, NL) *see* Gestrinone [INT] ... 962
Nemexin (AT, CH, DE, PL) *see* Naltrexone ... 1422
Nemmed (TH) *see* Meropenem ... 1299
Nemocid (IN) *see* Pyrantel Pamoate ... 1744
Nemozole (IN) *see* Albendazole ... 65
Nenoma (KR) *see* ClomiPRAMINE ... 475
Neoacotril (PH) *see* Glimepiride ... 966
NeoAlertop (PY) *see* Levocetirizine ... 1196
Neoalexil (MX) *see* Loratadine ... 1241
Neo-Allospasmin (BG) *see* Hyoscyamine ... 1026
Neo-B12 (AU) *see* Hydroxocobalamin ... 1020
Neobacigrin (MX) *see* Neomycin, Polymyxin B, and Dexamethasone ... 1437
Neobacigrin (MX) *see* Polymyxin B ... 1676
Neobacitracine (BE) *see* Bacitracin and Polymyxin B ... 222
Neobes (CR, DO, GT, HN, PA, SV) *see* Diethylpropion ... 624
Neobezeta (UY) *see* TOLBUTamide ... 2062
Neobloc (IL) *see* Metoprolol ... 1350
Neobon (KR) *see* Calcitriol ... 323
NeoCaf (KR) *see* Caffeine ... 319
Neocapil (CH, CZ) *see* Minoxidil (Topical) ... 1374
Neocare (ES) *see* Tretinoin (Topical) ... 2099
Neocef (PT) *see* Cefixime ... 380
Neoceptin-R (SG) *see* Ranitidine ... 1777
Neoclaritine (CL) *see* Desloratadine ... 594
Neoclarityn (AT, CH, CZ, DE, DK, EE, ES, FI, FR, GB, GR, IE, IT, MT, NL, NO, PL, PT, RU, SE, SK, TR) *see* Desloratadine ... 594
Neo-Clarosip (MX) *see* Clarithromycin ... 456
Neo-Codion[Sirup] (DE) *see* Codeine ... 497
Neoconal (KR) *see* Fluconazole ... 885
Neo-Cytamen (GB, IE, IT, NZ) *see* Hydroxocobalamin ... 1020
Neo Decapeptyl (BR) *see* Triptorelin ... 2107
Neo-Decapeptyl CR (PE) *see* Triptorelin ... 2107
Neodex-V (PH) *see* Neomycin, Polymyxin B, and Dexamethasone ... 1437
Neodexin (PH) *see* Neomycin, Polymyxin B, and Dexamethasone ... 1437
Neodrea (IN) *see* Hydroxyurea ... 1021
Neo-Ergo (TW) *see* Methylergonovine ... 1333
Neo-Fer (NO) *see* Ferrous Fumarate ... 870
Neofex (PH) *see* Fexofenadine ... 873

Neoflox (IN) *see* Flucloxacillin [INT] 885
Neoforge (KR) *see* Amlodipine and Valsartan 126
Neoform (PH) *see* MetFORMIN 1307
Neoftalm (AR) *see* Trimethoprim and Polymyxin B 2105
Neogaival (EC, UY) *see* Eszopiclone 793
Neograstim (LB) *see* Filgrastim 875
Neogynon 21 (DE) *see* Ethinyl Estradiol and Levonorgestrel 803
Neo Gynoxa (ID) *see* Metronidazole and Nystatin [CAN/INT] 1358
NEOHepatect (CZ) *see* Hepatitis B Immune Globulin (Human) 1002
Neointestin (ES) *see* Neomycin 1436
Neokay (GB) *see* Phytonadione 1647
Neokef (MY) *see* Cephalexin 405
Neo-K (ID) *see* Phytonadione 1647
Neolette (PY) *see* Ethinyl Estradiol and Desogestrel 799
Neo-Loridin (PH) *see* Desloratadine 594
Neolutin Forte (CZ) *see* Hydroxyprogesterone Caproate 1021
Neomas (AR) *see* Neomycin 1436
Neomazine (KR) *see* ChlorproMAZINE 429
Neomeladinine (AE) *see* Methoxsalen (Systemic) 1330
Neo-Mercazole (AE, AU, CH, DK, FR, GB, HN, ID, IE, IN, KW, NO, NZ, SA, VN, ZA) *see* Carbimazole [INT] 356
Neomercazole (CY, HK, PH, PK, QA, TR) *see* Carbimazole [INT] 356
Neomercazol (JO) *see* Carbimazole [INT] 356
Neomerdin (PH) *see* Carbimazole [INT] 356
Neometrin (PE) *see* Ergonovine [CAN/INT] 754
Neomicina Estersa (ES) *see* Neomycin 1436
Neomicina Roger (ES) *see* Neomycin 1436
Neomicina Salvat (ES) *see* Neomycin 1436
Neomicol (CR, DO, GT, HN, MX, NI, PA, SV) *see* Miconazole (Topical) 1360
Neomigran (HU, PL) *see* Dihydroergotamine 633
Neo-Mix (AT) *see* Neomycin 1436
Neomycin Drossapharm (CH) *see* Neomycin 1436
Neomycine (BE) *see* Neomycin 1436
Neomycine Diamant (BE, FR, LU) *see* Neomycin 1436
Neomycine Minims (NL) *see* Neomycin 1436
Neomycin (IL) *see* Neomycin 1436
Neomycin Polibisinbi Hydrocortison Kwanri M Ear Drop (KR) *see* Neomycin, Polymyxin B, and Hydrocortisone 1438
Neomycinsulfat Chevita (AT) *see* Neomycin 1436
Neomycinum (PL) *see* Neomycin 1436
Neo-Panlacticos (MX) *see* Thiamine 2028
Neophamid (KR) *see* Cyclophosphamide 517
Neophedan (ZA) *see* Tamoxifen 1971
Neophos (LB) *see* Cyclophosphamide 517
Neoplatin (ES) *see* CISplatin 448
Neoplatin (KR) *see* CARBOplatin 357
Neo-Polybacin (AE, BF, BH, BJ, CI, CY, EG, ET, GH, GM, GN, IQ, IR, JO, KE, KW, LB, LR, LY, MA, ML, MR, MU, MW, NE, NG, OM, QA, SA, SC, SD, SL, SN, SY, TN, TZ, UG, YE, ZA, ZM, ZW) *see* Bacitracin, Neomycin, and Polymyxin B 223
Neopra (HK) *see* Escitalopram 765
Neopral (PE) *see* Esomeprazole 771
Neopril (KR) *see* Enalapril 722
Neo Prodiar (ID) *see* Furazolidone [INT] 940
Neoprofen (BM) *see* Ibuprofen 1032
Neoquabin (PH) *see* Epirubicin 739
Neoral (FR, GB, IE, NZ, TW) *see* CycloSPORINE (Systemic) 522
Neorecormon (AT, BE, BG, CH, CZ, DE, DK, EE, ES, FI, FR, GB, GR, HN, IE, IT, MT, NL, NO, PL, PT, RU, SE, SK) *see* Epoetin Alfa 742
Neoresotyl (CL, PY) *see* Armodafinil 175
Neorisp (BG) *see* RisperiDONE 1818
Neorof (PH) *see* Propofol 1728
Neosechinbi (KR) *see* Chloramphenicol 421
Neosidantoina (ES) *see* Phenytoin 1640
Neo-Sinefrina (PT) *see* Phenylephrine (Systemic) 1638
Neosinicin (TW) *see* Phenylephrine (Systemic) 1638
Neo-Sintrom (CL) *see* Acenocoumarol [CAN/INT] 30
Neosolvon (AE) *see* Bromhexine [INT] 291
Neosporin (MX) *see* Polymyxin B 1676
Neosporin (AE, BH, KW, QA, SA) *see* Neomycin, Polymyxin B, and Gramicidin 1437
Neosporin Dermico (MX) *see* Bacitracin, Neomycin, and Polymyxin B 223
Neosporin-H (IN) *see* Bacitracin, Neomycin, Polymyxin B, and Hydrocortisone 223
Neosporin Oftalmico (MX) *see* Neomycin, Polymyxin B, and Gramicidin 1437
Neosporin Ophthalmic Ointment (AU, IN) *see* Bacitracin, Neomycin, and Polymyxin B 223
Neosporín Dérmico (MX) *see* Bacitracin and Polymyxin B 222
Neostigmina Braun (ES) *see* Neostigmine 1438
Neostigmin (HR, SE) *see* Neostigmine 1438
Neosulf (AU) *see* Neomycin 1436
Neosyd (ID) *see* Neomycin, Polymyxin B, and Gramicidin 1437
Neosynephrine Faure 10% (FR) *see* Phenylephrine (Systemic) 1638
Neo-Synephrine (IT) *see* Phenylephrine (Systemic) 1638
Neo-Synephrine Ophthalmic (BE, DE, PH) *see* Phenylephrine (Systemic) 1638
Neosynephrin-POS (CZ, DE) *see* Phenylephrine (Systemic) 1638
Neotalem (CL, CO, TH) *see* MitoXANtrone 1382
Neotalis (PH) *see* Neostigmine 1438
Neotasin (KR) *see* Clindamycin (Systemic) 460
Neoterb (AE, KW, QA) *see* Terbutaline 2004
Neo-Thyreostat (DE) *see* Carbimazole [INT] 356
Neotibi (ID) *see* Pyrazinamide 1745
Neotigason (AE, AR, AT, AU, BB, BE, BF, BG, BH, BJ, BM, BR, BS, BZ, CH, CI, CL, CN, CO, CY, CZ, DE, DK, EC, EE, EG, ET, FI, GB, GH, GM, GN, GR, GY, HK, HN, HR, IE, IL, IS, IT, JM, JO, KE, KR, KW, LR, LT, MA, ML, MR, MU, MW, MX, MY, NE, NG, NL, NO, NZ, PE, PH, PL, PT, PY, QA, RO, SA, SC, SD, SE, SG, SI, SK, SL, SN, SR, TH, TN, TR, TT, TW, TZ, UG, UY, VE, ZA, ZM, ZW) *see* Acitretin 43
Neo-Tiroimade (PT) *see* Liothyronine 1221
Neo-Tomizol (ES) *see* Carbimazole [INT] 356
Neotrex (MX) *see* ISOtretinoin 1127
Neotrexate (IN) *see* Methotrexate 1322
Neotri MR (BG) *see* Trimetazidine [INT] 2104
Neotrox (PH) *see* Carbimazole [INT] 356
Neo-Up (PH) *see* Sildenafil 1882
Neoxidil (AE, BE, BH, IL, KW, LB, SA, SG) *see* Minoxidil (Topical) 1374
Neox (PH) *see* Metoprolol 1350
NeOxyn (PH) *see* Oxytocin 1549
Neoxy Tape (JP) *see* Oxybutynin 1536
Neozine (BR) *see* Methotrimeprazine [CAN/INT] 1329
Nepatic (ID) *see* Gabapentin 943
Nepenthe (PH) *see* Diclofenac (Systemic) 617
Nepes (TW) *see* Donepezil 668
Nepezil (BR) *see* Donepezil 668
Nephro (KR) *see* Calcium Acetate 326
Nephron (AR) *see* Furosemide 940
N-Epi (TH) *see* Norepinephrine 1472
Neptazane (FR) *see* Methazolamide 1317
Nerapin (PY) *see* Nevirapine 1440
Neravir (TH) *see* Nevirapine 1440
Nerbloc (JP) *see* RimabotulinumtoxinB 1813
Nercon (MX) *see* Diazepam 613
Nerdipina (ES, PT) *see* NiCARdipine 1446
Nerelid (IT) *see* Nimesulide [INT] 1456
Nergart (JP) *see* Flurazepam 906

Neriderm (IL) *see* Diflucortolone [CAN/INT] 625
Neriforte (AT) *see* Diflucortolone [CAN/INT] 625
Nerilon (ID) *see* Diflucortolone [CAN/INT] 625
Neripros (ID) *see* RisperiDONE 1818
Nerisona (AR, AT, BE, BR, DE, GR, ID, IT, KR, MX, NL, PH, PT) *see* Diflucortolone [CAN/INT] 625
Nerisone (AE, EG, FR, GB, HK, NZ, PK, ZA) *see* Diflucortolone [CAN/INT] 625
Nerisone Forte (GB, ZA) *see* Diflucortolone [CAN/INT] 625
Nerispes (EE) *see* Nebivolol 1434
Nervan (VE) *see* Bromazepam [CAN/INT] 290
Nervinex (ES) *see* Brivudine [INT] 289
Nervistop L (AR) *see* LORazepam 1243
Nesacaine (CH) *see* Chloroprocaine 423
Nesdonal (HR, LU) *see* Thiopental [INT] 2029
Nesontil (AR) *see* Oxazepam 1532
NESP (JP, KR, MY, SG, TH, TW) *see* Darbepoetin Alfa 565
Nespo (SE) *see* Darbepoetin Alfa 565
Netaf (PE) *see* Domperidone [CAN/INT] 666
Neuart (JP) *see* Antithrombin 156
Neubalon (KR) *see* Thioridazine 2030
Neudexta (EE, HR, SE) *see* Dextromethorphan and Quinidine 611
Neufan (JP) *see* Allopurinol 90
Neugeron (MX) *see* CarBAMazepine 346
Neukine (TH) *see* Filgrastim 875
Neulactil (AU, DK, FI, GB, HK, NO, NZ, ZA) *see* Periciazine [CAN/INT] 1621
Neulasta (AT, AU, BE, BG, CH, CY, CZ, DE, DK, EE, ES, FI, FR, GB, GR, HN, HR, HU, IE, IS, IT, KR, LT, MT, NL, NO, PL, PT, RO, RU, SE, SI, SK, TR, TW) *see* Pegfilgrastim 1589
Neulastim (AE, AR, BR, CL, CO, EC, HK, ID, IL, IN, KW, LB, NZ, PE, PY, SA, SG, TH, UY, VN) *see* Pegfilgrastim 1589
Neulastim (AE, KW, SA) *see* Filgrastim 875
Neulastyl (PH) *see* Pegfilgrastim 1589
Neuleptil (AR, AT, BG, BR, CL, GR, IL, IT, LB, NL, PT, PY, RU, UY, VE) *see* Periciazine [CAN/INT] 1621
Neuleptol (KR) *see* Gabapentin 943
Neulin-SR (NZ, TW) *see* Theophylline 2026
Neumantine (TH) *see* Memantine 1286
Neumega (KR) *see* Oprelvekin 1519
Neumocort (PY) *see* Budesonide (Systemic) 293
Neupax (MX) *see* ALPRAZolam 94
Neupax (CR, DO, EC, GT, HN, NI, PA, PE, SV) *see* FLUoxetine 899
Neuperil (FI) *see* Periciazine [CAN/INT] 1621
Neupogen (AE, AR, AT, AU, BB, BE, BF, BG, BH, BJ, BM, BS, BZ, CH, CI, CL, CO, CY, CZ, DE, DK, EC, EE, EG, ES, ET, FI, FR, GB, GH, GM, GN, GR, GY, HK, HR, HU, ID, IE, IL, IN, IQ, IR, IS, IT, JM, JO, KE, KW, LB, LR, LT, LU, LY, MA, ML, MR, MT, MU, MW, MX, NE, NG, NL, NO, NZ, OM, PH, PK, PL, PT, PY, QA, RO, RU, SA, SC, SD, SE, SI, SK, SL, SN, SR, SY, TH, TN, TR, TT, TZ, UG, UY, VE, VN, YE, ZA, ZM, ZW) *see* Filgrastim 875
Neupopeg (AT, BE, BG, CH, CZ, DE, DK, EE, ES, FI, FR, GB, GR, HN, IE, IT, MT, NL, NO, PL, PT, RU, SE, SK, TR) *see* Pegfilgrastim 1589
Neupro (AR, AT, AU, BE, BH, BM, BR, CH, CL, CY, CZ, DE, DK, EE, ES, FR, GB, GR, HK, HR, IE, IT, KR, KW, LT, MY, NL, NO, PH, PL, PT, RO, SE, SG, SI, SK, TH, TR, TW) *see* Rotigotine 1851
Neupro Patch (ID, JP) *see* Rotigotine 1851
Neuractin (CO) *see* Valproic Acid and Derivatives 2123
Neuramin (FI) *see* Thiamine 2028
Neur-Amyl (AU) *see* Amobarbital 128
Neurazine (JO) *see* ChlorproMAZINE 429
Neuridon (LU) *see* Acetaminophen 32
Neuril (DK) *see* Gabapentin 943
Neuris (TH) *see* RisperiDONE 1818
Neurobene (CZ, HN) *see* Cyanocobalamin 515
Neurobiol (IT) *see* PHENobarbital 1632
Neurobloc (AT, BE, CZ, DE, DK, EE, FR, GB, HR, IE, IS, IT, LT, NL, NO, RO, SE, SI, SK, TR) *see* RimabotulinumtoxinB 1813
Neurocept (KR) *see* Donepezil 668
Neurocetam (MY, SG) *see* Piracetam [INT] 1661
Neurocil (DE) *see* Methotrimeprazine [CAN/INT] 1329
Neurocover-PG (KR) *see* Pregabalin 1710
Neurogel (UY) *see* ChlorproMAZINE 429
Neurolep (MX) *see* CarBAMazepine 346
Neurolepsin (AT) *see* Lithium 1230
Neuronova (ES) *see* Piracetam [INT] 1661
Neurontin (AE, AR, AT, AU, BE, BG, BH, BO, BR, CH, CN, CO, CR, CY, CZ, DE, DO, EC, EE, EG, ES, FI, FR, GB, GR, GT, HK, HN, HR, HU, ID, IE, IL, IN, IQ, IR, IS, IT, JO, KE, KR, KW, LB, LT, LY, MX, MY, NI, NL, NO, NZ, OM, PA, PE, PH, PL, PR, PT, QA, RU, SA, SE, SG, SI, SK, SV, SY, TH, TR, TW, UY, VE, VN, YE, ZA) *see* Gabapentin 943
Neuropam (TW) *see* LORazepam 1243
Neuroplus (EC) *see* Memantine 1286
Neurotol (FI) *see* CarBAMazepine 346
Neurotol (PY) *see* Amitriptyline 119
Neurotop (AT, BG, HU, LB) *see* CarBAMazepine 346
Neurox-250 (TH) *see* Cefuroxime 399
Neurtrol (TW) *see* OXcarbazepine 1532
Neurum (CL, EC) *see* Pregabalin 1710
Neuryl (EC) *see* ClonazePAM 478
Neusinol (BE) *see* Naphazoline (Nasal) 1426
Neu-Stam (VN) *see* Piracetam [INT] 1661
Neustatin-A (KR) *see* AtorvaSTATin 194
Neustatin-R (KR) *see* Rosuvastatin 1848
Neutapin (TH, TW) *see* QUEtiapine 1751
Neutoin (KR) *see* Donepezil 668
Neutracet (KR) *see* Acetaminophen and Tramadol 37
Neutrogin (JP, KR) *see* Lenograstim [INT] 1181
Neutromax (PE, PY, VN) *see* Filgrastim 875
Neutronorm (AT) *see* Cimetidine 438
Neutropain (HK) *see* Ibuprofen 1032
Nevanac (AE, AR, BR, CH, CL, CO, CR, CY, CZ, DE, DK, EE, GB, GR, GT, HK, HN, HR, IE, IL, IN, IS, JP, KW, LT, MY, NI, NL, NO, NZ, PA, PE, PH, PL, PT, QA, RO, SE, SG, SI, SK, SV, TH, TR, VN) *see* Nepafenac 1439
Neverpentin (TH) *see* Gabapentin 943
Nevetrol (KR) *see* Nebivolol 1434
Nevigramon (HN, HU, PL) *see* Nalidixic Acid [INT] 1418
Nevimune (IN) *see* Nevirapine 1440
Nevimuno (PY) *see* Nevirapine 1440
Neviolet (KR) *see* Nebivolol 1434
Neviran (HR) *see* Nevirapine 1440
Nevolmin (KR) *see* Nebivolol 1434
Newace (NL) *see* Fosinopril 932
New Azelan (VN) *see* Azelastine (Ophthalmic) 213
Newbutin SR (KR) *see* Trimebutine [CAN/INT] 2103
Newcef (KR) *see* CefTRIAXone 396
New Diatabs (ID, VN) *see* Attapulgite [CAN/INT] 204
New-GABA (KR) *see* Gabapentin 943
Newin (TW) *see* Oxybutynin 1536
Newitock (VN) *see* Formoterol 926
New-Lylo (TW) *see* Chloramphenicol 421
New-Nok (IL) *see* Permethrin 1627
Newpio (KR) *see* Pioglitazone 1654
Newpram (KR) *see* Escitalopram 765
Newquip (KR) *see* ROPINIRole 1844
New-Rexan (KR) *see* Methocarbamol 1320
Newropenem (KR) *see* Meropenem 1299
Newspar (ID) *see* Sparfloxacin [INT] 1930
Newtaxime (KR) *see* Cefotaxime 382
Newtolide (JP) *see* Hydrochlorothiazide 1009
Newtram (KR) *see* TraMADol 2074
Newtrazole (KR) *see* Itraconazole 1130

Newvast (KR) *see* AtorvaSTATin 194
Newzal (KR) *see* Levocetirizine 1196
Nexadron Oftal (AR) *see* Dexamethasone (Ophthalmic) 602
Nexadron Oftal (AR) *see* Dexamethasone (Systemic) 599
Nexa (ID) *see* Tranexamic Acid 2081
Nexavar (AE, AR, AT, AU, BE, BG, BR, CH, CL, CN, CO, CR, CY, CZ, DE, DK, DO, EC, EE, ES, FI, FR, GB, GR, GT, HK, HN, HR, HU, ID, IE, IL, IS, IT, JP, KR, KW, LB, LT, MT, MX, MY, NI, NL, NO, NZ, PA, PE, PH, PL, PT, PY, QA, RO, RU, SA, SE, SG, SI, SK, SV, TH, TR, TW, UY, VN) *see* SORAfenib 1923
Nexazin (HR) *see* Perindopril 1623
Nexazol (KR) *see* Esomeprazole 771
Nexen (FR) *see* Nimesulide [INT] 1456
Nexiam (BE) *see* Esomeprazole 771
Nexit (CL) *see* HydrOXYzine 1024
Nexito (PH) *see* Escitalopram 765
Nexium IV (MX) *see* Esomeprazole 771
Nexium (AE, AR, AT, AU, BB, BF, BG, BH, BJ, BM, BO, BR, BS, BZ, CH, CI, CL, CN, CO, CY, CZ, DE, DK, DO, EE, ES, ET, FI, GB, GH, GM, GN, GR, GY, HK, HN, HR, ID, IE, IL, IS, IT, JM, JO, JP, KE, KR, KW, LB, LR, LT, MA, ML, MR, MU, MW, MY, NE, NG, NI, NL, NO, NZ, PE, PH, PL, PR, PT, PY, QA, RO, RU, SA, SC, SD, SE, SG, SI, SK, SL, SN, SR, TH, TN, TR, TT, TW, TZ, UG, UY, VE, VN, ZA, ZM, ZW) *see* Esomeprazole 771
Nexium-MUPS (MX) *see* Esomeprazole 771
Nexodal (FI, IE, LT, NL, PT, SE, SI) *see* Naloxone 1419
Nexpro (IN) *see* Esomeprazole 771
Nexum (PK) *see* Esomeprazole 771
Nexxair (FR) *see* Beclomethasone (Nasal) 232
Neynna (ID) *see* Cyproterone and Ethinyl Estradiol [CAN/INT] 532
Nezalast (IN) *see* Azelastine and Fluticasone 214
Nezelex (KR) *see* Mometasone (Nasal) 1391
Nezkil (PK) *see* Linezolid 1217
Niacyn (PL) *see* Niacin 1443
Niagar (BE) *see* Chlorothiazide 426
Niar (BR, MX, PY) *see* Selegiline 1873
Niaspan (CH, DE, FI, GB, HK, IE, NL, PT, SE, TH) *see* Niacin 1443
Niaspan LP (FR) *see* Niacin 1443
Niaspanor (KR) *see* Niacin 1443
Nibelon (VN) *see* Flurbiprofen (Systemic) 906
Nibiol (FR, VN) *see* Nitroxoline [INT] 1469
Nibix (HR) *see* Imatinib 1047
Nicabate (AU) *see* Nicotine 1449
Nicabate Clear (AU) *see* Nicotine 1449
Nicabate CQ (NZ) *see* Nicotine 1449
Nicabate Lozenges (AU) *see* Nicotine 1449
Nicabate Soft Gum (AU) *see* Nicotine 1449
Nicangin (NO) *see* Niacin 1443
Nicardal (IT) *see* NiCARdipine 1446
Nicardia CD (TH) *see* NIFEdipine 1451
Nicardia Retard (TH) *see* NIFEdipine 1451
Nicardia (TH) *see* NIFEdipine 1451
Nicelate (JP) *see* Nalidixic Acid [INT] 1418
Nicene N (ZA) *see* Nitroxoline [INT] 1469
Nichistate (TW) *see* Ticlopidine 2040
Nichospor (ID) *see* Alendronate 79
Nichostan (ID) *see* Mefenamic Acid 1280
Nicizina (AR) *see* Isoniazid 1120
Nicobid (HK) *see* Niacin 1443
Nicobion (DE, FR, PY) *see* Niacinamide 1446
Nicolan TTS (AE) *see* Nicotine 1449
Nicoman (KR) *see* Nicotine 1449
Nicomen (VN) *see* Nicorandil [INT] 1449
Nicomild (TH) *see* Nicotine 1449
Nicopass sans sucre menthe fraicheur (FR) *see* Nicotine 1449
Nicopass sans sucre reghsse menthe (FR) *see* Nicotine 1449
Nicopatch (FR) *see* Nicotine 1449
Nicopion (KR) *see* BuPROPion 305
Nicorest (FR) *see* Nicotine 1449
Nicorette (AE, AT, AU, BE, BF, BG, BH, BJ, BR, CH, CI, CL, CN, CO, CR, CY, CZ, DE, DK, EC, EE, EG, ES, ET, FI, FR, GB, GH, GM, GN, GR, GT, HK, HN, HR, HU, IL, IQ, IR, IS, IT, JO, JP, KE, KW, LB, LR, LT, LU, LY, MA, ML, MR, MT, MU, MW, MY, NE, NG, NI, NL, NO, NZ, OM, PA, PL, QA, RO, RU, SA, SC, SD, SE, SG, SI, SK, SL, SN, SV, SY, TH, TN, TW, TZ, UG, VE, YE, ZA, ZM, ZW) *see* Nicotine 1449
Nicorette Fruit (FR) *see* Nicotine 1449
Nicorette Inhaler (AU) *see* Nicotine 1449
Nicorette Menthe (AE, BH, CY, EG, FR, IL, IQ, IR, JO, KW, LB, LY, OM, QA, SA, SY, YE) *see* Nicotine 1449
Nicorette Menthe Fraiche (FR) *see* Nicotine 1449
Nicorette Orange (FR) *see* Nicotine 1449
Nicorette Orange sans sucre (FR) *see* Nicotine 1449
Nicostop (PT) *see* Nicotine 1449
Nicostop (VN) *see* BuPROPion 305
Nicotab (SE) *see* Nicotine 1449
Nicotabs (TH) *see* Niacin 1443
Nicotibine (BE, IL, LU) *see* Isoniazid 1120
Nicotinamide (IT) *see* Niacinamide 1446
Nicotinell (AE, AT, AU, BE, BG, BH, CH, DE, DK, FI, FR, GB, GR, IE, IS, IT, KW, LT, NL, NO, PL, PT, SA, SE, SI, TR) *see* Nicotine 1449
Nicotinell Chewing Gum (HK) *see* Nicotine 1449
Nicotinell Fruit sans sucre (FR) *see* Nicotine 1449
Nicotinell Menthe sans sucre (FR) *see* Nicotine 1449
Nicotinell Mint Lozenge (KR) *see* Nicotine 1449
Nicotinell TTS (AE, AR, BB, BF, BH, BJ, BM, BS, BZ, CI, CL, CY, EE, EG, ET, FR, GH, GM, GN, GY, HK, HR, HU, IL, IQ, IR, JM, JO, KE, KR, KW, LB, LR, LU, LY, MA, ML, MR, MU, MW, MX, MY, NE, NG, NZ, OM, PH, PR, QA, SA, SC, SD, SL, SN, SR, SY, TH, TN, TT, TW, TZ, UG, UY, YE, ZM, ZW) *see* Nicotine 1449
Nicotinic Acid (AU) *see* Niacin 1443
Nicotinsaureamid Jenapharm (DE) *see* Niacinamide 1446
Nicotrans (IT) *see* Nicotine 1449
Nicotrol Gum (NZ) *see* Nicotine 1449
Nicovitol (AT) *see* Niacinamide 1446
Nicozid (IT) *see* Isoniazid 1120
Nidazea (BE) *see* MetroNIDAZOLE (Topical) 1357
Nidazole (AE, BH, JO, QA, SA) *see* MetroNIDAZOLE (Systemic) 1353
Nide (IT) *see* Nimesulide [INT] 1456
Nidem (AU) *see* Gliclazide [CAN/INT] 964
Nidil (TW) *see* Nicorandil [INT] 1449
Nidip (CO) *see* NiMODipine 1456
Nidipin (HU) *see* NIFEdipine 1451
Nidol (HK, HU, PK, TH) *see* Nimesulide [INT] 1456
Nidolid (PH) *see* Nimesulide [INT] 1456
Nidolium (TW) *see* Domperidone [CAN/INT] 666
Nidran (CN, JP, KR) *see* Nimustine [INT] 1457
Nidrane (UY) *see* Methotrimeprazine [CAN/INT] 1329
Nidrazid (CZ) *see* Isoniazid 1120
Nidrel (FR) *see* Nitrendipine [INT] 1463
Nifadil (HR) *see* NIFEdipine 1451
Nifangin (FI) *see* NIFEdipine 1451
Nifar (BF, BJ, CI, ET, GH, GM, GN, KE, LR, MA, ML, MR, MU, MW, NE, NG, SC, SD, SL, SN, TN, TZ, UG, ZM, ZW) *see* NIFEdipine 1451
Nifar-GB (MX) *see* NIFEdipine 1451
Nifdemin (FI) *see* NIFEdipine 1451
Nifebene (AT) *see* NIFEdipine 1451
Nifecard XL (SG) *see* NIFEdipine 1451
Nifecard (AE, AT, BH, HR, JO, SA) *see* NIFEdipine 1451
Nifecor (DE) *see* NIFEdipine 1451

Nifedepat (DE) *see* NIFEdipine 1451
Nifedicor (IT) *see* NIFEdipine 1451
Nifedigel (MX) *see* NIFEdipine 1451
NIfedilat (ZA) *see* NIFEdipine 1451
Nifedilong (IL) *see* NIFEdipine 1451
Nifedine (IN) *see* NIFEdipine 1451
Nifedin (IT) *see* NIFEdipine 1451
Nifedipin AL (HU) *see* NIFEdipine 1451
Nifedipin (HR) *see* NIFEdipine 1451
Nifedipin Pharmavit (HU) *see* NIFEdipine 1451
Nifedipin-ratiopharm (LU) *see* NIFEdipine 1451
Nifedipin Stada (LU) *see* NIFEdipine 1451
Nifedipresc MR (GB) *see* NIFEdipine 1451
Nifedix SR (KR) *see* NIFEdipine 1451
Nifehexal (AU, LU, VN) *see* NIFEdipine 1451
Nifelat (AR, HK, SG, TH) *see* NIFEdipine 1451
Nifelat-Q (TH) *see* NIFEdipine 1451
Nifelat Q (TR) *see* NIFEdipine 1451
Nifensar (PE) *see* NIFEdipine 1451
Nifensar Retard (PE) *see* NIFEdipine 1451
Niferon CR (KR) *see* NIFEdipine 1451
Nifeslow (LU) *see* NIFEdipine 1451
Nifestad (PH) *see* NIFEdipine 1451
Nifezzard (MX) *see* NIFEdipine 1451
Nificard (CY, EG, IQ, IR, KW, LB, LY, OM, QA, SY, YE) *see* NIFEdipine 1451
Nifipen (AE, BH, CY, EG, IQ, IR, JO, KW, LB, LY, OM, QA, SA, SY, YE) *see* NIFEdipine 1451
Niflactol (ES) *see* Niflumic Acid [INT] 1454
Niflam (IT) *see* Niflumic Acid [INT] 1454
Niflugel (BE, CH, CZ, FR) *see* Niflumic Acid [INT] 1454
Nifluril (BE, CH, CZ, FR, LU, PT) *see* Niflumic Acid [INT] 1454
Niften (IE) *see* NIFEdipine 1451
Nifuran (NZ) *see* Nitrofurantoin 1463
Nifurantin (CZ) *see* Nitrofurantoin 1463
Nifuroxazide EG (BE) *see* Nifuroxazide [INT] 1454
Nifuroxazide-Eurogenerics (LU) *see* Nifuroxazide [INT] 1454
Nifuroxazide-Ratiopharm (FR) *see* Nifuroxazide [INT] 1454
Nifuryl (EC) *see* Nitrofurantoin 1463
Nifutoin (TW) *see* Nitrofurantoin 1463
Niglinar (PE) *see* Nitroglycerin 1465
Nikofrenon (DE) *see* Nicotine 1449
Nikoril (PT) *see* Nicorandil [INT] 1449
Nilapur (ID) *see* Allopurinol 90
Nilatika (ID) *see* Metoclopramide 1345
Nildacin (ID) *see* Clindamycin (Systemic) 460
Nilgar M-15 (PH) *see* Pioglitazone and Metformin 1655
Nilgar M-30 (PH) *see* Pioglitazone and Metformin 1655
Nilgar (VN) *see* Pioglitazone 1654
Nilox (DE) *see* Nitroxoline [INT] 1469
Nilstat (AE) *see* Nystatin (Oral) 1481
Nimax (KR) *see* Nimesulide [INT] 1456
Nimbex (AE, AR, AT, AU, BB, BE, BH, BM, BS, BZ, CH, CL, CN, CR, CY, CZ, DE, DK, DO, EC, EG, ES, FI, FR, GB, GR, GT, GY, HK, HN, HU, IE, IL, IQ, IR, IT, JM, JO, KR, KW, LB, LT, LU, LY, MX, MY, NI, NL, NO, OM, PA, PE, PL, PR, PT, QA, RO, RU, SA, SE, SI, SR, SV, SY, TH, TR, TT, TW, YE) *see* Cisatracurium 447
Nimbisan (IT) *see* Brotizolam [INT] 293
Nimbium (BR, CO) *see* Cisatracurium 447
Nimed (BG, CZ, ID, PT) *see* Nimesulide [INT] 1456
Nimegen (MY, SG) *see* ISOtretinoin 1127
Nimelid (VE) *see* Nimesulide [INT] 1456
Nimel (IN) *see* Nimesulide [INT] 1456
Ni Meng Shu (CN) *see* Pipotiazine [CAN/INT] 1660
Nimenrix (AU, BE, CY, CZ, DE, DK, EE, ES, FR, GB, HK, HR, IS, LT, NL, NO, QA, SE, SI, SK) *see* Meningococcal Polysaccharide (Groups A / C / Y and W-135) Tetanus Toxoid Conjugate Vaccine [CAN/INT] 1290
Nimepast (CL) *see* Nimesulide [INT] 1456
Nimesil (IT, PL) *see* Nimesulide [INT] 1456
Nimesol (PY) *see* Nimesulide [INT] 1456
Nimesulene (IT) *see* Nimesulide [INT] 1456
Nimesulide Dorom (IT) *see* Nimesulide [INT] 1456
Nimesulide GNR (IT) *see* Nimesulide [INT] 1456
Nimesulide UCB (IT) *see* Nimesulide [INT] 1456
Nimicor (CL) *see* Simvastatin 1890
Nimicor (IT) *see* NiCARdipine 1446
Nimind (IN) *see* Nimesulide [INT] 1456
Nimm (HK, TR) *see* Nimesulide [INT] 1456
Nimobal (BR) *see* NiMODipine 1456
Nimodilat (AR) *see* NiMODipine 1456
Nimodin (PH) *see* NiMODipine 1456
Nimodipino Bayvit (ES) *see* NiMODipine 1456
Nimotop (AE, AT, AU, BB, BE, BG, BH, BM, BS, BZ, CH, CL, CN, CO, CR, CY, CZ, DE, DK, EC, EE, EG, ES, FI, FR, GB, GR, GT, GY, HK, HN, HR, HU, ID, IE, IL, IT, JM, JO, KR, KW, LB, LU, MX, MY, NI, NL, NO, NZ, PA, PE, PK, PL, PT, PY, QA, RO, RU, SA, SE, SG, SI, SR, SV, TH, TR, TT, TW, UY, VE, VN, ZA) *see* NiMODipine 1456
Nimotop (PT) *see* Nimesulide [INT] 1456
Nims (IT) *see* Nimesulide [INT] 1456
Nimulid (IN) *see* Nimesulide [INT] 1456
Nimus (CL) *see* Bezafibrate [CAN/INT] 261
Ninazo (VE) *see* Naphazoline (Nasal) 1426
Nincort (CN, TW) *see* Triamcinolone (Topical) 2100
Nincort (TW) *see* Triamcinolone (Systemic) 2099
Ninlium (TH) *see* Domperidone [CAN/INT] 666
Ninur (HR) *see* Nitrofurantoin 1463
Niofen Flu (PY) *see* Pseudoephedrine and Ibuprofen 1743
Niofen (PE) *see* Fusidic Acid (Topical) [CAN/INT] 943
Niotal (IT) *see* Zolpidem 2212
Nipatra (GB) *see* Sildenafil 1882
Nipent (BE, DE, ES, FR, GB, GR, IT, KR, NL) *see* Pentostatin 1618
Nipocin (HR) *see* Dibekacin [INT] 616
Nipresol (MX) *see* Metoprolol 1350
Nipride (BE, CH, FR, GB, IE, LU, NL, QA, SA) *see* Nitroprusside 1467
Niprina (ES) *see* Nitrendipine [INT] 1463
Niprusodio (UY) *see* Nitroprusside 1467
Nipruss (DE, EG, JO, LU) *see* Nitroprusside 1467
Nipurol (VE) *see* Allopurinol 90
Niquitin (BR, CO, MX) *see* Nicotine 1449
Niquitin Clear (HR, RO) *see* Nicotine 1449
Niquitin CQ Clear (IL) *see* Nicotine 1449
Niquitin CQ (HR, IL, SG) *see* Nicotine 1449
Niquitin Mint (TW) *see* Nicotine 1449
Niquitin sans sucre (FR) *see* Nicotine 1449
Nirapel (AR) *see* Nitrendipine [INT] 1463
Nirax (TW) *see* HydrOXYzine 1024
Nircadel (DK) *see* Lercanidipine [INT] 1181
Nirliv (TH) *see* Levofloxacin (Systemic) 1197
Nirmadil (ID) *see* Felodipine 850
Nirmet (TH) *see* MetroNIDAZOLE (Systemic) 1353
Nirocef (PH) *see* Cefdinir 376
Nirulid (DK) *see* AMILoride 113
Nirva (PH) *see* CloZAPine 490
Nirvaxal (IL) *see* Clidinium and Chlordiazepoxide 460
Nisal (IT) *see* Nimesulide [INT] 1456
Nise (PE) *see* Nimesulide [INT] 1456
Nisetron (CO) *see* Granisetron 983
Nisirol (PY) *see* Lisinopril 1226
Nisisco (FR) *see* Valsartan and Hydrochlorothiazide 2129
Nisis (FR) *see* Valsartan 2127
Nislev (ID) *see* Levofloxacin (Systemic) 1197
Nisodipen (AR) *see* Nisoldipine 1459
Nisoldin (KR) *see* Nisoldipine 1459
Nisolon-M (KR) *see* MethylPREDNISolone 1340

Nisom (CO) *see* NiMODipine ... 1456
Nisona (PE) *see* PredniSONE ... 1706
Ni Song (CN) *see* Ketorolac (Systemic) ... 1146
Nistaken (MX) *see* Propafenone ... 1725
Nistatina Metronidazol L.C.H. (CL) *see* Metronidazole and Nystatin [CAN/INT] ... 1358
Nistrom (IN) *see* Acenocoumarol [CAN/INT] ... 30
Nisulid (BR, CH) *see* Nimesulide [INT] ... 1456
Nisulin (TW) *see* Betahistine [CAN/INT] ... 252
Nisural (CL) *see* Nimesulide [INT] ... 1456
Nitan (MX) *see* Nitroprusside ... 1467
Nitanid (EC) *see* Nitazoxanide ... 1461
Nitarid (IN) *see* Nitazoxanide ... 1461
Nitavan (IN) *see* Nitrazepam [CAN/INT] ... 1461
Nitidex (AR) *see* DULoxetine ... 698
Nitidin (PY) *see* Ranitidine ... 1777
Nitoman (DE, DK, IE, PT, TW) *see* Tetrabenazine ... 2016
Nitracor (PL) *see* Nitroglycerin ... 1465
Nitradisc (LU, MX, PT) *see* Nitroglycerin ... 1465
Nitradisc TTS (GR) *see* Nitroglycerin ... 1465
Nitrados (NZ, SG) *see* Nitrazepam [CAN/INT] ... 1461
Nitral (ID) *see* Nitroglycerin ... 1465
Nitramin (GR) *see* Isosorbide Mononitrate ... 1126
Nitrapan (BR) *see* Nitrazepam [CAN/INT] ... 1461
Nitravet (IN) *see* Nitrazepam [CAN/INT] ... 1461
Nitrazepam (PL) *see* Nitrazepam [CAN/INT] ... 1461
Nitre AbZ (DE) *see* Nitrendipine [INT] ... 1463
Nitredon (TR) *see* Nitrazepam [CAN/INT] ... 1461
Nitregamma (DE) *see* Nitrendipine [INT] ... 1463
Nitren 1A Pharma (DE) *see* Nitrendipine [INT] ... 1463
Nitren acis (DE) *see* Nitrendipine [INT] ... 1463
Nitrencord (BR) *see* Nitrendipine [INT] ... 1463
Nitrendepat (DE) *see* Nitrendipine [INT] ... 1463
Nitrendi-BASF (DE) *see* Nitrendipine [INT] ... 1463
Nitrendil (AR) *see* Nitrendipine [INT] ... 1463
Nitrendimerck (DE) *see* Nitrendipine [INT] ... 1463
Nitrendipin AL (DE) *see* Nitrendipine [INT] ... 1463
Nitrendipin Apogepha (DE) *see* Nitrendipine [INT] ... 1463
Nitrendipin Atid (DE) *see* Nitrendipine [INT] ... 1463
!Nitrendipin Basics (DE) *see* Nitrendipine [INT] ... 1463
Nitrendipin beta (DE) *see* Nitrendipine [INT] ... 1463
nitrendipin corax (DE) *see* Nitrendipine [INT] ... 1463
Nitrendipin Heumann (DE) *see* Nitrendipine [INT] ... 1463
Nitrendipin Jenapharm (DE) *see* Nitrendipine [INT] ... 1463
Nitrendipin Lindo (DE) *see* Nitrendipine [INT] ... 1463
Nitrendipino Bayvit (ES) *see* Nitrendipine [INT] ... 1463
Nitrendipino Ratiopharm (ES) *see* Nitrendipine [INT] ... 1463
Nitrendipin-ratiopharm (DE) *see* Nitrendipine [INT] ... 1463
Nitrendipin Stada (DE) *see* Nitrendipine [INT] ... 1463
nitrendipin von ct (DE) *see* Nitrendipine [INT] ... 1463
Nitrendypina (PL) *see* Nitrendipine [INT] ... 1463
Nitren Lich (DE) *see* Nitrendipine [INT] ... 1463
Nitrensal (DE) *see* Nitrendipine [INT] ... 1463
Nitrepress (DE) *see* Nitrendipine [INT] ... 1463
Nitre-Puren (DE) *see* Nitrendipine [INT] ... 1463
Nitrest (IN) *see* Zolpidem ... 2212
Nit-Ret (CZ) *see* Nitroglycerin ... 1465
Nitriate (FR, VN) *see* Nitroprusside ... 1467
Nitriderm TTS (FR) *see* Nitroglycerin ... 1465
Nitrobaat (BE, NL) *see* Nitroglycerin ... 1465
Nitro-Bid (MY) *see* Nitroglycerin ... 1465
Nitrocard (PL) *see* Nitroglycerin ... 1465
Nitrocerin (GR) *see* Nitroglycerin ... 1465
Nitrocine 5 (AE, BH, CY, EG, IQ, IR, JO, KW, LB, LY, OM, QA, SA, SY, YE) *see* Nitroglycerin ... 1465
Nitrocine (CN, EE, ID, IE) *see* Nitroglycerin ... 1465
Nitrocontin (BF, BJ, CI, ET, GH, GM, GN, IE, IN, KE, LR, MA, ML, MR, MU, MW, NE, NG, SC, SD, SL, SN, TN, TW, TZ, UG, ZA, ZM, ZW) *see* Nitroglycerin ... 1465
Nitrocontin Continus (AE, BH, CY, EG, IQ, IR, JO, KW, LB, LY, OM, QA, SA, SY, YE) *see* Nitroglycerin ... 1465
Nitrocor (IT) *see* Nitroglycerin ... 1465
Nitroderm TTS-5 (NI) *see* Nitroglycerin ... 1465
Nitroderm TTS (AE, AR, AT, BB, BE, BF, BH, BJ, BM, BR, BS, BZ, CH, CI, CL, CY, DE, EC, EG, ES, ET, GH, GM, GN, GY, HR, HU, IL, IN, IQ, IR, IT, JM, JO, KE, KW, LB, LR, LU, LY, MA, ML, MR, MU, MW, NE, NG, NZ, OM, PL, PT, QA, SA, SC, SD, SL, SN, SR, SY, TN, TT, TW, TZ, UG, YE, ZA, ZM, ZW) *see* Nitroglycerin ... 1465
Nitroderm TTS Ext (CZ) *see* Nitroglycerin ... 1465
Nitroderm (VE) *see* Nitroglycerin ... 1465
Nitrodisc (BB, BM, BS, BZ, GY, JM, MY, SR, TT) *see* Nitroglycerin ... 1465
Nitrodom (AR) *see* Nitroglycerin ... 1465
Nitro-Dur 10 (IL) *see* Nitroglycerin ... 1465
Nitro-Dur (AE, AU, CH, ES, HU, IT, NO, PL, PT, SA) *see* Nitroglycerin ... 1465
Nitrodyl (GR, LU) *see* Nitroglycerin ... 1465
Nitrodyl TTS (GR) *see* Nitroglycerin ... 1465
Nitro (FI, HU) *see* Nitroglycerin ... 1465
Nitrofurantoin-ratiopharm (LU) *see* Nitrofurantoin ... 1463
Nitrofurantoin "Dak" (DK) *see* Nitrofurantoin ... 1463
Nitrogesic (UY) *see* Nitroglycerin ... 1465
Nitroglycerinum (PL) *see* Nitroglycerin ... 1465
Nitroglycerinum prolongatum (PL) *see* Nitroglycerin ... 1465
Nitrol (AE, BH, CY, EG, IQ, IR, JO, KW, LB, LY, OM, QA, SA, SY, YE) *see* Nitroglycerin ... 1465
Nitrolingual (AE, AT, BE, CH, DE, DK, GB, GR, HK, HU, IE, KR, LT, LU, NL, PH, PT, SE, SI, TW) *see* Nitroglycerin ... 1465
Nitrolingual Pumpspray (AU) *see* Nitroglycerin ... 1465
Nitrolingual Spray (KR, NZ, PH) *see* Nitroglycerin ... 1465
Nitrol R (JP) *see* Isosorbide Dinitrate ... 1124
Nitro Mack (LU) *see* Nitroglycerin ... 1465
Nitro-Mack (PL) *see* Nitroglycerin ... 1465
Nitro Mack Retard (AE, AT, BH, CY, CZ, EG, GR, IQ, IR, JO, KW, LB, LY, OM, QA, SA, SY, YE) *see* Nitroglycerin ... 1465
Nitromack Retard (PY) *see* Nitroglycerin ... 1465
Nitromex (NO, SE) *see* Nitroglycerin ... 1465
Nitromint Aerosol (BF, BJ, CI, ET, GH, GM, GN, KE, LR, MA, ML, MR, MU, MW, NE, NG, SC, SD, SL, SN, TN, TZ, UG, ZA, ZM, ZW) *see* Nitroglycerin ... 1465
Nitromint (HU, PL, SK, TH) *see* Nitroglycerin ... 1465
Nitromint Retard (AE, BB, BH, BM, BS, BZ, CY, EG, GY, IQ, IR, JM, JO, KW, LB, LY, OM, QA, SA, SR, SY, TT, YE) *see* Nitroglycerin ... 1465
Nitrom (TW) *see* Nitrazepam [CAN/INT] ... 1461
Nitronal Aqueous (PH) *see* Nitroglycerin ... 1465
Nitronal (FR) *see* Nitroglycerin ... 1465
Nitronal Spray (FR) *see* Nitroglycerin ... 1465
Nitrong (BE, LU) *see* Nitroglycerin ... 1465
Nitrong Retard (AT, GR) *see* Nitroglycerin ... 1465
Nitro-Pflaster (DE) *see* Nitroglycerin ... 1465
Nitro-Pflaster-ratiopharm (LU) *see* Nitroglycerin ... 1465
Nitroplast (ES) *see* Nitroglycerin ... 1465
Nitro Pohl (HU) *see* Nitroglycerin ... 1465
Nitroprus (BR) *see* Nitroprusside ... 1467
Nitroprusiato de sodio-ecar (CO) *see* Nitroprusside ... 1467
Nitroprusiato de sodio (PE, PY, VE) *see* Nitroprusside ... 1467
Nitroprussiat Fides (ES) *see* Nitroprusside ... 1467
Nitrosid (FI) *see* Isosorbide Dinitrate ... 1124
Nitrosid Retard (FI) *see* Isosorbide Dinitrate ... 1124
Nitrosorbide (BF, BJ, CI, ET, GH, GM, GN, IT, KE, LR, MA, ML, MR, MU, MW, NE, NG, SC, SD, SL, SN, TN, TZ, UG, ZM, ZW) *see* Isosorbide Dinitrate ... 1124
Nitrosorbon (DE, PH) *see* Isosorbide Dinitrate ... 1124
Nitrostat (TW) *see* Nitroglycerin ... 1465
Nitroxolin-MIP Forte (BG) *see* Nitroxoline [INT] ... 1469
Nitrozell Retard (AT, NL) *see* Nitroglycerin ... 1465

Nitrumon (BE, LU) *see* Carmustine ... 364
Nittyfor (HU) *see* Permethrin ... 1627
Niuliva (SG) *see* Hepatitis B Immune Globulin (Human) ... 1002
Nivadil (CH, DE, JP) *see* Nilvadipine [INT] ... 1456
Nivalen (AE, BF, BH, BJ, CI, CY, EG, ET, GH, GM, GN, IQ, IR, JO, KE, KW, LB, LR, LY, MA, ML, MR, MU, MW, NE, NG, OM, QA, SA, SC, SD, SL, SN, SY, TN, TZ, UG, YE, ZM, ZW) *see* Diazepam ... 613
Nivalin (BG, DE, HU, LT, PL, RU) *see* Galantamine ... 946
Nivaquine (AR, BE, FR, LB, LU) *see* Chloroquine ... 424
Nivelin (PY) *see* Clorazepate ... 487
Nivemycin (GB, IE) *see* Neomycin ... 1436
Nivestim (AU, GB, HK, MY, TR) *see* Filgrastim ... 875
Nix (BE, BG, DK, EE, FI, GR, IT, NO, PT, SE, SI) *see* Permethrin ... 1627
Nix Cream (BB, BM, BS, BZ, GY, JM, PR, SR, TT) *see* Permethrin ... 1627
Nix Creme Rinse (LU) *see* Permethrin ... 1627
Nix Dermal Cream (BB, BM, BS, BZ, GY, JM, PR, SR, TT) *see* Permethrin ... 1627
Nixtensyn (PH) *see* Diazepam ... 613
Nizac (AU) *see* Nizatidine ... 1471
Nizaractine (KR) *see* Nizatidine ... 1471
Nizatid (KR) *see* Nizatidine ... 1471
Nizax (DE, DK, FI, IT, NO) *see* Nizatidine ... 1471
Nizaxid (CL, FR, LU, PT) *see* Nizatidine ... 1471
Niz Creme (ZA) *see* Ketoconazole (Topical) ... 1145
Nizon (HR) *see* PredniSONE ... 1706
Nizoral 2% Cream (AU, NZ, PH) *see* Ketoconazole (Topical) ... 1145
Nizoral (AE, AT, BB, BE, BF, BG, BH, BJ, BM, BS, CH, CI, CN, CY, CZ, DE, DK, EE, EG, ET, FI, GH, GM, GN, GY, HK, ID, IE, IL, IQ, IR, IT, JM, JO, KE, KW, LB, LR, LT, LY, MA, ML, MR, MU, MW, MY, NE, NG, NL, OM, PH, PK, PL, PR, QA, RO, RU, SA, SC, SD, SG, SK, SL, SN, SR, SY, TH, TN, TR, TT, TZ, UG, UY, VE, VN, YE, ZA, ZM, ZW) *see* Ketoconazole (Topical) ... 1145
Nizoral (AE, AU, BB, BE, BH, BM, BS, CH, CN, CO, CY, CZ, DK, EC, EE, EG, FI, FR, GY, HK, ID, IL, IT, JM, JO, KW, LB, NL, NZ, PE, PH, PR, PY, QA, RU, SA, SG, SR, TH, TR, TT, TW, UY, VE, ZA) *see* Ketoconazole (Systemic) ... 1144
Nizoral Cream (GB, IE) *see* Ketoconazole (Topical) ... 1145
Nizoral Shampoo (DE, NZ, PH) *see* Ketoconazole (Topical) ... 1145
Niz Shampoo (ZA) *see* Ketoconazole (Topical) ... 1145
Noacid (BG) *see* Pantoprazole ... 1570
Noacid (UY) *see* Calcium Carbonate ... 327
Noac (UY) *see* Nabumetone ... 1411
Noalgos (IT) *see* Nimesulide [INT] ... 1456
Noan (BR, IT) *see* Diazepam ... 613
Noax (SI) *see* TraMADol ... 2074
Nobafon (TW) *see* Ibuprofen ... 1032
Nobelin (TW) *see* LevETIRAcetam ... 1191
Nobelzin (JP, KR) *see* Zinc Acetate ... 2199
Noberbar (JP) *see* PHENobarbital ... 1632
Nobiprox (KR) *see* Ciclopirox ... 433
Nobiten (BE) *see* Nebivolol ... 1434
Nobligan (NO, SE) *see* TraMADol ... 2074
Nobrium (AE) *see* Medazepam [INT] ... 1277
No-Burn (JO) *see* Silver Sulfadiazine ... 1887
Nobzol-1 (CO) *see* Fluconazole ... 885
Nobzol-2 (CO) *see* Fluconazole ... 885
Nocid (TH) *see* Omeprazole ... 1508
Noclaud (RO, SK) *see* Cilostazol ... 437
Noclot (PK) *see* Clopidogrel ... 484
Noctaderm (IN) *see* Doxepin (Topical) ... 678
Noctal (BR) *see* Estazolam ... 775
Noctamid (AT, BE, CH, CY, DE, EG, ES, GR, IE, NL, NZ, PT, TR, ZA) *see* Lormetazepam [INT] ... 1247
Noctamide (FR) *see* Lormetazepam [INT] ... 1247
Nocte (CR, GT, NI, PA, SV) *see* Zolpidem ... 2212
Nocte Sublingual (AR) *see* Zolpidem ... 2212
Noctilan (CL) *see* Brotizolam [INT] ... 293
Noctisson (AE, BG, BH, EG, IQ, IR, JO, LY, OM, QA, SY, YE) *see* Desmopressin ... 594
Noctofer (PL) *see* Lormetazepam [INT] ... 1247
Nocton (CL) *see* Lormetazepam [INT] ... 1247
Noctosom (IL) *see* Flurazepam ... 906
Nocturno (IL) *see* Zopiclone [CAN/INT] ... 2217
Nocutil (CH) *see* Desmopressin ... 594
Nodescrón (MX) *see* Vecuronium ... 2144
Nodict (IN, VN) *see* Naltrexone ... 1422
Nodik (GT) *see* Nitazoxanide ... 1461
Nodoff (TW) *see* OLANZapine ... 1491
Nodo (UY) *see* Nimesulide [INT] ... 1456
Nofat (PH) *see* Orlistat ... 1520
Nofaxin (KR) *see* Levofloxacin (Systemic) ... 1197
Noflam (NZ) *see* Naproxen ... 1427
Noflexin (ID) *see* Pefloxacin [INT] ... 1588
Nogerd (PK) *see* Itopride [INT] ... 1130
Nogermin (ES) *see* Nalidixic Acid [INT] ... 1418
Nograine (MX) *see* SUMAtriptan ... 1953
Nogram (DE) *see* Nalidixic Acid [INT] ... 1418
Nogrel (PH) *see* Clopidogrel ... 484
Nogren (ID) *see* Acetaminophen, Aspirin, and Caffeine ... 37
Noiafren (ES) *see* CloBAZam ... 465
Noken (JO) *see* Naproxen ... 1427
Noklot (PH) *see* Clopidogrel ... 484
Nolcer (PH) *see* Nizatidine ... 1471
Nolectin (PE) *see* Captopril ... 342
Nolicin (CZ, EE, HR, HU, LT, PL, RU, SI, SK) *see* Norfloxacin ... 1475
Noliprel (BG, CZ, EE, LT, PL, RU) *see* Perindopril and Indapamide [CAN/INT] ... 1626
Nolol (DO) *see* Atenolol ... 189
Nolotil (ES, PT) *see* Dipyrone [INT] ... 653
Nolpaza (EE, SK) *see* Pantoprazole ... 1570
Nolvadex-D (AU, CO, EE, HK, IE, MY, NZ, PY, SG, TH, UY) *see* Tamoxifen ... 1971
Nolvadex (AE, AT, AU, BB, BE, BF, BG, BH, BJ, BM, BR, BS, BZ, CI, CL, CR, CY, DE, DO, EG, ES, ET, FI, FR, GH, GM, GN, GR, GT, GY, HK, HN, HR, IE, IL, IN, IQ, IR, IT, JM, JO, KE, KR, KW, LB, LR, LU, LY, MA, ML, MR, MU, MW, MX, NE, NG, NI, NL, NO, NZ, OM, PA, PK, PL, PR, PT, QA, SA, SC, SD, SE, SG, SL, SN, SR, SV, SY, TN, TR, TT, TW, TZ, UG, VE, VN, YE, ZM, ZW) *see* Tamoxifen ... 1971
Nomactril (MX) *see* Octreotide ... 1485
Nomcramp (ZA) *see* Dicyclomine ... 622
Nomi-Nox (TW) *see* Donepezil ... 668
Nonafact (AT, BE, BG, CZ, EE, GR, HN, HR, ID, IE, IT, LT, MT, NL, PL, RO, RU, SE, SK, TR) *see* Factor IX (Human) ... 840
Nonasma (TW) *see* Metaproterenol ... 1307
Non-Preg (TH) *see* MedroxyPROGESTERone ... 1277
Nonsic (VN) *see* Fenoprofen ... 857
Noodis (BE, HU, LU) *see* Piracetam [INT] ... 1661
Noostan (AR, BE, PT) *see* Piracetam [INT] ... 1661
Nootron (BR) *see* Piracetam [INT] ... 1661
Nootrop (BE, DE, SE) *see* Piracetam [INT] ... 1661
Nootropicon (AR) *see* Piracetam [INT] ... 1661
Nootropil (AE, AT, BE, BG, BH, BR, CH, CY, CZ, DE, EC, EE, EG, ES, FI, GB, HK, HU, ID, IN, IT, KW, LB, LT, LU, MX, MY, NL, NO, PE, PH, PK, PL, PT, QA, RO, RU, SA, SE, SG, SI, SK, TH, TR, UY, ZA) *see* Piracetam [INT] ... 1661
Nootropyl (CL, FR, VN) *see* Piracetam [INT] ... 1661
Noottropil (JO) *see* Piracetam [INT] ... 1661
Nopatic (MX) *see* Gabapentin ... 943
Nopen (PH) *see* Naproxen ... 1427
Noperten (ID) *see* Lisinopril ... 1226

Nopil (AE, BH, CY, EG, IQ, IR, JO, KW, LB, LY, OM, QA, SA, SY, YE) *see* Sulfamethoxazole and Trimethoprim ... 1946
Nopral (AR) *see* Modafinil ... 1386
Nopreg Pill (VN) *see* Mifepristone ... 1366
Noprenia (ID) *see* RisperiDONE ... 1818
Nopres (ID) *see* FLUoxetine ... 899
Noprofen (TW) *see* Fenoprofen ... 857
Noprostol (ID) *see* Misoprostol ... 1379
Noptic (CL) *see* Eszopiclone ... 793
Norace (MX) *see* Norethindrone and Mestranol ... 1475
Noracin (QA) *see* Norfloxacin ... 1475
Noracod (QA) *see* Acetaminophen and Codeine ... 36
Noractone (AE, JO) *see* Spironolactone ... 1931
Noradrenalina (DO, GT, HN, PA) *see* Norepinephrine ... 1472
Noradrenalina Tartrato (IT) *see* Norepinephrine ... 1472
Noradrenaline Aguettant (FR) *see* Norepinephrine ... 1472
Noradrenaline (GB) *see* Norepinephrine ... 1472
Nor-Algifort (DO, GT, HN, SV) *see* Dexketoprofen [INT] ... 603
Noranat (AR, PY) *see* Indapamide ... 1065
Noranat SR (AR) *see* Indapamide ... 1065
Norapred (MX) *see* PredniSONE ... 1706
Noratak (CH, IL) *see* Nesiritide ... 1439
Norbactin (BF, BJ, CI, ET, GH, GM, GN, KE, LR, MA, ML, MR, MU, MW, NE, NG, SC, SD, SL, SN, TH, TN, TZ, UG, ZM, ZW) *see* Norfloxacin ... 1475
Norbactin Eye Drops (BF, BJ, CI, ET, GH, GM, GN, IN, KE, LR, MA, ML, MR, MU, MW, NE, NG, SC, SD, SL, SN, TN, TZ, UG, ZM, ZW) *see* Norfloxacin ... 1475
Norboral (DO, GT, HN, NI, SV) *see* GlyBURIDE ... 972
Norcetam (JO) *see* Piracetam [INT] ... 1661
Norcipen (JO) *see* Ampicillin ... 141
Norcolut (BB, BM, BS, BZ, EE, GY, HK, HU, JM, MY, PR, SR, TT, VN) *see* Norethindrone ... 1473
Norcuron (AE, AR, AT, AU, BE, BG, BH, CH, CL, CN, CY, CZ, DE, DK, EE, EG, ES, FI, FR, GB, GR, HK, HN, HR, HU, ID, IE, IL, IN, IQ, IR, IT, JO, KR, KW, LB, LU, LY, MT, MX, NL, NO, NZ, OM, PE, PH, PK, PL, PT, QA, RU, SA, SE, SI, SK, SY, TH, TR, VE, VN, YE) *see* Vecuronium ... 2144
Norcutin (MY, SG) *see* Norethindrone ... 1473
Nor-Dacef (AE, BH, CY, EG, IL, IQ, IR, JO, KW, LB, LY, OM, QA, SA, SY, YE) *see* Cefadroxil ... 372
Nordet (MX) *see* Ethinyl Estradiol and Levonorgestrel ... 803
Nordette 21 (NZ, TH) *see* Ethinyl Estradiol and Levonorgestrel ... 803
Nordette 28 (NZ, TH) *see* Ethinyl Estradiol and Levonorgestrel ... 803
Nordette (AE, AR, AU, BF, BH, BJ, CI, CL, CO, ET, GH, GM, GN, GR, HK, IL, KE, KW, LR, MA, ML, MR, MU, MW, MY, NE, NG, PH, QA, SA, SC, SD, SL, SN, TN, TZ, UG, ZA, ZM, ZW) *see* Ethinyl Estradiol and Levonorgestrel ... 803
Nordilet (JO, KR) *see* Somatropin ... 1918
Nordinet Infantil (MX) *see* Acetaminophen ... 32
Nordiol (GT, HN, NI, SV) *see* Carvedilol ... 367
Nordip (AU) *see* AmLODIPine ... 123
Nordipine (MY) *see* AmLODIPine ... 123
Norditropin (AE, AR, AT, BE, BG, BH, BR, CL, CN, CO, CZ, DK, EG, FI, GB, GR, HR, HU, IT, JO, JP, KR, KW, LB, MY, NL, NO, PT, QA, RO, RU, SA, SE, TW, VN) *see* Somatropin ... 1918
Norditropin Nordilet (SG, TH) *see* Somatropin ... 1918
Norditropin Simplex (KR) *see* Somatropin ... 1918
Norditropin Simplexx (DE, ES, IS, LT, SI, SK) *see* Somatropin ... 1918
Norditropin S (JP) *see* Somatropin ... 1918
Nordonil (PT) *see* Domperidone [CAN/INT] ... 666
Nordox (CL) *see* Phenazopyridine ... 1629
Norepine (TW) *see* Norepinephrine ... 1472
Norepin (PH) *see* Norepinephrine ... 1472
Norestin (BR) *see* Norethindrone ... 1473
Norfem (PH) *see* Ethinyl Estradiol and Norgestrel ... 812
Norfenon (MX) *see* Propafenone ... 1725
Norflex (AE, AU, BB, BE, BH, BM, BS, BZ, CH, CR, CY, DE, DO, EG, FI, GR, GT, GY, HK, HN, IE, IL, IQ, IR, JM, JO, KE, KW, LB, LU, LY, MU, MX, MY, NG, NL, NZ, OM, PA, PE, PK, PT, QA, SA, SE, SR, SV, SY, TH, TT, TW, UY, VE, YE, ZA) *see* Orphenadrine ... 1522
Norflogen (EC) *see* Norfloxacin ... 1475
Norflohexal (DE) *see* Norfloxacin ... 1475
Norflosal (CR, NI) *see* Norfloxacin ... 1475
Norflox (DE, IN) *see* Norfloxacin ... 1475
Norflox Eye (IN) *see* Norfloxacin ... 1475
Norfloxin (MY) *see* Norfloxacin ... 1475
Norgalax (AE, BE, BH, CH, CY, DE, EG, GB, IE, IQ, IR, JO, KW, LB, LU, LY, NL, OM, QA, RU, SA, SY, VN, YE) *see* Docusate ... 661
Norgalax Micro-enema (GB) *see* Docusate ... 661
Norglicem (ES) *see* GlyBURIDE ... 972
Noriday 28 (AU) *see* Norethindrone ... 1473
Noriday (AE, BF, BH, BJ, CI, ET, GB, GH, GM, GN, IE, KE, LR, MA, ML, MR, MU, MW, MY, NE, NG, NZ, QA, SC, SD, SL, SN, TN, TZ, UG, ZM, ZW) *see* Norethindrone ... 1473
Noriline (ZA) *see* Amitriptyline ... 119
Norimin (AE, AU, BF, BH, BJ, CI, CY, EG, ET, GB, GH, GM, GN, IQ, IR, JO, KE, KW, LB, LR, LY, MA, ML, MR, MU, MW, NE, NG, NZ, OM, QA, SA, SC, SD, SL, SN, SY, TN, TZ, UG, YE, ZM, ZW) *see* Ethinyl Estradiol and Norethindrone ... 808
Norinyl-1 28 (ZA) *see* Norethindrone and Mestranol ... 1475
Norinyl-1 (AU, BF, BJ, CI, ET, GH, GM, GN, KE, LR, MA, ML, MR, MU, MW, NE, NG, NZ, SC, SD, SL, SN, TN, TZ, UG, ZM, ZW) *see* Norethindrone and Mestranol ... 1475
Noripam (ZA) *see* Oxazepam ... 1532
Ñorispez (MX) *see* RisperiDONE ... 1818
Norit (IL) *see* Charcoal, Activated ... 416
Noritis (BF, BJ, CI, ET, GH, GM, GN, KE, LR, MA, ML, MR, MU, MW, NE, NG, SC, SD, SL, SN, TN, TZ, UG, ZM, ZW) *see* Ibuprofen ... 1032
Noritren (DK, EE, FI, IS, IT, LT, NO) *see* Nortriptyline ... 1476
Norivite-12 (ZA) *see* Cyanocobalamin ... 515
Norizec (PH) *see* Glimepiride ... 966
Norlevo (AU, CY, DK, ES, FI, FR, GR, IL, IN, IS, JP, KR, NO, PT, SE, SG, SI, TR, ZA) *see* Levonorgestrel ... 1201
NorLevo (NZ) *see* Levonorgestrel ... 1201
Norline (TH) *see* Nortriptyline ... 1476
Norlip (IL) *see* Bezafibrate [CAN/INT] ... 261
Nor-Lodipina (DO, GT, HN, NI, SV) *see* AmLODIPine ... 123
Norluten (FR) *see* Norethindrone ... 1473
Normabel (HR) *see* Diazepam ... 613
Normabrain (DE, IN, PH) *see* Piracetam [INT] ... 1661
Normadate (IN) *see* Labetalol ... 1151
Normaform (CH) *see* Phentermine ... 1635
Normalol (IL) *see* Atenolol ... 189
Normase (IL) *see* Lactulose ... 1156
Normaten (HK, MY) *see* Atenolol ... 189
Normaton (DO, GT, PA, SV) *see* BusPIRone ... 311
Normax Eye Ear Drops (IN) *see* Norfloxacin ... 1475
Normeg (EE) *see* LevETIRAcetam ... 1191
Normetec (ID, PH, TH) *see* Amlodipine and Olmesartan ... 126
Normison (AU, BE, CH, FI, FR, GB, IE, IT, LU, NL, NZ, PT) *see* Temazepam ... 1990
Normiten (IL) *see* Atenolol ... 189
Normix (AR, BG, CL, CZ, HN, IT, KR, LB, PH, SK, TR) *see* Rifaximin ... 1809

Normocard (PL) *see* Atenolol 189
Normodipine (HU, SG) *see* AmLODIPine 123
Normoglaucon (DE) *see* Metipranolol 1345
Normolax (AE, BH, CY, EG, IQ, IR, JO, KW, LB, LY, OM, QA, SA, SY, YE) *see* Lactulose 1156
Normolip (IN) *see* Gemfibrozil 956
Normopresan (IL) *see* CloNIDine 480
Normopresin (UY) *see* CloNIDine 480
Normopress (ZA) *see* Methyldopa 1332
Normorytmin (AR) *see* Propafenone 1725
Normotemp (EC) *see* Acetaminophen 32
Normoten (AE) *see* Atenolol 189
Normoten (PH) *see* Losartan 1248
Normpress (TH) *see* Propranolol 1731
Norodol (TR) *see* Haloperidol 993
Noroxin (AE, AR, AU, BB, BF, BH, BJ, BM, BS, BZ, CI, CN, CY, ET, FI, GH, GM, GN, GY, IT, JM, KE, KW, LB, LR, MA, ML, MR, MU, MW, MX, NE, NG, NL, PE, PK, PT, QA, SA, SC, SD, SL, SN, SR, TN, TR, TT, TZ, UG, VE, ZM, ZW) *see* Norfloxacin 1475
Noroxine (FR) *see* Norfloxacin 1475
Noroxin Oftalmico (MX) *see* Norfloxacin 1475
Norpace (AE, BB, BH, CH, DE, DK, HR, IE, IN, KR, MY, PH, QA, SR, TR, TT, ZA) *see* Disopyramide 653
Norpace Retard (HK, PH, ZA) *see* Disopyramide 653
Norpaso (AR) *see* Disopyramide 653
Norphed (PH) *see* Norepinephrine 1472
Norphin (IN) *see* Buprenorphine 300
Norpin (KR, TH) *see* Norepinephrine 1472
Norplant (LU, PH, TH, TW) *see* Levonorgestrel 1201
Norpramin (MX) *see* Desipramine 593
Norpress (NZ) *see* Nortriptyline 1476
Nor-Prilat (DO, GT, NI, SV) *see* Enalapril 722
Norprolac (AT, CA, CH, DE, ES, FI, FR, GB, GR, HK, IL, MX, NL, NO, SE, ZA) *see* Quinagolide [CAN/INT] 1755
Nor-Purinol (NI, SV) *see* Allopurinol 90
Nor-Sartan H (GT, HN, NI, SV) *see* Losartan and Hydrochlorothiazide 1250
Norset (FR) *see* Mirtazapine 1376
Norsol (CH) *see* Norfloxacin 1475
Norspan Patch (AU, CZ, DE, DK, EE, FI, HK, KR, NO, NZ, PH) *see* Buprenorphine 300
Norspan (SK) *see* Buprenorphine 300
Norspirinal (ID) *see* Aspirin 180
Norspor (TH) *see* Itraconazole 1130
Norswel (BF, BJ, CI, ET, GH, GM, GN, KE, LR, MA, ML, MR, MU, MW, NE, NG, SC, SD, SL, SN, TN, TZ, UG, ZM, ZW) *see* Naproxen 1427
Nortelol (HK) *see* Atenolol 189
Nortem (IE) *see* Temazepam 1990
Norten (PH) *see* Imidapril [INT] 1051
Nortens (ID) *see* Irbesartan 1110
Nortensin (AR) *see* Trandolapril 2080
Nor-Tenz (MX) *see* Brimonidine (Ophthalmic) 288
Norterol (PT) *see* Nortriptyline 1476
Nortimil (IT) *see* Desipramine 593
Nortin (TW) *see* Cyproterone and Ethinyl Estradiol [CAN/INT] 532
Nortrilen (AE, AT, BE, BF, BH, BJ, CH, CI, CY, CZ, DE, EG, ET, GH, GM, GN, GR, HK, ID, IQ, IR, JO, KE, KW, LB, LR, LU, LY, MA, ML, MR, MU, MW, NE, NG, NL, OM, QA, SA, SC, SD, SL, SN, SY, TN, TZ, UG, YE, ZA, ZM, ZW) *see* Nortriptyline 1476
Nortrilin (PK) *see* Nortriptyline 1476
Nortyline (TH) *see* Nortriptyline 1476
Nortylin (IL) *see* Nortriptyline 1476
Norum (TH) *see* Acyclovir (Systemic) 47
Noruxol (IT) *see* Collagenase (Topical) 507
Norvapine (AU) *see* AmLODIPine 123
Norvasc V (KR) *see* Amlodipine and Valsartan 126
Norvasc (AT, AU, BB, BF, BG, BJ, BM, BR, BS, BZ, CH, CI, CL, CN, CR, CY, CZ, DE, DK, DO, EC, EE, EG, ET, FI, GH, GM, GN, GR, GT, GY, HK, HN, HU, IL, IS, IT, JM, JO, JP, KE, KR, KW, LR, MA, ML, MR, MU, MW, MY, NE, NG, NI, NL, NO, NZ, PA, PE, PH, PK, PT, QA, RO, RU, SC, SD, SE, SG, SI, SK, SL, SN, SR, SV, TH, TN, TR, TT, TW, TZ, UG, UY, VE, ZA, ZM, ZW) *see* AmLODIPine 123
Norvas (CO, ES, MX) *see* AmLODIPine 123
Norvasc Protect (PH) *see* Amlodipine and Atorvastatin 124
Norvask (ID) *see* AmLODIPine 123
Nor-Vastina (DO, GT, HN, NI, PA, SV) *see* Simvastatin 1890
Norvastor (EC, PE) *see* Amlodipine and Atorvastatin 124
Norvetal (CO) *see* Ethinyl Estradiol and Levonorgestrel 803
Norvir (AE, AT, AU, BE, BG, BH, CH, CL, CN, CR, CY, CZ, DE, DK, EC, EE, EG, ES, FI, FR, GB, GR, GT, HK, HN, HR, HU, ID, IE, IL, IQ, IR, IS, IT, JO, KR, KW, LT, LU, LY, MT, MY, NI, NL, NO, NZ, OM, PA, PE, PL, PT, QA, RO, RU, SA, SE, SG, SI, SK, SV, SY, TH, TR, TW, VE, YE) *see* Ritonavir 1822
Norvom (ID) *see* Metoclopramide 1345
Norzetam (IT) *see* Piracetam [INT] 1661
Noscam (AE) *see* Naphazoline (Nasal) 1426
Noseling (TW) *see* Loratadine 1241
Nosemin (KR) *see* Cetirizine 411
Nosma (TW) *see* Theophylline 2026
Nostamin (PE) *see* Amiodarone 114
Noten (AU) *see* Atenolol 189
Notensyl (IL) *see* Dicyclomine 622
Notolac (VE) *see* Ketorolac (Systemic) 1146
No-Ton (TW) *see* Nabumetone 1411
No-Tos (AR) *see* Bromhexine [INT] 291
Notrixum (ID, TH) *see* Atracurium 198
No-Uric (AE, BH, CY, EG, IQ, IR, JO, KW, LB, LY, OM, QA, SA, SY, YE) *see* Allopurinol 90
Novaban (BE) *see* Tropisetron [INT] 2108
Novabritine (BE) *see* Amoxicillin 130
Novacalc (NO) *see* Calcium Gluconate 330
Novacef (AR) *see* Cefixime 380
Novacor (TH) *see* Bisoprolol 266
Novador (MX) *see* Cefuroxime 399
Novaflox (SG) *see* Ciprofloxacin (Ophthalmic) 446
Novaflox (SG) *see* Ciprofloxacin (Systemic) 441
Novahistex DM Decongestant (CA) *see* Pseudoephedrine and Dextromethorphan 1743
Novahistex DM Decongestant Expectorant (CA) *see* Guaifenesin, Pseudoephedrine, and Dextromethorphan 989
Novahistine DM Decongestant (CA) *see* Pseudoephedrine and Dextromethorphan 1743
Novahistine DM Decongestant Expectorant (CA) *see* Guaifenesin, Pseudoephedrine, and Dextromethorphan 989
Novalcina (VE) *see* Dipyrone [INT] 653
Novales (ID) *see* Pravastatin 1700
Novalgina (AR, CO, IT, PE, UY) *see* Dipyrone [INT] 653
Novalgin (AT, CH, CZ, DE, NL, PK) *see* Dipyrone [INT] 653
Novalgine (BE, VN) *see* Dipyrone [INT] 653
Noval (GR) *see* Timolol (Ophthalmic) 2043
Novamin (TW) *see* Prochlorperazine 1718
Novamox (BR) *see* Amoxicillin and Clavulanate 133
Novamox (PH) *see* Amoxicillin 130
Novanox (DE) *see* Nitrazepam [CAN/INT] 1461
Novantron (AT, CH, DE) *see* MitoXANtrone 1382
Novantrone (AE, BE, CN, DK, EG, ES, FI, FR, GB, GR, HN, HR, HU, IL, IT, JO, JP, KW, LU, NL, NO, NZ, PK, PL, PT, RO, RU, SA, SE, TR, TW, VN) *see* MitoXANtrone 1382
Nova-Pam (NZ) *see* ChlordiazePOXIDE 422
Novapressin (PK) *see* Terlipressin [INT] 2010
Novaprin (MX) *see* Danazol 558

Novarok (JP) *see* Imidapril [INT] 1051
Novasone Cream (AU) *see* Mometasone (Topical) 1391
Novasone Lotion (AU) *see* Mometasone (Topical) 1391
Novasone Ointment (AU) *see* Mometasone (Topical) 1391
Novaspin (KR) *see* AmLODIPine 123
Novastan (CN, DK, IT, JP, KR, NO, SE) *see* Argatroban 168
Novastep (DE) *see* Ethinyl Estradiol and Levonorgestrel 803
Novatec (BE, LU, NL) *see* Lisinopril 1226
Novatrex (FR) *see* Methotrexate 1322
Novaxen (MX) *see* Naproxen 1427
Novax (ID) *see* Amoxicillin 130
Novazole (BF, BJ, CI, ET, GH, GM, GN, KE, LR, MA, ML, MR, MU, MW, NE, NG, SC, SD, SL, SN, TN, TZ, UG, ZM, ZW) *see* MetroNIDAZOLE (Systemic) 1353
Novecin (AE, BH, CY, EG, IQ, IR, JO, KW, LB, LY, OM, QA, SA, SY, YE) *see* Ofloxacin (Systemic) 1490
Noveldexis (MX) *see* CISplatin 448
Novell-Eutropin (ID) *see* Somatropin 1918
Novellmycin (ID) *see* Fosfomycin 932
Novelon (IN) *see* Ethinyl Estradiol and Desogestrel 799
Novencil (EC) *see* Ampicillin 141
Noven (KR) *see* Fenoverine [INT] 857
Noventabedoce (ES) *see* Cyanocobalamin 515
Novepide (ID) *see* Rebamipide [INT] 1786
Noveron (ID) *see* Rocuronium 1838
Novertigo (PK) *see* Cinnarizine [INT] 440
Novertin (PY) *see* Betahistine [CAN/INT] 252
Novex (CO) *see* Fluticasone (Nasal) 910
Novhepar (GR) *see* LORazepam 1243
Novidat (AR) *see* Ciprofloxacin (Systemic) 441
Novidorm (AR) *see* Triazolam 2101
Novidroxin (DE) *see* Hydroxocobalamin 1020
Noviken LP (MX) *see* NIFEdipine 1451
Novina (MX) *see* Pravastatin 1700
Novirep (PK) *see* Nateglinide 1432
Novitropan (IL) *see* Oxybutynin 1536
Novlen (PY) *see* Etoricoxib [INT] 821
Novobedouze (BE, LU) *see* Hydroxocobalamin 1020
Novocef (HR) *see* Cefuroxime 399
Novocephal (AT) *see* Piracetam [INT] 1661
Novocortril (PE) *see* Hydrocortisone (Systemic) 1013
Novodil (IT) *see* Dipyridamole 652
Novodrin (DE) *see* Isoproterenol 1124
Novofem (CN, EE, GB, HK, IE) *see* Estradiol and Norethindrone 781
Novofem (EE, HK) *see* Ethinyl Estradiol and Norethindrone 808
Novofen-D (BB, BM, BS, BZ, GY, JM, NL, PR, SR, TT) *see* Tamoxifen 1971
Novofen (EC, HK, SG, TH, TW) *see* Tamoxifen 1971
Novofen Forte (BZ, GY, SR) *see* Tamoxifen 1971
Novogent (DE) *see* Ibuprofen 1032
Novo-Herklin 2000 (CR, DO, MX, NI, PA) *see* Permethrin 1627
Novolet N (KR) *see* Insulin NPH 1089
Novolin N (CN, JP, KR, MX) *see* Insulin NPH 1089
Novomin (HK, MY) *see* DimenhyDRINATE 637
Novomit (TW) *see* Prochlorperazine 1718
Novomix 30 (AE, AR, AT, AU, BE, BH, BR, CH, CL, CN, CO, CY, CZ, DE, DK, EE, ES, GB, GR, HK, HR, HU, ID, IE, IL, IN, JO, JP, KR, LB, MY, NO, NZ, PH, PK, PT, QA, RO, RU, SA, SG, TH, TR, TW, UY, VN) *see* Insulin Aspart Protamine and Insulin Aspart 1084
Novomix30 (KW) *see* Insulin Aspart Protamine and Insulin Aspart 1084
Novomix 50 (BE, CZ, EE, HR, IL, JP, RO) *see* Insulin Aspart Protamine and Insulin Aspart 1084
Novomix 70 (BE, CZ, EE, HR, IL, SE) *see* Insulin Aspart Protamine and Insulin Aspart 1084
Novommix 70 (RO) *see* Insulin Aspart Protamine and Insulin Aspart 1084
Novonordisk (MX) *see* Factor VIIa (Recombinant) 836
NovoNorm (AE, AR, AT, AU, BE, BF, BH, BJ, CH, CI, CL, CN, CO, CY, CZ, DE, DK, EE, EG, ES, ET, FI, FR, GB, GH, GM, GN, GR, HK, HN, HR, HU, IE, IL, IQ, IR, IS, IT, JO, KE, KR, KW, LB, LR, LT, LY, MA, ML, MR, MT, MU, MW, MX, MY, NE, NG, NL, NO, OM, PH, PK, PL, PT, PY, QA, RO, RU, SA, SC, SD, SE, SG, SI, SK, SL, SN, SY, TH, TN, TR, TW, TZ, UG, UY, VE, YE, ZA, ZM, ZW) *see* Repaglinide 1791
Novonorm (VN) *see* Repaglinide 1791
Novopulmon (DE, FR) *see* Budesonide (Systemic) 293
Novorapid (AE, AT, AU, BE, BH, BR, CH, CL, CN, CO, CY, CZ, DE, DK, EC, EE, ES, FI, FR, GB, GR, HN, HR, HU, ID, IE, IL, IS, IT, JO, JP, KR, KW, LB, LT, MT, MY, NL, NO, NZ, PE, PL, PT, QA, RO, RU, SA, SE, SG, SI, SK, TH, TR, TW, VN) *see* Insulin Aspart 1083
Novorapid Flexpen (PH) *see* Insulin Aspart 1083
Novorin (ID) *see* Leucovorin Calcium 1183
Novosef (AE, BH, CY, EG, IQ, IR, JO, KW, LB, LY, OM, PH, QA, RU, SA, SY, TR, YE) *see* CefTRIAXone 396
Novoseven (MX) *see* Factor VIIa (Recombinant) 836
NovoSeven (AE, AR, AT, BE, BG, BR, CH, CL, CN, CO, CY, CZ, DE, DK, EE, ES, FI, FR, GB, GR, HK, HN, HR, HU, ID, IE, IL, IN, IS, IT, JO, KR, LB, LT, MT, MY, NL, NO, NZ, PE, PL, PT, QA, RO, RU, SE, SG, SI, SK, TH, TR, TW, UY) *see* Factor VIIa (Recombinant) 836
Novoseven RT (AU, VN) *see* Factor VIIa (Recombinant) 836
NovoSeven RT (PH) *see* Factor VIIa (Recombinant) 836
Novosporina (PY) *see* Bacitracin, Neomycin, and Polymyxin B 223
Novoter (AE, BH, QA) *see* Fluocinonide 894
Novoxil (BR) *see* Amoxicillin 130
Novuxol (NL, TR) *see* Collagenase (Topical) 507
Novynette (BB, BM, BS, BZ, GY, HK, HR, JM, RO, SR, TH, TT, VN) *see* Ethinyl Estradiol and Desogestrel 799
Nowon Vaginal Supp. (KR) *see* Nonoxynol 9 1471
Noxafil (AE, AR, AT, AU, BE, BH, CH, CL, CN, CO, CY, CZ, DE, DK, EE, ES, FR, GB, GR, HK, HN, HR, IE, IL, IN, IS, IT, KR, KW, LT, MY, NL, NO, NZ, PE, PH, PL, PT, QA, RO, SE, SG, SI, SK, TH, TR) *see* Posaconazole 1683
Noxalide (IT) *see* Nimesulide [INT] 1456
Noxibel (EC, PY) *see* Mirtazapine 1376
Noxi (IN) *see* Lornoxicam [INT] 1248
Noxom (PY) *see* Nitazoxanide 1461
Noxon (IT) *see* Lornoxicam [INT] 1248
Noxrakin (TH) *see* Miconazole (Topical) 1360
Noyada (GB) *see* Captopril 342
Nozepam (RU) *see* Oxazepam 1532
Nozinan (AR, AT, BE, BG, CH, CZ, DK, EE, ES, FI, FR, GB, GR, HN, HR, ID, IE, IS, IT, LU, MT, NL, NO, NZ, PH, PL, PT, PY, RU, SE, SI, SK, TR, UY) *see* Methotrimeprazine [CAN/INT] 1329
Nplate (AR, AT, AU, BE, CH, CL, CY, CZ, DE, DK, EE, FR, GB, HK, HN, HR, IE, IL, IS, KR, LT, NL, NO, PL, PT, RO, SE, SI, SK, TR) *see* RomiPLOStim 1842
NT-Alergi (HK) *see* Loratadine 1241
NT-Diorea (HK) *see* Loperamide 1236
Nuardin (BE, LU) *see* Cimetidine 438
Nubaina (AR) *see* Nalbuphine 1416
Nubain (AE, AT, BF, BH, BJ, BR, CI, CY, CZ, DE, EE, EG, ET, GB, GH, GM, GN, GR, HN, HU, IE, IL, IQ, IR, JO, KE, KW, LB, LR, LY, MA, ML, MR, MU, MW, MY, NE, NG, NL, OM, PH, PK, PL, QA, SA, SC, SD, SI, SL, SN, SY, TN, TZ, UG, VE, YE, ZA, ZM, ZW) *see* Nalbuphine 1416
Nubral (AT, DE) *see* Urea 2114
Nucomyt (HK) *see* Acetylcysteine 40
Nuctalon (FR) *see* Estazolam 775
Nuctane (AR) *see* Triazolam 2101

Nuedexta (LT, NL, SI) *see* Dextromethorphan and Quinidine 611
Nuelin (AU, BB, BM, BS, BZ, DK, FI, GY, JM, NO, NZ, PH, PR, SG, SR, TT, VE) *see* Theophylline 2026
Nuelin SA (AE, BF, BH, BJ, CI, CR, CY, EG, ET, GH, GM, GN, IE, IQ, IR, JO, KE, KW, LB, LR, LY, MA, ML, MR, MU, MW, NE, NG, OM, PA, QA, SA, SC, SD, SL, SN, SY, TN, TZ, UG, YE, ZA, ZM, ZW) *see* Theophylline 2026
Nuelin SR (AE, AU, BH, CY, EG, HK, IQ, IR, JO, KW, LB, LY, MY, OM, QA, SA, SG, SY, TH, YE) *see* Theophylline 2026
Nufaclav (ID) *see* Amoxicillin and Clavulanate 133
Nufadol (ID) *see* Acetaminophen 32
Nufafloqo (ID) *see* Ofloxacin (Systemic) 1490
Nufalora (ID) *see* Loratadine 1241
Nufatrac (ID) *see* Itraconazole 1130
Nufex (IN) *see* Cephalexin 405
Nufloxib (AU) *see* Norfloxacin 1475
Nufolic (ID) *see* Folic Acid 919
Nuhair (TH) *see* Minoxidil (Topical) 1374
Nu-K (IE) *see* Potassium Chloride 1687
Nulartrin (AR) *see* Diacerein [INT] 613
Nulcer (ID) *see* Cimetidine 438
Nullatuss Clobutinol (DE) *see* Clobutinol [INT] 468
Nulobes (AR) *see* Diethylpropion 624
Nulojix (AR, AU, CH, CZ, DE, DK, EE, FR, GB, HR, IL, IT, LT, NL, NO, PL, RO, SE, SI, SK) *see* Belatacept 233
Nulox Forte (ID) *see* Meloxicam 1283
Nulox (ID) *see* Meloxicam 1283
Numbon (IL) *see* Nitrazepam [CAN/INT] 1461
Nuo Bin (CN) *see* Zolpidem 2212
Nuo Fei (CN) *see* Lafutidine [INT] 1157
Nuo Lan Pin (CN) *see* Nevirapine 1440
Nuo Shu An (CN) *see* Alfuzosin 84
Nuo Xin Shejg (CN) *see* Naltrexone 1422
Nuparin (PH) *see* Heparin 997
Nupentin (AU, NZ, SG) *see* Gabapentin 943
Nupic (IN) *see* Piracetam [INT] 1661
Nuril (ES) *see* Pipemidic Acid [INT] 1655
Nuril (IN) *see* Enalapril 722
Nurison (NL) *see* PredniSONE 1706
Nuro-B (MX) *see* Pyridoxine 1747
Nurofen (AT, AU, BE, BF, BG, BJ, CI, CY, CZ, DK, ET, FR, GB, GH, GM, GN, HR, IS, KE, LR, LT, MA, ML, MR, MU, MW, MY, NE, NG, NL, NZ, SC, SD, SE, SG, SI, SK, SL, SN, TN, TR, TZ, UG, VN, ZM, ZW) *see* Ibuprofen 1032
Nurofen Cold and Flu (AE, AU, BH, CY) *see* Pseudoephedrine and Ibuprofen 1743
Nurofen Cold & Flu (NZ, ZA) *see* Pseudoephedrine and Ibuprofen 1743
Nurofen for Children (TH) *see* Ibuprofen 1032
Nurofen Gel (IL, NZ) *see* Ibuprofen 1032
Nurofen Pro san sucre (FR) *see* Ibuprofen 1032
Nurona (JO, LB) *see* Gabapentin 943
Nu-Seals (AE, BF, BH, BJ, CI, CY, EG, ET, GH, GM, GN, IQ, IR, JO, KE, KW, LB, LR, LY, MA, ML, MR, MU, MW, NE, NG, OM, QA, SA, SC, SD, SL, SN, SY, TN, TR, TZ, UG, YE, ZM, ZW) *see* Aspirin 180
Nuspas (TW) *see* Hyoscyamine 1026
Nutracort (CO, CR, DO, GT, NI, PA, SV, VE) *see* Hydrocortisone (Topical) 1014
Nutralcon (PY) *see* Urea 2114
Nutram (PH) *see* Acetaminophen and Tramadol 37
Nutraplus (AE, AU, CH, MX, MY, NZ, SG, TH, TW) *see* Urea 2114
Nutrexon (ID) *see* Naltrexone 1422
Nutricee (PH) *see* Ascorbic Acid 178
Nutropin AQ (AT, AU, BE, BG, CH, CZ, DE, DK, EE, ES, FI, FR, GB, GR, IE, IT, MT, NL, NO, PL, PT, RU, SE, SK, TR) *see* Somatropin 1918
Nutropinaq (FR) *see* Somatropin 1918
Nuvacthen Depot (ES) *see* Cosyntropin 510
NuvaRing (AE, AR, AT, AU, BE, BR, CH, CL, CO, CR, CY, CZ, DE, DK, DO, EE, FI, FR, GB, GR, GT, HN, IE, IL, IS, IT, KR, KW, LB, LT, MX, MY, NI, NL, NO, NZ, PA, PE, PL, PT, QA, RU, SA, SE, SG, SI, SK, SV, TH, TW, UY) *see* Ethinyl Estradiol and Etonogestrel 802
Nuvaring (HR, RO, TR, VN) *see* Ethinyl Estradiol and Etonogestrel 802
Nuzak (ZA) *see* FLUoxetine 899
Nyclin (TW) *see* Niacin 1443
Nycoflox (EE) *see* FLUoxetine 899
Nycopren (AT, DK, FI) *see* Naproxen 1427
Nydrazide (PK) *see* Isoniazid 1120
Nyefax (AU) *see* NIFEdipine 1451
Nyefax Retard (NZ) *see* NIFEdipine 1451
Nymalize (BM) *see* NiMODipine 1456
Nyogel (AU, BE, FR, GB, IE, IS, ZA) *see* Timolol (Ophthalmic) 2043
Nyogel LP (FR) *see* Timolol (Ophthalmic) 2043
Nyolol (AE, BR, CH, CL, EE, FR, HK, IL, PT, PY, RU, SG, SK, TR, TW, UY, VE, VN) *see* Timolol (Ophthalmic) 2043
Nyrin (SG) *see* Leucovorin Calcium 1183
Nysa (VN) *see* Piroxicam 1662
Nysconitrine (LU) *see* Nitroglycerin 1465
Nyserin (PH) *see* Nitroglycerin 1465
Nystafar (VN) *see* Nystatin (Oral) 1481
Nystatin (AE) *see* Nystatin (Oral) 1481
Nystatin Gel (CH) *see* Nystatin (Topical) 1482
Nytaderm (QA) *see* Nystatin (Topical) 1482
Nytol (IL) *see* DiphenhydrAMINE (Systemic) 641
N-Zarevet (IL) *see* Calcium Carbonate 327
Oacerein (MX) *see* Diacerein [INT] 613
Oasil (ES, LU) *see* Meprobamate 1296
Oasil (GR) *see* ChlordiazePOXIDE 422
Oasil Simes (ES) *see* Meprobamate 1296
Obagi (VN) *see* Hydroquinone 1020
Obestat (EC) *see* Orlistat 1520
Obogen (PH) *see* Gentamicin (Systemic) 959
Obracin (BE, CH, NL) *see* Tobramycin (Systemic, Oral Inhalation) 2052
Obroxol (HK) *see* Ambroxol [INT] 109
Obutin (SG) *see* Oxybutynin 1536
OC-35 (TH) *see* Cyproterone and Ethinyl Estradiol [CAN/INT] 532
Occidal (TH) *see* Ofloxacin (Systemic) 1490
Oceral (AE, BR, CH, TR) *see* Oxiconazole 1536
Oceral GB (NZ) *see* Oxiconazole 1536
Ocid (IN, SG) *see* Omeprazole 1508
Ocillina (TW) *see* Oxacillin 1528
Ocina (VN) *see* Oxacillin 1528
Oclovir (AR) *see* Rimantadine 1813
O.C.M. (AR) *see* ChlordiazePOXIDE 422
Ocsaar (IL) *see* Losartan 1248
Ocsaar Plus (IL) *see* Losartan and Hydrochlorothiazide 1250
Octafix (FR) *see* Factor IX (Human) 840
Octagam (AT, AU, BE, BG, BH, BR, CH, CO, CZ, DE, DK, EE, FI, FR, GB, GR, HR, IN, LB, LT, MX, NL, NO, NZ, RO, SA, SE, SI, SK, TH, UY, VN) *see* Immune Globulin 1056
Octalbin (DK, FI, ID, MX) *see* Albumin 67
Octanine F (AE, SA, UY) *see* Factor IX (Human) 840
Octanyl (CO, CR, EC, GT, HN, NI, SV, UY) *see* Bromazepam [CAN/INT] 290
Octaplex (BE, DE, DK, EE, ES, FI, FR, IL, IS, LT, NL, SI, SK, TR, VE) *see* Prothrombin Complex Concentrate (Human) [(Factors II, VII, IX, X), Protein C, and Protein S] 1738
Octaplex (BR, CH, DK) *see* Protein C Concentrate (Human) 1738
Octaprin (AR) *see* Nimesulide [INT] 1456

Octasa (GB) *see* Mesalamine 1301
Octex (MX) *see* Sulfamethoxazole and Trimethoprim 1946
Octicaina (CO) *see* Benzocaine 246
Octide (ID, TW) *see* Octreotide 1485
Octim (FR) *see* Desmopressin 594
Octim Nasal Spray (GB, IE) *see* Desmopressin 594
Octocin (TH) *see* Oxytocin 1549
Octonativ-M (SE) *see* Antihemophilic Factor (Human) 152
Octonox (BE) *see* Lormetazepam [INT] 1247
Octostim (AE, AR, AT, AU, BH, CH, CL, CO, DE, EC, EE, EG, ES, FI, HK, HU, IL, IQ, IR, IS, KW, LT, LY, MX, NL, NO, NZ, OM, QA, SE, SG, SY, YE) *see* Desmopressin 594
Octostim Nasal Spray (KR) *see* Desmopressin 594
Octostin (AR) *see* Desmopressin 594
Octride (CO, EC, PH, TH) *see* Octreotide 1485
Ocu-Carpine (KR) *see* Pilocarpine (Ophthalmic) 1649
Ocuchloram (KR) *see* Chloramphenicol 421
Ocudol (VE) *see* Ketorolac (Ophthalmic) 1149
Ocudol (VE) *see* Ketorolac (Systemic) 1146
Ocufen (AU, BH, CL, CN, CO, DK, EC, FR, GB, IE, IT, KR, MY, PE, PH, QA, SA, TH, TW, VE, VN, ZA) *see* Flurbiprofen (Ophthalmic) 906
Ocuflam (ID) *see* Fluorometholone 896
Ocuflox (AU, KR, NZ) *see* Ofloxacin (Ophthalmic) 1491
Ocuflur (AT, BE, BG, CH, CZ, DE, GR, HN, IN, PL, PT, RU, VN) *see* Flurbiprofen (Ophthalmic) 906
Ocufridine (KR) *see* Trifluridine 2103
Ocugenta (KR) *see* Gentamicin (Systemic) 959
Ocuhomapine (KR) *see* Homatropine 1005
Oculast (IN) *see* Azelastine (Ophthalmic) 213
Oculpres-D (DO, HN) *see* Dorzolamide and Timolol 673
Oculten (DO, SV) *see* AcetaZOLAMIDE 39
Ocumetholone (KR, PH) *see* Fluorometholone 896
Ocuper (PH) *see* Timolol (Ophthalmic) 2043
Ocu-Pred (VE) *see* PrednisoLONE (Ophthalmic) 1706
Ocupres (BF, BJ, CI, ET, GH, GM, GN, IN, KE, LR, MA, ML, MR, MU, MW, NE, NG, SC, SD, SL, SN, TN, TZ, UG, ZM, ZW) *see* Timolol (Ophthalmic) 2043
Ocupres-E (BF, BJ, CI, ET, GH, GM, GN, KE, LR, MA, ML, MR, MU, MW, NE, NG, SC, SD, SL, SN, TN, TZ, UG, ZM, ZW) *see* Timolol (Ophthalmic) 2043
Ocuracin (KR) *see* Tobramycin (Ophthalmic) 2056
Ocusert Pilo-20 (GB) *see* Pilocarpine (Ophthalmic) 1649
Ocusert Pilo-40 (GB) *see* Pilocarpine (Ophthalmic) 1649
Ocusert Pilocarpine (GB) *see* Pilocarpine (Ophthalmic) 1649
Ocusyn (SG) *see* Tobramycin (Ophthalmic) 2056
Ocutropine (KR) *see* Atropine 200
Odace (ID) *see* Lisinopril 1226
Odace (PH) *see* Trandolapril 2080
Odaft (MY, PH) *see* Fluconazole 885
Odasyl (PH) *see* AmLODIPine 123
Odemase (DE) *see* Furosemide 940
Odemex (CR, DO, GT, HN, NI, PA, SV) *see* Furosemide 940
Odemin (FI) *see* AcetaZOLAMIDE 39
Odenil (ES) *see* Amorolfine [INT] 128
Odicoza (HK) *see* Dicloxacillin 621
Odipin (PH) *see* NIFEdipine 1451
OD Mac (PH) *see* Azithromycin (Systemic) 216
Odonazin (HR) *see* Mirtazapine 1376
Odontocromil (ES) *see* Fluoride 895
Odontol Plac (PY) *see* Chlorhexidine Gluconate 422
Odoxil (IN) *see* Cefadroxil 372
Odranal (CL) *see* Oxybutynin 1536
Odranal (AR, CO) *see* BuPROPion 305
Odrik (AE, AU, BH, DK, ES, FI, FR, GR, IE, KR, KW, LB, LU, PE, PT) *see* Trandolapril 2080
Oedemex (AE, BH, CH, CY, EG, IQ, IR, JO, KW, LB, LY, OM, QA, SA, SY, YE) *see* Furosemide 940
Oesclim (FR) *see* Estradiol (Systemic) 775
Oestring (SE) *see* Estradiol (Topical) 780
Oestrodidronel (BE) *see* Etidronate 813
Oestrodose (IL) *see* Estradiol (Systemic) 775
Oestrodose (PH) *see* Estradiol (Topical) 780
Oestro-Feminal (DE) *see* Estrogens (Conjugated/Equine, Systemic) 787
Ofal (AR) *see* Timolol (Ophthalmic) 2043
Ofcin (MY, TH, TW) *see* Ofloxacin (Systemic) 1490
Ofenac (KR) *see* Diclofenac (Systemic) 617
Ofenicol (PY) *see* Chloramphenicol 421
Ofertil (ID) *see* ClomiPHENE 473
Ofev (CZ, EE, LT, SE) *see* Nintedanib 1458
Oflacin (VN) *see* Ofloxacin (Ophthalmic) 1491
Ofla (TH) *see* Ofloxacin (Systemic) 1490
Oflaxsyn (CO) *see* Ofloxacin (Otic) 1491
Oflin (IN) *see* Ofloxacin (Systemic) 1490
Oflocee (TH) *see* Ofloxacin (Systemic) 1490
Oflocet (FR, NZ, PT) *see* Ofloxacin (Systemic) 1490
Oflocin (IT) *see* Ofloxacin (Systemic) 1490
Oflodal (TW) *see* Ofloxacin (Systemic) 1490
Oflodex (IL) *see* Ofloxacin (Systemic) 1490
Oflodura (DE) *see* Ofloxacin (Systemic) 1490
Oflovid (TW) *see* Ofloxacin (Ophthalmic) 1491
Oflox (AE, AR, BR, CL, CO, IL, PE, VE) *see* Ofloxacin (Ophthalmic) 1491
Ofloxin (BG) *see* Ofloxacin (Ophthalmic) 1491
Ofloxin (CZ, EE, LT, RO, SK, TH) *see* Ofloxacin (Systemic) 1490
Ofloxol (MY) *see* Ofloxacin (Systemic) 1490
Ofodex (MX) *see* Neomycin 1436
Oframax (BF, BJ, CI, ET, GH, GM, GN, IN, KE, LR, MA, ML, MR, MU, MW, NE, NG, SC, SD, SG, SL, SN, TH, TN, TZ, UG, VN, ZA, ZM, ZW) *see* CefTRIAXone 396
Oftacilox (PT) *see* Ciprofloxacin (Ophthalmic) 446
Oftacilox (PT) *see* Ciprofloxacin (Systemic) 441
Oftacon (CL, UY) *see* Cromolyn (Ophthalmic) 514
Oftadil (MX) *see* Chloramphenicol 421
Oftagen (PE) *see* Gentamicin (Systemic) 959
Oftal (CL) *see* Loteprednol 1251
Oftalbrax (AR) *see* Tobramycin (Ophthalmic) 2056
Oftalgesic (DO) *see* Ketorolac (Ophthalmic) 1149
Oftalmolets (AR) *see* Erythromycin (Ophthalmic) 764
Oftalmolosa Cusi Erythromycin (MY, SG) *see* Erythromycin (Ophthalmic) 764
Oftalmotrim (AE, EG, KW, QA, SA) *see* Trimethoprim and Polymyxin B 2105
Oftan-Akvakol (EE, FI) *see* Chloramphenicol 421
Oftan Atropin (FI) *see* Atropine 200
Oftan (CZ, NO, PH) *see* Timolol (Ophthalmic) 2043
Oftan Dexa (EE) *see* Dexamethasone (Systemic) 599
Oftan Dexa (EE, FI) *see* Dexamethasone (Ophthalmic) 602
Oftanex (PL) *see* Dipivefrin 651
Oftan-Metaoksedrin (FI) *see* Phenylephrine (Systemic) 1638
Oftan Mydrin (PL) *see* Tropicamide 2108
Oftan-Pilocarpin (FI) *see* Pilocarpine (Ophthalmic) 1649
Oftan-Syklo (FI, PL) *see* Cyclopentolate 517
Oftan Timolol (HK) *see* Timolol (Ophthalmic) 2043
Oftan-tropicamid (FI) *see* Tropicamide 2108
Oftaquix (BG, CZ, DE, DK, EE, FI, GB, GR, IE, IS, IT, LT, NL, PH, PL, PT, RO, SE, SK) *see* Levofloxacin (Ophthalmic) 1200
Oftarinol (PL) *see* Sodium Chloride 1902
Oftavir (UY) *see* Aciclovir (Ophthalmic) [INT] 43
Oft Cusi Atropina (ES) *see* Atropine 200
Oftlamotrim (MY) *see* Trimethoprim and Polymyxin B 2105
Oftol Forte (EC) *see* Loteprednol 1251
Ofus (HK) *see* Ofloxacin (Ophthalmic) 1491

Ofven (IN) *see* Ofloxacin (Ophthalmic) 1491
Ofven (IN) *see* Ofloxacin (Otic) 1491
Ogal (CO, PE) *see* Omeprazole 1508
Ogaran (KR) *see* Danaparoid [CAN/INT] 556
Ogast (FR) *see* Lansoprazole 1166
Ogastro (BB, BM, BS, BZ, CO, CR, EC, FR, GT, GY, HN, JM, MX, NI, PA, PE, PR, SR, SV, TT) *see* Lansoprazole 1166
Ogen (AU, BB, BM, BS, BZ, GY, ID, JM, NL, SR, TT) *see* Estropipate 793
OH B12 (IT) *see* Hydroxocobalamin 1020
OHB12 (PT) *see* Hydroxocobalamin 1020
Oikamid (CZ, HR) *see* Piracetam [INT] 1661
Oilezz (TH) *see* Ethinyl Estradiol and Desogestrel 799
Okacin (BE, BH, DK, JO, KW, LU, PH, PY, QA, SG, UY, VE) *see* Lomefloxacin [INT] 1233
Okacyn (ZA) *see* Lomefloxacin [INT] 1233
Okavax (HK, SG, TW, VN) *see* Varicella Virus Vaccine 2141
Okilon (JP) *see* Fluorometholone 896
Okinazole (JP) *see* Oxiconazole 1536
Okpine (TW) *see* OLANZapine 1491
Oksazepam (HR, PL) *see* Oxazepam 1532
Oksitocins (EE) *see* Oxytocin 1549
Olan (MX) *see* Lansoprazole 1166
Olandoz (ID) *see* OLANZapine 1491
Olane (PY) *see* PARoxetine 1579
Olanpin (KR) *see* OLANZapine 1491
Olanza OD (KR) *see* OLANZapine 1491
Olanzapro (PH) *see* OLANZapine 1491
Olapin-10 (KR, TH) *see* OLANZapine 1491
Olartan (TR) *see* Olmesartan 1496
Olatin (TW) *see* Oxaliplatin 1528
Olbetam (AT, BE, CH, CL, CN, DK, GB, GR, HK, HN, IL, IT, KR, KW, NL, NO, NZ, QA, SA, SG, SI, TH, TW, ZA) *see* Acipimox [INT] 43
Olcef (KR) *see* Cefuroxime 399
Oldan (ES) *see* Acemetacin [INT] 30
Oldeca (KR) *see* Barnidipine [INT] 227
Oldesar (KR) *see* Olmesartan 1496
Oldin (PY) *see* Warfarin 2186
Oldren (AR) *see* Eplerenone 740
Oldren (AR) *see* Metolazone 1348
Oleanz (IN) *see* OLANZapine 1491
Ole (KR) *see* Olmesartan 1496
Olena (GB) *see* FLUoxetine 899
Oleomycetin (DE) *see* Chloramphenicol 421
Oleptro (BM) *see* TraZODone 2091
Olexin (MX) *see* Omeprazole 1508
Olfen-75 SR (MY) *see* Diclofenac (Systemic) 617
Olfen (AE, BB, BM, BS, BZ, GY, HK, JM, JO, LB, MY, PR, SR, TT) *see* Diclofenac (Systemic) 617
Olfovel (TH) *see* Levofloxacin (Systemic) 1197
Olgotan (KR) *see* Olmesartan 1496
Olicard (BG, HR, HU, RO) *see* Isosorbide Mononitrate 1126
Olicide (PT) *see* Malathion 1268
Oliet (KR) *see* Orlistat 1520
Oliflox (PT) *see* Prulifloxacin [INT] 1742
Oligogranul Fluor (FR) *see* Fluoride 895
Oligogranul Magnesium (FR) *see* Magnesium Gluconate 1263
Oligosol F (BE) *see* Fluoride 895
Oligosol Mg (BE, CH, FR) *see* Magnesium Gluconate 1263
Oligostim Fe (BE) *see* Ferrous Gluconate 870
Oligostim Fluor (FR) *see* Fluoride 895
Oligostim Magnesium (FR) *see* Magnesium Gluconate 1263
Oligostim Mg (BE) *see* Magnesium Gluconate 1263
Olimestra (SK) *see* Olmesartan 1496
Olipcis (MX) *see* Oxaliplatin 1528
Olit (SG) *see* Omeprazole 1508
Olivin (HR) *see* Enalapril 722
Olmec (AR, LB) *see* Olmesartan 1496
Olmegan (IT) *see* Olmesartan and Hydrochlorothiazide 1498
Olmesta (BG) *see* Olmesartan 1496
Olmetec D (AR) *see* Olmesartan and Hydrochlorothiazide 1498
Olmetec (AE, AT, AU, BE, BR, CH, CN, CO, CZ, DE, DK, DO, EC, EE, ES, FI, FR, GB, GR, GT, HK, HN, ID, IL, IT, KR, KW, MY, NI, NL, NO, PE, PH, PT, QA, SA, SG, SV, TH, TW, UY, VE) *see* Olmesartan 1496
Olmetec Anlo (BR) *see* Amlodipine and Olmesartan 126
Olmetec-Anlo (EC) *see* Amlodipine and Olmesartan 126
Olmetec Comp (NO) *see* Olmesartan and Hydrochlorothiazide 1498
Olmetec HCT (BR, CO, EC) *see* Olmesartan and Hydrochlorothiazide 1498
Olmetec HCTZ (NL) *see* Olmesartan and Hydrochlorothiazide 1498
Olmetec Plus (AT, AU, BE, CH, CL, DE, DK, DO, EE, FI, GB, GR, GT, HK, HN, ID, KR, MY, NI, PE, PH, PT, QA, SA, SG, SV, TH, TR, TW, UY) *see* Olmesartan and Hydrochlorothiazide 1498
Olmetec Plus H (CZ) *see* Olmesartan and Hydrochlorothiazide 1498
Olmezar (PH) *see* Olmesartan 1496
Olmezar Plus (PH) *see* Olmesartan and Hydrochlorothiazide 1498
Olopa (KR) *see* Olopatadine (Ophthalmic) 1500
Olopanol (KR) *see* Olopatadine (Ophthalmic) 1500
Olopat (AR, JO, KW, QA) *see* Olopatadine (Ophthalmic) 1500
Olpin (KR) *see* Amlodipine and Atorvastatin 124
Oltrex (GT) *see* Ofloxacin (Systemic) 1490
Oltril (TH) *see* Valproic Acid and Derivatives 2123
Olvion (RO) *see* Sildenafil 1882
Olxarin (PH) *see* Enoxaparin 726
Olysio (AU, BE, CZ, DE, DK, EE, FR, GB, HR, IS, LT, NL, NO, RO, SE, SI, SK) *see* Simeprevir 1887
Olyster (IN) *see* Terazosin 2001
Olza (HK) *see* OLANZapine 1491
Omacor (AE, AR, AT, AU, BE, BG, BH, CR, CY, CZ, DE, DO, EE, FI, FR, GB, GR, GT, HN, HR, IE, IL, KR, KW, LT, MY, NI, NL, NO, PA, PL, PT, QA, RO, RU, SA, SI, SK, SV, TH) *see* Omega-3 Fatty Acids 1507
Omastin (SG) *see* Fluconazole 885
Omatropina (IT) *see* Homatropine 1005
Omca (DE) *see* FluPHENAZine 905
Omcet (AE, BH, JO, QA, SA) *see* Cetirizine 411
Omedar (AE, BH, CY, EG, IQ, IR, JO, KW, LB, LY, OM, QA, SA, SY, YE) *see* Omeprazole 1508
Omed (BF, BJ, CH, CI, ET, GH, GM, GN, ID, IN, KE, KR, LR, MA, ML, MR, MU, MW, NE, NG, SC, SD, SL, SN, TN, TZ, UG, ZM, ZW) *see* Omeprazole 1508
Omelon (MY, TW) *see* Omeprazole 1508
Omepac (PE) *see* Omeprazole, Clarithromycin, and Amoxicillin 1511
OMEP (DE) *see* Omeprazole 1508
Omep (HK) *see* Omeprazole 1508
Omepradex (IL) *see* Omeprazole 1508
Omepradex-Z (IL) *see* Omeprazole 1508
Omepra (IL) *see* Omeprazole 1508
Omepral (AU, JP) *see* Omeprazole 1508
Omepramix (BR) *see* Omeprazole, Clarithromycin, and Amoxicillin 1511
Omeprazon (JP) *see* Omeprazole 1508
Omepril (EC) *see* Omeprazole 1508
Omeq (KR) *see* Omeprazole 1508
Omertec (KR) *see* Olmesartan 1496
Omesar (IE) *see* Olmesartan 1496
Omesar Plus (IE) *see* Olmesartan and Hydrochlorothiazide 1498
Omesec (HK, MY, SG) *see* Omeprazole 1508

Omesel (VN) *see* Omeprazole 1508
Omex (CO) *see* Omeprazole 1508
Omexel LP (FR) *see* Tamsulosin 1974
Omezol (AE, BH, CY, EG, IN, IQ, IR, JO, KW, LB, LY, NZ, OM, QA, SA, SY, YE) *see* Omeprazole 1508
Omezole (HK, SG, TW) *see* Omeprazole 1508
Omez (VN) *see* Omeprazole 1508
Omezzol (EC) *see* Omeprazole 1508
Omic (BE, LU) *see* Tamsulosin 1974
Omicef (PH) *see* Cefdinir 376
Omicral (RO) *see* Itraconazole 1130
Omida (TW) *see* Midazolam 1361
Omifin (CO, MX) *see* ClomiPHENE 473
Omiflu (MY) *see* Oseltamivir 1523
Omilipis (AR, PY) *see* CARBOplatin 357
Omisec (AE, BH, CY, EG, IQ, IR, JO, KW, LB, LY, OM, QA, SA, SY, YE) *see* Omeprazole 1508
Omix Ocas (CH) *see* Tamsulosin 1974
Omizac (IN) *see* Omeprazole 1508
Omizec (HK) *see* Omeprazole 1508
Omnadren (PL) *see* Testosterone 2010
Omnalio (ES) *see* ChlordiazePOXIDE 422
Omnaris (AR, AU, BR, HK, MY, PH, SG, TH) *see* Ciclesonide (Nasal) 432
Omnatax (IN) *see* Cefotaxime 382
Omnexel (IE) *see* Tamsulosin 1974
Omniapharm (DE) *see* Bromhexine [INT] 291
Omnic (AE, AR, BH, BR, CL, CO, CZ, DE, DK, EE, ES, FI, GR, HR, HU, IL, IS, IT, JO, KW, LT, NL, NO, PE, PL, PT, QA, RO, RU, SA, SI, SK) *see* Tamsulosin 1974
Omnicef (AE, BB, BH, BM, BS, BZ, CY, EG, GY, ID, IL, IQ, IR, JM, JO, KR, KW, LB, LY, NL, OM, PR, QA, SA, SE, SR, SY, TH, TT, VN, YE) *see* Cefdinir 376
Omnic OCAS (CY, IL, KW, LB, QA, SA) *see* Tamsulosin 1974
Omnic Tocas (BG) *see* Tamsulosin 1974
Omnipen (AE, BH, CY, EG, IQ, IR, JO, KW, LB, LY, MX, OM, QA, SA, SY, YE) *see* Ampicillin 141
Omnitrope (AT, AU, BE, BG, CH, CZ, DE, DK, EE, ES, FI, FR, GB, GR, IE, IT, MT, NL, NO, NZ, PL, PT, RU, SE, SK, TR) *see* Somatropin 1918
Omnivox (PH) *see* Levofloxacin (Systemic) 1197
Omol (QA) *see* Acetaminophen 32
OMP (KR) *see* Omeprazole 1508
Omprazole (KR) *see* Omeprazole 1508
Omsat (BF, BJ, CI, DE, ET, GH, GM, GN, KE, LR, MA, ML, MR, MU, MW, NE, NG, SC, SD, SL, SN, TN, TZ, UG, ZM, ZW) *see* Sulfamethoxazole and Trimethoprim 1946
OMZ (ID) *see* Omeprazole 1508
Onabet (IN) *see* Sertaconazole 1877
Onacrine (SG) *see* Orphenadrine 1522
Onaven (KR) *see* Thiothixene 2031
Onbrez Breezhaler (AT, AU, BE, CH, CN, CY, CZ, DE, DK, EE, ES, FR, GB, HK, HN, HR, ID, IE, IL, IN, IS, KR, KW, LB, LT, MY, NL, NO, NZ, PH, PL, PT, QA, RO, SE, SG, SI, SK, TH, TR, TW, VN) *see* Indacaterol 1063
Onbrez (JP) *see* Indacaterol 1063
Onbrise Breezhaler (EC) *see* Indacaterol 1063
Onbrize (CL) *see* Indacaterol 1063
Onbrize Breezhaler (AR, BR, CO) *see* Indacaterol 1063
Oncaspar (DE) *see* Asparaginase (E. coli) 179
Oncaspar (DE, PL) *see* Pegaspargase 1588
Oncef (PH) *see* CefTRIAXone 396
Oncoblastin (CO, PE) *see* VinBLAStine 2160
Onco-Carbide (IT) *see* Hydroxyurea 1021
Oncocarbil (AR, PY) *see* Dacarbazine 549
Oncocarbin (IN) *see* CARBOplatin 357
Oncocarb (PE) *see* CARBOplatin 357
Oncocristin (CO, PE) *see* VinCRIStine 2163
Oncodocel (BR, CO) *see* DOCEtaxel 656
Oncodox (PE) *see* DOXOrubicin (Conventional) 679
Oncolis (BM) *see* FentaNYL 857
Oncoril (PH) *see* Gemcitabine 952
Oncostin (PH) *see* VinBLAStine 2160
Oncotaxel (AU, SG) *see* DOCEtaxel 656
Oncotecan (CO, EC, PE) *see* Topotecan 2069
OncoTICE (MX, PE, SE) *see* BCG 229
Oncotice (CY, DK, FI, IL, IN, IS, KR, NL, NO, PK, PL, SI) *see* BCG 229
OncoTice (VE) *see* BCG 229
Oncotin (PH) *see* CISplatin 448
Oncotiotepa (BE, ES, LU) *see* Thiotepa 2030
Oncotrone (BG) *see* MitoXANtrone 1382
Oncotron (IN) *see* MitoXANtrone 1382
Oncovin (AE, AT, AU, BF, BH, BJ, CH, CI, CZ, DE, DK, EE, EG, ES, ET, FI, FR, GB, GH, GM, GN, GR, HN, HR, IE, IT, KE, LR, LU, MA, ML, MR, MT, MU, MW, MX, NE, NG, NL, NO, PK, PL, PT, QA, RU, SA, SC, SD, SE, SK, SL, SN, TN, TR, TZ, UG, ZA, ZM, ZW) *see* VinCRIStine 2163
Ondak (CO) *see* Ondansetron 1513
Ondant (KR) *see* Ondansetron 1513
Ondarubin (MX) *see* IDArubicin 1037
Ondavell (ID, TH) *see* Ondansetron 1513
Ondaz (AU) *see* Ondansetron 1513
Onealfa (JP, KR, TW) *see* Alfacalcidol [CAN/INT] 82
One-Alpha (AE, BB, BF, BH, BJ, BM, BS, BZ, CI, CY, EG, ET, GH, GM, GN, GY, IL, IQ, IR, JM, JO, KE, KW, LB, LR, LY, MA, ML, MR, MU, MW, NE, NG, NL, OM, PR, QA, SA, SC, SD, SL, SN, SR, SY, TN, TT, TZ, UG, YE, ZA, ZM, ZW) *see* Ergocalciferol 753
One-Alpha (AE, CY, EG, GB, HK, IE, JO, KW, LB, MY, NZ, PL, QA, RO, RU, SA, SG, TH, TR, ZA) *see* Alfacalcidol [CAN/INT] 82
One Duro (JP) *see* FentaNYL 857
Oneflu (KR) *see* Fluconazole 885
Onelaxant-R (PH) *see* Baclofen 223
Onetic (ID) *see* Ondansetron 1513
Onexacin (PH) *see* Ofloxacin (Systemic) 1490
Onexid (PH) *see* Clarithromycin 456
Onfor (AR) *see* Nalbuphine 1416
Onglyza (AR, AT, AU, BE, BR, CH, CL, CN, CO, CY, CZ, DE, DK, EE, FR, GB, GR, HK, HN, HR, ID, IE, IL, IN, IT, JP, KR, KW, LT, MY, NL, NO, NZ, PH, PL, PT, QA, RO, RU, SA, SE, SG, SI, SK, TH, TR, TW, VN) *see* Saxagliptin 1867
Onic (ID) *see* Omeprazole 1508
Onicit (AR, BR, CL, CO, DO, GT, HN, MX, NI, PE, SV, VE) *see* Palonosetron 1561
Onirema (VE) *see* Nitrazepam [CAN/INT] 1461
Onkomet (TH) *see* Methotrexate 1322
Onkotrone (AU, EE, HU, LT, NZ, RO, SI, SK) *see* MitoXANtrone 1382
Onkovertin N (DE) *see* Dextran 607
Onquinin (JP) *see* Aprotinin 168
Onsenal (AT, DE, DK, FR, IE, TR) *see* Celecoxib 402
Onset-8 (PH) *see* Ondansetron 1513
Onsetron (KR) *see* Ondansetron 1513
Onsia (TH) *see* Ondansetron 1513
Onsleep (TW) *see* Zaleplon 2193
Onychomal (DE, LU) *see* Urea 2114
Onzapin (HK, ID, SG) *see* OLANZapine 1491
Onzapin OD (HK) *see* OLANZapine 1491
Onzapin ODT (SG) *see* OLANZapine 1491
Onzet (PH) *see* Ondansetron 1513
Onzet (TH) *see* Azithromycin (Systemic) 216
Onzod (TW) *see* Ondansetron 1513
Opalgyne (FR) *see* Benzydamine [CAN/INT] 249
Opal (PE) *see* Omeprazole 1508
Opamox (FI) *see* Oxazepam 1532
Opatanol (BE, CH, CZ, DE, DK, EE, FI, FR, GB, GR, HR, HU, IE, IS, IT, LT, MT, NL, NO, PL, PT, RO, RU, SE, SI, SK, TR) *see* Olopatadine (Ophthalmic) 1500
Opdivo (JP) *see* Nivolumab 1469

O.P.D. (TW) *see* Pilocarpine (Ophthalmic) 1649
Opel (PH) *see* Omeprazole 1508
Opeprim (JP) *see* Mitotane 1382
Operan (KR) *see* Ofloxacin (Ophthalmic) 1491
Opheryl (KR) *see* Orphenadrine 1522
Ophtagram (BE, CH) *see* Gentamicin (Systemic) 959
Ophtagram (CH) *see* Gentamicin (Ophthalmic) 962
Ophtamolol (HK) *see* Timolol (Ophthalmic) 2043
Ophtavit C (BE, LU) *see* Ascorbic Acid 178
Ophthaine (GB, IE) *see* Proparacaine 1728
Ophth-cyclovir (PK) *see* Aciclovir (Ophthalmic) [INT] 43
Ophth-fluorstrip (PK) *see* Fluorescein 894
Ophth-natamycin (PK) *see* Natamycin 1432
Ophtorenin (DE) *see* Bupranolol [INT] 300
Opigran (ID) *see* Granisetron 983
Opiodur (GB) *see* FentaNYL 857
Opizolam (ID) *see* ALPRAZolam 94
Opizole B (AE) *see* Betamethasone and Clotrimazole 256
Opizone (GB) *see* Naltrexone 1422
Oplat (CO) *see* Oxaliplatin 1528
Opnol (SE) *see* Dexamethasone (Ophthalmic) 602
Opnol (SE) *see* Dexamethasone (Systemic) 599
Oposim (AR) *see* Propranolol 1731
Oppvir (TW) *see* Acyclovir (Topical) 51
Oprad (MX) *see* Amikacin 111
Oprax (PE) *see* Omeprazole 1508
Oprazole (AE, BH, JO, KW, LB, QA, SA) *see* Omeprazole 1508
Oprestat (GT) *see* Irbesartan and Hydrochlorothiazide 1112
Opsacin (VN) *see* Neomycin, Polymyxin B, and Gramicidin 1437
Optaclor (PH) *see* Chloramphenicol 421
Optacrom (PH) *see* Cromolyn (Ophthalmic) 514
Optagen (PK) *see* Gentamicin (Ophthalmic) 962
Optagen (PK) *see* Gentamicin (Systemic) 959
Optaglo (PH) *see* Gatifloxacin 949
Optalgin (HU, IL) *see* Dipyrone [INT] 653
Optal-Pro (TH) *see* Ciprofloxacin (Ophthalmic) 446
Optal-Pro (TH) *see* Ciprofloxacin (Systemic) 441
Optal (TH) *see* Sulfacetamide (Ophthalmic) 1943
Optamide (PH) *see* AcetaZOLAMIDE 39
Optamol (PH) *see* Timolol (Ophthalmic) 2043
Optanac (KR) *see* Diclofenac (Ophthalmic) 621
Opthagen (PH) *see* Gentamicin (Ophthalmic) 962
Opthagen (PH) *see* Gentamicin (Systemic) 959
Opthavir (MX) *see* Aciclovir (Ophthalmic) [INT] 43
Opthazel (PE) *see* Azelastine (Ophthalmic) 213
Opthetic (NZ) *see* Proparacaine 1728
Opthmid (TR) *see* Sulfacetamide (Ophthalmic) 1943
Optibet (ID) *see* Betaxolol (Ophthalmic) 257
Optibet (ID) *see* Betaxolol (Systemic) 256
Optibex (PH) *see* Betaxolol (Ophthalmic) 257
Optichlor (AE, BH, KW, SA, SG) *see* Chloramphenicol 421
Opticide (TH) *see* Praziquantel 1702
Opticin (AE, JO, KW, QA) *see* Ciprofloxacin (Ophthalmic) 446
Opticle (KR) *see* Chloramphenicol 421
Opticrom (AU, BE, CH, EG, GB, HN, IE, NL, NZ, PT, SG, TR) *see* Cromolyn (Ophthalmic) 514
Opticron (FR) *see* Cromolyn (Ophthalmic) 514
Opticyclin (AE) *see* Tetracycline 2017
Optiderm Creme (DE) *see* Polidocanol 1672
Optidorm (DE) *see* Zopiclone [CAN/INT] 2217
Optifen (CH) *see* Ibuprofen 1032
Optiflox (BH, JO, KW, LB) *see* Ofloxacin (Ophthalmic) 1491
Optifluor Diba (MX) *see* Fluorescein 894
Optigen (SG) *see* Gentamicin (Ophthalmic) 962
Optigen (SG) *see* Gentamicin (Systemic) 959
Opti-Genta (IL) *see* Gentamicin (Ophthalmic) 962
Opti-Genta (IL) *see* Gentamicin (Systemic) 959
Optilast (IL) *see* Azelastine (Ophthalmic) 213
Optilone (AE, BH, QA, SA) *see* Fluorometholone 896
Optima (TH) *see* Irbesartan 1110
Optimin (ES) *see* Loratadine 1241
Optimol (AE, BH, DK, KW, MY, QA, SA, SE) *see* Timolol (Ophthalmic) 2043
Optimycin (BF, BJ, CI, ET, GH, GM, GN, KE, LR, MA, ML, MR, MU, MW, NE, NG, SC, SD, SL, SN, TN, TZ, UG, ZM, ZW) *see* Gentamicin (Systemic) 959
Optinate (DK, FI, IS, KR, NO, SE) *see* Risedronate 1816
Optinem (AT) *see* Meropenem 1299
Optipect (DE) *see* Codeine 497
Optipres (IN) *see* Betaxolol (Ophthalmic) 257
Optipres (IN) *see* Betaxolol (Systemic) 256
Optisulin (AT, BE, CH, CZ, DE, DK, EE, FI, FR, GB, GR, IE, IT, MT, NO, PL, PT, RU, SE, SK, TR) *see* Insulin Glargine 1086
Optocetine (QA) *see* Chloramphenicol 421
Optomycin (PH) *see* Chloramphenicol 421
Optovite B1 (ES) *see* Thiamine 2028
Optovite B12 (ES) *see* Cyanocobalamin 515
Optra (PK) *see* Ipratropium (Systemic) 1108
Optrex (NZ) *see* Cromolyn (Ophthalmic) 514
Optruma (AT, BE, BG, CH, CZ, DE, DK, EE, ES, FR, GB, GR, HN, IE, IT, LT, MT, NL, NO, PL, PT, RO, SE, SI, SK, TR) *see* Raloxifene 1765
Optryl (PH) *see* Erythromycin (Ophthalmic) 764
Opturem (DE) *see* Ibuprofen 1032
Opturma (HR) *see* Raloxifene 1765
Optycin (AU) *see* Tetracycline 2017
Opvero (AE, SA, TH) *see* Poliovirus Vaccine (Inactivated) 1673
OQ-Dilat (CO) *see* Phenylephrine (Systemic) 1638
Oqifresh (CO) *see* Naphazoline and Pheniramine 1426
OQ-Miot (CO) *see* Acetylcholine 40
Orabet (AT, DK, GB, IE) *see* MetFORMIN 1307
Orabet (DE) *see* TOLBUTamide 2062
Orabetic (PH) *see* GlyBURIDE 972
Oracaine (AU) *see* Cetylpyridinium and Benzocaine [CAN/INT] 415
Oracefal (FR) *see* Cefadroxil 372
Oracef (CZ) *see* Cephalexin 405
Oracillin VK (ZA) *see* Penicillin V Potassium 1614
Oracort (IL, NZ) *see* Triamcinolone (Systemic) 2099
Oracort (NZ) *see* Triamcinolone (Topical) 2100
Oraday (IN, TH) *see* Atenolol 189
Oradex (MY) *see* Chlorhexidine Gluconate 422
Oradexon (CL, FI, NL, PT, QA, SA) *see* Dexamethasone (Systemic) 599
Oradol (PH) *see* Ketorolac (Systemic) 1146
Oradroxil (IT) *see* Cefadroxil 372
Orafuran (BG) *see* Nitrofurantoin 1463
Orahex (PH) *see* Chlorhexidine Gluconate 422
Orajel (CH, PL) *see* Benzocaine 246
Oralcef (PY) *see* Cefixime 380
Oralcon (MY) *see* Ethinyl Estradiol and Levonorgestrel 803
Oralexin (LB) *see* Cephalexin 405
Oralfi (BR) *see* Darifenacin 568
Oralipin (CL) *see* Bezafibrate [CAN/INT] 261
Oralipin Retard (PY) *see* Bezafibrate [CAN/INT] 261
Oralsterone (TW) *see* Fluoxymesterone 903
Oramax (AE, KW, LB, QA, SA) *see* Fluconazole 885
Oramedy (HK, KR, SG) *see* Triamcinolone (Systemic) 2099
Oramedy (HK, KR, SG) *see* Triamcinolone (Topical) 2100
Oramorph (BE, FR, GB, IE, PT, SE) *see* Morphine (Systemic) 1394
Orandil (VN) *see* Nicorandil [INT] 1449
Oranor (MX) *see* Norfloxacin 1475

Orap (1 mg) (AE, BF, BH, BJ, CI, CY, EG, ET, GH, GM, GN, HK, IQ, IR, JO, KE, KW, LB, LR, LY, MA, ML, MR, MU, MW, NE, NG, OM, QA, SA, SC, SD, SL, SN, SY, TN, TZ, UG, YE, ZA, ZM, ZW) *see* Pimozide 1651
Orap (4 mg) (AE, BH, CY, EG, IL, IQ, IR, JO, KW, LB, LY, OM, QA, SA, SY, YE) *see* Pimozide 1651
Orap (AT, AU, BE, BR, CH, CZ, DE, DK, ES, FR, GB, HR, IE, IT, JP, LU, NL, NO, PL, VE) *see* Pimozide 1651
Orap Forte (4 mg) (AE, AR, BF, BH, BJ, CI, CY, EG, ET, GH, GM, GN, HK, ID, IL, IQ, IR, JO, KE, KW, LB, LR, LY, MA, ML, MR, MU, MW, NE, NG, OM, PT, QA, SA, SC, SD, SL, SN, SY, TN, TZ, UG, YE, ZM, ZW) *see* Pimozide 1651
Orap Forte (CL, PY, SI) *see* Pimozide 1651
Orapred (PE) *see* PredniSONE 1706
Oraqix (SE) *see* Lidocaine and Prilocaine 1213
Oratane (AE, AU, MY, NZ, SG) *see* ISOtretinoin 1127
Oratol F (PT) *see* Fluoride 895
Oravir (FR) *see* Famciclovir 843
Oraxim (AE, BH, CY, EG, IQ, IR, JO, KW, LB, LY, OM, QA, SA, SY, YE) *see* Cefuroxime 399
Orbachlor (PE) *see* Chloramphenicol 421
Orbatropin (PE) *see* Atropine 200
Orbenil (IL) *see* Cloxacillin [CAN/INT] 488
Orbenin (AE, BB, BD, BF, BH, BJ, BM, BS, BZ, CI, CY, EG, ET, GH, GM, GN, GR, GY, IE, IQ, IR, JM, JO, JP, KE, KR, KW, LB, LR, LU, LY, MA, ML, MR, MU, MW, NE, NG, NL, OM, PK, PR, QA, SA, SC, SD, SL, SN, SR, SY, TN, TT, TW, TZ, UG, YE, ZA, ZM, ZW) *see* Cloxacillin [CAN/INT] 488
Orbenine (FR) *see* Cloxacillin [CAN/INT] 488
Orbide (LB) *see* Glimepiride 966
Orbunol (PE) *see* Levobunolol 1194
Orcef-DS (PH) *see* Cefdinir 376
Oregan (ID) *see* Neomycin, Polymyxin B, and Dexamethasone 1437
Orelox (BB, BM, BS, BZ, CH, CZ, DE, EG, FI, FR, GR, GY, IT, JM, LB, LU, MX, NL, NO, PK, PL, PT, SR, TT, VN) *see* Cefpodoxime 388
Orencia (AE, AR, AT, AU, BE, BR, CH, CL, CO, CY, CZ, DE, DK, EE, FR, GB, GR, HK, HN, HR, IE, IL, IN, IS, IT, JP, KR, KW, LB, LT, NL, NO, NZ, PE, PL, PT, RO, SA, SE, SG, SI, SK, TR, TW) *see* Abatacept 23
Orencia SC (JP) *see* Abatacept 23
Orencia Subq PFS (KR) *see* Abatacept 23
Orfadin (AT, AU, BE, BG, BM, CH, CZ, DE, DK, EE, ES, FI, FR, GB, GR, HN, HR, IE, IL, IT, KR, LT, MT, NL, NO, PL, PT, RO, RU, SE, SI, SK, TR, TW) *see* Nitisinone 1461
Orfarin (JO, MY, TH, TW) *see* Warfarin 2186
Orfidal (ES) *see* LORazepam 1243
Orfidora (ES) *see* Indoramin [INT] 1070
Orfiril (CZ, DE, FI, HU) *see* Valproic Acid and Derivatives 2123
Orfiril Retard (SG) *see* Valproic Acid and Derivatives 2123
Orgalutran (AE, AR, AT, AU, BE, BG, BH, BR, CH, CL, CO, CY, CZ, DE, DK, EE, EG, ES, FI, FR, GB, GR, HK, HN, HR, ID, IE, IL, IQ, IR, IS, IT, JO, KR, KW, LB, LT, LY, MT, MX, MY, NL, NO, NZ, OM, PE, PK, PL, PT, QA, RO, RU, SA, SE, SG, SI, SK, SY, TH, TR, TW, UY, VE, VN, YE) *see* Ganirelix 949
Orgametril (AT, BE, CH, CZ, DE, DK, ES, FI, FR, HU, IN, LU, NL, PT, SE) *see* Lynestrenol [INT] 1261
Organoderm (DE) *see* Malathion 1268
Orgaran (AT, AU, BE, CH, DE, FI, FR, GB, GR, IT, LU, NL, NO, NZ, SE) *see* Danaparoid [CAN/INT] 556
Oributol (FI) *see* Ethambutol 798
Oricef (TW) *see* CeFAZolin 373
Oricyclin (FI) *see* Tetracycline 2017
Oridip (FI) *see* Lercanidipine [INT] 1181
Oridoxime (VN) *see* Pralidoxime 1694
Orinse (IN) *see* Chlorhexidine Gluconate 422
Oriphex (BF, BJ, CI, ET, GH, GM, GN, KE, LR, MA, ML, MR, MU, MW, NE, NG, SC, SD, SL, SN, TN, TZ, UG, ZM, ZW) *see* Cephalexin 405
Oripicin (VN) *see* Colchicine 500
Oriprim DS (KE, TZ, UG, ZW) *see* Sulfamethoxazole and Trimethoprim 1946
Oriprim (RU) *see* Sulfamethoxazole and Trimethoprim 1946
Oritaxim (BF, BJ, CI, ET, GH, GM, GN, KE, LR, MA, ML, MR, MU, MW, NE, NG, SC, SD, SL, SN, TN, TZ, UG, ZM, ZW) *see* Cefotaxime 382
Orivid (TH) *see* Ofloxacin (Systemic) 1490
Orixal (ID) *see* Clarithromycin 456
Orix (GR) *see* NIFEdipine 1451
Orizolin (BF, BJ, CI, ET, GH, GM, GN, KE, LR, MA, ML, MR, MU, MW, NE, NG, SC, SD, SL, SN, TN, TZ, UG, ZM, ZW) *see* CeFAZolin 373
Orizon (PY) *see* Eszopiclone 793
Orlifit (VN) *see* Orlistat 1520
Orlin (AE) *see* Ciprofloxacin (Systemic) 441
Orlist (PY) *see* Orlistat 1520
Orlobin (GR) *see* Amikacin 111
Ormidol (HR) *see* Atenolol 189
Ormodon (ZA) *see* Nitrazepam [CAN/INT] 1461
Orocal (FR) *see* Calcium Carbonate 327
Orocin (KR) *see* Ofloxacin (Systemic) 1490
Orodaxin (BR) *see* Ciprofibrate [INT] 441
Oroken (FR) *see* Cefixime 380
Oronazol (HR) *see* Ketoconazole (Topical) 1145
Oroperidys (FR) *see* Domperidone [CAN/INT] 666
Orosartan (KR) *see* Amlodipine and Valsartan 126
Orosept (ZA) *see* Chlorhexidine Gluconate 422
Orovas (PH) *see* Simvastatin 1890
Oroxine (AU, MY) *see* Levothyroxine 1205
Orpherin (KR) *see* Orphenadrine 1522
Orphipal (IN) *see* Orphenadrine 1522
Orpic (PH) *see* Ciprofloxacin (Systemic) 441
Orpidix (GR) *see* Ketotifen (Ophthalmic) 1150
Orpidix (GR) *see* Ketotifen (Systemic) [CAN/INT] 1149
Orprozil (IN) *see* Cefprozil 389
Orrepaste (MY, SG) *see* Triamcinolone (Systemic) 2099
Orrepaste (MY, SG) *see* Triamcinolone (Topical) 2100
Orsanac (PY) *see* Norfloxacin 1475
Orsanil (FI) *see* Thioridazine 2030
Orstanorm (FI, SE) *see* Dihydroergotamine 633
Ortanol (HR) *see* Omeprazole 1508
Ortho 7 7 7 (BB, BM, BS, BZ, GY, JM, NL, PR, SR, TT) *see* Ethinyl Estradiol and Norethindrone 808
Ortho-Creme (AU) *see* Nonoxynol 9 1471
Ortho Cyclen (IL) *see* Ethinyl Estradiol and Norgestimate 810
Ortho-Est (ZA) *see* Estropipate 793
Orthonase (TH) *see* Calcitonin 322
Ortho-Novin (AE, BH, CY, EG, IL, IQ, IR, JO, KW, LB, LY, OM, QA, SA, SY, YE) *see* Norethindrone and Mestranol 1475
Ortho-Novum 1 35 (CO, FR) *see* Ethinyl Estradiol and Norethindrone 808
Ortho-Novum 1/35 (FR) *see* Ethinyl Estradiol and Norethindrone 808
Ortho-Novum 1 50 (AE, AT, BH, CY, EG, IL, IQ, IR, JO, KW, LB, LY, OM, QA, SA, SY, YE) *see* Norethindrone and Mestranol 1475
Ortho-Novum (MX) *see* Norethindrone 1473
Ortopsique (MX) *see* Diazepam 613
Ortoton (DE) *see* Methocarbamol 1320
Ortrel (VE) *see* Ethinyl Estradiol and Norgestimate 810
Ortrip (TH) *see* Nortriptyline 1476
Orudis (AE, BH, CY, DK, EG, ES, FI, IQ, IR, IS, IT, JO, KW, LB, LY, NO, OM, QA, SA, SE, SY, UY, YE) *see* Ketoprofen 1145
Orudis EC (PH) *see* Ketoprofen 1145
Orudis Gel (AU) *see* Ketoprofen 1145

Orudis R-PR (BB, BM, BS, BZ, GY, JM, NL, PR, SR, TT) *see* Ketoprofen ... 1145
Orudis SR (AU) *see* Ketoprofen ... 1145
Orugal (LT) *see* Itraconazole ... 1130
Orungal (BG, EE, HR, HU, PL, RU) *see* Itraconazole ... 1130
Oruvail (AE, BF, BH, BJ, CI, CY, EG, ET, GB, GH, GM, GN, GR, IE, IQ, IR, JO, KE, KW, LB, LR, LY, MA, ML, MR, MU, MW, NE, NG, NZ, OM, PK, QA, SA, SC, SD, SG, SL, SN, SY, TN, TZ, UG, YE, ZM, ZW) *see* Ketoprofen ... 1145
Oruvail SR (AU, NZ) *see* Ketoprofen ... 1145
Orvakline (HK) *see* AtorvaSTATin ... 194
Orvek (AE, BH, CY, EG, IQ, IR, JO, KW, LB, LY, OM, QA, SA, SY, YE) *see* Penicillin V Potassium ... 1614
Orzol (PY) *see* Itraconazole ... 1130
Osan (HR) *see* Telmisartan ... 1988
Osartan Plus (KR) *see* Losartan and Hydrochlorothiazide ... 1250
Osartil (HK) *see* Losartan ... 1248
Osbone (KR) *see* Etidronate ... 813
Os-Cal 500 + D (HK) *see* Calcium and Vitamin D ... 326
Os-Cal + D (SG) *see* Calcium and Vitamin D ... 326
Oscal (NZ) *see* Calcium Carbonate ... 327
Oseban (EC) *see* Ibandronate ... 1028
Oseotenk (AR) *see* Alendronate ... 79
Osetron (AU) *see* Ondansetron ... 1513
Oseum (MX) *see* Calcitonin ... 322
Osficar (CO) *see* Alendronate ... 79
Osficar Plus (CO) *see* Alendronate and Cholecalciferol ... 81
Osflex (ID) *see* Hyaluronate and Derivatives ... 1006
Osiren (AT) *see* Spironolactone ... 1931
Osmanil (GB) *see* FentaNYL ... 857
Osmitrol (AU, IN, NL, NZ, SA, SG) *see* Mannitol ... 1269
Osmo-Adalat (IL) *see* NIFEdipine ... 1451
Osmofundina (PT) *see* Mannitol ... 1269
Osmofundin (AT, SG) *see* Mannitol ... 1269
Osmofusin-M (BG) *see* Mannitol ... 1269
Osmohale (DK, IT) *see* Mannitol ... 1269
Osmosteril (NL) *see* Mannitol ... 1269
Osmycin (ID) *see* Spiramycin [CAN/INT] ... 1931
Osnervan (DE) *see* Procyclidine [CAN/INT] ... 1721
Ospa-V (AE, BH, CY, EG, IQ, IR, JO, KW, LB, LY, OM, QA, SA, SY, YE) *see* Penicillin V Potassium ... 1614
Ospamox (AE, AT, BG, BH, CR, CY, DE, DO, EG, GT, HR, ID, IQ, IR, JO, KW, LB, LY, MY, NI, NZ, OM, PA, PL, PT, QA, RO, RU, SA, SK, SV, SY, UY, YE) *see* Amoxicillin ... 130
Ospen (AE, AT, EG, FR, JO, KW, LB, MY, QA, SA, SG, UY, VE) *see* Penicillin V Potassium ... 1614
Ospexina (CO) *see* Cephalexin ... 405
Ospexin (AT, BG, BH, CY, CZ, EG, IQ, IR, JO, KW, LB, LY, MY, OM, QA, SA, SY, YE) *see* Cephalexin ... 405
Osporin (PH) *see* CycloSPORINE (Systemic) ... 522
Ospronim (ZA) *see* Pentazocine ... 1616
Ospur F (DE) *see* Fluoride ... 895
Osseor (CN, EE) *see* Strontium Ranelate [INT] ... 1938
Ossin (CZ, DE) *see* Fluoride ... 895
Ossmax (AU) *see* Alendronate ... 79
Ostedron (PL) *see* Etidronate ... 813
Ostelin (AU, IT) *see* Ergocalciferol ... 753
Ostelox (ID) *see* Meloxicam ... 1283
Osteluc (JP) *see* Etodolac ... 815
Osteo-D (TW) *see* Calcitriol ... 323
Osteocal 500 (FR, ID) *see* Calcium Carbonate ... 327
Osteocal (PH) *see* Calcitonin ... 322
Osteocap (MY) *see* Calcitriol ... 323
Osteoclax (CO) *see* Risedronate ... 1816
Osteocor (PH) *see* Alendronate ... 79
Osteodron (PH) *see* Alendronate ... 79
Osteofar (ID) *see* Alendronate ... 79
Osteoflam (IN) *see* Diclofenac (Systemic) ... 617
Osteoflam (PH) *see* Meloxicam ... 1283
Osteofluor (AT, FR) *see* Fluoride ... 895
Osteofort Plus (DO) *see* Alendronate and Cholecalciferol ... 81
Osteofos (HK, IN) *see* Alendronate ... 79
Osteol (PY) *see* Alendronate ... 79
Osteomax (PH) *see* Alendronate ... 79
Osteomin (MX) *see* Calcium Carbonate ... 327
Osteonate OD (ID) *see* Risedronate ... 1816
Osteoplus D (EC) *see* Alendronate and Cholecalciferol ... 81
Osteo-Plus (PH) *see* Alendronate ... 79
Osteopor (UY) *see* Alendronate ... 79
Osteosan (CL) *see* Alendronate ... 79
Osteotop (PE) *see* Etidronate ... 813
Osteotriol (DE) *see* Calcitriol ... 323
Osteovan (CR) *see* Alendronate ... 79
Osteum (ES) *see* Etidronate ... 813
Osteve (LB) *see* Alendronate ... 79
Ostex (CO) *see* Alendronate ... 79
Ostidil-D3 (IT) *see* Alfacalcidol [CAN/INT] ... 82
Ostiral (TR) *see* Raloxifene ... 1765
Ostirein (GR) *see* Diacerein [INT] ... 613
Osyrol (DE, JP) *see* Spironolactone ... 1931
Otalex (VE) *see* Ciprofloxacin and Hydrocortisone ... 446
Otarex (IL) *see* HydrOXYzine ... 1024
Otaxem (MX) *see* Methotrexate ... 1322
Otede (ID) *see* DiphenhydrAMINE (Systemic) ... 641
Otedram (MX) *see* Bromazepam [CAN/INT] ... 290
Otenol (MY) *see* Terbinafine (Topical) ... 2004
Otex HC (CL, PY, UY) *see* Ciprofloxacin and Hydrocortisone ... 446
Otidin (IL) *see* Tetracaine (Topical) ... 2017
Otisyn (FI) *see* Benzocaine ... 246
Otoclear (PH) *see* Docusate ... 661
Otodrops (EC) *see* Ciprofloxacin and Hydrocortisone ... 446
Otodyne (EC) *see* Antipyrine and Benzocaine ... 156
Oto Eni (MX) *see* Ciprofloxacin and Hydrocortisone ... 446
Otoflox (AR, DO, EC) *see* Ofloxacin (Otic) ... 1491
Otofluor (IN) *see* Fluoride ... 895
Otogesic (AE, BH, CY, EG, IL, IQ, IR, JO, KW, LB, LY, OM, QA, SA, SY, YE) *see* Antipyrine and Benzocaine ... 156
Otonil (PY) *see* Ofloxacin (Otic) ... 1491
Otosec (CO, PE) *see* Ciprofloxacin (Otic) ... 446
Otosec (CO, PE) *see* Ciprofloxacin (Systemic) ... 441
Otosec HC (CO, DO, GT, PA, PE) *see* Ciprofloxacin and Hydrocortisone ... 446
Otowax (PH) *see* Docusate ... 661
Otreon (AT, ES, IT) *see* Cefpodoxime ... 388
Otrivin (CH, IS) *see* Azelastine (Nasal) ... 213
Otrivine Anti-Allergie (BE) *see* Azelastine (Nasal) ... 213
Otsu-manitol (ID) *see* Mannitol ... 1269
Ouliting (CN) *see* Rizatriptan ... 1836
Ouyi (CN) *see* Cefadroxil ... 372
Ova-Mit (BB, BM, BS, BZ, GY, JM, PR, SR, TR, TT) *see* ClomiPHENE ... 473
Ovamit (EC, JO, KW, MY, TH) *see* ClomiPHENE ... 473
Ovastar (HK) *see* Lovastatin ... 1252
Overal (IT) *see* Roxithromycin [INT] ... 1853
Ovidrel (AR, AU, BR, CL, CN, CO, EC, HK, ID, IN, KR, MX, MY, NZ, PE, PH, SG, TW, VE) *see* Chorionic Gonadotropin (Recombinant) ... 432
Ovipreg (IN) *see* ClomiPHENE ... 473
Oviskin (ID) *see* Betamethasone (Topical) ... 255
Ovitrelle (BE, BH, CH, CY, CZ, DE, DK, EE, ES, FR, GB, GR, HN, HR, IE, IL, IS, IT, KW, LB, LT, NL, NO, PL, PT, RO, RU, SA, SE, SI, SK, TR) *see* Chorionic Gonadotropin (Recombinant) ... 432
Ovoplex 30-150 (ES) *see* Ethinyl Estradiol and Levonorgestrel ... 803
Ovral (AR, BB, BF, BJ, BM, BS, BZ, CI, ET, GH, GM, GN, GR, GY, IN, JM, KE, LR, MA, ML, MR, MU, MW, MX, NE, NG, NL, PE, PK, SC, SD, SL, SN, SR, TN, TT, TZ,

UG, ZA, ZM, ZW) *see* Ethinyl Estradiol and Norgestrel ... 812
Ovranette (AT, GB) *see* Ethinyl Estradiol and Levonorgestrel ... 803
Ovulen 50 (NL) *see* Ethinyl Estradiol and Ethynodiol Diacetate ... 801
Ovulet (PH) *see* ClomiPHENE ... 473
Ovurila (ID) *see* Ketoprofen ... 1145
Ovysmen 0.5 35 (AT, BE, DE) *see* Ethinyl Estradiol and Norethindrone ... 808
Ovysmen 1 35 (AT, CH, DE) *see* Ethinyl Estradiol and Norethindrone ... 808
Ovysmen (AE, BE, BF, BH, BJ, CI, CY, EG, ET, GB, GH, GM, GN, IQ, IR, JO, KE, KW, LB, LR, LY, MA, ML, MR, MU, MW, NE, NG, OM, QA, SA, SC, SD, SL, SN, SY, TN, TZ, UG, YE, ZM, ZW) *see* Ethinyl Estradiol and Norethindrone ... 808
Oxacilina (CO) *see* Oxacillin ... 1528
Oxacillin (PL) *see* Oxacillin ... 1528
Oxacin (TW) *see* Ofloxacin (Systemic) ... 1490
Oxaflox (ID) *see* Pefloxacin [INT] ... 1588
Oxair (MY) *see* Montelukast ... 1392
Oxalatin (AU) *see* Oxaliplatin ... 1528
Oxalee (PH) *see* Oxaliplatin ... 1528
Oxalem (PH) *see* Oxaliplatin ... 1528
Oxalepsy (PK) *see* OXcarbazepine ... 1532
Oxalept (HR) *see* OXcarbazepine ... 1532
Oxalip (TH, TW) *see* Oxaliplatin ... 1528
Oxaltic (AR) *see* Oxaliplatin ... 1528
Oxaltie (EC, LB, PK) *see* Oxaliplatin ... 1528
Oxanon (BR) *see* Oxacillin ... 1528
Oxan (PH) *see* Oxacillin ... 1528
Oxapen (PH) *see* Oxacillin ... 1528
Oxapla (KR) *see* Oxaliplatin ... 1528
Oxaplat (TH) *see* Oxaliplatin ... 1528
Oxaprim (IT) *see* Sulfamethoxazole and Trimethoprim ... 1946
Oxaprost (AR) *see* Misoprostol ... 1379
Oxatadine (KR) *see* Oxatomide [INT] ... 1532
Oxatalis (PH) *see* Oxacillin ... 1528
Oxatokey (ES) *see* Oxatomide [INT] ... 1532
Oxazepam Efeka (LU) *see* Oxazepam ... 1532
Oxazepam-Eurogenerics (LU) *see* Oxazepam ... 1532
Oxazepam (PL) *see* Oxazepam ... 1532
Oxazepam-ratiopharm (LU) *see* Oxazepam ... 1532
Oxcap (IN) *see* Amoxapine ... 128
Oxcar (PY) *see* OXcarbazepine ... 1532
Oxedep (CN) *see* FLUoxetine ... 899
Oxeno (AR) *see* Loxoprofen [INT] ... 1255
Oxeol (DK, FR) *see* Bambuterol [INT] ... 227
Oxerin (CO) *see* Oxaliplatin ... 1528
Oxetal (HR) *see* Oxatomide [INT] ... 1532
Oxetine (AE, JO, LB, SA) *see* FLUoxetine ... 899
Oxetol (MX) *see* OXcarbazepine ... 1532
Oxibron (AR) *see* Clenbuterol [INT] ... 460
Oxicone (TW) *see* Oxiconazole ... 1536
Oxiflux (RO) *see* Pentoxifylline ... 1618
Oxifungol (MX) *see* Fluconazole ... 885
Oxigen (BR) *see* NiMODipine ... 1456
Oxiklorin (FI, KR) *see* Hydroxychloroquine ... 1021
Oximag (PL) *see* Magnesium Oxide ... 1265
Oxipelle (BR) *see* Oxiconazole ... 1536
Oxiplus (PY) *see* Beclomethasone (Nasal) ... 232
Oxiplus SF (UY) *see* Beclomethasone (Nasal) ... 232
Oxis (AE, AR, AU, BB, BF, BH, BJ, BM, BS, BZ, CH, CI, CN, CR, CY, DE, DO, ET, GH, GM, GN, GT, GY, HN, HU, IE, IL, IS, JM, KE, KW, LB, LR, MA, ML, MR, MU, MW, MY, NE, NG, NI, NL, NZ, PA, PH, PR, QA, SA, SC, SD, SE, SG, SI, SK, SL, SN, SR, SV, TN, TR, TT, TZ, UG, ZA, ZM, ZW) *see* Formoterol ... 926
Oxistat (AR, MX) *see* Oxiconazole ... 1536
Oxis Turbuhaler (MX) *see* Formoterol ... 926
Oxis turbuhaler (PL) *see* Formoterol ... 926
Oxitan (TH) *see* Oxaliplatin ... 1528
Oxitel (PH) *see* Oxaliplatin ... 1528
Oxitol (PY) *see* Oxytocin ... 1549
Oxitone (AE, BH, CY, IL, IQ, IR, JO, KW, LB, LY, OM, PH, QA, SA, SY, YE) *see* Oxytocin ... 1549
Oxitosona (ES) *see* Oxymetholone ... 1546
Oxitrin (PY) *see* Rifampin ... 1804
Oxivent (BE, CH, DE, GB, IE, IT, LU) *see* Oxitropium [INT] ... 1536
Oxizole (TW) *see* Oxiconazole ... 1536
Oxleti (ES) *see* Oxatomide [INT] ... 1532
Oxocin (TW) *see* Oxytocin ... 1549
Oxogina (VE) *see* Naloxone ... 1419
Oxole (AU) *see* Fluconazole ... 885
Oxol (PH) *see* Betaxolol (Ophthalmic) ... 257
Oxol (TH) *see* Oxaliplatin ... 1528
Oxopurin 400 SR (IL) *see* Pentoxifylline ... 1618
Ox-Pam (NZ) *see* Oxazepam ... 1532
Oxpin (KR) *see* OXcarbazepine ... 1532
OXP (KR) *see* Oxaliplatin ... 1528
Oxrate (IN) *see* OXcarbazepine ... 1532
Oxsoralen (AE, AR, BR, CL, CZ, HK, JO, JP, KW, LB, NO, SA) *see* Methoxsalen (Systemic) ... 1330
Oxsoralen (AE, AT, BH, CH, CY, EG, HK, HN, IQ, IR, JO, JP, KR, KW, LB, LY, NL, OM, PK, PL, QA, SA, SG, SY, YE) *see* Methoxsalen (Topical) ... 1331
Oxsoralen Lotion (ID) *see* Methoxsalen (Topical) ... 1331
Oxsoralen Ultra (AE, BH) *see* Methoxsalen (Systemic) ... 1330
Oxsoralen Ultra (SG) *see* Methoxsalen (Topical) ... 1331
Oxtercid (ID) *see* Cefuroxime ... 399
Oxtin (ID) *see* Oxatomide [INT] ... 1532
Oxyal (AE) *see* Hyaluronate and Derivatives ... 1006
Oxyban (TW) *see* Oxybutynin ... 1536
Oxycod (IL) *see* OxyCODONE ... 1538
OxyContin (AR, AT, AU, BR, CH, CL, CN, CO, CR, CY, CZ, DK, EC, EE, ES, FI, GB, GT, HK, HN, IE, IL, IT, MY, NI, NL, NO, NZ, PA, PE, PH, PL, PT, SE, SG, SV, VE) *see* OxyCODONE ... 1538
Oxycontin CR (KR) *see* OxyCODONE ... 1538
Oxycontin (HR, HU, IS, RO, SI, SK, TR) *see* OxyCODONE ... 1538
Oxycontin LP (FR) *see* OxyCODONE ... 1538
Oxyfast (JP) *see* OxyCODONE ... 1538
Oxyflux (MX) *see* Clenbuterol [INT] ... 460
Oxygesic (DE) *see* OxyCODONE ... 1538
Oxylone (SG) *see* Oxymetholone ... 1546
Oxynorm IV (SG) *see* OxyCODONE ... 1538
Oxynorm (AT, AU, BE, CH, CY, DK, ES, FI, FR, GB, HK, IS, MY, NO, NZ, PH, SE, SG, TR) *see* OxyCODONE ... 1538
OxyNorm (JP) *see* OxyCODONE ... 1538
Oxypine (TW) *see* OXcarbazepine ... 1532
Oxytrol (AU, NZ) *see* Oxybutynin ... 1536
Oxzin (KR) *see* Oxaprozin ... 1532
Oxzoralen (QA) *see* Methoxsalen (Systemic) ... 1330
Ozadep (VN) *see* CloZAPine ... 490
Ozapex (KR) *see* OLANZapine ... 1491
Ozcef (AU) *see* Cefaclor ... 372
Ozen (ID) *see* Cetirizine ... 411
Oziclide MR (AU) *see* Gliclazide [CAN/INT] ... 964
Ozidal (AU) *see* RisperiDONE ... 1818
Ozidia (FR) *see* GlipiZIDE ... 967
Ozin (AU) *see* OLANZapine ... 1491
Ozlodip (AU) *see* AmLODIPine ... 123
Ozmep (AU) *see* Omeprazole ... 1508
Ozolan (RO) *see* Anastrozole ... 148
Ozpan (AU) *see* Pantoprazole ... 1570
Ozurdex (BE, CH, CO, CZ, DE, DK, EE, FR, GB, HK, HR, IL, IN, IS, KR, LT, NL, NO, PL, PT, RO, SE, SG, SI, SK, TH) *see* Dexamethasone (Ophthalmic) ... 602
Ozvir (AU) *see* Acyclovir (Systemic) ... 47

Pabal (AE, AT, BE, CH, DE, DK, EE, FI, FR, GB, GR, HN, IE, KW, LT, NL, NO, PL, PT, QA, SA, SE, SK) *see* Carbetocin [CAN/INT] 350
Pacancer (KR) *see* DOCEtaxel 656
Paceco (MY, SG) *see* Acetaminophen and Codeine 36
Pacemol (KR) *see* Acetaminophen 32
Pacetin (KR) *see* CefOXitin 386
Paceum (CH) *see* Diazepam 613
Pacifen (GT, HN, NI, SV) *see* Bromazepam [CAN/INT] 290
Pacifen (NZ, TW) *see* Baclofen 223
Pacif (JP) *see* Morphine (Systemic) 1394
Pacisulide (HK) *see* Nimesulide [INT] 1456
Pacitane (IN) *see* Trihexyphenidyl 2103
Pacitran (PE) *see* Diazepam 613
Paclimedac (ID) *see* PACLitaxel (Conventional) 1550
Paclitaxin (TH) *see* PACLitaxel (Conventional) 1550
Pacovanton (MX) *see* Nitazoxanide 1461
Pactens (GR) *see* Bisoprolol 266
Pacxel (KR) *see* PACLitaxel (Conventional) 1550
Pacyl (IN) *see* ALPRAZolam 94
Padexol (KR) *see* PACLitaxel (Conventional) 1550
Padonil (ID) *see* GlyBURIDE 972
Padrin (JP) *see* Prifinium [INT] 1712
Paesumex (AE, BH, CY, EG, IQ, IR, JO, KW, LB, LY, OM, QA, SA, SY, YE) *see* Atenolol 189
Paferxin (MX) *see* Cephalexin 405
Pagavit (MX) *see* Thiamine 2028
Painnox (TH) *see* Mefenamic Acid 1280
Painoff (TW) *see* Ketorolac (Systemic) 1146
Painstop (TW) *see* Mefenamic Acid 1280
Pain Will Pass (TW) *see* Tiaprofenic Acid [CAN/INT] 2034
Pai Tong Xin (CN) *see* Reteplase 1794
Pakinol (KR) *see* ROPINIRole 1844
Palatrin (MX) *see* Lansoprazole 1166
Palexia (BG, CH, CZ, DK, EE, FI, GB, HR, IE, IL, LT, NL, SI, SK, TR) *see* Tapentadol 1975
Palexia Depot (DK, FI, NO, SE) *see* Tapentadol 1975
Palexia IR (AU) *see* Tapentadol 1975
Palexia PR (CY, TR) *see* Tapentadol 1975
Palexia Retard (BG, DE, EE, HR, LT, NL, RO, SK) *see* Tapentadol 1975
Palexia SR (GB, IE, IL, SG) *see* Tapentadol 1975
Paliadon Retardkaps (DE) *see* HYDROmorphone 1016
Palin (PL, RU) *see* Pipemidic Acid [INT] 1655
Palitrex (ID) *see* Cephalexin 405
Palladon (CH, DK, FI, IS, NL, NO, SE, SI) *see* HYDROmorphone 1016
Palladone (BE, CZ, EE, ES, GB, GR, HN, IE, IL, PT) *see* HYDROmorphone 1016
Palladone SR (GB, IE, SK) *see* HYDROmorphone 1016
Palladone-SR (HU) *see* HYDROmorphone 1016
Palladon OD (SE) *see* HYDROmorphone 1016
Palladon Retard (CH) *see* HYDROmorphone 1016
Pallagicin (HU) *see* DOXOrubicin (Conventional) 679
Pallidone (NZ) *see* Methadone 1311
Pal Mucil Polvo Vegetal Fino (PY) *see* Psyllium 1744
Palon (TH) *see* Propranolol 1731
Paloxi (ID, IL, KR) *see* Palonosetron 1561
Palpal Chew Tab (KR) *see* Sildenafil 1882
Palpasin (PH) *see* Piroxicam 1662
Palpitin (HN, HU, PL) *see* Disopyramide 653
Palux (JP) *see* Alprostadil 96
Paluxon (HR) *see* PARoxetine 1579
Palzen (IN) *see* Palonosetron 1561
Pamacid (AU) *see* Famotidine 845
Pam-A (SG, VN) *see* Pralidoxime 1694
Pamcl (TW) *see* Pralidoxime 1694
Pamecil (BF, BJ, CI, ET, GH, GM, GN, HK, JO, KE, LR, MA, ML, MR, MU, MW, MY, NE, NG, RO, SC, SD, SL, SN, TN, TZ, UG, ZM, ZW) *see* Ampicillin 141
Pamelor (BR) *see* Nortriptyline 1476
Pamid (IL) *see* Indapamide 1065
Pamidria (LB) *see* Pamidronate 1563
Pamidrom (BR) *see* Pamidronate 1563
Pamidron (JO) *see* Pamidronate 1563
Pamigen (CR, EC, GT, HN, NI, SV) *see* Gemcitabine 952
Pamisol (AU, MX, MY, NZ, SG, TW) *see* Pamidronate 1563
Pamitor (HR, TR) *see* Pamidronate 1563
Pamizep (PH) *see* Diazepam 613
Pam (NL) *see* Penicillin G Procaine 1613
PAM (NZ) *see* Pralidoxime 1694
Pamocil (IT) *see* Amoxicillin 130
Pamol (BH, DK, JO, NZ, QA) *see* Acetaminophen 32
Pamorelin (NO) *see* Triptorelin 2107
Pamoxicillin (TW) *see* Amoxicillin 130
Pamoxin (KR) *see* Amoxicillin 130
Pampara (MY, TW, VN) *see* Pralidoxime 1694
Pamu (KR) *see* Pralidoxime 1694
Panacef (IT) *see* Cefaclor 372
Panacta (PH) *see* Ampicillin 141
Panadeine (BB, BM, BS, BZ, CZ, GY, HK, HN, JM, MY, NL, NZ, PR, SR, TT) *see* Acetaminophen and Codeine 36
Panadeine Co (AE, BH, CY, EG, IQ, IR, JO, KW, LB, LY, OM, QA, SA, SY, YE) *see* Acetaminophen and Codeine 36
Panadeine Forte (AU) *see* Acetaminophen and Codeine 36
Panadiene (AU, BB, BS, HK, JM, JP, MY, NL, NZ) *see* Acetaminophen and Codeine 36
Panadiene Extra (AU) *see* Acetaminophen and Codeine 36
Panado-Co Caplets (ZA) *see* Acetaminophen and Codeine 36
Panadol Actifast (MY, SG) *see* Acetaminophen 32
Panadol (AE, AU, BE, BF, BG, BH, BJ, CH, CI, CL, CY, CZ, EE, EG, ET, FI, FR, GB, GH, GM, GN, GR, HK, HU, ID, IE, IL, IQ, IR, IT, JO, KE, KR, KW, LB, LR, LU, LY, MA, ML, MR, MU, MW, NE, NG, NL, NZ, OM, PE, PK, PL, PT, QA, RO, RU, SA, SC, SD, SG, SK, SL, SN, SY, TH, TN, TW, TZ, UG, YE, ZM, ZW) *see* Acetaminophen 32
Panadol Duo (FI) *see* Acetaminophen and Codeine 36
Panadol Extend (SG) *see* Acetaminophen 32
Panadol for Children (SG) *see* Acetaminophen 32
Panadol Night (NZ) *see* Acetaminophen and Diphenhydramine 36
Panadon (HR) *see* Acetaminophen 32
Panafcort (AU, ZA) *see* PredniSONE 1706
Panafen (NZ) *see* Ibuprofen 1032
Panafox (PH) *see* CefOXitin 386
Panagrel (PE) *see* Clopidogrel 484
Panaldine (JP) *see* Ticlopidine 2040
Panalene (AR) *see* Adapalene 54
Panamax (AU) *see* Acetaminophen 32
Panamicyn (CO) *see* Erythromycin (Systemic) 762
Panamor (ZA) *see* Diclofenac (Systemic) 617
Panataxel (EC) *see* PACLitaxel (Conventional) 1550
Panaxid (BE, LU) *see* Nizatidine 1471
Pan-Benzathine Pen G (HK) *see* Penicillin G Benzathine 1609
Panbesy (BE, HK, LU, SG, TH) *see* Phentermine 1635
Panbicin (TW) *see* Epirubicin 739
Panbicort (JO) *see* Triamcinolone (Systemic) 2099
Pancef (BG) *see* Cefixime 380
Panconium (IN) *see* Pancuronium 1567
Pancrease (BE, DK, ES, FI, NL, NO, NZ, SE) *see* Pancrelipase 1566
Pancrease HL (GB) *see* Pancrelipase 1566
Pancrex (IT) *see* Pancrelipase 1566
Pancuron (BR, PY) *see* Pancuronium 1567
Pancuronio (CO) *see* Pancuronium 1567
Pancuronium Bromide (AU) *see* Pancuronium 1567
Pancuronium (PL) *see* Pancuronium 1567

Pandel (CL, JP, PE, PY, UY) *see* Hydrocortisone (Topical) ... 1014
Pandiuren (AR) *see* AMILoride ... 113
Pan-Fungex (PT) *see* Clotrimazole (Topical) ... 488
Panfurex (FR, LU) *see* Nifuroxazide [INT] ... 1454
Pangavit Pediátrico (MX) *see* Cyproheptadine ... 529
Pangest (BR) *see* Bromopride [INT] ... 292
Pangetan NF (CO) *see* Loperamide ... 1236
Pangraf (IN) *see* Tacrolimus (Systemic) ... 1962
Panimycin (JP) *see* Dibekacin [INT] ... 616
Panloc (ID) *see* Pantoprazole ... 1570
Panmicol (AR) *see* Clotrimazole (Topical) ... 488
Panmycin (AE, BH, CY, EG, IQ, IR, JO, KW, LB, LY, MY, OM, QA, SA, SY, YE) *see* Tetracycline ... 2017
Pannox (PH) *see* Cloxacillin [CAN/INT] ... 488
Panodil (DK, NO, SE) *see* Acetaminophen ... 32
Panolin (KR) *see* Pamidronate ... 1563
Panoral (DE) *see* Cefaclor ... 372
Panoral Forte (DE) *see* Cefaclor ... 372
Panorin (KR) *see* Pamidronate ... 1563
Panos (FR) *see* Tetrazepam [INT] ... 2020
Panprax (CH) *see* Pantoprazole ... 1570
Panraf (JO) *see* Tacrolimus (Systemic) ... 1962
Panrazol (HK) *see* Pantoprazole ... 1570
Pansida (KR) *see* Sulfadoxine and Pyrimethamine [INT] ... 1946
Pantaxin (PH) *see* Cefotaxime ... 382
Pantazol (PH) *see* Pantoprazole ... 1570
Pantec (IN) *see* Pantoprazole ... 1570
Pantecta (CR, DO, ES, GT, HN, IT, NI, NL, PA, SV) *see* Pantoprazole ... 1570
Pantelmin (AT, BR, CO, EC, PE, PT, PY, UY, VE) *see* Mebendazole [CAN/INT] ... 1274
Pantemon (JP) *see* Hydrochlorothiazide ... 1009
Pantenol (PY) *see* Dexpanthenol ... 606
Panteon (KR) *see* Pantoprazole ... 1570
Pantex (PY) *see* Albendazole ... 65
Panthenol (CZ, DE, HN, HU) *see* Dexpanthenol ... 606
Pantinol (AT) *see* Aprotinin ... 168
Pantoavenir IV (IL) *see* Pantoprazole ... 1570
Panto-Byk (LU) *see* Pantoprazole ... 1570
Pantocar (PH) *see* Pantoprazole ... 1570
Pantocid (NZ, TH, ZA) *see* Pantoprazole ... 1570
Pantoc (PT) *see* Pantoprazole ... 1570
Pantocycline (TH) *see* Tetracycline ... 2017
Pantodac (IN) *see* Pantoprazole ... 1570
Pantodar (AE, BH, CY, EG, IQ, IR, JO, KW, LB, LY, OM, QA, SA, SY, YE) *see* Pantoprazole ... 1570
Pantolax (DE) *see* Succinylcholine ... 1939
Pantoloc (AT, AU, CN, DK, EG, FR, HK, JO, KR, LT, PH, SE, TW, VN) *see* Pantoprazole ... 1570
Pantomed (KR) *see* Pantoprazole ... 1570
Pantomicina (AR, CL, PE, VE) *see* Erythromycin (Systemic) ... 762
Pantopan (IN, IT) *see* Pantoprazole ... 1570
Pantop (AR, PK, VE) *see* Pantoprazole ... 1570
Pantoprix (PH) *see* Pantoprazole ... 1570
Pantoprol (TH) *see* Pantoprazole ... 1570
Pantopump (ID) *see* Pantoprazole ... 1570
Pantor (PH) *see* Pantoprazole ... 1570
Pantostac (KR) *see* Pantoprazole ... 1570
Panto (TR) *see* Pantoprazole ... 1570
Pantozol (AE, BE, BH, CH, CY, DE, EG, ID, IQ, IR, JO, KW, LB, LU, LY, MX, NL, OM, PH, SA, SE, SY, YE) *see* Pantoprazole ... 1570
Pantozole (QA) *see* Pantoprazole ... 1570
Pantrixon (PH) *see* CefTRIAXone ... 396
Pantul (EE) *see* Pantoprazole ... 1570
Pantul (PE) *see* Thiopental [INT] ... 2029
Panwarfin (GR) *see* Warfarin ... 2186
Panzole (MY, SG) *see* Pantoprazole ... 1570
Panzor (FI) *see* Pantoprazole ... 1570
Panzytrat (AU) *see* Pancrelipase ... 1566
Paparin (IN) *see* Papaverine ... 1573
Papaverini (ID) *see* Papaverine ... 1573
Papaverinum Hydrochloricum (PL) *see* Papaverine ... 1573
Papaverol (EC) *see* Papaverine ... 1573
Papilock (JP) *see* CycloSPORINE (Ophthalmic) ... 529
Papulex (GB) *see* Niacinamide ... 1446
Para-IV (PH) *see* Acetaminophen ... 32
Paracefan (BE) *see* CloNIDine ... 480
Paracetamol (HR) *see* Acetaminophen ... 32
Paracetamol Pharmavit (HU) *see* Acetaminophen ... 32
Paracetamol-ratiopharm (LU) *see* Acetaminophen ... 32
Paracet (IS, NO) *see* Acetaminophen ... 32
Paracid (BE) *see* Lindane ... 1217
Paracodina (ES, IT, PT) *see* Dihydrocodeine, Aspirin, and Caffeine ... 632
Paracodin (AT, AU, CH, DE, IE) *see* Dihydrocodeine, Aspirin, and Caffeine ... 632
Paracodin[gtt.] (AT, CH, DE, IE) *see* Dihydrocodeine, Aspirin, and Caffeine ... 632
Paracodine (BE) *see* Dihydrocodeine, Aspirin, and Caffeine ... 632
Paracodol (ZA) *see* Acetaminophen and Codeine ... 36
Paracort (TW) *see* Fluocinolone (Topical) ... 893
Para-Co (TH) *see* Codeine ... 497
Paradeine (TH) *see* Acetaminophen and Codeine ... 36
Paradine (MY) *see* Acetaminophen and Codeine ... 36
Paraflex (HR, NO, SE, TR, ZA) *see* Chlorzoxazone ... 430
Parafon DSC (IN) *see* Chlorzoxazone ... 430
Parafon Forte (MX, TH) *see* Chlorzoxazone ... 430
Paragin (TH) *see* Acetaminophen ... 32
Paralgin (AU) *see* Acetaminophen ... 32
Paramax (EE) *see* Acetaminophen and Codeine ... 36
Paramet (KR) *see* RABEprazole ... 1762
Paramix (MX) *see* Nitazoxanide ... 1461
Paramol (IL, LB, RO, TW) *see* Acetaminophen ... 32
Paramol Kat Drops (IL) *see* Acetaminophen ... 32
Paranausine (BE, LU) *see* DimenhyDRINATE ... 637
Paranthil (ZA) *see* Albendazole ... 65
Parapaed (DE) *see* Acetaminophen ... 32
Parapaed Junior (NZ) *see* Acetaminophen ... 32
Parapaed Six Plus (NZ) *see* Acetaminophen ... 32
Paraplatin (AT, BE, BG, CH, EC, EE, EG, ES, FI, FR, GB, HK, HN, HR, HU, IE, IT, JO, LU, NL, PH, PT, QA, RU, SE, TH, TR, TW, UY) *see* CARBOplatin ... 357
Parapoux (FR) *see* Permethrin ... 1627
Paraqueimol (BR) *see* Sulfacetamide (Ophthalmic) ... 1943
Parareg (ES) *see* Cinacalcet ... 439
Paratabs (IS) *see* Acetaminophen ... 32
Paratram (BR) *see* Acetaminophen and Tramadol ... 37
Paratropina (PY) *see* Homatropine ... 1005
Parcemol Forte (HK) *see* Acetaminophen ... 32
Parcemol (HK) *see* Acetaminophen ... 32
Parcono (TH) *see* Acetaminophen and Codeine ... 36
Parcoten (HK) *see* Acetaminophen and Codeine ... 36
Pardopa (IN) *see* Carbidopa and Levodopa ... 351
Pardopa [+ Levidopa] (PL) *see* Carbidopa ... 351
Parexel (CO, PY) *see* PACLitaxel (Conventional) ... 1550
Pargitan (SE) *see* Trihexyphenidyl ... 2103
PARI CR (IN) *see* PARoxetine ... 1579
Paride (ID) *see* Glimepiride ... 966
Pariet (AE, AR, AT, AU, BB, BE, BG, BH, BM, BO, BR, BS, CH, CN, CO, CR, CY, DE, DK, DO, EC, EG, ES, FI, FR, GB, GR, GT, GY, HK, HN, ID, IE, IL, IQ, IR, IS, IT, JM, JO, JP, KR, KW, LB, LT, LY, MX, MY, NI, NL, NZ, OM, PA, PE, PH, PL, PR, PT, PY, QA, RU, SA, SE, SG, SR, SV, SY, TH, TR, TT, TW, UY, VE, VN, YE, ZA) *see* RABEprazole ... 1762
Parilac (IL) *see* Bromocriptine ... 291
Parizac (ES) *see* Omeprazole ... 1508
Parkan (HN, HU) *see* Trihexyphenidyl ... 2103
Parkemed (AT) *see* Mefenamic Acid ... 1280

Parken (CO) *see* Carbidopa and Levodopa ... 351
Parkilyne (ZA) *see* Selegiline ... 1873
Parkinal (ID) *see* Trihexyphenidyl ... 2103
Parkinane LP (FR) *see* Trihexyphenidyl ... 2103
Parkintrel (KR) *see* Amantadine ... 105
Parkirop (IN) *see* ROPINIRole ... 1844
Parkomet (AE, BH, CY, EG, IQ, IR, JO, KW, LY, OM, QA, SY, YE) *see* Carbidopa and Levodopa ... 351
Parkopan (DE, EE, PL) *see* Trihexyphenidyl ... 2103
Parlodel (AE, AR, AT, AU, BD, BE, BF, BH, BJ, BR, CH, CI, CL, CO, CY, CZ, DK, EC, EE, EG, ES, ET, FI, FR, GB, GH, GM, GN, GR, HK, HN, HR, HU, ID, IE, IN, IQ, IR, IT, JO, JP, KE, KR, KW, LB, LR, LY, MA, ML, MR, MT, MU, MW, MX, MY, NE, NG, NL, NO, NZ, OM, PE, PH, PK, PL, PT, PY, QA, RU, SA, SC, SD, SK, SL, SN, SY, TN, TR, TW, TZ, UG, UY, VE, VN, YE, ZM, ZW) *see* Bromocriptine ... 291
Parmenison (AT) *see* PredniSONE ... 1706
Parmol (HK) *see* Acetaminophen ... 32
Parnate (AE, AR, AU, BF, BH, BJ, BR, CI, CY, DE, EG, ES, ET, GB, GH, GM, GN, IE, IL, IQ, IR, JO, KE, KW, LB, LR, LY, MA, ML, MR, MU, MW, NE, NG, OM, QA, SA, SC, SD, SL, SN, SY, TN, TZ, UG, YE, ZA, ZM, ZW) *see* Tranylcypromine ... 2083
Parocline (FR) *see* Minocycline ... 1371
Paromon (HK) *see* Acetaminophen ... 32
Paronal (BE, NL) *see* Asparaginase (E. coli) ... 179
Paroten (EC) *see* PARoxetine ... 1579
Parotin (HK) *see* PARoxetine ... 1579
Parotin (TW) *see* Dipyridamole ... 652
Paroxat (LB, SA) *see* PARoxetine ... 1579
Paroxil CR (KR) *see* PARoxetine ... 1579
Parsel (MX) *see* Dihydroergotamine ... 633
PARS (IN) *see* Rabies Immune Globulin (Human) ... 1764
Parten-50 (PH) *see* Losartan ... 1248
Partobulin (CZ, GB, HK, IT, TR) *see* Rh_o(D) Immune Globulin ... 1794
Partocon INJ (FI) *see* Oxytocin ... 1549
Partogamma (IT) *see* Rh_o(D) Immune Globulin ... 1794
Partogloman (AT) *see* Rh_o(D) Immune Globulin ... 1794
Partusisten (CH, CZ, DE, HR, HU, NL, PL) *see* Fenoterol [INT] ... 857
Partusisten intrapartal (PL) *see* Fenoterol [INT] ... 857
Parvid (PH) *see* Acetaminophen ... 32
Parvolex (GB, IE, NZ) *see* Acetylcysteine ... 40
Pasconeural-Injektopas (DE) *see* Procainamide ... 1716
Pasedol (CO, EC) *see* DimenhyDRINATE ... 637
Pasetocin (JP) *see* Amoxicillin ... 130
Paspertin (HU) *see* Metoclopramide ... 1345
Paspirin (KR) *see* Triflusal [INT] ... 2103
Pasport (TR) *see* Tadalafil ... 1968
Pasquam (ID) *see* Dexpanthenol ... 606
Pasrin (ZA) *see* BusPIRone ... 311
Passifuril (BR) *see* Nifuroxazide [INT] ... 1454
Passiva (PE) *see* AtoMOXetine ... 191
Passton (TW) *see* Mefenamic Acid ... 1280
Pasta de Lassar (MX) *see* Zinc Oxide ... 2200
Pastaron (JP) *see* Urea ... 2114
Pasta Zinci (PL) *see* Zinc Oxide ... 2200
Pataday (AE, BH, IL, KW, QA, SA, SG, VN) *see* Olopatadine (Ophthalmic) ... 1500
Patanol (AE, AR, AU, BH, BO, BR, CL, CN, CO, CR, DO, GT, HK, HN, ID, IL, IN, JO, JP, KR, KW, LB, MY, NI, NZ, PA, PE, PH, PY, QA, SA, SG, SV, TH, TW, UY, VE, VN, ZA) *see* Olopatadine (Ophthalmic) ... 1500
Patanol GV (JP) *see* Olopatadine (Ophthalmic) ... 1500
Patanol S (CO, CR, DO, GT, HN, NI, PA, SV, UY) *see* Olopatadine (Ophthalmic) ... 1500
Patir (IL) *see* Terbinafine (Systemic) ... 2002
Patir (IL) *see* Terbinafine (Topical) ... 2004
Patrex (SE) *see* Sildenafil ... 1882
Patricin (JP) *see* FlavoxATE ... 881
Patryl (PH) *see* MetroNIDAZOLE (Systemic) ... 1353
Pauly (MX) *see* Pantoprazole ... 1570
Pavacol-D (GB) *see* Pholcodine [INT] ... 1646
Pavedal (CL) *see* Metolazone ... 1348
Pavulon (AE, AT, AU, BD, BE, BG, BH, CH, CN, CY, CZ, DE, DK, EE, EG, ES, FI, FR, GB, GR, HK, HN, HR, HU, ID, IE, IN, IQ, IR, IT, JO, JP, KW, LB, LU, LY, MT, MY, NL, NO, OM, PH, PK, PL, PT, QA, RU, SA, SE, SG, SI, SK, SY, TH, TR, TW, VE, VN, YE) *see* Pancuronium ... 1567
Pavulone (IL) *see* Pancuronium ... 1567
Paxadorm (ZA) *see* Nitrazepam [CAN/INT] ... 1461
Paxam (AU, NZ) *see* ClonazePAM ... 478
Paxan (CO) *see* PARoxetine ... 1579
Paxel (KR, PH) *see* PACLitaxel (Conventional) ... 1550
Paxene (AT, BE, BG, CH, CZ, DE, DK, EE, ES, FI, FR, GB, GR, HN, IE, IT, MT, NL, NO, PL, PT, RU, SE, SK, TR) *see* PACLitaxel (Conventional) ... 1550
Paxetil (KR) *see* PARoxetine ... 1579
Paxicam (ID) *see* Meloxicam ... 1283
Paxil (BB, BM, BS, BZ, CR, DO, EC, GT, GY, HN, JM, MX, NI, PA, PR, RU, SR, SV, TR, TT, VE) *see* PARoxetine ... 1579
Paxil CR (BB, BM, BS, BZ, CR, DO, EC, GT, GY, HN, JM, KR, MX, NI, PA, PR, SR, SV, TT) *see* PARoxetine ... 1579
Paxilfar (PT) *see* TraMADol ... 2074
Paximol (SG) *see* Acetaminophen ... 32
Paxirasol (CZ, HU) *see* Bromhexine [INT] ... 291
Paxistil (BE) *see* HydrOXYzine ... 1024
Paxium (PT) *see* ChlordiazePOXIDE ... 422
Paxon (CL) *see* BusPIRone ... 311
Paxtibi (ES) *see* Nortriptyline ... 1476
Paxtine (AU) *see* PARoxetine ... 1579
Paxum (IN) *see* Diazepam ... 613
Paxus (ID) *see* PACLitaxel (Conventional) ... 1550
Paxxet (IL) *see* PARoxetine ... 1579
Pax (ZA) *see* Diazepam ... 613
Pazeadin (JP) *see* Diltiazem ... 634
Pazergicel (GR) *see* Etofenamate [INT] ... 815
Pazidium (PY) *see* Clorazepate ... 487
Pazolam (LB) *see* ALPRAZolam ... 94
PC-20 (TH) *see* Piroxicam ... 1662
P-Cin (IN) *see* Pefloxacin [INT] ... 1588
P.D.T. Vax Purified (KR) *see* Diphtheria and Tetanus Toxoids, and Acellular Pertussis Vaccine ... 649
Peace (MY, TW) *see* Triprolidine and Pseudoephedrine ... 2105
Peast C (JP) *see* ChlordiazePOXIDE ... 422
Pebact (PK) *see* Pefloxacin [INT] ... 1588
PecFent (GB) *see* FentaNYL ... 857
Pectal Expectorant (AE, BH) *see* GuaiFENesin ... 986
Pectal (QA, SA) *see* GuaiFENesin ... 986
Pectinfant (LU) *see* Codeine ... 497
Pectite (JP) *see* Mecysteine [INT] ... 1277
Pectocil (ID) *see* Acetylcysteine ... 40
Pectodrill (CZ, ES, PL) *see* Carbocisteine [INT] ... 357
Pectolin (AU) *see* Pholcodine [INT] ... 1646
Pectomucil (LU) *see* Acetylcysteine ... 40
Pectoral Edulcor (LU) *see* Codeine ... 497
Pectox (AR, CH) *see* Carbocisteine [INT] ... 357
Pectril (PH) *see* Cephalexin ... 405
Pedea (AT, BE, BG, CH, CZ, DE, DK, EE, ES, FI, FR, GB, GR, IE, IT, KR, MT, NL, NO, PL, PT, RU, SE, SK, TR) *see* Ibuprofen ... 1032
Pediafer (LB) *see* Ferrous Sulfate ... 871
Pediaphyllin PL (LU) *see* Theophylline ... 2026
Pediazole (AE, BH, CY, EC, EG, FR, GR, IQ, IR, JO, KW, LB, LY, MX, MY, OM, PE, PH, PK, QA, SA, SY, TW, VE, YE) *see* Erythromycin and Sulfisoxazole ... 765
Pedipan (KR) *see* Acetaminophen ... 32
Pedipur (PL) *see* Methenamine ... 1317
Pedovex (AE) *see* Clopidogrel ... 484

Pedvax HIB (BR) *see* Haemophilus b Conjugate Vaccine ... 991
Pefaxin (TW) *see* Pefloxacin [INT] ... 1588
Pefcin (IN) *see* Pefloxacin [INT] ... 1588
Pef (IN) *see* Pefloxacin [INT] ... 1588
Peflacine (AE, FR, GR, ID, LB, PT, SA, TR, VN) *see* Pefloxacin [INT] ... 1588
Peflacin (EG, HU, IT, NZ) *see* Pefloxacin [INT] ... 1588
Pegasys (AE, AR, AT, AU, BE, BG, BH, BR, CH, CL, CN, CO, CY, CZ, DE, DK, EC, EE, ES, FI, FR, GB, GR, HK, HN, HR, HU, ID, IE, IL, IS, IT, JO, JP, KR, LB, LT, MT, MX, MY, NL, NO, NZ, PE, PH, PK, PL, PT, PY, QA, RO, RU, SA, SE, SG, SI, SK, TH, TR, TW, UY, VE, VN) *see* Peginterferon Alfa-2a ... 1590
Pegasys PFS (KR) *see* Peginterferon Alfa-2a ... 1590
Pegfel (RO) *see* Lercanidipine [INT] ... 1181
Peg-Intron (AE, BH, CY, JO, KW, LB, QA, SA) *see* Peginterferon Alfa-2b ... 1596
PEG-Intron (AT, AU, BE, BG, BR, CH, CL, CN, CO, CR, CZ, DE, DK, DO, EC, EE, ES, FI, FR, GR, GT, HN, ID, IE, IL, IS, IT, KR, LT, MT, MY, NI, NL, NO, NZ, PA, PE, PH, PK, PL, PT, RU, SE, SG, SI, SK, SV, TH, TR, TW, VE) *see* Peginterferon Alfa-2b ... 1596
Peg-Intron (HK, KR) *see* Interferon Alfa-2b ... 1096
PegIntron (HR, HU, RO) *see* Peginterferon Alfa-2b ... 1596
Peg Intron (JP, VN) *see* Peginterferon Alfa-2b ... 1596
Peglasta (MY, SG, TH) *see* Pegfilgrastim ... 1589
Pegtron (MX) *see* Peginterferon Alfa-2b ... 1596
Pehacort (ID) *see* PredniSONE ... 1706
Peitel Crema (CR, DO, EC, GT, HN, NI, PA, PE, SV) *see* Prednicarbate ... 1703
Peitel (ES, LB, MX) *see* Prednicarbate ... 1703
Pekiron (TW) *see* Amorolfine [INT] ... 128
Pelascap (ID) *see* Imipenem and Cilastatin ... 1051
Pelastin IV (ID) *see* Imipenem and Cilastatin ... 1051
Peldacyn (PH) *see* Clindamycin (Systemic) ... 460
Pelitin (TW) *see* Ampicillin ... 141
Pelmain (JP) *see* Mecysteine [INT] ... 1277
Pelmec Duo (AR) *see* Amlodipine and Benazepril ... 125
Peloxin (TW) *see* Pefloxacin [INT] ... 1588
Peltazon (JP) *see* Pentazocine ... 1616
Pelzont (RO) *see* Nicotine ... 1449
Pemar (CL) *see* Piroxicam ... 1662
Pemax (SG) *see* Pefloxacin [INT] ... 1588
Pemine (IT) *see* PenicillAMINE ... 1608
Pen V (HK) *see* Penicillin V Potassium ... 1614
Penaderm (DE) *see* Urea ... 2114
Penadur (CH, LU) *see* Penicillin G Benzathine ... 1609
Penadur - LA (BB, BM, BS, BZ, GY, JM, PR, SR, TT) *see* Penicillin G Benzathine ... 1609
Penadur LA (BF, BJ, CI, ET, GH, GM, GN, KE, LR, MA, ML, MR, MU, MW, NE, NG, SC, SD, SL, SN, TN, TZ, UG, ZM, ZW) *see* Penicillin G Benzathine ... 1609
Penadur L.A. (GR, PT) *see* Penicillin G Benzathine ... 1609
Penalgin (CO) *see* Nimesulide [INT] ... 1456
Penamine (JO) *see* PenicillAMINE ... 1608
Penamox (AE, BH, JO, MX, QA, SA) *see* Amoxicillin ... 130
Penam (PH) *see* Imipenem and Cilastatin ... 1051
Penbiosyn (PH) *see* Amoxicillin ... 130
Penbrex (KR) *see* Ampicillin ... 141
Penbritin (AE, BF, BH, BJ, CI, CY, EG, ET, GH, GM, GN, HK, IE, IQ, IR, JO, KE, KW, LB, LR, LY, MA, ML, MR, MU, MW, MX, MY, NE, NG, OM, PE, QA, SA, SC, SD, SL, SN, SY, TN, TZ, UG, YE, ZA, ZM, ZW) *see* Ampicillin ... 141
Pencarv (PH) *see* Penicillin G (Parenteral/ Aqueous) ... 1611
Pencil (PH) *see* Cilostazol ... 437
Pencor (HK, MY, SG, TH) *see* Doxazosin ... 674
Pendepon (CZ) *see* Penicillin G Benzathine ... 1609
Pender (KR) *see* Phentermine ... 1635
Pen Di Ben (AR, CR, DO, GT, HN, NI, PA, SV) *see* Penicillin G Benzathine ... 1609
Pendine (AU) *see* Gabapentin ... 943
Pendysin (DE) *see* Penicillin G Benzathine ... 1609
Penedil (IL) *see* Felodipine ... 850
Penegra (BF, BJ, CI, ET, GH, GM, GN, IN, KE, LR, MA, ML, MR, MU, MW, NE, NG, PH, SC, SD, SL, SN, TN, TZ, UG, ZM, ZW) *see* Sildenafil ... 1882
Pengatine (KR) *see* Gabapentin ... 943
Pengesic (SG) *see* TraMADol ... 2074
Pengesic SR (HK) *see* TraMADol ... 2074
Pengesod (MX) *see* Penicillin G (Parenteral/ Aqueous) ... 1611
Penhance (PH) *see* Amoxicillin and Clavulanate ... 133
Penibrin (IL) *see* Ampicillin ... 141
Penicilamin (CZ) *see* PenicillAMINE ... 1608
Penicilina Northia (AR) *see* Penicillin G (Parenteral/ Aqueous) ... 1611
Penicillamin (FI, SE) *see* PenicillAMINE ... 1608
Penicillin G (BG) *see* Penicillin G (Parenteral/ Aqueous) ... 1611
Penicillin G- Natrium (AT) *see* Penicillin G (Parenteral/ Aqueous) ... 1611
Penicillinum procainicum (PL) *see* Penicillin G Procaine ... 1613
Penicomb (GR) *see* Econazole ... 703
Penid (KR) *see* Methylphenidate ... 1336
Penidural (NL) *see* Penicillin G Benzathine ... 1609
Penidure LA 6 (IN) *see* Penicillin G Benzathine ... 1609
Penidure LA 12 (IN) *see* Penicillin G Benzathine ... 1609
Penidure LA 24 (IN) *see* Penicillin G Benzathine ... 1609
Peniern (ES) *see* Penicillin G Procaine ... 1613
Penifasa 900 (ES) *see* Penicillin G Procaine ... 1613
Penilente (BF, BJ, CI, ET, GH, GM, GN, KE, LR, MA, ML, MR, MU, MW, NE, NG, SC, SD, SL, SN, TN, TZ, UG, ZM, ZW) *see* Penicillin G Benzathine ... 1609
Penilevel (ES) *see* Penicillin V Potassium ... 1614
Peniroger Procain (ES) *see* Penicillin G Procaine ... 1613
Peniroger Retard (ES) *see* Penicillin G Benzathine ... 1609
Penlac (BM) *see* Ciclopirox ... 433
Penles (PH) *see* Naproxen ... 1427
Penodil (TR) *see* Ampicillin ... 141
Penoxil (MY) *see* Penicillin V Potassium ... 1614
Penphylline (TW) *see* Pentoxifylline ... 1618
Penpol (KR) *see* Pentosan Polysulfate Sodium ... 1617
Pen-Rafa V-K (IL) *see* Penicillin V Potassium ... 1614
Penral-Night (KR) *see* Acetaminophen ... 32
Penrazole (SG) *see* Omeprazole ... 1508
Pensodital (MX) *see* Thiopental [INT] ... 2029
Pensodril (GR) *see* Isosorbide Dinitrate ... 1124
Penstapho (BE, IT) *see* Oxacillin ... 1528
Penstapho N (BE) *see* Cloxacillin [CAN/INT] ... 488
Pentacard (BE, ID) *see* Isosorbide Mononitrate ... 1126
Pentacarinat (AT, BB, BE, BG, BM, BS, BZ, CH, CZ, DE, DK, EE, ES, FI, FR, GB, GY, HK, HN, IE, IT, JM, MT, NL, NO, NZ, PR, PT, RU, SE, SI, SK, SR, TH, TR, TT) *see* Pentamidine ... 1616
Pentacarinate (GR) *see* Pentamidine ... 1616
Pentacrin (GR) *see* Diacerein [INT] ... 613
Pentagin (JP) *see* Pentazocine ... 1616
Pentaglobin (AT, DE, SG, TH, VN) *see* Immune Globulin ... 1056
Pentajin (JP) *see* Pentazocine ... 1616
Pental (KR) *see* Pentazocine ... 1616
Pental (TR) *see* Thiopental [INT] ... 2029
Pentam 300 (MX) *see* Pentamidine ... 1616
Pentamon (HR) *see* Pentoxifylline ... 1618
Pentarim (MX) *see* Thiopental [INT] ... 2029
Pentasa (AE, AU, BE, BH, CH, CN, CY, DK, EG, FR, GB, HK, HR, HU, IQ, IR, IS, JO, JP, KW, LB, LU, LY, MY, NL, NO, OM, PH, QA, RO, RU, SA, SE, SG, SI, SK, SY, TH, TR, TW, VN, YE) *see* Mesalamine ... 1301

Pentasa Enema (NZ) *see* Mesalamine 1301
Pentasa SR (AE, BH, CY, EG, IL, IQ, IR, JO, KR, KW, LB, LY, OM, QA, SA, SY, YE) *see* Mesalamine 1301
Pentasa Tab (NZ) *see* Mesalamine 1301
Pentasol (CO) *see* Clobetasol 468
Pentavir (AR) *see* Famciclovir 843
Pentawin (IN) *see* Pentazocine 1616
Pentazocina[inj.] (ES) *see* Pentazocine 1616
Pentazocinum (PL) *see* Pentazocine 1616
Pentazol (PH) *see* Thiopental [INT] 2029
Pentcillin (JP) *see* Piperacillin [CAN/INT] 1656
Penthal (PH) *see* Thiopental [INT] 2029
Penthotal (CN) *see* Thiopental [INT] 2029
Pentilin (HR) *see* Pentoxifylline 1618
Pentixol (TW) *see* Flupentixol [CAN/INT] 903
Pentocur (DK, FI, NO) *see* Thiopental [INT] 2029
Pentofuryl (DE) *see* Nifuroxazide [INT] 1454
Pentolate (JO, SA) *see* Cyclopentolate 517
Pentone (AU) *see* PENTobarbital 1617
Pentorel (IN) *see* Buprenorphine 300
Pentostam (AE, EG, GB, IL, KW, QA, SA, SI) *see* Sodium Stibogluconate [INT] 1913
Pentotal (KR) *see* Thiopental [INT] 2029
Pentotex (MY) *see* Thiopental [INT] 2029
Pentothal (AU, BB, BM, BS, BZ, CH, FR, GR, GY, ID, IT, JM, LU, MX, NL, NZ, PH, PT, PY, SE, SG, SR, TT, TW, UY) *see* Thiopental [INT] 2029
Pentothal Sodico (ES) *see* Thiopental [INT] 2029
Pentothal Sodium (ES, PL) *see* Thiopental [INT] 2029
Pentowin (HK) *see* Pantoprazole 1570
Pentoxal (PH) *see* Pentoxifylline 1618
Pentoxi (CH) *see* Pentoxifylline 1618
Pentoxifilina (CO) *see* Pentoxifylline 1618
Pentoxifyllin AL (HU) *see* Pentoxifylline 1618
Pentoxifyllin-B (HU) *see* Pentoxifylline 1618
Pentoxifyllin Pharmavit (HU) *see* Pentoxifylline 1618
Pentoxifyllin-ratiopharm (LU) *see* Pentoxifylline 1618
Pentoxine (JO) *see* Pentoxifylline 1618
Pentoxin SR (KR) *see* Pentoxifylline 1618
Pentox (PH) *see* Pentoxifylline 1618
Pentox von ct (LU) *see* Pentoxifylline 1618
Pentrexyl (BE, BF, BJ, CI, DK, ET, GB, GH, GM, GN, GR, IT, KE, LR, MA, ML, MR, MU, MW, MX, NE, NG, NO, SC, SD, SL, SN, TH, TN, TZ, UG, ZM, ZW) *see* Ampicillin 141
Pentrexyl (QA) *see* Amoxicillin 130
Pentrexyxl (KW) *see* Amoxicillin 130
Pentrxyl (QA) *see* Ampicillin 141
Pentyllin (AE, BH, CY, EG, IQ, IR, JO, KW, LB, LY, OM, QA, SA, SY, YE) *see* Pentoxifylline 1618
Pen Ve Oral (BR) *see* Penicillin V Potassium 1614
Pen-Vi-K (MX) *see* Penicillin V Potassium 1614
Penvir Labia (BR) *see* Penciclovir 1608
Penzathine (KR) *see* Penicillin G Benzathine 1609
Pepcid AC (CH, IE) *see* Famotidine 845
Pepcidac (FR) *see* Famotidine 845
Pepcid (BB, BM, BS, BZ, GB, GY, JM, SE, SR, TT) *see* Famotidine 845
Pepcidina (PT) *see* Famotidine 845
Pepcidin (DK, FI, JO, NL, NO, SE) *see* Famotidine 845
Pepcidine (AT, BE, CH, LU, MX, NZ, PE, VN) *see* Famotidine 845
Pepcidin Rapitab (NO) *see* Famotidine 845
Pepdif (TR) *see* Famotidine 845
Pepdine (BF, BJ, CI, ET, FR, GH, GM, GN, KE, LR, MA, ML, MR, MU, MW, NE, NG, SC, SD, SL, SN, TN, TZ, UG, ZM, ZW) *see* Famotidine 845
Pepevit (MX) *see* Niacin 1443
Pepfamin (TH) *see* Famotidine 845
Peprazom (PH) *see* Esomeprazole 771
Pepridon (PH) *see* Domperidone [CAN/INT] 666
Pepsamar (BF, BJ, BR, CI, CN, CO, ES, ET, GH, GM, GN, GR, KE, LR, MA, ML, MR, MU, MW, NE, NG, PE, PT, SC, SD, SL, SN, TN, TZ, UG, VE, ZM, ZW) *see* Aluminum Hydroxide 103
Pepsytoin-100 (TH) *see* Phenytoin 1640
Peptax (PY) *see* Magaldrate and Simethicone 1261
Peptazol (AR, MY, SG) *see* Pantoprazole 1570
Peptazole (HK) *see* Pantoprazole 1570
Pepticus (PY) *see* Pantoprazole 1570
Peptifam (AE, BH, CY, EG, IQ, IR, JO, KW, LB, LY, OM, QA, SA, SY, YE) *see* Famotidine 845
Peptizole (TH) *see* Omeprazole 1508
Peptoci (TH) *see* Famotidine 845
Peptomet (CY) *see* Domperidone [CAN/INT] 666
Peptonorm (GR) *see* Sucralfate 1940
Peptoran (HR) *see* Ranitidine 1777
Pepzan (AU, MY, NZ) *see* Famotidine 845
Pepzol (ID) *see* Pantoprazole 1570
Peracillin (KR) *see* Piperacillin [CAN/INT] 1656
Peracin (TH) *see* Piperacillin [CAN/INT] 1656
Peragit (DK, NO) *see* Trihexyphenidyl 2103
Peramiflu (KR) *see* Peramivir 1619
Perasian (TH) *see* Loperamide 1236
Peratam (KR) *see* Cefoperazone and Sulbactam [INT] 382
Peratsin (FI) *see* Perphenazine 1627
Peraxin (PH) *see* Pefloxacin [INT] 1588
Perazodin (SG, TR) *see* Dipyridamole 652
Perciclina (PT) *see* Demeclocycline 589
Percocet-5 (IL) *see* Oxycodone and Acetaminophen 1541
Percodan (IL) *see* Oxycodone and Aspirin 1542
Perderm (AE, BH, CY, EG, HK, HN, IL, IQ, IR, JO, KW, LB, LY, OM, QA, SA, SY, YE) *see* Alclometasone 72
Perdipina (IT) *see* NiCARdipine 1446
Perdipine (CN, ID, JP, KR, PH, TW) *see* NiCARdipine 1446
Perdipine LA (JP) *see* NiCARdipine 1446
Perdix (GB, LB) *see* Moexipril 1388
Perdolan codeine (BE) *see* Acetaminophen and Codeine 36
Perdolan Mono (LU) *see* Acetaminophen 32
Perencal (KR) *see* Pentoxifylline 1618
Perennum (PY) *see* Potassium Chloride 1687
Perfalgan (AE, AT, AU, BG, CH, CZ, DE, DK, EE, FI, FR, GB, GR, HR, IE, IL, IN, IS, IT, JO, KR, KW, LB, LT, MT, NL, NO, NZ, PL, PT, RO, RU, SA, SE, SI, SK, TR, VN, ZA) *see* Acetaminophen 32
Perfan (BE, DE, GB, IE, IT, NL) *see* Enoximone [INT] 730
Perfane (FR, IT, LU) *see* Enoximone [INT] 730
Perfen (TW) *see* Ibuprofen 1032
Perfudal (ES) *see* Felodipine 850
Perfusalgan (BE) *see* Acetaminophen 32
Pergamid (AR) *see* Aniracetam [INT] 150
Pergogreen (NZ) *see* Menotropins 1292
Pergonal 75 75 (AT) *see* Menotropins 1292
Pergonal 500 (AE, BG, BH, CY, EG, IL, IQ, IR, JO, KW, LB, LY, OM, QA, SA, SY, YE) *see* Menotropins 1292
Pergonal (AR, CZ, DE, ES, GR, HN, HR, HU, NL, RU, UY) *see* Menotropins 1292
Pergotime (BE, DK, FR, NO, SE) *see* ClomiPHENE 473
Periactin (AE, AT, AU, BE, BF, BH, BJ, CH, CI, CO, CY, DK, EC, EE, EG, ES, ET, FI, GB, GH, GM, GN, IE, IL, IQ, IR, IT, JO, KE, KW, LB, LR, LU, LY, MA, ML, MR, MT, MU, MW, MY, NE, NG, NL, NO, OM, PK, PL, PT, QA, RU, SA, SC, SD, SE, SK, SL, SN, SY, TH, TN, TR, TZ, UG, VE, YE, ZM, ZW) *see* Cyproheptadine 529
Periactine (FR) *see* Cyproheptadine 529
Periafin (TW) *see* Terbinafine (Systemic) 2002
Periafin (TW) *see* Terbinafine (Topical) 2004
Pericate (IL) *see* Haloperidol 993
Pericephal (AT) *see* Cinnarizine [INT] 440
Peridane (MX) *see* Pentoxifylline 1618
Peridon (IT, JO) *see* Domperidone [CAN/INT] 666
Peridys (FR) *see* Domperidone [CAN/INT] 666

Periflux (ID) *see* Domperidone [CAN/INT] 666
Perigard (MY, PH) *see* Perindopril 1623
Perilax (DK, ZA) *see* Bisacodyl 265
Perinace (MY, SG) *see* Perindopril 1623
Perindal (HK) *see* Perindopril 1623
Perindo (AU) *see* Perindopril 1623
Perindo Combi (AU) *see* Perindopril and Indapamide [CAN/INT] 1626
Perinorm (IN, RU, ZA) *see* Metoclopramide 1345
Perio-Aid (CL) *see* Chlorhexidine Gluconate 422
Perio Chip (IL) *see* Chlorhexidine Gluconate 422
Periochip (NO) *see* Chlorhexidine Gluconate 422
PerioChip (SG) *see* Chlorhexidine Gluconate 422
Periocline (JP) *see* Minocycline 1371
Periogard (PT) *see* Chlorhexidine Gluconate 422
Periostat (GB, IE) *see* Doxycycline 689
Perioxidin (MX) *see* Chlorhexidine Gluconate 422
Periplum (IT) *see* NiMODipine 1456
Peripress (FI) *see* Prazosin 1703
Peripril Plus (PH) *see* Perindopril and Indapamide [CAN/INT] 1626
Perisafe (TW) *see* Enalapril 722
Peritol (BB, BM, BS, BZ, CZ, DE, GY, HN, HU, IN, JM, PL, PR, RO, RU, SK, SR, TT, VN) *see* Cyproheptadine 529
Perivasc (AU) *see* AmLODIPine 123
Perjeta (AR, AU, BR, CH, CY, CZ, DE, DK, EE, FR, GB, HK, HR, IE, IL, IS, JP, KR, LT, MX, NL, NO, NZ, PH, QA, RO, SE, SI, SK, TH, TR) *see* Pertuzumab 1627
Perketan (IT) *see* Ketanserin [INT] 1144
Perkin (KR) *see* Carbidopa and Levodopa 351
Perlinganit (BG, HU, KR, LU, PL) *see* Nitroglycerin 1465
Perlutex (AE, BB, BM, BS, BZ, DK, GY, JM, NO, SR, TT) *see* MedroxyPROGESTERone 1277
Perlutex Leo (CR, DO, GT, NI, PA, SV) *see* MedroxyPROGESTERone 1277
Permadoze oral (PT) *see* Cyanocobalamin 515
Permadoze (PT) *see* Cyanocobalamin 515
Permicren (UY) *see* Permethrin 1627
Permid (PH) *see* Loperamide 1236
Permite (IN) *see* Permethrin 1627
Pernamed (TH) *see* Perphenazine 1627
Pernazine (TH) *see* Perphenazine 1627
Perofen (BB, BM, BS, BZ, GY, JM, SG, SR, TT) *see* Ibuprofen 1032
Perone (TW) *see* Metoclopramide 1345
Perphenan (IL) *see* Perphenazine 1627
Perry (TW) *see* Nalidixic Acid [INT] 1418
Persantin 75 (CO) *see* Dipyridamole 652
Persantin 100 (AU) *see* Dipyridamole 652
Persantin (AE, AR, AT, AU, BB, BD, BF, BH, BJ, BM, BR, BS, BZ, CH, CI, CL, CY, CZ, DK, EE, EG, ES, ET, FI, GB, GH, GM, GN, GR, GY, HK, HN, HR, ID, IN, IQ, IR, IS, IT, JM, JO, KE, KR, KW, LB, LR, LY, MA, ML, MR, MT, MU, MW, MX, MY, NE, NG, NL, NO, NZ, OM, PE, PH, PK, PL, PR, PT, QA, RU, SA, SC, SD, SE, SG, SI, SK, SL, SN, SR, SY, TN, TR, TT, TW, TZ, UG, UY, VE, YE, ZM, ZW) *see* Dipyridamole 652
Persantin Depot (AT, FI) *see* Dipyridamole 652
Persantine (BE, FR, VN) *see* Dipyridamole 652
Persantin Forte (DE) *see* Dipyridamole 652
Persantin PL (NZ) *see* Dipyridamole 652
Persantin Prolonguets (PT) *see* Dipyridamole 652
Persantin Retard (IE, IS, NL) *see* Dipyridamole 652
Persantin SR (AU) *see* Dipyridamole 652
Persidal-2 (ID) *see* RisperiDONE 1818
Pertacilon (SG) *see* Captopril 342
Perti (VE) *see* Pefloxacin [INT] 1588
Pertofran (RU) *see* Desipramine 593
Pertranquil (BE, LU) *see* Meprobamate 1296
Pervasum (ES) *see* Cinnarizine [INT] 440
Peryndopryl Anpharm (PL) *see* Perindopril 1623
Pesatril (MX) *see* Lisinopril 1226
Pe-Tam (LU) *see* Acetaminophen 32
Petercillin (ZA) *see* Ampicillin 141
Peterkaien (ZA) *see* Lidocaine (Systemic) 1208
Peterkaien (ZA) *see* Lidocaine (Topical) 1211
Peteyu (TH) *see* Propylthiouracil 1735
Pethidin (CH) *see* Meperidine 1293
Pethidine (GB, HK, IN, KR, PK, TW) *see* Meperidine 1293
Pethidine Injection (AU, NZ) *see* Meperidine 1293
Pethidine Roche (ZA) *see* Meperidine 1293
Pethidine Tablet (NZ) *see* Meperidine 1293
Petidina (CL) *see* Meperidine 1293
Petidin (DK, NO, SE) *see* Meperidine 1293
Petilin (AE, BF, BH, BJ, CI, CY, EG, ET, GH, GM, GN, IQ, IR, JO, KE, KW, LB, LR, LY, MA, ML, MR, MU, MW, NE, NG, OM, QA, SA, SC, SD, SL, SN, SY, TN, TZ, UG, YE, ZA, ZM, ZW) *see* Valproic Acid and Derivatives 2123
Petimid (TR) *see* Ethosuximide 813
Petina (MY) *see* Cyproheptadine 529
Petinimid (AT, CH, CZ, PL, RO) *see* Ethosuximide 813
Petnidan (DE, HU, LU) *see* Ethosuximide 813
Petralar (JO) *see* Fluocinolone (Topical) 893
Petylyl (PL) *see* Desipramine 593
Peucetol (MX) *see* Pantoprazole 1570
Pevalon (CY) *see* PHENobarbital 1632
Pevaryl (AE, AT, AU, BE, BF, BG, BH, BJ, CH, CI, CY, CZ, DK, EE, EG, ES, ET, FI, FR, GB, GH, GM, GN, GR, HN, HU, IE, IS, IT, JO, KE, KW, LB, LR, LU, MA, ML, MR, MT, MU, MW, MY, NE, NG, NL, NO, NZ, PH, PL, PT, SA, SC, SD, SE, SK, SL, SN, TN, TR, TZ, UG, VE, VN, ZM, ZW) *see* Econazole 703
Pevaryl Lipogel (HU, MX) *see* Econazole 703
Pevaryl P.v. (HU) *see* Econazole 703
Pexacin (TW) *see* Pefloxacin [INT] 1588
Pexal (BM, BZ, GY, SR) *see* Pentoxifylline 1618
Pexid (AU, BE, ES, FR, LU) *see* Perhexiline [INT] 1621
Pexola (CO, UY) *see* Pramipexole 1695
Pexol (PE) *see* Pentoxifylline 1618
Pexsig (AU) *see* Perhexiline [INT] 1621
Peyona (GB, IE) *see* Caffeine 319
Pezide (TH) *see* GlipiZIDE 967
P Guard (JP) *see* Morphine (Systemic) 1394
Phaltrexia (ID) *see* Naltrexone 1422
Pharcal (TH) *see* Calcium Carbonate 327
Phardex (ID) *see* TiZANidine 2051
Pharflox (ID) *see* Ofloxacin (Systemic) 1490
Pharmacen-M (MX) *see* Acetaminophen 32
Pharmacetin Otic (TH) *see* Chloramphenicol 421
Pharmachem (PH) *see* GuaiFENesin 986
Pharmaclor (AE, BH, CY, EG, IL, IQ, IR, JO, KW, LB, LY, OM, QA, SA, SY, YE) *see* Cefaclor 372
Pharmafer (LB) *see* Ferrous Sulfate 871
Pharmafil (MX) *see* Theophylline 2026
Pharma-Fluor (NL) *see* Fluoride 895
Pharmaplatin (PK) *see* CARBOplatin 357
Pharmapress (HK) *see* Enalapril 722
Pharmarubicin RD (CN) *see* Epirubicin 739
Pharmaton (MX) *see* Pyridoxine 1747
Pharmaton (MX) *see* Thiamine 2028
Pharmaton Complex (MX) *see* Ergocalciferol 753
Pharmauracil (PK) *see* Fluorouracil (Systemic) 896
Pharmet (ZA) *see* Methyldopa 1332
Pharmexin (BH, CY, EG, IQ, IR, JO, KW, LB, LY, OM, QA, SA, SY, YE) *see* Cephalexin 405
Pharmix (PH) *see* Furosemide 940
Pharmorubicin (AU, GB, HK, IE, MY, NZ, PH) *see* Epirubicin 739
Pharmorubicin CS (SG, TH) *see* Epirubicin 739
Pharmorubicin PDF (KR) *see* Epirubicin 739
Pharmorubicin PFS (KR, TW) *see* Epirubicin 739
Pharmotidine (PH) *see* Famotidine 845

Pharmyork (GR) *see* Metoclopramide 1345
Pharnax (TH) *see* ALPRAZolam 94
Pharnazine (TH) *see* FluPHENAZine 905
Pharodime (ID) *see* CefTAZidime 392
Pharothrocin (ID) *see* Erythromycin (Systemic) 762
Pharozepine (ID) *see* OXcarbazepine 1532
Pharquinon (VE) *see* Hydroquinone 1020
Pharynx (HK, MY, SG) *see* Cetylpyridinium and Benzocaine [CAN/INT] 415
Pheburane (GB) *see* Sodium Phenylbutyrate 1908
Phemax (TH) *see* Orphenadrine 1522
Phenaemal (EE, SK) *see* PHENobarbital 1632
Phenasen (AU) *see* Arsenic Trioxide 177
Phenazol (PH) *see* Naphazoline and Pheniramine 1426
Phenergan (AE, AT, AU, BB, BE, BF, BH, BJ, BM, BS, BZ, CH, CI, CY, DK, EG, ET, FI, FR, GB, GH, GM, GN, GR, GY, IE, IN, IQ, IR, IS, JM, JO, KE, KW, LB, LR, LU, LY, MA, ML, MR, MU, MW, MY, NE, NG, NL, NO, NZ, OM, PK, QA, SA, SC, SD, SL, SN, SR, SY, TN, TR, TT, TZ, UG, YE, ZA, ZM, ZW) *see* Promethazine 1723
Phenerzin (PH) *see* Promethazine 1723
Phenhydan (AT, CH, DE, EE, HU, LU) *see* Phenytoin 1640
Phenicol (IL, JO) *see* Chloramphenicol 421
Phenilep (ID) *see* Phenytoin 1640
Phenkin (KR) *see* Phentermine 1635
Phenlin (TW) *see* Phenytoin 1640
Phenobarbitone (AU, NZ) *see* PHENobarbital 1632
Phenobarbitone Injection (GB) *see* PHENobarbital 1632
Phenobarbiton (HR) *see* PHENobarbital 1632
Phenobarbiton-natrium (HR) *see* PHENobarbital 1632
Phenotal (JO, TH) *see* PHENobarbital 1632
Phenpro Abz (DE) *see* Phenprocoumon [INT] 1635
Phenprogamma (DE) *see* Phenprocoumon [INT] 1635
Phental (ID) *see* PHENobarbital 1632
Phentolep (JO) *see* Phenytoin 1640
Phentolmin (KR) *see* Phentolamine 1636
Phentosol (IN) *see* Phentolamine 1636
Phepix (TW) *see* Econazole 703
Phinev (ID) *see* EPINEPHrine (Systemic, Oral Inhalation) 735
Pholcodine Linctus (GB) *see* Pholcodine [INT] 1646
Pholcodin (HR) *see* Pholcodine [INT] 1646
Pholcolin (IE) *see* Pholcodine [INT] 1646
Pholcotussin (CN) *see* Pholcodine [INT] 1646
Pholtex Forte (AU) *see* Pholcodine [INT] 1646
Pholtrate (AU) *see* Pholcodine [INT] 1646
Phosbine (KR) *see* Calcium Acetate 326
Phos-Ex (DE) *see* Calcium Acetate 326
PhosEx (GB) *see* Calcium Acetate 326
PhosLo (CL, GB, KR) *see* Calcium Acetate 326
Phospholine Iodide (IL) *see* Echothiophate Iodide 703
Phospholine Jodide (HN) *see* Echothiophate Iodide 703
Phospholinjodid (AT) *see* Echothiophate Iodide 703
Phosphosorb (DE) *see* Calcium Acetate 326
Phostat (IN) *see* Calcium Acetate 326
Photobarr (CZ, EE, RO) *see* Porfimer 1682
Photoderm Max Bio (MX) *see* Mannitol 1269
Photofrin (AR, BG, DE, FI, FR, GB, GR, HN, IE, IL, JP, NL, PL, PT, SE, TW, VN) *see* Porfimer 1682
Phudicin (CN, HK) *see* Fusidic Acid (Topical) [CAN/INT] 943
Phylobid (BF, BJ, CI, ET, GH, GM, GN, IN, KE, LR, MA, ML, MR, MU, MW, NE, NG, SC, SD, SL, SN, TN, TZ, UG, ZA, ZM, ZW) *see* Theophylline 2026
Phymet DTF (IE) *see* Methadone 1311
Phymet DTF Syrup (AU) *see* Methadone 1311
Physeptone (AE, AU, GB) *see* Methadone 1311
Physiodose (PL) *see* Sodium Chloride 1902
Physostigmine Salicylate (AU) *see* Physostigmine 1647
Physostigminum Salicylicum (PL) *see* Physostigmine 1647
Piax (AU, NZ) *see* Clopidogrel 484
Pibaksin (ID) *see* Mupirocin 1404
Picain (FI) *see* Bupivacaine 299
Picamic (ID) *see* Ketoconazole (Systemic) 1144
Picato (AU, BE, CH, CZ, DE, DK, EE, ES, FR, GB, HR, IE, IL, KR, LT, NO, NZ, RO, SE, SI, SK) *see* Ingenol Mebutate 1083
Picetam (SG) *see* Piracetam [INT] 1661
Picillina (TW) *see* Piperacillin [CAN/INT] 1656
Piclodin (ID) *see* Ticlopidine 2040
Picolax (GB, HK, IE) *see* Sodium Picosulfate, Magnesium Oxide, and Citric Acid 1911
Picolight Powder (KR) *see* Sodium Picosulfate, Magnesium Oxide, and Citric Acid 1911
Picoprep (BE, BG, CZ, DK, EE, FR, HN, IS, LT, NL, NO, NZ, PH, PT, RO, SE, SK, TH, VN, ZA) *see* Sodium Picosulfate, Magnesium Oxide, and Citric Acid 1911
Picoprep Powder (CY, KR, QA, SA) *see* Sodium Picosulfate, Magnesium Oxide, and Citric Acid 1911
Picoprep Powder for Oral Solution (HK) *see* Sodium Picosulfate, Magnesium Oxide, and Citric Acid 1911
PicoPrep Powder for Solution (AU) *see* Sodium Picosulfate, Magnesium Oxide, and Citric Acid 1911
Pico-Salax (IL) *see* Sodium Picosulfate, Magnesium Oxide, and Citric Acid 1911
Picosalax (NZ) *see* Sodium Picosulfate, Magnesium Oxide, and Citric Acid 1911
Picosalax Powder for Oral Administration (AU) *see* Sodium Picosulfate, Magnesium Oxide, and Citric Acid 1911
Pidilat (DE) *see* NIFEdipine 1451
Pidogul (KR) *see* Clopidogrel 484
Pidopidon (JP) *see* Pyridoxine 1747
Pigmentasa (ES) *see* Hydroquinone 1020
Pikangwang (CN) *see* Ketoconazole (Topical) 1145
Piladex (PY) *see* Minoxidil (Topical) 1374
Pilian (MY, TW) *see* Cyproheptadine 529
Pill 72 (HK) *see* Levonorgestrel 1201
Pillozen (KR) *see* Piroxicam 1662
Pilo (BE, FR, NO) *see* Pilocarpine (Ophthalmic) 1649
Pilocan (BR) *see* Pilocarpine (Ophthalmic) 1649
Pilocarpol (DE) *see* Pilocarpine (Ophthalmic) 1649
Pilocar (VE) *see* Pilocarpine (Ophthalmic) 1649
Pil Ofteno (GT, SV) *see* Pilocarpine (Ophthalmic) 1649
Pilogan (CO) *see* Minoxidil (Topical) 1374
Pilogel (GB, IE, TW) *see* Pilocarpine (Ophthalmic) 1649
Pilogel HS (CL, CZ, SG, SI) *see* Pilocarpine (Ophthalmic) 1649
Pilokarpin (DK, SI, SK) *see* Pilocarpine (Ophthalmic) 1649
Pilomann (DE) *see* Pilocarpine (Ophthalmic) 1649
Pilomin (BG) *see* Pilocarpine (Ophthalmic) 1649
Pilopine-HS (AE, BF, BH, BJ, CI, CY, EG, ET, GH, GM, GN, IQ, IR, JO, KE, KW, LB, LR, LY, MA, ML, MR, MU, MW, NE, NG, OM, QA, SA, SC, SD, SL, SN, SY, TN, TZ, UG, YE, ZM, ZW) *see* Pilocarpine (Ophthalmic) 1649
Pilopos (CZ) *see* Pilocarpine (Ophthalmic) 1649
Pilopt Eye Drops (AU, NZ) *see* Pilocarpine (Ophthalmic) 1649
Piloral (JP) *see* Clemastine 459
Pilotina (QA) *see* Pilocarpine (Ophthalmic) 1649
Pilotonina (IT) *see* Pilocarpine (Ophthalmic) 1649
Pima-Biciron (DE) *see* Natamycin 1432
Pimafucin (BE, CZ, DE, FI, HU, LU, PL, PT) *see* Natamycin 1432
Pimaryl (ID) *see* Glimepiride 966
Pimax (PH) *see* Tamsulosin 1974
Pimcef (PE) *see* Cefepime 378
Pime (TH) *see* Cefepime 378
Pimidel (RU) *see* Pipemidic Acid [INT] 1655
Pimodac (IN) *see* Pimozide 1651
Pinar (PE, PY) *see* Pinaverium [CAN/INT] 1651

Pinavalt (CO, MX) *see* Ebastine [INT] ... 702
Pinden (IL) *see* Pindolol ... 1652
Pindomex (FI) *see* Pindolol ... 1652
Pinex (NO) *see* Acetaminophen ... 32
Pinfetil (ID) *see* ClomiPHENE ... 473
Pingfu (CN) *see* Nadifloxacin [INT] ... 1411
Ping Te (CN) *see* Salmeterol ... 1860
Pink (AR) *see* Desogestrel [INT] ... 597
Pinloc (FI) *see* Pindolol ... 1652
Pinox (HR) *see* Lercanidipine [INT] ... 1181
Pinsaun (TW) *see* Amitriptyline ... 119
Pioglite (VN) *see* Pioglitazone ... 1654
Pioglit G (IN) *see* Pioglitazone and Glimepiride ... 1654
Pioglit (IN, PY) *see* Pioglitazone ... 1654
Pioglit-MF15 (IN) *see* Pioglitazone and Metformin ... 1655
Pio (HR) *see* Pioglitazone ... 1654
Piokil Plus (VE) *see* Permethrin ... 1627
Piolidone (KR) *see* Pioglitazone ... 1654
Piomax (KR) *see* Pioglitazone ... 1654
Piomed (UY) *see* Pioglitazone ... 1654
Piomin (KR) *see* Pioglitazone ... 1654
Pionix-M (ID) *see* Pioglitazone and Metformin ... 1655
Pionix (ID) *see* Pioglitazone ... 1654
Pioplus (PH) *see* Pioglitazone and Metformin ... 1655
Piosugar (TW) *see* Pioglitazone ... 1654
Piota (TW) *see* Pioglitazone ... 1654
Piouno (PH) *see* Pioglitazone ... 1654
Piovalen (GR) *see* Cimetidine ... 438
Piozone (PH, TH) *see* Pioglitazone ... 1654
Pipamperon-neuraxpharm (DE) *see* Pipamperone [INT] ... 1655
Pipcil (LU) *see* Piperacillin [CAN/INT] ... 1656
Pipeacid (IT) *see* Pipemidic Acid [INT] ... 1655
Pipedac (IT) *see* Pipemidic Acid [INT] ... 1655
Pipefort (IT) *see* Pipemidic Acid [INT] ... 1655
Pipemid (IT, UY) *see* Pipemidic Acid [INT] ... 1655
Piperacillin (PL) *see* Piperacillin [CAN/INT] ... 1656
Piperonil (IT) *see* Pipamperone [INT] ... 1655
Pipertaz (TH) *see* Piperacillin and Tazobactam ... 1657
Piperzam (ES) *see* Piperacillin [CAN/INT] ... 1656
Pipetecan (AR) *see* Irinotecan ... 1112
Pipolphen (HN, HU, VN) *see* Promethazine ... 1723
Piportil (BR, EG, FR, HN, NO, NZ, PL, RU, SG) *see* Pipotiazine [CAN/INT] ... 1660
Piportil Depot (AU, GB, ZA) *see* Pipotiazine [CAN/INT] ... 1660
Piportil L4 (AR, BR, CL, CO, FR, MX, PE, PL, PY, QA, UY) *see* Pipotiazine [CAN/INT] ... 1660
Pipracil (IN) *see* Piperacillin [CAN/INT] ... 1656
Pipracin (IL) *see* Piperacillin [CAN/INT] ... 1656
Pipraks (CY, EG, IQ, IR, JO, KW, LB, LY, OM, SY, YE) *see* Piperacillin [CAN/INT] ... 1656
Pipram (BR, FR, GR, IT, NL, UY) *see* Pipemidic Acid [INT] ... 1655
Pipril (AE, BH, ES, GR, HN, HR, IE, PK, QA, SA) *see* Piperacillin [CAN/INT] ... 1656
Piptaz (PH, VN) *see* Piperacillin and Tazobactam ... 1657
Pipurin (IT) *see* Pipemidic Acid [INT] ... 1655
Pipurol (BR) *see* Pipemidic Acid [INT] ... 1655
Pira (AR) *see* GlyBURIDE ... 972
Pirabene (AT, DE, HU) *see* Piracetam [INT] ... 1661
Piracas (IN) *see* Piracetam [INT] ... 1661
Piracebral (BG, DE, LU) *see* Piracetam [INT] ... 1661
Piracemed (BE) *see* Piracetam [INT] ... 1661
Piracetam AbZ (DE) *see* Piracetam [INT] ... 1661
Piracetam AL (DE) *see* Piracetam [INT] ... 1661
Piracetam EG (BE) *see* Piracetam [INT] ... 1661
Piracetam-Elbe-Med (DE) *see* Piracetam [INT] ... 1661
Piracetam-Farmatrading (PT) *see* Piracetam [INT] ... 1661
Piracetam Faro (AT) *see* Piracetam [INT] ... 1661
Piracetam Heumann (DE) *see* Piracetam [INT] ... 1661
Piracetam Interpharm (AT) *see* Piracetam [INT] ... 1661
Piracetam-neuraxpharm (DE) *see* Piracetam [INT] ... 1661
Piracetam Prodes (ES) *see* Piracetam [INT] ... 1661
Piracetam-ratiopharm (DE, LU, PT) *see* Piracetam [INT] ... 1661
Piracetam-RPh (DE) *see* Piracetam [INT] ... 1661
Piracetam Stada (DE) *see* Piracetam [INT] ... 1661
Piracetam Verla (DE) *see* Piracetam [INT] ... 1661
piracetam von ct (DE) *see* Piracetam [INT] ... 1661
Piracetan (PY) *see* Piracetam [INT] ... 1661
Piracetop (BE) *see* Piracetam [INT] ... 1661
Piracetrop (DE) *see* Piracetam [INT] ... 1661
Pirac (PY) *see* Piroxicam ... 1662
Piraldina (AE, BG, BH, CY, EG, IL, IN, IQ, IR, IT, JO, KW, LB, LY, OM, QA, SA, SY, YE) *see* Pyrazinamide ... 1745
Piram-D (NZ) *see* Piroxicam ... 1662
Piramil (EE) *see* Ramipril ... 1771
Piramox (AE, BF, BH, BJ, CI, CY, EG, ET, GH, GM, GN, IQ, IR, JO, KE, KW, LB, LR, LY, MA, ML, MR, MU, MW, NE, NG, OM, QA, SA, SC, SD, SL, SN, SY, TN, TZ, UG, YE, ZM, ZW) *see* Amoxicillin ... 130
Piram (TH) *see* Piroxicam ... 1662
Pirantelina (PY) *see* Pyrantel Pamoate ... 1744
Piratam (SG) *see* Piracetam [INT] ... 1661
Piratin (HK) *see* Piracetam [INT] ... 1661
Piratropil (RU) *see* Piracetam [INT] ... 1661
Pirax (CH) *see* Piracetam [INT] ... 1661
Pirax (TH) *see* Piroxicam ... 1662
Pirazetam-Eurogenerics (LU) *see* Piracetam [INT] ... 1661
Pirazimida (ES) *see* Pyrazinamide ... 1745
Pirazinamida (PE) *see* Pyrazinamide ... 1745
Pirazinamida Prodes (ES) *see* Pyrazinamide ... 1745
Pirazinid (TR) *see* Pyrazinamide ... 1745
Piridon (UY) *see* Donepezil ... 668
Piridoxina Austral (AR) *see* Pyridoxine ... 1747
Piriglutina (ES) *see* Pyridoxine ... 1747
Pirilene (FR) *see* Pyrazinamide ... 1745
Pirimir (MX) *see* Phenazopyridine ... 1629
Pirium (GR) *see* Pimozide ... 1651
Pirkam (DK) *see* Piroxicam ... 1662
Pirocam (TW) *see* Piroxicam ... 1662
Pirocutan (DE) *see* Piroxicam ... 1662
Pirocutan Gel (DE) *see* Piroxicam ... 1662
Pirom (DK) *see* Piroxicam ... 1662
Piroxedol (CO) *see* Piroxicam ... 1662
Piroxicam (CO) *see* Piroxicam ... 1662
Piroxim (AE, BF, BH, BJ, CI, CO, CY, EC, EG, ET, GH, GM, GN, IQ, IR, JO, KE, KW, LB, LR, LY, MA, ML, MR, MU, MW, NE, NG, OM, QA, SA, SC, SD, SL, SN, SY, TN, TZ, UG, YE, ZM, ZW) *see* Piroxicam ... 1662
Pirox (IN, MX) *see* Piroxicam ... 1662
Pisaben L-A (EC) *see* Penicillin G Benzathine ... 1609
Pisacaina (EC) *see* Lidocaine and Epinephrine ... 1212
Pisacaina (EC) *see* Lidocaine (Topical) ... 1211
Pisacilina (CO) *see* Penicillin G (Parenteral/Aqueous) ... 1611
Pitaduce (KR) *see* Pravastatin ... 1700
Pitava (VN) *see* Pitavastatin ... 1663
Pithiorol (TW) *see* Pindolol ... 1652
Pitocin (EC) *see* Oxytocin ... 1549
Pitocin INJ (IN) *see* Oxytocin ... 1549
Pitogin (ID) *see* Oxytocin ... 1549
Piton S INJ (AE, BH, CY, EG, IQ, IR, JO, KW, LB, LY, NL, OM, QA, SA, SY, YE) *see* Oxytocin ... 1549
Pitressin (AU, CZ, DE, GR, HK, ID, IE, NZ, TW) *see* Vasopressin ... 2142
Pitrex (IL) *see* Tolnaftate ... 2063
Pitrion (IL) *see* Miconazole (Topical) ... 1360
Pivepol (PL) *see* Dipivefrin ... 651
Pixelon (UY) *see* Pipemidic Acid [INT] ... 1655
Pixicam (ZA) *see* Piroxicam ... 1662
Piyeloseptyl (TR) *see* Nitrofurantoin ... 1463

Pizaccord (AU) *see* Pioglitazone 1654
Pizide (TH) *see* Pimozide 1651
Pizofen (JO) *see* Pizotifen [CAN/INT] 1664
Pizogran (TR) *see* Pizotifen [CAN/INT] 1664
Pizomed (TH) *see* Pizotifen [CAN/INT] 1664
Pizzard (MX) *see* Desmopressin 594
PK-Merz (AE, AT, BF, BG, BH, BJ, CH, CI, CL, CR, CY, CZ, DE, DO, EC, EE, EG, ET, GH, GM, GN, GT, HK, HN, HR, HU, IL, IQ, IR, JO, KE, KR, KW, LB, LR, LU, LY, MA, ML, MR, MU, MW, MX, MY, NE, NG, NI, OM, PA, PH, PK, PT, PY, QA, SA, SC, SD, SK, SL, SN, SV, SY, TN, TW, TZ, UG, YE, ZA, ZM, ZW) *see* Amantadine 105
Plabic (KR) *see* Clopidogrel 484
Placet (PY, UY) *see* OLANZapine 1491
Placidel (ES) *see* Amobarbital 128
Placidox 2 (IN) *see* Diazepam 613
Placidox 5 (IN) *see* Diazepam 613
Placidox 10 (IN) *see* Diazepam 613
Placil (AU) *see* ClomiPRAMINE 475
Placis (ES, JO, TH, TR) *see* CISplatin 448
Plac-Out (AR) *see* Chlorhexidine Gluconate 422
Placta (ID, SG) *see* Clopidogrel 484
Pladizol (RO, SK) *see* Cilostazol 437
Pladogrel (ID) *see* Clopidogrel 484
Plagril (SG) *see* Clopidogrel 484
Plak Out (CH) *see* Chlorhexidine Gluconate 422
Plamed (KR) *see* Clopidogrel 484
Plamet (BR) *see* Bromopride [INT] 292
Plan B (DO, HN, NI, SV) *see* Levonorgestrel 1201
Plancol (KR) *see* Hydrocortisone (Topical) 1014
Plander (IT) *see* Dextran 607
Plander R (IT) *see* Dextran 607
Planipart[vet.] (FR) *see* Clenbuterol [INT] 460
Planovar (JP) *see* Ethinyl Estradiol and Norgestrel 812
Plantassel (GT, HN, NI, PA, SV) *see* Nitazoxanide 1461
Planum (DE) *see* Temazepam 1990
Plaqacide Mouthrinse (AU) *see* Chlorhexidine Gluconate 422
Plaquemax (BR) *see* Oprelvekin 1519
Plaquenil (CN, CY, IS, KW, LT, LU, MX, QA, RO, SA, VN) *see* Hydroxychloroquine 1021
Plaquenil Sulfate (AR, AT, AU, BB, BE, BF, BG, BJ, BM, BS, BZ, CH, CI, CZ, DK, EE, ES, ET, FI, FR, GB, GH, GM, GN, GR, GY, HK, HN, IE, IL, IT, JM, KE, LR, MA, ML, MR, MT, MU, MW, MY, NE, NG, NL, NO, NZ, PH, RU, SC, SD, SE, SK, SL, SN, SR, TH, TN, TR, TT, TW, TZ, UG, ZA, ZM, ZW) *see* Hydroxychloroquine 1021
Plaquetasa (CR, GT, SV) *see* Aspirin 180
Plaquetil (PY) *see* Ticlopidine 2040
PlaquEx (BG) *see* Clopidogrel 484
Plaquinol (BR, CL, CO, CR, DO, EC, GT, HN, NI, PA, PE, PT, PY, SV, VE) *see* Hydroxychloroquine 1021
Plasbumin (AE, ID, LB, SG) *see* Albumin 67
Plasil (AE, BF, BH, BJ, BR, CI, CO, CY, EG, ET, GH, GM, GN, IQ, IR, IT, JO, KE, KW, LB, LR, LY, MA, ML, MR, MU, MW, MX, NE, NG, OM, PY, QA, SA, SC, SD, SL, SN, SY, TH, TN, TZ, UG, YE, ZM, ZW) *see* Metoclopramide 1345
Plaslloid (TW) *see* Aminocaproic Acid 113
Plasmasteril (BE, PL, TR) *see* Hetastarch 1004
Plasmex (IN) *see* Dextran 607
Plasmodin (ID) *see* Sulfadoxine and Pyrimethamine [INT] 1946
Plasmotrim (BR) *see* Artesunate 178
Plastin (PH) *see* Imipenem and Cilastatin 1051
Plastufer (DE) *see* Ferrous Sulfate 871
Platamine (AE, BH, CY, HR, IQ, IR, IT, JO, KW, LB, LY, OM, QA, SA, SY, YE) *see* CISplatin 448
Platecil (PH) *see* Cilostazol 437
Platiblastin (CH, DE) *see* CISplatin 448
Platidiam (BG, CZ, HN, HU, PL, RU) *see* CISplatin 448
Platimit (HR) *see* CISplatin 448
Platinex (HR, IT, QA) *see* CISplatin 448
Platinol (AR, AT, BE, CH, EE, EG, FI, GR, LU, NO, SE, UY) *see* CISplatin 448
Platinox (PH) *see* Oxaliplatin 1528
Platin (PH) *see* CISplatin 448
Platistil (ES, PT) *see* CISplatin 448
Platistine (LU) *see* CISplatin 448
Platistin (FI, NO, SE) *see* CISplatin 448
Platof (ID) *see* Pentoxifylline 1618
Platogrix (ID) *see* Clopidogrel 484
Platosin (GB, KR, MY, NL, PK, RO, TH) *see* CISplatin 448
Platout (TW) *see* Clopidogrel 484
Plato (ZA) *see* Dipyridamole 652
Platsul-A (AR, CL) *see* Silver Sulfadiazine 1887
Plaucina (ES) *see* Enoxaparin 726
Plavitor (KR) *see* Clopidogrel 484
Plavix (AE, AR, AT, AU, BB, BD, BE, BF, BG, BH, BJ, BM, BO, BR, BS, BZ, CH, CI, CL, CN, CO, CR, CY, CZ, DE, DK, DO, EE, EG, ES, ET, FI, FR, GB, GH, GM, GN, GR, GT, GY, HK, HN, ID, IE, IL, IS, IT, JM, JO, JP, KE, KR, KW, LB, LR, LT, MA, ML, MR, MT, MU, MW, MX, MY, NE, NG, NI, NL, NO, NZ, PA, PE, PH, PK, PL, PR, PT, PY, QA, RU, SA, SC, SD, SE, SG, SK, SL, SN, SR, SV, TH, TN, TR, TT, TW, TZ, UG, UY, VE, VN, ZA, ZM, ZW) *see* Clopidogrel 484
Plavos (ID) *see* Clopidogrel 484
Plecaz MR (MY) *see* Gliclazide [CAN/INT] 964
Plegomazin (BB, BM, BS, BZ, CZ, GY, IQ, JM, PR, SR, SY, TT) *see* ChlorproMAZINE 429
Plegomazine (HU) *see* ChlorproMAZINE 429
Plegridy (AU, CZ, DE, DK, EE, HR, LT, NO, SE, SI, SK) *see* Peginterferon Beta-1a 1602
Plenacor (BR, CO, EC) *see* Atenolol 189
Plenactol (CN) *see* Orphenadrine 1522
Plendil (AE, AR, BB, BE, BF, BG, BH, BJ, BM, BS, BZ, CH, CI, CN, CR, CY, CZ, DK, DO, EC, EE, EG, ES, ET, FI, GB, GH, GM, GN, GR, GT, GY, HK, HN, HR, HU, IE, IN, IQ, IR, IS, IT, JM, JO, KE, KW, LB, LR, LT, LU, LY, MA, ML, MR, MU, MW, MX, MY, NE, NG, NI, NL, OM, PA, PE, PK, PL, PR, PY, QA, RO, RU, SA, SC, SD, SE, SK, SL, SN, SR, SV, SY, TH, TN, TT, TW, TZ, UG, VN, YE, ZA, ZM, ZW) *see* Felodipine 850
Plendil Depottab (NO) *see* Felodipine 850
Plendil ER (AU, NZ, PH) *see* Felodipine 850
Plendil PR (TR) *see* Felodipine 850
Plendil Retard (AT) *see* Felodipine 850
Plenidon (CL, PE) *see* Zaleplon 2193
Plenum (UY) *see* Psyllium 1744
Plenur (ES) *see* Lithium 1230
Pleoxtin (KR) *see* Oxaliplatin 1528
Pleroxi (ID) *see* Piroxicam 1662
Pletaal (AE, AR, CN, JP, MY, PE, PH, PK, TH, TW, VN) *see* Cilostazol 437
Pletal (AU, DE, GB, IE, IT, SE, TR) *see* Cilostazol 437
Pletoz (IN) *see* Cilostazol 437
Pletzolyn (PH) *see* Piperacillin and Tazobactam 1657
Plexafer (BF, BJ, CI, ET, GH, GM, GN, KE, LR, MA, ML, MR, MU, MW, NE, NG, SC, SD, SL, SN, TN, TZ, UG, ZA, ZM, ZW) *see* Ferrous Sulfate 871
Plexicodim (MX) *see* OxyCODONE 1538
Pleya (TW) *see* Cilostazol 437
Pliaglis (AR, GB) *see* Lidocaine and Tetracaine 1214
Plicet (HR) *see* Acetaminophen 32
Plidan (AR) *see* Diazepam 613
Plivit C (HR) *see* Ascorbic Acid 178
Plivit B1 (HR) *see* Thiamine 2028
Plivit B6 (HR) *see* Pyridoxine 1747
Plumarol (ES) *see* Miglitol 1367
Pluriamin (CL) *see* Doxylamine and Pyridoxine 693
Plurimen (ES) *see* Selegiline 1873
Pluscal (AR) *see* Calcium Carbonate 327

Pluserix (BB, BF, BJ, BM, BS, BZ, CI, ET, GH, GM, GN, GY, JM, KE, LR, MA, ML, MR, MU, MW, NE, NG, NL, SC, SD, SL, SN, SR, TN, TT, TZ, UG, ZA, ZM, ZW) *see* Measles, Mumps, and Rubella Virus Vaccine ... 1273
Plusplatin (EC) *see* Oxaliplatin ... 1528
Plusssz balance calcium (PL) *see* Calcium Carbonate ... 327
Plusssz Magnez (PL) *see* Magnesium Oxide ... 1265
9 PM eye drops (IN) *see* Latanoprost ... 1172
PMQ-INGA (IN) *see* Primaquine ... 1713
Pneumera (RO) *see* Formoterol ... 926
Pneumo 23 (AE, AR, AT, BE, BG, CL, CN, CO, CR, CY, CZ, DO, EC, EE, ES, FR, GT, HK, HN, HR, ID, IN, IT, JO, LB, LT, MY, NZ, PA, PE, PH, PK, PL, PY, RO, SA, SE, SG, SI, SK, SV, TH, TR, TW, UY, VN) *see* Pneumococcal Polysaccharide Vaccine (23-Valent) ... 1671
Pneumo 23 Imovax (IL) *see* Pneumococcal Polysaccharide Vaccine (23-Valent) ... 1671
Pneumocal (PH) *see* Levofloxacin (Systemic) ... 1197
Pneumo Novum (DK) *see* Pneumococcal Polysaccharide Vaccine (23-Valent) ... 1671
Pneumovax II (GB, IE) *see* Pneumococcal Polysaccharide Vaccine (23-Valent) ... 1671
Pneumovax 23 (AE, AR, AU, CH, HK, NL, PH, TW) *see* Pneumococcal Polysaccharide Vaccine (23-Valent) ... 1671
Pneumovax (CN, IS, JP, SE, SG) *see* Pneumococcal Polysaccharide Vaccine (23-Valent) ... 1671
Pnu-Imune 23 (GR) *see* Pneumococcal Polysaccharide Vaccine (23-Valent) ... 1671
Pocral (KR) *see* Chloral Hydrate [CAN/INT] ... 418
Podevta (SG) *see* Insulin Glargine ... 1086
Podofilia NRO (MX) *see* Podophyllum Resin ... 1672
Podofilm (CL, HK, SG) *see* Podophyllum Resin ... 1672
Podomexef (CH, DE) *see* Cefpodoxime ... 388
Podowart Paint (IN) *see* Podophyllum Resin ... 1672
Poen-Caina (UY) *see* Proparacaine ... 1728
Poenfenicol (AU) *see* Chloramphenicol ... 421
Poenflox (VE) *see* Ofloxacin (Ophthalmic) ... 1491
Poengatif (PE, UY) *see* Gatifloxacin ... 949
Poenkerat (PY) *see* Ketorolac (Ophthalmic) ... 1149
Poenkerat (PY) *see* Ketorolac (Systemic) ... 1146
Pofol (KR, SG, TH) *see* Propofol ... 1728
Pogetol (TH) *see* ChlorproMAZINE ... 429
Polaramin (AT, DK, IT, NO, SE) *see* Dexchlorpheniramine ... 603
Polaramine (AE, BB, BE, BF, BH, BJ, BM, BR, BS, BZ, CH, CI, CO, EG, ES, ET, FR, GH, GM, GN, GY, HK, ID, JM, KE, KW, LR, LU, MA, ML, MR, MU, MW, MX, NE, NG, NL, PR, QA, SA, SC, SD, SG, SL, SN, SR, TN, TT, TW, TZ, UG, VN, ZA, ZM, ZW) *see* Dexchlorpheniramine ... 603
Polaramine (non-prescription) (AU) *see* Dexchlorpheniramine ... 603
Polaramine Repetabs (FR, GR) *see* Dexchlorpheniramine ... 603
Polaramin Prolongatum (SE) *see* Dexchlorpheniramine ... 603
Polaramin Prolong Depottab (NO) *see* Dexchlorpheniramine ... 603
Polarax (SG) *see* Dexchlorpheniramine ... 603
Polcotec (MX) *see* Metoclopramide ... 1345
Poldomet [+ Levidopa] (PL) *see* Carbidopa ... 351
Poleon (JP) *see* Nalidixic Acid [INT] ... 1418
Polibroxol (SG) *see* Ambroxol [INT] ... 109
Polibutin (ES) *see* Trimebutine [CAN/INT] ... 2103
Policor (UY) *see* Cilostazol ... 437
Polidocasklerol (JP) *see* Polidocanol ... 1672
Poli-Flunarin (SG) *see* Flunarizine [CAN/INT] ... 892
Polio Salk "Sero" (AT) *see* Poliovirus Vaccine (Inactivated) ... 1673
Polisulfade (PT) *see* Bacitracin and Polymyxin B ... 222
Politone (TW) *see* Pioglitazone ... 1654
Polixin (MX) *see* Polymyxin B ... 1676
Polixin Ungena (MX) *see* Bacitracin and Polymyxin B ... 222
Polixin Ungena (MX) *see* Bacitracin, Neomycin, and Polymyxin B ... 223
Pollakisu (JP) *see* Oxybutynin ... 1536
Polomigran (PL) *see* Pizotifen [CAN/INT] ... 1664
Polo (TW) *see* Felodipine ... 850
Polpressin (PL) *see* Prazosin ... 1703
Polstigminum (PL) *see* Neostigmine ... 1438
Polyanion (AT) *see* Pentosan Polysulfate Sodium ... 1617
Polybamycin (MY, SG, VN) *see* Bacitracin, Neomycin, and Polymyxin B ... 223
Poly-B con Vitamina C (MX) *see* Pyridoxine ... 1747
Polybon (TH) *see* Amitriptyline and Perphenazine ... 122
Polycain (JP) *see* Econazole ... 703
Polyfax (MY) *see* Bacitracin and Polymyxin B ... 222
Polymagma (PH) *see* Attapulgite [CAN/INT] ... 204
Polymox (MX) *see* Amoxicillin ... 130
Polymyxin B Pfizer (DE) *see* Polymyxin B ... 1676
Polymyxine B FNA (NL) *see* Polymyxin B ... 1676
Polynovate (TH) *see* Betamethasone (Topical) ... 255
Polypen (PH) *see* Ampicillin ... 141
Polypress (TH) *see* Prazosin ... 1703
Polyquin Forte (SG) *see* Hydroquinone ... 1020
Polysporin (BR) *see* Bacitracin, Neomycin, and Polymyxin B ... 223
Polysporin Ophthalmic (ZA) *see* Bacitracin and Polymyxin B ... 222
Polytanol (TH) *see* Amitriptyline ... 119
Polytrim (AT, BE, BH, NL, PT) *see* Trimethoprim and Polymyxin B ... 2105
Polyxit (TH) *see* Gemfibrozil ... 956
Polyzalip (TH) *see* Bezafibrate [CAN/INT] ... 261
Pomalyst (AU, CZ, KR, SG) *see* Pomalidomide ... 1677
Ponaltin (KR) *see* Ranitidine ... 1777
Ponaris (PE) *see* Levofloxacin (Systemic) ... 1197
Poncofen (ID) *see* Mefenamic Acid ... 1280
Poncohist (ID) *see* Cyproheptadine ... 529
Pondactone (TH) *see* Spironolactone ... 1931
Pondex (ID) *see* Mefenamic Acid ... 1280
Pondnadysmen (TH) *see* Mefenamic Acid ... 1280
Pondnoxcill (TH) *see* Amoxicillin ... 130
Pondtroxin (TH) *see* Levothyroxine ... 1205
Pongyl V (KR) *see* Griseofulvin ... 985
Ponmel (HN) *see* Mefenamic Acid ... 1280
Ponser (PH) *see* Mefenamic Acid ... 1280
Ponstan-500 (MX) *see* Mefenamic Acid ... 1280
Ponstan (AE, AU, BD, BH, BR, CH, CO, CY, EC, EG, FI, GB, GH, GR, HK, ID, IE, IL, IN, IQ, IR, JO, JP, KE, KW, LB, LY, MU, MY, NZ, OM, PK, PT, QA, SA, SG, SY, TH, TR, TW, TZ, UG, VE, YE, ZA, ZW) *see* Mefenamic Acid ... 1280
Ponstan Forte (AE, BH, CY, EG, IL, IQ, IR, JO, KW, LB, LY, OM, QA, SA, SY, YE, ZA) *see* Mefenamic Acid ... 1280
Ponstil (UY) *see* Mefenamic Acid ... 1280
Ponstyl (FR, MU) *see* Mefenamic Acid ... 1280
Pontacid (MY) *see* Mefenamic Acid ... 1280
Pontal (KR) *see* Mefenamic Acid ... 1280
Pontalon (SG) *see* Mefenamic Acid ... 1280
Ponzyr V (KR) *see* Griseofulvin ... 985
Popscaine (JP) *see* Levobupivacaine [INT] ... 1194
Por-8 (DE, HR, HU, LU) *see* Ornipressin [INT] ... 1522
POR-8 Ferring (AT, CH) *see* Ornipressin [INT] ... 1522
POR-8 (NZ, ZA) *see* Ornipressin [INT] ... 1522
POR 8 Sandoz (AU) *see* Ornipressin [INT] ... 1522
Porazine (TH) *see* Perphenazine ... 1627
Poro (ID, MY, PH, SG, TH) *see* Acetaminophen ... 32
Porosal (VE) *see* Alendronate ... 79
Portalak (HR) *see* Lactulose ... 1156

Portal (HR, HU) *see* FLUoxetine 899
Portora (CZ) *see* Trimetazidine [INT] 2104
Posanol (TW) *see* Posaconazole 1683
Poscal (KR) *see* Calcitriol 323
Poshuin (KR) *see* Calcium Acetate 326
Posid (PH) *see* Etoposide 816
Posiject (GB, IE) *see* DOBUTamine 654
Posipen (MX, PE) *see* Dicloxacillin 621
Positon (TR) *see* Triamcinolone (Topical) 2100
Pospargin (ID, VN) *see* Methylergonovine 1333
Pospenem (KR) *see* Meropenem 1299
Posprand (BR) *see* Repaglinide 1791
Possia (EE, PL, PT) *see* Ticagrelor 2035
Postafen (DK, FI, IS, NO, SE) *see* Meclizine 1277
Postafene (BE) *see* Meclizine 1277
Postiline (AR) *see* Sevelamer 1881
Postinor-1 (AU, NZ) *see* Levonorgestrel 1201
Postinor-2 (AU, CN, HK, MX, PE, SG, TW, VE) *see* Levonorgestrel 1201
Postinor (BE, CH, CL, CN, EE, HU, IS, LT, PL, SE) *see* Levonorgestrel 1201
Postinor Uno (BR) *see* Levonorgestrel 1201
Postmenop (TH) *see* Estradiol (Systemic) 775
Posyd (ID) *see* Etoposide 816
Posyd (ID) *see* Etoposide Phosphate 820
Potarlon (TW) *see* Mefenamic Acid 1280
Pota-Vi-Kin (MX) *see* Penicillin V Potassium 1614
Potecin (PH) *see* Clindamycin (Systemic) 460
Potekam (PY) *see* Topotecan 2069
Potendol SR (KR) *see* TraMADol 2074
Povanil (TH) *see* ClonazePAM 478
Poviral (AR) *see* Acyclovir (Systemic) 47
Poviral (AR) *see* Acyclovir (Topical) 51
Powegon (TW) *see* Cimetidine 438
Power Gel (KR) *see* Lidocaine (Topical) 1211
Poxidium (AE, BH, CY, EG, IL, IQ, IR, JO, KW, LB, LY, OM, QA, SA, SY, YE) *see* Clidinium and Chlordiazepoxide 460
Pozapam (TH) *see* Prazepam [INT] 1702
Pozhexol (TH) *see* Trihexyphenidyl 2103
Pozola (TW) *see* Pantoprazole 1570
Ppar (PH) *see* Pioglitazone 1654
P.P.V. (AE) *see* Penicillin V Potassium 1614
Prabetic (ID) *see* Pioglitazone 1654
Pracetam (VN) *see* Piracetam [INT] 1661
Pradaxa (AE, AR, AT, AU, BE, BH, CH, CL, CN, CO, CY, CZ, DE, DK, EC, EE, FR, GB, GR, GT, HK, HN, HR, ID, IE, IL, IN, IS, IT, JP, KR, KW, LB, LT, MY, NL, NO, NZ, PE, PH, PL, PT, QA, RO, RU, SA, SE, SG, SI, SK, SV, TH, TR, TW, UY, VN) *see* Dabigatran Etexilate 542
Pradif (PT) *see* Tamsulosin 1974
Praecicalm (DE) *see* PENTobarbital 1617
Pragmarel (FR) *see* TraZODone 2091
Prakten (TR) *see* Cyproheptadine 529
Pralax (ID) *see* Lactulose 1156
Pralia (JP) *see* Denosumab 589
Pralifan (ES) *see* MitoXANtrone 1382
Praline (TW) *see* Ethinyl Estradiol and Desogestrel 799
Praloxin (KR) *see* Pefloxacin [INT] 1588
Pramace (SE) *see* Ramipril 1771
Pramide (PT) *see* Pyrazinamide 1745
Pramidin (PL) *see* Metoclopramide 1345
Pramil (PY) *see* Sildenafil 1882
Pramin (AU, IL, TW) *see* Metoclopramide 1345
Prandase (IL) *see* Acarbose 29
Prandin (AT, BE, BG, CH, CZ, DE, DK, EE, ES, FI, FR, GB, GR, HN, IE, IT, MT, NL, NO, PL, PT, RU, SE, SK, TR) *see* Repaglinide 1791
Prandin E2 (ZA) *see* Dinoprostone 640
Prandin (KR) *see* Deflazacort [INT] 587
Pranex LP (PE) *see* Acemetacin [INT] 30
Pranex (PE) *see* Acemetacin [INT] 30
Pranidol (MX) *see* Propranolol 1731
Praol (GR) *see* Meprobamate 1296
Prasone (TW) *see* Pramoxine and Hydrocortisone 1698
Prastan (KR) *see* Pravastatin 1700
Prasudoc (IN) *see* Prasugrel 1699
Pratin (MY, TW) *see* Pravastatin 1700
Pratisol (NZ, TW, ZA) *see* Prazosin 1703
Pratsiol (BG, FI) *see* Prazosin 1703
Prava (CH) *see* Lomustine 1235
Pravachol (AT, AU, BB, BM, BS, BZ, DK, FI, GR, GY, HK, JM, NO, NZ, PE, PK, SE, SR, TR, TT, VE) *see* Pravastatin 1700
Pravacol (AR, BR, CL, EC, MX, PE, PT) *see* Pravastatin 1700
Pravalip (IL) *see* Pravastatin 1700
Pravaselect (IT) *see* Pravastatin 1700
Pravasin (DE, LU) *see* Pravastatin 1700
Pravasine (BE) *see* Pravastatin 1700
Pravator (IN, QA, RO) *see* Pravastatin 1700
Prava (ZA) *see* Pravastatin 1700
Pravaz (PH) *see* Pravastatin 1700
Pravidel (DE, SE) *see* Bromocriptine 291
Pravyl (CO) *see* Pravastatin 1700
Praxel (CL, MX, TH) *see* PACLitaxel (Conventional) 1550
Praxilene (BE, CH, ES, FR, GB, IE, IT, LU, PT) *see* Naftidrofuryl [INT] 1416
Praxin (HU) *see* FLUoxetine 899
Praxin (PY, UY) *see* Prazosin 1703
Praxiten (AT, HR) *see* Oxazepam 1532
Prayanol (CL) *see* Amantadine 105
Prazac (KR) *see* FLUoxetine 899
Prazene (IT) *see* Prazepam [INT] 1702
Prazex (VN) *see* Lansoprazole 1166
Prazidec (MX) *see* Omeprazole 1508
Prazide (VN) *see* Pyrazinamide 1745
Prazine (IN) *see* Praziquantel 1702
Prazinil (FR) *see* Carpipramine [INT] 367
Prazin (JO) *see* ALPRAZolam 94
Praziquin (AE, BH, CY, EG, IL, IQ, IR, JO, KW, LB, LY, OM, QA, SA, SY, YE) *see* Praziquantel 1702
Prazite (TH) *see* Praziquantel 1702
Prazitral (AR) *see* Praziquantel 1702
Prazol (AE, BH, CY, EG, IQ, IR, JO, KW, LB, LY, OM, QA, SA, SY, YE) *see* ALPRAZolam 94
Prazole (TH) *see* Omeprazole 1508
Prazone-S (TH) *see* Cefoperazone and Sulbactam [INT] 382
Prazopress (IN) *see* Prazosin 1703
Prazovex (MY) *see* ALPRAZolam 94
Precedex (AE, AR, AU, BH, BR, CZ, HK, ID, KR, KW, LB, MX, MY, NZ, PE, PH, PL, QA, SA, SG, TH, TW, UY, VN) *see* Dexmedetomidine 604
Precoce (AR) *see* Dapoxetine [INT] 561
Precose (MY, TW) *see* Acarbose 29
Precoxi (MY) *see* Nimesulide [INT] 1456
Preda (KR) *see* Estradiol (Systemic) 775
Predalone (LB) *see* PrednisoLONE (Systemic) 1703
Pred Forte (AE, BE, BR, CH, CL, CN, EG, FI, GB, HK, IE, IL, JO, KR, KW, LB, NL, NZ, PH, QA, SA, SG, TH, TR, TW, VN, ZA) *see* PrednisoLONE (Ophthalmic) 1706
Predial (DO, GT, HN, NI, SV) *see* MetFORMIN 1307
Predicor (LB) *see* PredniSONE 1706
Predlitem (MX) *see* MethylPREDNISolone 1340
Predmet (IN) *see* PrednisoLONE (Ophthalmic) 1706
Predmet (IN) *see* PrednisoLONE (Systemic) 1703
Pred Mild (AE, BR, HK, JO, LB, MY, NZ, PH, SA, SG, TH, ZA) *see* PrednisoLONE (Ophthalmic) 1706
Prednefrin (CO, PE) *see* PrednisoLONE (Ophthalmic) 1706
Prednefrin Forte (AU, PE, VE) *see* PrednisoLONE (Ophthalmic) 1706
Prednicort (BE, LU, PY) *see* PredniSONE 1706
Prednidib (MX) *see* PredniSONE 1706

Prednimax (EC) *see* PrednisoLONE (Systemic) 1703
Predniment (NL) *see* PredniSONE 1706
Prednimut (NL) *see* PredniSONE 1706
Predniocil (PT) *see* PrednisoLONE (Ophthalmic) 1706
Predni-Ophtal (DE) *see* PrednisoLONE (Ophthalmic) 1706
Predni-POS (CZ) *see* PrednisoLONE (Ophthalmic) 1706
Prednisone (CY) *see* PredniSONE 1706
Prednison (FI, NO) *see* PredniSONE 1706
Prednison Galepharm (CH) *see* PredniSONE 1706
Prednison Streuli (CH) *see* PredniSONE 1706
Prednison "Dak" (DK) *see* PredniSONE 1706
Prednitop (AT, CH, TR) *see* Prednicarbate 1703
Prednol (TR) *see* MethylPREDNISolone 1340
Prednox (PH) *see* MethylPREDNISolone 1340
Predonium DS (NZ) *see* Perindopril and Indapamide [CAN/INT] 1626
Predonium (HK, NZ) *see* Perindopril and Indapamide [CAN/INT] 1626
Predon (MY) *see* PrednisoLONE (Ophthalmic) 1706
Pre Dopa (JP) *see* DOPamine 669
Predoral (PH) *see* PredniSONE 1706
Predozone (BG) *see* Trimetazidine [INT] 2104
Predsol-Forte (DO, HN) *see* PrednisoLONE (Ophthalmic) 1706
Predsol (GB) *see* PrednisoLONE (Ophthalmic) 1706
Predsone (PH) *see* PredniSONE 1706
Preductal (HN, PL, RO) *see* Trimetazidine [INT] 2104
Preductal MR (EE, HR) *see* Trimetazidine [INT] 2104
Preduxl (HK) *see* Trimetazidine [INT] 2104
Predxal (MX) *see* Telmisartan 1988
Predxal (VN) *see* TraMADol 2074
Prefamone (CH, FR, LU) *see* Diethylpropion 624
Prefamone Chronule (BE) *see* Diethylpropion 624
Prefrin (AE, AR, AU, BH, CY, EC, EG, IL, IQ, IR, JO, KW, LB, LY, NZ, OM, QA, SA, SY, YE, ZA) *see* Phenylephrine (Systemic) 1638
Pregabadin (PY) *see* Pregabalin 1710
Pregalin (KR) *see* Pregabalin 1710
Pregnyl (AE, AR, AT, AU, BE, BG, BH, CH, CL, CO, CY, CZ, DE, DK, EC, EG, ES, FI, GB, GR, HU, ID, JO, KR, KW, LB, LT, MX, MY, NL, NO, NZ, PH, PK, PL, PT, QA, RO, RU, SA, SE, SG, SI, SK, TH, TR, TW, UY, VE, ZA) *see* Chorionic Gonadotropin (Human) 431
Pregyl (PE) *see* Chorionic Gonadotropin (Human) 431
Prelar Depot (MX) *see* Leuprolide 1186
Prelat (PH) *see* Captopril 342
Prelod (TH) *see* AmLODIPine 123
Premarin CD (AR) *see* Estrogens (Conjugated/Equine, Systemic) 787
Premarin (AU, BF, BG, BH, BJ, BR, CI, CN, CO, CR, EC, EG, ET, GB, GH, GM, GN, GT, HK, HN, IE, IL, IN, IT, JO, KE, LR, MA, ML, MR, MU, MW, MY, NE, NG, NI, NZ, PA, PE, PH, PK, QA, RU, SA, SC, SD, SG, SL, SN, SV, TH, TN, TR, TW, TZ, UG, VE, VN, ZM, ZW) *see* Estrogens (Conjugated/Equine, Systemic) 787
Premarin Crema (PY) *see* Estrogens (Conjugated/Equine, Systemic) 787
Premarin Crema Vaginal (CO) *see* Estrogens (Conjugated/Equine, Systemic) 787
Premarin Creme (ZA) *see* Estrogens (Conjugated/Equine, Systemic) 787
Premarin Vaginal (AE, BH, CY, EG, IQ, IR, JO, KW, LB, LY, OM, QA, SA, SY, YE) *see* Estrogens (Conjugated/Equine, Systemic) 787
Premarin Vaginal Creme (AE, BB, BH, BM, BS, BZ, CY, EG, GY, HK, IL, IQ, IR, JM, JO, KR, KW, LB, LY, MY, NL, OM, PK, PR, QA, SA, SR, SY, TH, TT, TW, YE) *see* Estrogens (Conjugated/Equine, Systemic) 787
Premid (DK) *see* Balsalazide 226
Premina (KR) *see* Estrogens (Conjugated/Equine, Systemic) 787
Preminent HD (JP) *see* Losartan and Hydrochlorothiazide 1250
Preminent (JP) *see* Losartan and Hydrochlorothiazide 1250
Premosan (AE, BH, KW, QA, SA) *see* Metoclopramide 1345
Prena (KR) *see* MethylPREDNISolone 1340
Prencoid (VN) *see* PrednisoLONE (Systemic) 1703
Prenessa (EE) *see* Perindopril 1623
Prenolol (SG, TH) *see* Atenolol 189
Prenol (VN) *see* PrednisoLONE (Systemic) 1703
Prenormine (AR) *see* Atenolol 189
Prenoxad (GB) *see* Naloxone 1419
Prent (CH, DE, IT, PT, TR) *see* Acebutolol 29
Prepadine (GB) *see* Dosulepin [INT] 673
Prepenem (HK, KR, TH) *see* Imipenem and Cilastatin 1051
Prepidil (AE, AT, BE, BG, BH, CO, CY, CZ, EG, ES, FR, HN, HR, HU, IL, IQ, IR, IT, JO, KW, LB, LU, LY, MY, NL, OM, PK, PL, QA, SA, SK, SY, YE, ZA) *see* Dinoprostone 640
Prepram (MX) *see* Citalopram 451
Presacor (EC) *see* PredniSONE 1706
Pres (DE) *see* Enalapril 722
Preservex (GB, IE) *see* Aceclofenac [INT] 30
Presiam (AR) *see* Zofenopril [INT] 2206
Presilam (CL) *see* AmLODIPine 123
Presil (CO) *see* Enalapril 722
Presinex (BG, GB, IE, IL) *see* Desmopressin 594
Presinex Nasal Spray (SG) *see* Desmopressin 594
Presinol 500 (DE) *see* Methyldopa 1332
Presinol (AT, DE) *see* Methyldopa 1332
Presin (PY) *see* Propranolol 1731
Presiten (DO) *see* Lisinopril 1226
Preslow (ES, PT) *see* Felodipine 850
Presmin (BR) *see* Betaxolol (Systemic) 256
Presolin (HK, TH) *see* Irbesartan 1110
Presolol (AU, TW) *see* Labetalol 1151
Presomen (DE) *see* Estrogens (Conjugated/Equine, Systemic) 787
Presopril-D (DO) *see* Enalapril and Hydrochlorothiazide 725
Pressocard (PL) *see* Labetalol 1151
Pressolat (IL) *see* NIFEdipine 1451
Prestarium (EE) *see* Perindopril and Indapamide [CAN/INT] 1626
Prestarium (HR, PL) *see* Perindopril 1623
Prestole (FR) *see* Hydrochlorothiazide and Triamterene 1012
Prestoral (ID) *see* Propranolol 1731
Prestoril (IL) *see* Perindopril 1623
Pretanix (HU) *see* Indapamide 1065
Pretenol (MY) *see* Atenolol 189
Preterax (AR, AT, BB, BH, BM, BS, BZ, CH, CO, CR, DO, EG, FR, GR, GT, GY, HN, IT, JM, MX, NI, NL, PA, PE, PH, PK, PR, PY, QA, SG, SR, SV, TR, TT, TW, VE) *see* Perindopril and Indapamide [CAN/INT] 1626
Preterax Arginine (AE, KW, LB, SA) *see* Perindopril and Indapamide [CAN/INT] 1626
Preterax Forte (CH) *see* Perindopril and Indapamide [CAN/INT] 1626
Pretilon (ID) *see* MethylPREDNISolone 1340
Preto (KR) *see* Clopidogrel 484
Prevacid (CN, MY, PH, PK, SG, TH) *see* Lansoprazole 1166
Prevecilina (CO) *see* Penicillin V Potassium 1614
Prevenar 13 (AE, AR, AT, AU, BE, CH, CL, CO, CR, CY, CZ, DE, DK, DO, EC, EE, FR, GB, GT, HK, HN, HR, ID, IE, IL, IS, KR, LB, LT, MY, NI, NL, NO, NZ, PA, PH, PL, PT, QA, RO, SA, SE, SG, SI, SK, SV, TH, TW) *see* Pneumococcal Conjugate Vaccine (13-Valent) 1670
Previscan (FR) *see* Fluindione [INT] 892
Prevoc (AE, BH, JO, SA) *see* Ticlopidine 2040

Prewell (TW) *see* BuPROPion 305
Prexal (JO) *see* OLANZapine 1491
Prexanil Combi (HR) *see* Perindopril and Indapamide [CAN/INT] 1626
Prexan (IT) *see* Naproxen 1427
Prexaton (AU) *see* BuPROPion 305
Prex (KR) *see* Baclofen 223
Prezal (NL) *see* Lansoprazole 1166
Prezista (AE, AR, AT, AU, BB, BE, BH, BM, BR, BS, BZ, CH, CL, CN, CO, CY, CZ, DE, DK, DO, EC, EE, FR, GB, GR, GY, HK, HN, HR, IE, IL, IS, IT, JM, JP, KR, KW, LT, MY, NL, NO, NZ, PL, PR, PT, QA, RO, RU, SA, SE, SG, SI, SK, SR, TH, TR, TT, TW, UY) *see* Darunavir 569
Priacin (SG) *see* Simvastatin 1890
Priadel (BE, GB, LU, NL, NO, NZ, PT, TR) *see* Lithium 1230
Priadel Retard (CH) *see* Lithium 1230
Prialta-Met (PH) *see* Pioglitazone and Metformin 1655
Prialta (PH) *see* Pioglitazone 1654
Prialt (AT, BE, BG, CH, CZ, DE, DK, EE, ES, FI, FR, GB, GR, HN, HR, IE, IT, MT, NL, NO, PL, PT, RO, RU, SE, SK, TR) *see* Ziconotide 2196
Priaxen (BB, BF, BJ, BM, BS, BZ, CI, ET, GH, GM, GN, GY, JM, KE, LR, MA, ML, MR, MU, MW, NE, NG, SC, SD, SL, SN, SR, TN, TR, TT, TZ, UG, ZM, ZW) *see* Naproxen 1427
Priciasol (BE) *see* Naphazoline (Nasal) 1426
Pridax (RO) *see* Alprostadil 96
Pridecil (BR) *see* Bromopride [INT] 292
Prifinial[vet.] (AT, CH, FR) *see* Prifinium [INT] 1712
Priftin (CA) *see* Rifapentine 1807
Prilace (AU) *see* Ramipril 1771
Prilace (EC) *see* Enalapril 722
Prilen Plus (HR) *see* Ramipril and Hydrochlorothiazide [CAN/INT] 1773
Priligy (AT, BE, BG, BR, CH, CN, CO, CZ, DE, DK, EE, ES, FI, FR, GB, HK, HR, IT, KR, LB, LT, MX, MY, NL, PH, PT, RO, SE, SG, SI, SK, TH) *see* Dapoxetine [INT] 561
Prilosan (MX) *see* Lansoprazole 1166
Prilox (IN) *see* Lidocaine and Prilocaine 1213
Primacef (PE) *see* CeFAZolin 373
Primace (PH) *see* Captopril 342
Primacin (AU) *see* Primaquine 1713
Primacor (AU, BR, GB, HK, IL, IN, KR, MX, MY, NZ, PH, TH, TW) *see* Milrinone 1370
Primaderm (AR) *see* Prednicarbate 1703
Primapen (ID) *see* Ampicillin 141
Primax (CO) *see* Ciclopirox 433
Primaxin IV (BB, BM, BS, BZ, GY, JM, SR, TT) *see* Imipenem and Cilastatin 1051
Primaxin (AU, GB, GR, NZ) *see* Imipenem and Cilastatin 1051
Primera 30 (BR) *see* Ethinyl Estradiol and Desogestrel 799
Primeral (IT) *see* Naproxen 1427
Primet (ID) *see* Pyrimethamine 1749
Primid (BR) *see* Primidone 1714
Primidon (HR) *see* Primidone 1714
Primiprost (IN) *see* Dinoprostone 640
Primocef (AE) *see* Cefotaxime 382
Primodex (UY) *see* Piracetam [INT] 1661
Primogonyl (DE) *see* Chorionic Gonadotropin (Human) 431
Primogyn Depot (ZA) *see* Estradiol (Systemic) 775
Primolut Depot (EC) *see* Hydroxyprogesterone Caproate 1021
Primolut (EG, PK) *see* Norethindrone 1473
Primolutin (DE) *see* Norethindrone 1473
Primolut N (AE, BB, BD, BF, BH, BJ, BM, BS, BZ, CH, CI, CL, CY, DE, EG, ET, FI, GB, GH, GM, GN, GY, ID, IE, IL, IQ, IR, IS, JM, JO, JP, KE, KR, KW, LB, LR, LY, MA, ML, MR, MU, MW, NE, NG, NL, NO, OM, PH, PK, PL, PR, QA, SA, SC, SD, SG, SL, SN, SR, SY, TH, TN, TR, TT, TZ, UG, YE, ZA, ZM, ZW) *see* Norethindrone 1473
Primolut-N (KR) *see* Norethindrone 1473
Primolut Nor (AR, BE, BG, CZ, EC, GR, IT, PT, PY, RU, SE, SI, UY, VN) *see* Norethindrone 1473
Primoniat Depot (CL) *see* Testosterone 2010
Primosept (CH) *see* Trimethoprim 2104
Primoteston Depot (AU, BF, BJ, CI, EC, ET, GH, GM, GN, KE, KR, LR, MA, ML, MR, MU, MW, NE, NG, SC, SD, SL, SN, TN, TZ, UG, ZM, ZW) *see* Testosterone 2010
Primotestone Depot (AE, KW) *see* Testosterone 2010
Primperan (AE, AT, BE, BF, BH, BJ, CH, CI, CO, CR, CY, CZ, DK, DO, EE, EG, ES, ET, FI, FR, GH, GM, GN, GR, GT, HK, HN, JO, JP, KE, KW, LB, LR, LU, MA, ML, MR, MT, MU, MW, MY, NE, NG, NI, NL, PA, PE, PT, QA, RU, SA, SC, SD, SE, SG, SK, SL, SN, SV, TN, TR, TW, TZ, UG, VE, VN, ZM, ZW) *see* Metoclopramide 1345
Primperil (AR) *see* Metoclopramide 1345
Primzole (SG) *see* Sulfamethoxazole and Trimethoprim 1946
Prinac AC (MX) *see* Folic Acid 919
Prindex (MX) *see* Carbinoxamine 356
Prinil (CH) *see* Lisinopril 1226
Prinivil (AT, AU, BB, BG, BM, BR, BS, BZ, CZ, FR, GR, GY, HR, HU, IT, JM, MX, PL, SR, TT, VE) *see* Lisinopril 1226
Prink (KR) *see* Alprostadil 96
Prinox (AR) *see* ALPRAZolam 94
Prinox (PY) *see* Amiodarone 114
Prinparl (JP) *see* Metoclopramide 1345
Prinwin (TW) *see* Perindopril 1623
Prinzide (AT, BG, BR, CH, FR, GR, IT, MX, NZ) *see* Lisinopril and Hydrochlorothiazide 1229
Prioderm (AE, BE, BF, BH, BJ, CH, CI, CY, DK, EG, ET, FI, FR, GH, GM, GN, IE, IL, IQ, IR, IS, JO, KE, KW, LB, LR, LU, LY, MA, ML, MR, MU, MW, NE, NG, NL, NO, OM, QA, SA, SC, SD, SE, SL, SN, SY, TN, TZ, UG, YE, ZA, ZM, ZW) *see* Malathion 1268
Priorheum (DE) *see* Piroxicam 1662
Priorix (AE, AU, BB, BM, BS, BZ, CY, GB, GY, IE, IL, JM, KR, KW, NL, NO, PH, RO, SA, SE, SR, TT, TW) *see* Measles, Mumps, and Rubella Virus Vaccine 1273
Priorix Tetra (AE, CY, SA) *see* Measles, Mumps, Rubella, and Varicella Virus Vaccine 1274
Priper (AR, PY) *see* Pipemidic Acid [INT] 1655
Prism (IN) *see* Deflazacort [INT] 587
Pristine (HK, MY) *see* Ketoconazole (Topical) 1145
Pristinex (HK) *see* Ketoconazole (Topical) 1145
Pristinex (MY) *see* Ketoconazole (Systemic) 1144
Pristiq (AE, AR, AU, BR, CL, CO, CR, EC, GT, HK, HN, IL, KW, MY, NI, PA, QA, SA, SG, SV, TH) *see* Desvenlafaxine 598
Pristiq SR (PH) *see* Desvenlafaxine 598
Prisutomycin (TW) *see* Piperacillin [CAN/INT] 1656
Pritanol (ID) *see* Allopurinol 90
Pritoral (CL) *see* Telmisartan 1988
Pritor (AR, KR, PE, PH, VE) *see* Telmisartan 1988
Pritorplus (AT, BE, BG, CH, CZ, DE, DK, EE, ES, FI, FR, GB, GR, IE, IT, KR, MT, NL, NO, PH, PL, PT, RU, SE, SK, TR) *see* Telmisartan and Hydrochlorothiazide 1990
PritorPlus (HR, HU, RO) *see* Telmisartan and Hydrochlorothiazide 1990
Privent DPS (IN) *see* Ketotifen (Ophthalmic) 1150
Privigen (IL) *see* Immune Globulin 1056
Privina (BR) *see* Naphazoline (Nasal) 1426
Privin (AT) *see* Naphazoline (Nasal) 1426
Prixina (PL) *see* Prulifloxacin [INT] 1742
Prixin (AR, PY) *see* Ampicillin and Sulbactam 145
Prixlae (PH) *see* Cetirizine 411

Prizma (IL) *see* FLUoxetine 899
Prizma (QA) *see* Piperacillin and Tazobactam 1657
Pro-C (AU) *see* Ascorbic Acid 178
Proalgin (BG) *see* Dipyrone [INT] 653
Proanes (ID) *see* Propofol 1728
Probamato (PT) *see* Meprobamate 1296
Probamyl (BE) *see* Meprobamate 1296
ProBanthine (AE, EG, KW) *see* Propantheline 1727
Pro-Banthine (AU, BB, BE, BF, BJ, BM, BS, BZ, CI, CY, ET, FR, GB, GH, GM, GN, GY, HK, ID, IE, IN, JM, KE, LR, LU, MA, ML, MR, MU, MW, NE, NG, NL, QA, SC, SD, SL, SN, SR, TN, TT, TW, TZ, UG, ZA, ZM, ZW) *see* Propantheline 1727
Probat (ID) *see* GuaiFENesin 986
Probecid (FI, NO, SE) *see* Probenecid 1716
Probecilin (BR) *see* Probenecid 1716
Probelin (PH) *see* Clobetasol 468
Probenecid Weimer (DE) *see* Probenecid 1716
Probenecid "Dak" (DK) *see* Probenecid 1716
Probenecid "Medic" (DK) *see* Probenecid 1716
Probenil (AR) *see* Bepotastine 250
Pro-Bextra IM/IV (CL) *see* Parecoxib [INT] 1576
Probi RHO (D) (MX) *see* Rh_o(D) Immune Globulin 1794
Probirina (MX) *see* Ribavirin 1797
Probitor (AU, BG, MY, SG) *see* Omeprazole 1508
Probitor HP7 (AU) *see* Omeprazole, Clarithromycin, and Amoxicillin 1511
Procadex (IN) *see* Ceftibuten 394
Procainamid Duriles (DE) *see* Procainamide 1716
Procainamide Cloridrato (IT) *see* Procainamide 1716
Procainamide Durules (NZ) *see* Procainamide 1716
Procainamid (PL) *see* Procainamide 1716
Procainamidum (PL) *see* Procainamide 1716
Procaine Penicillin. G (FI) *see* Penicillin G Procaine 1613
Procain-Penicillin Streuli (CH) *see* Penicillin G Procaine 1613
Procal (BE, LU, NL) *see* Fluoride 895
Procalmadiol (BE, LU) *see* Meprobamate 1296
ProCalm (AU) *see* Prochlorperazine 1718
Procal (TW) *see* Calcium Acetate 326
Procamid depot (FI) *see* Procainamide 1716
Procamide (BR, IT) *see* Procainamide 1716
Procapen (FI) *see* Penicillin G Procaine 1613
Procarbizol (PK) *see* Propylthiouracil 1735
Procardin (SG) *see* Dipyridamole 652
Proca (TW) *see* Calcium Acetate 326
Procefa (ID) *see* Cefotaxime 382
Procef (AR, AT, CH, CO, EC, HK, MX, MY, PH, PT, SG, TH, TR, VE) *see* Cefprozil 389
Procepim (ID) *see* Cefepime 378
Proceptin (SG) *see* Omeprazole 1508
Prochic (TH) *see* Colchicine 500
Prochlor (MY) *see* Prochlorperazine 1718
Pro-Cid (AU) *see* Probenecid 1716
Procid (TW) *see* Probenecid 1716
Procil (TW) *see* Propylthiouracil 1735
Procip (NZ) *see* Ciprofloxacin (Systemic) 441
Prociralan (RO) *see* Ivabradine [INT] 1134
Procirex (IT) *see* Bromopride [INT] 292
Proclose (MX) *see* Octreotide 1485
Proclozine (TH) *see* Prochlorperazine 1718
Procomvax (AT, BE, BG, CH, CZ, DE, DK, ES, FI, FR, GB, GR, HN, IE, IT, NL, NO, PT, RU, SE, TR) *see* Haemophilus b Conjugate and Hepatitis B Vaccine 991
Procoralan (AE, AR, AT, BE, BH, BR, CH, CL, CO, CY, CZ, DE, DK, EC, EE, FR, GR, HN, HR, IE, IS, IT, KR, KW, LB, LT, NL, PL, PT, QA, SA, SE, SI, SK, TR, VN) *see* Ivabradine [INT] 1134
Procor (IL) *see* Amiodarone 114
Procren Depot (DK, FI, NO, SE) *see* Leuprolide 1186
Procrin (ES) *see* Leuprolide 1186
Proctofoam (GB) *see* Pramoxine and Hydrocortisone 1698
Proctofoam HC (AE, IL, QA) *see* Pramoxine and Hydrocortisone 1698
Proculin (RO) *see* Naphazoline (Ophthalmic) 1426
Procur (AU, NZ, SG) *see* Cyproterone [CAN/INT] 530
Pro-Cure (IL) *see* Finasteride 878
Procuta Ge (FR) *see* ISOtretinoin 1127
Procythol (GR) *see* Selegiline 1873
Prodafem (AT, CH) *see* MedroxyPROGESTERone 1277
Prodeine-15 (AU) *see* Acetaminophen and Codeine 36
Prodeine Forte (AU) *see* Acetaminophen and Codeine 36
Prodent Fluor (PY) *see* Fluoride 895
Prodep (IN) *see* FLUoxetine 899
Prodexin (AE, BH, CY, EG, IQ, IR, JO, KW, LB, LY, OM, QA, SA, SY, YE) *see* Naproxen 1427
ProDilantin (FR) *see* Fosphenytoin 934
Prodinam (AR) *see* Strontium Ranelate [INT] 1938
Prodol (ZA) *see* Cetylpyridinium and Benzocaine [CAN/INT] 415
Prodopa (NZ) *see* Methyldopa 1332
Prodormol (IL) *see* PENTobarbital 1617
Proemend (JP) *see* Fosaprepitant 929
Pro-Epanutin (AT, AU, DK, FI, GB, GR, IE, IS, NL, NO, SE, SI) *see* Fosphenytoin 934
Profamid (DK) *see* Flutamide 907
Profasi (AE, AT, BH, DK, EG, FI, GB, GR, HU, IN, NL, NO, NZ, PK, PL, QA, RU, SA, SI) *see* Chorionic Gonadotropin (Human) 431
Profasi HP (ES, IT, PT) *see* Chorionic Gonadotropin (Human) 431
Profast (RO) *see* Propofol 1728
Profat (ID) *see* Sucralfate 1940
ProFeme 3.2 (AU) *see* Progesterone 1722
ProFeme 10 (AU) *see* Progesterone 1722
Profemina (CL) *see* Estrogens (Conjugated/Equine, Systemic) 787
Profenac (AE, BH, CY, EG, IQ, IR, JO, KW, LB, LY, OM, QA, SA, SY, YE) *see* Diclofenac (Systemic) 617
Profen (HK) *see* Ibuprofen 1032
Profenid (AE, AT, BB, BG, BH, BS, CO, CZ, EC, EE, FR, ID, IL, JM, KW, LB, MX, NL, PE, PL, PT, PY, QA, SA, TR, VE, VN) *see* Ketoprofen 1145
Profenid Gel (ID) *see* Ketoprofen 1145
Profenil (HK, HN) *see* Alverine [INT] 104
Profergan (BR) *see* Promethazine 1723
Profertil (ID) *see* ClomiPHENE 473
Profex (IL) *see* Propafenone 1725
Profiben (MX) *see* Pentoxifylline 1618
Profika (ID) *see* Ketoprofen 1145
Profilar (AE, BH, CY, EG, IQ, IR, JO, KW, LB, LY, OM, QA, SA, SY, YE) *see* Ketotifen (Systemic) [CAN/INT] 1149
Profilnine SD (AE, MY, PH, SG, TH) *see* Factor IX (Human) 840
Profinal (AE, BH, KW, LB, MY, QA, SA) *see* Ibuprofen 1032
Profiten (IL) *see* Ketotifen (Systemic) [CAN/INT] 1149
Proflam (BR) *see* Aceclofenac [INT] 30
Proflox (EC, TH) *see* Ciprofloxacin (Systemic) 441
Proflox (PT) *see* Moxifloxacin (Systemic) 1401
Profurex (PH) *see* Cefuroxime 399
Profuzosin (PH) *see* Alfuzosin 84
Progandol (ES) *see* Doxazosin 674
Progandol Neo (ES) *see* Doxazosin 674
Progeffik (TW) *see* Progesterone 1722
Progendo (CL) *see* Progesterone 1722
Progen (KR) *see* MedroxyPROGESTERone 1277
Progering (PE) *see* Progesterone 1722
Progesic (AE, GB, QA) *see* Fenoprofen 857
Progesic (HK) *see* Acetaminophen 32
Progestan (NL) *see* Progesterone 1722

Progesterone Retard Pharlon (FR) *see* Hydroxyprogesterone Caproate 1021
Progestin (PA, SV) *see* Progesterone 1722
Progestogel (HK, LU) *see* Progesterone 1722
Progevera (ES) *see* MedroxyPROGESTERone 1277
Proglicem (AR, CH, DE, FR, IT, NL, NO, SG) *see* Diazoxide 616
Proglycem (GR, KR, TW) *see* Diazoxide 616
Progonadyl (AR) *see* Menotropins 1292
Progor (LB, TH, TW) *see* Diltiazem 634
Progout (AU, SG) *see* Allopurinol 90
Prograf XL (AU, CO) *see* Tacrolimus (Systemic) 1962
Prograf (AE, AR, AT, AU, BE, BH, BR, CH, CL, CN, CO, CR, CY, CZ, DE, DK, DO, EE, EG, FI, FR, GB, GR, GT, HK, HN, HR, ID, IE, IL, IQ, IR, IS, IT, JO, JP, KR, KW, LB, LY, MY, NI, NL, NZ, OM, PA, PE, PH, PL, PY, QA, RO, RU, SA, SE, SG, SK, SV, SY, TH, TR, TW, UY, VE, VN, YE) *see* Tacrolimus (Systemic) 1962
Progras (AR) *see* Sorbitol 1927
Progyl (ID) *see* MetroNIDAZOLE (Systemic) 1353
Progynon (CH, DE, DK, IT, SE) *see* Estradiol (Systemic) 775
Progynon Depot (IN, TW) *see* Estradiol (Systemic) 775
Progynova (AR, AT, AU, BE, BZ, CL, CN, CO, CR, DO, FI, FR, GT, HN, ID, IL, IN, KR, MY, NI, NO, NZ, PA, PE, PH, PL, RU, SE, SG, SV, UY, VE, ZA) *see* Estradiol (Systemic) 775
Prohem (ID) *see* Phytonadione 1647
Prohessen (ID) *see* Cyproheptadine 529
Prohiper (ID) *see* Methylphenidate 1336
Prohytens (ID) *see* Ramipril 1771
Proimer (KR) *see* Procyclidine [CAN/INT] 1721
Proinfark (ID) *see* DOPamine 669
Proken (AE, BH, JO, LB, QA, SA) *see* Naproxen 1427
Prokinyl (LU) *see* Metoclopramide 1345
Proladone (AU) *see* OxyCODONE 1538
Prolanzo (PH) *see* Lansoprazole 1166
Prolastat (CO, EC) *see* Cabergoline 319
Prolaxan (ID) *see* Bisacodyl 265
Prolax (TW) *see* Chlorzoxazone 430
Prolepsi (ID) *see* OXcarbazepine 1532
Proleukin (AE, AR, AT, BE, BR, CH, CO, CZ, DE, DK, EC, EG, ES, FI, FR, GB, GR, HK, HN, HU, IE, IL, IS, IT, KR, LB, NL, NZ, PE, PL, PT, RU, SG, SI, TR, TW, UY) *see* Aldesleukin 72
Prolia (AR, AT, AU, BE, BR, CH, CL, CY, CZ, DE, DK, EE, ES, FR, GB, GR, HK, HN, HR, IL, IS, LT, MX, MY, NL, NO, NZ, PE, PH, PL, QA, RO, SA, SE, SG, SK, TH, TR, TW) *see* Denosumab 589
Prolid (RU) *see* Nimesulide [INT] 1456
Prolift (BR, CL) *see* Reboxetine [INT] 1786
Prolipase (AT, CH, CZ, HR, PL) *see* Pancrelipase 1566
Prolisina E2 (AR) *see* Dinoprostone 640
Prolix 20 (PH) *see* PredniSONE 1706
Prolixan (AT, CH, CZ, HU, IT, NL, PT) *see* Azapropazone [INT] 210
Prolixin-D (CO) *see* FluPHENAZine 905
Prolol (IL) *see* Propranolol 1731
Prolong 1000 (CL, PE) *see* Lidocaine (Topical) 1211
Prolongal (AR) *see* Dapoxetine [INT] 561
Prolon (ID) *see* MethylPREDNISolone 1340
Prolopa (BE, BR, PY, UY) *see* Benserazide and Levodopa [CAN/INT] 244
Prolopar (CL) *see* Benserazide and Levodopa [CAN/INT] 244
Prolutin (IT) *see* Hydroxyprogesterone Caproate 1021
Proluton Depot (AR, AT, BH, CO, DE, GR, LB, MY, PE, PK, QA, SA, TH, TR) *see* Hydroxyprogesterone Caproate 1021
Promactil (ES, PE) *see* ChlorproMAZINE 429
Promazine (PH) *see* ChlorproMAZINE 429
Promecilina (MX) *see* Ampicillin 141
Promedes (JP) *see* Furosemide 940
Prome (ID) *see* Promethazine 1723
Promel (VE) *see* Dipyrone [INT] 653
Prometazina Cloridrato (IT) *see* Promethazine 1723
Prometazina (IT) *see* Promethazine 1723
Prometil (PH) *see* Prochlorperazine 1718
Promet (JO, PH) *see* Promethazine 1723
Prometrium (BM) *see* Progesterone 1722
Prometrium (KR) *see* Trospium 2108
Promexin (JP) *see* ChlorproMAZINE 429
Promezine (MY) *see* Promethazine 1723
Promezol (ID) *see* Omeprazole 1508
Promiced (MX) *see* Metoprolol 1350
Promit (CH, DE) *see* Dextran 607
Promiten (LU, NO) *see* Dextran 607
Promixin (DE, DK, GB, IE, NO) *see* Colistimethate 504
Promnix (IL) *see* Tamsulosin 1974
Promostan (TW) *see* Alprostadil 96
Pronaxen (SE) *see* Naproxen 1427
Pronax (PH) *see* Finasteride 878
Pronestyl (AU, BE, CH, CL, EG, ET, GB, IE, IN, KE, LU, MY, NL, NO, QA, SG, TW, TZ, UG, ZA) *see* Procainamide 1716
Proneurax (VE) *see* Galantamine 946
Proneurin (DE) *see* Promethazine 1723
Pronicy (ID) *see* Cyproheptadine 529
Pronid (TW) *see* Probenecid 1716
Pronoctan (DK) *see* Lormetazepam [INT] 1247
Pronon (JP) *see* Propafenone 1725
Pronoran (BG, PL, RU) *see* Piribedil [INT] 1662
Pronta (PY) *see* Levonorgestrel 1201
Prontovent (IT) *see* Clenbuterol [INT] 460
Propafen (CO) *see* Propafenone 1725
Propafenon Genericon (HR) *see* Propafenone 1725
Propafenon Pharmavit (HU) *see* Propafenone 1725
Propalong (AR) *see* Propranolol 1731
Propamide (MY, SG) *see* ChlorproPAMIDE 429
Propam (NZ) *see* Diazepam 613
Propanline (TW) *see* Propantheline 1727
Propaphenin (DE) *see* ChlorproMAZINE 429
Proparakain-POS (DE) *see* Proparacaine 1728
Proparin (MX) *see* Heparin 997
Propavent (AR) *see* Beclomethasone (Nasal) 232
Propavent (AR) *see* Beclomethasone (Systemic) 230
Propayerst (AR) *see* Propranolol 1731
Propecia (AE, AR, AU, BB, BH, BR, BS, BZ, CN, CO, CY, DO, EC, ES, GT, HK, HN, HR, IL, IS, JM, JP, KW, MY, NI, NL, NZ, PA, PE, PH, QA, RO, SA, SE, SG, SV, TH, TT, TW) *see* Finasteride 878
Propect (ID) *see* Ambroxol [INT] 109
Properil (CL) *see* Captopril 342
Propeshia (MX) *see* Finasteride 878
Propess (AE, BR, CN, FI, FR, HK, IL, SA, SE) *see* Dinoprostone 640
Propess Vag SR (KR) *see* Dinoprostone 640
Propexol (PE) *see* Periciazine [CAN/INT] 1621
Propine (AU, FI, FR, GB, IE, IN, IT, KR, PT, TH, TR) *see* Dipivefrin 651
Propinorm (IE) *see* Propiverine [INT] 1728
Propofol-Lipuro (EC) *see* Propofol 1728
Propovan (PY) *see* Propofol 1728
Propoven (EE) *see* Propofol 1728
Propra (EE) *see* Propranolol 1731
Propral (FI) *see* Propranolol 1731
Propranolol Eurogenerics (LU) *see* Propranolol 1731
Propra-Ratiopharm (PL) *see* Propranolol 1731
Proprin (GB) *see* Aspirin 180
Propycil (BG, CH, CZ, DE, HN, HU, PT, SK, TR) *see* Propylthiouracil 1735
Propyl (TH) *see* Propylthiouracil 1735
Propylthiocil (IL) *see* Propylthiouracil 1735
Propyl-Thiouracil (CH) *see* Propylthiouracil 1735
Propylthiouracile (BE) *see* Propylthiouracil 1735
Propylthiouracil "Dak" (DK) *see* Propylthiouracil 1735

Propyltiouracil "Medic" (DK) *see* Propylthiouracil 1735
ProQuad (AU, CZ, ES, HR, IE, IT, LT, NL, NZ, PL, PT, RO, SG, SK) *see* Measles, Mumps, Rubella, and Varicella Virus Vaccine 1274
Proquin (AU) *see* Ciprofloxacin (Systemic) 441
Proracyl (FR) *see* Propylthiouracil 1735
Proris (ID) *see* Ibuprofen 1032
Prorynorm (LU) *see* Propafenone 1725
Proscar (AE, AR, AT, AU, BE, BG, BH, BM, BO, BR, CH, CL, CN, CR, CY, CZ, DE, DK, DO, EC, EE, EG, ES, FI, GB, GR, GT, GY, HK, HN, HR, HU, ID, IE, IT, JO, KR, KW, LB, LU, MT, MX, MY, NI, NO, NZ, PA, PE, PH, PK, PL, PR, PT, QA, RO, RU, SA, SE, SG, SK, SR, TH, TR, TW, VE, VN) *see* Finasteride 878
Prosedar (PT) *see* Quazepam 1751
Prosertin (MX) *see* Sertraline 1878
Prosinal (ID) *see* Ibuprofen 1032
Prosmide (LB) *see* Bicalutamide 262
Prosogan fd (ID) *see* Lansoprazole 1166
Prospera (HR) *see* RisperiDONE 1818
Prostacare (LB) *see* Finasteride 878
Prostacur (ES) *see* Flutamide 907
Prostaden (UY) *see* Cyproterone [CAN/INT] 530
Prostafilina-A (CO) *see* Cloxacillin [CAN/INT] 488
Prostafilina A (PE) *see* Cloxacillin [CAN/INT] 488
Prostafilina (VE) *see* Oxacillin 1528
Prostaglandina E2 (ES) *see* Dinoprostone 640
Prostandin (JP, KR) *see* Alprostadil 96
Prostanus (PH) *see* Finasteride 878
Prostap (GB, IE) *see* Leuprolide 1186
Prostaphlin-A (PH) *see* Cloxacillin [CAN/INT] 488
Prostaphlin (CZ, EE, HN) *see* Oxacillin 1528
Prostarmon E (TW) *see* Dinoprostone 640
Prostasil (PE) *see* Dutasteride 702
Prostavasin (AE, AR, BR, CN, CY, EG, HU, JO, KW, LU, MX, PH, SK, UY) *see* Alprostadil 96
Prostenon (EE) *see* Dinoprostone 640
Prostera (PH) *see* Terazosin 2001
Prosteride (HK, PH, TH) *see* Finasteride 878
Prosterid (HU) *see* Finasteride 878
Prostica (DE) *see* Flutamide 907
Prostide (ID) *see* Finasteride 878
Prostigmin (AE, AT, BB, BF, BH, BJ, BM, BS, BZ, CH, CI, CY, CZ, DE, EC, EG, ET, GH, GM, GN, GY, ID, IL, IQ, IR, JM, JO, KE, KW, LB, LR, LY, MA, ML, MR, MU, MW, NE, NG, NL, NO, OM, PK, PR, PY, QA, SA, SC, SD, SG, SI, SL, SN, SR, SY, TH, TN, TT, TZ, UG, YE, ZA, ZM, ZW) *see* Neostigmine 1438
Prostigmina (IT) *see* Neostigmine 1438
Prostigmine (BE, BR, CL, CO, ES, FR, GR, LU, MX, PE, PT, UY, VN) *see* Neostigmine 1438
Prostigmin[inj.] (GB, HR, IE) *see* Neostigmine 1438
Prostigmin INJ (AU) *see* Neostigmine 1438
Prostig (PH) *see* Neostigmine 1438
Prostin 15m (BE, BG, CZ, HN, NL, NZ) *see* Carboprost Tromethamine 360
Prostin/15M (HR, LU) *see* Carboprost Tromethamine 360
Prostin (CZ) *see* Alprostadil 96
Prostin E2 (AE, AT, BE, BF, BG, BH, BJ, CH, CI, CY, EG, ET, GB, GH, GM, GN, GR, HK, HN, HR, HU, ID, IE, IL, IQ, IR, IT, JO, KE, KW, LB, LR, LU, LY, MA, ML, MR, MU, MW, MY, NE, NG, NL, OM, PT, QA, SA, SC, SD, SG, SL, SN, SY, TH, TN, TR, TW, TZ, UG, YE, ZA, ZM, ZW) *see* Dinoprostone 640
Prostin E2 Vaginal Cream (AU) *see* Dinoprostone 640
Prostin E2 Vaginal Gel (NZ) *see* Dinoprostone 640
Prostine E2 (VN) *see* Dinoprostone 640
Prostine (FR) *see* Dinoprostone 640
Prostine VR (FR) *see* Alprostadil 96
Prostinfenem (DK, NO, SE) *see* Carboprost Tromethamine 360
Prostin Pediatrico (CL) *see* Alprostadil 96
Prostin VR (AE, AU, BE, BH, CH, CO, CY, EG, GB, GR, HN, HR, HU, IL, IN, IQ, IR, IT, JO, KW, LB, LY, NL, NZ, OM, PL, QA, SA, SY, TH, TW, YE, ZA) *see* Alprostadil 96
Prostin VR (LU) *see* Dinoprostone 640
Prostin VR Paedeatric (MY) *see* Alprostadil 96
Prostivas (DK, FI, NO, SE) *see* Alprostadil 96
Prostodin (IN, VN) *see* Carboprost Tromethamine 360
Prostop (UY) *see* Finasteride 878
Prosu 2 (TW) *see* Estradiol (Systemic) 775
Prosulf (GB) *see* Protamine 1737
Protalgine (MX) *see* LamoTRIgine 1160
Protamina (ES) *see* Protamine 1737
Protamina solfato (IT) *see* Protamine 1737
Protamine Choay (FR) *see* Protamine 1737
Protamine Sulfate Injection (AU) *see* Protamine 1737
Protamine Sulphate (GB) *see* Protamine 1737
Protamine Sulphate Injection BP (AU) *see* Protamine 1737
Protamini Sulfas (FI) *see* Protamine 1737
Protaminsulfat (NO) *see* Protamine 1737
Protaminsulfat Novo (AT) *see* Protamine 1737
Protaminsulfat "Leo" (DE, DK) *see* Protamine 1737
Protaminum Sulfuricum (PL) *see* Protamine 1737
Protan (KR) *see* Latanoprost 1172
Protanol (BR) *see* Amitriptyline 119
Protaphane HM (AE, BF, BH, BJ, CI, CY, EG, ET, GH, GM, GN, HK, IL, IQ, IR, JO, KE, KW, LB, LR, LY, MA, ML, MR, MU, MW, MY, NE, NG, OM, PH, QA, SA, SC, SD, SL, SN, SY, TH, TN, TZ, UG, YE, ZA, ZM, ZW) *see* Insulin NPH 1089
Protaxos (MY, TH) *see* Strontium Ranelate [INT] 1938
Protazine (MY) *see* Prochlorperazine 1718
Protec (AE, KW, QA, SA) *see* Cefepime 378
Protec (PH) *see* Ethinyl Estradiol and Levonorgestrel 803
Protectfluor (NL) *see* Fluoride 895
Protelos (AE, AT, BE, BH, CL, CR, CY, CZ, DE, DK, DO, EE, FR, GB, GR, GT, HN, HR, IE, IL, IT, KW, LT, NI, NL, PA, PE, PL, PT, QA, RO, SA, SE, SI, SK, SV, TR, UY, VN) *see* Strontium Ranelate [INT] 1938
Proterenal (AR) *see* Isoproterenol 1124
Proternol L (TW) *see* Isoproterenol 1124
Proteside (JO) *see* Finasteride 878
Protexel (FR) *see* Protein C Concentrate (Human) 1738
Protha (TW) *see* Promethazine 1723
Prothazin (CZ) *see* Promethazine 1723
Prothiaden (AU, BE, BH, CZ, DK, EG, ES, FR, GB, HK, IE, IN, KR, MY, NL, NZ, PK, QA, SA, SG, SK, TH, VN, ZA) *see* Dosulepin [INT] 673
Prothiazine (IL) *see* Promethazine 1723
Prothin (HK) *see* Diethylpropion 624
Prothiucil (AT) *see* Propylthiouracil 1735
Prothrombinex-VF (AU, NZ) *see* Factor IX Complex (Human) [(Factors II, IX, X)] 838
Prothuril (GR) *see* Propylthiouracil 1735
Protiaden (CH, IT) *see* Dosulepin [INT] 673
Protiadene (PT) *see* Dosulepin [INT] 673
Protinal (IN) *see* Bromocriptine 291
Protium (GB, IE) *see* Pantoprazole 1570
Protocort (ID) *see* Betamethasone (Topical) 255
Protonexa (BG) *see* Lansoprazole 1166
Protonix (PH) *see* Omeprazole 1508
Protopan (PY) *see* Pantoprazole 1570
Protopec (JO) *see* Tacrolimus (Topical) 1968
Protopic (AE, AR, AT, BE, BH, BR, CH, CL, CN, CO, CY, CZ, DE, DK, EC, EE, FI, FR, GB, GR, HK, HR, ID, IE, IL, IT, KR, KW, LT, MT, MY, NL, NO, PE, PH, PL, PT, QA, RO, RU, SA, SE, SG, SK, TH, TR, TW, UY, VE, VN) *see* Tacrolimus (Topical) 1968
Protopis (IS) *see* Tacrolimus (Topical) 1968
Protopy (AT, BE, CH, CZ, DE, DK, EE, FI, FR, GB, GR, IE, IT, MT, NL, NO, PL, PT, RU, SE, SK, TR) *see* Tacrolimus (Topical) 1968

Protos (AR, AU, BR, CO, HK, ID, NZ, PH, SG, TW) *see* Strontium Ranelate [INT] 1938
Protosol (IL) *see* Aprotinin 168
Protozol (BF, BJ, CI, ET, GH, GM, GN, KE, LR, MA, ML, MR, MU, MW, NE, NG, SC, SD, SL, SN, TN, TZ, UG, ZM, ZW) *see* MetroNIDAZOLE (Systemic) 1353
Protozole (PH) *see* MetroNIDAZOLE (Systemic) 1353
Provagen (PH) *see* Progesterone 1722
Provagin (ID) *see* Metronidazole and Nystatin [CAN/INT] 1358
Provake (IN) *see* Modafinil 1386
Provames (FR) *see* Estradiol (Systemic) 775
Provasc (PH) *see* AmLODIPine 123
Provas (DE) *see* Valsartan 2127
Provelyn (ID) *see* Pregabalin 1710
Proven (AU) *see* Ibuprofen 1032
Provenge (CZ, EE, LT, NL, SE, SK) *see* Sipuleucel-T 1893
Provera (AE, AU, BE, BF, BG, BH, BJ, BR, CI, CL, CN, CO, CY, CZ, DK, EC, EE, EG, ET, FI, GB, GH, GM, GN, GR, HK, HN, HR, ID, IE, IL, IN, IQ, IR, IT, JO, KE, KR, KW, LB, LR, LY, MA, ML, MR, MU, MW, MX, NE, NG, NL, NO, NZ, OM, PE, PH, PL, PT, QA, SA, SC, SD, SE, SG, SI, SK, SL, SN, SY, TH, TN, TW, TZ, UG, VE, VN, YE, ZA, ZM, ZW) *see* MedroxyPROGESTERone 1277
Provera LD (MY) *see* MedroxyPROGESTERone 1277
Provexel NS (PH) *see* Albuterol 69
Provic (KR) *see* Clopidogrel 484
Provigil (BE, GB, IE, IL, IT, KR, PY, SG, TW, ZA) *see* Modafinil 1386
Provimicina (ES) *see* Demeclocycline 589
Provinace (HK) *see* Perindopril 1623
Provipen Benzatina (ES) *see* Penicillin G Benzathine 1609
Provipen Procaina (ES) *see* Penicillin G Procaine 1613
Proviron (AT, AU, BE, BR, CH, CL, CZ, DE, ES, FI, FR, GB, HR, HU, IT, LU, MX, NL, PT) *see* Mesterolone [INT] 1307
Proviron Depot (VE) *see* Testosterone 2010
Provironum (IN) *see* Mesterolone [INT] 1307
Provisc (LU, ZA) *see* Hyaluronate and Derivatives 1006
Provisual (AR) *see* Gentamicin (Ophthalmic) 962
Provisual (AR) *see* Gentamicin (Systemic) 959
Provitina Magnesium (PL) *see* Magnesium Gluconate 1263
Provive (AU, HK, KR, LB, NZ) *see* Propofol 1728
Provocholine (IL) *see* Methacholine 1310
Provokit (DE) *see* Methacholine 1310
Provon (PE) *see* Ibuprofen 1032
Provula (ID) *see* ClomiPHENE 473
Prowel (TW) *see* Metoclopramide 1345
Proxacin (BR) *see* Ciprofloxacin (Systemic) 441
Proxalyoc (FR) *see* Piroxicam 1662
Proxen (AE, AT, BH, CH, CY, EG, IQ, IR, JO, KW, LB, LY, OM, QA, SA, SY, TW, VN, YE) *see* Naproxen 1427
Proxicef (HR) *see* Cephalexin 405
Proximax (PH) *see* Piroxicam 1662
Proxuric (ID) *see* Allopurinol 90
Prox (UY) *see* Zaleplon 2193
Prozac 20 (KR, MY, PH, TW) *see* FLUoxetine 899
Prozac (AE, AR, AU, BE, BF, BH, BJ, BR, CI, CL, CN, CZ, ES, ET, FR, GB, GH, GM, GN, HK, HR, HU, IE, IL, IT, JO, KE, KR, KW, LB, LR, LU, MA, ML, MR, MU, MW, NE, NG, NL, NZ, PE, PK, PT, QA, RO, RU, SA, SC, SD, SG, SK, SL, SN, TH, TN, TR, TZ, UG, VE, VN, ZM, ZW) *see* FLUoxetine 899
Prozac Dispersible (KR) *see* FLUoxetine 899
Prozac Weekly (KR) *see* FLUoxetine 899
Prozef (ZA) *see* Cefprozil 389
Prozelax (PH) *see* Tamsulosin 1974
Prozepam (ID) *see* Diazepam 613
Prozil (DK) *see* ChlorproMAZINE 429
Prozine (JO) *see* ALPRAZolam 94
Prozin (IT) *see* ChlorproMAZINE 429
Prozit (TR) *see* FLUoxetine 899
Prozolan (MX) *see* Pantoprazole 1570
PrroQuad (EE) *see* Measles, Mumps, Rubella, and Varicella Virus Vaccine 1274
Prulif (IN) *see* Prulifloxacin [INT] 1742
Prurid (PY) *see* HydrOXYzine 1024
Pruritrat (BR) *see* Lindane 1217
Pryleugan (DE) *see* Imipramine 1054
Prysoline (IL) *see* Primidone 1714
Pseudocef (AT, DE, JP) *see* Cefsulodin [INT] 391
Pseudono (TH) *see* Pseudoephedrine 1742
Psicodex (LB) *see* ChlordiazePOXIDE 422
Psiconor (UY) *see* Citalopram 451
Psilo Balsam (CZ, RU) *see* DiphenhydrAMINE (Systemic) 641
Psiquium (CO) *see* Amitriptyline 119
Psoradexan (BG) *see* Anthralin 150
Psorcutan (AT, DE, PL, TR) *see* Calcipotriene 321
Psoriderm (IT) *see* Anthralin 150
Psorinol (IN) *see* Anthralin 150
Psychopax (AT, CH) *see* Diazepam 613
Psycoton (IT) *see* Piracetam [INT] 1661
Psynor (PH) *see* ChlorproMAZINE 429
P.T.B. (AE, BH, CY, EG, IL, IQ, IR, JO, KW, LB, LY, OM, QA, SA, SY, YE) *see* Pyrazinamide 1745
Pterin (PH) *see* Methotrexate 1322
Ptinolin (GR) *see* Ranitidine 1777
PTU (AU, IN, UY, VN) *see* Propylthiouracil 1735
Pucaine (KR) *see* Bupivacaine 299
P&U Carboplatin (ZA) *see* CARBOplatin 357
P&U Cisplatin (ZA) *see* CISplatin 448
Pu Hui Zhi (CN) *see* Pravastatin 1700
Pu Ke (CN) *see* Mannitol 1269
Pulcet (BG) *see* Pantoprazole 1570
Pu Le Xin (CN) *see* Propranolol 1731
Pulin (MY, SG) *see* Metoclopramide 1345
Pulmicon Susp for Nebulizer (KR) *see* Budesonide (Systemic) 293
Pulmicort (AE, AT, BE, BG, BH, BR, CH, CL, CO, CR, CY, CZ, DE, DK, DO, EE, EG, FI, FR, GB, GR, GT, HN, HR, HU, ID, IN, IS, JO, JP, KW, LB, NI, NL, NO, PA, PK, PL, PT, QA, RO, RU, SA, SE, SK, SV, TR, TW, UY, VE, VN) *see* Budesonide (Systemic) 293
Pulmicort Nasal (KR, PL, TW) *see* Budesonide (Nasal) 296
Pulmicort Nasal Turbohaler (KE, MU, NG) *see* Budesonide (Systemic) 293
Pulmicort Turbohaler (CN) *see* Budesonide (Systemic) 293
Pulmicort Turbuhaler (KE, MU, NG) *see* Budesonide (Systemic) 293
Pulmison (ZA) *see* PredniSONE 1706
Pulmitropic (SA) *see* Bromhexine [INT] 291
Pulmocodeina (EC) *see* Codeine 497
Pulmodual (PH) *see* Ipratropium and Albuterol 1109
Pulmo-Rest (ID) *see* Bromhexine [INT] 291
Pulmoxel (PH) *see* Terbutaline 2004
Pulmozyme (AR, AT, AU, BB, BE, BG, BM, BR, BS, BZ, CH, CO, CY, CZ, DE, DK, EC, EE, ES, FI, FR, GB, GR, GY, HN, HR, HU, IE, IL, IS, IT, JM, JP, KW, LB, LT, LU, MT, MX, NL, NO, NZ, PE, PL, PT, RO, RU, SE, SI, SK, SR, TR, TT, UY) *see* Dornase Alfa 672
Pulsamin (JP) *see* Etilefrine [INT] 815
P&U Methotrexate (ZA) *see* Methotrexate 1322
Pumpitor DI (ID) *see* Omeprazole 1508
Pumpitor (ID, SG) *see* Omeprazole 1508
Puraid (KR) *see* Bromopride [INT] 292
Purata (ZA) *see* Oxazepam 1532
Purazine (ZA) *see* Cinnarizine [INT] 440
Purbal (ZA) *see* Sulfamethoxazole and Trimethoprim 1946

Purbloka (ZA) *see* Propranolol 1731
Purderal (ZA) *see* Ethambutol 798
Puregon (AE, AR, AT, BE, BH, BR, CH, CL, CN, CO, CY, CZ, DE, DK, EC, EG, FR, GB, GR, HK, HN, HR, ID, IE, IL, IS, IT, KR, KW, LB, LT, MX, MY, NL, NO, PE, PH, PK, PL, PT, QA, RO, SA, SE, SG, SI, SK, TH, TR, TW, VE) *see* Follitropin Beta 921
Purgeron (JP) *see* Docusate 661
Purgo-Pil (LU) *see* Bisacodyl 265
Purgoxin (ZA) *see* Digoxin 627
Puribact (IN) *see* Prulifloxacin [INT] 1742
Puribel 300 (MX) *see* Allopurinol 90
Puricemia (ID) *see* Allopurinol 90
Puricos (ZA) *see* Allopurinol 90
Purid (CL) *see* Pipemidic Acid [INT] 1655
Puri-Nethol (AE, AT, BE, BF, BG, BH, BJ, CH, CI, CY, CZ, DE, EE, EG, ET, FI, GB, GH, GM, GN, HK, HR, ID, IE, IL, IN, IQ, IR, IS, JO, KE, KR, KW, LB, LR, LT, LU, LY, MA, ML, MR, MU, MW, NE, NG, NO, NZ, OM, QA, SA, SC, SD, SE, SG, SI, SK, SL, SN, SY, TH, TN, TR, TZ, UG, UY, VN, YE, ZA, ZM, ZW) *see* Mercaptopurine 1296
Purinethol (AR, CL, FR, GR, IT, MX, NL, PH, PL, RU) *see* Mercaptopurine 1296
PuriNethol (AU) *see* Mercaptopurine 1296
Purinetone (PK, SG) *see* Mercaptopurine 1296
Purinol (AE, JO, MY, RU) *see* Allopurinol 90
Puritrid (FI) *see* AMILoride 113
Puromylon (ZA) *see* Nalidixic Acid [INT] 1418
Puroxan (CO, PH, TH) *see* Doxofylline [INT] 679
Purtraline (TW) *see* Sertraline 1878
Pusarat (MX) *see* Simvastatin 1890
Pusili (CN) *see* Ornidazole [INT] 1522
Pu Wei (CN) *see* Nimesulide [INT] 1456
P-Vate (TH) *see* Clobetasol 468
P.V. Carpine Liquifilm Ophthalimic Solution (AU, NZ) *see* Pilocarpine (Ophthalmic) 1649
Pyassan (HN) *see* Cephalexin 405
Pybactam (ID) *see* Piperacillin and Tazobactam 1657
Pycazide (GB) *see* Isoniazid 1120
Pycip (MY) *see* Ciprofloxacin (Systemic) 441
Pyderma (ID) *see* Desoximetasone 598
Pylor (ID) *see* Loratadine 1241
Pylorid (HR, HU, LU, PH) *see* Ranitidine 1777
Pylorid (PL) *see* Bismuth 265
PyloriPac (BR) *see* Lansoprazole, Amoxicillin, and Clarithromycin 1169
Pyndale (PH) *see* Pindolol 1652
Pyocefal (FR) *see* Cefsulodin [INT] 391
Pyoredol (AR, FR) *see* Phenytoin 1640
Pyostacine (BE, LU) *see* Quinupristin and Dalfopristin 1762
Pyrafat (AT, DE, HK) *see* Pyrazinamide 1745
Pyralfin (BF, BJ, CI, ET, GH, GM, GN, KE, LR, MA, ML, MR, MU, MW, NE, NG, SC, SD, SL, SN, TN, TZ, UG, ZA, ZM, ZW) *see* Sulfadoxine and Pyrimethamine [INT] 1946
Pyralin EN (AU) *see* SulfaSALAzine 1950
Pyramen (BG, HU) *see* Piracetam [INT] 1661
Pyramide (TH) *see* Pyrazinamide 1745
Pyraminol (GB) *see* Piracetam [INT] 1661
Pyramin (PH) *see* Pyrazinamide 1745
Pyramistin (JP) *see* Trihexyphenidyl 2103
Pyramox (TH) *see* Amoxicillin 130
Pyrantelum (PL) *see* Pyrantel Pamoate 1744
Pyrapam (TH) *see* Pyrantel Pamoate 1744
Pyrazid (PK) *see* Pyrazinamide 1745
Pyrazinamide (TH) *see* Pyrazinamide 1745
Pyrazinamid (HR, HU, PL) *see* Pyrazinamide 1745
Pyrazinamid Lederle (CH) *see* Pyrazinamide 1745
Pyrazinamid "Dak" (DK) *see* Pyrazinamide 1745
Pyrazinamid "Medic" (DK) *see* Pyrazinamide 1745
Pyrazine (JO) *see* Pyrazinamide 1745
Pyreazid (ES) *see* Isoniazid 1120
Pyredal (NO) *see* Phenazopyridine 1629
Pyrethia (JP) *see* Promethazine 1723
Pyricontin Continus (IN) *see* Pyridoxine 1747
Pyridam (ID) *see* Piroxicam 1662
Pyridium (AE, BF, BH, BJ, BR, CI, CR, CY, DE, EG, ES, ET, FR, GH, GM, GN, GT, HN, IN, IQ, IR, JO, KE, KW, LB, LR, LY, MA, ML, MR, MU, MW, NE, NG, NI, OM, PA, PE, QA, SA, SC, SD, SL, SN, SV, SY, TN, TZ, UG, UY, VE, YE, ZA, ZM, ZW) *see* Phenazopyridine 1629
Pyridoxine Aguettant (FR) *see* Pyridoxine 1747
Pyridoxine-Labaz (LU) *see* Pyridoxine 1747
Pyridoxine Renaudin (FR) *see* Pyridoxine 1747
Pyridoxin Recip[Tab.] (SE) *see* Pyridoxine 1747
Pyridoxin "Dak" (DK) *see* Pyridoxine 1747
Pyrifoam (AU, NZ) *see* Permethrin 1627
Pyrilax (PL) *see* Bisacodyl 265
Pyrimine (TH) *see* Pyridostigmine 1746
Pyrinol (KR) *see* Pyridostigmine 1746
Pyrinon (PH) *see* Pyridostigmine 1746
Pyrisept (BR) *see* Phenazopyridine 1629
Pyrisone (SG) *see* Dapsone (Systemic) 561
Pyrivitol (AT) *see* Pyridoxine 1747
Pyrolate (PK) *see* Glycopyrrolate 975
Pyronium (BE) *see* Phenazopyridine 1629
Pyroxin (AU) *see* Pyridoxine 1747
Pyroxy (TH) *see* Piroxicam 1662
Pysolan (ID) *see* Lansoprazole 1166
Pytazen SR (NZ) *see* Dipyridamole 652
PZA (CH) *see* Pyrazinamide 1745
PZA-Ciba (IN, SG) *see* Pyrazinamide 1745
P.Z.A. (TW) *see* Pyrazinamide 1745
P-Zide (BF, BJ, CI, ET, GH, GM, GN, IN, KE, LR, MA, ML, MR, MU, MW, NE, NG, SC, SD, SL, SN, TN, TZ, UG, ZA, ZM, ZW) *see* Pyrazinamide 1745
Pzocin XL (KR) *see* Doxazosin 674
Pzoret (CO) *see* Tazarotene 1980
Q200 (HK, NZ) *see* QuiNINE 1761
Q300 (HK, NZ) *see* QuiNINE 1761
Qari (CN, IT, PK) *see* Rufloxacin [INT] 1855
Qian Bai (CN) *see* Hydroquinone 1020
Qian Er Fen (CN) *see* Rifaximin 1809
Qi Ke (CN) *see* Ornidazole [INT] 1522
Qilaflox (ID) *see* Ciprofloxacin (Systemic) 441
Qinda (CN) *see* Lornoxicam [INT] 1248
Qing Da (CN) *see* Piracetam [INT] 1661
Qinosyn (PH) *see* Ciprofloxacin (Systemic) 441
Qiquan (CN) *see* Pentoxifylline 1618
Qitai (CN) *see* Salmeterol 1860
Qiu Lu (CN) *see* Ciprofloxacin (Ophthalmic) 446
Qlaira (AR, AU, BE, BR, CH, CL, CO, CY, CZ, DE, DK, EC, EE, FI, FR, GB, HK, HR, IE, IS, KR, LT, MY, NL, NZ, PE, PH, RO, SE, SG, SI, SK) *see* Estradiol and Dienogest 780
Qlair (IL) *see* Estradiol and Dienogest 780
Q.O.L. (KR) *see* Clopidogrel 484
Qpime (AE) *see* Cefepime 378
Qpril (AU, NZ) *see* Quinapril 1756
Q-Pril (IN) *see* Quinapril 1756
Qrazol (KR) *see* Omeprazole 1508
Qtipine (PH) *see* QUEtiapine 1751
QTR-Alfa (IN) *see* Alfacalcidol [CAN/INT] 82
Quadrax (MX) *see* Ibuprofen 1032
Quadropril (AT, DE, HU) *see* Spirapril [INT] 1931
Qualiaden (HK) *see* Dosulepin [INT] 673
Qualiceclor (HK) *see* Cefaclor 372
Qualiclinda (HK) *see* Clindamycin (Systemic) 460
Qualiclovir (HK) *see* Acyclovir (Systemic) 47
Qualiclovir (HK) *see* Acyclovir (Topical) 51
Qualidrox (HK) *see* Cefadroxil 372
Qualidrozine (HK) *see* HydrOXYzine 1024
Qualigyl (HK) *see* MetroNIDAZOLE (Systemic) 1353
Quali-Itrazole (HK) *see* Itraconazole 1130

Quali-Mentin (HK) *see* Amoxicillin and Clavulanate 133
Qualiphor (HK) *see* Cefaclor 372
Qualipid (HK) *see* Gemfibrozil 956
Qualiquan (HK) *see* Doxepin (Systemic) 676
Qualisac (HK) *see* FLUoxetine 899
Qualisone (PH) *see* PredniSONE 1706
Qualitriptine (HK) *see* Amitriptyline 119
Qualixamin (HK) *see* Tranexamic Acid 2081
Quamatel (HU) *see* Famotidine 845
Quamox (PE) *see* Ivermectin (Systemic) 1136
Quamtel (BB, BM, BS, BZ, GY, JM, SR, TT) *see* Famotidine 845
Quaname (BE, LU) *see* Meprobamate 1296
Quanil (IT) *see* Meprobamate 1296
Quanox Gotas (CO) *see* Ivermectin (Systemic) 1136
Quanox Locion (CO) *see* Ivermectin (Topical) 1137
Quantalan (CH, PT) *see* Cholestyramine Resin 431
Quantalan Zuckerfrei (AT) *see* Cholestyramine Resin 431
Quantia (HK, TW) *see* QUEtiapine 1751
Quantrel (VE) *see* Pyrantel Pamoate 1744
Quark (IT) *see* Ramipril 1771
Quasar (IT) *see* Verapamil 2154
Quasym LP (FR) *see* Methylphenidate 1336
Quazium (IT) *see* Quazepam 1751
Quelicin Chloride (ID, PH) *see* Succinylcholine 1939
Quellada-M (GB) *see* Malathion 1268
Quellada (BE, IE, LU) *see* Lindane 1217
Quellada Cream (AU) *see* Lindane 1217
Quellada Creme Rinse (AU) *see* Lindane 1217
Quellada Head Lice Treatment (AU) *see* Lindane 1217
Quellada Head Lice Treatment (AU, NZ) *see* Permethrin 1627
Quellada Lotion (AU) *see* Lindane 1217
Quemiciclina-S (PE) *see* Tetracycline 2017
Quemicitina (AR, BR) *see* Chloramphenicol 421
Quemox (MY, TH) *see* Mebendazole [CAN/INT] 1274
Quenobilan (ES) *see* Chenodiol 417
Quensyl (DE) *see* Hydroxychloroquine 1021
Quentan[vet.] (FR) *see* Bromhexine [INT] 291
Queritan (PY) *see* Clindamycin (Systemic) 460
Querto (DE) *see* Carvedilol 367
Questran (BE, BG, DK, EC, EG, FI, FR, GB, GR, HK, HN, IE, IS, IT, KR, MX, NL, NO, NZ, SA, SE, SI, TH, VN) *see* Cholestyramine Resin 431
Questran Light (AR, BR, CZ, MY) *see* Cholestyramine Resin 431
Questran Lite (AU, NZ, PH, ZA) *see* Cholestyramine Resin 431
Questran Loc (DK, SE) *see* Cholestyramine Resin 431
Quetapel (NZ) *see* QUEtiapine 1751
Quetapin (KR) *see* QUEtiapine 1751
Quetiap RD (PH) *see* QUEtiapine 1751
Quetiazic (CR, EC, GT, HN, NI, PA, SV) *see* QUEtiapine 1751
Quetidin (CO, PY) *see* QUEtiapine 1751
Quety (KR) *see* QUEtiapine 1751
Que Wei (CN) *see* Tazarotene 1980
Quexel (CR, DO, EC, GT, HN, PA, SV) *see* MetFORMIN 1307
Quibron T SR (ID) *see* Theophylline 2026
Quicktra (HR) *see* Meloxicam 1283
Quiedorm (ES) *see* Quazepam 1751
Quietiline (FR) *see* Bromazepam [CAN/INT] 290
Quilaxin (MY) *see* Pefloxacin [INT] 1588
Quilonium-R (PH) *see* Lithium 1230
Quilonorm (AT) *see* Lithium 1230
Quilonorm Retardtabletten (CH) *see* Lithium 1230
Quilonum Retard (DE) *see* Lithium 1230
Quilonum retard (LU) *see* Lithium 1230
Quilonum SR (AU) *see* Lithium 1230
Quilox (PH) *see* Ciprofloxacin (Systemic) 441
Quimocyclar (MX) *see* Tetracycline 2017
Quimoral Plus (PE) *see* Nimesulide [INT] 1456
Quimotus (AR) *see* DOXOrubicin (Conventional) 679
Quinacris (BR) *see* Chloroquine 424
Quinaglute Dura-tabs (ZA) *see* QuiNIDine 1759
Quinapro (IE) *see* Quinapril 1756
Quinaspen (ZA) *see* Quinapril 1756
Quinate (AU) *see* QuiNINE 1761
Quinazil (IT) *see* Quinapril 1756
Quinbisu (AU) *see* QuiNINE 1761
Quinbloc (MY) *see* Hydroquinone 1020
Quinicardine (PE) *see* QuiNIDine 1759
Quiniduran (IL) *see* QuiNIDine 1759
Quinimax (BF, BJ, CI, ET, GH, GM, GN, KE, LR, MA, ML, MR, MU, MW, NE, NG, SC, SD, SL, SN, TN, TZ, UG, ZA, ZM, ZW) *see* QuiNINE 1761
Quininga (IN) *see* QuiNINE 1761
Quinobiotic (ID, PE) *see* Ciprofloxacin (Systemic) 441
Quinocort (VE) *see* Ciprofloxacin and Dexamethasone 446
Quinomed L (AR) *see* Levofloxacin (Systemic) 1197
Quinoryl (PH) *see* Ciprofloxacin (Ophthalmic) 446
Quinos (KR) *see* Ciprofloxacin (Systemic) 441
Quinotic HC (VE) *see* Ciprofloxacin and Hydrocortisone 446
Quinsil (TH) *see* Quinapril 1756
Quipine (AU) *see* QUEtiapine 1751
Quiprex (CO) *see* Quinapril 1756
Quiralam (ES) *see* Clobutinol [INT] 468
Quitaxon (BF, BJ, CI, ET, FR, GH, GM, GN, KE, LR, MA, ML, MR, MU, MW, NE, NG, SC, SD, SL, SN, TN, TZ, UG, ZM, ZW) *see* Doxepin (Systemic) 676
Quitulcer (TW) *see* Lansoprazole 1166
QuitX (AU) *see* Nicotine 1449
Quixidar (AT, BE, BG, CH, CZ, DE, DK, EE, FR, GB, IE, IT, MT, NL, NO, PL, RU, SE, SK, TR) *see* Fondaparinux 924
Quomen (TH) *see* BuPROPion 305
Quotavil (HK) *see* Ofloxacin (Systemic) 1490
Quoxol (ES) *see* Oxatomide [INT] 1532
Qupron (KR) *see* Ciprofloxacin (Systemic) 441
Qura Nasal (AR) *see* Phenylephrine (Systemic) 1638
Qutacin (TW) *see* Gentamicin (Systemic) 959
Qutipin (KR) *see* QUEtiapine 1751
Qvar (AU, CH, CR, DO, FR, GB, GT, HN, HR, IE, IL, MY, NI, NZ, PA, PT, SV, TH) *see* Beclomethasone (Systemic) 230
Qvar Autohaler (AU, FR) *see* Beclomethasone (Nasal) 232
Q Var (CH, CR, DO, GB, GT, HN, MY, NI, NZ, PA, PT, SV, TH) *see* Beclomethasone (Nasal) 232
Qvar Inhaler (AU) *see* Beclomethasone (Nasal) 232
Q-Win (PH) *see* QUEtiapine 1751
R-A (KR) *see* Leflunomide 1174
Rabaphen (PH) *see* DiphenhydrAMINE (Systemic) 641
Rabeact-20 (HK) *see* RABEprazole 1762
Rabec (AR, LB) *see* RABEprazole 1762
Rabecid (PK) *see* RABEprazole 1762
Rabegen (KR) *see* RABEprazole 1762
Rabeloc (IN, VN) *see* RABEprazole 1762
Rabeol (KR) *see* RABEprazole 1762
Raberin (KR) *see* RABEprazole 1762
Rabestad (HK) *see* RABEprazole 1762
Rabesta (KR) *see* RABEprazole 1762
Rabet (KR) *see* RABEprazole 1762
Rabetra (HK) *see* RABEprazole 1762
Rabezole (QA, SA) *see* RABEprazole 1762
Rabies-Imovax (FI, NO, SE) *see* Rabies Vaccine 1764
Rabies MIRV Vaccine (NZ) *see* Rabies Vaccine 1764
Rabiesvax (PH) *see* Rabies Vaccine 1764
Rabiet (KR) *see* RABEprazole 1762
Rabigam (ZA) *see* Rabies Immune Globulin (Human)....1764
Rabipur (AT, AU, BG, CZ, DE, FR, GB, HR, ID, IE, IN, NL, PH, RO, SE, SG, TH) *see* Rabies Vaccine 1764

Rabister (KR) *see* RABEprazole 1762
Rabugen-M (HK, MY) *see* Domperidone [CAN/INT] 666
Rabugen (HK, MY) *see* Domperidone [CAN/INT] 666
Rabuman Berna (PH, TH) *see* Rabies Immune Globulin (Human) 1764
Rabzole (AU) *see* RABEprazole 1762
Raceca (VN) *see* Racecadotril [INT] 1765
Race-F (IN) *see* Racecadotril [INT] 1765
Racetam (SG) *see* Piracetam [INT] 1661
Raciper (IN) *see* Esomeprazole 771
Racovel (MX) *see* Carbidopa and Levodopa 351
Racser (MY) *see* Lidocaine and Prilocaine 1213
Radedorm (BG, EE) *see* Nitrazepam [CAN/INT] 1461
Radepur (AE, BH, CY, DE, EG, IQ, IR, JO, KW, LB, LY, OM, QA, SA, SY, YE) *see* ChlordiazePOXIDE 422
Radicortin (AE, BF, BH, BJ, CI, CY, EG, ET, GH, GM, GN, IQ, IR, JO, KE, KW, LB, LR, LY, MA, ML, MR, MU, MW, NE, NG, OM, QA, SA, SC, SD, SL, SN, SY, TN, TZ, UG, YE, ZM, ZW) *see* Hydrocortisone (Systemic) 1013
Radikal (BE, LU) *see* Malathion 1268
Radinat (EC) *see* Ranitidine 1777
Radiocillina (AE, BF, BH, BJ, CI, CY, EG, ET, GH, GM, GN, IL, IQ, IR, JO, KE, KW, LB, LR, LY, MA, ML, MR, MU, MW, NE, NG, OM, QA, SA, SC, SD, SL, SN, SY, TN, TZ, UG, YE, ZM, ZW) *see* Ampicillin 141
Radiocin (AE, BF, BH, BJ, CI, CY, EG, ET, GH, GM, GN, IQ, IR, JO, KE, KW, LB, LR, LY, MA, ML, MR, MU, MW, NE, NG, OM, QA, SA, SC, SD, SL, SN, SY, TN, TZ, UG, YE, ZM, ZW) *see* Fluocinolone (Topical) 893
Radisemide (AE, BF, BH, BJ, CI, CY, EG, ET, GH, GM, GN, IQ, IR, JO, KE, KW, LB, LR, LY, MA, ML, MR, MU, MW, NE, NG, OM, QA, SA, SC, SD, SL, SN, SY, TN, TZ, UG, YE, ZM, ZW) *see* Furosemide 940
Radizepam (AE, BF, BH, BJ, CI, CY, EG, ET, GH, GM, GN, IQ, IR, JO, KE, KW, LB, LR, LY, MA, ML, MR, MU, MW, NE, NG, OM, QA, SA, SC, SD, SL, SN, SY, TN, TZ, UG, YE, ZM, ZW) *see* Diazepam 613
Radol (ID) *see* TraMADol 2074
Radouna (JP) *see* Furosemide 940
Radox (BF, BH, BJ, CI, CY, EG, ET, GH, GM, GN, IQ, IR, JO, KE, KW, LB, LR, LY, MA, ML, MR, MU, MW, NE, NG, OM, QA, SA, SC, SD, SL, SN, SY, TN, TZ, UG, YE, ZM, ZW) *see* Doxycycline 689
Rafax XR (TW) *see* Venlafaxine 2150
Rafen (AU) *see* Ibuprofen 1032
Rafofer (CL) *see* Iron Sucrose 1118
Rafree (PH) *see* Meloxicam 1283
Rafton (FR) *see* Budesonide (Systemic) 293
Ragitar (CO) *see* Rasagiline 1781
Ralenost (TH) *see* Alendronate 79
Ralgec (PH) *see* Mefenamic Acid 1280
Ralopar (PT) *see* Cefotaxime 382
Ralovera (AU) *see* MedroxyPROGESTERone 1277
Raloxiqueen (KR) *see* Raloxifene 1765
Ralox (VN) *see* Raloxifene 1765
Ralozam (AU) *see* ALPRAZolam 94
Ralsin (MY) *see* Terazosin 2001
Raltiva (CN) *see* Fexofenadine 873
Ralydan (DK) *see* Lidocaine and Tetracaine 1214
Ralzal (IN) *see* Rupatadine [INT] 1855
Ramace (AU, BE, DK, FI, LU, MY, NZ, SG) *see* Ramipril 1771
Ramace H (IN) *see* Ramipril and Hydrochlorothiazide [CAN/INT] 1773
Ramado Retard (KR) *see* TraMADol 2074
Ramaxir (TR) *see* Flucloxacillin [INT] 885
Ramey (TW) *see* Ramipril 1771
Ramezol (KR) *see* Omeprazole 1508
Ramicard (DE) *see* Ramipril and Hydrochlorothiazide [CAN/INT] 1773
Ramicin (ID) *see* Rifampin 1804
Ramickin (KR) *see* Amikacin 111
Ramicor (PY) *see* Ramipril 1771
Ramily (TW) *see* Ramipril 1771
Ramimed HCT (TR) *see* Ramipril and Hydrochlorothiazide [CAN/INT] 1773
Ramipres (CL) *see* Ramipril 1771
Ramipril Comp (EE) *see* Ramipril and Hydrochlorothiazide [CAN/INT] 1773
Ramipril Plus (IL) *see* Ramipril and Hydrochlorothiazide [CAN/INT] 1773
Ramiprin (KR) *see* Ramipril 1771
Ramipro (PH) *see* Ramipril 1771
Ramitace (TW) *see* Ramipril 1771
Ramitens (IL) *see* Ramipril and Hydrochlorothiazide [CAN/INT] 1773
Ramixal (ID) *see* Ramipril 1771
Ramlac (LB) *see* Lactulose 1156
RA-Morph (NZ) *see* Morphine (Systemic) 1394
Ramoxin (JO) *see* Cephalexin 405
Rampil (ZA) *see* Ramipril 1771
Ramset (KR) *see* Ramosetron [INT] 1774
Ramset OD (KR) *see* Ramosetron [INT] 1774
Ramtrex (PH) *see* Tobramycin and Dexamethasone 2056
Ranacid (BH, JO, KW, LB, SA) *see* Ranitidine 1777
Ranacox (BE) *see* Etoricoxib [INT] 821
Rancef (AU) *see* Cephalexin 405
Rancil (TH) *see* Amoxicillin 130
Ranclav (TH, ZA) *see* Amoxicillin and Clavulanate 133
Ranclazide MR (TH) *see* Gliclazide [CAN/INT] 964
Ranclor (MX) *see* Cefaclor 372
Randa (JP) *see* CISplatin 448
Randin (AE, BH, CY, EG, IQ, IR, JO, KW, LB, LY, OM, QA, SA, SY, YE) *see* Ranitidine 1777
Ranemax (UY) *see* Strontium Ranelate [INT] 1938
Ranexa (AT, CH, CY, CZ, DE, EE, FR, GB, GR, HR, IE, IL, LT, NL, PL, PT, RO, SE, SI, SK, TR) *see* Ranolazine 1779
Ranexid (PH) *see* Tranexamic Acid 2081
Ranfuzosin (SG) *see* Alfuzosin 84
Rangin (HU) *see* Isosorbide Mononitrate 1126
Rani 2 (AU) *see* Ranitidine 1777
Ranial (IN) *see* Ranitidine 1777
Raniben (IT) *see* Ranitidine 1777
Raniberl (CZ) *see* Ranitidine 1777
Ranicux (DE) *see* Ranitidine 1777
Ranidil (IT) *see* Ranitidine 1777
Ranidin (ES) *see* Ranitidine 1777
Ranidine (TH) *see* Ranitidine 1777
Ranimex (FI) *see* Ranitidine 1777
Ranin (ID, TH) *see* Ranitidine 1777
Ranione (KR) *see* Ranitidine 1777
Raniplex (FR) *see* Ranitidine 1777
Ranisan (AE, BH, CY, CZ, EG, IQ, IR, JO, KW, LB, LY, OM, QA, SA, SY, YE) *see* Ranitidine 1777
Ranisen (MX) *see* Ranitidine 1777
Ranisulin-N (PH) *see* Insulin NPH 1089
Ranitab (EC) *see* Ranitidine 1777
Ranital (CZ, HR) *see* Ranitidine 1777
Ranitic (LU) *see* Ranitidine 1777
Ranitidin-B (HU) *see* Ranitidine 1777
Ranix (HR) *see* Ranitidine 1777
Ranmark (JP) *see* Denosumab 589
Ranmoxy (AU, ZA) *see* Amoxicillin 130
Ranofen (ZA) *see* Ibuprofen 1032
Ranolip (RO) *see* Lisinopril 1226
Ranoxyl Heartburn Relief (AU) *see* Ranitidine 1777
Ranoxyl (TH) *see* Amoxicillin 130
Ransilun 30/70 (PH) *see* Insulin NPH and Insulin Regular 1090
Ransim (AU) *see* Simvastatin 1890
Ranspa (KR) *see* Fenoverine [INT] 857
Ranstar (MX) *see* Stavudine 1934

Rantac (AE, BH, CY, EG, IN, IQ, IR, JO, KW, LB, LY, OM, QA, SA, SY, YE) *see* Ranitidine 1777
Rantacid (FI) *see* Ranitidine 1777
Rantag (AE, QA, SA) *see* Ranitidine 1777
Rantin (ID) *see* Ranitidine 1777
Rantric (CO) *see* Tazarotene 1980
Rantudal (GR) *see* Acemetacin [INT] 30
Rantudil (CN, DE, HU, LU, MX, PL, PT, TR, VN) *see* Acemetacin [INT] 30
Rantudil Forte (RO, SA) *see* Acemetacin [INT] 30
Rantudil Retard (MX, RO, SA) *see* Acemetacin [INT] 30
Ranvir (TH) *see* Acyclovir (Systemic) 47
Ranx (IN) *see* Ranolazine 1779
Ranzepam (AU) *see* Diazepam 613
Raost (ID) *see* Diclofenac (Systemic) 617
Rapacan (IN) *see* Sirolimus 1893
Rapamune (AE, AR, AT, AU, BE, BG, BH, BR, CH, CL, CN, CO, CR, CY, CZ, DE, DK, EC, EE, ES, FI, FR, GB, GR, GT, HK, HN, HR, IE, IL, IS, IT, JO, KR, KW, LB, LT, MT, MX, MY, NI, NL, NO, NZ, PA, PE, PH, PL, PT, QA, RO, RU, SA, SE, SG, SI, SK, SV, TH, TR, TW, VE, VN) *see* Sirolimus 1893
Rapeed (PH) *see* RABEprazole 1762
Raperon (KR) *see* Acetaminophen 32
Rapiacta (JP) *see* Peramivir 1619
Rapicet (KR) *see* Acetaminophen and Tramadol 37
Rapidocain (CH) *see* Lidocaine (Systemic) 1208
Rapidol (CL) *see* Acetaminophen 32
Rapifen (AE, AT, AU, BE, BG, BH, BR, CH, CL, CY, CZ, DE, DK, EE, EG, ES, FI, FR, GB, GR, HK, HN, HR, HU, IE, IL, IQ, IR, IT, JO, KW, LB, LU, LY, MT, NL, NO, NZ, OM, PL, PT, PY, QA, RU, SA, SE, SG, SI, SK, SY, TR, TW, UY, VE, YE, ZA) *see* Alfentanil 83
Rapilin (IN) *see* Repaglinide 1791
Rapilysin (AE, AT, AU, BE, BG, BH, CH, CY, CZ, DE, DK, EE, ES, FI, FR, GB, GR, HN, HR, IE, IS, IT, LT, MT, NL, NO, NZ, PL, PT, QA, RO, RU, SE, SG, SI, SK, TR) *see* Reteplase 1794
Rapime (ID) *see* Cefepime 378
Rapison (JP, KR) *see* Hydrocortisone (Systemic) 1013
Rapivir (MX, UY) *see* ValACYclovir 2119
Rapril (KR) *see* Enalapril 722
Rapydan (BE, GR, IE, NL, NO, PT, SE) *see* Lidocaine and Tetracaine 1214
Rapyden (CZ) *see* Lidocaine and Tetracaine 1214
Raquiferol (AR) *see* Ergocalciferol 753
Raquiferol BC (PY) *see* Ergocalciferol 753
Raquiferol D2 (PE) *see* Ergocalciferol 753
Raquitriol (AR) *see* Calcitriol 323
Rasalect (IN) *see* Rasagiline 1781
Rasal (ES) *see* Olsalazine 1500
Rasax (AR) *see* Rasagiline 1781
Rasedon 500 (JP) *see* Hydroxocobalamin 1020
Rashfree (PH) *see* Zinc Oxide 2200
Rasilamlo HCT (AU, CH) *see* Aliskiren, Amlodipine, and Hydrochlorothiazide 87
Rasilez D (AR, CL) *see* Aliskiren and Hydrochlorothiazide 87
Rasilez (AE, AR, AT, AU, BE, BR, CH, CL, CN, CO, CR, CZ, DE, DK, EC, EE, FR, GB, GR, GT, HK, HN, HR, ID, IE, IL, IN, IS, IT, JP, KR, KW, LB, LT, MY, NI, NL, NO, NZ, PA, PE, PH, PL, PT, QA, RO, RU, SA, SE, SG, SI, SK, SV, TH, TR, TW) *see* Aliskiren 85
Rasilez Fc (BH, CY) *see* Aliskiren 85
Rasilez HCT (AE, AT, AU, BE, BR, CH, CO, CZ, DE, DK, EC, EE, FR, GR, HK, HR, ID, IE, IN, KW, LB, LT, MY, NL, NO, PE, PH, PT, QA, SA, SE, SI, SK, TR) *see* Aliskiren and Hydrochlorothiazide 87
Rasilez HCT Fc (CY) *see* Aliskiren and Hydrochlorothiazide 87
Rasitol (MY, PH, SG, TW) *see* Furosemide 940
Rastinon (AE, AT, AU, BE, BH, CH, CY, EG, ES, GR, IE, IN, IQ, IR, IT, JO, KW, LB, LU, LY, MX, OM, SA, SY, YE) *see* TOLBUTamide 2062
Rastocin (HR) *see* DOXOrubicin (Conventional) 679
Rasuritek (JP) *see* Rasburicase 1783
Ratic (HK, TH) *see* Ranitidine 1777
Ratinal (ID) *see* Ranitidine 1777
ratio-Cotridin (CA) *see* Triprolidine, Pseudoephedrine, and Codeine [CAN/INT] 2105
Ratiograstim (GB) *see* Filgrastim 875
ratio-Magnesium (CA) *see* Magnesium Glucoheptonate [CAN/INT] 1262
Ratiopharm (DE) *see* Nitroglycerin 1465
Raupasil (BG, PL) *see* Reserpine 1793
Rauracid (JP) *see* Fluocinonide 894
Rauserpine (TW) *see* Reserpine 1793
Rauverid (PH) *see* Reserpine 1793
Ravalgen (EC) *see* Clopidogrel 484
Ravimed (MY) *see* MedroxyPROGESTERone 1277
Ravotril (CL) *see* ClonazePAM 478
Raxeto (AR) *see* Raloxifene 1765
Raxide (PH) *see* Ranitidine 1777
Rayor (TW) *see* Dihydroergotamine 633
Rayzon (ZA) *see* Parecoxib [INT] 1576
Razene (NZ) *see* Cetirizine 411
Razex (JO) *see* Spiramycin [CAN/INT] 1931
Razlin (JP) *see* Cinnarizine [INT] 440
Razon (LB) *see* Pantoprazole 1570
R Calm (BE) *see* DiphenhydrAMINE (Systemic) 641
RCOL (IN) *see* Charcoal, Activated 416
Reactine (FR, MX) *see* Cetirizine 411
Realdiron (BG) *see* Interferon Alfa-2b 1096
Realfa (IN) *see* Interferon Alfa-2b 1096
Reapam (NL) *see* Prazepam [INT] 1702
Reasec (CH, CZ, DE, HN, VN) *see* Diphenoxylate and Atropine 644
Rebacip (LB) *see* RABEprazole 1762
Rebagen (IN) *see* Rebamipide [INT] 1786
Rebamol (TW) *see* Methocarbamol 1320
Rebaten LA (BR) *see* Propranolol 1731
Rebetol (AE, AT, AU, BE, BG, BH, CH, CN, CY, CZ, DE, DK, DO, EE, ES, FI, FR, GB, GR, ID, IE, IL, IS, IT, JO, LB, LT, MT, MY, NL, NO, NZ, PA, PE, PH, PL, PT, QA, RU, SE, SG, SI, SK, TH, TR, VE) *see* Ribavirin 1797
Rebif (AE, AR, AU, BH, BR, CH, CN, CY, CZ, DE, DK, EE, ES, FR, GB, HK, HR, HU, ID, IE, IL, IN, IS, JO, KR, KW, LB, LT, MX, MY, NL, NZ, PE, PH, PL, RO, SA, SE, SG, SI, SK, TH, TW) *see* Interferon Beta-1a 1100
Rebis (KR) *see* Rebamipide [INT] 1786
Reboot (IN) *see* Reboxetine [INT] 1786
Rebose (IN) *see* Acarbose 29
Reboxxin (IN) *see* Reboxetine [INT] 1786
Rebozet (ID) *see* Eltrombopag 714
Recain (ID) *see* Bupivacaine 299
Recansa (ID) *see* Rosuvastatin 1848
Recessan (PY) *see* Polidocanol 1672
Rechol (ID) *see* Simvastatin 1890
Recita (IN) *see* Escitalopram 765
Recital (IL) *see* Citalopram 451
Recit (AR) *see* AtoMOXetine 191
Recivit (GB) *see* FentaNYL 857
Reclide (VE) *see* Gliclazide [CAN/INT] 964
Reclor (IN) *see* Chloramphenicol 421
Reclovax (TH) *see* Acyclovir (Systemic) 47
Recodryl (ID) *see* DiphenhydrAMINE (Systemic) 641
Recofol (AE, BH, CH, CY, HU, ID, IL, JO, MX, SG, TH) *see* Propofol 1728
Reco (ID) *see* Chloramphenicol 421
Recolfar (ID) *see* Colchicine 500
Recombicyte (PH) *see* Filgrastim 875

Recombinate (AR, AT, AU, BE, BG, BR, CH, CZ, DE, DK, EE, FI, FR, GB, IE, IL, IT, NL, NZ, SE, TH) *see* Antihemophilic Factor (Recombinant) 152
Recostar (KR) *see* Rebamipide [INT] 1786
Recovir-Em (TH) *see* Emtricitabine and Tenofovir 721
Recozin (PH) *see* Cetirizine 411
Recrea Forte (NO) *see* Minoxidil (Topical) 1374
Recrea (SE) *see* Minoxidil (Topical) 1374
Rectodelt (HU) *see* PredniSONE 1706
Rectogesic (AU, BE, CH, CZ, DE, DK, FI, FR, GB, IE, IL, IT, NL, NO, NZ, PT, SE, SG, SK) *see* Nitroglycerin 1465
Recutin (KR) *see* Trimebutine [CAN/INT] 2103
Recycline (IL) *see* Tetracycline 2017
Redaflam (MX) *see* Nimesulide [INT] 1456
Redap (DK) *see* Adapalene 54
Redevant (MX) *see* Pitavastatin 1663
Reditux (IN, VN) *see* RiTUXimab 1825
Red Off (UY) *see* Naphazoline (Ophthalmic) 1426
Redomex (BE) *see* Amitriptyline 119
Redotex (MX) *see* Atropine 200
Redoxon C (BB, BF, BJ, BM, BS, BZ, CI, ET, GH, GM, GN, GY, JM, KE, LR, MA, ML, MR, MU, MW, NE, NG, PR, SC, SD, SL, SN, SR, TN, TT, TZ, UG, ZM, ZW) *see* Ascorbic Acid 178
Redoxon (AE, AR, AT, AU, BE, BH, BR, CH, CO, CY, CZ, EC, EG, ES, FI, GB, GR, IE, IL, IQ, IR, IT, JO, KW, LB, LU, LY, OM, PE, PT, PY, QA, SA, SY, TR, UY, VE, YE) *see* Ascorbic Acid 178
Redoxon Forte (EC, IN) *see* Ascorbic Acid 178
Reducar (HK) *see* ISOtretinoin 1127
Reducel (PH) *see* Gemfibrozil 956
Redufast (PY) *see* Rimonabant [INT] 1814
Reduff (PH) *see* Ketoconazole (Topical) 1145
Redusa Forte (HK) *see* Phentermine 1635
Redusa (HK) *see* Phentermine 1635
Redustat (DO, GT, PA, SV) *see* Orlistat 1520
Redutens (ID) *see* Ramipril 1771
Reedvit 10000 (AR) *see* Cyanocobalamin 515
Refacto AF (BE, CH, DE, DK, EE, FR, GB, NO, SE) *see* Antihemophilic Factor (Recombinant) 152
Refacto (AT, CY, CZ, GR, HU, IT, NL, PL) *see* Antihemophilic Factor (Recombinant) 152
Refador (CZ) *see* MitoXANtrone 1382
Reflex (JP) *see* Mirtazapine 1376
Reflin (IN, JO, LT) *see* CeFAZolin 373
Reflux (NL) *see* Methenamine 1317
Refobacin (DE) *see* Gentamicin (Ophthalmic) 962
Refobacin (DE) *see* Gentamicin (Systemic) 959
Refolinon (GB, LU) *see* Leucovorin Calcium 1183
Refractyl Ofteno (CR, DO, GT, HN, PA, PE, SV) *see* Cyclopentolate 517
Refraxol (PE) *see* CloZAPine 490
Reftax (ZA) *see* Cefotaxime 382
Refusal (NL) *see* Disulfiram 654
Regad (MX) *see* Pantoprazole 1570
Regadrin B (VN) *see* Bezafibrate [CAN/INT] 261
Regaine (AE, AT, BG, BH, CH, CY, CZ, DK, EE, EG, GR, HK, HN, HR, IL, IQ, IR, IT, JO, KW, LB, LT, LY, NL, OM, PL, PT, QA, RU, SA, SI, SK, SY, TH, TR, TW, VE, VN, YE) *see* Minoxidil (Topical) 1374
Regaine Extra Strength For Men (HK) *see* Minoxidil (Topical) 1374
Regaine For Men (HK) *see* Minoxidil (Topical) 1374
Regaine For Unisex (HK) *see* Minoxidil (Topical) 1374
Regaine For Women (HK) *see* Minoxidil (Topical) 1374
Regamen (ID) *see* Norethindrone 1473
Regelan (PK) *see* Metoclopramide 1345
Regenon (AT, BE, DK, LU) *see* Diethylpropion 624
Regenon Retard (DE) *see* Diethylpropion 624
Regental (UY) *see* Naltrexone 1422
Regitina (AR, BR, VE) *see* Phentolamine 1636
Regitin (CH, CZ, DK, HN) *see* Phentolamine 1636
Regitine (AU, BE, CN, EG, GR, HK, HU, IL, LU, NL, NZ) *see* Phentolamine 1636
Reglan (BG, HR, IN, SI) *see* Metoclopramide 1345
Reglinide (TW) *see* Repaglinide 1791
Reglin (TR) *see* Repaglinide 1791
Reglit (PE) *see* Rosiglitazone 1847
Reglomar (PH) *see* Metoclopramide 1345
regnyl (HK) *see* Chorionic Gonadotropin (Human) 431
Regpara (HK, JP, KR, SG, TH, TW) *see* Cinacalcet 439
Regranex (AT, BE, BG, CH, CZ, DE, DK, EE, ES, FI, FR, GB, GR, HN, IE, IL, IT, KR, MT, MX, NL, NO, PL, PT, RO, RU, SE, SK, TR) *see* Becaplermin 230
Regroe (PH) *see* Minoxidil (Topical) 1374
Regro (SG) *see* Minoxidil (Topical) 1374
Regrou (ID) *see* Minoxidil (Topical) 1374
Regrowth (TH) *see* Minoxidil (Topical) 1374
Regtect (JP) *see* Acamprosate 28
Regubeat (IN) *see* Disopyramide 653
Regulact (MX) *see* Lactulose 1156
Regulane AF (AR) *see* Loperamide and Simethicone 1237
Regulane (AR) *see* Loperamide 1236
Regulan (GB, IE) *see* Psyllium 1744
Regulip (AE, BH, CY, EG, IL, IQ, IR, JO, KW, LB, LY, OM, QA, SA, SY, YE) *see* Gemfibrozil 956
Regulon (BG, MY) *see* Ethinyl Estradiol and Desogestrel 799
Regurin (GB, IE) *see* Trospium 2108
Regutol (AE, BH, CY, EG, IQ, IR, JO, KW, LB, LY, OM, QA, SA, SY, YE) *see* Docusate 661
Reinin (PH) *see* Gabapentin 943
Reisevit (AT) *see* Pyridoxine 1747
Reizer (TW) *see* ChlorproMAZINE 429
Rekawan (DE) *see* Potassium Chloride 1687
Rekawan Retard (AT) *see* Potassium Chloride 1687
Rekaxime (MY) *see* Cefotaxime 382
Relac (TW) *see* BusPIRone 311
Relacum (MX) *see* Midazolam 1361
Relafen (CN, KR, VN) *see* Nabumetone 1411
Relaflex (GT, HN, NI, SV) *see* Orphenadrine 1522
Relanium (LT, PL, RU) *see* Diazepam 613
Relatrac (CO, MX, PE) *see* Atracurium 198
Relaxan (DK) *see* Gallamine Triethiodide [INT] 948
Relax (EC) *see* BusPIRone 311
Relaxil-G (HU) *see* GuaiFENesin 986
Relaxin (PH) *see* Cephalexin 405
Relaxin (TW) *see* Succinylcholine 1939
Relefact (CZ, GR, IE) *see* Gonadorelin [CAN/INT] 980
Relefact LH-RH (AT, KR, NL) *see* Gonadorelin [CAN/INT] 980
Relenza (AE, AR, AT, AU, BE, BG, BH, BR, CH, CL, CN, CY, CZ, DE, DK, EE, ES, FI, FR, GB, GR, HK, HN, HR, IE, IL, IS, IT, KR, KW, LT, MX, MY, NL, NO, NZ, PH, PL, PT, QA, RO, SA, SE, SG, SI, SK, TH, TR, TW, VN) *see* Zanamivir 2194
Relert (BE, CR, DO, FI, GT, IL, NI, PA, PT, SV) *see* Eletriptan 711
Relexa (SK) *see* Celecoxib 402
Relexil (MX) *see* Pioglitazone 1654
Relieva (BG) *see* Frovatriptan 938
Relifen (JP, ZA) *see* Nabumetone 1411
Reliferon (PH) *see* Interferon Alfa-2b 1096
Relifex (AE, BB, BF, BG, BH, BJ, BM, BR, BS, BZ, CI, CY, CZ, DE, DK, EE, EG, ET, FI, GB, GH, GM, GN, GR, GY, HN, IE, IQ, IR, IS, IT, JM, JO, KE, KW, LB, LR, LT, LY, MA, ML, MR, MU, MW, MX, NE, NG, NO, NZ, OM, PH, PK, PL, QA, SA, SC, SD, SE, SL, SN, SR, SY, TN, TR, TT, TW, TZ, UG, YE, ZM, ZW) *see* Nabumetone 1411
Religrast (PH) *see* Filgrastim 875
Relinide (VN) *see* Repaglinide 1791
Relisan (ZA) *see* Nabumetone 1411
Relisorm L (BR, HU) *see* Gonadorelin [CAN/INT] 980

Relistor (AR, AT, AU, BE, BR, CH, CL, CY, CZ, DE, DK, EE, FR, GB, GR, HN, HR, IE, IT, MX, NL, NO, PL, PT, RO, SE, SI, SK, TR) *see* Methylnaltrexone 1334
Relitaz (RO) *see* RABEprazole 1762
Relitone (ZA) *see* Nabumetone 1411
Relivan (ID) *see* Terbutaline 2004
Reliveran (AR) *see* Metoclopramide 1345
Reliv (SE) *see* Acetaminophen 32
Reloc (KR) *see* Loxoprofen [INT] 1255
Relpax (AE, AT, AU, BG, BH, BR, CH, CL, CO, CZ, DE, DK, EE, ES, FR, GB, GR, HN, IE, IS, IT, JO, KW, MX, NL, NO, NZ, PL, QA, RO, RU, SA, SE, SG, SI, SK, TH, TR, ZA) *see* Eletriptan 711
Reltebon (GB) *see* OxyCODONE 1538
Relvar Ellipta (CH, CY, CZ, DE, DK, EE, GB, HK, HR, IL, IS, JP, LT, NL, NO, RO, SE, SI, SK, TR) *see* Fluticasone and Vilanterol 914
Remaltin (TW) *see* Gabapentin 943
Remantadin (BG) *see* Rimantadine 1813
Remecin (TW) *see* Donepezil 668
Remedacen (DE) *see* Dihydrocodeine, Aspirin, and Caffeine 632
Remedium (TR) *see* Diazepam 613
Remedol (PR, TR) *see* Acetaminophen 32
Remember (TW) *see* Galantamine 946
Remergil (DE) *see* Mirtazapine 1376
Remergon (BE) *see* Mirtazapine 1376
Remeron (AE, AR, AT, BH, BR, CH, CN, CO, CR, CY, CZ, DK, DO, EE, EG, FI, GR, GT, HN, ID, IL, IQ, IR, IS, IT, JO, JP, KR, KW, LB, LT, LY, MX, MY, NI, NL, NO, OM, PA, PE, PK, PL, PT, QA, RO, RU, SA, SE, SG, SI, SK, SV, SY, TR, TW, UY, VE, VN, YE, ZA) *see* Mirtazapine 1376
Remeron SolTab (CO, HK, PH, SG) *see* Mirtazapine 1376
Remestyp (BG, CZ, IN, KR, PL, RU) *see* Terlipressin [INT] 2010
Remethan (DE, MY, SG) *see* Diclofenac (Systemic) 617
Remex (FR) *see* Acyclovir (Systemic) 47
Remex (FR) *see* Acyclovir (Topical) 51
Remicade (AE, AR, AT, AU, BE, BG, BH, BR, CH, CL, CN, CO, CR, CY, CZ, DE, DK, DO, EC, EE, ES, FI, FR, GB, GR, HK, HN, HR, HU, ID, IE, IL, IN, IS, IT, JO, JP, KR, LT, MT, MX, MY, NI, NL, NO, NZ, PA, PE, PH, PL, PT, QA, RO, RU, SA, SE, SG, SI, SK, SV, TH, TR, UY, VE, VN) *see* InFLIXimab 1070
Remid (DE, PY) *see* Allopurinol 90
Remide (KR) *see* Rebamipide [INT] 1786
Remin (AE) *see* Aspirin 180
Reminy ERI (CL) *see* Galantamine 946
Reminyl XL (GB, IE) *see* Galantamine 946
Reminyl (AE, AR, AT, AU, BE, BH, BR, CH, CN, CO, CR, CY, CZ, DE, DK, DO, EE, EG, ES, FI, FR, GB, GR, GT, HN, ID, IE, IL, IS, IT, JP, KW, LB, MX, MY, NI, NL, NO, NZ, PA, PH, PT, QA, RO, SA, SE, SG, SI, SV, TH, TR, TW, UY, VN) *see* Galantamine 946
Reminyl ER (AR, BR, CO, EC, PE) *see* Galantamine 946
Reminyl LP (FR) *see* Galantamine 946
Reminyl PRC (HK, IL, QA) *see* Galantamine 946
Remirta (BG) *see* Mirtazapine 1376
Remirta OD (HK) *see* Mirtazapine 1376
Remital (ID) *see* OLANZapine 1491
Remixil ODT (KR) *see* Mirtazapine 1376
Remmicade (LB) *see* InFLIXimab 1070
Remniq (AU) *see* Alemtuzumab 75
Remodulin (AR, AT, AU, BE, BM, CH, CL, CZ, DE, DK, EE, FI, FR, GR, IL, IS, IT, KR, LT, NL, NO, PT, SE, SI, SK, TW) *see* Treprostinil 2093
Remofen (AE, BH, JO, QA) *see* Ibuprofen 1032
Remontal (ES) *see* NiMODipine 1456
Remopain (ID) *see* Ketorolac (Systemic) 1146
Remotil (PT) *see* Domperidone [CAN/INT] 666
Removchol (ID) *see* AtorvaSTATin 194
Remov (IT) *see* Nimesulide [INT] 1456
Remox (UY) *see* Minoxidil (Topical) 1374
Remsima (KR) *see* InFLIXimab 1070
Remstin (KR) *see* Clemastine 459
Remwestyp (CN) *see* Terlipressin [INT] 2010
Remycin (TR, TW) *see* Doxycycline 689
Renabetic (ID) *see* GlyBURIDE 972
Renacardon (ID) *see* Enalapril 722
Renacet (GB) *see* Calcium Acetate 326
Renacor (DE) *see* Enalapril and Hydrochlorothiazide 725
Renagas (ID) *see* Clidinium and Chlordiazepoxide 460
Renagel (AE, AU, BR, CY, ES, FI, GR, HR, IT, JP, KR, KW, LB, LT, PE, PL, RO, SA, SI, SK, TR, TW, UY) *see* Sevelamer 1881
Renallapin (KR) *see* Enalapril 722
Renamid (HR) *see* AcetaZOLAMIDE 39
Renaquil (ID) *see* LORazepam 1243
Renatriol (DE) *see* Calcitriol 323
Renax (TR) *see* ALPRAZolam 94
Renborin (JP) *see* Diazepam 613
Renedil (BE, LU) *see* Felodipine 850
Renelate (IN) *see* Strontium Ranelate [INT] 1938
Renezide (ZA) *see* Hydrochlorothiazide and Triamterene 1012
Ren (HK) *see* Diclofenac (Systemic) 617
Renidac (MX) *see* Sulindac 1953
Renidur (PT) *see* Enalapril and Hydrochlorothiazide 725
Renitec (AE, AR, AT, AU, BE, BF, BG, BH, BJ, BR, CI, CN, CO, CY, CZ, EC, EE, EG, ES, ET, FI, FR, GH, GM, GN, GR, HK, HN, HU, JO, KE, KW, LB, LR, LU, MA, ML, MR, MU, MW, MY, NE, NG, NL, NO, NZ, PE, PH, PK, PT, QA, SA, SC, SD, SE, SL, SN, TN, TR, TW, TZ, UG, VE, VN, ZM, ZW) *see* Enalapril 722
Renitec Comp (FI, NO) *see* Enalapril and Hydrochlorothiazide 725
Renitec Plus 20/6 (AU) *see* Enalapril and Hydrochlorothiazide 725
Renitec Plus (EE) *see* Enalapril and Hydrochlorothiazide 725
Renitek (RU) *see* Enalapril 722
Reniten (CH) *see* Enalapril 722
Renitol (PH) *see* Mannitol 1269
Renivace (JP) *see* Enalapril 722
Renogen (PH, TH) *see* Epoetin Alfa 742
Renogram (HR) *see* Nalidixic Acid [INT] 1418
Renormax (ES, IT) *see* Spirapril [INT] 1931
Renova (ZA) *see* Tretinoin (Topical) 2099
Renovia (BG) *see* Lercanidipine [INT] 1181
Renpress (ES, NL, NO) *see* Spirapril [INT] 1931
Rentibloc (KR) *see* Sotalol 1927
Rentylin (LU) *see* Pentoxifylline 1618
Renuvie (PH) *see* RisperiDONE 1818
Renvela (AT, BE, CH, CL, CR, CY, CZ, DE, DK, EE, FR, GB, GT, HK, HN, HR, IE, IL, IS, KR, KW, LT, MY, NL, NO, PA, PH, PT, RO, SE, SG, SI, SK, SV, TH, TR) *see* Sevelamer 1881
Renzat (PH) *see* AzaTHIOprine 210
Reodon (HR) *see* Repaglinide 1791
Reodyn (FI) *see* Carbocisteine [INT] 357
Reoflen (GR) *see* Triflusal [INT] 2103
Reolin (IL) *see* Acetylcysteine 40
Reomax (IT) *see* Ethacrynic Acid 797
ReoPro (AR, AT, AU, BE, BG, BR, CH, CL, CO, CZ, DE, DK, ES, FI, FR, GB, GR, HK, IE, IL, IN, IS, IT, KR, LU, MX, MY, NL, NO, NZ, PE, PK, PL, PT, RU, SE, SG, SI, TH, TW, ZA) *see* Abciximab 24
Reosil (VE) *see* Bromhexine [INT] 291
Repafet (MX) *see* Rupatadine [INT] 1855
Repaglid (PY) *see* Repaglinide 1791
Repampia (VN) *see* Rebamipide [INT] 1786
Repanorm (TW) *see* Repaglinide 1791
Repinox (CR, DO) *see* Nitazoxanide 1461
Repitend (EE) *see* LevETIRAcetam 1191

Repivate (ZA) *see* Betamethasone (Topical) 255
Replagal (AT, AU, BE, CH, CZ, DK, EE, ES, FI, FR, GB, GR, HN, HR, HU, IE, IL, IS, IT, JP, LT, NL, NO, NZ, PY, RO, SE, SI, SK, TW) *see* Agalsidase Alfa [CAN/INT] 63
Replenine VF (IL, MY) *see* Factor IX (Human) 840
Reposo-Mono (BE) *see* Meprobamate 1296
Repreve (AU, NZ) *see* ROPINIRole 1844
Reprostom (ID) *see* Finasteride 878
Repulson (JP) *see* Aprotinin 168
Requip XL (CY) *see* ROPINIRole 1844
Requip (AE, AR, AT, BE, BG, CH, CL, CZ, DE, DK, EE, ES, FI, FR, GB, GR, HK, HN, HR, HU, IE, IL, IT, JP, KW, LT, MY, NL, NO, NZ, PK, PL, PT, QA, SA, SE, SG, SK, TR, TW) *see* ROPINIRole 1844
Requip CR (JP) *see* ROPINIRole 1844
Requip Depot (IS) *see* ROPINIRole 1844
Requip PD (HK, ID, KR, MY, PH, SG, TH, TW) *see* ROPINIRole 1844
requip (SI) *see* ROPINIRole 1844
Rescufolin (NO) *see* Leucovorin Calcium 1183
Rescuvolin (BE, CH, DK, GR, KR, LU, SE, TH, TW) *see* Leucovorin Calcium 1183
Resdone (AU) *see* RisperiDONE 1818
Reseril (IT) *see* Nefazodone 1435
Reset (IT) *see* Aniracetam [INT] 150
Resflox (ID) *see* Sparfloxacin [INT] 1930
Resibron (ID) *see* Piracetam [INT] 1661
Resical (CZ, PT) *see* Calcium Polystyrene Sulfonate [CAN/INT] 333
Resikali (FR) *see* Calcium Polystyrene Sulfonate [CAN/INT] 333
Resincalcio (AR, MY) *see* Calcium Polystyrene Sulfonate [CAN/INT] 333
Resincolestiramina (SG, UY) *see* Cholestyramine Resin 431
Resinsodio (MY, SG) *see* Sodium Polystyrene Sulfonate 1912
Reskuin (ID) *see* Levofloxacin (Systemic) 1197
Reslin (JP) *see* TraZODone 2091
Resmin (JP) *see* DiphenhydrAMINE (Systemic) 641
Resochin (AE, AT, BF, BG, BH, BJ, CI, CY, DE, EG, ES, ET, GH, GM, GN, HR, ID, IL, IN, IQ, IR, IT, JO, KE, KW, LB, LR, LY, MA, ML, MR, MU, MW, NE, NG, NL, OM, QA, SA, SC, SD, SL, SN, SY, TN, TZ, UG, YE, ZA, ZM, ZW) *see* Chloroquine 424
Resochina (PT) *see* Chloroquine 424
Resolor (BE, BR, CH, CN, CO, CY, CZ, DE, DK, EE, FR, GB, HK, HR, IL, KR, LT, NL, NO, PE, PH, PL, PT, QA, RO, SE, SG, SK, TH, TR, VN) *see* Prucalopride [CAN/INT] 1741
Resolve Jock Itch (AU) *see* Miconazole (Topical) 1360
Resolve Solution (AU, SG) *see* Miconazole (Topical) 1360
Resolve Tinea (AU, MY, SG) *see* Miconazole (Topical) 1360
Resonium A (AT, AU, GB, HK, HN, MY, NL, TR, TW) *see* Sodium Polystyrene Sulfonate 1912
Resonium (DK, FI, PT, SE) *see* Sodium Polystyrene Sulfonate 1912
Resonium (VN) *see* Calcium Polystyrene Sulfonate [CAN/INT] 333
Resorcal (CL) *see* Racecadotril [INT] 1765
Resotrans (AU, MX, NZ) *see* Prucalopride [CAN/INT] 1741
Resotyl (CL, PE) *see* Modafinil 1386
Respal (LB) *see* RisperiDONE 1818
Respidual (VE) *see* Ipratropium and Fenoterol [CAN/INT] 1109
Respigen (NZ) *see* Albuterol 69
Respilene (FR) *see* Pholcodine [INT] 1646
Respine (MY) *see* Reserpine 1793
Resplamin (JP) *see* Aminocaproic Acid 113
Respocort (NZ) *see* Beclomethasone (Nasal) 232
Respocort (NZ) *see* Beclomethasone (Systemic) 230
Resprim (AU) *see* Sulfamethoxazole and Trimethoprim 1946
Resprim Forte (AU) *see* Sulfamethoxazole and Trimethoprim 1946
Restamine (AE, BH, CY, EG, IQ, IR, JO, KW, LB, LY, OM, QA, SA, SY, YE) *see* Loratadine 1241
Restasis (AR, BR, CN, CO, GR, HK, IL, KR, LB, MY, PE, PH, SI, TH, TW, VE) *see* CycloSPORINE (Ophthalmic) 529
Resteclin (IN) *see* Tetracycline 2017
Restenil (DK, NO) *see* Meprobamate 1296
Restinil (PY, UY) *see* Remifentanil 1789
Restoril (PK) *see* Temazepam 1990
Resulax (SE) *see* Sorbitol 1927
Resulin (IT) *see* Nimesulide [INT] 1456
Result (KR) *see* Omeprazole 1508
Resyl (AT, BG, CH, SE) *see* GuaiFENesin 986
Retacnyl (CR, DO, GT, KR, MX, MY, PA, PE, PH, SG, SV, VE) *see* Tretinoin (Topical) 2099
Retadox (LB) *see* Doxycycline 689
Retafer (FI, HR, MY) *see* Ferrous Sulfate 871
Retafyllin (EE, HU) *see* Theophylline 2026
Retardillin (HU) *see* Penicillin G Procaine 1613
Retarpen (AT, BH, CY, CZ, EG, HR, IL, IQ, IR, JO, KW, LB, LY, MY, OM, PL, QA, SA, SG, SY, YE) *see* Penicillin G Benzathine 1609
Retarpen LA (AE) *see* Penicillin G Benzathine 1609
Retavit (IL) *see* Tretinoin (Topical) 2099
Retaxim (HR) *see* Tamoxifen 1971
Retcol (JP) *see* ChlordiazePOXIDE 422
Retensin (PH) *see* Captopril 342
Retep (AR) *see* Furosemide 940
Reteven (PE, VE) *see* Oxybutynin 1536
Reticrem (CO) *see* Tretinoin (Topical) 2099
Reticulogen (ES) *see* Cyanocobalamin 515
Reticus (IT) *see* Desonide 597
Retidex B12 (ES) *see* Cyanocobalamin 515
Retigel (CO) *see* Tretinoin (Topical) 2099
Retin-A (AE, AU, BH, BR, CH, CO, FR, ID, IE, JO, KW, LB, MX, PE, PH, PK, QA, SA, TH, UY, ZA) *see* Tretinoin (Topical) 2099
Retin A (AT, GR, IT, PT) *see* Tretinoin (Topical) 2099
Retino-A (IN) *see* Tretinoin (Topical) 2099
Retinofluor (AU) *see* Fluorescein 894
Retinova (SE) *see* Tretinoin (Topical) 2099
Retinyl (GR) *see* Maprotiline 1271
Retirides (ES) *see* Tretinoin (Topical) 2099
Retonel (ID) *see* Risedronate 1816
Retrieve Cream (AU) *see* Tretinoin (Topical) 2099
Retrieve (NZ, SG) *see* Tretinoin (Topical) 2099
Retrokor (PH) *see* CefTRIAXone 396
Retrovir (AE, AR, AT, AU, BB, BE, BG, BH, BM, BS, BZ, CH, CY, CZ, DE, DK, EE, EG, ES, FI, FR, GB, GR, GY, HK, HN, ID, IE, IL, IN, IQ, IR, IT, JM, JO, KW, LB, LY, MT, MY, NL, NO, NZ, OM, PH, PL, PT, PY, QA, RO, RU, SA, SE, SG, SI, SK, SR, SY, TH, TR, TT, TW, UY, VE, VN, YE) *see* Zidovudine 2196
Retrovir AZT (CL) *see* Zidovudine 2196
Retrovir-AZT (MX, PE) *see* Zidovudine 2196
Reugast (PT) *see* Fenbufen [INT] 852
Reumacid (AE, BH, CY, EG, IQ, IR, JO, KW, LB, LY, OM, QA, SA, SY, YE) *see* Indomethacin 1067
Reumacillin (FI) *see* PenicillAMINE 1608
Reumatrex (PE) *see* Methotrexate 1322
Reumon (PT) *see* Etofenamate [INT] 815
Reumophan (MX) *see* Chlorzoxazone 430
Reumophan Alka (MX) *see* Chlorzoxazone 430
Reumophan Vit (MX) *see* Chlorzoxazone 430
Reusin (ES) *see* Indomethacin 1067
Reutenox (ES) *see* Tenoxicam [INT] 2001
Reuxen (RO) *see* Naproxen 1427

Revanin (BF, BJ, CI, ET, GH, GM, GN, KE, LR, MA, ML, MR, MU, MW, NE, NG, SC, SD, SL, SN, TN, TZ, UG, ZM, ZW) *see* Acetaminophen ... 32
Revapol (MX) *see* Mebendazole [CAN/INT] ... 1274
Revasc (AT, CZ, EE, FR, GB, GR, HN, IE, IT, MT, NL, NZ, PL, PT, RO, RU, SK, TR) *see* Desirudin ... 593
Revatio (AT, AU, BE, CH, CZ, DE, DK, EE, ES, FI, FR, GB, GR, HK, HR, IE, IL, IS, IT, JP, KR, LT, MT, MY, NL, NO, NZ, PL, PT, RO, RU, SE, SI, SK, TH, TR, TW) *see* Sildenafil ... 1882
Revcid (ID) *see* Allopurinol ... 90
Revectina (BR) *see* Ivermectin (Systemic) ... 1136
Revelin (TW) *see* Rivastigmine ... 1833
Revellex (ZA) *see* InFLIXimab ... 1070
Reventa (PH) *see* Alendronate ... 79
Revestine (DE, DK, FI, GB, HR, NO, PT, SK) *see* Teduglutide ... 1982
Revestive (CZ, EE, LT, NL, SE) *see* Teduglutide ... 1982
Revez (AR) *see* Naltrexone ... 1422
Re-Via (MX) *see* Naltrexone ... 1422
ReVia (AU) *see* Naltrexone ... 1422
Revia (BR, CZ, DK, EE, EG, FI, FR, HK, HN, HU, KR, NO, NZ, RO, SE, TW) *see* Naltrexone ... 1422
Reviderm (ID) *see* Tretinoin (Topical) ... 2099
Revivan (IT) *see* DOPamine ... 669
Revlimid (AE, AT, AU, BE, CH, CL, CR, CY, CZ, DE, DK, EC, EE, FR, GB, GR, GT, HK, HN, HR, IE, IL, IS, IT, JP, KR, KW, LB, LT, MX, MY, NI, NL, NO, NZ, PA, PE, PH, PT, RO, RU, SE, SG, SI, SK, SV, TH, TR) *see* Lenalidomide ... 1177
Revocon (IN) *see* Tetrabenazine ... 2016
Revolade (AR, AT, AU, BE, BR, CH, CL, CZ, DK, EE, FR, GB, GR, HK, HR, IE, IL, IS, JP, KR, KW, LT, MX, MY, NL, NO, NZ, PE, PH, PL, PT, QA, RO, RU, SA, SE, SG, SI, SK, TH, TR, TW) *see* Eltrombopag ... 714
Rewise (TW) *see* Donepezil ... 668
Rewodina (DE, MY, RU) *see* Diclofenac (Systemic) ... 617
Rexacrom (NZ) *see* Cromolyn (Nasal) ... 514
Rexalgan (IT) *see* Tenoxicam [INT] ... 2001
Rexambro (NL, SE) *see* Ambroxol [INT] ... 109
Rexamide (IL) *see* Loperamide ... 1236
Rexavin (ID) *see* Griseofulvin ... 985
Rexidil (TW) *see* Minoxidil (Topical) ... 1374
Rexidron (ID) *see* Amiodarone ... 114
Rexifine (KR) *see* Doxofylline [INT] ... 679
Rexigen (ZA) *see* Propranolol ... 1731
Reximide (MY) *see* Loperamide ... 1236
Rexipin (KR) *see* Doxofylline [INT] ... 679
Rexivin (MX) *see* Methocarbamol ... 1320
Rexocef (HR) *see* Cefpodoxime ... 388
Rexta (ID) *see* Oxaliplatin ... 1528
Rexulti (AU) *see* Vortioxetine ... 2183
Reyataz (AE, AR, AT, AU, BE, BG, BH, CH, CL, CN, CO, CY, CZ, DE, DK, EE, ES, FI, FR, GB, GR, HK, HN, HR, HU, ID, IE, IL, IS, IT, KR, KW, LB, LT, MT, MX, MY, NL, NO, NZ, PE, PL, PT, QA, RO, RU, SA, SE, SG, SI, SK, TH, TR, TW, UY) *see* Atazanavir ... 185
Rezolsta (CZ, EE, GB, HR, NL, PT, SE, SK) *see* Darunavir and Cobicistat ... 572
Rezostatin (TW) *see* Simvastatin ... 1890
Rezult (IN) *see* Rosiglitazone ... 1847
R-Glucagon Lilly (MX) *see* Glucagon ... 970
Rhelafen Forte (ID) *see* Ibuprofen ... 1032
Rhelafen (ID) *see* Ibuprofen ... 1032
Rheodextran Infusia (CZ) *see* Dextran ... 607
Rheodextran Spofa (CZ) *see* Dextran ... 607
Rheomacrodex 10% (AT, DK, GB) *see* Dextran ... 607
Rheomacrodex (BR, CZ, DE, EC, FR, LU, NL, NO, SE) *see* Dextran ... 607
Rheo-Ma Inj (KR) *see* Piroxicam ... 1662
Rhesogam (DE) *see* $Rh_o(D)$ Immune Globulin ... 1794
Rhesogamma P (AR) *see* $Rh_o(D)$ Immune Globulin ... 1794
Rhesogamma (SE) *see* $Rh_o(D)$ Immune Globulin ... 1794
Rhesonativ (AE, BH, CY, DE, DK, EE, EG, IL, IQ, IR, IS, JO, KW, LB, LT, LY, NL, NO, OM, QA, SA, SE, SI, SK, SY, YE) *see* $Rh_o(D)$ Immune Globulin ... 1794
Rhesugam (ZA) *see* $Rh_o(D)$ Immune Globulin ... 1794
Rhesuman Berna (CO, HK, IL, MY, TH) *see* $Rh_o(D)$ Immune Globulin ... 1794
Rhesuman (CH, ES, GR, IN, IT, PK, TR) *see* $Rh_o(D)$ Immune Globulin ... 1794
Rhetoflam (ID) *see* Ketoprofen ... 1145
Rheudenolone (KR) *see* Triamcinolone (Systemic) ... 2099
Rheugasin (VN) *see* Acemetacin [INT] ... 30
Rheugesic (ZA) *see* Piroxicam ... 1662
Rheumacid (BF, BJ, CI, ET, GH, GM, GN, KE, LR, MA, ML, MR, MU, MW, NE, NG, SC, SD, SL, SN, TN, TZ, UG, ZM, ZW) *see* Indomethacin ... 1067
Rheumagel-Dr. Schmidgall (AT) *see* Diethylamine Salicylate [INT] ... 624
Rheuma-Gel-ratiopharm (DE) *see* Etofenamate [INT] ... 815
Rheumanox (TH) *see* Ibuprofen ... 1032
Rheumetan (KR) *see* Acemetacin [INT] ... 30
Rheumide (KR) *see* Leflunomide ... 1174
Rheumon (AT, CH, DE, LU, PT) *see* Etofenamate [INT] ... 815
Rheumox (GB, IE) *see* Azapropazone [INT] ... 210
Rheuna PAP (KR) *see* Ketoprofen ... 1145
Rheutrop (AT) *see* Acemetacin [INT] ... 30
Rhilor D (PK) *see* Loratadine and Pseudoephedrine ... 1242
Rhinaf (EC) *see* Naphazoline (Nasal) ... 1426
Rhinal (PY) *see* Naphazoline (Nasal) ... 1426
Rhinapen elixir (KR) *see* Acetaminophen ... 32
Rhinathiol (AE, BH, CY, HU, ID, KR, KW, LB, NL, QA, SA) *see* Carbocisteine [INT] ... 357
Rhinathiol Antirhinitis (BE) *see* Chlorpheniramine and Phenylephrine ... 426
Rhinex (DE) *see* Naphazoline (Nasal) ... 1426
Rhinil (HK) *see* Cetirizine ... 411
Rhiniramine SR (HK) *see* Dexchlorpheniramine ... 603
Rhino Clenil (AE, BH, CY, EG, IQ, IR, JO, KW, LB, LY, OM, QA, SA, SY, YE) *see* Beclomethasone (Nasal) ... 232
Rhinocort (AE, AU, BB, BE, BH, BM, BS, CH, CL, CN, CO, CR, CY, DK, DO, EE, EG, FI, FR, GB, GT, HK, HN, HR, HU, ID, IE, IN, IS, IT, JM, KW, LB, NI, NL, NO, NZ, PA, PE, PL, PR, QA, RO, SA, SE, SK, SV, TH, TR, TT, VE) *see* Budesonide (Nasal) ... 296
Rhinocort Aqua (HK) *see* Budesonide (Systemic) ... 293
Rhinocort Aqua (VN) *see* Budesonide (Nasal) ... 296
Rhinocort Hayfever (AU) *see* Budesonide (Nasal) ... 296
Rhinogan (PH) *see* Fexofenadine ... 873
Rhinolast (IL, PK) *see* Azelastine (Nasal) ... 213
Rhinomaxil (FR) *see* Beclomethasone (Nasal) ... 232
Rhinopront (LU) *see* Norepinephrine ... 1472
Rhinoside (GR) *see* Budesonide (Systemic) ... 293
Rhinos SR (ID) *see* Loratadine and Pseudoephedrine ... 1242
Rhinovent (CH, KR) *see* Ipratropium (Nasal) ... 1109
Rhinureflex (FR) *see* Pseudoephedrine and Ibuprofen ... 1743
Rhodiasectral (AR) *see* Acebutolol ... 29
Rhogam (BE, HK, HU) *see* $Rh_o(D)$ Immune Globulin ... 1794
Rhomustin (BG) *see* Bendamustine ... 241
Rhomuz (ID) *see* Loperamide ... 1236
Rhonal (VE) *see* Aspirin ... 180
Rhoneparina (PY) *see* Heparin ... 997
Rhophylac (AE, FR, GB, IL, KW, LB, SA) *see* $Rh_o(D)$ Immune Globulin ... 1794
Rhumagel (SG) *see* Piroxicam ... 1662
Rhythmonorm (IN) *see* Propafenone ... 1725
Riabal (FR, IT) *see* Prifinium [INT] ... 1712

Riabroxol (AE, SA) *see* Ambroxol [INT] 109
Riacetamid (AE) *see* Sulfacetamide (Ophthalmic) 1943
Riachol (AE) *see* Chloramphenicol 421
Rialac (AE, BH, JO, KW, QA) *see* Lactulose 1156
Rialol (AE) *see* Betaxolol (Ophthalmic) 257
Riamet (AT, AU, BE, CH, CZ, DE, FR, GB, GR, MY, NL, NZ, PT, SE, SG, SI) *see* Artemether and Lumefantrine 177
Riamide (AE, QA) *see* Metoclopramide 1345
RiaSTAP (AU, NZ) *see* Fibrinogen Concentrate (Human) 874
Riastap (BE, CY, DK, FR, GB, IS, NO, SE, SI, SK) *see* Fibrinogen Concentrate (Human) 874
Riatropine (AE) *see* Atropine 200
Riaxine (AE, SA) *see* Bromhexine [INT] 291
Riazolin (AE, QA) *see* Naphazoline (Ophthalmic) 1426
Ribafit (IN) *see* Rimonabant [INT] 1814
Riball (JP) *see* Allopurinol 90
Ribastamin (AR) *see* Risedronate 1816
Ribavin (IN, LB) *see* Ribavirin 1797
Ribeca (KR) *see* Difluprednate 626
Ribeca (KR) *see* Difluprednate (Topical) [INT] 627
Ribobis (JP) *see* Riboflavin 1803
Ribobutin (JP) *see* Riboflavin 1803
Ribodoxo (DE) *see* DOXOrubicin (Conventional) 679
Ribofluor (DE) *see* Fluorouracil (Systemic) 896
Ribomustin (AR, CH, CO, CZ, DE) *see* Bendamustine 241
Ribone (IL) *see* Risedronate 1816
Ribon (LU) *see* Riboflavin 1803
Ribonne (KR) *see* Ibandronate 1028
Riboract (JP) *see* Riboflavin 1803
Ribotine (KR) *see* Ranitidine 1777
Ribovact (SE) *see* Bendamustine 241
Ributin (IN) *see* Rifabutin 1803
Riclasip (MX) *see* Amoxicillin and Clavulanate 133
Ricovir (TH) *see* Tenofovir 1998
Ridal (SG) *see* RisperiDONE 1818
Ridamin (SG) *see* Loratadine 1241
Ridaq (ZA) *see* Hydrochlorothiazide 1009
Ridaura (AE, AR, AT, AU, BE, BF, BG, BH, BJ, BR, CH, CI, CN, CY, CZ, DE, DK, EE, EG, ES, ET, FI, GB, GH, GM, GN, GR, IE, IL, IQ, IR, IT, JO, JP, KE, KR, KW, LB, LR, LU, LY, MA, ML, MR, MT, MU, MW, NE, NG, NL, NO, NZ, OM, PT, QA, RU, SA, SC, SD, SE, SK, SL, SN, SY, TN, TR, TW, TZ, UG, YE, ZA, ZM, ZW) *see* Auranofin 204
Ridauran (FR) *see* Auranofin 204
Ridaura Tiltab (AE, BH, CY, EG, HK, IL, IQ, IR, JO, KW, LB, LY, MY, OM, QA, SA, SY, YE) *see* Auranofin 204
Ridazine (CN, TH) *see* Thioridazine 2030
Ridazin (IL, IN) *see* Thioridazine 2030
Ridene (MX) *see* NiCARdipine 1446
Ridonra (TW) *see* Allopurinol 90
Ridroqueen (KR) *see* Risedronate 1816
Ridworm (AU) *see* Mebendazole [CAN/INT] 1274
Rienso (CH, CZ, DK, EE, GB, HR, LT, NL, RO, SE, SI, SK) *see* Ferumoxytol 871
Rifabutin "Pharmacia" (DK) *see* Rifabutin 1803
Rifacilin (IN) *see* Rifampin 1804
Rifacin (AE, PH, QA, SA) *see* Rifampin 1804
Rifadex (EC) *see* Rifampin 1804
Rifadin (AE, AR, AU, BF, BH, BJ, CI, CY, CZ, EG, ET, GB, GH, GM, GN, GR, HK, IE, IQ, IR, IT, JO, KE, KW, LB, LR, LY, MA, ML, MR, MU, MW, MX, NE, NG, NL, NZ, OM, PK, PT, QA, SA, SC, SD, SE, SL, SN, SY, TN, TR, TW, TZ, UG, YE, ZA, ZM, ZW) *see* Rifampin 1804
Rifadine (BE, FR, LU, VN) *see* Rifampin 1804
Rifadom (AR) *see* Rifaximin 1809
Rifagen (ES) *see* Rifampin 1804
Rifaldin (BR, CL, ES) *see* Rifampin 1804
Rifaldin[inj.] (ES) *see* Rifampin 1804
Rifamcin (TH) *see* Rifampin 1804
Rifamed (HN, HU) *see* Rifampin 1804
Rifampicin Labatec (CH) *see* Rifampin 1804
Rifampicin (PL) *see* Rifampin 1804
Rifampin (KR) *see* Rifampin 1804
Rifapin (AE, BH, CY, EG, IQ, IR, JO, KW, LB, LY, OM, QA, SA, SY, YE) *see* Rifampin 1804
Rifaprodin (ES) *see* Rifampin 1804
Rifarad (AE, BF, BH, BJ, CI, CY, EG, ET, GH, GM, GN, IQ, IR, JO, KE, KW, LB, LR, LY, MA, ML, MR, MU, MW, NE, NG, OM, QA, SA, SC, SD, SL, SN, SY, TN, TZ, UG, YE, ZA, ZM, ZW) *see* Rifampin 1804
Rifaren (SG, TR) *see* Rifampin 1804
Rifarm (FI) *see* Rifampin 1804
Rifasynt (CY, JO, MY) *see* Rifampin 1804
Rifater (MX) *see* Pyrazinamide 1745
Rifatime (IN) *see* Rifaximin 1809
Rifocina (PE) *see* Rifampin 1804
Rifocina Spray (CO) *see* Rifampin 1804
Rifodex (KR) *see* Rifampin 1804
Rifoldin (AT) *see* Rifampin 1804
Rifoldine (CH) *see* Rifampin 1804
Rifonilo (ES) *see* Rifampin 1804
Riforal (ES) *see* Rifampin 1804
Rifun 40 (DE) *see* Pantoprazole 1570
Rigaminol (PE) *see* Gentamicin (Systemic) 959
Rigesoft (HU) *see* Levonorgestrel 1201
Rigevidon 21+7 (HK, MY) *see* Ethinyl Estradiol and Levonorgestrel 803
Rigevidon 21 + 7 (VN) *see* Ethinyl Estradiol and Levonorgestrel 803
Rigevidon (AE, BH, CY, EG, GB, IQ, IR, JO, KW, LB, LY, MY, OM, QA, SA, SY, YE) *see* Ethinyl Estradiol and Levonorgestrel 803
Rigix (PY) *see* Sildenafil 1882
Rikaparin (TW) *see* Tranexamic Acid 2081
Riklinak (AR) *see* Amikacin 111
Riklona (ID) *see* ClonazePAM 478
Rikodeine (AU) *see* Dihydrocodeine, Aspirin, and Caffeine 632
Rilamir (DK, FI) *see* Triazolam 2101
Rilan Nasal (BR) *see* Cromolyn (Nasal) 514
Rilaquin (PY) *see* Warfarin 2186
Rilatine (LU) *see* Methylphenidate 1336
Rilax (PH) *see* Lactulose 1156
Rilcapton (SG) *see* Captopril 342
Rileptid (HK, RO) *see* RisperiDONE 1818
Rilex (DE) *see* Tetrazepam [INT] 2020
Rilox (ID) *see* Ofloxacin (Systemic) 1490
Rilutek (AR, AT, AU, BE, BO, BR, CH, CL, CN, CO, CR, CY, CZ, DE, DK, DO, EC, ES, FI, FR, GB, GR, GT, HK, HN, HR, HU, IE, IL, IS, IT, KR, LB, LT, LU, MX, NI, NL, NO, PA, PE, PH, PL, PR, PT, PY, RO, RU, SE, SI, SK, SV, TH, TR, TW, UY, VE) *see* Riluzole 1812
Rimacillin (AE, BB, BF, BH, BJ, BM, BS, BZ, CI, CY, EG, ET, GH, GM, GN, GY, IQ, IR, JM, JO, KE, KW, LB, LR, LY, MA, ML, MR, MU, MW, NE, NG, NL, OM, PR, QA, SA, SC, SD, SL, SN, SR, SY, TN, TT, TZ, UG, YE, ZM, ZW) *see* Ampicillin 141
Rimactan (AT, BG, CH, DK, ES, FR, HR, IS, LU, MX, NL, NO, SE, SI, UY, VE, VN) *see* Rifampin 1804
Rimactan[inj.] (CH) *see* Rifampin 1804
Rimactane (BB, BF, BH, BJ, BM, BS, BZ, CI, ET, GB, GH, GM, GN, GY, ID, IL, IN, JM, KE, LR, MA, ML, MR, MU, MW, MY, NE, NG, QA, SA, SC, SD, SL, SN, SR, TN, TT, TZ, UG, ZA, ZM, ZW) *see* Rifampin 1804
Rimafed (PH) *see* Rifampin 1804
Rimapen (FI) *see* Rifampin 1804
Rimarex (IN) *see* Moclobemide [CAN/INT] 1384
Rimatet (AE, BB, BF, BH, BJ, BM, BS, BZ, CI, CY, EG, ET, GH, GM, GN, GY, IQ, IR, JM, JO, KE, KW, LB, LR, LY, MA, ML, MR, MU, MW, NE, NG, OM, PR, QA, SA,

SC, SD, SL, SN, SR, SY, TN, TT, TZ, UG, YE, ZM, ZW) *see* Tetracycline 2017
Rimecin (TH) *see* Rifampin 1804
Rimexel (LU) *see* Rimexolone 1814
Rimicid (BG) *see* Isoniazid 1120
Rimifon (CH, ES, FR, GB) *see* Isoniazid 1120
Rimodar (IN) *see* Sulfadoxine and Pyrimethamine [INT] 1946
Rimogras (PY) *see* Rimonabant [INT] 1814
Rimoslim (IN) *see* Rimonabant [INT] 1814
Rimpacin (AE, BF, BH, BJ, CI, CY, EG, ET, GH, GM, GN, IQ, IR, JO, KE, KW, LB, LR, LY, MA, ML, MR, MU, MW, NE, NG, OM, QA, SA, SC, SD, SL, SN, SY, TN, TZ, UG, YE, ZA, ZM, ZW) *see* Rifampin 1804
Rimpin (IN) *see* Rifampin 1804
Rimycin (AU) *see* Rifampin 1804
Rinafed (CR, GT, HN, PA, SV) *see* Pseudoephedrine 1742
Rinalin (DO, GT, NI, PA, SV) *see* Azelastine (Nasal) 213
Rinalix (MY, SG) *see* Indapamide 1065
Rinatec (GB, IE) *see* Ipratropium (Systemic) 1108
Rinepan (PE) *see* Rupatadine [INT] 1855
Rinex (LB) *see* Triamcinolone (Nasal) 2100
Ringworm Ointment (AU) *see* Tolnaftate 2063
Rinialer (ES, PT) *see* Rupatadine [INT] 1855
Rinityn (PH, SG) *see* Loratadine 1241
Rinobudex (EC, PE) *see* Mometasone (Nasal) 1391
Rino-Clenil (KR, TH) *see* Beclomethasone (Nasal) 232
Rinoclenil (RO) *see* Beclomethasone (Nasal) 232
Rinofed (AE) *see* Triprolidine and Pseudoephedrine 2105
Rinofer (ID) *see* Iron Sucrose 1118
Rinofug (RO) *see* Naphazoline (Nasal) 1426
Rinolast D (CO) *see* Fexofenadine and Pseudoephedrine 874
Rino-Lastin (BR) *see* Azelastine (Nasal) 213
Rinolic (ID) *see* Allopurinol 90
Rinol (IT) *see* Naphazoline (Nasal) 1426
Rinomar (BE) *see* Pseudoephedrine 1742
Rinoral (CH) *see* Pseudoephedrine 1742
Rinosol (PY, TR) *see* Beclomethasone (Nasal) 232
Rintal (PE) *see* Naphazoline (Nasal) 1426
Rinvox (ID) *see* Levofloxacin (Systemic) 1197
Riobant (IN) *see* Rimonabant [INT] 1814
Riomont (IN) *see* Rimonabant [INT] 1814
Riotol (TW) *see* Ethambutol 798
Riperidon (KR) *see* RisperiDONE 1818
Riper (TW) *see* RisperiDONE 1818
Ripin (TW) *see* Rifampin 1804
Ripol (CL) *see* Sildenafil 1882
Riptam (MX) *see* Oxaliplatin 1528
Riptam (PE) *see* MitoMYcin (Systemic) 1380
Ripunin (TW) *see* Allopurinol 90
Risal (KR) *see* Triflusal [INT] 2103
Riscom (CH) *see* Etofenamate [INT] 815
Risdin (PH) *see* RisperiDONE 1818
Risdon (TW) *see* RisperiDONE 1818
Risedro (AU) *see* Risedronate 1816
Risek (AE, BH, JO, KW, LB, MY, PH, QA, SA) *see* Omeprazole 1508
Riseto (KR) *see* Risedronate 1816
Risfree (KR) *see* RisperiDONE 1818
Risidon (PT) *see* MetFORMIN 1307
Risnel (KR) *see* Risedronate 1816
Risnia (HR) *see* RisperiDONE 1818
Risofos (IN) *see* Risedronate 1816
Risolid (DK, FI) *see* ChlordiazePOXIDE 422
Risonato (EC) *see* Risedronate 1816
Rison (RO) *see* RisperiDONE 1818
Risopent (VE) *see* Clenbuterol [INT] 460
Risoperin (KR) *see* RisperiDONE 1818
Risordan (FR, GR) *see* Isosorbide Dinitrate 1124
Risordan LP (FR) *see* Isosorbide Dinitrate 1124
Rispa (AU) *see* RisperiDONE 1818
Risperdal (AE, AR, AT, AU, BD, BE, BF, BH, BJ, BO, BR, CH, CI, CL, CN, CO, CY, CZ, DE, DK, DO, EC, EE, EG, ES, ET, FI, FR, GB, GH, GM, GN, GR, HK, HN, ID, IE, IL, IQ, IR, IS, IT, JO, KE, KR, KW, LB, LR, LY, MA, ML, MR, MT, MU, MW, MX, MY, NE, NG, NO, NZ, OM, PE, PH, PK, PT, QA, SA, SC, SD, SE, SG, SI, SK, SL, SN, SY, TH, TN, TR, TW, TZ, UG, UY, VE, VN, YE, ZA, ZM, ZW) *see* RisperiDONE 1818
Risperdal Consta (AE, AU, BH, CH, CN, CY, DE, DO, EC, GB, HK, ID, IE, IL, IS, JO, JP, KR, KW, LB, MY, NZ, PE, PH, QA, SA, SE, SG, SI, SK, TH, TW) *see* RisperiDONE 1818
Risperdalconsta LP (FR) *see* RisperiDONE 1818
Risperdal Const (BB, BM, BS, BZ, GY, JM, NL, PR, SR, TT) *see* RisperiDONE 1818
Risperdal Quicklet (AU, BB, BM, BS, BZ, DE, DO, GB, GY, HK, IE, JM, NL, NZ, PH, PR, SG, SI, SR, TH, TT) *see* RisperiDONE 1818
Risperidex (IL) *see* RisperiDONE 1818
Risperigamma (HK) *see* RisperiDONE 1818
Risperon (VN) *see* RisperiDONE 1818
Rispid (IN) *see* RisperiDONE 1818
Rispolept (RU) *see* RisperiDONE 1818
Rispolet (EE, PL) *see* RisperiDONE 1818
Rispolux (CR, GT, NI, PA, SV) *see* RisperiDONE 1818
Rispond (IL, PH) *see* RisperiDONE 1818
Rispons (HK) *see* RisperiDONE 1818
Risset (HR) *see* RisperiDONE 1818
Ristaben (EE) *see* SitaGLIPtin 1897
RISTIDIC (BG) *see* Rivastigmine 1833
Ristonat (ID) *see* Risedronate 1816
Ritalina (AR, BR, PY, UY) *see* Methylphenidate 1336
Ritalin (AE, AT, AU, BF, BH, BJ, CH, CI, CL, CO, CY, CZ, DE, DK, EG, ET, GB, GH, GM, GN, HK, HN, ID, IE, IL, IQ, IR, IS, JO, JP, KE, KW, LB, LR, LY, MA, ML, MR, MU, MW, MX, MY, NE, NG, NO, NZ, OM, PE, PK, QA, SA, SC, SD, SE, SG, SI, SL, SN, SY, TN, TW, TZ, UG, VE, YE, ZM, ZW) *see* Methylphenidate 1336
Ritalina LA (BR, UY) *see* Methylphenidate 1336
Ritaline (BE, FR, GR) *see* Methylphenidate 1336
Ritaline LP (FR) *see* Methylphenidate 1336
Ritalin LA (AU, CO, HK, ID, IL, MY, PE, PT, TR) *see* Methylphenidate 1336
Ritalin LP (VE) *see* Methylphenidate 1336
Ritalin-SR (CH, HK, ID, MY, NZ, SG) *see* Methylphenidate 1336
Ritalin SR (NO, VE) *see* Methylphenidate 1336
Ritalmex (HU) *see* Mexiletine 1359
Rithmik (AU) *see* Amiodarone 114
Ritmetol (HU) *see* Metoprolol 1350
Ritmocor (CL) *see* Propafenone 1725
Ritmocor (IT) *see* QuiNIDine 1759
Ritmodan (IT, PT) *see* Disopyramide 653
Ritmoforine (NL) *see* Disopyramide 653
Ritmonorm (BR, PY) *see* Propafenone 1725
Ritomune (LB) *see* Ritonavir 1822
Ritovir (IN, UY) *see* Ritonavir 1822
Rityne (TH) *see* Loratadine 1241
Rivadem (IN, VN) *see* Rivastigmine 1833
Rivamensa Patch (KR) *see* Rivastigmine 1833
Rivameron Patch (KR) *see* Rivastigmine 1833
Rivapress (TW) *see* Methyldopa 1332
Rivastach (JP) *see* Rivastigmine 1833
Rivasta (TH) *see* Rivastigmine 1833
Rivast (TW) *see* Rivastigmine 1833
Rivatril (FI) *see* ClonazePAM 478
Rivilina (AR, PE) *see* Aprotinin 168
Rivoleve (CH) *see* LevETIRAcetam 1191
Rivopam (SG) *see* ClonazePAM 478
Rivoram (JO) *see* ClonazePAM 478
Rivotril (AE, AR, AT, AU, BD, BE, BG, BH, BO, BR, CH, CR, CY, CZ, DE, DK, DO, EC, EE, EG, ES, FR, GB,

GH, GR, GT, HK, HN, HR, HU, IL, IQ, IR, IS, IT, JO, JP, KE, KR, KW, LB, LT, LU, LY, MX, MY, NI, NL, NO, NZ, OM, PA, PE, PH, PK, PL, PR, PT, PY, QA, RO, SA, SG, SI, SK, SV, SY, TH, TR, TW, TZ, UG, UY, VE, VN, YE, ZM) *see* ClonazePAM 478
Rixadone (AU) *see* RisperiDONE 1818
Rixia (TW) *see* Metolazone 1348
Rizact (IN) *see* Rizatriptan 1836
Rizalt (IL) *see* Rizatriptan 1836
Rizamelt (NZ) *see* Rizatriptan 1836
Rizan (ES) *see* Pimecrolimus 1650
Rizatan (TW) *see* Rizatriptan 1836
R-Loc (BF, BJ, CI, ET, GH, GM, GN, KE, LR, MA, ML, MR, MU, MW, NE, NG, SC, SD, SL, SN, TN, TZ, UG, ZM, ZW) *see* Ranitidine 1777
RND (TW) *see* Ranitidine 1777
Roaccutan (AR, CO, DK, EC, FI, HU, IT, MX, PE, PT, PY, UY, VE) *see* ISOtretinoin 1127
Roaccutane (AE, AU, BB, BE, BG, BH, BS, BZ, CH, CY, CZ, EE, EG, FR, GB, GH, GR, GY, HK, HR, IE, IL, IQ, IR, JM, JO, KE, KR, KW, LB, LT, LU, LY, NL, OM, PH, PK, PR, QA, SA, SI, SK, SR, SY, TH, TR, TT, TW, TZ, UG, YE, ZM) *see* ISOtretinoin 1127
Roaccutane (BH, KW, QA, SA) *see* Tretinoin (Topical) 2099
Roaccuttan (CO) *see* ISOtretinoin 1127
Roacnetan (CN) *see* ISOtretinoin 1127
RoActemra (AT, BE, CH, CZ, DE, DK, EE, FR, GB, HN, HR, IE, IS, LT, NL, NO, PL, PT, RO, RU, SE, SI, SK, TR) *see* Tocilizumab 2057
Roacutan (BR) *see* ISOtretinoin 1127
Roacuttan (HN) *see* ISOtretinoin 1127
Roar (IN) *see* Doxofylline [INT] 679
RoatTeq (CY) *see* Rotavirus Vaccine 1851
Ro-A-Vit (GH, KE, TZ, UG, ZM) *see* Vitamin A 2173
Robatrol (TW) *see* Ribavirin 1797
Robavin (KR) *see* Ribavirin 1797
Robaxin-750 (GB) *see* Methocarbamol 1320
Robaxin (AE, BB, BH, BM, BS, BZ, CH, CO, CY, EG, ES, FI, GY, IL, IQ, IR, JM, JO, KR, KW, LB, LY, NL, OM, QA, SA, SR, SY, TT, YE, ZA) *see* Methocarbamol 1320
Robaz (GR, PH, TH) *see* MetroNIDAZOLE (Topical) 1357
Robicillin VK (AE, BH, CY, EG, IQ, IR, JO, KW, LB, LY, OM, QA, SA, SY, YE) *see* Penicillin V Potassium 1614
Robinax (IN) *see* Methocarbamol 1320
Robin (KR) *see* Leucovorin Calcium 1183
Robinul (AE, EG, JP) *see* Glycopyrrolate 975
Robinul Inj. (AT, AU, BE, CH, DE, DK, FI, GB, GR, IE, NL, NO, NZ, SE, ZA) *see* Glycopyrrolate 975
Robitessin (VE) *see* GuaiFENesin 986
Robitussin (AE, AR, BH, CO, CR, CY, DO, EC, EG, ES, GB, GT, HN, IE, IL, IQ, IR, IT, JO, KW, LB, LU, LY, MX, MY, NI, OM, PA, PH, PL, QA, SA, SV, SY, TH, TW, YE) *see* GuaiFENesin 986
Robitussin Chesty Cough (AU, NZ) *see* GuaiFENesin 986
Robitussin Childrens Cough & Cold (CA) *see* Pseudoephedrine and Dextromethorphan 1743
Robitussin Cough & Cold (CA) *see* Guaifenesin, Pseudoephedrine, and Dextromethorphan 989
Robitussin DM (MX) *see* Guaifenesin and Dextromethorphan 987
Robitussin EX (HK) *see* GuaiFENesin 986
Robitussin Plain (VN) *see* GuaiFENesin 986
Roboral (IL) *see* Oxymetholone 1546
Roburol (IN) *see* Bambuterol [INT] 227
Rocaltriol (DK) *see* Calcitriol 323
Rocaltrol (AE, AT, AU, BB, BE, BG, BH, BM, BR, BS, BZ, CH, CL, CN, CO, CY, CZ, DE, EC, EE, EG, ES, FI, FR, GB, GH, GY, HK, HN, HR, HU, IE, IL, IQ, IR, IT, JM, JO, JP, KE, KR, KW, LB, LU, LY, MT, MX, NL, NO, NZ, OM, PE, PH, PK, PL, PT, QA, RO, RU, SA, SE, SG, SI, SK, SR, SY, TH, TR, TT, TW, TZ, UG, UY, VE, VN, YE, ZM) *see* Calcitriol 323
Rocatan (KR) *see* Losartan 1248
Rocefalin (ES) *see* CefTRIAXone 396
Rocefin (BR, CO, IT) *see* CefTRIAXone 396
Rocefort (GT, HN, NI, SV) *see* CefTRIAXone 396
Rocephalin (DK, FI, IS, NO, SE) *see* CefTRIAXone 396
Rocephin (AE, AT, AU, BH, CH, CN, CY, DE, EC, EG, GB, GH, GR, HK, HR, HU, IE, IL, IQ, IR, JO, JP, KE, KR, KW, LB, LY, MX, NL, OM, PE, PH, PK, PL, PT, PY, QA, RO, SA, SG, SY, TH, TW, TZ, UG, UY, VE, VN, YE, ZM) *see* CefTRIAXone 396
Rocephine (BE, FR, LU) *see* CefTRIAXone 396
Rocephin "Roche" (CZ) *see* CefTRIAXone 396
Rocgel (FR) *see* Aluminum Hydroxide 103
Rocidar (AE, BH, CY, EG, IQ, IR, JO, KW, LB, LY, OM, QA, SA, SY, YE) *see* CefTRIAXone 396
Rocmaline (FR) *see* Arginine 171
Roco (KR) *see* Simvastatin 1890
Rocornal (AT, DE, JP, KR) *see* Trapidil [INT] 2085
Rocta (AU) *see* ISOtretinoin 1127
Roculax (ID) *see* Rocuronium 1838
Rocumeron (KR) *see* Rocuronium 1838
Rocuronio (CO) *see* Rocuronium 1838
Rocur (UY) *see* Rocuronium 1838
Rocy Gen (PH) *see* Gentamicin (Systemic) 959
Rodanol (RU) *see* Nabumetone 1411
Rodazid (PH) *see* MetroNIDAZOLE (Systemic) 1353
Rofatuss (DE) *see* Clobutinol [INT] 468
Rofenid (BE) *see* Ketoprofen 1145
Roflual (FR) *see* Rimantadine 1813
Rofucal (MX) *see* Hydrochlorothiazide 1009
Rogaine (AU, FI, IE, NO, NZ, SE) *see* Minoxidil (Topical) 1374
Rogasti (IL) *see* Famotidine 845
Rogitine (GB) *see* Phentolamine 1636
Rohypnol (PL) *see* Nitrazepam [CAN/INT] 1461
Roical (MY) *see* Calcitriol 323
Roin (JP) *see* Cinnarizine [INT] 440
Rojamin (EC) *see* Cyanocobalamin 515
Rojazol (HR) *see* Miconazole (Topical) 1360
Rokamol Plus (IL) *see* Acetaminophen and Codeine 36
Rolan (AE, BH, CY, EG, IQ, IR, JO, KW, LB, LY, OM, QA, SA, SY, YE) *see* Ranitidine 1777
Rolesen (EC) *see* Ketorolac (Systemic) 1146
Rolicytin (MX) *see* Clarithromycin 456
Rolip (PK) *see* Rosuvastatin 1848
Rolsical (IN) *see* Calcitriol 323
Romacef (PH) *see* CefTAZidime 392
Romenem (TH) *see* Meropenem 1299
Romergon (RO) *see* Promethazine 1723
Romeron (KR) *see* Rocuronium 1838
Romilar rood (NL) *see* Bromhexine [INT] 291
Romiplate (JP) *see* RomiPLOStim 1842
Romisan (ID) *see* Irinotecan 1112
Ronalin (AE, BH, CY, EG, IQ, IR, JO, KW, LB, LY, OM, QA, SA, SY, YE) *see* Bromocriptine 291
Ronasil Derm Gel (KR) *see* Terbinafine (Systemic) 2002
Ronasil Derm Gel (KR) *see* Terbinafine (Topical) 2004
Ronazol (ID) *see* MetroNIDAZOLE (Systemic) 1353
Ronem (ID) *see* Meropenem 1299
Ronex (ID) *see* Tranexamic Acid 2081
Ronexine (IL) *see* Methotrimeprazine [CAN/INT] 1329
Ronox (TH) *see* Gemfibrozil 956
Ronsen Yipu (CN) *see* Tetanus Immune Globulin (Human) 2015
Rontadol (AR) *see* SUMAtriptan 1953
Rontafur (AR) *see* Leucovorin Calcium 1183
Rontin (TH) *see* Gabapentin 943
Ropaccord (AU) *see* ROPINIRole 1844

Ropen (PH) *see* Meropenem 1299
Ropibam (AU) *see* Ropivacaine 1846
Ropica (TW) *see* Ropivacaine 1846
Ropimax (KR) *see* ROPINIRole 1844
Ropion (JP) *see* Flurbiprofen (Systemic) 906
Ropiva (KR) *see* Ropivacaine 1846
Ropril (AE, BH, CY, EG, IQ, IR, JO, KW, LB, LY, OM, QA, SA, SY, TR, YE) *see* Captopril 342
R.O.R. Vax (FR) *see* Measles, Mumps, and Rubella Virus Vaccine 1273
Rosaced gel (BE, FR) *see* MetroNIDAZOLE (Topical) 1357
Rosa (KR) *see* Losartan 1248
Rosa Plus F (KR) *see* Losartan and Hydrochlorothiazide 1250
Roscillin (IN) *see* Ampicillin 141
Rosiced (PT) *see* MetroNIDAZOLE (Topical) 1357
Rosiden (KR, MY, SG) *see* Piroxicam 1662
Rosilan (PT) *see* Deflazacort [INT] 587
Rosil (TH) *see* Clindamycin (Topical) 464
Rosis (TW) *see* Furosemide 940
Rosix (CO) *see* Rosiglitazone 1847
Rossitrol (IT) *see* Roxithromycin [INT] 1853
Rostal (KR) *see* Cilostazol 437
Rosucard (SG) *see* Rosuvastatin 1848
Rosucol (PH) *see* Rosuvastatin 1848
Rosulfant (CO) *see* SulfaSALAzine 1950
Rosup (TW) *see* Loxapine 1255
Rosuterol (KR) *see* Rosuvastatin 1848
Rosuvas (LB) *see* Rosuvastatin 1848
Rosuvaz (PH) *see* Rosuvastatin 1848
Roswin (PH) *see* Rosuvastatin 1848
Rotamax (KR) *see* Losartan 1248
Rotaqor (MY) *see* AtorvaSTATin 194
Rotarix (AE, AR, AT, AU, BE, BG, BH, BR, CH, CL, CO, CY, CZ, DE, DK, DO, EC, EE, ES, FI, FR, GB, GR, HK, HR, ID, IE, IN, IT, JM, JP, KW, LB, LT, MT, MX, MY, NL, NO, NZ, PA, PE, PH, PL, PT, PY, QA, RO, RU, SA, SE, SG, SI, SK, TH, TR, TT, TW, VE, VN) *see* Rotavirus Vaccine 1851
RotaTeq (AE, AU, BH, CO, CR, EC, GT, HK, HN, ID, IL, IN, JP, KR, KW, LB, LT, MY, NI, NZ, PH, QA, SG, SI, SK, SV, TH, TW) *see* Rotavirus Vaccine 1851
Rotateq (BR, HR, RO, VN) *see* Rotavirus Vaccine 1851
Rotaver (ID) *see* Betahistine [CAN/INT] 252
Rotelol (PH) *see* Atenolol 189
Rotesan (ES) *see* Roxithromycin [INT] 1853
Rothacin (AE) *see* Indomethacin 1067
Rotifar (HK, MY) *see* Loratadine 1241
Rotip (TW) *see* Rosuvastatin 1848
Rotopar (EC) *see* Albendazole 65
Rotram (BR) *see* Roxithromycin [INT] 1853
Rotramin (ES) *see* Roxithromycin [INT] 1853
Roug-mycin (GR) *see* Erythromycin (Systemic) 762
Roumin (TW) *see* Prochlorperazine 1718
Rovacor (IN) *see* Lovastatin 1252
Rovadin (ID) *see* Spiramycin [CAN/INT] 1931
Rovalcyte (FR) *see* ValGANciclovir 2121
Rovamax (PH) *see* Spiramycin [CAN/INT] 1931
Rovamicina (BR, CO, IT) *see* Spiramycin [CAN/INT] 1931
Rovamycin (AT, EG, IL, KW, NO, TH) *see* Spiramycin [CAN/INT] 1931
Rovamycine (AE, AR, BE, BG, BH, CH, CZ, DE, EE, ES, FR, GR, HK, HN, HU, ID, JO, KR, LB, LT, LU, MY, NL, PK, PL, PT, PY, QA, RO, RU, SG, SI, SK, VN) *see* Spiramycin [CAN/INT] 1931
Rovamycin Forte (IN) *see* Spiramycin [CAN/INT] 1931
Rovartal (PY) *see* Rosuvastatin 1848
Rovatim (PH) *see* Cefepime 378
Rovatitan (KR) *see* Rosuvastatin 1848
Rovetin (KR) *see* Rosuvastatin 1848
Rovicine (CH) *see* Neomycin 1436
Rovista (PH, PK) *see* Rosuvastatin 1848
Rovixida (AR) *see* Gentamicin (Systemic) 959
Roxcef (BF, BJ, CI, ET, GH, GM, GN, KE, LR, MA, ML, MR, MU, MW, NE, NG, SC, SD, SL, SN, TN, TZ, UG, ZM, ZW) *see* CefTRIAXone 396
Roxet (AU) *see* PARoxetine 1579
Roxi 1A Pharma (DE) *see* Roxithromycin [INT] 1853
Roxi Basics (DE) *see* Roxithromycin [INT] 1853
Roxibeta (DE) *see* Roxithromycin [INT] 1853
Roxibion (FI) *see* Roxithromycin [INT] 1853
Roxicaina (CO) *see* Lidocaine (Topical) 1211
Roxicam (AE, BH, CY, EG, IQ, IR, JO, KW, LB, LY, OM, QA, SA, SY, YE) *see* Piroxicam 1662
Roxid (IN) *see* Roxithromycin [INT] 1853
roxidura (DE) *see* Roxithromycin [INT] 1853
Roxifen (SG) *see* Piroxicam 1662
Roxigamma (DE) *see* Roxithromycin [INT] 1853
Roxigrun (DE) *see* Roxithromycin [INT] 1853
Roxihexal (DE) *see* Roxithromycin [INT] 1853
Roxiklinge (DE) *see* Roxithromycin [INT] 1853
Roxil (AE, BH, LB, QA, SA) *see* Cefadroxil 372
Roximol (IN) *see* Roxithromycin [INT] 1853
Roxin (AU) *see* Norfloxacin 1475
Roxi-paed 1A Pharma (DE) *see* Roxithromycin [INT] 1853
Roxi-Puren (DE) *see* Roxithromycin [INT] 1853
Roxi-saar (DE) *see* Roxithromycin [INT] 1853
Roxithro-Lich (DE) *see* Roxithromycin [INT] 1853
Roxithromycin AZU (DE) *see* Roxithromycin [INT] 1853
Roxithromycin Heumann (DE) *see* Roxithromycin [INT] 1853
Roxithromycin-ratiopharm (DE) *see* Roxithromycin [INT] 1853
Roxithromycin Stada (DE) *see* Roxithromycin [INT] 1853
Roxithromycin "UNP" (DK) *see* Roxithromycin [INT] 1853
Roxium (TH) *see* Piroxicam 1662
roxi von ct (DE) *see* Roxithromycin [INT] 1853
Roxi-Wolff (DE) *see* Roxithromycin [INT] 1853
Roxol (KR) *see* Ambroxol [INT] 109
Roxonin (AE, BH, KW, LB, QA, SA) *see* Loxoprofen [INT] 1255
Roxon (PH) *see* CefTRIAXone 396
Roxorin (PY, UY) *see* DOXOrubicin (Conventional) 679
Roxyrol (IN) *see* Roxithromycin [INT] 1853
Royen (AR, CO, UY) *see* Calcium Acetate 326
Rozac (IN) *see* Adapalene 54
Rozacreme (FR) *see* MetroNIDAZOLE (Topical) 1357
Rozagel (FR) *see* MetroNIDAZOLE (Topical) 1357
Rozamet (HR) *see* MetroNIDAZOLE (Topical) 1357
Roza Plus (KR) *see* Losartan and Hydrochlorothiazide 1250
Rozasaltan (KR) *see* Losartan 1248
Rozataplus (KR) *see* Losartan and Hydrochlorothiazide 1250
Roza (TR) *see* MetroNIDAZOLE (Topical) 1357
Rozerem (ID, JP) *see* Ramelteon 1770
Rozex (AR, AT, AU, BE, BR, CH, CO, CZ, DK, EE, FI, FR, GB, HK, IE, IL, IT, KR, LB, MY, NL, NO, NZ, PE, PL, PY, SA, SE, SG, UY, VE, ZA) *see* MetroNIDAZOLE (Topical) 1357
Rozgra (ID) *see* Sildenafil 1882
Rozinin (TW) *see* Rosuvastatin 1848
Rozoxin (TW) *see* Levofloxacin (Systemic) 1197
Rualba (KR) *see* Leflunomide 1174
Rubex (BR) *see* DOXOrubicin (Conventional) 679
Rubicin (PH) *see* DOXOrubicin (Conventional) 679
Rubidexol (MX) *see* Methadone 1311
RubieFol (DE) *see* Folic Acid 919
RubieMen (DE) *see* DimenhyDRINATE 637
RubieNex (DE) *see* Ergotamine 754

Rubifen (AR, ES, MY, NZ, PT, SG, TH, UY) *see* Methylphenidate ... 1336
Rubilem (MX, PE) *see* DAUNOrubicin (Conventional) ... 577
Rubimycin (ZA) *see* Erythromycin (Systemic) ... 762
Rubisandin (ID) *see* Epirubicin ... 739
Rubocort (GR) *see* Clobetasol ... 468
Rubophen (HU) *see* Acetaminophen ... 32
Rubramin (PH) *see* Cyanocobalamin ... 515
Rubranova (BR) *see* Hydroxocobalamin ... 1020
Rucef (PH) *see* Cefuroxime ... 399
Ruconest (CZ, DE, DK, EE, FI, FR, GB, IL, LT, NL, NO, PL, PT, SE, SI, SK) *see* C1 Inhibitor (Recombinant) ... 316
Rudakol (HR) *see* Mebeverine [INT] ... 1275
Rudotel (DE, HU, LT, PL, RU, SK) *see* Medazepam [INT] ... 1277
Ruflam (CO) *see* Rufloxacin [INT] ... 1855
Rufull (JP) *see* Fluocinonide ... 894
Rui Di (CL) *see* Ribavirin ... 1797
Rui Jei (CN) *see* Remifentanil ... 1789
RuiLi (CN) *see* Nimesulide [INT] ... 1456
Rui Na Ti (CN) *see* Ketotifen (Systemic) [CAN/INT] ... 1149
Rui Nuo Sai (CN) *see* Tobramycin (Systemic, Oral Inhalation) ... 2052
Rui Tong Li (CN) *see* Reteplase ... 1794
Rui Yang (CN) *see* Febuxostat ... 848
Rukasyn (KR) *see* Ampicillin and Sulbactam ... 145
Rulid (AR, BE, BR, CH, CZ, DE, FR, HR, HU, IT, JP, LU, MX) *see* Roxithromycin [INT] ... 1853
Rulide (AT, AU, ES, NL, PT) *see* Roxithromycin [INT] ... 1853
Rulivan (ES) *see* Nefazodone ... 1435
Rulofer G (DE) *see* Ferrous Gluconate ... 870
Rulofer N (DE) *see* Ferrous Fumarate ... 870
Rumafluor (FR) *see* Fluoride ... 895
Rumaterin (KR) *see* Diacerein [INT] ... 613
Rumicil (LU) *see* Acetylcysteine ... 40
Rumorf (IN) *see* Morphine (Systemic) ... 1394
Runbao (CN) *see* Urea ... 2114
Runbo (CN) *see* Cromolyn (Ophthalmic) ... 514
Run Rui (CN) *see* CloNIDine ... 480
Runzheng (CN) *see* Tropicamide ... 2108
Ruo Mai (CN) *see* Loxoprofen [INT] ... 1255
Rupafin (AR, BR, CY, DE, EE, ES, GB, GR, HR, IT, LT, NL, SG, SI, SK, TH, TR) *see* Rupatadine [INT] ... 1855
Rupahjist (IN) *see* Rupatadine [INT] ... 1855
Rupan (AE, BH, CY, EG, IQ, IR, JO, KW, LB, LY, OM, QA, SA, SY, YE) *see* Ibuprofen ... 1032
Rupastar (IN) *see* Rupatadine [INT] ... 1855
Rupatall (BE, SE) *see* Rupatadine [INT] ... 1855
Rupatal (NZ) *see* Rupatadine [INT] ... 1855
Rupax (CR, DO, GT, HN, NI, PA, SV) *see* Rupatadine [INT] ... 1855
Rupegen (AR) *see* Gentamicin (Systemic) ... 959
Rupilip (MX) *see* Rosuvastatin ... 1848
Rupiz (IN) *see* Rupatadine [INT] ... 1855
Ruprofen (TH) *see* Ibuprofen ... 1032
Rusedal (DE) *see* Medazepam [INT] ... 1277
Rustin (IE) *see* AmLODIPine ... 123
Rustor (PH) *see* Rosuvastatin ... 1848
Ruvamed (GR) *see* Piroxicam ... 1662
Rydene (BE, LU) *see* NiCARdipine ... 1446
Ryebact (PH) *see* Erythromycin (Systemic) ... 762
Rynacrom (AU, GB, IE) *see* Cromolyn (Nasal) ... 514
Rysmon TG (KR) *see* Timolol (Ophthalmic) ... 2043
Rythma (PH) *see* Amiodarone ... 114
Rythmex (IL) *see* Propafenone ... 1725
Rythmical (IL) *see* Disopyramide ... 653
Rythmodan (AE, AT, AU, BE, BH, CY, CZ, EG, FR, GB, GR, IE, IQ, IR, JO, KW, LB, LU, LY, NL, NZ, OM, PL, QA, RU, SA, SY, YE, ZA) *see* Disopyramide ... 653
Rythmodan Retard (PL, ZA) *see* Disopyramide ... 653
Rythmodul (DE) *see* Disopyramide ... 653
Rythmol (CO, FR, VN, ZA) *see* Propafenone ... 1725
Rythmonorm (GR) *see* Propafenone ... 1725
Rythocin (TH) *see* Erythromycin (Systemic) ... 762
Rytmilen (BG, CZ, PL, RU) *see* Disopyramide ... 653
Rytmocard (BG, PH) *see* Propafenone ... 1725
Rytmol (UY) *see* Propafenone ... 1725
Rytmonorma (AT) *see* Propafenone ... 1725
Rytmonorm (AE, AU, BE, CH, CN, CY, CZ, DE, DK, EE, EG, ES, FI, HK, HN, HR, HU, ID, IT, JO, KR, KW, LT, LU, MY, NL, NZ, PE, PL, PT, QA, RU, SE, SG, SI, SK, TH, TR, TW, VE) *see* Propafenone ... 1725
Ryvel (ID) *see* Cetirizine ... 411
Ryytmonorm (RO) *see* Propafenone ... 1725
Ryzen (ID) *see* Cetirizine ... 411
SAAZ (IN) *see* SulfaSALAzine ... 1950
Sabima (MX) *see* Secnidazole [INT] ... 1872
Sabril (AE, AR, AT, AU, BE, BH, BR, CH, CL, CO, CY, CZ, DE, EG, FR, GB, GR, HK, HN, HR, HU, IE, IT, KR, KW, LB, LU, NL, NZ, PL, PT, PY, QA, SA, SG, SI, SK, TH, TR, TW, UY, VN, ZA) *see* Vigabatrin ... 2158
Sabrilan (IL) *see* Vigabatrin ... 2158
Sabrilex (DK, ES, FI, IS, NO, SE) *see* Vigabatrin ... 2158
Sabrinin (AT) *see* Niflumic Acid [INT] ... 1454
Sabutal (TW) *see* Albuterol ... 69
Sadoxol (UY) *see* Cilostazol ... 437
Safemar (MX) *see* Lansoprazole ... 1166
Safe Pill (PH) *see* Ethinyl Estradiol and Levonorgestrel ... 803
Safe Plan (TW) *see* Levonorgestrel ... 1201
Safepril (TW) *see* Lisinopril ... 1226
Safe (TW) *see* Loperamide ... 1236
Safol (ID) *see* Propofol ... 1728
Safrosyn S (MY) *see* Naproxen ... 1427
Sagalon (ID) *see* Doxepin (Systemic) ... 676
Sagalon (ID) *see* Doxepin (Topical) ... 678
Sagal (PY) *see* Remifentanil ... 1789
Sagestam Eye Drops (ID) *see* Gentamicin (Ophthalmic) ... 962
Sagestam Eye Drops (ID) *see* Gentamicin (Systemic) ... 959
Saifulong (CN) *see* Cefotaxime ... 382
Saifuning (CN) *see* CeFAZolin ... 373
Saikel (AR) *see* Rufinamide ... 1854
Sai Lai De (CN) *see* Balsalazide ... 226
Saitan (CN) *see* Telmisartan ... 1988
Saizen (AE, AR, AT, AU, BH, BR, CH, CL, CN, CO, CR, CY, CZ, DE, DO, EC, EE, ES, FI, FR, GR, GT, HK, HN, HU, ID, IL, IS, IT, JO, KR, KW, MY, NI, NO, NZ, PA, PH, PT, QA, SA, SE, SG, SK, SV, TH, TR, TW, VN) *see* Somatropin ... 1918
Salac (PY) *see* Clobetasol ... 468
Salagen (AT, CH, CO, DE, ES, FI, FR, GB, GR, HK, IL, IT, JP, KR, NO, PT, SE, SG, TH, TW, VN) *see* Pilocarpine (Systemic) ... 1649
Salalin (TW) *see* Chlorzoxazone ... 430
Salamol (CH, MY) *see* Albuterol ... 69
Salarizine (JP) *see* Cinnarizine [INT] ... 440
Sala (TW) *see* Salsalate ... 1862
Salazine (TH, TW) *see* SulfaSALAzine ... 1950
Salazodin (UY) *see* SulfaSALAzine ... 1950
Salazopirina (PT) *see* SulfaSALAzine ... 1950
Salazopyrin (AE, AT, AU, BH, CH, CY, DK, EG, ES, FI, GB, HN, HU, IE, IL, IQ, IR, IS, IT, JO, KW, LB, LY, NO, NZ, OM, PK, PL, QA, SA, SE, SY, TR, YE, ZA) *see* SulfaSALAzine ... 1950
Salazopyrina (ES) *see* SulfaSALAzine ... 1950
Salazopyrine (BE, FR, LU, NL, VN) *see* SulfaSALAzine ... 1950
Salazopyrine EC (BE) *see* SulfaSALAzine ... 1950
Salazopyrin-EN (AU, BG, CH, CO, CZ, EE, FI, GB, HK, IL, IT, KR, MY, NO, NZ, SE, TH, TW, ZA) *see* SulfaSALAzine ... 1950

Salazopyrin EN (HR, RO) *see* SulfaSALAzine 1950
Salazopyrin Entabs (AE, BH, CY, DK, EG, IQ, IR, JO, KW, LB, LY, OM, QA, SA, SY, YE) *see* SulfaSALAzine 1950
Salbetol (IN) *see* Albuterol 69
Salbron (ID) *see* Albuterol 69
Salbuflo (PH) *see* Albuterol 69
Salbulin (LU) *see* Albuterol 69
Salbutalan (MX) *see* Albuterol 69
Salbutamol-GW (HU) *see* Albuterol 69
Salbutamol (HU) *see* Albuterol 69
Salbutan (VE) *see* Albuterol 69
Salbutin (AE, BH, CY, EG, IQ, IR, JO, KW, LB, LY, OM, QA, SA, SY, YE) *see* Albuterol 69
Salbutol (KR) *see* Albuterol 69
Salbuven (ID) *see* Albuterol 69
Salbuvent (PE) *see* Albuterol 69
Salimag (PL) *see* Magnesium Salicylate 1265
Salinex (IN) *see* Furosemide 940
Salipax (BB, BM, BS, BZ, GY, JM, MY, PL, SR, TT) *see* FLUoxetine 899
Salisalido (AE, BH, CY, EG, IQ, IR, JO, KW, LB, LY, OM, QA, SA, SY, YE) *see* Aspirin 180
Salivon (ID) *see* SulfaSALAzine 1950
Salmaplon (IN) *see* Albuterol 69
Salmed (PH) *see* Fluticasone and Salmeterol 912
Salmeflo (PH) *see* Fluticasone and Salmeterol 912
Salmocalcin (AR) *see* Calcitonin 322
Salmocin (TH) *see* Calcitonin 322
Salofalk (AT, AU, BG, CH, CL, CN, CO, CR, CZ, DE, EE, GB, GT, HK, HN, HR, HU, ID, IE, LT, MY, NL, PA, PE, PH, PL, RO, SG, SI, SK, SV, TH, TR, UY) *see* Mesalamine 1301
Salofalk Foam Enema (AU) *see* Mesalamine 1301
Salomol (TW) *see* Albuterol 69
Salongo (ES) *see* Oxiconazole 1536
Salopyr (FI) *see* SulfaSALAzine 1950
Salopyrine (GR) *see* SulfaSALAzine 1950
Salospir (GR) *see* Aspirin 180
Salpraz (AU) *see* Pantoprazole 1570
Saltam (ID) *see* Albuterol 69
Salterprim (ZA) *see* Allopurinol 90
Saluretil (ES) *see* Chlorothiazide 426
Saluretin (BG) *see* Chlorthalidone 430
Saluric (GB, IE) *see* Chlorothiazide 426
Salurin (AE, KW, SA) *see* Furosemide 940
Salutrid (FI) *see* Chlorothiazide 426
Salutyl (IN) *see* Collagenase (Topical) 507
Salvacam (CR, DO, GT, HN, NI, PA, SV) *see* Piroxicam 1662
Salvacolina (DO, ES, GT, HN, PA, SV) *see* Loperamide 1236
Salvacyl (GB) *see* Triptorelin 2107
Salymbra (EE) *see* Tianeptine [INT] 2033
Salzone (BF, BJ, CI, ET, GH, GM, GN, KE, LR, MA, ML, MR, MU, MW, NE, NG, SC, SD, SL, SN, TN, TZ, UG, ZM, ZW) *see* Acetaminophen 32
Samixon (AE, BH, CY, EG, IQ, IR, JO, KW, LB, LY, OM, QA, SA, SY, YE) *see* CefTRIAXone 396
Samnir (TH) *see* Cefdinir 376
Samsca (AU, CZ, DE, DK, EE, FR, GB, HK, HR, ID, JP, KR, LT, NL, NO, PH, PL, PT, RO, SE, SK, TH) *see* Tolvaptan 2064
Samtirel (JP) *see* Atovaquone 197
Sanaprav (AT, IT) *see* Pravastatin 1700
Sanaxin (AT) *see* Cephalexin 405
Sanbenafil (ID) *see* Sildenafil 1882
Sancoba (JP) *see* Cyanocobalamin 515
Sancos (TW) *see* Lovastatin 1252
Sancotec (KR) *see* Cetirizine 411
Sancuso Patch (GB, HK, KR, LT, SK) *see* Granisetron 983
Sanda (TH) *see* CycloSPORINE (Systemic) 522
Sandel (TW) *see* Dipyridamole 652
Sandepril (ID) *see* Maprotiline 1271
Sandimmun (AT, AU, BE, BF, BJ, CH, CI, CL, CZ, DE, DK, EE, EG, ET, FI, FR, GB, GH, GM, GN, GR, HK, HN, ID, IE, IL, IS, IT, JP, KE, KR, LR, MA, ML, MR, MT, MU, MW, MY, NE, NG, NO, NZ, PE, PH, PK, PL, PT, RU, SC, SD, SE, SI, SK, SL, SN, TN, TR, TW, TZ, UG, UY, VE, ZM, ZW) *see* CycloSPORINE (Systemic) 522
Sandimmune (NL) *see* CycloSPORINE (Systemic) 522
Sandimmun Neoral (AE, AR, AT, AU, BH, BR, CH, CL, CY, CZ, EE, EG, FI, GB, GR, HK, HR, ID, IL, IQ, IR, IS, JO, KR, KW, LB, LY, MY, NO, OM, PE, PH, PL, PY, QA, RO, SA, SE, SI, SK, SY, TH, TR, UY, VE, VN, YE, ZA) *see* CycloSPORINE (Systemic) 522
Sandmigrin (IS) *see* Pizotifen [CAN/INT] 1664
Sandobicin (ID) *see* DOXOrubicin (Conventional) 679
Sandocal (PT) *see* Calcium Glubionate 330
Sandoglobulina (CO, IT, PE) *see* Immune Globulin 1056
Sandoglobulin (AE, BH, CZ, DK, EG, FI, GR, IL, KW, LB, NO, NZ, PK, QA) *see* Immune Globulin 1056
Sando-K (GB) *see* Potassium Bicarbonate and Potassium Chloride 1687
Sando-K (GB) *see* Potassium Chloride 1687
Sandomigran (AR, AT, AU, BE, BR, CZ, DE, ES, FR, GB, HK, HU, IE, IL, IT, JO, LU, MY, NL, NZ, SK, VE) *see* Pizotifen [CAN/INT] 1664
Sandomigrin (DK, NO, SE, TR) *see* Pizotifen [CAN/INT] 1664
Sandopril (AT, LU) *see* Spirapril [INT] 1931
Sandostatin (AE, AR, AT, AU, BD, BG, BH, BR, CH, CL, CN, CY, CZ, DE, DK, EE, EG, ES, FI, GB, GR, HK, HN, HR, ID, IE, IL, IN, IQ, IR, IS, JO, JP, KR, KW, LB, LT, LY, MT, MY, NO, NZ, OM, PE, PH, PK, PL, PY, QA, RO, RU, SA, SE, SG, SI, SK, SY, TH, TR, TW, UY, VE, VN, YE) *see* Octreotide 1485
Sandostatina (IT, MX, PT) *see* Octreotide 1485
Sandostatina LAR (CO) *see* Octreotide 1485
Sandostatine (BE, FR, NL) *see* Octreotide 1485
Sandostatin LAR (AE, AR, AU, BG, BH, BR, CH, CL, CN, CY, EC, EE, HR, ID, IL, IS, JP, KR, LB, LT, MY, NO, NZ, PE, PH, PY, RO, SA, SE, SG, SI, SK, TH, TW, UY, VN) *see* Octreotide 1485
Sandoz Fenezal (AU) *see* Promethazine 1723
Sandrena (CL) *see* Estradiol (Topical) 780
Sandrena (BR, CH) *see* Estradiol (Systemic) 775
Sandrena Gel (AU, DE) *see* Estradiol (Systemic) 775
Sanelor (LU) *see* Loratadine 1241
Sanexon (ID) *see* MethylPREDNISolone 1340
Sanifer (UY) *see* Ivermectin (Systemic) 1136
Saniter (CL) *see* Carbidopa and Levodopa 351
Sanmasu (TW) *see* Butenafine 314
Sanmetidin (ID) *see* Cimetidine 438
Sanmol Infusion (ID) *see* Acetaminophen 32
Sanobamat (BE) *see* Meprobamate 1296
Sanogyl (FR) *see* Fluoride 895
Sanoma (DE) *see* Carisoprodol 363
Sanoral (EE) *see* Amlodipine and Olmesartan 126
Sanoral HCT (EE) *see* Olmesartan, Amlodipine, and Hydrochlorothiazide 1498
Sanorin (CZ, EE) *see* Naphazoline (Ophthalmic) 1426
Sanorin (CZ, EE, RU) *see* Naphazoline (Nasal) 1426
Sanor (MY) *see* Clorazepate 487
Sanotrexat (ID) *see* Methotrexate 1322
Sanpicillin (ID) *see* Ampicillin 141
Sanpime (PH) *see* Cefepime 378
Sanpo (TW) *see* Loperamide 1236
Sanprima Forte (ID) *see* Sulfamethoxazole and Trimethoprim 1946
Sanprima (ID) *see* Sulfamethoxazole and Trimethoprim 1946
Sanroxa (ID) *see* Oxaliplatin 1528
Sansibast (MX) *see* Montelukast 1392

Sanspen (PH) *see* Bupivacaine ... 299
Santesar (ID) *see* Losartan ... 1248
Santeson (PH) *see* Dexamethasone (Ophthalmic) ... 602
Santimin (TW) *see* Carbinoxamine ... 356
Santiten (TW) *see* Ketotifen (Systemic) [CAN/INT] ... 1149
Santocyn (ID) *see* Oxytocin ... 1549
Santotaxel (ID) *see* PACLitaxel (Conventional) ... 1550
Santrone (HK) *see* MitoXANtrone ... 1382
Santuril (CH) *see* Probenecid ... 1716
Sanval (RU) *see* Zolpidem ... 2212
Saphris (AU, BR, CL, CO, IL, MY, NZ, PH, SG) *see* Asenapine ... 179
Sapofen (AE, BH, JO, KW, QA, SA) *see* Ibuprofen ... 1032
Sapofen Plus (BH, KW, QA, SA) *see* Pseudoephedrine and Ibuprofen ... 1743
Sapratol (JP) *see* Cinnarizine [INT] ... 440
Sapril (PH) *see* Fosinopril ... 932
Sarcoderma (PT) *see* Lindane ... 1217
Sarcoton (BR) *see* Disulfiram ... 654
Sarex (TH) *see* Lactulose ... 1156
Saridine-E (HK, TH) *see* SulfaSALAzine ... 1950
Saridon (CO) *see* Acetaminophen ... 32
Sarlotan Plus (KR) *see* Losartan and Hydrochlorothiazide ... 1250
Sarnol (EC) *see* Permethrin ... 1627
Saropram (KR) *see* Escitalopram ... 765
Sarotard (KR) *see* Amitriptyline ... 119
Sarotena (IN) *see* Amitriptyline ... 119
Saroten (BF, BJ, CI, CY, DE, DK, EE, ET, GH, GM, GN, GR, IR, JO, KE, LR, MA, ML, MR, MU, MW, NE, NG, PT, RU, SA, SC, SD, SE, SL, SN, TN, TR, TZ, UG, ZA, ZM, ZW) *see* Amitriptyline ... 119
Saroten Retard (CH, MY) *see* Amitriptyline ... 119
Sarotex (NL, NO, UY) *see* Amitriptyline ... 119
Sarotex Retard (NO) *see* Amitriptyline ... 119
Sarpul (JP) *see* Aniracetam [INT] ... 150
Sartan-8 (PH) *see* Candesartan ... 335
Sartan-16 (PH) *see* Candesartan ... 335
Sativex (AU, CZ, DE, DK, ES, FI, GB, IS, NL, NO, NZ, SE, SK) *see* Tetrahydrocannabinol and Cannabidiol [CAN/INT] ... 2018
Satolax-10 (JP) *see* Bisacodyl ... 265
Satoren (CO, DO, EC, GT, HN, NI, PA, SV) *see* Losartan ... 1248
Satoren H (CO) *see* Losartan and Hydrochlorothiazide ... 1250
Satural (PL) *see* Calcium Glubionate ... 330
Savacol Mouth and Throat Rinse (AU) *see* Chlorhexidine Gluconate ... 422
Savador (IN) *see* Doripenem ... 671
Savene (AT, BE, BG, CH, CZ, DE, DK, EE, FR, GB, GR, HN, HR, IE, IT, JP, LT, MT, NL, NO, PL, PT, RO, RU, SE, SI, SK, TR) *see* Dexrazoxane ... 606
Saventrine (AE, FI, GB, GR, IE, QA, SG) *see* Isoproterenol ... 1124
Savilen (GR) *see* Ciprofibrate [INT] ... 441
Savlon (AE) *see* Chlorhexidine Gluconate ... 422
Savox (TW) *see* Amikacin ... 111
Sawatal (JP) *see* Propranolol ... 1731
Saxobin (TW) *see* Doxazosin ... 674
Sayana (IL) *see* MedroxyPROGESTERone ... 1277
Sayana Press (GB) *see* MedroxyPROGESTERone ... 1277
Sayomol (ES) *see* Promethazine ... 1723
SBT (IL) *see* Buprenorphine ... 300
Scabecid (FR) *see* Lindane ... 1217
Scabene (PK) *see* Lindane ... 1217
Scabicin (IL) *see* Crotamiton ... 514
Scabimite (ID) *see* Permethrin ... 1627
Scabisan (MX) *see* Permethrin ... 1627
Scabi (TW) *see* Lindane ... 1217
Scabix (BR) *see* Lindane ... 1217
Scaboma (MY, VN) *see* Lindane ... 1217
Scaflam (BR, CO, VE) *see* Nimesulide [INT] ... 1456
Scalid (BR) *see* Nimesulide [INT] ... 1456
Scalpmad (KR) *see* Minoxidil (Topical) ... 1374
Scandicain (AT, CH) *see* Mepivacaine ... 1295
Scandicaine (BE, LU, NL, SA) *see* Mepivacaine ... 1295
Scandinibsa (ES, PT) *see* Mepivacaine ... 1295
Scandonest (AE, AU, BG, EE, EG, FI, KR, KW, LT, NZ, RO, SI, SK) *see* Mepivacaine ... 1295
Scandonest Sans Vasoconstricteur (PL) *see* Mepivacaine ... 1295
Scarda (TH) *see* Piracetam [INT] ... 1661
S-Celepra (PH) *see* Escitalopram ... 765
Scelto (ID) *see* Ketorolac (Systemic) ... 1146
Scene (VN) *see* Azelaic Acid ... 213
Scepos (TW) *see* Calcipotriene ... 321
Schmerz Spray (DE) *see* Indomethacin ... 1067
Scilin M30 (PH) *see* Insulin NPH and Insulin Regular ... 1090
SciLin N (CN) *see* Insulin NPH ... 1089
Scilin N (HK, PH) *see* Insulin NPH ... 1089
Scilin R (PH) *see* Insulin Regular ... 1091
SciLocyte (PH) *see* Filgrastim ... 875
Scitropin A (AU, TH) *see* Somatropin ... 1918
Scitropina (SG) *see* Somatropin ... 1918
Scitropin (PH) *see* Somatropin ... 1918
Sclefic (BG) *see* Riluzole ... 1812
Sclerol (IN) *see* Polidocanol ... 1672
Sclerovein (SE) *see* Polidocanol ... 1672
Scoburen (FR) *see* Scopolamine (Systemic) ... 1870
Scoline (IN) *see* Succinylcholine ... 1939
Scolmin (PH) *see* Scopolamine (Systemic) ... 1870
Scopamin (ID) *see* Scopolamine (Systemic) ... 1870
Scopma (ID) *see* Scopolamine (Systemic) ... 1870
Scopoderm (AT, DK, FI, GB, IS, SE) *see* Scopolamine (Systemic) ... 1870
Scopoderm TTS (AE, FR, NL, NZ, QA, SI) *see* Scopolamine (Systemic) ... 1870
Scopolamine Dispersa (CH) *see* Scopolamine (Systemic) ... 1870
Scorbex (ZA) *see* Ascorbic Acid ... 178
Scutamil C (CZ) *see* Carisoprodol ... 363
SD-Hermal (DE) *see* Clotrimazole (Topical) ... 488
Sea-Legs (NZ) *see* Meclizine ... 1277
Seaze (AU) *see* LamoTRIgine ... 1160
Sebexol (DE) *see* Urea ... 2114
Sebifin (IN) *see* Terbinafine (Systemic) ... 2002
Sebifin (IN) *see* Terbinafine (Topical) ... 2004
Sebiprox (KR) *see* Ciclopirox ... 433
Sebizole (AU, NZ) *see* Ketoconazole (Topical) ... 1145
Sebo-Lenium (CH) *see* Selenium Sulfide ... 1877
Sebosel (IL, TH) *see* Selenium Sulfide ... 1877
Sebrinal (PY) *see* Hydroquinone ... 1020
Sebron (KR) *see* Acetylcysteine ... 40
Secagyn (IL) *see* Ergotamine ... 754
Secapine (ZA) *see* Cimetidine ... 438
Secfar (BR) *see* Secnidazole [INT] ... 1872
Sechvitan (JP) *see* Pyridoxine ... 1747
Secnidal (CO, EC, PE) *see* Secnidazole [INT] ... 1872
Secnil (IN) *see* Secnidazole [INT] ... 1872
Secnol (FR, VN) *see* Secnidazole [INT] ... 1872
Seconal Sodium (GB) *see* Secobarbital ... 1872
Secotex (AR, BR, CL, CO, CR, DO, GT, HN, MX, NI, PA, PE, PY, SV, UY, VE) *see* Tamsulosin ... 1974
Secotex OCAS (CR, DO, EC, GT, HN, NI, PA, SV) *see* Tamsulosin ... 1974
Sectral (AT, BB, BE, BM, BR, BS, BZ, CH, CZ, EG, ES, FR, GB, GY, HK, IE, IL, IN, IQ, IR, IT, JM, JP, KR, LU, LY, PL, SG, SR, SY, TT, TW, VN, YE, ZA) *see* Acebutolol ... 29
Sectral LP (FR) *see* Acebutolol ... 29
Securo (AR) *see* Ivermectin (Systemic) ... 1136
Securon (GB, IE) *see* Verapamil ... 2154
Seczol (VE) *see* Secnidazole [INT] ... 1872
Sedaben (BE) *see* Lormetazepam [INT] ... 1247

Sedacoron (AT, HK, JO, LB, SA, TW, VN) *see* Amiodarone ... 114
Sedacum (ID, PH) *see* Midazolam ... 1361
Sedalito (MX) *see* Acetaminophen ... 32
Sedamax (PE) *see* Bromazepam [CAN/INT] ... 290
Sedanium-R (GR) *see* Famotidine ... 845
Sedansol Iso (JP) *see* Isoproterenol ... 1124
Sedans Tranquilizante (ES) *see* Meprobamate ... 1296
Sedarest (PE) *see* Estazolam ... 775
Sedatival (CL, PE) *see* Ketazolam [INT] ... 1144
Sedatival (AR) *see* LORazepam ... 1243
Sedergine (BE) *see* Aspirin ... 180
Sederlona (ES) *see* CloBAZam ... 465
Sedium (PY) *see* Diazepam ... 613
Sedlingtus (AU) *see* Pholcodine [INT] ... 1646
Sedofan II (AE) *see* Pseudoephedrine ... 1742
Sedofan (AE, BH, KW, LB, QA, SA) *see* Triprolidine and Pseudoephedrine ... 2105
Sedolox (AT) *see* Zopiclone [CAN/INT] ... 2217
Sedorm (CO) *see* Zopiclone [CAN/INT] ... 2217
Sedotime (ES, PE) *see* Ketazolam [INT] ... 1144
Sedoz (PH) *see* Midazolam ... 1361
Sedrena (JP) *see* Trihexyphenidyl ... 2103
Sedron (KR) *see* Risedronate ... 1816
Sedural (IL) *see* Phenazopyridine ... 1629
Seduxen (BB, BM, BS, BZ, EE, GY, HN, HU, JM, NL, PR, SR, TT, VN) *see* Diazepam ... 613
Sefaclor (MY) *see* Cefaclor ... 372
Sefdene (HK) *see* Piroxicam ... 1662
Sefdin (IN) *see* Cefdinir ... 376
Sefloc (TH) *see* Metoprolol ... 1350
Sefmal (HK, SG, VN) *see* TraMADol ... 2074
Sefmex (HK, MY) *see* Selegiline ... 1873
Sefmic (HK) *see* Mefenamic Acid ... 1280
Sefnac (TH) *see* Diclofenac (Systemic) ... 617
Sefnor (TH) *see* Norfloxacin ... 1475
Sefotak (AE, BH, CY, CZ, EG, IQ, IR, JO, KW, LB, LY, OM, QA, SA, SY, YE) *see* Cefotaxime ... 382
Sefpime (PH, TH) *see* Cefepime ... 378
Sefson (PE) *see* Dorzolamide ... 673
Sefson T (PE) *see* Dorzolamide and Timolol ... 673
Seftem (JP, KR, TW) *see* Ceftibuten ... 394
SEF (TR) *see* Cephalexin ... 405
Sefuxim (HK) *see* Cefuroxime ... 399
Seglor (AR, FR, IT, LU, TW) *see* Dihydroergotamine ... 633
Seglor Retard (PT) *see* Dihydroergotamine ... 633
Segregam (CO) *see* Pantoprazole ... 1570
Seguril (ES) *see* Furosemide ... 940
Seibule (JP) *see* Miglitol ... 1367
Seif (PH) *see* Ethinyl Estradiol and Levonorgestrel ... 803
Seladin (MY, SG) *see* Naproxen ... 1427
Selars (TW) *see* Oxazepam ... 1532
Selaxa (GR) *see* Amikacin ... 111
Seldepar (TR) *see* Selegiline ... 1873
Seldiar (HR) *see* Loperamide ... 1236
Seldron (SG) *see* Selenium Sulfide ... 1877
Selectan (HK) *see* Valsartan ... 2127
Selectin (IT) *see* Pravastatin ... 1700
Selectol (AE, AT, BE, CH, CL, CY, DE, FI, GR, HR, IE, KR, LU, TR) *see* Celiprolol [INT] ... 404
Selecturon (AT) *see* Celiprolol [INT] ... 404
Selegesic (PH) *see* Acetaminophen ... 32
Selegil (CO, PE) *see* Selegiline ... 1873
Selegos (PH, RO, SG) *see* Selegiline ... 1873
Selektine (NL) *see* Pravastatin ... 1700
Selektine (SA) *see* Meloxicam ... 1283
Selemycin (AE, BH, CY, EG, IL, IQ, IR, JO, KW, LB, LY, OM, QA, SA, SY, YE) *see* Amikacin ... 111
Selenium Microsol (FR) *see* Selenium ... 1876
Selenix (PT) *see* Selenium Sulfide ... 1877
Seler (PY) *see* Benserazide and Levodopa [CAN/INT] ... 244
Selexa (PT) *see* Celecoxib ... 402
Selezin (TW) *see* Selegiline ... 1873
Selfide (TH) *see* Selenium Sulfide ... 1877
Selgene (AU) *see* Selegiline ... 1873
Selgina (CL) *see* Selegiline ... 1873
Selgin (IN, PK) *see* Selegiline ... 1873
Selipran (AT, CH) *see* Pravastatin ... 1700
Sellon (HK, MY, TH) *see* Selenium Sulfide ... 1877
Selokeen (NL) *see* Metoprolol ... 1350
Seloken (BE, DK, FI, FR, ID, IS, IT, JP, NO, SE) *see* Metoprolol ... 1350
Seloken Retard (AT, IT) *see* Metoprolol ... 1350
Seloken Zoc (FI, SE) *see* Metoprolol ... 1350
Seloken-Zok (MX) *see* Metoprolol ... 1350
Seloken Zok (IS) *see* Metoprolol ... 1350
Selopral (FI) *see* Metoprolol ... 1350
Selozok (BE, DK, LU) *see* Metoprolol ... 1350
Selo-zok (DK, NO) *see* Metoprolol ... 1350
Selozok LP (FR) *see* Metoprolol ... 1350
Selson (KR) *see* Selenium Sulfide ... 1877
Selsun (AE, AR, AT, BB, BE, BH, BM, BR, BS, BZ, CH, CO, CY, DK, EG, FI, FR, GB, GR, GY, ID, IE, IN, IQ, IR, JM, JO, KW, LB, LU, LY, NL, NO, NZ, OM, PK, PL, QA, SA, SE, SG, SR, SY, TT, VN, YE) *see* Selenium Sulfide ... 1877
Selsun Amarillo (PE) *see* Selenium Sulfide ... 1877
Selsun Azul (PE) *see* Selenium Sulfide ... 1877
Selsun Blue (AE, AU, BH, CL, CY, EG, FI, ID, IQ, IR, JO, KW, LB, LY, NO, OM, QA, SA, SE, SY, YE) *see* Selenium Sulfide ... 1877
Selsun Blu (IT) *see* Selenium Sulfide ... 1877
Selsun R (NL) *see* Selenium Sulfide ... 1877
Seltouch (JP) *see* Felbinac [INT] ... 850
Seltra (KR) *see* Sertraline ... 1878
Selukos (AT, DE, FI, NO, SE) *see* Selenium Sulfide ... 1877
Sembrina (BF, BJ, CI, ET, FI, GH, GM, GN, KE, LR, MA, ML, MR, MU, MW, NE, NG, SC, SD, SL, SN, TN, TZ, UG, ZM, ZW) *see* Methyldopa ... 1332
Semicillin (HN) *see* Ampicillin ... 141
Semicillin (TH) *see* Penicillin V Potassium ... 1614
Semi-Daonil (AE, AR, AU, BH, CH, CY, EG, GB, IE, IQ, IR, JO, KW, LB, LY, MA, OM, PT, QA, SA, SY, YE) *see* GlyBURIDE ... 972
Semide (TW) *see* Cholestyramine Resin ... 431
Semi-Euglucon (AR, AT, AU, NZ) *see* GlyBURIDE ... 972
Seminac Continus (ID) *see* TraMADol ... 2074
Seminac (ID) *see* TraMADol ... 2074
Sempera (DE) *see* Itraconazole ... 1130
Semprex-D (BM) *see* Acrivastine and Pseudoephedrine ... 46
Sendoxan (DK, FI, NO, SE) *see* Cyclophosphamide ... 517
Seniere (AU) *see* Betahistine [CAN/INT] ... 252
Seniran (JP) *see* Bromazepam [CAN/INT] ... 290
Senorm L.A. (IN) *see* Haloperidol ... 993
Senpivac (PH) *see* Bupivacaine ... 299
Senro (ES) *see* Norfloxacin ... 1475
Sensamol (IL) *see* Acetaminophen ... 32
Sensaval (SE) *see* Nortriptyline ... 1476
Sensibit (MX) *see* Loratadine ... 1241
Sensibit (MX) *see* Loratadine and Pseudoephedrine ... 1242
Sensifluor (IT) *see* Fluoride ... 895
Sensinil (CO) *see* Lidocaine (Systemic) ... 1208
Sensipar (AU, NZ) *see* Cinacalcet ... 439
Sensitin (PH) *see* Levocetirizine ... 1196
Sensitive Eyes Saline Solution (PL) *see* Sodium Chloride ... 1902
Sensitram (BR) *see* TraMADol ... 2074
Sensival (IN, KR) *see* Nortriptyline ... 1476
Sensorcaine (IN, PH) *see* Bupivacaine ... 299
Senta (TW) *see* Diflunisal ... 626
Sentil (KR) *see* CloBAZam ... 465
Sentionyl (PH) *see* GlyBURIDE ... 972

Senzulin (TH) *see* Pioglitazone 1654
Sepamit (JP) *see* NIFEdipine 1451
Sepan (DK) *see* Cinnarizine [INT] 440
Separin (JP) *see* Tolnaftate 2063
Sepex (AR) *see* Ceftibuten 394
Sepexin (IN) *see* Cephalexin 405
Sephros (MY) *see* CefOXitin 386
Sepibest (MX) *see* CarBAMazepine 346
Sepidrin (KR) *see* Doxepin (Topical) 678
Sepime (PH) *see* Cefepime 378
Sepirone (TW) *see* BusPIRone 311
Seporin (KR) *see* Cefaclor 372
Sepram (FI) *see* Citalopram 451
Septalone (IL) *see* Chlorhexidine Gluconate 422
Septax (IL) *see* CefTAZidime 392
Septidiaryl (FR) *see* Nifuroxazide [INT] 1454
Septidron (ZA) *see* Pipemidic Acid [INT] 1655
Septilisin (MX) *see* Polymyxin B 1676
Septilisin (AR) *see* Cephalexin 405
Septipan (PH) *see* Cefixime 380
Septofervex (PL) *see* Chlorhexidine Gluconate 422
Septofort (BG, HU) *see* Chlorhexidine Gluconate 422
Septolete Plus (EE) *see* Cetylpyridinium and Benzocaine [CAN/INT] 415
Septol (IL) *see* Chlorhexidine Gluconate 422
Septran Forte (CR, DO, GT, HN, NI, PA, SV) *see* Sulfamethoxazole and Trimethoprim 1946
Septran (IN, PK, PY) *see* Sulfamethoxazole and Trimethoprim 1946
Septrin (AE, AU, BF, BH, BJ, CI, CY, EG, ES, ET, GB, GH, GM, GN, ID, IE, IQ, IR, JO, KE, KR, KW, LB, LR, LY, MA, ML, MR, MU, MW, MX, NE, NG, OM, PE, PH, QA, SA, SC, SD, SG, SL, SN, SY, TN, TZ, UG, VN, YE, ZM, ZW) *see* Sulfamethoxazole and Trimethoprim 1946
Septrin DS (HK) *see* Sulfamethoxazole and Trimethoprim 1946
Septrin Forte (AU) *see* Sulfamethoxazole and Trimethoprim 1946
Sepvadol[vet.] (FR) *see* Niflumic Acid [INT] 1454
Sequase (AU, CH) *see* QUEtiapine 1751
Sequax (PY) *see* Thioridazine 2030
Sequest (ID) *see* Cholestyramine Resin 431
Sequinan (AR) *see* RisperiDONE 1818
Seralbumin (CR, DO, GT, HN, PA, PY, SV) *see* Albumin 67
Seramar (CO) *see* Levalbuterol 1189
Seranace (GB, IE, ZA) *see* Haloperidol 993
Serat (VN) *see* Sucralfate 1940
Serc (AU, GB, HR, IE, MX, NZ, PK, TH, ZA) *see* Betahistine [CAN/INT] 252
Serdolect (AE, AR, AT, AU, BE, BG, CH, CZ, DE, DK, EE, ES, FI, GR, HR, HU, IE, IL, IS, KW, LB, MY, NL, NO, PH, PL, PT, QA, RO, RU, SE, SK, TR) *see* Sertindole [INT] 1878
Serecid (NZ) *see* HydrOXYzine 1024
Seredol Deca (PH) *see* Haloperidol 993
Serefar (UY) *see* Oxazepam 1532
Serefrex (AR) *see* Ketanserin [INT] 1144
Seremig (ID) *see* Flunarizine [CAN/INT] 892
Serenace (AE, BD, BH, CY, GB, JP, QA, SA, SG, TR) *see* Haloperidol 993
Serenada (IL) *see* Sertraline 1878
Seren (AE, BH, CY, EG, IL, IQ, IR, JO, KW, LB, LY, OM, QA, SA, SY, YE) *see* ChlordiazePOXIDE 422
Serenal (PT) *see* Oxazepam 1532
Serenase Dekanoat (DK) *see* Haloperidol 993
Serenase (FI) *see* Haloperidol 993
Serenata (PH) *see* Sertraline 1878
Serene (TH) *see* Clorazepate 487
Serenzin (JP) *see* Diazepam 613
Serepax (AU, IN, NZ, QA, ZA) *see* Oxazepam 1532
Serepress (IT) *see* Ketanserin [INT] 1144
Seresta (BE, CH, FR, LU, NL) *see* Oxazepam 1532
Seretaide (PT) *see* Fluticasone and Salmeterol 912
Seretide Accuhaler (AU) *see* Fluticasone and Salmeterol 912
Seretide (AR, AT, BB, BE, BG, BM, BR, BS, BZ, CH, CL, CN, CO, CR, DK, DO, EC, EE, ES, FI, FR, GB, GT, GY, HK, HN, HR, ID, IE, IL, IN, IS, IT, JM, KR, LT, MX, MY, NI, NL, NZ, PA, PE, PH, PL, PY, RO, SE, SG, SI, SK, SR, SV, TH, TT, TW, VE, VN) *see* Fluticasone and Salmeterol 912
Seretide Diskus (AE, CY, KW, LB, QA, SA) *see* Fluticasone and Salmeterol 912
SeretideDiskus (BH) *see* Fluticasone and Salmeterol 912
Seretide Evohaler (BH) *see* Fluticasone and Salmeterol 912
Seretide (PH) *see* Salmeterol 1860
Serevent (AE, AR, AT, BB, BE, BF, BG, BH, BJ, BM, BO, BR, BS, BZ, CH, CI, CL, CO, CR, CY, CZ, DE, DK, DO, EC, EE, EG, ES, ET, FI, FR, GB, GH, GM, GN, GR, GT, GY, HK, HN, HR, HU, ID, IE, IL, IQ, IR, IS, IT, JM, JO, KE, KR, KW, LB, LR, LT, LU, LY, MA, ML, MR, MT, MU, MW, MX, MY, NE, NG, NI, NL, NO, NZ, OM, PA, PE, PK, PL, PR, PT, PY, QA, RU, SA, SC, SD, SE, SG, SI, SK, SL, SN, SR, SV, SY, TH, TN, TR, TT, TW, TZ, UG, UY, VE, VN, YE, ZA, ZM, ZW) *see* Salmeterol 1860
Serevent Inhaler and Disks (AU) *see* Salmeterol 1860
Serevent Rotadisks (HU) *see* Salmeterol 1860
Serflu (UY) *see* Fluticasone and Salmeterol 912
Serfoxide (ES) *see* Pyridoxine 1747
Sergen (TW) *see* Butenafine 314
Serivia Gran (KR) *see* Sildenafil 1882
Serlain (BE) *see* Sertraline 1878
Serlect (MX) *see* Sertindole [INT] 1878
Serlife (ZA) *see* Sertraline 1878
Serlift (TH, VN) *see* Sertraline 1878
Serlin (TH) *see* Sertraline 1878
Sermonil (TH) *see* Imipramine 1054
Sernade (ID, PH) *see* Sertraline 1878
Serobid (IN) *see* Salmeterol 1860
Serocryptin (AE, BH, CY, EG, HU, IQ, IR, IT, JO, KW, LB, LY, MY, OM, PE, QA, SA, SY, YE) *see* Bromocriptine 291
Serofene (AR, MX, VE) *see* ClomiPHENE 473
Seroflo (HK) *see* Fluticasone and Salmeterol 912
Serolox (CR, GT, HN, NI, PA, SV) *see* Sertraline 1878
Serolux (MX) *see* Sertraline 1878
Seronex (MX) *see* Domperidone [CAN/INT] 666
Seronil (FI) *see* FLUoxetine 899
Serophene (AE, AT, AU, BH, CH, CY, CZ, EG, HK, IQ, IR, JO, KR, KW, LB, LY, NL, NZ, OM, PH, QA, SA, SG, SY, TH, TW, UY, VN, YE) *see* ClomiPHENE 473
Seroplex (FR) *see* Escitalopram 765
Seropram (AT, BG, CH, CZ, ES, FR, GR, HN, HU, IT, MX, VE) *see* Citalopram 451
Seroquel (AE, AR, AT, BB, BE, BG, BH, BM, BO, BR, BS, BZ, CH, CL, CN, CO, CY, CZ, DE, DK, DO, EC, EE, ES, FI, GB, GR, GY, HK, HR, ID, IE, IL, IS, IT, JM, JO, KR, KW, LB, LT, MX, MY, NL, NO, NZ, PE, PH, PK, PL, PR, PT, PY, QA, RO, RU, SA, SE, SI, SR, TH, TR, TT, TW, UY, VE, VN) *see* QUEtiapine 1751
Seroquel IR (HK) *see* QUEtiapine 1751
Seroquel Prolong (IS) *see* QUEtiapine 1751
Seroquel SR (SI) *see* QUEtiapine 1751
Seroquel XR (AU, CH, CN, CY, GB, HK, HR, ID, IE, IL, KW, LB, LT, MY, PH, QA, RO, SG, SK, TH, VN) *see* QUEtiapine 1751
Sero-Tet (MY, PH) *see* Tetanus Immune Globulin (Human) 2015
Serotia (PH) *see* QUEtiapine 1751
Seroxat (AE, AT, BD, BF, BH, BJ, CI, CN, CO, CY, CZ, DE, DK, EE, EG, ES, ET, FI, GB, GH, GM, GN, GR,

HK, HR, HU, ID, IE, IL, IQ, IR, IS, IT, JO, JP, KE, KR, KW, LB, LR, LT, LU, LY, MA, ML, MR, MU, MW, MY, NE, NG, NL, NO, OM, PE, PH, PK, PL, PT, QA, RO, SA, SC, SD, SE, SG, SI, SK, SL, SN, SY, TH, TN, TW, TZ, UG, YE, ZM, ZW) *see* PARoxetine 1579
Seroxat CR (AE, BH, CN, HK, KW, QA, SA, SG, TH) *see* PARoxetine 1579
Serpafar (GR) *see* ClomiPHENE 473
Serpalan (BM) *see* Reserpine 1793
Serpasil (ID, IN) *see* Reserpine 1793
Serroquel XR (AE) *see* QUEtiapine 1751
Sertacream (IT) *see* Sertaconazole 1877
Sertan (HN, HU) *see* Primidone 1714
Serten (PH) *see* Atenolol 189
Sertex (MX) *see* Sertraline 1878
Sertra (AU, TH) *see* Sertraline 1878
Sertranex (AE, BH, CO, CY, EG, IL, IQ, IR, JO, KW, LB, LY, OM, QA, SA, SY, YE) *see* Sertraline 1878
Sertranquil (CO) *see* Sertraline 1878
Servambutol (PE) *see* Ethambutol 798
Servamox (MX) *see* Amoxicillin and Clavulanate 133
Servicef (MX) *see* Cephalexin 405
Serviclor (MX) *see* Cefaclor 372
Servicor (UY) *see* Deflazacort [INT] 587
Servidipine (MY) *see* NIFEdipine 1451
Servidoxine (EC) *see* Doxycycline 689
Serviflox (MY, SG) *see* Ciprofloxacin (Systemic) 441
Servigenta (MY) *see* Gentamicin (Systemic) 959
Servipen-G Forte (CH) *see* Penicillin G Procaine 1613
Servispor (TW) *see* Cephalexin 405
Servitet (MY) *see* Tetracycline 2017
Servitrim (MX) *see* Sulfamethoxazole and Trimethoprim 1946
Serzone (AU, BB, BH, BM, BR, BS, BZ, GY, JM, KW, NL, NZ, PL, QA, SR, TT, ZA) *see* Nefazodone 1435
Sesaren XR (EC) *see* Venlafaxine 2150
Sestrine (AR) *see* Repaglinide 1791
Setacol (AU) *see* Scopolamine (Systemic) 1870
Setaloft (HK) *see* Sertraline 1878
Setamol (HK) *see* Acetaminophen 32
Setegis (HU) *see* Terazosin 2001
Setine (TW) *see* PARoxetine 1579
Setinin (HK) *see* QUEtiapine 1751
Setin (TH) *see* Cetirizine 411
Setin (ZA) *see* Metoclopramide 1345
Setisin (MY) *see* Neostigmine 1438
Setofilm (GB) *see* Ondansetron 1513
Seton (TW) *see* Phenoxybenzamine 1635
Setopain ER (KR) *see* Acetaminophen 32
Setopain (KR) *see* Acetaminophen 32
Setoral (TW) *see* Ramosetron [INT] 1774
Setoram (KR) *see* Torsemide 2071
Setrax (CO) *see* Sertraline 1878
Setrilan (IT) *see* Spirapril [INT] 1931
Setrof (HK) *see* Sertraline 1878
Setrol (IN) *see* Sodium Tetradecyl Sulfate 1914
Setrona (AU, NZ) *see* Sertraline 1878
Setronax (HK, MY, SG, VN) *see* Ondansetron 1513
Setron (IL, TW) *see* Granisetron 983
Setrovel (ID) *see* Tropisetron [INT] 2108
Sevenal (HN, HU) *see* PHENobarbital 1632
Severin (MX) *see* Nimesulide [INT] 1456
Sevikar (AU, BE, CH, DE, DK, FI, GB, GR, KR, NL, PT, RO, TW) *see* Amlodipine and Olmesartan 126
Sevikar Comp (FI) *see* Olmesartan, Amlodipine, and Hydrochlorothiazide 1498
Sevikar HCT (BE, BG, CH, CZ, DE, GB, KR, NL, RO, SI, TW) *see* Olmesartan, Amlodipine, and Hydrochlorothiazide 1498
Sevredol (AU, CH, CZ, HR, NZ, RO, SI, SK, TR) *see* Morphine (Systemic) 1394
Sevredol (RO) *see* Chloramphenicol 421
Sha Ba Ke (CL) *see* Secnidazole [INT] 1872
Shacillin (AE, BH, CY, EG, IQ, IR, JO, KW, LB, LY, OM, QA, SA, SY, YE) *see* Ampicillin 141
Shamoxil (AE, BH, CY, EG, IQ, IR, JO, KW, LB, LY, OM, QA, SA, SY, YE) *see* Amoxicillin 130
Shanamef (HK) *see* Mefenamic Acid 1280
Shanleting (CN) *see* AtorvaSTATin 194
Shanvac-B (PH, TW) *see* Hepatitis B Vaccine (Recombinant) 1002
Sharizole (AE, BH, CY, EG, IQ, IR, JO, KW, LB, LY, OM, QA, SA, SY, YE) *see* MetroNIDAZOLE (Systemic) 1353
Sharonim (HK) *see* Nimesulide [INT] 1456
Sharox-500 (ID) *see* Cefuroxime 399
Shengda (CN) *see* Dipyridamole 652
Sheng Jun (CN) *see* Isoniazid 1120
Shepherd (CN) *see* Azithromycin (Systemic) 216
Shilova (AU) *see* ValACYclovir 2119
Shilshul X2 (IL) *see* Loperamide 1236
Shinasyn (MY) *see* Ampicillin and Sulbactam 145
Shincef (KR) *see* Cefuroxime 399
Shinclop (VN) *see* Clopidogrel 484
Shincort (HK, MY, PH, TH) *see* Triamcinolone (Systemic) 2099
Shinoxol (SG) *see* Ambroxol [INT] 109
Shintamet (MY, PH) *see* Cimetidine 438
Shiton (TW) *see* Norethindrone 1473
Shorant (MX) *see* Insulin Glulisine 1086
Showmin (TW) *see* Cyproheptadine 529
Shu Lan Xin (CN) *see* Rifampin 1804
Shumeifen (CN) *see* Buprenorphine 300
Shun Song (CN) *see* Acemetacin [INT] 30
Shuntan (CN) *see* Aniracetam [INT] 150
Shuweixin (CN) *see* Doxofylline [INT] 679
Siadocin (TH) *see* Doxycycline 689
Sialexin (TH) *see* Cephalexin 405
Siamdopa (TH) *see* Methyldopa 1332
Siamformet (TH) *see* MetFORMIN 1307
Siamidine (TH) *see* Cimetidine 438
Sia-mox (TH) *see* Amoxicillin 130
Siaten (ES) *see* Zopiclone [CAN/INT] 2217
Sibelium (AE, AR, AT, BE, BG, BH, CH, CN, CZ, DK, EC, EG, ES, FR, GR, ID, IE, IN, IT, JO, KR, KW, LB, MX, NL, PH, PK, PT, PY, QA, SA, TH, TR, UY, VE, VN, ZA) *see* Flunarizine [CAN/INT] 892
Siblix (AR) *see* ARIPiprazole 171
Sicadol (CL, PY) *see* Mefenamic Acid 1280
Sical (AU) *see* Calcitriol 323
Sicatem (PY) *see* CISplatin 448
Sicco (DE) *see* Indapamide 1065
Sicmylon (JP) *see* Nalidixic Acid [INT] 1418
Sicolitio (UY) *see* Lithium 1230
Sicorten (AT, BE, CH, CZ, DE, ES, HU, LU, NL) *see* Halometasone [INT] 993
Sicovit C (RO) *see* Ascorbic Acid 178
Sidegra (TH) *see* Sildenafil 1882
Sidelg (CO, CR, DO, HN, NI, PA, SV) *see* Orlistat 1520
Sidenar (AR) *see* LORazepam 1243
Sidevar (MX) *see* Lovastatin 1252
Sidomon (TW) *see* Fluoxymesterone 903
Sifaclor (TH) *see* Cefaclor 372
Sifloks (AE, BH, CY, EG, IQ, IR, JO, KW, LB, LY, OM, QA, SA, SY, YE) *see* Ciprofloxacin (Systemic) 441
Siflox (ID) *see* Ciprofloxacin (Systemic) 441
Sifrol (AE, AR, AT, BE, BG, BH, BR, CH, CL, CN, CY, CZ, DE, DK, EG, FI, FR, GB, GR, HN, HR, ID, IE, IL, IQ, IR, IS, IT, JO, KW, LB, LT, LY, MX, MY, NL, NO, OM, PE, PH, PT, PY, QA, RO, RU, SA, SE, SG, SK, SY, TR, VE, VN, YE) *see* Pramipexole 1695
Sifrol ER (KW, LB) *see* Pramipexole 1695
Sigadoc-Spray (DE) *see* Indomethacin 1067
Sigadoxin (PT) *see* Doxycycline 689
Sigamsporin (AE) *see* CycloSPORINE (Systemic) 522

Sigaprim (DE) *see* Sulfamethoxazole and Trimethoprim 1946
Sigmacort (AU, HK) *see* Hydrocortisone (Topical) 1014
Sigmart (CN, JP, KR, TW) *see* Nicorandil [INT] 1449
Sigmasporin (KW, QA) *see* CycloSPORINE (Systemic) 522
Sigmaxin (AU) *see* Digoxin 627
Signifor (AU, CH, CZ, DE, DK, EE, FR, GB, HR, IS, KR, LT, NL, NO, RO, SE, SG, SI, SK, TR) *see* Pasireotide 1583
Signopam (HU, PL) *see* Temazepam 1990
Signopharm (HU) *see* Temazepam 1990
Si Jin (CN) *see* Ebastine [INT] 702
Sikacin (TW) *see* Amikacin 111
Siklos (FR, GB, TR) *see* Hydroxyurea 1021
Sikzonoate (ID) *see* FluPHENAZine 905
Silax (ID) *see* Furosemide 940
Silbron (AR) *see* Bromhexine [INT] 291
Sildefil (AR) *see* Sildenafil 1882
Sildegra (SG) *see* Sildenafil 1882
Silence (HK, TW) *see* LORazepam 1243
Silex (PH) *see* Cefepime 378
Silgram (PH) *see* Ampicillin and Sulbactam 145
Silica (KR) *see* Pregabalin 1710
Siligaz (CL) *see* Domperidone [CAN/INT] 666
Si LiMeng (CN) *see* Acipimox [INT] 43
Silkis (ES, FR, GB, GR, HK, IE, KR, MX, NO, SG, TW, VN) *see* Calcitriol 323
Silmazin (KR) *see* Silver Sulfadiazine 1887
Silodyx (BE, CZ, EE, FR, GR, LT, NL, PL, PT, SE, SK) *see* Silodosin 1885
Silomat (AR, AT, BE, BR, CZ, DE, FI, FR, IT, LU, PT) *see* Clobutinol [INT] 468
Siltin (TW) *see* Selegiline 1873
Silvadene (MX, TR, TW) *see* Silver Sulfadiazine 1887
Silvadiazin (AE, KW) *see* Silver Sulfadiazine 1887
Silvadin (EC) *see* Silver Sulfadiazine 1887
Silvazine (AU) *see* Silver Sulfadiazine 1887
Silvederma (ES, PH, VE) *see* Silver Sulfadiazine 1887
Silvercept (KR) *see* Donepezil 668
Silverderm (TH) *see* Silver Sulfadiazine 1887
Silverdiazina (PE) *see* Silver Sulfadiazine 1887
Silverin (BH, JO, QA, SA) *see* Silver Sulfadiazine 1887
Silverol (IL) *see* Silver Sulfadiazine 1887
Silverstar (KR) *see* Cilostazol 437
Silvex (HK) *see* Silver Sulfadiazine 1887
Silvie (KR) *see* Sildenafil 1882
Silvirin (IN, VN) *see* Silver Sulfadiazine 1887
Simaglen (HK) *see* Cimetidine 438
Simarc-2 (ID) *see* Warfarin 2186
Simaron (JP) *see* Fluocinonide 894
Simaspen (ZA) *see* Simvastatin 1890
Simazepan (PY) *see* Oxazepam 1532
Simbado (ID) *see* Simvastatin 1890
Simcard (HK) *see* Simvastatin 1890
Simchol (ID) *see* Simvastatin 1890
Simclovix (ID) *see* Clopidogrel 484
Simdak (IS, SI, SK) *see* Levosimendan [INT] 1205
Simdax (AE, AR, AT, BG, BR, CY, CZ, ES, FI, GR, HR, HU, IL, IT, KW, MX, NO, NZ, PE, PT, QA, RO, RU, SE, SG, TR, UY) *see* Levosimendan [INT] 1205
Simenda (IN) *see* Levosimendan [INT] 1205
Simextam (ID) *see* Cefoperazone and Sulbactam [INT] 382
Simfix (ID) *see* Cefixime 380
Si Mi An (CN) *see* Mifepristone 1366
Simikan (ID) *see* Amikacin 111
Simlo (MX) *see* Simvastatin 1890
Simovil (IL) *see* Simvastatin 1890
Simpiox (CO) *see* Ivermectin (Systemic) 1136
Simplaqor (MX) *see* Simvastatin 1890
Simponi (AR, AT, AU, BE, BR, CH, CL, CN, CO, CY, CZ, DE, DK, EE, FR, GB, GR, HK, HN, HR, IE, IL, IS, JP, KR, LT, MY, NL, NO, NZ, PH, PL, PT, RO, SE, SG, SI, SK, TH, TR, TW) *see* Golimumab 977
Simprofen (ID) *see* Dexketoprofen [INT] 603
SimStatin (NZ) *see* Simvastatin 1890
Simtec (MY) *see* Cetirizine 411
Simtin (HK, MY, SG) *see* Simvastatin 1890
Simucil (ID) *see* Acetylcysteine 40
Simucin (TH) *see* Acetylcysteine 40
Simulect (AE, AR, AT, AU, BE, BG, BH, BR, CH, CL, CN, CO, CY, CZ, DE, DK, EC, EE, ES, FI, FR, GB, GR, HK, HN, HR, HU, ID, IE, IL, IN, IS, IT, JP, KR, LT, MT, MX, MY, NL, NO, NZ, PE, PH, PK, PL, PT, PY, QA, RO, RU, SA, SE, SG, SI, SK, TH, TR, TW, UY, VE, VN) *see* Basiliximab 228
Simultan (CL) *see* Thioridazine 2030
Simultan D (EC) *see* Valsartan and Hydrochlorothiazide 2129
Simultan A (AR) *see* Amlodipine and Valsartan 126
Simultan (EC) *see* Valsartan 2127
Simvacor (IL, KW, MY, SG) *see* Simvastatin 1890
Simva (CR, DO, GT, HN, NI, PA, SV) *see* Simvastatin 1890
Simvahexal (TW) *see* Simvastatin 1890
Simvahex (PH) *see* Simvastatin 1890
Simvalord (KR) *see* Simvastatin 1890
Simvar (AU) *see* Simvastatin 1890
Simvast (AE, BH, QA) *see* Simvastatin 1890
Simvastan (KR) *see* Simvastatin 1890
Simvastar (KR) *see* Simvastatin 1890
Simvata (KR) *see* Simvastatin 1890
Simvatin (AE, BH, CY, EG, IQ, IR, JO, KR, KW, LB, LY, OM, QA, SA, SY, YE, ZA) *see* Simvastatin 1890
Simvaxon (IL) *see* Simvastatin 1890
Simvor (TH, VN) *see* Simvastatin 1890
Sinaler (PY) *see* Loratadine 1241
Sinalfa (DK, NO) *see* Terazosin 2001
Sinalgen (CO) *see* Hydrocodone and Acetaminophen 1012
Sinalgia (PY) *see* Dipyrone [INT] 653
Sinalgico (AR) *see* Piroxicam 1662
Sinapsan (DE) *see* Piracetam [INT] 1661
Sinarest-AF (IN) *see* Chlorpheniramine and Pseudoephedrine 427
Sincer (TW) *see* Acebutolol 29
Sinclote (TW) *see* Clodronate [CAN/INT] 469
Sincronex (UY) *see* Diazepam 613
Sincrosa (MX) *see* Acarbose 29
Sindaxel (BG, HK, HR, ID, RO) *see* PACLitaxel (Conventional) 1550
Sindol (UY) *see* Ketoprofen 1145
Sindopa (NZ) *see* Carbidopa and Levodopa 351
Sindoxplatin (HK, PH) *see* Oxaliplatin 1528
Sindroxocin (HK, HR, PH, RO, RU) *see* DOXOrubicin (Conventional) 679
Sinedin (PH) *see* Carbidopa and Levodopa 351
Sinedol (DO, MX) *see* Acetaminophen 32
Sinedopa (HK, MY) *see* Carbidopa and Levodopa 351
Sinedopa Mite (MY) *see* Carbidopa and Levodopa 351
Sine-Fluor (ES) *see* Desonide 597
Sinemet 25 100 (HK, MY, PH) *see* Carbidopa and Levodopa 351
Sinemet (AT, AU, BE, BR, CH, CR, CY, CZ, DE, DK, DO, EC, EE, EG, ES, FI, FR, GB, GR, GT, HK, HN, IE, IS, IT, JO, KR, KW, LB, LT, MT, MX, MY, NI, NL, NO, NZ, PA, PK, PL, PT, PY, QA, RU, SA, SE, SK, SV, TH, TR, TW, UY, VE) *see* Carbidopa and Levodopa 351
Sinemet CR (AU, BE, BG, CH, CN, CR, CY, CZ, DO, GB, GR, GT, HK, HN, IL, IT, KR, KW, LT, MY, NI, NL, NZ, PA, PE, PH, PT, QA, SV) *see* Carbidopa and Levodopa 351
Sinemet [+ Levodopa] (PL) *see* Carbidopa 351
Sinemet Retard (ES) *see* Carbidopa and Levodopa 351

Sinequan (AE, AT, AU, BE, BH, CY, EG, ES, GR, HK, IQ, IR, JO, KW, LB, LY, NL, NO, OM, QA, SA, SY, TH, TW, YE) *see* Doxepin (Systemic) 676
Sinergina (ES) *see* Phenytoin 1640
Sinersul (HR) *see* Sulfamethoxazole and Trimethoprim 1946
Sinersul (HR) *see* Trimethoprim 2104
Sinetens (AR) *see* Prazosin 1703
Sinflo (TW) *see* Ofloxacin (Systemic) 1490
Singkalus Chewable (KR) *see* Montelukast 1392
Singloben (MX) *see* GlipiZIDE 967
Singulair (AE, AR, AT, AU, BB, BE, BG, BH, BM, BO, BR, BS, BZ, CH, CL, CN, CR, CY, CZ, DE, DK, DO, EC, EE, EG, ES, FI, FR, GB, GR, GT, GY, HK, HN, HR, HU, IE, IL, IS, IT, JM, JO, JP, KR, KW, LB, LT, MX, MY, NI, NL, NO, NZ, PA, PE, PH, PK, PL, PR, PT, QA, RO, RU, SA, SE, SG, SI, SK, SR, SV, TH, TR, TT, TW, UY, VE, VN) *see* Montelukast 1392
Singular Chew (KR) *see* Montelukast 1392
Sinkast (JO, TW) *see* Montelukast 1392
Sinlip (PY) *see* Rosuvastatin 1848
Sinmaron (TW) *see* Mirtazapine 1376
Sinnorvapin (KR) *see* AmLODIPine 123
Sinocort (ID) *see* Triamcinolone (Systemic) 2099
Sinocort (ID) *see* Triamcinolone (Topical) 2100
Sinofuan Implant (CN) *see* Fluorouracil (Systemic) 896
Sinogan (CL, CO, MX, PE, VE) *see* Methotrimeprazine [CAN/INT] 1329
Sinop (AR) *see* AmLODIPine 123
Sinopren (ZA) *see* Lisinopril 1226
Sinopril (AE, BH, CY, EG, IQ, IR, JO, KW, LB, LY, OM, QA, SA, SY, YE) *see* Lisinopril 1226
Sinoric (ID) *see* Allopurinol 90
Sinotic (JO) *see* Fosinopril 932
Sinoxal (HR) *see* Oxaliplatin 1528
Sinozol (MX) *see* Itraconazole 1130
Sinpebac (MX) *see* Mupirocin 1404
Sinpet (MX) *see* Phentermine 1635
Sinplatin (BG, RO) *see* CISplatin 448
Sinquan (CH, DK) *see* Doxepin (Systemic) 676
Sinral (ID) *see* Flunarizine [CAN/INT] 892
Sintalgin (BR) *see* Nimesulide [INT] 1456
Sintec (TW) *see* Enalapril 722
Sinthrome (GB) *see* Acenocoumarol [CAN/INT] 30
Sintodian (IT) *see* Droperidol 695
Sintonal (ES) *see* Brotizolam [INT] 293
Sintopozid (HK) *see* Etoposide 816
Sintrex (TW) *see* CefTRIAXone 396
Sintrom (AR, AT, BE, BG, CH, FR, GR, IL, IT, MX, PT, PY, RO, VN) *see* Acenocoumarol [CAN/INT] 30
Sintropic (TW) *see* Tropicamide 2108
Sinty (TW) *see* Simvastatin 1890
Sinufin (MX) *see* Amoxicillin and Clavulanate 133
Sinvacor (IT) *see* Simvastatin 1890
Sinver (VE) *see* Cinnarizine [INT] 440
Sinzac (TW) *see* FLUoxetine 899
Sioban (IN) *see* Albendazole 65
Siofor (BG, DE, PL, SI, SK) *see* MetFORMIN 1307
Siozole (IN) *see* Omeprazole 1508
Sipam (TH) *see* Diazepam 613
Sipentin (ID) *see* Gabapentin 943
Sipla (ID) *see* GuaiFENesin 986
Sipo (TW) *see* Ramipril 1771
Sipralexa (BE) *see* Escitalopram 765
Siproxan (TW) *see* Ciprofloxacin and Hydrocortisone 446
Siptazin (JP) *see* Cinnarizine [INT] 440
Siqualone (DK, FI, NO, SE) *see* FluPHENAZine 905
Siquent Hycor Eye Ointment (AU) *see* Hydrocortisone (Topical) 1014
Siraliden (PL) *see* Nitrofurantoin 1463
Siramid (ID) *see* Pyrazinamide 1745
Siran 200 (IL) *see* Acetylcysteine 40
Sirdalud (AE, AR, AT, BB, BE, BF, BH, BJ, BM, BR, BS, BZ, CH, CI, CL, CO, CY, CZ, DE, DK, EE, EG, ES, ET, FI, FR, GH, GM, GN, GR, GY, HN, ID, IL, IN, IQ, IR, IT, JM, JO, KE, KR, KW, LB, LR, LT, LY, MA, ML, MR, MT, MU, MW, MX, NE, NG, NL, NO, OM, PE, PH, PL, PR, PT, PY, QA, RU, SA, SC, SD, SE, SI, SK, SL, SN, SR, SY, TH, TN, TR, TT, TW, TZ, UG, VE, VN, YE, ZA, ZM, ZW) *see* TiZANidine 2051
Sirdalud MR (CH, MX, NL) *see* TiZANidine 2051
Sirdalud Retard (DK, FI) *see* TiZANidine 2051
Sirdalum (UY) *see* TiZANidine 2051
Sirop des Vosges (FR) *see* Pholcodine [INT] 1646
Siroxyl (BE, GR) *see* Carbocisteine [INT] 357
Sirtal (DE) *see* CarBAMazepine 346
Sirturo (BE, CZ, DE, DK, EE, GB, HR, KR, LT, NL, RO, SE, SI, SK) *see* Bedaquiline 233
Sisare Gel (DE) *see* Estradiol (Systemic) 775
Sistopress (MX) *see* AmLODIPine 123
Si Tai (CN) *see* Piracetam [INT] 1661
Siterone (NZ) *see* Cyproterone [CAN/INT] 530
Sitran (CO) *see* SUMAtriptan 1953
Situroxime (ID) *see* Cefuroxime 399
Sivas (KR) *see* Simvastatin 1890
Sivastin (IT) *see* Simvastatin 1890
Sivkort (MY) *see* Triamcinolone (Systemic) 2099
Siweitan (CN) *see* Zaleplon 2193
Sixacin (PY) *see* Piperacillin and Tazobactam 1657
Sixanol (PY, UY) *see* Fluconazole 885
Sixime (TH) *see* Cefixime 380
Sixol (MX) *see* Colchicine 500
Sizopin (IN) *see* CloZAPine 490
Sizoril (ID) *see* CloZAPine 490
Sizzle (PK) *see* Fexofenadine 873
Skabicid (CZ) *see* Lindane 1217
Skelaxin (CA) *see* Metaxalone 1307
Skelid (AT, AU, BE, CH, DE, ES, FI, FR, GB, HN, HU, LU, NL, NZ, SE) *see* Tiludronate 2042
Skiacol (FR, VN) *see* Cyclopentolate 517
Skindure (TH) *see* Miconazole (Topical) 1360
Skinfect (TH) *see* Gentamicin (Systemic) 959
Skinoderm (IL) *see* Azelaic Acid 213
Skinorem (IQ, IR, JO, LB, LY, OM, SY, YE) *see* Azelaic Acid 213
Skinoren (AE, AT, BE, BH, CH, CY, CZ, DE, DK, EE, EG, ES, FI, GB, GR, HK, HN, HR, IE, IS, IT, KW, LT, MY, NO, NZ, PH, PK, PL, PT, QA, RO, RU, SA, SE, SI, SK, TH, TR, TW, ZA) *see* Azelaic Acid 213
Skinpred (CO) *see* Prednicarbate 1703
Skirax (TW) *see* Acyclovir (Systemic) 47
Skopolamin (NO) *see* Scopolamine (Systemic) 1870
Skopryl (HR) *see* Lisinopril 1226
Skopryl Plus (RO) *see* Lisinopril and Hydrochlorothiazide 1229
Skyton (TW) *see* Spironolactone 1931
Sladial (HR) *see* Sorbitol 1927
Slakin (KR) *see* Orphenadrine 1522
Sleepeze-PM (ZA) *see* DiphenhydrAMINE (Systemic) 641
Sleepin (TW) *see* Nitrazepam [CAN/INT] 1461
Sleepman (TW) *see* Zolpidem 2212
Slepzol (ID) *see* Zolpidem 2212
Slo-Phyllin (AE, BH, CY, EG, GB, IQ, IR, JO, KW, LB, LY, OM, QA, SA, SY, YE) *see* Theophylline 2026
Slo-Theo (HK) *see* Theophylline 2026
Slow-Apresoline (AE, BB, BF, BJ, BM, BS, BZ, CI, EG, ET, GH, GM, GN, GY, IL, IQ, IR, JM, JO, KE, KW, LB, LR, LY, MA, ML, MR, MU, MW, NE, NG, NL, OM, PR, SC, SD, SL, SN, SR, SY, TN, TT, TZ, UG, YE, ZM, ZW) *see* HydrALAZINE 1007
Slow Deralin (IL) *see* Propranolol 1731
Slow-Fe (AE, BB, BH, BM, BS, BZ, CY, EG, GY, IQ, IR, JM, JO, KW, LB, LY, OM, QA, SA, SR, SY, TT, YE) *see* Ferrous Sulfate 871

Slow-K (AE, AR, AU, BB, BF, BH, BJ, BM, BR, BS, BZ, CI, EG, ET, GH, GM, GN, GY, HK, IL, IQ, IR, JM, JO, KE, KW, LB, LR, LY, MA, ML, MR, MU, MW, MY, NE, NG, NL, NZ, OM, PR, QA, SA, SC, SD, SL, SN, SR, SY, TN, TT, TW, TZ, UG, UY, YE, ZA, ZM, ZW) *see* Potassium Chloride 1687
Slow-K MR (CY, TR) *see* Potassium Chloride 1687
Slow-Lopresor (LU, NZ) *see* Metoprolol 1350
Slow-Mag (PL) *see* Magnesium Chloride 1261
Slow-Nifine (LU) *see* NIFEdipine 1451
Sluxdin (TW) *see* Losartan 1248
Smarten (TW) *see* Captopril 342
Smizole (KR) *see* Cilostazol 437
Smoodipin (KR) *see* QUEtiapine 1751
Smood (MY) *see* Domperidone [CAN/INT] 666
S-Morphine (KR) *see* Morphine (Systemic) 1394
Snafi (AE, BH, KW, QA, SA) *see* Tadalafil 1968
Sno Phenicol (AE) *see* Chloramphenicol 421
Sno Pilo (AE, IE) *see* Pilocarpine (Ophthalmic) 1649
Snuzaid (AU) *see* DiphenhydrAMINE (Systemic) 641
Sobril (NO, SE) *see* Oxazepam 1532
Sobrium (MY) *see* Zolpidem 2212
Socalm (IN) *see* QUEtiapine 1751
Socef (ID) *see* CefTRIAXone 396
Soclaf (ID) *see* Cefotaxime 382
Socliden (PY) *see* Oxybutynin 1536
Soclor (ID) *see* Cefaclor 372
Soden (SG) *see* Naproxen 1427
Sodibic (AU) *see* Sodium Bicarbonate 1901
Sodio Fluoruro (IT) *see* Fluoride 895
Sodio Nitroprussiato (IT) *see* Nitroprusside 1467
Sodipen (MX) *see* Penicillin G (Parenteral/ Aqueous) 1611
Sodipryl (CH) *see* Naftidrofuryl [INT] 1416
Sodium Amytal (GB) *see* Amobarbital 128
Sodium Chloride (PL) *see* Sodium Chloride 1902
Sodium Nitroprusside BP (AU) *see* Nitroprusside 1467
Sodium Nitroprusside (GB) *see* Nitroprusside 1467
Sodolac (PT) *see* Etodolac 815
Sofargen (IT) *see* Silver Sulfadiazine 1887
Sofasin (GR) *see* Norfloxacin 1475
Soficlor (HK, MY) *see* Cefaclor 372
Sofidrox (MY, SG) *see* Cefadroxil 372
Sofilex (HK, MY, SG) *see* Cephalexin 405
Sofix (ID) *see* Cefixime 380
Soflax (AE, SA) *see* Lactulose 1156
Soframycin Ear/Eye Drops (AU, NZ) *see* Framycetin [INT] 937
Soframycine (BE) *see* Framycetin [INT] 937
Soframycin (IN, ZA) *see* Framycetin [INT] 937
Sofra-Tulle (IN, SA, TH, ZA) *see* Framycetin [INT] 937
Softan (CN) *see* Rosuvastatin 1848
Soft Mate Consept 2 (PL) *see* Sodium Thiosulfate 1915
Soft U Derm Forte (ID) *see* Urea 2114
Solac (ID) *see* Lactulose 1156
Solanax (JP) *see* ALPRAZolam 94
Solantin (TW) *see* Dipyridamole 652
Solaquin (AE, BH, BR, CY, EG, HK, IQ, IR, JO, KW, LB, LY, MY, OM, QA, SA, SY, YE) *see* Hydroquinone 1020
Solaquin Forte (AE, BH, CY, EG, IQ, IR, JO, KW, LB, LY, MY, OM, QA, SA, SY, YE) *see* Hydroquinone 1020
Solara (JP) *see* Eplerenone 740
Solarcaine (HK) *see* Lidocaine (Topical) 1211
Solart (IT) *see* Acemetacin [INT] 30
Solasic (ID) *see* Mefenamic Acid 1280
Solatran (BE, CH, ZA) *see* Ketazolam [INT] 1144
Sola (TW) *see* Chlorzoxazone 430
Solavert (AU) *see* Sotalol 1927
Solaxin (HK, ID, JP) *see* Chlorzoxazone 430
Solax (PY) *see* Furosemide 940
Solciclina (MX) *see* Amoxicillin 130
Soldrin Oftálmico (MX) *see* Neomycin, Polymyxin B, and Dexamethasone 1437
Solfluor (CN) *see* Fluoride 895
Solgol (AT, DE, ES) *see* Nadolol 1411
Solia (TH) *see* Albuterol 69
Soliris (AU, IL, JP, KR, NZ) *see* Eculizumab 703
Solirus (AT, BE, CH, CZ, DE, DK, EE, FR, GB, HK, HR, IE, IT, NL, NO, PL, PT, RO, SE) *see* Eculizumab 703
Soliten (IN) *see* Solifenacin 1917
Soliwax (GB) *see* Docusate 661
Solmin (TW) *see* Zaleplon 2193
Solmucol (HU, LU, SG) *see* Acetylcysteine 40
Solmux (HK) *see* Carbocisteine [INT] 357
Solnasin (PL) *see* Sodium Chloride 1902
Solofen (TW) *see* Baclofen 223
Sologen (KR) *see* MethylPREDNISolone 1340
Solomet (FI) *see* MethylPREDNISolone 1340
Solone (AE) *see* PrednisoLONE (Systemic) 1703
Solonex (CO) *see* Isoniazid 1120
Solosa (ID, PH) *see* Glimepiride 966
Solosin (DE) *see* Theophylline 2026
Solotik (LB) *see* Sertraline 1878
Solotrate (TH) *see* Isosorbide Mononitrate 1126
Solotrim (AT, IL) *see* Trimethoprim 2104
Solox (NZ) *see* Lansoprazole 1166
Solpadeine (AE, BH, CY, EG, IQ, IR, JO, KW, LB, LY, OM, QA, SA, SY, YE) *see* Acetaminophen and Codeine 36
Solpadol (GB, IE) *see* Acetaminophen and Codeine 36
Solpenox (ID) *see* Amoxicillin 130
Solplex 40 (IT) *see* Dextran 607
Solplex 70 (IT) *see* Dextran 607
Soltamox (GB) *see* Tamoxifen 1971
Soltrim (MX) *see* Sulfamethoxazole and Trimethoprim 1946
Solubron (PE) *see* Bromhexine [INT] 291
Solu Celestan (AT, DE) *see* Betamethasone (Systemic) 253
Solucis (IT) *see* Carbocisteine [INT] 357
Solu Cortef (AE, BD, BE, BF, BH, BJ, BR, CH, CI, CL, CO, CY, DK, EC, EE, EG, ET, FI, GB, GH, GM, GN, GR, HK, HN, HR, IE, IQ, IR, IS, IT, JO, KE, KR, KW, LB, LR, LY, MA, ML, MR, MU, MW, MY, NE, NG, NL, NO, OM, PE, PH, PK, QA, RU, SA, SC, SD, SE, SG, SL, SN, SY, TH, TN, TR, TW, TZ, UG, YE, ZA, ZM, ZW) *see* Hydrocortisone (Systemic) 1013
Solu-Cortef (AU, CN, EC, NZ, VE, VN) *see* Hydrocortisone (Systemic) 1013
Solu Cortef M.O.V. (AE, BH, CY, EG, IQ, IR, JO, KW, LB, LY, OM, QA, SA, SY, YE) *see* Hydrocortisone (Systemic) 1013
Soludeks 1 (HR) *see* Dextran 607
Soludeks 40 (HR) *see* Dextran 607
Soludeks 70 (HR) *see* Dextran 607
Soludril Rhinites (LU) *see* Pseudoephedrine 1742
Solulexin (MY) *see* Cephalexin 405
Solu-Medrol (AE, AU, BG, BH, CL, CN, CY, EG, HK, HR, IS, KW, LB, LT, MX, MY, PK, QA, RO, SA, SI, SK, TH, TR, UY, VN) *see* MethylPREDNISolone 1340
Solu Medrol (BF, BJ, CI, ET, GH, GM, GN, KE, LR, MA, ML, MR, MU, MW, NE, NG, SC, SD, SL, SN, TN, TZ, UG, ZM, ZW) *see* MethylPREDNISolone 1340
Solunim (JP) *see* Fluocinonide 894
Solupred (FR) *see* PrednisoLONE (Systemic) 1703
Solu-Pred (MY) *see* MethylPREDNISolone 1340
Solural (MX) *see* Calcium Chloride 328
Solural (MX) *see* Magnesium Chloride 1261
Solu-Tisone (TW) *see* Hydrocortisone (Systemic) 1013
Solutricine Maux de Gorge tetracaine (FR) *see* Tetracaine (Topical) 2017
Soluwax Ear Drops (MY, SG) *see* Docusate 661
Solvazinc (GB) *see* Zinc Sulfate 2200
SolvEasy Tinea (AU, NZ) *see* Terbinafine (Topical) 2004

SolvEasy Tinea Cream (AU, NZ) *see* Terbinafine (Systemic) ... 2002
Solvetan (GR) *see* CefTAZidime ... 392
Solvex (AE) *see* Carbocisteine [INT] ... 357
Solvex (DE) *see* Reboxetine [INT] ... 1786
Solvex (IL, QA, SA) *see* Bromhexine [INT] ... 291
Solvexin (JO, KW) *see* Bromhexine [INT] ... 291
Solvezink (NO, SE) *see* Zinc Sulfate ... 2200
Solvin (EC) *see* Beta-Carotene ... 251
Solvinex (ID) *see* Bromhexine [INT] ... 291
Solving (IT) *see* Nimesulide [INT] ... 1456
Solvolan (BG, SK) *see* Ambroxol [INT] ... 109
Solvolin (CH) *see* Bromhexine [INT] ... 291
Solvoxine (PH) *see* Oxytocin ... 1549
Somac (AU, CZ, FI, NO, NZ) *see* Pantoprazole ... 1570
Somadril (DK, NO, SE) *see* Carisoprodol ... 363
Soma (GR) *see* Carisoprodol ... 363
Somalium (BR) *see* Bromazepam [CAN/INT] ... 290
Somatonorm (HR) *see* Somatropin ... 1918
Somatran (CL) *see* SUMAtriptan ... 1953
Somatuiline LP (LB) *see* Lanreotide ... 1165
Somatulina (ES) *see* Lanreotide ... 1165
Somatuline (AT, BE, CN, CZ, EE, GR, HN, HR, JO, JP, LT, NL, PL, RO, RU, SI, SK, TR) *see* Lanreotide ... 1165
Somatuline Autogel (AR, AU, BG, CH, CL, CO, CY, DE, GB, IE, IL, KR, NZ, SE, TH) *see* Lanreotide ... 1165
Somatuline LA (AU) *see* Lanreotide ... 1165
Somatuline LP (BH, FR) *see* Lanreotide ... 1165
Somatuline P.R. (CZ, FI, HK, IL, SG, TW) *see* Lanreotide ... 1165
Somavert (AR, AT, BE, BG, BR, CH, CZ, DE, DK, EE, ES, FI, FR, GB, GR, HN, HR, IE, IL, IT, JP, LT, MT, NL, NO, PE, PT, RO, RU, SE, SG, SI, SK, TR) *see* Pegvisomant ... 1604
Sombutol (FI) *see* PENTobarbital ... 1617
Somese (CL, CO, EC, MY, PE, VE) *see* Triazolam ... 2101
Somidem (AU, MY) *see* Zolpidem ... 2212
Somidex (TH) *see* MethylPREDNISolone ... 1340
Somin (TW) *see* Dexchlorpheniramine ... 603
Somit (AR, PY, UY) *see* Zolpidem ... 2212
Somlan (AR) *see* Flurazepam ... 906
Somnatrol (AR) *see* Estazolam ... 775
Somnil (CO) *see* Zolpidem ... 2212
Somnol (HN) *see* Zopiclone [CAN/INT] ... 2217
Somnols (EE) *see* Zopiclone [CAN/INT] ... 2217
Somno (PE) *see* Zolpidem ... 2212
Somnosan (DE) *see* Zopiclone [CAN/INT] ... 2217
Somnovit (ES) *see* Loprazolam [INT] ... 1241
Somofillina (IT) *see* Theophylline ... 2026
Somol (CL) *see* DiphenhydrAMINE (Systemic) ... 641
Sompraz (IN) *see* Esomeprazole ... 771
Sona (HR) *see* Adapalene ... 54
Sonata (AE, AT, AU, BE, BG, BH, CH, CZ, DE, DK, EE, ES, FI, FR, GB, GR, HN, HR, IE, IT, KW, LT, MT, MX, NL, NO, NZ, PL, PT, QA, RO, SE, SK, TR) *see* Zaleplon ... 2193
Sone (AU) *see* PredniSONE ... 1706
Songar (IT) *see* Triazolam ... 2101
Sonias (JP) *see* Pioglitazone and Glimepiride ... 1654
Sonicor (ID) *see* MethylPREDNISolone ... 1340
Sonide (IN) *see* Nitroprusside ... 1467
Sonin (DE) *see* Loprazolam [INT] ... 1241
Soniphen (PH) *see* DiphenhydrAMINE (Systemic) ... 641
Soni-Slo (AE, BF, BH, BJ, CI, CY, EG, ET, GH, GM, GN, IE, IQ, IR, JO, KE, KW, LB, LR, LY, MA, ML, MR, MU, MW, NE, NG, OM, QA, SA, SC, SD, SL, SN, SY, TN, TZ, UG, YE, ZM, ZW) *see* Isosorbide Dinitrate ... 1124
Sonlax (BG) *see* Zopiclone [CAN/INT] ... 2217
Soolda (CN) *see* FlavoxATE ... 881
Sooner (JP) *see* Isoproterenol ... 1124
Soonway (TW) *see* Scopolamine (Systemic) ... 1870
Soother (TW) *see* Ketotifen (Systemic) [CAN/INT] ... 1149
Sopental (ZA) *see* PENTobarbital ... 1617
Soperam (ID) *see* Cefoperazone and Sulbactam [INT] ... 382
Sophiamin (JP) *see* ChlordiazePOXIDE ... 422
Sophidone LP (FR) *see* HYDROmorphone ... 1016
Sophipren Ofteno (CL, CR, DO, GT, HN, NI, PA, SV) *see* PrednisoLONE (Ophthalmic) ... 1706
Sophixin DX Ofteno (CR, DO, GT, HN, NI, PA, SV) *see* Ciprofloxacin and Dexamethasone ... 446
Sophixin Ofteno (CR, DO, GT, HN, NI, PA, SV, VE) *see* Ciprofloxacin (Ophthalmic) ... 446
Sophixin Ofteno (CR, DO, GT, HN, NI, PA, SV, VE) *see* Ciprofloxacin (Systemic) ... 441
Sophos (PY) *see* AtoMOXetine ... 191
Sopralan-30 (ID) *see* Lansoprazole ... 1166
Sopranix (SE) *see* Lansoprazole ... 1166
Soprol-5 (PH) *see* Bisoprolol ... 266
Soprol (DO, IE) *see* Bisoprolol ... 266
Soproxen (TH) *see* Diclofenac (Systemic) ... 617
Sorbangil (NO, SE) *see* Isosorbide Dinitrate ... 1124
Sorbevit B12 (ES) *see* Cyanocobalamin ... 515
Sorbidilat (CH) *see* Isosorbide Dinitrate ... 1124
Sorbidin (AU, VN) *see* Isosorbide Dinitrate ... 1124
Sorbilac (HK) *see* Lactulose ... 1156
Sorbilande (IT) *see* Sorbitol ... 1927
Sorbilax (AU) *see* Sorbitol ... 1927
Sorbimon (HU) *see* Isosorbide Mononitrate ... 1126
Sorbinate SR (TH) *see* Isosorbide Mononitrate ... 1126
Sorbisterit (AT, BE, CH, CL, DE, DK, EE, FI, GB, LT, NL, SE, SI, SK) *see* Calcium Polystyrene Sulfonate [CAN/INT] ... 333
Sorbit Fresenius (AT) *see* Sorbitol ... 1927
Sorbit Leopold (AT) *see* Sorbitol ... 1927
Sorbit Mayrhofer (AT) *see* Sorbitol ... 1927
Sorbitol Aguettant (FR) *see* Sorbitol ... 1927
Sorbitol Baxter (LU) *see* Sorbitol ... 1927
Sorbitol Delalande (BE, FR) *see* Sorbitol ... 1927
Sorbitol-Infusionslosung (DE) *see* Sorbitol ... 1927
Sorbitrate (IN, LU) *see* Isosorbide Dinitrate ... 1124
Sorbon (IL) *see* BusPIRone ... 311
Sorbonit (HN, HU, PL) *see* Isosorbide Dinitrate ... 1124
Sorgoa (LU) *see* Tolnaftate ... 2063
Sorialen (TW) *see* Methoxsalen (Systemic) ... 1330
Soriatane (FR, VN) *see* Acitretin ... 43
Sorifran (MX) *see* Lansoprazole ... 1166
Sorlex (PH) *see* Cephalexin ... 405
S-Oropram (HK) *see* Escitalopram ... 765
Sortis (AT, BG, CH, CZ, DE, HR, PL, SE, SI, SK) *see* AtorvaSTATin ... 194
Sosegon (AE, BF, BH, BJ, CI, CY, EC, EG, ES, ET, GH, GM, GN, IL, IQ, IR, JO, JP, KE, KW, LB, LR, LY, MA, ML, MR, MU, MW, NE, NG, OM, PK, PT, QA, SA, SC, SD, SL, SN, SY, TN, TZ, UG, YE, ZM, ZW) *see* Pentazocine ... 1616
Sosegon[inj./rect.] (ES, JP) *see* Pentazocine ... 1616
Sosser (CO) *see* Sertraline ... 1878
Sostril (DE) *see* Ranitidine ... 1777
Sotacor (AR, AT, AU, BF, BJ, BR, CI, CN, CO, DK, ET, FI, GB, GH, GM, GN, HK, ID, IE, KE, LR, MA, ML, MR, MU, MW, MY, NE, NG, NL, NO, NZ, SC, SD, SE, SL, SN, TH, TN, TZ, UG, ZA, ZM, ZW) *see* Sotalol ... 1927
Sotagard (IN) *see* Sotalol ... 1927
Sotahexal (DE, HU, SG, VN, ZA) *see* Sotalol ... 1927
Sotalex (BE, CH, CZ, DE, FR, GR, HN, HU, IT, LU, PH, PL, PT, RU, SI, VN) *see* Sotalol ... 1927
Sotalex Mite (EE) *see* Sotalol ... 1927
Sotalol Knoll (HU) *see* Sotalol ... 1927
Sotalon (KR) *see* Sotalol ... 1927
Sotalon (TW) *see* Zaleplon ... 2193
Sotapor (ES) *see* Sotalol ... 1927
Sotatic-10 (ID) *see* Metoclopramide ... 1345
Sotax (TR) *see* Sotalol ... 1927
Sotilen (AE, BF, BH, BJ, CI, CY, EG, ET, GH, GM, GN, HK, IQ, IR, JO, KE, KW, LB, LR, LY, MA, ML, MR, MU,

MW, NE, NG, OM, QA, SA, SC, SD, SL, SN, SY, TN, TZ, UG, YE, ZM, ZW) *see* Piroxicam 1662
Sotrel (TW) *see* Benazepril 238
Sotret (IN, TH) *see* ISOtretinoin 1127
Sotrexe (MX) *see* ISOtretinoin 1127
Sotropil (ID) *see* Piracetam [INT] 1661
Sovarel (ES) *see* Almitrine [INT] 92
Sovenor (MY, SG) *see* Buprenorphine 300
Sovriad (JP) *see* Simeprevir 1887
Soxietas (ID) *see* ALPRAZolam 94
Sozol (AU) *see* Pantoprazole 1570
SP54 (HU, MY) *see* Pentosan Polysulfate Sodium 1617
Spaderizine (JP) *see* Cinnarizine [INT] 440
Spagerin (KR) *see* FlavoxATE 881
Spamilan (PL) *see* BusPIRone 311
Span-K (AU, HK, MY, NZ, PH) *see* Potassium Chloride 1687
Spara (CN, JP, KR, TW) *see* Sparfloxacin [INT] 1930
Spardac (IN) *see* Sparfloxacin [INT] 1930
Sparflo (VN) *see* Sparfloxacin [INT] 1930
Sparlox (IN) *see* Sparfloxacin [INT] 1930
Sparos (ID) *see* Sparfloxacin [INT] 1930
Sparx (BF, BJ, CI, ET, GH, GM, GN, KE, LR, MA, ML, MR, MU, MW, NE, NG, SC, SD, SL, SN, TN, TZ, UG, ZA, ZM, ZW) *see* Sparfloxacin [INT] 1930
Spasdon Drops (PH) *see* Dicyclomine 622
Spashi (ID) *see* Scopolamine (Systemic) 1870
Spasium (TH) *see* Trospium 2108
Spaslax (TW) *see* TiZANidine 2051
Spasmaverine (FR) *see* Alverine [INT] 104
Spasmed (EE) *see* Trospium 2108
Spasmex (AR, CL, HR, IL, KR, KW, LB, PY, QA, RU, SI, TH, TR, TW) *see* Trospium 2108
Spasmine (BE) *see* Alverine [INT] 104
Spasmolina (PL) *see* Alverine [INT] 104
Spasmo-Lyt (AE, BG, BH, CN, CY, CZ, DK, EG, FI, HK, IL, IQ, IR, JO, KW, LB, LY, OM, QA, SA, SY, YE) *see* Trospium 2108
Spasmolyt (AT, DE, KR, MY, SG, TH) *see* Trospium 2108
Spasmonal (AE, BE, BH, CN, CY, GB, HK, HN, IE, KW, LB, PK, SA, SG) *see* Alverine [INT] 104
Spasmonal (BE, LU) *see* Mebeverine [INT] 1275
Spasmonal Forte (CY, GB, IE, LB) *see* Alverine [INT] 104
Spasmoplex (PT) *see* Trospium 2108
Spasmopriv (CO, IN, MX, PH, PK, SG, TH, TW, VN) *see* Fenoverine [INT] 857
Spasmopriv (FR) *see* Mebeverine [INT] 1275
Spasmotalin (SA) *see* Mebeverine [INT] 1275
Spasmo-Urgenin Neo (CH) *see* Trospium 2108
Spasmoverine (VN) *see* Alverine [INT] 104
Spastec (TW) *see* Pinaverium [CAN/INT] 1651
Spasuret (DE) *see* FlavoxATE 881
Spasuri (TH) *see* FlavoxATE 881
Spatam (SG) *see* Acetylcysteine 40
Spatomin (KR) *see* Dicyclomine 622
Spaxim (ID) *see* Cefixime 380
Spazol (TH) *see* Itraconazole 1130
Spectracef (GR, PT) *see* Cefditoren 378
Spectra (IN) *see* Doxepin (Systemic) 676
Spectroderm (PE) *see* Mupirocin 1404
Spectrum (IT) *see* CefTAZidime 392
Spedifen (FR) *see* Ibuprofen 1032
SP Edonal (VN) *see* Erdosteine [INT] 753
Spedra (BE, CZ, DE, EE, ES, FR, GB, HR, LT, NL, RO, SE, SI, SK) *see* Avanafil 205
Speeda (PH, TH) *see* Rabies Vaccine 1764
Speedifen (TH) *see* Ibuprofen 1032
Spektracef (TR) *see* Cefditoren 378
Spektramox (SE) *see* Amoxicillin and Clavulanate 133
Spektrel (PH) *see* Gemifloxacin 957
Spersacarpin (DE) *see* Pilocarpine (Ophthalmic) 1649
Spersacarpine (CH, MY, PK, SE, TW) *see* Pilocarpine (Ophthalmic) 1649
Spersadex (CH, DE, HK, NO, ZA) *see* Dexamethasone (Ophthalmic) 602
Spersadex (CH, DE, HK, NO, ZA) *see* Dexamethasone (Systemic) 599
Spersanicol (HK, KR) *see* Chloramphenicol 421
Spersin (NZ) *see* Bacitracin, Neomycin, and Polymyxin B 223
Spica Spinal (ID) *see* Bupivacaine 299
Spifen (FR) *see* Ibuprofen 1032
Spike (KR) *see* Ketoconazole (Systemic) 1144
Spinax (TW) *see* Baclofen 223
Spinolac (VN) *see* Spironolactone 1931
Spirabiotic (ID) *see* Spiramycin [CAN/INT] 1931
Spiractin (AU, ZA) *see* Spironolactone 1931
Spiradan (ID) *see* Spiramycin [CAN/INT] 1931
Spiranter (ID) *see* Spiramycin [CAN/INT] 1931
Spirapril Sanabo (AT) *see* Spirapril [INT] 1931
Spiraxin (ES) *see* Rifaximin 1809
Spiriva (AE, AR, AT, AU, BE, BG, BH, BO, BR, CH, CL, CN, CO, CR, CY, CZ, DE, DK, DO, EC, EG, ES, FI, FR, GB, GR, GT, HK, HN, HR, ID, IE, IL, IQ, IR, IS, IT, JO, JP, KR, KW, LB, LT, LY, MX, MY, NI, NL, NO, NZ, OM, PA, PE, PH, PL, PR, PT, PY, QA, RO, RU, SA, SE, SG, SI, SK, SV, SY, TH, TR, TW, UY, VE, VN, YE) *see* Tiotropium 2046
Spiriva Respimat (AE, CN, CY, ID, KR, MY, PH, SG, TH, VN) *see* Tiotropium 2046
Spirix (DK, FI, NO) *see* Spironolactone 1931
Spiroctan (FR, LU) *see* Spironolactone 1931
Spirolac (PY) *see* Fluconazole 885
Spirolacton (ID) *see* Spironolactone 1931
Spirola (ID) *see* Spironolactone 1931
Spirolair (BE, LU) *see* Pirbuterol 1662
Spirolon (BF, BJ, CI, EC, ET, GH, GM, GN, KE, LR, MA, ML, MR, MU, MW, MY, NE, NG, SC, SD, SL, SN, TN, TZ, UG, ZM, ZW) *see* Spironolactone 1931
Spiron (DK, HU) *see* Spironolactone 1931
Spirone (PE) *see* Spironolactone 1931
Spirono-Isis (DE) *see* Spironolactone 1931
Spironolactone-Eurogenerics (LU) *see* Spironolactone 1931
Spironolactone-Searle (LU) *see* Spironolactone 1931
Spironolacton-ratiopharm (LU) *see* Spironolactone 1931
Spironol (IL) *see* Spironolactone 1931
Spiropent (AT, CO, CY, CZ, DE, ES, GR, HU, ID, IT, JP, MX, PE, PH, TR) *see* Clenbuterol [INT] 460
Spirosine (GR) *see* Cefotaxime 382
Spirotone (NZ, TW) *see* Spironolactone 1931
Spitomin (BG, HU, LT, RO, SK) *see* BusPIRone 311
Spiva with MCT-LCT (PH) *see* Propofol 1728
Splendil (BR, CL, JP) *see* Felodipine 850
Splendil ER (KR) *see* Felodipine 850
SP-Mucosov (SG) *see* Bromhexine [INT] 291
Spondylon (DE) *see* Ketoprofen 1145
Sponex (KR) *see* Itraconazole 1130
Sporacid (ID) *see* Itraconazole 1130
Sporal (CY, JO, TH, VN) *see* Itraconazole 1130
Sporanox IV (HK, PH) *see* Itraconazole 1130
Sporanox (AE, AR, AT, AU, BB, BE, BF, BH, BJ, BM, BR, BS, BZ, CH, CI, CL, CN, CO, CY, CZ, DK, EC, EE, EG, ES, ET, FI, FR, GB, GH, GM, GN, GR, GY, HK, ID, IE, IL, IQ, IR, IS, IT, JM, JO, KE, KR, KW, LB, LR, LU, LY, MA, ML, MR, MT, MU, MW, MX, MY, NE, NG, NL, NO, NZ, OM, PE, PH, PK, PR, PT, PY, QA, RU, SA, SC, SD, SE, SI, SK, SL, SN, SR, SY, TN, TR, TT, TW, TZ, UG, UY, VE, VN, YE, ZA, ZM, ZW) *see* Itraconazole 1130
Sporavast (JO) *see* Itraconazole 1130
Sporaxyl (TH) *see* Ketoconazole (Systemic) 1144
Sporaxyl (TH) *see* Ketoconazole (Topical) 1145

Sporicef (TH) *see* Cephalexin ... 405
Sporidex (AE, IN, PH) *see* Cephalexin ... 405
Sporidin AF (TH) *see* Cephalexin ... 405
Sporidin (TH) *see* Cephalexin ... 405
Sporiline (FR) *see* Tolnaftate ... 2063
Sporium (CO) *see* Ketoconazole (Topical) ... 1145
Spornar (TH) *see* Itraconazole ... 1130
Sportflex (BE) *see* Indomethacin ... 1067
Spray-Pax (FR, RU) *see* Pyrethrins and Piperonyl Butoxide ... 1746
Sprimeo (GR, NL) *see* Aliskiren ... 85
S-Pro 600 (TH) *see* Ibuprofen ... 1032
Sprycel (AE, AR, AT, AU, BE, BG, BH, BR, CH, CL, CN, CO, CY, CZ, DE, DK, EE, ES, FI, FR, GB, GR, HK, HN, HR, HU, ID, IE, IL, IN, IS, IT, JO, JP, KR, KW, LB, LT, MT, MY, NL, NO, NZ, PE, PL, PT, QA, RO, RU, SA, SE, SG, SI, SK, TH, TR, TW, UY) *see* Dasatinib ... 574
Sputopur (HU) *see* Acetylcysteine ... 40
Spy (IN) *see* Artesunate ... 178
Spyrocon (ID) *see* Itraconazole ... 1130
Sratop (AU) *see* CeFAZolin ... 373
Srilane (BE, FR, LU) *see* Idrocilamide [INT] ... 1040
SRK (CH) *see* Albumin ... 67
Stabilanol (IL) *see* Fluconazole ... 885
Stabin (KR) *see* Cinnarizine [INT] ... 440
Stable (TW) *see* HydrALAZINE ... 1007
Stablon (AR, AT, BH, BR, EG, FR, ID, IN, KW, MX, MY, PK, PT, QA, SA, SG, TH, TR, VE, VN) *see* Tianeptine [INT] ... 2033
Staborin (KR) *see* Tianeptine [INT] ... 2033
Staclazide 30 MR (HK) *see* Gliclazide [CAN/INT] ... 964
Stadaglicin (KR) *see* Cromolyn (Ophthalmic) ... 514
Stadalax (CZ) *see* Bisacodyl ... 265
Stada Uno (SG) *see* NIFEdipine ... 1451
Stadin (KR) *see* Famotidine ... 845
Stadol (JP, PL) *see* Butorphanol ... 314
Stadovas (HK, MY) *see* AmLODIPine ... 123
Staflocil (FI) *see* Cloxacillin [CAN/INT] ... 488
Stagid (PT) *see* MetFORMIN ... 1307
Stalene (TH) *see* Fluconazole ... 885
Stalevo (AE, AR, AT, AU, BE, BG, BH, BR, CH, CL, CN, CO, CY, CZ, DE, DK, EC, EE, ES, FI, FR, GB, GR, HK, HN, ID, IE, IL, IS, IT, JO, KR, KW, LB, LT, MT, MY, NL, NO, NZ, PE, PL, PT, QA, RU, SA, SE, SG, SI, SK, TH, TR, TW, UY, VE, VN) *see* Levodopa, Carbidopa, and Entacapone ... 1196
Stalev (PH) *see* Levodopa, Carbidopa, and Entacapone ... 1196
Stalip-A (PH) *see* Amlodipine and Atorvastatin ... 124
Stamaril (AE, AR, AU, BE, BG, CH, CL, CO, CY, CZ, DE, DK, EC, EE, FI, FR, GB, HK, HN, HR, IE, IL, IN, IS, IT, KR, LT, MY, NO, NZ, PE, PK, PL, PY, RO, SE, SG, SI, SK, TR, UY) *see* Yellow Fever Vaccine ... 2192
Stambutol (FI) *see* Ethambutol ... 798
Stamcor (IN) *see* Amlodipine and Atorvastatin ... 124
Stamlo (SG) *see* AmLODIPine ... 123
Stammin (GR) *see* Piracetam [INT] ... 1661
Stancef (PH) *see* CeFAZolin ... 373
Standacillin (AE, BG, BH, CY, EE, EG, IQ, IR, JO, KW, LB, LY, OM, QA, RO, SA, SY, YE) *see* Ampicillin ... 141
Standcillin (MY) *see* Ampicillin ... 141
Stapam (TW) *see* LORazepam ... 1243
Stapenor (AT) *see* Oxacillin ... 1528
Staphlex (NZ) *see* Flucloxacillin [INT] ... 885
Staphycid (BE) *see* Flucloxacillin [INT] ... 885
Staphylex (AU, DE) *see* Flucloxacillin [INT] ... 885
Stapin ER (KR) *see* Felodipine ... 850
Starasid (JP) *see* Cytarabine (Conventional) ... 535
Starcef (ID) *see* Cefixime ... 380
Starcef (IT) *see* CefTAZidime ... 392
Starcitin (HR) *see* Citalopram ... 451
Starhal (VN) *see* Haloperidol ... 993
Staril (AE, BH, GB, JO, KW, LB, QA, SA) *see* Fosinopril ... 932
Starin (TH) *see* Sertraline ... 1878
Starlix (AE, AR, BE, BH, BR, CH, CL, CO, CY, CZ, DE, DK, EE, EG, ES, FI, FR, GB, GR, HN, HR, HU, ID, IE, KW, LT, MT, MX, MY, NL, NO, PE, PH, PT, QA, RO, RU, SE, SG, SI, SK, TR, TW, UY, VE) *see* Nateglinide ... 1432
StarQuin (NZ) *see* Hetastarch ... 1004
Starsis (JP) *see* Nateglinide ... 1432
Starstat-EZ (IN) *see* Ezetimibe and Simvastatin ... 834
stas Hustenstiller N (DE) *see* Clobutinol [INT] ... 468
Statex (SG) *see* Morphine (Systemic) ... 1394
Statin (CO) *see* Simvastatin ... 1890
Statol (TR) *see* AtorvaSTATin ... 194
Stator (ID) *see* AtorvaSTATin ... 194
Stator (IL) *see* Rosuvastatin ... 1848
Statrol (AE, BF, BH, BJ, CI, CY, EG, ET, GH, GM, GN, IL, IQ, IR, JO, KE, KW, LB, LR, LY, MA, ML, MR, MU, MW, NE, NG, OM, QA, SA, SC, SD, SL, SN, SY, TN, TW, TZ, UG, YE, ZA, ZM, ZW) *see* Neomycin and Polymyxin B ... 1437
Staurodorm (AT, DE, LU) *see* Flurazepam ... 906
Stavid (MY) *see* Simvastatin ... 1890
Stavigile (BR) *see* Modafinil ... 1386
Stavinor (ID) *see* AtorvaSTATin ... 194
Stavir (IN, LB, TH) *see* Stavudine ... 1934
Stazepine (HU) *see* CarBAMazepine ... 346
Stazol (ID) *see* Cilostazol ... 437
Stazolin (TW) *see* CeFAZolin ... 373
Stazol (PY) *see* AcetaZOLAMIDE ... 39
Stazol (TW) *see* Econazole ... 703
S.T.D. (ZA) *see* Sodium Tetradecyl Sulfate ... 1914
Stecin (KR) *see* Acetylcysteine ... 40
Steclin V (ZA) *see* Tetracycline ... 2017
Stediril 30 (BE, CZ, NL) *see* Ethinyl Estradiol and Levonorgestrel ... 803
Stediril (BE, FR) *see* Ethinyl Estradiol and Norgestrel ... 812
Stei (TH) *see* Betahistine [CAN/INT] ... 252
Stelara (AR, AT, AU, BE, BR, CH, CL, CO, CR, CY, CZ, DE, DK, DO, EE, FR, GB, GT, HK, HN, HR, ID, IE, IL, IS, JP, KR, LT, MY, NI, NL, NO, NZ, PA, PH, PL, PT, RO, RU, SA, SE, SG, SI, SK, SV, TH, TR, TW) *see* Ustekinumab ... 2117
Stelax (AU, HK) *see* Baclofen ... 223
Stelazine (AE, AR, AU, BB, BF, BH, BJ, BM, BR, BS, BZ, CI, CO, CY, EG, ET, GH, GM, GN, GR, GY, HK, ID, IL, IQ, IR, JM, JO, KE, KW, LB, LR, LY, MA, ML, MR, MU, MW, MX, NE, NG, NL, NZ, OM, PH, PK, PL, QA, SA, SC, SD, SL, SN, SR, SY, TN, TR, TT, TZ, UG, YE, ZM, ZW) *see* Trifluoperazine ... 2102
Stelazine Forte Solution (GB, IE) *see* Trifluoperazine ... 2102
Stelazine MR (TR) *see* Trifluoperazine ... 2102
Stellasil (QA) *see* Trifluoperazine ... 2102
Stellatropine (LU) *see* Atropine ... 200
Stelosi (ID) *see* Trifluoperazine ... 2102
Stemetil (AE, AU, BB, BF, BH, BJ, BM, BS, BZ, CI, CY, DK, EG, ET, FI, GB, GH, GM, GN, GY, ID, IE, IL, IN, IQ, IS, IT, JM, KE, KW, LR, MA, ML, MR, MU, MW, NE, NG, NL, NO, NZ, OM, PK, QA, SC, SD, SE, SG, SL, SN, SR, TN, TR, TT, TZ, UG, YE, ZA, ZM, ZW) *see* Prochlorperazine ... 1718
Stemflova (FI, NO) *see* Terlipressin [INT] ... 2010
Stemgen (ZA) *see* Ancestim [INT] ... 150
Stemzine (AU) *see* Prochlorperazine ... 1718
Stenac (MY) *see* Acetylcysteine ... 40
Stenvix (JO) *see* Clopidogrel ... 484
Sterax (BE, CH, DE, LU) *see* Desonide ... 597
Stercia-5 (TH) *see* Finasteride ... 878
Stericort (PH) *see* Hydrocortisone (Systemic) ... 1013

Sterilid-V (PH) *see* Sulfacetamide and Prednisolone ... 1944
Sterimox (PH) *see* Amoxicillin ... 130
Sterizol (PH) *see* Silver Sulfadiazine ... 1887
Stermin (TW) *see* Atenolol ... 189
Sterodex (IL) *see* Dexamethasone (Ophthalmic) ... 602
Sterodex (IL) *see* Dexamethasone (Systemic) ... 599
Sterogyl-15 (FR) *see* Ergocalciferol ... 753
Sterogyl (BE, LU) *see* Ergocalciferol ... 753
Steronase AQ (IL) *see* Triamcinolone (Systemic) ... 2099
Steron (TH) *see* Norethindrone ... 1473
Sterotop (IN) *see* Prednicarbate ... 1703
Sterzar (TH) *see* Finasteride ... 878
Stesolid (AE, BH, CH, CY, DE, DK, EG, FI, HN, ID, IL, IQ, IR, IS, JO, LY, NO, OM, QA, SA, SE, SY, TW, YE) *see* Diazepam ... 613
Stesolid Rectal Tube (DE, HK) *see* Diazepam ... 613
Stidine (TW) *see* TiZANidine ... 2051
Stiedex (GB) *see* Desoximetasone ... 598
Stiemycin (AE, BR, CY, GB, IE, JO, KR, LB, NZ, SG, TH, UY, ZA) *see* Erythromycin (Topical) ... 765
Stieprox (AU, FI, GR, IE, MY, NO, PH, SG, SK, TH, TW) *see* Ciclopirox ... 433
Stieva-A (AU, CL, CO, CR, DO, GT, HN, KR, MX, MY, PY, SG, SV, TH, UY) *see* Tretinoin (Topical) ... 2099
Stieva-A Forte (MY) *see* Tretinoin (Topical) ... 2099
Stigmin (KR) *see* Neostigmine ... 1438
Stigmosan (HU) *see* Neostigmine ... 1438
Stilaze (BE) *see* Lormetazepam [INT] ... 1247
Stildem (AU) *see* Zolpidem ... 2212
Stilnix (IL) *see* Zolpidem ... 2212
Stilnoct (BE, DK, FI, GB, IE, IS, LU, NL, NO, SE) *see* Zolpidem ... 2212
Stilnox (AU, BF, BG, BJ, BR, CH, CI, CL, CN, CO, CR, CY, CZ, DE, DO, EE, ES, ET, FR, GH, GM, GN, GR, GT, HK, HN, HU, ID, IT, JO, KE, KR, KW, LB, LR, LT, MA, ML, MR, MU, MW, MX, MY, NE, NG, NI, PA, PE, PH, PK, PL, PT, PY, QA, RO, SA, SC, SD, SK, SL, SN, SV, TN, TR, TW, TZ, UG, VE, VN, ZA, ZM, ZW) *see* Zolpidem ... 2212
Stilnox CR (AU, BR, CO, HK, KR, MY, SG) *see* Zolpidem ... 2212
Stimu-ACTH (FR) *see* Corticorelin ... 509
Stimubral (PT) *see* Piracetam [INT] ... 1661
Stimuloton (BB, BM, BS, BZ, GY, JM, SR, TT) *see* Sertraline ... 1878
Stimycine (BE, FR) *see* Erythromycin (Topical) ... 765
Stiprox (MX, PE) *see* Ciclopirox ... 433
Stiron (KR) *see* Tianeptine [INT] ... 2033
Stivarga (AR, AU, CH, CL, CY, CZ, DE, DK, EE, ES, FR, GB, HK, HR, IL, IS, JP, KR, LT, MY, NL, NO, RO, SE, SG, SI, SK, TH, TR) *see* Regorafenib ... 1787
Stobiol (ID) *see* Bismuth ... 265
Stocpium (KR) *see* Trospium ... 2108
Stocrin (AE, AT, AU, BE, BG, BH, BR, CH, CL, CN, CO, CR, CY, CZ, DE, DK, EC, EE, FI, FR, GB, GR, GT, HK, HN, HR, HU, IE, IL, IS, IT, KR, KW, LT, MT, MX, MY, NI, NL, NO, NZ, PA, PE, PL, PT, QA, RO, RU, SE, SG, SI, SK, SV, TH, TR, TW, UY, VE, VN, ZA) *see* Efavirenz ... 707
Stodine (KR) *see* Lafutidine [INT] ... 1157
Stogamet (TW) *see* Cimetidine ... 438
Stogar (JP, KR) *see* Lafutidine [INT] ... 1157
Stolax (ID) *see* Bisacodyl ... 265
Stomacer (ID) *see* Omeprazole ... 1508
Stomax (AE, BH, CY, EG, IQ, IR, JO, KW, LB, LY, OM, QA, SA, SY, YE) *see* Famotidine ... 845
Stomec (TH) *see* Omeprazole ... 1508
Stomedine (FR, TH) *see* Cimetidine ... 438
Stomet (IT) *see* Cimetidine ... 438
Stomica (ID) *see* Scopolamine (Systemic) ... 1870
Stoparen (GR, LB) *see* Cefotaxime ... 382
Stopen (CO) *see* Piroxicam ... 1662
Stopit (IL) *see* Loperamide ... 1236
Stoppot (PL) *see* Methenamine ... 1317
Storan (KR) *see* Lafutidine [INT] ... 1157
Storvas (IN, MY) *see* AtorvaSTATin ... 194
Stotidin (KR) *see* Lafutidine [INT] ... 1157
Stratasin (MX) *see* Indomethacin ... 1067
Strattera (AE, AR, AT, AU, BE, BG, BH, CH, CL, CN, CO, CR, CY, CZ, DE, DK, DO, EC, EE, FI, FR, GB, GR, GT, HK, HN, HR, IE, IS, IT, JO, JP, KR, KW, LB, LT, MX, MY, NI, NL, NO, NZ, PA, PE, PH, PL, PT, QA, RO, SA, SE, SG, SI, SK, SV, TH, TR, TW, ZA) *see* AtoMOXetine ... 191
Strefen (FR) *see* Flurbiprofen (Systemic) ... 906
Strepfen (DK, GB, PT, TR) *see* Flurbiprofen (Systemic) ... 906
Strepsils Chesty Cough Lozenge (SG) *see* Ambroxol [INT] ... 109
Strepsils (EE, FI, IE) *see* Flurbiprofen (Systemic) ... 906
Strepsils Intensive (BG) *see* Flurbiprofen (Systemic) ... 906
Streptocin (MY) *see* Streptomycin ... 1937
Strepto-Hefa (DE) *see* Streptomycin ... 1937
Streptomycinum (PL) *see* Streptomycin ... 1937
Strepto (TH) *see* Streptomycin ... 1937
Stribild (AU, BE, CH, CZ, DE, DK, EE, ES, FR, GB, HK, HR, IL, IS, JP, KR, LT, NL, NO, NZ, SE, SK) *see* Elvitegravir, Cobicistat, Emtricitabine, and Tenofovir ... 718
Strimox (SG) *see* Amoxicillin ... 130
Stripole (TH) *see* Pantoprazole ... 1570
Striverdi Respimat (AU, CH, CZ, DE, DK, EE, FI, GB, IS, LT, NL, NO, RO, SE, SG, SK) *see* Olodaterol ... 1498
Striverdi Respipmat (SI) *see* Olodaterol ... 1498
Strodin (KR) *see* Glycopyrrolate ... 975
Strokan FC (MY) *see* Ticlopidine ... 2040
Stromectol (AU, FR, GR, NL, NO, NZ, SG, SI, VN) *see* Ivermectin (Systemic) ... 1136
Stronat (IN) *see* Strontium Ranelate [INT] ... 1938
Strumazol (BE, LU, NL) *see* Methimazole ... 1319
STS (IL) *see* Sodium Tetradecyl Sulfate ... 1914
Stud 100 (AU, IL) *see* Lidocaine (Topical) ... 1211
Stugeron (AR, BE, BH, BR, CH, CL, CO, CY, CZ, EE, EG, ES, GB, GR, HK, HN, HR, HU, ID, IE, IN, IT, JO, KW, LB, LT, LU, MX, MY, PE, PH, PK, PT, PY, QA, RO, SA, SG, SI, SK, TH, TR, UY, VE, VN, ZA) *see* Cinnarizine [INT] ... 440
Stugeron Forte (EC, GB, HR) *see* Cinnarizine [INT] ... 440
Stunarone (IL) *see* Cinnarizine [INT] ... 440
Stutgeron (AT, DE, HU, IE) *see* Cinnarizine [INT] ... 440
Styptin 5 (IN) *see* Norethindrone ... 1473
Suadian (IT) *see* Naftifine ... 1416
Suallergic (TW) *see* Cromolyn (Nasal) ... 514
Subamycin (IN) *see* Tetracycline ... 2017
Subcuvia (FR, GB) *see* Immune Globulin ... 1056
Suben (TW) *see* Bisacodyl ... 265
Subgam (GB, IE) *see* Immune Globulin ... 1056
Sublimaze (AR, AU, GB, IE, NZ, PH, ZA) *see* FentaNYL ... 857
Suboxone (AT, AU, BE, BG, CH, CY, CZ, DE, DK, EE, FI, FR, GB, GR, HK, HN, HR, HU, ID, IE, IS, IT, LT, MT, MY, NL, NO, NZ, PL, PT, RO, RU, SE, SG, SI, SK, TR, TW) *see* Buprenorphine and Naloxone ... 304
Subsalicilato de Bismuto (MX) *see* Bismuth ... 265
Sub Tensin (ES) *see* Nitrendipine [INT] ... 1463
Subulin (TW) *see* Pseudoephedrine ... 1742
Subutex (AE, AT, AU, BE, BG, CH, CZ, DE, DK, EE, FI, FR, HR, ID, IE, IL, IS, NO, PT, QA, SE, SG, TW) *see* Buprenorphine ... 300
Succi (AR) *see* Succinylcholine ... 1939
Succicaptal (FR) *see* Succimer ... 1939
Succicholine (KR) *see* Succinylcholine ... 1939
Succinil (BR) *see* Succinylcholine ... 1939
Succinyl Asta (HU, LU) *see* Succinylcholine ... 1939
Succinyl Forte (IL) *see* Succinylcholine ... 1939

Sucedal (EC) *see* Zolpidem ... 2212
Sucee (MY) *see* Cyproterone and Ethinyl Estradiol [CAN/INT] ... 532
Suclari (KR) *see* Clarithromycin ... 456
Suclear (HK) *see* Gliclazide [CAN/INT] ... 964
Sucrabest (LU) *see* Sucralfate ... 1940
Sucrafilm (BR) *see* Sucralfate ... 1940
Sucraid (TW) *see* Sacrosidase ... 1860
Sucralfin (IT) *see* Sucralfate ... 1940
Sucralose (AE) *see* Sucralfate ... 1940
Sucral (PY) *see* Sucralfate ... 1940
Sucramal (CR, DO, GT, HN, IT, NI, PA, SV) *see* Sucralfate ... 1940
Sucrate (CN, HK, LB) *see* Sucralfate ... 1940
Sucrate Gel (SG) *see* Sucralfate ... 1940
Sucrazide (AE, BH, CY, EG, IL, IQ, IR, JO, KW, LB, LY, OM, QA, SA, SY, YE) *see* GlipiZIDE ... 967
Sucrox (AR) *see* Iron Sucrose ... 1118
Sudafed (AE, BB, BH, BM, BS, BZ, CY, EE, EG, FR, GB, GY, IE, IN, IQ, IR, IT, JM, JO, KR, KW, LB, LT, LY, MX, NL, OM, PL, PT, QA, SA, SR, SY, TT, YE) *see* Pseudoephedrine ... 1742
Sudafed Sinus 12 Hour Relief (AU, NZ) *see* Pseudoephedrine ... 1742
Sude (CN) *see* Sucralfate ... 1940
Sudomyl (NZ) *see* Pseudoephedrine ... 1742
Sudosian (TH) *see* Pseudoephedrine ... 1742
Suduvax (KR) *see* Varicella Virus Vaccine ... 2141
Su Fen Ni (CN) *see* SUFentanil ... 1941
Sufenta (AR, AT, BE, CH, CL, CZ, DE, DK, EG, FI, FR, HR, ID, IS, LU, NL, NO, PL, PT, SA, SE, SI, TR, TW, UY, ZA) *see* SUFentanil ... 1941
Sufenta Forte (LB, SA, ZA) *see* SUFentanil ... 1941
Sufental (KR) *see* SUFentanil ... 1941
Sufentil (IN) *see* SUFentanil ... 1941
Sufen (TW) *see* Tiaprofenic Acid [CAN/INT] ... 2034
Sufisal (DO, GT, HN, MX, NI, SV) *see* Pentoxifylline ... 1618
Sufortanon (ES) *see* PenicillAMINE ... 1608
Sufrexal (BE, CZ, IT, LU, MX, NL, NO, PT) *see* Ketanserin [INT] ... 1144
Suftrex (EC) *see* Sulfamethoxazole and Trimethoprim ... 1946
Sugiran (ES) *see* Alprostadil ... 96
Sugril (TH) *see* GlyBURIDE ... 972
Suifac (MX) *see* Omeprazole ... 1508
Suismycetin (BB, BM, BS, BZ, GY, JM, PR, SR, TT) *see* Chloramphenicol ... 421
Sui Yue (CN) *see* Valsartan ... 2127
Sukit (TW) *see* Aluminum Hydroxide ... 103
Sukolin (FI, HN) *see* Succinylcholine ... 1939
Sulam (TH) *see* Ampicillin and Sulbactam ... 145
Sulbaccin (TH) *see* Ampicillin and Sulbactam ... 145
Sulbacin (IN, KR, PH) *see* Ampicillin and Sulbactam ... 145
Sulbazone (KR) *see* Cefoperazone and Sulbactam [INT] ... 382
Sulbazon (PH) *see* Cefoperazone and Sulbactam [INT] ... 382
Sulcef (RO) *see* Cefoperazone and Sulbactam [INT] ... 382
Sulcolon (ID) *see* SulfaSALAzine ... 1950
Sulconar (PE) *see* Carbidopa and Levodopa ... 351
Sulcran (CL) *see* Sucralfate ... 1940
Sulcrate (JP) *see* Sucralfate ... 1940
Suldisyn (GR) *see* Sulconazole ... 1943
Suldox (ID) *see* Sulfadoxine and Pyrimethamine [INT] ... 1946
Sulfacet (DE) *see* Sulfamethoxazole and Trimethoprim ... 1946
Sulfacet-R (CA) *see* Sulfur and Sulfacetamide ... 1953
Sulfacet Sodium (VE) *see* Sulfacetamide (Ophthalmic) ... 1943
SulfacidE (IL) *see* Sulfacetamide (Ophthalmic) ... 1943
Sulfaclan (KR) *see* Sulfacetamide (Ophthalmic) ... 1943
Sulfactin (PL) *see* Dimercaprol ... 638
Sulfadiacina de Plata (PY) *see* Silver Sulfadiazine ... 1887
Sulfadiazina (IT) *see* SulfADIAZINE ... 1944
Sulfadiazina Reig Jofre (ES) *see* SulfADIAZINE ... 1944
Sulfadiazine (GB) *see* SulfADIAZINE ... 1944
Sulfadiazine Suspensie FNA (NL) *see* SulfADIAZINE ... 1944
Sulfadiazin-Heyl (DE) *see* SulfADIAZINE ... 1944
Sulfadiazin Streuli (CH) *see* SulfADIAZINE ... 1944
Sulfadin (PH) *see* Silver Sulfadiazine ... 1887
Sulfamylon (BM, KR) *see* Mafenide ... 1261
Sulfaplata (CO, DO, EC, GT, HN, PA, SV) *see* Silver Sulfadiazine ... 1887
Sulfargin (EE) *see* Silver Sulfadiazine ... 1887
Sulfasalazin (HR) *see* SulfaSALAzine ... 1950
Sulfas-Chinidin (ID) *see* QuiNIDine ... 1759
Sulfast (PH) *see* Glimepiride ... 966
Sulfate d'Atropine-Chauvin (LU) *see* Atropine ... 200
Sulfate de Neomycine-Chauvin (LU) *see* Neomycin ... 1436
Sulfato de Efedrina Klinos (VE) *see* EPHEDrine (Systemic) ... 734
Sulfato de Efedrina (UY) *see* EPHEDrine (Systemic) ... 734
Sulfex (HK, SG) *see* Sulfacetamide (Ophthalmic) ... 1943
Sulfidrin (IN) *see* EPHEDrine (Systemic) ... 734
Sulfitis (ID) *see* SulfaSALAzine ... 1950
Sulfoid Trimetho (MX) *see* Sulfamethoxazole and Trimethoprim ... 1946
Sulfomyl (GB) *see* Mafenide ... 1261
Sulfotrimin (DE) *see* Sulfamethoxazole and Trimethoprim ... 1946
Sulidamor (IT) *see* Nimesulide [INT] ... 1456
Sulide (IT) *see* Nimesulide [INT] ... 1456
Sulidene[vet.] (FR) *see* Nimesulide [INT] ... 1456
Sulidin (PH) *see* Nimesulide [INT] ... 1456
Sulidor (PT) *see* Nimesulide [INT] ... 1456
Sulimax (PY) *see* Cefoperazone and Sulbactam [INT] ... 382
Sulimed (ES) *see* Nimesulide [INT] ... 1456
Sulindal (ES) *see* Sulindac ... 1953
Sulinda (TW) *see* Sulindac ... 1953
Sulindec (TW) *see* Sulindac ... 1953
Sulingqiong (CN) *see* Granisetron ... 983
Sullivan (PH) *see* Amoxicillin and Clavulanate ... 133
Sulmycin (DE) *see* Gentamicin (Systemic) ... 959
Suloril (TW) *see* Sulindac ... 1953
Sulosin (KR) *see* Tamsulosin ... 1974
Sulotrim (HR) *see* Sulfamethoxazole and Trimethoprim ... 1946
Sulotrim (HR) *see* Trimethoprim ... 2104
Sulperason (RU) *see* Cefoperazone and Sulbactam [INT] ... 382
Sulperazon (BG, CL, CO, CZ, HK, LT, MY, PE, PL, SK, TH, TR, UY, VE, VN) *see* Cefoperazone and Sulbactam [INT] ... 382
Sulperazone (PH) *see* Cefoperazone and Sulbactam [INT] ... 382
Sultamicilina (AR) *see* Ampicillin and Sulbactam ... 145
Sultam (PH) *see* Tamsulosin ... 1974
Sultanol (DE, JP) *see* Albuterol ... 69
Sulvina (ES) *see* Griseofulvin ... 985
Suma-B (MX) *see* Thiamine ... 2028
Sumagran (AU) *see* SUMAtriptan ... 1953
Sumamed (BG, CN, CZ, EE, PL, SK) *see* Azithromycin (Systemic) ... 216
Sumapen (PH) *see* Penicillin V Potassium ... 1614
Sumatab (AU) *see* SUMAtriptan ... 1953
Sumatran (SG) *see* SUMAtriptan ... 1953
Sumatridex (IL) *see* SUMAtriptan ... 1953
Sumavel DosePro (DE, DK) *see* SUMAtriptan ... 1953
Sumax (BR) *see* SUMAtriptan ... 1953
Sumaytene (TW) *see* Tazarotene ... 1980
Sumeth (PK) *see* Succinylcholine ... 1939

Sumial (ES) *see* Propranolol 1731
Sumig (PH) *see* SUMAtriptan 1953
Sumiko (VN) *see* PARoxetine 1579
Sumitran (MY, SG) *see* SUMAtriptan 1953
Sumitrex (IN, MX) *see* SUMAtriptan 1953
Sundiol (SK) *see* Alfacalcidol [CAN/INT] 82
Sunet Hton (TW) *see* Acetaminophen and Codeine 36
Sunglizide (HK, MY) *see* Gliclazide [CAN/INT] 964
Sunglucon (HK) *see* GlipiZIDE 967
Sunizine (SG) *see* Cetirizine 411
Sunpla (KR) *see* Eptaplatin [INT] 751
Sunpraz (RU) *see* Pantoprazole 1570
Suntrim Forte (TH) *see* Sulfamethoxazole and Trimethoprim 1946
Suntrim (TH) *see* Sulfamethoxazole and Trimethoprim 1946
Sunzepam (MX) *see* Diazepam 613
Supadol mono (LU) *see* Acetaminophen 32
Supecef (TW) *see* Cefepime 378
Superace (TR) *see* Captopril and Hydrochlorothiazide 345
Supercet (PE) *see* Acetaminophen and Tramadol 37
Supercillin (TW) *see* Amoxicillin 130
Superin (IN) *see* Parecoxib [INT] 1576
Supernem (TW) *see* Imipenem and Cilastatin 1051
Supernide (TW) *see* Repaglinide 1791
Superocin (TW) *see* Ciprofloxacin (Systemic) 441
Supertidine (TW) *see* Famotidine 845
Supirocin (MY, SG) *see* Mupirocin 1404
Suplac (TH) *see* Bromocriptine 291
Suplasyn (DE, ID) *see* Hyaluronate and Derivatives 1006
Suposin (PY) *see* Nonoxynol 9 1471
Supplin (AE, BH, CY, EG, IQ, IR, JO, KW, LB, LY, OM, QA, SA, SY, YE) *see* MetroNIDAZOLE (Systemic) 1353
Suppojuvent Sedante (ES) *see* Chloral Hydrate [CAN/INT] 418
Supra (AE, BH, CY, EG, IQ, IR, JO, KW, LB, LY, OM, QA, SA, SY, YE) *see* Sildenafil 1882
Supracef (FI) *see* Cefixime 380
Supracyclin (AT, CH, PE) *see* Doxycycline 689
Supradol (DO, PA, SV) *see* Ketorolac (Systemic) 1146
Suprafen (KR) *see* Acetaminophen and Tramadol 37
Supraflox (TH) *see* Ciprofloxacin (Systemic) 441
Supraler D (PY) *see* Desloratadine and Pseudoephedrine 594
Supraler (PY) *see* Desloratadine 594
Supral (IN) *see* Iron Dextran Complex 1117
Supramycina (CR, DO, EC, GT, HN, NI, PA, PY, SV) *see* Doxycycline 689
Supran (IL) *see* Cefixime 380
Suprarenin (AT, DE) *see* EPINEPHrine (Systemic, Oral Inhalation) 735
Suprasec (AR) *see* Loperamide 1236
Supraviran (JO, LB) *see* Acyclovir (Systemic) 47
Suprax (AE, BH, CZ, DE, EG, GB, HU, IE, IT, JO, KR, KW, LB, QA, RU, SA, SK, TR) *see* Cefixime 380
Suprefact® [CA] *see* Buserelin [CAN/INT] 309
Suprefact® Depot [CA] *see* Buserelin [CAN/INT] 309
Suprekof (PH) *see* GuaiFENesin 986
Supremin (PH) *see* Phentermine 1635
Supressin (AT) *see* Doxazosin 674
Supretic (PY) *see* Hydroxychloroquine 1021
Supricort (PE) *see* Fluocinolone (Topical) 893
Suprimal (EC) *see* Mesalamine 1301
Suprimal (NL) *see* Meclizine 1277
Suprim (PE) *see* Sulfamethoxazole and Trimethoprim 1946
Suprimun (CL) *see* Mycophenolate 1405
Suprin (IT) *see* Sulfamethoxazole and Trimethoprim 1946
Suqi (CN) *see* Mometasone (Topical) 1391
Sural (CZ, HN, HU) *see* Ethambutol 798
Surazem (LU) *see* Diltiazem 634
Surbronc (BE, FR) *see* Ambroxol [INT] 109
Surecef (PH) *see* Cefaclor 372
Sure Cure (QA) *see* Adapalene 54
Surepost (JP) *see* Repaglinide 1791
Suretin (CH, IT, MX) *see* Tazarotene 1980
Surfacten (JP, KR) *see* Beractant 250
Surfont (DE) *see* Mebendazole [CAN/INT] 1274
Surgam (AU, BE, BH, CH, CZ, DE, EG, FR, GB, GR, HN, HR, HU, IE, KR, KW, LB, LU, MX, NL, NZ, PK, PL, PT, QA, SA, SG, SK, TR, TW, VN, ZA) *see* Tiaprofenic Acid [CAN/INT] 2034
Surgamic (ES) *see* Tiaprofenic Acid [CAN/INT] 2034
Surgam SR (KR) *see* Tiaprofenic Acid [CAN/INT] 2034
Surgamyl (DK, FI, IT) *see* Tiaprofenic Acid [CAN/INT] 2034
Suring (TW) *see* Acetaminophen and Codeine 36
Surishia (TW) *see* Phenazopyridine 1629
Surixime (PH) *see* Cefixime 380
Surlid (DK, FI, SE) *see* Roxithromycin [INT] 1853
Survanta (AE, AR, AT, AU, BB, BE, BG, BH, BM, BR, BS, BZ, CH, CL, CO, CR, CY, CZ, DE, DO, EC, EG, ES, FR, GB, GR, GT, GY, HK, HN, HU, ID, IE, IL, IQ, IR, JM, JO, KW, LB, LU, LY, MX, MY, NI, NL, NO, NZ, OM, PA, PE, PH, PK, PL, PR, PY, QA, SA, SG, SR, SV, SY, TH, TT, TW, UY, VE, VN, YE, ZA) *see* Beractant 250
Survanta-Vent (SE) *see* Beractant 250
Suspen ER (KR) *see* Acetaminophen 32
Sustac (AE, BB, BH, BM, BS, BZ, CY, EG, GY, HR, HU, IQ, IR, JM, JO, KW, LB, LY, OM, QA, SA, SR, SY, TT, YE) *see* Nitroglycerin 1465
Sustanon (EG, JO, KW, SA) *see* Testosterone 2010
Sustemial (IT) *see* Ferrous Gluconate 870
Sustiva (AT, BE, BG, CH, CZ, DE, DK, EE, FR, GB, GR, HN, HR, IE, IT, MT, NL, NO, PL, RO, RU, SE, SK, TR) *see* Efavirenz 707
Sustonit (PL) *see* Nitroglycerin 1465
Sutac (TH) *see* Cetirizine 411
Sutene (KR) *see* SUNItinib 1957
Sutent (AE, AR, AT, AU, BE, BG, BH, BR, BZ, CH, CL, CN, CO, CR, CY, CZ, DE, DK, DO, EC, EE, ES, FI, FR, GB, GR, GT, HK, HN, HR, HU, ID, IE, IL, IS, IT, JP, KW, LB, LT, MT, MY, NI, NL, NO, NZ, PA, PE, PH, PL, PT, QA, RO, RU, SA, SE, SG, SI, SK, SV, TH, TR, TW, UY, VE, VN) *see* SUNItinib 1957
Sutolin (TW) *see* Naproxen 1427
Suton (TW) *see* Mefloquine 1280
Sutran X (PY) *see* Haloperidol 993
Sutril (ES) *see* Torsemide 2071
Suxamethonium (AU, NZ) *see* Succinylcholine 1939
Suxameton (DK) *see* Succinylcholine 1939
Suxametonio cloruro (CL) *see* Succinylcholine 1939
Suxametonio Cloruro (PY) *see* Succinylcholine 1939
Suxidina (ES) *see* Oxazepam 1532
Suxilep (BG, DE, HU, RU) *see* Ethosuximide 813
Suximal (PT) *see* Ethosuximide 813
Suxin (CN) *see* BusPIRone 311
Suxinutin (AT, CL, FI, HN, HU, SE) *see* Ethosuximide 813
Su Ya (CN) *see* Celiprolol [INT] 404
Suym Otico (PE) *see* Acetic Acid 39
Suzin (TW) *see* Flunarizine [CAN/INT] 892
Suzutolon (JP) *see* Betahistine [CAN/INT] 252
Svedocain (ES) *see* Bupivacaine 299
Sweetcee (TH) *see* Ascorbic Acid 178
Swelcid (PH) *see* Celecoxib 402
Swich (PH) *see* Cefpodoxime 388
Swiflor (TW) *see* Cefaclor 372
Swiss Relief Dual Release (IL) *see* Diclofenac (Systemic) 617
Swityl (TW) *see* Dicyclomine 622
Sycara (EE) *see* Azelastine and Fluticasone 214

Syclop (PH) *see* CloZAPine ... 490
Sycrest (BE, CH, CY, CZ, DE, DK, EE, GB, HR, IS, NO, PL, PT, QA, RO, SE, SK, TR) *see* Asenapine ... 179
Sydepres (PH) *see* FluPHENAZine ... 905
Sydnaginon (ID) *see* Ethinyl Estradiol and Levonorgestrel ... 803
Sydolil (MX) *see* Ergotamine ... 754
Syklofosfamid (TR, TW) *see* Cyclophosphamide ... 517
Sykofen (TH) *see* Ketotifen (Systemic) [CAN/INT] ... 1149
Sylomet (PH) *see* Promethazine ... 1723
Sylos Vaginal Tab (KR) *see* Oxiconazole ... 1536
Sylvant (CZ, DE, HR, LT, SE, SI, SK) *see* Siltuximab ... 1885
Sylvite (PH) *see* Potassium Chloride ... 1687
Symbenda (KR, SG) *see* Bendamustine ... 241
Symbicort Forte (TH) *see* Budesonide and Formoterol ... 297
Symbicort (HR, IS, LT, SI, SK) *see* Budesonide and Formoterol ... 297
Symbicort Rapihaler (AU) *see* Budesonide and Formoterol ... 297
Symbicort Turbohaler (BE, DE, GB, IE) *see* Budesonide and Formoterol ... 297
Symbicort Turbuhaler (AE, AR, AT, AU, BB, BG, BH, BM, BR, BS, BZ, CH, CL, CN, CO, CR, CY, CZ, DK, DO, EE, FI, FR, GR, GT, GY, HK, HN, ID, IL, IT, JM, JO, JP, KR, KW, LB, MY, NI, NL, NO, NZ, PA, PE, PH, PL, PR, PT, PY, RU, SA, SE, SG, SR, SV, TH, TR, TT, TW, UY, VE, VN) *see* Budesonide and Formoterol ... 297
Symbiocort Turbuhaler (ES, MX) *see* Budesonide and Formoterol ... 297
Symbyax (MX) *see* FLUoxetine ... 899
Symitec (TW) *see* Cetirizine ... 411
Symmetrel (AE, AU, BH, CH, CY, EG, GR, HR, IE, IQ, IR, JO, KW, LB, LY, NL, NO, NZ, OM, QA, SA, SY, VE, YE) *see* Amantadine ... 105
Symoron (NL) *see* Methadone ... 1311
Sympal (DE) *see* Clobutinol [INT] ... 468
Sympal (DE) *see* Dexketoprofen [INT] ... 603
Synacthen (AR, AT, AU, BE, CH, CZ, DE, DK, GB, IE, IT, KR, LU, NO, NZ, PL, RO, RU, SE, SI) *see* Cosyntropin ... 510
Synacthen Deposito (CO, VE) *see* Cosyntropin ... 510
Synacthen Depot (AE, AT, AU, BF, BG, BH, BJ, CH, CI, CL, CY, CZ, DK, EG, ET, FI, GB, GH, GM, GN, GR, HN, HR, IE, IL, IQ, IR, IT, JO, KE, KR, KW, LB, LR, LY, MA, ML, MR, MU, MW, NE, NG, NL, NO, NZ, OM, PL, PT, QA, SA, SC, SD, SE, SL, SN, SY, TN, TR, TZ, UG, UY, YE, ZA, ZM, ZW) *see* Cosyntropin ... 510
Synacthene (FR, GR, IN, VN) *see* Cosyntropin ... 510
Synagis (AE, AR, AT, AU, BE, BG, BH, BO, BR, CH, CL, CO, CR, CY, CZ, DE, DK, DO, EC, EE, EG, ES, FI, FR, GB, GR, GT, HK, HN, HR, HU, IE, IQ, IR, IT, JO, JP, KR, KW, LB, LT, LY, MT, MX, MY, NI, NL, NO, NZ, OM, PA, PE, PL, PR, PT, QA, RO, RU, SA, SE, SG, SI, SK, SV, SY, TR, TW, UY, VE, YE) *see* Palivizumab ... 1560
Synalar (MX) *see* Polymyxin B ... 1676
Synalar (AE, AT, BE, BF, BH, BJ, CH, CI, CY, DK, EE, EG, ES, ET, FR, GB, GH, GM, GN, GR, HK, IQ, IR, IS, JO, KE, KW, LB, LR, LY, MA, ML, MR, MT, MU, MW, NE, NG, NO, NZ, OM, PK, PT, QA, SA, SC, SD, SE, SI, SK, SL, SN, SY, TN, TR, TZ, UG, YE, ZM, ZW) *see* Fluocinolone (Topical) ... 893
Synalar Simple (UY) *see* Fluocinolone (Topical) ... 893
Synarela (DK, FI, IS, NO, SE) *see* Nafarelin ... 1414
Synarel (AU, BE, BF, BG, BJ, BR, CI, CZ, DE, ES, ET, FR, GB, GH, GM, GN, GR, HN, HU, IE, KE, LR, LU, MA, ML, MR, MU, MW, MX, NE, NG, NL, PL, PT, RU, SC, SD, SG, SI, SL, SN, TN, TR, TW, TZ, UG, ZA, ZM, ZW) *see* Nafarelin ... 1414
Synasteron (BE) *see* Oxymetholone ... 1546
Synaze (HR, RO) *see* Azelastine and Fluticasone ... 214
Synbicort (RO) *see* Budesonide and Formoterol ... 297
Synbicort Turbuhaler (QA) *see* Budesonide and Formoterol ... 297
Synbrozil (HK) *see* Gemfibrozil ... 956
Synclar (HK) *see* Clarithromycin ... 456
Syncon (MY) *see* Gliclazide [CAN/INT] ... 964
Syncrospas (IN) *see* Fenoverine [INT] ... 857
Syncumar (HN, PL, RU) *see* Acenocoumarol [CAN/INT] ... 30
Syndopa (VN) *see* Carbidopa and Levodopa ... 351
Synephron (JP) *see* Furosemide ... 940
Synercid (FR, GR, HN, IT, KR) *see* Quinupristin and Dalfopristin ... 1762
Synermox (NZ) *see* Amoxicillin and Clavulanate ... 133
Syneudon (DE) *see* Amitriptyline ... 119
Synflex (AU, IE) *see* Naproxen ... 1427
Synflorix (AE, AR, AT, AU, BE, CL, CY, CZ, DE, EC, EE, ES, GB, HK, HR, ID, IL, IS, LB, LT, MY, NL, NO, NZ, PE, PH, PL, PT, QA, RO, SA, SE, SG, SI, SK, TH, TR, TW, VN) *see* Pneumococcal Conjugate Vaccine (10-Valent) [CAN/INT] ... 1668
Syn M.D. (BE, CH, LU) *see* Sorbitol ... 1927
Synomax (IN) *see* AcetaZOLAMIDE ... 39
Synox (IN) *see* Levothyroxine ... 1205
Synphase-2 (AE) *see* Ethinyl Estradiol and Norethindrone ... 808
Synphasic 28 (AU, NZ) *see* Ethinyl Estradiol and Norethindrone ... 808
Synrelina (CH) *see* Nafarelin ... 1414
Synrelin (AR) *see* Nafarelin ... 1414
Synsul (CO) *see* Sulfacetamide (Ophthalmic) ... 1943
Syntace (TW) *see* Ramipril ... 1771
Syntaris (AE, BE, BH, DE, IN, KW, NL, QA) *see* Flunisolide (Nasal) ... 893
Syntarpen (PL) *see* Cloxacillin [CAN/INT] ... 488
Syntarpen (PL) *see* Oxacillin ... 1528
Syntesor (PH) *see* Hydrocortisone (Systemic) ... 1013
Syntex (MX) *see* Polymyxin B ... 1676
Synthetic Oxytocin INJ (IN) *see* Oxytocin ... 1549
Synthocilin (IN) *see* Ampicillin ... 141
Synthomycin (RU) *see* Chloramphenicol ... 421
Synthroid (BR, CO, KR, KW, NZ, QA) *see* Levothyroxine ... 1205
Synthyroxine (KR) *see* Levothyroxine ... 1205
Syntocil (TR) *see* Ampicillin ... 141
Syntocinon (CL, DK, EG, HR, IS, LU, PT, SI, TR, VN) *see* Oxytocin ... 1549
Syntocinon INJ (AR, AT, AU, BE, BF, BJ, BR, CH, CI, DE, ES, ET, FI, FR, GB, GH, GM, GN, HK, ID, IE, IT, KE, LR, MA, ML, MR, MU, MW, MX, MY, NE, NG, NL, NZ, PE, PH, PK, PL, PY, SC, SD, SE, SG, SL, SN, TN, TZ, UG, UY, VE, ZA, ZM, ZW) *see* Oxytocin ... 1549
Syntocinon Spray (AT, CH, NO, PL, SE) *see* Oxytocin ... 1549
Syntofene (FR) *see* Ibuprofen ... 1032
Syntometrine (AU, NZ) *see* Oxytocin and Ergometrine Maleate [INT] ... 1550
Syntostigmin (BG) *see* Neostigmine ... 1438
Syntrend (TW) *see* Carvedilol ... 367
Synvisc (AE, AR, AU, BR, CH, EC, GB, HK, IE, JP, MX, NZ, PE, PH, PY, SE, SG, TH, UY, VE) *see* Hyaluronate and Derivatives ... 1006
Synvisc One (HK, SG) *see* Hyaluronate and Derivatives ... 1006
Synvisc-One (PH) *see* Hyaluronate and Derivatives ... 1006
Synvodex (PH) *see* Silver Sulfadiazine ... 1887
Synzar (TW) *see* Losartan and Hydrochlorothiazide ... 1250
Syollone (KR) *see* Econazole ... 703
Syprine (KR, SG, TW) *see* Trientine ... 2102
Syrea (DE) *see* Hydroxyurea ... 1021

Syrop acidi e-aminocapronici (PL) *see* Aminocaproic Acid 113
Syscan (IN) *see* Fluconazole 885
Syscor CC (BB, BM, BS, BZ, GY, JM, NL, NZ, SR, TT) *see* Nisoldipine 1459
Syscor (AT, BE, CH, ES, FI, GR, IT, LU, NL, NZ, PL, TW) *see* Nisoldipine 1459
Syscor ER (KR) *see* Nisoldipine 1459
Syscor MR (GB) *see* Nisoldipine 1459
Sysmuco (ID) *see* Rebamipide [INT] 1786
S.Z. (TW) *see* Clobetasol 468
T3 Actin (MY, VN) *see* Tretinoin (Topical) 2099
T3Actin (PH, SG) *see* Tretinoin (Topical) 2099
T3ADA (MY) *see* Adapalene 54
T3 (GR, PY) *see* Liothyronine 1221
T3Mycin (HK, PH, SG) *see* Clindamycin (Topical) 464
T4KP (TH) *see* Levothyroxine 1205
T4 (PY) *see* Levothyroxine 1205
Tabalon 400 (MX) *see* Ibuprofen 1032
Tabaxin (KR) *see* Piperacillin and Tazobactam 1657
Tabcin (AR) *see* Ambroxol [INT] 109
Tabel (KR) *see* Ketorolac (Systemic) 1146
Tabellae Ephedrini (TW) *see* EPHEDrine (Systemic) 734
Tabine (PH) *see* Cytarabine (Conventional) 535
Tabitral (MX) *see* Halobetasol 993
Tabloid (UY) *see* Thioguanine 2029
Tabocine (AE) *see* Doxycycline 689
Tabphyn MR (GB) *see* Tamsulosin 1974
Tabrin (GR) *see* Ofloxacin (Systemic) 1490
Tabulin (KR) *see* Glycopyrrolate 975
Taceedo (PH) *see* DOCEtaxel 656
Tacex (MX) *see* CefTRIAXone 396
Tachydaron (DE) *see* Amiodarone 114
Tacirel LM (PT) *see* Trimetazidine [INT] 2104
Tacrobell (KR) *see* Tacrolimus (Systemic) 1962
Tacrol (PK) *see* Tacrolimus (Topical) 1968
Tacrotec (PH) *see* Tacrolimus (Systemic) 1962
Tadex (FI, TW) *see* Tamoxifen 1971
Tadilor (DO) *see* Metoprolol 1350
Tadim (AU, GR, NL, SE) *see* Colistimethate 504
Tadol (SI) *see* TraMADol 2074
Tador (RO) *see* Dexketoprofen [INT] 603
Taesun Cream (KR) *see* Diflorasone 625
Tafenil (MX) *see* Flutamide 907
Tafil D (MU) *see* ALPRAZolam 94
Tafil (DE, DK, IS, MX, VE) *see* ALPRAZolam 94
Tafinlar (AU, BE, BM, CH, CZ, DE, DK, EE, FR, GB, HR, IL, IS, LT, NL, NO, RO, SE, SI, SK) *see* Dabrafenib 546
Tafirol Flex (MX) *see* Chlorzoxazone 430
Tafirol (PE) *see* Acetaminophen 32
Tafloc (ZA) *see* Ofloxacin (Systemic) 1490
Tagal (MX) *see* CefTAZidime 392
Tagamet (AE, AU, BB, BF, BH, BJ, BM, BR, BS, BZ, CI, CN, CY, EG, ES, ET, FR, GB, GH, GM, GN, GR, GY, IE, IL, IQ, IR, IT, JM, JO, KE, KR, KW, LB, LR, LU, LY, MA, ML, MR, MU, MW, MX, MY, NE, NG, NL, OM, PK, PT, QA, SA, SC, SD, SE, SG, SL, SN, SR, SY, TN, TT, TW, TZ, UG, VN, YE, ZM, ZW) *see* Cimetidine 438
Tagidine (KR) *see* Trimetazidine [INT] 2104
Tagocin (KR) *see* Teicoplanin [INT] 1983
Tagonis (DE) *see* PARoxetine 1579
Tagraf (PH) *see* Tacrolimus (Systemic) 1962
Tagra (LB) *see* Tadalafil 1968
Tagremin (RO) *see* Sulfamethoxazole and Trimethoprim 1946
Tagren (EE, HR) *see* Ticlopidine 2040
Tahor (FR, MU) *see* AtorvaSTATin 194
Taigalor (IT) *see* Lornoxicam [INT] 1248
Takadol (FR) *see* TraMADol 2074
Takanarumin (JP) *see* Allopurinol 90
Takepron (AE, BF, BH, BJ, CI, CN, ET, GH, GM, GN, JO, JP, KE, KW, LB, LR, MA, ML, MR, MU, MW, NE, NG, QA, SA, SC, SD, SL, SN, TN, TW, TZ, UG, ZA, ZM, ZW) *see* Lansoprazole 1166
Takepron OD (HK) *see* Lansoprazole 1166
Takesulin (JP) *see* Cefsulodin [INT] 391
Taks (AE, BH, CY, EG, IQ, IR, JO, KW, LB, LY, OM, QA, SA, SY, YE) *see* Diclofenac (Systemic) 617
Talam (AU) *see* Citalopram 451
Talavir (IT) *see* ValACYclovir 2119
Talcef (PE) *see* Cefotaxime 382
Talcom (CN) *see* Clopidogrel 484
Talema (VE) *see* Diazepam 613
Talion (CN, ID, JP, KR) *see* Bepotastine 250
Talispenem (VN) *see* Imipenem and Cilastatin 1051
Talliton (BB, BM, BS, BZ, GY, HK, JM, SR, TT) *see* Carvedilol 367
Talopram (PY) *see* Escitalopram 765
Talorat (NI) *see* Loratadine 1241
Taloxa (AT, BE, CH, CZ, DE, ES, FR, HN, HU, IT, LU, NL, NO, PL, PT, SE) *see* Felbamate 850
Talpramin (MX) *see* Imipramine 1054
Talusin (LB) *see* Tamsulosin 1974
Talval (CH) *see* Idrocilamide [INT] 1040
Talwin Lactate (IT, PE) *see* Pentazocine 1616
Talymus (JP) *see* Tacrolimus (Topical) 1968
Tamalis (CZ) *see* Rupatadine [INT] 1855
Tamate (AU) *see* Topiramate 2065
Tambocor (AE, AU, BE, BF, BH, BJ, BM, CH, CI, CL, CR, CY, DE, DK, EE, EG, ET, FI, GB, GH, GM, GN, GR, GT, HK, HN, IE, IL, IQ, IR, IS, JO, JP, KE, KR, KW, LB, LR, LU, LY, MA, ML, MR, MU, MW, MX, MY, NE, NG, NI, NL, NO, NZ, OM, PA, PH, QA, RO, SA, SC, SD, SE, SL, SN, SV, SY, TH, TN, TW, TZ, UG, UY, YE, ZA, ZM, ZW) *see* Flecainide 882
Tambocor CR (NZ, PH) *see* Flecainide 882
Tambutol (KR) *see* Ethambutol 798
Tambux (AR) *see* Rifabutin 1803
Tamdura (IN) *see* Dutasteride and Tamsulosin 702
Tamec (CH) *see* Tamoxifen 1971
Tametil (HR) *see* Domperidone [CAN/INT] 666
Tamifen (AE, BH, CY, EG, IQ, IR, JO, KW, LB, LY, OM, QA, SA, SY, YE) *see* Tamoxifen 1971
Tamifine (VN) *see* Tamoxifen 1971
Tamiflu (AE, AR, AT, AU, BE, BG, BH, BR, CH, CL, CN, CO, CY, CZ, DE, DK, EC, EE, ES, FI, FR, GB, GR, HK, HN, HR, HU, IE, IL, IS, IT, JP, KR, KW, LB, LT, MT, MX, NL, NO, NZ, PE, PH, PK, PL, PT, PY, QA, RO, RU, SA, SE, SG, SI, SK, TH, TR, TW, UY, VN) *see* Oseltamivir 1523
Tamik (FR, VN) *see* Dihydroergotamine 633
Tamin (ES) *see* Famotidine 845
Tamirin SR (KR) *see* Galantamine 946
Tamizam (BE, LU) *see* Tamoxifen 1971
Tamlosin SR (KR) *see* Tamsulosin 1974
Tamlosin (TW) *see* Tamsulosin 1974
Tamofen (CN, DK, FI, HK, ID, IL, NO, TW) *see* Tamoxifen 1971
Tamofon (AE, JO) *see* Tamoxifen 1971
Tamolan (TH) *see* TraMADol 2074
Tamoliv (ID) *see* Acetaminophen 32
Tamophar (AE, BH, KW, SA) *see* Tamoxifen 1971
Tamoplex (KR, PE, PH) *see* Tamoxifen 1971
Tamorex (KR) *see* Tamoxifen 1971
Tamosin (AU) *see* Tamoxifen 1971
Tamoxen (AU) *see* Tamoxifen 1971
Tamoxifen-Eurogenerics (LU) *see* Tamoxifen 1971
Tamoxifen-Hexal (LU) *see* Tamoxifen 1971
Tamoxifen-ratiopharm (LU) *see* Tamoxifen 1971
Tamoxifen-Teva (HU) *see* Tamoxifen 1971
Tamoxifen-Zeneca (LU) *see* Tamoxifen 1971
Tamoxi (IL) *see* Tamoxifen 1971
Tamoxit (LB) *see* Tamoxifen 1971
Tamsil (AU) *see* Terbinafine (Systemic) 2002
Tamsnal SR (KR) *see* Tamsulosin 1974

Tamsulin (IL, KW) *see* Tamsulosin 1974
Tamsulo (KR) *see* Tamsulosin 1974
Tamsulon (CR, DO, EC, GT, HN, NI, SV) *see* Tamsulosin 1974
Tamunal (KR) *see* Tamsulosin 1974
Tanapress (ID) *see* Imidapril [INT] 1051
Tanatril (AE, AR, AT, CN, CZ, DE, FR, GB, GR, HK, IN, IT, JP, KR, LB, MY, PK, PL, SG, VN) *see* Imidapril [INT] 1051
Tanattril (SA, SK, TH) *see* Imidapril [INT] 1051
Tancofeto (MY) *see* Vancomycin 2130
Tancore (TW) *see* Acetylcysteine 40
Tandegyl (PK) *see* Clemastine 459
Tandemact (AT, BE, BG, CH, CZ, DE, DK, EE, ES, FI, FR, GB, GR, HN, HR, IE, IT, LT, MT, NL, NO, PL, PT, RO, RU, SE, SK, TR) *see* Pioglitazone and Glimepiride 1654
Tandiur (AR) *see* Hydrochlorothiazide 1009
Tandix (PT) *see* Indapamide 1065
Tanflex (ID) *see* Benzydamine [CAN/INT] 249
Tang Rui (CN) *see* Nateglinide 1432
Tanidina (ES) *see* Ranitidine 1777
Tanston (PE) *see* Mefenamic Acid 1280
Tantum (AT, BG, CZ, DE, EG, GR, ID, IN, IT, LB, PK, PL, PT, TR, VE) *see* Benzydamine [CAN/INT] 249
Tantum Gargle (KR) *see* Benzydamine [CAN/INT] 249
Tantum Verde (IL, RU, UY) *see* Benzydamine [CAN/INT] 249
Tanvimil-C (AR) *see* Ascorbic Acid 178
Tanvimil B6 (AR) *see* Pyridoxine 1747
Tanyl (CO) *see* CloZAPine 490
Tanyl (IL) *see* FentaNYL 857
Tanzal (ES) *see* Oxatomide [INT] 1532
Tanzaril (TH) *see* Losartan 1248
Tapazol (BR, CO, PE, VE) *see* Methimazole 1319
Tapazole (CH, IT, LB, PH, TH) *see* Methimazole 1319
Tapclob (GB) *see* CloBAZam 465
Tapcynta (IN) *see* Tapentadol 1975
Tapdin (PH) *see* Methimazole 1319
Tapenta (JP) *see* Tapentadol 1975
Tapocin (CN, KR) *see* Teicoplanin [INT] 1983
Taporin (MX) *see* Cefotaxime 382
Tapram (KR) *see* Doxapram 673
Tapros 3M (ID) *see* Leuprolide 1186
Tapros (ID) *see* Leuprolide 1186
Taquidine (TW) *see* Lansoprazole 1166
Tarabutine (KR) *see* Trimebutine [CAN/INT] 2103
Tarac (TW) *see* Tazarotene 1980
Taradyl (BE) *see* Ketorolac (Systemic) 1146
Taraten (TH) *see* Clotrimazole (Topical) 488
Taravid (AE, BH, CY, EG, IQ, IR, JO, KW, LB, LY, OM, QA, SA, SY, YE) *see* Ofloxacin (Systemic) 1490
Tarceva (AR, AT, AU, BE, BG, BH, BR, CH, CL, CN, CO, CY, CZ, DE, DK, EC, EE, ES, FI, FR, GB, GR, HK, HN, HR, HU, ID, IE, IL, IS, IT, JP, KR, KW, LB, LT, MT, MX, MY, NL, NO, NZ, PE, PH, PL, PT, PY, QA, RO, RU, SE, SG, SI, SK, TH, TR, TW, UY, VN) *see* Erlotinib 756
Tarcum (PH) *see* Atracurium 198
Tardensone (TW) *see* Acarbose 29
Tardocillin (DE) *see* Penicillin G Benzathine 1609
Tardyferon (AE, BH, CY, ES, FR, HU, IL, LU, QA) *see* Ferrous Sulfate 871
Tareg (CL, FR, IT, KR, PH) *see* Valsartan 2127
Tareg D (CL) *see* Valsartan and Hydrochlorothiazide 2129
Tarein (TW) *see* Ibuprofen 1032
Targaxan (GB) *see* Rifaximin 1809
Targinact (BE, CY, EE, GB, HR, NL, SI) *see* Oxycodone and Naloxone 1542
Targin (AT, AU, CH, CZ, DE, DK, IE, IL, IS, MY, NZ, PH, RO, SG, SK) *see* Oxycodone and Naloxone 1542
Targiniq (FI, NO, SE) *see* Oxycodone and Naloxone 1542
Targin PR (KR) *see* Oxycodone and Naloxone 1542
Targocid (AE, AR, AT, AU, BE, BG, BH, BR, CH, CL, CN, CZ, DE, DK, ES, FI, FR, GB, GR, HK, HN, HR, HU, ID, IE, IL, IN, JO, KR, KW, LB, LU, MX, MY, NL, NO, NZ, PE, PK, PL, PY, QA, RO, SA, SE, SG, SI, SK, TH, TR, TW, UY, VE, VN, ZA) *see* Teicoplanin [INT] 1983
Targoplanin (JO) *see* Teicoplanin [INT] 1983
Targosid (IT, PT) *see* Teicoplanin [INT] 1983
Targretin (AT, BE, CL, CZ, DE, DK, EE, ES, FR, GB, GR, HR, HU, IT, LT, NL, NO, PL, RO, SE) *see* Bexarotene (Systemic) 261
Targrettin (SK) *see* Bexarotene (Systemic) 261
Tariflox (ID) *see* Ofloxacin (Systemic) 1490
Tarimus (KR) *see* Tacrolimus (Systemic) 1962
Tariol (KR) *see* Calcitriol 323
Taripel Gel (CL) *see* Clindamycin and Tretinoin 464
Tarisin (PK) *see* Flunisolide (Nasal) 893
Tari-S (KR) *see* Bepotastine 250
Tarivid (AT, BE, BF, BJ, CH, CI, CL, DK, EE, ET, FI, GB, GH, GM, GN, HN, ID, IE, IL, IN, JP, KE, KR, LR, MA, ML, MR, MT, MU, MW, MY, NE, NG, NO, PK, PL, PT, RU, SC, SD, SE, SG, SK, SL, SN, TH, TN, TR, TW, TZ, UG, ZA, ZM, ZW) *see* Ofloxacin (Systemic) 1490
Tarivid (CN, HK, ID, KR, MY, SG, TW) *see* Ofloxacin (Otic) 1491
Tarivid (CN, ID, KR, QA, TH) *see* Ofloxacin (Ophthalmic) 1491
Tarjod (PL) *see* Potassium Iodide 1690
Tarka (AE, AR, AU, BG, BH, CH, CO, CR, CZ, DE, EC, EE, EG, ES, GR, GT, HN, HR, HU, IE, IT, KR, KW, LB, LT, NI, NL, PA, PE, PH, PK, PL, QA, RO, RU, SE, SI, SK, SV, TR, VE, ZA) *see* Trandolapril and Verapamil 2080
Tarka LP (FR) *see* Trandolapril and Verapamil 2080
Tarka Retard (BH) *see* Trandolapril and Verapamil 2080
Tarocine (BH) *see* Doxycycline 689
Tarocin (KW) *see* Doxycycline 689
Tarocort (IL) *see* Hydrocortisone (Topical) 1014
Taroctyl (IL) *see* ChlorproMAZINE 429
Taroflex (SK) *see* Ofloxacin (Systemic) 1490
Tarontal (GR, ID, TR) *see* Pentoxifylline 1618
Taronystatin (KR) *see* Nystatin (Topical) 1482
Taropen (PL) *see* Penicillin G Benzathine 1609
Tarpan (PY) *see* Famotidine 845
Tarunal (KR) *see* Tamsulosin 1974
Tarupain (KR) *see* Hydroxocobalamin 1020
Tasigna (AE, AR, AT, AU, BE, BH, BR, CH, CL, CN, CO, CY, CZ, DE, DK, EC, EE, FR, GB, GR, HK, HN, HR, ID, IE, IL, IS, IT, JO, JP, KR, KW, LB, LT, MY, NL, NO, NZ, PE, PH, PL, PT, QA, RO, RU, SA, SE, SG, SI, SK, TH, TR, TW, VN) *see* Nilotinib 1454
Taskine (AE, BH, CY, EG, IQ, IR, JO, KW, LB, LY, OM, QA, SA, SY, YE) *see* Ibuprofen 1032
Tasmar (AR, AT, BB, BE, BG, BM, BR, BS, BZ, CH, CL, CR, CY, CZ, DE, DK, DO, EE, EG, ES, FI, FR, GB, GR, GT, GY, HN, HR, IE, IT, JM, LT, MT, MX, NI, NL, NO, NZ, PA, PE, PH, PL, PT, QA, RO, RU, SE, SI, SK, SR, SV, TR, TT, UY, VN) *see* Tolcapone 2062
Tasmen (KR) *see* Acetaminophen 32
Tasovak (MX) *see* Piperacillin and Tazobactam 1657
Tatig (NZ) *see* Sertraline 1878
Tatinol (CN) *see* Tianeptine [INT] 2033
Taural (AR) *see* Ranitidine 1777
Taurolite (CN) *see* Ursodiol 2116
Tauxib (SE) *see* Etoricoxib [INT] 821
Tavanic (AE, AR, AT, BE, BG, BH, BM, BS, CH, CL, CR, CY, CZ, DE, DO, EE, EG, FI, FR, GB, GT, HN, IE, IL, JM, JO, KW, LB, LT, NI, NL, PA, PE, PT, PY, QA, RO, SA, SE, SK, SV, VE) *see* Levofloxacin (Systemic) 1197
Tavan-SP (ZA) *see* Pentosan Polysulfate Sodium 1617
Tavegil (BB, BM, BS, BZ, DE, ES, GB, GY, IE, IT, JM, LU, NL, SR, TT) *see* Clemastine 459

Tavegyl (AE, AT, BF, BG, BH, BJ, CH, CI, CO, CZ, DK, EC, EE, EG, ET, GH, GM, GN, HN, HU, ID, IN, IS, KE, KW, LR, LT, MA, ML, MR, MU, MW, NE, NG, NO, PT, QA, RO, RU, SA, SC, SD, SE, SI, SL, SN, TH, TN, TR, TZ, UG, ZA, ZM, ZW) *see* Clemastine 459
Taver (MY, TR, VN) *see* CarBAMazepine 346
Tavetine (MY) *see* Clemastine 459
Tavidan (TH) *see* Fenoverine [INT] 857
Tavinex (AR) *see* Ambroxol [INT] 109
Tavor (MX) *see* Oxybutynin 1536
Tavor (BG, CZ, DE, GR, IT, TR) *see* LORazepam 1243
Tavor (EC) *see* Fluconazole 885
Taxagon AC (UY) *see* TraZODone 2091
Taxagon (AR) *see* TraZODone 2091
Taxanit (MX) *see* DOCEtaxel 656
Taxelo (KR) *see* DOCEtaxel 656
Taxenil (AR) *see* Dipyrone [INT] 653
Taxilan (ID) *see* Sucralfate 1940
Taximax (ID) *see* Cefotaxime 382
Taxime (AE, BH, CY, EG, IQ, IR, JO, KW, LB, LY, OM, QA, SA, SY, YE) *see* Cefotaxime 382
Taxim (PH) *see* Cefotaxime 382
Taxinsheng (CN) *see* Nimotuzumab [INT] 1457
Taxocef-O (PH) *see* Cefixime 380
Taxocris (UY) *see* PACLitaxel (Conventional) 1550
Taxol (AE, AR, AT, AU, BE, BH, BR, CH, CN, CO, CZ, DE, DK, EE, EG, ES, FI, FR, GR, HK, HN, IT, JO, KR, KW, LB, NL, NO, NZ, PK, PL, QA, RU, SE, SI, TH, TR, VN, ZA) *see* PACLitaxel (Conventional) 1550
Taxomed (PE) *see* DOCEtaxel 656
Taxotere (AE, AR, AT, AU, BD, BE, BF, BG, BH, BJ, BO, BR, CH, CI, CL, CN, CO, CR, CY, CZ, DE, DK, DO, EC, EE, EG, ET, FI, FR, GB, GH, GM, GN, GR, GT, HK, HN, HR, HU, ID, IE, IL, IS, IT, JO, JP, KE, KR, LB, LR, LT, MA, ML, MR, MT, MU, MW, MX, MY, NE, NG, NI, NL, NO, NZ, PA, PE, PH, PK, PL, PR, PT, PY, QA, RO, RU, SA, SC, SD, SE, SG, SI, SK, SL, SN, SV, TH, TN, TR, TW, TZ, UG, UY, VE, VN, ZA, ZM, ZW) *see* DOCEtaxel 656
Taxozen (KR) *see* DOCEtaxel 656
Taxus (EC, PE) *see* Tamoxifen 1971
Tazac (AU, TW) *see* Nizatidine 1471
Tazicef (KR, PH) *see* CefTAZidime 392
Tazidan (PH) *see* CefTAZidime 392
Tazidem (PH) *see* CefTAZidime 392
Tazime (CN, KR, SG) *see* CefTAZidime 392
Tazobac (CH, DE) *see* Piperacillin and Tazobactam 1657
Tazobact (HR) *see* Piperacillin and Tazobactam 1657
Tazobak (PH) *see* Piperacillin and Tazobactam 1657
Tazocel (ES) *see* Piperacillin and Tazobactam 1657
Tazocilline (FR) *see* Piperacillin and Tazobactam 1657
Tazocillin (IL) *see* Piperacillin and Tazobactam 1657
Tazocin (AE, BE, BG, BH, BR, CN, CO, CR, CY, CZ, EC, EE, EG, GB, GT, HK, HN, HR, ID, IE, IL, IQ, IR, IT, JO, KR, KW, LB, LT, LY, MX, NI, NL, NO, OM, PA, PE, PH, PK, PL, QA, RO, SA, SE, SG, SI, SK, SV, SY, TH, TR, TW, YE) *see* Piperacillin and Tazobactam 1657
Tazocin EF (AU, DO, MY, NZ) *see* Piperacillin and Tazobactam 1657
Tazodac (IN) *see* TraZODone 2091
Tazoderm Forte (IN) *see* Tazarotene 1980
Tazomax (UY) *see* Piperacillin and Tazobactam 1657
Tazonam (AR, AT, CL, PY) *see* Piperacillin and Tazobactam 1657
Tazopen (PH) *see* Piperacillin and Tazobactam 1657
Tazoperan (KR) *see* Piperacillin and Tazobactam 1657
Tazopip (AU, IL) *see* Piperacillin and Tazobactam 1657
Tazopril (VE) *see* Piperacillin and Tazobactam 1657
Tazorac (CZ) *see* Tazarotene 1980
Tazorex (IL) *see* Piperacillin and Tazobactam 1657
Tazoten (TW) *see* Tazarotene 1980
Tazpen (MY, SG) *see* Piperacillin and Tazobactam 1657
Tazret (PH) *see* Tazarotene 1980
Tazrobida (MY, TH) *see* Piperacillin and Tazobactam 1657
Taz (SK) *see* Ethinyl Estradiol and Drospirenone 801
Tazun (MX) *see* ALPRAZolam 94
TB Rif (ID) *see* Rifampin 1804
TBSF (AU) *see* Factor IX Complex (Human) [(Factors II, IX, X)] 838
TBZet (ID) *see* Pyrazinamide 1745
3TC (AE, AR, AU, BB, BH, BM, BS, BZ, GY, HK, ID, JM, KW, MX, NZ, QA, SR, TT, UY) *see* LamiVUDine 1157
3TC-HBV (ID) *see* LamiVUDine 1157
Tc (PL) *see* Tetracycline 2017
Td-pur (PH) *see* Diphtheria and Tetanus Toxoid 645
TD Spray Iso Mack (HU, LU) *see* Isosorbide Dinitrate 1124
Tebantin (VN) *see* Gabapentin 943
Tebegran (MX) *see* SUMAtriptan 1953
Tebilon (AT) *see* Isoniazid 1120
Tebranic (TH) *see* Piperacillin and Tazobactam 1657
Tebraxin (IT) *see* Rufloxacin [INT] 1855
Tebrazid (BE, CH, LU) *see* Pyrazinamide 1745
Tebruxim (MX) *see* Cefotaxime 382
Tecfidera (AU, CZ, DE, DK, EE, FR, GB, HR, LT, NL, NO, RO, SE, SI, SK, TR) *see* Dimethyl Fumarate 639
Tecnid (BR) *see* Secnidazole [INT] 1872
Tecnocris (BR) *see* VinCRIStine 2163
Tecnofen (MX) *see* Tamoxifen 1971
Tecnoplatin (MX) *see* CISplatin 448
Tecnosal (PT) *see* Triflusal [INT] 2103
Tecnovorin (BR) *see* Folic Acid 919
Tecnovorin (BR, EC) *see* Leucovorin Calcium 1183
Tecomax (BR) *see* Terconazole 2006
Tecovel (PH) *see* Levocetirizine 1196
Tecta (CO, CR, DO, EC, GT, HN, MX, NI, PA, SV) *see* Pantoprazole 1570
Teddy-C (TH) *see* Ascorbic Acid 178
Tedicumar (ES) *see* Warfarin 2186
Tedigaster (ES) *see* Cimetidine 438
Tediprima (ES) *see* Trimethoprim 2104
Tedocad (BG) *see* DOCEtaxel 656
Tedoxy (PH) *see* Doxycycline 689
Tedral (CO) *see* Ephedrine and Theophylline [INT] 734
Teeth Tough (IL) *see* Fluoride 895
Tefal (PY) *see* Ibandronate 1028
Tefilin (DE) *see* Tetracycline 2017
Tefodine (AU) *see* Fexofenadine 873
Tegeline (LB) *see* Immune Globulin 1056
Tegol (TW) *see* CarBAMazepine 346
Tegral (PK) *see* CarBAMazepine 346
Tegrepin (PH) *see* CarBAMazepine 346
Tegretal (CL, DE) *see* CarBAMazepine 346
Tegretol (AE, AR, AU, BB, BD, BE, BF, BH, BJ, BM, BR, BS, BZ, CH, CI, CN, CO, CR, CY, CZ, DK, EC, EE, EG, ES, ET, FI, FR, GB, GH, GM, GN, GR, GT, GY, HK, HN, HR, HU, ID, IE, IL, IQ, IR, IS, IT, JM, JO, JP, KE, KR, KW, LB, LR, LT, LU, LY, MA, ML, MR, MU, MW, MX, MY, NE, NG, NI, NL, NO, NZ, OM, PA, PE, PH, PK, PL, PT, PY, QA, RO, RU, SA, SC, SD, SE, SG, SI, SL, SN, SR, SV, SY, TH, TN, TR, TT, TW, TZ, UG, UY, VE, VN, YE, ZM, ZW) *see* CarBAMazepine 346
Tegretol CR (CZ, EE, EG, HR, HU, IL, KR, NZ, PE, QA, RO, SA, SG, SI, SK, TR) *see* CarBAMazepine 346
Tegretol Retard (FI) *see* CarBAMazepine 346
Teicocid (PY, UY) *see* Teicoplanin [INT] 1983
Teicod (TW) *see* Teicoplanin [INT] 1983
Teicoin (TW) *see* Teicoplanin [INT] 1983
Teicon (BR) *see* Teicoplanin [INT] 1983
Teicosin (KR) *see* Teicoplanin [INT] 1983
Teicox (AR) *see* Teicoplanin [INT] 1983
Teikeden (HK) *see* Cefuroxime 399

Tekam (AE, BH, CY, EG, IQ, IR, JO, KW, LB, LY, OM, QA, SA, SY, YE) *see* Ketamine 1143
Tekamen (MY) *see* Irinotecan 1112
Tekast (PH) *see* Montelukast 1392
Tekturna (EE) *see* Aliskiren 85
Telacort (KR) *see* Deflazacort [INT] 587
Telalgin (GR) *see* Dipyrone [INT] 653
Telavic (JP) *see* Telaprevir 1983
Telavist (FR) *see* Nedocromil 1435
Telbit (KR) *see* Ofloxacin (Ophthalmic) 1491
Telbit (KR) *see* Ofloxacin (Systemic) 1490
Tele-Stulin (DE) *see* Naphazoline (Ophthalmic) 1426
Telfast-D (HK, MY, SG, TH) *see* Fexofenadine and Pseudoephedrine 874
Telfast (AE, AT, AU, BE, BF, BG, BH, BJ, CH, CI, CY, CZ, DE, DK, EE, EG, ES, ET, FI, FR, GB, GH, GM, GN, HK, HR, ID, IE, IL, IS, IT, JO, KE, KW, LB, LR, MA, ML, MR, MU, MW, MY, NE, NG, NO, NZ, PH, PL, PT, QA, RO, RU, SA, SC, SD, SE, SG, SI, SK, SL, SN, TH, TN, TR, TZ, UG, VN, ZA, ZM, ZW) *see* Fexofenadine 873
Telfast BD 60 (ID) *see* Fexofenadine and Pseudoephedrine 874
Telfast Decongestant (AU) *see* Fexofenadine and Pseudoephedrine 874
Telfast HD 180 (ID) *see* Fexofenadine and Pseudoephedrine 874
Telfast HD (ID) *see* Fexofenadine 873
Telfast OD 120 (ID) *see* Fexofenadine and Pseudoephedrine 874
Telfast OD (ID) *see* Fexofenadine 873
Telfast Oral Solution (MY) *see* Fexofenadine 873
Telfast (PH) *see* Fexofenadine and Pseudoephedrine 874
Telfast Plus (ID) *see* Fexofenadine and Pseudoephedrine 874
Telfex-d (PK) *see* Fexofenadine and Pseudoephedrine 874
Telgin-G (JP) *see* Clemastine 459
Te Li Da (CN) *see* Butenafine 314
Telisid-H (IN) *see* Telmisartan and Hydrochlorothiazide 1990
Telma-20 (IN) *see* Telmisartan 1988
Telmican (KR) *see* Telmisartan 1988
Telmican Plus (KR) *see* Telmisartan and Hydrochlorothiazide 1990
Telmicard (LB) *see* Telmisartan 1988
Telminovo (KR) *see* Telmisartan and Amlodipine 1989
Telmione Plus (KR) *see* Telmisartan and Hydrochlorothiazide 1990
Telmisar (PY) *see* Telmisartan 1988
Telmito (KR) *see* Telmisartan 1988
Telmito Plus (KR) *see* Telmisartan and Hydrochlorothiazide 1990
Telmitrend (KR) *see* Telmisartan 1988
Telmitrend Plus (KR) *see* Telmisartan and Hydrochlorothiazide 1990
Telmotens (SG) *see* Telmisartan 1988
Telnase (AU, NZ) *see* Triamcinolone (Systemic) 2099
Telos (DE) *see* Lornoxicam [INT] 1248
Telzer (MX) *see* Fosamprenavir 928
Telzir (AR, AT, AU, BB, BE, BG, BM, BR, BS, CH, CL, CO, CR, CY, CZ, DE, DK, DO, EE, ES, FI, FR, GB, GR, GT, GY, HN, HR, HU, IE, IS, IT, JM, LT, MT, NI, NL, NO, PA, PE, PL, PR, PT, RO, RU, SE, SK, SV, TR, TT, UY) *see* Fosamprenavir 928
Temador (BE) *see* Temazepam 1990
Temaze (AU) *see* Temazepam 1990
Temazepam "NM" (DK) *see* Temazepam 1990
Temerit (FR) *see* Nebivolol 1434
Temesta (AT, BE, CH, DK, FI, FR, LU, NL, SE) *see* LORazepam 1243
Temetex (AE, TR) *see* Diflucortolone [CAN/INT] 625
Temgesic (AE, AT, BE, BF, BH, BJ, BR, CH, CI, CY, CZ, DE, DK, EE, EG, ES, ET, FI, FR, GB, GH, GM, GN, GR, HK, IQ, IR, IT, JO, KE, KW, LB, LR, LU, LY, MA, ML, MR, MT, MU, MW, MX, NE, NG, NL, NO, NZ, OM, PK, PL, QA, RU, SA, SC, SD, SE, SG, SK, SL, SN, SY, TH, TN, TR, TW, TZ, UG, YE, ZA, ZM, ZW) *see* Buprenorphine 300
Temiral (ID) *see* Aciclovir (Ophthalmic) [INT] 43
Temizol (PY) *see* Albendazole 65
Temobela (VN) *see* Temozolomide 1991
Temodal IV (SG) *see* Temozolomide 1991
Temodal (AE, AR, AT, AU, BE, BG, BH, BO, BR, CH, CL, CN, CO, CY, CZ, DE, DK, DO, EE, EG, ES, FI, FR, GB, GR, HK, HR, HU, ID, IE, IL, IN, IQ, IR, IT, JO, JP, KR, KW, LB, LT, LY, MT, MX, MY, NL, NO, NZ, OM, PA, PE, PH, PL, PR, PT, PY, QA, RO, RU, SA, SE, SG, SI, SK, SY, TH, TR, TW, UY, VE, VN, YE) *see* Temozolomide 1991
Temo (IL) *see* Temozolomide 1991
Temomedac (IS) *see* Temozolomide 1991
Temo (TW) *see* Hetastarch 1004
Temovex (PH) *see* Temozolomide 1991
Temozam (PH) *see* Temozolomide 1991
Temozol (PH) *see* Temozolomide 1991
Tempol (MY) *see* Acetaminophen 32
Temporol (HU, ZA) *see* CarBAMazepine 346
Tempovate (ID) *see* Clobetasol 468
Tempra (ID, JP, LU, MX) *see* Acetaminophen 32
Tempte (TW) *see* Acetaminophen 32
Tempus (PY) *see* Formoterol 926
Temrevac-HB (PH) *see* Hepatitis B Vaccine (Recombinant) 1002
Temserin (GR) *see* Timolol (Ophthalmic) 2043
Temtabs (AU) *see* Temazepam 1990
Tenace (ID) *see* Enalapril 722
Tenacid (IT) *see* Imipenem and Cilastatin 1051
Tenaten (ID) *see* Enalapril 722
Tenazide (ID) *see* Enalapril and Hydrochlorothiazide 725
Tencilan (AR) *see* Clorazepate 487
Tendiol (EC) *see* Atenolol 189
Tendolon (MY) *see* Calcitonin 322
Tenesmin (UY) *see* Nimesulide [INT] 1456
Tenoblock (FI) *see* Atenolol 189
Tenocor (TH) *see* Atenolol 189
Teno-Em (TH) *see* Emtricitabine and Tenofovir 721
Tenofir (CO) *see* Tenofovir 1998
Tenof (TH) *see* Tenofovir 1998
Tenoloc (CZ, SK) *see* Celiprolol [INT] 404
Tenolol (BF, BJ, CI, ET, GH, GM, GN, KE, LR, LU, MA, ML, MR, MU, MW, NE, NG, NZ, SC, SD, SG, SL, SN, TH, TN, TZ, UG, ZA, ZM, ZW) *see* Atenolol 189
Tenol (SA) *see* Atenolol 189
Tenomal (GR) *see* Propranolol 1731
Tenomet (TR) *see* Cimetidine 438
Tenopress (AE, BH, CY, EG, IQ, IR, JO, KW, LB, LY, OM, QA, SA, SY, YE) *see* Atenolol 189
Tenoprin (FI) *see* Atenolol 189
Tenopt (AU) *see* Timolol (Ophthalmic) 2043
Tenormin (AE, AT, AU, BB, BD, BE, BF, BG, BH, BJ, BM, BS, BZ, CH, CI, CL, CO, CR, CY, CZ, DE, DK, DO, EE, EG, ES, ET, GB, GH, GM, GN, GR, GT, GY, HK, HN, HR, HU, ID, IE, IN, IQ, IR, IT, JM, JO, JP, KE, KR, KW, LB, LR, LU, LY, MA, ML, MR, MT, MU, MW, MX, MY, NE, NG, NI, NL, NO, OM, PA, PE, PH, PK, PT, QA, RU, SA, SC, SD, SE, SI, SK, SL, SN, SR, SV, SY, TH, TN, TR, TT, TZ, UG, UY, VE, VN, YE, ZM, ZW) *see* Atenolol 189
Tenormine (FR) *see* Atenolol 189
Tenormin ICN (HU) *see* Atenolol 189
Tenorvas (PH) *see* Atenolol 189
Tenovate (IN) *see* Clobetasol 468
Tenoxen (BR) *see* Tenoxicam [INT] 2001
Tenox (FI, IE) *see* Temazepam 1990

Tenozet (JP) *see* Tenofovir 1998
Tensan (AT) *see* Nilvadipine [INT] 1456
Tensaprin (CR) *see* Carisoprodol 363
Tensarten-HCT (CO) *see* Losartan and Hydrochlorothiazide 1250
Tens (CO) *see* Lacidipin [INT] 1154
Tensen (TW) *see* Finasteride 878
Tensiber (SG, VN) *see* Irbesartan 1110
Tensicap (ID) *see* Captopril 342
Tensidox (ID) *see* Doxazosin 674
Tensig (AU) *see* Atenolol 189
Tensil D (PY) *see* Enalapril and Hydrochlorothiazide 725
Tensilo (ID) *see* NiCARdipine 1446
Tensinor (TR) *see* Atenolol 189
Tensiobas (ES) *see* Doxazosin 674
Tensiomen (BG, HN, SK, VN) *see* Captopril 342
Tensiomin (HU) *see* Captopril 342
Tensiphar (ID) *see* Lisinopril 1226
Tensivask (ID) *see* AmLODIPine 123
Tensobon (DE) *see* Captopril 342
Tensocardil (ES) *see* Fosinopril 932
Tensodox (EC, PE, PY) *see* Cyclobenzaprine 516
Tensogradal (ES) *see* Nitrendipine [INT] 1463
Tensolisin D (DO, HN) *see* Lisinopril and Hydrochlorothiazide 1229
Tensopril (AR, IL) *see* Lisinopril 1226
Tensoril (PH) *see* Captopril 342
Tenso Stop (ES) *see* Fosinopril 932
Tensotec (GR) *see* Moexipril 1388
Tensotin (QA) *see* Atenolol 189
Tensuril (BR) *see* Diazoxide 616
Tensyn (CO) *see* Lisinopril 1226
Tentalux (ID) *see* Dexpanthenol 606
Tenualax (AR) *see* Lactulose 1156
Tenuate (AU, FR, KR) *see* Diethylpropion 624
Tenuate Dospan (AE, BH, CY, EG, IL, IQ, IR, JO, KW, LB, LY, NZ, OM, PE, QA, SA, SY, YE) *see* Diethylpropion 624
Tenuatina (ES) *see* Dihydroergotamine 633
Tenutan (BB, BM, BS, BZ, GY, JM, SR, TT) *see* Doxycycline 689
Tenvalin (EC) *see* Ibuprofen 1032
Tenvor (LB) *see* Tenofovir 1998
Tenzar (SK) *see* Olmesartan 1496
Tenzipin (HR) *see* Isradipine 1130
Teoclear (KR) *see* Theophylline 2026
Teoclear LA (AR) *see* Theophylline 2026
Teoden (BR) *see* Albuterol 69
Teofilina Retard (CO, EC) *see* Theophylline 2026
Teolin (HR) *see* Theophylline 2026
Teolong (BR, PY) *see* Theophylline 2026
Teonim (IT) *see* Nimesulide [INT] 1456
Teoplus (DO, GT, HN, NI, SV) *see* Theophylline 2026
Teosona (AR) *see* Theophylline 2026
Teotard (BG, EE, HR, RO, RU) *see* Theophylline 2026
Teoula (FR) *see* Zofenopril [INT] 2206
Tepadina (GB, HR, KR, TR) *see* Thiotepa 2030
Tepam-BASF (DE) *see* Tetrazepam [INT] 2020
Teperin (HN, HU, IQ, JO) *see* Amitriptyline 119
Tequin (AU, BR, MX, MY, SG, ZA) *see* Gatifloxacin 949
Teracin (AE) *see* Tetracycline 2017
Teracorte (TH) *see* Desoximetasone 598
Teradi (ID) *see* Attapulgite [CAN/INT] 204
Teradrin (TW) *see* Terazosin 2001
Teralfa (IN) *see* Terazosin 2001
Teralithe (FR) *see* Lithium 1230
Teramol Forte (PH) *see* Acetaminophen 32
Teramol (PH) *see* Acetaminophen 32
Teramoxyl (PH) *see* Amoxicillin 130
Terapam (KR) *see* Terazosin 2001
Terap (AR) *see* Foscarnet 931
Terasin (MY) *see* Terazosin 2001
Terasma (ID) *see* Terbutaline 2004
Terastat (JO) *see* Terazosin 2001
Terazoflo (DE) *see* Terazosin 2001
Terazol (DK, FI) *see* Terconazole 2006
Terbac (MX) *see* CefTRIAXone 396
Terbasmin (ES, IT) *see* Terbutaline 2004
Terbifin (HK) *see* Terbinafine (Systemic) 2002
Terbihexal (AU) *see* Terbinafine (Systemic) 2002
Terbron (MY) *see* Terbutaline 2004
Terbu Expectorant (TH) *see* Terbutaline 2004
Terbulin (IL) *see* Terbutaline 2004
Terbul (LU) *see* Terbutaline 2004
Terburop (CO, EC) *see* Terbutaline 2004
Terbutalin AL (HU) *see* Terbutaline 2004
Terbutalin Stada (PL) *see* Terbutaline 2004
Terbutil (BR) *see* Terbutaline 2004
Tercef (BG) *see* CefTRIAXone 396
Terclodine (PH) *see* CloNIDine 480
Terconal (IT) *see* Terconazole 2006
Terconer (TW) *see* Terconazole 2006
Terekol (AR) *see* Terbinafine (Systemic) 2002
Terekol (AR) *see* Terbinafine (Topical) 2004
Terfamex (CR, DO, EC, GT, HN, PA, SV) *see* Phentermine 1635
Terfex (VE) *see* Terbinafine (Systemic) 2002
Terfex (VE) *see* Terbinafine (Topical) 2004
Terfine (TW) *see* Terbinafine (Systemic) 2002
Terfine (TW) *see* Terbinafine (Topical) 2004
Terflurazine (ZA) *see* Trifluoperazine 2102
Terfluzine (FR, HU, PL) *see* Trifluoperazine 2102
Terfung (TW) *see* Terbinafine (Systemic) 2002
Terfung (TW) *see* Terbinafine (Topical) 2004
Tergecef (PH) *see* Cefixime 380
Teribone (JP) *see* Teriparatide 2008
Terican (MX) *see* Irinotecan 1112
Teril (AU, IL, NZ) *see* CarBAMazepine 346
Teril-CR (IL) *see* CarBAMazepine 346
Teripin (KR) *see* Terlipressin [INT] 2010
Terix (MX) *see* Amphotericin B (Conventional) 136
Terizin (SG) *see* Cetirizine 411
Terlissin (TW) *see* Terlipressin [INT] 2010
Terlistat (IN) *see* Terlipressin [INT] 2010
Terloc Duo (AR) *see* Amlodipine and Benazepril 125
Terloc (PY) *see* AmLODIPine 123
Terlomexin (FR) *see* Fenticonazole [INT] 868
Ternafast (VN) *see* Fexofenadine 873
Ternelin (JP) *see* TiZANidine 2051
Terolut (DK, FI, NO) *see* Dydrogesterone [INT] 702
Teromac (PH) *see* Ketorolac (Systemic) 1146
Teromar (CO) *see* Tiotropium 2046
Terramycin Plus (PH) *see* Bacitracin, Neomycin, and Polymyxin B 223
Tersigan (JP) *see* Oxitropium [INT] 1536
Tersigat (DE, FR) *see* Oxitropium [INT] 1536
Tertensif (BG, CZ, EE, ES, FI, HR, HR, PL, RO) *see* Indapamide 1065
Tertensif SR (LT, SI, SK) *see* Indapamide 1065
Tertroxin (AU, CZ, GB) *see* Liothyronine 1221
Terzolin (DE) *see* Ketoconazole (Topical) 1145
TESAA (TW) *see* Telmisartan 1988
Tesacof (MX) *see* Bromhexine [INT] 291
Tesavel (EE) *see* SitaGLIPtin 1897
Tesoprel (DE, KR) *see* Bromperidol [INT] 292
Tesoprel Tropfen (DE) *see* Bromperidol [INT] 292
Tespadan (BG) *see* Amlodipine and Olmesartan 126
Tespamin (JP, TW) *see* Thiotepa 2030
Tespral (PK) *see* Itopride [INT] 1130
Tess (BR) *see* Cyproterone and Ethinyl Estradiol [CAN/INT] 532
Tess (IN) *see* Triamcinolone (Topical) 2100
Testex (ES) *see* Testosterone 2010
Testim (BE, GB, IE, IS, NO, SI, SK) *see* Testosterone 2010
Testoderm (AT) *see* Testosterone 2010

Testogel (BG, IS, TR) *see* Testosterone 2010
Testo Gel (IE) *see* Testosterone 2010
Testom (RO) *see* Testosterone 2010
Testopatch (FR) *see* Testosterone 2010
Testormon (PT) *see* MethylTESTOSTERone 1345
Testosteron Ferring (AT) *see* Testosterone 2010
Testosteronum propionicum (PL) *see* Testosterone 2010
Testotonic B (IL) *see* MethylTESTOSTERone 1345
Testotop (LU) *see* Testosterone 2010
Testoviron (BH, CY, JO, LB, PK, SI, TR) *see* Testosterone 2010
Testoviron-Depot (AR, CH, CO, DE, DK, IL, PE, PT, PY, SE, UY) *see* Testosterone 2010
Testoviron Depot (QA, SA) *see* Testosterone 2010
Testovis (IT) *see* MethylTESTOSTERone 1345
Tetabulin (AT, CZ, IE, IT, KR, PL) *see* Tetanus Immune Globulin (Human) 2015
Tetabuline (BE) *see* Tetanus Immune Globulin (Human) 2015
Tetabulin S/D (AR) *see* Tetanus Immune Globulin (Human) 2015
Tetagam (AT, CH, HK, ID, PT, ZA) *see* Tetanus Immune Globulin (Human) 2015
Tetagam P (DE, PH) *see* Tetanus Immune Globulin (Human) 2015
Tetagam-P (GR, TH) *see* Tetanus Immune Globulin (Human) 2015
Tetaglobuline (BF, BJ, CI, ET, GH, GM, GN, KE, LR, MA, ML, MR, MU, MW, NE, NG, SC, SD, SL, SN, TN, TZ, UG, ZM, ZW) *see* Tetanus Immune Globulin (Human) 2015
Tetaglobulin (IN) *see* Tetanus Immune Globulin (Human) 2015
Tetanobulin S/D (DE) *see* Tetanus Immune Globulin (Human) 2015
Tetanobulin (TW) *see* Tetanus Immune Globulin (Human) 2015
Tetanogamma (BR, DO) *see* Tetanus Immune Globulin (Human) 2015
Tetanogamma P (MX) *see* Tetanus Immune Globulin (Human) 2015
Tetesept Calcium (AT) *see* Calcium Carbonate 327
Tetgam (LB) *see* Tetanus Immune Globulin (Human) 2015
Tethexal (DE) *see* Tetrazepam [INT] 2020
Tetidis (HR) *see* Disulfiram 654
Tetmodis (HR, RO) *see* Tetrabenazine 2016
Tetrabiotico (EC) *see* Tetracycline 2017
Tetracilin (PY) *see* Tetracycline 2017
Tetracyclinum (PL) *see* Tetracycline 2017
Tetradar (BH, QA, SA) *see* Tetracycline 2017
Tetradin (PT) *see* Disulfiram 654
Tetra Flam (DE) *see* Tetrazepam [INT] 2020
Tetrahes (ID, KR) *see* Tetrastarch 2019
Tetralgin Haler (AR) *see* Ergotamine 754
Tetramdura (DE) *see* Tetrazepam [INT] 2020
Tetramig (FR) *see* Tetracycline 2017
Tetrana (TH) *see* Tetracycline 2017
Tetrarco (AE, NL) *see* Tetracycline 2017
Tetrarelax (DE) *see* Tetrazepam [INT] 2020
Tetra-saar (DE) *see* Tetrazepam [INT] 2020
Tetraseptin (CH) *see* Tetracycline 2017
Tetraspan (DK, EE, HK, PH, TW) *see* Tetrastarch 2019
Tetrasuiss (AE, BB, BF, BH, BJ, BM, BS, BZ, CI, CY, EG, ET, GH, GM, GN, GY, IQ, IR, JM, JO, KE, KW, LB, LR, LY, MA, ML, MR, MU, MW, NE, NG, OM, PR, QA, SA, SC, SD, SL, SN, SR, SY, TN, TT, TZ, UG, YE, ZM, ZW) *see* Tetracycline 2017
Tetrazep 1A Pharma (DE) *see* Tetrazepam [INT] 2020
Tetrazep AbZ (DE) *see* Tetrazepam [INT] 2020
Tetrazepam AL (DE) *see* Tetrazepam [INT] 2020
Tetrazepam beta (DE) *see* Tetrazepam [INT] 2020
Tetrazepam Heumann (DE) *see* Tetrazepam [INT] 2020
Tetrazepam-neuraxpharm (DE) *see* Tetrazepam [INT] 2020
Tetrazepam-ratiopharm (DE) *see* Tetrazepam [INT] 2020
Tetrazepam Stada (DE) *see* Tetrazepam [INT] 2020
Tetrazepam-Teva (DE) *see* Tetrazepam [INT] 2020
tetrazep von ct (DE) *see* Tetrazepam [INT] 2020
Tetrecu (EC) *see* Tetracycline 2017
Tetrex (AE, AU, BH, BR, CY, EG, IQ, IR, JO, JP, KW, LB, LY, MX, OM, QA, SA, SY, YE, ZA) *see* Tetracycline 2017
Tetronine (KR) *see* Liothyronine 1221
Tetuman berna (HK, PE, TH, TW) *see* Tetanus Immune Globulin (Human) 2015
Tetuman (NL) *see* Tetanus Immune Globulin (Human) 2015
Tevacidol (DE) *see* Alfacalcidol [CAN/INT] 82
Tevacycline (IL) *see* Tetracycline 2017
Tevagastrim (IL) *see* Filgrastim 875
Teva Grastim (AU) *see* Filgrastim 875
Tevagrastim (HK) *see* Filgrastim 875
Tevalamotrigine Chew Tab (KR) *see* LamoTRIgine 1160
Tevanate (BG, TW) *see* Alendronate 79
Tevapirin (IL) *see* Aspirin 180
Teveten (AE, AT, AU, BE, BG, BH, CH, CN, CY, CZ, DE, DK, EE, FI, FR, GB, GR, HK, HN, HR, HU, IE, JO, KR, KW, LB, LT, NL, NO, PH, PK, PL, PT, QA, SA, SE, TH, TR, TW, VN) *see* Eprosartan 748
Teveten Comp (DK, FI, NO, SE) *see* Eprosartan and Hydrochlorothiazide 750
Teveten Plus (AE, AT, AU, BE, BG, BH, CH, CY, DE, EE, GR, HK, HR, IE, KR, KW, NL, PH, PT, QA, RU, SA, TR) *see* Eprosartan and Hydrochlorothiazide 750
Teveten Plus H (CZ) *see* Eprosartan and Hydrochlorothiazide 750
Tevetens (ES) *see* Eprosartan 748
Tevetens Plus (ES) *see* Eprosartan and Hydrochlorothiazide 750
Tevetenz (IT) *see* Eprosartan 748
Texa (BE) *see* Lindane 1217
Texate (MX) *see* Methotrexate 1322
Texicam (AR) *see* Tenoxicam [INT] 2001
Texorate (ID) *see* Methotrexate 1322
Texot (AR, LB, UY) *see* DOCEtaxel 656
Texzine (PH) *see* Cetirizine 411
TEZEO (BG) *see* Telmisartan 1988
TFT (BE, NL) *see* Trifluridine 2103
TFT Ophtiole (PH, TW) *see* Trifluridine 2103
6-TG (IN) *see* Thioguanine 2029
Thacapzol (SE) *see* Methimazole 1319
Thaden (ZA) *see* Dosulepin [INT] 673
Thado (TW) *see* Thalidomide 2022
Thais (FR) *see* Estradiol (Systemic) 775
Thaled (JP) *see* Thalidomide 2022
Thalix (IN, PH) *see* Thalidomide 2022
Thalomid (AU) *see* Thalidomide 2022
Tham (DE, GR) *see* Tromethamine 2107
Thamesol (IT) *see* Tromethamine 2107
Thelban (MY) *see* Albendazole 65
Theo-2 (BE, LU) *see* Theophylline 2026
Theo-24 (IT) *see* Theophylline 2026
Theo-Bros (GR) *see* Theophylline 2026
Theoclear (KR) *see* Theophylline 2026
Theocodil (ID) *see* Ephedrine and Theophylline [INT] 734
Theo-Dur (AR, CZ, DK, FI, GR, IT, JP, LU, MY, NO, PK, SA, SE, TR) *see* Theophylline 2026
Theolair (CH, ES, IT, LU, NL) *see* Theophylline 2026
Theolair S (PE) *see* Theophylline 2026
Theolan (KR) *see* Theophylline 2026
Theolin (AE, BH, CY, EG, IQ, IR, JO, KW, LB, LY, OM, QA, SA, SY, YE) *see* Theophylline 2026

Theolin SR (SG) *see* Theophylline 2026
Theolong (JP) *see* Theophylline 2026
Theo PA (IN) *see* Theophylline 2026
Theophar (AE, BH, KW, QA, SA) *see* Theophylline 2026
Theophtard (HU) *see* Theophylline 2026
Theophylline Bruneau (LU) *see* Theophylline 2026
Theophyllin-ratiopharm (LU) *see* Theophylline 2026
Theoplus Retard (AT, GR) *see* Theophylline 2026
Theoral (JP) *see* Etilefrine [INT] 815
Theospirex (HU) *see* Theophylline 2026
Theospirex Retard (AT) *see* Theophylline 2026
Theostat LP (FR) *see* Theophylline 2026
Theostat (LU) *see* Theophylline 2026
Theotard (IL) *see* Theophylline 2026
Theovix (GR) *see* Erdosteine [INT] 753
Theracim (ID, PH, TH) *see* Nimotuzumab [INT] 1457
Theraflu (MX) *see* Loratadine and Pseudoephedrine 1242
Theralite (CO) *see* Lithium 1230
Theramatic (GR) *see* Chenodiol 417
TherCIM (AR, CO, CU, IN) *see* Nimotuzumab [INT] 1457
Therodel (ID) *see* Clopidogrel 484
Thevier (DE) *see* Levothyroxine 1205
Thiabet (DE) *see* MetFORMIN 1307
Thiamazol Henning (AT, DE) *see* Methimazole 1319
Thiamine Injection (AU) *see* Thiamine 2028
Thidim (ID) *see* CefTAZidime 392
Thilodexine (GR) *see* Dexamethasone (Ophthalmic) 602
Thilol (TR) *see* Trifluridine 2103
Thilonium (GR) *see* Befunolol [INT] 233
Thimelon (ID) *see* MethylPREDNISolone 1340
Thinin (TW) *see* Thioridazine 2030
Thioguanine Wellcome (IT) *see* Thioguanine 2029
Thioguanin Glaxo Wellcome (AT, DE) *see* Thioguanine 2029
Thiojex (PE) *see* Thiopental [INT] 2029
Thiomed (TH) *see* Thioridazine 2030
Thiooplex (GR, IT) *see* Thiotepa 2030
Thiopen (PK, TH) *see* Thiopental [INT] 2029
Thiopental (AE, BH, CY, EG, IQ, IR, JO, KW, LB, LY, OM, PL, QA, SA, SY, YE) *see* Thiopental [INT] 2029
Thiopental Biochemie (AT) *see* Thiopental [INT] 2029
Thiopentax (BR, PY) *see* Thiopental [INT] 2029
Thioprine (AU) *see* AzaTHIOprine 210
Thioridazin (PL) *see* Thioridazine 2030
Thioridazin prolongatum (PL) *see* Thioridazine 2030
Thioril (IN) *see* Thioridazine 2030
Thiosia (TH) *see* Thioridazine 2030
Thio-Tepa (AR, CZ) *see* Thiotepa 2030
Thiotepa Lederle (AT, CH, DE, FR) *see* Thiotepa 2030
Thiozine (PH) *see* Thioridazine 2030
Thomaedex 40 (DE) *see* Dextran 607
Thomasin (DE) *see* Etilefrine [INT] 815
Thombran (DE) *see* TraZODone 2091
Thromaxin (PH) *see* Azithromycin (Systemic) 216
Thrombo-Aspilets (ID) *see* Aspirin 180
Thrombo-ASS (EE) *see* Aspirin 180
Thrombocid (CH, ES) *see* Pentosan Polysulfate Sodium 1617
Thrombophob (DE) *see* Heparin 997
Thromboreduct (DE) *see* Heparin 997
Thromboreductin (AT, BG, CH, CZ, HK, HN, HR, MY, PH, RO, TH, TR) *see* Anagrelide 147
Thrombotrol-VF (AU, NZ) *see* Antithrombin 156
Thrupas (KR) *see* Silodosin 1885
Thybon Henning (DE) *see* Liothyronine 1221
Thycaprol (DK) *see* Methimazole 1319
Thydin (PH) *see* Levothyroxine 1205
Thymazole (MY) *see* Carbimazole [INT] 356
Thymeol (JP) *see* Melitracen [INT] 1283
Thymicol (KR) *see* Guaifenesin, Pseudoephedrine, and Dextromethorphan 989
Thymogam (PH) *see* Antithymocyte Globulin (Equine) 157
Thymoglobuline (AU, BG, CN, DK, FI, GB, GR, HK, KR, MY, NO, SI, TH) *see* Antithymocyte Globulin (Rabbit) 158
Thyradin S (JP) *see* Levothyroxine 1205
Thyrax (BE, CZ, ID, PH, PT) *see* Levothyroxine 1205
Thyrax Duotab (BF, BJ, CI, ET, GH, GM, GN, KE, LR, MA, ML, MR, MU, MW, NE, NG, SC, SD, SL, SN, TN, TZ, UG, ZM, ZW) *see* Levothyroxine 1205
Thyreotom (CY, EG, IQ, JO, LY, SY) *see* Liotrix 1221
Thyreotom Forte (AE, BH, CY, EG, IL, IQ, IR, JO, KW, LB, LY, OM, QA, SA, SY, YE) *see* Liotrix 1221
Thyrex (AT) *see* Levothyroxine 1205
Thyro-4 (GR) *see* Levothyroxine 1205
Thyrogen (AT, AU, BE, BR, CH, CL, CY, CZ, DE, DK, EE, FI, FR, GR, HK, HN, HR, IE, IL, IS, IT, JP, KR, LB, LT, MY, NL, NO, PE, PL, PT, RO, SE, SG, SI, SK, TH, TR, TW, UY) *see* Thyrotropin Alfa 2031
Thyroid-S (TW) *see* Levothyroxine 1205
Thyronine (JP) *see* Liothyronine 1221
Thyroprotect (DE) *see* Potassium Iodide 1690
Thyrosan (PL) *see* Propylthiouracil 1735
Thyrosit (TH) *see* Levothyroxine 1205
Thyrostat (GR) *see* Carbimazole [INT] 356
Thyrotardin inject. (DE) *see* Liothyronine 1221
Thyroxin (FI) *see* Levothyroxine 1205
Thyroxin-Natrium (NO) *see* Levothyroxine 1205
Thyrozol (BG, CL, DE, LU, PL, VN) *see* Methimazole 1319
Tiabine (TW) *see* TiaGABine 2032
Tiadil (PT) *see* Diltiazem 634
Tiadyl (AR) *see* Candesartan 335
Tiadyl Plus (AR) *see* Candesartan and Hydrochlorothiazide 338
Tiamacon (TW) *see* Magaldrate and Simethicone 1261
Tiamidexal (MX) *see* Thiamine 2028
Tiamina (CO) *see* Thiamine 2028
Tiaminal (MX) *see* Thiamine 2028
Tiamin "Dak" (DK) *see* Thiamine 2028
Tiamon (DE) *see* Dihydrocodeine, Aspirin, and Caffeine 632
Tian Di Da (CN) *see* Amifostine 109
Tianeurax (DE) *see* Tianeptine [INT] 2033
Tianli Runzhu (CN) *see* Chloramphenicol 421
Tiarix (PY) *see* PARoxetine 1579
Tiaryt (ID) *see* Amiodarone 114
Tiazid (PE) *see* Hydrochlorothiazide 1009
Tiazomet A (CO, EC) *see* Ezetimibe and Atorvastatin 833
Tiazomet-S (CO) *see* Ezetimibe and Simvastatin 834
Tiberal (AE, BE, CH, EC, FR, QA, RU, SA) *see* Ornidazole [INT] 1522
Tibicel (ID) *see* Pyrazinamide 1745
Tibigon (ID) *see* Ethambutol 798
Tibinide (SE) *see* Isoniazid 1120
Tibitol (ID, IN) *see* Ethambutol 798
Tibofem (UY) *see* Tibolone [INT] 2035
Tibolux (EC) *see* Tibolone [INT] 2035
Tibona (UY) *see* Tibolone [INT] 2035
Tibutol (PE) *see* Ethambutol 798
Ticarcin (PH) *see* Ticarcillin and Clavulanate Potassium [CAN/INT] 2038
Ticard (TH) *see* Ticlopidine 2040
Ticlid (AE, AR, BB, BE, BH, BM, BO, BR, BS, BZ, CL, CO, CR, CY, CZ, DO, EC, EG, FR, GB, GR, GT, GY, HN, HU, IQ, IR, IS, JM, JO, KW, LB, LU, LY, MX, MY, NI, NL, NO, OM, PA, PE, PK, PL, PR, PY, QA, SA, SE, SR, SV, SY, TH, TR, TT, UY, VE, YE) *see* Ticlopidine 2040
Ticlidil (IL) *see* Ticlopidine 2040

Ticlodin (RO) *see* Ticlopidine 2040
Ticlodix (PT) *see* Ticlopidine 2040
Ticlodone (GR, IT, KR) *see* Ticlopidine 2040
Ticlod (TW) *see* Ticlopidine 2040
Ticlopid (BG) *see* Ticlopidine 2040
Ticlopine (TH) *see* Ticlopidine 2040
Ticlop (JO) *see* Ticlopidine 2040
Ticlo (RU) *see* Ticlopidine 2040
Ticopar (AE, KW, SA) *see* Ticlopidine 2040
Ticuring (ID) *see* Ticlopidine 2040
Tidact (PH, TW) *see* Clindamycin (Systemic) 460
Tidigesic (IN) *see* Buprenorphine 300
Tidilor (AE, BH, CY, EG, IQ, IR, JO, KW, LB, LY, OM, QA, SA, SY, YE) *see* Loratadine 1241
Tidomet CR (PH) *see* Carbidopa and Levodopa 351
Tidomet Forte (IN) *see* Carbidopa and Levodopa 351
Tidomet L.S. (IN) *see* Carbidopa and Levodopa 351
Tidomet (PH, TH) *see* Carbidopa and Levodopa 351
Tidomet Plus (IN) *see* Carbidopa and Levodopa 351
Tidorzak (PE) *see* Dorzolamide and Timolol 673
Tienam (AE, BD, BE, BG, BH, BR, CH, CL, CN, CO, CR, CY, CZ, DK, EC, EE, EG, ES, FI, FR, GT, HK, HN, HR, ID, IE, IL, IN, IT, JP, KW, LB, LT, MT, MX, MY, NI, NL, NO, PA, PE, PH, PK, PT, QA, RO, RU, SA, SE, SG, SK, SV, TH, TR, TW, VN) *see* Imipenem and Cilastatin 1051
Tiersil Once (KR) *see* Terbinafine (Systemic) 2002
Tiersil Once (KR) *see* Terbinafine (Topical) 2004
Tiesilan (CO, EC) *see* Imipenem and Cilastatin 1051
Tiferomed (MX) *see* Dacarbazine 549
Tifis (JP) *see* Tofisopam [INT] 2061
Tigalin (ID) *see* Bacitracin, Neomycin, and Polymyxin B 223
Tigein (TW) *see* Teicoplanin [INT] 1983
Tigerfil (HK, PH) *see* Sildenafil 1882
Tigna (CO) *see* Econazole 703
Tigreat (FR, NO) *see* Frovatriptan 938
Tikleen (IN, VN) *see* Ticlopidine 2040
Tiklid (AT, ES, IT) *see* Ticlopidine 2040
Tiklyd (DE) *see* Ticlopidine 2040
Tikpid (PH) *see* Ticlopidine 2040
Tilade (AR, AT, BR, CZ, DE, DK, ES, FI, GB, GR, HU, ID, IE, IT, LU, NL, PL, SK) *see* Nedocromil 1435
Tilade CFC Free (AU, NZ) *see* Nedocromil 1435
Tilade Mint (AE, BH, CY, EG, IQ, IR, JO, KW, LB, LY, OM, QA, SA, SG, SY, YE) *see* Nedocromil 1435
Tilad (ES) *see* Nedocromil 1435
Tilarin (AT, FI, IT, PL) *see* Nedocromil 1435
Tilatep (VN) *see* Teicoplanin [INT] 1983
Tilatil (AR, BR) *see* Tenoxicam [INT] 2001
Tilavist (AT, CH, DK, ES, IL, IT, NL, NO, PL, PT, SE) *see* Nedocromil 1435
Tilazem 90 (ZA) *see* Diltiazem 634
Tilazem (AR, CL, CO, MX, PE, UY, ZA) *see* Diltiazem 634
Tilcotil (AT, AU, BE, CH, CZ, DE, DK, ES, FI, FR, HU, IT, LU, MX, NL, PT) *see* Tenoxicam [INT] 2001
Tilcotil "Roche" (HU) *see* Tenoxicam [INT] 2001
Tildiem (BE, BH, CH, CL, FR, GB, GR, IE, IT, JO, KW, LU, MY, NL, SA, VN) *see* Diltiazem 634
Tildiem CR (NL) *see* Diltiazem 634
Tildiem LA (GB) *see* Diltiazem 634
Tildiem Retard (GR) *see* Diltiazem 634
Tilidon (ID) *see* Domperidone [CAN/INT] 666
Tilodene (AU) *see* Ticlopidine 2040
Tilol (TW) *see* Timolol (Ophthalmic) 2043
Tiloptic (IL) *see* Timolol (Ophthalmic) 2043
Tilstigmin (IN) *see* Neostigmine 1438
Tilur (CH) *see* Acemetacin [INT] 30
Timabak (BE, HK) *see* Timolol (Ophthalmic) 2043
Timacor (FR) *see* Timolol (Ophthalmic) 2043
Timalen (HR) *see* Timolol (Ophthalmic) 2043
Timat (CO) *see* Budesonide (Nasal) 296
Timazol (TH) *see* Methimazole 1319
Timenten (AT) *see* Ticarcillin and Clavulanate Potassium [CAN/INT] 2038
Timentin (AE, AU, BE, BF, BH, BJ, BR, CI, CN, CY, CZ, EG, ET, GB, GH, GM, GN, GR, HK, ID, IE, IL, IQ, IR, IT, JO, KE, KR, KW, LB, LR, LY, MA, ML, MR, MU, MW, MX, NE, NG, NL, NZ, OM, PE, PL, QA, RO, RU, SA, SC, SD, SL, SN, SY, TN, TW, TZ, UG, VN, YE, ZA, ZM, ZW) *see* Ticarcillin and Clavulanate Potassium [CAN/INT] 2038
Timet (AE, BH, CY, EG, IQ, IR, JO, KW, LB, LY, OM, QA, SA, SY, YE) *see* Cimetidine 438
Timexole (MX) *see* Sulfamethoxazole and Trimethoprim 1946
Timicolid (IT) *see* Anthralin 150
Timipen (ID) *see* Imipenem and Cilastatin 1051
Timivudin (MX) *see* Zidovudine 2196
Timo-COMOD (KR) *see* Timolol (Ophthalmic) 2043
Timohexal (DE) *see* Timolol (Ophthalmic) 2043
Timolast (TW) *see* Timolol (Ophthalmic) 2043
Timol (TW) *see* Timolol (Ophthalmic) 2043
Timolux (NZ) *see* Timolol (Ophthalmic) 2043
Timonil (DE, HU) *see* CarBAMazepine 346
Timonil Retard (CH, DE, IL) *see* CarBAMazepine 346
Timonol SR (KR) *see* CarBAMazepine 346
Timoptic (AT, BG, CH, PE, PL, RO, SK) *see* Timolol (Ophthalmic) 2043
Timoptic-XE (KR) *see* Timolol (Ophthalmic) 2043
Timoptol (AE, AU, BE, BF, BH, BJ, CI, CN, CZ, DE, ET, FR, GB, GH, GM, GN, HK, IE, IT, JO, KE, KW, LB, LR, MA, ML, MR, MU, MW, MY, NE, NG, NL, NZ, PH, PK, PT, SA, SC, SD, SL, SN, TH, TN, TW, TZ, UG, VN, ZA, ZM, ZW) *see* Timolol (Ophthalmic) 2043
Timoptol-XE (AU, CL, NZ, PE, SG, TW) *see* Timolol (Ophthalmic) 2043
Timosan (EE, FI, SE) *see* Timolol (Ophthalmic) 2043
Timox (DE) *see* OXcarbazepine 1532
Timpilo (BE, CH, CZ, DE, DK, FR, GR, RU, SE) *see* Dorzolamide and Timolol 673
Tinacef (AR, PY) *see* CefTAZidime 392
Tinactin (PH) *see* Tolnaftate 2063
Tinaderm M (CO) *see* Tolnaftate 2063
Tinaderm (AE, AR, AU, BH, CL, CR, DO, EC, ES, GR, GT, HN, IE, IN, IT, MX, NI, NZ, PA, PE, QA, SA, SV, VE, ZA) *see* Tolnaftate 2063
Tinaderme (PT) *see* Tolnaftate 2063
Tinatox (DE) *see* Tolnaftate 2063
Tinazole (KR) *see* Fluconazole 885
Tindurin (HN, HU) *see* Pyrimethamine 1749
Tineafax (AU) *see* Tolnaftate 2063
Tinidil (HR) *see* Isosorbide Dinitrate 1124
T-Inmun (PY) *see* Tacrolimus (Systemic) 1962
Tinnic (ID) *see* Loratadine 1241
Tinox (CO, PE, PY, VE) *see* Tibolone [INT] 2035
Tinseet (UY) *see* Oxatomide [INT] 1532
Tinset (AR, AT, BE, CZ, DE, FR, GB, GR, HU, ID, IT, LU, MX, NL, PT, TH, ZA) *see* Oxatomide [INT] 1532
Tinset Gel (IT) *see* Oxatomide [INT] 1532
Tintel (KR) *see* Pinaverium [CAN/INT] 1651
Tintus (FI) *see* GuaiFENesin 986
Tinuvin (TW) *see* Ketoconazole (Systemic) 1144
Tiobarbital (ES) *see* Thiopental [INT] 2029
Tiodin (SG) *see* Ticlopidine 2040
Tiof (EC) *see* Timolol (Ophthalmic) 2043
Tiof Plus (PY) *see* Dorzolamide and Timolol 673
Tioguanina (ES) *see* Thioguanine 2029
Tiopental (CO, CR, GT, HN, HR, NI, PY, VE) *see* Thiopental [INT] 2029
Tiopental Sodico (AR) *see* Thiopental [INT] 2029
Tiopex (GB) *see* Timolol (Ophthalmic) 2043
Tiopnetal (UY) *see* Thiopental [INT] 2029
Tiorfan (BR, DE, ES, FR, PT) *see* Racecadotril [INT] 1765

Tiorfix (BE, IT) *see* Racecadotril [INT] 1765
Tiotal (PY) *see* Phenazopyridine 1629
Tiotil (EE, SE) *see* Propylthiouracil 1735
Tiova Rotacaps (IN) *see* Tiotropium 2046
Tipem (KR) *see* Imipenem and Cilastatin 1051
Tipidine (TH) *see* Ticlopidine 2040
Tipidin (HK, MY, SG) *see* Ticlopidine 2040
Tiptipot (IL) *see* Pseudoephedrine 1742
Tiramate (NZ) *see* Topiramate 2065
Tirdicef (ID) *see* Cefotaxime 382
Tiren (MY) *see* Tranexamic Acid 2081
Tirgon N (LU) *see* Bisacodyl 265
Tirizine (HK) *see* Cetirizine 411
Tirocal (MX) *see* Calcitriol 323
Tirodril (ES) *see* Methimazole 1319
Tiroidine (MX) *see* Levothyroxine 1205
Tirolaxo (ES) *see* Docusate 661
Tiromax (KR) *see* Trospium 2108
Tirostat (CO, EC) *see* Propylthiouracil 1735
Tirotax (MX, PL) *see* Cefotaxime 382
Tiroxin (CO, EC) *see* Levothyroxine 1205
Tisamid (CZ, FI) *see* Pyrazinamide 1745
Tiscerin (KR) *see* Methotrimeprazine [CAN/INT] 1329
Tisercin (HU, RU, VN) *see* Methotrimeprazine [CAN/INT] 1329
Tismafam (ID) *see* Famotidine 845
Tismalin (ID) *see* Terbutaline 2004
Tisolon-4 (ID) *see* MethylPREDNISolone 1340
Tisopt (KR) *see* Dorzolamide and Timolol 673
Tissulest (MX) *see* Pravastatin 1700
Titralac (NO) *see* Calcium Carbonate 327
Ti-Tre (IT) *see* Liothyronine 1221
Titus (AE, BF, BH, BJ, CI, CY, EG, ET, GH, GM, GN, GR, IQ, IR, JO, KE, KW, LB, LR, LY, MA, ML, MR, MU, MW, NE, NG, OM, QA, SA, SC, SD, SL, SN, SY, TN, TZ, UG, YE, ZM, ZW) *see* LORazepam 1243
Tixteller (NL) *see* Rifaximin 1809
Tizalin (TW) *see* TiZANidine 2051
Tizan (TH) *see* TiZANidine 2051
TMS (DE) *see* Sulfamethoxazole and Trimethoprim 1946
Tobacin (IN) *see* Tobramycin (Ophthalmic) 2056
Toban F (PE) *see* Loperamide 1236
Toban F Plus (PE) *see* Loperamide and Simethicone 1237
Toban (PE) *see* Loperamide 1236
Toberan (KR) *see* Tobramycin (Ophthalmic) 2056
Tobesyn Eye Drop (KR) *see* Tobramycin and Dexamethasone 2056
Tobi (AR, CY, CZ, DK, FR, GB, HR, IE, IL, IS, JP, LT, PE, PY, RO, SI, SK) *see* Tobramycin (Systemic, Oral Inhalation) 2052
Tobitil (IN) *see* Tenoxicam [INT] 2001
Tobra-V (PH) *see* Tobramycin (Ophthalmic) 2056
Tobrabiotic Soft (AR) *see* Loteprednol and Tobramycin 1251
Tobracin (EG) *see* Tobramycin (Systemic, Oral Inhalation) 2052
Tobracin (JO) *see* Tobramycin (Ophthalmic) 2056
Tobracort (MX, PE) *see* Tobramycin and Dexamethasone 2056
Tobra-Day (AU) *see* Tobramycin (Ophthalmic) 2056
Tobra-Day (AU) *see* Tobramycin (Systemic, Oral Inhalation) 2052
Tobradex (AE, AR, BE, BF, BG, BH, BJ, BR, CH, CI, CL, CN, CO, CR, CY, DK, EE, EG, ES, ET, FR, GB, GH, GM, GN, GR, GT, HK, HN, HR, HU, ID, IL, IN, IQ, IR, IS, IT, JO, KE, KR, KW, LB, LR, LT, LY, MA, ML, MR, MU, MW, MY, NE, NG, NI, NL, NZ, OM, PA, PE, PH, PK, PY, QA, RO, SA, SC, SD, SI, SK, SL, SN, SV, SY, TN, TW, TZ, UG, UY, VE, VN, YE, ZA, ZM, ZW) *see* Tobramycin and Dexamethasone 2056
Tobragan D (CO) *see* Tobramycin and Dexamethasone 2056
Tobragan (BR, CL) *see* Tobramycin (Ophthalmic) 2056
Tobra-gobens (DO) *see* Tobramycin (Systemic, Oral Inhalation) 2052
Tobra (KR) *see* Tobramycin (Ophthalmic) 2056
Tobral D (EC) *see* Tobramycin and Dexamethasone 2056
Tobral (EC, IT) *see* Tobramycin (Ophthalmic) 2056
Tobramaxin (DE) *see* Tobramycin (Ophthalmic) 2056
Tobramex (PH) *see* Tobramycin (Ophthalmic) 2056
Tobramex (PH) *see* Tobramycin (Systemic, Oral Inhalation) 2052
Tobraneg (IN) *see* Tobramycin (Systemic, Oral Inhalation) 2052
Tobrasix (AT) *see* Tobramycin (Systemic, Oral Inhalation) 2052
Tobrasol (VE) *see* Tobramycin (Ophthalmic) 2056
Tobrasone (NO, SE) *see* Tobramycin and Dexamethasone 2056
Tobravisc (GB) *see* Tobramycin (Ophthalmic) 2056
Tobraxona (PE) *see* Tobramycin and Dexamethasone 2056
Tobre (KR) *see* Tobramycin (Ophthalmic) 2056
Tobrex (AE, AT, AU, BE, BF, BG, BH, BJ, BR, CH, CI, CL, CN, CO, CY, CZ, DK, EE, EG, ET, FI, FR, GH, GM, GN, GR, HK, HN, HR, IL, IQ, IR, JO, KE, KW, LB, LR, LT, LY, MA, ML, MR, MU, MW, MY, NE, NG, NL, NO, NZ, OM, PE, PK, PL, PT, PY, QA, RO, RU, SA, SC, SD, SE, SI, SK, SL, SN, SY, TH, TN, TR, TW, TZ, UG, UY, VE, VN, YE, ZA, ZM, ZW) *see* Tobramycin (Ophthalmic) 2056
Tobrimin (DO) *see* Tobramycin (Ophthalmic) 2056
Tobrin (AE, BH, CY, EG, IQ, IR, JO, KW, LB, LY, OM, QA, SA, SY, YE) *see* Tobramycin (Ophthalmic) 2056
Tobrin (EG) *see* Tobramycin (Systemic, Oral Inhalation) 2052
Tobucin (TW) *see* Tobramycin (Systemic, Oral Inhalation) 2052
Tobumide (SG) *see* TOLBUTamide 2062
Tobutol (TH) *see* Ethambutol 798
Tobymet (ID) *see* Cimetidine 438
Tobyprim (ID) *see* Trimethoprim 2104
Tocalm (CL) *see* Ambroxol [INT] 109
Tocarlol (TH) *see* Carvedilol 367
Tocef (ID) *see* Cefixime 380
Tocin (TW) *see* Tobramycin (Ophthalmic) 2056
Tocopin (VN) *see* Teicoplanin [INT] 1983
Tocrat (AR) *see* Nitrendipine [INT] 1463
Toctino (AT, BG, CH, DE, DK, EE, FI, FR, GB, IS, LT, NO, RO, SI, SK) *see* Alitretinoin (Systemic) [CAN/INT] 88
Todacin (TH) *see* Clindamycin (Systemic) 460
Todesaar (TH) *see* Candesartan 335
Todolac (DK) *see* Etodolac 815
Todo (TW) *see* Etodolac 815
Tofedex (ID) *see* Dexketoprofen [INT] 603
Tofexo (TH) *see* Fexofenadine 873
Tofranil (AE, AR, AT, AU, BB, BE, BF, BG, BH, BJ, BM, BR, BS, BZ, CH, CI, CO, CY, DE, DK, EE, EG, ES, ET, FI, FR, GB, GH, GM, GN, GR, GY, HK, ID, IE, IL, IQ, IR, IT, JM, JO, KE, KW, LB, LR, LU, LY, MA, ML, MR, MT, MU, MW, MX, MY, NE, NG, NL, NO, NZ, OM, PH, PK, PL, PT, PY, QA, RU, SA, SC, SD, SE, SK, SL, SN, SR, SY, TN, TR, TT, TW, TZ, UG, UY, VE, YE, ZA, ZM, ZW) *see* Imipramine 1054
Tofranil-PM (AR, PY) *see* Imipramine 1054
Tohsino (JP) *see* Fluocinonide 894
Toilax (DK, FI, IE, NO, SE) *see* Bisacodyl 265
Tolanase (GB) *see* TOLAZamide 2062
Tolbutamid R.A.N. (DE) *see* TOLBUTamide 2062
Tolcamin (CO) *see* Ifosfamide 1040
Tolchicine (TH) *see* Colchicine 500

Tolectin (BF, BH, BJ, CI, CY, EG, ET, GH, GM, GN, JO, KE, LB, LR, MA, ML, MR, MU, MW, NE, NG, OM, PL, SC, SD, SL, SN, SY, TN, TZ, UG, ZA, ZM, ZW) *see* Tolmetin ... 2062
Tolectin-gel (PL) *see* Tolmetin ... 2062
Tolerade (AU) *see* Imipramine ... 1054
Tolerane (AR, PY) *see* Flurbiprofen (Ophthalmic) ... 906
Tolexine (FR, HK) *see* Doxycycline ... 689
Tolexine Ge (FR) *see* Doxycycline ... 689
Tolima (DE) *see* Thiamine ... 2028
Toliman (IT) *see* Cinnarizine [INT] ... 440
Tolinase (AE, BH, CY, EG, ES, IL, IQ, IR, JO, KW, LB, LY, NL, OM, QA, SA, SY, YE) *see* TOLAZamide ... 2062
Tolmex (EC) *see* Cetirizine ... 411
Tolmicen (CZ, IT, PT) *see* Tolciclate [INT] ... 2062
Tolmide (SG) *see* TOLBUTamide ... 2062
Tolnadem (IN) *see* Tolnaftate ... 2063
Tolnaderm (MY, SG) *see* Tolnaftate ... 2063
Tolnate (PH) *see* Tolnaftate ... 2063
Toloxim (PT) *see* Mebendazole [CAN/INT] ... 1274
Toloxin (TH) *see* Digoxin ... 627
Tolsiran (JP) *see* TOLBUTamide ... 2062
Tolsol (IN) *see* Tolnaftate ... 2063
Toltem (AR) *see* Tolterodine ... 2063
Tolterox (UY) *see* Tolterodine ... 2063
Toltin (UY) *see* Tolterodine ... 2063
Tolumide (JP) *see* TOLBUTamide ... 2062
Tolyprin (DE) *see* Azapropazone [INT] ... 210
Tomizol (KR) *see* Ornidazole [INT] ... 1522
Tomudex (AR, AT, AU, BE, BG, BR, CH, CZ, EE, ES, FR, GB, HN, HU, IE, IS, IT, KR, LU, MX, NL, NO, PL, PT, RU, SG, TR, UY, VE) *see* Raltitrexed [CAN/INT] ... 1769
Tonafil (TH) *see* Sildenafil ... 1882
Tonaf (TH) *see* Tolnaftate ... 2063
Tonavir (PY, UY) *see* Stavudine ... 1934
Tonec (TW) *see* Aceclofenac [INT] ... 30
Toniker (TW) *see* Acetaminophen ... 32
Tonixan (PY) *see* Folic Acid ... 919
Tonizep 5 (TH) *see* Donepezil ... 668
Tonlief (TW) *see* Aceclofenac [INT] ... 30
Tonlin (TW) *see* FlavoxATE ... 881
Tonocalcin (MY) *see* Calcitonin ... 322
Tonocardin (HR) *see* Doxazosin ... 674
Tonokardin (HR) *see* Doxazosin ... 674
Tonolyte 2 (TH) *see* TiZANidine ... 2051
Tonolyte 4 (TH) *see* TiZANidine ... 2051
Tonopan (MX) *see* Dihydroergotamine ... 633
Tonotil (UY) *see* Benserazide and Levodopa [CAN/INT] ... 244
Tonsaric (TW) *see* Allopurinol ... 90
Tonstop (TW) *see* Orphenadrine ... 1522
Tontec (TW) *see* Nabumetone ... 1411
Tontin (TW) *see* Tolmetin ... 2062
Tonus-Forte (DE) *see* Etilefrine [INT] ... 815
Tonustab (DE) *see* Etilefrine [INT] ... 815
Tonval (PE) *see* Pantoprazole ... 1570
Topalgic (FR) *see* TraMADol ... 2074
Topamac (AR, CO, EC, IN, PE, PY, UY) *see* Topiramate ... 2065
Topamax (AE, AT, AU, BE, BG, BH, BR, CH, CL, CN, CY, CZ, DE, EE, EG, ES, FI, GB, HK, HR, IE, IL, IQ, IR, IT, JM, JO, KR, KW, LB, LT, LY, MX, MY, NL, NZ, OM, PH, PK, PL, PT, QA, RO, RU, SA, SG, SI, SK, SY, TH, TR, TW, VE, VN, YE, ZA) *see* Topiramate ... 2065
Topamax Sprinkle (AE, BH, CY, HK, IL, KR, KW, NZ, SA) *see* Topiramate ... 2065
Topazol (ID) *see* Pantoprazole ... 1570
Topcid (IN) *see* Famotidine ... 845
Topcort (HK) *see* Mometasone (Topical) ... 1391
Topcort (ID) *see* Desoximetasone ... 598
Topicaine (AU) *see* Benzocaine ... 246
Topicaine (NZ) *see* Tetracaine (Topical) ... 2017
Topicil (MY, NZ) *see* Clindamycin (Topical) ... 464
Topicorte (AE, BE, BH, CY, EG, FR, IL, IQ, IR, JO, KW, LB, LU, LY, MY, NL, OM, PT, QA, SA, SY, TH, YE) *see* Desoximetasone ... 598
Topicorten V (IL) *see* Clioquinol and Flumethasone [CAN/INT] ... 465
Topicrem (ES) *see* Magnesium Salicylate ... 1265
Topictal (CR, EC, GT, HN, NI, PA, PY, SV) *see* Topiramate ... 2065
Topidil (TH) *see* Felodipine ... 850
Topifort (IN) *see* Clobetasol ... 468
Topifug (DE) *see* Desonide ... 597
Topimax (CR, DK, DO, GT, HN, IS, NI, NO, PA, SE, SV) *see* Topiramate ... 2065
Topimicyn (PE) *see* Bacitracin, Neomycin, and Polymyxin B ... 223
Topimide (TW) *see* Tropicamide ... 2108
Topimo (TW) *see* Pimozide ... 1651
Topina (JP) *see* Topiramate ... 2065
Topinmate (TW) *see* Topiramate ... 2065
Topirol (PH) *see* Topiramate ... 2065
Topiron (KR) *see* Topiramate ... 2065
Topisolon (AT, BB, BM, BS, BZ, CH, DE, GY, IE, JM, PR, SE, SR, TT, ZA) *see* Desoximetasone ... 598
Topistin (SG) *see* Ciprofloxacin (Systemic) ... 441
Topitrim (IL) *see* Topiramate ... 2065
Topizide (TH) *see* GlipiZIDE ... 967
Topmate (KR) *see* Topiramate ... 2065
Topodria (CO) *see* Topotecan ... 2069
Topogyne (GB, RO) *see* Misoprostol ... 1379
Topokebir (AR) *see* Topotecan ... 2069
Topomac (GR) *see* Topiramate ... 2065
Topotecin (JP) *see* Irinotecan ... 1112
Topotel (IN, PH, TH) *see* Topotecan ... 2069
Topo (TH) *see* Etoposide ... 816
Topoxy (TH) *see* Desoximetasone ... 598
Topramine (TH) *see* Imipramine ... 1054
Toprazole (MY) *see* Pantoprazole ... 1570
Toprazol (KR) *see* Pantoprazole ... 1570
Toprec (FR) *see* Ketoprofen ... 1145
Toprol XL (AU) *see* Metoprolol ... 1350
Topron (MX) *see* Nifuroxazide [INT] ... 1454
Topsy (ID) *see* Lidocaine and Prilocaine ... 1213
Topsym (AE, AT, BH, CH, CY, DE, EC, EG, IL, IQ, IR, JO, JP, KW, LB, LY, OM, PE, PT, QA, SA, SY, TW, YE) *see* Fluocinonide ... 894
Topsym F (AT) *see* Fluocinonide ... 894
Topsym Polyol (PY) *see* Fluocinonide ... 894
Topsyne (FR, NL) *see* Fluocinonide ... 894
Topsyn (IT, MX) *see* Fluocinonide ... 894
Toradol (AE, AU, BH, CY, DK, EC, EG, FI, HK, ID, IQ, IR, IS, IT, JO, KW, LB, LY, NO, OM, PH, PK, QA, SA, SE, SY, YE) *see* Ketorolac (Systemic) ... 1146
Tora-Dol (CH) *see* Ketorolac (Systemic) ... 1146
Toral (ID) *see* Torsemide ... 2071
Toramate (TW) *see* Topiramate ... 2065
Toranax (VN) *see* ALPRAZolam ... 94
Torasic (ID) *see* Ketorolac (Systemic) ... 1146
Torem (BG, CH, DE, EE, GB, KR, SE) *see* Torsemide ... 2071
Torendo (BG) *see* RisperiDONE ... 1818
Torental (BE, FR, LU) *see* Pentoxifylline ... 1618
Toricam Gel (TW) *see* Piroxicam ... 1662
Toricard-5 (PH) *see* Nebivolol ... 1434
Torid (IL) *see* AtorvaSTATin ... 194
Torio (TH) *see* Simvastatin ... 1890
Torisel (AR, AU, BE, BR, CH, CL, CO, CY, CZ, DE, DK, EE, FR, GB, HK, HN, HR, IE, IL, IS, IT, JP, KR, KW, LT, MY, NL, NO, PH, PL, PT, QA, RO, SA, SE, SG, SI, SK, TH, TR, TW) *see* Temsirolimus ... 1994
Torizin (JP) *see* Cinnarizine [INT] ... 440
Torleva (IN, VN) *see* LevETIRAcetam ... 1191
Torolac (JO) *see* AtorvaSTATin ... 194

Torolan (VN) *see* OLANZapine ... 1491
Torospar (IN) *see* Sparfloxacin [INT] ... 1930
Torpain (ID) *see* Ketorolac (Systemic) ... 1146
Torpas (VE) *see* Tiaprofenic Acid [CAN/INT] ... 2034
Torpezil (PH) *see* Donepezil ... 668
Torq (IN) *see* Tolterodine ... 2063
Torq SR (IN) *see* Tolterodine ... 2063
Torrem (BE) *see* Torsemide ... 2071
Torsem (KR) *see* Torsemide ... 2071
Torsix (TW) *see* Torsemide ... 2071
Torvalipin (SG) *see* AtorvaSTATin ... 194
Torvast (IT) *see* AtorvaSTATin ... 194
Torymycin (TH) *see* Doxycycline ... 689
Tosadex (TR) *see* Bicalutamide ... 262
Tosan (TH) *see* Losartan ... 1248
Toselac (KR) *see* Etodolac ... 815
Tosidrin (ES) *see* Dihydrocodeine, Aspirin, and Caffeine ... 632
Tosma (ID) *see* Ketotifen (Systemic) [CAN/INT] ... 1149
Tospin (TW) *see* Trospium ... 2108
Tosse (GR) *see* Ambroxol [INT] ... 109
Tosseque (PT) *see* Bromhexine [INT] ... 291
Tossimex (CH) *see* Bromhexine [INT] ... 291
Tostop (AR, PY) *see* Bromhexine [INT] ... 291
Tostran (GB) *see* Testosterone ... 2010
Tostrex Gel (KR) *see* Testosterone ... 2010
Tostrex (ID) *see* Testosterone ... 2010
Tosumin (TW) *see* Triprolidine and Pseudoephedrine ... 2105
Totacef (EE, HN, HU) *see* CeFAZolin ... 373
Totapen (FR) *see* Ampicillin ... 141
Totasedan (CL) *see* Bromazepam [CAN/INT] ... 290
Totect (BM) *see* Dexrazoxane ... 606
Totinal (AE, BH, CY, EG, IQ, IR, JO, KW, LB, LY, OM, QA, SA, SY, YE) *see* Ketotifen (Systemic) [CAN/INT] ... 1149
Touxium Mucolyticum (LU) *see* Acetylcysteine ... 40
Tovanor (AU) *see* Glycopyrrolate ... 975
Tovast (KR) *see* AtorvaSTATin ... 194
Toviaz (AT, BE, CH, CZ, DE, DK, EE, GB, GR, HK, HR, ID, IE, IL, IS, IT, JP, KR, LT, MY, NL, NO, PH, PL, PT, RO, SE, SI, SK, TR) *see* Fesoterodine ... 872
Toviaz PR (CY) *see* Fesoterodine ... 872
Tovincocard (IT) *see* Dipyridamole ... 652
Toxopirin (DO) *see* Pyrimethamine ... 1749
Tozaar (IN) *see* Losartan ... 1248
Trabilin (BB, BM, BS, BZ, CR, GT, GY, HN, JM, NI, PA, SR, SV, TT) *see* TraMADol ... 2074
Tracan (KR) *see* Acetaminophen and Tramadol ... 37
Tracefusin (MX) *see* Zinc Chloride ... 2200
Tracetate (ID) *see* Megestrol ... 1281
Traceton (TW) *see* Acetaminophen and Tramadol ... 37
Trachisan (BH, JO, KW) *see* Chlorhexidine Gluconate ... 422
Trachon (ID) *see* Itraconazole ... 1130
Tracil (AR) *see* Nitrendipine [INT] ... 1463
Tracin (KR) *see* Terazosin ... 2001
Tracleer (AT, AU, BE, BR, CH, CN, CO, CZ, DE, DK, EC, EE, ES, FI, FR, GB, GR, HK, HN, HR, IE, IL, IS, IT, JP, KR, LT, MY, NL, NO, NZ, PT, RO, SE, SG, SI, SK, TH, TW, VN) *see* Bosentan ... 280
Tracne (HK) *see* Tretinoin (Topical) ... 2099
Trac (PH) *see* Atracurium ... 198
Tracrium (AE, AR, AT, AU, BB, BD, BE, BF, BG, BH, BJ, BM, BR, BS, BZ, CH, CI, CL, CN, CY, CZ, DE, DK, EC, EE, EG, ES, ET, FI, FR, GB, GH, GM, GN, GR, GY, HK, HN, HU, ID, IE, IL, IN, IQ, IR, IT, JM, JO, JP, KE, KW, LB, LR, LT, LY, MA, ML, MR, MT, MU, MW, MX, NE, NG, NL, NO, NZ, OM, PH, PK, PL, PT, PY, QA, RO, RU, SA, SC, SD, SE, SG, SK, SL, SN, SR, SY, TH, TN, TR, TT, TW, TZ, UG, UY, VN, YE, ZA, ZM, ZW) *see* Atracurium ... 198
Tracrrium (SI) *see* Atracurium ... 198
Tractocile (AE, AR, AT, BE, BH, CH, CN, CY, CZ, DE, DK, EE, FI, FR, GB, GR, HK, HR, HU, IE, IS, IT, JO, KR, LB, LT, MY, NL, NO, NZ, PH, PL, PT, QA, RO, SA, SE, SI, SK, TH, TR, VN, ZA) *see* Atosiban [INT] ... 197
Tracur (BR) *see* Atracurium ... 198
Tracurix (AR, JO, PY) *see* Atracurium ... 198
Tradaxin (MX) *see* Cetirizine ... 411
Tradea (MX) *see* Methylphenidate ... 1336
Tradelia (DE) *see* Estradiol (Systemic) ... 775
Tradolan (AE, BH, CY, EG, IQ, IR, JO, KW, LB, LY, OM, QA, SA, SE, SY, YE) *see* TraMADol ... 2074
Tradol-Puren (DE) *see* TraMADol ... 2074
Tradonal (PH) *see* TraMADol ... 2074
Tradorec XL (GB, IE) *see* TraMADol ... 2074
Trafloxal (BE, NL) *see* Ofloxacin (Ophthalmic) ... 1491
Trajenta (AU, BE, CH, CN, CZ, DK, EE, FR, GB, HK, HR, ID, IL, KR, LT, MY, NL, NO, PH, QA, RO, SA, SE, SG, SI, SK, TH, TW, VN) *see* Linagliptin ... 1215
Trajenta Duo (HK, ID, KR, MY, PH, SG) *see* Linagliptin and Metformin ... 1217
Trajentamet (AU) *see* Linagliptin and Metformin ... 1217
Trakipearl (JP) *see* ChlordiazePOXIDE ... 422
Traldiar (GT, HN, PA, SV) *see* Acetaminophen and Tramadol ... 37
Tralenta (IS) *see* Linagliptin ... 1215
Traler (AR) *see* Bepotastine ... 250
Tralgit SR (SK) *see* TraMADol ... 2074
Tral (PH) *see* Ketorolac (Systemic) ... 1146
Tramacet (BB, BM, BS, BZ, CO, DO, GB, GY, IE, JM, MX, PR, SR, TT) *see* Acetaminophen and Tramadol ... 37
Tramada (MY) *see* TraMADol ... 2074
Tramadex (IL) *see* TraMADol ... 2074
Tramadolor (LT) *see* TraMADol ... 2074
Tramadol Slovakofarma (HU) *see* TraMADol ... 2074
Tramagetic (DE) *see* TraMADol ... 2074
Tramagit (DE) *see* TraMADol ... 2074
Tramahexal (ZA) *see* TraMADol ... 2074
Trama Inj (IL) *see* TraMADol ... 2074
Tramake (IE) *see* TraMADol ... 2074
Tramal (AE, AT, AU, BF, BH, BJ, CH, CI, CN, CO, CR, CY, CZ, DE, DO, EC, EE, EG, ET, FI, GH, GM, GN, GR, GT, HN, HR, IQ, IR, JO, JP, KE, KW, LB, LR, LU, LY, MA, ML, MR, MU, MW, NE, NG, NI, NL, NZ, OM, PA, PE, PH, PK, PL, PT, QA, RU, SA, SC, SD, SK, SL, SN, SV, SY, TH, TN, TW, TZ, UG, VE, YE, ZA, ZM, ZW) *see* TraMADol ... 2074
Tramalgin (BG) *see* TraMADol ... 2074
Tramal Retard (AE, BH, KW, LB, SA) *see* TraMADol ... 2074
Tramal SR (NZ) *see* TraMADol ... 2074
Tramazac (BF, BJ, CI, ET, GH, GM, GN, IN, KE, LR, MA, ML, MR, MU, MW, NE, NG, SC, SD, SL, SN, TH, TN, TZ, UG, ZM, ZW) *see* TraMADol ... 2074
Tramaze (PH) *see* TraMADol ... 2074
Tramcontin (CN) *see* TraMADol ... 2074
Tramedo (AU) *see* TraMADol ... 2074
Tramedo SR (AU) *see* TraMADol ... 2074
Tramed (TW) *see* TraMADol ... 2074
Tramic (TH) *see* Tranexamic Acid ... 2081
Tramiphen (KR) *see* Acetaminophen and Tramadol ... 37
Tramsone (KR) *see* Triamcinolone (Systemic) ... 2099
Tramsone (SG) *see* Triamcinolone (Topical) ... 2100
Tramundin Retard (AE, KW) *see* TraMADol ... 2074
Tramundin retard (BH) *see* TraMADol ... 2074
Tramus (ID) *see* Atracurium ... 198
Tranalpha (AU) *see* Trandolapril ... 2080
Tranarest (IN) *see* Tranexamic Acid ... 2081
Trancon (TH) *see* Clorazepate ... 487
Trandate (AE, AT, AU, BB, BE, BF, BH, BJ, BM, BS, BZ, CH, CI, CL, CY, CZ, DK, EE, EG, ES, ET, FR, GB, GH, GM, GN, GR, GY, HK, HN, HU, IE, IL, IQ, IR, IS, IT, JM, JO, KE, KR, KW, LB, LR, LU, LY, MA, ML, MR, MU, MW, MY, NE, NG, NL, NO, NZ, OM, PT, QA, SA, SC,

SD, SE, SG, SI, SL, SN, SR, SY, TN, TR, TT, TW, TZ, UG, VE, VN, YE, ZA, ZM, ZW) *see* Labetalol 1151
Trane (AR) *see* ChlorproPAMIDE 429
Tranexam (EC, RU, TW) *see* Tranexamic Acid 2081
Tranexic (TW) *see* Tranexamic Acid 2081
Tranexid (ID) *see* Tranexamic Acid 2081
Tranex (IT) *see* Tranexamic Acid 2081
Trangorex (ES, VE) *see* Amiodarone 114
Trankimazin Retard (ES) *see* ALPRAZolam 94
Tranmix (VN) *see* Tranexamic Acid 2081
Tranqipam (ZA) *see* LORazepam 1243
Tranquilin (LU) *see* Meprobamate 1296
Tranquinal (BR, CR, DO, EC, GT, HN, NI, PA, PY, SV, UY) *see* ALPRAZolam 94
Tranquirit (IT) *see* Diazepam 613
Tranquo (LU) *see* Oxazepam 1532
Transamina (UY) *see* Tranexamic Acid 2081
Transamin (BR, CN, HK, JP, KR, MY, PE, PK, TH, TW, VN) *see* Tranexamic Acid 2081
Transene (IT) *see* Clorazepate 487
Transic (TH) *see* Tranexamic Acid 2081
Transiderm Nitro (AU, FI, IE, NL, NO, SE) *see* Nitroglycerin 1465
Transilane (TW) *see* Psyllium 1744
Transimune (IN) *see* AzaTHIOprine 210
Transital (ES) *see* Amobarbital 128
Transpulmin G (PH) *see* GuaiFENesin 986
Transtec (BE, CH, CL, CO, DE, EC, ES, GB, HN, HR, HU, IE, MX, NO, PE, PT, SK) *see* Buprenorphine 300
Trantalol (MY, SG) *see* Labetalol 1151
Tranxa (ID) *see* Tranexamic Acid 2081
Tranxen (DK, VE) *see* Clorazepate 487
Tranxene (AE, BB, BE, BH, BM, BS, BZ, CY, CZ, EC, EG, FR, GB, GR, GY, HK, HN, IE, IL, IQ, IR, JM, JO, KR, KW, LB, LT, LU, LY, MX, MY, NL, OM, PH, PK, PL, PR, PT, QA, SA, SG, SR, SY, TH, TR, TT, TW, VN, YE) *see* Clorazepate 487
Tranxilene (TR) *see* Clorazepate 487
Tranxilium (AR, AT, CH, DE, ES) *see* Clorazepate 487
Trapanal (DE, HU) *see* Thiopental [INT] 2029
Trapax (AR, PY) *see* LORazepam 1243
Trapex (IN) *see* LORazepam 1243
Trappen (JP) *see* Fluocinonide 894
Trarium (KR) *see* Atracurium 198
Trasik (ID) *see* TraMADol 2074
Traskolan (PL) *see* Aprotinin 168
Trastal (CN) *see* Piribedil [INT] 1662
Trastocir (AR) *see* Cilostazol 437
Trastoner (AR) *see* Piribedil [INT] 1662
Trasylol (AE, AT, AU, BE, BG, BH, BR, CH, CO, CY, CZ, DE, DK, EG, FI, FR, GB, GR, HK, HN, HR, ID, IE, IL, IQ, IR, IT, JO, KW, LB, LU, LY, MX, MY, NL, NO, OM, PE, PH, PL, SA, SE, SY, TW, UY, VE, YE, ZA) *see* Aprotinin 168
Traumalix (CH) *see* Etofenamate [INT] 815
Traumon (AT, DE, LU) *see* Etofenamate [INT] 815
Travamin (IL) *see* DimenhyDRINATE 637
Travastal (AR, BR, DE, EG, FR, GR, IN, MY, PT, SG, TH) *see* Piribedil [INT] 1662
Travastal Retard (EG) *see* Piribedil [INT] 1662
Travastan (IT) *see* Piribedil [INT] 1662
Travatan (AE, AR, AT, AU, BE, BG, BO, BR, CH, CL, CN, CO, CR, CY, CZ, DE, DK, DO, EC, EE, ES, FI, FR, GB, GR, GT, HK, HN, ID, IE, IL, IS, IT, JO, KR, KW, LB, LT, MT, MX, MY, NI, NL, NO, NZ, PA, PE, PH, PK, PL, PR, PT, PY, QA, RU, SA, SE, SG, SI, SK, SV, TH, TR, TW, UY, VE, VN, ZA) *see* Travoprost 2089
Travatanz (JP) *see* Travoprost 2089
Travel-Gum (CZ, IT, TR) *see* DimenhyDRINATE 637
Travel Well (ES) *see* DimenhyDRINATE 637
Travin (HR) *see* BusPIRone 311
Travisco (BR, IT) *see* Trapidil [INT] 2085
Travital Folic Acid (BE) *see* Folic Acid 919
Travogen (AE, AT, BE, BH, CH, CY, EE, EG, GR, HK, JO, KW, LB, LT, MY, PH, PL, QA, RO, RU, SA, SG, SI, TH, TR) *see* Isoconazole [INT] 1120
Trawell (CH) *see* DimenhyDRINATE 637
Traxam (GB, IE, IT) *see* Felbinac [INT] 850
Trayebta Duo (MX) *see* Linagliptin and Metformin 1217
Trayenta (AR, BR, CL, CO, MX) *see* Linagliptin 1215
Trayenta Duo (AR, CL) *see* Linagliptin and Metformin 1217
Trazec (AT, BE, BG, CH, CZ, DE, DK, EE, ES, FI, FR, GB, GR, HN, IE, IT, MT, NL, NO, PL, PT, RU, SE, SK, TR) *see* Nateglinide 1432
Trazenta (JP) *see* Linagliptin 1215
Trazidex Ofteno (DO, GT, HN, NI, PA, SV) *see* Tobramycin and Dexamethasone 2056
Trazinine (JP) *see* Aprotinin 168
Trazodil (IL) *see* TraZODone 2091
Trazodone-Continental (LU) *see* TraZODone 2091
Trazolan (BE, IN, LU, NL) *see* TraZODone 2091
Trazole (JO) *see* Itraconazole 1130
Trazone (PT, TW) *see* TraZODone 2091
Trazonil (IN) *see* TraZODone 2091
Trazo (TH) *see* TraZODone 2091
TRD-Contin (IN) *see* TraMADol 2074
Treakisym (JP) *see* Bendamustine 241
Treanda (HK) *see* Bendamustine 241
Trebanol (MX) *see* Atenolol 189
Trebon (HK) *see* Acetylcysteine 40
Treclinac (EE, ES, LT, NL) *see* Clindamycin and Tretinoin 464
Treclinax (BE) *see* Clindamycin and Tretinoin 464
Treclin (GB) *see* Clindamycin and Tretinoin 464
Tredol (AE, BH, CY, EG, IQ, IR, JO, KW, LB, LY, OM, QA, SA, SY, YE) *see* Atenolol 189
Tredum (PY) *see* Bromazepam [CAN/INT] 290
Treflucan (AE, BH, CY, EG, IQ, IR, JO, KW, LB, LY, OM, QA, SA, SY, YE) *see* Fluconazole 885
Trefpod (HR) *see* Cefpodoxime 388
Tremesal (VE) *see* Doxycycline 689
Trenaxin (PH) *see* Tranexamic Acid 2081
Trenazin (AR) *see* Tetrabenazine 2016
Trendinol (ES) *see* Nitrendipine [INT] 1463
Trenelone (PT) *see* Dexchlorpheniramine 603
Trenfyl (ID) *see* Pentoxifylline 1618
Trenlin (HK) *see* Pentoxifylline 1618
Trenlin SR (SG) *see* Pentoxifylline 1618
Trenstad (VN) *see* Emtricitabine and Tenofovir 721
Trentadil (BE, FR, KR, LU) *see* Bamifylline [INT] 227
Trental (AE, AR, AT, AU, BB, BD, BG, BH, BM, BO, BR, BS, BZ, CH, CL, CO, CR, CY, CZ, DE, DK, DO, EC, EE, EG, ES, FI, GB, GT, GY, HK, HN, HR, HU, ID, IE, IL, IN, IQ, IR, IS, IT, JM, JO, JP, KR, KW, LB, LT, LY, MT, MX, MY, NI, NL, NO, NZ, OM, PA, PE, PH, PK, PL, PR, PT, PY, QA, RU, SA, SE, SG, SI, SK, SR, SV, SY, TR, TT, TW, UY, VE, YE) *see* Pentoxifylline 1618
Trental SR (EG) *see* Pentoxifylline 1618
Trentina (ES) *see* Trimethoprim 2104
Trentin (ID) *see* Tretinoin (Topical) 2099
Treonam (PE) *see* Aztreonam 220
Trepal-400 (TH) *see* Pentoxifylline 1618
Treparasen (GR) *see* Pindolol 1652
Trepar (PH) *see* DACTINomycin 551
Trepiline (ZA) *see* Amitriptyline 119
Trepina (MX) *see* CarBAMazepine 346
Treprost (JP) *see* Treprostinil 2093
Trerief (JP) *see* Zonisamide 2215
Tretin (KR) *see* ISOtretinoin 1127
Trevilor (DE) *see* Venlafaxine 2150
Trewilor (AT) *see* Venlafaxine 2150
Trexan (AE, EG, PK) *see* Naltrexone 1422
Trexan (EE, FI, HN, HU, LT, PL, RU, TR, TW) *see* Methotrexate 1322
Trexapin (IL) *see* OXcarbazepine 1532

Trexate (TH) *see* Methotrexate 1322
Trexofin (SG) *see* CefTRIAXone 396
Trexol (MX) *see* TraMADol 2074
TRIAcelluvax (DE) *see* Diphtheria and Tetanus Toxoids, and Acellular Pertussis Vaccine 649
Triafemi (FR) *see* Ethinyl Estradiol and Norgestimate 810
Triaken (MX) *see* CefTRIAXone 396
Trialam (TW) *see* Triazolam 2101
Trialmin (ES) *see* Gemfibrozil 956
Tri-Alzor (PH) *see* Olmesartan, Amlodipine, and Hydrochlorothiazide 1498
Triam-Denk (HK) *see* Triamcinolone (Systemic) 2099
Triampur Compositum (BG, EE) *see* Hydrochlorothiazide and Triamterene 1012
Trianil (JO) *see* ClomiPRAMINE 475
Trianol (PH) *see* Allopurinol 90
Triapten (PL) *see* Foscarnet 931
Triatec (BR, CH, CN, DK, FR, GR, ID, IL, IT, NO, PT, SE, VN) *see* Ramipril 1771
Triatec Comp (CH, DK, PT, SE) *see* Ramipril and Hydrochlorothiazide [CAN/INT] 1773
Triatec HCT (IT) *see* Ramipril and Hydrochlorothiazide [CAN/INT] 1773
Triateckit (FR) *see* Ramipril 1771
Triatec Plus (GR, TR) *see* Ramipril and Hydrochlorothiazide [CAN/INT] 1773
Triatop Lotion (CN) *see* Ketoconazole (Topical) 1145
Triax-1 (PH) *see* CefTRIAXone 396
Triax (IL) *see* CefTRIAXone 396
Triaxone (AE, KW, LB, QA, SA, SG) *see* CefTRIAXone 396
Triazide (TW) *see* Hydrochlorothiazide and Triamterene 1012
Tribedoce DX (MX) *see* Cyanocobalamin 515
Tribedoce (MX) *see* Thiamine 2028
Tribiot (MX) *see* Bacitracin and Polymyxin B 222
Tribiot (MX) *see* Bacitracin, Neomycin, and Polymyxin B 223
Tribiot (MX) *see* Polymyxin B 1676
Tributin (CO, KR) *see* Trimebutine [CAN/INT] 2103
Tribux (PL) *see* Trimebutine [CAN/INT] 2103
Tricalma (CL) *see* ALPRAZolam 94
Tricef (CL, PT, SE, TR) *see* Cefixime 380
Tricefin (SG) *see* CefTRIAXone 396
Tricef (TW) *see* CefTRIAXone 396
Tricel-D (EC) *see* Loratadine and Pseudoephedrine 1242
Tricel (EC) *see* Loratadine 1241
Trichex (AT) *see* MetroNIDAZOLE (Systemic) 1353
Triciclor (ES) *see* Ethinyl Estradiol and Levonorgestrel 803
Tricil (BF, BJ, CI, ET, GH, GM, GN, KE, LR, MA, ML, MR, MU, MW, NE, NG, SC, SD, SL, SN, TN, TZ, UG, ZM, ZW) *see* Ampicillin 141
Tricilest (FR, TH) *see* Ethinyl Estradiol and Norgestimate 810
Tricil (PY) *see* Metoclopramide 1345
Tricin (PH) *see* Triamcinolone (Topical) 2100
Tricivir (AR, CL) *see* Abacavir, Lamivudine, and Zidovudine 22
Triclazone (IN) *see* Rosiglitazone and Glimepiride 1847
Tricodein (DE) *see* Codeine 497
Tricodein Solco (AT, CH) *see* Codeine 497
Tricor (CL) *see* Adenosine 55
Tricort (FI, PH) *see* Triamcinolone (Systemic) 2099
Tricort (FI, PH) *see* Triamcinolone (Topical) 2100
Tricortone (AU) *see* Triamcinolone (Systemic) 2099
Tricortone (AU) *see* Triamcinolone (Topical) 2100
Tricoxane (CL) *see* Minoxidil (Topical) 1374
Tridep (BG) *see* Amitriptyline 119
Tridesilon (CO, CR, DE, DO, GB, GT, HN, NI, PA, SV) *see* Desonide 597
Tridesonit (FR) *see* Desonide 597
Tridezibarbitur (AT) *see* PHENobarbital 1632
Tridil (BR) *see* Nitroglycerin 1465
Tridol (KR) *see* TraMADol 2074
Tridyl (TH) *see* Trihexyphenidyl 2103
Triella (FR) *see* Ethinyl Estradiol and Norethindrone 808
Trifalicina (AR) *see* Ampicillin 141
Trifamox (AR, PY) *see* Amoxicillin 130
Trifed (AE, BH, CY, EG, ID, IQ, IR, JO, KW, LB, LY, OM, QA, SA, SY, YE) *see* Triprolidine and Pseudoephedrine 2105
Trifeme (AU, NZ) *see* Ethinyl Estradiol and Levonorgestrel 803
Triflucan (FR, IL, TR) *see* Fluconazole 885
Triflumann (DE, LU) *see* Trifluridine 2103
Triflumed (TH) *see* Trifluoperazine 2102
Tri Fluoro Timidina Poen (AR) *see* Trifluridine 2103
Trifluridin Thilo (AT) *see* Trifluridine 2103
Triflux (IT) *see* Triflusal [INT] 2103
Trifolget (PE) *see* Ciprofibrate [INT] 441
Trifosfaneurina (ES, PT) *see* Thiamine 2028
Trigan (RU) *see* Dicyclomine 622
Trigastronol (ES) *see* Bismuth 265
Triglizil (CO) *see* Gemfibrozil 956
Trigoa (DE) *see* Ethinyl Estradiol and Levonorgestrel 803
Trigynon (AT, BE) *see* Ethinyl Estradiol and Levonorgestrel 803
Triherpine (CH, GR, HU, IT, PL, VN) *see* Trifluridine 2103
Trihexifenidilo (CO) *see* Trihexyphenidyl 2103
Trihexin (KR) *see* Trihexyphenidyl 2103
Tri-Iodo-Tironina (AR) *see* Liothyronine 1221
Trijec (ID) *see* CefTRIAXone 396
Trijodthyronin (AT, PL) *see* Liothyronine 1221
Trijodthyronin BC (DE) *see* Liothyronine 1221
Trilac (ID) *see* Triamcinolone (Systemic) 2099
Trilafon (BE, CH, DK, ID, IS, IT, LU, NL, NO, PL, SE) *see* Perphenazine 1627
Trilaxant (PH) *see* Baclofen 223
Trilaxin (PH) *see* Ampicillin 141
Trileptal (AE, AR, AT, AU, BE, BG, BH, BO, BR, CH, CL, CN, CO, CR, CY, CZ, DE, DK, DO, EC, EE, EG, ES, FI, FR, GB, GR, GT, HK, HN, HR, ID, IE, IQ, IR, IS, IT, JO, KW, LB, LT, LY, MX, MY, NI, NL, NO, NZ, OM, PA, PE, PH, PL, PR, PY, QA, RO, RU, SA, SE, SI, SK, SV, SY, TH, TR, TW, UY, VE, VN, YE) *see* OXcarbazepine 1532
Trileptin (IL) *see* OXcarbazepine 1532
Trilifan (FR) *see* Perphenazine 1627
Trilin (ID) *see* Amitriptyline 119
Trilizin (TW) *see* Perphenazine 1627
Trilombrin (EC, ES) *see* Pyrantel Pamoate 1744
Triltec (LB) *see* Ramipril 1771
Tri-Luma (AR, BR, CL, CO, HK, MX, MY, PE, PH, SG, TH, VE) *see* Fluocinolone, Hydroquinone, and Tretinoin 894
Triluma (UY) *see* Fluocinolone, Hydroquinone, and Tretinoin 894
Trimaxazole (SG) *see* Sulfamethoxazole and Trimethoprim 1946
Trimaze (ZA) *see* Clotrimazole (Topical) 488
Trimcort (TW) *see* Trimethoprim 2104
Trimedat (LB) *see* Trimebutine [CAN/INT] 2103
Trimelasin (PK) *see* Fluocinolone, Hydroquinone, and Tretinoin 894
Trimepranol (CZ) *see* Metipranolol 1345
Trimesan (PL) *see* Trimethoprim 2104
Trimetabol (CO) *see* Cyproheptadine 529
Trimetin (FI) *see* Trimethoprim 2104
Trimetin (TW) *see* Trimebutine [CAN/INT] 2103
Trimetoger (MX) *see* Sulfamethoxazole and Trimethoprim 1946
Trimetop (EE) *see* Trimethoprim 2104

Trimetoprim (NO) *see* Trimethoprim ... 2104
Trimet (PE) *see* Trimebutine [CAN/INT] ... 2103
Trimexazol (MX) *see* Sulfamethoxazole and Trimethoprim ... 1946
Trimexazole (TH) *see* Sulfamethoxazole and Trimethoprim ... 1946
Trimezol (BG) *see* Sulfamethoxazole and Trimethoprim ... 1946
Trimez (PK) *see* Trimetazidine [INT] ... 2104
Trimin (AE, BH, CY, EG, IL, IQ, IR, JO, KR, KW, LB, LY, OM, QA, SA, SY, YE) *see* Perphenazine ... 1627
Trimin (TW) *see* DimenhyDRINATE ... 637
Trim (IT, ZA) *see* Sulfamethoxazole and Trimethoprim ... 1946
Trimol-A (AE) *see* Trimethoprim ... 2104
Trimonit (PL) *see* Nitroglycerin ... 1465
Trimopan (DK, GB) *see* Trimethoprim ... 2104
Trimoprim (HK) *see* Sulfamethoxazole and Trimethoprim ... 1946
Trimovax (AE, BG, HK, IT, PK, TH, TW) *see* Measles, Mumps, and Rubella Virus Vaccine ... 1273
Trimoxis (PH) *see* Sulfamethoxazole and Trimethoprim ... 1946
Trimox (TH) *see* Amoxicillin ... 130
Trimox (TW) *see* Sulfamethoxazole and Trimethoprim ... 1946
Trim (PY) *see* Trimebutine [CAN/INT] ... 2103
Trinergot (MX) *see* Ergotamine ... 754
Trineurovita (MX) *see* Pyridoxine ... 1747
Trinicalm (IN) *see* Trifluoperazine ... 2102
Trinipatch (LU) *see* Nitroglycerin ... 1465
Trinordiol 21 (DE) *see* Ethinyl Estradiol and Levonorgestrel ... 803
Trinordiol (AE, AR, AT, BE, BF, BH, BJ, BR, CI, CL, CZ, DE, DK, ET, FI, GH, GM, GN, GR, HK, IE, IT, KE, KW, LR, MA, ML, MR, MU, MW, MX, MY, NE, NG, NL, PH, PL, QA, RU, SC, SD, SE, SL, SN, TN, TZ, UG, ZM, ZW) *see* Ethinyl Estradiol and Levonorgestrel ... 803
Trinovum (AT, BE, BF, BJ, CH, CI, CO, DE, DK, ET, GB, GH, GM, GN, HR, IE, IS, IT, KE, LR, MA, ML, MR, MU, MW, NE, NG, PL, RU, SC, SD, SI, SL, SN, TN, TZ, UG, ZA, ZM, ZW) *see* Ethinyl Estradiol and Norethindrone ... 808
Trinsica 20 (MX) *see* Omeprazole and Sodium Bicarbonate ... 1511
Trinsica 40 (MX) *see* Omeprazole and Sodium Bicarbonate ... 1511
Trinter (IE) *see* Nitroglycerin ... 1465
Triocalcit (PE) *see* Calcitriol ... 323
TRIOFLEN (BG) *see* Triflusal [INT] ... 2103
Trioftín (MX) *see* Neomycin ... 1436
Trioftín (MX) *see* Polymyxin B ... 1676
Triomar (IL) *see* Omega-3 Fatty Acids ... 1507
Triomax (JO) *see* Sulfamethoxazole and Trimethoprim ... 1946
Triosules (AR) *see* Fluorouracil (Systemic) ... 896
Triox (MX) *see* CefTRIAXone ... 396
Triozine (TH) *see* Trifluoperazine ... 2102
Tripacel (AU, TH, TW) *see* Diphtheria and Tetanus Toxoids, and Acellular Pertussis Vaccine ... 649
Tripavac (PH) *see* Diphtheria and Tetanus Toxoids, and Acellular Pertussis Vaccine ... 649
Tripenem (ID) *see* Meropenem ... 1299
Tripgen (PH) *see* Amitriptyline ... 119
Triphasil (AU, NZ, ZA) *see* Ethinyl Estradiol and Levonorgestrel ... 803
Triphenidyl (CZ) *see* Trihexyphenidyl ... 2103
Tripril (MY) *see* Ramipril ... 1771
Triprim (AU, CZ, TW) *see* Trimethoprim ... 2104
Tri-Profen Cold and Flu (AU) *see* Pseudoephedrine and Ibuprofen ... 1743
Triptafen (GB) *see* Amitriptyline and Perphenazine ... 122
Tripta (MY, SG, TH) *see* Amitriptyline ... 119
Triptanol (MX) *see* Amitriptyline ... 119
Triptil (PY) *see* Amitriptyline ... 119
Triptizol (IT) *see* Amitriptyline ... 119
Triptyl (FI) *see* Amitriptyline ... 119
Tripvac (IN) *see* Diphtheria and Tetanus Toxoids, and Acellular Pertussis Vaccine ... 649
Triquilar (AE, BH, CY, CZ, DE, DO, EC, EG, GR, IN, IQ, IR, IS, JO, KR, KW, LB, LY, MX, OM, PY, QA, SA, SK, SY, UY, VE, YE) *see* Ethinyl Estradiol and Levonorgestrel ... 803
Triquilar ED (AU, ID, MY, NZ, TH) *see* Ethinyl Estradiol and Levonorgestrel ... 803
Triram (KR) *see* Triazolam ... 2101
TriRegol (GB) *see* Ethinyl Estradiol and Levonorgestrel ... 803
Trisekvens (SE) *see* Estradiol and Norethindrone ... 781
Trisekvens (SE) *see* Ethinyl Estradiol and Norethindrone ... 808
Trisenox (AT, BE, BG, CH, CZ, DE, DK, EE, ES, FI, FR, GB, GR, HN, HR, IE, IL, IT, JP, KR, LT, MT, NL, NO, PL, PT, RO, RU, SE, SK, TR) *see* Arsenic Trioxide ... 177
Trisequens (BF, BG, BJ, CH, CI, CL, CY, EC, ET, FR, GH, GM, GN, HR, KE, LB, LR, MA, ML, MR, MU, MW, NE, NG, SC, SD, SL, SN, TN, TR, TZ, UG, UY, ZM, ZW) *see* Estradiol and Norethindrone ... 781
Trisequens (BR, PE, PY, UY) *see* Ethinyl Estradiol and Norethindrone ... 808
Trisequens Forte (IL) *see* Estradiol and Norethindrone ... 781
Trisequens Forte (IL) *see* Ethinyl Estradiol and Norethindrone ... 808
Tri-Sequens (KR, SG) *see* Ethinyl Estradiol and Norethindrone ... 808
Tri-Sequens (KR, SG, VN) *see* Estradiol and Norethindrone ... 781
Trisolvat (CO) *see* Sulfamethoxazole and Trimethoprim ... 1946
Trisorcin (HR) *see* PenicillAMINE ... 1608
Trisul (NZ) *see* Sulfamethoxazole and Trimethoprim ... 1946
Tritace (AE, AR, AT, AU, BB, BE, BF, BG, BH, BJ, BM, BS, BZ, CI, CL, CO, CR, CZ, DK, DO, EC, EG, ET, GB, GH, GM, GN, GT, GY, HK, HN, HR, HU, IE, JM, JO, KE, KR, KW, LB, LR, LU, MA, ML, MR, MU, MW, MX, NE, NG, NI, NL, NZ, PA, PH, PK, PL, PR, PY, QA, SC, SD, SI, SK, SL, SN, SR, SV, TH, TN, TT, TW, TZ, UG, UY, ZM, ZW) *see* Ramipril ... 1771
Tritace Comp (IL) *see* Ramipril and Hydrochlorothiazide [CAN/INT] ... 1773
Tritace-HCT (AR, BB, BS, CR, DO, GT, HN, JM, NI, NL, PA, PY, SV, TT) *see* Ramipril and Hydrochlorothiazide [CAN/INT] ... 1773
Tritace Plus (BG, KR, RO) *see* Ramipril and Hydrochlorothiazide [CAN/INT] ... 1773
Tritazide (AT, BE, CZ, HR, MX, TH) *see* Ramipril and Hydrochlorothiazide [CAN/INT] ... 1773
Trittico AC (CL, CO, CZ, RO) *see* TraZODone ... 2091
Trittico (AE, AT, BG, BH, CH, CL, CO, CY, EG, GR, HK, HN, IL, IQ, IR, IT, JO, KR, KW, LB, LY, OM, PE, PL, PY, QA, RU, SA, SG, SI, SK, SY, VE, YE) *see* TraZODone ... 2091
Trittico CR (KR) *see* TraZODone ... 2091
Trittico Prolonged-Release (HK) *see* TraZODone ... 2091
Triumeq (CZ, DE, DK, EE, GB, HR, IS, LT, SE, SI, SK) *see* Abacavir, Dolutegravir, and Lamivudine ... 22
Trivam (ID) *see* Propofol ... 1728
Trivanex (TH) *see* Griseofulvin ... 985
Trivastal (PH, PY, QA, TR, VE) *see* Piribedil [INT] ... 1662
Trivastal Retard (AE, KW, SA, VN) *see* Piribedil [INT] ... 1662
Trivedon (HK) *see* Trimetazidine [INT] ... 2104
Triviraten Berna (HK, MY, NZ, PH, TH) *see* Measles, Mumps, and Rubella Virus Vaccine ... 1273

Trivirina (CO) *see* Trifluridine ... 2103
Trivorin (MX) *see* Ribavirin ... 1797
Trivudin (AR) *see* Abacavir, Lamivudine, and Zidovudine ... 22
Trixilem (CL, MX, TH) *see* Methotrexate ... 1322
Trixone (MY) *see* CefTRIAXone ... 396
Triyodotironina (ES) *see* Liothyronine ... 1221
Triyotex (CR, DO, GT, HN, MX, PA, SV) *see* Liothyronine ... 1221
Trizedon MR (ID) *see* Trimetazidine [INT] ... 2104
Trizef (PH) *see* Cefpodoxime ... 388
Trizele (KR) *see* MetroNIDAZOLE (Systemic) ... 1353
Trizidine (TH) *see* Trimetazidine [INT] ... 2104
Triz (IN) *see* Cetirizine ... 411
Trizivir (AE, AT, AU, BE, BG, BH, CH, CN, CO, CR, CZ, DE, DK, EC, FI, FR, GB, GR, HK, HN, HR, HU, IE, IL, IS, IT, LT, MX, NL, NO, PE, PT, QA, RU, SA, SE, SK, TR, TW, UY, VE) *see* Abacavir, Lamivudine, and Zidovudine ... 22
Trizole (PH) *see* Sulfamethoxazole and Trimethoprim ... 1946
Trobalt (AU, BE, CH, CY, CZ, DK, EE, FR, GB, HK, HR, HU, IE, IL, LT, NL, NO, PL, RO, SE, SI, SK) *see* Ezogabine ... 835
Trobenide (VN) *see* Tiaprofenic Acid [CAN/INT] ... 2034
Trocal (AR) *see* Prasugrel ... 1699
Trofentyl (IN, PH) *see* FentaNYL ... 857
Trofurit (HU) *see* Furosemide ... 940
Trogiar (ID) *see* MetroNIDAZOLE (Systemic) ... 1353
Troken (LB, MY) *see* Clopidogrel ... 484
Trolac (ID, KR) *see* Ketorolac (Systemic) ... 1146
Trolise (FR) *see* Pitavastatin ... 1663
Trolit (PE) *see* Ethinyl Estradiol and Levonorgestrel ... 803
Trolovol (FR, HR) *see* PenicillAMINE ... 1608
Trombex (SK) *see* Clopidogrel ... 484
Trombocil (PH) *see* Cilostazol ... 437
Tromboject (KR) *see* Sodium Tetradecyl Sulfate ... 1914
Trombovar (FR, NL, RU, SG) *see* Sodium Tetradecyl Sulfate ... 1914
Tromcor (PH) *see* Aspirin ... 180
Tromix (CO) *see* Azithromycin (Systemic) ... 216
Tronamycin (KR) *see* Tobramycin (Systemic, Oral Inhalation) ... 2052
Troncel (AR) *see* Strontium Ranelate [INT] ... 1938
Tropamid (TR) *see* Tropicamide ... 2108
Tropan (IN) *see* Oxybutynin ... 1536
Trophires (ES) *see* Pholcodine [INT] ... 1646
Tropicamet (IN) *see* Tropicamide ... 2108
Tropicamid (BG) *see* Tropicamide ... 2108
Tropicamidum (PL) *see* Tropicamide ... 2108
Tropicee (PH) *see* Ascorbic Acid ... 178
Tropicol (BE, LU, PT) *see* Tropicamide ... 2108
Tropicur (AR) *see* Mefloquine ... 1280
Tropidene (ID) *see* Piroxicam ... 1662
Tropidrol (ID) *see* MethylPREDNISolone ... 1340
Tropikacil (PE) *see* Tropicamide ... 2108
Tropikamid (HR, NO) *see* Tropicamide ... 2108
Tropimil (IT) *see* Tropicamide ... 2108
Tropin (KR, PK, SG) *see* DOPamine ... 669
Tropixal (GR, JO) *see* Tropicamide ... 2108
Tropocer (CO, PY, VE) *see* NiMODipine ... 1456
Trovas (AU) *see* AtorvaSTATin ... 194
Trozet (PH, TH, TW) *see* Letrozole ... 1181
Trozolet (CL, EC, PY, UY, VE) *see* Anastrozole ... 148
Trozolite (AR) *see* Anastrozole ... 148
Trubloc (PH) *see* Atenolol ... 189
Tructum (CO) *see* Terazosin ... 2001
Tructum (PE) *see* Ofloxacin (Otic) ... 1491
Trudexa (AT, BE, BG, CH, CZ, DE, DK, EE, FI, FR, GB, GR, HN, IE, IT, MT, NL, NO, PL, PT, RU, SE, SK, TR) *see* Adalimumab ... 51
Trulicity (CZ, EE, SE) *see* Dulaglutide ... 697
Trusopt (AE, AR, AT, AU, BB, BE, BG, BH, BM, BO, BR, BS, BZ, CH, CL, CO, CR, CY, CZ, DE, DK, DO, EC, EE, EG, FI, FR, GB, GR, GT, GY, HK, HN, HR, HU, IE, IL, IS, IT, JM, JO, KR, KW, LB, LT, MT, MX, MY, NI, NL, NO, NZ, PA, PE, PH, PK, PL, PR, PT, QA, RO, RU, SA, SE, SG, SI, SK, SR, SV, TH, TR, TT, TW, UY, VE, VN) *see* Dorzolamide ... 673
Truvada (AR, AT, AU, BE, BG, CH, CL, CY, CZ, DE, DK, EE, ES, FI, FR, GB, GR, HK, HN, HR, IE, IL, IS, IT, JP, KR, LT, MT, MX, NL, NO, NZ, PL, PT, RO, RU, SE, SG, SI, SK, TH, TR) *see* Emtricitabine and Tenofovir ... 721
Truvast (PH) *see* AtorvaSTATin ... 194
Truvaz (ID) *see* AtorvaSTATin ... 194
Truxa (EC, UY) *see* Levofloxacin (Systemic) ... 1197
Tryasol (DE) *see* Codeine ... 497
Trycam (TH) *see* Triazolam ... 2101
Trynol (TW) *see* Amitriptyline ... 119
Tryptanol (AR, BR, EC, JP, PE) *see* Amitriptyline ... 119
Tryptizol (AE, AT, BH, CH, EG, ES, GB, JO, KW, LB, NL, PT, QA, SE) *see* Amitriptyline ... 119
Trytomer (IN) *see* Amitriptyline ... 119
Tryzan (AU) *see* Ramipril ... 1771
Ttmycin (TW) *see* Tetracycline ... 2017
Tubilysin (FI) *see* Isoniazid ... 1120
Tubocin (HU) *see* Rifampin ... 1804
Tugaldin (ES) *see* Rifampin ... 1804
Tukol D (MX) *see* Guaifenesin and Dextromethorphan ... 987
Tulip (MX) *see* Simvastatin ... 1890
Tulip (SG, SK, TW) *see* AtorvaSTATin ... 194
Tulotract (DE) *see* Lactulose ... 1156
Tulupressin (DE) *see* Etilefrine [INT] ... 815
Tumetil (VE) *see* Mexiletine ... 1359
Tums EX Sugar Free (IL) *see* Calcium Carbonate ... 327
Tums (IL) *see* Calcium Carbonate ... 327
Tums Smoothies EX Peppermint (IL) *see* Calcium Carbonate ... 327
Tums Ultra Assorted Berries (IL) *see* Calcium Carbonate ... 327
Tums Ultra Spearmint (IL) *see* Calcium Carbonate ... 327
Tuosai (CN) *see* Torsemide ... 2071
Turfa (DE) *see* Hydrochlorothiazide and Triamterene ... 1012
Turixin (DE) *see* Mupirocin ... 1404
Turoptin (CH, IT) *see* Metipranolol ... 1345
Turox (GR, PT, SE) *see* Etoricoxib [INT] ... 821
Turpan (ID) *see* Acetaminophen ... 32
Tusben (IT) *see* Dimemorfan [INT] ... 637
Tusitato (MX) *see* Benzonatate ... 247
Tussamag-Codeinsaft (DE) *see* Codeine ... 497
Tussamed (DE) *see* Clobutinol [INT] ... 468
Tussed (DE) *see* Clobutinol [INT] ... 468
Tussine (JO) *see* Bromhexine [INT] ... 291
Tussipect Codein Tropfen Mono (DE) *see* Codeine ... 497
Tussoretard (DE) *see* Codeine ... 497
Tussoret (DE) *see* Codeine ... 497
Tuxi (NO) *see* Pholcodine [INT] ... 1646
TWC 30 (IN) *see* Acetaminophen and Codeine ... 36
Twelvmin-s (JP) *see* Hydroxocobalamin ... 1020
Twinrix (AE, AR, AU, BB, BE, BH, BM, BO, BR, BS, BZ, CH, CL, CN, CO, CR, CZ, DE, DK, DO, EC, EE, ES, FI, FR, GB, GR, GT, GY, HK, HN, HR, HU, IE, IL, IN, IS, IT, JM, LT, MT, MX, MY, NI, NL, NO, NZ, PA, PE, PH, PL, PR, PT, PY, QA, RO, SA, SE, SG, SI, SK, SR, SV, TH, TR, TT, TW, UY, VE, VN) *see* Hepatitis A and Hepatitis B Recombinant Vaccine ... 1000
Twynsta (AU, BE, CY, CZ, DE, EE, FR, GR, HK, HR, HU, ID, IE, KR, KW, LT, MY, NL, PH, PL, PT, RO, SE, SG, SI, SK, TH, TW, VN) *see* Telmisartan and Amlodipine ... 1989
Tyavax (FR) *see* Typhoid and Hepatitis A Vaccine [CAN/INT] ... 2111
Tybikin (TH) *see* Amikacin ... 111
Tybost (AU, CZ, DE, DK, EE, FI, GB, HR, LT, NL, SE, SK) *see* Cobicistat ... 495

Tydadex (ZA) *see* TOLBUTamide 2062
Tygacil (AE, AR, AT, AU, BE, BG, BH, BR, CH, CL, CN, CO, CR, CY, CZ, DE, DK, EC, EE, ES, FI, FR, GB, GR, GT, HK, HN, HR, HU, ID, IE, IL, IN, IS, IT, JP, KR, KW, LB, LT, MT, MX, MY, NI, NL, NO, NZ, PA, PE, PH, PL, PT, QA, RO, RU, SA, SE, SG, SI, SK, SV, TH, TR, TW, VE, VN) *see* Tigecycline 2040
Tykerb (AE, AR, AU, BH, BR, CL, CO, CR, DO, HK, HN, ID, IL, IN, JP, KR, KW, LB, MY, NZ, PA, PE, PH, QA, SA, SG, SV, TH, TW, UY) *see* Lapatinib 1169
Tyklid (IN) *see* Ticlopidine 2040
Tylenol 8-hour (TH) *see* Acetaminophen 32
Tylenol Acetaminophen Extended Relief (CN) *see* Acetaminophen 32
Tylenol (BR, CH, DE, JP, KR, MX, PH, PT, TH, VE) *see* Acetaminophen 32
Tylenol ER (KR) *see* Acetaminophen 32
Tylenol Extra Fuerte (PY) *see* Acetaminophen 32
Tylenol Forte (AE, BH, CY, EG, IQ, IR, JO, KW, LB, LY, OM, QA, SA, SY, YE) *see* Acetaminophen 32
Tylenol Oxy (KR) *see* Oxycodone and Acetaminophen 1541
Tylenol PM (CL) *see* Acetaminophen and Diphenhydramine 36
Tylex CD (MX) *see* Codeine 497
Tylex CD (CR, DO, GT, MX, NI, PA, SV) *see* Acetaminophen and Codeine 36
Tylex (BB, BM, BS, BZ, GY, JM, MX, SR, TT) *see* Acetaminophen 32
Tylonic (ID) *see* Allopurinol 90
Tymelyt (AT, BE, CZ, DK, LU, SE) *see* Lofepramine [INT] 1232
Tymer (LB, QA) *see* Gatifloxacin 949
Tynept (IN) *see* Tianeptine [INT] 2033
Typbar (TH) *see* Typhoid Vaccine 2112
Typherix (HK, PH, VN) *see* Typhoid Vaccine 2112
Typhim VI (AU, BG, CO, CR, DO, EE, FI, GT, HK, ID, KR, MY, NZ, PE, PH, PK, SG, SV, TH, TW) *see* Typhoid Vaccine 2112
Typhim Vi (AE, CN, HR, IL, IS, LT, RO, SA, SI, SK, VN) *see* Typhoid Vaccine 2112
Typhoral (IN) *see* Typhoid Vaccine 2112
Typhovax (KR) *see* Typhoid Vaccine 2112
Typh-Vax (NZ) *see* Typhoid Vaccine 2112
Tyran (ID) *see* Ranitidine 1777
Tyraq (HR) *see* Levothyroxine 1205
Tyrazol (FI) *see* Carbimazole [INT] 356
Tyrix Vi (KR) *see* Typhoid Vaccine 2112
Tysabri (AE, AT, AU, BE, BG, BH, BR, CH, CY, CZ, DE, DK, EE, ES, FI, FR, GB, GR, HK, HN, HR, HU, IE, IL, IS, IT, JP, KR, KW, LB, LT, MT, NL, NO, NZ, PL, PT, QA, RO, RU, SE, SG, SI, SK, TR) *see* Natalizumab 1432
Tyvaso (BM) *see* Treprostinil 2093
Tyverb (BE, CH, CY, CZ, DE, DK, EE, FR, GB, GR, HR, IE, IS, IT, LT, NL, NO, PL, PT, RO, SE, SI, SK, TR) *see* Lapatinib 1169
Tyxan (TW) *see* DOCEtaxel 656
Tzarevet X (IL) *see* Calcium Carbonate 327
Ubactam (KR) *see* Ampicillin and Sulbactam 145
Ucecal [salmon] (LU) *see* Calcitonin 322
Ucefa (TW) *see* Cefadroxil 372
Ucemine PP (BE, LU) *see* Niacinamide 1446
Ucerax (IE, KR) *see* HydrOXYzine 1024
Ucerom (KR) *see* Cefpirome [INT] 388
Ucetam (PK) *see* Piracetam [INT] 1661
Ucholine (TH) *see* Bethanechol 257
U-Clor (TW) *see* Cefaclor 372
Udihep (TH) *see* Ursodiol 2116
Udilol (TW) *see* Carvedilol 367
Udopa (ID) *see* DOPamine 669
Udoxan (MY) *see* Oxytocin 1549
Udrik (DE) *see* Trandolapril 2080
Ufarin (CL) *see* Isoconazole [INT] 1120
Ufo (TW) *see* Fosfomycin 932
Ulcafate (PK) *see* Sucralfate 1940
Ulcaid (AU, ZA) *see* Ranitidine 1777
Ulcar (AE, BH, CY, EG, FR, IQ, IR, JO, KW, LB, LY, OM, QA, SA, SY, YE) *see* Sucralfate 1940
Ulcatif (AE, BH, CY, EG, IQ, IR, JO, KW, LB, LY, OM, QA, SA, SY, YE) *see* Famotidine 845
Ulcedex (LB) *see* Clidinium and Chlordiazepoxide 460
Ulcedin (IT) *see* Cimetidine 438
Ulcelac (AR) *see* Famotidine 845
Ulcemex (CL, PY) *see* Pantoprazole 1570
Ulcenol (VE) *see* Famotidine 845
Ulceran (AE, BG, BH, CY, EG, IQ, IR, JO, KW, LB, LY, OM, QA, SA, SG, SY, TR, YE) *see* Famotidine 845
Ulceran (HU, PE) *see* Ranitidine 1777
Ulcerase (PT) *see* Collagenase (Topical) 507
Ulcerfate (IN) *see* Sucralfate 1940
Ulcerfen (AR) *see* Cimetidine 438
Ulcerin (HK) *see* Cimetidine 438
Ulcerlmin (JP, KR) *see* Sucralfate 1940
Ulcermin (PT) *see* Sucralfate 1940
Ulcertec (MY) *see* Sucralfate 1940
Ulcetab (ZA) *see* Sucralfate 1940
Ulcex (IT) *see* Ranitidine 1777
Ulcicure (QA, SA) *see* Sucralfate 1940
Ulcidine (MY) *see* Cimetidine 438
Ulcimet (EC, ID, PE, UY) *see* Cimetidine 438
Ulcim (ZA) *see* Cimetidine 438
Ulcinorm (VN) *see* Ranitidine 1777
Ulcin (PH) *see* Ranitidine 1777
Ulciran (PY) *see* Ranitidine 1777
Ulcium (EC) *see* Esomeprazole 771
Ulcodin (HR) *see* Ranitidine 1777
Ulcogant (AT, BE, CH, CZ, DE, HU, LU, NL, PE) *see* Sucralfate 1940
Ulcolind Wismut (DE) *see* Bismuth 265
Ulcomedina (IT) *see* Cimetidine 438
Ulcomet (EE) *see* Cimetidine 438
Ulcosal (ES) *see* Nizatidine 1471
Ulcosan (CZ) *see* Ranitidine 1777
Ulcozol (EC, PE) *see* Omeprazole 1508
Ulcumaag (ID) *see* Sucralfate 1940
Ulcuprazol (DO) *see* Omeprazole 1508
Ulcyte (AU) *see* Sucralfate 1940
Uldapril (MX) *see* Lansoprazole 1166
UL Ergometrine (PH) *see* Ergonovine [CAN/INT] 754
Ulex (TW) *see* Crotamiton 514
Ulfadin (CO) *see* Famotidine 845
Ulfagel (EC) *see* Famotidine 845
Ulfamid (HR, HU, PL) *see* Famotidine 845
Ulfaret (ES, GR) *see* Cefsulodin [INT] 391
Ulmo (ID) *see* Famotidine 845
Ulnor (DE) *see* Omeprazole 1508
Ulpax (MX) *see* Lansoprazole 1166
Ulpraz (ID) *see* Omeprazole 1508
Ulprix (BG) *see* Pantoprazole 1570
Ulremif (BG) *see* Remifentanil 1789
Ulsaheal (AE, BH, IQ, JO, QA, SA) *see* Sucralfate 1940
Ulsal (AT) *see* Ranitidine 1777
Ulsanic (ID, IL, JP, TH, TW, ZA) *see* Sucralfate 1940
Ulsen (MX) *see* Omeprazole 1508
Ulsicral (ID) *see* Sucralfate 1940
Ulsikur (ID) *see* Cimetidine 438
Ultibro Breezhaler (AU, CZ, DE, DK, EE, ES, GB, HR, IE, LT, NL, NO, SE, SG, SI, SK) *see* Indacaterol and Glycopyrronium [CAN/INT] 1063
Ultibro (JP) *see* Indacaterol and Glycopyrronium [CAN/INT] 1063
Ulticer (HK) *see* Ranitidine 1777
Ultipus (HK) *see* Cimetidine 438
Ultiva (AE, AR, AT, AU, BB, BE, BH, BM, BR, BS, BZ, CH, CL, CO, CR, CY, CZ, DE, DK, DO, EC, EG, ES, FI, FR,

GB, GR, GT, GY, HK, HN, IE, IL, IQ, IR, IT, JM, JO, JP, KR, KW, LB, LT, LY, MX, MY, NI, NL, NO, NZ, OM, PA, PE, PL, PT, QA, RO, SA, SE, SG, SI, SK, SR, SV, SY, TR, TT, VE, YE) *see* Remifentanil 1789
Ultop (HR) *see* Omeprazole 1508
Ultra Carbon (AE, CY, EG, QA) *see* Charcoal, Activated 416
Ultracarbon (MY, SG, TR) *see* Charcoal, Activated 416
Ultracare (IL) *see* Benzocaine 246
Ultracef (IE) *see* Cefadroxil 372
Ultracef (UY) *see* Cefotaxime 382
Ultracet (BR, CN, HK, ID, KR, MY, SG, TH, TW, VE) *see* Acetaminophen and Tramadol 37
Ultracillin (AE) *see* Ampicillin 141
Ultracloxam (LB) *see* Ampicillin and Cloxacillin [INT] 144
Ultracortenol (AE, AR, PY, SE, TW, VN) *see* PrednisoLONE (Ophthalmic) 1706
Ultracortenol (AR, NO, PY, SE) *see* PrednisoLONE (Systemic) 1703
Ultra-K (BE) *see* Potassium Gluconate 1690
Ultramac Semi (KR) *see* Acetaminophen and Tramadol 37
Ultra-Mag (AT) *see* Magnesium Gluconate 1263
Ultra-Mg (BE) *see* Magnesium Gluconate 1263
Ultra Mg (LU) *see* Magnesium Gluconate 1263
Ultramox (AE) *see* Amoxicillin 130
Ultramox (PH) *see* Ampicillin and Sulbactam 145
Ultran (PH) *see* Ranitidine 1777
Ultraxime (PH) *see* Cefixime 380
Ultreon (DE) *see* Azithromycin (Systemic) 216
Ulxit (AT) *see* Nizatidine 1471
Ulzec (ZA) *see* Omeprazole 1508
Ulzol (ID) *see* Omeprazole 1508
Umaren (HU) *see* Ranitidine 1777
Umbral (EC) *see* Acetaminophen 32
U-Mirtaron (TW) *see* Mirtazapine 1376
U-Miso (TW) *see* Misoprostol 1379
Umprel (AT) *see* Bromocriptine 291
Umuline NPH (FR) *see* Insulin NPH 1089
Umuline Profil 30 (FR) *see* Insulin NPH and Insulin Regular 1090
Umuline Protamine Isophane (FR) *see* Insulin NPH 1089
Umuline Rapide (FR) *see* Insulin Regular 1091
Unacid (DE) *see* Ampicillin and Sulbactam 145
Unacim (FR) *see* Ampicillin and Sulbactam 145
Unacor (RO) *see* Milrinone 1370
Unacron (KR) *see* Pancuronium 1567
Unakalm (ES, NL, PT) *see* Ketazolam [INT] 1144
Un Alfa (FR) *see* Alfacalcidol [CAN/INT] 82
Unaserus (JP) *see* Nalidixic Acid [INT] 1418
Unasyn (AE, AT, BF, BG, BH, BJ, BR, CI, CL, CN, CO, CR, CY, CZ, EC, EE, EG, GN, GT, HK, HN, HU, ID, IL, IQ, IR, IT, JO, KR, KW, LB, LT, LY, MA, ML, MR, MY, NE, NI, OM, PA, PE, PH, PK, PL, QA, RO, SA, SD, SG, SI, SK, SN, SV, SY, TH, TN, UY, VN, YE, ZA) *see* Ampicillin and Sulbactam 145
Unat (AT, DE, HK, PT, TH) *see* Torsemide 2071
Unava (PY) *see* Gliclazide [CAN/INT] 964
Unazid (HR) *see* Hydrochlorothiazide 1009
Undiarrhea (TW) *see* Loperamide 1236
Unex (EC) *see* Ciprofloxacin (Systemic) 441
Unguentum Neomycini (PL) *see* Neomycin 1436
Unguentum Zinci Oxydati (PL) *see* Zinc Oxide 2200
Unibenestan (ES) *see* Alfuzosin 84
Unibron (MX) *see* Albuterol 69
Unicam (AE, BH, CY, EG, IQ, IR, JO, KW, LB, LY, OM, QA, SA, SY, YE) *see* Piroxicam 1662
Unicast (JO) *see* Montelukast 1392
Unicil 1 Mega (CO) *see* Penicillin G (Parenteral/Aqueous) 1611
Unicil (CO) *see* Penicillin G Benzathine 1609
Uniclar (CO) *see* Mometasone (Nasal) 1391
Uniclor (PE) *see* Chloramphenicol 421
Uniclox (CO) *see* Dicloxacillin 621
Unicontin-400 Continus (IN) *see* Theophylline 2026
Unicontin (PT) *see* Theophylline 2026
Unicort (CO) *see* Hydrocortisone (Topical) 1014
Unicycline (AE) *see* Demeclocycline 589
Uniderm (CO, MX) *see* Fusidic Acid (Topical) [CAN/INT] 943
Uniderm (HK, KR, TH) *see* Clobetasol 468
Unidipin (HU, LU) *see* NIFEdipine 1451
Unidox (BH, CY, EG, IQ, IR, JO, KW, LB, LY, OM, PL, QA, RO, SA, SY, YE) *see* Doxycycline 689
Unidoxy (KR) *see* Doxycycline 689
Unidrox (AT, CZ, HK, HU, IT) *see* Prulifloxacin [INT] 1742
Unidur (AE) *see* Theophylline 2026
Uni-Dur (HR) *see* Theophylline 2026
Unifed (AE, BH, CY, EG, IQ, IR, JO, KW, LB, LY, OM, QA, SA, SY, YE) *see* Triprolidine and Pseudoephedrine 2105
Unifedrine (BR) *see* EPHEDrine (Systemic) 734
Uni-Feno (HK) *see* PHENobarbital 1632
Uniflex (MY) *see* Betamethasone (Topical) 255
Uniflox (FR) *see* Ciprofloxacin (Systemic) 441
Uniflox (HR) *see* Ofloxacin (Ophthalmic) 1491
Unifyl Retard (CH) *see* Theophylline 2026
Unigastrozol (MX) *see* Pantoprazole 1570
Uniglit (JO) *see* Pioglitazone 1654
Unigo (HK, TH) *see* MetroNIDAZOLE (Systemic) 1353
Unihep (AE, QA) *see* Heparin 997
Uniket (ES) *see* Isosorbide Mononitrate 1126
Unilactone (AE, BH, CY, EG, IQ, IR, JO, KW, LB, LY, OM, QA, SA, SY, YE) *see* Spironolactone 1931
Unilat (HR, RO) *see* Latanoprost 1172
Unimetone (KR) *see* Nabumetone 1411
Uninaltrex (BR) *see* Naltrexone 1422
Uninechol (KR) *see* Bethanechol 257
Uninex (HR) *see* Fosfomycin 932
Uni-Pholco (HK) *see* Pholcodine [INT] 1646
Uniphyllin Continus (AE, BF, BH, BJ, CI, CY, EG, ET, GB, GH, GM, GN, KE, LR, MA, ML, MR, MU, MW, NE, NG, SC, SD, SL, SN, TN, TZ, UG, ZA, ZM, ZW) *see* Theophylline 2026
Uniphylline (JO) *see* Theophylline 2026
Uniphyllin (TW) *see* Theophylline 2026
Unipiren (VN) *see* Cefpirome [INT] 388
Unipres (CZ, HR, HU, PL) *see* Nitrendipine [INT] 1463
Unipril (CO) *see* Enalapril 722
Unipril (IT) *see* Ramipril 1771
Uniquin (AT) *see* Lomefloxacin [INT] 1233
Unireda (VN) *see* Rebamipide [INT] 1786
Uniretic (PH) *see* Moexipril and Hydrochlorothiazide 1388
Unisom Sleepgels (AU, NZ) *see* DiphenhydrAMINE (Systemic) 641
Unitax (TW) *see* Cefotaxime 382
Unitf (KR) *see* Trifluridine 2103
Unitrac (SG) *see* Itraconazole 1130
Unitral (PH) *see* TraMADol 2074
Uni-Tranxene (LU) *see* Clorazepate 487
Unitrexates (VN) *see* Methotrexate 1322
Unitten (VN) *see* Ketotifen (Ophthalmic) 1150
Unival (MX) *see* Sucralfate 1940
Univasc (ID, KR, PH, TR) *see* Moexipril 1388
Univasc Plus (KR) *see* Moexipril and Hydrochlorothiazide 1388
Univate (MY) *see* Clobetasol 468
Univitan K1 (HK) *see* Phytonadione 1647
UniWarfin (IN) *see* Warfarin 2186
Unizuric 300 (MX) *see* Allopurinol 90
Unocef (MY) *see* CefTRIAXone 396
Unoximed (PH) *see* Cefuroxime 399
Unwanted (IN) *see* Mifepristone 1366
Upfen (FR) *see* Ibuprofen 1032

Upha C (MY) *see* Ascorbic Acid ... 178
Uphageron (MY) *see* Cinnarizine [INT] ... 440
Uphalexin (MY, SG) *see* Cephalexin ... 405
Uphamol Plus Codeine (MY) *see* Acetaminophen and Codeine ... 36
Upixon (ID) *see* Pyrantel Pamoate ... 1744
Uplyso (FR) *see* Taliglucerase Alfa ... 1971
Upostelle (GB) *see* Levonorgestrel ... 1201
Uprofen (TW) *see* Ibuprofen ... 1032
Upsa-C (AE, BE, BH, CY, EG, IL, IQ, IR, JO, KW, LB, LY, OM, QA, SA, SY, YE) *see* Ascorbic Acid ... 178
Uracare (TW) *see* Trospium ... 2108
Uracil (TH) *see* Propylthiouracil ... 1735
Uracin (KR) *see* Crotamiton ... 514
Uractone (LU) *see* Spironolactone ... 1931
Uractonum (SG, TR) *see* Spironolactone ... 1931
Uramin (TW) *see* DOPamine ... 669
Uramol (CL, PE) *see* Urea ... 2114
Uramox (IL) *see* AcetaZOLAMIDE ... 39
Urantoin (EC) *see* Nitrofurantoin ... 1463
Uraplex (ES, GR, IT) *see* Trospium ... 2108
Urbadan (CO, EC, PE) *see* CloBAZam ... 465
Urbal (ES) *see* Sucralfate ... 1940
Urbanil (BR) *see* CloBAZam ... 465
Urbanol (ZA) *see* CloBAZam ... 465
Urbanyl (CH, FR) *see* CloBAZam ... 465
Urbason (AT, CZ, DE, ES, HR, NL) *see* MethylPREDNISolone ... 1340
Urbason Retard (BE, IT) *see* MethylPREDNISolone ... 1340
Urdafalk (ID) *see* Ursodiol ... 2116
Ureadin (ES) *see* Urea ... 2114
Urealeti (EC) *see* Urea ... 2114
Ureativ (BR) *see* Urea ... 2114
Urecare (HK, SG) *see* Urea ... 2114
Urecholine (FI) *see* Bethanechol ... 257
Urederm (AU) *see* Urea ... 2114
Uregyt (CZ, DE, HN, HU, RU) *see* Ethacrynic Acid ... 797
Urelac (CO) *see* Urea ... 2114
Urem (DE) *see* Ibuprofen ... 1032
Uremide (AU, NZ) *see* Furosemide ... 940
Uremin (KR) *see* Desmopressin ... 594
Uremol (AR) *see* Urea ... 2114
Urenide (TW) *see* Bumetanide ... 297
Ureotop (DE) *see* Urea ... 2114
Urepyrin (TW) *see* Phenazopyridine ... 1629
Uresix (ID) *see* Furosemide ... 940
Uretin (KR) *see* Azosemide [INT] ... 220
Uretol SR (KR) *see* Tolterodine ... 2063
Urex-M (AU) *see* Furosemide ... 940
Urex (AU, HK, JP) *see* Furosemide ... 940
Urex (EC) *see* FlavoxATE ... 881
Urex Forte (HK) *see* Furosemide ... 940
Urginol (AR) *see* Tolterodine ... 2063
Uribac (MX) *see* Pipemidic Acid [INT] ... 1655
Uriben (GB) *see* Nalidixic Acid [INT] ... 1418
Uribeta (CR, DO, GT, HN, PA, SV) *see* Interferon Beta-1b ... 1103
Uricad (TH) *see* Allopurinol ... 90
Uric (JP) *see* Allopurinol ... 90
Uriconorm (CH) *see* Allopurinol ... 90
Uricrim (VE) *see* Urea ... 2114
Uridin (TW) *see* Tolterodine ... 2063
Uridon (PY) *see* Norfloxacin ... 1475
Uridoz (FR) *see* Fosfomycin ... 932
Uriduct (DE) *see* Doxazosin ... 674
Uridyne (PK) *see* Tolterodine ... 2063
Urief (CN, JP, TH, TW) *see* Silodosin ... 1885
Uriflow (PH) *see* Bethanechol ... 257
Urigen (CO) *see* Norfloxacin ... 1475
Urihexal (ZA) *see* Oxybutynin ... 1536
Uriken (MX) *see* Pipemidic Acid [INT] ... 1655
Urilzid (PH) *see* Hydrochlorothiazide ... 1009
Urimax-D (IN) *see* Dutasteride and Tamsulosin ... 702
Urimax (IN) *see* Tamsulosin ... 1974
Urimeg (PY) *see* Furosemide ... 940
Urimor (AU) *see* Methyclothiazide ... 1331
Urinal (BH, JO) *see* Furosemide ... 940
Urineg (ID) *see* Nalidixic Acid [INT] ... 1418
Urinex (FI) *see* Chlorothiazide ... 426
Urinol (MY) *see* Allopurinol ... 90
Urinorm (PH) *see* Febuxostat ... 848
Urion (FR) *see* Alfuzosin ... 84
Uripax (MY, PE) *see* FlavoxATE ... 881
Uripiser (MX) *see* Pipemidic Acid [INT] ... 1655
Urisan (ES) *see* Pipemidic Acid [INT] ... 1655
Urisept (EG, QA) *see* Phenazopyridine ... 1629
Urispadol (DK) *see* FlavoxATE ... 881
Urispas (200 mg) (NL) *see* FlavoxATE ... 881
Urispas (AE, AT, BE, BF, BG, BH, BJ, CH, CI, CY, EG, ET, FR, GB, GH, GM, GN, HK, IE, IL, IN, IQ, IR, JO, KE, KW, LB, LR, LT, LY, MA, ML, MR, MU, MW, MY, NE, NG, OM, PT, PY, QA, RU, SA, SC, SD, SG, SL, SN, SY, TH, TN, TR, TZ, UG, YE, ZA, ZM, ZW) *see* FlavoxATE ... 881
Uritin-D (IN) *see* Dutasteride and Tamsulosin ... 702
U-Ritis (TW) *see* Naproxen ... 1427
Urivesc (TH) *see* Trospium ... 2108
Urivox (PK) *see* FlavoxATE ... 881
Urixin (MY) *see* Pipemidic Acid [INT] ... 1655
Urnal (TW) *see* Tamsulosin ... 1974
Uro-Beniktol N (CH) *see* Neomycin ... 1436
Urocal (PY) *see* Phenazopyridine ... 1629
Urocarb (AU) *see* Bethanechol ... 257
Uro Cefasabal (PE) *see* Pipemidic Acid [INT] ... 1655
Urocitra-C Pwd (KR) *see* Potassium Citrate and Citric Acid ... 1689
Uroclar (PH) *see* Rufloxacin [INT] ... 1855
Uroctal (AE, BH, CY, EG, IQ, IR, JO, KW, LB, LY, OM, QA, SA, SY, YE) *see* Norfloxacin ... 1475
Urocuad (CO) *see* Allopurinol ... 90
Uroden (IT) *see* Pipemidic Acid [INT] ... 1655
Urodolox (AR) *see* Aceclofenac [INT] ... 30
Uroflax (PY) *see* Oxybutynin ... 1536
Uroflow (CZ, EE) *see* Tolterodine ... 2063
Uroflox (MX, TH) *see* Rufloxacin [INT] ... 1855
Uroflox (IN, PT) *see* Norfloxacin ... 1475
Urofuran (FI) *see* Nitrofurantoin ... 1463
Urogen (TW) *see* Phenazopyridine ... 1629
Urogesic (SG) *see* Phenazopyridine ... 1629
Urogetix (ID) *see* Phenazopyridine ... 1629
Urogquad (AR) *see* Allopurinol ... 90
Urogram (HR) *see* Nalidixic Acid [INT] ... 1418
Uroin (KR) *see* Nitrofurantoin ... 1463
Urokit Doxo-cell (DE) *see* DOXOrubicin (Conventional) ... 679
Uromedin (PY) *see* Finasteride ... 878
Uromitexan (AE, AT, AU, BE, BG, BH, CH, CL, CN, CZ, DE, DK, EE, EG, ES, FI, FR, GB, GR, HK, HN, HR, HU, ID, IE, IN, IS, IT, JO, KR, LB, LT, LU, MT, NL, NO, NZ, PK, PL, PT, QA, RO, RU, SA, SE, SG, SI, SK, TH, TR, TW, UY, VN) *see* Mesna ... 1305
Uro-Nebacetin N (DE) *see* Neomycin ... 1436
Uronid (ES) *see* FlavoxATE ... 881
Uronor (UY) *see* Norfloxacin ... 1475
Uronovag (MX) *see* Pipemidic Acid [INT] ... 1655
U-Ron (TW) *see* CefTRIAXone ... 396
Uropan (TR) *see* Oxybutynin ... 1536
Uropimide (CL, IT, PY) *see* Pipemidic Acid [INT] ... 1655
Uropipedil (ES) *see* Pipemidic Acid [INT] ... 1655
Uropipemid (MX) *see* Pipemidic Acid [INT] ... 1655
Uroprin (TW) *see* Phenazopyridine ... 1629
Uroprot (MX, TH) *see* Mesna ... 1305
Uropyrine (BE) *see* Phenazopyridine ... 1629
Uropyrine (LU) *see* FlavoxATE ... 881
Uropyrin (TW) *see* Phenazopyridine ... 1629

Uro-Q (KR) *see* Tolterodine 2063
Uroquad (AE, BB, BF, BJ, BM, BS, CI, ET, GH, GM, GN, GY, JM, KE, LR, MA, ML, MR, MU, MW, NE, NG, SC, SD, SL, SN, SR, TN, TT, TZ, UG, ZM, ZW) *see* Allopurinol 90
Urorec (EE, FR, GR, HR, IE, LT, NL, PL, PT, RO, RU, SE, SI, SK, TR) *see* Silodosin 1885
Urosan (IT) *see* Pipemidic Acid [INT] 1655
Urosan (JP) *see* Ursodiol 2116
Uroseptal (EC) *see* Norfloxacin 1475
Urosetic (IT) *see* Pipemidic Acid [INT] 1655
Urosin (AT, DE, EC, LU) *see* Allopurinol 90
Urosin (MY, TW) *see* Atenolol 189
Urositol (KR) *see* Tolterodine 2063
Urostop (KR) *see* Propiverine [INT] 1728
Uro-Tablinen (DE) *see* Nitrofurantoin 1463
Urotams SR (KR) *see* Tamsulosin 1974
Uro Tarivid (AE, BH, CY, EG, IQ, IR, JO, KW, LB, LY, OM, QA, SA, SY, YE) *see* Ofloxacin (Systemic) 1490
Urotin S SR (KR) *see* Tolterodine 2063
Urotoina (PY) *see* Nitrofurantoin 1463
Urotone (IN) *see* Bethanechol 257
Urotractan (DE) *see* Methenamine 1317
Urotractin (HK, ID, IT, MY, SG, TH) *see* Pipemidic Acid [INT] 1655
Urotrim (HR) *see* Trimethoprim 2104
Urotrol (TW) *see* Propiverine [INT] 1728
Uroverine (KR) *see* Propiverine [INT] 1728
Uroxacin (AR) *see* Norfloxacin 1475
Uroxacin (CO) *see* Phenazopyridine 1629
Uroxal (HU) *see* Oxybutynin 1536
Uroxal (ID) *see* FlavoxATE 881
Uroxate (TH, TW) *see* FlavoxATE 881
Uroxatral (CL) *see* Alfuzosin 84
Uroxatral OD (AR, PY, UY) *see* Alfuzosin 84
Uroxatral uno (CH, DE) *see* Alfuzosin 84
Uroxina (BR) *see* Pipemidic Acid [INT] 1655
Uroxin (AE, BH, KW, LB, SA) *see* Norfloxacin 1475
Uroxin (HK, SG) *see* Ciprofloxacin (Systemic) 441
Ursacol (BR, CO, IT) *see* Ursodiol 2116
Ursa-Fenol (GR) *see* Chloramphenicol 421
Ursa (JO, PH) *see* Ursodiol 2116
URSA (TH) *see* Ursodiol 2116
Ursilon (VN) *see* Ursodiol 2116
Ursnon (JP) *see* Fluorometholone 896
Ursobilane (ES) *see* Ursodiol 2116
Ursochol (BE, CH, ES, ID, IS, LU, NL) *see* Ursodiol 2116
Ursodamor (IT) *see* Ursodiol 2116
Ursofalk (AR, AT, AU, BG, CL, CN, CO, CR, CY, CZ, DE, EC, EE, EG, GR, GT, HK, HN, HR, HU, IE, IL, KR, KW, LB, LU, MX, MY, NI, NZ, PA, PE, PH, PK, PT, RO, SA, SE, SI, SK, SV, TH, TR, UY) *see* Ursodiol 2116
Ursogal (GB) *see* Ursodiol 2116
Urso (IN) *see* Ursodiol 2116
Ursolic (TW) *see* Ursodiol 2116
Ursolin (TH) *see* Ursodiol 2116
Ursolite (ES) *see* Ursodiol 2116
Ursolit (IL) *see* Ursodiol 2116
Ursoliv (PH) *see* Ursodiol 2116
Ursolvan (FR) *see* Ursodiol 2116
Ursopol (PL) *see* Ursodiol 2116
Ursosan (JP, RU) *see* Ursodiol 2116
Urso Vinas (ES) *see* Ursodiol 2116
Urticef (ID) *see* Cefixime 380
Urutal (HR) *see* Betahistine [CAN/INT] 252
Usanimals (MX) *see* Magnesium Citrate 1262
Usenta (AR, CL, PE) *see* Bosentan 280
Usix (VN) *see* Furosemide 940
Utamine (TW) *see* DOBUTamine 654
Utapine (TW) *see* QUEtiapine 1751
Utergin (ID) *see* Methylergonovine 1333
Uterine (PH) *see* Methylergonovine 1333
Uteronovin (PY) *see* Ergonovine [CAN/INT] 754
Utinor (PH) *see* Norfloxacin 1475
UT-in (ZA) *see* Norfloxacin 1475
Utisept (TH) *see* Trimethoprim 2104
Utmos (TH) *see* Pioglitazone 1654
Utoin (TH) *see* Phenytoin 1640
Utoral (PH) *see* Fluorouracil (Systemic) 896
Utovlan (GB) *see* Norethindrone 1473
Utrogestan (AT, BE, BG, BR, CH, CZ, EC, ES, FR, GB, HR, HU, ID, JO, KR, LB, LU, MX, MY, PH, PT, RO, SG, SK, TR, UY, VN) *see* Progesterone 1722
Uvadex (CZ, FR) *see* Methoxsalen (Topical) 1331
Uvamin (IL) *see* Nitrofurantoin 1463
Uvamin Retard (CH, GT, HN, LB, NI, PA, SV, TT) *see* Nitrofurantoin 1463
Uvesterol D (FR) *see* Ergocalciferol 753
Uxen (AR) *see* Amitriptyline 119
U-Zet (TW) *see* FLUoxetine 899
Uzolam (TW) *see* Midazolam 1361
Uzolin (TW) *see* CeFAZolin 373
Uzol (TW) *see* Fluconazole 885
Vaben (IL) *see* Oxazepam 1532
Vabon (TH) *see* Danazol 558
Vaccin Varilrix (FR) *see* Varicella Virus Vaccine 2141
Vaciclor (SG) *see* ValACYclovir 2119
Vacillin (TH) *see* Ampicillin 141
Vaclo (ID) *see* Clopidogrel 484
Vaclovir (AU) *see* ValACYclovir 2119
Vacontil (AE, BF, BH, BJ, CI, CY, EG, ET, GH, GM, GN, IQ, JO, KE, KW, LB, LR, MA, ML, MR, MU, MW, MY, NE, NG, OM, QA, SC, SD, SL, SN, TN, TZ, UG, VN, ZM, ZW) *see* Loperamide 1236
Vacopan (MY, TH) *see* Scopolamine (Systemic) 1870
Vacrax (MY) *see* Acyclovir (Systemic) 47
Vacyless (TW) *see* ValACYclovir 2119
Vadiral (CO) *see* ValACYclovir 2119
Vagicillin (DE) *see* Neomycin 1436
Vagifem (AT, AU, BE, BG, CH, CL, CN, CZ, DE, DK, EE, FI, GB, GR, HK, HN, IE, IL, IT, KR, NL, NO, NZ, PH, PL, PT, SE, SG, TR, UY) *see* Estradiol (Topical) 780
Vagimen (CR, DO, GT, HN, NI, PA, SV) *see* Clotrimazole (Topical) 488
Vagistin (ID) *see* Metronidazole and Nystatin [CAN/INT] 1358
Vagizol (PH) *see* Clotrimazole (Topical) 488
Vagomine (BE, LU) *see* DimenhyDRINATE 637
Vagostin (TW) *see* Neostigmine 1438
Vagran (VE) *see* Vancomycin 2130
Vaksan (AR) *see* Ambroxol [INT] 109
Vaksin Jerap Bio-Td (ID) *see* Diphtheria and Tetanus Toxoid 645
Valatan (TH) *see* Valsartan 2127
Valaxam (EC) *see* Amlodipine and Valsartan 126
Valaxona (DK) *see* Diazepam 613
Valazyd-H (PH) *see* Valsartan and Hydrochlorothiazide 2129
Valazyd (PH) *see* Valsartan 2127
Valbazen Vet (NO) *see* Albendazole 65
Valcivir (IN) *see* ValACYclovir 2119
Valcote (CO, EC) *see* Valproic Acid and Derivatives 2123
Valcyclor (CO) *see* ValACYclovir 2119
Valcyte (AE, AT, AU, BE, BG, BH, BR, CH, CN, CY, CZ, DE, DK, EE, ES, FI, GB, GR, HK, HN, HR, ID, IE, IL, IS, IT, KR, KW, LB, LT, MX, MY, NL, NO, NZ, PH, PL, QA, RO, SA, SE, SG, SI, SK, TH, TR, TW, VN) *see* ValGANciclovir 2121
Valdefer (MX) *see* Ferrous Sulfate 871
Valdimex (ID) *see* Diazepam 613
Valdocef (SK) *see* Cefadroxil 372
Valdres (ID) *see* DiphenhydrAMINE (Systemic) 641
Valdure IM (BZ, CR, DO, GT, HN, NI, PA, SV) *see* Parecoxib [INT] 1576

Valdyne (CR, DO, GT, HN, NI, PA, SV) *see* Celecoxib 402
Valeans (IT) *see* ALPRAZolam 94
Valemia (ID) *see* Simvastatin 1890
Valenor 2 (ID) *see* Levonorgestrel 1201
Valent-H (IN) *see* Valsartan and Hydrochlorothiazide 2129
Valeptol SR (KP) *see* Valproic Acid and Derivatives 2123
Valeric (CN) *see* Allopurinol 90
Valetta (PK) *see* Risedronate 1816
Valette (AT, AU, DE) *see* Estradiol and Dienogest 780
Valifol (MX) *see* Isoniazid 1120
Valiquid (DE) *see* Diazepam 613
Valisanbe (ID) *see* Diazepam 613
Valium (AE, AR, AT, AU, BE, BF, BG, BH, BJ, BR, CH, CI, CY, DE, DK, EC, EE, EG, ES, ET, FR, GH, GM, GN, GR, HR, ID, IE, IN, IQ, IR, IT, JO, KE, KR, KW, LB, LR, LU, LY, MA, ML, MR, MT, MU, MW, MX, MY, NE, NG, NO, OM, PE, PH, PK, PL, PT, PY, QA, SA, SC, SD, SK, SL, SN, SY, TN, TR, TZ, UG, UY, VN, YE, ZM, ZW) *see* Diazepam 613
Valiuzam (AE, BH, CY, EG, IQ, IR, JO, KW, LB, LY, OM, QA, SA, SY, YE) *see* Diazepam 613
Valixa (AR, CL, CO, EC, PE, PY, UY, VE) *see* ValGANciclovir 2121
Vallixa (JP) *see* ValGANciclovir 2121
Valnoc (PE) *see* Eszopiclone 793
Valontan (ES, IT) *see* DimenhyDRINATE 637
Valopride (IT) *see* Bromopride [INT] 292
Valora (HR) *see* Alendronate 79
Valoran (EE) *see* Cefotaxime 382
Valosartan (KR) *see* Valsartan 2127
Valosine SR (TH) *see* Venlafaxine 2150
Valosine (TW) *see* Venlafaxine 2150
Valpakine (BR, EC) *see* Valproic Acid and Derivatives 2123
Valpam (AE, AU, BH, CY, EG, HK, IQ, IR, JO, KW, LB, LY, OM, QA, SA, SY, YE) *see* Diazepam 613
Valparin (TH) *see* Valproic Acid and Derivatives 2123
Valpax (PY) *see* ClonazePAM 478
Valporal (IL) *see* Valproic Acid and Derivatives 2123
Valprax (PE) *see* Valproic Acid and Derivatives 2123
Valpro (AU, HK) *see* Valproic Acid and Derivatives 2123
Valpron (VE) *see* Valproic Acid and Derivatives 2123
Valraci (KR) *see* ValACYclovir 2119
Valsaone (KR) *see* Valsartan 2127
Valsaprex-H (CO) *see* Valsartan and Hydrochlorothiazide 2129
Valsarect (KR) *see* Valsartan 2127
Valstar (CA, IL) *see* Valrubicin 2127
Valsup (CO) *see* Valproic Acid and Derivatives 2123
Valtan H (PE) *see* Valsartan and Hydrochlorothiazide 2129
Valtan Plus (KR) *see* Valsartan and Hydrochlorothiazide 2129
Valtaxin (CA) *see* Valrubicin 2127
Valtcro (KR) *see* ValACYclovir 2119
Valtec-CR (IN) *see* Valproic Acid and Derivatives 2123
Valtens H (GT) *see* Valsartan and Hydrochlorothiazide 2129
Valtensin (BG, HK) *see* Valsartan 2127
Valtensin HCT (HK) *see* Valsartan and Hydrochlorothiazide 2129
Valtra (KR) *see* ValACYclovir 2119
Valtrex (AE, AR, AT, AU, BB, BD, BG, BH, BM, BR, BS, BZ, CH, CL, CN, CO, CR, CY, CZ, DE, DO, EC, EE, EG, ES, FI, GB, GR, GT, GY, HK, HN, ID, IE, IL, IQ, IR, IS, JM, JO, JP, KR, KW, LB, LT, LY, MY, NI, NO, NZ, OM, PA, PH, PK, PL, PR, PT, PY, QA, RO, RU, SA, SE, SG, SI, SK, SR, SV, SY, TH, TR, TT, TW, VE, YE) *see* ValACYclovir 2119
Valtropin (AT, BE, BG, CH, CZ, DE, DK, EE, ES, FI, FR, GB, GR, IE, IT, MT, NL, NO, PL, PT, RU, SE, SK, TR) *see* Somatropin 1918
Valved (ID) *see* Triprolidine and Pseudoephedrine 2105
Valvex (PH) *see* Valsartan 2127
Valvir (AU, ID) *see* ValACYclovir 2119
Valzepam (PH) *see* Diazepam 613
Vamcee (PH) *see* Ascorbic Acid 178
Vamcloxil (PH) *see* Cloxacillin [CAN/INT] 488
Va-Mengoc-BC (AR) *see* Meningococcal (Groups A / C / Y and W-135) Diphtheria Conjugate Vaccine 1289
Vanafen (HK) *see* Chloramphenicol 421
Vanafen Otologic (TH) *see* Chloramphenicol 421
Vanafen S (TH) *see* Chloramphenicol 421
Vanbiotic (CO) *see* Vancomycin 2130
Vancel (BR, PY) *see* CARBOplatin 357
Vancep (ID) *see* Vancomycin 2130
Vancin-S (TH) *see* Vancomycin 2130
Vancocina CP (CL) *see* Vancomycin 2130
Vancocin (AE, AT, AU, EG, JO, RU, SA, SI, VN) *see* Vancomycin 2130
Vancocina (IT) *see* Vancomycin 2130
Vancocin CP (AU, CN, CZ, IN, MX, MY, PK, PL, TW) *see* Vancomycin 2130
Vancocin HCl (AR, BE, BF, BJ, CH, CI, DK, ET, FI, GB, GH, GM, GN, HK, KE, LR, MA, ML, MR, MU, MW, NE, NG, NZ, PH, SC, SD, SE, SL, SN, TN, TW, TZ, UG, ZA, ZM, ZW) *see* Vancomycin 2130
Vanco (DE) *see* Vancomycin 2130
Vancoled (AE, EG, KR, KW, MY, VN) *see* Vancomycin 2130
Vancolon (AE, BH, KW, LB, QA, SA) *see* Vancomycin 2130
Vancomax (PY) *see* Vancomycin 2130
Vancomet (PH) *see* Vancomycin 2130
Vancomicina (CR, DO, GT, HN, NI, PA, SV) *see* Vancomycin 2130
Vanconin (TW) *see* Diazepam 613
Vancor (AE) *see* Pefloxacin [INT] 1588
Vancorin (TR) *see* Vancomycin 2130
Vancosan (LT) *see* Vancomycin 2130
Vanco-Teva (IL) *see* Vancomycin 2130
Vancotex (MY) *see* Vancomycin 2130
Vancotil (SG) *see* Loperamide 1236
Vancotrat (BR) *see* Vancomycin 2130
Vancozin (KR) *see* Vancomycin 2130
Vandral (ES) *see* Venlafaxine 2150
Vanesten (TH) *see* Clotrimazole (Topical) 488
Vanid (HK, TH) *see* Flunarizine [CAN/INT] 892
Vaniqa (AU, BE, CZ, DE, ES, FR, GB, HR, IE, IL, IS, IT, LB, LT, NL, NZ, PT, RO, SK) *see* Eflornithine 710
Vanish (CL, PY) *see* Desogestrel [INT] 597
Vanlyo (TW) *see* Vancomycin 2130
Vannair (BR, CL, HK, NZ, PE) *see* Budesonide and Formoterol 297
Vanoran (PY) *see* Rosiglitazone and Metformin 1847
Vanoxide-HC (CA) *see* Benzoyl Peroxide and Hydrocortisone 248
Vanox (PY) *see* Candesartan 335
Vansilar (TH) *see* Sulfadoxine and Pyrimethamine [INT] 1946
Vantal (CR, DO, GT, HN, NI, PA, SV) *see* Benzydamine [CAN/INT] 249
Vantas (AR, BG, CH, CZ, DE, DK, EE, FI, FR, IE, LT, MY, NO, PL, RO, SE, SG, SI, TH) *see* Histrelin 1005
Vantasse (BE, NL) *see* Histrelin 1005
Vanter (LT) *see* Sucralfate 1940
Vantocil (ID) *see* Vancomycin 2130
Vantoxyl (MX) *see* Pentoxifylline 1618
Vantril (PY) *see* Ibuprofen 1032
Vantydin (TW) *see* Fexofenadine and Pseudoephedrine 874

Vaqta (AE, AU, BH, CN, DE, GB, IE, MX, NZ, QA, SA, SG, TH, TW) *see* Hepatitis A Vaccine 1001
Varcor (CO) *see* Valsartan 2127
Varedet (UY) *see* Vancomycin 2130
Varfarin (HR) *see* Warfarin 2186
Varfine (PT) *see* Warfarin 2186
Vargatef (CZ, DE, EE, HR, IE, LT, NL, SE) *see* Nintedanib 1458
Varicela Biken (EC) *see* Varicella Virus Vaccine 2141
Varilrix (AE, AR, AU, BB, BE, BH, BM, BS, BZ, CH, CL, CN, CO, CR, CY, CZ, DK, DO, EE, EG, ES, FI, GB, GT, GY, HK, HN, HU, IL, IN, IS, JM, KR, KW, LB, LT, MX, MY, NI, NL, NO, PA, PE, PH, PY, QA, RO, SA, SE, SI, SR, SV, TT, TW, UY, VN) *see* Varicella Virus Vaccine 2141
Varimer (PE, PY) *see* Mercaptopurine 1296
Varipox (IN) *see* Varicella Virus Vaccine 2141
Variquel (BE, DK, GB, SE) *see* Terlipressin [INT] 2010
Varitect (HK, TH, TW) *see* Varicella-Zoster Immune Globulin (Human) 2142
Varivax (DE, ES, FR, GB, HK, IE, LT, PH, SI, SK, TH, TR) *see* Varicella Virus Vaccine 2141
Varnoline (FR) *see* Ethinyl Estradiol and Desogestrel 799
Vartalan AM (CL) *see* Amlodipine and Valsartan 126
Vartelon (HK) *see* Diclofenac (Systemic) 617
Varteral (CO) *see* Amlodipine and Valsartan 126
Vascace (BR, GB, IE, PH) *see* Cilazapril [CAN/INT] 434
Vascal (DE) *see* Isradipine 1130
Vascardin (AE, BB, BF, BH, BJ, BM, BS, BZ, CI, CY, EG, ET, GH, GM, GN, GY, ID, IQ, IR, JM, JO, KE, KW, LB, LR, LY, MA, ML, MR, MU, MW, NE, NG, OM, QA, SA, SC, SD, SL, SN, SR, SY, TN, TT, TZ, UG, YE, ZM, ZW) *see* Isosorbide Dinitrate 1124
Vascoman (IT) *see* Manidipine [INT] 1269
Vascon (ID) *see* Norepinephrine 1472
Vascon (IN) *see* EPINEPHrine (Systemic, Oral Inhalation) 735
Vascord (CH) *see* Amlodipine and Olmesartan 126
Vascord HCT (CH) *see* Olmesartan, Amlodipine, and Hydrochlorothiazide 1498
Vascor (JO, QA) *see* AmLODIPine 123
Vascor (MY, SG) *see* Simvastatin 1890
Vascor (PH) *see* Imidapril [INT] 1051
Vascotasin (BG) *see* Trimetazidine [INT] 2104
Vascoten (MY, SG) *see* Atenolol 189
Vaseretic (CO, EC) *see* Enalapril and Hydrochlorothiazide 725
Vasetic (KR) *see* Enalapril and Hydrochlorothiazide 725
Vasexten (BE, CZ, GR, NL, SA) *see* Barnidipine [INT] 227
Vasican (HN, SG) *see* Bromhexine [INT] 291
Vasilip (HK) *see* Simvastatin 1890
Vaslan (ES) *see* Isradipine 1130
Vasoactin (EC) *see* NiMODipine 1456
Vasocal EK (EC) *see* Amlodipine and Benazepril 125
Vasocardin (BG) *see* Metoprolol 1350
Vasocardol CD (AU) *see* Diltiazem 634
Vasocedine (BE) *see* Pseudoephedrine 1742
Vasoclear-V (PH) *see* Naphazoline (Ophthalmic) 1426
Vasodilren (KR) *see* Carvedilol 367
Vasodip (IL) *see* Lercanidipine [INT] 1181
Vasoflex (CL) *see* NiMODipine 1456
Vasogeron (PY) *see* Cinnarizine [INT] 440
Vasomet (JP) *see* Terazosin 2001
Vasomil (ZA) *see* Verapamil 2154
Vasomotal (DE, PY) *see* Betahistine [CAN/INT] 252
Vasonal (HK) *see* Enalapril 722
Vasonase (ES) *see* NiCARdipine 1446
Vasonit (RO) *see* Pentoxifylline 1618
Vasopentox (PE) *see* Pentoxifylline 1618
Vasopin (IN) *see* Vasopressin 2142
Vasopress (PH) *see* Enalapril 722
Vasopril (AE, JO) *see* Enalapril 722
Vasopten (IN) *see* Verapamil 2154
Vasorel (CN) *see* Trimetazidine [INT] 2104
Vasorel MR (CN) *see* Trimetazidine [INT] 2104
Vasoretic (IT) *see* Enalapril and Hydrochlorothiazide 725
Vasosan P-Granulat (DE) *see* Cholestyramine Resin 431
Vasosan (PL) *see* Cholestyramine Resin 431
Vasosan S-Granulat (DE, FR) *see* Cholestyramine Resin 431
Vasoserc Forte (LB) *see* Betahistine [CAN/INT] 252
Vasoserc (LB) *see* Betahistine [CAN/INT] 252
Vasosin (TW) *see* Vasopressin 2142
Vasosta (PH) *see* Captopril 342
Vasotal (UY) *see* Betahistine [CAN/INT] 252
Vasotenal EZ (PE) *see* Ezetimibe and Simvastatin 834
Vasotenal (PE) *see* Simvastatin 1890
Vasoten (MY) *see* Bisoprolol 266
Vasotin (ID) *see* Dipyridamole 652
Vasotop (EC) *see* AmLODIPine 123
Vasotop (IN) *see* NiMODipine 1456
Vasotrate-60 OD (PH) *see* Isosorbide Mononitrate 1126
Vasotrate (IN, PH) *see* Isosorbide Mononitrate 1126
Vasotrate-OD (SG) *see* Isosorbide Mononitrate 1126
Vasotrol (VN) *see* Isosorbide Mononitrate 1126
Vaspine ER (KR) *see* Felodipine 850
Vasran (GB) *see* Alfuzosin 84
Vassapro (PH) *see* Trimetazidine [INT] 2104
Vastarel (AE, AR, CY, DK, EG, FR, GR, IE, IT, JO, LB, NO, PK, PT, QA, SA, SG, TR, VN) *see* Trimetazidine [INT] 2104
Vastarel LM (PT) *see* Trimetazidine [INT] 2104
Vastarel LP (AR) *see* Trimetazidine [INT] 2104
Vastarel MR (AE, BH, BR, CL, CO, CY, EG, HK, KW, PE, PH, PY, QA, SA, SG, TH, UY, VE, VN) *see* Trimetazidine [INT] 2104
Vastat Flas (ES) *see* Mirtazapine 1376
Vasten (CO) *see* AmLODIPine 123
Vasten (FR) *see* Pravastatin 1700
Vastensium (ES) *see* Nitrendipine [INT] 1463
V-AS (TH) *see* Aspirin 180
Vastia (HK, KR) *see* Donepezil 668
Vastinan (KR) *see* Trimetazidine [INT] 2104
Vastinan MR (KR) *see* Trimetazidine [INT] 2104
Vastin (AU) *see* Fluvastatin 915
Vastinol (TH) *see* Trimetazidine [INT] 2104
Vastoran (AU) *see* Pravastatin 1700
Vastor (JO) *see* AtorvaSTATin 194
Vastus (AR) *see* Albendazole 65
Vatran (IT) *see* Diazepam 613
Vavo (AE, BH, KW, QA, SA) *see* Ketoconazole (Systemic) 1144
Vaxar (KR) *see* Lacidipin [INT] 1154
Vaxcel Cefobactam (MY) *see* Cefoperazone and Sulbactam [INT] 382
Vaxdil (CO) *see* Minoxidil (Systemic) 1374
Vaxigel (PE) *see* Metronidazole and Nystatin [CAN/INT] 1358
Vaxol (PH) *see* Cilostazol 437
Vaxor (JO) *see* Venlafaxine 2150
Vazidin (HR) *see* Trimetazidine [INT] 2104
Vazigam (ZA) *see* Varicella-Zoster Immune Globulin (Human) 2142
Vaztor (PH) *see* AtorvaSTATin 194
V-Bloc (ID) *see* Carvedilol 367
V-Cil-K (AE, BB, BF, BJ, BM, BS, BZ, CI, ET, GH, GM, GN, GY, JM, KE, LR, MA, ML, MR, MU, MW, NE, NG, NL, PR, SC, SD, SL, SN, SR, TN, TT, TZ, UG, ZM, ZW) *see* Penicillin V Potassium 1614
V-Cillin K (BF, BJ, CI, ET, GH, GM, GN, KE, LR, MA, ML, MR, MU, MW, NE, NG, SC, SD, SL, SN, TN, TZ, UG, ZM, ZW) *see* Penicillin V Potassium 1614
V-Dalgin (IL) *see* Dipyrone [INT] 653
Vebac (ID) *see* Aztreonam 220
Veclam (IT) *see* Clarithromycin 456

Vectarion (BR, EC, ES, FR, NO, VN) *see* Almitrine [INT] ... 92
Vectavir (AE, AT, AU, BB, BE, BH, BM, BS, BZ, CZ, DE, DK, EE, ES, FI, GR, GY, HN, IE, IS, IT, JM, NL, NO, PL, SE, SG, SK, SR, TR, TT) *see* Penciclovir ... 1608
Vectavir (LU) *see* Famciclovir ... 843
Vectibix (AR, AT, AU, BE, BR, CH, CL, CY, CZ, DE, DK, EE, FR, GB, GR, HK, HN, HR, IE, IL, IS, IT, JP, KR, LT, MX, MY, NL, NO, PL, PT, QA, RO, RU, SE, SI, SK, TR) *see* Panitumumab ... 1568
Vector (IL) *see* Valsartan ... 2127
Vector Plus (IL) *see* Valsartan and Hydrochlorothiazide ... 2129
Vectrine (FR, ID, VN) *see* Erdosteine [INT] ... 753
Vecural (PY, UY) *see* Vecuronium ... 2144
Vecure (AU) *see* Vecuronium ... 2144
Vecuron (BR, PH) *see* Vecuronium ... 2144
Vedilma (VN) *see* Carbidopa and Levodopa ... 351
Vedilol (AU, KR) *see* Carvedilol ... 367
Veedol (TH) *see* Nimesulide [INT] ... 1456
Veemycin (TH) *see* Doxycycline ... 689
Vefarol (PH) *see* Cefaclor ... 372
Vegevit B12 (PL) *see* Cyanocobalamin ... 515
Vekfazolin (GR) *see* Cefuroxime ... 399
Velacom (ID) *see* Glimepiride ... 966
Velamox (PE) *see* Amoxicillin ... 130
Velapax (RU) *see* Venlafaxine ... 2150
Velaral (EC) *see* Loperamide ... 1236
Velaxin (HK) *see* Venlafaxine ... 2150
Velbastine (HK, KR, PH, SG) *see* VinBLAStine ... 2160
Velbe (AE, AR, AT, AU, BE, BF, BH, BJ, CH, CI, CZ, DE, DK, EE, EG, ES, ET, FI, FR, GB, GH, GM, GN, GR, HN, HR, IE, IT, KE, LR, LU, MA, ML, MR, MT, MU, MW, MY, NE, NG, NL, NO, PK, PL, PT, QA, RU, SA, SC, SD, SE, SK, SL, SN, TN, TR, TZ, UG, ZA, ZM, ZW) *see* VinBLAStine ... 2160
Velcade (AE, AR, AT, AU, BB, BE, BG, BH, BM, BR, BS, BZ, CH, CL, CN, CO, CR, CY, CZ, DE, DK, DO, EC, EE, ES, FI, FR, GB, GR, GT, GY, HK, HN, HR, HU, ID, IE, IL, IN, IS, IT, JM, JO, JP, KR, KW, LB, LT, MT, MX, MY, NL, NO, NZ, PA, PE, PH, PL, PR, PT, PY, QA, RO, RU, SA, SE, SG, SI, SK, SR, TH, TR, TT, TW, VE, VN) *see* Bortezomib ... 276
Veletri (GB) *see* Epoprostenol ... 746
Vellios (ID) *see* Scopolamine (Systemic) ... 1870
Vellofent (RO) *see* FentaNYL ... 857
Velmetia (AT, CH, CZ, DE, EE, FR, HR, IT, LT, NL, PH, PL, PT, RO, SK) *see* Sitagliptin and Metformin ... 1898
Velodan (ES) *see* Loratadine ... 1241
Velonarcon (PL) *see* Ketamine ... 1143
Velorin (MY) *see* Atenolol ... 189
Velphoro (AU, CZ, DE, DK, EE, FI, GB, HR, NL, PT, SE, SG, SK) *see* Sucroferric Oxyhydroxide ... 1941
Veltam Plus (IN) *see* Dutasteride and Tamsulosin ... 702
Velutine (ID) *see* Albuterol ... 69
Vematina (MX) *see* Valproic Acid and Derivatives ... 2123
Vemetis-10 (HK) *see* Domperidone [CAN/INT] ... 666
Vemizol (MY) *see* Albendazole ... 65
Vena (JP) *see* DiphenhydrAMINE (Systemic) ... 641
Venalax (PH) *see* Albuterol ... 69
Venapas Oint (TW) *see* DiphenhydrAMINE (Systemic) ... 641
Venasmin (JP) *see* DiphenhydrAMINE (Systemic) ... 641
VENBIG (DK, TH) *see* Hepatitis B Immune Globulin (Human) ... 1002
Vencel (PY) *see* Donepezil ... 668
Vencid (MY) *see* Pantoprazole ... 1570
Vendal (UY) *see* Morphine (Systemic) ... 1394
Venderol (SG) *see* Albuterol ... 69
Venetlin (JP) *see* Albuterol ... 69
Venexor (HK, JO) *see* Venlafaxine ... 2150
Venexor XR SR (KR) *see* Venlafaxine ... 2150
Venitrin (IT) *see* Nitroglycerin ... 1465
Veniz-XR (IN) *see* Venlafaxine ... 2150
Venlafact SR (KR) *see* Venlafaxine ... 2150
Venla (IL) *see* Venlafaxine ... 2150
Venlalic XL (GB) *see* Venlafaxine ... 2150
Venla RBX (AU) *see* Venlafaxine ... 2150
Venlax (CL) *see* Venlafaxine ... 2150
Venlax Retard (CL) *see* Venlafaxine ... 2150
Venlax XR (LB) *see* Venlafaxine ... 2150
Venlor XR (HK) *see* Venlafaxine ... 2150
Venodenol (ID) *see* Polidocanol ... 1672
Venofer (AR, AU, BE, BG, CH, CL, CN, CO, CR, CY, CZ, DE, DK, DO, FI, FR, GB, GR, GT, HK, HN, HR, ID, IL, IS, JO, LB, LT, MY, NI, NL, NO, NZ, PA, PE, PK, PL, PT, PY, RO, SE, SG, SI, SK, SV, TR, UY, VE, ZA) *see* Iron Sucrose ... 1118
Venofer (DK) *see* Ferrous Sulfate ... 871
Venoferrum (KR) *see* Iron Sucrose ... 1118
Venohem (PY) *see* Acenocoumarol [CAN/INT] ... 30
Venoscler (UY) *see* Polidocanol ... 1672
Venoxil (MX) *see* Cinnarizine [INT] ... 440
Venozol (ID) *see* CeFAZolin ... 373
Ventamol (HK, ID) *see* Albuterol ... 69
Ventavis (AR, AT, AU, BE, BG, CH, CL, CN, CO, CY, CZ, DE, DK, FI, FR, GB, GR, HK, HN, HR, HU, ID, IE, IL, IT, LT, MY, NL, NO, PE, PT, RO, RU, SE, SG, SI, SK, TH, TR, TW, UY, VN) *see* Iloprost ... 1046
Ventavis RES (KR) *see* Iloprost ... 1046
Ventaxin OR (KR) *see* Venlafaxine ... 2150
Venter (EE, HR, HU, PL, RO, RU, SK) *see* Sucralfate ... 1940
Venterol (TH) *see* Albuterol ... 69
Venteze (ZA) *see* Albuterol ... 69
Vent FB Inhaler (IN) *see* Budesonide and Formoterol ... 297
Ventilan (CO, PT) *see* Albuterol ... 69
Ventilar (EC) *see* Montelukast ... 1392
Ventilastin Novolizer (DE, FR) *see* Albuterol ... 69
Ventilat (DE) *see* Oxitropium [INT] ... 1536
Ventipulmin[vet.] (CH, DE, FR) *see* Clenbuterol [INT] ... 460
Ventodisk (LU) *see* Albuterol ... 69
Ventol (AE, BH, CY, EG, IQ, IR, JO, KW, LB, LY, OM, QA, SA, SY, YE) *see* Albuterol ... 69
Ventolair (DE) *see* Beclomethasone (Nasal) ... 232
Ventolair (DE) *see* Beclomethasone (Systemic) ... 230
Ventolase (ES) *see* Clenbuterol [INT] ... 460
Ventolin (AE, AR, AU, BB, BE, BF, BG, BH, BJ, BM, BS, BZ, CH, CI, CL, CY, CZ, DO, EC, EE, EG, ES, ET, GH, GM, GN, GT, GY, HK, HN, HR, HU, ID, IE, IL, IQ, IR, IS, IT, JM, JO, KE, KR, KW, LB, LR, LU, LY, MA, ML, MR, MU, MW, MX, MY, NE, NG, NI, NL, NZ, OM, PA, PE, PH, PK, PL, PR, PY, QA, RU, SA, SC, SD, SI, SK, SL, SN, SR, SV, SY, TH, TN, TR, TT, TW, TZ, UG, UY, YE, ZM, ZW) *see* Albuterol ... 69
Ventolin CFC-Free (AU) *see* Albuterol ... 69
Ventoline (DK, FI, FR, NO, SE) *see* Albuterol ... 69
Ventor (GR) *see* Nimesulide [INT] ... 1456
Ventox (FI) *see* Oxitropium [INT] ... 1536
Ventrisol (PL) *see* Bismuth ... 265
Venxor (HK) *see* Venlafaxine ... 2150
Vepan (IN) *see* Cefadroxil ... 372
Vepesid (AR, AT, BE, BR, CH, CN, CZ, DE, DK, EE, ES, FI, GB, GR, HN, IE, IT, JP, LB, MT, NL, NO, PH, PK, PL, PT, RO, RU, SE, SI, SK, TR, TW, UY, ZA) *see* Etoposide ... 816
VePesid (AU, HR, LU) *see* Etoposide ... 816
Vepeside (FR) *see* Etoposide ... 816
Veracaps SR (AU) *see* Verapamil ... 2154
Veracol (NZ) *see* CefTRIAXone ... 396
Veradol (AR) *see* Naproxen ... 1427
Verahexal (DE, LU) *see* Verapamil ... 2154
Veraloc (DK) *see* Verapamil ... 2154
Veramex (DE) *see* Verapamil ... 2154
Veramil (IN) *see* Verapamil ... 2154
Veramina (AR) *see* Fosfomycin ... 932

Verapamil Hydrochloride (AE, BH, CY, IQ, IR, JO, KW, LB, LY, OM, QA, SA, SY, YE) *see* Verapamil 2154
Verapamil Pharmavit (HU) *see* Verapamil 2154
Veraplex (ID, RU, TH) *see* MedroxyPROGESTERone 1277
Verapress 240 SR (IL) *see* Verapamil 2154
Veratad (CO) *see* Verapamil 2154
Veraxin (HR) *see* Nitrendipine [INT] 1463
Verboril (AR) *see* Doxycycline 689
Verboril (AT, GR) *see* Diacerein [INT] 613
Vercef (AE, BF, BH, BJ, CI, ET, GH, GM, GN, KE, KW, LR, MA, ML, MR, MU, MW, MY, NE, NG, SC, SD, SL, SN, TN, TZ, UG, ZA, ZM, ZW) *see* Cefaclor 372
Verdix (ID) *see* Amikacin 111
Verdiz (PH) *see* Betahistine [CAN/INT] 252
Verelan (PH) *see* Verapamil 2154
Vergo (NZ) *see* Betahistine [CAN/INT] 252
Vericin (VE) *see* Cinnarizine [INT] 440
Vericlar (GT, HN, SV) *see* Naphazoline (Ophthalmic) 1426
Vericordin (AR) *see* Atenolol 189
Verimed (VN) *see* Mebeverine [INT] 1275
Verine (AE, SA) *see* Mebeverine [INT] 1275
Verine SR (QA) *see* Mebeverine [INT] 1275
Verisop (IE) *see* Verapamil 2154
Verispasmin (GR) *see* FlavoxATE 881
Verladyn (DE) *see* Dihydroergotamine 633
Verlost (GR) *see* Ranitidine 1777
Vermaqpharma Vet (NO) *see* Praziquantel 1702
Vermazol (TR) *see* Mebendazole [CAN/INT] 1274
Vermectil (BR) *see* Ivermectin (Systemic) 1136
Vermectin (TH) *see* Ivermectin (Systemic) 1136
Vermid (KR) *see* Mebendazole [CAN/INT] 1274
Vermin-Dazol (MX) *see* Mebendazole [CAN/INT] 1274
Vermine (TH) *see* Verapamil 2154
Vermin Plus (MX) *see* Albendazole 65
Vermis (TH) *see* Acyclovir (Systemic) 47
Vermokill (PY) *see* Ivermectin (Systemic) 1136
Vermox (AE, AU, BB, BE, BF, BG, BH, BJ, BM, BS, BZ, CH, CI, CN, CY, CZ, DE, DK, EE, EG, GB, GH, GM, GN, GR, GY, HK, HN, HR, HU, ID, IE, IL, IQ, IR, IS, IT, JM, JO, KE, KW, LB, LR, LT, LU, LY, MA, ML, MR, MU, MW, MX, NE, NG, NL, NO, NZ, OM, PK, PL, PR, QA, RO, RU, SA, SC, SD, SE, SI, SK, SL, SN, SR, SY, TN, TR, TT, TZ, UG, YE, ZA, ZM, ZW) *see* Mebendazole [CAN/INT] 1274
Verof (BR) *see* Fusidic Acid (Topical) [CAN/INT] 943
Verorab (BG, CN, CO, CR, DO, GT, HN, KR, MY, PA, PE, SV, VN) *see* Rabies Vaccine 1764
Verospiron (BG, CZ, EE, HN, HU, LT, SK) *see* Spironolactone 1931
Verpamil (AE, BH, CY, EG, HU, IL, IQ, IR, JO, KW, LB, LY, OM, QA, SA, SY, YE) *see* Verapamil 2154
Versacid (PH) *see* Lansoprazole 1166
Versant XR (PH) *see* Felodipine 850
Versatis (BE, CL, CO, CR, DO, EE, GT, HN, HR, NI, PA, PE, RO, RU, SE, SK, SV) *see* Lidocaine (Topical) 1211
Versatis Plaster (GB, IE) *see* Lidocaine (Topical) 1211
Versed (FR) *see* Midazolam 1361
Versef (PH) *see* Cefaclor 372
Versibet (ID) *see* Glimepiride 966
Versigen (TH) *see* Gentamicin (Systemic) 959
Verstadol (ES) *see* Butorphanol 314
Verstran (PK) *see* Prazepam [INT] 1702
Verte (PE) *see* Orlistat 1520
Vertigal (HR) *see* Betahistine [CAN/INT] 252
Vertigmine (AR) *see* DimenhyDRINATE 637
Vertigol (PY) *see* Meclizine 1277
Vertigon (ID, SG) *see* Cinnarizine [INT] 440
Vertimed (RO, TR) *see* Betahistine [CAN/INT] 252
Vertine (GB) *see* Salmeterol 1860
Vertinex (LB) *see* Betahistine [CAN/INT] 252
Vertin (IN) *see* Betahistine [CAN/INT] 252
Vertirosan (AT) *see* DimenhyDRINATE 637
Vertisal (DO, GT, HN, NI, SV) *see* MetroNIDAZOLE (Systemic) 1353
Vertisin (UY) *see* Lovastatin 1252
Vertivom (ID) *see* Metoclopramide 1345
Vertizole (MX) *see* Mebendazole [CAN/INT] 1274
Vert (PH) *see* Betahistine [CAN/INT] 252
Vertrol (PH) *see* Betahistine [CAN/INT] 252
Verum (CO) *see* Betahistine [CAN/INT] 252
Verutex (BR) *see* Fusidic Acid (Topical) [CAN/INT] 943
Vesanoid (AE, AR, AT, AU, BE, BH, BR, CH, CN, CO, CY, CZ, DE, FI, FR, GB, HK, HR, IE, IL, IT, JO, JP, KR, KW, MX, NL, NO, NZ, PE, PH, PK, PL, PT, PY, QA, SI, SK, TH, TW, VE, VN) *see* Tretinoin (Systemic) 2096
Vesconac (TH) *see* Diclofenac (Systemic) 617
Vesdil (DE) *see* Ramipril 1771
Vesicare (AR, AU, BE, BR, CH, CL, CN, CY, CZ, DK, EE, ES, FI, FR, GB, GR, HK, HN, HR, ID, IL, IS, JO, JP, KR, KW, LB, LT, MY, NL, NO, NZ, PE, PH, PL, PT, QA, RO, RU, SA, SE, SG, SI, SK, TH, TR, TW, VN) *see* Solifenacin 1917
Vesiker (IT) *see* Solifenacin 1917
Vesikur (DE) *see* Solifenacin 1917
Vesilac (PH) *see* Bisacodyl 265
Vesitab (ID) *see* Betahistine [CAN/INT] 252
Vesitrim (IE) *see* Solifenacin 1917
Vesnon-V (TH) *see* TraMADol 2074
Vessel (BR) *see* Cinnarizine [INT] 440
Vestaclav (MY) *see* Amoxicillin and Clavulanate 133
Vestein (ID) *see* Erdosteine [INT] 753
Vesyca (SG) *see* Ranitidine 1777
Vetio (AR) *see* MitoMYcin (Systemic) 1380
Vetoben (TH) *see* Albendazole 65
Vetrimil (TW) *see* Verapamil 2154
Vetubia (HR, RO) *see* Everolimus 822
Vewon (TW) *see* Fluoxymesterone 903
Vexal-A (PH) *see* Anastrozole 148
Vexazone (AU) *see* Pioglitazone 1654
Vexel (PH) *see* PACLitaxel (Conventional) 1550
Vexepam (PH) *see* Diazepam 613
Vexer (PH) *see* Pregabalin 1710
Vexlev (PH) *see* LevETIRAcetam 1191
Vexol (AE, AT, CH, CY, DE, DK, ES, FI, FR, GB, GR, HK, IE, IT, KR, LB, MX, NL, NO, NZ, PT, QA, SA, SE, SG, TR) *see* Rimexolone 1814
Vexolon (BE) *see* Rimexolone 1814
Vexonib-4 (PH) *see* Zoledronic Acid 2206
Vexpinem (PH) *see* Imipenem and Cilastatin 1051
VFEND (AE, AR, AT, AU, BE, BG, BH, BM, BR, BZ, CH, CL, CN, CO, CR, CY, CZ, DE, DK, EC, EE, ES, FI, FR, GB, GR, GT, HK, HN, HR, HU, ID, IE, IL, IN, IS, IT, JO, JP, KR, KW, LB, LT, MT, MX, MY, NI, NL, NO, NZ, PA, PE, PH, PL, PT, QA, RO, RU, SA, SE, SG, SI, SK, SV, TH, TR, TW, ZA) *see* Voriconazole 2176
Vherdex (PH) *see* Dexamethasone (Systemic) 599
Viaclav (ID) *see* Amoxicillin and Clavulanate 133
Viagra (AE, AT, AU, BE, BF, BH, BJ, BR, CH, CI, CL, CN, CO, CR, CY, CZ, DE, DK, DO, EC, EE, EG, ES, ET, FI, FR, GB, GH, GM, GN, GR, GT, HK, HN, HR, HU, ID, IE, IL, IQ, IR, IS, IT, JO, JP, KE, KR, KW, LB, LR, LT, LY, MA, ML, MR, MT, MU, MW, MX, MY, NE, NG, NI, NL, NO, NZ, OM, PA, PE, PH, PL, PT, QA, RO, RU, SA, SC, SD, SE, SG, SI, SK, SL, SN, SV, SY, TH, TN, TR, TW, TZ, UG, UY, VE, VN, YE, ZA, ZM, ZW) *see* Sildenafil 1882
Vialebex (FR) *see* Albumin 67
Viamox (PH) *see* Amoxicillin and Clavulanate 133
Viani (DE) *see* Fluticasone and Salmeterol 912
Viarex (AE, BF, BH, BJ, CI, CY, EG, ET, GH, GM, GN, IL, IQ, IR, JO, KE, KW, LB, LR, LY, MA, ML, MR, MU, MW, NE, NG, OM, QA, SA, SC, SD, SL, SN, SY, TN, TZ, UG, YE, ZA, ZM, ZW) *see* Beclomethasone (Nasal) 232

Viasin Powder (KR) *see* Sildenafil 1882
Viatim (AT, DE, FI, GB, IE, NL) *see* Typhoid and Hepatitis A Vaccine [CAN/INT] 2111
Viatrex (PH) *see* CefTRIAXone 396
Viaxol (MX) *see* Ambroxol [INT] 109
Vibativ (CZ, DE, EE, FI, GB, HR, LT, NL, PT, SE, SK) *see* Telavancin 1986
Vibeden (DK) *see* Hydroxocobalamin 1020
Vibradox (DK, PT) *see* Doxycycline 689
Vibramicina (AR, CL, CO, MX, PE, PT, UY, VE) *see* Doxycycline 689
Vibramycin (AE, AT, AU, BB, BF, BG, BH, BJ, BM, BS, BZ, CH, CI, CY, DE, EG, ET, GB, GH, GM, GN, GR, GY, HK, HU, ID, IE, IQ, IR, JM, JO, KE, KW, LB, LR, LY, MA, ML, MR, MU, MW, MY, NE, NG, NL, NO, OM, PH, PK, QA, RU, SA, SC, SD, SE, SL, SN, SR, SY, TH, TN, TT, TZ, UG, YE, ZA, ZM, ZW) *see* Doxycycline 689
Vibramycine (FR) *see* Doxycycline 689
Vibramycin N (KR) *see* Doxycycline 689
Vibratab (BE) *see* Doxycycline 689
Vibraveineuse (FR) *see* Doxycycline 689
Vibravenos (DE) *see* Doxycycline 689
Vicafidt (MX) *see* Clopidogrel 484
Vicalud (KR) *see* Bicalutamide 262
Vicalvit (PL) *see* Calcium Carbonate 327
Vicapan N (DE) *see* Cyanocobalamin 515
Vicard (AT) *see* Terazosin 2001
Viccillin (ID) *see* Ampicillin 141
Vicef (BF, BJ, CI, ET, GH, GM, GN, KE, LR, MA, ML, MR, MU, MW, NE, NG, SC, SD, SL, SN, TN, TZ, UG, ZM, ZW) *see* Ascorbic Acid 178
Vicknox (HK) *see* Zolpidem 2212
Vicks expectorant adulte (FR) *see* GuaiFENesin 986
Vicks Vaposyrup (BE) *see* GuaiFENesin 986
Vick-Thiaden (HK) *see* Dosulepin [INT] 673
Viclorax (PE) *see* Doxycycline 689
Vicorax (TW) *see* Acyclovir (Topical) 51
Victanyl (GB) *see* FentaNYL 857
Victoza (AE, AR, AT, AU, BE, BR, CH, CL, CN, CY, CZ, DE, DK, EE, FR, GB, HK, HR, HU, IE, IL, IN, IS, JP, KR, KW, LB, LT, MY, NL, NO, NZ, PH, PL, PT, QA, RO, RU, SE, SG, SI, SK, TH, TR, VN) *see* Liraglutide 1222
Victrelis (AR, AU, BE, BR, CH, CO, CY, CZ, DE, DK, EE, FR, GB, HK, HR, HU, ID, IE, IL, IS, LT, MX, MY, NL, NO, NZ, PE, PL, QA, RO, SE, SG, SI, SK, TH, TR, VN) *see* Boceprevir 273
Vidanovir (HN) *see* Didanosine 622
Vidan (RO) *see* Mefenamic Acid 1280
Vidastat (PH) *see* Simvastatin 1890
Vidaxil (MX) *see* Digoxin 627
Vidaza (AR, AT, AU, BE, CH, CL, CO, CR, CY, CZ, DE, DK, DO, EE, FR, GB, GR, GT, HK, HN, HR, IE, IL, IS, JP, KR, LB, LT, MX, MY, NI, NL, NO, NZ, PA, PE, PH, PL, PT, RO, SE, SG, SI, SK, SV, TH, TR, TW, ZA) *see* AzaCITIDine 209
Vidcef (KR) *see* Cefadroxil 372
Videx DDI (CO) *see* Didanosine 622
Videx (AT, AU, BE, CL, CN, CY, CZ, DE, DK, EC, EE, EG, ES, FR, GB, GR, HR, ID, IE, IT, LB, MT, MY, NL, PL, PT, RU, SE, SI, TR, TW, UY, VE, VN, ZA) *see* Didanosine 622
Videx EC (AU, BG, CH, EE, FI, HK, HU, IE, MX, MY, NO, NZ, PE, RO, SE, SG, SI, SK, TH, TW, VN) *see* Didanosine 622
Videx EC SR (KR) *see* Didanosine 622
Videx Pediatric (HK) *see* Didanosine 622
Vidopen (GB, IE) *see* Ampicillin 141
Vidora (FR) *see* Indoramin [INT] 1070
Vidox (UY) *see* Mupirocin 1404
Vidya (TW) *see* Rosiglitazone 1847
Viepax (IL) *see* Venlafaxine 2150
Viepax XR (IL, SG) *see* Venlafaxine 2150
Viergyt-K (RO) *see* Amantadine 105
Vifas (TH) *see* Fexofenadine 873
Viflox (ID) *see* Ciprofloxacin (Systemic) 441
Vifolin (AE, BH, CY, EG, IL, IQ, IR, JO, KW, LB, LY, OM, QA, SA, SY, YE) *see* Folic Acid 919
Vigamox (AE, AR, BG, BR, CH, CL, CO, CR, CY, CZ, DE, DK, EE, FI, GT, HK, HN, ID, IE, IL, IN, IS, JP, KR, KW, LT, MY, NI, NZ, PA, PE, PH, RO, SA, SE, SG, SK, SV, TH, TR, TW, UY, VE, VN, ZA) *see* Moxifloxacin (Ophthalmic) 1403
Vigam (TH) *see* Immune Globulin 1056
Vigantol (ES) *see* Ergocalciferol 753
Vigantolo (IT) *see* Ergocalciferol 753
Vi-Gel (PH) *see* Indomethacin 1067
Vigia (CO) *see* Modafinil 1386
Vigicer (AR) *see* Modafinil 1386
Vigil (CZ, DE) *see* Modafinil 1386
Vigiten (LU) *see* LORazepam 1243
Vigocid (PH) *see* Piperacillin and Tazobactam 1657
Vijomikin (GT, HN, PA, SV) *see* Amikacin 111
Vikadar (AE, BH, JO, SA) *see* Penicillin V Potassium 1614
Viken (MX) *see* Cefotaxime 382
Vilimen (TR) *see* Memantine 1286
Vilne (EC) *see* Vinorelbine 2168
Vilona (MX) *see* Ribavirin 1797
Vimax (ID) *see* Sildenafil 1882
Vimizim (CZ, DE, DK, EE, FR, HR, LT, NL, SE, SK) *see* Elosulfase Alfa 714
Vimpat (AR, AU, BE, CH, CO, CY, CZ, DE, DK, EE, FR, GB, GR, HK, HR, IE, IL, IS, KR, LT, MY, NL, NO, NZ, PH, PL, PT, RO, RU, SE, SI, SK, TH, TR) *see* Lacosamide 1154
Vinacil (MX) *see* Neomycin 1436
Vinafluor (ID) *see* Fluoride 895
Vinatin (BR) *see* VinBLAStine 2160
Vinbine (IN) *see* Vinorelbine 2168
Vinblastina (CO) *see* VinBLAStine 2160
Vinblastine Sulfate Injection (AU) *see* VinBLAStine 2160
Vinblastin (HU, PL) *see* VinBLAStine 2160
Vinces (AR) *see* VinCRIStine 2163
Vincidal (MX) *see* Loratadine 1241
Vincran (KR) *see* VinCRIStine 2163
Vincrina (PY) *see* VinCRIStine 2163
Vincrisin (BE) *see* VinCRIStine 2163
Vincristina (IT) *see* VinCRIStine 2163
Vincristine-David Bull (LU) *see* VinCRIStine 2163
Vincristine Delta West (HR) *see* VinCRIStine 2163
Vincristine Sulfate (PL) *see* VinCRIStine 2163
Vincristin (HU, PL) *see* VinCRIStine 2163
Vincrisul (ES) *see* VinCRIStine 2163
Vindacin (MX) *see* Sulindac 1953
Viner (HR) *see* Sildenafil 1882
Vingraf (PH) *see* Tacrolimus (Systemic) 1962
Vinorgen (PE, PY) *see* Vinorelbine 2168
Vinotel (PH) *see* Vinorelbine 2168
Vinracine (HK, MY, SG) *see* VinCRIStine 2163
Vintec (MX) *see* VinCRIStine 2163
Vioflox (KR) *see* Ofloxacin (Systemic) 1490
Vioson (PH) *see* Ofloxacin (Systemic) 1490
Viotisone (TH) *see* Ofloxacin (Systemic) 1490
Viplena (EC) *see* Orlistat 1520
Viprazo (PH) *see* Omeprazole 1508
Viracept (AE, AT, AU, BB, BE, BF, BG, BH, BJ, BM, BR, BS, BZ, CH, CI, CN, CO, CZ, DE, DK, EC, EE, ES, ET, FI, FR, GB, GH, GM, GN, GR, GY, HN, HU, IE, IL, IT, JM, JP, KE, KR, KW, LR, MA, ML, MR, MT, MU, MW, MX, MY, NE, NG, NL, NO, PH, PL, PT, PY, QA, RO, RU, SC, SD, SE, SG, SI, SK, SL, SN, SR, TH, TN, TR, TT, TZ, UG, UY, VE, VN, ZA, ZM, ZW) *see* Nelfinavir 1436

Viraferon (AT, BE, BG, CH, CZ, DE, DK, EE, ES, FI, GR, HN, IE, IT, MT, NL, NO, PL, PT, RU, SE, SK, TR) *see* Interferon Alfa-2b 1096
ViraFeronPEG (AT, BE, BG, CH, CZ, DE, DK, EE, ES, FI, FR, GB, HN, IE, IT, MT, NL, NO, PL, PT, RU, SE, SK, TR) *see* Peginterferon Alfa-2b 1596
Viralex-DS (PH) *see* Acyclovir (Systemic) 47
Viramid (KR) *see* Ribavirin 1797
Viramune (AE, AR, AT, AU, BE, BF, BG, BH, BJ, BR, CH, CI, CL, CN, CO, CY, CZ, DE, DK, EE, EG, ES, ET, FI, FR, GB, GH, GM, GN, GR, HK, HN, HR, HU, ID, IE, IL, IQ, IR, IS, IT, JO, KE, KR, KW, LB, LR, LT, LY, MA, ML, MR, MT, MU, MW, MX, MY, NE, NG, NL, NO, NZ, OM, PE, PL, PT, PY, QA, RO, RU, SA, SC, SD, SE, SG, SI, SK, SL, SN, SY, TN, TR, TW, TZ, UG, UY, VE, YE, ZA, ZM, ZW) *see* Nevirapine 1440
Viramune XR (HK) *see* Nevirapine 1440
Viranet (AR) *see* ValACYclovir 2119
Viratop (BE) *see* Acyclovir (Systemic) 47
Viratop (BE) *see* Acyclovir (Topical) 51
Virax (KR) *see* Acyclovir (Systemic) 47
Virazide (AU, MX, PK) *see* Ribavirin 1797
Virazin (KR) *see* Ribavirin 1797
Virazole (AE, BE, BH, BR, CR, CY, EG, GB, GT, HN, IQ, IR, JO, KW, LB, LY, NI, NL, OM, QA, SA, SE, SV, SY, YE) *see* Ribavirin 1797
Virbez (PH) *see* Irbesartan 1110
Virdual (CO) *see* Lamivudine and Zidovudine 1160
Viread (AR, AT, AU, BE, BG, BR, CH, CL, CN, CY, CZ, DE, DK, EE, ES, FI, FR, GB, GR, HK, HN, HR, HU, IE, IL, IS, IT, KR, LT, MT, MX, NL, NO, NZ, PL, PT, RO, RU, SA, SE, SG, SI, SK, TH, TR, TW, UY, VN) *see* Tenofovir 1998
Viregyt-K (BG, HU) *see* Amantadine 105
Virenza (IN) *see* Zanamivir 2194
Virest (HK, SG) *see* Acyclovir (Systemic) 47
Virex (CO) *see* Aciclovir (Ophthalmic) [INT] 43
Virex (CO) *see* Acyclovir (Systemic) 47
Virex (CO) *see* Acyclovir (Topical) 51
Virgan (AR, BE, CZ, DE, FR, GB, HK, KR, PH, PT) *see* Ganciclovir (Systemic) 948
Viridal (DE, IE) *see* Alprostadil 96
Viridin (PT) *see* Trifluridine 2103
Virilit (DE) *see* Cyproterone [CAN/INT] 530
Virless (MY, SG, TW) *see* Acyclovir (Systemic) 47
Virless (SG) *see* Acyclovir (Topical) 51
Virlix (BF, BJ, CI, ES, ET, FR, GH, GM, GN, KE, LR, MA, ML, MR, MU, MW, NE, NG, PH, PT, SC, SD, SL, SN, TN, TZ, UG, ZM, ZW) *see* Cetirizine 411
Virobron (AR) *see* Nimesulide [INT] 1456
Viroclear (HK) *see* Acyclovir (Systemic) 47
Virofral (DK) *see* Amantadine 105
Virogon (TH) *see* Acyclovir (Systemic) 47
Virogon (TH) *see* Acyclovir (Topical) 51
Virolex (HU, RO) *see* Acyclovir (Systemic) 47
Virolex (SK) *see* Aciclovir (Ophthalmic) [INT] 43
Virol (IN) *see* Abacavir 20
Virolox (HR) *see* Acyclovir (Systemic) 47
Virolox (HR) *see* Acyclovir (Topical) 51
Viromed (TH) *see* Acyclovir (Systemic) 47
Viromidin (ES) *see* Trifluridine 2103
Virophta (FR) *see* Trifluridine 2103
Virormone (AE, BH, CY, EG, IQ, IR, JO, KW, LB, LY, OM, QA, SA, SY, YE) *see* Testosterone 2010
Virorrever (AR, PY) *see* Efavirenz 707
Virosol (AR) *see* Amantadine 105
Virostav (MY) *see* Stavudine 1934
Virpes (AE, JO) *see* Acyclovir (Systemic) 47
Virucid (TR, VN) *see* Acyclovir (Systemic) 47
Virucil (CO) *see* Ampicillin 141
Virxit (CO) *see* Indinavir 1066
Virzen (CO) *see* Efavirenz 707
Virzin (DE) *see* Acyclovir (Systemic) 47
Virzin (DE) *see* Acyclovir (Topical) 51
VisaBelle (IL) *see* Dienogest [CAN/INT] 623
Visacor (AU, NZ) *see* Rosuvastatin 1848
Visadron (AT, BE, DE, NL, PT) *see* Phenylephrine (Systemic) 1638
Visalmin (BR) *see* Chloramphenicol 421
Visanette (CY) *see* Dienogest [CAN/INT] 623
Visanne (AR, AT, AU, CH, CO, CZ, DE, DK, EC, FI, FR, HK, HN, HR, IS, KR, MY, NL, NO, PT, QA, RO, SA, SE, SG, SI, SK, TH) *see* Dienogest [CAN/INT] 623
Visannette (BE, EE, LT, MX, TR) *see* Dienogest [CAN/INT] 623
Visano (DE) *see* Meprobamate 1296
Visclair (GB, IE) *see* Mecysteine [INT] 1277
Viscoat (AU, DE, GR, IN, IT, NZ, PH, TH, TR, TW, VN, ZA) *see* Sodium Chondroitin Sulfate and Sodium Hyaluronate 1905
Viscolyt (DK) *see* Bromhexine [INT] 291
Viscoseal (DE, MY) *see* Hyaluronate and Derivatives 1006
Visine Allergy (NZ) *see* Naphazoline and Pheniramine 1426
Visine Allergy with Antihistamine (AU) *see* Naphazoline and Pheniramine 1426
Visiokan (IT) *see* Kanamycin 1142
Visiol (MY) *see* Hyaluronate and Derivatives 1006
Viskeen (NL) *see* Pindolol 1652
Viskeen Retard (NL) *see* Pindolol 1652
Visken (AT, AU, BE, BF, BG, BJ, BR, CH, CI, CZ, DE, DK, EE, EG, ES, ET, FI, FR, GB, GH, GM, GN, GR, HK, HN, HU, IE, IN, IS, IT, KE, LR, LU, MA, ML, MR, MT, MU, MW, MX, NE, NG, NO, NZ, PH, PL, PT, QA, RU, SA, SC, SD, SE, SK, SL, SN, TN, TR, TZ, UG, UY, VE, ZA, ZM, ZW) *see* Pindolol 1652
Viskene (PT) *see* Pindolol 1652
Viskoferm (SE) *see* Acetylcysteine 40
Visonest (BR) *see* Proparacaine 1728
Vistachlor (PH) *see* Chloramphenicol 421
Vistaflox (PH) *see* Ciprofloxacin (Ophthalmic) 446
Vistaflox (PH) *see* Ciprofloxacin (Systemic) 441
Vistagan (AT, CH, CO, CZ, DE, GR, HN, HR, HU, IT, PL, RU, VE) *see* Levobunolol 1194
Vistagan (PK) *see* Betaxolol (Ophthalmic) 257
Vistagan (PK) *see* Betaxolol (Systemic) 256
Vista (JP) *see* OnabotulinumtoxinA 1512
Vistallerg (PH) *see* Naphazoline and Pheniramine 1426
Vistamethasone (TR) *see* Betamethasone (Systemic) 253
Vistamin (PK) *see* PenicillAMINE 1608
Vistapred (PH) *see* PrednisoLONE (Ophthalmic) 1706
Vistapred (PH) *see* PrednisoLONE (Systemic) 1703
Vistaril (KE, SE, TR, TW) *see* HydrOXYzine 1024
Vistide (AT, AU, BE, BG, CH, CZ, DE, DK, ES, FI, FR, GR, HN, IE, IT, NL, NO, PL, PT, RO, RU, SE, SI, TR) *see* Cidofovir 433
Vistimon (DE) *see* Mesterolone [INT] 1307
Visuanestetico (IT) *see* Proparacaine 1728
Visumetazone (IT) *see* Dexamethasone (Ophthalmic) 602
Visumetazone (IT) *see* Dexamethasone (Systemic) 599
Visumidriatic (IT) *see* Tropicamide 2108
Vit'C (BE) *see* Ascorbic Acid 178
Vita-C (JO) *see* Ascorbic Acid 178
Vita-B1 (FI) *see* Thiamine 2028
Vita-B2 (FI, PL) *see* Riboflavin 1803
Vita-B6 (FI) *see* Pyridoxine 1747
Vitac (CL) *see* Ascorbic Acid 178
Vitacalcin (PL) *see* Calcium Carbonate 327
Vita-Cedol Orange (BB, BM, BS, BZ, GY, JM, PR, SR, TT) *see* Ascorbic Acid 178
Vitacid Acne (BR) *see* Clindamycin and Tretinoin 464
Vitacilina (MX) *see* Neomycin 1436
Vitacon (PL) *see* Phytonadione 1647

Vita-E 400 (EC) *see* Vitamin E 2174
Vitaferro Brause (DE) *see* Ferrous Gluconate 870
Vitak (JP) *see* Phytonadione 1647
Vitalen (MX) *see* Cyanocobalamin 515
Vitam-Doce (AR) *see* Cyanocobalamin 515
Vitamet (PH) *see* Metoclopramide 1345
Vitamin C (HR, HU) *see* Ascorbic Acid 178
Vitamin A (AU) *see* Vitamin A 2173
Vitamina B1 Biol (AR) *see* Thiamine 2028
Vitamina B12-Ecar (CO) *see* Cyanocobalamin 515
Vitamina D2 Salf (IT) *see* Ergocalciferol 753
Vitamina PP Angelini (IT) *see* Niacinamide 1446
Vitamin B!1!2-Depot-Injektopas (DE) *see* Hydroxocobalamin 1020
Vitamin B!1!2 (HR, HU) *see* Cyanocobalamin 515
Vitamin B!1!2 Lannacher (AT) *see* Cyanocobalamin 515
Vitamin B!1-Hevert (DE) *see* Thiamine 2028
Vitamin B!1 (HU) *see* Thiamine 2028
Vitamin B!1-Injektopas (DE) *see* Thiamine 2028
Vitamin B!1 Jenapharm (DE) *see* Thiamine 2028
Vitamin B 1 Kattwiga (DE) *see* Thiamine 2028
Vitamin B!1-ratiopharm (DE) *see* Thiamine 2028
Vitamin B!2-Injektopas (DE) *see* Riboflavin 1803
Vitamin B!2 Jenapharm (DE) *see* Riboflavin 1803
Vitamin B2 (PE) *see* Riboflavin 1803
Vitamin B!2 Streuli[Ampullen] (CH) *see* Riboflavin 1803
Vitamin B3 (AU) *see* Niacinamide 1446
Vitamin B!6 (HU) *see* Pyridoxine 1747
Vitamin B!6 Streuli (CH) *see* Pyridoxine 1747
Vitamin B12 Depot (NO) *see* Hydroxocobalamin 1020
Vitamin B12 Recip (SE) *see* Cyanocobalamin 515
Vitamine C Lambo (BE) *see* Ascorbic Acid 178
Vitamine C OJG (BE) *see* Ascorbic Acid 178
Vitamine-C-Qualiphar (LU) *see* Ascorbic Acid 178
Vitamine C Repha (BE) *see* Ascorbic Acid 178
Vitamine C Roter (LU) *see* Ascorbic Acid 178
Vitamine B!6 Richard (FR) *see* Pyridoxine 1747
Vitamine B12-Dulcis (LU) *see* Cyanocobalamin 515
Vitamine K!1 Roche (FR) *see* Phytonadione 1647
Vitamin K1 (KR) *see* Phytonadione 1647
Vitamin K (HK) *see* Phytonadione 1647
Vitaminol (GR) *see* Ergocalciferol 753
Vitaminum B1 (PL) *see* Thiamine 2028
Vitaminum B2 (PL) *see* Riboflavin 1803
Vitaminum B6 (PL) *see* Pyridoxine 1747
Vitaminum B12 (PL) *see* Cyanocobalamin 515
Vitaminum PP (PL) *see* Niacinamide 1446
Vitamon Fluor (BE) *see* Fluoride 895
Vitanon[inj.] (JP) *see* Thiamine 2028
Vitantial (ES) *see* Thiamine 2028
Vitaros (GB) *see* Alprostadil 96
Vitarubin (CH) *see* Cyanocobalamin 515
Vitarubin-Depot (CH) *see* Hydroxocobalamin 1020
Vitascorbol (FR) *see* Ascorbic Acid 178
Vitasul (PH) *see* Sulfacetamide (Ophthalmic) 1943
Vitaverán Fólico (MX) *see* Folic Acid, Cyanocobalamin, and Pyridoxine 921
Vit. B1 Agepha (AT) *see* Thiamine 2028
Vit. B6 Agepha (AT) *see* Pyridoxine 1747
Vitekta (AU, CZ, EE, FI, HR, LT, NL, SE, SK) *see* Elvitegravir 717
Vitera (RO) *see* LevETIRAcetam 1191
Vitka Infant (ID) *see* Phytonadione 1647
Vitodex Eye Drop (KR) *see* Tobramycin and Dexamethasone 2056
Vitonic (LU) *see* Ascorbic Acid 178
Vitozid (HR) *see* Lisinopril and Hydrochlorothiazide 1229
Vitupen (KR) *see* Phentermine 1635
Vivacor (KR) *see* Rosuvastatin 1848
Vivadex (GB) *see* Tacrolimus (Systemic) 1962
Vivanza (BG, ES) *see* Vardenafil 2138
Vivasartan Plus (PH) *see* Losartan and Hydrochlorothiazide 1250
Vivatec (DK, FI, NO) *see* Lisinopril 1226
Vivaxim (AU, HK, MY, NZ, PE) *see* Typhoid and Hepatitis A Vaccine [CAN/INT] 2111
Vivelle-Dot (BE, DK) *see* Estradiol (Systemic) 775
Vivelledot (FR) *see* Estradiol (Systemic) 775
Vivelon (PH) *see* Clopidogrel 484
Vivial (KR) *see* Hyaluronate and Derivatives 1006
Vividrin (KR, TH, TR) *see* Cromolyn (Ophthalmic) 514
Vividrin (PH) *see* Cromolyn (Nasal) 514
Vividyl (IT) *see* Nortriptyline 1476
Vivinox (DE) *see* DiphenhydrAMINE (Systemic) 641
Vivioptal Junior (MX) *see* Magnesium Sulfate 1265
Vivir (KR) *see* Acyclovir (Systemic) 47
Vivir (KR) *see* Acyclovir (Topical) 51
Vivitar (GT, MX, SV) *see* Spironolactone 1931
Vivotif Berna (AE, AT, CH, DK, ES, HK, IT, KR, MY, NL, PH, QA, SA) *see* Typhoid Vaccine 2112
Vivotif Berna Capsule (NO) *see* Typhoid Vaccine 2112
Vivotif (DE, GB, IE) *see* Typhoid Vaccine 2112
Vivotif Oral (AU) *see* Typhoid Vaccine 2112
Vivotif Oralt Vaccin (SE) *see* Typhoid Vaccine 2112
Vivradoxil (MX) *see* Doxycycline 689
Vivrone (PH) *see* Testosterone 2010
Viza (CL) *see* ARIPiprazole 171
Vizendo (RO) *see* Montelukast 1392
Vizerul (AR) *see* Ranitidine 1777
Vizol (HR) *see* Naphazoline (Ophthalmic) 1426
Vizomet (MY) *see* Mometasone (Topical) 1391
VM 26-Bristol (DE) *see* Teniposide 1997
Vocado HCT (DE) *see* Olmesartan, Amlodipine, and Hydrochlorothiazide 1498
Vocefa Forte (ID) *see* Cefadroxil 372
Vocefa (ID) *see* Cefadroxil 372
Vodin (ID) *see* Diazepam 613
Voker (MY) *see* Famotidine 845
Volar (JO, LB) *see* Gabapentin 943
Volataren Oftalmico (CL) *see* Diclofenac (Ophthalmic) 621
Voldic (AE, BH, CY, EG, IQ, IR, JO, KW, LB, LY, OM, QA, SA, SY, YE) *see* Diclofenac (Systemic) 617
Voldic Emulgel (AE, BH, CY, EG, IL, IQ, IR, JO, KW, LB, LY, OM, QA, SA, SY, YE) *see* Diclofenac (Systemic) 617
Volequin (ID) *see* Levofloxacin (Systemic) 1197
Volibris (AT, AU, BE, CH, CN, CO, CY, CZ, DE, DK, EE, FR, GB, GR, HN, HR, HU, IE, IL, IS, IT, JP, KR, LT, MY, NL, NO, NZ, PL, PT, RO, SE, SI, SK, TR, TW) *see* Ambrisentan 107
Volirop (AU) *see* Carvedilol 367
Volmax (AE, BH, CY, EC, EG, HU, IQ, IR, JO, KW, LB, LY, OM, QA, SA, SY, YE) *see* Albuterol 69
Volmizolin (SK) *see* CeFAZolin 373
Volna-K (TW) *see* Diclofenac (Systemic) 617
Volog (AE, BF, BH, BJ, CI, CY, EG, ET, GH, GM, GN, IL, IQ, IR, JO, KE, KW, LB, LR, LY, MA, ML, MR, MU, MW, NE, NG, OM, PK, QA, SA, SC, SD, SL, SN, SY, TN, TR, TZ, UG, YE, ZA, ZM, ZW) *see* Halcinonide 992
Volon A 10 (DE) *see* Triamcinolone (Systemic) 2099
Volon A 40 (DE) *see* Triamcinolone (Systemic) 2099
Volon A Antibiotikafrei (AT, DE) *see* Triamcinolone (Systemic) 2099
Volon A Antibiotikafrei (AT, DE) *see* Triamcinolone (Topical) 2100
Volon A (AT, DE) *see* Triamcinolone (Systemic) 2099
Volone (HR) *see* Nebivolol 1434
VoLox (ID) *see* Levofloxacin (Systemic) 1197
Voltaflam (PK) *see* Diclofenac (Systemic) 617
Voltaflex (BR) *see* Diclofenac (Systemic) 617
Voltalen Emulgel (NZ) *see* Diclofenac (Systemic) 617
Voltalen (HK, NZ) *see* Diclofenac (Systemic) 617
Voltaren Acti-Go (IL) *see* Diclofenac (Systemic) 617

Voltaren (AE, AR, AT, BE, BF, BG, BH, BJ, BR, CH, CI, CL, CO, CY, CZ, DE, DK, EE, EG, ET, FI, GH, GM, GN, HK, HR, HU, ID, IL, IQ, IR, IS, IT, JO, KE, KW, LB, LR, LT, LY, MA, ML, MR, MU, MW, MY, NE, NG, NL, NO, NZ, OM, PH, PL, PT, PY, QA, RO, RU, SA, SC, SD, SE, SI, SK, SL, SN, SY, TH, TN, TR, TW, TZ, UG, UY, VE, VN, YE, ZA, ZM, ZW) *see* Diclofenac (Systemic) 617
Voltaren (BH, EG, HU, QA, RO, TR) *see* Diclofenac (Ophthalmic) 621
Voltaren Colirio (BR) *see* Diclofenac (Ophthalmic) 621
Voltaren Dolo (FR) *see* Diclofenac (Systemic) 617
Voltarene (FR) *see* Diclofenac (Ophthalmic) 621
Voltarene (FR, GR) *see* Diclofenac (Systemic) 617
Voltaren Forte (MX) *see* Codeine 497
Voltaren Forte (PH) *see* Diclofenac (Systemic) 617
Voltaren Ofta (IT) *see* Diclofenac (Ophthalmic) 621
Voltaren Oftalmico (PY, UY) *see* Diclofenac (Ophthalmic) 621
Voltaren Ophtha (AE, AT, AU, CH, CO, CZ, DE, DK, EE, FI, HK, ID, IL, IS, KW, LB, MY, NO, NZ, PE, PH, PT, SA, SE, SG, TH, TW, VN) *see* Diclofenac (Ophthalmic) 621
Voltaren Rapid (AU, NZ) *see* Diclofenac (Systemic) 617
Voltaren SR (BH, CY, EG, HK, LB, NZ, PH, SA) *see* Diclofenac (Systemic) 617
Voltarol (IE) *see* Diclofenac (Systemic) 617
Voltarol Ophtha (GB) *see* Diclofenac (Ophthalmic) 621
Volta (TH) *see* Diclofenac (Systemic) 617
Voltfast (SG) *see* Diclofenac (Systemic) 617
Voltine (AE, BH, CY, EG, IQ, IR, JO, KW, LB, LY, OM, QA, SA, SY, YE) *see* Diclofenac (Systemic) 617
Volton-CR (HK) *see* Diclofenac (Systemic) 617
Volulyte (CZ, DK) *see* Tetrastarch 2019
Volumin (IN) *see* Albumin 67
Voluven (AR, AU, BH, CH, CL, CN, CY, EE, FI, FR, GR, HK, HN, HR, ID, IL, IS, JP, KR, LT, MY, NL, NO, NZ, PH, QA, RO, SA, SE, SG, SI, SK, TH, TW, UY) *see* Tetrastarch 2019
Vomaine (PH) *see* Metoclopramide 1345
Vomceran (ID) *see* Ondansetron 1513
Vomerin (ID) *see* Domperidone [CAN/INT] 666
Vometa FT (MY) *see* Domperidone [CAN/INT] 666
Vometa (ID, PH) *see* Domperidone [CAN/INT] 666
Vometron (ID) *see* Ondansetron 1513
Vomidrine (PT) *see* DimenhyDRINATE 637
Vomina (VN) *see* DimenhyDRINATE 637
Vomiof (IN) *see* Ondansetron 1513
Vomiseda (TW) *see* Meclizine 1277
Vomisin (MX) *see* DimenhyDRINATE 637
Vomitil-M (TH) *see* Domperidone [CAN/INT] 666
Vomitil (PK) *see* Domperidone [CAN/INT] 666
Vomizole (ID) *see* Pantoprazole 1570
Vomiz (TW) *see* Ondansetron 1513
Voncento (CZ, DE, EE, GB, SE) *see* Antihemophilic Factor/von Willebrand Factor Complex (Human) 154
Voncon (GR) *see* Vancomycin 2130
Vopar (HK, TH) *see* Benserazide and Levodopa [CAN/INT] 244
V-Optic (IL) *see* Timolol (Ophthalmic) 2043
Vorange (HK, MY, SG) *see* Ascorbic Acid 178
Voraxaze (SG) *see* Glucarpidase 971
Vorcum (VE) *see* Voriconazole 2176
Voren (PH, TW) *see* Diclofenac (Systemic) 617
Vornal (HR) *see* Voriconazole 2176
Vorotal (TW) *see* Levofloxacin (Systemic) 1197
Vorth-TP (IN) *see* Tapentadol 1975
Vosol (NZ) *see* Acetic Acid 39
Votalen SR (NZ) *see* Diclofenac (Systemic) 617
Votalin (CN) *see* Diclofenac (Systemic) 617
Votan (PH) *see* Diclofenac (Systemic) 617
Votan SR (PH) *see* Diclofenac (Systemic) 617
Votmine (MY) *see* DimenhyDRINATE 637
Votrex (AE) *see* Diclofenac (Systemic) 617
Votrient (AR, AT, AU, BE, BR, CH, CL, CY, CZ, DE, DK, EE, FR, GB, HK, HR, ID, IE, IL, IN, IS, JP, KR, LT, MX, MY, NL, NO, NZ, PE, PH, PL, PT, QA, RO, SA, SE, SG, SK, TH, TR) *see* PAZOPanib 1584
Vottrient (SI) *see* PAZOPanib 1584
Votubia (CH, CY, CZ, DE, DK, EE, ES, FR, GB, NO, SE) *see* Everolimus 822
Votum (CH, DE) *see* Olmesartan 1496
Voveran (IN) *see* Diclofenac (Ophthalmic) 621
Voveran (IN) *see* Diclofenac (Systemic) 617
Voxam (AU) *see* FluvoxaMINE 916
Voxamin (CO) *see* FluvoxaMINE 916
Voxamine (PH) *see* FluvoxaMINE 916
Voxitin (AE, BH, CY, EG, IL, IQ, IR, JO, KW, LB, LY, OM, QA, SA, SY, YE) *see* CefOXitin 386
Voxytane (MY) *see* Oxybutynin 1536
VP-Gen (EC, PY) *see* Etoposide 816
VPRIV (AU) *see* Velaglucerase Alfa 2147
Vpriv (BE, CH, CY, CZ, DE, DK, EE, FR, HR, IE, IL, LT, NL, NO, PL, PT, SE, SI, SK, TR) *see* Velaglucerase Alfa 2147
VP-TEC (MX) *see* Etoposide 816
Vrinone (AE) *see* Progesterone 1722
Vuclodir (PY) *see* LamiVUDine 1157
Vulamox (ID) *see* Amoxicillin and Clavulanate 133
Vulcasid (MX) *see* Omeprazole 1508
Vulketan[vet.] (AT, CH) *see* Ketanserin [INT] 1144
Vulmizolin (CZ) *see* CeFAZolin 373
Vulsivan (CO) *see* CarBAMazepine 346
Vultin 600 (TH) *see* Gabapentin 943
Vultin (HK, TH) *see* Gabapentin 943
Vuminix (MX) *see* FluvoxaMINE 916
Vumon (AR, AT, AU, BE, BG, CH, CN, CZ, ES, GR, HN, HU, IT, KR, LU, MX, NL, NO, PL, PT, UY, VN, ZA) *see* Teniposide 1997
Vurdon (AE, BF, BH, BJ, CI, CY, EG, ET, GH, GM, GN, IQ, IR, JO, KE, KW, LB, LR, LY, MA, ML, MR, MU, MW, NE, NG, OM, QA, SA, SC, SD, SL, SN, SY, TN, TZ, UG, YE, ZM, ZW) *see* Diclofenac (Systemic) 617
V-Van Plus (KR) *see* Valsartan and Hydrochlorothiazide 2129
Vytorin (AR, AT, AU, BR, CN, CR, EC, ES, GR, GT, HK, HN, ID, IS, KR, MX, MY, NI, NZ, PA, PE, PH, SG, SI, SK, SV, TH, TW, UY, VE, VN) *see* Ezetimibe and Simvastatin 834
Vytral (MX) *see* Folic Acid, Cyanocobalamin, and Pyridoxine 921
Vytral (MX) *see* Zinc Sulfate 2200
Vyview Top (HK) *see* Chloramphenicol 421
V-Z Vax (PH) *see* Varicella Virus Vaccine 2141
Wakaflavin-L (JP) *see* Riboflavin 1803
Waklert (IN) *see* Armodafinil 175
Walacort (IN) *see* Betamethasone (Systemic) 253
Walaphage (IN) *see* MetFORMIN 1307
Walix (IT) *see* Oxaprozin 1532
Wanidine (TW) *see* QuiNIDine 1759
Waran (SE) *see* Warfarin 2186
Warazix (JP) *see* HydrOXYzine 1024
Warca (TH) *see* Mebendazole [CAN/INT] 1274
Warfant (TR) *see* Warfarin 2186
Warfar (CO, KR) *see* Warfarin 2186
Warfarina (PE) *see* Warfarin 2186
Warfil 5 (DO) *see* Warfarin 2186
Warfin (PL) *see* Warfarin 2186
Warik (PH) *see* Warfarin 2186
Wasserlax (ES) *see* Docusate 661
Waucoton (GR) *see* Propranolol 1731
Wax-Eze (HK) *see* Docusate 661
Waxsol (AU, GB, IE, LB, NZ) *see* Docusate 661
Wazole (TW) *see* Isoconazole [INT] 1120
Wecoli (TW) *see* Bethanechol 257
Weibamycin (TW) *see* Doxycycline 689
Weichilin (TW) *see* Ranitidine 1777

Weidos (TW) *see* Ranitidine 1777
Weifacodine (NO) *see* Pholcodine [INT] 1646
Weifa-Kalsium (NO) *see* Calcium Carbonate 327
Weihong (CN) *see* Azithromycin (Systemic) 216
Weijiangzhi (CN) *see* Gemfibrozil 956
Wei Lun (CN) *see* Gentamicin (Ophthalmic) 962
Weimok (TW) *see* Famotidine 845
WeiPing (CN) *see* Alfuzosin 84
Weisdin (TW) *see* Cimetidine 438
Weisida (CN) *see* Lafutidine [INT] 1157
Weisu (TW) *see* Sulindac 1953
Wei Tai (CN) *see* Itopride [INT] 1130
Weitul (TW) *see* Domperidone [CAN/INT] 666
Welchol (NO) *see* Colesevelam 503
We Li Ang (CL) *see* Phenylephrine (Systemic) 1638
Wellbutrin XL (BB, BH, BM, BS, CO, CR, EC, GT, HN, JM, KR, KW, PA, PE, TH, TW) *see* BuPROPion 305
Wellbutrin (MX, PE, PY, TW, VE) *see* BuPROPion 305
Wellbutrin Retard (IS, SK) *see* BuPROPion 305
Wellbutrin SR (AR, BB, BM, BS, CL, CR, DO, EC, GT, HK, HN, HU, JM, KR, MY, NI, PA, SG, SV, UY) *see* BuPROPion 305
Wellbutrin XR (CY, HR, IL, SI, TR) *see* BuPROPion 305
Wellcoprim (BE, FR, LU) *see* Trimethoprim 2104
Welldorm (GB) *see* Chloral Hydrate [CAN/INT] 418
Wellnara (JP) *see* Estradiol and Levonorgestrel 781
Wellparin (VN) *see* Heparin 997
Wellvone (AT, AU, BE, CH, DE, DK, ES, FR, GB, GR, IE, IT, NL, PT, SE, SI, ZA) *see* Atovaquone 197
Weltmine (KR) *see* Phentermine 1635
Wendica (VN) *see* Carbidopa and Levodopa 351
Wen Fei (CN) *see* Eszopiclone 793
Werdo (DE) *see* Riboflavin 1803
Wergen (TW) *see* Cimetidine 438
Wesfalin (AR) *see* Acebutolol 29
Wesipin (TW) *see* Atenolol 189
Westcort (KR) *see* Hydrocortisone (Topical) 1014
Westenicol (MX) *see* Chloramphenicol 421
Westhidroxo (MX) *see* Hydroxocobalamin 1020
White-C (PH) *see* Filgrastim 875
Wick Formula 44 Plus L (PL) *see* GuaiFENesin 986
Widahes-130 (ID) *see* Hetastarch 1004
Widahes (ID) *see* Hetastarch 1004
Widecillin (ID) *see* Amoxicillin 130
Wilate (AU, EE, MX, UY) *see* Antihemophilic Factor/von Willebrand Factor Complex (Human) 154
Willlong (LU) *see* Nitroglycerin 1465
Willmon-100 (HK) *see* Sildenafil 1882
Wilnativ (DK) *see* Antihemophilic Factor/von Willebrand Factor Complex (Human) 154
Wilopres Plus (PH) *see* Losartan and Hydrochlorothiazide 1250
Wilovex (PH) *see* Levofloxacin (Systemic) 1197
Wilprafen (CZ, DE, HU, LU, RU) *see* Josamycin [INT] 1141
Wilzin (AT, BE, CH, CZ, DE, DK, EE, FI, FR, GB, GR, HN, HR, IE, IT, MT, NL, NO, PL, PT, RO, RU, SE, SK, TR, TW) *see* Zinc Acetate 2199
Wimotin (KR) *see* Mosapride [INT] 1401
Winadeine (EC) *see* Acetaminophen and Codeine 36
Winadeine F (EC) *see* Acetaminophen and Codeine 36
Winadol (CO, VE) *see* Acetaminophen 32
Winadol Forte (CO) *see* Acetaminophen and Codeine 36
Winaflox (PH) *see* Norfloxacin 1475
Winasorb (CR, DO, GT, HN, NI, PA, SV) *see* Acetaminophen 32
Winbutol (TW) *see* Ethambutol 798
Wincef (TW) *see* Cefadroxil 372
Wincocef (PH) *see* Cefadroxil 372
Windol (TW) *see* Nalidixic Acid [INT] 1418
Winex (AE, KW, LB, QA, SA) *see* Cefixime 380
Winglore (AU) *see* Ipilimumab 1106
Wingora (PH) *see* Sildenafil 1882
Winiful (TW) *see* Famotidine 845
Winleril (TW) *see* Thioridazine 2030
Winlex (TW) *see* Cephalexin 405
Winlomylon (BF, BJ, CI, ET, GH, GM, GN, KE, LR, MA, ML, MR, MU, MW, NE, NG, SC, SD, SL, SN, TN, TZ, UG, ZA, ZM, ZW) *see* Nalidixic Acid [INT] 1418
Winobanin (DE) *see* Danazol 558
Winpen (BF, BJ, CI, ET, GH, GM, GN, KE, LR, MA, ML, MR, MU, MW, NE, NG, SC, SD, SL, SN, TN, TZ, UG, ZM, ZW) *see* Amoxicillin 130
Winpicillin (TW) *see* Ampicillin 141
Winpress (TW) *see* CloNIDine 480
WinRho SDF (AU, IL, PH) *see* Rh_o(D) Immune Globulin 1794
Winsepal (TW) *see* Rosiglitazone 1847
Winstop 30 (TW) *see* Ethinyl Estradiol and Levonorgestrel 803
Winstop T/28 (TW) *see* Ethinyl Estradiol and Levonorgestrel 803
Winsumin (TW) *see* ChlorproMAZINE 429
Wintel (TW) *see* Tetracycline 2017
Wintomilon (PT) *see* Nalidixic Acid [INT] 1418
Wintomylon (AR, BF, BJ, BR, CI, CO, EC, ET, GH, GM, GN, KE, LR, MA, ML, MR, MU, MW, MX, MY, NE, NG, PE, SC, SD, SL, SN, TH, TN, TZ, UG, ZM, ZW) *see* Nalidixic Acid [INT] 1418
Wintron (JP) *see* Nalidixic Acid [INT] 1418
Wintyl (TW) *see* Dicyclomine 622
Witgen (TW) *see* Memantine 1286
Withamycin (TW) *see* Doxycycline 689
Woncare (PH) *see* Fusidic Acid (Topical) [CAN/INT] 943
Wonclor (KR) *see* Cefaclor 372
Wonmp (KR) *see* Omeprazole 1508
Wormazol (AE, BH, QA, SA) *see* Mebendazole [CAN/INT] 1274
Wormgo (ZA) *see* Mebendazole [CAN/INT] 1274
Wormicide (TH) *see* Praziquantel 1702
Wormin (AE, BF, BH, BJ, CI, CY, EG, ET, GH, GM, GN, IN, IQ, IR, JO, KE, KW, LB, LR, LY, MA, ML, MR, MU, MW, NE, NG, OM, QA, SA, SC, SD, SL, SN, SY, TN, TZ, UG, YE, ZM, ZW) *see* Mebendazole [CAN/INT] 1274
Wosulin 30/70 (PH) *see* Insulin NPH and Insulin Regular 1090
Wosulin 70/30 (BR) *see* Insulin NPH and Insulin Regular 1090
Wosulin-N (PH) *see* Insulin NPH 1089
Wosulin R (BR) *see* Insulin Regular 1091
Wycillina A P (IT) *see* Penicillin G Benzathine 1609
Wydora (DE) *see* Indoramin [INT] 1070
Wydox (PH) *see* Oxacillin 1528
Wyeth-Ayerst HRF (AU) *see* Gonadorelin [CAN/INT] 980
Wymesone (IN) *see* Dexamethasone (Systemic) 599
Wypresin (AT) *see* Indoramin [INT] 1070
Wystamm (FR) *see* Rupatadine [INT] 1855
Wytens (FR) *see* Bisoprolol and Hydrochlorothiazide 267
Xacin (TH) *see* Norfloxacin 1475
Xadosin XL (TW) *see* Doxazosin 674
Xadosin (TW) *see* Doxazosin 674
Xafon (CN) *see* Lornoxicam [INT] 1248
Xagrid (AT, BE, CH, CZ, DE, DK, EE, ES, FI, FR, GB, GR, HN, HR, IE, IS, IT, LT, MT, NL, NO, PL, PT, RO, RU, SE, SK, TR) *see* Anagrelide 147
Xalacom (AE, AR, AT, AU, BE, BH, BR, BZ, CH, CL, CN, CO, CY, CZ, DE, DK, EE, FR, GB, GR, HK, HN, HR, ID, IE, IL, IN, IT, JO, JP, KR, KW, LB, LT, MY, NL, NZ, PE, PH, PL, PT, QA, RU, SA, SE, SG, SI, SK, TH, TR, TW, UY, VE, VN, ZA) *see* Latanoprost and Timolol [CAN/INT] 1172
Xalar (DO, GT, PA, SV) *see* Montelukast 1392
Xalatan (AE, AR, AT, AU, BE, BG, BH, BO, BR, CH, CL, CN, CO, CY, CZ, DE, DK, EC, EE, EG, ES, FI, FR, GB, GR, HK, HR, HU, ID, IE, IL, IN, IQ, IR, IS, IT, JO, KR,

KW, LB, LT, LY, MX, MY, NL, NO, NZ, OM, PE, PH, PK, PL, PR, PT, QA, RO, RU, SA, SE, SG, SI, SK, SY, TH, TR, TW, VE, VN, YE, ZA) *see* Latanoprost ... 1172
Xalavist (PH) *see* Latanoprost ... 1172
Xalavist Plus (PH) *see* Latanoprost and Timolol [CAN/INT] ... 1172
Xalcom (FI, IS, RO) *see* Latanoprost and Timolol [CAN/INT] ... 1172
Xalecin (TH) *see* Levofloxacin (Systemic) ... 1197
Xalexa (VN) *see* PARoxetine ... 1579
Xalgetz (VN) *see* Tamsulosin ... 1974
Xaliplat (PY) *see* Oxaliplatin ... 1528
Xalkori (AR, AU, BE, CH, CN, CY, CZ, DE, DK, EE, ES, FR, GB, HK, HR, ID, IE, IL, IS, JP, KR, MY, NL, NO, QA, RO, SA, SE, SG, SI, SK, TH, TR) *see* Crizotinib ... 511
Xaluprine (GB, HR) *see* Mercaptopurine ... 1296
Xalvobin (HR) *see* Capecitabine ... 339
Xalyn-Or (MX) *see* Amoxicillin ... 130
Xamamina (IT) *see* DimenhyDRINATE ... 637
Xambrex (PH) *see* Ambroxol [INT] ... 109
Xamiol (AT, AU, BE, BG, CH, CN, CY, CZ, DE, DK, EE, ES, FI, FR, GR, HK, IL, IT, KR, KW, LB, LT, MY, NL, PH, PL, PT, QA, SE, SG, SI, SK, TH, TW, VN) *see* Calcipotriene and Betamethasone ... 321
Xamiol (GB) *see* Calcipotriene ... 321
Xanacine (TH) *see* ALPRAZolam ... 94
Xanaes (AR) *see* Azelastine (Ophthalmic) ... 213
Xanagis (IL) *see* ALPRAZolam ... 94
Xanax (AE, AR, AU, BB, BE, BF, BG, BH, BJ, BM, BS, BZ, CH, CI, CO, CY, CZ, DE, EE, EG, ET, FR, GB, GH, GM, GN, GR, GY, HK, HR, HU, IE, IQ, IR, IT, JM, JO, KE, KW, LB, LR, LT, LU, LY, MA, ML, MR, MU, MW, MY, NE, NG, NL, NZ, OM, PE, PK, PL, PT, QA, RO, RU, SA, SC, SD, SI, SK, SL, SN, SR, SY, TH, TN, TR, TT, TW, TZ, UG, VN, YE, ZM, ZW) *see* ALPRAZolam ... 94
Xanax SR (BG, SG) *see* ALPRAZolam ... 94
Xanax XR (IL, KW, LT, RO, TH, TW) *see* ALPRAZolam ... 94
Xandase (TH) *see* Allopurinol ... 90
Xanef (DE) *see* Enalapril ... 722
Xanidine (SG, TH) *see* Ranitidine ... 1777
Xanol (TH) *see* Allopurinol ... 90
Xanomel (HU) *see* Ranitidine ... 1777
Xanor (AT, FI, NO, PH, SE, ZA) *see* ALPRAZolam ... 94
Xanor XR (PH) *see* ALPRAZolam ... 94
Xanthium (LU) *see* Theophylline ... 2026
Xantomicin Forte (PY) *see* Indomethacin ... 1067
Xantor (PH) *see* AtorvaSTATin ... 194
Xantromid (PY) *see* Methotrexate ... 1322
Xanturenasi (IT) *see* Pyridoxine ... 1747
Xanurace (PH) *see* Allopurinol ... 90
Xarelto (AE, AR, AU, BB, BE, BM, BR, BS, BZ, CH, CL, CN, CO, CR, CY, CZ, DE, DK, DO, EC, EE, FR, GB, GR, GT, GY, HK, HN, HR, ID, IE, IL, IN, IS, IT, JM, JP, KR, KW, LB, LT, MY, NI, NL, NO, NZ, PA, PE, PH, PL, PR, PT, QA, RO, SA, SE, SG, SI, SK, SR, SV, TH, TR, TT, TW, UY, VN) *see* Rivaroxaban ... 1830
Xarope 44E (BR) *see* Guaifenesin and Dextromethorphan ... 987
Xasmun (ES) *see* Nitrendipine [INT] ... 1463
Xasmun (ES) *see* Norfloxacin ... 1475
Xatalin (SE) *see* Azelastine and Fluticasone ... 214
Xatosin XL (KR) *see* Alfuzosin ... 84
Xatral XL (AE, BH, ID, IL, JO, KR, KW, LB, QA, TH, TR, TW) *see* Alfuzosin ... 84
Xatral XL PR (CY) *see* Alfuzosin ... 84
XAtral XL (SA) *see* Alfuzosin ... 84
Xatral (AE, AT, BE, BF, BH, BJ, CH, CI, CN, CZ, DK, ET, FI, FR, GB, GH, GM, GN, GR, IE, IL, IT, KE, KW, LB, LR, MA, ML, MR, MU, MW, NE, NG, NL, NO, PH, QA, SA, SC, SD, SE, SL, SN, TN, TR, TZ, UG, VN, ZA, ZM, ZW) *see* Alfuzosin ... 84
Xatral LP (BG, FR, HK, RO) *see* Alfuzosin ... 84
Xatral OD (BR, CO, CR, DO, EC, GT, HN, MX, NI, PA, PE, PH, PY, SE, SV, VE) *see* Alfuzosin ... 84
Xatral PR (LB) *see* Alfuzosin ... 84
Xatral SR (AE, AU, BH, CY, EE, EG, IL, LT, PK, RO, SA, SG, SK, TR) *see* Alfuzosin ... 84
Xatral XR 10 (SG) *see* Alfuzosin ... 84
Xazal (ES) *see* Levocetirizine ... 1196
Xebramol (TH) *see* Acetaminophen ... 32
Xedin (MX) *see* Cefotaxime ... 382
Xefo (AE, AR, AT, BG, BR, CH, DK, EG, GR, HU, IE, IL, KR, LB, LT, PL, RO, SA, SE, SI, SK, TH, TR, ZA) *see* Lornoxicam [INT] ... 1248
Xefocam (RU) *see* Lornoxicam [INT] ... 1248
Xefo Rapid (AR, BG, CZ, LT, RO, SI, SK) *see* Lornoxicam [INT] ... 1248
Xelent (PH) *see* Cefaclor ... 372
Xelevia (CZ, DE, EE, FR, GR, HR, LT, NL, PH, PT, RO, SK) *see* SitaGLIPtin ... 1897
Xeljanz (AR, CH, IL, JP, KR, MY, PH) *see* Tofacitinib ... 2059
Xelobig (KR) *see* Capecitabine ... 339
Xelocan (KR) *see* Capecitabine ... 339
Xeloda (AE, AR, AT, AU, BB, BE, BF, BG, BH, BJ, BM, BR, BS, BZ, CH, CI, CL, CN, CO, CY, CZ, DE, DK, EC, EE, ES, ET, FI, FR, GB, GH, GM, GN, GR, GY, HK, HN, HR, HU, ID, IE, IL, IS, IT, JM, JO, KE, KR, KW, LB, LR, LT, LU, MA, ML, MR, MT, MU, MW, MX, MY, NE, NG, NL, NO, NZ, PH, PK, PL, PT, PY, QA, RO, RU, SA, SC, SD, SE, SG, SI, SK, SL, SN, SR, TH, TN, TR, TT, TW, TZ, UG, UY, VE, VN, ZA, ZM, ZW) *see* Capecitabine ... 339
Xeltic (HK) *see* GlyBURIDE ... 972
Xeltic (TH) *see* GlipiZIDE ... 967
Xenalon Lactabs (DO) *see* Spironolactone ... 1931
Xenar (IT) *see* Naproxen ... 1427
Xenazina (IT) *see* Tetrabenazine ... 2016
Xenazine (FR, GB, IL, KR, LT, NL, NZ, SI, SK) *see* Tetrabenazine ... 2016
Xenical (AE, AR, AT, AU, BB, BE, BF, BG, BH, BJ, BM, BO, BR, BS, BZ, CH, CI, CL, CN, CO, CY, CZ, DE, DK, EC, EE, ES, ET, FI, FR, GB, GH, GM, GN, GR, GY, HK, HR, HU, ID, IE, IL, IS, IT, JM, KE, KR, KW, LB, LR, LT, MA, ML, MR, MT, MU, MW, MX, NE, NG, NL, NO, NZ, PE, PH, PK, PL, PR, PT, PY, QA, RO, RU, SA, SC, SD, SE, SG, SI, SK, SL, SN, SR, TH, TN, TR, TT, TW, TZ, UG, UY, VE, VN, ZA, ZM, ZW) *see* Orlistat ... 1520
Xenidate XL (GB) *see* Methylphenidate ... 1336
Xenifar (ID) *see* Naproxen ... 1427
Xenista (PH) *see* Orlistat ... 1520
Xenocy (ID) *see* AtoMOXetine ... 191
Xenoflox (PH) *see* Ciprofloxacin (Systemic) ... 441
Xenoma (RO) *see* RisperiDONE ... 1818
Xentor (PH) *see* AtorvaSTATin ... 194
Xeomeen (MX) *see* IncobotulinumtoxinA ... 1062
Xeomin (AR, AT, AU, BG, BR, CH, DE, DK, ES, FI, FR, GB, IT, KR, LT, NL, NO, PL, PT, RO, RU, SE, SG, SI, SK) *see* IncobotulinumtoxinA ... 1062
Xepabet (ID) *see* Gliclazide [CAN/INT] ... 964
Xepacycline (SG) *see* Tetracycline ... 2017
Xepafen (ID) *see* Ibuprofen ... 1032
Xepagan (MY) *see* Promethazine ... 1723
Xepalium (ID) *see* Flunarizine [CAN/INT] ... 892
Xepamet (ID, MY, SG) *see* Cimetidine ... 438
Xepanicol (HK, ID, SG) *see* Chloramphenicol ... 421
Xepaprim Forte (ID) *see* Sulfamethoxazole and Trimethoprim ... 1946
Xepaprim (ID) *see* Sulfamethoxazole and Trimethoprim ... 1946
Xepin (GB) *see* Doxepin (Topical) ... 678
Xeplion (CH, CY, CZ, DK, EE, GB, HR, IE, IL, IS, LT, RO, SE, SI, SK, TR) *see* Paliperidone ... 1556
Xeradin (ID) *see* Ranitidine ... 1777
Xerenal (AT) *see* Dosulepin [INT] ... 673

Xerendig (MX) *see* Somatropin 1918
Xergic (AU, NZ) *see* Fexofenadine 873
Xeristar (AT, BE, BG, CH, CZ, DE, DK, EE, ES, FI, FR, GB, HN, HR, IE, IT, MT, NL, NO, PL, RO, RU, SE, SK, TR) *see* DULoxetine 698
Xerxes (ID) *see* Imipenem and Cilastatin 1051
Xet 20 (PH) *see* PARoxetine 1579
Xetanor (BG) *see* PARoxetine 1579
Xetine-P (TW) *see* PARoxetine 1579
Xetin (PY) *see* Carvedilol 367
XET (TW) *see* PARoxetine 1579
Xevolac (PH) *see* Ketorolac (Systemic) 1146
Xex (EC) *see* Sildenafil 1882
Xfen Flashtab (PH) *see* Ibuprofen 1032
Xgeva (AR, AU, BE, CH, CY, CZ, DE, DK, EE, ES, FR, GB, HK, HR, IE, LT, MX, MY, NL, NO, NZ, PH, RO, SE, SG, SI, SK, TR) *see* Denosumab 589
Xiaflex (AU) *see* Collagenase (Systemic) 506
Xiapex (CH, CY, CZ, DK, EE, ES, FR, GB, HR, IE, NO, SE, TR) *see* Collagenase (Systemic) 506
Xibra-90 (PH) *see* Etoricoxib [INT] 821
Xicalom (ID) *see* Piroxicam 1662
Xicam (TH) *see* Piroxicam 1662
Xicard (PH) *see* Carvedilol 367
Xi Er Sheng (CN) *see* Selenium Sulfide 1877
Xiety (ID) *see* BusPIRone 311
Xie Yi Li (CN) *see* Riluzole 1812
Xifaxan (AU, DE, HK, NL, NZ, PL) *see* Rifaximin 1809
Xifaxanta (GB) *see* Rifaximin 1809
Xifen (PH) *see* Tamoxifen 1971
Xifia (RO) *see* Cefixime 380
Xigduo (CZ, DE, DK, EE, GB, HR, LT, NL, NO, SE, SI, SK) *see* Dapagliflozin and Metformin 561
Xigduo XR (AU) *see* Dapagliflozin and Metformin 561
Xilan (PY) *see* Rosiglitazone 1847
Xilbac (CO, EC) *see* Ampicillin and Sulbactam 145
Xilep XL (KR) *see* Fluvastatin 915
Xilep (KR) *see* Fluvastatin 915
Xilonest (PE) *see* Lidocaine and Epinephrine 1212
Xilonest (PE) *see* Lidocaine (Systemic) 1208
Xilonest (PE) *see* Lidocaine (Topical) 1211
Xilopar (DE) *see* Selegiline 1873
Xilotane Oral (PT) *see* Lidocaine (Topical) 1211
Xilox (HU) *see* Nimesulide [INT] 1456
Ximede (ID) *see* Nimesulide [INT] 1456
Ximino (BM) *see* Minocycline 1371
Ximovan (DE) *see* Zopiclone [CAN/INT] 2217
Xin Hong Kang (CN) *see* Erythromycin (Systemic) 762
Xin Ke Fei (CN) *see* Nadifloxacin [INT] 1411
Xin Luo Shu (CN) *see* Emtricitabine 720
Xintoprost (AR) *see* VinBLAStine 2160
Xin Yu Sen (CN) *see* Labetalol 1151
Xipamid (IN) *see* Xipamide [INT] 2191
Xipen (MX) *see* Pentoxifylline 1618
Xismox XL (GB) *see* Isosorbide Mononitrate 1126
Xithrone (AE, BH, CY, EG, IQ, IR, JO, KW, LB, LY, OM, QA, SA, SY, YE) *see* Azithromycin (Systemic) 216
Xitocin (MX) *see* Oxytocin 1549
Xizhixin (CN) *see* Lansoprazole 1166
XL-Dol Infantil (MX) *see* Acetaminophen 32
Xola (AE, BH, KW, SA) *see* Dorzolamide 673
Xolair (AE, AR, AT, AU, BE, BG, BR, CH, CL, CO, CY, CZ, DE, DK, EC, EE, ES, FI, FR, GB, GR, HK, HN, HR, HU, ID, IE, IL, IS, IT, JO, JP, KR, KW, LB, LT, MT, MY, NL, NO, NZ, PE, PH, PL, PT, QA, RO, RU, SA, SE, SG, SI, SK, TH, TR, TW, VE) *see* Omalizumab 1503
Xolamin (JP) *see* Clemastine 459
Xolamol (AE, BH, JO, KW, SA) *see* Dorzolamide and Timolol 673
Xolof D (EC) *see* Tobramycin and Dexamethasone 2056
Xolvax (VE) *see* Ambroxol [INT] 109
Xon-ce (ID) *see* Ascorbic Acid 178
Xoprin (PE) *see* Omeprazole 1508
Xorimax (HK, LB, MY, PH, SG) *see* Cefuroxime 399
Xorim (LB) *see* Cefuroxime 399
Xorufec (MX) *see* Cefuroxime 399
Xotepic (PL) *see* Pantoprazole 1570
Xozal (GR) *see* Levocetirizine 1196
Xpandyl (GT) *see* Tadalafil 1968
XSM (CN) *see* Loratadine 1241
Xsom (PH) *see* Esomeprazole 771
X'Tac (MY) *see* Ranitidine 1777
Xtandi (CH, CY, CZ, DE, DK, EE, FR, GB, HR, IS, JP, LT, NL, NO, RO, SE, SI, SK, TR) *see* Enzalutamide 733
Xtandi SC (KR) *see* Enzalutamide 733
Xtane (IN) *see* Exemestane 828
Xtenda (PH) *see* CefTRIAXone 396
X-Trant (IN) *see* Estramustine 782
Xue Qing (CN) *see* Lovastatin 1252
Xun Ao (CN) *see* Prulifloxacin [INT] 1742
Xusal (DE, MX) *see* Levocetirizine 1196
Xuzal (EC) *see* Levocetirizine 1196
Xycam (ZA) *see* Piroxicam 1662
Xyclomed (PH) *see* Cyclophosphamide 517
Xydap (IN) *see* Dapoxetine [INT] 561
Xydep (AU) *see* Sertraline 1878
Xylanaest Mit Epinephrin (AT) *see* Lidocaine and Epinephrine 1212
Xylistin (IN) *see* Colistimethate 504
Xylocain-Adrenalin (DK, NO) *see* Lidocaine and Epinephrine 1212
Xylocain Adrenalin (FI, IS, SE) *see* Lidocaine and Epinephrine 1212
Xylocain Aerosol (DK, SE) *see* Lidocaine (Topical) 1211
Xylocaina Ointment (IT) *see* Lidocaine (Topical) 1211
Xylocaina Pomada (AR) *see* Lidocaine (Topical) 1211
Xylocaina Spray (CO, IT) *see* Lidocaine (Topical) 1211
Xylocaine IV (TW) *see* Lidocaine (Systemic) 1208
Xylocaine Adrenaline (AE, BH, EG, JO, NL, SA, SK) *see* Lidocaine and Epinephrine 1212
Xylocaine (AE, BH, CY, JO, KW, NZ, QA, SA) *see* Lidocaine (Systemic) 1208
Xylocaine Aerosol (AU, HK, NL) *see* Lidocaine (Topical) 1211
Xylocaine Gel (AE, BE, BH, CY, EG, FR, GR, IE, IQ, IR, JO, KW, LB, LY, OM, PK, QA, SA, SY, YE) *see* Lidocaine (Topical) 1211
Xylocaine Jalea (UY) *see* Lidocaine (Topical) 1211
Xylocaine Jelly (BF, BJ, CI, ET, GH, GM, GN, HK, ID, IN, KE, LR, MA, ML, MR, MU, MW, NE, NG, NZ, PH, SC, SD, SG, SL, SN, TH, TN, TW, TZ, UG, VN, ZM, ZW) *see* Lidocaine (Topical) 1211
Xylocaine met Adrenaline (BE) *see* Lidocaine and Epinephrine 1212
Xylocaine Ointment (AE, AU, BF, BH, BJ, CI, CY, EG, ET, GH, GM, GN, GR, IN, IQ, IR, JO, KE, KW, LB, LR, LY, MA, ML, MR, MU, MW, MY, NE, NG, NL, NZ, OM, PH, QA, SA, SC, SD, SL, SN, SY, TN, TZ, UG, YE, ZM, ZW) *see* Lidocaine (Topical) 1211
Xylocain-Epinephrin (AT) *see* Lidocaine and Epinephrine 1212
Xylocaine Pump Spray (AU, EE) *see* Lidocaine (Topical) 1211
Xylocaine (SI) *see* Lidocaine (Topical) 1211
Xylocaine Spray (BE, BF, BJ, CI, ET, GB, GH, GM, GN, GR, HK, ID, IL, KE, KR, LR, MA, ML, MR, MU, MW, MY, NE, NG, NL, PH, PL, SC, SD, SG, SL, SN, TH, TN, TW, TZ, UG, ZA, ZM, ZW) *see* Lidocaine (Topical) 1211
Xylocaine Topical Solution (AE, BH, CY, EG, IQ, IR, JO, KW, LB, LY, OM, QA, SA, SY, YE) *see* Lidocaine (Topical) 1211
Xylocaine Viscosa (PY) *see* Lidocaine (Topical) 1211

Xylocaine Viscous (GB, IE, IN, MY, TH) *see* Lidocaine (Topical) 1211
Xylocaine Viscous Topical Solution (AU, GB) *see* Lidocaine (Topical) 1211
Xylocaine Viscus (GR) *see* Lidocaine (Topical) 1211
Xylocaine Viskeus Topical Solution (NL) *see* Lidocaine (Topical) 1211
Xylocaine w Adrenaline (HK) *see* Lidocaine and Epinephrine 1212
Xylocaine with Adrenaline (AU, BF, BJ, CI, ET, GH, GM, GN, IN, KE, LR, MA, ML, MR, MU, MW, NE, NG, SC, SD, SL, SN, TN, TZ, UG, ZM, ZW) *see* Lidocaine and Epinephrine 1212
Xylocain Gel (AT, CH, DE, DK, FI, NO, SE) *see* Lidocaine (Topical) 1211
Xylocain (IS) *see* Lidocaine (Topical) 1211
Xylocain Liniment (DK) *see* Lidocaine (Topical) 1211
Xylocain Ointment (AT, CH, DE, FI) *see* Lidocaine (Topical) 1211
Xylocain Salve (DK) *see* Lidocaine (Topical) 1211
Xylocain Spray (AT, CH, DE, NO) *see* Lidocaine (Topical) 1211
Xylocain Viscous (AT, CH) *see* Lidocaine (Topical) 1211
Xylocain Viskos (DE, SE) *see* Lidocaine (Topical) 1211
Xylocain Visks (FI) *see* Lidocaine (Topical) 1211
Xylocard (AT, AU, BE, FR, IN, IS, NO, NZ, SE, SG, VN) *see* Lidocaine (Systemic) 1208
Xylodent (IL) *see* Chlorhexidine Gluconate 422
Xyloderm (MX) *see* Neomycin 1436
Xylo-Efa 10% Cardiologica (UY) *see* Lidocaine (Systemic) 1208
Xylonol (TW) *see* Allopurinol 90
Xylorane (MX) *see* Citalopram 451
Xyntha (AR, AU, CL, KR, NZ, SA, SG, TW) *see* Antihemophilic Factor (Recombinant) 152
Xyrem (AT, BE, BG, CH, CY, CZ, DE, DK, EE, ES, FI, FR, GB, GR, HN, IE, IT, MT, NL, NO, PL, PT, RU, SE, SK, TR) *see* Sodium Oxybate 1908
Xyvion (AU) *see* Tibolone [INT] 2035
Xyzal (AE, AU, BG, BH, CH, CN, CY, CZ, DE, DK, EE, FI, FR, GB, HK, HR, HU, ID, IE, IT, JP, KR, KW, LB, LT, MY, NL, NO, PH, PL, PT, QA, RO, RU, SA, SE, SG, SI, SK, TH, TR, TW, VN) *see* Levocetirizine 1196
Xyzall (AT, BE) *see* Levocetirizine 1196
Xyzine (TW) *see* Levocetirizine 1196
8Y (ID) *see* Antihemophilic Factor (Human) 152
Yadim (HK) *see* CefTAZidime 392
Yafix (ID) *see* Cefixime 380
Yaila (KR) *see* Vardenafil 2138
Yal (CZ) *see* Docusate 661
Ya Li (CN) *see* Azosemide [INT] 220
Yalone (ID) *see* MethylPREDNISolone 1340
Yamatetan (JP, KR) *see* CefoTEtan 385
Yantil (NL) *see* Tapentadol 1975
Yantil Retard (NL) *see* Tapentadol 1975
Yaridon (ID) *see* Domperidone [CAN/INT] 666
Yarina (RU) *see* Ethinyl Estradiol and Drospirenone 801
Yarox (ID) *see* Cefpirome [INT] 388
Yasmin (AR, AT, AU, BB, BH, BM, BR, BS, BZ, CH, CL, CN, CO, CR, CY, DE, DK, DO, EC, ES, FI, GB, GT, GY, HK, HN, HR, ID, IE, IL, IN, IS, IT, JM, KR, KW, LB, MX, MY, NI, NL, NO, NZ, PA, PE, PH, PL, PR, PT, PY, QA, RO, SA, SE, SG, SR, SV, TH, TR, TT, TW, UY, VE, VN, ZA) *see* Ethinyl Estradiol and Drospirenone 801
Yasminelle (BE, CH, CZ, DE, EE, LT, NO, PL, PT, SI, SK) *see* Ethinyl Estradiol and Drospirenone 801
Yasmin IQ (PE) *see* Ethinyl Estradiol and Drospirenone 801
Yasnal (HR) *see* Donepezil 668
Yax Femicare (GT) *see* Ethinyl Estradiol and Drospirenone 801
YAZ (AU, BB, BG, BM, BS, BZ, CR, DO, EC, GT, GY, HK, HN, ID, IL, JM, KR, MY, NI, NL, NZ, PA, PH, PR, SG, SR, SV, TH, TT, TW) *see* Ethinyl Estradiol and Drospirenone 801
Yaz (CY, HR, IS, JP, KW, LB, LT, PY, QA, RO, SI, VN) *see* Ethinyl Estradiol and Drospirenone 801
Yaz Metafolin (AR) *see* Ethinyl Estradiol, Drospirenone, and Levomefolate 812
Yeastazol (PH) *see* Clotrimazole (Topical) 488
Yectamid (MX) *see* Amikacin 111
Yellox (CH, CZ, DE, DK, EE, ES, FR, GB, HR, LT, NL, NO, RO, SE, SI, SK) *see* Bromfenac 291
Yeloshu (CN) *see* Reboxetine [INT] 1786
Yentreve (AE, AT, BE, BG, CH, CL, CZ, DE, DK, EE, ES, FI, FR, GB, HN, HR, IE, IL, IT, MT, MX, NL, NO, NZ, PL, RU, SE, SK, TR) *see* DULoxetine 698
Yentuogin (TW) *see* Bacitracin, Neomycin, and Polymyxin B 223
Yervoy (AR, AU, BE, CH, CL, CY, CZ, DE, DK, EE, FR, GB, HR, IE, IL, IS, LT, MX, NL, NO, NZ, RO, SE, SI, SK, TR) *see* Ipilimumab 1106
Yesan (GR) *see* Timolol (Ophthalmic) 2043
Yi Du (CN) *see* Phenazopyridine 1629
Yifen (CN) *see* Flucloxacillin [INT] 885
Yi Han Ning (CN) *see* DimenhyDRINATE 637
Yiheng (CN) *see* Quinapril 1756
Yihfu (TW) *see* Clobetasol 468
Yi Ke Long (CN) *see* Docusate 661
Yilin (CN) *see* Etidronate 813
Yingtaiqing (CN) *see* Diclofenac (Systemic) 617
YiPing (CN) *see* Acipimox [INT] 43
Yi Pu Li (CN) *see* Epoetin Alfa 742
Yi Sheng Bao Er (CN) *see* Rabies Immune Globulin (Human) 1764
Yi Shuang (CN) *see* Enalapril and Hydrochlorothiazide 725
YiTing (CN) *see* Piracetam [INT] 1661
Yi Xing (CN) *see* Oprelvekin 1519
Yi You Ning (CN) *see* Nadifloxacin [INT] 1411
Ylox (AR) *see* Minoxidil (Topical) 1374
Ymana (HR) *see* Memantine 1286
Yo'Come Penney (TW) *see* Charcoal, Activated 416
Yong Xi (CN) *see* Doxycycline 689
Yonistib (RO) *see* Bicalutamide 262
Youbaifen (CN) *see* Dexketoprofen [INT] 603
Youbiqing (CN) *see* Imiquimod 1055
You Care (TW) *see* Imiquimod 1055
Youfei (CN) *see* Oxazepam 1532
You-Jet (TW) *see* Sertraline 1878
You Jia (CN) *see* AtorvaSTATin 194
You Ke Xin (CL) *see* Secnidazole [INT] 1872
Youlifu (CN) *see* Crotamiton 514
Youngproma (KR) *see* Procyclidine [CAN/INT] 1721
Youtong (CN) *see* Leflunomide 1174
Youzhouer (CN) *see* Hydrocortisone (Topical) 1014
Ysomega (FR) *see* Omega-3 Fatty Acids 1507
Yucomy (MY, VN) *see* Ketoconazole (Topical) 1145
Yuhan-Zid (KR) *see* Isoniazid 1120
Yuma (KR) *see* Hydroxychloroquine 1021
Yungken (TW) *see* FlavoxATE 881
Yunir (MX) *see* Pinazepam [INT] 1652
Yuredol (MX) *see* Cyclobenzaprine 516
Yurelax (ES, MX) *see* Cyclobenzaprine 516
Yuren (TW) *see* Diclofenac (Systemic) 617
Yvermil (PY) *see* Ivermectin (Systemic) 1136
Yylofen (VN) *see* Baclofen 223
Zaart-H (IN) *see* Losartan and Hydrochlorothiazide 1250
Zaart (HK) *see* Losartan 1248
Zabak (RO) *see* Ketotifen (Ophthalmic) 1150
Zabel (AU) *see* Terbinafine (Systemic) 2002
Zacafemyl (MX) *see* Mifepristone 1366
Zacetin (KR) *see* ALPRAZolam 94
ZAC (ID) *see* FLUoxetine 899

Zactin (AU, SG, TW) *see* FLUoxetine 899
Zactos (MX) *see* Pioglitazone 1654
Zadec (PH) *see* Ketotifen (Systemic) [CAN/INT] 1149
Zadec SRO (PH) *see* Ketotifen (Systemic) [CAN/INT] 1149
Zadim (PH) *see* CefTAZidime 392
Zadin (KR) *see* Ketotifen (Systemic) [CAN/INT] 1149
Zaditen (AE, AR, AT, AU, BB, BF, BG, BH, BJ, BM, BR, BS, BZ, CH, CI, CL, CO, CY, CZ, DE, DK, EC, EE, EG, ES, ET, FI, FR, GB, GH, GM, GN, GY, HK, HN, HU, IE, IL, IQ, IR, IS, IT, JM, JO, KE, KW, LB, LR, LU, LY, MA, ML, MR, MT, MU, MW, MX, MY, NE, NG, NL, NO, NZ, OM, PE, PH, PL, PT, PY, QA, RO, RU, SA, SC, SD, SE, SG, SI, SK, SL, SN, SR, SY, TH, TN, TR, TT, TW, TZ, UG, UY, VN, YE, ZM, ZW) *see* Ketotifen (Ophthalmic) 1150
Zaditen (AE, AR, AT, AU, BE, BF, BG, BH, BJ, BR, CH, CI, CO, CY, CZ, DE, DK, EC, EG, ET, FI, FR, GB, GH, GM, GN, GR, HK, HN, ID, IE, IL, IQ, IR, IT, JO, KE, KR, KW, LB, LR, LY, MA, ML, MR, MT, MU, MW, MY, NE, NG, NL, NO, NZ, OM, PE, PH, PL, PT, PY, QA, RU, SA, SC, SD, SE, SG, SK, SL, SN, SY, TH, TN, TR, TW, TZ, UG, UY, VE, YE, ZM, ZW) *see* Ketotifen (Systemic) [CAN/INT] 1149
Zaditen SDU (HK, TH) *see* Ketotifen (Systemic) [CAN/INT] 1149
Zadolina (MX) *see* CefTAZidime 392
Zadomen (MY) *see* Mebendazole [CAN/INT] 1274
Zadorin (BB, BF, BH, BJ, BM, BS, BZ, CI, CY, EG, ET, GH, GM, GN, GY, IQ, IR, JM, JO, KE, KW, LB, LR, LY, MA, ML, MR, MU, MW, NE, NG, OM, QA, SA, SC, SD, SL, SN, SR, SY, TN, TT, TZ, UG, YE, ZM, ZW) *see* Doxycycline 689
Zafibral (JO, SG) *see* Bezafibrate [CAN/INT] 261
Zafin (EC, PY) *see* Acetaminophen and Tramadol 37
Zafiron (PL) *see* Formoterol 926
Zafular (VN) *see* Bezafibrate [CAN/INT] 261
Zagam (CH, DE, FR, HK, LU, NZ, PH, PL) *see* Sparfloxacin [INT] 1930
Zaike (CN) *see* Cefaclor 372
Zakol (PE) *see* Latanoprost 1172
Zakol T (PE) *see* Latanoprost and Timolol [CAN/INT] 1172
Zalain (AR, BG, BO, CL, CN, CO, CR, CZ, DE, DO, EC, GT, HK, HN, MX, NI, PA, PE, PL, PR, PY, RU, SG, SV, TH, TR, TW, UY, VE) *see* Sertaconazole 1877
Zalain Cream (SG) *see* Sertaconazole 1877
Zalconex (KR) *see* Mometasone (Nasal) 1391
Zaldem (LB) *see* Diltiazem 634
Zaldiar (AT, BE, CH, CL, CO, CR, CZ, DE, DO, EE, ES, FR, GT, HN, HR, ID, IL, MX, NI, NL, PA, PE, PL, RO, RU, SI, SK, SV, VE) *see* Acetaminophen and Tramadol 37
Zalopram (DO) *see* Citalopram 451
Zalox (CL) *see* Modafinil 1386
Zalpen (PH) *see* Penicillin G Benzathine 1609
Zaltrap (CH, CZ, DE, DK, EE, ES, GB, HK, IS, LT, NL, SE, SI, SK) *see* Ziv-Aflibercept (Systemic) 2204
Zaltrap (ES, HR, NL, RO) *see* Aflibercept (Ophthalmic) 63
Zalvor (LU) *see* Permethrin 1627
Zamadol (BR, GB) *see* TraMADol 2074
Zamene (ES) *see* Deflazacort [INT] 587
Zamudol (FR) *see* TraMADol 2074
Zamur (CR, GT, HN, NI, PA, SV, TT) *see* Cefuroxime 399
Zanaflex (GB, IE) *see* TiZANidine 2051
Zanapam (AE, BH, CY, EG, IL, IQ, IR, JO, KW, LB, LY, OM, QA, SA, SY, YE) *see* ALPRAZolam 94
Zandil (PH) *see* Diltiazem 634
Zanedip (IT, KR, VN) *see* Lercanidipine [INT] 1181
Zan (HR) *see* Zaleplon 2193
Zanicor (PT) *see* Lercanidipine [INT] 1181
Zanidip (AT, AU, BE, CH, CN, DK, ES, FI, FR, GB, GR, HU, NL, NO, NZ, PT, SE, TH) *see* Lercanidipine [INT] 1181
Zanipress (DK) *see* Enalapril and Hydrochlorothiazide 725
Zanlan (GT, HN, NI, PA, SV) *see* Cetirizine 411
Zanocin (IN, ZA) *see* Ofloxacin (Systemic) 1490
Zanprex (PH) *see* OLANZapine 1491
Zantac (AE, AU, BB, BE, BF, BG, BH, BJ, BM, BS, BZ, CI, CN, CO, CR, CY, CZ, DK, DO, EC, EE, EG, ET, FI, GB, GH, GM, GN, GR, GT, GY, HK, HN, HU, ID, IE, IL, IQ, IR, IS, IT, JM, JO, KE, KR, KW, LB, LR, LT, LU, LY, MA, ML, MR, MU, MW, MY, NE, NG, NI, NL, NO, NZ, OM, PA, PE, PH, PK, PL, PR, PT, PY, QA, RO, RU, SA, SC, SD, SE, SI, SL, SN, SR, SV, SY, TH, TN, TR, TT, TW, TZ, UG, UY, VE, VN, YE, ZA, ZM, ZW) *see* Ranitidine 1777
Zantadin (ID) *see* Ranitidine 1777
Zantic (CH, DE) *see* Ranitidine 1777
Zanuric (JO) *see* Allopurinol 90
Zapain (GB, IE) *see* Acetaminophen and Codeine 36
Zapen (CO) *see* CloZAPine 490
Zapilux (BG) *see* OLANZapine 1491
Zapine (TW) *see* CloZAPine 490
Zaplon (IN) *see* Zaleplon 2193
Zappa (IL) *see* OLANZapine 1491
Zaprace (CN) *see* Benazepril 238
Zapril (NZ) *see* Cilazapril [CAN/INT] 434
Zaprine (ZA) *see* AzaTHIOprine 210
Zapros XL (KR) *see* Alfuzosin 84
Zapto-Co (ZA) *see* Captopril and Hydrochlorothiazide 345
Zapto (ZA) *see* Captopril 342
Zarator (AR, CL, DK, ES, PT) *see* AtorvaSTATin 194
Zarator Plus (AR) *see* Ezetimibe and Atorvastatin 833
Zarbin (MX) *see* Gemcitabine 952
Zaret (CO) *see* Azithromycin (Systemic) 216
Zarin (MY) *see* Miconazole (Topical) 1360
2Zaris (PH) *see* Losartan and Hydrochlorothiazide 1250
Zariviz (IT) *see* Cefotaxime 382
Zarom (ID) *see* Azithromycin (Systemic) 216
Zarondan (DK, NO) *see* Ethosuximide 813
Zarontil (KR) *see* Ethosuximide 813
Zarontin (AE, AR, AU, BE, BH, CY, EG, ES, FR, GB, GR, IE, IL, IQ, IR, IT, JO, KE, KW, LB, LU, LY, MY, NZ, OM, QA, SA, SI, SY, UY, YE, ZA, ZW) *see* Ethosuximide 813
Zaroxolyn (CH, DE, HK, IL, IT, KR) *see* Metolazone 1348
Zartan (KR, ZA) *see* Losartan 1248
Zarzio (GB, HK, HR, MY, RO, TR) *see* Filgrastim 875
Zastidin (VN) *see* Nizatidine 1471
Zatamil (AU) *see* Mometasone (Topical) 1391
Zatin (AE, BH, CY, EG, IQ, IR, JO, KW, LB, LY, OM, QA, SA, SY, YE) *see* Ketotifen (Systemic) [CAN/INT] 1149
Zatofen (PK) *see* Ketotifen (Ophthalmic) 1150
Zatofen (PK) *see* Ketotifen (Systemic) [CAN/INT] 1149
Zatrol (CL) *see* Omeprazole 1508
ZA (TW) *see* Azelaic Acid 213
Zavedos (AE, AR, AT, AU, BE, BG, BH, BR, CH, CL, CN, CO, CY, CZ, DE, DK, EC, EE, EG, ES, FI, FR, GB, GR, HK, HN, HR, HU, IE, IL, IN, IQ, IR, IS, IT, JO, KR, KW, LB, LT, LU, LY, MT, MY, NL, NO, NZ, OM, PE, PH, PK, PL, PT, QA, RO, RU, SA, SE, SI, SK, SY, TH, TR, TW, UY, VE, YE, ZA) *see* IDArubicin 1037
Zavedos CS (SG) *see* IDArubicin 1037
Zavel (KR) *see* IDArubicin 1037
Zaverucin (VN) *see* IDArubicin 1037
Zavesca (AT, AU, BE, BG, BR, CH, CL, CO, CZ, DE, DK, EE, FI, FR, GB, GR, HN, HR, IE, IL, IT, KR, LT, MT, NL, NO, NZ, PT, RO, RU, SE, SI, SK, TR, TW) *see* Miglustat 1367
Zaxem (AT) *see* Butenafine 314
Zaxine (ES) *see* Rifaximin 1809

Zaxter (TH) *see* Meropenem 1299
Zayasel (CR, GT, HN, NI, PA, SV) *see* Terazosin 2001
Zcure (PH) *see* Pyrazinamide 1745
Z-Dorm (ZA) *see* Zopiclone [CAN/INT] 2217
Zeben (TH) *see* Albendazole 65
Zebet (PH) *see* Gliclazide [CAN/INT] 964
Zebron (PY) *see* Ambroxol [INT] 109
Zeclar (FR) *see* Clarithromycin 456
Zecovir (IT) *see* Brivudine [INT] 289
Zecroxil (PH) *see* Celecoxib 402
Zedace (AU) *see* Captopril 342
Zedan (PK) *see* ARIPiprazole 171
Zedbac (GB) *see* Azithromycin (Systemic) 216
Zedd (AU) *see* Azithromycin (Systemic) 216
Zedott (IN) *see* Racecadotril [INT] 1765
Zefei (PH) *see* Gemcitabine 952
Zeferom (PH) *see* Cefpirome [INT] 388
Zeffix (AE, AT, AU, BE, BG, BH, CH, CY, CZ, DE, DK, EE, ES, FI, FR, GB, GR, HN, HR, HU, IE, IL, IT, JO, KR, KW, LB, LT, MT, MY, NL, NO, NZ, PH, PK, PL, PT, QA, RO, RU, SA, SE, SG, SI, SK, TH, TR, TW, VN) *see* LamiVUDine 1157
Zeflodan (PH) *see* Cloxacillin [CAN/INT] 488
Zeflomed (PK) *see* Pefloxacin [INT] 1588
Zeflox (LB) *see* Cefaclor 372
Zefocent (PH) *see* Cefotaxime 382
Zefone 250 (BF, BJ, CI, ET, GH, GM, GN, KE, LR, MA, ML, MR, MU, MW, NE, NG, SC, SD, SL, SN, TN, TZ, UG, ZM, ZW) *see* CefTRIAXone 396
Zefotax (PH) *see* Cefotaxime 382
Zefral (PH) *see* Cefixime 380
Zefxon (MY, TH) *see* Omeprazole 1508
Zegacid (PH) *see* Omeprazole and Sodium Bicarbonate 1511
Zegen (PH) *see* Cefuroxime 399
Zehu-Ze (IL) *see* Permethrin 1627
Zeid (MX) *see* Simvastatin 1890
Zeisin Autohaler (DE) *see* Pirbuterol 1662
Zeite (PY) *see* Imatinib 1047
Zela (TH) *see* Albendazole 65
Zelax (LB) *see* Escitalopram 765
Zelboraf (AU, BE, BR, CH, CL, CY, CZ, DE, DK, EE, FR, GB, HK, HR, IL, IS, KR, LT, MX, NL, NO, NZ, PH, QA, RO, SE, SG, SI, SK, TH, TR) *see* Vemurafenib 2148
Zeldox (AE, AR, AT, AU, BG, BH, CL, CN, CZ, DE, DK, EE, ES, FI, HK, HR, IS, JO, KR, KW, LB, LT, MY, NO, NZ, PE, PH, PL, PT, QA, RO, RU, SE, SG, SI, SK, TH, UY, VN) *see* Ziprasidone 2201
Zelface (ID) *see* Azelaic Acid 213
Zeliris (ID) *see* Azelaic Acid 213
Zelitrex (AU, BE, DK, FR, NL) *see* ValACYclovir 2119
Zelleta (GB) *see* Desogestrel [INT] 597
Zelta (CO, DO, GT, HN, PA, SV) *see* OLANZapine 1491
Zema (TH) *see* Clotrimazole (Topical) 488
Zemil (LB) *see* Ezetimibe 832
Zemitra (PK) *see* Ezetimibe 832
Zemplar (AE, AR, AT, AU, BG, BH, BR, CH, CL, CO, CY, CZ, DE, DK, EC, EE, FI, GB, GR, HK, HN, HR, HU, ID, IE, IL, IT, KR, KW, LT, MX, MY, NL, NO, PE, PT, QA, RO, SE, SG, SI, SK, TR, TW, UY, VE) *see* Paricalcitol 1577
Zemtrial (PH) *see* Diltiazem 634
Zemuron (AR) *see* Rocuronium 1838
Zemyc (ID) *see* Fluconazole 885
Zenalb 20 (CO) *see* Albumin 67
Zenalb (GR, ID, SG, TH, VN) *see* Albumin 67
Zenalosyn (NL) *see* Oxymetholone 1546
Zenapax (CZ, DK) *see* DACTINomycin 551
Zenaro (RO) *see* Levocetirizine 1196
Zenavan (ES) *see* Etofenamate [INT] 815
Zendal (MY) *see* Albendazole 65
Zendhin (HK, MY) *see* Ranitidine 1777
Zendol (IN) *see* Danazol 558
Zenhale (BR, CO, MX, MY, SG, TH) *see* Mometasone and Formoterol 1392
Zenibrax (VN) *see* Clidinium and Chlordiazepoxide 460
Zenith (PH) *see* Azithromycin (Systemic) 216
Zenmolin (AE, BH, CY, EG, HK, IL, IQ, IR, JO, KW, LB, LY, OM, QA, SA, SY, YE) *see* Albuterol 69
Zenpro (MY, SG) *see* Omeprazole 1508
Zenra (RO) *see* Ramipril 1771
Zenriz (ID) *see* Cetirizine 411
Zensil (TH) *see* Cetirizine 411
Zental (RO) *see* Albendazole 65
Zentel (AE, AU, BB, BF, BG, BH, BJ, BM, BR, BS, BZ, CH, CI, CL, CN, CO, CR, CY, CZ, DO, EC, EG, ET, FR, GH, GM, GN, GR, GT, GY, HN, IQ, IR, IT, JM, JO, KE, KR, KW, LB, LR, LY, MA, ML, MR, MU, MW, MX, MY, NE, NG, NI, OM, PA, PE, PL, PR, PT, QA, SA, SC, SD, SG, SI, SK, SL, SN, SR, SV, SY, TH, TN, TT, TZ, UG, VE, VN, YE, ZA, ZM, ZW) *see* Albendazole 65
Zentius (AR, CL, EC) *see* Citalopram 451
Zentro (PH) *see* Cefotaxime 382
Zenusin (AE, BF, BH, BJ, CI, CY, EG, ET, GH, GM, GN, IQ, IR, JO, KE, KW, LB, LR, LY, MA, ML, MR, MU, MW, NE, NG, OM, QA, SA, SC, SD, SL, SN, SY, TN, TZ, UG, YE, ZM, ZW) *see* NIFEdipine 1451
ZepAllergy (AU) *see* Cetirizine 411
Zepanc (TW) *see* ClonazePAM 478
Zepax (PH) *see* CefOXitin 386
Zepilen (BG, HR, LT, NZ, SG, TR) *see* CeFAZolin 373
Zepime (PH) *see* Cefepime 378
Zepim (PH) *see* Cefepime 378
Zepotin (PH) *see* CefOXitin 386
Zepradon (VN) *see* Ziprasidone 2201
Zeprex (PH) *see* OLANZapine 1491
Zepril (AR) *see* Abacavir 20
Zeptrigen (PH) *see* CefTAZidime 392
Zepym (PH) *see* Cefepime 378
Zequin (PK) *see* Gatifloxacin 949
Zeraffic (KR) *see* LamiVUDine 1157
Zeran (BF, BJ, CI, ET, GH, GM, GN, KE, LR, MA, ML, MR, MU, MW, NE, NG, SC, SD, SL, SN, TN, TZ, UG, ZM, ZW) *see* Cetirizine 411
Zerdin (PH) *see* Ranitidine 1777
Zerene (BG, ES, FI, NO) *see* Zaleplon 2193
Zerit (AR, AT, AU, BE, BG, BH, CH, CL, CN, CO, CY, CZ, DE, DK, EC, EE, ES, FI, FR, GB, GR, HK, HN, HR, HU, ID, IE, IT, KR, KW, LB, LT, LU, MT, MX, NL, NO, NZ, PE, PL, PT, QA, RO, RU, SA, SE, SG, SI, SK, TR, TW, VE, VN, ZA) *see* Stavudine 1934
Zerlin (ID) *see* Sertraline 1878
Zero-X (KR) *see* Orlistat 1520
Zerodol (BR) *see* Ketorolac (Systemic) 1146
Zerodol CR (PE) *see* Aceclofenac [INT] 30
Zerodol (PE) *see* Aceclofenac [INT] 30
Zerodown (KR) *see* Orlistat 1520
Zerogen (IN) *see* Desogestrel [INT] 597
Zeropenem (AR) *see* Meropenem 1299
Zerosma (IN) *see* Ketotifen (Systemic) [CAN/INT] 1149
Zerotyph (KR) *see* Typhoid Vaccine 2112
Zerpex (BE) *see* Brivudine [INT] 289
Zerrsox (PH) *see* Amoxicillin 130
Zertine (HK, TH) *see* Cetirizine 411
Zertin (PH) *see* Erdosteine [INT] 753
Zestaval (TR) *see* Albendazole 65
Zestoretic (AE, BB, BE, BF, BH, BJ, BM, BS, BZ, CH, CI, CR, CY, DK, DO, EG, ES, ET, GB, GH, GM, GN, GR, GT, GY, HK, HN, ID, IE, IL, IQ, IR, JM, JO, KE, KW, LB, LR, LY, MA, ML, MR, MU, MW, MX, NE, NG, NI, NL, NO, OM, PA, PE, PK, PT, QA, SA, SC, SD, SE, SL, SN, SR, SV, SY, TN, TR, TT, TZ, UG, VN, YE, ZA, ZM, ZW) *see* Lisinopril and Hydrochlorothiazide 1229
Zestril (AE, AU, BB, BE, BF, BH, BJ, BM, BR, BS, BZ, CH, CI, CL, CN, CR, CY, DK, DO, EG, ES, ET, FR, GB, GH, GM, GN, GR, GT, GY, HK, HN, ID, IE, IQ, IR, JM,

JO, KE, KR, KW, LB, LR, LU, LY, MA, ML, MR, MU, MW, MX, MY, NE, NG, NI, NL, OM, PA, PE, PH, PK, PT, QA, SA, SC, SD, SE, SL, SN, SR, SV, SY, TH, TN, TR, TT, TW, TZ, UG, VN, YE, ZM, ZW) *see* Lisinopril 1226
Zesunate (IN) *see* Artesunate 178
Zeta (AE, BH, JO, KW, LB, QA, SA) *see* Fusidic Acid (Topical) [CAN/INT] 943
Zetaler (PE) *see* Cetirizine 411
Zetam (IN) *see* Piracetam [INT] 1661
Zetavim (UY) *see* Ezetimibe 832
Zetavudin (PY) *see* Lamivudine and Zidovudine 1160
Zeteze (AU) *see* Ezetimibe and Atorvastatin 833
Zetia (BR, CR, DO, GT, JP, NI, PA, PE, SV) *see* Ezetimibe 832
Zetina (EC) *see* Simvastatin 1890
Zetix (CL, EC) *see* Zopiclone [CAN/INT] 2217
Zeto (IL) *see* Azithromycin (Systemic) 216
Zetop (NZ) *see* Cetirizine 411
Zetran-5 (TH) *see* Clorazepate 487
Zetrix (PH, TH) *see* Cetirizine 411
Zetron (LB) *see* Azithromycin (Systemic) 216
Zetron (TH) *see* Ondansetron 1513
Zetropil (ID) *see* Piracetam [INT] 1661
Zeven (MY) *see* Acyclovir (Topical) 51
Zevin (TH) *see* Acyclovir (Systemic) 47
Zevin (TH) *see* Acyclovir (Topical) 51
Zexate (PH, UY, VE, VN) *see* Methotrexate 1322
Zhenrui (CN) *see* Pilocarpine (Ophthalmic) 1649
Zhiruo (CN) *see* Palonosetron 1561
Zhoulixin (CN) *see* Ketoconazole (Topical) 1145
Zhu Ning (CN) *see* Gatifloxacin 949
Ziac (AR, BB, BS, CL, CO, CR, DO, EC, GT, JM, NI, NL, PA, PE, PH, SV, TT, VE) *see* Bisoprolol and Hydrochlorothiazide 267
Ziagel (AU) *see* Lidocaine (Topical) 1211
Ziagen (AE, AT, AU, BB, BE, BG, BH, BM, BS, BZ, CH, CL, CN, CO, CR, CY, CZ, DE, DK, DO, EC, EE, ES, FI, FR, GB, GR, GT, GY, HK, HN, HR, HU, IE, IL, IS, IT, JM, KR, LT, MT, MY, NI, NL, NO, NZ, PA, PE, PL, PT, QA, RO, RU, SA, SE, SG, SK, SR, SV, TR, TT, TW, VE, VN) *see* Abacavir 20
Ziagenavir (AR, BR, MX, TH, UY) *see* Abacavir 20
Ziak (ZA) *see* Bisoprolol and Hydrochlorothiazide 267
Ziaxel (NZ) *see* Trandolapril and Verapamil 2080
Zibac (ID) *see* CefTAZidime 392
Zibil (MX) *see* Albuterol 69
Zicho (ID) *see* Azithromycin (Systemic) 216
Ziclar (PY) *see* Carvedilol 367
Ziclin (ZA) *see* Gliclazide [CAN/INT] 964
Zidalex (ID) *see* Levofloxacin (Systemic) 1197
Zidime (AE, JO, KW, QA) *see* CefTAZidime 392
Zidomax (EC) *see* Lamivudine and Zidovudine 1160
Zidon-DT (IN) *see* Domperidone [CAN/INT] 666
Zidoval (AU) *see* MetroNIDAZOLE (Systemic) 1353
Zidoval (IL) *see* MetroNIDAZOLE (Topical) 1357
Zidovir (IN, LB, PY) *see* Zidovudine 2196
Zidronic (EC) *see* Zoledronic Acid 2206
Ziefmycin (TW) *see* Dicloxacillin 621
Zienam (AR, AT, DE, PY, UY, VE) *see* Imipenem and Cilastatin 1051
Zient (MX) *see* Ezetimibe 832
Zifluvis (CO) *see* Acetylcysteine 40
Zigat (PH) *see* Moxifloxacin (Systemic) 1401
Zilarex (AU) *see* Cetirizine 411
Zilden (PH) *see* Sildenafil 1882
Zildon (RO) *see* Donepezil 668
Zildox (PH) *see* Oxaliplatin 1528
Zilfujim (AU) *see* Ondansetron 1513
Zilium (BE) *see* Domperidone [CAN/INT] 666
Zilpro (PK) *see* Cefprozil 389
Zilroz (VN) *see* Cefprozil 389
Zilutra (CZ) *see* Trimetazidine [INT] 2104
Zimac (SA) *see* Azithromycin (Systemic) 216
Zimaquin (CL, PE, TH) *see* ClomiPHENE 473
Zimax (LB) *see* Azithromycin (Systemic) 216
Zimericina (CO) *see* Azithromycin (Systemic) 216
Zimerz (PH) *see* Memantine 1286
Zimmex (TH) *see* Simvastatin 1890
Zimoclone (IE) *see* Zopiclone [CAN/INT] 2217
Zimor (MY, SG) *see* Omeprazole 1508
Zimovane (GB) *see* Zopiclone [CAN/INT] 2217
Zimox (IT) *see* Amoxicillin 130
Zimstat (AU) *see* Simvastatin 1890
Zimulti (SE) *see* Rimonabant [INT] 1814
Zinacef (AE, BE, BG, BH, CH, CN, CO, CY, CZ, DK, EE, ES, FI, GB, GR, HU, IE, IS, JO, KW, LB, LT, LU, MT, NL, NO, NZ, PH, PT, QA, RU, SA, SE, SK, TR, VN) *see* Cefuroxime 399
Zinamide (AU, GB, IE, NZ) *see* Pyrazinamide 1745
Zinasen (LB, PE) *see* Flunarizine [CAN/INT] 892
Zinat (CH) *see* Cefuroxime 399
Zinavin (CO) *see* Vinorelbine 2168
Zinca (TW) *see* Zinc Acetate 2199
Zincef (KR) *see* Cefuroxime 399
Zincfrin (AU, BE, CO, DK, FI, GR, NZ, PK, SE) *see* Phenylephrine and Zinc Sulfate [CAN/INT] 1640
Zincfrin (GR, PK) *see* Disulfiram 654
Zincol (IL) *see* Zinc Sulfate 2200
Zincteral (CZ, PL) *see* Zinc Sulfate 2200
Zincun (PY) *see* Piroxicam 1662
Zindaclin (AU, BE, CZ, GB, HK, IL, MY, PL, PT, TR) *see* Clindamycin (Topical) 464
Zindacline (FR) *see* Clindamycin (Topical) 464
Zindolin (TR) *see* Ciprofloxacin (Systemic) 441
Zinebi (IN) *see* Nebivolol 1434
Zineryt (SI) *see* Erythromycin (Topical) 765
Zinetac (IN) *see* Ranitidine 1777
Zinetron (MX) *see* Citalopram 451
Zinex (PH) *see* Cetirizine 411
Zinfect (TR) *see* Azithromycin (Systemic) 216
Zinforo (AR, AU, BE, CH, CZ, DE, DK, EE, ES, GB, HK, HR, IE, IL, IS, LT, MY, NL, NO, NZ, RO, SE, SG, SI, SK) *see* Ceftaroline Fosamil 391
Zinnat (AE, AT, AU, BB, BE, BF, BG, BH, BJ, BM, BR, BS, BZ, CH, CI, CL, CO, CR, CY, CZ, DE, DK, DO, EC, EE, EG, ES, ET, FI, FR, GB, GH, GM, GN, GT, GY, HK, HN, HR, HU, ID, IE, IL, IQ, IR, IS, IT, JM, JO, KE, KR, KW, LB, LR, LT, LU, LY, MA, ML, MR, MU, MW, MX, MY, NE, NG, NI, NL, NZ, OM, PA, PE, PH, PK, PL, PR, PY, QA, RO, SA, SC, SD, SK, SL, SN, SR, SV, SY, TH, TN, TR, TW, TZ, UG, UY, VE, VN, YE, ZA, ZM, ZW) *see* Cefuroxime 399
Zintergia (CO) *see* Amantadine 105
Zintrepid (CL, MX) *see* Ezetimibe and Simvastatin 834
Zinvel (TH) *see* Zoledronic Acid 2206
Ziohex (PH) *see* Zolpidem 2212
Ziorel (LB) *see* Irbesartan 1110
Ziphanol (PH) *see* Butorphanol 314
Ziproc (PH) *see* CloZAPine 490
Zircol (AU) *see* Lercanidipine [INT] 1181
Zirid (EE) *see* Itopride [INT] 1130
Zirtec (IT) *see* Cetirizine 411
Zirtek (GB, IE) *see* Cetirizine 411
Zirtraler (DO, GT, HN, NI, PA, SV) *see* Cetirizine 411
Ziruvate (JP) *see* Diltiazem 634
Zispin (GB, IE) *see* Mirtazapine 1376
Zistic (ID) *see* Azithromycin (Systemic) 216
Zitadim (ID) *see* CefTAZidime 392
Zitanid (ID) *see* TiZANidine 2051
Zita (PK) *see* TiZANidine 2051
Zitazonium (CZ, HK, HU, PH, RU) *see* Tamoxifen 1971
Zithrax (ID) *see* Azithromycin (Systemic) 216
Zithromac SR (JP) *see* Azithromycin (Systemic) 216
Zithromax IV (MY, SG) *see* Azithromycin (Systemic) 216

Zithromax (AE, AT, AU, BD, BF, BH, BJ, CH, CI, CL, CN, CY, EG, ET, FI, FR, GB, GH, GM, GN, GR, HK, ID, IE, IL, IQ, IR, JO, KE, KW, LB, LR, LY, MA, ML, MR, MU, MW, MY, NE, NG, NL, NZ, OM, PH, PK, PT, PY, QA, SA, SC, SD, SE, SG, SL, SN, SY, TH, TN, TR, TW, TZ, UG, YE, ZA, ZM, ZW) *see* Azithromycin (Systemic) ... 216
Zithrox (AE, BH, CY, EG, IQ, IR, JO, KW, LB, LY, OM, QA, SA, SY, YE) *see* Azithromycin (Systemic) ... 216
Zitoxin (VE) *see* Minoxidil (Topical) ... 1374
Zitrim (CO) *see* Azithromycin (Systemic) ... 216
Zitrocin (PY) *see* Azithromycin (Systemic) ... 216
Zitromax (AR, BE, BR, CR, DK, EC, GT, HN, IS, IT, NI, PA, PE, SV, TR, UY, VE) *see* Azithromycin (Systemic) ... 216
Zitumex (GR) *see* Piroxicam ... 1662
Ziverone (MX) *see* Acyclovir (Systemic) ... 47
Zix (PY) *see* Clarithromycin ... 456
Zmax (HK, IL, SG) *see* Azithromycin (Systemic) ... 216
Zmax One Dose (PH) *see* Azithromycin (Systemic) ... 216
Z-Mol (PY) *see* Acetaminophen ... 32
Zoamcton (PE) *see* Somatropin ... 1918
Zobonic (TW) *see* Zoledronic Acid ... 2206
Zobral (TR) *see* Levocetirizine ... 1196
Zocardis (RU) *see* Zofenopril [INT] ... 2206
Zocef (TH) *see* Cefuroxime ... 399
Zocin (AE, JO) *see* Azithromycin (Systemic) ... 216
Zocor (AE, AR, AU, BB, BE, BF, BG, BH, BJ, BM, BR, BS, BZ, CH, CI, CL, CN, CO, CR, CY, CZ, DE, DK, EC, EE, EG, ES, ET, FI, FR, GB, GH, GM, GN, GR, GT, GY, HK, HN, HR, HU, ID, IE, IT, JM, JO, KE, KR, KW, LB, LR, LU, MA, ML, MR, MU, MW, MX, MY, NE, NG, NI, NL, NO, PA, PE, PH, PK, PL, PT, QA, RO, SA, SC, SD, SK, SL, SN, SR, SV, TH, TN, TR, TT, TW, TZ, UG, UY, VE, VN, ZM, ZW) *see* Simvastatin ... 1890
Zocord (AT, SE) *see* Simvastatin ... 1890
Zocor HP (PH) *see* Simvastatin ... 1890
Zodac (AU) *see* Cetirizine ... 411
Zoderm (IN) *see* Oxiconazole ... 1536
Zodiac (KR) *see* Acyclovir (Systemic) ... 47
Zodol (CL, PY) *see* TraMADol ... 2074
Zodonrel (TH) *see* TraZODone ... 2091
Zodorm (IL) *see* Zolpidem ... 2212
Zofaden (MX) *see* Zoledronic Acid ... 2206
Zofadep (PH) *see* CeFAZolin ... 373
Zofecard (HR) *see* Zofenopril [INT] ... 2206
Zofen (AE, SA) *see* Pizotifen [CAN/INT] ... 1664
Zofen (BG) *see* Zofenopril [INT] ... 2206
Zofenil (AT, BE, DE, DK, ES, FI, FR, GB, IE, IS, KR, LU, NO, PT, SE) *see* Zofenopril [INT] ... 2206
Zofen (MY) *see* Ibuprofen ... 1032
Zofepril (GR, IT) *see* Zofenopril [INT] ... 2206
Zofil (NL) *see* Zofenopril [INT] ... 2206
Zofistar (EE, LT) *see* Zofenopril [INT] ... 2206
Zoflut (IN) *see* Fluticasone (Oral Inhalation) ... 907
Zoflut (IN) *see* Fluticasone (Topical) ... 911
Zofran (AE, AR, AT, AU, BB, BE, BF, BG, BH, BJ, BM, BR, BS, BZ, CH, CI, CN, CY, CZ, DE, DK, EC, EE, EG, ES, ET, FI, GB, GH, GM, GN, GY, HK, HN, HR, HU, ID, IE, IL, IQ, IR, IS, IT, JM, JO, JP, KE, KR, KW, LB, LR, LT, LU, LY, MA, ML, MR, MT, MU, MW, MX, MY, NE, NG, NL, NO, NZ, OM, PE, PH, PK, PL, PT, PY, QA, RU, SA, SC, SD, SE, SI, SK, SL, SN, SR, SY, TH, TN, TR, TT, TW, TZ, UG, VE, VN, YE, ZM, ZW) *see* Ondansetron ... 1513
Zofran Melt (AE, BH, KW, QA, SA) *see* Ondansetron ... 1513
Zofran Zydis (CR, DO, GT, KR, NI, NZ, PA, SV, TH) *see* Ondansetron ... 1513
Zofredal (ID) *see* RisperiDONE ... 1818
Zofron (GR) *see* Ondansetron ... 1513
Zoiral (TR) *see* ClomiPRAMINE ... 475
Zolacos CP (AU) *see* Bicalutamide ... 262
Zoladex (AE, AR, AT, BB, BD, BE, BF, BG, BJ, BM, BR, BS, BZ, CH, CI, CL, CN, CR, CY, CZ, DE, DK, DO, EC, EE, EG, ES, ET, FI, FR, GB, GH, GM, GN, GR, GT, GY, HK, HN, HR, HU, ID, IE, IL, IN, IQ, IR, IS, IT, JM, JO, JP, KE, KR, KW, LR, LT, LU, LY, MA, ML, MR, MT, MU, MW, MY, NE, NG, NI, NL, NO, OM, PA, PE, PH, PK, PL, PR, PT, RO, RU, SC, SD, SE, SG, SK, SL, SN, SR, SV, SY, TH, TN, TR, TT, TW, TZ, UG, UY, VE, VN, YE, ZA, ZM, ZW) *see* Goserelin ... 981
Zoladex Depot (AE, BH, KR, LB, QA, SA) *see* Goserelin ... 981
Zoladex Implant (AT, AU, BE, BG, CH, CZ, DE, DK, EE, ES, FI, FR, GB, GR, HN, IE, IT, MT, NO, PL, PT, RU, SE, SK, TR) *see* Goserelin ... 981
Zoladex Inj. (NZ) *see* Goserelin ... 981
Zoladex LA (AR, BB, BH, BM, BS, CO, EC, HR, ID, IL, IN, JM, LB, MY, NL, PH, PR, QA, RO, SG, TH, TT, TW, UY) *see* Goserelin ... 981
Zoladin (KR) *see* AcetaZOLAMIDE ... 39
Zolam (IN, JO) *see* ALPRAZolam ... 94
Zolaram (TR) *see* ALPRAZolam ... 94
Zolarem (AE, BF, BH, BJ, CI, CY, EG, ET, GH, GM, GN, IQ, IR, JO, KE, KW, LB, LR, LY, MA, ML, MR, MU, MW, NE, NG, OM, QA, SA, SC, SD, SL, SN, SY, TN, TZ, UG, YE, ZA, ZM, ZW) *see* ALPRAZolam ... 94
Zolasatin (MX) *see* Anastrozole ... 148
Zolastin (ID) *see* ALPRAZolam ... 94
Zolcer (ID) *see* Lansoprazole ... 1166
Zoldac (BF, BJ, CI, ET, GH, GM, GN, KE, LR, MA, ML, MR, MU, MW, NE, NG, SC, SD, SL, SN, TN, TZ, UG, ZM, ZW) *see* ALPRAZolam ... 94
Zoldem (AT, DE) *see* Zolpidem ... 2212
Zoldicam (MX) *see* Fluconazole ... 885
Zoldox (TW) *see* Zolpidem ... 2212
Zoldron-4 (PH) *see* Zoledronic Acid ... 2206
Zolecef (AE, BH, CY, EG, IQ, IR, JO, KW, LB, LY, OM, QA, SA, SY, YE) *see* CeFAZolin ... 373
Zole (IN) *see* Miconazole (Topical) ... 1360
Zolennic (TH) *see* Zoledronic Acid ... 2206
Zoleshot (PH) *see* Fluconazole ... 885
Zoletalis (PH) *see* Zoledronic Acid ... 2206
Zolgen (PH) *see* ALPRAZolam ... 94
Zolidina (PY) *see* CeFAZolin ... 373
Zolid (PK) *see* Pioglitazone ... 1654
Zolid Plus (PH) *see* Pioglitazone and Metformin ... 1655
Zoliget (PH) *see* Pioglitazone and Glimepiride ... 1654
Zolim (DE) *see* Mizolastine [INT] ... 1384
Zolinox (IN) *see* Zopiclone [CAN/INT] ... 2217
Zolinza (AR, AU, CL, CO, KR) *see* Vorinostat ... 2182
Zolistam (IT) *see* Mizolastine [INT] ... 1384
Zolmia (ID) *see* Zolpidem ... 2212
Zolmide (PH) *see* AcetaZOLAMIDE ... 39
Zolmiles (BG) *see* ZOLMitriptan ... 2210
Zolmin (KR) *see* Triazolam ... 2101
Zolnite (IN) *see* Eszopiclone ... 793
Zolnox (PY, UY) *see* Zolpidem ... 2212
Zolodin (PH) *see* Sertraline ... 1878
Zoloft (AE, AR, AU, BB, BF, BG, BH, BJ, BM, BR, BS, BZ, CH, CI, CN, CY, CZ, DE, DK, EC, EE, EG, ET, FI, FR, GH, GM, GN, GR, GY, HK, HR, ID, IQ, IR, IS, IT, JM, JO, JP, KE, KR, KW, LB, LR, LT, LY, MA, ML, MR, MU, MW, MY, NE, NG, NL, NO, NZ, OM, PE, PH, PK, PL, PT, QA, RO, RU, SA, SC, SD, SE, SI, SK, SL, SN, SR, SY, TH, TN, TT, TW, TZ, UG, UY, VE, VN, YE, ZA, ZM, ZW) *see* Sertraline ... 1878
Zolon (MY, TW) *see* Zopiclone [CAN/INT] ... 2217
Zolotem-250 (TH) *see* Temozolomide ... 1991
Zolotral (PH) *see* Sertraline ... 1878
Zol (PH) *see* MetroNIDAZOLE (Systemic) ... 1353
Zolpibell (AU) *see* Zolpidem ... 2212
Zolpicin (TW) *see* Zolpidem ... 2212
Zolpid (KR) *see* Zolpidem ... 2212
Zolpinox (DE) *see* Zolpidem ... 2212

Zolpirest (PH) *see* Zolpidem 2212
Zolpitop (BE) *see* Zolpidem 2212
Zolpra (MX) *see* Pantoprazole 1570
Zolpra (CO) *see* Cefadroxil 372
Zolsana (BG) *see* Zolpidem 2212
Zolterol (MY) *see* Diclofenac (Systemic) 617
Zolterol SR (SG) *see* Diclofenac (Systemic) 617
Zoltrim (EC) *see* Sulfamethoxazole and Trimethoprim 1946
Zoltum (CR, EC, GT, HN, NI, PA, PE, SV) *see* Pantoprazole 1570
Zolvera (GB, IE) *see* Verapamil 2154
Zomacton (AR, AT, AU, BE, BG, CZ, DK, EE, ES, FI, GR, HK, KR, LT, NL, NO, RO, SE, SG, SK) *see* Somatropin 1918
Zomax (AE, BH, CY, EG, IQ, IR, JO, KW, LB, LY, OM, QA, SA, SY, YE) *see* Azithromycin (Systemic) 216
Zomegoal (MX) *see* Zoledronic Acid 2206
Zomen (RO) *see* Zofenopril [INT] 2206
Zomera (IL) *see* Zoledronic Acid 2206
Zometa (AE, AR, AT, AU, BE, BG, BH, BO, BR, CH, CL, CN, CY, CZ, DE, DK, EC, EE, ES, FI, FR, GB, GR, HK, HR, HU, ID, IE, IT, JO, JP, KR, KW, LB, LT, MT, MX, MY, NL, NO, NZ, PE, PH, PK, PL, PR, PT, PY, QA, RO, RU, SA, SE, SG, SI, SK, TH, TR, TW, UY, VE, VN, ZA) *see* Zoledronic Acid 2206
Zometic (CL) *see* Zopiclone [CAN/INT] 2217
Zomianne (TW) *see* Zopiclone [CAN/INT] 2217
Zomig (AE, AT, AU, BB, BE, BF, BH, BJ, BM, BR, BS, BZ, CH, CI, CN, CR, CY, CZ, DK, DO, ES, ET, FR, GB, GH, GM, GN, GT, GY, HK, HN, HR, HU, IE, IL, IS, IT, JM, KE, KR, KW, LR, LT, MA, ML, MR, MU, MW, MX, NE, NG, NI, NL, NO, NZ, PA, PE, PH, PK, PL, PR, PT, QA, RU, SC, SD, SE, SG, SI, SK, SL, SN, SR, SV, TH, TN, TR, TT, TZ, UG, VE, ZA, ZM, ZW) *see* ZOLMitriptan 2210
Zomigon (AR, GR, UY) *see* ZOLMitriptan 2210
Zomigoro (FR) *see* ZOLMitriptan 2210
Zomig Rapimelt (AE, EE, FI, IL, KW, SE) *see* ZOLMitriptan 2210
Zomm (PY) *see* Albuterol 69
Zonac (PY) *see* Hydrocortisone (Systemic) 1013
Zondar (FR) *see* Diacerein [INT] 613
Zonegran (AT, AU, BE, BG, CH, CY, CZ, DE, DK, EE, ES, FI, FR, GB, GR, HN, HR, HU, ID, IE, IN, IS, IT, LT, MT, MY, NL, NO, PH, PT, RO, RU, SE, SI, SK, TH, TR) *see* Zonisamide 2215
Zopam (TH) *see* Diazepam 613
Zopax (ZA) *see* ALPRAZolam 94
Zopercin (VN) *see* Piperacillin and Tazobactam 1657
Zophren (FR) *see* Ondansetron 1513
Zopidem (TW) *see* Zolpidem 2212
Zopimed (ZA) *see* Zopiclone [CAN/INT] 2217
Zopim (TW) *see* Zolpidem 2212
Zopinox (FI) *see* Zopiclone [CAN/INT] 2217
Zopistad (VN) *see* Zopiclone [CAN/INT] 2217
Zopitran (IN) *see* Zopiclone [CAN/INT] 2217
Zopivane (ZA) *see* Zopiclone [CAN/INT] 2217
Zopral (AU) *see* Lansoprazole 1166
Zopranol (BE, ES, GR, IT, LU, NL, PT) *see* Zofenopril [INT] 2206
Zopraz (PE) *see* Lansoprazole 1166
Zopyrin (HK, KR) *see* SulfaSALAzine 1950
Zorac (AT, AU, BE, BG, BR, DE, ES, FR, GB, GR, HR, IE, IL, IT, LB, NZ, PL, SE) *see* Tazarotene 1980
Zorac Gel (IL) *see* Tazarotene 1980
Zoradine (MY) *see* Carbocisteine [INT] 357
Zorafen (MY) *see* Ibuprofen 1032
Zoral (HK, MY, SG) *see* Acyclovir (Systemic) 47
Zoral (HK, MY, SG) *see* Acyclovir (Topical) 51
Zoralin (ID) *see* Ketoconazole (Systemic) 1144
Zoranate (MY) *see* DimenhyDRINATE 637
Zoratadine-P (MY) *see* Loratadine and Pseudoephedrine 1242
Zora (TH) *see* LORazepam 1243
Zorax (SG) *see* Acyclovir (Systemic) 47
Zorax (SG) *see* Acyclovir (Topical) 51
Zorced (MX) *see* Simvastatin 1890
Zoref (PT) *see* Cefuroxime 399
Zorep-1 (PE) *see* Pioglitazone and Glimepiride 1654
Zorep-2 (PE) *see* Pioglitazone and Glimepiride 1654
Zorexin (MY) *see* Acyclovir (Systemic) 47
Zoria (TW) *see* Urea 2114
Zorimin (TW) *see* Zolpidem 2212
Zoroxin (AT, LU) *see* Norfloxacin 1475
Zosaar (MY) *see* Losartan 1248
Zosert (IN) *see* Sertraline 1878
Zosfam (KR) *see* Famciclovir 843
Zostavax (AT, AU, CH, CZ, DE, EE, HR, IE, IL, KR, LT, NL, NZ, PL, PT, RO, SE, SI, SK, TH) *see* Zoster Vaccine 2218
Zostavax (HK, MY) *see* Varicella Virus Vaccine 2141
Zostevir (CZ) *see* Brivudine [INT] 289
Zostex (CN, DE, TR) *see* Brivudine [INT] 289
Zostydol (AR) *see* Brivudine [INT] 289
Zosvir (EC) *see* ValACYclovir 2119
Zosyn (IN, JP) *see* Piperacillin and Tazobactam 1657
Zotaline (TH) *see* Sertraline 1878
Zotan (TW) *see* Tamsulosin 1974
Zotax (HK) *see* Azithromycin (Systemic) 216
Zoteon (CL) *see* Tobramycin (Systemic, Oral Inhalation) 2052
Zoter (ID) *see* Acyclovir (Systemic) 47
Zotinar (PT) *see* Desonide 597
Zoton (AU, GB, IE, IL, IT) *see* Lansoprazole 1166
Zoton Fastab (GB, IE) *see* Lansoprazole 1166
Zotran (CL) *see* ALPRAZolam 94
Zovast (PH) *see* Simvastatin 1890
Zovilam (TH) *see* Lamivudine and Zidovudine 1160
Zovirax (AE, AR, AT, AU, BB, BD, BE, BF, BG, BH, BJ, BM, BO, BR, BS, CH, CI, CR, CY, CZ, DO, EC, EE, EG, ET, FI, FR, GB, GH, GM, GN, GR, GT, GY, HK, HN, HU, ID, IE, IL, IN, IQ, IR, IT, JM, JO, JP, KE, KR, KW, LB, LR, LY, MA, ML, MR, MT, MU, MW, MY, NE, NG, NI, NL, NO, NZ, OM, PA, PE, PH, PK, PL, PR, PT, PY, QA, RU, SA, SC, SD, SE, SK, SL, SN, SV, SY, TN, TR, TT, TW, TZ, UG, UY, YE, ZA, ZM, ZW) *see* Acyclovir (Systemic) 47
Zovirax (AE, AR, AU, BB, BE, BH, BM, BR, BS, CH, CL, CN, CY, CZ, EC, EE, EG, FI, FR, GB, GY, HK, HR, ID, IE, IL, IS, JM, JO, KR, KW, LB, LT, MY, NL, NO, NZ, PE, PR, PT, PY, QA, RO, SA, SE, SK, TH, TR, TT, TW, UY, VN, ZA) *see* Acyclovir (Topical) 51
Zovirax (AU, BE, BR, CH, CL, CZ, EE, EG, ES, FI, FR, GB, HK, ID, IE, IL, IN, KR, MX, MY, NO, NZ, RO, SE, SG, TH, TR, UY) *see* Aciclovir (Ophthalmic) [INT] 43
Zovirax Eye Ointment (SA) *see* Aciclovir (Ophthalmic) [INT] 43
Zovir (DK, IS) *see* Acyclovir (Systemic) 47
Zovir (DK, IS) *see* Acyclovir (Topical) 51
Zovir (IS) *see* Aciclovir (Ophthalmic) [INT] 43
Zoxanid (GT, HN, NI, PA, SV) *see* Nitazoxanide 1461
Zoxan LP (FR) *see* Doxazosin 674
Zoxan (VN) *see* Doxazosin 674
Zoxin (JO) *see* CefOXitin 386
Zoxon (HK) *see* CefTRIAXone 396
Zoylex (PE) *see* Acyclovir (Systemic) 47
Zpladex (SI) *see* Goserelin 981
Z Span (AE) *see* Zinc Sulfate 2200
Zudaw (TW) *see* Metoclopramide 1345
Zudenina (CO, EC) *see* Adapalene 54
Zudenina F (CO) *see* Adapalene 54
Zulbex (HR, RO) *see* RABEprazole 1762
Zulida (CN) *see* Sulindac 1953
Zulin (RO) *see* Mirtazapine 1376
Zultracet (PK) *see* Acetaminophen and Tramadol 37

Zultrop Forte (ID) *see* Sulfamethoxazole and Trimethoprim ... 1946
Zultrop (ID) *see* Sulfamethoxazole and Trimethoprim ... 1946
Zumaflox (ID) *see* Ciprofloxacin (Systemic) ... 441
Zumenon (AT, BE, GB) *see* Estradiol (Systemic) ... 775
Zunden (IT) *see* Piroxicam ... 1662
Zuolexin (CN) *see* Reboxetine [INT] ... 1786
Zuparex (MX) *see* Piroxicam ... 1662
Zurcal (AT, BR, CH, CL, CO, EC, MX, PE, PT) *see* Pantoprazole ... 1570
Zurcale (BE) *see* Pantoprazole ... 1570
Zurcamed (BE) *see* Pantoprazole ... 1570
Zurcazol (GR) *see* Pantoprazole ... 1570
Zurig (IN) *see* Febuxostat ... 848
Zurma (VN) *see* Mosapride [INT] ... 1401
Zutectra (GB) *see* Hepatitis B Immune Globulin (Human) ... 1002
Zutura (EC) *see* Esomeprazole ... 771
Zuvair (IN) *see* Zafirlukast ... 2192
Zu Zu Ton (TW) *see* Bisacodyl ... 265
Zwagra (AE, BH, CY, EG, IQ, IR, JO, KW, LB, LY, OM, QA, SA, SY, YE) *see* Sildenafil ... 1882
Zyban (AE, AT, BB, BE, BG, BM, BR, BS, BZ, CH, CY, CZ, DE, DK, FI, FR, GB, GR, GY, IE, IL, IN, IS, IT, JM, NL, NO, NZ, PL, PR, PT, RO, SA, SE, SI, SR, TR, TT) *see* BuPROPion ... 305
Zyban LP (FR) *see* BuPROPion ... 305
Zyban SR (BH, KW, QA, SG) *see* BuPROPion ... 305
Zyban Sustained Release (AU) *see* BuPROPion ... 305
Zycalcit (IN) *see* Calcitonin ... 322
Zyclara (GB) *see* Imiquimod ... 1055
Zydac (AE, QA) *see* Ranitidine ... 1777
Zydalis (IN) *see* Tadalafil ... 1968
Zydarin (TH) *see* Warfarin ... 2186
Zydelig (CZ, DE, DK, EE, GB, HR, NL, NO, PT, SE, SK) *see* Idelalisib ... 1038
Zydol XL (GB) *see* TraMADol ... 2074
Zydol (AU, GB, IE) *see* TraMADol ... 2074
Zydol SR (AU) *see* TraMADol ... 2074
Zydom (PH) *see* Domperidone [CAN/INT] ... 666
Zydowin (BF, BJ, CI, ET, GH, GM, GN, KE, LR, MA, ML, MR, MU, MW, NE, NG, SC, SD, SL, SN, TN, TZ, UG, ZA, ZM, ZW) *see* Zidovudine ... 2196
Zyklolat-Edo (DE) *see* Cyclopentolate ... 517
Zyklolat EDO (LU) *see* Cyclopentolate ... 517
Zyklomat (MY) *see* Gonadorelin [CAN/INT] ... 980
Zylap (AU) *see* OLANZapine ... 1491
Zylapour (GR) *see* Allopurinol ... 90
Zylet (AR, BR, IL, PH, TH) *see* Loteprednol and Tobramycin ... 1251
Zylexx SR (PK) *see* BuPROPion ... 305
Zylium (BR) *see* Ranitidine ... 1777
Zyllergy (IL) *see* Cetirizine ... 411
Zyloprim (AU, BB, BM, BS, CR, DO, GY, JM, MX, PA, PH, PR, PY, SR, TT) *see* Allopurinol ... 90
Zyloric (AE, BE, BF, BH, BJ, BR, CH, CI, CL, CY, DE, EE, EG, ES, ET, FI, FR, GB, GH, GM, GN, HK, ID, IE, IN, IQ, IR, IT, JO, KE, KR, KW, LB, LR, LU, LY, MA, ML, MR, MT, MU, MW, MY, NE, NG, NL, NO, OM, PK, PL, PT, QA, RU, SA, SC, SD, SE, SG, SK, SL, SN, SY, TH, TN, TR, TZ, UG, UY, VE, VN, YE, ZM, ZW) *see* Allopurinol ... 90
Zylovaa-H (MY) *see* Losartan and Hydrochlorothiazide ... 1250
Zylovaal (MY) *see* Losartan ... 1248
Zymafluor (AE, AT, BE, BG, BH, CH, CY, DE, EG, ES, FR, HU, IL, IQ, IR, IT, JO, KW, LB, LU, LY, NL, OM, PL, QA, SA, SY, TH, TW, YE) *see* Fluoride ... 895
Zymanta (MX) *see* ClonazePAM ... 478
Zymar (AE, BR, CL, IL, IN, KW, LB, MX, MY, PH, SA, SG, TH, TR, ZA) *see* Gatifloxacin ... 949
Zymaran (AR, CO, EC, PE, VE) *see* Gatifloxacin ... 949
Zymar XD (BR) *see* Gatifloxacin ... 949
Zymed (TH) *see* Cetirizine ... 411
Zyngot (PE) *see* Allopurinol ... 90
Zynicor (IN) *see* Nicorandil [INT] ... 1449
Zynoc (TW) *see* Sulconazole ... 1943
Zynootrop (PH) *see* Piracetam [INT] ... 1661
Zynor (HK, MY) *see* AmLODIPine ... 123
Zynox (ZA) *see* Naloxone ... 1419
Zyntabac (ES) *see* BuPROPion ... 305
Zypadhera (CZ, DE, DK, EE, FR, GB, HR, IE, IL, IS, LT, NL, NO, PT, RO, SE, SI, SK, TR) *see* OLANZapine ... 1491
Zypeace OD (KR) *see* OLANZapine ... 1491
Zypine (AU) *see* OLANZapine ... 1491
Zypine ODT (AU) *see* OLANZapine ... 1491
Zypraz (ID) *see* ALPRAZolam ... 94
Zyprexa (AE, AR, AT, AU, BE, BF, BH, BJ, BR, CH, CI, CL, CN, CO, CR, CY, CZ, DE, DK, EE, EG, ES, ET, FI, FR, GB, GH, GM, GN, GR, HK, HR, ID, IE, IL, IS, IT, JO, JP, KE, KW, LB, LR, LT, MA, ML, MR, MT, MU, MW, MX, MY, NE, NG, NI, NL, NO, NZ, PE, PK, PL, PT, QA, RO, RU, SA, SC, SD, SE, SG, SI, SK, SL, SN, TH, TN, TR, TW, TZ, UG, VE, VN, ZA, ZM, ZW) *see* OLANZapine ... 1491
Zyprexa Velotab (AE, AT, BE, BG, CH, CY, CZ, DE, DK, EE, ES, FI, FR, GB, GR, IE, IT, KW, LB, MT, NL, NO, PL, PT, QA, RU, SE, SK, TR) *see* OLANZapine ... 1491
Zyprexa Zydis (AR, CN, HK, ID, MY, NZ, SG, TH, TW) *see* OLANZapine ... 1491
Zyrac (TH) *see* Cetirizine ... 411
Zyren (KR) *see* ALPRAZolam ... 94
Zyrepin (KR) *see* OLANZapine ... 1491
Zyrlex (SE) *see* Cetirizine ... 411
Zyrona (SE) *see* Cyproterone and Ethinyl Estradiol [CAN/INT] ... 532
Zyroric (KR) *see* Allopurinol ... 90
Zyrova (PH) *see* Rosuvastatin ... 1848
Zyrtec (AE, AT, AU, BE, BG, BH, BR, CH, CL, CO, CR, CY, CZ, DE, DK, DO, EE, EG, ES, FI, FR, GT, HK, HN, HU, IN, JO, KR, KW, LB, LT, LU, MT, MY, NL, NO, NZ, PA, PE, PH, PK, PL, PT, QA, RO, RU, SA, SI, SK, SV, TH, TR, TW, UY, VE, VN, ZA) *see* Cetirizine ... 411
Zytaz (IN) *see* CefTAZidime ... 392
Zythrocin (TW) *see* Azithromycin (Systemic) ... 216
Zytiga (AR, AU, BE, BR, BZ, CH, CL, CO, CY, CZ, DE, DK, EE, FR, GB, HK, HR, HU, ID, IE, IL, IS, KR, LT, MX, MY, NL, NO, NZ, PH, PL, QA, RO, SA, SE, SG, SI, SK, TH, TR, VN) *see* Abiraterone Acetate ... 26
Zytofen (TH) *see* Ketotifen (Systemic) [CAN/INT] ... 1149
Zytram XL (NZ) *see* TraMADol ... 2074
Zytram XL SR (KR) *see* TraMADol ... 2074
Zytram BD (NZ) *see* TraMADol ... 2074
Zytrim (DE) *see* AzaTHIOprine ... 210
Zytrin (IN) *see* Terazosin ... 2001
Zyven-OD (IN) *see* Desvenlafaxine ... 598
Zyverin (TW) *see* Ribavirin ... 1797
Zyvir (KE) *see* Acyclovir (Systemic) ... 47
Zyvox (AE, AR, AU, BH, BR, CL, CN, CR, CY, DO, EC, EG, GB, GT, HK, HN, ID, IE, IQ, IR, JO, KR, KW, LB, LY, MY, NI, NZ, OM, PA, PE, PH, QA, RU, SA, SG, SV, SY, TH, TW, UY, VE, YE) *see* Linezolid ... 1217
Zyvoxam (MX) *see* Linezolid ... 1217
Zyvoxid (AT, BE, BG, CH, CO, CY, CZ, DE, DK, EE, FI, FR, GR, HR, IL, IS, IT, LT, NL, NO, PL, RO, SE, SI, SK, TR, ZA) *see* Linezolid ... 1217
Zyxem (MX) *see* Levocetirizine ... 1196
Zyzyx (PH) *see* Pregabalin ... 1710

NOTES

NOTES

NOTES

NOTES

NOTES

NOTES

NOTES

NOTES

Other Offerings by Lexicomp

Anesthesiology & Critical Care Drug Handbook

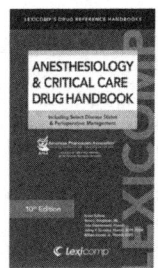

Designed for anesthesiologists, critical care practitioners, and all healthcare professionals involved in the treatment of surgical or ICU patients.

Includes: Extensive drug information to help ensure appropriate clinical management of patients; intensivist and anesthesiologist perspective; over 2000 medications most commonly used in the preoperative and critical care setting; Special Topics/Issues addressing frequently encountered patient conditions.

Drug Information Handbook

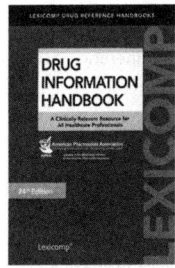

This easy-to-use drug reference is for the pharmacist, physician, or other healthcare professional requiring fast access to relevant drug information.

Over 1500 drug monographs are detailed with up to 39 fields of information per monograph. A valuable appendix offers charts and reviews of special topics such as guidelines for treatment and therapy recommendations. A pharmacologic category index is also provided.

Drug Information Handbook for Advanced Practice Nursing

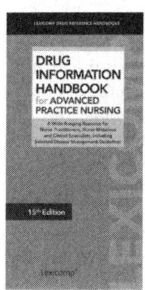

Designed to assist the advanced practice nurse with prescribing, monitoring and educating patients.

Includes: Over 4800 generic and brand names cross-referenced by page number; generic drug names and cross-references highlighted in RED; labeled and investigational indications; adult, geriatric, and pediatric dosing; and up to 75 fields of information per monograph.

Drug Information Handbook for Nursing

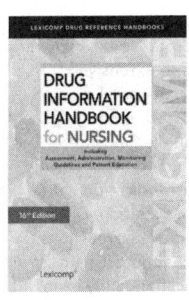

Designed for registered professional nurses and upper-division nursing students requiring dosing, administration, monitoring and patient education information.

Includes: Over 4800 generic and brand name drugs, cross-referenced by page number; drug names and specific nursing fields highlighted in RED for easy reference, Nursing Actions field includes Physical Assessment and Patient Education guidelines.

To order, call Customer Service at 1-866-397-3433 or visit www.lexi.com.
Outside of the U.S., call +1-330-650-6506 or visit www.lexi.com.

Other Offerings by Lexicomp

Drug Information Handbook for Oncology

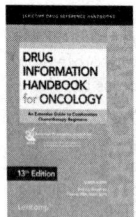

Designed for oncology professionals requiring information on combination chemotherapy regimens and dosing protocols.

Includes: Monographs containing warnings, adverse reaction profiles, drug interactions, dosing for specific indications, vesicant, emetic potential, combination regimens, and more; where applicable, a special Combination Chemotherapy field links to specific oncology monographs; Special Topics such as Cancer Treatment Related Complications, Bone Marrow Transplantation, and Drug Development.

Geriatric Dosage Handbook

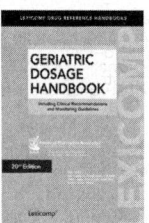

Designed for healthcare professionals managing geriatric patients.

Includes: A wide range of adult and geriatric dosing; special geriatric considerations; up to 44 key fields of information in each monograph, including Medication Safety Issues; extensive information on drug interactions, as well as dosing for patients with renal/hepatic impairment.

Pediatric & Neonatal Dosage Handbook

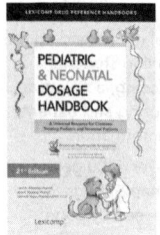

This book is designed for healthcare professionals requiring quick access to extensive pediatric and neonatal drug information. Each monograph contains multiple fields of content, including usual dosage by age group, indication, and route of administration. Drug interactions, adverse reactions, extemporaneous preparations, pharmacodynamics/ pharmacokinetics data, and medication safety issues are covered.

Pediatric & Neonatal Dosage Handbook with International Trade Names Index

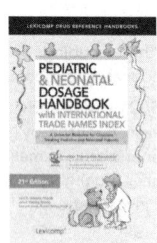

The *Pediatric & Neonatal Dosage Handbook with International Trade Names Index* is the trusted pediatric drug resource of medical professionals worldwide. The international edition contains content from the Lexicomp *Pediatric & Neonatal Dosage Handbook*, plus an International Trade Names Index including trade names from over 100 countries.

Other Offerings by Lexicomp

Lexicomp® Online™

Wolters Kluwer Clinical Drug Information applications – including Lexicomp – are used in more than 96% of the hospitals achieving Honor Roll status as ranked by U.S. News & World Report's Best Hospitals 2014-2015 and Best Children's Hospitals 2014-2015.

Lexicomp Online integrates industry-leading databases and enhanced searching technology, delivering time-sensitive clinical information at the point of care. Our easy-to-use interface and concise information eliminate the need to navigate through multiple pages or make unnecessary mouse clicks.

Lexicomp Online includes multiple databases and modules covering the following topic areas:

- Core Drug Information with Specialty Fields
- Pediatrics and Geriatrics
- Interaction Analysis
- Pharmacogenomics
- Infectious Diseases
- Laboratory Tests and Diagnostic Procedures
- Natural Products
- Patient Education
- Drug Identification
- Calculations
- I.V. Compatibility: *King® Guide to Parenteral Admixtures™*
- Toxicology

Register for a FREE 45-day trial

Visit www.lexi.com/institutions

Academic and institutional licenses available.

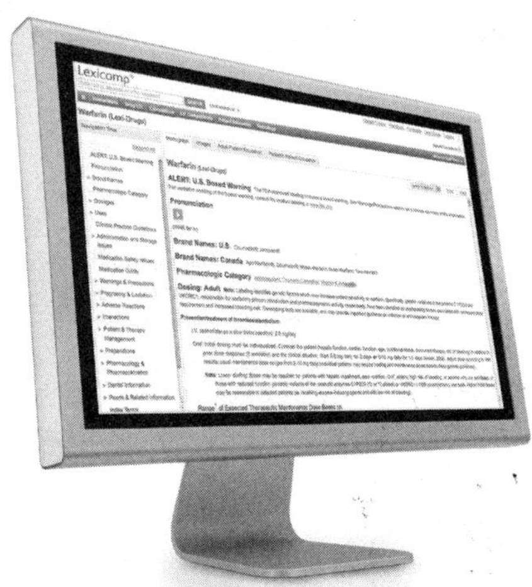

To order, call Customer Service at 1-866-397-3433 or visit www.lexi.com.
Outside of the U.S., call +1-330-650-6506 or visit www.lexi.com.

Lexicomp® Mobile Apps

Apps for smartphones and tablets

The Clinical Drug Information unit of Wolters Kluwer takes pride in creating quality drug information for use at the point of care. Our content is not subject to third-party recommendations, but based on the contributions of our respected authors and editors, internal clinical team, and thousands of professionals within the healthcare industry who continually review and validate our data.

With our Lexicomp Mobile Apps, you can be confident you are accessing the most timely drug information available for mobile devices. All updates are included with your annual subscription.

Lexicomp Mobile Apps databases include:

- Adult Drug Information
- Pediatric & Neonatal Drug Information
- Pediatric Drug Information (Spanish Version)
- Drug Interactions
- Natural Products
- Toxicolgy
- Household Products
- Infectious Diseases
- Lab & Diagnostic Procedures
- Nursing Drug Information
- Dental Drug Information
- Oral Soft Tissue Diseases
- Pharmacogenomics
- Patient Education
- Drug I.D.
- Medical Calculators
- I.V. Compatibility*
- Drug Allergy & Idiosyncratic Reactions
- Pregnancy & Lactation
- The 5-Minute Clinical Consult
- The 5-Minute Pediatric Consult
- AHFS DI® Essentials™
- Stedman's Medical Dictionary for the Health Professions and Nursing
- Stedman's Medical Abbreviations

* I.V. compatibility information © copyright King Guide Publications, Inc.

Visit www.lexi.com for more information and device compatibility!

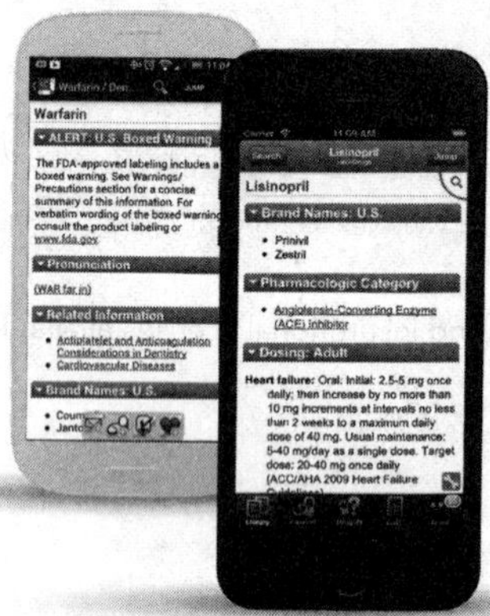

To order, call Customer Service at 1-866-397-3433 or visit www.lexi.com.
Outside of the U.S., call +1-330-650-6506 or visit www.lexi.com.